U0301094

主 译 赫 捷
王红阳
石远凯

第 9 版

HOLLAND-FREI 癌症医学 CANCER MEDICINE

主 编 Robert C. Bast Jr. · Carlo M. Croce · William N. Hait
Waun Ki Hong · Donald W. Kufe · Martine Piccart-Gebhart
Raphael E. Pollock · Ralph R. Weichselbaum
Hongyang Wang · James F. Holland

人民卫生出版社
·北 京·

Holland-Frei Cancer Medicine, 9e by Robert C. Bast Jr., Carlo M. Croce, William Hait, Waun Ki Hong, Donald W. Kufe, Martine Piccart-Gebhart, Raphael E. Pollock, Ralph R. Weichselbaum, Hongyang Wang, James F. Holland.

ISBN: 978-1-118-93469-2

图书在版编目（CIP）数据

Holland-Frei 癌症医学/（美）小罗伯特·C. 巴斯特（Robert C. Bast Jr）主编；赫捷，王红阳，石远凯主译. —北京：人民卫生出版社，2021. 12

ISBN 978-7-117-31656-9

Ⅰ. ①H… Ⅱ. ①小…②赫…③王…④石… Ⅲ. ①癌-诊疗 Ⅳ. ①R73

中国版本图书馆 CIP 数据核字(2021)第 099937 号

人卫智网	www. ipmph. com	医学教育、学术、考试、健康，购书智慧智能综合服务平台
人卫官网	www. pmph. com	人卫官方资讯发布平台

图字:01-2019-3236 号

Holland-Frei 癌症医学

Holland-Frei Aizheng Yixue

主　　译：赫　捷　王红阳　石远凯

出版发行：人民卫生出版社（中继线 010-59780011）

地　　址：北京市朝阳区潘家园南里 19 号

邮　　编：100021

E - mail：pmph @ pmph. com

购书热线：010-59787592　010-59787584　010-65264830

印　　刷：北京盛通印刷股份有限公司

经　　销：新华书店

开　　本：889×1194　1/16　　**印张**：111

字　　数：4710 千字

版　　次：2021 年 12 月第 1 版

印　　次：2021 年 12 月第 1 次印刷

标准书号：ISBN 978-7-117-31656-9

定　　价：1198. 00 元

打击盗版举报电话：010 - 59787491　E - mail：WQ @ pmph. com

质量问题联系电话：010 - 59787234　E - mail：zhiliang @ pmph. com

主译

赫　捷　王红阳　石远凯

副主译

高树庚

译者（按姓氏笔画排序）

于　晗　于乐兴　于晶琳　马　帅　马光辉　马福海　王　龙　王　旭　王　彤　王　杰　王　栋
王　莹　王　健　王　睿　王　镇　王义平　王先火　王海月　王海娟　王甜甜　王朝阳　王鲁强
王婷婷　王嘉炜　井莹莹　毛　宇　文　文　邓　垒　邓　婷　左赋兴　叶　菲　叶　慧　由婷婷
史幼梧　付　静　白元松　丛　丹　冯轲昕　毕林涛　吕　铮　吕岩霖　吕洪伟　吕桂帅　朱一鸣
朱镇星　向　阳　向　威　危晏平　刘　飞　刘　昊　刘　欣　刘　曼　刘　婷　刘天舒　刘玉秀
刘康栋　刘蒙蒙　刘嘉琦　关有彦　安菊生　许宋锋　许金芳　孙　文　孙阳春　寿建忠　李　亮
李　洋　李　勇　李　楠　李　懿　李　鑫　李一帆　李亚健　李志铭　李佩东　李玲玉　李敏娟
李维坤　李嘉根　杨　文　杨　杨　杨　晰　杨飞亚　杨长良　吴　彤　吴　忧　吴建中　何　倩
佐　晶　谷俊杰　邹宝华　辛　影　沈　皓　宋玉婷　宋永平　张　帆　张　良　张　爽　张文龙
张宁宁　张杨倩雯　张利平　张兵雷　张晓伟　张培霖　张梦璐　张清媛　张婷婷　张新佶　张鑫鑫
陈　东　陈　竺　陈　艳　陈　瑶　陈　磊　陈　羲　陈先凯　陈耐飞　陈淑桢　陈新焕　陈赛娟
陈馨蕊　邵欣欣　邵禹铭　范　阳　林　华　林泽晓　郑　博　岳　圆　金　鹏　金立超　周　迪
周光飚　周城城　郑　凯　郑　博　宗倩妮　孟令俊　孟肖利　孟祥志　赵　燕　赵四敏　赵亚男
赵自然　赵羽西　赵振国　赵继敏　赵善民　胡海涛　柳菁菁　钟巧凤　钟宇新　段晶晶　洪振亚
宣云东　姚　晨　贺　佳　贺宇飞　秦婴逸　袁　华　袁光文　袁筑慧　夏结来　顾宗廷　顾桂颖
钱海利　钱海鹏　徐　泉　徐立斌　郭　威　郭　曦　郭晓晶　郭献灵　唐丽丽　陶　丹　桑铭辰
黄慧强　曹传振　曹军宁　曹琦琪　龚　涛　龚彩凤　崔久嵬　康文哲　寇芙蓉　彭　攀　葛　阳
董亚萍　韩　冷　韩　瑜　韩　颖　韩苏军　韩贺东　韩鑫坤　程　敏　程　颖　程宁涛　曾　瑄
曾　嘉　雷呈志　雷群英　路　静　廖理达　谭紫雯　颜晓菁　瞿　望　瞿慧敏

审校（按姓氏笔画排序）

刁建东　于　晗　于乐兴　于胜吉　万经海　卫立辛　王　旭　王　彤　王　昕　王　翔　王　睿
王大力　王义平　王天有　王成锋　王华庆　王红阳　王孟昭　王鲁强　毛友生　文　文　巴　一
石远凯　田艳涛　付　静　代恩勇　白元松　白春梅　丛　丹　丛明华　冯继锋　邢念增　毕林涛
吕桂帅　朱镇星　向　阳　危晏平　刘　曼　刘　巍　刘玉秀　刘绍严　安菊生　祁雪伟　孙　文
孙　恺　孙阳春　李　印　李　宁　李　军　李　肖　李　亮　李　鑫　李晓阳　杨　文　杨　杨
吴　宁　吴　彤　吴世凯　吴令英　何　倩　何慧斯　张　旭　张文龙　张会来　张艳华　张培霖
陈　瑶　陈　磊　陈淑桢　陈新焕　林冬梅　罗志国　周　迪　周　健　周宗玫　周剑峰　周爱萍
郑　博　孟令俊　赵　峻　赵方辉　赵四敏　赵亚男　赵继敏　胡夕春　胡南均　姜文奇　姚　晨
贺　佳　贺宇飞　夏结来　顾桂颖　高树庚　高禹舜　郭晓晶　唐丽丽　曹琦琪　崔久嵬　葛　阳
董亚萍　蒋　芳　韩　冷　韩志鹏　韩贺东　程　敏　程　颖　程宁涛　雷群英　路　静　赫　捷
谭紫雯　谭锋维　薛　奇　魏文强

主译助理

陈淑桢

献辞

从第 1 版的准备到接下来的 8 个版次,Emil Frei III, Tom 对我们和他的队友们来说都是一位杰出的主编。他对癌症的深入了解、他广泛的职业和个人修养以及他的远见,都为这本书及其相关作品注入了力量。他是一个站在世界肿瘤学学科塔尖的人,正是因为他的参与促进了肿瘤学作为一门医学学科的创立。他是个完美的临床医生,在他管理美国国家癌症研究所、得克萨斯大学安德森癌症研究中心和哈佛大学 Dana-Farber 癌症研究所期间,为美国培训出了大量伟大的肿瘤学家。他是翻译研究的先驱。他的著作、演讲和奔放的友谊使他成为每一位肿瘤专家的良师益友。他的影响永垂后世。

我们这些珍视他的博爱的编辑们非常想念他,并将第 9 版《Holland-Frei 癌症医学》献给这位伟人。

James F. Holland
Robert C. Bast Jr.
Donald W. Kufe
Ralph R. Weichselbaum
Raphael E. Pollock
William N. Hait
Waun Ki Hong

前言

我们对于癌症的理解，无论从分子、细胞还是临床水平，都在不断加深。随着数十种新型靶向药物、抗体和预测性生物标志物的开发和批准应用，分子诊断和治疗向临床的转化，让我们开始逐步实现精准医学。如何吸收这些知识，对学生、住院医师、研究员和肿瘤学专家，都是严峻的挑战。如果实验室研究人员想将他们的发现转化为人类应用的话，需要根据癌症生物学对临床肿瘤学进行准确概述。由于新疗法和诊断可能适用于多种部位的肿瘤，因此制药和生物技术公司必须了解整个肿瘤学领域的新进展和未满足的需求。

第 9 版《Holland-Frei 癌症医学》从检测、诊断和癌症管理等方面，全面综述了临床肿瘤学的基本原则。书中介绍了癌症的生物学特征和肿瘤疾病的临床表现。肿瘤学专家现在必须熟悉能揭示肿瘤起源和发病机制的通路和过程。书中也深入讨论转化医学，让肿瘤学专家了解技术程序，比如二代测序、DNA 和组蛋白的表观遗传修饰、转录体测序、非编码 RNA、具有特殊功能的 RNA、蛋白组学和代谢组学等。书中介绍了癌症及其转移灶之间的异质性，并讨论了异质性对临床管理的影响。利用定量肿瘤学来解释肿瘤发生发展是合理的，它不仅介绍了生物统计学和新的试验设计，还介绍了生物信息学和系统生物学。

这项工作包括常规和新型药物使用的简明指南。与过去的版本一样，本书强调多学科诊疗，包括外科学、放射肿瘤学、肿瘤心理学和流行病学。这本书对每个学科的肿瘤学专家都是有价值的。第 9 版《Holland-Frei 癌症医学》，包括基于网络的电子访问，链接到相关的参考文献，都将定期更新。

主编们挑选了一些专家，由他们撰写关于各自章节所涵盖的学科和疾病。鉴于肿瘤学的全球重要性，现在已纳入来自欧洲和亚洲的主编。随着科学界和医学界对癌症过程及其预防和治疗的未知性逐渐消失，我们相信这项工作内容可以帮助读者了解目前肿瘤学状况，以及为读者对未来进行批判性探索提供平台。

致谢

我们衷心感谢 Jene' Reinartz 的杰出贡献，她的不懈努力对《Holland-Frei 癌症医学》的组织至关重要。我们也非常感谢我们的助手 Cheryl Ashorn、Michelle Denney、Guishuai Lv、Kate Charlesworth-Miller、Sharon Palko、Kathy Profrock、Ruby Robinson、Catherine Rotsaert、Mary Werowinski 和 Elizabeth Wilkins，他们帮助完成了这本书。我们感谢 Nancy Hubener 为完成本书所做的努力。我们感谢 Michael Ewer 博士在审阅多个章节方面的努力和专业知识。

与 John Wiley 公司合作是一种特别的乐趣。我们的初始编辑 Thom Moore 在建立该项目和获得《Holland-Frei 癌症医学》版权方面发挥了重要作用。他的远见和毅力至关重要。Claire Bonnet 在完成这本书方面确实非常出色。Wiley 的工作人员一直非常乐于助人。

我们的作者利用他们非凡的知识、经验和判断力，捕捉了每个主题和疾病部位的关键点。我们感谢他们的努力，并为每一章感到骄傲。

最后，我们必须承认，这些知识都是我们从病人身上学到的。正是他们的勇气、平和及应对疾病的力量，每天都激励着我们。我们希望第 9 版《Holland-Frei 癌症医学》能提升我们的诊疗水平，以帮助以后的患者。

作者名单

Stuart A. Aaronson, MD
Aron Professor
Department of Oncological Sciences
Icahn School of Medicine at Mount Sinai
New York, NY
USA

Amy Abernethy, MD, PhD
Professor of Medicine, Division of Medical Oncology
Director, Center for Learning Health Care
Duke University Medical Center & Duke Clinical Research Institute
Durham, NC
USA

David H. Abramson, MD
Chief
Ophthalmic Oncology Service, Department of Surgery
Memorial Sloan Kettering Cancer Center
New York, NY
USA

Jeremy S. Abramson, MD, MMSc
Assistant Professor, Medicine, Harvard Medical School
Dana-Farber Cancer Institute
Boston, MA
USA

Ala Abudayyeh, MD
Assistant Professor, Division of Internal Medicine
Section of Nephrology
The University of Texas MD Anderson Cancer Center
Houston, TX
USA

Mario Acunzo, PhD
Research Scientist
James Comprehensive Cancer Center
The Ohio State University
Columbus, OH
USA

Roberto Adachi, MD
Associate Professor
Department of Pulmonary Medicine
The University of Texas MD Anderson Cancer Center
Houston, TX
USA

Ranjana H. Advani, MD
The Saul A. Rosenberg, MD, Professor of Lymphoma
Department of Medicine/Medical Oncology
Stanford University
Stanford, CA
USA

Judy U. Ahrar, MD
Associate Professor
Department of Interventional Radiology, Division of Diagnostic Imaging
The University of Texas MD Anderson Cancer Center
Houston, TX
USA

Jaffer A. Ajani, MD
Professor
Department of Gastrointestinal (GI) Medical Oncology
Division of Cancer Medicine
The University of Texas MD Anderson Cancer Center
Houston, TX
USA

James P. Allison, PhD
Professor and Chair
Department of Immunology
The University of Texas MD Anderson Cancer Center
Houston, TX
USA

Edward P. Ambinder, MD
Tisch Cancer Institute
Clinical Professor of Medicine
Icahn School of Medicine at Mount Sinai
New York, NY
USA

Kenneth C. Anderson, MD
Professor of Medicine
Medical Oncology
Dana-Farber Cancer Institute/Harvard Medical School
Boston, MA
USA

Ana Aparicio, MD
Associate Professor
Genitourinary Medical Oncology
The University of Texas MD Anderson Cancer Center
Houston, TX
USA

James Armitage, MD
Professor, Internal Medicine
Division of Hematology & Oncology
UNMC Oncology-Hematology Division
Omaha, NE
USA

Sarah T. Arron, MD, PhD
Associate Professor
Department of Dermatology
University of California
San Francisco, CA
USA

Rony Avritscher, MD
Associate Professor
Department of Interventional Radiology
The University of Texas MD Anderson Cancer Center
Houston, TX
USA

Diwakar D. Balachandran, MD
Associate Professor
Department of Pulmonary Medicine
The University of Texas MD Anderson Cancer Center
Houston, TX
USA

Jacqueline C. Barrientos, MD
Assistant Professor
Medicine
Hofstra Northwell School of Medicine
New Hyde Park, NY
USA

Lara Bashoura, MD
Associate Professor
Department of Pulmonary Medicine
The University of Texas MD Anderson Cancer Center
Houston, TX
USA

Robert C. Bast Jr., MD
Vice President for Translational Research
The University of Texas MD Anderson Cancer Center
Houston, TX
USA

Susan Bates, MD
Professor of Medicine
Division of Hematology/Oncology
Columbia University Medical Center
New York, NY
USA

Stephen B. Baylin, MD
Deputy Director
The Sidney Kimmel Comprehensive Cancer Center
Johns Hopkins University
Baltimore, MD
USA

Georgia M. Beasley, MD
Duke University Medical Center
Durham, NC
USA

Jonathan S. Berek, MD, MMS, FASCO
Laurie Kraus Lacob Professor
Fellow, Stanford Distinguished Careers Institute
Director, Special Programs, Stanford Cancer Institute
Director, Stanford Women's Cancer Center
Director, Stanford Health Care Communication Program
Stanford University School of Medicine
Stanford, CA
USA

Ross S. Berkowitz, MD
William H. Baker Professor of Gynecology
Director of Division of Gynecologic Oncology at Brigham and Women's Hospital and Dana Farber Cancer Institute
Director of New England Trophoblastic Disease Center
Harvard Medical School
Boston, MA
USA

Leslie Bernstein, PhD
Professor and Director
Division of Cancer Etiology, Department of Population Sciences
Beckman Research Institute and the City of Hope Comprehensive Cancer Center
Duarte, CA
USA

Donald A. Berry, PhD
Professor
Department of Biostatistics
The University of Texas MD Anderson Cancer Center
Houston, TX
USA

Joseph R. Bertino, MD
Professor
Medicine and Pharmacology
Robert Wood Johnson Medical School
Rutgers, The State University of New Jersey
New Brunswick, NJ
USA

Teena Bhatla, MD
Assistant Professor of Pediatrics
Division of Pediatric Hematology-Oncology
New York University Medical Center
The Stephen D. Hassenfeld Children's Center for Cancer and Blood Disorders
New York, NY
USA

Boris Blechacz, MD, PhD
Assistant Professor
Department of Gastroenterology, Hepat, & Nutr
Division of Internal Medicine
The University of Texas MD Anderson Cancer Center
Houston, TX
USA

Mark Bloomston, MD, FACS
Professor
Division of Surgical Oncology
Department of Surgery
The Ohio State University
Wexner Medical Center
Columbus, OH
USA

Otis W. Brawley, MD, MACP
Chief Medical Officer
American Cancer Society, Inc.
Atlanta, GA
USA

Freddie Bray, PhD
Head
Section of Cancer Surveillance
International Agency for Research on Cancer
Lyon
France

Malcolm Brenner, MB, PhD
Professor
Center for Gene Therapy
Baylor College of Medicine
Houston, TX
USA

Robert S. Bresalier, MD
Professor, Gastroenterology, Hepatology & Nutrition
Division of Internal Medicine
The University of Texas MD Anderson Cancer Center
Houston, TX
USA

Kristin Brogaard, PhD
Project Manager
Institute for Systems Biology
Seattle, WA
USA

Lionel Brookes, 3rd, PhD
Postdoctoral student
Department of Dermatology
University of California
San Francisco, CA
USA

Kristoffer W. Brudvik, MD, PhD
Postdoctoral Fellow
Department of Surgical Oncology
The University of Texas MD Anderson Cancer Center
Houston, TX
USA

Alan H. Bryce, MD
Assistant Professor of Medicine
Department of Hematology/Oncology
Mayo Clinic Arizona
Scottsdale, AZ
USA

Earle F. Burgess, MD
Attending Physician, Medical Oncology
Levine Cancer Institute, Carolinas HealthCare System
Charlotte, NC
USA

Meredith Buxton, PhD
Assistant Professor
Department of Surgery
UCSF School of Medicine
San Francisco, CA
USA

Aman U. Buzdar, MD, FACP
Professor of Medicine and Internist
Department of Breast Medical Oncology, Division of Cancer Medicine
The University of Texas MD Anderson Cancer Center
Houston, TX
USA

Maria E. Cabanillas, MD
Associate Professor
Department of Endocrine Neoplasia and Hormonal Disorders
The University of Texas MD Anderson Cancer Center
Houston, TX
USA

Guangwen Cao, MD, PhD
Professor
Department of Epidemiology
Second Military Medical University
Shanghai
China

William L. Carroll, MD
Julie and Edward J. Minskoff Professor of Pediatrics and Pathology
Chief, Division of Pediatric Hematology-Oncology at NYU Langone Medical Center
Stephen D. Hassenfeld Children's Center for Cancer and Blood Disorders
New York, NY
USA

Tina Cascone, MD, PhD
Fellow, Cancer Medicine
The University of Texas MD Anderson Cancer Center
Houston, TX
USA

A. P. Chahinian, MD
Professor
Department of Medicine
Mount Sinai School of Medicine
New York, NY
USA

Richard Champlin, MD
Chair, Professor of Medicine
Department of Stem Cell Transplantation and Cellular Therapy
The University of Texas MD Anderson Cancer Center
Houston, TX
USA

Martin C. Chang, MD, PhD, FCAP, FRCPC
Assistant Professor
Lab Med and Pathobiology
Mount Sinai Hospital
Toronto, ON
Canada

Joe Y. Chang, MD, PhD
Director, Stereotactic Radiotherapy Program
Department of Radiation Oncology
The University of Texas MD Anderson Cancer Center
Houston, TX
USA

Alejandro Chaoul, PhD
Assistant Professor
Department of Palliative, Rehabilitation & Integrative Medicine
The University of Texas MD Anderson Cancer Center
Houston, TX
USA

Brian F. Chapin, MD
Assistant Professor
Department of Urology, Division of Surgery
The University of Texas MD Anderson Cancer Center
Houston, TX
USA

Sai-Juan Chen, MD, PhD
Professor of Hematology
State Key Laboratory of Medical Genomics
Shanghai Institute of Hematology
Rui-Jin Hospital affiliated to Shanghai Jiao Tong University School of Medicine
Shanghai
China

Zhu Chen, PhD
Vice-Chairman, 12th Standing Committee of the National People's Congress
President, Chinese Medical Association
Beijing
China

Anne Chiang, MD, PhD
Assistant Professor
Department of Medicine, Section of Medical Oncology
Yale School of Medicine, Yale Cancer Center, and Smilow Cancer Hospital
New Haven, CT
USA

Steven J. Chmura, MD, PhD
Associate Professor of Radiation and Cellular Oncology
The University of Chicago Pritzker School of Medicine
Chicago, IL
USA

James E. Cleaver, PhD
Professor Emeritus
Department of Dermatology
University of California
San Francisco, CA
USA

Steven K. Clinton, MD, PhD
Professor
Department of Internal Medicine
College of Medicine
The Ohio State University Comprehensive Cancer Center
Arthur G. James Cancer Hospital and Richard J. Solove Research Institute (OSUCCC – James)
Columbus, OH
USA

Jeffrey I. Cohen, MD
Chief, Laboratory of Infectious Diseases
National Institute of Allergy and Infectious Diseases
National Institutes of Health
Bethesda, MD
USA

Carmel J. Cohen, MD
Professor, Division of GYN Oncology
Department of Obstetrics and Gynecology
Ruttenberg Cancer Center, Icahn School of Medicine at Mount Sinai Medical Center
New York, NY
USA

Harvey J. Cohen, MD
Division Chief of Geriatrics, Director of the Center for the Study of Aging and Human Development
Duke University Medical Center
Durham, NC
USA

Lorenzo Cohen, PhD
Professor and Director
Integrative Medicine Program
Department of Palliative, Rehabilitation and Integrative Medicine
The University of Texas MD Anderson Cancer Center
Houston, TX
USA

Peter D. Cole, MD
Associate Professor
Pediatrics
Albert Einstein College of Medicine
The Children's Hospital at Montefiore
Bronx, NY
USA

Elizabeth Comen, MD
Medical Oncologist
Breast Medicine Service
Memorial Sloan Kettering Cancer Center
New York, NY
USA

Philip P. Connell, MD
Associate Professor
Department of Radiation and Cellular Oncology
University of Chicago Hospital
Chicago, IL
USA

Laurence J. Cooper, MD, PhD
Visiting Scientist
Pediatrics Research
The University of Texas MD Anderson Cancer Center
Houston, TX
USA

Carlos Cordon-Cardo, MD, PhD
Professor and Chair
Department of Pathology
Icahn School of Medicine at Mount Sinai
New York, NY
USA

Christopher L. Corless, MD, PhD
Medical Director of the Cancer Pathology Share Resource
Oregon Health & Science University
Portland, OR
USA

Jorge Cortes, MD
Professor of Medicine
Chair CML and AML Section
Department of Leukemia
The University of Texas MD Anderson Cancer Center
Houston, TX
USA

David Cosgrove, MB, BCh
Assistant Professor, Department of Oncology
Johns Hopkins University
Baltimore, MD
USA

Richard Cote, MD, FRCPath
Professor & Joseph R. Coulter Jr. Chair, Department of Pathology
Professor, Department of Biochemistry and Molecular Biology
Chief of Pathology
Jackson Memorial Hospital
University of Miami Miller School of Medicine
Miami, FL
USA

Kenneth H. Cowan, MD, PhD
Director, Fred and Pamela Buffett Cancer Center
University of Nebraska Medical Center
Omaha, NE
USA

Christopher H. Crane, MD
Professor with Tenure
Department of Radiation Oncology
The University of Texas MD Anderson Cancer Center
Houston, TX
USA

Carlo M. Croce, MD
Distinguished University Professor
The John W. Wolfe Chair in Human Cancer Genetics
Professor and Chair
Department of Molecular Virology, Immunology and Medical Genetics
The Wexner Medical Center
The Ohio State University
Columbus, OH
USA

Christopher P. Crum, MD, FRCP
Professor of Pathology, Harvard Medical School
Department of Pathology
Brigham and Women's Hospital
Boston, MA
USA

William Cruz-Munoz, PhD
Postdoctoral Fellow
Biological Sciences Platform
Sunnybrook Research Institute
Toronto, ON
Canada

Steven A. Curley, MD, FACS
Professor of Surgery and Chief
Division of Surgical Oncology
Baylor College of Medicine
Houston, TX
USA

Timothy A. Damron, MD, FACS
Professor of Orthopedic Surgery
Upstate University Hospital
Syracuse, NY
USA

Siamak Daneshmand, MD
Associate Professor of Urology (Clinical Scholar)
Director of Urologic Oncology, USC Institute of Urology
Los Angeles, CA
USA

John W. Davis, MD, FACS
Associate Professor, Department of Urology
Division of Surgery
The University of Texas MD Anderson Cancer Center
Houston, TX
USA

Shaheenah Dawood, MD, MBBch, FACP, FRCP, MPH, CPH
Head of Medical Oncology
Dubai Hospital
Dubai
United Arab Emirates

Lisa M. DeAngelis, MD, FAAN
Neuro-Oncologist
Chair, Department of Neurology
Lillian Rojtman Berkman Chair in Honor of Jerome B. Posner
Memorial Sloan Kettering Cancer Center
New York, NY
USA

Yadwinder S. Deol, PhD
Postdoctoral Research Fellow
University of Michigan Comprehensive Cancer Center
Ann Arbor, MI
USA

Maria T. De Sancho, MD, MSc
Associate Professor of Clinical Medicine
Non-Malignant Hematology Program at Weill Cornell Medicine's Center for Blood Disorders
New York, NY
USA

Summer B. Dewdney, MD
Assistant Professor
Division of Gynecologic Oncology
Rush University Medical Center
Chicago, IL
USA

Radwa G. Diab, MD, MBBCH, PhD
Lecturer of Medical Parasitology
Faculty of Medicine, Alexandria University
Alexandria
Egypt

Robert B. Diasio, MD
Director, Mayo Clinic Cancer Center
William J. and Charles H. Mayo Professor
Departments of Molecular Pharmacology & Experimental Therapeutics and Oncology
Rochester, MN
USA

Burton F. Dickey, MD
Professor
Department of Pulmonary Medicine
The University of Texas MD Anderson Cancer Center
Houston, TX
USA

Zeliha Gunnur Dikmen, MD, PhD
Faculty of Medicine
Department of Biochemistry
Hacettepe University
Ankara
Turkey

Michaela A. Dinan, PhD
Medical Instructor, Division of Medical Oncology
Duke University Medical Center
Durham, NC
USA

Nicholas C. Dracopoli, PhD
Vice President and Head of Oncology Biomarkers
Janssen Research & Development, LLC.
Raritan, NJ
USA

Anthony Dragun, MD
Assistant Professor
Department of Radiation Oncology
James Graham Brown Cancer Center
Louisville, KY
USA

Madeleine M. Duvic, MD
Professor, Dermatology
The University of Texas MD Anderson Cancer Center
Houston, TX
USA

George A. Eapen, MD
Professor
Department of Pulmonary Medicine
The University of Texas MD Anderson Cancer Center
Houston, TX
USA

John M. L. Ebos, PhD
Assistant Professor of Oncology
Department of Cancer Genetics
Department of Medicine
Department of Pharmacology and Therapeutics (Graduate Program)
Roswell Park Cancer Institute
Buffalo, NY
USA

Joseph P. Eder, MD
Professor of Medicine (Medical Oncology)
Yale-New Haven Hospital
New Haven, CT
USA

Eleni Efstathiou, MD, PhD
Associate Professor, Department of Genitourinary Medical Oncology, Division of Cancer Medicine
The University of Texas MD Anderson Cancer Center
Houston, TX
USA

Suhendan Ekmekcioglu, PhD
Professor
Melanoma Medical Oncology – Research
The University of Texas MD Anderson Cancer Center
Houston, TX
USA

Mervat Z. El Azzouni, MD, PhD
Professor of Medical Parasitology
Faculty of Medicine
Alexandria University
Alexandria
Egypt

Lawrence Einhorn, MD
Professor of Medicine, Division of Hematology-Oncology/Department of Urology
Indiana University School of Medicine
Melvin and Bren Simon, Cancer Center, IN
USA

Carmen P. Escalante, MD
Professor and Chairman
Department of General Internal Medicine, Ambulatory Treatment and Emergency Care
The University of Texas MD Anderson Cancer Center
Houston, TX
USA

Laura Esserman, MD, MBA
Professor, Departments of Surgery and Radiology, and Affiliate Faculty, Institute for Health Policy Studies
University of California
San Francisco, CA
USA

David S. Ettinger, MD, FACP, FCCP
Alex Grass Professor of Oncology
The Sidney Kimmel Comprehensive Cancer Center at Johns Hopkins
Baltimore, MD
USA

Douglas B. Evans, MD
Ausman Family Foundation Professor of Surgery
Chairman, Department of Surgery
Medical College of Wisconsin
Milwaukee, WI
USA

Scott E. Evans, MD
Associate Professor
Department of Pulmonary Medicine
The University of Texas MD Anderson Cancer Center
Houston, TX
USA

Steven M. Ewer, MD
Division Cardiovascular Medicine
University of Wisconsin School of Medicine of Public Health
Madison
WI, USA

Michael S. Ewer, MD, MPH, JD, LLM, MBA
Special Assistant to the Vice President of Medical Affairs
The University of Texas MD Anderson Cancer Center
Houston, TX
USA

Stefan Faderl, MD
Chief
John Theurer Cancer Center's Leukemia Division
Hackensack, NJ
USA

Saadia A. Faiz, MD
Associate Professor
Department of Pulmonary Medicine
The University of Texas MD Anderson Cancer Center
Houston, TX
USA

Mark K. Ferguson, MD
Professor of Surgery
Department of Surgical Oncology
University of Chicago Medical Center
Chicago, IL
USA

Jacques Ferlay, MSc, ME
Informatics Officer
Section of Cancer Surveillance
International Agency for Research on Cancer
Lyon
France

Renata Ferrarotto, MD
Assistant Professor of Medicine
Department of Thoracic-Head and Neck Medical Oncology
The University of Texas MD Anderson Cancer Center
Houston, TX
USA

William D. Figg Sr, Pharm D
Deputy Chief
Genitourinary Malignancies Branch Center for Cancer Research, National Cancer Institute, National Institutes of Health
Bethesda, MD
USA

Lisa Figueiredo, MD
Assistant Professor
Pediatrics
Albert Einstein College of Medicine
The Children's Hospital at Montefiore
Bronx, NY
USA

Tito Fojo, MD, PhD
Professor of Medicine
Division of Hematology/Oncology
Columbia University Medical Center
New York, NY
USA

Patrick M. Forde, MD, MBBCh
Assistant Professor of Oncology
Sidney Kimmel Comprehensive Cancer Center
Johns Hopkins
Baltimore, MD
USA

Adolfo Firpo-Betancourt, MD, MPA
Professor of Pathology
The Mount Sinai Hospital
New York, NY
USA

Jasmine H. Francis, MD
Assistant Attending
Ophthalmic Oncology Service, Department of Surgery
Memorial Sloan-Kettering Cancer Center
New York, NY
USA

Arthur E. Frankel, MD
Professor in the Department of Internal Medicine
UT Southwestern Medical Center
Dallas, TX
USA

Milo Frattini, MD, PhD
Head
Laboratory of Molecular Pathology
Institute of Pathology
Locarno
Switzerland

Arnold S. Freedman, MD
Professor of Medicine
Harvard Medical School
Dana Farber Cancer Institute
Boston, MA
USA

Michael L. Friedlander, MD, MBChB, PhD
Conjoint Professor of Medicine
Director of Medical Oncology
The Prince of Wales Hospital
Consultant Medical Oncologist
Royal Hospital for Women
Sydney, NSW
Australia

Emil Frei III, MD (deceased)
Director and Physician-in-Chief
Dana-Farber Cancer Institute
Boston, MA
USA

Jing Fu, MD, PhD
Research Assistant
International Lab on Signaling Transduction
Eastern Hepatobiliary Surgery Hospital
Shanghai
China

Valentin Fuster, MD, PhD
Professor, Icahn School of Medicine
Physician-in-Chief
Mount Sinai Hospital
New York, NY
USA

Robert F. Gagel, MD
Head, Division of Internal Medicine
The University of Texas MD Anderson Cancer Center
Houston, TX
USA

Robert C. Gallo, MD
Homer & Martha Gudelsky Distinguished Professor in Medicine & Director, Institute of Human Virology
University of Maryland School of Medicine
Baltimore, MD
USA

Jianjun Gao, MD, PhD
Assistant Professor, Department of Genitourinary Medical Oncology, Division of Cancer Medicine
The University of Texas MD Anderson Cancer Center
Houston, TX
USA

M. Kay Garcia, DrPH, MSN, LAc
Associate Professor
Department of Palliative, Rehabilitation and Integrative Medicine
The University of Texas MD Anderson Cancer Center
Houston, TX
USA

Adam S. Garden, MD
Professor, Department of Radiation Oncology
The University of Texas MD Anderson Cancer Center
Houston, TX
USA

Chirag D. Gandhi, MD, FACS, FAANS
Associate Professor of Neurosurgery, Neurology, and Radiology
Program Director, Neurointerventional Fellowship
Associate Program Director, Neurosurgical Residency
Rutgers University – New Jersey Medical School
Chief and Division Director, Neurological Surgery
Newark Beth Israel Medical Center
Newark, NJ
USA

Teresa A. Gilewski, MD
Professor of Clinical Medicine
Weill Cornell Medical College
Memorial Sloan-Kettering Cancer Center
New York, NY
USA

Edward L. Giovannucci, MD, ScD
Professor of Nutrition and Epidemiology
Department of Nutrition & Department of Epidemiology
Harvard T.H. Chan School of Public Health
Boston, MA
USA

Donald P. Goldstein, MD
Founder and Director Emeritus
Brigham and Women's Hospital
Boston, MA
USA

Daniel R. Gomez, MD
Assistant Professor
Radiation Oncology Department
The University of Texas MD Anderson Cancer Center
Houston, TX
USA

Sangeeta Goswami, MD, PhD
Internal Medicine Resident
University of Pittsburg Medical Center
Pittsburg, PA
USA

Elizabeth M. Grainger, PhD, RD
Professor, Department of Emergency Medicine
Division of Internal Medicine
The University of Texas MD Anderson Cancer Center
Houston, TX
USA

Jill Granger, BSc, MSc
Research Supervisor
Cancer Stem Cell Laboratory
Department of Internal Medicine-Hematology/Oncology
University of Michigan
Ann Arbor, MI
USA

Joe W. Gray, PhD
Professor and Gordon Moore Endowed Chair, Department of Biomedical Engineering
Director, OHSU Center for Spatial Systems Biomedicine
Associate Director for Biophysical Oncology, Knight Cancer Institute
Oregon Health & Science University
Portland, OR
USA

David J. Grdina, PhD
Professor of Radiation and Cellular Oncology
Department of Radiation and Cellular Oncology
The University of Chicago
Chicago, IL
USA

F. Anthony Greco, MD
Director, Sarah Cannon Cancer Center
Senior Investigator
Department of Oncology
Sarah Cannon Research Institute and Tennessee Oncology, PLLC
Nashville, TN
USA

Iqbal Grewal, PhD, DSc, FRCPath
Vice President, Head of Immuno-Oncology in the Oncology Therapeutic Area
Janssen Research & Development, LLC
Raritan, NJ
USA

Elizabeth A. Grimm, PhD
Professor, Department of Melanoma Medical Oncology
Waun Ki Hong Distinguished Chair in Translational Oncology
The University of Texas MD Anderson Cancer Center
Houston, TX
USA

Horiana B. Grosu, MD
Assistant Professor
Department of Pulmonary Medicine
The University of Texas MD Anderson Cancer Center
Houston, TX
USA

Luca Grumolato, PhD
Associate Professor
INSERM U982-Department of Biology
University of Rouen Normandie
Mont Saint Aignan
France

Jian Gu, PhD
Associate Professor
Department of Epidemiology, Division of OVP, Cancer Prevention and Population Sciences
The University of Texas MD Anderson Cancer Center
Houston, TX
USA

Eric Guerin, MD
Scientist
Laboratoire de Biochimie et Biologie Moléculaire
Hôpital de Hautepierre - Hôpitaux Universitaires de Strasbourg
Strasbourg
France

Jose G. Guillem, MD
Colorectal Service, Department of Surgery
Memorial Sloan Kettering Cancer Center
New York, NY
USA

Radhika Gulhar, BA
Medical student
Department of Dermatology
University of California
San Francisco, CA
USA

James L. Gulley, MD, PhD, FACP
Chief
Genitourinary Malignancies Branch
Center for Cancer Research
National Cancer Institute
National Institutes of Health
Bethesda, MD
USA

Michael Haake, MD
Medical Director
Department of Radiation Oncology
Levine Cancer Institute at Carolinas Medical Center and Senior Physician
Southeast Radiation Oncology
Charlotte, NC
USA

John D. Hainsworth, MD
Senior Investigator
Department of Oncology
Sarah Cannon Research Institute and Tennessee Oncology, PLLC
Nashville, TN
USA

William N. Hait, MD, PhD
Global Head, Research and Development
Janssen Pharmaceutical Companies of Johnson and Johnson
Raritan, NJ
USA

Douglas Hanahan, PhD
Director, Swiss Institute for Experimental Cancer Research
Professor, Department of Molecular Oncology
Swiss Federal Institute of Technology
Lausanne
Switzerland

Axel-R. Hanauske, MD, PhD, MBA
Senior Medical Fellow, Medical Oncology, Global Early Drug Development
Eli Lilly and Company
Indianapolis, IN
USA

Eric K. Hansen, MD
Radiation Oncologist
The Oregon Clinic
Portland, OR
USA

Curtis C. Harris, MD
Chief
Laboratory of Human Carcinogenesis
National Cancer Institute, National Institutes of Health
Bethesda, MD
USA

Harold A. Harvey, MD
Director, Hematology/Oncology Fellowship Program
Penn State Hershey Cancer Institute
Hershey, PA
USA

Saima Hassan, MD, PhD, FRCSC
Postdoctoral Research Fellow
Department of Biomedical Engineering
Oregon Health & Science University
Portland, OR
USA

Laura M. Heiser, PhD
Assistant Professor
Department of Biomedical Engineering
Affiliated Faculty
OHSU Center for Spatial Systems Biomedicine
Oregon Health & Science University
Portland, OR
USA

William P. D. Hendricks, PhD
Assistant Professor
Integrated Cancer Genomics Division
Translational Genomics Research Institute
Phoenix, AZ
USA

Bryan T. Hennessy, MD
Senior Lecturer
RCSI and Consultant Medical Oncologist
Beaumont Hospital
Our Lady of Lourdes Hospital
Dublin
Ireland

Roy S. Herbst, MD, PhD
Professor (Ensign Professor of Medicine)
Department of Medicine, Section of Medical Oncology
Yale School of Medicine, Yale Cancer Center, and
Smilow Cancer Hospital
New Haven, CT
USA

Michael F. Herfs, PhD
Principal Investigator
GIGA-Cancer
Laboratory of Experimental Pathology
Department of Pathology
University of Liege
Liege
Belgium

H. Franklin Herlong, MD
Professor of Medicine
Department of Gastroenterology, Hepatology and Nutrition
The University of Texas MD Anderson Cancer Center
Houston, TX
USA

James G. Herman, MD
Professor of Medicine
Co-Leader, UPCI Lung Cancer Program
University of Pittsburgh Cancer Institute
Pittsburgh, PA
USA

John V. Heymach, MD, PhD
Chair, Department of Thoracic Head and Neck
The University of Texas MD Anderson Cancer Center
Houston, TX
USA

Teru Hideshima, MD, PhD
Institute Scientist
Department of Medical Oncology
Dana-Farber Cancer Institute
Principal Associate in Medicine
Harvard Medical School
Boston, MA
USA

Bradford R. Hirsch, MD, MBA
Department of Medicine
Adjunct Assistant Professor
Duke University Medical Center
Durham, NC
USA

James W. Hodge, PhD, MBA
Senior Investigator
Laboratory of Tumor Immunology and Biology
Center for Cancer Research
National Cancer Institute
National Institutes of Health
Bethesda, MD
USA

Lorne J. Hofseth, PhD
Professor and Graduate Director, College of Pharmacy
University of South Carolina
Professor, Drug Discovery & Biomedical Sciences
South Carolina College of Pharmacy
Columbia, SC
USA

James F. Holland, MD, ScD (hc)
Distinguished Professor of Neoplastic Diseases
Director Emeritus of Derald H. Rutttenberg Cancer Center
Icahn School of Medicine at Mount Sinai
New York, NY
USA

Jimmie C. Holland, MD
Wayne E. Chapman Chair in Psychiatric Oncology
Memorial Sloan-Kettering Cancer Center
New York, NY
USA

Waun Ki Hong, MD, DMSc (Hon)
Professor of Thoracic/Head and Neck Medical Oncology
American Cancer Society
Professor, Samsung Distinguished University Chair in Cancer Medicine Emeritus
The University of Texas MD Anderson Cancer Center
Houston, TX
USA

Leroy Hood, MD, PhD
Providence Health & Services
Institute for Systems Biology
Seattle, WA
USA

Richard T. Hoppe, MD
The Henry S. Kaplan-Harry Lebeson Professor in Cancer Biology
Department of Radiation Oncology
Stanford University
Stanford, CA
USA

Neil S. Horowitz, MD
Assistant Professor
Obstetrics and Gynecology
Brigham and Women's Hospital
Boston, MA
USA

Arti Hurria, MD
Professor, Department of Medical Oncology and Therapeutics Research
City of Hope
Altadena, CA
USA

Ilya Iofin, MD
Assistant Professor of Orthopedics
Mount Sinai Hospital
New York, NY
USA

Nitin Jain, MD, MSPH
Associate Professor, Physical Medicine and Rehabilitation and Orthopaedics, Director of PM&R Research and Co-Director of Orthopaedic Sports Medicine Research
Vanderbilt Stallworth Rehabilitation Hospital
Nashville, TN
USA

Anuja Jhingran, MD
Professor
Department of Radiation Oncology
Section of Gynecology
The University of Texas MD Anderson Cancer Center
Houston, TX
USA

Carlos A. Jimenez, MD
Professor
Department of Pulmonary Medicine
The University of Texas MD Anderson Cancer Center
Houston, TX
USA

Roy Jones, MD, PhD
Professor, Cancer Medicine, Department of Stem Cell Transplantation & Cellular Therapy
The University of Texas MD Anderson Cancer Center
Houston, TX
USA

Virgil Craig Jordan, OBE, PhD, DSc, FMedSci
Professor of Breast Medical Oncology and Professor of Molecular and Cellular Oncology
The University of Texas MD Anderson Cancer Center
Houston, TX
USA

Roshni D. Kalachand, MBBCh, MD
Specialist Registrar in Medical Oncology
Beaumont Hospital and Royal College of Surgeons
Dublin
Ireland

Hagop M. Kantarjian, MD
Professor and Chairman, Department of Leukemia
The University of Texas MD Anderson Cancer Center
Houston, TX
USA

Michael Karin, PhD
Distinguished Professor of Pharmacology
Pharmacology
University of California, San Diego
La Jolla, CA
USA

Ahmed O. Kaseb, MD
Associate Professor, Department of Gastrointestinal (GI) Medical Oncology, Division of Cancer Medicine
The University of Texas MD Anderson Cancer Center
Houston, TX
USA

Richard M. Kaufman, MD
Assistant Professor of Pathology
Harvard Medical School
Medical Director, Adult Transfusion Service
Brigham and Women's Hospital
Boston, MA
USA

Ronan J. Kelly, MD
Director of the Gastroesophageal Cancer Therapeutics Program
Johns Hopkins University School of Medicine
Baltimore, MD
USA

Robert S. Kerbel, PhD
Senior Scientist, Biological Sciences Platform
Sunnybrook Research Institute
Professor, Department of Medical Biophysics
University of Toronto
Toronto, ON
Canada

Merrill S. Kies, MD
Professor of Medicine
Department of Thoracic–Head and Neck Medical Oncology
The University of Texas MD Anderson Cancer Center
Houston, TX
USA

Youn H. Kim, MD
The Joanne and Peter Haas, Jr., Professor for Cutaneous Lymphoma Research
Department of Dermatology
Stanford University
Stanford, CA
USA

Jeri Kim, MD
Associate Professor, Department of Genitourinary Medical Oncology, Division of Cancer Medicine
The University of Texas MD Anderson Cancer Center
Houston, TX
USA

Catherine E. Klein, MD
Professor of Medicine
Division of Medical Oncology
University of Colorado
Aurora, CO

Chief, Hematology/Oncology
Eastern Colorado Health Care
Denver Veterans Affairs
Denver, CO
USA

Justin M. Ko, MD, MBA, FAAD
Clinical Associate Professor, Dermatology
Stanford Medical
Redwood City, CA
USA

Christian Kollmannsberger, MD, FRCPC
Clinical Associate Professor of Medicine
Division of Medical Oncology
University of British Columbia
BCCA Vancouver Cancer Centre
Vancouver, BC
Canada

Ritsuko K. Komaki, MD
Professor
Department of Radiation Oncology
The University of Texas MD Anderson Cancer Center
Houston, TX
USA

Scott Kopetz, MD, PhD
Associate Professor, GI Medical Oncology
The University of Texas MD Anderson Cancer Center
Houston, TX
USA

Michael Kroll, MD
Professor
Department of Pulmonary Medicine
The University of Texas MD Anderson Cancer Center
Houston, TX
USA

Deborah Kuban, MD, FACR, FASTRO
Professor, Department of Radiation Oncology
The University of Texas MD Anderson Cancer Center
Houston, TX
USA

Donald W. Kufe, MD
Distinguished Physician, Dana-Farber Cancer Institute
Professor of Medicine, Harvard Medical School
Leader, Translational Pharmacology and Early Therapeutic Trials Program
Dana-Farber/Harvard Cancer Center
Boston, MA
USA

Anita Kumar, MD
Assistant Attending, Lymphoma Service
Department of Medicine
Memorial Sloan-Kettering Cancer Center and
Instructor of Clinical Medicine
Weill Cornell Medical College
New York, NY
USA

Michael E. Kupferman, MD
Associate Professor
Department of Head and Neck Surgery
The University of Texas MD Anderson Cancer Center
Houston, TX
USA

Ann S. LaCasce, MD
Assistant Professor of Medicine
Harvard Medical School
Boston, MA
USA

Stephen Y. Lai, MD, PhD
Associate Professor
Department of Head and Neck Surgery
The University of Texas MD Anderson Cancer Center
Houston, TX
USA

Raymond S. Lance, MD
Urologist
Deaconess Medical Center-Spokane
Spokane, WA
USA

Robert S. Langer, ScD
David H. Koch Institute Professor
Department of Chemical Engineering
Massachusetts Institute of Technology
Cambridge, MA
USA

Peter F. Lebowitz, MD, PhD
Global Therapeutic Area Head, Oncology
Janssen Research & Development, LLC.
Raritan, NJ
USA

Michelle M. Le Beau, PhD
Arthur and Marian Edelstein Professor of Medicine
Director, University of Chicago Comprehensive Cancer Center
Chicago, IL
USA

J. Jack Lee, PhD, MS, DDS
Associate Vice Provost, Quantitative Research
The University of Texas MD Anderson Cancer Center
Houston, TX
USA

Richard T. Lee, MD
Assistant Professor
Department of Medicine
University Hospitals and Case Western Reserve University
Cleveland, OH
USA

Donghui Li, PhD
Professor of Medicine
Department of Gastrointestinal Medical Oncology
The University of Texas MD Anderson Cancer Center
Houston, TX
USA

Scott M. Lippman, MD
Professor
Moores Cancer Center
University of California San Diego
La Jolla, CA
USA

Virginia R. Litle, MD
Associate Professor of Surgery
Boston University School of Medicine
Boston, MA
USA

Jennifer K. Litton, MD
Associate Professor
Breast Medical Oncology
The University of Texas MD Anderson Cancer Center
Houston, TX
USA

Danny Liu
Research Assistant
Brigham and Women's Hospital
Harvard Medical School
Boston, MA
USA

Yanlan Liu, PhD
Post-doctoral Researcher
Brigham and Women's Hospital
Harvard Medical School
Boston, MA
USA

Christopher J. Logothetis, MD
Chairman & Professor
Genitourinary Medical Oncology
The University of Texas MD Anderson Cancer Center
Houston, TX
USA

Gabriel Lopez, MD
Assistant Professor
Department of Palliative, Rehabilitation and Integrative Medicine
The University of Texas MD Anderson Cancer Center
Houston, TX
USA

Charles Lu, MD, SM
Professor, Department of Thoracic/Head and Neck Medical Oncology, Division of Cancer Medicine
The University of Texas MD Anderson Cancer Center
Houston, TX
USA

Karen Lu, MD
Chair, Department of Gynecologic Oncology and Reproductive Medicine, Division of Surgery
The University of Texas MD Anderson Cancer Center
Houston, TX
USA

Guishuai Lv, MD
Research Assistant
International Lab on Signaling Transduction
Eastern Hepatobiliary Surgery Hospital
Shanghai
China

Donald F. Lynch, Jr., MD
Urologist
Eastern Virginia Medical School
Norfolk, VA
USA

Anirban Maitra, MD
Professor of Pathology
Department of Pathology
The University of Texas MD Anderson Cancer Center
Houston, TX
USA

Melanie Majure, MD
HS Clinical Instructor
UCSF School of Medicine
San Francisco, CA
USA

Robert G. Maki, MD, PhD, FACP
Professor of Medicine, Pediatrics, and Orthopaedics
Mount Sinai Medical School
New York, NY
USA

Shan Man, BSc
Senior Technician/Lab Manager
Biological Sciences Platform
Sunnybrook Research Institute
Toronto, ON
Canada

Alberto M. Marchevsky, MD
Director, Pulmonary and Mediastinal Pathology
Cedars-Sinai Medical Center
West Hollywood, CA
USA

Kim A. Margolin, MD
Director, Multi-disciplinary Melanoma Program
City of Hope Department of Medical Oncology and Comprehensive Cancer Center
Duarte, California
USA

Megan E. McNerney, MD, PhD
Assistant Professor of Pathology
Department of Pathology
University of Chicago
Chicago, IL
USA

Jeffrey I. Mechanick, MD
Clinical Professor of Medicine
Division of Endocrinology, Diabetes, and Bone Disease
Icahn School of Medicine at Mount Sinai
New York, NY
USA

Stephanie C. Melkonian, PhD
Postdoctoral Research Fellow
Department of Epidemiology
The University of Texas MD Anderson Cancer Center
Houston, TX
USA

Ilgen Mender, PhD
Postdoctoral Researcher
Department of Cell Biology
The University of Texas Southwestern Medical Center
Dallas, TX
USA

Department of Biochemistry
Faculty of Medicine, Hacettepe University
Ankara
Turkey

Matthew Meyerson, MD, PhD
Professor
Department of Pathology
Dana-Farber Cancer Institute
Boston, MA
USA

Eric A. Millican, MD
Fellow, Procedural Dermatology
Vanderbilt University
Nashville, TN
USA

Gordon B. Mills, MD, PhD
Professor
Department of Systems Biology
The University of Texas MD Anderson Cancer Center
Houston, TX
USA

Bruce D. Minsky, MD
Professor of Radiation Oncology
Frank T. McGraw Memorial Chair
Department of Radiation Oncology
The University of Texas MD Anderson Cancer Center
Houston, TX
USA

David L. Mitchell, PhD
Professor
Department of Carcinogenesis
Science Park-Research Division
Department of Carcinogenesis
The University of Texas MD Anderson Cancer Center
Smithville, TX
USA

Francesca Molinari, PhD
Scientific collaborator
Laboratory of Molecular Pathology
Institute of Pathology
Locarno
Switzerland

Daniel Morgensztern, MD
Associate Professor
Department of Medicine, Division of Medical Oncology
Washington University School of Medicine St. Louis
Missouri, MO
USA

Rodolfo C. Morice, MD
Professor
Department of Pulmonary Medicine
The University of Texas MD Anderson Cancer Center
Houston, TX
USA

Donald L. Morton, MD, FACS (deceased)
Chief of the Melanoma Program and Co-Director of the Surgical Oncology Fellowship Program
John Wayne Cancer Institute (JWCI)
Santa Monica, CA
USA

Jeffrey A. Moscow, MD
Pediatric Hematologist-Oncologist
Senior Investigator, National Cancer Institute
Bethesda, MD
USA

Judy S. Moyes, MA (Cantab), MB, BChir, FRCPC, FRCPCH
Technical Writer
Pediatrics Research
The University of Texas MD Anderson Cancer Center
Houston, TX
USA

Mariela Blum Murphy, MD
Assistant Professor
Department of Gastrointestinal Medical Oncology
The University of Texas MD Anderson Cancer Center
Houston, TX
USA

Muhammed Murtaza, MBBS, PhD
Assistant Professor
Co-Director, Center for Noninvasive Diagnostics
Translational Genomics Research Institute
Phoenix, AZ
USA

Hyman B. Muss, MD
Mary Jones Hudson Distinguished Professorship in Geriatric Oncology
School of Medicine
UNC-Chapel Hill
Chapel Hill, NC
USA

Serge Patrick Nana-Sinkam, MD
Associate Professor
Division of Pulmonary, Allergy, Critical Care and Sleep Medicine
Department of Molecular Virology, Immunology & Medical Genetics
James Comprehensive Cancer Center
The Ohio State University
Columbus, OH
USA

Vignesh Narayanan, MD
Fellow, Hematology-Oncology
University of Colorado
Aurora, CO
USA

Victor A. Neel, MD, PhD
Assistant Professor, Department of Dermatology
Harvard Medical School
Boston, MA
USA

Lior Nesher, MD
Infectious Disease Institute
Soroka University Medical Center
Senior lecturer, Faculty of Health Sciences
Ben-Gurion University of the Negev
Beersheba
Israel

Craig R. Nichols, MD
Director-Testicular Cancer Commons
Co-Director Testicular Cancer Multidisciplinary Clinic
Virginia Mason Medical Center
Seattle, WA
USA

Monique Nilsson, PhD
Senior Research Scientist, Department of Thoracic Head and Neck
The University of Texas MD Anderson Cancer Center
Houston, TX
USA

Larry Norton, MD
Deputy Physician-in-Chief for Breast Cancer Programs
Memorial Sloan Kettering Cancer Center
New York, NY
USA

Daniel P. Nussbaum, MD
Resident, General Surgery
Department of Pharmacology and Cancer Biology
Duke University Medical Center
Durham, NC
USA

Susan O'Brien, MD
Professor
Department of Leukemia
Division of Cancer Medicine
The University of Texas MD Anderson Cancer Center
Houston, TX
USA

Takao Ohnuma, MD, PhD
Professor of Medicine
Division of Hematology and Oncology
Tisch Cancer Institute
Icahn School of Medicine at Mount Sinai
New York, NY
USA

Amir Onn, MD
Head, Institute of Pulmonary Medicine
Sheba Medical Center
Ramat Gan
Israel

Susana Ortiz-Urda, MD, PhD, MBA
Assistant Professor
Department of Dermatology
University of California
San Francisco, CA
USA

Brian O'Sullivan, MD, FRCPI, FRCPC
Professor, Department of Radiation Oncology
University of Toronto
Head, Radiation Oncology Sarcoma Site Group
Princess Margaret Cancer Centre
Toronto, ON
Canada

Jamie S. Ostroff, PhD
Chief, Behavioral Sciences Service
Director, Tobacco Treatment Program
Memorial Sloan Kettering Cancer Center
New York, NY
USA

Marta Paez-Ribes, PhD
Research Associate
Department of Pathology
University of Cambridge
Cambridge
UK

Margaret Pain, MD
Neurosurgical Resident
Icahn School of Medicine at Mount Sinai
New York, NY
USA

Ben Ho Park, MD, PhD
Professor, Department of Oncology, Johns Hopkins University
Professor of Oncology, Breast and Ovarian Cancer Program
Associate Director, Hematology/Oncology Fellowship Training Program
Associate Director for Research Training and Education
The Sidney Kimmel Comprehensive Cancer Center at Johns Hopkins
Baltimore, MD
USA

Harvey I. Pass, MD
Stephen E. Banner Professor of Thoracic Oncology
Professor of Surgery and Cardiothoracic Surgery
Director, General Thoracic Division
Chief, Thoracic Oncology
NYU Langone Medical Center
New York, NY
USA

Anisha B. Patel, MD
Assistant Professor of Dermatology
The University of Texas MD Anderson Cancer Center
Houston, TX
USA

Krina K. Patel, MD
Assistant Professor
Stem Cell Transplantation and Cellular Therapy
The University of Texas MD Anderson Cancer Center
Houston, TX
USA

Natalya N. Pavlova, PhD
Postdoctoral Research Fellow
Cancer Biology and Genetics Program
Memorial Sloan Kettering Cancer Center
New York, NY
USA

Karl Peggs, MD, MA, MRCP, FRCPath
Senior Lecturer in Stem Cell Transplantation and Immunotherapy
University College Hospital London
London
UK

Errol J. Philip, PhD
Chief Clinical Research Fellow in the Department of Psychiatry and Behavioral Sciences
Memorial Sloan Kettering Cancer Center
New York, NY
USA

Martine Piccart-Gebhart, MD, PhD
Professor of Oncology
Université Libre de Bruxelles (ULB)
Head of the Medicine Department
Jules Bordet Institute
Brussels
Belgium

Marco A. Pierotti, PhD
Scientific Directorate
Fondazione Istituto Ricerche Pediatriche Città della Speranza
Padova
Italy

Head
Molecular Genetics of Cancer Unit
Fondazione Istituto FIRC di Oncologia Molecolare
Milan
Italy

Raphael E. Pollock, MD, PhD, FACS
Professor and Director, Division of Surgical Oncology
Surgeon in Chief, James Comprehensive Cancer Center
Surgeon in Chief, The Ohio State University Health System
The Ohio State University Wexner Medical Center
Columbus, OH
USA

Yves Pommier, MD, PhD
Chief
Developmental Therapeutics Branch, National Cancer Institute, National Institutes of Health
Bethesda, MD
USA

Carol S. Portlock, MD
Attending Physician
Lymphoma Service, Department of Medicine
Memorial Sloan-Kettering Cancer Center and
Professor of Clinical Medicine
Weill Cornell Medical College
New York, NY
USA

Kalmon D. Post, MD, FACS, FAANS
Chairman Emeritus Department Neurosurgery
Professor Neurosurgery & Medicine
Icahn School of Medicine at Mount Sinai
Program Director Department Neurosurgery
Mount Sinai Health System
New York, NY
USA

Selvaraj E. Pravinkumar, MD, FRCP
Associate Professor
Department of Critical Care
The University of Texas MD Anderson Cancer Center
Houston, TX
USA

Nathan D. Price, PhD
Professor and Associate Director
Institute for Systems Biology
Seattle, WA
USA

Xia Pu, PhD
Instructor
Department of Epidemiology
The University of Texas MD Anderson Cancer Center
Houston, TX
USA

Sergio Quezada, PhD
Professorial Research Fellow
UCL Cancer Institute
London
UK

Derek Raghavan, MD, PhD, FACP, FRACP, FASCO
President, Levine Cancer Institute &
Professor-Medicine, UNC School of Medicine,
Charlotte Campus, Carolinas HealthCare System
Charlotte, NC
USA

Kristjan T. Ragnarsson, MD
Professor and Chairman
Department of Rehabilitation Medicine
Icahn School of Medicine at Mount Sinai
New York, NY
USA

Jamal Rahaman, MD
Associate Clinical Professor
The Mount Sinai Hospital
New York, NY
USA

Kanti R. Rai, MD
Professor of Medicine and Professor of Molecular Medicine
Joel Finkelstein Cancer Foundation
Hofstra Northwell School of Medicine
New Hyde Park, NY
USA

Noopur Raje, MD
Director, Center for Multiple Myeloma
Rita Kelley Chair in Oncology
Massachusetts General Hospital Cancer Center
Associate Professor of Medicine
Harvard Medical School
Boston, MA
USA

Pilar Ramos, PhD
Postdoctoral Fellow
Integrated Cancer Genomics Division
Translational Genomics Research Institute
Phoenix, AZ
USA

Jacob H. Rand, MD
Hematologist
Montefiore Medical Center
Bronx, NY
USA

Mark J. Ratain, MD
Leon O. Jacobson Professor of Medicine
Department of Medicine and Committee on Clinical Pharmacology and Pharmacogenomics
University of Chicago
Chicago, IL
USA

Chandrajit P. Raut, MD, MSc, FACS
Associate Surgeon, General and Gastrointestinal Surgery
Brigham and Women's Hospital
Harvard Medical School
Boston, MA
USA

John C. Reed, MD, PhD
Pharmaceutical Research & Early Development
Roche Innovation Center
Basel
Switzerland

Marvin S. Reitz, PhD
Adjunct Professor
School of Medicine
Institute of Human Virology
Baltimore, MD
USA

David C. Rice, MB, BCh, BAO, FRCSI
Professor
Department of Thoracic and Cardiovascular Surgery
Division of Surgery
The University of Texas MD Anderson Cancer Center
Houston, TX
USA

Stephen B. Riggs, MD
Attending Surgeon, Department of Urology and Levine Cancer Institute
Carolinas HealthCare System
Charlotte, NC
USA

Brian I. Rini, MD, FACP
Professor of Medicine
Department of Solid Tumor Oncology
Cleveland Clinic Taussig Cancer Institute
Cleveland, OH
USA

Ana M. Rodriguez, MD, MPH, FACOG
Assistant Professor
Department of Obstetrics & Gynecology
University of Texas Medical Branch
Galveston, TX
USA

Kenneth V. I. Rolston, MD, FACP
Adjunct Professor, Department of Medicine/Infectious Diseases Section
The University of Texas MD Anderson Cancer Center
Houston, TX
USA

Bruce J. Roth, MD
Professor of Medicine
Division of Oncology, Section of Medical Oncology
Washington University School of Medicine
Missouri, MO
USA

Jacob Rotmensch, MD
Oncologist
Department of Gynecologic Oncology
Rush University Medical Center
Chicago, IL
USA

Eric K. Rowinsky, MD
Adjunct Professor, Department of Medicine
NYU School of Medicine
New York, NY
USA

Julia H. Rowland, PhD
Director, Office of Cancer Survivorship
Division of Cancer Control and Population Sciences, National Cancer Institute, NIH-DHHS
Bethesda, MD
USA

Hope S. Rugo, MD
Clinical Professor, Department of Medicine (Hematology/Oncology)
University of California San Francisco School of Medicine
San Francisco, CA
USA

Rachel A. Sanford, MD
Fellow, Division of Cancer Medicine Fellowship Program
The University of Texas MD Anderson Cancer Center
Houston, TX
USA

David T. Scadden, MD
Massachusetts General Hospital
Director, MGH Center for Regenerative Medicine
Boston, MA
USA

Amy C. Schefler, MD, FACS
Attending
Retina Consultants of Houston
Houston, TX
USA

Charles A. Schiffer, MD
Professor of Medicine and Oncology
Joseph Dresner Chair for Hematologic Malignancies
Department of Oncology
Karmanos Cancer Center
Wayne State University School of Medicine
Detroit, MI
USA

Jeffery Schlom, PhD
Chief
Laboratory of Tumor Immunology and Biology
National Cancer Institute
National Institutes of Health
Bethesda, MD
USA

Carl Schmidt, MD
Associate Professor
Department of Surgery
The Ohio State University Wexner Medical Center
Columbus, OH
USA

Leslie R. Schover, PhD
Professor of Behavioral Science
The University of Texas MD Anderson Cancer Center
Houston, TX
USA

Lawrence H. Schwartz, MD
James Picker Professor of Radiology
Department of Radiology
University of Columbia
Columbia, OH
USA

Aleksandar Sekulic, MD, PhD
Associate Professor of Dermatology
Vice Chair, Department of Dermatology
Chair, Cutaneous Oncology Disease Group
Mayo Clinic Arizona
Scottsdale, AZ
USA

Boris Sepesi, MD
Assistant Professor
Thoracic and Cardiovascular Surgery
The University of Texas MD Anderson Cancer Center
Houston, TX
USA

Vickie R. Shannon, MD
Professor
Department of Pulmonary Medicine
The University of Texas MD Anderson Cancer Center
Houston, TX
USA

Padmanee Sharma, MD, PhD
Professor, Department of Genitourinary Medical Oncology, Division of Cancer Medicine
The University of Texas MD Anderson Cancer Center
Houston, TX
USA

Manish R. Sharma, MD
Assistant Professor of Medicine
Department of Medicine and Committee on Clinical Pharmacology and Pharmacogenomics
University of Chicago
Chicago, IL
USA

Jerry W. Shay, PhD
Professor, Department of Cell Biology
UT Southwestern Medical Center
Dallas, TX
USA

Professor
Center for Excellence in Genomics Medicine Research
King Abdulaziz University
Jeddah
Saudi Arabia

Steven I. Sherman, MD
Associate Vice Provost, Clinical Research
Chair and Naguib Samaan Distinguished Professor in Endocrinology
Department of Endocrine Neoplasia and Hormonal Disorders
The University of Texas MD Anderson Cancer Center
Houston, TX
USA

Jinjun Shi, PhD
Assistant Professor of Anaesthesia
Department of Anaesthesia
Brigham and Women's Hospital
Harvard Medical School
Boston, MA
USA

Junichi Shindoh, MD, PhD
Associate Professor
Department of Hepatobiliary and Pancreatic Surgery
The University of Tokyo
Tokyo
Japan

Elizabeth Shpall, MD
Professor, Department of Stem Cell Transplantation and Cellular Therapy
The University of Texas MD Anderson Cancer Center
Houston, TX
USA

Zahid H. Siddik, PhD
Professor of Medicine (Pharmacology)
The University of Texas MD Anderson Cancer Center
Houston, TX
USA

Branimir I. Sikic, MD
Professor of Medicine (Oncology)
Stanford Medicine
Stanford, CA
USA

Richard T. Silver, MD
Professor of Medicine, Division of Hematology-Oncology
Department of Medicine
Weill Cornell Medical College
New York, NY
USA

Lewis R. Silverman, MD
Associate Professor
Department of Medicine, Hematology and Medical Oncology
Mount Sinai Hospital
New York, NY
USA

Richard Simon, DSc
Associate Director
Division of Cancer Treatment and Diagnosis
National Cancer Institute
Bethesda, MD
USA

Cardinale B. Smith, MD, MSCR
Assistant Professor of Medicine
Associate Program Director of Research, Internal Medicine Residency
Division of Hematology/Medical Oncology and Brookdale Department of Geriatrics and Palliative Medicine
Icahn School of Medicine at Mount Sinai
New York, NY
USA

Vernon K. Sondak, MD
Chief of the Division of Cutaneous Oncology and Director of Surgical Education
H. Lee Moffitt Cancer Center and Research Institute
Tampa, FL
USA

Stephen T. Sonis, DMD, DMSc
Clinical Professor of Oral Medicine and Diagnostic Sciences
Harvard School of Dental Medicine
Brigham and Women's Hospital
Boston, MA
USA

Gabriella Sozzi, PhD
Head
Tumor Genomics Unit
Department of Experimental Oncology and Molecular Medicine
Fondazione IRCCS Istituto Nazionale dei Tumori
Milan
Italy

Margaret R. Spitz, MD, MPH
Professor
Dan L. Duncan Cancer Center
Baylor College of Medicine
Houston, TX
USA

William G. Stebbins, MD
Assistant Professor of Dermatology
Vanderbilt University
Nashville, TN
USA

Richard M. Stone, MD
Chief of Staff
Program Director, Adult Leukemia
Professor of Medicine
Harvard Medical School Center/Program
Boston, MA
USA

Michael D. Stubblefield, MD
National Medical Director for Cancer Rehabilitation
Select Medical
Medical Director for Cancer Rehabilitation
Kessler Institute for Rehabilitation
West Orange, NJ
USA

Sumit K. Subudhi, MD, PhD
Assistant Professor
Department of Genitourinary Medical Oncology
Division of Cancer Medicine
The University of Texas MD Anderson Cancer Center
Houston, TX
USA

Zhifei Sun, MD
Research Assistant
Department of Leukemia
University of Texas Medical Center
Dallas, TX
USA

Max W. Sung, MD
Associate Professor of Medicine, Hematology and Medical Oncology
The Mount Sinai Hospital
New York, NY
USA

Thomas Suter, MD
Professor of Medicine
Department of Cardiology
University Hospital Bern
Basel
Switzerland

Susan M. Swetter, MD
Professor of Dermatology
Palo Alto Veterans Affairs Health Care System and the Stanford University Medical Center
Stanford, CA
USA

Stephen G. Swisher, MD, FACS
Division Head, Division of Surgery
The University of Texas MD Anderson Cancer Center
Houston, TX
USA

Chris H. Takimoto, MD, PhD, FACP
Vice President, Translational Medicine Early Development
Janssen Research & Development, LLC.
Raritan, NJ
USA

Kenneth K. Tanabe, MD, FACS
Associate Professor
Director, Mesothelioma Program
Director, Thoracic Chemo-Radiation Program
The University of Texas MD Anderson Cancer Center
Department of Thoracic-Head & Neck Medical Oncology
Houston, TX
USA

Koji Taniguchi, MD, PhD
Assistant Project Scientist
Pharmacology
University of California, San Diego
La Jolla, CA
USA

Nizar M. Tannir, MD, FACP
Professor and Deputy Chairman
Department of Genitourinary Medical Oncology
The University of Texas MD Anderson Cancer Center
Houston, TX
USA

Haruko Tashiro, MD, PhD
Post-doctoral fellow
Baylor College of Medicine
Houston, TX
USA

Ayalew Tefferi, MD
Professor of Medicine and Hematology
Department of Internal Medicine Mayo Clinic
Rochester, MN
USA

Anish Thomas, MBBS, MD
Staff Clinician
Thoracic and Gastrointestinal Oncology Branch, Center for Cancer Research
National Cancer Institute
National Institutes of Health
Bethesda, MD
USA

Melanie B. Thomas, MD, MS
Associate Center Director for Experimental Therapeutics
Gibbs Cancer Center & Research Institute – Spartanburg
Spartanburg, SC
USA

David C. Thomas, MD, MHPE
Professor of Medicine, Medical Education and Rehabilitation Medicine
Vice Chair for Education
Samuel Bronfman Department of Medicine

Associate Dean for CME
Icahn School of Medicine at Mount Sinai
New York, NY
USA

Craig B. Thompson, MD
President and CEO-Member
Cancer Biology and Genetics Program
Memorial Sloan Kettering Cancer Center
New York, NY
USA

Jelena Todoric, MD, PhD
Postdoctoral Researcher
Pharmacology
University of California, San Diego
La Jolla, CA
USA

Jeffrey M. Trent, PhD
Professor
Integrated Cancer Genomics Division
Translational Genomics Research Institute
Phoenix, AZ
USA

Susan Tsai, MD
Assistant Professor of Surgery
Department of Surgery
Medical College of Wisconsin
Milwaukee, WI
USA

Anne S. Tsao, MD
Associate Professor
Department of Thoracic-Head & Neck Medical Oncology
The University of Texas MD Anderson Cancer Center
Houston, TX
USA

David A. Tuveson, MD, PhD
Professor
Cold Spring Harbor Laboratory
Cold Spring Harbor, NY
USA

Douglas S. Tyler, MD
John Woods Harris Distinguished Chair in Surgery
University of Texas Medical Branch
Galveston, TX
USA

Marc Uemura, MD
Fellow in Hematology and Medical Oncology
Anderson Cancer Center
Houston, TX
USA

Atsushi Umemura, MD, PhD
Assistant Professor
Department of Molecular Gastroenterology and Hepatology, Graduate School of Medical Science
Kyoto Prefectural University of Medicine
Kyoto
Japan

David J. Vander Weele, MD, PhD
Section of Hematology-Oncology, Department of Medicine
Comprehensive Cancer Center
University of Chicago
Chicago, IL
USA

Ara A. Vaporciyan, MD
Professor and Chairman
Director of Clinical Education and Training
Department of Thoracic and Cardiovascular Surgery
M.G. & Lillie A. Johnson Chair for Cancer Treatment & Research
The University of Texas MD Anderson Cancer Center
Houston, TX
USA

Jean-Nicolas Vauthey, MD
Professor, Department Surgical Oncology
Chief, Hepato-Pancreato-Biliary Section
The University of Texas MD Anderson Cancer Center
Houston, TX
USA

Michael A. Via, MD
Assistant Professor of Medicine
Associate Fellowship Director
Director of Metabolic Support
Division of Endocrinology, Diabetes, and Bone Disease
Mount Sinai Beth Israel Medical Center
Icahn School of Medicine at Mount Sinai
New York, NY
USA

Srinivas R. Viswanathan, MD, PhD
Director
Department of Gynecologic Radiation Oncology
Dana-Farber Cancer Institute
Boston, MA
USA

Bert Vogelstein, MD
Professor, Department of Oncology
Johns Hopkins University
Baltimore, MD
USA

Daniel D. Von Hoff, MD, FACP
Director, AHSC Cancer Therapeutics Program
Department of Medicine
University of Arizona College of Medicine
Physician in Chief and Distinguished Professor
Translational Genomics Research Institute
Phoenix, AZ
USA

Evan Vosburgh, MD
Clinical Associate Professor of Medicine
Department of Medicine
Yale University School of Medicine
New Haven, CT
USA

Michael J. Wallace, MD
Professor
Department of Interventional Radiology
The University of Texas MD Anderson Cancer Center
Houston, TX
USA

Hongyang Wang, MD
Professor and Director
National Center for Liver Cancer
China

Eastern Hepatobiliary Surgery Hospital
Shanghai
China

Ralph R. Weichselbaum, MD
Daniel K. Ludwig Distinguished Service Professor of Radiation and Cellular Oncology
Chair, Department of Radiation and Cellular Oncology
University of Chicago
Hospital Director, Chicago Tumor Institute
Chicago, IL
USA

Robert A. Weinberg, PhD
Professor of Biology
Whitehead Institute
Massachusetts Institute of Technology
Cambridge, MA
USA

John N. Weinstein, MD, PhD
Professor and Chair, Department of Bioinformatics and Computational Biology, Division of Quantitative Sciences
The University of Texas MD Anderson Cancer Center
Houston, TX
USA

Ainsley Weston, PhD
Associate Director for Science
Division of Respiratory Disease Studies
Centers for Disease Control and Prevention (CDC)
Morgantown, WV
USA

Max S. Wicha, MD
Madeline and Sidney Forbes Professor of Oncology
University of Michigan Comprehensive Cancer Center
Ann Arbor, MI
USA

Talia W. Wiesel, PhD
Assistant Professor
Psychiatry
Icahn School of Medicine at Mount Sinai
New York, NY
USA

Christopher P. Wild, PhD
Director, International Agency for Research on Cancer
Lyon
France

William N. William, Jr., MD
Associate Professor
Department of Thoracic / Head and Neck Medical Oncology
The University of Texas MD Anderson Cancer Center
Houston, TX
USA

Ignacio I. Wistuba, MD
Professor and Chair
Department of Translational Molecular Pathology
Anderson Clinical Faculty Chair for Cancer Treatment and Research
The University of Texas MD Anderson Cancer Center
Houston, TX
USA

Robert A. Wolff, MD
Professor of Medicine
Department of Gastrointestinal Medical Oncology
The University of Texas MD Anderson Cancer Center
Houston, TX
USA

Scott E. Woodman, MD, PhD
Assistant Professor
Department of Melanoma Medical Oncology, Division of Cancer Medicine
The University of Texas MD Anderson Cancer Center
Houston, TX
USA

Woodring E. Wright, MD, PhD
Department of Cell Biology
University of Texas Southwestern Medical Center
Dallas, TX
USA

Xifeng Wu, MD, PhD
Professor and Department Chair
Department of Epidemiology
The University of Texas MD Anderson Cancer Center
Houston, TX
USA

Ping Xu, PhD
Research Associate
Biological Sciences Platform
Sunnybrook Research Institute
Toronto, ON
Canada

Xiao-Jing Yan, MD
Physician and Research Fellow
Shanghai Institute of Hematology
Rui Jin Hospital
Shanghai Jiao Tong University School of Medicine
Shanghai
China

Haining Yang, PhD
Associate Professor
Cancer Biology Program
University of Hawaii Cancer Center
Honolulu, HI
USA

James C. Yao, MD
Professor with Tenure
Department of Gastrointestinal Medical Oncology
The University of Texas MD Anderson Cancer Center
Houston, TX
USA

Andrew J. Yee, MD
Instructor in Medicine
Massachusetts General Hospital Cancer Center
Harvard Medical School
Boston, MA
USA

Sai-Ching Jim Yeung, MD, PhD, FACP
Professor, Department of Emergency Medicine, Division of Internal Medicine
The University of Texas MD Anderson Cancer Center
Professor, Department of Emergency Medicine and Department of Endocrine Neoplasia and Hormonal Disorders
The University of Texas MD Anderson Cancer Center
Houston, TX
USA

Anthony F. Yu, MD
Cardiologist
Memorial Sloan Kettering Cancer Center
Department of Medicine, Cardiology Service
New York, NY
USA

Anna Yuan, DMD
Oral Medicine Fellow
Brigham and Women's Hospital
Boston, MA
USA

Jonathan S. Zager, MD
Professor
Moffitt Cancer Center
Tampa, FL
USA

Michael R. Zalutsky, PhD, MA
Professor of Radiology
Department of Research
Duke University School of Medicine
Durham, NC
USA

Sarina van der Zee, MD
Fellow, The Zena and Michael A. Wiener Cardiovascular Institute
The Mount Sinai Medical Center
New York, NY
USA

Guang-Biao Zhou, MD
Professor of Institute of Zoology
State Key Laboratory of Biomembrane and Membrane Biotechnology
Institute of Zoology
Chinese Academy of Sciences
Beijing
China

Amado Zurita-Saavedra, MD
Assistant Professor, Genitourinary Medical Oncology
The University of Texas MD Anderson Cancer Center
Houston, TX
USA

目录

第一篇

绪　　论

第 1 章　癌症的主要表现

James F. Holland, MD, ScD (hc) ■ Waun Ki Hong, MD, DMSc (Hon) ■ Donald W. Kufe, MD ■ Robert C. Bast Jr., MD ■ William N. Hait, MD, PhD ■ Raphael E. Pollock, MD, PhD, FACS ■ Ralph R. Weichselbaum, MD

概述

癌症在早期是无症状的。然而，当导管受损、癌细胞侵犯到神经纤维并引起疼痛或功能障碍，肿瘤分泌物引起全身症状，如发烧、体重减轻或疲劳，当发生溃疡和出血，或当肿块被发现时，症状就会出现。事实上，癌症可以模拟其他疾病的常见症状，任何持续两周的症状，即使是间歇性的，都有可能是癌症的表现。因此，癌症需要进行鉴别诊断。

癌症是任何动物的任何器官均可发生的多种疾病的集合。癌症的特征即为细胞的增殖，而这类细胞与构成机体器官的细胞有着不同程度的差异。癌细胞的增殖有快有慢，细胞组成的肿块有大有小。癌症实际上是异常细胞的出现和累积，而这类细胞的进化方式不同于普通细胞。因此，癌症不同于肥大和增生，后两者主要是正常细胞的病变。

癌细胞不遵循组织中细胞结构和功能调控的复杂规则。各种各样的细胞和组织和谐共存构成了人类的各种器官，如眼睛、手指或肾脏，每个器官都有其特定的解剖学定位，它们相互协作完成被赋予的任务，这就是我们称之为生命的奇迹。人们也在孜孜不倦地探索多细胞生物中这种精妙调控的机制以解析生命的神奇构造。

癌症不同于其他良性肿瘤中的异常细胞，不会像正常组织细胞那样生长受限。良性肿瘤也会扩增和积聚成团，但不会攻击或侵犯邻近组织。癌细胞积聚而成的新生物可以突破邻近的细胞膜和基底膜间的解剖屏障。通过化学和物理作用的方式，癌细胞植入到正常细胞的间隙，再用类似的方式破坏、取代正常细胞。哺乳动物的胎盘也有类似的行为，但胎盘侵袭的位置和生长都具有自限性。白细胞也会渗出浸润组织，但它们不具有癌症的其他特征。癌细胞对正常的生长限制信号不太敏感或完全不敏感，因此可以进行无限侵袭。

当癌细胞到达循环系统（淋巴管或毛细血管），通常会穿透管壁，这一过程并不完全是偶然的，而是癌症侵袭的一部分。随后，在通过淋巴管或静脉循环被带到远端组织的过程中，癌细胞可能会发生粘连、外渗和定植，从而形成转移灶。如前所述，在缺乏干预的情况下，如果给予足够的时间，癌症的进展几乎会毫无例外地引起解剖学或功能紊乱，最终导致机体死亡。

癌症并非起源于一个具有完全侵袭性的癌细胞。蛋白质合成信号紊乱是常见的癌前病变，几乎都是由脱氧核糖核酸（DNA）转录的核糖核酸（RNA）在质量或数量上的异常引起的。DNA 突变、编码促进增殖重要蛋白质的特定基因过表达，或者抑制细胞生长的蛋白编码基因缺失均可引起上述异常。一些基因也可能发生丢失、移位或扩增。事实上，染色体的异常删失、复制或融合均可能发生。这些 DNA 的异常变化都会导致 RNA 信息异常或失衡，引起蛋白质的性质或数量的差异，从而导致细胞功能紊乱。某些情况下这些功能性异常极其严重，对细胞是致命的，导致细胞启动凋亡程序进行自我清除。在其他非致死的情况下，细胞功能异常会导致疾病，有些疾病会表现出癌症的特征。一系列内因和外因均可引起细胞内基因的突变、过表达或者低表达，继而通过不同的信号通路，使其演变为具有肿瘤表型的细胞。当局限于基底膜的上皮层时，这些细胞被称为原位癌或上皮内瘤变。间质组织中也有可能发生类似的变化，但较难识别。即使癌细胞没有穿透基底膜，未表现出癌细胞的侵袭性，也会出现一系列的分子异常，最终发展为光学下可识别的细胞变化。此外，这些不断演变的癌细胞通常是侵袭性癌症的前体细胞。

在癌症的早期，细胞还处于增殖积累阶段，其症状较为隐匿。随着癌症的进展，由于癌细胞形成肿块的上皮表面溃烂，或受影响的机体结构或器官的功能发生了改变，症状就出现了。但几乎所有癌症能引起的症状，其他非癌性疾病中也会出现。尽管一些症状通常可以用良性疾病来解释，谨慎的临床医生也会将癌症纳入这些症状的鉴别诊断中，因为他们不可能做出从来没有考虑过的诊断。癌症可以发生在任何年龄段。但是，随着年龄增长，机体器官的疾病发生率也随之升高，接触到环境致癌物的风险更高，最初的 DNA 突变发展为侵袭性癌症的机会也更大。因此，年龄是大多数癌症的主要危险因素。

常见的症状，如咽喉痛、流涕或支气管炎，也可能是由咽喉癌、鼻窦癌或支气管癌引起的。事实上，出现这些症状的患者由于医生在鉴别诊断中没有考虑到癌症，也没有进行适当的观察，通常在诊断为癌症前就已经作为良性疾病接受了反复、长期的治疗。癌症的症状，如腹泻、便秘或轻微疼痛，通常看起来很平常；同时也可能是间歇性的，可能会出现短暂的自发缓解，这种现象通常会导致患者和医生误诊。事实上，反复或长期出现某种症状也是良性疾病的常见特征，这大大增加了癌症的隐匿性。

癌症症状可由以下明确的病因引起：

肿瘤可导致重要导管发生部分或者全部梗阻。肿瘤生长到一定程度，会部分或完全堵塞重要的导管。这一症状的典型表现为支气管癌，癌细胞会阻塞部分支气管引起咳嗽，使纤毛清除分泌物的能力下降，部分情况下会导致支气管肺炎。完全支气管阻塞可导致肺不张和慢性肺炎。肿瘤包块压迫或渗透引起的肌肉功能障碍对食管腔的损害会导致吞咽困难，在症状出现的早期，常常被误诊为良性疾病。胃癌很少引起完全梗阻,但会引起其动力学改变。症状可能表现为容易产生饱腹感、厌食、消化不良和恶心。肿瘤引起的横结肠、降结肠、乙状结肠或直肠狭窄可导致排便习惯的改变,包括排便变细、便秘、近端肠蠕动引起的一过性痉挛和/或腹泻。胰头癌或胆管癌而导致的胆总管受损会引起梗阻性黄疸,这一症状在轻微消化不良或不明原因的瘙痒(归因于胆盐淤积)之后也常发生。

腹膜后肿物或膀胱肿瘤压迫输尿管会引起输尿管梗阻,进一步导致输尿管积水和肾积水,通常无症状,或表现为腰部及侧腰的轻度不适,也可能表现为尿路感染。输尿管双侧梗阻则会导致尿毒症,症状复杂多变。尿道在前列腺段狭窄时,表现为尿流减少、膀胱排空不足、尿频、尿急、夜尿,严重时还会导致阻塞性尿路疾病和尿毒症。

由于盲肠、升结肠和膀胱并非实体,且腔径较大,其内的肿瘤通常不会引起梗阻,但会造成正常功能障碍,导致排便排尿习惯改变。触诊或X光发现肿块也是癌症的一种表现,如乳腺癌。肿瘤取代实质器官导致的功能不全是肿块出现的典型症状。原发性肿瘤或更为常见的转移性脑瘤,常因为脑功能异常而被发现。癫痫、麻痹、感觉或协调异常、记忆功能缺陷和性格改变都可能是肿瘤占位的表现。这些症状的出现不仅是因为大脑的一个特殊区域受到了影响,还可能是因为颅骨不能扩张导致了颅内压升高所致。脊髓的类似功能障碍与远端运动和感觉现象可以反映肿瘤占位以及对脊髓或马尾的侵犯情况。原发性或转移性肿瘤占位导致的肝功能异常,常伴有肝内胆管受压,并会引起黄疸。如果肝脏肿瘤过大,会导致消化系统紊乱,疼痛,在上腹部可见并可触及肿块。甲状旁腺癌通常以肿块的形式出现,少量患者实验室检查显示甲状腺功能减退,但肿块在甲状腺功能减退症中极其少见,可用于鉴别诊断。

软组织肉瘤通常表现为可触诊的肿块。睾丸癌通常也表现为肿块,睾丸增大或许不太明显,但触诊时更硬更重。卵巢癌也可作为附件肿块被检出。

当出现肿块或有形态变化的团块时,需要根据临床检查、影像学或活检结果排除癌症。通常大多数脂肪瘤和自检发现的剑状突起在临床上可忽略。明显的乳房肿块,即使是疑似肿块,都需要通过适当的细胞学或组织学检查来评估。以下这些肿块同样需要通过检查进一步确诊,如甲状腺结节、质硬的肿大淋巴结、无感染情况下持续肿大2周的结节、具有黑色素瘤或癌变特点的皮肤肿块,尤其是出现溃烂时,新发的皮下、腹部或阴囊肿块,这些肿块都需要考虑癌症的可能。

皮肤或上皮表面的溃疡可导致失血,成为感染的源头。持续数周或数月的皮肤溃疡也容易被忽视,通常被当作是某次受伤未愈的普通伤口。支气管溃疡可导致咯血,常表现为痰中带血,很少大量出血。任何一种上消化道癌症都可能引起溃疡和出血,出血通常具有缓慢,间歇性,症状隐匿的特点,导致缺铁性贫血。呕血或大量黑便并不多见。盲肠癌和升结肠癌常因溃疡和出血而出现贫血症状。

膀胱癌和肾癌常表现为血尿,有时在尿常规检查中,通过显微镜镜检或由于生化检测异常而偶然发现。肾出血引起的血块可导致输尿管绞痛。血尿症状通常较少预示前列腺癌,但血精症则提示良性或恶性前列腺疾病,因为精囊癌极为罕见。

子宫内膜癌多表现为绝经后阴道出血,但任何正常月经周期外的阴道出血均值得注意。性交中接触性出血提示宫颈溃疡,最常见的原因就是癌症。

疼痛通常被认为是早期癌症的表现,然而事实并非如此。大多数癌症最初是无痛的。当肿瘤侵犯、压迫或牵拉神经时,或当近端平滑肌收缩以试图绕过管道阻塞或功能失调的远端时,疼痛就发生了。大多数自行缓解的短暂疼痛不是由癌症引起的。然而,当不明原因、非典型的疼痛反复出现或持续发生时,就应该考虑将癌症纳入鉴别诊断。新出现的疼痛,即使并不严重也要认真鉴别。腹痛以及与关节疼痛症状不同的骨骼痛值得特别关注,应尽早确定病因。痛性乳房肿块也不应该排除癌症的可能。

体重减轻可能是尚未排查的癌症的早期指征,当伴随轻度不适、乏力、疲劳时,应当特别注意。其他很多疾病也会引起这些常见症状,但不应最后才考虑癌症。如果在初步检查后仍不能确诊,则必须在短期间隔后进行第二次完整病史采集和体格检查。

癌症引起的胸腔、心包或腹腔积液可导致呼吸困难和不适。腹围增大,常伴有不适、少尿、便秘和体重增加,是腹水的主要症状。在胸腔内,支气管肺癌、间皮瘤、转移性乳腺癌或卵巢癌、原发浆膜癌是恶性积液的常见原因。腹水是卵巢癌和浆膜癌的特征性症状。胰腺癌、间皮瘤、腹膜和肝脏的转移癌以及一些非肿瘤性疾病也应进行鉴别诊断。

空腔脏器壁被侵袭导致的穿孔会引起突发疼痛。这种罕见的症状出现时,大多数情况下并不会优先考虑到癌症的可能。由原发或转移性的肺部肿瘤所致的胸膜穿孔会导致气胸,这种急症不太常见。胃癌向横结肠化生,引起腹部轻度不适,这种症状易被误诊或忽视,而后会突然出现腹泻和明显的胃绞痛反射。阑尾癌是一种罕见的肿瘤,常因肿瘤破裂而表现为急性阑尾炎合并腹膜炎。结肠穿孔多由憩室炎引起,而非结肠癌。绒毛膜癌致宫外孕破裂已有报道。食管癌或支气管癌在晚期可能会导致气管食管瘘。

持续一周以上不明原因的发热需考虑癌症的可能。霍奇金病、其他淋巴瘤、急性白血病、肾癌和肝癌均有可能引起发热。某些癌症由于溃疡、阻塞或白细胞生成紊乱而易发生感染。

癌症也可能引起内分泌亢奋综合征。肾上腺功能亢进,初始可表现为多毛症,有可能是肾上腺癌的表现。小细胞肺癌也可导致库欣综合征。甲状旁腺癌很少引起甲状旁腺功能亢进,但卵巢癌和鳞癌可能会引起该症状。分泌甲状腺激素、雌激素、胰岛素、胰高血糖素、醛固酮、肾上腺素或去甲肾上腺素的肿瘤通常是相应内分泌器官的良性肿瘤,但也必须始终将癌症纳入其鉴别诊断。功能性神经内分泌肿瘤可能分泌血清素和其他血管活性物质,导致类癌综合征。

副癌综合征可能是癌症的早期症状。重症肌无力、雷诺综合征、肥大性骨关节病和杵状指以及难治性贫血可分别提示胸腺瘤、骨髓瘤、肺癌和血液恶病质(以及胸腺瘤),因此这些症状的病因必须谨慎判断。

一些肿瘤缺少标志性症状,需通过巴氏涂片、人乳头瘤病毒(HPV)鉴定、乳房X光检查、前列腺特异性抗原检测、结肠镜检查、计算机断层扫描、肺部扫描和全身皮肤检查进行筛查。这些需要借助检测方法才能发现的无症状癌症通常比有典型症状的癌症进展更加缓慢。少数情况下,无症状患者的常规化学或血液学检查数据也能提示癌症或白血病。这些偶然发现的肿瘤也印证了前文提到的观点，即大多数癌症在发病早期是无症状的。

多种疾病、危险因素暴露和生活方式都可导致人群对癌症易感。易感高危人群包括：炎症性肠病、宫颈HPV感染、乙型或丙型肝炎感染的患者；曾接受辐射照射、早期接受过烷基化剂、蒽环类药物或鬼臼毒素衍生物治疗，或接触石棉等特殊环境的人士；吸烟、酗酒或日晒过度的人群；有癌症易感家族史的人群，尤其是其肿瘤具有家族遗传性。以上人群中特定癌症发生的频率显著高于普通人群，需要密切监控。

对癌症的恐惧并不会导致癌症易感。然而，与胃癌相比，胰腺癌更容易发生抑郁，抑郁也有可能是胰腺肿瘤形成的早期症状。

现状

癌症确诊时往往已经错过了容易治愈的早期阶段。癌症的早期症状常被忽视或误诊。影像学、早期手术、激素治疗、化疗和免疫治疗技术的进步降低了乳腺癌的死亡率；病毒鉴定、细胞学和早期治疗降低了宫颈癌的死亡率；结肠镜检查和息肉切除降低了结肠癌的死亡率。其他的筛查项目有望在癌症症状出现之前对其进行诊断。像梅毒一样，癌症取而代之成为症状多变的混淆视听者。许多有症状的癌症患者仍然可以用现有的方法治愈。然而，一旦癌症早期症状出现，拖延治疗有害无益。因此，将癌症纳入鉴别诊断可以挽救更多的生命。

展望未来

基于基因组学和蛋白质组学的诊断技术的发展将为癌症的早期诊断带来新的机遇。实验室方法不仅可以加速临床诊断，基因组和蛋白质组学的发现也会改变我们对癌症进程的理解。这一认识对癌症预防和治疗的影响将是革命性的。未来，在临床症状出现之前，我们就可以借助仪器检测实验室指标从而发现癌症，而通过主要症状来诊断癌症可能会成为历史。实际上，个体的蛋白质谱偏离群体指标并不那么重要，如果偏离了自身健康时的蛋白质谱，则应该引起重视。如果未来要实现癌症的预防和早期诊断，公众的意识和依从性仍是关键的决定因素。

（陈淑桢 译　王红阳 审）

第 2 章　肿瘤的生物学特性

Douglas Hanahan, PhD ■ Robert A. Weinberg, PhD

概述

肿瘤医学的一个难解之谜在于其各个层面的复杂性和多变性。肿瘤的特性为从肿瘤的多样性表现中凝练出疾病的复杂特点提供了一种总体原则，可以帮助人们更好地理解肿瘤。肿瘤的理论模型涉及八种生物学能力（即肿瘤的特性），是癌细胞在长期的肿瘤发生和恶性进展中形成的。癌细胞的两个典型的特点有助于其获得这些生物学能力。这八个显著特性包括：持续的增殖信号、逃避生长抑制、抵抗细胞死亡、实现复制永生化、诱导血管新生、激活侵袭和转移、细胞能量和代谢紊乱，以及逃避免疫清除。基因组的不稳定性及其伴随的基因突变和促肿瘤炎症反应是肿瘤获得这些生物学特征的主要促进因素。这些特征能力的整合涉及"肿瘤微环境"（tumor microenvironment, TME）里的多种细胞类型间的相互作用，肿瘤微环境由肿瘤细胞和肿瘤相关间质组成，肿瘤相关间质包含了三种经典的支持细胞：血管生成细胞（angiogenic vascular cell, AVC）、成纤维细胞的多种亚型和浸润其中的免疫细胞（infiltrating immune cell, IIC）。此外，由于在肿瘤发展过程中，癌细胞要经历各种不同的表型变化及基因多样化的复杂环境，因此构成肿瘤个体的肿瘤细胞本身往往也具有异质性。综上所述，肿瘤的特征——必要的能力及其促进因素——可被用于探索和阐明多种类型人类肿瘤的发生机制和共性，在肿瘤治疗中也具有潜在的应用价值。

从极其复杂的肿瘤表型中提炼共性

正如前一章和这本百科全书式教科书的其他章节所系统描述的那样，癌症的表现形式复杂多样，令人困惑。在遗传学、组织病理学、对系统生理的影响，预后以及对治疗干预的反应等方面，不同部位的肿瘤存在显著的差异，这也是肿瘤学总体上是按器官分门别类的原因，而本书也是按器官特异性对肿瘤进行分类并罗列章节的。

面对肿瘤所表现出的高度多样性和复杂性，人们可能会问：在复杂的遗传和表型掩盖下，是否存在某种潜在的规律（共性机制）适用于多种类别和分型的肿瘤。我们相继在 2000 年和 2011 年提出假设，人类癌症的复杂性反映了机体应对癌症挑战的不同方式，也就是说我们观察到的不同症状的肿瘤性疾病必然需要借助各种策略获得一些共有的特性，以维持细胞长期的异常增殖以及肿瘤细胞群或集中或播散的生长。我们将肿瘤获得的特性称为"肿瘤的特征"[1,2]，并进一步提出肿瘤生长的两个显著特征——癌细胞基因组突变水平的升高和免疫细胞复杂互作所导致的炎症反应，是原发性肿瘤获得必要标志性特征的关键促进因素。我们近来提出的关于癌症的生物学特征理论中的八大特征和两种促进因素都归纳体现在图 2-1 中。

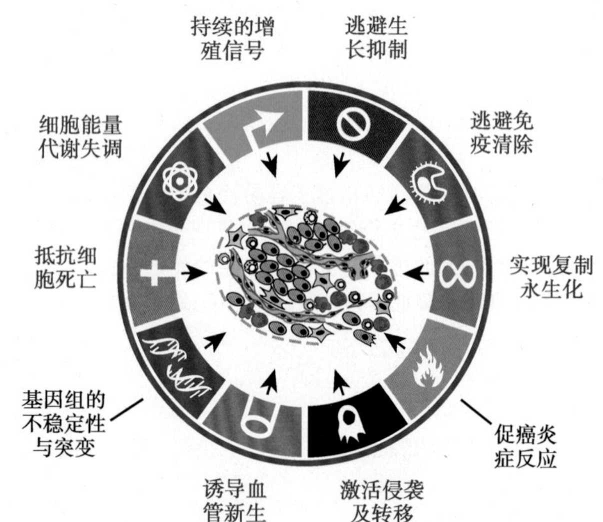

图 2-1　癌症的生物学特性。该示意图说明了恶性疾病发生的必要条件——癌症的特征——包括八种不同的互补功能和两种促进因素（黑色文字）[1,2]。这些特性可能是在癌症的不同发展阶段获得的，不同癌症获得这些特性的机制也相差甚远。癌症病变的两个异常特征参与了肿瘤发生过程中这些特性的获得：基因组的不稳定性和随之发生的调节基因的突变，以及免疫炎性细胞的生理浸润，例如伤口愈合，这两种因素均可促进一种或者多种癌症特性的产生。不同形式的癌症对某种特性的依赖性不同。腺瘤性肿瘤通常缺乏侵袭和转移的能力。白血病可能不需要血管新生或侵袭能力，但是进展到淋巴瘤则同时需要以上两种能力。在某些癌症中，逃避肿瘤免疫可能没那么必要，但我们也日益意识到这种现象是广泛存在的

接下来的章节我们首先描述上述肿瘤病理生理学的 10 个关键因素，再介绍癌细胞如何通过招募正常细胞并以多种方式帮助自身获得上述特性。最后，我们将简要探讨肿瘤特性这一理论的潜在临床意义。如需了解更多的相关细节和背景，读者可参考提出肿瘤特性理论[1,2]的文献和阐述间质细胞在促进肿瘤特性形成中的作用[3]的原始文献。但请读者注意，本篇只将上述 3 篇参考文献中没有引用的最新文献列入在本书的参考文献中。癌症生物学的教科书[4]也可以为本章所概述的癌症发病机制提供更多的细节。

获得的功能体现了癌症的生物学特性

在我们目前的理论体系中，不是每种肿瘤都具备上述 8 种

特性,但在多数人类癌症中这些特性是普遍存在的(图 2-1)。每种特性在辅助肿瘤及其组成细胞的形成、进展和生存上均有不同的作用,下文将简要阐述。

特性 1:持续的增殖信号

癌症的定义标准是机体内正常情况下调控细胞生长的信号发生紊乱并引起的慢性、非正常性的细胞增殖,例如在胚胎发育、生理性增殖和全身稳态维持中协调(短暂的)细胞分裂和增殖的信号出现了失控。这些调控细胞分裂和增殖的信号既有正向调控信号(诱导性信号)也有负向调控信号(抑制性信号)。因此,癌症的第一种特性囊括了一组复杂的感应信号,来指导细胞生长——分裂周期的开始和进展以产生子代细胞。与正常情况下短期的增殖信号激活不同,肿瘤疾病中的增殖刺激信号是长期持续的。

关于持续增殖信号的机制,最被广为接受的理论是癌细胞的基因突变,使其转变为驱动细胞增殖的激活基因。这些被激活的基因被定义为癌基因,使临时的促增殖信号得以持续激活。与正常细胞相比,这些癌基因通常编码结构、功能或丰度改变的蛋白质,从而可以接收细胞外的增殖信号并通过复杂的调节网络在细胞内传递。

肿瘤中突变基因维持增殖信号的典型通路包括表皮生长因子(epidermal growth factor,EGF)受体及其下游 KRAS-RAF-MEK-MAPK 通路,该通路通过一系列蛋白磷酸化,将生长刺激信号传递给核内细胞分裂元件。在多种人类肿瘤中,均发现同一种或几种上述信号通路的蛋白质存在持续激活,包括表皮生长因子受体(EGFR)和相关酪氨酸激酶受体,如 HER2 和 ALK,此类突变会导致下游信号转导分子 KRAS、BRAF 和 MEK 的长期活化。然而,我们注意到有丝分裂主要通路的激活并不完全依赖在肿瘤发生发展中癌细胞获得的基因组的改变。某些情况下,即使没有明显的体细胞基因突变,自分泌(细胞自身刺激)和旁分泌(细胞对细胞的刺激)信号转导网络的表观遗传失调也可为癌细胞提供长期的促生长信号。

特性 2:逃避生长抑制

维持正常细胞中增殖信号平衡的关键在于制动机制,要么阻止增殖信号起始,要么在启动后及时阻断增殖信号启动的细胞分裂过程。编码“制动”蛋白质的基因通常被称为抑癌基因(tumor suppressor gene,TSG)。典型的抑癌基因是细胞生长-分裂周期的直接调控因子,包括视网膜母细胞瘤蛋白(retinoblastoma protein,pRb)和几种细胞周期蛋白依赖性激酶抑制蛋白。分子制动系统自身的活性受控于细胞表面受体转导的胞外促生长和抑生长信号,以及对胞内生理状态的监测,以维持组织稳态和协调短暂的生理性增殖。

以 p53 蛋白为主导的细胞内监测系统确保细胞仅在正常的生理状态下完成增殖和分裂循环。因此,p53 不仅可以检测到细胞基因组未修复的损伤,也可检测到可能损害基因组精准复制、染色体分离和细胞分裂的应激性生理紊乱。随后作为细胞应激警报的响应,p53 激活细胞周期元件的抑制因子。若存在严重的基因组损伤或应激性生理异常,p53 及相关蛋白可诱导程序性细胞死亡——一种抑制细胞增殖极端形式(见下文)。

Rb 和 *p53* 这两种常见抑制通路中的许多基因也被归类为抑癌基因,这些基因的缺失或突变而导致的功能丧失表明其具有抑制增殖的作用,或者通过表观遗传(例如 DNA 和组蛋白甲基化修饰)下调这些基因的表达也可达到类似的效果。因此,*p53* 基因突变出现在约 40% 的人类肿瘤中,而在其余 *p53* 基因未突变的肿瘤中,或多或少都有基因异常或表观遗传改变,也可导致 p53 信号通路异常。

基因组和转录组的分析表明,大多数人类肿瘤的 Rb 和 p53 肿瘤抑制通路均含有基因组或表观遗传缺陷。此外,在大量针对肿瘤起始、生长和恶性进展的癌细胞培养和小鼠模型的功能实验中,研究者们也证实了这些通路中的 TSG 对抑制肿瘤进展至关重要。正常情况下,制动系统通常通过限制细胞无限增殖来维持组织稳态。因此,逃避增殖抑制,确保癌细胞的持续增殖和肿瘤生长不受制动机制控制显然是肿瘤的一种标志性特征。

特性 3:抵抗细胞死亡

机体内还存在另一种抑制细胞异常增殖的机制,即在正常发育和内稳态异常或过剩情况下,胞内信号参与调控细胞程序性死亡。程序性细胞死亡的典型形式是凋亡,即基因编码的程序性细胞碎解、死亡。在多种形式的损伤下,正常细胞可启动凋亡程序,例如:细胞错误定位或异常增殖迁移。当细胞检测到各种异常的、来自细胞的或非细胞的自发信号时,均可触发凋亡程序。

细胞程序性凋亡步骤包括特定的酶(例如半胱天冬酶)导向性降解染色体和其他关键细胞器,细胞固缩和破碎,最后被邻近细胞或组织特异性吞噬细胞吞噬,尤其是巨噬细胞。在哺乳动物组织中,细胞凋亡级联反应可以在不到一个小时内完成,因此即使通过细胞毒性化疗或血管功能不全引起急性缺氧等手段诱导细胞凋亡,在组织切片中依然难以观察到凋亡细胞。

对凋亡小体的快速吞噬可避免将可能触发免疫反应的亚细胞成分释放到组织间隙中,这种“免疫沉默”区别于另一种程序性细胞死亡——坏死性凋亡。长期以来,坏死性凋亡也被称为细胞坏死,即死细胞的被动降解过程,然而,细胞坏死也可以是一种主动的程序化过程,由与凋亡程序不同的细胞调节因子和效应分子调控。多种条件可诱发坏死性凋亡,例如氧气和能量缺乏、病毒感染和炎症[5]。坏死性凋亡(或者被动的坏死)时,细胞破裂释放的内容物和免疫原性细胞碎片会诱发(或加剧)免疫炎症反应,兼有促进和拮抗肿瘤的作用,这点将在下文中讨论。

第三种可诱导的程序性细胞死亡称为自噬,在细胞营养缺乏的条件下,自噬通过降解不太重要的细胞器并回收其组分完成细胞器的循环。因此,自噬帮助细胞获取生存和生长所必需的、无法从周围环境中获得的代谢物和营养物。虽然细胞自噬通常是促进细胞生存的方式,然而,在极端营养缺乏或其他急性细胞应激环境下可能会导致自噬再循环的过度活化,使细胞走上细胞器的补充低于生存所需最低水平的单行道,细胞会发生不同于细胞程序性凋亡和坏死性凋亡的“自噬相关”死亡。换句话说,根据肿瘤细胞的生理状态,自噬可以促进细胞存活并进一步增殖,也可以通过自噬相关细胞死亡来清除肿瘤细胞[6]。

若肿瘤细胞自身及其衍生细胞要维持增殖性扩增并向恶性程度更高的肿瘤表型转化，就必须采取多种方式规避或削弱上述三种细胞死亡的触发机制。

特性 4：实现无限复制

肿瘤细胞持续增殖的第三个固有障碍暗藏在哺乳动物染色体的线性结构中——染色体末端的端粒长度随着细胞分裂次数的增加而逐渐减少，端粒记录了细胞谱系中持续分裂的细胞世代数。端粒由数千个串联拷贝的六核苷酸序列组成，位于每个染色体的末端，与特定的 DNA 结合蛋白结合。这些核蛋白复合物共同作用，保护染色体末端免遭监测 DNA 损伤的 DNA 修复复合体的降解，同时避免裸 DNA 末端催化的染色体端对端融合。

值得注意的是，当端粒重复的数量减少至某一阈值以下时，会触发"保险丝"，p53 抑癌蛋白将会发挥感知 DNA 损伤的作用，介导细胞周期停滞或细胞凋亡。肿瘤细胞通过绕过这些 p53 诱导的抗增殖反应（例如通过 *p53* 基因的失活突变）允许具有较短端粒的癌细胞短暂的规避短端粒检查点并继续增殖。但是端粒 DNA 的持续缩短最终将导致染色体末端的保护性核蛋白帽丧失，使染色体发生端对端融合，并在有丝分裂期间发生"断裂—融合—桥循环"的染色体畸变，最终引起核型混乱导致细胞走向死亡而非分裂。

正常的胚胎和组织干细胞可激活端粒保护及延伸系统，以维持细胞的复制能力，许多发展成熟的肿瘤中的癌细胞则借助这一系统，绕开有丝分裂中端粒截短和端粒功能障碍所造成的有丝分裂抑制。这个系统需要表达一种延伸端粒的酶，即端粒酶。另一种不太常见的维持端粒长度的机制为选择性染色体间重组。因此，癌细胞通过多种方式获得维持其端粒长度的能力，逾越了端粒过短带来的增殖鸿沟，从而获得无限复制潜能（即细胞永生），保障了癌细胞群的持续扩增。

特性 5：诱导血管新生

与正常器官一样，为了维持细胞的活力和增殖，肿瘤需要稳定的氧气、葡萄糖和其他营养素的供应和代谢废物的排出，肿瘤相关脉管系统正起到了这样的作用。临床和实验研究已证实了缺血在正常组织中的危害性：细胞通过不同形式的程序性死亡导致组织和器官的破坏和功能障碍。同样的，通常当扩张中的癌细胞巢距离最近的毛细血管超过 200μm 时，癌细胞会无法获得充足的血源性营养素，其生长便会停止。在许多肿瘤类型中，血管新生的激活有利于癌细胞的增殖。

当细胞处于扩散极限时，会激活临近毛细血管的多种应激反应系统，其中最典型的是缺氧诱导转录因子（hypoxia-inducible transcription factor，HIF），它可以调节数百种基因，包括直接或间接诱导血管新生和适应应激的基因。与缺血组织中的细胞相似，缺乏足够氧气和葡萄糖的癌细胞会死于坏死/坏死性凋亡、程序性细胞凋亡或广泛自噬。这也是多数生长旺盛的肿瘤血管丰富，且伴有持续血管新生的原因。

值得注意的是，肿瘤相关的新生血管通常有异常的形态和功能。肿瘤血管曲折、扩张和渗透性高，具有不稳定的血流模式和没有血流的"死区"，与正常脉管系统中稳定持续的血流形成鲜明对比。此外，不同类型肿瘤的血管分布差异很大，例如肾癌往往高度血管化，而胰腺导管腺癌的新生血管则不明显。

最后，我们注意到，尽管持续血管新生是大多数实体瘤的标志，但某些肿瘤有替代的方法：在某些情况下，肿瘤利用侵袭和转移的特性来接入正常组织的脉管系统。因此，特定类型的癌细胞可以沿着正常组织毛细血管增殖和生长，产生限制在 200μm 扩散半径内的套管。虽然在某些肿瘤（例如胶质母细胞瘤）和对强效血管新生抑制剂有反应的肿瘤中，血管融合很显著，但大多数肿瘤仍依赖于持续的血管新生来维持其侵袭性生长；另外，还有些肿瘤适应了低氧的环境，具有了大多数肿瘤不具备的在低氧环境中存活的能力。

特性 6：激活侵袭和转移能力

上面详述的 5 个特征是癌细胞持续增殖所必需的，第 6 种则不太直观——高度恶性的癌细胞变得具有侵袭性和转移性。侵袭性生长程序使癌细胞入侵邻近的组织、血液和淋巴管内部，借此播散到周围和远处的解剖部位。组织引流的淋巴管系统可以将癌细胞转运到淋巴结，形成转移性生长（淋巴结转移），这些细胞集落反过来可以作为血源播散的源头。直接通过肿瘤血管或间接通过淋巴结进入血流的细胞很快会到达远处器官的微血管中，并通过血管壁渗出到附近的组织实质，这些种子一样的微转移灶在异位组织中或死亡或处于休眠状态，或以极低的效率产生肉眼可见的转移，也就是所谓的"定植"过程。

肿瘤入侵和转移作用的调节极其复杂，涉及细胞的固有程序和组织微环境中辅助细胞的协助。癌细胞内在的典型调节机制是上皮癌细胞的上皮—间质转化（epithelial-mesenchymal transition，EMT），该作用在正常器官起始中发挥细胞转移和组织扩张的作用。肿瘤微环境可以诱导上文所述的缺氧应答系统，并调控肿瘤的侵袭转移，该系统可以激活 HIF（HIF1α 和 HIF2α），从而调控包括 EMT 过程相关基因在内的数百种基因的表达[7,8]。这两种转录调控系统都可以调节血液、淋巴系统和异位组织中促侵袭迁移及细胞存活的基因。

值得注意的是，从肿瘤起始细胞到高侵袭性恶性肿瘤，这种标志性特征的获得可以发生在肿瘤发生和进展的各个阶段。在某些情况下，侵袭和转移的能力出现较晚，反映了癌细胞的遗传或表观遗传的进化过程，只有原发性肿瘤内的少数细胞亚群能够通过进化成为具有侵袭性或转移性的癌细胞。在其他情况下，肿瘤在早期就获得了这种能力，即肿瘤内的许多癌细胞已具备侵袭和转移的能力。此外，有研究表明 EMT 在某些情况下可能出现短暂的激活，有助于细胞的播散和定植，但随后 EMT 在形成的转移灶中又被关闭了[9,10]。目前尚不明确原发性肿瘤是否在进化中主动地选择并获得这些使之受益的侵袭和转移特征；也有可能这些影响肿瘤恶性程度的能力只是整个细胞调节网络激活（例如增殖信号传导、EMT 和 HIF）的副产物——肿瘤细胞选择性地启动这些功能，以帮助癌细胞获得其他标志性特性来促进原发肿瘤的形成。

特性 7：细胞能量和代谢紊乱

大约 90 年前 Otto Warburg 提出了癌症细胞改变能量利用

(特别是葡萄糖)以维持自身增殖的理论,他观察到即使在氧气水平有利于氧化磷酸化的条件下,一些癌细胞在培养环境下依然提高对葡萄糖的摄取能力用于糖酵解。这一现象是违反常理的,因为糖酵解产生ATP(细胞内能量的主要载体)的效率要低得多。现在我们已经认识到,Warburg所描述的"有氧糖酵解"除了ATP之外还产生了细胞生长和分裂所必需的许多大分子。实际上,癌细胞的代谢模式并非新的发明,而是类似于分裂活跃的正常细胞。此外,我们还要认识到癌细胞中的氧化磷酸化和有氧糖酵解并不是全或无的关系,相反,癌细胞继续利用氧化磷酸化,并且掺入不同速率的糖酵解,二者的比例在时间上是动态变化的,在肿瘤内不同的亚区域和不同的组织微环境中也是可动态变化的。

通过使用放射性标记的类似物作为示踪剂,有氧糖酵解可以通过正电子发射断层成像(positronemission tomography,PET)间接监测。PET所用的^{18}F-氟脱氧葡萄糖被广泛用于可视化高糖酵解肿瘤的位置,通常这类肿瘤的葡萄糖转运蛋白的表达升高,由此葡萄糖摄取也增加。虽然葡萄糖是多数癌细胞的主要能量来源,但谷氨酰胺也是另一种主要的血运能量来源,同时也是脂质和氨基酸的前体。在少数情况下,谷氨酰胺的摄取和代谢能够补偿葡萄糖的匮乏,然而大多数情况下,谷氨酰胺倾向于补充和增强葡萄糖的功能,为癌细胞的生长和增殖提供能量和生物材料[11]。

细胞代谢供能的第三个参与者是乳酸,虽然长期以来乳酸被认为是细胞在有氧代谢和无氧糖酵解过程中分泌的有毒废物,但目前乳酸具有多样的促肿瘤能力的观点已成为共识[12]。在某些癌细胞中,特别是葡萄糖匮乏的细胞,细胞外的乳酸可通过特定的转运蛋白转向胞内,作为生成ATP和生物材料的能量来源。与此相似,一些肿瘤相关的成纤维细胞(cancer-associated fibroblast,CAF)也可以利用乳酸。因此,在某些肿瘤中可能存在代谢共生的关系,葡萄糖输入/乳酸输出细胞和乳酸输入细胞之间存在相互协作的关系。

最后,我们还注意到一个未解之谜,即肿瘤的代谢特征是否相对独立于前述六个调节机制,还是受其他特性的调控。诸如*KRAS*和*cMYC*等原癌基因的激活以及*p53*等抑癌基因功能的丧失可能对癌细胞能量代谢重编程起到一定的作用。由于上述原因,细胞能量和新陈代谢重编程最初被定义为肿瘤的"新兴特征"[2]。但无论这一"新兴特征"是否实至名归,它毫无疑问也是癌细胞一个重要的表型[13]。

特性8:逃避免疫清除

第8个特征已经讨论了几十年,最初认为原发肿瘤必须找到规避免疫系统主动监测的方法,否则异常增殖的癌前细胞会被免疫系统清除。虽然这一猜想在具有高度抗原性的小鼠肿瘤模型和病毒诱导的人类肿瘤中已证实,但免疫监视阻碍早期肿瘤进展的普遍机制尚不明确。一个因素是免疫的自身耐受——自发产生的癌细胞大多数表达与正常组织中起始细胞相同的抗原,因此常被免疫系统忽略,这反映了免疫系统对自身抗原的耐受。然而,免疫系统对另一些癌细胞表达的抗原未产生耐受性,包括胚胎抗原,以及基因组高频突变产生的新抗原,这些抗原可以诱发抗肿瘤免疫应答,成为备受关注的抗肿瘤疗法的新策略。

相比之下,约20%由病毒诱发的肿瘤,其免疫应答机制较为明确:致癌病毒会表达免疫系统不耐受的外来抗原(包括驱动细胞恶性转化的原癌蛋白),诱发体液和细胞免疫反应以杀死感染病毒的癌前细胞,从而在肿瘤形成的初期将其根除。实际上,病毒转化的细胞可以成功地逃避免疫消除而产生肿瘤,这证明了肿瘤病毒在进化中或在病毒转化的癌细胞中选择性地获得免疫逃逸能力。尽管如此,免疫系统可能是病毒诱发肿瘤的重要屏障,在各种原因所致的免疫受损人群中,例如器官移植和艾滋病患者的癌症发病率更高。

尽管存在免疫缺陷,但非病毒诱导的人类癌症的发病率没有明显的增加,间接表明其他80%的人类肿瘤的形成是由于机体缺乏对早期肿瘤的免疫监视所致。多种证据表明在肿瘤进展的后期,一些肿瘤必须应对免疫识别和免疫攻击,进而进化出获得性免疫逃逸的策略。人类肿瘤的组织病理揭示了免疫攻击和免疫逃逸的潜在作用。例如,在接受了肿瘤切除手术的结直肠癌患者中,有大量细胞毒性T淋巴细胞(cytotoxic T lymphocyte,CTL)浸润的患者,与肿瘤分级和大小类似但T淋巴细胞浸润较少的患者相比,前者的预后更佳[14]。这些数据表明免疫系统是阻碍癌细胞持续生长和播散的重要屏障,然而在高侵袭性的肿瘤中,这种屏障必已相应减弱或丧失[14]。实际上,肿瘤及其相关间质的免疫表型,被认为是新的肿瘤诊断指标,如果与传统标准相结合,或许可以更准确地评估预后,并更有效的指导治疗[15,16]。因此,我们可将抗肿瘤免疫反应视为各种肿瘤在长期多阶段的进展过程中需要规避的重要屏障。

然而,纵观各种人类肿瘤,免疫系统发挥作用的方式尚不明确。在各种器官特异性肿瘤的发生发展中,免疫系统何时激活、免疫反应确切的特征及效应、以及患者的遗传背景如何影响抗肿瘤免疫,以上这些问题我们知之甚少。然而,逃避免疫破坏的确是肿瘤发展的必要条件,因此被列为癌症的特征之一。

综上所述,我们认为这8种标志性特征,以及下文所述的两种获取肿瘤特征的能力是恶性肿瘤发生的必要条件(图2-1)。然而,我们不能忽视这种简单理论背后的复杂机制:不同肿瘤可通过整合、利用和操控多种原本用于维持正常细胞、组织和器官内稳态的机制;同时值得我们注意的是,不同肿瘤获得以上特性的方式也不尽相同。

有助于必要功能获得的变异

长期以来,我们认为肿瘤长期进展和恶性转化的过程涉及一系列的限速步骤,反映了不断进展的肿瘤细胞需要获得上述讨论的8种特征性能力。那么如何获得这些能力?目前,可通过以下两种较为明确的方式获得:①基因组不稳定性和肿瘤细胞中随之发生的促肿瘤发生的基因突变;②由免疫系统细胞所致的炎症反应协同上述促肿瘤效应。

基因组的不稳定性及相应的促肿瘤特征形成的基因突变

基因组不稳定性和随之而来的相关基因突变是癌症获得标志性能力的首要方式。细胞基因组极易遭受DNA损伤,例如来自正常代谢的各种化学反应产物、环境暴露以及细胞分裂的复制过程。上述产生的基因缺陷，如果不加修复，将成为细胞可遗传的突变，这表明细胞需要一套复杂的蛋白质系统连续监测 DNA 完整性，对损伤做出应答，并且进行修复。一旦损伤无法修复将会启动细胞清除，由抑癌基因 *p53* 精密调控，因此 *p53* 也被称为“基因组卫士”。

这种高效的基因组完整性维护机制通常将基因突变和基因组重排维持在较低水平，这与肿瘤细胞通过遗传进化和表型选择来获得特征性功能的方式并不兼容。这种一分为二的观点为频繁观察到的癌细胞基因组不稳定性提供了令人信服的解释。实际上，许多肿瘤的癌细胞都携带了一些缺陷，这些缺陷容易被监测和修复基因组损伤的系统识别。最典型的高频突变是 *p53* 等位基因突变，出现在约 40% 的癌症中；正常 *p53* 监视出现缺失，受损的 DNA 持续得不到修复，将使突变细胞得以存活并将受损基因组遗传给后代。在许多肿瘤中也发现 DNA 修复酶和基因组维护酶存在缺陷，同样的，DNA 修复元件的遗传性家族缺陷将导致促肿瘤突变的形成，增加细胞癌变风险。

肿瘤中细胞谱系进行着持续快速地增殖，相比正常组织中的普通细胞，肿瘤细胞的连续性生长和分裂循环显著增多，DNA 复制过程中发生致突变错误的可能性也进一步增加，所导致的就是前文所述的结果：DNA 严重缩短并功能失调，端粒触发染色体重排和融合，会以多种方式影响基因的功能。在这种核型混乱中幸存下来的突变癌细胞就有可能获得有利的表型，由此具备克隆扩增的能力。

高通量 DNA 测序技术使得大规模、系统分析独立癌细胞的基因组数据成为可能，该技术也进一步证实了基因突变是癌症发生的基础。通过联合其他基因组解析的方法，例如运用比较基因组杂交以识别拷贝数变异、利用“染色体图谱”以检测易位，癌细胞基因组紊乱的全貌第一次呈现在了我们面前[17~20]。结果表明，癌细胞普遍存在染色体重排或局部的基因突变，或二者兼而有之，因此几乎所有形式的癌症都涉及癌细胞基因组的突变。基因变异的密度在不同肿瘤中的量级不同，在某些儿科癌症中检测到的变异数量非常低，而在紫外线诱导的黑色素瘤和烟草导致的肺癌基因组中则存在数量巨大的突变。因此，基因突变差异范围极大，可以从几十个点突变到数十万个点突变，从二倍体染色体核型到不同的非整倍染色体核型、易位乃至多处大规模扩增和缺失。

高通量基因组技术产生了指数级的数据，也向科学家提出了新的挑战，癌细胞基因组中大量的突变究竟哪些与上述标志性特征的获得相关。许多癌细胞中记录到的突变数量已大大超过了可能参与重塑细胞表型的突变的数量。相同癌症类型或亚型的患者队列中，特定突变的重复出现提示其可能在癌症中具有一定功能。然而，许多突变可能仅仅出现在某些个体的肿瘤中，重复出现的频率较低。还有一些突变虽然在癌细胞基因组中普遍存在，但它们可能仅仅是基因组不稳定的附带产物，伴随其他造成肿瘤选择优势的突变而产生，并协助这些基因促进克隆的扩增和肿瘤的发生及发展。因此，也有理论认为癌症细胞包含两类突变：驱动突变和伴随突变。未来研究的当务之急是分析这些基因组数据来识别驱动基因突变及其对获得标志性特征的作用，不仅要分析特定癌症类型中常见的突变，还要关注其他虽不常见但在功能上影响个体肿瘤生长和进展的关键基因。第二个要务是阐明常见和罕见驱动突变作为不同肿瘤类型治疗靶点的潜力。某些肿瘤中驱动突变带来的优势性特征在其他肿瘤中可能是通过表观基因组的变化获得的，也就是说染色质中细胞的遗传变化并不表现为核苷酸序列的改变，这无疑增加了分析的复杂性[21~22]。也有观点认为，以上 8 种标志性特征都可以通过调控基因的表观遗传变化来实现，且既可发生在癌细胞中，也可发生在促肿瘤的相关间质细胞中[23]。对于表观遗传机制作为肿瘤发生主要协同者的观点，目前学界的认识还不统一，在某些肿瘤中基因组不稳定性也可能并未发挥很大的作用，在这些肿瘤中 DNA 突变有可能是肿瘤特征性功能的结果而并非驱动因素。

癌症遗传学领域将迎来快速发展的时代，成千上万的癌细胞基因组将会得到全面多维的解析，包括 DNA 序列和拷贝数的改变，基因转录、剪接和翻译的变化，以及染色质结构调节区域的变异，调控基因转录可及性的组蛋白和 DNA 甲基化的重编程等。从大量的数据集中提炼及定位出特定的基因改变，以及它们在遗传和表观遗传上对获得标志性功能的作用，并利用这些知识来提高人类癌症检测、评估和治疗的水平，对我们来说既是巨大的挑战也是机遇。

促肿瘤的免疫细胞浸润(炎症)

促肿瘤的免疫细胞浸润是癌症获得标志性能力的第 2 种形式。值得注意的是，大多数肿瘤存在免疫系统多种类型细胞（所谓的浸润型免疫细胞，或 IIC[3]）的共同浸润。虽然浸润型免疫细胞引起的炎症常被认为是试图清除肿瘤的失败尝试，但最近的证据提出了一个更加令人担忧的观点：浸润型免疫细胞可以旁分泌方式帮助肿瘤细胞实现多种功能，包括上述 8 种肿瘤特性中的 7 种。IIC 可以提供多种增殖和存活信号、促血管生成因子、促进局部侵袭和血源性转移。此外，这些 IIC（T 调节细胞和髓源性抑制细胞）可以积极地抑制免疫系统用来消灭癌细胞的细胞毒性 T 淋巴细胞的功能。

在不同类型的肿瘤和肿瘤发生的不同时期，肿瘤可以通过多种途径募集促进肿瘤生长的 IIC。招募信号包括趋化因子和细胞因子等，目前信号分子仍然没有被完全阐明。在某些情况下，肿瘤病变的发生可能引发组织异常或损伤信号，吸引 IIC，激活适应性和先天性免疫系统。在其他情况下，通过激活转录网络，致癌信号诱导细胞因子和趋化因子的表达从而招募 IIC。在早期病变中，所募集的 IIC 可帮助早期癌细胞增殖、存活、逃避抗生长调控或激活血管新生。在进展的后期，肿瘤边缘的 IIC 可促进侵袭。有研究表明，当癌细胞在血液循环中迁移并在远处定植时，IIC 也可以与之配合[24]。此外，某些 IIC，如巨噬细胞，可以使癌细胞受到 DNA 损伤活性氧的影响，从而导致癌细胞基因组的突变和进化。这些后天获得的特征表明肿瘤细胞已获得了特征性能力，也进一步支持了在炎症组织微环境中，IIC 可能无意中促进了早期癌细胞的形成和/或进展的观点。

癌症组织病理学的复杂性——肿瘤微环境

病理学家早就认识到实体肿瘤具有复杂的组织学结构，其不仅包括癌细胞，还包括各种不同形态的细胞，这些细胞与非癌组织的成分相似,既存在于正常组织中也受到感染或伤口愈合损伤修复等情况的影响。与许多正常组织中支持上皮细胞的间质相似,肿瘤的非癌成分也被称之为肿瘤间质。与正常组织间质一样,肿瘤相关的间质包含了血管、成纤维细胞的集合,在许多情况下还可见到 IIC。长期以来,我们把对肿瘤间质作用的理解做如下简化:内皮细胞通过产生新生血管为肿瘤提供氧气和营养,而癌症相关的成纤维细胞(CAF)作为递质或者提供结构支撑,IIC 如前文所述,介导无效的抗肿瘤免疫反应。如上所述,我们现在认识到,肿瘤内多种多样的间质细胞可以在功能上协助肿瘤获得 8 种肿瘤特性中的 7 种[3]。

如图 2-2 所示,与正常组织相似,肿瘤通常在概念上划分为实质(由癌细胞组成)和间质(由表面正常的支持细胞组成);这两个部分的组合加上细胞外成分(包括细胞外基质 ECM 和基底膜 BM)越来越多的被称为"肿瘤微环境"(tumor microenvironment,TME);有些人也将 TME 称为非癌性的间质部分,尽管微环境这一说法在概念上包含了整个肿瘤,即肿瘤实质以及间质部分。

这三种间质细胞包含了肿瘤微环境中的大部分间质成分:由内皮细胞和辅助性周细胞组成的血管生成细胞(AVC)、CAF 以及 IIC[3]。然而,这些简单的分类方法掩盖了细胞间质成分和细胞表型的多样性。CAF 具有多种亚型,其中最常见的两种类型来源于表达 α-平滑肌肌动蛋白肌成纤维细胞、间充质干细胞和组织星状细胞,或者来源于 α-平滑肌肌动蛋白阴性结缔组织来源的成纤维细胞。这两种亚型都是通过 TME 发出的旁分泌信号,对各自正常来源的细胞进行表观遗传重编程而产生的;这些诱导信号与损伤修复或炎症反应中成纤维细胞参与的信号通路类似。IIC 也有越来越多的亚型被发现,每一种都有独特的功能和特征;有些或可追踪到谱系来源(例如表达骨髓中招募的免疫细胞祖细胞标志),而另一些则是通过 TME 中特定的诱导信号进行"局部驯化"的结果。促肿瘤的 IIC 包括不同亚型的细胞,例如巨噬细胞、中性粒细胞、部分分化的骨髓祖细胞,在某些情况下还包括 B 淋巴细胞和 T 淋巴细胞的特殊亚型。尽管内皮细胞和周细胞的表位和基因表达谱表现出了组织和肿瘤类型特异性的特征,肿瘤血管系统的内皮细胞和周细胞的多样性则相对局限,可能与肿瘤的生物学特性有一定的关联。另一种不同类型的内皮细胞形成淋巴管网络,随着肿瘤附近的淋巴管生成而扩大,并与淋巴转移有关。

最近的研究对间质细胞的功能做出了更细致的探索,通过解析其帮助肿瘤获取特征性功能的作用,揭示了间质细胞在疾病发病机制中的重要性[2,3]。作为一个之前没有讨论过的例子,CAF 可以在不同的肿瘤背景下分泌蛋白酶、增殖信号配体

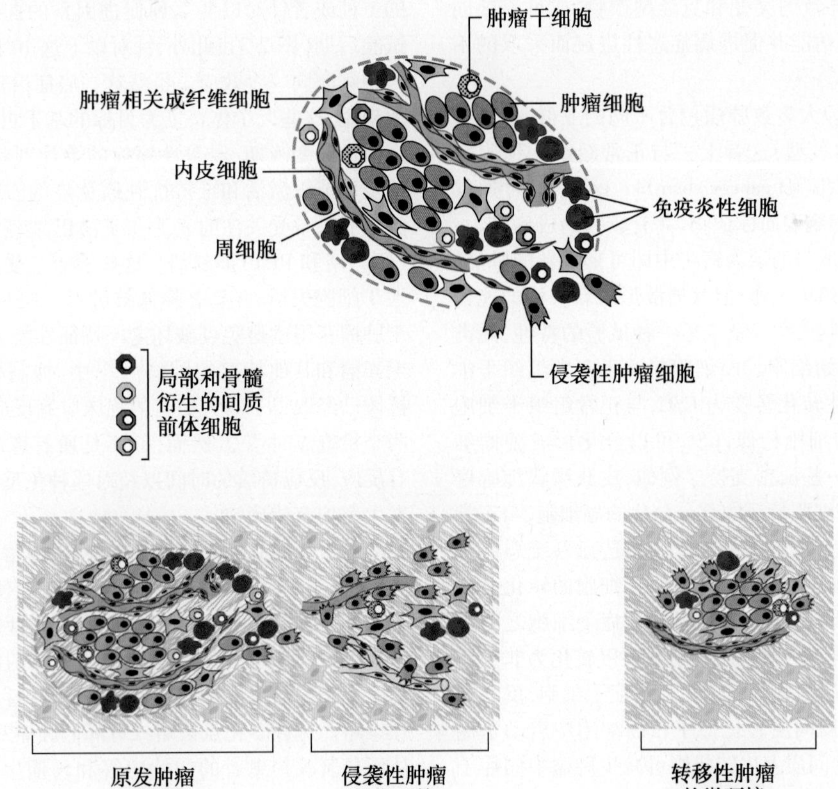

图 2-2　促进肿瘤特性产生的肿瘤微环境的构成。大多数实体肿瘤的微环境都是由不同类型的细胞集合构成的,包括两个不同的部分——癌细胞实质和支持细胞构成的间质。这两个部分都包含了不同的细胞和亚细胞类型,它们共同促进了肿瘤的生长和进展[2,3]。值得注意的是,肿瘤中存在的免疫炎性细胞既可包括促和/或抑肿瘤的免疫抑制细胞,也可包括肿瘤杀伤细胞。靠下的一组图示意了一个重要的特点:肿瘤微环境是动态变化的,其成分和组成的细胞类型(亚型)不同,在肿瘤发生不同阶段,即癌变前的阶段(图中未显示)和恶性阶段对组织学的影响也不同,这些差异部位包括原发性肿瘤的核心、侵袭性的肿瘤边缘、侵入性病灶以及转移部位

和/或其他生物活性分子，造成不同的肿瘤表型。多种文献记载，CAF 可将上皮细胞从正常组织结构施加的生长抑制中解放出来，诱导促肿瘤的炎症反应，促进局部侵袭和转移灶的播散，并为癌细胞提供代谢能量。CAF 还可以诱导血管新生，并可以显著削弱 CTL 的免疫抑制作用。

展望未来，在不同癌症类型和不同进展阶段中，继续绘制不同类型间质细胞及其亚型的多维图谱仍是一项重要的目标。

TME 还涉及癌细胞亚群的遗传和功能异质性。事实上，人们早就认识到，单个肿瘤病变内的癌细胞在形态和遗传上是异质的。基因组测序技术（核型分析、比较基因组杂交、等位基因缺失分析、外显子组（基因）测序，以及目前已处于单细胞水平的全基因组测序）记录了基因组突变的进化过程，早期肿瘤中初生的癌细胞最终会发展为具有基因多样性的更高分级的肿瘤中共存的亚群。

瘤内异质性的第二个明显表现体现在表观遗传水平上。因此，在许多癌症中，侵袭性肿瘤边缘的癌细胞具有明显的表型差异，它们经历了 EMT，纤维化更明显，也随之获得了侵袭能力。另一些则保留了它们起源细胞类型不同程度的分化特征，例如，鳞状上皮。此外，目前认为不同类型肿瘤的区域组织学的变化特征（至少在某些情况下）可以反映基因型不同的癌细胞克隆；基因组不稳定导致的突变和克隆副产物，或可反映同一肿瘤为了获得特征性功能并促进癌症恶性进展而采取的不同应对措施。

此外，现在普遍认为大多数肿瘤包含不同的亚群，极少有癌细胞表现出的类似的表型，这看上去与正常组织干细胞相似。这些癌症干细胞样细胞（cancer stem-like cells，CSC）通常增殖较慢，表达组织干细胞表面标记物，具有较强的成瘤能力，将少量细胞异位移植到适当的动物宿主中即可形成新的肿瘤，虽然其他的肿瘤细胞增殖更迅速，但其播散形成新肿瘤的能力却逊于癌症干细胞样细胞[9,25]。基于后一种试验的特性，此类细胞也被定义为肿瘤起始细胞。癌细胞起源于正常组织干细胞或前体细胞，经过恶性转化转变为 CSC，与正常组织干细胞会分化产生不同类型的细胞相似，CSC 可以分化形成肿瘤细胞，这一假设也得到了一些证据支持。例如，皮肤鳞状细胞癌中的 CSC 产生具有鳞状细胞特征的部分分化的癌细胞，与正常皮肤干细胞产生的鳞状上皮细胞相似。许多造血系统恶性肿瘤，明显是由正常的干细胞/祖细胞向造血干细胞的转化而来的。然而，在其他情况下，癌症干细胞与非癌症干细胞之间似乎存在一种动态的相互转化，即癌症干细胞可以转化为非癌症干细胞，反之亦然，例如癌细胞可以转化为癌症干细胞，反之也可以；在一些病例中，上皮间质转化似乎在癌细胞中启动了癌症干细胞表型，而反向的间质上皮转化则可减少肿瘤中癌症干细胞的数量[9,25]。有研究提示增殖能力相对较弱的癌症干细胞可能对某些基因毒性抗癌药物有更强的耐药性，这为耐药性和临床复发研究提供了新的思路。因此，针对 CSC 的治疗可能是实现长期有效的癌症治疗的关键。

靶向癌症特性的治疗（协同治疗）

癌症医学面临的一个重要问题：是否可以将癌症特性概念化并应用于临床。将癌症特性概念化可能带来的好处是帮助癌症研究者建立通用的原则，从而为人类癌症发生和进展找到合理的分子和细胞机制。通过多平台对肿瘤细胞及病变组织全基因组测序数据、RNA 转录本、蛋白质和磷酸蛋白、DNA 以及组蛋白甲基化图谱进行剖析，产生了海量的数据（见参考文献[26]以及本书的其他章节）。此外，这些日益强大的分析技术还能外推出其他结论，包括肿瘤发生和肿瘤进展中的损伤图谱，尤其是肿瘤转移过程中的损伤分析；另外，这些技术还有可能为了解肿瘤在个性化靶向治疗的应答期和复发期分别产生的适应性和反应机理提供思路。如何整合所有信息以确定特定的致癌通路，如何利用这些信息确定新的治疗靶点，如何确定适应性耐药的模式，然后利用这些数据进行诊断、预后和治疗的优化，这些都是我们面临的巨大挑战。尽管这些假设尚未证实，但癌症的特征可能对于信息的整合和过滤有所裨益。我们或许可以根据日益增长的调控通路库来过滤癌症基因组、转录组、蛋白质组、磷酸蛋白质组以及甲基化组等生物组学数据，并基于以上分析明确肿瘤获取各种癌症特性所依赖的遗传和表观遗传特征，进而对疾病进行更精确的处理。

我们还预想未来肿瘤特性这一概念也会有助于临床治疗方案的设计。值得注意的是，已经有一些针对 8 个癌症特性中的 1 种或者针对以上 2 种促进因素的药物获批或已处于临床试验后期（图 2-3）；此外，针对以上这 10 种机制，有许多不同的药物靶向同一个效应。虽然这一癌症治疗进展振奋人心，但总地来说，这些以个体特征为目标的基于机制的治疗方法并没有实质性改变晚期、侵袭性癌症的治疗现状。但也有例外，通过免疫调节以激活和维持抗肿瘤免疫的方法表现出了明显的优势，例如，备受关注的表达在 T 淋巴细胞上的免疫检查点受体（CTLA4 和 PD1）抑制剂。这些检查点受体激活后可使细胞毒性 T 细胞失活，并显著降低抗肿瘤免疫应答的效能，从而有助于肿瘤获得逃避免疫破坏这一特征性能力。值得注意的是，在黑素瘤和其他特定的肿瘤[27,28]中，抑制检查点活化的治疗性抗体已经取得了令人振奋的临床应答反应，特别是同时靶向这两个检查点时[29]。然而，并不是所有患者都对这种免疫疗法有反应，反应持续的时间以及对这种免疫疗法的适应性抵抗的发生率均有待确定。

对于靶向其他癌症特性的疗法，通常会看到肿瘤对治疗有反应，但一段时间后，适应性耐药机制会使存活的癌细胞（肿瘤干细胞）绕过治疗带来的阻滞，恢复恶性生长。研究者也提出了多种方案来解决目前靶向治疗失败的问题。我们认为靶向功能上不同的特性，即同时靶向多个特性可能是效能更高的治疗策略。这种多靶点策略或可降低肿瘤对治疗的获得性耐药，从而显著改善患者的初始应答和长期生存[30]。当然，有效地控制这些组合的毒性也是一个重要的问题。因此，除了简单的组合疗法外，也有必要进行靶向肿瘤特性的序贯性、间歇性或分层疗法；在控制毒性和适应性耐药的同时，对药物进行微调以最大限度地提高疗效。进一步，可以利用基因工程从头构建的动物模型以及来源于患者的异体种植模型（PDX），来对备选的临床试验方案进行测试，将模型预测的可能性调整到临床可接受的范围内，进而把最佳的试验方案从临床前试验推进到临床试验及个体化治疗[31~33]。

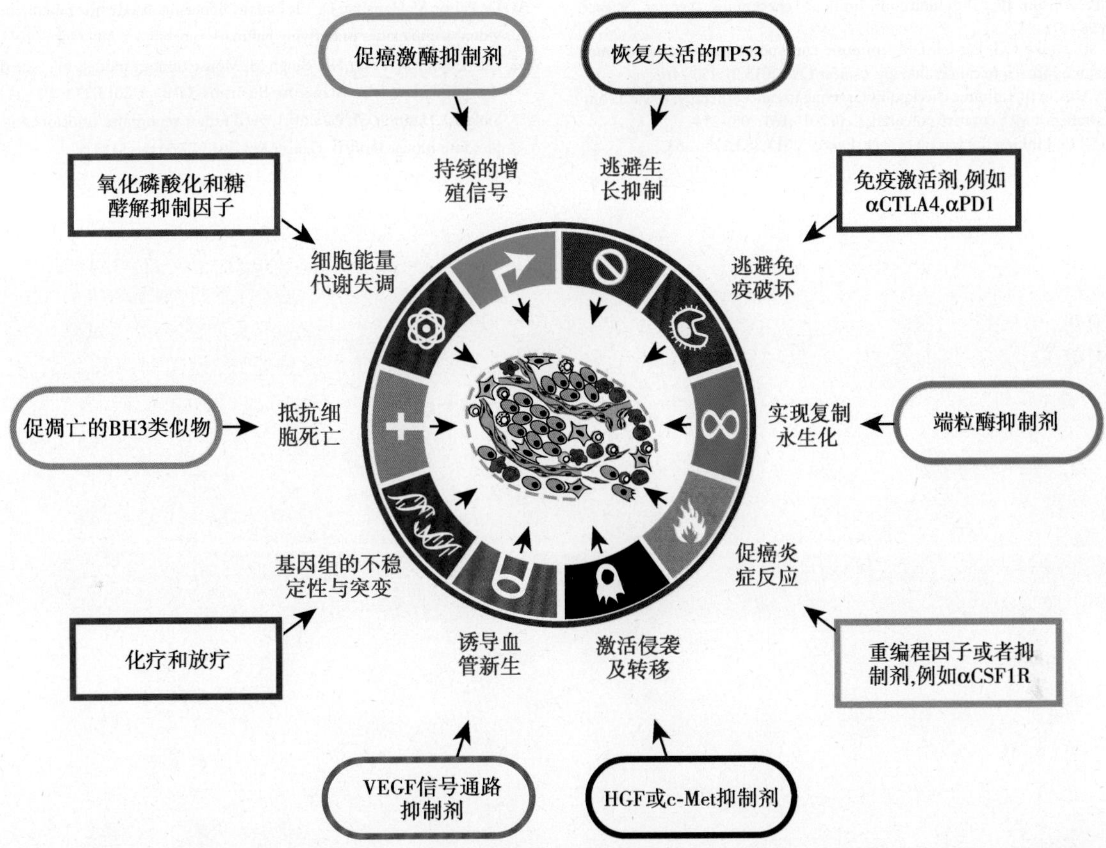

图 2-3　针对癌症特性的治疗靶点。针对 8 种癌症特性以及 2 种有效地促进因素(基因组不稳定性和肿瘤促进炎症),均已研发出对其功能进行破坏或干扰的药物。其中一些靶向药物已获批临床使用,还有一些正在进行临床试验;此外,还有一系列新的靶向药物正在进行研发和临床前评估。我们也认识到肿瘤最终均会对这些靶向药产生适应性耐药,由此提出了一种假设:通过同时靶向多个单独的癌症特性,或许可以控制乃至避免单药治疗出现的适应性耐药问题[30];临床和临床前试验正在评估以上假设的可能性

总之,肿瘤的生物学特性可以为现代肿瘤学学生提供理解本书后续专题章节的基础和框架;宏观上来说,本章节也为探索和解读癌症致病机制,并将这些知识更有效地应用于人类癌症诊断和治疗策略的开发奠定了理论基础。

(陈淑桢　曹琦琪 译　王红阳 审)

参考文献

1 Hanahan D, Weinberg RA. The hallmarks of cancer. *Cell*. 2000;**100**:57–70.
2 Hanahan D, Weinberg RA. Hallmarks of cancer: the next generation. *Cell*. 2011;**144**:346–674.
3 Hanahan D, Coussens LM. Accessories to the crime: functions of cells recruited to the tumor microenvironment. *Cancer Cell*. 2012;**21**:309–322.
4 Weinberg RA. *The Biology of Cancer*. New York: Garland Press; 2013.
5 Vanden Berghe T, Linkermann A, Jouan-Lanhouet S, et al. Regulated necrosis: the expanding network of non-apoptotic cell death pathways. *Nat Rev Mol Cell Biol*. 2014;**15**:135–147.
6 Rebecca VW, Amaravadi RK. Emerging strategies to effectively target autophagy in cancer. *Oncogene*. 2015. doi: 10.1038/onc.2015.99 (Epub ahead of print).
7 Keith B, Johnson RS, Simon MC. HIF1α and HIF2α: sibling rivalry in hypoxic tumour growth and progression. *Nat Rev Cancer*. 2011;**12**:9–22.
8 Semenza GL. Hypoxia-inducible factors: mediators of cancer progression and targets for cancer therapy. *Trends Pharmacol Sci*. 2012;**33**:207–214.
9 Baccelli I, Trumpp A. The evolving concept of cancer and metastasis stem cells. *J Cell Biol*. 2012;**198**:281–293.
10 Savagner P. Epithelial-mesenchymal transitions: from cell plasticity to concept elasticity. *Curr Top Dev Biol*. 2015;**112**:273–300.
11 Daye D, Wellen KE. Metabolic reprogramming in cancer: unraveling the role of glutamine in tumorigenesis. *Semin Cell Dev Biol*. 2012;**23**:362–369.
12 Dhup S, Dadhich RK, Porporato PE, Sonveaux P. Multiple biological activities of lactic acid in cancer: influences on tumor growth, angiogenesis and metastasis. *Curr Pharm Des*. 2012;**18**:1319–1330.
13 Ward PS, Thompson CB. Metabolic reprogramming: a cancer hallmark even Warburg did not anticipate. *Cancer Cell*. 2012;**21**:297–308.
14 Fridman WH, Pagès F, Sautès-Fridman C, Galon J. The immune contexture in human tumours: impact on clinical outcome. *Nat Rev Cancer*. 2012;**12**:298–306.
15 Galon J, Mlecnik B, Bindea G, et al. Towards the introduction of the 'Immunoscore' in the classification of malignant tumours. *J Pathol*. 2014;**232**:199–209.
16 Galon J, Angell HK, Bedognetti D, Marincola FM. The continuum of cancer immunosurveillance: prognostic, predictive, and mechanistic signatures. *Immunity*. 2013;**39**:11–26.
17 https://tcga-data.nci.nih.gov/tcga/tcgaHome2.jsp
18 http://www.sanger.ac.uk/research/projects/cancergenome/
19 http://icgc.org/
20 http://www.ncbi.nlm.nih.gov/sky/
21 You JS, Jones PA. Cancer genetics and epigenetics: two sides of the same coin? *Cancer Cell*. 2012;**22**:9–20.
22 Easwaran H, Tsai HC, Baylin SB. Cancer epigenetics: tumor heterogeneity, plasticity of stem-like states, and drug resistance. *Mol Cell*. 2014;**54**:716–727.
23 Azad N, Zahnow CA, Rudin CM, Baylin SB. The future of epigenetic therapy in solid tumours – lessons from the past. *Nat Rev Clin Oncol*. 2013;**10**:256–266.
24 Labelle M, Hynes RO. The initial hours of metastasis: the importance of cooperative host-tumor cell interactions during hematogenous dissemination. *Cancer Discov*. 2012;**2**:1091–1099.
25 Visvader JE, Lindeman GJ. Cancer stem cells: current status and evolving complexities. *Cell Stem Cell*. 2012;**10**:717–728.
26 The Cancer Genome Atlas Network. Comprehensive molecular portraits of human breast tumours. *Nature*. 2012;**490**:61–70.

27 Sharma P, Allison JP. The future of immune checkpoint therapy. *Science*. 2015;**348**:56-61.
28 Topalian SL, Drake CG, Pardoll DM. Immune checkpoint blockade: a common denominator approach to cancer therapy. *Cancer Cell*. 2015;**27**:450-461.
29 Sharma P, Allison JP. Immune checkpoint targeting in cancer therapy: toward combination strategies with curative potential. *Cell*. 2015;**161**:205-214.
30 Hanahan D. Rethinking the war on cancer. *Lancet*. 2013;**383**:558-563.
31 De Palma M, Hanahan D. The biology of personalized cancer medicine: facing individual complexities underlying hallmark capabilities. *Mol Oncol*. 2012;**6**:111-127.
32 Das Thakur M, Pryer NK, Singh M. Mouse tumour models to guide drug development and identify resistance mechanisms. *J Pathol*. 2014;**232**:103-111.
33 Siolas D, Hannon GJ. Patient-derived tumor xenografts: transforming clinical samples into mouse models. *Cancer Res*. 2013;**73**:5315-5319.

第二篇

肿瘤生物学

第 3 章 人类肿瘤分子生物学、基因组学、蛋白质组学与小鼠动物模型

Srinivas R. Viswanathan, MD, PhD ■ David A. Tuveson, MD, PhD ■ Matthew Meyerson, MD, PhD

概述

癌症是一种基因相关的疾病。控制细胞增殖基因的异常会导致恶性细胞的无限生长。因此，为了诊断和治疗癌症，我们需要了解肿瘤的分子基础：基因、信使核糖核酸（messenger ribonucleic acids, mRNA）以及产生的蛋白质，并应对分子生物学工具有足够的了解。

本章内容主要针对希望了解分子生物学基础知识的临床医生或实习医师。它是“方法导向”的，为本书其他章节搭建基本框架。本章将概述分子生物学家最常用方法的基本原理，并列举相关技术用于临床的实例。无论在诊断（如分析肿瘤预后和病理资料）还是治疗方面（如生产药物、类似重组生长因子和单克隆抗体的生物制剂），分子生物学已经在临床肿瘤学中发挥了重要的作用。

我们首先将概述基因、基因表达和基因克隆。随后对技术的讨论将遵循遗传信息的传递过程：从 DNA、RNA 到蛋白质。关于本部分的详细介绍可以参考其他书籍[1~3]。

概述：基因结构

基因与基因表达

基因是遗传的最小单位和所有表型的最终决定因素。正常人类的基因组 DNA 含有 20 000~25 000 个蛋白质编码基因，但在特定的时间只有一部分在细胞中表达。例如，在红细胞中特异性表达的血红蛋白基因，在脑细胞中并不表达。在某时刻、特定细胞中所表达的所有基因转录产物及其表达水平的集合称为“转录组”。

根据分子生物学的中心法则，基因首先被转录成 mRNA，然后被翻译成蛋白质，蛋白质作为效应分子行使功能。因此，分子生物学家分析基因表达或活化，通常指的是 DNA 转录成 RNA 和 RNA 翻译成蛋白质的过程。转录过程包括以基因 DNA 作为模板产生基因的 RNA 拷贝（“转录物”）。然后核糖体将 mRNA 包含的序列信息翻译成由氨基酸组成的蛋白质。

基因的功能元件

每个基因都由几个功能元件组成，参与基因表达的各个过程（图 3-1）。一般说来基因包含 2 大类功能元件：启动子区和编码区。

启动子主要控制基因在何时何组织中表达。例如血红蛋白基因的启动子决定其基因在红细胞中表达而不在脑细胞中表达。那么，在组织中如何实现基因的特异性表达？基因启动子区的 DNA 含有特定的结构和核苷酸序列（见下面的“结构部分”），使基因在特定的细胞中表达，正是这些元件指导血红蛋白基因在红细胞中转录成 mRNA。由于这些元件位于和基因相同的 DNA 上，因此称之为“顺式作用元件”。另外，增强子也属于组织特异性顺式作用元件，它们虽然和基因处在相同的 DNA 分子上，但远离基因的编码区域[4,5]。在这些细胞中，顺式作用元件通过结合特异的蛋白分子来起始基因转录。这些蛋白分子与编码基因的 DNA 同处于细胞核中，称为“反式作用因子”。例如，脑细胞中不含有结合血红蛋白基因启动子的反式作用因子，所以其无法表达，但脑细胞中含有与神经元特异性启动子结合的反式作用因子。

基因编码蛋白的结构信息包含在基因编码区中。编码区包含了指导红细胞将氨基酸以正确顺序装配成血红蛋白的序列信息。那么基因编码区如何能决定蛋白的氨基酸顺序？如后文所述，DNA 是由四种不同的核苷酸按特定的顺序组合而成的，是线性的多聚核苷酸结构。在基因的编码区中，核苷酸编码了蛋白的氨基酸序列。遗传密码以三联子的形式进行编码，每 3 个核苷酸编码一个氨基酸，4 种核苷酸可有 64 种三联子编码方式，足以满足构成蛋白质的 20 种氨基酸的需要；也使遗传密码具有简并性，即多种密码子可以编码同一个氨基酸[6]。在“核苷酸测序”部分将讲到，通过一些方法可以测出任意基因的序列（见下文）。

因此，通过三联子编码方式可以预测基因编码蛋白质的氨基酸序列。

结构分析

精确结构

核苷酸是 DNA 的基本单位（图 3-2）。它是由不可变部分（带有磷酸基团的脱氧核糖）和可变部分（碱基）组成。出现在 DNA 核苷酸中的 4 种碱基中有两种嘌呤：腺嘌呤（adenine, A）和鸟嘌呤（guanine, G），另外两种是嘧啶：胞嘧啶（cytosine, C）和胸腺嘧啶（thymine, T）。核苷酸通过磷酸基团按一定的顺序相连，碱基则通过氢键发生相互作用。碱基配对遵循特定的规则，即 A 与 T 配对、G 与 C 配对。DNA 通常为双链，即由两条线性的链并排排列，链上的碱基正好相互配对，使 DNA 链与其配对的 DNA 链完全互补，这种互补性使得每条 DNA 链上的信息都能被精确的复制。

每条 DNA 链中，前一个脱氧核苷酸的 5′磷酸与后一个脱氧核苷酸的羟基以磷酸二酯键相连。因此，DNA 具有方向性：遗传密码是从 5′向 3′方向编码的。双链 DNA 中与翻译方向

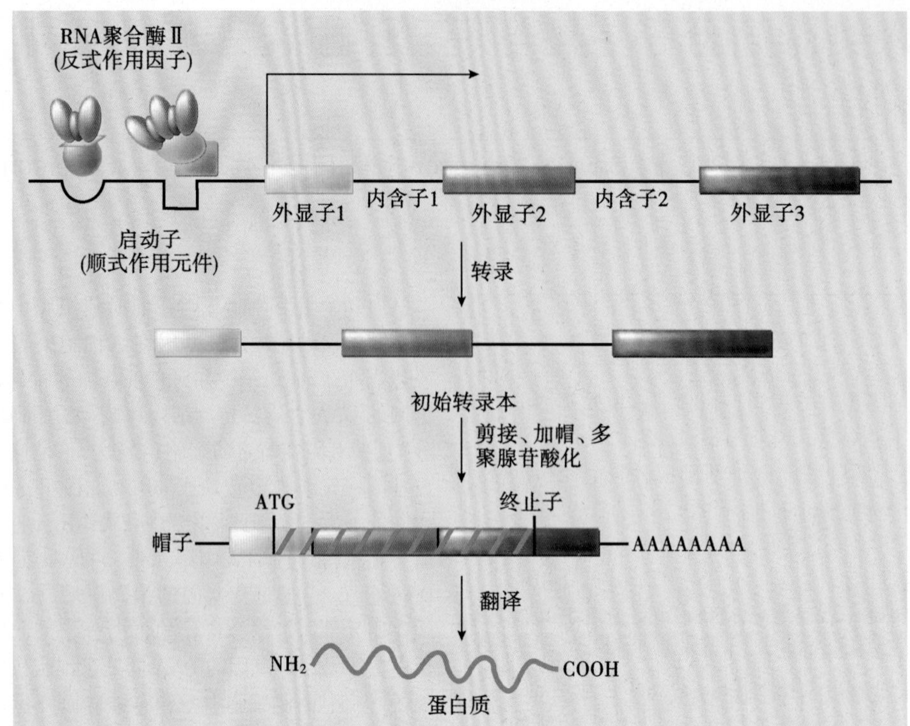

图 3-1 基因表达。基因 DNA 转录为信使核糖核酸(mRNA),而 mRNA 又被翻译成蛋白质。图示基因的各种功能元件。外显子(exon)是最后出现在成熟 RNA 中的基因序列,分开的外显子之间的非编码 DNA 片段称为内含子(intron)。启动子(promoter)控制着基因的转录及表达。启动子区的特定核苷酸序列(顺式作用元件)与蛋白质(反式作用因子)结合,即启动子与 RNA 聚合酶Ⅱ结合,启动基因转录。由 RNA 聚合酶Ⅱ转录的初产物与基因的 DNA 链完全互补。但在出核时,转录初产物中的外显子经过剪接加工后相连(去除内含子),同时在 5′端加帽、3′端加上多聚腺苷酸化的尾巴,成为成熟的 mRNA,并在胞质翻译成蛋白质

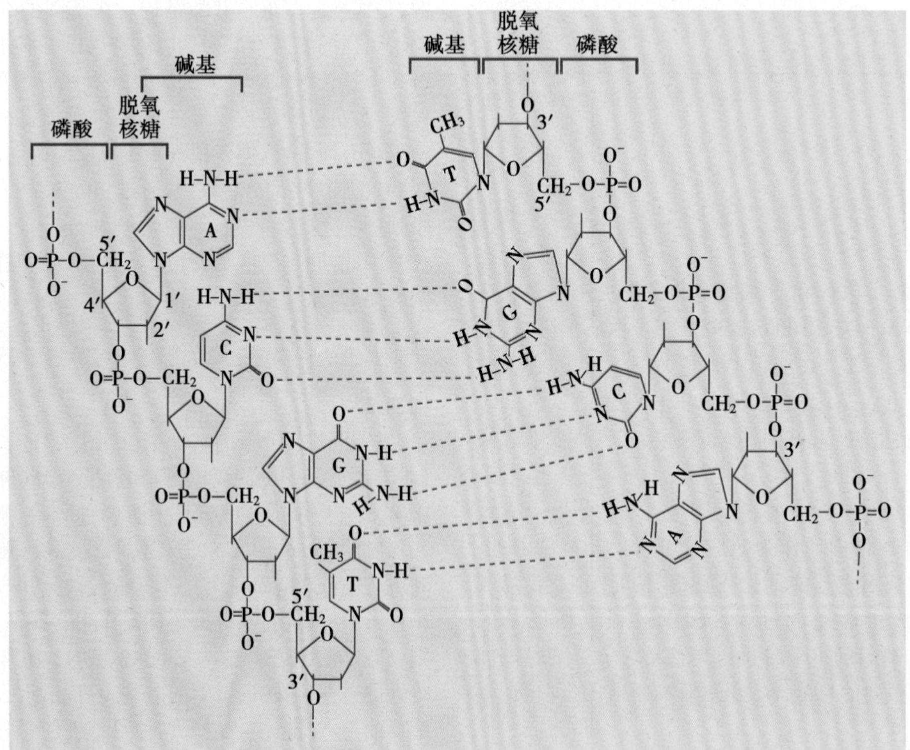

图 3-2 双链 DNA 结构。五碳脱氧核糖通过磷酸键交替连接构成 DNA 链的基本骨架。图中所示,左边的 DNA 链按照脱氧核糖 5′到 3′碳原子顺序,碱基顺序为 A-C-G-T,这就是 DNA 的阅读顺序。嘌呤(purine)和嘧啶(pyrimidine)碱基与脱氧核糖 1′碳原子相连。处于 DNA 双链内侧的碱基之间以氢键(虚线)相连构成碱基对。碱基 A 与 T 配对,G 与 C 配对,具有特异性

一致(5′—3′)的单链称为正义链,它的互补链则称为反义链[7]。

总体结构

在真核生物中,多数基因的编码区域是不连续的,它们由转录成熟 mRNA 的外显子(exon)和分割外显子的内含子(intron)区域组成,内含子不会出现在成熟的 mRNA 中(图 3-1)。内含子的确切功能尚不清楚,可能含有进化中保守的调节序列。然而多数内含子的序列没有外显子保守,提示内含子的整体结构可能比其特定的核苷酸顺序更重要。总而言之,最终参与编码蛋白质的 DNA 仅占总 DNA 的很少一部分,而基因之间大量的非转录 DNA 可能起着某种重要的结构性作用。还有许多区域会转录"非编码"RNA,虽然这些调节性 RNA 不能被翻译成蛋白质,但其转录和功能都较活跃[8~10]。

在细胞核中,DNA 也并非单独存在,DNA 与称之为组蛋白的辅助蛋白质形成染色质[11]。多种辅助蛋白质帮助 DNA 进行正确的包装。例如,双螺旋 DNA 在细胞内通常是以超螺旋的结构存在[12],在 DNA 复制和转录中必须进行部分解螺旋[13],这就需要拓扑异构酶和组蛋白乙酰化酶等辅助蛋白的参与。

总结

基因决定对应蛋白质的序列和结构。尽管人类每个细胞核中都含有 20 000~25 000 个基因,但在特定的时间,只有小部分基因在特定的细胞中表达。启动子(或和增强子一起)决定了基因表达的时间和地点。基因的编码区决定了其编码蛋白质的氨基酸序列。除了编码蛋白质的基因序列,基因组还包含了大量调节序列和非编码 RNA 序列。DNA 是线性的多聚核苷酸链,它通常与其互补链通过碱基配对原则(A 与 T 配对,C 与 G 配对)形成 DNA 双链。在细胞核中,DNA 与辅助蛋白结合形成染色质。

分子生物学技术

限制性核酸内切酶和 DNA 重组

真核生物染色体中单个的 DNA 分子长达数百万个碱基对,由于难以直接分析,科学家通常将 DNA 切割成较小的片段。分子生物学家可以借助细菌进化出的一组高度多样化的酶——限制性内切酶,从内部特异性切割 DNA 链[14]。

自然情况下,这套进化出来的内切酶系统可以保护细菌免受外源 DNA 分子(例如噬菌体)的侵袭。这些内切酶通过识别特异的核苷酸序列来区别 DNA 究竟是"自己的"还是"外来的",即不含有特定序列的 DNA 是不会被这些内切酶降解的。但当这些内切酶遇到特定的序列时会结合并切割这些双链 DNA。一般来说限制性内切酶所识别的特定序列为 4~6 个碱基的回文序列,即每条单链从任一方向阅读时都与另一条链从相同的方向(例如都从 5′向 3′阅读)阅读时的序列是一致的(图 3-3)[15]。

尽管限制性内切酶可以将 DNA 切成相对较小的片段,但用于分析的 DNA 片段不能太短(否则 DNA 所带的部分信息会丢失)。如果将 DNA 切得过小,每个 DNA 碎片的信息量会少到被忽略。从统计意义上说,限制性内切酶识别的序列越长,该序列在基因组 DNA 中出现的频率就越低。通常识别序列为 6 个碱基长度的限制性内切酶(因此被称为"六碱基内切酶")所切成的 DNA 片段的长度即可符合分析的要求。比如从大肠埃希菌(escherichia coli)中分离的内切酶 EcoRI 所识别的序列为"GAATTC"。不管该序列位于基因组何处,EcoRI 都会在 G 与 A 之间将 DNA 双链分子切开(图 3-3)(注意,反义链在 3′—5′方向读取 CTTAAG,也会在 5′—3′方向读取 GAATTC,即回文序列的特征)。

基因克隆

机制

目前,有多种强大的技术可以进行基因分析,其中"基因克隆"技术是其他各项技术的基石(图 3-3)。我们可以利用克隆技术在实验室中使 DNA 得到高保真的复制,为生物学分析和其他技术操作,如外源 DNA 连接等,提供充足的 DNA 材料。20 世纪 70 年代早期,Cohen 及其同事[16]在细菌与噬菌体中发现了两种重要的工具:质粒和连接酶,从而使分子克隆技术成为现实。

质粒是一种独立于细菌自身 DNA 之外的环状 DNA 分子,可在胞质中复制。天然的质粒常常带有对宿主细胞有用的遗传信息,比如赋予抗生素抗性的基因。质粒对于基因克隆有着非常重要的作用,因为质粒具有利用宿主细胞的酶系统来复制自身所需的必需信息,而且可产生上千个拷贝。

DNA 连接酶是一种由细菌(或噬菌体感染细菌)产生的酶,可以将不同的 DNA 片段连接在一起。核苷酸序列并不影响 DNA 连接酶的连接效率,因此即使那些在自然界中通常不相连的 DNA,连接酶也可将其连接在一起。实际上,克隆的优势在于能够按需"混合和匹配"DNA 片段。

限制性核酸内切酶法克隆质粒

在基因克隆中,可以利用限制性内切酶在质粒复制必需区以外的序列中将其切开(图 3-3)。假如我们用 EcoRI 在质粒的非复制区进行切割,其将识别 DNA 中的 GAATTC 序列并在两条核苷酸链中的 G 与 A 间将质粒切开。这就会在切口末端处形成具有突出单链序列的 AATT"尾巴"(注意,当在 5′—3′方向读取核苷酸时,有义链中的尾部序列与反义链中的序列相同)。而另外一条外源 DNA 链也被相同的内切酶 EcoRI 切割产生具有同样突出单链序列的 AATT"尾巴",质粒 DNA 的末端单链 AATT 序列与另一条 DNA 的末端单链 TTAA 序列(从 3′—5′阅读)之间由于互补而形成配对。这样外源 DNA 就可以结合于质粒的缺口,再次形成闭合的 DNA 环(对于质粒复制是必需的)。

尽管质粒可以和外源 DNA 末端通过碱基互补相连,但这种连接并不是共价连接。DNA 连接酶可以将质粒与外源 DNA 共价连在一起,形成永久的重组环形 DNA,就能消除重组环的不稳定性。该质粒不但带有在细菌中复制所需的信息,同时还带有外源的 DNA。虽然 EcoRI 切割质粒产生的两个黏性末端之间也可以互补重新形成天然质粒,但分子生物学家已经设计了多种方法来避免这种情况的发生。需要指出的是,重组的 DNA 并不一定必须要具有单链黏性末端,DNA 连接酶也可以将两条不带单链尾的平末端共价连接在一起。

将重组质粒重新导入到宿主细菌中[称之为"转化"(trans-

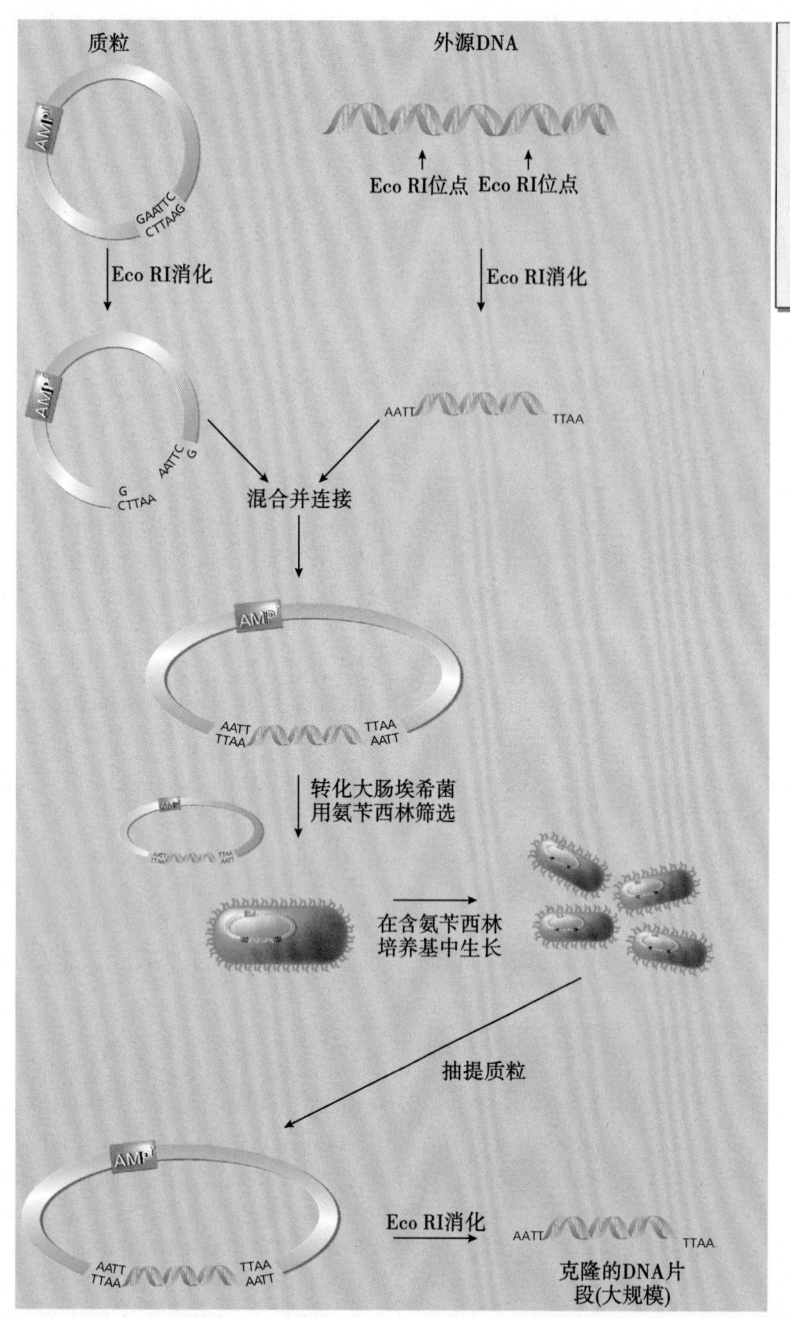

图 3-3　限制性内切酶 EcoRI 切割 DNA 与基因克隆。图例中所示少量的外源 DNA（纳克级）被 EcoRI 切割。DNA 序列中含有 EcoRI 内切酶的识别位点 GAATTC（见框中所示），EcoRI 在识别序列处将双链 DNA 切开，产生 5′单链序列的“尾巴”。只要 DNA 含有内切酶识别位点即可被识别，不受来源的限制。同时质粒载体也可以用相同的 EcoRI 消化成线性的 DNA 分子。具有 5′单链“尾巴”的外源 DNA 可以与载体黏性末端互补配对，通过 DNA 连接酶共价连接。将重组 DNA 导入到大肠埃希菌的过程称为转化。由于细菌本身对氨苄西林（ampicillin）没有抗性，所以只有含有质粒 DNA（带有氨苄西林抗性基因）的细菌才能在氨苄西林培养基中生长。同时质粒 DNA 带有复制起点位点，可以在细菌中不断复制产生多个拷贝。当培养物中细菌达到一定浓度时，可用生化方法分离出质粒 DNA。再用 EcoRI 内切酶将外源 DNA 从质粒上切下，就能得到扩增 10^6 倍的产物

formation）］时，被插入的外源 DNA 会随着质粒一起被复制，同时转化的细菌可以在液体培养基中大量繁殖。随着宿主细胞的分裂，其所携带的质粒就会被不断地复制。当培养液中的质粒累积到一定量时（一般 1 升培养基中约含几毫克），就可进行纯化，得到纯度较高的质粒。然后用限制性内切酶（EcoRI）将外源 DNA 从质粒上剪切下来，用于进一步的分析或其他操作。采用相同的方法，我们也可以利用细菌病毒（噬菌体）来获取大量的重组外源 DNA 的噬菌体。在上述实验中，质粒或者噬菌体就像车辆一样将外源 DNA 运载入宿主细菌，因此称其为“载体（vector）”。

这些极其强大的工具现已成为所有分子生物学实验室标准设备的一部分，它极大地推动了我们随后提到的一些分析技

术的发展。目前已有多篇技术手册详细介绍了这些技术[17,18]。

Gateway 法克隆质粒

Gateway 是一种克隆质粒的商业系统,因其易于在质粒之间转移 DNA 片段而受到研究人员的广泛欢迎。在 Gateway 克隆中,首先在目标 DNA 片段的 5′和 3′末端添加特定的 Gateway 序列(分别称为“attB1”和“attB2”)。然后使用识别这些 Gateway 序列的名为 BP Clonase 的特有重组酶将该片段重组为 Gateway 供体载体,以产生克隆,其中称为“attL1”和“attL2”的序列位于目标片段的两端。一旦进入 Gateway 供体载体,可以使用另一种称为“LR Clonase”的重组酶混合物将该片段(现称为“入门克隆”)转移到数千种的 Gateway 目标载体中的任意一种中[19]。因此这种基于重组酶的技术允许基因片段在质粒之间穿梭,而不需要限制性消化和纯化的步骤(图 3-4a)。

Gibson 法克隆质粒

克隆发展最新的技术称为 Gibson 组装法,该方法可以轻松组装多个末端重叠的 DNA 片段。在该方法中,将两种或更多种待组装的片段与三种 DNA 酶——核酸外切酶、聚合酶和连接酶混合在一起。核酸外切酶去除待连接片段的 5′末端,从而暴露 3′的单链 DNA 末端。然后这些末端重叠的串联片段通过 3′端退火,由 DNA 聚合酶和 DNA 连接酶分别填充间隙和空缺。这些片段可以通过一步等温反应连接在一起。常规情况下,这种强大的合成生物学方法可以组装多达数百千碱基的多个 DNA 片段[20]。例如,最近 Gibson 组装法使用 600 个末端重叠的串联片段,合成了大小为 16.3k 碱基的完整小鼠线粒体基因组(图 3-4b)[21]。

基因探针和杂交

从这部分开始我们将重点介绍如何在细胞或组织中的全部基因组 DNA 或 RNA 中来检测某一特定基因的 DNA 或 mRNA。完成这一任务的前提是我们已获得目的基因 DNA 的片段。目前获得基因 DNA 的方法有多种,可以从基因组 DNA 构建的基因文库或 cDNA 文库中获得,也可以通过 PCR 的方法(将在随后的章节中详细介绍)得到。这些 DNA 片段可以是任何大小,从基因的少部分(几百甚至更少的核苷酸)到整个基因(几千个核苷酸)都可以。我们正是用这些克隆片段来检测目的基因的 DNA 或 RNA,这些片段称为探针(probe)。

BP反应:attB底物(attB-PCR产物或线性化attB表达克隆)与attP底物(供体载体)重组,组建包含attL的进入克隆(参见下图)。该反应由BP Clonase™混合物催化

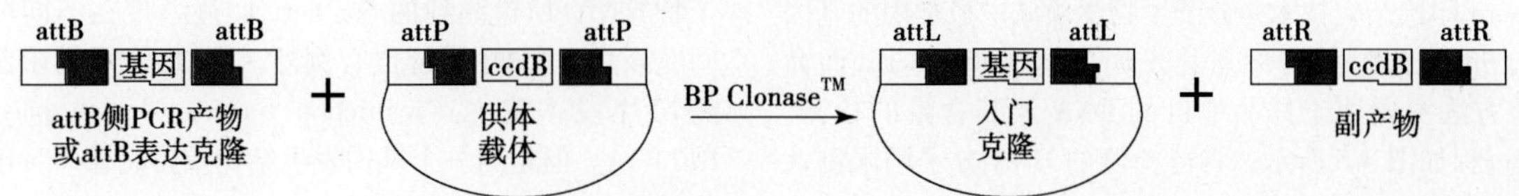

LR反应:促进attL底物(进入克隆)与attR底物(目标载体)重组以组建包含attB的表达克隆(参见下图)。该反应由LR Clonase™混合物催化

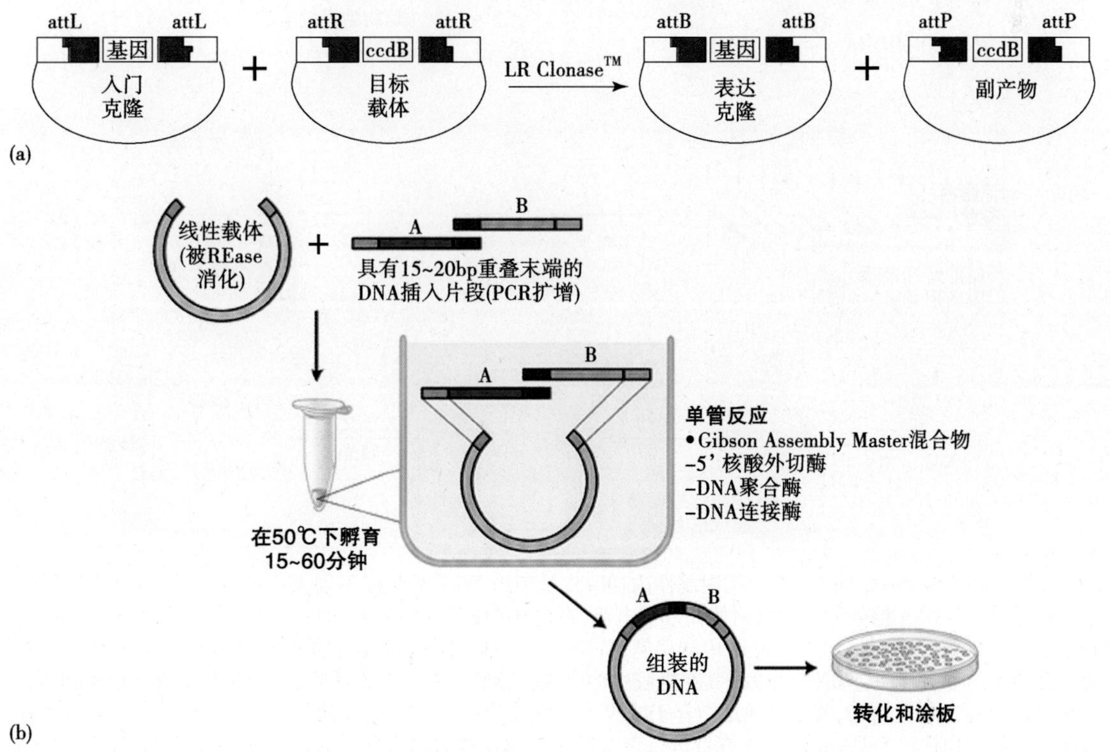

图 3-4　(a)Gateway 法。(b)Gibson 法

基因探针的长度不能太短，必须有足够长的碱基对才能与目的基因进行特异性识别。探针识别目的基因的过程称为分子杂交（nucleic acid hybridization）。分子杂交的基础是两条DNA链通过碱基互补配对形成较稳定的双链区（退火），即A与T配对，G与C配对（图3-2）。两条完全互补的DNA链之间配对的作用力大于部分互补的DNA链，而且配对的DNA链越长，其配对的作用力也越大。目前在分子杂交基础之上已开发出多种生物技术，如Southern杂交、基因芯片和PCR等（见下文）。

总结

利用识别特异性位点的限制性内切酶，我们可以从基因组DNA将目的基因片段切下，同时将其大量扩增用于随后的生物学分析，该过程称为克隆，而用于克隆基因的细菌质粒和噬菌体称为载体。DNA连接酶可以将外源DNA连接到细菌质粒和噬菌体上，外源DNA可以随载体一起扩增。扩增的外源基因DNA可被用做探针在细胞或组织基因组的DNA或RNA中检测相应的基因。

基因分析：DNA

Southern 印迹杂交

Southern印迹杂交技术是分子生物学领域中最常用的基因组DNA分析方法之一，为纪念其发明者E. M. Southern，而命名[22]。该方法主要用于样品中目的DNA及其含量的检测。具体实验过程如图3-5所示。将待检测的DNA分子用限制性内切酶消化成不同大小的片段后，通过琼脂糖凝胶电泳进行分离（DNA的磷酸基团使DNA带负电荷，所以DNA在电场中向正极移动；线状双链DNA分子的迁移速率与分子量成反比，分子越大则所受阻力越大，也越难在凝胶孔隙中通过，因而迁移越慢。因此在电场中分子越小，越靠近正极）。

Southern印迹的最终目标是使用核酸杂交鉴定切割DNA的特定片段。由于电泳中使用的琼脂糖凝胶很厚，DNA片段可以在其中移动，因此凝胶中的DNA并不适合做进一步的分析。因此必须将DNA片段转移到可以与之不可逆结合的固体支持物上以进行核酸杂交研究。因此，在电泳后，将纸薄膜微过滤器（由硝酸纤维素或尼龙制成）置于凝胶的平坦部分上。然后在垂直于DNA电泳移动的方向上使液体通过琼脂糖凝胶，当液体灌注凝胶时，DNA片段沉积并黏附在滤膜上，DNA片段将按大小转移到固相支持物上。

接着通过多种技术中的任何一种对克隆的DNA片段（探针）进行放射性显影。含有DNA的膜浸泡在含有放射性核素的探针中。如果待检物中含有与探针互补的序列，则二者通过碱基互补进行结合，游离的探针经洗涤后会去除，特异性结合的部分可以用X线放射自显影技术进行检测。

经过X线放射自显影，最后将得到含有一条或多个条带的X光片。每条对应于一条限制性核酸内切酶所切割产生的DNA片段，并含有与所标记探针互补的序列。正常情况下，一个特异探针所检测到的Southern印迹条带在不同个体样品之间应该是相同的［尽管也有例外，见随后介绍的限制性核酸内酶切片段多态性（restriction fragment length polymorphisms，RFLP）］。但是当一个基因发生结构重排时，Southern条带的模式就会改变。

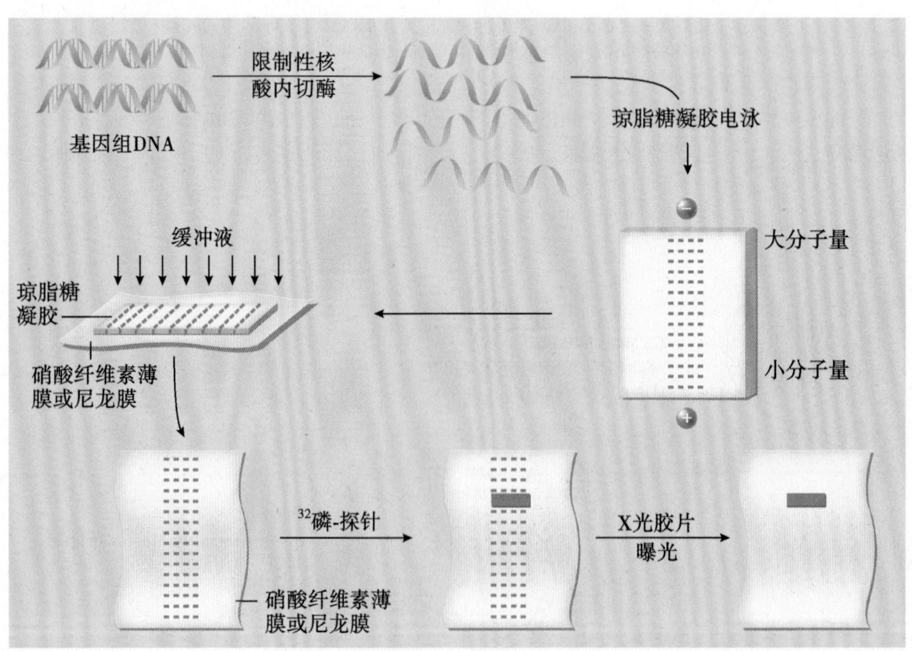

图3-5 基因组Southern印迹杂交。用限制性内切酶将基因组DNA消化成不同大小的片段，通过琼脂糖凝胶电泳进行分离。DNA携带的磷酸基团使其带负电荷，在电场中向正极移动。但这一运动受到琼脂糖的阻碍，分子越小则所受阻力越小，在凝胶孔隙中迁移越快；反之分子越大则所受阻力越大，迁移越慢。当电泳结束后通过缓冲液的垂直移动将DNA片段按其在凝胶中的位置转移到硝酸纤维素薄膜或尼龙膜上。利用毛细运动，DNA片段从凝胶转运出来，并不可逆地结合于滤膜上。仍按片段大小排列在滤膜上的DNA片段与放射性核素或其他标志物标记的DNA或RNA探针进行杂交反应。经X线放射自显影后，含有与探针互补序列的DNA片段所在的位置将会显示一条杂交带

例如，c-abl探针通常在正常基因组DNA中识别2 000bp的EcoRI片段。如果慢性粒细胞白血病（CML）患者的易位断点发生在该片段内，部分c-abl基因和一个EcoRI位点会从9号染色体移至22号染色体。分析患者DNA的Southern印迹可能发现：①如果受体染色体的EcoRI位点比原先的EcoRI位点更远，则会检测到更大的片段；或者②如果受体染色体的EcoRI位点比原先的EcoRI位点更近，则会检测到更小的片段。因此，Southern印迹杂交是一种可以灵敏地检测染色体大范围重排的技术，例如与恶性肿瘤相关的染色体重排。

由于在Southern印迹中杂交在膜上的探针信号的强弱与所检测到的目的基因的拷贝数成正比，因此该方法也可以用于对目的基因进行定量分析。例如采用Southern印迹杂交技术可在30%乳腺肿瘤中检测到癌基因*HER-2/neu*扩增[23]。

聚合酶链反应（PCR）

用Southern印迹杂交技术测定基因序列时，至少需要1~2mg的基因组DNA，相应的就需要约几个毫克的新鲜或新鲜冷冻的组织。PCR是一种强大的可用于扩增特定片段DNA的技术，理论上讲甚至可以测定单个DNA分子。因此，如果所检测DNA的序列是已知的话，那么微量的组织、甚至单个细胞所含的DNA经过PCR扩增后，得到的DNA数量就足够用于后续的分析，甚至保存的石蜡块与石蜡组织切片也能用于PCR分析[24]。PCR的反应原理如图3-6所示。两种单链寡核苷酸序列是引物，与模板所扩增的目的片段两端的序列互补。引物与模板DNA混合物经过加热后，模板DNA完全解链，然后降低到一定温度使引物与模板DNA的互补区结合，这个过程称为“退火”。这时加入的DNA聚合酶将以目的DNA为模板在引物的3′端不断地增加核苷酸，形成一条新的目的DNA拷贝链。混合物再次被加热使模板DNA完全解链后退火，更多引物会结合到原始的模板DNA链和新生成的DNA链上。这时新加入的DNA聚合酶将会产生4条DNA拷贝链。随着这一过程不断地重复，目的DNA的数量会以指数形式增加。研究者在嗜热古细菌的嗜热水生菌（thermus aquaticus）发现并克隆了耐

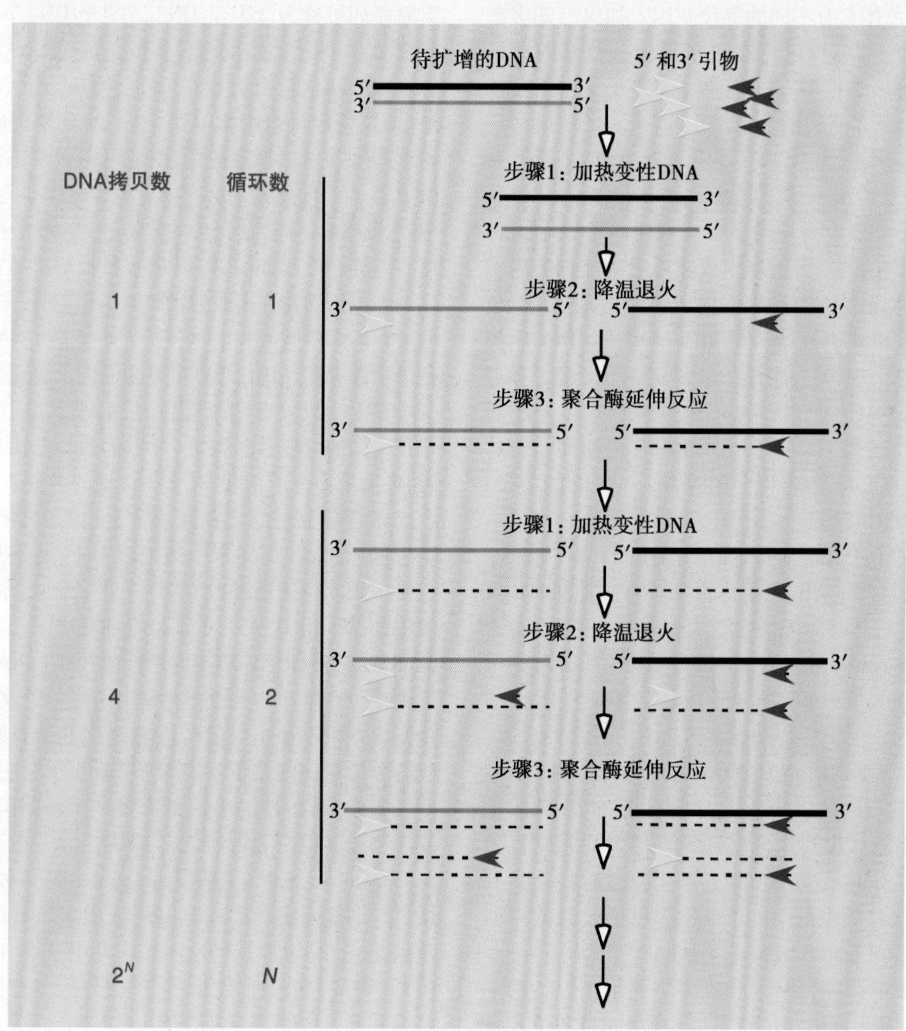

图3-6　聚合酶链反应。将含有模板DNA、与靶序列两端互补的寡核苷酸引物（10~20个碱基）的混合物加热变性成单链后，将温度降至一定程度后，引物与模板DNA单链互补序列会配对：5′引物与下链配对，而3′引物与上链退火配对。在反应混合物中所加的耐热DNA聚合酶（Taq酶）将从与模板上的退火引物部位开始合成新的DNA链。最后将生成一条与模板序列完全一致的双链DNA。在经过加热变性、退火等过程后，DNA聚合酶又将产生一对新的双链DNA分子。这时反应混合物就含有四条双链DNA分子。经几轮循环（通常20~50个）后，就可获得2^n个DNA拷贝产物

热的 DNA 聚合酶(Taq),由于其能够耐受 95℃的高温,因此 DNA 加热变性后,该酶并不会失活,整个 PCR 反应只需加一次酶即可[25,26],从而使 PCR 可以自动化进行。现在每个分子生物学实验室与许多临床实验室都备有 PCR 仪,将 PCR 反应混合物在其上运行 20~50 个循环后就能从微量的起始样品扩增得到大量的目的 DNA 产物并用于后续分析。

DNA 多态性

基因多态性(字面意思是"存在多种形式")是指 DNA 区域中的一个位点存在两种或两种以上形式的等位基因。基因多态性与突变的区别就是基因多态性在正常人群中更常发生,具有正常表型。通常,差异基因在人群中出现的频率大于等于 1%才称做多态性,例如血型和组织相容性复合物分子等。

基因多态性并不会导致个体表型的改变。例如在基因的内含子区域或两基因之间的核苷酸序列发生改变都不会导致蛋白质改变,因此这种改变是"沉默"的。如果这些变化具有多态性和多频性,那么个体的多态性很可能是杂合的。换句话说,个体中的双倍染色体含有不同的等位基因。如果已知多态性变化的染色体位置,那么可以将它用来定位其他基因的标记。目前已发现多种多态性 DNA 的位置,这为开发癌相关基因的定位鉴定技术打下了坚实的基础。

限制性片段长度多态性(RFLP)是用单克隆 DNA 探针和 Southern 印迹杂交法来检测个体之间基因组 DNA 的差异。采用 Southern 印迹杂交法来检测基因多态性主要基于以下两种机制。首先,单核苷酸的改变可能产生或破坏限制性核酸内切酶的识别位点,当用特定的限制性核酸内切酶消化 DNA 时,该基因的 Southern 印迹模式会改变。例如,某个体的 DNA 序列是……AGGATTTCGA……,另一个体的单个核苷酸出现了多态性,使该序列变为……AGGAATTCGA……,这就会产生一个新的 EcoRI 位点(GAATTC)(图 2-3)。当用 EcoRI 内切酶切割这两个个体的基因组 DNA 时,后者将会比前者少一条旧的条带,并多出两条新条带(图 3-3)。

第二种机制则是由于真核细胞中的基因组 DNA 具有一个神秘的特征,整个基因组充满了大量功能未知的重复序列。这些序列在基因组 DNA 上以头尾相串联的方式相连,因此称之为串联重复序列(tandem repeat)。Alu 序列(由于其含有一个限制性内切酶 AluI 的特异性识别位点)是人类基因组 DNA 中比较典型的重复序列。由于其是人类基因组 DNA 中特有的序列,因此可以作为多物种 DNA 混合物中人类基因组 DNA 的鉴定标志。许多情况下,串联 Alu 重复序列的数量因个体而异[27]。因此,如果用能够识别包含串联重复序列的限制性片段的 DNA 探针进行 Southern 印迹,那么个体间最后将会得到不同的杂交图谱。这种类型的 RFLP 也称为可变数目的串联重复(variable number of tandem repeat,VNTR)。

由于这两种机制的限制性片段长度多态性均可以孟德尔方式遗传给下一代,因此可用其进行基因定位。RFLP 位点常常存在基因组 DNA 的特定位置(基因座)。如果在特定遗传疾病的家庭中,所有受影响的个体都继承了相同的 RFLP,则表明该疾病的基因可能与 RFLP 基因座接近(或"连锁")。利用 RFLP 多态性进行遗传病基因定位是克隆致病基因的第一步。因此这些多态性位点是我们进行致病基因鉴定的反向遗传分析工具,可用来鉴定许多与恶性转化相关的基因。一个典型的例子是 17 号染色体上 BRCA1 基因,该基因突变是可遗传性乳腺癌发生的一个重要因素[28]。

RFLP 同时也可用于发现肿瘤中的基因缺失(图 3-7a),但前提是被分析个体在这一位点为杂合状态,即在某条染色体上具有一种多态性而在另一条上具有其他多态性(如果被分析个体为纯合体,则其肿瘤组织与正常组织的 Southern 印迹杂交图谱相同)。如果患有癌症的个体特定的 RFLP(称为信息个体)是杂合的,则可以使用识别多态性的探针通过 Southern 印迹分析其的肿瘤,并以相同的方式与正常组织进行比较。如果杂合个体的肿瘤细胞 DNA 丢失了正常 DNA 中的一个 RFLP,称之为纯合性增加或杂合性丢失(loss of heterozygosity,LOH)。LOH 一般是抑癌基因的标志,如视网膜母细胞瘤基因 Rb 或 TP53[29,30]。

另一种有趣的基因多态性标记称为微卫星 DNA。整个人类基因组大约散布着 5 万个由 dC-dA 组成的短重复序列(串联重复 10~60 次)拷贝,其原因不明[31]。由于相对较长的重复序列(前面提过的 VNTR)被称为小卫星 DNA,因此更短的 dC-dA 重复序列被称为微卫星 DNA("卫星 DNA"一词的来源是由于重复 DNA 的浮力密度与大多数基因组 DNA 不同,当通过密度梯度离心纯化基因组 DNA 时,会出现与主 DNA 带不同的小卫星带)。特定位置中微卫星 DNA 的重复次数具有多态性。由于这些序列可以稳定遗传,因此可用做多态性标记。两个多态微卫星之间的重复单元的数量差异可以小至几个核苷酸,而传统的 Southern 印迹杂交法的分辨率为 100 个核苷酸,无法检测到这些差异。然而,PCR 可以很容易地解决这些差异。在短重复序列中设计引物并用放射性核素标记,通过 PCR 扩增产物,然后通过聚丙烯酰胺凝胶电泳分析。小卫星 DNA 与微卫星 DNA 在基因定位中的作用比 RFLP 更为强大,这是因为不同于 RFLP 在一个基因座只具有两个等位基因,小卫星 DNA 与微卫星 DNA 重复序列的可变数量很大,可以为每个基因座创建多个等位基因,极大地提高了杂合体(作为标记的必要条件)的出现概率。

尽管微卫星的重复数通常是稳定的,但在一些肿瘤,比如结直肠癌中,肿瘤样本中微卫星 DNA 的重复次数明显不同于正常组织。由于这种改变存在于整个肿瘤基因组中,提示肿瘤组织的基因组 DNA 处于不稳定的状态[32,33]。这可能是由于人类细胞维持基因组 DNA 均一性的校正(proofreading)基因发生了突变。在酵母中突变这些基因后,会导致 dCdA 重复序列的重复次数极不稳定。遗传性非息肉性结直肠癌就是由于定位于 2 号染色体的校正基因 *MSH2* 发生了突变所致[34,35]。

当然,多态性的出现不需要产生新的限制性位点、串联重复序列或其他明显的标志。单核苷酸多态性(single nucleotide polymorphism,SNP)是基因组 DNA 中另一种常见的 DNA 多态性[36],是基因编码区或非编码区中单核苷酸的变异。在人类基因组中平均每 1 350 个碱基对中就有 1 个 SNP[37~39]。与 RFLP 和微卫星多态性相似,单核苷酸多态性可用于定位致癌基因并确定人类癌症中染色体的杂合性丢失(loss of heterozygosity,LOH)。

通过 SNP 分析检测 LOH 的方法主要是通过微阵列或测序(见下文)。微阵列方法中,基因组 DNA 经过 PCR 扩增,其产物与含有大量的 SNP 位点的微阵列进行杂交,来检测 LOH 的染色体区域(即含有肿瘤抑制因子的区域)以及扩增区域(即含有癌基因的区域)(图 3-7b)。SNP 阵列使大规模的拷贝数

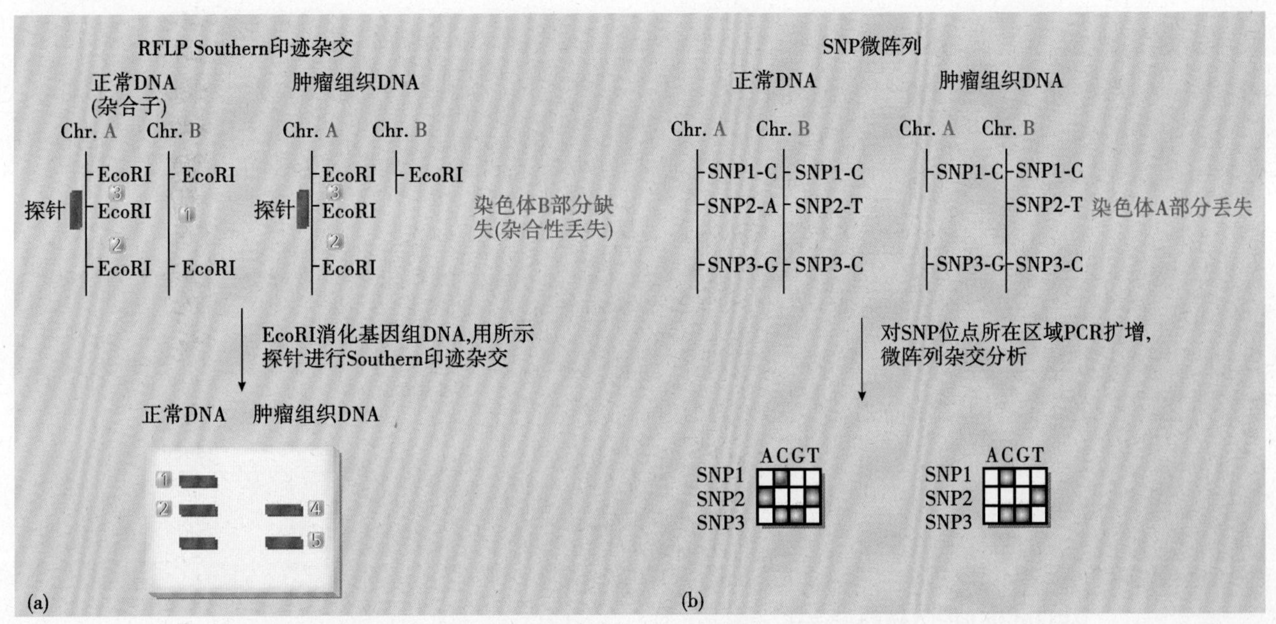

图3-7 在肿瘤组织中检测杂合性丢失(loss of heterozygosity,LOH)的方法。(a)限制性片段长度多态性(restriction fragment length polymorphism,RFLP)与Southerm印迹杂交。图中所示的样本基因组EcoRI识别位点为杂合:A染色体中的第二个EcoRI位点在另外一条双倍染色体B中缺失。肿瘤细胞起源于丢失B染色体的单个细胞。对正常DNA样本和肿瘤DNA样本在琼脂糖凝胶中分别进行Southern印迹杂交分析。用图中所示的探针对正常DNA样本探测后显示出杂合的带型(在两条染色体上具有多态性),而肿瘤DNA则丢失其中一种带型,丢失的正是抑癌基因。(b)单核苷酸多态性(single nucleotide polymorphism,SNP)微阵列。图中所示的个体基因组中2和3号位置的SNP为杂合,而1号SNP为纯合。对每个SNP位点PCR扩增并进行微阵列杂交分析。在微阵列杂交分析中杂合SNP信号出现丢失说明包含SNP位点的染色体片段丢失了

分析实现了高通量自动化[40,41]。下一代核苷酸测序方法(下面详细讨论)也允许推断拷贝数的改变,两者的区别在于对比的测序深度[42]。这两种技术均可用于石蜡包埋组织样本,使利用病理标本进行基因组研究成为现实[43]。

核酸测序

Sanger 测序法

基因编码区内的核苷酸序列编码其相应蛋白质的氨基酸序列。因此,基因的核苷酸序列可用于预测其蛋白质产物的结构和功能。回顾历史,用于DNA测序的主要方法是Sanger及其同事发明的"酶链终止"法[44]。链终止方法依赖于DNA聚合酶的特性(图3-8),DNA聚合酶是从单个核苷酸开始产生新DNA聚合物的酶。但是DNA聚合酶需要一个单链DNA作为模板才能发挥作用并产生新的聚合物。DNA聚合酶在延伸的DNA链的3′末端添加新的核苷酸,但新核苷酸的碱基必须能够与聚合酶所在模板上的碱基配对(即互补配对)。加入该核苷酸后,聚合酶移至模板上的下一个核苷酸,并将新的核苷酸添加到延伸链的3′末端。同样,新核苷酸必须与模板中的下一个碱基互补。当该过程完成时,DNA聚合酶将产生新的DNA链,其核苷酸序列与模板DNA完全互补。

核苷酸测序基于以下发现:当DNA聚合酶将异常核苷酸添加到生长链中时,聚合会停止。最常用的合成"终止"核苷酸是双脱氧核苷酸,它们的脱氧核糖基团的3′碳上缺少1个羟基,一旦加入DNA链,该双脱氧核糖核酸就不能和下一个核苷酸以磷酸二酯键相连(图3-2)。例如,存在双脱氧腺苷三磷酸(ddATP)的情况下,DNA聚合反应就会终止在新生链中任何出

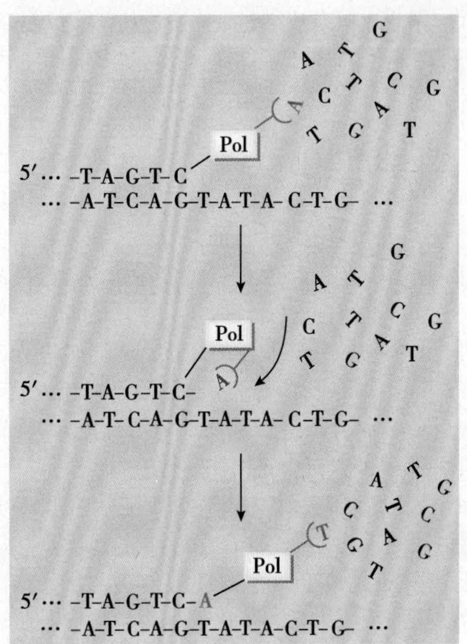

图3-8 DNA聚合酶。示意图中,DNA聚合酶正利用模板(下方链)创建一条新的DNA链(上方链)。根据模板链的下一个核苷酸,DNA聚合酶在新生链上按5′-3′方向连接特定核苷酸。Pol,DNA聚合酶

现A的位置(对应于模板中T的位置)(图3-9)。因此当我们在体外试管中进行这种聚合反应时,一次就会产生成千上万个新生的DNA链。当正常的腺嘌呤脱氧三磷酸核苷酸(dATP)混有适量比例的腺嘌呤双脱氧三磷酸核苷酸(ddATP)时,就会

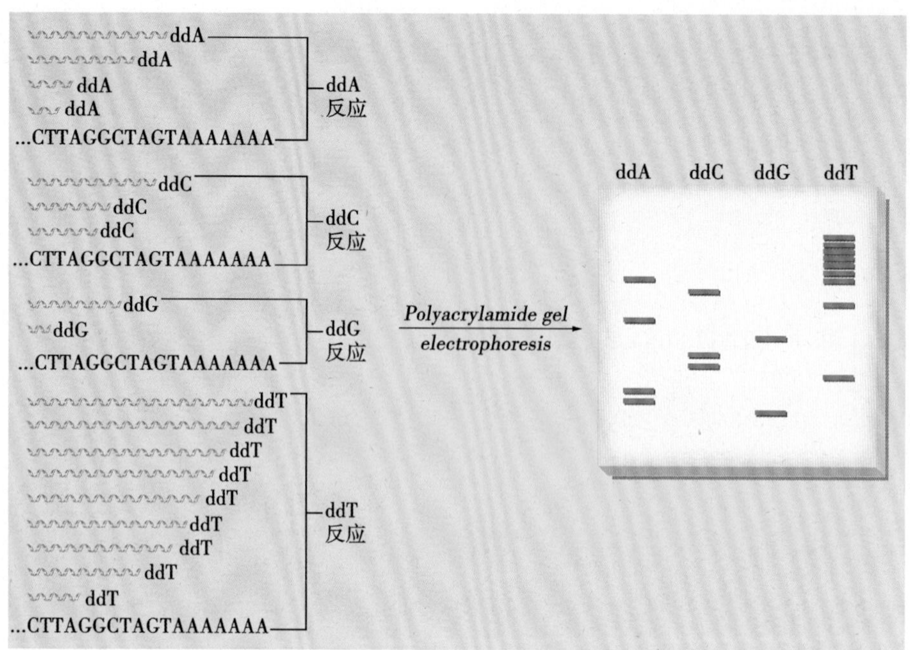

图 3-9 链终止法对 DNA 进行测序。图示例子是对末端为 CTTAGGCTAGTAAAAAAA 的 DNA 进行测序分析。利用这一模板 DNA，同时进行 4 个独立的 DNA 聚合反应，每个反应体系中分别含有四种双脱氧核糖核苷酸（ddATP、ddCTP、ddGTP 和 ddTTP）。在每一个反应中，当与模板中相应位置互补的双脱氧核糖核苷酸加入到正在合成中的 DNA 链上时，会终止 DNA 聚合反应。这样就会合成成千上万个对应不同终止位置且片段大小不同的新 DNA 链。而这些不同大小的 DNA 链可通过尿素聚丙烯酰胺凝胶电泳分离，DNA 链越长越靠近胶的顶端，相反 DNA 链越短越靠近胶的底端。如果新生 DNA 链被放射性核素标记，那么放射自显影后可在 X 线片呈现出测序结果。对于测序电泳图谱的识读，应从胶片底部逐个向顶部读取。根据相应位置和双脱氧核糖核苷酸的种类，对应的互补核苷酸就是模板的序列。从图中所示的测序图谱底端开始读出的序列为“GAATCCGATCATTTTTTT”，其对应的互补序列“CTTAGGCTAGTAAAAAAA”就是待测序列。用荧光标记的毛细管电泳测序结果的判读与上述方法基本类似

有一部分新生链分子终止在模板上含有 T 的位置。这就形成一种全部具有相同起始端和以 A 残基为 3′端结尾（对应于模板为 T）的一系列长短不一片段的混合物。如果将双脱氧核糖核苷酸用不同的荧光标记，然后就可以在聚丙烯酰胺凝胶或毛细管凝胶中进行电泳分离（见下文）。每一条带代表着一条从起始端到一个含有 A 残基位置的片段。当同时进行四种双脱氧核糖核苷酸链式反应时，由于每个双脱氧核苷酸的荧光标记不同，4 种反应的混合物进行毛细管电泳分离时，计算机可自动根据颜色判读 DNA 链中这四种碱基的顺序。

Sanger 测序已经成为生物技术的基石，并帮助顺利完成了人类基因组计划，该项目于 1990 年启动并于 2003 年完成。随着人类基因组序列图谱的完成，基因组研究者的工作重心已经从测定新的物种基因组转移到比较基因组测序。通过对正常人群与患病人群进行高通量测序来探索基因变异与疾病的关系。

最活跃的比较测序领域是癌症基因组学，针对特定基因或基因家族的早期测序研究确定了癌症与正常基因组之间的关键差异，这些发现为靶向治疗提供了基础。例如，对胃肠道间质瘤（GIST）的 DNA 测序发现其存在 c-kit 蛋白酪氨酸激酶基因突变[45]，后续研究表明用 c-kit 抑制剂 STI-571 或 Gleevec 可成功对 GIST 进行治疗[46]。酪氨酸激酶表皮生长因子受体（*EGFR*）激活型突变普遍存在于肺腺癌组织中，尤其在东亚人群中[47~49]。这些激活突变可预测对激酶抑制剂吉非替尼和厄洛替尼的反应[47~49]。超过一半的黑素瘤携带了 *BRAF* 丝氨酸—苏氨酸激酶基因激活突变[50]，随后在其他癌症类型（结肠直肠癌、肺癌和甲状腺癌）中也发现了该突变。*BRAF* 抑制剂 Vemurafenib 可改善携带 *BRAF* V600E 活化突变的转移性黑色素瘤患者的总体生存率[51]。在结直肠癌、胶质母细胞瘤[52]和乳腺癌中发现了磷脂酰肌醇 3-激酶催化亚基基因 *PIK3CA* 的突变。而在真性红细胞增多症等骨髓增生性疾病中发现了 *JAK2* V617F 这种特异性的激活突变[53~55]。

高通量测序

最新的癌症基因组学研究采用了“下一代”测序技术，该技术远远超过了传统的 Sanger 测序的规模和分辨率。新一代测序方法可以同时进行数百万个短片段测序反应[56~59]。癌症基因组学高通量测序的最大优势之一是不需要对克隆 DNA 模板进行纯化，也能够对含有众多突变的癌症样本进行有效检测[60]。实际上，高通量测序分析已经成为癌症突变研究领域的首选技术，也逐渐开始被纳入临床诊断测试中。

2008 年，科学家首次采用高通量测序对急性髓细胞白血病的基因组进行了检测[61]。此后，研究者对其他许多类型肿瘤的编码区（外显子组）或全基因组也进行了测序。这些工作大都是在癌症基因组图谱（the Cancer Genome Atlas，TCGA）和国际癌症基因组联盟（International Cancer Genome Consortium，ICGC）

的倡议和协调下进行的[64]。

大多数商业测序平台属于“循环阵列测序”，是在大量 DNA 分子上并行完成基于酶组的测序和基于成像的序列检测的迭代循环[58]。目前存在许多循环阵列测序方法，包括 Illumina(Solexa)、Pacific Bio、454/Roche、SOLiD 和 Ion Torrent。

上述所有方法中，待测序的 DNA 样品首先被剪切成小 DNA 片段的文库。然后将常见的衔接子序列连接到每个片段，并将这些衔接子用作 PCR 扩增的起始点，使每个片段克隆扩增。扩增产物在每个循环结束时在整个阵列上完成成像测序。通过这种方式，可以高通量测序大量的 DNA 片段[58]。

每种循环阵列测序方法各有不同，主要不同点是：产生不同空间的 PCR 扩增 DNA 片段的方法和测序所采用的生物化学技术。不同方法之间的读取长度、规模、成本和精度也存在差异。目前，Illumina 测序平台的应用最为广泛[62]。Illumina 测序通过“桥式 PCR”的方法产生克隆扩增。在该方法中，与衔接子序列互补的正向和反向引物被固定到一张玻璃片。PCR 扩增产生约 1 000 个拷贝空间簇的 DNA 片段，然后进行循环测序。在每个测序循环中，DNA 聚合酶掺入具有可逆 3′终止部分的荧光标记的 dNTP。与 Sanger 测序概念类似，仅允许将单个碱基添加到每个片段的 3′末端，然后将所有片段(或“特征”)用四种颜色成像，每种颜色对应于一种 dNTP 种类，再切割可逆的 3′终止部分，之后重新开始下一个测序循环。由于所有片段的测序都是平行的，因此在整个过程结束时，该方法能够获得每一个片段中的 DNA 序列(图 3-10)[58]。

靶标富集和临床测试

虽然上述方法可对整个基因组进行测序，但有些测序在技术或计算上并不一定可行，经济上也未必划算或必要。“靶标富集”是指在测序之前在核苷酸文库中富集特定的目的基因组区域。靶标富集可以通过多种方法进行，包括 PCR、分子倒置(molecular inversion)和杂交捕获(hybrid capture)；在大多数情况下，杂交捕获技术已成为最广泛使用的方法。关于这一点，有非常好的综述供参考[63]。

在用杂交捕获技术进行靶标富集时，将感兴趣的基因组区域的寡核苷酸探针与片段化的 DNA 文库杂交，并洗掉非结合的片段。杂交反应可以发生在载玻片表面或溶液中。在癌症基因组学中，杂交捕获技术常用于将全基因组文库减少到仅对应于“外显子组”或蛋白质编码基因组区域的那些片段。全外显子组测序将待测序的 DNA 总量从 3Gb 减少到 30Mb。该方法可以减少计算的需求、成本和测序时间，同时仍然可以阐明人类癌症中的大多数体细胞突变[63,64]。

随着高通量测序成本的降低和可靠性的提高，该技术也越来越多地被纳入临床检测。目前若干机构和商业公司在销售靶向基因组检测项目，他们使用靶向富集和高通量测序技术对一组选定的肿瘤驱动基因进行测序，从而提供基因组数据进行预后或治疗选择。

生物信息学方法

对上述测序技术产生的数据进行分析的生物信息学方法同样重要。一旦从肿瘤样品和对照中获得了 DNA 序列，第一步就是通过去除低质量序列(通常在读取末端)并去除与衔接子一致的序列来控制初始读数。然后使用几种序列比对算法将肿瘤和正常样品的读数与参考基因组进行比对并鉴定差异。随后生物信息学工具一般用于评估三种主要类型的改变：单核苷酸取代或小片段插入缺失、拷贝数改变和结构重排(图 3-11)[42,64]。

单核苷酸取代和小片段插入缺失

肿瘤与对照种系和参考基因组相比，其特定序列的改变频率不同，即单核苷酸取代或小片段插入缺失(“indel”)。例如，种系通常是以 50%(如果是杂合的)或 100%(如果是纯合的)的频率突变，但肿瘤样品中存在一定频率范围的单碱基取代，这取决于肿瘤突变的等位基因、样品纯度和染色体倍数。最终，突变研究是一门统计学，癌症序列中突变计数的统计学意义是其基础[42,64]。目前有很多体细胞突变的查询工具，包括 MuTect[65]、Varscan2[66]、JointSNVMix[67] 和 MutSigCV[68]。和其他精准的发现突变的方法不同，这些突变查询系统的总体目标是应用统计方法来检测具有高度特异性的低等位基因部分的体细胞突变。遗漏突变的主要原因包括肿瘤与正常组织的混合、肿瘤内异质性和染色体倍数差异。高通量测序相比 Sanger 测序的一个基本优势为前者是数字化的，而非模拟的。这意味着可以多次读取相同的 DNA 片段，允许“重复采样”或具有足够的覆盖深度，以便在统计学显著水平上提供可信的体细胞改变情况[42,64]。

拷贝数变化

新一代测序提供了在单核苷酸水平上研究拷贝数变化的能力，与基于阵列的技术相比显著提高了分辨率。简单来说，通过比较肿瘤样本中基因座与正常对照中的读数，就可以通过高通量测序数据推断出拷贝数，已有一些生物信息学工具可以进行这种分析。这些工具均考虑到给定窗口内的拷贝数读取必须针对该区域中的序列覆盖进行标准化。这一点是至关重要的，基因组的覆盖范围可能会因为 GC 含量、模糊映射读取和其他因素而不同[64,69]。

结构重排

通常情况下我们是从序列的两端获得测序序列。末端配对测序允许人们确定测序片段的两端是否以预期的距离对应参考的基因组。当测序的序列“分裂”时，序列的两端映射到基因组的不同部分。阐释序列“分裂”可用于识别染色体内和染色体间的重排、倒置、重复和其他结构变化[42,70,71]。

总结

基因组 DNA 是巨大的生物大分子，为其分析带来了一定的困难。从细菌中分离纯化的核酸内切酶能将 DNA 分子切割成易于检测的片段，通过琼脂糖凝胶电泳按照 DNA 片段的大小进行分离分析，我们可以通过 Southern 印迹检测携带对应于目的基因的核苷酸序列片段。DNA 测序可以确定产生稳定遗传差异的特定核苷酸变化(突变)，测序既可以通过传统的“Sanger”方法也可以用高通量方法来完成。PCR 技术使检测极少量组织中的特定基因成为可能。在全基因组 DNA 中存在多种类型的多态性位点：产生或破坏限制性核酸内切酶位点会导致 RFLP；产生包含可变数量的串联重复序列的微卫星；还有 SNP 所代表的单碱基变异。研究者通过微阵列技术或高通量测序的方法来研究核苷酸的多态性，并用于基因图谱绘制和癌症诊断。高通量测序可以高通量、高分辨率地对癌症样品进行

DNA

接头序列

随机片段化的基因组DNA，将接头序列加在片段两端

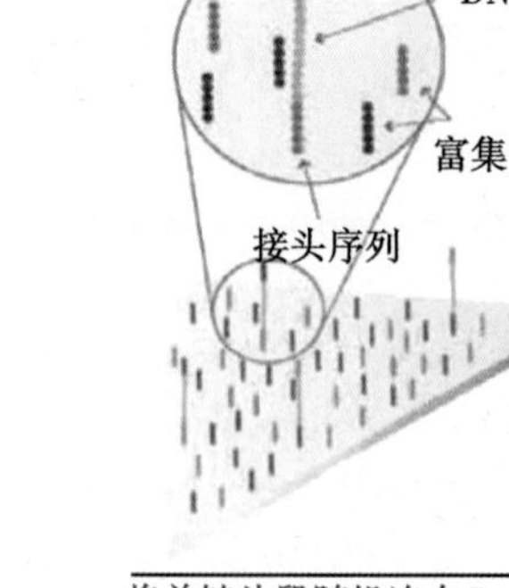

将单链片段随机连在flow cell通道上

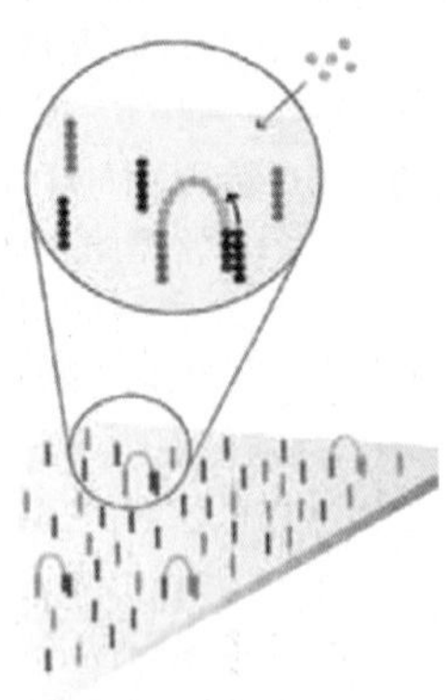

添加未标记的核苷酸和酶以启动固相桥式扩增

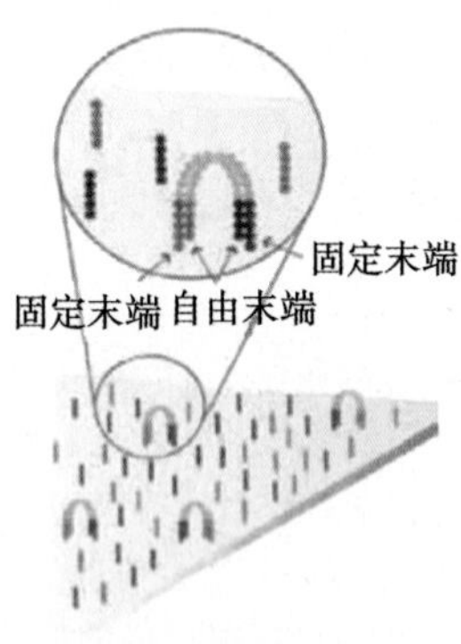

将酶掺入核苷酸，并在固相底物上建立双链桥

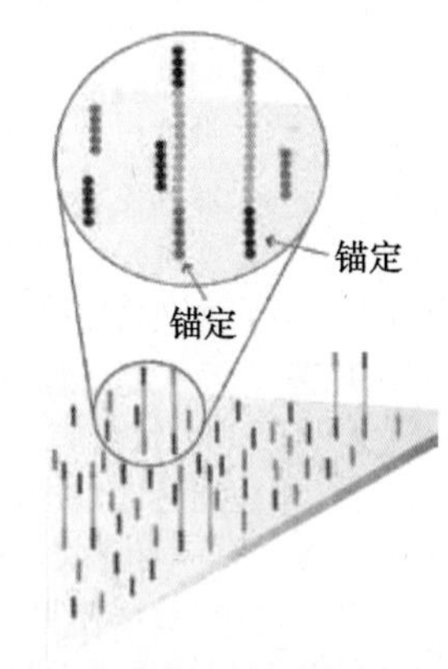

通过变性使单链模板锚定在基质上

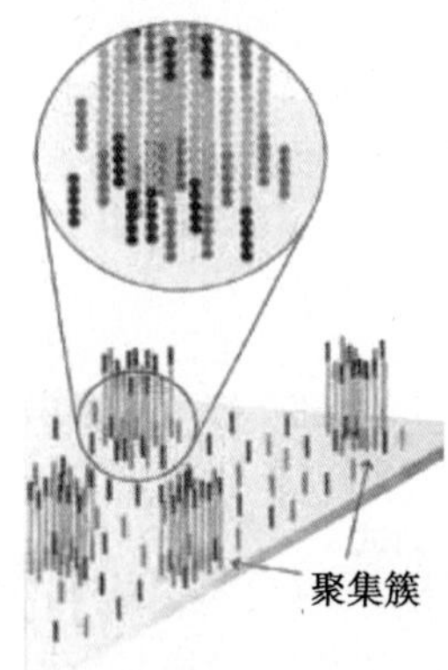

在流通池的每个通道中产生数百万个密集的双链DNA簇

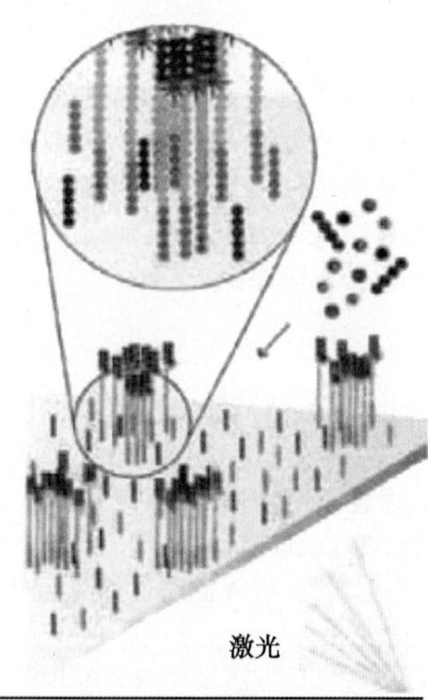

通过添加四个标记的可逆终止子、引物和DNA聚合酶开始第一个测序循环

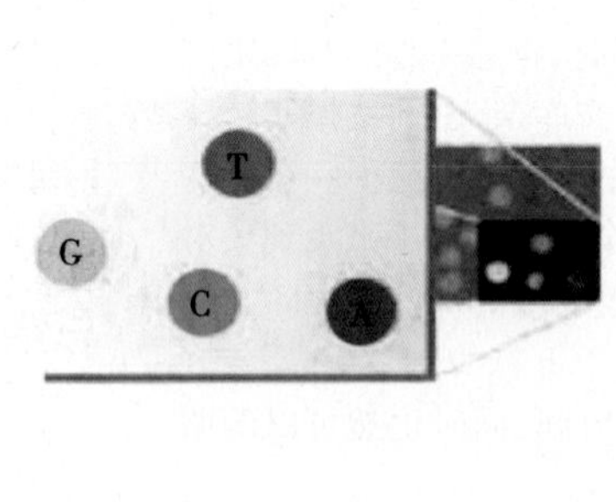

激光激发下捕获每个簇发出的荧光，识别第一个碱基

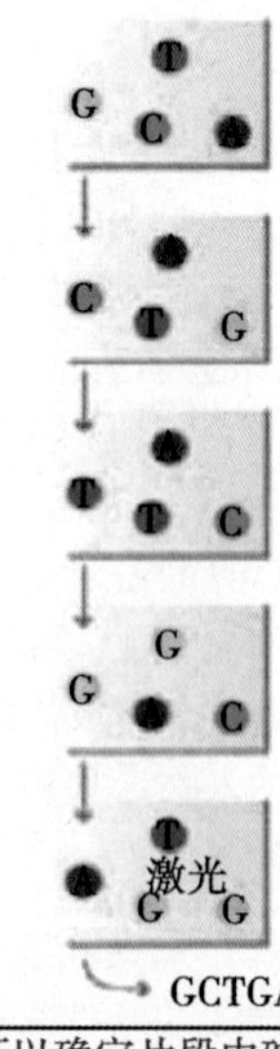

重复测序循环以确定片段中碱基的序列，每次确定一个碱基

图 3-10 用 Illumina platform 进行下一代测序（next generation sequencing，NGS）

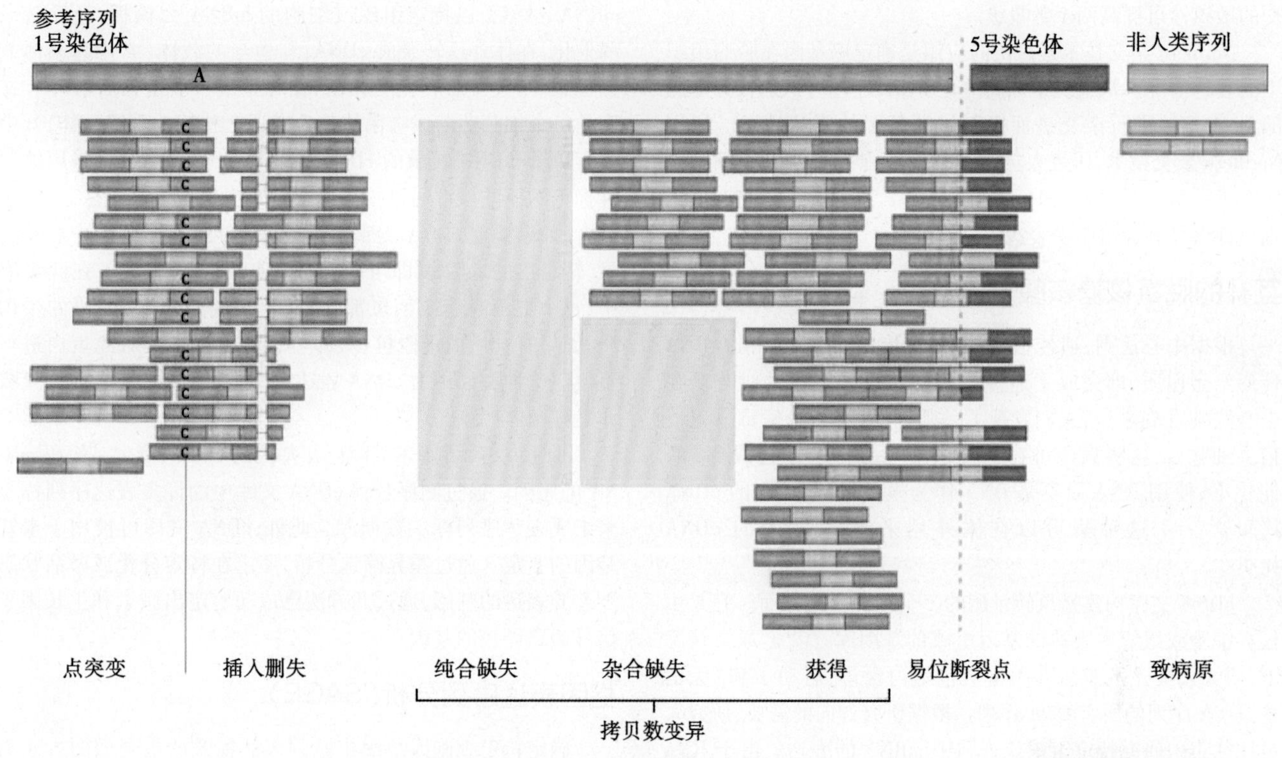

图 3-11　通过第二代测序检测基因组的改变类型

测序，从而检测异质肿瘤组织中的低频突变、拷贝数改变和结构重排。

基因表达：mRNA 转录物分析

结构分析

基因表达的第一步是将 DNA 携带的遗传信息转录成 RNA。核糖核苷酸是组成 RNA 的基本单位，与 DNA 分子的脱氧核糖核苷酸类似，区别为：①核糖的 2′碳被羟基基团取代而不是氢原子；②核糖核苷酸的碱基中没有胸腺嘧啶，只有尿嘧啶（去甲基化的胸腺嘧啶），通过氢键与腺嘌呤配对。与前述的 DNA 聚合酶类似，RNA 聚合酶 Ⅱ 以基因的 DNA 序列为模板，通过与模板 DNA 互补的方式合成多聚核糖核苷酸。

为了确保转录的正确性，RNA 聚合酶 Ⅱ 必须具备以下条件：①使用 DNA 的反义链作为模板；②在基因的起始点启动转录；③在基因的终止点终止转录。确保正确转录的信号经由基因启动子区特定的核苷酸序列传递给 RNA 聚合酶 Ⅱ。经过读取和转译这些信号，在 RNA 聚合酶 Ⅱ 的作用下，产生了与模板 DNA 完全互补的从转录起始至终止点的 RNA 转录本。然而，并不是所有转录出来的 RNA 都能进入细胞质成为 mRNA，内含子序列在转录本中会被剪切掉，其机制有待阐明，外显子的末端连接在一起形成剪切体[72]。mRNA 除了发生剪切外，基本的转录本进一步通过加帽和加尾修饰，即在 5′端[73]加入甲基三磷酸鸟苷，在 3′端加入 20~40 poly（A）尾[74]。这些修饰可能促进了蛋白质的翻译效率[75,76]和 mRNA 从细胞核向细胞质的转运，并可以增强 mRNA 在细胞质中的稳定性。

Northern 印迹

在 RNA 水平分析基因表达的前提是细胞或组织中必须含有目的基因的转录产物（mRNA）。相对于检测 DNA 表达的 Southern 杂交，检测特定基因转录产物的方法被命名为 Northern 杂交。RNA 易于从细胞中完整地分离[77]，与基因组 DNA 相比，信使 RNA 分子要小很多，因此可以直接通过琼脂糖电泳进行分析，无需对其进行高分子量 DNA 分析所必需的酶切消化。

RNA 是单链并具有自身折叠的倾向，因此可通过碱基互补配对原则在链内形成二级结构。由于二级结构会导致 RNA 在非变性凝胶上电泳异常，因此 RNA 需要在变性剂（甲醛、乙二醛/二甲基亚砜）的作用下进行电泳分析。经过变性的琼脂糖凝胶电泳分离，RNA 以与 DNA 相同的方式转移到硝酸纤维素或尼龙基膜上进行 Southern 印迹（图 3-5）。Northern 印迹的杂交方案和印迹洗涤基本上与 Southern 印迹相同。通过 Northern 杂交，基因特异的 RNA 即可被鉴定分析。

由于 Northern 杂交敏感性的限制，只有 RNA 丰度相对较高的情况下才能够通过该技术进行检测。对 mRNA 进行富集是增加 Northern 杂交敏感性的一种方法。通常，在细胞或组织中，mRNA 在总 RNA 中的比例低于 10%，其他 RNA 包括核糖体 RNA（rRNA）和转运 RNA（tRNA）。通过去除缺少 3′ poly（A）尾部的所有 RNA 分子，可以富集 mRNA[78]。将与多聚 A 尾互补的多聚 U 或多聚 T 固定于固相支持介质如塑料珠上，经过反应，具有多聚 A 尾的 mRNA 将会结合于此介质上，而不具多聚 A 的 RNA 将会被洗脱，再将结合在固相介质上的 mRNA 进行洗脱用于 Northern 杂交。经过 mRNA 的纯化，Northern 杂交的敏感性可提高两个数量级。

Northern 杂交技术最广泛的应用是确定癌基因在肿瘤组织中的表达情况。从组织中分离纯化 RNA，经过与识别特异基因的 DNA 探针进行杂交进而确定目的基因的表达情况。运用 Northern 杂交技术，研究人员在人肿瘤细胞系和白血病细胞中鉴定了最早的原癌基因 c-abl 和 c-myc[79,80]。随后研究者们发现了许多在肿瘤组织中表达的原癌基因。

互补的脱氧核糖核酸

根据中心法则，遗传信息从 DNA 传递给 RNA，再从 RNA 传递给蛋白质，即完成了遗传信息的转录和翻译的过程。在中心法则发现之后，人们发现了一则例外：逆转录病毒。入侵宿主细胞后，这些病毒可在逆转录酶（一种 DNA 合成酶）的催化下，使用 RNA 而不是 DNA 作为模板形成 RNA 的 cDNA 拷贝[81,82]。这种酶可以在体外用来制造 RNA 的 cDNA 拷贝。

cDNA 文库构建是反转录酶的一个重要应用方面。它是由仅在细胞或组织中表达的基因组成的基因库[83,84]。通常情况下，研究人员并不关注基因组上包括内含子、启动子和“无信息”DNA 序列的所有 DNA 序列。根据研究方向的需要，研究人员往往集中研究特定组织或细胞中 mRNA 的表达。由于 RNA 单链的特点决定了无法将其直接连接到克隆载体上，cDNA 文库构建技术应运而生。

为了制备 cDNA 文库，需从细胞或组织中分离出所有的 mRNA。然后，以特定组织或细胞的 mRNA 为模板，经反转录酶催化，在体外反转录成 cDNA，与适当的载体（常用噬菌体或质粒载体）连接后转化受体菌，在琼脂平板上生长后，cDNA 文库的每个细菌菌落或噬菌体都含有一个独特的重组载体，其中含有单个 mRNA 转录的 cDNA 拷贝（图 3-3）。然后，采用放射性标记的核酸探针通过核酸杂交对 cDNA 文库进行鉴定[85,86]。或者，如果构建 cDNA 文库的克隆载体能够在宿主菌中启动转录，转录出的 mRNA 即可翻译成其编码的蛋白质。在此文库中，每个细菌菌落或菌斑都含有一个特异 mRNA 编码的蛋白质，如果有合适的蛋白抗体，即可通过抗体杂交对此蛋白进行鉴定。这种文库称为 cDNA 表达文库，表达文库常用的克隆载体是噬菌体（λgt11）[87]。

cDNA 文库可用于克隆已知基因的 cDNA，确定其编码 mRNA 的序列。通过测序获得 cDNA 文库中的许多表达序列标签来组成表达序列标签数据库。此外，cDNA 文库可被用于未知基因的鉴定。通过差异筛选分析，鉴定在特定分化或激活状态下差异表达的基因，通过此方法已成功鉴定出激素和生长因子信号通路调控的基因[88]。

基因表达序列分析（SAGE）

确定特定细胞或组织中基因表达模式的最全面的方法为建立 cDNA 文库并对每个克隆进行测序。最初这被认为是一项不可能完成的任务，研究者曾开发了一种称为基因表达系列分析（SAGE）的技术来完成这一目标。在 SAGE 中，研究者对

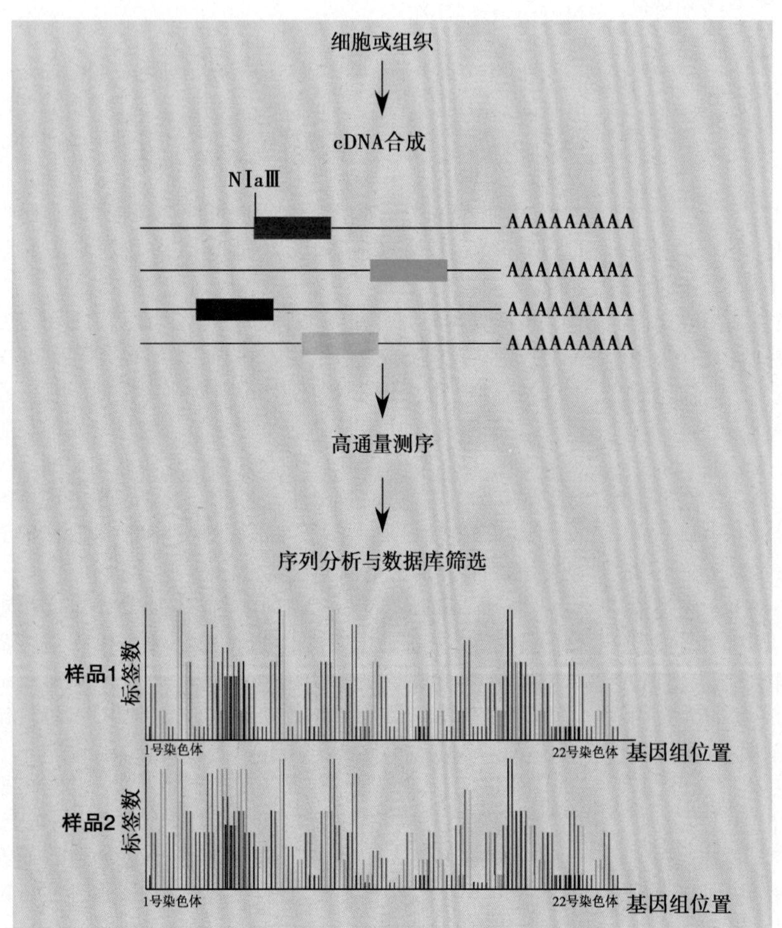

图 3-12 基因表达序列分析文库（SAGE）的构建及分析。第一步，从组织或细胞中调取 cDNA，构建 cDNA 文库，然后用磁珠固定双链 cDNA 的 3′端。第二步，选择锚定酶（通常是 NⅠaⅢ）对 cDNA 进行酶切，几乎能对所有的 cDNA 分子进行酶切。随后，连接另一个包含标签酶识别位点的接头到 cDNA 末端，此标签酶是一种 2 型限制性核酸内切酶（通常为 MmeI），会切开识别序列附近的 3 个位点。之后直接将这些标签用于单分子 DNA 测序平台，通过软件分析数据读取获得的序列和标签，与同源 cDNA 匹配，并以数字形式给出基因表达谱

每个表达基因上特定区域的寡核苷酸序列（称为 SAGE 标签）进行测序，并量化其出现次数（称为 SAGE 标签数）。因此，SAGE 标签出现的频率正好确定了基因的表达丰度。

SAGE 的灵敏度和定量准确度在理论上是无限的。构建 SAGE 文库不需要事先知道什么基因在目标细胞中表达。因此，SAGE 能够检测和量化先前未表征的基因表达。

以往构建 SAGE 文库在技术上存在一定的挑战[89]。单个分子测序平台的建立使得 SAGE 和其他序列标签为基础的方法更易于完成（并且在许多情况下甚至替代原方法）。图 3-12 对此方法进行了概括总结。

应用 SAGE 文库可比较来源于正常和肿瘤组织的不同类型细胞的基因表达差异[90]。SAGE 是国际癌症研究中心（National Cancer Institute，NCI）资助的肿瘤基因解剖工程（Cancer Gene Anatomy Project，CGAP）中的一项技术[91]。这一计划的目标是建立各种组织来源的正常和肿瘤组织中基因差异表达的目录。迄今为止，已经有 120 多个 SAGE 文库收录于美国国家生物技术教育中心/CGAP SAGE 图谱网站（http://cgap.nci.nih.gov/SAGE）[91,92]。

DNA 表达谱分析

DNA 微阵列（又称 DNA 芯片）是另一种检测基因表达差异的方法，目前有两种基本类型：寡核苷酸芯片[93,94]和 cDNA 芯片[95,96]。两种方法都将 DNA 序列固定在固体支持物（例如玻璃显微镜载玻片或硅晶片）表面的网格阵列中。在寡核苷酸阵列的情况下，使用类似于光刻的一系列光导耦合反应，在芯片表面上原位合成一段 25nt 的已知 DNA 序列的片段。运用这种方法，在 1.3cm×1.3cm 的芯片上可涵盖包括 18 000 多个基因的 400 000 个 DNA 序列。在 cDNA 芯片中，cDNA 探针通过点样机器人设备在玻璃片上进行点样，制成芯片。下一步是从样本中（例如肿瘤）纯化 RNA，对 RNA 进行酶促荧光标记，将荧光标记的材料与微阵列杂交。所以通过激光共聚焦扫描对微点阵每一位点的荧光强度进行检测，阵列上每个斑点的荧光强度与该斑点代表的基因的表达水平成正比，便可对样品进行定性及定量分析。图 3-13 对此过程进行了概括。

微阵列分析是分析人类癌症和癌症分类中基因表达模式的有效方法。基因表达谱分析是对肿瘤进行分类预测、鉴定肿瘤的特定亚型和发现新的肿瘤类型的方法。应用这种技术已经成功准确地将急性髓系白血病和急性淋巴白血病加以区分[97]。此后，借助该技术，一些新的癌症特定亚型也得以鉴定发现，如白血病[98]、淋巴瘤[99,100]、脑癌[101]、乳腺癌[102,103]、前列腺癌[104,105]、肺癌[106,107]等。

解读微阵列数据的挑战在于识别有意义的基因表达模式并将其与噪声区分开来。噪声（随机基因表达水平）主要由以下几个方面产生：①芯片之间的变异；②RNA 标记和杂交方法的变异；③检测样品的生物学变异是噪声产生的最主要来源。通过使用下文"转录组测序"部分中描述的方法，可避免阵列技术的许多问题。因此，随着不断改进，测序技术将变得更加经济实惠被广泛推广，逐渐取代微阵列技术。

反转录聚合酶链反应（RT-PCR）

cDNA 技术的另一个重要用途是将 PCR 应用于 RNA。由于 Taq 聚合酶是 DNA 聚合酶（见上文），无法直接以 RNA 为模

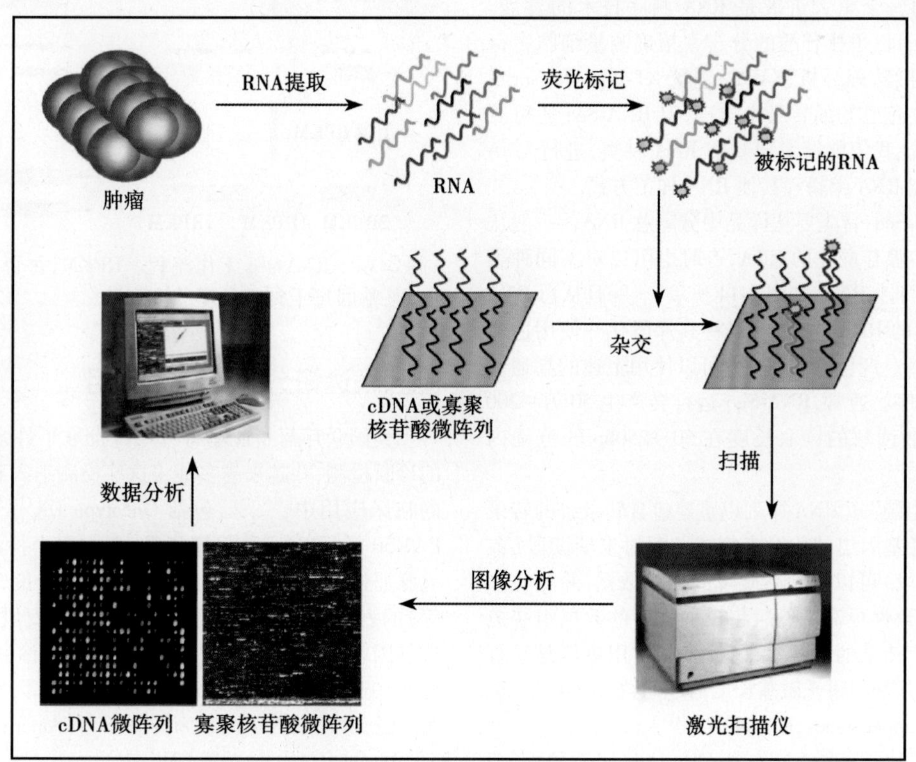

图 3-13　DNA 表达谱分析。从肿瘤组织或细胞中提取 RNA，对其末端进行荧光标记，然后与 cDNA 芯片或寡聚核苷酸芯片进行杂交，通过激光扫描仪收集杂交信号。由于芯片上的每个点代表一个独立的基因克隆，因此可以确定特定序列同源 RNA 的表达

板进行扩增。然而,将 RNA 反转成 cDNA 解决了 RNA 的检测问题。

通过 PCR 反应检测 RNA 表达的第一步是以目的 mRNA 为模板产生 cDNA 拷贝。这可以由长链 T[与 poly(A)尾互补]或与 mRNA 的 3′区序列部分互补的引物来完成。一旦产生单链 cDNA,就可以用 Taq 聚合酶在标准 PCR 反应中将其扩增(图 3-6)。RT-PCR 一个成功的应用实例是在慢性粒细胞白血病的临床标本中检测到了 bcr-abl 的融合基因,此基因融合是由于染色体易位导致的,由于其首先在美国费城发现,因此被命名为费城染色体。自那以后,逆转录聚合酶链反应(RT-PCR)在临床和实验室中的应用得更加广泛。

通过 PCR 检测 mRNA 表达的一个关键问题是如何对扩增的 PCR 产物进行定量分析。在 Northern 杂交和核酸保护分析中,杂交信号的强度直接反映了 mRNA 的表达水平,从而可以对 mRNA 的表达量进行比较。在 PCR 反应中,聚合酶效率的轻微改变都会导致扩增样品的偏差以指数级增加,反应达到的饱和度也可能有较大差异。然而,一些可以将 PCR 产物标准化的技术也应运而生,实现了可量化的比较。

值得注意的是,实时定量 PCR[109]是一种连续监测扩增的方法,在无偏移的线性范围内对持续增加的扩增进行定量比较。常用的实时定量 PCR 方法在扩增区域内设计荧光探针,一端含有荧光标签,另一端含有猝灭剂;扩增导致探针被消化,从而释放出游离的荧光分子,荧光信号与扩增次数成比例,以此利用荧光信号的积累实时监测整个 PCR 进程。

转录组测序

转录组分析的一个重大进展是 RNA 测序技术的发展。RNA 测序(RNA-Seq)以单核苷酸的分辨率精确测量细胞中存在的转录本。虽然微阵列分析、SAGE、定量 RT-PCR 和 Northern 印迹均可用于量化已知的转录本丰度,但 RNA-Seq 还可发现新的转录物。这让我们能够发现新的 RNA 种类,进行 RNA 剪接模式分析,研究 RNA 编辑和其他 RNA 加工方式。

为了进行 RNA-Seq,首先要从样品中分离总 RNA。一般从总 RNA 群中选择多腺苷酸化的 RNA,有时也可以对不同种类的 RNA 进行富集(即小 RNA,如图 3-14 所示)。一旦从总 RNA 群中选择了感兴趣的 RNA 亚型,可以将其片段化并使用逆转录酶逆转录成 cDNA。产生的 cDNA 就可以使用上述的高通量平台进行扩增和测序。通常,RNA-Seq 运行会产生 50 万~200 万个短读数,大多数读数的读取长度在 50~250bp 的范围内(图 3-14)[110]。

接下来必须"组装"短 RNA 序列以重建包含转录组的转录本,一般通过与参考基因组的比对来完成。配对末端读段(或者从两端测序的片段)可以得到高质量的测序数据,并且与参考基因组比对的一致性更高。然后将读取比对的数据组装成转录模型,量化各个转录的表达水平,此步骤常用单位是每百万碱基读长中来自某基因每千碱基长度的序列数(reads per kilobase per million mapped reads,RPKM)[111~113]。

RNA-Seq 可以量化转录本丰度、识别未注释的转录本、剪接变体、基因融合、非人类转录本和体细胞突变等,明显优于微阵列分析(受到预先设计探针数量的限制)。因此,RNA-Seq 将逐步取代微阵列技术作为转录组研究的常规方法。

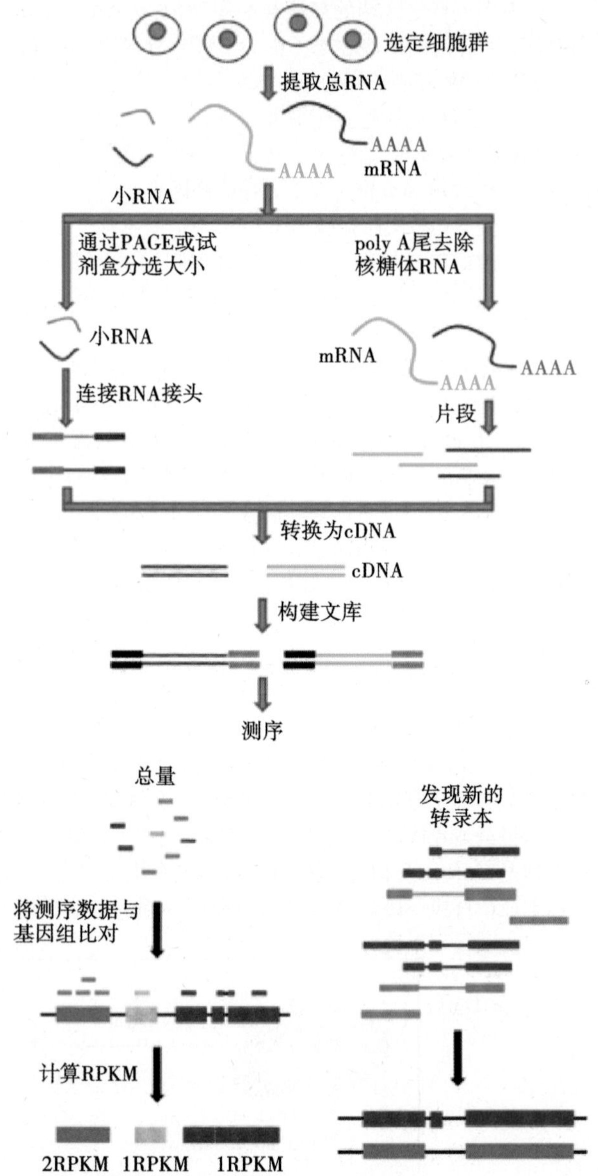

图 3-14 RNA-seq 工作流程。RPKM,每百万碱基读长中来自某基因每千碱基长度的序列数

基因表达谱分析的临床应用

美国联邦药品管理局(FDA)批准了许多基于基因表达谱的诊断检测,并越来越多地将这些检测纳入到早期乳腺癌患者的临床应用中[114,115],包括 Oncotype DX[116]、Mammaprint[117]、PAM50[118]和 H:I 乳腺癌指数[119]。每个检测用一组基因(从乳腺癌指数中的两个基因到 Mammaprint 的 70 个基因,数量不等)的表达水平提供相关患者乳腺癌复发风险的预后信息,这些基因表达检测在临床效果、适应证和诊断有效性上各不相同。在这些检测中,Oncotype DX 或 21 基因复发评分的使用最为广泛,并已纳入美国临床肿瘤学会(American Society of Clinical Oncology,ASCO)的管理指南。

Oncotype DX 评分基于三个不同的数据集,是通过实时定量 PCR 在大量患者的石蜡固定组织中检测候选基因组(250 个癌症相关基因)的表达而开发出来的。之后通过一个独立的数据集对该评分进行验证，该数据集源自 NSABP B-14 试验（一项大型前瞻性随机临床试验），这项试验旨在测试他莫昔芬在激素受体阳性、淋巴结阴性乳腺癌患者中的疗效[116]，结果发现由 21 个基因组成的基因标记可以预测患者 10 年内乳腺癌的复发率。根据 21 个基因的表达水平设计算法，并产生 0 到 100 之间的数字，称为复发评分。复发分数分为低（分数<18）、中（≤18 分数<30）和高（分数≥30）。各个队列的随访研究证实，基于 Oncotype DX 复发评分的预后分析是最可靠的。该评分目前被用于指导淋巴结阴性、雌激素受体（ER）阳性乳腺癌患者的预后，并可以告知这些女性是否能从辅助化疗中获益。复发评分低的女性预后一般较好，从辅助化疗获益较少。

随着越来越多的基因组和转录组学数据的产生，人们更多地致力于开发各种肿瘤的分子预后检测。但我们要仔细考虑这些检测在应用时的临床效果、确切的适应证和适用的患者人群。目前，肿瘤分子的预后分析可以补充但仍不能取代传统的临床预后因素。

总结

DNA 分子携带的遗传信息在 RNA 聚合酶Ⅱ的作用下转录成信使 RNA（mRNA），转录出的 mRNA 经过 5′加帽和 3′加尾修饰后由细胞核转运至细胞质。在反转录酶的作用下，mRNA 可被转录成 cDNA，进行 cDNA 文库的构建，进而成为分析基因表达的有力工具。有多种技术可以研究细胞质 mRNA 的表达水平，包括 Northern 印迹、RT-PCR、微阵列分析和 RNA-Seq。随着微阵列和 RNA-Seq 技术的快速发展，研究者需要生物信息学家的专业知识进行表达谱分析以阐明遗传学网络。肿瘤的基因表达谱可以个性化地指导癌症患者的治疗计划。

表观遗传调控

近几十年来，对肿瘤发生相关基因的研究集中于遗传信息发生改变的基因。然而，近来抑癌基因和癌基因的表观遗传调控研究进展表明，表观遗传修饰在肿瘤进展中具有非常重要的作用。表观遗传修饰影响基因的表达而不引起任何 DNA 序列的改变。表观遗传调节主要包括 DNA 甲基化、组蛋白修饰和非编码 RNA 的调节，这些修饰在细胞分化和肿瘤发生扮演着重要的角色。例如，研究已表明 DNA 甲基化在沉默基因表达、印记和 X 染色体失活中起着重要作用[120~122]。DNA 甲基化和印记的遗传缺陷导致发育缺陷并增加了肿瘤发生的风险。最近的研究表明，组蛋白修饰和 DNA 甲基化是肿瘤发生的驱动事件[123~125]。小鼠实验表明，通过在生殖细胞中引入 DNA 甲基转移酶基因 DNMT1 的一个等位基因亚型，可以导致 DNA 甲基化的程度降低 90%，进而促进肿瘤的发生[126]。

伴随着表观遗传学的发展，更加全面、高通量的检测方法应运而生。这些技术包括甲基化敏感性随机引物 PCR（MS-AP-PCR）[127]、CpG 岛扩增结合代表性差异分析技术（MCA-RDA）[128]、基于 CpG 岛芯片的差异甲基化杂交（DMH）[129]、限制性标记基因组扫描（MCARDA）[130]、甲基-CpG 结合域亲和层析[131]以及经去甲基化和去乙酰化处理后的基因表达谱分析[132]等，这些技术都已成功用于鉴定不同类型癌症的新甲基化基因座[133]。甲基化—特异性数字核型分析（MSDK）是一种基于序列的分析技术，可实现全面和无偏倚的全基因组 DNA 甲基化分析[134]。该技术利用对甲基化敏感的酶（如 EagI）和对 DNA 进行片段化的酶（如 NⅠaⅢ）对基因组 DNA 进行处理，从而获得短序列标签，通过对这些标签进行测序以确定其在全基因组上的分布并评价其发生甲基化的水平。

DNA 甲基化和染色质修饰是紧密相关的过程，非编码 RNA 可能在介导两者的关联中发挥着重要的作用[133,135]。近几年，研究发现组蛋白修饰的数量和类型越来越多，同时也鉴定了更多在组蛋白修饰过程中起关键作用的酶类。四种核心组蛋白（H2A、H2B、H3 和 H4）存在多种翻译后修饰如乙酰化、甲基化、磷酸化、泛素化、SUMO 化、ADP-核糖基化、瓜氨酸化和脯氨酸异构化等。大部分修饰通过影响其他蛋白的募集而发挥功能，其中一些分子与 DNA 修复和染色质凝集有关。利用特异性识别甲基化组蛋白 H3-lys9 的抗体和新开发的 ChIP-on-chip 技术[136]、全基因组映射技术（GMAT）[137]以及 ChIP-seq 技术[138]可以在全基因组范围内分析异染色质的变化。

最新一些研究表明，癌症存在广泛的全基因组表观遗传失调。一些大规模癌症基因组测序项目也揭示了表观遗传修饰蛋白的体细胞突变[139]。这些突变包括急性髓细胞白血病中 DNA 甲基转移酶 DNMT3A 的突变[140,141]、骨髓性白血病和胶质瘤中 DNA 去甲基化酶（例如，TET2，IDH1，IDH2）的突变[142~144]，肾细胞中组蛋白甲基转移酶 SETD2 的突变[145]、膀胱癌中组蛋白去甲基化酶 KDM6A 的突变[146]等。以上发现表明异常的表观遗传修饰和基因突变协同可以促进肿瘤的发生，而表观遗传修饰因子本身也有可能发生遗传突变。

总结

表观遗传修饰在肿瘤发生、发展中的作用日渐明确，表观遗传改变事件的发生先于遗传变异。研究的不断深入和分子生物学技术的飞速发展，为表观遗传学及表观基因组学的发展提供了强有力的技术支持。癌症基因组测序计划已经确定了一些表观遗传修饰蛋白的高频突变。由于表观遗传过程是可逆的并且可以用 DNA 和组蛋白修饰酶的抑制剂靶向抑制，目前研究人员正在尝试用一些靶向表观遗传改变的方法治疗不同类型的肿瘤。

基因表达：蛋白质分析

蛋白质结构

蛋白质是由氨基酸分子连接而成的聚合物。编码蛋白质的核苷酸序列决定了其氨基酸序列。由于氨基酸彼此连接形成线性聚合物，因此如 DNA 转录成 RNA 一样，蛋白质也具有方向性，mRNA 的 5′端对应蛋白质的氨基端，3′端对应蛋白质的羧基端（图 3-1）。

许多蛋白质翻译后必须经过修饰才具有生物学活性，称为翻译后修饰。例如，许多分泌蛋白的氨基端具有 20~30 个氨基酸组成的前导肽序列，高度疏水的结构嵌入到内质网膜和分泌颗粒中，引导蛋白穿膜，当蛋白质分泌后，前导肽会被剪切掉，即成为成熟的有活性的蛋白质分子。

蛋白质的另一种修饰是在氨基酸侧链上加入非肽类基团，包括糖基化、磷酸化修饰和二硫键。磷酸化修饰通常发生在丝氨酸、苏氨酸和酪氨酸磷酸化位点上，在蛋白质的功能调节中具有重要的作用。细胞表面有许多生长因子受体，包括血小板衍生生长因子（PDGF）受体[147]、巨噬细胞集落刺激因子（M-CSF）受体[148,149]等，M-CSF本身就是酪氨酸激酶蛋白，当受体与配体结合后，受体发生构象改变从而使自身发生磷酸化，再经过一系列的级联酶促反应把磷酸基团从一个化合物转移到另一个化合物上，从而实现反应的级联放大。蛋白质的磷酸化修饰是生物体内一种普遍的调节方式，在细胞信号传递过程中占有极其重要的地位。酪氨酸激酶受体通路在细胞增殖过程中起到非常重要的促进作用，因此，酪氨酸激酶抑制剂甲磺酸伊马替尼（imatinib mesylate）和格列卫（gleevec）可阻断c-abl和c-kit酪氨酸激酶的活性，从而成为有效的抗肿瘤药物[46,150]。

SDS-聚丙烯酰胺凝胶电泳

与核酸分离方法类似，蛋白质也可通过电泳进行分离。然而，与核酸不同，并不是所有的蛋白质都带有负电荷，而且它们也不具有统一的核质比。在电场作用下，自然构象的蛋白质将会以一种未知的方式进行迁移。为了克服上述问题，研究者在电泳体系中加入了阴离子去垢剂十二烷基硫酸钠（SDS）。SDS以一个分子对应两个氨基酸的方式与蛋白质分子结合从而使蛋白质带上负电荷，负电荷的数量对应于蛋白质的分子量大小，从而可以按照分子量对蛋白质进行分离。

因为蛋白质分子比核酸分子小，电泳在对小分子量分子有更高分辨率的聚丙烯酰胺凝胶上进行。SDS消除了蛋白质原有的电荷差别，使蛋白质分子电泳的迁移率主要取决于其本身的分子量，而与蛋白质所带的电荷无关。在电场作用下，蛋白质分子量的对数与电泳迁移率呈负相关[151]。因为β-巯基乙醇可减少半胱氨酸上巯基的形成从而使蛋白质多聚体得以解离，所以当β-巯基乙醇存在时，SDS-PAGE可对蛋白亚单位进行分析；当缺乏β-巯基乙醇时，可对蛋白的多聚体结构进行分析。SDS-PAGE也是检测蛋白纯度的一种方法，其广泛应用于免疫共沉淀实验和蛋白质免疫印记杂交（western blot）中，如下所述。

免疫印迹

免疫印迹是蛋白质分析最流行和最成熟的技术之一（图3-15a）[152]。蛋白质的混合物可以通过SDS-PAGE电泳分离，分离的蛋白质通过电泳转移到硝酸纤维素膜或尼龙膜中，方向垂直于第一次电泳的方向，蛋白质可与膜可以稳定结合。与检测DNA的Southern杂交和检测RNA的Northern杂交类似，检测蛋白质的杂交技术称为蛋白免疫印迹杂交（western blot）。可以将蛋白质印迹浸泡在含有靶向目标蛋白的特异性抗体的溶液中。如果抗体被标记，则可以检测印迹上结合的抗体。后续可通过酶催化显色或发光反应或者通过放射性核素（例如^{125}I）和放射自显影来检测标记的蛋白。也可以通过在含有标记的抗免疫球蛋白抗体的溶液中洗涤印迹来检测未标记的抗体。通过WB可检出经Southern杂交未发现扩增的可验证乳腺癌患者中HER2蛋白的过表达[23]。此外，由于蛋白质是细胞活性和生物功能的最终执行者，蛋白水平的过表达意义更加重要，因此研究者将其作为判定基因过表达的“金标准”。

免疫沉淀

分子生物学一个最基本的方法是用探针检测特定的DNA或RNA复合物中特定基因的表达情况。与此类似，用特异的抗体作为探针也可检测蛋白复合物中是否有特定的目标蛋白存在。免疫沉淀是利用在混合物中加入识别特定蛋白的抗体，使其在一定条件下与其靶蛋白进行结合（图3-15b），之后可以通过添加与免疫球蛋白结合的蛋白质（例如抗免疫球蛋白抗体或葡萄球菌蛋白A）来收集该混合物中的所有免疫球蛋白。这些蛋白质通常与固体支持物结合，例如聚苯乙烯珠，可以通过低速离心从溶液中富集。当珠子被离心到离心管底部时，即得到附着的免疫球蛋白和靶蛋白。当在SDS和β-ME中煮沸时，蛋白质复合物会解离，并可以通过SDS-PAGE电泳将其分离，这个过程称为免疫沉淀。为了验证抗体的特异性，通常在免疫反应中加入不能识别目标蛋白的抗体作为研究的对照。两次沉淀的产物可以同时在SDS-PAGE上进行电泳，通过是否在对照泳道或者实验泳道中检测到目标蛋白质来对其进行鉴定。蛋白质可以通过染色反应来鉴定，如果蛋白质是放射性制剂标记的，则可通过放射自显影来鉴定。

研究者通过上述方法成功发现视网膜母细胞瘤易感基因（Rb）的表达产物与病毒编码的蛋白间存在相互作用。利用针对腺病毒蛋白的抗体在腺病毒转化或感染细胞的蛋白质混合物中进行免疫沉淀。除了腺病毒蛋白外，沉淀中还含有另一种蛋白质，这种蛋白质被证实是由视网膜母细胞瘤易感基因编码的蛋白质[153]。当用SV40病毒大T抗原的抗体进行免疫共沉淀时，在沉淀复合物中发现了Rb蛋白的存在，从而确定了T抗原蛋白与Rb蛋白之间存在相互作用[154]。上述研究揭示了病毒蛋白在诱导宿主细胞转化过程中的作用机制。

酶联免疫吸附试验（ELISA）

检测血清中的蛋白含量已成为肿瘤筛查、诊断和疗效评价的有效工具。其中最经典的实例是检测前列腺癌患者血清中前列腺特异抗原（PSA）的表达，可以用于前列腺癌的诊断和随访[155,156]。酶联免疫吸附试验（ELISA）是用来检测PSA和血清中其他蛋白质的一种方法[157]。该方法的描述见图3-15c。ELISA是采用酶标记的抗体（或抗原）在固相支持物表面检测未知抗原（或抗体）的含量。酶与抗体（或抗原）交联后，再与结合在固相支持物表面的相应抗原或抗体反应，形成荧光标记或化学发光标记的抗体—抗原复合物，此时加入酶、底物和显色剂，在酶催化底物后液体会呈现显色反应，液体显色的强弱和标记的抗体—抗原复合物的量成正比，以此反映待测的抗原或抗体量。如果ELISA体系中存在两个独立的结合不同抗原表位的抗体，即可应用此方法检测血清中小分子的含量（如药物水平）。

蛋白质测序

鉴定蛋白质最直接的方法是对蛋白质中的氨基酸序列进行分析，自动测序仪的应用已经使氨基酸序列的分析过程大大简化，而且由于技术的发展仅仅需要皮摩尔级的蛋白即可进行测序。通过蛋白免疫印记获得的少量蛋白经过染色后即可进

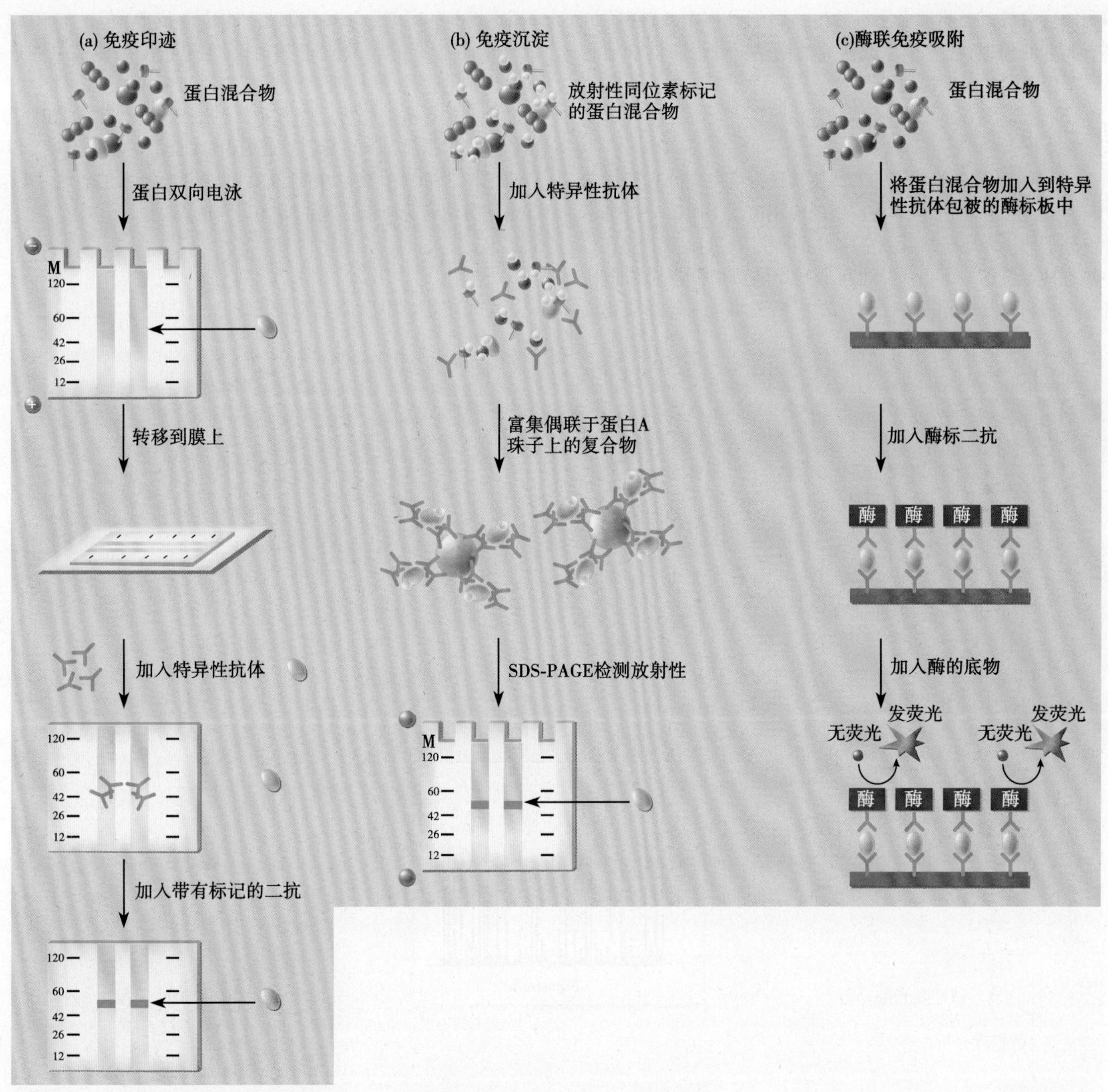

图 3-15　鉴定和检测蛋白质的方法。(a)蛋白免疫印记(Western blot)。将蛋白样品通过聚丙烯酰胺凝胶电泳按分子量大小进行分离。然后在电场作用下将分离好的蛋白质转移到杂交膜(硝酸纤维素膜或尼龙膜)上,用抗特异蛋白的抗体(图中灰色的椭圆球表示)进行杂交反应,再与放射性标记和酶标的抗免疫球蛋白的二抗进行杂交反应。(b)免疫沉淀。蛋白特异性抗体(图中灰色的椭圆球表示)与放射性标记的细胞裂解液或表达上清中相应的蛋白(图中以不同的几何形状代表)结合后,再与蛋白 A/G(Protein A/G)或二抗偶联的 agarose 或 Sepharose 珠子孵育,通过离心得到珠子—蛋白 A/G 或二抗—抗体—目的蛋白复合物,沉淀经洗涤后,去除未结合的蛋白,重悬于电泳上样缓冲液,在高温及还原剂的作用下,抗原与抗体解离,离心收集上清,通过聚丙烯酰胺凝胶电泳对蛋白进行分离,然后通过放射自显影进行检测。(c)酶链免疫反应(ELISA)。为了进行酶链免疫反应,必须有高特异性和高亲和力的可识别不同抗原表位的两株抗体。将其中一株抗体包被于酶标板上,然后与待分析的样品(组织、血液或体液标本)进行孵育。用酶标或放射性核素标记的第二株抗体检测结合于反应板上的蛋白并对其进行定量分析。ELISA 是非常敏感的蛋白检测方法,可对皮摩尔级的蛋白进行检测

行氨基酸序列分析[158]。

蛋白质测序技术引领分子肿瘤学进入了一个新时代。癌基因 v-sis 存在于猴肉瘤病毒中，经过蛋白序列分析发现 v-sis 编码的蛋白与一个驱动血小板的生长因子（PDGF B 链基因）具有高度的相似性[159,160]。此研究为阐述癌基因和正常细胞增殖基因之间的关联提供了重要的依据。

质谱分析

近年来，质谱技术的飞速发展使其成为蛋白质分析的优选工具，其在疾病诊断分析中有广阔的应用前景。质谱分析是一种将分子转换为离子然后测量其质量的技术，可以鉴定混合物中具有特定质量的蛋白质。也可通过串联质谱分析对蛋白质进行更精确的鉴定分析。在此方法中，首先将蛋白质片段化成肽段，再对肽段进一步片段化，之后进行测序分析[161,162]。质谱方法简要总结在图 3-16 中。最近，出现了一种新的称为细胞培养中氨基酸的稳定同位素标记（stable isotope labeling by amino acids in cell culture，SILAC）的质谱技术[163]。在 SILAC 中，细胞在含有正常或重（非放射性）氨基酸的培养基中培养。随着细胞的生长，氨基酸被细胞掺入到其合成的蛋白质中，将样品合并进行质谱分析。含有重氨基酸或轻氨基酸的相同蛋白质可以根据质量来区分，从而测定两个样品的蛋白丰度。SILAC 已成为癌症生物学中定量蛋白质组学研究的有力手段。详情请参阅有关质谱[164]和 SILAC[165]的综述。

工程蛋白表达

分子生物学中许多实验的最终目标是运用生物学技术合

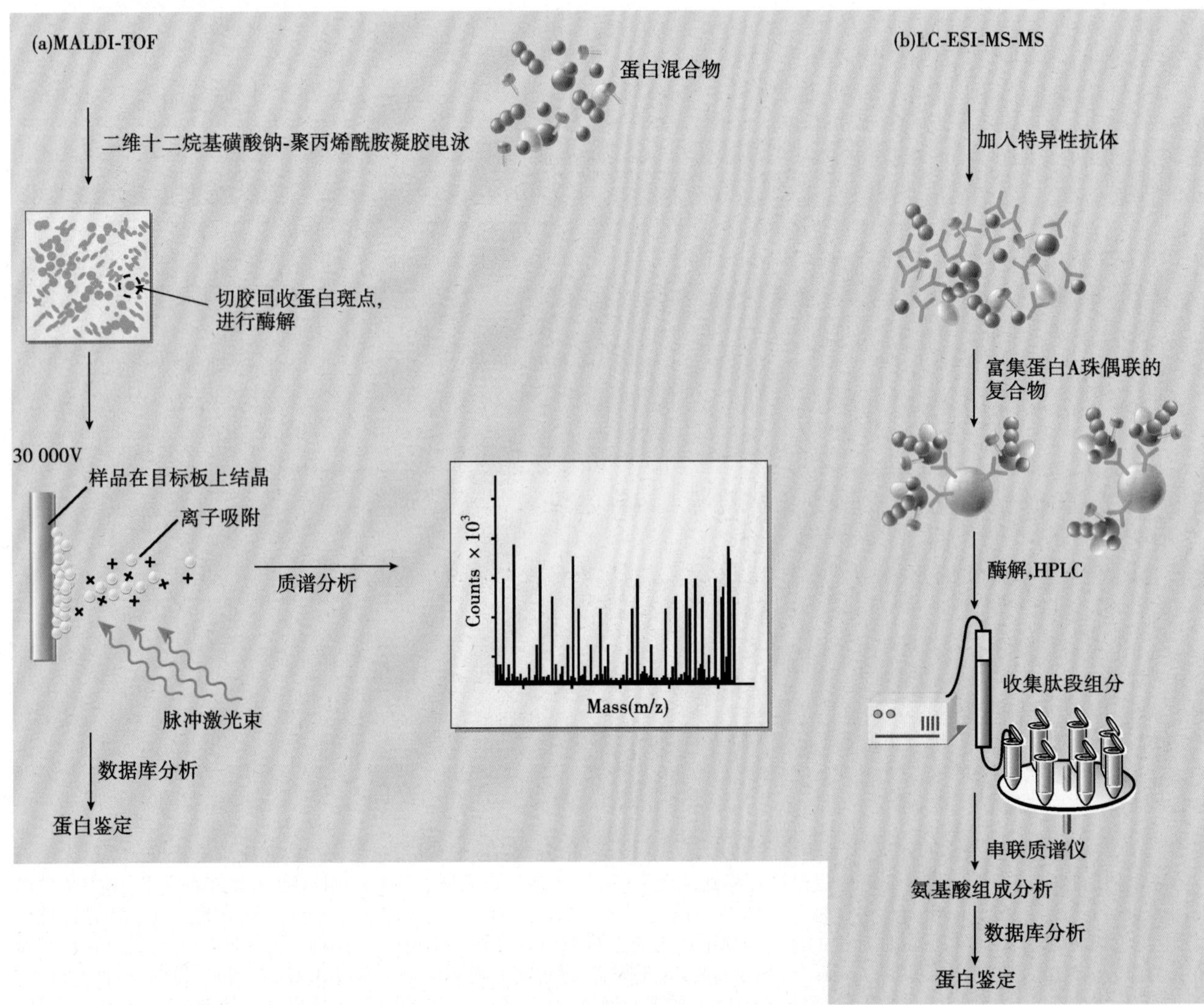

图 3-16 质谱分析。(a)基质辅助激光解析电离化/飞行时间质谱（MALDI-TOF）。对于基因序列已知的生物，从蛋白质双向电泳中分离得到的目标蛋白斑点可通过基质辅助激光解析电离化/飞行时间质谱来进行解析。蛋白样品在二维电泳中按照分子量大小和所带电荷进行分离。切胶得到的蛋白斑点经过蛋白酶消化与基质溶液混合并且在目标板上形成结晶。当电子束通过目标板时，基质吸收激光能量后挥发，携带一些样品进入真空。在激光发射时，对靶板施加高压以加速电离样品向飞行时间（TOF）质谱分析仪的移动。由此产生的多态指纹可用于进行数据库搜索，以明确蛋白质的类型。(b)液相色谱串联电喷雾正离子源质谱（LC-ESIMS-MS）技术应用于蛋白质中氨基酸序列的解析，以达到对蛋白的精确分析。此种方法结合毛细管高效液相色谱分析（HPLC）技术，可以保证很低的离子流速从而达到多肽离子流分析的敏感度。经过液相色谱和电喷雾电离后，再通过线性与串联质谱仪分析来获得氨基酸的序列信息

成基因编码的蛋白质，这个过程称为工程蛋白表达。如果用 DNA 重组的方法表达出的蛋白具有天然蛋白的特性，那么说明编码此蛋白的基因被成功克隆。如果特定的蛋白质很难通过天然来源获得，也可以通过蛋白表达工程的方式来获得。

体外翻译

体外翻译系统是一种简单、快速的体外蛋白表达系统，可以全部在试管中进行。mRNA 翻译需要得所有原料可以从高效合成蛋白的细胞中提取，例如需要兔网织红细胞和小麦胚芽。在反应体系中加入 20 种氨基酸、合成或纯化的 RNA，在适当的反应条件下，即可翻译成蛋白质。如果反应体系中的氨基酸经过放射性物质标记（如^{35}S 甲硫氨酸），则可通过聚丙烯酰胺凝胶电泳和放射自显影进行鉴定分析。可利用蛋白特异性抗体并通过 Western 杂交的方法，来确定目的蛋白是否被成功翻译。

大规模生产重组蛋白

体外翻译系统只能满足小规模研究分析的需要，为了得到大量的蛋白质，必须采用体内蛋白翻译系统。最简单的方法是将目的蛋白的 cDNA 克隆至含有启动子的原核表达载体或噬菌体中，然后转化至合适的宿主菌中，大量的 mRNA 即可被转录并翻译成蛋白质。对菌体蛋白进行纯化便可获得目的蛋白，临床上使用的干扰素[166-168]就是通过这种方法生产的。

如前所述，许多真核生物的蛋白质需要经过翻译后修饰才能具有活性。真核表达系统能够实现蛋白质的修饰，细菌表达系统缺乏完成复杂修饰如糖基化修饰的体系，且真核蛋白结构和功能维持所必需的二硫键在原核细胞环境中也无法形成。与原核表达系统类似，cDNA 被克隆至真核表达载体，然后将其转染至哺乳动物细胞中即可实现外源蛋白的表达[169]。然而，应用此系统获得大量蛋白质的成本较高。酵母、昆虫和植物细胞是介于哺乳动物细胞和细菌表达系统之间的更简单、更经济的选择，这些真核表达细胞可以成功实现外源表达蛋白的翻译后修饰如二硫键形成。这里描述的细菌和动物细胞类似的表达系统正在研发中，我们期待该系统可以替代真核表达宿主细胞进行蛋白的表达和修饰，感兴趣的读者可进一步了解[170,171]。

分析蛋白—蛋白相互作用的方法

后基因组时代研究的重要任务是揭示蛋白质的功能，阐明其参与的信号通路和调控网络。研究蛋白功能的方法之一是寻找与其相互作用的功能已知的蛋白质。通过全基因组水平的分析来揭示在生理条件下蛋白—蛋白相互作用的信号网络[172]，将其与基因表达数据和其他的数据相结合，从而在细胞水平上得到蛋白质分子参与的信号通路和调控网络。研究大规模蛋白质相互作用的方法包括：蛋白芯片、酵母双杂、Pull-down 实验等方法。Pull-down 实验是将免疫共沉淀和质谱分析相结合的检测蛋白相互作用的方法，而蛋白质芯片是将最初用于 DNA 或 RNA 分析（见上文）的微阵列技术应用于分析蛋白质相互作用。

经典的酵母双杂交系统是在酵母细胞中进行的。该系统需要利用酵母生长转录因子 Gal4 的两个不同的结构域——DNA 结合（DNA binding，DB）和反式激活因子（trans-activator，TA）结构域，以及一段 DNA 靶序列。在双杂交筛选中，待分析的两种蛋白质分别与 Gal4 的 DB 和 TA 结构域融合，得到的融合蛋白被称为“诱饵”和“猎物”。如果这两种蛋白质相互作用，则 DB 和 TA 结构域将会紧密接触并产生功能性的转录激活因子，其活性可通过报告基因进行检测。酵母双杂交实验可以在以下几个水平上进行：①检测两个已知蛋白的相互作用；②寻找鉴定与已知蛋白相互作用的蛋白；③检测多种蛋白之间的相互作用。与其他检测蛋—蛋白相互作用的方法不同，酵母双杂交并不需要重组蛋白的表达和纯化等过程。因此，在全基因组范围内进行酵母双杂交是相当简单的，并且几乎适用于所有蛋白质相互作用的研究。蛋白质相互作用组学（interactome）研究方法的发展促进了后基因组时代的基因组功能注释[173~175]。

总结

DNA 携带的遗传信息通过转录为 RNA 进而翻译成蛋白质，翻译出的蛋白与 DNA 和 RNA 一样具有方向性，其 5′端和 3′端分别为氨基和羧基端，蛋白质需要经过翻译后修饰才能发挥功能。

蛋白质可通过在聚丙烯酰胺凝胶电泳（PAGE）中加入阴离子去垢剂十二烷基磺酸钠（SDS）加以分离。SDS-PAGE 也是进行蛋白质免疫共沉淀和蛋白质印记实验的必需步骤。蛋白质测序技术目前已经能够利用微量的蛋白通过测序进行氨基酸序列分析。我们可以使用诸如 SILAC 方法的质谱进行大规模的定量蛋白质组学检测。

体外实验可利用兔网织红细胞和麦胚提取物系统对蛋白质进行翻译合成。将编码蛋白质的 DNA 序列连接至表达载体后转染至宿主细胞内，可将其转录为 mRNA 进而翻译成蛋白质。原核表达系统是简单、经济的外源蛋白表达系统，但其无法完成维持生物学活性必需的蛋白质翻译后修饰过程。真核表达系统是更加高效的蛋白表达系统，可实现蛋白的翻译后修饰从而维持蛋白的生物学活性，包括作为宿主的酵母、昆虫和植物细胞表达系统。

蛋白质相互作用的整体分析可以帮助我们描绘蛋白相互作用图谱，并揭示调控和功能网络，有助于我们更好地在系统水平理解细胞的功能。

癌症治疗靶点的筛选和鉴定

人类基因组测序计划的成功实施使我们对蛋白编码基因有了全面的认识。癌症基因组测序工作也为我们提供了癌症中最常见的突变基因的列表。但更具挑战性的任务是如何从大量的突变中鉴定出影响肿瘤发生、发展的功能性突变。高新技术的发展为系统鉴定肿瘤发展相关的基因提供了强有力的支持。概括地说，这些技术可分为功能丧失的方法（抑制基因表达后对细胞的表型进行评估）或功能获得的方法（使基因过表达后对细胞的表型进行评估）。

基因功能缺失技术

RNA 干扰

RNA 干扰（RNAi）是一种古老的生物学途径，其作用机制为短（18~21nt）双链 RNA（dsRNA）分子以序列特异性的方式催化诱导互补的 mRNA 分子降解。天然存在两种能够诱导

RNAi 的 dsRNA。植物和其他一些低等真核生物具备将较长的 dsRNA 底物内源加工成短链的干扰 RNA(siRNA)的能力;在实验室中,可以将合成的 siRNA 导入培养的细胞中[176,177]。微小 RNA(miRNA)代表了第二种小 dsRNA。miRNA 是真核基因组的组成部分,在进化过程中(包括在人类中)非常保守[178,179]。miRNA 在基因组的转录非常像 mRNA,其会被加工成长度约 22nt 的成熟形式。加工完成后的 siRNA 和 miRNA 的功能类似,都可以通过序列特异性负调节基因表达。

miRNA 和 dsRNA 具有序列特异性内源性沉默的特性,表明可以通过设计不同的 siRNA 用以抑制任何基因的表达[180]。事实上,在过去的 15 年中,RNAi 技术已成为实验室功能缺失研究的主要方法。从抑制培养细胞的单个基因的功能到体内基因治疗技术(特异性靶向疾病相关的等位基因)的开发,RNAi 技术已获得了广泛的应用。

化学合成的 siRNA 和通过将 shRNA 构建于真核表达载体并经过 Dicer 酶剪切出的 siRNA,都可以诱导哺乳动物细胞中的特定靶基因的表达沉默[181,182]。shRNA 可以在含有 RNA 聚合酶Ⅲ启动子的质粒中表达,或者可以在 RNA 聚合酶Ⅱ启动子的控制下,作为较长转录物的一部分,以 miRNA 样的形式进行表达[183]。在任何一种情况下,siRNA 会被纳入 RNA 诱导的沉默复合物(RISC)并指导靶 mRNA 进行序列特异性降解或翻译抑制,导致蛋白质表达降低[184]。尽管 siRNA 的合成方法简单,能高效地抑制靶基因的表达,但其成本相对较贵且在实验应用中有一定的局限性。以载体为基础的 shRNA 系统具有可携带耐药标签、稳定表达 RNAi 构建体以及可通过细菌繁殖成为可再生资源等优点。最近,研究者还开发了可诱导的 RNAi 载体,允许精细时空调节 RNAi 诱导的基因敲除[185]。

siRNA 和 shRNA 文库已成功用于基于转染的阵列筛选,观察基因抑制后发生的表型,如细胞凋亡、细胞信号或细胞周期改变[186~188]。对于其他许多癌症相关的表型,例如不依赖于锚定的集落形成、衰老旁路或肿瘤异种移植物,长期的基因抑制是必要的,因此需要 RNAi 载体的稳定整合和表达。基于逆转录病毒的文库能够在难以转染的细胞中进行研究,这是其显著优点。基于慢病毒的系统尤其如此,该系统甚至可用于感染有丝分裂后和其他难以转染的细胞,包括原代细胞或已分化的细胞[189,190]。

CRISPR/CAS9

过去 5 年的一项重大发现是观察到微生物获得性免疫系统可用于改造哺乳动物细胞的基因组。多年来,研究者已经观察到微生物基因组包含了具有间隔序列的重复元件簇[191,192],这些簇被称为 CRISPR(clustered regularly interspaced short palindromic repeats),或者成簇规则间隔的短回文序列,与这些重复元件相邻的是 CRISPR 相关(CRISPR-associated, Cas)基因。干扰 CRISPR 的许多重复间隔序列是噬菌体起源的,表明 CRISPR-Cas 系统代表了细菌针对噬菌体感染的适应性免疫。实际上,机制研究表明 CRISPR 阵列被转录为非编码 RNA 转录物(称为 crRNA),经加工后与 Cas 蛋白复合物结合。广泛研究的 CRISPR/Cas 系统类型是Ⅱ型 CRISPR,crRNA 与另一种反式激活 RNA(称为 tracrRNA)以及 Cas9 DNA 核酸酶结合。crRNA 和 tracrRNA 形成 RNA 杂合体,识别含有原型间隔区相邻基序(protospacer-adjacent motif, PAM)的 DNA,并介导识别位点附近的切割。CRISPR/Cas 系统现在已被确立为许多古细菌和细菌中获得性免疫系统的基础,可以保护其免受外来遗传元件(即噬菌体或质粒)的影响。读者可以阅读相关综述作更细致的了解[193,194]。

该领域的一个分水岭是,研究者们认识到Ⅱ型 CRISPR/Cas9 系统可以被修饰并转移到其他细胞,因此该系统可作为一种强大的基因组编辑工具。tracrRNA:crRNA 杂合体可以被设计为单个 RNA 嵌合体[195]、sgRNA 和可修饰间隔区(或指导)序列,来靶向切割目标 DNA 序列。这种可编程的 RNA 分子工具在引导下,几乎可以在基因组中任何位点附近进行切割。实际上,CRISPR/Cas9 切割以高度通用的方式改造哺乳动物细胞[196,197]。由 Cas9 诱导的双链断裂通常由非同源末端连接修复(nonhomologous end joining, NHEJ),这种修复通常在切割部位引入小的插入缺失(因此可能会诱导基因移位)。因此,CRISPR/Cas9 技术是诱导目的基因沉默的有力手段。此外,当 Cas9 与同源定向修复模板结合使用时,Cas9 诱导的切割可以通过同源重组进行修复,从而实现精确的基因组编辑。

最近的研究报道了基因组规模的 sgRNA 慢病毒文库,类似于上面讨论的全基因组 RNAi 文库[198]。这些 CRISPR 文库可以用以评估基因组中任何基因以及其引起的表型变化。与 shRNA 相比,CRISPR 介导的基因表达抑制通常更稳健,"脱靶"效应可能更少。因此,基于 CRISPR/Cas9 文库进行基因组规模筛选很可能成为功能基因组学的基石,并可进一步完善前期 shRNA 筛选所取得进展(图 3-17)。

基因功能获得性技术

cDNA 文库是基因功能获得研究最常用的技术,该技术将 cDNA 文库瞬时或稳定转染导入细胞使文库内包含的基因高度激活进而发挥生物学活性。目前,已有大型的克隆 cDNA 成功应用的实例[200,201],而且其中一些与其他需要重组导入的系统具有相容性,可以将目标基因开放阅读框(open reading frames, ORF)在不同载体之间成功转换,从而满足不同的研究需要。

基因功能获得的方法已有广泛应用,包括鉴定信号转导途径的调节剂,如转录报告基因评估[202]、鉴定可以逃逸衰老的基因[201]和赋予抗药性的基因表型[203]。根据筛选的目标,cDNA 既可以通过转染瞬时表达(一种适用于转录报告驱动的系统,时间短),也可以通过病毒 cDNA 表达载体进行稳定整合(许多与致癌转化相关的筛选经常用到该方法,需要长期表达和选择)。

另外一种基因功能获得的方法是通过 miRNA 文库来筛选与特定表型相关的 miRNA。如上所述,miRNA 是一类内源性的小 RNA,通过诱导 mRNA 靶标降解或抑制其翻译,从而抑制蛋白质的表达。与癌症有关的 miRNA 包括 let-7、RAS、c-Myc 和其他癌基因的负调节因子[204];在淋巴瘤中上调的 miR-17-92 簇,可促进淋巴瘤的发生[205];BCL2 的负调节因子 miR-15 和 miR-16,在慢性淋巴细胞白血病中的表达下调[206]。这表明 miRNA 在肿瘤发生中的角色尚不明确,还需要进一步的深入研究。最近研究人员通过反转录病毒介导的 miRNA 表达文库鉴定出 miR-372 和 miR-373,发现它们在 Ras 介导的抗凋亡通路中发挥着重要的作用,表明这些 miRNA 可能具有致癌功能[207]。未来我们有望鉴定出更多与肿瘤发生相关的 miRNA

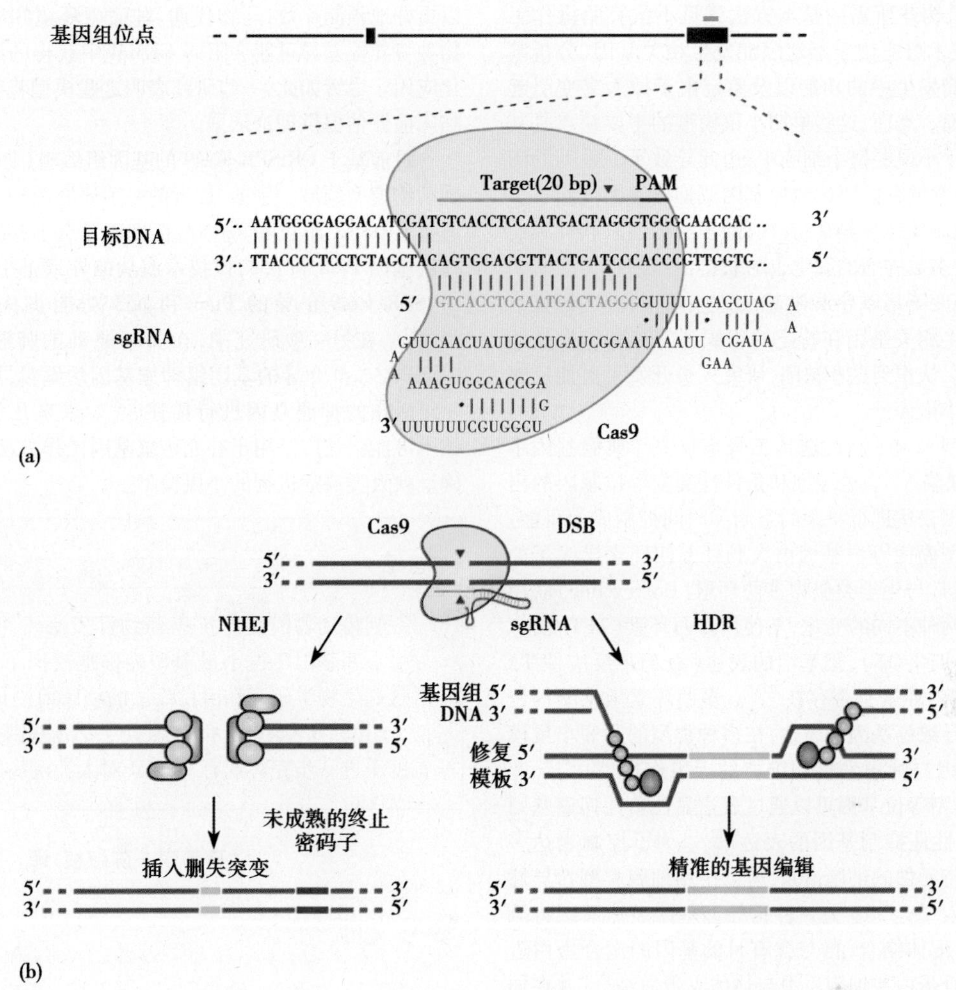

图 3-17 (a)图示 RNA 引导的 Cas9 核酸酶,通过 20nt 的引导序列(蓝色)指向目标 DNA。红色三角形代表 Cas9 将启动 DSB 的大致位置。(b)Cas9 创建的 DSB 可以通过容易出错的 NHEJ 或同源重组来修复

和其调控的靶基因,从而为进一步阐明肿瘤发生相关的机制提供新的思路。

总结

无偏倚的全基因组功能筛选越来越多地被用来鉴定和验证新的肿瘤治疗靶点。这些筛选大多数在细胞培养模型中进行,而后通过肿瘤组织样本进行验证。RNA 干扰和 CRISPR/Cas9 筛选是主要的功能缺失研究方法,而 ORF 筛选则代表了主要的功能获得研究方法。部分筛选已经发现了一些在肿瘤发生中有关键作用的基因。细胞培养模型的发展和以上新技术在动物模型中的应用,使得这些基础研究的发现更有可能在肿瘤患者身上得到验证。

人类癌症的小鼠模型

尽管癌症生物学在分子水平上得到了迅速的发展,但这些研究成果离临床应用还有很长的距离。实验室研究向临床应用研究转化的一个限制性因素是,能否获得可以准确模拟人类肿瘤的体内动物模型。在过去几十年的癌症研究中,动物模型特别是模式小鼠发挥了重要的作用,为开发有效的抗肿瘤治疗方法奠定了重要的基础[208]。最初,这种啮齿类动物模型的应用很大程度上局限于自发性或致癌性肿瘤,或者更常见的是,将小鼠或人类肿瘤细胞异位或原位移植到同源小鼠或免疫缺失小鼠中。尽管这些方法都不能准确地反映人类癌症的复杂性,但在研究抗肿瘤药物的监管批准过程中,传统上仍需要使用这些模型进行临床前研究。

伴随着 20 世纪 80 年代早期分子生物学和胚胎学的发展,基因工程鼠模型(genetically engineered mouse models, GEMM)应运而生。GEMM 的发展使得直接在体内进行肿瘤发生相关基因的研究成为可能,目前几乎所有的人类肿瘤都有相应的基因工程鼠[209]。第一代基因工程鼠是通过导入肿瘤发生相关的癌基因构建的,这些基因鼠证实了癌基因 c-Myc、Ras 和一些病毒癌基因的功能,研究者成功创建了淋巴瘤、乳腺癌和胰腺癌的动物模型[210]。虽然许多早期的肿瘤模型提供了丰富的信息,但由于异位表达盒和组织嵌合所固有的非生理特性,大多数人类癌症无法用这种方法精确建模。另一种建立人类癌症模型的早期方法是通过破坏或“敲除”(knockout, KO)内源性肿瘤抑制基因的等位基因,这些基因往往被认为是癌症易感基因。尽管这种 KO 小鼠的肿瘤谱与同源的人类肿瘤的情况显著不同,但 KO 小鼠证实了 Knudsen 对抑癌基因功能的假设。

转基因和KO小鼠构建所需的基本方法详见小鼠胚胎操作工具书[211]。上述技术可应用于鉴定癌症发生相关基因、分析基因联合作用在肿瘤发生中的功能以及鉴定由于插入突变引起的遗传变异等方面。然而，这些早期小鼠模型的主要缺点是基因工程突变存在于小鼠的每个细胞中，由此导致了一系列的问题。首先，如果正常发育需要的致癌基因或抑癌基因受到了影响，可能会引起胚胎致死或异常；其次，除了遗传性家族性肿瘤综合征外，由于大多数肿瘤的发生也与获得性体细胞突变密切相关，因此多数突变不足以导致肿瘤的发生；第三，上述研究不足以发现肿瘤发生相关基因在特定的组织器官和肿瘤发生特定时期中的作用。认识到这些缺陷，研究人员开发了更能反映人类疾病状态的小鼠模型。

目前小鼠模型采用了新的遗传工具来解决经典癌基因小鼠和KO小鼠的缺陷[212]。诱导型和条件性突变等位基因的出现使得对癌症基因表达进行复杂的空间和时间控制成为可能。常见类型的诱导型癌症等位基因由大肠杆菌四环素操纵子的变体转录调节，通常与化学类似物多西环素（Doxycycline）联用调控表达。它有两种不同的变化，不使用多西环素（TET-OFF）和使用多西环素（TET-ON），靶基因的表达（由TET反应性TA调节）则取决于多西环素是否存在[213]。多西环素敏感型等位基因可以用于诱导致癌基因的表达，在多种类型的肿瘤小鼠模型中证明致癌基因与肿瘤发展和维持的因果作用[209,214]。此外，多西环素依赖型等位基因可以通过表达显性负性抑癌基因和shRNA来可逆性地抑制基因的表达[215]。为了控制表达多西环素依赖性遗传元件的细胞谱系，可以使用细胞类型特异性启动子编码四环素TA[213]。另一种诱导型基因表达系统将雌激素受体（ER）与配体结合，再与含有目的基因的嵌合蛋白进行融合。这种融合蛋白在细胞质中与热休克蛋白结合，并在加入雌激素类似物（如他莫昔芬）后释放。ER与Myc和P53的融合蛋白已被用于构建多种癌症的小鼠模型[216,217]。条件性等位基因突变可以直接调节基因的表达，主要是通过删除抑癌基因，或借助内源启动子激活癌基因的单个等位基因的表达。条件突变等位基因由噬菌体P1 Cre/loxP系统控制，其中Cre重组酶将指导两端34bp LoxP位点的DNA元件的环化和切除。因此，条件性抑癌基因的等位基因由含有内含子LoxP的外显子基因组成，并且这些等位基因在二倍体水平表达，直到引入Cre重组酶并导致基因敲除，从而使其mRNA和蛋白质表达缺失。条件致癌基因通常是沉默的，直到Cre重组酶去除了它的转录沉默或“终止”元件后，致癌基因才开始表达，在这种情况下，染色体从单倍体变为二倍体，其中一半染色体由致癌的等位基因组成。目前其他重组酶也被用于小鼠构建，配合多种控制条件基因表达的相关策略使用。诱导型癌症等位基因可以单独使用，也可以与条件性突变等位基因联用，从而使添加的配体可以控制Cre重组酶的表达，进而实现癌症基因表达时间和空间的精细调控[218,219]。利用这些最先进的技术，研究者目前已经开发出更好的模拟侵袭性和浸润性癌进展的GEMM，包括肺癌、胰腺癌、前列腺癌、卵巢癌和乳腺癌[209]。这些模型通常表现出病理生理性疾病，包括恶病质、转移、体细胞生化和基因组的改变，这在同源的人类恶性肿瘤中很常见。目前研究正在开发GEMM在癌症诊断和治疗中的作用。GEMM未解答的问题包括：与异种肿瘤移植模型相比，尚无证据表明GEMM可以更好地预测疗效；药物代谢、肿瘤微环境和细胞内在通路的物种特异性差异可能会阻碍GEMM中获得的成果向临床的转化应用。尽管如此，一些研究表明这些模型将为抗肿瘤药物的临床前评估提供理论依据。

目前基于CRISPR/Cas9的基因组编辑（见上文）也已扩展到动物模型领域。例如，最近的一项研究就通过流体动力学注射将CRISPR质粒和sgRNA直接递送至小鼠肝脏以靶向肿瘤抑制基因Pten和p53，该技术成功的导致了小鼠肝脏成瘤，且CRISPR/Cas9介导的Pten和p53功能丧失与KO小鼠相当[221]。在另一项研究中，在kras驱动的肺癌模型上使用了CRISPR/cas9介导的基因组抑癌基因的编辑，可以从功能上对一组潜在的抑癌基因进行描述[222]。未来几年，CRISPR/Cas9技术可能会被广泛用于补充传统基因操作方法，以构建能够准确反映人类癌症进程的小鼠模型。

总结

啮齿动物模型是抗癌药物开发必不可少的组成部分。一些基因工程小鼠模型准确地模拟了人类的疾病，对疾病生物学研究和潜在疗法的临床前测试有很大的帮助。CRISPR/Cas9技术补充了传统的基因操作方法，并有助于进一步完善现有GEMM对人类疾病的模拟。

（曹琦琪　陈淑桢　译　文文　孙文　校）

参考文献

The complete reference list can be found on the Wiley Companion Digital Edition of this title (see inside front cover for login instructions).

2 Alberts B (ed). *Molecular Biology of the Cell*, 5th ed. New York: Garland Science; 2008.

6 Nirenberg M, Leder P. RNA codewords and protein synthesis. The effect of trinucleotides upon the binding of sRNA to ribosomes. *Science.* 1964;**145(3639)**:1399–1407.

7 Watson JD, Crick FH. Molecular structure of nucleic acids; a structure for deoxyribose nucleic acid. *Nature.* 1953;**171(4356)**:737–738.

16 Cohen SN, Chang AC, Boyer HW, Helling RB. Construction of biologically functional bacterial plasmids in vitro. *Proc Natl Acad Sci U S A.* 1973;**70(4594039)**:3240–3244.

18 Green MR. *Molecular Cloning: A Laboratory Manual*, 4th ed. Cold Spring Harbor, NY: Cold Spring Harbor Laboratory Press; 2012. 3 p.

20 Gibson DG, Young L, Chuang R-Y, Venter JC, Hutchison CA, Smith HO. Enzymatic assembly of DNA molecules up to several hundred kilobases. *Nat Methods.* 2009;**6(5)**:343–345.

22 Southern EM. Detection of specific sequences among DNA fragments separated by gel electrophoresis. *J Mol Biol.* 1975;**98(1195397)**:503–517.

23 Slamon DJ, Godolphin W, Jones LA, et al. Studies of the HER-2/neu proto-oncogene in human breast and ovarian cancer. *Science.* 1989;**244(2470152)**:707–712.

26 Mullis KB, Faloona FA. Specific synthesis of DNA in vitro via a polymerase-catalyzed chain reaction. *Methods Enzymol.* 1987;**155**:335–350.

27 Nakamura Y, Leppert M, O'Connell P, et al. Variable number of tandem repeat (VNTR) markers for human gene mapping. *Science.* 1987;**235(3029872)**:1616–1622.

28 Miki Y, Swensen J, Shattuck-Eidens D, et al. A strong candidate for the breast and ovarian cancer susceptibility gene BRCA1. *Science.* 1994;**266(5182)**:66–71.

36 Wang DG, Fan JB, Siao CJ, et al. Large-scale identification, mapping, and genotyping of single-nucleotide polymorphisms in the human genome. *Science.* 1998;**280(9582121)**:1077–1082.

37 Sachidanandam R, Weissman D, Schmidt SC, et al. A map of human genome sequence variation containing 1.42 million single nucleotide polymorphisms.

Nature. 2001;**409**(**6822**):928–933.

38 Altshuler D, Pollara VJ, Cowles CR, et al. An SNP map of the human genome generated by reduced representation shotgun sequencing. *Nature*. 2000;**407**(**6803**):513–516.

44 Sanger F, Nicklen S, Coulson AR. DNA sequencing with chain-terminating inhibitors. *Proc Natl Acad Sci U S A*. 1977;**74**(**12**):5463–5467.

46 Joensuu H, Roberts PJ, Sarlomo-Rikala M, et al. Effect of the tyrosine kinase inhibitor STI571 in a patient with a metastatic gastrointestinal stromal tumor. *N Engl J Med*. 2001;**344**(**11287975**):1052–1056.

47 Lynch TJ, Bell DW, Sordella R, et al. Activating mutations in the epidermal growth factor receptor underlying responsiveness of non-small-cell lung cancer to gefitinib. *N Engl J Med*. 2004;**350**(**21**):2129–2139.

48 Pao W, Miller V, Zakowski M, et al. EGF receptor gene mutations are common in lung cancers from "never smokers" and are associated with sensitivity of tumors to gefitinib and erlotinib. *Proc Natl Acad Sci U S A*. 2004;**101**(**36**):13306–13311.

49 Paez JG, Jänne PA, Lee JC, et al. EGFR mutations in lung cancer: correlation with clinical response to gefitinib therapy. *Science*. 2004;**304**(**5676**):1497–1500.

51 Chapman PB, Hauschild A, Robert C, et al. Improved survival with vemurafenib in melanoma with BRAF V600E mutation. *N Engl J Med*. 2011;**364**(**26**):2507–2516.

56 Hodges E, Xuan Z, Balija V, et al. Genome-wide in situ exon capture for selective resequencing. *Nat Genet*. 2007;**39**(**17982454**):1522–1527.

61 Ley TJ, Mardis ER, Ding L, et al. DNA sequencing of a cytogenetically normal acute myeloid leukaemia genome. *Nature*. 2008;**456**(**7218**):66–72.

65 Cibulskis K, Lawrence MS, Carter SL, et al. Sensitive detection of somatic point mutations in impure and heterogeneous cancer samples. *Nat Biotechnol*. 2013;**31**(**3**):213–219.

66 Koboldt DC, Zhang Q, Larson DE, et al. VarScan 2: somatic mutation and copy number alteration discovery in cancer by exome sequencing. *Genome Res*. 2012;**22**(**3**):568–576.

68 Lawrence MS, Stojanov P, Polak P, et al. Mutational heterogeneity in cancer and the search for new cancer-associated genes. *Nature*. 2013;**499**(**7457**):214–218.

72 Sharp PA. Split genes and RNA splicing. *Cell*. 1994;**77**(**7516265**):805–815.

81 Baltimore D. RNA-dependent DNA polymerase in virions of RNA tumour viruses. *Nature*. 1970;**226**(**5252**):1209–1211.

82 Temin HM, Mizutani S. RNA-dependent DNA polymerase in virions of Rous sarcoma virus. *Nature*. 1970;**226**(**5252**):1211–1213.

89 Velculescu VE, Zhang L, Vogelstein B, Kinzler KW. Serial analysis of gene expression. *Science*. 1995;**270**(**7570003**):484–487.

95 Schena M, Shalon D, Davis RW, Brown PO. Quantitative monitoring of gene expression patterns with a complementary DNA microarray. *Science*. 1995;**270**(**5235**):467–470.

97 Golub TR, Slonim DK, Tamayo P, et al. Molecular classification of cancer: class discovery and class prediction by gene expression monitoring. *Science*. 1999;**286**(**10521349**):531–537.

113 Trapnell C, Williams BA, Pertea G, et al. Transcript assembly and quantification by RNA-Seq reveals unannotated transcripts and isoform switching during cell differentiation. *Nat Biotechnol*. 2010;**28**(**5**):511–515.

122 Herman JG, Baylin SB. Gene silencing in cancer in association with promoter hypermethylation. *N Engl J Med*. 2003;**349**(**21**):2042–2054.

126 Gaudet F, Hodgson JG, Eden A, et al. Induction of tumors in mice by genomic hypomethylation. *Science*. 2003;**300**(**12702876**):489–492.

138 Mikkelsen TS, Ku M, Jaffe DB, et al. Genome-wide maps of chromatin state in pluripotent and lineage-committed cells. *Nature*. 2007;**448**(**17603471**):553–560.

150 Druker BJ, Sawyers CL, Kantarjian H, et al. Activity of a specific inhibitor of the BCR-ABL tyrosine kinase in the blast crisis of chronic myeloid leukemia and acute lymphoblastic leukemia with the Philadelphia chromosome. *N Engl J Med*. 2001;**344**(**11287973**):1038–1042.

176 Fire A, Xu S, Montgomery MK, Kostas SA, Driver SE, Mello CC. Potent and specific genetic interference by double-stranded RNA in Caenorhabditis elegans. *Nature*. 1998;**391**(**9486653**):806–811.

178 Lee RC, Feinbaum RL, Ambros V. The C. elegans heterochronic gene lin-4 encodes small RNAs with antisense complementarity to lin-14. *Cell*. 1993;**75**(**5**):843–854.

179 Wightman B, Ha I, Ruvkun G. Posttranscriptional regulation of the heterochronic gene lin-14 by lin-4 mediates temporal pattern formation in C. elegans. *Cell*. 1993;**75**(**5**):855–862.

195 Jinek M, Chylinski K, Fonfara I, Hauer M, Doudna JA, Charpentier E. A programmable dual-RNA-guided DNA endonuclease in adaptive bacterial immunity. *Science*. 2012;**337**(**6096**):816–821.

197 Cong L, Ran FA, Cox D, et al. Multiplex genome engineering using CRISPR/Cas systems. *Science*. 2013;**339**(**6121**):819–823.

198 Shalem O, Sanjana NE, Hartenian E, et al. Genome-scale CRISPR-Cas9 knockout screening in human cells. *Science*. 2014;**343**(**6166**):84–87.

214 Chin L, Tam A, Pomerantz J, et al. Essential role for oncogenic Ras in tumour maintenance. *Nature*. 1999;**400**(**6743**):468–472.

第 4 章　癌基因

Marco A. Pierotti, PhD ■ Milo Frattini, MD, PhD ■ Francesca Molinari, PhD ■
Gabriella Sozzi, PhD ■ Carlo M. Croce, MD

概述

肿瘤的发生发展是一个复杂连续的过程，主要由体细胞的基因突变累积效应所导致。肿瘤中典型的基因突变包括癌基因的激活和抑癌基因的失活，这两种机制决定了肿瘤的表型。癌基因是正常细胞基因中的原癌基因的一种变体，通常参与细胞的生长调控，可通过基因突变、染色体重排或者基因扩增等方式激活。本章将首先介绍发现和识别癌基因的方法；其次，举例说明原癌基因激活的遗传机制（点突变，基因扩增，染色体重排）；最后，阐述癌基因在各种肿瘤发生发展中的作用。

识别癌基因的异常改变为癌症的分子检测诊断提供了行之有效的方法。更重要的是，癌基因的发现为各种肿瘤新疗法提供了潜在的靶点，部分靶点已经在临床试验中得到了验证。此类靶向癌基因药物的目标在于选择性地杀伤肿瘤细胞而非正常细胞。靶向疗法在一些原本难以治愈的肿瘤中表现出了令人振奋的疗效。但是，由于继发性耐药的存在，这些治疗方法也无法 100% 地杀灭肿瘤细胞。在本章的最后一部分，总结了所有已研发的相关治疗靶点。

早在一个多世纪以前，Boveri 就提出，从分子水平来看，癌症是由细胞 DNA 损伤引起的，这一观点已经被多项研究证实。首先，癌细胞可以将“癌性”状态的性状传递给子代细胞；其次，大部分公认的诱变剂也有致癌的作用；最后，通过对几种人类肿瘤，尤其是造血系统相关肿瘤的核型进行分析，研究者发现肿瘤细胞均存在多发性的染色体畸变以及细胞基因组的病理性重排。综上所述，人类肿瘤发生的分子机制是由于特定基因结构和/或基因功能的改变，而这些基因在正常情况下调控着细胞的生长和分化，即调控着细胞的分裂和凋亡[1,2]。

在过去的几十年里 DNA 重组技术，尤其是人类全基因组测序的发展，使科学家们得以探查和分析影响癌症发生的重要遗传因素。其中，研究者通过 RNA 病毒（反转录病毒）转染细胞，确认了“病毒性癌基因”的细胞起源，这一发现具有里程碑式的意义；但同时发现，并非所有基因转化的细胞都存在相应的病毒[3,4]。这种促进细胞转化的遗传物质，根据其最初来源被称为病毒或细胞基因组，在正常生理状态下被称作原癌基因，在肿瘤组织中发生改变后称其为癌基因[5]。第二项技术是对癌细胞（主要是造血系统来源）的克隆增殖和复发性遗传异常（包括易位、倒位等）的识别和鉴定。研究者通过染色体区域的染色，分析调控基因扩增区域的异常染色情况，如均染区，发现了其他的致癌基因[6]。此外，染色体缺失的检测技术可以鉴定和克隆另一种类型的癌症相关基因——抑癌基因，正常细胞中抑癌基因负调控细胞的生长，而在肿瘤细胞中它的负调控功能被抑制[5,6]。高通量测序技术发现，基因点突变是癌基因激活的一种常见机制[7]。除了以上技术，我们还可通过蛋白激酶组学分析蛋白激酶[8]、通过磷酸酶组学分析磷酸酶[9]以及其他参与癌症发展的多种蛋白的异构体（如 PI3K）[10]。

本章将简要介绍癌基因的发现方法，细胞原癌基因的功能，原癌基因激活的遗传机制。探讨影响肿瘤发生发展的一些特异的癌基因，并简述一些具有潜在药靶价值的新靶点。

癌基因的发现和鉴定

第一个癌基因是通过对逆转录病毒的研究发现的。逆转录病毒（RNA 肿瘤病毒）的基因组在被其感染的动物细胞中可以被逆转录成 DNA[11]。在感染过程中，经过逆转录过程的病毒 DNA 可以插入宿主细胞的染色体中，这种整合的逆转录病毒 DNA，被称为前病毒，其可以跟随宿主的细胞 DNA 一起复制，通过宿主细胞膜出芽的方式产生子代病毒，进而感染其他细胞[11]。当将这些逆转录病毒注射进实验动物体内后，急性转化型逆转录病毒可在注射后几天内迅速引起肿瘤，而慢性或弱致瘤性逆转录病毒则需经过数月的潜伏期后，才能在易感种系的实验动物中形成组织特异性肿瘤。

关于劳斯肉瘤病毒（Rous sarcoma virus，RSV）的一项研究（图 4-1）发现了一个奇特的现象，即逆转录病毒癌基因是变异了的宿主细胞的原癌基因，逆转录病毒癌基因通过与宿主 DNA 重组，整合到逆转录病毒的基因组中，这一过程被称为逆转录病毒转导[5]。该研究揭示了 RSV 的转化基因并不是病毒复制必需的[12]。分子杂交实验进一步表明，RSV 转化基因（*v-src*）与真核生物中广泛保守的宿主细胞基因（*c-src*）同源[13]。通过对来源于禽类、啮齿类、猫科动物和非人类灵长类的大量急性转化型逆转录病毒的研究，研究者成功地发现了几十种不同的逆转录病毒癌基因（表 4-1）。每一个逆转录病毒癌基因都具有快速促瘤和高效体外转化的特性，这也正是急性转化型逆转录病毒成瘤的主要特点。

与急性转化型逆转录病毒不同，弱致癌性逆转录病毒不携带病毒致癌基因。包括小鼠乳腺肿瘤病毒（mouse mammary tumor virus，MMTV）和多种动物白血病病毒在内的逆转录病毒，通过插入突变来诱发肿瘤（图 4-2）[6]。该过程是将前病毒 DNA 整合到受感染细胞的宿主基因组中。在少数细胞中，前病毒插入到原癌基因附近，随后，在长末端重复序列内的转录调控元件的驱动下，原癌基因的表达出现异常[6]。由此可见，前病毒的整合导致了突变，进而激活了原癌基因。而弱致癌性逆转录病毒形成肿瘤需要一个较长的潜伏期。因为通过前病毒

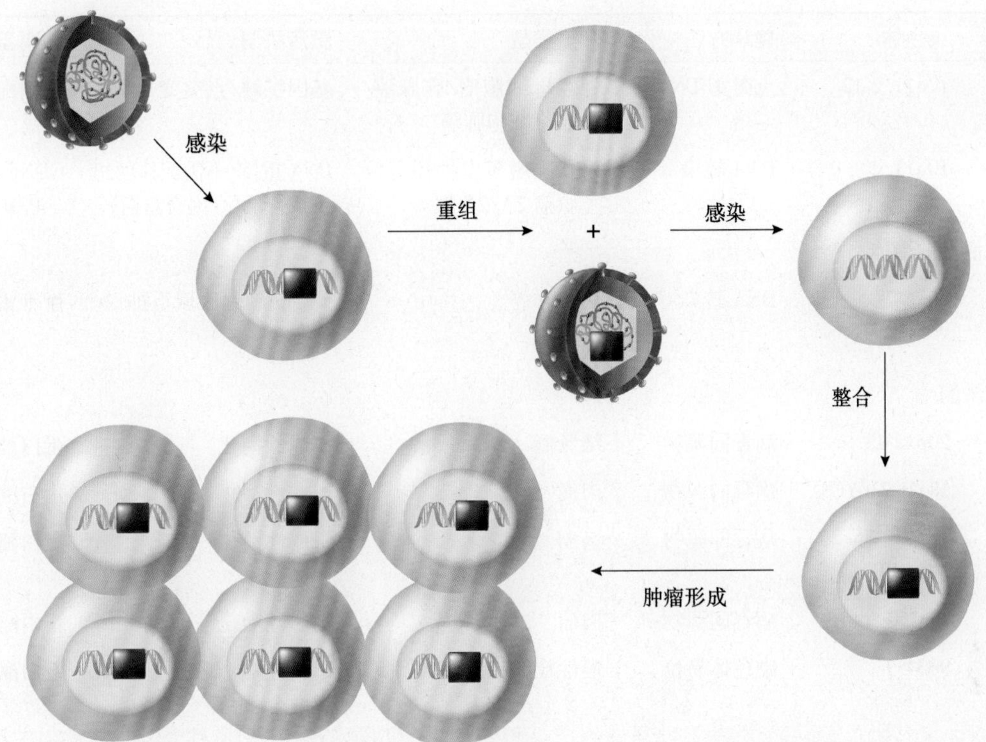

图 4-1　逆转录病毒转导。RNA 肿瘤病毒感染携带活化 *src* 基因的人类细胞（红框）。在逆转录病毒基因组与宿主 DNA 进行重组后，癌基因 *c-src* 被命名为 *v-src*。当携带 *v-src* 的逆转录病毒感染人类细胞时，病毒癌基因被迅速转录，并由此诱发肿瘤快速形成

表 4-1　癌基因

癌基因	染色体	确认方法	肿瘤类型	激活机制	编码蛋白功能
生长因子					
V-SIS	22q12.3-13.1	同源序列	神经胶质瘤/纤维肉瘤	组成性产生	β 链 PDGF
*INT*2	11q13	前病毒插入	乳癌	组成性产生	FGF 家族成员
*KS*3	11q13.3	DNA 感染	卡波西肉瘤	组成性产生	FGF 家族成员
HST	11q13.3	DNA 感染	胃癌	组成性产生	FGF 家族成员
生长因子受体					
酪氨酸激酶:跨膜蛋白					
EGFR	7p1.1-1.3	DNA 扩增/DNA 测序	鳞状细胞癌/非小细胞肺癌	基因扩增/蛋白/点突变	EGF 受体
v-FMS	5q33-34(FMS)	病毒同源物	肉瘤	组成性活化	CSFI 受体
v-KIT	4q11-21(KIT)	病毒同源物/DNA 测序	肉瘤/胃肠间质瘤	组成性活化/点突变	干细胞因子受体
v-ROS	6q22(ROS)	病毒同源物	肉瘤	组成性活化	嵌入型蛋白
MET	7p31	DNA 转染	MNNG 处理过的人骨肉瘤细胞株	DNA 重排/不需配体的组成性活化（融合蛋白）	HGF/SF 受体
TRK	1q32-41	DNA 转染	结肠癌/甲状腺癌	DNA 重排/不需配体的组成性活化（融合蛋白）	NGF 受体

续表

癌基因	染色体	确认方法	肿瘤类型	激活机制	编码蛋白功能
NEU	17q11.2-12	点突变/DNA 扩增	神经母细胞瘤/乳腺癌/非小细胞肺癌	基因扩增/点突变	未知配体
RET	10q11.2	DNA 转染	甲状腺癌多发性内分泌腺瘤 2A/2B 型	DNA 重排/不需配体的组成性活化(融合蛋白)	GDNF/NTT/ART/PSP 受体
缺乏蛋白激酶活性的受体					
MAS	6q24-27	DNA 转染	表皮样癌	5′端非编码区域重排	血管紧张素受体
信号转导分子					
细胞质酪氨酸激酶					
SRC	20p12-13	病毒同源物	结肠癌	组成性活化	蛋白酪氨酸激酶
v-YES	18q21-23(YES)	病毒同源物	肉瘤	组成性活化	蛋白酪氨酸激酶
v-FGR	1p36.1-36.2(FGR)	病毒同源物	肉瘤	组成性活化	蛋白酪氨酸激酶
v-FES	15q25-26(FES)	病毒同源物	肉瘤	组成性活化	蛋白酪氨酸激酶
ABL	9q34.1	染色体易位	慢性粒细胞白血病	DNA 重排(组成性活化/融合蛋白)	蛋白酪氨酸激酶
膜相关 G 蛋白					
HRAS	11p15.5	病毒同源物/DNA 转染	结肠癌、肺癌、胰腺癌	点突变	GTP 酶
KRAS	12p11.1-12.1	病毒同源物/DNA 转染	急性髓细胞白血病、甲状腺癌、黑色素瘤/结肠/肺	点突变	GTP 酶
NRAS	1p11-13	DNA 转染	癌、黑色素瘤	点突变	GTP 酶
BRAF	6	DNA 测序	黑色素瘤、甲状腺、结肠、卵巢	点突变	丝氨酸/苏氨酸激酶
GSP	20	DNA 测序	甲状腺瘤	点突变	Gs-α
GIP	3	DNA 测序	卵巢、肾上腺癌	点突变	Gi-α
GTP 酶交换因子(GEF)					
DBL	Xq27	DNA 转染	弥漫性 B 细胞淋巴瘤	DNA 重排	Rho 和 Cdc42Hs 的 GEF
VAV	19p13.2	DNA 转染	造血细胞	DNA 重排	Ras 的 GEF
丝氨酸/苏氨酸激酶:细胞质					
v-MOS	8q11(MOS)	病毒同源物	肉瘤	组成性活化	蛋白激酶(丝氨酸/苏氨酸)
v-RAF	3p25(RAF-1)	病毒同源物	肉瘤	组成性活化	蛋白激酶(丝氨酸/苏氨酸)
PIM-1	6p21(PIM-)	插入突变	T 细胞淋巴瘤	组成性活化	蛋白激酶(丝氨酸/苏氨酸)
细胞质调节因子					
v-CRK	17p13(CRK)	病毒同源物	—	细胞底物组成性酪氨酸磷酸化(如:桩蛋白)	SH-2/SH-3 衔接蛋白

续表

癌基因	染色体	确认方法	肿瘤类型	激活机制	编码蛋白功能
转录因子					
v-MYC	8q24.1(MYC)	病毒同源物	癌、髓细胞瘤病	解除限制性活性	转录因子
N-MYC	2p24	DNA 扩增	肺部神经母细胞瘤	解除限制性活性	转录因子
L-MYC	1p32	DNA 扩增	肺癌	解除限制性活性	转录因子
v-MYB	6q22-24	病毒同源物	成髓细胞过多症	解除限制性活性	转录因子
v-FOS	14q21-22	病毒同源物	骨肉瘤	解除限制性活性	转录因子 API
v-JUN	p31-32	病毒同源物	肉瘤	解除限制性活性	转录因子 API
v-SKI	1q22-24	病毒同源物	癌	解除限制性活性	转录因子
v-REL	2p12-14	病毒同源物	淋巴细胞白血病	解除限制性活性	突变 NF-κB
v-ETS-1	11p23-q24	病毒同源物	红细胞增多症	解除限制性活性	转录因子
v-ETS-2	21q24.3	病毒同源物	红细胞增多症	解除限制性活性	转录因子
v-ERB A1	17p11-21	病毒同源物	红细胞增多症	解除限制性活性	T3 转录因子
v-ERB A2	3p22-24.1	病毒同源物	红细胞增多症	解除限制性活性	T3 转录因子
其他					
BCL2	18q21.3	染色体易位	B 细胞淋巴瘤	组成性活化	抗凋亡蛋白
MDM2	12q14	DNA 扩增	肉瘤	基因扩增/增加蛋白	P53 复合体

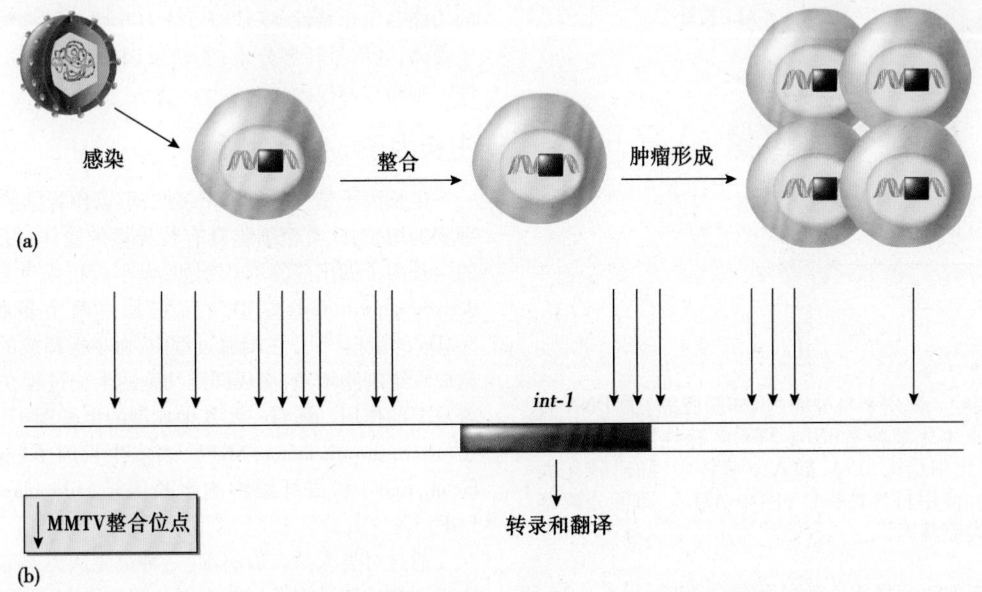

图 4-2 插入突变。(a)该过程独立于逆转录病毒携带的基因。逆转录病毒,例如 MMTV,感染人类细胞后,前病毒 DNA 整合到受感染细胞的宿主基因组中,极少数情况下,前病毒插入原癌基因(例如 *int-1*)附近并激活原癌基因。活化的原癌基因导致细胞转化并形成肿瘤。(b)MMTV 逆转录病毒在原癌基因 *int-1* 附近的整合位点。所有位点都受 *int-1* 控制

插入导致细胞突变,并从单个转化细胞发展到肿瘤的概率较低。在对鸡的法氏囊淋巴瘤的研究中,首次发现了弱致瘤性逆转录病毒的插入突变,这类基因通常与急性转化型逆转录病毒携带的癌基因(如 *myc*、*myb* 和 *erb B*)相同[6,14]。然而,在许多情况下,插入突变常被当作一种手段,用于鉴定新发现的癌基因,例如 *int-1*、*int-2*、*pim1* 和 *lck*[6]。

通过 DNA 介导的转化技术,研究者首次证实了人类肿瘤中存在活化的原癌基因[15,16]。该技术也被称为基因转移或转染,可以用肿瘤的供体 DNA 转化啮齿类动物细胞受体株 NIH 3T3(一种永生化小鼠细胞系)(图 4-3)[17]。这种检测方法十

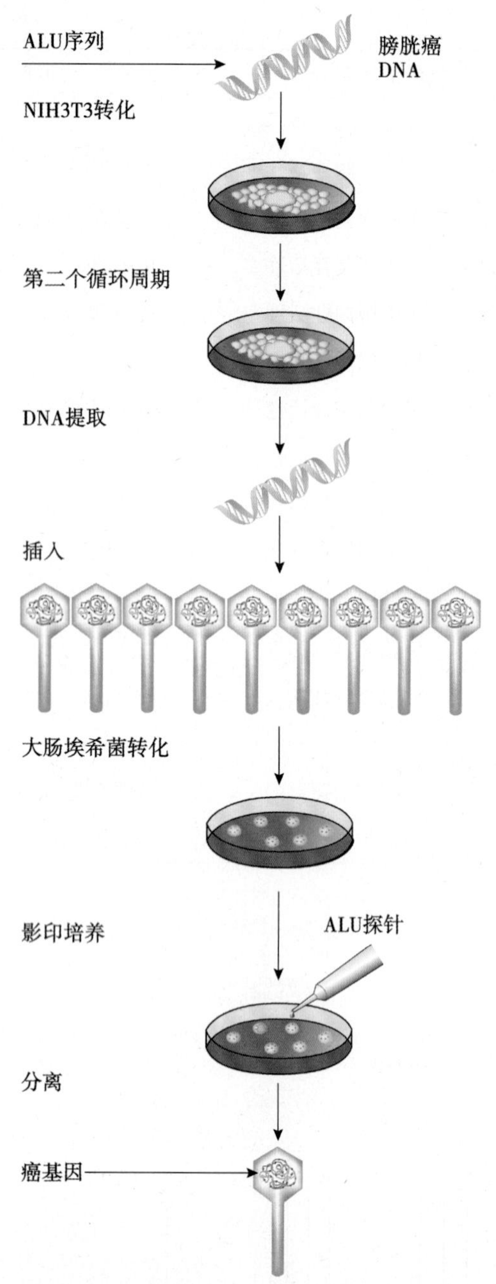

图 4-3 转染实验。使用来自肿瘤(例如膀胱癌)的 DNA 转化啮齿动物的永生化细胞系(NIH 3T3)。在连续若干循环后,提取来自转化细胞的 DNA,插入 p 载体中,随后转化大肠埃希菌菌株。使用特异性探针(图中 ALU),即可分离鉴定所涉及的人类癌基因

分灵敏,可以检测到肿瘤样本中的单拷贝癌基因,也可以通过分子克隆技术分离转化癌基因[18]。总的来说,在基因转移实验中,约有 20%的人类肿瘤中的基因能诱导 NIH 3T3 细胞转化。Weinberg 实验室发现,将异位表达端粒酶催化亚基(hTERT)、猿猴病毒 SV40 大 T 产物和突变的癌基因 H-ras 蛋白三者结合,可直接导致正常人类上皮细胞和成纤维细胞产生致瘤性转化,这进一步证实了转染试验的价值[19]。基因转移技术鉴定的许多癌基因与逆转录病毒转导的癌基因完全一致或密切相关[20]。与此同时,基因转移技术也发现了大量新的致癌基因(如 *neu*、*met* 和 *trk*)[21]。然而,多数情况下,通过基因转移鉴定的癌基因在作为供体 DNA 来源的人体肿瘤中并未活化,而是在实验过程中通过基因重排被激活。最知名的例子就是在甲状腺乳头状癌中,*ret* 基因由于基因重组而活化[22]。

染色体易位已经成为新癌基因发掘的风向标,尤其是在很多血液和实质肿瘤中[23,24]。这些异常主要包括染色体重排以及整条染色体或染色体片段的增加或缺失。在人类肿瘤中首次发现的结构性染色体组型异常是慢性粒细胞白血病(chronic myelogenous leukemia,CML)患者细胞中的特征性小染色体[23],后来被确定为第 22 号染色体的衍生物。这种异常染色体以其发现的城市被命名为费城染色体。在 20 世纪 70 年代早期,染色体显带技术的广泛应用,使得许多染色体易位在人类白血病、淋巴瘤和实体肿瘤中的细胞遗传学特性得以被精确描述[25]。随后,分子克隆技术的发展,使得在各种肿瘤的染色体断点处或附近鉴定原癌基因成为可能。虽然其中一部分原癌基因此前已经通过逆转录病毒得以鉴定,如 *myc* 和 *abl*,但是,通过染色体断点克隆技术,更多新的癌基因被发现和鉴定。近年来,通过高通量测序技术和人类基因组计划中的生物信息学技术,许多与癌症发展有关的新基因被发现,如 *BRAF* 和 *PIK3CA*[7,10]。

癌基因、原癌基因及其功能

癌基因编码了参与细胞生长调控的蛋白质。癌基因的结构和/或表达的改变可以使其激活并成为致癌基因,进而诱导易感细胞出现肿瘤表型。根据正常基因(原癌基因)蛋白产物的功能和生化特性,癌基因可分为五类:①生长因子;②生长因子受体;③信号转导分子;④转录因子;⑤其他,其中包括程序性细胞凋亡调控因子。

生长因子

生长因子是一种分泌型多肽,可以作为细胞外信号刺激靶细胞的增殖,此类靶细胞具有特异性的受体,可以对特定类型的生长因子做出应答[2]。例如,血小板衍生生长因子(platelet-derived growth factor,PDGF),它是由两个多肽链组成的约 30kDa 的蛋白[26]。在凝血过程中,血小板释放的 PDGF 可以刺激成纤维细胞增殖,而成纤维细胞的生长过程在伤口愈合中起着重要的作用。还有一些其他典型的生长因子,如神经生长因子(nerve growth factor,NGF)、表皮生长因子(epidermal growth factor,EGF)和成纤维细胞生长因子(fibroblast growth factor,FGF)等。

通过对类人猿肉瘤病毒(一种最先从类人猿纤维肉瘤中分离得到的逆转录病毒)的 *sis* 癌基因的研究,研究者发现了生长因子与逆转录病毒癌基因之间的联系。序列分析结果显示,*sis* 编码 PDGF 的 β 链[26]。由此可见,异常表达的生长因子可以持续性激活其受体,导致持续、异常的细胞增殖,从而发挥致癌基因的作用。这种机制称为自分泌刺激(图 4-4)[26]。这一来源于实验动物的模型进一步在人类隆突性皮肤纤维肉瘤(dermatofibrosarcoma protuberans,DP)中得到证实。DP 是一种浸润性皮肤肿瘤,其特异的细胞遗传学特征是在第 17 号和第 22 号染色体上存在相互易位和过量环状染色体[26]。对该断裂点进行分子克隆后发现,I 型胶原 α1 链(*COL1A1*)基因与 *PDGF-β*

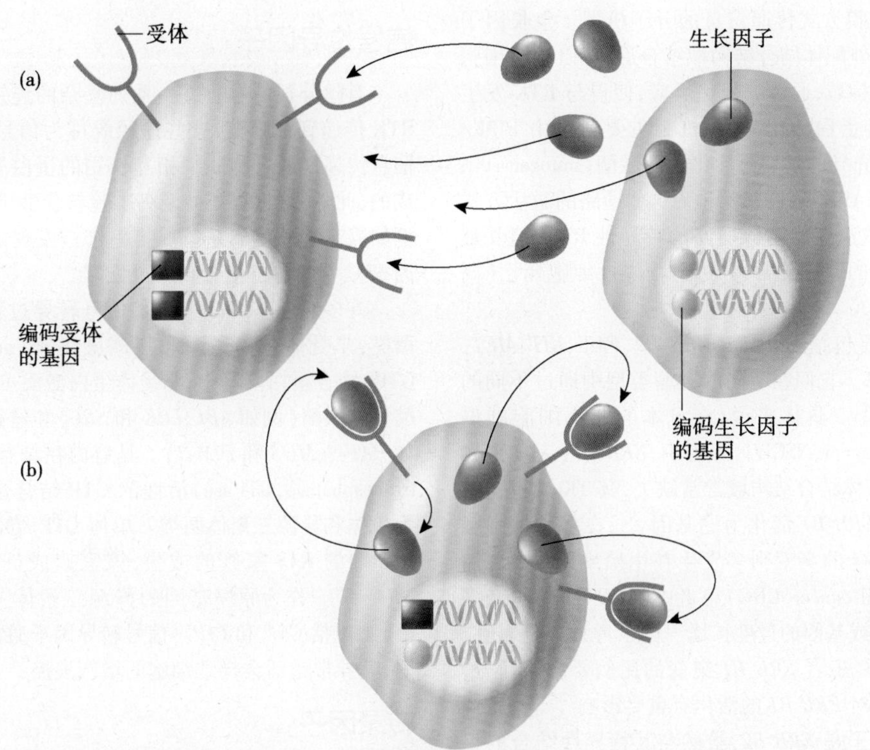

图 4-4　旁分泌和自分泌刺激。(a)右侧细胞产生的生长因子刺激左侧细胞，其细胞膜上携带有与其合适的受体。该过程被称为旁分泌刺激。(b)细胞分泌的生长因子与同一细胞上的相应受体结合的过程被称为自分泌刺激

基因的融合导致了 *PDGF-β* 外显子的缺失和该生长因子的持续性释放。后续实验中，通过基因转移技术将 DP 的基因组 DNA 转移到 NIH 3T3 细胞内，证实了人类重组 *PDGF-β* 基因参与了内源性 PDGF 受体的活化，进而导致自分泌机制的发生[26]。另一个生长因子作为癌基因发挥作用的例子是成纤维细胞生长因子家族的成员 *int-2*，其在小鼠乳腺癌中可以通过 MMTV 插入突变激活[27]。

生长因子受体

一些病毒癌基因是由具有内在酪氨酸激酶(tyrosine kinase，TK)活性的正常生长因子受体变异而来的[28]，这些生长因子受体统称为酪氨酸激酶受体(receptor tyrosine kinase，RTK)，具有以下三个主要结构域的特征性蛋白结构：①细胞外配体结合结构域；②跨膜结构域；③细胞内酪氨酸激酶催化结构域(图 4-5)。

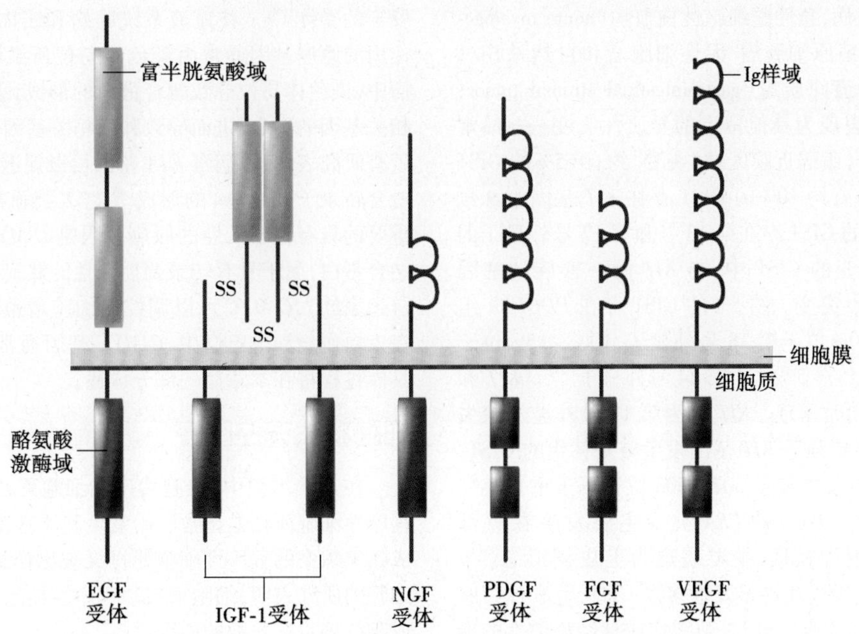

图 4-5　代表性酪氨酸激酶受体家族的示意图

RTK 是以单向跨细胞膜方式传递信息的分子机器。生长因子与其特异性受体的胞外配体结合结构域结合后,可以激活细胞内酪氨酸激酶催化结构域,通过二聚化反应,使得与 RTK 发生物理相互作用的下游蛋白活化,这一机制主要通过由 PI3K/AKT 轴和 STAT 蛋白介导的丝裂原活化蛋白激酶(mitogen-activated protein kinase,MAPK)通路来实现。这些通路的激活方式并不完全相同,具体取决于参与该通路的特异性 RTK,但其最终结果都会导致细胞的复制异常,并逃避程序性细胞死亡(凋亡)[28]。

常见的 RTK 主要包括 *ERB B1*、*ERB B2*、*FMS*、*KIT*、*MET*、*RET*、*ROS*、*ALK* 和 *TRK*。它们在不同的肿瘤类型中通过不同的机制转化为癌基因[28]。具体来说,在日本的非小细胞肺癌(non-small cell lung cancer,NSCLC)患者中,*ERB B1*(表皮生长因子受体 EGFR)的配体结合结构域常常缺失,其 TK 域也会发生点突变,从而导致 *ERB B1* 活化为癌基因[29];在多发性肺腺癌患者人群中,*ERB B1* 的突变则多发生在生殖细胞中[30];而在结直肠癌(colorectal cancer,CRC)患者中,*ERB B1* 的突变多表现为配体的过表达或基因的过度扩增[31,32]。除此以外,还应注意到,日本的 NSCLC 患者 *ERB B1* 突变的比例要高于西方,这表明种族差异可能对 *ERB B1* 的活化有重要影响[29]。

另一个典型的例子是 *ERB B2*,虽然与其特异性结合的生长因子尚不清楚,但其在不同肿瘤中也表现出不同的突变机制。在乳腺癌和胃癌中 *ERB B2* 的突变主要表现为基因扩增,在胃癌、结直肠癌和乳腺癌中则主要表现为点突变。然而,*ERB B2* 的免疫组化染色显示,无论 *ERB B2* 是否突变,其在肿瘤组织内的表达水平并没有差异,这表明 *ERB B2* 的过表达不一定伴随突变[33]。

同样,原癌基因 *KIT* 在肿瘤细胞中的激活也表现为三种不同的机制:①通过自分泌和/或旁分泌的干细胞因子(stem cell factor,SCF)刺激;②通过其他激酶的交叉活化和/或磷酸酶活性调节的丧失;③*KIT* 基因若干个不同外显子突变所导致的活化[34]。*KIT* 突变,尤其是第 17 号外显子突变,常见于肥大细胞增生症/肥大细胞白血病,急性髓细胞性白血病(acute myelogenous leukemia,AML),精原细胞瘤/无性细胞瘤和自然杀伤/T 细胞淋巴瘤。在胃肠道间质瘤(gastrointestinal stromal tumor,GIST)中,*KIT* 突变多表现为其他位点的异质性突变——最常见的是第 11 号外显子(编码近膜区域)突变,约有 65%的 GIST 存在此位点的突变,另有约 10%的 GIST 存在 *KIT* 基因第 9 号外显子的突变,约 2%的 GIST 存在第 13 号和第 17 号外显子的突变。在 *KIT* 基因突变的 GIST 中,与 *KIT* 同一家族的基因 *PDGFRA* 也可能存在点突变。约 5%的 GIST 存在 *PDGFRA* 组成性活化突变,其中 80%位于第 18 号外显子,10%~15%位于第 12 号外显子,其余 1%~5%位于第 14 号外显子[34]。*KIT* 和 *PDGFRA* 的突变不会同时出现。*KIT* 基因第 11 号外显子缺失的胃部 GIST 的侵袭性要强于 *KIT* 基因发生碱基替代的 GIST,另一种罕见的 *KIT* 第 9 号外显子 502—503 位密码子重复突变主要发生在小肠 GIST 中。*PDGFRA* 突变主要发生在胃部 GIST,此类肿瘤恶性程度较低,主要表现为上皮样形态[34]。*KIT* 基因的胚系突变主要发生在早发性多发 GIST,色素性荨麻疹,黑色素细胞痣,黑色素瘤,贲门失弛缓症或神经丛增生的患者中。

信号传导因子

有丝分裂信号通过一系列复杂的连锁途径从细胞表面的 RTK 传递到细胞核,这些途径统称为信号转导级联[28]。这种信息传递是通过胞质中相互作用的蛋白质的逐步磷酸化来完成的,此外,该过程还涉及鸟嘌呤核苷酸结合蛋白和第二信使,例如腺苷酸环化酶系统。第一个被发现的逆转录病毒致癌基因 *SRC* 就参与了信号转导过程[13,28]。

许多原癌基因都参与了信号转导过程[35],主要分为以下两类:非受体蛋白激酶和三磷酸鸟苷(guanosine triphosphate,GTP)结合蛋白。其中,非受体蛋白激酶可进一步细分为两类:酪氨酸激酶(例如 *ABL*、*LCK* 和 *SRC*)和丝氨酸/苏氨酸激酶(例如 *RAF-1*、*MOS* 和 *PIM-1*)。具有内在鸟苷三磷酸酶(guanosine triphosphatase,GTPase)活性的 GTP 结合蛋白也可进一步细分为单体和异源三聚体两类。单体 GTP 结合蛋白属于原癌基因中重要的 *RAS* 家族的成员,该家族成员包括 *HRAS*、*KRAS* 和 *NRAS*[36]。作为原癌基因的异源三聚体 GTP 结合蛋白(G 蛋白)则包括 *GSP* 和 *GIP*。信号转导因子通常经突变转化为癌基因,其异常激活会导致细胞的增殖失控[36]。

转录因子

转录因子是调节靶基因或基因家族表达的核蛋白[37]。转录调控过程由转录因子和特定的 DNA 序列或 DNA 结构域(例如锌指结构)结合所介导,该类序列或结构域通常位于靶基因的上游。此外,转录因子还可以通过与其他蛋白结合来发挥作用,比如与特定关联体形成异源二聚体复合物。转录因子将胞外信号转化为基因表达的改变,是信号转导途径中的最后一环。

许多作为转录因子的原癌基因是通过其逆转录病毒的同源体发现的[37],例如 *ERB A*、*ETS*、*FOS*、*JUN*、*MYB* 和 *C-MYC*。由 *FOS* 和 *JUN* 共同形成的 AP-1 转录因子可以正向调控多个促进细胞分裂的靶基因[38]。*ERB A* 是 T3 甲状腺激素和碘塞罗宁的受体[39]。在血液系统肿瘤和实体肿瘤中,起转录因子作用的原癌基因通常由染色体易位所激活。在某些类型的肉瘤中,染色体易位导致融合蛋白的形成,表现为 *EWS* 基因与其相关基因的融合,进而导致肿瘤相关基因转录活性的异常。最近有研究表明,腺病毒 *E1A* 基因可以促进正常人成纤维细胞中融合转录子 fli1/ews 的形成[40]。人类血液系统肿瘤中另一个重要的具有转录活性的原癌基因是 *C-MYC* 基因(编码核 DNA 结合蛋白,属于具有转录调控活性的螺旋-环状-螺旋/亮氨酸拉链超家族),*C-MYC* 可以调控促细胞增殖相关基因的表达[41]。在人白血病和淋巴瘤中,*C-MYC* 基因通常由染色体易位激活,具体过程将在本章后一部分详述。

细胞凋亡调控因子

在正常组织中,细胞增殖和细胞死亡之间是动态平衡的。程序性细胞死亡是正常胚胎发生和器官发育的重要组成部分。成熟组织中的程序性细胞死亡又被称作细胞凋亡[42]。对肿瘤细胞的研究表明,细胞增殖和程序性细胞死亡的失控是肿瘤形成和抗癌治疗失败的原因之一。

研究者在人淋巴瘤中首次发现了原癌基因 *BCL-2* 可以调

控程序性细胞死亡。实验研究表明，在显性性状下，*BCL-2* 的激活可以抑制淋巴细胞群的程序性细胞死亡。*BCL-2* 基因编码的蛋白质位于线粒体内膜，内质网和核膜。尽管 BCL-2 蛋白的作用机制尚未完全阐明，但研究提示，BCL-2 蛋白不仅可以作为抑制细胞膜脂质过氧化的抗氧化剂[43]，还可以通过蛋白质-蛋白质的相互作用与其同源蛋白结合而发挥功能。比如，BAX 是 BCL-2 家族中促进细胞凋亡的分子，其与 BCL-2 的相互作用对于细胞凋亡调控是必须的。BH1 和 BH2 是 BCL-2 蛋白上的两个结构域，对两者的定点突变显示，此区域对于 *BCL-2* 与 *BAX* 基因的结合非常重要（图 4-6）。尽管染色体易位是 *BCL-2* 基因活化的主要机制，但仍有研究表明，*BCL-2* 的点突变

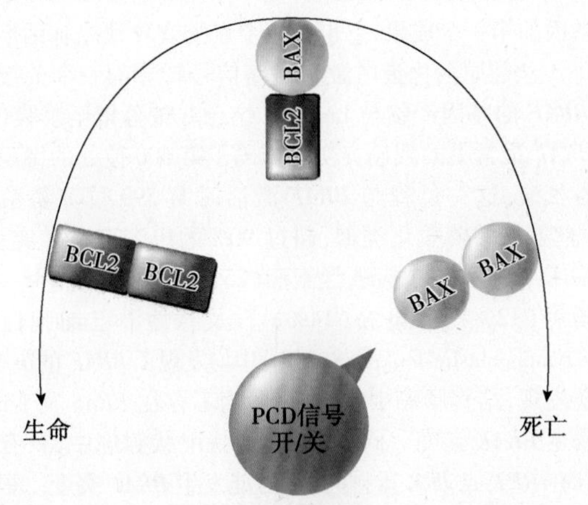

图 4-6　*BCL-2* 对细胞周期的调控作用。如果只存在 *BAX*，细胞则进入凋亡。*BCL-2* 通过与 *BAX* 相互作用调控细胞周期。当 *BCL-2* 过表达，细胞周期失去调控，凋亡受到抑制，结果会导致肿瘤形成。这是肿瘤发生的一个重要原因。PCD，程序性细胞死亡（program cell death or apoptosis）

（在高级别 B 细胞淋巴瘤中）和基因扩增（在约 30% 不存在 *BCL-2* 易位的高分化弥漫性大细胞淋巴瘤中）也是其发挥功能的重要作用机制[44]。不仅如此，在乳腺癌、前列腺癌、甲状腺癌和肺癌等多种实体肿瘤中，*BCL-2* 的表达与临床的相关性也已被证实[45,46]。

另一个参与凋亡调控的癌基因是凋亡蛋白酶-9（*caspase-9*），其主要通过以下途径被激活：细胞色素 c 释放到细胞质中，导致凋亡蛋白酶适配体 APAF-1 和凋亡蛋白酶-9 前体（pro-caspase-9）的活化，而后两者结合形成一种叫凋亡小体的全酶复合物[47]。凋亡蛋白酶-9 进一步激活下游的凋亡蛋白酶-3 以及凋亡蛋白酶-6，凋亡蛋白酶-7，凋亡蛋白酶-8 等其他凋亡蛋白酶，引起 DNA 的片段化和细胞凋亡。其中，*AKT* 可以通过对凋亡蛋白酶-9 的第 196 位丝氨酸的磷酸化水平进行调控来凋亡小体的功能[48]。这种磷酸化可以导致凋亡蛋白酶-9 介导的细胞凋亡被抑制，而且这种抑制是特异性的，可能与 *AKT* 使凋亡蛋白酶-9 的内在催化作用失活有关。最近的研究还表明，*BAX* 可以通过 APAF-1 来刺激凋亡蛋白酶-9，进而参与细胞的凋亡过程，从而对线粒体膜损伤做出应答[49]。

癌基因激活机制

细胞原癌基因的遗传变化是癌基因激活的基础。这些基因水平的改变使细胞获得了生长优势。人类肿瘤中癌基因激活的四种机制包括：①基因突变；②基因扩增；③染色体重排以及④基因的过表达。其中，前三种机制可以导致原癌基因结构的改变或表达的增加（图 4-7）。由于肿瘤的发生是一个多步骤的过程，因此这一过程可能会包括两种或两种以上的机制，通常会联合原癌基因的激活和抑癌基因的丢失或失活。

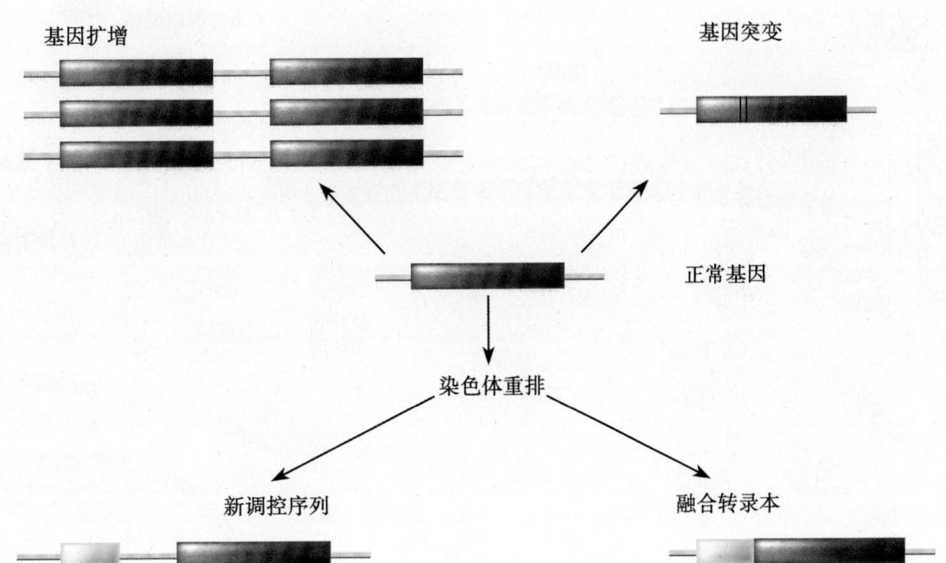

图 4-7　癌基因激活（从原癌基因到癌基因）的主要机制示意图。正常基因（原癌基因）及其被转录部分（长方形）。基因扩增的情况下，后者能被复制 100 倍，导致正常蛋白表达过量，染色体重排，如易位后，该基因的转录可能会受到另一个基因的新调控序列所调控。点突变情况下，单个氨基酸的替换能改变基因产物的生物化学特征，比如能导致细胞中的酶出现组成性活化等。染色体重排比如易位或倒置，会产生基因融合转录本，从而形成嵌合的癌蛋白

基因突变

基因突变通过改变其编码蛋白的结构来激活原癌基因，这些改变通常涉及关键蛋白的调控区域或催化结构域，可以导致突变蛋白出现不受调控的持续性活化。碱基替换，缺失和插入等各种类型的基因突变，都能够激活原癌基因[50]，例如，*ERB B*、*KIT*、*ROS*、*MET* 和 *TRK* 等逆转录病毒癌基因经常因为其氨基末端配体结构域的碱基缺失而被激活。但是，在人类肿瘤中最具代表性的癌基因突变依然是碱基替换（点突变），碱基替换的发生可以使蛋白质中的单一氨基酸发生改变。

点突变在原癌基因 *RAS* 家族（*KRAS*、*HRAS* 和 *NRAS*）中非常常见。人类 *RAS* 基因编码一个参与信号转导的 21kDa（189 个氨基酸）大小的膜结合蛋白，该蛋白具有鸟嘌呤核苷酸结合活性以及内在的 GTPase 活性。RAS 蛋白被激活后，可以将酪氨酸激酶和其下游的丝氨酸/苏氨酸激酶（例如 RAF 和 MAPK）进行偶联，从而进行信号转导（图 4-8）[51]。RAS 蛋白的长期激活状态会持续地刺激该信号通路而导致恶性转化。这种状态通常由第 12 位密码子（*KRAS* 基因）或第 13、61 位密码子（*NRAS* 基因）的点突变导致，还有极少一部分突变会发生在第 59、117 或 146 位密码子[52]。人类肿瘤中 *RAS* 基因的突变被证实与致癌物的暴露有关，例如非小细胞肺癌中 *KRAS* 突变可能与吸烟有关，尤其是与苯并芘的暴露有关[53]。据估计，*RAS* 基因突变在所有人类肿瘤中的比例高达 15%～20%。由于促进内胚层干/祖细胞的扩增并阻断其分化的主要是 *KRAS* 基因，而不是 *HRAS* 或 *NRAS*[54]，因此 *KRAS* 突变主要发生于内胚层起源的肿瘤，包括胰腺癌（90%）、结直肠癌（40%）和肺癌[36,51]。*NRAS* 突变则多见于血液系统恶性肿瘤，其在急性髓细胞性白血病和骨髓增生异常综合征中的发生率高达 25%，在黑素瘤和结直肠癌中也不罕见[55]。虽然甲状腺癌中 *RAS* 的突变比例很高，但并未发现出某一种 *RAS*（*KRAS*、*HRAS* 或 *NRAS*）突变占主导；同时 *RAS* 突变已被证明与高分化甲状腺癌的滤泡表型有关。此外，有研究发现粪便样品中 *KRAS* 突变的检测可用于结直肠癌的早期诊断[56]，而检测血浆样品中的 *KRAS* 突变的情况则可以用于患者的随访监测[57]。

除癌症外，其他疾病中也存在 *RAS* 突变，如 *NRAS* 突变可以导致人类自身免疫性淋巴增生综合征[58]，而 *HRAS* 和 *KRAS* 突变则在努南综合征突变谱中较为常见[51]。有趣的是，很少发现以上疾病的患者罹患癌症，因此，*RAS* 基因在癌症发生中所起的作用仍需重新评估。

BRAF 基因是人类基因组计划中采用高通量基因技术来筛选癌基因的第一个成果，它也是一个点突变导致癌基因激活的例子[7]。丝裂原活化蛋白激酶通路信号转导的一个关键环节就是 *BRAF* 的基因产物与 ras-GTP 结合并被募集至浆膜（图 4-8）。*BRAF* 最常见的致癌突变是密码子第 600 位处的缬氨酸突变成谷氨酸，这一过程与 *BRAF* 激活时第 599 位苏氨酸和第 602 位丝氨酸的磷酸化类似，超过 90% 的患者存在此突变[7]。通过临床组织标本的检测，黑素瘤（75%）、甲状腺癌（45%）、结肠直肠癌（12%）、卵巢癌（14%）[59] 及急性淋巴细胞白血病（acute lymphoblastic leukemia，ALL）中均发现了 *BRAF* 的突变[60]。此外还发现，结直肠癌中，只有当肿瘤不存在 *KRAS* 突变时，才可能发生 *BRAF* 突变。同样，在乳头状甲状腺癌中，只有当肿瘤不存在 *RET* 或 *TRK* 重排时，才可能发生 *BRAF* 突变。根据这些互斥现象，研究者推测，*BRAF* 和 *K-RAS* 的改变，或 *BRAF*、*RET* 和 *TRK* 的改变，分别可能在结直肠癌和甲状腺癌的发生中具有相同的功能[59,61]。另一方面，在结直肠癌中，*BRAF* 突变常发生于存在 *hMLH1* 启动子甲基化的散发病例中，而遗传性

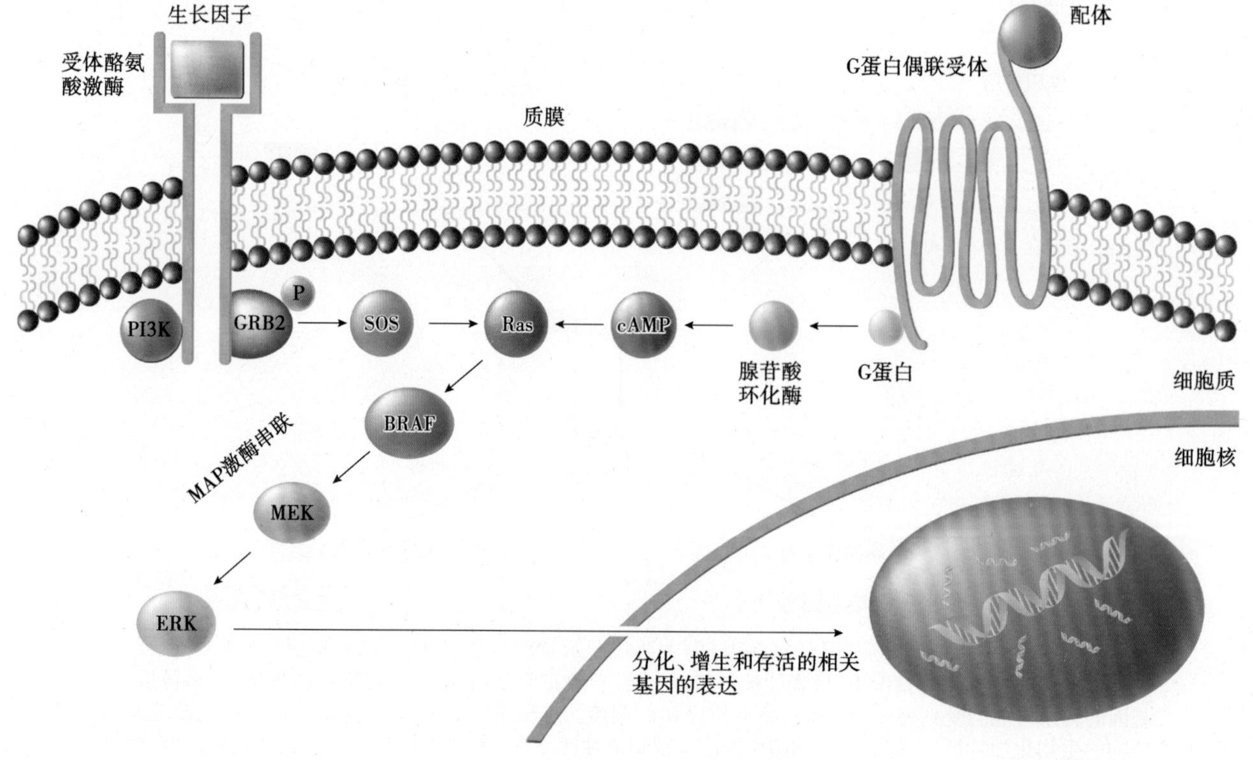

图 4-8 RAS-RAF-MAPK 信号通路

非息肉病相关的结直肠癌中则不存在这样的突变。因此，*BRAF*有可能作为遗传性非息肉病相关性结直肠癌的一个诊断标志物[62]。此外，*BRAF*突变还常见于增生性息肉和锯齿状腺瘤[63]，这可能和这些疾病癌变过程中的早期或关键事件有关。根据不同的肿瘤类型和生长部位，*BRAF*突变对患者预后的影响也有不同：例如在卵巢癌中，*BRAF*突变与Ⅰ型卵巢癌相关，此类卵巢癌生长缓慢，通常仅局限于卵巢[64]；而在乳头状甲状腺癌和结直肠癌中，*BRAF*突变通常意味着肿瘤的高侵袭性[59]。*BRAF*突变，特别是V600E突变，非常容易被检测到，现在已成为早期诊断或患者随访中的一种监测手段。这种手段可以提高穿刺活检细胞学检查时，可疑乳头状甲状腺癌的检出率[65]。但是，该检测并不能用于皮肤黑色素瘤的早期诊断，而只能用于接受过生物学化疗患者的随访监测[66]。这是因为，包括Spitz痣和蓝痣在内的所有皮肤痣在发生成瘤性转化前，均存在高频率的*BRAF*突变[67]。

另一个点突变引起基因活化的典型例子是*RET*原癌基因，该突变常见于Ⅱ型多发性内分泌肿瘤（multiple endocrine neoplasia，MEN）综合征（ⅡA和ⅡB型）以及家族性髓样甲状腺癌（familial medullary thyroid carcinomas，FMTC）中，其中ⅡA型MEN与*RET*第634位密码子的突变相关度最高（85%），特别是C634R。该胚系点突变影响了位于RET受体近膜区的一个半胱氨酸残基，通过形成异常的分子间二硫键进而激活受体酪氨酸激酶，这种活化不依赖于配体，也不会引起受体持续性二聚体化，但该受体被激活后同样具有致癌潜能。大多数ⅡB型MEN患者在激酶结构域中携带了M918T突变，这通常意味着更具侵袭性的亚型。大约有50%的髓样甲状腺癌存在V804、M918和E768的零星突变，而FMTC突变则均匀分布在细胞外半胱氨酸富集区的各型半胱氨酸中，偶尔也存在于酪氨酸激酶区。同C634R一样，M918T突变也可以导致激酶的配体非依赖性激活。最近有研究表明，在ⅡB型MEN中还发现了两个可以影响激酶片段铰链区运动的串联突变（V804和E805）[68]。

基因扩增

基因扩增是指细胞基因组内基因拷贝数的增加。基因扩增的最初发现是由于它可作为一些肿瘤细胞系获得耐药性，生长不受药物抑制的机制。该过程是通过基因组DNA的冗余复制发生的，通常会导致双微体（double-minute chromosome，DM）和均染区（homogeneously staining region，HSR）等核型异常[69]。DM是没有着丝粒的特征性微型染色体结构；HSR是一种缺乏正常染色条带的明暗交替结构的染色体片段。DM和HSR均代表着大片发生扩增的基因组DNA区域，其内含有多达数百个拷贝的基因。这种基因扩增导致基因表达增加，赋予了细胞生长的选择优势。

人类肿瘤中DM和HSR较为常见，表明特异性原癌基因的扩增可能是肿瘤中的普遍现象[69]。研究表明，*MYC*、*ERB B*和*RAS*这三个原癌基因家族在大量的人类肿瘤中存在扩增（表4-2）。*C-MYC*的扩增存在于20%～30%的乳腺癌和卵巢癌中[69]；*MYC*原癌基因家族的新成员——*N-MYC*，在神经母细胞瘤中存在扩增[70]，该扩增还与神经母细胞瘤的晚期阶段密切相关（表4-3），表明*N-MYC*在肿瘤进展中发挥了重要作用[70]；而*L-MYC*在小细胞肺癌和膀胱癌中存在扩增[71]。此外，在一些肿瘤中，*C-MYC*的活化还可以由APC和/或β-catenin的改变来介导，β-catenin在胞质和核内的积聚会导致*C-MYC*转录的增加[72]。c-myc的核内积聚可以作为四肢滑膜肉瘤高危人群的诊断标志物[73]。有研究表明，*ERB B2*改变和*C-MYC*的扩增和过表达，与乳腺癌由非侵袭性向侵袭性转变以及患者的预后不良有关[74]。在黑素瘤和髓母细胞瘤中[75,76]，c-myc是一个可有效识别高危患者的预后标志物。约50%的胶质母细胞瘤[77]、10%～20%的头颈部鳞状细胞癌以及约50%的结直肠癌存在*ERB B*的扩增[78]，其中胶质母细胞瘤的*ERB B*扩增通常伴随着第2～7号外显子的缺失，导致*ERB B*被组成性激活为*ERB B1*的变体Ⅲ[77]。除此以外，大约25%的乳腺癌、卵巢癌、子宫内膜癌、胃癌和唾液腺癌[33]，16%的非小细胞肺癌以及一部分恶性胰腺内分泌肿瘤（胃泌素瘤）中均存在*ERB B2*基因的扩增和过表达。厚黑色素瘤，胰腺癌和前列腺肿瘤的免疫组化结果也提示了*ERB B2*的过表达[33]。

表4-2 人类肿瘤中的癌基因扩增

肿瘤类型	扩增基因	频率(%)
神经母细胞瘤	*MYCN*	20～25
小细胞肺癌	*MYC*	15～20
胶质母细胞瘤	*ERB B1*(*EGFR*)	33～50
乳腺癌	*MYC*	20
	ERB B2(*EGFR2*)	约20
	FGFR1	12
	FGFR2	12
	CCND1(*cyclin d1*)	15～20
食管癌	*MYC*	38
	CCND1(*cyclin d1*)	25
胃癌	*KRAS*	10
	CCNE(*cyclin e*)	15
肝癌	*CCND1*(*cyclin d1*)	13
肉瘤	*MDM2*	10～30
	CDK4	11
宫颈癌	*MYC*	25～50
卵巢癌	*MYC*	20～30
	ERB B2(*EGFR2*)	15～30
	AKT2	12
头颈癌	*MYC*	7～10
	ERB B2(*EGFR2*)	10
	CCND1(*cyclin d1*)	约50
结直肠癌	*MYB*	15～20
	HRAS	29
	KRAS	22

表 4-3　N-myc 拷贝数与神经母细胞瘤的分期及生存率的相关性

肿瘤类型	病例数	频率(%)
良性星形胶质细胞瘤	0/64	0
低期别	31/772	4
4-S 期	15/190	8
进展期	612/1 974	31
合计	658/3 000	22

在乳腺癌中，*ERB B2* 扩增预示着肿瘤晚期和预后不良。一些肿瘤中，*RAS* 基因家族的成员，包括 *KRAS* 和 *NRAS*，存在偶发性的扩增[33]。

染色体重排

高频染色体重排常见于恶性血液病和一些实体瘤中，主要包括染色体易位和少数的染色体反转[79]。染色体重排导致恶性血液病的发生可通过两种不同的机制：①原癌基因的转录激活；②形成融合基因。转录激活是由于染色体重排，导致一个原癌基因移动至免疫球蛋白或 T 细胞受体(TCR)基因附近(图 4-7)。因此引起血细胞中原癌基因的持续激活，导致细胞发生恶性转化。

当染色体断裂点位于两个不同的基因时，染色体重排会产生融合基因，形成由一个基因的头部和另一个基因的尾部组成的复合结构。一般来说，参与融合的两个基因对嵌合蛋白的转化活性均有一定作用。在恶性血液病中，免疫球蛋白或 TCR 基因的生理重排中的错误，被认为是高频染色体重排的原因[80]。表 4-4 列举了一些恶性血液病及实体瘤染色体重排的分子特征。在一些情况下，同一个原癌基因参与几种不同的易位，如 *C-MYC*、*EWS* 和 *RET*。

基因活化

大约 85%的 Burkitt 淋巴瘤中存在 t(8;14)(q24;q32)易位，这是典型的原癌基因转录活化的例子。这种染色体重排将

表 4-4　肿瘤的染色体重排的分子特征

影响的基因	重排	疾病	蛋白类型
恶性血液病			
基因融合			
C-ABL(9q34)	t(9;22)(q34;q11)	慢性髓性白血病和急性白血病	BCR 激活的酪氨酸激酶
BCR(22q11)			
ALK(2p23)	t(2;5)(p23;q35)	间变性大细胞淋巴瘤	NPM 激活的酪氨酸激酶
NPM(5q35)			
PDGFR-B(5q33)	t(5;12)(q33;p13)	慢性髓单核细胞白血病	tel 激活的酪氨酸激酶
TEL(12p13)			
PBX1(1q23)	t(1;19)(q23;p13.3)	急性前 B 细胞白血病	同源异形结构域(HLH 结构域)
E2A(19p13.3)			
PML(15q21)	t(15;17)(q21;q11-22)	急性髓性白血病	锌指结构
RAR(17q21)			
CAN(6p23)	t(6;9)(p23;q34)	急性髓性白血病	无同源性
DEK(9q34)			
REL	ins(2;12)(p13;p11.2-14)	非霍奇金淋巴瘤	NF-κB 家族
NRG		无同源性	
IG 位点的癌基因			
C-MYC	t(8;14)(q24;q32)	Burkitt 淋巴瘤，BL-ALL	HLH 结构域
	t(2;8)(p12;q24)		
	t(8;22)(q24;q11)		
BCL-1(*PRADI*?)	t(11;14)(q13;q32)	慢性 B 细胞淋巴细胞白血病	PRADI-GI 细胞周期蛋白
BCL-2	t(14;18)(q32;21)	滤泡型淋巴瘤	线粒体内膜
BCL-3	t(14;19)(q32;q13.1)	慢性 B 细胞白血病	CDC10 模体
IL-3	t(5;14)(q31;q32)	急性前 B 细胞白血病	生长因子

续表

影响的基因	重排	疾病	蛋白类型
TCR 位点的癌基因			
C-MYC	t(8;14)(q24;q11)	急性T细胞白血病	HLH 结构域
LYLA	t(7;19)(q35;p13)	急性T细胞白血病	HLH 结构域
TALA/SCL/TCL-5	t(1;14)(q32;q11)	急性T细胞白血病	HLH 结构域
TAL-2	t(7;9)(q35;q34)	急性T细胞白血病	HLH 结构域
Rhombotin 1/TTG-1	t(11;14)(p15;q11)	急性T细胞白血病	LIM 结构域
Rhombotin 2/TTG-2	t(11;14)(p13;q11)	急性T细胞白血病	LIM 结构域
	t(7;11)(q35;p13)		
HOX 11	t(10;14)(q24;q11)	急性T细胞白血病	同源异型结构域
	t(7;10)(q35;q24)		
TAN-1	t(7;9)(q34;q34.3)	急性T细胞白血病	Notch 同系物
TCL-1	t(7q35-14q32.1)	慢性B淋巴细胞白血病	
	t(14q11-14q32.1)		
实体瘤			
肉瘤中的基因融合			
FLI1,EWS	t(11:22)(q24:q12)	尤文肉瘤	ETS 转录因子家族
ERG,EWS	t(21:22)(q22:q12)	尤文肉瘤	ETS 转录因子家族
ATV1,EWS	t(7:21)(q22:q12)	尤文肉瘤	ETS 转录因子家族
ATF1,EWS	t(12:22)(q13:q12)	软组织透明细胞肉瘤	转录因子
CHN,EWS	t(9:22)(q22 31:q12)	黏液样软骨肉瘤	类固醇受体家族
WT1,EWS	t(11:22)(p13:q12)	促纤维增生性小圆细胞肿瘤	Wilms 肿瘤基因
SSX1,SSX2,SYT	t(X:18)(p11.2:q11.2)	滑膜肉瘤	HLH 结构域
PAX3,FKHR	t(2:13)(q37:q14)	腺泡状肉瘤	同源异型框同系物
PAX7,FKHR	t(1:13)(q36:q14)	横纹肌肉瘤	同源异型框同系物
CHOP,TLS	t(12:16)(q13:p11)	黏液样脂肉瘤	转录因子
VAR,HMG1-C	t(var:12)(var:q13-15)	脂肪瘤	HMG DNA 结合蛋白
HMG1-C?	t(12:14)(q13-15)	子宫肌瘤	HMG DNA 结合蛋白
甲状腺癌中的基因融合			
RET/PTC1	inv(10)(q11.2:q2.1)	甲状腺乳头状癌	H4 激活的酪氨酸激酶
RET/PTC2	t(10:17)(q11.2:q23)	甲状腺乳头状癌	Rla(PKA)激活的酪氨酸激酶
RET/PTC3	inv(10)(q11.2)	甲状腺乳头状癌	ELE1 激活的酪氨酸激酶
TRK	inv(1)(q31:q22-23)	甲状腺乳头状癌	TPM3 激活的酪氨酸激酶
TRK-T1(T2)	inv(1)(q31:q25)	甲状腺乳头状癌	TPR 激活的酪氨酸激酶
TRK-T3	t(1q31:3)	甲状腺乳头状癌	TFG 激活的酪氨酸激酶
血液病和实体瘤			
其他位点癌基因			
PTH 失控调控 *PRAD1*	inv(11)(p15:q13)	甲状旁腺腺瘤	PRADI-GI 细胞周期蛋白
BTG1 失控调控 *MYC*	t(8:12)(q24:q22)	慢性B淋巴细胞白血病	MYC-HLH 结构域

IG:免疫球蛋白;TCR:T细胞受体;HLH:螺旋-环-螺旋结构域;HMG:高迁移基因;H4:组蛋白H4;ELE1:核受体共激活因子4;TPR和TFG:具有二聚体的螺旋区域的部分不典型基因;Rla:PKA的调控亚基;TPM3:非肌肉拓扑霉素异型体。

位于染色体 8q24 的 *C-MYC* 基因易位至 14q32，使其在此受到免疫球蛋白重链基因调节元件的调控。在另外一些 Burkitt 淋巴瘤病例中，*C-MYC* 基因也可通过免疫球蛋白轻链基因的易位而活化。如位于 2p12 内 k 位点的 t(2;8)(p12;q24)，和位于 22q11 内 λ 位点的 t(8;22)(q24;q11)(图 4-9)。尽管与 *C-MYC* 基因有关的染色体断裂点的位置在不同 Burkitt 患者个体中可能差异很大，但易位后的效果相同。基因突变同样可引起 *C-MYC* 基因的改变，*C-MYC* 基因在易位到 Ig 基因后，可在 *C-MYC* 反式激活区和编码区发生突变[81]，或者在伴随或不伴随 *C-MYC* 基因易位的情况下，在非编码基因 1 号外显子和 1 号外显子/1 号内含子边界发生突变[82]。在一些 T 细胞 ALL(T-ALL) 中，*C-MYC* 基因因 t(8;14)(q24;q11)易位而活化，此时其受到 TCR 基因调控元件的控制[83]。在 T-ALL 中，除 *C-MYC* 基因外，一些编码核蛋白的原癌基因，也可因 T 细胞受体 α 或 β 的不同染色体易位而活化，其中包括 *HOX11*，*TAL1*，*TAL2* 和 *RBTN1/TGT1*[84]。这些基因编码的蛋白可通过 DNA 结合及蛋白与蛋白间的相互作用起到转录因子的功能，其表达异常可导致细胞的增殖失去控制。

在白血病和淋巴瘤中，许多其他的原癌基因也可通过染色体易位而被激活。

基因融合

通过对 CML 中费城染色体断裂点的克隆，研究者首次发现了基因融合[25]。CML 中的 t(9;22)(q34;q11)易位，使正常位于 9q34 的 *C-ABL* 基因与位于 22q11 的 *BCR* 基因发生了融合(图 4-10)。*BCR/ABL* 融合形成了 der(22)染色体，此融合基因可编码一个 210kD 的嵌合蛋白，其可以增强酪氨酸激酶活性且造成异常的细胞定位[25]。但目前 *BCR/ABL* 融合蛋白影响肿瘤髓系克隆扩增的具体机制仍不明确。多达 20% 的 ALL 的病例中也发现存在 t(9;22)易位，但在这些病例中，*BCR* 基因的断裂点与在 CML 中有所不同，BCR 断裂后会编码一个 185kDa 的 *BCR/ABL* 融合蛋白[85]。这个分子量较小的 *BCR/ABL* 融合蛋白可以导致完全不同的肿瘤表型，但目前原因尚不明确。抑制 BCR/ABL 酪氨酸激酶活性已作为一种新的针对 CML 患者的治疗手段。伊马替尼疗法能在常规化疗失败的 CML 患者中达到抗白血病的效果[86]。然而，目前已经出现伊马替尼耐药的案例[87]。伊马替尼治疗失败的原因，可能是 *BCR/ABL* 基因扩增，或单个氨基酸替换影响了位于 ATP 结合域或位于 ABL 激酶结构域 ATP 口袋中的残基，导致其结构发生了改变，从而影响了伊马替尼对 BCR/ABL 酪氨酸激酶活性的抑制效果。因此，目前正在讨论利用 BCR/ABL 融合蛋白依赖的分子伴侣——热休克蛋白 90 来克服伊马替尼耐药[87]。

在恶性血液病中，除 *C-ABL* 外，另外 2 个编码酪氨酸激酶的基因也可发生基因融合，导致肿瘤的形成。退行性大细胞淋巴瘤中的 t(2;5)(p23;q35)易位使 *NPM* 基因(5q35)和 *ALK* 基因(2p23)[88]发生融合。*ALK* 编码一个与胰岛素生长因子受体家族类似的跨膜酪氨酸激酶，而 NPM 蛋白是一个核仁磷酸蛋

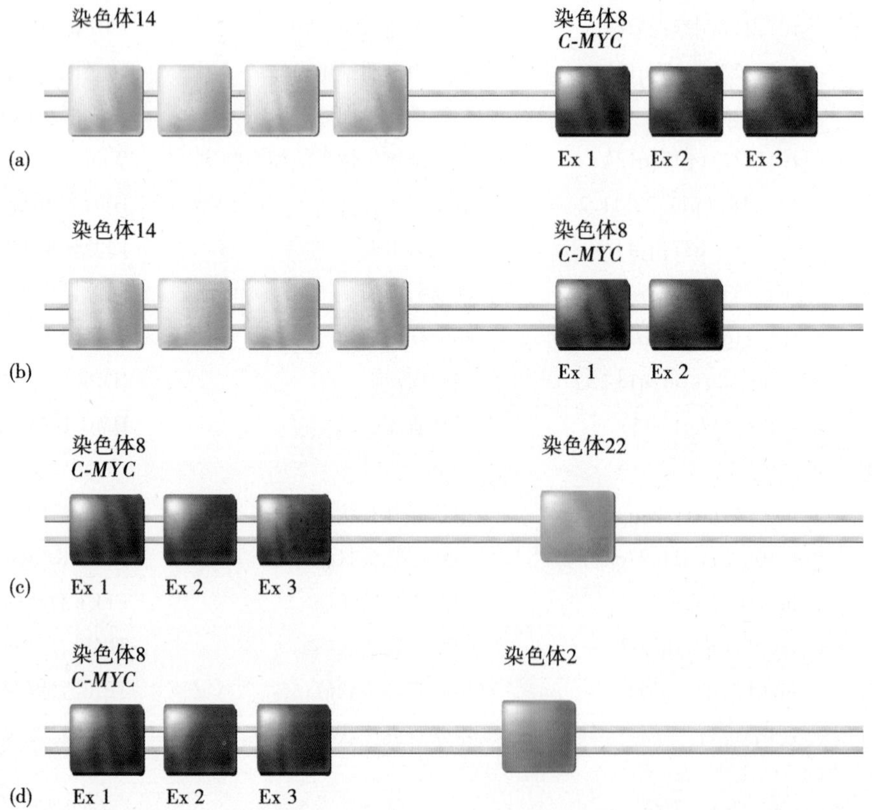

图 4-9　Burkitt 淋巴瘤中的 *C-MYC* 基因易位。(a)t(8;14)(q24;q32)易位，位于 14q32 的免疫球蛋白重链基因的易位。(b)t(8;14)(q24;q32)易位，只有 *C-MYC* 的两个外显子易位到 14q32 免疫球蛋白重链基因的调控因子下。(c)t(8;22)(q24;q11)易位，位于 22q11 的免疫球蛋白轻链基因的 1 位点的易位。(d)t(2;8)(p12;q24)易位，位于 2p12 的免疫球蛋白轻链基因 k 位点的易位

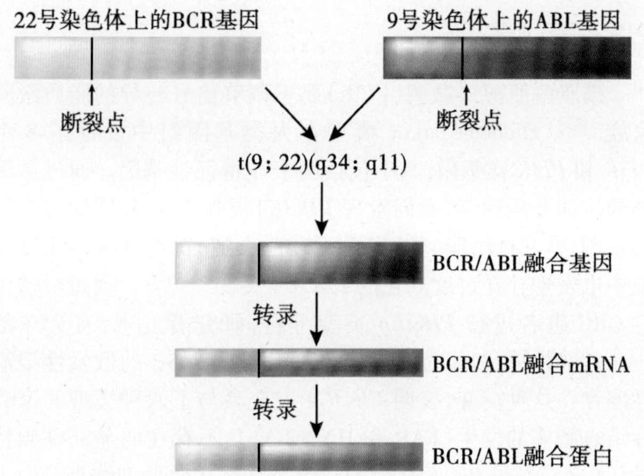

图 4-10　基因融合。CML 中的 t(9;22)(q34;q11)易位决定了 *ABL* 与 *BCR* 基因的融合，并由此编码一个 210KD 大小的融合癌蛋白

白，主要参与核糖体的装配。NPM/ALK 融合产生了一个嵌合癌蛋白，其可以持续地表达，并具有 ALK 酪氨酸激酶的活性。而 t(5;12)(q33;p13)易位，特别是在慢性粒细胞白血病(CMML)中，可导致 *tel* 基因(12p13)与酪氨酸激酶区域血小板源生长因子受体 b 基因(5q33 位的 PDGFR-B 基因)相融合(表 4-4)[89]。

基因融合有时也可形成嵌合转录因子[90]。在儿童前 B 细胞 ALL 中发现的 t(1;19)(q23;p13)易位，可以造成 *E2A* 转录因子基因(19p13)与 *PBX1* 同源结构域基因(1q23)融合[91]，E2A/PBX1 融合蛋白由 E2A 蛋白氨基末端反式激活结构域和 PBX1 蛋白的 DNA 结合同源结构域构成。在急性早幼粒白血病中，t(15;17)(q22;q21)易位使位于 15q22 的 *PML* 基因与位于 17q21 的 *RARA* 基因融合[92]。具有 *PML/RARA* 融合基因的白血病患者，对类维生素 A 治疗有较好的反应。在这些病例中，反式维生素 A 治疗可以诱导早幼粒白血病细胞的分化。

位于染色体 11q23 的 *ALL1* 基因，在大约 5%～10%的成人和儿童急性白血病中都存在[93]。特别的是，*ALL1* 基因可与不同染色体上的很多伴侣基因相融合。已有报道，存在 20 多种 *ALL1* 基因的交互易位，其中最常见的是在 4,6,9 和 19 号染色体上。研究者发现在大约 5%的成人急性白血病中，*ALL1* 基因与其自身的一部分出现了融合，称为自身融合[94]。人们认为 *ALL1* 基因的自身融合是通过体细胞的重组机制完成的，在细胞遗传学异常的 11 三体综合征的急性白血病人群中有很高的发生率。*ALL1* 基因编码一个大分子量蛋白，其包含一个 DNA 结合模体，一个反式激活结构域和一个果蝇 trithorax 蛋白(三空腔结构蛋白)同源区域(同源基因表达的调控子)。*ALL1* 融合基因的多种伴侣基因可编码多种蛋白，其中一些是具有 DNA 结合模体的核蛋白[94]。ALL1 融合蛋白含有 ALL1 的氨基末端与不同融合伴侣基因的羧基末端，包括自融合在内的所有 ALL1 融合蛋白的重要特征是，ALL1 蛋白的氨基末端结构域与 ALL1 蛋白剩余的部分解离。

实体瘤，尤其是肉瘤，具有与肿瘤特异组织类型相关的染色体易位特征[95]。通常，实体瘤中的基因易位会导致基因融合，编码产生嵌合的癌蛋白[96]。目前研究显示，在肉瘤中，由基因易位产生的大部分融合基因都编码转录因子。表 4-4 总结了实体瘤中的基因易位，其中最具有代表性的，即在黏液性脂肪肉瘤中，t(12;16)(q13;p11)易位使位于 16p11 的 *FUS*(*TLS*)基因与位于 12q12 的 *CHOP* 基因相融合[97]，以及在尤文肉瘤中，t(11;22)(q24;q12)易位使得位于 22q12 的 *EWS* 基因与位于 11q24 的 *FLI1* 基因融合[98]。

在 DP 中，已发现存在 t(17;22)(q22;q13)的交互易位，以及来源于 t(17;22)的过多的环状染色体产生[99]。

尽管如前所述，在淋巴瘤和白血病中，融合基因的研究已经取得了初步的成功，但在实体瘤中，首例从分子水平被定义为融合蛋白的染色体异常是在乳头状甲状腺癌中发现的 10 号染色体的倒位[100]。在这种肿瘤中，两种主要的结构变化反复出现，即 inv(10)(q112.2;q21.2)和 t(10;17)(q11.2;q23)，其中前者的发生频率更高。这两种异常体现了 10 号染色体上的原癌基因 *RET* 激活的细胞遗传学机制，并分别形成了癌基因 *RET/PTC1* 和 *RET/PTC2*。此外，导致 ret 活化的其他染色体重排机制近期也有报道，这特别常见于切尔诺贝利污染地区的儿童中[101,102]。实际上，*RET* 基因中的所有断点都在 11 号内含子内，所以受体的 TK 结构域完整，并使 *RET/PTC* 癌蛋白可以通过 Y1062 与 SHC 结合从而激活下游级联反应[103]。涉及 *RET* 基因的体细胞染色体重排是 *PTC* 中最常见的遗传改变，尽管在不同的地理区域中观察到的这种改变的发生频率范围跨度很大(从 5%到 70%)[104]。最近的研究结果表明，*RET/PTC* 重排发生频率的差异部分是由于不同的检测方法和肿瘤遗传异质性造成的[105]。相同类型的肿瘤中 1 号染色体的改变与 NTRK1(一号染色体)的激活相关，NTRK1 是一种 NGF 受体，与 *RET* 一样，可在 PTC 中形成嵌合的融合癌蛋白[106]。对这两种源于 TK 受体激活的癌基因进行比较分析，可以发现表征癌基因激活的普遍细胞遗传学和分子机制。在所有情况下，染色体重排是将两个受体的 TK 部分融合到不同基因的 5′末端，后者由于它们的广泛作用被称为“活化基因”。在大多数情况下，后者与相关受体位于同一染色体，RET 在 10 号染色体，NTRK1 在 1 号染色体。

此外，虽然功能不同，但各种活化基因有以下三个共同的特性：

1. 表达普遍化。
2. 具有或可能具有能够形成二聚体或多聚体的结构域。
3. 将生物信号从膜传递到细胞质。

这些特征可以解释 *RET* 和 *NTRK1* 原癌基因的激活机制。事实上，在将其 TK 结构域与活化基因融合后，①*RET* 和 *NTRK1* 原本仅特异性表达于神经细胞亚群，其发生融合后会在甲状腺上皮细胞中表达；②它们的二聚化引发了细胞质结构域持续性的、配体非依赖性的反式自磷酸化，因此，其可以募集含有 SH2 和 SH3 的细胞质效应蛋白，如 Shc 和 Grb2 或磷脂酶 C gamma(PLC)，从而持续诱导有丝分裂；③*RET* 和 *NTRK1* 的酶活性在细胞质中的重新定位可以使它们与不常见的底物相互作用，这可能会改变它们的功能特性。*RET* 重排、*NTRK1* 重排以及 *BRAF* 突变之间相互排斥，并且在 PTC 中显示出相似但不同的基因表达模式[59]。总体而言，具有 *RET/PTC* 重排的乳头状癌通常发病年龄较小，并且如果转移，多为淋巴结转移，临床病理多为乳头状且一般预后较好。

蛋白过表达和组成性磷酸化

蛋白质过表达本质上是一种表达失调，其机制尚不清楚。其中一个例子是 Akt，它包含三种丝氨酸—苏氨酸激酶，是调节生存信号的主要作用因子。一般来说，Akt 蛋白有六个磷酸化位点：Ser124 和 Thr450 是基本的磷酸化位点，Tyr315 和 Tyr316 依赖于 Src，Thr308 是调节的主要位点并被 3-磷酸肌醇依赖性蛋白激酶 1 磷酸化，Ser473 磷酸化可使 Akt 活性最大化，但其磷酸化机制仍存在争议。不同的生长因子和白细胞介素刺激可使细胞中的 Akt 磷酸化活化，PTEN 则抑制其活性。Akt 一旦被激活，就会从胞膜中分离并移位到细胞质和细胞核中。Akt 可以通过 Bad 和 caspase-9 的磷酸化直接发挥作用，或通过诱导 IKK 蛋白激酶和转录因子从头表达间接发挥作用。Akt 还可以通过参与细胞周期进程来确保细胞存活[107]。对组织样本的分析显示，*AKT3* 编码的蛋白质在低分化的乳腺癌和前列腺癌中过度表达，可促进散发性黑色素瘤进展[108]。Akt1 主要与散发性甲状腺癌的发病相关，而 Akt2 是在卵巢癌、胰腺癌、甲状腺癌和 CRC 中发挥关键的作用。*AKT* 基因的突变很少见[109]。

大规模基因组分析发现的新的标志物

激酶

最近一项研究将人类基因组中编码蛋白激酶的基因（统称为激酶组）划分成一个系统的树图，其含有九大群基因。利用高通量测序技术和人类基因组计划的生物信息学方法，研究者对其中九大群中的三群进行了突变分析[110]。这其中包含了 90 个酪氨酸激酶基因（TK 组），43 个酪氨酸激酶样蛋白基因（TKL 组）和 5 个受体型鸟苷酸环化酶基因（RGC 组）。该分析涵盖了 35 个 CRC 细胞系和 147 个结直肠标本中所有可能编码激酶结构域的外显子[8]。该分析在 7 个基因（TK 组的 *NTRK3*、*FES*、*KDR*、*EPHA3*、*NTRK2*，TKL 组的 *MLK4* 和 RGC 组的 *GUCY2F*）中发现了 35 种不同类型的体细胞突变，这些突变可以作为化疗干预的潜在靶标[8]。

磷酸酶

蛋白酪氨酸磷酸酶（PTP）基因超家族（即磷酸酶组）由三个主要家族组成：①经典的 PTP，包括受体型蛋白酪氨酸磷酸酶（RPTP）和非受体型蛋白酪氨酸磷酸酶（NRPTP）；②双特异性磷酸酶（DSP），这种磷酸酶除了可以将酪氨酸残基去磷酸化，还可使丝氨酸和苏氨酸去磷酸化；③低分子量磷酸酶（LMP）[111]。研究者使用高通量技术，对 175 个 CRC 中的 53 个经典 PTP（21 个 RPTP 和 32 个 NRPTP），32 个 DSP 和 1 个 LMP 的所有编码外显子进行了突变分析[9]，发现了 6 个含有体细胞突变的基因，包括 RPTP 亚家族三个成员（*PTPRF*、*PTPRG* 和 *PTPRT*）和 NRPTP 亚家族的三个成员（*PTPN3*、*PTPN13* 和 *PTPN14*）。总体而言，研究分析鉴定了 77 个突变，影响了 26% 的结直肠肿瘤[9]。绝大多数突变会导致蛋白质丧失磷酸酶活性。鉴定出蛋白磷酸酶突变位点后，可以通过新的靶向药物使其再活化，更有甚者，可以将突变的磷酸酶相应的激酶失活，进而调控其底物水平。

PI3K 异构体

磷脂酰肌醇 3-激酶（PI3K）属于调节信号转导的脂质激酶家族[112]。Hidden-Markov 模型在人类基因组中发现了 8 个 *PI3K* 和 *PI3K* 样基因，其中包括两个非特征性基因。通过激酶结构域的分析预测，人们发现 *PIK3CA* 是唯一具有体细胞突变的基因[10]。在结肠、肺、卵巢、肝脏、大脑、胃和乳房等几种癌症中也发现存在过度活化的 *PIK3CA* 突变[113~115]。通过对遗传性 CRC 患者进行 *PIK3CA* 突变分析，研究者发现，有 21% 的 FAP 侵袭性癌，21% 的 HNPCC 侵袭性癌和 15% 的散发性浸润性癌存在这种突变，表明 *PIK3CA* 突变参与了两种类型的家族性结直肠癌的发生（FAP 和 HNPCC），且不存在明显的种族特异性（这一点与 *BRAF* 基因不一致）；并且在散发型结直肠癌患者中，*PIK3CA* 突变的频率相差不大[116]。除了点突变，*PIK3CA* 还存在基因拷贝数的增加，特别在卵巢癌中更为常见。

肿瘤起始和进展中的癌基因

人类肿瘤形成是一个复杂的多步骤过程，涉及原癌基因（激活）和抑癌基因（失活）的连续改变。按年龄对人类实体瘤的发病率进行统计分析，发现五个或六个独立的突变事件就有可能会导致肿瘤形成。在人类白血病中，则可能只需要三到四个不同基因的突变事件。

化学致癌动物模型的研究，为我们理解肿瘤多步骤发生的本质提供了基础[118]。在小鼠皮肤癌模型中，肿瘤的形成涉及三个阶段，称之为起始，促进和进展。皮肤癌的起始可以通过化学诱变剂如 7,12-二甲基-苯并蒽（DMBA）诱导（图 4-11）。使用 DMBA 处理后的小鼠皮肤看起来是正常的。但如果使用促进剂（例如佛波醇酯 TPA）连续处理皮肤，则会形成癌前乳头状瘤。化学促进剂如 TPA 等可以刺激肿瘤生长，但不是诱癌物质。在连续使用促进剂数月后，一些乳头状瘤将发展成皮肤癌。但单独使用 DMBA 或 TPA 则不会诱发皮肤癌。用 DMBA 诱导的小鼠乳头状瘤通常有 *HRAS* 癌基因突变，突变发生在 61 位密码子处。小鼠皮肤肿瘤模型表明乳头状瘤的起始是由化学诱变剂 DMBA 在个体皮肤细胞中诱导 *HRAS* 基因突变的结

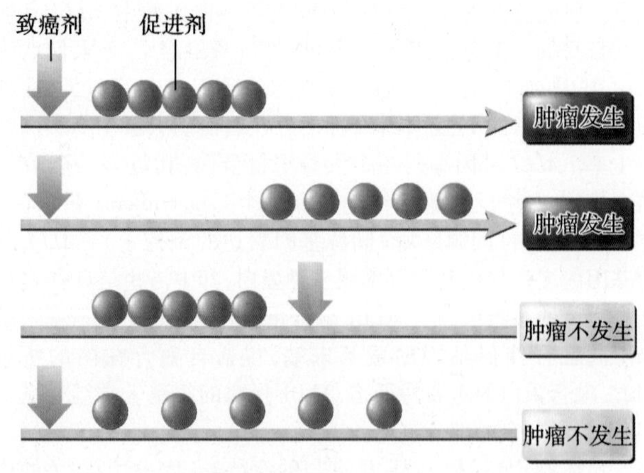

图 4-11 一些可能的诱变剂和肿瘤促进剂的暴露方式及其效果。只有当先后暴露于致癌剂（如 DMBA 等诱变剂）和促进剂，且暴露的促进剂浓度高于阈值时才会导致肿瘤发生

果。然而,为了使皮肤上形成乳头状瘤,必须通过促进剂持续刺激突变细胞的生长,而要使乳头状瘤发展成癌则还需其他尚未明确的遗传变化。

虽然单个癌基因足以引起肿瘤形成,但由单个癌基因导致的肿瘤通常不会出现在肿瘤实验模型中[119]。相反,不同癌基因通常协同作用促进肿瘤的产生。癌基因之间的协同作用也可以通过使用非永生化细胞系的体外转化研究来证明。例如,研究证实了核内的MYC蛋白与细胞质膜相关RAS蛋白在大鼠胚胎成纤维细胞转化中的协同作用[120]。

两种不同类别的癌基因(如核内和细胞质中)之间可以通过协作促进肿瘤转化,但协同作用并不是肿瘤转化所严格必需的[121]。事实上,这些转基因小鼠品系通常具有更高的肿瘤发生率,且肿瘤多为克隆性,由此暗示肿瘤发生有其他因素参与[122]。

人类血液系统恶性肿瘤克隆进化的细胞遗传学研究有助于人们理解人类肿瘤发生和发展的多个步骤[123]。CML从慢性期到急性白血病的演变中,最重要的特征是在恶性细胞克隆的核型中存在遗传改变的累积。CML的早期慢性期的定义是存在单个费城染色体。t(9;22)易位而形成的*BCR/ABL*基因融合被认为是CML的起始事件。而在CML向更恶性表型的生物学进展中,会对应出现另外的细胞遗传学异常,例如会产生第二个费城染色体、17号等臂染色体或8号染色体三体[124]。尽管恶化CML的核型变化在患者之间有所不同,但遗传改变的累积总是与低恶性分化细胞向高恶性去分化细胞的转化有关。

人类肿瘤的发生和发展涉及原癌基因的激活和抑癌基因的失活或缺失。然而,原癌基因激活的机制和时间进程取决于不同的肿瘤类型。在血液系统恶性肿瘤、软组织肉瘤和乳头状甲状腺癌中,恶性过程主要开始于染色体重排引起的多种癌基因的激活[90]。白血病和淋巴瘤中的许多染色体重排,被认为是正常B细胞和T细胞发育过程中免疫球蛋白或TCR生理性基因重排发生错误引起的。血液系统恶性肿瘤进展到晚期会出现癌基因突变(主要是*RAS*家族),抑癌基因如*TP53*的失活,以及偶尔会出现的染色体易位[125]。

在肺癌中,肿瘤起始涉及原癌基因和抑癌基因的突变。这些突变通常被认为是由化学致癌因素引起的,特别是在与烟草相关的肺癌中。研究者发现在大多数肺癌,特别在吸烟者的肿瘤中,一种新的抑癌基因(称为*FHIT*)出现了失活[126]。随后,*KRAS*(尤其在腺癌亚型中)和*TP53*突变驱动了肺癌的恶性转化[127]。

就CRC而言,遗传学变异的集中筛查明确了CRC的两种主要类型,它们的致癌过程是不同的。其中一种类型称为RER(复制错误表型)阳性肿瘤,是以正常核型、正常DNA指数和微卫星位点(MSI)的遗传不稳定性为特征,现在也称为MSI阳性肿瘤[128]。第二种类型是以*APC*、*KRAS*和*TP53*基因的变异以及MSI的遗传缺失为特征[129]。后者肿瘤的发生经历了从正常上皮、异常增生上皮、再逐渐进展到恶性肿瘤的过程,这期间累积了多种同源选择的遗传学改变[130]。该模型最早在1990年由Vogelstein提出,表明APC(或称为APC-β-catenin信号途径更为合适)突变代表了肿瘤的起始突变事件,它会导致增生增殖并形成早期腺瘤。K-ras蛋白的稳定化则会使腺瘤进入晚期阶段。染色体18q的抑癌基因(例如*DCC*)的缺失和TP53基因的突变则会导致原位癌形成(图4-12)[128~130]。

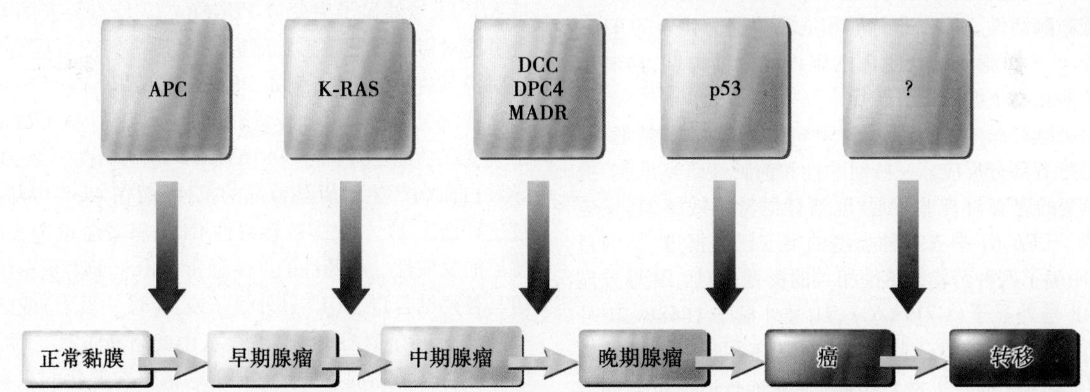

图4-12 结直肠癌的发生发展。结直肠癌来源于正常结肠上皮细胞向侵袭性肿瘤转化进程中的一系列生理学改变,在这一多步骤的过程中,伴随有特异性的遗传物质的改变(以垂直箭头表示)

在黑色素瘤中,绝大多数病例存在*BRAF*突变,这表明肿瘤处在早期阶段,因为这种突变在诸如Spitz和蓝痣等癌前病变中也可检测到[7,67]。

虽然人类肿瘤的发生和发展途径存在差异,但各种类型恶性肿瘤的研究已经清楚地表明:人类肿瘤发生是一个多步骤的过程。

作为新药靶点的癌基因

一些癌基因在细胞生存中发挥着关键的作用。事实上,它们中的大多数都编码了生长因子受体或参与了信号转导。因此,它们是新药研发的天然靶标,这些新的药物能够选择性地阻断其靶标,使得原本失调的细胞功能得以恢复。以下是对靶向治疗最新的认识总结。

ERB B2

*ERB B2*基因扩增发生在一部分乳腺癌中。针对erb B2受体的单克隆抗体(MoAb),曲妥珠单抗,是第一种进入临床试验的抗erb B2药物,对*ERB B2*基因扩增/过表达患者的疗效明显。曲妥珠单抗适用于转移性乳腺癌患者,最近也被用于辅助

和新辅助治疗。目前,新型靶向治疗,如 MoAb(帕妥珠单抗和第二代曲妥珠单抗,名为 T-DM1,曲妥珠单抗与美坦新联用)和小分子酪氨酸激酶抑制剂(TKI)(拉帕替尼),已常规用于转移患者的治疗和新辅助治疗。不幸的是,并非所有 *ERB B2* 基因扩增的患者都可受益于曲妥珠单抗,这可能是由于 *ERB B2* 下游成员存在异常表达。实际上,临床前研究显示,突变引起的 *PIK3CA* 基因激活以及 PTEN 蛋白表达的缺失会导致肿瘤对曲妥珠单抗产生抗性[33]。

最近,研究发现 *ERB B2* 在其他实体瘤中表达失调,可能会影响临床治疗。在多达 34%的晚期胃癌或胃食管连接癌患者中检测到 *ERB B2* 基因存在扩增或蛋白质过度表达,曲妥珠单抗被批准用于 erb B2 阳性患者(通过荧光原位杂交或免疫组织化学评估)的治疗[33]。在 CRC 中,*ERB B2* 基因扩增是一种罕见现象(<5%),这与 EGFR 靶向治疗耐药有关[131]。然而,在肿瘤异种移植的体内模型中,曲妥珠单抗在 CRC 中的功效需要更多实验加以证明。最近的一项回顾性研究显示,在肺腺癌中 *ERB B2* 基因突变的患者(约 1%)可能从曲妥珠单抗治疗中获益。此外,*ERB B2* 基因突变或扩增可能会导致 EGFR 靶向治疗的继发性耐药[33]。

ERB B1

ERB B1 编码受体型酪氨酸激酶,在肿瘤细胞的增殖、血管生成和转移中起重要的作用。因此,靶向 erb B1 是一种非常有价值的肿瘤治疗方式。临床使用的两类 erb B1 拮抗剂 MoAb 和 TKI,目前已成功进入Ⅲ期临床试验。以西妥昔单抗和帕尼单抗为代表的 MoAb 在 *ERB B1* 无活性状态时结合其受体的胞外结构域,可以通过与受体的竞争性结合来阻断配体诱导的受体型酪氨酸激酶活性。以吉非替尼和厄洛替尼为代表的 TKI,可以与 ATP 可逆的竞争结合受体的胞内催化结构域,抑制受体的自身磷酸化和下游的信号转导[77]。

在非小细胞肺癌中,只有 10%~20%的患者对吉非替尼/厄洛替尼的治疗有部分反应。一些回顾性和前瞻性研究证实,携带 *EGFR* 突变的患者对吉非替尼/厄洛替尼特别敏感,其反应率高达 80%。*ERB B1* 中有多种类型的突变已被报道,但到目前为止,仅明确了四种药物敏感性相关的突变,包括 19 号外显子缺失和 18 号外显子(G719A/C)、21 号外显子 L858R、21 号外显子 L861Q 的置换突变。此外,*ERB B1* 基因拷贝数的增加(7 号染色体多体或基因扩增)也逐渐成为选择适用患者的另一种方式[132]。对吉非替尼/厄洛替尼敏感的患者具有以下特征:无吸烟史、亚洲人种、女性和腺癌的病理类型。部分患者在接受了吉非替尼/厄洛替尼治疗后,开始对药物敏感,后来发生了耐药,通过对这部分病例的研究发现,肿瘤 *ERB B1* 基因的 20 号外显子中出现了继发性特异体细胞突变(T790M)。此外,*MET* 和 *ERB B2* 基因扩增也是肿瘤对酪氨酸激酶抑制剂耐药的另一种机制。目前有研究者正在评估特异性针对 T790M 突变的新型抑制剂,这种药物被称为"不可逆抑制剂"[134,135]。

在结直肠癌中,以单克隆抗体 MoAb 为代表的 erb B1 抑制剂表现出很好的临床效果。西妥昔单抗或帕尼单抗单药治疗时只有 9%~12%的有效率,但当这些药物与伊立替康联用时,对之前使用伊立替康单药治疗无效的患者,其治疗有效率可增加至 20%~30%。与早期研究的结论不同,最近的数据表明,通过免疫组织化学和荧光原位杂交确定 erb B1 蛋白的表达情况并不能用于预测 EGFR 靶向疗法的疗效,这主要是由于这两种检测方法实际上很难被重复。与之相反,可以通过检测 *KRAS* 和 *NRAS* 基因突变来预测 EGFR 靶向治疗的效果(有突变的患者疗效通常较差),并且必须在施用 MoAb 之前检测突变的情况[136]。此外,通过对其他 *ERB B1* 下游成员的基因或蛋白水平的检测,研究者发现,诸如 *BRAF* 和 *PIK3CA* 点突变以及 PTEN 蛋白表达缺失,也可能促进了肿瘤对西妥昔单抗/帕尼单抗的耐药,但到目前为止这一问题仍然存在争议,因此在使用 MoAb 治疗之前并没有强制要求对这些突变进行检测[137]。

西妥昔单抗和帕尼单抗也在 10%~13%的头颈部鳞状细胞癌患者中有效,EGFR 靶向治疗是第一个也是唯一一个可以改善复发或转移性肿瘤患者生存期的靶向疗法[138]。

KIT 和 *PDGFRA*

研究者发现,原本作为酪氨酸激酶抑制剂用于治疗 bcr-abl 阳性白血病的伊马替尼,在治疗胃肠道间质瘤(GIST)时仍然有效(图 4-13)。病理上,可以用 *KIT* 和 *PDGFRA* 的突变情况来预测这种其靶向药物的有效性。肿瘤 *KIT* 11 号外显子突变的患者对其部分反应率高达 85%~90%的,而 *KIT* 9 号外显子突变的患者也有约 50%的部分反应率。最近的数据指出,对于 *KIT* 9 号外显子突变的患者,更好的治疗方法是使用双倍剂量的伊马替尼。与携带其他类型突变的 *GIST* 患者相比,*KIT* 11 号外显子突变的 *GIST* 患者到治疗失败的中位时间更长。没有 *KIT* 或 *PDGFRA* 突变的患者对伊马替尼的反应率要低于携带 11 号外显子突变的患者,但仍有 39%的患者对其有反应。极少数携带 *KIT* 13 号外显子突变或 *PDGFRA* 17 位点突变的 *GIST* 患者也可能对伊马替尼敏感。研究发现某些突变可能会使肿瘤产生对伊马替尼的抗性,例如 D842V *PDGFRA* 18 号外显子突变,但这种情况极为少见。有意思的是,D842V *PDGFRA* 18 号外显子突变在功能上等同于 D816V *KIT* 17 号外显子突变,后者可导致白血病产生对伊马替尼的抗性,而在 *GIST* 中却从未发现过这种情况[139]。大多数转移性 GIST 患者会逐渐丧失对伊马替尼的反应性。耐药性的产生通常是由于 KIT 蛋白内的 ATP/伊马替尼结合口袋(13 号外显子或 14 号外显子)或活化环(17 号外显子)中产生了继发性突变,由此阻断了其与伊马替尼的结合。伊马替尼剂量虽已增加但病情仍在恶化的患者,可以选择尝试其他酪氨酸激酶抑制剂。舒尼替尼(SU11248)是 KIT、PDGFRA、FMS 样酪氨酸激酶 3 和血管内皮生长因子受体 2 的抑制剂,已被 FDA 批准用于治疗对伊马替尼耐药或无法耐受的 GIST 患者。

最近发现,*KIT* 突变在黑色素瘤诊疗中也具有重要的临床指导意义。有研究表明,黑素瘤患者的 *KIT* 突变存在于特定的亚型中,大多数是葡萄膜黑色素瘤,39%是黏膜型,36%是肢端型,28%是皮肤经受长期日光照射引起的黑色素瘤,但在没有慢性日光损伤的皮肤黑色素瘤中则没有此突变(0%)[140]。L576P 点突变是 *KIT* 典型的突变类型。临床病例报告和人葡萄膜黑色素瘤细胞系的研究结果提示,伊马替尼可以抑制黑色素瘤细胞增殖并降低其侵袭率[141]。但葡萄膜黑色素瘤对伊马替尼的体内反应性尚待临床试验评估(目前已开展)

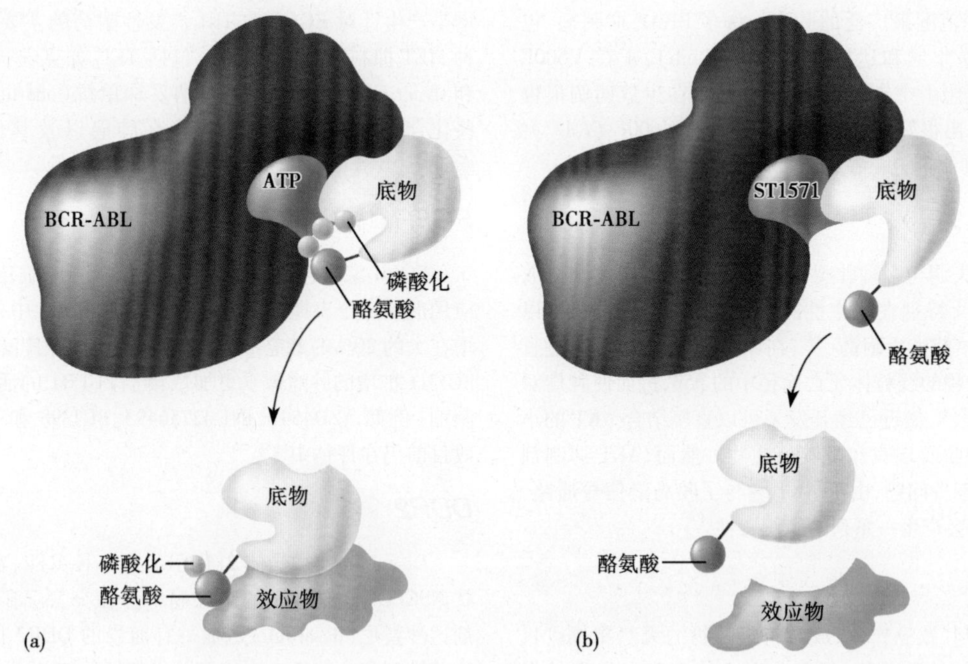

图 4-13　伊马替尼的作用方式。(a)ATP 结合 BCR-ABL 融合蛋白后的效果。ATP 结合于融合蛋白的激酶口袋,磷酸化底物可以作用于下游效应分子。(b)伊马替尼存在时,其可以代替 ATP 结合于融合蛋白的激酶口袋

RET

近来相继开发出了 *RET* 相关的各种治疗方法,包括 TKI,显性失活 *RET* 突变体的基因治疗,单克隆抗体,可以识别并抑制 RET 的核酸酶抗性的适配体。此类策略相关的临床前研究显示,RET 可作为肿瘤精准治疗的潜在靶点。临床病例研究发现,*RET* 重排在乳头状甲状腺癌中发挥了一定的作用,同时还发现一小部分肺癌(1%~2%)存在 *RET* 重排。目前关于 *RET* 重排,已经发现了两种特异性的基因融合(*CCDC6-RET* 和 *KIF5B-RET*)机制。*RET* 重排似乎仅存在于腺癌类型中,并且不与 *ERB B1* 或 *KRAS* 突变或 *ALK* 重排同时出现。目前市售的针对 RET 的 TKI 至少有六种[凡德他尼(vandetanib],索拉非尼(sorafenib),舒尼替尼(sunitinib),卡博替尼(cabozantinib),瑞格菲尼(regorafenib)和普纳替尼(ponatinib)],但这些药物在 RET 重排肺癌中的疗效尚不清楚[81,142]。

RAS

临床试验检测了许多靶向 *K-RAS* 活性的治疗方法。通常,直接针对 *K-RAS* 的抑制剂对人体细胞也会有很强的毒性。目前,最有前景的药物是氨基二磷酸酯,该药物已进入临床试验,用于多种肿瘤(包括乳腺癌和前列腺腺癌)骨转移的治疗。

此外,*K-RAS* 突变还可预测靶向其上游活化 RTK(例如 EGFR)疗法的效果。实际上,*K-RAS* 突变可作为独立因素预测西妥昔单抗或帕尼单抗在晚期 CRC 患者中的治疗效果[137]。直到 2013 年,临床上才要求在使用 EGFR 靶向治疗之前必须明确 *K-RAS* 2 号外显子的 12 和 13 位密码子的突变情况。然而,研究发现在 CRC 中可以检测出其他不同位点的 *K-RAS* 突变(位于 3 号和 4 号外显子的 59、61、117 和 146 位处的密码子,这些突变在高达 5%的患者中出现),这些区域对 K-RAS 的活性至关重要,大型队列研究表明,*K-RAS* 3-4 号外显子突变可以预测 MoAb 对 EGFR 治疗时的疗效(突变的患者疗效较差)[136,143,144]。此外,*N-RAS* 突变也可发生在 CRC 中(高达 5%的病例存在突变,且其突变发生在与 *K-RAS* 基因突变相同的密码子中),并且最近已经有研究证明携带该基因突变的患者对 EGFR 靶向治疗不敏感[55,136,145]。因此,总体而言,在发生转移的 CRC 患者中使用 EGFR 靶向治疗之前,必须对 *K-RAS* 和 *N-RAS* 的基因突变情况进行综合分析。*K-RAS* 突变在预测肺腺癌患者中 EGFR TKI 的临床疗效方面的作用,与临床前模型和少数特定队列中的初步结果并不一致,目前的假设是 *K-RAS* 突变不能预测这些药物的实际功效。

BRAF

BRAF 为恶性黑素瘤的药物治疗提供了一个关键的新靶点,靶向 BRAF 的药物包括反义寡核苷酸和小分子抑制剂。这些抑制剂可以抑制 BRAF 蛋白的表达,阻断 BRAF/ras 的相互作用,阻断其或下游靶蛋白 MAPK 的激酶活性。除了以上方法,维罗非尼(vemurafenib)是一种选择性的 BRAF TKI,已被批准用于黑色素瘤患者的治疗。美国 FDA 批准该药用于治疗携带 V600E 特异性突变的黑色素瘤患者,而欧洲药品管理局批准其用于所有携带密码子 600 突变的患者(突变包括 V600K、V600D 和 V600G,总计有超过 10%的黑色素瘤患者)。维罗非尼可使携带 *BRAF* 突变的黑色素瘤患者的肿瘤迅速消退,但 10~12 个月后,BRAF 会发生继发性改变(出现异常剪接的 BRAF 蛋白或其他 BRAF 体细胞突变),并导致患者很快出现转移性病变[146]。

最近有研究发现,*BRAF* 突变也可影响 NSCLC。在一小部分病例中(可达 2%),*BRAF* 突变不仅发生在密码子 600,也可以发生在其他重要的密码子(466、469 和 594)中;因此,肺癌是

BRAF 密码子突变范围最广泛的肿瘤。许多 BRAF 抑制剂，包括索拉非尼、维罗非尼和达拉非尼（dabrafenib），正在 V600E *BRAF* 突变的肺癌患者中进行临床研究；其中在少数病例报告中，维罗非尼表现出很好的疗效。对于携带非 V600E *BRAF* 突变的肺癌，MEK 抑制剂也正在进行临床试验[81,147]。

AKT

AKT 表达的失调与多种肿瘤对 AKT 药物的反应性和对放疗的耐受有关[148]，特别在化生性肿瘤中，AKT 表达失调可以促进肿瘤对激素治疗产生耐药[149]，在卵巢癌中，它可以通过直接调节 caspase 依赖的线粒体死亡途径中的 p53，进而使肿瘤对顺铂耐药[150]。此外，最近已经开发了可以直接结合 AKT 的小分子抑制剂，例如曲西瑞宾和吡啶衍生物。然而，AKT 抑制剂的临床应用也有不少问题，由于 AKT 参与了胰岛素信号通路，因此 AKT 抑制剂会产生一系列的组织毒性[108]。

PIK3CA

PIK3CA 由于其致癌作用，成为特定药物的天然靶标。目前已开发了多种相关的药物，但药物对人体细胞有很强的毒性。一些 PIK3CA 抑制剂已进入临床试验评估阶段。*PIK3CA* 突变，至少在临床前阶段，被发现与转移性乳腺癌对曲妥珠单抗的耐药性有关[151]，同时也有一种说法，只有特定位点的突变（即在 20 号外显子发生的突变）可以使转移性 CRC 产生对西妥昔单抗或帕尼单抗的耐药，但还需进一步实验确认[137]。此外，研究者们也正在开展临床试验，以研究特异性抑制剂在 *PIK3CA* 突变型卵巢癌中的疗效。然而，*PIK3CA* 突变在临床诊断中的主要应用还是在接受阿司匹林辅助治疗的 CRC 患者中。实际上，阿司匹林可以有效地预防结直肠腺瘤和结直肠癌，其可能的机制是抑制环氧合酶。但这种抗癌作用仅限于环氧合酶过表达的患者。两项大型前瞻性研究表明，阿司匹林对携带 *PIK3CA* 突变的患者有更好的疗效，这可能是因为 *PIK3CA* 基因突变的产物会进一步诱导环氧合酶的表达。一项基于回顾性分析的最新研究证实了 *PIK3CA* 突变对阿司匹林辅助治疗患者的疗效预测价值。有趣的是，在服用另一种特异性环氧合酶抑制剂罗非昔布的患者中未观察到这种作用[152,153]。

BCL-2

许多研究小组一直致力于开发阻断抗凋亡分子 BCL-2 成员功能的抗癌药物，希望以此杀伤肿瘤。方法包括通过反义寡核苷酸下调 BCL-2 的表达，或在 BCL-2 的结合袋中使用多肽或有机小分子，使之不能结合促凋亡蛋白。这些小分子抑制剂在癌症治疗中的优势在于它们的作用靶点和机制不同于细胞毒性药物和放疗。因此，将小分子抑制剂与其他治疗方法联用，可以产生协同作用而不会导致交叉耐药或增加毒性[154]。

MET

MET 是由肝细胞生长因子激活的受体型酪氨酸激酶。在多种肿瘤中可以观察到 MET 蛋白的过表达，MET 过表达通常与患者的预后不良有关。仅有一部分 MET 阳性肿瘤的 MET 过表达是由 *MET* 基因扩增引起的。在 NSCLC 中，2%～4%的肺鳞状和非鳞状细胞癌中存在 *MET* 基因扩增。有趣的是，*MET* 扩增是产生针对 EGFR 的 TKI 继发性耐药的主要机制之一。多种 MET 抑制剂已相继问世，包括 TKI［如克唑替尼（crizotinib）和 tivantinib］和 MoAb［如奥纳妥珠单抗（onartuzumab）］，但这些化合物的疗效仍需进一步在肺癌以及其他癌症中进行验证[81,155]。

FGFR

FGFR 家族包括四个成员，其中 FGFR1 临床肿瘤诊疗中的应用前景最令人期待。特别的是，在 NSCLC 中，*FGFR1* 基因扩增在大约 20%的鳞癌中发生，但在腺癌中，其发生率小于 2%。FGFR1 扩增的肿瘤似乎更加依赖于 FGFR1 的活性。FGFR1 抑制剂（例如 AZD4547、JNJ-42756493、BGJ398 和 ponatinib）的疗效目前仍在评估中[81,156]。

DDR2

Discoidin 死亡受体 2（DDR2）是一种 RTK，在大约 4%的鳞状 NSCLC 和大约 1%的肺腺癌中存在突变。多靶点激酶抑制剂达沙替尼（dasatinib）是唯一有前景的 DDR2 抑制剂，其在临床前模型和少数患者中均显示出良好的疗效[81,157]。

ALK

ALK 的重排主要会导致其与 *EML4* 发生基因融合。在大约 3%～7%的肺腺癌中可以发现此融合蛋白。目前已经在 EML4-ALK 融合蛋白中发现存在多个 *EML4* 基因断裂点。在极少数情况下，ALK 也可与其他基因融合，比如 *TFG* 和 *KIF5B* 基因[81]。第一种 ALK 选择性抑制剂以多靶点抑制剂克唑替尼为代表。在第一个入组了 ALK 阳性患者的临床试验中，克唑替尼疗效显著：总生存率为 61%，疾病控制率为 71%，无进展生存期显著增长。因此 FDA 迅速批准了克唑替尼用于治疗 ALK 易位的肺腺癌（*ALK* 易位可通过荧光原位杂交确定）[158]。可惜的是，由于多种系统性耐药机制的出现，克唑替尼只能在短时间内有效，其耐药机制包括：ALK 活性位点继发性突变，erb B 基因家族通路激活，*ALK* 拷贝数增加，*KIT* 基因扩增和 *KRAS* 突变。当前，人们正积极研发第二代 ALK 抑制剂，以治疗对克唑替尼产生耐药的肺腺癌患者[81]。在 *ERB B1* 突变型肺腺癌中，ALK 重排也被认为是肿瘤对 EGFR TKI 产生获得性耐药的机制之一（但不是最常见的）[81]。

ROS1

在约 1%～2%的肺腺癌中存在 *ROS1* 癌基因的重排。*ROS1* 与 *ALK* 基因具有高度的同源性（TK 结构域内同源性 49%，ATP 结合位点同源性 77%），*ROS1* 基因重排和 *ALK* 基因易位可在患者中产生叠加的临床病理特征[81]。多靶点抑制剂克唑替尼已在 *ROS1* 重排患者中显示出疗效，其初步缓解率为 57%，疾病控制率为 79%。因此，肺腺癌患者的临床诊断中需同时检测 *ROS1* 基因重排[159]。

总结

人类肿瘤的发生发展是一个多步骤过程，涉及体细胞中遗传变化的累积。这些遗传改变包括原癌基因的激活和抑癌基因的失活，两者决定了肿瘤的发生发展。癌基因是从正常细胞的原癌基因转变而来的。原癌基因是一类调节细胞正常生长的基因，包括生长因子、生长因子受体、信号转导分子、转录因子和调节程序性细胞死亡的基因。原癌基因可以通过突变、染色体重排或基因扩增被激活。染色体重排，包括易位和倒置，可以通过基因的异常转录调控（例如，转录激活）或基因融合来激活原癌基因。抑癌基因也参与了正常细胞的生长调节，其失活通常是因点突变或其蛋白序列截短以及正常等位基因的缺失造成的。

癌基因的发现是肿瘤分子和遗传学基础研究的一个重大突破，加深了我们对正常细胞增殖、分化和程序性细胞死亡调控的认识。鉴别癌基因的异常为癌症的分子诊断和监测提供了工具，更为癌症治疗提供了潜在靶标。新药研发的目标是选择性地杀死癌细胞，同时保留正常细胞。靶向特定的癌基因来触发程序性细胞死亡的治疗方法具有广阔前景。第一个例子就是采用伊马替尼抑制 CML 中肿瘤特异性 BCR/ABL 酪氨酸激酶。伊马替尼在其他不同类型的肿瘤中也可发挥作用，在 GIST 中抑制酪氨酸激酶受体 *c-KIT*，在脊索瘤中则可以阻断 PDGFR 信号通路。另一个实例是吉非替尼和西妥昔单抗的应用，它们分别抑制 ERB B1 酪氨酸激酶的细胞内结构域和细胞外结构域。此后，大量新的靶向药物进入了临床试验，在一些难治性肿瘤中取得了较好疗效。高通量技术的应用，为新的癌基因鉴定，深入认识肿瘤的分子机制，将来开发更好的联合疗法奠定了基础。

（沈皓 于晗 陈瑶 译 陈磊 孙文 陈淑桢 校）

参考文献

The complete reference list can be found on the Wiley Companion Digital Edition of this title (see inside front cover for login instructions).

1 Bernards R, Weinberg RA. A progression puzzle. *Nature*. 2002;**418**:823.

2 Hanahan D, Weinberg RA. Hallmarks of cancer: the next generation. *Cell*. 2011;**144**:646–674.

3 Bishop JM. Retroviruses and oncogenes II. In: *Les Prix Nobel*. Stockholm: Almqvist and Wiksell; 1989:220–238.

4 Varmus HE. Retroviruses and oncogenes I. In: *Les Prix Nobel*. Stockholm: Almqvist and Wiksell; 1989:194–212.

5 Todd R, Wong DT. Oncogenes. *Anticancer Res*. 1999;**19**:4729–4746.

8 Bardelli A, Parsons DW, Silliman N, et al. Mutational analysis of the tyrosine kinome in colorectal cancers. *Science*. 2003;**300**:949.

9 Wang Z, Shen D, Parsons DW, et al. Mutational analysis of the tyrosine phosphatome in colorectal cancers. *Science*. 2004;**304**:1164–1166.

11 Mahalingam S, Meanger J, Foster PS, Lidbury BA. The viral manipulation of the host cellular and immune environments to enhance propagation and survival: a focus on RNA viruses. *J Leukoc Biol*. 2002;**72**:429–439.

12 Rubin H. The early history of tumor virology: Rous, RIF, and RAV. *Proc Natl Acad Sci U S A*. 2011;**108**:14389–14396.

14 Sanchez-Beato M, Sanchez-Aguilera A, Piris MA. Cell cycle deregulation in B-cell lymphomas. *Blood*. 2002;**101**:1220–1235.

15 Krontiris TG, Cooper GM. Transforming activity of human tumor DNAs. *Proc Natl Acad Sci U S A*. 1981;**78**:1181–1184.

16 Dayaram T, Marriott SJ. Effect of transforming viruses on molecular mechanisms associated with cancer. *J Cell Physiol*. 2008;**216**:309–314.

20 Macaluso M, Russo G, Cinti C, et al. Ras family genes: an interesting link between cell cycle and cancer. *J Cell Physiol*. 2002;**192**:125–130.

23 Falini B, Mason DY. Proteins encoded by genes involved in chromosomal alterations in lymphoma and leukemia: clinical value of their detection by immunocytochemistry. *Blood*. 2002;**99**:409–426.

27 Grimm SL, Nordeen SK. Mouse mammary tumor virus sequences responsible for activating cellular oncogenes. *J Virol*. 1998;**72**:9428–9435.

29 Paez JG, Janne PA, Lee JC, et al. EGFR mutations in lung cancer: correlation with clinical response to gefitinib therapy. *Science*. 2004;**304**:1497–1500.

35 Cantley LC, Auger KR, Carpenter C, et al. Oncogenes and signal transduction. *Cell*. 1991;**64**:281–302.

36 Malumbres M, Barbacid M. RAS oncogenes: the first 30 years. *Nat Rev Cancer*. 2003;**3**:459–465.

37 Darnell JE Jr. Transcription factors as targets for cancer therapy. *Nat Rev Cancer*. 2002;**2**:740–749.

41 Boxer LM, Dang CV. Translocations involving c-myc and cmyc function. *Oncogene*. 2001;**20**:5595–5610.

42 Konopleva M, Zhao S, Xie Z, et al. Apoptosis. Molecules and mechanisms. *Adv Exp Med Biol*. 1999;**457**:217–236.

43 Danial NN. BCL-2 family proteins: critical checkpoints of apoptotic cell death. *Clin Cancer Res*. 2007;**13**:7254–7263.

46 Mazaris E, Tsiotras A. Molecular pathways in prostate cancer. *Nephrourol Mon*. 2013;**5**:792–800.

57 Frattini M, Gallino G, Signoroni S, et al. Quantitative and qualitative characterization of plasma DNA identifies primary and recurrent colorectal cancer. *Cancer Lett*. 2008;**263**:170–181.

69 Storlazzi CT, Lonoce A, Guastadisegni MC, et al. Gene amplification as double minutes or homogeneously staining regions in solid tumors: origin and structure. *Genome Res*. 2010;**20**:1198–1206.

77 Ciardiello F, Tortora G. EGFR antagonists in cancer treatment. *N Engl J Med*. 2008;**358**:1160–1174.

81 Gerber DE, Gandhi L, Costa DB. Management and future directions in non-small cell lung cancer with known activating mutations. *Am Soc Clin Oncol Educ Book*. 2014:e354–e365. doi: 0.14694/EdBook_AM.2014.34.e353.

95 Skapek SX, Chui CH. Cytogenetics and the biologic basis of sarcomas. *Curr Opin Oncol*. 2000;**12**:315–322.

97 Xia SJ, Barr FG. Chromosome translocations in sarcomas and the emergence of oncogenic transcription factors. *Eur J Cancer*. 2005;**41**:2513–2527.

103 Ciampi R, Nikiforov YE. RET/PTC rearrangements and BRAF mutations in thyroid tumorigenesis. *Endocrinology*. 2007;**148**:936–941.

104 Arighi E, Borrello MG, Sariola H. RET tyrosine kinase signaling in development and cancer. *Cytokine Growth Factor Rev*. 2005;**16**:441–467.

118 Weinberg RA. Oncogenes and multistep carcinogenesis. In: Weinberg RA, ed. *Oncogenes and the Molecular Origins of Cancer*. New York, NY: Cold Spring Harbor; 1989:307–326.

120 Land H, Parada LF, Weinberg RA. Tumorigenic conversion of primary embryo fibroblasts requires at least two cooperating oncogenes. *Nature*. 1983;**304**:596–602.

122 Pelengaris S, Khan M, Evan G. c-MYC: more than just a matter of life and death. *Nat Rev Cancer*. 2002;**2**:764–776.

123 Nowell PC. The clonal evolution of tumor cell populations. *Science*. 1976;**194**:23–28.

130 Fearon ER, Vogelstein B. A genetic model for colorectal tumorigenesis. *Cell*. 1990;**61**:759–767.

136 Douillard JY, Oliner KS, Siena S, et al. Panitumumab-FOLFOX4 treatment and RAS mutations in colorectal cancer. *N Engl J Med*. 2013;**369**:1023–1034.

137 Custodio A, Feliu J. Prognostic and predictive biomarkers for epidermal growth factor receptor-targeted therapy in colorectal cancer: beyond KRAS mutations. *Crit Rev Oncol Hematol*. 2013;**85**:45–81.

146 Tronnier M, Mitteldorf C. Treating advanced melanoma: current insights and opportunities. *Cancer Manag Res*. 2014;**6**:349–356.

153 Domingo E, Church DN, Sieber O, et al. Evaluation of PIK3CA mutation as a predictor of benefit from nonsteroidal anti-inflammatory drug therapy in colorectal cancer. *J Clin Oncol*. 2013;**31**:4297–4305.

第 5 章　抑癌基因

David Cosgrove, MB, BCh ■ Ben Ho Park, MD, PhD ■ Bert Vogelstein, MD

概述

癌症是一种遗传性疾病。促生长基因(癌基因)和抑癌基因的突变以及其他变异可在细胞的一生中积累,从而导致癌症。与癌基因不同,抑癌基因通常需要双等位基因的失活才能使细胞具有癌的表型。导致家族性癌症的遗传性抑癌基因突变的发现,很大程度地揭示了抑癌基因的功能。这些发现提示有癌症家族史的个体有必要进行相应的临床筛查,同时也有助于开发靶向特定抑癌基因失活的癌细胞的新疗法。

一个多世纪以来,家族谱系研究、流行病学和细胞遗传学研究一直支持癌症具有遗传基础的假设。然而,直到最近 40 年才有确凿的证据表明癌症是一种遗传性疾病。现在我们知道癌症的产生是一个多阶段的过程。在这个过程中,细胞基因的遗传性突变和体细胞突变导致了细胞的多次克隆选择,具有最强生长能力和侵袭性生长特性的细胞才能占据优势。突变的主要靶点包括癌基因和抑癌基因两大类,它们控制着细胞增殖和死亡的比率。在成年人的所有正常组织中,这个比率正好是 1.0;而突变会使这个比率增加。此外,还有第三类基因,称之为基因组稳定性基因,它们在发生突变时不会改变细胞增殖和死亡的比率,而是通过增加癌基因和抑癌基因的突变频率,间接促进肿瘤的发生。

癌细胞内绝大多数与肿瘤发展和肿瘤细胞生物学行为相关的突变是体细胞突变(即在肿瘤发展过程中产生的),这种突变只存在于肿瘤细胞内。只有很小一部分突变是组成型的,存在于受影响个体的所有体细胞内。这种突变是可遗传的,增加了后代罹患癌症的风险。

本书已在其他章节详述了癌基因的定义及功能。在此我们简单总结它们的一般特征,以便同抑癌基因进行比较。一般而言,癌基因在多种生长调控通路中具有关键作用,其蛋白产物分布于许多亚细胞单位中。肿瘤细胞内的原癌基因位点由于点突变、染色体重排、基因扩增或其他基因序列的变化而产生了获得性的功能改变(活化)。尽管在家族性甲状腺髓样癌患者中发现 *RET*(在转染过程中发生了重排)的胚系突变,在遗传性肾乳头状细胞癌患者中发现了 *MET*(转移)的胚系突变,但在绝大多数肿瘤中原癌基因的突变都是体细胞突变。

与癌基因的等位基因位点存在激活突变不同,突变使抑癌基因在肿瘤细胞中呈失活状态。同癌基因一样,抑癌基因在细胞内的功能也是多种多样的。

基因组稳定性基因的缺陷也与多种人类癌症有关。与抑癌基因类似,基因组稳定性基因在人类癌症中呈失活状态。然而,与抑癌基因的突变不同的是,基因组稳定性基因的突变常遗传给子代。例如,乳腺癌易感基因 1(*BRCA1*)或乳腺癌易感基因 2(*BRCA2*)的遗传性突变在遗传性乳腺癌和卵巢癌的发生中发挥着关键的作用,但这些基因很少在非家族形式的乳腺癌中发生体细胞突变。

目前,科学家在人类癌症的癌基因、抑癌基因和基因组稳定性基因的遗传性突变和体细胞突变的鉴定方面已经取得了巨大的进展。通过对小鼠、果蝇、蠕虫和其他生物体等多种模型系统的分析,以及对人类癌细胞系的研究和人类癌细胞的测序,已经在一定程度上阐明了这些基因的功能。本章的主要目的是对确立抑癌基因存在的体细胞遗传学和流行病学研究进行综述;并描述一些代表性抑癌基因的鉴定和克隆方法;重点介绍几项抑癌基因在细胞增殖和死亡调控中作用的研究;并举例说明基因组稳定性基因与常见人类癌症的因果关系。

肿瘤发展的遗传学基础

近 150 年来人类癌症的遗传基础一直都是研究的重点。1866 年,Broca 描述了一个家族,该家族中的多名成员罹患乳腺癌或肝癌。他由此提出,受影响组织内的遗传异常促进了肿瘤的发展[1]。孟德尔的工作被重新发现之后,Haaland 在研究了多种近交系小鼠自发性乳腺肿瘤的发生率后提出,肿瘤发生可能遵循孟德尔遗传特征[2]。同样,Warthin 通过对 1895 年至 1913 年间密歇根大学医院癌症患者的家族谱系分析确定了四个对特定类型癌症敏感的多代家系,这些癌症的传播似乎符合孟德尔学说的常染色体显性遗传的特征(图 5-1)[3]。虽然这些研究和其他研究表明某些癌症存在遗传基因基础,但也可能存在癌症家族聚集现象的其他解释(例如,暴露于相似环境或饮食中的致癌物质)。此外,需要强调的是,人类的大多数癌症似乎是散发的、孤立的事件。

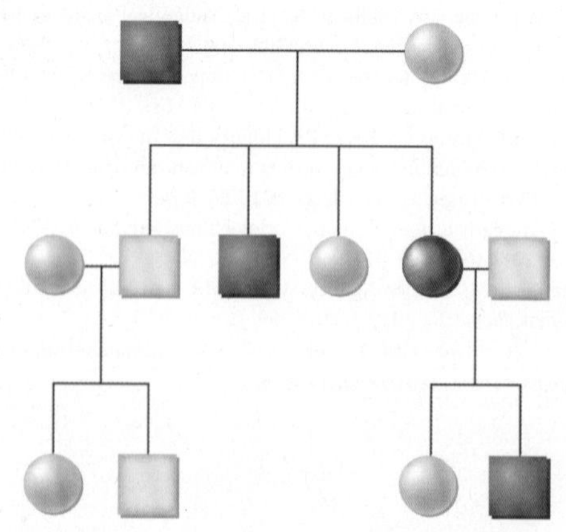

图 5-1　癌症的家族遗传谱。患癌症的成员用带阴影的方块(男性)或圆形(女性)表示。这个癌症家系展示了一个显性遗传模式,这意味着每个后代都有 50% 的机会继承一个高患癌风险的胚系突变

Boveri首先提出了体细胞突变在肿瘤发展中的作用[4]。他发现,在由两个精子受精的海胆卵细胞中异常有丝分裂会导致子细胞的染色体丢失,在由此形成的原肠胚中可观察到异常的组织团块。他认为这些异常组织在物理形态上与肿瘤中所见的低分化组织相似,并提出假设——癌症是由产生异常有丝分裂的细胞畸变引起的。但限于当时的条件,因为无法获得动物和人类肿瘤核型的直接的实验数据支持,Boveri的假设在当时显然没有得到承认。尽管几十年后的核型研究似乎支持了Boveri的假设,但因为无法确定肿瘤中染色体数量的变化是肿瘤形成的原因还是结果,这一假说仍然受到质疑。

1911年,Rous发表了一项在癌症遗传基础研究史上具有里程碑意义的发现。他发现,鸡身上产生的肉瘤的无细胞滤液可在正常鸡的体内中诱发相同的肉瘤[5]。这一现象强有力地证明了肿瘤可以由病毒诱发,也支持了癌症可以归因于特定的遗传因素的观点。在Rous首次报告的60年后,科学家确定了Rous肉瘤病毒的致癌区域。对相应转化序列的进一步鉴定和克隆表明,病毒的致癌性依赖于*vsrc*——细胞内原癌基因*csrc*转导和突变的拷贝。之后,又发现所有急性转化RNA肿瘤病毒的致癌基因都是转导的细胞基因(事实上,它们被定义为致癌基因。)病毒癌基因可引起细胞恶性转化,原因在于它们是细胞癌基因的突变形式,或在细胞内异常高表达。在人类肿瘤中,体细胞突变可在原癌基因位点产生致癌的等位基因。

癌基因在大多数类型的人类癌症中都发挥着作用,但在"液体"肿瘤如白血病和淋巴瘤以及肉瘤中,这种作用尤为突出。这类肿瘤通常具有特征性的染色体易位,染色体断点处的原癌基因与无关基因融合可产生具有增加细胞增殖或减少细胞死亡特性的融合产物。

细胞致瘤性的体细胞遗传学研究

Ephrussi等人[6]和Harris[7]的研究提供了令人信服的证据证明了细胞形成肿瘤的能力在细胞水平上表现为隐性性状。他们观察到,恶性细胞与非恶性细胞的融合可抑制小鼠肿瘤细胞在同种系小鼠体内的生长;但当杂交细胞在体外培养传代一段时间后,致瘤性又可恢复。恶性肿瘤特征的再现与特定染色体的丢失有关。研究者对这一现象的解释为:体细胞杂交可抑制肿瘤细胞的恶性特征。之后,进一步的小鼠、大鼠和仓鼠种内体细胞的杂交研究,以及啮齿动物肿瘤细胞与正常人类细胞的种间杂交研究都支持了这一观点[8,9]。然而,啮齿动物—人杂交细胞的核型不稳定性,使对参与抑制作用的人染色体的分析变得很复杂。Stanbridge和他的同事通过研究人肿瘤细胞系与人正常二倍体成纤维细胞融合而形成的杂交细胞,成功地解决了这个问题[10,11]。他们的分析证实,保留两组亲本染色体的杂交细胞的恶性特征明显受到了抑制,只有极少量的杂交细胞因染色体丢失才会形成致瘤变异体。此外,研究表明,特定染色体的丢失(而不仅仅是一般的染色体丢失)与细胞致瘤性的恢复有关。杂交细胞即使表达活化的癌基因(如突变的*ras*基因),其致瘤性也可能受到抑制[11,12]。

特定染色体的丢失与肿瘤恶性特征的恢复之间存在关联,表明一条染色体(甚至可能是单一基因)就足以抑制细胞的致瘤性。为了直接验证这一假设,人们应用微细胞介导的染色体转移技术将单个染色体从正常细胞转移到肿瘤细胞。研究发现,将11号染色体转入HeLa细胞(人宫颈癌细胞系)可抑制细胞的致瘤表型[13]。同样,将11号染色体转入Wilms肿瘤细胞也可抑制细胞的致瘤性,而转入其他几条染色体则没有作用[14]。许多研究表明,即使是非常小的染色体片段的转移,也可以特异性地抑制某些癌细胞系的致瘤特性。

尽管恶性细胞与正常细胞融合产生的杂交细胞或者转入特定染色体片段形成的杂交细胞在免疫缺陷动物体内的生长经常受到抑制,但它们仍保留了其亲代肿瘤细胞的其他性状特征,如永生化和体外锚定非依赖性生长等。这一现象与大多数恶性肿瘤的发生是源于多种基因的改变的观点相一致。细胞融合或微细胞染色体转移后对细胞致瘤性的抑制,可能只是校正了恶性细胞中众多变异中的一种。

总之,体细胞遗传学研究方法为正常细胞中存在关键性生长调节基因的理论提供了早期和有说服力的证据,这些关键基因可以抑制永生化甚至完全癌变细胞的表型特征。

视网膜母细胞瘤:抑癌基因功能的范例

Harris等进行最初的细胞融合实验的同时,Knudson通过分析视网膜母细胞瘤年龄特异性的发病率,提出了二次"打击"或突变事件是视网膜母细胞瘤发展所必需的[15]。视网膜母细胞瘤在大多数情况下是散发的,但在某些家系中表现为常染色体显性遗传。Knudson提出,在具有遗传性视网膜母细胞瘤的个体中,第一次打击出现在生殖系细胞中,因此该突变将出现在身体的所有细胞中。但是,此易感位点的突变尚不足以形成肿瘤,第二次体细胞突变被认为是促进肿瘤形成的必要条件。由于在发育过程中,至少有一个视网膜细胞发生一次体细胞突变的可能性很高,因此这就可以解释某些家系中视网膜母细胞瘤的显性遗传模式。在非遗传性视网膜母细胞瘤中,这两种突变都是在同一细胞内发生的。虽然理论上这两次打击都可能发生于不同的基因,但随后的研究(见下文)得出的结论是,这两次打击都位于同一个基因位点,最终导致视网膜母细胞瘤1(RB1)易感基因的两个等位基因失活。Knudson的假说不仅阐明了遗传性和体细胞的遗传变化在肿瘤发生过程中的协同作用机制,而且还将人类癌症的隐性遗传决定因素的概念与体细胞遗传学中肿瘤发生存在隐性特征的发现联系了起来。

通过对视网膜母细胞瘤患者进行核型分析,研究人员发现了可能与遗传性视网膜母细胞瘤有关的基因位点的第一条线索。研究人员在某些病例中发现13号染色体存在组成型缺失[16]。随后对视网膜母细胞瘤患者进行的细胞遗传学研究发现只有约5%的患者可检测到13号染色体的胚系缺失。在这些患者中,常见的缺失区域集中在染色体带13q14周围[17]。与核型正常的家庭成员相比,缺失13q14的患者体内酯酶D(esterase D,一种生理功能未知的酶)的水平降低[18]。这一发现提示酯酶D基因可能存在于13q14染色体带内。通过分析遗传性视网膜母细胞瘤家系中酯酶D同工酶的分离模式和视网膜母细胞瘤的发生情况,也确定了酯酶D和*RB1*位点是遗传连锁的[19]。

随后,研究人员发现一名特殊的遗传性视网膜母细胞瘤患儿，其酯酶D水平大约是正常值的一半，但对他的血细胞和皮肤成纤维细胞进行的核型研究却没有发现13号染色体的缺失[20]。有趣的是，尽管该患儿似乎有一个13号染色体的完整拷贝，其肿瘤细胞内酯酶D的活性却完全丧失。这些发现提示肿瘤细胞中的13号染色体拷贝存在酯酶D和*RB1*位点的亚显微缺失。此外，研究人员还得出结论，该患儿*RB1*的初始突变在细胞水平上是隐性的（即一个*RB1*等位基因失活的细胞具有正常表型）。然而，第二次事件（如携带野生型*RB1*等位基因的13号染色体丢失）可使*RB1*突变的致癌效应完全显现。这与Knudson的两次打击假说完全一致[15,21]。

为了验证这些发现的普遍性，Cavenee和他的同事们利用13号染色体的DNA探针对遗传性和散发性视网膜母细胞瘤进行了研究。使用检测DNA多态性的探针可将患者正常组织和肿瘤组织中13号染色体的两个亲本拷贝区分开来。Cavenee小组通过使用这些标记物来比较每位患者成对的正常组织样本和肿瘤样本，证明在超过60%的研究病例中，13号染色体等位基因的杂合性丢失（LOH-亦即一组亲本标记物的丢失）发生在肿瘤形成的过程中[22]。13号染色体尤其是包含*RB1*基因区域的LOH可通过多种不同的机制产生（图5-2）。

此外，通过研究遗传性病例，研究人员发现肿瘤细胞内的13号染色体的拷贝来源于受影响的亲本，其携带野生型*RB1*基因的染色体已丢失[22,23]。这些数据证实，无论最初的突变是遗传获得，还是在发育中的视网膜母细胞中产生的，*RB1*基因的致病性突变都是通过相同的染色体机制发生的。遗传性视网膜母细胞瘤患者患其他类型癌症尤其是骨肉瘤的风险要高于正常人群。含*RB1*基因座的染色体13q区域的LOH同样可见于遗传性视网膜母细胞瘤患者发生的骨肉瘤细胞内，表明*RB1*等位基因的失活对这些患者骨肉瘤的发生至关重要[24,25]。染色体13q的LOH也常见于散发性骨肉瘤。这些关于视网膜母细胞瘤和骨肉瘤的分子研究为Knudson的“两次打击”假说提供了强有力的证据，并提示肿瘤可能是由于各种抑癌基因的失活而造成的[11,21,23]。此外，这些研究还表明，某一特定类型的肿瘤，无论是遗传性还是散发性的，似乎都是由同一基因的遗传改变引起的。

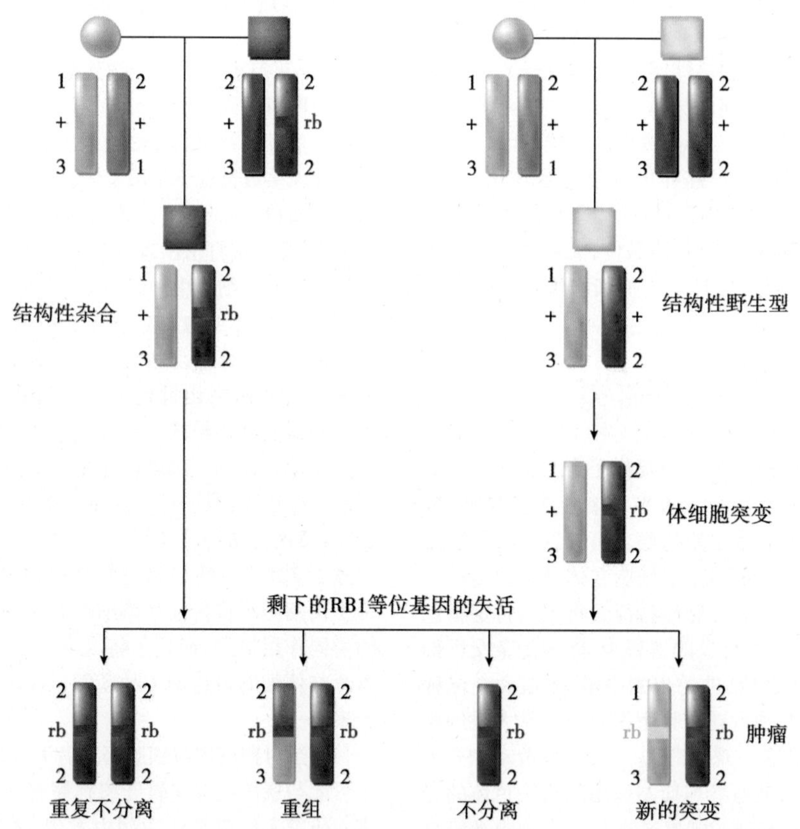

图5-2 导致染色体13q14带的视网膜母细胞瘤易感基因（*RB1*）位点等位基因杂合性缺失的染色体机制。在遗传性视网膜母细胞瘤中（左上角），子代从受影响的父亲那里遗传了一个突变的*RB1*等位基因（*rb*），从他的母亲那里遗传了一个正常的*RB1*等位基因（+）。因此，他的所有细胞中都有一个野生型和一个突变的*RB1*等位基因（即*RB1*的结构性基因型为rb/+）。在其正常细胞中，13号染色体的两个拷贝（分别来自双亲各一个）可以通过*RB1*基因位点侧翼的DNA多态性标记物（多态性等位基因以数字命名）来区分。所保留的野生型*RB1*等位基因失活后可发生视网膜母细胞瘤。现已发现在肿瘤发展过程中，保留的野生型*RB1*等位基因失活的遗传机制包括：染色体不分离和13号染色体剩余基因拷贝的复制、有丝分裂重组、不分离和使保留的*RB1*等位基因失活的新的*RB*突变。右上角显示的是非遗传性（散发性）视网膜母细胞瘤的情况。发育中的视网膜细胞发生体细胞突变，使其中一个*RB1*等位基因失活。如果剩余的*RB1*等位基因通过图示的机制之一发生失活，视网膜母细胞瘤就会发生

RB1 基因的克隆与分析

RB1 基因的分子克隆得益于一种定位于染色体 13q14 区的 DNA 标记物，这种 DNA 标记物可用于检测视网膜母细胞瘤中的 DNA 重排[26]。通过分析该 DNA 标记物两侧的序列，研究人员发现了一个具有 RB1 特性的基因[27~29]。*RB1* 基因的结构较为复杂，它的 27 个外显子分布于超过 200kb 的 DNA 序列中，其 RNA 转录本约为 4.7kb。*RB1* 基因在机体内广泛表达，而不是仅局限于视网膜母细胞和成骨细胞。

RB1 被克隆之后，研究者就可以研究使其失活的突变。虽然在一小部分视网膜母细胞瘤和骨肉瘤病例中存在 *RB1* 序列的严重缺失，但大多数肿瘤可能表达了全长的 *RB1* 转录本，在使用 Southern blotting 分析时并未检测到其有基因重排[30~33]。因此，在大多数情况下，*RB1* 基因的遗传性和体细胞突变检测需要详细描述它的序列。对突变的 *RB1* 等位基因的深入分析为 Knudson 的二次打击模型提供了明确的分子证据。

正如预测的那样，在遗传性视网膜母细胞瘤患者的结构性细胞（血液）中发现了一个突变的等位基因和一个正常的等位基因。在这类个体的视网膜母细胞瘤中，剩余的 *RB1* 等位基因通过体细胞突变失活。这通常是由严重的染色体事件引起的（图 5-2），但在某些情况下也可由点突变引起。同一个遗传性视网膜母细胞瘤患者体内的多个肿瘤均含有相同的胚系突变，但不同的体细胞突变影响了剩余的 *RB1* 等位基因。绝大多数单纯患有视网膜母细胞瘤且无家族史的患者，其肿瘤中有两种体细胞突变，但在结构性细胞中两种等位基因都正常。

令人困惑的是，尽管观察到 *RB1* 广泛表达，但具有 *RB1* 胚系突变的患者仅会罹患有限的几种肿瘤。*RB1* 胚系突变的患者有较高的发生为数不多的几种肿瘤类型的风险，包括儿童视网膜母细胞瘤、骨肉瘤、软组织肉瘤和老年黑色素瘤。尽管 *RB1* 体细胞突变存在于包括乳腺癌、小细胞肺癌、膀胱癌、胰腺癌和前列腺癌等多种类型的癌症中，但 *RB1* 胚系突变并未增加个体对大多数常见癌症的易感性[34]。视网膜母细胞瘤蛋白在视网膜上皮细胞中的功能可能不同于其在其他类型细胞中的功能，因此 *RB1* 基因在视网膜细胞中扮演"看门人"的角色，而在其他类型的细胞中则不是。

视网膜母细胞瘤蛋白 P105-RB 的功能

RB1 基因的蛋白产物是一个核磷酸化蛋白，称为 p105-Rb，或者经常被称为 pRB，其分子量为 105kD。Whyte 和同事的研究为 pRB 的功能提供了重要的见解，他们成功地将人类肿瘤的发生与 DNA 肿瘤病毒引起的实验性肿瘤联系了起来。他们证明了 pRB 可与 5 型小鼠 DNA 肿瘤病毒编码的癌蛋白 E1A 形成复合体[35]。之前关于 E1A 的研究已经证实，它对细胞生长有多种影响，包括细胞永生化、在肿瘤恶性转化中与其他癌基因（例如突变的 *ras* 癌基因等位基因）协同作用。因此，E1A 通过与 pRB 的相互作用而使 pRB 功能失活，这可能与 E1A 的某些转化功能有关。使 E1A 与 pRB 结合能力失活的突变也使 E1A 的转化功能失活[36,37]，这一数据支持了这个假设。

其他 DNA 肿瘤病毒癌蛋白如 SV40 T 抗原和 16 型和 18 型人类乳头瘤病毒（HPV）的 E7 蛋白等也可与 pRB 形成复合物（图 5-3）[38,39]，这些结果进一步证实了 pRB 与 DNA 肿瘤病毒癌蛋白之间的物理相互作用的重要性。许多使这些病毒癌蛋白失去转化活性的突变也使其丧失了与 pRB 相互作用的能力。此外，来自"高风险"HPV（即与肿瘤进展相关的 HPV，如 HPV16 和 HPV18）的 E7 蛋白与 pRB 的结合能力显著高于来自"低风险"HPV 的 E7 蛋白。这些对 pRB 的研究为 DNA 肿瘤病毒可能部分通过灭活抑癌基因产物而使细胞发生转化的理论提供了令人信服的证据。此外，由于 DNA 肿瘤病毒依赖于细胞内成分进行病毒基因组的复制，上述实验还为 pRB 可能通过与细胞内蛋白［如调控细胞进入细胞周期的 DNA 合成期（S 期）的蛋白］的相互作用来调控正常细胞生长的假说提供了依据。

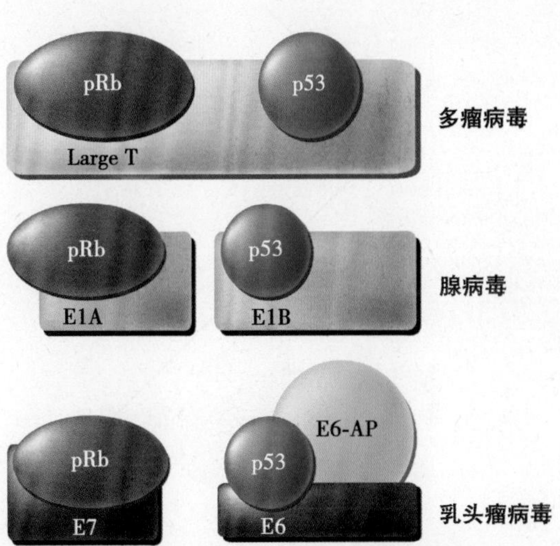

图 5-3 抑癌基因产物与 DNA 肿瘤病毒编码蛋白的相互作用示意图。来自多瘤病毒的大 T 抗原［如类人猿病毒 40（SV40）］结合视网膜母细胞瘤（pRB）和 p53 蛋白。对于腺病毒和高危人类乳头瘤病毒（16 型 HPV 和 18 型 HPV），多种病毒蛋白产物可与 pRB 和 TP53 形成复合物。一种被称为 E6 相关蛋白（E6-AP）的细胞蛋白与 HPV E6 蛋白形成复合物，协同降解 TP53

在细胞周期的正常进程中 pRB 的功能活性受磷酸化的调控。因此，pRB 在细胞周期的 G1 期主要是未磷酸化或低磷酸化状态，在 G2 期磷酸化水平达到峰值（图 5-4）。调节 pRB 功能最重要的磷酸化事件发生在 G1 与 S 期的交界阶段，由细胞周期蛋白和细胞周期依赖性蛋白激酶（CDK）复合物介导[34,40]。未磷酸化的 pRB 可与 E2F 家族的蛋白形成复合体，通过募集转录抑制蛋白抑制基因转录[40]。一旦被磷酸化，pRB 将不能与 E2F 有效结合（图 5-4）。E2F 则可与受分化调节的转录因子伴侣蛋白（DP）形成二聚体，激活一系列基因的表达，包括可调节或促进周期进入 S 期的蛋白如 DNA 聚合酶、胸腺嘧啶苷酸合成酶、核苷酸还原酶、细胞周期蛋白 E、二氢叶酸还原酶等[40]。在条件敲除小鼠模型中，E2F 蛋白可直接影响细胞的增殖[41]。现在也已经鉴定了其他一些与 pRB 结合的细胞蛋白，但与 pRB 与 E2F 的相互作用相比，它们的功能及其与 pRB 相互作用的意义尚不明确。毫无疑问，进一步的研究将会更好地揭示 pRB 和其同源蛋白 p107 和 p130[42] 的功能失活是如何影响肿瘤生长的。

TP53 基因

20 世纪 70 年代后期的研究发现了一种相对分子量约为

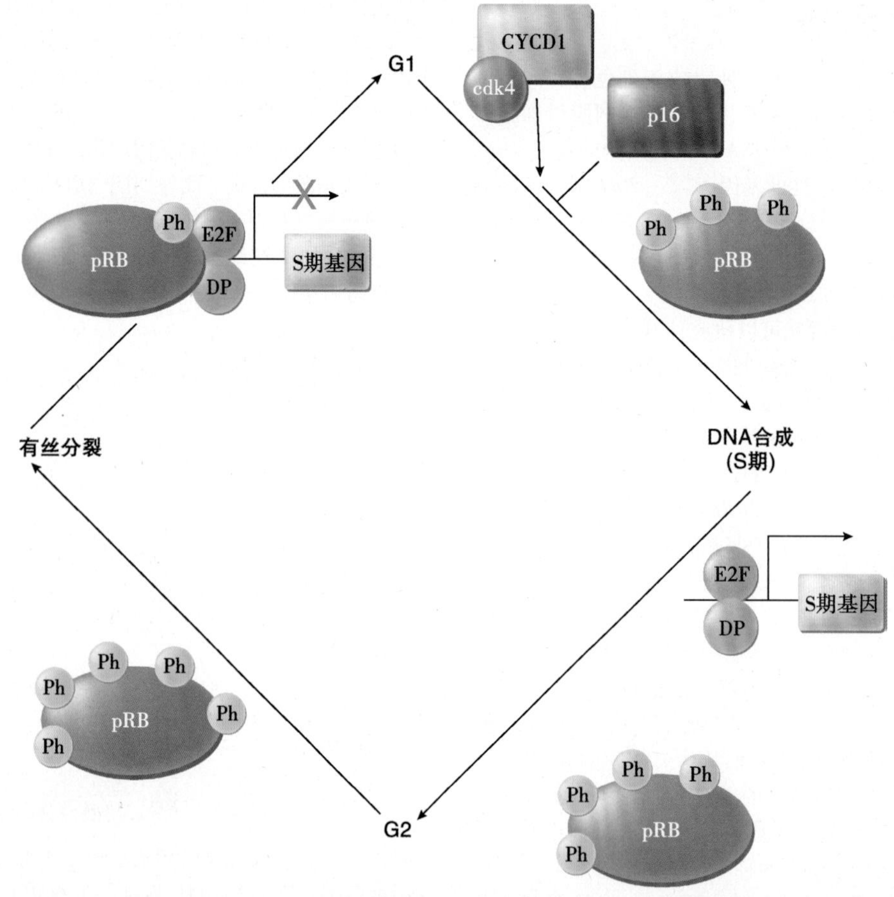

图 5-4　视网膜母细胞瘤蛋白(pRB)的功能在细胞周期中受磷酸化调控。pRB 蛋白在细胞周期的 G1 期为低磷酸化状态,在整个细胞周期的进程中特定位点的磷酸化(Ph)逐渐增加。在 DNA 合成(S 期)之前使 pRB 发生磷酸化的蛋白复合物包括一个周期蛋白(Cyc)和一个周期蛋白依赖的激酶(Cdk),例如周期蛋白 D1 和 Cdk4。CycD1/Cdk4 复合物受 p16 抑制蛋白调控,p16 抑制蛋白本身就是染色体 9p 上一个抑癌基因 *CDKN2* 的产物(见文)。低磷酸化的 pRB 可与转录调控蛋白 E2F 结合。当 pRB 通过与 E2F 蛋白的相互作用被带到基因启动子区,pRB 抑制 E2F/DP 靶基因的表达。pRB 的磷酸化将其从 E2F/DP 蛋白复合物中释放出来,导致包括参与 DNA 合成的基因在内的一系列基因活化。此图也表明,pRB 在 G2 期磷酸化增加,而在细胞周期的后期或接近后期 pRB 去磷酸化

53kD 的细胞磷蛋白,可与 SV40 的 T 抗原形成紧密复合物,此蛋白因而被命名为 p53 蛋白[43~45]。进一步的研究发现,TP53 也可与其他病毒癌基因产物如腺病毒 E1B 蛋白等形成复合物。*TP53* 在正常细胞中表达水平较低,但在许多肿瘤和肿瘤细胞系中呈高水平表达[43,46~48]。这些初步发现表明 *TP53* 水平的升高可能与癌症有关。与这一观点相一致的是,基因转移研究表明,*TP53* 在体外实验中具有癌基因的功能[49~51]。然而,随后对人类肿瘤的研究发现 *TP53* 实际上是一种抑癌基因[52]。

在多种类型的肿瘤如结肠直肠癌、膀胱癌、乳腺癌和肺癌中,常见染色体 17p 的杂合性丢失[53,54]。详细的基因定位显示,结直肠癌中所缺失的 17p 区域包含 *TP53* 基因[52]。对这些伴随 17p LOH 的肿瘤中保留的 *TP53* 等位基因序列的分析表明,此 *TP53* 等位基因发生了突变[52]。这与 Knudson 二次打击学说中关于抑癌基因预期变化的假设完全一致。很快,其他类型的肿瘤也观察到相同的结果,这些结果解释了许多以前 *TP53* 被认为是癌基因时出现的困惑[55~59]。基因转移研究提供了 *TP53* 在人类癌症中是抑癌基因的更多证据。但这种过表达研究并不容易解释,因为许多与肿瘤发生无关的基因也可以抑制转染细胞的生长[60~63]。基于对多种类型肿瘤的全基因组测序的结果,*TP53* 被认为是人类癌症中最常发生突变的基因[64]。

在 Li-Fraumeni 综合征(LFS)患者和小部分罹患肉瘤或骨肉瘤但不符合更严格的 LFS 诊断标准的儿科患者中存在着 *TP53* 的胚系突变[65~67]。LFS 患者罹患多种类型肿瘤的风险要高于正常人群,包括软组织肉瘤、骨肉瘤、脑肿瘤、乳腺癌和白血病。在 1/2~2/3 的 LFS 患者中,*TP53* 的胚系突变发生于编码序列的中心核心区域,这种突变类似于散发性癌症中常见的体细胞突变[68]。一些 LFS 患者及具有 LFS 表型特征的家系中,一种被称为 *hCHK2* 的基因中存在胚系突变,该基因可以磷酸化 TP53 并控制细胞对 DNA 损伤事件的应答反应[69]。

除了体细胞突变和遗传性突变外,*TP53* 的功能还可通过其他机制失活。前已述及,大多数宫颈癌患者含有高风险或者癌相关 HPV 的基因组(如 HPV 16 型或 18 型)。高风险而非低

风险型 HPV 的 *E6* 基因产物可与一种被称为 E6-AP（E6 相关蛋白）的细胞蛋白结合，促进 TP53 的降解[70~74]。在一部分软组织肉瘤患者中，染色 12q 区域的相关基因异常扩增[75]，导致称为小鼠双微基因 2（MDM2）的 TP53 结合蛋白发生过表达。最近许多研究发现，染色体 1q 区域的基因扩增，导致了另一种 TP53 结合蛋白 MDM4 在多种类型的肿瘤中过表达[76]。DNA 转染研究表明，*MDM2* 和 *MDM4* 基因在过表达时均可作为癌基因发挥作用，其可能是通过结合 TP53 并使其失活来发挥致癌功能的。这两种蛋白都能遮蔽 TP53 的转录激活域，促进 TP53 发生泛素化并加速其被蛋白酶体降解[77~79]。与 MDM2 是 TP53 的关键抑制因子的观点一致的是，*MDM2* 扩增和过表达的肉瘤很少存在 *TP53* 的体细胞突变[80]。在小鼠胚系细胞中破坏 *MDM2* 和 *MDM4* 基因会导致小鼠死亡，可能是因为这会引起 TP53 的活性失控。相应地，破坏小鼠 *TP53* 基因可使 MDM2 缺陷和 *MDM2* 缺陷小鼠不出现胚胎致死[81,82]。还有其他一些调节 TP53 功能的机制，包括一种称为核磷蛋白的核浆穿梭蛋白的突变，除急性早幼粒细胞白血病外，几乎 100%的成人急性髓系白血病细胞的胞质中均含有此蛋白[83]。

TP53 的功能

尽管 p53 的非转录功能也有报道（参考新近发表的综述），p53 蛋白的主要功能是一种转录调控蛋白[84,85]。野生型 p53 蛋白可通过其中央核心结构域与特定的 DNA 序列结合（图 5-5）。p53 的氨基末端序列是转录激活域，羧基端序列则是 p53 形成自体二聚体或四聚体所必需的。TP53 可激活一系列细胞周期调控基因的转录，包括 *WAF1/p21/CIP1*（编码调控 Cdk 活性的蛋白）[86]，*MDM2*（如上所述，编码 TP53 的负调控蛋白），和 14-3-3（调控 G2/M 进展的蛋白）[87]，和多种在细胞凋亡过程中起作用的基因，如 *PUMA* 和 *NOXA* 等。通过靶向同源重组来实验性地破坏这些基因，可模拟与 *TP53* 失活相关的一些表型[88,89]。

TP53 的绝大多数体细胞突变都是错义突变，导致蛋白质中心部分（第 5-9 号外显子）的氨基酸替换[90]。这些错义突变通过以下两种机制之中的一种，显著影响 p53 蛋白与相应 DNA 识别序列的结合能力[91]。有些突变（例如，248 或 273 位编码子的突变）改变了直接与序列特异性 DNA 结合的 *TP53* 的序列。其他突变（如 175 位密码子）可影响 TP53 的折叠，从而间接影响其与 DNA 的结合能力。通过"敲入"小鼠模型表明，这些错义突变能够带来"功能获得"（gain of function），而不是显性负效应（dominant negative effect），从而将精确的错义突变引入到内源性 *TP53* 基因[92~96]。

尽管 TP53 对 G2/M 期具有关键作用，在某些情况下，TP53 可在 G1/S 检查点起作用，调控细胞是否进入 DNA 合成期[97,98]。在其他情况下，TP53 可以决定细胞是否凋亡或程序性死亡[85]。对癌症治疗特别有意义的是，有数据表明，一些 TP53 功能缺失的肿瘤细胞对放疗和化疗药物（如顺铂等）不太敏感[92,99,100]。然而，对其他肿瘤细胞的研究表明，*TP53* 状态与细胞对化疗反应的关系正好相反，TP53 功能缺失的细胞对 DNA 损伤因子非常敏感，但对 5-氟尿嘧啶耐药[101]。迄今为止，对人类原发肿瘤的研究发现，*TP53* 突变状态与癌细胞对化疗和/或放疗的反应性之间可能存在非常复杂的关系。尤其很难区分 *TP53* 的突变对疾病自然进程的影响，与其对治疗和其他细胞压力反应的影响[102,103]。希望对 TP53 的进一步研究能够阐明它的正常功能，明确它在许多不同肿瘤中频繁失活的原因，以及其失活对肿瘤生长和治疗反应的影响。

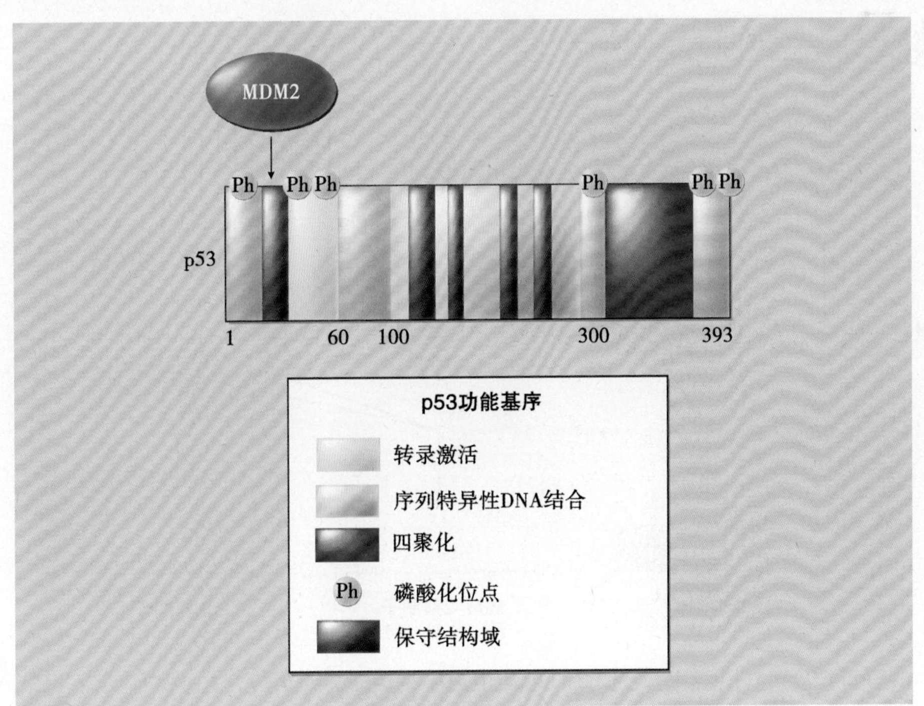

图 5-5　TP53 功能基序。该图展示了 *TP53* 参与转录激活、序列特异性 DNA 结合、四聚体化以及与 MDM2 蛋白结合的序列。该图标出了不同物种 p53 蛋白之间高度保守的 TP53 序列的五个不同区域。此外，此图还标明了 p53 蛋白中几个磷酸化（Ph）位点和调节 TP53 功能的位点的位置

周期蛋白依赖性激酶抑制剂 2A 位点

对染色体 9p 上细胞周期蛋白依赖性激酶抑制子 2A(*CDKN2A*)位点的研究很好地说明了，从多个方面对于一个特定的位点进行研究，如果结果趋向于一致，则该位点很可能是癌症发展的一个关键因素。9p 染色体的 LOH 常出现于多种不同类型的肿瘤中，包括黑色素瘤、胶质瘤、非小细胞肺癌、膀胱癌、头颈部癌和白血病等[104~107]。令人非常感兴趣的是，在一部分肿瘤中存在影响染色体 9p21 区域的纯合(完全)缺失[108~110]，这有力地说明该区域存在抑癌基因。除了肿瘤中染色体 9p 序列的频繁体细胞改变外，对一些遗传性黑色素瘤家族的连锁研究表明，一个黑色素瘤易感性基因也存在于相同的 9p 区域[111]。这些数据引起了人们对染色体 9p 区域的极大兴趣，该区域被认为含有一个或多个抑癌基因。研究者通过定位克隆的方法，获得了一个基因，其最初被称为多重肿瘤抑制因子 1(MTS1)[112]。对 *MTS1* 的序列分析表明，它与之前发现的 Cdk 抑制蛋白 p16 的编码基因的序列相同[113]。p16 蛋白通过抑制 Cdk4 和 Cdk6 发挥作用，因此又被称为细胞周期蛋白依赖性激酶 4 抑制蛋白(INK4)。另一个高度相关的基因可编码被称为 p15 的第二个 INK4 蛋白，其紧邻染色体 9p 上的 *p16/MTS1* 基因(图 5-6)。编码 p16 蛋白的基因通常被称为 *INK4A*，而编码 p15 的基因通常被称为 *INK4B*[114,115]。目前两者被批准的通用缩写分别为 *CDKN2A* 和 *CDKN2B*。

随后的研究表明，*CDKN2A* 的杂合突变存在于一些具有黑色素瘤或胰腺癌遗传易感性的家族中[116~119]。*CDKN2A* 的体细胞突变存在于多种不同类型的肿瘤中，包括但不限于黑色素瘤、胶质瘤、胰腺癌和膀胱癌以及白血病。在一些肿瘤中，影响 *CDKN2A* 基因的缺失也会影响 *CDKN2B* 基因[120]。在某些罕见的肿瘤中，缺失仅使 *CDKN2B* 失活，对 *CDKN2A* 无影响[120]。*CDKN2A* 突变的发生率和特异性在不同类型肿瘤之间存在显著的差异。与 *RB1*、*TP53* 等其他抑癌基因不同，纯合缺失是肿瘤中 *CDKN2A* 失活的一种较常见的机制[121]。

研究人员对 *CDKN2A* 位点的详细研究发现了一种新的转录产物。该转录产物包含与 $p16^{INK4A}$ 蛋白转录本相同的核苷酸序列，但具有独特的 5′序列(图 5-6)[114,115,122]。它编码一种称为 p14 替代阅读框蛋白($p14^{ARF}$)。值得注意的是，人类 $p14^{ARF}$ 与最初鉴定的小鼠蛋白 $p19^{ARF}$ 是相同的，$p19^{ARF}$ 因其分子量被命名为 p19。

$p14^{ARF}$ 转录本包含一个特殊的第一外显子(外显子 1β)。外显子 1α 是第一个出现在 p16 转录本中的外显子(图 5-6)。$p14^{ARF}$ 的转录本中外显子 1β 与外显子 2、外显子 3 依次拼接。$p14^{ARF}$ 和 $p16^{INK4A}$ 蛋白的转录本都含有外显子 2 与外显子 3，但两者的蛋白序列完全不同，原因是 $p14^{ARF}$ 的翻译始自外显子 1β 的一个特殊甲硫氨酸密码子，并延续到外显子 2，采用了与 $p16^{INK4A}$ 完全不同的开放读码框。对 *CDKN2A* 位点的体细胞突变和遗传突变的深入研究表明，使 $p16^{INK4A}$ 蛋白失活的局部突

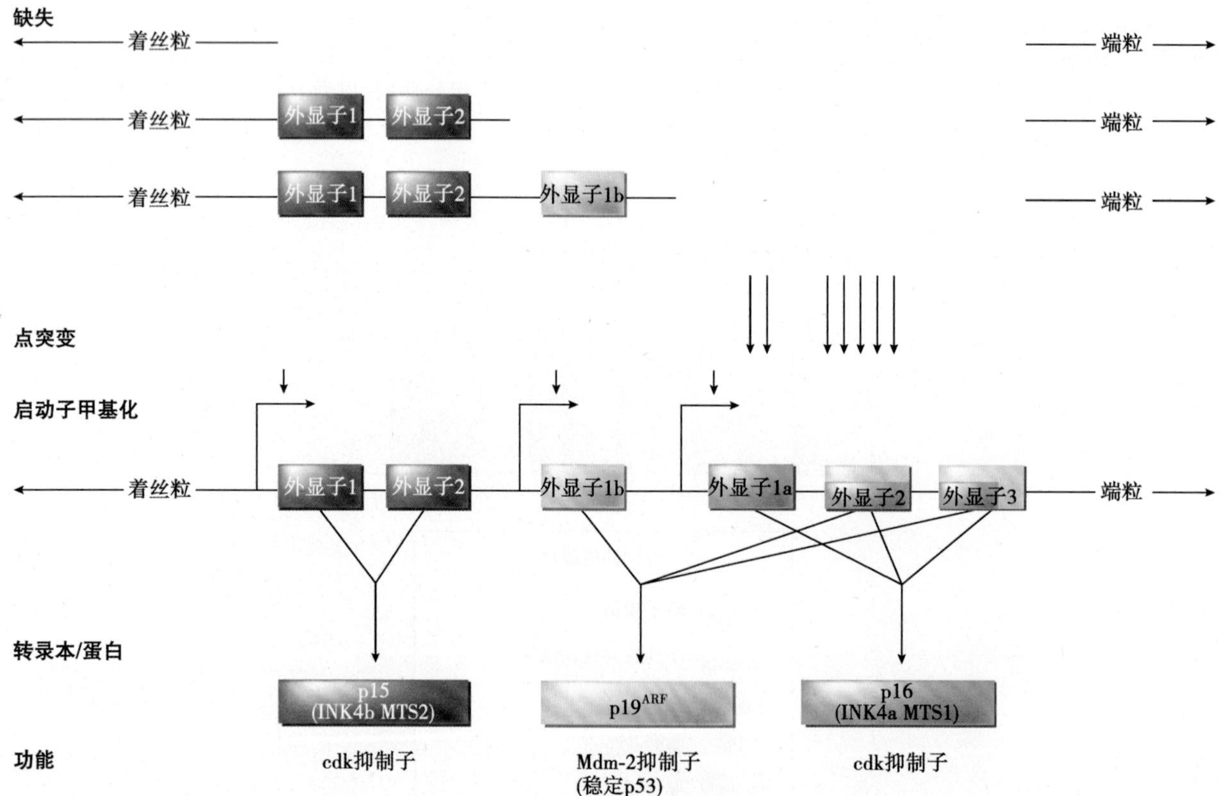

图 5-6 *CDKN2B*(p15)和 *CDKN2A*(p16/$p19^{ARF}$)位点的基因组结构、突变位点和转录产物。图中显示了 p15、p16 和 p19ARF 转录产物的来源，以及人类癌症中具有代表性的基因组缺失、点突变(长箭头)和启动子甲基化(短箭头)。*CDKN2B* 和 *CDKN2A* 位点的外显子以矩形表示。该图还标出了它们的转录产物/蛋白及其可能的功能。棕色矩形表示编码 *p15* 的转录产物中的开放阅读框；黄色矩形表示编码 p19ARF 的转录产物中的开放阅读框；橘色矩形表示编码 p16 的转录产物中的开放阅读框。图中基因位点、外显子和转录产物的大小并未按比例显示

变在人类癌症中很常见——已鉴定出 60 多个胚系突变，但使 p14ARF 失活的局部突变并不常见[114,115]。然而，频繁发生的 *CDKN2A* 位点的纯合缺失意味着突变失活的 p14ARF、p16INK4A 以及 p15INK4B 可能在肿瘤发生的过程中有很强的选择性（图 5-6）。其他研究表明，在某些类型的肿瘤中，p16INK4A 分子和 p14ARF 的表达丢失是由 *CDKN2A* 位点处 DNA 调控序列的甲基化导致的（图 5-6）[123~125]。最近的研究表明，DNA 甲基转移酶在启动和维持 p16 抑癌基因的表观遗传沉默中有重要的作用[126,127]。此外，对胚系 p14ARF 和 p16INK4A 失活小鼠的研究表明，这些蛋白在体内有抑癌基因的功能[128~130]。

p16INK4A 蛋白通过抑制 Cdk4 的活性来调控细胞的致瘤性生长。如前所述，pRB 磷酸化可以影响其在转录水平调控 E2F 靶基因的能力（图 5-4）。周期蛋白 D1/Cdk4 复合物在调节 pRB 磷酸化和功能方面发挥着关键的作用[124]。因此，p16INK4A 蛋白通过调节 Cdk4 的活性，反过来影响 pRB 的磷酸化。据推测，p16INK4A 的失活会导致 pRB 的异常磷酸化，并导致高度磷酸化的 pRB 无法结合 E2F，从而使 pRB 无法适当调控 G1-S 转化过程中相关基因的表达。p14ARF 通过直接与 MDM2 蛋白结合，抑制 MDM2 诱导的 TP53 降解，从而维持 TP53 在细胞中的适当功能[115]。p14ARF 发挥抑癌基因作用的模式与 p16INK4A 维持正常 pRB 功能的机制类似。

然而，与这一解释相反的是，p14ARF 和 TP53 的改变在癌细胞中经常共存，这表明它们不会改变同一通路；而 Rb 和 p16INK4A 的改变在细胞内是互斥的，支持了它们影响着相同通路的事实[131]。这些发现强调了癌基因和抑癌基因不能单独起作用的概念。相反，它们是在错综复杂的级联或网络中发挥作用，而这些级联或网络对肿瘤的发生和治疗都有重要的影响[85,132]（图 5-7）。

结肠腺瘤样息肉病基因

结肠腺瘤样息肉病基因的鉴定及胚系突变

少数遗传性综合征中出现的结肠癌是由息肉引起的。一种息肉病综合征被称为家族性腺瘤样息肉病（FAP）或结肠腺瘤样息肉病（APC）。FAP 是一种常染色体显性遗传病。在美国，每 8 000 人中就有 1 人罹患 FAP。该综合征的特征是在青年患者的结肠和直肠中出现大量腺瘤样息肉。典型的 FAP 患者，其一生中患结肠癌的风险极高，到 60 岁时几乎 100%的患者会罹患结肠癌。

有 FAP 特征但无家族病史的患者，其染色体 5q 会出现中间缺失，这一发现极大地帮助了 APC 基因的定位[133]。后续的

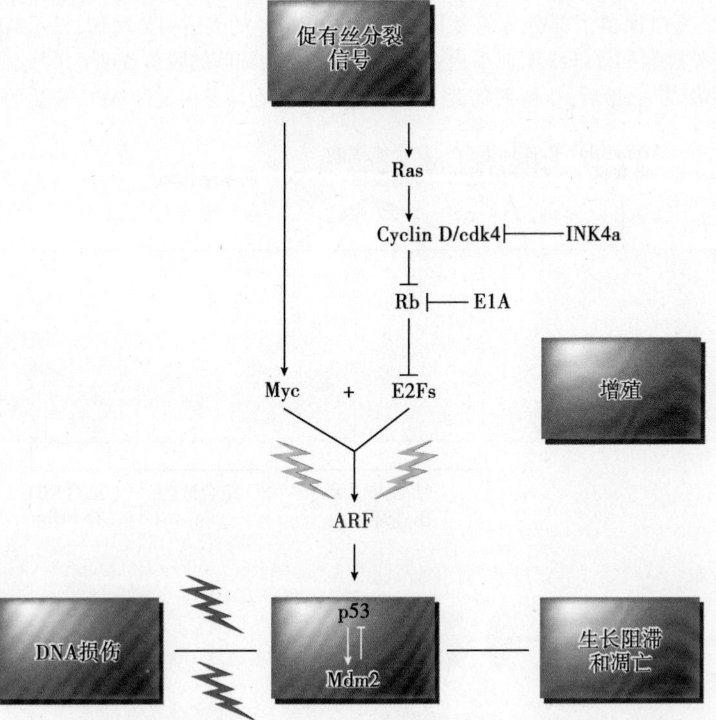

图 5-7　p19*RF 蛋白在检查点控制中的作用。p19ARF 蛋白（ARF）会对细胞增殖通常所需的增殖信号做出反应。当这些信号超过一个临界阈值时，ARF 依赖的检查点（黄色闪电）被激活，ARF 引起 TP53 依赖的反应，诱导细胞生长停滞和/或凋亡。目前已知的引起 ARF-TP53 信号通路活化的因子包括 Myc、E1A 和 E2F-1。总的来说，"上游"癌蛋白，如突变的 *RAS* 等位基因的产物、组成型激活的受体或细胞质内信号转导癌蛋白等，也可能通过周期蛋白 D-Cdk4-RBE2F 或 MYC 依赖通路（这两信号通路通常都是细胞进入 S 期所必需的）激活 ARF。p16INK4A 可通过抑制细胞周期蛋白 d 依赖性激酶抑制促有丝分裂信号的活性。在图中，E1A 通过拮抗（至少是部分拮抗）RB 的功能而发挥作用。简言之，Myc 和 E2F-1 被证明只能通过影响 ARF 而激活 TP53，尽管外源性过表达这些蛋白可以在 ARF 阴性细胞中以比较低的效率激活 TP53。ARF 对 TP53 的激活可能依赖于 Mdm2 特定功能的失活。DNA 损伤信号（如电离和紫外线辐射、低氧应激）通过多种信号通路激活（蓝色闪电）TP53

DNA 连锁研究证实,在多个罹患 FAP 或相关的被称 Gardner 综合征的家系中,其息肉病表型与 DNA 标记物在染色体 5q21 附近出现分离[134,135]。1991 年,研究人员应用定位克隆的方法明确了 *APC* 基因为 FAP 的致病基因[136~139]。*APC* 基因很大,有超过 15 个外显子,可变剪接会影响其转录产物的 5′非翻译区。*APC* 的主要转录产物编码了一种成人多种组织中表达的含 2 843 个氨基酸残基的蛋白。

绝大多数 FAP 患者的 *APC* 基因中都能发现杂合性胚系突变[140~142]。在 FAP 患者中,所有的胚系 *APC* 突变都可使 APC 蛋白功能失活。绝大部分胚系突变是 *APC* 基因编码区近 5′端的无义或移码突变(图 5-8)。与 Knudson 的二次打击学说相一致,在相关肿瘤中可以发现剩余的野生型 *APC* 等位基因会因体细胞突变而失活[143,144]。虽然在家族性腺瘤性息肉病的患者中,其肠外肿瘤(如颌骨骨瘤和硬纤维瘤)易感性的具体分子机制尚不明确,*APC* 基因特定位点的胚系突变的确与临床特征存在相关性[145]。然而,现在我们对息肉病家系中息肉数量不同的原因也有一定的了解[143,146]。*APC* 基因 5′端的突变,与 APC 成瘤能力减弱有关。后者是因为核糖体重新进入了 APC 转录产物中提前终止密码子的下游,导致翻译而成的 APC 蛋白保留了部分正常功能[146]。与 *APC* 基因中三分之一段的突变相比,3′端三分之一段的突变与较轻的息肉表型相关,这一结果可能也是由于突变后的 APC 蛋白保留了部分抑癌基因的功能[146]。出乎意料的是,结肠外肿瘤如硬纤维瘤似乎更常见于 *APC* 基因 3′端存在突变的患者[143]。最后,在德系犹太人家庭中发现了发生于 *APC* 基因的中间部位的可增加结直肠癌易感性的错义突变[147]。这种突变不会改变基因产物的功能,但会制造一个高度可变的"热点",导致在其周围核苷酸中发生体细胞性缺失或插入,从而产生截短体。

散发性结肠肿瘤中的体细胞突变

在普通人群中由胚系 *APC* 突变引起的结直肠癌十分罕见(只存在于约 0.5%的结肠癌中),*APC* 基因的体细胞突变存在于绝大多数散发性结直肠腺瘤和结直肠腺癌中[148]。在很多散发的结直肠腺瘤和癌中,含有 *APC* 基因的染色体 5q 区域可能会受到杂合性丢失的影响。这一发现提示 *APC* 基因的失活可能在结肠肿瘤中普遍存在[54,149]。自 *APC* 基因被鉴定以来,研究人员对结直肠肿瘤中可导致 *APC* 基因失活的体细胞突变进行了详细的分析。散发性肿瘤中 *APC* 基因的体细胞突变与 FAP 患者中 *APC* 基因的胚系突变在性质上和位置上是类似的(图 5-8)。目前的研究结果表明,在不同大小或病理特征的结直肠肿瘤中,多达 90%的肿瘤都含有可导致 APC 基因失活的体细胞突变[143~150]。

功能

APC 基因编码一种大小约为 300kD 的庞大蛋白,该蛋白被认为可以调控结肠隐窝处细胞的黏附、迁移或凋亡。APC 蛋白定位于结肠上皮细胞基底侧的细胞膜,在接近隐窝顶部的细胞中 APC 的表达明显增加,提示 APC 可能在细胞到达隐窝顶点时调控细胞的脱落或凋亡[151]。与这一观点相一致的是,有报道称,在缺乏内源性 APC 表达的结直肠癌细胞中恢复 APC 蛋

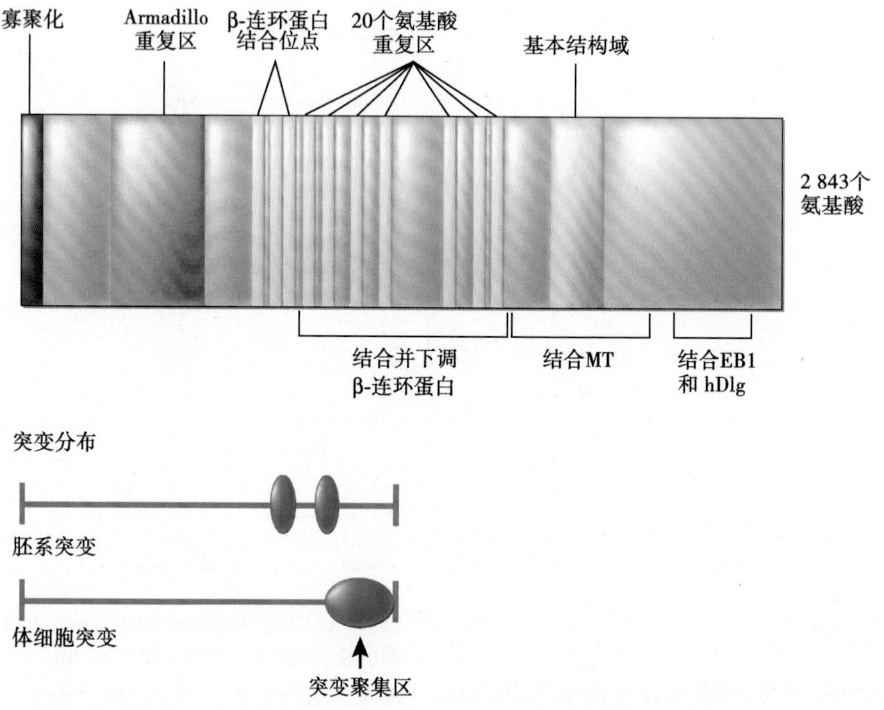

图 5-8 Apc 蛋白结构域与突变分析结果的示意图。不同 Apc 结构域的相对位置。在 Apc 蛋白的氨基端存在一个参与同源寡聚化的假定结构域。该图还标出了与果蝇 armadillo 蛋白相似但功能未知的重复序列、介导与 β-连环蛋白结合并下调其功能的序列、位于羧基端 1/3 处的基本结构域(可易化 Apc 蛋白与微管(MT)形成复合体)),以及位于羧基末端的序列(可与 EB1 和 hDlg 相互作用)。*APC* 基因(主要是终止链)的胚系突变分布在序列的 5′端的一半序列中,在 1061 和 1309 密码子处有两个明显的"热点"。结直肠癌中 *APC* 基因的体细胞突变似乎集中在一个被称为"突变簇区域"的区域,而在 1309 和 1450 密码子处的突变最为常见

白表达可促进其凋亡[152,153]。

APC 蛋白可与多种蛋白质结合，包括 β 连环蛋白（β-catenin）、Y 连环蛋白（Y-catenin，也称为斑珠蛋白）、糖原合成酶激酶 3β（GSK3β）、末端结合蛋白 1（EB1）、人类果蝇大光盘（hDLG）、微管及相关蛋白轴蛋白（axin）和行为素（conductin）[154]。除 β-连环蛋白、GSK3β、行为素和轴蛋白外，现在 APC 与其他蛋白的相互作用的意义还不是很清楚。很多证据提示 APC 蛋白对 β-连环蛋白有很重要的调控作用[154,155]。β-连环蛋白是一种细胞内高表达的蛋白。它通过结合 α-连环蛋白，使细胞间黏附分子 E-cadherin 的胞质区和皮层肌动蛋白的细胞骨架相连接。在很多结直肠癌中截短的（突变的）APC 蛋白缺少某些或者全部的与 β-连环蛋白结合的关键重复模序。除了可与 β-连环蛋白结合外，APC 蛋白还可以与 GSK3β 一起，和其他蛋白如轴蛋白和行为素协同，通过磷酸化调节 β-连环蛋白在细胞质中的含量。在 APC 突变或者 APC 不能有效调控 β-连环蛋白的结直肠癌中，β-连环蛋白在细胞内聚集并与 T 细胞转录因子 4（TCF-4）形成复合物并进入细胞核（图 5-9）。β-连环蛋白入核后将作为转录共激活因子，活化受 Tcf-4 调控的基因如 Wnt 的表达，而由 APC 失活引起的 β-连环蛋白活化可以绕过其调节蛋白如 Wnt。与 β-连环蛋白是 APC 调控的重要靶点的观点一致，在少数缺少 *APC* 突变的结直肠癌患者中发现存在 β-连环蛋白的体细胞突变[156-158]。这些突变都可改变 β-连环蛋白氨基端的 GSk3β 共有磷酸化位点，可能会使 β-连环蛋白耐受 APC 与 GSK3β 介导的降解，使其具有致癌性。尽管 APC 体细胞突变在结肠和直肠以外的肿瘤中很少见，但 β-连环蛋白氨基端的致癌性突变却存在于多种不同类型的癌症中[159,160]。

Wilms 肿瘤基因

Wilms 肿瘤是儿童最常见的肾脏肿瘤，约占所有儿童癌症的 6%[161]。Wilms 肿瘤在许多方面与视网膜母细胞瘤类似：均可发生在双侧或单侧，有单个或多个病灶，并以散发性或遗传性的方式发生。也可以用视网膜母细胞瘤的两次突变模型来解释 Wilms 肿瘤[162]。然而，Wilms 肿瘤患者中遗传性病例并不像在视网膜母细胞瘤患者中那样常见。几乎所有携带遗传性 *RB1* 基因位点突变的患者都可能罹患视网膜母细胞瘤，但是只有大约 50% 携带肾母细胞瘤致病基因胚系突变的患者会罹患肾母细胞瘤（即低外显率）[161]。

最早有关 Wilms 肿瘤遗传学基础的发现来自 1964 年的一篇报道。该报道介绍了同时患有 Wilms 肿瘤和散发性无虹膜畸形（即先天性无虹膜）的 6 位患者[163]。研究者认为可能是影响一个或多个基因位点的染色体异常（现在常称为相邻基因综合征）导致了这两种非常罕见的情况同时发生，即一个位点突变可能导致无虹膜，另外一个位点的突变则会导致 Wilms 肿瘤。在随后的研究中发现在患有 WAGR 综合征（伴无虹膜畸形的 Wilms 肿瘤、泌尿生殖系统异常、智力低下）的儿童中，其外周血样本中存在染色体 11p13 中间缺失[164]，从而证实了这一假说。对少数散发性 Wilms 肿瘤组织进行的细胞遗传学研究发现，这些肿瘤中染色体 11p13 带存在缺失或易位[165,166]。随后研究人员使用限制性片段长度多态性（RFLP）探针对来自 Wilms 肿瘤患者的肿瘤及配对的正常细胞进行研究，发现在遗传性和散发性 Wilms 肿瘤患者中常存在染色体 11p 的杂合性丢失[167~170]。

通过分析 WAGR 综合征患者肿瘤的基因失活突变，以及一小部分患有单侧 Wilms 肿瘤但无相关先天畸形患者的肿瘤

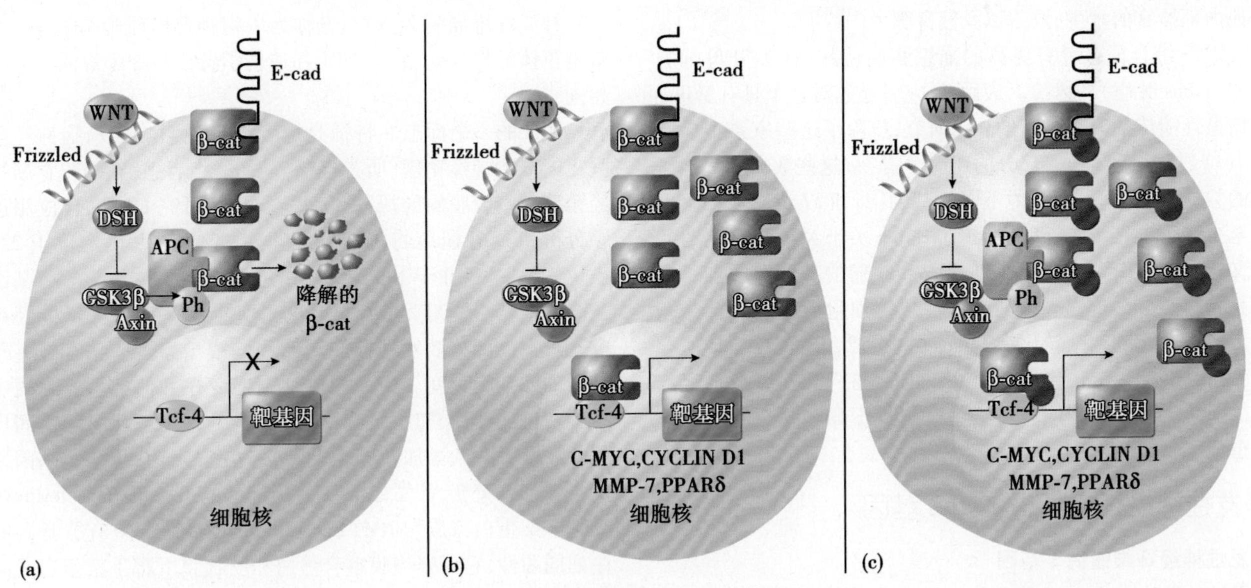

图 5-9　Apc、轴蛋白和 Gsk3β 蛋白在正常细胞中调节 β-连环蛋白（β-cat）的功能，以及 Apc 或 β-cat 缺陷对肿瘤细胞影响的模式图。β-Cat 是一种含量丰富的细胞蛋白，大部分 β-Cat 与细胞黏附蛋白 E-cadherin（E-cad）的胞质结构域结合。（a）在正常细胞中，糖原合成酶激酶 3β（Gsk3β）、Apc 和轴蛋白促进胞质内游离的 β-cat 的降解（可能是 Gsk3β 引起 β-cat N 端序列发生磷酸化的结果）。激活的 Wnt 通路可抑制 Gsk3β 的活性和 β-cat 降解，这是 Frizzled 受体和 Dsh 信号蛋白作用的结果。（b）在结直肠癌等肿瘤细胞内 Apc 突变导致 β-cat 积累并与转录因子 Tcf-4 结合，引起 Tcf-4 靶基因 *c-myc*、周期蛋白 D1、*MMP-7*、PPARS 等的转录激活（见文中所述）。（c）癌细胞中 β-cat 的点突变和微小缺失抑制 Gsk3β 和 Apc 引起的 β-cat 的磷酸化和降解，从而导致 *c-myc* 等 Tcf-4 靶基因的激活

的体细胞突变，研究人员于 1990 年鉴定了 Wilms 肿瘤基因（*WT1*）[171]。*WT1* 基因包含 10 个外显子，其转录本易被选择性剪接[172,173]。相对于 *RB1*、*P53* 和 *APC* 等基因相对广泛的表达，*WT1* 基因的表达似乎仅限于胚胎肾组织和少部分其他组织[174,175]。*WT1* 基因的 mRNA 编码的蛋白分子量约为 45-49kD，具有 4 个锌指结构域。一开始研究人员根据其氨基酸序列推测，WT1 蛋白具有转录调控功能[174]。尽管一些 WT1 亚型可能在 RNA 加工过程中起作用而非发挥转录调控的功能，但是有几项研究证实了 WT1 的确具有转录调节功能[173,174]。WT1 蛋白可抑制许多生长诱导基因启动子元件的转录活性，包括早期生长反应基因-1（EGR1）、胰岛素样生长因子 2（IGF-2）和血小板衍生生长因子 A 链（PDGFA），这表明 WT1 基因可能在基因抑制中起作用[176]。其他一些研究表明，根据细胞种类和启动子环境的不同，WT1 基因能激活或抑制基因表达[177]。近期研究表明，WT1 能激活表皮生长因子家族成员之一——双调蛋白（amphiregulin）的表达[178]，这与 WT1 可能具有转录激活生理功能的观点相一致。Amphiregulin 表达的缺失可能会导致 Wilms 肿瘤进展时去分化。近期的研究显示，某些 *WT1* 基因差异剪接体具有完全不同的调节基因表达的作用，这也增加了 WT1 作为转录调节因子的复杂特性[179,180]。

在 WAGR 综合征患者中，*WT1* 基因的失活可明显促进 Wilms 肿瘤的进展。此外，在将近 10% 的散发性肾母细胞瘤患者中能检测到 *WT1* 基因的体细胞突变[181]。然而，大量证据表明，其他基因的突变也可引起 Wilms 肿瘤。首先，在 Wilms 肿瘤患者中，染色体 11p 区等位基因缺失通常涉及 11p15，而非含有 *WT1* 基因的 11p13 带[181~183]。其次，染色体 11p15 区域包含一个可导致 Beckwith-Wiedemann 综合征（BWS，一种先天性异常）的基因。BWS 综合征患者表现为肾脏、胰腺内分泌部以及其他内部器官的增生，巨舌以及偏身肥大[184,185]。

BWS 综合征患者有更高的罹患胚胎性肿瘤（如肝母细胞瘤和 Wilms 肿瘤）的风险。最后，研究者通过对三个具有 Wilms 肿瘤显性遗传的家系进行的连锁研究，排除了这些家系中易感位点与 11p 染色体任何部分的连锁[186,187]。这些数据和其他研究的数据表明，至少有三种不同的基因[即 *WT1*、*BWS* 基因，以及至少一个不在 11p 染色体上（在 Haber 关于 X 染色体基因的论文提及）的基因]的胚系突变使 Wilms 瘤的易感性增加。最终是否需要多个这样基因的遗传性和体细胞突变的组合才能将发育中的肾脏细胞转化为 Wilms 肿瘤，或者是否存在其他导致 Wilms 肿瘤的遗传途径，仍有待确定。在 Wilms 肿瘤中观察到的遗传异质性与视网膜母细胞瘤明显不那么复杂的遗传途径形成了重要的对比。

多发性神经纤维瘤病 1 和 2 基因

多发性神经纤维瘤病 1 基因

Von Recklinghausen 病又称神经纤维瘤病 1（NF1），是一种显性遗传性综合征，具有多种疾病表现。神经纤维瘤病 1 的共性特征是病变会累及来自神经嵴的组织。NF1 患者除了几乎全部发生神经纤维瘤外，罹患嗜铬细胞瘤、神经鞘瘤、神经纤维肉瘤和原发性脑瘤的风险也较高[188~190]。通过连锁分析，NF1 基因最初定位于染色体 17q 的近着丝粒区[191,192]。后来，通过对 2 例 NF1 患者的核型研究发现了涉及染色体 17q11 带的胚系染色体重排[193,194]。在进一步的工作中，发现这两例患者均有染色体 17q11 带的局灶性遗传改变。研究人员针对该染色体区域进行了大量的定位克隆工作，最终在 1991 年鉴定出了 *NF1* 基因[195~197]。*NF1* 基因是很大，其 DNA 跨越 350kb，编码一个分子量约为 300kD 的蛋白。尽管 *NF1* 基因的胚系突变被认为是所有或几乎所有 NF1 患者相关疾病特征的基础，但只在大约一半至三分之二的 NF1 患者中发现了特定的 *NF1* 胚系突变[188,190,198,199]。针对如此庞大的一个基因，其突变检测方法存在不同程度的缺陷和不敏感性，使得在其余 NF1 患者中检测 *NF1* 基因胚系突变很困难。到目前为止，已经发现了超过 1 500 种关于此基因不同的突变。

除了在 NF1 患者存在 *NF1* 基因的胚系突变外，在一部分结直肠癌、黑色素瘤、神经母细胞瘤和来自骨髓增生异常综合征患者的骨髓细胞中，*NF1* 基因也存在体细胞突变[188,198,200~202]。与预期的抑癌基因作用一致，这些突变使 *NF1* 失活。对神经纤维瘤病患儿中出现的白血病的研究清楚地表明，与 Knudson 模型的预测一致，在肿瘤形成过程中，*NF1* 基因的两个拷贝都发生了失活[203]。同 *RB1*、*TP53* 和 *APC* 基因类似，*NF1* 基因的表达也十分广泛。因此，和其他遗传性肿瘤综合征一样，多发性神经纤维瘤病患者的恶性肿瘤组织特异性的原因令人费解。*NF1* 基因编码的蛋白被称为神经纤维瘤蛋白（neurofibromin），是鸟苷三磷酸（GTP 酶）活化蛋白家族（GAP）的一个成员[188,204~206]。RAS-GAP 可能是研究得最充分的 GAP，它能明显增强野生型 K-Ras、H-Ras 和 N-Ras 蛋白的 GTP 酶活性。虽然目前 *NF1* 基因缺陷影响细胞生长的机制尚未完全阐明，但推测很可能是由于神经纤维瘤蛋白功能的失活，导致了小 Ras 样 GTP 酶所调控的信号通路发生了改变所致[207]。

神经纤维瘤病 2 基因

神经纤维瘤病 2（NF2，也称为中枢神经纤维瘤病）是一种常染色体显性疾病，它与 NF1 在遗传学特征和临床特征上均不相同[188,208,209]。

NF2 的一个标志性特征是患者会出现影响第八脑神经前庭支的双侧神经鞘瘤（听神经瘤）。NF2 患者患脑膜瘤、脊髓神经鞘瘤和室管膜瘤的风险也明显增加。研究人员联合应用连锁分析和 LOH 研究将神经纤维瘤病 2（NF2）基因定位于 22q 染色体[210~212]，并于 1993 年采用定位克隆的方法将 *NF2* 基因克隆[213,214]。在 NF2 患者中可检测到使 *NF2* 基因失活的胚系突变。在一部分散发性神经鞘瘤和脑膜瘤患者中也存在 *NF2* 基因的体细胞突变。*NF2* 的体细胞突变在其他类型的肿瘤中并不常见。然而，初步研究表明，尽管在 NF2 患者中恶性间皮瘤的发生率并未增加[209]，但在恶性间皮瘤患者中 *NF2* 基因常发生体细胞突变[215,216]。NF2 基因编码的一种蛋白质 Merlin 与细胞骨架蛋白家族[ERM（Ezrin/Radixin/Moesin）]有非常高的序列同源性，它可充当膜整合蛋白和丝状膜下脚手架蛋白之间的连接蛋白[214]。因此，*NF2* 基因的改变可能（至少在一定程度上）通过对细胞形状、细胞间相互作用和/或细胞运动的影响促进了肿瘤的发展。

Von Hippel-Lindau 基因

Von Hippel-Lindau（VHL）综合征是一种罕见的显性疾病，受累个体易患中枢神经系统和视网膜血管网织细胞瘤、透明细胞型肾癌和嗜铬细胞瘤[217~219]。连锁分析发现 *VHL* 基因定位于染色体 3p 区段。与许多其他遗传性癌症相关基因一样，LOH 研究表明 *VHL* 基因是典型的抑癌基因，在肿瘤发生过程中其两个等位基因都会出现失活[218,220]。*VHL* 基因在 1993 年经定位克隆被鉴定[221]。

在表现出 VHL 综合征特征的家族中，大多数个体含有使一个 VHL 等位基因失活的胚系突变[217~219]。与其他一些遗传性癌症综合征一样，研究者已初步观察到 VHL 基因型与表型的关系。具体来说，某一类的 *VHL* 胚系突变只与肾癌的发生有关；第二类突变与肾癌和嗜铬细胞瘤的易感性有关；而第三类突变只与嗜铬细胞瘤有关[218]。80%以上的散发性透明细胞型肾细胞癌患者存在 *VHL* 基因的体细胞突变，但在其他病理学类型的肾细胞癌（如乳头状癌）中未发现此类突变[218,219]。大约 20%的散发性透明细胞肾癌未检测到 *VHL* 基因突变。然而，在许多这样的病例中，*VHL* 基因可能由于表观遗传学因素而沉默失活[222]，这一失活机制与本章前面提到的 *CDKN2A* 位点失活有关。*VHL* 基因的失活在除透明细胞型肾癌以外的其他类型肿瘤中并不常见的[218]。

VHL 基因编码一个由 213 种氨基酸组成的蛋白，其主要功能是通过蛋白降解来调控血管生成。*VHL* 编码的蛋白是泛素连接酶复合物的一部分，该复合物在氧气存在下可以降解缺氧诱导因子 1a（HIF-1a）。正常细胞缺氧或肿瘤细胞发生 *VHL* 突变，会稳定 HIF-1a 转录因子，导致血管内皮生长因子等细胞因子表达，从而刺激血管生成。血管生成是与肿瘤形成相关的最重要的间质过程之一，对 *VHL* 和肾细胞癌的生物化学和细胞生物学的进一步研究可能有助于我们加深对肿瘤血管生成机制的理解[223,224]。

基因组稳定性相关基因

已经发现一些由 DNA 损伤识别和修复相关的基因失活而导致的隐性癌症易感综合征，包括共济失调毛细血管扩张症（ataxia telangiectasia，AT）、Bloom 综合征、着色性干皮病和 Fanconi 贫血。在以上不同的综合征中，癌症的类型和增加患癌风险的 DNA 损伤因子都各不相同。AT 杂合子可轻微增加罹患乳腺癌的风险[225]，但在其他隐性癌症综合征中，只有纯合子才能显著增加罹患癌症的风险。此研究结果与前面描述的显性癌症易感性综合征（即：遗传性视网膜母细胞瘤、FAP、NF1 和 NF2）形成鲜明的对比——在这些综合征中，杂合子能显著增加个体的患癌风险。可能由于这种纯合子具有胚胎致死性，因此抑癌基因突变纯合体即使存在，也会非常罕见。需要注意的很重要的一点是，抑癌基因不仅可抑制癌症的发生，其主要的功能是调控正常细胞的平衡；它们的失活和正常的胚胎发育是不相容的。

由于隐性癌症综合征十分罕见，因此，对肿瘤中基因组稳定性调控基因功能的讨论重点将集中于常染色体显性遗传综合征。这些综合征包括家族性癌症中最常见的类型，主要是结肠、乳腺和其他器官肿瘤。

DNA 错配修复基因缺陷和遗传性非息肉性结直肠癌

结肠癌的家族聚集性很早已被人们所认识，大约 5%的结肠癌可归因于对癌症风险有很强影响的遗传性基因缺陷，另外 10%～15%的结肠癌则含有对癌症风险有中度影响的遗传性基因缺陷。在西方社会，由 *APC* 基因的胚系突变引起的结直肠癌病例约占全部病例的 0.5%～1%，而遗传性非息肉病性结直肠癌（hereditary nonpolyposis colorectal cancer，HNPCC）则占 2%～4%[226~228]。

尽管患者在癌症确诊前没有明显的临床症状，或者结肠癌在一个家族中聚集可能是偶然的，但目前已经建立了一套诊断标准，可以鉴别那些最有可能患 HNPCC 的个人和家族[226~229]。典型的诊断标准包括：①排除家族性息肉病；②至少有三个亲属罹患结直肠癌，其中一个是其他亲属的一级亲属；③连续两代或以上患病；④至少有一人在确诊时未满 50 周岁。虽然并非所有 HNPCC 患者都符合这些标准，但该标准可以排除有显著不同遗传基础的家族聚集性结直肠癌[226,228]。

已经鉴定出几个与 HNPCC 相关的基因，包括染色体 2p 上的 mutS 同源物 2 和 6（*MSH2*，*MSH6*），染色体 3p 上的 mutS 同源物 1（*MLH1*），染色体 7p 上的减数分裂后分离 2（*PMS2*）[226,228~231]。几乎所有典型的 HNPCC 病例中都会检测到这四个基因的胚系突变。*MSH2* 和 *MLH1* 基因的蛋白产物在 DNA 错配的识别和修复中起着关键作用（图 5-10）。细胞中 DNA 错配修复（*MMR*）基因的两个等位基因一个正常而另一个突变时，DNA 修复几乎不受影响。然而，在正常的上皮细胞，这个正常的等位基因会因为体细胞突变而失活。这种“第二次打击”破坏了 MMR 的功能，因此细胞在随后的分裂周期中可能会产生大量的突变。由于这些突变优先发生在单核苷酸、二核苷酸和三核苷酸重复序列（如微卫星序列区）中，因此这种表型通常被称为微卫星不稳定性（MSI）表型[226]。

尽管大约 15%～20%的结肠癌具有 MSI 表型，但只有 2%～4%的结直肠癌患者中存在已知的 MMR 基因胚系突变[226,229~234]。显然，只有一小部分具有 MSI 表型的散发性结直肠癌是由已知的 MMR 基因的胚系突变引起的。MMR 基因的体细胞突变存在于某些具有 MSI 表型的散发性结直肠癌中[235]。然而，在大多数散发病例中，*MLH1* 基因的失活是由表观遗传失活所致[236,237]。

MMR 缺陷细胞中产生的许多突变可能对细胞生长有害。少部分突变有可能激活癌基因或使抑癌基因失活。在 MMR 缺陷的肿瘤细胞中，一些基因是优先突变的，可能是因为这些突变会赋予细胞选择性生长的优势。例如，在这些癌症中，含有重复 DNA 序列的基因如微卫星束有可能成为突变的靶点。这一预测已获得了数据的支持。

BRCA1 和 BRCA2 基因

与结直肠癌一样，家族病史一直是乳腺癌的主要危险因素。一级亲属中多人罹患乳腺癌的人群，其患癌风险最高。然而，直到 20 世纪 80 年代末才有证据表明，某些家族乳腺癌的易感性可归因于高外显率的常染色体显性等位基因。在 1990 年，Hall 和他的同事发现了一个乳腺癌易感基因 *BRCA1*，其定位于染色体 17q21[238]。其他人发现，*BRCA1* 的胚系突变会大大增加罹患乳腺癌和卵巢癌的风险[239,240]。随着对 *BRCA1* 定位的染色体 17q 区域的深入研究，研究者最终于 1994 年通过定位克隆技术对该基因进行了鉴定[241,242]。

乳腺癌患者 *BRCA1* 基因胚系突变的研究取得了令人瞩目的进展。通过对有四个或更多 60 岁之前就确诊为乳腺癌或/

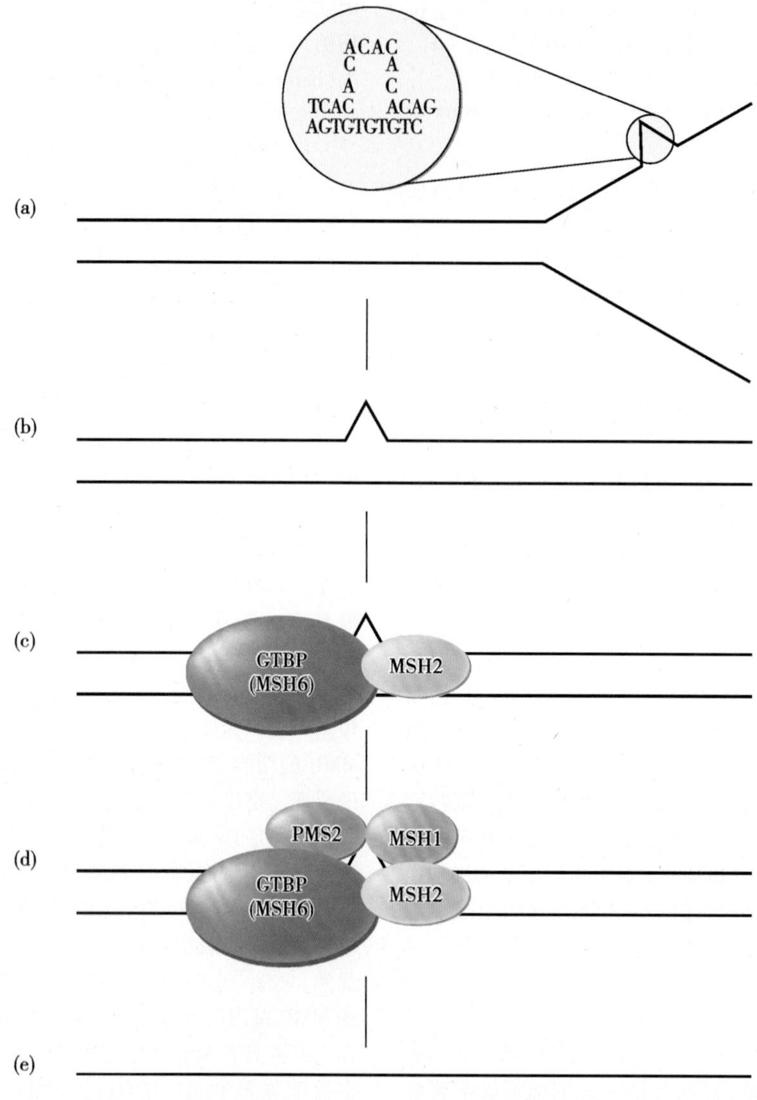

图 5-10 人类细胞中的错配修复途径。(a,b)DNA 复制过程中可能会发现 DNA 的错配,比如链滑动(图中显示)或碱基的错误插入(图中未显示)。(c)DNA 错配可被 MutS 同源物识别。最常执行此功能的是 Msh2 和 GTBP/Msh6。但在某些情况下,另外一种 MutS 同源物 Msh3 可替代 GTBP/Msh6。(d,e)MutL 同源物,比如 Mlh1 和 Pms2 被募集到 Msh2/Msh6 复合体。DNA 错配在一系列蛋白的作用下被修复,这些蛋白包括核酸外切酶、解旋酶、DNA 聚合酶以及 DNA 连接酶

和卵巢癌的家庭成员的家系进行研究,研究者发现近 50%的家系有 *BRCA1* 基因的胚系突变[243~245]。事实上,在同时罹患乳腺癌和卵巢癌的家系中,约有 75%的家系存在 *BRCA1* 基因的胚系突变,这可能是导致其癌症易感的原因[243,244]。目前已经鉴定出多种不同的 *BRCA1* 基因胚系突变,大多数突变会导致该基因合成截短的 BRCA1 蛋白[243,244]。大多数 *BRCA1* 基因的胚系突变只在一个或几个家系中被发现,有一些突变则频繁地出现。目前 11 种最常见的 *BRCA1* 基因突变,约占观察到的全部突变的 45%[244,245]。事实上,*BRCA1* 基因两个最常见的突变(185 delAG 和 5382 insC)约占突变总数的 10%。值得注意的是,位于 *BRCA1* 基因 185 位密码子的移码突变涉及两个碱基(腺嘌呤和鸟嘌呤)的缺失(185 delAG),20 多个家族性乳腺癌或卵巢癌的犹太人家系中存在该突变。此外,不考虑癌症家族史的情况下,对德系犹太人的人口调查表明,大约有 1%的人群携带了 185 delAG 基因突变[244~246]。*BRCA1* 基因胚系突变的家系研究表明,携带失活突变的人群,其一生中患乳腺癌和卵巢癌的风险分别为 85%和 50%[243,244,247]。目前尚不确定相比携带其他 *BRCA1* 基因突变的人群,携带某些特定的 *BRCA1* 基因胚系突变的人群的罹患乳腺癌和卵巢癌的风险是否更高。

对大多数抑癌基因而言,存在很多与其相关的家族性癌症综合征,同样,*BRCA1* 基因的胚系突变也可导致机体细胞内存在一个突变的等位基因。然后,通过图 5-2 所示的机制,第二个野生型等位基因失活后就会产生癌症。在 *BRCA1* 基因(和 *BRCA2*)相关的病例中,引起 *BRCA1* 基因失活的第二次"打击"通常是剩余野生型等位基因的杂合性丢失。此外,研究者在大约 50%的未经筛选的乳腺癌患者和 65%~80%的未经筛选的卵巢癌患者中都发现了 *BRCA1* 基因位点的杂合性丢失[244,248]。由于大多数乳腺癌和卵巢癌并无遗传易感性(即它们是散发

的)，因此以上研究提示 BRCA1 在散发性乳腺癌和卵巢癌的发病中发挥了重要的作用。然而，尽管有这些 LOH 的数据，但散发性乳腺癌和卵巢癌病例中很少出现 *BRCA1* 基因突变，这表明大多数散发性肿瘤至少仍有一个野生型的等位基因[244,248]。令人意外的是，这一发现提示 BRCA1 基因在较常见的、非家族性的乳腺癌和卵巢癌的发生中并不起作用。但是，在散发性乳腺癌和卵巢癌患者中，BRCA1 蛋白的下游效应分子仍有可能发生改变，从而提示在这类癌症发生中起重要作用的是信号通路，而不是基因本身[249]。

虽然在大约 40%～50% 的有多个乳腺癌患者的家系中，*BRCA1* 基因的胚系突变是癌症易感性的基础，但另一种称为 *BRCA2* 的高外显率常染色体显性易感基因，在很多无 *BRCA1* 突变的多乳腺癌患者家系中也有重要的作用。1994 年发现 *BRCA2* 基因定位于染色体 13q12-q13 区[250]，并于 1995 年通过定位克隆的方法鉴定了该基因[251]。尽管 *BRCA1* 和 *BRCA2* 基因的胚系突变引起女性患乳腺癌的风险相似(终生患癌的风险约为 80%)，但相对于 *BRCA1* 突变会导致 40%～50%的卵巢癌患病风险而言，*BRCA2* 突变导致的卵巢癌患病风险只有约 10%。男性 *BRCA1* 突变携带者的终生乳腺癌患病风险仅为 1%[252]，与之不同的是，男性 *BRCA2* 突变携带者患乳腺癌的风险则会显著升高，终生风险约为 7%。男性和女性 *BRCA2* 突变携带者患胰腺癌和其他几种癌症的风险也会有所增加[244]。和 *BRCA1* 的情况一样，在一些散发的乳腺癌、胰腺癌、头颈部和其他部位的癌症中已经观察到染色体 13q12 区处的 *BRCA2* 位点的杂合性缺失，而不是在 13q14 区的 *RB1* 位点处，这表明 *BRCA2* 可能是肿瘤中体细胞突变的目标。然而，与 *BRCA1* 一样，在散发性癌症中很少检测到体细胞 BRCA2 的突变[244]。这再次表明，在这些散发性癌症中，遗传学改变的靶点是信号通路，而不是基因本身。

BRCA1 和 *BRCA2* 基因各自编码一个很大的核蛋白。这两种蛋白质的氨基酸序列彼此之间或与其他已知蛋白质之间只有很短的相似区域。由于它们缺乏明显的功能基序，因此早期很难阐明 BRCA1 和 BRCA2 基因在细胞中的功能。但一些证据表明，这两个蛋白都可直接或间接与酵母 Rad51 的同源蛋白发生相互作用(Rad51 具有修复断裂双链 DNA 的功能)[253～260]。此外，BRCA1、BRCA2 和 Rad51 蛋白都存在于细胞核内一个稳定的多蛋白复合体中。因此，有人认为 BRCA1 和 BRCA2 可能在 DNA 损伤(特别是双链 DNA 断裂)修复反应中发挥了作用[261]。其他研究结果则提示 BRCA1 和 BRCA2 可能在转录调控中发挥了作用[262]。虽然 DNA 修复和转录调控是截然不同的两种功能，但两者可能被一个称为转录偶联 DNA 修复的过程联系起来[255]。这一观点已有先例，因为某些引起着色性干皮病的一些核苷酸切除修复基因也能在转录中发挥作用[263]，修复某些类型的 DNA 损伤确实需要与转录相偶联[264]。

候选抑癌基因

表 5-1 总结了前面讨论的抑癌基因和其他抑癌基因。它们的区别在于前者的胚系失活性突变与遗传性癌症的易感性有关。胚系突变与罹患癌症风险升高之间的相关性为基因在肿瘤发生中的作用提供了毋庸置疑的证据。其他的发现，例如在散发性癌症中发现的某一抑癌基因等位基因位点的杂合性缺失伴随着另一位点的体细胞突变，为很多遗传性癌症易感基因可能有更广泛作用的观点提供了证据。虽然表 5-1 中的抑癌基因确实与遗传性癌症综合征有关，但正如 *APC* 基因 I1307K 突变的发现一样，其他抑癌基因的胚系突变引起癌症发生的风险可能没那么高。本章节末列出了所有已报道的抑癌基因的完整列表，实际上该列表也随着癌症深入测序研究中不断出现的新数据而不断地在更新。根据这些测序研究中发现的基因失活突变率，研究者估计在各种类型的人类癌症中大约有 100 个抑癌基因在发挥作用[64]。这些基因中的大多数只是体细胞性失活，不会引起遗传性癌症易感综合征。

表 5-1　与遗传性肿瘤易感综合征相关的部分抑癌基因和稳定性基因

基因[a]	综合征	遗传模式	信号通路[b]	主要遗传性肿瘤类型[c]
APC	FAP	显性	APC	结肠、甲状腺、胃、小肠
AXIN2	息肉病	显性	APC	结肠
CDH1(E-cadherin)	家族性胃癌	显性	APC	胃
GPC3	Simpson-Golabi-Behmel 综合征	X-连锁	APC	胚胎
CYLD	家族性圆柱瘤	显性	APOP	Pilotrichomas
EXT1，*EXT2*	遗传性多发性骨软骨瘤	显性	GLI	骨
PTCH	Gorlin	显性	GLI	皮肤，成神经管细胞瘤
SUFU	成神经管细胞瘤易感体质	显性	GLI	皮肤，成神经管细胞瘤
FH	遗传性副神经节瘤	显性	HIF1	平滑肌瘤
SDHB，*SDHC*，*SDHD*	家族性副神经节瘤	显性	HIF1	副神经节瘤、嗜铬细胞瘤
VHL	von Hippel-Lindau	显性	HIF1	肾
TP53(*p53*)	Li-Fraumeni	显性	TP53	乳腺、肉瘤、肾上腺、脑等

续表

基因[a]	综合征	遗传模式	信号通路[b]	主要遗传性肿瘤类型[c]
WT1	家族性 Wilms 肿瘤	显性	TP53	Wilms 瘤
STK11(*LKB1*)	黑斑息肉综合征	显性	PI3K	小肠、卵巢、胰腺
PTEN	Cowden	显性	PI3K	错构瘤、胶质瘤、子宫
TSC1,*TSC2*	结节性硬化	显性	PI3K	错构瘤、肾
CDKN2A(*p16INK4A*,*p14ARF*)	家族性恶性黑色素瘤	显性	RB	黑色素瘤、胰腺
CDK4	家族性恶性黑色素瘤	显性	RB	黑色素瘤
RB1	遗传性视网膜母细胞瘤	显性	RB	眼
NF1	神经纤维瘤	显性	RTK	神经纤维瘤
BMPR1A	青年型多发性息肉病	显性	SMAD	胃肠道
MEN1	Ⅰ型多发内分泌肿瘤	显性	SMAD	甲状旁腺、垂体、胰岛细胞、类癌
SMAD4(*DPC4*)	青年型多发性息肉病	显性	SMAD	胃肠道
BHD	Birt-Hogg-Dube	显性	?	肾、毛囊
HRPT2	甲状旁腺功能亢进-颌肿瘤	显性	?	甲状旁腺、颌纤维瘤
NF2	神经纤维瘤	显性	?	脑膜瘤、听神经瘤
MUTYH	息肉病	隐性	BER	结肠
ATM	共济失调毛细血管扩张	隐性	CIN	白血病、淋巴瘤、脑
BLM	Bloom	隐性	CIN	白血病、淋巴瘤、皮肤
BRCA1,*BRCA2*	遗传性乳腺癌	显性	CIN	乳腺、卵巢
FANCA, *FANCC*, *FANCD2*, *FANCE*,*FANCF*,*FANCG*	范可尼贫血 A,C,D2,E,F,和 G 型	隐性	CIN	白血病
NBS1	Nijmegen 断裂综合征	隐性	CIN	淋巴瘤、脑
RECQL4	Rothmund-Thomson 综合征	隐性	CIN	骨、皮肤
WRN	Werner 综合征	隐性	CIN	骨、脑
MSH2,*MLH1*,*MSH6*,*PMS2*	HNPCC	显性	MMR	结肠、子宫
XPA,*XPC*;*ERCC2*,*ERCC3*,*ERCC4*,*ERCC5*;*DDB2*	着色性干皮病	隐性	NER	皮肤

[a] 该表列出了所有主要的信号通路和遗传性易感性肿瘤的代表性基因。所列名称为通用基因缩写，括号内是其他名称。

[b] 在很多情况下，一种基因参与了多条信号通路。此表为每个基因列出了单独的信号通路，此通路代表了该基因“最可能”涉及的通路，但不排除还有其他信号通路。

[c] 在大多数情况下，由基因的体细胞突变引起的非家族性肿瘤谱包括了发生在家族性病例中的肿瘤和其他类型肿瘤。例如，*TP53* 和 *CDKN2A* 突变除了分别在易患 Li-Fraumeni 综合征和家族性恶性黑色素瘤的人群中存在，很多其他的肿瘤也存在 *TP53* 和 *CDKN2A* 突变。

APC，结肠腺瘤样息肉病；APOP，细胞凋亡信号通路；BER，碱基剪切修复；CIN，染色体不稳定性；FAP，家族性腺瘤样息肉病；GLI，胶质瘤相关癌基因；HIF1，缺氧诱导因子 1；MMR，错配修复；NER，核苷酸剪切修复；PI3K，磷脂酰肌醇 3 激酶；RB，视网膜母细胞瘤；RTK，受体酪氨酸激酶；SMAD，SMA-和 MAD 相关蛋白 4；WT；野生型。

对 RNA 的研究已经发现了大量在癌症中转录水平降低的基因。一些此类基因最初被称为抑癌基因仅仅是基于其表达的减少。这些基因中的少部分可能确实在生长调控中发挥着关键的作用，但基因表达数据提供的证据不足以与癌症的发生建立因果关系。基因在癌症中表达的改变更多地反映了癌症的影响（即与发生癌症的组织或器官中的正常细胞相比，癌细胞生长和分化特性的改变及其微环境的异常），而不是肿瘤发生的原因。此外，非生理性、高水平的外源性表达许多在癌症中不起作用的基因可能会显著改变细胞的生长，从而导致对我们无法对这些候选基因的功能进行正确的分析。最后，研究者在定义某个基因在肿瘤发生中具有因果作用并将其认定为抑癌基因之前，应仔细权衡相关的功能证据。目前唯一公认的鉴定抑癌基因的方法是：在特定类型的癌症中，该基因存在大量统计学上高度显著的失活突变[64]。

总结

大量的证据表明，抑癌基因的突变是大多数常见人类癌症的主要分子决定因素。目前，利用分子克隆技术已鉴定出数十种抑癌基因。某些情况下，这些基因是胚系失活的，它们的失活容易导致癌症。更多的情况下，这些抑癌基因在肿瘤发展过程中会因体细胞突变而失活。

尽管我们对于抑癌基因的了解已经比较深入，但仍然有大量工作需要去做。随着对抑癌基因的正常细胞功能以及这些正常功能如何被基因突变所破坏的研究不断深入，我们对肿瘤发生机制的理解也将不断深入。有必要指出的是，抑癌基因与癌基因不同，通常不会成为药物的直接靶点：所有药物都旨在使其靶蛋白失活，而抑癌基因在癌症中已经失活。因此，对癌症中抑癌基因突变进行临床应用最好的策略可能是靶向其相应的上调的下游通路。所以，了解这些基因发挥作用的信号通路至关重要。

（于乐兴 译 杨文 孙文 校）

参考文献

The complete reference list can be found on the Wiley Companion Digital Edition of this title (see inside front cover for login instructions).

1 Broca P. Etiologie des productions accidentelles. *Traite des Tumerus*. 1866: 147–157.

4 Boveri T. *The Origin of Malignant Tumors*. Baltimore, MD: Williams and Wilkins; 1929.

10 Stanbridge EJ, Der CJ, Doersen CJ, et al. Human cell hybrids: analysis of transformation and tumorigenicity. *Science*. 1982;**215**(**4530**):252–259.

15 Knudson AGJ. Mutation and cancer: statistical study of retinoblastoma. *Proc Natl Acad Sci U S A*. 1971;**68**(**4**):820–823.

19 Sparkes RS, Murphree AL, Lingua RW, et al. Gene for hereditary retinoblastoma assigned to human chromosome 13 by linkage to esterase D. *Science*. 1983;**219**(**4587**):971–973.

21 Knudson AG Jr. Hereditary cancer, oncogenes, and antioncogenes. *Cancer Res*. 1985;**45**(**4**):1437–1443.

22 Cavenee WK, Dryja TP, Phillips RA, et al. Expression of recessive alleles by chromosomal mechanisms in retinoblastoma. *Nature*. 1983;**305**(**5937**):779–784.

26 Dryja TP, Rapaport JM, Joyce JM, Petersen RA. Molecular detection of deletions involving band q14 of chromosome 13 in retinoblastomas. *Proc Natl Acad Sci U S A*. 1986;**83**(**19**):7391–7394.

35 Whyte P, Buchkovich KJ, Horowitz JM, et al. Association between an oncogene and an anti-oncogene: the adenovirus E1A proteins bind to the retinoblastoma gene product. *Nature*. 1988;**334**(**6178**):124–129.

43 DeLeo AB, Jay G, Appella E, Dubois GC, Law LW, Old LJ. Detection of a transformation-related antigen in chemically induced sarcomas and other transformed cells of the mouse. *Proc Natl Acad Sci U S A*. 1979;**76**(**5**):2420–2424.

52 Baker SJ, Fearon ER, Nigro JM, et al. Chromosome 17 deletions and p53 gene mutations in colorectal carcinomas. *Science*. 1989;**244**(**4901**):217–221.

54 Vogelstein B, Fearon ER, Hamilton SR, et al. Genetic alterations during colorectal-tumor development. *N Engl J Med*. 1988;**319**(**9**):525–532.

69 Bartek J, Falck J, Lukas J. CHK2 kinase—a busy messenger. *Nat Rev Mol Cell Biol*. 2001;**2**(**12**):877–886.

75 Oliner JD, Kinzler KW, Meltzer PS, George DL, Vogelstein B. Amplification of a gene encoding a p53-associated protein in human sarcomas. *Nature*. 1992;**358**(**6381**):80–83.

76 Marine JC, Jochemsen AG. Mdmx and Mdm2: brothers in arms? *Cell Cycle*. 2004;**3**(**7**):900–904.

85 Vogelstein B, Lane D, Levine AJ. Surfing the p53 network. *Nature*. 2000;**408**(**6810**): 307–310.

86 el-Deiry WS, Tokino T, Velculescu VE, et al. WAF1, a potential mediator of p53 tumor suppression. *Cell*. 1993;**75**(**4**):817–825.

88 Waldman T, Kinzler KW, Vogelstein B. p21 is necessary for the p53-mediated G1 arrest in human cancer cells. *Cancer Res*. 1995;**55**(**22**):5187–5190.

89 Yu J, Wang Z, Kinzler KW, Vogelstein B, Zhang L. PUMA mediates the apoptotic response to p53 in colorectal cancer cells. *Proc Natl Acad Sci U S A*. 2003;**100**(**4**):1931–1936.

90 Hollstein M, Hergenhahn M, Yang Q, Bartsch H, Wang ZQ, Hainaut P. New approaches to understanding p53 gene tumor mutation spectra. *Mutat Res*. 1999;**431**(**2**):199–209.

92 Jeffers JR, Parganas E, Lee Y, et al. Puma is an essential mediator of p53-dependent and -independent apoptotic pathways. *Cancer Cell*. 2003;**4**(**4**):321–328.

101 Bunz F, Hwang PM, Torrance C, et al. Disruption of p53 in human cancer cells alters the responses to therapeutic agents. *J Clin Invest*. 1999;**104**(**3**): 263–269.

112 Kamb A, Gruis NA, Weaver-Feldhaus J, et al. A cell cycle regulator potentially involved in genesis of many tumor types. *Science*. 1994;**264**(**5157**): 436–440.

121 Cairns P, Polascik TJ, Eby Y, et al. Frequency of homozygous deletion at p16/CDKN2 in primary human tumours. *Nat Genet*. 1995;**11**(**2**):210–212.

124 Jacobs JJ, Kieboom K, Marino S, DePinho RA, van Lohuizen M. The oncogene and Polycomb-group gene bmi-1 regulates cell proliferation and senescence through the ink4a locus. *Nature*. 1999;**397**(**6715**):164–168.

126 Bachman KE, Park BH, Rhee I, et al. Histone modifications and silencing prior to DNA methylation of a tumor suppressor gene. *Cancer Cell*. 2003;**3**(**1**):89–95.

131 Vogelstein B, Kinzler KW. Cancer genes and the pathways they control. *Nat Med*. 2004;**10**(**8**):789–799.

132 Schmitt CA, Fridman JS, Yang M, et al. A senescence program controlled by p53 and p16INK4a contributes to the outcome of cancer therapy. *Cell*. 2002;**109**(**3**):335–346.

136 Groden J, Thliveris A, Samowitz W, et al. Identification and characterization of the familial adenomatous polyposis coli gene. *Cell*. 1991;**66**(**3**):589–600.

143 Kinzler KW, Vogelstein B. Lessons from hereditary colorectal cancer. *Cell*. 1996;**87**(**2**):159–170.

145 Nieuwenhuis MH, Vasen HF. Correlations between mutation site in APC and phenotype of familial adenomatous polyposis (FAP): a review of the literature. *Crit Rev Oncol Hematol*. 2007;**61**(**2**):153–161.

152 Morin PJ, Vogelstein B, Kinzler KW. Apoptosis and APC in colorectal tumorigenesis. *Proc Natl Acad Sci U S A*. 1996;**93**(**15**):7950–7954.

162 Knudson AG Jr, Strong LC. Mutation and cancer: a model for Wilms' tumor of the kidney. *J Natl Cancer Inst*. 1972;**48**(**2**):313–324.

167 Fearon ER, Vogelstein B, Feinberg AP. Somatic deletion and duplication of genes on chromosome 11 in Wilms' tumours. *Nature*. 1984;**309**(**5964**):176–178.

171 Call KM, Glaser T, Ito CY, et al. Isolation and characterization of a zinc finger polypeptide gene at the human chromosome 11 Wilms' tumor locus. *Cell*. 1990;**60**(**3**):509–520.

181 Haber DA, Housman DE. The genetics of Wilms' tumor. *Adv Cancer Res*. 1992;**59**:41–68.

188 Gutman D. Neurofibromatosis type 1. In: Kinzler KW, ed. *The Genetic Basis of Human Cancer*. New York, NY: McGraw-Hill; 1998:423–442.

203 Shannon KM, O'Connell P, Martin GA, et al. Loss of the normal NF1 allele from the bone marrow of children with type 1 neurofibromatosis and malignant myeloid disorders. *N Engl J Med*. 1994;**330**(**9**):597–601.

207 Patrakitkomjorn S, Kobayashi D, Morikawa T, et al. NF1 tumor suppressor, neurofibromin, regulates the neuronal differentiation of PC12 cells via its associating protein, collapsin response mediator protein-2. *J Biol Chem*. 2008;**283**(**14**):9399–9413.

218 Linehan WM. Renal carcinoma. In: Kinzler KW, ed. *The Genetic Basis of Human Cancer*. New York, NY: McGraw-Hill; 1998:455–474.

226 Boland CR. Hereditary nonpolyposis colorectal cancer. In: Kinzler KW, ed. *The Genetic Basis of Human Cancer*. New York, NY: McGraw-Hill; 1998:333–346.

229 Lynch HT, de la Chapelle A. Genetic susceptibility to non-polyposis colorectal cancer. *J Med Genet*. 1999;**36**(**11**):801–818.

236 Herman JG, Umar A, Polyak K, et al. Incidence and functional consequences of hMLH1 promoter hypermethylation in colorectal carcinoma. *Proc Natl Acad Sci U S A*. 1998;**95**(**12**):6870–6875.

238 Hall JM, Gryfe R, Kim H, et al. Linkage of early-onset familial breast cancer to chromosome 17q21. *Science*. 1990;**250**(**4988**):1684–1689.

243 Collins FS. BRCA1—lots of mutations, lots of dilemmas. *N Engl J Med*. 1996;**334**(**3**):186–188.

第 6 章　表观遗传在人类癌症中发挥的作用

James G. Herman, MD ■ Stephen B. Baylin, MD

概述

在过去的 20 年中,我们对癌症发生发展机制的理解取得了令人兴奋的进展:我们逐渐认识到,这类疾病不仅是由遗传变化驱动,而且也由表观遗传变化驱动[1~4]。严格地说,表观遗传是指在分裂的体细胞中可遗传的基因表达的改变,这种改变不依赖于 DNA 碱基序列的变化[5~7]。该定义包含了两条与癌症中表观遗传改变及其临床重要性的重要信息。首先,癌症表观遗传变化时其编码和非编码基因的 DNA 序列保持不变,不依赖不可逆的碱基突变。其次,与此密切相关的是,这些表观遗传变化是可能被逆转的,如此则能够恢复正常的基因表达,使野生型基因的固有功能得以重现[1,2,4,7~10]。

表观遗传变化对癌症的发生发展至关重要,这一认识来源于我们对人类基因组如何正确地控制基因表达的理解—人类基因组通过 DNA 的染色质组装,能够在不同的组织和发育过程中调控基因的表达[5~7,11]。例如,表观遗传过程在正常胚胎发育和成体细胞更新过程中起着重要作用,尽管细胞具有一样的 DNA 序列,表观遗传决定了在发育和分化期间不同的细胞表型。随着我们对基因调控的认知不断增长,我们对癌症发生发展的关键表观遗传变化的全面理解也在迅速加深,但相对而言,这种理解可能仍处于早期阶段。然而,我们已经学到了很多,包括从表观遗传学角度出发对基本的癌症生物学和癌症发生发展的理解,这些知识具有明显的转化应用前景,本章将对此进行讨论。

基因表达的表观遗传调控机制

染色质的形成

虽然基因表达的所有基本信息都存在于 DNA 的主要碱基序列中,我们可将 DNA 序列视为存储这种基本编码的"硬盘",但细胞中基因表达的模式取决于 DNA 在合成和复制后是如何被修饰的,以及它是如何在细胞核中被蛋白质或染色质包裹起来进行排列的[5~7,11]。因此后一种包装过程可以看作是"软件",它可以读出 DNA 序列中包含的"硬盘"信息。DNA 修饰和染色质包装的主要作用是平衡基因组,使大多数 DNA 处于沉默或低转录状态,以防止在进化过程中累积的重复序列、潜在转座因子和病毒插入序列的不必要表达[5,6,12]。DNA 包装的第一个要素是它与组成染色质的蛋白质的相互作用。染色质的基本支架蛋白是组蛋白,组蛋白与 DNA 组装形成核心部件即核小体(图 6-1),核小体的形成对于细胞核中 DNA 的排列至关重要[13,14]。

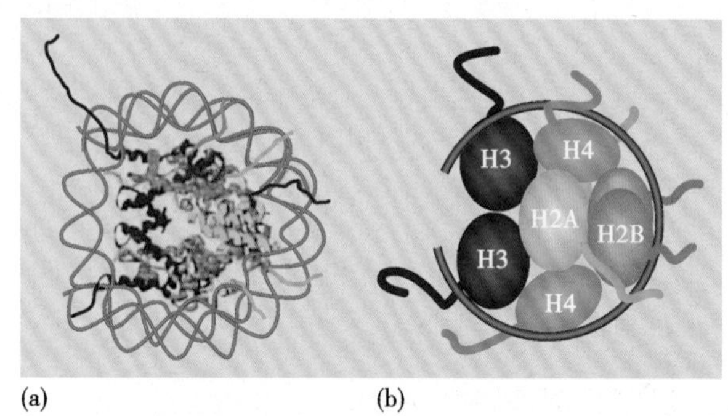

图 6-1　核小体的结构。(a)DNA 双螺旋缠绕在组成性组蛋白的蛋白质结构周围的模式图,如文中所述。(b)示意图显示了 DNA 上组蛋白 H3/H4 四聚体的构架,两组 H2A/H2B 二聚体形成的组蛋白核心与 DNA(黑线)缠绕在一起。可以看到组蛋白尾部的氨基末端从八个组蛋白组成的核小体核心中突出

核小体由约 146bp 的 DNA 缠绕核心组蛋白 H2A、H2B、H3 和 H4 组成的八聚体两圈组成[13,14]。在 DNA 基因表达谱的功能调控中,不仅核小体必须正确地沿 DNA 线性分布,还必须排列成更高阶的多核小体结构[13,14](图 6-2)。这些动态变化是由染色质重塑蛋白介导的。沿着 DNA 线性排列的核小体,其分布越广、排列越不规则,高级结构的致密程度越低,染色质越"开放",DNA 越容易进行基因转录(图 6-2),这种情况常常出现在活化基因启动子的内部及周围区域。相反,核小体分布越规则、越均匀,其高级结构越致密(图 6-2),染色质越"闭合",对基因转录的抑制作用越强。后一种构像在人类基因组中占主导地位,正如前所述,可以防止不必要的基因表达并保持染色质的结构稳定。

核小体的功能依赖于染色质的状态,这与上述染色质的动态结构密切相关。染色质状态取决于活化和抑制性的组蛋白"修饰"的不同比例[6,7,11,14,15]。这些修饰主要位于从核小体组装体突出的组蛋白尾部的关键氨基酸上,包括赖氨酸乙酰化、赖氨酸和精氨酸甲基化、丝氨酸和苏氨酸磷酸化、谷氨酸 ADP-核糖基化、赖氨酸泛素化和类泛素化这些形式[6,7,11,14,15]。

这些修饰标记间的平衡形成了最初被称为的"组蛋白代码",现在人们意识到这要比预想的更复杂。这些修饰与核小体的定位一并参与基因组的组装,使得组成型和细胞类型依赖的特定染色质模式在不停的细胞分裂过程中保持开放和/或封闭的构象,并确保这些模式在非分裂细胞中保持稳定[6,7,11]。正是通过这种方式,细胞得以维持基因表达模式和染色体结构的"记忆",促进正常的发育并维持成熟细胞的更新和分化状态[14,15]。

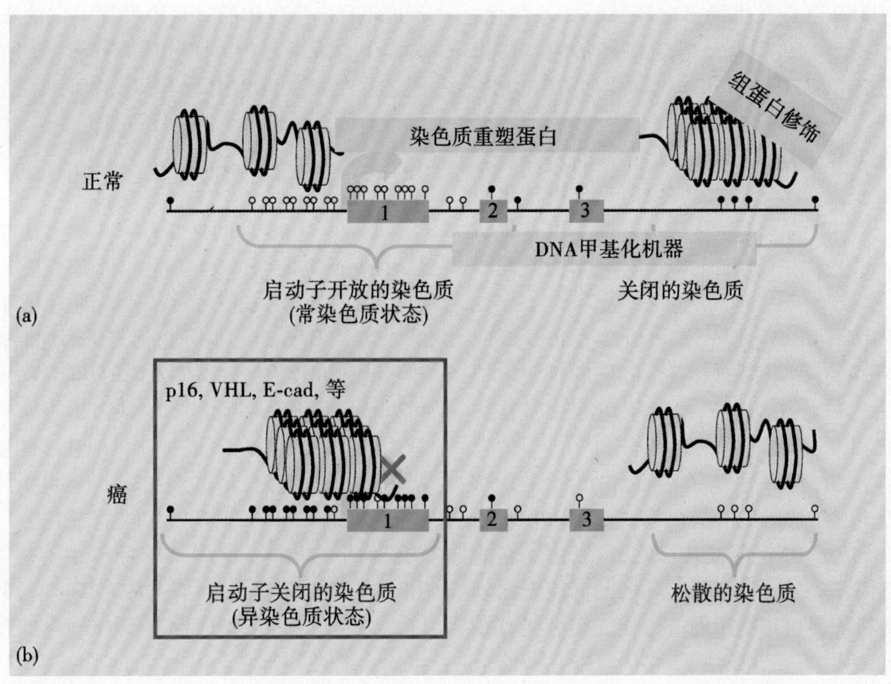

图 6-2　人类 DNA(直黑线)的组装排列。(a)对于正常细胞,核小体的排列更为线性(黄色圆圈,DNA 缠绕如图 6-1 所示),大多数含有 CpG 岛的基因启动子周围的染色质为"开放"排列(未甲基化的 CpG 位点显示为白色棒棒糖),它们正在进行转录或可以被诱导转录(大的浅蓝色箭头)。模型基因的外显子 1-3 由编号的浅蓝色框表示。基因内和延伸超出第三外显子的 DNA 区域被呈现为典型的闭合的转录抑制构象,正如大多数正常人类基因组中的基因一样。该封闭结构由核小体的更紧凑的三维组织构架表示,并且封闭区域中的 CpG 位点被显示为甲基化(黑色棒棒糖)。黄色方块中的文字描述了染色质重塑蛋白复合物、组蛋白修饰酶和进行 DNA 甲基化的酶(DNA 甲基化机器),它们负责 DNA 组装,如正文中所述。(b)癌细胞中存在的典型的染色质变异模式,基因组中正常闭合和开放染色质区域的位置发生了转变。许多封闭区域现在都有一个开放的染色质,其 DNA 甲基化丢失;而一大群基因,其启动子本应是封闭的染色质,现在已具有异常的 CpG 岛 DNA 甲基化和转录抑制状态(标示转录起始位点的亮蓝箭头被大红色 X 覆盖)

组蛋白修饰最经典的方式是前面提到的赖氨酸甲基化和乙酰化,其与基因转录的高低状态密切相关。这些修饰依次由催化甲基化的组蛋白甲基转移酶(histone methyltransferase,HMT)、去除这些甲基基团的组蛋白去甲基化酶,以及分别添加和去除乙酰基团的组蛋白乙酰化酶(histone acetylase,HAT)和组蛋白去乙酰化酶(histone deactylase,HDAC)家族完成[7,11,15~17]。对于这些动态修饰,与基因状态相关的关键甲基化标记有:组蛋白 3 的第 4 位赖氨酸的甲基化(H3K4me3),这与开放染色质的活化转录特征有关;以及第 9 位赖氨酸或第 27 位赖氨酸的甲基化(H3K9me3,H3K27me3),这是基因表达被抑制的特征[6,15]。赖氨酸的甲基化修饰可以携带更多的信息,因为它可以以单甲基化、二甲基化或三甲基化的状态存在[6,7,11,15]。组蛋白乙酰化也存在调节平衡,其中 HAT 和 HDAC 的酶活性决定了组蛋白的状态:组蛋白赖氨酸乙酰化是开放、转录活化染色质的典型特征,而去乙酰化则更多的与染色质封闭和转录抑制相关[7,11,15]。在基因启动子上这种转录活化修饰的例子是 H3K9 的乙酰化和 H4K16 的乙酰化[7,11,15]。

DNA 甲基化

虽然不是在所有的多细胞生物中广泛存在,人类、其他哺乳动物和其他高等生物中还拥有另一层面的表观遗传调节方式。在包装人类基因组时,与染色质状态紧密协同的一个关键修饰是把甲基直接添加到复制后的 DNA 中[7,10,17,18]。当胞嘧啶正好位于鸟嘌呤之前或"CpG"二核苷酸中时,通过 DNA 甲基转移酶(DNA methyltransferase,DNMT)家族蛋白的催化,即可将甲基基团从 S-腺苷甲硫氨酸转移连接到 DNA 胞嘧啶的第 5 位碳原子(C5)上完成这一过程[17~19]。

DNA 甲基化的作用[19]与 CpG 二核苷酸在人类和其他基因组中的分布密切相关。这是一种非随机和不均匀的分布,在进化过程中,由于甲基化 CpG 的脱氨作用导致胞嘧啶(C)变为胸腺嘧啶(T),CpG 随着进化而逐渐消失[7,17,18]。如果不能修复这些胸腺嘧啶,就会导致 C 转向 T。然而,仍有一些未删除的富含 CpG 的片段(~0.4 至数千 kb)或所谓的"CpG 岛"被零星地保存下来,这对 DNA 的甲基化特别重要[17,18]。这些 CpG 岛,特别在约 50%~60%的人类基因的 5′末端[17,18],是非 DNA 甲基化的,而其余 DNA 中的大多数 CpG 位点是甲基化的[4,7,17,18](图 6-2)。

DNA 甲基化的模式如图 6-2 所示。DNA 甲基化与前面提及的核小体定位和组蛋白修饰紧密配合,决定了基因组的表观遗传调控。因此,甲基化的 DNA 有助于维持严格的遗传状态,这种状态下大部分基因组处于相对的转录抑制,这在封闭染色质或在染色体中心体周围的"异染色区"中最为明显。与此相反,与基因启动位点相关的非 DNA 甲基化 CpG 岛,则可以反映或促进待转录和/或转录活化的状态[4,7,17]。DNA 甲基化与组蛋白修饰紧密协作,与转录抑制相关,维持许多封闭染色质的抑制状态。因此，如 H3K9 位点发生组蛋白赖氨酸去乙酰化，并出现抑制性甲基化标记如 H3K9me3，则与 DNA 的甲基化相关[17~19]。相应的，这些标记尤其是 H3K9me，对靶向 DNA 甲基化有着重要作用[17~19]。

值得注意的是，相对于上述 DNA 甲基化在抑制基因转录中的作用，近来的研究发现了一个重要的例外：5mC 甲基化会出现在活跃而非抑制性基因的基因主体区域。这类甲基化与组蛋白标记 H3K36me3 协同作用，允许转录延伸并增强基因的表达[7,10,20,21]。

在表观基因组中 DNA 甲基化模式是如何建立和维持的呢？最近的一些重要进展有助于我们对这个问题的理解。长期以来，人们一直认为三种生物活性酶，即三种 DNA 甲基转移酶（DNMT），负责建立和维持 DNA 位点的甲基化[19]。具体来说，DNMT1 主要是维持性的 DNA 甲基转移酶，它负责在 DNA 复制期间保持原来已建立的 DNA 甲基化模式。DNMT3A 和 DNMT3B 主要是从头合成的 DNA 甲基转移酶，可以建立新的 DNA 甲基化位点。然而，许多数据表明，实际情况可能更加复杂，三种 DNA 甲基转移酶和相互作用的蛋白质之间可能存在协同作用，在某些情况特别是应激条件下，它们可以在功能上相互替代[22]。例如，DNMT3A 和 DNMT3B 可以修复 DNMT1 在 DNA 合成过程中产生的错误[14]。

虽然上述建立 DNA 甲基化模式的理论已经得到认可，但长期以来人们一直认为，去除这种修饰是一个被动的事件，只有在 DNA 复制过程中，在甲基化位点未被保留的情况下才能实现。然而，令人兴奋的是，如今我们认识到，如同组蛋白的修饰一样，DNA 甲基化也存在不同的主动去甲基化过程。一种被称为 TET（ten-eleven translocation）的蛋白酶家族，可以通过一系列的氧化步骤，将 5mC（5-methyl cytosine，5mC）转化为 5-羟甲基胞嘧啶（5-hydroxylmethyl cytosine，5hmC）及其他氧化产物，并通过随后的 DNA 修复步骤，将 5mC 转化为胞嘧啶[19,23,24]。这些转化在正常发育过程和成体细胞功能中都非常重要，稍后我们将概述它们对癌症的重要性[25~27]。

癌症中 DNA 甲基化和染色质的改变或“癌症表观基因组”

DNA 甲基化丢失

事实上，所有的癌症类型的表观遗传模式都与前几节中描述的正常细胞明显不同[4,7,8]（图 6-2）。迄今为止，癌症 DNA 甲基化的研究已经较为透彻，目前至少有两个主要的甲基化变化已经得到了广泛的认可。首先，在正常细胞基因组 DNA 中的甲基化在癌症基因组中广泛丢失，表现为整体低甲基化[1,2,7,8,10]（图 6-2）。事实上，这是第一个研究较为透彻的癌症染色质异常[28]，但是这种变化的后果还有待进一步阐明。这些低甲基化通常发生在封闭的染色质区域，由于这些区域的 DNA 甲基化有助于维持 DNA 的转录抑制，因此低甲基化可能与转录异常相关[1~4]。实际上，据报道，许多具有致癌潜力并且通常在正常细胞中低表达的基因，其在癌症中的表达上调与启动子区域 DNA 甲基化变化有关[1]。此外，中心体周围区域是多种类型的癌症中 DNA 甲基化丢失高发位点，可能在肿瘤形成不稳定染色体的过程中发挥一定的作用[1~4,29]。最近，在肿瘤中也观察到基因体区域 DNA 甲基化的缺失，这可能对基因表达产生与上述相反的影响，如前所述，这些区域的甲基化可以通过增强转录延伸来促进基因表达[7,20,21]。

基因启动子的 DNA 高甲基化

启动子 CpG 岛的局部 DNA 甲基化增加，是迄今为止最被认可的、研究最深入的与癌症表观遗传异常相关的染色质变化。如前所述，CpG 岛在正常细胞中不受这种变化的影响[1~4,7,8]（图 6-2）。这种变化与基因的转录完全抑制有关，对于那些研究较为深入抑癌基因的功能缺失，这种甲基化的变化可以替代基因突变所产生的基因功能缺失作用[1~4,7,8]。除了这些经典的抑癌基因，通过随机地在癌细胞 DNA 中筛选 DNA 高甲基化的基因，例如在癌症基因组图谱项目（Cancer Genome Atlas Project，TCGA）中进行筛选，可以发现在多种类型的癌症中，一个特定病人的肿瘤中有数百个这样的基因存在[1~4,7,8,30~33]。虽然所有这些基因变化可能不是驱动特定癌症发生或发展的关键因素，但包括经典抑癌基因在内的许多基因确实编码了一些至关重要的基因，这些基因的功能丧失会对肿瘤发展产生重要的影响[3,4,7,8]。许多在癌症中很少或从未发生突变的基因，仍可以在肿瘤进展过程中发生启动子 DNA 的高甲基化和表达沉默，从而在肿瘤发生过程中发挥重要作用[4,7,8]。在这方面，几乎所有已知的在肿瘤发生过程中起作用的关键通路，在一种或多种肿瘤类型中，都与具有癌症特异的 DNA 高甲基化的基因有关[3,4,7,8]（表 6-1）。此外，许多相关基因在具有恶变倾向的癌前病变中表现出 DNA 甲基化改变，比如“良性”结肠息肉[1,2,4,7,8,34]。在这些恶变前的结肠病变中，存在多个高甲基化的基因，这些基因一旦失活，就会使关键通路的调控失调，比如 Wnt 通路。众所周知，Wnt 通路会驱动结肠癌的发生和发展[1,2,4,7,8,34]。这些发现形成了一种假说，即在许多情况下表观遗传变化可能对肿瘤的发生和细胞的异常增殖至关重要，这些异常增殖的细胞通常出现在有癌症风险的环境中，比如慢性炎症中[4,7,34~36]。除了上述发现，现在人们越来越认识到，DNA 甲基化差异的增加可能会影响基因启动子区以外的关键基因组区域[3,4,7,14,19,37,38]。正常组织和癌组织中，位于启动子 CpG 岛远端称为“CpG 岛岸”区域的甲基化程度也是不一样的[37,38]。

表 6-1 癌症中基因启动子高甲基化和基因沉默导致信号通路活性异常的例子

通路	3~5 个基因
Wnt 通路	APC，SFRP 家族，SOX17
细胞周期调控	Rb，p16，p15，p14，p73
DNA 损伤修复	MLH1，O6-MGMT，GST-Pi，BRCA1
凋亡	DAP 激酶，caspase 8，TMS-1
肿瘤细胞侵袭，血管生成	THBS1，E-cadherin*，VHL，APC，LKB1，TIMP3
肿瘤结构	Growth-factor response ER**，RAR-β，SOCS-1

* E-钙黏蛋白。

** 生长因子反应的雌激素受体。

上述岛岸区域在正常组织中也存在甲基化的差异，因此对癌症本身来说，特别是用来反应相关基因的表达变化，不如近端启动子 CpG 岛区域的意义明确。类似地，越来越多的证据显示在基因增强子区域或 DNA 调节序列中存在着甲基化的增加，它们通过结合关键蛋白以及组蛋白的修饰，调控基因的表达。这些序列与基因近端启动子之间的距离是可变的，而且往往相距很远[39~41]。增强子的从头 DNA 甲基化变化也可能导致癌症中的关键基因表达异常，尤其是可能增加癌症的风险状态[42,43]。虽然癌症中增强子 DNA 差异甲基化的研究越来越多，但这些变化的作用及其与基因启动子 CpG 岛高甲基化之间的平衡仍有待阐明。

癌症中 DNA 甲基化和染色质的远程变化

对整个基因组中 CpG 甲基化和染色质的深入分析取得了令人振奋的进展，研究发现在癌症和正常细胞之间存在甲基化可以改变的非随机区域，它们在许多染色体中占据兆碱基的区域(100kb 至 10Mb)[3,4,7,8,44~46]。这些区域基本上 CpG 贫乏，存在的 CpG 则高度甲基化，但在不同的正常组织中，甲基化的程度存在显著差异，因而产生了“部分甲基化区域”这个术语[3,4,7,8,44~46]。癌症的特征是在这些区域中出现正常 DNA 甲基化的丢失，产生所谓低甲基化的兆碱基岛或谷，如迄今在结肠癌和其他癌症中的发现[3,4,7,8,44~46]。在这些序列区域中，癌症可以建立远程的抑制性组蛋白修饰状态，如 H3K9 甲基化[3,4,7,8,44~46]。在某些区域，可能有较远的非抑制性或较开放的染色质区域[45,47~50]。有趣的是，嵌入在这些大区域中的许多包含启动子 CpG 岛的小基因，可以获得 DNA 从头甲基化(见前面详述)[3,4,7,8,45]。因此，从本质上讲，癌症中的低甲基化峡谷经常表现出许多与癌症相关的甲基化丢失及局部 CpG 岛的甲基化增高[3,4,45]。此外，这些大区域可能含有比预期高得多的基因，这些基因参与了胚胎和成体干细胞的染色质调控，特别容易受到异常的启动子 CpG 岛 DNA 高甲基化的影响[3,4,7,8,35,45,51,52]。

癌症中遗传和表观遗传改变之间的联系越来越紧密

过去几年中最有趣的一个发现是，在几乎所有肿瘤类型中，最常见的突变类型发生在编码建立和维持表观基因组的蛋白质的基因中[3,4,7,53,54]。虽然这些基因突变的确切意义仍有待确定，但这些基因突变与肿瘤发生、DNA 甲基化异常或染色质变化之间存在一些关键联系。一个相关的重要例子是 IDH1/IDH2 基因突变、TET 基因突变和 DNA 高甲基化这三者之间的关系，与在年轻患者低度恶性胶质瘤和在血癌中的发现一致[55~57]，这些突变与 DNA 和组蛋白去甲基化通路的改变有关。其中包括组蛋白甲基化水平的变化和启动子区域 CpG 岛 DNA 高甲基化频率的增加，类似于之前在一部分结肠癌中明确的 CpG 岛甲基化表型(CpG Island Methylator Phenotype，CIMP)[56~59]。我们还需要进一步了解 IDH 突变，尤其是其导致的染色质和 DNA 甲基化变化的原因。突变的 IDH 基因导致由酮戊二酸生成的 2-羟基戊二酸的大量积累，并导致酮戊二酸的消耗[60~62]。后者是多种酶的关键辅助因子，这些酶包括那些有助于调节和维持关键染色质标记的蛋白质，以及前面提到的可以防止异常 DNA 甲基化的 TET 蛋白[63,64]。随着时间的推移，这些变化被认为会促进抑制性组蛋白标记的增加和随后的 DNA 高甲基化[60~62]。最近在小鼠中的研究表明，IDH 突变是早期肿瘤进展事件的驱动因素[65]，它可以通过阻断正常干/祖细胞的正常分化，促进异常的自我更新并减少谱系的形成和分化[57,60,66]。重要的是，直接靶向 IDH 突变的药物已经开发出来，目前正在 AML 和脑瘤中进行临床实验。

另一组有趣的突变发生在一种儿童脑瘤亚型的关键抑制性组蛋白标记上。H3K27 的突变，仅存在于组蛋白 H3 多个拷贝的一个等位基因中，阻遏了催化 H3K27 甲基化的酶 EZH2 的活性。相应的，这些肿瘤 H3K27me3 出现了显著的缺失[3,3,67,68]，可能会诱导基因的异常激活并驱动肿瘤的起始和/或进展。

癌症中 DNA 甲基化改变的临床意义

尽管 DNA 甲基化对癌症中染色质变化的全面影响仍有待深入研究，但至少在两大类的转化应用中，已经取得了重要的研究进展。首先是将 DNA 高甲基化的基因启动子序列作为肿瘤生物标志物；其次是使用表观遗传疗法来靶向可逆的异常基因沉默，这一方法可能会有疗效[1,2,9,69~71]。

癌症的 DNA 甲基化生物标志物

与其他分子检测方法相比，检测癌症中的 DNA 甲基化变化有一些显著的优势。首先，在许多情况下甲基化变化的总体频率比突变的变化更大[3,7,30,69]。到目前为止，这一结论可能适用于大多数实体瘤和血液癌症，尽管不同肿瘤类型中发生改变的特定基因是不同的。第二个检测 DNA 甲基化变化的优点与基因沉默有关，基因沉默仅限于许多基因的启动子区域，使得这种改变容易成为癌症分子标志物检测的靶标。这些基因的庞大数量使得构建检测基因组合成为可能，其中 DNA 高甲基化标记物基本覆盖了癌症基因组，因此提高了在特定患者中检出标志物的概率[72]。事实上，在癌症的早期或侵袭前阶段以及其他癌症后期进展中，许多基因都出现了异常，这使得 DNA 甲基化标志物在癌症风险评估、早期诊断、肿瘤的再次分子分期和肿瘤生物学行为预测方面具有潜在的应用价值。因此，由于 DNA 甲基化发生的频率高、出现时间早并且用单一测定法就可以测定每种基因的甲基化特性，使得 DNA 甲基化检测在癌症的早期诊断中得到推广。表 6-2 中列出了前面提到的每种可能作为肿瘤标志物的部分实例。对于肺癌的风险评估，目前检测痰液 DNA 中的高甲基化基因序列有很大的应用前景，在肺癌发生高危个体中该方法可以在标记物监测开始后的特定时间内预测肺癌的发生[2,73]。另外有研究通过检测血液或粪便中 DNA 甲基化的改变来检测结肠癌，在突变检测时加入这种方法可以提高检测的效能[74~79]。在尿液中检测此类基因的甲基化可以对膀胱癌的风险进行分层或为膀胱癌的早期诊断提供依据[80]，并在前列腺活检中提高前列腺癌的诊断水平[81,82]。目前，临床医生应用美国 CLIA 实验室批准的检测方法，可以对粪便和前列腺活检组织进行检测。

研究发现发生甲基化变化的基因参与了癌症发展的一些关键信号通路，因此癌症 DNA 甲基化变化的第二个应用领域是可以把它们作为潜在的预后或预测性生物标志物（表 6-2）。通常，大多数基因的 DNA 甲基化与患者的不良预后有关，因此它们可以作为预后生物标志物。这与关键抑癌基因的沉默会导致关键信号通路发生变化的现象是一致的。因此，具有单个或多个基因改变的肿瘤的恶性程度更高、或分子水平上更加趋于晚期，从而导致更差的预后[83,84]。最近，研究通过在肺癌和纵隔淋巴结 DNA 中同时检测一个小型的 DNA 高甲基化基因组合，可以准确地将 1 期肺癌患者重新分期到 3 期，并预测哪些患者具有快速复发的风险[85]。

表 6-2 基因启动子 DNA 高甲基化序列作为肿瘤生物标志物的应用实例：接近临床应用

高危状态的早期诊断和/或检测：
肺癌高危人群痰中 CpG 岛 DNA 高甲基化检测[5,22]
前列腺癌活检组织和尿液 GSTP1 DNA 甲基化检测[27,28]
预后：
检测肺癌肿瘤和淋巴结基因队列中的 DNA 高甲基化，来重新分期 1 期非小细胞肺癌并预测早期复发[31]
检测 DNA 高甲基化预测胶质母细胞瘤对替莫唑胺的敏感性[32-34]
特定基因的高甲基化
全基因组 DNA 甲基化谱
组蛋白修饰图谱
预测：
CpG 岛高甲基化作为化疗、激素治疗和靶向治疗反应的标志物，例如胶质瘤患者的 MGMT 和替莫唑胺治疗

特定基因的 DNA 甲基化可能影响癌细胞对不同疗法的敏感性，这一点也可被肿瘤学家应用于患者的临床处理。例如，某个基因的作用是修复损伤的 DNA，它的沉默可能会增加肿瘤对 DNA 损伤药物的反应。一个最明显例子是恶性脑瘤—胶质母细胞瘤，如果这类患者肿瘤中 DNA 损伤修复基因 *O6MGMT* 出现高甲基化，那么患者对 DNA 烷化剂替莫唑胺（temazolamide）的反应更好，并且治疗后的无瘤期更长[86-88]。其他研究表明，卵巢癌对顺铂的敏感性可能是由 *FANCF* 基因的沉默介导的[89,90]；结肠癌对拓扑异构酶抑制剂的敏感性可能是由 Werner 综合征基因（*WRN*）的沉默介导的[91]。最近，有研究报道 SMAD1 的启动子甲基化可以预测弥漫性大 B 细胞淋巴瘤（DBCL）患者对阿霉素的耐药性[92]，而低剂量的 DNMT 抑制剂则可以逆转 SMAD1 的表达抑制，缓解化疗耐药性[92]。这些临床前研究的发现正在进行 I 期临床试验，前期的数据表明 DNMT 抑制剂可以诱导更好的化疗反应[92]。在临床使用之前，所有这些研究发现都需要在其他队列中进行确认，并且最好在前瞻性评估的患者中进行。然而，对于仅适用于一线治疗的患者，这些研究可能非常有助于患者治疗选择的优化。越来越多的大型临床试验试图对这些基于标志物的方法进行验证，并将其纳入肿瘤学的标准实践中。最后，其他 DNA 甲基化的变化，如肿瘤 DNA 中正常 DNA 甲基化的缺失、以及代表活化或抑制性基因功能的染色质标记的变化，非常有望成为潜在的癌症分子标志物。

癌症的“表观遗传”治疗

这种类型的治疗是指通过将异常的基因表达模式恢复正常来对癌症进行治疗的手段。迄今为止，可以实现这一目标的药物有两类：能够在实验中诱导 DNA 去甲基化的药物如 5-氮杂-胞苷或氮杂胞苷和 5-氮杂-2-脱氧胞苷或地西他滨，以及抑制组蛋白去乙酰化酶的药物 SAHA。这些药物已被 FDA 分别批准用于治疗白血病前期病变、骨髓增生异常和皮肤 T 细胞淋巴瘤。阿扎胞苷（azacitidine）[93] 和地西他滨（decitabine）[7,94-96] 在临床上都有一定的治疗效果。在最近的一项随机Ⅲ期试验中，阿扎胞苷治疗的患者显示出了一定的生存获益[97]。尽管这两类药物在以往难治性肿瘤中的反应率和持久的反应性令人印象深刻，但必须注意的是，它们发挥作用的确切模式仍有待证明，也就是说，尽管有相应的实验证据，它们可能不仅仅在临床上单独或部分地通过表观遗传效应来发挥作用[70,95,98,99]。因此，许多临床试验正在其他血液系统恶性肿瘤中测试这些药物，尤其是利用 DNA 去甲基化药物治疗急性髓性白血病和慢性髓性白血病的临床试验，很有可能取得不错的结果[94,100]。此外，还有实验室证据表明 DNA 去甲基化和组蛋白去乙酰化酶的活性抑制之间存在协同作用，可以使癌症中 DNA 高甲基化的基因重新表达[101]。因此，多项临床试验正在探索这些药物联合治疗的临床潜力。这些临床试验大多数都与相关的研究一起进行，在试验中检测 DNA 去甲基化和异常沉默基因的重新表达是否与治疗的反应一致、是否能够预测治疗反应。在未来几年里，所有这些临床研究将明确这些药物的治疗效果和起效机制。

在实体肿瘤中，以往表观遗传疗法的研究较少[102,103]。目前，实体瘤的表观遗传治疗正成为一个焦点，并取得了一些有前景的重要结果[70,71]。本章其他部分多处提到，就像在血液恶性肿瘤中一样，由于治疗靶点的普遍存在，表观遗传疗法在这些癌症中有很大的潜力。最近的临床前研究探索了低剂量的 DNMT 抑制剂对实体肿瘤细胞的影响，发现纳摩尔剂量的阿扎胞苷（商品名 Vidaza）和地西他滨（商品名 Dacogen）就可以产生抗肿瘤效应，这一定程度上反映了这些药物不仅可以“重编程”癌细胞，而且几乎没有脱靶效应[104]。越来越多的临床试验正在使用这种低剂量的治疗方法，并联合新出现的 DNA 去甲基化药物如作为 5-氮杂-2-脱氧胞苷前药的 SGI-110[105,106]。这些临床试验还将这些药物与其他表观遗传治疗药物如组蛋白去乙酰化酶抑制剂（histone deactylase inhibitor，HDACi）进行联合。例如，在最近开展的一项 65 例前期接受过治疗的晚期非小细胞肺癌患者试验中，这种联合疗法在一小部分患者中产生了强劲、持久的反应[107]。此外，这些试验结果表明，表观遗传疗法可以诱导更多的患者对后续的治疗产生更好的反应[107]，包括标准化疗和新型免疫疗法[108,109]。在免疫治疗方面，临床前研究表明，DNA 甲基化抑制剂可以在肺癌和其他实体肿瘤中活化涉及数百个基因的复杂通路，通过这些通路募集免疫细胞[110]。目前正在进行更大规模的临床试验，以检测上述 DNA 甲基化药物对非小细胞肺癌患者化疗和免疫治疗的增敏作用。除了在非小细胞肺癌中的这些研究，其他研究还发现，DNA 甲基化抑制剂诱导可以使晚期浆液性卵巢癌患者接受后续的化疗[111]。

可以肯定的是，在未来的几年里，正如血液肿瘤一样，实体肿瘤中将出现很多基于表观遗传学治疗方法的临床试验，这些试验中也会包括阐明表观遗传疗法确切机制的研究。实体肿瘤及血液恶性肿瘤中的研究，不仅将指导目前现有药物的应用，而且还将促进新的、更有效、更特异药物的开发。随着针对异常 DNA 甲基化发生精确机制研究的不断深入，以及对参与启动和维持这种变化的染色质成分的不断了解，将会鉴定出新的分子靶点，同时也会随之开发出基于这些靶点的联合疗法。目前已开发出针对染色质组装中几个关键步骤的小分子抑制剂，其中一些已经进入临床试验[4,70,71,112-116]。

总结

过去十多年的研究，特别是 DNA 甲基化方面的研究，已经充分表明癌症从发生发展到晚期，不仅是一种基因病，同时也是表观遗传疾病。这些研究与染色质成分如何包装人类基因组以调节基因表达模式的基本知识紧密相关，将有助于开发新的癌症生物标志物以及新型治疗策略。在未来十年内，这些策略有进入癌症临床应用的巨大潜力。

（贺宇飞 译　孙文　陈淑桢 校　王红阳 审）

参考文献

The complete reference list can be found on the Wiley Companion Digital Edition of this title (see inside front cover for login instructions).

1 Esteller M. Epigenetics in cancer. *N Engl J Med*. 2008;**358(11)**:1148–1159.

3 Shen H, Laird PW. Interplay between the cancer genome and epigenome. *Cell*. 2013;**153(1)**:38–55.

4 Baylin SB, Jones PA. A decade of exploring the cancer epigenome - biological and translational implications. *Nat Rev Cancer*. 2011;**11(10)**:726–734.

5 Allis C, Jenuwein T, Reinberg D (eds) Caparros M (associate editor). *Epigenetics*. Cold Spring Harbor, NY: Cold Spring Harbor Laboratory Press; 2007.

8 Jones PA, Baylin SB. The epigenomics of cancer. *Cell*. 2007;**128(4)**:683–692.

9 Egger G, Liang G, Aparicio A, Jones PA. Epigenetics in human disease and prospects for epigenetic therapy. *Nature*. 2004;**429(6990)**:457–463.

13 Kornberg RD, Lorch Y. Twenty-five years of the nucleosome, fundamental particle of the eukaryote chromosome. *Cell*. 1999;**98(3)**:285–294.

14 Jones PA. Functions of DNA methylation: islands, start sites, gene bodies and beyond. *Nat Rev Genet*. 2012;**13(7)**:484–492.

15 Allis CD, Jenuwein T, Reinberg D. Overview and concepts. In: Allis CD, Jenuwein T, Reinberg D, eds. *Epigenetics*. Cold Spring Harbor, NY: Cold Spring Harbor Laboratory Press; 2007.

18 Li E, Bird A. DNA methylation in mammals. In: Allis CD, Jenuwein T, Reinberg D, eds. *Epigenetics*. Cold Spring Harbor, NY: Cold Spring Harbor Laboratory Press; 2007.

22 Rhee I, Bachman KE, Park BH, et al. DNMT1 and DNMT3b cooperate to silence genes in human cancer cells. *Nature*. 2002;**416(6880)**:552–556.

23 Tahiliani M, Koh KP, Shen Y, et al. Conversion of 5-methylcytosine to 5-hydroxymethylcytosine in mammalian DNA by MLL partner TET1. *Science*. 2009;**324(5929)**:930–935.

31 Hammerman PS, Hayes DN, Wilkerson MD, et al. Comprehensive genomic characterization of squamous cell lung cancers. *Nature*. 2012;**489(7417)**:519–525.

35 Ohm JE, McGarvey KM, Yu X, et al. A stem cell-like chromatin pattern may predispose tumor suppressor genes to DNA hypermethylation and heritable silencing. *Nat Genet*. 2007;**39(2)**:237–242.

36 Feinberg AP, Ohlsson R, Henikoff S. The epigenetic progenitor origin of human cancer. *Nat Rev Genet*. 2006;**7(1)**:21–33.

45 Berman BP, Weisenberger DJ, Aman JF, et al. Regions of focal DNA hypermethylation and long-range hypomethylation in colorectal cancer coincide with nuclear lamina-associated domains. *Nat Genet*. 2012;**44(1)**:40–46.

50 Timp W, Feinberg AP. Cancer as a dysregulated epigenome allowing cellular growth advantage at the expense of the host. *Nat Rev Cancer*. 2013;**13(7)**:497–510.

51 Schlesinger Y, Straussman R, Keshet I, et al. Polycomb-mediated methylation on Lys27 of histone H3 pre-marks genes for de novo methylation in cancer. *Nat Genet*. 2007;**39(2)**:232–236.

52 Widschwendter M, Fiegl H, Egle D, et al. Epigenetic stem cell signature in cancer. *Nat Genet*. 2007;**39(2)**:157–158.

53 You JS, Jones PA. Cancer genetics and epigenetics: two sides of the same coin? *Cancer Cell*. 2012;**22(1)**:9–20.

54 Garraway LA, Lander ES. Lessons from the cancer genome. *Cell*. 2013;**153(1)**:17–37.

56 Noushmehr H, Weisenberger DJ, Diefes K, et al. Identification of a CpG island methylator phenotype that defines a distinct subgroup of glioma. *Cancer Cell*. 2010;**17(5)**:510–522.

58 Issa JP. Aging and epigenetic drift: a vicious cycle. *J Clin Invest*. 2014;**124(1)**:24–29.

60 Lu C, Ward PS, Kapoor GS, et al. IDH mutation impairs histone demethylation and results in a block to cell differentiation. *Nature*. 2012;**483(7390)**:474–478.

67 Chan K-M, Fang D, Gan H, et al. The histone H3.3K27M mutation in pediatric glioma reprograms H3K27 methylation and gene expression. *Genes Dev*. 2013;**27(9)**:985–990.

68 Lewis PW, Muller MM, Koletsky MS, et al. Inhibition of PRC2 activity by a gain-of-function H3 mutation found in pediatric glioblastoma. *Science*. 2013;**340(6134)**:857–861.

69 Laird PW. The power and the promise of DNA methylation markers. *Nat Rev Cancer*. 2003;**3(4)**:253–266.

70 Ahuja N, Easwaran H, Baylin SB. Harnessing the potential of epigenetic therapy to target solid tumors. *J Clin Invest*. 2014;**124(1)**:56–63.

71 Azad N, Zahnow CA, Rudin CM, Baylin SB. The future of epigenetic therapy in solid tumours-lessons from the past. *Nat Rev Clin Oncol*. 2013;**10(5)**:256–266.

79 Imperiale TF, Ransohoff DF, Itzkowitz SH, et al. Multitarget stool DNA testing for colorectal-cancer screening. *N Engl J Med*. 2014;**370(14)**:1287–1297.

85 Brock MV, Hooker CM, Ota-Machida E, et al. DNA methylation markers and early recurrence in stage I lung cancer. *N Engl J Med*. 2008;**358(11)**:1118–1128.

86 Esteller M, Garcia-Foncillas J, Andion E, et al. Inactivation of the DNA-repair gene MGMT and the clinical response of gliomas to alkylating agents. *N Engl J Med*. 2000;**343(19)**:1350–1354.

87 Hegi ME, Diserens AC, Gorlia T, et al. MGMT gene silencing and benefit from temozolomide in glioblastoma. *N Engl J Med*. 2005;**352(10)**:997–1003.

93 Silverman LR, Demakos EP, Peterson BL, et al. Randomized controlled trial of azacitidine in patients with the myelodysplastic syndrome: a study of the cancer and leukemia group B. *J Clin Oncol*. 2002;**20(10)**:2429–2440.

96 Issa JP. Optimizing therapy with methylation inhibitors in myelodysplastic syndromes: dose, duration, and patient selection. *Nat Clin Pract Oncol*. 2005;**2(Suppl 1)**:S24–S29.

101 Cameron EE, Bachman KE, Myohanen S, Herman JG, Baylin SB. Synergy of demethylation and histone deacetylase inhibition in the re-expression of genes silenced in cancer. *Nat Genet*. 1999;**21(1)**:103–107.

104 Tsai HC, Li H, Van Neste L, et al. Transient low doses of DNA-demethylating agents exert durable antitumor effects on hematological and epithelial tumor cells. *Cancer Cell*. 2012;**21(3)**:430–446.

107 Juergens RA, Wrangle J, Vendetti FP, et al. Combination epigenetic therapy has efficacy in patients with refractory advanced non-small cell lung cancer. *Cancer Discov*. 2011;**1(7)**:598–607.

108 Brahmer JR, Tykodi SS, Chow LQ, et al. Safety and activity of anti-PD-L1 antibody in patients with advanced cancer. *N Engl J Med*. 2012;**366(26)**:2455–2465.

109 Topalian SL, Hodi FS, Brahmer JR, et al. Safety, activity, and immune correlates of anti-PD-1 antibody in cancer. *N Engl J Med*. 2012;**366(26)**:2443–2454.

第 7 章　癌症基因组及其演化

William P. D. Hendricks, PhD ■ Aleksandar Sekulic, MD, PhD ■ Alan H. Bryce, MD ■ Muhammed Murtaza, MBBS, PhD ■ Pilar Ramos, PhD ■ Jeffrey M. Trent, PhD

概述

100 多年前，Paul Ehrlich 教授凭借“魔法子弹”这一假说被授予诺贝尔生理学和医学奖，他认为“魔法子弹”能够基于其独特的分子特征特异性地靶向并杀死癌细胞等细胞。目前已完成的人类基因组计划和癌症基因组学革命已经绘制了许多常见恶性肿瘤潜在的特定基因突变。然而，癌症在临床表现、病程、病理甚至分子层面都存在很大的异质性，正是由于这种异质性的存在，使我们需要对病人进行个体化的治疗。因此，我们不仅仅需要一粒神奇的子弹，更需要一个可以精确打击的武器库。虽然肿瘤间和肿瘤内的基因组异质性对癌症管理和药物发现提出了巨大挑战，但最近的一些进展为战胜癌症带来了希望。这些进展主要体现在：首先，针对不同癌症的靶基因目录正在迅速增加；其次，我们开始了解多种突变如何聚集在少数药靶通路；再次，越来越多的药物和生物制剂被开发出来针对更多癌症基因组亚型（例如，免疫检查点抑制剂）；最后，借助下一代测序技术能比以往更早地监测疾病复发。本章将重点介绍这些新进展以及它们的整合是如何帮助“魔法子弹”对肿瘤实施精确打击。

摘要

癌症是一种遗传性疾病，癌基因和抑癌基因（TSG）的突变在克隆性扩增的细胞中逐步累积，从而驱动了细胞的恶性转化。在整个 20 世纪，大量证据不断支持上述观点，与此同时，对癌症突变亚型的日益了解也加速了临床癌症诊疗方式的创新。21 世纪初开始的基因组学革命，通过建立详尽的癌症突变目录以及明确不同个体肿瘤之间和同一肿瘤内部存在的巨大基因组异质性，加深了我们对癌症的认识。这些数据的使用极大推动了靶向药物的开发，基于基因组学的临床肿瘤治疗方案的制订，同时也催生了疾病早期检测新方法的建立。然而，我们在诸如：对不同癌症致病突变的认识、对已发现突变相关生物学功能的理解，如何开发靶向不同突变的药物，以及如何应对肿瘤耐药发生等方面仍存在明显的不足。本章中，我们将回顾癌症遗传学和基因组学的历史及研究方法，总结目前癌症突变谱研究的进展，探讨癌症演化和基因组异质性的最新观点，另外还将以黑色素瘤基因组学研究为例介绍癌症基因组学研究如何影响肿瘤的临床诊疗。

引言

正如前面章节所详述的，癌症是一种遗传性疾病，逐步积累的突变赋予了细胞选择性生长优势，从而诱发细胞癌变[1]。当细胞经历克隆扩增的波动时，这类突变会改变细胞增殖和死亡的速率以及细胞基因组的稳定性。随着癌基因突变的积累，细胞会在不断增殖过程中获得越来越多恶性表型。这些标志性的癌症表型主要包括：细胞过度增殖，丧失生长抑制，逃避免疫监视，促进炎症反应，侵袭和转移能力增强，基因组不稳定增加，细胞永生化，诱导血管生成，细胞能量稳态失衡和抵抗细胞死亡[2]。通过突变赋予细胞生长优势的癌症基因被称为癌基因或抑癌基因。当癌基因通过热点部位的突变被激活时，会驱动细胞信号转导途径的持续激活，从而加速细胞的增殖。当抑癌基因发生突变失活时，则不再促进细胞死亡，从而降低细胞的凋亡率。该模型已在结直肠癌中得到充分证实，*APC* 肿瘤抑癌基因的突变在大多数结直肠癌病例中都被发现能够诱发腺瘤形成。而其他参与细胞增殖，细胞周期和细胞凋亡过程的癌相关基因发生突变则可进一步诱发恶性肿瘤的高侵袭性和高转移能力等表型[3,4]。许多其他类型的癌症也被证明遵循类似演化模式，与此同时我们也发现在相同类型癌症中仍存在许多不同的恶性演化途径（图 7-1）。

虽然癌基因中的一些突变发生在胚系中并且是可遗传的，绝大多数突变（约 90%）散发于组织中，通常由于长期的复制错误、基因毒性应激，和/或环境损伤引起。这些突变可能是由于细微的序列改变（单碱基替换和一个或几个碱基的插入或缺失），染色体拷贝数的变化（扩增，缺失，染色体丢失或重复），或者是染色体结构的变化（染色体间和染色体内易位，反转或其他类型的重排）导致的。在本章的其余部分，我们将这些改变称为体细胞单核苷酸变异（SNV），拷贝数变异（CNV）或结构变异（SV）。SNV、CNV 和 SV 的典型例子如图 7-2 所示，包括 *NRAS*（一种最常发现突变的癌基因）中激活型的错义 SNV、*TP53*（一种最常见的肿瘤抑制因子）中引起功能失活的纯合缺失 CNV，以及涉及 *BCR* 和 *ABL* 激活的易位 SV。癌基因的表观遗传学修饰也可显著改变基因的功能，这些修饰虽然不直接改变 DNA 序列本身，但能够改变 DNA 甲基化水平、染色质修饰或依赖于非编码 RNA 的基因表达从而参与肿瘤发生。这个日益重要的研究领域将在其他章节中讨论。本章中，我们将重点关注 DNA 序列改变引发的突变[6~9]，通过列举当前基因组分析中的方法，汇集具有里程碑意义的癌症基因组研究结果，以及评估癌症演化在临床管理中的作用来展示癌症基因组学研究的进展。最后我们以黑色素瘤为例探讨基因组学、肿瘤演化如何指导临床诊疗。

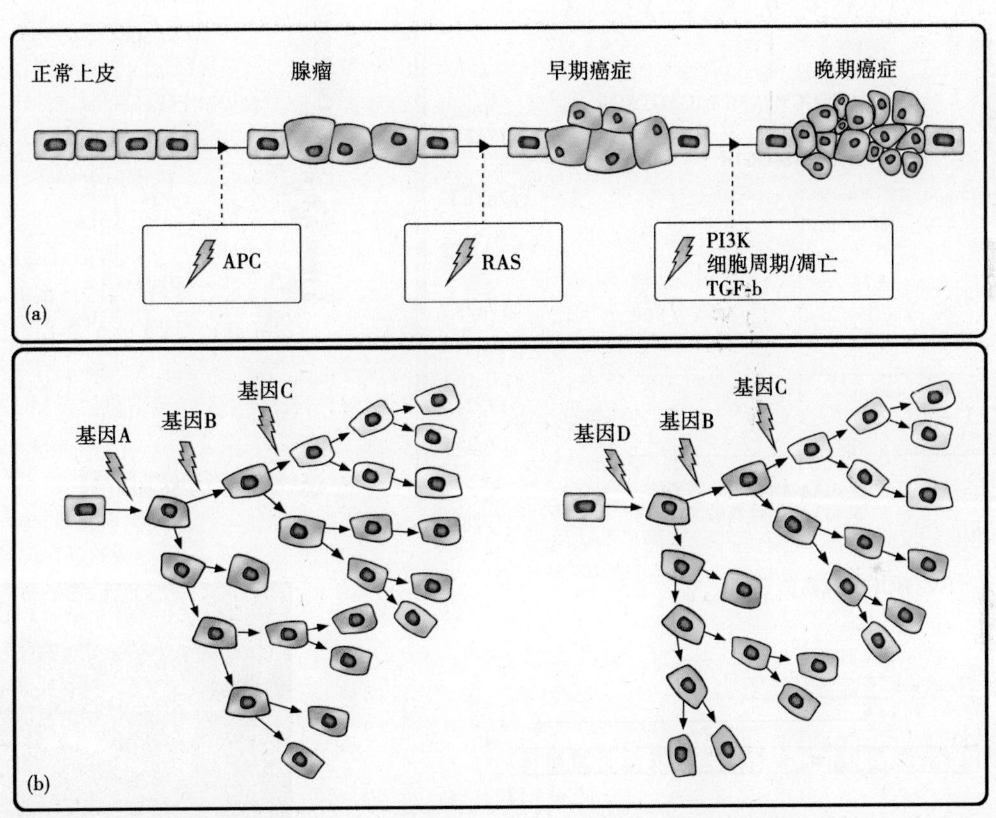

图 7-1　癌症是由多样化的分支突变逐步积累引起的。(a)结直肠癌逐渐发展的“Vogelgram”模型[3]。肿瘤抑制因子 *APC* 的失活通常在结直肠癌前病变中首先发现。随后 *RAS* 致癌基因的突变激活与早期腺瘤向早期癌症的转变相关。分子改变的逐渐积累最终导致恶性肿瘤侵入基底膜并转移至淋巴结和远端器官。(b)扩增模型描绘了不同的癌症起始突变以及癌细胞的分支演化。具体表现为伴随着癌细胞克隆性生长,细胞内不断累积的次级突变导致了肿瘤间和肿瘤内异质性

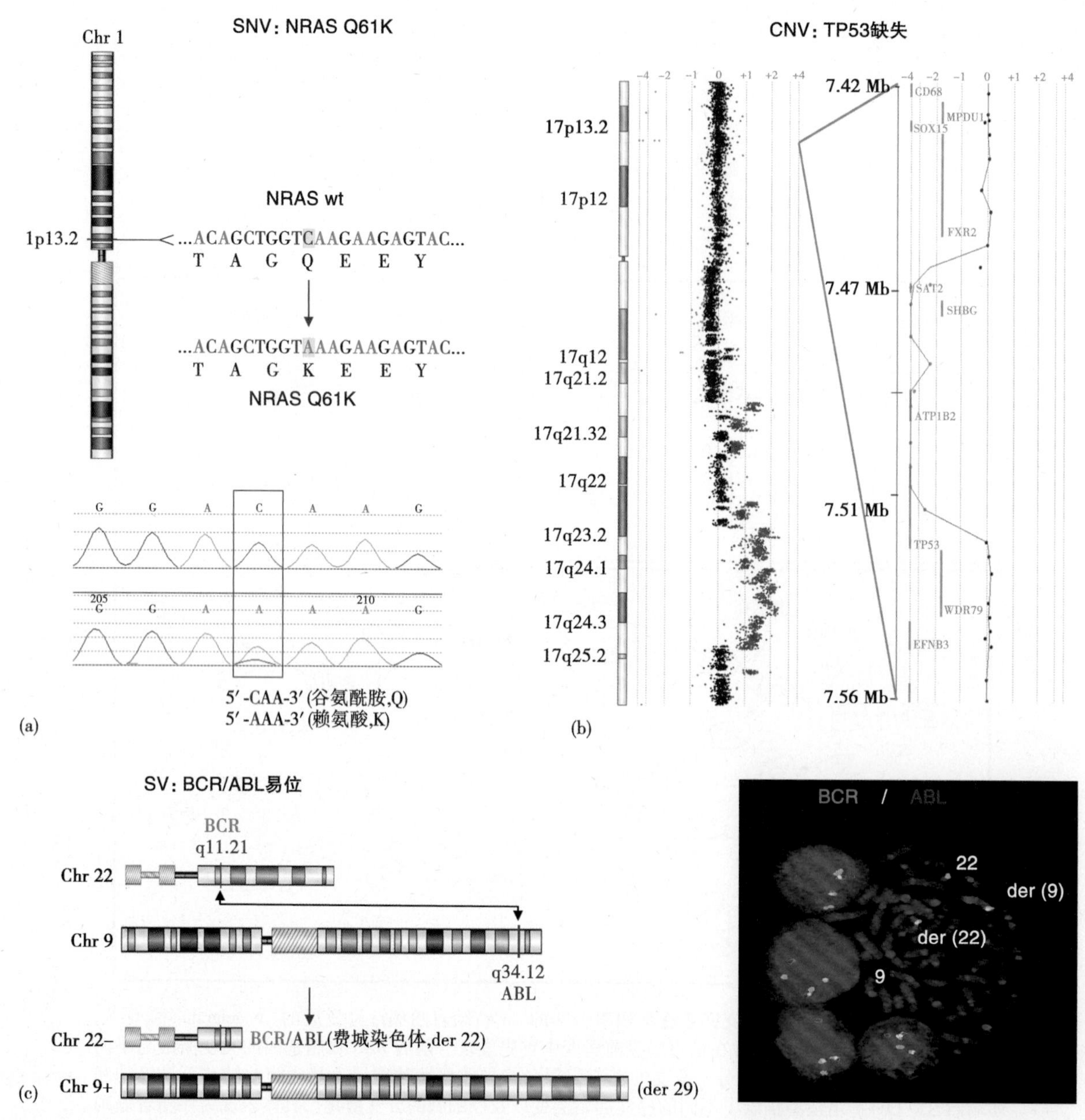

图 7-2 癌症突变类型(a)位于 1 号染色体上的 *NRAS* 癌基因在多种癌症中都发现激活型突变。单核苷酸变异(SNV)会导致密码子改变,即氨基酸 61-Q61K 处的谷氨酰胺(Q)取代赖氨酸(K)(上图)。下图显示的是携带 *NRAS Q61K* 突变的肿瘤样品 Sanger 测序图。(b)第 17 号染色体的 CGH log2 比率图(左),第 17 号染色体上一段纯和缺失的区域,该区域的断裂位点位于 *TP53* 肿瘤抑制因子内(右)。DNA 拷贝数发生丢失的区域绘制在轴的左侧,相应的发生染色体扩增的区域绘制在右侧。每个 log2 比率数据(点)和 log2 比率移动平均值(线)已标出。(c)*BCR* 和 *ABL* 基因之间发生 DNA 易位,形成的 *BCR-ABL* 融合基因被称为费城染色体(左)。右图是使用识别 *BCR*(绿色)和 *ABL*(红色)基因的荧光探针标记处于有丝分裂间期和有丝分裂期的 BCR-ABL 融合基因 t(9;22)。BCR 和 ABL 探针信号重合会产生黄色信号,这提示了相应细胞内染色体发生了 t(9;22)易位。资料来源:*BCR-ABL* 显微照片由 St. Jude 儿童研究医院的 Susana Raimondi 博士提供

癌症基因组学的历史和研究方法

癌症遗传学的早期历史

癌症遗传病因学研究领域的不断扩展和深入与遗传学和遗传技术的开创性进展紧密相关(图 7-3a)。19 世纪末和 20 世纪初的许多具有里程碑意义的研究奠定了癌症基因组学的基础——自然选择演化论的发展[10],可遗传生物单位的发现[11],染色体[12]、染色体遗传[13,14]和染色体基因[15]的鉴定,以及连接生物学、遗传学和演化理论的现代演化合成[16]。随后发现的 DNA 结构为理解遗传密码和遗传信息分子传递机制提供了框架[17]。同时,由于可遗传乳腺癌和结直肠癌的报道增多[18],人们越来越多地认识到癌症可以由化学因素(如煤焦油[19]和香烟烟雾[20]),物理因素(如辐射[21])和生物制剂(如病毒[22])引发。这些致癌物质也具有致突变性,这一发现使人们开始推测癌症是一种突变疾病。虽然有人很早就认为癌症是一种染色体疾病或一种突变疾病,但癌症作为一种遗传性疾病的概念直到 20 世纪后期才被确立。这主要归功于细胞遗传学和测序技术,以及携带癌基因的正常细胞系等突破性的实验进展,这些实验能够在分子水平上评估癌基因的突变,并明确肿瘤发生中的因果作用。其中一些具有里程碑意义的研究如图 7-3a 所示。

分子细胞遗传学:癌症中常见染色体变异的鉴定

20 世纪中期,通过对外周血中固定的白细胞染色体进行染色等细胞遗传学的新技术,人类开始对细胞染色体进行经验性观察[23,24]。借助这种方法,Nowell 首次发现了与癌症类型相关的常见的特异性遗传变异——几乎在所有慢性粒细胞白血病(CML)评估病例中都出现的"费城染色体"片段[25]。十多年后,Rowley 用染色体条带绘制了该片段的成分,确定费城染色体为染色体 9 和 22 之间的平衡相互易位[26,27]。这些发现促使人们寻找癌症内部和癌症之间的常见结构畸变,并在肉瘤、白血病和淋巴瘤中都鉴定出了特征性易位。然而,大多数癌症在染色体畸变的数量和类型上差异很大,很少有固定的类型[28]。

在 Nowell 和 Rowley 的发现之后,染色体条带和光谱核型分析(SKY)的快速发展使得利用荧光原位杂交(FISH)的技术逐步探寻癌细胞中的染色体畸变成为可能,这种技术主要依靠与特定染色体杂交的荧光 DNA 探针[29~38]。已开发的全基因组细胞遗传学分析方法还包括 SKY[29],多重荧光原位杂交(M-FISH)[39],染色体显微切割[38]和比较基因组杂交(CGH)[40]。CGH 是特别强大的荧光分子细胞遗传学技术,用于筛选肿瘤基因组中全基因组染色体拷贝数的变化。

在载玻片(微阵列)上印刷核酸的新方法通过降低成本和增加通量,很快彻底改变了分子细胞遗传学。阵列比较基因组杂交(aCGH)最初用于在染色体区域间隔(1-3Mb 分辨率)将大探针(大片段插入克隆或人工染色体)[41,42]点样到载玻片上。现在,由小型、可定制的寡核苷酸探针[43,44]组成的高分辨率全基因组平台在乳腺癌[45~47]、黑色素瘤[48~50]、B 细胞淋巴瘤[51,52]等癌症的鉴定上具有更高的通量和敏感性。同样的,针对成千上万个单核苷酸多态性(SNP)设计的寡核苷酸阵列也可用于肿瘤基因组复杂性的研究,目前已经可以对数百万个 SNP 进行快速基因分型(Affymetrix,Illumina)。与 CGH 阵列类似,SNP 微阵列对特异性杂交信号的定量分析,可用于拷贝数或杂合性丢失(LOH)的评估[53~55]。SNP 微阵列的重要癌症研究应用包括 NCI-60 细胞系组的基因分型[56]以及肺癌[57]、AML[55,58]、神经母细胞瘤[59]、黑色素瘤[56,60,61]、基底细胞癌[54]、乳腺癌[62]、结肠直肠癌[62~64]、胶质母细胞瘤[65,66]和胰腺癌[67]。

SV 和 CNV 都可以使用分子细胞遗传学和细胞基因组学工具进行鉴定。易位是癌症中最常见的 SV 之一,与在 CML 中的费城染色体的情况相同,是许多血液肿瘤和肉瘤的特征性畸变。它们发生在同一染色体内(染色体内)或不同染色体(染色体间)中,表现为染色体片段从一个位置移动到另一个位置。其他类型的 SV 包括染色体缺失、重复、倒位、插入、成环及等染色体。这些 SV 可能是由于双链断裂(DSB)修复或其他染色体内或染色体间重组的错误引起的[68]。易位和其他 SV 可以激活癌基因(例如当 *ABL* 酪氨酸激酶通过与 *BCR* 基因融合进行激活)或使 TSG 失活(例如当易位时涉及 *TP53* 肿瘤抑制因子基因的中断并导致功能丧失)。肿瘤细胞中最简单也是最常见的染色体畸变是整条染色体的增益或缺失的 CNV。它们是由染色体分离缺陷引起的。CNV 的功能目前难以确定,因为畸变区通常延伸超过数万兆碱基并且可能影响数百至数千个基因。现在已经可以将由染色体扩增(amplification)或缺失(deletion)造成的肿瘤相关的染色体改变缩小至比整条染色体的增益(gain)或丢失(loss)更精确的范围,这些小范围的异常可以改变已知癌基因或抑癌基因的拷贝数。通过分子细胞遗传学发现的实体肿瘤癌基因扩增的经典例子是乳腺癌中的 *ERBB2* 基因和多种肿瘤中的 *MYC* 基因,而基因组特定区域的丢失通常伴随抑癌基因的缺失,例如 *TP53*、*RB1*、*PTEN* 和 *CDKN2A*。抑癌基因的这种缺失对于促进遗传性肿瘤的发生至关重要,在遗传性肿瘤中,单个 TSG 等位基因的胚系突变一定伴随着野生型等位基因的缺失,同样,在散发性癌症中两个等位基因也同时失活。

分子遗传学:癌症中常见序列改变的鉴定

尽管一些分子细胞遗传学技术能够检测染色体断裂点的碱基对,但对于 DNA 本身细微序列变化的检测仍需要分子遗传学技术的进一步发展。分子克隆技术的发展和聚合酶链式反应(PCR)技术的发明使得检测这些突变所需的数百万份 DNA 拷贝成为可能[69]。再加上基于双脱氧核苷酸链终止和琼脂糖凝胶电泳的 Sanger 测序方法的进步[70],比如荧光标记核苷酸、毛细管电泳、配对端测序、鸟枪测序和改进的实验室自动化等,使得人类可以进行整个基因组规模的测序。该技术使人类基因组计划(HGP)——这一价值 30 亿美元的公共资助国际合作项目于 1990 年正式启动。覆盖 94%基因组的人类基因组草图于 2001 年发表[71,72],而完整的基因图谱则在 2003

1902 1910 1911 1918 1925 1927 1942 1950 1953 1956 1960 1970 1971 1973 1976 1977 1979 1982 1989

Morgan将基因定位于染色体上

煤焦油具有致癌性

Lockhart-Mummery对可遗传癌症的早期观察

Huxley发现的现代综合进化理论

Doll/Hill将吸烟与肺癌联系在一起

Tjio/Levan发明了染色体分离技术,并鉴定出人类染色体数目是46条

Ludwig Gross——癌症的病毒起源

Knudson提出了癌症形成的“二次打击”假说

Varmus/Bishop在正常DNA中发现了原癌基因

Sanger发明了双脱氧DNA测序技术

鉴定*RAS*癌基因和Myc基因的扩增和易位

Boveri定义了染色体可遗传性以及癌症的遗传学基础理论

Rous证明了鸡肉瘤病毒的致癌性

Muller证明X射线可诱发突变

Watson/Crick发现了DNA双螺旋结构

Nowell/Hungerford发现了首个癌症遗传学改变——费城染色体

Rowely运用细胞遗传学确定费城染色体发生了*BCR-ABL*易位

Weinberg证明导入肿瘤DNA能够将正常细胞转化为肿瘤细胞

发现*TP53*基因

1990 1991 1994 1999 2000 2001 2002 2003 2004 2005 2006 2007 2008 2009 2010 2011 2012 2013 2014

关于癌症进展和遗传学“Vogelgram”模型的提出

首个家族性乳腺癌易感基因*BRCA1*的鉴定

癌症中BRAF突变的鉴定；HapMap计划正式启动

大规模平行测序技术的发展

COSMIC数据库的建立；首个商业用途下一代测序仪的发明(454生命科学公司)

癌症中PIK3CA和EGFR突变的鉴定

Solexa(Illumia)测序仪的上市；首个采用NGS分析的美国实验

首个癌症全基因组数据发布—AML；可逆的末端终止法测序

癌症中IDH1突变的鉴定；首个配对的肿瘤原发灶和转移灶测序

黑色素瘤的分子靶向治疗

单细胞测序技术

228 000人类基因组测序

人类基因组计划(HGP)

结直肠癌中*APC*抑癌基因的鉴定

dbSNP数据库的建立

人类基因组图谱初稿完成

人类基因组(build34版)完成；ENCODE计划开始

实体瘤中*ETS-ETV4*基因易位的鉴定

完成乳腺癌和结直肠癌外显子组测序；EML4-ALK基因易位的鉴定；SOLID测序仪的上市

肿瘤内基因组异质性的检测

千人基因组测序计划第一阶段工作完成

循环肿瘤DNA(ctDNA)的测序

(a)

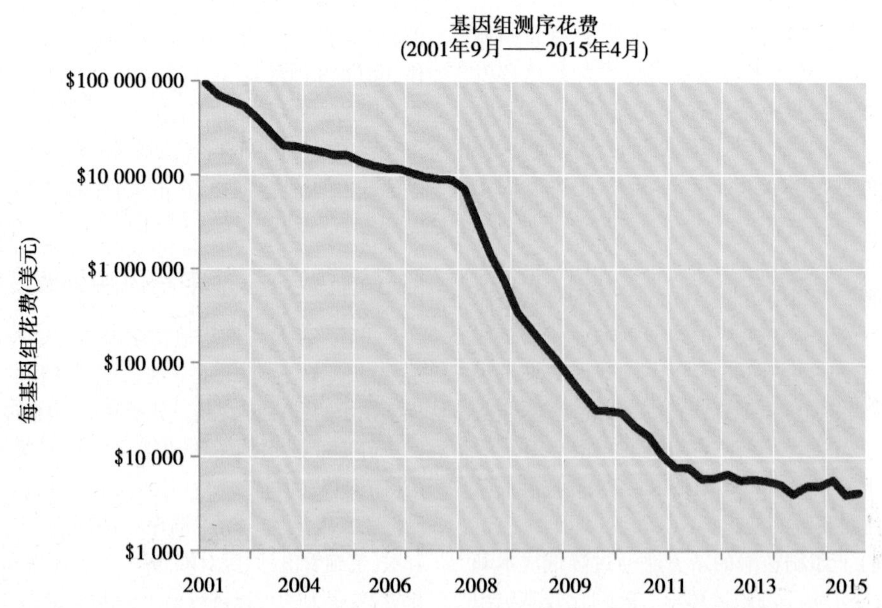

(b)

图 7-3 癌症基因组学的历史。(a)癌症遗传学和基因组学研究里程碑事件时间表,从 1902 年 Boveri 发现癌症染色体异常到 2014 年完成 228 000 人的基因组测序。(b)每 3 000Mb 基因组(即人类基因组的大小)测序的成本随着时间推移不断下降

年提前完成[73]。除了建立全基因组规模人类基因的位置、组织和序列，在该项目过程中学到的技术和信息经验使得在整个基因家族[74~77]和大多数蛋白质编码基因组水平上的首个癌症突变筛选成为可能[62,65~67]。尽管如此，但基于 Sanger 法的测序技术需要数目庞大的插入片段才能完整覆盖整个基因组，所以费用较高且技术复杂，因此在大规模平行测序技术出现之前，该方法在癌症基因组大规模鉴定中的应用依然受到一定限制。

基因表达微阵列：癌症的特征与通路

在 aCGH 研究中使用的微阵列最初是为高通量基因表达研究而开发的。互补 DNA（RNA 逆转录形成的 cDNA）和后来的寡核苷酸微阵列则被用于 mRNA 转录的高通量定量研究。这些技术进步可以与 20 世纪 90 年代的自动化 Sanger 测序技术相媲美。通过这些技术，人类对一些特定癌症亚型的基因特征和相关通路有了初步认识。基因表达系列分析（SAGE）作为另一种实用的方法，被用于对转录本进行高通量数字量化[78]。基因表达谱分析方法虽然最初是被设计用于测定单个基因的表达，但该方法后来被扩展用于分析研究外显子和基因组水平的转录[79]，以及成熟的人类微 RNA（miRNA）的表达[80]。通过分析基因表达模式，可以将传统组织病理学或细胞遗传学技术不易区分的同一种癌症细分为不同亚型，例如，弥漫性大 B 细胞淋巴瘤（DLBCL）[81,82]、肺癌[83]、黑色素瘤[84]和乳腺癌[85,86]。在某些情况下，不同的亚型会表现出不同的临床特征，并且对标准疗法的反应也各不相同。因此，基因表达谱的分析还被广泛用于鉴定可以预测疾病进展、治疗反应或转移的特定基因组合[87~89]，以及发现特定的细胞遗传学异常[90~92]或基因突变[93~96]。尽管微阵列在灵敏度和稳定性上已经被大规模平行测序技术所超越，但受限于成本和临床实际，基因表达谱仍然在癌症生物学和医学中发挥重要作用。目前，基于微阵列（OncoType DX 和 MammaPrint）的乳腺癌临床试剂盒已经上市。

大规模平行测序：绘制癌症基因组全貌

得益于 21 世纪初人类基因组计划的完成，人类对癌症基因组学的认识突飞猛进。通过这些技术进步，完成一个基因组测序的成本从一开始预计的 10 亿美元已经降低到人类基因组计划完成时的 100 万美元大关，但这种巨额的成本仍然阻碍了大规模的基因组研究[97]。因此，美国国家人类基因组研究所发起了一项价值 7 000 万美元的测序技术计划，希望通过这个计划将完成一个基因组测序的成本降至 1 000 美元大关。人类基因组测序的成本现在略低于 2 000 美元，并且正在稳步接近 1 000 美元（图 7-3b）。

对 1 000 美元基因组的追求需要从根本上重新思考 DNA 的测序方法。即使在最专业的实验条件中，Sanger 测序也面临着难以克服的瓶颈，包括①需要分子克隆步骤和/或单独的 PCR 反应以产生测序模板，以及②每个测序反应只能容纳相对较小的基因组区域。因此，即使在多孔板中平行操作，克隆/扩增和多区域的测序也需要大量的材料、设备和分析时间。测序成本和通量的范式转换无需通过克隆或单独的 PCR 反应即可生成测序模板，将整个测序文库固定在单个反应室中，并在反应室中对数百万个模板进行大规模平行测序。该方法不仅可以对单个 DNA 分子进行测序，还可以灵敏的检测到来自异质性肿瘤样本中的稀有突变。这种快速，精准且廉价的方法被称为下一代测序（NGS）。

20 世纪 90 年代和 21 世纪初的关键发明，如合成测序、焦磷酸测序、菌落测序和乳液 PCR，为第一批 NGS 平台的开发提供了技术保障[98~101]。第一个 NGS 平台在 2000 年由 Lynx Therapeutics（后来被 Solexa 收购）开发，但它并没有得到广泛应用[102]。第一个商用系统是 454 生命科学公司于 2004 年开发的 454 FLX 焦磷酸测序仪[103]，随后是 2006 年的 Solexa（现为 Illumina）基因组分析仪，以及 2007 年 Applied Biosystems 研发的寡核苷酸连接和检测（SOLiD）系统，其中也包含了 polony 测序[104,105]。2008 年，Solexa 系统在一个实验室中仅用 2 个月就完成了 James Watson 的基因组测序[106]。这些平台可以对多个癌症基因组进行测序和组装，并且运用该方法对两个肺癌基因组中全基因组的 SV 进行鉴定[107]。该研究利用配对末端法，发现了非常复杂的基因组重排，包括以前从未报告的融合转录本。重要的是，该研究还证明 DNA 拷贝数可以通过被测基因组片段的相对局部丰度进行估计，其敏感度与 aCGH 平台相当，并且还能提供 DNA 的序列信息。大规模平行测序方法在极大地提高测序通量的同时，降低了测序成本。目前，一台常规的商用测序仪器在 6 天的工作周期中可以对 5 000 亿个碱基（相当于 156 个人类基因组或平均 156 倍基因组覆盖度）进行测序，而且其通量仍然在稳步提高。

目前存在许多大规模平行测序平台，这些内容在其他地方有更详细的评述[108]。表 7-1 概述了目前使用的一些最常见的平台。它们在 DNA 序列、拷贝数和结构的分析以及转录组学和表观基因组学等多个不同研究领域得到广泛应用。DNA 测序主要包括从头测序和重复测序，从头测序的经典应用是确定了鲍氏不动杆菌的基因组序列[109]。重测序主要应用于在人类基因组中鉴定正常变异或癌症等疾病状态，其主要原理是通过将 NGS 测序读数对应到参考基因组来鉴定样品和对照之间的差异[65]。当然，很多研究和应用并不需要对全基因组进行测序，因此，通过富集靶基因，对其进行重点测序分析可以有效降低成本。最开始是将确定的基因组区域与生物素化的 BAC 杂交，并通过链霉抗生物素蛋白珠收集这些序列进行测序[110]，后来出现了很多新的富集方法，例如杂交富集（寡核苷酸溶液或寡核苷酸微阵列），高度多重 PCR 和微滴 PCR[111~114]。人类基因组中有一小部分已经在功能上进行了鉴定，因此，对含有编码区的 1%的基因组（即所有外显子）进行测序价值最高，这就是外显子组测序。因此，目前已经上市很多具有实用价值的人外显子组和其他靶向基因富集试剂盒（主要包括常见的癌症基因）。这种靶向特定基因的方法能够实现快速、精准、低成本的测序，不仅有助于生物学发现，在临床检测中也发挥了重要的作用。

表 7-1 大规模平行测序平台

公司	系统平台[a]	最新发布	模板准备	测序化学	最大读取长度	每次运行的通量（Gb）	精确度	运行时间	应用
Illumina	Illumina HiSeq 400	2015	乳液 PCR	可逆终止子	150	1 500	>99%	<1~3. 5 天	WGS, E-S, RNA-S, T-S, C-S, MG
	Illumina HiSeq 3000	2015	乳液 PCR	可逆终止子	150	750	>99%	<1~3. 5 天	WGS, E-S, RNA-S, T-S, C-S, MG
	llumina HiSeq 2500	2014	固相	可逆终止子	125	500	>99%	6 天	WGS, E-S, RNA-S, T-S, C-S, MG, DN-S
	Illumina HiSeq X（Ten/Five）	2014	固相	可逆终止子	150	1 800	>99%	<3 天	WGS
	Illumina MiSeq	2014	固相	可逆终止子	300	15	>99%	4h	E-S, RNA-S, T-S, C-S, DN-S
	Illumina NextSeq 500	2014	固相	可逆终止子	150	120	>99%	30h	WGS, E-S, RNA-S, T-S, C-S, MG
Life Technologies	IonTorrent Personal Genome Machine	2014	乳液 PCR	质子检测	400	2	>99%	2h	Microbial WGS, E-S, RNA-S, T-S, C-S, MG
	IonTorrent Proton	2014	乳液 PCR	质子检测	200	10	>99%	2~4h	Microbial WGS, E-S, RNA-S, T-S, C-S, MG
	SOLiD	2014	乳液 PCR	连接测序	75	120	99. 99%	8 天	WGS, DN-S, E-S, RNA-S, T-S, C-S, MG
Pacific Biosciences	PacBio RS Ⅱ	2014	单分子	实时测序	15 000	3	85%	20min	DN-S, T-S
Roche	454 GS Junior	2014	乳液 PCR	焦磷酸测序	400	0. 07	>99%	10h	Microbial DN-S, E-S
	454 GS FLX	2014	乳液 PCR	焦磷酸测序	700	0. 7	100%	24h	Microbial DN-S, E-S

WGS，全基因组测序；E-S，外显子组测序；RNA-S，RNA；测序；T-S，靶向测序；C-S，ChIP 测序；MG，宏基因组学；和 DN-S，从头测序。[a] 某些型号可以使用其他版本。

癌症基因组图谱

标志性的癌症基因组研究

尽管在过去的遗传学研究中发现了不同类型癌症之间的共性，但过去十年的高通量基因组研究为此提供了更为复杂的观点。第一个大规模癌症突变基因的筛选主要是针对单个基因（如 *BRAF*）进行高通量 Sanger 测序[115,116]，或者对不同癌症中的蛋白激酶等基因家族进行测序[74~77,117,118]。值得注意的是，通过筛选在绝大多数人类黑色素瘤[115]和痣[119]中鉴定出活化的 *BRAF* 突变，并且在人类乳腺癌中鉴定出 *ERBB2* 突变[118]。2003 年，通过对 140 例急性髓性白血病（AML）样本的筛选，建立了第一个癌症基因组（包括 12 个靶基因的 110 个外显子）[120]。该研究鉴定了 6 个先前已知的编码突变，并且惊人地发现了 7 个先前未知的 AML 基因组中的编码突变。不久之后，对 11 例乳腺癌和 11 例结直肠癌中 13 023 种基因进行 Sanger 外显子组测序的结果于 2006 年发表[121]。该研究发现，每个肿瘤平均有 90 个突变基因，共发现了 189 个频繁突变的基因，但只有一个亚组（平均每个肿瘤有 11 个突变基因）被认为与肿瘤发生或进展有关。在对相同肿瘤的另外 7 000 个基因的后续分析中发现，在大量不太频繁变异的基因群中确实存在少数频繁突变的基因（这一现象类似丘陵中突起的山峰）。2008 年，四个 Sanger 外显子组测序项目进一步在多形性胶质母细胞瘤[62,65,66]和胰腺癌[67]中对 20 000 多个基因进行了鉴定。结果显示，在每个胰腺癌或胶质母细胞瘤中的平均突变数为 63 和 47，并且在胶质母细胞瘤中发现了具有低频突变的新基因，如 *IDH1* 和 *PIK3R1* 突变。更引人注目的是，该研究发现很少有未知基因发生高频突变。之后的研究也进一步证明，过去几十年的低通量基因技术已经鉴定出了绝大部分高频突变。癌症基因组研究领域以后的挑战是如何对许多不频繁突变在癌症中的作用做出解释和分析。然而，这些研究同时也发现，在癌症中发生突变的通常是核心信号通路内的多个基因而不是单个基因，这说明肿瘤治疗的切入点应该是异常通路而不是单个异常基因。

在这些具有里程碑意义的研究之后，随着大规模平行测序技术的成熟，癌症基因组计划的数量，广度和规模迅速增加。2008 年，第一次采用大规模平行测序技术分析了两例肺癌[107]，此后，2008 年和 2009 年又分别对独立的 AML 病例进行了癌症全基因组测序[122,123]。这些研究侧重于对全基因组 SV 的评估和错义突变。2009 年，通过对原发性乳腺癌和其相对应的转移性肿瘤进行测序，确定了每对样本中共有的和排他的突变，进而对乳腺癌的演化进行了全基因组评估[124]。2010 年在黑色素瘤细胞系 COLO-829[125]和小细胞肺癌细胞系[126]中第一次对所有类别全基因组突变进行了系统评估。这些研究发现在紫外线相关性黑色素瘤和烟草相关性肺癌中，突变负荷（黑色素瘤超过 33 000 个突变，肺部突变 23 000 个）远远大于一般肿瘤。此后，类似研究层出不穷，目前已经在所有常见癌症，许多罕见癌症，原发/复发/转移匹配群组，甚至正在接受治疗的癌症中完成了相关的大型基因组分析。

大规模癌症基因组的研究也得到了国家和国际组织的支持。美国国家癌症研究所（NCI）和美国国家人类基因组研究所（NHGRI）于 2005 年启动了一项大型合作项目，即癌症基因组图谱（TCGA；见 http://cancergenome. nih. gov/），其目的是运用多种先进的基因组技术，全面识别与多种癌症类型相关的所有基因组改变。TCGA 的研究范围从一开始的多形性胶质母细胞瘤[65]、卵巢癌[127]和鳞状细胞肺癌[128]逐渐扩展至结直肠[129]、乳腺[130]、子宫内膜[131]、AML[132]、透明细胞肾细胞[133]、扩张的胶质母细胞瘤[134]、尿道上皮细胞[135]、肺腺癌[136]、胃[137]、嫌色细胞肾细胞[138]、乳头状甲状腺[139]、头颈部鳞状细胞[140]、低级别胶质瘤[141]、皮肤黑色素瘤[142]和其他 18 项泛癌研究[143]。其数据从 11 000 多个病例中收集，涵盖了 34 种癌症类型。国际癌症基因组联盟（ICGC；见 http://icgc. org）成员在 2010 年开始了来自另一项雄心勃勃的研究[144]，计划全面记录与至少 50 种不同癌症相关的所有基因组畸变。该联盟目前包括 55 个项目，涵盖 33 种癌症类型，纳入了超过 13 000 名的病例，并已经出版了关于亚硫酸氢盐测序技术[145,146]、DLBCL[147]、伯基特淋巴瘤[148]、X 染色体超突变[149]、突变过程的特征[150]和原发性中枢神经系统淋巴瘤[151]的出版物。这些全面的大型项目的最终成功将持续快速推进我们对癌症遗传学和基因组学的理解，并可能彻底改变癌症诊断和治疗的方法。

癌症基因组数据库和分析工具

虽然 TCGA、ICGC 和其他基因组数据库的数据是公开的，但是，对这些数据进行系统分析仍然是一项具有挑战性的工作。不过，得益于网络分析软件的不断进步，不管是基因组学研究领域的新手还是经验丰富的生物信息学家，都可以较轻松的进行癌症基因组学研究（表 7-2）。由维康信托桑格研究院癌症基因组计划开发维护的癌症体细胞突变目录（COSMIC；见 http://www. sanger. ac. uk/genetics/CGP/cosmic）是最早且功能最全面的用于挖掘此类数据的的软件之一[152]。COSMIC 包含的数据是从出版物中人工收集的，目前一共纳入了 2 万多个相关靶向研究和基因研究。当前版本（2014 年 8 月）中收录了 100 多万个样本中的 200 多万个突变，包括 12 000 个癌症基因组。除 SNV 外，它还详细介绍了 600 多万个非编码突变，10 000 个融合突变，61 000 个 SV、70 万个 CNV 和 6 000 万个表达变异。使用关键词、基因或癌症类型可以轻松查询这些数据。COSMIC 还包括很多高级工具，这些工具通过与其他数据库的关联，可以进行人类癌症基因的详细普查（癌症基因普查；见 http://www. sanger. ac. uk/genetics/CGP/Census）[5,153]以及突变特征和药物敏感性的评估。另一个高度通用的数据门户网站是由 Memorial Sloan-Kettering 癌症研究所维护的癌症基因组学 cBioPortal[154]。该门户网站主要包含高度加工的癌症细胞系百科全书（CCLE）和 TCGA 数据集，不仅提供了功能强大且直观的网络界面，可以通过基因名称或癌症类型进行查询，还可以通过应用程序编程接口进行更高级分析，与 R 和 MATLAB 进行集成分析。ICGC 数据库也有类似的门户网站（见 http://dcc. icgc. org）。

表 7-2 癌症基因组学数据库

名称	详情	链接
canEvolve	分析来自 TCGA、GEO 和 Array Express 的 10 000 个患者样品中的 mRNA、miRNA、蛋白质表达和 CNV 数据	www. canevolve. org
canSAR	来自 COSMIC、chEMBl、UniProt、BindingDB、Array Express 和 STRING 的生物、化学和药理学数据的综合分析	https://cansar. icr. ac. uk
cBioPortal	TCGA 数据门户；图形可视化和分析	http://www. cbioportal. org
CGAP	基因表达的图形汇总和分析；整合细胞遗传学数据	http://cgap. nci. nih. gov
CGHub	安全、全面的数据存储库；TCGA、CCLE 和 TARGET 项目	https://cghub. ucsc. edu
CPRG	用于癌症研究的综合分析工具	http://www. broadinstitute. org/software/cprg
COSMIC	最大的基因组数据库；手动策划的出版物和大型测序研究的输出	http://www. sanger. ac. uk/genetics/CGP/cosmic
EBI Array Express	带注释的功能基因组学数据；通过微阵列和高通量测序项目生成的数据	http://www. ebi. ac. uk/microarray-as/ae
EGA	综合数据存储库；禁止进入；ICGC 输出；SNV 和 CNV 数据	https://www. ebi. ac. uk/ega
GDAC	用于基因组分析的管道；用户友好的界面	http://gdac. broadinstitute. org
GEO	基因表达微阵列和功能基因组数据库	http://www. ncbi. nlm. nih. gov/geo
ICGC	可视化工具；50 种肿瘤类型的基因组学、转录组学和表观基因组学表征	http://dcc. icgc. org
MethylCancer	甲基化数据库；解释甲基化，基因表达和癌症生物学的相关性	http://methycancer. psych. ac. cn
SomamiR	存储经过实验验证的非编码 RNA 中的体细胞突变	http://compbio. uthsc. edu/SomamiR
UCSC Cancer Genome Browser	多用途数据查看器包含多种数据类型，包括临床信息	https://genome-cancer. soe. ucsc. edu

上述门户网站用户只要通过简单的生物信息学培训即可以实现高级分析，但对数据要求更高的用户也可以通过另外的数据库来获得各种级别的原始数据。由加州大学圣克鲁兹分校（UCSC）负责的癌症基因组学中心（CGHub）是一个储存美国国家癌症研究所（NCI）数据的安全中央数据库，包括 TCGA、CCLE 和有效治疗临床试验数据库（TARGET）[155]。欧洲基因组-表型数据库（见 http://ega. crg. eu）同样收集并提供测序和基因分型数据，主要是 ICGC 中的癌症数据。相关数据存储库和分析工具还可以用于其他数据类型的分析存储。目前，在 65 000 多个人类肿瘤中观察到的细胞遗传学畸变和融合已经可以通过 NCI 癌症基因组解剖项目[CGAP]网站上的癌症染色体畸变的 Mitelman 数据库获得（http://cgap. nci. nih. gov）[28]。而来自众多基因表达微阵列研究的数据则由多个单位同时存储，包括美国国家生物技术信息中心（NCBI Gene Expression Omnibus；见 http://www. ncbi. nlm. nih. gov/geo/）和欧洲生物信息学研究所（EBI Array Express；见 http://www. ebi. ac. uk/microarray-as/ae/）。其他的数据存储库和网络资源见表 7-2。

大量且多样化的人类癌症基因图谱

尽管过去 10 年很少发现新的频繁且重要的突变，但对癌症基因组的系统研究揭示了许多新的不频繁突变以及相关突变过程和失调的通路。总突变负荷本身可以反映癌症病因并且与临床过程有关。这种负荷比最初的预期的变化更大。在一些儿科癌症例如横纹肌样瘤[156]和卵巢的小细胞癌中，已发现仅具有单一编码 SNV 的病例[157]，而诸如 AML 的白血病平均每个病例具有 9 个编码 SNVs（图 7-4）。相反，具有诱变病因的癌症如膀胱癌，肺癌和黑色素瘤的突变率要高得多，分别含有 148 217 和 254 个编码 SNV，而具有错配修复缺陷的肿瘤可包含数千个编码 SNV。不同的突变特征也可以反映这些外部和内部诱变因素，比如紫外线损伤部位的癌症中存在二嘧啶 C>T 转换的富集[150]。虽然癌症中存在 CNV 和 SV 谱的广泛变异，但最常见的变异依旧是编码 SNV。37%的癌症存在全基因组倍增，其中四分之一的实体瘤基因组包含大规模染色体变异和 10%局部 CNV。目前，已经有超过 140 个基因组区域被发现

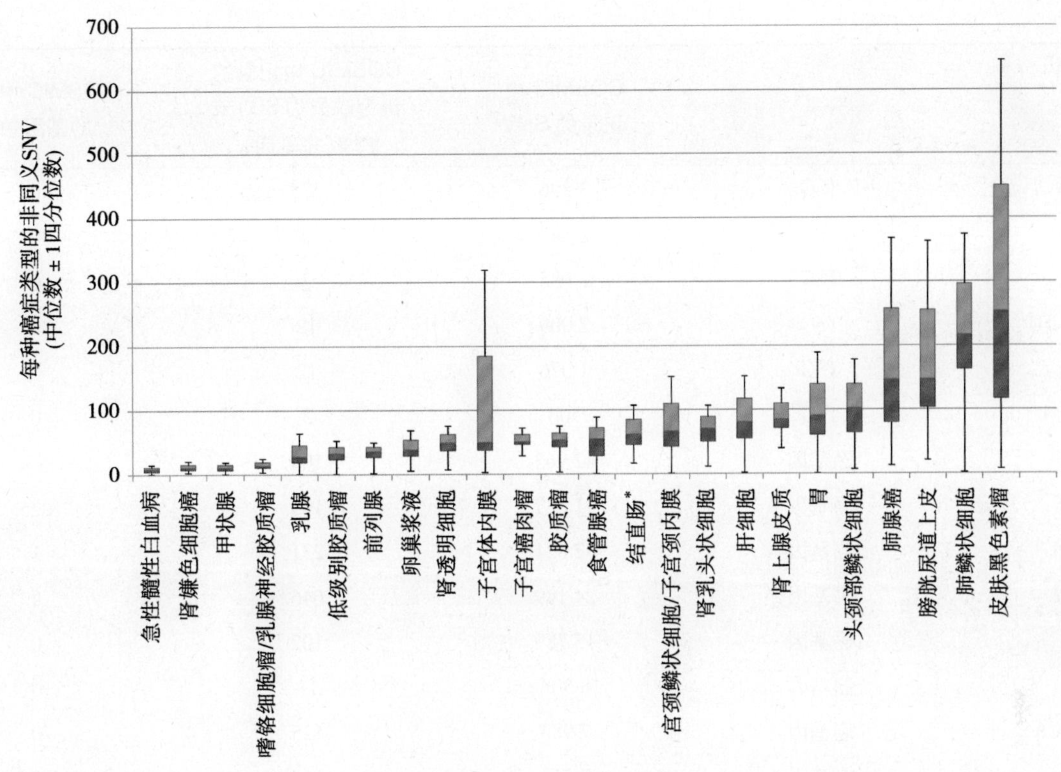

图 7-4　在选择的人类癌症类型中，每种肿瘤类型编码单核苷酸变异（SNV）的数量。从公布的 TCGA 研究获得的 DNA 测序数据用于计算每种癌症类型中编码 SNV 突变的分布和中位数。彩色条形图表示 25%和 75%的四分点。离群值（低于 Q1−1. 5×IQR 或高于 Q3+1. 5×IQR 的值）未显示，星号表示超过 10%离群值的研究

含有常见的 CNV，但其中只有 38 个含有已知的癌基因[158~160]。大多数实体瘤也含有数十个 SV，但其中大部分仅仅只是携带 SV，主要分布在不含基因的区域上。全基因组测序最近还在 2%~3%的癌症中[161~163]发现了“染色体碎裂”现象，即有丝分裂间期染色体分离的错误导致单个或几个染色体的破碎以及单个细胞中的染色体大规模重排。

“间断演化”模型认为，除诱变病因外，突变负荷的变异还可能与突变时间，患者年龄和前体细胞中发生的分裂数量有关[164~166]。最终，只有少数可以赋予细胞选择性生长优势的突变可以“驱动”癌症，我们称其为驱动型突变。其他突变仅仅只是被携带，对细胞生长没有表型效应[167]。根据突变在癌症中出现的模式和频率，可以将突变分为驱动型突变或携带型突变[4,168,169]，但这些突变在癌症中的作用需要在实验中进一步验证。

据估计，存在超过 138 种癌症驱动基因[4]，其中 571 种与癌症基因普查中的癌症存在因果关系（见 http://cancer. sanger. ac. uk/census）[5]。表 7-3 给出了前 10 个最常见的突变癌症基因，而表 7-4 中给出了与美国最致命的癌症相关的癌症基因。虽然突变看起来非常复杂，但其对癌症的治疗却带来了潜在的希望。例如，在高度复杂的癌症（例如黑色素瘤和肺癌中的突变 BRAF 和 ALK）中靶向突变蛋白的药物可以看到显著的临床反应[194,195]。此外，多种癌症基因通常会聚集在一个共同的通路上，这些突变基因对通路造成的影响可能是相同的。因此，特定通路受基因组畸变影响的概率可能远高于任何单个基因突变的频率。实际上，大多数驱动基因会聚集在标志性通路上，并且最终影响到细胞分化，细胞增殖，细胞死亡和基因组的维持[2]。因此，需要整合多种类型的基因组数据去阐明体细胞癌症遗传学的复杂性。

表 7-3　COSMIC 数据库中十种最常发生突变的癌基因和抑癌基因（TSG）

基因	分类[a]	COSMIC 中记录的 SNV	COSMIC 中记录的纯合缺失（TSG）或扩增（癌基因）[b]	COSMIC 中记录的基因融合
TP53	TSG	28 253	17	1
NPM1	TSG	5 224	1	319
CDKN2A	TSG	4 836	1 046	0
APC	TSG	4 351	10	0

续表

基因	分类[a]	COSMIC 中记录的 SNV	COSMIC 中记录的纯合缺失(TSG)或扩增(癌基因)[b]	COSMIC 中记录的基因融合
PTEN	TSG	3 296	275	0
VHL	TSG	2 443	2	0
TET2	TSG	2 085	3	0
NOTCH1	TSG	2 009	12	0
NF2	TSG	1 076	12	0
CEBPA	TSG	706	3	0
JAK2	癌基因	42 963	109	35
BRAF	癌基因	41 637	105	625
KRAS	癌基因	32 021	231	1
EGFR	癌基因	24 189	646	0
FLT3	癌基因	15 789	102	0
IDH1	癌基因	8 508	11	0
PIK3CA	癌基因	7 983	425	0
KIT	癌基因	7 413	106	0
CTNNB1	癌基因	5 372	12	22
NRAS	癌基因	4 278	31	0

[a] 使用 COSMIC 数据库中的样本数据，通过 20/20 rule[4] 确定致癌基因和 TSG 状态（参见 http://www.sanger.ac.uk/genetics/CGP/cosmic/）。
[b] 显示平均基因组倍性≤2.7 和总基因拷贝数≥5 或平均基因组倍性>2.7 且总基因拷贝数≥9 的样品的扩增。显示平均基因组倍性≤2.7 和总基因拷贝数=0 或平均基因组倍性>2.7 且总拷贝数<（平均基因组倍性-2.7）的样品的纯合缺失。

表 7-4 致死率较高的癌症类型中常见的突变基因

癌症[a]	家族性癌症基因	常见的体细胞突变基因	参考文献
乳房	BRCA1,BRCA2,PTEN,TP53	PIK3CA, TP53, MAP3K1, GATA3, MLL3, CDH1, PTEN,ERBB2,MAPK2K4、CDKN2A、PTEN、RB1	62,121,130,170~172
结直肠	APC, MSH2, MLH1, MSH6, PMS2, MUTYH, LKB1, SMAD4, BMPR1A, PTEN, KLLN	APC, TP53, KRAS, PIK3CA, FBXW7, SMAD4, TCF7L2, NRAS, ARID1A, SOX9, FAM123B, ERBB2, IGF2, NAV2, TCF7L1	62,121,129,173,174
肝	HFE, SLC25A13, ABCB11, FAH, HMBS, UROD	TP53, CTNNB1, AXIN1, RPS6KA3, RB1, FAM123A, CDKN2A, MYC, RSPO2, CCND1, FGF19, ARID1A, ARID1B, ARID2, MLL, MLL3	175~178
肺	EGFR,BRAF,KRAS,TP53	TP53, KRAS, STK11, EGFR, ALK, BRAF, AKT1, DDR2, HER2, MEK1, NRAS, PIK3CA, PTEN, RET, ROS1, EML4, NTRK1, FHIT, FRA3B, FGFR1, HER2	57,75,116,118,126,128, 136,179
胰腺	BRCA2,PALB2	KRAS, TP53, CDKN2A, SMAD4, MLL3, TGFRB2, ARID1A, SF3B1, ROBO2, KDM6A, PREX2	67,180~183
前列腺	BRCA2,BRCA1,HOXB13	EPHB2, ERG, TMPRSS2, PTEN, TP53, SPOP, FXA1, MED12, NKX3-1	166,184~188
卵巢	STK11,BRCA1,BRCA2	FBXW7, AKT2, ERBB2, TGFBR1, TGFBR2, BRAF, KRAS, PIK3CA, PTEN, ARID1A, BRCA1, MMP-1, BRCA1, BRCA2, MLPA, MAPH	127,189~192

[a] 据估计，2015 年导致美国死亡人数最多的 7 种癌症[193]。

虽然现在似乎已经发现了大多数的癌症基因,但与癌症有关的新基因仍时有发现,这些新基因在许多癌症中突变频率较低,但在罕见且以前未发现的癌症中突变频率较高。流行病学研究[196]证明,大多数癌症需要5~8个驱动型突变,但现实中除了儿科病例等例外(仅发现三个,甚至更少的驱动因子),大多数癌症中仅发现3~6个驱动因子[4]。这些缺少的驱动型突变可能是由于测序技术和研究设计的技术限制以及我们对DNA非编码区域或表观遗传学机制的理解有限所致。显然,癌症驱动型突变的目录仍不完整,在目前已有的癌症基因组全貌的基础上,仍然需要做很多工作来详细描述这些更为广阔的内容,以指导临床癌症管理。

癌症基因组景观的临床意义

现在,从癌症基因组工程获得的详尽信息极大地加深了我们对人类肿瘤的发生、发展和临床表现的理解。这些数据和运用的技术也影响癌症筛查、诊断和治疗。随着测序成本的持续下降,外显子组和全基因组的群体筛查变得越来越可行,并且每个患者的个人基因组序列可能构成其医疗记录的关键组成部分。这种筛查可能发现一些在疾病表现出临床症状之前难以被发现的新的突变,并且当我们将遗传变异与疾病表型相联系,筛查的作用将指数性增长。美国国立卫生研究院通过建立精准医学计划已经认识到这种新的医疗保健方法的重要性[197]。小基因组的靶向Sanger测序已经普遍用于家族性癌症筛查。在例如胚系*BRCA1/2*或*MLH1/MSH2*突变的情况下,其显著增加了乳腺/卵巢或结直肠癌的终身风险,基因组测试可指导关于监测和预防性手术的临床决策。现在,基于NGS的数百个基因的测序能够以相似的成本完成,从而能够检测较低外显率的罕见变异,这些变异在较小的面板中是不可检测的。例如,在一项对141名患有乳腺癌家族或个人史的*BRCA1/2*阴性患者的研究中,除了*BRCA1/2*之外,在16个病人中检测到一组40个额外基因,其中在9个基因中包含致病性变异,例如*TP53*和*PTEN*[198]。这些研究结果形成了国家综合癌症网络的新指南,建议对具有乳腺癌或卵巢癌家族史但常见遗传性突变为阴性的病人建立针对性检查项目[199]。在家族性癌基因的基因检测中,有针对性的NGS小组比传统诊断工具也表现出更为敏感和更为特异的性质,例如在其他研究中的*BRCA1/2*、*TP53*和*APC*[170,200~202]。鉴于NGS组、外显子组甚至全基因组的诊断率已在多项研究中显示出优于小型的Sanger组[203,204],NGS组也可能会促进鉴别诊断和患者分层。

自首次报道染色体常见异常——CML中的*BCR-ABL*易位以来,癌症遗传学的发现推动了靶向药物的发展。选择性酪氨酸激酶抑制剂伊马替尼,旨在靶向BCR-ABL融合基因及其在CML中的组成型活性酪氨酸激酶蛋白产物,是第一个成功的靶向治疗药物[205~207]。靶向癌症特异性突变的范例极大地改善了化疗的治疗指标,现在已经取得了巨大的成功。成功的案例包括伊马替尼对*PDGFR*和*KIT*突变的胃肠道间质瘤(GIST)和嗜酸性粒细胞综合征[208~210]的影响;达沙替尼和尼罗替尼治疗原发性和伊马替尼耐药的CML[211~213];曲妥珠单抗,一种靶向Her2/ErbB2酪氨酸激酶受体的中和抗体,该受体的编码基因*ERBB2*在25%~30%的乳腺癌中被扩增和过表达[214,215];舒尼替尼治疗肾细胞癌、GIST和胰腺神经内分泌肿瘤[216~218];吉非替尼和厄洛替尼在5%~10%的欧洲血统型肺腺癌患者和在25%~30%的具有EGFR活化突变的日本患者中具有显著疗效[219,220];克唑替尼治疗ALK重排肺癌[221,222];vismodegib在带有hedgehog通路突变的基底细胞癌中的作用[223];vemurafenib在*BRAF*突变的黑色素瘤中的作用[224]。癌症基因突变也与这些靶向治疗的先天或获得性耐药有关。例如,*BCR-ABL*基因的扩增在对伊马替尼耐药的CML患者中是常见的[205,225]。除了能够规避或治疗耐药性的药剂之外,针对癌症中的基因组靶标的许多新型治疗剂正在进行临床前研究和临床试验。

肿瘤学实践的基本目标是为个体患者推荐有科学证据支持的最有效的治疗方法。基因组数据预计可以提供这样的数据。然而,尽管HGP在2003年完成,但基因组医学进入医疗流程的速度却非常缓慢。2010年,发表了首次使用个性化分子谱分析指导难治性转移性癌症治疗选择的试点研究结果。尽管存在相当大的挑战,包括缺乏先前的新型试验设计、整体患者损耗和药物使用的多样化,但在68名患者中发现,27%的患者通过分子谱分析(基因表达微阵列分析)引导的治疗选择相较于当前的患者进展方案,具有更长的无进展生存期[226]。为患者提供基因组工具的下一个主要进展是结合全基因组测序和全面的RNA测序,对转移性三阴性乳腺癌(TNBC)患者进行个体化的治疗[227]。TNBC的特征在于不存在雌激素受体(ER)、黄体酮受体(PR)和HER-2的表达。该研究鉴定了RAS/RAF/MEK和PI3K/AKT/mTOR信号通路中的体细胞突变,这些通路导致临床试验将靶向*MEK*和*mTOR*基因的药物结合起来,获得了令人振奋的治疗结果。

新的试验设计,例如上述试验设计,包括适应性试验、篮式试验和伞式试验,旨在将个体化治疗扩展到所有癌症患者中。多个大型学术观察性和干预性临床试验现已经发表[228~233]或正在进行中(见 http://clinicaltrials.gov)。这些研究包括适应性试验,如I-SPY 2(通过影像和分子分析预测治疗反应的系统研究),在研究过程中根据患者的反应改善治疗方法[234]。篮式试验,如NCI MATCH试验根据突变谱将患有各种晚期癌症的患者分配到治疗组中,然后使用与其肿瘤突变相匹配的药物进行治疗[231]。伞式试验也在单个疾病中进行多项药物研究的试验中应用。例如,进行中的Stand Up To Cancer和黑色素瘤研究梦之队临床试验正在对单一组织学特征的缺失通用治疗靶点的非V600 BRAF转移性黑色素瘤患者群体中评估分子指导治疗的效果。在一项非治疗试验研究(现为随机治疗研究)中,全基因组和全转录组测序的组合被用于鉴定与临床药物治疗相匹配的分子变异,这些药物都是符合药典标准、FDA批准和研究的药物[230]。在临床相关时间段内返回可操作信息的挑战是相当大的。这包括患者同意、肿瘤活检、质量DNA/RNA提取、DNA和RNA测序、数据整合、报告生成以及肿瘤委员会审查,以制定治疗计划(图7-5)。简化这一过程对于将这些工具扩展应用到主要学术研究中心至关重要。

在临床试验的背景下,大规模肿瘤基因组特征已经可以鉴定出预测性的生物标志物——常见的基因组改变可以区分最可能从特定药物中受益的患者。这些标志物利于患者分组到最合适的治疗选择并且已经快速商业化,提供了巨大的临床价值。现在,肿瘤学家及其患者可以进行更广泛的测序,可能有助于诊断和治疗的决策。超过100个学术中心和50个商业实

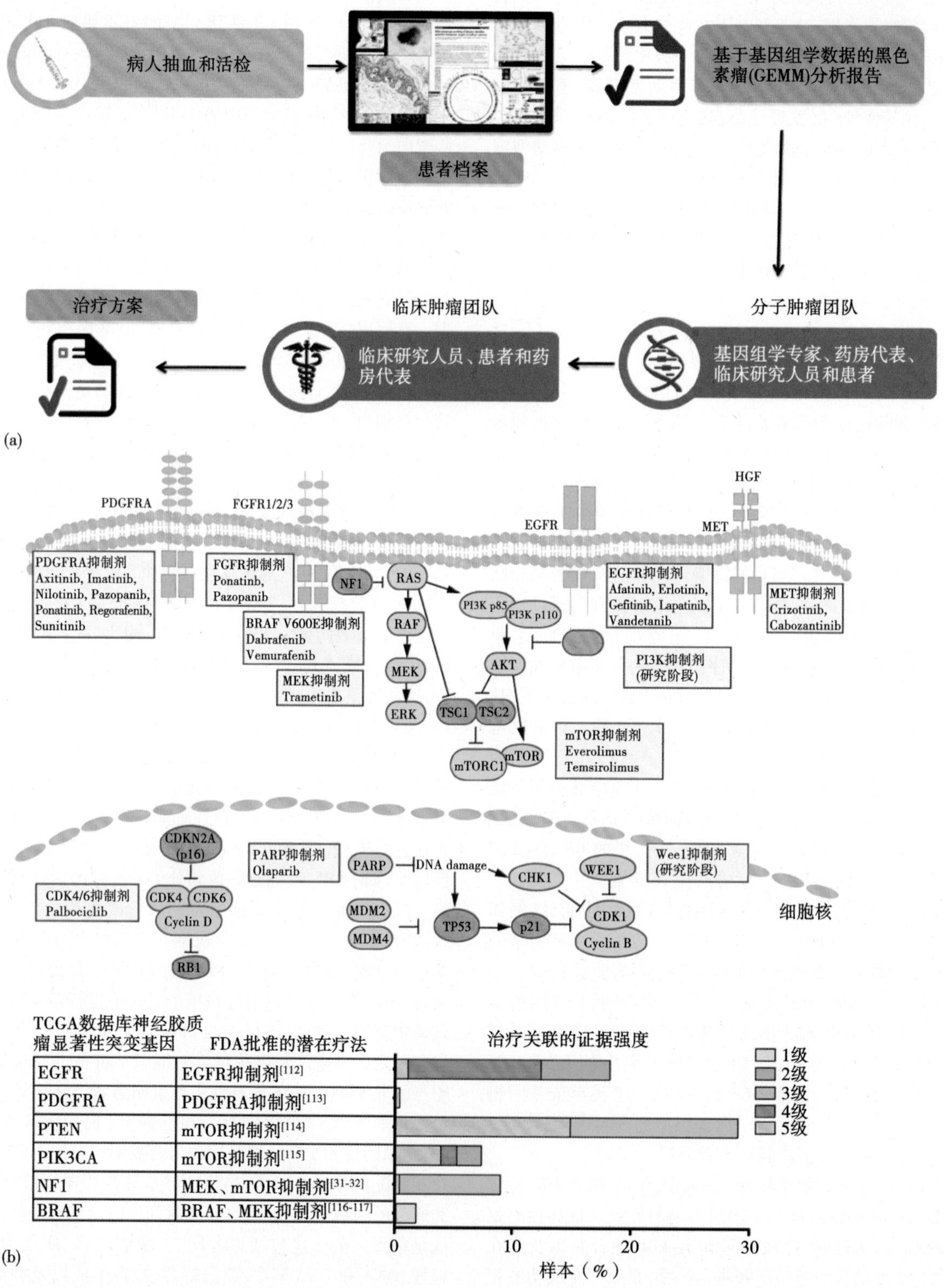

图 7-5　精准医学临床实践路径。(a)流程图描述了从患者知情同意到基因组学分析，再到形成治疗方案整个过程中的关键步骤。从组织活检到制定治疗方案整个过程计划在 5 周内完成。资料来源：LoRusso，P，等。携带非 V600 BRAF 突变的转移性黑色素瘤患者选择性分子治疗方案的先导研究：来自 SU2C/MRA 黑色素瘤梦想团队的经验。Molecular Cancer Therapeutics. 2015 Aug 14(8)：1962-1971.（经授权使用）。(b)在原发性胶质母细胞瘤 TCGA 数据集中发现的显著突变基因的潜在治疗意义。(上图)发生高频突变的主要信号通路及其潜在治疗药物。(下左图)来自 TCGA 的高频突变的基因列表及其对应的 FDA 批准的潜在靶向治疗药物。(下右图)柱形图反映了基因层面变异与临床治疗意义之间关联性的强度

验室已经提供了这种检测服务。表 7-5 中提供了此类商业检测的示例。虽然成本仍然不能广泛使用，但扩展组、外显子组或全基因组的测序将在未来几年继续改变筛查和诊断的模式。然而，常规临床使用不仅需要进一步降低成本，而且还需要更全面的数据支持基因组学相关的临床结果，以说明此类检测和标签外药物使用的益处。因此，商业测序实验室将需要获得 FDA 和 Medicare 批准。这些数据将确保保险公司涵盖这些检测。一些迹象已经表明前景乐观，其中包括程序术语代码的增加和医疗保险和医疗补助服务中心费用表中包含的 21 个测序的初步清单。最后，胚系基因组分析（无论是遗传性癌症检测的一部分还是在肿瘤匹配的正常组织中进行）都需要偶然发现具有不明确的疾病关联的假定病原性基因组变异体，因此仍面临挑战。关于患者自主权与患者对这些信息的了解会导致身体或精神伤害的看法之间的平衡，存在着广泛的争议[235]。

表 7-5　商业化的癌症基因组检测产品

提供商	产品	说明[a]
Ambry Genetics	Exome Next	全外显子组+线粒体基因组，SNV，CNV
Ambry Genetics	*BRCA1* 和 *BRCA2* 基因测序	SNV，CNV，BRCA1/2 SV
Arup Laboratories	胃肠道遗传性癌症 panel	15 个基因+内含子/外显子连接，SNV，CNV
Ashion Analytics	GEM Cancer panel	562 基因，肿瘤/胚系，SNV，CNV
	GEM GW	全外显子组，肿瘤/胚系，SNV，CNV，SV
	RNA Sequencing	RNA，肿瘤/胚系。基因表达，融合基因，可变剪接，SNV
Cancer Genetics Incorporated（CGI）	FOCUS：CLL	七个明确的 CLL 靶点
	FOCUS：Myeloid	54 个基因，预后和治疗评估
Caris	MI Profile	47 个基因，SNVs
Foundation Medicine	Foundation One	236 个基因，19 个基因的 47 个内含子及相关的 SNV、CNV、SV
	Foundation One Heme	405 基因，31 个内含子相关的 SV，265 个基因的 RNA-seq。血液肿瘤中的 SNV、CNV、SV，融合基因和基因表达
GeneDx	XomeDx	全外显子组，SNV
	XOMEDX Plus	全外显子组+线粒体基因组，SNV
	XOMEDX Slice	靶向外显子组，SNV
	Comprehensive cancer panel	29 个基因，SNV，CNV
GPS@ WUSTL	Comprehensive Cancer Gene Set Analysis	42 个基因测序及突变分析
Agendia	Mammaprint	70 个基因的微阵列基因表达分析。预测化疗效果和乳腺癌复发风险
Myriad Genetics	BRACAnalysis	Sanger 法，BRCA1/2，乳腺癌和卵巢癌
	COLARIS	Sanger 法，六种基因，遗传性结直肠癌
	COLARIS AP	Sanger 法，APC 和 MYH 基因，腺瘤性息肉病结肠癌风险
	MELARIS	Sanger 法，CDKN2A，遗传性黑色素瘤
	PANEXIA	Sanger 法，PALB2+BRCA2 基因，胰腺癌风险评估
	Myriad myRisk Hereditary Cancer	Sanger 法，25 个基因，乳腺癌、卵巢癌、胃癌、结肠直肠癌、胰腺癌、黑色素瘤、前列腺癌和子宫内膜癌风险评估
NeoGenomics Laboratories	NeoTYPE Cancer Exome Profile	4 813 个基因，SNV
	NeoTYPE Profiles	定制基因组合，SNV
OncotypeDX	OncotypeDX Breast Cancer Assay	RT-PCR，21 种基因，基因表达，化疗疗效和浸润性乳腺癌复发风险

续表

提供商	产品	说明[a]
	OncotypeDX Colon Cancer Assay	RT-PCR,18 个基因,基因表达,Ⅱ期和Ⅲ期结肠癌复发风险
	OncotypeDX Prostate Cancer Assay	RT-PCR<17 基因,基因表达,前列腺癌的治疗方案选择
Paradigm	PCDx	未明确说明检测基因数目,DNA 和 RNA 分析,SNV,CNV,SV,基因表达,基因融合,可变剪接
Personal Genome Diagnostics(PGDX)	全基因组分析	全基因组,肿瘤或 ctDNA 和胚系,SNV,CNV,SV
	CancerXome	全外显子组,SNV,CNV,SV
	Cancer Select(R88,R203)	88 或 203 个基因,SNV,CNV,SV
	ImmunoSelect-R	外显子,预测新抗原评估免疫治疗效果
	PlasmaSelect-R	ctDNA 中的 58 个基因,SNV
Quest Diagnostics	OncoVantage	34 个基因,SNVs

[a] 上述描述源自公司网站,可能不完整。同时也不构成对任何特定产品的认可。

在肿瘤和正常组织之间 mRNA 或蛋白质表达的相对差异不同,癌症基因中的体细胞突变是癌细胞的排他性和特异性标记。最近利用这一事实在血浆中使用无细胞肿瘤特异性 DNA(ctDNA),作为肿瘤负荷的精准循环生物标志物。用于监测肿瘤负荷、治疗反应和复发的 ctDNA 值首先在结直肠癌中被识别[236]。该研究鉴定了反复突变的结直肠癌基因(*TP53*、*PIK3CA*、*APC* 和 *KRAS*)在患者肿瘤中的体细胞突变,并使用针对每位患者专门设计的高灵敏度检测回顾性分析血浆样品。结果显示,与影像和癌胚抗原相比,ctDNA 水平反映了治疗期间肿瘤负荷的变化。实施 ctDNA 作为肿瘤监测的常规生物标志物的挑战包括需要识别每个患者的体细胞改变,患者特异性分子测定的设计以及特别是在疾病的早期阶段循环中低丰度的突变。最近的另一项研究使用肿瘤 NGS 和数字 PCR,发现治疗期间的 ctDNA 水平反映了转移性乳腺癌的疾病进展[237]。在这些结果中,与循环肿瘤细胞或 CA-125(乳腺癌的糖蛋白生物标志物)相比,ctDNA 被发现更具响应性,适用于最大规模的患者。在肺癌[238,239],黑色素瘤[240],和骨肉瘤[241]中支持 ctDNA 系列分析监测肿瘤负荷的相似结果已经发表。

分子方法的进展包括使用高深度经过噪声校正的靶向 NGS 检测可以对局部、潜在可切除的癌症患者进行研究[242,243]。最近在局部乳腺癌方面的研究表明,ctDNA 可以预测癌症术后复发,中位数为 8 个月,之后肿瘤可在成像中检测到[244]。这项研究和其他在局部癌症中描述 ctDNA 的论文中,证明了通过个体化治疗策略展示了通过治疗意图优化癌症治疗的新机会[245]。

使用 ctDNA 作为生物标志物指导临床癌症管理的益处仍需要进行前瞻性试验来确定。然而,与许多循环肿瘤细胞或糖蛋白生物标志物相比,迄今为止报道的观察性研究显示 ctDNA 具有优异的监测肿瘤负荷的表现[246]。在癌症类型之间存在一些差异,ctDNA 在患者中具有广泛的适用性,如最近一项针对 640 名患者进行的综合调查所示[246]。同一项研究发现,55%的可治愈疾病患者可检测到 ctDNA。这些结果表明,通过改进分子检测方法可以在癌症患者表现出症状之前检测 ctDNA,有望产生比传统方法具有更高特异性的筛选检测[247~250]。

癌症进化

对癌症基因组进行测序的能力揭示了分子进化过程及其对于理解癌症生物学和治疗的重要性。虽然这一概念不是新的,但这一概念的历史考虑主要局限于肿瘤日益恶化是一种线性克隆进化过程的观念[1]。然而,越来越清楚的是,癌症进化通过不断产生克隆多样性导致巨大的异质性。因此,多个相关但不同的克隆谱系可能在一个患者中共存[251]。这些谱系在进展和转移的能力[252]以及对治疗的反应性或抵抗方面存在差异[253]。这种复杂的分支进化模型对于理解癌症生物学和开发更好的治疗方法至关重要。

癌症进化的基石在于基因组突变的积累,最终影响细胞表型。虽然大多数获得性癌症突变可能是携带突变,但少部分将影响关键的细胞途径和过程,从而充当疾病的驱动因素。然而,导致癌症诱变增加确切的分子机制尚不完全清楚。最近对数以千计的癌症基因组进行的分析确定了至少 20 种不同的突变特征,在各种癌症中这些特征会通过不同过程导致肿瘤突变,大多数癌症都具有多种不同的诱变过程[150]。尽管一些确定的导致突变的因素,例如紫外线、吸烟或接触化学治疗剂,是众所周知的,但许多与已知的致病过程无关。阐明这种新的诱变机制对于促进更好的预防和治疗策略的发展至关重要。

突变的积累提供了癌症进化的原料(种群多样性)。然而,这种积累通常有助于时间和空间约束内的克隆进化过程。获得突变的顺序可以显著影响细胞命运。例如,*BRCA1* 或 *BRCA2* 的缺失会在 *TP53* 正常情况下导致细胞周期停滞,但在 *TP53* 缺失的情况下不会出现此类情况[254]。与此观察结果一致,乳腺癌中 *BRCA1* 的第二拷贝的丢失通常发生在 *TP53* 缺失之后。突变事件的顺序还可以取决于细胞类型和分化状态。*KRAS* 或 *NRAS* 突变可见于结肠癌发展早期,而类似的 *NRAS* 突变主要见于骨髓增生异常综合征的晚期[255,256]。另一方面,克隆多样化的空间限制已在透明细胞肾细胞癌和非小细胞肺癌引起关注[257,258]，其中不同的克隆在肿瘤的特定空间位置发展。事实上，这种空间分离可能导致“平行进化”，其特征在于在各个克隆中独立出现的不同突变，但靶向相同的基因或相同的途径，如在多种癌症中观察到的[259]。这种平行进化的一个重要现实意义是，有效的靶向治疗必须能够同时抑制单个患者体内独立的分子上的不同克隆。

虽然克隆多样化至关重要，但最近的数据表明，最具攻击性的克隆的简单生长不会完全解释癌症中克隆进化的程度。实际上，类似于一般的进化生物学原理，没有物种孤立地进化，癌症似乎不仅在与宿主相互作用的生态系统内发展，而且与其他共存的肿瘤克隆相互作用。例如，在胶质母细胞瘤的实验模型中，携带 *EGFR* 突变的次要克隆似乎通过旁分泌机制支持主要的 *EGFR-wt* 克隆[260]。同样，在斑马鱼黑色素瘤异种移植模型的异质肿瘤中，观察到了“合作入侵”的现象。在这里，侵入性克隆的存在使得能够侵入另一个，否则是非侵入性克隆[261]。这种克隆合作不仅适用于肿瘤存活和进展，而且还延伸到治疗抗性领域。例如，在结肠癌模型中，*EGFR* 抑制剂抗性 *KRAS* 突变的小克隆的存在似乎通过涉及转化生长因子 α 和双调蛋白的旁分泌机制支持药物敏感的 *KRAS-wt* 克隆的存活[253]。

基于上述时间和空间约束以及克隆相互作用，已经提出了几种克隆进化模型[259]。这些模型的范围从①线性进化的简单模型，其中突变的连续累积导致越来越具有侵袭性的克隆，超越其原先的克隆，②异域物种形成模型，其中亚群体在肿瘤位置上不同的区域发展，包括克隆相互作用的模型，包括③克隆竞争的模型与不同的克隆竞争拮抗进化形式的增长优势和④个体克隆之间共生关系的克隆合作模型（图 7-6）。

了解癌症进化的分子谱和机制能够帮助我们更好地治疗癌症。分子异质性和克隆进化限制了靶向治疗的益处。在每个患者的肿瘤内的不同分子特征的克隆的组合使得在肿瘤治疗过程中得到筛选，即使在最初对治疗有反应的患者中也表现为获得性治疗抗性。先前存在的体细胞突变（甚至是突变携带事件）或在治疗期间获得的新突变可以导致治疗抗性。虽然实验模型的改进增强了我们对实验室中复杂克隆进化的理解和干扰能力，但是在靶向治疗取得进展的患者中，血浆中 ctDNA 分析等方法的开发可以监测临床中的克隆进化[262]。多项研究表明，在血浆中可检测到驱动抗性的体细胞突变。例如，用厄洛替尼或吉非替尼（EGFR 抑制剂）治疗的肺癌患者最常发生获得性治疗抗性，这是由于 *EGFR p. T790M* 中的第二突变影响药物结合。在常规成像显示疾病进展前 16 周，可在 ctDNA 中检测到这种耐药驱动突变[239]。相似的数据已在结直肠癌患者中报道，他们在西妥昔单抗（一种抗 EGFR 的抗体）上取得进展，其中 *KRAS* 突变在疾病进展的前几周出现[263]。最近一项对结直肠癌患者的研究证实，如果靶向治疗在疾病进展（药物假期）后被取消，并被化疗取代，那么 ctDNA 中 *Kras* 突变的循环水平就会下降（这表明 *Kras* 突变携带肿瘤亚克隆的衰退）[264]。虽然这些研究使用了深层靶向测序策略来研究导致

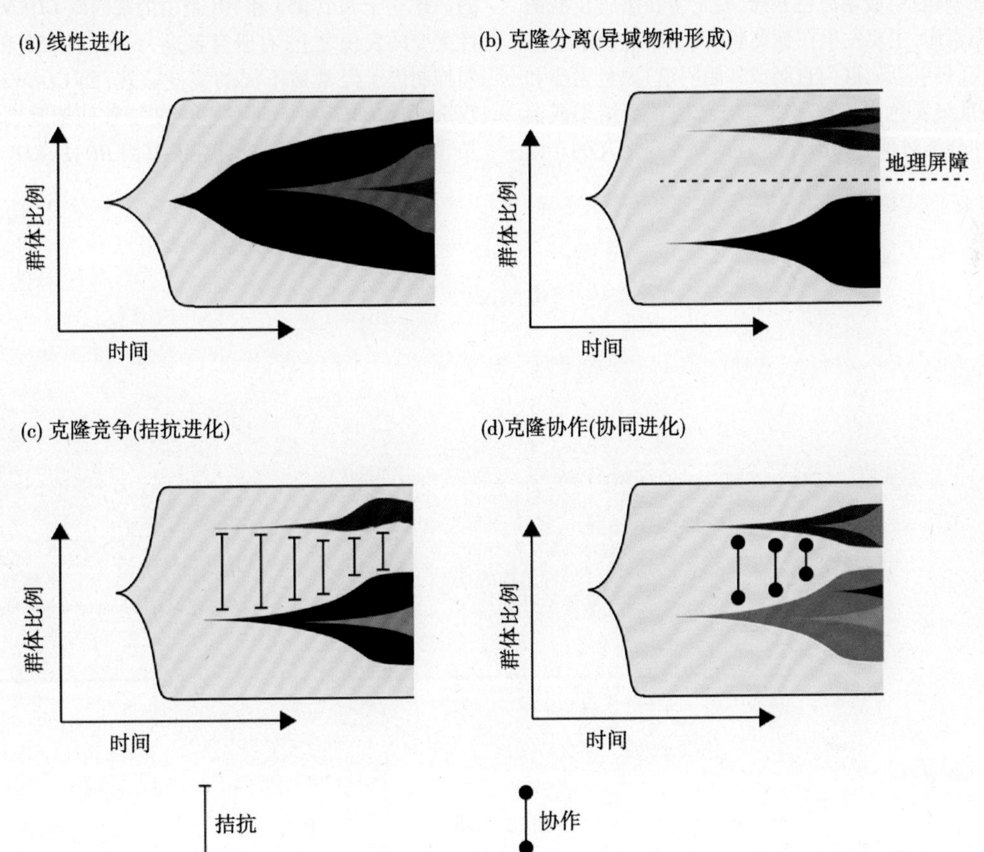

图 7-6 （a）伴随着长时间突变不断累积的线性进化理论。可以看出，如果亚克隆未能获得完全超越其祖克隆的能力，线性进化将导致异质性的发生。（b）当亚克隆分布在肿瘤内不同位置时，肿瘤亚克隆可以通过类似于异域物种形成的过程单独进化。（c）克隆竞争可能发生在不同亚克隆之间，不同亚克隆之间互相拮抗以获得足够的生长优势。（d）亚克隆之间也存在着互相协作的关系

治疗抵抗的假设基因，但也描述了无假设全基因组分析来发现治疗抵抗的新驱动因素[265]。这些描述ctDNA分析追踪克隆进化的原则性证明结果保证了对基于ctDNA的、个性化的适应性、顺序或组合治疗策略的研究。

癌症基因组学和临床实践的演变：黑色素瘤的案例研究

背景

恶性黑色素瘤是美国第六大常见癌症，也是少数几种发病率上升的癌症之一[266]。尽管在疾病的早期阶段发现并手术切除即可治愈，但仅4mm的肿瘤厚度即预示着疾病的转移性和不良的预后。最近在黑色素瘤的精准医疗方面取得的巨大进展有力地说明了基因组学影响临床癌症管理的潜力。在本节中，我们将重点介绍这一进展及其对黑色素瘤治疗的影响，而黑色素瘤的临床特征将在第111章详细讨论。黑色素瘤是一种恶性变化的黑素细胞疾病，临床上根据其解剖位置、组织病理学、是否暴露于阳光、TNM分期等将其进一步细分[267]。从部位上说，皮肤黑色素瘤最常见于暴露在阳光下的皮肤。根据受阳光照射的主要部位进一步分类，包括长期暴露于阳光的区域（例如面部和前臂）和断断续续受阳光照射的部位（例如背部）。不常见的亚型包括：肢端黑色素瘤，易发生在手脚皮肤的非毛发区域；眼黑素瘤，主要发生在葡萄膜上，结膜黑色素瘤所占比例较小；黏膜（鼻咽，肠，肛门直肠或外阴阴道）黑色素瘤和原发性中枢神经系统黑色素瘤。尽管有时无法预测结果或治疗后的反应，这种分类对预后和治疗还是具有一定意义的。此外，过去十年中，转移性黑素瘤均使用细胞毒性化学疗法统一进行治疗，而人们日益发现其效果有限[268]。

黑色素瘤的遗传基础

在不同的临床过程中，黑色素瘤的各组织病理学亚型之间容易混淆，而基因组特征有助于分辨其病因，生物学类型以及最佳治疗方法。正如乳腺癌可以根据ER，PR和Her2的状态进行最佳表征一样，基因型由于其对治疗的意义，现如今也应该在治疗黑色素瘤的临床方法中发挥出重要作用。尽管对黑色素瘤的生成仍然知之甚少，但已知黑素细胞中癌基因突变的逐步积累是其原因之一（图7-7）[269]。大多数黑色素瘤是散发性的，其中5%～10%的病例源于家族性倾向，即主要由第一个被鉴定出的家族性黑色素瘤基因——肿瘤抑制子*CDKN2A*的胚系变异引起（40%的家族性病例）[270～272]。其他癌症基因如*CDK4*、*BRCA2*、*BAP1*、*TERT*启动子，*MITF*和*POT1*的罕见变异，也在家族性病例中被发现[273～278]。除了遗传，紫外线辐射也被认为是皮肤黑色素瘤的最大危险因素，但非阳光直射部位的黏膜、肢端或眼等部位黑色素瘤的形成非此原因[279]。与紫外线辐射的病因相一致，黑色素瘤的其他风险因素包括皮肤白皙、雀斑和良性痣数量增多、*MC1R*胚系变异以及过度暴晒等[280～283]。

黑色素瘤的早期遗传和功能特征表明，它的发生是由细胞周期控制基因的失活突变以及细胞增殖通路的激活突变驱动的。建立于调节p53和RB蛋白的基因座*CDKN2A*易发生家族性突变的发现之上，有研究者进一步发现p53和RB蛋白等肿瘤抑制因子经常被不同的突变破坏，如*CDKN2A*、*CDK4*、*RB1*、*TP53*和*MDM2*突变，而这些突变能够使细胞实现无约束地生长[284～288]。同时，增殖通路相关基因*BRAF*、*KIT*、*NRAS*和*PTEN*

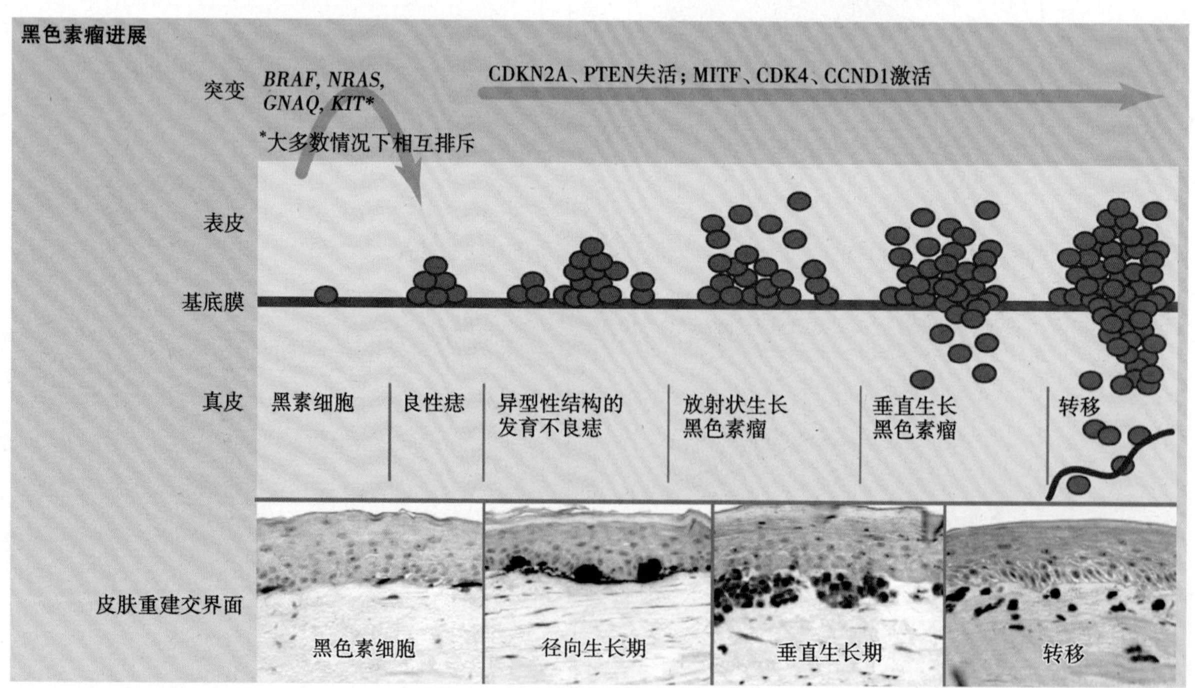

图7-7　皮肤黑色素瘤的遗传基础。黑色素瘤是最致命的皮肤癌，是由黑素细胞（色素生成细胞）的恶性转化引起的。这些细胞会累积遗传改变，导致异常的增殖和散播。临床上，黑色素瘤病变可以根据位置和进展程度进行分类，范围从良性痣到转移性黑素瘤。黑色素瘤中重要的驱动基因如图所示。MAPK信号通路经常由于膜受体的改变或*RAS/BRAF*基因的突变而发生组成型激活

也被证明发生频繁突变，与细胞周期肿瘤抑制因子的失活相互作用以促进恶性肿瘤发生[1115,119,289~302]。细胞遗传学和分子学研究进一步指出在染色体 1p、6q、7p 和 11q 的反复变化区域中存在尚未鉴定的基因或许也与此相关[288,303~311]。与许多人类癌症的早期遗传分析相一致，这些研究通常在不同的小群组或模型系统中进行，仅关注单个临床亚型中的一个或几个基因，并且经常产生非决定性的结果。

黑色素瘤基因组景观

通过一系列基因组研究，各亚型之间和个体肿瘤基因组内的显著遗传复杂性很快就通过上述分析被揭示了出来。在 126 个肿瘤中进行全基因组 aCGH 分析并对 *BRAF* 和 *NRAS* 靶向测序，揭示了基于亚型的体细胞突变的不同模式。*BRAF* 和 *NRAS* 突变被证明在间歇性暴露于阳光的部位和皮肤的黑色素瘤中富集，但在长期暴露于阳光的部位，黏膜和肢端的黑色素瘤中很少见。突变的模式也因黏膜黑色素瘤的亚型中 CNV 的富集程度而变化。随后的分析确证了 CNV 模式与预后不良以及亚型特异性的 *KIT* 突变相关[49,289]。在晒伤部位的皮肤黑色素瘤和 10%~20%的黏膜和肢端黑色素瘤中，亚型特异性的 *KIT* 突变发生频率很低[48,312]。疾病分子亚群的存在通过基因表达微阵列研究已被证实[84,313,314]，临床上黑色素瘤的分子亚群分类预示着这些类型可能与临床结果相关或被作为治疗靶点使用[315]。

2011 年开始的一系列大规模平行测序研究使人们对皮肤黑色素瘤基因组的理解有了爆炸性的增长，并且在最近的两个涉及超过 500 例的大型多项研究中达到了顶峰[142,275,315~325]。这些研究不仅证实了之前提及的 *BRAF*、*NRAS*、*NF1*、*TP53*、*CDKN2A* 和 *RB1* 确实是重要的黑色素瘤的驱动因子，并且也指出了之前未被提及与该疾病相关的新基因，包括 *RAC1*、*PREX2*、*PPP6C*、*ARID2*、*TACC1*、*GRM3*、*MAP3K4*、*MAP3K9*、*IDH1*、*MRPS31*、*RPS27* 和 *TERT* 启动子。黑色素瘤现在主要根据 *BRAF*、*RAS* 和 *NF1* 的状态进行分类，这些基因突变后，能够构成性地激活细胞增殖的中枢调节因子促分裂原活化蛋白激酶(MAPK)通路(图 7-8)[142]。在 10%以上的病例中，这些突变往往是相互排斥的，这就表明有四种基因组亚型：BRAF、NRAS、NF1 和三重野生型(TWT)。全基因组测序还能够表征黑色素瘤中的突变特征，进一步阐明紫外线辐射在各种亚型中的作用。暴露于阳光下的皮肤黑色素瘤的特征在于紫外线特征突变，即在二嘧啶中发生的胞嘧啶取代胸腺嘧啶(C>T)占总突变负荷的 60%以上[142,318,326]。奇怪的是，尽管 *BRAF* 和 *NRAS* 在大多数暴露于阳光的黑色素瘤发生中起作用，但其中最常见的突变并不是 C>T 取代。虽然黑色素瘤的平均突变负荷在所有癌症类型中最高，但突变频率的范围为每兆碱基 0.1~100 个突变[169]。这种显著的异质性伴随疾病的临床异质性，体现在从突变率最高的暴露在阳光下的皮肤上的黑色素瘤>100/Mb，中等突变率的黏膜黑色素瘤的 2~5/Mb，到最低突变率的葡萄膜和中枢神经

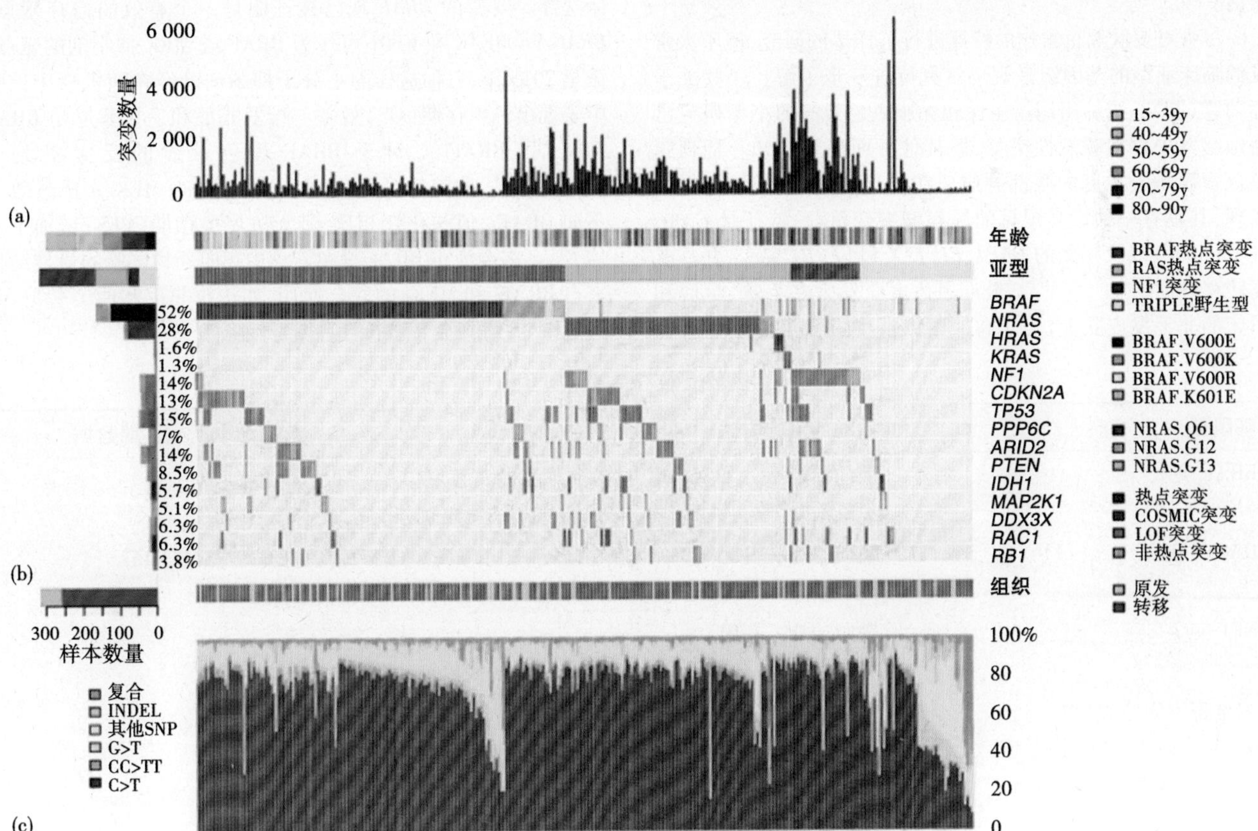

图 7-8　皮肤黑色素瘤基因组概览。(a)每个样本的突变总数、发病年龄和突变亚型[BRAF、RAS(N/H/K)、NF1 和 Triple-WT](一例超突变患者以及一例 NRAS 和 BRAF 同时发生热点突变的患者未展示出来)。(b)每例样本中发生突变的基因(不同颜色代表不同突变类型，其中 BRAF 和 NRAS 的热点突变被特殊颜色标记)。(c)所有黑色素瘤样本(原发或转移)的突变类型和突变谱。对于配对的原发和转移样品，只展示出其转移灶的突变信息

系统黑色素瘤的<0.1/Mb之中[316,327,328]。

在各种黑色素瘤中，皮肤BRAF黑色素瘤占比50%以上。尽管其他激活*BRAF*的突变、扩增甚至融合确实也有所发生，皮肤BRAF黑色素瘤的病因主要还是源于热点错义突变V600E，其特征在于：多发于年轻患者；91%的UV特征；与TWT相比相对较少的CNV；*BRAF*、*MITF*、*PD-1*和*PD-L1*的扩增；*TP53*突变的富集以及更为频繁的*PTEN*缺失等。第二常见的是RAS黑色素瘤（30%），其病因通常是*NRAS* Q61R/K/L发生突变，偶尔也会发生在*K*-或*H-RAS*上。尽管该类别的分子特征与*BRAF*亚型相似，但这些突变几乎总是与*BRAF*突变相互排斥。NF1黑色素瘤占比15%，其中大部分含有*NF1*失活突变。该亚型发生在老年患者中，具有最高的SNV负荷且包含UV特征。它可与*BRAF*和*NRAS*突变共同发生，并倾向于表现出与其他突变的"RAS病"基因（如*RASA2*）共存的模式[319]。与*BRAF*和*RAS*突变类似，大多数NF1突变可以激活RAS和MAPK通路。TWT黑色素瘤是一种缺乏频发性驱动突变的异质性亚型，其中*KIT*、*CTNNB1*、*GNAQ*、*GNA11*和*EZH2*突变的频率不高。该亚型的显著特征包括：更多数量的SV、融合和CNV；仅30%含有UV特征；含有*KIT*、*PDGFRA*、*KDR*、*CDK4*、*CCND1*、*MDM2*和*TERT*的扩增；只有少数（7%）包含*TERT*启动子突变[142]。要强调的是，尽管基因组亚型存在多样性，但绝大多数黑色素瘤的驱动突变最终都汇聚在MAPK和PI3K通路上，大约91%的皮肤黑色素瘤依赖于这一单一通路的异常激活[329]。

尽管对皮肤黑色素瘤的特征进行了详尽的研究，但不太常见的临床亚型的基因组景观仍然有待进一步了解。一些关于葡萄膜、肢端、结缔组织增生性和黏膜黑色素瘤的小型研究已经确定其中存在频发性突变，但其他方面尚且未知。葡萄膜黑色素瘤是最常见的眼部肿瘤。在对近80个病例的研究中发现，其具有一种极其罕见的黑素瘤突变负荷，特征是*GNAQ*突变（50%）以及频繁的*BAP1*、*EIF1AX*和*SF3B1*突变，并具有高转移倾向[324,325,330~332]。肢端黑色素瘤发生在手掌、足底和甲床的非毛发皮肤上，是非高加索人群中最常见的黑色素瘤亚型，并且由于其诊断较晚，预后较皮肤黑色素瘤差[333]。虽然近十年来主要研究的是*BRAF*野生型，但在较大的皮肤基因组学研究中很少涉及其相关内容，并且可用的数据集有限。共有38个肢端黑色素瘤在6项研究中得到鉴定，并确定了以下特征：约30%的*KIT*突变，20%的*BRAF*突变，10%的*NRAS*突变，低SNV负荷，高CNV和SV负荷，以及UV特征缺失[49,316~318,332,334,335]。另一种罕见的侵袭性亚型黏膜黑色素瘤主要是*BRAF*野生型。关于它的数据更为稀缺，仅有10例在一项研究中得到了综合评估[327]。该研究主要证实了先前的靶向和细胞基因组学分析，在两个或更少的样本中显示出低SNV频率、高CNV和SV负荷、UV特征的缺失以及*KIT*、*PTEN*和其他推定的癌症基因的频发突变。结缔组织增生性黑色素瘤是一种罕见的侵袭性纤维形式的真皮黑色素瘤。最近也有研究它的特征（62例），初步结果显示SNV负荷明显高（迄今为止最高的62个突变/Mb之一），具有UV特征，缺乏*BRAF*或*NRAS*突变，以及激活MAPK和PI3K通路的多种突变[336]。这些罕见的肿瘤类型之间显著的相似和差异支撑了其潜在的独特病因，可能有助于指导治疗管理。

黑色素瘤基因组学的临床意义

尽管未能确定上述基因组亚型或黑素瘤中的其他分子分类与结果确实具有相关性，但这些基因组亚型与晚期转移性黑素瘤的治疗有直接关系（表7-6）。BRAF亚型则具有最多的临床选择。突变的*BRAF*现已被证明是一个有效的治疗靶点，*BRAF* V600E/K和K601可作为BRAF或MEK抑制剂的靶点。截至2015年，三种这样的小分子抑制剂已经在随机临床试验中表现出总生存期（OS）效益。维罗非尼和达拉非尼是BRAF抑制剂（BRAFi），对于BRAF黑色素瘤的反应率大于90%[244,337]。曲美替尼是一种MEK抑制剂（MEKi），虽然效果不如BRAFi，但与化疗相比，其无进展生存期（PFS）增加了三倍[338]。迄今为止BRAF黑色素瘤中靶向药物试验的最佳结果来自BRAFi和MEKi的联合使用，如达拉非尼和曲美替尼，其PFS和OS得到显著增长且总体毒性降低[339,340]。

表7-6 黑色素瘤不同基因型的治疗方案

基因型	批准的治疗方法	选择的Ⅰ期或Ⅱ期数据
BRAF突变	靶向治疗——维罗非尼、达拉非尼和曲美替尼 免疫治疗[a]——伊匹单抗、派姆单抗和纳武单抗	考比替尼
RAS突变	靶向治疗——无 免疫治疗[a]——伊匹单抗、派姆单抗和纳武单抗	曲美替尼、MEK162
NF1突变	靶向治疗——无 免疫治疗[a]——伊匹单抗、派姆单抗和纳武单抗	无
三重野生型（TWT）[b]	靶向治疗——无 免疫治疗[a]——伊匹单抗、派姆单抗和纳武单抗	无
TWT——KIT突变或过表达	靶向治疗——无 免疫治疗[a]——伊匹单抗、派姆单抗和纳武单抗	伊马替尼、尼罗替尼
TWT——GNAQ/GNA11突变	靶向治疗——无 免疫治疗[a]——伊匹单抗、派姆单抗和纳武单抗	司美替尼、曲美替尼、MEK162

[a] 免疫治疗的Ⅲ期研究未包括除BRAF以外的基因分型。FDA的批准不针对特定基因型，因此所有基因型可用。

[b] 迄今为止没有一项试验明确界定了TWT患者，但KIT和GNAQ/GNA11病例确实发生在这一类患者中。

针对 RAS、NF1、TWT 以及罕见组织等黑色素瘤亚型的靶向药物的研发还没有完成临床Ⅲ期研究，已落后于 BRAF 黑素瘤的研究进度。尽管如此，目前的成果也已显示出显著功效，激励研究者们持续努力研发药剂。RAS 黑色素瘤在临床试验中已经开始使用各种 MEK 抑制剂进行治疗，包括曲美替尼[341]、MEK162[342]和司美替尼[343]。其中，只有 MEK162 显示出了显著的反应率（约 20%），而其他药物则最佳只能稳定病情。目前尚未针对 NF1 黑色素瘤进行特异性试验，部分原因在于对该亚型的新认识层出不穷以及其与 RAF 和 RAS 亚型存在一定的重叠。相互矛盾的临床前报告表明 NF1 突变和损失既可产生对 MEKi 的敏感性，也可导致抗性，而这种关系也依赖于 RAF/RAS 状态[319,344~346]。在两项对 TWT 皮肤、肢端和黏膜中很常见的 *KIT* 突变的黑色素瘤随机进行的Ⅱ期研究中发现，伊马替尼的总体反应率为 19%~29%，在经典 *KIT* SNV 而不是扩增的情况下反应最佳[286,347]。*GNAQ/GNA11* 突变疾病中最有力的数据来自使用 MEKi 司美替尼的随机Ⅱ期研究[348]。在 49%的患者中，司美替尼成功诱导肿瘤消退，并且，虽然不具有统计学意义，但是可使 OS 从 9.1 个月显著改善至 11.8 个月。除了在临床前研发中的 ERK、IDH1、EZH2 和光激酶抑制剂之外，临床试验中还包括 CDK、MDM2 和 PI3K/Akt/mTOR 抑制剂，它们可能与许多亚型相关和/或可能应用于另外的亚型[142]。

基因组学对免疫疗法的影响目前知之甚少。即使在晚期疾病中，使用 CTLA-4 抑制剂伊匹单抗（ipilimumab）和 PD1 抑制剂派姆单抗（pembrolizumab）和纳武单抗（nivolumab）进行免疫治疗，也可以彻底改变黑色素瘤治疗的长期存活率，但基因组学对免疫疗法的预测或预后的作用仍有待充分阐明[349~351]。基于免疫原性是与总突变负荷成比例增加的概率性聚集的假设，突变负荷作为免疫治疗反应的预测因素得到关注，但迄今为止没有任何预期数据证实这一点。然而这一假设得到了以下事实的支持：PD1 抑制剂首先被批准用于黑色素瘤，然后是肺癌（两种具有最高突变负荷的癌症），而肾细胞癌的突变负荷非常低，但在二期研究中已证实其对 PD1 抑制剂有反应性。在关于派姆单抗和纳武单抗的研究中，只有少数患有非皮肤黑色素瘤和眼黑素瘤的患者被排除在外。虽然 20%~35%的患者有 *BRAF* V600 突变，但并未按照常规进行基因分型，因此 *NRAS* 突变异和 TWT 患者的比率尚且未知。

黑色素瘤的耐药性和进展

尽管在 BRAF 黑色素瘤中靶向药物具有效果，但不论是先天的还是继发产生的耐药性，都仍然是黑色素瘤研究中一个关键的挑战。只有约 50%的患者对 BRAFi 有反应，而这些有反应的患者对 BRAFi 的获得性抗性总在发展[244]。BRAFi 抗性由多种机制驱动，其中大多数机制是通过 PI3K 通路重激活 MAPK 活性或重定向增殖信号传导。通过 *NRAS*[352]、*MEK1*[353,354]、*MEK2*[354]、*NF1*[344]或 *BRAF*（通过扩增）中的进一步突变可以产生抗性[355]。*BRAF* 剪接变异[356]、*EGFR* 激活[357,358]和 *COT* 激活[359]也牵涉其中。其他受体酪氨酸激酶如 *PDGFR-β* 和 *IGF-1R* 的激活或 *PTEN* 的缺失也已在实验室模型中得到证实[344,360~364]。为了检验在临床环境中确定这些抗性的机制是否可以找出有针对性的治疗方法且规避对 BRAFi 的抵抗，相关的临床试验正在进行中。表 7-7 中给出了在用 BRAFi 和 MEKi 双重抑制后来规避特异性抗性机制的假设方法。

表 7-7　获得性 BRAFi/MEKi 抗性的可能治疗方案

抗性机制	治疗策略
EGFR 激活	EGFR 抑制剂——厄洛替尼、吉非替尼、阿法替尼和达沙替尼 PIK3 抑制剂——试验中
IGF-1R 激活 *PTEN* 缺失 *PTEN* 突变 PIK3CA 激活	PIK3Ca 抑制剂——试验中
cMET 激活	cMET 抑制剂——克里唑蒂尼
PDGFR-β 激活	RTK 抑制剂——达沙替尼、舒尼替尼
FGFR 激活	FGFR 抑制剂——普纳替尼、达沙替尼
COT 激活	ERK 抑制剂——试验中

随着最近转移性疾病新的靶向和免疫疗法的批准，临床医生准确识别患者疾病的遗传特征以优化结果目前变得至关重要。同样，基因组检测可以加速新药研发，准确识别不太常见的黑色素瘤亚型，并可能通过鉴定抗性通路以指导个体化的药物选择。因此，黑色素瘤的基因组景观与其临床异质性是相一致的，不同位置的黑色素瘤具有明显不同的基因型特征，表明不同的病因。当前的挑战在于如何在实际临床环境中使用可用的基因组技术。理论上说，可以通过识别个体患者中活跃的进化机制来指导治疗选择。

黑色素瘤亚型有分子多样性，甚至患有相同疾病亚型的个体患者之间也有分子多样性，其中的复杂程度明显越来越高。如前一节关于癌症进化的概述，最近的数据表明，黑色素瘤的发展无法通过累积突变导致日益恶化的表型的线性模型完全解释。相反，一种新兴观点认为癌症是由分支克隆进化过程驱动的复杂生态系统。因此，单个患者中可能存在多个相关但不同的克隆谱系[251]，而其中一些谱系更可能发展和转移[252]。此外，这种多样性可能提供导致耐药的逃避机制。这一点很好地说明了黑色素瘤中 BRAF 抑制作用的普遍发展，其中快速复发的疾病可能具有多个不同的耐药机制，甚至在单个患者中也存在不同的个体亚克隆[365]。这一挑战因以下事实而得到加强：抗性由突变驱动，其他似乎是通过表观遗传或翻译后过程介导的[366]。这些观察结果提出的一个明显而关键的问题是，转移性环境中的单个肿瘤活检是否能够捕获疾病异质性的全部谱、其驱动因素以及潜在的治疗靶点。这个难题的解决方案可能是在更大范围内监测克隆复杂性的方法，例如试图在分子层面研究患者血液中的循环肿瘤 DNA，即“液体活检”。新兴数据描述 ctDNA 的检测和肿瘤与血浆样本之间 BRAF 突变状态具有一致性是令人鼓舞的结果[246,367,368]。此外，另有证据表明连续 ctDNA 分析可能是对免疫治疗有用的治疗反应的标志物。

总结

癌症基因组病变的详细特征已经确定了驱动肿瘤发生的生物学通路，通过分子分型，不仅癌症诊断得到改善，药物研发治疗靶标的选择进一步扩增，而且促进了使用靶向药物和复杂生物标志物的更快和更有效的临床试验开发，创建了早期检测和复发监测的标志。然而，我们在对某些癌症致病突变的认识、对已经发现突变的生物学功能的理解，开发能够靶向许多不同突变的药物，以及抵御不可避免的耐药性出现等方面，仍然存在差距。如本章所述，基因组学已经为我们对癌症生物学和癌症医学的理解做出了非凡的贡献。癌症基因组学的巨大潜力才刚刚开始展现。

致谢

作者感谢为这些研究提供支持的患者们。我们还要感谢 Matthew Taila 和 Victoria Zismann 在准备时的帮助和对本章节的校对以及 Jeffrey Watkins 对于图表制作的协助。WPDH、AS、AHB 和 JMT 获得了癌症-黑色素瘤研究联盟/黑色素瘤梦想团队转化癌症研究基金（SU2C-AACR-DT0612）的研究支持。Stand Up To Cancer 是由美国癌症研究协会（AACR）管理的娱乐产业基金会的一个项目。NIH R01CA195670 支持 WPDH、AS、PR 和 JMT。另外，Pardee Foundation、NIH R01CA179157 和 NIHR01CA185072 也支持 AS。MM 还得到了亚利桑那州科学基金会的资助。JMT 还得到了 Komen 乳腺癌基金会 KG111063、黑色素瘤研究联盟 VUMC42693-R、戴尔公司的筑梦成真计划以及耶鲁癌症中心 UM1 CA186689 的慷慨支持。

本章名词表

阵列比较基因组杂交（CGH）——微阵列平台经过优化，可识别全基因组 DNA 拷贝数变化。

染色体碎裂——在一个或几个染色体中的单个事件中发生广泛染色体重排的现象。

拷贝数目变异（CNV）——DNA 拷贝数的变化，例如相对于参考序列的扩增或缺失。

驱动突变——一种突变，赋予发生该突变的细胞选择性生长优势。

表观基因组学——对整个基因组中表观遗传变化的全面研究。

外显子组测序——NGS 在许多外显子（基因组的编码区域）的平行测序中的应用。

荧光原位杂交（FISH）——使用荧光探针检测染色体上特定 DNA 序列的细胞遗传学技术。

基因表达阵列——寡核苷酸微阵列平台设计用于探测转录组范围内丰富的 RNA 信息。

基因组学——研究基因组的结构、功能、进化和序列。

胚系突变——生殖细胞谱系中的突变存在于身体的所有细胞中并传递给后代。

杂合性缺失——通过缺失或其他突变事件丧失杂合基因座上的正常功能性等位基因。

大规模并行测序（也称为下一代测序或 NGS）——基于大量基因或整个基因组的同时测序的高通量测序方法。

突变丘陵——低频率发生的突变。

突变山——BRAF V600E 等突变，常见于单一癌症类型或多种癌症类型。

单核苷酸多态性（SNP）阵列——微阵列平台探测全基因组 SNP，用于表征癌症中的等位基因变异、LOH 或 CNV。

原癌基因——当此类基因被突变激活时促进癌症表型。

过客突变——一种突变，不能赋予发生该突变的细胞选择性生长优势。

Sanger 测序——使用双脱氧链终止和琼脂糖凝胶电泳对单个基因或基因组进行靶向 DNA 测序的方法。

单核苷酸多态性（SNP）——单个核苷酸序列差异发生在群体中个体的胚系中。

单核苷酸变异（SNV）——相对于参考序列的 DNA 序列的变化，包括点突变和小的插入和缺失。

体细胞突变——在细胞子群中体细胞获得突变（例如在癌症中）。

结构变异（SV）——结构 DNA 变化，如重排，易位，倒位等。

转录组学——研究细胞或细胞群中的所有 RNA 转录物。

肿瘤抑制子——一种保护细胞过程的基因，当其失活时，促进肿瘤发生。

（陈磊 赵燕 张杨倩雯 译 陈瑶 孙文 审）

参考文献

The complete reference list can be found on the Wiley Companion Digital Edition of this title (see inside front cover for login instructions).

2 Hanahan D, Weinberg RA. Hallmarks of cancer: the next generation. *Cell*. 2011;**144(5)**:646–674.

3 Fearon ER, Vogelstein B. A genetic model for colorectal tumorigenesis. *Cell*. 1990;**61(5)**:759–767.

4 Vogelstein B, Papadopoulos N, Velculescu VE, Zhou S, Diaz LA, Kinzler KW. Cancer genome landscapes. *Science*. 2013;**339(6127)**:1546–1558.

8 Jones PA, Baylin SB. The fundamental role of epigenetic events in cancer. *Nat Rev Genet*. 2002;**3(6)**:415–428.

9 Calin GA, Croce CM. MicroRNA signatures in human cancers. *Nat Rev Cancer*. 2006;**6(11)**:857–866.

25 Nowell P. A minute chromosome in human granulocytic leukemia. *Science*. 1960;**132**:1497.

27 Rowley JD. Letter: a new consistent chromosomal abnormality in chronic myelogenous leukaemia identified by quinacrine fluorescence and Giemsa staining. *Nature*. 1973;**243(5405)**:290–293.

42 Pinkel D, Segraves R, Sudar D, et al. High resolution analysis of DNA copy number variation using comparative genomic hybridization to microarrays. *Nat Genet*. 1998;**20(2)**:207–211.

71 Lander ES, Linton LM, Birren B, et al. Initial sequencing and analysis of the human genome. *Nature*. 2001;**409(6822)**:860–921.

84 Bittner M, Meltzer P, Chen Y, et al. Molecular classification of cutaneous malignant melanoma by gene expression profiling. *Nature*. 2000;**406(6795)**:536–540.

87 van't Veer LJ, Dai H, van de Vijver MJ, et al. Gene expression profiling predicts clinical outcome of breast cancer. *Nature*. 2002;**415(6871)**:530–536.

107 Campbell PJ, Stephens PJ, Pleasance ED, et al. Identification of somatically acquired rearrangements in cancer using genome-wide massively parallel paired-end sequencing. *Nat Genet*. 2008;**40(6)**:722–729.

115 Davies H, Bignell GR, Cox C, et al. Mutations of the BRAF gene in human cancer. *Nature*. 2002;**417(6892)**:949–954.

119 Pollock PM, Harper UL, Hansen KS, et al. High frequency of BRAF mutations in nevi. *Nat Genet*. 2003;**33(1)**:19–20.

142 The Cancer Genome Network. Genomic classification of cutaneous melanoma. *Cell*. 2015;**161(7)**:1681–1696.

157 Ramos P, Karnezis AN, Hendricks WP, et al. Loss of the tumor suppressor SMARCA4 in small cell carcinoma of the ovary, hypercalcemic type (SCCOHT). *Rare Dis*. 2014;**2(1)**:e967148.

165 Tomasetti C, Vogelstein B. Variation in cancer risk among tissues can be explained by the number of stem cell divisions. *Science*. 2015;**347(6217)**:78–81.

174 Lipson D, Capelletti M, Yelensky R, et al. Identification of new ALK and RET gene fusions from colorectal and lung cancer biopsies. *Nat Med*. 2012;**18(3)**:382–384.

197 Collins FS, Varmus H. A new initiative on precision medicine. *N Engl J Med*. 2015;**372(9)**:793–795.

206 Druker BJ, Talpaz M, Resta DJ, et al. Efficacy and safety of a specific inhibitor of the BCR-ABL tyrosine kinase in chronic myeloid leukemia. *N Engl J Med*. 2001;**344(14)**:1031–1037.

219 Paez JG, Janne PA, Lee JC, et al. EGFR mutations in lung cancer: correlation with clinical response to gefitinib therapy. *Science*. 2004;**304(5676)**:1497–1500.

223 Sekulic A, Migden MR, Oro AE, et al. Efficacy and safety of vismodegib in advanced basal-cell carcinoma. *N Engl J Med*. 2012;**366(23)**:2171–2179.

226 Von Hoff DD, Stephenson JJ, Rosen P, et al. Pilot study using molecular profiling of patients' tumors to find potential targets and select treatments for their refractory cancers. *J Clin Oncol*. 2010;**28(33)**:4877–4883.

230 LoRusso PM, Boerner SA, Pilat MJ, et al. Pilot trial of selecting molecularly guided therapy for patients with non–V600 BRAF-mutant metastatic melanoma: experience of the SU2C/MRA melanoma dream team. *Mol Cancer Ther*. 2015;**14(8)**:1962–1971.

231 Conley BA, Doroshow JH. Molecular analysis for therapy choice: NCI MATCH. Seminars in oncology; 2014: Elsevier.

246 Bettegowda C, Sausen M, Leary RJ, et al. Detection of circulating tumor DNA in early- and late-stage human malignancies. *Sci Transl Med*. 2014;**6(224)**: 224ra24.

263 Diaz LA Jr, Williams RT, Wu J, et al. The molecular evolution of acquired resistance to targeted EGFR blockade in colorectal cancers. *Nature*. 2012;**486(7404)**: 537–540.

265 Murtaza M, Dawson SJ, Tsui DW, et al. Non-invasive analysis of acquired resistance to cancer therapy by sequencing of plasma DNA. *Nature*. 2013;**497(7447)**: 108–112.

272 Kamb A, Gruis NA, Weaver-Feldhaus J, et al. A cell cycle regulator potentially involved in genesis of many tumor types. *Science*. 1994;**264(5157)**:436–440.

278 Zuo L, Weger J, Yang Q, et al. Germline mutations in the p16INK4a binding domain of CDK4 in familial melanoma. *Nat Genet*. 1996;**12(1)**:97–99.

287 Albino A, Vidal M, McNutt N, et al. Mutation and expression of the p53 gene in human malignant melanoma. *Melanoma Res*. 1994;**4(1)**:35–45.

323 Huang FW, Hodis E, Xu MJ, Kryukov GV, Chin L, Garraway LA. Highly recurrent TERT promoter mutations in human melanoma. *Science*. 2013;**339(6122)**: 957–959.

339 Flaherty KT, Infante JR, Daud A, et al. Combined BRAF and MEK inhibition in melanoma with BRAF V600 mutations. *N Engl J Med*. 2012;**367(18)**:1694–1703.

349 Hodi FS, O'Day SJ, McDermott DF, et al. Improved survival with ipilimumab in patients with metastatic melanoma. *N Engl J Med*. 2010;**363(8)**:711–723.

351 Weber JS, D'Angelo SP, Minor D, et al. Nivolumab versus chemotherapy in patients with advanced melanoma who progressed after anti-CTLA-4 treatment (CheckMate 037): a randomised, controlled, open-label, phase 3 trial. *Lancet Oncol*. 2015;**16(4)**:375–384.

第 8 章　癌症的染色体畸变

David J. Vander Weele，MD，PhD ■ Megan E. McNerney，MD，PhD ■ Michelle M. Le Beau，PhD

概述

大多数白血病、淋巴瘤或实体肿瘤患者的恶性肿瘤细胞中都有克隆性染色体异常，对这些染色体异常的鉴定有助于正确的诊断、评估预后以及选择合适的治疗方案。如今，我们通常集中于几个关键基因，结合病理学评估、细胞遗传学分析和分子研究等方法对个体恶性疾病进行分析和评估。高通量方法的出现，如新一代测序技术，使得测量整个基因组或大量与癌症相关的基因成为可能，为我们诊断、表征和治疗癌症的方式带来了革命性的变化。未来对于肿瘤的研究需要建立一个集成分子模式，即联合染色体型、基因/微小核糖核酸（miRNA）表达、脱氧核糖核酸（DNA）甲基化/表观遗传基因组改变、基因突变状态和每个患者肿瘤的化学敏感性，以及疾病的易感性等，以利于开发降低毒性和延长生存期的个体化治疗方案。

简介

癌症是一种在复杂的细胞和组织微环境中，由于大量遗传和表观遗传异常的逐步积累而引起的异质性疾病，这些变异改变了调节基因组稳定性、细胞增殖和分化、细胞死亡、黏附、血管生成、侵袭和转移的基因的功能。对中期染色体（metaphase chromosome）的分析使我们首次对恶性细胞的遗传解剖有了更广泛的了解，并确定了许多癌症的异常遗传特征，如缺失、易位和基因扩增。特定的细胞遗传学异常，与白血病、淋巴瘤或实体瘤形态学上不同的亚群密切、并且有时特异性的相关[1,2]。检测这些反复出现的异常有助于明确诊断并完善与预后相关的重要信息。在血液系统恶性肿瘤中，具有良好预后遗传特征的患者会更受益于已知毒性谱的标准疗法，而那些临床和细胞遗传学特征较差的患者可以通过更强化或试验性疗法收获更佳的效果。异常克隆的消失是治疗后完全缓解的重要指标，而新异常的出现则表明克隆的进化，并且肿瘤通常表现出更具侵袭性的行为。类似地，在实体瘤中，检测到反复发生的细胞遗传学异常或遗传改变可以为选择靶向治疗或研究性临床试验提供帮助。鉴于基因组分析的快速进展，人们可以设想一种新的方法来治疗癌症患者，这种方法基于恶性细胞以及宿主因子的分子谱分析，而宿主因子能够影响疾病的发展和治疗[3]。本章重点介绍细胞遗传学分析在人类肿瘤诊断、预后和分子病理学中的重要作用。

基因组重排的遗传后果

反复染色体易位（recurring chromosomal translocation）导致位于断裂点的基因发生改变，并在恶性转化过程中发挥不可或缺的作用[2]。受影响的基因可分为几个功能类别，包括酪氨酸或丝氨酸蛋白激酶、细胞表面受体、生长因子和转录调节因子。其中转录调节因子是受影响最大的一类，它们通过诱导或抑制基因转录来调节生长和分化。染色体易位以显性方式导致基因功能改变的机制主要有两种：第一种是基因表达失调，其是淋巴肿瘤中易位（translocation）的特征，包括 B 细胞系肿瘤中的免疫球蛋白基因和 T 细胞系肿瘤中的 T 细胞受体基因，这种失调导致癌基因的无序或组成型表达。第二种机制是新的融合蛋白的表达，它是由位于不同染色体上的两个基因的编码序列并列而产生的。这些肿瘤特异性的融合蛋白是治疗的新靶点。例如慢性粒细胞白血病（chronic myelogenous leukemia，CML）中 t(9;22) 产生的 BCR-ABL1 嵌合蛋白，或者肺癌中的间变性淋巴瘤激酶（anaplastic lymphoma kinase，ALK）融合蛋白。

许多人类肿瘤，特别是实体肿瘤，是由纯合隐性突变引起的。这些基因被称为“抑癌基因”（tumor suppressor gene，TSG），其正常的作用是限制细胞增殖、促进分化或修复 DNA。抑癌基因的特征是由于染色体丢失或缺失以及其他遗传机制造成的遗传物质丢失[2]。越来越多的 TSG 被证实通过单倍不足（haploinsufficiency）发挥作用，即其中一个等位基因的丢失导致蛋白质产物水平降低一半，从而扰乱正常的细胞加工[4]。这种机制在骨髓肿瘤的反复性缺失中很常见。相反，整体或部分染色体的获得或来自基因扩增（例如乳腺癌中的 *ERBB2/HER2*）会造成拷贝数的改变，会导致一种或多种关键基因的表达增加。

人类肿瘤的发病需要一种以上的突变。由于染色体和分子突变在导致疾病的途径中相互作用，因此，癌症生物学的一个重要研究领域是阐明染色体和分子突变的谱系。我们在此描述了目前已知的与白血病、淋巴瘤或实体瘤特定细胞遗传学亚群相关的协同突变作用。

染色体命名法

染色体异常的描述根据国际人类细胞遗传学命名系统（表 8-1）进行[5]。首先列出染色体总数目，然后是性染色体，数字和结构异常按升序排列。观察到至少两个具有相同结构重排的细胞，例如，易位、缺失或倒位，或获得相同染色体，或三个细胞各显示相同染色体丢失，这些被认为是存在异常克隆的证据。细胞具有正常核型被认为是正常细胞系的证据，有一个例外是反复发生结构异常的单细胞，这可能代表了恶性细胞的核型。

表 8-1　细胞遗传学和遗传学专业术语词汇表[2]

术语	定义
扩增(Amplification)	DNA 片段的拷贝数增加
非整倍体(Aneuploidy)	因得到或缺失而产生的异常染色体数目
带状染色体(Banded chromosomes)	由于特殊染色或在染色前用酶预处理,每个染色体对都具有明暗片段交替的独特图案
断点(Breakpoint)	染色体上参与结构重排的某个特定位点,例如易位或缺失
着丝粒(Centromere)	染色体收缩的部分,是纺锤体纤维附着的位置,在有丝分裂期间通过缩短附着在对极上的纺锤体纤维使染色单体分离
克隆(Clone)	克隆被定义为具有相同的附加或结构重排染色体的两个细胞,或具有相同染色体缺失的三个细胞
缺失(Deletion)	染色体的一段丢失,通常是由于两次断裂和中间片段丢失(中间缺失)造成的
二倍体(Diploid)	正常染色体数目和染色体组分
表观遗传学(Epigenetics)	对基因组修饰改变导致的可遗传变化的基因功能的研究,这种修饰如 DNA 或组蛋白甲基化,它不是原 DNA 序列的改变
荧光原位杂交(Fluorescence in situ hybridization)	一种分子细胞遗传学技术,基于荧光标记的 DNA 探针与中期或间期细胞的互补 DNA 序列杂交,用于检测数量和结构异常
单倍体(Haploid)	只有正常组成的一半,即 23 条染色体
超二倍体(Hyperdiploid)	含有附加染色体;因此,染色体数目为 47 或更大
亚二倍体(Hypodiploid)	染色体丢失,染色体数目小于等于 45
倒位(Inversion)	在同一染色体上发生两处断裂,中间部分发生旋转
等臂染色体(Isochromosome)	染色体由一条染色体臂的相同拷贝组成(由着丝粒分开),另一条臂丢失
核型(Karyotype)	根据国际上建立的系统排列细胞中的染色体,使得最大的染色体是第一个,最小的染色体是最后一个。正常的雌性或雄性核型分别被描述为 46,XX 或 46,XY
杂合性缺失(Loss of heterozygosity, LOH)	通常是由于染色体的严重异常,如缺失,导致失去一个位点或片段的亲本(也称为半合子状态)。拷贝中性 LOH 是指一个染色体(或片段)的两个拷贝来自一个亲本,而另一个拷贝的缺失(也称为单亲二体)
单核苷酸多态性(Single nucleotide polymorphisms, SNP)	这是一种常见的、可遗传的 DNA 序列变异,每 100~300 碱基对发生一次的单个核苷酸(A、T、C 或 G)改变
假二倍体(Pseudodiploid)	二倍体染色体数量伴随结构异常
反复性异常(Recurring abnormality)	见于多个有类似肿瘤的病人的一种数量上或结构上的异常
易位(Translocation)	至少有两条染色体断裂,并发生物质交换
符号命名	
p	短臂
q	长臂
+	表示整条染色体的增加(例如,+8)
-	表示整条染色体的缺失(例如,-7)
t	易位
del	缺失
inv	倒位
i	等臂染色体
mar	标记染色体
r	环状染色体

染色体组分核型分析方法

荧光原位杂交

荧光原位杂交(fluorescence in situ hybridization,FISH)广泛应用于对癌症的诊断,其基础是标记的DNA探针与附着于显微镜玻璃载玻片上的转位期染色体或分裂间期细胞中的互补DNA结合[6]。FISH可以在骨髓或血涂片、固定的切片组织上进行。例如,福尔马林固定石蜡包埋(FFPE)组织,因为它不需要分离的细胞。探针现在可用于大多数临床相关的异常检测,例如着丝粒特异性的探针用于检测干细胞移植环境中的数值异常和性染色体组分;基因座的特异性探针用于检测易位、缺失和扩增(图8-1a~e)。FISH的优点包括:①快速检测;②在常规细胞遗传学分析显示正常的样本中,FISH表现出高灵敏度和特异性的细胞遗传学异常;③能够从低有丝分裂指数或终末分化细胞样本中获得细胞遗传学数据。主要的缺点是无法鉴定一些特殊的异常情况。FISH一般通过评价诊断时的核型异常来评估治疗效果,例如,检测口服酪氨酸激酶抑制剂(tyrosine kinase inhibitor,TKI)治疗后CML患者的*BCR-ABL1*融合。在实体肿瘤中的应用包括检测基因扩增,例如乳腺癌中的*ERBB2*基因和肺癌中的*EGFR*或*ALK*基因,或膀胱癌中的UroVysion™检测。

其他低通量方法

除了FISH之外,其他低通量检测方法,如原位杂交(ISH),逆转录聚合酶链反应(reverse transcription polymerase chain reaction,RT-PCR)和免疫组织化学(immunohistochemistry,IHC),是临床上检测易位或拷贝数畸变(copy number aberration,CNA)的主要分子检测方法。例如,它们能够帮助急性早幼粒细胞白血病(acute promyelocytic leukemia,APL)进行快速诊断,以及乳腺癌中ER/PR和ERBB2表达状况的检测。低通量检测也存在一定的缺点,比如由于目前肿瘤的基因改变愈加复杂,使用高通量检测会更加高效实惠。

单核苷酸多态性阵列

单核苷酸多态性(single nucleotide polymorphism,SNP)阵列探针能够广泛地探测基因组中常见的SNP。它们提供敏感的CNA检测,按千碱基的顺序,提供比核型分析更高的分辨率(3-5M分辨率)(图8-1f)。与核型分析不同,它们不需要分离细胞,这对实体瘤样本来说是个优势。SNP阵列还能够检测拷贝数中性杂合子缺失(copy-number neutral loss-of-heterozygosity,CN-LOH),但不能检测出平衡易位。SNP阵列可用于对白血病和淋巴瘤的核型分析及FISH分析的辅助检测,并且在相当比例的核型正常的病例中,SNP阵列有助于检测基因组异常。

下一代测序

下一代测序(next-generation sequencing,NGS)是以大规模并行的方式测序,同时分析超过10亿个DNA片段,它使临床癌症诊断发生了革命性的变化。NGS能够进行最全面的检测,提供有关基因改变谱的数据,包括CNA、LOH、易位、单核苷酸突变、小插入和缺失(插入缺失)、种系易感性变异、药物基因组信息和致癌病毒鉴定。由于仪器、设计、软件的进步和成本的降低,下一代测序分析正在迅速发展。NGS在某些中心是常规使用的,并且有望在肿瘤学中得到广泛应用。

DNA或RNA可以从新鲜组织、FFPE组织、载玻片刮片或活组织检查获得。NGS通常只需要少量材料,并且一些测试甚至可以用细针抽吸。尽管较低的细胞结构(cellularity)可以通过更大的测序深度来弥补,高肿瘤细胞结构仍是首选的[7]。将提取的核酸转化为测序文库并产生75~250bp配对的末端读数,然后将其与参考基因组比对。

通过计数与区域对齐的读数的数量来检测CNA,并将该数量与从正常二倍体样品中收集的数据进行比较(图8-2a)。LOH的区域是通过检测该区域内的SNP等位基因频率来确定的。与IHC和FISH相比,NGS检测7个以上的纯合缺失和扩增具有99%的敏感性和100%的特异性[7]。值得注意的是,NGS提供类似于阵列的平均DNA含量。相反,ISH是在逐个细胞的基础上进行的;因此,对于具有低肿瘤细胞结构的样品,ISH可能具有更高的灵敏度。易位可以通过以下两点来读取:①映射到基因组的不一致部分的读取;②直接映射到断点的读取来表征(图8-2b)。虽然NGS可以达到与FISH相当的灵敏度和特异性,并提供更精细的信息[8],但FISH目前仍是鉴定易位的黄金标准。

靶基因组合

靶基因组合覆盖小于0.05%的基因组,由数十到数百个具有临床意义的基因组成。有些组合是综合性的,而另一些是为肿瘤类型量身定做的。与全基因组测序相比,它们具有成本效益高、测序深度大、灵敏度高、周转时间短、低生物信息学负担以及规避偶然发现问题等优点。

为了鉴定CNA,通常通过探针从DNA中杂交富集靶基因。靶向易位不太容易直接获得,因为大多数易位在内含子中具有断点,其可能比NGS的读长(reads)更长。因此,DNA的捕获探针必须靶向内含子,这增加了被测DNA的区域(图8-2a)。基于RNA的测序避免了插入内含子的问题,但仅限于检测有表达的嵌合融合转录本,并且无法检测常见的易位,例如IGH/MYC。此外,RNA在FFPE样本中也会发生降解。

外显子测序

外显子捕获是通过杂交捕获所有蛋白质编码DNA(约1%的基因组)来富集的。一些临床研究实验室将此作为所有潜在致病基因中的突变和CNA的无偏倚测定方法。其成本低于全基因组测序,但其缺点是在检测易位方面的应用有限。

全基因组测序

全基因组测序(whole genome sequencing,WGS)是对整个肿瘤基因组的测序,无需预先进行富集步骤,可识别编码区和非编码区的所有结构变化。虽然应用于科学研究和一些临床试验[9],WGS却受限于成本、数据大小和计算的要求难以广泛应用。但是,随着测序成本的降低和实验室对NGS数据的经验积累,WGS可得到更广泛的应用。

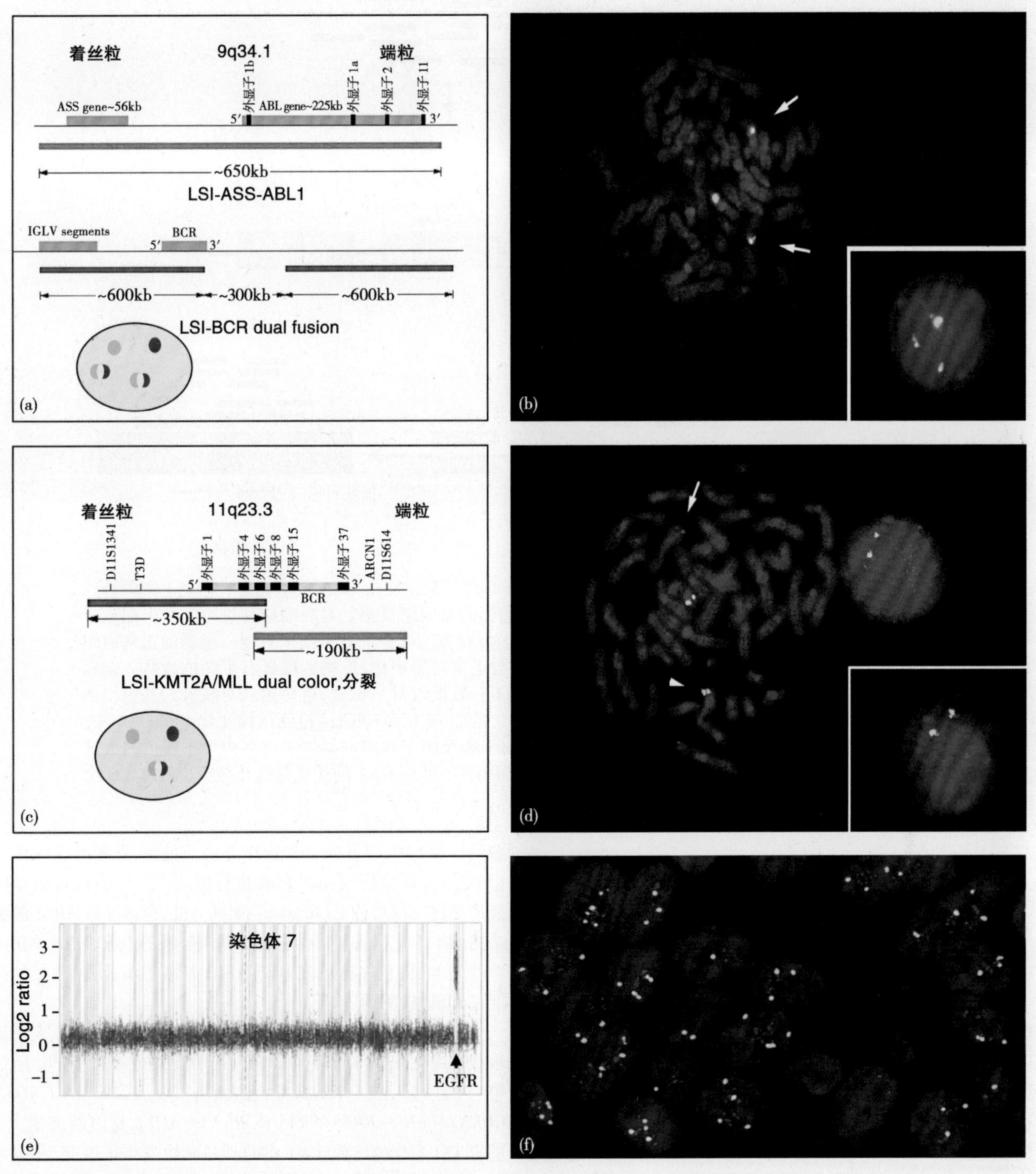

图 8-1　荧光原位杂交和 SNP 阵列分析。分图(b)、(d)和(e)代表分裂中期或分裂间期细胞的 FISH 检测图像；细胞用 4,6-二脒基-2-苯基吲哚-二盐酸盐(DAPI)复染。(a)BCR 和 ABL1 双重融合探针(雅培分子)检测序列的基因组起源示意图，以及分裂间期细胞中信号的构型示意图。(b)在具有 t(9;22)的细胞中，正常的 9 和 22 同源物上观察到一个绿色和一个红色信号，并且在 der(9)和 der(22)费城染色体(Ph chromosome)上观察到两个黄色融合信号(箭头)，这是 ABL1 和 BCR 序列并置的结果。(c)KMT2A/MLL 分裂探针(雅培分子)示意图，以及分裂间期细胞中信号的构型示意图。(d)在 11q23.3 易位的细胞中，观察到正常 11 号染色体同源物上种系结构的一个黄色融合信号，在 der(11)染色体上观察到绿色信号，并且在伴侣染色体上观察到红色信号。(e,f)基因扩增的检测。(e)胶质母细胞瘤中 DNA 拷贝数畸变的 SNP 阵列分析揭示了 EGFR 基因座的扩增。(f)乳腺癌中 ERBB2/HER2 扩增的 FISH 分析。用光谱绿(绿色信号)标记的探针是 17 号染色体(CEP17)的着丝粒特异性探针。大多数细胞具有 17 号染色体着丝粒的两个拷贝；然而，多倍体细胞具有更多拷贝。用光谱橙(红色信号)标记的探针是 ERBB2/HER2 基因的基因座特异性探针，估计平均每个细胞 10~20 个拷贝(雅培分子)。ERBB2/HER2:CEP17 比率≥2.0。资料来源：芝加哥大学病理学系 Carrie Fitzpatrick 博士

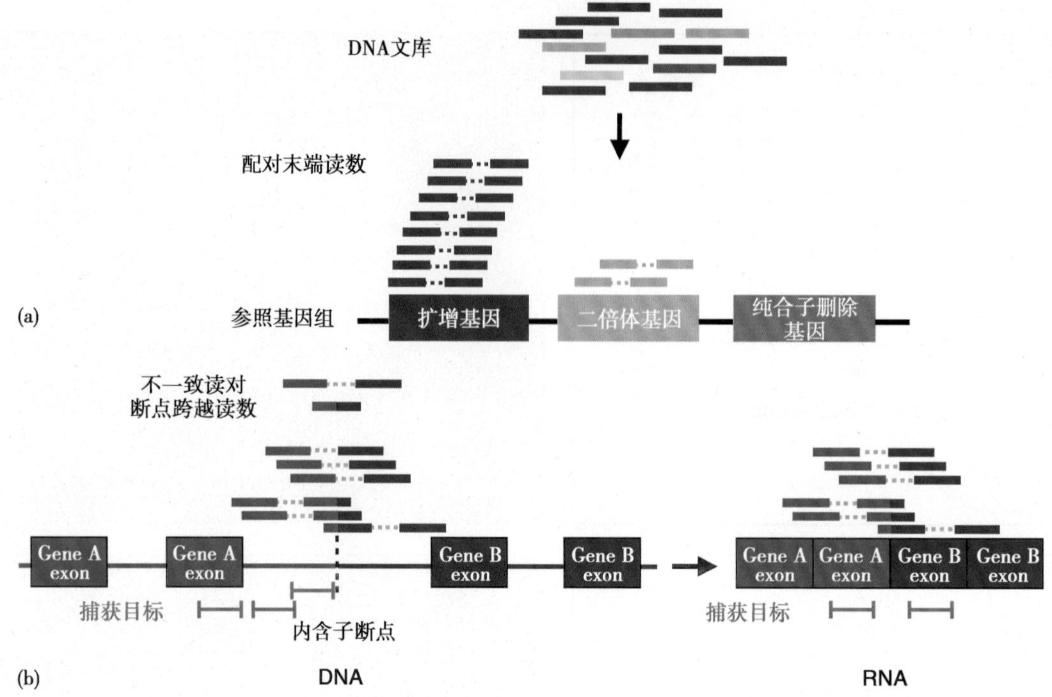

图 8-2 通过下一代测序技术(NGS)检测染色体畸变。(a)拷贝数改变由 DNA 文库确定,该 DNA 文库可以来源于全基因组 DNA,或通过外显子组捕获,或自较小的靶向基因组富集。对肿瘤样品进行配对末端或单端(未显示)NGS,并将读数与参考人类基因组比对。将区域对齐的读数的数量与来自同一患者的正常组织进行比较,或者比较正常二倍体患者样本数据库资料。与正常对照相比,扩增区域具有更高的读数。杂合或纯合缺失区域的读数比预期更少。(b)易位可以通过不一致读取对来识别,这些读取对映射到基因组的两个不同区域,或者来自跨越断点的读取。可以从 DNA(左图)或 RNA(右图)检测结构变化。在 DNA 中,可通过全基因组测序或通过初始捕获步骤鉴定易位。由于涉及两个基因的易位通常在内含子序列的大区域中发生异质断裂,因此必须设计捕获探针以跨越该中间序列。使用 RNA 的优点是比外显子长的内含子会被剪切,仅外显子需要捕获探针

特定的克隆性疾病

慢性粒细胞白血病

在所有恶性疾病中,第一个染色体异常是在慢性粒细胞白血病(chronic myelogenous leukemia,CML)中被发现的[10]。费城(Ph)染色体由倒位 t(9;22)(q34.1;q11.2)(图 8-1a,8-1b,8-4a)产生,其在多能干细胞中产生淋巴和骨髓系细胞。标准 t(9;22)存在于约 92%的 CML 患者中,而 7% CML 患者的变异易位同时涉及第三条染色体。产生的遗传学后果是将 9 号染色体 ABL1 癌基因的 3′端部分移到 22 号染色体 BCR 基因的 5′端部分旁边。缺乏 t(9;22)的罕见 CML 患者具有仅在分子水平上才可检测到的 ABL1 和 BCR 的重排(约 0.5%的病例)[11]。t(9;22)和由此产生的 BCR-ABL1 融合是 CML 的必要条件[11]。BCR-ABL1 融合蛋白通过 RAS/MAPK、PI3K/AKT 和 JAK/STAT 途径向细胞核传递生长调控信号而获得了新的功能。几种市售的口服 TKI 可抑制 BCR-ABL1 的酪氨酸激酶活性:甲磺酸伊马替尼(Gleevec/STI571,诺华制药)、达沙替尼(Sprycel,BMS-354825,百时美施贵宝)和尼罗替尼(Tasigna,AMN107,诺华制药)[12,13]。另外一些口服药物正在临床试验中进行测试[14]。伊马替尼在 CML 的各个阶段都表现出显著的活性,这是大多数新诊断 CML 患者的首选治疗方法,而这些患者的反应性可以通过 FISH 分析或 qRT-PCR 进行监测[15,16]。有几种类型的遗传变化与伊马替尼(Imatinib)耐药有关,包括导致 ABL1 激酶结构域中干扰伊马替尼结合的氨基酸替换的点突变,以及获得额外的 Ph 染色体拷贝或 BCR-ABL1 基因扩增,这两种变异都能被 FISH 检测到[15]。

以往大多数处于加速或急性期的 CML 患者(80%)表现出核型的进化,通常是染色体 8 或 19 的增加,或第二个 Ph(通过第一个获得),或一个等臂染色体(17q),以及 *TP53*、*RB1*、*MYC*、*CDKN2A*(*p16*)、*KRAS*/*NRAS* 或 *RUNX1*/*AML1* 基因的突变[11]。随着 TKI 治疗的出现,CML 的自然进化史发生了改变,在爆发期的核型也有所不同,但尚未进行准确的描述。

有趣的是,除了 ABL1 外,每一种口服 TKI 都能阻断激酶的活性,因此已有证据表明它们对其他血液系统恶性肿瘤有效,包括有 PDGFRB 重排的骨髓增生性肿瘤(MPN)。PDGFRB 是一种骨髓增生性高嗜酸性粒细胞综合征的变体,还包括表达 FIP1L1-PDGFRA 融合蛋白的嗜酸性粒细胞增多综合征骨髓增生性变体,以及 KIT 激活的肥大细胞恶性肿瘤。在一些实体瘤中同样如此,例如 KIT 突变的黑色素瘤和 GIST[17]。

其他骨髓增生性肿瘤

有 15% 未经治疗的和 40% 经治疗的真性红细胞增多症

(polycythemia vera, PV)患者存在异常的细胞遗传学克隆,而当该病发展为急性髓样白血病(acute myeloid leukemia, AML)时,这一异常出现的比例为 100%(表 8-2)[18,19]。一种常见的变化是在 30%的患者中可见+8 或+9、del(13q)或 del(20q)。白血病期常出现 del(5q)(40%)或-7(20%)。细胞遗传学分析显示 60%的原发性骨髓纤维化(myelofibrosis, MF)存在克隆异常,通常为+8、-7 或有 del(7q)、del(11q)、del(13q)和 del(20q)[18]。核型的改变可能标志着 AML 的进化。导致 STAT、PI3K 和 MAPK 信号通路激活的 JAK2^{V617F} 突变出现在 PV(90%~95%)、原发性血小板增多症(essential thrombocythemia, ET, 50%~70%)和 MF(40%~50%)的患者中[20,21]。JAK2 未突变的 ET 和 MF 患者中,多数携带钙网蛋白基因(CALR)的体细胞突变[22,23]。

表 8-2 恶性骨髓疾病中反复发生的染色体异常

疾病[a]	染色体异常	频率	相关基因[b]		结果
慢性粒细胞白血病(CML)	t(9;22)(q34.1;q11.2)	约 99%[c]	*ABL1*	*BCR*	融合蛋白——改变细胞因子信号通路,基因组不稳定性
真性红细胞增多症(PV)	+8	20%(合并)	—	—	—
	+9				
	del(20q)				
	del(13q)				
	部分三体 1q				
原发性骨髓纤维化(MF)	+8	30%(合并)	—	—	—
	+9				
	-7/del(7q)				
	del(5q)/t(5q)				
	del(20q)				
	del(13q)				
	部分三体 1q				
急性髓性白血病(AML)	t(8;21)(q22;q22.1)	10%	*RUNX1T1/ETO*	*RUNX1/AML1*	融合蛋白——改变转录调控
	t(15;17)(q24.1;q21.2)	9%	*PML*	*RARA*	融合蛋白——改变转录调控
	inv(16)(p13.1q22)或者 t(16;16)(p13.1;q22)	5%	*MYH11*	*CBFB*	融合蛋白——改变转录调控
	t(9;11)(p21.3;q23.3)	全部的 5%~8%	*MLLT3/AF9*	*KMT2A/MLL*	融合蛋白——改变的染色质结构和转录调控
	t(10;11)(p12;q23.3)	t(11q23.3)	*MLLT10/AF10*	*KMT2A*	
	t(11;19)(q23.3;p13.3)		*KMT2A*	*MLLT1/ENL*	
	t(11;19)(q23.3;p13.1)		*KMT2A*	*ELL*	
	t(6;11)(q27;q23.3)		*MLLT4/AF6*	*KMT2A*	
	其他 t(11q23.3)		*KMT2A*		
	del(11)(q23)				
	+8	8%			
	-7 or del(7q)	14%			
	del(5q)/t(5q)	12%			

续表

疾病[a]	染色体异常	频率	相关基因[b]		结果
	t(6;9)(p23;q34.1)	1%	*DEK*	*NUP214/CAN*	融合核孔蛋白
	inv(3)(q21.3q26.2) or t(3;3)	2%	*MECOM/EVI1*		过表达 *MECOM*
	del(20q)	5%			
治疗相关的髓系肿瘤(therapy-related MN)	-7 or del(7q)	45%			
	del(5q)/t(5q)	40%			
	der(1;7)(q10;p10)	2%			
	dic(5;17)(q11.1-13;p11.1-13)	5%		*TP53*	功能丧失——DNA损伤反应
	t(9;11)(p21.3;q23.3)/t(11q23)	3%	*MLLT3*	*KMT2A*	融合蛋白——改变的转录调控
	t(11;16)(q23.3;p13.3)	2%(t-MDS)	*KMT2A*	*CREBBP*	
	t(21q22.1)	2%	*RUNX1/AML1*		
	t(3;21)(q26.2;q22.3)	3%	*MECOM*	*RUNX1*	过表达 MECOM
骨髓增生异常综合征(不平衡)	+8	10%			
	-7/del(7q)[d]	12%			
	del(5q)/t(5q)[d]	15%			
	del(20q)	5%~8%			
	-Y	5%			
	i(17q)/t(17p)[d]	3%~5%	*TP53*	—	功能丧失,DNA损伤反应
	-13/del(13q)[d]	3%			
	del(11q)[d]	3%			
	del(12p)/t(12p)[d]	3%			
(平衡)	t(1;3)(p36.3;q21.2)[d]	1%	*MMEL1*	*RPN1*	MMEL1——转录激活的失调?
	(2;11)(p21;q23.3)/t(11q23.3)[d]	1%		*KMT2A*	KMT2A 融合——改变转录
	inv(3)(q21.3;q26.2)/t(3;3)[d]	1%	*RPN1*	*MECOM/EVI1*	通过 MECOM 改变转录调节
慢性髓细胞性白血病(CMML)	t(5;12)(q32;p13.2)	约 2%	*PDGFRB*	*ETV6/TEL*	融合蛋白——改变信号通路

[a]AML,急性髓性白血病;CML,慢性粒细胞白血病;CMML,慢性髓细胞白血病;MDS,骨髓增生异常综合征。
[b]基因按核型中的引用顺序列出,例如,对于 CML,ABL1 为 9q34.1,BCR 为 22q11.2。
[c]患有 CML 的稀有患者在正常出现的 22 号染色体中具有与 BCR 相邻的 ABL1 插入。
[d]在 2008 年世界卫生组织(WHO)分类中被认为是持续性细胞减少症患者中 MDS 的推定证据,但没有发育不全或细胞增多。

原发性骨髓增生异常综合征

骨髓增生异常综合征(myelodysplastic syndrome,MDS)是一组异质性疾病[24,25]。在诊断时,40%~60%的原发性 MDS 患者的骨髓细胞中可检测到克隆性染色体异常,包括难治性血细胞减少症伴单系发育不良(25%),难治性贫血伴环状铁粒幼细胞增多(refractory anemia with ring sideroblasts,RARS,10%),难治性血细胞减少症伴多系发育异常(refractory cytopenia with multilineage dysplasia,RCMD,50%),母细胞过量的难治性贫血(refractory anemia with excess blasts,RAEB-1,2,50%~70%),具有

分离的 del(5q)的 MDS(100%),无法分类 MDS 和儿童期 MDS(表 8-2)[26~28]。常见的改变是+8、del(5q)、-7/del(7q)和 del(20q),这些类似于新发的急性髓性白血病中所见的变化(图 8-3a)。在 MDS 中几乎从未见过与新生儿 AML 的独特形态学亚群密切相关的复发性易位。

具有独立的 del(5q)的 MDS 发生在患有 RA 的老年患者中(通常是女性),他们通常伴有未成熟细胞计数的下降,血小板计数正常或升高[30]。这些患者常有单一的或者伴随的 5q 中间缺失,疾病相对良性,病程持续数年[29]。编码 40S 核糖体亚基必需成分的 RPS14 的单倍体不足可能是造成红细胞生成缺陷的原因[31],而两个相邻的微小核糖核酸 miR-145 和 miR-146a 与 RPS14 的缺失相关,并介导该疾病中可见的巨核细胞发育不良[32,33]。

SNP 微阵列可以检测出 10%~15%核型正常的病例的异常。其中,7q、11q 和 17p 的 LOH 与预后不良相关[34,35]。根据国际预后评分系统的修订,其中"非常好的结果(very good outcome)"患者具有单一的-Y 或 del(11q)异常;"结果良好(good outcome)"者核型正常,具有单独 del(5q)或具有一个额外异常,单独 del(12p)或单独 del(20q);具有"中间结果(intermediate outcome)"的那些患者具有 del(7q)、+8、+19、i(17q)或任何其他单一或双重异常;结果"差(poor outcome)"的患者有-7、inv(3q)/t(3;3)双重异常,包括-7/del(7q)以及 3 种异常的复杂核型;那些"结果非常差(very poor outcome)"的患者核型更加复杂,有大于 3 个异常,并且通常伴随染色体异常[5,26,36,37]。

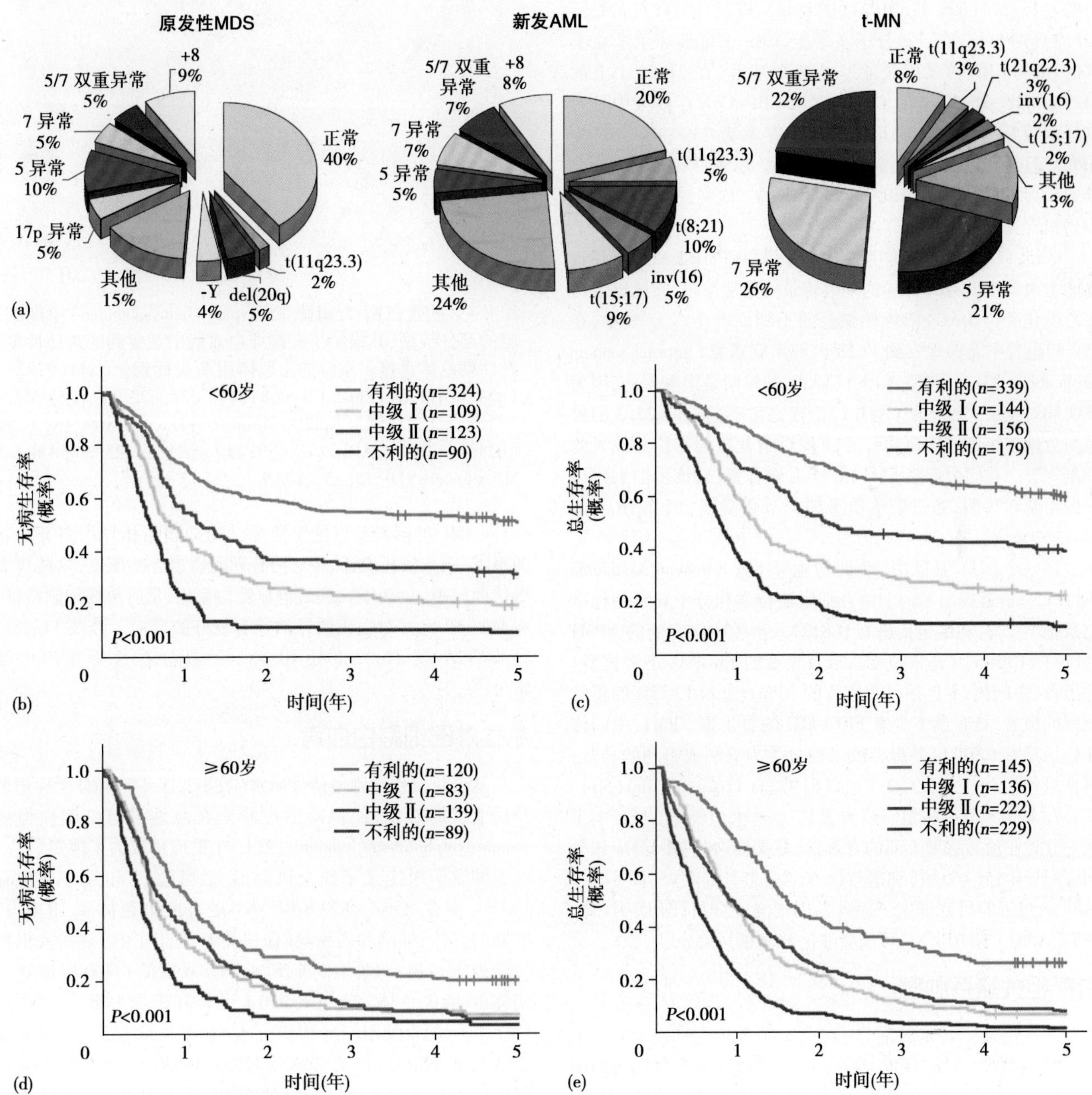

图 8-3 (a)MDS,新发 AML 和 t-MN 中反复出现的染色体异常的频率。(b~e)根据四个欧洲白血病网络组分类的患者结果。(b)无病生存率和(c)年龄小于 60 岁的 AML 患者的总体生存率。(d)无病生存率和(e)60 岁或以上患者的总体生存率。资料来源:Mrozek 等[29]经美国临床肿瘤学会许可转载

新发急性髓性白血病

大约75%的急性髓性白血病(acute myeloid leukemia, AML)患者可检测到染色体克隆异常,且具有指导预后和治疗的意义[38~41],其中最常见的异常是+8和-7(图8-3a)[2]。复发性易位发生在年龄较小的患者,中位年龄在30岁;而其他异常,如del(5q)或-7/del(7q),发生在中位年龄超过50岁的患者中。现在,世界卫生组织将特定的复发性异常及其分子对应物识别为AML中的独立疾病实体(表8-2)[2]。这些实体包含核结合因子(core-binding factor,CBF)白血病,其特征包括发生在5% AML中的t(8;21)(q22;q22.1)(图8-4b)和发生在5% AML(25% of AMMoL)中的inv(16)(p13.1q22)(图8-4c)、APL中的t(15;17)(q24.1;q21.2)(图8-4d),以及t(9;11)(p21.3;q23.3)(图8-4e)[2]。在分子水平上,CBF重排破坏了造血必需的、编码CBF转录因子亚基的两个基因(在21q22.1上的RUNX1和在16q22上的CBFB)[42]。CBF-AML在成人中具有良好的预后(t(8;21)的总体5年生存率为70%;inv(16)为60%),但是t(8;21)在儿童中预后较差。尽管只有KIT突变会导致预后不良,但KIT、KRAS和NRAS的二次突变在CBF-AML中仍很常见[42]。

t(15;17)产生融合维甲酸受体-α蛋白(PML-RARA),其致癌能力来源于RARA介导的基因转录的异常抑制,通过组蛋白去乙酰化酶(HDAC)依赖性染色质重塑而产生[43]。其中,在35%的患者中能够观察到FLT3内部串联重复(internal tandem duplication,ITD)。典型t(15;17)APL的诊断是很重要的,因为该疾病对全反式维甲酸(ATRA)治疗是敏感的。11q23.3的易位与急性单核细胞白血病有关,1岁以下儿童的易位是成人的4倍[41,44]。它们会产生KMT2A/MLL融合蛋白,该蛋白编码组蛋白甲基转移酶,通过染色质重塑调节靶基因(例如HOX基因)的转录[45]。

在一个国际项目中,欧洲白血病网(European Leukemia Net,ELN)最近提出了一个整合细胞遗传学和分子异常的标准化系统[38]。有利组包括患有t(8;21),inv(16),突变的NPM1而没有FLT3-ITD(正常核型),以及突变的CEBPA(正常核型)的患者;中间体-Ⅰ包括具有突变的NPM1和FLT3-ITD的正常核型的患者,具有或不具有FLT3-ITD的野生型NPM1;中间体Ⅱ包括具有t(9;11)的患者或未被分类为有利或不利的异常;不良组包括inv(3q)/t(3;3),t(6;9),t(11q23.3),del(5q),-7,17p缺失或复杂核型(≥3异常)。一些大型研究已经证实了这一分类在预测结果方面的有效性,并支持这些基因群应该分别应用于年轻(<60岁)和老年(>60岁)患者的观点(图8-3b~e)[39]。最近的研究证实了额外基因的突变分析,即DNMT3A、TET2、ASXL1和RUNX1,可能会细化ELN的风险分层[46~49]。

治疗相关髓系肿瘤

治疗相关的髓系肿瘤(therapy-related myeloid neoplasm,t-MN)由t-MDS/t-AML组成,是用于治疗恶性和非恶性疾病的细胞毒性治疗的晚期并发症[50]。5号染色体的部分缺失,即del(5q)(图8-4f),和/或部分或全部的7号染色体的缺失[-7/del(7q)],在接受烷化剂处理的患者中是特征性的(图8-3a)。在临床上,存在MDS的这些患者具有较长的潜伏期(5年),并且有些患者快速发展为具有多系发育不良和预后不良(中位存活8个月)的AML。根据我们的经验,92%的t-MN患者核型异常,70%的染色体存在染色体5或7或两者同时的异常[51],这些观察结果已在其他系列研究中得到证实[52]。相比之下,只有约20%的新发AML患者具有相似的染色体5或7或两者同时异常[2]。对5号染色体缺失段(5q31.2带)内基因的分子分析符合单倍性不全模型,在该模型中,HSC中5q上多个基因的协同丢失在疾病发病过程中起协同作用,并且多个单倍体不足的髓系白血病基因(EGR1、APC、RPS14、miR-145/miR-146a)已被鉴定出[53~54]。

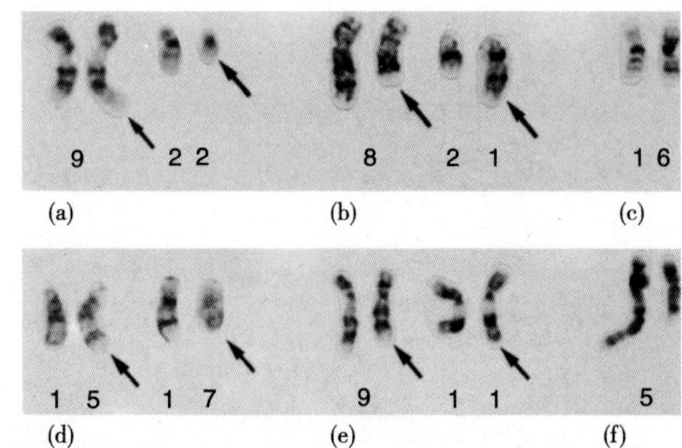

图8-4 胰蛋白酶-吉姆萨带(trypsin-Giemsa-banded)中期细胞的部分核型,其描绘了在髓样白血病中观察到的选择性复发性染色体重排。重排的染色体用箭头标识。(a)t(9;22)(q34.1;q11.2),CML.(b)t(8;21)(q22;q22.1),AML-M2.(c)inv(16)(p13.1q22),AMMoL-M4Eo.(d)t(15;17)(q24.1;q21.1),APL.(e)t(9;11)(p21.3;q23.3),AMoL-M5.(f)del(5)(q15q35),t-MN

t-AML的第二亚型见于接受已知抑制拓扑异构酶Ⅱ药物的患者,例如依托泊苷、替尼泊苷和阿霉素。临床上,这些患者潜伏期较短(1~2年),表现为显性白血病,常有单核细胞特征、无前驱MDS,并对强化诱导治疗有较好的反应。涉及11q23.3处KMT2A或21q22.1处RUNXL的易位在这个亚组中很常见[50]。

急性淋巴细胞白血病

基于复发性细胞遗传学异常(表8-3,图8-5)和分子标记的预后亚组的确定,使风险适应疗法在急性淋巴细胞白血病(acute lymphoblastic leukemia,ALL)中的应用成为了现实[55,56]。儿童肿瘤学组定义了四个风险组:低风险[5年无事件生存(EFS),至少85%],ETV6-RUNX1融合或染色体4、10和17的同时三体;标准和高风险(保留在各自的国家癌症研究机构风险组中);极高风险(5年EFS,45%或更低)具有极端亚二倍体(<44染色体)或BCR-ABL1融合和诱导失败[57]。使用CMA进行的全基因组分析研究表明,在儿童ALL中,亚显微CNA的频率很高,包括PAX5(32%)、IKZF1(IKAROS,29%)、CDKN2A/B(50%)、BTG1和EBF1(8%)的缺失,这些缺失扰乱了控制B细胞发育和分化的基因和途径[58]。IKZF1的遗传改变与B细胞起源ALL(B cell progenitor ALL)的极差预后有关[59]。

表 8-3　恶性淋巴系统疾病的细胞遗传学与免疫表型的关系

疾病[a]	染色体异常	频率[b]	涉及基因[c]		结果[d]
急性淋巴细胞白血病					
前体 B(Precursor B)	t(12;21)(p13.2;q22.1)	25%	*ETV6/TEL*	*RUNX1/AML1*	融合蛋白——转录因子(TF)
	t(9;22)(q34.1;q11.2)	10%[e]	*ABL1*	*BCR*	融合蛋白——细胞因子信号通路改变
	t(4;11)(q21.3;q23.3)	5%	*AFF4*	*KMT2A*	融合蛋白——转录因子
Pre-B	t(1;19)(q23;p13.3)	6%(30%)	PBX1	TCF3(E2A)	融合蛋白——转录因子
B(SIg+)	t(8;14)(q24.2;q32.3)或变异体	7%(100%)	MYC	IGH	失调表达——转录因子
其他	超二倍性(50~60)	10%	—	—	—
	del(12p),t(12p)	10%			
T	t(11;14)(p15.4;q11.2)	1%	LMO1	TRA	失调表达——转录因子
	t(11;14)(p13;q11.2)	3%	LMO2	TRA	失调表达——转录因子
	t(10;14)(q24.3;q11.2)	3%	TLX1	TRA	失调表达——转录因子
	del(9p),t(9p)	<1%(10%)	CDKN2A,CD-KN2B		肿瘤抑制基因——细胞周期调控
非霍奇金淋巴瘤					
B 细胞 NHL					
Burkitt	t(8;14)(q24.2;q32.3)	95%	MYC	IGH	失调表达——转录因子
	t(2;8)(p12;q24.2)	1%	IGK	MYC	失调表达——转录因子
	t(8;22)(q24.2;q11.2)	4%	MYC	IGL	失调表达——转录因子
滤泡性 SNCL DLBCL	t(14;18)(q32.3;q21.3)	80%	IGH	BCL2	失调表达——抗凋亡蛋白
		20%			
DLBCL	t(3;22)(q27;q11.2)	全部 45%	BCL6	IGL	失调表达——转录因子
	t(3;14)(q27;q32.3)	t(3q27)	BCL6	IGH	失调表达——转录因子
MCL	t(11;14)(q13.3;q32.3)	约 100%	CCND1	IGH	失调表达——转录因子
LPL	t(9;14)(p13.2;q32.3)	—	PAX5	IGH	失调表达——转录因子
MALT	t(11;18)(q22.2;q21.3)	40%~50%	BIRC3/API2	MALT1	融合蛋白——NFkB 活化
	t(1;14)(p22.3;q32.3)	10%	BCL10	IGH	失调表达——增加的 NFkB 活化
	t(14;18)(q32.3;q21.3)	10%~20%	IGH	MALT1	失调表达——增加的 NFkB 活化
	t(3;14)(p13;q32.3)	10%	FOXP1	IGH	失调表达——转录因子
PCFCL	t(14;18)(q32.3;q21.3)	40%	IGH	BCL2	失调表达——抗凋亡蛋白
T 细胞 NHL					
ALK+ALCL	t(2;5)(p23.2;q35.1)	75%	ALK	NPM1	酪氨酸激酶失调表达
ALK-ALCL	t(6;7)(p25.3;q32.3)	10%~15%	IRF4,DUSP22	—	TF(IRF4)和磷酸酶(DUSP22)失调表达
鼻型/NK 细胞型(Nasal/NK cell)	i(1q),i(7q),i(17q)	—	—	—	—
肝脾型	i(7q)	>95%	—	—	—
外周型	t(5;9)(q33.3;q22.2)	15%	ITK	SYK	组成型活化酪氨酸激酶(SYK)
慢性淋巴细胞白血病					
B	t(11;14)(q13.3;q32.3)	10%[b]	CCND1	IGH	失调表达——细胞周期调控

续表

疾病[a]	染色体异常	频率[b]	涉及基因[c]		结果[d]
	t(14;19)(q32.3;q13.2)	5%	IGH	BCL3	失调表达——增加的 NFkB 活化
	t(2;14)(p13;q32.3)	5%		IGH	
	t(14q32.3)	15%	IGH		
	del(13q)	30%			
	+12	25%			
T	t(8;14)(q24.2;q11.2)	5%	MYC	TRA	失调表达——转录因子
	inv(14)(q11.2q32.3)	5%	TRA/TRD	IGH	失调表达
	inv(14)(q11.2q32.1)	5%	TRA/TRD	TCL1A	失调表达——转录因子
多发性骨髓瘤					
B	-13/del(13q)	40%			
	t(4;14)(p16.3;q32.3)	15%	FGFR3	IGH	失调表达——生长因子受体和组蛋白甲基转移酶
			WHSC1/MMSET	IGH	
	t(14;16)(q32.3;q23)	5%	IGH	MAF	失调表达——转录因子
	t(6;14)(p21;q32.3)	4%	CCND3	IGH	失调表达——细胞周期调控
	t(11;14)(q13.3;q32.3)	15%	CCND1	IGH	失调表达——细胞周期调控
	t(14q32.3)	50%	IGH		
	del(17p)/t(17p)	30%	TP53		DNA 损伤反应丧失
	获得 1q	20%			
	超二倍性:+3,+5,+7,+9,+11				
成人 T 细胞白血病/淋巴瘤					
—	t(14;14)(q11.2;q32.3)	—	TRA	IGH	失调表达
	inv(14)(q11.2;q32.3)		TRA/TRD	IGH	失调表达
	+3				

[a]DLBCL,弥漫性大 B 细胞淋巴瘤;MCL,套细胞淋巴瘤;LPL,淋巴浆细胞样淋巴瘤;MALT,黏膜相关淋巴肿瘤;PCFCL,原发性皮肤滤泡中心性淋巴瘤;ALCL,间变性大细胞淋巴瘤。

[b]百分比指的是疾病的总体频率。括号内的数字表示疾病形态学或免疫学亚型内的频率。

[c]基因在核型中是按引文顺序排列的,例如,对于前体 B 急性淋巴细胞白血病(precursor B ALL),ETV6 在 12p13.2,RUNX1 在 21q22.3。

[d]TF,转录因子。

[e]通过细胞遗传学分析,儿童发病率约为 5%,成人发病率约为 25%;使用分子探针检测,这一频率在成年人中为 30%,在 60 岁以上的成年人中为 50%。

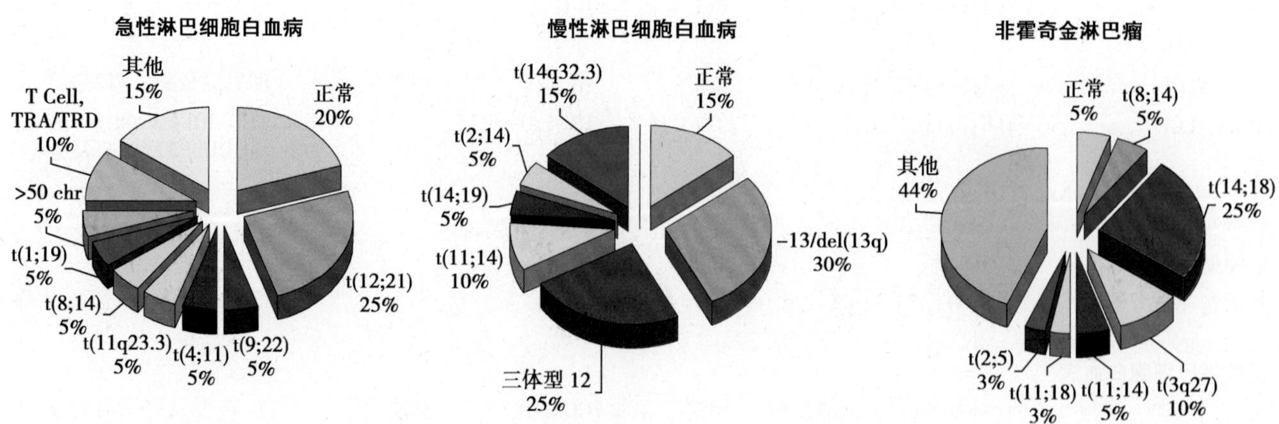

图 8-5 在 ALL、CLL 和 NHL 中复发性染色体异常发生的频率

易位 9;22

ALL 中 t(9;22)的发生率在成年人总体中为 30%,在 60 岁以上的成年人中为 50%,在儿童中为 5%,并且与极差的预后相关。约 70%的患者携带其他异常,通常伴有+der(22)t(9;22)、+21 或-7(与较差的预后相关)[60]。大多数病例具有 B 系表型(CD10+、CD19+和 TdT+),但也经常表达髓系相关抗原(CD13 和 CD33)。在超过半数的患者中,BCR 的断裂更为接近,导致 BCR-ABL1 融合蛋白更小,酪氨酸激酶活性更强(BCR-ABL1^{p190})。高达 80%的 Ph+ ALL 病例中可检测到 IKZF1 基因的遗传改变,此类患者即使使用 TKI 治疗,也会导致不良的预后[61]。

涉及 11q 的易位

KMT2A 基因在 11q23.3 位点的易位在所有患者中占 5%,但在所有婴儿中占 80%。其中,最常见的是 t(4;11)(q21.3q23.3)(图 8-6a),其次是 t(11;19)(q23;p13.3)。t(4;11)患者具有 pro B 表型(CD10-,CD19+),共表达单核细胞(CD15+)或较少见的 T 细胞标志物,对常规化疗的反应较差(成人:缓解率为 75%,EFS 仅为 7 个月)[62]。

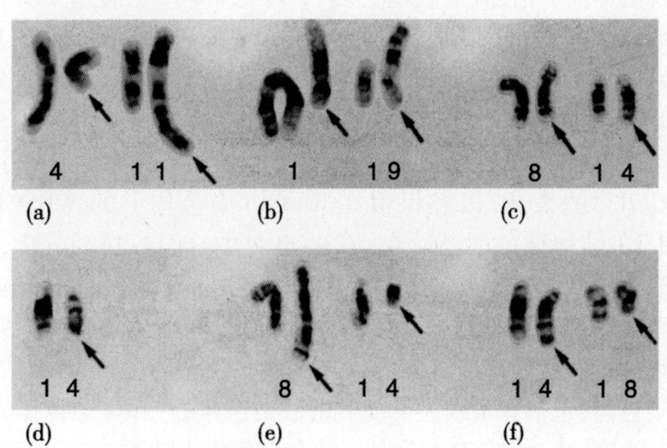

图 8-6　胰蛋白酶-吉姆萨带(trypsin-Giemsa-banded)中期细胞的部分核型,描述淋巴系肿瘤中所观察到的反复发生的染色体重排。重排的染色体用箭头标识。(a)ALL 中 t(4;11)(q21.3;q23.3)。(b)pre-B 细胞 ALL 中 t(1;19)(q23;p13.3)。(c)B 细胞 ALL 和 Burkitt 淋巴瘤中 t(8;14)(q24.2;q32.3)。(d)T 细胞白血病/淋巴瘤中 inv(14)(q11.2;q32.3)。(e)T 细胞白血病/淋巴瘤中 t(8;14)(q24.2;q11.2)。(f)B 细胞淋巴瘤中 t(14;18)(q32.3;q21.3)

易位 12;21

t(12;21)(p13.2;q22.3)在儿童早期 B 白血病中占很高的比例(约 25%),但在成人中并不常见(约 4%)[63]。这种隐性易位不能通过细胞遗传学分析检测,但可以通过 RT-PCR 或 FISH 分析可靠地检测到。t(12;21)定义了 1~10 岁患者的一个独特的亚组,具有 B 系免疫表型(CD10+,CD19+,HLA-DR+)和良好的预后(5 年无事件生存率高达 91%,而其他 ALL 患者为 65%)。t(12;21)染色体异位产生的融合蛋白,包含 ETS 家族转录抑制因子 ETV6/TEL 的 N 端,以及转录因子 RUNX1 的大部分氨基酸序列。

超二倍性

一些 ALL 患者的白血病细胞的特征是获得了多条染色体。其中包含两个不同的亚组:一组有 1-4 条额外的染色体[47~50],更常见的组有>50 条染色体(通常是 51~60 条染色体)。后一种亚组在儿童中很常见(约 30%),但在成人中很少见(<5%)。某些附加染色体是常见的(X 染色体,染色体 4、6、10、14、17、18 和 21)。>50 条染色体的患者中+4、+10、+17 的患者如果具有以下临床特征则预后更好,这些特征包括年龄 1~9 岁,白细胞计数低(中位数 6700/L),免疫表型良好(早期 pre-B 或 pre-B)[64]。

易位 1;19 和易位 8;14

t(1;19)(q23;p13.3)的预后良好,该染色体易位存在于约 6%的 B 系白血病患儿中(图 8-6b)。白血病细胞具有胞浆免疫球蛋白,分别为 CD10+、CD19+、CD34-和 CD9+。t(8;14)(q24.2;q32.3)染色体易位存在于成熟 B 细胞 ALL 中(图 8-6c)。这些病人在诊断时有较高的中枢神经系统受累和/或腹腔淋巴结受累的发生率。在过去,其预后一直很差,但高强度化疗的使用显著改善了预后(儿童的 EFS 占 80%)。

Ph 样急性淋巴细胞白血病

Ph 样急性淋巴细胞白血病(Ph 样 ALL)是一种新型的 ALL 高危亚群(儿童占 15%,成人占 30%),其特征是 HSC 基因表达增加,与 Ph 阳性 ALL 相似的基因表达谱,以及 IKZF1 的高频率缺失和突变,这些会导致预后不良。在 Ph 样 ALL 中负责活化激酶和细胞因子受体信号特征的基因改变包括影响 *CRLF2*、*JAK2*、*ABL1*、*PDGFRB*、*EPOR*、*EBF1*、*FLT3*、*IL7R*、*SH2B3* 等基因的点突变和基因融合[65,66]。

T 细胞急性淋巴细胞性白血病

T 淋巴细胞白血病/淋巴瘤有明显的反复异常模式,包括 14q11.2 处的 T 细胞受体位点(图 8-6d,e)和 7 号染色体(7q34)和(7p14)两个区域(表 8-3)[67,68]。最常见的是 t(10;11)(q24.3;q11.2)(7%的儿童和 30%的成人患者,TLX1 基因)和隐睾 t(5;14)(q35.1;q32.1)(TLX3,20%的儿童和 10%~15%的成人病例)。大约 30%的患者伴随着 *NOTCH1* 基因的突变。T 细胞患者大多为年轻男性,通常有纵隔肿瘤肿块,白细胞计数高,脑脊液中有白血病细胞。

慢性淋巴细胞性白血病

只有 50%的慢性淋巴细胞白血病(chronic lymphocytic leukemia,CLL)患者可通过细胞遗传学分析检测到异常,使用 FISH 分析可将检测率提高到 80%(表 8-3,图 8-5)[69]。FISH 最常检测到的变化是:-13/del(13q)(55%),11q 上 ATM 缺失(18%),+12(16%),17p 上 TP53 缺失,6q 缺失(6%)[70]。17p(32 个月)或 11q(79 个月)患者的中位生存期,对比无明显异常(111 个月)、+12(114 个月)或-13/del(13q)(133 个月)患者更短。ZAP-70 是 T 细胞活化的关键酶,在含有未突变 IGH 基因的 CLL 细胞中上调,导致预后不良[71]。CLL 细胞发生 IGH 突变,以及缺乏 ZAP-70 和 CD38 表达的患者,诊断后无治疗期最长[72]。

T 细胞白血病和大颗粒淋巴细胞白血病是罕见的疾病。在 T-CLL 和 T 细胞淋巴瘤中均有报道涉及 14q11.2 的重排,无论是否伴有 14q32.3 的突变(表 8-3)[67]。最常见的是 inv(14)(q11.2q32.3)(图 8-6d)。

非霍奇金淋巴瘤

90%以上的非霍奇金淋巴瘤(non-Hodgkin lymphoma, NHL)以克隆性染色体异常为特征,其与组织学和免疫表型相关(表8-3,图8-5)[73,74]。例如,t(14;18)在滤泡小裂细胞淋巴瘤中占很高比例(70%~90%)。大多数有t(3;22)(q27;q11.2)或t(3;14)(q27;q32.3)的病人都有t(8;14)(q24.2;q32.3)。在B细胞肿瘤(约70%)中,IGH(14q32.3)经常参与易位。同样,很大比例的T细胞肿瘤的特征是TCR基因在14q11.2、7q34或7p14的重排。基因表达谱已被证明在区分淋巴瘤的独特基因亚型方面是有用的[75]。例如,基因表达谱显示DLBCL(弥漫性大B细胞淋巴瘤)至少包括三种不同的亚型(生发中心B细胞样淋巴瘤、活化B细胞样淋巴瘤和原发性纵隔B细胞淋巴瘤),每一种都有独特的致癌机制、预后和治疗反应[76]。

T(8;14)或变异t(2;8)或t(8;22),是地方性和非地方性Burkitt肿瘤以及EB病毒阴性和阳性肿瘤的特征(图8-6c)。此外,t(8;14)在其他淋巴瘤中也有发现,尤其是小的无核裂细胞(非Burkitt)和大细胞免疫母细胞淋巴瘤,以及HIV相关的BL(100%)和HIV相关的DLBCL(30%)[77]。t(8;14)通过将编码外显子与IGH序列(14q32.3)并置得到MYC(8q24.2)的组成型表达。MYC是一种转录因子,在DNA复制、增殖和凋亡等许多细胞生物学功能中发挥着关键作用。

70%~90%的滤泡性淋巴瘤和20%的DLBCL都具有t(14;18)(图8-6f),其中18q21.3处的BCL2基因与IGH J段并置,导致抗凋亡线粒体膜蛋白BCL2表达失调[78]。常见的继发性异常包括-7、+18和del(6q)。由滤泡性淋巴瘤发展为DLBCL引起的双发性淋巴瘤同时具有BCL2和MYC易位[79]。

T(11;14)(q13.3;q32.3)在几乎所有的被套细胞淋巴瘤(mantle cell lymphoma, MCL)病例中均可观察到,MCL通常预后不良,中位生存期为3年,同时也可在3%的骨髓瘤和高达20%的淋巴细胞前白血病中观察到[80]。这种易位导致细胞周期蛋白D1(Cyclin D1, CCND1)基因被IGH基因激活,该基因位于离断点100~130kb的位置。D型细胞周期蛋白作为生长因子传感器,通过磷酸化和RB1失活调控细胞分裂。

在40%的DLBCL和高达10%的滤泡性淋巴瘤中可发生导致BCL6在3q27过表达的重排,最常见的原因是t(3;22)(q27;q11.2)或t(3;14)(q27;q32.3)[73]。BCL6是一种96kD的POZ/Zn手指转录抑制因子,可抑制淋巴细胞活化、分化、细胞周期阻滞和凋亡相关基因。在未发生易位的DLBDL中,约20%的BCL6的5′端调控区域已经发现了体细胞突变,这表明BCL6的过表达比最初认识到的更为广泛[81]。

黏液相关淋巴组织(mucosa associated lymphoid tissue, MALT)结外边缘区B细胞淋巴瘤(MALT淋巴瘤)由几个基因亚群组成,一个以+3+其他异常(60%)为特征,另一个以t(11;18)(q21.2;q21.3)(25%~50%)及其变异为特征[82]。t(11;18)导致凋亡抑制基因BIRC3(API2)与一个18q21.3的新基因MALT1融合,其产物能够激活NFkB通路。

间变性大细胞淋巴瘤(anaplastic large cell lymphoma, ALCL)的特点是发病时年龄较轻、皮肤和/或淋巴结被大的特异性淋巴瘤细胞浸润,这种浸润常常倾向于累及皮质旁区和淋巴结窦。大多数此类肿瘤表达一种或多种T细胞抗原,少数表达B细胞抗原,有些同时表达T-和B细胞抗原(无表型)。t(2;5)(p23.2;q35.1)、t(1;2)(q25;p23)或涉及ALK酪氨酸激酶基因2p23的变异重排在T细胞或无表型的ALCL中发生频率很高[83]。肿瘤细胞在细胞膜和高尔基体区域CD30呈阳性,在60%~85%的病例中可检测到ALK的表达,在这些病例中,ALK+的五年存活率为80%,而ALK-肿瘤的五年存活率为40%。

多发性骨髓瘤

FISH与浆细胞富集技术的联合应用导致发现了高比例的骨髓瘤、滤泡后B细胞(post-follicular B cells)的单克隆恶性肿瘤,以及恶化前意义不明的单克隆丙种球蛋白病(monoclonal gammopathy of undetermined significance, MGUS)(表8-3)[84,85]。MGUS以染色体非整倍性、IGH易位(45%)、高二倍体和13q缺失(15%~50%)为特征,其导致细胞周期蛋白D/RB1通路失调,也被认为是浆细胞骨髓瘤中最早的改变[84,86~88]。

骨髓瘤的分子细胞遗传学分类可分为三大类:①具有IGH易位的非高二倍体(骨髓瘤患者占40%,MGUS患者占10%);②超二倍体;③其他异常[84,86]。在15%的病例中发现t(11;14)(q13.3;q32.2),这导致了CCND1过表达。另外,在大约15%的患者中可以检测到t(4;14)(p16.3;q32.3),这种突变解除了转位到der(14)的成纤维细胞生长因子受体3基因(FGFR3)的表达,以及保留在der(4)染色体上的WHSC1/MMSET结构域的表达。在5%的患者中,t(14;16)(q32.3;q23)会导致MAF转录因子基因的过表达。t(4;14)和t(14;16)均与较差的临床结局相关,而t(11;14)患者的预后较好。将近一半的骨髓瘤患者是高二倍体(45%),最常见的是49~56条染色体,包括3条或3条以上奇数染色体的三体(染色体3、5、7、9、11、15、19或21),这是一个与老年患者和更有利预后相关的遗传亚群。

在10%的骨髓瘤中,FISH检测发现17p上的TP53缺失与预后不良有关(这些患者中37%也有TP53突变)。1号染色体异常经常导致1q的增加和1p(CDKN2C)的丢失,这与较短的存活时间有关[89]。因此,骨髓瘤综合FISH检测手段应该包括1p探针,特别是1q探针。

随着骨髓瘤疾病的进展,还会发生包括NRAS和KRAS的突变(30%~40%)、MYC失调和表观遗传学改变。在MGUS和多发性骨髓瘤中,有几个基因通过异常启动子高甲基化而沉默,包括DAPK1(67%)、SOCS1、CDKN2B(p15)和CDKN2A(p16)[86]。

实体瘤

与血液恶性肿瘤相比,由于技术上的限制,我们对实体肿瘤染色体改变的认识较为落后。然而,随着基因分析的最新进展,染色体的改变显然在实体肿瘤中起着更重要作用(表8-4)。虽然具有疾病特异性基因融合的简单核型是血液病恶性肿瘤和肉瘤的常见表型,但其他实体肿瘤的染色体畸变往往涉及更大比例基因组的改变。事实上,实体肿瘤中体细胞CNA的中位数为39,远高于血液恶性肿瘤[90]。CNA的极端病例被描述为"染色体碎裂"和"染色体丛",涉及高度复杂的重新排列[91,92]。这通常与 TP53 突变和预后不良有关[93]。与血液恶性肿瘤一样,实体肿瘤中许多反复发生的异常涉及编码转录调节因子或酪氨酸激酶的基因,后者可产生潜在的可用药蛋白。除了提供潜在的治疗靶点外,染色体改变还可以阐释实体肿瘤生物学改变,改善疾病分类,预测治疗反应并提示预后。代表性疾病和相关反复出现的染色体畸变将在以下章节中讨论。

表 8-4　实体瘤中反复出现的染色体异常

肿瘤类型	染色体异常	频率	融合产物或候选基因受影响[a]		结果
膀胱癌	t(4;4)(p16.3;p16.3)	3%	FGFR3	TACC3	激酶激活
	t(12;17)(q13.1;q12)	3%	DIP2B	ERBB2	激酶激活
	add(6p22.3)	20%	E2F3/SOX4		
	add(7p12)	10%~15%	EGFR		激酶激活
	add(3q26.3)	20%	PIK3CA		
	add(12q13.2)	10%~15%	ERBB3		激酶激活
	del(9p21.3)	50%	CDKN2A		
	del(17p11.2)	25%	NCOR1		
	del(10q23.3)	10%~15%	PTEN		激酶激活
	del(13q14.2)	15%	RB1		
	del(9q34.1)	5%~10%	TSC1		激酶激活
乳腺癌	t(1;1)(p12;q44)	2%	MAGI3	AKT3	激酶激活
	add(11q13.3)	15%	CCND1		Luminal 亚型
	add(8p11.23)	15%	ZNF703		Luminal 亚型
	add(8q24.2)	20%	MYC		基底细胞样型
	add(17q12)	15%	ERBB2		激酶激活
	add(7p12)	3%	EGFR		激酶激活
	del(8q23.2)	10%	CSMD1		
	del(13q14.2)	5%	RB1		
	del(10q23.3)	5%	PTEN		激酶激活
宫颈癌	add(8q24.2)	8%	MYC	—	
	add(11q13.3)	3%	CCND1		
	add(7p12)	3%	EGFR		激酶激活
	add(17q12)	3%	ERBB2		激酶激活
结肠癌	t(2;11)(p11.2;p15.1)	3%	TCF7L1	NAV2	
	t(10;10)(q25.2;25.3)	3%	VTI1A		
	add(17q12)	5%	ERBB2	TCF7L2	激酶激活
	add(8q24.2)	6%	MYC		
	add(11p15.5)	4%	IGF2,miR-483		
	add(1q)	17%			
	del(3p14.2)	10%	FHIT		
	del(16p13.3)	25%	RBFOX1		
	del(6q26)	10%	PARK2		
	del(5q22.2)	2%	APC		

续表

肿瘤类型	染色体异常	频率	融合产物或候选基因受影响[a]		结果
	del(14q)	30%			
	del(15q)	30%			
子宫内膜癌	i(1)(q10)			—	
	add(15q26.3)	2%	IGF1R		预后不良
	add(8q24.2)	5%	MYC		上皮浆液性
	add(17q12)	4%	ERBB2		上皮浆液性
	add(19q12)	4%	CCNE1		上皮浆液性
食管癌	add(11q13.3)	—	CCND1	—	—
头颈癌	t(4;4)(p16.3;p16.3)	<5%	FGFR3	TACC3	
	add(3q26.3)	20%	SOX2		
	add(7p12)	15%	EGFR		激酶激活
	add(11q13.3)	35%	CCND1		
	del(9p21.3)	25%	CDKN2A		
肺癌(小细胞)	inv(1)(p32p34.3)	10%	RLF	MYCL1	—
	add(3q26.2)	25%~30%	SOX2		
	add(1p34.3)		MYCL		
	add(8q24.2)		MYC		
	add(6p22.3)		SOX4		
	add(19q12)		URI1		
	del(13q14.2)		RB1		
	del(8p21.1)		ESCO2		
	del(5q31.3)		ANKHD1		
	del(5q12.1)		KIF2A		
肺癌(非小细胞)	inv(2)(p21p23.2)	5%	EML4	ALK	激酶激活
	t(4;6)(p15.2;q22.1)	全部 ROS1 2%	SLC34A2	ROS1	激酶激活
	t(6;20)(q22.1;q12)		ROS1	SDC4	激酶激活
	t(5;6)(q32;q22.1)		CD74	ROS1	激酶激活
	inv(10)(p11.2q11.2)	全部 RET 1%	KIF5B	RET	激酶激活
	inv(6)(q22.1q25)		ROS1	EZR	激酶激活
	inv(10)(q11.2q21.2)		RET	CCDC6	激酶激活
	add(12q15)	5%~10%	MDM2		
	add(7p12)	8%	EGFR		激酶激活
	del(9p21.3)	25%	CDKN2A		
前列腺癌	t(1;7)(q32.1;p21)	1%	SLC45A3	ETV1	
	t(7;7)(q32;q34)	1%	NRF1	BRAF	激酶激活
	t(1;17)(q32.1;q21.3)	1%	SLC45A3	ETV4	

续表

肿瘤类型	染色体异常	频率	融合产物或候选基因受影响[a]		结果
	t(21;21)(q22.3;q22.3)	全部 TMPRSS2-ERG	TMPRSS2	ERG	ETS 家族成员
	del(21)(q22.3q22.3)	45%	TMPRSS2	ERG	融合——转录改变
	t(1;21)(q32.1;q22.3)	1%	SLC45A3	ERG	
	t(3;21)(q27.2;q22.3)	1%	ETV5	TMPRSS2	
	t(7;21)(p21;q22.3)	1%	ETV1	TMPRSS2	
	t(17;21)(q21;q22)	1%	ETV4	TMPRSS2	
	t(1;7)(q32.1;q34)	1%	SLC45A3	BRAF	激酶激活
	7 号染色体三体型				
	8 号染色体单体型				
肾细胞	t(X;17)(p11.2;q23.1)	所有 TFE	TFE3	CLTC	
	t(X;1)(p11.2;p34.3)	易位	TFE3	SFPQ	
	inv(X)(p11.2q13.1)	约 2%	TFE3	NONO	
	t(X;17)(p11.2;q25)		TFE3	ASPSCR1	
	add(5q)	69%			
	add(7q)	20%			
	del(3p25.3)	95%	VHL		
	del(14q)	42%			
	del(8p)	32%			
	del(9p)	29%			
甲状腺癌	inv(10)(q11.2;q21)	25%	RET	CCD6	激酶激活
	Inv(10)(q11.2;q11.2)	10%	RET	NCOA4	激酶激活
	t(10;17)(q11.2;q24.2)	2%	RET	PRKAR1A	激酶激活
	inv(1)(q21.3;q23.1)		TPM3	NTRK1	
	t(1;3)		NTRK1	TPR/TFG	
	inv(7q21.2;q34)		AKAP9	BRAF	激酶激活
唾液腺黏液样癌	t(11;19)(q21;p13.2)	35%~70%	MAML2	MECT1/CRTC1	预后良好
脂肪瘤	add(12q)	80%~90%	HMGA2,MDM2	—	—
滑膜肉瘤	t(X;18)(p11.2;q11.2)	—	SSX1	SS18/SYT	染色质重塑改变
横纹肌肉瘤(肺泡类型)	t(2;13)(q36.1;q14.1)	—	PAX3	FOXO1	—
	t(1;13)(p36.1;q14.1)		PAX7	FOXO1	
骨外黏液样软骨肉瘤	t(9;22)(q22;q12.2)	50%~60%	NR4A3	EWSR1	—
	t(9;17)(q22;q12)	15%~20%	NR4A3	TAF15	
黏液炎性成纤维细胞性肉瘤	t(1;10)(p22.1;q24.3)	约 95%	TGFBR3	MGEA5	—
	add(3p12.1)		VGLL3		

续表

肿瘤类型	染色体异常	频率	融合产物或候选基因受影响[a]		结果
先天性纤维肉瘤	t(12;15)(p13.2;q25.3)	约95%	ETV6	NTRK3	转录改变
纤维黏液样肉瘤	t(7;16)(q34;p11.2)	约95%	CREB3L2	FUS	—
间变性星形细胞瘤	7号染色体三体型	30%	—	—	—
	del(9p)	30%			
	del(10q)	30%~40%			
胶质母细胞瘤	7号染色体三体型	50%~60%	—	—	—
	del(9p)	30%~40%			
	10号染色体单体型	50%~60%			
	13号染色体单体型	30%~40%			
神经鞘瘤	del(22q12.2)	45%	NF2	—	—
	add(9q34)	10%			
	add(17q)	5%			
尤因肉瘤	t(11;22)(q24.3;q12.2)	85%	FLI1	EWSR1	转录改变
	t(21;22)(q22.3;q12.2)	10%	ERG	EWSR1	转录改变
髓母细胞瘤	6号染色体单体型	—	—	—	预后良好
	add(8q24)				预后不良
	i(17q)				
成神经细胞瘤	add(2p24.3)	60%	MYCN	—	—
	add(2p23.2)	10%	ALK		
Wilms瘤	add(1q)	25%~30%		—	预后不良
	del(11p13)	10%~30%	WT1		
	del(Xq11.1)	13%	AMER1		
	del(16q)	10%~15%			
中胚层肾瘤	t(12;15)(p13.2;q25.3)	—	ETV6	NTRK3	细胞性亚型
视网膜母细胞瘤	del(13q14.2)	约3%	RB1	—	—
软组织透明细胞肉瘤	t(12;22)(q13.1;q12.2)	—	ATF1	EWSR1	转录改变
	t(2;22)(q33.3;q12.2)		CREB1	EWSR1	转录改变
睾丸肿瘤	i(12p)	合计接近	—	—	—
	add(12p)	100%			
隆突性皮肤纤维肉瘤	t(17;22)(q21.3;q13.1)	—	COL1A1	PDGFB	激酶激活

[a] 基因在核型中按引文顺序排列，如膀胱癌中，DIP2B为12q13.1，ERBB2为17q12。

肉瘤

肉瘤(sarcomas)是一组异质性的疾病，随着时间的推移，目前认为肉瘤由多种不同的实体组成。组织学相似性并不总是表现为相似的临床行为，这些疾病的遗传基础知识有助于优化疾病分类，并有助于我们理解这些不同的疾病之间的关系。

1983年，t(11;22)(q24.3;q12.2)染色体异常在尤因肉瘤(Ewing sarcomas)中被发现[94,95]。这种易位导致尤因肉瘤断点区1(Ewing sarcoma breakpoint region 1，EWSR1)与Friend白血病病毒整合位点1(friend leukemia virus integration site 1，FLI1)的框内融合，前者属于FET家族，后者属于ETS转录因子家族。由此得到的EWS-FLI1融合蛋白由EWS的N端反活化域与FLI1的DNA结合域融合而成，其形成一种致癌转录因子，能够上调或下调数千个基因，这是肿瘤发生所必需的[96~98]。融合断点是可变的，不同融合产物的功能意义也不尽相同[99]。

10年后，在约10%的尤因肉瘤中发现了EWSR1和ETS相关基因(ERG)融合。ERG编码的另一个ETS家族成员在DNA结合ETS域中与FLI1具有98%的同源性[100]。加上EWS-FLI1，这些肿瘤占尤因肉瘤的95%。其余5%包含FET家族成员的其他融合,特别是 EWSR1 或 FUS 与 ETS 家族成员的融合,包括 FLI1、ERG、ETV1、ETV4 或 FEV[101]。这些融合相互排斥,表明其产生的蛋白质功能相似。

尤因样肉瘤(Ewing-like sarcomas)在组织学上与尤因肉瘤相似,但不包含可检测到的 FET/ETS 染色体重排。他们的特点是其他的重排,包括 EWSR1 和非 ETS 家庭成员[102]。随着我们对融合基因和相关疾病理解的加深,这些疾病的诊断定义可能会发生改变。EWSR1 与其他肉瘤(包括 EWSR1-ATF1 和透明细胞肉瘤、EWSR1-WT1 和结缔性圆形细胞瘤、EWSR1-NR4A3 和骨外黏液样软骨肉瘤、EWSR1-DDIT3 和黏液样脂肪肉瘤、EWSR1-ZNF278 和小圆形细胞肉瘤)的重排关系使诊断变得更加困难。与尤因肉瘤一样,每个诊断最常见的是单一的重排,但一个或两个相关基因也可以与其他基因形成融合伴侣。1986 年在滑膜肉瘤中发现了一个涉及 SS18(18q11.2)和 SSX1(Xp11.23)的易位[103]。大量的基因和伪基因与 SSX1 同源,其中许多可以与 SS18 形成融合癌基因。由此产生的融合蛋白通过与 SWIF-SNF 染色质重构复合物和多囊群蛋白复合物(polycomb group protein complex)的相互作用来调控转录[104~106]。不同的融合基因产物似乎具有细微的功能差异,并导致形态学上不同的肿瘤变异。

肾细胞癌

传统的肾细胞癌(renal cell carcinoma,RCC)是指透明细胞癌,约占全部肾癌病例的 85%。几乎所有的透明细胞 RCC 都与 VHL 通过缺失、突变和/或表观遗传沉默等破坏有关。通常在肿瘤的每个细胞中都会发生 VHL 基因改变,这表明基因变化发生在亲本克隆中,可能对肿瘤的发生起着至关重要的作用[107]。除了 VHL 的丢失,90%或更多的透明细胞 RCC 还含有位于 3p 上的其他基因的缺失,包括 PBRM1、SETD2 和 BAP1[108]。

通常认为嗜酸细胞瘤和嗜铬细胞癌起源于集合管的夹层细胞,在组织学上很难区分。然而,嗜酸细胞瘤很少发生转移,这表明先前关于嗜酸细胞瘤转移的报道可能是由于误诊[109]。两者都可能存在多种染色体异常;嗜酸细胞瘤经常有重排导致的 CCND1(11q13)过表达,而嗜色细胞癌则无此种重排。识别这些变化可以预测转移的潜在风险,进而影响疾病的临床处理[110]。

神经胶质瘤

少突胶质细胞瘤(oligodendrogliomas)是一种分化良好的肿瘤,它与 1q 和 19p 的不平衡易位有关,随后会导致 1p 和 19q 的丢失。间变性少突胶质细胞瘤和少星形细胞瘤的分化程度较低,它们的预后可能与共缺失的存在有关。在少突胶质细胞瘤中,存在这种协同缺失的肿瘤对化疗很敏感,患者的中位生存期超过 10 年。相反,没有这些变化的肿瘤更可能具有星形细胞特征,生存期更短(2~3 年)[111]。因此建议在诊断时对所有的少突胶质细胞瘤进行共缺失评估。

非小细胞肺癌

除了预测对细胞毒性治疗的反应外,许多染色体改变所产生的蛋白产物已成为药物靶点。十年前,EGFR 的小分子抑制剂被发现对约 10%的非小细胞肺癌(non-small-cell lung cancer,NSCLC)患者有效。NSCLC 是一个亚群,从不吸烟的腺癌患者居多,尤其是亚洲患者[112~113]。大多数治疗应答者有 EGFR 突变,突变等位基因频繁扩增。在这一发现之前,KRAS 突变是在非小细胞肺癌中唯一被确定的驱动因素[114],这一发现提供了一个具有挑战性的药物靶点。2007 年,EML4-ALK 融合癌基因在约 5%的患者中被发现,尤其是年轻、从不吸烟或轻度吸烟者[115]。仅仅 4 年后,克里唑替尼(Crizotinib)就被 FDA 批准用于 EML4-ALK 易位患者。在有能预测治疗反应的遗传学改变的患者中,EGFR 和 ALK 的靶向抑制剂比细胞毒性治疗更有效。

虽然携带每种驱动癌基因的患者比例较低,但在腺癌中驱动癌基因的数量在不断增加(图 8-7)。这些包括 ALK 与其他

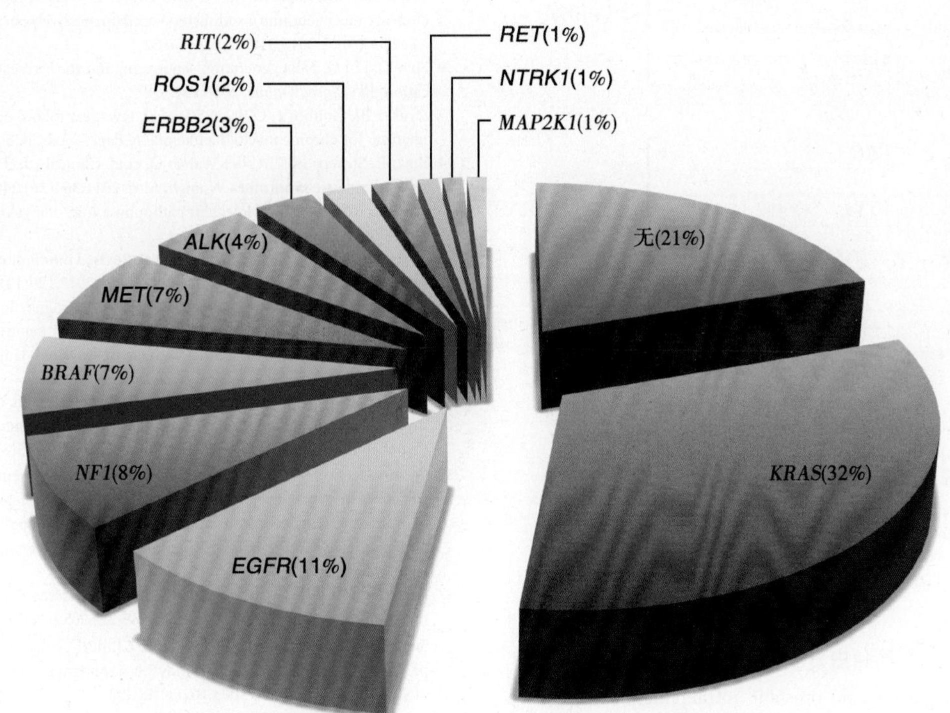

图 8-7 肺腺癌驱动基因改变的频率,与染色体异常有关的基因用粗体标记

基因的融合；CD74-ROS1、SLC34A2-ROS1 及其他涉及 ROS1 的融合；KIF5B-RET 和其他 RET 融合体；涉及 NTRK1 的融合；以及其他方式的融合。最近的测序工作已经明确了 MET 和 ERBB2 的扩增[116]。最初在胶质母细胞瘤中发现了 FGFR3-TACC3 突变，后续在肺鳞癌和尿路上皮癌中也有类似发现[117]。合并 ALK、ROS1 和 NTRK1 的患者可能对克里唑替尼有反应。目前正在对携带 RET 融合基因的患者进行多种 RET 抑制剂的临床试验，携带 FGFR 家族融合基因的肿瘤可能对 FGFR 抑制剂更加敏感。对于新诊断的 NSCLC 患者，特别是腺癌患者或诊断时年龄较轻的患者，建议进行驱动基因变异检测。随着已识别的驱动突变数量的增加，多重评估或更全面的测序技术已经取代了基于 PCR 的单个基因检测。

前列腺癌

考虑到前列腺癌的高患病率，TMPRSS2-ERG 融合可能是人类肿瘤中最常见的基因融合了，大约 40%～50% 的前列腺癌患者存在该基因融合[118,119]。ERG 正常状态下表达水平非常低，该融合导致了 ERG 的高表达，这种高表达由雄激素受体调控的 TMPRSS2 启动子驱动。与肉瘤中的 EWSR1 融合基因相似，其他多个 ETS 家族成员也在前列腺癌中形成融合基因，包括 ETV1、ETV4、ETV5、ELK4，这些融合相互排斥。这些 ETS 家族成员均可与 5′端融合伙伴形成融合，包括 TMPRSS2 或 SCL45A3 或其他融合者。总的来说，60%的前列腺癌存在 ETS-家族融合（图 8-8）。

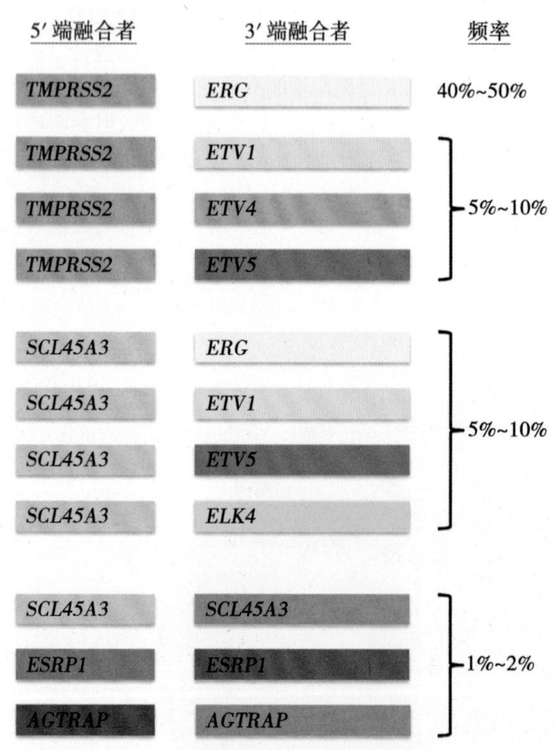

图 8-8 前列腺癌融合基因鉴定

ETS 家族重排似乎是肿瘤发生的早期事件，并已在前列腺癌前上皮内肿瘤（preneoplastic prostatic intraepithelial neoplasm，PIN）病变中得到证实[120]。最初，ETS 家族重排与预后不良有关，随后的报告又驳斥了这一发现，所以这仍然是一个有争论的话题。近来，临床前数据显示了 ETS 重组细胞系和异种移植模型对 PARP1 抑制剂的敏感性，目前这类抑制剂正在临床试验中进行评估[121]。

大约 1%的前列腺癌具有 CRAF 和 BRAF 的融合，并且对索拉非尼敏感[122]。据估计，100% 的晚期前列腺癌都存在 PTEN-PI3K-AKT 通路的改变，而 PTEN 在局限性前列腺癌中的缺失预示着更差的预后[123]。PTEN 的缺失和 MYC 的扩增预示着前列腺癌的死亡率将比没有这两种异常的情况增加 50 倍[124]。然而，到目前为止，PI3K 和 AKT 抑制剂还没有显示出临床疗效。

大约 5%的局限性前列腺癌有 AURKA 或 MYCN 的扩增。然而，在侵袭性神经内分泌变异体中，扩增率可高达 40%[125]。临床前模型显示神经内分泌肿瘤对 AURKA 抑制剂的敏感性，正在进行的临床试验在测试这些药物对这种侵袭性亚型的敏感性。虽然很少有通过临床试验之外的方式对前列腺癌染色体畸变进行评估，但随着下一代测序技术和融合特异性检测方法的普及，相信相关的评估会得到更广泛的应用。

（李亮 译 郑博 陈淑桢 校）

参考文献

The complete reference list can be found on the Wiley Companion Digital Edition of this title (see inside front cover for login instructions).

1 Heim S, Mitelman F. *Cancer Cytogenetics: Chromosomal and Molecular Genetic Aberrations of Tumor Cells*. New York: Wiley; 2011.

2 Ouyang KJ, Le Beau MM. Role of cytogenetic analysis in the diagnosis and classification of hematopoietic neoplasms. In: Orazi A, Weiss LM, Foucar K, Knowles DM, eds. *Knowles' Neoplastic Hematopathology*. Philadelphia: Lippincott Williams & Wilkins; 2014:232–264.

3 Godley LA, Cunningham J, Dolan ME, et al. An integrated genomic approach to the assessment and treatment of acute myeloid leukemia. *Semin Oncol*. 2011;**38(2)**:215–224.

7 Frampton GM, Fichtenholtz A, Otto GA, et al. Development and validation of a clinical cancer genomic profiling test based on massively parallel DNA sequencing. *Nat Biotechnol*. 2013;**31(11)**:1023–1031.

9 Shyr D, Liu Q. Next generation sequencing in cancer research and clinical application. *BiolProced Online*. 2013;**15(1)**:4.

12 Druker BJ, Guilhot F, O'Brien SG, et al. Five-year follow-up of patients receiving imatinib for chronic myeloid leukemia. *N Engl J Med*. 2006;**355(23)**:2408–2417.

24 Bejar R, Stevenson K, Abdel-Wahab O, et al. Clinical effect of point mutations in myelodysplastic syndromes. *N Engl J Med*. 2011;**364(26)**:2496–2506.

25 Lindsley RC, Ebert BL. Molecular pathophysiology of myelodysplastic syndromes. *Annu Rev Pathol*. 2013;**8**:21–47.

26 Greenberg PL, Tuechler H, Schanz J, et al. Revised international prognostic scoring system for myelodysplastic syndromes. *Blood*. 2012;**120(12)**:2454–2465.

29 Mrozek K, Marcucci G, Nicolet D, et al. Prognostic significance of the European LeukemiaNet standardized system for reporting cytogenetic and molecular alterations in adults with acute myeloid leukemia. *J Clin Oncol*. 2012;**30(36)**:4515–4523.

38 Dohner H, Estey EH, Amadori S, et al. Diagnosis and management of acute myeloid leukemia in adults: recommendations from an international expert panel, on behalf of the European LeukemiaNet. *Blood*. 2010;**115(3)**:453–474.

39 Grimwade D, Hills RK, Moorman AV, et al. Refinement of cytogenetic classification in acute myeloid leukemia: determination of prognostic significance of rare recurring chromosomal abnormalities among 5876 younger adult patients treated in the United Kingdom Medical Research Council trials. *Blood*. 2010;**116(3)**:354–365.

48 Network TCGAR. Genomic and epigenomic landscapes of adult de novo acute myeloid leukemia. *N Engl J Med*. 2013;**368(22)**:2059–2074.

51 Smith SM, Le Beau MM, Huo D, et al. Clinical-cytogenetic associations in 306 patients with therapy-related myelodysplasia and myeloid leukemia: the University of Chicago series. *Blood*. 2003;**102(1)**:43–52.

55 Harrison CJ. Acute lymphoblastic leukemia. *Clin Lab Med*. 2011;**31(4)**:631–647, ix.

58 Mulligan CG. Genomic characterization of childhood acute lymphoblastic

leukemia. *Semin Hematol*. 2013;**50**(**4**):314–324.
68 Van Vlierberghe P, Ferrando A. The molecular basis of T cell acute lymphoblastic leukemia. *J Clin Invest*. 2012;**122**(**10**):3398–3406.
74 Dave BJ, Nelson M, Sanger WG. Lymphoma cytogenetics. *Clin Lab Med*. 2011;**31**(**4**):725–761, x–xi.
76 Alizadeh AA, Eisen MB, Davis RE, et al. Distinct types of diffuse large B-cell lymphoma identified by gene expression profiling. *Nature*. 2000;**403**(**6769**):503–511.
85 Hartmann L, Biggerstaff JS, Chapman DB, et al. Detection of genomic abnormalities in multiple myeloma: the application of FISH analysis in combination with various plasma cell enrichment techniques. *Am J Clin Pathol*. 2011;**136**(**5**):712–720.
87 Morgan GJ, Walker BA, Davies FE. The genetic architecture of multiple myeloma. *Nat Rev Cancer*. 2012;**12**(**5**):335–348.
91 Baca SC, Prandi D, Lawrence MS, et al. Punctuated evolution of prostate cancer genomes. *Cell*. 2013;**153**(**3**):666–677.
92 Stephens PJ, Greenman CD, Fu B, et al. Massive genomic rearrangement acquired in a single catastrophic event during cancer development. *Cell*. 2011;**144**(**1**):27–40.
96 Delattre O, Zucman J, Plougastel B, et al. Gene fusion with an ETS DNA-binding domain caused by chromosome translocation in human tumours. *Nature*. 1992;**359**(**6391**):162–165.
97 Ouchida M, Ohno T, Fujimura Y, et al. Loss of tumorigenicity of Ewing's sarcoma cells expressing antisense RNA to EWS-fusion transcripts. *Oncogene*. 1995;**11**(**6**):1049–1054.
102 Ordonez JL, Osuna D, Herrero D, et al. Advances in Ewing's sarcoma research: where are we now and what lies ahead? *Cancer Res*. 2009;**69**(**18**):7140–7150.
108 Cancer Genome Atlas Research Network. Comprehensive molecular characterization of clear cell renal cell carcinoma. *Nature*. 2013;**499**(**7456**):43–49.
111 Cairncross G, Wang M, Shaw E, et al. Phase III trial of chemoradiotherapy for anaplastic oligodendroglioma: long-term results of RTOG 9402. *J Clin Oncol*. 2013;**31**(**3**):337–343.
115 Soda M, Choi YL, Enomoto M, et al. Identification of the transforming EML4-ALK fusion gene in non-small-cell lung cancer. *Nature*. 2007;**448**(**7153**):561–566.
116 Cancer Genome Atlas Research Network. Comprehensive molecular profiling of lung adenocarcinoma. *Nature*. 2014;**511**(**7511**):543–550.
121 Brenner JC, Ateeq B, Li Y, et al. Mechanistic rationale for inhibition of poly(ADP-ribose) polymerase in ETS gene fusion-positive prostate cancer. *Cancer Cell*. 2011;**19**(**5**):664–678.
123 Taylor BS, Schultz N, Hieronymus H, et al. Integrative genomic profiling of human prostate cancer. *Cancer Cell*. 2010;**18**(**1**):11–22.
125 Beltran H, Rickman DS, Park K, et al. Molecular characterization of neuroendocrine prostate cancer and identification of new drug targets. *Cancer Discov*. 2011;**1**(**6**):487–495.

第 9 章　癌症中 miRNA 的表达

Serge Patrick Nana-Sinkam, MD ■ Mario Acunzo, PhD ■ Carlo M. Croce, MD

概述

在过去的二十年中，研究人员根据功能和大小确定了一组新型的非编码 RNA(ncRNA)，其中研究最深入的是称之为 microRNA(miRNA)的短链非编码 RNA。miRNA 长度约为 22 个核苷酸，在包括癌症在内的大量生物过程和疾病的调控中发挥了关键的作用。自 2002 年首次发现 miRNA 与癌症之间的关联以来，miRNA 已成为癌症发生和发展基本过程的中心调节因子。最近，研究人员在包括血液、痰液和尿液等体液中检测到了 miRNA，使得 miRNA 成为潜在的非侵入性疾病的诊断和预后生物标志物。将 miRNA 应用于癌症治疗已经成为研究的热点，是癌症治疗研究的最新前沿之一。尽管如此，我们对这些小分子及其在癌症中应用的理解仍有很大的提高空间。在本章中，我们概述了 miRNA 与癌症之间的联系，重点阐述如何推进其向临床应用转化。

背景

随着对肿瘤复杂性认识的不断深入，研究人员也不断地在癌症中寻找可用于开发新型生物标志物和疗法的新型分子途径，以达到拯救生命的最终目标。几十年来，研究人员一直认为，大部分人类基因组由无法编码蛋白质的“垃圾 DNA”或“暗物质”组成。在过去的二十年中，研究人员发现了以前被认为无用的人类基因组区域是有功能的。位于这些区域的一些基因编码了非编码 RNA(ncRNA)，其中研究得最多的是 miRNA。自二十年前在秀丽隐杆线虫中首次被发现以来，miRNA 已逐渐被认为是癌症发生发展基本生物过程的关键调节因子[1,2]。miRNA 的长度大约为 22 个核苷酸(nt)，往往在物种间高度保守，并且通常在实体瘤和血液系统恶性肿瘤中表现出广泛的失调[3,4]。通过直接结合靶标 mRNA 的 3′或 5′非翻译区(UTR)，miRNA 可以降解靶 mRNA 或抑制靶 mRNA 的翻译。此外，由于 miRNA 相对短小，它们可以同时调节数十至数百个基因，由此阻断许多生物途径。miRNA 能够调节多达 60%的人类基因组的估计可能是错误的，但 miRNA 确实能够调节超过 90%的蛋白编码基因[4,5]。miRNA 通常位于染色体的脆弱区域，因此易于通过染色体扩增、缺失或重排被调节[6]。miRNA 在肿瘤环境中的调节机制很复杂，目前只揭示了部分机制。越来越多的研究表明，可以通过多种机制对 miRNA 进行调控，包括加工过程关键组分的改变，表观遗传沉默，以及会干扰 miRNA 结合和调节的 miRNA 或靶 mRNA 的多态性[7]。肿瘤和细胞的特异性使 miRNA 调控和发挥作用的机制进一步复杂化。目前已经鉴定的 miRNA 接近 3 000 种。对于不同类型的肿瘤和细胞，miRNA 可起到抑癌或促癌的作用，调控肿瘤发生的基本过程(肿瘤的特征)，包括分化、增殖和血管生成[8]。肿瘤中 miRNA 的调节机制，以及 miRNA 在肿瘤发生和发展中的作用，才刚刚开始被阐释。尽管高通量分析方法可以用于鉴定临床相关的 miRNA 生物标志物，但仍然存在重复性差的问题，同时还受到 miRNA 靶标预测和验证算法不成熟的限制。因此，将 miRNA 转化为临床决策标志物仍然需要相当多的工作，同时还必须考虑实现特异性肿瘤 miRNA 递送的困难。可喜的是，随着 miRNA 生物学特性向临床的转化，在不久的将来有望实现 miRNA 的应用，尤其在治疗方面。例如基于纳米技术递送 miRNA 的载体，是一种典型的在人体中实现 miRNA 有效穿梭的新型可用工具。Santaris/miRNA Therapeutics 公司已经测试了一种经人工递送的针对 miR-122 的拮抗剂，用于治疗丙型肝炎。最近，研究人员已经启动了在肝细胞癌中人工递送 miR-34 的临床试验，还启动了一项检测复发性恶性间皮瘤中的 miR-16 替代物的 I 期临床试验。这些研究预示着未来一系列 miRNA 有望应用于人类癌症的治疗。

microRNA 的合成与产生

miRNA 是由进化上保守的基因编码的具有约 22 个核苷酸长度的短链非编码 RNA。miRNA 更常位于蛋白质编码基因的内含子或外显子内(约 70%)，或位于基因间的区域(30%)。基因间 miRNA 的表达与其宿主基因的表达有关，所有基因内的 miRNA 都具有独立的转录单位[9]。miRNA 通过一系列相互关联的精密协同步骤进行加工和合成，其每一步过程的调控原理都处于研究中(图 9-1)。在第一步中，称为初始 miRNA(pri-miRNA)的长链初级转录本由 RNA 聚合酶Ⅱ催化转录。然后 pri-miRNA 与称为脊椎动物 DiGeorge 综合征关键区基因 8(DGCR8)的双链 RNA 结合域(dsRBD)蛋白结合[10]。一种称为 Drosha/DGCR8 复合物的核糖核酸内切酶-Ⅲ将 pri-miRNA 切割成约含 70 个核苷酸(nt)的较小的茎环结构，称为前体 miRNA(pre-miRNA)。然后双链 RNA 结合蛋白 Exportin 5(XPO5)将前体 miRNA 从细胞核转运到细胞质[11]。一旦进入细胞质，前体 miRNA 被由核糖核酸内切酶-Ⅲ Dicer、Argonaute 2(Ago 2)和反式激活应答 RNA 结合蛋白(TRBP)组成的复合物切割成含 18~25 个核苷酸的成熟 miRNA。Ago2 蛋白属于 Argonaute 蛋白家族，它能将片段结合到向导 RNA(包括 miRNA)上。由两条链组成的 miRNA 随后被装配到 RNA 诱导沉默复合物(RISC)中，成熟链被保留而互补链被降解。剩余的链具有与靶基因 3′或 5′UTR 的互补性，通过内切酶活性或翻译抑制导致靶基因降解。最近，研究人员证实了 miRNA 也可以与转录产物的编码序列结合，导致翻译抑制[12]。成熟 miRNA 的“种子”序列与靶标之间的互补程度是 miRNA 生物学效应的主要决定因素。研究人员现也发现了 miRNA 生物合成的一些

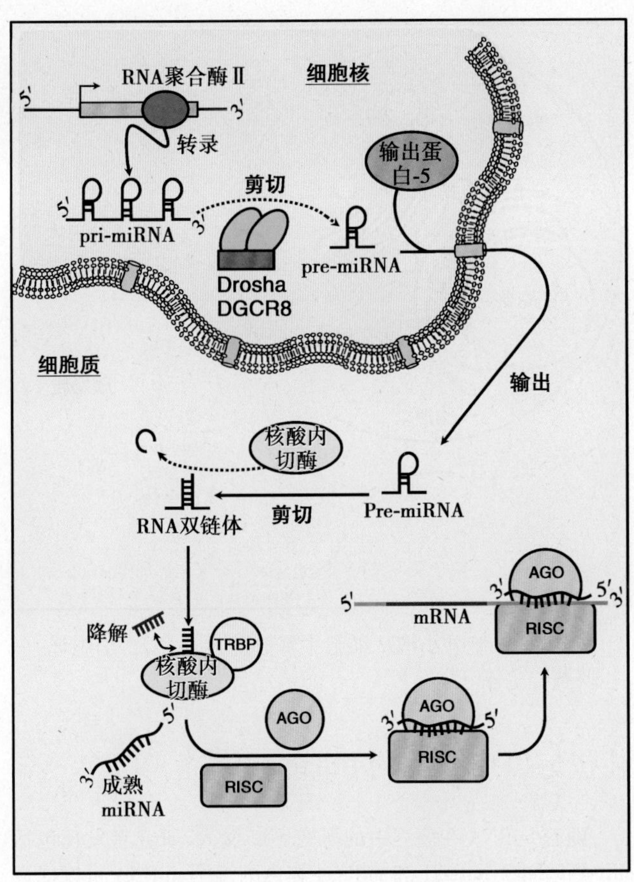

图9-1　MicroRNA生物合成

其他机制，表明我们开始认识到这一过程的复杂性。

癌症中的microRNA失调

Calin等人[13]在一项研究中首次将miRNA失调与癌症联系起来。他们在研究慢性淋巴细胞性白血病（CLL）的发病机制时，惊奇的发现在68%的CLL患者中，一对miRNA——miR-15a/16-1以及缺失的白血病基因（DLEU）均位于染色体13q14.3区域，这对miRNA要么被删除，要么被下调[13]。另外，这两种miRNA在正常的CD5$^+$B细胞中均高表达。这两个发现表明，这些miRNA实际上对疾病的发生有重要的作用。其他研究者证实了这一初步的观察结果，他们发现miR-15a/16-1与促存活分子Bcl2之间存在功能联系。他们在体外证实miR-15a/16-1可以靶向Bcl2，从而诱导细胞发生凋亡。自从在CLL中首次发现miRNA以来，研究者已经观察到miRNA在实体瘤和血液恶性肿瘤中存在广泛的表达失调。在过去的几年里，研究人员已经证实导致这种失调的原因是多方面的。例如，Drosha和Dicer等与miRNA生物发生有关蛋白质的表达和或功能可能会发生改变并导致miRNA的异常表达，从而导致癌症[14]。在很大一部分卵巢癌患者中发现Drosha和Dicer的表达水平降低[15]。此外，miRNA启动子的表观遗传改变，如其甲基化的改变，也可导致miRNA表达水平的改变[16]。与其他发挥促癌或抑癌作用的失调基因一样，单个miRNA的表观遗传表达失调可能是致癌的触发事件。例如研究的较为深入的miR-155，转基因小鼠中miR-155的失调可能会诱发白血病[17]。Bcl6是miR-127的直接靶点，原发性前列腺癌和膀胱肿瘤中抑癌性的miR-127能上调原癌基因Bcl6的表达。另一方面，miRNA也可以通过作用于表观遗传调控相关的酶，影响细胞整体的甲基化状态。例如，在肺癌中，miR-29家族可以通过影响DNA甲基转移酶DNMT3a和DNMT3b的从头合成来调节细胞的甲基化水平[18]。miRNA的另一个重要而复杂的调节机制与基因的转录调控有关[19]。MYC癌基因诱导的miR-17/92簇激活可调节E2F1的抗凋亡作用，从而介导MYC的增殖效应[20]。最近，有研究探索了膜酪氨酸激酶受体对miRNA表达的影响。例如，肝细胞生长因子受体c-MET能够通过转录因子AP1诱导促癌miR-221/222簇的表达，这表明，c-MET失调在癌症中的重要作用至少部分与失调的miRNA表达有关[21]。最后，鉴于p53的丢失是癌症中最具代表性的基因异常之一，miR-34a家族与p53之间的关系是miRNA参与肿瘤相关基因转录调控的另一个重要例子[22]。p53可以刺激miR-34家族的转录，诱导细胞的凋亡和衰老。在很多p53突变的卵巢癌患者中，p53功能的丧失诱导了miR-34家族的下调[23]。因此在癌症中，miRNA的广泛失调可能既是造成癌症的原因，也是癌症的结果。癌症中miRNA的广泛失调会显著影响多种细胞信号通路的下游靶标。

最近，研究人员还发现miRNA功能可能通过其靶基因种子序列的突变而发生改变。此类突变可使miRNA失去对相应mRNA的调控作用，这类突变也可以作为判断临床结局的生物标志物。在几种实体恶性肿瘤中已发现了3′UTR的突变，包括卵巢癌、肺癌、乳腺癌和结肠癌。反之，miRNA基因序列中的单核苷酸多态性（SNP）也可以改变miRNA的功能。miRNA对mRNA功能的调节对miRNA第2-8核苷酸内的碱基错配高度敏感，这段核苷酸序列被定义为种子区域[24]。因此，miRNA基因上的单点突变或转录后修饰（如RNA编辑）可以改变miRNA的功能或修饰miRNA的靶标[25,26]。例如，Kras 3′UTR中let-7（lethal-7）miRNA互补位点的SNP会增加人群罹患非小细胞肺癌的风险[27]。在幼年型髓单核细胞白血病（JMML）中也可以检测到Kras 3′UTR中let-7结合位点的突变[28]。

MicroRNA可作为癌症的生物标志物

在过去几年中，研究人员发现miRNA几乎与所有类型的癌症都有关。早期研究的重点是应用高通量平台，将miRNA失调模式与临床参数联系起来。最初的方法之一由Volinia等人在2005年提出，他们描述了六种人类实体瘤的miRNA特征，检测到miR-21、miR-17-5p和miR-191在某些肿瘤中过表达[29]。自最初的研究以来，研究人员进行了多项类似的研究，其主要目标是鉴定与预后相关的miRNA特征。Yanaihara等人对1期肺腺癌病例进行了高通量分析，鉴定出了40多个可以区分肺肿瘤和瘤旁未受侵袭肺组织的miRNA[30]。一项更广泛的研究在22种不同类型的肿瘤中，探索了如何根据不同组织来源的miRNA表达谱对肿瘤进行高度准确的分类[31]。还有些研究关注能作为潜在预后标志物的预选miRNA，例如Nadal等人[32]探究了肿瘤抑制性miR-34作为早期肺腺癌的预后生物标志物的可能性。他们发现miR-34b/c在近一半（46%）的早期肺腺癌存在甲基化和表达下调，而且明确了miR-34b/c表达下调及 miR-34b/c 甲基化与患者的不良预后有关。例如，另一项独立的研究表明，miRNA 表达水平可能与慢性粒细胞白血病（CML）中的 BCR-ABL 激酶活性相关[33]，表明在治疗中可以利用 miRNA 来调整治疗以改善患者的临床结局。miRNA 另一个非常有趣的应用是可以综合考虑其与编码和非编码基因的表达，将其作为癌症早期阶段的预后特征性标志物。Akagi 等人[34]在 148 例 1 期肺腺癌中探究了 42 个预选基因作为预测性生物标志物的可能性。研究人员通过独立队列的测试及随后的验证，开创了一种与 1 期肺腺癌生存率相关的四基因分类法（DLC1，XPO1，HIF1A，BRCA1）。此外，他们还证实了在同一队列中 miR-21 的表达与存活率之间存在独立的相关性。最后，他们证实将四基因分类法和 miR-21 表达结合可以预测癌症的预后，效能优于以上任何单一的生物标志物。尽管 miRNA 表达谱的研究取得了振奋人心的进展，但研究人员尚未就哪些 miRNA 能提供最准确的预后信息达成共识。缺乏可重复性的一个主要原因是 miRNA 分析研究容易受到某些偏差的影响，其他高通量分析也存在类似的问题，包括队列规模小、平台间的差异（阵列、测序、RT-pPCR）和数据解读的多样性。

MicroRNA 可作为癌症中的非侵入性生物标志物

癌症中无创性生物标志物可为临床决策提供必要的信息，但其发展依然不明朗，仍需要持续性的研究和深入。多项研究表明，miRNA 在不同的 pH 和温度条件下以相对稳定的形式存在于体液（血清，血浆，尿液，痰，脑脊液和支气管肺泡灌洗液）中[35~37]。miRNA 也存在于血液中，在血浆、血小板、红细胞和有核血细胞中都能够检测到。最早的一项研究表明，可以在前列腺癌患者的循环系统中检测到 miRNA[38]。Shen 等人[39]证实，血浆中的 miRNA 可以作为鉴别孤立性肺结节的生物标志物。随后的一项更大规模的研究进一步证实了循环 miRNA 可以用于肺癌的早期检测[40]。

学界对 miRNA 在血液循环中的具体定位仍然存在很大的争议。然而，有研究发现循环 miRNA 被包装在细胞外囊泡（EV）中，并与 RNA 结合蛋白（如 Argonaute 2 或脂蛋白复合物）相结合，从而阻止了它们的降解（图 9-2）[41~44]。EV 是一种小的膜包裹的流体颗粒，是通过完全独立的机制，由多种类型细胞释放的脱落囊泡和外泌体组成[45]。目前，研究人员主要关注的是外泌体，即 40~100 纳米的囊泡，这些颗粒由脂质双层组成，由分泌性多囊体（MVB）产生，与质膜融合后释放到细胞外环境。外泌体包含其来源细胞的多种分子成分，包括脂质，蛋白质，信使 RNA（mRNA）和 miRNA，它们可以从供体细胞转移到受体靶细胞，使细胞间可以直接通讯，以重编程肿瘤微环境[42]。在诸如癌症的病理状态下，外泌体通过交互来影响主要的肿瘤相关通路，例如上皮间质转化（EMT）、癌症干性、血管生成和肿瘤微环境内多种类型细胞的转移[46~49]。在包括血浆、尿液、母乳、羊水、恶性腹水和支气管肺泡灌洗液在内的多种体液中也可以检测到外泌体，表明它们可以作为潜在的疾病生物标志物[50]。

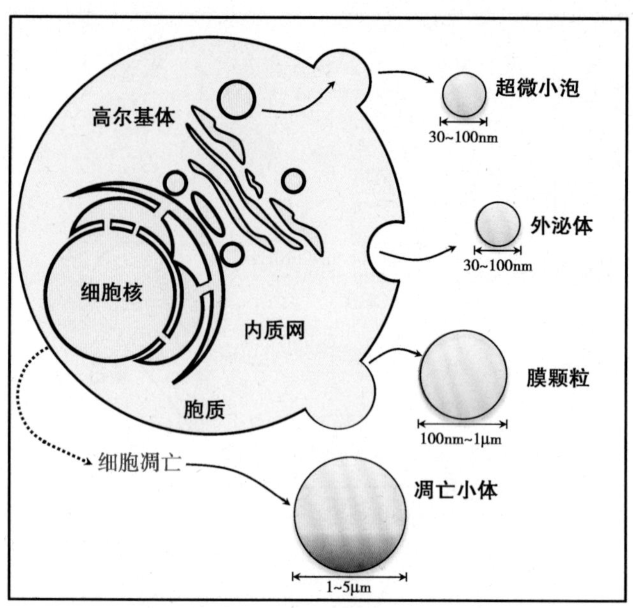

图 9-2 细胞外小泡从细胞中释放的过程，凋亡细胞释放凋亡小体

某些与癌症有关的 miRNA

随着 miRNA 在癌症中的研究不断深入，研究者发现包括 miR-155、let-7、miR-21 和 miR-34 在内的多个 miRNA 可以促进肿瘤的发生发展，临床试验正研究这些 miRNA 作为临床诊断和治疗的生物标志物的可行性。

LET-7

let-7 基因最初是在秀丽隐杆线虫中被发现的，它是发育的关键调节因子[51]。在各个物种中，let-7 家族成员的成熟形式高度保守。let-7 miR 家族在不同物种发育过程中细胞增殖和分化的调节中起着至关重要的作用。此外，let-7 是完全分化细胞的标志物，在干细胞中无法检测到[52]。let-7 家族包含 12 个成员，位于 9 个不同染色体，它们定位的脆弱位点与不同类型的实体肿瘤有关[53]。这些 miR 的失调已被证明是多种类型癌症的特征[54~56]。let-7 的靶基因和调节因子中，研究最多的是 c-Myc 癌基因，此外还发现它们之间存在着双重负反馈。

MiR-21

MiR-21 是目前研究最多的肿瘤 miRNA 之一，因为它的大多数靶基因是肿瘤抑制因子（例如 PTEN、Bcl2 以及 Sprouty1 和 2）。这种 miRNA 可能是最活跃的 miRNA 之一，因为它参与正反馈和负反馈循环，对各种刺激都有反应。miR-21 是乳腺、卵巢、宫颈、结肠、肺、肝、脑、食道、前列腺、胰腺和甲状腺等实体肿瘤中最常改变的 miRNA 之一[29,57~59]。miR-21 在白血病中的表达上调[60]，表明它在肿瘤发展和进展中起着重要的作用。此外，最近的一项研究将 miR-21 作为多种肿瘤的生物标志物，揭示了其作为癌症诊断工具的潜力[61]。

MiR-34

miR-34 家族由三个高度相关的 miRNA 组成：miR-34a、

miR-34b 和 miR-34c。在除肺以外的所有组织(尤其是大脑)中,miR-34a 的表达水平均高于 miR-34b/c[62]。这些 miRNA 由 p53 直接诱导产生,会对 DNA 损伤或致癌应激[63]产生应答,并通过靶向 c-Myc、Bcl2、C-Met 和 Src 对 p53 下游效应产生影响[64]。miR-34a 不仅在肿瘤抑制中有重要的作用,还在多种细胞模型中影响细胞对药物的反应,包括 HCC、乳腺癌、膀胱癌、HNSCC 和 NSCLC(例如,miR-34a 的过表达会下调 PDGFR,进而恢复 TRAIL 诱导的 NSCLC 细胞系的凋亡)[65]。

MiR-200 家族

miR-200 家族由五个成员组成:miR-200a、miR-200b、miR-200c、miR-141 和 miR-429。这些 miR 在上皮组织中高表达,并通过抑制 EMT、迁移、侵袭、肿瘤细胞黏附和转移参与抑制肿瘤[66]。在 miR-200 家族的靶基因中,研究最多的是 EMT 的两个核心介导因子,ZEB1 和 ZEB2。ZEB1 能抑制 miR-200 家族成员的表达,因此存在双重 ZEB/miR-200 负反馈回路[67]。此外,有证据表明乳腺癌转移可能受 Akt-miR200-E-钙粘蛋白轴的调控。具体而言,三种 Akt 亚型的平衡可以调控原发性和转移性人类乳腺癌中 miR-200 和 E-cadherin mRNA 的表达[68]。

靶向治疗与 miRNA

鉴于单个或一组 miRNA 的失调可以诱发恶性肿瘤,因此可以假设,至少在体外,通过定向靶向它们的失调,可以控制癌变。此外,miRNA 的失调可能会诱发肿瘤细胞对传统化疗药物的耐药。例如,利用选择性创建的耐药细胞系的全 miRNA 表达谱,研究人员鉴定了特定的会导致细胞获得性耐药的 miRNA。这些发现已经将 miRNA 转化为直接的靶点和化疗药物反应性的预测因子。重要的是,特定 miRNA 对化疗耐药性的作用可能具有高度的肿瘤特异性。如前所述,miRNA 具有同时靶向和调节多种生物途径的能力。就 CLL 而言,特定的 miRNA 表达模式可以在临床上预测哪些患者会对氟达拉滨有反应[69]。在诸如肺癌的实体瘤中,包括 miR-21、miR-30、miR-221 和 miR-222 在内的 miRNA 都与肿瘤细胞对化疗药物的反应性有关。最近,Vecchione 等人[70]分析了一个 miRNA 的表达特征,该特征能用于判断卵巢癌的化疗耐药性。据报道,miRNA 表达特征分析可用于鉴定对替莫唑胺耐药的胶质母细胞瘤亚型[71]。

近几年,miRNA 作为定向疗法已应用于人类疾病的研究,并已在体外和小鼠疾病模型中开展。定向治疗的主要目标是操纵肿瘤中失控的 miRNA,从而调控其下游的靶基因和生物学途径。该方法可以通过靶向特定的 miRNA,或增强现有药物的疗效来实现。通过选择性功能补益(例如类似物),或沉默(例如拮抗剂)的方式来操纵 miRNA 可以得到多种结果。miRNA 可以通过多种方式进行传递,包括病毒载体和纳米颗粒(NP)。基于病毒的载体已在实体肿瘤中被有效地用于传递 miRNA,包括肺癌的 let-7[72]。然而,用于传递小分子的病毒载体存在局限性,包括载体对宿主的潜在免疫原性和毒性。最近,研究人员已将脂基的 NP 用作小分子(包括 miRNA)的载体。NP 是小型工程化颗粒的代表,特别适合用于药物传递,因其组成成分可变,所以能使结合和吸收最优化。近期有研究证实了 NP 作为 miRNA 体内递送载体的效能。例如,Wu 等人最近的研究表明,在肺癌中,脂基的 NP 可以有效地在体内外进行 miR-29 的递送[73]。在一项独立研究中,Trang 等人表明递送 let-7 可以抑制肿瘤的生长和多种癌基因的表达[74]。miRNA 治疗同样也需要考虑脱靶效应、载体的稳定性和毒性等问题。miRNA 海绵是 miRNA 拮抗剂的替代策略。RNA 海绵能够同时抑制大量的 miRNA 分子。环状 RNA(circRNA)是一种天然存在的、具有代表性的 miRNA 海绵。circRNA 是一类可形成共价闭合连续环的 RNA,其 3′和 5′末端连接在一起形成环形的 RNA 分子。这种结构特征保证了 circRNA 在细胞质中的稳定性,同时还赋予了 circRNA 结合多种 miRNA 分子的能力,从而可以抑制 miRNA 的功能。circRNA 源自蛋白质编码基因,但不编码任何蛋白质,因此被分类为 ncRNA[75]。最近,研究人员证实了一种名为 R1as/CiRS-7 的 circRNA 可以充当 miR-7 的海绵。这种 circRNA 能够通过 63 个 miR-7 结合位点充当其特异性的海绵,从而下调 miR-7[76]。模仿天然 circRNA 作用的合成海绵是一种调节癌症中异常 miRNA 表达的新方法,可满足同时下调多个 miRNA 或 miRNA 家族的需求[77]。

最近,研究人员开发了新的计算工具,用于设计合成 miRNA。这些 miRNA 能够同时有效地靶向多种特定的 mRNA(多靶点,多位点靶向)。Lagana 等人[78]在 2014 年开发并验证了一种称为"miR-Synth"的生物信息学工具,该工具是一种能够同时靶向 MET 和 EGFR 的合成 miRNA。有趣的是,该工具可为多种不同的靶标组合合成 miRNA。通过重新引入 miRNA,或使用合成技术调节 miRNA 的表达(miRNA 海绵)以抑制失调的 miRNA,以及使用能够同时调节不同基因表达的合成 miRNA,来调节癌症中 miRNA 的理念是可行的,但并不意味着该策略毫无问题。以 miRNA 为核心的癌症疗法有着广阔的前景,但因其脱靶问题和传递困难,目前尚无法将其应用到临床。

MiRNA 在人类中的应用

虽然大多数以 miRNA 为中心的研究都基于实验室探索,但越来越多的临床试验已将 miRNA 作为预测或治疗的生物标志物,或作为定向疗法。目前,有超过 100 项包含 miRNA 的临床试验正在积极招募或已完成招募。这些研究大多将 miRNA 作为潜在的临床生物标志物。过去的几年里,我们目睹了 miRNA 开始被用于临床治疗研究。此类研究中最受认可的是使用针对 miR-122 的拮抗剂来治疗丙型肝炎[79]。SPC3649(米雷韦森)治疗健康志愿者和慢性丙型肝炎患者的Ⅰ期和Ⅱ期临床试验已经结束[80]。目前,检测米雷韦森在慢性丙型肝炎无应答患者中疗效的研究正在进行。在癌症领域,有两项激动人心的研究有望进入临床应用。第一项研究是一项正在进行的多中心Ⅰ期临床试验,拟研究 miR-34 脂质体制剂(MRX34)在不可切除的原发性肝癌患者或晚期转移性实体恶性肿瘤(有或无转移)患者中的疗效。第二项研究的药物是 MesomiR-1,该Ⅰ期临床试验将在先前治疗失败的恶性胸膜间皮瘤患者或晚期非小细胞肺癌患者中研究 EGFR 靶向递送载体递送 miR-16 对肿瘤的治疗效果。

(吴彤 译　危晏平 校　孙文　陈淑桢 审)

部分参考文献

1 Lee RC, Feinbaum RL, Ambros V. The *C. elegans* heterochronic gene lin-4 encodes small RNAs with antisense complementarity to lin-14. *Cell*. 1993;**75**:843-854.

2 Ambros V. The functions of animal microRNAs. *Nature*. 2004;**431**:350-355.

3 Croce CM. Causes and consequences of microRNA dysregulation in cancer. *Nat Rev Genet*. 2009;**10**:704-714.

4 Lagos-Quintana M, Rauhut R, Lendeckel W, Tuschl T. Identification of novel genes coding for small expressed RNAs. *Science*. 2001;**294**:853-858.

5 Miranda KC, Huynh T, Tay Y, et al. A pattern-based method for the identification of MicroRNA binding sites and their corresponding heteroduplexes. *Cell*. 2006;**126**:1203-1217.

6 Calin GA, Croce CM. MicroRNA signatures in human cancers. *Nat Rev Cancer*. 2006;**6**:857-866.

7 Nana-Sinkam SP, Hunter MG, Nuovo GJ, et al. Integrating the MicroRNome into the study of lung disease. *Am J Respir Crit Care Med*. 2009;**179**:4-10.

8 Nana-Sinkam SP, Croce CM. Non-coding RNAs in cancer initiation and progression and as novel biomarkers. *Mol Oncol*. 2011;**5**:483-491.

9 Rodriguez A, Griffiths-Jones S, Ashurst JL, Bradley A. Identification of mammalian microRNA host genes and transcription units. *Genome Res*. 2004;**14**:1902-1910.

10 Gregory RI, Yan KP, Amuthan G, et al. The Microprocessor complex mediates the genesis of microRNAs. *Nature*. 2004;**432**:235-240.

11 Bohnsack MT, Czaplinski K, Gorlich D. Exportin 5 is a RanGTP-dependent dsRNA-binding protein that mediates nuclear export of pre-miRNAs. *RNA*. 2004;**10**:185-191.

12 Helwak A, Kudla G, Dudnakova T, Tollervey D. Mapping the human miRNA interactome by CLASH reveals frequent noncanonical binding. *Cell*. 2013;**153**:654-665.

13 Calin GA, Dumitru CD, Shimizu M, et al. Frequent deletions and down-regulation of micro- RNA genes miR15 and miR16 at 13q14 in chronic lymphocytic leukemia. *Proc Natl Acad Sci U S A*. 2002;**99**:15524-15529.

14 Karube Y, Tanaka H, Osada H, et al. Reduced expression of Dicer associated with poor prognosis in lung cancer patients. *Cancer Sci*. 2005;**96**:111-115.

15 Merritt WM, Lin YG, Han LY, et al. Dicer, Drosha, and outcomes in patients with ovarian cancer. *N Engl J Med*. 2008;**359**:2641-2650.

16 Fabbri M, Garzon R, Cimmino A, et al. MicroRNA-29 family reverts aberrant methylation in lung cancer by targeting DNA methyltransferases 3A and 3B. *Proc Natl Acad Sci U S A*. 2007;**104**:15805-15810.

17 Costinean S, Sandhu SK, Pedersen IM, et al. Src homology 2 domain-containing inositol-5-phosphatase and CCAAT enhancer-binding protein beta are targeted by miR-155 in B cells of Emicro-MiR-155 transgenic mice. *Blood*. 2009;**114**:1374-1382.

18 Saito Y, Liang G, Egger G, et al. Specific activation of microRNA-127 with downregulation of the proto-oncogene BCL6 by chromatin-modifying drugs in human cancer cells. *Cancer Cell*. 2006;**9**:435-443.

19 Lee Y, Kim M, Han J, et al. MicroRNA genes are transcribed by RNA polymerase II. *EMBO J*. 2004;**23**:4051-4060.

20 O'Donnell KA, Wentzel EA, Zeller KI, Dang CV, Mendell JT. c-Myc-regulated microRNAs modulate E2F1 expression. *Nature*. 2005;**435**:839-843.

21 Garofalo M, Romano G, Di Leva G, et al. EGFR and MET receptor tyrosine kinase-altered microRNA expression induces tumorigenesis and gefitinib resistance in lung cancers. *Nat Med*. 2012;**18**:74-82.

22 He L, He X, Lowe SW, Hannon GJ. microRNAs join the p53 network—another piece in the tumour-suppression puzzle. *Nat Rev Cancer*. 2007;**7**:819-822.

23 Corney DC, Flesken-Nikitin A, Godwin AK, Wang W, Nikitin AY. MicroRNA-34b and microRNA-34c are targets of p53 and cooperate in control of cell proliferation and adhesion-independent growth. *Cancer Res*. 2007;**67**:8433-8438.

24 Brennecke J, Stark A, Russell RB, Cohen SM. Principles of microRNA-target recognition. *PLoS Biol*. 2005;**3**:e85.

25 Nigita G, Alaimo S, Ferro A, Giugno R, Pulvirenti A. Knowledge in the investigation of A-to-I RNA editing signals. *Front Bioeng Biotechnol*. 2015;**3**:18.

26 Kawahara Y, Zinshteyn B, Sethupathy P, Iizasa H, Hatzigeorgiou AG, Nishikura K. Redirection of silencing targets by adenosine-to-inosine editing of miRNAs. *Science*. 2007;**315**:1137-1140.

27 Chin LJ, Ratner E, Leng S, et al. A SNP in a let-7 microRNA complementary site in the KRAS 3' untranslated region increases non-small cell lung cancer risk. *Cancer Res*. 2008;**68**:8535-8540.

28 Steinemann D, Tauscher M, Praulich I, Niemeyer CM, Flotho C, Schlegelberger B. Mutations in the let-7 binding site - a mechanism of RAS activation in juvenile myelomonocytic leukemia? *Haematologica*. 2010;**95**:1616.

29 Volinia S, Calin GA, Liu CG, et al. A microRNA expression signature of human solid tumors defines cancer gene targets. *Proc Natl Acad Sci U S A*. 2006;**103**:2257-2261.

30 Yanaihara N, Caplen N, Bowman E, et al. Unique microRNA molecular profiles in lung cancer diagnosis and prognosis. *Cancer Cell*. 2006;**9**:189-198.

31 Rosenfeld N, Aharonov R, Meiri E, et al. MicroRNAs accurately identify cancer tissue origin. *Nat Biotechnol*. 2008;**26**:462-469.

32 Nadal E, Chen G, Gallegos M, et al. Epigenetic inactivation of microRNA-34b/c predicts poor disease-free survival in early-stage lung adenocarcinoma. *Clin Cancer Res*. 2013;**19**:6842-6852.

33 Ferreira AF, Moura LG, Tojal I, et al. ApoptomiRs expression modulated by BCR-ABL is linked to CML progression and imatinib resistance. *Blood Cells Mol Dis*. 2014;**53**:47-55.

34 Akagi I, Okayama H, Schetter AJ, et al. Combination of protein coding and noncoding gene expression as a robust prognostic classifier in stage I lung adenocarcinoma. *Cancer Res*. 2013;**73**:3821-3832.

35 Creemers EE, Tijsen AJ, Pinto YM. Circulating microRNAs: novel biomarkers and extracellular communicators in cardiovascular disease? *Circ Res*. 2012;**110**:483-495.

36 Shen J, Liao J, Guarnera MA, et al. Analysis of microRNAs in sputum to improve computed tomography for lung cancer diagnosis. *J Thorac Oncol*. 2014;**9**:33-40.

37 Xing L, Todd NW, Yu L, Fang H, Jiang F. Early detection of squamous cell lung cancer in sputum by a panel of microRNA markers. *Mod Pathol*. 2010;**23**:1157-1164.

38 Mitchell PS, Parkin RK, Kroh EM, et al. Circulating microRNAs as stable blood-based markers for cancer detection. *Proc Natl Acad Sci U S A*. 2008;**105**:10513-10518.

39 Shen J, Liu Z, Todd NW, et al. Diagnosis of lung cancer in individuals with solitary pulmonary nodules by plasma microRNA biomarkers. *BMC Cancer*. 2011;**11**:374.

40 Boeri M, Verri C, Conte D, et al. MicroRNA signatures in tissues and plasma predict development and prognosis of computed tomography detected lung cancer. *Proc Natl Acad Sci U S A*. 2011;**108**:3713-3718.

第 10 章　肿瘤中的异常信号通路

Luca Grumolato, PhD ■ Stuart A. Aaronson, MD

概论

绝大多数人类肿瘤都存在一种或多种异常激活的信号通路，这些激活的信号通路导致了肿瘤的发生和/或进展。本章节讲述了生长因子如何将信号传递给具有内源酪氨酸激酶活性的受体，进而激活下游的磷脂酰肌醇-3′-激酶（PI-3-K）/Akt 和 Ras/MAP 激酶通路，并促进细胞的增殖与存活。本章节通过介绍不同的生长因子信号通路致癌变化的范例，进一步讨论这些通路与人类肿瘤之间的关系及其对肿瘤的影响。同时，还将介绍正常细胞与肿瘤细胞内一般的细胞信号转导规律，并简要讨论一些特定信号通路的失调对特定类型肿瘤的发生及进展的影响，包括细胞因子、转化生长因子 β（TGFβ）家族、Wnt、Hedgehog、Notch 及核受体等介导的信号通路。本章节还将阐述癌基因成瘾与靶向治疗的概念，并通过代表性的例子来阐释如何将我们对肿瘤信号通路异常机制不断加深的认知转化并应用于临床。

多细胞生物体内的很多过程需要细胞与细胞间的交流来完成，比如胚胎发育、组织分化及机体对创伤与感染的反应等。这些复杂的信号网络交流主要是由生长因子、细胞因子及激素介导的。这些因子正向或反向的影响细胞的增殖，同时在相应的靶细胞内诱发一系列的差异应答。介导这些反应的细胞质分子被称为第二信使，生物化学信号经第二信使最终转导入细胞核来诱导相关基因的表达，参与细胞的有丝分裂和分化反应。

生长因子信号通路中关键基因的致病性表达同样可以促进细胞的恶性生长。此类基因的典型代表是类人猿肉瘤病毒的 *v-sis* 癌基因，该基因可编码一种与人类血小板衍生生长因子 β 链（PDGF-β）同源的生长因子[1]。后续的研究表明其他逆转录病毒癌基因的正常副本可编码跨膜生长因子受体[2,3]。此外，其他在细胞内生长因子信号转导过程早期发挥作用的基因也被认为是癌基因。目前的研究表明，这些基因的变异导致了生长因子信号通路的组成性激活，进而促进了人类大多数肿瘤的发生发展。

由于篇幅有限，本章将主要介绍具有酪氨酸（Tyr）激酶活性的受体所介导的生长因子信号通路。此外，本章还将简要介绍其他由配体激活的肿瘤生物学相关信号通路。

具有酪氨酸激酶活性的生长因子受体

多年来，激素由于可以在远离分泌细胞的远处发挥生物学功能而被人们熟知。激素是一种信号分子，来源于组织液，在体内发挥效应。生长因子研究最初的发现表明其有更多微妙的功能，比如神经生长因子（NGF）[4]能够刺激鸡胚神经细胞的生长，上皮生长因子（EGF）可以促进门齿萌发与眼睑张开[5]。生长因子相关研究的一项重要发现是：EGF 与其受体结合后，其受体会产生独特的酶活性[5]。病毒癌基因产物的研究证实了 *v-src* 可发挥蛋白激酶的作用[6,7]。虽然以往也鉴定了许多的蛋白激酶，但这些蛋白激酶具有的是磷酸化丝氨酸（Ser）和/或苏氨酸（Thr）残基的活性。此外，已有充分的证据表明磷酸化与去磷酸化作用会影响许多蛋白的活性。随后的研究发现 *src* 的产物也是一种独特的蛋白激酶，其可以特异性地磷酸化 Tyr 残基[8]。科恩而后发现 EGF 可导致其纯化受体的 Tyr 残基发生磷酸化[5]。后续的研究证实，Tyr 激酶活性对很多有丝分裂信号分子的功能至关重要。

已知的 50 多种受体 Tyr 激酶（RTK）属于至少 18 个不同的受体家族[9,10]（图 10-1）。所有的受体 Tyr 激酶均单次跨膜，包含一个较大的胞外糖基化配体结合域，细胞质部分包含一个保守的蛋白 Tyr 激酶区域。细胞质内除了催化区域，还包括一个近膜区与一个羧基端尾。鉴于上述结构，RTK 也被看作是含有跨胞膜的配体结合域和蛋白酪氨酸激酶域的膜相关变构酶，它可催化三磷酸腺苷（ATP）γ 磷酸基团转移到外源性底物的 Tyr 残基及其自身的多肽链。因此，Tyr 的磷酸化表明这些受体成功转导了生长因子携带的信息。

RTK 可以通过其配体导致的受体寡聚化而激活，受体寡聚化可以稳定相邻细胞质结构域之间的相互作用并控制激酶活性的激活[10]。二聚化可发生在两个相同受体之间（同源二聚化）、同一受体家族不同成员之间或受体和辅助蛋白之间（异二聚化），这扩展了每种受体识别的配体库，增加了特定受体刺激效应通路的多样性[10]。

每一类 RTK 结合配体并发生寡聚化的方式不同[10,11]。例如，PDGF 凭借其二聚体的结构特点诱导受体二聚化[12]。EGF 诱导表皮生长因子受体（EGFR）胞外结构域的构象变化，导致二聚化结构域暴露，而在缺乏 EGF 的情况下此结构被掩盖[10]。成纤维细胞生长因子，和 EGF 一样是单体配体，需要借助辅助分子硫酸乙酰肝素蛋白多糖，以诱导受体二聚化[13,14]。相比之下，胰岛素受体家族的受体亚单位是由以二硫键结合的同源或异源二聚体构成，通过与配体结合，导致预先形成的二聚体受体发生构象变化，进而激活受体[15,16]。

内源性蛋白激酶的激活导致 RTK 胞质中特定 Tyr 残基的自磷酸化。此外，激酶结构域中的 Tyr 磷酸化会刺激受体的内在催化活性。生物化学与结构学的研究揭示了一些介导 RTK 激活的分子机制。已有充分的证据表明，配体结合引起受体二聚化后，第二个 RTK 会以反式的形式发生自磷酸化。在非磷酸化状态时，激酶域特殊结构域的特异构象会影响磷酸基团的转移，此时的受体处于低催化活性状态。激酶域的磷酸化可以解除对激酶的抑制，增强其催化活性，并使其可以不依赖于配体而持续激活一段时间。尽管在单体状态，激酶活性维持在较

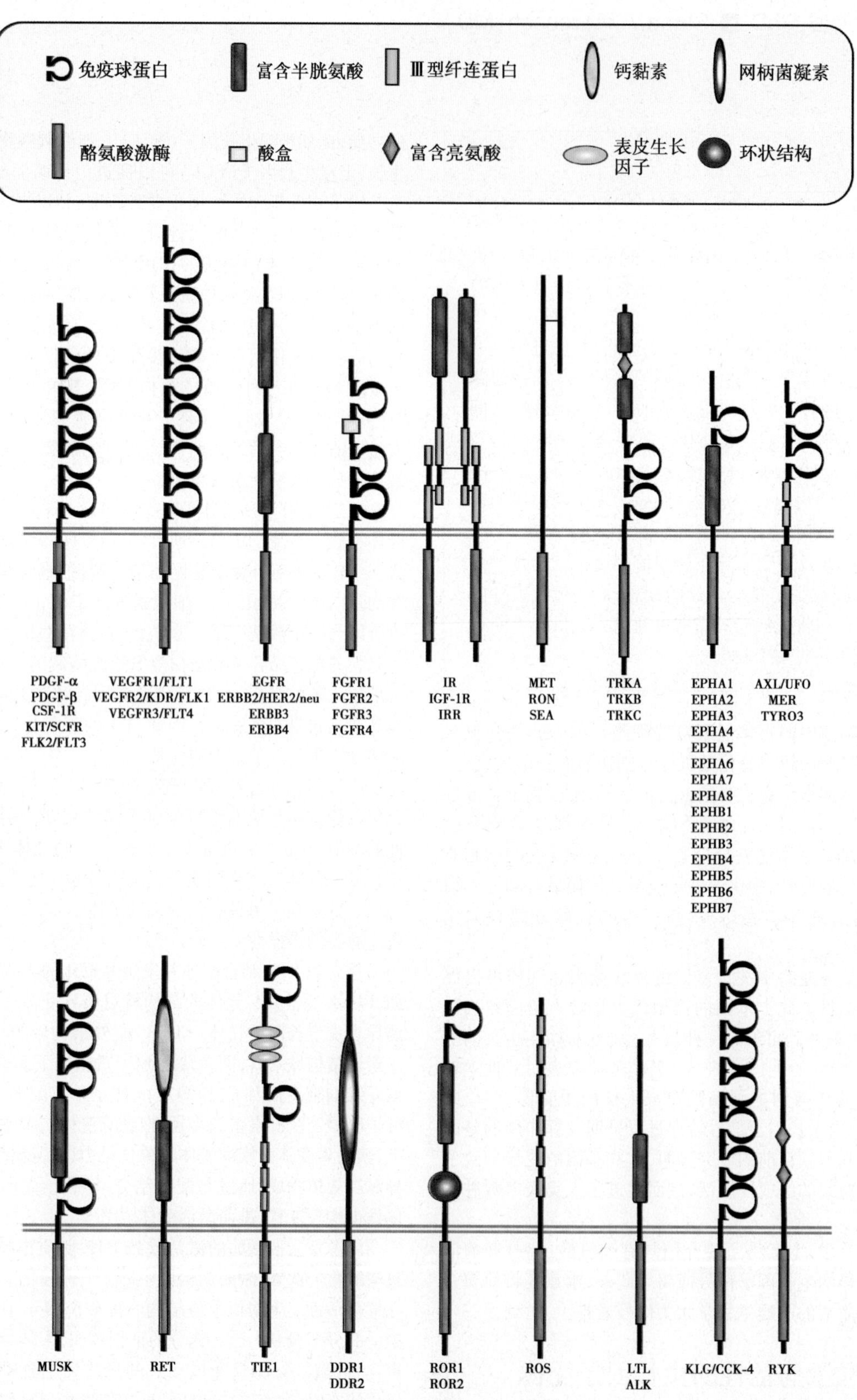

图 10-1 受体酪氨酸激酶家族

低的基础水平，然而一旦二聚体形成，其活性足以诱导反式自磷酸化。除此机制外，不同的 RTK 包含激酶域外的顺式—抑制元件，例如在近膜域（例如 KIT 和 MuSK）或 C-端尾（例如 Tie2），它们在受体的二聚化后可被反式—磷酸化破坏。除了调节受体催化活性，RTK 自磷酸化还可以为下游分子参与信号转导创造特殊的锚定位点（见下一节）。

肿瘤细胞内影响生长因子受体的变异

尽管自分泌或旁分泌环路可以组成型地激活生长因子受体，但由于其可变性，还存在很多其他的激活机制。此类变异的典型是禽红细胞增多症病毒癌基因 *v-erbB*，它相当于 EGFR 的截短型，因其配体结合域被删除而变异为组成型激活受体[2]。在人类多种恶性肿瘤中有很多会影响 RTK 的变异。其中一种类型的变异是由于正常受体发生了扩增或过表达，例如 EGFR，ErbB-2 与 MET[17~20]。ErbB-2 基因最初在原发性人乳腺癌和唾液腺肿瘤中被发现存在扩增[21,22]。临床研究表明，正常的 ErbB-2 基因在人乳腺癌和卵巢癌中经常被扩增和/或过表达[23]，并且可以通过检测乳腺癌中 ErbB-2 的高表达来提示患者预后不良[17,18]。虽然 ErbB-2 过度表达主要存在于腺癌中，但也有研究在鳞状细胞癌和胶质母细胞瘤中检测到正常 EGFR 的过度表达[17,24]。在很多情况下，EGFR 可被某个配体的自分泌刺激所激活，其中最常见的配体便是转化生长因子-α。

基因变异，例如突变或重排，同样可以激活不同恶性肿瘤中 RTK 的转化能力[25]。例如，部分恶性胶质瘤、肺癌和乳腺癌存在 EGFR 的组成型激活，这与 EGFR 受体的胞外域发生删除或 Tyr 激酶域[26,27]发生突变有关[17,24]。大约三分之一的甲状腺乳头状癌存在体细胞 *ret* 基因的重排激活，而甲状腺乳头状癌胞外域半胱氨酸残基的胚系突变会影响其受体二聚化，引发多发性内分泌瘤病（MEN）2A 和家族性甲状腺髓样癌。值得注意的是，RET 激酶域的点突变与 MEN 2B 的发病有关[28]，表明癌基因变异影响了不同的受体区域，从而上调了 RTK 的催化功能。肝细胞生长因子受体 MET 是胚系突变激活 RTK 的另一个例子，并与遗传性乳头状肾癌的发生密切相关。研究者在各种散发性肿瘤（包括肾癌、肝癌和胃癌）中也发现扩增/过表达或突变均可异常激活 MET[20]。另外，其他几种受体，包括间变性淋巴瘤激酶（ALK）、ROS1 和 TrkA，也可以通过染色体重排产生含有活化 TK 结构域的融合产物，进而导致其在人类恶性肿瘤中发生恶性激活[25]。

要点

- 生长因子通过受体二聚化及随后的反式磷酸化来激活 RTK。
- Tyr 磷酸化是受体传递信号的标志，可特异性募集不同的效应分子或接头蛋白。
- 肿瘤细胞内 RTK 可通过不同机制发生组成型激活。其中包括受体/配体过表达、RTK 扩增/突变以及由染色体易位导致的组成型活性融合蛋白的形成。

Tyr 激酶受体信号通路

被称为接头蛋白和支架蛋白的分子在细胞内信号转导中发挥不可或缺的作用[29]，它们将各种蛋白募集到特定位置并组装形成 RTK 级联反应的蛋白网络。这些接头蛋白通常包含各种结构域，用来介导蛋白与蛋白之间的相互作用，包括 Src 同源物 2（SH2）结构域和能与特定的含有磷酸化 Tyr 的序列相结合的结构域，或可识别并结合富含脯氨酸序列的目标蛋白的 SH3 结构域[29,30]。Grb2 是接头蛋白的一员，它对小 G 蛋白 Ras 的激活至关重要（图 10-2）。

PDGF 系统已成为识别信号级联成分的原型。PDGF 受体（PDGFR）激酶的激活使某些分子变得可连接和/或被磷酸化。这些分子包括磷脂酶 C-γ[31]，PI-3-K 调节亚单位（p85）[32]，NCK[33]，磷酸酶 SHP-2[34]，Grb2[35]，CRK[36]，RAS p21 GTP 酶激活蛋白（GAP）[37]，SRC 和 SRC 样酪氨酸激酶[38]。这些分子中很多都包含了 SH2 或 SH3 结构域。

PI-3-K 与细胞存活信号

细胞存活和死亡的调节对于成年生物个体的正常发育和组织稳态都是必不可少的，机体必须去除受损细胞并维持细胞的终末分化状态。一旦出现异常，可能会导致突变积累进而引发肿瘤或退行性疾病。

PI-3-K 是一种脂质激酶，催化 γ-磷酸从 ATP 转移到磷酸肌醇（PtdIns）的 D3 位置，产生 PtdIns（3，4，5）P3。这些脂质分子可以在多种级联反应中起作用，促进多种蛋白质的活化（图 10-2）。研究表明，在不同类型的细胞中，PI-3-K 的激活对细胞生存信号的维持至关重要[39,40]。经典的 Ⅰ 型 PI-3-K 由两个紧密关联的调节亚基和催化亚基组成，二者由两个不同的基因座编码。PI-3-K 活化的经典模式涉及 SH2 结构域将调节亚基与 RTK 的磷酸化 Tyr 残基结合，导致其构象变化进而促进催化亚基活化。PI-3-K 有几种已知的下游效应元件，包括 Rac、蛋白激酶 C 的某些异构体、Akt 以及病毒癌基因 *v-Akt* 的细胞同源物，其效应大部分与细胞存活相关[39,40]。三个人类同源序列编码了一个分子量为 57kDa 的丝/苏氨酸激酶，该激酶包含一个 N 端普列克底物蛋白同源（PH）结构域，可与激活的 PI-3-K 的 Ptdlns 产物结合。目前认为这些脂质分子可以介导 Akt 定位于质膜。此外，Akt 蛋白的 308 位苏氨酸残基与 473 位丝氨酸残基的磷酸化是其完全激活所必需的[39,40]。

通过调节下游不同的信号通路与效应分子[41]（图 10-2），Akt 可以在不同类型的细胞内促进增殖并抑制凋亡。Akt 可以磷酸化促凋亡蛋白 BAD（BCL2 相关的细胞死亡激动剂），从而为胞质蛋白 14-3-3 创建一个锚定位点，该位点可以隔离 BAD 并抑制其活性。Akt 还可以使 FOXO 转录因子磷酸化，形成 14-3-3 的结合位点，从而将它们保留在胞质并抑制其转录靶点的表达，靶点包括促凋亡蛋白（例如配体 BIM 和 FAS）。此外，Akt 通过磷酸化 MDM2 增加 p53 的降解，也有证据显示 Akt 可以促进核因子-κB（NF-κB）转录因子复合体的促存活功能，同时抑制 c-Jun N 端激酶（JNK）与 p38 通路的促凋亡效应[41]。除了促进细胞存活，Akt 还可以抑制结节性硬化复合物 2 的磷酸化，从而激活 mTOR 或 GSK3 并发挥促进细胞生长的作用，而 GSK3 通常可靶向降解细胞周期蛋白 D1[41,42]（图 10-2）。

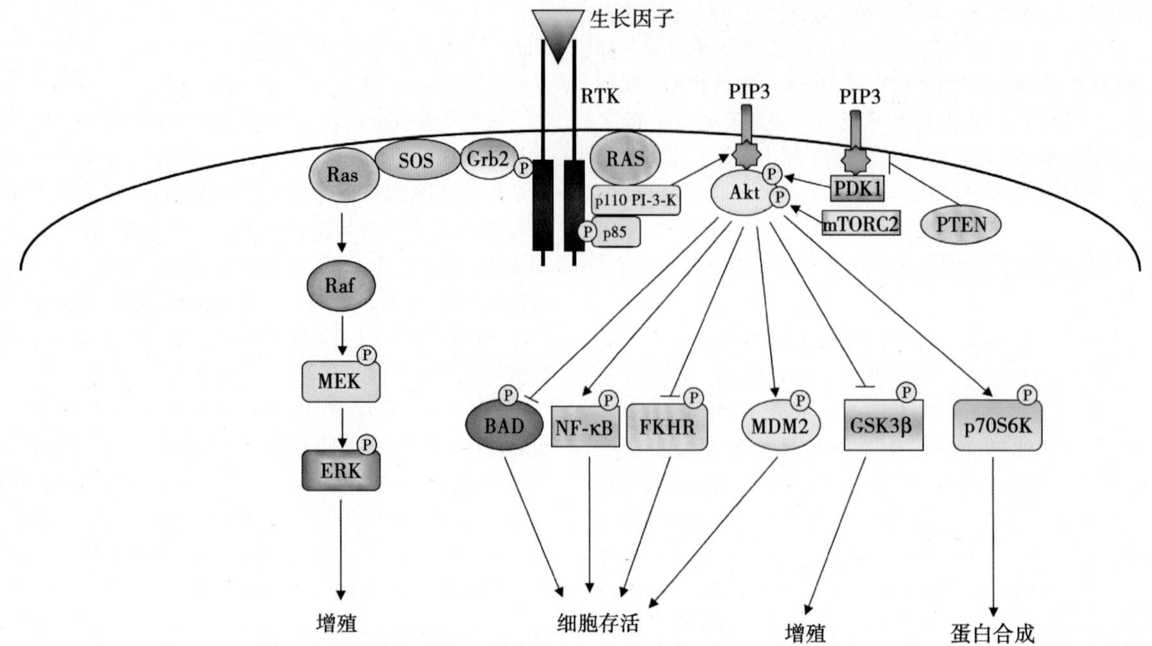

图 10-2 受体酪氨酸激酶的胞内效应器

PI-3-K 信号与肿瘤

早期的研究发现，编码 p110α 催化亚基的 *PIK3CA* 基因在大多数卵巢肿瘤和卵巢肿瘤细胞系中存在扩增的情况[43]。随后的研究表明，*PIK3CA* 是人类肿瘤中最常见的突变癌基因之一，其突变广泛存在于结肠癌、乳腺癌、子宫内膜癌、脑癌和胃癌中[44,45]。尽管 Akt 在癌症中的突变频率较低，但它依旧在人类恶性肿瘤中发挥了重要的作用。研究发现，*Akt1* 基因在原发性胃腺癌中可扩增 20 倍[46]。另有研究表明，在胰腺癌和卵巢癌细胞系以及部分卵巢癌和乳腺癌组织中，*Akt2* 基因也呈扩增和过表达的状态[47]。Akt2 的过表达在有较强侵袭性的未分化肿瘤中更常见。乳腺癌、结肠癌和卵巢癌中存在 Akt1 PH 区域的错义突变，该突变会导致其病理性地定位在质膜上并长时间激活[48]。

PI-3-K/Akt 通路参与肿瘤进展的进一步证据来自抑癌基因同源性磷酸酶—张力蛋白（PTEN）的发现，该基因在大部分神经胶质瘤、子宫内膜肿瘤、黑色素瘤、前列腺癌、肾癌及小细胞肺癌中存在突变失活[42,45,49]。通过使磷脂酰肌醇的三个位点去磷酸化，PTEN 直接对抗 PI-3-K 的活性，从而抑制 Akt 活化。

Ras

Ras 蛋白是 RTK 信号转导的主要结点，并且是细胞外信号转导所必需的重要组成元件（图 10-2）。这些小 GTP 结合蛋白是膜结合的细胞内信号分子，介导多种细胞功能，包括增殖、分化和存活。Ras 作为一种分子开关，可以从失活的 GDP 结合状态转换为活化的 GTP 结合状态。典型的 Ras 激活包括鸟嘌呤核苷酸交换因子（GEF）向膜的募集，以响应生长因子的结合及随后的 RTK 激活[50]。GEF 促进了 Ras 催化结构域中 GDP 的释放，与 GDP 相比，细胞内 GTP 的相对丰度确保了 GTP 的优先结合。SOS（son of sevenless）是 Ras GEF 的最经典范例，它通过与接头蛋白 Grb2 的稳定结合而被带到胞膜处[51]。尽管 Ras 是 GTP 酶，但实际上其固有的 GTP 酶活性很低，需要额外的蛋白 GAP 来促进 GTP 水解。GAP 可以将 GTP 水解加速多个数量级，从而负调节 Ras 的功能[50,52]。神经纤维蛋白是一种 Ras GAP，由 *NF1* 基因编码，在不同类型的肿瘤中存在突变失活，包括成胶质细胞瘤、肺癌以及家族性肿瘤综合征的 I 型神经纤维瘤[50,53]。Ras 通过许多下游效应因子介导多种生物效应。目前已发现多种以 GTP 依赖性方式直接结合 Ras 的蛋白，包括 Raf、Ral 和 PI-3-K[52]。事实上，Ras 可以不依赖 RTK 来激活 PI-3-K，从而为 Ras 和 PI-3-K 的生存信号提供直接的连接[50]。

Ras 与肿瘤

研究表明，在超过 15% 的人类肿瘤中，Ras 被致癌激活。在某些肿瘤中，例如胰腺癌，其激活频率高达 60%[52,54]。Ras 与肿瘤相关的最初证据是从转化逆转录病毒——Harvey 和 Kirsten 肉瘤病毒中发现的，二者的基因与细胞源的癌基因 *H-ras* 和 *K-ras* 类似。通过将人肿瘤细胞系基因组 DNA 转染到 NIH3T3 小鼠成纤维细胞中，并从转化的基因座中分离得到了 DNA 片段，由此研究者鉴定出了第一批人类癌基因，这些癌基因被证实是病毒 *ras* 基因的人类同源物[55]。

导致 Ras 激活的主要热点突变会降低 Ras 水解 GTP 的固有速率，使该分子对 GAP 刺激的 GTP 水解的敏感性明显降低。因此，该效应最终会导致 Ras 组成型激活，这种激活方式基本不依赖生长因子刺激的 GTP 结合[52,54]。

Ras 信号通路的下游：Ras>Raf>MAPK 激酶级联网络

Ras 最著名的效应分子是丝/苏氨酸激酶 Raf。大多数情况下，Raf 可与 Ras 结合，Raf 对于 Ras 的功能发挥必不可少，例如细胞转化[56,57]。目前哺乳动物的 Raf 有三种亚型，分别为 A-Raf，B-Raf 和 C-Raf（也称为 Raf-1），三种亚型有不同的表达模式[57]。Ras-GTP 与 Raf 的氨基末端结合并促进其活化，从而导致参与 Raf 活性调节的 Raf 同源或异源二聚化以及不同 Ser/Thr 和 Tyr 残基的磷酸化[57,58]。一旦被激活，Raf 可以磷酸化有丝分裂原/细胞外信号调节激酶（MEK）并导致其活化。MEK

也被称为 MAP 激酶(MKK),是一种双重特异性激酶[56,58](图 10-2)。然后,MEK 可以通过 Thr 183 位点和 Tyr 185 位点上的协同磷酸化来激活 MAP 激酶或细胞外信号调节激酶(ERK)。ERK 会易位到细胞核,通过磷酸化 Ser 或 Thr 位点激活多种蛋白质,包括 ETS 家族的转录因子和参与蛋白质翻译的激酶 p90 RSK[58,59]。Ras-Raf-MAPK 信号通路的激活会促进 DNA 的合成与细胞增殖,如诱导细胞周期蛋白 D1 表达[60]。该蛋白在早期细胞周期进程中起主要的调节作用,同时其也是肿瘤中扩增最频繁的基因之一[61]。

Raf 与肿瘤

Raf 对人类肿瘤直接影响的发现较晚,一半以上的黑色素瘤细胞系和原发性肿瘤中存在 B-Raf 的突变[62]。B-Raf 突变通常只发生在少数特定的残基,例如缬氨酸 600(valine 600),随后在其他恶性肿瘤中也发现存在此位点的突变,包括甲状腺癌(60%)、结直肠癌(10%)和肺癌(6%)[56]。B-Raf 是最常见的癌基因之一,在所有肿瘤中其突变比例是 8%,而 A-Raf 与 C-Raf 的突变远低于此频率,这可能是由于相比于 B-Raf,后者的基础酶活性较弱[56]。值得注意的是,癌基因 B-Raf 的激活同样可以由染色体易位产生,易位会产生包含 B-Raf 催化羧基末端的融合蛋白。此类易位已经在小儿星形细胞瘤、神经胶质瘤和甲状腺癌中发现[56]。

其他 MAP 激酶

除了 ERK,还有其他 MAP 激酶属于不同的 MAPK 级联,具有不同的上游激活剂和下游效应分子。JNK 和 p38 是应激激活的激酶,参与细胞应对一系列的胞外刺激,包括有丝分裂原、炎性因子和紫外线辐射等[63]。与激活 MAPK/ERK 级联的能力相比,Ras 仅能最低程度地干扰 JNK 和 p38,它们的活性主要由小 G 蛋白 Rho 家族(包括 Rac1、Cdc42 和 RhoA)诱导。与 ERK 相似,导致 JNK 或 p38 激活的信号通路包括多种可磷酸化 JNK 亚型的 MKK[63]。

与 ERK 一样,激活的 JNK 与 p38 最终会磷酸化不同的转录因子,促进相应靶基因的表达。转录因子 ATF2、ELK1、JUN、MYC 和 MEF2 等可被 JNK/p38 或两者直接磷酸化[63,64]。值得注意的是,其中一些转录因子最初是作为逆转录病毒致癌基因被发现的。

关键点

- 活化后的 RTK 促进 PI-3-K 介导合成 Ptdlns3P,进一步招募并激活 Akt 激酶。Akt 可调节下游不同的效应分子,在各种类型细胞中促进细胞的存活。
- RTK 主要通过激活 Ras/Raf/MAPK 信号通路刺激细胞的增殖。
- 在人类肿瘤中,由于编码不同关键效应分子的基因发生了突变,例如 PI-3-K、Ras 和 Raf,导致下游通路经常可以不依赖于 RTK 而发生活化。

肿瘤中异常失调的其他信号通路

虽然大多数(即使不是全部)类型的肿瘤都普遍存在 RTK 通路的激活,但其他信号通路也在肿瘤的发生和发展中发挥了重要作用。在胚胎发育过程和成年期,这些通路发挥着多种生理功能,与 RTK 信号转导类似,由于突变、染色体重排或其他机制,它们可能在肿瘤中被异常激活(或失活)。

尽管 RTK 代表了有酶活性的细胞表面受体的最大家族,仍然有其他类别的受体具有酶活功能。例如,转化生长因子-β(TGFβ)可以诱导四聚体复合物的形成,该四聚体包含两个Ⅰ型和两个Ⅱ型 TGFβ 受体,均为 Ser/Thr 激酶。Ⅱ型受体磷酸化Ⅰ型受体,后者通过结合并磷酸化 SMAD 转录因子将信号传递,最终激活 SMAD[65]。依据细胞环境的不同,TGFβ 信号通路可对肿瘤发挥抑制或促进作用。在癌前细胞,TGFβ 信号促进细胞凋亡,因此可以解释为什么某些肿瘤(包括结直肠癌和胰腺癌)存在频繁的 TGFβ 受体或 SMAD 失活突变。另有一些肿瘤,包括神经胶质瘤、黑素瘤和乳腺癌,可以通过不同的机制规避 TGFβ 的肿瘤抑制活性,同时维持一条有功能的通路,因此,在较晚期的肿瘤中,TGFβ 可以通过肿瘤细胞与微环境之间的相互干扰来促进肿瘤的进展和转移[65]。

其他表面受体缺乏一种固有的催化活性,但却可以直接与酶接头蛋白相互作用进而介导信号播散,例如,某些细胞因子受体就可以与具有 Tyr 激酶活性的 Janus 激酶(JAK)家族结合[66]。细胞因子诱导受体二聚化后,JAK 相互之间以及受体的 C 端都会发生磷酸化,因此为转录因子家族、信号转导分子和转录激活子(STAT)提供了停靠位点。被 JAK 磷酸化,STAT 通过其 SH2 结构域形成同型或异型二聚体,并转移至细胞核以转录激活其靶基因[66,67]。在患有不同类型的骨髓增生性肿瘤(包括真性红细胞增多症和原发性血小板增多症)的患者中,JAK2 的激活突变很常见,突变增强了细胞因子超敏性和细胞因子非依赖性的增殖[68]。尽管 STAT 突变很少见,研究发现不同的肿瘤可以通过不同的机制激活 STAT3 与 STAT5,进而影响肿瘤的生长、侵袭以及与免疫系统之间的相互作用[67]。另一个受体直接与酶活蛋白发生相互作用的例子是 G 蛋白偶联受体(GPCR),它是一个含有七次跨膜域的蛋白大家族,可以被不同类型的配体激活,包括激素、神经递质和细胞因子[69]。尽管某些肿瘤的 GPCR 或 G 蛋白中含有突变,但肿瘤中异常激活该信号通路的最常见机制是通过受体过表达和自分泌刺激[69]。GPCR 信号通路主要与内分泌系统肿瘤相关,例如某些细胞因子配体信号也是肿瘤微环境的主要调节器[70]。

肿瘤中其他公认信号通路的激活主要是通过更加复杂的机制,涉及不同的共受体、适配蛋白和有或无酶活性的细胞质复合体。Wnt、Hedgehog、Hippo、Notch 和肿瘤坏死因子(TNF)/NF-κB 信号通路就是这种情况。这些不同的信号通路有一个共同的特点:

配体与受体结合后会导致转录因子或共转录因子在细胞膜上或附近区域稳定或活化,例如 NF-κB(TNF)[71]、GLI(Hedgehog)[72]、YAP/TAZ(Hippo)[73] 和 β-catenin(Wnt)[74]。Notch 通路可以代表这一特征性变化,Delta/Jagged 配体与 NOTCH 结合后,会诱导 Notch 受体发生裂解并释放其胞质结构域,后者入核并激活 CBF1、Su(H)(Suppressor of Hairless)及转录因子 Lag-1[75]。这些高度保守的信号通路调节基础的生理过程，是成体正常胚胎发育以及维持干细胞或前体细胞状态所必需的。以上信号通路具有调节细胞的增殖、存活及分化等功能，这也是为什么这些信号通路频繁参与肿瘤发生的原因。例如，在多数结直肠癌中，不同基因的突变会导致 Wnt/β-catenin 信号通路的变异激活[74,76,77]。值得注意的是，不同机制引起的 Wnt 信号异常激活在乳腺癌、肾上腺皮质癌和肝细胞癌等多种类型的肿瘤中均很常见[74,78~80]。

不同种类的信号分子可以穿过细胞膜，并在细胞质或细胞核中与大量的转录因子家族结合，后者可作为此类配体的受体。一旦与它们的配体结合，核受体通过与不同的共刺激因子相互作用，并以同源或异源二聚体的方式激活特定靶基因的表达[81]。核受体家族大约有 50 个成员，它们调节不同的生理过程，在某些类型的肿瘤中发挥关键的作用。例如，大部分乳腺和前列腺肿瘤的增殖和生长分别依赖于雌激素/孕激素和雄激素受体。这些研究有力地推动了对性激素拮抗剂或性激素合成抑制剂敏感的肿瘤的治疗[82~84]。核受体影响肿瘤的另一个例子是早幼粒细胞白血病（PML）与维 A 酸受体 α（RARα）基因的染色体易位产生的 PML-RAR 融合蛋白。PML-RAR 可以招募更多的共抑制因子到 RARα 靶基因调节区域，进而抑制髓系细胞的正常分化。这使未成熟的粒细胞前体细胞积聚，并诱发致命的血液恶性肿瘤——急性早幼粒细胞白血病（APL）。研究者将这种致癌机制成功转化成一种基于全反式维 A 酸（RA）的新型治疗方法，该疗法对 70%～80% 的 APL 患者有效[85]。APL 的例子阐述了在临床中如何通过特异地靶向肿瘤内异常激活的信号通路来阻断或限制肿瘤的生长和/或扩散，这一概念将在下文中进一步讨论。

要点

- 其他配体家族信号通过受体激活不同的下游效应通路。
- 大多数情况下，此类受体在细胞表面或附近直接或间接激活特定的转录因子，进而调节特定靶基因的表达。
- 某些配体穿过细胞膜与作为转录因子的同源受体结合。
- 这些通路调控了一系列的生理过程，不同机制导致的通路变异失调在各种肿瘤的起始和/或进展过程中发挥着重要的作用。

生长因子信号与肿瘤治疗

随着与癌基因细胞转化功能相关的很多信号通路被阐明，研究者继而致力于研究靶向癌变激活的信号通路或下游分子的治疗策略。基于靶基因的一个重要优势在于这些方法一般可以有效地监测体内靶点分子的抑制情况。这种治疗策略将临床反应与药物动力学的靶点抑制分析相关联，从而加快了临床试验的进程。此类药物的另一个优点是一些药物的固有毒性似乎比标准化疗方案要小。这类方法都基于“癌基因成瘾”的观点，这种观点认为尽管肿瘤细胞具有复杂的突变事件模式，但其细胞的生长和/或存活可能特别依赖于一种或几种信号通路[86]。这些通路被认为可以抗衡肿瘤内其他同样也可由癌基因变异引发的促凋亡信号，一旦促存活信号被阻断，肿瘤细胞会遭受所谓的“致癌性休克”并死亡[87]。对肿瘤细胞系及转基因小鼠的研究支持了这一想法[88]，研究通过关闭癌基因的表达使癌基因（如 K-Ras）诱导的肿瘤完全消退[89]。靶向变异激活信号通路的治疗，无论单独使用还是与传统的化疗或放疗结合，都已对某些类型的恶性肿瘤产生了很好的治疗效果。

然而，很多情况表明，其他基因的变异通常会激活同一信号通路，最终会导致在靶向治疗时，该通路会绕开被靶向的癌基因而继续保持通路活性，并会伴有相关疾病的进展（请参阅以下部分）。

单克隆抗体

肿瘤细胞表面生长因子信号的启动是一个潜在的治疗干预靶点。单克隆抗体可特异性中和生长因子的活性或干扰配体受体间的相互作用。单克隆抗体已被用于干扰特定类型肿瘤中过表达的受体[90]（表 10-1）。曲妥珠单抗（赫赛汀，基因泰克公司）是抗 ErbB2 的人源化单克隆抗体，它是临床上第一个被批准用来靶向癌基因产物的抗肿瘤药物。实验证据进一步表明曲妥珠单抗增强了过表达 ErbB2 乳腺癌对紫杉烷类化合物、蒽环类药物及铂类化合物的反应性[91]。西妥昔单抗（爱必妥，英克隆公司）是一种针对 EGFR 的单克隆嵌合抗体，已被批准与化疗和放疗联合治疗结直肠癌和头颈癌[91~93]。值得注意的是，研究表明西妥昔单抗可显著改善野生型 K-Ras 结直肠癌患者的生存。然而，在 40% K-Ras 突变的肿瘤中，它并没有表现出疗效优势[94]。因此，为了治疗干预能够成功，需要对肿瘤进行必要的特定遗传背景检测。

表 10-1 靶向异常信号通路的肿瘤治疗

肿瘤药物	靶点	疾病
单克隆抗体		
贝伐单抗（安维汀）	VEGF	结直肠癌，非小细胞肺癌，肾细胞癌，恶性胶质瘤，宫颈癌
西妥昔单抗（爱必妥）	EGFR	结直肠癌，头颈癌
地诺单抗（Xgeva）	RANKL	骨巨细胞瘤
帕尼单抗（Vectibix）	EGFR	结直肠癌
帕妥珠单抗（Perjeta）	ErbB2	乳腺癌

续表

肿瘤药物	靶点	疾病
拉米单抗(Cyramza)	VEGFR2	胃腺癌
西妥昔单抗(西尔万特)	IL-6	淋巴细胞瘤
曲妥单抗(赫赛汀)	ErbB2	乳腺癌和胃癌
融合蛋白		
阿柏西普(Zaltrap)	VEGFA,VEGFB,PGF	结直肠癌
小分子抑制剂		
阿比特龙(Zytiga)	睾酮生成	前列腺癌
阿法替尼(Gilotrif)	EGFR,ERBB2,ERBB4	非小细胞肺癌
阿那曲唑(Arimidex)	雌激素合成	乳腺癌
阿西替尼(Inlyta)	VEGFR,PDGFR,c-KIT	肾细胞癌
博舒替尼(Bosulif)	Abl,Src	慢性髓性白血病
卡波替尼(Cometriq)	c-Met, RET, VEGFR, c-KIT, FLT-3, TIE-2,TRKB,AXL	甲状腺癌
塞立替尼(Zykadia)	ALK	非小细胞肺癌
克唑替尼(Xalkori)	ALK 和 c-Met	非小细胞肺癌
达布拉非尼(Tafinlar)	B-Raf	黑色素瘤
达沙替尼(Sprycel)	Abl 和 Src	慢性髓性白血病,急性淋巴细胞白血病
恩杂鲁胺(Xtandi)	AR	前列腺癌
厄洛替尼(Tarceva)	EGFR	非小细胞肺癌,胰腺癌
依维莫司(Afinitor)	mTOR	肾细胞癌,星形细胞瘤,原始神经外胚层肿瘤,乳腺癌
依西美坦(Aromasin)	雌激素合成	乳腺癌
氟维司群(Faslodex)	ER	乳腺癌
吉非替尼(易瑞沙)	EGFR	非小细胞肺癌
依鲁替尼(Imbruvica)	BTK	慢性淋巴细胞性白血病,套细胞淋巴瘤
艾代拉里斯(Zydelig)	PI-3-K	慢性淋巴细胞性白血病
拉帕替尼(Tykerb)	EGFR 和 ERBB2	乳腺癌
来曲唑(Femara)	雌激素合成	乳腺癌
伊马替尼(格列卫)	Abl,PDGFR,c-Kit	慢性髓性白血病,胃肠道间质瘤,急性淋巴细胞白血病,隆凸性皮肤纤维肉瘤
尼洛替尼(达西那)	Abl,PDGFR,c-Kit	慢性髓性白血病
帕唑帕尼(Votrient)	VEGFR,PDGFR,c-KIT	肾细胞癌,软组织肉瘤
瑞戈非尼(Stivarga)	VEGFR,Ret,Kit,PDGFR,Raf	结直肠癌,胃肠道间质瘤,
索拉非尼(Nexavar)	VEGFR,PDGFR,FLT3,c-Kit,Raf,Ret	肾细胞癌,肝细胞癌,甲状腺癌
舒尼替尼(Sutent)	VEGFR,PDGFR,FLT3,c-Kit,Ret	胃肠道间质瘤,肾细胞癌,原始神经外胚层肿瘤
他莫昔芬	ER	乳腺癌
替米罗莫司(Torisel)	mTOR	肾细胞癌

续表

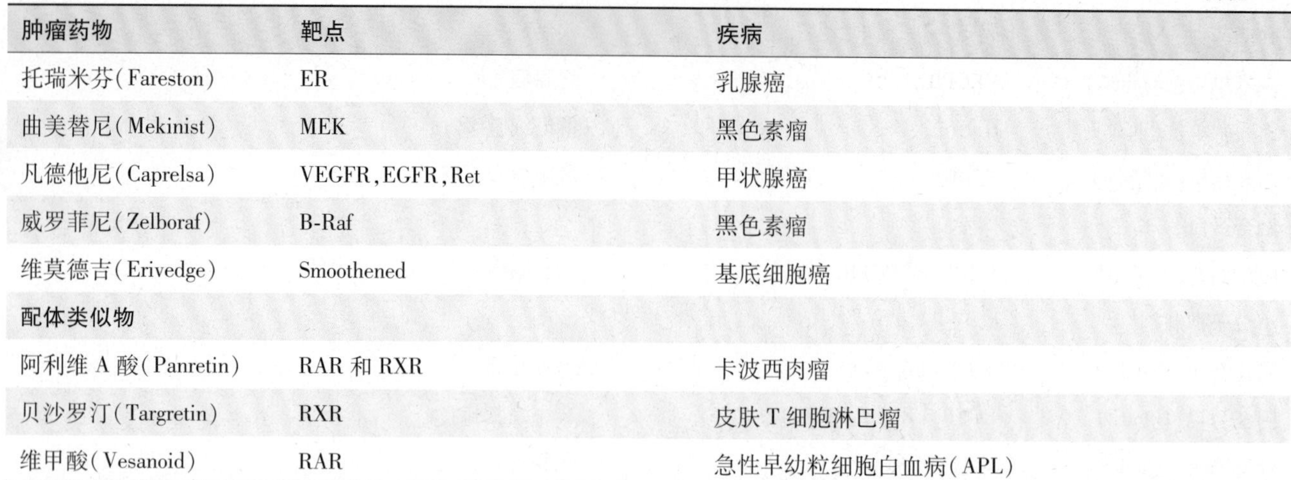

肿瘤药物	靶点	疾病
托瑞米芬(Fareston)	ER	乳腺癌
曲美替尼(Mekinist)	MEK	黑色素瘤
凡德他尼(Caprelsa)	VEGFR,EGFR,Ret	甲状腺癌
威罗菲尼(Zelboraf)	B-Raf	黑色素瘤
维莫德吉(Erivedge)	Smoothened	基底细胞癌
配体类似物		
阿利维 A 酸(Panretin)	RAR 和 RXR	卡波西肉瘤
贝沙罗汀(Targretin)	RXR	皮肤 T 细胞淋巴瘤
维甲酸(Vesanoid)	RAR	急性早幼粒细胞白血病(APL)

另一个例子是贝伐单抗(安维汀,基因泰克公司),它是靶向血管内皮生长因子(VEGF)的单克隆抗体,VEGF 是一个可以促进血管新生的配体。FDA 已经批准贝伐单抗用于治疗恶性胶质瘤、结直肠癌、肾癌和肺癌。与曲妥珠单抗和西妥昔单抗相反,贝伐单抗靶向的是肿瘤微环境中的血管内皮细胞。它的优点包括:与遗传不稳定的肿瘤细胞相比,这种正常细胞不太可能产生耐药性,并且可能这种疗法适用的肿瘤类型更广泛[95]。值得注意的是,最近的研究表明靶向 VEGF 也可能直接影响某些表达 VEGF 受体的肿瘤细胞[96]。

酪氨酸激酶抑制剂

随着对肿瘤中生长因子信号转导重要作用的日益了解,研究者们继而致力于开发组成型激活 Tyr 激酶的小分子抑制剂(表 10-1)。其中,最引人注目的例子是伊马替尼(格列卫,诺华制药),一种非 RTK 的 Abl 小分子抑制剂。Abl 作为费城染色体的一部分在慢性粒细胞性白血病(CML)中发生易位,从而产生 *Bcr-Abl* 融合癌基因[97]。伊马替尼与 Abl 激酶域的 ATP 结合口袋相互作用并稳定 Abl 产物的催化失活构象[98]。临床试验快速明确了伊马替尼对 CML 及其治疗靶点 *Bcr-Abl* 的作用。伊马替尼在疾病的慢性期疗效显著,其中 95%经标准疗法治疗失败的患者的循环 Ph+细胞被完全清除。在中位随访 18 个月后,仅 9%的患者出现复发[99],伊马替尼因此获得了监管部门的批准。对处于慢性期的患者,伊马替尼的治疗效果最好,且副作用少,而髓母细胞瘤的患者在接受伊马替尼治疗后则容易复发。然而,在疾病的进展期,肿瘤细胞往往会对伊马替尼产生耐药,既可以通过突变来干扰伊马替尼与 Abl 的结合,也可以促使 *Bcr-Abl* 基因的扩增[98]。研究发现伊马替尼可以抑制相关的 RTK,特别是 Kit 和 PDGFR,这两个激酶在胃肠道间质瘤(GIST)中存在激活突变,因此 FDA 批准了伊马替尼用于此类肿瘤的治疗。

靶向 RTK 的其他小分子还有吉非替尼(易瑞沙,阿斯利康)和厄洛替尼(特罗凯,OSI/Genentech)等,已被批准用于治疗 EGFR 突变的肺癌[100]。在肺癌和成神经细胞瘤等肿瘤中,ALK 是一种由染色体易位或突变激活的受体,克唑替尼(赛可瑞,辉瑞)可抑制 ALK 的活性[101]。还有更多其他的小分子抑制剂可以靶向不同的 Tyr 激酶,这些激酶与肿瘤发生和血管新生有关,例如索拉菲尼(多吉美,拜耳)和舒尼替尼(索坦,辉瑞),已被批准用于治疗某些特定的肿瘤,包括晚期肾细胞癌、肝细胞癌和伊马替尼难治性 GIST(表 10-1)。

生长因子下游信号抑制

在肿瘤细胞内激活的生长因子信号通路的下游成分也是潜在的治疗靶点。尽管目前尚无有效和特异的 Ras 抑制剂进入临床,但最近批准的靶向 RTK 信号下游成分的新的小分子,证实了靶向下游效应分子策略的有效性(表 10-1)。一个典型的例子是威罗菲尼(*Vemurafenib*,泽波拉夫,Plexxikon/罗氏公司),该药物在 2011 年被批准用于治疗携带 B-Raf V600E 突变的黑色素瘤。由于威罗菲尼选择性地阻断突变型而非野生型 B-Raf,其因此成为研究的范例。与其他靶向治疗药物相似,经过最初的反应期,肿瘤往往会逐渐失去对药物的反应性。威罗菲尼获得性耐药的若干机制已有报道,包括 Ras 突变、B-Raf 剪接变异体的特殊表达或 RTK 的过表达,例如 PDGFR[56]。最近的证据表明,在不使用 B-raf 抑制剂的情况下,对威罗菲尼耐药的黑色素瘤细胞的适应性可能会降低。因此,威罗菲尼间歇性给药可以阻止耐药细胞的克隆扩增,从而预防或延迟耐药性复发[102]。

最新研究进展表明,生长因子信号异常在肿瘤中的重要作用正在引领肿瘤治疗的新时代。随着对靶向药物分子基础认知的增强以及对其获得性抵抗机制了解的深入,我们有充足的理由相信未来将会出现基于肿瘤基因谱的个体化治疗。十年前,个体化治疗还处于畅想阶段,然而随着基因测序的进展[103]、原代及循环肿瘤细胞的分离及 DNA 测序的实现[104,105],个体化治疗指日可待。

要点

- 肿瘤细胞为了生存会对某一特殊的信号通路产生依赖性或成瘾性。
- 在临床上可以通过不同的治疗策略来特异靶向肿瘤细胞中异常失调的通路,包括单克隆抗体,Tyr 激酶抑制剂和下游效应子抑制剂。

总结

多细胞机体的生理过程是通过复杂的相互连接的信号通路网络来调节的，而生理过程通常由激素、细胞因子和生长因子介导。这些分子以即时、精细的方式特异调控某一特定细胞群的表型，包括增殖、分化、存活及活力。当信号转导通路出现问题时，这种精确的调节就会失控，从而产生异常的细胞行为，导致细胞发生转化。大多数（如果不是全部）人类肿瘤包含多种通路的异常激活（或是抑制），从而导致细胞增殖、存活、侵袭和转移扩散能力的增强。这些变异由不同的机制介导，包括自分泌/旁分泌失调或影响某一通路特定成分基因的改变。在本章节，我们讨论通过受体酪氨酸激酶介导的生长因子信号通路，并聚焦这些受体促进细胞增殖和存活的两个主要下游通路，即 PI-3-K/Akt 和 Ras/MAP 激酶通路。我们提供了不同的范例，特别强调了这些异常对肿瘤发生的影响。本章讨论了正常细胞和肿瘤细胞中细胞信号转导的一般原理，还简要讨论了特定类型肿瘤的起始和进展如何受到其他几种信号转导通路失调的影响，包括细胞因子、TGFβ 配体家族、Wnt、Hedgehog、Notch 和核受体调控的信号通路。

最后，我们讨论了癌基因成瘾和靶向治疗的概念，通过典型的例子来说明如何进一步将我们对于癌症中特定信号通路异常失调机制的认识转化到临床实践中。

致谢

L. G. 受 INSERM 和鲁昂大学精英项目主席及“鲁昂抗癌联盟”的基金资助。SAA 受 NCI、NICHD 及乳腺癌研究基金会资助。

（吕桂帅　吕洪伟　译　付静　校　陈淑桢　审）

参考文献

The complete reference list can be found on the Wiley Companion Digital Edition of this title (see inside front cover for login instructions).

9 Aaronson SA. Growth factors and cancer. *Science*. 1991;**254**(**5035**):1146–1153.

10 Lemmon MA, Schlessinger J. Cell signaling by receptor tyrosine kinases. *Cell*. 2010;**141**(**7**):1117–1134.

16 Pollak M. The insulin and insulin-like growth factor receptor family in neoplasia: an update. *Nat Rev Cancer*. 2012;**12**(**3**):159–169.

17 Citri A, Yarden Y. EGF-ERBB signalling: towards the systems level. *Nat Rev Mol Cell Biol*. 2006;**7**(**7**):505–516.

18 Arteaga CL, Engelman JA. ERBB receptors: from oncogene discovery to basic science to mechanism-based cancer therapeutics. *Cancer Cell*. 2014;**25**(**3**):282–303.

19 Trusolino L, Bertotti A, Comoglio PM. MET signalling: principles and functions in development, organ regeneration and cancer. *Nat Rev Mol Cell Biol*. 2010;**11**(**12**):834–848.

20 Gherardi E, Birchmeier W, Birchmeier C, Vande WG. Targeting MET in cancer: rationale and progress. *Nat Rev Cancer*. 2012;**12**(**2**):89–103.

24 Tebbutt N, Pedersen MW, Johns TG. Targeting the ERBB family in cancer: couples therapy. *Nat Rev Cancer*. 2013;**13**(**9**):663–673.

25 Shaw AT, Hsu PP, Awad MM, Engelman JA. Tyrosine kinase gene rearrangements in epithelial malignancies. *Nat Rev Cancer*. 2013;**13**(**11**):772–787.

26 Lynch TJ, Bell DW, Sordella R, et al. Activating mutations in the epidermal growth factor receptor underlying responsiveness of non-small-cell lung cancer to gefitinib. *N Engl J Med*. 2004;**350**(**21**):2129–2139.

27 Paez JG, Janne PA, Lee JC, et al. EGFR mutations in lung cancer: correlation with clinical response to gefitinib therapy. *Science*. 2004;**304**(**5676**):1497–1500.

29 Wagner MJ, Stacey MM, Liu BA, Pawson T. Molecular mechanisms of SH2- and PTB-domain-containing proteins in receptor tyrosine kinase signaling. *Cold Spring Harb Perspect Biol*. 2013;**5**(**12**):a008987.

39 Engelman JA, Luo J, Cantley LC. The evolution of phosphatidylinositol 3-kinases as regulators of growth and metabolism. *Nat Rev Genet*. 2006;**7**(**8**):606–619.

40 Vanhaesebroeck B, Stephens L, Hawkins P. PI3K signalling: the path to discovery and understanding. *Nat Rev Mol Cell Biol*. 2012;**13**(**3**):195–203.

41 Manning BD, Cantley LC. AKT/PKB signaling: navigating downstream. *Cell*. 2007;**129**(**7**):1261–1274.

42 Fruman DA, Rommel C. PI3K and cancer: lessons, challenges and opportunities. *Nat Rev Drug Discov*. 2014;**13**(**2**):140–156.

44 Samuels Y, Wang Z, Bardelli A, et al. High frequency of mutations of the PIK3CA gene in human cancers. *Science*. 2004;**304**(**5670**):554.

45 Kandoth C, McLellan MD, Vandin F, et al. Mutational landscape and significance across 12 major cancer types. *Nature*. 2013;**502**(**7471**):333–339.

50 Karnoub AE, Weinberg RA. Ras oncogenes: split personalities. *Nat Rev Mol Cell Biol*. 2008;**9**(**7**):517–531.

52 Pylayeva-Gupta Y, Grabocka E, Bar-Sagi D. RAS oncogenes: weaving a tumorigenic web. *Nat Rev Cancer*. 2011;**11**(**11**):761–774.

56 Holderfield M, Deuker MM, McCormick F, McMahon M. Targeting RAF kinases for cancer therapy: BRAF-mutated melanoma and beyond. *Nat Rev Cancer*. 2014;**14**(**7**):455–467.

62 Davies H, Bignell GR, Cox C, et al. Mutations of the BRAF gene in human cancer. *Nature*. 2002;**417**(**6892**):949–954.

63 Wagner EF, Nebreda AR. Signal integration by JNK and p38 MAPK pathways in cancer development. *Nat Rev Cancer*. 2009;**9**(**8**):537–549.

65 Massague J. TGFbeta signalling in context. *Nat Rev Mol Cell Biol*. 2012;**13**(**10**):616–630.

66 Stark GR, Darnell JE Jr. The JAK-STAT pathway at twenty. *Immunity*. 2012;**36**(**4**):503–514.

70 Lappano R, Maggiolini M. G protein-coupled receptors: novel targets for drug discovery in cancer. *Nat Rev Drug Discov*. 2011;**10**(**1**):47–60.

71 Perkins ND. The diverse and complex roles of NF-kappaB subunits in cancer. *Nat Rev Cancer*. 2012;**12**(**2**):121–132.

72 Briscoe J, Therond PP. The mechanisms of Hedgehog signalling and its roles in development and disease. *Nat Rev Mol Cell Biol*. 2013;**14**(**7**):416–429.

73 Harvey KF, Zhang X, Thomas DM. The Hippo pathway and human cancer. *Nat Rev Cancer*. 2013;**13**(**4**):246–257.

74 Clevers H, Nusse R. Wnt/beta-catenin signaling and disease. *Cell*. 2012;**149**(**6**):1192–1205.

75 Guruharsha KG, Kankel MW, Artavanis-Tsakonas S. The Notch signalling system: recent insights into the complexity of a conserved pathway. *Nat Rev Genet*. 2012;**13**(**9**):654–666.

81 Evans RM, Mangelsdorf DJ. Nuclear receptors, RXR, and the big bang. *Cell*. 2014;**157**(**1**):255–266.

82 Jordan VC. Chemoprevention of breast cancer with selective oestrogen-receptor modulators. *Nat Rev Cancer*. 2007;**7**(**1**):46–53.

84 Mills IG. Maintaining and reprogramming genomic androgen receptor activity in prostate cancer. *Nat Rev Cancer*. 2014;**14**(**3**):187–198.

87 Sharma SV, Settleman J. Oncogene addiction: setting the stage for molecularly targeted cancer therapy. *Genes Dev*. 2007;**21**(**24**):3214–3231.

96 Goel HL, Mercurio AM. VEGF targets the tumour cell. *Nat Rev Cancer*. 2013;**13**(**12**):871–882.

98 Druker BJ. Translation of the Philadelphia chromosome into therapy for CML. *Blood*. 2008;**112**(**13**):4808–4817.

100 Sharma SV, Bell DW, Settleman J, Haber DA. Epidermal growth factor receptor mutations in lung cancer. *Nat Rev Cancer*. 2007;**7**(**3**):169–181.

101 Hallberg B, Palmer RH. Mechanistic insight into ALK receptor tyrosine kinase in human cancer biology. *Nat Rev Cancer*. 2013;**13**(**10**):685–700.

103 Vogelstein B, Papadopoulos N, Velculescu VE, Zhou S, Diaz LA Jr, Kinzler KW. Cancer genome landscapes. *Science*. 2013;**339**(**6127**):1546–1558.

第 11 章　诱导分化治疗

Sai-Juan Chen, MD, PhD ■ Xiao-Jing Yan, MD ■ Guang-Biao Zhou, MD ■ Zhu Chen, PhD

概述

分化异常是人类恶性肿瘤的主要特征之一，特别是在血液系统恶性肿瘤中。目前认为，多种基因和表观遗传学调节异常可以影响各种肿瘤细胞的分化过程，并在肿瘤发生中起重要作用。诱导分化治疗是指应用针对细胞分化过程中关键调节因子的靶向药物，从而恢复正常细胞的稳态，并最终清除肿瘤细胞的治疗方法。在过去的四十年中，通过研究肿瘤细胞分化受阻或者停滞的分子机制，发现了一系列的药物作用靶点；同时通过体内或者体外研究筛选了多种能够诱导肿瘤细胞分化成熟的药物。该领域的转化研究逐渐将诱导分化治疗从一个“概念”转向了真正的临床实践。最成功的肿瘤诱导分化治疗的典范是应用全反式视黄酸(all-trans-retinoic acid，ATRA)和三氧化二砷(arsenic trioxide，ATO)协同靶向治疗急性早幼粒细胞白血病(acute promyelocytic leukemia，APL)。本章讨论了诱导分化治疗的基础理论和该治疗方法的临床成果。

肿瘤分化阻滞的分子机制

目前已知，肿瘤的临床侵袭性与其分化状态之间存在一定的相关性，低分化肿瘤通常具有更高的侵袭性。为了更好地了解肿瘤分化停滞或者受阻的生物学行为，必须阐明正常细胞分化的相关调节机制以及它们在癌细胞分化过程中出现怎样的异常，这些研究对于发现有意义的治疗靶点非常重要。众所周知，多能胚胎干细胞能够自我更新并分化成具有生物体特定功能的各种细胞。这些细胞在精确的调节下，以非常有序的方式发育成不同类型的细胞、组织和器官。大量证据表明，干细胞分化机制需要细胞/组织特异性或时间特异性转录因子的连续作用，这些转录因子在特定条件下可以激活或抑制分化相关基因[1-3]。基因的转录表达也可以通过表观遗传学的多种机制来共同调节。值得注意的是，在正常发育过程中调节细胞分化的多种途径和网络都在肿瘤发生中存在遗传学和表观遗传学的异常。因此，调节胚胎形态发生和维持干细胞特性的调节因子在癌细胞中存在异常表达。同时，维持细胞处于分化状态的调节程序通常在癌细胞中表现为功能缺失(图 11-1)。

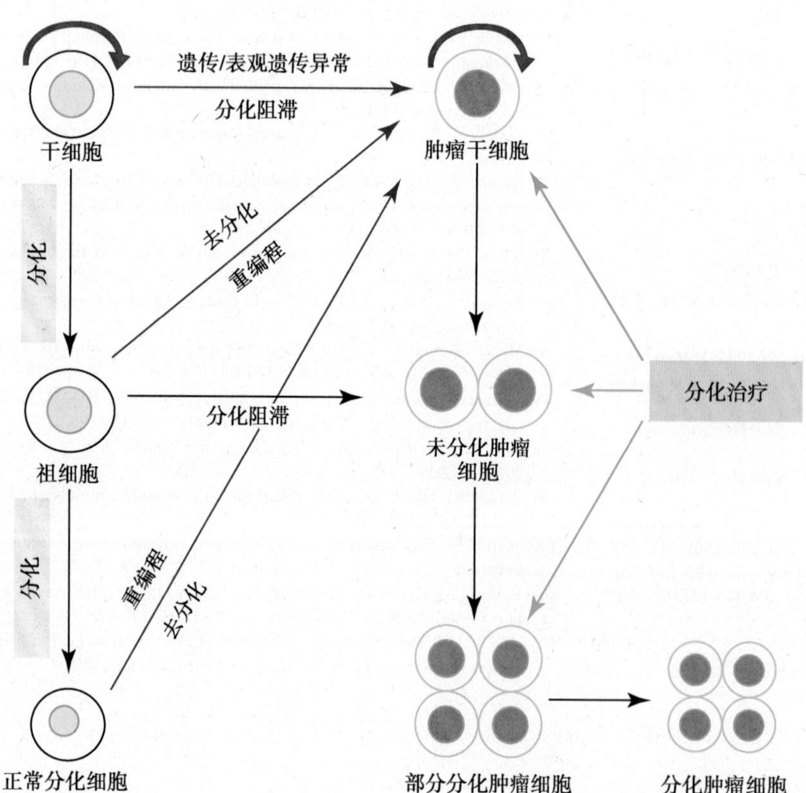

图 11-1　癌症的分化阻滞和分化治疗。除自我更新外，正常干细胞能够分化为特定的成熟细胞，而分化阻滞可能导致癌症的发生。肿瘤干细胞可能源自遗传学和/或表观遗传异常的正常干细胞，也可能源自遗传学和/或表观遗传异常而导致去分化和重编程的正常祖细胞或分化细胞。诱导分化治疗通过诱导癌症干细胞和未分化癌细胞的分化来发挥治疗效果

转录因子

细胞分化可以认为是一个获得不同功能的连续过程，细胞最终命运的确定主要通过转录因子（transcription factors，TF）和表观遗传修饰因子的共同作用来调控基因表达来实现[3,4]。TF 是能与 DNA 结合并反式激活或反式抑制靶基因转录的胞核蛋白，它们通常与辅因子（激活剂或抑制剂）组装成多蛋白复合物，从而在调节干/祖细胞基因表达谱和决定细胞分化成熟为特定细胞系的过程中起关键调节作用[5]。TF 为细胞增殖和程序性死亡（如细胞凋亡）所必需。近来，研究发现通过让细胞过表达特定的 TF，能够让细胞重编程，诱导分化成熟的细胞转分化为具有多能干性的细胞，这些结果为 TF 在细胞命运中发挥关键作用提供了强有力的证据[6-11]。此外，已经有大量的实验数据表明细胞分化受到系列特异性的 TF 调控[3,5,12]。因此，基因突变或基因异常融合造成的基因表达或功能异常，可以导致分化相关的 TF 出现异常，进而会干扰正常干/祖细胞的分化程序[5]，最终可能会产生具有生长和存活优势的未成熟的子代细胞，促进癌症的发生。

肿瘤相关的 TF 可根据结构和/或功能特征分为不同类别[12]，例如亮氨酸拉链因子（bZIP，例如 c-JUN）、螺旋-环-螺旋因子（bHLH，例如 MYC）、Cys4 锌指［例如核受体（nuclear receptors，NR）、GATA 转录因子］、螺旋-转角-螺旋因子（HTH，例如 HOX 家族、OCT-1/2）和 Rel 同源区域［例如核因子（nuclear factor，NF）-κB］。这些 TF 是细胞增殖、分化和凋亡的关键调节因子，它们的突变和/或异常表达在细胞恶性转化中起重要作用。其中特别值得关注的是一类特殊的配体激活锌指蛋白——NR 超家族，因为它们是多种细胞/组织类型分化状态起始和/或维持的主要调节因子[13]。该家族包含多种受体，可以作用于不同类型的配体，包括类固醇/甲状腺激素、视黄酸、维生素 D3 和某些脂肪酸。值得注意的是，这些受体很多会在各种癌症中出现表达水平或蛋白质结构的异常，这些异常以激素非依赖性方式引起正常激素调节基因的异常活化，甚至激活与激素调节无关的一些基因，进而在肿瘤发生过程中起重要作用，具体内容将会在标题为“靶向异常 TF 的药物”部分中详细讨论。

长期以来，由于造血相关的激素和信号通路以及调节造血干/祖细胞（hematopoietic stem/progenitor cells，HSPC）命运的特异性 TF 的发现，对造血功能的认知一直处于正常和异常细胞分化生物学研究的前沿（图 11-2）[5,14,15]。髓系和淋系分化的每个阶段，具有特征性的 TF 在调节网络中发挥作用。例如，RUNX1、GATA1、C/EBPα、C/EBPβ、MYB、E2A、PAX5、TAL1/SCL 或 PU. 1 均会精准规律地开放或关闭，以确保血细胞分化的特异性[3,15]。这些 TF 最初是在白血病的分子异常中（包括基因突变或基因融合）被识别的，例如：通过 *CEBPA* 突变的急

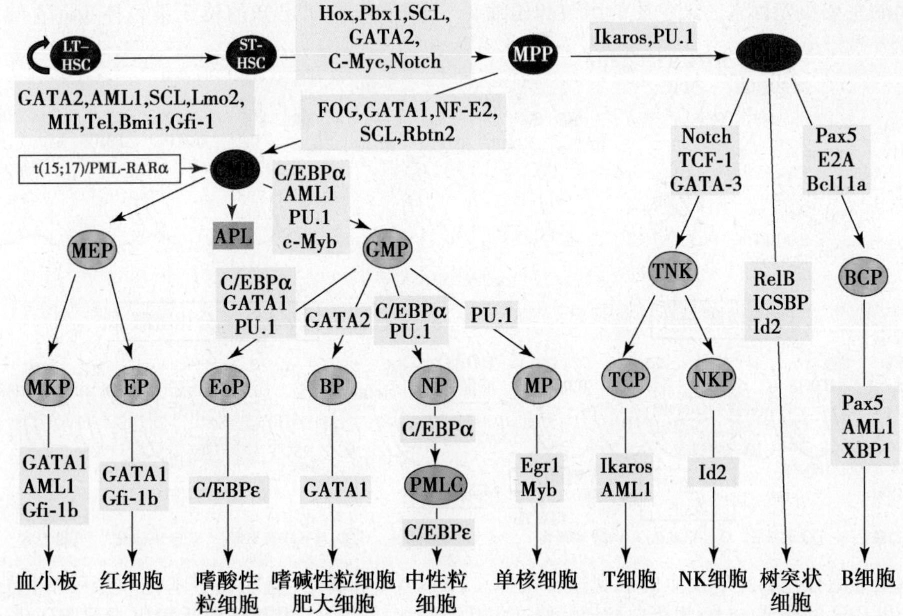

图 11-2　信号传导通路和转录因子（TF）调节造血干/祖细胞（HSPC）的分化。分化阻滞可能会导致白血病，例如急性早幼粒细胞白血病（APL）是一种特殊类型的急性髓细胞性白血病（AML）的亚型，其特征是骨髓/外周血中异常早幼粒细胞分化停滞而聚集、具有 t（15；17）染色体易位和 PML-RARα 融合基因，以及严重出血综合征。实际上，几乎所有正常造血细胞发育过程中的信号分子和 TF 都在血液恶性肿瘤中发生遗传学异常（基因融合、点突变、基因扩增/缺失）和/或表达失调。APL，急性早幼粒细胞白血病；BCP，B 细胞祖细胞；BP，嗜碱性粒细胞祖细胞；CLP，共同淋系祖细胞；CMP，共同髓系祖细胞；EoP，嗜酸性粒细胞祖细胞；EP，红系祖细胞；GMP，粒细胞-巨噬细胞祖细胞；HSC，造血干细胞；LT，长期；LT-HSC，长期造血干细胞；MEP，巨核细胞-红细胞祖细胞；MKP，巨核细胞祖细胞；MP，单核细胞祖细胞；MPP，多潜能祖细胞；NKP，NK 细胞祖细胞；NP，中性粒细胞祖细胞；PMLC，早幼粒细胞；ST，短期；ST-HSC，短期造血干细胞；TCP，T 细胞祖细胞；TNK，T/NK 细胞祖细胞

性髓细胞性白血病（acute myeloid leukemia，AML）发现了 C/EBPα，通过 t(8;21) 易位的 AML 发现了 RUNX1（*AML1*），通过 t(1;14) T 细胞急性淋巴细胞白血病（acute lymphoblastic leukemia，ALL）发现了 SCL（*TAL1*）[16-18]。白血病中这些造血 TF 的异常使得造血细胞停滞在了早期分化阶段。

目前已经证实了异常 TF 干扰细胞分化是肿瘤发生中的“驱动因素”，因此研发靶向这些蛋白的药物用于治疗是肿瘤研究的热点之一。目前大多数抗癌药物研究都集中在细胞表面受体上，因为药物通过这种方式作用于细胞相对容易，然而在转录水平起作用的药物需要穿过胞膜并进入胞核，因此研发通过影响癌症相关转录模式以重建分化的相关药物需要投入更多的努力。诱导分化药物研发可以针对转录机制中 TF 和 DNA 之间或 TF 与其他蛋白质之间具有明确相互作用位点的小分子药物，以调节关键的 TF 靶基因；另一方面通过基因治疗重新导入分化相关的野生型 TF 也可以作为肿瘤分化治疗的策略。

表观遗传修饰

表观遗传调控是灵活调控基因表达的关键机制之一，可通过有丝分裂和潜在的减数分裂进行遗传，而不改变基因组序列[19,20]。生物体的所有细胞具有同样的基因组信息，但表现为不同的表型，具有不同的功能。这种表型的多样性是由于不同细胞类型之间具有不同的基因表达模式。众所周知，染色质状态是基因开放或关闭的主要决定因素。染色质的组装和压缩受到多种机制调节，包括 DNA 甲基化（胞嘧啶甲基化和羟甲基化）或去甲基化，组蛋白的翻译后修饰（磷酸化、乙酰化、甲基化和泛素化），以及非编码 RNA 介导的途径[20-22]。目前已经确定了多种酶为表观遗传学调节机制中的调节因子（图 11-3a 和 b），如 DNA 甲基转移酶（DNA methyltransferases，DNMT）和 DNA 去甲基化酶，组蛋白脱乙酰酶（histone deacetylases，HDAC）和组蛋白乙酰转移酶（histone acetyltransferases，HAT），以及组蛋白甲基转移酶（histone methyltransferases，HMT）和组蛋白去甲基化酶（histone demethylases，HDM）。DNA 或组蛋白的各种修饰是紧密相关的，它们可以相互增强或相互抑制。许多组蛋白修饰酶是辅因子复合物的组分，并且与 TF 协同作用以调节基因表达（图 11-3c）。

近来，新的技术平台可以在多能干以及分化细胞中建立全面的表观遗传学组图谱，可以进一步支持细胞分化伴随着染色质状态动态变化的这一理论[22-25]。不同模式生物的遗传学研究表明，染色质调节因子在关键的发育分化和决定细胞命运中具有重要作用。癌细胞往往在全基因组水平发生了特征性的表观遗传调节异常，例如低甲基化、特定启动子区域的高甲基化、组蛋白去乙酰化、微小 RNA（microRNA、miRNA）分子的下调，以及表观遗传学调节机制中某些组分的失调[20,21,26]。目前，在某些肿瘤中确定了多种常见的表观遗传修饰调节因子的体细胞改变，包括实体瘤和造血系统恶性肿瘤[27-30]。例如，在急性白血病和骨髓增生异常综合征（myelodysplastic syndrome，MDS）中，除了已知的位于染色体 11q23 的 *MLL1* 基因（mixed

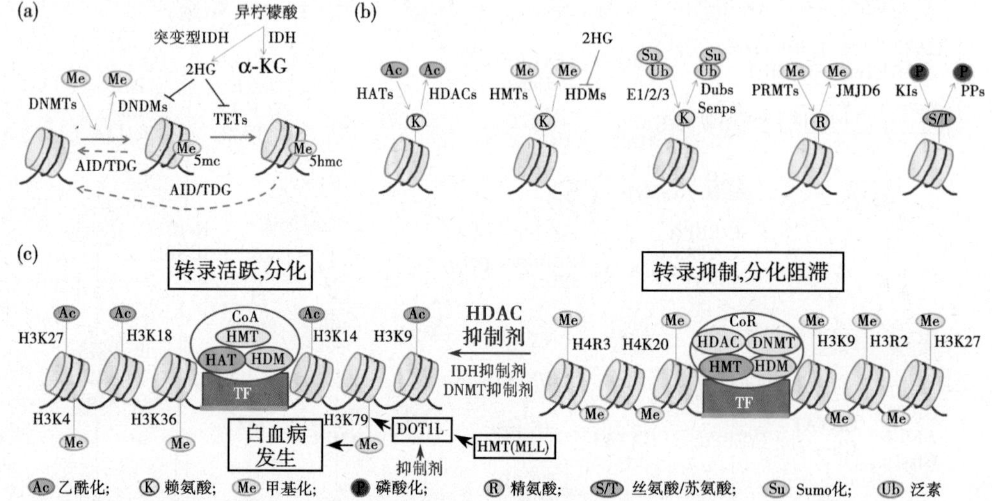

图 11-3 涉及细胞分化和肿瘤发生的表观遗传调控。(a) DNA 甲基化（胞嘧啶甲基化和羟甲基化）受不同酶 DNMT、TET 和 IDH 的调节。(b) 组蛋白翻译后修饰包括磷酸化、乙酰化、甲基化和泛素化或 SUMO 化，这些修饰受多种因素调节，如 HAT、HDAC、HMT、HDM 等。值得注意的是，已发现这些表观遗传修饰的基因多数在人类的癌症中发生了突变，包括实体瘤和血液系统恶性肿瘤。(c) 染色质修饰和转录因子（TF）均可通过启动子区域调节基因表达。在肿瘤细胞中，通过染色质浓缩、DNA 甲基化和组蛋白脱乙酰化使基因表达沉默，从而导致分化阻滞。抑制 HDAC、DNMT 和 IDH 可以诱导癌细胞的主动转录和分化。某些 HMT（例如 MLL 和相关的融合蛋白）可以通过 DOT1L 增强 H3K79 甲基化而激活某些白血病致病基因的转录，而 DOT1L 抑制剂可能会抑制白血病致病基因以治疗白血病。2HG，2-羟基戊二酸；5hmc，5-羟甲基胞嘧啶；5mc，5-甲基胞嘧啶；α-KG，α-酮戊二酸；AID，激活诱导脱氨酶；CoA，辅助活化因子；CoR，辅助抑制因子；DNDMs，DNA 去甲基化酶；DNMT，DNA 甲基转移酶；Dubs，去泛素化酶；E1/2/3，泛素活化酶 E1、泛素交联酶 E2、泛素蛋白连接酶 E3；H，组蛋白；HAT，组蛋白乙酰转移酶；HDAC，组蛋白去乙酰化酶；HDM，组蛋白去甲基酶；HMT，组蛋白甲基转移酶；IDH，异柠檬酸脱氢酶；JMJD6，铁（Ⅱ）和 2-酮戊二酸依赖性双加氧酶 Jumonji 结构域-6 蛋白；KIs，激酶；PPs，磷酸酶；PRMTs，蛋白精氨酸甲基转移酶；Senps，SUMO-特异性蛋白酶；TDG，胸腺嘧啶-DNA 糖苷酶；TET，10-11 号染色体易位；TF，转录因子

lineage leukemia,混合细胞白血病基因 1)的异常,还发现了其他表观遗传学调节因子的突变,包括含有 SET 结构域的蛋白质(*MLL2*,*SETD2*)[31]、tet 甲基胞嘧啶双加氧酶 2(*TET2*)[32-34]、异柠檬酸脱氢酶(*IDH1*/*IDH2*)[35]、zeste 同源增强子 2(*EZH2*)[38,39]、DNA 甲基转移酶 3A(*DNMT3A*)[40,41]、附加性梳状因子 1(*ASXL1*)[36,37]等。这些突变不仅可以促进白血病的发生,还可以作为临床预后判定的分子标志物,其突变状态可能与患者的总体生存率相关。表观遗传修饰与基因的异常共同促使基因表达模式发生持续性变化,使得细胞因分化阻滞、凋亡异常或生长失控而获得选择性优势,导致肿瘤的发生。由于表观遗传修饰通常是可逆的,因此针对表观遗传修饰调节因子的治疗方法在临床应用上更具前景。

肿瘤干细胞

大多数癌症在细胞增殖和分化状态方面具有异质性。近年来,大量证据表明在实体肿瘤(肺癌、结肠癌、前列腺癌、卵巢癌、脑肿瘤、黑色素瘤等)和白血病的癌细胞中存在低分化的干细胞样细胞[42-45]。这些细胞能够自我更新并形成肿瘤包块,现在被称为肿瘤干细胞(cancer stem cell,CSC)[46]。事实上,人类单个白血病启动细胞(leukemia-initiating cell,LIC;或称白血病干细胞)即可以在动物模型中导致 AML 的发生[47]。因此,肿瘤细胞群体内亦有明确的分级,具有特定自我更新能力的 CSC 是肿瘤起始细胞,而所有其他肿瘤细胞都来自于进一步分化的 CSC(图 11-1)。

目前,CSC 的特性及其在肿瘤发生中作用机制的相关研究仍是肿瘤研究的焦点。一般而言,CSC 相当于肿瘤始动、进展、转移、复发和耐药性的驱动力[43,48]。然而,由于 CSC 表型在不同肿瘤之间有所区别,且受到起始转化以及肿瘤发展不同阶段的影响,所以对其严格定义并不容易。使用细胞表面标志物或细胞内分子通过流式细胞分析技术分选 CSC,然后进行鉴定,是目前 CSC 研究的常用方法[42,43]。但仍有很多问题需待进一步解决,如某些肿瘤缺乏特异性的 CSC 分子标志物,某些 CSC 不表达这些标志物,某些分化的癌细胞也表达与 CSC 相似的分子标志物,部分 CSC 分子标志物在正常组织的干/祖细胞也有表达,因而缺乏特异性。值得注意的是,在 CSC 中存在的某些分子途径或网络的失调,而分化的癌细胞没有这些异常,提示基因表达谱具有一定的研究价值,它们最终可能可以作为新的 CSC 标志物。目前发现 PI3K/Akt、PTEN、JAK/STAT、TGF-β、Wnt/β-联蛋白(catenin)、Hedgehog、Notch、NF-κB 和 Bcl-2 等信号通路均与 CSC 的自我更新和分化调控有关[42,43]。传统的细胞毒性化疗(cytotoxic chemotherapy)或放疗作用于具有快速增殖或分裂能力的癌细胞,而 CSC 处于相对静止的状态并且分裂缓慢,因而传统疗法通常无法对其进行清除,从而导致肿瘤细胞的再生与疾病的复发[48-50]。目前普遍认为只有当 CSC 被完全清除时,肿瘤患者才能真正被治愈。近年来科学和医学领域均关注 CSC 特性的研究,因为这些细胞为癌症治疗提供了独特的靶标。干细胞特定的表面分子、信号传导通路或肿瘤微环境的变化能够通过诱导 CSC 进入分化度更高的状态,为 CSC 干细胞性维持的重要因素。因此,CSC 靶向治疗策略致力于通过作用于这些表面分子、信号传导通路或调节肿瘤微环境以达到清除 CSC 的目的[44,45,48,49]。目前已经进行了大量的研究工作,其成果一部分已经应用到肿瘤治疗中,同时研究者们还在致力于高通量的化合物筛选以发现新的 CSC 靶向药物[51,52]。

癌细胞分化诱导药物

肿瘤诱导分化治疗是指应用特异性的药物诱导肿瘤细胞发生细胞周期停滞,或者重新启动肿瘤细胞向终末细胞分化的程序,使肿瘤细胞获得特定的功能,最终发生凋亡[53]。这一概念比较适用于血液系统恶性肿瘤,但对于实体瘤诱导分化治疗有时难以定义,通常指将恶性细胞转化为相对良性表型的过程,伴随着增殖和转移能力的降低以及出现成熟细胞标志物的表达[4]。有意思的是,一些最初被认为是分化诱导剂的药物已经被证明是直接靶向了癌蛋白,而一些新研发的靶向药物已被发现可以引发癌细胞的显著分化。迄今为止,已经鉴定了约 80 种分化诱导剂并对其进行了生物合成和改建,其中大部分试剂正在进行体外或动物模型的研究,一小部分已经用于临床治疗。

靶向于异常转录因子的药物

如前所述,TF 在正常细胞分化中起着重要作用,而在肿瘤中可能受到异常调节或存在功能异常。调节分化相关 TF 的功能和/或使其恢复正常是肿瘤诱导分化治疗的主要策略之一。在这里,我们介绍一些可以特异性靶向 TF 的诱导分化剂。

视黄酸类似化合物

视黄酸类似化合物(retinoids)是一组维生素 A 衍生物。视黄酸(retinoic acid,RA)是视黄醇的生理性活性代谢产物,可以调节正常或癌细胞的多种生物学功能,包括发育、分化、增殖和凋亡[13,54-56]。RA 最重要的异构体是全反式视黄酸(all-trans-retinoic acid,ATRA),13-顺式视黄酸(13-cRA)和 9-顺式视黄酸(9-cRA),它们具有不同的生物活性和亲和性配体[57,58]。合成的视黄酸类似化合物包括贝沙罗汀和芬维 A 胺。RA 主要通过其核受体来影响细胞分化。视黄酸受体(retinoic acid receptors,RAR;具有三个主要亚型 RAR-α/-β/-γ)和视黄酸 X 受体(retinoid X receptors,RXR;具有三个主要亚型 RXR-α/-β/-γ)以异二聚体 RAR/RXR 的形式介导 RA 的信号传导[13,56]。这些受体异二聚体能够在基因组水平与靶基因启动子上被称为视黄酸反应元件(retinoic acid response elements,RARE)的特定基序结合。RAR/RXR 在募集共激活因子(CoA)或共抑制因子(CoR)复合体的同时,分别激活或抑制基因转录。作用模式的不同取决于配体 RA 的存在与否。生理浓度的 RA(10^{-9}mol/L)能够使 RAR/RXR 释放 CoR(例如 N-CoR/SMRT 复合物和染色质重塑复合物,如 HDAC、DNMT 等)并募集 CoA(例如具有 HAT 活性的 p300/CBP 复合物),从而导致参与细胞分化(例如 C/EBPα 和 PU.1)、生长和凋亡的基因被转录激活[56,56-65]。

视黄酸类似化合物信号传导通常在癌变过程中被干扰,这表明该途径的恢复可能是一种癌症治疗潜在的选择[54,55,58,66]。有意思的是,在急性早幼粒细胞白血病(APL)细胞系(例如 NB4 和 HL60)或新鲜的原代 APL 细胞中,能够观察到 RA 诱导的分化作用[67,68]。用药理浓度(10^{-7}~10^{-6}mol/L)的 RA,特别是 ATRA 处理 APL 细胞后,这些细胞可以终末分化为形态和功能成熟的粒细胞[67]。而其他类型的急性髓细胞性白血病

(AML)细胞通常不受RA影响,类维生素A的诱导分化作用不明显,对于一部分细胞系如THP-1和U937(单核细胞白血病细胞系)、K562(CML急变期细胞系)和HEL(红白血病细胞系)有一定的诱导分化作用[59,68]。迄今为止,诱导分化治疗最成功的临床实践是在APL中使用ATRA,这将在下一节中详细讨论。

研究表明,视黄酸类似化合物可以在体外诱导多种实体肿瘤细胞系的分化,并在多种肿瘤动物模型(畸胎瘤、黑色素瘤、成神经细胞瘤、骨肉瘤和横纹肌肉瘤)中抑制肿瘤生长[57,69,70]。在甲状腺癌细胞系中,视黄酸可以诱导Ⅰ型碘甲状腺原氨酸-5′-脱碘酶和钠/碘共转运体的表达,它们是甲状腺细胞分化的标志物[71-73]。在前期临床研究中,对碘缺乏或碘摄取不足的低分化甲状腺癌,而无法行手术治疗的患者,在给予0.3~1.5mg/(kg·d)剂量的13-cRA口服5周至9个月,结果显示20%~40%的患者有放射性碘摄取的增加[73-75]。使用了^{18}F-FDG正电子放射断层成像(PET)对13-cRA治疗甲状腺癌的疗效进行评估,结果表明视黄酸类似化合物是治疗甲状腺癌具应用前景的诱导分化药物。

除了诱导分化外,类维生素A还通过其他作用方式发挥抗肿瘤作用,如抑制细胞增殖、促进细胞凋亡以及抑制血管生成和肿瘤转移[56,57]。值得注意的是,视黄酸类似化合物可以有效治疗某些皮肤癌前病变和恶性肿瘤,且效果良好[76],贝沙罗汀是首个人工合成的高选择性RXR激动剂,已被证实可以诱导皮肤T细胞淋巴瘤(cutaneous T-cell lymphoma,CTCL)细胞的凋亡,并下调凋亡抑制因子生存素(survivin)及其受体[77],因此,口服类维生素A药物已经被美国食品药品监督管理局(FDA)批准用于治疗APL和CTCL。

维生素D化合物

维生素D在细胞增殖和分化中具有多种作用[78],主要是由NR超家族成员——维生素D受体(vitamin D receptor,VDR)介导的,1,25二羟基维生素D_3(1,25D)是维生素D生理活性形式。在正常生理情况下,VDR与RXR形成VDR/RXR异二聚体,与靶基因启动子区域的维生素D反应元件(vitamin D response elements,VDRE)结合,调节靶基因的转录。当1,25D缺乏时,VDR/RXR异二聚体会募集包括HDAC在内的共抑制因子,导致转录抑制[66];而当1,25D存在时,配体可以和VDR/RXR结合,导致受体异二聚体构象发生变化,激活靶基因的转录,而在这一过程中,招募转录共激活因子是必不可少的步骤。VDR还可以直接与其他多种蛋白质(例如β-联蛋白)相互作用并调节其活性[80]。1,25D亦可以通过激活膜信号转导通路,如MAPK通路、脂质信号通路或PI3K/AKT通路,引发"快速反应"[79,81,82]。

与类维生素A的诱导分化作用相似,1,25D可以诱导多种类型的人AML细胞系(HL-60、U937、NB4、THP-1和KG-1)分化[78]。研究表明,1,25D可以在动物模型中促进白血病细胞的分化,从而显著延长了白血病移植小鼠的生存期。但是该药物的临床试验结果并不令人满意,1,25D和维生素D类似物(vitamin D analogs,VDA)在AML或MDS患者中均未使患者获益[83,84],其临床无效的重要原因可能是疾病存在异质性。另外,1,25D的治疗剂量较大而毒副作用较严重也限制了该药的临床应用,主要是药物诱发的致死性高钙血症[85]。

PPARγ激动剂

过氧化物酶体增殖物激活受体γ(peroxisome proliferator-activated receptor gamma,PPARγ)也是NR超家族的成员[89]。PPARγ与RXR形成异二聚体,然后与靶基因启动子区域中的PPARγ反应元件结合。目前已知PPARγ在多种类型细胞的增殖、分化和凋亡中发挥重要的调节作用[89]。PPARγ激动剂已被研发合成出来,包括用于治疗2型糖尿病的药物(例如曲格列酮、罗格列酮)和非甾体抗炎药(例如吲哚美辛)[59,69]。

应用激动剂激活PPARγ可以在体外和动物模型中抑制多种类型肿瘤的生长并诱导其分化,包括结肠癌、乳腺癌、前列腺癌、甲状腺癌、脂肪肉瘤、垂体腺瘤和急性白血病等[90-92]。PPARγ激动剂也可能通过影响细胞周期、细胞凋亡和肿瘤抑制基因(例如*PTEN*和*BRCA1*)的表达发挥抗肿瘤作用[59,93,94]。此外,PPARγ激动剂具有一定的"脱靶"效应,与PPARγ受体活性无关[59]。

PPARγ激动剂的临床试验已在多种恶性肿瘤中进行。早期的研究表明,在少数中度或高度恶性的脂肪肉瘤患者中罗格列酮可以诱导肿瘤向终末脂肪细胞分化[95],但该结果未能在后期的临床试验中得到证实[96]。而在乳腺癌、前列腺癌、结肠癌、肺癌和甲状腺癌的临床研究中,均未能证明TGZ治疗使得患者获益[59,73,96-98]。尽管PPARγ激动剂的临床效果并不理想,但其低毒性和与其他抗癌药物的潜在协同作用,仍促使研究者对其继续进行探索,该药仍可能是联合治疗的潜在药物。

靶向表观遗传修饰的药物

目前已知调控分化的表观遗传修饰和转录因子在多种肿瘤中存在异常,且在实体瘤和血液系统恶性肿瘤中发现了一系列调节表观遗传修饰的基因出现重现性的体细胞突变。因此,靶向调节表观遗传修饰的因子从而诱导肿瘤细胞分化的临床前和临床研究一直备受关注[99],目前大量的药物研究正在进行中,其中少数药物在某些类型的肿瘤中已经产生了可喜的结果,获得了FDA的批准。

DNMT制剂

DNA甲基化是最具特征的表观遗传修饰,是稳定的表观遗传学标记[100],其过程由DNA甲基转移酶(DNA methyltransferase,DNMT)催化介导。肿瘤抑制基因的高甲基化和DNMT的过表达被认为是肿瘤发生的关键因素,因此DNMT抑制剂也称去甲基化药物(HMA)作为抗肿瘤药物具有良好的应用前景[101,102]。迄今为止,5-氮杂胞苷[阿扎胞苷(5-Aza)]和5-氮杂-2′-脱氧胞苷[地西他滨(Dec)]是最成功的HMA,已被FDA批准用于治疗MDS或AML患者,同时5-Aza也已被FDA和欧洲药品管理局(EMA)批准用于慢性粒单核细胞白血病(CMML)的治疗[101]。HMAs的作用具有"双重机制",呈剂量依赖性,大剂量时具有细胞毒性和/或增殖抑制作用,低剂量时具有DNA去甲基化作用[101,102]。许多研究发现应用5-Aza或Dec治疗后AML细胞会发生终末分化[102-104],而Dec杀伤髓细胞性白血病细胞的作用与DNA损伤和细胞凋亡无关[102]。在某些实体肿瘤细胞中,5-Aza或Dec可以通过多种机制诱导癌细胞凋亡和衰老[105]。

临床研究表明,低剂量多次使用HMA药物(Dec 20mg/m^2,连用5天;5-Aza 75mg/m^2,连用7天;每28天一个疗程)可以发挥 DNA 去甲基作用，较高剂量治疗（Dec 45mg/m^2，连续 3 天，每 42 天一个疗程）显示更好的抗肿瘤作用[102,106-109]。在 MDS 患者中，5-Aza 治疗的总体反应率为 20%～30%，与标准治疗相比显著提高了患者生存率；而 Dec 在最佳剂量下细胞遗传学缓解率（Cyto-CR）可以达到 35%～50%，较历史对照比患者生存期明显延长[102,106-108,110,111]。在非小细胞肺癌和难治性卵巢癌等实体瘤中，HMA 与其他药物联合治疗方案的临床试验也取得了较好的结果[105,112,113]。因此，合理使用现有的 HMA 并继续努力研发针对性更强且毒性更小的新型 DNMT 抑制剂值得鼓励。

HDAC 抑制剂

作为催化组蛋白脱乙酰化的酶，HDAC 参与了细胞生长和分化的调控。研究发现，在多种癌症中存在 HDAC 的异常表达或突变以及组蛋白乙酰化修饰状态的异常[114]。因此，HDAC 已成为一类新的癌症治疗靶点（图 11-3c）。目前已经发现了一系列组蛋白脱乙酰酶抑制剂（histone deacetylase inhibitors，HDACI），如亚磺酰苯胺异羟肟酸（suberoylanilide hydroxamic acid，SAHA；伏立诺他）或丙戊酸（valproic acid，VPA）。HDACI 可促进多种实体瘤细胞（例如肺癌、前列腺癌、甲状腺癌、乳腺癌，软骨肉瘤和胶质母细胞瘤）和造血系统恶性肿瘤细胞系的生长停滞、细胞分化和凋亡，而对正常组织作用很小[69,115-121]。例如，SAHA 和 VPA 能够诱导表达 AML1-ETO 的 AML 细胞系 Kasumi-1 在体外发生分化和早期凋亡，在小鼠白血病异种移植模型中也具有类似的作用。

基于临床前的研究结果，多项 HDACI 的临床试验也在开展。前期研究结果显示，SAHA 在一系列血液系统恶性肿瘤中有效[122]，尤其是在难治性皮肤 T 细胞淋巴瘤（CTCL）患者中疗效显著，因此成为 FDA 批准的首个 HDACI 药物。另外一项临床试验中，应用 VPA 和 ATRA 联合治疗 8 例难治性或高危 AML 患者，初步研究结果显示，7 例患者临床获益，并出现外周血白血病细胞向粒-单核细胞分化。尽管在血液系统恶性肿瘤治疗方面 HDACI 取得了较好的结果，但实体瘤患者中 HDACI 治疗的临床数据仍不足[123]。今后，HDACI 与常规抗肿瘤治疗的联合用药在实体瘤中还需进一步探索。

DOT1L 抑制剂

MLL 基因定位于 11q23 染色体，该基因编码 SET 结构域的组蛋白甲基转移酶，在特定基因催化组蛋白 H3 的赖氨酸 4 位点（H3K4）发生甲基化[124]。*MLL* 对于胎儿和成人的造血功能至关重要，因为它调节 HOX 基因以及一些造血干/祖细胞（HSPC）扩增和分化的关键调节基因的表达[125-127]。*MLL* 基因异常往往与患者预后不良有关，在婴儿白血病中的发生率占 70%以上，而在成人 AML 约为 10%的发生率[128]。*MLL* 基因异常包括 MLL 蛋白水平表达异常、*MLL* 部分串联重复（PTD）、累及 *MLL* 的染色体易位（MLL 重排）而形成融合基因。融合基因被翻译成融合蛋白，其 MLL 的催化结构域（SET 结构域）丢失，与之融合的伙伴基因部分能够与组蛋白 H3K79 甲基转移酶 DOT1L 相互作用[129,130]，因此融合蛋白在 MLL 部分保留了基因特异性识别元件，同时获得了将 DOT1L 募集到这些位置的能力。由于招募 DOT1L 而引起的异位 H3K79 甲基化导致白血病相关基因（例如 *HOXA9* 和 *MEIS1*）的表达增强[131]，DOT1L 促进了 MLL 融合蛋白的恶性转化能力，在白血病发生过程中发挥了催化驱动作用。

因此，有人提出抑制 DOT1L 可能是 MLL 相关白血病的治疗策略之一（图 11-3c）。体外和体内实验证明，DOT1L 的特异性抑制剂 EPZ-5676 可以通过引起细胞周期停滞并促进细胞分化来选择性杀死携带 *MLL* 融合基因的细胞[132]。1 期临床试验数据表明，EPZ-5676 用于治疗复发难治性 *MLL* 重排的急性白血病患者，总体上安全性和耐受性良好（NCT01684150），34 名患者有 8 名获得生物学或临床缓解，包括 2 名完全缓解和 1 名部分缓解[133]。其他 DOT1L 抑制剂（例如 EPZ4777 和 SYC-522）也已被证明可促进 MLL 相关白血病细胞的分化和凋亡[134-136]。有趣的是，生物信息学分析表明 DOT1L 可能在乳腺癌的发病机制中亦发挥作用，体外研究表明 DOT1L 抑制剂可选择性抑制乳腺癌细胞的增殖、自我更新和转移能力并诱导细胞分化[137]。

异柠檬酸脱氢酶抑制剂

近来，在人类神经胶质瘤、黑色素瘤、甲状腺癌、软骨肉瘤和 AML 中都发现了异柠檬酸脱氢酶（isocitrate dehydrogenase，IDH）的体细胞突变，IDH 有两种酶即 IDH1 和 IDH2，突变位点集中在 IDH1 的 132 位精氨酸（R132）或 IDH2 的 140 位、172 位精氨酸（R140 和 R172），这些精氨酸位点位于酶的催化口袋中，因此赋予了这些蛋白酶新的活性，即将 α-酮戊二酸（α-KG）催化为 2-羟基戊二酸（2- HG）[140,141]。高浓度的 2-HG，是一种“竞争性合成代谢物”，已被证明可以抑制 α-KG 依赖性双加氧酶，包括组蛋白和 DNA 去甲基化酶，如上所述，这些都是表观遗传学调节的主要因子（图 11-3a）[140-143]。研究发现，癌症相关的 IDH 突变可以诱导细胞分化阻滞，从而促进肿瘤发生，因此可能成为诱导分化治疗的潜在靶点[143,144]。与此一致的是，选择性的 IDH1 突变 R132H 抑制剂（AGI-5198）可以诱导与胶质细胞分化相关的基因表达，并促进携带 IDH1 突变 R132H（mIDH1）细胞向星形胶质细胞分化[145]，而在 mIDH1 胶质瘤异种移植小鼠中，阻断 mIDH1 可以抑制具有 ID 神经胶质瘤细胞的生长，但对于野生型 IDH1 神经胶质瘤细胞的生长没有作用。另外，AGI-6780 是一种新研发的能有效选择性抑制 IDH2 突变 R140Q 的小分子化合物，能够在体外诱导红白血病细胞系 TF-1 和 AML 原代细胞的分化[146]。这些发现都表明针对肿瘤相关的突变类型的 IDH1 或 IDH2 靶向抑制药物能够诱导肿瘤细胞的分化，为癌症靶向诱导分化治疗的临床应用进一步提供了有力的证据。

最近有了 AG-120（IDH1 突变的抑制剂）和 AG-221（IDH2 突变的抑制剂）前期临床研究取得进展的报道（https://www.clinicaltrials.gov/）[144]。AG-120 具有良好的耐受性，在进展期 IDH1 突变阳性的 AML 患者中显示出令人鼓舞的临床疗效，似乎能够将患者体内白血病细胞中的 2-HG 降低至正常水平，并使白血病细胞分化为成熟粒细胞。17 例患者中有 14 例可评估疗效，其中 7 例患者对药物有反应，4 例获得了完全缓解（Daniel Pollyea 于第 26 届欧洲癌症研究与治疗组织专题讨论会发表）。与临床观察的结果一致，AG-120 在体外降低了细胞内 2-HG 水平并诱导了携带 IDH1 突变 R132H 的 TF-1 细胞系和 IDH1 突变的 AML 患者原代细胞的分化（第 56 届美国血液学会的年会（ASH）会议，摘要 70455）。在第 56 届 ASH 会议上公示了 AG-221 单药治疗 IDH2 突变阳性的进展期血液系统恶性肿瘤患者的1期临床试验初步结果，AG-221具有良好的安全性，并且使得患者得到了持久性的临床获益（摘要70721），该研究仍在进行中，已经入组的48例患者中，有20例患者达到了客观缓解，包括12例完全缓解和8例部分缓解，且疗效持续时间可长达8个月。有意思的是，在IDH2突变的白血病小鼠模型和原代人AML异种移植动物模型中，AG-221亦可以诱导白血病细胞分化并损伤IDH2突变的白血病细胞的自我更新能力（第56届ASH会议，摘要70656和76334）。

事实上，肿瘤诱导分化治疗药物的研究逐渐取得了进展。APL作为诱导分化治疗的经典疾病模型备受关注，大量临床数据证实了诱导分化药物可使绝大部分患者得以治愈。此外，其他的一些诱导分化的药物在临床前和临床试验中也显示出较好的治疗效果，肿瘤诱导分化治疗虽然仍处于起步阶段，但却为数以百万的癌症患者带来了希望。

APL——肿瘤诱导分化治疗的成功典范

APL是AML的M3亚型，不仅具有特殊的临床表现，而且具有独特的分子生物学发病机制和有效的靶向诱导分化治疗方法。

APL的临床治疗策略

APL在1957年首次被描述，是急性白血病中最为凶险的一种类型[147]。APL患者的骨髓存在异常早幼粒细胞的积聚，疾病进展迅速，如不进行治疗患者在数周时间内即可能死亡，患者具有特征性的临床表现，为弥散性血管内凝血（disseminated intravascular coagulation，DIC）或纤溶亢进引起的严重出血综合征。在ATRA治疗之前的时代，应用联合化疗的APL患者的5年生存率仅有23%~35%[148]。受中国传统理念“改邪归正”和西方医学诱导癌细胞分化的启发，20世纪70年代末开始，上海血液研究所（SIH）的科学家开始了对白血病诱导分化治疗的研究[148]。

1980年，美国的一个研究组报道了13-cRA作用于HL-60细胞系体外诱导细胞终末分化的结果[67]，在少数几例APL个案中，用13-cRA治疗后患者获得了临床改善或完全缓解，并伴有早幼粒细胞的分化成熟和凝血功能障碍的改善[149-151]。与此同时，SIH研究组在专注于ATRA治疗作用的研究，并首次报道了ATRA治疗APL的临床试验研究结果[152]，令人振奋的是，接受ATRA单药治疗的24例APL患者（16例新诊断和8例蒽环类耐药的病例）均获得了完全缓解，同时研究者观察到患者体内的早幼粒细胞分化成为成熟的中性粒细胞，这一结果很快得到了大量来自世界各地其他临床数据的证实[59,148]。ATRA治疗已经成为新诊断APL患者诱导治疗的标准方案，随后联合ATRA与化疗可以使APL的疗效进一步提高。此外，ATRA和化疗在APL的巩固和维持治疗中可以降低复发率的作用亦得到证实。通过应用该治疗策略，APL患者的5年总体生存率（overall survival，OS）提升至约70%~80%[69,148,153-155]。ATRA常规剂量为45mg/（m^2·d），而SIH的ATRA推荐剂量为25mg/（m^2·d），因为减少ATRA初始剂量可以降低ATRA的副作用，且获得了与常规剂量相同的治疗效果[156]。

尽管ATRA/化疗的联合方案已被证实是非常有效的APL治疗方法，但仍有约20%~30%的APL患者复发[157-159]。自20世纪90年代初以来，三氧化二砷（ATO）的应用进一步改善了APL的临床疗效。体外研究表明，ATO可以同时诱导APL细胞的分化和凋亡，其作用是剂量依赖性的，与ATRA诱导分化治疗相比，ATO诱导细胞分化的作用相对较弱，分化是部分性的[160]。临床上，经ATRA/化疗联合治疗后仍难治或复发的APL与新诊断的APL应用ATO治疗均可达到完全缓解，表明ATRA与ATO之间无交叉耐药性[161]。临床试验的结果也证实了与单独使用ATRA或ATO相比，ATRA/ATO的联合方案治疗新诊断APL患者，其生存期更长[148,162,163]，其疗效不受FLT3突变状态的影响，而在接受ATRA/化疗治疗的APL患者中FLT3突变是不良预后因素[164]。因此，目前APL治疗新的策略尽量减少化疗的应用，而将ATRA联合ATO作为主要治疗方案。ATRA和ATO联合治疗方案的完全缓解率约95%，5年OS达92%[162]。值得注意的是，根据Sanz评分（表11-1），APL患者可以分成不同危险度的组别，不含化疗的联合方案治疗非高危APL患者的2年EFS和OS率非常高，分别为97%和99%[158,165]。基于以上研究结果，在一些新近更新的权威指南中，基于ATRA/ATO的治疗方案已成为APL治疗的一线方案。尽管巩固或维持治疗的具体细节尚未达成共识，但普遍认为应该依次给予ATRA、ATO和基于蒽环类药物的化疗。APL治疗的建议列于表11-2和表11-3中。

表11-1 APL危险分层的Sanz积分

特征	低危	中危	高危
白细胞/（$\times10^9$/L）	≤10	≤10	>10
血小板/（$\times10^9$/L）	>40	≤40	≤40

表11-2 APL的推荐治疗方案（中国）

	非高危APL	高危APL
诱导治疗	ATRA 25mg/（m^2·d）×（28~42d）或直到临床缓解 ATO 0.16mg/（kg·d）×（28~35d）或直到骨髓缓解 HU 20~40mg/（kg·d）（当白细胞>10×10^9/L）	ATRA 25mg/（m^2·d）×（28~42d）或直到临床缓解 ATO 0.16mg/（kg·d）×（28~35d）或直到骨髓缓解 IDA 6~8mg/（m^2·d）×3d或DNR 45mg/（m^2·d）×3d
巩固治疗	DA：DNR 45mg/（m^2·d）×3d+Ara-C 100~200mg/（m^2·d）×7d MA：MTZ 6~8mg/（m^2·d）×3d+Ara-C 100~200mg/（m^2·d）×7d HA：HHT 2~3mg/（m^2·d）×3d+Ara-C 100~200mg/（m^2·d）×7d	DA或［DNR+Ara-C 1.5~2.5g/（m^2·d）×3d］ MA或［MTZ+Ara-C 1.5~2.5g/（m^2·d）×3d］ HA或［HHT+Ara-C 1.5~2.5g/（m^2·d）×3d］

续表

	非高危 APL	高危 APL
维持治疗	ATRA 25mg/m²×28d ATO 0.16mg/kg×28d 6-MP+MTX:6-MP 100mg/d,第 1~7、15~21 天 MTX 20mg/d,第 1、8、15、21 天 5 周期连续使用 ATRA、ATO 和化疗	ATRA 25mg/m²×28d ATO 0.16mg/kg×28d 6-MP+MTX:6-MP 100mg/d,第 1~7、15~21 天 MTX 20mg/d,第 1、8、15、21 天 5 周期连续使用 ATRA、ATO 和化疗

Ara-C,阿糖胞苷;ATO,三氧化二砷;ATRA,全反式维甲酸;HU,羟基脲;IDA,去甲氧柔红霉素;DNR,柔红霉素;MTZ,米托蒽醌;HHT,高三尖杉酯碱;6-MP,6-巯基嘌呤;MTX,甲氨蝶呤。

表 11-3　APL 的推荐治疗方案(2015 年 NCCN 指南)

	诱导治疗	巩固治疗
高危 APL	ATRA 45mg/(m²·d)直到临床缓解+DNR 50mg/(m²·d)×4+Ara-C 200mg/(m²·d)×7d ATRA 45mg/(m²·d)直到临床缓解+DNR 60mg/(m²·d)×3d+Ara-C 200mg/(m²·d)×7d ATRA 45mg/(m²·d)直到临床缓解+ IDA 12mg/(m²·d),第 2、4、6、8 天	ATO 0.15mg/(kg·d)×5d/周×5 周×2 周期,然后[ATRA 45mg/(m²·d)×7d+DNR 50mg/(m²·d)×3d]×2 周期 [DNR 60mg/(m²·d)×3d+Ara-C 200mg/(m²·d)×7d],然后(DNR 45mg/(m²·d)×3d+Ara-C 1.5~2g/m² q12h×3) [ATRA 45mg/(m²·d)×15+IDA 5mg/(m²·d)×3d+Ara-C 1g/(m²·d)×4d],然后[ATRA 45mg/(m²·d)×15d+MTZ 10mg/(m²·d)×5d],然后[ATRA 45mg/(m²·d)×15d+IDA 12mg/(m²·d)×1d+Ara-C 150mg/m² q8h×4]
非高危 APL	ATRA 45mg/(m²·d)×(1~36d)+IDA 6~12mg/(m²·d)第 2、4、6、8 天+ATO 0.15mg/(kg·d)×(9~26d) ATRA 45mg/(m²·d)直到临床缓解+ATO 0.15mg/(kg·d) 直到骨髓缓解 ATRA 45mg/(m²·d)直到临床缓解+DNR 50mg/(m²·d)×4d+Ara-C 200mg/(m²·d)×7d ATRA 45mg/(m²·d)直到临床缓解+DNR 60mg/(m²·d)×3d+Ara-C 200mg/(m²·d)×7d ATRA 45mg/(m²·d)直到临床缓解+ IDA 12mg/(m²·d)第 2、4、6、8 天	[ATRA 45mg/(m²·d)×28d+ATO 0.15mg/(kg·d)×28d],然后[ATRA 45mg/(m²·d)×7d/2 周×3 + ATO 0.15mg/(kg·d)×5d/周×5 周] ATO 0.15mg/(kg·d)×5d/周×4 周/8 周×4 周期+ATRA 45mg/(m²·d)×2 周/4 周×7 周期 ATO 0.15mg/(kg·d)×5d/周×5 周×2 周期,然后[ATRA 50mg/(m²·d)×7d+DNR 50mg/(m²·d)×3d]×2 周期 [DNR 60mg/(m²·d)×3d+Ara-C 200mg/(m²·d)×7d]×1 周期,然后[DNR 45mg/(m²·d)×3d+Ara-C 1g/m² q12h×4]×1 周期 [ATRA 45mg/(m²·d)×15d+IDA 5mg/(m²·d)×3d],然后[ATRA 45mg/(m²·d)×15d+MTZ 10mg/(m²·d)×5d],然后[ATRA 45mg/(m²·d)×15d+IDA 12mg/(m²·d)×1d]

Ara-C,阿糖胞苷;ATO,三氧化二砷;ATRA,全反式维甲酸;HU,羟基脲;IDA,去甲氧柔红霉素;DNR,柔红霉素;MTZ,米托蒽醌;HHT,高三尖杉酯碱;6-MP,6-巯基嘌呤;MTX,甲氨蝶呤;NCCN,美国国家综合癌症网。

ATO 的常规给药方式是静脉途径,研究发现口服剂型在复发性 APL 中亦具有活性,其疗效在随后的前期临床研究中得以评估。复方黄黛片(Realgar-Indigo naturalis formula,RIF)是一种口服中药复方制剂,其主要成分为四硫化四砷(As_4S_4),As_4S_4 是砷剂的另外一种存在形式,目前已有报道显示传统中医应用 RIF 治疗 APL 临床有效[167,168]。且临床随机对照研究也表明 RIF 和静脉 ATO 治疗 APL,两组的完全缓解率、3 年 OS 或 2 年无病生存率均无显著差异[169-170]。这些研究证实了长期口服砷剂的可行性和安全性,但其安全性数据仍需要更长的随访时间,目前在美国或欧洲尚无口服的砷剂用于治疗 APL。

随着 APL 的预后逐渐提高,患者早期死亡(与出血、分化综合征或感染有关)和复发(包括中枢神经系统复发)的问题变得越来越重要。对于具有 APL 临床和病理特征的患者,应在首次疑诊 APL 时就开始应用 ATRA,无需等待遗传学结果[166]。尽早应用 ATRA 可以预防致命性的出血并发症。分化综合征(differentiation syndrome,DS)是 ATRA 或 ATO 治疗中的常见并发症,在美国和欧洲的发病率约为 25%[171,172],但在东亚人群中相对较少(5%~10%)[154,162]。DS 的体征和症状包括白细胞增高,伴间质性肺浸润引起的呼吸困难,外周性水肿,不明原因发热,体重增加,低血压和急性肾衰竭等。及早发现 DS 并立即应用化疗和地塞米松(10mg,每日两次)治疗,死亡率可降至 3%甚至更低[172,173],诊断时伴有白细胞计数高(WBC>30 ×10⁹/L)的患者给予糖皮质激素预防 DS 可能会使患者受益。另外,对于高危 APL 患者,推荐常规性预防中枢神经系统(CNS)白血病,给予甲氨蝶呤 5~10mg、阿糖胞苷 40~50mg 和地塞米松 5mg,一般 6~8 次[166]。另一个问题是 ATO 的副作用,因为长期以来砷剂都被认为是烈性毒药。实际上,包含 ATO 的治疗方案被证明是非常安全的,常见的不良反应包括轻微的骨髓抑制、肝毒性、胃肠道反应和神经毒性,均可以控制并且通常是可逆的,一般不需要停药[162,166]。在极少数情况下,可观察到由于心电图 QT 间隔延长而导致的心律不齐，可以通过采取适当的预防措施和停药来控制[174]。ATO 维持治疗后停止治疗 2 年时患者的尿液砷浓度低于一些国家或地区政府机构建议的安全限值，但血浆、指甲和头发中的砷含量略高于健康对照组[162]。

APL 的发生和治疗机制

目前已经明确，t(15;17)(q22;q21)染色体易位引起的 PML-RARα 基因融合是 APL 发生的关键驱动力，它对 RARα 和 PML 相关途径通路起主要的负向调节作用[175]。融合蛋白可以抑制造血分化所需靶基因的转录表达，并导致白血病干细胞(LIC)的增殖和自我更新增加[175-177]。通过募集 CoR，PML-RARα 融合蛋白与 RXR 受体结合，在靶基因的 RARE 处起组成型转录抑制因子的作用，从而导致特征性的分化阻滞[148,176,178]。在正常细胞中，PML 蛋白多聚化形成多蛋白亚核结构，称为 PML 核体(PML-NB)[179]，PML-NB 已被证明在 DNA 损伤修复、凋亡、生长、衰老和血管生成中起着重要作用，最近发现其在 HSPC 维持中也同样重要。在 APL 细胞中，由于 PML/PML-RARα 异源复合物的形成，导致 PML-NB 被破坏，从而干扰了 PML 的正常生物学功能[180]。该机制可能与 RAR/RXR 通路异常共同起作用，使得 APL 患者的造血细胞发生特异性的分化阻滞并获得自我更新能力，从而将具有定向分化的 HSPC 转化为永生化的白血病干细胞(图 11-4)。

APL 发病机制中 PML-RARα 起关键作用，而 ATRA 和 ATO 对于 APL 的治疗特异性强且疗效好，提示 PML-RARα 是 APL 治疗特异性的潜在分子基础。大量研究证实了 ATRA 和 ATO 可以通过不同但互补的机制发挥作用，为两种药物联合使用以实现协同功效和降低毒性提供了生物学依据。在药理学水平(10^{-7}～10^{-6} mol/L)，ATRA 与融合蛋白中 RARα 部分的配体结合域(ligand-binding domain，LBD)相结合，并诱导嵌合受体的构象变化[181,182]，这导致 CoR 复合体的置换和 CoA 复合体的募集并从靶基因启动子结合区域将 PML-RARα 解离，从而恢复了野生型 RARα 的功能并逆转了细胞分化阻滞[148,63,178,183]。ATRA 还可以引起 PML-RARα 癌蛋白降解并导致细胞核结构的恢复和 PML-NB 的重组，RARα 信号传导途径的重新恢复使 APL 细胞分化，疾病得以控制。尽管 ATRA 和蒽环类药物是非常有效的 APL 治疗方法，但 APL 患者仍可能复发，这可能是由于 ATRA 无法清除 LIC。最初的细胞和分子机制研究发现，ATO 对 APL 细胞的作用呈剂量依赖性[160,187]。在低浓度时 ATO 诱导 APL 细胞部分分化，而在高浓度时主要诱导细胞凋亡的发生，这两种作用都与 PML-RARα 的降解有关。ATO 通过直接结合 PML 部分的 RBCC 结构域来降解

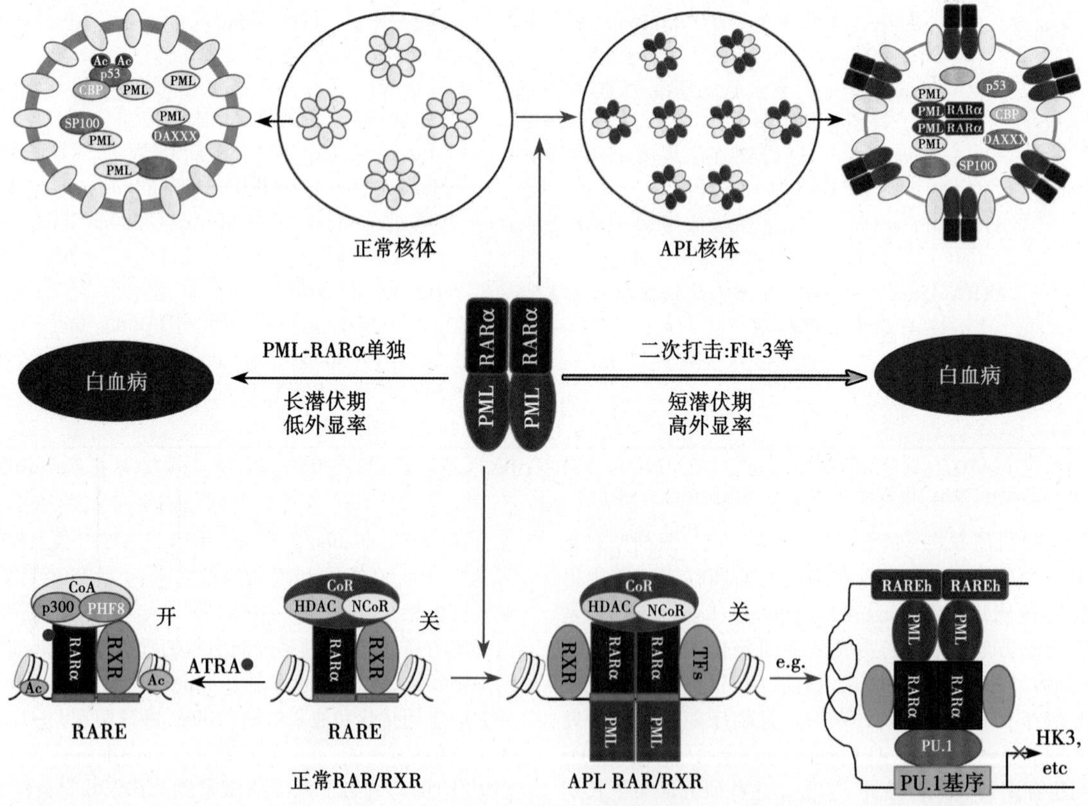

图 11-4 APL 发病的分子机制。PML-RARα 在 APL 白血病发生过程中起着关键作用，它对 RARα-和 PML 相关途径起主要的负向调节作用。在生理条件下，RAR/RXR 异二聚体与靶基因启动子上名为视黄酸反应元件(RARE)的特定基序结合，并招募共激活因子(CoA)或共抑制因子(CoR)复合物差异性地激活或抑制基因转录，招募过程取决于配体的存在与否，例如 ATRA。通过招募 CoR，与 RXR 共受体结合的融合蛋白在靶基因的 RARE 处起组成型转录抑制因子的作用。另一方面，PML 蛋白在正常细胞中多聚化形成多蛋白亚核结构，被称为 PML 核体(PML-NB)。在 APL 细胞中，由于 PML/PML-RARα 异源复合物的形成，PML-NB 被破坏。RAR，视黄酸受体；RARE，视黄酸反应元件；RXR，视黄酸 X 受体

PML-RARα 和 PML，其具体机制为 ATO 的结合导致 PML 的构象变化，PML-RARα 和 PML 发生蛋白质-蛋白质聚集和 SUMO 化（sumoylation）[188]。同时，ATO 诱导的氧化应激使 PML 通过二硫键交联，从而促进 PML 同源二聚化[189]。SUMO 化的 PML 和 PML-RARα 募集泛素连接酶 RNF4，最终通过蛋白酶体降解[190,191]。此外，砷还可以通过与 PML-RARα 以外的其他机制发挥作用，例如由线粒体介导的途径起促凋亡作用、诱导 DNA 损伤、影响端粒酶活性，促进自噬等[148,192]。值得注意的是，ATO 可以通过多种途径清除 LIC，这可能是 APL 患者用 ATO 治疗获得最终成功的关键因素[148,177,183,192,193]。PML 和 PML-

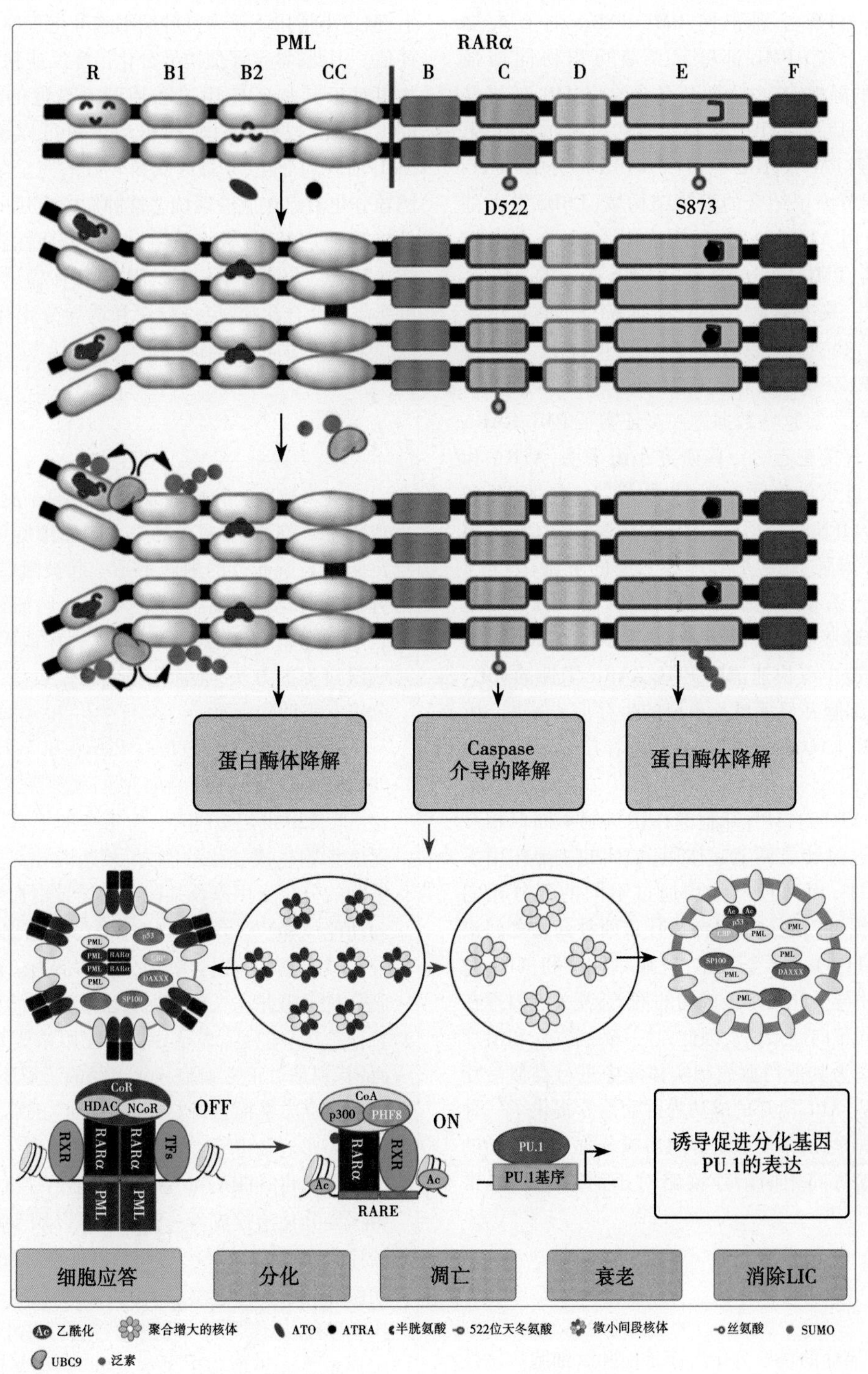

图 11-5　APL 的治疗机制。ATRA 和 ATO 分别靶向 PML-RARα 的 C-末端和 N-末端，从而促进 PML-RARα 癌蛋白的降解。ATRA 结合癌蛋白 RARα 部分的配体结合域（LBD），而 ATO 结合 PML 部分的 RBCC 结构域，从而诱发融合蛋白的构象变化和降解。PML-RARα 的降解导致核结构的恢复和 PML-NB 的重组。ATRA 的结合还导致 CoR 复合物的置换和 CoA 复合物的募集，并从靶基因的启动子中解除 PML-RARα 的结合，从而恢复了野生型 RARα 的功能。ATRA 和 ATO 的协同作用导致多种细胞效应，包括白血病细胞的分化、凋亡和衰老，重要的是消除了白血病干细胞（LIC）。ATO，三氧化二砷；ATRA，全反式维甲酸；SUMO，SUMO 化；UBC9，泛素结合酶 9

RARα 充分快速的降解是 LIC 清除从而疾病得以治愈所必需的[194,195]，而 ATO 可以达到此效应。砷还可以通过抑制 Notch 通路、拮抗 Hedgehog-Gli 通路以及抑制 NF-κB 和 β-catenin 来促进 LIC 的清除。作用机制的多样性可能是砷剂在 APL 中作为单药或联合药物具有很强活性的原因。

由于 ATRA 和 ATO 分别靶向 PML-RARα 的 C-末端（RARα 部分）和 N-末端（PML 部分），两者可以协同增强 PML-RARα 癌蛋白的降解，这也为两药联合治疗 APL 效果最优提供合理的解释。应用 ATRA/化疗治疗后复发的 APL 患者中约 40%能检测到 PML-RARα 癌蛋白 RARα 部分中与 ATRA 结合或共同核调节因子结合的配体结构域（LBD）发生基因突变[196-198]，而使用 ATRA/ATO/化疗治疗后，少数 APL 患者会出现复发/耐药，PML-RARα 癌蛋白 PML 部分的基因突变可能是其原因之一，突变后 PML-RARα 与 ATO 的直接结合位点被破坏[199,200]。另外，少数 APL 患者携带由 t(11;17)(q23;q21)产生的 PLZF-RARα 融合基因，这些患者对 ATRA 和 ATO 治疗耐药[201,202]。这些数据进一步证实了 PML-RARα 是 ATRA 和 ATO 的直接靶点。一些研究小组表明，ATRA 和 ATO 在多种途径中显示出协同作用[148,176,203,204]，包括 TF 和辅因子、钙信号激活、IFN 途径活化、蛋白酶体系统激活、细胞周期阻滞、细胞凋亡增强、端粒酶和端粒长度的下调，cAMP/PKA 活性上调和通过诱导细胞膜砷转运蛋白（AQP9）的表达来增强 APL 细胞对砷吸收等。最近的研究表明，ATRA/ATO 联合在小鼠 APL 模型中可快速清除 PML-RARα 阳性的 LIC，从而完全杀灭 APL 细胞并显著延长小鼠的生存期[177,194]。所有这些都在 ATRA 和 ATO 联合治疗 APL 患者疗效显著的治疗机制中发挥作用。

总之，ATRA 和 ATO 对 APL 细胞的作用机制不同但相互有交叉，ATRA 主要通过转录调节起作用，ATO 的主要作用发生在蛋白质调节水平，而两种药物均通过不同的部分靶向 PML-RARα，这些数据可以进一步解释为什么两种药物之间没有交叉耐药性（图 11-5）。迄今为止，应用 ATRA 和 ATO 对 APL 的治疗是癌症诱导分化治疗最成功的例子，其关键因素在于两种药物能够协同靶向癌蛋白。因此，这一疾病发病和治疗机制研究历史可以作为其他白血病和实体瘤中进行类似治疗的范例。更重要的是，APL 治疗的成功为肿瘤治疗提供了一种新的思路，诱导分化治疗从本质上是针对影响分化途径分子的靶向治疗，而联合或协同靶向治疗策略对于消除 CSC 非常有效。

展望

综上所述，针对癌症的诱导分化治疗是使肿瘤细胞从恶性转变为良性的过程，其成功为科学家和临床医生获得更好的肿瘤治疗效果带来了希望。然而，对于除 APL 以外的其他实体瘤和血液恶性肿瘤，诱导分化治疗的研究和应用才刚刚起步，其中一个主要的挑战是癌症的组织病理学分型和临床阶段的复杂性，导致缺乏一个理想的反映肿瘤进展的模型。建立表型上具有肿瘤起始组织类型特征，而形态上能够体现肿瘤细胞向良性细胞转化的肿瘤模型可能有助于肿瘤诱导分化治疗研究的成功。另外，目前对于大多数肿瘤缺乏有效的能用于评估诱导分化治疗效果的明确标志物，在体内往往难以评估药效是通过细胞毒性还是诱导细胞分化实现的，这也是诱导分化研究滞后的原因。经典的治疗反应评估主要集中在肿瘤团块的缩小上，但这不适用于仅恢复肿瘤细胞分化程序的分化疗法的反应评估。因此，鉴定评估诱导分化治疗反应精准的新型生物标志物组对于其临床应用迫在眉睫。最近的证据表明，靶向除 PML-RARα 以外的白血病驱动蛋白可以诱导一些其他类型 AML 细胞的分化，并最终获得较好的完全缓解，进一步拓宽了诱导分化治疗在血液系统恶性肿瘤中应用的道路。尽管如此，目前看来实体瘤比大多数白血病的异质性要强得多，并且其发病涉及更复杂的分子机制。因此，实体瘤诱导分化治疗的发展可能需要联合化疗、免疫疗法和诱导分化药物多方位的方法，以产生多重协同靶向作用。

总结

大多数人类肿瘤表现出异常的细胞分化特征，通常伴随着增殖和/或凋亡的失调。癌细胞可以在分化的特定阶段与所涉及的细胞谱系一起被阻滞，否则它们可能分化为不恰当的细胞类型。因此，肿瘤诱导分化治疗代表了旨在重新激活内源性分化程序或阻滞癌细胞分化/成熟过程的方法，通常伴随着恶性表型的消失和至少部分正常表型的恢复。

诱导分化的概念是由 Pierce 和 Verneyin 在 1961 年的研究中首次提出，当时他们观察到畸胎瘤细胞的分化[205]。20 世纪 70 年代，有重要的报道证明了 DMSO 对促红细胞生成分化的能力，某些诱导剂对神经母细胞瘤细胞的分化作用以及某些药物诱导白血病细胞出现形态和功能成熟[59,67,206-208]。因此，在体外细胞实验中，许多分子被证明具有诱导癌症分化的潜力。触发肿瘤细胞克服分化受阻并进入凋亡途径已成为杀死恶性细胞的理想替代疗法。但是，诱导分化治疗历来受到许多因素的阻碍，特别是对正常细胞分化途径的了解不足，而且较细胞毒性治疗方案而言，诱导癌细胞向“正常”细胞/组织的转变过程要复杂得多[69]。

直到将 ATRA 和 ATO 应用于治疗 APL 的成功，才使得诱导分化治疗成为一种真正可以用于临床实践的肿瘤治疗方法[53]。这一突破使 APL 从曾经的恶性程度最高的疾病转变为治愈率最高的人类癌症之一，其 5 年 OS 率达到 90%以上[148]。另外，在过去几年中，对于分化途径的理解方面也取得了进展，这些途径与调节细胞增殖和存活的途径相互影响，并且对其他类型白血病的分子靶向治疗亦表现出了诱导分化作用，其应用潜能需要在临床上进一步探索。

本章重点介绍了诱导分化治疗的基本理论以及这种新型疗法的临床成果。

致谢

这项工作得到了中国国家重点基础研究项目（973：2013CB966803）、“十二五”科研重大项目（2013ZX09303302）、卫生部项目（201202003）、国家重点实验室优秀项目（81123005）、国家自然科学基金（81170519）和教育部高校新世纪优秀人才计划（NCET-13-1037）的部分支持。

（陈赛娟 颜晓菁 周光飚 陈竺 译）

参考文献

The complete reference list can be found on the Wiley Companion Digital Edition of this title (see inside front cover for login instructions).

3 Regalo G, Leutz A. Hacking cell differentiation: transcriptional rerouting in reprogramming, lineage infidelity and metaplasia. *EMBO Mol Med*. 2013;**5**:1154–1164.

4 Xu WP, Zhang X, Xie WF. Differentiation therapy for solid tumors. *J Dig Dis*. 2014;**15**:159–165.

5 Sive JI, Gottgens B. Transcriptional network control of normal and leukaemic haematopoiesis. *Exp Cell Res*. 2014;**329**:255–264.

20 Taby R, Issa JP. Cancer epigenetics. *CA Cancer J Clin*. 2010;**60**:376–392.

22 Chen T, Dent SY. Chromatin modifiers and remodellers: regulators of cellular differentiation. *Nat Rev Genet*. 2014;**15**:93–106.

28 Shih AH, Abdel-Wahab O, Patel JP, Levine RL. The role of mutations in epigenetic regulators in myeloid malignancies. *Nat Rev Cancer*. 2012;**12**:599–612.

42 Pattabiraman DR, Weinberg RA. Tackling the cancer stem cells – what challenges do they pose? *Nat Rev Drug Discov*. 2014;**13**:497–512.

43 Chen K, Huang YH, Chen JL. Understanding and targeting cancer stem cells: therapeutic implications and challenges. *Acta Pharmacol Sin*. 2013;**34**:732–740.

53 Pettersson F, Miller WH Jr, Nervi C, et al. The 12th international conference on differentiation therapy: targeting the aberrant growth, differentiation and cell death programs of cancer cells. *Cell Death Differ*. 2011;**18**:1231–1233.

56 Ablain J, de The H. Retinoic acid signaling in cancer: the parable of acute promyelocytic leukemia. *Int J Cancer*. 2014;**135**:2262–2272.

57 Connolly RM, Nguyen NK, Sukumar S. Molecular pathways: current role and future directions of the retinoic acid pathway in cancer prevention and treatment. *Clin Cancer Res*. 2013;**19**:1651–1659.

59 Nowak D, Stewart D, Koeffler HP. Differentiation therapy of leukemia: 3 decades of development. *Blood*. 2009;**113**:3655–3665.

69 Cruz FD, Matushansky I. Solid tumor differentiation therapy – is it possible? *Oncotarget*. 2012;**3**:559–567.

73 Haugen BR. Redifferentiation therapy in advanced thyroid cancer. *Curr Drug Targets Immune Endocr Metabol Disord*. 2004;**4**:175–180.

79 Hughes PJ, Marcinkowska E, Gocek E, Studzinski GP, Brown G. Vitamin D3-driven signals for myeloid cell differentiation – implications for differentiation therapy. *Leuk Res*. 2010;**34**:553–565.

86 Deeb KK, Trump DL, Johnson CS. Vitamin D signalling pathways in cancer: potential for anticancer therapeutics. *Nat Rev Cancer*. 2007;**7**:684–700.

90 Grommes C, Landreth GE, Heneka MT. Antineoplastic effects of peroxisome proliferator-activated receptor gamma agonists. *Lancet Oncol*. 2004;**5**:419–429.

99 Azad N, Zahnow CA, Rudin CM, Baylin SB. The future of epigenetic therapy in solid tumours—lessons from the past. *Nat Rev Clin Oncol*. 2013;**10**:256–266.

101 Gnyszka A, Jastrzebski Z, Flis S. DNA methyltransferase inhibitors and their emerging role in epigenetic therapy of cancer. *Anticancer Res*. 2013;**33**:2989–2996.

102 Saunthararajah Y. Key clinical observations after 5-azacytidine and decitabine treatment of myelodysplastic syndromes suggest practical solutions for better outcomes. *Hematol Am Soc Hematol Educ Prog*. 2013;**2013**:511–521.

123 Ververis K, Hiong A, Karagiannis TC, Licciardi PV. Histone deacetylase inhibitors (HDACIs): multitargeted anticancer agents. *Biologics*. 2013;**7**:47–60.

129 Bernt KM, Zhu N, Sinha AU, et al. MLL-rearranged leukemia is dependent on aberrant H3K79 methylation by DOT1L. *Cancer Cell*. 2011;**20**:66–78.

130 Neff T, Armstrong SA. Recent progress toward epigenetic therapies: the example of mixed lineage leukemia. *Blood*. 2013;**121**:4847–4853.

145 Rohle D, Popovici-Muller J, Palaskas N, et al. An inhibitor of mutant IDH1 delays growth and promotes differentiation of glioma cells. *Science*. 2013;**340**:626–630.

146 Wang F, Travins J, DeLaBarre B, et al. Targeted inhibition of mutant IDH2 in leukemia cells induces cellular differentiation. *Science*. 2013;**340**:622–626.

148 Wang ZY, Chen Z. Acute promyelocytic leukemia: from highly fatal to highly curable. *Blood*. 2008;**111**:2505–2515.

151 Flynn PJ, Miller WJ, Weisdorf DJ, et al. Retinoic acid treatment of acute promyelocytic leukemia: in vitro and in vivo observations. *Blood*. 1983;**62**:1211–1217.

152 Huang ME, Ye YC, Chen SR, et al. Use of all-trans retinoic acid in the treatment of acute promyelocytic leukemia. *Blood*. 1988;**72**:567–572.

155 Tallman MS, Andersen JW, Schiffer CA, et al. All-trans retinoic acid in acute promyelocytic leukemia: long-term outcome and prognostic factor analysis from the North American Intergroup protocol. *Blood*. 2002;**100**:4298–4302.

156 Chen GQ, Shen ZX, Wu F, et al. Pharmacokinetics and efficacy of low-dose all-trans retinoic acid in the treatment of acute promyelocytic leukemia. *Leukemia*. 1996;**10**:825–828.

160 Chen GQ, Shi XG, Tang W, et al. Use of arsenic trioxide (As_2O_3) in the treatment of acute promyelocytic leukemia (APL): I. As_2O_3 exerts dose-dependent dual effects on APL cells. *Blood*. 1997;**89**:3345–3353.

162 Hu J, Liu YF, Wu CF, et al. Long-term efficacy and safety of all-trans retinoic acid/arsenic trioxide-based therapy in newly diagnosed acute promyelocytic leukemia. *Proc Natl Acad Sci U S A*. 2009;**106**:3342–3347.

166 Mi JQ, Li JM, Shen ZX, Chen SJ, Chen Z. How to manage acute promyelocytic leukemia. *Leukemia*. 2012;**26**:1743–1751.

175 Lallemand-Breitenbach V, Zhu J, Kogan S, Chen Z, de The H. Opinion: how patients have benefited from mouse models of acute promyelocytic leukaemia. *Nat Rev Cancer*. 2005;**5**:821–827.

176 de The H, Chen Z. Acute promyelocytic leukaemia: novel insights into the mechanisms of cure. *Nat Rev Cancer*. 2010;**10**:775–783.

177 Dos Santos GA, Kats L, Pandolfi PP. Synergy against PML-RARa: targeting transcription, proteolysis, differentiation, and self-renewal in acute promyelocytic leukemia. *J Exp Med*. 2013;**210**:2793–2802.

180 de The H, Le Bras M, Lallemand-Breitenbach V. The cell biology of disease: acute promyelocytic leukemia, arsenic, and PML bodies. *J Cell Biol*. 2012;**198**:11–21.

183 Nichol JN, Garnier N, Miller WH Jr. Triple A therapy: the molecular underpinnings of the unique sensitivity of leukemic promyelocytes to anthracyclines, all-trans-retinoic acid and arsenic trioxide. *Best Prac Res Clin haematol*. 2014;**27**:19–31.

188 Zhang XW, Yan XJ, Zhou ZR, et al. Arsenic trioxide controls the fate of the PML-RARalpha oncoprotein by directly binding PML. *Science*. 2010;**328**:240–243.

192 Chen SJ, Zhou GB, Zhang XW, et al. From an old remedy to a magic bullet: molecular mechanisms underlying the therapeutic effects of arsenic in fighting leukemia. *Blood*. 2011;**117**:6425–6437.

第 12 章　肿瘤干细胞

Yadwinder S. Deol, PhD ■ Jill Granger, BSc ■ MSc, Max S. Wicha, MD

概述

大量证据表明，在许多肿瘤中都存在拥有干细胞特性的细胞亚群。这些"肿瘤干细胞"(cancer stem cell，CSC)在肿瘤的发生和发展中起着重要的作用。此外，这群细胞可能介导了抗肿瘤药物的耐药性，因此对肿瘤复发起着重要作用。这更突显了研发针对肿瘤干细胞的癌症治疗方法的重要性。在本章中，我们将回顾组织干细胞在癌变中的作用、调控这些细胞的信号通路以及靶向 CSC 治疗药物的研究进展。最后，我们将回顾 CSC 模型的临床意义。

肿瘤干细胞假说

癌症起源于"原始胚胎样细胞"的观点可以追溯到一百多年前[1]。然而，直到最近几十年，细胞和分子技术才能直接验证这些观点。"肿瘤干细胞(CSC)假说"由两个独立但相互关联的概念组成：其一为癌症的细胞起源，其二则是癌症的细胞组成。

癌变模型与癌症细胞起源

目前，学界已经提出了两种主要的致癌模型，如图 12-1。经典的"随机"模型认为，肿瘤可能起源于任何细胞，癌变通过随机突变和克隆选择进行。如(图 12-1b)所示，在癌变过程中积累突变，由达尔文理论选择最适合的癌细胞克隆驱动疾病发展。相较于随机模型，CSC 模型则假定癌变起源于那些具有或获得自我更新等干细胞特性的细胞。必须强调的是，CSC 模型并非认为组织干细胞是癌症发生的唯一细胞来源。虽然正常组织干细胞可能会发展为癌症[2,3]，但有证据表明，一些癌症是通过组织祖细胞突变使其获得自我更新能力而产生[4]。肿瘤形成过程中会呈现一定程度的等级结构，在这种等级的顶端是 CSC，其被定义为拥有维持自我更新能力的癌细胞(图 12-1a)。将 CSC 移植到小鼠模型时能产生肿瘤，并再现原代肿瘤的表型异质性。

虽然"随机"和"CSC 模型"最初被认为相互排斥，但更多的研究表明汲取两种理论的精华能更好地描述肿瘤的发展。Vogelstein 的报道认为，许多器官的癌症发病率与其组织干细胞分裂数目成正比[5]，后者反映器官干细胞频率和分裂率。由于组织干细胞突变是随机的，这便提供了统一的致癌模型，即干细胞可能是突变和随后克隆选择的功能单元。除此之外，

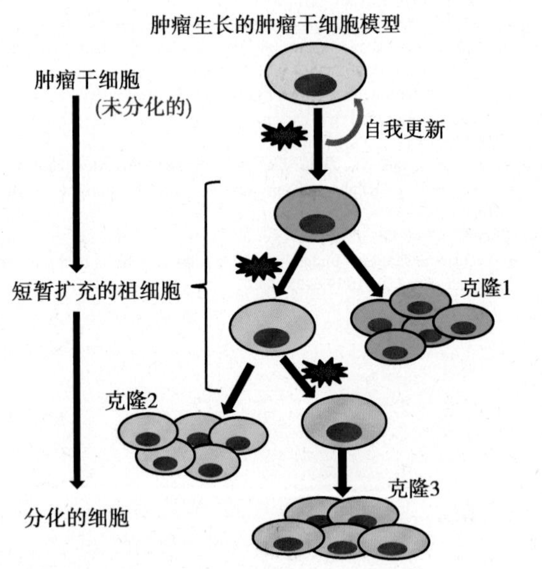

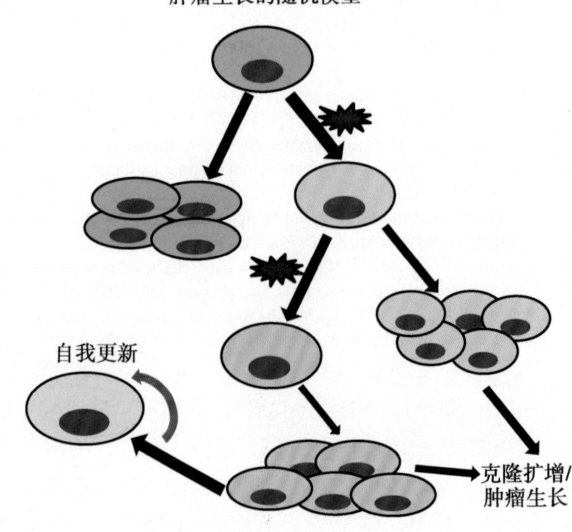

图 12-1　两种肿瘤发生模式的示意图。(a)描述"肿瘤干细胞"模型，肿瘤发生在具有干细胞特性的细胞中，由位于细胞层级顶端的"肿瘤干细胞"驱动，产生组织层次分明的肿瘤。然后这些细胞产生分化的克隆后代，形成肿瘤。(b)描述肿瘤发生的随机或经典模型，任何细胞的随机突变都会产生癌性克隆群体，这些克隆群体通过突变进一步演化

CSC 可能在肿瘤演化过程中发生突变,形成含有多种 CSC 及其克隆后代的肿瘤。两种致癌模型概念的结合,为肿瘤内异质性的产生提供分子解释,这个现象对治疗具有重大意义。

肿瘤干细胞在多种肿瘤中的统一概念

CSC 于 1997 年在人类白血病中被首次发现[6]。在这个开创性研究中,John Dick 等人证明只有少部分人原代白血病细胞移植到免疫抑制的非肥胖糖尿病/严重免疫缺陷(nonobese diabetic/severely compromised immunodeficient, NOD/SCID)小鼠体内后能够出现白血病[6]。此外,通过 CD34+/CD38-表型特征,肿瘤起始白血病细胞被前瞻性地识别,这是一种类似于正常造血干细胞的表型。虽然发现这些白血病起始细胞的频率约为 1/250 000,但小鼠移植模型产生的白血病可展现原代肿瘤的表型异质性。利用类似的肿瘤移植技术,研究者随后在多种实体肿瘤中发现了 CSC,其中包括乳腺癌[7]、脑癌[8]、前列腺癌[9,10]、结肠癌[11,12]、胰腺癌[13]、肝癌[14,15]、肺癌[16]、黑色素瘤[17]和头颈部癌[18]。事实上,研究证据表明大多数肿瘤都是呈等级结构,且具有表现出干细胞特性的细胞群。

CSC 的分选、鉴定和特征化

为了研究 CSC 的基本属性,首先有必要借助技术手段对这些细胞进行分选、鉴定、纯化和特征化,使其能够与大部分肿瘤细胞区分开来。CSC 功能特性包括自我更新能力和分化潜能,可以通过各种体内外实验来识别和表征这一重要细胞群体。

目前已有几种方法或技术来鉴定和分离干细胞样癌细胞:流式细胞术检测 CSC 相关标记的表达、染料排斥试验、乙醛脱氢酶(aldehyde dehydrogenase, ALDH)测定、标记滞留(PKH 染色)以及在核黄素存在下使用自体荧光。利用这些技术富集的 CSC 可通过成球实验或体内连续移植实验进行功能验证,以评估其肿瘤发生和自我更新能力。以下各节列出这些方法的详细信息。

CSC 表面标志物表达

基于细胞表达 CD44 而缺乏 CD24 的特征(即 CD44+/CD24-),人们首次在人类实体肿瘤乳腺癌中发现 CSC[7]。有趣的是,这些标记物也有助于从其他多种实体肿瘤中分离 CSC。同时,CD133 已被证明可用于富集脑癌和肺癌中的 CSC[8,16]。另一种干细胞标志物 ALDH 也可与 CD44/CD24 或 CD133 联合运用于识别一些肿瘤中的 CSC 群。ALDH 是一类参与维生素 A 氧化合成维 A 酸的酶家族[19],ALDH 已被证实是乳腺癌[20]、卵巢癌[21]、结肠癌[22]、头颈部癌[23]和黑色素瘤[24]中可用的 CSC 标志物,其活性可用商品化的乙醛脱氢酶干细胞检测试剂测定。

染料排斥试验

染料排斥试验基于干细胞高表达 ABCG2/BCRP1 等 ATP 结合转运蛋白,具有外排若丹明(Rhodamine)或烟酸己可碱(Hoechst)等亲脂性染料的能力[25]。利用流式细胞仪分析,观察到一群不保留染料的侧群细胞[26]。一些研究表明,这种侧群在具有肿瘤起始能力的细胞中富集,且能向不同类型的细胞群分化[27]。除了在几种类型的癌症中,在骨髓和正常实体组织中也可观察到这种干细胞样侧群[28,29]。Hoechst 染料的细胞毒性限制其用于功能性研究。

标记滞留

利用荧光 PKH 染料在细胞膜进行标记滞留实验是另一种体外鉴定 CSC 的染色方法。这种染料由能够结合细胞膜脂质双层结构的荧光团组成[30]。细胞分裂后,染料可在子代细胞间均匀分布,荧光强度随连续的细胞分裂而减弱[31]。干细胞和 CSC,通常会经历一个非对称的自我更新过程,产生一个干细胞和一个子代细胞。产生的干细胞处于休眠状态,因此 PKH 染料可保留较长的时间,而子代细胞的 PKH 染色强度则随增殖和分化降低。利用流式细胞术可对这些子代细胞进行鉴定和分类,该方法已成功应用于小鼠造血干细胞和乳腺干细胞的分离[32]。

最近有报道称,在核黄素存在时,CSC 表现出自身荧光[33]。研究人员利用流式细胞术从侧群中分离出这些细胞,并证明这些 CSC 具有较强的成球能力,更强的耐药性,较高的转移性,且具有长期体内致瘤作用。此外,已在几种癌症中检测到这种自发荧光的 CSC 样细胞群,这些证据均支持肿瘤干细胞模型[33]。

成球实验

成球实验是另一种体外实验,已被证明可用于鉴定 CSC 群。这个实验基于正常和恶性干细胞共同的特性:悬浮培养时可存活单个细胞克隆形成的细胞球[34]。这些细胞球可连续传代并在每一代都显示干细胞特性。成球实验还可结合一些体外 CSC 实验,例如在球体形成过程中添加 PHK 染料,会形成含有单一标记的起始细胞克隆球体[35]。

体内 CSC 连续稀释实验

虽然已证明 CSC 标志物和体外检测有助于 CSC 的分离鉴定,但这些技术具有局限性。CSC 标志物表达是变化的,可受培养条件或肿瘤微环境的影响[36]。此外,成球实验不涉及肿瘤起始能力[37]。鉴于这些方法的局限性,免疫抑制小鼠移植瘤实验则是鉴定 CSC 的"金标准"[37]。在小鼠体内接种有限稀释的细胞悬液,以能否成瘤来评估该细胞的致瘤性。因此,"肿瘤干细胞"是一个可操作的定义。

值得注意的是,免疫抑制小鼠模型也有其局限性。在人类黑色素瘤中,小鼠模型免疫功能的强弱对肿瘤起始细胞频率有强烈影响[38]。最近研究表明,免疫系统可能对 CSC 的调节发挥重要作用[39,40],并通过将肿瘤移植到同源免疫小鼠中来阐明这些作用。这类研究通过连续移植实验证实 CSC 的存在[41]。

谱系示踪研究

对所有移植研究的一种质疑是,它们会扰乱肿瘤发展的正常微环境。为了克服这个局限,研究者利用细胞标记和谱系示踪进行了一系列的研究。这些研究证实了皮肤肿瘤[42],脑肿瘤[43]和结肠肿瘤[44]中存在 CSC。

EMT/MET 和肿瘤干细胞

上皮—间质转化(epithelial-mesenchymal transition, EMT)是胚胎发育过程中一个特别重要的生理过程,发生 EMT 时上皮细胞获得间质表型,其特点是丧失细胞黏附能力并获得侵袭性。EMT 最初是在发育过程中被发现的,其在原肠胚形成期诱导中胚层细胞迁移,或神经嵴细胞从神经管背侧分离[45]。在癌症中，EMT与转移过程有关，来自原发肿瘤的上皮细胞获得间质表型进而侵入其他组织[46]。

EMT受微环境信号的调控，这些信号可介导核心转录因子驱动的表观遗传改变。微环境因素包括：组织缺氧，转化生长因子-β（transforming growth factor-β，TGF-β）和其他炎症分子，随后诱导EMT相关转录因子表达，如TWIST1、TWIST2、SNAI1、SNAI2、ZEB1和ZEB2等[47,48]。这些转录因子的过表达将通过抑制E-钙黏蛋白等细胞黏附分子，诱导间质特征和侵袭性表型[49]。TWIST1在胚胎发育过程中参与间充质发育，且被证明能诱发乳腺癌转移[50]。研究表明EMT过程中会产生CSC样细胞[51,52]。而且，SNAI1或TWIST1过表达可在MCF10A和永生化人乳腺上皮细胞中诱导EMT[53]。此外，这些细胞中干细胞标志物CD44表达升高，CD24表达降低，这表明诱导产生CSC样表型。在HRAS-g12V致癌模型中，TWIST1与增强乳腺癌细胞形成微球体和继发肿瘤的能力有关[54]。根据乳腺癌分子分型，紧密连接蛋白低表达型乳腺癌具有EMT样基因表达特征。这些癌症中有较高比例的CD44+/24-细胞处于间质状态，肿瘤表现出高侵袭性，并有更大的转移倾向。除此之外，TWIST1可上调BMI表达，当TWIST1被miR-200簇抑制时，CSC的自我更新和细胞分化减少。类似地，BMP通过诱导MET关键调节因子miR-205和miR-200家族来调控MET[55]。

上述研究显示EMT在获得干细胞表型中的作用。CSC可能具有不同的表型，一种与肿瘤的侵袭转移有关，而另一种状态则维持肿瘤生长。近期有研究利用基因表达，分析比较不同亚型乳腺癌中分离的ALDH+和CD44+/24-乳腺癌干细胞。该基因表达分析表明，尽管两种细胞群能独立地在NOD/SCID小鼠体内致瘤，但在原代肿瘤中它们的功能和解剖有着很大区别。ALDH+CSC通常在肿瘤内部以较快速度自我更新和增殖，反之CD44+/24-CSC多为间质状态，位于肿瘤边缘或浸润前沿展现出EMT表型，处于更加静息的状态[56]。这两类细胞另一特征为，CD44+/24-细胞波形蛋白呈强阳性且E-钙黏蛋白阴性，而ALDH+细胞中E-钙黏蛋白呈强阳性而波形蛋白阴性。因此，这些CD44+/24-细胞多为EMT样细胞，在缺氧、转化生长因子-β等炎症因子刺激下可能侵袭血管。

这些研究还表明，乳腺癌干细胞在受肿瘤微环境调控过程中，可维持EMT与MET状态之间的可塑性转变。乳腺癌干细胞从EMT样到MET样状态的相互转换被证明是由microRNA网络调控。这类网络包括诱导EMT的miR-9、miR-100、miR-221和miR-155，以及诱导MET的miR-200、miR-205和miR-9[57]。乳腺癌干细胞从静止的间质样状态转化为增生的上皮样状态对形成肿瘤远处转移至关重要。在自发性鳞状细胞癌模型中敲除TWIST1可逆转EMT，使细胞增殖并形成转移[58]。同样，EMT诱导物Prrx1缺失是肺癌转移形成的必要条件[59]。此外，研究发现MET促进因子，如miR-200家族成员，能促进乳腺癌细胞转移，并诱导上皮细胞分化[60]。与此同时，乳腺癌细胞Id1基因通过下调TWIST1将细胞从EMT转化为MET，这是建立宏转移（macrometastasis）的必要条件[61]。上述研究证明CSC两种状态之间具有可塑性，且CSC受微环境因子调控，微环境因子能调节遗传调控因子和多种转录因子。由于根除CSC可能需要靶标多种CSC群体，因此研发针对多种CSC状态的治疗方案具有重要意义。

肿瘤干细胞的信号转导通路及其治疗靶点

与正常细胞的调控一样，在多种肿瘤中一些进化保守的发育通路对CSC的调控起着重要作用。不同肿瘤类型中保留的这些CSC调控通路将进一步完善肿瘤干细胞模型。此外，无论肿瘤类型如何，这些通路都可提供共同的潜在治疗靶点。

Hedgehog 信号通路

Hedgehog（Hh）家族蛋白质控制着细胞生长、存活以及干细胞/祖细胞的维持。Hh信号调控异常与多种癌症类型有关，包括由体细胞突变引起的信号调节异常。Hh蛋白与Patched（Ptc）受体结合激活信号级联反应，诱导锌指转录因子Gli1-3及其下游靶点基因上调[62-64]。在哺乳动物中有三种Hh配体，分别为sonic hedgehog（SHH），Indian hedgehog（IHH）和desert hedgehog（DHH），其中SHH是表达量最高的Hh信号分子，参与许多上皮组织信号调控。Hh信号异常激活与基底细胞癌[65,66]、髓母细胞瘤[67,68]、横纹肌肉瘤[69]、胶质瘤、乳腺癌、食管癌、胃癌、胰腺癌、前列腺癌和小细胞肺癌相关[70]，胶质瘤中也存在Gli1扩增[71]。

Hh信号通路在人和小鼠的乳腺发育中起着重要作用。在小鼠中，Gli1结构激活或Gli3的失活导致乳腺芽发育缺陷[72]。Gli1异位表达可诱导核内Snail表达，导致妊娠期小鼠乳腺组织中E-钙黏蛋白表达缺失[73]。此外，转录因子FOXC2还通过上调Hh信号通路和Snail促进间充质分化[74]。同样，SHH在小鼠乳腺中过表达也会导致乳腺芽发育缺陷[75]。干扰Hh通路中其他分子，如SMO激活或PTCH1缺失可导致末端乳腺芽畸形[76]。正常乳腺干细胞在形成微球体过程中表达PTCH1、Gli1和Gli2，该通路在分化时表达下调。Hh信号通路在干细胞调控中发挥了重要作用，Hh配体或Gli1/Gli2过表达激活Hh信号通路，激活多梳基因家族成员BMI-1，增加微球体的形成和大小[77]。小鼠乳腺肿瘤病毒（mouse mammary tumor virus，MMTV）启动子驱动SMO激活，可增强转基因小鼠体内原代乳腺上皮细胞微球体形成[76]。Hh配体可通过旁分泌影响乳腺干细胞的有丝分裂，这个过程可能受TP63调控，并参与对孕期乳腺分化的调控[78]。除了TP63，转录因子Runx2也被证明可调控Hh配体的表达[79]。

Hh信号通路成员SHH、PTCH1和GLI1在侵袭性乳腺癌中高表达，这提示该通路在人类乳腺癌中发挥重要作用[80]。此外，Hh配体表达与基底样（basal-like）乳腺癌相关，基底样乳腺癌是一种预后较差的侵略性表型。这些发现在小鼠模型中得到证实，Hh配体异位表达可在BLBC小鼠体内诱导高侵袭性肿瘤[81]。同样，在乳腺癌中观察到SHH启动子低甲基化导致SHH上调，乳腺癌临床样本中NF-κB的表达也与之相关[82]。Hh信号通路也与乳腺癌骨转移相关，在骨转移中，肿瘤细胞分泌Hh配体激活破骨细胞转录骨桥蛋白（osteopontin，OPN）。这个过程参与破骨细胞的成熟和骨吸收激活，促进肿瘤转移[83]。

Hh通路最常用的拮抗剂是植物生物碱环巴胺，它与SMO结合并下调Gli1[84]。其他与SMO结合的拮抗剂包括，SANT1-4[85]、KAAD-环巴胺（KAAD-cyclopamine）[84]、复合物-5（compound-5）、复合物-Z（compound-Z）[86]和Cur-61414[87]。此外，

5E1 单克隆抗体可靶向 SHH 治疗小细胞肺癌[88]。GDC-0449(Vismodegib,商品名:Erivedge)为 FDA 第一个批准的 Hh 通路抑制剂,在临床试验中与 Notch 信号通路抑制剂 RO4929097(γ-分泌酶抑制剂,GSI)联用[89]。

Notch 信号通路

Notch 是另一种进化保守的信号通路,参与许多组织细胞的命运决定、增殖和分化调控。Notch 信号级联的核心成员包括配体 Delta-like-1、-3 和-4(DLL1、DLL3 和 DLL4),Jagged-1 和-2(JAG1 和 JAG2),以及四个跨膜受体(Notch1-4)。Notch 受体与配体结合后,受体经历两次蛋白水解过程。首先,解离发生在靠近细胞膜的胞外侧。随后 γ-分泌酶复合物介导的跨膜结构域发生第二次裂解,导致受体胞内结构域从膜上释放。水解后,胞内的 Notch 结构域转入细胞核,与广泛表达的转录因子 CSL 形成复合物,并招募共同激活因子,如核转录激活蛋白家族(mastermind-like-1,-2,-3;MAML-1,-2,-3)[90]。Notch 信号的转录靶点不仅有分化相关因子,如发状分裂相关增强因子(Hairy/enhancer of split,Hes)和 Hes 相关家族(HRT/HRP/Hey),还包括细胞周期调节因子(p21 和 cyclin D1)和凋亡调节因子[90,91]。

Notch 1 的致癌作用最早是在急性淋巴细胞白血病(T cell acute lymphoblastic leukemia,T-ALL)中发现的,其中 t(7;9)(q34;q34.3)易位导致 Notch1 与 T 细胞抗原受体 β(T cell receptor-β,TCR-β)并置。这种易位导致配体非依赖性激活和胞内 Notch 1 异常表达,该过程由调节 T 细胞分化的 TCR-β 调控[92]。利用 MMTV 启动子使小鼠乳腺过表达 Notch 4 可阻止细胞分化,从而导致异常泌乳,低分化乳腺癌和唾液腺癌发生在小鼠 2~7 月龄之间[93]。该研究再次强调了 Notch 信号在多种组织分化和肿瘤发生中的作用。已有文献报道 Ras 过表达与 Notch 1 水平升高相关[94]。此外,约 50%原发性人乳腺癌中 Notch 信号抑制调控因子 Numb 丢失,这些肿瘤的 Notch 1 活性增加[95]。文献报道 Notch 信号分子在胰腺癌、肾癌、前列腺癌、多发性骨髓瘤、霍奇金淋巴瘤和间变性淋巴瘤等肿瘤中过表达[96~100]。在肺癌中,Notch 信号的作用因细胞类型而异:在小细胞肺癌中,Notch 信号不活跃,但 Hes1 和 Hash1 激活[101],持续活化的胞内 Notch 受体诱导 Notch 信号通路激活,导致生长停滞[102]。相比之下,Notch 信号在非小细胞肺癌中激活,其中 Hes1 和 Hey1 表达水平较高[101]。

研究报道 CD24+/24-乳腺 CSC 的 Notch 通路被激活[103]。通过 SAGE 分析发现,正常乳腺和乳腺癌中 CD44+细胞群的 Notch 3 被上调[104]。其他研究表明,Notch 4 是乳腺癌干细胞最重要的调控因子[105]。此外,Notch 信号异常激活是乳腺癌发生的早期事件,并已在导管内原位癌(ductal carcinoma in situ,DCIS)中观察到。利用 γ-分泌酶抑制剂治疗原发性 DCIS 可显著减少微球体的形成[103]。同样,在体外微球体培养系统中,通过 DSL 肽激活 Notch 信号可促进在三维基质凝胶中培养的微球体自我更新和分支化形态形成[106],这个过程可被 Notch 4 封闭抗体或 γ-分泌酶抑制剂所抑制。因此,激活 Notch 信号可使上皮细胞保持增殖状态,而非分化成癌。

Notch 通路调节也被归因于通过高甲基化和低甲基化的表观遗传调控。Notch 的配体 DLL1 基因高甲基化导致 NOTCH1 表达降低[107]。同样,与癌旁组织相比,肿瘤中 *NOTCH4* 基因启动子甲基化程度降低[108]。多发性骨髓瘤细胞中 *JAG2* 过表达与多发性骨髓瘤患者和细胞系来源的恶性细胞低甲基化有关[109]。敲低乳腺干细胞中经典的 Notch 效应因子 Cbf-1 可增加干细胞活性,而持续性的 Notch 信号将增加管腔祖细胞数目,导致增生和肿瘤发生[110]。此外,*JAG1* 和 *NOTCH1* 的共表达与较差的总生存率有关[111]。在 ESA+CD24-CD44+的 BCSC 中,Notch 4 和 Notch 1 活性比大部分已分化的肿瘤细胞分别高 8 倍和 4 倍,抑制其活性可减缓肿瘤生长[105]。

Notch 与其他致癌途径如 ErbB2、Jak/Stat、TGF-β、NF-κB、Wnt 和 Hh[112] 的互相作用会增加 Notch 通路的复杂程度。ErbB2 通过细胞周期蛋白 D1 诱导 Notch 1 活化[113],DAPT 和拉帕替尼联用靶向治疗体内外的 DCIS 祖细胞[114]。Wnt 通路借助 Jagged-1(WNT/TCF 通路靶点)和 Mel-18(Bmi-1 负调控因子)与 Notch 通路相互作用。研究表明,敲低 Mel-18 可上调 Jagged-1,增强 BCSC 的自我更新能力,从而激活 Notch 通路[115]。Notch 的活化进一步激活 Hh 通路,并增加 Ptch 和 Gli 的表达[77]。综上所述,针对多个干细胞通路靶点的治疗能为靶向治疗提供一种新的策略。许多抑制 Notch 信号通路的药物尚处于早期临床试验阶段,这些药物包括阻断 Notch 合成的 γ-分泌酶抑制剂[116],特异性拮抗 Notch 受体的抗体[117,118]和特异性拮抗 Notch 配体 DLL4 的抗体[119,120]。

Wnt 信号通路

Wnt/β-catenin/TCF 信号通路是另一个复杂的进化保守的通路,不但参与成体组织稳态发育和维持,还涉及细胞增殖、分化、迁移和凋亡[121]。它也参与调节胚胎干细胞和组织特异性干细胞的自我更新和维持[122~124]。Wnt 信号调节异常是几种癌症的特征,在这些癌症中,参与信号通路的分子作为肿瘤抑制因子还是增强因子取决于其激活状态[125~127]。Wnt 信号通路包括经典通路和非经典通路。经典 Wnt 通路包括激活 β-catenin/TCF 复合体,导致其与 APC(adenomatous polyposis coli,腺瘤性结肠息肉)蛋白解离随后转入细胞核,从而激活转录 TCF/LEF[128]。这进而导致 c-myc 和 cyclin D1 等致癌靶点上调。这一经典途径已被广泛研究,并被发现在许多癌症中表达异常。非经典 Wnt 信号通路包括调节细胞骨架的平面细胞极性通路和调控细胞内钙水平的 Wnt 钙依赖通路[129,130]。APC 突变(Wnt 通路分子参与调节 β-catenin 稳定)与大多数的散发性结直肠癌相关[131,132]。APC 种系突变已被证明与家族性息肉病综合征有关,这种疾病与多发肠道息肉发展有关,有较高的致癌倾向。除了结肠癌,在肝癌、黑色素瘤、甲状腺癌和卵巢癌中也已发现 β-catenin 致癌性突变[133]。在结肠癌、乳腺癌、前列腺癌、肺癌和其他癌症中,Wnt 拮抗基因如分泌卷曲相关蛋白(secreted frizzled-related protein,SFRP)被甲基化导致该基因沉默[121]。

Wnt 信号在一些癌症中参与 CSC 的维持。在转基因小鼠模型中,敲降 LRP5(Wnt 共受体关键成分)可显著减少干/祖细胞[134]。此外,过表达 Wnt-1 的转基因小鼠乳腺富集表达乳腺干细胞标志物角蛋白 6 和 Sca1 的上皮细胞,这表明乳腺癌可能与 Wnt 激活后的干细胞扩增有关。Wnt/β-catenin 通过下调 E-钙黏蛋白及上调 Snail 与 Twist 参与 EMT 调控[135],EMT 被证明可诱导乳腺癌细胞的干细胞样表型[52]。Wnt 信号可维持胚胎干细胞的多能性和神经分化[136],还参与肿瘤缺氧诱导的干细胞扩增,该过程由乏氧诱导因子 1-α(hypoxia-inducible factor 1α,Hif1-α)介导[137]。

目前,一些抑制 Wnt 信号通路的药物正在研发中。在临床前模型中,发现两种非甾体抗炎药(nonsteroidal anti-inflammatory drug,NSAID)舒林酸[138]和塞来昔布[139,140],分别通过靶向散乱蛋白(Dishevelled,Dvl)和环氧化酶来抑制 Wnt 信号,目前正在对舒林酸进行二期临床试验研究[141]。此外,一些非 NSAID 抑制剂,如 NSC668036 和 PCN-N3 等被证明通过抑制 Dvl 降低β-catenin,以此稳定破坏复合体[142,143]。除此之外,针对 Wnt 通路成员的抗体也在开发中。Wnt3A 中和抗体在小鼠前列腺癌模型中具有抑制增殖和促进凋亡的作用[144]。另一种单克隆抗体 omp-54F28 可通过特异性靶向 CSC 来抑制人源肿瘤异体移植模型(patient-derived xenograft,PDX)的肿瘤生长。Wnt 诱骗受体[145]和针对 Wnt 共调节因子 R 脊椎蛋白的抗体也在研制中。目前,上述这些抑制 Wnt 信号通路的药物正在进行早期临床试验。

肿瘤干细胞临床意义及展望

大量证据表明,CSC 不仅在肿瘤增殖和转移中起作用,还在化疗药物耐药中发挥重要作用,CSC 对细胞毒性药物耐药最初出现在临床前模型中[146,147],后来在临床试验中得到证实[148]。CSC 对放射治疗的抵抗在多种肿瘤中得到确认,研究表明,患者在接受化疗或放疗后表达 CSC 标志的细胞相对比例上升[148]。目前已发现若干造成 CSC 抵抗的机制,这些机制包括细胞周期动力学改变,抗凋亡蛋白表达增加,细胞转运蛋白增加以及 DNA 修复效率提高[149]。除了 CSC 相对耐药外,化疗还可能激活细胞因子活化 CSC,包括 IL-8 和 IL-6。针对这些细胞因子及其受体的抑制剂已被开发,一些正在进入临床试验。

CSC 模型具有重要的临床意义。除了强调靶向 CSC 的重要性外,它们的存在还意味着其在肿瘤微环境中发挥着关键作用,因此未来在设计治疗试验和设置临床终点时需要更加深思熟虑。目前,实体瘤反应评价标准(response evaluation criteria in solid tumors,RECIST)评估的肿瘤缩小率被认为是评价治疗效果的重要终点。然而,在各种肿瘤类型中,肿瘤缩小率与患者的最终生存期相关性很低[150]。肿瘤缩小是衡量治疗对肿瘤影响的一个指标,由于 CSC 只占肿瘤体积的一小部分,成功靶向这些细胞并不一定导致肿瘤缩小。因此,目前开发针对 CSC 药物的方法包括在一期试验中获取 CSC 毒性,然后将 CSC 靶向药物与传统化疗药相结合。由于 CSC 与正常组织干细胞共享许多信号通路,因此在临床引入此类疗法时需要谨慎评估其安全性。图 12-2 中总结了一些目前处于早期临床试验阶段的 CSC 靶向药物。有趣的是,初步数据表明这些药物具有良好的耐受剂量,且在此剂量下可降低连续活检中 CSC 的数量[151]。上述研究表明,CSC 可能比正常组织干细胞更依赖这些通路,这为癌症治疗提供了一个有利窗口。目前,正在开发更直接地检测 CSC 靶向药物效果的新方法,包括检测循环肿瘤细胞(circulating tumor cell,CTC)中标志物的表达来获得 CSC。CTC 中富集的 CSC,在介导肿瘤转移中发挥着重要作用[152~154]。

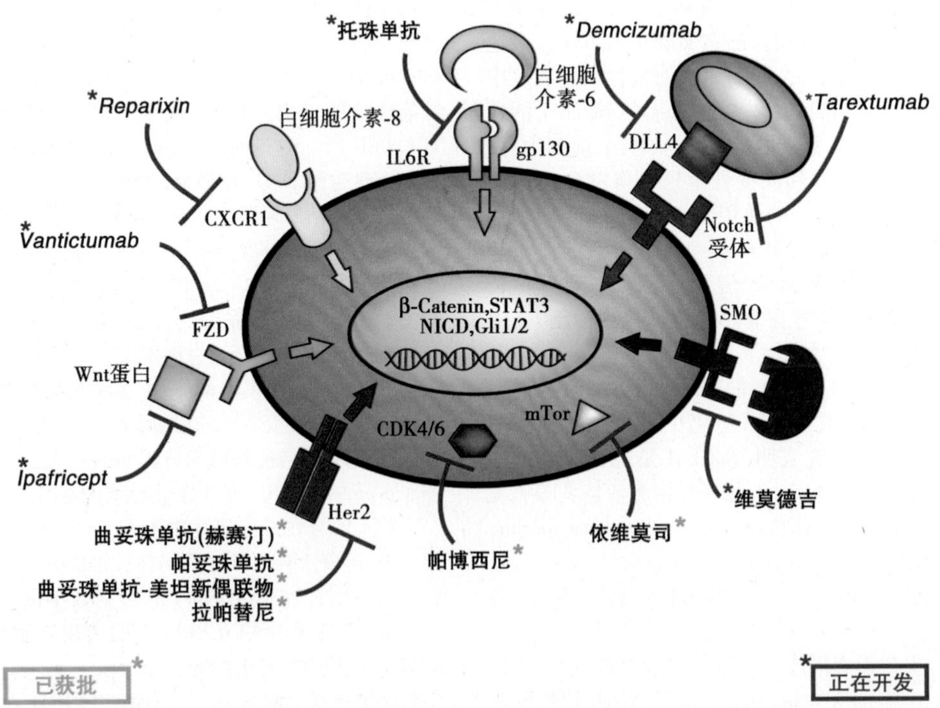

图 12-2 肿瘤干细胞靶向药物及目前正处于早期临床试验阶段或已被 FDA 批准的肿瘤干细胞靶向药及其细胞靶点。IL6R,白细胞介素-6 受体;gp130,IL6 家族细胞因子共用受体;Her2,人类表皮生长因子受体 2;DLL4,Notch 受体配体 4;β-Catenin,β-连环蛋白;STAT3,信号传导及转录激活蛋白 3;NICD,Notch 的胞内段;Gli1/2,锌指转录因子 1/2;CXCR1,G 蛋白偶联受体超家族;FZD,Wnt 信号通路的跨膜受体;SMO,Hedgehog 信号通路细胞表面受体;CDK4/6,周期蛋白依赖性激酶 4/6;mTor,西罗莫司靶蛋白

CSC 模型预测 CSC 靶向疗法应用于辅助治疗，可获得最佳的疗效。因为 CSC 具有足够的自我更新能力，能通过微转移产生临床意义上的病灶。因此，辅助治疗的效果直接关系到其消除微转移的能力。研究表明，Her2 靶向药物如曲妥珠单抗，用于 Her2+乳腺癌辅助治疗时，具有明显预防复发的效果[148]。Her2 作为 CSC 重要的调节因子，在乳腺癌中有重要临床意义[155]。

免疫治疗发展是癌症治疗中最令人兴奋的领域之一，例如免疫检查点阻滞剂等。有趣的是，有证据表明 CSC 可能特别擅长逃避免疫监视。免疫逃避的机制包括高表达 PDL-1 和分泌免疫抑制的 TGF-β。目前正在开发一些调节免疫系统并靶向 CSC 的方案，例如基于 CSC 的疫苗和多肽。未来这种方法可能与免疫检查点阻滞剂相结合，以更有效地靶向 CSC。

在世界范围内，目前有超过 70 个临床试验使用新的 CSC 靶向药。这些研究大多处于早期阶段，未来几年有望产生令人兴奋的重要成果。最后，研究者需要进行严谨的临床随机对照试验，以确定成功靶向 CSC 是否能改善患者预后。

结论

尽管目前在研究癌症分子基础方面已取得相当大的进展，但这种不断深入的理解尚未带来晚期癌症患者存活率的显著提高。对于大多数常见癌症，肿瘤转移使得疾病无法根治。大量证据表明，许多癌症具有等级结构，并由具有干细胞特征的细胞群驱动。这些特性包括自我更新和分化能力，并能形成肿瘤组织。这些细胞被称为“肿瘤起始细胞”或“肿瘤干细胞”，它们可能介导肿瘤转移，并造成治疗抵抗。靶向干细胞群体的辅助治疗能限制肿瘤转移并显著提高患者的生存，因此认识和理解调控肿瘤干细胞的分子机制具有重要的临床意义。

（董亚萍 译　陈淑桢　吴彤　吕桂帅 校）

参考文献

The complete reference list can be found on the Wiley Companion Digital Edition of this title (see inside front cover for login instructions).

1 Huntly BJ, Gilliland DG. Cancer biology: summing up cancer stem cells. *Nature*. 2005;**435**(**7046**):1169–1170. PubMed PMID: 15988505.

2 Sell S. On the stem cell origin of cancer. *Am J Pathol*. 2010;**176**(**6**):2584–2594. PubMed PMID: 20431026. Pubmed Central PMCID: 2877820.

3 Reya T, Morrison SJ, Clarke MF, Weissman IL. Stem cells, cancer, and cancer stem cells. *Nature*. 2001;**414**(**6859**):105–111. PubMed PMID: 11689955.

4 Pattabiraman DR, Weinberg RA. Tackling the cancer stem cells - what challenges do they pose? *Nat Rev Drug Discov*. 2014;**13**(**7**):497–512. PubMed PMID: 24981363. Pubmed Central PMCID: 4234172.

5 Tomasetti C, Vogelstein B. Cancer etiology. Variation in cancer risk among tissues can be explained by the number of stem cell divisions. *Science*. 2015;**347**(**6217**):78–81. PubMed PMID: 25554788. Pubmed Central PMCID: 4446723.

6 Bonnet D, Dick JE. Human acute myeloid leukemia is organized as a hierarchy that originates from a primitive hematopoietic cell. *Nat Med*. 1997;**3**(**7**):730–737. PubMed PMID: 9212098.

7 Al-Hajj M, Wicha MS, Benito-Hernandez A, Morrison SJ, Clarke MF. Prospective identification of tumorigenic breast cancer cells. *Proc Natl Acad Sci U S A*. 2003;**100**(**7**):3983–3988. PubMed PMID: 12629218. Pubmed Central PMCID: 153034.

8 Singh SK, Hawkins C, Clarke ID, Squire JA, Bayani J, Hide T, et al. Identification of human brain tumour initiating cells. *Nature*. 2004;**432**(**7015**):396–401. PubMed PMID: 15549107.

9 Collins AT, Berry PA, Hyde C, Stower MJ, Maitland NJ. Prospective identification of tumorigenic prostate cancer stem cells. *Cancer Res*. 2005;**65**(**23**):10946–10951. PubMed PMID: 16322242.

10 Patrawala L, Calhoun T, Schneider-Broussard R, Li H, Bhatia B, Tang S, et al. Highly purified CD44+ prostate cancer cells from xenograft human tumors are enriched in tumorigenic and metastatic progenitor cells. *Oncogene*. 2006;**25**(**12**):1696–1708. PubMed PMID: 16449977.

11 O'Brien CA, Pollett A, Gallinger S, Dick JE. A human colon cancer cell capable of initiating tumour growth in immunodeficient mice. *Nature*. 2007;**445**(**7123**):106–110. PubMed PMID: 17122772.

12 Ricci-Vitiani L, Lombardi DG, Pilozzi E, Biffoni M, Todaro M, Peschle C, et al. Identification and expansion of human colon-cancer-initiating cells. *Nature*. 2007;**445**(**7123**):111–115. PubMed PMID: 17122771.

13 Li C, Heidt DG, Dalerba P, Burant CF, Zhang L, Adsay V, et al. Identification of pancreatic cancer stem cells. *Cancer Res*. 2007;**67**(**3**):1030–1037. PubMed PMID: 17283135.

14 Ma S, Chan KW, Hu L, Lee TK, Wo JY, Ng IO, et al. Identification and characterization of tumorigenic liver cancer stem/progenitor cells. *Gastroenterology*. 2007;**132**(**7**):2542–2556. PubMed PMID: 17570225.

16 Kim CF, Jackson EL, Woolfenden AE, Lawrence S, Babar I, Vogel S, et al. Identification of bronchioalveolar stem cells in normal lung and lung cancer. *Cell*. 2005;**121**(**6**):823–835. PubMed PMID: 15960971.

17 Schatton T, Murphy GF, Frank NY, Yamaura K, Waaga-Gasser AM, Gasser M, et al. Identification of cells initiating human melanomas. *Nature*. 2008;**451**(**7176**):345–349. PubMed PMID: 18202660. Pubmed Central PMCID: 3660705.

18 Prince ME, Sivanandan R, Kaczorowski A, Wolf GT, Kaplan MJ, Dalerba P, et al. Identification of a subpopulation of cells with cancer stem cell properties in head and neck squamous cell carcinoma. *Proc Natl Acad Sci U S A*. 2007;**104**(3):973–978. PubMed PMID: 17210912. Pubmed Central PMCID: 1783424.

20 Ginestier C, Hur MH, Charafe-Jauffret E, Monville F, Dutcher J, Brown M, et al. ALDH1 is a marker of normal and malignant human mammary stem cells and a predictor of poor clinical outcome. *Cell Stem Cell*. 2007;**1**(**5**):555–567. PubMed PMID: 18371393. Pubmed Central PMCID: 2423808.

21 Silva IA, Bai S, McLean K, Yang K, Griffith K, Thomas D, et al. Aldehyde dehydrogenase in combination with CD133 defines angiogenic ovarian cancer stem cells that portend poor patient survival. *Cancer Res*. 2011;**71**(**11**):3991–4001. PubMed PMID: 21498635. Pubmed Central PMCID: 3107359.

22 Huang EH, Hynes MJ, Zhang T, Ginestier C, Dontu G, Appelman H, et al. Aldehyde dehydrogenase 1 is a marker for normal and malignant human colonic stem cells (SC) and tracks SC overpopulation during colon tumorigenesis. *Cancer Res*. 2009;**69**(**8**):3382–3389. PubMed PMID: 19336570. Pubmed Central PMCID: 2789401.

23 Clay MR, Tabor M, Owen JH, Carey TE, Bradford CR, Wolf GT, et al. Single-marker identification of head and neck squamous cell carcinoma cancer stem cells with aldehyde dehydrogenase. *Head Neck*. 2010;**32**(**9**):1195–1201. PubMed PMID: 20073073. Pubmed Central PMCID: 2991066.

24 Luo Y, Dallaglio K, Chen Y, Robinson WA, Robinson SE, McCarter MD, et al. ALDH1A isozymes are markers of human melanoma stem cells and potential therapeutic targets. *Stem Cells*. 2012;**30**(**10**):2100–2113. PubMed PMID: 22887839. Pubmed Central PMCID: 3448863.

34 Dontu G, Abdallah WM, Foley JM, Jackson KW, Clarke MF, Kawamura MJ, et al. In vitro propagation and transcriptional profiling of human mammary stem/progenitor cells. *Genes Dev*. 2003;**17**(**10**):1253–1270. PubMed PMID: 12756227. Pubmed Central PMCID: 196056.

35 Pece S, Tosoni D, Confalonieri S, Mazzarol G, Vecchi M, Ronzoni S, et al. Biological and molecular heterogeneity of breast cancers correlates with their cancer stem cell content. *Cell*. 2010;**140**(**1**):62–73. PubMed PMID: 20074520.

38 Quintana E, Shackleton M, Sabel MS, Fullen DR, Johnson TM, Morrison SJ. Efficient tumour formation by single human melanoma cells. *Nature*. 2008;**456**(**7222**):593–598. PubMed PMID: 19052619. Pubmed Central PMCID: 2597380.

46 Kang YB, Massague J. Epithelial-mesenchymal transitions: twist in development and metastasis. *Cell*. 2004;**118**(**3**):277–279. PubMed PMID: WOS: 000223353100004. English.

56 Liu S, Cong Y, Wang D, Sun Y, Deng L, Liu Y, et al. Breast cancer stem cells transition between epithelial and mesenchymal states reflective of their normal counterparts. *Stem Cell Rep*. 2014;**2**(**1**):78–91. PubMed PMID: 24511467. Pubmed Central PMCID: 3916760.

71 Kinzler KW, Bigner SH, Bigner DD, Trent JM, Law ML, O'Brien SJ, et al. Identification of an amplified, highly expressed gene in a human glioma. *Science*. 1987;**236**(**4797**):70–73. PubMed PMID: 3563490.

77 Liu S, Dontu G, Mantle ID, Patel S, Ahn NS, Jackson KW, et al. Hedgehog signaling and Bmi-1 regulate self-renewal of normal and malignant human mammary stem cells. *Cancer Res*. 2006;**66**(**12**):6063–6071. PubMed PMID: 16778178. Pubmed Central PMCID: 4386278.

83 Kang Y, Siegel PM, Shu W, Drobnjak M, Kakonen SM, Cordon-Cardo C, et al.

A multigenic program mediating breast cancer metastasis to bone. *Cancer Cell*. 2003;**3**(**6**):537-549. PubMed PMID: 12842083.

103 Farnie G, Clarke RB, Spence K, Pinnock N, Brennan K, Anderson NG, et al. Novel cell culture technique for primary ductal carcinoma in situ: role of Notch and epidermal growth factor receptor signaling pathways. *J Natl Cancer Inst*. 2007;**99**(**8**):616-627. PubMed PMID: 17440163.

105 Harrison H, Farnie G, Howell SJ, Rock RE, Stylianou S, Brennan KR, et al. Regulation of breast cancer stem cell activity by signaling through the Notch4 receptor. *Cancer Res*. 2010;**70**(**2**):709-718. PubMed PMID: 20068161. Pubmed Central PMCID: 3442245.

106 Dontu G, Jackson KW, McNicholas E, Kawamura MJ, Abdallah WM, Wicha MS. Role of Notch signaling in cell-fate determination of human mammary stem/progenitor cells. *BCR*. 2004;**6**(**6**):R605-R615. PubMed PMID: 15535842. Pubmed Central PMCID: 1064073.

137 Conley SJ, Gheordunescu E, Kakarala P, Newman B, Korkaya H, Heath AN, et al. Antiangiogenic agents increase breast cancer stem cells via the generation of tumor hypoxia. *Proc Natl Acad Sci U S A*. 2012;**109**(**8**):2784-2789. PubMed PMID: 22308314. Pubmed Central PMCID: 3286974.

150 Reddy RM, Kakarala M, Wicha MS. Clinical trial design for testing the stem cell model for the prevention and treatment of cancer. *Cancer*. 2011;**3**(**2**):2696-2708. PubMed PMID: 24212828. Pubmed Central PMCID: 3757438.

151 Schott AF, Landis MD, Dontu G, Griffith KA, Layman RM, Krop I, et al. Preclinical and clinical studies of gamma secretase inhibitors with docetaxel on human breast tumors. *Clin Cancer Res*. 2013;**19**(**6**):1512-1524. PubMed PMID: 23340294. Pubmed Central PMCID: 3602220.

155 Korkaya H, Paulson A, Iovino F, Wicha MS. HER2 regulates the mammary stem/progenitor cell population driving tumorigenesis and invasion. *Oncogene*. 2008;**27**(**47**):6120-6130. PubMed PMID: 18591932. Pubmed Central PMCID: 2602947.

第 13 章　癌症和细胞死亡

John C. Reed, MD, PhD

概述

细胞死亡是一种人体正常的生理现象，机体通过细胞死亡与细胞新生的平衡来保持组织稳态。肿瘤的出现在一定程度上就是由于这种生理性细胞死亡机制出现缺陷，遗传或表观遗传学的改变使癌前或癌细胞具有选择性的生存优势，最终导致细胞出现病理性扩增。不仅如此，这种正常细胞死亡途径缺陷还可以促进癌细胞的恶性发展、逃脱免疫系统攻击、对放疗或化疗不敏感等特征。目前已有研究发现了多种与人类恶性肿瘤细胞死亡缺陷有关的机制，这些研究结果有助于我们更加深入地认识癌症发病的新机制，同时也为探索以诱导肿瘤细胞自然死亡为目标的靶向治疗提供新靶点。

简介

逃避内源性细胞死亡过程是癌症的主要特征之一[1]。人体每天都会有大量细胞死亡，成人平均每天大约有 500 亿~700 亿个细胞死亡，而每年死亡的细胞量则相当于一个人的体重。生理条件下，这种“程序性”的细胞死亡与每日因细胞分裂产生新生细胞数量相当，从而实现了组织的稳态。细胞死亡机制多样，除了凋亡和坏死这两种最为常见的途径之外，其他特殊的死亡方式也曾被报道过，包括坏死性凋亡、细胞焦亡、细胞铁死亡及自噬性细胞死亡等。在维持正常组织稳态及哺乳动物发育过程中，细胞凋亡是细胞死亡中最常见的非病理死亡途径[2~4]。

近年来的研究表明，癌细胞内源性的死亡机制出现障碍，从而获得了一定的选择性生存优势。而介导癌细胞死亡障碍的诸多分子机制也已被证实，这不但明确了人类肿瘤和癌症的致病机制，还可以提供药物治疗靶点，以重启细胞自然死亡过程，达到癌细胞“自我毁灭”的目的[5,6]。此外，也有报道称，癌细胞还可以通过沉默或中和内源性细胞死亡激活剂以逃脱死亡，而替换或重启这些内源性程序性细胞死亡（programmed cell death，PCD）激活因子的策略对于根治肿瘤具有一定潜在价值[7,8]。

调节细胞死亡机制的缺陷可以通过多种途径促进癌症发展[2,5,6]。第一，激活的癌基因（如 C-MYC 等）不但可以调控恶性转化细胞的增殖，还能促进细胞凋亡，而这种促凋亡效应又会被促进细胞生存蛋白的作用所抵消，进而形成癌基因的“互补”形式[9]。第二，各种细胞周期“监测点”会启动异常复制或分裂的细胞凋亡，但是凋亡缺陷或其他死亡机制缺陷则可以促进异常细胞分裂，最终发展成肿瘤。第三，由于 DNA 复制错误和染色体分离紊乱都会引发细胞自杀，而细胞死亡机制缺陷将会导致基因组不稳定。第四，死亡机制缺陷导致生长因子（或激素）非依赖型细胞存活，从而有助于恶性转化的细胞逃脱正常的旁分泌和内分泌生长控制机制。第五，在大多数生长较快的实体肿瘤中，由于微环境缺氧和代谢压力会引起细胞死亡，但死亡机制缺陷的细胞则可以逃脱死亡从而在上述环境中生存。第六，上皮细胞失去由整合素介导的对细胞外基质附着时，便会发生凋亡，所以细胞死亡机制缺陷也可以导致实体瘤的侵袭和转移[10]。第七，细胞死亡机制缺陷可以使肿瘤细胞逃脱免疫监视，避免被细胞毒性 T 细胞（cytolytic T-cell，CTL）和自然杀伤细胞（natural killer，NK）所攻击。

本章将介绍细胞死亡的主要途径，并举例说明这些途径在癌症中的缺陷，包括死亡相关基因的低表达（低活性）和细胞生存基因的过表达（高活性）。此外，随着对癌症死亡机制缺陷的深入研究，许多肿瘤药物的研发和进展情况也将会在本章中进行概述。为了简洁起见，本章仅引用有代表性的参考文献，并因此向研究细胞死亡生物学领域的贡献者们致歉。

细胞死亡途径

为了研究细胞死亡途径，研究者们采用多种方法对这些细胞死亡机制进行分类，目前已明确了几种内源性细胞死亡途径[11,12]。其中最重要的一类是细胞内蛋白酶半胱氨酸依赖的天冬氨酸特异性蛋白酶（cysteine-dependent aspartate-specific protease，Caspase）家族[13]，因此，细胞死亡机制可以广泛地分成 Caspase 依赖途径及 Caspase 非依赖途径两种，但在很多情况下这两种机制会共同出现。

Caspase 依赖性细胞死亡

Caspase 依赖性细胞死亡的形态变化完全符合“凋亡”的标准——细胞脱离外基质、变圆、缩小、核染色质凝集、核破碎、包膜出泡形成凋亡小体。Caspase 介导的级联蛋白水解最终会直接或间接引起这些细胞形态学变化，目前采用蛋白质组学法对该方面的全面研究仍在继续[14]。

Caspase 在级联调控网络中既是上游的“启动者”，又是下游的“效应者”，通过剪切、激活，形成蛋白水解级联反应[15,16]。这些蛋白酶均以无活性酶原形式存在于动物细胞胞浆中，大部分 Caspase 激活主要是通过这些聚集的无活性酶原蛋白相互作用[16]。一旦激活，这些上游 Caspase 起始因子便会裂解，激活下游 Caspase 效应因子。上游 Caspase 起始因子含有介导蛋白相互作用的 N-末端功能结构域，即 Caspase 相关募集结构域（Caspase-associated recruitment domain，CARD）和死亡效应结构域（death effector domain，DED）（表 13-1）。虽然 Caspase 编码基因失活突变的总量相对较少，但研究证实在多种癌症中均存在上述情况。

表 13-1　细胞死亡蛋白相关结构域

结构域	蛋白名称(举例)
Caspase 催化结构域	Caspase 蛋白酶家族半胱氨酸蛋白酶
Caspase 相关募集结构域(CARD)	Caspase-1,-4,-5,-9;Apaf1;ASC;NLRP1,4
死亡结构域(DD)	TNFR1, FAS, DR4, DR5, TRADD, RAIDD,RIP1
死亡效应结构域(DED)	Caspase-8,-10;FADD;c-FLIP
杆状病毒 IAP 重复结构域(BIR)	XIAP,c-IAP1,c-IAP2,Livin,Apollon,ML-IAP,NAIP
Bcl-2 同源性结构域(BH)	Bcl-2,Bcl-XL,Mcl-1,Bax,Bak,Bim,Bid

研究表明多种途径可以激活 Caspase,进而诱导凋亡或类似凋亡的事件发生(图 13-1)。例如,CTL 和 NK 细胞通过穿孔素依赖机制,将凋亡诱导蛋白酶,主要是颗粒酶 B(一种丝氨酸蛋白酶),引入靶细胞,激活 Caspase[17]。与半胱氨酸蛋白酶不同,颗粒酶 B 是一种丝氨酸蛋白酶,但其功能类似于 Caspase,也能在天冬酰胺残基处特异性水解剪切底物[18],剪切和激活多个 Caspase。肿瘤细胞则通过表达各种免疫配体,与 T 细胞受体(PD1、Tim3、LAG3 等)结合以抑制其激活,或与 NK 抑制受体-杀伤性免疫球蛋白样受体(killer immunoglobulin-like receptor,KIR)结合等途径来逃脱这种细胞死亡机制。

另外一条 Caspase 活化通路是由肿瘤坏死因子(tumor necrosis factor,TNF)受体所介导。30 个已知的 TNF 受体家族中有 8 个胞内区含有所谓的"死亡结构域(death domain, DD)"[19,20]。这些包含 DD 的 TNF 受体均可以转导 Caspase 活化信号,主要包括 TNFR1/CD120a、Fas/APO1/CD95、死亡受体(death receptor-3, DR3)/Apo2/Weasle、DR4/TrailR1、DR5/

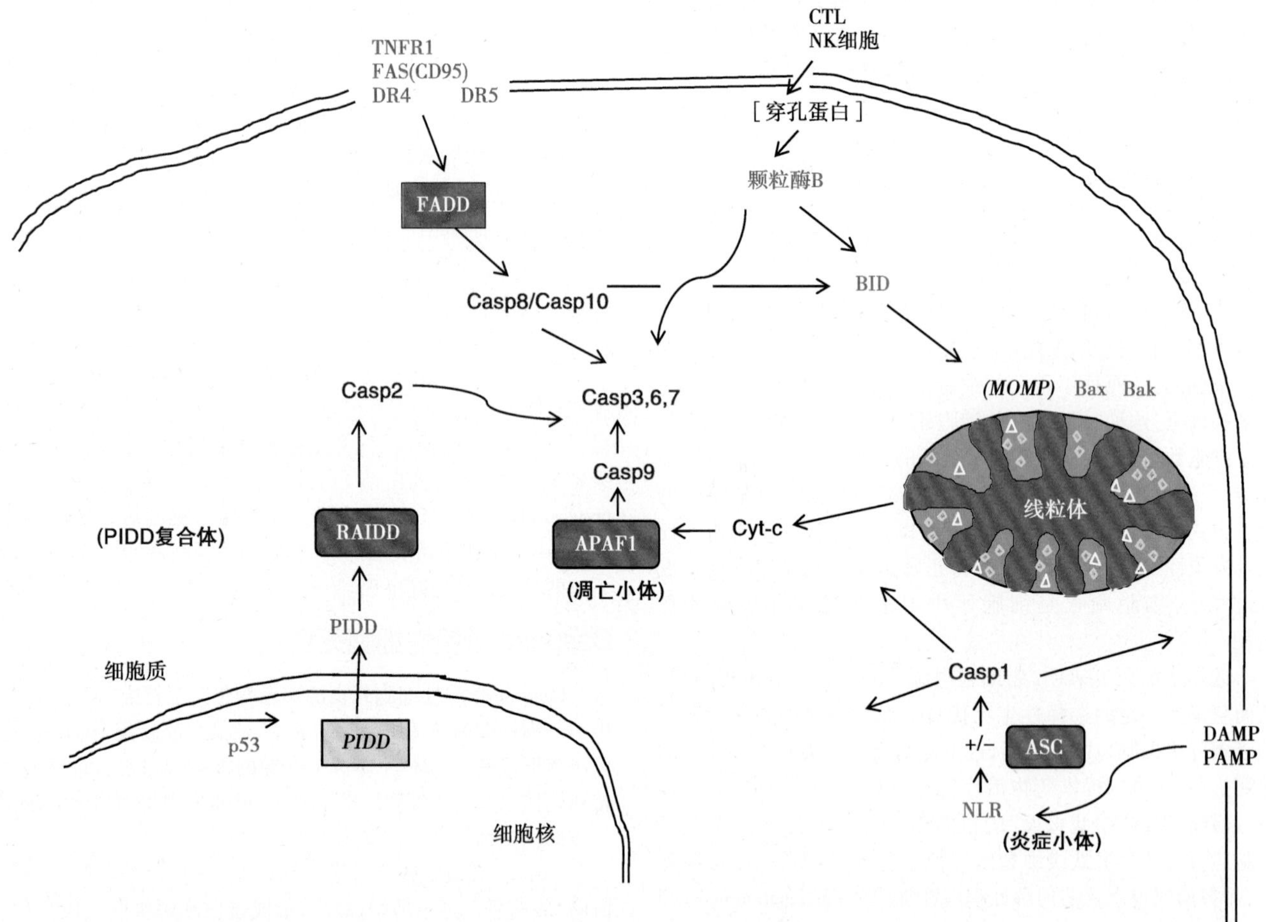

图 13-1　Caspase 激活途径。该图介绍了在哺乳动物细胞中 Caspase 主要激活途径。上述示意图简要展示了体内相关事件的过程。如图所示,外源性途径起始于 TNF 家族细胞因子受体(TNFR1、FAS)和 TRAIL 受体(DR4 和 DR5)。这些蛋白质在细胞质死亡结构域中招募衔接蛋白(包括 FADD),组装形成死亡诱导信号复合物(DISC),该复合物能够结合含 DED 的半胱天冬酶原(pro-Caspase)特别是 pro-Caspase-8,并诱导其活化。Caspase-8 分解下游效应蛋白酶,如 Caspase-3、-6、-7 以及促凋亡 Bcl-2 家族成员 Bid,Bid 能够调控 MOMP 诱导的 Bax 和 Bak。CTLS 和 NK 细胞可以使颗粒酶 B 进入靶细胞(左上所示)。这种蛋白酶能够剪切并激活 Caspase 家族的多个成员以及 Bid。内源性途径(左下所示)起始于各种刺激引起线粒体释放 Cyt-c,这些刺激包括促凋亡 Bcl-2 家族蛋白水平升高(如 Bax 和 Bak 蛋白)。在细胞质中,Cyt-c 结合并激活 Apaf-1,使其与结合并激活 Caspase-9,进而形成凋亡小体。活化的 Caspase-9 直接剪切并激活效应蛋白酶,Caspase-3 和 Caspase-7。外源性病原相关的分子模式(PAMP)和内源性损伤相关分子模式(DAMP)激活 NLR 家族蛋白,使其寡聚化,并能导致炎症小体的组装。在许多情况下,炎症小体可能含有接头蛋白 ASC。ASC 具有 PYD 结构域能够与 Caspase-1 结合。活化的 Caspase-1 可分解多种细胞蛋白,包括细胞因子以及能够导致渗透压和细胞死亡的质膜蛋白

TrailR2 及 DR6 等。当配体与这些细胞表面受体结合后，导致受体聚集，一些胞内蛋白，包括特定的 pro-Caspase，被募集到这些受体的胞内结构域，共同形成“死亡诱导信号复合物”(death-inducing signaling complex，DISC)，触发 Caspase 活化，诱导细胞凋亡[21]。募集至 DISC 的特异性 Caspase 主要是 Caspase-8，在某些情况下是 Caspase-10。这些 Caspase 的 N 末端前结构域均含有 DED，能够结合 fas 相关死亡域(fas associated death domain，FADD)中相应的 DED。FADD 是含有 DD 和 DED 两个结构域的二分体衔接蛋白。FADD 的主要作用是桥接 DD 与 DED 两个家族的蛋白。*fadd* 基因敲除小鼠细胞能够耐受 TNF 家族细胞因子及其受体诱导的细胞凋亡；而 Caspase-8 基因敲除小鼠细胞，在 TNF 家族死亡受体活化因子的诱导下，同样不发生细胞凋亡，表明 Caspase-8 在此细胞凋亡通路中是不可缺少的[22,23]。但是有研究发现小鼠缺失的 Caspase-10 基因，在人类 2 号染色体上呈现明显的基因复制扩增[15]。因此，Caspase-8 与 Caspase-10 在人类细胞中可能是冗余基因。编码 TNF 家族配体或受体基因突变已在多种癌症中得到证实。例如，在淋巴恶性肿瘤中发现了 *FAS*(*CD95*)基因的体细胞突变[24,25]。Fas(CD95)DD 内的错义突变同时常保留野生型等位基因，这是一种显性负向机制，而在 DD 外的错义突变则常伴有等位基因丢失。

在细胞凋亡中，线粒体也发挥着重要作用。线粒体释放细胞色素 c(Cyt-c)于胞质中，引发多蛋白 caspase 活化复合物的组装，即形成“凋亡小体”(apoptosome)[26~29]。“凋亡小体”的核心成分是 Apaf1，是一种 Caspase 激活蛋白，能够结合 Cyt-c 而发生寡聚化，并特异性地结合 pro-Caspase-9。Apaf1 和 pro-Caspase-9 通过各自 CARD 相互作用。CARD-CARD 这种相互作用在凋亡通路的许多环节中发挥重要作用。当小鼠来源细胞的 *apaf2* 或 *pro-Caspase-9* 基因被敲除后，利用药物触发线粒体释放 Cyt-c，细胞却不能发生凋亡，这进一步证实了上述通路在凋亡中的核心作用[30,31]。然而，这些细胞死亡还能够以非凋亡的方式发生[32]，表明线粒体能够调节 Caspase 依赖性和非依赖性两条细胞死亡通路(见下文)。线粒体还可以通过与 Bid 等蛋白相互作用参与 TNF 家族死亡受体介导的细胞死亡通路。当 Caspase-8 蛋白裂解时 Bid 激活，进一步促进线粒体释放 Cyt-c[33]。但是在大多数细胞类型中，线粒体(“内源性”)与死亡受体(“外源性”)的 Caspase 活化通路是完全相互独立的[34]。肿瘤细胞可以通过多种机制来抵抗线粒体依赖性凋亡，如下所述。

在有感染和炎症的情况下，激活的 Caspase-1 启动 Caspase 依赖的细胞死亡形式被称为焦亡[35]。Caspase-1 含有 CARD 前域，可以直接与 NLR(nucleotide binding domain and leucine-rich repeat domain)蛋白的 CARD 结合，如 NLRP1(NALP1)。或者与双向接头蛋白 ASC(Pycard)的 CARD 结合，ASC 还含有一个 PRYIN 结构域(PYD)，可以与 NLRP3(NALP3)等 NLR 家族蛋白或 AIM2 等蛋白结合。NLR 寡聚体与病原体成分或组织损伤过程中相关分子的结合过程“炎症小体”，可以招募并激活 Caspase-1[36~38]。焦亡和癌症的关系目前还仍不明确。

Caspase-2 是 Caspase 家族另一个携带 CARD 的成员，可以特异性与带有 DD 区的双向接头蛋白 RAIDD(receptor-interacting protein-associated ICH-1/CED-3 homologous protein with a death domain)结合[39]。Caspase-2 激活与基因毒性应激有关，主要通过抑癌基因 p53 诱导 PIDD(p53-induced protein with a death domain)表达，PIDD 含有的 DD 蛋白与 RAIDD 的 DD 区结合，形成寡聚体，并组装成一个多蛋白复合物，称为“PIDD 复合体”[40]。

另外，还有些 Caspase 激活机制也被报道过，但其在细胞死亡的病理生理学中所起的作用目前仍不清楚[41~44]。

Caspase 非依赖性细胞死亡

多种 Caspase 非依赖性细胞死亡机制已被明确，这里列举一些典型例子(图 13-2)。坏死可由多种刺激因素引起。当细胞渗透压无法维持平衡时，细胞膜完整性受损，最终导致细胞肿胀和破裂。在细胞坏死过程中一些细胞器(包括线粒体和溶酶体)通常也会膨胀和破裂，释放出促细胞死亡的分子。破坏细胞生物能的因素都可以诱发细胞坏死，如缺氧和低血糖等，导致为细胞膜离子泵提供能量的三磷酸腺苷(adenosine triphosphate，ATP)浓度不足，并对细胞膜上形成跨膜通道的血清补体因子等造成损伤。坏死与癌症生物学密切相关，当肿瘤生长迅速，远超过其血管供应(即血管生成不足)，造成组织缺氧和营养不足，这时往往伴随坏死现象。

除了上述依赖 Caspase 途径的细胞色素 C(Cyt-c)，线粒体还可以启动 Caspase 非依赖途径的细胞死亡[45]。除了细胞色素 Cyt-c，线粒体还释放与凋亡相关的其他几种蛋白，包括内切酶 G、AIF(核内切酶激活剂)、Smac(Diablo)和 Omi(HtrA2)，它们是 Caspase 抑制蛋白家族的拮抗剂，被称为凋亡蛋白抑制剂(IAP)(见下文)[46,47]。此外，线粒体调节的凋亡和非凋亡性死亡在很多情况下是很难区分的，这可能是由于这些细胞器释放的一些蛋白质(如 EndoG 和 AIF)均可以促进染色质凝聚和 DNA 分裂，导致细胞形态学相似。很多刺激都可以引起线粒体调节的凋亡和非凋亡性细胞死亡，包括生长因子缺乏、氧化剂、Ca^{2+}超载、DNA 损伤剂、微管修饰药物等。从这个意义上讲，线粒体有时被认为是决定细胞生死的压力信号“集中营”[48~50]。

线粒体细胞死亡机制均涉及线粒体膜完整性的破坏，但膜通透性的改变可以通过不同的机制介导[51]。在缺血-再灌注损伤(活性氧 ROS 和硝基自由基诱导的氧化应激)和 Ca^{2+} 失调损伤(细胞膜完整性受损或内质网 ER 逃逸)等情况下，跨越细胞内外膜的 MPTP 复合物开放，线粒体的渗透稳态受到干扰[52~54]。线粒体内膜通透性的改变使水和电解质进入富含蛋白质的线粒体基质，导致细胞器膨胀，含有广泛折叠嵴的内膜表面积远大于外膜，最终使线粒体外膜爆裂。在 MPTP 复合物病理性开放过程中，对 ATP 产生至关重要的电化学梯度(质子梯度)丢失，细胞生物学功能受到严重损害。目前认为，引起线粒体通透性改变的主要原因是 MPTP 复合物重要组成部分腺嘌呤核苷酸转位体(adenine nucleotide translocator，ANT)。

此外，细胞死亡机制可能还涉及线粒体外膜透化(mitochondrial outer membrane permeabilization，MOMP)，即外膜选择性地通透，从而释放位于膜间隙的 Cyt-c 等蛋白[51,55,56]。在 MOMP 作用下，细胞才可形成电化学梯度，并维持线粒体渗透稳态。MOMP 主要由 Bcl-2 家族(见下文)中促凋亡成员 Bax 和 Bak(也可能是 Bok)所调控[57~60]。目前已明确的触发 MOMP 机制是促凋亡蛋白(如 Bid、Bim)与 PUMA(p53 upregulated

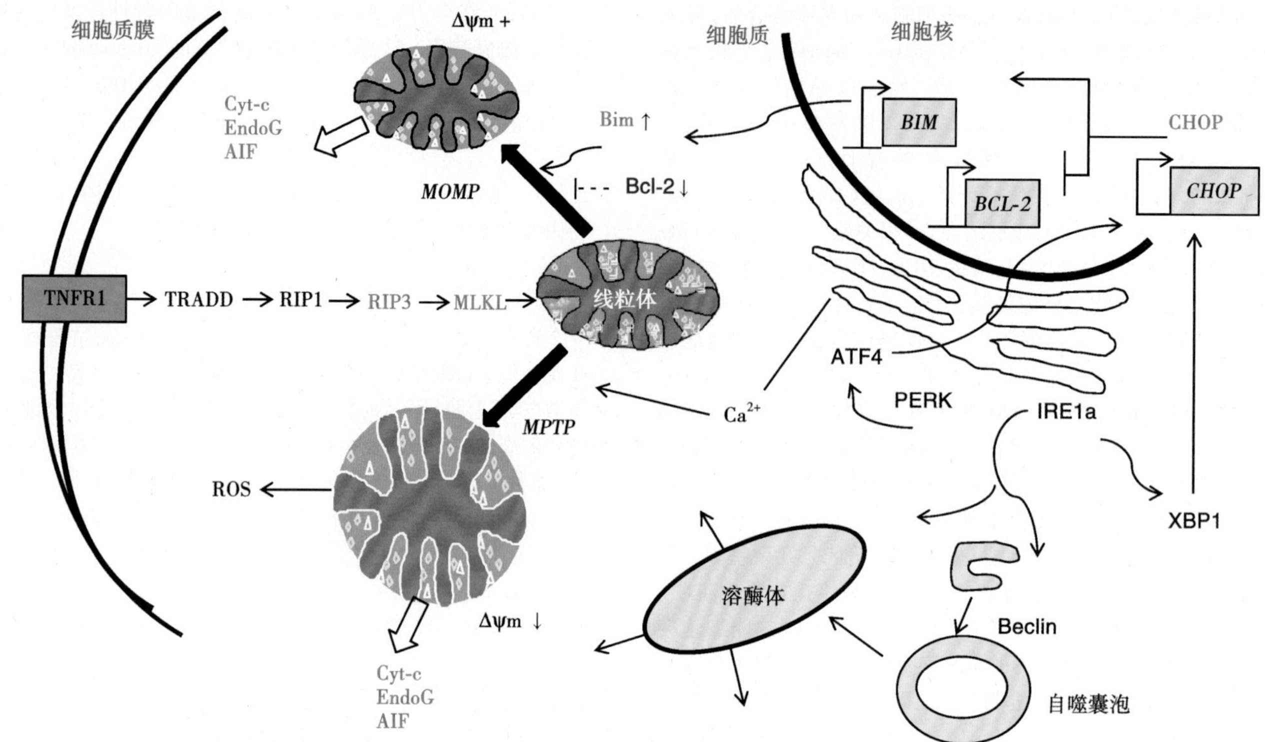

图 13-2 Caspase 依赖性细胞死亡途径。该图介绍了 TNFR1 介导的坏死途径(程序性坏死)涉及一系列的事件,包括 RIP1(receptor-interacting serine/threonine-protein kinase 1)的招募,进而激活 RIP3,激活混合谱系激酶结构域样(mixed lineage kinase domain-like,MLKL),并引起线粒体及溶酶体变化,刺激活性氧类物质(reactive oxygen species,ROS)形成并导致坏死。细胞质中的 TNFR1 死亡结构域与含有死亡结构域结合蛋白 TRADD(tumor necrosis factor receptor type 1-associated DEATH domain protein)结合,后者再与 RIP1 死亡结构域结合。激酶级联反应先传递到 RIP1,随后是 RIP3,然后是 MLKL。线粒体释放蛋白,包括 Cyt-c、endoG 和 AIF(apoptosis-inducing factor),储存在膜间隙。线粒体外膜透化(mitochondrial outer membrane permeabilization,MOMP)可引发线粒体释放(图中上方),该过程受到 Bcl-2 家族蛋白调节,但 Bcl-2 家族蛋白并不参与细胞器肿胀调节。线粒体膜通透性转换孔(mitochondrial permeability transition pore,MPTP)复合物开放也可引发线粒体释放,导致线粒体肿胀和电化学梯度降低(ΔΨm)。MPTP 开放可由 Ca^{2+} 内流和氧化应激等刺激引起。内质网中未折叠蛋白的积累可传导未折叠蛋白反应信号,包括 IRE1α 的激活,IRE1α 激活可导致 Xbp1 mRNA 剪接生成 Xbp1 蛋白(转录因子)和激酶 PERK 的激活,PERK 磷酸化促进 ATF4 mRNA 的翻译和转录因子形成。未折叠蛋白反应转录因子(XBP1、ATF4、ATF6)集中于 CHOP 基因的启动子,编码一种上调促凋亡基因 Bim,下调抗凋亡基因 Bcl-2 的转录因子。自噬小泡形成起始于内质网中,形成双层膜小泡与溶酶体融合(图中右下方)

modulator of apoptosis)对 Bax 和/或 Bak 的作用,可以诱导线粒体外膜上的 Bax 和 Bak 聚集,形成病理性通道,导致 Cyt-c 等蛋白流失。Bax 和/或 Bak 调控的 MOMP 通过释放 Cyt-c 引发 Caspase 依赖性细胞死亡和凋亡线粒体途径,其次,它还可以诱导 Caspase 非依赖性的细胞坏死途径,当 Cyt-c 较少时,MOMP 促进氧化磷酸化解偶联,导致呼吸链上的电子形成有毒自由基[61]。

由于线粒体介导的细胞死亡机制具有多样性,因此肿瘤中涉及这些细胞器及其调控机制也会有多种变化。目前已明确的肿瘤能量代谢方式由依赖有氧呼吸转变为非依赖氧的糖酵解(Warburg 效应),这样使肿瘤细胞更少地依赖线粒体。事实上,与同一正常细胞系相比,这些肿瘤细胞中线粒体数量会更少些[62]。

CTC(circulating tumor cell)和 NK 细胞诱导的细胞死亡也可以通过 Caspase 非依赖途径。颗粒酶 B 可以直接裂解与 Caspase 类似的底物[63,64],从而避免引起 Caspase 诱导的凋亡相关蛋白水解。除了颗粒酶 B,CTC 和 NK 细胞还含有其他的细胞毒性颗粒[17]。此外,CTL 和 NK 细胞在靶细胞膜上形成穿孔素通道也可以导致细胞渗透失衡,诱发 Caspase 非依赖性细胞死亡。利用 CTL 和 NK 细胞所激活细胞死亡机制的多样性,可以尝试利用免疫系统攻击肿瘤细胞,因为肿瘤细胞的死亡障碍(见下文)可以被这些免疫细胞所介导的细胞毒性作用所逆转。

坏死是由 TNFR1 启动的 Caspase 非依赖性细胞死亡机制。当 Caspase-8 功能失活时,TNFR1 可以激活细胞非凋亡性死亡信号通路,该通路涉及丝氨酸/苏氨酸蛋白激酶 Rip1、Rip3 和混合谱系激酶结构域样蛋白(mixed lineage kinase domain-like,MLKL)[65~67]。Rip3 依赖性坏死主要是线粒体产生 ROS 的过程。坏死的发现始于 TNF-α 通过 Caspase 非依赖性机制杀伤肿瘤细胞,这种细胞死亡途径为癌症治疗提供了一个渠道。

Caspase 依赖与非依赖性细胞死亡机制都与内质网(endoplasmic reticulum,ER)应激有关。多种微环境(包括肿瘤相关微环境)均可导致 ER 中未折叠蛋白的积累,从而触发一种自适应信号转导反应,称为未折叠蛋白反应(unfolded protein response,UPR)[68~70]。在 UPR 发生过程中,编码促凋亡转录因子CHOP的基因转录增加,进而刺激编码DR5(death receptor 5、TRAIL受体2)表达,进而导致Caspase-8依赖性凋亡发生。此外,据报道CHOP还可以直接刺激编码Bim基因转录,Bim是Bcl-2家族中促凋亡基因(见下文),它可以刺激线粒体膜中Bax/Bak寡聚体形成,并诱导MOMP从线粒体中释放Cyt-c等蛋白。因此,ER应激可以通过多种途径激活Caspase依赖及非依赖性细胞死亡,并因细胞类型和病理生理环境的不同而不同。

此外,ER在调节细胞内Ca^{2+}稳态中发挥重要作用,它可以改变细胞内游离Ca^{2+}浓度,与细胞死亡存在潜在联系[70~72]。因为在一些极端情况下,内质网腔中Ca^{2+}释放可以触发多条下游信号通路,促进细胞死亡。此外,ER与线粒体紧密相连,既可以促进细胞生存,也可以导致细胞死亡。ER膜与线粒体紧密接触后会形成特殊结构,使Ca^{2+}从内质网外排到线粒体,协助能量传递。但是,过多的Ca^{2+}进入线粒体则会触发MPTP复合物开放,从而导致线粒体膨胀,最终破裂。

自噬(自我吞噬)是细胞的一种分解代谢机制,是指衰老的蛋白质和细胞器被包裹在双层膜囊泡中,与内质网分离,然后被运送到溶酶体中降解其中内容物。自噬的生理作用包括维持蛋白质稳态,补充泛素-蛋白酶体系统,清除未展开、有缺陷及老化蛋白质,以及在营养缺乏期间提供代谢底物等[73,74]。在缺营养情况下,自噬可以促进细胞存活,并被认为有助于肿瘤形成。但在一些极端情况下,依赖于自噬组成部分的细胞死亡机制被报道为自噬性细胞死亡,并且是Caspase非依赖性细胞死亡[75]。毒性化疗药物处理后的肿瘤细胞会出现自噬性细胞死亡[76]。

还有些其他的Caspase非依赖性细胞死亡机制曾被报道,包括溶酶体依赖性细胞死亡、铁依赖性细胞死亡(铁中毒)等[11,77,78],本章节就不详细阐述了。以上这些细胞死亡机制都有可能与癌症生物学相关。

癌症的死亡抵抗机制

研究证实癌细胞能够抑制Caspase,从而抑制细胞凋亡发生,其中至少有三个机制参与其中:①抑制Caspase酶原的激活(前体酶);②中和活化的Caspase(活性酶);③抑制编码Caspase或Caspase激活蛋白基因的表达(见下文)。癌细胞产生出多种抵抗Caspase依赖性细胞死亡的机制。在此,我们总结了部分比较典型的作用机制。

IAP

IAP家族是Caspase的内源性抑制因子(在人体细胞中包括其8个家族成员)[15,79,80]。IAP蛋白质家族在进化上高度保守,可以直接结合活化的Caspase,抑制其蛋白酶活性,或者靶向地破坏活化的Caspase结构[79,81,82]。癌症和白血病发生时伴有IAP的过度表达,使其更难介导Caspase依赖性蛋白水解过程,此过程是凋亡性细胞死亡的前提。

IAP的特征是存在称为杆状病毒内重复序列(baculovirus internal repeats,BIR)的蛋白相互作用域,每个蛋白编号在1~3之间(表13-1)[83]。大部分IAP也携带RING(really interesting new gene)结构,其通过与泛素结合酶(ubiquitin-conjugating enzymes,UBC)相互作用发挥E3连接酶活性。线粒体释放的一些凋亡蛋白,特别是SMAC和HtrA2[84,85],能够结合特定的BIR,从而在IAP表面与竞争性蛋白发生相互作用。在许多情况下,SMAC与IAP结合诱导其发生泛素化和蛋白酶体降解。因此,引发MOMP的因子可清除多种IAP家族蛋白,进而起到抑制Caspase反应的作用。

IAP家族成员中最常见的Caspase抑制剂是XIAP(命名原则是其编码基因位于X染色体上)。XIAP蛋白含有3个BIR蛋白结构域。XIAP蛋白(及其邻近片段)的BIR2结构结合下游效应蛋白酶Caspase-3和Caspase-7,能够有效抑制远端细胞凋亡。XIAP蛋白的BIR3结构结合上游启动蛋白酶Caspase-9,则可抑制线粒体凋亡途径的上游步骤。有研究证实在癌症和白血病中,XIAP在mRNA和蛋白质水平均过量表达,这显然是由表观遗传机制引起的,而并非XIAP基因损伤引起。在AKT高活性的肿瘤中,XIAP蛋白的稳定性也可能增加[86]。

虽然c-IAP1(BIRC2)和c-IAP2(BIRC3)蛋白直接作为酶抑制剂的作用很小,但其也能与Caspase-3、Caspase-7和Caspase-9结合,依赖自身的E3连接酶活性来控制Caspase的降解。这些IAP家族成员也可以通过影响TNF家族受体的信号转导的方式,参与其他细胞死亡相关机制[65,66,87]。细胞因子TNF-α与TNFR1的结合可触发至少三种不同的信号途径,每种途径都涉及受体上蛋白复合物的重叠[88]。除了参与上述Caspase依赖和Caspase非依赖的细胞信号途径,TNFR1还能参与c-IAP1和c-IAP2参与的细胞生存途径。在这方面,c-IAP1和c-IAP2的BIR3结构域可直接结合激酶Rip1。在TNFR1介导的生存途径中,Rip1形成包含E3连接酶c-IAP1、c-IAP2和TRAF2的蛋白复合物,刺激RIP1发生非典型的泛素化(Lys 63连接,而非Lys-48连接),从而启动信号转导途径,激活转录因子NF-κB[89,90]。NF-κB能够影响许多参与宿主防御和免疫调节的靶基因表达,其中有些基因能够抑制凋亡(见下文)[91]。因此,NF-κB通路不仅能够抵消Caspase通路功能,发挥抑制细胞凋亡的作用,而且还能解释TNF-α炎症反应的不良作用。此外,c-IAP1和c-IAP2能够抑制RIP3依赖的细胞程序性坏死,这可能是由于它们具有E3连接酶作用,这个过程可能涉及泛素/蛋白酶体介导的Rip3蛋白水平的降低。在人类癌症中,染色体易位能够产生黏膜相关淋巴组织嵌合蛋白(MALT-c-IAP2),从而使c-IAP2功能丧失,这一点在淋巴瘤研究中已有报道[92,93]。此外,一些癌症的基因组对TRAF2编码基因及与TNF家族受体信号相关的c-IAP1/c-IAP2结合蛋白具有扩增作用。此外,也有报道通过表观遗传机制解释c-IAP1和c-IAP mRNA和蛋白质的过度表达。c-IAP2是NF-κB的直接转录靶点之一,在多种类型的人类恶性肿瘤中已经明确了其经典途径(RelA)及替代途径(RelB)活性过强。

IAP家庭的其他成员(Survivin、Apollon/Bruce、ML-IAP等)也存在与细胞死亡途径相关的作用机制。另外,这些蛋白也具有细胞死亡调节之外的其他作用,例如,Survivin蛋白在染色体分离和细胞分裂中发挥基础作用[94]。

c-FLIP

c-FLIP蛋白是另外一种类型的Caspase内源性调节剂。在癌症中,c-FLIP蛋白的过表达也十分常见[95,96]。c-FLIP结构类似于某些 Caspase，含有一对类似于 Caspase-8 和 Caspase-10 的死亡效应结构域。在 TNF 家族死亡受体信号传导中，c-FLIP 可以直接结合并抑制 Caspase-8 和 Caspase-10 激活。然而，c-FLIP 作用不仅仅局限于抑制 Caspase-8 和 Caspase-10 的激活，它还可能与这些 Caspase 蛋白协同促进 NF-κB 的激活，其相应的作用机制目前还不明确[97]。这种复杂相互作用在小鼠研究中得到证实，敲除 c-Flip 或 Caspase-8 基因的小鼠表现出类似胚胎致死表型。c-Flip 除了能够促进 NF-κB 活化外，本身也是 NF-κB 的直接转录靶标，其表达显著上调（正反馈）[98]。

Bcl-2

Bcl-2 家族蛋白是线粒体外膜透化的主要调节者。Bcl-2 家族分子属于进化保守蛋白质，该家族成员可以促进（如 Bax、Bak 等）或抑制（如 Bcl-2、Bcl-XL）线粒体外膜透化的作用[99~101]。人类有 26 个 Bcl-2 家族蛋白成员，成员之间相互作用形成复杂的同二聚体和异二聚体网络，介导细胞生存或者死亡[102,103]。在癌症发生中，许多 Bcl-2 家族蛋白表达和功能发生改变，这就解释了为什么癌细胞面对多种引起细胞死亡刺激（包括大多数具有细胞毒性的抗癌药物和 X 射线照射、生长因子剥夺和针对生长因子受体信号转导途径的治疗性抑制剂）会产生内在抵抗力。

许多 Bcl-2 家族成员在羧基末端附近有一个疏水性氨基酸，将其固定在线粒体外膜中。相比之下，其他 Bcl-2 家族成员如 Bid、Bim 和 Bad 则缺乏这些膜锚定域。但是，在某些特定刺激下，Bcl-2 家族成员能够动态靶向线粒体。此外，还有一些成员（如 Bax）虽然具有膜锚定域，但其正常情况下保持锁定状态，避免与蛋白结合，只有在受到刺激时才能暴露膜锚定域。

根据预测的或实验证明的三维结构，Bcl-2 家族蛋白质可大致分为两大亚群。一类亚群的结构类似于细菌毒素（如大肠杆菌素和白喉毒素）的穿孔结构域[104~106]。这些 α-螺旋孔样蛋白包括抗凋亡蛋白（Bcl-2、Bcl-XL、Mcl-1、Bfl-1、Bcl-W、Bcl-B）和促凋亡蛋白（Bax、Bak、Bok 和 Bid）。这一亚群的大多数蛋白质可以通过氨基酸序列同源性的保守区来识别，包括 Bcl-2 同源结构域 BH1、BH2、BH3 和 BH4（表 13-1）。然而还有其他情况，Bid 蛋白虽然仅包含 BH3 结构域，但其具有与 Bcl-XL、Bcl-2 和 Bax 相同的蛋白折叠构象。迄今为止，这些蛋白（Bcl-XL、Bcl-2、Bax 及 Bid）在体外合成膜实验中均能形成离子传导通道[107]，但该功能的意义目前尚不明确。Bcl-2 家族的另一亚群蛋白仅存在 BH3 结构域，包括 Bad、Bik、Bim、HrK、Bcl-Gs、p193、APR（Noxa）和 PUMA，它们均属于促凋亡蛋白。在许多情况下，其细胞死亡诱导活性取决于与抗凋亡的 Bcl-2 家族蛋白形成二聚体的能力，作为 Bcl-2 和 Bcl-XL 等蛋白的转显性抑制因子发挥作用[101,102]。然而，一些蛋白（如 Bim、Bid 和 Puma）也可以与促凋亡蛋白 Bax 和 Bak 相互作用，发挥凋亡激动剂的作用。他们能够嵌入膜结构并发生寡聚化，作为激动剂诱导线粒体膜中的寡聚化反应，引起线粒体外膜透化增加。

BH3 结构域能够介导 Bcl-2 家族蛋白间的二聚化作用（图 13-3）。BH3 结构域由约 16 个氨基酸长度的两性 α-螺旋结构构成，其可以嵌入抗凋亡蛋白（如 Bcl-2、Bcl-XL）表面的疏水性空隙中[104,105]。仅含有 BH3 结构域的 Bcl-2 家族蛋白是一系列环境刺激信号与线粒体诱导细胞凋亡通路之间的关联点（见下文）。

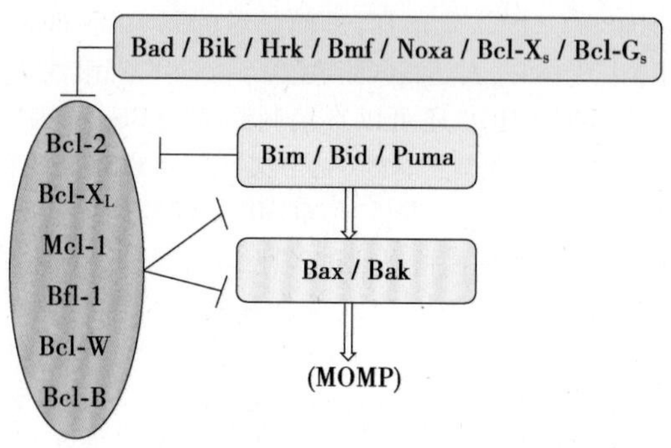

图 13-3 Bcl-2 家族蛋白相互作用网络。该图介绍了 Bcl-2 家族促凋亡和抗凋亡蛋白之间的功能和物理作用与线粒体外膜透化调节有关

Bcl-2 家族成员能够调节线粒体外膜透化，也有人认为它们能够调节线粒体其他生物学功能。例如，组成 MPTP 复合物的成分，包括 ANT 和电压依赖性阴离子通道（voltage-dependent anion channel，VDAC），与 Bcl-2 家族成员相互作用能够促进 MPTP 的开放，而与抗凋亡蛋白相互作用则抑制 MPTP 的开放[108]。此外，VDAC 被认为是线粒体释放 Cyt-c 的促进剂，Bcl-XL 通过对 ANT 的作用[109]，增强 ATP 向胞质中的传递作用，从而支持细胞在缺乏生长因子的情况下继续存活[110]。抗凋亡 Bcl-XL 也能调节线粒体代谢，从而减少乙酰辅酶 A 的产生，具体机制尚不清楚[111]。乙酰辅酶 A 的减少会使凋亡相关蛋白（包括某些 Caspase）的 N-乙酰化减少，从而导致这些蛋白酶的激活更加困难。Bcl-2 也被认为能够调节线粒体氧化还原代谢，其机制亦不明确[112]。

除了影响线粒体，也有研究报道了 Bcl-2 家族蛋白与内质网应激之间的联系[113]。例如，Bax 和 Bak 可以结合 ER 应激信号蛋白 IRE-1α（UPR 信号通路的核心成分）[114]。IRE-1α 是一种定位于内质网的跨膜蛋白，含有一个胞质蛋白激酶结构域和一个内切核糖核酸酶结构域。Bax 和 Bak 刺激 IRE-1α 的内在自身激酶活性和核糖核酸酶活性，从而刺激 CHOP 诱导转录因子 XBP-1（通过 RNA 剪接机制）的产生，同时刺激应激酶激活（Ask1、p38MAPK、JNK1 等）。促凋亡蛋白（Bak/Bax）和抗凋亡蛋白（Bcl-2/Bcl-XL）对内质网 Ca^{2+} 的调节具有相反作用，这可能是由于对内质网中的 Ca^{2+} 通道蛋白（IP3Rs、BI-1、TmBim3）不同作用导致的[72]。

除了参与线粒体和内质网引发的细胞死亡，Bcl-2 家族蛋白也参与自噬性细胞死亡的控制。抗凋亡蛋白 Bcl-2 与自噬相关蛋白 Beclin 结合，阻止其与下游自噬蛋白（如 ATG5）形成复合物，从而阻碍 Beclin 参与的自噬发生[115]。当营养缺乏时，Bcl-2 可以抑制细胞死亡，此过程依赖自噬途径[116]。Beclin 最近被认为是"单倍型不足"的抑癌基因[117]，这提示抑制自噬有助于肿瘤的发生。自噬、肿瘤发生和抗凋亡 Bcl-2 家族蛋白之间联系的最新研究表明，Bcl-2 家族蛋白在控制细胞生死过程中起主要开关作用。

在人类癌症中关于 Bcl-2 家族成员的基因组病变已有大量记载[6,118~120]。其相关机制之一是染色体易位引发转录及翻译过度（Bcl-2），基因扩增（Bcl-2、Bcl-X、Mcl-1），使抑制 Bcl-2 家族基因表达的 microRNA（miR）基因缺失或突变失活（miR15-16

靶向 Bcl-2mRNA)，从而引发 Bcl-2 家族成员过度活化。此外，在某些人类癌症中，Bcl-2 家族的促凋亡成员(Bax)也会发生突变失活。在癌症和白血病中，广泛多样的表观遗传机制也能导致 Bcl-2 家族基因表达失调，其中的部分机制概述如下。

癌症信号转导通路的改变对细胞死亡机制的影响

如前所述，多种受体介导的信号转导途径是细胞死亡的核心机制，包括酪氨酸激酶生长因子受体及其下游通路，在很多类型的癌症发生中这些通路处于失调状态。在此，主要阐述了生长因子受体介导的信号转导和细胞死亡途径之间的联系(图 13-4)。

蛋白激酶

蛋白酪氨酸激酶(protein tyrosine kinase，PTK)通过催化其身或各种底物上酪氨酸磷酸化进一步传递信号，导致磷脂酰肌醇 3′激酶(PI3K)和 AKT 通路的激活，及 Raf/MEK/Erk 通路的激活(见本书其他部分)。此外，大多数的非受体 PTK(Src 家族、Jak 家族、c-Abl 等)和 Ras 家族 GTP 酶也能激活上述两个信号通路。

编码 AKT 的小鼠基因与一些小鼠白血病病毒中发现的 v-akt 癌基因相似。在胸腺瘤中，在 c-akt 基因邻近插入逆转录病毒可引起的 c-akt 的激活[122]。人类有三种 AKT 基因。AKT 能够磷酸化核心凋亡机制中的大量蛋白[123]。例如，AKT 能够靶向 Bcl-2 家族中的促凋亡蛋白 Bad，促使 Bad 发生磷酸化，抑制 Bad 与 Bcl-XL 形成异二聚体[124]。AKT 还可使 Bax 的 184 位点的丝氨酸磷酸化，抑制其从胞质转移到线粒体膜上[125]，此外，AKT 还能够抑制 Bim 的促凋亡活性[126]。在人类，AKT 也能够使 pro-Caspase-9 磷酸化，从而阻断线粒体凋亡通路下游信号的转导[127]。另一个与凋亡相关的 AKT 的底物是叉头转录因子(forkhead transcription factor，FKHD)。FKHD 家族中的某些成员(如 Foxo-3)具有调控细胞凋亡的能力，这可能与影响编码 FASL 基因的转录有关[128]。AKT 促使 FKHD 磷酸化，进而抑制后者入核。AKT 也能引起 XIAP 的磷酸化，通过减少泛素依赖性蛋白酶体降解，来提高 XIAP 蛋白的稳定性[86]。

多种生长因子受体和淋巴因子受体能够通过 Jak/STAT 通路传递信号。STAT 家族转录因子可以刺激 Bcl-X 基因的转录，这可能是其抑制凋亡的机制之一[129]。另外，Jak 家族的非受体 PTK 能够激活 PI3K，从而导致 AKT 家族激酶的激活。这些信号机制也与各种癌基因相关，如 BCR-ABL 及某些类型白血病的致瘤因子[130]。

Raf/MEK/Erk 信号通路与细胞死亡具有重要联系。例如，Erk 能够使前凋亡蛋白 Bim 丝氨酸 69 位点发生磷酸化，通过蛋白酶体依赖的机制促进 Bim 蛋白降解[131]。Raf/MEK/Erk 通路能够导致 Bim 蛋白积累，从而促进细胞凋亡发生。MEK 能够

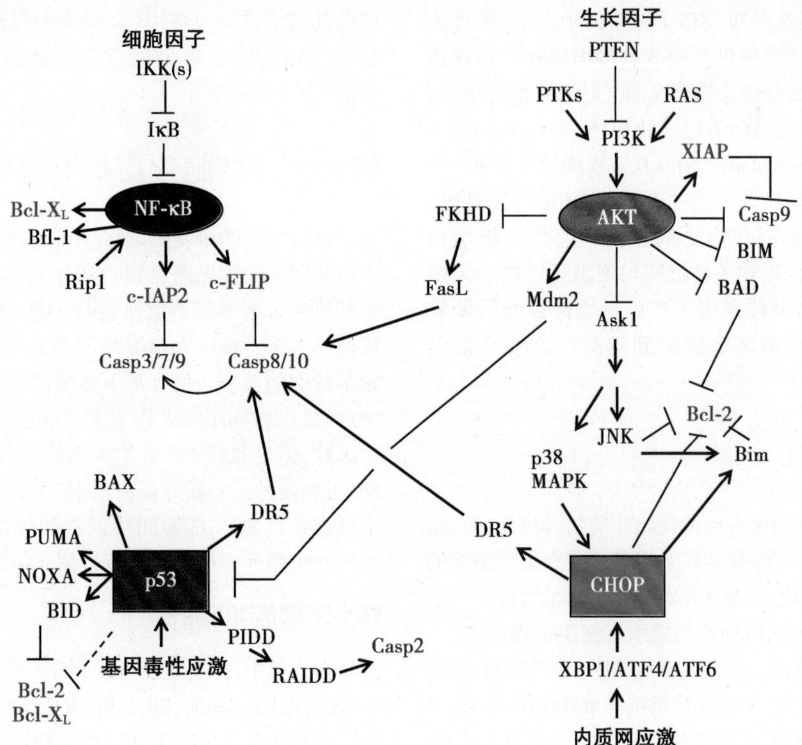

图 13-4　信号转导与细胞死亡调节。该图介绍了一些转录因子和激酶在细胞凋亡调控中发挥重要作用，包括蛋白激酶 AKT(PKB)和转录因子 p53、NF-κB 和 CHOP。图中显示了细胞凋亡调节蛋白和基因相互之间关联的部分实例。多种生长因子受体和癌蛋白激活 PI3K，产生第二信使，进而激活蛋白激酶 AKT(PKB)。PTEN 是一种脂蛋白磷酸酶，可防止上述第二信使的积累。在许多肿瘤中，由于基因缺失、基因突变或其他机制使 PTEN 不能表达[89]。AKT 发生磷酸化可使与细胞凋亡直接或间接相关的多个蛋白质激活(箭头所示)或失活(⊥所示)[121]。转录因子 CHOP 的表达受内质网应激产生的转录因子(包括 XBP1、ATF4 和 ATF6)的调控，相关信息见正文

促进抗凋亡蛋白 Bcl-2 蛋白的磷酸化,增强其促生存功能[132]。

蛋白质乙酰化

组蛋白赖氨酸残基的乙酰化能够控制染色质结构,进而影响基因转录。该机制目前研究已经比较成熟。但是,越来越多的研究认为非组蛋白的乙酰化可通过多种机制影响生理过程。在细胞死亡调控方面,已有研究发现蛋白乙酰化失调能够影响细胞死亡核心蛋白装置的关键组分。如用组蛋白脱乙酰基酶(HDAC)抑制剂处理癌细胞时,只有转录因子 FOXO1 发生乙酰化才能诱导 Bim 表达[133]。此外,乙酰化还可通过其他转录因子(STAT、NF-κB、p53)的赖氨酸修饰,间接影响多种凋亡和细胞死亡相关基因[134]。抑癌基因 p53 的乙酰化依赖一种与转录无关的 Bax 激活[135]。DNA 损伤修复蛋白 Ku70 发生乙酰化可通过影响细胞死亡中核心蛋白组分的相互作用,中和其抗凋亡功能。如前所述,Bcl-XL 也可影响线粒体乙酰辅酶 A 的产生,进而使有些蛋白质发生 N-α-乙酰化,例如某些依赖该种翻译后修饰介导下游反应的 Caspase 蛋白酶[111]。

转录因子

正如所料,在人类癌症中常见到细胞死亡相关基因发生表观遗传失调,但其机制十分复杂。其中与癌症密切相关的是类固醇激素受体,包括雌激素、雄激素和维生素 D 受体,它们能够调节各种细胞死亡和细胞存活基因的表达。例如,在乳腺上皮细胞或者雌激素受体(estrogen receptor,ER)表达阳性的乳腺腺癌中,ER 是 Bcl-2 基因表达的重要转录调节因子[136]。视黄醇受体和其他核受体也通过转录机制调节各种细胞死亡和存活基因的表达[137]。此外,部分转录因子在前文已经介绍过了,例如 FKHD 家族成员(FOXO3、FOXO1)、CHOP(CCAAT/enhancer-binding protein homologous protein)、NF-κB 家族成员及 p53。当转录因子离开细胞核与线粒体表面的 Bcl-2 家族成员接触时,细胞死亡蛋白的非转录机制开始发挥主导作用[138]。组蛋白乙酰化和去乙酰化的染色质相关修饰酶与细胞死亡核心蛋白组分也有关联。因此,如果转录因子和染色质修饰酶的调控在癌变过程中发生畸变,最终会影响到细胞死亡核心蛋白组分。

癌症化疗药物毒性

尽管越来越多的靶向药物有望替代化疗药物,但目前而言,化疗药物的应用仍然是治疗癌症的基本手段。这些化学药物的作用原理是抑制 DNA 合成、诱导 DNA 损伤或破坏微管。一些经典的癌症化疗药物和 X 射线照射均能引起细胞损伤,其进一步触发的分子事件与细胞死亡核心装置有关联。一些细胞保护性蛋白能够阻断细胞死亡途径,对化疗抵抗有重要作用。

p53 是基因毒性应激诱导细胞凋亡的主要介质之一。放疗和 DNA 损伤抗癌药物能有效刺激肿瘤抑制因子 p53 的激活。p53 蛋白作为一种四聚体转录因子,其水平由 E3 连接酶 Mdm2 控制。p53 能够直接诱导仅有一个 BH3 结构域蛋白(Bim、Bid 和 PUMA)及直接诱导线粒体外膜透化的 Bax 蛋白的表达[139~142]。活化的 p53 也能刺激 TNF 家族死亡受体 5(DR5)的转录,从而使肿瘤细胞对其配体反应更加敏感[143]。在许多类型的人类癌症中,多种机制可以导致 p53 的失活,如基因缺失、基因突变(突变使其丧失转录活性)和 Mdm2 基因的扩增。在血液学癌症的临床试验中,采用小分子药物阻断 MDM2 蛋白与 p53 相互作用具有良好的治疗效果[144],并且这些小分子药物与 Bcl-2 抑制剂具有协同作用[145]。

有证据表明 p53 除了发挥核转录因子的作用外,还可通过非转录机制促进细胞凋亡。有报道称 p53 的细胞质库与线粒体有关,其能够直接诱导 Bax 的活化,抑制 Bcl-2 和 Bcl-XL 活化[146,147]。更为重要的是即使 p53 发生突变也能激活细胞死亡途径,这进一步增加了针对这一途径寻找药物干预的希望。

DNA 损伤也可通过 p53 非依赖性调节机制与细胞死亡核心蛋白装置建立联系。例如,Ku70 在修复断裂 DNA 中发挥重要作用。Ku70 与 Bax 结合并抑制其易位到线粒体,但当 DNA 损伤时,Ku70 发生乙酰化可释放出结合的 Bax[148,149]。Ku70 还能与 c-FLIP 相互作用并抑制其泛素化和蛋白酶体降解,而 Ku70 乙酰化可促进 c-FLIP 释放,导致其自身降解,促进细胞凋亡[150]。另外一种 DNA 修复蛋白 RAD9 在 DNA 损伤后,从细胞核转移到线粒体,并在线粒体上结合并中和抗凋亡蛋白 Bcl-2 和 Bcl-XL,从而促进细胞死亡[151]。

抗微管药物也可通过多种机制影响细胞死亡途径。通常情况下,Bcl-2 家族促凋亡蛋白 Bmf-1 被隔离在微管上。当抗癌药物破坏微管结构时,Bmf-1 被释放出来,进而结合并中和 Bcl-2 家族的抗凋亡成员[152]。研究证实 Bim 参与微管靶向药物诱导的细胞死亡,而其他仅含 BH3 的蛋白质 Bmf 和 Puma 可能促进了这一过程[153]。微管靶向药物也刺激 Caspase 级联反应,导致 Bcl-2 多个部位发生磷酸化,从而破坏其抗凋亡功能[154,155]。

借助靶向细胞死亡机制开发抗癌药物

在抗癌药物研发中,通过中和抗凋亡或激活细胞死亡核心蛋白装置的治疗思路已经取得了很大的进展。所有的药物靶点都可通过至少三个层次进行干预:基因水平、mRNA 水平和蛋白质水平。相应干预策略的差异主要取决于靶基因及其生物学特性的差别。尽管基于核酸的治疗手段(RNA 治疗、基因治疗)已经在临床前进行了大量探索,有些甚至还被纳入了临床试验,但是此处主要介绍了调控蛋白质靶点的治疗策略。此外,尽管多种信号转导蛋白(例如:蛋白激酶、转录因子)参与上述细胞死亡途径,能够间接促进肿瘤细胞死亡,此处重点介绍了核心细胞死亡机制直接调控因子。

Bcl-2 家族抑制剂

在人类中,已鉴定出 6 个 Bcl-2 家族的抗凋亡成员(Bcl-2、Bcl-XL、Mcl-1、Bcl-W、Bfl-1、Bcl-B),这些基因在多种类型的部分癌症患者体内呈现高表达。在某些癌症病例中,甚至同时存在两个或两个以上的 Bcl-2 家族抗凋亡成员的过度表达。Bcl-2 或 Bcl-2 家族的其他抗凋亡成员的过度表达与化疗耐药有关,原因是这些蛋白质能够阻碍 DNA 损伤剂、微管修饰药物和抗代谢产物诱导的细胞死亡。因此,通过使 Bcl-2 和相关蛋白失活来恢复细胞的化疗敏感性,已经成为非常有前景的癌症治疗策略。

目前已经鉴定了能够结合抗凋亡的 Bcl-2 家族蛋白,并能中和其活性的化学物质，相应药物进入了临床开发阶段。例如性腺激素（venetoclax）在人类临床试验中取得了理想的效果，现已被美国食品和药物管理局（FDA）批准用于某些类型的白血病治疗。有研究报道了能够靶向抗凋亡Bcl-2家族蛋白表面的（立体结构）缝隙的化合物，这些化合物可以作为抗凋亡Bcl-2家族蛋白质内源性拮抗剂中BH3基序的受体[6,104,120]。这些模拟BH3肽基结构的化合物抑制抗凋亡的Bcl-2家族蛋白，防止Bcl-2蛋白的过度增加。据报道，有多种天然产物和合成化学物质能够靶向Bcl-2或Bcl-XL上的BH3结合位点，其中有些物质已被证实能够促进体外培养的肿瘤细胞凋亡，抑制小鼠模型的肿瘤生长[156~162]。开发抗凋亡Bcl-2家族蛋白化学拮抗剂有两种策略，一种是利用高特异性抑制剂（仅中和抗凋亡Bcl-2家族中的6种蛋白），另一种是利用能够结合多个家族成员的广谱抑制剂。这两种策略可以相互平衡，从而有效保障药物的安全性。例如，抑制Bcl-2、Bcl-XL、Bcl-W活性的化学抑制剂（navitoclax）的研发陷于停滞，原因是Bcl-XL有助于维持血小板的寿命，而该抑制剂能够导致血小板减少[163~165]。相比之下，特异性Bcl-2抑制剂（venetoclax）没有血小板减少的副作用，但其作用范围较窄，可能仅对Bcl-2是主要致病因素的癌症有治疗效果。

目前也提出了一些其他的针对Bcl-2家族蛋白的癌症治疗方法，但这些方法多数没有效果。例如，有设想通过模拟Bid、Bim、PUMA活性，研发Bax、Bak的直接抑制剂[166]，但是该设想一直没有实现。另外，也应积极探索上调Bcl-2家族成员表达的间接机制。Mdm2的小分子拮抗剂（idasanutlin）能够引起p53蛋白的累积，进而刺激包括Bax、NOXA、BID、PUMA在内的几个Bcl-2家族促凋亡基因的转录。Mdm2拮抗剂现已进入临床试验，其对某些类型的恶性肿瘤（如急性白血病）有比较理想的治疗效果。Mdm2抑制剂是否仅适用于p53未发生突变的癌症，其对某些含有p53突变体（这些突变体仍然保留了退出细胞核的能力，并能直接调节Bcl-2家族蛋白的活性）的恶性肿瘤患者是否有益有待进一步的研究。此外，MEK的化学抑制剂（曲美替尼、考比替尼等）可以通过降低其泛素化和降解蛋白酶体来提高Bim蛋白的水平。另外，Akt小分子抑制剂有望恢复由这种蛋白激酶磷酸化的促凋亡Bcl-2家族蛋白（如Bad、Bax等）的活性，目前该小分子也抑制剂正处于临床试验阶段。最后，也有人报道了针对核受体家族"孤儿成员"Nur77的化合物，这类化合物能够使转录因子从细胞核转移到线粒体中，并与线粒体中的Bcl-2、Bfl-1和Bcl-B相互作用促进细胞死亡[138,167~169]。

TRAIL

目前也广泛开展了TNF家族细胞因子的抗癌活性的临床前评价。这些研究主要是基于内源性细胞凋亡机制开发的两种治疗策略，分别是注射重组蛋白（构成细胞因子配体的功能片段）或者激动剂型的单克隆抗体（结合并激活TNF家族死亡受体）。

TNF-α是TNF家族成员，由于其具有促炎作用，能够直接杀伤肿瘤细胞，大量研究尝试将TNF-α用于癌症治疗。但到目前为止，TNF-α仅用于治疗四肢的黑色素瘤和软组织肉瘤等比较少见的癌症治疗[170]。TNF相关凋亡诱导配体（TNF-related apoptosis-inducing ligand，TRAIL）能够诱导肿瘤细胞凋亡，但不会诱导炎症信号，有可能作为TNF-α的替代物用于肿瘤治疗。包括灵长类动物在内的临床前研究数据表明TRAIL的可溶性片段能够进入机体组织，对机体正常组织没有毒性，同时对小鼠异种移植瘤具有明显的抑制效果[171]。在小鼠模型中，TRAIL与细胞毒性抗癌药物联合使用，可起到协同抗肿瘤活性的作用。基于这些研究数据，有研究团队对一种重组的TRAIL开展了临床试验，但试验结果最终未能达到理想的效果。TRAIL在临床疗效不佳的原因有很多，如肿瘤发生时下游凋亡信号通路受到阻断，肿瘤细胞"诱饵"受体（与TRAIL竞争结合死亡受体）的表达，DR4（TRAIL-R1）和DR5（TRAIL-R2）的表达水平不足等[171]。

有研究报道了DR4、DR5或两者的激动剂抗体用于临床试验[172,173]。研究结果显示作为单一的治疗药物，这些抗体的临床效果很差，其中一些抗体还具有肝脏毒性[174,175]，这可能是由于FcR与肝内Kuppfer细胞结合所致。激动剂抗体均借助FcR结合来实现与肿瘤细胞受体的联系，因此，这一过程依赖巨噬细胞、NK细胞或其他表达FcR的免疫细胞，来实现凋亡信号的传递。近来，利用FcR非依赖性机制来实现与死亡受体联系的工程抗体已进入临床研究阶段。

TRAIL及其受体可以通过两种途径诱导细胞凋亡，即线粒体依赖性途径和线粒体非依赖性途径，具体哪种途径取决于特定肿瘤中的细胞凋亡类型[176]。线粒体依赖的信号传导途径通过激活Caspase-8和Bid，从而激活能够与Bax和Bak相互作用蛋白，诱导线粒体外膜透化。线粒体非依赖性的凋亡优势在于绕过了生存蛋白（如Bcl-2）造成的细胞凋亡障碍。化疗中，难以治疗的癌症往往具有线粒体通路缺陷，借助线粒体非依赖性凋亡机制开展这一类型的癌症治疗具有很大优势。然而，由于没有可靠的预测性生物标志物，在癌症发生中TRAIL是通过线粒体依赖性机制，还是非依赖性机制，仅能通过经验判断。

c-FLIP能够阻遏TRAIL诱导的凋亡，其与正常招募到TRAIL受体复合物的Caspase有关联。由于mRNA剪接作用，c-FLIP蛋白存在短型和长型两种亚型。长型的c-FLIP蛋白在许多癌症中过度表达，通过调节Caspase激活抑制TNF家族死亡受体介导的信号传导[95]。目前已经鉴定出了多种能够降低c-FLIP蛋白水平的化合物，包括亚过氧苯胺羟肟酸（SAHA）[177]、三萜类化合物（Bardoxolone）及其类似物。Bardoxolone即2-氰基-3,12-二氧代齐墩果烷-1,9(11)-二烯-28-羧酸（CDDO）[178~183]。研究表明人肿瘤细胞对TRAIL单独治疗有抵抗力，但是CDDO与重组TRAIL联合使用可以抑制移植到小鼠体内的人类肿瘤组织的生长[184]。因此，CDDO等化合物可恢复癌细胞对TRAIL（或抗TRAIL受体抗体激动剂）的敏感性，可作为TRAIL治疗的辅助药物。在小鼠实验中，TRAIL和CDDO类似物的联合使用并没有毒性反应[184]，这两种靶向疗法的联合使用具有很好的研究前景。

IAP抑制剂

针对IAP抑制剂的研发，最常用的策略是模拟IAP内源性拮抗剂（特别是SMAC、HtrA2）的作用。SMAC、HtrA2模拟物结合多个IAP家族成员的BIR结构域，从而破坏它们与Caspase（Caspase-3、-7、-9）和激酶（RIP1、RIP2）的相互作用[185]。要结合IAP家族成员取代Caspase和激酶功能，促进细胞凋亡或抑制信号转导，必须将 SMAC 和 HtrA2 活性区被还原为 4 个氨基酸肽[186]。目前已经报道了几种能够占据 IAP 上四聚体结合位点的肽基化合物[187~189]以及天然产物，其中有些已经进入临床试验。SMAC 模拟复合物作为凋亡诱导物用于体外培养的肿瘤细胞系时，仅能偶尔表现出单体活性，这也是终止这类药物研发的原因之一。然而，SMAC 模拟物通常可以使肿瘤细胞对细胞毒性抗癌药物和 TNF 家族死亡受体（如 TRAIL 和靶向 TRAIL 受体的激动剂）介导的细胞凋亡更加敏感。从这个意义上说，IAP 拮抗剂有利于 TNF 家族死亡受体诱导的细胞死亡通路发挥作用，这为联合治疗提供了坚实的理论基础。

另一类开发 IAP 化学抑制剂的方法是采用酶活性抑制分析从化合物文库中筛选化合物，在这个系统中重组 IAP 化合物与活化的 Caspase 混合，形成一种抑制酶复合物，如果化合物能够替代 Caspase 活性，就能通过含氟底物的分解体现出来[190,191]。然而，通过这种方法筛选化合物，还没有获得具有足够亲和力的分子进入临床试验。

还有一种策略是通过线粒体凋亡蛋白 ARTS 的释放破坏 IAP[192]。ARTS 蛋白能够结合某些 IAP，如 XIAP、c-IAP1、c-IAP2。现已证明 ARTS 蛋白能够将 E3 连接酶（Siah-1）招募到 IAP，并促进其降解[193]。据报道源自 ARTS 的短肽可以诱导细胞凋亡，但目前还未转化出类药物分子。另外，ARTS 在 IAP 上结合位点的结构特征也有待明确，该问题的深入研究可能为蛋白-蛋白相互作用界面的"成药性"提供新的见解。

一些肿瘤存在两个及以上 IAP 家族成员的过度表达，这表明采用同时针对多个 IAP 成员的广谱抑制剂可能比单独的选择性药物效果更好。同时选择性药物和广谱抑制剂的治疗指标还需要更加广泛的比较，从而揭示最佳的药物研发方向。

结论

在癌症的发生发展中，程序性细胞死亡机制的失调发挥着关键作用。尽管许多机制细节仍有待进一步揭示。对细胞死亡途径和调节这些途径的蛋白质网络的阐述，有助于我们了解细胞死亡决策机制。在某些领域，研究人员正在努力开展基础理论向治疗策略的转化研究，甚至已经完成了癌症新治疗药物的开发。

（赵善民 井莹莹 译 韩志鹏 校 卫立辛 审）

缩略语列表

BH	Bcl-2 同源结构域
CARD	Caspase 富集功能域
Caspase	半胱氨酸天冬氨酸蛋白酶
Cyt-c	细胞色素 c
CTL	细胞毒性 T 细胞
DD	死亡结构域
DED	死亡效应结构域
DISC	死亡诱导信号复合体
DR	死亡受体
ER	内质网
FasL	Fas 配体
FKHD	叉头转录因子
IAP	细胞凋亡抑制剂
miR	微小 RNA
MOMP	线粒体外膜透化
MPTP	线粒体膜通透性转换孔
MLKL	混合系列蛋白激酶样结构域
MALT	黏膜相关淋巴组织
MM	多发性骨髓瘤
NK	自然杀伤细胞
NHL	非霍奇金淋巴瘤
PI3K	磷脂酰肌醇 3-激酶
PCD	程序性细胞死亡
ROS	活性氧
TNFR1	TNF 受体 1
TNF	肿瘤坏死因子
UBC	泛素结合酶

参考文献

The complete reference list can be found on the Wiley Companion Digital Edition of this title (see inside front cover for login instructions).

2 Green DR, Evan G. A matter of life and death. *Cancer Cell*. 2002;**1**:19–30.
3 Danial NN, Korsmeyer SJ. Cell death: critical control points. *Cell*. 2004;**116(2)**:205–219.
5 Reed JC. Apoptosis-targeted therapies for cancer. *Cancer Cell*. 2003;**3**:17–22.
11 Kroemer G, El-Deiry WS, Golstein P, et al. Classification of cell death: recommendations of the nomenclature committee on cell death. *Cell Death Differ*. 2005;**12(Suppl 2)**:1463–1467.
12 Galluzzi L, Maiuri MC, Vitale I, et al. Cell death modalities: classification and pathophysiological implications. *Cell Death Differ*. 2007;**14(7)**:1237–1243.
15 Reed JC, Doctor KS, Godzik A. The domains of apoptosis: a genomics perspective. *Sci STKE*. 2004;**2004(239)**:re9.
20 Kersse K, Verspurten J, Vanden Berghe T, Vandenabeele P. The death-fold superfamily of homotypic interaction motifs. *Trends Biochem Sci*. 2011;**36(10)**:541–552.
21 Peter ME, Krammer PH. The CD95(APO-1/Fas) DISC and beyond. *Cell Death Differ*. 2003;**10(1)**:26–35.
28 Adams JM, Cory S. Apoptosomes: engines for caspase activation. *Curr Opin Cell Biol*. 2002;**14**:715–720.
33 Korsmeyer SJ, Wei MC, Saito M, Weiler S, Oh KJ, Schlesinger PH. Pro-apoptotic cascade activates BID, which oligomerizes BAK or BAX into pores that result in the release of cytochrome *c*. *Cell Death Differ*. 2000;**7**:1166–1173.
35 Bergsbaken T, Fink SL, Cookson BT. Pyroptosis: host cell death and inflammation. *Nat Rev Microbiol*. 2009;**7(2)**:99–109.
46 Green DR, Galluzzi L, Kroemer G. Mitochondria and the autophagy-inflammation-cell death axis in organismal aging. *Science*. 2011;**333(6046)**:1109–1112.
48 Kroemer G, Reed JC. Mitochondrial control of cell death. *Nat Med*. 2000;**6**:513–519.
53 Marzo I, Brenner C, Zamzami N, et al. The permeability transition pore complex: a target for apoptosis regulation by caspases and Bcl-2-related proteins. *J Exp Med*. 1998;**187**:1261–1271.
55 Green DR, Kroemer G. The pathophysiology of mitochondrial cell death. *Science*. 2004;**305**:626–629.
58 Vaux D, Korsmeyer S. Cell death in development. *Cell*. 1999;**96**:245–254.
69 Kaufman RJ. Orchestrating the unfolded protein response in health and disease. *J Clin Invest*. 2002;**110**:1389–1398.
70 Kim I, Xu W, Reed JC. Cell death and endoplasmic reticulum stress: disease relevance and therapeutic opportunities. *Nat Rev Drug Discov*. 2008;**7(12)**:1013–1030.
71 Giorgi C, Romagnoli A, Pinton P, Rizzuto R. Ca2+ signaling, mitochondria and cell death. *Curr Mol Med*. 2008;**8(2)**:119–130.
72 Sano R, Reed J. ER stress-induced cell death mechanisms. *Biochim Biophys Acta*. 2013;**1833(12)**:3460–3470.
73 Mizushima N, Levine B, Cuervo AM, Klionsky DJ. Autophagy fights disease through cellular self-digestion. *Nature*. 2008;**451(7182)**:1069–1075.
75 Kroemer G, Marino G, Levine B. Autophagy and the integrated stress response. *Mol Cell*. 2010;**40(2)**:280–293.
79 Deveraux QL, Reed JC. IAP family proteins: suppressors of apoptosis. *Genes Dev*.

1999;**13**:239–252.

80 LaCasse EC, Mahoney DJ, Cheung HH, Plenchette S, Baird S, Korneluk RG. IAP-targeted therapies for cancer. *Oncogene*. 2008;**27**(**48**):6252–6275.

91 Baud V, Karin M. Is NF-kappaB a good target for cancer therapy? Hopes and pitfalls. *Nat Rev Drug Discov*. 2009;**8**(**1**):33–40.

96 Yu JW, Shi Y. FLIP and the death effector domain family. *Oncogene*. 2008;**27**(**48**):6216–6227.

101 Chipuk JE, Moldoveanu T, Llambi F, Parsons MJ, Green DR. The BCL-2 family reunion. *Mol Cell*. 2010;**37**(**3**):299–310.

102 Strasser A. The role of BH3-only proteins in the immune system. *Nat Rev Immunol*. 2005;**5**:189–200.

104 Fesik SW. Insights into programmed cell death through structural biology. *Cell*. 2000;**103**:273–282.

116 Shimizu S, Kanaseki T, Mizushima N, et al. Role of Bcl-2 family proteins in a non-apoptotic programmed cell death dependent on autophagy genes. *Nat Cell Biol*. 2004;**6**(**12**):1221–1228.

119 Calin GA, Croce CM. Chromosomal rearrangements and microRNAs: a new cancer link with clinical implications. *J Clin Invest*. 2007;**117**(**8**):2059–2066.

120 Huang J, Fairbrother W, Reed J. Therapeutic targeting of Bcl-2 family for treatment of B-cell malignancies. *Expert Rev Hematol*. 2015;**8**(**3**):283–297.

121 Testa JR, Bellacosa A. AKT plays a central role in tumorigenesis. *Proc Natl Acad Sci U S A*. 2001;**98**(**20**):10983–10985.

132 Konopleva M, Contractor R, Tsao T, et al. Mechanisms of apoptosis sensitivity and resistance to the BH3 mimetic ABT-737 in acute myeloid leukemia. *Cancer Cell*. 2006;**10**(**5**):375–388.

166 Czabotar P, Westphal D, Dewson G, et al. Bax crystal structures reveal how BH3 domains activate Bax and nucleate its oligomerization to induce apoptosis. *Cell*. 2013;**152**(**3**):519–531.

171 Ashkenazi A. Targeting death and decoy receptors of the tumour-necrosis factor superfamily. *Nat Rev Cancer*. 2002;**2**:420–430.

173 Lemke J, von Karstedt S, Zinngrebe J, Walczak H. Getting TRAIL back on track for cancer therapy. *Cell Death Differ*. 2014;**21**(**9**):1350–1364.

185 Fesik SW, Shi Y. Structural biology. Controlling the caspases. *Science*. 2001;**294**:1477–1478.

186 Shi Y. A conserved tetrapeptide motif: potentiating apoptosis through IAP-binding. *Cell Death Differ*. 2002;**9**:93–95.

191 Wu TY, Wagner KW, Bursulaya B, Schultz PG, Deveraux QL. Development and characterization of nonpeptidic small molecule inhibitors of the XIAP/caspase-3 interaction. *Chem Biol*. 2003;**10**:759–767.

第 14 章　肿瘤细胞永生化：靶向端粒酶

Ilgen Mender, PhD ■ Zeliha Gunnur Dikmen, MD, PhD ■ Woodring E. Wright, MD, PhD ■ Jerry W. Shay, PhD

概述

寻找肿瘤治疗的特定靶向药物仍然是一项挑战。肿瘤细胞的无限增殖(永生化)是肿瘤的一个特征,这与核糖核蛋白酶复合物组成的端粒酶激活相关。约 85%~90%的人类原发性肿瘤表达端粒酶活性,而大多数正常细胞却不表达。端粒酶被认为是一种独特而几乎通用的肿瘤治疗靶点。虽然目前已经开展了有关端粒酶靶向治疗的多项研究,但仍然没有得到批准的药物。本章重点介绍不同靶向端粒酶方法的优缺点和总结临床前和临床试验结果。我们还将回顾由端粒酶介导的端粒脱帽的新方法,其靶向表达端粒酶的肿瘤细胞而不针对正常细胞。

端粒酶：肿瘤治疗的广谱靶点

端粒$(TTAGGG)_n$是在线性染色体末端发现的六聚体核苷酸重复序列。端粒在不同生物体中长度不同:如人类(2~15kb)和小鼠(高达 100kb)[1]。端粒受到特殊的蛋白质复合物的保护,以防止被识别为受损或破损的染色体。这种特殊的蛋白质复合物被称为 shelterin 复合体,用于稳定染色体末端,这一复合体包括 6 种蛋白质成分(TRF1, TRF2, Rap1, TIN2, TPP1 和 POT1),主要保护端粒 DNA 末端免受外切核酸酶破坏和被 DNA 损伤机制识别[1~3]。Shelterin 复合体有助于形成每个端粒末端被称为端粒 T 环结构(T-loop)的特殊套索状环样结构。每条染色体末端单链端粒 DNA 悬突区可以反转插入到端粒 DNA 双链结构中,中断双链 TTAGGG 重复序列后形成三链结构,这也称为替代环(D-loop)。D-loop 与单链 TTAGGG 结合蛋白 POT1 相结合,整个 T 环和 D 环结构的基本作用是隐藏或掩蔽单链和双链端粒 DNA,防止其被识别为损伤的 DNA,因此在端粒维持中发挥重要作用[4]。

G-四联体是在端粒 DNA 鸟嘌呤碱基之间产生的二级结构,保护染色体末端免于降解[5]。正常体细胞在培养中分裂的能力有限,在细胞分裂达到极限数后停止增殖(这是所谓的 Hayflick 限制),这与 DNA 复制周转率有关[6]。因为 DNA 聚合酶不能复制 DNA 后随链的 3′末端(通常称为末端复制问题),在没有维持机制的情况下,端粒会随着每次细胞分裂而缩短,直到端粒消失殆尽为止[7]。除了末端复制问题,体内外氧化应激和/或其他未知的过程可能都会加速端粒缩短。只有少数无帽状态的短端粒可以诱导依赖 p53 的 G1/S 细胞周期停滞,也被称为复制型衰老。当细胞进入衰老,正常细胞即停留在一个静止阶段。如果重要的细胞周期检查点基因如 TP53 或 pRB 发生改变,则细胞可越过衰老得以继续增殖(细胞生存期延长),直到许多端粒末端严重缩短引起染色体末端的融合和促进染色体断裂融合桥循环(也被称为危机)。衰老和危机是两个保护细胞免于向早期癌症发展的根本机制。逃离危机的细胞几乎普遍表达端粒酶,即核糖核蛋白细胞逆转录酶(图 14-1a),其中有两个延长端粒的必需成分:催化成分 hTERT(端粒酶逆转录酶)和端粒酶 RNA 组分(hTR 或 hTERC)(图 14-1b)[8,9]。端粒酶在人类早期胚胎发育中表达,随后仅在胚胎干细胞和部分增殖祖细胞(例如雄性生殖精母细胞、激活的淋巴细胞和其他一些瞬时扩增细胞)中表达,而在其他大多数组织中不表达(图 14-2a)[10]。端粒酶不是细胞恶性转化绝对必需的因素;然而,约 85%~90%的原发性人类肿瘤都具有端粒酶活性(图 14-2a),而绝大多数正常组织没有检测到端粒酶活性[9]。也存在一种少见的(约占 3%~10%)维持端粒长度的机制称为端粒替代延长(alternative lengthening of telomeres, ALT),其涉及端粒内同源重组和 T 环解离。

已有几项关于正常细胞和肿瘤细胞中端粒酶表达/活化变化的研究报道。某些癌症中 TERT 启动子区域内 DNA 重排断点与 TERT 表达增加相关[11]。此外,在永生化的非致瘤性成纤维细胞中,TERT 启动子突变可导致端粒酶激活[12]。不同的研究表明 TERT 启动子突变[13]和 TERT 基因扩增[14,15]与 TERT 转录活化和端粒酶的激活相关。尽管对具有极低丰度转录本的基因如 TERT 难以调节,但有研究报道另一种调控端粒酶的机制是替代性拼接。DNA 直接转录来的前体 mRNA(pre-mRNA)经过剪切过程切除其中的内含子(非编码序列)并连接外显子(编码序列),以产生用于成熟蛋白质翻译的 mRNA。但是,在 RNA 剪接期间,在前 mRNA 中可以切除或者保留外显子以合成具有多功能作用的多种不同蛋白质。这个过程是已知的可变剪接[16],可能对端粒酶的调节很重要。

将 hTERTcDNA 导入大多数正常细胞会导致端粒酶的再激活和无限的细胞增殖[17,18],上述现象表明端粒酶活性的抑制主要受到转录机制调节,而全长 hTERT 的产生可能参与端粒酶激活[19,20]。然而,转录后调节以及表观遗传改变可能在这个动态过程中发挥着重要作用[19]。在人类发育过程中抑制端粒酶以及在肿瘤进程中重新激活端粒酶的机制目前仍不明确。选择性剪接是抑制或重新激活端粒酶可能的机制之一。研究发现有不同的 hTERT 剪切变异体,例如 α-、β-、αβ-[16,21,23,24],它们都可能在调节端粒酶活性中发挥作用[16,20]。hTERTα 是其中一个已知的剪切变异体,其可以作为显性失活抑制剂来抑制端粒酶活性。因此,hTERTα 和全长 hTERT 以及其他剪切变异体可能对端粒酶活性发挥重要调节作用[19,25]。最近的论文研究表明,38bp 的可变数目串联重复序列的一段 1.1kb 区域(在旧大陆灵长类动物中高度保守)是排除外显子 7 和 8 以外产生 β-剪切变异体的必不可少的位点,并且在这些重复序列之间的 RNA 配对决定是否进行 hTERT 剪接[26,27]。重要的是,选择性剪接的错误调节是几乎所有肿瘤的标志。另外,我们最

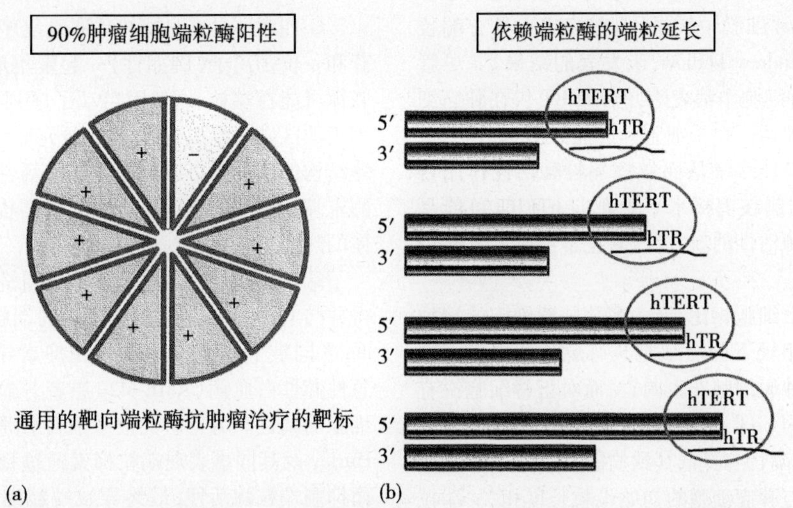

图 14-1　正常细胞由于缺少端粒酶活性而不能延长其端粒,因此导致细胞寿命缩短,而肿瘤细胞(约 90%的肿瘤细胞,a)可以通过端粒酶(包括 hTERT 和 hTR 亚基,b)延长其端粒导致其无限增殖(癌症的标志)。正常细胞和肿瘤细胞之间端粒酶的差异表达使端粒酶成为几乎通用的治疗靶标

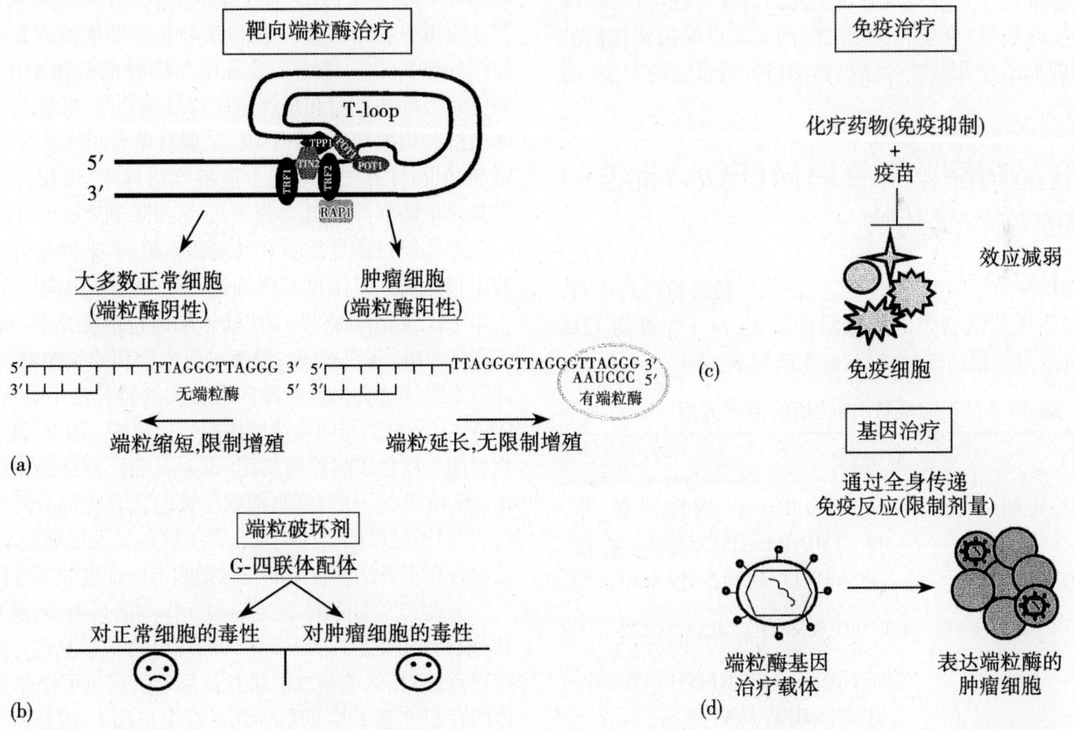

图 14-2　端粒 T-loop 结构示意图。这种结构在正常细胞和肿瘤细胞中相似,但正常细胞通常不表达端粒酶,端粒逐渐缩短,而表达端粒酶的肿瘤细胞可以维持其端粒长度(a)。G-四联体稳定剂(b),免疫疗法(c)和基因治疗方法(d)皆存在一定的缺点。G-四联体稳定剂存在一定的毒性效应,其除了可以结合和稳定端粒 T 环结构以外,还可以结合在除端粒以外染色体的其他区域。因此,这些药物对正常细胞和肿瘤细胞都具有毒性(b)。免疫疗法最重要的缺点之一是当化疗和靶向癌症患者的疫苗联合使用时,由于大多数化疗药物都具有免疫抑制作用,化疗药物可以阻断免疫效果(c)。基因治疗面临的挑战是如何将基因载体高效率转染进入全身的肿瘤细胞(d)。此外,针对治疗的免疫反应可以限制剂量。基因疗法通常需要更多侵入性基因传递方案,并且通常不能以口服方式全身给药

近对端粒酶调节有新的认识。这一领域以往的共识认为hTERT在正常分化的人体组织中转录沉默。然而，有越来越多的证据表明hTERT在正常细胞中转录，但剪接成不具有端粒酶活性的剪切变异体（Andrew Ludlow，未发表的结果）。尽管hTR（hTERC）几乎在所有细胞中都表达，但hTERT仅在肿瘤细胞中检测到极低水平的表达。在干细胞和肿瘤细胞中，什么机制调节TERT表达至其最佳水平从而发挥端粒酶活性作用目前仍然未知，然而可以推测在剪接水平上靶向hTERT可能是一种降低肿瘤细胞端粒酶活性的新方法，对正常细胞的毒性可能很小。

与具有长端粒的正常细胞相比，绝大多数肿瘤细胞的端粒相对较短。正常干细胞相较于肿瘤细胞具有更长的端粒。靶向端粒酶给药可能促进肿瘤细胞发生凋亡，而对正常细胞没有显著影响[28]。例如，将hTERT显性阴性突变体导入肿瘤细胞系中，可以导致肿瘤细胞凋亡和降低其致瘤能力[29,30]。肿瘤细胞凋亡途径发生的死亡与肿瘤细胞的初始端粒长度相关，端粒较短的肿瘤细胞会在端粒较长的肿瘤细胞之前死亡[31]。此外，与其他肿瘤靶点相比，肿瘤细胞极少对靶向端粒酶的治疗产生抵抗[32]。但是，在ALT或其他端粒维持机制中并没有得到相关的实验证据。所有这些因素表明端粒酶不仅是一种独特和几乎普遍的癌症靶点，而且靶向端粒酶可能是副作用相对较少，比标准化疗方案更具有安全性的治疗方法。因此，深入理解端粒、端粒酶、衰老和肿瘤之间的关系可以拓宽我们的认知，并为肿瘤治疗和基础肿瘤生物学研究提供新的方法（图14-1）。

尚未有食品药品监督管理局（FDA）批准的靶向端粒/端粒酶药物

基于端粒酶的不同治疗方法虽然在临床前实验得到证明，但是目前在临床前试验中的端粒酶抑制剂，没一个获得FDA批准。最有潜力的靶向端粒/端粒酶策略见表14-1。

表14-1　靶向端粒/端粒酶的治疗方案

治疗方案	抑制剂
G-四联体稳定剂	BRACO19，RHPS4，端粒抑素，卟琳，TMPyP4，CX-3543/喹氟拉辛，AS1411/阿糖胞苷/Ara-C
免疫治疗	GV1001，VX-001，GRNVAC1/2
基因治疗	Telomelysin，Ad-hTERT-NTR/CB1954，hTERTp-HRP/IAA
端粒和端粒酶相关的蛋白质	格尔德霉素，姜黄素
T-oligo方案	PARP抑制剂
小分子抑制剂	BIBR1532
寡核苷酸	GRN163L
端粒酶介导的端粒脱帽方法	慢病毒突变hTERC，6-硫代-2′脱氧鸟苷

G-四联体稳定剂

G-四联体是在鸟嘌呤串联重复序列存在条件下，鸟嘌呤核苷和一价阳离子（例如钾）一起聚集形成的四联体形态。G-四联体可能在端粒、癌基因启动子序列，和其他生物学相关的基因组的区域中形成[33]。已有研究证明靶向人类端粒中G-四联体结构的小分子可以抑制端粒酶活性（可能间接作用）和端粒酶末端断裂[34]。因此，这个二级结构的特征是设计小分子配体的热门靶点。

端粒抑素是目前报道的从环圈链霉菌3533-SV4中分离获得并与G-四联体结构相互作用的端粒酶抑制剂[35,36]。Nakajima和同事[37]的研究表明端粒抑素导致端粒酶抑制并诱导从急性髓性白血病（AML-M2）患者骨髓分离出的原发性白血病细胞的凋亡。另有研究报道了G-四联体的配体称为TMPyP4。Hurley及其同事表现端粒抑素通过稳定分子内G-四联体结构而抑制端粒酶活性，最终导致端粒缩短，而TMPyP4促进分子间G-四联体的形成诱导后期桥的产生，从而抑制ALT阳性细胞以及端粒酶阳性细胞的增殖。他们研究报道还指出相较于其他G-四联体化合物例如TMPyP4[38]，端粒抑素与分子内G-四联体结构结合更紧密和更特异。另一项研究报道了端粒G4配体RHPS4（五环吖啶），RHPS4通过稳定由单链端粒DNA形成的G-四联体结构，从而在亚微摩尔水平降低端粒酶活性[39]。其他报道也指出RHSP4能以端粒长度不依赖的方式引起端粒加帽的改变[40]。体内实验证明与抗肿瘤药物相比，RHSP4具有更有效的抗肿瘤和抗肿瘤转移效应[41]。尽管基于其体外和体内抗肿瘤效应，BRACO19（三取代吖啶）归类为G-四联体稳定剂，但在体外气管或肠上皮细胞培养中，该化合物的有效性因其对生物屏障的低渗透性而受到限制[42]。在体外实验中，一些配体通过诱导细胞衰老或细胞凋亡，来抑制各种肿瘤细胞的生长。这些配体也发挥端粒脱帽的短期效应[43]。在过去的十年中，已经出现许多G-四联体配体包括荧光素、双取代吖啶、阳离子卟啉、苝四羧酸二酰亚胺衍生物和吲哚喹啉。然而，研究证据表明这一类化合物靶向端粒酶的特异性十分有限，与双链DNA相比，它们与四联体结构的结合较差。因此，许多这些化合物可能不仅会影响肿瘤细胞，也会影响正常细胞中的四联体结构（图14-2b）。任何抑制细胞生长的化合物都会降低端粒酶活性，所以不足以证明这些化合物能够特异性地抑制端粒酶，尤其是没有在不表达端粒酶的正常细胞上验证过的那些化合物。

一些与G-四联体稳定剂相互作用的蛋白质，具有诱导衰老和/或凋亡的能力。尽管G-四联体结构似乎是很好的抗肿瘤治疗靶点，但在除端粒外的染色体复制区域也可以观察到G-四联体的存在。基于G-四联体还具有由末端G-四分体形成的大面积平面表面，到目前为止设计的大多数小分子都是针对这种普遍的结构而不是针对一个特定G-四联体。因此，对这些化合物的普遍关注是其安全性问题：靶向G-四联体结构的小分子配体影响肿瘤细胞的同时，也可能影响正常细胞的端粒结构[44,45]（图14-2b）。

虽然有两个已经进入临床试验的四联体相关的小分子，但是目前并没有直接的证据证明这些小分子是针对端粒酶的靶向治疗。第一个药物CX-3543（quarfloxin/quarfloxacin，Cylene Pharmaceuticals，SanDiego，CA，USA）是一种氟喹诺酮衍生物，可在核仁中通过抑制 Pol1 转录,选择性地破坏核仁素/rDNA 中的 G-四联体结构,导致肿瘤细胞增殖减少并诱导肿瘤细胞凋亡[46,47]。但是,由于 CX-3543 与 MYC G-四联体结构相互影响[46],所以其体外抗增殖能力和体内异种移植物模型中的抗肿瘤效应,可能与端粒的 G-四联体不具有相关性。另外,CX-3543 有选择性靶向 Pol1 而不是靶向端粒功能,这进一步提示 CX-3543 对端粒功能可能是有间接影响或者甚至没有影响[47]。临床试验中的另一种可以形成稳定的 G-四联体结构的药物是 AS1411(Cytarabine/Ara-C, Antisoma Research, London, UK),其特异性针对核仁素[48]。

免疫治疗

近几十年来,研究人员对肿瘤相关抗原(TAA)特异性免疫治疗开展了相关研究。然而,作为大多数 TAA 免疫疗法仅限于少数肿瘤类型,基于端粒酶在大多数肿瘤细胞中的广泛表达,靶向端粒酶的免疫疗法理论上是一种有效的治疗方案[49]。hTERT 在蛋白酶体中通过 E3 泛素连接酶降解产生的蛋白质片段/肽,可以在肿瘤细胞表面由主要组织相容性复合物 MHC Ⅰ类途径递呈。因此,通过患者自身免疫系统($CD8^+$T 淋巴细胞)特异性识别靶向此类抗原,是杀伤表达端粒酶的肿瘤细胞的直接方法[50,51](见参考文献[52])。目前已经开发出几种 hTERT 疫苗,但是 GV1001 和 GRNVAC1 都是临床试验中最有希望的疫苗(表 14-2)。GV1001 是 16 个氨基酸残基组成的 TERT 肽(aa 611~626),可以与多态性的 HLA Ⅱ类分子相结合。最近的研究表明转染 hTERT 基因的树突状细胞接种有助于诱导端粒酶特异性 $CD4^+$ 和 $CD8^+$ T 细胞应答[53],以及在不可切除的胰腺癌患者和非小肺癌癌症患者中和 GV1001 一起接种可以诱导 hTERT 特异性 T 细胞反应[54,55]。应用 GV1001 和环磷酰胺联合治疗的肝细胞癌患者对Ⅱ期临床试验表现为部分或完全无反应[56]。在Ⅲ期临床试验中,GV1001 联合化疗应用没有改善晚期或转移性胰腺患者的总生存期[57]。GRNVAC1 主要用于诱导 $CD4^+$ 和 $CD8^+$ T 细胞产生免疫反应。GRNVAC1 是通过在体外将编码近全长 hTERT 蛋白的 mRNA 导入自体树突细胞制备的。这类树突状细胞被重新引入患者体内,进而可以特异识别患者肿瘤中表达的任何 hTERT 肽[32]。目前,在急性髓性白血病患者中 GRNVAC1 已进入Ⅱ期临床试验阶段。由于单药疗法可能疗效有限,组合治疗可能是一种杀死具有异质性的肿瘤细胞的更有效的方法。但是,大多数化疗药物具有免疫抑制作用,可能会妨碍免疫效果。基于此原因,疫苗可能不应当与化学治疗药物联合使用[58](图 14-2c)。因此,需要研究新的策略来改善和增强化疗期间端粒酶疫苗的免疫应答效果。

表 14-2 靶向端粒酶疫苗的临床试验

疫苗	政府临床试验标识符/阶段	条件	药物干预	状态
GV1001	NCT01223209/1 期	癌症	GV1001,LTX-315	已完成
	NCT01247623/1/2 期	晚期恶性黑色素瘤	GV1001	已完成
	NCT01342224/1 期	局部晚期胰腺癌	Tadalafil 和疫苗	激活,但未招募
	NCT00425360/3 期	局部晚期或转移性胰腺癌	Gemcitabine, capecitabine, GV1001	已完成
	NCT01579188/3 期	不可手术的 3 期非小细胞肺癌	GV1001	未招募
	NCT00509457/未提供	非小细胞肺癌	GV1001	已完成
	NCT00444782/2 期	肝细胞癌	GV1001	已完成
	NCT00358566/3 期	晚期不可切除胰腺癌	GV1001, gemcitabine	终止
GRNVAC1	NCT00510133/2 期	急性髓性白血病	GRNVAC1	激活,但未招募
VX001	NCT01935154/2 期	非小细胞肺癌转移	VX001	招募

基因治疗

肿瘤基因治疗主要通过将治疗性 DNA 导入患者细胞中,从而达到治疗肿瘤的目的。编码具有治疗效应的 DNA 导入靶细胞后,在细胞器的协调配合下完成 DNA 表达最终形成诱导靶细胞凋亡的蛋白产物。基因可以通过溶瘤病毒载体导入,导入基因包括催化药物前体的代谢酶或者自杀基因[59]。尽管基因治疗具有靶向肿瘤的高度特异性,但目前其仍面临诸多挑战,包括制备工艺和配方较为复杂,以及临床试验需要专业技术人员的通力合作[60](图 14-2d)。一些研究表明,基因治疗是肿瘤治疗的有效方案,但其易产生脱靶效应。成功的抗肿瘤治疗需要靶向肿瘤细胞,缩小肿瘤病灶并实现持久的抗肿瘤效应[61,62]。工程技术改造的腺病毒载体可以针对性进入具有端粒酶活性的肿瘤细胞从而杀死肿瘤细胞。这些腺病毒载体具有端粒酶逆转录酶(TERT)启动子,可以驱动腺病毒的复制。在这种情况下,病毒在端粒酶阳性的细胞中特异性复制[63],而在大多数正常细胞中不能复制[63]。病毒复制扩增可以导致肿瘤细胞裂解,裂解释放的病毒颗粒又可以感染邻近的肿瘤细胞[63-66]。这就是目前已知的具有肿瘤特异性复制能力的腺病毒(hTERTp-TRAD)的基因治疗方案[61,67]。其中包括端粒酶介导的病毒治疗产品 Telomelysin(OBP-301),其是 hTERT 启动子驱动的改进型溶瘤腺病毒。临床前期研究表明 Telomelysin 以及其他类似修饰的腺病毒对多种肿瘤细胞具有显著的治疗效果[64,66,68,69]。Ⅰ期临床试验结果显示其无明显毒副作用,但存在众多可控的毒副作用，包括发热、畏寒和注射部位疼痛。部分实体瘤患者会出现无症状的淋巴细胞短暂下降[70]。而且系统性治疗方案对端粒酶阳性的处于增殖状态的正常干细胞具有潜在的毒性，因此 hTERTp-TRAD 可能短暂影响增殖性细胞包括肠隐窝处增殖细胞、血液细胞以及一群表皮基底层和表皮基底上层细胞[8,60]。另外值得关注的是，瘤内注射不足以使肿瘤病灶完全消退[71]。

自杀基因疗法也被称为“基因导向的酶前体药物治疗”，类似溶瘤基因治疗，可以特异性作用于肿瘤细胞，而对正常细胞几乎无影响[32,72]。自杀基因治疗包括三个基本步骤：首先是靶向载体；其次将载体携带的由 hTERT 驱动的酶编码基因转染到细胞中；最后，形成被酶激活的药物前体，进而导致毒素释放到细胞质中引发端粒酶阳性细胞死亡[72]。尽管基因治疗（自杀基因或者溶瘤载体）具有治疗前景，但不如疫苗或者寡核苷酸治疗效果显著[73]。未来的方向在于制备多功能病毒载体，譬如仅在表达端粒酶的 p53 突变细胞中特异性复制的载体，这样可能潜在地减少对正常增殖干细胞的毒性作用。

小分子抑制剂和反义寡核苷酸

最近十年，研究人员通过筛选数以万计的化合物用于寻找抑制端粒酶活性的小分子抑制剂，除了候选化合物 BIBR1532 以外，目前没有发现高效特异的小分子抑制剂。BIBR1532 虽然在临床前研究模型中取得了良好结果[74,75]，但可能由于其与端粒酶较低的结合及解离效率使其无法进入到临床试验阶段[76,77]。经过多年的新药的筛选，Geron 公司研发生产的 GRN163L（Imetelstat）是与小分子抑制剂类似的药物，它是一种靶向端粒酶的脂肪修饰的 N3′→P5′硫代氨基磷酸酯寡聚核苷酸，能与识别端粒的端粒酶 RNA 亚单位（hTR）互补结合，从而显著抑制端粒酶活性，因此，GRN163L 是一类竞争性端粒酶抑制剂[78]。GRN163L 是第二代改良型 GRN163，拥有 13bp 的非反义寡核苷酸，可以通过 5′末端偶联亲脂的棕榈油酰基 C16 增加细胞摄入[28]。GRN163L 对不同的肿瘤细胞系和异种移植物模型均有显著的端粒酶活性抑制作用，体内外实验证明其在肝癌[79]、肺癌[80]、乳腺癌[81,82]、膀胱癌[71]、多发性骨髓瘤[83]、胰腺癌[84]、结直肠癌[85]、恶性胶质瘤[86]以及食管腺癌[87]细胞系中均可以显著抑制端粒酶活性进而导致端粒长度的进行性缩短。在肿瘤异种移植瘤模型中，GRN163L 能够减少肿瘤的转移。研究人员采用裸鼠尾静脉注射肺腺癌 A549 细胞建立人肺腺癌转移瘤模型，实验组给予每周三次并持续三周腹腔注射 15mg/kg GRN163L，结果发现实验组肺腺癌转移瘤小鼠中未发现肺部肿瘤[80]。在肝癌细胞移植瘤小鼠模型中，GRN163L 可以抑制肿瘤生长并提高肿瘤细胞对传统化疗药物的敏感性[79]。在乳腺癌肺转移移植瘤模型中，给予 12 次 GRN163L 处理（每周三次持续四周，30mg/kg），可以有效抑制乳腺癌细胞的增殖和减少乳腺癌细胞的肺转移[82]。在人骨髓瘤细胞移植瘤模型中，GRN163L 可以减少肿瘤大小以及延长肿瘤小鼠的生存期[83]。尽管体内外实验研究提示 GRN163L 具有良好的抗肿瘤作用，但由于其导致的血液系统和肝脏功能障碍等副作用，目前 GRN163L 尚未通过临床试验。临床上出现 GRN163L 所致的剂量限制性毒性时，例如血小板减少症，就需要中断 GRN163L 药物剂量直到患者血小板回升到正常水平，这就可能导致停药期间端粒重新延长。

GRN163L（Imetelstat）是第一个进入临床试验的端粒酶活性抑制剂，目前包括 10 项Ⅰ期临床试验和 6 项Ⅱ期临床试验在内的 17 项研究已经完成。相关临床试验总结见表 14-3。50~74 岁的晚期实体瘤患者（结直肠癌 6 人，肺癌 3 人，间皮瘤 2 人，胰腺癌 2 人，其他癌症 7 人）表现为活化部分促凝血酶原激酶时间（active prolonged thromboplastin，aPTT）延长、胃肠副反应、乏力、贫血、GGT 升高以及周围神经病变。尽管 GRN163L 导致血小板减少症的限制性毒性剂量是 4. 8mg/kg，但 1 人在给予 GRN163L（3. 2mg/kg）出现不明原因死亡[88]。14 例局部复发或转移性乳腺癌（MBC）病例（再次转移性乳腺癌病例 3 人，先前接受新佐剂紫杉烷治疗的乳腺癌病例 6 人）在 GRN163L 联合紫杉醇和贝伐单抗治疗时，Ⅰ期临床试验结果显示最常见的药物毒性是血细胞减少。大多数患者由于出现治疗引起的中性粒细胞减少和血小板缺少等副作用，减少或延迟了 GRN163L 和/或者紫杉醇药物使用剂量[73]。儿科实体肿瘤患者Ⅰ期临床试验结果显示外周血单核细胞端粒酶活性降低，Ⅱ期临床试验推荐的端粒酶阳性肿瘤患者的最大耐受剂量为 285mg/m^2（MTD）。在该项研究中，在 21 天治疗周期的第 1 天和第 8 天给予两小时的静脉输注，结果显示剂量限制性毒性水平（DLT；360mg/m^2）引起的骨髓功能抑制导致治疗延迟超过 14 天。在治疗过程中，由于病理分级和治疗循环数等原因，部分患者出现贫血、淋巴细胞减少、中性粒细胞减少、血小板减少症和导管相关性感染[89]。由于给予 GRN163L 治疗的病人总生存期较差，晚期乳腺癌Ⅱ期试验（NCT01256762）因此终止[49]。在 21 天治疗周期的第 1 天和第 8 天给予 GRN163L，在此治疗周期中 GRN163L 可能不能有效抑制端粒酶活性，因而肿瘤细胞可以产生新的端粒平衡长度。

表 14-3　GRN163L 相关临床试验

临床试验·政府标识符/期	病例类型	药物干预	状态
NCT01568632/1 期	难治性或复发性实体瘤/淋巴瘤	GRN163L	撤回
NCT01273090/1 期	难治性或复发性实体瘤/淋巴瘤	GRN163L	已完成
NCT01243073/2 期	原发性血小板增多症/真性红细胞增多症（ET/PV）	GRN163L，标准治疗	暂停
NCT00594126/1 期	难治性或复发性多发性骨髓瘤	GRN163L	已完成

续表

临床试验·政府标识符/期	病例类型	药物干预	状态
NCT01916187/1 期	神经母细胞瘤	GRN163L,13-顺式维 A 酸	撤回
NCT00732056/1 期	复发或转移性乳腺癌	GRN163L,紫杉醇,贝伐单抗	已完成
NCT00310895/1 期	难治性或复发性恶性实体瘤	GRN163L	已完成
NCT00718601/1 期	多发性骨髓瘤	GRN163L,硼替佐米,地塞米松	已完成
NCT01242930/2 期	多发性骨髓瘤	GRN163L,标准治疗	启动,未招募
NCT00510445/1 期	晚期或转移性非小细胞肺癌	GRN163L,紫杉醇,卡铂	已完成
NCT01265927/1 期	Her2 阳性乳腺癌	GRN163L,曲妥珠单抗	启动,未招募
NCT00124189/1 期	慢性淋巴组织增生性疾病(CLD)	GRN163L	已完成
NCT02011126/2 期	复发或难治性实体瘤	GRN163L	撤回
NCT01137968/2 期	非小细胞肺癌	GRN163L,贝伐单抗	已完成
NCT01731951/未提供	原发性或继发性骨髓纤维化	GRN163L	启动,未招募
NCT01256762/2 期	复发或转移性乳腺癌	GRN163L,紫杉醇,包括/未包括贝伐单抗	已完成
NCT01836549/2 期	复发性或难治性脑肿瘤	GRN163L	招募中

开发端粒酶抑制剂的挑战

端粒酶抑制剂的开发研究还存在其他潜在挑战。以 GRN163L 为例,诱导细胞衰老或者坏死的响应时间和细胞复制循环后端粒磨损出现时间一样长。因此,这种延迟响应限制了其可以作为晚期癌症患者一线治疗方案的实用性。因此也有研究提示可在传统治疗之后应用端粒酶抑制剂来抑制残留肿瘤细胞生长[65]。在一项已完成的Ⅱ期临床研究中,将标准化双联化疗方案后使用 GRN163L 作为晚期非小细胞肺癌(NSCLC)的维持治疗(clinicaltrials. gov:NCT01137968)。此研究主要用于观察 GRN163L 是否可以作为维持方案延长 NSCLC 患者无进展生存期(PFS)。将符合条件的Ⅳ期 NSCLC 或晚期局部复发 NSCLC 患者分为两组,一组为 21 天治疗周期的第 1 天和第 8 天接受静脉滴注 2 小时 GRN163L(9.4mg/kg),结合 21 天治疗周期的第 1 天给予或不给予贝伐单抗,另一组为患者接受传统治疗方案(接受贝伐单抗的患者随机分配继续维持治疗或无贝伐单抗维持治疗)。研究发现,虽然与对照组相比 GRN163L 治疗组的 PFS 无统计学意义,但在临床试验初始,端粒长度最短的患者治疗效果最为明显[90]。此种类型试验研究的经验对于推动未来基于抑制端粒酶活性的肿瘤治疗新策略的发展具有重要意义。

慢病毒载体构建的突变型 hTERC 过表达和靶向野生型 hTERC 的 siRNA 是针对端粒酶靶向治疗的不同类型的基因治疗策略

另一种以破坏肿瘤细胞中端粒维持机制为目的的新策略是在模板区域表达突变体 hTR(hTERC)(人端粒酶 RNA 突变模板;MT-hTERC)。野生型端粒重复序列包含 DNA 结合位点,能与端粒结合蛋白质如 POT1,TRF1 和 TRF2 相结合[91,92]。推测 MT-hTERC 直接合成的突变 DNA 可以破坏端粒蛋白与 DNA 的结合[93~95],进而导致染色体端粒的脱帽。研究发现 TRF2 突变诱导的人端粒脱帽可以诱导细胞生长停滞(p53 依赖)和凋亡[96,97]。通过慢病毒载体将 MT-hTERC 导入端粒酶阳性的人肿瘤细胞中,可以导致肿瘤细胞的表型改变以及在肿瘤细胞移植瘤模型中显著抑制肿瘤生长[94,95]。另一种方法,通过靶向野生型人端粒酶 RNA(WT-hTERC)的慢病毒载体表达 siRNA(发夹结构的小干扰 RNA)可以抑制细胞生长和诱导凋亡(这些效应不依赖于端粒长度)。MT-hTERC 和 anti-WT-hTERC-siRNA 共表达对肿瘤细胞具有叠加或者协同作用。因此,由于不需要依赖 p53、初始端粒长度或者端粒进行性缩短,突变 hTERC 和 siRNA 成为有前途的抗肿瘤靶向治疗策略[98]。然而,在临床中,这些基因治疗方案需要实现靶向肿瘤细胞的高效率转染方可提高肿瘤基因治疗的有效性。

以端粒酶为基础靶向端粒脱帽的小分子化合物 6-硫代-2′-脱氧鸟苷(6-thio-dG)可以克服基因治疗存在的问题

理想的肿瘤靶点是仅在肿瘤细胞表达,而正常组织细胞不表达。与其他肿瘤靶点相比,端粒酶是几乎存在于所有肿瘤细胞中最广泛的靶点,而正常细胞除一些增殖性祖细胞外,都不具有端粒酶活性。因此,以端粒酶为靶点可以为肿瘤治疗提供新策略。

到目前为止，在端粒生物学方面有两种不同的治疗策略：靶向端粒策略或靶向端粒酶策略。靶向抑制端粒酶的策略与端粒长度相关，而靶向端粒的策略与起始的端粒长度无关（图14-3）。这导致了两种策略之间最主要的区别。如果仅仅抑制端粒酶，可能存在长的停滞期（从端粒酶抑制到发挥生物学效应之间的时间差）。因此，靶向端粒酶治疗在端粒长度显著缩短后方能观察到肿瘤的生长抑制、衰老和凋亡现象，导致靶向端粒酶的治疗周期一般很长[29,30]。

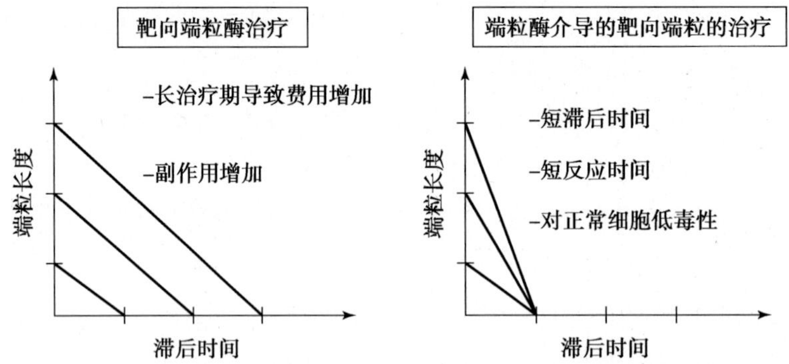

图14-3 靶向端粒酶治疗效应（例如 Imetelstat/GRN163L）取决于最初的肿瘤细胞端粒长度。肿瘤细胞具有可变的端粒长度。因此，与端粒较短的细胞相比，端粒长的细胞预估需要更长的端粒酶抑制剂的治疗时间才能获得更好的治疗效果（左侧）。所以靶向端粒酶的长期治疗将可能导致不良的副反应、高昂的治疗费用以及可能重建稳定的新端粒长度的反馈回路。与靶向端粒酶治疗相反，端粒酶介导的靶向端粒治疗（例如6-thio-dG 或 MT-hTERC 基因治疗）由于与初始端粒长度无关，因此治疗时间大大缩短，在较短的时间内降低肿瘤负荷是这类方法的关键优势（右侧）。这类治疗方法另一个最重要的优点是对大多数不表达端粒酶的正常细胞毒性较小。然而，MT-hTERC 治疗方案具有所有基因治疗所涉及的局限性，包括基因治疗可感染几乎所有细胞和目的基因转染效率不高的局限。然而，例如6-thio-dG 核苷的新方案可以口服使用并且副作用小，共有所有小分子具备的显著优势

一些靶向端粒而非端粒酶的方法（例如，G-四联体）可以导致端粒脱帽，其不依赖于 p53 状态和初始端粒长度。由于正常细胞和基因组其他区域中也存在形成的四联体结构，所以 G-四联体可能对正常组织造成损害[99]。因此，非靶向端粒酶的方法可能缺少有效的治疗窗口。此外，端粒酶抑制剂或端粒靶向治疗可能需要与其他细胞毒性药物联合使用，从而降低肿瘤细胞异质性导致的抵抗治疗的能力[99]。例如，来自 mTR 敲除小鼠的细胞表现为端粒功能障碍，从而使细胞对一些抗肿瘤药物（例如阿霉素）敏感[100]。该研究结果表明靶向端粒酶的治疗与化疗药物相结合可能提高细胞对化疗药物敏感性，导致细胞耐药能力降低。

在最近的研究工作中，我们聚焦一种新方法来筛选可以特异性地使端粒酶阳性细胞端粒脱帽的小分子。理论上讲，这种小分子的靶向治疗消除了基因治疗带来的一些问题，同时也可以减少从治疗开始到肿瘤减小的滞后期。为了验证这个想法，我们决定聚焦于核苷类似物，其是端粒酶的良好底物（不是端粒酶抑制剂），也更特异性地靶向端粒酶而非其他聚合酶。6-硫代-2′-脱氧鸟苷（6-thio-dG）是一种新的靶向端粒核苷类似物，可以被端粒酶识别并被端粒酶用作底物[101]。我们最近的研究结果表明，在具有不同长度端粒的端粒酶阳性的肿瘤细胞中，6-thio-dG 通过引起端粒结构改变形成端粒功能障碍诱导损伤灶（TIF），从而导致细胞的端粒功能障碍，并将这些细胞与正常细胞和 ALT 细胞相比较。有趣的是，除了短期细胞杀伤效应，在存活的肿瘤细胞而非正常细胞中 6-thio-dG 导致快速进行性的端粒缩短。这些研究表明，6-thio-dG 主要靶向优先被端粒酶用作底物的端粒。在免疫缺陷小鼠人移植瘤模型中，研究发现，6-thio-dG 抑制肺癌生长（没有观察到明显的副作用，例如，没有死亡，没有体重减轻）以及引起端粒功能障碍。长期使用 6-thio-dG，未观察到对正常组织的副作用，而且血液、肝脏和肾脏功能指标都在可接受的范围内。因此，6-thio-dG 通过利用端粒酶作为催化剂来改变端粒，使其被识别为 DNA 损伤，是一种有潜力的靶向端粒的“端粒毒药”。此外，开发更多有效的核苷类似物将成为未来靶向肿瘤细胞永生化肿的新方向。

总结

端粒是线性染色体末端的保护结构。因为存在末端复制问题，端粒随着细胞分裂而缩短，然而，端粒维持机制和端粒长度的进行性缩短相互制衡。大多数正常细胞不表达端粒酶活性，而几乎所有人类原发性肿瘤中都可以检测到明显的端粒酶活性，因此，端粒是针对肿瘤特异性和广谱性的靶点。

尽管针对端粒酶的肿瘤治疗有很多有前景的方案，目前仍没有药物被批准上市。靶向人类端粒中富含 G 的 DNA 序列的 G-四联体稳定剂，可以抑制端粒酶活性并导致端粒末端结构被破坏。然而，这些化合物的特异性不足，在影响肿瘤细胞的同时也不可避免地会影响正常细胞中的四联体结构。

免疫疗法可利用 TERTGV1001（肽疫苗）和 GRN-VAC1（体外树突细胞激活）进行临床试验。由于化疗药物的免疫抑制作用，这些疫苗与传统肿瘤的化学治疗方案相结合的有效性受到限制。

GRN163L(Imetelstat)是靶向端粒酶的寡核苷酸药物。GRN163L 能够抑制端粒酶的活性,引起肿瘤细胞端粒长度的进行性缩短。由于其对血细胞的毒副作用,GRN163L 治疗实体瘤的临床试验尚未取得进展。GRN163L 面临的一个潜在挑战是其诱导细胞衰老或者凋亡所需(长滞后)的响应时间。

基因疗法是一种通过向细胞中导入治疗性 DNA 的靶向肿瘤的成熟技术。突变 hTERT(显性阴性方案)或针对 hTERT 的 siRNA 是一些临床前研究中的不同的基因治疗方法。另外,伴随慢病毒引入突变体 hTERC 是依赖端粒酶的端粒"脱帽"方法。基因疗法是一种很有前景的抗肿瘤治疗方法,但需要较高转染效率以靶向大多数肿瘤细胞。

端粒酶抑制剂的典型代表 GRN163L 在发挥其酶抑制效应和生物效应之间存在很长的滞后期。相反,端粒酶介导的靶向端粒治疗滞后期将大幅缩短。其中一个例子是一种核苷类似物 6-thio-dG,其是靶向端粒的新方法,它可以优先被端粒酶识别并掺入端粒中导致 TIFs。这种小分子治疗方案主要对表达端粒酶的细胞具有短期细胞杀伤效应(短滞后时间),而对端粒酶沉默的正常细胞(例如,静息干细胞)的影响则很小。

(叶菲 郭献灵 译 韩志鹏 校 卫立辛 审)

参考文献

The complete reference list can be found on the Wiley Companion Digital Edition of this title (see inside front cover for login instructions).

1 de Lange T. How shelterin solves the telomere end-protection problem. *Cold Spring Harb Symp Quant Biol*. 2010;**75**:167–77.

2 Shay JW. Are short telomeres predictive of advanced cancer? *Cancer Discov*. 2013;**3**:1096–8.

4 Palm W, de Lange T. How shelterin protects mammalian telomeres. *Annu Rev Genet*. 2008;**42**:301–34.

5 Gilson E, Geli V. How telomeres are replicated. *Nat Rev Mol Cell Biol*. 2007;**8**:825–38.

9 Shay JW, Wright WE. Role of telomeres and telomerase in cancer. *Semin Cancer Biol*. 2011;**21**:349–53.

11 Davis CF, Ricketts CJ, Wang M, *et al*. The somatic genomic landscape of chromophobe renal cell carcinoma. *Cancer Cell*. 2014;**26**:319–30.

12 Zhao Y, Wang S, Popova EY, *et al*. Rearrangement of upstream sequences of the hTERT gene during cellular immortalization. *Genes Chromosomes Cancer*. 2009;**48**:963–74.

13 Huang FW, Hodis E, Xu MJ, *et al*. Highly recurrent TERT promoter mutations in human melanoma. *Science*. 2013;**339**:957–9.

16 Wong MS, Wright WE, Shay JW. Alternative splicing regulation of telomerase: a new paradigm? *Trends Genet*. 2014;**30**:430–8.

18 Bodnar AG, Ouellette M, Frolkis M, *et al*. Extension of life-span by introduction of telomerase into normal human cells. *Science*. 1998;**279**:349–52.

28 Herbert BS, Gellert GC, Hochreiter A, *et al*. Lipid modification of GRN163, an N3′—>P5′ thio-phosphoramidate oligonucleotide, enhances the potency of telomerase inhibition. *Oncogene*. 2005;**24**:5262–8.

31 Gowan SM, Harrison JR, Patterson L, *et al*. A G-quadruplex-interactive potent small-molecule inhibitor of telomerase exhibiting in vitro and in vivo antitumor activity. *Mol Pharmacol*. 2002;**61**:1154–62.

32 Harley CB. Telomerase and cancer therapeutics. *Nat Rev Cancer*. 2008;**8**:167–79.

35 Kim MY, Vankayalapati H, Shin-Ya K, *et al*. Telomestatin, a potent telomerase inhibitor that interacts quite specifically with the human telomeric intramolecular G-quadruplex. *J Am Chem Soc*. 2002;**124**:2098–9.

38 Kim MY, Gleason-Guzman M, Izbicka E, *et al*. The different biological effects of telomestatin and TMPyP4 can be attributed to their selectivity for interaction with intramolecular or intermolecular G-quadruplex structures. *Cancer Res*. 2003;**63**:3247–56.

39 Gowan SM, Heald R, Stevens MF, *et al*. Potent inhibition of telomerase by small-molecule pentacyclic acridines capable of interacting with G-quadruplexes. *Mol Pharmacol*. 2001;**60**:981–8.

40 Leonetti C, Amodei S, D'Angelo C, *et al*. Biological activity of the G-quadruplex ligand RHPS4 (3,11-difluoro-6,8,13-trimethyl-8H-quino[4,3,2-kl]acridinium methosulfate) is associated with telomere capping alteration. *Mol Pharmacol*. 2004;**66**:1138–46.

42 Taetz S, Baldes C, Murdter TE, *et al*. Biopharmaceutical characterization of the telomerase inhibitor BRACO19. *Pharm Res*. 2006;**23**:1031–7.

43 Kelland L. Targeting the limitless replicative potential of cancer: the telomerase/telomere pathway. *Clin Cancer Res Off J Am Assoc Cancer Res*. 2007;**13**:4960–3.

49 Mocellin S, Pooley KA, Nitti D. Telomerase and the search for the end of cancer. *Trends Mol Med*. 2013;**19**:125–33.

52 Liu JP, Chen W, Schwarer AP, *et al*. Telomerase in cancer immunotherapy. *Biochim Biophys Acta*. 1805;**2010**:35–42.

56 Greten TF, Forner A, Korangy F, *et al*. A phase II open label trial evaluating safety and efficacy of a telomerase peptide vaccination in patients with advanced hepatocellular carcinoma. *BMC Cancer*. 2010;**10**:209.

57 Middleton G, Silcocks P, Cox T, *et al*. Gemcitabine and capecitabine with or without telomerase peptide vaccine GV1001 in patients with locally advanced or metastatic pancreatic cancer (TeloVac): an open-label, randomised, phase 3 trial. *Lancet Oncol*. 2014;**15**:829–40.

58 Kyte JA, Gaudernack G, Dueland S, *et al*. Telomerase peptide vaccination combined with temozolomide: a clinical trial in stage IV melanoma patients. *Clin Cancer Res Off J Am Assoc Cancer Res*. 2011;**17**:4568–80.

60 Shay JW, Keith WN. Targeting telomerase for cancer therapeutics. *Br J Cancer*. 2008;**98**:677–83.

61 Keith WN, Bilsland A, Hardie M, *et al*. Drug insight: cancer cell immortality-telomerase as a target for novel cancer gene therapies. *Nat Clin Pract Oncol*. 2004;**1**:88–96.

63 Fujiwara T, Urata Y, Tanaka N. Therapeutic targets and drugs IV: telomerase-specific gene and vector-based therapies for human cancer. In: Hiyama K, ed. *Telomeres and Telomerase in Cancer*. Menlo Park, CA: Geron Corporation; 2009:293–312.

65 Ouellette MM, Wright WE, Shay JW. Targeting telomerase-expressing cancer cells. *J Cell Mol Med*. 2011;**15**:1433–42.

67 Keith WN, Thomson CM, Howcroft J, *et al*. Seeding drug discovery: integrating telomerase cancer biology and cellular senescence to uncover new therapeutic opportunities in targeting cancer stem cells. *Drug Discov Today*. 2007;**12**:611–21.

70 Nemunaitis J, Tong AW, Nemunaitis M, *et al*. A phase I study of telomerase-specific replication competent oncolytic adenovirus (telomelysin) for various solid tumors. *Mol Ther*. 2010;**18**:429–34.

73 Ruden M, Puri N. Novel anticancer therapeutics targeting telomerase. *Cancer Treat Rev*. 2013;**39**:444–56.

84 Burchett KM, Yan Y, Ouellette MM. Telomerase inhibitor Imetelstat (GRN163L) limits the lifespan of human pancreatic cancer cells. *PLoS One*. 2014;**9**:e85155.

86 Marian CO, Cho SK, McEllin BM, *et al*. The telomerase antagonist, imetelstat, efficiently targets glioblastoma tumor-initiating cells leading to decreased proliferation and tumor growth. *Clin Cancer Res*. 2010;**16**:154–63.

88 Molckovsky A, Siu LL. First-in-class, first-in-human phase I results of targeted agents: highlights of the 2008 American society of clinical oncology meeting. *J Hematol Oncol*. 2008;**1**:20.

89 Thompson PA, Drissi R, Muscal JA, *et al*. A phase I trial of imetelstat in children with refractory or recurrent solid tumors: a Children's Oncology Group Phase I Consortium Study (ADVL1112). *Clin Cancer Res*. 2013;**19**:6578–84.

98 Li S, Rosenberg JE, Donjacour AA, *et al*. Rapid inhibition of cancer cell growth induced by lentiviral delivery and expression of mutant-template telomerase RNA and anti-telomerase short-interfering RNA. *Cancer Res*. 2004;**64**:4833–40.

99 Kelland LR. Overcoming the immortality of tumour cells by telomere and telomerase based cancer therapeutics—current status and future prospects. *Eur J Cancer*. 2005;**41**:971–9.

100 Lee KH, Rudolph KL, Ju YJ, *et al*. Telomere dysfunction alters the chemotherapeutic profile of transformed cells. *Proc Natl Acad Sci U S A*. 2001;**98**:3381–6.

101 Mender I, Gryaznov S, Dikmen ZG, et al. Induction of telomere dysfunction by the telomerase substrate precursor, 6-thio-2′ deoxyguanosine. *Cancer Discov*. 2015;**5**:82–95.

第 15 章　肿瘤代谢

Natalya N. Pavlova, PhD ■ Craig B. Thompson, MD

概述

细胞的高效增殖依赖于细胞代谢的重塑，这样可以维持细胞生长时的生物合成需求。癌基因异常激活产生的持续信号可活化促生长的代谢通路，将细胞锁定在生物大分子净合成和抵抗细胞死亡的状态。促癌信号传递促进细胞摄取代谢底物，例如葡萄糖和谷氨酰胺，也可以促使细胞利用非经典的营养物质。非增殖的组织选择性地将吸收的代谢底物在线粒体中氧化以维持氧化磷酸化和能量生成。与之不同，肿瘤细胞优先将代谢底物用于生物合成过程，包括脂肪酸、胆固醇、非必需氨基酸和核苷酸的生物合成。这些累积的前体被用来维持细胞生长所必需的生物大分子合成。癌基因介导特定代谢物水平的升高也会影响代谢通路外的细胞过程，不仅导致细胞表观遗传状态的变化，也会改变肿瘤微环境中的长距离效应。近期的研究表明肿瘤细胞代谢的变化可被用于改善多种肿瘤的诊断和治疗。

邪恶的建设者

肿瘤的统一特征是失去了对细胞增殖的外在控制。正常组织中细胞的数量和细胞间相互位置由细胞外信号所维持，包括组织特异的可溶生长因子以及从细胞外基质到黏附细胞的信号。这些机制共同调控细胞生存和增殖的时机和程度。本底水平的信号调控日常的组织维持。组织的异常变化引起生长信号上调从而增强终末分化细胞的形成，例如皮肤损伤状态时的表皮角质细胞和皮肤成纤维细胞，又如应对感染状态的 T 细胞。因此只有在应对细胞类型特异的、有足够强度和持续时间的信号时，细胞增殖才会发生。这保证了多细胞生物在结构和生物化学完整性上的总体稳定。

与正常细胞不同，肿瘤细胞在遗传学和表观遗传上的变异使其以不依赖于外界生长信号刺激的方式在组织中增殖和累积，同时能够抵抗抑制生长的信号[1]。这些适应性的变化使得肿瘤细胞能够在正常细胞生长受到严格调控的条件下存活和增殖。发生于生长因子受体的基因突变、拷贝数扩增和基因转位是肿瘤中最为常见的促生长遗传变异，也因此被称为“驱动变异”。例如在美国和日本的非小细胞肺癌病人中表皮生长因子受体（epidermal growth factor receptor，EGFR）激活突变的发生频率分别是 10%和 35%[2]。人表皮生长因子受体 2（erb-b2 receptor tyrosine kinase 2，HER2）的基因扩增则存在于 25%～30%的乳腺癌[3]。除了生长因子受体，生长因子和基质黏附信号下游的信号整合蛋白在肿瘤中常被异常激活。例如高达 70%的乳腺癌中存在磷脂酰肌醇 3-激酶（phosphoinositide 3-kinase，PI3K）通路的突变[4]；高达 90%的胰腺肿瘤由鼠肉瘤病毒原癌基因同源体（kirsten rat sarcoma viral oncogene homolog，KRAS）激活突变驱动[5]；细胞型骨髓细胞瘤病毒癌基因（cellular-myelocytomatosis viral oncogene，c-Myc）基因的扩增则出现于高达 50%的不同组织来源的人类肿瘤中[6]。

在接收适当的生长信号后，细胞将进行分裂产生两个子代细胞。为此，细胞需合成一系列足够的生物分子来构建一个有功能的新细胞。这些生物分子具有高度的多样性，不仅包括许多类型的蛋白质，也包括脂类及用于生成细胞膜和细胞器膜的脂类及其衍生物、用于糖基化蛋白的己糖、用于基因组复制的戊糖和碱基。为了保证细胞不会在缺乏充足生物分子供应的状态下进行自我复制，控制细胞增殖的信号同时调控着营养物质的摄取和生物大分子前体的生物合成。在受生长因子刺激后，细胞进行代谢重塑以维持所需的生物合成。代谢重塑一方面包括从所在环境中摄取足够多的生物合成原料；另一方面，正在增殖的细胞将这些原料优先用于生物合成，而非用于产生能量的分解代谢。

要点

生理状态下，正常组织中的促生长信号是瞬时的。癌基因异常激活介导连续的信号传递，使得细胞能够持续接收促生长的刺激信号。肿瘤代谢因此被持续改变以维持细胞增殖。

本章将会介绍恶性转化重塑细胞代谢来促进营养物质摄取和生物合成的机制。此外，本章会探讨肿瘤细胞的异常代谢状态促进肿瘤扩增和散播，及其对细胞表观遗传状态和肿瘤微环境的显著调控效应。基于此我们将进一步讨论如何将肿瘤代谢异常用于肿瘤的检测和治疗。

从酵母到哺乳动物——相同手段不同目的

代谢通路和驱动代谢活动的代谢酶在进化中是显著保守的，然而多细胞生物的代谢调控方式与单细胞生物具有根本的不同。单细胞生物，特别是细菌或酵母，利用外界营养物质的充盈程度作为启动细胞增殖的信号[7]。依据环境条件协调细胞增殖，这种策略使得单细胞生物最大限度地取得进化优势。而对于多细胞生物来说，进化的目标不仅是扩增更多的细胞—细胞的过度增殖反而导致生理紊乱—而且要维持器官和组织的功能及结构完整性、协助损伤修复和对抗感染。为此，多细胞生物发展出了复杂的组织特异性调控机制来调节细胞存活和增殖，并在需要时能够快速介导特定细胞类群的增殖。而肿瘤中组织特异调控机制的缺失则使代谢呈现促进细胞增殖的状态。这种代谢状态可以从多细胞生物和单细胞生物的代谢调控差异中找到解析的方式。

细胞代谢以还原态的碳和氮等物质的获取和逐步的生物化学转换为中心。葡萄糖是主要的代谢底物，可被所有的活细胞利用并作为①生物能量的来源，以三磷酸腺苷（adenosine triphosphate，ATP）中高能磷酸键的形式存在；②许多生物分子碳骨架的来源。葡萄糖分子不能提供氮元素这个重要的化学组分，而氨基酸和碱基的合成需要氮。因此对单细胞和多细胞生物来说，获取含还原态氮的原料至关重要。尽管某些细菌可以将大气中的氮气还原为氨，大部分物种必须从环境中摄取还原态的氮。单细胞生物可以使用游离氨作为还原态氮的来源。例如野生或原养型酵母可在合成型完全培养基中增殖，该培养基仅含有葡萄糖作为唯一碳源以及氨作为唯一氮源。酵母细胞含有从该培养基提供原料中合成所有种类生物大分子的全部代谢酶。

多细胞生物依赖葡萄糖作为主要的碳源，并以氨基酸作为还原态氮的主要来源。与单细胞生物不同，在构成蛋白的二十种氨基酸中，多细胞生物丧失了合成其中九种氨基酸的能力（这九种氨基酸被称为必需氨基酸，其他被称为非必需氨基酸）。谷氨酰胺这种氨基酸是两个氮原子的载体，也是多细胞生物主要的"氮货币"。谷氨酰胺是还原态氮来源，因为其特殊的重要性，多细胞生物中谷氨酰胺是绝大多数正在增殖细胞的"条件性必需"氨基酸[8]。

葡萄糖和谷氨酰胺作为多细胞生物关键代谢底物的重要性体现为，哺乳动物血浆中这两种营养物质的浓度持续保持在几乎恒定的水平：葡萄糖水平介于 4~6mM；谷氨酰胺作为血浆中丰度最高的氨基酸位于 0.6~0.9mM 范围内[9]。葡萄糖和谷氨酰胺水平的稳定是多种机制共同维持的，包括激素介导的肌糖原和肝糖原储备和利用、葡萄糖和谷氨酰胺的从头合成以及摄食行为调控。

单细胞生物生存环境中不存在持续恒定的碳源和氮源。它们依赖营养物质感知的机制来评估环境中营养物质的可利用程度。例如在酵母中葡萄糖限制可激活蔗糖非发酵 1 激酶（sucrose nonfermenting 1，Snf1），即哺乳动物中单磷酸腺苷激活的蛋白激酶（5′ adenosine monophosphate-activated protein kinase，AMPK）的同源蛋白，进而促进能量的生成并抑制生物合成过程[10]。在酵母培养物中加入葡萄糖能够促发细胞向合成代谢和细胞增殖转变[11,12]。在葡萄糖充足时，与哺乳动物 RAS 蛋白同源的鸟苷三磷酸（guanosine triphosphate，GTP）酶 Ras1 和 Ras2 被激活并促进细胞周期进程。葡萄糖下游的另一个信号传递蛋白是 Sch9 激酶，与哺乳动物中的蛋白激酶 B（protein kinase B，又称 AK strain transforming，Akt）和核糖体蛋白 S6 激酶（ribosomal protein S6 kinase，S6K）相关。Sch9 能够促进葡萄糖进入生物合成过程[13]。同时，酵母细胞通过与哺乳动物一般性调控阻遏蛋白 2（general control nonderepressible 2，GCN2）同源的丝氨酸/苏氨酸激酶 Gcn2 衡量氨基酸状态。空载转运 RNA（transfer RNA，tRNA）在氨基酸水平不足时会在细胞内累积，进而激活 Gcn2。激活后的 Gcn2 可降低蛋白翻译速率并诱导一般性调控阻遏蛋白 4［general control nonderepressible 4，Gcn4；哺乳动物中为激活转录因子 4（activating transcription factor 4，ATF4）］表达。Gcn4 作为转录因子可以控制多个氨基酸从头合成相关酶的表达[14]。葡萄糖缺乏时，活化的 Snf1 抑制 Gcn4 表达，从而协调氮代谢和碳代谢[15]。当细胞内氨基酸水平升高时，西罗莫司靶点 1 或 2［target of rapamycin1/2，TOR1/2；哺乳动物中为 mTOR（mammalian target of rapamycin）］可被激活并协调多个合成代谢过程，包括蛋白翻译和脂肪酸生物合成。如果此时营养来源依然充足，细胞生长将进一步转变为细胞分裂。该过程不断重复直至细胞外的营养供给降低到增殖必需的阈值以下。

对于多细胞生物，血浆或细胞间隙中含有充足的葡萄糖和谷氨酰胺可供细胞使用。与酵母细胞相比，这些细胞仅有存在合适外源生长信号的条件下才会进行增殖。首先，细胞获取胞外葡萄糖和谷氨酰胺的能力被受体酪氨酸激酶控制。单细胞生物没有受体酪氨酸激酶，故而多细胞生物中细胞因子或生长因子的刺激向细胞发出摄取营养物质用于代谢底物的生成过程的指令。来源于受体酪氨酸激酶的信号汇集于 PI3K/Akt 并将其激活，不仅促发胞浆中囊泡上的葡萄糖转运蛋白（glucose transporter，GLUT）向细胞膜转位[16,17]，而且刺激 GLUT 基因表达[18]以驱动葡萄糖进入细胞。故此在被诱导增殖的细胞中，PI3K/Akt 信号可以促进葡萄糖的摄取。这种现象可见于免疫反应中激活的 T 细胞[19]，也见于被诱导合成大量生物大分子的细胞，如乳腺中的泌乳细胞[20]。

除了葡萄糖转运受生长因子调控外，哺乳动物细胞在受生长因子刺激后会快速启动一类立早基因的转录，其中即包括转录因子 c-Myc。c-Myc 驱动许多代谢基因的表达并调控谷氨酰胺这一主要氮源的摄取[21]。c-Myc 促进谷氨酰胺转运精氨酸转运载体 2（alanine-serine-cysteine transporter 2，ASCT2）和系统 N 转运载体 2（system N transporter SN2，SN2）的表达[22]；谷氨酰胺酶（glutaminase 1，GLS1）将谷氨酰胺降解成谷氨酸和游离氨，c-Myc 也增强 GLS1 的表达[23]。通过增加谷氨酰胺的吸收，c-Myc 也会间接影响细胞对必需氨基酸的摄取。必需氨基酸向细胞内的输入与谷氨酰胺向细胞外空间的输出相偶联[24]，这种机制使得细胞能够依据细胞内谷氨酰胺水平协调必需氨基酸的摄取。

葡萄糖吸收不仅被受体酪氨酸激酶信号增强，细胞锚定于细胞外基质也是该过程的重要条件。细胞在失去基质黏附时，即使存在可溶的生长因子葡萄糖摄取仍是被抑制的[25]。这确保了细胞的增殖及其在组织中的位置都在代谢水平受到调控。

综上所述，受体酪氨酸激酶介导的促生长信号转导是营养物质摄取过程中的调控节点。尽管 RAS 从酵母到哺乳动物都是保守的，哺乳动物的 RAS 蛋白不再受葡萄糖丰度的调节，而是受组织特异受体的调控。与之相似，尽管哺乳动物的 TOR 蛋白保留了对氨基酸水平的敏感性，但也受生长信号的调控。结节性硬化症蛋白 2（tuberous sclerosis complex 2，TSC2）是 mTOR 的负调控蛋白，Akt 依赖的 TSC2 磷酸化导致 TSC2 失活和生长信号传递。下面将对生长信号传递通路的遗传变异如何影响肿瘤细胞营养摄取展开讨论。

要点

丰富的营养物质能够充分刺激单细胞生物生长，但是对多细胞生物没有作用，因为后者摄取环境中营养物质的能力是由外界生长刺激信号控制的。

肿瘤细胞的不良摄食习惯

现代肿瘤研究最早的发现之一是肿瘤和未转化组织在营养物质摄取上的基本差异，随后才发现癌基因和致癌物质在肿瘤发生中的角色。在19世纪20年代，德国生理学家奥托·沃伯格对腹水瘤和正常非增殖组织的切片进行生化分析发现肿瘤细胞的葡萄糖摄入速率远远超过正常组织[26]。在约30年之后，美国病理学家哈里·伊格尔发现培养的HeLa细胞对谷氨酰胺的需求超过其他氨基酸10到100倍，远超蛋白合成所需的量[27]。

在信号转导层面，细胞葡萄糖摄取受PI3K/Akt调控。PI3K/Akt将GLUT蛋白靶向细胞膜，同时在转录水平增强GLUT蛋白的表达[17]。因此，PI3K/Akt信号通路在肿瘤中的特异变化使得肿瘤细胞持续地摄取葡萄糖。RAS和鸡肉瘤病毒同源型基因(cellular homolog of Rous sarcoma oncogene，c-Src)在激活后也可以促进GLUT1的表达[28]。为了将碳供给和氮供应相匹配，肿瘤细胞同时增强对谷氨酰胺的摄取。如前所述，哺乳动物细胞中谷氨酰胺摄取和利用的关键驱动因素是c-Myc[22,29]。随着c-Myc水平的异常升高，肿瘤细胞持续地摄入并利用谷氨酰胺以支持能量代谢、核苷酸生物合成，同时协调必需氨基酸的摄取和非必需氨基酸的生物合成以维持蛋白生成。

肿瘤起源于完整的正常组织，这种环境并不能维持无序的细胞增殖。因此，肿瘤经常缺乏足够的血管系统，因为组织内血管新生受组织特异因子的负调控[30]。肿瘤细胞分泌促血管生成分子确实会引起毛细血管的生成，但这些血管倾向于发育不完全而且不能充分地供给肿瘤生长需要的氧气和营养物质。由于肿瘤细胞的增殖不断消耗所在微环境中的氨基酸和葡萄糖，生长中的肿瘤会面临不断恶化的增殖环境。自噬是肿瘤细胞适应营养限制采用的方式之一。自噬是细胞饥饿时临时采用的一种手段，用一种可调控的方式将自身的蛋白质、脂类甚至整个细胞器进行分解代谢以维持存活[31]。AMPK是细胞内主要的生物能量感受器，应对ATP/AMP比率的下降启动自噬的过程。相应地，mTOR是自噬的抑制蛋白[32]。肿瘤体内生长过程中自噬的重要性可见于Kras的G12D突变和鼠肉瘤病毒癌基因同源基因B(v-Raf murine sarcoma viral oncogene homolog B，Braf)的V600E突变引发的肺肿瘤中。敲除自噬分子机器关键组分自噬相关蛋白7(autophagy related 7，Atg7)基因可显著限制肿瘤细胞的增殖和侵袭性[33,34]。

尽管自噬可以作为应对营养短缺维持细胞能量的临时手段，但是自噬并不能作为新生物质/生物量的来源。除了从细胞内的蛋白回收氨基酸，最近的研究显示KRAS和c-Src转化的细胞可从细胞外可溶蛋白中获取氨基酸。这些蛋白在细胞膜皱褶处以大型囊泡(直径长达1～2μm)形式摄入[35]。这些囊泡也被称作巨胞饮小体(源自拉丁语)。在营养物质缺乏条件下，巨胞饮小体被运送至溶酶体，其中吞入的物质则被降解。这种替代性的回收营养物质的形式使得细胞能够解锁通常不可用的氨基酸存储来源以度过氨基酸缺乏。RAS驱动的巨胞饮是在进化过程中古老的获取营养的机制。事实上，在黏菌中，例如网柄菌，巨胞饮是主要的营养摄取通路[36]。因此，在癌基因转化的细胞中巨胞饮的重新激活可以被看做是肿瘤细胞如何利用进化过程中古老的营养摄取机制的另一范例。

肿瘤中不充分的血管网络导致的另一问题是氧气供给减少，即低氧。氧气不充足会对细胞代谢造成显著的影响，抑制耗氧的生物化学反应。在低氧条件下受抑制的反应之一是硬脂酰辅酶A去饱和酶(stearoyl-CoA desaturase 1，SCD1)催化的反应。SCD1将脂肪酸碳键去饱和，产生不饱和脂肪酸。不饱和脂肪酸对细胞膜和细胞器膜适度的流动性非常重要。为了避免这一问题，Ras转化的细胞被发现从细胞外环境中利用不饱和脂类以绕过细胞对SCD1催化去饱和反应的需求[37]。

要点

癌基因信号传递使得细胞能够不受限制地利用葡萄糖和谷氨酰胺这些传统的代谢原料，同时使得细胞能够获取非经典的生物分子来源。

行走的电子

活细胞中大部分生化反应在能量上都是不利的，需要特别的代谢酶进行催化。代谢反应可被分为两种类型：①分解反应—复杂的生物分子被降解为简单的组分；②合成反应—简单的组分用来生成氨基酸、脂肪酸、核苷酸等复杂的生物分子。分解代谢过程包括底物发生氧化的反应。在这些氧化步骤中产生的电子以氢化物阴离子(:H^-)的形式被捕捉，并被特殊的辅酶荷载，包括烟酰胺腺嘌呤二核苷酸(nicotinamide adenine dinucleotide，NAD^+)和黄素腺嘌呤二核苷酸(flavin adenine dinucleotide，FAD)，还原形式为NADH和$FADH_2$；或者烟酰胺腺嘌呤二核苷酸磷酸(nicotinamide adenine dinucleotide phosphate，$NADP^+$)，还原形式为NADPH。NADH和$FADH_2$中电子的化学能被位于线粒体内膜的电子传递链中一系列酶复合体所利用。NADH/$FADH_2$来源的电子经由电子传递链运输直至遇到氧气产生水分子。被传递的电子所带有的化学能由电子传递链运输，用于产生线粒体基质和膜间腔的质子浓度梯度。该过程产生的跨线粒体内膜的电化学势能维持着ATP合酶的活性。ATP合酶是一个超分子复合物并在二磷酸腺苷(adenosine diphosphate，ADP)上再生高能磷酸键产生ATP。电子传递链与ADP向ATP转化相耦联，被称作氧化磷酸化。

活细胞中ATP与ADP的比例为无数能量上不利进行的细胞过程提供了热力学驱动力，也驱动了激酶介导的蛋白和脂类磷酸化——广泛调控多种蛋白功能和细胞内传递信号的模式。

通过电子传递链维持电化学质子浓度梯度依赖于氧气和ADP的可利用度。氧气是电子的终末受体，而ADP是ATP合酶的底物。从NADH/$FADH_2$来源电子的过度内流会耗竭氧气和ADP的供应，停止氧化磷酸化反应。电子因此会停留在电子传递链，进而脱离位于内膜内的载体蛋白，与细胞内水溶的环境反应形成活性氧簇(reactive oxygen species，ROS)。ROS是活泼的氧化剂，可以广泛地和生物分子反应，如脂类、蛋白和核酸。为了控制氧化还原状态，细胞产生多种多样的中和ROS的分子，也被称为抗氧化剂。然而，当ROS水平升高至超过细胞抗氧化能力时，它们会导致细胞器和DNA的广泛损伤。

如前所述，绝大多数的分解代谢反应将底物的氧化和 NAD^+/FAD 至 NADH/$FADH_2$ 的还原相偶联。与之不同，某些代谢反应可将电子传递至另一个结构相关的辅因子 $NADP^+$，将其还原为 NADPH，而 NADH 和 $FADH_2$ 主要用于产生能量，NADPH 通过维持谷胱甘肽和相关含巯基分子的还原状态来补充细胞抗氧化剂池。另外，NADPH 的还原力也被用于复杂生物分子的合成，例如需要一系列还原反应进行生物合成的脂肪酸和核苷酸。细胞如何优先进行某一类的还原反应而非其余的反应呢？研究表明，很多促生长信号不仅能够增强细胞摄取生化反应底物，也会协调将底物分配给生物产能途径还是生物合成过程。

要点

活细胞通过氧化从环境中摄取的生化反应底物维持存活。分解代谢反应生成简单的结构单元，进而在生物合成反应中被持续使用。此外，分解代谢反应作为还原力的来源维持细胞能量生成，促进生物合成反应，增强抗氧化抵抗过程。

沃伯格效应——如何外松内紧

细胞内葡萄糖分解代谢发生在两个区室：第一阶段糖酵解发生于细胞质，而第二阶段位于线粒体，包括一系列的三羧酸循环反应（tricarboxylic acid cycle，TCA 循环，也被称为柠檬酸循环或克雷布斯循环）。己糖激酶（hexokinase，HK）磷酸化葡萄糖产生 6-磷酸葡萄糖，即糖酵解首个限速步骤（图 15-1a）。己糖激酶介导的反应能够阻止葡萄糖返回细胞外的空间。糖酵解第二个限速步骤是磷酸果糖激酶（phosphofructokinase 1，PFK1）催化的不可逆磷酸化。Akt 不仅可以将 GLUT1 转运蛋白靶向至细胞膜，也可以增强 HK 和 PFK1 的活力，从而调节葡萄糖参与糖酵解代谢[38,39]。实际上在移除生长因子后 Akt 对细胞凋亡的抑制作用就依赖于葡萄糖[40]。而仅仅过表达 GLUT1 和己糖激酶 HK 就足够抑制生长因子移除导致的细胞死亡[39]。2,6-二磷酸果糖由 6-磷酸果糖-2-激酶/果糖-2,6-二磷酸酶 3（6-phosphofructo-2-kinase/fructose-2,6-biphosphatase 3，PFKFB3）产生，是 PFK1 的别构激活剂。肿瘤细胞中 PFKFB3 高频率的过表达可以进一步增强 PFK1 的活力[41]。

在葡萄糖捕获和降解的下游，糖酵解和 TCA 循环的各种中间体为细胞从头合成几乎所有氨基酸、脂酰基和核苷酸提供骨架，支持大分子的合成。当发现致癌突变能够促进葡萄糖涌入细胞来维持生物合成前体的供应时，也就明确了肿瘤生成过程中为何选择沃伯格效应。一旦能够摄取过量葡萄糖并抵抗凋亡，肿瘤细胞就基本拥有了无限的大分子前体供应，并将任何超过所需的碳通过糖酵解的终产物丙酮酸转化为乳酸从细胞中排出。肿瘤中的突变促进葡萄糖摄取进而使肿瘤体现出的这种贪婪的代谢行为也称为有氧糖酵解。有氧糖酵解能将肿瘤与正常细胞的无氧糖酵解相区分，即缺氧时葡萄糖摄入增加。

最近研究表明有氧糖酵解并不局限于肿瘤细胞。正常细胞在受生长因子刺激后也会体现出类似沃伯格效应的代谢状态[42]。沃伯格效应是生长因子驱动的现象，而非肿瘤细胞特定的“异常状态”。这也提示沃伯格效应可能是为了增强细胞生物合成能力对代谢进行的部分重编程。生长因子刺激后，将葡萄糖分解代谢产能最大化可能不是促进生物合成的最佳方式，这一点逐渐得到接受[43]。

糖酵解如何促进生物合成？糖酵解中间物可作为多个通路生物合成前体和 NADPH 生成的底物（图 15-1a）。其中便是从 6-磷酸葡萄糖起始的磷酸戊糖途径（pentose phosphate pathway，PPP）。6-磷酸葡萄糖氧化后可产生两个 NADPH 分子，进而经过一系列的相互转化生成 5-磷酸核糖—核苷酸的结构组分。值得注意的是，磷酸戊糖途径中的转酮酶类似蛋白（transketolase like 1，TKTL1）是一些肿瘤细胞系生长所需的，也是病人预后差的指标[44]。

糖酵解的另一个关键分支点在 3-磷酸甘油酸。3-磷酸甘油酸经三步连续反应转换为丝氨酸。代谢研究表明，丝氨酸的生物合成在肿瘤中被高度上调，超过了蛋白生物合成的需求量[45]。而且编码丝氨酸生物合成限速酶的基因磷酸甘油酸脱氢酶（3-phosphoglycerate dehydrogenase，PHGDH）在乳腺癌和黑色素瘤中频繁扩增，不仅预示着肿瘤的侵袭性，而且是肿瘤体内生长所需的[46,47]。为什么肿瘤细胞要产生过量的丝氨酸呢？丝氨酸不仅是蛋白翻译的基本元件，也是一碳循环或叶酸循环的关键底物。在该循环中，丝氨酸中的碳被传递至四羟叶酸（tetrahydrofolate，THF）分子。叶酸循环包括一系列复杂的氧化还原转换，其中即涉及丝氨酸提供的甲基。该循环在调控细胞生长和增殖的许多过程中都是不可或缺的[48]。特别值得注意的是，丝氨酸来源的碳可作为：①嘌呤合成的碳供体；②组蛋白和 DNA 甲基转移酶的底物 S-腺苷甲硫氨酸的甲基供体；③生成 NADPH 时还原力的供体。正如近期研究显示，细胞内超过 50%的 NADPH 是由一碳通路产生[49]。综上所述，糖酵解中间物向磷酸戊糖途径和丝氨酸生物合成途径分流不仅提供 NADPH，也为核苷酸合成提供了结构组分。

细胞如何分流糖酵解中间物进而控制生物合成速率呢？对生长因子信号通路互作的研究做出了有启示性的重要发现。具体而言，肿瘤细胞表达丙酮酸激酶 M（pyruvate kinase M，PKM）的 M2 剪接变体。而正常细胞则选择性地表达 M1 变体[50]。丙酮酸激酶是一个限速酶，催化磷酸烯醇式丙酮酸（phosphoenolpyruvate，PEP）向丙酮酸的转化（图 15-1a）。引人注意的是，与 PKM1 相比，PKM2 亚型是丙酮酸激酶活性较低的形式。而且 PKM2 通过其 C 端序列与磷酸化的酪氨酸残基结合可被进一步抑制[51]。将 PKM2 替换为 PKM1 亚型可降低肿瘤细胞的成瘤潜力，促进氧耗，抑制乳酸生成[50]。PKM2 的低催化效率产生的“交通堵塞”导致 PEP 累积，进而促进累积的糖酵解中间物进入前述的两条通路[52]。此外，磷酸戊糖途径的下游产物 5-磷酸琥珀酰亚胺咪唑羧胺核糖（phosphoribosylaminoimidazolesuccinocarboxamide，SAICAR）[53]和丝氨酸合成通路的下游产物（丝氨酸本身）[54]作为 PKM2 的别构激活剂使得细胞能够平衡糖酵解在生物合成和生物产能中的代谢模式。PKM2 除了控制糖酵解流量，还在基因表达水平促进葡萄糖代谢。在表皮细胞生长因子（epidermal growth factor，EGF）处理的细胞中，PKM2 被细胞外调节蛋白激酶 1 或 2（extracellular regulated protein kinase，Erk1/2）磷酸化并转位至细胞核，进而直接

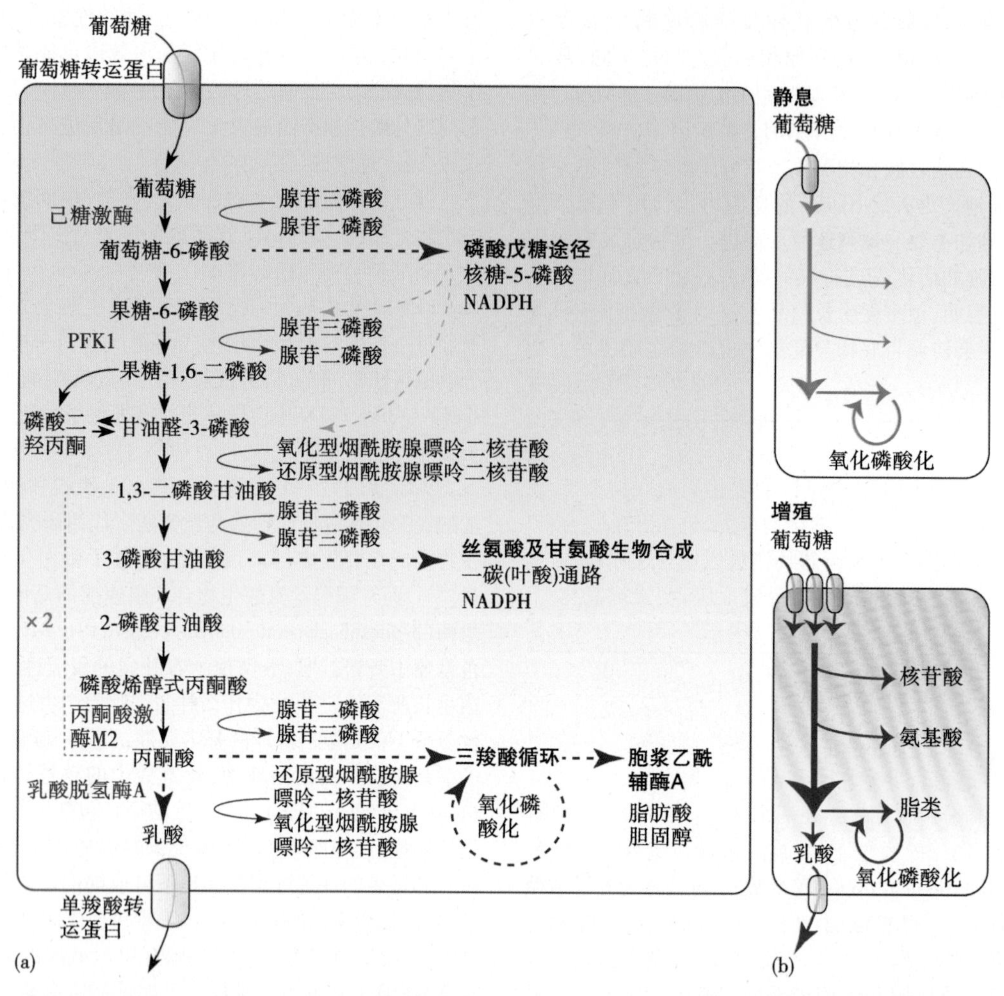

图 15-1 糖酵解。(a)通过糖酵解,一分子葡萄糖经分解代谢产生两分子丙酮酸,进而被转运至线粒体作为 TCA 循环中乙酰辅酶 A 的来源。另外,丙酮酸可被转变成乳酸并分泌出细胞。除了产能,糖酵解也参与细胞生物合成。6-磷酸葡萄糖可进入磷酸戊糖途径产生 NADPH 和 5-磷酸核糖,用于核苷酸生物合成;其中间代谢物也可回流至糖酵解(灰色虚线箭头所示)。此外,3-磷酸甘油酸可被转变为丝氨酸,进而作为叶酸(一碳)循环的碳供体。叶酸循环不仅产生 NADPH,而且为核苷酸生物合成和甲基化反应提供一碳单位。PFK1,磷酸果糖激酶 1。(b)静息的细胞消耗适量葡萄糖并选择性地将其分解为丙酮酸提供给线粒体中的氧化磷酸化反应。在增殖细胞中,生长因子信号或持续激活的癌基因促进葡萄糖摄取。不同于静息细胞,细胞在生长因子刺激后所消耗的绝大部分葡萄糖进入生物合成反应产生核苷酸、氨基酸和脂类,或者以乳酸排出

调控 GLUT1 和乳酸脱氢酶 A 基因的表达,促进沃伯格效应[55]。

糖酵解流量增强使得增殖细胞能够动态调控多种生物合成中间体的生成,同时将多余的碳以乳酸的形式分泌出细胞(图 15-1b)。这些发现能够解释为何生长因子能够增强葡萄糖摄取并促进葡萄糖进入糖酵解通路,但为何糖酵解产生的丙酮酸被选择性转变为乳酸而不是进入 TCA 循环呢?这个现象的解释之一是,在高速摄取葡萄糖时细胞需防止 TCA 循环过度产生 NADH/FADH2[56]。因为过量的电子供体会快速消耗可用的 ADP,导致电子传递链过载,超量生成 ROS。为避免这种情况发生,NADH 和 ATP 均为线粒体关键代谢酶丙酮酸脱氢酶的别构抑制剂,减少丙酮酸依赖的乙酰辅酶 A 合成,使电子传递链不至于产生超出细胞所需的 ATP。

除了受 ATP 和 NADH 别构调控,丙酮酸脱氢酶(pyruvate dehydrogenase,PDH)也被丙酮酸脱氢酶激酶 1(pyruvate dehydrogenase kinase 1,PDK1)磷酸化负调控。当细胞内参与电子传递链的电子供体生成速率超过氧气的吸收能力时,PDK1 的表达被诱导。尤其是 PDK1 转录可被缺氧诱导因子 1α(hypoxia inducible factor 1α,HIF1α)上调,HIF1α 是缺氧时被诱导表达的转录因子[57,58]。HIF1α 激活乳酸脱氢酶 A(lactate dehydrogenase A,LDHA)的转录,重新引导碳流量从 TCA 循环转向生成乳酸[59]。尽管 HIF1α 经典的激活方式是缺氧,转化的细胞在正常氧含量仍可诱导 HIF1α,其糖酵解也较活跃[60]。HIF1α 并不是唯一可以转录激活 PDK1 的蛋白。另一个在肿瘤中被经常激活的 Wnt/β-catenin 通路也可上调 PDK1 和乳酸转运蛋白(monocarboxylate transporter 1, MCT1)的表达,介导沃伯格效应[61]。

从代谢的角度,癌基因介导衰老(oncogene-induced senescence,OIS)的发生机制可能是丙酮酸代谢失控。在 OIS 这种现象中,癌基因如 RAS 或 BRAF 突变体过表达诱发生长停滞、

ROS 过量生成和 DNA 损伤应激反应[62]。有趣的是，OIS 的发生依赖于 PDH 的活力。通过表达 PDK1 或者抑制 PDH 磷酸酶 2(pyruvate dehyrogenase phosphatase 2，PDP2)的方式调控 PDH 活性可以帮助细胞逃避 OIS[63]。

十年前发现，在真核细胞进化过程中线粒体的作用更多是合成生物大分子，而非生成 ATP。从进化的角度，线粒体之所以成为关键细胞器是因为它们提供了多种多样的生物合成前体，也就是消耗反应。TCA 循环中间物离开线粒体用作许多合成反应的前体，包括糖、非必需氨基酸和脂肪酸生物合成。此外线粒体维持铁硫簇的合成，对许多位于线粒体和胞浆酶类的功能至关重要。

胞浆中脂肪酸和胆固醇的生物合成对增殖细胞尤为重要。脂肪酸和胆固醇生物合成的通用前体是乙酰辅酶 A。由于辅酶 A 分子较大不能穿过线粒体膜，细胞不能将线粒体乙酰辅酶 A 库直接用于生物合成。不过 TCA 中间物柠檬酸能从线粒体穿梭至胞浆，被 ATP-柠檬酸裂酶(ATP-citrate lyase，ACL)剪切形成乙酰辅酶 A(图 15-2)。ACL 对肿瘤生成至关重要，抑制 ACL 可在小鼠中抑制肿瘤生长[64,65]。值得注意的是，ACL 酶在 Akt 诱导后被激活[66]。因此 Akt 不仅能够增强葡萄糖摄取和分解代谢，也会将碳流从线粒体中分拨至脂肪酸生物合成。

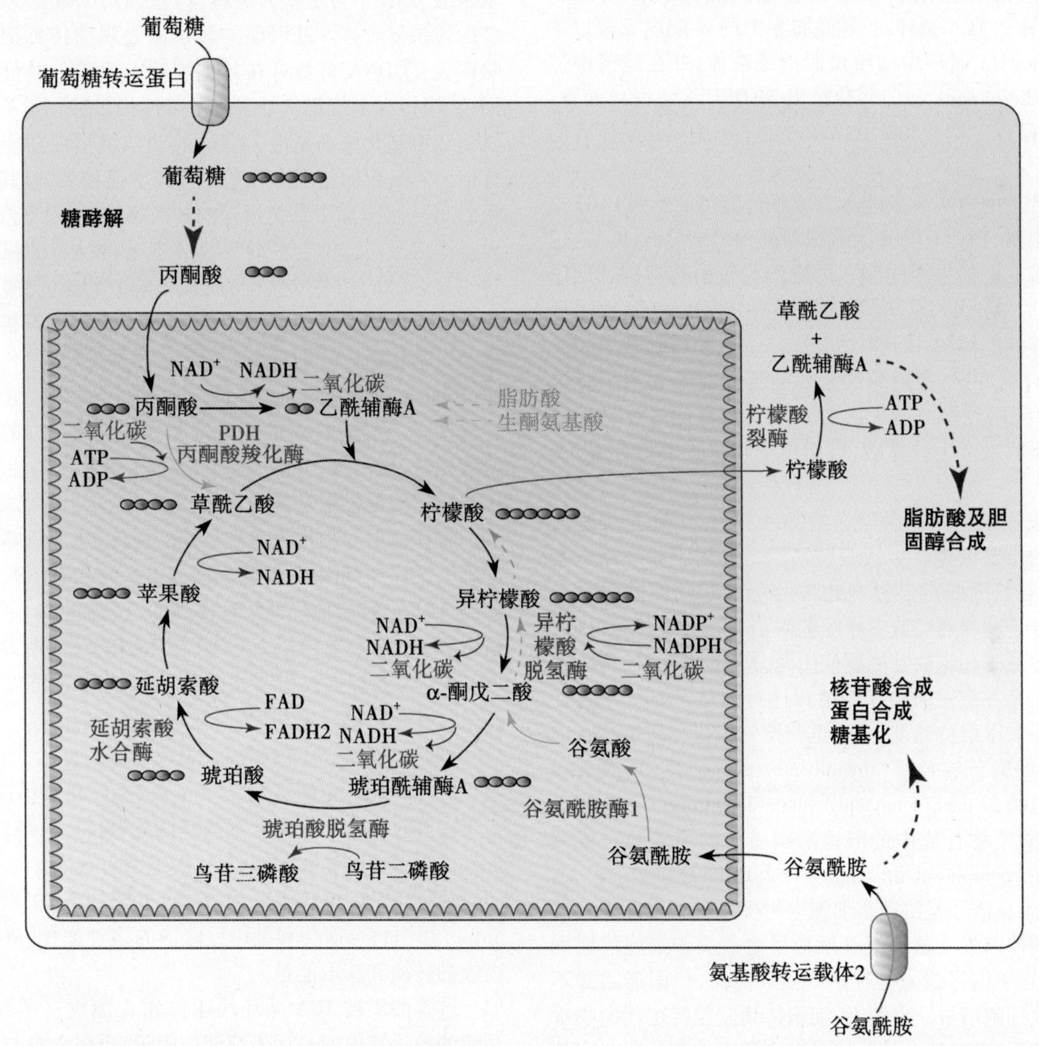

图 15-2　线粒体中的碳代谢。糖酵解来源的丙酮酸可作为三羧酸(TCA)循环中乙酰辅酶 A 的供体。柠檬酸消耗性外流进入胞浆(褐色箭头所示)能够维持线粒体外的乙酰辅酶 A 库，用于脂肪酸和胆固醇的生物合成。谷氨酰胺和丙酮酸可作为补给性的底物补充 TCA 循环中间体(绿色实线箭头所示)。在乙酰辅酶 A 不足的条件下，谷氨酰胺来源的 α-酮戊二酸经还原性羧化反应可产生柠檬酸(绿色虚线箭头所示)。粉红圆圈标示分子中的碳原子。NAD⁺，氧化型烟酰胺腺嘌呤二核苷酸；NADH，还原型烟酰胺腺嘌呤二核苷酸；PDH，丙酮酸脱氢酶；ATP，腺苷三磷酸；ADP，腺苷二磷酸；NADP⁺，氧化型烟酰胺腺嘌呤二核苷酸磷酸；NADPH，还原型烟酰胺腺嘌呤二核苷酸磷酸

要点

促生长信号增强葡萄糖摄取并重塑糖酵解以满足细胞生长时增强的生物合成需求。

谷氨酰胺和合成代谢——援兵降临

许多肿瘤细胞(包括接收了生长信号的正常细胞)活跃地利用谷氨酰胺。谷氨酰胺摄取和水解成谷氨酸的过程被称为

谷氨酰胺分解。该过程由转录因子 c-Myc 协调。事实上 c-Myc 扩增使细胞特别依赖谷氨酰胺供给。为什么谷氨酰胺对增殖细胞如此重要呢？首先，在 TCA 循环中间体离开线粒体参与合成反应时，谷氨酰胺的碳骨架可用于补足 TCA 循环。因为增殖细胞从 TCA 循环不断借用中间体，例如柠檬酸，来维持生物合成。中间体的消耗必须由别处来源的碳流补足，即补给反应过程。已知的两个主要补给输入途径有：谷氨酰胺来源的 α-酮戊二酸；经由丙酮酸羧化酶（pyruvate carboxylase，PC）催化丙酮酸羧化反应形成的草酰乙酸（图 15-2）。尽管谷氨酰胺是肿瘤细胞喜好的补给物，具有高 PC 活性的细胞可利用 PC 产生的草酰乙酸应对谷氨酰胺缺乏或谷氨酰胺酶被抑制的状态[67]。除了补充 TCA 循环，谷氨酰胺来源的 α-酮戊二酸以苹果酸的形式在 TCA 循环中间阶段脱离线粒体，并在胞浆中被苹果酸酶（malic enzyme，ME）氧化产生 NADPH[68]。总体而言，苹果酸酶、磷酸戊糖途径和叶酸循环产生了细胞内几乎所有的 NADPH。

糖酵解产生的丙酮酸在进入 TCA 循环时可能受到 PDH 负调控因素的限制，例如 HIF1α 上调或 Wnt 信号通路激活。这也同时制造了难题—如果丙酮酸在丙酮酸脱氢酶被抑制、LDHA 和 MCT 被激活双重作用下从 TCA 循环中分流出去，TCA 循环如何产生足够的柠檬酸用于生物合成？一些肿瘤细胞采用了令人意外的解决方案：在丙酮酸来源的乙酰辅酶 A 水平受限时，肿瘤细胞利用谷氨酰胺来源的 α-酮戊二酸通过反转 TCA 循环的部分反应来产生柠檬酸，进而用于脂肪酸生物合成（图 15-2）[69,70]。

谷氨酰胺除了将其碳骨架供给 TCA 循环外，还是细胞所需还原态氮的主要供体。尽管其胺基氮主要用于非必需氨基酸生物合成，谷氨酰胺的胺基氮也参与嘌呤和嘧啶的生物合成。合成一分子胸腺嘧啶或者尿嘧啶需消耗一分子谷氨酰胺，合成一分子腺嘌呤和胞嘧啶则要使用两分子谷氨酰胺，鸟嘌呤合成则需要三个谷氨酰胺分子。值得注意的是，c-Myc 不仅促进谷氨酰胺摄取以维持碱基合成，也调控一些核苷酸生物合成酶的表达，例如胸苷酸合酶（thymidylate synthase，TS）、次黄嘌呤单磷酸脱氢酶 2（inosine monophosphate dehydrogenase 2，IMPDH2）和核苷酸生物合成中的限速酶磷酸核糖焦磷酸合成酶（phosphoribosyl pyrophosphate synthetase 2，PRPS2）[71,72]。

总之，促生长信号是协调多细胞生物摄取和利用外界营养物质的核心调控因素。这一概念颠覆了之前关于细胞代谢网络自调控、独立于信号输入存在的观点。然而，代谢通路并不仅仅被动接收细胞信号。事实上，细胞持续监控特定代谢物水平的升高和降低，进而整合相关信息以协调生长和分化在内的多种细胞过程。

要点

谷氨酰胺通过两种方式维持合成代谢，既可作为碳源补充 TCA 循环中间体，维持生物合成，又可以为核苷酸和非必需氨基酸的生物合成提供还原态氮。

细胞核闻香知味

已知代谢物可作为特定代谢酶的别构调控因子，为细胞应对代谢物水平波动、调整分解和合成反应间的平衡提供反馈调控机制。其例证之一是糖酵解生物合成分支出的两个产物 SAICAR 和丝氨酸对糖酵解关键代谢酶 PKM2 的别构激活调控。

引人注意的是，一些代谢物的信号传递能力远超对代谢通路的调控。代谢物可作为辅因子或底物参与代谢活动之外的许多酶促反应，并且通过其丰度变化向这些过程传递调控信息[73]。特定代谢物的水平调控表观遗传标记的沉积和去除，使细胞能够应对营养状态变化协调的改变其基因表达程式[74]。

真核细胞染色质由基因组 DNA 缠绕组蛋白八聚体构成。基因组 DNA 中特定基因座进行转录时，DNA 必须临时解开以装配转录复合体。基因座的转录由表观遗传标记的沉积和移除调控：①DNA 自身可在其胞嘧啶 5 位碳上共价结合甲基基团；②组蛋白上特定氨基酸残基可连接多种化学基团。其中乙酰化和甲基化修饰是最为多样的调控组蛋白功能的表观遗传标记。乙酰化标记大多和基因转录增强相关，且其转换效率较快（以分钟计）。甲基化标记的转换率较低，根据修饰残基的差异会体现激活或抑制的效果。表观遗传标记的组合不仅指导转录复合体的招募和装配，而且影响 DNA 基因座在转录时总体的可接近程度，因此对基因转录具有显著的调控效应。乙酰化和甲基化标记分别直接来源于乙酰辅酶 A 和 S-腺苷甲硫氨酸（S-adenosylmethionine，SAM）这两种代谢物。组蛋白乙酰基转移酶将乙酰辅酶 A 的乙酰基团标记到组蛋白的赖氨酸和精氨酸残基，而一碳（叶酸）循环的产物 SAM 则为组蛋白和 DNA 甲基转移酶提供甲基基团。

将代谢中间物作为表观标记的前体，这一策略使细胞能够准确上调代谢基因以应对“营养充足”的状态。通过遗传手段抑制 ACL 会特定地降低线粒体外的乙酰辅酶 A，并显著影响组蛋白乙酰化状态，导致 GLUT、HK、PFK1 和 LDHA 表达减弱[75]。通过这种方式，高水平的乙酰辅酶 A 可以改变组蛋白乙酰化并促进葡萄糖利用，增强沃伯格效应。

细胞代谢状态不仅调控着表观标记的标示，而且影响着乙酰化和甲基化标记的移除。Sirtuin 去乙酰化酶借助 NAD^+ 催化组蛋白和许多非组蛋白上乙酰基团的移除[76]；与之类似，氧化形式的 FAD 是组蛋白去甲基化酶 1（lysine-specific histone demethylase 1，LSD1）的辅因子[77]。通过感知 NAD^+/NADH 比例，Sirtuin 蛋白整合遗传和翻译后修饰的多种变化，进而在代谢中高效的转换和获取能量。

许多酶类被 TCA 循环代谢物如 α-酮戊二酸、琥珀酸和富马酸调控。其中即包括表观调控因子，也包含参与非组蛋白翻译后修饰的酶类。值得一提的是，α-酮戊二酸可作为一些酶的辅因子，如含有 Jumonji C 结构域的组蛋白去甲基化酶、TET（ten-eleven translocation）家族甲基胞嘧啶羟化酶以及调控 HIF1α 水平等过程的脯氨酰羟化酶。α-酮戊二酸在这些酶促过程中被转变为琥珀酸。重要的是，琥珀酸和其下游产物富马酸可作为 α-酮戊二酸依赖酶类的抑制剂[78]。通过这种方式，α-酮戊二酸丰度相对于琥珀酸和富马酸水平的变化在许多细胞过程中产生广泛的影响。特定类型肿瘤也确实以代谢酶突变的方式利用 TCA 循环代谢物的信号传递潜能。这些突变导致传递信号代谢物水平的异常升高。这些代谢物由于其和癌基因的相似性而被称作致癌代谢物[79]。

在肿瘤中迄今发现了三类代谢酶的重复突变。TCA 循环代谢酶琥珀酸脱氢酶(succinate dehydrogenase,SDH)和富马酸水合酶(fumarate hydratase,FH)的功能缺失突变分别导致琥珀酸和富马酸累积。SDH 的双等位缺失支持遗传性副神经节瘤和嗜铬细胞瘤的发展[80],而 FH 缺失能够促进罕见的家族性肿瘤综合征遗传性平滑肌瘤和肾细胞癌(hereditary leiomyomatosis and renal cell cancer,HLRCC)[81]。异柠檬酸脱氢酶 1 和 2(isocitrate dehydrogenase,IDH1 和 IDH2)的功能获得突变则存在于大多数低级别脑胶质瘤病例中,也存在于急性髓性白血病(acute myeloid leukemia,AML)、软骨肉瘤和胆管癌[82~85]。发生于 IDH1 和 IDH2 的突变赋予了该代谢酶非同寻常的新功能:尽管野生型异柠檬酸脱氢酶催化异柠檬酸转化为 α-酮戊二酸,其突变体则将 α-酮戊二酸还原为 2-羟戊二酸的 D 型对映异构体[86,87]。尽管细胞中 D-2-羟戊二酸水平一般非常低,但是带有 IDH 突变的细胞则会将该代谢物积累至毫摩量级。由于 D-2-羟戊二酸与 α-酮戊二酸的结构相似性,D-2-羟戊二酸可作为 α-酮戊二酸依赖酶类的竞争性抑制剂[88]。

由于许多 α-酮戊二酸依赖酶类参与表观重塑,致癌代谢物驱动的肿瘤中表观遗传组具有显著改变。例如在 SDH 驱动的副神经节瘤和散发的胃肠道基质肿瘤中,SDH 缺失与 DNA 甲基化水平上升(称为高甲基化因子表型)相关[89,90]。类似的,IDH1 和 IDH2 突变与脑胶质瘤和急性髓性白血病的高甲基化因子表型具有很强的相关性[91,92]。在急性髓性白血病中,IDH 突变与甲基胞嘧啶羟化酶 TET2 的功能缺失突变是互斥的,进一步加强了这两个酶的机制性联系[92]。在不同细胞类型中引入 IDH 突变体或者用 D-2-羟戊二酸处理细胞足够引发 DNA 和组蛋白甲基化的变化并抑制细胞分化[93,94]。相应地,在脑胶质瘤和急性髓性白血病细胞模型中靶向抑制 IDH 突变体能够促进细胞分化[95,96]。总之,致癌代谢物对 DNA 和组蛋白甲基化组进行整体重塑并可能通过将细胞锁定在未分化状态以促进肿瘤发生。

要点

肿瘤细胞的代谢适应不仅促进大分子生物合成,也能对细胞命运体现出显著的非代谢效应。

从小偷小摸到罪魁祸首——肿瘤细胞如何带坏邻居

一般认为组织中的微环境在遗传上具有稳定的细胞构成。肿瘤发生过程中肿瘤附近的微环境发生显著的改变。最突出的是其组成成分—成纤维细胞、血管内皮细胞以及先天和获得性免疫相关细胞—从维持稳态转变成为促进肿瘤生长的活跃分子[97]。肿瘤采用多样的信号异化正常细胞,包括分泌因子、细胞和细胞相互作用以及代谢物水平的变化。下述两个肿瘤代谢异常影响微环境的例子。

肿瘤摄取营养物质的增加与胞外液体环境中的被分泌的大量乳酸密切相关,这对肿瘤微环境产生了广泛的效应。乳酸通过稳定内皮细胞中的 HIF1α 参与促进血管新生的过程[98]。除了激活促进血管生成的核因子激活 B 细胞的 κ-轻链增强因子(nuclear factor kappa-light-chain-enhancer of activated B cells,NF-κB)和 PI3K 信号通路[99~101],乳酸还促进巨噬细胞分泌血管内皮生长因子(vascular endothelial growth factor,VEGF)[102]。此外乳酸通过抑制单核细胞迁移[103]、阻碍 T 细胞和树突状细胞激活来减弱所在部位的抗肿瘤免疫反应[104,105],同时也会影响肿瘤相关巨噬细胞的极化状态和定位模式[106,107]。肿瘤相关巨噬细胞存在两种功能亚型:M1 型,与促炎细胞因子分泌相关;M2 型,参与免疫抑制和损伤修复。肿瘤相关巨噬细胞绝大部分是 M2 极化形式,而乳酸可以直接诱导 M2 亚型[106]。最后,乳酸累积导致肿瘤细胞外基质 pH 的下降,进而增加大量降解基质酶类的活性以促进侵袭[108,109]。

肿瘤细胞采用的另一策略是从微环境中选择性消耗色氨酸这种氨基酸,进而降低抗肿瘤免疫反应[110]。为此,肿瘤细胞上调色氨酸降解酶类吲哚胺 2,3-双加氧酶(indoleamine 2,3-dioxygenase,IDO)和色氨酸 2,3-双加氧酶(tryptophan 2,3-dioxygenase,TDO)的表达。这两个酶均将色氨酸降解为犬尿氨酸。色氨酸水平不足引发效应 T 细胞的凋亡[111]。此外,犬尿氨酸的累积能够促进免疫抑制性调节 T 细胞的出现[112]。最后,犬尿氨酸介导的信号转导能够增强肿瘤细胞自身的侵袭性和降解细胞外基质的能力[113]。

要点

肿瘤细胞利用特定代谢物的信号传递能力来影响其微环境中细胞的状态并促进肿瘤发生。

肿瘤代谢走进临床

肿瘤细胞葡萄糖摄取增加这一代谢特征已在肿瘤成像中成功应用超过三十年。氟的放射性同位素 ^{18}F 标记 2-脱氧葡萄糖后可被细胞摄入,由正电子放射断层扫描(positron emission tomography,PET)检测[114]。^{18}F-氟代脱氧葡萄糖(^{18}F-fluorodeoxyglucose,^{18}F-FDG)以和葡萄糖相同的方式被转运进细胞并被 HK 磷酸化,但其不能被进一步分解代谢,所以会在细胞内累积。作为非侵入式的肿瘤检测手段,^{18}F-FDG-PET 被广泛用于肿瘤的临床检测和分型以及疗效监测。然而 ^{18}F-FDG-PET 也具有局限性,包括免疫细胞(例如自免疫性甲状腺炎)组织浸润产生的假阳性,不能有效检测糖酵解活性低的肿瘤(常见于前列腺癌)。另外,某些组织特别是脑,体现出持续高水平的葡萄糖摄取。这也阻碍了脑肿瘤的检测。紧随 ^{18}F-FDG 的成功应用,更多的示踪代谢物,例如 ^{18}F-氟代谷氨酰胺[115]、^{11}C-乙酸[116]、α-^{11}C-甲基-L-色氨酸[117,118]正在开发过程中。其他代谢成像手段例如 ^{1}H 磁共振波谱(magnetic resonance spectroscopy,MRS)也正在开发以用于临床。MRS 可以在特定组织中检测内源代谢物的丰度。例如 MRS 利用 D-2-羟戊二酸累积作为标志物已经用于 IDH1 突变的脑胶质瘤的检测[119]。

不仅限于肿瘤成像,至少两种代谢治疗肿瘤的方式已在临床上取得几十年的成功应用。来源于细菌的重组 L-天冬酰胺酶可以降解天冬酰胺这个氨基酸,并于 1978 年被美国食品药品管理局批准用于治疗儿童急性淋巴细胞白血病[120]。白血病细胞不能合成足够的天冬酰胺,因此清除血浆中的天冬酰胺

(对谷氨酰胺也可能如此)使细胞更容易死亡。核苷酸生物合成抑制剂是另一代谢治疗成功案例。这些药物包括胸腺嘧啶合成抑制剂5-氟尿嘧啶、缺氧核苷酸合成阻断剂吉西他滨和羟基脲,以及抗叶酸药物甲氨蝶呤。甲氨蝶呤能够干扰二羟叶酸还原酶介导的四羟叶酸合成过程,阻碍叶酸循环驱动的核苷酸合成。悉尼·法伯在20世纪40年代在波士顿首次揭示抗叶酸药物的疗效[121],其作用机制在1958年被发现[122]。

肿瘤细胞对葡萄糖代谢的依赖性推动了大量靶向葡萄糖摄取或糖酵解不同步骤的治疗试验。然而抗糖酵解的干预手段,例如通过葡萄糖类似物2-脱氧葡萄糖或者药物氯尼达明抑制HK,未显示出一致的临床试验结果[123]。氯尼达明产生了系统性不良反应[123],而2-脱氧葡萄糖则引发补偿性的胰岛素样生长因子I(insulin-like growth factor-I,IGF-I)受体介导信号通路的激活[124]。表15-1所示为正在开发的靶向代谢通路治疗药物的简况。

表15-1 正在进行临床开发的肿瘤代谢疗法

酶靶点	靶点复合物	代谢通路
葡萄糖转运子的GLUT家族	根皮素和水飞蓟宾	葡萄糖摄取
MCT(乳酸转运子)	AZD3965	糖酵解
PDK1	二氯乙酸盐	丙酮酸分解代谢
线粒体复合体I	二甲双胍	氧化磷酸化
谷氨酰胺酶(GLS1)	CB-839	谷氨酰胺分解
脂酸合成酶	TVB-2640	脂酸合成
HMGCR	他汀类	固醇合成
IDH1*	AG-120	肿瘤代谢物产生
IDH2*	AG-221	肿瘤代谢物产生
IDO/TDO	INCB024360和indoximod	色氨酸降解

*译注:已于2019年被FDA批准用于AML。

糖尿病标准治疗药物二甲双胍作为治疗性和化学预防性抗癌药体现出了治疗希望。多个回顾性研究提示,服用二甲双胍不仅降低糖尿病病人的肿瘤风险,而且体现较好的肿瘤治疗效果。二甲双胍的疗效在非糖尿病患者中也被进一步证实[125]。二甲双胍的抗肿瘤活性机制可能是复杂的。二甲双胍可抑制电子传递链复合体I从而抑制线粒体氧化磷酸化,导致AMP/ATP比率升高以活化AMPK[126]。二甲双胍也可能通过减少ROS生成降低DNA损伤体现其肿瘤预防效果[127]。最后二甲双胍的系统性效应可能介导了其抗肿瘤功能,例如二甲双胍能降低肝脏糖异生以及血液IGF-I水平。

要点

肿瘤细胞对多种代谢异常的依赖性为成像和治疗策略构建了基础。

结论

近期肿瘤代谢的诸多发现已阐明肿瘤细胞如何重编程其代谢以维持生长,解决营养和供氧限制,改变肿瘤细胞和相邻细胞的命运。可预见的是还有许多问题有待研究:细胞如何感知和估量众多代谢物水平;细胞如何将代谢物的复杂丰度信息转变成摄取营养、执行细胞死亡和分化的程式;细胞如何与微环境和生物整体相互通讯。除去宏量营养物质外,微量营养物质如维生素、金属离子在肿瘤细胞代谢和信号传递中的作用刚开始被揭示。我们对肿瘤代谢日益了解已经转变成创新性的成像和治疗工具,可以预见这些工具库在未来将继续扩大。

总结

多细胞生物中细胞增殖被外界刺激所控制,包括可溶生长因子以及细胞对细胞外基质的黏附。促生长信号导致细胞代谢状态的显著改变,增强其从头合成生长所需大分子——蛋白质、脂类和核酸——的能力。促生长的信号直接增强对周围环境中代谢底物的吸收,保证增殖细胞有充足的大分子前体供给以维持生长。促生长信号也会改变底物的下游代谢命运,将其用于前体物质生成以维持多种生物合成反应,包括脂肪酸、胆固醇、非必需氨基酸和核苷酸的生物合成。促生长信号在自然状态下是瞬时的。与正常组织相比,肿瘤细胞累积异常激活的癌基因,将细胞代谢锁定在持续获取营养物质和进行大分子生物合成的状态。

尽管促生长信号影响代谢底物的摄取及其在细胞代谢通路中的代谢模式,细胞中特定代谢物水平的变化也调节多种非代谢过程。例如细胞内代谢物可作为多种表观遗传酶类的底物或辅因子。特定代谢物水平的变化因此能够改变细胞表观遗传状态。某些类型肿瘤通过代谢酶突变的方式利用这种调控模式。近期研究基于此发现了促肿瘤的代谢中间物并将其命名为致癌代谢物。此外,肿瘤细胞代谢异常能够影响肿瘤微环境中其他细胞,促进肿瘤的生长和扩散。

基于肿瘤特异的代谢变化,多个用于成像和治疗的药剂在临床上已得到应用。我们对肿瘤特异代谢变化的深入理解为未来拓展更多的此类应用提供了希望。

(王义平 雷群英 译 王旭 雷群英 校)

参考文献

The complete reference list can be found on the Wiley Companion Digital Edition of this title (see inside front cover for login instructions).

1 Hanahan D, Weinberg RA. Hallmarks of cancer: the next generation. *Cell*. 2011;**144**(**5**):646–674.

7 Broach JR. Nutritional control of growth and development in yeast. *Genetics*. 2012;**192**(**1**):73–105.

9 Hensley CT, Wasti AT, DeBerardinis RJ. Glutamine and cancer: cell biology, physiology, and clinical opportunities. *J Clin Invest*. 2013;**123**(**9**):3678–3684.

12 Zaman S, Lippman SI, Schneper L, Slonim N, Broach JR. Glucose regulates transcription in yeast through a network of signaling pathways. *Mol Syst Biol*. 2009;5:245.

17 Wieman HL, Wofford JA, Rathmell JC. Cytokine stimulation promotes glucose uptake via phosphatidylinositol-3 kinase/Akt regulation of Glut1 activity and trafficking. *Mol Biol Cell*. 2007;**18**(**4**):1437–1446.

19 Jacobs SR, Herman CE, Maciver NJ, et al. Glucose uptake is limiting in T cell acti-

vation and requires CD28-mediated Akt-dependent and independent pathways. *J Immunol*. 2008;**180(7)**:4476-4486.
20 Boxer RB, Stairs DB, Dugan KD, et al. Isoform-specific requirement for Akt1 in the developmental regulation of cellular metabolism during lactation. *Cell Metab*. 2006;**4(6)**:475-490.
22 Wise DR, DeBerardinis RJ, Mancuso A, et al. Myc regulates a transcriptional program that stimulates mitochondrial glutaminolysis and leads to glutamine addiction. *Proc Natl Acad Sci U S A*. 2008;**105(48)**:18782-18787.
25 Schafer ZT, Grassian AR, Song L, et al. Antioxidant and oncogene rescue of metabolic defects caused by loss of matrix attachment. *Nature*. 2009;**461(7260)**:109-113.
26 Warburg O. On the origin of cancer cells. *Science*. 1956;**123(3191)**:309-314.
27 Eagle H. The minimum vitamin requirements of the L and HeLa cells in tissue culture, the production of specific vitamin deficiencies, and their cure. *J Exp Med*. 1955;**102(5)**:595-600.
29 Yuneva M, Zamboni N, Oefner P, Sachidanandam R, Lazebnik Y. Deficiency in glutamine but not glucose induces MYC-dependent apoptosis in human cells. *J Cell Biol*. 2007;**178(1)**:93-105.
32 Kim J, Kundu M, Viollet B, Guan KL. AMPK and mTOR regulate autophagy through direct phosphorylation of Ulk1. *Nat Cell Biol*. 2011;**13(2)**:132-141.
35 Commisso C, Davidson SM, Soydaner-Azeloglu RG, et al. Macropinocytosis of protein is an amino acid supply route in Ras-transformed cells. *Nature*. 2013;**497(7451)**:633-637.
39 Rathmell JC, Fox CJ, Plas DR, Hammerman PS, Cinalli RM, Thompson CB. Akt-directed glucose metabolism can prevent Bax conformation change and promote growth factor-independent survival. *Mol Cell Biol*. 2003;**23(20)**:7315-7328.
40 Elstrom RL, Bauer DE, Buzzai M, et al. Akt stimulates aerobic glycolysis in cancer cells. *Cancer Res*. 2004;**64(11)**:3892-3899.
43 Vander Heiden MG, Cantley LC, Thompson CB. Understanding the Warburg effect: the metabolic requirements of cell proliferation. *Science*. 2009;**324(5930)**: 1029-1033.
45 Locasale JW, Grassian AR, Melman T, et al. Phosphoglycerate dehydrogenase diverts glycolytic flux and contributes to oncogenesis. *Nat Genet*. 2011;**43(9)**:869-874.
46 Possemato R, Marks KM, Shaul YD, et al. Functional genomics reveal that the serine synthesis pathway is essential in breast cancer. *Nature*. 2011;**476(7360)**: 346-350.
50 Christofk HR, Vander Heiden MG, Harris MH, et al. The M2 splice isoform of pyruvate kinase is important for cancer metabolism and tumour growth. *Nature*. 2008;**452(7184)**:230-233.
51 Christofk HR, Vander Heiden MG, Wu N, Asara JM, Cantley LC. Pyruvate kinase M2 is a phosphotyrosine-binding protein. *Nature*. 2008;**452(7184)**:181-186.
57 Kim JW, Tchernyshyov I, Semenza GL, Dang CV. HIF-1-mediated expression of pyruvate dehydrogenase kinase: a metabolic switch required for cellular adaptation to hypoxia. *Cell Metab*. 2006;**3(3)**:177-185.
60 Lum JJ, Bui T, Gruber M, et al. The transcription factor HIF-1alpha plays a critical role in the growth factor-dependent regulation of both aerobic and anaerobic glycolysis. *Genes Dev*. 2007;**21(9)**:1037-1049.
63 Kaplon J, Zheng L, Meissl K, et al. A key role for mitochondrial gatekeeper pyruvate dehydrogenase in oncogene-induced senescence. *Nature*. 2013; **498(7452)**:109-112.
64 Bauer DE, Hatzivassiliou G, Zhao F, Andreadis C, Thompson CB. ATP citrate lyase is an important component of cell growth and transformation. *Oncogene*. 2005;**24(41)**:6314-6322.
65 Hatzivassiliou G, Zhao F, Bauer DE, et al. ATP citrate lyase inhibition can suppress tumor cell growth. *Cancer Cell*. 2005;**8(4)**:311-321.
69 Wise DR, Ward PS, Shay JE, et al. Hypoxia promotes isocitrate dehydrogenase-dependent carboxylation of alpha-ketoglutarate to citrate to support cell growth and viability. *Proc Natl Acad Sci U S A*. 2011;**108(49)**:19611-19616.
70 Metallo CM, Gameiro PA, Bell EL, et al. Reductive glutamine metabolism by IDH1 mediates lipogenesis under hypoxia. *Nature*. 2012;**481(7381)**:380-384.
73 Wellen KE, Thompson CB. A two-way street: reciprocal regulation of metabolism and signalling. *Nat Rev Mol Cell Biol*. 2012;**13(4)**:270-276.
74 Lu C, Thompson CB. Metabolic regulation of epigenetics. *Cell Metab*. 2012;**16(1)**:9-17.
75 Wellen KE, Hatzivassiliou G, Sachdeva UM, Bui TV, Cross JR, Thompson CB. ATP-citrate lyase links cellular metabolism to histone acetylation. *Science*. 2009;**324(5930)**:1076-1080.
76 Imai S, Armstrong CM, Kaeberlein M, Guarente L. Transcriptional silencing and longevity protein Sir2 is an NAD-dependent histone deacetylase. *Nature*. 2000;**403(6771)**:795-800.
86 Ward PS, Patel J, Wise DR, et al. The common feature of leukemia-associated IDH1 and IDH2 mutations is a neomorphic enzyme activity converting alpha-ketoglutarate to 2-hydroxyglutarate. *Cancer Cell*. 2010;**17(3)**:225-234.
87 Dang L, White DW, Gross S, et al. Cancer-associated IDH1 mutations produce 2-hydroxyglutarate. *Nature*. 2010;**465(7300)**:966.
92 Figueroa ME, Abdel-Wahab O, Lu C, et al. Leukemic IDH1 and IDH2 mutations result in a hypermethylation phenotype, disrupt TET2 function, and impair hematopoietic differentiation. *Cancer Cell*. 2010;**18(6)**:553-567.
93 Lu C, Ward PS, Kapoor GS, et al. IDH mutation impairs histone demethylation and results in a block to cell differentiation. *Nature*. 2012;**483(7390)**:474-478.
95 Rohle D, Popovici-Muller J, Palaskas N, et al. An inhibitor of mutant IDH1 delays growth and promotes differentiation of glioma cells. *Science*. 2013;**340(6132)**:626-630.
106 Colegio OR, Chu NQ, Szabo AL, et al. Functional polarization of tumour-associated macrophages by tumour-derived lactic acid. *Nature*. 2014;**513(7519)**: 559-563.
113 Opitz CA, Litzenburger UM, Sahm F, et al. An endogenous tumour-promoting ligand of the human aryl hydrocarbon receptor. *Nature*. 2011;**478(7368)**:197-203.
119 Choi C, Ganji SK, DeBerardinis RJ, et al. 2-hydroxyglutarate detection by magnetic resonance spectroscopy in IDH-mutated patients with gliomas. *Nat Med*. 2012;**18(4)**:624-629.
125 Rizos CV, Elisaf MS. Metformin and cancer. *Eur J Pharmacol*. 2013;**705(1-3)**: 96-108.

第16章　晚期或早期转移性疾病的小鼠治疗模型

Robert S. Kerbel, PhD ■ Marta Paez-Ribes, PhD ■ Shan Man, BSc ■ Ping Xu, PhD ■ Eric Guerin, MD ■ William Cruz-Munoz, PhD ■ John M. L. Ebos, PhD

概述

临床前治疗模型的频发失败是肿瘤药物开发中始终存在的问题，其中也包括在荷瘤小鼠中显示阳性结果的治疗，却在临床试验入组病人中得不到预期的效果。有多种可能的原因会造成高发的假阳性结果。一种可能性是在全身转移性疾病的治疗中，临床前治疗模型无论在微观还是宏观，尤其是在宏观层面，都无法准确模拟临床情况。因此，在小鼠体内建立原发性肿瘤的模型，肿瘤为移植瘤或自发成瘤，可以是鼠源或人源的，也可以来自细胞系或是包括人源组织异种移植（patient-derived xenograft, PDX）的肿瘤组织移植，通过治疗荷瘤小鼠来预测药物临床效果仍然是肿瘤药物开发中普遍的方式。在本章中，我们总结了肿瘤自发转移小鼠模型建立的最新进展，特别是原发性肿瘤手术切除后仍然进展到晚期的小鼠模型，包括使用人肿瘤细胞系、PDX和基因工程小鼠模型（genetically engineered mouse model, GEMM）。本章讨论该类模型已取得的有限的治疗研究结果，以及它们与相应Ⅲ期临床试验结果回顾性或前瞻性地的联系。已有的结果表明，利用此类模型预测在临床转移性疾病患者的治疗效果可能有一定的益处。此外，此类模型的一些局限性也在本章讨论范畴。

引言

新型抗癌药物的开发是一项艰苦复杂、费力且昂贵的工程，其最终失败率远高于其他治疗领域；据报道，在肿瘤学的所有Ⅲ期临床试验中，超过60%是失败的，未能达到其主要终点[1]。通常来讲，这种长期且昂贵的临床试验都先在小鼠临床前模型进行评估，且在随后的小范围Ⅰ期/Ⅱ期临床试验中取得了令人满意的结果，之后才会进一步开展关键的双盲随机安慰剂对照Ⅲ期临床试验。因此，Ⅲ期临床试验的高失败率引发了很多关键问题，其中包括：①为什么在肿瘤治疗的小鼠临床前模型中容易出现过高的假阳性结果，如何改进模型以便更好的预测临床试验的结果？②为什么Ⅲ期临床试验无法重现Ⅱ期临床试验的阳性结果，如何改进小范围的Ⅱ期临床试验设计以便更好地预测Ⅲ期临床试验的结果？

本章将针对第一个问题，首先讨论导致小鼠治疗模型中如此高“假阳性”的可能原因，随后分析一些克服当前小鼠肿瘤治疗模型局限性的策略，并将重点研究提高小鼠肿瘤模型的临床相关性的方法，即与临床治疗全身转移性疾病早期（微观的）或晚期（宏观的）阶段，尤其是晚期阶段的相关性。

影响小鼠肿瘤治疗模型临床相关性和预测效能的因素

在临床相关性和预测效能等方面，已有很多综述和评述报道了使用临床前小鼠肿瘤治疗模型评估肿瘤药物活性的局限性[2~4]。其中一些因素广为人知，另一些鲜为人知的因素则未能引起重视，其中包括：①癌症患者的高发年龄段为中年或老年，但是我们对于相应年龄段小鼠的肿瘤治疗研究认识几乎为零[5]。相反的，治疗研究（至少涉及肿瘤移植模型时）一般在6~10周龄小鼠体内开展。从这个角度上讲，这大体相当于开展了小儿肿瘤临床试验。然而，因为一些影响肿瘤药物活性的关键指标，比如药物代谢、药物动力学，在儿童和成年人之间存在差异，肿瘤药物对二者的作用可能会相差甚远。②相比较于典型的临床试验中，入组患者的基因差异显著，小鼠研究多采用近交小鼠品系，使得研究组群中具有高度的基因同质性。这基本上消除或严重降低了人类基因组异质性对药物半衰期和代谢等重要指标的影响，而这些指标可能对治疗结果产生重大影响[6]。③在小鼠和人类之间，药物的最适剂量或最大耐受剂量（maximum tolerated dose, MTD）都有很大差异。例如，相较于人体，很多化疗药物的最大耐受剂量在小鼠体内要高很多[6]。这可能会造成肿瘤对药物应答良好的假象，尤其是在治疗人类移植肿瘤的研究中。④许多常用的小鼠移植肿瘤模型的小鼠免疫原性高，因此会出现免疫系统活化（假设免疫活性小鼠被用作治疗研究的宿主）对治疗结果的影响，这会扭曲或夸大药物本身的功能效果[7]。⑤临床前研究中经常使用不合适的终点，脱离临床实际[8]。例如，基于影像学检测的无进展生存期（progression free survival, PFS）作为一个常见的临床终点越来越多地在Ⅲ期临床试验中被用作主要或次要终点，却很少用于评估小鼠体内的疗效。相反的，尤其在使用肿瘤移植的原发性肿瘤模型中，我们通常仅检测治疗对肿瘤生长本身的影响。在肿瘤没有明显消退的情况下，经常会发现肿瘤生长延迟。从临床角度来看，生长延迟被视为“治疗失败”或是疾病进展，然而，在肿瘤研究人员眼中，治疗组相较于对照组出现肿瘤生长延迟通常被看作效果良好。⑥检索近来肿瘤研究文献就会发现，肿瘤药物在小鼠体内的研究方式跟半世纪或更久之前几乎一致：肿瘤细胞经常以皮下注射的方式移植入小鼠体内，等肿瘤长至一定尺寸就建立起了“异位”原发肿瘤模型，随后就可以对荷瘤小鼠进行治疗。肿瘤组织可以是鼠源或者人源的。在这两种情况下，特别是鼠源肿瘤移植时，肿瘤细胞增殖快，肿瘤倍增时间可以很短。这使得肿瘤对多种癌症药物敏感，尤其是细胞毒性化疗药物，其可以优先靶向处于DNA复制期或者微管等胞内结构和多种DNA复制相关酶激活的细胞。此外，增殖中的肿瘤细胞也会对其他类型药物(例如信号转导抑制剂)敏感。然而,这种高增殖率并不是大多数人类自发性肿瘤的典型特征。⑦临床上对晚期多器官转移性疾病(例如肺、肝、脑和骨等)的治疗很少在小鼠临床前模型上实施[4]。无论肿瘤是移植的还是自发的,治疗已经发生明显肿瘤转移的小鼠都比小鼠原发性肿瘤的治疗更加复杂、昂贵且周期更长。然而,人类常见的恶性实体肿瘤进展到晚期,发生全身转移时是难以成功治疗的。实际上,这种情况基本上是不可治愈的,即使在一些Ⅲ期临床试验中得到阳性结果,患者无进展生存期以及总生存期的延长也很有限。虽然数据上可能具有统计学意义且具有可观的风险比率,但是这些结果的临床意义和相关成本效益往往很小[9]。

接下来我们将讨论目前对小鼠全身转移性疾病模型治疗的一些尝试;这些方法利用了人肿瘤细胞系或 PDX 建立的移植肿瘤以及 GEMM 中的自发肿瘤,重点讨论疾病晚期阶段,也涉及对疾病早期微转移阶段的论述。

利用肿瘤细胞系建立晚期内脏转移的人类肿瘤术后异种移植模型

大约十年前,人们首次尝试建立原发灶切除后的肿瘤自发转移模型,基本方法演变自 Fidler 的开创性研究[11]。Fidler 首次报道了在 B16 小鼠黑色素瘤细胞中获得转移能力(尤其是肺向转移)更强的变异亚系的方法,其中涉及一系列体内筛选,包括连续多次的静脉 B16 小鼠黑色素瘤细胞接种,并从形成“人造的”或“实验性”肺转移。研究进行了连续 10 次的静脉接种以筛选细胞,从而产生了转移性依次增强的连续亚系,例如 B16F1 和 B16F10 亚系[11]。在我们的实验中,我们尝试从切除的原发肿瘤灶中[10]筛选出具有自发转移扩散能力的类似细胞亚系,这些转移细胞需要具有完成远处转移所需的所有早期和晚期步骤的能力。为了实现这一目标,我们将人乳腺癌细胞系(例如“三阴性”MBA-MD-231 细胞系)植入雌性免疫缺陷(SCID)小鼠的乳腺脂肪垫中,这种做法与异位皮下注射相比,更能增加远处转移到肺等部位的速度和程度[12,13]。一旦原发肿瘤达到预定的体积/大小(例如 500mm^3),将原发灶手术切除。这可以延长小鼠存活时间,从而使来源于原发灶的肿瘤细胞有足够的时间可以在远处器官如肺中形成宏观转移。在原发灶肿瘤切除大约 4 个月后就可以观察到转移形成[10]。随后取多个肺转移瘤建立细胞系,再次注射到小鼠乳腺脂肪垫中,4 周后切除原发灶肿瘤。这会使得肿瘤形成肺转移的速度加快、程度加深(有时候也会形成肺外转移)。取单个肺转移灶,从中建立一种亚系,比如侵袭性更强的转移亚系 LM2.4[10]。将其用于实验性治疗研究,在原位注射细胞,肿瘤长大后切除原发灶,大约一个月后可以出现显性转移,转移灶大多局限于肺,有时也会转移至淋巴结或肝等部位[10]。实验性治疗开始于肿瘤进展的晚期阶段,将生存情况作为评估治疗功效的主要终点[10]。此外,可以用标记物对这种高转移性的细胞亚群进行标记,以此来检测随时间变化的肿瘤负荷和治疗效应。此类标记物包括可以进行全身光学/生物发光成像的荧光素酶[14],以及可以转导人绒毛膜促性腺激素蛋白 β 亚基(β-hCG)的基因,β-hCG 可以在尿液中检测到以此作为肿瘤负荷的分子标志[15]。采用上述方法多种晚期转移性疾病模型已成功建立,不仅是人类乳腺癌,还包括人类恶性黑色素瘤[16]、肾细胞癌[17]和结直肠癌[18]的模型。此外,不经过先前体内的连续筛选,晚期腹膜内转移性卵巢癌[19]和局灶性晚期原位肝细胞癌[20]的模型也已建立。

晚期转移性疾病模型建立的根本原因是,相比对小鼠原发性肿瘤的治疗,大多数实验性疗法在治疗晚期转移性疾病时效果会大打折扣。然而,例外情况也可能偶有发生,即特定药物或疗法在治疗晚期转移情况时比治疗原发性肿瘤效果更好,或者在两种情况下效果都很显著。这种疗法在对临床晚期转移患者的治疗中更有可能取得好的效果(尽管效果程度可能不同)。我们还用类似的方法来研究更早期微观肿瘤的辅助治疗[14]。因此,一旦原发肿瘤被切除,治疗就应该尽快开始,虽然此时全身影像显示没有显性的系统性转移,但是有一部分小鼠有形成后续转移的风险[14,17,18]。

已有的证据表明,利用晚期转移模型可以更好地评估药物活性以预测特定药物或疗法对患者的疗效。但局限性仍然存在,因此利用该方法预测疗效时,两次观察尤为重要。

第一次观察,观察对象是一系列结果,包括重复先前的失败的Ⅲ期临床试验,很多已经在常规原发性肿瘤的小鼠模型中取得良好的疗效,却在Ⅲ期临床试验中以失败告终[21]。一个著名的Ⅲ期临床试验失败的例子是口服抗血管生成酪氨酸激酶抑制剂(tyrosine kinase inhibitor,TKI)加常规化疗的联合疗法[21]。目前有超过 15 项此类Ⅲ期试验在乳腺癌、结肠直肠癌和肺癌等肿瘤的治疗中是失败的,未能达到其主要或次要终点[22~24]。最令人失望的例子是 Guerin 等人回顾的四项独立的Ⅲ期试验,这些试验评估了舒尼替尼在联合不同的化疗药物,或单独使用时的疗效[24]。试验都采用了一线或二线的治疗方案。且一线治疗试验都是在多个不同原发性肿瘤模型中治疗取得阳性的临床前结果之后开始的[25]。如图 16-1 所示,三种不同的抗血管生成药物,即舒尼替尼,另一种口服 TKI(帕唑帕尼)或靶向血管内皮生长因子(vascular endothelial growth factor,VEGF)受体-2 的抗体(DC101),在治疗 MDA-MB-231 乳腺癌细胞系来源的 LM2.4 转移亚系形成的原位肿瘤[24,25]时均可以造成肿瘤显著的生长延迟[25]。然而,在另一组中,对原发肿瘤切除后进展到肿瘤晚期转移阶段的小鼠进行治疗,疗效为阴性,中位总生存期缺乏统计学差异[24]。并且,将抗血管生成药物(例如舒尼替尼)联合标准紫杉醇化疗,结果仍为阴性[24]。如果替换口服 TKI,将 VEGFR-2 抗体与相同的化疗药物联合使用,则与未治疗的对照小鼠相比,可以观察到中位总生存时间的延长。虽然与紫杉醇治疗组相比,总生存期的延长并不具有统计学意义[24],但是可能会发现 PFS 的延长。因此,这一结果似乎代表了许多 VEGF 抗体例如贝伐单抗联合化疗(尤其是紫杉醇)取得阳性结果的Ⅲ期临床试验,其中观察到 PFS 延长的幅度不大,但具有统计学意义[24]。

第二次观察主要关注全身性转移的小鼠中自发脑转移瘤的形成,这些小鼠患恶性黑色素瘤或乳腺癌,并在特定治疗策略下延长了其生存期。在生存期延长的全身性转移患者中发生中枢神经系统转移在临床上越来越多见,例如采用曲妥珠单抗加化疗治疗的转移性乳腺癌的女性[26]。在这种情况下出现较高脑转移复发率的基础是由于患者生存期的延长,使得脑中的微转移有足够时间发展成为肉眼可见的病变,产生明显的症

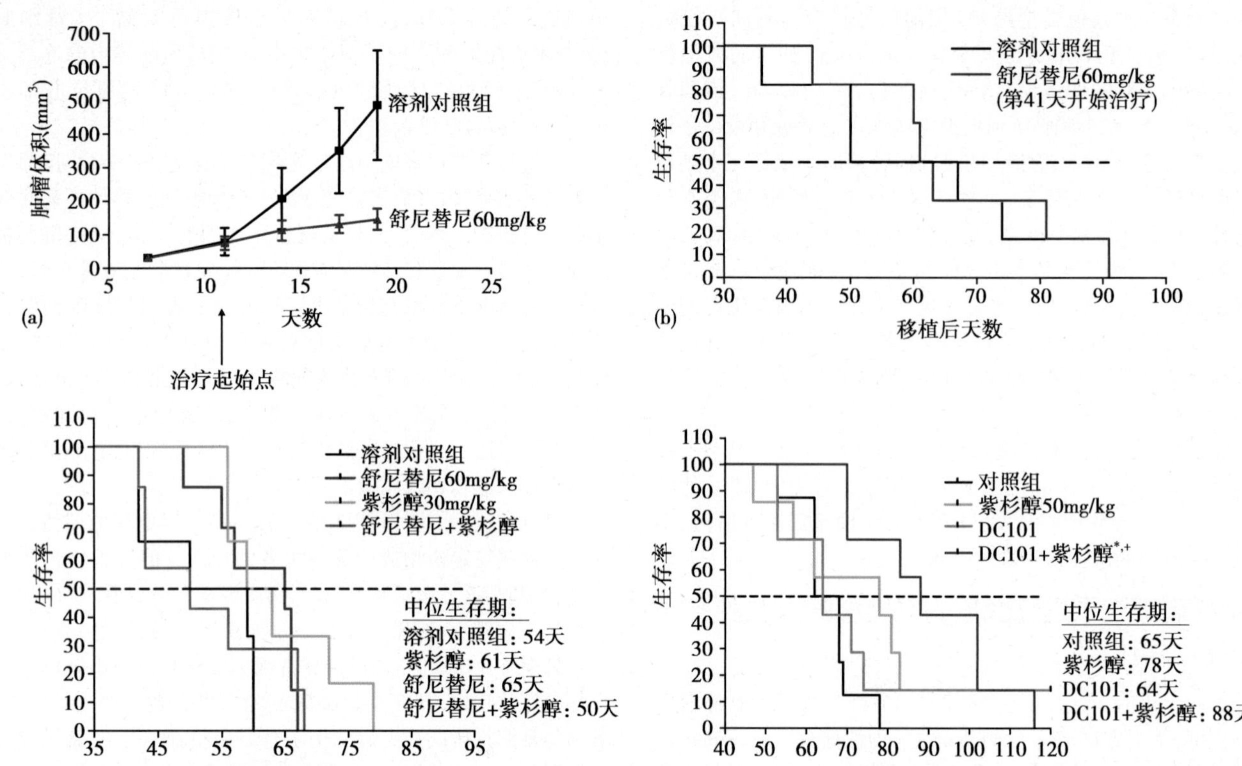

图 16-1 舒尼替尼与 DC101(一种靶向 VEGF 受体 2 的抗体,治疗原发性肿瘤与显性转移,伴或不伴有化疗方案)的结果对比。LM2. 4[10]是 MDA-MB-231 肿瘤可自发转移的亚系,将其注射到小鼠的乳腺脂肪垫中,建立原发性肿瘤(a),或切除肿瘤并使小鼠发生转移,同时通常在肿瘤切除后约 20 天(b~d)开始治疗。(a)开始治疗后,舒尼替尼可有效治疗原发性肿瘤(箭头),而(b)舒尼替尼采用相同剂量和治疗时间治疗术后晚期转移进展的小鼠,生存率无变化。舒尼替尼与标准紫杉醇联用不能改善紫杉醇的疗效,实际上会使结果恶化(c)。相反,DC101 VEGFR-2 抗体可提高紫杉醇的疗效(d)。帕唑帕尼可产生与舒尼替尼相似的效果,此处未显示。统计结果和实验细节由 Guerin 等提供

状。小鼠治疗模型中自发性脑转移的出现使得建立起了自发性脑转移模型,此过程中,黑色素瘤脑转移瘤中建立的细胞系再次移植可以维持其自发脑转移的特性,并且可以在生存期未延长的情况下发生脑转移[16]。这表示筛选出了能够自发脑转移的转移性肿瘤细胞亚群[16]。其他研究揭示了自发性脑转移的一些可能的分子驱动因素,其中涉及内皮素受体 B(endothelin receptor B)的表达增加[27]。有趣的是,内皮素受体和内皮素被认为是促进脑肿瘤和转移瘤生长的生存机制,并且可以产生对 Fidler 团队治疗方法的耐受[28]。因此,内皮素受体拮抗剂现在被认为是脑肿瘤的潜在治疗策略,如胶质母细胞瘤,并且可能在未来用于 CNS 转移性疾病的治疗中。

肿瘤转移治疗临床前模型的“前瞻性”研究:类似疗法与其临床效果的关联性

两种类型的研究分别用于评估试验疗法对晚期转移或早期微肿瘤灶(辅助疗法)的疗效,并随后在Ⅲ期临床试验中对其评估。这至少在一定程度上可以对肿瘤转移术后的药物疗效进行前瞻性分析。其中一项研究使用抗血管生成药物(舒尼替尼)作为辅助疗法治疗早期乳腺癌,其中舒尼替尼治疗是在手术切除 LM2. 4 原发性乳腺肿瘤不久,全身影像未检测到显性转移时开始的[14]。在原发性肿瘤的治疗中使用短疗程高剂量的抗血管生成药物辅助治疗已被证明可以抑制肿瘤生长,但是对治疗转移疾病没有益处。实际上,该辅助疗法与对照组相比反而加速了转移过程,减少了生存时间[14]。由此,我们建议在没有更多临床前数据表明抗血管药物辅助治疗对临床患者有益之前,要谨慎开展大型、昂贵且耗时的抗血管生成药物辅助治疗的临床试验[14]。之后,许多辅助治疗的Ⅲ期临床试验开始开展,这些实验包括在乳腺癌和直肠癌中采用贝伐单抗联合化疗药物,随后使用贝伐单抗维持治疗[29,30],在肝细胞癌中使用索拉非尼和在肾细胞癌中单用索拉非尼或舒尼替尼而不联合化疗药物。所有这些试验都没有增加无病生存期,并且在一次试验中,含有贝伐单抗的治疗组与仅化疗组相比结果更差[30]。因此,虽然不能证明辅助治疗有害,但这些结果仍支持我们最初的观点,基于临床前辅助治疗模型的结果,特别是在没有临床前试验结果支持抗血管生成辅助疗法可以成功的前提下,进行此类辅助疗法临床试验还为时过早。

前瞻性有效性研究的第二个例子来自评估低剂量节律性化疗单独或与抗血管生成药物联用治疗晚期转移性疾病的疗效。许多临床前研究表明基于节律化疗的方案在治疗小鼠晚期转移疾病时取得了令人惊讶的良好效果,尽管同一种化疗方案在治疗原发性肿瘤时效果并不显著[4,10],或者在原发性肿瘤小鼠和晚期转移小鼠中疗效相似[4]。这些结果促使随后的Ⅱ期甚至是随机对照Ⅲ期临床试验的启动,以评估节律化疗方案的疗效。第一个报道的该类Ⅲ期试验,称为 CAIRO3。该试验

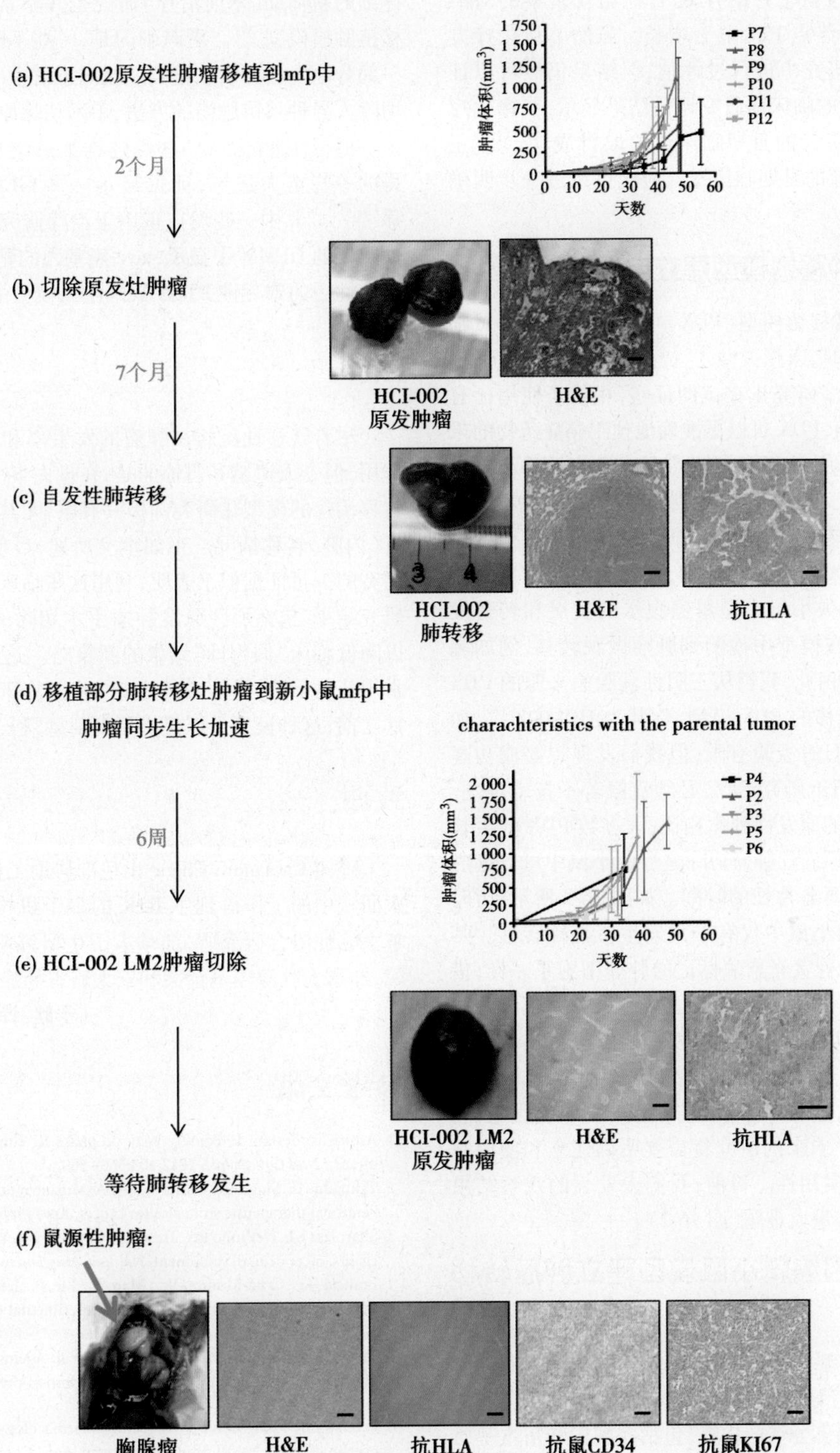

图 16-2　由乳腺癌 PDX 建立自发转移模型。(a)将三阴性乳腺癌 PDX 肿瘤 HCI-00235 的部分植入 SCID 小鼠的乳腺脂肪垫(mammary fat pads, mfp)中。连续传代后，肿瘤的生长速率保持相似。(b)2 个月后，切除原发肿瘤，维持小鼠生存以观察远处显性转移灶的形成。(c)7 个月后，1 只小鼠(55 只被检测小鼠)发生了肺转移，该转移灶呈人类白细胞抗原(human leukocyte antigen, HLA)阳性，其大小足以植入新小鼠的 mfp 中。(d)将这种肺转移的部分肿瘤灶植入新的 SCID 小鼠的 mfp 中。与亲本 HCI-002 相比，新肿瘤生长速率加快(6 周后大小达到 1 000mm^3)。(e)新肿瘤的组织结构与亲本肿瘤的组织结构相似。在连续传代后，可以维持生长速率。(f)15.9%植入 PDX 肿瘤的小鼠中也出现了鼠源性胸腺淋巴瘤。这些肿瘤(HLA 阴性，无人类成分)显示出较高的增殖率，而造血祖细胞抗原 CD34 阳性。箭头显示了小鼠胸腺瘤。比例尺为 150μm。因此，结果表明，使用 PDX 发生远处转移的可能性很小，明显的自发转移发生的时间较长，并且在较老的 SCID 小鼠中可以发生复杂的小鼠胸腺瘤[36]

评估了每日低剂量卡培他滨加贝伐单抗节律化疗作为一线转移性结直肠癌患者的维持治疗的疗效[31]。与仅观察的对照组相比,实验组的主要终点 PFS 显著增长。虽然节律化疗方案未在之前的临床前研究中进行过评估,但结果仍然可以证明,在晚期转移背景下的临床前研究评估结果显示,节律化疗有望在未来治疗转移患者的Ⅲ期临床试验取得成功[32]。正在进行的其他节律化疗的Ⅲ期临床试验应该可以进一步明确其作用。

利用人源肿瘤异种移植模型建立自发转移模型

使用人源肿瘤异种移植模型(PDX)可以大大提高小鼠临床前模型的预测能力和临床相关性[33]。正如前面所述或其他模型所发现的,目前许多研究正在试图证实,相较于使用已有的细胞系进行肿瘤移植,PDX 可以更准确地预测癌症药物的未来临床效果[33]。然而,所有 PDX 研究都是在免疫缺陷小鼠中研究原发性肿瘤的生长和治疗反应。我们还不清楚 PDX 应用于治疗肿瘤(微观的或宏观的)转移的研究结果。只有少数研究报道了 PDX 模型中发生转移性疾病,例如人源化免疫缺陷型 NOD-SCID-IL2Rγ 缺失小鼠中卵巢癌腹水的发展和转移发生[34]。一些研究报道在模型中检测到肿瘤微观转移,例如乳腺癌 PDX 模型中[35]。由此,我们从三阴性乳腺癌来源的 PDX 开始,尝试建立显性转移的 PDX 模型,称其为 HCI-002[35],如图 16-2 所示。虽然我们的经验有限,但我们发现想要成功建立这种模型并合理应用于研究治疗,必须克服若干技术难题。首先,与来源于细胞系的原发性肿瘤相比,大多数 PDX 的生长非常缓慢。因此,即使原发灶肿瘤切除之后的小鼠中可以形成显性转移,这也可能需要非常长的时间。如图 16-2 所示,历时 9 个月的时间,在 55 只小鼠中仅有一只发生了显性转移。其次,使用 PDX 组织不能像荧光素酶标记的肿瘤细胞系一样,借助全身生物发光成像等技术轻松完成远处转移的检测。因此,这将需要其他复杂的成像方法,例如,使用能够进行小动物成像的专用 MRI 设备,但是这种设备通常位于动物饲养设施之外,由于可能引起感染,这意味着一旦将小鼠拿离饲养设施,它们就不能再返回饲养。未来的研究将需要明确建立和使用基于 PDX 的转移模型的实用性。目前,我们未发表的观察结果表明这还必须克服一些重大难题(图 16-2)。

利用肿瘤自发基因编辑小鼠模型建立肿瘤转移模型

基因工程小鼠模型(genetically engineered mouse model, GEMM)用于临床前治疗研究是早期肿瘤药物开发的一项重大创新。这种模型具有很多公认的优势,包括在肿瘤和宿主基质之间没有物种差异,以及这种小鼠具有免疫能力,相较于之前在免疫抑制小鼠中建立肿瘤移植模型,可使肿瘤免疫治疗研究更好地开展。鉴于最近使用免疫检查点抑制抗体如伊匹单抗或纳武单抗的显著临床效果,这被认为是与异种移植模型相比的一个主要优势。使用"人源化"免疫抑制小鼠可能作为在没有自身免疫系统的免疫缺失小鼠中进行免疫疗法研究的新策略[34]。然而,GEMM 至少在目前还存在一些缺点。先前大多数此类模型是非转移性的;而且,多个原发性肿瘤发生时间不一致,这使得围手术期新辅助治疗或辅助治疗研究难以开展。全球关于术后辅助治疗或转移治疗[37]的研究文献数量有限,详细的新辅助(术前治疗)研究也并不常见[38],而且可能需要移植肿瘤模型[38]。更讽刺的是,一些 GEMM 转移模型还需将一部分原发性肿瘤移植到二级同系宿主中,然后用之前所述的切除人异种移植肿瘤的方法,手术切除原发性肿瘤[39]。

值得注意的是,一些综述详细总结了最近 GEMM 模型取得的一些重大进展,证据显示一些 GEMM 可以自发远处转移[40,41]。其中一些现在正用于治疗研究,例如,"RapidCap"前列腺癌的 GEMM 中显示,myc 癌基因的靶向治疗可以在产生去势抗性后的致死性 PTEN 缺陷小鼠模型中抑制转移的发生[42]。

结论

尽管转移性疾病在肿瘤的发生率和死亡率中发挥关键的作用,但令人遗憾和震惊的是,在过去半个世纪中,对临床肿瘤转移治疗的模型化研究却极其有限,尤其是针对晚期显性的全身(内脏)转移情况。正如本文所述,目前情况已经开始改变,已有的少量证据似乎表明,利用这些临床相关的转移模型治疗研究结果,包括那些原发肿瘤手术切除的模型,可能是一种可以降低临床"假阳性"结果的新策略。这些模型可能不能用于常规药物筛选,但是在药物进一步的临床开发以及临床试验设计之前,这种模型可以提供更多信息,利于决策更加明智。

致谢

感谢 Cassandra Cheng 出色的协助工作。资助基金信息:本次回顾中的工作得到了 RSK 的多个机构基金的支持,包括加拿大癌症协会研究所,加拿大卫生研究院,美国国立卫生研究院,加拿大乳腺癌基金会和安大略省癌症研究所。

(于晗 译 危晏平 李亮 校)

参考文献

1 Amiri-Kordestani L, Fojo T. Why do phase III clinical trials in oncology fail so often? *J Natl Cancer Inst*. 2012;**104**:568–569.

2 Talmadge JE, Singh RK, Fidler IJ, Raz A. Murine models to evaluate novel and conventional therapeutic strategies for cancer. *Am J Pathol*. 2007;**170**:793–804.

3 Sharpless NE, DePinho RA. The mighty mouse: genetically engineered mouse models in cancer drug development. *Nat Rev Drug Discov*. 2006;**5**:741–754.

4 Francia G, Cruz-Munoz W, Man S, Xu P, Kerbel RS. Mouse models of advanced spontaneous metastasis for experimental therapeutics. *Nat Rev Cancer*. 2011;**11**:135–141.

5 Meehan B, Garnier D, Dombrovsky A, et al. Ageing-related responses to antiangiogenic effects of sunitinib in atherosclerosis-prone mice. *Mech Ageing Dev*. 2014;**140**:13–22.

6 Peterson JK, Houghton PJ. Integrating pharmacology and in vivo cancer models in preclinical and clinical drug development. *Eur J Cancer*. 2004;**40**:837–844.

7 Hewitt HB, Blake ER, Walder AS. A critique of the evidence for active host defence against cancer, based on personal studies of 27 murine tumours of spontaneous origin. *Br J Cancer*. 1976;**33**:241–259.

8 Singh M, Lima A, Molina R, et al. Assessing therapeutic responses in Kras mutant cancers using genetically engineered mouse models. *Nat Biotechnol*. 2010;**28**:585–593.

9 Ocana A, Tannock IF. When are "positive" clinical trials in oncology truly positive? *J Natl Cancer Inst*. 2011;**103**:16–20.

10 Munoz R, Man S, Shaked Y, et al. Highly efficacious non-toxic treatment for advanced metastatic breast cancer using combination UFT-cyclophosphamide metronomic chemotherapy. *Cancer Res*. 2006;**66**:3386–3391.

11 Fidler IJ. Selection of successive cell lines for metastasis. *Nat New Biol*. 1973;**242**:148–149.

12 Kubota T. Metastatic models of human cancer xenografted in the nude mouse: the importance of orthotopic transplantation. *J Cell Biochem*. 1994;**56**:4–8.

13 Morikawa K, Walker SM, Jessup JM, Fidler IJ. In vivo selection of highly metastatic cells from surgical specimens of different primary human colon carcinomas implanted into nude mice. *Cancer Res*. 1988;**48**:1943–1948.

14 Ebos JML, Lee CR, Cruz-Munoz W, Bjarnason GA, Christensen JG, Kerbel RS. Accelerated metastasis after short-term treatment with a potent inhibitor of tumor angiogenesis. *Cancer Cell*. 2009;**15**:232–239.

15 Francia G, Emmenegger U, Lee CR, et al. Long term progression and therapeutic response of visceral metastatic disease non-invasively monitored in mouse urine using beta-hCG choriogonadotropin secreting tumor cell lines. *Mol Cancer Ther*. 2008;**7**:3452–3459.

16 Cruz-Munoz W, Man S, Xu P, Kerbel RS. Development of a preclinical model of spontaneous human melanoma CNS metastasis. *Cancer Res*. 2008;**68**:4500–4505.

17 Jedeszko C, Paez-Ribes M, Di Desidero T, et al. Orthotopic primary and post-surgical adjuvant or metastatic renal cell carcinoma therapy models reveal potent anti-tumor activity of minimally toxic metronomic oral topotecan with pazopanib. *Sci Transl Med*. 2015;**7**:282ra50.

18 Hackl C, Man S, Francia G, Milsom C, Xu P, Kerbel RS. Metronomic oral topotecan prolongs survival and reduces liver metastasis in improved preclinical orthotopic and adjuvant therapy colon cancer models. *Gut*. 2013;**62**:259–271.

19 Hashimoto K, Man S, Xu P, et al. Potent preclinical impact of metronomic low-dose oral topotecan combined with the antiangiogenic drug pazopanib for the treatment of ovarian cancer. *Mol Cancer Ther*. 2010;**9**:996–1006.

20 Tang TC, Man S, Lee CR, Xu P, Kerbel RS. Impact of UFT/cyclophosphamide metronomic chemotherapy and antiangiogenic drug assessed in a new preclinical model of locally advanced orthotopic hepatocellular carcinoma. *Neoplasia*. 2010;**12**:264–274.

21 Kerbel RS. A decade of experience in developing preclinical models of advanced or early stage spontaneous metastasis to study antiangiogenic drugs, metronomic chemotherapy and the tumor microenvironment. *Cancer Journal*. 2015;**21**:274–283.

22 Gori B, Ricciardi S, Fulvi A, Del Signore E, de Marinis F. New oral multitargeted antiangiogenics in non-small-cell lung cancer treatment. *Future Oncol*. 2012;**8**:559–573.

23 Mackey JR, Kerbel RS, Gelmon KA, et al. Controlling angiogenesis in breast cancer: a systematic review of anti-angiogenic trials. *Cancer Treat Rev*. 2012;**38**:673–688.

24 Guerin E, Man S, Xu P, Kerbel RS. A model of postsurgical advanced metastatic breast cancer more accurately replicates the clinical efficacy of antiangiogenic drugs. *Cancer Res*. 2013;**73**:2743–2748.

25 Abrams TJ, Murray LJ, Pesenti E, et al. Preclinical evaluation of the tyrosine kinase inhibitor SU11248 as a single agent and in combination with "standard of care" therapeutic agents for the treatment of breast cancer. *Mol Cancer Ther*. 2003;**2**:1011–1021.

26 Lin NU, Winer EP. Brain metastases: the HER2 paradigm. *Clin Cancer Res*. 2007;**13**:1648–1655.

27 Cruz-Munoz W, Jaramillo ML, Man S, et al. Roles for endothelin receptor B and BCL2A1 in spontaneous CNS metastasis of melanoma. *Cancer Res*. 2012;**72**:4909–4919.

28 Kim SW, Choi HJ, Lee HJ, et al. Role of the endothelin axis in astrocyte- and endothelial cell-mediated chemoprotection of cancer cells. *Neuro Oncol*. 2014;**16**:1585–1598.

29 Cameron D, Brown J, Dent R, et al. Adjuvant bevacizumab-containing therapy in triple-negative breast cancer (BEATRICE): primary results of a randomised, phase 3 trial. *Lancet Oncol*. 2013;**14**:933–942.

30 de Gramont A, Van Cutsem E, Schmoll HJ, et al. Bevacizumab plus oxaliplatin-based chemotherapy as adjuvant treatment for colon cancer (AVANT): a phase 3 randomised controlled trial. *Lancet Oncol*. 2012;**13**:1225–1233.

31 Simkens LHJ, van Tinteren H, May A, et al. Maintenance treatment with capecitabine and bevacizumab in metastatic colorectal cancer, the phase 3 CAIRO3 study of the Dutch Colorectal Cancer Group (DCCG). *Lancet*. 2015 [Epub head of print].

32 Kerbel RS, Grothey A. Gastrointestinal cancer: Rationale for metronomic chemotherapy in phase III trials. *Nat Rev Clin Oncol*. 2015;**12**:313–314.

33 Tentler JJ, Tan AC, Weekes CD, et al. Patient-derived tumour xenografts as models for oncology drug development. *Nat Rev Clin Oncol*. 2012;**9**:338–350.

34 Bankert RB, Balu-Iyer SV, Odunsi K, et al. Humanized mouse model of ovarian cancer recapitulates patient solid tumor progression, ascites formation, and metastasis. *PLoS ONE*. 2011;**6**:e24420.

35 DeRose YS, Wang G, Lin YC, et al. Tumor grafts derived from women with breast cancer authentically reflect tumor pathology, growth, metastasis and disease outcomes. *Nat Med*. 2011;**17**:1514–1520.

36 Paez-Ribes M, Man S, Xu P, et al. Development of patient derived Xenograft models of overt spontaneous breast cancer metastasis: a cautionary note. *PLoS One*. 2016;**11**:e0158034.

37 Ebos JML, Kerbel RS. Impact of antiangiogenic therapy on invasion, disease progression, and metastasis. *Nat Rev Clin Oncol*. 2011;**8**:210–221.

38 Ebos JM, Mastri M, Lee CR, et al. Neoadjuvant antiangiogenic therapy reveals contrasts in primary and metastatic tumor efficacy. *EMBO Mol Med*. 2014;**6**:1561–1576.

39 Doornebal CW, Klarenbeek S, Braumuller TM, et al. A preclinical mouse model of invasive lobular breast cancer metastasis. *Cancer Res*. 2013;**73**:353–363.

40 Rampetsreiter P, Casanova E, Eferi R. Genetically modified mouse models of cancer invasion and metastasis. *Drug Discov Today Dis Models*. 2011;**9**:67–74.

41 Saxena M, Christofori G. Rebuilding cancer metastasis in the mouse. *Mol Oncol*. 2013;**7**:283–296.

42 Cho H, Herzka T, Zheng W, et al. RapidCaP, a novel GEM model for metastatic prostate cancer analysis and therapy, reveals myc as a driver of Pten-mutant metastasis. *Cancer Discov*. 2014;**4**:318–333.

第17章 肿瘤血管新生

John V. Heymach, MD, PhD ■ Amado Zurita-Saavedra, MD ■ Scott Kopetz, MD, PhD ■ Tina Cascone, MD, PhD ■ Monique Nilsson, PhD

概述

血管新生是指新毛细血管的生长过程，是肿瘤生长和转移的核心，也是肿瘤治疗的潜在靶点。目前，抗血管新生药物已成为许多实体肿瘤标准治疗方案的一部分，在某些癌症（如肾细胞癌和结肠直肠癌）中，抗血管新生治疗已取得了显著的成功，而在其他肿瘤中的疗效则较弱，甚至没有疗效。本章将重点阐述人类癌症内在的生物学行为——肿瘤血管新生的基本原理，并总结目前血管新生抑制剂相关的临床试验和临床应用中的经验教训。

肿瘤血管新生

血管新生，即新毛细血管的生长过程，是肿瘤生长和转移扩散的核心。四十多年前，血管新生被认为是肿瘤治疗的潜在靶点[1]。自此之后，血管新生研究领域经历了爆炸式的发展，已经从理论研究进入以血管新生为治疗靶点的临床验证阶段，现在抗血管新生治疗已是常规的临床治疗方案。贝伐单抗（Bevacizumab）是一种靶向血管内皮生长因子（vascular endothelial growth factor，VEGF）的单克隆抗体，它通过了目前最严格的临床验证，并成为治疗结直肠癌、肺癌、肾细胞癌和其他恶性肿瘤的标准药物。其他几种抗血管新生药物也已成为某些肿瘤的常规治疗用药，包括靶向VEGF受体-2的抗体雷莫芦单抗（ramucirumab）、靶向VEGF和胎盘生长因子（placental-growth factor，PlGF）的蛋白阿柏西普（aflibercept），还有一些靶向血管新生通路的酪氨酸激酶抑制剂包括舒尼替尼（sunitinib）、帕唑帕尼（pazopanib）、索拉菲尼（sorafenib）、凡德他尼（vandetanib）和阿昔替尼（axitinib）。

虽然该领域已经取得了令人鼓舞的进展，但迄今为止，抗血管新生药物的临床疗效仍不尽人意，许多关键问题仍未得到解答：抗血管新生治疗应如何与其他治疗方案和治疗方式相结合？抗血管新生治疗适用于什么类型的肿瘤？适用于哪个阶段？是否可以研发标志物来筛选最有可能从治疗中获益、或可能对治疗产生严重不良反应的患者？基础研究人员和临床医生解决这些问题的能力一定程度上决定了肿瘤抗血管新生治疗的最终疗效。

因此，对临床医生而言，在肿瘤的诊断和治疗中，了解肿瘤血管新生的细胞和分子基础有重要的意义。本章将重点阐述人类癌症内在的生物学行为——肿瘤血管新生的基本原则，并总结目前血管新生抑制剂相关的临床试验和临床应用中的经验教训。

靶向肿瘤血管的理论基础

近年来，我们对正常细胞向癌细胞转化的分子和遗传事件的理解有了的巨大的进步，对此本书的许多章节都有提及。意料之中的是，在这类研究中出现的大多数治疗方法也都是针对癌细胞的。这些疗法确实取得了一些令人瞩目的成绩，例如在慢性粒细胞白血病中靶向癌基因BCR-ABL或在胃肠道间质肿瘤中靶向突变的c-KIT的疗法。在这些成功的例子中，细胞的存活和其他关键细胞过程似乎都高度依赖于某个单一信号通路的活化。对于绝大多数实体肿瘤，靶向癌细胞中的单一分子通路，其疗效相对来说非常有限。在本章中总结的实验和临床证据表明，作为靶点，癌细胞和微血管内皮细胞并不相互排斥，因此开发靶向微血管内皮细胞的疗法也是一种明智的选择。

肿瘤细胞通过一系列的基因突变，导致了某些特定致癌基因的活化以及抑癌基因的丢失，使肿瘤细胞获得能够自给自足的生长信号，并对抑制生长的信号不敏感、对凋亡信号无应答，最终获得无限复制的潜能并具备成瘤性[2]。目前的证据表明，肿瘤的这些特性可能是必要的，但不足以支撑肿瘤细胞扩增为一个有症状、临床上能够检测到的、具有转移性和致死性的细胞群体。肿瘤要具备转移性和/或致死性的表型，必须首先招募血管并能够维持自身的血供，这一过程即肿瘤血管新生[2]。

肿瘤至少可通过四种机制招募血管：①挟持（co-option）现有血管；②从现有血管中萌发新血管（即血管新生，angiogenesis）；③从头产生新血管，通常通过成体骨髓来源的细胞来产生（即血管发生，vasculogenesis）；④血管套叠，将间质组织柱插入先前已有的血管腔内[3]。

非血管新生性肿瘤是无害的

在肿瘤发展的早期，肿瘤还不能募集新的微血管内皮细胞，也不能诱导血管新生。因此，在这个阶段，大多数人类肿瘤以微小的体积停留在原位并处于休眠状态，对宿主是无害的[4]。

非致病性癌症：患有非血管新生性休眠肿瘤的患者生存期更长

人类的非血管新生性肿瘤在直径约为1mm或更小时便停止了扩增。100多年来，病理学家通过对意外死亡的人进行尸检发现，在特定年龄阶段的人群中，大量的个体患有原位肿瘤，而终其一生，只有很少一部分人被诊断出患有癌症[5]。例如，在40~50岁死于创伤的女性中，39%的人的乳房中发现有原位肿瘤，但只有1%的人被诊断出患有癌症。在60~70岁死于创伤的男性中，46%的人被发现患有前列腺原位癌，但只有15%的人被明确诊断出患有癌症。抑制原位肿瘤发展的一种机制可能是宿主源性因子阻止了肿瘤向血管新生表型的转换。生理水平的内源性血管新生抑制因子(详见后续内容)可能在这一过程中发挥了重要作用[6]。

肿瘤组织的扩增是癌症产生致病性的必要条件

肿瘤组织的扩增超出了非血管新生性肿瘤的初始显微尺寸,从而导致了癌症的致病性,该过程通常依赖于肿瘤对内皮细胞的募集作用。当肿瘤细胞向血管新生表型转变时,其对内皮细胞的募集就开始了[7~9]。肿瘤细胞获得血管新生表型需要经历一系列的改变,可能包括:①肿瘤细胞的血管新生蛋白表达增加,如 VEGF、碱性成纤维细胞生长因子(basic fibroblast growth factor,bFGF)等;②间质细胞的血管新生蛋白表达增加(如间质成纤维细胞),这一过程是由肿瘤自身诱导的;③内源性的血管新生抑制因子(如肿瘤和间质成纤维细胞分泌的血小板反应蛋白-1(thrombospondin-1,TSP-1)表达的减少;④招募骨髓来源的内皮前体细胞(血管新生表型转换的阐述详见下文)。同时,随着研究的不断深入,其他的机制也将会被逐渐揭示。肿瘤缺乏血管新生可以阻止其体积扩大,从而避免了肿瘤的转移扩散和肿瘤相关症状的出现,即"非致病性癌症"[6]。这个概念对于肿瘤治疗意义重大。阻断血管新生不仅可以减缓临床上有明显症状肿瘤的生长,还可以防止微小病灶演变为临床上有明显症状的肿瘤。

正常组织和器官的扩增也需要募集微血管内皮细胞,例如在肝部分切除手术后[10]。事实上,血管新生是生殖、发育和修复的基础,但生理性血管新生以短暂的毛细血管生长为主,通常只持续数天(排卵血管新生)、数周(伤口愈合血管新生)或数月(胎儿和胎盘血管新生),之后毛细血管生长便会在一个相对固定的时间段内自动减弱[11,12]。血管新生的生理作用也有助于解释血管新生抑制剂临床应用时所产生的一些毒副反应。

历史背景

100 多年前,在手术过程中医生观察到相比于正常组织,肿瘤的血管更多[13]。这一现象被认为是源于宿主现有血管的简单舒张反应[14]。血管舒张被认为是代谢产物或肿瘤坏死产物从肿瘤中逃逸时产生的副作用。后续有三篇报告提出肿瘤充血可能与新血管形成有关,而不仅仅是血管舒张反应引起的,但这些观点在当时并没有引起重视[15,16]。虽然如此,学界关于肿瘤是否可以仅仅依靠现存的血管系统就能扩增到厘米级大小的争论又持续了 20 多年[17]。即使是少数接受肿瘤能够诱导血管新生这一观点的研究者,也普遍认为这只是一种炎症反应,是肿瘤生长的副作用,而不是肿瘤生长的必要条件[18]。现在人们已经认识到,炎症反应和肿瘤血管新生通常是相互联系的,炎症细胞的募集在启动和促进肿瘤血管新生中起着关键作用。

血管新生研究的开始

假说:肿瘤的生长依赖于血管新生

1971 年,Folkman 提出了肿瘤生长依赖于血管新生的新假说[1]。该假说认为肿瘤细胞和肿瘤内的血管内皮细胞可能构成高度整合的生态系统,通过肿瘤细胞发出的"扩散性的"化学信号,内皮细胞可能从静止状态转变为快速生长阶段。另一种推测是血管新生可能是肿瘤治疗的一个靶点(如抗血管新生疗法)。这些想法是基于 Folkman 和 Frederick Becker 在 20 世纪 60 年代早期进行的实验,该实验揭示了在没有肿瘤血管新生的情况下,肿瘤在离体灌注器官中的生长受到严重限制(图 17-1)[19~23]。

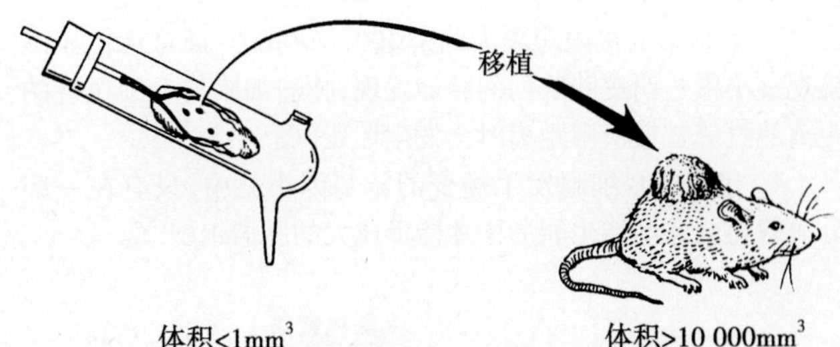

图 17-1 在离体灌注器官内,肿瘤的生长停留在无血管期[20]。整个器官由灌注支持,允许肿瘤从宿主中分离后,可以在由灌注支持的器官内生长。在无血管的环境中,肿瘤的体积小于 1mm^3,而在小鼠体内肿瘤体积可超过 10 000mm^3

这些概念在当时并没有被广泛接受。研究肿瘤血管新生的另一个障碍是当时的传统观念,即任何由肿瘤诱导产生的新血管,会像伤口中的新血管一样,一旦形成后就不能退化了。根据这一假设,科学家们得出结论,抗血管新生疗法永远无法使肿瘤消退,因此,研究血管新生抑制剂将是徒劳的。直到科学家能够可再生性地对血管内皮细胞进行培养,发现了内源性的血管新生蛋白质,并鉴定了能在体内外抑制血管新生的药物,人们才最终广泛接受 Folkman 在 1971 年提出的假说,血管新生才成为一个新的研究领域[24~28]。

整个 20 世纪 70 年代,实验室都致力于研究并证明肿瘤血管是新增殖的毛细血管;血管新生过程的具体步骤是可以被鉴定的;可以建立针对血管新生的定性和定量生物测定方法;辐射抑制肿瘤细胞增殖后,有活力的肿瘤细胞仍可释放可扩散的、能在体内刺激新毛细血管生长和内皮细胞有丝分裂的血管新生因子;坏死肿瘤的产物自身不能促进血管新生;血管新生可以被抑制[29~32]。迄今本领域已经扩展为涉及包括从发育生物学到分子遗传学的广泛的基础科学学科,以及各种临床专业,包括肿瘤学、心脏病学、皮肤病学、妇科学、眼科学和风湿病学。

实验证据

到 20 世纪 80 年代中期,已经有大量的实验证据支持肿瘤生长依赖于血管新生的假说,它可以简单地表述为:"肿瘤一旦发生,肿瘤细胞群每一次扩增前,聚集在肿瘤中的新毛细血管的数量都必然先增多[33]。"该假说的前提是如果血管新生能被完全抑制,肿瘤就会在一个很小,甚至可能是显微级别大小的状态下保持休眠状态[22]。该假说推测新血管的形成虽然是肿瘤扩增的必要不充分条件,但缺乏新血管形成仍会使体积超过 1~2mm^3 的原发肿瘤的扩增受到抑制,并将转移灶限制在显微水平的休眠病变状态(图 17-1)。

大量临床前证据同样支持肿瘤依赖血管新生的假说[34],包括药理学和遗传学的研究,以及后续章节中讨论的临床研究。支持血管新生假说的一些发现包括:

1. 皮下荷瘤在血管形成前生长缓慢，肿瘤体积呈线性增长。血管形成后，肿瘤生长迅速，肿瘤体积呈指数增长[35,36]。

2. 生长在兔眼玻璃体内的肿瘤仍然存活，但在长达 100 天的时间内，其直径限制在 0.50mm 以下。一旦这样的肿瘤到达视网膜表面，它就会产生新的血管，其体积在 2 周内可以达到无血管肿瘤的 19 000 倍[37]。

3. 氧扩散的极限距离大约是 100~200μm。通过活体显微镜观察小鼠透明皮肤腔内的肿瘤发现，肿瘤细胞与毛细血管的距离超过氧扩散极限距离时会发生坏死（图 17-2）[38]。

4. 在胰岛 β 细胞发生癌变的转基因小鼠中，只有在一部分血管化的癌前增生胰岛中才能形成大的肿瘤组织[8]。

5. 致癌物诱导大鼠自发结肠癌的过程中，存在一个早期阶段（肿瘤直径<3.5mm），在此期间，肿瘤暂时由已经存在的宿主微血管扩张后供应能量[39]。该阶段类似于血管挟持（co-option）[40]。随后，新的毛细血管萌发和增殖（血管新生），导致微血管密度增加、肿瘤快速生长。

6. 在仅由 VEGF 诱导血管新生的小鼠中给予 VEGF 中和抗体后[41]，小鼠所荷肿瘤的生长抑制率达 90%以上。而该抗体对体外培养的肿瘤细胞没有影响[42]。通过其他方法阻断 VEGF，包括根据 VEGF 受体设计的融合蛋白（VEGF trap）可以达到同样的效果[43]。此外，使用抗体中和另一种血管新生因子 bFGF 也可以得到类似的结果[44]。

人黑色素瘤

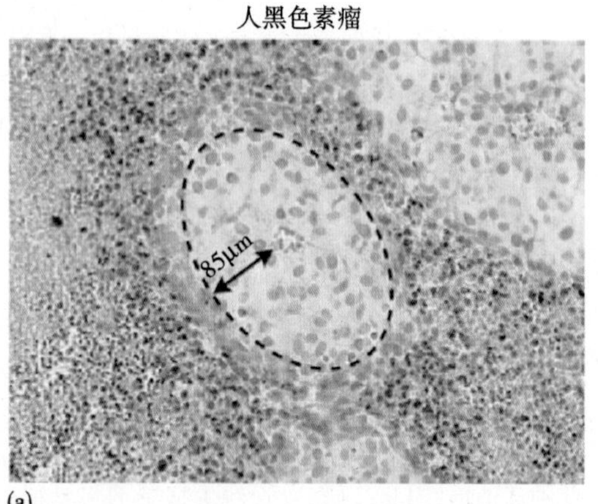

(a)

大鼠前列腺癌

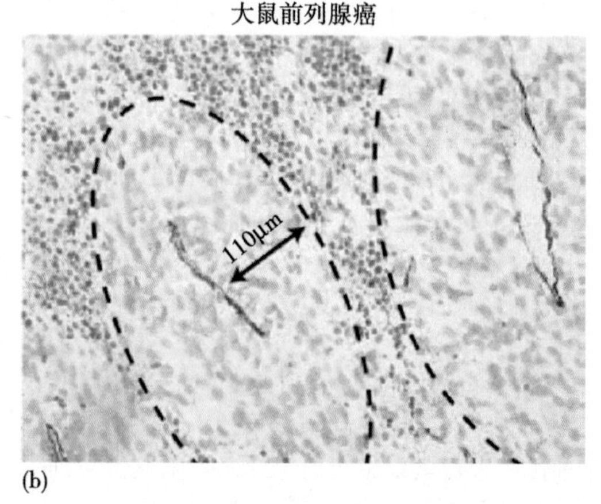

(b)

图 17-2 （a）在种植于 SCID 小鼠的人黑色素瘤组织中，肿瘤细胞生长在微血管周围平均半径约为 85μm 的圆形区域内。椭圆结构是由切割方式所致。（b）大鼠前列腺癌细胞生长在微血管周围平均半径约为 110μm 的圆形区域内

肿瘤血管新生生物学

血管新生在癌前病变和早期肿瘤发生中的作用

四十多年前，Folkman 和他的同事用离体灌注器官进行实验时发现，由于缺乏血管新生，肿瘤的生长受到了严重的限制[20,45]。这项研究和其他研究都提出实体肿瘤的生长依赖于新的毛细血管芽（即血管新生），没有血管新生的实体肿瘤可能会进入完全休眠状态[1]。该理论的提出，表明血管新生不仅可以作为晚期肿瘤的潜在治疗靶点，还可以作为化学药物预防的靶点。近年来，越来越多的临床前和临床研究证实了血管新生确实是晚期肿瘤的治疗靶点。尽管临床前研究对这一理念提供了强有力的支持，但针对阻断癌症早期发展的血管新生抑制剂（化学药物预防）的研究仍然是滞后的[46,47]。

临床前研究揭示了血管新生在早期肿瘤发生中的作用

在 20 世纪 70 年代，Gullino[48]研究发现癌前组织表现出早期血管新生的迹象，并提出阻断这一过程可以用于预防癌症。后来，Hanahan 和他的同事利用转基因小鼠肿瘤发生模型，证明一些癌前病变在早期的癌变中经历了“血管新生转换（angiogenic switch）”的过程，这一过程表明血管新生刺激因子和抑制因子之间的平衡发生了变化[8,9]。研究发现，在这些模型中，VEGF 和基质金属蛋白酶-9（matrix metalloproteinase-9，MMP-9）在血管新生转换中发挥了重要的作用[49~51]。在小鼠胰岛细胞癌模型中，四种不同的抗血管新生药物（TNP-470、内皮抑制素、血管抑素、MMP 抑制剂 BB-94）在预防肿瘤形成（化学药物预防）、迟滞小肿瘤生长（早期干预）以及使已形成的肿瘤消退方面展现出截然不同的活性[8,52,53]。在另一项研究中，将乳腺癌细胞（例如体外转化而来的肿瘤细胞，非原发肿瘤细胞）植入大鼠背部皮肤窗室中，发现在肿瘤组织生长到非新生血管化肿瘤的极限大小（0.2~2mm）之前，肿瘤的血管新生就早已开始了。这些研究和其他临床前研究表明，血管新生是肿瘤发生早期的、关键的步骤，抗血管新生药物可能会抑制肿瘤的进展和生长。

在人肿瘤中癌前病变与血管新生增加有关

来自人临床标本的研究也支持血管新生发生在肿瘤进展早期的假设，尤其在癌前阶段。在宫颈癌中，在早期不典型增生［宫颈上皮内瘤变，cervical intraepithelial neoplasia，CIN Ⅰ］阶段就发现血管密度出现轻微增加。宫颈上皮内瘤变中晚期异常增生（CIN Ⅱ~Ⅲ）阶段表现出明显的血管新生转换，新生血管沿着异常增生上皮下的基底膜密集排列[54,55]。肺癌患者和高危人群的肺活检显示，增生、化生、原位癌等这些癌前病变都与病变周围黏膜的微血管密度增加有关[56~58]。同时，还发现

了一种被称为血管新生性鳞状细胞增生异常[57]的独特血管新生模式。在支气管癌前病变中虽尚未发现特异性的血管新生刺激因子,但可以观察到 VEGF[56]、表皮生长因子受体(epidermal growth factor receptor,EGFR)[59]和 COX-2[60]的水平升高。

血管新生在癌症转移扩散中的作用

血管新生除了能促进小的癌前或恶性病变生长外,还能促进肿瘤的血源性转移扩散。这种扩散可能是由于肿瘤中的"马赛克(mosaic)"血管的作用。在马赛克血管中内皮细胞和肿瘤细胞一起形成血管腔表面,从而促进肿瘤细胞脱落进入循环。有研究发现,在结肠癌移植模型中,约 15%的血管是马赛克血管,其中肿瘤细胞似乎直接接触管腔血管表面,而没有内皮细胞作为屏障[61]。在人肿瘤活检中也检测到类似数目的马赛克血管。这些结果提示肿瘤血管的不规则结构和功能可能促进了肿瘤细胞脱落进入循环并发生转移扩散。

微小转移灶也依赖于血管新生,以便进展为临床症状明显的肿瘤。微小转移灶可能在较远的部位长期休眠,但当其中一小部分获得足够的血液供应时,肿瘤就可以进行扩增;血管新生抑制剂可以在多种小鼠模型中抑制这一过程[62~67]。原发性肿瘤和转移瘤的持续生长依赖于足够的血液供应。因此,从理论上来说,血管新生抑制剂在化学药物预防、在早期及隐匿性转移癌或晚期肿瘤的治疗中都可能有一定的疗效[46,68,69]。

综上所述,这些临床前和临床研究表明,诱导血管新生是肿瘤进展早期的、重要的步骤,不仅参与了癌前病变,还参与了肿瘤的转移扩散。因此,血管新生是化学药物预防一个可靠的靶标。目前仍需要进一步研究阐明早期血管新生的关键调控因子,并研发不同类型的抗血管新生药物,以满足化学药物预防、晚期肿瘤治疗等不同应用场景的需求。

血管新生的调控因子

促进肿瘤血管新生的可扩散因子的发现

20 世纪 70 年代的一项研究发现,肿瘤植入无血管性角膜或带血管蒂的鸡绒毛膜可诱导新毛细血管的生长,表明肿瘤释放了可扩散的血管新生因子[9]。该结果推动了体内外生物检测技术的发展,促进了肿瘤血管新生因子的研究[70]。

成纤维细胞生长因子

bFGF(或 FGF-2)是第一个从肿瘤中分离纯化的血管新生蛋白(1982 年),之后又发现了酸性 FGF(aFGF 或 FGF-1)[28,71,72]。酸性和 bFGF 可以在体外刺激内皮细胞有丝分裂和迁移,是体内最有效的血管新生蛋白之一。它们对肝素和硫酸肝素有很高的亲和性[73]。bFGF 受体的表达水平非常低。多种类型的肿瘤均可分泌 bFGF,包括中枢神经系统肿瘤、肉瘤、泌尿生殖系统肿瘤,甚至肿瘤血管系统中的内皮细胞。鉴定肿瘤分泌到细胞外基质中 FGF 的结合蛋白,可以阐明肿瘤细胞动员其储存的 FGF 的机制[74~76]。此外,一些肿瘤能够募集巨噬细胞[77]并激活它们分泌 bFGF[78],而另一些肿瘤通过募集肥大细胞,利用肥大细胞含有的大量肝素来俘获 bFGF。在自发性肿瘤的转基因小鼠中,在肿瘤进展的早期阶段,aFGF 和 bFGF 是由具有促血管新生特性的肿瘤细胞分泌进入条件培养基的,而不是由血管新生前体细胞分泌的[38,79]。bFGF 还能够干扰白细胞与内皮细胞的黏附作用,有研究表明,分泌 bFGF 的肿瘤可能产生局部免疫耐受[80~82]。在小鼠肿瘤模型中,抑制 FGFR 信号通路导致肿瘤血管新生受阻、肿瘤生长缓慢[83]。

在癌症患者的血清和尿液中,以及不同类型的脑肿瘤患者的脑脊液中,bFGF 水平出现异常的升高[84,85]。肾癌中高水平的 bFGF 与患者预后不良密切相关[86]。此外,Wilms 肿瘤患儿尿液中 bFGF 水平与疾病分期和肿瘤分级有关[87]。

除促进肿瘤血管新生外,在各种肿瘤中还发现了多种 FGFR 融合蛋白,包括肺鳞状细胞癌、膀胱癌、胶质母细胞瘤和甲状腺癌;由于抑制 FGFR 能够阻碍 FGFR 融合蛋白阳性肿瘤模型的生长,因此 FGFR 融合蛋白可能是一种致癌驱动因子[88]。还有报道显示,一部分小细胞肺癌中存在 FGFR1 扩增,携带 FGFR 扩增的肿瘤细胞对 FGFR 靶向抑制敏感[89]。在这些情况下,抑制 FGFR 将产生直接的抗肿瘤细胞效应以及通过靶向肿瘤血管系统产生的间接抗肿瘤效应。

血管内皮生长因子家族

Dvorak 首次提出肿瘤血管新生与微血管通透性增加有关[90]。这导致了血管通透性因子(vascular permeability factor,VPF)的发现[91~93]。随后 Ferrara 和他的同事对 VPF 进行了测序并在 1989 年提出 VPF 是一种血管新生特异性诱导剂,并将其命名为血管内皮生长因子(VEGF)[92~94]。与此同时,Folkman 实验室从一种肿瘤(sarcoma 180)中分离纯化出一种新的血管新生蛋白,并与 Ferrara 合作表明其为 VEGF[94]。迄今为止已发现了 40 多种血管新生诱导物,其中大多数为肿瘤产物(表 17-1)[3,95]。VEGF 是一种内皮细胞有丝分裂原和运动原,具有在体内促进血管新生的作用[96~98]。其表达与胚胎发生中血管的生长有关,对胚胎血管系统的发育起着至关重要的作用[99,100]。在女性生殖系统和肿瘤中,VEGF 表达也与血管新生相关[49,101~103]。VEGF 是一种 40~45kDa 的同源二聚体蛋白,并带有一个信号序列,可由多种细胞和大多数肿瘤细胞分泌。VEGF 有五种亚型,分别含有 121、145、165、189 和 206 个氨基酸,其中 $VEGF_{165}$ 是多种正常细胞和肿瘤细胞产生的主要分子亚型。在血管内皮细胞上主要存在 VEGF 的两种受体,即 180kDa 的 fms 样酪氨酸激酶(fms-like tyrosine kinase,Flt-1)[104]和 200kDa 的人激酶插入结构域受体(human kinase insert domain-containing receptor,KDR)及其小鼠同源蛋白 Flk-1[105]。VEGF 与两种受体都可结合,但 KDR/Flk-1 二聚体转导的是内皮细胞增殖和趋化的信号[106~109]。VEGF 家族的其他结构同源物包括 VEGF-B、VEGF-C、VEGF-D 和 VEGF-E[110,111]。VEGF-C 和 VEGF-D 与主要表达在淋巴管内皮细胞的 Flt-4 结合[112,113]。

Klagsbrun 等人发现,神经引导分子 neuropilin-1 是 $VEGF_{165}$ 而非 VEGF 的共受体[114,115]。这一发现为血管系统与神经系统的协调生长提供了一个分子介质。其他神经引导蛋白和/或其受体也是血管新生调节因子。例如 neuropilin 是 VEGF 和信号素的受体。信号素抑制神经轴突的生长,同时也是一种血管新生抑制剂。Ephrins 是一种神经引导分子,也是胚胎发生过程中决定动脉和静脉发育的遗传因子。肿瘤血管内皮细胞表达 EphrinB2。可能由于神经系统和血管系统的调节因子存在重叠，因此脑肿瘤的血管新生具有独特的特征，如与这些肿瘤恶性表型相关的高间质液压（interstitial fluid pressure，IFP）和低氧张力等特性[116]。

表 17-1 血管新生调控因子例举

促进血管新生的分子	抑制血管新生的分子	转录因子、癌基因和其他调控因子
血管内皮生长因子（VEGF）	干扰素-α，β，γ	缺氧诱导因子（HIF）-1α，2α
碱性成纤维细胞生长因子（bFGF）	血小板反应蛋白-1，2	核因子-κB（NF-κB）
转化生长因子-α（TGF-α）	血管生成素 2	表皮生长因子受体（EGFR）
血小板生长因子（PDGF）	基质金属蛋白酶组织抑制因子（TIMP）	Ras
表皮生长因子（EGF）	内皮抑素	p53
血管生成素	血管抑素	von Hippel-Lindau
白介素-6	白介素-12	钙黏蛋白
白介素-8	内皮抑素	整合蛋白
基质金属蛋白酶（MMP）	血小板反应蛋白-1	导向蛋白
肝细胞生长因子（HGF）		Id1，Id2
基质细胞衍生因子-1α（SDF-1α）		脯氨酰羟化酶
Delta 样配体 4（DLL4）		myc
Ephrin 家族		
单核细胞趋化蛋白-1 及其他趋化因子		

Neuropilin 不是酪氨酸激酶受体，包括肿瘤细胞在内的非内皮细胞都可以表达这种受体。因此肿瘤细胞合成的 VEGF 能够结合到表达 Neuropilin 的细胞的表面。表面结合的 VEGF 可使内皮细胞向肿瘤细胞趋化，也可近距离介导肿瘤细胞对微血管的挟持。Neuropilin 还能与胎盘生长因子-2（placenta growth factor-2，PlGF-2）结合，而肝素对于 $VEGF_{165}$ 及 PlGF-2 与 neuropilin-1 的结合至关重要[40,117]。在体内存在的天然细胞表面多糖是硫酸肝素，而不是肝素。硫酸肝素可以促进 VEGF 或 PlGF-2 与 VEGF 的相互作用。肿瘤坏死区周围由于缺氧，肿瘤表达的 VEGF 会增多[118~121]。缺氧能够激活缺氧诱导因子-1（hypoxia-inducible factor-1，HIF-1），HIF-1 可与 VEGF 启动子中的缺氧反应元件（hypoxia response element，HRE）结合，导致 VEGF mRNA 的转录[106,120]。此外，缺氧还可以增强 VEGF mRNA 的稳定性。

VEGF 的信号转导

尽管 VEGF-A 与 VEGFR1 结合的亲和力高于 VEGFR-2，但 VEGF-A 对肿瘤内皮细胞的大部分生物学作用被认为是由 VEGFR-2 介导的。与配体结合后，VEGFR-2 发生二聚化，导致酪氨酸激酶的活化和包括 Tyr951、Tyr996、Tyr1054、Tyr1175、Tyr1214 在内的氨基酸位点发生自磷酸化[122]。这些位点的磷酸化会进一步活化 PI3K、磷脂酶 C-γ（phospholipase C-γ，PLC-γ）、Akt、Src、Ras、MAPK 等下游信号分子（图 17-3）。Tyr1175 位点的磷酸化可介导 VEGFR-2 与 PLC-γ 的结合并导致其磷酸化，进而促进 Ca^{2+} 释放并激活蛋白激酶 C（protein kinase C，PKC）。PKC 的活化和 Ca^{2+} 的动员对 VEGF-A 诱导的细胞增殖和一氧化氮的产生至关重要[123]。

PI3K 通路在细胞增殖、存活和迁移的调控中有重要的作用。VEGF-A 具有促进 PI3K 的 p85 亚基磷酸化和增强 PI3K 酶活性的功能。已有研究发现 Src 激酶、β-catenin、VE-cadherin 参与了 VEGF-A 对 PI3K 的激活过程，但具体机制仍不清楚[124,125]。VEGFR-2 诱导的 PI3K 活化可导致磷脂酰肌醇-3，4，5-三磷酸（phosphatidylinositol-3，4，5-trisphosphate，PIP3）的蓄积，从而引起 Akt/PKB 磷酸化。Akt/PKB 一旦被磷酸化激活，则会抑制促凋亡蛋白 BAD 和 caspase-9 的活性。

Src 家族激酶成员 Src、Fyn 和 Yes 都在内皮细胞中表达。在 VEGFR-2 自磷酸化后，T 细胞特异性接头蛋白（T cell-specifc adapter，TSAd）与 Tyr951 位点结合，然后与 Src 发生相互作用。Src 激酶控制肌动蛋白应激纤维组织，可能介导了 VEGF-A 诱导的 PI3K 活化。配体与 VEGFR-2 结合后也可活化 Ras 通路，进一步通过多种途径激活在细胞增殖中起重要作用的 Raf-1-MEK-ERK 信号通路[122,126]。

VEGF 的生物学功能

最初的研究认为 VEGF 是调节血管通透性的物质[110,127]。使小静脉和微静脉高渗是 VEGF 的一个重要功能。VEGF 确实是血管通透性最有效的调节因子之一，肿瘤相关血管具有高通透性也主要是由肿瘤分泌的 VEGF 造成的。虽然 VEGF 增加微血管通透性的机制尚不完全清楚，但至少部分是由于：VEGF 诱导的内皮细胞开孔[100]、相邻内皮细胞间连接的开放[128]、以及与一氧化氮产生有关的钙依赖途径[129~131]。

除了可以影响血管通透性，VEGF 还可以调控内皮细胞的存活，可以通过激活 PI3K-Akt 通路[132]、促进抗凋亡蛋白 bcl-2 的表达[133]抑制内皮细胞凋亡。体内研究表明，阻断 VEGF 可导致未成熟、无周细胞覆盖血管的凋亡增加[134]。VEGF 是一种内皮细胞有丝分裂原，但内皮细胞的增殖主要还是依赖 VEGFR-2 及其下游的 Erk1/2、JNK/SAPK、PKC 信号通路[133,135]。虽然 VEGF 作为内皮细胞有丝分裂原的活性不如 bFGF 等其他因子，但它在血管新生的关键过程中具有更广泛的活性。VEGF 能够诱导参与基底膜降解的 MMP 和丝氨酸蛋白酶的表达，这是内皮细胞发芽和侵袭的必要条件[133]。此外，VEGF 还可以通过 FAK 和 p38 MAPK 诱导肌动蛋白重组，促进内皮细胞迁移[3,128,133,136]。

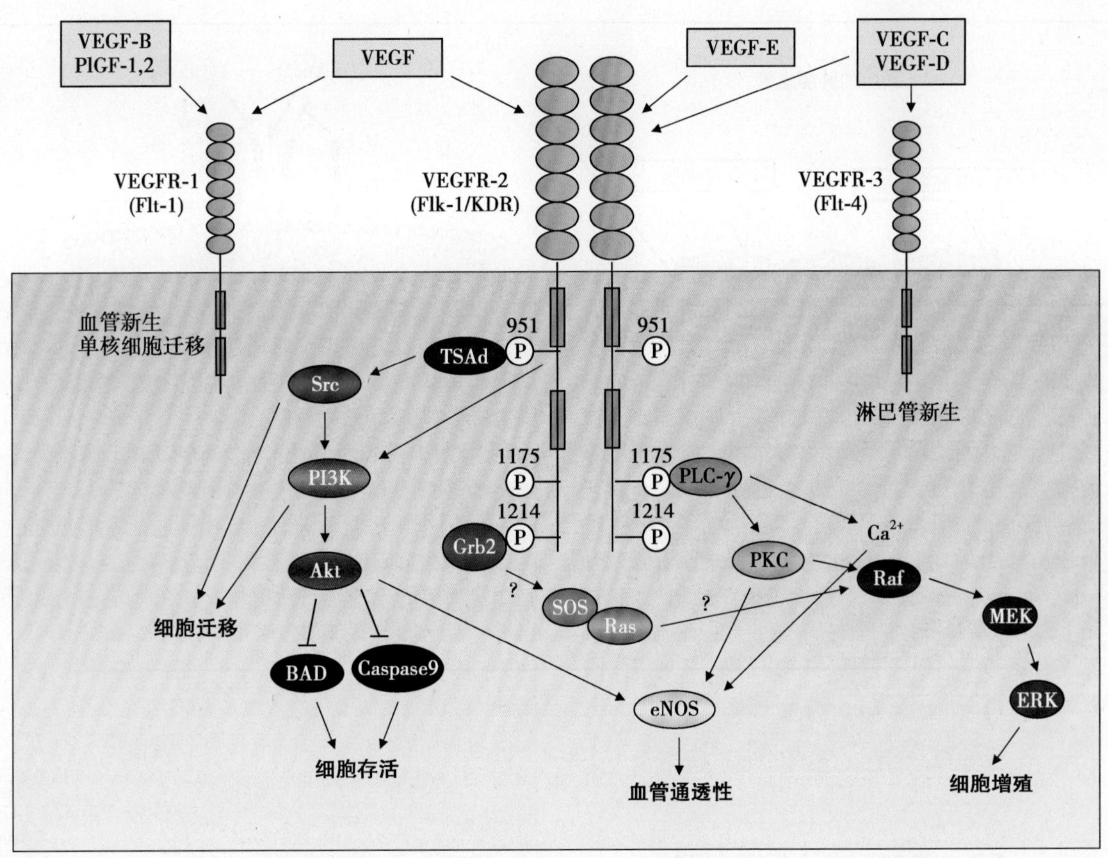

图 17-3 VEGFR 的信号转导。VEGF 家族成员 VEGF、VEGF-B、VEGF-C、VEGF-D、VEGF-E 和 PlGF 可与三种 VEGFR 酪氨酸激酶结合,导致二聚化、受体自磷酸化和下游通路的激活。图中展示了 VEGFR-2 介导的信号通路。配体结合 VEGFR-2 激活信号转导分子 PLC-(γ)、PI3K、Akt、Ras、Src 和 MAPK,调控细胞增殖、迁移、生存和血管通透性

循环 VEGF 可能是肿瘤用来招募骨髓源性细胞的血管新生信号之一,这些骨髓源性细胞包括内皮祖细胞和髓样细胞,这些招募过程被认为分别是由 VEGFR-2 和 VEGFR-1 介导的[137~141]。尽管也存在不依赖 VEGFR-1 的机制,但越来越多的证据表明,表达 VEGFR 的骨髓源性细胞通过创造"转移巢(metastatic niche)"促进肿瘤的形成,并/或促进肿瘤血管新生[142~147]。循环内皮细胞和髓细胞作为潜在的生物标志物正在被进一步研究,如本章后续所述,它们可能参与了肿瘤对 VEGF 通路抑制剂的耐药性[148,149]。值得注意的是,并不是所有的血管内皮生长因子都来源于肿瘤。癌症患者血清 VEGF 的浓度与其血小板计数密切相关。VEGF 储存在血小板中,并由血小板运输和释放[150]。此外,Pinedo 和他的同事发现,血小板计数越高,癌症患者的预后越差[151,152]。因此,对于那些可以招募骨髓源性内皮细胞的肿瘤,肿瘤与骨髓之间的交流通信可能部分是由循环血小板中的 VEGF 介导的。

血管生成素

血管生成素-1(angiopoietin-1,Ang1)是一种大小为 70kDa 的蛋白配体,它可与一种只在内皮细胞上表达的特异的酪氨酸激酶结合,这种激酶被称为 Tie2(也称为 Tek)。Ang1 与内皮细胞上表达的 Tie2 结合,Tie2 随后发生二聚化并磷酸化。活化的 Tie2 能够激活 PI3K 和 Ras/Raf/MEK 通路,促进内皮细胞的存活和增殖/迁移(图 17-4)[153]。Tie1 的配体尚不明确[114,154~157]。与 VEGF 一样,Ang1 是一种内皮细胞特异的生长因子。然而,Ang1 在体外并不是直接的内皮细胞有丝分裂原,而是通过诱导内皮细胞招募周细胞和平滑肌细胞进入血管壁来发挥作用的。当 Tie2 被 Ang1 激活后,内皮细胞产生的 PDGF-BB(可能还有其他因子)引起了周细胞和平滑肌的募集[158]。在过度表达 Ang1 的小鼠皮肤中,血管新生增多[157]。同时,血管明显增大,小鼠皮肤发红。与过度表达 VEGF 的小鼠不同,这类小鼠的血管无渗漏,无皮肤水肿。在皮肤中同时表达 Ang1 和 VEGF 的双转基因小鼠中,表皮血管新生以累加的方式增加,但血管并不出现渗漏[159]。这个模型与伤口愈合时的血管新生非常相似,包括相对无渗漏的血管、血管壁含有周细胞和一些血管周围的平滑肌细胞。与此相反,肿瘤的血管有渗漏,血管壁薄,含有的周细胞少。血管生成素-2(angiopoietin-2,Ang2)是由癌巢内的血管内皮细胞产生的,能够封闭 Tie-2 受体,具有抑制周细胞和平滑肌的作用[154]。尽管肿瘤中的一些微血管达到了小静脉的直径,肿瘤血管仍然是很薄的"单层内皮细胞脉管(endothelium-lined tubes)"。高水平的 Ang2 与黑色素瘤患者的转移有关,在临床前模型中,Ang2 可以促进转移形成[160,161]。值得注意的一点是,血管新生素和 VEGF 在血管新生中是共同发挥作用的,两者的活性都与环境有关;在新生或成熟的血管中,血管新生素和 VEGF 的活性是不同的。由于 VEGF 对 Ang2 的促血管新生活性有很大的影响,因此联合使用靶向 Ang/Tie2 和

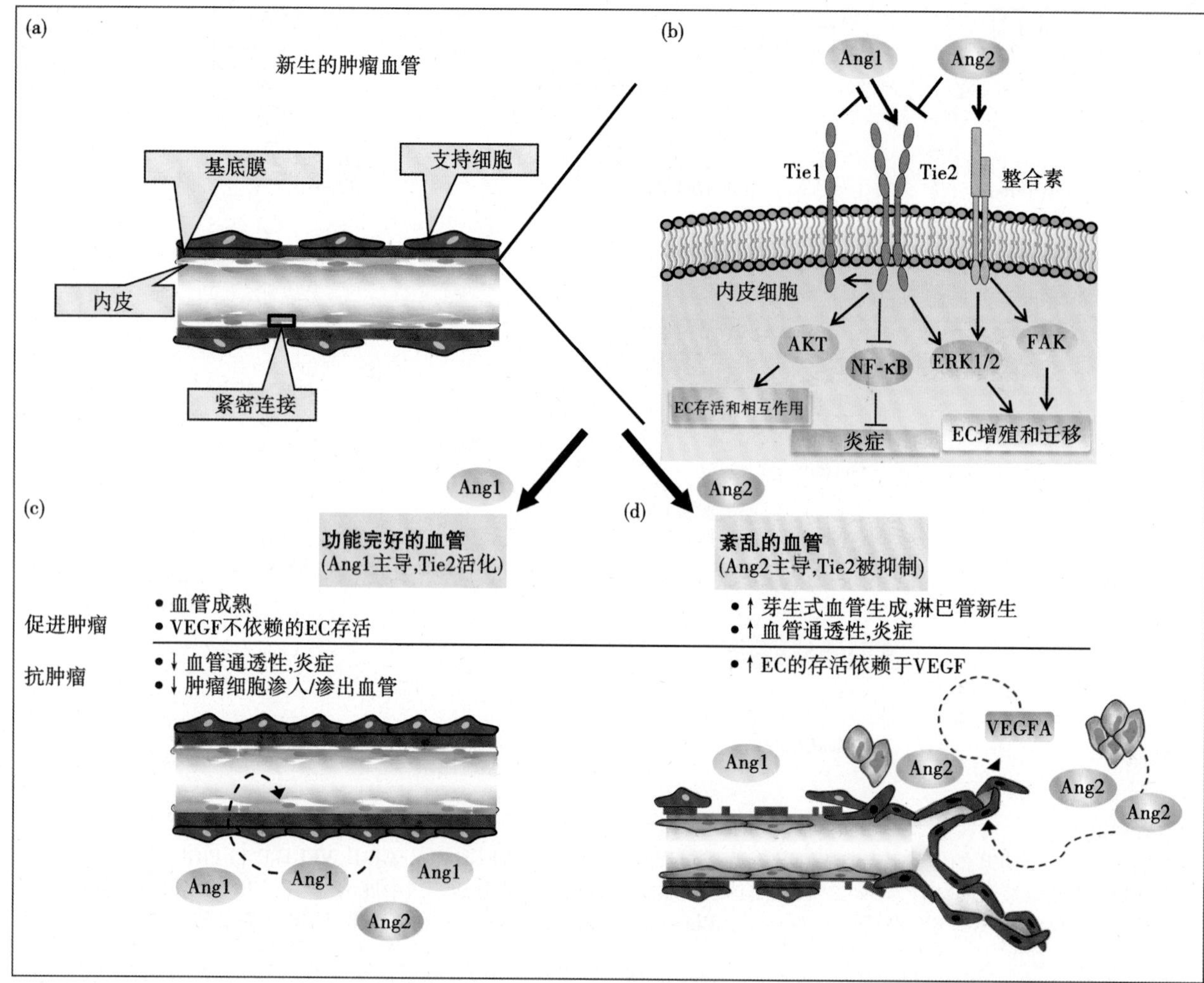

图 17-4 Ang/Tie2 信号通路。(a)静止状态下新生肿瘤血管结构的示意图。内皮细胞(绿色)形成管腔,与周围的血管细胞紧密连接(蓝色),并由基底膜分离。(b)Ang1 与定位于内皮细胞上的 Tie2 结合;Tie2 随后二聚化并磷酸化。活化的 Tie2 激活 PI3K 和 Ras/Raf/MEK 通路,促进内皮细胞的存活和增殖/迁移。一般情况下,Ang2 具有拮抗 Ang1 的作用,诱导血管通透性增加,发生血管化。自磷酸化的 Tie2 激活 Tie1,而 Tie1 的胞外结构域又干扰 Ang1/Tie2 结合,从而拮抗 Ang1 信号。Ang1 具有抗炎作用,而 Ang2 具有促炎作用。Ang1 活化的 Tie2 能够抑制 NF-κB 介导的炎症因子表达,而 Ang2 通过阻断 Ang1 功能促进炎症因子表达。(c)血管周细胞分泌 Ang1,与内皮细胞表达的 Tie2 结合。在这种相互作用中,Ang1 有助于血管的完整性,降低血管通透性,维持血管系统的稳态。(d)Ang2 通过介导周细胞的解离和破坏细胞间连接,在血管生成中发挥重要作用。在其他促血管生成因子(如 VEGF)存在的情况下,内皮细胞增殖和/或迁移形成新血管芽,导致血管生成紊乱。在缺乏促血管生成因子的情况下,Ang2 信号通路导致内皮细胞的凋亡和消退。资料来源:经许可转载自 Cascone 和 Heymach 2012。153© 2012 美国临床肿瘤学会

VEGF 受体通路的抑制剂,可能会有较好的临床治疗效果,目前这种联合的临床试验正在进行。然而,由于血管新生素既有促肿瘤作用,也有抗肿瘤作用,这主要取决于特定的条件和环境,因此目前仍然没有靶向血管新生素的最佳方法[153]。

其他调控血管新生的因子

白细胞介素-8(Interleukin-8,IL-8)是由单核细胞、巨噬细胞和肿瘤细胞产生的促炎趋化因子[162]。IL-8 诱导内皮细胞的增殖和趋化,也促进内皮细胞存活[162,163]。IL-8 与细胞表面的 G 蛋白偶联受体 CXCR1 和 CXCR2 相互作用,激活包括 PI3K 和 MAPK 在内的下游信号分子[164]。肝细胞生长因子/扩散因子(hepatocyte growth factor/scatter factor,HGF/SF)是 c-Met 的配体[165]。HGF 最初被认为是用于原代肝细胞培养的有丝分裂原,后来被证实可以促进肿瘤血管新生。c-Met 在内皮细胞上表达,被肿瘤分泌的 HGF/SF 激活后可以促进基质降解和内皮细胞的侵袭。NOTCH 蛋白及其配体的表达在某些癌症中升高;NOTCH 信号通路已被证明既能促进又能抑制肿瘤生长,这主要取决于肿瘤的类型[166]。NOTCH 与其配体 DLL4 之间可以产生相互作用,进一步通过 NOTCH 与 VEGF/VEGFR 通路的复杂交叉调控促进肿瘤血管的新生[167,168]。

内源性血管新生抑制剂

一系列促血管新生蛋白,包括 VEGF、bFGF、IL-8、PDGF 和 PD-ECGF。天然的血管新生抑制剂包括干扰素(interferon-α,IFN-α)、IL-12、血小板因子 4(platelet factor 4)、TSP-1、血管抑素(angiostatin)、内皮抑制素(endostatin)、抑制蛋白(arrestin)、血

管能抑素(canstatin),肿瘤抑素(tumstatin),PEX(MMP-2),色素上皮衍生因子(pigment epithelium-derived factor,PEDF),抗血管新生抗凝血酶Ⅲ(抗凝血酶Ⅲ的片段,名为 aaAT),可以引起血管内皮细胞的增殖、迁移或增加其存活率;而内源性血管新生抑制剂可以抑制这一过程[27,169~175]。

有研究发现干扰素-α 能够抑制内皮细胞迁移,血小板因子 4 可以抑制内皮细胞增殖,从而首次提示内源性血管新生抑制剂的存在[176~178]。后续研究发现,这两种因子都有抑制血管新生的作用[176~180]。然而,Bouck 和她的同事首次发现肿瘤也可以产生血管新生抑制剂,他们随后提出,血管新生表型是由内源性抑制因子和血管新生刺激因子之间的平衡决定的[181]。非致瘤性仓鼠细胞系能够通过丢失抑癌基因并同时启动血管新生而获得致瘤性。非致瘤性细胞分泌高水平的血管新生抑制剂即 TSP-1 的截短体,而相对于非致瘤细胞,该因子在致瘤细胞中的表达水平则降低了大约 96%[182]。在成纤维细胞和乳腺上皮细胞中,TSP-1 受野生型抑癌基因 p53 的调控[183,184]。这些细胞被转化后,p53 功能缺失显著降低了血管新生抑制剂的水平。恢复 p53 的功能则可以上调肿瘤细胞 TSP-1 的表达,引起肿瘤细胞的抗血管新生活性。在自发乳腺癌的转基因小鼠模型中,TSP-1 的缺失能够加速乳腺癌的生长[185]。研究表明,血管新生表型的转换涉及一种由肿瘤产生的血管新生负调控因子,而 Folkman 认为这是一种普遍的血管新生机制,并且能够用来解释一种公认的、但尚未阐明的临床和实验现象:肿瘤块抑制肿瘤的生长。在这种现象中,“某些肿瘤被切除后,例如乳腺癌、结肠癌和成骨肉瘤,远处的转移灶会加速增长”[186,187]。术后化疗主要是为了预防或延缓继发性转移瘤的生长。几项针对终末期患者的研究表明,原发肿瘤可以抑制继发性肿瘤[188]。在黑色素瘤中,原发肿瘤部分自发消退后,转移瘤会出现快速的生长,当使用电离辐射使小细胞肺癌消退时,远处的转移瘤可能会迅速生长[173,189]。一旦证实肿瘤可以产生血管新生的负调控因子,那么很明显,原发肿瘤在自身血管床上刺激血管新生的同时,也可能抑制远处转移灶血管床的血管新生[182]。然而,以上情况的发生至少有两个条件是必须的:第一,原发肿瘤(即第一个生长的肿瘤)在其自身的血管床上能产生比抑制因子更多的血管促进因子;第二,相比血管新生促进因子,血管抑制因子在循环中的半衰期必须更长。在 1991 年进入 Folkman 实验室之后,O'Reilly 和他的同事们在接下来的 8 年里发现了血管抑制素、内皮抑制素和抗血管新生型抗凝血酶,并验证了这个假设[171~173,190,191]。

血管抑素

血管抑素(angiostatin)是一种大小为 38kDa 的纤溶酶原片段,是从皮下荷有 Lewis 肺癌的小鼠的血清和尿液中分离纯化而获得的,它能够通过抑制肺癌转移灶的血管新生来抑制其生长(图 17-5)[171]。血管抑素不是由肿瘤细胞分泌的,而是由肿瘤细胞释放的一系列酶水解循环纤溶酶原而产生的。这些肿瘤产生的酶中至少有一种,尿激酶纤溶酶原激活剂(urokinase plasminogen activator,uPA),能将纤溶酶原转化为纤溶酶,而低氧肿瘤细胞中的磷酸甘油激酶则能降低纤溶酶原,使其能被几

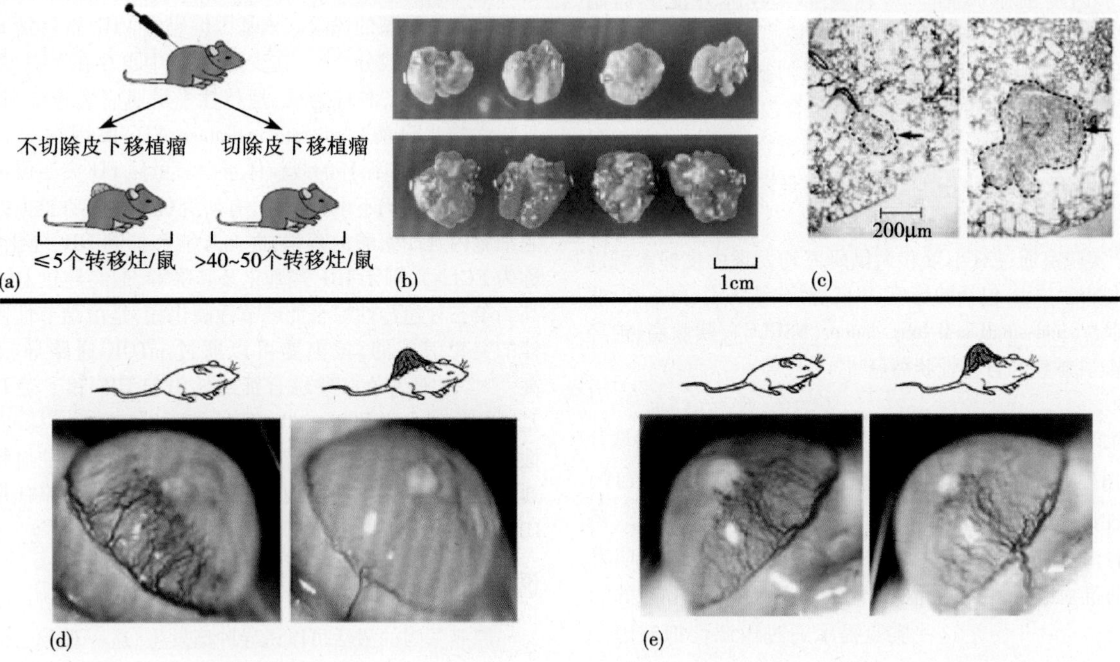

图 17-5　(a)Lewis 肺癌荷瘤小鼠[499]。当肿瘤大小达到 1.5~2cm^2 时切除肿瘤,5 天或 15 天后处死动物。(b)上图:带有原发肿瘤的小鼠的肺组织。下图:切除肿瘤并在 15 天后处死的小鼠的肺组织。(c)左图:显微镜下观察到的小鼠未切除原发肿瘤的肺转移。通过 von Willebrand 因子染色只发现了单一的中心微血管,表明没有血管新生。这种休眠的转移灶最长的直径为 200μm。右图:切除原发肿瘤 5 天后处死的小鼠肺上较大的转移灶,其中有 8 或 9 条新血管。(d)在 SCID 小鼠的背部接种人前列腺癌(LNCaP)细胞可以抑制由植入的 bFGF(80ng)缓释颗粒诱导的角膜新生血管形成(右图)。左图显示在没有移植原发肿瘤的情况下,植入 bFGF 缓释颗粒 5 天后即可诱导角膜新生血管形成。表明 LNCaP 前列腺癌可以产生血管抑素。(e)在 SCID 小鼠背部种植一种不产生血管生成抑制因子的人结肠癌,作为(d)的阴性对照

种不同的金属蛋白酶转化为血管抑素[192]。有研究报道了血管抑素抗血管新生的几种可能机制：诱导内皮细胞凋亡[193~195]；抑制血纤维蛋白溶酶结合 $\alpha_v\beta_3$-integrin 引起的内皮细胞迁移[196,197]；抑制 HGF 诱导的 c-MET、Akt 和 ERK-1/2 通路活化[198]；下调 VEGF 在肿瘤细胞中的表达[199]。这些发现表明血管抑素可以通过直接或间接的方式来抑制血管新生。相应的，对荷有不同肿瘤的小鼠单独用血管抑素治疗、或以血管抑素和内皮抑素融合蛋白的形式联合治疗、或与 IL-12 联合进行治疗，确实可以有效地抑制肿瘤[199~202]。

内皮抑素

与发现血管抑素的策略一样（如肿瘤肿块抑制肿瘤生长的现象），通过对小鼠血管内皮瘤和人小细胞肺癌的研究，发现了内皮抑素（endostatin）和抗血管新生型抗凝血酶-Ⅲ AT[172,173,191]。内皮抑素和 aaAT 都是由肿瘤细胞释放的酶将较大的初始蛋白分解而产生的。内皮抑素是胶原酶ⅩⅧ内部一段大小为 20~22kDa 的片段[172,191,203,204]。它是首个被鉴定的细胞外来源的内源性血管新生抑制因子，通常需要经过蛋白水解加工才能发挥作用[3,205]。内皮抑素与血管抑素一样，对肿瘤内皮细胞有直接和间接的作用，并存在多种不同的作用机制。它是一种内皮细胞增殖和迁移的特异性抑制剂[206~207]，可阻断 $VEGF_{121}$ 和 $VEGF_{165}$ 与 KDR/Flk-1 受体的结合，进而抑制下游的信号通路[208]。虽然内皮抑素不与 VEGF 结合[208]，但它确实下调了 VEGF 在肿瘤细胞中的表达。在 bFGF 处理过的内皮细胞中，内皮抑素部分通过激活 Shb 接头蛋白的酪氨酸激酶信号，诱导了内皮细胞凋亡[209]。内皮抑素在体外能够抑制 VEGF 诱导的主动脉环新生微血管的形成[210]，并抑制 MMP-2 的催化活性[211,212]。因此，内皮抑素可以抑制内皮细胞和肿瘤细胞的侵袭特性。内皮抑素还能通过结合内皮细胞表面的 α_5 和 α_v 整合素，尤其是 $\alpha_5\beta_1$ 整合素，抑制整合素依赖的内皮细胞迁移[213]。有人提出 $\alpha_5\beta_1$ 整合素可能是内皮抑素的功能型受体[34]。

多个实验室通过对小鼠和大鼠研究均发现内皮抑素可以抑制多种肿瘤[214]。包括肺腺癌、甲状腺癌、结肠癌、白血病、非小细胞肺癌（non-small cell lung cancer，NSCLC）、胰腺癌、神经母细胞瘤、乳腺癌和自发性胰岛癌[215~222]。

肿瘤抑素

肿瘤抑素（Tumstatin）（28kDa）是 α_3 胶原的 NC1 结构域片段，在体内外具有抗血管新生的活性[223~227]。肿瘤抑素[α_3(Ⅳ) NC1]通过 $\alpha_v\beta_3$ 和 $\alpha_6\beta_1$ 整合素与内皮细胞结合[223,224,226,227]，诱导增殖的内皮细胞发生凋亡[225]。细胞生物学实验证明肿瘤抑素的抗血管新生活性依赖于 $\alpha_v\beta_3$ 整合素与增殖的内皮细胞的结合[223,227]。这些实验提示通过内源性抑制因子如肿瘤抑素的作用，$\alpha_v\beta_3$ 整合素也可以作为血管新生的负性调控因子[223,228~230]。

抗血管新生型抗凝血酶Ⅲ

人小细胞肺癌能抑制免疫缺陷小鼠远端血管的新生和肿瘤生长。这些细胞在体外产生了一种酶，将 58kDa 的循环抗凝血酶Ⅲ分解为 53kDa 的蛋白，其中抗凝血酶外部的应力环被缩回到分子体内。53kDa 的抗凝血酶Ⅲ的“剪切”形式是一种特异性的内皮细胞抑制剂，即抗血管新生型抗凝血酶Ⅲ（antiangiogenic conformation of antithrombin Ⅲ），能有效抑制血管新生，但没有凝血酶结合活性。抗凝血酶Ⅲ没有抗内皮或抗血管新生活性。尚不清楚是何种酶引起了这种构象变化。人胰腺癌也能产生 53kDa 的抗血管新生型抗凝血酶剪切体[215]。

其他调控血管新生的通路

低氧诱导因子 1

缺氧环境可以通过稳定转录因子低氧诱导因子 1（hypoxia-inducible factor 1，HIF-1），促进包括 VEGF 在内的血管新生因子的表达[231,232]。HIF-1 由两个亚基构成，分别为 HIF-1α 和 HIF-1β。HIF-1β 是组成性表达的，而 HIF-1α 的表达则受到其他因素的严格调控。HIF-1α 的稳定性主要是由缺氧控制。当氧充足时，脯氨酰羟化酶可以修饰 HIF-1α 402 位和 564 位的脯氨酸残基，使其与抑癌基因 VHL 结合并促 HIF-1α 的降解[232]。HIF-1α 和-β 亚基结合后，HIF-1 转位至细胞核，调节血管新生、细胞存活、侵袭和糖代谢的相关基因表达[232]。事实上，在包括 VEGF 在内的强效血管新生促进因子的调控中，HIF-1α 处于核心的地位。

虽然最初 HIF-1 被认为主要受缺氧调控，但最近的研究揭示了一些非缺氧调节因子，包括受体酪氨酸激酶，如 EGFR[233]、PI3K/AKT/mTOR 通路，以及包括三羧酸循环在内的代谢通路[234,235]。这些通路的改变已被证明可能导致遗传性癌症综合征的发生，进一步突出了它们在癌症发生中的作用。例如，von Hippel-Lindau 病中 VHL 基因的胚系突变会显著增加患肾细胞癌（renal cell carcinoma，RCC）、中枢神经系统血管母细胞瘤和其他肿瘤的风险。该基因编码的 VHL 蛋白是 HIF 降解复合物的组成成分[234]。在少数 RCC 中也存在 VHL 基因的散发性突变。第二种综合征，遗传性平滑肌瘤病和肾细胞癌，由延胡索酸水合酶（fumarate hydratase，FH）基因突变引起[236]。FH 是参与 TCA 循环的线粒体蛋白。虽然 FH 突变促进肿瘤发生的机制目前仍不十分清楚，有研究提出 FH 功能丧失可能引起细胞内延胡索酸的蓄积，进一步能够抑制 HIF 羟化酶（也被称为 EGLN），抑制 HIF 羟基化及其降解，最终导致 HIF 水平升高。第三种遗传性综合征结节性硬化症，是由结节性硬化复合体的突变引起的，该突变可以通过 mTOR 通路导致 HIF 升高[237,238]。还存在一些综合征能够引起 HIF 和下游 HIF 调控基因产物的水平升高，产生“假缺氧”的状态[235,237]。多种遗传性癌症综合征的发生均与 HIF 通路有关，提示调控血管新生的通路失调可能在早期肿瘤形成中发挥作用。目前有几种针对 HIF 的药物正在临床开发中。

调控血管新生的癌基因

原癌基因的激活可以诱导肿瘤发生，这一观点已被广泛证实。在组织培养中，活化的癌基因可以促进细胞增殖、抑制细胞凋亡[239]。虽然这些变化是通过改变细胞增殖和凋亡之间的平衡来促进肿瘤的发生，但相当多的证据表明，仅凭这些变化不足以引起扩张性肿瘤的生长[240,241]。肿瘤必须获得足够的血管，才能使其生长到直径超过 1~2mm 大小。已有的研究表明，用癌基因转染肿瘤细胞可以使细胞促血管新生分子的产生增加[242]，体内研究也表明血管新生抑制剂可以限制癌基因驱使的肿瘤生长[243]。例如在肺癌患者中，K-Ras、p53 和 EGFR 等癌基因的突变就与血管新生相关。对血管新生因子有调控作用的癌基因包括以下基因：

Ras

Ras 是最常见的致癌基因之一，在 17%～25% 的人类肿瘤中存在活化[244]。在组织培养研究中，用 Ras 致癌基因转染转化小鼠内皮细胞后，VEGF 的表达水平增加，而用 PI3K 抑制剂渥曼青霉素（wortmannin）处理这些细胞后，VEGF 的表达被抑制，表明突变的 Ras 以 PI3K 依赖的方式调控 VEGF 的表达[245]。在人非小细胞肺癌[246]和其他疾病类型中，K-Ras 基因突变与 VEGF 的高表达呈正相关。在黑色素瘤的转基因模型中，通过四环素下调肿瘤中 Ras 基因的表达，6 小时后即可观察到肿瘤癌巢内大量微血管内皮细胞凋亡。几天后肿瘤细胞开始死亡，12 天时较大的肿瘤完全消失[247]。

P53

除了调控细胞周期和凋亡外，新近研究表明 p53 通过改变促血管新生和抗血管新生分子的表达，间接促进肿瘤血管新生。在组织培养研究中，表达野生型 p53 的成纤维细胞分泌高水平的抗血管新生糖蛋白 TSP-1。然而，野生型 p53 的缺失和突变体的表达会导致 TSP-1 mRNA 和蛋白表达减少。对 73 例 NSCLC 临床样本进行免疫组化评分，发现 p53 的核定位与微血管数目之间存在显著的统计学相关性[248]。此外，在对 107 例 NSCLC 患者的分析中发现，p53 与 VEGF 的表达水平及微血管的数目之间有显著相关性[249]。NSCLC 中野生型 p53 的缺失可能促进肿瘤细胞表达其他促血管新生因子。野生型 p53 已被证实能促进 Mdm2 介导的 HIF-1α 的泛素化和降解[250]。在组织培养中，野生型 p53 的缺失不仅与 HIF-1α 的升高有关，还可以促进低氧诱导的 VEGF 的表达[250]。

Myc

Myc 是一种多能性转录因子，在多种类型的肿瘤中表达升高，其在调节血管新生、炎症等方面发挥了重要作用。Myc 的活性受到 RAS 通路的调控[242]，Myc 活化后又部分通过影响 TSP-1 来调控血管新生。Myc 还可以与 HIF-1α 通路相互作用，不仅可以通过不依赖缺氧的方式诱导血管新生[251]，还可以在 Myc 驱使的肿瘤发生转基因小鼠模型中，通过调控肥大细胞的募集来影响肿瘤发生[252]。

EGFR 家族

EGFR 是受体酪氨酸激酶 erbB 家族的成员之一，该家族还包括 HER2/Neu、HER3（ErbB3）和 HER4（ErbB4）。越来越多的证据表明，EGFR 的激活会导致促血管新生分子的产生。最初在前列腺癌细胞系中的实验表明，给予肿瘤细胞 EGF 处理可以上调 HIF-1α 的表达[253]。EGF 已被证明可以增加某些肿瘤细胞系中 VEGF 的生成[254,255]，相反，用 EGFR 抑制剂处理肿瘤细胞可以降低 VEGF 在各种肿瘤中的表达[233,255～257]。在 NSCLC 细胞系中，EGF 能够激活 HIF-1α 并在组织培养时可以诱导趋化因子受体 CXCR4 的表达[258]。此外，对 172 名 NSCLC 患者样本的免疫组化染色发现，EGFR 的表达与 HIF-1α 的水平呈正相关[259]，EGFR 突变导致受体持续活化，引起 HIF-1α 和 VEGF 表达水平的升高[260]。

与 EGFR 一样，HER2/Neu 在调节血管新生中也发挥了作用。在人乳腺癌小鼠模型中利用单克隆抗体曲妥珠单抗（Herceptin）抑制 HER2，可阻断多种血管新生因子的产生，诱导血管正常化和消退，并增强 VEGF 通路阻断的效果[261,262]。

靶向肿瘤血管系统的治疗方法

血管新生抑制剂与血管靶向药物

血管新生是指从原有的血管系统中形成新的血管。因此，血管新生抑制剂通常针对这一过程的早期阶段，包括内皮的发芽和存活过程，这些过程通常要依赖于 VEGF。血管靶向药物（vascular targeting agent，VTA）也被称为血管阻断剂（vascular disrupting agent，VDA），与血管新生抑制剂不同，VTA 靶向的是已建立的异常肿瘤血管系统[263]。VTA 可诱导肿瘤血管迅速崩溃，对正常脉管系统也会产生一系列的副作用，包括急性冠状动脉综合征、血栓性静脉炎和肿瘤疼痛。目前这些药物尚未进入癌症的常规临床应用，但有几种正在进行临床试验。最初在Ⅱ期临床试验中，Vadimezan（ASA404）与化疗联合治疗肺癌患者得到了阳性的结果[264]。不幸的是，这些发现并没有在随后的Ⅲ期临床试验中得到验证，该试验评估了 vadimezan 与卡铂/紫杉醇联用作为一线治疗方案在 NSCLC 中的疗效，结果显示实验组与对照组的总体生存期（overall survival，OS）并没有显著的差异［中位 OS 分别为 13.4 个月和 12.7 个月（HR = 1.01；P = 0.535）］。由于缺乏临床效果，诺华公司终止了 vadimezan 在肺癌中的研发[265]。ABT-751 是另一种具有临床前抗癌活性的 VDA，但在 ABT-751 与多西紫杉醇联用作为二线方案治疗 NSCLC 的Ⅰ/Ⅱ期临床研究中，它未能提高患者的无进展生存期（progression-free survival，PFS）[266]。

化疗药和其他药物的抗血管新生作用

多项临床前研究表明，几种“经典”的化疗药物也可能有强大的抗血管新生或血管靶向作用，而低剂量、频繁给药（节律给药）可能会增强这种作用[267～269]。其中几个类似的方案正在进行临床评估。此外，某些化疗药物，特别是紫杉烷类和长春花生物碱，可能比其他药物具有更强的抗血管新生作用，这可能有助于解释为什么在化疗中添加贝伐单抗等抗血管新生药物时，疗效的增强程度有所不同。这促使人们进一步研究各种最初被认为主要针对肿瘤细胞的药物。这些药物中有许多后续被发现也有抗血管新生的作用，因此“意外抗血管新生”的概念就应运而生[270]。

靶向 VEGF 通路

VEGF 属于结构相似的一组由同源二聚体组成的生长因子家族的成员，该家族还包括 PlGF、VEGF-B、VEGF-C、VEGF-D 和 VEGF-E。如前所述，VEGF 家族成员与跨膜受体酪氨酸激酶结合，包括 VEGFR-1（Flt-1）、VEGFR-2（KDR Flk-1）和 VEGFR-3（Flt-4）（图 17-3）。VEGF 或 VEGFR 对血管通透性、内皮细胞的增殖、迁移和存活的影响主要是由 VEGFR-2 介导的，而 VEGFR-3 主要表达在淋巴内皮上[122,129]。靶向 VEGF 通路的药物包括与配体结合的单克隆抗体（如贝伐单抗）或阻断受体的抗体（雷莫芦单抗）。此外，许多小分子受体酪氨酸激酶抑制剂（receptor tyrosine kinase inhibitor，RTKI）已被开发用于靶向血管新生过程中的关键信号通路。这些 RTK 包括瓦他拉尼

[vatalanib(PTK787)]、凡德他尼[vandetanib(ZD6474)]、舒尼替尼[sunitinib(SU11248)]、阿西替尼[axitinib(AG-013736)]和尼达尼布[nintedanib(BIBF 1120)],这些抑制剂已成为许多临床前和临床研究的重点。由于不同受体酪氨酸激酶的结构域高度相似,除了抑制 VEGFR 外,RTKI 通常还抑制 PDGFR、c-KIT、FGFR 和 Axl 等多种受体。与单靶点药物相比,这些多靶点药物具有更高的抗癌活性。此外,这些药物可以口服,对患者来说更为方便。相反,这些抑制剂的脱靶效应可能导致额外的毒副作用。每个抑制剂靶向受体的特异性、它们的药代动力学指标以及抑制受体的能力,可能是其临床活性的关键决定因素。表 17-2 列出了目前 FDA 批准的针对 VEGF 通路的代表性药物。

表 17-2 临床获批的 VEGF 通路抑制剂

类型	药物	靶点	批准情况
单克隆抗体	贝伐单抗(avastin)	VEGF-A	FDA 批准用于结直肠癌、乳腺癌、非小细胞肺癌、铂类耐受的卵巢癌及晚期宫颈癌
	IMC-1121B 雷莫芦单抗	VEGFR-2 胞外结构域	FDA 批准用于晚期胃癌和食管胃交界部腺癌,转移性非小细胞肺癌
可溶性诱饵受体	VEGF 诱饵(aflibercept)	VEGF-A,VEGF-B,PlGF	FDA 批准用于转移性结直肠癌
受体酪氨酸激酶抑制剂	凡德他尼[vandetanib(ZD6474)]	VEGFR-2,EGFR,RET	FDA 批准用于进行性甲状腺髓样癌
	索拉菲尼(sorafenib)	VEGFR-2,3,PDGFR-β,Flt-3,c-Kit,B-Raf	FDA 批准用于肾细胞癌、肝细胞癌及转移性分化甲状腺癌
	舒尼替尼[sunitinib(SU11248)]	VEGFR-1,2,PDGFR,c-Kit,RET,Flt-3	FDA 批准用于肾细胞癌、胃肠间质瘤及胰腺神经内分泌瘤
	阿西替尼[AG-013736(axitinib)]	VEGFR-1,2,3,PDGFR	FDA 批准用于肾细胞癌
	仑伐替尼(Lenvatinib)	VEGFR-2,3	FDA 批准用于甲状腺癌
	尼达尼布[BIBF 1120(nintedanib)]	VEGFR-1,2,3,PDGFR,FGFR-1/3	FDA 和 EU 批准用于特发性肺纤维化,EU 批准用于非小细胞肺癌
	帕唑帕尼[GW786034(pazopanib)]	VEGFR2	FDA 批准用于肾细胞癌和软组织肉瘤

VEGF,血管内皮生长因子;VEGFR,血管内皮生长因子受体;PlGF,胎盘生长因子;EGFR,表皮生长因子受体;PDGFR,血小板源生长因子受体;FDA,美国食品和药品管理局;EU,欧盟。

抗血管新生药物联合化疗:增强抗肿瘤活性的机制

临床前和临床研究表明,抗血管新生治疗能够提高细胞毒性治疗的效果[271,272]。这一发现与先前的预期是矛盾的。最初科学家们预期,靶向肿瘤血管系统将大大减少向实体肿瘤的氧气和药物输送,从而导致缺氧,并减弱许多化疗药物以及放疗的治疗效果[271,272]。肿瘤血管系统由弯曲和高通透性的血管组成,其结构和功能是异常的。这些瘤内血管内的血流情况并不一致。增殖的肿瘤细胞压迫血液和淋巴管,造成以间质高血压(血管外静压升高)、酸中毒和缺氧为典型特性的微环境[273,274]。这种异常的血管网络和间质性高血压会阻碍向肿瘤细胞的药物传递。此外,缺氧使肿瘤细胞对辐射和多种细胞毒性药物产生耐药性,并增加了基因不稳定性,使得有更大转移潜能的肿瘤细胞得以生存。除对肿瘤细胞的直接作用外,缺氧还能通过 PHD2 在肿瘤内皮细胞中传递信号导致血管异常[275],并且随着肿瘤微环境中 pH 值的降低,缺氧还会减弱肿瘤浸润免疫细胞的细胞杀伤功能。总体而言,实体肿瘤内异常的血管系统极大地阻碍了药物的输送和疗效。

抗血管新生治疗提高化疗效果的一种解释是,这些药物可能使肿瘤血管"正常化"。在癌症动物模型中,VEGF 信号的抑制导致癌症的血管网络更接近于正常组织中的血管。这种"正常化"的血管系统更少渗漏,更少扩张,有更少的弯曲血管,基底膜更为正常,周细胞覆盖率更高。除血管形态变化外,肿瘤内的间质液压(IFP)减少,氧化作用增加,并可以改善化疗药物向肿瘤的输送(图 17-6)[276~284]。Ⅰ/Ⅱ期临床试验的结果显示,晚期直肠癌患者接受贝伐单抗和化疗(同时还接受了放疗)的疗效与临床前研究的发现基本一致。贝伐单抗治疗可以降低肿瘤的 IFP,并增加肿瘤中成熟的、被周细胞覆盖血管的数量[285,286]。

抗血管新生药物联合放疗

越来越多的证据表明,抗血管新生治疗可以提高实体瘤放疗的疗效。其机制可以包括以下几个方面。首先,放疗可能促使肿瘤组织中紊乱的和高通透性的血管系统"正常化"[271,287]。血管正常化使向肿瘤组织的氧气输送更加有效,缓解肿瘤缺氧状况,并通过增加氧自由基的形成,在一定程度上增强辐射诱导的细胞毒性。然而,这种缺氧的缓解可能是暂时的,因为长

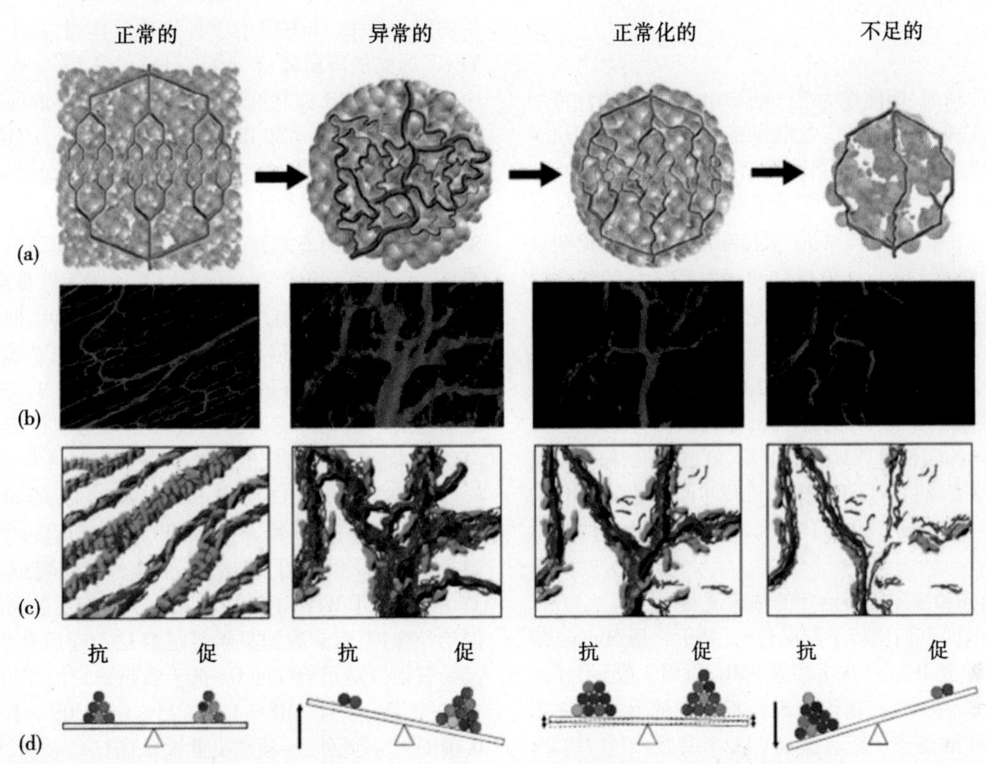

图 17-6　抗血管新生药物治疗期间肿瘤血管系统的变化[271]。(a)肿瘤血管网络结构和功能异常。抗血管新生治疗可以改善肿瘤血管的结构和功能。持续或积极的抗血管新生治疗方案可能最终导致血管供应无法支持肿瘤生长。(b)抑制 VEGFR2 使血管正常化。左边是双光子图像,展示的是正常的骨骼肌血管;随后的代表性图像显示的是用 VEGR2 特异性抗体治疗后第 0 天、第 3 天和第 5 天的小鼠结肠癌血管系统。(c)血管正常化过程中基底膜(蓝色)和周细胞(红色)覆盖的变化。(d)这些血管系统的变化可能反映了微环境中促血管新生因子和抗血管新生因子之间平衡的变化

期使用抗血管新生药物最终也会减少肿瘤内"正常化"的血管,影响肿瘤内的血管供应,从而使肿瘤再次缺氧,并导致肿瘤对放疗的敏感性降低。这一假说在小鼠荷瘤模型中得到了验证,该模型显示在某段时间内("正常化时间窗"),放疗和抗血管新生药物联用的效果最显著[283,288]。

抗血管新生治疗可以增强放疗的抗内皮细胞作用。虽然最初认为放疗的抗肿瘤作用是通过直接作用于肿瘤细胞实现的,但最近的证据表明,放疗也可诱导内皮细胞凋亡[288~290]。其他研究也证实了这些发现[291]。但抗血管新生药物与辐射间相互作用的确切机制仍不清楚。

然而,一些临床前研究表明,抗血管新生药物可以协同或增强放疗的效果[292~296]。阻断血管内皮细胞中 VEGF 信号通路可以使肿瘤相关的血管对放疗更加敏感。此外,放疗可以诱导 VEGF 的表达,而 VEGF 则通过阻断放疗诱导的内皮细胞凋亡来促进肿瘤对放疗的耐受[297,298]。

抗血管新生治疗与放疗联合还需进一步研究,其可能原因之一是,研究者在临床前研究中发现,放射治疗引起的部分毒副作用如肠道辐射损伤,可能也是由内皮细胞凋亡引起的[299]。在接受了贝伐单抗、化疗和放疗联合治疗后,部分肺癌患者出现了食管瘘的副作用[300]。显然,还需要进行更多的研究来评估这些组合的可行性和有效性。

抗血管新生治疗的临床进展

肿瘤血管新生作为癌症治疗靶点的假说,已在多种类型肿瘤的Ⅲ期随机临床试验中得到证实。贝伐单抗是一种靶向 VEGF 的单克隆抗体,目前已成为转移性结直肠癌、非小细胞肺癌和其他类型肿瘤的标准治疗药物[301,302];VEGFR 酪氨酸激酶抑制剂(tyrosine kinase inhibitor,TKI)如舒尼替尼(sunitinib)、帕唑帕尼(pazopanib)、阿昔替尼(axitinib)和索拉菲尼(sorafenib)已被批准用于 RCC 和其他疾病的治疗[303,304]。这些进展,加上我们对肿瘤血管新生生物学通路的深入了解,以及对这些通路靶向药物的开发和优化,使得基于抗血管新生药物单用或联合其他治疗的临床试验数量急剧增加。由于 VEGF 是肿瘤血管新生的关键调控因子,目前大多数药物都以靶向 VEGF 通路为主。

VEGF 通路抑制剂用于抗癌治疗的临床经验。贝伐单抗是最早的 VEGF 通路抑制剂之一,它的临床试验开始于 1997 年。当作为单药来治疗晚期实体瘤时,从肿瘤的客观反应来讲,除 RCC 外,VEGF 通路抑制剂的临床活性一般都较低。例如,在一项包含 25 例患者的贝伐单抗Ⅰ期临床试验中,患者的肿瘤无一出现部分或完全缓解反应[305]。此外,在 243 例既往接受过治疗的结直肠癌患者中,贝伐单抗治疗的客观有效率(objective response rates,ORR)仅为 3%,而 FOLFOX4 化疗(氟尿嘧啶、奥沙利铂、亮氨酸)的客观有效率为 9.2%,联合应用的客观有效率为 21.8%。VEGFR TKI 作为单一药物使用时反应率也较低(将在下文中具体讨论)。因此,VEGF 通路抑制剂常被作为化疗或其他靶向药物联合治疗方案的一部分。现就 VEGF 通路抑制剂在几种常见肿瘤中的临床应用现状进行综述。

肾细胞癌

VEGF 通路抑制剂,即使作为单一药物治疗,在转移性肾细胞癌中的疗效也是非常不错的。这些肿瘤一般常以 von Hippel-Lindau 基因的失活为标志,该基因失活会导致 VEGF 和其他血管新生调节因子的表达升高[306]。随机临床试验的结果显示,与安慰剂对照组相比,贝伐单抗、索拉菲尼和帕唑帕尼明显延缓了肿瘤的进展[307~309]。舒尼替尼和阿西替尼在转移性肾细胞癌中也显示出明显的抗肿瘤活性,它们在Ⅲ期临床试验中的客观有效率为 25%~45%[304,310,311]。

细胞因子疗法(以 IFN-α 和 IL-2 为基础的治疗法)一直是治疗 RCC 的主要方法,可以作为评价抗血管治疗疗效的阳性对照。VEGF 受体的四种 RTKI(索拉菲尼、舒尼替尼、帕唑帕尼和阿西替尼)和单克隆抗 VEGF 抗体(贝伐单抗)治疗 RCC 的Ⅲ期试验结果都分别显示,相比于干扰素,抗 VEGF 疗法的治疗效果更好。

对比抗 VEGF 治疗和细胞因子治疗的临床试验

Motzer 和他的同事们比较了舒尼替尼(每天口服 50mg 共 4 周,之后 2 周停药)或 IFN-α(皮下注射 9MU,每周 3 次)治疗初治转移性 RCC 的疗效[304]。他们发现经舒尼替尼治疗的患者的 PFS(研究的首要终点)显著提高(11 个月比 5 个月,$P<0.001$)。接受舒尼替尼治疗的患者治疗反应率更高、OS 更长、生活质量更高[310]。

细胞因子治疗联合或不联合抗 VEGF 治疗的临床试验

Escudier 等人[312]和癌症与白血病研究 B 组机构(Cancer and Leukemia Group B)开展了安慰剂对照的随机Ⅲ期试验,比较 IFNα-2a 与 IFNα-2a 联合贝伐单抗在初治转移性 RCC 患者中的治疗作用[313]。结果显示,接受联合生物治疗的患者的 PFS 明显延长,其 OS 也有改善的趋势[314,315]。由于超过 50% 的患者接受了包括 VEGF 靶向药物在内的二线治疗,因此不同治疗组间的生存差异可能受到了影响[315,316]。

细胞因子治疗后接受抗 VEGF 治疗的临床试验

Escudier 等[303]以接受一线细胞因子治疗后进展的晚期 RCC 患者为对象,开展了一项索拉菲尼(400mg 每次,每日 2 次)对比安慰剂的Ⅲ期临床试验。结果显示,索拉菲尼组的中位 PFS 为 5.5 个月,安慰剂组的中位 PFS 为 2.8 个月($P<0.01$)。OS 分析显示索拉菲尼降低了患者的死亡风险(HR=0.88;95% CI 0.74~1.04;$P=0.146$)[317]。虽然该结果没有统计学差异,但将安慰剂组中交叉到索拉菲尼组的患者截尾后,二组间的 OS 存在显著差异(索拉菲尼组 17.8 个月,安慰剂组 14.3 个月;HR=0.78;95%CI 0.62~0.97;$P=0.0287$)。

抗 VEGF 治疗后的治疗

抗 VEGF 对 RCC 的良好治疗效果从根本上改变了这种疾病的治疗模式。然而,抗 VEGF 治疗并不能完全消除肿瘤,只能一定程度上延长患者的生存,因此这种疾病的治疗仍有很大的提高空间。对一种 VEGF 靶向药物耐药的患者可能还会对另一种 VEGF 靶向药物反应[318~320]。尚不清楚这种交叉敏感性是否与 RTKI 的混杂性、药物的药代动力学或药物与 VEGF 受体亲和性的不同有关。

mTOR 抑制在 RCC 中的研究

两项临床试验[321,322]研究了抑制 mTOR 在晚期肾癌患者中的治疗效果。mTOR 有多种生物学作用,其中之一便是作为 VEGF 通路的下游效应分子。Hudes 等人[321]在一项临床试验中比较了 mTOR 抑制剂替西罗莫司(temsirolimus)单药与 IFN-α 单药、替西罗莫司和 IFN-α 联用作为一线方案治疗 RCC 的效果,结果显示与 IFN-α 相比,替西罗莫司可显著延长患者的 OS(10.9 个月比 7.3 个月,$P=0.008$);联合用药组与干扰素单药治疗组相比无明显差异。此外,替西罗莫司组发生的严重不良事件少于 IFN-α 组。在一项安慰剂对照随机Ⅲ期试验中,作为 VEGF TKI 的后续治疗,与安慰剂相比,mTOR 抑制剂依维莫司可显著延长患者的 PFS(4 个月比 1.9 个月,$P<0.001$)[322]。但两组间的 OS 并没有显著差异,这可能是由于安慰剂组的患者肿瘤进展后被允许交叉进入依维莫司组进行治疗。虽然依维莫司的毒性通常较轻,但部分严重(3 级或 4 级)毒性反应的数量明显增加,包括:口腔炎,$P=0.03$;感染,$P=0.03$;高胆固醇血症,$P=0.03$;高血糖,$P<0.0001$;淋巴细胞减少,$P=0.002$;血磷过低,$P=0.01$。目前还没有前瞻性数据可以直接比较依维莫司和 VEGF RTKI 在 VEGF 抑制剂治疗后肿瘤进展的患者中的治疗作用,但有数据显示舒尼替尼治疗后肿瘤进展的患者,接受替西罗莫司治疗的 OS 低于索拉菲尼治疗组(12.3 个月比 16.6 个月;分层 HR=1.31;95% CI 1.05~1.63;双侧 $P=0.01$)[323]。此外,一项随机Ⅱ期临床试验表明,依维莫司治疗患者的 PFS 要劣于舒尼替尼,尤其是作为一线用药时[324]。与序贯治疗相比,目前没有证据支持联合使用不同作用机制的药物,同时这种药物联合的毒性可能会增加,如贝伐单抗与替西罗莫司的药物联合(相比于贝伐单抗和干扰素)[325]。

抗血管新生作为 RCC 的辅助治疗

多种抗血管新生药物的出现促进了 RCC 辅助治疗临床试验的发展。早期的 E2805 临床试验,将患者随机分配至索拉菲尼组(400mg,每日 2 次)、舒尼替尼组(50mg/d,每 6 周 4 次)或安慰剂组治疗 1 年,结果发现索拉菲尼和舒尼替尼均不能延迟患者术后肿瘤的复发时间(索拉菲尼或舒尼替尼组患者术后至肿瘤复发的时间为 5.6 年,安慰剂组为 5.7 年)[326]。

抗血管新生治疗 RCC 的疗效预测

已有研究表明,较高的 VEGF 水平与较差的肿瘤分期、分级、患者的状态表现和总体预后有关[317,327,328]。此外,在索拉菲尼对比安慰剂治疗 RCC 的Ⅲ期临床试验中,VEGF 浓度处于最高四分位的患者接受索拉菲尼治疗的获益要大于那些浓度较低的患者[327]。然而,VEGF 是否能作为预测标志物来筛选可能从 VEGF 靶向治疗中获益的 RCC 患者,目前的研究结果并不一致[329]。最近,一项研究利用来自两项后续的临床Ⅱ期和Ⅲ期试验的样本,发现 IL-6 可以预测 RCC 患者接受帕唑帕尼治疗后的 PFS 获益[330]。然而,目前能够在 RCC 中预测已上市药物和活性药物之间疗效差异的生物标志物都没有经过临床验证。

抗血管新生治疗 RCC 的未来方向

对接受 VEGF 和 mTOR 抑制剂治疗后肿瘤依然进展的患者,采用 FGF 和 VEGF 受体抑制剂多韦替尼作为三线方案进行治疗,尽管与索拉菲尼治疗相比,这未能提高患者的 PFS[331],但它很可能会抑制其他帮助肿瘤逃脱 VEGF 信号阻断的通路,如 cMET 通路。鉴于免疫检查点抑制剂等新型免疫药物在 RCC 临床试验中令人振奋的结果,多项临床试验正在评估免疫药物与血管新生抑制剂联用的效果。

结肠直肠癌

晚期结直肠癌是第一个在Ⅲ期临床试验中证明了抗血管新生治疗疗效的癌症,至今仍是抗血管新生治疗研究的最好的实体肿瘤之一。2004 年,一项Ⅲ期随机安慰剂对照研究在初治转移性结直肠癌患者中比较了单纯标准 IFL 化疗(伊立替康、氟尿嘧啶和甲酰四氢叶酸)或化疗联合贝伐单抗的疗效[301]。接受 IFL 和贝伐单抗联合治疗患者的 OS 和 PFS 显著延长,客观反应率也更高。这项试验提供了明确的证据,表明将血管新生抑制剂加入化疗方案可以延长患者的生存期,正是基于该临床试验的结果,美国 FDA 批准了贝伐单抗联合含氟尿嘧啶化疗作为一线方案治疗转移性结直肠癌。

后续的研究以此发现为基础相继展开。在一项针对既往接受过治疗的结直肠癌患者的临床试验中,研究者发现接受了贝伐单抗和 FOLFOX4 化疗联合治疗的患者的生存期要长于仅接受 FOLFOX4 治疗的患者[332],尽管该生存获益(2.1 个月)低于该药物组合在一线临床试验中的结果(4.7 个月)。造成这种结果的原因可能是该临床实验中患者的肿瘤分期更晚。

在贝伐单抗或安慰剂联合 FOLFOX 或 XELOX 作为一线治疗结直肠癌的临床研究中,尽管患者的 PFS 有所延长(9.4 个月比 8.0 个月),但 OS 并没有提高(21.3 个月比 19.9 个月)[333]。该研究和 IFL 研究之间的差异可能是由于两种化疗药之间存在不同的细胞毒性基础,或是由于 IFL 研究采用的是疾病进展才停药的治疗模式,而该研究中的治疗会因奥沙利铂的毒性累积而中断。一些研究评估了患者在接受奥沙利铂和氟嘧啶的一线化疗初始疗程后再使用贝伐单抗治疗的效果。这些“维持”方案已经证明了贝伐单抗联合氟嘧啶的治疗效果。CAIRO-3 随机临床研究表明,与仅做观察处理的组相比,贝伐单抗单药或与卡培他滨联合使用均可改善患者生存。

队列研究表明,贝伐单抗一线治疗疾病进展后继续抑制 VEGF 对结直肠癌仍有一定的疗效。TML 研究在先前接受过含贝伐单抗的一线方案治疗并进展的患者中评估了 FOLFIRI 或 FOLFOX(由医师决定)化疗或化疗联合贝伐单抗的二线治疗方案的疗效。该研究证实了联合贝伐单抗的方案可以延长患者的生存期,虽然只延长了 1.4 个月,但其统计学差异显著,贝伐单抗的持续治疗也因此被加入了结直肠癌的治疗指南。

研究者对 ziv-aflibercept 也进行了类似的研究。ziv-aflibercept 是一种含有 VEGFR1 和 VEGFR2 胞外结构域的融合蛋白,因此对 VEGF-A 和 PlGF 都有抑制作用。先前接受过奥沙利铂治疗(可能同时也接受了贝伐单抗治疗)的患者被随机分配到 FOLFIRI 联合贝伐单抗组或 FOLFIRI 联合安慰剂组[334]。该研究达到了首要的研究终点,联合贝伐单抗组患者的 OS 延长了 1.4 个月(13.5 个月比 12.1 个月),PFS 和反应率也得到了提高。ziv-aflibercept 组的患者中,3 级、4 级腹泻以及口腔炎的发生率显著高于对照组,这与 PlGF 在被覆黏膜修复中的作用是一致的[335]。除抗血管新生联合化疗的二线方案外,这两项研究的结果为那些接受了基于贝伐单抗的一线方案并出现疾病进展的患者提供了新的治疗选择。

目前,针对结直肠癌临床试验数据的分析并未能发现有效的生物标志物。在针对早期 Hurwitz 临床试验的一个分组分析中,VEGF-A、血小板反应蛋白的表达水平以及微血管密度都与患者的预后无关[336]。类似的,研究者通过对影响结直肠癌进展的癌基因(如 K-Ras、b-raf 和 p53)进行分析,也未能发现其与患者的临床转归有关联[337]。与转移性乳腺癌一样,通过对一项Ⅱ期临床试验的数据进行分析,研究者发现在治疗期间显著高血压症状的出现与患者的临床转归有关[338]。

在晚期结直肠癌中虽然单克隆抗体是研究的最为透彻的抗血管新生剂,但研究者们也在随机Ⅲ期临床试验中检测了对 VEGFR 有不同选择性的 TKI 的疗效。一项早期的随机Ⅲ期临床试验比较了仅 FOLFOX4 化疗或化疗联合口服小分子 RTKI 瓦他拉尼作为一线方案治疗转移性结直肠癌的疗效。这项研究发现联合治疗不能改善患者的 PFS 或 OS[339]。其他包括舒尼替尼和塞地拉尼布在内的一些药物,也进行了类似的临床研究,但都没有发现有治疗效果。一种抑制 VEGFR 的多激酶抑制剂——瑞戈非尼(Regorafenib)是个例外,由于与安慰剂相比,其在 CORRECT 研究中可以将 OS 延长 1.4 个月,因此被获批用于治疗结直肠癌[340]。虽然 TKI 的毒副作用一般比较严重,但目前尚不清楚大分子抑制剂的疗效通常较好而 TKI 联合化疗却效果欠佳的原因。

胃癌和胃食管交界癌

AVAGAST 研究初步评估了抗血管新生治疗在晚期胃癌中的疗效,该研究还评估了贝伐单抗联合顺铂-卡培他滨作为一线方案的治疗效果[341]。结果显示,尽管 PFS 和反应率有所提高,但 OS 没有差异,因此贝伐单抗在胃癌或胃食管交界(gastroesophageal junction,GEJ)癌中的临床研究就没有继续开展。

相反,一项针对 355 名胃腺癌或胃食管交界腺癌患者的二线研究显示,与安慰剂相比,雷莫芦单抗具有一定的疗效,因此其获得了美国 FDA 的批准并进入临床应用。雷莫芦单抗是一种结合于 VEGFR2 的 N 端并可以阻止受体与配体的结合及受体构象变化的单克隆抗体[342],它最初是从噬菌体展示文库中鉴定出来的,其结合 VEGFR2 的亲和力达到了惊人的皮摩尔级[343,344]。REGARD 研究表明,与安慰剂相比,雷莫芦单抗作为二线治疗能够改善患者的生存获益,其 OS 中位数为 5.2 个月,而对照组为 3.8 个月[345]。该药物的耐受性良好,虽然 3 级高血压的风险略有增加(8%比 3%),但血栓栓塞事件的风险没有加重。

随后进行了另外两项研究,进一步评估了抗血管新生治疗在晚期胃食管癌中的疗效。由于许多肿瘤学家的临床实践是在二线采用细胞毒性化疗,因此 RAINBOW 试验就被设计为在先前接受过一线基于铂类和氟嘧啶化疗并出现进展的患者中评估紫杉醇联合雷莫芦单抗或安慰剂的疗效[346]。这项包含了 655 例患者的国际临床研究达到了其设计的主要终点——OS 得到了改善(9.6 个月比 7.3 个月)。对该研究的亚组分析发现,高加索地区患者的生存获益明显高于亚洲患者。AVAGAST 研究中也发现存在同样的地域差异现象,这表明亚洲和高加索地区的患者在疾病生物学或治疗模式上存在差异。这种差异的潜在生物学机制目前还不清楚。

一项Ⅱ期临床研究评估了雷莫芦单抗或安慰剂联合 FOLFOX 化疗对初治晚期胃食管癌患者的治疗作用。结果显示,尽管疾病控制率有所提高,但 OS 和 PFS 没有差异。因此,雷莫芦单抗的使用目前仅限于接受含氟嘧啶或铂类化疗后肿瘤进展的晚期胃癌或胃食管交界腺癌患者。

也有临床试验研究了 VEGFR TKI 在胃癌中的疗效。一项随机临床研究评估了多烯紫杉醇联合舒尼替尼或安慰剂作为二线治疗胃癌的疗效。这项小规模的Ⅱ期临床试验虽然发现反应率增加了很多(41% vs 14%),但患者的 TTP(Time To Progression)或 OS 没有明显的改善[347]。相反,一项随机Ⅲ期研究在接受了两种或两种以上前期治疗并进展的患者中,评估了两种不同剂量的 VEGFR TKI——阿帕替尼对胃癌的治疗效果。结果显示,两种剂量的阿帕替尼在 PFS(3.7/3.2 个月比 1.4 个月)和 OS(4.8/4.3 个月比 2.5 个月)方面的改善均优于安慰剂[348]。阿帕替尼的毒副反应包括高血压和手足综合征,符合其作用机制。该结果仍需后续研究确认。

非小细胞肺癌

血管新生抑制剂作为单药治疗晚期非小细胞肺癌

靶向 VEGF 的抑制剂作为单药治疗晚期非小细胞肺癌时,其客观肿瘤反应率通常较低。在一项化疗单药或联合贝伐单抗治疗非小细胞肺癌(NSCLC)的Ⅱ期临床试验中,对照组的 19 名患者在疾病进展后接受了高剂量贝伐单抗单药治疗,虽然其中 5 名患者病情稳定,但并没有肿瘤出现客观反应[349]。尽管到目前为止还没有研究表明与化疗或其他靶向药相比 VEGFR TKI 能够延长患者的 OS,但 VEGFR TKI 作为单药在 NSCLC 中有明显的抗肿瘤活性。

凡德他尼(Vandetanib)是一种 VEGFR/EGFR 双靶向抑制剂,是迄今为止研究最为透彻的药物之一。在一项包含 168 例局部晚期或转移性的、对铂类耐受的 NSCLC 患者的随机Ⅱ期临床试验中,接受凡德他尼治疗与接受吉非替尼(gefitinib)治疗的患者相比中位 PFS 有一定的改善,并且差异具有统计学意义(11.0 周比 8.1 周,$P=0.011$)[350]。一项Ⅱ期临床研究在 181 例初治 NSCLC 患者中直接比较了凡德他尼与化疗(卡铂和紫杉醇)或凡德他尼联合化疗的疗效[351]。与单纯化疗相比,凡德他尼组患者的 PFS 有下降的趋势(11.5 周比 23.1 周,P 值无统计学意义)。凡德他尼治疗 NSCLC 患者的Ⅲ期临床试验已经完成[352]。另一项Ⅲ期研究比较了凡德他尼与标准二线药物厄罗替尼(erlotinib)的疗效,发现凡德他尼治疗的患者与厄罗替尼相比 PFS 没有显著改善(PFS 中位数为 2.6 个月比 2.0 个月)。次要研究终点包括 OS(HR=1.01;$P=0.83$)、ORR(均为 12%)疼痛症状恶化时间(HR=0.92;$P=0.28$)均无显著性差异。在非劣效性分析中,两种药物的 PFS 和 OS 相似[353]。

索拉菲尼在晚期复发性 NSCLC 中也显示出了单药活性。在一项随机停药的Ⅱ期临床试验(ECOG2501)中,经索拉菲尼治疗病情稳定的 NSCLC 患者(N=97)被随机分为索拉菲尼继续治疗组和安慰剂组[354]。索拉菲尼组的 PFS 明显长于安慰剂组(3.6 个月比 1.9 个月,$P=0.01$)。有趣的是,只有一个病人的肿瘤有客观反应,这说明 NSCLC 与 RCC 类似[303],其客观肿瘤反应率可能不是早期药物研究中最合适的疗效判定指标。

舒尼替尼在复发性 NSCLC 患者中也显示出令人鼓舞的单药活性[355]。在 63 例患者中有 7 例发生了客观肿瘤反应(ORR 11.1%),70%患者的肿瘤出现了一定程度的缩小。总的来说,舒尼替尼的安全性是可以接受的,但仍有两名鳞状细胞癌患者死于治疗相关的肺出血。患者在接受其他血管新生抑制剂治疗时也出现了这种毒副作用,导致贝伐单抗和其他几种药物的适应证中剔除了肺鳞状细胞癌。

帕唑帕尼(Pazopanib,葛兰素史克公司)是一种靶向 VEGFR、PDGFR、FGFR-1 和 FGFR-3 的 TKI,其作为新辅助治疗在Ⅰ/Ⅱ期 NSCLC 中表现出了令人鼓舞的疗效[356],其可耐受的毒副反应包括高血压、腹泻和疲劳。该药物在 NSCLC 辅助治疗和晚期 NSCLC 治疗中的活性和有效性目前正在研究中[357]。其他 VEGFR TKI 包括瓦他拉尼、阿西替尼[358]和 XL647 在晚期 NSCLC 中也显示出了单药活性[359]。

贝伐单抗联合化疗治疗晚期 NSCLC

由于血管新生抑制剂的单药活性较弱,因此其通常与化疗联合用于 NSCLC 的治疗。最初Ⅱ期临床试验表明,在未接受过化疗的晚期 NSCLC 患者中,贝伐单抗联合标准的卡铂和紫杉醇双重化疗方案可以改善患者的 ORR 和 TTP[349]。在这项研究中还出现了一个意想不到且令人担忧的副作用:严重的肺出血——贝伐单抗治疗组的 67 例患者中 6 例发生了肺出血,其中 4 例死亡。与严重咯血相关的肿瘤特征包括:肿瘤位于中心位置、肿瘤靠近主要血管、治疗前或治疗中肿瘤出现坏死和空腔化以及鳞状组织亚型。由于鳞状细胞癌通常位于肺中央,且比腺癌更容易空腔化,因此尚不清楚鳞状组织亚型是否是咯血的主要危险因素,还是仅仅是其他危险因素的一个替代品。

基于上述Ⅱ期临床试验中贝伐单抗的良好疗效,美国东部肿瘤协作团体(Eastern Cooperative Oncology Group,ECOG)开展了一项编号为 E4599 的随机Ⅱ/Ⅲ期临床试验,在 878 名初治的晚期(肿瘤分期ⅢB 或Ⅳ期)非鳞状 NSCLC 患者中,比较了标准的卡铂和紫杉醇六个疗程化疗或化疗联合贝伐单抗的疗效[302]。与单纯接受卡铂-紫杉醇化疗相比,接受卡铂-紫杉醇和贝伐单抗联合治疗的患者的中位 OS(12.3 个月比 10.3 个月,HR=0.77,$P=0.003$)、中位 PFS(6.2 个月比 4.5 个月,$P<0.0001$)和反应率(35%比 15%,$P<0.001$)均显著改善。与贝伐单抗相关的主要 3 级或更高级别的毒副作用是出血(贝伐单抗组 4.4%,标准化疗组 0.7%)、发热性中性粒细胞减少症和高血压。在排除了肺鳞状细胞癌患者后,贝伐单抗组致死性咯血的总发生率约为 1%。考虑到贝伐单抗组患者的 1 年和 2 年生存率分别提高了 7% 和 8%,上述毒副反应风险还是可以接受的。

有趣的是,通过对 E4599 研究的分组分析,研究者意外发现尽管女性患者接受贝伐单抗治疗后确实在肿瘤反应率和 PFS 方面有所受益,但贝伐单抗组的生存获益主要还是来源于男性患者[360]。出现这种明显性别差异的原因还不清楚。在老年患者(>70 岁)中,贝伐单抗治疗组的毒副反应发生率似乎有所增加,但其 OS 并没有明显的改善[361]。

E4599 是首个表明靶向治疗与标准化疗联合可以显著改善晚期 NSCLC 患者 OS 的随机Ⅲ期研究。另一项类似的随机Ⅲ期临床试验(AVAIL)测试了贝伐单抗联合另一种标准化疗方案(顺铂+吉西他滨)在 NSCLC 中的治疗效果[362]。该研究共纳入了 1 043 名患者,患者被随机分配到联合用药组——低剂量(7.5mg/kg)或高剂量(15mg/kg)贝伐单抗+顺铂-吉西他滨化疗(每 3 周 1 次)及对照组(单用顺铂-吉西他滨)。与单用顺铂-吉西他滨组相比,贝伐单抗联合化疗组患者的 PFS 和

ORR 得到了明显的改善,但 OS 并没有提高。低剂量和高剂量的贝伐单抗在疗效和毒副反应方面没有显著差异。该临床试验结果与抗血管新生药物促进血管正常化的假说是一致的[363]。

目前,临床试验正在检测贝伐单抗联合化疗在 NSCLC 新辅助或辅助治疗中的作用。Ⅱ期临床试验——BEACON 正在研究在基于顺铂化疗的治疗方案中加入贝伐单抗是否能够提高 NSCLC 新辅助治疗的反应率。ECOG 的临床试验 E1505 是一项Ⅲ期随机研究,该研究在接受手术切除治疗的 IB～ⅢA 期 NSCLC 患者中,对比了术后接受辅助化疗或辅助化疗联合贝伐单抗治疗的疗效,目前该研究已经结束,后续将公布结果。

基于以上这些结果,一些肿瘤学家认为贝伐单抗联合卡铂-紫杉醇是一种新的针对非鳞状 NSCLC 的标准治疗方案。虽然有前述 AVAIL 研究的结果作为参考,但对于初治的 NSCLC 患者,贝伐单抗联合任何含铂类治疗是否能获得类似的治疗效果,以及在患者选择时是否应参考额外的临床标准如性别或年龄,目前仍没有定论。

雷莫芦单抗联合化疗治疗难治性 NSCLC

FDA 最近批准了雷莫芦单抗联合二线多烯紫杉醇治疗复发性 NSCLC。批准的依据是Ⅲ期 REVEL 试验的结果。REVEL 试验是一项包含了 1 253 名非鳞状细胞和鳞状细胞 NSCLC 患者的国际研究,这些局部晚期或肿瘤转移的患者在接受了基于铂类的化疗后,疾病发生了进展[364]。这些患者被随机分配到雷莫芦单抗联合多烯紫杉醇治疗组或安慰剂联合多烯紫杉醇组。与安慰剂组相比,雷莫芦单抗治疗组患者的中位 OS(10.5 个月比 9.1 个月;HR=0.857;P=0.235)和中位 PFS(4.5 个月比 3.0 个月;HR=0.762;P<0.000 1)均显著改善。雷莫芦单抗治疗组的 ORR 也有所改善(23%比 14%;P<0.000 1)。相比于安慰剂组,雷莫芦单抗治疗组患者更常见的≤3 级毒副反应是中性粒细胞减少(48.8%比 39.8%)、发热性中性粒细胞减少(15.9%比 10.0%)、疲劳(14.0%比 10.5%)、白细胞减少(13.7%比 12.5%)和高血压(5.6%比 2.1%)。与安慰剂组相比,雷莫芦单抗治疗组的出血事件更多,但两组中 3 级或更高级别出血事件的发生率类似。

VEGFR TKI 联合化疗一线治疗 NSCLC

随机临床试验也正在评估 VEGFR TKI/化疗联合作为一线方案治疗晚期 NSCLC 的效果。Ⅲ期临床试验 ESCAPE(Evaluation of Sorafenib, Carboplatin and Paclitaxel Efficacy in NSCLC——评估索拉菲尼、卡铂和紫杉醇对 NSCLC 的疗效)在 926 名患者中比较了卡铂-紫杉醇化疗或化疗联合索拉菲尼治疗 NSCLC 的效果,结果发现索拉菲尼的加入未能显著提高非鳞状细胞癌患者的 OS,并且在亚组分析中还发现索拉菲尼的加入会对鳞状细胞癌患者产生不利的影响[365]。Ⅲ期临床试验 NexUS (NCT00449033)评估了顺铂-吉西他滨化疗或化疗联合索拉菲尼治疗 NSCLC 的疗效,由于未能达到研究设计的 OS 主要终点,试验被提前终止。

西地尼布(cediranib)是一种口服的靶向 VEGFR、PDGFR 和 KIT 的 TKI。加拿大国家癌症研究所(National Cancer Institute of Canada, NCIC)开展了编号为 BR24 的Ⅱ/Ⅲ期临床试验,检测了西地尼布联合卡铂-紫杉醇在 296 名肺癌患者中的治疗效果[366]。虽然在西地尼布组中观察到患者的 PFS 和 ORR 有所改善,但按照预先的计划,在Ⅱ期试验结束时通过对试验情况的分析,研究者发现了大量的与剂量相关的副作用(脱水、腹泻和疲劳等),因此终止了该临床试验。类似的Ⅱ期试验 N0528 评估了吉西他滨-卡铂化疗或化疗联合西地尼布(每日 45mg 口服)治疗肺癌的安全性和有效性。结果显示,联合组和单纯化疗组相比,反应率(20%比 18%;P=1.0)、中位 PFS(6.3 个月比 4.5 个月;HR=0.69;p=0.15)和中位 OS(11.8 个月比 9.9 个月;HR=0.66;P=0.16)均无明显差异,西地尼布治疗组患者 3 级及以上毒副反应的发生率有所提高(71%比 45%;P=0.01)[367]。

考虑到严重的毒副反应,NCIC 设计了与上述研究类似的 BR29 Ⅲ期临床试验,进一步评估了西地尼布(20mg)联合卡铂-紫杉醇在 NSCLC 中的疗效。但研究的中期分析显示,联合用药的疗效不足,因此研究被终止[368]。

如前所述,有研究在 181 例肺癌患者中评估了凡德他尼联合卡铂-紫杉醇(vandetanib with carboplatin-paclitaxel, VCP)对比卡铂-紫杉醇或凡德他尼单药的疗效[351]。结果显示,VCP 即使在鳞状细胞组织亚型和肺癌脑转移接受过治疗的患者中也可以安全使用。与卡铂-紫杉醇相比,接受 VCP 治疗的患者 ORR (32%比 25%)和 PFS(24 周比 23 周;HR=0.76,单侧 P=0.098)有改善的趋势。

尼达尼布除了对 VEGFR 有活性外,还对 PDGFR 和 FGFR 有抑制活性。一项Ⅱ期临床研究显示,在接受过治疗的 NSCLC 中,尼达尼布作为单药有一定的抗肿瘤活性,48%的患者在接受治疗后疾病稳定[369]。尼达尼布联合化疗的二期临床试验目前正在进行中。综上所述,目前为止,VEGFR TKI 联合化疗作为一线方案治疗 NSCLC 的临床试验结果并不尽人意,其疗效的进展十分有限,在某些情况下还有很大的毒副作用。

VEGFR TKI 联合化疗治疗复发性 NSCLC

凡德他尼也被用于联合多烯紫杉醇治疗既往接受过含铂类药物化疗的 NSCLC 患者[370]。127 名患者被随机分配至多烯紫杉醇联合低剂量(100mg,每日 1 次)或高剂量(300mg,每日 1 次)凡德他尼组。该研究达到了其设计的主要终点,凡德他尼治疗延长了患者的中位 PFS,但有趣的是,低剂量组患者的获益趋势更大(低剂量组、高剂量组和对照组的 PFS 分别为 19 周、17 周和 12 周)。在这些结果的基础上,研究者进行了一项随机Ⅲ期临床试验(ZODIAC),比较了凡德他尼(100mg 每天)联合多烯紫杉醇与多烯紫杉醇单药在 NSCLC 中的疗效。该研究达到了其主要的终点,凡德他尼延长了患者 PFS(HR=0.79, P<0.001),但患者的 OS 并未得到显著改善[352]。基于该研究的一项生物标志物分析表明,EGFR 拷贝数增加的患者在接受凡德他尼治疗后获益更大[371]。

最近的一项随机Ⅲ期临床试验——LUME-Lung 1 检测了尼达尼布在铂类耐受型 NSCLC 患者中的治疗效果。该临床试验比较了多烯紫杉醇联合尼达尼布或安慰剂在 NSCLC 患者中的疗效,结果显示无论在哪种组织类型中,与对照组相比,尼达尼布组患者的 PFS 都显著延长(HR=0.79;P=0.001 9;鳞状细胞癌 HR=0.77, P=0.02;腺癌 HR=0.77, P=0.001 9)[372]。此外,接受尼达尼布治疗的肺腺癌患者的 OS 也明显延长(HR=0.83;P=0.035 9;中位 OS 为 12.6 个月比 10.3 个月),但鳞状细胞癌患者中未出现这种情况。LUME-Lung 2A 研究旨在检测尼达尼布联合培美曲塞的疗效,初步的结果表明,尼达尼布联合治疗可以显著改善铂类耐受型非鳞状细胞癌患者的 PFS,而对 OS 的影响不大[373]。基于以上结果,欧盟(European Union, EU)最近批准了尼达尼布用于 NSCLC 的治疗。此外,基于两个随机Ⅲ期临床试验的数据,FDA 和 EU 还批准了尼达尼布用于特发性肺纤维化的治疗[374,375]。

抗血管新生药物联合其他靶向药物治疗 NSCLC

调控肿瘤血管新生和肿瘤细胞存活的分子通路十分复杂,两者间还存在一定程度的交互[241,376]。因此,靶向单一通路的治疗方法通常不能长期控制肿瘤,并不可避免的会产生肿瘤耐药。靶向药物的联合使用则不仅可以提高临床治疗效果,同时还可以避免化疗相关的毒副作用。由于 EGFR 和 VEGF 是已知的相互关联的有效治疗靶点,因此研究者正在 NSCLC 和其他一些疾病中开展同时阻断这两条通路的临床研究。抑制 EGFR 可能通过 HIF-α 依赖和非依赖的机制下调 VEGF[233,257,259,260,377~379],同时 EGFR 与 VEGFR-2 一样,可能也在肿瘤相关内皮细胞上表达[380~382]。临床前的研究发现,肿瘤对 EGFR 抑制剂产生获得性耐药与 VEGF 水平升高和肿瘤血管新生增加有关[383]。

临床上已经开展了同时抑制 VEGF 和 EGFR 的研究,其中既包括单一靶向药物的联合应用,也包括同时靶向两个靶点的多靶点 TKI(如上文提到的凡德他尼)作为单药进行治疗。一项随机Ⅱ期临床试验比较了贝伐单抗和厄洛替尼联合与单纯化疗(多烯紫杉醇或培美曲塞)或化疗联合贝伐单抗在难治性或复发性 NSCLC 患者中的治疗作用[384]。与化疗相比,贝伐单抗-厄洛替尼组患者的 PFS 和耐受性有提高的趋势。研究者们随后开展了一项随机Ⅲ期临床研究——BETA(BEvacizumab/TArceva,贝伐单抗/特罗凯)试验,在 636 名二线患者中比较了贝伐单抗-厄洛替尼联合与厄洛替尼单药的治疗效果。与厄洛替尼组相比,贝伐单抗-厄洛替尼联合组患者的 PFS(3.4 个月比 1.7 个月)和 ORR 有所改善,但 OS 并没有延长(9.3 个月比 9.2 个月)。然而,在携带 EGFR 突变的患者中,这种组合的疗效似乎更显著。另一项针对 EGFR 突变型 NSCLC 的Ⅲ期临床研究(厄洛替尼单药对比厄洛替尼联合贝伐单抗)证实了上述发现[385]。携带 EGFR 突变的 NSCLC 对贝伐单抗高度敏感的分子机制还不完全清楚,可能是由于这些肿瘤存在 HIF-1α 组成型激活,从而对 VEGFR 信号通路更加依赖[260]。此外,有研究在临床前模型中发现,EGFR TKI 耐药与 VEGF 的升高有关[386]。最后,ATLAS Ⅲ期临床研究在接受过一线治疗的 NSCLC 患者中对比了贝伐单抗-厄洛替尼联合与贝伐单抗-安慰剂联合作为维持方案的治疗效果,由于中期分析显示贝伐单抗-厄洛替尼联合可显著改善患者的 PFS,因此该实验被提前终止[387]。总之,这些数据支持采用联合抑制 VEGF 和 EGFR 的方法来治疗携带 EGFR 突变的 NSCLC。

可手术 NSCLC 的抗血管新生治疗

临床试验同样也在研究血管新生抑制剂作为新辅助或辅助治疗方案在可手术的 NSCLC 中的疗效。一项术前的临床试验发现 VEGFR TKI 帕唑帕尼具有显著的抗肿瘤活性,可以使 87% 患者的肿瘤体积缩小[388]。Ⅲ期随机试验(ECOG1505)正在接受了完全手术切除的ⅠB~ⅢA 期 NSCLC 患者中检测与四个周期的标准化疗相比,化疗联合贝伐单抗是否能够改善患者的预后。

乳腺癌

抗血管新生药物对转移性乳腺癌患者 OS 的改善作用未能通过临床试验的验证,因而目前 FDA 还没有批准任何抗血管新生药物用于乳腺癌的治疗。一项随机临床研究在 715 名初治转移性 HER2 阴性乳腺癌患者中比较了紫杉醇单药或联合贝伐单抗的疗效,基于该研究的结果,贝伐单抗于 2008 年获得了 FDA 的加速批准[389]。该研究显示贝伐单抗联合治疗显著提高了反应率(21%提高至 37%)和患者的 PFS(5.9 个月提高至 11.8 个月),但对 OS 无明显影响。加速批准是有条件的,需要进一步开展研究以提供更多贝伐单抗可以改善生存的证据。AVADO 研究检测了多烯紫杉醇单药或联合贝伐单抗的疗效,数据显示贝伐单抗联合治疗组的反应率和患者的 PFS 也有类似的改善,但 HER2 阴性患者的 OS 没有改善[390]。同样,RIBBON-1 研究也显示,化疗联合贝伐单抗与化疗单药治疗相比,反应率和 PFS 有所提高,但 OS 没有改善[391]。在 HER2 阳性患者的研究中,与多烯紫杉醇联合曲妥珠单抗治疗相比,贝伐单抗联合治疗能提高反应率(77%比 66%),但未能改善患者的 PFS 或 OS[392]。基于以上结果,FDA 于 2011 年撤销了对贝伐单抗治疗乳腺癌的批准。同样令人失望的结果也出现在 ROSE 研究中,该研究评估了雷莫芦单抗联合多烯紫杉醇的疗效,联合治疗未能改善患者的 PFS[393]。

AVADO 研究的后续分析表明,患者血浆的高 VEGF-A 水平有可能成为预测贝伐单抗疗效的生物标志物[394]。前瞻性研究 MERiDiAN 正在验证上述假设,该研究的主要疗效终点是血浆高 VEGF-A 水平人群的 PFS。

肝癌

肝癌(肝细胞癌)是一种全球性的恶性肿瘤,几十年来其预后一直较差,并且缺乏有效的治疗药物。抗血管新生疗法的出现为肝癌治疗带来了新的希望。

在一项随机安慰剂对照的Ⅲ期临床试验中,与对照相比,索拉菲尼延长了患者的 OS(5.5 个月比 2.5 个月)[395]。目前临床试验正在检测多种抗血管新生药物的疗效。

其他恶性肿瘤

其他多种恶性肿瘤都开展了抗血管新生治疗(特别是抗 VEGF 治疗)的临床试验,并在某些肿瘤中取得了初步的阳性结果(也有一部分试验失败)。本书的其他章节已介绍了这些临床研究的情况,在此仅作简要总结。

胰腺癌:一项大型Ⅲ期临床试验比较了吉西他滨联合贝伐单抗与吉西他滨联合安慰剂在胰腺癌中的疗效,结果是阴性的。胰腺癌仍是抗血管新生治疗的难点。

软组织肉瘤:2012 年,Ⅲ期临床研究——PALETTE(NCT00753688)取得了阳性结果,FDA 因此批准了帕唑帕尼治疗转移性非脂肪细胞性软组织肉瘤[396]。

卵巢癌:Ⅲ期临床研究——AURELIA 显示,化疗联合贝伐单抗可以显著改善铂类耐药型卵巢癌患者的 PFS 和 ORR,因此 2014 年贝伐单抗获 FDA 批准用于卵巢癌的治疗[397]。

宫颈癌:Ⅲ期临床试验(GOG 240)检测了贝伐单抗和非铂类化疗组合对晚期宫颈癌患者的疗效,基于该研究的结果,

FDA 批准了贝伐单抗用于持续性、复发性或晚期宫颈癌的治疗[398]。

胶质母细胞瘤：虽然早期的临床研究显示贝伐单抗似乎对胶质母细胞瘤有不错的疗效[399,400]，但在进一步的Ⅲ期临床试验中，贝伐单抗并没有改善新发胶质母细胞瘤患者的 OS[401]。Ⅲ期临床研究（REGAL）在复发性胶质母细胞瘤患者中对比了西地拉尼单药或联合洛莫司汀（lomustine）与洛莫司汀单药的疗效，结果也是阴性的[402]。

胶质瘤：一些研究抗 VEGF 治疗的Ⅱ期临床试验表明贝伐单抗单药对晚期胶质瘤有一定的治疗效果。基于这些阳性结果，研究者已将数据提交 FDA 以获得加速批准，并开展了概念验证性的Ⅲ期临床试验。

非霍奇金淋巴瘤：几个Ⅱ期临床试验报道了抗 VEGF 治疗的早期阳性结果，并因此启动了Ⅲ期临床试验，目前正在进行中。

抗血管新生治疗的毒副作用

开发血管新生抑制剂是希望能够提供一种相对无毒的方法来减缓或阻止肿瘤的生长，并且这种方法可以长期使用，目的是将癌症转化为一种可控的慢性疾病。根据已有的临床经验，似乎血管新生抑制剂的副作用确实总体上是可以接受的，与化疗的副作用也并不重叠。然而，某些毒副反应似乎是各类抗血管新生药物所特有的，在某些情况下甚至会威胁患者的生命。

单纯的 VEGF 拮抗剂（如贝伐单抗）为研究阻断 VEGF 后产生的生理和病理生理效应提供了一个重要的渠道；同时阻断 VEGF 和其他激酶（如索拉非尼和舒尼替尼）的药物会产生与被阻断的激酶相关的特异的副作用。还可能发生额外的药物特异的异质性副作用。此外，在多种疾病的治疗中，由于抗血管新生药物通常是与化疗药物联合使用的，而且常常会延长患者的 PFS，因而化疗相关的副作用可能会随着药物使用时间的延长而增加。例如，在 E2100 Ⅲ期乳腺癌临床试验中，在接受了贝伐单抗和基于紫杉醇的化疗联合治疗后，患者受到了 VEGF 相关副作用的严重困扰，如高血压、脑血管缺血、头痛和蛋白尿，以及 3 级和 4 级的毒性反应如感染、疲劳和感觉神经病变[389]。感染和疲劳等毒性反应很可能是患者长期化疗的结果，因为接受贝伐单抗治疗的患者在 PFS 延长的同时，其接受紫杉醇化疗的时间也相应延长了。

多项Ⅲ期临床试验的开展使我们能够在大规模人群中评估这些毒副反应，而较小的临床研究则侧重于评估个体的毒副反应。在本节中，我们将重点讨论与 VEGF 直接相关及与 VEGF 拮抗基本原理（如在正常组织中配体-受体相互作用）有关的毒副反应。这些副作用包括在大多数疾病中使用抗 VEGF 治疗时出现的毒性，以及一些虽然机制上与 VEGF 拮抗相关、但在某些特定疾病中更常见的副作用（如肠穿孔和肺出血）。非特异性 RTKI 治疗时出现的与 VEGF 抑制无关的副作用将不在这里讨论。

高血压

在接受抗 VEGF 治疗的患者中最常见的毒副反应是高血压。通常是轻度到中度，很少有严重（恶性）高血压的报道。高血压被认为与血管内皮功能的改变有关，而 VEGF 受体下游一氧化氮通路的阻断会影响血管内皮的功能[403]。与抗 VEGF 治疗相反，VEGF 输注与血压降低有关。尽管抗 VEGF 相关高血压似乎对标准的降压药物有反应，并且在抗 VEGF 治疗停止后是可逆的，但临床上并未仔细研究如何处理抗 VEGF 相关的高血压。对于出现轻度至中度高血压副作用的患者，可以在适当的降压药物治疗下继续抗 VEGF 治疗。最近的数据表明，出现高血压副作用可能与患者预后的改善有关，高血压可能是预测肿瘤反应的一种药代动力学或药效动力学的替代标志物[404]。对 E2100 Ⅲ期乳腺癌临床试验的分析发现，高血压与 VEGF 特定的单核苷酸多态性之间存在关联，这还有待进一步证实[405]。最近一项研究对贝伐单抗和化疗治疗 NSCLC 的Ⅲ期试验（ECOG 4599）进行了亚组分析，结果显示在贝伐单抗治疗的患者中，高血压副作用的出现与患者临床预后改善正相关[406]。同样，通过对六项评估阿西替尼在不同类型实体肿瘤患者中疗效的Ⅱ期临床试验数据进行分析，研究者发现舒张压>90mmHg 可能作为患者生存期延长的生物标志物[325]。目前仍需要进一步的前瞻性研究来验证高血压作为临床反应生物标志物是否可靠。

动脉血栓栓塞

在一部分 VEGF 抑制剂的临床试验中，患者血栓栓塞和心血管事件的发生率有所增加。这些毒副反应虽然不常见，但可能十分严重并危及生命。5 个贝伐单抗的Ⅲ期临床试验（所有试验均排除了近期有中风或心脏病发作史的患者）所汇总的数据显示，血栓栓塞和心血管事件的 HR 为 2.0，患者的绝对风险从对照组的 1.7%增加到贝伐单抗治疗组的 3.8%。而静脉血栓栓塞事件并没有出现相应的增加。贝伐单抗引起的脑血管缺血可能包括短暂性缺血发作或中风；心肌梗死和心绞痛的发生率也有所增加[407]。这些毒副反应在老年（>65 岁）和有动脉血栓栓塞病史的患者中更为常见。这些毒副反应的处理与未接受抗 VEGF 治疗的患者类似。患者在接受抗 VEGF 治疗时出现高血压，通常可以通过抗高血压治疗来处理，相比之下，如果出现动脉血栓栓塞事件，停止 VEGF 靶向治疗则可能更合适。

接受 VEGF 靶向治疗的患者经常出现头痛症状，在Ⅲ期试验中大约 3%的时间会出现严重头痛。这些头痛本质上是典型的偏头疼，而且似乎对血清素受体活性药物等抗偏头痛药物的治疗有反应。头痛可能会复发，如果肿瘤持续对抗 VEGF 治疗有反应并需继续接受治疗时，患者可能需要长期使用慢性抗偏头痛药物如 β 受体阻断剂等来缓解症状。这种头痛与更严重的中枢神经系统缺血事件之间的关系尚不清楚。

可逆性脑后部白质病变综合征

可逆性脑后部白质病变综合征（reversible posterior leukoencephalopathy syndrome，RPLS）是抗 VEGF 治疗的一种罕见性中枢神经系统并发症。RPLS 是一种亚急性神经综合征，典型的症状包括头痛、皮质盲和癫痫，有报道在接受 VEGF 靶向治疗的患者中出现过该症状。尽管有研究表明脑后动脉的血管痉挛可能导致了 RPLS，但目前 RPLS 的病因及其与 VEGF 抑制的关系均不清楚。RPLS 发生后应立即停止抗 VEGF 治疗并进行适当的抗高血压处理（高血压是 RPLS 一个潜在的诱发因素）[408,409]。

肾毒性

肾毒性通常以蛋白尿的形式出现，在长期接受抗 VEGF 治疗的患者中很常见，多达40%的患者至少有一定程度的蛋白尿症状。更严重的蛋白质损失（如肾病综合征）在患者中较为罕见，发生率约1%~2%。虽然研究还不透彻，但研究者发现停止抗VEGF治疗后蛋白尿症状是可以逆转的，并且患者后续还可以继续接受抗VEGF治疗。一种标准的处理方法是，当尿蛋白排出≥2g/24h时，暂时停用贝伐单抗，当蛋白排出<2g/24h时，恢复使用贝伐单抗。若出现了肾病性的蛋白尿，则应当停止贝伐单抗治疗。从机制的角度看，VEGF在肾小球内环境稳定中起着重要作用，因此抗VEGF治疗产生肾毒性并不令人惊讶[410]。最近的一项研究将贝伐单抗引起的蛋白尿与肾血栓性微血管病联系起来，表明VEGF在预防肾血栓性微血管病中有重要的作用[411]。

肺出血

在一项肺癌早期Ⅱ期临床试验中，患者出现了肺出血的毒性副反应，该试验还观察到了致命的出血事件[349]。这个试验表明鳞状细胞癌患者发生该并发症的风险会增加，因而概念验证性的NSCLC Ⅲ期临床试验（E4599）排除了出现咯血症状（每次咯血量等于或超过1/2茶匙）以及接受抗凝治疗或非甾体类抗炎药物治疗的患者。尽管如此，危及生命的肺出血的发生率仍高达1.9%（1.2%是致死事件），表明我们仍不能很好地预测哪些患者将发生这种并发症[302]。应当将肺出血事件作为知情同意的一部分，并告知所有接受贝伐单抗或其他VEGF靶向药物治疗的肺癌患者。这种副作用的机制例如它的量效关系尚不清楚。肺出血常见于鳞状细胞肺癌患者可能与这类癌症容易发生中央坏死有关；同时中心空腔化在接受抗VEGF治疗的肺癌中也很常见。

肠穿孔

肠穿孔常见于晚期结直肠癌和卵巢癌患者，但据报道，尽管在非腹部或骨盆的癌症中发生率较低，但几乎所有接受贝伐单抗治疗的癌症类型都出现过肠穿孔。近期的一项分析表明，发生这种并发症的患者30天内的死亡率为12.5%，可见其严重性[412]。有综述提出，原发肿瘤完整、近期接受过乙状结肠镜或结肠镜检查、或既往接受过腹部或盆腔放疗的患者发生肠穿孔的概率更高。有趣的是，既往消化性溃疡史、憩室病史或使用过非甾体抗炎药与肠穿孔并没有明显的关联[413]。目前，我们还没有有效的排除指标来防止患者发生这种并发症。虽然临床前证据表明抗VEGF治疗可能会大大降低正常小肠绒毛的血管密度，但肠穿孔的确切病因仍不清楚[414]。当抗VEGF治疗与放疗联合使用时，肠穿孔可能会加剧[294]。

控制肠穿孔的关键在于对其症状的认知和识别以及紧急的手术干预。在抗VEGF治疗时进行手术干预可能会增加患者术后并发症的风险，例如进一步的肠穿孔和腹部瘘。然而，患者有生命危险时，即使有并发症风险，实施外科干预仍然是必要的[191,415]。

抗血管新生治疗相关临床研究的经验教训和未来方向

缩小抗血管新生治疗临床前研究和临床应用之间疗效的差异

虽然在临床前动物模型中，单一的抗血管新生药物就可以显著影响肿瘤的生长，但在针对患者的临床试验中，大多数抗血管新生药物必须与其他治疗方案联合使用才能有效。这种抗肿瘤活性的不同主要是因为小鼠肿瘤模型和癌症患者之间存在一些关键的差异。与实验模型相比，患者在肿瘤异质性和遗传背景方面的差异更大。此外，在小鼠癌症模型中，肿瘤的生长速度往往很快，这可能会提高肿瘤对抗血管新生药物的敏感性。在临床前模型中，通常在肿瘤发展的早期就开始进行治疗，而在临床上，患者在接受治疗时肿瘤可能已经存在多年，并且临床试验通常包含了晚期、转移性的肿瘤患者[416]。

VEGF通路抑制剂的耐药机制

对大多数实体肿瘤来说，传统化疗的治疗效果在一定程度上受限于肿瘤细胞快速突变产生的耐药性。由于抗血管新生药物是针对肿瘤内皮细胞的，而肿瘤内皮细胞是二倍体且基因稳定，因此最初研究者认为肿瘤不会像对细胞毒性化疗那样对抗血管新生治疗产生耐药性[191,415]。然而，迄今为止的临床经验表明，几乎所有肿瘤在VEGF抑制剂治疗后最终都会进展。已有研究提出了肿瘤对VEGF通路抑制剂产生原发性或获得性耐药、或至少对VEGF通路抑制剂敏感性降低的几种可能机制[149,417]。

靶点抑制不彻底

药物可能无法在足够长的时间内维持足够高的浓度，从而不能持续地抑制VEGF受体信号通路和肿瘤血管的新生。在检测VEGFR抑制剂SU5416和SU6668疗效的临床试验中，治疗前和治疗中的肿瘤活检显示，所有病例中VEGFR磷酸化的抑制率都<50%，这可能是导致这些试验得不到阳性结果的原因之一[418,419]。对于其他TKI，如吉非替尼和伊马替尼，靶点抑制不彻底已经被证明是由基因变异造成的，例如EGFR或BCR-ABL的继发性突变，或是由于表观遗传改变降低了细胞内抑制剂的浓度[420~422]。目前尚不清楚肿瘤内皮细胞是否存在VEGFR突变。

通过表达其他血管新生因子绕开VEGF通路

肿瘤基因突变或HIF-1等通路的激活可能会导致肿瘤细胞表达其他血管新生因子（或血管新生抑制因子表达降低）[232,423]。反过来，即使在VEGF阻断的情况下，这些变化仍可能会促进肿瘤内皮细胞的增殖和生存。例如，相比早期乳腺癌，晚期乳腺癌会表达更多的促血管新生因子[424]，这可能有助于解释为什么相比于先前接受过治疗的患者，贝伐单抗联合标准化疗对初治转移性乳腺癌患者的疗效更佳[425,426]。

最近，Cascone等[427]在人类肺腺癌的小鼠移植瘤模型中发现，与贝伐单抗获得性耐药相关的基因表达变化主要发生在间质细胞而非肿瘤细胞中。其中，EGFR和FGFR信号通路在间质中上调，在对VEGF抑制剂产生获得性耐药的移植瘤的周细胞中、以及对VEGF抑制剂原发性耐药的肿瘤内皮细胞中，活化EGFR的表达增加。此外，血管系统模式的改变也体现了肿瘤的耐药表型。对贝伐单抗产生获得性耐药的人NSCLC小鼠模型的特征是出现周细胞覆盖的、正常化的血管重建，而原发性耐药动物模型的特征则是曲折、无周细胞覆盖的血管。同时抑制VEGF和EGFR两条通路降低了血管周细胞的覆盖率，并延长了荷瘤动物的PFS，提示肿瘤间质通路的改变可能导致NSCLC对VEGF抑制剂产生耐药，而靶向这些通路则可能提高治疗的效果。评估 FOLFIRI 联合贝伐单抗治疗结直肠癌的Ⅱ期临床试验发现，IL-8 基线水平较高患者的 PFS 较差。在同一研究中，在肿瘤出现影像学进展之前，相比于基线，循环中与血管新生和髓细胞募集相关的几种促血管新生细胞因子（如 FGF、HGF、PlGF、SDF 和 MCP）的水平出现了升高[428]。

大量的研究表明肿瘤可以通过增加其他血管新生因子的表达来逃避对 VEGFR 通路的抑制。在临床前模型中，抑制 FGFR 通路可以恢复肿瘤对 VEGF 靶向药物的敏感性[83]。有研究发现 Galectin-1（Gal1）参与了肿瘤对抗血管新生治疗的抵抗。在低氧条件下，Gal1 的表达上调并调节 EGFR 和 VEGF 的转运，促进肿瘤血管新生。在培养的内皮细胞中，GAL1 与 VEGF3R2 上的中性分支 N-聚糖结合，导致 VEGFR2 发生信号转导并停留在细胞表面。在动物实验中，与对抗 VEGF 治疗敏感的肿瘤相比，抗 VEGF 难治性肿瘤的缺氧和 Gal1 表达水平都较高。因而同时靶向 Gal1 和 VEGF 能够提高抗肿瘤活性[429]。

髓细胞的浸润增加也与肿瘤对抗血管新生治疗的耐药性有关[430]。与对抗血管新生药物敏感的肿瘤相比，难治性肿瘤中 CD11b+Gr1+的骨髓源性抑制细胞（myeloid-derived suppressor cell，MDSC）的数量增加[148]。最近的研究发现，Th17（T helper type 17）细胞产生的 IL-17 通过上调 G-CSF 促进 IL-17 依赖、VEGF 不依赖的血管新生，从而导致骨髓和脾脏的 MDSC 向肿瘤动员和募集[431]。在小鼠中，IL-17 被抑制后，抗 VEGF 治疗对难治性肿瘤的疗效得到改善。

缺氧诱导的细胞凋亡阈值改变

抗血管新生治疗会引起血管供给不足而导致肿瘤缺氧，但肿瘤细胞内的某些变化可能使其抵抗这种缺氧。例如，在小鼠异种移植模型中，携带 p53 突变的肿瘤细胞对缺氧不敏感，对 VEGFR2 抑制剂的反应也不理想[432]。有研究在接受了贝伐单抗和伊立替康治疗的复发性高级胶质瘤患者的肿瘤活检样本中检测了碳酸酐酶 9（carbonic anhydrase 9，CAIX）（缺氧的标志物）的表达，结果发现 CAIX 高表达患者的 1 年生存率较差[433]。同样，另一项研究在接受节律性依托泊苷和贝伐单抗联合治疗的恶性胶质瘤患者中，检测了肿瘤组织中 CAIX 和 VEGF 的表达，发现 CAIX 低表达且 VEGF 高表达患者的 PFS 更好[434]。

肿瘤内皮细胞的遗传变异

肿瘤内皮细胞是正常的二倍体细胞，因此可以推断其基因稳定，而近年来小鼠动物模型的研究结果对这一假设提出了挑战[435]。此外，有研究通过对具有特定遗传变异的 B 细胞非霍奇金淋巴瘤患者的肿瘤组织活检，发现肿瘤微血管系统的内皮细胞具有相同的特异性染色体易位[436]。基因不稳定的肿瘤内皮细胞可能来源于一个共同的内皮祖细胞[437]，也可能是肿瘤微环境中血管新生因子压力下肿瘤细胞向内皮表型分化的产物。也有假设认为这是由于肿瘤细胞和内皮细胞发生了融合。总的来说，这一发现的意义及与其他类型肿瘤的关联尚不清楚，但这和其他越来越多的发现是一致的，都表明肿瘤内皮细胞和肿瘤细胞一样，是一个复杂的治疗靶点。

宿主的遗传多样性

最近的研究表明，VEGF 基因的多态性与罹患癌症的风险有关[438~440]，并可能影响乳腺癌[405]和胶质母细胞瘤患者[441]在接受贝伐单抗和化疗联合治疗时的反应。也有研究报道了其他调节血管新生的基因（如 IL-8 和 HIF 家族基因）存在多态性。全基因组水平分析多态性的高通量方法的出现，有助于分析宿主的遗传差异及其对血管新生抑制剂反应的影响。

指导 VEGF 通路抑制剂应用的潜在生物标志物

对 VEGF 通路抑制剂相关生物标志物的迫切需求

尽管抗血管新生治疗在临床上取得的进展有目共睹，但迄今为止其疗效依然有限，仅在少数患者中有效，而且肿瘤会不可避免地对其产生耐药性。肿瘤对 VEGF 抑制剂产生耐药性的机制尚不完全清楚，解析这些机制是筛选易耐药的患者并建立联合治疗方案以克服耐药的关键。此外，这些药物的生物活性仍然难以评估，因为作为单药治疗时通常不会使肿瘤缩小，因此无法用客观反应来判定其疗效。例如，在一项贝伐单抗的Ⅰ期临床试验中，25 名患者中无一对治疗有客观反应[442]。因此，迫切需要生物标志物来识别最有可能对治疗产生反应或产生耐药的患者，选择最佳药物剂量，并确定药物靶点是否被有效抑制[443~445]。理想情况下，这种标志物的检测方法应该是无创的，并易于在常规临床中操作。目前还没有生物标志物经过验证并进入临床应用，但研究人员正在临床试验和临床前研究中对很多标志物进行测试（表 17-3）。这些标志物可分为：直接评估组织或血管系统变化的侵入性标志物；可在血液或尿液中检测到的循环标志物；影像学标志物。下面将讨论部分代表性的标志物。

表 17-3　目前在研的用于评估抗血管新生药物疗效的候选标志物

标志物	评估参数	评价/局限	参考文献
基于肿瘤的标志物			
组织活检	免疫组化检测： • 以蛋白表达作为标志物 • 微血管密度 • 肿瘤血管的血管周细胞包绕情况 • 细胞增殖/凋亡及基因组分析	在一些肿瘤中很难应用	285，286，358，418，486，487
组织间隙液压测定	肿瘤间隙液压	只可应用于某些特定肿瘤	285，286，488，489
组织氧含量测定	肿瘤氧压	在某些肿瘤中难以检测	490

续表

标志物	评估参数	评价/局限	参考文献
皮肤损伤修复	损伤修复时间	可以作为判断疗效的标志物及反应副作用的指征	491
血液和尿液中的循环标志物			
血液中的 CEC、CPC 或 CEP	存活的 CEC、CPC 或 CEP 的浓度	循环细胞的来源、活力、表面分型尚不明确	285 ~ 288,458,463,470,471,475,492
血液循环中的蛋白(细胞因子,促新生血管生成因子等)	血液中细胞因子、促新生血管生成因子、缺氧标志物、内皮细胞损伤及其他因子的浓度	可以用商业化的多通道试剂盒或 ELISA 来检测	288,453,458 ~ 460,462,493,494
尿液中的蛋白水平	尿液中的 MMP,VEGF 等	仅能检测分泌型蛋白,治疗引起的肾功能改变也会影响检测结果(如蛋白尿)	495
基于放射成像的标志物			
CT 成像	血流量和血容量、渗透表面积乘积、平均通过时间	分辨率,复合参数的测定	285,286,496
PET 成像	示踪剂的摄取	分辨率,复合参数的测定	285~287,496
MRI	血流量、通透性	分辨率,复合参数的测定	288,481,497,498

CEC,循环内皮细胞;CEP,循环前体内皮细胞;CT,计算机断层扫描;MMP,基质金属蛋白酶;MRI,磁共振成像;PET,正电子放射断层造影;VEGF,血管内皮细胞生长因子。

侵入性标志物

治疗前和治疗中进行系列活检有可能在细胞和分子水平上直接证明药物对肿瘤和其他组织的疗效,但在临床试验之外时这种方法就显得很不切实际。该方法已在直肠癌患者中证明了贝伐单抗可导致微血管密度、肿瘤细胞凋亡和增殖的变化[285,286,446]。肿瘤间质液压(interstitial fluid pressure,IFP)是影响血管功能的一个关键参数,其变化也被证实可以作为标志物[286,287]。这种方法也可能有助于解释某些药物缺乏显著临床疗效的原因。例如,在 VEGFR TKI SU5416 和 SU6668 的临床试验中,研究者在治疗后的肿瘤活检样本中发现 VEGFR 和其他关键靶点的活性未被完全抑制[418,419],表明可能需要更高的药物浓度或更强效的抑制剂。此外,在直肠癌患者接受贝伐单抗治疗后,通过分析其肿瘤细胞和肿瘤相关巨噬细胞(tumor-associated macrophage,TAM)基因表达的变化发现,SDF1α-CXCR4 通路和 VEGF 受体 NRP1 的表达都发生了上调[447]。

抗 VEGF 治疗后肿瘤微环境中 TAM 的表达与患者的预后相关。一项对复发性胶质母细胞瘤患者(接受过包括贝伐单抗在内的多种 VEGF 抑制剂的治疗)的回顾性尸检研究显示,肿瘤中 CD68+、CD11+TAM 表达的增加与患者的不良预后有关,提示 CD68+、CD11+TAM 可能作为肿瘤逃逸治疗的生物标志物[448]。

血液或尿液中的循环标志物

肿瘤血管新生受到促血管新生因子、抗血管新生因子和细胞因子(这些因子由肿瘤细胞、间质细胞和炎性细胞释放)之间的平衡调节。这些因子很多都能在循环血和其他体液中检测到,并可以作为监测抗 VEGF 治疗的生物标志物[417,443~445]。

研究已经评估了血浆和血清中 VEGF 和可溶性 VEGF-2 的水平作为 VEGF 抑制剂活性的药效学生物标志物、预后标志物和临床效益的预测标志物的可行性。在临床前模型中,VEGF 抑制剂在非荷瘤和荷瘤的小鼠中均可导致血浆中 VEGF 水平的迅速升高和可溶性 VEGF-2 的下降[449~451]。同时,血浆 VEGF 的升高存在剂量依赖性,并与 VEGF 抑制剂的疗效相关,提示其可能有助于合适药物剂量的选择。

这些标志物也在临床试验中进行了评价。贝伐单抗(单药或联合细胞毒性药物)可以提高患者血清和血浆中总 VEGF 的水平[285,287,305,307]。有趣的是,其中的一项研究显示,即使是低剂量的贝伐单抗也可以使患者血清中游离 VEGF 的浓度下降到无法检测的水平[305]。大多数 VEGFR TKI 都有类似的作用。研究最多的是马来酸舒尼替尼(SU11248,Sutent®,辉瑞制药),它与其他 TKI 一样,都能在治疗中引起血浆 VEGF 水平的升高,以及可溶性 VEGFR-2(soluble VEGFR-2,sVEGFR-2)的减少,而停药时,这些变化会被快速逆转[288,452~457]。另一项研究发现,sVEGFR-2 的变化与血浆中药物的水平有关[458]。总之,这些发现表明 VEGF 和 sVEGFR-2 可能是有效的抗 VEGF 治疗药效学标志物。

VEGF 的基线水平也可以预测某些药物的疗效,尽管不同研究的结果尚不一致。与单纯化疗相比,VEGF 表达高的 NSCLC 患者更有可能对贝伐单抗和化疗的联合治疗产生反应[459]。有趣的是,TKI 凡德他尼出现了相反的趋势:在三项随机Ⅱ期临床研究中,相比于对照组,VEGF 较低的患者从凡德他尼治疗中的获益更大[460]。因此 VEGF 等标志物的预测价值可能取决于特定的药物和疾病类型。

新技术的出现，如多重微珠分析，使研究人员能够分析更多种类的因子。一项随机Ⅱ期临床研究鉴定了一个包含 35 种细胞因子和血管新生因子的特征谱，该特征谱可以预测凡德他尼的疗效[461]。在这些循环生物标志物中，肿瘤患者的 PlGF 水平在抗 VEGF 治疗后出现了一致的上升，并且不依赖于肿瘤或抗 VEGF 药物的类型，表明 PlGF 可能是一种新的抗血管新生治疗的药效学生物标志物[285,287,288,453,462,463]。后续的研究将确定 PlGF 水平是否可以预测抗 VEGF 治疗的疗效。最后，多重微珠分析也可用于解析耐药性产生的潜在机制。目前已发现一些候选的耐药分子，包括 SDF1α-CXCR4 通路、bFGF、IL-6、HGF 和 IL-8[287,288,461,463,464]。

VEGF 的单核苷酸多态性

研究也评估了 VEGF 基因型和 VEGF 单核苷酸多态性(single-nucleotide polymorphism，SNP)作为潜在标志物来预测肿瘤对 VEGF 靶向药物反应的可行性。SNP 可能通过改变基因的表达或转录后修饰来影响肿瘤对药物的反应。在 ECOG 4599 临床试验中，通过对 133 例晚期 NSCLC 患者的分析，研究者发现 VEGFA-634GG、ICAM1 469T/C 和 IL8-251T/A 这些 SNP 特征是患者 OS 和 PFS 的最佳预测因子[465]。E2501 随机Ⅱ期临床研究在转移性 NSCLC 患者中比较了索拉菲尼与安慰剂的疗效，通过对收集到的 88 份血样进行 DNA 分析，研究人员发现 VEGFA-1498CC 和 VEGFA-634CC 基因型与患者 PFS 的改善有关[466]。在晚期乳腺癌患者中，贝伐单抗的疗效与患者 *VEGF* 和 *VEGFR-2/KDR* 特定的基因多态性有关[405]。

最近，在一项贝伐单抗和索拉菲尼治疗复发性胶质母细胞瘤的Ⅱ期临床研究中，*VEGF* 和 *VEGFR-2* 启动子中的 SNP 与患者的 6 个月 PFS 有关。此外，该研究还发现 *VEGF* 启动子中的 SNP 与患者更严重的毒性反应有关[441]。

循环内皮细胞和循环内皮祖细胞

成熟的循环内皮细胞(circulating endothelial cell，CEC)(来源于现有血管)和骨髓来源的循环前体细胞(circulating precursor cell，CPC)或循环内皮祖细胞(circulating endothelial progenitor，CEP)可分化为成熟的内皮细胞，促进新生血管的形成。已有研究探索了这些细胞作为生物标志物在抗血管新生治疗中的作用[139,140,143,288,458,467~470]。与临床前模型一致的是[471,472]，在治疗过程中，某些患者成熟 CEC 细胞(其中一大部分是凋亡细胞，可能是脱落的肿瘤内皮细胞)的数量会出现增加，这种增加可能与接受抗血管新生或 VTA 治疗后患者的获益有关[458,473~475]。在一项转移性乳腺癌研究中，通过包含环磷酰胺和甲氨蝶呤的低剂量米洛诺明化疗方案对患者进行两个月的连续治疗，在随后两年多的随访中，患者的 CEC 计数都与 DFS 和 OS 相关[475]。相反，患者在接受贝伐单抗[285~287]或舒尼替尼治疗后，其 CPC 会出现下降[463]。尽管这些结果是令人鼓舞的，但是将循环细胞作为生物标志物进行临床应用仍然需要进行标准化并对细胞群进行表型鉴定[476~478]。

成像

目前正在研究多种不同的技术以评估与肿瘤血管系统相关的影像学参数，如灌注、通透性、低氧和代谢活性。这些技术包括动态增强 MRI(DCE-MRI)、CT 和正电子发射断层扫描[444,445,479~485]。这些方法具有非侵入性、可连贯性评估的重要优势。然而，每种方法都有很多的局限。肿瘤内血流和血管通透性存在显著的异质性，目前的方法普遍缺乏空间分辨率来对此进行精确评估。此外，大多数方法评估的都是复合参数，参数则同时依赖于肿瘤的血流和血管通透性[417]。这些研究的成本也会限制它们的应用，特别在大型随机临床试验中对其实用性进行验证时。

结论

40 多年前，科学家们提出肿瘤血管新生是癌症治疗的一个潜在靶点[1]。自此开创性发现之后，该领域已经从一个概念发展到有数十种新药正在进行临床试验的时代。现在，血管新生抑制剂是肺癌、结直肠癌、肾癌、乳腺癌和其他几种癌症的标准治疗方案的一部分。尽管这些近期的进展已经表明抗血管新生作为一种治疗肿瘤的方式是可行的，并且无数患者已从中获益，但到目前为止，这种治疗在临床上取得的进展仍然是有限的。随着该领域从最初的婴儿期发展到现在的青少年时期，有一些关键问题亟待解决以便充分释放抗血管新生疗法治疗癌症的潜力。这些问题包括：理解抗血管新生治疗提高化疗和放疗疗效的机制并设计适当的联合治疗方案；鉴定除 VEGF 外的其他驱动血管新生的关键信号通路，并开发能够抑制这些通路的药物；探索生物标志物来筛选哪些患者会从特定药物的治疗中获益(或产生毒副作用)；探索血管新生抑制剂在极早期癌症中的应用，从而使处于显微体积的肿瘤休眠。

致谢

感谢医学博士 Judah Folkman 在肿瘤血管新生研究中的开创性工作以及他慷慨的指导。我们还要感谢 Rakesh Jain 博士和 George Sledge 博士对本章早期版本的贡献。

(孙文 译　张培霖 校　吕桂帅　李亮 审)

参考文献

The complete reference list can be found on the Wiley Companion Digital Edition of this title (see inside front cover for login instructions).

1 Folkman J. Tumor angiogenesis: therapeutic implications. *N Engl J Med*. 1971;**285**:1182–1186.

2 Hanahan D, Weinberg RA. The hallmarks of cancer. *Cell*. 2000;**100**:57–70.

3 Carmeliet P, Jain RK. Angiogenesis in cancer and other diseases. *Nature*. 2000;**407**:249–257.

4 Achilles EG, Fernandez A, Allred EN, et al. Heterogeneity of angiogenic activity in a human liposarcoma: a proposed mechanism for "no take" of human tumors in mice. *J Natl Cancer Inst*. 2001;**93**:1075–1081.

8 Folkman J, Watson K, Ingber D, Hanahan D. Induction of angiogenesis during the transition from hyperplasia to neoplasia. *Nature*. 1989;**339**:58–61.

9 Hanahan D, Folkman J. Patterns and emerging mechanisms of the angiogenic switch during tumorigenesis. *Cell*. 1996;**86**:353–364.

18 Folkman J. Toward an understanding of angiogenesis: search and discovery. *Perspect Biol Med*. 1985;**29**:10–36.

19 Folkman J, Long DM Jr, Becker FF. Growth and metastasis of tumor in organ culture. *Cancer*. 1963;**16**:453–467.

20 Folkman J, Cole P, Zimmerman S. Tumor behavior in isolated perfused organs: in vitro growth and metastases of biopsy material in rabbit thyroid and canine intestinal segment. *Ann Surg*. 1966;**164**:491–502.

21 Folkman J. Anti-angiogenesis: new concept for therapy of solid tumors. *Ann Surg*. 1972;**175**:409–416.

40 Holash J, Maisonpierre PC, Compton D, et al. Vessel cooption, regression, and growth in tumors mediated by angiopoietins and VEGF. *Science*. 1999;**284**:1994–1998.

47 Williams WN, Kim ES, Heymach JV, Lippman SL. Molecular Targets for Cancer Chemoprevention. *Nat Rev Drug Discov*. 2009;**8**(**3**):213–225.

53 Parangi S, O'Reilly M, Christofori G, et al. Antiangiogenic therapy of transgenic mice impairs de novo tumor growth. *Proc Natl Acad Sci U S A*. 1996;**93**:2002–2007.

67 Naumov GN, Bender E, Zurakowski D, et al. A model of human tumor dormancy: an angiogenic switch from the nonangiogenic phenotype. *J Natl Cancer Inst*. 2006;**98**:316–325.

68 Herbst RS, Hidalgo M, Pierson AS, Holden SN, Bergen M, Eckhardt SG. Angiogenesis inhibitors in clinical development for lung cancer. *Semin Oncol*. 2002;**29**:66–77.

123 Nilsson M, Heymach JV. Vascular endothelial growth factor (VEGF) pathway. *J Thorac Oncol*. 2006;**1**:768–770.

139 Asahara T, Murohara T, Sullivan A, et al. Isolation of putative progenitor endothelial cells for angiogenesis. *Science*. 1997;**275**:964–967.

144 Lyden D, Young AZ, Zagzag D, et al. Id1 and Id3 are required for neurogenesis, angiogenesis and vascularization of tumour xenografts. *Nature*. 1999;**401**:670–677.

153 Cascone T, Heymach JV. Targeting the angiopoietin/Tie2 pathway: cutting tumor vessels with a double-edged sword? *J Clin Oncol*. 2012;**30**:441–444.

154 Maisonpierre PC, Suri C, Jones PF, et al. Angiopoietin-2, a natural antagonist for Tie2 that disrupts in vivo angiogenesis. *Science*. 1997;**277**:55–60.

173 O'Reilly MS, Pirie-Shepherd S, Lane WS, Folkman J. Antiangiogenic activity of the cleaved conformation of the serpin antithrombin. *Science*. 1999;**285**:1926–1928.

174 Moses MA, Sudhalter J, Langer R. Identification of an inhibitor of neovascularization from cartilage. *Science*. 1990;**248**:1408–1410.

241 Nilsson M, Hanrahan E, Heymach J. Angiogenesis inhibitors for the Treatment of Lung Cancer. In: Teicher BA, Ellis LM, eds. *Antiangiogenic Agents in Cancer Therapy*, 2nd ed. Totowa, NJ: Humana Press; 2008.

260 Xu L, Nilsson MB, Saintigny P, et al. Epidermal growth factor receptor regulates MET levels and invasiveness through hypoxia-inducible factor-1α in non-small cell lung cancer cells. *Oncogene*. 2010;**29**(**18**):2616–2627.

265 Lara PN Jr, Douillard JY, Nakagawa K, et al. Randomized phase III placebo-controlled trial of carboplatin and paclitaxel with or without the vascular disrupting agent vadimezan (ASA404) in advanced non-small-cell lung cancer. *J Clin Oncol*. 2011;**29**:2965–2971.

266 Rudin CM, Mauer A, Smakal M, et al. Phase I/II study of pemetrexed with or without ABT-751 in advanced or metastatic non-small-cell lung cancer. *J Clin Oncol*. 2011;**29**:1075–1082.

271 Jain RK. Normalization of tumor vasculature: an emerging concept in antiangiogenic therapy. *Science*. 2005;**307**:58–62.

273 Jain RK. Normalizing tumor vasculature with anti-angiogenic therapy: a new paradigm for combination therapy. *Nat Med*. 2001;**7**:987–989.

301 Hurwitz H, Fehrenbacher L, Novotny W, et al. Bevacizumab plus irinotecan, fluorouracil, and leucovorin for metastatic colorectal cancer. *N Engl J Med*. 2004;**350**:2335–2342.

304 Motzer RJ, Hutson TE, Tomczak P, et al. Sunitinib versus interferon α in metastatic renal-cell carcinoma. *N Engl J Med*. 2007;**356**:115–124.

310 Motzer RJ, Hutson TE, Tomczak P, et al. Overall survival and updated results for sunitinib compared with interferon α in patients with metastatic renal cell carcinoma. *J Clin Oncol*. 2009;**27**:3584–3590.

312 Escudier B, Pluzanska A, Koralewski P, et al. Bevacizumab plus interferon α-2a for treatment of metastatic renal cell carcinoma: a randomised, double-blind phase III trial. *Lancet*. 2007;**370**:2103–2111.

330 Tran HT, Liu Y, Zurita AJ, et al. Prognostic or predictive plasma cytokines and angiogenic factors for patients treated with pazopanib for metastatic renal-cell cancer: a retrospective analysis of phase 2 and phase 3 trials. *Lancet Oncol*. 2012;**13**:827–837.

351 Heymach JV, Paz-Ares L, De Braud F, et al. Randomized phase II study of vandetanib alone or with paclitaxel and carboplatin as first-line treatment for advanced non-small-cell lung cancer. *J Clin Oncol*. 2008;**26**:5407–5415.

352 Herbst RS, Sun Y, Eberhardt WE, et al. Vandetanib plus docetaxel versus docetaxel as second-line treatment for patients with advanced non-small-cell lung cancer (ZODIAC): a double-blind, randomised, phase 3 trial. *Lancet Oncol*. 2010;**11**:619–626.

370 Heymach JV, Johnson BE, Prager D, et al. Randomized, placebo-controlled phase II study of vandetanib plus docetaxel in previously treated nonsmall-cell lung cancer. *J Clin Oncol*. 2007;**25**:4270–4277.

371 Heymach JV, Lockwood SJ, Herbst RS, Johnson BE, Ryan AJ. EGFR biomarkers predict benefit from vandetanib in combination with docetaxel in a randomized phase III study of second-line treatment of patients with advanced non-small cell lung cancer. *Ann Oncol*. 2014;**25**:1941–1948.

376 Byers LA, Heymach JV. Dual targeting of the vascular endothelial growth factor and epidermal growth factor receptor pathways: rationale and clinical applications for non-small-cell lung cancer. *Clin Lung Cancer*. 2007;**8**(**Suppl 2**): S79–S85.

384 Herbst RS, O'Neill VJ, Fehrenbacher L, et al. Phase II study of efficacy and safety of bevacizumab in combination with chemotherapy or erlotinib compared with chemotherapy alone for treatment of recurrent or refractory non small-cell lung cancer. *J Clin Oncol*. 2007;**25**:4743–4750.

386 Naumov GN, Nilsson MB, Cascone T, et al. Combined vascular endothelial growth factor receptor and epidermal growth factor receptor (EGFR) blockade inhibits tumor growth in xenograft models of EGFR inhibitor resistance. *Clin Cancer Res*. 2009;**15**:3484–3494.

418 Heymach JV, Desai J, Manola J, et al. Phase II Study of the Antiangiogenic Agent SU5416 in Patients with Advanced Soft Tissue Sarcomas. *Clin Cancer Res*. 2004;**10**:5732–5740.

427 Cascone T, Herynk MH, Xu L, et al. Upregulated stromal EGFR and vascular remodeling in mouse xenograft models of angiogenesis inhibitor-resistant human lung adenocarcinoma. *J Clin Invest*. 2011;**121**:1313–1328.

428 Kopetz S, Hoff PM, Morris JS, et al. Phase II trial of infusional fluorouracil, irinotecan, and bevacizumab for metastatic colorectal cancer: efficacy and circulating angiogenic biomarkers associated with therapeutic resistance. *J Clin Oncol*. 2010;**28**:453–459.

443 Zurita A, Wu H, Heymach J. Blood-based biomarkers for VEGF inhibitors. In: Davis D, Herbst R, Abbruzzese J, eds. *Antiangiogenic Cancer Therapy*. Boca Raton, FL: CRC Press; 2007:517–531.

444 Jain RK, Duda DG, Clark JW, Loeffler JS. Lessons from phase III clinical trials on anti-VEGF therapy for cancer. *Nat Clin Pract Oncol*. 2006;**3**:24–40.

474 Heymach J, Kulke M, Fuchs C, et al. Circulating endothelial cells as a surrogate marker of antiangiogenic activity in patients treated with endostatin. *Proc Am Soc Clin Oncol*. 2003;**22**:979.

第三篇

定量肿瘤学

第 18 章　癌症生物信息学

John N. Weinstein, MD, PhD

概述

生物信息学是一个快速发展的科学领域，其计算方法被应用于生物数据的分析和解释。生物数据大多来源于细胞或分子水平，通常是大型多变量数据集的形式。在癌症研究中，最常见的情况是DNA、RNA、蛋白质和/或代谢物水平的分子表达谱分析，用于探索生物学，鉴定潜在的治疗靶标和/或用于临床预测。新的大规模并行测序技术造成了目前的数据泛滥，这给我们的计算机硬件、分析软件和生物信息学人力资源造成了巨大压力。因此，目前测序项目的计算方面比实验室工作更昂贵、更耗时。

生物信息学分析可以提出假设也可以验证假设。当作为提出假设的手段时，研究人员需要过滤大量的假阳性结果，以便识别一个或几个有用的发现；当作为验证假设的手段时，严格的统计推断是必需的。目前大量的统计和机器学习算法，脚本和软件包可以用来进行数据分析，并且数据分析的手段还在快速的增加。然而，由于数据集通常很大，所以生物信息学的一个重要方面是数据可视化，例如沿着基因组长度排列的数据展示，或者是以最常见的聚类热图的形式。

癌症生物学家和临床研究人员应该领导大规模数据集的生物学分析，但统计分析应该由信息学专业人士（或在其辅助下）进行。当存在比病例（例如患者）更多的变量（例如基因）时，非专业人士倾向于获得显著的 P 值甚至在随机化数据集中看到错误模式。此外，在数据管理和预处理过程中出现的细微错误往往会导致数据产生误导或错误结论。

随着高通量分子表达谱分析项目变得更便宜更易于操作，它们已逐步被纳入学术或商业的个人机构研究中。此外，在该领域的大型公共项目也在不断增加。在细胞系的水平上，第一个大型公共项目是NCI-60，研究人员把1990年以来美国国家癌症研究所使用过的60个癌症系用来筛选超过100 000种化合物和天然产品的抗癌活性。该研究最近收到了癌细胞系百科全书（Cancer Cell Line Encyclopedia），癌症药物敏感性基因组学项目（Genomics of Drug Sensitivity in Cancer project）以及其他项目的关注。在临床水平上，癌症基因组图谱项目（Cancer Genome Atlas project）受到了广泛的关注，该项目分析了超过10 000例33种不同类型的人类癌症，并且有大量的类似项目正在进行中或处于起草阶段。这些需要大量生物信息学支持的项目催生了强大的生物信息学专业知识社区，并用来作为开发新算法、软件和可视化手段的测试平台。

我可以向你保证数据分析的这股狂热持续不过今年。

——1957 年某主流出版社编辑语

对于上一代人，大多数关于癌症的实验室研究结果可以容纳在一个简单的电子表格中或者写入实验室笔记本。实验数据通常由实验者自己使用非常基本的统计算法进行分析。随着20世纪90年代中期微阵列的出现，以及十年之后大规模并行“第二代”测序技术的诞生，这种情况逐渐发生变化。在千禧年之际，有一个半开玩笑的语言——大多数生物医学研究人员很快会放弃传统实验室转而扑到计算机上，挖掘“生物工厂”生成的数据。当然这一切还没有发生，目前传统实验室还在蓬勃发展。但我们确实看到越来越多的生物工厂，其中突出的是高通量测序中心。总的来说，计算机化的趋势是明确无误的。这种趋势很大程度上是新的机器人增强技术的结果，使得它能够更快、更便宜、更可靠地执行实验室部分的大规模分子表达谱分析项目和筛选分析。因此，大型中心和小型实验室可以生成越来越强大的数据流。这些趋势共同产生了大量的数据集，这些数据集通常包含数十亿或数万亿的条目，需要更复杂、更大规模、通常更微妙的统计分析和“生物解释”资源。

就像“光年”这个概念被引入天文距离，因为天文距离太大而无法以英里或公里来理解，“Huge”（Human Genome Equivalent，人类基因组当量；约33亿碱基对）这个概念被引入基因组学。莎士比亚的所有著作（戏剧、十四行诗和诗歌）包含500多万个字母，仅相当于不到0.002Huge。现在，数据的存储、管理、传输、分析和解释通常是研究的瓶颈，而不是传统实验室数据生成这一过程本身。数据泛滥已被不同程度地比喻为雪崩、洪水、洪流或海啸。生物信息学是一个基于统计学、计算机科学、生物学和医学的多学科领域，是对当前生物医学研究和临床进展至关重要的领域，虽然目前生物信息学领域日新月异，但其仍处于未成熟阶段。

本章的目的不是为庞大、快速发展的癌症生物信息学提供全面的解析。因为在有限的篇幅我们无法做到这一点。有关一些子领域，例如蛋白质和核酸的代谢组分析和结构分析的篇幅也会较为简短。

本章的目的也不是盘点该领域先驱研究人员的功劳，或引用所有值得一提的生物信息学工具和资源。相反，本章的目的是：①阐明癌症生物信息学在当前和未来的广泛应用；②突出强调目前可用的统计算法、计算工具和数据资源；③提示非专业人士在浏览生物信息学文献、了解生物信息学家的工作、使用生物信息学更好地了解癌症并为癌症患者提供直接帮助时应该记住的一些问题。

生物信息学的定义和范围

生物信息学的定义

“生物信息学”这个术语并不新鲜。它首次出现在1970年并具有非常广泛的含义[1]，但其目前适用的定义是一个几乎是塔木德争论的问题。多个学术委员会、学术调查和出版物一直在努力解决这个问题，甚至试图区分"bioinformatician"和"bioinformatic"[2]。就目前而言，美国国家生物技术信息中心(NCBI)的生物信息学的扩展定义是最准确的："生物信息学是一个科学领域，是生物学、计算机科学和信息技术合并为一的学科。生物信息学中有三个重要的子学科：开发新的算法和统计数据，用以评估大数据集之间的关系；分析和解释各种类型的数据，包括核苷酸和氨基酸序列，蛋白质结构域和蛋白质结构；以及能够有效访问和管理不同类型信息的工具的开发和使用。

"生物信息学与相关或重叠学科(如计算生物学和医学信息学)之间不存在明确的界限。计算生物学包括数据分析和理论方法的开发和应用，数学建模和计算模拟技术，以及生物，行为和社会系统的研究[3]。"它包括但远远超出了对生物信息学的生物分子特征的关注。医学信息学被定义为"通过将计算机应用于医疗保健和医学的各个方面来分析和传播医学数据的信息科学领域"[4]。医学信息学与临床研究和临床实践的实际需求密切相关。而生物信息学与临床前研究更紧密地联系在一起。然而这两者在如生物标志物的临床试验项目中应该协同作用。

人们的共识会赋予一个词的最终含义，了解该领域范围的最佳方式是列出与其相关的一些关键词。正如美国最高法院大法官波特斯图尔特的名言："当我看到它时，我就知道它是怎么回事了。"大多数生物信息学项目包括生物分子、大型数据库、多变量统计分析、高性能计算、分子数据图形可视化、生物学或生物医学解释。生物信息学分析的典型数据来源包括微阵列、DNA 测序、RNA 测序、蛋白质和代谢物的质谱以及组织病理学描述和临床记录。一些突出的数据集源于在特定实验室中进行的研究，但是大型公共数据库和搜索资源正在发挥着越来越大的作用。

生物信息学能够解决的典型问题

生物信息学分析能够阐释的问题涉及生物学机制、通路、网络、生物标志物和生物印记、大分子结构、癌症的亚类、早期检测以及临床结果变量的预测，例如风险、存活、转移、对治疗的反应和复发。本章引用的范例生物信息学项目包括分子表达谱的设计，统计分析和生物学解释。图 18-1 显示了通用测序项目中样本和信息流的示意图，其目的是将突变和/或 DNA 拷贝数异常鉴定为可能的生物标志物。来自此类研究的数据还可用于对癌症进行分组或进行直接比较，例如比较肿瘤与成对的正常组织，肿瘤类型对比肿瘤类型，应答者对比无应答者，转移性对比非转移性，或原发性对比复发性癌症。

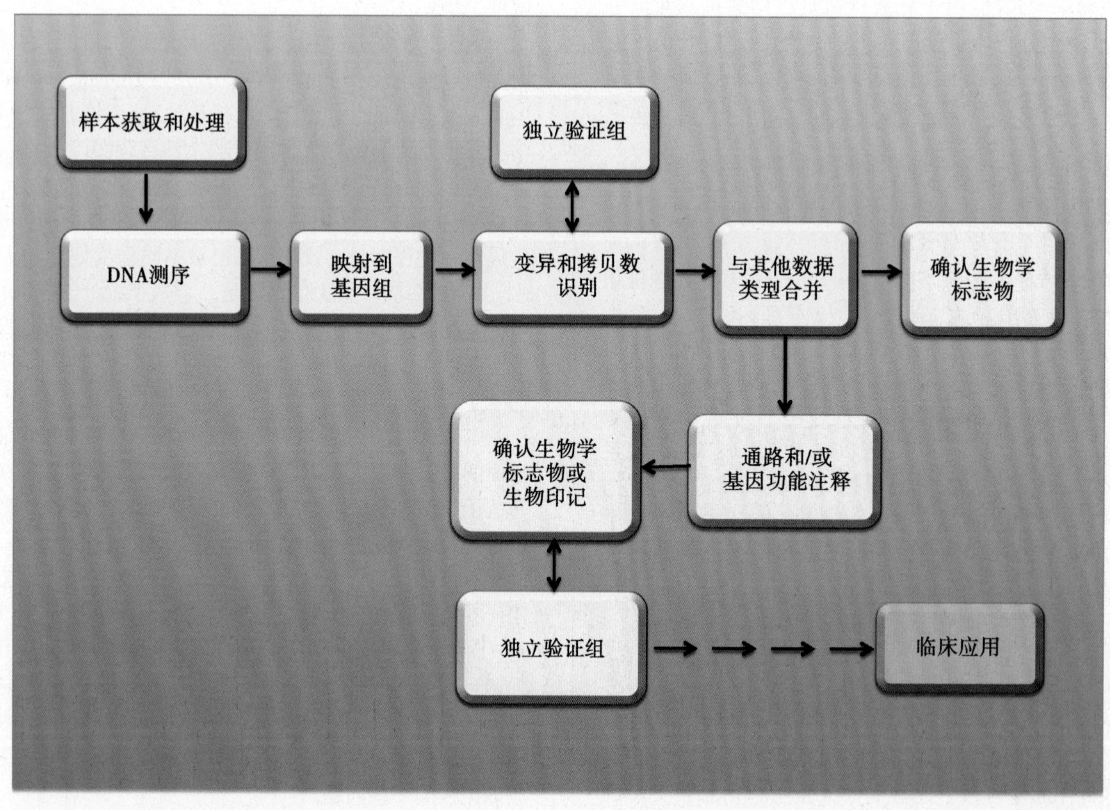

图 18-1 基于癌症测序的标本和信息流，以探索突变和/或拷贝数异常作为临床应用的可能生物标志物的流程图。黄色框表示流程图的"生物学解释"方面。如四个连续箭头所示，在达到临床应用之前必须克服许多障碍(科学方面，技术方面，计算方面，道德方面和监管方面)。可以针对 DNA、RNA、蛋白质和代谢组水平的其他数据类型绘制类似的示意图(包括基于微阵列的研究，而不是测序)

一个常见的目标是预测生存时间、复发时间或转移的“预后型”生物标志物。然而，对这些生物标记物的研究热度一直在下降，一部分原因是它们无法指导治疗，还有是因为癌症治疗发生了迅速的变化，以至于疾病的自然病史已经失去了很多意义。相反，研究的焦点转向了“预测型”生物标志物。该术语的涵盖面是广泛的，其词源学尚不清楚，它包含了一类分子标记物，这些分子标记物能够预测哪些患者会对特定疗法具有反应性。与其紧密关联的另一个概念是“可作用的”生物标志物。可作用的预测性生物标志物可以是治疗的靶点，也可以仅与患者的治疗反应性相关。到目前为止，生物信息学能够确认的更多是关联和相关性而不是因果关系，但是诸如 siRNA，shRNA，CRISPR 的生物干扰技术和随后出现的合成性致死药理学筛选正在产生具有直接因果关系的大数据集。

模拟化（微阵列）到数字化（测序）的转变

我们正在见证从微阵列（基础模拟技术）到 DNA 和 RNA 测序（基本数字技术）的转变。数字革命首先发生在计算机领域，随后到了电视机、手表、照相机和汽车，以及现在的生物医学研究。与微阵列相比，DNA 和 RNA 测序提供了关于癌症分子表达谱的更精确、更深入、更广泛的信息。例如，对肿瘤中的 mRNA 混合物（RNA-seq）进行测序可以产生关于 mRNA 剪接、mRNA 编辑、克隆异质性和进化、病毒插入、融合基因表达和整体表达水平的等位基因组分的信息。与之相比，表达微阵列通常仅提示样品中存在的 mRNA 种类的相对量。当然，这个转型也伴随着问题的出现。截至 2015 年，测序平均比基因表达微阵列更昂贵。大规模并行的第二代测序目前在硬件、软件和“湿件”（即人员）上对生物信息学界提出了新的挑战。

硬件挑战

摩尔定律[5]广为人知。它是关于大型集成电路上单位表面区域可容纳晶体管的数量。这个数字以一种非常稳定的速度增加，自 20 世纪 60 年代以来每两年增加两倍。结果是由于晶体管的速度增加，计算能力的成本每 18 个月减少一半。然而，摩尔定律未能准确的预言测序成本的下降，从 2007 年末到 2011 年底，随着第二代测序面世，测序成本下降了 1 000 倍（从每个人类基因组大约 1 000 万美元减少到大约 1 万美元）（图 18-2）。自此，由于我们在等待“第三代”测序技术（例如基于单分子测序的技术）的成本效益，测序价格的下跌已经大幅放缓。尽管如此，即使我们装备有大量内存和数千个 CPU 的高性能计算机每天运行 24 小时，但还是常常被基因组计算所困扰，主要是基因组的序列比对，计算需求非常大，以至于对散热和电力供应通常有很高的要求。一些大型数据中心需要自己的发电站。另一个大数据问题是，即使沿着高速线传输大量序列和相关注释也可能需要很长时间。云计算可以帮助解决我们的电力和存储空间的限制，但仍然需要向云端上传和下载大量数据。目前越来越多的计算工具被开发出来用于处理数据。

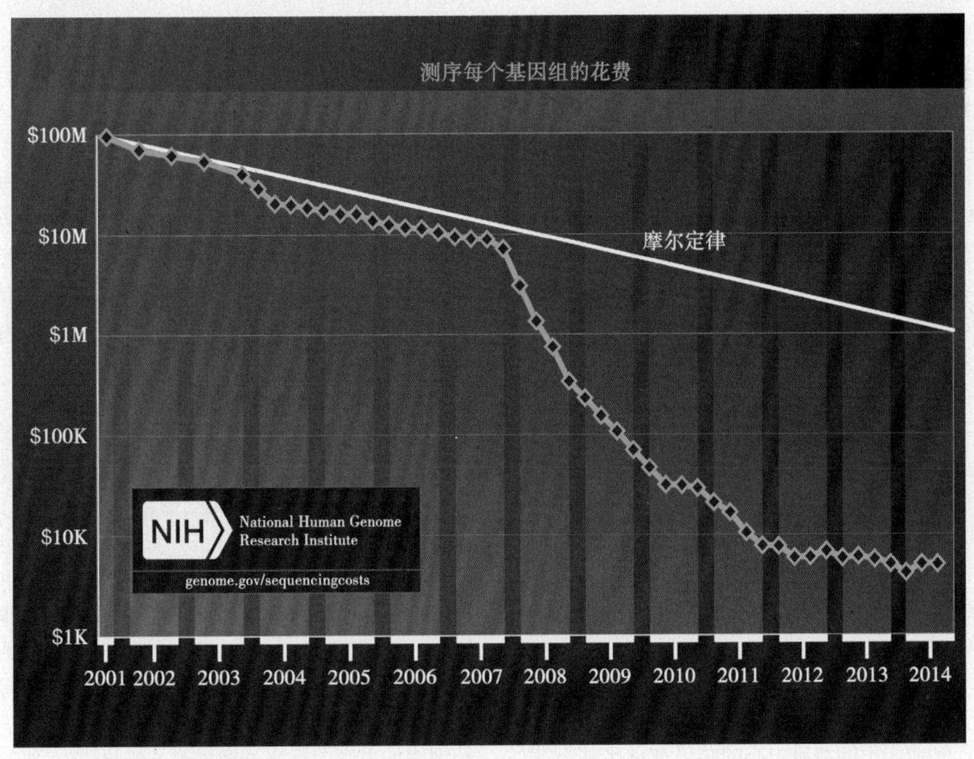

图 18-2　人类全基因组测序的每个基因组的成本。该图显示了 2007 年末的一个拐点，此时大规模并行测序被广泛应用。我们正在等待主要基于单分子测序的“第三代”技术的成熟和成本效益

人们不太熟悉但更严重的问题是 Kryder 定律[6]，类似于摩尔定律，但它描述的是数据存储的成本，而不是计算能力。2004 年 Kryder 定律预测，存储成本将每 6 个月减少到原来的二分之一。2009 年，该定律修正为存储成本每年下降 40%，但从 2009 年到 2014 年的实际减少幅度仅为每年 15%。标准全基因组 BAM 文件（二进制比对图谱文件/序列）所需的存储空间具有 30 倍的基因组平均覆盖率"仅"约 100GB，但是鉴定肿瘤内少数克隆的突变可能需要数以百计的基因组覆盖率冗余（如果可以识别的话）。通过仅编码与参考标准的差异可以压缩所需的存储空间，但是这种压缩会受到质控信息记录和其他类型的注释需要的限制。即使是大型机构也会耗尽存储空间。重新测序样本可能比长时间存储测序数据更便宜。

然而大规模存储有新的可能性，而这个突破就是 DNA 本身。DNA 可能是最紧凑的存储介质。一克 DNA 可以编码大约 700 000GB 的数据（大约 7 000 个全基因组 BAM 文件）。一个团队将所有莎士比亚的十四行诗编码在 DNA 中，另一个团队编码了整本书——其内在错误率仅为每百万比特两个，远远优于磁性硬盘驱动器或人类校对者[7]。然后他们通过复制 DNA 生产了 700 亿本书——足以让世界上每个人拥有 10 本（不占用书架上的空间）。在适当的储存条件下，即使在室温下，DNA 仍可保持稳定，可以稳定保存数十万年。如果您面临将知识传递到未来文明的挑战，那么 DNA 存储将是您最好的选择。目前大规模将信息写入和导出 DNA 的技术还是过于昂贵，但价格在快速的下降。

软件挑战

生物信息学软件开发领域日新月异。目前正在开发和部署的功能强大的软件包就有数百个，其中一些是商业软件包，但大多数都是学术软件包，是开源、公开的。对于任何计算功能的需求，目前的选择都是多得惊人。这导致了用户社区的碎片化，他们在很大程度上还没有围绕特定的算法，软件或网站进行合并。在生物信息学家中，"非这里开发"综合征时有发生。其结果是生物信息学领域变成了经典的巴别塔，不同软件包的开发人员通常无法良好地交流。尽管国际上在标准化方面做出了重大努力，但各种注释方案和数据格式仍然互不兼容。

特别是在测序方面，在算法上还存在着重大挑战[8]。如果大规模并行测序技术及其数据真正是数字化的，那么应该能够确定某一特定 DNA 碱基对是否存在突变。然而情况并非如此，如图 18-3 所示，三个大型测序中心对相同测序数据的体细胞突变识别一致性的差异很大，可能与克隆异质性、肿瘤细胞占比过低、基因组某些区域的覆盖率差和/或 DNA 降解有关。另一个原因是概率性的。如果任一个测序中心对于包含 30 亿个碱基的基因组中识别给定碱基对的突变的准确率为 99.999%，那么他们仍然会对成千上万的识别产生分歧。重要的突变，例如驱动突变和其他癌症生物标记的识别，必须通过独立技术进行验证。三种验证的策略是：①对相同样品的 DNA 和 RNA 相互验证，②使用不同测序中心的结果进行比对[9]，以及③使用另一种不同技术如 PCR 进行后续验证。

人力挑战

目前，人员（湿件）和专业知识方面的问题甚至比硬件或软件问题更严重。生物信息学是多学科的交叉领域，涉及计算机科学、统计学、生物学和医学。拥有以上所有学科专业知识并且能够灵活交叉应用的人才并不是很多。尽管一些必要分析有着约定俗成的流程（通常是原始数据到映射序列这一过程），生物信息学项目的大部分步骤通常需要定制分析和多学科团队的共同努力。

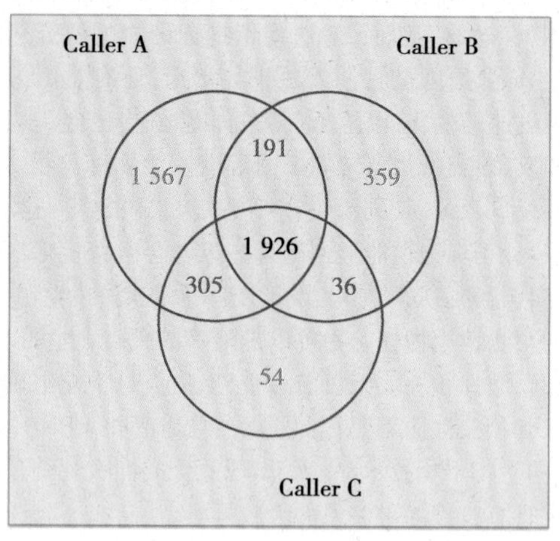

图 18-3 维恩图显示了 20 个 TCGA 子宫内膜癌及癌旁样本由 3 个不同测序中心根据统一外显子测序结果分析出的体细胞点突变识别的差异。点突变的差别还算较小，插入缺失或者结构变异将会产生各大的中心差异[9]

典型的大型分子表达谱分析项目的生物信息学部分可以大致分为数据管理、统计分析和生物解释三大块。数据管理听起来很简单，但对于包含来自多种分子技术和临床数据源的数据的项目，它可能极具挑战性。当哈勃望远镜于 1990 年投入使用时，它最初因其镜子中的 1.3mm 误差而无法正常工作，因为在最终测试期间，定制的"零校正器"取代了传统的零校正器。1999 年，火星气候轨道飞行器丢失了，因为计算机软件以磅-秒而不是牛顿-秒（公制单位）产生输出；轨道飞行器的不正确轨迹使它太靠近火星，使它在大气中解体。类似的数据不匹配问题是生物信息学领域所特有的。缺失或不小心编写的注释经常会导致关于数据字段的确切含义的疑惑或错误的结论。

多学科生物信息学团队中的角色

与简单实验室实验不同，高度多变量数据的统计分析通常需要计算分析方面的专业知识。生物医学研究人员也应参与统计分析，对所采用的方法和潜在的问题有基本的了解。研究人员应该准备好向数据分析师提供：①要求数据解决的问题，②生物医学领域信息，③可能影响分析的技术和实验设计的特性信息。如果数据分析师没有获得这些信息，他们可能会根据错误的前提生成错误的答案，或者为错误的问题找到了正确答案。然而，对于未经训练的人来说，单独或没有非常严密的监督下执行数据管理任务和统计分析是很危险的。经验表明，未经训练的人倾向于犯过度乐观的错误[10]。他们往往取得非常积极的，甚至是突破性的结果，后来证明这些结果毫无意义。"非自然选择"在这种现象中发挥作用；人类受主观思想的影响有一种倾向，既不同的分析方式直到其中一种得到理想的结果。除此之外，人类还倾向于在数据中找到不存在的模式或规律。正如允许统计学家进行脑部手术或让脑外科医生进行统计分析。

相反,在生物医学阐释中,生物医学研究人员应起带头作用,灵活运用在特定领域和癌症生物学的专业知识。每个基础、转化或临床癌症研究人员都应该能够使用一系列可用的生物学解释工具来探索基于大规模分子数据集的基因、途径、网络、细胞生物学实体和临床相关指标。培训研究人员使用这些工具是生物信息学家的主要责任。生物信息学家应该能够用图形、非数学的方式来解释他们正在使用的统计或机器学习算法的原理。生物信息学家还应具有为项目选择最佳工具和数据资源所必需的更广泛知识,并且具有定制算法或数据的图形可视化所必需的编程能力。

生物信息学的分析、可视化和阐释

表 18-1 列出了一些在癌症分析中可能具有重要意义的分子数据类型和现象,通常用于早期检测或预测癌症风险、诊断、预后、对治疗的反应、复发或转移。“组学(omic)”这个术语看起来有些不自然,但它使用起来方便,并且在词源学上是合理的。后缀“-ome”来自希腊语,用于“抽象实体、群体或群体”,因此,组学是对实体的总体研究[11]。有趣的是在基因组学的单基因层面我们有其对应的遗传学,但对于蛋白组学和代谢组学的单分子层面我们却没有对应学科。

许多统计学原理、算法和软件对数据的类型是不敏感的,但每种类型的数据都有其自身的特点,需要定制的分析。比如数据的背景级别、规范化、变异过滤、分布属性、阈值以及表示为连续或二分值的问题都需要特别注意。针对这些问题,如果程序选择不当可能导致分析出现完全错误的结果。事实上,生物信息学中最重要、最具挑战性、通常无法解决的问题来自最单调,最不显眼的任务:预处理数据以最大限度地减少噪声而不消除信号。同样重要的是,如果数据集和分析程序无法在数月或数年后再次进行交叉检查和独立分析,则会出现巨大的机会损失和未纠正或无法纠正的错误。

“数据整合”这个词朗朗上口,但它代表了一个需要深入研究的领域。有许多方法可以使不同的数据类型相互匹配,因此可以集成,但它们的表现都不是完全令人满意的。表 18-2 列出了许多网络上的分析工具,这些工具可用于生物信息数据的分析、可视化、整合和解释。

视觉模式识别是人类的强项,即使是很有数学天赋的人,他们也可以在呈现为图形的数据中更好的解释数据的模式。因此,图形表示法是生物信息学中的核心工具。分层聚类分析是最常使用的数据挖掘方法。它构建了类似于系统发育学中相似和差异的树干。例如,对一组患者样本进行的基因表达谱分析研究产生的一个矩阵,其中每列代表一个患者,每行代表一个基因,矩阵中的每个条目都是基因的表达水平。特定患者的肿瘤。将患者聚类可以显示其基因表达特征相似性和差异性,聚类基因可以显示不同基因在患者样品中表达模式的相似性和差异性。

表 18-1　生物信息数据类型、现象和数据源

数据类型

基因组学——种系,体细胞(DNA 水平)
- 单个核苷酸变异(SNV)
- 插入/缺失(Indel)
- 拷贝数变异
- 杂合缺失(LOH)
- 易位
- 重复元件
- 功能模体
- 域结构
- 融合基因
- 病毒插入
- 假性基因

表观组学
- DNA 甲基化(CpG 岛)
- DNA 甲基化(非 CpG 岛)
- DNA 修饰(其他)
- 组蛋白修饰(乙酰化,甲基化等)

转录组学(RNA 水平)
- mRNA 表达谱
- microRNA 表达谱
- lncRNA 表达谱
- 转录本剪接突变
- RNA 编辑
- 等位基因指标

蛋白组学
- 蛋白表达谱
- 转录后修饰
- 蛋白复合体和互作

代谢组学
- 代谢物流动
- 代谢物表达水平
- 靶向识别(MRM)

染色体组学
- 转录因子靶点
- 组蛋白修饰物靶点
- 复制起始位点及其动力学
- 转录起始位点及其动力学
- 染色体位置的可接近性
- 微卫星不稳定性(MSI)
- 染色体不稳定性(CIN)
- 3D 染色体排列
- 长期基因调控
- 有丝分裂/减数分裂编排

药物组学
- 治疗反应性
- 天然和获得性耐药
- 药物动力学

免疫组学
- 表位映射
- 免疫细胞分析
- 免疫调节网络模型

连接组学
- 同时发生又互不干扰的元素
- 中心节点
- 随机与无标度特性
- 非同配性

病理学
- 分组,亚分组
- 分级
- 肿瘤细胞占比
- 克隆异质性(微观/宏观)
- 标志物研究(免疫组化/原位杂交等)

临床研究
- 生存
- 无病生存
- 复发时间
- 治疗反应性

数据源

大批检测
- 全外显子测序(WES)
- 全基因组测序(WGS)
- 亚硫酸氢钠测序
- 低覆盖度拷贝数测序
- 反相蛋白质阵列
- 质谱分析法
- 抗体阵列
- 核酸微阵列

单细胞检测

单细胞测序(DNA/RNA)
- 流式细胞学(荧光标签,金属标签)

临床研究
- 病例记录
- 临床试验

其他
- siRNA,shRNA
- CRISPR
- 质谱分析法
- 显微切割,分离肿瘤细胞
- 显微镜
- 影像学
- 循环外泌体,循环肿瘤细胞(CTC)

表 18-2 在线应用的生信分析工具和数据源

UCSC 基因组浏览器[12]——提供对基因组序列数据库的交互式在线访问，以及多种生物的丰富注释数据。基因组序列水平显示，并附一系列注释标记（可由用户选择）。例如，有些标记可以提供预测基因，转录因子靶标，DNA 重复元件，微小 RNA 以及跨物种比较基因组信息。一个与其相关的癌症基因组学浏览器，用于显示和分析癌症基因组数据以及相关的临床数据[13]（http://genome.ucsc.edu/）。

cBioportal[14]——用于直观，交互式探索多种癌症基因组数据集的资源以及来自许多不同公共分子表达谱分析项目的相关信息，包括 TCGA（http://www.cbioportal.org/）。

Cytoscape —— 一个灵活的开源软件平台，用于分析，可视化和注释复杂的交互网络（http://www.cytoscape.org/）。

Bioconductor —— 一个大型的开源，开放式的开发程序集合（截至 2015 年 3 月，包含 934 个），主要用 R 编写，用于分析，图形可视化和生物信息数据的注释[15]（http://www.bioconductor.org）。

Ingenuity 通路分析——信号通路，调节网络和疾病数据的综合分析（可在公共和商业版本中获得）（http://www.ingenuity.com）。

Pathway studio——分子相互作用和相关工具的资源整合，部分基于生物和医学文献（商业产品）的自然语言处理（http://www.elsevier.com/solutions/pathway-studio）。

Oncomine——包含数百种公共癌症微阵列基因表达研究的数据库，以及用于 meta 数据分析的相关工具，例如用于鉴定肿瘤亚型，生物标志物和治疗靶标（可在公共和商业版本中获得）[16]（http://www.lifetechnologies.com/us/en/home/life-science/cancer-research/cancer-genomics/cancer-genomics-data-analysis-compendia-bioscience/oncomine-cancer-genomics-data-analysis-tools/oncomine-genebrowser.html）。

基因本体论（GO）[17]——通过运用规范的词汇和类别（或术语）的层次结构来统一注释基因和基因产物的国际计划。形式上，该结构是“非循环图”，其中层次结构中的每个类别可以具有多个父类别。有三种独立的本体：生物过程，分子功能和细胞成分。在两种基因表达谱的比较中，GO 经常用于鉴定相对过表达或表达不足的基因的类别。用于富集统计评估的工具包括 AmiGo，David，GoMiner 和 OBO-Edit（http://geneontology.org/）。

TCGA 二代聚集热图（NG CHM）简介——聚类热图是生物信息学中常用的可视化图形，常用于展示分子表达谱数据库中的规律。但是它们一般是静态的图像。NG-CHM 是一个高度互动的版本，人们可以使用类似谷歌地图技术进行缩放和探索；链接到相关的公共数据资源，包括 pathway program，UCSC 基因组浏览器和 cBio Portal；在运行中重新着色热图；运用统计工具箱以进行详细的数据分析；生成高分辨率的图片；并存储重现地图所需的所有元数据达数月数年之久。（http://bioinformatics。mdanderson.org/main/TCGA/NGCHM）。

癌症基因组图谱（TCGA）数据门户——访问非限制性 TCGA 数据的主要门户（http://cancergenome.nih.gov）。

Firehose——一种分析基础设施，通过数十种分析算法来处理吉比特或太比特规模的数据集，数据集主要是包括 TCGA 在内的癌症基因组计划。附加组件 Nozzle 提供了便捷的结果格式（http://gdac.broadinstitute.org）。

Regulome Explorer——一套用于探索和可视化大型复杂数据集的工具，具有机器学习算法（随机森林）和圆形表意图布局，线性多轨浏览器和 2D 绘图（http://explorer.cancerregulome.ORG）。

Paradigm——基于基因之间的信号通路相互作用推断患者特异性基因活动的程序。它结合了肿瘤样本的多组学数据，并可以根据概率推断预测一条通路的活动水平（http://sbenz.github.com/Paradigm）[18]。Paradigm Shift（http://github.org/paradigm-shift）是其相关程序，它使用置信传播算法从通路相互作用背景下的基因表达和拷贝数数据中推断基因活性。

NCI 基因组数据共享-正在开发的综合计算基础设施，用于存储和协调通过 NCI 资助的研究计划产生的癌症基因组数据。

GenBank——NIH/NLM 基因序列数据库，所有可公开获得的 DNA 序列的注释集合（http://www.ncbi.nlm.nhi.gov/genbank）。

GEO（Gene Expression Omnibus）——基于微阵列的功能基因组数据库和基于测序的基因表达数据集（http://www.ncbi.nlm.nih.gov/geo）。

Cancer Genomics Hub（CGHub）——一个安全的数据存储库，用于存储、编目和访问来自癌症基因组图谱联盟和相关项目的癌症基因组序列，比对和突变信息（包括限制访问的个人可识别数据）（https://cghub.ucsc.edu/）。

聚类热图

聚类热图(CHM)是最常用的总结生信数据模式的方式。行和列的分层聚类用于突出数据中的模式。聚类热图在 20 世纪 90 年代早期被引入生物信息学[19]，目前它们已经成为组学数据分析可视化中最常用的图形。聚类热图出现在成千上万的出版物中，第一个已知影响医疗实践的聚类热图出现在 1993 年，如图 18-4 所示，它反映了在 NCI-60 抗癌细胞系中筛选含铂化合物的药物活性的相关性。它推进了奥沙利铂的临床应用和开发，目前奥沙利铂是治疗结肠直肠癌的标准化疗药物。

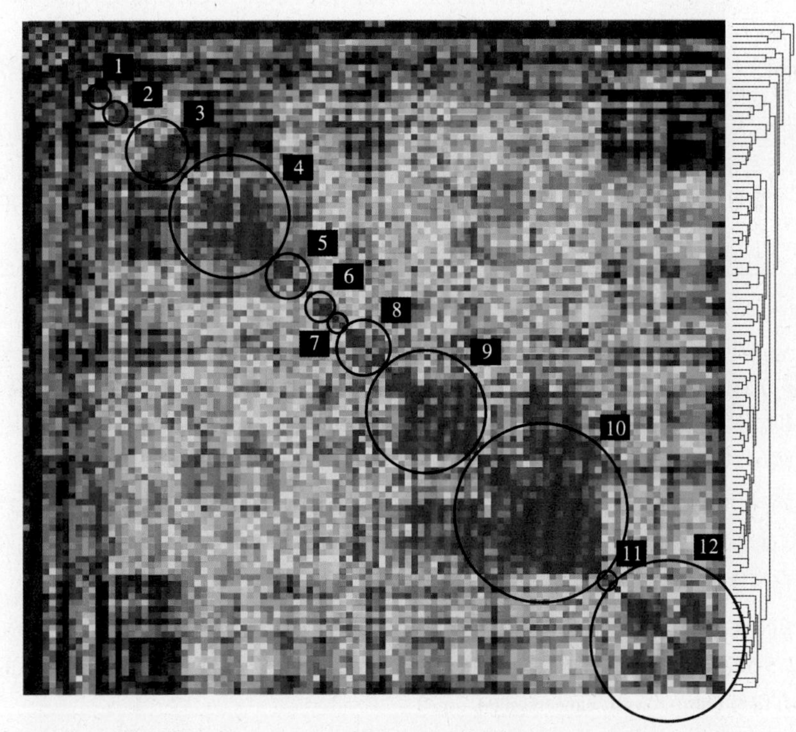

图 18-4 药物对比聚类热图显示了含铂化合物对 NCI-60 人癌细胞系组的作用活性。药物在两个轴上以相同的聚类顺序列出，因此热图在对角线两侧是对称的。红色表示药物作用的高相关性，蓝色表示低相关性。数据定义了 12 个家族(与化合物的化学结构高度相关)。第 4 组药物完全由二氨基环己基衍生物(包括奥沙利铂)组成，对结直肠细胞系具有特异作用活性。这些信息促进了奥沙利铂的临床开发，奥沙利铂现已成为治疗结直肠癌的标准药物(T Fojo，T Myers，J N Weinstein)

产生假设和假设引导的研究

纵观历史，生物学主要是一门观察类科学。达尔文通过对加拉帕戈斯雀类和其塔群岛物种进行客观的观察，而不是通过试验，提出了自然选择的假说。到了 20 世纪中叶，生物学中占主导地位的研究模式已转为严密观察。然而随后受到物理学中重要实验提出的概念影响，生物学实验再次退回观察实验为主的学科。直到 20 世纪 90 年代，随着微阵列和其他高通量分子技术的成熟，生物学的研究模式再度转型为假设引导的实验和提出假设的组学研究。2000 年公布的人类基因组序列草案巩固了这一趋势，并促进产生了癌症基因组图谱(TCGA)和国际癌症基因组联盟(ICGC)等其他大规模分子表达谱分析项目。正如引言中所指出的，高通量组学研究的趋势是生物信息学成为生物医学科学中重要组成部分的主要原因。

多重假设测试陷阱

这是未经统计学培训的人员在生物信息学分析中最常见的错误。在利用大型分子或临床数据库开发生物标记物时，$P<0.05$ 并不难发现。例如，通过微阵列或通过 RNA 测序产生的 20 000 个基因表达值的数据库，该数据库来自对特定药物有反应的 50 名肿瘤患者和 50 名没有反应的肿瘤患者。如果目的是探索肿瘤中与药物反应正相关的基因(预测性生物标志物)，则需要同时测试约 20 000 种不同的假设，每个基因是一种。由于 P 值(拒绝零假设没有差异)有 1/20 的概率小于 0.05，所以即使数据是随机的，也会出现大约 1 000 个潜在的生物标志物。另外，在分析多个统计算法、基因子集或样本子集的时候，出现多个假设问题的概率会升高。如果为了 P 值小于 0.05 而尝试五种不同的算法，那么即便 P 值是极小的，它也是有误导性的。理论上，最简单但过于保守的补救措施是 Bonferroni 校正，其中临界 P 值(例如 0.05)除以独立假设的数量以获得校正的临界值。对于 20 000 个独立的基因，P 值要达到 $P=0.05/20\,000=2.5\times10^{-6}$ 才能被认为具有统计学意义。最常用于校正的是基于错误发现率(FDR)的算法，显然为阳性结果的部分(即零假设的明显拒绝)实际上会被判为假阳性。统计细微差别很复杂，单是校正算法就被提出了 10 余种[20]。生物信息学中一种流行的方法是微阵列统计分析(SAM)算法，它将数据中的相关结构考虑在内[21]。

多重假设问题突出了生物信息学中假设生成和假设检验之间的重要差异。对于后者，必须遵守严格的统计推断规则否则结果是不正确的。例如，如果研究者仅仅挖掘未修正的 $P<0.05$ 的基因，则上述情况下约 1 000 个基因将被虚假地鉴定为

生物标记物。然而，如果研究者在查看数据之前开始，只关注20 000个中的一个单基因，那么无论有多少其他基因存在于数据集，该基因的临界水平将是$P=0.05$。

假设提出包括核查每个基因是否是足够合理的候选生物标记，以保证进一步的研究。FDR提供了该合理性的度量。人们可以按照FDR值的顺序排列基因，从最低到最高，并保留列表顶部所有基因作为候选基因，并根据需要将列表向下延伸。与通常的P值标准类比，倾向于选择0.05的FDR截止值，但这可能过于保守。在生物学或医学科学中，我们也不会奢望20次中有19次是正确的。实际上，接受为阳性候选的数量应取决于独立验证候选的"成本"与错失阳性候选的"成本"之间的平衡。如果验证步骤是一个简单的实验，那么我们可以容忍更多的假阳性结果；如果验证步骤很复杂，如大手术，那么我们则不能容忍任何假阳性。假阳性、真阳性和"阳性预测值"的问题在公共卫生和临床实践的许多领域中常被提及，例如在PSA筛查的争议中。这些问题在整个生物信息学分析中反复出现。因此重要的是，进行统计分析的人员需要了解被问到的问题，被问及的原因以及后续行动的成本/效益比。

大型分子表达谱项目的分析和生物学解释

大规模的分子表达谱分析项目为生物信息学的应用提供了重要的舞台，也为该领域的创新提供了丰富的测试平台。表18-3列出了一些较为突出的大型公开赞助的分子表达谱分析

表18-3 人类癌症、正常组织以及细胞系的大型分子表达谱项目

可培养肿瘤细胞
NCI-60——自1990年以来，NCI用于筛选超过100 000种化合物和天然产物抗癌活性的60个人类细胞系[22]。这是第一个将药理学与多种癌细胞的多方面分子表达谱分析联系起来的大型公共项目。该项目促进了生物信息学新工具的开发，包括聚类热图[19]和统计学以及机器学习方面的创新[23]。NCI-60为CCLE，GDSC的设计提供了一个模板，并促进了TCGA的诞生（见下文）。该项目仍在继续（数据来自 http://discover.nci.nih.gov/cellminer/home.do）。
癌细胞系百科全书（CCLE）——947种不同人类癌细胞系的基因表达，DNA拷贝数和测序数据以及在479种细胞系中对24种抗癌药物进行代谢抑制试验的相关数据。Naïve Bayes和弹性网络算法可以根据细胞谱系、遗传缺陷和基因表达预测其药物反应谱[24]。该项目仍在继续（http://www.broadinstitute.org/ccle）。
癌症药物敏感性基因组学（GDSC）——639种人类癌细胞系中点突变、插入缺失、微卫星不稳定性和DNA重排的基因表达谱，以及130个抗癌剂在275-507细胞系上进行的代谢抑制实验相关数据。弹性网络回归可根据细胞系的分子表达谱预测药物敏感性[25]。该项目仍在继续（http://www.cancerrxgene.org/）。
临床肿瘤和组织
人类基因组计划——计划于1986年发起[26]，宣布序列草案的文章发表于2001年[27,28]。当时许多研究人员惊讶地发现，生物信息学分析显示只有大约23 000个人类基因，而不是预期的大于50 000个。该项目在2004年完成度达到了99%[29]，但是生物信息学的一个主要难点是软件和数据库的更新，以便与参考序列的持续改进保持同步。目前的参考序列是第38版（http//www.cancerrxgene.org/）。
国际HapMap项目——于2002年启动，用于定义人群子集中的常见DNA序列变异。不相关的个体在序列上具有约99.9%的同一性，但剩余的序列和拷贝数多态性对生物信息学分析来说既是有用的信息又是数据处理上的难题[30]（http://hapmap.ncbi.nlm.nih.gov/）。
癌症基因组图谱（TCGA）——始于2005年，在基因组学、表观基因组学、转录组学、病理学和临床水平对25种类型的10 000个人类癌组织样本进行分子表达谱分析。于2008年发表的第一个项目是胶质母细胞瘤[31]。来自33种癌症类型的超过10 000个肿瘤的分子表达谱得到了收录，超过了最初的目标。"泛癌症"项目[32,33]总结了所研究的前12种肿瘤类型之间的相似性和差异。它解决了①跨多种肿瘤类型的特定功能主题（例如驱动突变、异常信号途径和耐药基因）的共性，以及②肿瘤类型可以通过多种方式细分为更加精细的类别，这会促进更加精确、靶向的临床治疗方式。TCGA最初专注于DNA和RNA谱，但后来添加了反相蛋白质阵列（RPPA）和质谱法的蛋白质研究[34,35]。涵盖所有33种TCGA肿瘤类型的综合泛癌症分析计划于2016年完成（http://cancergenome.nih.gov/）。
国际癌症基因组联盟（ICGC）[36]——于2008年推出，对50种不同的人类癌症类型进行分子表达谱分析，其方式类似于TCGA。TCGA研究网络和ICGC正在合作进行全基因组测序和分析来自2 000名患者的各种癌症（https://icgc.org/）。
辅助性肺癌富集标志物鉴定和测序试验（ALCHEMIST）——由NCI的国家临床试验网络（National Clinical Trials Network）于2014年发起，用于鉴定具有遗传变化（EGFR突变或ALK重排）的早期肺癌患者，以评估针对这些变化的靶向药物的疗效（http://www.cancer.gov/types/lung/research/alchemist）。
治疗特殊反应人群倡议——由NCI于2014年发起，旨在探索对治疗具有特殊反应性的人群的独特分子基础。使用的主要技术是全外显子测序和mRNA测序（http://www.nih.gov/news/health/sep2014/nci 24.htm）。

续表

基因型-组织表达项目(GTEx)——由美国国立人类基因组研究所于 2006 年启动,以评估来自多达 900 名尸体志愿捐献者的多个正常组织中基因型和表达水平之间的相关性,以辅助全基因组的关联研究和作为癌症和其他疾病研究的正常背景数据(http://www.gtexportal.org/home/)。
1 000 个基因组项目——于 2008 年启动,旨在建立关于人类种系基因组变异的最详细目录[37](http://www.gtexportal.org/home)。
DNA 元件百科全书(ENCODE)——由 NHGRI 发起,作为人类基因组计划的后续行动。其最终目的是识别人类基因组中的所有功能元件,特别是那些不位于 RNA 编码区域的功能元件[38](https://www.encodeproject.org)。
促进发展有效治疗的治疗适用性研究(TARGET)—— 影响儿科癌症的起始,进展和治疗反应性的遗传变化(基因表达、DNA 拷贝数、DNA 甲基化和 microRNA 表达)的多机构分子表达谱分析(https://ocg.cancer.gov/programs/target)。

项目。大规模项目的“第一波浪潮”主要集中在癌细胞系和大量的原发肿瘤样本以及血液或正常组织对照。然而,其他项目待解决的问题更加尖锐,需要基于显微切割、单细胞测序[39]、福尔马林固定石蜡包埋样本、治疗前/治疗后配对样本、原发肿瘤/转移灶配对样本,以及比较来自同一原发肿瘤不同部位的样本,来自同一患者的不同转移灶的比较,原发/复发配对样本,以及来自应答者和非应答者的样本。“第二波浪潮”项目利用了许多当前的算法和程序进行数据分析和解释,也推动了新型生物信息学工具的开发。例如,单细胞测序,特别是在 DNA 水平上,为生物信息学提出了一系列新的要求,但同时也为精辟的分析提供了新的机会。由于复发性肿瘤可以反映原发性肿瘤中的微小克隆,对治疗选择很重要,所以对于越来越多的肿瘤类型和临床情况,二次活检可能会越来越多被接受。

图 18-5 示意性地显示了迄今为止最突出的分子表达谱分析项目 TCGA 中组织和信息的流动。超过 50 个临床中心提供了成对的肿瘤和正常样本(血液和/或肿瘤相邻的“正常”组织)以及 33 种肿瘤类型的病理学和临床病史信息。具有特定肿瘤专业知识的一组病理学家对样本进行分析是至关重要的。样本在 Biospecimen Core Resource 处理以产生 DNA、RNA 和蛋白质制备物,然后在基因组测序和基因组表征中心中对其进行分析(主要通过微阵列或测序)。数据收集于 2015 年完成,但数据分析和解释将是延续多年的工作。数据协调中心组织并进一步对数据进行质量控制,然后在 TCGA 数据门户网站上尽快公布“非限制性”数据集。“受限制的”数据(可能足以识别个体患者的数据)只有经过注册和审查程序以确保机密性和适当使用的研究人员才能访问。例如,原始的 DNA 和 RNA 测序数据是受限制数据,因为它们可以识别到个体。数据分析和解释的重任落在七个指定的基因组数据分析中心(GDAC),它们已经成为一个 TCGA 社区,共享生物信息学专业知识。

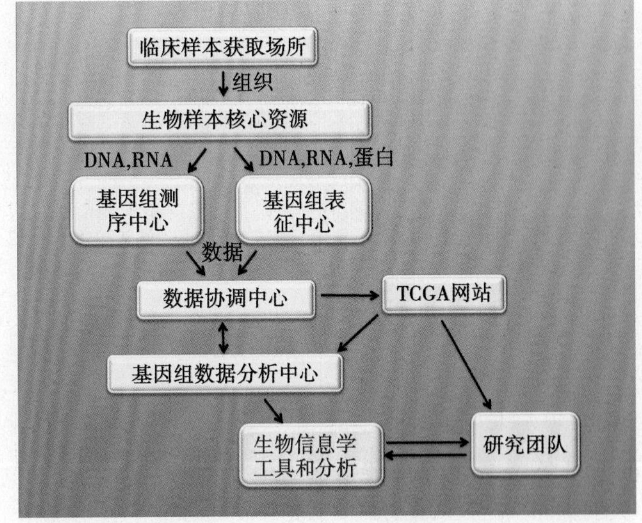

图 18-5 《癌症基因组图谱项目》中样本收集和信息应用流程图。项目中的肿瘤组织样本、正常血样以及癌旁组织样本取样自不同的临床中心,并根据既定的方案进行预处理。Biospecimen Core Resource 负责审查临床样本质量、随附的临床数据以及其对应的 DNA,RNA 和蛋白质样品,在对样品进行了质量控制后,将它们发送到了基因组测序中心和基因组表征中心。这些中心通过测序、微阵列分析或其他技术对样本进行了分析,然后将数据发送至数据协调中心。处理完成后,非限制形式的数据就会在 TCGA 网站上公开并供研究团队使用,其中就包括 TCGA 的基因组数据分析中心。为简单起见,该流程图省略了信息处理的很多详细组分,例如 Broad Institute 的 Firehose,它对数据进行了大量分析;Sage Bionetics 的 Synapse,它提供了分析环境和分析工具,能够促进数据的广泛协作使用;Memorial Sloan-Kettering 的 cBio,将数据转换为非专业人员也可以访问的形式;MD Anderson 的聚类热图,用于将 DNA、RNA 和蛋白质数据集中进行模式识别。临床数据和病理学的专家评论也没有展示

TCGA 的主要衍生产品是围绕疾病特异性和泛癌分析工作组(PCAWG)的大型生物信息学社区的整合。每个分析工作组(AWG)集合了数据分析和生物/医学解释所需的多学科专业知识的人才。位于数据分析中心的是 GDAC,但许多其他个人和机构也加入进来。因为 AWG 中的每个人都在深入研究相同的数据集和数据类型,这行程了一个强大的创造性环境,用于开发数据分析、可视化、解释的新型工具。图 18-6 是基于 TCGA 的多层面尿路膀胱癌分析。图 18-6a 显示了 DNA 测序数据的紧凑图形可视化,图 18-6b 显示了 RNA 表达水平的“二代”交互式聚类热图,图 18-6c 显示了关键的信号通路。

TCGA 最初被设计为一系列以疾病为重点的项目,但 PCAWG 发现的不同肿瘤类型间的相似性和差异是更加宝贵的数据。图 18-7 将泛癌症项目示意性地表示为的 3D 矩阵。

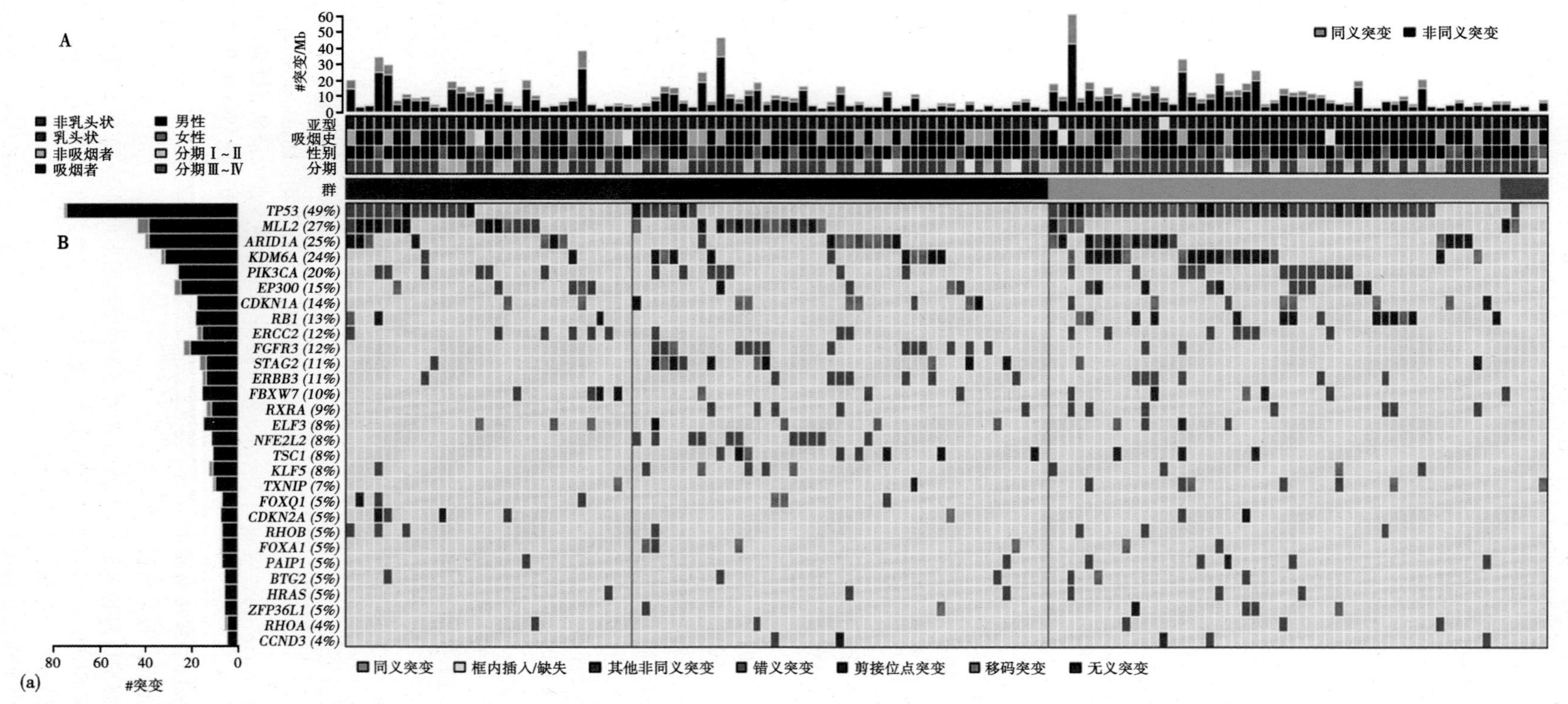

图 18-6 TCGA 尿路膀胱癌项目中的数据可视化。来源:癌症基因组图谱研究网络 2014[40]。131 名患者的肿瘤标本被纳入分析。(a)膀胱癌标本中基因突变谱的可视化,用 MutSig 1.5 算法评分评估显著突变的基因(来自 J. Kim, A. Cherniack, G. Getz, D. Kwiatkowski)。(b)mRNA 表达谱数据在交互式二代聚类热图上显示。基因标注于纵轴;患者标本标注于横轴(来自 B. Broom, R. Akbani, D. Kane, M. Ryan, C. Wakefield, J. Weinstein)。(c)在尿路上皮膀胱癌中发现在 DNA 水平上发生改变的四个信号通路。在 p53/Rb 通路、RTK/RAS/PI3K 通路、组蛋白修饰系统和 SWI/SNF 复合物中发现了体细胞突变和拷贝数改变(CNA)。红色,激活型遗传改变;蓝色,失活型遗传改变。显示的百分比表示至少一个等位基因的激活或失活

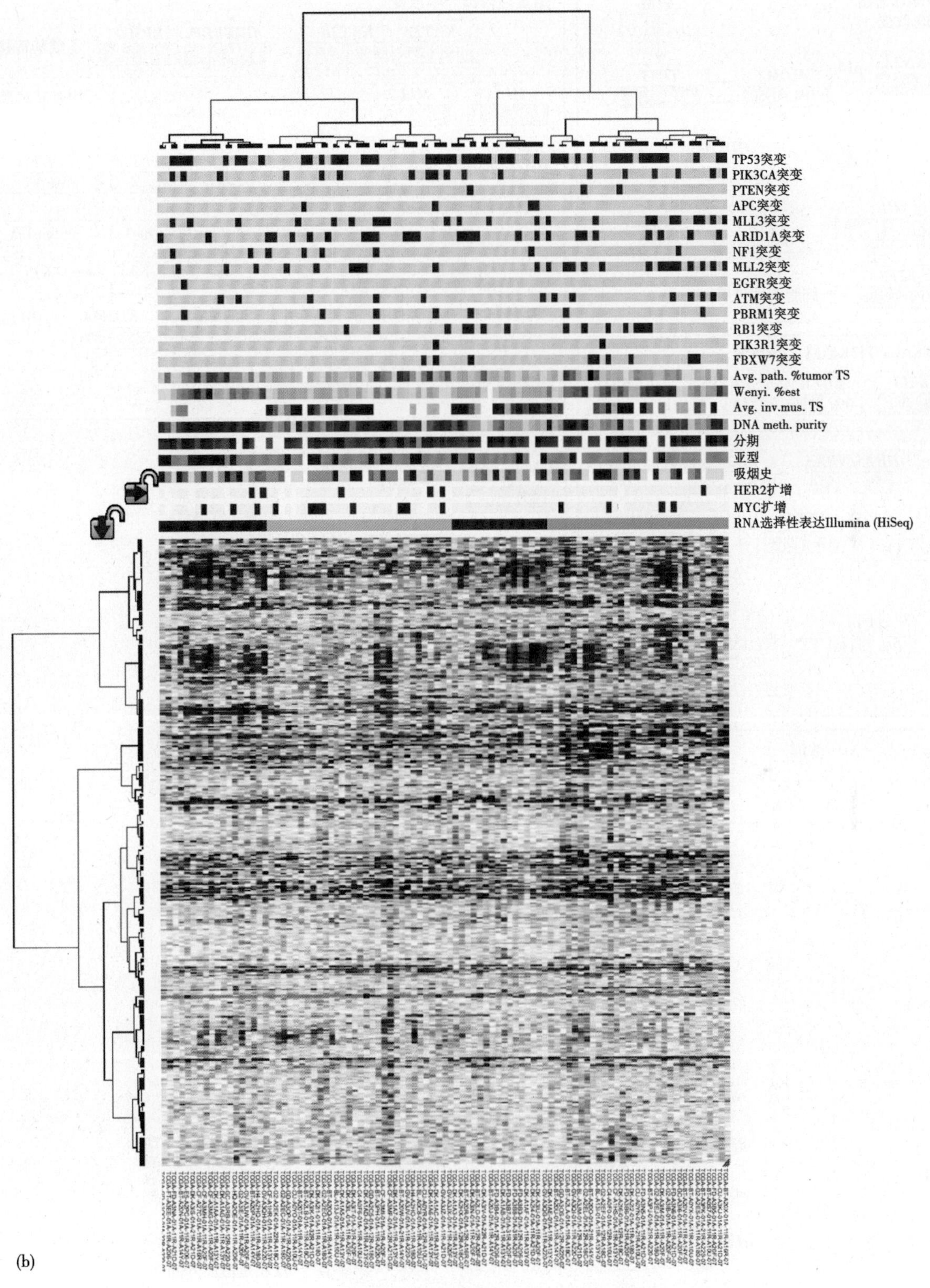
TP53突变
PIK3CA突变
PTEN突变
APC突变
MLL3突变
ARID1A突变
NF1突变
MLL2突变
EGFR突变
ATM突变
PBRM1突变
RB1突变
PIK3R1突变
FBXW7突变
Avg. path. %tumor TS
Wenyi. %est
Avg. inv.mus. TS
DNA meth. purity
分期
亚型
吸烟史
HER2扩增
MYC扩增
RNA选择性表达Illumina (HiSeq)
(b)

图 18-6(续)

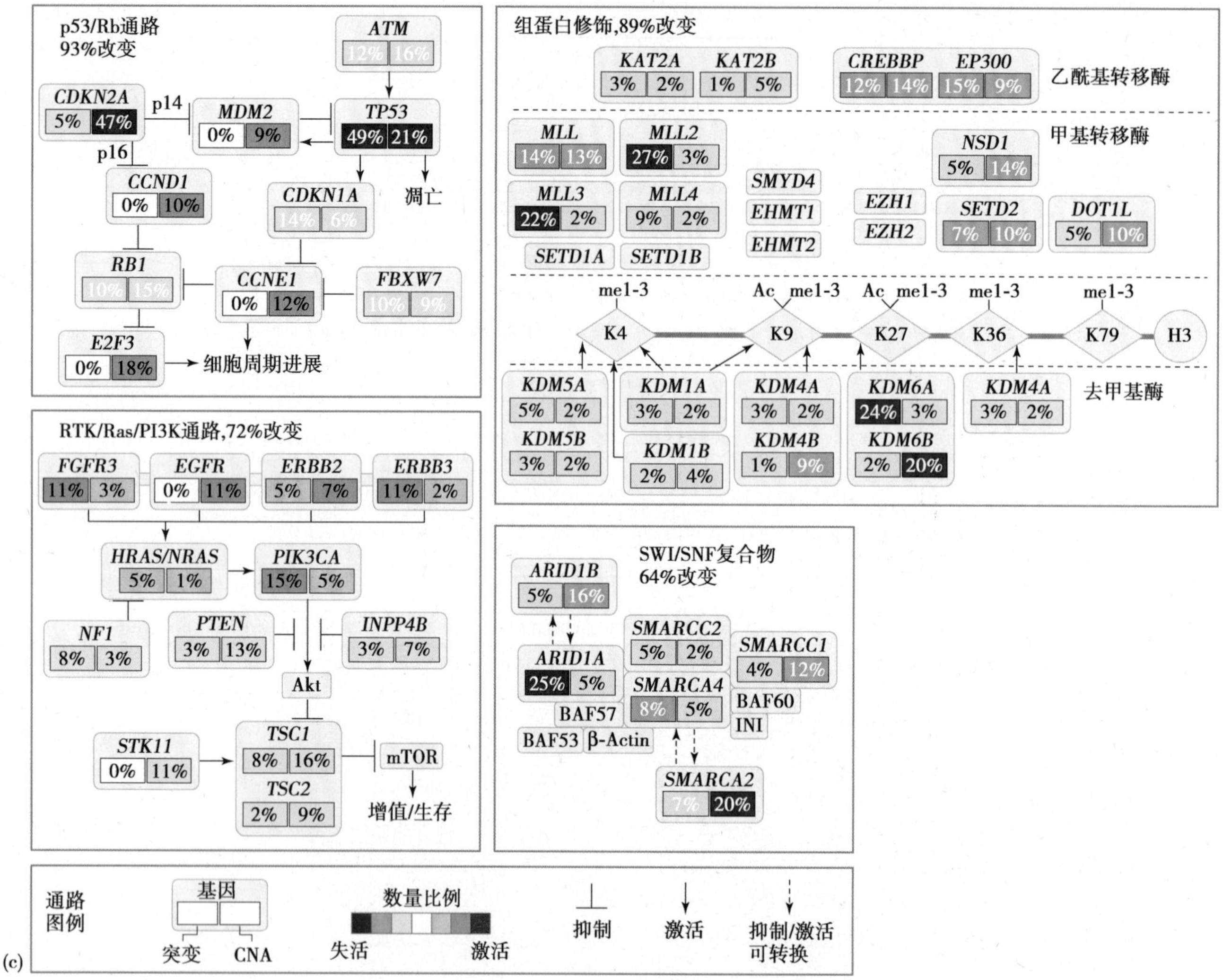

p53/Rb通路
93%改变
ATM
12% 16%
CDKN2A
5% 47%
p14
MDM2
0% 9%
TP53
49% 21%
p16
CCND1
0% 10%
CDKN1A
14% 6%
凋亡
RB1
10% 15%
CCNE1
0% 12%
FBXW7
10% 9%
E2F3
0% 18%
细胞周期进展
RTK/Ras/PI3K通路,72%改变
FGFR3
11% 3%
EGFR
0% 11%
ERBB2
5% 7%
ERBB3
11% 2%
HRAS/NRAS
5% 1%
PIK3CA
15% 5%
NF1
8% 3%
PTEN
3% 13%
INPP4B
3% 7%
Akt
STK11
0% 11%
TSC1
8% 16%
mTOR
TSC2
2% 9%
增值/生存
组蛋白修饰,89%改变
KAT2A
3% 2%
KAT2B
1% 5%
CREBBP
12% 14%
EP300
15% 9%
乙酰基转移酶
MLL
14% 13%
MLL2
27% 3%
NSD1
5% 14%
甲基转移酶
SMYD4
EHMT1
EHMT2
MLL3
22% 2%
MLL4
9% 2%
EZH1
EZH2
SETD2
7% 10%
DOT1L
5% 10%
SETD1A
SETD1B
me1-3
Ac
me1-3
Ac
me1-3
me1-3
me1-3
K4
K9
K27
K36
K79
H3
KDM5A
5% 2%
KDM1A
3% 2%
KDM4A
3% 2%
KDM6A
24% 3%
KDM4A
3% 2%
去甲基酶
KDM5B
3% 2%
KDM1B
2% 4%
KDM4B
1% 9%
KDM6B
2% 20%
SWI/SNF复合物
64%改变
ARID1B
5% 16%
SMARCC2
5% 2%
SMARCC1
4% 12%
ARID1A
25% 5%
SMARCA4
8% 5%
BAF60
BAF57
INI
BAF53
β-Actin
SMARCA2
7% 20%
通路
图例
基因
突变
CNA
数量比例
失活
激活
抑制
激活
抑制/激活
可转换
(c)

图 18-6(续)

突变
拷贝数
基因表达
DNA甲基化
微小RNA
反相蛋白质阵列
临床数据
数据类型
BRCA
BLCA
COAD
GBM
HNSC
KIRC
LAML
LUAD
LUSC
OV
READ
UCEC
肿瘤类型
基因/位点

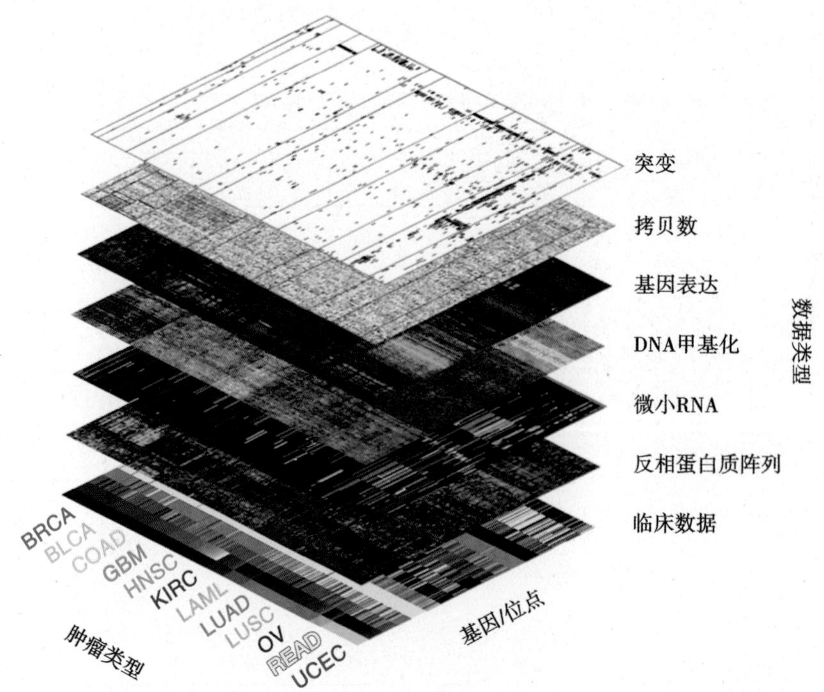

图 18-7 将 Pan-Cancer TCGA 项目表示为三维矩阵,其中坐标轴分别是肿瘤类型,数据类型和基因/位点

统计学方法及相关隐患

表 18-4 列出了一些生物信息学中常用的统计学方法和机器学习算法。表中的描述旨在向读者提供关于如何在生物信息学中使用该算法的一般了解，而不是针对有统计学基础人员。在本节中将会详细介绍两个最常用的统计学方法，主要目的是指出这两种方法在它们的使用和对生物信息学数据的解释中的限制和容易出现的错误。即使是最简单的单变量统计数据也经常被误用或产生误导。如表 18-4 所示，该节将集中强调生物学家和临床研究人员应该考虑的问题，而不是生物统计学家想要考虑的更加复杂的情况。

表 18-4　生物信息学中常用的统计学算法

单变量分析
非配对 t 检验：两个样本均值的统计检验。双样本 t 检验用于检查两个样本是否不同，通常用于两组数据正态分布方差未知，而且样本量较小。
配对 t 检验：样本配对，例如：治疗前后的肿瘤样本。
置换 t 检验：两组数据可以不服从正态分布，但分布要相同。几乎所有的参数统计学检验都有其对应的非参数的检验方法，可以通过改变数据形式获得 P 值。
Wilcoxon 符号秩检验：配对 t 检验的非参数版本。（基于等级资料，正态非必要）。
Wilcoxon 秩和检验：非配对 t 检验的非参数版本。（基于等级资料，正态非必要）。
多变量分析
差异分析（ANOVA）：不同形式的 ANOVA 将 t 检验的应用拓展到符合正态分布的多变量数据集（例如，超过 2 种肿瘤组织参与比较）。
多变量差异分析（MANOVA）：类似 ANOVA，但是考虑到了变量之间的相互作用（依赖）。
交叉验证：可用于基于一组样品中一种或多种基因的表达预测结果（例如，存活）。对 90% 的患者进行预测模型训练，然后对其他 10% 进行测试。然后迭代地省略不同组的 10%，以便在特定轮次的训练和测试期间堆积关于模型在患者样本上成功的统计数据。但是，如果模型以任何方式“调整”以在交叉验证的基础上对其进行优化，则必须需要一组单独的样本对其进行验证，以避免对算法产生过于乐观的结论。在大多数情况下，无论如何都必须使用独立的数据集验证模型。
Bootstrap：找出计算统计量的统计置信界限（例如，基于 N 个基因的表达模式的相似性和差异，两个患者的肿瘤之间的 Pearson 或 Spearman 相关系数）。接下来，我们从基因组中选择大小为 N 的随机样本，以产生具有 N 个值的“伪样本”，然后计算该样本的 Pearson 相关系数。我们这样做了很多次，比如 10 000 次，建立 Pearson 相关系数的直方图，并根据该直方图选择 95% 置信区间。因为采样是通过替换进行的，所以任何给定的基因可能在给定样本中出现 0，1，2，3 或更多次（根据 Poisson 分布，平均值为 1）。
接收者操作特征曲线（Receiver-Operator Characteristic，ROC）：当鉴别阈值从低到高变化时，灵敏性与 1-特异性的关系图体现了二元分类器的性能（例如特定基因的表达作为复发的预测因子）。ROC 曲线下面积与（非参数）Wilcoxon 秩和检验直接相关。
分层聚类分析：聚类将类似的概况表现在树状结构中（例如，肿瘤标本间或不同基因间）以阐明它们之间的相似性和差异的模式。聚类（监督或无监督）通常用于定义肿瘤类型的子类别。
Fisher 精确检验：列联表中变量独立性的置换检验。例如，如果临床试验中的每位患者被标记为治疗的应答者或非应答者，并且针对特定基因标记为野生型或突变体，则研究结果可以表示为 2×2 的列联表。Fisher 精确检验（单尾或双尾）给出零假设的 P 值，即基因的状态对响应没有影响。“确切”表示即使非常小的样本量，P 值也是准确的。该检验可以扩展应用到更大的列联表（即 m×n）。
Bayesian 方法：在分析数据之前基于指定的先前的经验或最佳猜测，将概率或分布分配给（后续的）结果或参数的统计方法。然后应用贝叶斯定理来修正后续的概率。贝叶斯方法在概念上与更常见的“频率学派”方法不同。一个例子是多臂，生物标志物探索的临床试验，其中累积经验用于重新评估特定生物标志物预测治疗反应的可能性-然后使用该信息让更多的病人收益。

Student t 检验

Student t 检验的命名并非因为它迎合了新手学员的需要。相反，它是由一名啤酒厂化学家/学者于 1908 年提出的，因为受到当时的公司政策的限制故只能以笔名“Student”发表。t 检验被广泛用于癌症生物信息学。例如，用于评估治疗和未治疗患者之间血液或肿瘤中基因的平均表达水平是否不同。如果治疗和未治疗的样本来自同一患者，则可以调用配对 t 检验（具有更高的统计学效力）。每个实验室生物学家都非常熟悉 t 检验，但 t 检验有两个限制值得注意，因为它们经常被忽略：

- （配对或非配对）t 检验经常被用于检验样本集之间的差异，但如果样本量不够大时，则仅当两组样本值近似正态分布时才能计算正确的 P 值。原始 Student t 检验的扩展应用允许两组的标准差不同，但是要得到正确的 P 值，两组的数据分布仍要满足正态。但生物信息学中的数据很少是正态分布的，因此 t 检验得到的 P 值通常是不正确的。例如，微阵列数据通常在分析之前进行对数转换，但这种使它们的数据分布更接近正常的行为是徒劳的。这导致了在随后的分析中，有噪音的低表达数据被赋予太多的权重，这会严重扭曲获得的结果。唯一令人满意的程序是滤除低噪声，低幅度数据。但究竟如何在不丢弃太多数据或引入偏差的情况下做到这一点是一项极其复杂的挑战。
- 如果样本在必要的意义上不是彼此独立的，那么 t 检验得到的 P 值也可能是错误的。一个常见的错误是将技术重复（例如，测定中的三次重复）视为独立的。例如，如果一项检测在 10 名患者的一式三份样本中测量治疗前后基因的表达，则每组中的实际样本数量将为 30。但是如果患者之间的表达差异远大于同一患者不同样本之间的差异（通常情况下），那么治疗前组合治疗后组实际上都各只有 10 个独立值。t 检验的统计效力取决于 N，即样本数。因此，如果 t 检验过程中使用 N = 30，则得到的 P 值将过于乐观；治疗无效的假设可能被虚假地拒绝。

Wilcoxon 秩和检验和 Wilcoxon 符号秩检验

Wilcoxon 秩和检验和 Wilcoxon 符号秩检验分别是 t 检验和配对 t 检验的非参数数据的对应检验算法。也就是说它们具有 t 检验类似的功能，但他们的分析是基于数据的等级分布，而不是实际的数值分布。因此它们不依赖于正态分布的假设。但是这两种检验通常具有独立性，因此它们会遇到与上述重复 t 检验相同的问题。当样本处于正态时，它们的检验效能略低于 t 检验，但它们对离群值和其他类型的非正态性不太敏感，因此他们的检验效能不太会受到数据分布的干扰。但是选择这两种检验也要付出相应的代价。想象一下，一组样本中基因的表达水平在 1 到 2 个单位范围内，而另一组样本中相同基因的表达水平与第一组样本的表达水平相差很大，范围是 101 到 102 个单位。非参数测试不会受到这种分布差异的影响，就好像第二组的值范围只是 2.1 到 2.2 单位，仅与第一组的那些略有不同。在非参数检验中只有数据分级最重要，所以非常大的差异不会比相对较小的差异造成更大的影响。虽然在一些情况下 t 检验的 P 值不可靠，但 t 检验可以更真实地反映数据情况。因此除了 P 值与 P 值相关的参数，应该始终考虑数据实际值和差异；具有统计学意义并不意味着具有生物学意义。

t 检验及其对应的非参数检验是生物信息学中最简单的统计检验。它们在原理和实践上比多变量和机器学习分析简单得多。尽管如此，前面的例子指出了在使用它们时可能犯的严重错误以及专业知识对于生物信息学中大多数数据的统计分析的重要性。

（郑博 译 李亮 校 陈磊 审）

参考文献

1 Hesper B, Hogeweg P. Bioinformatica: een werkconcept. *Kameleon*. 1970;**1**:28-29.
2 Luscombe NM, Greenbaum D, Gerstein M. What is bioinformatics? A proposed definition and overview of the field. *Methods Inf Med*. 2001;**40(4)**:346-358.
3 http://bioinformaticsweb.tk. Bioinformatics definition - a review 2015
4 Mosby. *Mosby's Dental Dictionary*, 2nd ed. Maryland Heights: Elsevier B.V.; 2008.
5 Moore GE. Cramming more components onto integrated circuits. *Electronics*. 1965;**38(8)**:114-117.
6 Kryder MH, Kim CS. After hard drives - What comes next? *IEEE T MAGN*. 2009;**45(10)**:3406-3413.
7 Church GM, Gao Y, Kosuri S. Next-generation digital information storage in DNA. *Science*. 2012;**337(6102)**:1628.
8 Lawrence MS, Stojanov P, Polak P, et al. Mutational heterogeneity in cancer and the search for new cancer-associated genes. *Nature*. 2013;**499(7457)**:214-218.
9 Kim SY, Speed TP. Comparing somatic mutation-callers: beyond Venn diagrams. *BMC Bioinformatics*. 2013;**14**:189.
10 Baggerly KA, Coombes KR. Deriving chemosensitivity from cell lines: forensic bioinformatics and reproducible research in high-throughput biology. *Ann Appl Stat*. 2009;**3**:1309-1334.
11 Weinstein JN. Fishing expeditions. *Science*. 1998;**282(5389)**:628-629.
12 Kent WJ, Sugnet CW, Furey TS, et al. The human genome browser at UCSC. *Genome Res*. 2002;**12(6)**:996-1006.
13 Goldman M, Craft B, Swatloski T, et al. The UCSC Cancer Genomics Browser: update 2013. *Nucleic Acids Res*. 2013;**41(Database issue)**:D949-D954.
14 Cerami E, Gao J, Dogrusoz U, et al. The cBio cancer genomics portal: an open platform for exploring multidimensional cancer genomics data. *Cancer discovery*. 2012;**2(5)**:401-404.
15 Huber W, Carey VJ, Gentleman R, et al. Orchestrating high-throughput genomic analysis with Bioconductor. *Nat Methods*. 2015;**12(2)**:115-121.
16 Rhodes DR, Kalyana-Sundaram S, Mahavisno V, et al. Oncomine 3.0: genes, pathways, and networks in a collection of 18,000 cancer gene expression profiles. *Neoplasia*. 2007;**9(2)**:166-180.
17 Ashburner M, Ball CA, Blake JA, et al. Gene ontology: tool for the unification of biology. The Gene Ontology Consortium. *Nat Genet*. 2000;**25(1)**:25-29.
18 Vaske CJ, Benz SC, Sanborn JZ, et al. Inference of patient-specific pathway activities from multi-dimensional cancer genomics data using PARADIGM. *Bioinformatics*. 2010;**26(12)**:i237-i245.
19 Weinstein JN, Myers TG, O'Connor PM, et al. An information-intensive approach to the molecular pharmacology of cancer. *Science*. 1997;**275(5298)**:343-349.
20 Farcomeni A. A review of modern multiple hypothesis testing, with particular attention to the false discovery proportion. *Stat Methods Med Res*. 2008;**17(4)**:347-388.
21 Tusher VG, Tibshirani R, Chu G. Significance analysis of microarrays applied to the ionizing radiation response. *Proc Natl Acad Sci U S A*. 2001;**98(9)**:5116-5121.
22 Shoemaker RH, Monks A, Alley MC, et al. Development of human tumor cell line panels for use in disease-oriented drug screening. *Prog Clin Biol Res*. 1988;**276**:265-286.
23 Weinstein JN, Kohn KW, Grever MR, et al. Neural computing in cancer drug development: predicting mechanism of action. *Science*. 1992;**258(5081)**:447-451.
24 Barretina J, Caponigro G, Stransky N, et al. The Cancer Cell Line Encyclopedia enables predictive modelling of anticancer drug sensitivity. *Nature*. 2012;**483(7391)**:603-607.
25 Garnett MJ, Edelman EJ, Heidorn SJ, et al. Systematic identification of genomic markers of drug sensitivity in cancer cells. *Nature*. 2012;**483(7391)**:570-575.
26 DeLisi C. Meetings that changed the world: Santa Fe 1986: Human genome baby-steps. *Nature*. 2008;**455(7215)**:876-877.
27 McPherson JD, Marra M, Hillier L, et al. A physical map of the human genome. *Nature*. 2001;**409(6822)**:934-941.
28 Venter JC, Adams MD, Myers EW, et al. The sequence of the human genome. *Science*. 2001;**291(5507)**:1304-1351.
29 International Human Genome Sequencing C. Finishing the euchromatic sequence of the human genome. *Nature*. 2004;**431(7011)**:931-945.
30 International HapMap C, Altshuler DM, Gibbs RA, et al. Integrating common and rare genetic variation in diverse human populations. *Nature*. 2010;**467(7311)**:52-58.
31 Cancer Genome Atlas Research N. Comprehensive genomic characterization defines human glioblastoma genes and core pathways. *Nature*. 2008;**455(7216)**:1061-1068.
32 Cancer Genome Atlas Research N, Weinstein JN, Collisson EA, et al. The Cancer Genome Atlas Pan-Cancer analysis project. *Nat Genet*. 2013;**45(10)**:1113-1120.
33 Hoadley KA, Yau C, Wolf DM, et al. Multiplatform analysis of 12 cancer types reveals molecular classification within and across tissues of origin. *Cell*. 2014;**158(4)**:929-944.
34 Li J, Lu Y, Akbani R, et al. TCPA: a resource for cancer functional proteomics data.

Nat Methods. 2013;**10(11)**:1046–1047.

35 Akbani R, Ng PKS, Werner HMJ, et al. *Nat Commun*. 2014;5(**3887**). doi: 10.1038/ncomms4887 PMID: 24871328.

36 International Cancer Genome C, Hudson TJ, Anderson W, et al. International network of cancer genome projects. *Nature*. 2010;**464(7291)**:993–998.

37 Genomes Project C, Abecasis GR, Altshuler D, et al. A map of human genome variation from population-scale sequencing. *Nature*. 2010;**467(7319)**:1061–1073.

38 Consortium EP. The ENCODE (ENCyclopedia Of DNA Elements) Project. *Science*. 2004;**306(5696)**:636–640.

39 Navin N, Kendall J, Troge J, et al. Tumour evolution inferred by single-cell sequencing. *Nature*. 2011;**472**:90–94.

40 Cancer Genome Atlas Research Network. Comprehensive molecular characterization of urothelial bladder carcinoma. *Nature*. 2014;**507(7492)**:315–322.

第19章　系统生物学和基因组学

Saima Hassan, MD, PhD, FRCSC ■ Laura M. Heiser, PhD ■ Joe W. Gray, Ph. D.

概述

癌症是复杂的适应性系统，包括癌细胞，近端和远端细胞，以及影响癌细胞行为的可溶性和不溶性蛋白质。与癌症有关的特征被称为癌症的固有特征，而包括近端和远端微环境的特征被称为癌症的外在特征。基因组学研究旨在全面探索癌症在细胞和分子层面的表达谱，而癌症系统生物学致力于开发实验和理论方法用于理解不同组分如何协同调节癌症功能。这些研究的总体目标是通过分析癌症内在和外在的分子和细胞组分来预测癌症行为-包括进展和对治疗的反应性。在这里，我们回顾了国际上对于不同肿瘤类型的基因组学、表观基因组学和蛋白质组学特征（多组学）研究的最新进展。我们总结了建立原子特征与癌症行为之间关联的工作。最后，我们总结了目前用于理解和操纵复杂癌症系统行为的计算和实验模型。

引言

生物系统行为的研究传统上是简化论，侧重于特定的基因或信号通路。目前，研究人员致力于探索癌症的分子表达谱，并以此建立了癌症特征与生物医学行为之间的联系，另外机械理论模型的建立也开始起步。癌症的系统生物学研究方法包括研究癌细胞的内在分子特征，以及外来微环境的信号如何影响癌细胞信号传导和表型反应（图19-1）。

内在癌症系统生物学，原以研究肿瘤实质内的恶性细胞为主，现随着基因组和表观基因组分析技术的进步而发展。这些技术可以对个体肿瘤内基因组变异以及转录和蛋白质组进行全面测量。近期的研究发现了与复发关系紧密的癌症亚群；对癌症异质性有了更深的理解；区分了预后亚组并发现了一系列治疗反应性的预测因子；促进了新治疗靶点的开发[1,2]。

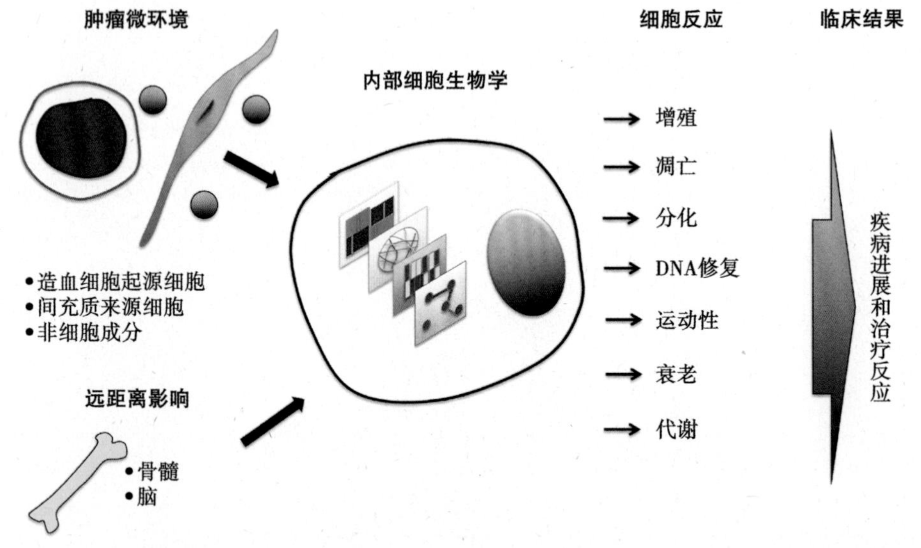

图19-1　外在和内在系统生物学对细胞功能影响的示意图，具有提示患者病情进展和治疗反应的潜力。外部系统生物学组分由肿瘤微环境组成，包括造血细胞来源细胞、间充质来源细胞和非细胞成分，以及来自骨髓和其他多个器官的远距离影响。结合系统生物学方法，可以使用各种终点研究细胞功能，包括细胞增殖、细胞凋亡、分化、DNA修复、运动、衰老和代谢。我们的实验室正在努力将这些终点结合起来，以更好地了解肿瘤进展和对治疗的反应，以及其临床意义

外在系统生物学主要关注的是改变肿瘤细胞行为的外部信号。外在信号可能来自靠近肿瘤细胞的微环境（例如，浸润的免疫细胞，癌症相关成纤维细胞（CAF）和血管内皮细胞）[3]以及来自远端器官，尤其是大脑[4,5]。最近的研究指出肿瘤微环境（肿瘤微环境）的临床重要性即肿瘤间质成分可以预测病人预后[6]，肿瘤微环境可以调节肿瘤的治疗反应性和耐药性[7]，并且免疫微环境已被证明可介导肿瘤的发生、发展[8]和治疗反应性[9~11]。

总的来说，内在和外在的系统生物学致力于探索癌细胞及其与环境的相互作用。本章将涵盖内在和外在系统生物学两方面的内容。内在系统生物学部分将关注高通量基因组学的临床影响和癌细胞系作为患者治疗反应的预测模型的使用。外在系统生物学部分将讨论肿瘤微环境不同的组分，及其临床意义，以及如何将微环境纳入临床前模型。

要点

组学的意义

- TCGA 研究已经开始使用患者样本来明确具有预后意义和新治疗靶标的新肿瘤分类
- 癌细胞系被用于鉴定可预测治疗反应性并存在于患者样品中的基因标签
- 数据分析工具的开发和验证使多组学数据整合成为可能

癌症的内在系统生物学和基因组学

自从人类基因组图谱以来，众多技术进步已经实现了“组学”时代，其中高通量分析工作实现了对癌症发生、进展、药物反应期间出现的肿瘤和相关基质中 DNA、RNA 和蛋白质水平变化的全面评估[12]。目前，许多研究旨在使用这些数据来改善癌症的临床诊断和治疗。其瓶颈在于数据处理和解释[13]。消除瓶颈将需要新的生物信息学方法，可以有效地识别可调节的分子事件和药物治疗靶点。虽然平台的稳健性和基因标签的验证是影响其临床应用的主要问题[14,15]，但是为了更好地将基因组平台整合到临床中，更多的实用性问题需要解决。例如，目前下一代肿瘤库需要更完备的基础设施，更大的医疗服务团队来收集和管理相关组织和其对应的临床大数据[16]。用于研究的组织包括手术标本、组织活检和血液样本，每种样本的采样和处理步骤都不相同。尽管还存在着诸多问题，目前一些机构已经开始使用基因组平台来指导临床试验，特别是以目前治疗手段效果很差的疾病，如病因不明的肿瘤[12,17,18]。

本节分为三个部分：①患者样本的基因组分析，以更好地了解癌症生物学，并有助于推动未来的临床试验。②临床前模型有助于筛选治疗反应性更好的癌症亚型。③生物信息学方法整合不同的基因组平台。

高通量基因组学

高分辨率基因组分析技术正被用于国际癌症基因组分析工作，以汇总驱动几乎所有主要类型癌症的病理生理学的畸变。总之，癌症基因组图谱[19]（TCGA，http://cancergenome.nih.gov/）项目和国际癌症基因组联盟[20,21]（ICGC，http://www.icgc.org/）已经评估了 55 个样本中超过 12 000 个样本的畸变[22]。这些努力的主要目标是提高癌症患者的预防、诊断和治疗水平[19]。在这些项目中，患者样本已经在多个平台上进行了分析，这些平台检查了全基因组和整个外显子组[23~26]，mRNA，DNA 甲基化[27]，miRNA 谱[28,29]，蛋白质和磷酸化蛋白水平[30]。几种癌症的结果已经公开可用[25,31~33]，最近几篇论文描述了十几种人类癌症类型特征的综合分析[34~36]。人类癌症中重要的基因组畸变[37]包括：①DNA 拷贝数的体细胞突变，其增加或降低重要编码和非编码 RNA 的转录水平；②改变基因表达，蛋白质结构和蛋白质稳定性和/或改变转录本剪接方式的体细胞突变；③通过改变基因启动子关联或创建新的融合基因来影响转录水平的结构性变异[38,39]；④影响基因表达的表观基因组修饰[40,41]。

对这些丰富数据集的分析已经产生了深刻的临床影响，使得我们可以更好地治疗不同的癌症。例如，尿路上皮膀胱癌富含染色质调节基因的突变，表明可针对染色质修饰进行治疗的可能[23]。高级别浆液性卵巢癌中有一半具有同源重组缺陷，表明了他们可能对聚（ADP-核糖）聚合酶（PARP）抑制剂更加的敏感[25]。现在出现了将肿瘤分层为生物学不同亚型的分类系统，并且与常用的组织学分类相比，新分型具有更大的预后和预测意义。目前已经有针对乳腺癌[42,43]、结肠癌[44]、胰腺癌[45]、卵巢癌[25]、肺癌[46]、胃癌的说明性分类系统[24]。METABRIC 队列由近 2 000 例乳腺肿瘤组成，包含了拷贝数和基因表达变化的相关信息[49]。分析拷贝数概况确定了 10 个乳腺癌亚群，每个亚群具有其独特的基因谱改变和生存曲线。

我们对乳腺癌分子表达谱的理解尤为深刻。TCGA 乳腺癌研究[33]的一个重要观察结果是，在>5%的肿瘤中发生了一些常见的突变（例如：TP53，PIK3CA，CDH1，MLL3，GATA3 和 MED12），此外还有数百种发生在<1%乳腺癌个体肿瘤中。个体肿瘤中的基因组变异通常由“驱动”和“伴随”变异混合组成。在肿瘤进展期间驱动变异发挥了重要作用，因为它们可以调控癌症的发生，发展和多种恶性表型，以及癌症对治疗反应性[48]。伴随突变对癌症病理生理学没有调控作用，是在癌症进展期间偶然发生在基因组不稳定的肿瘤中。

最近对胶质母细胞瘤的研究说明了基因组与治疗之间的强相关性。最初的 TCGA 研究[31,50]证实了在替莫唑胺治疗的胶质母细胞瘤中由于错配修复缺陷导致 MGMT 启动子甲基化和超突变表型之间的联系。Johnson 等[51]对初始和复发性低级别胶质瘤进行了全外显子测序。在用替莫唑胺治疗的 10 个肿瘤中，6 个高度突变的复发肿瘤携带涉及 AKT-mTOR 通路相关的驱动突变。这表明对使用替莫唑胺治疗的复发性低级别胶质瘤患者可以考虑使用靶向 AKT-mTOR 途径的药物。在许多情况下，复发性肿瘤与原发性肿瘤在基因组层面有着显著的差异，所以在患者治疗期间要密切的监测。

2012 年启动的泛癌方法，分析了 TCGA 不同癌症中的基因组变异[36]，其目的是确定多种癌症类型共有的基因组特征。最初的研究集中于 13 种癌症[52,53]，基因组和蛋白质组学平台的综合分析确定了与生存相关的全新癌症亚型[34]。有趣的是，泛癌蛋白质组学分析方法揭示了 HER2 在几种癌症中表达升高，包括子宫内膜癌，膀胱癌和肺腺癌[30]。由于子宫内膜癌与乳腺癌相比具有更高的 HER2 表达，这表明抗 HER2 药物，如 T-DM1，可能对子宫内膜癌更加有效[30]。泛癌方法适用于篮式临床试验，这些试验以不同肿瘤的特定分子突变为指导，而传统临床试验设计则使用基于组织学分类的大量人群[54]。

对这些大规模数据进行有效的可视化和计算分析是至关重要的。大量的分析软件层出不穷，表 19-1 列出了一些最受欢迎的工具。

表 19-1　公共计算与可视化分析工具

工具	网址(Url)
UCSC Cancer Genome Browser	https://genome-cancer.ucsc.edu/
cBioPortal for Cancer Genomics	http://www.cbioportal.org
Sage Synapse	https://www.synapse.org
Catalog of Somatic Mutations in Cancer	http://cancer.sanger.ac.uk/cosmic
The Cancer Proteome Atlas	http://app1.bioinformatics.mdanderson.org/tcpa/_design/basic/index.html

基因标签——评估患者预后，预测治疗反应性

癌症的组织学特性和局部侵袭仍然常被用作远处转移性扩散的标志和预后指标。然而在过去十年中，传统的癌症分类策略已经通过对基因组学的相关研究得到了补充。在1999年，研究证明基因表达谱可用于区分急性髓系白血病和急性淋巴细胞白血病[55]。随后的研究对乳腺癌的基因表达进行了分析，确定了乳腺癌的全新亚型，包括激素受体阳性管腔A型和管腔B型、HER2富集型、基底型和正常型。这些亚型的分类在几个独立的队列中得到验证，并被发现具有很强的预后意义[56]。

目前研究人员正在努力使用这些来开发临床预后基因标签。例如，在乳腺癌中，van' t Veer等[57]发现了由70个基因组成的基因标签，可以预测年轻乳腺癌患者的复发情况。这个标签现在由Agendia BV代理以商品名MammaPrint上市，并且在独立的病人队列中得到验证，效果优于"Adjuvant!"临床病理学风险评估在线软件[58,59]。另外有小型回顾性研究表明MammaPrint可以作为乳腺癌预后标志物[59,60]，但尚无前瞻性数据证明其在辅助治疗中的益处。另一项由Genomic Health代理以商品名OncotypeDx上市的检测是于2004年开发的，研究人员使用RT-PCR技术，测定了福尔马林固定的石蜡包埋肿瘤组织中提取的RNA。研究人员在两项临床试验中回顾性地测试了这种21个基因测定，发现其具有预后意义。它现在被广泛用于临床，以预测患有雌激素受体阳性和早期乳腺癌患者的远端复发风险和化疗的潜在益处[61,62]。其他几个预后型、预测型基因标签也进入了人们的视线[63,64]，其中包括由17个基因组成的雌激素受体阳性乳腺癌、淋巴结阴性乳腺癌的基因标签[65]，由50个基因组成的(PAM50)复发风险标签[66]，由44基因组成的Rotterdam签名[67]。

其他癌症的亚型基因标签也被陆续报道出来。例如在结肠癌中，研究人员已经确定了三种独特的基因标签：Oncotype Dx结肠癌检测(Genomic Health, Inc.)、ColoPrint(Agendia)和ColDx(Almac)[71]。尽管这些检测已被证明是独立的预后生物标志物，它们的预测价值仍然是未知的[72]。目前学术界正在努力，以对应基于多种结直肠癌分类方案的基因表达标签[44]。例如，基因表达分析确定了基底样和管腔样结直肠癌亚型与预后密切相关[73]。据报道，新发现的三种胰腺导管腺癌亚型显示出对治疗反应的差异[45]。目前正在进行的整个肿瘤学范围内的分类工作正在尝试整合基因组和蛋白质组学谱，以确定超越肿瘤起源的全新亚型。最近的研究表明他们成功将肿瘤统一分类为11种主要亚型[34]。随着其他肿瘤类型被添加到分析中，这种方法将变得更加强大。

药物基因组学中患者肿瘤的实验模型

探索与临床结果(例如癌症进展或对治疗的响应)有因果关系的分子特征需要实验模型，其中包括可以携带异常基因和调控网络的细胞系。来自患者肿瘤的细胞系被广泛用作癌症的实验室模型[74]。细胞系是用于研究细胞内在生物学强有力的模型系统，原因有几个：①可再生资源；②可在实验室环境中操作；③适合基因组分析；④可用于评估治疗反应[74,75]。尽管第一批肿瘤来源的细胞系建立于20世纪50年代，但随着NCL60平台的发展，它们作为实验工具的应用获得了关注[76,77]。NCI60由60个人类肿瘤细胞系组成，代表9种癌症类型，并已被用于筛选超过100 000种化合物的治疗效果[78]。使用COMPARE算法分析这些数据提供了一种定量方法用于鉴定细胞分子特征与对特定化合物的敏感性之间的关联[78]。

自从NCI60的实用性被证明以来，其他几个小组已经开发了癌细胞系组，包括泛癌[79~81]和组织特异性集合(例如，乳腺、[82]肺[83,84]和黑素瘤[85])。最完善的癌细胞系组之一，是由约70个乳腺癌细胞系组成的组，已被用于评估基因功能和确定治疗反应和耐药的机制[82,86,87]。最近，包含多个肿瘤的大型细胞系集合已经被用于探索癌症的分子特征与分子扰动剂效果之间的关联[80,81,88]。癌症细胞系与原发肿瘤的基因组和表观基因组特征的对比表明癌症细胞系能够反映原发性肿瘤的组学多样性，而这一特性可能会影响治疗反应。癌症细胞系和原发肿瘤的相似性包括：①复发拷贝数变化和突变[82,86,89]，②转录亚型[86,89]，③信号通路活性[86]。当然也有重要的例外。例如，据报道在塑料器皿上生长的细胞系发生了表观基因组的改变[90]，并且一些细胞系不能保留存在于它们来源的肿瘤中的基因组变异。胶质母细胞瘤是后者的一个典型的例子，因为在塑料器皿上生长的胶质母细胞瘤通常不能保留原发性肿瘤中常见的EGFR致癌基因的扩增区域。

在乳腺癌中，药物敏感性和分子特征之间的相关性分析显示，大约30%的测试化合物与癌症亚型或基因组拷贝数异常相关[86]，并且可以确定预测药物敏感性基因标签对约50%化合物有着稳健的效果[86,87]。更重要的是，在原发性患者样本中可以观察到许多体外培养细胞内出现的基因特征[80,81,87]，这表明细胞系研究可用于指导可用于对临床患者进行分层的基因特征。来自其他组织类型的证据也支持这样的观点，即细胞系是研究治疗反应分子基础的强大模型系统。例如，体外模型系统准确对应了几个临床现象，其中包括：①EGFR突变的肺癌对吉非替尼有良好反应性[92]，②乳腺癌HER2/ERBB2扩增对曲妥珠单抗和/或拉帕替尼有良好反应性[82,93]，③具有突变或扩增的BCR-ABL的肿瘤对甲磺酸伊马替尼有良好反应性。当然，在塑料器皿上生长的细胞系不能模拟人类癌症的每一个方面。一个突出的不足是他们没有模拟微环境对癌细胞行为的影响。如何建立可以模拟来自微环境影响的模型会在本章后面阐述。

整合分析的原则

几种计算工具可以识别与生物行为相关的分子标签。其中第一个是基因集富集分析(GSEA)[95]。GSEA 的基本原理是分析预定义基因组的表达,它们具有共同生物功能、染色体位置或调节功能,以确定它们是否在不同群体中显示出表达的差异。例如,GSEA 分析确定 RAS、NGF 和 IGF1 通路在 TP53 突变体与 TP53 野生型癌症中存在差异表达[95]。

网络分析工具 PARADIGM[96]可以识别在不同群体之间存在活性差异的信号通路。PARADIGM 整合了多种组学数据类型,包括 DNA 拷贝数和基因表达,以计算来自公开数据库(例如,NCI 通路互作数据库 KEGG、Reactome 数据库以及 BioCarta 数据库)的 1 300 多种信号转导,转录和代谢通路的整合通路水平(IPL)。然后可以利用 IPL 来识别群体之间不同的子网络(例如,治疗反应性肿瘤与治疗抗性肿瘤)。子网络由相互关联的通路特征(基因,蛋白质,复合物,家族,过程等)组成,这些特征在一类肿瘤中与另一类肿瘤相比具有独特的活性。例如,对 TCGA 乳腺癌样本进行 PARADIGM 分析可以发现 HIF1-α/ARNT 通路活性在基底样乳腺癌中升高,表明这些恶性肿瘤可能对血管生成抑制剂和/或在低氧条件下被激活的生物还原药物敏感[33]。

包含通路信息的分析工具存在着一个重要问题,即不同的基因和网络存在着研究深度的区别,因此在分析所得的通路结果中存在固有的偏差。HotNet2 是一种使用试图避免策展偏差(curation bias)的策略来查找异常网络的算法。HotNet2 使用了改进的扩散过程,并在识别子网络时考虑热流的来源或方向性,以减少策展偏差的影响。该工具最近被应用于泛癌网络分析,以确定影响已知癌症表型的 16 个频繁突变的网络[97]。

多团队协作推动了系统生物学的发展

不断发展的谱系分析技术和随后产生的大型复杂数据集需要强大的分析方法,以促进“大数据到知识”的转换(http://bd2k.nih.gov/)。这项工作仍处于起步阶段;大量的分析方法不断出现,因此难以确定哪种方法表现最佳。一种评估算法表现的新方法是学科内多研究小组共同评估的新模式。DREAM 项目(http://dreamchallenges.org)就是这种方法的一个例子。DREAM 将研究人员团结在一起,以解决系统生物学中的复杂问题,同时遴选出分析表现最佳的新算法。其中的一个关键方面是消除“自我评估陷阱”,即数据生成、数据分析和模型验证都是在同一研究中完成[98]。此外,通过这种协作模式获得的进步比传统的单一团队要快得多。

最近的两个 DREAM 项目证明了这种协作方法的高效。在 NCI-DREAM7 项目中,未经发表的一组乳腺癌细胞系的药物敏感性以及转录和蛋白表达谱被免费提供给科学界[99]。超过 40 个国际组织通过使用各种机器学习和统计算法开发了药物反应的预测因子。对所有结果的荟萃分析表明,建模非线性关系和整合现有知识是生成稳健预测生物标记的要点。另一个 DREAM 项目试图评估计算策略从乳腺癌的临床特征,基因表达和拷贝数概况预测乳腺癌存活的能力[100]。这个项目使用来自 METABRIC 乳腺癌队列的数据[49],在多轮盲法中评估超过 1 400 个模型的性能。该项目评估出的性能最佳的预后模型明显优于第一代 70 基因风险预测器[58]。有趣的是,这项研究还证明了所有模型的集合预测优于最好的独立模型。这些结果证明了多团队协作在推动算法开发和识别临床相关生物标记方面的高效性。

要点

肿瘤微环境(TME)

- TME 由多种细胞和非细胞成分组成
- TME 成分影响癌症进展和患者预后
- TME 与患者治疗反应性和耐药性高度相关
- TME 的临床前建模具有挑战性,但现在适用于高通量平台
- PDX 可以预测患者的治疗反应性,并且可以用于临床试验

肿瘤微环境

肿瘤微环境的成分

肿瘤微环境有着不同的分类方法[7],一种方法将肿瘤微环境分为三大类:造血细胞类细胞,间充质类细胞和非细胞成分[101]。造血类细胞包含淋巴系来源细胞和髓系来源细胞。淋巴系细胞由 T 细胞、B 细胞和天然杀伤细胞组成,而髓系细胞由巨噬细胞、嗜中性粒细胞和髓源抑制细胞组成。间充质类细胞包括成纤维细胞、肌成纤维细胞、间充质干细胞、脂肪细胞和内皮细胞。其中两个主要组成部分是肿瘤相关性成纤维细胞(CAF)和内皮细胞。CAF 是受肿瘤细胞调控并促进肿瘤生长、血管生成和远处转移的成纤维细胞[102,103]。内皮细胞和周细胞也被证明在肿瘤进展所需的血管生长形成中起重要作用[104]。非细胞成分中最重要的是细胞外基质(ECM)。ECM 可以进一步细分为两部分:基底膜,由Ⅳ型胶原、层粘连蛋白和纤连蛋白组成;间质基质,由纤维状胶原蛋白、蛋白多糖和糖蛋白组成。ECM 在维持组织结构、细胞侵袭、肿瘤进展和血管生成方面发挥作用[105]。

肿瘤微环境和癌症的特征

Hanahan 和 Weinberg[106]定义了六种癌症的特征,在肿瘤生长中至关重要。其包括:①逃避细胞凋亡,②生长信号的自给自足,③对抗生长信号的不敏感性,④组织侵袭和转移,⑤无限的复制潜力,⑥持续的血管生成。11 年后,六个癌症特征的概念得到了更新,研究人员确认肿瘤微环境是肿瘤生长的重要参与者,并增加了两个癌症特征:能量代谢的重编程和免疫逃逸。然而,将癌症特征分为两个不同类别的起源(肿瘤细胞和肿瘤微环境)是一种人为的分类,因为大多数癌症标志(7/8)实际上是间质细胞和癌细胞之间相互作用的产物[107]。

肿瘤微环境在调节治疗反应和预测复发预后中的作用

肿瘤微环境可以从正反两个方面调节肿瘤治疗药物的作用。一个典型的例子是血管正常化,其中可以通过调节肿瘤血管系统以改善化疗药物的运输[7,108]。肿瘤的血管系统是异常的并具有高渗透性的未成熟血管,其在运输营养物质和药物的能力受损。抗血管生成药物可以改造未成熟血管,恢复“正常化的血管系统”,使化疗药物可以更好地抵达肿瘤组织[108]。此外,肿

瘤微环境可以作为局部和长期治疗反应性的预测生物标志物。例如,黑色素瘤具有一种独特类型的转移,指患者在距离原发病灶超过 2cm 但未超出区域淋巴结盆的皮肤和皮下组织中发生局部转移。对这类疾病的治疗方法之一是门诊治疗,在病灶内注射白介素 2。我们的共同作者之一(SH)研究了治疗后 6~8 周的活检组织在疾病部位的免疫反应,发现对治疗有着良好反应的患者表现出 CD8 阳性 T 细胞在肿瘤周围浸润增加并有着更好的预后。这与其他研究一起提示,肿瘤微环境中的局部反应可能是调节系统反应的重要因素,反过来又会影响整体生存[109,110]。

癌症对化疗的抗性既可能是由肿瘤微环境介导的内在过程,也可以是获得性过程,即对治疗干预的适应性宿主反应[7,111]。对于内在抗性,目前已经提出了几种机制来解释这一现象:①肿瘤微环境中释放的保护性生存信号,②血管损伤和渗漏引起的药物输送受损,③间质细胞分泌趋化因子的旁分泌信号,④免疫抑制[7,112]。免疫应答是介导获得性治疗耐药的重要因素。对紫杉醇的抗性已被证明部分是由于 IL-34,集落刺激因子(CSF)-1 表达增强和巨噬细胞浸润增加[113]。目前已开发出一种单克隆抗体 RG7155(Roche),其靶向巨噬细胞和 CSF-1 受体,并已证实在弥漫型巨细胞肿瘤患者有着良好效果[114]。与获得性耐药有关的其他机制包括诱导衰老相关的分泌表型和细胞分化的变化。

肿瘤微环境的相关研究已经发现了小鼠模型中局部复发的预测标志物和肿瘤患者的预后标志物。另外,还有研究报道了一种炎症特征,其与临床可检测的疾病的复发相关,但不与晚期复发性疾病相关。该炎症特征的特点在于血清 IL-6 和血管内皮生长因子(VEGF)的增加。癌细胞的免疫逃逸机制可以使微小的残留灶进展至复发性肿瘤[115,116]。Park 等发现肿瘤微环境在乳腺癌中有着重要的预后意义[6]。他们使用激光捕获显微切割技术从患者原发肿瘤中分离出间质细胞。一个来源于间质的基因标签是总体存活和无复发存活的强预后标志物。免疫细胞是该基因标签的重要组成部分,在预后较好的患者中表现出 T 细胞和 NK 细胞标记物的富集,表明其处于 TH1 型免疫应答。原发肿瘤中间质含量的预后意义,称为肿瘤/间质比例,也已在结肠癌和乳腺癌中得到证实[117]。此外,免疫细胞的预后价值也在乳腺癌和结肠癌中得到了探讨[118~121]。在两项三阴性乳腺癌患者的随机对照试验中,研究人员发现间质淋巴细胞浸润是与总生存期相关的独立预后标志物[120]。在结肠癌中,测量某些淋巴细胞群存在的评分,称为免疫评分(immunescore),与目前的 AJCC(美国癌症联合委员会)预后标志物(T 期-肿瘤深度和 N 期-淋巴结受累)相比,它显示出更强的预后提示意义[122]。有趣的是,免疫评分在局部结直肠癌患者中可能具有巨大的临床意义,这部分患者在成像病理学上没有可检测到的扩散或淋巴结受累,但其中 25%的患者会复发[123]。在两个独立的队列中,免疫评分能够确定复发风险较高的患者,这部分患者可能会在辅助治疗中获益[123,124]。鉴于间质基因标签的预后意义,当肿瘤起源的基因标签被发现时要重点考虑肿瘤样本中间质的组成成分和占比。

模拟肿瘤微环境

大多数实验室开发的靶向肿瘤微环境的药物在临床试验中尚未获得成功[126,127]。这可能是受到了内在肿瘤因素或临床前模型的局限性的影响。临床前模型的常见争议是癌细胞系本身无法模拟癌细胞与其微环境相互作用的信号通路。表 19-2 总结了一些化疗敏感性模型,这些模型可以更好地模拟肿瘤与其微环境之间的复杂相互作用。

表 19-2 药物敏感性模型的优缺点

模型	优点	缺点
细胞系	• 资源可自我复制 • 易于使用 • 适合高通量筛选	• 细胞系通常来源于强侵略性的肿瘤 • 无法模拟复杂的旁分泌和内分泌对肿瘤生长的影响
2D 模型	• 易于使用 • 适合高通量筛选	• 2D 单层细胞和体内条件下的细胞在形态,极性,受体表达,癌基因表达上存在差异[128]
3D 模型	• 3D 球体可以更好地模拟实体肿瘤中的缺氧核心和药物扩散模式 • 与 2D 模型相比,对治疗具有不同的反应	• 可能会受到细胞大小和形状变化的影响 • 可能需要更专业的设备和更高的成本 • 需要更大的人力资源 • 如果使用基质胶,需要考虑批次之间的差异[129]
微环境微阵列	• 适合高通量筛选 • 可评估不同微环境蛋白质对治疗反应和抵抗力的影响	• 难以模拟肿瘤异质性 • 相关统计分析方法不够完备[130] • 方法仍需要验证[130]
老鼠模型	• 可用于评估药物对原发性肿瘤生长和远处转移的治疗效果 • 转基因小鼠和异种移植物均可用于观察临床试验的反应[131,132]	• 难以在更大规模上使用以测试多种治疗药物
异种移植物	• 易于使用,因为癌细胞系可以很容易地注射或移植	• 使用通常代表强侵袭性肿瘤的癌细胞系和免疫缺陷小鼠
转基因技术	• 可以更好地模拟人体肿瘤进展[133]	• 难以在临床前研究中使用,因为小鼠的年龄需要同步才能对尺寸类似的肿瘤进行治疗研究
患者来源的异种移植物(PDX)	• 可再生组织资源[134,135] • 与患者肿瘤相似的基因组特性[131] • PDX 模型的治疗反应更加类似于患者[131]	• 需要获取患者肿瘤样本并在小鼠中种植 • 需要免疫缺陷小鼠[131] • 种植失败率高,在某些肿瘤类型中的治疗时间长[131]

癌细胞在塑料培养皿上单层生长的二维(2D)模型通常被用于评估药物反应性[128]。这些 2D 模型已经在很多临床药物的开发中起到了巨大的作用。目前对于肿瘤微环境信号的模拟也有了几种方法。一种方法是采用 2D 共培养,使癌细胞系与间质细胞一块培养。共培养模型可以探索受肿瘤微环境影响的肿瘤基因型,表型和治疗反应性的变化[136,137]。或者,癌症细胞可以培养在来自癌细胞的不同微环境中的可溶性和不溶性蛋白质组成的底物上,这些底物会有利于癌症细胞的播散。这可以通过安排由携带一种或多种微环境蛋白质的数千个单独阵列元件组成的微阵列来有效地完成。这些在下文中被称为微环境微阵列(MEArrays)。MEArray 是通过将细胞外基质,生长因子和其他蛋白质组合加到培养底物上而制备的,其为约 200μm 直径斑点,能够支持细胞黏附和生长。随后活细胞被种植到 MEArray 以评估外加物质对细胞生长的影响[130,138]。在 MEArray 上生长的细胞也可以用药物进行处理以评估微环境蛋白质对治疗反应的影响。通常,研究人员会使用亲和试剂对生长的细胞进行免疫荧光染色,来监测感兴趣的癌症相关表型(例如,增殖、凋亡、分化状态和衰老),然后使用高内容成像技术进行量化[130,139](图 19-2)。

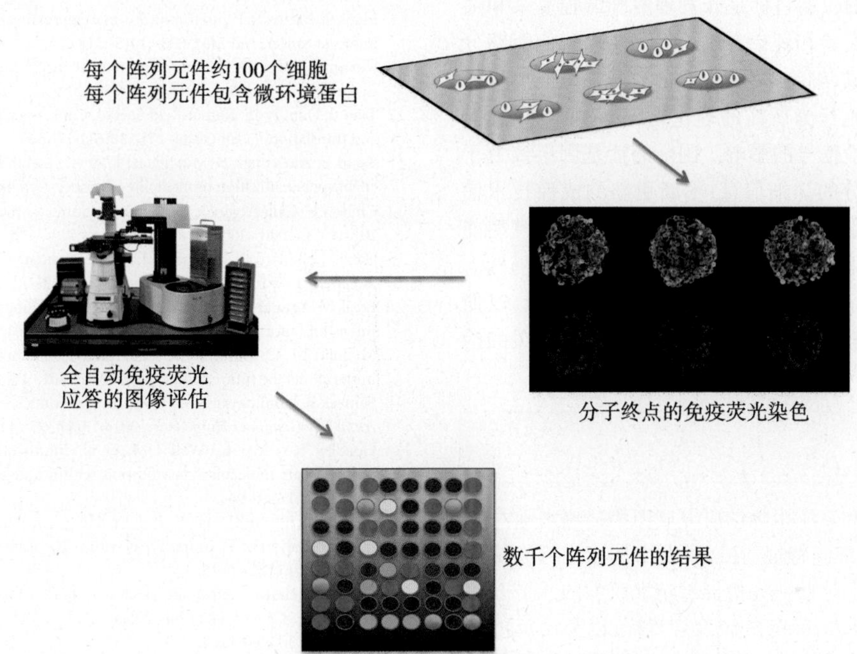

图 19-2　使用微环境微阵列评估不同微环境对癌细胞生长影响的示意图。数千个微环境蛋白质被富集于直径为约 250μm 的面积上,以促进癌细胞的生长。荧光图像分析记录下了由微环境蛋白诱导的免疫荧光染色模式的变化

三维(3D)培养方法是在由细胞外蛋白质和其他种类细胞组成的 3D 环境中培养细胞[7,128,140]。基质组分如基质(例如,基质胶)或支架(例如,胶原蛋白、层粘连蛋白和藻酸盐)可以添加到 3D 模型中,以便更好地模拟组织结构。从小鼠肉瘤细胞中分离出的基质胶是基底膜衍生的水凝胶,其通常被用于癌症模型并能够支持肿瘤生长和血管生成[141,142]。然而,使用基质胶的挑战之一是其相对不确定的分子组成和不同批次间的差异性[129]。除了高通量平台之外,微流体系统包括 3 个相连的小室,一个是入口水库,一个细胞培养室还有一个出口水库,可用于 2D 和 3D 模型[128]。3D 共培养模型也在开发之中。有研究团队已经成功利用 3D 共培养技术体外 24 小时内培养出了一个大型乳腺癌肿瘤[143]。随着 3D 细胞打印技术[144,145]可以将多种类型细胞"安放"在实验室构建的癌症组织框架中,3D 共培养模型对体内微环境的还原度正在增加。

肿瘤微环境的重要性也已在小鼠模型中得到了很好的证实。在异体移植小鼠模型中,癌细胞系被注射到免疫功能缺陷的小鼠中。当异位皮下注射癌细胞时,转移很少发生。而当肿瘤细胞处于有利的微环境中时,原位种植模型中肿瘤细胞生长的比异位种植模型更快并且具有更大的转移倾向[146]。尽管异种移植模型是研究肿瘤生长和转移抑制的有用工具,但它们受到宿主免疫缺陷状态的限制和使用来自侵袭性更强肿瘤的细胞系的限制[131]。异种移植模型中药物的疗效尚未显示与临床试验中的疗效相关[147]。因此,基因工程或转基因小鼠是更为实际可靠的模型。该模型的优点在于小鼠具有免疫活性,肿瘤从预侵袭性、侵袭性到远处转移,更类似于人类肿瘤的进展[133]。一些转基因小鼠模型诱发肿瘤周期短,并已用作测试化疗敏感性[127,132,148]。然而,这些模型难以大规模使用,因为需要同步幼崽的出生时间,肿瘤的诱发时间和后续的治疗[148]。

最近,患者来源的异种移植物(PDX)模型被用于研究肿瘤治疗效果。PDX 是把患者肿瘤组织植入免疫缺陷小鼠中建立的[131]。植入成功率从低至 13%[149]到高达 71%不等[150]。PDX 模型使人体组织从小鼠到小鼠的移植性成为可能,是一种可再生组织资源[134]。全基因组测序结果揭示 PDX 肿瘤与人类肿瘤在拷贝数和结构变异方面的高度相似性。目前已经有

研究用PDX更好地了解乳腺癌生长中的克隆进化[151]。PDX目前被用于评估乳腺癌，肺癌，黑色素瘤和胰腺癌的化学敏感性[131,152]。初步研究表明PDX模型的治疗反应性和临床预后有着良好的相关性[150,152]。因此，PDX模型逐渐被整合到治疗药物的临床前开发的后期阶段。PDX模型在共同临床试验中也得到了使用，其中药物的效果在病人和小鼠中共同评估，以便更好地制定对抗耐药性的策略[131]。

结论

癌症系统生物学的长期目标是开发理解和调控复杂和适应性癌症行为所需的实验和理论方法。这将要求我们能够分析这些癌症的分子组成、细胞排列和解剖位置，并且需要我们开发出能够预测癌细胞行为所需的理论框架，包括调控肿瘤行为的近端和远端环境信号的影响。国际癌症基因组致力于提供关于癌症分子成分的详细信息；不断更新的成像技术使得癌组织的多尺度测量成为可能；越来越精确的生物模型能够更准确地识别与癌细胞行为相关的分子特征。现在仍然需要开发可用于预测复杂适应系统行为的癌症相关分析，以便于这些信息可用于更准确地预测癌症行为并设计更持久的治疗策略。

总结

癌症基因组学和系统生物学研究试图描述癌细胞内在和外在的分子和细胞特征，并以预测个体癌症行为的方式解释所得数据。这些研究指导着精准医学的几个方面，包括预测癌症行为，确定最佳治疗目标，以及制定可持久控制个体癌症的策略。目前，国际组学分析工作已经产生了数百至数千种主要癌症类型的组学数据，并且这些数据被免费提供给科学界使用。计算科学家在建立癌症组学特征与癌症行为之间的关联方面正在取得良好进展——尤其是在癌症进展和治疗反应方面。系统生物学家现在正在开发实验策略和理论策略来理解和预测复杂系统的行为。这些研究主要关注癌细胞本身的行为以及远端和近端环境对癌细胞行为的影响。本章重点介绍了所有这些领域的工作，并提供了各方面最新进展的说明性例子。

（郑博 译　李亮 校　陈磊 审）

致谢

作者感谢以下研究资助组织：SH，加拿大乳腺癌基金，美国临床肿瘤学会（ASCO）征服癌症基金会青年研究者奖，乳腺癌研究基金会和Evelyn H. Lauder家族捐赠，加拿大卫生研究院（CIHR）班廷（Banting）博士后奖学金，以及安大略癌症研究所的安大略政府资助。JG和LH，Susan G. Komen乳腺癌基金支持，NIH/NCI U54 CA112970项目及俄勒冈健康与科学大学（OHSU）Knight癌症研究所。

参考文献

The complete reference list can be found on the Wiley Companion Digital Edition of this title (see inside front cover for login instructions).

1 Werner HM, Mills GB, Ram PT. Cancer systems biology: a peek into the future of patient care? *Nat Rev Clin Oncol*. 2014;**11(3)**:167–176.
2 Zou J, Zheng MW, Li G, Su ZG. Advanced systems biology methods in drug discovery and translational biomedicine. *Biomed Res Int*. 2013;**2013**:742835.
3 Hanahan D, Coussens LM. Accessories to the crime: functions of cells recruited to the tumor microenvironment. *Cancer Cell*. 2012;**21(3)**:309–322.
5 Antoni MH, Lutgendorf SK, Cole SW, et al. The influence of bio-behavioural factors on tumour biology: pathways and mechanisms. *Nat Rev Cancer*. 2006;**6(3)**:240–248.
6 Finak G, Bertos N, Pepin F, et al. Stromal gene expression predicts clinical outcome in breast cancer. *Nat Med*. 2008;**14(5)**:518–527.
7 Klemm F, Joyce JA. Microenvironmental regulation of therapeutic response in cancer. *Trends Cell Biol*. 2015;**25(4)**:198–213.
12 Tran B, Dancey JE, Kamel-Reid S, et al. Cancer genomics: technology, discovery, and translation. *J Clin Oncol*. 2012;**30(6)**:647–660.
13 Good B, Ainscough B, McMichael J, Su A, Griffith O. Organizing knowledge to enable personalization of medicine in cancer. *Genome Biol*. 2014;**15(8)**:438.
14 Chibon F. Cancer gene expression signatures – the rise and fall? *Eur J Cancer*. 2013;**49(8)**:2000–2009.
15 Hatzis C, Bedard PL, Birkbak NJ, et al. Enhancing reproducibility in cancer drug screening: how do we move forward? *Cancer Res*. 2014;**74(15)**:4016–4023.
16 Basik M, Aguilar-Mahecha A, Rousseau C, et al. Biopsies: next-generation biospecimens for tailoring therapy. *Nat Rev Clin Oncol*. 2013;**10(8)**:437–450.
17 Manolio TA, Chisholm RL, Ozenberger B, et al. Implementing genomic medicine in the clinic: the future is here. *Genet Med*. 2013;**15(4)**:258–267.
18 Sameek R, Chinnaiyan AM. Translating genomics for precision cancer medicine. *Annu Rev Genomics Hum Genet*. 2014;**15(1)**:395–415.
34 Hoadley KA, Yau C, Wolf DM, et al. Multiplatform analysis of 12 cancer types reveals molecular classification within and across tissues of origin. *Cell*. 2014;**158(4)**:929–944.
35 Omberg L, Ellrott K, Yuan Y, et al. Enabling transparent and collaborative computational analysis of 12 tumor types within The Cancer Genome Atlas. *Nat Genet*. 2013;**45(10)**:1121–1126.
36 Cancer Genome Atlas Research Network, Weinstein JN, Collisson EA, et al. The Cancer Genome Atlas Pan-Cancer analysis project. *Nat Genet*. 2013;**45(10)**:1113–1120.
37 Collisson EA, Cho RJ, Gray JW. What are we learning from the cancer genome? *Nat Rev Clin Oncol*. 2012;**9(11)**:621–630.
48 Vogelstein B, Papadopoulos N, Velculescu VE, Zhou S, Diaz LA Jr, Kinzler KW. Cancer genome landscapes. *Science*. 2013;**339(6127)**:1546–1558.
54 Sleijfer S, Bogaerts J, Siu LL. Designing transformative clinical trials in the cancer genome era. *J Clin Oncol*. 2013;**31(15)**:1834–1841.
56 Perou CM, Børresen-Dale A-L. Systems biology and genomics of breast cancer. *Cold Spring Harb Perspect Biol*. 2011;**3(2)**:a003293. doi:10.1101/cshperspect.a003293.
74 Sharma SV, Haber DA, Settleman J. Cell line-based platforms to evaluate the therapeutic efficacy of candidate anticancer agents. *Nat Rev Cancer*. 2010;**10(4)**:241–253.
78 Holbeck SL, Collins JM, Doroshow JH. Analysis of FDA-approved anti-cancer agents in the NCI60 Panel of human tumor cell lines. *Mol Cancer Ther*. 2010;**9(5)**:1451–1460.
80 Barretina J, Caponigro G, Stransky N, et al. The cancer cell line encyclopedia enables predictive modelling of anticancer drug sensitivity. *Nature*. 2012;**483(7391)**:603–607.
81 Garnett MJ, Edelman EJ, Heidorn SJ, et al. Systematic identification of genomic markers of drug sensitivity in cancer cells. *Nature*. 2012;**483(7391)**:570–575.
82 Neve RM, Chin K, Fridlyand J, et al. A collection of breast cancer cell lines for the study of functionally distinct cancer subtypes. *Cancer Cell*. 2006;**10(6)**:515–527.
86 Heiser LM, Sadanandam A, Kuo WL, et al. Subtype and pathway specific responses to anticancer compounds in breast cancer. *Proc Natl Acad Sci U S A*. 2012;**109(8)**:2724–2729.
87 Daemen A, Griffith O, Heiser L, et al. Modeling precision treatment of breast cancer. *Genome Biol*. 2013;**14(10)**:R110.
88 CTD2 Data Portal: National Cancer Institute, Office of Cancer Genomics, 6 April 2015. Available from: https://ctd2.nci.nih.gov/dataPortal/CTD2_DataPortal.html.
100 Margolin AA, Bilal E, Huang E, et al. Systematic analysis of challenge-driven improvements in molecular prognostic models for breast cancer. *Sci Transl Med*. 2013;**5(181)**:181re1.
107 Hanahan D, Weinberg RA. Hallmarks of cancer: the next generation. *Cell*.

2011;**144(5)**:646–674.

120 Adams S, Gray RJ, Demaria S, et al. Prognostic value of tumor-infiltrating lymphocytes in triple-negative breast cancers from two phase III randomized adjuvant breast cancer trials: ECOG 2197 and ECOG 1199. *J Clin Oncol*. 2014;**32(27)**:2959–2966.

121 Pages F, Berger A, Camus M, et al. Effector memory T cells, early metastasis, and survival in colorectal cancer. *N Engl J Med*. 2005;**353(25)**:2654–2666.

126 Kelland LR. Of mice and men: values and liabilities of the athymic nude mouse model in anticancer drug development. *Eur J Cancer*. 2004;**40(6)**:827–836.

127 Sharpless NE, Depinho RA. The mighty mouse: genetically engineered mouse models in cancer drug development. *Nat Rev Drug Discov*. 2006;**5(9)**:741–754.

128 Breslin S, O'Driscoll L. Three-dimensional cell culture: the missing link in drug discovery. *Drug Discov Today*. 2013;**18(5–6)**:240–249.

130 Labarge MA, Parvin B, Lorens JB. Molecular deconstruction, detection, and computational prediction of microenvironment-modulated cellular responses to cancer therapeutics. *Adv Drug Deliv Rev*. 2014;**69–70**:123–131.

131 Hidalgo M, Amant F, Biankin AV, et al. Patient-derived xenograft models: an emerging platform for translational cancer research. *Cancer Discov*. 2014;**4(9)**:998–1013.

132 Lunardi A, Pandolfi PP. A co-clinical platform to accelerate cancer treatment optimization. *Trends Mol Med*. 2015;**21(1)**:1–5.

138 Rantala J, Kwon S, Korkola J, Gray J. Expanding the diversity of imaging-based RNAi screen applications using cell spot microarrays. *Microarrays*. 2013;**2(2)**: 97–114.

140 Bissell MJ, Rizki A, Mian IS. Tissue architecture: the ultimate regulator of breast epithelial function. *Curr Opin Cell Biol*. 2003;**15(6)**:753–762.

第 20 章 癌症研究中的统计学新方法

J. Jack Lee, PhD, MS, DDS ■ Donald A. Berry, PhD

概述

随着癌症靶点和抗肿瘤药物研究的快速增长，癌症研究正在前所未有地迅猛发展。基因组学、蛋白组学和表观遗传学的发展为我们提供了个体患者详尽的肿瘤学特征资料，我们可以将每位患者视作独立的个体，从而为他们提供个性化的精准治疗方案。然而，后期肿瘤临床试验的低成功率及新药成功上市的高成本，迫使药物研发过程发生改变。统计学新方法可以帮助设计和开展临床试验，促进生物标记物的发现和验证，并精简试验流程。贝叶斯统计的应用提供了良好的理论基础，该理论基础能够支持适应性设计的发展并提高试验的灵活性和效率，同时保持理想的统计操作性特征。

本章介绍新方法的主要目的：①在对治疗效果下结论时，更有效地利用临床试验信息；②在对参与临床试验的患者尽可能有效治疗的同时，要更有效地利用患者资源；③更快地识别出较好的药物和治疗方案，快速推进研发过程。基本的前提是利用所有可用的证据，从正在进行的临床试验中收集信息并将其放入已知的知识背景中去。本章介绍的新方法具有直观的吸引力，但是其中一些仍然有争议。一些已经应用到了实际临床试验中，而其他一些方法是否可用于临床试验仍处于发展或被评价过程中。

本章将讨论两类新方法：一类是传统频率论统计方法在应用中的自然推广，另一类是基于贝叶斯统计思想的方法。贝叶斯方法是按实时的信息积累（数据逐渐累积）来不断进行调整，频率法则依附于特定的试验及其设计。但是，这些互补的方法间存在许多重叠。

本章主要包括以下内容：通过实例介绍和解释基础的概率理论和贝叶斯方法，比较频率学派和贝叶斯方法的异同点，讨论了通过应用适应性随机化、预测概率、期中和外延分析、析因设计等适应性设计的发展。此外，还讨论了可用于综合试验及外部信息的分层模型、可用于缩短药物开发周期的Ⅰ/Ⅱ期和Ⅱ/Ⅲ期临床试验无缝连接试验设计、可同时评价多种药物的平台设计（platform design），并通过 BATTLE 和 I-SPY2 试验说明这些新统计学方法的应用。最后，给出了新的试验设计及其实施的计算资源信息。

随着癌症靶点和抗肿瘤药物研究的快速增长，癌症研究正在前所未有地迅猛发展。基因组学、蛋白组学和表观遗传学的发展为我们提供了个体患者详尽的肿瘤学特征资料，我们可以将每位患者视作独立的个体，从而为他们提供个性化的精准治疗方案。现代的计算机技术允许统计学家模拟复杂的试验设计并评价设计特征，如检验效能和假阳性率。其基本要求是提前给定设计方案。

后期肿瘤临床试验的低成功率[1-3]及将新药推向市场的高成本[4]迫使药物研发过程发生改变。认识到现代化的需求，FDA 于 2006 年 3 月发布了关键路径分析报告，确定发展生物标记物和精简试验流程为该过程中两个必须要变化的领域[5]。随后，FDA 各中心发布了进一步的指导原则：医疗器械与放射健康中心（Center for Devices and Radiological Health，CDRH）于 2006 年发布了医疗器械临床试验中使用贝叶斯统计的初步指南，并于 2010 年发布了最终指南[6]。生物制剂评估和研究中心（Center for Biologics Evaluation and Research，CBER）及药物评估与研究中心（Center for Drug Evaluation and Research，CDER）发布了一份联合指导文件，用于规划和实施临床试验中的适应性设计[7]。此外，CDRH 于 2015 年发布了医疗器械临床研究适应性设计指导原则草案[8]。

本章所介绍的新方法的主要目的是：①在对治疗效果下结论时，更有效地利用临床试验信息；②在对参与临床试验的患者尽可能有效治疗的同时，要更有效的利用患者资源；③更快地识别出较好的药物和治疗方案，快速推进研发过程。基本的前提是利用所有可用的证据，从正在进行的临床试验中收集信息并将其放入我们已知的知识背景中去。本章介绍的新方法具有直观的吸引力，但是其中一些仍然有争议。一些已经应用到了实际临床试验中，而其他一些方法是否可用于临床试验仍处于发展或被评价过程中。

本章将讨论两类新方法：一类是传统频率论统计方法在应用中的自然推广，另一类是基于贝叶斯统计思想的方法。熟悉贝叶斯思想的读者也许想跳过一些贝叶斯相关小节。贝叶斯方法专门是按实时的信息积累（数据逐渐累积）来不断进行调整，频率法则依附于特定的试验及其设计。但是，这些互补的方法间存在许多重叠。本章许多临床试验设计的开发利用贝叶斯方法作为一种工具，以便在临床试验中更有效地治疗患者和更迅速地识别出更好的药物。但是，我们总能找到由此得出的试验设计的频率派性质（例如假阳性率和检验效能），通常需要模拟得出。确保一项设计预设的频率特征意味着贝叶斯方法可以用于具有好的频率特征的试验。

引言

对照是实验研究的基本原则之一。在临床试验中，一个治疗方案的结果需要与受试者接受的其他方案的结果进行对比才能评估其是否有效。解决这个问题最好的方法就是将患者随机分配到试验组和对照组。尽管有些不采用随机化方法的研究也能评估治疗方案的效应，但是非随机化研究都有其局限性。而且，随机化并不要求对需要比较的各组或治疗方案间采用等比例分配。临床试验中是可以采取非等比例随机化分配的,这种非等比例分配既可以是固定的比率(ratio)也可以采取适应性比率(即分配概率取决于试验中已累积的数据)。(后一种可能性是本章的重点)。

大部分临床试验是根据方案进行的,临床试验的方案旨在评估治疗的整体效应[9]。方案可能会涉及回顾性的或者零星的数据收集,但它们通常是前瞻性的。前瞻性的方案对试验如何实施进行了描述,包括患者如何分组以及这项试验将何时结束。偏离了方案可能将很难或者几乎不可能从试验中得出科学的推断(即使是为了避免受试者暴露在不必要的风险下)。只有按试验方案正确地执行试验,才能基于合理的统计理论做出有效的推断。

贝叶斯方法

本节主要介绍贝叶斯方法的思想以及贝叶斯方法如何与传统的频率派方法联系起来。这部分介绍确实是很浅显的。想进一步了解其内容可阅读对贝叶斯思想和方法全面而基本的介绍[10],或关于贝叶斯方法在医学研究[11]尤其是临床试验中[12~15]作用的讨论,以及其他描述了更高级的贝叶斯方法[16~17]的论著。

贝叶斯修正

任何统计方法的本质是看它如何处理不确定性。在贝叶斯方法里,不确定性是以概率来量化的。任何未知事件的发生都有一个概率。频率派的方法也用到概率,但是却以一种更受限制的方式,如后文所述。一些"概率"会在贝叶斯方法中使用而在频率派方法中却没有对应的定义,例如某药物有效的概率、特定的化疗对患者起作用的概率以及某种特定疗法在后续的临床试验结果中显示出有统计学意义获益的概率。

贝叶斯理论框架就是一种学习方式。随着可用的信息增加,一个人可以不断更新自己在某个方面原来并不了解的知识,而这个过程本身就在不断产生信息。在存在不确定性情况下进行学习的基本工具就是贝叶斯法则,该法则涉及逆概率。许多读者所熟知的一个例子是计算诊断试验中的阳性预测值(positive predictive value,PPV):得到一个阳性检验结果时,被检验的个体患病的概率是多少?逆概率就是确实患有某种疾病的情况下出现阳性检验结果的概率,即检验的灵敏度。PPV还依赖于特异度,即个体不患病情况下出现阴性检验结果的概率。同样 PPV 依赖于人群中疾病的患病率。在应用贝叶斯法则进行统计推断时,与 PPV 相类似的"后验概率"就是在给定试验结果后原假设成立的概率。与疾病患病率类似的就是原假设为真的"先验概率"。

下面来考虑一个非常简单的例子,一个受试者只有两个可能的反应率(r):$r=0.75$ 和 $r=0.5$。如果你习惯于思考诊断试验中的 PPV,那么可将其中之一认为是患者有病的概率,而另一个认为是患者无病的概率。现在的问题就是:r 是等于 0.75 还是 0.5?在任何试验开始前,认为这两个反应率发生的可能性是相同的:$P(r=0.75)=P(r=0.50)=1/2$。

贝叶斯方法的重点是学习。一旦有可用的新信息,概率值就被重新计算,计算后的概率就又被认为是"给定"的。统计学家们用一种符号来帮助他们思考和计算随着新信息积累而变化的概率。他们用竖线将感兴趣的未知事件与已知的(或者是给定的)条件分开:$P(A|B)$ 读作"给定了 B 后 A 的概率。"假定 R 为"肿瘤反应"(tumor response),N 代表"不反应"(nonresponse),使用上述符号就可表示为 $P(R|r=0.75)=0.75$。更有趣的是,假设存在肿瘤反应,则 $r=0.75$ 的概率就表示为:$P(r=0.75|R)$。这两个表达式是互逆的,分别表示感兴趣的事件和被假设的事件。贝叶斯法则就是这两个表达式之间的关系。即,$r=0.75$ 的更新或修正后(后验)概率如下:

$$P(r=0.75|R)=P(R|r=0.75)P(r=0.75)/P(R)$$

等号右边的分母遵循全概率法则:

$$\begin{aligned}P(R)&=P(R|r=0.75)P(r=0.75)+P(R|r=0.50)P(r=0.50)\\&=(0.75)(1/2)+(0.5)(1/2)\\&=5/8\end{aligned}$$

也就是说,$P(R)$ 是所考虑的两个反应率 0.75 和 0.5 的平均值,这里的平均值是关于相应的先验概率的,这个例子里是各占一半。把数值代入贝叶斯公式,$r=0.75$ 的后验概率为:

$$P(r=0.75|R)=(0.75)(1/2)/(5/8)=3/5$$

因此,新的证据使 $r=0.75$ 的概率从 1/2(或 50%)增加到了 60%。由于总概率是 100%,在单次反应里前述证据使 $r=0.50$ 的概率从 50%降低到 40%。接下来考虑第二个独立的观察对象。第二个观察对象的信息获取之前,r 的概率就是第一个观察对象的后验概率。如果第二个观察对象也发生反应,那么第二次应用贝叶斯法则就得到 $P(r=0.75|R,R)=9/13=69\%$,进一步使之前为 50%和 60%的概率增高。一方面,如果第二个观察对象没有反应,那么 $P(r=0.75|R,N)=3/7=43\%$,$r=0.75$ 的概率从 60%降到了 43%。这个过程可以无限地进行下去,可以在每次有了一个观察对象之后就更新,也可以在已有的所有证据基础上利用所有观察对象信息进行一次性更新。反应率 r 取各种可能值的当前概率在任何时候都可以得到。这些概率取决于原始的先验概率和中间数据。这些更新和实时学习的过程是利用贝叶斯方法设计和实施临床试验的一个重大优势。前述例子只考虑了 r 的两个可能值。更实际些的话,反应率 r 可能取 0 到 1 之间的任何值。图 20-1a 左侧显示一条固定的或者是平直的曲线,代表备选的先验分布。这条平直的曲线表示在 r 的取值范围内其概率都是相同的,这也许可以称之为"开放的先验分布",因为后验分布几乎全部依据当前实验得到的信息。在一个单个的肿瘤反应发生之后,贝叶斯更新就将概率分布变成图 20-1a 右侧所显示的分布,即当先验分布是图中左侧所显示的那样时,那么右侧就是在观测到 R 发生之后的后验分布。当观察到 R 发生后,r 的分布偏向更大的值转移,对应着较大反应率更可能发生。贝叶斯法则量化了这种可能。

除了图 20-1a 中第一个图显示的,还有许多候选的先验分布。如图 20-1b~d 所示另外三对先验/后验分布。每一对图的左侧是先验分布,右侧即为观察到 R 后的后验分布。此外,图 20-1b~d 的左侧曲线本身分别都是图 20-1a~c 右侧曲线的后验分布,但这是在观察结果是 N(nonresponse,不反应)的情况下得到的。直观上,若出现一个无肿瘤反应结果,r 值概率的集中趋势将变得更小。从数学角度看，观察到 R 意味着将当前的分布乘以 r（反应率）并将之重新正态化以便使曲线下面积为1。同样地，观察到 N 意味着乘以 $(1-r)$，也就是未反应率。图 20-1 的一个含义是，以图 20-1a 左侧图为先验开始，图 20-1 从左到右从上到下依次观察到 RNRNRNR。图 20-1 中所示的八条曲线分别与以下几个函数形式成正比：$1, r, r(1-r), r^2(1-r), r^2(1-r)^2, r^3(1-r)^2, r^3(1-r)^3$ 和 $r^4(1-r)^3$。每一个有反应的观察对象（R）使 r 的指数增加了1，而每个没有反应的（N）则使 $(1-r)$ 的指数增加了1。从图中明显可以看到增加的观察对象导致分布变得更窄。随着观察对象数量的增加，分布趋向于集中在一个单独的点上，这个点就是"真正"的 r 值，即产生观察对象的反应率。网页 https://biostatistics. mdanderson. org/SofwareDownload/SingleSofware/Index/96 提供了在 beta-binomial 分布环境中贝叶斯修正的可视化演示的免费软件。这一节的主要内容并不是关于后验分布计算方法，而是强调通过使用贝叶斯方法，我们在临床试验的任何时候都可以找到后验分布。

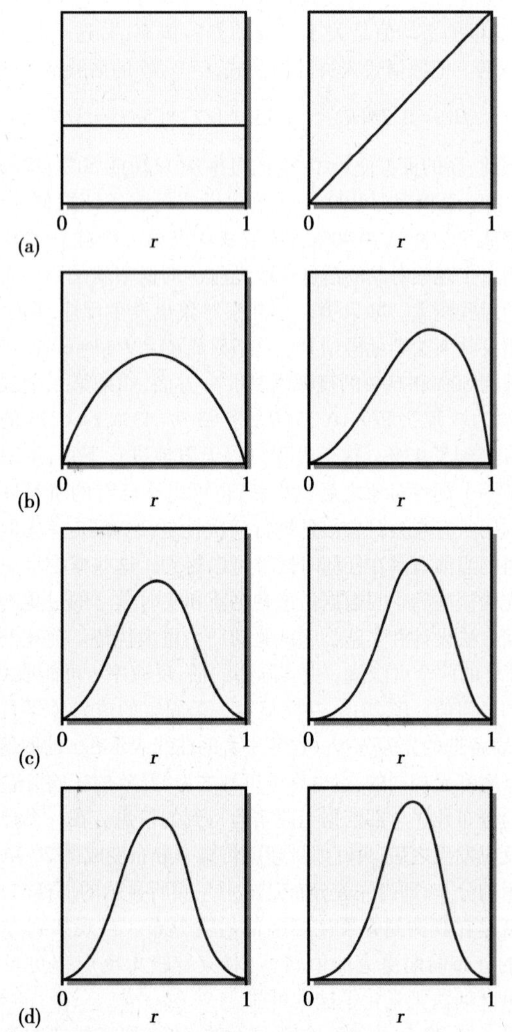

图 20-1　反应率 r 的先验分布。每一对图的左侧是反应率 r 的先验分布，右侧图是在观察到一个患者的反应后 r 的后验分布。左侧每个图反应的（预测）概率是 0.500，在（a）、（b）、（c）、（d）四种情况下，右侧图的相应概率分别增加到了 0.667、0.600、0.571 和 0.556。当先验分布反映了更大的不确定性时，变化越大，学习也更快速

先验概率

贝叶斯方法需要一个起点即各种参数的先验分布。前例中，我们必须提前或独立于所进行的试验知道反应率 r 的概率分布。这个先验分布可以是主观判定的也可以是明确地基于之前试验的结果。例如在一些常见情况下，一个合适的默认分布就是无信息的或者开放的[10,13]，在此情形上参数的所有可能取值都被赋予相同的先验概率。图 20-1a 的左侧分布就是一个例子。

无信息或者均匀先验分布（flat prior distribution）忽略了可从实验外部获得的信息从而局限了使用贝叶斯方法的优势。然而，即使从一开始就使用先验信息不能反映任何判定的均匀分布，贝叶斯方法的好处也是很大的。均匀先验分布起了一些重要的作用：其中之一就是它可以区分当前研究中数据提供的证据和研究之前信息提供的证据；另一个就是使用均匀先验分布得出的贝叶斯方法分析结论通常与对应的频率派方法结果相同。

先验分布通常要基于历史数据。假设一种相似的药物（或者同样的药物用于可能不同的患者群体）在 20 个患者中得到的反应率是 50%：10 个反应者，10 个未反应者。反应率 r 所对应的似然值（参见后述"频率学派和贝叶斯学派的比较"）是 $r^{10}(1-r)^{10}$。假定历史情况和当前实验情况可能有些不同，那么没有任何调整地直接使用历史数据作为 r 的先验分布并不合理，但是采用某种方式来利用这些相关信息产生先验分布是合适的。一个可能性（将会在"时间风险"的章节中讲述）就是将历史信息折扣后应用到当前试验的背景下。例如，权衡出一个历史观测数据的信息只相当于当前观测值 30% 的权重，这就意味着可利用一个与 $r^3(1-r)^3$ 成比例的先验分布。这个分布如图 20-1d 的左侧所示。

稳健性

若存在足够的数据，基本上所有的观察值都有相似的后验分布，这就是稳健性。这意味着对于适中样本或是大样本，假定何种特殊先验分布都不会影响很大。我们以图 20-1 中的 8 个分布为例，依次考虑每一个分布作为不同个体的先验分布。参数 r 是某种药的反应率。假设试验中有 40 个患者经过治疗，20 个发生反应。根据稳健性原则，这项研究中上述提到的 8 个个体的药物反应率将会非常接近。图 20-2 是 8 个后验分布，这些曲线几乎重叠，这 8 个 95% 概率区间也将非常接近。观测到的样本数据比图 20-1 中的各种先验分布对结果的影响更大。

若两个先验分布明显不同且先验分布中包含的相应信息较强，稳健原则依然适用，但是需要大量的数据才能让两个不同的分布靠拢。

频率学派和贝叶斯学派的比较

在频率学派方法中，检验假设和参数中不涉及概率。相反，概率分配只针对数据，对给定未知参数赋予一个特定值时计算概率。例如，常见的 P 值就是当原假设为真时，已观察到数据或更极端数据的概率值。用符号表示就是：

- 频率派 P 值：P（已观察到或更极端的数据 $\mid H_0$）
- 贝叶斯后验概率：$P(H_0\mid$ 已观察到数据）

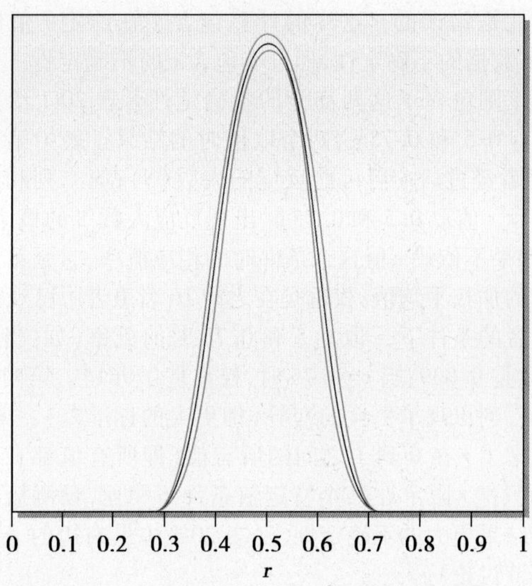

图 20-2　基于一个实验(20 个反应,20 个未反应)的反应率 r 的后验分布。这里的 8 个先验分布就是图 20-1 中所示的 8 个分布,除了比例常数它们分别是 $1, r, r(1-r), r^2(1-r), r^2(1-r)^2, r^3(1-r)^2, r^3(1-r)^3, r^4(1-r)^3$。相应的后验分布与 $r^{20}(1-r)^{20}, r^{21}(1-r)^{20}, r^{21}(1-r)^{21}, r^{22}(1-r)^{21}, r^{22}(1-r)^{22}, r^{23}(1-r)^{22}, r^{23}(1-r)^{23}$ 和 $r^{24}(1-r)^{23}$ 成正比。这 8 个非常相似的后验分布显示了稳健性原则

这两个概念很容易混淆。P 值常被解释为无效的概率,而 $1-P$ 则解释为有效的概率。这种解释是错误的。这相当于在没有先验概率的情况下试图得到贝叶斯后验概率,这是不可能的。

频率派 P 值和贝叶斯后验概率之间存在两个重要的差异。一是条件的倒置:在频率派中的假设(H_0)是在贝叶斯派中是以一定概率存在的;二是频率派的 P 值除了包含已观察到数据的概率,还包含了观察值以外更极端情况的概率。

例如,在一个单臂Ⅱ期试验中,检验假设为 $H_0: r=0.5$ 和 $H_1: r=0.75$,假设Ⅰ类错误 $\alpha=5\%$,样本量 $n=33$,检验效能为 90%。假如最终结果是 33 名患者中有 22 名发生反应,频率派认为单侧 P 值就是在原假设($H_0: r=0.5$)成立的条件下,33 名患者中有 22 名或更多人发生反应的概率。在原假设成立的情况下,观察到 22、23、24 名……反应者的概率就是 $P=0.022\,5+0.010\,8+0.004\,5+\cdots\cdots=0.040\,1$。由于此时 P 值小于 5%,观察到 22 名患者就被称为有统计学意义”。

在已知 33 名患者中有 22 名发生反应的情况下,贝叶斯方法算的是假设($H_1: r=0.75$)的后验概率(即 $1-H_0$ 的概率)。(如前所述,贝叶斯计算仅依赖于实际观察到数据的概率值,即 33 名患者中有 22 名发生反应,但频率派的计算还包括 23、24 名……的反应概率)应用贝叶斯定理:

$$P(H_1|22\text{ of }33)=P(22\text{ of }33|H_1)P(H_1)/P(22\text{ of }33)$$

如等式中所述,假设在观察数据之前 H_0 和 H_1 成立的概率是相同的,分母遵循全概率定律:

$$P(22\text{ of }33)=P(22\text{ of }33|H_1)P(H_1)+P(22\text{ of }33|H_0)P(H_0)$$
$$=(0.082\,3)(0.5)+(0.022\,5)(0.5)=0.052\,4$$

因此,

$$P(H_1|22\text{ of }33)=(0.082\,3)(0.5)\ /\ 0.052\,4=0.785$$
$$P(H_0|22\text{ of }33)=(0.022\,5)(0.5)\ /\ 0.052\,4=0.215$$

这种算法只考虑了两种假设,$r=0.5$ 和 $r=0.75$。再考虑 r 的其他取值时,贝叶斯法则通过 $P(22\text{ of }33|r)$ 来衡量它们,被称为 r 的似然函数。似然函数的图示如图 20-3,它表示由观测数据所表现出的对反应率 r 的支持度。有相同似然函数值的 r 值得到数据相同的支持度。只有相对的似然值才是重要的。例如,$r=0.5$ 与 $r=0.75$ 比较的结果只依赖于它们的似然(0.082 3 和 0.022 5)之比,即图 20-3 中标出的似然值之比。由于 0.082 3/0.022 5=3.66,因此数据提供给 $r=0.75$ 的支持是 $r=0.5$ 的 3.66 倍。

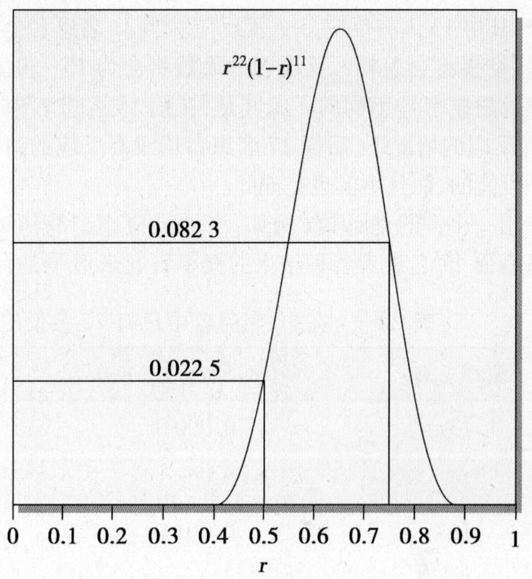

图 20-3　33 名患者中 22 名反应率 r 的似然值。此似然值为 $P(22\text{ of }33|r)$,与 $r^{22}(1-r)^{11}$ 成正比。$r=0.5$ 和 0.75 的似然值被标出,是文章例子中计算涉及的值

这两种方法的结论从概念和数值上都不同。在频率派方法中,P 值为 0.040 1,结果被认为“有统计学意义”。一些研究人员把“有统计学意义”解释成“H_0 不太可能成立”的意思,然而这并不是它本来的含义,其含义为“H_0 为真时,不太可能观察到当前及其更极端数据”。H_0 的贝叶斯后验概率则直接回答了:H_0 成立的概率是 0.215。尽管它比先验概率 0.50 小(因为数据更偏向于支持 H_1 而不是 H_0),但它是频率派 P 值的 5 倍。

这两种方法在区间估计方面也有不同的解释。在贝叶斯方法中,可以计算出一个参数落在任意给定区间内的概率。而在频率派中,对于给定的固定参数,置信区间则有一个大样本极限意义下的频率解释。所以“95%置信区间有 95%的概率包含待估参数”的说法是不正确的。尽管有不同的解释,但是两种方法间仍有一点是一致的。也就是说,若先验分布是均匀的(如图 20-1a 左侧的分布),那么一个置信区间的贝叶斯后验概率基本上与频率派置信区间的置信度水平是一样的。比如,如果先验分布是均匀的,那么表示一个参数落在它的 95%置信区间的贝叶斯后验概率事实上就是 95%。对于非平直的先验分布,一个 95%置信区间的后验概率可以大于或小于 95%。如果

先验分布所依据的历史数据与当前实验中的数据一致，那么表示参数落在95%置信区间内的后验概率将会大于95%。如果历史数据与当前实验的数据不一致，那么95%置信区间包含真实参数的概率将明显小于95%。

预测概率

对于试验设计和试验监测而言，预测未来(伴随着必然的不确定性)的能力是重要的。贝叶斯方法可以不必假定任何假设成立就能计算未来的结果概率。即使不是在数学上，至少在逻辑上看，其过程很直接。对于一个指定的实验设计，我们可以找到每个参数值观察到未来数据的条件概率，并根据各参数值的当前概率对其取加权平均。本节将会详细探讨预测概率。

再来看前述33名患者的试验。假定已经有16名患者经过治疗，其中13人有反应，3人无反应。当33名患者全部经过治疗后，结果将会怎样？反应者的人数将会为13~30，但这些事件发生的概率是不同的。尤其是，在前16名患者中已经有13名有反应的情况下，后面17名患者均没有反应的情况似乎是很不可能的，而且事实也是如此。

使用一个r的估计值(例如，当前反应率，13/16=0.81)去计算后面17名患者各种结果的概率看起来似乎是合理的，但这可能是错误的。这样的计算包含了在给定r值的情况下，未来数据的不确定性，但没有包含r的不确定性。贝叶斯预测概率则包含了这两部分的不确定性。表20-1给出了假定r只有0.5和0.75这两个取值时的结果。表中第一列为33名患者经过治疗后可能反应的人数(S)；第二列和第三列分别表示r值取0.5和0.75时出现反应人数S的概率；第四列为，如果不依赖r值这个条件时的相应概率，它是第二列和第三列的加权平均值，权重是在之前16名患者中已观察到13名反应者的条件下，r取0.5和0.75时的概率(如：当r=0.5时，权重是0.039；当r=0.75时，权重是0.961)。第四列比第二和第三列出现了更大的变异(即更大的标准差)。典型的，如果考虑了r在0到1之间的所有值(即所有值都有阳性概率)，与只把r限定在某个特定值条件下相比，预测概率反映了未来结果更大的不确定性。(表20-1中最右边的一列将会在下一节讨论)。

为了方便起见，假设先验概率是相等的：$P(H_1)=P(H_0)=0.5$。尽管这些表达式中没有竖线"|"，但这些概率可以依赖于其他现有的证据信息，比如，以往的临床试验和临床前试验的结果。生物评价中也可能有额外的信息，比如考虑靶向性治疗时。在设定$P(H_0)$和$P(H_1)$时，全部这些情况都会被考虑进去。

表20-1 在16名患者中已有13名反应的前提下，33名患者全部接受治疗后反应数S的预测概率

S(of 33)	$P(S\|r=0.5)$	$P(S\|r=0.75)$	$P(S)$	$P(H_1)$
13	0.000 0	0.000 0	0.000 0	0.000 2
14	0.000 1	0.000 0	0.000 0	0.000 6
15	0.001 0	0.000 0	0.000 0	0.001 7
16	0.005 2	0.000 0	0.000 2	0.005 0
17	0.018 2	0.000 0	0.000 7	0.014 8
18	0.047 2	0.000 1	0.001 9	0.043 2
19	0.094 4	0.000 5	0.004 2	0.119 2
20	0.148 4	0.002 5	0.008 2	0.288 7
21	0.185 5	0.009 3	0.016 2	0.549 1
22	0.185 5	0.027 9	0.034 1	0.785 1
23	0.148 4	0.066 8	0.070 1	0.916 4
24	0.094 4	0.127 6	0.126 3	0.970 5
25	0.047 2	0.191 4	0.185 7	0.990 0
26	0.018 1	0.220 9	0.212 9	0.996 6
27	0.005 2	0.189 3	0.182 0	0.998 9
28	0.001 0	0.113 6	0.109 1	0.999 6
29	0.000 1	0.042 6	0.040 9	0.999 9
30	0.000 0	0.007 5	0.007 2	1.000 0

注：第二列$P(S|r=0.5)$列和第三列$P(S|r=0.75)$列是在r值为0.5和0.75时计算出的概率值。第四列$P(S)$列是第二和第三列的加权平均值，其各自的权重分别为0.039和0.961。最后一列给出了$P(H_1)$，它表示33名患者中有S名反应者的情况下$H_1(r=0.75)$的概率。

贝叶斯与频率派期中分析的比较

贝叶斯方法与频率派方法之间,既有许多共同点,也有一些不同之处。这一节就介绍一个主要的不同之处。在贝叶斯方法中,可以得到一个观测结果就来更新各种假设的概率。这个简单的过程意味着一定程度的灵活性,而这点却是频率派很难做到的。

再来考虑前述试验设计:患者人数为 $n=33$,检验 $H_0:r=0.5$ 与 $H_1:r=0.75$。如果观察到 22 名或者更多的反应者,将会有足够的证据来拒绝 H_0,而倾向于 H_1(单侧检验,Ⅰ类错误率取 5%)。但是,安排 33 名患者进行试验性治疗而没有评估期中结果则存在一个伦理问题,并将会受到机构审查委员会的质疑。如果在试验期间得到一个确定性结论(要么是阳性,明确支持 $r>0.5$;或者阴性,支持 $r\leqslant 0.5$),那么这项试验应该终止。假定 16 名患者经过治疗后,我们发现 13 名发生反应,3 名未反应,从贝叶斯角度讲,更新后的 H_1 概率是 96.1%(假设先验概率 $P(H_0)=0.5$)。

这个概率是否是"确定性"还不清楚。关于是否要继续进行一项试验的决定是复杂的。有了当前和未来的结果后,它将取决于试验的预期影响。在贝叶斯方法中,可以通过它们的预测概率来衡量未来结果的影响。例如,当 33 名患者全部经过治疗后的结果已知时,假定试验的预期影响取决于 H_1 的后验概率是否大于 95%,那么就可以计算该事件的预测概率。表 20-1 的最右侧一列表示 33 名患者中有 S 名发生反应时,H_1 的后验概率。为了使后验概率大于 95%,33 名患者中至少需要有 24 名反应者。该事件的预测概率是反应人数 $S\geqslant 24$ 的预测概率之和(表 20-1 的第四列)等于 0.864 2。尽管 H_1 的当前概率确实是大于 95%,但由于 S 和 r 的不确定性,观察到 H_1 的后验概率大于 95%的可能性将降低 1-0.864 2=0.135 8。这就是说还是有一定的概率表示当前结论只是暂时性的结论。当前结论会发生变化的可能性将被综合考虑到是否继续试验的决定当中。

如果当前结论仍可维持足够高的预测概率,那么我们有理由来终止试验。这对于无论是主张无效还是优效都是成立的。根据预测概率及早终止一项试验的可能性应该在试验方案中明确说明。

频率派观点的重点是Ⅰ类错误率 α。它是当 H_0 成立的情况下拒绝 H_0 的概率,并依赖于试验设计。对于样本例数固定为 33 名患者的样本,计算很明确,大于等于 22 名反应者时,拒绝 H_0 的概率为 $\alpha=0.040\,1$(见前一节)。当可能提前终止试验时,计算就变得更复杂。在前例中,当前 16 名患者中有 12 名或更多反应者时,如果试验终止且 H_0 被拒绝,那么,由于有更多的可能性拒绝 H_0,导致 α 增加。假设 $r=0.5$,那么拒绝 H_0 的概率现在变为 0.064 0。由于这个概率大于 0.05,所以习惯上就要调整终止标准和拒绝标准使 α 减少到 0.05。例如,只有在经过治疗的 16 名患者中有 13 名或更多反应者,或者在经过治疗的 33 名患者中有 22 名或更多的反应者的情况下拒绝 H_0,才会得到总的Ⅰ类错误为 0.045 0。

因此当进行期中分析时,得到有统计学意义的结论会更困难。原因就在于Ⅰ类错误率是在假定某个检验假设为真的前提下计算出的(药物无效的原假设)。从某种意义上说,一个研究者会由于使用频率派的期中分析而受到惩罚。而从贝叶斯观点看就不会由于期中分析而产生这样的惩罚。原因就是贝叶斯概率不依赖任何给定的原假设。

尽管Ⅰ类错误率不是贝叶斯统计量,但是无论多复杂的贝叶斯设计都能对它进行估计。如果设计中有期中分析,那么这样的计算就包含对Ⅰ类错误适当的惩罚。这种计算就像之前给出的例子中的一样,是很简单的。在更复杂的情况下,需要采用蒙特卡罗模拟。

一项乳腺癌试验说明了贝叶斯设计的一些优势[18]。该试验将 65 岁以上患有乳腺癌的妇女随机分成两组,一组接受标准化疗,另一组接受卡培他滨(抗肿瘤药)治疗。样本大小预计为 600~1 800。在第 600 名患者纳入试验后,遵循试验方案,计算预测概率。在给定现有样本以及在当前样本基础上持续随访的情况下,计算出有统计学意义的预测概率。如果达到了预定的界值,将停止增加其他患者,但仍将继续观察已纳入的患者。在第一次期中分析时,研究达到了预测概率的界值点,所以不再入组患者(最终样本量为 633)。事实上,后来的研究表明,在这个研究人群中,接受标准化疗的女性比接受卡培他滨治疗的女性乳腺癌复发和死亡的风险更低[19]。

分析问题

本节的目的是考虑两类统计分析问题:第一类是前序章节的延伸;第二类与第一类无关,涉及的是生存分析一个特定的方面。

分层模型:综合信息

在分析临床试验的数据时,通常可以获得关于当前治疗的其他信息。本节将讨论一种称为分层建模的方法,它的用途之一是综合不同来源的信息。该方法适用于多种情形,包括 meta 分析和历史资料的综合。分层模型是一种随机效应模型。在 meta 分析中,有两个水平,一个水平是某试验内的个体患者,另一个水平是试验。分层模型可用在研究设计方面,如对不同疾病或疾病亚型的结果进行合并。也可应用在看似无联系的方面,如整群随机。分层模型在研究设计方面的应用将在下一节阐述。

考虑一个Ⅱ期临床试验,该试验 33 例患者中 21 例有反应。按原假设 $H_0:r=0.50$ 获得的单侧 P 值为 0.08,所以该结果在 5%的检验水准下无统计学意义。现在考虑一个早Ⅰ期临床试验,使用相同的疗法,20 例患者中 15 例有反应。尽管接受治疗的人群或试验实施的机构可能有所不同,这些信息看起来似乎是有关联的。但是,如何在分析中综合考虑这些信息并非易事。频率学派的方法是就某一特定试验而言的,它假想这上述两个试验是某个较大试验的一部分。如果假定整个数据是从 53 例患者中 36 例有反应的一次试验中得到的,那么从频率学派角度,得到的 P 值为 0.006 3,具有显著的统计学意义。然而这一结论是错误的,因为前提假设是错误的。并且,频率学派尚不清楚如何解决这一问题。

任何假定两项试验的反应率相同的贝叶斯分析也会犯类似的错误。我们有理由认为反应率 r 在不同试验中是不同的。即使两项试验的受试者纳排标准相同,且给予相同的治疗,两试验的反应率也有可能不同。一方面，入选标准在不同试验场景下的应用会有差别。然而，即使患者具有高度的相似性，其结果也会随时间、地点的不同而不同。我们对癌症的了解和诊断方式随着时间的推移也在发生变化。另一方面，伴随治疗的应用及临床和实验室指标的评估上也会有不同。完善的分析方法是要明确地考虑两个 r 值，第一项试验的 $r1$ 和第二项试验的 $r2$。

概括来说，有两个极端的假设使得分析更容易进行，但均是错误的。其中一种假设 $r1$ 和 $r2$ 无关，任何关于 $r2$ 的推断仅依据第二项试验的数据；另一种假设是 $r1=r2$，然后合并这两项试验的结果。

两个 r 值可能相同，也可能不同。在贝叶斯分层模型中，两种可能性都是允许的，且都不需要进行假设。换句话说，$r1$ 和 $r2$ 被认为是来自 r 值的总体。该总体可能具有较小的变异（同质性），也可能有很大的变异（异质性）。观测到的反应率提供了异质性程度的信息，反应率差别越大则提示异质性越大。当观测到的反应率相近时，$r1$ 和 $r2$ 的估计精度要高于两者相去甚远的情形。前一种情况下，试验之间具有较强的信息可借用度；如果不同试验的结果差别很大，则其信息可借用度较低，而且任何单项试验的信息很难应用于其他试验中。

更为普遍的是，对于某一特定的疗效，能够提供支持信息的相关研究或数据集的数目可以有很多个。这些研究可能是异质的，可能考虑了不同的患者群体。下面的例子具有一般性，但比前面的例子更复杂，因为它包含了 9 项研究[20]。这些研究唯一的共同点是它们都关注了同一种治疗策略的效力。

反应率可以是 0 到 1 之间的任何值。表 20-2 和图 20-4 显示了每项研究的反应例数 S 和样本例数 n。每项研究对应一个反应率，从 $r1$，$r2$ 一直到 $r9$ 共 9 个。9 个研究中的每一个样本反应率（S/n）都是相应 r 的估计值。150 例患者中有 106 例发生反应。如果假设 9 个反应率相等，则其共同反应率 r（假设是一个均匀的先验分布）的后验分布如图 20-4 所示，标有“汇总分析”。

表 20-2 各研究的观测反应率（包括其标准误）和调整反应率的估计值，S 为反应例数，n 为样本例数

研究编号	反应例数（S）	样本大小（n）	观测反应率（标准误）	贝叶斯估计（标准差）
1	11	16	0.69（1.116）	0.69（0.094）
2	20	20	1.00（0.000）	0.90（0.064）
3	4	10	0.40（0.155）	0.53（0.121）
4	10	19	0.53（0.115）	0.57（0.094）
5	5	14	0.36（0.128）	0.48（0.109）
6	36	46	0.78（0.061）	0.77（0.058）
7	9	10	0.90（0.095）	0.80（0.097）
8	7	9	0.78（0.139）	0.73（0.110）
9	4	6	0.67（0.192）	0.68（0.125）
总计	106	150	0.71（0.037）	0.68（0.064）

注：贝叶斯估计值一列在文中有描述。

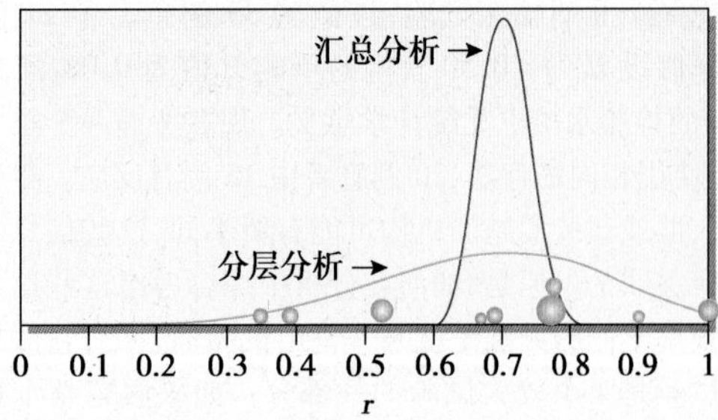

图 20-4 反应率比较。r 轴上的点代表了表 20-2 中列出的所观测到的反应率。点的面积大小与样本例数 n 近似成比例。汇总分析曲线显示了假设无研究效应时反应率 r 的分布情况。分层分析曲线显示了考虑各研究间存在异质性后反应率分布的贝叶斯估计

虽然该汇总分析是错误的，但 106/150 的总体估计可能还是相对合理的。然而，这一估计值的精度太高了（相当于其标准误太小）。相比较而言，图 20-4 中的“分层分析”曲线则是研究总体中反应率分布的贝叶斯估计（该曲线为假定 r 值服从的 beta 分布的参数具有无信息先验分布条件下的平均后验分布）。由于是典型的分层分析，该曲线比同质性假设条件下的类似曲线具有更大的变异性。

在分层分析中，单项研究 r 的分布由该研究的数据而定，但它也受其他研究的影响。表 20-2 最右边的一列显示了每项研究的反应率分布的后验均值。它也是该研究新纳入患者反应性的预测概率。单项研究的概率向总体平均值的方向压缩。研究例数越少，观测到的反应率越远离总体平均值，则压缩的程度越大。分层借用是合理的，因为它并不假定所有研究都具有相同的真实反应率，而且信息借用的程度大小是由数据本身所决定。

图 20-5 提供了表 20-2 最右侧两列数据的图示比较，表明了估计值的压缩。贝叶斯估计值居于简单汇总（完全压缩）和

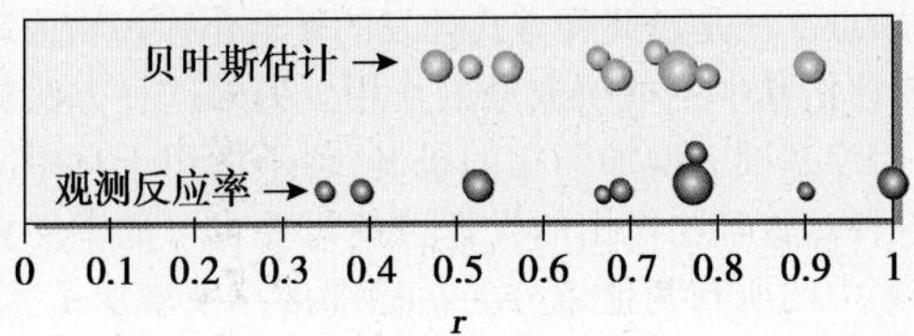

图 20-5　观测反应率与贝叶斯估计值比较。有关数值在表 20-2 中最右边两列给出。绘制在 r 轴上的点表示所观测到的反应率，与图 20-4 类似，点的面积大小与样本例数 n 近似成比例。贝叶斯估计假定了一个分层模型，并显示出向总体平均值压缩的倾向

每项单独研究之间。压缩量-包括前文提到的两个极端情形-取决于试验总体的先验分布。这种先验分布应该事先设定。设定多种先验分布可以用来总体结论的敏感性。

压缩是分层建模的结果。建立这种模型的目的是合理地利用所获得的信息来提高研究精度或减少所需的样本例数。以表 20-2 中的 1 号研究为参照。将其他 8 项研究的数据进行简单汇总，会大大提高反应率估计的精度。例如，标准误将由 0.116 减少到 0.037。但是，考虑到研究间存在可能的异质性后，这种汇总就不合理了。分层地利用信息也会提高估计的精度，但提高的幅度较小。贝叶斯估计的标准差从 0.116 减小到 0.094，只减少了约 20%。尽管减小量小于简单汇总的，但这却意味着，在保持同样精度的条件下，实施这项临床试验（按表 20-2 中研究 1 进行设定）可以节约 50% 以上的样本例数：$(0.116/0.094)^2-1=52\%$。例如，为了在一次独立研究中获得相同的标准误，将需要 25 例患者，而不是表 20-2 中的研究 1 的 16 例。

分层分析还可以考虑患者的协变量，在考虑未知效应的同时调整研究间已知的差异。在这个例子中和更复杂的分层背景下[21]，建立模型时允许借用其他研究和数据库的信息。如果研究间的结果是一致的，则借用的程度就较大。如果结果有很大不同（考虑协变量后），则意味着研究间存在异质性，这时借用的程度会较低。

试验设计中的分层模型

在许多情况下，研究者可以从相关但不一定完全相同的试验中获取信息进行试验设计。

考虑设计治疗某疾病的一项试验，且该疾病有多个亚型，例如某肿瘤有几种不同的组织学亚型。不同亚型间的反应率很有可能不同。该背景与上节的例子实际上是一致的。关注点是不同亚型的肿瘤反应率。就像上一节描述的一样，这涉及一个分布问题。认识到亚型之间的信息可以相互借用后，则能更准确地估算每一单个亚型的反应率，进而降低每个亚型内的样本量。

信息借用的程度取决于研究结果，就像前述章节描述的一样。换句话说，样本量的节省是无法准确预测的。然而，如果可以监测到期中结果就可以解决这个问题。期中结果可用于确定与各种反应率估计相关的精确度。如果必须决定停止试验而期中结果又无法获得时，在认识到最终的精确度不能被完美预测的前提下，应在试验设计阶段评估有关亚型间异质性的不确定性，并相应地选择合适的样本量。

时间风险

时间-事件分析（time-to-event，TITE）或生存分析普遍应用于癌症研究中。本节将重点放在生存分析更窄的一个方面，以便更好地了解癌症及其治疗。在下文中，我们使用癌症与白血病 B 组（cancer and leukemia group B，CALGB）的 8541 号方案临床试验的数据进行举例说明[22]。

这项试验考虑了环磷酰胺、多柔比星、5-氟尿嘧啶（cyclophosphamide、doxorubicin、and 5-fluorouracil；CAF）化疗方案治疗淋巴结阳性乳腺癌的三种不同剂量：高、中、低剂量，分别对应的是按 600mg/m^2、60mg/m^2 和 600mg/m^2 服药 4 个周期，按 400mg/m^2、40mg/m^2 和 400mg/m^2 服药 6 个周期，以及按 300mg/m^2、30mg/m^2 和 300mg/m^2 服药 4 个周期。主要终点是无病生存期（disease-free survival），图 20-6 显示了三个剂量组的 Kaplan-Meier 曲线。我们没有提供组间的比较（高剂量 vs. 中剂量组；高剂量 vs. 低剂量组）P 值，因为其是否有统计学意义与本文目的无关。

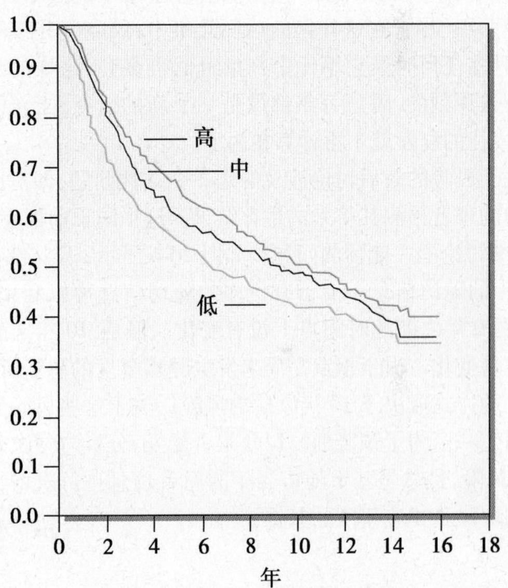

图 20-6　CALGB 8541 试验三个 CAF 剂量组的无病生存率曲线

尽管图 20-6 是标准的生存曲线，但它未能提供增加剂量或不同剂量强度下患者获益的全部情况。这在时间-风险曲线图中更清楚一些。风险是指某特定时间段里事件发生数占该时间段初始时面临风险人数的比例。例如，假设事件为复发，在第一年风险集中有 100 名患者，如果第一年中这些患者有 10 例出现疾病复发，则第一年的复发风险为 10%。进入第二年将有 90 名患者面临风险。如果第二年有另外 18 名患者出现复发，则第二年的复发风险为 18/90＝20%。如果要从图 20-6 的生存曲线图计算风险度，则用上一年的生存率减去当年的生存率，再除以上一年的生存率。各年的风险度如图 20-7 所示。

图 20-7 中引人注意的是，三个治疗组的风险度都随时间推移而减少（第二年以后）。由此反映了这种疾病的异质性。最有侵袭性的肿瘤复发早，在刚开始的几年风险度明显偏高。一旦患者的肿瘤复发，他们便不再是风险人群。余下的患者肿瘤侵袭性较弱，因此复发率较低。

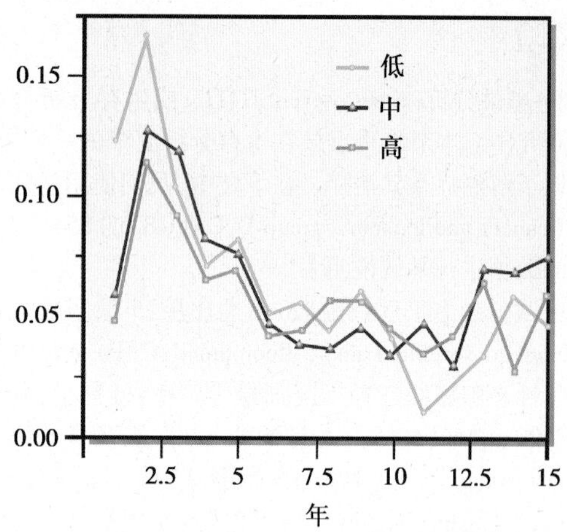

图 20-7 CALGB 8541 试验三个 CAF 剂量组的风险度。由图 20-6 衍生而来

就一个治疗组的效果来看,高剂量组的显著获益局限于前5年左右。实际上,在前6年,高剂量组患者每年的风险度都低于其他两组(尽管在这6年的后面几年中,风险度并没降低多少,而且在任何时候它不比中剂量组低很多)。这样的结果是令人印象深刻的,因为每年都像是一个新的研究,当新的一年开始,以往的复发就不再计算在内了。

关于风险的最后讨论涉及的是一个共性问题,即对已经在试验中的患者预测其将来的生存结果。这不同于前面在"预测概率"中讨论的一般预测问题。如图 20-6 所示,不少患者有至少10年的随访信息。由于有更多的随访信息可以利用,这些曲线在10年之前的时间点上没有变化。但是,10年之后的曲线则容易变化。由于重点是尚未发生肿瘤复发的患者,因此曲线变化的方式取决于10年以后的风险。关于这些风险的信息可见图 20-7。为了预测何时以及是否复发,分析时每次仅考虑1年的风险,且总是基于随访当年的患者信息。每次增加的风险预测取决于相应年度的数据。

统计设计原则:决策分析和析因试验

决策分析

临床实践与临床研究均涉及决策的制定。列出每个决策可能导致的结果、概率及后果,从正反两方面罗列各个决策的利弊,从而选择合适的决策。由于预测概率在决策过程中起着至关重要的作用,因此利用贝叶斯方法制定决策会比较理想。试验设计和最佳样本量的选择就是获益于决策分析的决定,详细做法可参见其他参考文献[23~32]。

析因试验

大多数的肿瘤药物比较试验,检验的都是一个试验组相对于一个对照组的效应。两组患者在接受了按肿瘤分型和分期确定的标准治疗和既往治疗的基础上,可能会接受一些额外的治疗。他们可能会开展手术或接受伴随的放疗和可能包含多种药物的其他化疗。如果新的试验处理显示出充分的效果,则其将会被纳入肿瘤的标准治疗。该方法简单明了,但也有一些缺点。一是以此种方式开发的复合化疗药物或联合治疗,不能评估其中各单项成分的作用。另外这种方法提供了在标准治疗基础上增加药物的机制,但不适用于从中减少的情况,一种试验药物作用的发挥可能需要也可能不需要标准治疗方案中的所有其他组分。在标准治疗中增加试验药物,可能会使方案的一些成分变成多余,但是,我们无法鉴别出这些成分。

从某种程度上讲,这样的难题无法避免。虽然某些成分从来没有证明过其对综合疗效有贡献,但要从标准化疗中去除这些成分是非常困难的,其中还有伦理的考虑。然而,较好的药物开发方法应该能减少这些问题,并且好的治疗应该得到更快的发展。统计学上理想试验设计的基本原则是改变各种相关因素,以便充分地了解它们对试验结果的影响。这种影响可能涉及各因素之间的交互作用,研究它们之间的交互作用也是一项重要的工作。我们所需要做的是利用现有的数据建立这些因素之间关系的模型。

其中一种可选的方法为析因设计,每次改变一个因素展开不同的研究[33]。举个最简单的例子,将患者随机分配到四种不同的处理:单独A、单独B、A和B合用以及两者都不用(最后一种并不意味着"无治疗",因为所有患者都接受标准治疗)。这四种可能性的示意图见图 20-8,"A"表示患者接受A,"非A"表示患者不接受A。这个因素可以是药物或其他干预因素(例如,A可能是放射治疗、化疗前而非化疗后的手术治疗,或者是相对于低剂量的高剂量药物等)。图 20-8 从左向右显示的不是时间顺序。这两种药物可能同时给予或按先后顺序给予,A先B后或B先A后。事实上,先后或同时用药可以是析因设计中另外一个考虑因素[34,35]。

析因设计的一个优点是它们能够估计单个药物的"主效应",因此一个试验可以回答两个(或更多)问题,且与二臂试验样本量相同。另一个优点是可以评估各因素之间的交互作用。例如,将图 20-8 中上面两种不同处理的差别与下面两种不同处理的差别进行比较,探讨在使用药物A时和不使用药物A时B的作用是否相同。表 20-3 给出了图 20-8 中所考虑的药物A和药物B的四种可能组合的交互作用类型,这里假设终点指标为反应率。对于负交互作用,联合用药的作用低于单独给药的作用之和。对于正交互作用,联合用药的作用大于单独给药的作用之和。

析因设计的一个局限是,一些治疗的组合可能不符合伦理或实际中不可能。例如图 20-8 中有一组合是既不给予药物A也不给予药物B。在一些肿瘤治疗中不可能设立这样的治疗组。试验设计中设立三个组优于两个组,但是这样就无法评价单个药物的作用,同时也丧失了析因设计在样本量上的优点。

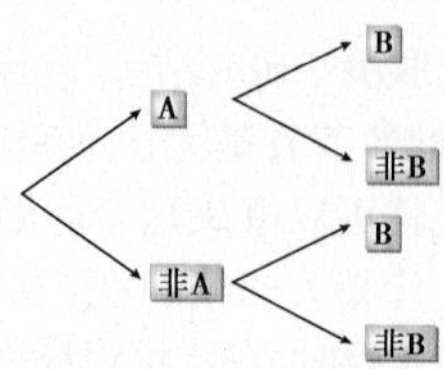

图 20-8 药物A、B及两药物组合的 2×2 析因设计。有4种可能的治疗组合

表 20-3　析因设计 4 种治疗组合的反应率(%)，以标准治疗为基础增加药物 A 和药物 B(假设的效应)

治疗组合	均无效	A 有效 B 无效	B 有效 A 无效	叠加效果	负交互作用	正交互作用 (例 1)	正交互作用 (例 2)
A 和 B	20	30	30	40	30	50	40
A 非 B	20	30	20	30	30	30	20
B 非 A	20	20	30	30	30	30	20
非 A 非 B	20	20	20	20	20	20	20

当设计一项具有特定检验效能的双臂试验时，在不增加样本量的情况下，可以加入第二个因素。评估各因素间交互作用的检验效能达不到评估主效应的检验效能，但会获得一些关于交互作用的信息。如果要求提高评估交互作用的检验效能，则需要增加样本量。然而，合理的通常也是更实际的做法是保持样本量不变，而接受评估交互作用的中等检验效能。在临床和统计上理解交互作用都是必不可少的，并且交互作用无法通过单个双臂试验确定。析因设计可以考虑两个以上的因素，并且每个因素可以考虑两个以上的水平。图 20-9 显示了一个更复杂的 2×2×3 的析因设计的例子，药物 C 有三个剂量。每位患者的数据对分别估计 A、B、C 的主效应都有贡献，故不需要增加样本量。估计三阶交互效应的检验效能低于估计二阶交互效应的检验效能，但图 20-9 中析因设计的结果也会包含一些关于药物 A、B 和 C 的三阶交互作用的信息。

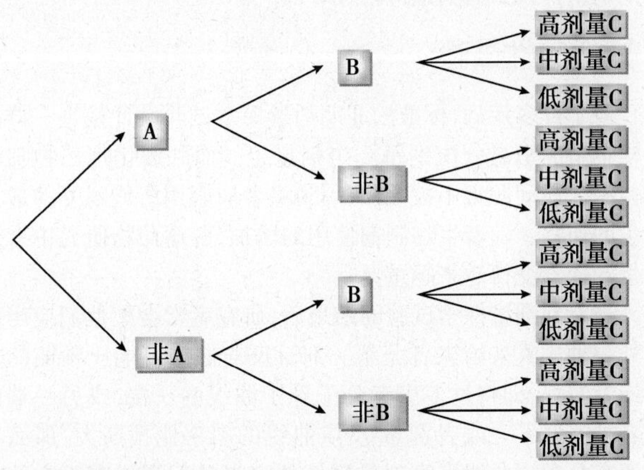

图 20-9　考虑药物 A、B 以及三个水平药物 C 的 2×2×3 析因设计及其组合。有 12 种可能的治疗组合

对于大型析因设计，一种修正的方案是采用适应性随机化方法，本章接下来的一节中将进行讨论。不同组合的疗效和毒性可以用非平衡分配予以研究，随着数据的累积将有希望得到某些有明显偏向的组合。如果不管联合使用或未使用其他药物，某种药物都是无效的，则放弃该药物。

在许多肿瘤药物的考虑上，毒性和疗效一样重要。析因设计有办法同时纳入两方面内容。例如，可以根据毒性建立容许组合(admissible combination)的概念，在试验开始时就只能允许全部因子组合的某些特定的组合。随着相关毒性经验的累积，其他的组合可以成为容许组合，或者原有的容许组合的数目减少。在设定的容许组合中，可以根据有关疗效的累积信息来随机地或适应性地将患者分配到不同的治疗组合中。

临床试验的适应性设计

本部分主要关注于一系列适应性或动态试验设计方法，即试验过程中所观察到的结果会影响到后续试验的进行。关注的重点是临床试验，但这种思想也可以应用到临床前研究中。

临床试验设计方法通常是静态的、固定的，即试验的样本量、给药方法以及随机化方案都要事先确定，试验过程中观察到的试验结果并不用于指导试验的进程。但亦有例外：一些肿瘤药物的Ⅱ期临床试验采用两阶段设计，当第一阶段分析结果显示药物已没有足够希望在试验结束得到有效结论时即终止该试验。此外，大部分的Ⅲ期临床试验也设计进行期中分析，以发现是否具有足够的证据揭示不同治疗组间的差异以提前结束试验。然而，传统的提前结束试验标准是非常保守的，以至于很少有试验能够提前结束。

静态试验设计以其简单的设计方法成为获得可靠的统计推断的手段。静态试验设计的样本量与本部分所要讨论的试验设计方法的样本量相比往往较大。此外，静态试验设计通常仅考虑两个治疗组从而可以直接进行组间比较。这也并不是说静态试验设计总能明确给出两组的优劣，而是说它通常能将哪一组更优的不确定度进行明确量化。尽管静态试验设计方法具有上述优点，但它往往会减缓药物研发的速度并增加不必要的费用。目前可供研发的肿瘤药物数量成指数级增长，所以一次仅关注一种药物而将其他无数药物放在一边等待评价的做法十分低效。制药企业和医学研究人员一般需要考虑同时研发数百种、甚至数千种药物，而静态试验设计方法阻碍了多种药物的同时研发进程。而且在同时研发多种药物时，静态试验设计方法不能有效地解决药物的剂量反应问题。因此，与药物研发过程紧密结合的动态试验设计方法成为医学研究合理发展的必然。适应性设计的使用要以调整试验设计为目的，对不断累积的试验数据进行定期或持续的监查，而调整的依据在于试验数据能否揭示未知检验假设。这些可能出现的调整包括提前结束试验、限制入组标准、增加试验研究中心或纳入特定亚组的患者、当试验结论不明确时增加样本量、舍去或增加一些组别/剂量等，而所有这些可能出现的调整则都依赖于已观察到的试验数据。同时，适应性设计还包括根据累积的试验数据进行不均衡的随机化调整，例如，对于能够更好地反映检验假设信息或疗效较好的组别，我们可以增大其样本量比例[36]。适应性调整不仅仅局限于利用本试验进行过程中所观察到的数据，其他正在进行的临床试验所报道的信息亦可加以利用。应用贝叶斯方法将使这些信息的利用更加方便，例如采用贝叶斯分层模型。

适应性设计已越来越多地应用于肿瘤药物临床试验中。不仅应用于制药企业所申办的临床试验,更多地也应用于一般的肿瘤临床试验。例如:美国得克萨斯大学 MD 安德森癌症研究中心(MD Anderson Cancer Center,MDACC)所展开的一系列临床试验均为前瞻适应性设计[37],下面给出常用的适用性设计实例。

Ⅰ期临床试验中连续再评估方法

肿瘤药物Ⅰ期临床试验的目的是确定最大耐受剂量(maximum-tolerated dose,MTD),Ⅰ期试验设计一般使用严格的、基于算法的加减设计(up-and-down design)或基于统计模型的适应性设计。3+3 设计的衍生方法[38]和加速滴定设计[39]是Ⅰ期试验中加减设计常用的两种形式。连续再评估方法(continual reassessment method,CRM)及其一系列变形是基于模型的剂量探索设计的具体形式。

3+3 设计的主要思想为:先入组 3 例患者,若 3 个患者中没有人发生毒性事件,则增加一个剂量水平再入组 3 例患者;若 3 个患者中有 2~3 例发生了毒性事件,则以目前剂量低一级的剂量水平作为 MTD,要求至少 6 例患者接受过该剂量水平。若 3 个患者中有 1 例发生了毒性事件,则在该剂量水平上再纳入 3 例患者,如果 6 名患者中 2 例或更多发生了毒性事件,则也以目前剂量低一级的至少 6 例患者使用过的剂量水平作为 MTD[40]。这种试验设计方法是适应性的,但其所做的调整是非常粗糙的。它倾向于将患者分到较低的剂量水平,并选择到无效的 MTD,并且下一剂量的选择只基于当前剂量的结果而忽略了该试验中其他剂量累积的信息。换句话说,该设计中剂量分配是短视的,没有以充分的统计推断为基础[41]。

CRM 及其衍生方法[42~44]使用了贝叶斯修正,它假定剂量和毒性之间存在某一特定的函数关系(如 logistic 函数关系)。将患者分配到与已指定目标毒性最为接近的剂量组,根据该时间点所累积数据计算得到的贝叶斯后验概率来衡量其接近程度。因此,CRM 设计是以充分的统计推断为基础的。CRM 的改进包括控制过量用药的剂量递增设计(escalation with overdose control design,EWOC)[45]以及贝叶斯模型平均连续再评估方法(Bayesian model averaging continual reassessment method,BMA-CRM)[46]。

与 3+3 设计相比,CRM 设计可以更有效地找到 MTD。尽管 CRM 类型的设计已成为 MD 安德森癌症中心Ⅰ期试验的首选设计,它在许多方面还在改进中。其中一个方面的改进是确定一个基本原则:忽略试验中任何信息都是错误的(当然,需要注意的是,分析利用信息是一项工作,且可能需要建模)。Ⅰ期临床试验中同样会累积一些药物的有效性信息,这些信息非常有限,尤其对建立剂量-效应关系而言。但是至少在进入Ⅱ期临床试验的某一特定剂量水平(通常为 MTD)上,可以利用药物在该剂量水平Ⅰ期临床试验中的有效性信息。这一观点促进了Ⅰ/Ⅱ期临床试验无缝连接设计的应用,这种设计可以同时考察药物的有效性和安全性,或者在重点关注药物的毒性之后继而转向有效性的评价。这一方法无论从缩短试验时间还是节省患者资源方面都非常高效。

3+3 和 CRM 的试验实施都不是最优的,因为研究者需要暂停患者入组以等待药物的毒性信息,这种暂停是非常低效率的,而且会导致逻辑问题。临床试验的暂停或者终止应当由于发生安全性问题,而非由于试验设计。在累积试验患者的毒性(或有效性)信息时,很少会有某一非预期的剂量水平是下一个患者必须要入组的,而且每一个剂量水平都有潜在的可能提供有用的信息。因此,应当利用一种根据前瞻性原则建立药物剂量-反应(包括毒性和有效性)关系模型的设计,或者使用 TITE-CRM 设计,他们能在前面患者没有得到充分评价时入组下一剂量组的患者[47~48],而不是暂停试验。当新药的毒性效应不是在给药后很快观察到而是在给药一段时间后才可观察到时,可采用其他设计,包括期望最大化 CRM(expectation-maximization CRM)[49]和数据增强 CRM(data augmentation CRM)[50]方法。基于模型选择的剂量探索设计也可用于评价联合药物试验[51~55]。

Ⅰ期试验设计的另一个限制,也是 3+3 和 CRM 设计的另外一个缺陷,是它们假定毒性事件是二分类的,且不考虑有效性。而更好的方法(同样是由于使用了所有可用信息)是在Ⅰ/Ⅱ阶段设计中同时考虑药物的毒性的严重程度和有效性[56~62]。

随着越来越多的生物制剂进行临床试验,剂量探索试验从确定 MTD(基于高毒性化疗药物的使用)转向为确定最佳生物剂量(optimal biological dose,OBD)。生物制剂在治疗剂量范围内预期有较低毒性,最佳剂量一般定义为靶向制剂具有最高有效率的最低安全剂量。目前已经有多种方法用于确定Ⅰ期剂量探索试验的 OBD[52,62~64]。读者可参阅 Braun[65]来全面了解Ⅰ期剂量探索试验的适应性设计。

Ⅱ期适应性试验

对于许多疾病,标准的Ⅱ期剂量探索试验设计是将一群固定样本量的患者分配到每一个剂量组。而肿瘤化疗药物临床试验中上述问题常不被关注,因为患者应服用所能耐受的最大剂量的药物。随着生物制剂使用的增加,肿瘤药物研究中有效剂量的探索变得越来越重要。

当看到剂量探索试验的结果后,研究者常会想他们应当用另外一种方式来给患者分组。剂量反应曲线可能比预期的左偏或者右偏,即将过多患者分配到了曲线的一端,或另一端的患者被浪费了。或者剂量-反应曲线的斜率比预期大,那么若把原来分配到曲线平直剂量区域的患者分配到斜率很大的剂量区域就会获得更多信息。或者早期患者的试验结果已经清楚表明剂量反应曲线整个范围内都很平直,那完全可以提前结束试验。又或者试验中主要观察指标的标准差比预期值大(或者小),则应增大(或减小)试验的样本量。

Ⅱ期研究的序贯设计已用于评估在特定剂量范围内的新疗法的疗效。当研究者做出决定,认为药物没有足够的疗效,不需进一步的试验,或者已选出最优剂量进行Ⅲ期确证性试验时,剂量探索即可终止。早期的单臂设计使用两个阶段来达到预定的有效率,同时控制Ⅰ类和Ⅱ类错误[66,67]。有研究提出了包含有效性和/或无效终止规则的针对二分类结局的贝叶斯适应性试验设计方法[68]。Berry 等人进行了随着试验数据的不断积累,序贯地开展试验和分析数据(参见其他方法[70,71])的Ⅱ期设计,并通过预测概率早期有效终止试验[72]。关于成组序贯设计可参见 Jennison 和 Turnbull 的相关著作[73]。

Berry 等[69]以某一治疗脑卒中的生物神经保护剂临床试验为例对该方法进行了阐述，该方法也可用于肿瘤研究。根据目前已观察结果，将每个进入试验的患者分配至 16 个剂量组(包括安慰剂组)中的一个，以最大限度地获取药物剂量反应关系信息。这个被分配的剂量组可能在剂量反应曲线上斜率最大的区域，也可能是安慰剂组或高剂量组。但随着信息积累，若已证明某剂量组剂量反应曲线平直，则之后新入组病例不会被分配到该剂量组。

在剂量探索试验阶段，总样本量和每个剂量组的样本量事先都不确定。当数据显示该药物可使患者中度获益、剂量反应曲线轻度倾斜或者数据的标准差比较大时，剂量探索试验的样本量会比较大。而当数据显示该药物可以使患者获益较大或根本无法获益、剂量反应曲线在较窄的剂量范围内上升或者数据的标准差较小时，剂量探索试验的样本量一般会较小。另外，当数据的标准差非常大时，剂量探索试验的样本量往往会比较小。这是因为非常大的标准差意味着试验需要非常大的样本量来确证药物的疗效，而如此大的样本量在药物研发中往往是不太可能的，所以只能在试验的剂量探索阶段即停止试验以免造成巨大的资源浪费。

Berry 等的脑卒中临床试验[69]，其终点疗效指标是服药 13 周脑卒中量表得分相对基线的变化。如果患者的入组速度较快，而得到终点疗效指标又存在时间上的滞后，那适应性分组的优点就不能完全发挥(注：可以找到优化入组速度和疗效指标评估时间的“最佳点”[74])。为了使试验终点疗效指标评价滞后的影响最小化，从基线到服药 13 周，研究者每周都对患者进行脑卒中量表评价。考虑到每个患者在不同时间点的观察结果具有相关性，且观察时间点越接近，相关系数越大，研究者建立纵向模型，根据患者当前的观察信息对其终点疗效指标进行贝叶斯预测，并据此对药物治疗效果的概率分布进行调整。

与剂量探索试验的标准设计方法相比，适应性剂量探索方法可以更有效地确定有效剂量组，并节约样本量。此外，还可以在一个试验中考虑多个剂量组，即使一些剂量组在试验过程中很少、甚至不会被用到。因此，适应性剂量探索方法具有区分邻近剂量组的疗效、估计剂量反应曲线中细微差别的能力。

该脑卒中临床试验的情形与其他许多临床试验都非常相似。寻找药物的有效剂量是药物研发中的普遍问题，但却很少能被很好或高效地完成。在脑卒中试验中，如果没有观察试验的早期疗效指标，则该试验适应性设计的优势就会大打折扣。同样，在肿瘤药物的临床试验中，在观察到试验的主要疗效指标之前，研究者可以对试验早期可利用的信息(如疾病的局部控制、生物标记物等)进行评价。此外，贝叶斯适应性设计可用于在Ⅱ期临床试验中筛选联合治疗方案，通过将选择过程转化为贝叶斯假设检验问题，利用当前的后验概率适应性地将患者分配到联合治疗组中[75]。最后，许多类型的药物都有可能从Ⅰ期试验无缝地连接到Ⅱ期或从Ⅱ期无缝地连接到Ⅲ期。这也是下一部分要讲的内容。

Ⅰ/Ⅱ期和Ⅱ/Ⅲ期临床试验无缝连接设计

将药物研发设置成不同阶段是有问题的。我们认定了某个试验阶段的结果之后，再进入下一阶段，例如在Ⅰ期临床试验得到 MTD，或者按Ⅱ期临床试验的剂量治疗的终点疗效会转变为Ⅲ期试验的临床获益。与此相反的是，贝叶斯方法认为不可能确切地获知某一个量，无论有多少可利用的信息，这种不确定性是一直存在的。药物研发过程是一个持续的过程，而对药物研发过程的阶段划分是非常武断的。

将药物研发过程划分成不同阶段的一个后果是阶段之间的停顿导致药物研发周期的延长。例如，在Ⅱ期和Ⅲ期临床试验之间需要暂停以启动一个或多个关键性研究。而上述脑卒中临床试验在设计上则避免了这样的间断，它在每一个时间点(一般为每周)，根据一定的算法进行决策分析，从而建议试验选择：①继续剂量探索阶段试验；②因缺乏疗效而结束试验(剂量-反应曲线斜率不足，或者更准确地说，剂量-反应呈阳性的证据不足以证明继续试验的合理性)；③转向确证性试验阶段。而试验转向Ⅲ期临床试验阶段是无缝连接的，患者的入组不会中断。甚至从理论上讲，它可以在双盲临床试验中不必告知研究者直接转向Ⅲ期确证性试验阶段，即研究者只是继续随机入组患者，而不知道组别已经变为了Ⅲ期剂量组和安慰剂组。

许多试验设计都同时包括Ⅰ期和Ⅱ期试验[37,57~61,64,76~80]，在试验中对药物有效性和毒性进行考察。试验中只可应用准许的剂量组或不同剂量组的联合，并随着剂量组的不断被准许，剂量水平不断提高。同时，这些设计也考察药物的剂量毒性关系和剂量疗效关系。

旨在同时包含Ⅱ和Ⅲ期的试验设计使用的是从Ⅱ期无缝转换到Ⅲ期试验[81~85]。无缝连接是指：患者入组试验，可以将其视为Ⅱ期；若累积的数据强烈表明药物/治疗对局部控制或生存没有效果，则结束试验；若数据结果显示该药物可能对局部控制产生一定作用，且这种作用可转化为生存获益，则试验将会扩大，入组速度也将相应提高。在试验扩大过程中，在其他中心准备加入试验时，初始中心持续入组患者以保证当地的患者入组不出现中断。由于早期入组患者数据也将用于计算生存率，因此该方法可以高效的利用患者资源；且由于拥有最长的随访期，这些患者也是所有入组患者中信息量最为丰富的。

该试验继续进行直到发生以下情况之一时停止：①根据预测概率判定继续进行试验也是无用的；②达到了试验的最大样本量；③最终得到有统计学意义的预测概率足够大。当第 3 种情况发生时，试验停止入组，制药企业可以为进一步药品上市做准备。

例如，预期情况下，传统Ⅲ期临床试验样本量为 900 例。这也是无缝连接设计的最大样本量。实际入组病例数很可能远远小于这个样本量，特别是当试验结果非常有前景或根本没有前景时。相比较而言，相同期中分析次数且使用传统终止试验规则的传统Ⅲ期临床试验的样本量也只是稍微少一点。贝叶斯设计有时候会需要相对较大的样本量(接近于 900 例)，但这种设计的好处在于只有在必需的时候才需要大的样本量。传统临床试验可能在完成预设样本量的试验后仍只得出含糊不清的结论，而贝叶斯设计则可以选择继续进行试验以解决这一问题(从最大样本量角度来讲这一问题，也许在完成 900 例患者结束试验时仍无法得到任何结论，但是从逻辑上来讲，还是要事先指定一个最大样本量)。在无缝适应性设计中，可以利用试验中积累的数据重新估计样本量，从而减小样本量[86~90]。

传统的药物研发策略包括开展Ⅰ期试验以确定MTD，然后在此基础上进行Ⅱ期临床试验以评价疾病的局部控制；如果评价结果为阳性，则开展以生存率为主要疗效指标的Ⅲ期临床试验。与传统策略相比，无缝连接方法大幅度减小样本量，并最大限度地减少了阶段之间的中断时间，从而大大缩短了药物研发的整体时间。

适应性随机化

到目前为止，讨论适应性设计的目的是希望尽可能快速高效的完成试验。另一种适应性设计的目的是尽可能高效地完成受试者分配。适应性随机化包括两种主要方法：协变量调整适应性随机化（covariate-adjusted adaptive randomization）和结果-适应性随机化（outcome-adaptive randomization）。协变量调整适应性随机化方案可根据与预后相关的特定特征的基线测量（预后标记物）给患者分配治疗组，这样均衡了不同治疗组间的重要因素[91,92]。相反，结果-适应性随机化方案根据已经参加试验的患者对治疗的反应给患者分配治疗组，该方案倾向于将更多的患者分配到治疗效果较好的组中[93,94]。结果-适应性随机化增加了更多患者接受更有效治疗的可能性，这种策略有利于参与试验的个体，增强了试验的"个体伦理"[95]。另外，均衡设计的随机化最大限度地提高了统计效能，强调试验的"群体"或"集体伦理"，目的是从试验中确定有效的治疗方法，从而为后面患者群体带来益处。除了可以吸引更多的患者参与临床试验外，结果-适应性随机化策略还具有高效、快速得出结论的重要优点。

适应性随机化的目的是随着试验的进行和结果的积累，不断增大患者分配到试验结果较好组的概率权重。还可以考虑采用其他的分配算法，如贝叶斯概率成正比分配算法。很多试验设置了两个以上的治疗组，这些组间可能是完全不相关的，也可能是密切相关的。例如，一项在接受骨髓移植的白血病患者中，确定一种抑制急性排斥反应（GVHD）的附加预防制剂的剂量[96]。该试验评价了在标准预防用药基础上加上5个喷司他丁剂量组（包括零剂量组）的效果。而问题在于不同剂量水平的药物有可能影响到移植器官的成功移植，从而影响到患者的存活，且这种抑制作用可能与剂量有关试验采用了联合终点指标：100天内无排斥反应存活时间。移植器官的移植成功和无排斥反应的分歧意味着试验的剂量-反应曲线并不一定是单调的，即曲线有可能在小剂量时上升，然后随着剂量的增加而下降。起初可以逐渐、缓慢增大剂量水平来分配患者，但当剂量水平都成为可容许剂量时，更多的患者将会被分配到疗效较好的剂量组。

假定一位患者符合该临床试验的入组标准。可根据当前试验结果所积累的信息计算该患者分配到每一个可容许剂量组优于安慰剂组的贝叶斯概率，以决定该患者被分配到哪一个剂量组。患者被随机分配到每一个剂量组，但其分配到每一组的权重与所计算的贝叶斯概率成正比。疗效很差的剂量组将不会被分入，也就是说分入该剂量组的权重变为了0。当发现试验药物有效时，试验结束；当发现试验药物无效时，试验也同样结束。试验中患者从已累积的试验数据中获益，其目的不仅是为了使患者获得更好的治疗，还可以使试验更有效、快速地得出结论。每一种试验设计方法的频率学论中的特征可以通过蒙特卡罗模拟试验的方法进行估计，并通过对分配算法中的参数调整满足试验期望的操作特征。

结果-适应性随机化可以在频率学或贝叶斯框架下构建。采用频率学方法获得各种标准下的最佳随机概率[97,98]，且在患者分配时可用期中数据来估计反应率[99]。"双重适应性偏币"设计[100,101]拓展了这个方法，该设计通过综合考虑已分配给各组患者的比例和当前期望的分配比例，从而计算出实现具有较小变异的最佳设计的随机概率。

最直观的方法是标准贝叶斯适应性随机化，当 $\Phi_1=\text{Prob}(\theta_1>\theta_2)$，将患者分配到组1，其中 $\theta_i(i=1,2)$ 表示随机化时 p_i 的后验概率。该方法通过使用幂变换进行了扩展，$\Phi_1=Prob(\theta_1>\theta_2)^c/(Prob(\theta_1>\theta_2)^c+Prob(\theta_1<\theta_2)^c)$，其中 $c=n/(2N)$，n 是当前入组的患者数量，N 是试验中的最大患者数量，目的是降低随机概率的变异性[102]。因此，随机化概率在试验开始时约为0.5，随着数据的累积而改变，尤其是当数据显示治疗组间的反应率有很大差异时。随机化概率可以限制在0.5左右，以减小其变异性。其他方案使用治疗效果的后验平均值（或中位数）来确定随机化概率：$\Phi_1=\hat{\theta}_1/(\hat{\theta}_1+\hat{\theta}_2)$，其中 $\hat{\theta}_i$ 是 $i=1,2$ 时 θ_i 的后验平均值（或中位数）[103,104]。

可以设计一个临床试验，从一个等概率的随机方案开始，然后在观察到患者对治疗效果的反应后再过渡到一个适应性随机方案。适应性随机化策略可与基于预测概率的无效性和/或有效性的早期停止规则相结合。这种形式使药物研发过程合理化。①试验开始时，由于疗效信息不多，采用等概率随机化。②在累积了适量的数据后，可以切换到适应性随机化，在现有数据的基础上，将更多的患者分配到疗效较好的组别。③继续入组患者至最大样本量，但允许进行期中监察，以便在有足够证据推断治疗效果时尽早停止试验。这样灵活的试验形式是贝叶斯适应性临床试验设计的优点[105]。

使用适应性随机化评价多个治疗方法，需要试验统计学家仔细审查人群的变动情况，以防止不同治疗的有偏比较。这是在使用倾向于将更多的患者分配给疗效较好的治疗组的适应性随机化方案时应当注意的问题，因为该方案可能导致治疗组间的患者特征不均衡[106]。可以通过确定对照组的最小随机分配概率来控制各组的随机分配比例，从而在一定程度上控制研究出现人群的不均衡。大量的分配人群的变动会使研究的推断不合理，当治疗组间的预后协变量不均衡时，可以通过回归分析来解决。Marchenko等人提出了监测适应性试验的建议[107]。

将结果-适应性随机化策略纳入临床试验的优缺点已经引发了大量的讨论，且可能取决于应用该策略的具体情况。在二分类终点的双臂试验中首选等概率随机化，因为它更容易实现、样本量少且无应答者少[106]。最近一项结果-适应性随机化的分析质疑了在双臂试验中使用这种策略的伦理学问题[108]。当不同治疗组的效应之间存在较大差异时，适应性随机化策略可以提高患者反应率，并获得较好的统计检验效能[109]。在试验设计中加入早期终止规则将在一定程度上降低这一优势。与等概率随机化策略相比，适应性随机化策略在评价罕见疾病的试验中可能更有优势。在一个多组多阶段的研究中，特别是其中一种治疗方式较其他组更有效时，适应性随机化将更加适合[69,104,109]。

外延分析

临床试验结束时不能得出明确的结论是比较常见的。例如,药物注册时要求试验主要疗效指标的统计检验水准为 5%,而实际得到的 P 值为 6%,药监部门认为该试验的检验效能不够,建议重新展开一项临床试验。此时,在现有试验的基础上增加样本量可以是更为有效的办法(扩充试验),但这样做会导致试验的Ⅰ类错误增大,其道理与期中分析相同。

要解决这一问题的策略是在方案设计阶段就应考虑到根据试验结果进一步继续试验的可能性,从而对检验水准做适当调整。与期中分析中检验水准的调整相比,外延分析(extraim analysis)中检验水准的调整是反向的,它需要把总检验水准的大部分分配到原来计划好样本量的试验上。例如,在每一个可能的时点取相同检验水准的方法要比 O' Brein-Fleming 设计更合适,这是因为后者在外延分析中太过保守。扩充试验将会导致试验的最大样本量和平均样本量的增加,但是适度的增加平均样本量(如 20%)可以大幅度的提高试验的检验效能(从 80%提高到 95%),因此,只有当扩充试验是值得做的,才会考虑进行试验。

在这种设计中,对试验检验水准的"惩罚"可以用将无效分析作为设计的一部分来部分或全部的抵消。也就是说,在所设定期中分析时间点,试验可以由于阴性结果的证据充足而结束。因为试验因无效而结束时,不会拒绝原假设,所以无效分析可以抵消因外延分析带来的检验水准的惩罚。增补样本量的多少取决于在做出继续试验的决定时现有的数据信息,以及外延分析的次数。在所设计的试验中,根据预测效能来设计每一次的外延。通常对效能的定义会假定取特定参数值 r,而预测效能会考虑到 r 的所有可能取值。用于外延分析的数据起到两个作用:一是用于试验的最终结果分析,二是用于调整 r 的贝叶斯概率分布。给定样本量 n,计算 r 每一个可能取值下的效能,并对依据不同 r 的概率分布条件下的效能求平均,从而得到在给定样本量 n 时的预测效能。这样做能够确保在额外入组适量病例使总样本量达到 n 的情况下,试验的预测效能仍能达到预定值。如果试验没有设定最终的总样本量 n 时,这样的继续试验将不可取。

因部分终点信息暂无法获得而终止试验是大可不必的。某些与主要疗效指标相关的早期信息(如生物标记物、功能状态等)则可以为主要疗效指标的预测提供信息。凡是可以通过完整、精确描述的过程,都可以被模拟。模拟试验的一个优点是每次迭代重复,它都可以提供完全入组的试验数据,据此可以计算试验设计的各种特征,包括检验效能、实际样本量和外延试验的可能性等。

贝叶斯框架非常适合于整合试验外部的信息以进行推断。例如,可以采用分层相称先验和效能先验将历史信息自适应地整合入临床试验[110,111]。类似疗法或器械的历史数据可在许多研究中轻松获取。有效和适当地使用历史信息来加强对新试验的推断已在医疗器械的发展中证实[112]。

过程还是试验? 在有无适应性分配的平台试验中同时评价多种药物

在药物研发过程中最大的创新是对大量具有潜在研发能力的药物进行有效的处理。一次研发一种药物的观点正在改变。是否能够同时和有效地对多种药物进行筛选成为一个制药企业生存的重要条件。

基于平台的临床试验设计是开发新药和疗法过程中的一个创新[113,114]。平台设计是针对特定疾病而不是针对某个临床方案的操作和统计框架。可将每种新的药物或疗法视为一个"模块",可以从特定的疾病"平台"中进入和退出。可以同时筛选多种新的疗法,它是替代多个独立Ⅱ期试验来评价多个治疗组的方法。贝叶斯建模和随机化的方法可以方便地融入平台设计中,并且平台设计比多个单独的试验更有效。一旦在Ⅰ期试验中确定了新药的合适剂量,就可以将该新药添加到该平台中。如果筛选过程中累积的数据表明某药物没有产生预期的结果,则还可以将其从平台中剔除。从平台剔除的药物可以返回到Ⅰ期研究中,以重新确定最佳治疗剂量或剂量方案。如果该Ⅰ期试验确定的变化后的剂量可能是有益的,则之前从平台除去的药物可以重新进入筛选过程。

基于平台的设计为筛选试验的开展带来了重要的统计学挑战。贝叶斯后验分布和预测概率需要集约计算;但是,在计算预测概率之后,可以为平台设计的持续监测指定边界。在保持预定的Ⅰ类错误率的同时,必须正确实施序贯适应性策略以监测大部分试验药物的无效性。平台设计是基于在试验获得成功的后验预测概率建立无效终止规则。该设计使用贝叶斯模型来解释模型参数的期中估计所产生的不确定性,并使用模拟来校正设计参数。贝叶斯模型还用于解释试验中未来患者的治疗反应的变异性。

许多关于多臂/或多阶段试验设计的研究包含类似的提高药物开发效率的策略[115~119]。Berry[120]讨论了基于平台的设计和相关的主方案、伞式试验(umbrella trial)和篮式试验(basket trial),特别适用于生物标记物研究。基于平台的设计具有潜在的优势,包括减少治疗筛选过程的总时间;大幅减少分配给对照组的患者数量;增加可筛选的治疗方法的数量,从而扩展了试验中患者可用的治疗方案;减少因不同独立试验间的异质性所产生的偏倚;改善对内在多重性的控制;更好地为后续确证性试验的决策提供信息。

统计学新方法在临床肿瘤试验的应用

该部分简述两项应用统计学新方法的肿瘤临床试验:"整合生物标记物的肺癌消除靶向治疗方法"(biomarker-integrated approaches of targeted therapy of lung cancer elimination, BATTLE)以及"通过影像和分子分析预测治疗效果的系列研究"(Investigation of serial studies to predict your therapeutic response with imaging and molecular analysis, I-SPY2)试验。BATTLE 试验[121,122]评价了Ⅳ期复发性非小细胞肺癌患者中 4 种靶向治疗的效果,根据患者的生物标记物特点(包括基因表达、基因突变、拷贝数和免疫组化测定的蛋白质含量)从四种靶向治疗方式中选择一个最合适的。终点指标是 8 周疾病控制率。该试验采用了结果-适应性随机化和基于 probit 分层模型的无效性终止规则。当生物标记物特征表明患者不会从某药物中获益时,按照终止规则,将该药物从特定患者的随机化分配中排除。BATTLE-2 试验使用第一次试验的结果筛查 10~15 个候选生物标记物。它将适应性随机化融入两阶段设计,以评估非小细胞肺癌的四种治疗方法。该试验是一个包括训练、测试和验证的过程,以选择最佳的生物标记物。该设计采用了分组 lasso 和适应性 lasso 方法来识别预后和预测标记物[123,124]。

多中心 I-SPY2 试验[125]在每个基于生物标记物的患者组内采用适应性随机化,并使用无效或有效终止规则。I-SPY2 试验评价了乳腺癌中新辅助治疗同多达 12 种试验药物联用的效果[126]。该试验随机分组了 700 多名患者,将两种试验药物转化入确诊性研究阶段,并成功证明了这种适应性试验设计可以降低药物开发成本,提高新药筛选效率[125~127]。

临床试验软件

我们可以从网上获取许多用于设计和实施临床试验的软件,其中包括专利产品和免费产品[128]。在 MD 安德森软件下载站点可以找到许多有用的创新试验设计、实施和分析的软件程序(https://biostatistics.mdanderson.org/SoftwareDownload/)。用于 I 期剂量探索试验中 CRM[129]的软件包括 CRM 模拟器、BMA-CRM 和 TITE-CRM。CRM 模拟器使用毒性先验信息选择最佳剂量水平,并允许用户改变参数直到达到期望的输出。BMA-CRM[46]通过设置多组毒性反应先验信息的概率来选择最佳剂量。针对 TITE-CRM[48]开发的软件当延迟毒性反应存在时仍可确定最佳剂量。

在肿瘤剂量探索试验中,用于确定剂量的 EWOC 方法[45,130]的软件使用了适应性学习。同 CRM 法相比,该方法可让更少的患者接受亚治疗或严重毒性反应剂量,使更多患者使用的剂量接近 MTD,并且所估计的剂量的平均偏差和均方误差较低。另一种方法使用修正后的毒性后验区间(mTPI)和贝叶斯决策理论来确定肿瘤药物的最佳剂量[131]。

另外一种可以降低患者接受亚治疗或过度毒性剂量可能性的方法是贝叶斯最优区间(BOIN)设计[132]。在 I 期临床试验中,R 函数(BOIN.r)通过计算最优概率区间来确定 MTD,优化每个参加试验的患者的剂量分配。当指定设计参数后,BOIN 设计使用了一种算法,与传统 3+3 设计的实施类似。在确定 MTD 方面,BOIN 设计与 CRM 类似,但 BOIN 设计将患者分配到亚治疗或过度毒性剂量的风险要低得多。

预测概率设计[72]可以根据设定的 I 型和 II 类错误率确定预测概率的截断值和计算连续试验监测所需的终止界限。BFDesigner[133]可用于建立有效的终止规则。在采用适应性设计时可用的其他计算工具有参数求解器,它可在给定随机变量的两个分位数或均数和方差时计算该随机变量的分布参数;还有针对终点指标为二分类的双臂试验的计算工具预测概率,它能够计算一组疗效优于另一组疗效或因为无效终止的后验预测概率[16]。随着越来越多的软件用于设计和实施创新临床试验,统计学新方法从理论转化到实际应用的速度也会越来越快。

致谢

感谢癌症和白血病 B 组允许使用来自 CALGB 8541 和 LeeAnn Chastain 的数据。这项工作得到了国家癌症研究所的基金(CA016672)的部分支持。

(贺佳 郭晓晶 姚晨 刘玉秀 夏结来 王彤 秦婴逸 张新佶 许金芳 何倩 王睿 韩贺东 刘曼 谭紫雯 译、校)

部分参考文献

12 Berry DA. Introduction to Bayesian methods III: use and interpretation of Bayesian tools in design and analysis. *Clin Trials*. 2005;**2**:295–300.

13 Berry DA. Bayesian clinical trials. *Nat Rev Drug Discov*. 2006;**5**:27–36.

14 Lee JJ, Chu CT. Bayesian clinical trials in action. *Stat Med*. 2012;**31**:2955–2972.

15 Speigelhalter DJ, Abrams KR, Myles JP. *Bayesian Approaches to Clinical Trials and Healthcare Evaluation*. Chichester, UK: John Wiley & Sons, Ltd; 2004.

16 Berry SM, Carlin BP, Lee JJ, Muller P. *Bayesian Adaptive Methods for Clinical Trials*. Boca Raton: Chapman and Hall/CRC Press; 2010.

31 Ventz S, Trippa L. Bayesian designs and the control of frequentist characteristics: a practical solution. *Biometrics*. 2015;**71**:218–226.

33 Simon R, Freedman LS. Bayesian design and analysis of two x two factorial clinical trials. *Biometrics*. 1997;**53**:456–464.

37 Biswas S, Liu DD, Lee JJ, Berry DA. Bayesian clinical trials at the University of Texas MD Anderson Cancer Center. *Clin Trial*. 2009;**6**:205–216.

46 Yin G, Yuan Y. Bayesian model averaging continual reassessment method in phase I clinical trials. *J Am Stat Assoc*. 2009;**104**:954–968.

48 Cheung YK, Chappell R. Sequential designs for phase I clinical trials with late-on-set toxicities. *Biometrics*. 2000;**56**:1177–1182.

52 Mandrekar SJ, Cui Y, Sargent DJ. An adaptive phase I design for identifying a biologically optimal dose for dual agent drug combinations. *Stat Med*. 2007;**26**:2317–2330.

59 Zhang W, Sargent DJ, Mandrekar SJ. An adaptive dose-finding design incorporating both toxicity and efficacy. *Stat Med*. 2006;**25**:2365–2383.

62 Zang Y, Lee JJ, Yuan Y. Adaptive designs for identifying optimal biological dose for molecularly targeted agents. *Clin Trials*. 2014;**11**:319–327.

64 Hoering A, LeBlanc M, Crowley J. Seamless phase I-II trial design for assessing toxicity and efficacy for targeted agents. *Clin Cancer Res*. 2011;**17**:640–646.

65 Braun TM. The current design of oncology phase I clinical trials: progressing from algorithms to statistical models. *Chin Clin Oncol*. 2014;**3**:1.

69 Berry DA, Mueller P, Grieve AP, et al. Adaptive Bayesian designs for dose-ranging drug trials. In: Gatsonis C, Carlin B, Carriquiry A, eds. *Case Studies in Bayesian Statistics V*. New York, NY: Springer-Verlag; 2001:99–181.

72 Lee JJ, Liu DD. A predictive probability design for phase II cancer clinical trials. *Clin Trials*. 2008;**5**:93–106.

74 Gajewski BJ, Berry SM, Quintana M, et al. Building efficient comparative effectiveness trials through adaptive designs, utility functions, and accrual rate optimization: finding the sweet spot. *Stat Med*. 2015;**34**:1134–1149.

75 Cai C, Yuan V, Johnson VE. Bayesian adaptive phase II screening design for combination trials. *Clin Trials*. 2013;**10**:353–362.

78 Yin G, Li Y, Ji Y. Bayesian dose-finding in phase I/II trials using toxicity and efficacy odds ratio. *Biometrics*. 2006;**62**:777–784.

79 Huang X, Biswas S, Oki Y, et al. A parallel phase I/II clinical trial design for combination therapies. *Biometrics*. 2007;**63**:429–436.

80 Yuan Y, Yin G. Bayesian phase I/II drug-combination trial design in oncology. *Ann Appl Stat*. 2011;**5**:924–942.

81 Inoue LYT, Thall P, Berry DA. Seamlessly expanding a randomized phase II trial to phase III. *Biometrics*. 2002;**58**:264–272.

97 Hu F, Rosenberger W. Optimality, variability, power: evaluating response-adaptive randomization procedures for treatment comparisons. *J Am Stat Assoc*. 2003;**98**:671–678.

102 Thall PF, Wathen KJ. Practical Bayesian adaptive randomisation in clinical trials. *Eur J Cancer*. 2007;**43**:859–866.

103 Lee JJ, Gu X, Liu S. Bayesian adaptive randomization designs for targeted agent development. *Clin Trials*. 2010;**7**:584–597.

105 Yin G, Chen N, Lee JJ. Phase II trial design with Bayesian adaptive randomization and predictive probability. *J R Stat Soc: Ser C: Appl Stat*. 2012;**61**:219–235.

107 Marchenko O, Fedorov V, Lee JJ, Nolan C, Pinheiro J. Adaptive clinical trials: overview of early-phase designs and challenges. *Ther Innov Regul Sci*. 2014;**48**:20–30.

108 Hey SP, Kimmelman J. Are outcome-adaptive allocation trials ethical? *Clin Trials*. 2015;**12**:102–106.

109 Lee JJ, Chen N, Yin G. Worth adapting? Revisiting the usefulness of outcome-adaptive randomization. *Clin Cancer Res*. 2012;**18**:4498–4507.

110 Hobbs BP, Carlin BP, Mandrekar SJ, Sargent DJ. Hierarchical commensurate and power prior models for adaptive incorporation of historical information in clinical trials. *Biometrics*. 2011;**67**:1047–1056.

112 Campbell G. Bayesian statistics in medical devices: innovation sparked by the FDA. *J Biopharm Stat*. 2011;**21**:871–887.

117 Wason JMS, Jaki T. Optimal design of multi-arm multi-stage trials. *Stat Med*. 2012;**31**:4269–4279.

118 Wason JM, Trippa L. A comparison of Bayesian adaptive randomization and multi-stage designs for multi-arm clinical trials. *Stat Med*. 2014;**33(13)**:2206–2221.

119 Parmar MKB, Carpenter J, Sydes MR. More multiarm randomised trials of superiority are needed. *Lancet*. 2014;**384**:283–284.
120 Berry DA. The brave new world of clinical cancer research: adaptive biomarker-driven trials integrating clinical practice with clinical research. *Mol Oncol*. 2015;**9**:951–959.
121 Zhou X, Liu S, Kim ES, et al. Bayesian adaptive design for targeted therapy development in lung cancer—a step toward personalized medicine. *Clin Trial*. 2008;5:181–193.
122 Kim ES, Herbst RS, Wistuba II, et al. The BATTLE trial: personalizing therapy for lung cancer. *Cancer Discov*. 2011;**1**:44–53.
124 Gu X, Chen N, Wei C, et al. Bayesian two-stage biomarker-based adaptive design for targeted therapy development. *Stat Biosci* 2015. http://link.springer.com/article/10.1007/s12561-014-9124-2.
127 Quantum Leap. *I-SPY 2 Breast Cancer Clinical Trial Graduates Two Promising Drugs*. 2013. Available at: http://www.quantumleaphealth.org/spy-2-trial-graduates-2-new-drugs-press-release/ (accessed 17 July 2015).
128 Lee JJ, Chen N. Software for design and analysis of clinical trials. In: Crowley J, Hoering A, eds. *Handbook of Statistics in Clinical Oncology*, 3rd ed. Boca Raton, FL: Chapman & Hall/CRC Press; 2012:305–324.
132 Liu S, Yuan Y. Bayesian optimal interval designs for phase I clinical trials. *J R Stat Soc: Ser C: Appl Stat*. 2015;**64**:507–523.

第 21 章　基因组医学时代基于生物标志物的临床试验设计

Richard Simon, DSc ■ Martine Piccart-Gebhart, MD, PhD

概述

人们日益认识到癌症的分子异质性，同时越来越多的强大工具描绘出了这种异质性的"分子画像"，这就要求开发新的研究范式，为"个性化"医学的发展提供可靠的基础。我们对临床试验设计和分析的新方法进行回顾，以便在开发"靶向性"的治疗和诊断方法中应用。

引言：为什么我们需要新的生物标志物驱动的临床试验设计和分析范式

随机临床试验使可靠的循证医学得以发展。通常是对一种相对于对照方案的治疗方案进行评估，受试患者群体是根据原发部位、组织学、分期和既往治疗的次数大致确定的。近年来，人类肿瘤 DNA 测序已经证实，原发部位的癌症往往由一组具有高度异质性的病灶组成，导致这些病灶发生和侵袭的基因组变异不同[1]。肿瘤的驱动基因和通路往往是异质性的，可以通过不同的分子靶向治疗。普适性的临床试验难以筛选出对新药效果最好的肿瘤患者亚组。在普适性临床试验中，由于样本量已经增加到即使平均治疗效果改善程度很小，也能获得统计上的显著性差异，只有一小部分受试者实际上从治疗中获益，而对没有受益的患者产生毒性，并且过度治疗为该类人群带来巨大的社会经济负担。

今天，我们有强大的工具能够从生物学的角度表征肿瘤，并利用这种特征来前瞻性构建设计和分析信息更丰富的临床试验，从而为接受治疗的患者带来更好的治疗效果。在这一章中，我们讨论这些现代设计和分析，更好地满足"个性化"肿瘤学的需要。

结合辅助诊断的分子靶向药物的Ⅱ期临床试验

目前，大多数抗癌药物都是针对特定的分子靶点开发的。在某些情况下，这些靶点已经被很好地研究和理解，并且有令人信服的生物学基础和来自Ⅰ期临床试验的证据，后续开发将锁定具有该药物靶标异常的患者亚组。对于其他一些药物，有多个靶点，并且难以确定某个药物靶点是否驱动特定患者的肿瘤生物学特征[2]。

在前一种情况下，理想和稳妥的方法是和药物一起共同开发可以检测药靶异常的伴随诊断方法。

在分子肿瘤学时代，Ⅱ期临床试验不仅必须确定该药物在特定组织学类型肿瘤治疗中是否总体上有效，而且还必须确定后续Ⅲ期临床试验是否会受限于候选的伴随诊断。Freidlin 等人[3]描述了单一候选生物标志物用于随机Ⅱ期临床试验的设计。该设计使人们能够确定该药物是否应该：①在Ⅲ期富集试验中开发，②在对所有受试者进行分层的试验分析中开发，③在不检测生物标志物的情况下在所有受试者试验中开发，或④不再进一步开发。该设计见图 21-1。通过确定样本量，使得在 0.10 的单侧显著性水平下，标志物阳性亚组的中位无进展生存期(PFS)翻倍的治疗效果的检出效率为 0.9。这通常会需要至少同样的样本量来评估标志物阴性亚组的治疗效果。如果标志物阳性亚组治疗效果不显著，则在单侧 0.05 显著性水平下，检测整体治疗效果。如果该治疗效果在统计学上不显著，则不推荐该药物用于Ⅲ期开发。如果整体治疗效果显著，则建议采用传统的Ⅲ期试验，不测量候选生物标志物。如果标志物阳性亚组的治疗效果是显著的，则检查标志物阴性亚组治疗效果的危险比的 80% 置信区间。如果置信区间上限低于 1.3，则说明该治疗在标志物阴性患者中效果不明显，建议进行富集Ⅲ期临床试验。如果置信下限高于 1.5，则认为该治疗在标志物阴性患者中效果良好，并推荐使用传统的Ⅲ期试验，在Ⅲ期试验中甚至可以不测量生物标志物。否则，建议进行生物标志物分层Ⅲ期试验。

Pusztai 和 Hess[4]以及 Jones 和 holmgren[5]报道了用于评估单臂Ⅱ期研究中标志物亚组内治疗效果的Ⅱ期临床试验设计。这些设计主要为了确保不会错过只在测试阳性患者中才会表现出活性的药物，并且在药物活性足够广泛以至于不需要标志物分层的情况下，过多的患者数量是不需要的。

还有更为复杂的Ⅱ期临床试验设置，即事先不知道生物标志物的阈值，或存在多个候选生物标志物。非小细胞肺癌(NSCLC)的 BATTLE Ⅰ试验是一个使用反应自适应随机化的Ⅱ期临床试验的例子[6]，这将在本书的另一章中讨论。值得注意的是，一些统计学家对这种自适应随机化设计的有效性提出了质疑[7]。

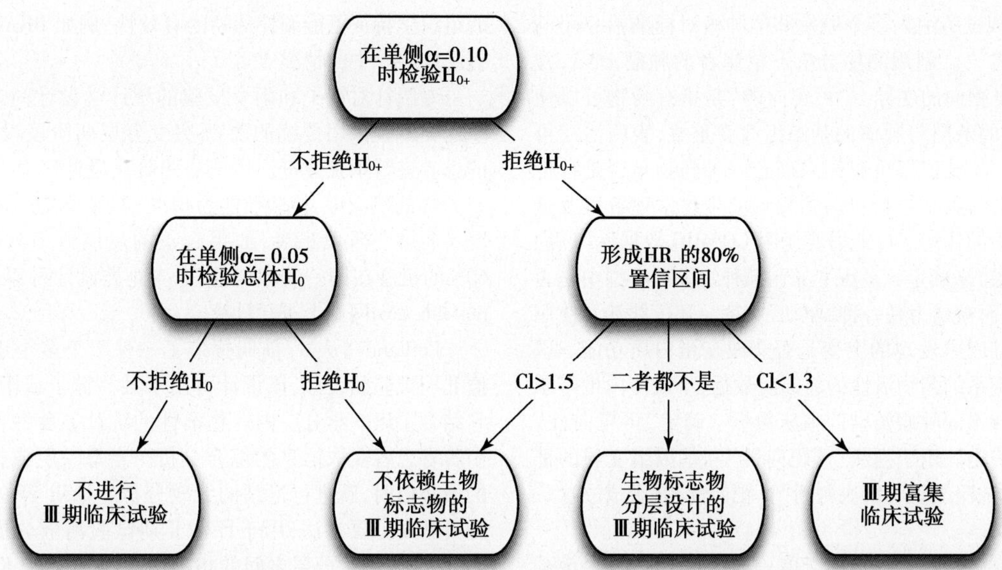

图 21-1　随机化Ⅱ期的分析策略被设计用于决定Ⅲ期试验是否应该仅限于生物标志物阳性的人群，或同时包括阳性和阴性，是否不应该测量生物标志物，或者Ⅱ期结果是否支持进行Ⅲ期试验。数据来自文献[3]。HR_+是治疗手段在生物标志物阳性组的危险比。HR_-是治疗手段在生物标志物阴性组的风险比。H_{0+}是 $HR_+ = 1$ 的零假设。H_0 是总体 HR = 1 的零假设

Ⅱa 期“雨伞”和“篮子”发现临床试验

大型肿瘤测序研究，如英国的癌症基因组计划和美国的癌症基因组图谱（TCGA），已经在多种原发肿瘤位点发现了重现性的基因组变异[1]。这些数据为基于肿瘤生物学特征的个体化治疗提供了科学依据。然而，在将肿瘤基因学发现转化为临床肿瘤学应用仍面临许多挑战，第一个挑战是肿瘤基因组整体的巨大异质性，这意味着在既定的肿瘤类型中存在多个罕见的基因组片段。

针对一种肿瘤的单个小基因组片段异常，开发单一靶向药物是一项漫长、低效和昂贵的工作。我们以 HER2 突变为例，与 HER2 基因扩增相反，在晚期乳腺癌中，HER2 突变发生频率低至 1%～2%。有初步证据表明，使用强效不可逆酪氨酸激酶抑制剂如 neratinib 可以靶向这些突变[8]。对大约 40 名患者进行“验证性”Ⅱ期试验，需要筛查 2 000～4 000 名晚期乳腺癌患者。此外，在这项研究结束时，这种新药相对于标准治疗或其他具有类似突变的肿瘤类型的潜在价值仍不得而知。图 21-2 突出显示了这种药物在携带“小”基因组变异的乳腺癌（BC）人群中发挥作用所面临的挑战。因此，这种基因组变异将在“雨伞”发现试验的背景下，找到与其最佳匹配的候选药物，在该试验中，一组基因组变异将在多个乳腺癌Ⅱ期分组中被筛选和研究。另外，一项篮子试验可以检测几种肿瘤类型中的 HER2 突变，研究酪氨酸激酶抑制剂（TKI）的活性，如果缺乏抗肿瘤活性则适用“早期停止规则”。这些日益流行的临床试验形式将在后面介绍。

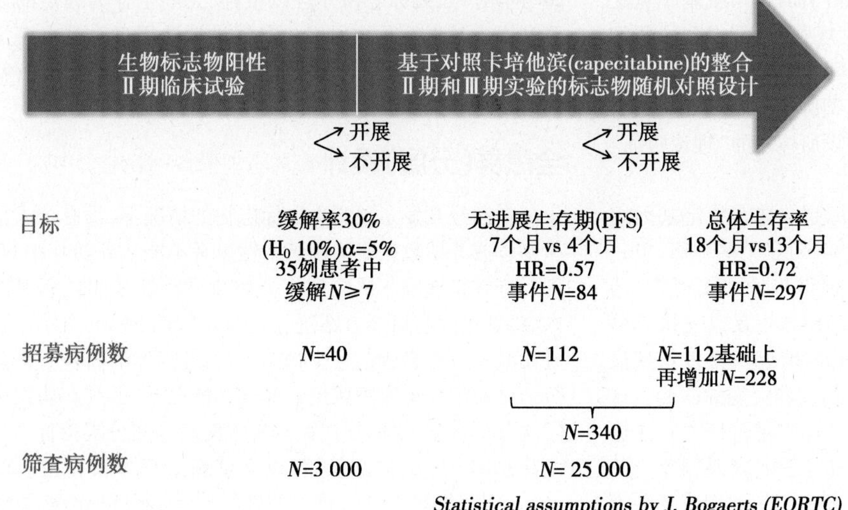

图 21-2　第二阶段和第三阶段临床试验的模式，开发一种抑制某靶点的药物，该靶点在 1%～2%的病例中发生突变。虽然临床试验所需的患者数量是合理的，但筛选的患者数量非常大。将此类药物的开发纳入针对多个目标的国家和国际通用筛选计划中，然后对符合条件的患者进行临床试验。HR，风险比；N，例数

"篮子"发现试验纳入多个原发部位肿瘤对标准治疗耐药的晚期癌症患者[9]。利用测序分析评估患者的肿瘤 DNA,并确定是否存在可靶向的变异。"可靶向的"是指有药物可以使用,其分子靶点的范围与肿瘤的基因组改变重叠,表明治疗可能对患者有益。多种证据可以用来确定一种药物是否是特定突变的理想候选药物。包括对药物靶点的生物学理解以及这些靶点在疾病中的作用。可能需要使用 COSMIC 数据库(癌症体细胞突变目录)来确定该基因变异在某种组织学类型中是否频繁地发生,从而被认为是一种"驱动"突变。还可能涉及使用算法来预测在基因中发现的突变是否会改变蛋白质功能。以及使用基于细胞系的药物活性的临床前数据、小鼠体内携带该突变的移植瘤或不同肿瘤类型的临床数据。确定"可靶向性"的规则应预先确定。用于判断"可靶向性"和基因组变异的证据,可能有助于试验组织者解决判断"可靶向性"是否成立这一两难的问题。

"篮子试验"一词通常特定用于单一药物的临床试验,该药物针对具有多种组织学类型的患者和单一或多个基因的多种突变类型。涉及多种药物的试验通常被称为"雨伞试验"。这两种类型的试验都是早期发现试验,并试图确定有证据表明某种药物对具有特定肿瘤的基因组特征具有显著抗肿瘤活性。这些阳性线索应在以后扩大的Ⅱ期或Ⅱ/Ⅲ期试验中得到证实。

一些雨伞试验是随机设计的;对于接受符合"可靶向性"规则的药物的患者,将其与对照药物或基于医生选择的药物的结果进行比较,而不考虑基因组特征。

国立癌症研究所实施的 MPACT(molecular profiling based assignment of cancer therapeutics)和 Stand-Up-To-Cancer 在 $BRAF^{WT}$ 黑色素瘤患者中开展的临床试验,都是用 2∶1的随机对照方案[10]。随机对照的雨伞试验需要回答两个明确的问题。一个是检验试图将药物与肿瘤基因组学特征匹配的策略并不比未考虑任何基因组学特征的标准治疗方案有效这一零假设。既往随机对照临床试验往往评估一种药物或者治疗方案,而此处零假设涉及将一组药物和生物标志物进行匹配这样的策略。因此针对某一特定靶点获得足够多的有效抑制剂这一目标显得尤为重要。匹配策略效果将取决于基因组特征的类型和将药物与肿瘤进行匹配的"规则"。如果肿瘤类型较多且未基于"规则"匹配,或者"规则"经常发生变化,该临床试验的实用意义就会受到限制。对于监管部门而言,审批基于宽泛肿瘤类型筛选得到的药物比审批基于"规则"匹配得到的药物更为困难。随机确定的对照组使我们可以用无进展生存期作为终点事件。然而,针对单一组织学类型肿瘤的临床试验相对于包含多种类型肿瘤的临床试验,零假设所体现的"理论验证"显得意义更为丰富。

随机设计的雨伞试验的第二个目标是筛选在特定基因组和组织学特征条件下个体化应用的药物。对于某些肿瘤,单一基因,比如"NRAS"的突变频率足够高,使得Ⅱ期试验能够对药物进行充分评估。而许多情况下入组病例数不足以支持充分的Ⅱ期评估。然而,由于相对于传统的Ⅱ期试验,可以看到显著的有效性,该临床试验能够用于筛选药物和突变的匹配。这些先导药物应该在 follow-up 试验中扩大样本量验证[8]。在这样的发现性试验中,在评估药物针对携带某种特定基因突变的肿瘤的有效性时,必须考虑发生这种突变的细胞类型或者肿瘤的组织学特征可能调控药物的有效性,例如 BRAF 抑制剂在结直肠癌治疗中的情况[11]。

专门针对篮子和雨伞试验的统计学设计尚未见报道。许多此类试验采用传统的药物-突变分层两阶段设计,将有足够的患者进行单独分析。传统的两阶段设计区分 10%的反应率与 35%的反应率,检验效能为 85%,Ⅰ型错误概率为 10%,只需要 5 名第一阶段患者,如果真正的反应概率只有 10%,则有 60%的机会在第一阶段终止[12]。此类设计可以在 http://brb.nci.nih.gov 网站上进行计算。

LeBlanc 等人[13]前期报道了一种用于多个组织学类型肿瘤Ⅱ期试验的设计,该设计可用于某些篮子或雨伞临床试验。它结合了组织学分层内药物活性的统计显著性检验和从研究中所有患者获取信息的综合分析。当每一层或整体达到指定的最小值时,就进行连续的无效分析。Thall 等人[14]开发了一种贝叶斯分层方法,用于评估Ⅱ期试验离散分层中处理的效果,同时考虑了分层之间的相关性。Freidlin 和 Korn[15]批评了这种方法,他们认为,"在结果数据中,似乎没有足够的证据来确定借用不同亚组的信息是正确的"。

使用单个二元生物标志物的Ⅲ期设计

靶向(富集)设计

只有那些被认为最有可能从实验药物中获益的患者才有资格参与的设计称为"靶向设计"或"富集设计",如图 21-3a 所示。在富集设计中,利用已获分析验证的诊断判断入组随机临床试验的资格,比较包含新药的方案和对照方案。这种方法现在已经被用于许多药物的关键试验,这些药物的分子靶点在疾病的背景下生物学作用已经被很好地理解。例如曲妥珠单抗(trastuzumab)[16],维穆拉菲尼(vemurafenib)[17],和克瑞唑替尼(crizotinib)[18]。

富集设计对曲妥珠单抗的开发是非常有效的,尽管当初试验并不完善,但后来得到了改进。Simon and Maitournam[19,20]开发了一个通用公式来比较富集设计和标准设计在随机入组和筛选入组的病例数方面的差别。他们发现富集设计非常高效,并将富集试验设计的样本量规划方法上传 http://brb.nci.nih.gov 网站。二元标志物并且以生存/无病生存为终点的设计都可利用该基于 web 的程序。富集设计适用于对靶点有深入生物学基础理解的情况,即认为检测阴性的患者不会从新药中获益。

全患群(分层)设计

在已经开发了预测生物标志物的情况下,没有令人信服的生物学或Ⅱ期数据表明测试阴性患者不能从新治疗中获益,通常最好在Ⅲ期临床试验中将分类指标阳性和阴性病例同时纳入,将新治疗与对照方案进行比较。如图 21-3b 所示。在试验开始时对所有患者进行生物标志物检测,然后将所有患者随机分为试验治疗组或对照组。在这种情况下,必须在协议中预先定义分析计划,说明如何在分析中使用预测分类指标。分析计划将总体上定义测试策略,以评估新治疗方案在检测阳性患者、检测阴性患者和总体上的效果[21]。测试策略必须控制试

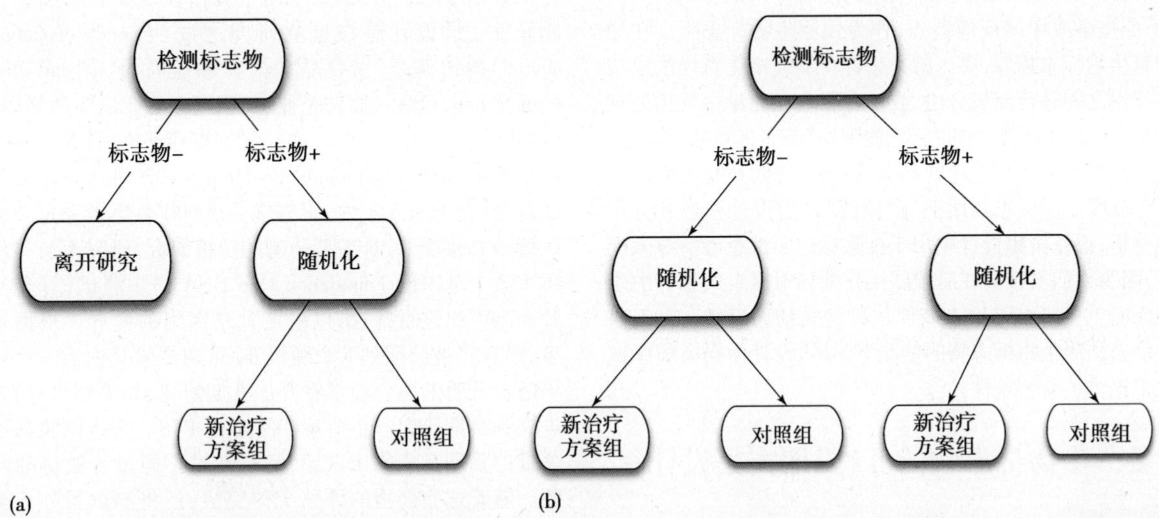

图 21-3 (a)靶向富集设计用于评估一种新的治疗方法,该方法用于使用预测标志物检测方法确定为最有可能收益的患者群体。主要用于那些有令人信服的理由相信"标志物阴性"患者不会从新治疗中获益,并且有经分析验证的检测方法可用的情况下。(b)"全患群"设计和"标志物分层"设计用于评估一种新的治疗方法与对照方法在以二元标志物为预判的人群中的有效性。一个完整的前瞻性分析计划应该包括在标志物阳性、阴性和总体人群中治疗组与对照组的比较。通过将整个研究范围的Ⅰ型错误限制在传统的5%水平的重点分析计划内,对标志物阳性患者的治疗有效性的判断不必局限于总体是否有效或存在显著交互作用的情况

验的总体Ⅰ型错误。总体Ⅰ型错误是指实际上治疗效果在总体上和在生物标志物特异性亚组内都是相等的,但比较得出统计上有显著差异的错误结论。对Ⅰ型总体误差的控制通常要求使用显著性阈值<0.05 来解释单个显著性检验。临床试验的规模也应适当,以便为这些试验提供足够的统计效能。仅仅对分类指标进行分层是不够的,也就是说,在不指定完整分析计划的情况下,对分类器进行平衡、随机化。"分层"的主要价值(例如,平衡)随机化是确保只有测试结果足够充分的患者才会进入试验。随机化的预分层对于在检测阳性或阴性亚组中对治疗效果进行推断的有效性是不必要的[22]。如果在试验开始时没有一个已经分析验证的检测,但在分析时将可用,那么最好不要对随机化过程进行预分层。

已有报道描述了几种基本的分析方案,基于网页的样本量计算工具可以在 http://brb.nci.nih.gov 上找到。如果有一定的证据表明如果这种治疗总体有效,很可能在检测呈阳性的病例中更有效,那么可以首先使用5%的显著性阈值来比较治疗组与对照组。只有当检测阳性患者的治疗与对照比较阈值为5%时有显著性,才会将新治疗与检测阴性患者的对照进行比较,并再次使用5%的统计显著性阈值。这种序贯方法能将Ⅰ型的总体错误控制在5%[23]。在人们对预测指标信心有限的情况下,它可以作为有效的"回退"分析方法。新治疗组的结果首先与对照组的总体结果进行比较。如果这种差异在更低显著性阈值(如 0.03)时不显著,则仅对检测阳性患者与对照组进行比较。后一种比较使用的显著性阈值为 0.02,或者初始测试没有使用传统 0.05 以下任一阈值[23]。在对候选生物标志物有中等信心的情况下,可以使用 MAST 分析计划[24]。在最后的分析中,首先要检验的是对标志物阳性患者没有治疗效果的零假设。显著性的阈值预设为低于 0.05 的Ⅰ型错误的某个值 α_+。例如,α_+ 可能为 0.04。如果该零假设被拒绝,则使用 0.05 的显著性阈值检验标记阴性患者的零假设。如果标志物阳性患者零假设未被拒绝,则使用 $0.05-\alpha_+$ 的显著性阈值检验总体患者人群的零假设测试,该案例中为 0.01。

Freidlin 等人[25]和 Mandrekar 以及 Sargent[26]报道了利用分层和富集设计"真实世界"的研究。Wang 等人[27]和 Rosenblum, VanDerLaan[28]以及 Simon N, Simon R. 报道了富化设计的自适应形式,其以"全患群"开始,并自适应地限制入组资格。

前瞻性-回顾性设计

在某些情况下,一项包含存档肿瘤标本的完整随机临床试验可用于评估由新的候选生物标志物确定的亚组的治疗效果。例如,抗 EGFR 抗体在结直肠癌中的有效性假设将仅限于肿瘤不包含 K-RAS 突变的患者,这一假设是在其他研究者提出这一假设之前已有的随机对照临床试验中评估的。Simon 等[30]描述了一种前瞻性回顾性方法,使用存档的肿瘤标本对一项关于预测生物标志物的随机Ⅲ期试验进行重点再分析。该方法要求大多数患者都能获得存档标本,并在进行双盲检测前制定一项以单个标志物为重点的分析计划。为了被认作Ⅰ型证据,结果还必须在两项这样的前瞻性回顾性试验中进行评估。没有必要在随机化过程中使用标志物作为分层变量。这与标记阳性患者治疗效果分析的有效性无关[22]。Simon[22]还指出,对于回顾性前瞻性研究方法来说,没有必要限定最小的肿瘤存档数量比例。关键因素是治疗组之间在可用的存档标本方面不应存在偏倚。如果在随机化分组之前病人和医生就组织标本档案达成一致,就可以确保没有这种偏倚。

导入设计

预测生物标志物通常被认为是在治疗开始前从肿瘤或患者身上获得的生物测量值。Hong 和 Simon[31]开发了一种导入

设计，该设计允许在新治疗或对照组的短时导入期后测量药物动力学、免疫学或中间反应终点，作为预测生物标志物。在导入期测量生物标志物后，要么所有患者在继续接受新疗法或切换到对照组之间进行随机分组，或仅对那些在测量中与预处理基线测量相比有显著变化的“标志物阳性”患者进行随机分组。生物标记物不作为比较治疗的终点，直到标志物被检测后才进行随机化分组。该标志物用于“全患群”分层设计中患者分层和独立分析，或在富集设计中用于排除标记阴性患者。导入期应较短，因为人们不希望在后续随机分配到对照组的患者的生存期或无病生存期由于导入期使用试验药物而延长。在无法确定治疗前预测生物标志物的情况下，导入设计为提高临床试验的效率提供了有利条件。

包括多个生物标志物的Ⅱ/Ⅲ期富集设计

图 21-4 显示了一个新的 Lung-MAP 生物标志物驱动的临床试验原型的结构，该原型用于难治性晚期肺鳞癌患者的药物开发。该设计是在癌症研究之友（Friends of Cancer Research）的协调下，由食品和药物管理局（Food and Drug Administration，FDA）、制药企业、美国国家临床试验网络（US National Clinical Trials Network）、国家癌症研究所（National Cancer Institute，NCI）和 Foundation Medicine 公司共同开发的。根据计划，在未来 5 年内，将有多达 5 000 名患者通过 200 多个医疗中心接受Ⅱ/Ⅲ期新药物的随机研究，研究人员将使用分析 182 个基因的 Foundation One DNA 测序测试，对参与者的肿瘤基因组进行筛选，以确定其基因组的变异。根据筛选结果，患者将被分配到 5 个随机Ⅱ/Ⅲ期试验其中的一个。这五项随机试验的每一项都将开展Ⅱ期研究，如果结果有希望，将进展到Ⅲ期研究。主要观察终点是 PFS。这些试验都可能是关键的Ⅲ期富集临床试验，具有针对不同患者亚群的伴随诊断。随着这些药物的评估工作完成，还将测试另外 5 至 7 种药物。

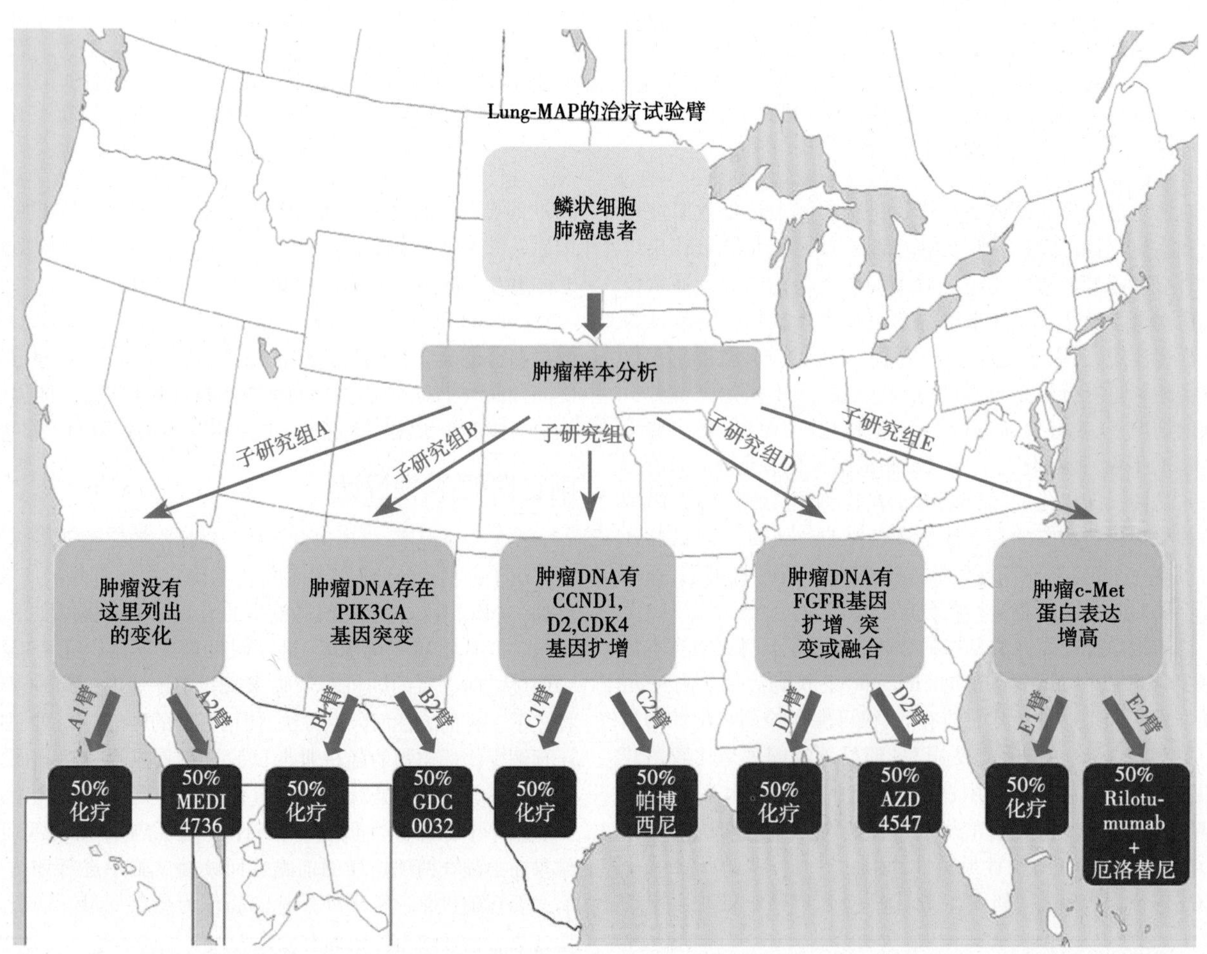

图 21-4 Lung-MAP 临床试验主设计。筛选肺鳞状细胞癌患者肿瘤基因组的突变。根据所发现的基因组变异，患者被纳入 6 项随机临床试验中的一项。每一项分试验都将相同的对照治疗与专门为一类基因组改变患者设计的治疗进行比较。每个组成部分的临床试验都是随机的Ⅱ/Ⅲ期临床试验，这可能是为选定的患者群体批准试验药物的关键依据

“基因组时代”的临床试验所需新的合作模式和未来的挑战

在为了治疗而对癌症进行分子分型方面，我们仍处于“学习曲线”的起点。很有可能，我们很快就会从依赖于 DNA 水平变异的简单分类转向更复杂的分类，也包括 RNA 测序和(磷酸化)蛋白平台生成的关键信息。我们也可以预见“通路导向”的治疗策略将取代单靶点导向的治疗策略，因为考虑到癌细胞的可塑性，单靶点导向的治疗策略很可能失败。将“基因组学”转移到“治疗”意味着要处理不确定性，统计学家将继续在这方面发挥关键作用。

同时，实现“个性化”肿瘤治疗的优势需要改变临床学术研究范式，在药物开发行业设置大型的合作团队，破除药物开发路径之间的壁垒，实现组合研究策略，在监管评价方面对于新的化合物和创新药物组合采用更灵活机动的审批路径。

结论

在肿瘤学中，由于分子靶向药开发成本高昂，使用对大多数患者没有益处的方案治疗宽泛的患者群体，在经济学上的可持续性较差，故难以获得成功。人类疾病分子异质性已经得到公认，这就要求开发新的设计和分析范式，利用随机临床试验为预测医学提供可靠的基础。

(文文 译　于晗　李亮 校)

参考文献

1 Stratton MR, Campbell PJ, Futreal PA. The cancer genome. *Nature*. 2009;**458**:719–724.

2 Sawyers CL. The cancer biomarker problem. *Nature*. 2008;**452**:548–552.

3 Freidlin B, McShane LM, Polley MY, Korn EL. Randomized phase II trial designs with biomarkers. *J Clin Oncol*. 2012;**30**:3304–3309.

4 Pusztai L, Hess KR. Clinical trial design for microarray predictive marker discovery and assessment. *Ann Oncol*. 2004;**15**:1731–1737.

5 Jones CL, Holmgren E. An adaptive Simon two-stage design for phase 2 studies of targeted therapies. *Contemp Clin Trials*. 2007;**28**:654–661.

6 Kim ES, Herbst JJ, Wistuba II, et al. The BATTLE trial: personalizing therapy for lung cancer. *Cancer Discov*. 2011;**1**:44–53.

7 Korn EL, Freidlin B. Outcome-adaptive randomization: is it useful? *J Clin Oncol*. 2011;**29**:771–776.

8 Bose R, Kavuri S, Searleman A, et al. Activating HER2 mutations in HER2 gene amplification negative breast cancer. *Cancer Discov*. 2013;**3**(**2**):224–237.

9 Simon R, Roychowdhury S. Implementing personalized cancer genomics in clinical trials. *Nat Rev Drug Discov*. 2013;**12**:358–369.

10 Simon R, Polley E. Clinical trials for precision oncology using next generation sequencing. *Pers Med*. 2013;**10**:485–495.

11 Prahallad A, Sun C, Huang S, et al. Unresponsiveness of colon cancer to BRAF (V600E) inhibition through feedback activation of EGFR. *Nature*. 2012;**483**:100–103.

12 Simon R. Optimal two-stage designs for phase II clinical trials. *Control Clin Trials*. 1989;**10**:1–10.

13 LeBlanc M, Rankin C, Crowley J. Multiple histology phase II trials. *Clin Cancer Res*. 2009;**15**:4256–62.

14 Thall PF, Wathen JK, Bekele BN, Champlin RE, Baker LO, Benjamin RS. Hierarchical Bayesian approaches to phase II trials in diseases with multiple subtypes. *Stat Med*. 2003;**22**:763–80.

15 Freidlin B, Korn EL. Borrowing information across subgroups in phase II trials: Is it useful? *Clin Cancer Res*. 2013;**19**:1326–34.

16 Shak S. Overview of the trastuzumab (Herceptin) anti-HER2 monoclonal antibody clinical program in HER2-overexpressing metastatic breast cancer. *Semin Oncol*. 1999;**26**:71–77.

17 Chapman PB, Hauschild A, Robert C, et al. Improved survival with vemurafenib in melanoma with BRAF V600E mutation. *N Engl J Med*. 2011;**364**:2507–2516.

18 Shaw AT, Yeap BY, Solomon BJ, et al. Effect of crizotinib on overall survival in patients with advanced non-small-cell lung cancer harbouring ALK gene rearrangement: a retrospective analysis. *Lancet Oncol*. 2011;**12**:1004–1012.

19 Simon R, Maitournam A. Evaluating the efficiency of targeted designs for randomized clinical trials. *Clin Cancer Res*. 2005;**10**:6759–6763.

20 Maitournam A, Simon R. On the efficiency of targeted clinical trials. *Stat Med*. 2005;**24**:329–339.

21 Simon RM. *Genomic Clinical Trials and Predictive Medicine*. Cambridge, MA: Cambridge University Press; 2013.

22 Simon R. Stratification and partial ascertainment of biomarker value in biomarker driven clinical trials. *J Biopharm Stat*. 2014;**2**(**5**):1011–1021.

23 Simon R. Using genomics in clinical trial design. *Clin Cancer Res*. 2008;**14**:5984–5993.

24 Freidlin B, Korn EL. Biomarker enrichment strategies: matching trial design to biomarker credentials. *Nat Rev Clin Oncol*. 2014;**11**:81–90.

25 Freidlin B, McShane LM, Korn EL. Randomized clinical trials with biomarkers: design issues. *J Natl Cancer Inst*. 2010;**102**:152–160.

26 Mandrekar SJ, Sargent DJ. Predictive biomarker validation in practice: lessons from real trials. *Clin Trials*. 2010;**7**:567–573.

27 Wang SJ, Hung HMJ, O'Neill RT. Adaptive patient enrichment designs in therapeutic trials. *Biom J*. 2009;**51**:358–374.

28 Rosenblum M, VanDerLaan MJ. Optimizing randomized trial designs to distinguish which subpopulations benefit from treatment. *Biometrika*. 2011;**98**:845–860.

29 Simon N, Simon R. Adaptive enrichment designs in clinical trials. *Biostatistics*. 2013;**14**:613–625.

30 Simon RM, Paik S, Hayes DF. Use of archived specimens in evaluation of prognostic and predictive biomarkers. *J Natl Cancer Inst*. 2009;**101**:1–7.

31 Hong F, Simon R. Run-in phase III trial designs with pharmacodynamic predictive biomarkers. *J Natl Cancer Inst*. 2013;**105**:1628–1633.

第 22 章　临床信息学

Edward P. Ambinder, MD

概述

医学信息学是信息技术与医疗保健的结合。对于肿瘤学而言，对信息的深入理解是至关重要的，因为需要及时跟进快速变化的基础、转化和临床癌症研究等发现，基于泛组学技术发展而来的精准医学干预手段、最新的实践指南、不断变化的医疗偿付方式，以及占主导地位但有时却令人失望的储存了我们的健康数据且作为医疗保健系统窗口的电子健康记录（electronic health record, EHR）。所有这一切都必须在一个价值提升的实践环境中进行，该环境可以在一个协调良好的体系中不断衡量我们的医疗服务质量，体系中的患者被多方位地数字化连接起来，包括他们的医院、智能手机和医疗设备、个人健康记录和多个电子病历。肿瘤学家很快就会有一个清晰、适用的"肿瘤学数字化健康信息技术系统"，通过获取每个癌症患者的有意义、可操作的数据，这将重新定义癌症研究。它仍将涉及对医学具有革新性意义的移动计算变革，计算机将完成我们的工作、应用程序（App）之间以及 EHR 协同工作以进行患者教育，和实现真正意义上的电子医疗数据共享和再利用。当今，大多数病人的癌症治疗被记录在电子病历系统中。像 ASCO 的 CancerLinQ 这样的快速学习系统（rapid learning system, RLS），其能够获取所有数据，并使用大数据分析工具来捕捉和比较类似癌症患者的最佳治疗方法和结果，据此我们将实现真正的精准医疗。随着癌症治疗发展成为快速学习系统，在不断发展的"物联网"中，医疗设备和医疗保健平台会给我们前所未有的、实现 24 小时实时掌握化疗病人健康状况的能力，这将为卫生系统节省大量开支，提高医疗服务质量，促进医学研究的创新发展。

前言

肿瘤学家和他们的患者正面临着医疗保健实践、研究、政府监管、商业实践、沟通和医疗偿付方面的颠覆性变化——这些变化是由单个领域的进步和信息技术与医疗技术、医疗实践、生物学和物理学等多个领域的融合所带来的。我们在大的医院系统或负责任的医疗组织而非小的团体中开展实践；在从按服务收费过渡到捆绑支付和与明确的医疗服务接触的过程中，应对不断变化的偿付方式；用电子媒介而不是纸来记录病人的治疗过程；看到医患关系变得更加以患者为中心；等等。我们越来越多地与包括患者在内的所有医疗保健相关方进行线上沟通。

计算机的使用带来了信息数量、质量和查找便捷性的显著提高，而互联网使得人们毫不费力地将所有人和事联系在一起，这一切都永远地改变了我们的生活。然而，我们仍然对与医疗保健系统交互的电子设备感到失望，因为它们仍然需要输入或口述数据，而输入的数据不容易被计算机理解，或者由于缺乏无缝的数据交互（输入的数据可以在另一个设备中被有效地理解、使用和再使用），而无法轻松地共享、再使用或报告。

1997 年，Clayton Christensen 预示了这种革命性的转变[1]，2008 年，他还特别提醒我们这种转变对医疗保健领域的影响[2]。随着信息的电子化、廉价化、人人可得化以及以消费者为导向，几乎所有最近的硬件和软件的信息技术进步都是从消费者开始，而不是从企业开始，从而首次给这个新的、颠覆性的医学数字化世界下了定义。肿瘤学家和他们的患者必须开始理解这一革命性的变化，它将直接解决我们目前所面临的问题。

肿瘤数字化健康信息技术系统

通用数据元和值集

通用数据元通过明确标识每个数据字段的标签和为数据输入选择的适当值来定义要在医疗记录中收集的数据。在可能的情况下，值集的选择应该参考一个标准的代码系统，例如用于描述门诊谈话的临床医学术语表（例如 SNOMED-CT）、实验室数据（例如 LOINC）、描述基础和临床研究的术语[例如癌症生物医学信息学网格（caBIG）]，以及为了计费和报告而定义的特定疾病分类的元素和代码（例如 ICD-9 和 ICD-10 代码）。

数据类型

计算机捕获电子结构化和电子非结构化数据。使用机器可读、可再利用、可共享、可操作、多用户和多用途的数据元和值集对数据进行结构化。非结构化或叙述性数据通过打字或听写来输入，并添加上下文，使其为人类所理解，而不是为计算机所理解（除非使用复杂的自然语言处理工具，或通过元数据进行标记，使其可搜索）。可搜索或机器可读的数据将允许 EHR 提供临床决策支持（clinical decision support, CDS）、用户教育和二次报告。实际上，这两种类型的数据对于获取完整的患者健康记录都很重要。

软件性能和文档编制

软件性能是指软件程序应该提供的功能。对所有电子医疗记录而言，电子处方软件是必需的，而临床肿瘤学需用电子医疗记录管理化疗。表 22-1 列出了 ASCO 的 EHR 工作组定义的 EHR 功能要素，表 22-2 列出了肿瘤 EHR 中所需的肿瘤学特定的资料内容。

表 22-1　由 ASCO 电子健康记录工作组定义的 EHR 功能

EHR 功能单元	如何在医疗实践中使用
查看患者信息	检查患者的症状或主诉、用药清单、检测结果和其他临床资料
收集数据	建立可搜索的电子病历。利用可自定义的模板建立病历
编制资料	将患者与实践对象的人口、病史信息汇总，并绘制图表供分析使用。生成报告。
查询患者或医疗数据以生成标准和/或自定义的报告	协助评估、诊断和复审急性或慢性疾病和治疗方案，并根据已制定的指南提供适当的临床警报和提醒。与其他系统兼容
临床决策支持	与内部工作管理和其他内部信息系统（如实验室信息系统，laboratory information system，LIS）进行交互；与其他医院、实验室、影像、药房和付款人沟通
搜索功能	查询数据库以获得关于临床问题和费用的报告
患者管理	管理个别患者的急、慢性疾病和病情
医疗服务市场营销	关于最常提供的医疗服务类型的信息。提供对患者的临床情况、转诊机构和患病人群的分析
标准化	给所诊治患者制订标准化疾病管理目标和治疗方案
计费和编码	使用 ICD 和 CPT 代码对患者的详细情况进行内部检查和平衡；集成 E&M 代码和 HCPCS 代码。医嘱录入，实验室检查、影像学检查、转诊等的预约，和其他非药物治疗
制订化疗方案	经适当授权和确认的化疗启动、相关辅助治疗和剂量修改
电子处方	授权和管理处方续药。访问药品的信息。在线把新处方传送到药房
信息交流	与患者、同事、付款人、医院和药房进行在线交流
提供内置的合规的、有监管的指导	保证合规合法
临床试验	进行研究、注册和临床试验
患者互动	整合来自患者的信息，包括来自个人健康记录（personal health record，PHR）、医院及患者医疗设备的数据
质量检测	使用数据参与质量检测程序

表 22-2　肿瘤 EHR 中需要的肿瘤特定文档

提供按菜单编排的部位/组织学/病理结果
在流程图上管理病人对治疗的反应
记录辅助/根治性治疗与姑息治疗的意图和目标
根据标准指南记录患者的表现状况
列出并发症情况及化疗可能发生的主要毒副反应
制订和管理化疗/生物治疗方案
管理和自动化调整体表面积（body surface area，BSA）、开始和维持剂量
管理化疗给药——静脉和口服，周期数，持续时间
记录给药过程
跟踪治疗的持续时间和计划的周期数
计划和记录放射治疗和/或维持效果
评估疼痛和关爱支持的需求
管理临床试验中的患者
临床肿瘤治疗计划、总结和生存报告

互联网

互联网是数字化医疗保健系统的通信和消息传递的组件。互联网的发展可以分为四个阶段。最初，互联网被用来“搜索”信息，并利用文本、文件、图片和其他媒体进行“交流”。用户主要是学术界人士和商界人士。电子邮件和论坛很受欢迎。随后，我们能够使用 web 站点做更多的事。消费者发现了互联网，商业也爆炸式增长。再有，我们能够使用 Facebook 这样的社交媒体网站进行“社交”和“协作”。随着移动计算主导互联网，应用程序暴增。现在，我们正在进入“物联网”时代，任何医疗设备都可以通过互联网与其他设备和计算机进行便捷的通信。

计算机交互性和数据交换

计算机交互性和数据交换或共享要求一个 EHR 系统中创建的数据被发送到另一个 EHR 系统中，并具有完整的解读和逻辑关系，以便将其放置在接收程序的适当数据字段中。ASCO 和国家癌症研究所的 caBIG 和社区癌症中心项目建立的 EHR 临床肿瘤学规范（Clinical Oncology Requirements for the EHR，CORE）规定了肿瘤学中核心通用的数据元、功能和交互标准，用于帮助定义医疗卫生信息技术认证委员会（Certification Commission for Healthcare Information Technology, CCHIT)所使用的最初的肿瘤学EHR认证标准[3]。无缝交互标准通过定义和传输医疗信息起着最重要的作用,使我们的数据输入、计算机化工作流程和结果报告变得十分简化和高效。

我们在医学中使用的大多数数据元已经定义、标准化并统一为代码集和临床词汇表(SNOMED-CT)。第1阶段电子病历有效使用为公共卫生报告带来了一定交互性。第2阶段电子病历有效使用中明确定义的内容、词汇和转运标准为患者转移管理提供更多的交互性支持。业内领先的标准开发组织(Standards Developing Organization, SDO) Health Level Seven International(HL7®)定义并标准化了临床摘要文档的使用,这些称为整合临床文档体系结构(consolidated clinical document architecture, C-CDA)文档。

笔者主持的ASCO数据标准和交互性工作组(ASCO's Data Standards and Interoperability Task Force)已经开发了两套肿瘤学专用的交互技术标准[4,5]。我们选择为辅助乳腺癌和辅助结直肠癌[6~8]而开发的ASCO治疗方案和摘要论文模板,并将其转化为实施指南(implementation guide, IG)。IG可用于创建交互性文档,该文档可在任何遵循HL7 C-CDA标准的计算机系统之间进行电子交互传输[9]。CDA定义文档的内容和传输,文档可以很大。该文件标准[题为《临床肿瘤治疗计划和总结》(Clinical Oncology Treatment Plan and Summary, COTPS)]总结了几乎所有由医生、医院、实验室、影像中心、药房和癌症患者在患癌过程中创建的医疗报告中的癌症数据,并对患者及其医疗提供者进行审查和指导。我们计划为其他常见癌症创建类似的C-CDA文档、患者报告的结果和癌症幸存者康复计划。

在2014年HIMSS交互性展示上,ASCO的COTPS被用来演示如何使用通用数据元,标准化的报告,遵循交互性标准,并使用创新的数据输入工具可以使医疗服务提供者工作流程效率更高,且使批注和报告得以共享、更具可操作性和实现多个目标。这样,10个供应商都可使用这些标准来实时交换数据。新型的数据输入工具(包括语音识别转录为文本、数据、结构化数据的工具),医护计划管理器,各类医疗装置(可在患者家中实现数据获取和警报功能),患者教育,患者自报告结果和问卷,关于质量、研究、人口健康的可行性报告,及多个大数据分析注册中心都已涌现。一个健康信息交换系统实时捕获并显示临床报告的汇编,并将其提供给所有供应商系统,与此同时记录一名接受乳腺癌辅助治疗的妇女的癌症治疗过程。医护计划管理系统能够在电子系统中为患者、护理人员和所有服务提供者创建ASCO的COTPS。

HL7即将批准一种新的、灵活的、更简单的交互性和数据交换标准,称为快速医疗交互资源(Fast Healthcare Interoperability Resources, FHIR)[10]。FHIR可以表示粒状或离散的数据元和文档。FHIR优势部分来自技术的优雅简洁。它结合了HL7 V2、HL7 V3和CDA的最佳特性,同时利用了最新的web服务技术。FHIR中包含的主要技术变化是从以文档为中心的方法,向使用应用程序编程接口(API)的数据级访问方法的根本性转变。该接口能够使用公共API与包括EHR在内的任何软件交换数据,这可以促进健康IT系统之间的交互性生态系统。具体地说,FHIR提供了一个称为资源的模块化概念,可以使用一组非常基本的结构化数据(如药物列表或实验室结果)对其进行扩展和调整,使之成为当今基于文档的交换体系结构的一个进步。FHIR提供了一个即插即用的平台,可以在系统内部和系统之间工作,在概念上类似于Apple app系统。FHIR还允许开发人员通过使用公共API和遵循一组定义明确的规则来创建新的应用程序。大多数供应商可能会采用公共API,提供统一的方法来与任何应用程序共享数据。系统可以使用与其他资源相同的框架轻松地读取扩展,当FHIR和智能平台结合在一起时,我们就有了一个灵活的交互标准,可以捕捉苹果公司应用程序的功能。最近,在ANSI认证的HL7标准开发组织协调下,许多EHR供应商和医疗保健组织启动了Argonaut Project项目,加速查询或响应的交互性,共享电子医疗保健信息,这些措施令过去一直鼓励私有化的集团发生了积极的改变[11]。

对于肿瘤学家来说,我们将拥有真正的交互性和数据交换,这使得小型灵活的应用程序将能够接受来自另一个应用程序或企业范围内的EHR的数据,有效地使用这些数据并将其发送到另一个应用程序,最终将更新后的数据返回到原始应用程序源,而更新后的数据可以被理解并纳入原始程序的数据库。高效的数据录入工具、为肿瘤学家或其患者而设的教育链接(如CDS)、整合健康数据和创建有用的个人健康记录(personal health record, PHR)、重要的实时和有效的提醒,以及数据的自动二级使用并报告用于质量监测、州注册数据和快速学习系统(rapid learning system, RLS)。企业范围内的EHR需要数年时间进行更新,而且在教育用户方面收效甚微,因此可以依赖上述这些来自可信来源的灵活应用程序来改进其产品。医疗保险和医疗补助服务中心(Centers for Medicare and Medicaid Service, CMS)在其最近的报告《为国家连接医疗和保健》(Connecting Health and Care for the Nation)中将交互性作为国家的一个主要目标[12]。

电子健康记录数据库和存储库

EHR是一个系统的数据库,它收集纵向的、可追溯的、安全的、不可修改的关于单个患者或人群的数字化健康信息和数据。它能够在所有医疗保健机构、提供者和患者之间共享信息。它应该展示数据资料,准确地获取和显示病人的最新健康状况和他们的临床情况。EHR应该在其所定义的临床活动和管理要求中做到完善的归档工作,但是目前这个系统在高效的数据输入、教育和安全性、服务提供者工作流程辅助、CDS支持、EHR之间的无缝交互、即插即用模块设计和自动注册以及其他二次报告生成等需求方面还难以令人满意。这是因为最初的EHR创建者是根据纸质图表来建模的,该过程是被动的,并且不参与到医疗保健中。缺乏对临床工作流程、提供者或医疗保健系统需求的理解。今天,政府对购买EHR和满足需要交互性、质量改进、CDS和注册报告来实现的有意义的功能而采取财政激励,已经说服了大多数肿瘤学家采用它们。不幸的是,他们并不满意,因为这些有意义的功能在当今的EHR中设计得很差。EHR数据不仅需要以前纸质系统就能完成的简洁记录密切相关和符合逻辑的临床活动,而且还要能够实现更高的目标如临床和人口研究、质量检测、注册管理机构报告、报销文件,但是目前EHR尚不能有效满足这些需求。我们与癌症患者面对面交流的时间减少了,更多的时间是在电脑屏幕上使用菜单、界面和提醒[13]。由于使用 EHR，我们的工作日平均延长了 48 分钟[14]。

EHR 必须变得更加擅长进行数据输入，提供语音到文本到数据的功能（口述，并让计算机使用自然语言和机器阅读技能，将口述的材料放入相应的数据字段）。通过开放他们的软件，EHR 供应商可以释放出一支有创造力的开发者大军，帮助他们的用户和改进产品。

美国医师学会医学信息学委员会（The Medical Informatics Committee of the American College of Physicians）最近研究了 EHR 文档问题，并撰写了一篇出色的立场文件，对表 22-3 中列出的更改提出了令人信服的建议。然而，在可预见的未来，电脑仍将是我们个人与医疗系统的纽带。我们必须找到更有效的方法来捕获和再利用数据，并让计算机做更多的工作。

表 22-3　美国医师学会提出电子健康档案的基本文件[15]

临床文档的主要目的应该是通过加强沟通来给患者治疗提供支持和改善临床结果
医生应该为文档制定标准，由各个专科医师制定的标准设置来促进信息交流
EHR 应促进治疗疗效的提高和实现价值导向医疗的数据分析之间的无缝连接
只有在对医护工作和质量改进有重要价值时才收集结构化数据
预先授权不做唯一的数据和格式要求
当病人能够查看他们的病程记录和其他记录时，病人的参与度和医护质量将得到提高
需要进行研究以改善记录护理的流程并使技术进步，以便更好、更准确地记录观察结果
EHR 的开发应针对纵向的基于团队的医护进行优化
在再利用数据时，应该包含嵌入式标记来标识原始来源
应该删除用于指示已经记录的内容的复选框
患者生成的数据应纳入他们的医疗记录，并保持源标识

个人健康档案

患者将继续在医疗保健中发挥更积极的作用，因为他们将承担更大比例的医疗保健费用，使人们了解他们的价值观和愿望，并帮助做出关键决定。有了互联网上无限的教育资源，我们的病人可以接触到和我们一样的医学文献和教科书。在为患者提供更易理解的电子报告使用要求下，CMS 提议病人可以访问他们的实验室检测结果，患者与肿瘤学家之间的电子邮件往来变得普遍（可偿付部分支付者），而且随着大部分医疗报告都以数字化形式呈现，患者将可以控制他们的医疗记录。MD 安德森癌症中心已经成功实施了一个试点项目，使几乎所有的医疗记录都可以通过电子方式提供给患者。大多数病人非常满意，对大多数医生而言，其中许多人最初持怀疑态度，不过现已经转变为"开放获取"医疗的支持者[16]。非常成功的 OpenNotes 项目就是一个例子，说明病人是多么渴望获得更多与他们相关的医疗信息[17]。

知识和教育

肿瘤学知识库

在使用数据收集和输入工具将癌症患者的可操作健康数据整合到我们的 EHR 中之后，我们需要 EHR 与 CDS 工具帮助搜索目前可用的知识库，并且服务于肿瘤学的 RLS 系统，为我们提供一种"可汇集所有具有共同特征（一种健康状态）的人群中的个体患者数据，以生成新知识的技术"，来改善患者的疗效、医护质量以及如 Yu 等所述的利用实践指南或算法的医疗保健服务价值[18]。我们的肿瘤学知识库包括临床试验数据、系统生物学数据、病人来源的数据（健康和保健）以及关于操作过程和疗效的卫生系统数据。

临床试验数据来自发表在同行评审期刊的论文，或者来自由专业协会召集的专家审查和权衡过质量和不足之处，并作为临床实践指南发表的医学文献的系统性综述。

肿瘤学中的系统生物学数据帮助我们描述在不同癌症进展过程中发现的分子、细胞生长调控和免疫变化，使我们能够了解它们的原因、分类和治疗方法。随着计算生物学及其分析工具能够处理泛组学的 TB 级数据，不久以后，从个体患者得到的基因组、转录组、蛋白质组和代谢物可以常规进行分析评估。灵活便捷的资源，比如癌症基因组图谱（Cancer Genome Atlas）[19]和全球基因组和健康联盟（Global Alliance for Genomics and Health）[20]将支持服务提供者和研究人员为患者提供个体化治疗并改善治疗效果。这些知识基础数据库协同工作，将通过确定与特定泛基因组异常相关的癌症对治疗的反应，加速靶向药物的评估和批准过程。

最后，数字化健康信息技术系统将使用我们的 EHR 临床数据、患者报告数据、实验室信息系统和数据库、行政索赔数据、癌症登记处、健康、活动和营养数据，以及上市后的监测数据，以获取反映真实世界接受了我们治疗的患者群体的医疗系统数据。

临床决策支持系统（CDSS）

临床决策支持系统（clinical decision support system，CDSS）是用户选择的或情景感知调用的应用程序工具，这些应用程序工具可以访问 EHR 使用的知识库或实践指南，以教育和/或提醒用户有关特定于患者的临床决策和服务点的健康管理。Musen 等人描述了以下三种类型的 CDSS[21]：

- 信息管理（直接链接到教科书章节或 Internet 站点或信息按

钮等工具,它是嵌入在 EHR 中的上下文敏感的链接,允许方便地检索 EHR 或 Internet 链接中的相关信息,并在随后进行电子化再利用)[22]

- 情景感知(警报或患者指示板)
- 基于患者特定逻辑的诊断和治疗选择指导,这些可以从知识库或 RLS(如 CancerLinQ)中获得[18]。

快速学习系统

随着癌症患者越来越多地将他们的医疗记录数字化,很明显,这些记录中有一个宝贵的临床数据库,通过开放 97%没有进行临床试验的癌症患者的情况,这些数据有可能造福社会。通过了解我们的新治疗方法和程序在获得监管批准后对非临床试验患者的相对益处或危害,我们可以持续不断地应用新发现和改进治疗。医学研究所研讨会的国家癌症政策论坛(National Cancer Policy Forum of the Institute of Medicine workshop)题为"循证实践的基础:癌症护理的快速学习系统"的报告,审查了癌症 RLS 的要素[23]。委员会建议,这样一个系统的要素包括登记和数据库、新出现的信息技术、以病人为中心和病人驱动的 CDS 和病人参与的工具、适应文化变化的方法、临床实践指南、临床肿瘤学的医护需求、联邦政策问题和影响。ASCO 和其他组织已开始为癌症定义 RLS,称为 CancerLinQ[24,25]。它将使用这些工具来加深对癌症生物学的理解,从而基于分子驱动诊断来定义癌症;还将纳入一个治疗开发系统,使用肿瘤 EHR 注册,以发展更智能和更快的临床试验。由于它将临床研究和转化研究更无缝地结合在一起,有潜力确保每一位癌症患者的经验都能为研究提供信息,并改善医护水平。

RLS 将要求计算工具从结合了机器学习、数据可视化、统计和编程的大型数据库中做出数据编译和分析。对于癌症患者来说,这个大数据操作可以整合所有来自医疗设备的临床数据、基因组数据、保健和健康数据,以及来自医疗保险和私人支付者的医疗支付数据。ASCO 的 CancerLinQ 希望从我们的办公室、癌症中心和医院获得所有居住在美国的癌症患者的 EHR 和临床知识库数据。肿瘤学家可以输入患者的所有临床信息,并要求 CancerLinQ 通过电子方式将患者与最接近的一组具有相似临床特征的患者进行匹配,从而揭示出对这些相似患者产生最佳疗效的治疗方法。此外,它可以生成提高质量和成本效益的医疗知识。其过程如 Sim 等人[26]最初描述的那样,通过为基于实践的研究网络创建一个信息学基础设施,使用内置在 EHR 中的 CDSS 功能来收集基于实践的证据,从而链接机器可读的肿瘤知识库和指南库。

移动计算革命

如今,通用 Windows 和 Mac OS X 电脑是电子病历最常用的设备,但它们承担着 30 年来快速、计划外变化的负担。许多医生和患者对许多现有的 EHR 软件选择感到失望,这些软件依赖于现有的 PC 和 Mac 范例,使用 windows、图标、菜单和指针进行人机交互。

随着苹果公司在 2007 年推出 iPhone,苹果公司推出了一个自然的类人界面,可以感知触摸、触摸力、声音、视觉、听觉、位置、身体位置、身高和方向。它可以通过 Wi-Fi、蓝牙、蜂窝和近场通信(Near Field Communication,NFC)进行通信。它已经成为最容易学习和最有效的移动操作系统。目前,大多数 EHR 供应商都在通过 iPhone、iPad 和 Android 设备提供对其程序的访问,而有人则呼吁为 EHR 开发一个类似苹果的应用程序平台[27]。

管理和医疗领导对移动 HIT 进化的共识

这是第一次,我们的卫生信息技术(health information technology,HIT)的思想领导者,负责卫生信息和 EHR 技术的政府团体、国会,美国总统和他的专家小组,医学学科带头人和专业组织,医疗标准组织,信息专家,医疗保健行业,甚至很多供应商/开发者都达成共识,技术基础设施,以及最近在硬件、软件和服务方面的进步可以在医生和他们的计算机之间提供一种新的关系。在这种关系中,计算机可作为我们高效、最新、个性化、可定制、安全、可共享和知识渊博的助手。Halamka 在 2011 年提出并推广了"电子医疗(Electronic Medicine)"一词[28],以敦促 EHR 采用这些先进的移动计算技术。我冒昧地将过去 4 年开发的其他项目纳入,这些项目将帮助肿瘤学家参与到真正的肿瘤学数字化健康信息技术系统中。

云计算

云计算是指将患者数据存储在连接到 Internet 的集中式服务器中,而不是存储在我们的办公室中。云计算提供了扩展复杂软件的能力,这些复杂软件可以与不同站点的所有软件用户同时频繁更新,从而消除了我们的办公室处理数据库管理、服务器托管和数据安全的需求,从而节省了大量资金。通过互联网连接,EHR 可以更容易地与患者和其他医生共享数据,向外部注册中心发送报告,并拥有成熟的工具来帮助初学者学习该软件,随后进行更新。

应用程序

应用程序(App)是基于 web 使用的 API 多功能小型程序,具有扩展性,可以处理从其他应用程序或 EHR 程序传递的数据。应用程序可以为 EHR 提供新的功能或者从 EHR 收集数据并将其发送到注册中心或 RLS 中,这些注册中心或 RLS 可以分析这些新数据并为 EHR 程序提供 CDS。API 只是程序员可以调用以使用其他程序服务和数据功能的集合。API 包含很小的、原子数据块,这些数据块必须使用一致的单元和术语,以便更有效地处理数据。自然语言处理被用来从我们的叙述口述中提取这些微小的数据块,并创建结构化的机器可读内容,这些内容可以被计算机更有效地用于任何目的。这是一种理想的方法,允许医学专业协会为难以从其软件符合专科医师需求的 EHR 提供专门的更新工具。

模块化软件和应用程序编程接口(API)

Mandl 和 Kohane[27]设计的可替代医学应用和可再利用技术(substitutable medical apps and reusable technology,SMART)平台是将苹果应用模型系统引入 EHR 生态系统的理想平台。Mandl 最近指出该平台如何在紧急情况下工作,从而允许疾病控制和预防中心(CDC)创建一个应用程序,该应用程序可以与任何合作的 EHR 一起工作,并重塑急诊室分流工作流程,以强调转运历史,并推荐快速更新的评估和隔离指南,以处理出现在急诊室的发烧患者和最近前往埃博拉疫区旅行的患者[29]。该 App 可被所有 EHR 立即使用且易于更新，并可将医院隔离的所有患者的具体数据发送回 CDC 用于国家层面的监测和报告。他指出，这个假想的应用程序可以快速编写一次，并在几乎所有地方运行。

主动参与的、数字化连接的数字化患者、医疗设备和物联网

在这段时间里，我们的卫生系统已经发生了变化，病人不再是医疗保健系统的被动参与者，而是非常积极地参与进来，因为他们可以获得与我们在互联网上拥有的相同的医学文献，他们完整的医疗记录允许他们与提供者共同决策，从而获得更好的结果和更少的医疗事故诉讼。通过使用 web 站点或应用程序中现有的数字化教育工具，患者可以更好地了解他们的疾病、治疗方法、即将进行的程序、合适的临床试验、知情同意，并可以将他们的价值观、愿望和误解直接提供给某些机构中共享的电子病历。

随着我们进入物联网时代，伴随着廉价、准确、智能的医疗设备的产生、疾病预防和早期医疗的干预以及人们对患者健康的日益关注，这些医疗设备和可穿戴电子装置将迅速被普及，它们可以与我们的智能手机无线连接，提供便利有偿的远程医疗咨询，为在家中的患有慢性疾病的患者提供咨询，并对我们的治疗方案或疾病的不良事件进行早期监测。测量生命体征的数字化设备和数字化心电图、听诊器、照相机、眼镜、耳镜和连接在我们智能手机上的超声波设备，可以远程完成身体检查[30]。监测和分析这些数字化数据将需要大数据工具，而这些工具正在迅速发展，以改变目前的医疗实践。在使用医疗设备时，会出现某些监管和合规问题，如安全性、可审核性以及溯源等问题，正在得到解决。

精准医学

精准医疗是一种预防和治疗策略，使用大规模生物数据库（如人类基因组序列）、功能强大的方法（如蛋白质组学、代谢组学、基因组学、多种细胞分析甚至移动卫生等技术）和计算工具来分析大量数据，并考虑到个体差异。全基因组测序已达到 1 000 美元的门槛，我们正快速接近对“数字化”患者生殖系 DNA、RNA、微生物、表观基因组及其环境、解剖学和临床特征进行测序的能力[31]。这种数字化人体数据的广度将使奥巴马总统能够启动精准医疗计划，支持一个共同的医疗数据集，提供一个真正的医疗数据交互、保持私密和安全的，以及基于价值和质量的支付系统[32,33]。

“苹果化”医学（Apple-ization of medicine）

苹果公司凭借其独特的能力，创造、营销和整合最好的硬件、软件和计算机服务，并与许多不同领域的其他领先公司合作，促成了许多行业的革命性变革。现在，凭借其最新的移动操作系统、平台工具包、移动计算架构和应用软件模型，以及它们最近与许多大的医疗保健行业相关方的联盟，它有能力为医疗保健做同样的事情。Apple 的 HealthKit 能够同步健康和健康数据、个人健康记录和医疗设备数据，它是一个驻留在 iPhone 上与医疗设备协作交互的平台。iPhone 通过加速度计、麦克风、陀螺仪和 GPS（全球定位系统）传感器收集生命体征、身体位置、活动、行为、营养、肺功能和睡眠等信息，并与其他医疗设备连接，了解患者的步态、运动障碍、健康状况、语言、营养、记忆力、哮喘吸入器使用情况，以及葡萄糖和氧气等生物医学分析。数据安全可靠，符合 HIPPA 要求，并以愉快、图形化的方式提供给患者。它是一个由患者控制的双向医疗交流平台。它的数据可以通过电子方式发送到任何合作的 EHR、分析仓库存储库或提供商集团，苹果公司不能出售、误用或查看这些数据。

苹果的医学研究工具包平台是一个开源软件工具，消费者和患者能够决定他们是否愿意参与医学研究，以及他们的数据如何与研究人员共享。目的是为医学研究人员提供一种新的方法，通过使用他们的 iPhone 和 Apple Watch 收集世界各地患者的信息。研究工具包平台是为与苹果的 HealthKit 软件协同工作而设计。患者可以数字注册，签署同意书以进行试验，可以直接与研究中心联系，获得有关该研究的最新信息以及获得单项或汇总结果。创新的研究应用程序能够监测疾病对生理、心理和行为的影响，同时监视治疗的不良事件。斯坦福大学的一项心脏病研究在 3 天内登记了 1 万多名患者，而他们的预期是在 1 年内每个机构能纳入 50 名患者。

对于肿瘤学家而言，这些创新的发展将使我们的患者能够佩戴可用于通过互联网测量和发送数据到其智能手机的设备，这些智能手机将具有用于 HIPAA 兼容存储、分析和图形表示的健康平台软件，然后可以被发送到患者选择的个人提供者、医院或医疗警报捕获站点。

由无缝交互性标准和肿瘤学 RLS 提供的移动计算、可操作和共享的数据将继续为我们提供支持，以有效、迅速地生成一个对所有利益相关者“很有效”的医疗保健系统。

（文文 译 于晗 吕桂帅 校）

参考文献

1 Christensen CM. *The Innovator's Dilemma: When New Technologies Cause Great Firms to Fail*. Boston, MA: Harvard Business School Press; 1997.

2 Christensen CM, Grossman JH, Hwang J. *The Innovator's Prescription: A Disruptive Solution for Health Care*. New York, NY: McGraw-Hill; 2008.

3 American Society of Clinical Oncology. Clinical oncology requirements for the EHR (CORE). October 6, 2009. Available from: http://www.asco.org/sites/default/files/oct_2009_-_asco_nci_core_white_paper.pdf. Accessed October 15, 2015.

4 http://www.hl7.org

5 https://en.wikipedia.org/wiki/Clinical_Document_Architecture

6 Hewitt M, Greenfield S, Stovall E. *From Cancer Patient to Cancer Survivor: Lost in Transition*. Washington, DC: The National Academies Press; 2006.

7 American Society of Clinical Oncology. Chemotherapy treatment plan and summary resources. Available from: http://www.instituteforquality.org/chemotherapy-treatment-plan-and-summaries. Accessed October 18, 2015.

8 Salz T, Oeffinger KC, McCabe MS, et al. Survivorship care plans in research and practice. *CA Cancer J Clin*. 2012;**62**:101–117.

9 HL7 CDA® R2 Implementation Guide: Clinical Oncology Treatment Plan and Summary, Release 1 Clinical Oncology Treatment Plan and Summary, DSTU Release 1 2013 [cited September 5, 2014]. http://www.hl7.org/implement/standards/product_brief.cfm?product_id=327. Accessed October 15, 2015.

10 http://www.hl7.org/implement/standards/fhir/

11 http://mycourses.med.harvard.edu/ec_res/nt/6209858F-CDDD-4518-ADF8-F94DF98B5ECF/Argonaut_Project-12_Dec_2014-v2.pdf

12 http://www.healthit.gov/sites/default/files/nationwide-interoperability-roadmap-draft-version-1.0.pdf

13 Electronic Health Records (EHRs) in the Oncology Clinic: How Clinician Interaction with EHRs Can Improve Communication with the Patient http://jop.ascopubs.org/content/early/2014/07/15/JOP.2014.001385.extract.

14 McDonald CJ, Callaghan FM, Weissman A. Use of Internist's free time by ambulatory care electronic medical record systems. *JAMA Intern Med*. 2014; **174(11)**:1860–1863.

15 Kuhn T, Basch P, Barr M, Yackel T. For the medical informatics committee of the American college of physicians. Clinical documentation in the 21st century: executive summary of a policy position paper from the American college of physicians. *Ann Intern Med*. 2015;**162**:301–303.

16 Merrill M. Patients, referring docs at MD Anderson making good use of Web portal. Healthcare IT News July 6, 2010. Available from: http://www.healthcareitnews.com/news/patients-referring-docs-md-anderson-making-good-use-web-portal. Accessed March 15, 2012.

17 http://www.myopennotes.org

18 Yu PP. Knowledge bases, clinical decision support systems, and rapid learning in oncology. *J Oncol Pract*. 2015;**11**:1–4.

19 http://cancergenome.nih.gov

20 http://www.genomicsandhealth.org

21 Musen MA, Greenes RA, Middleton B: Clinical decision-support systems, in Shortliffe EH, Cimino JJ (eds): *Biomedical Informatics: Computer Applications in Health Care and Biomedicine*. London, UK, Springer London, 2014.

22 http://www.hl7.org/implement/standards/product_brief.cfm?product_id=208

23 Institute of Medicine. A foundation for evidence-driven practice: a rapid learning system for cancer. Available from: http://www.nap.edu/openbook.php?record_id=12868. Accessed March 12, 2012.

24 Abernethy AP, Etheredge LM, Ganz PA, et al. Rapid-learning system for cancer care. *J Clin Oncol*. 2010;**28**:4268–4274.

25 Accelerating Progress Against Cancer: ASCO's blueprint for transforming clinical translational cancer research. November 2011. Available at http://www.cancerprogress.net/blueprint.html. Accessed March 12, 2012.

26 Sim I, Gorman P, Greenes RA, et al. Clinical decision support systems for the practice of evidence-based medicine. *J Am Med Inform Assoc*. 2001;**8**:527–534.

27 Mandl KD, Kohane IS. No small change for the health Information economy. *N Engl J Med*. 2009;**360**:1278–1281.

28 Halamka JD The rise of electronic medicine. http://www.technologyreview.com/news/425298/the-rise-of-electronic-medicine/.

29 Mandl KD. Ebola in the United States: EHRs as a public health tool at the point of care. *JAMA Published online October*. 2014;**20**. doi: 10.1001/jama.2014.15064.

30 Sinofsky S. Patience, IoT is the new electronic. http://blog.learningbyshipping.com/2015/02/02/patience-iot-is-the-new-electronic/.

31 Topol EJ. Individualized medicine from prewomb to tomb. *Cell*. 2014;**157(1)**: 241–253.

32 Proposed Shared Nationwide Interoperability Roadmap http://www.healthit.gov/sites/default/files/nationwide-interoperability-roadmap-draft-version-1.0.pdf.

33 Francis S, Collins FS, Varmus H. A new initiative on precision medicine. *N Engl J Med*. 2015;**372**:793–795.

第四篇

致 癌 作 用

第 23 章　化学物致癌

Lorne J. Hofseth, PhD ■ Ainsley Weston, PhD ■ Curtis C. Harris, MD

概述

人类暴露于化学致癌物会引发癌症。诱发癌症的因素是相对可预测的，但也是高度变化的。这些决定因素包括：暴露的类型、暴露的量、暴露的时间和宿主（如人类）的遗传构成。遗传构成包括基因的单核苷酸变异（如脱氧核糖核酸修复基因的单核苷酸多态性）和个体的代谢组、蛋白组、微生物组、转录组、表观基因组背景。越来越多证据表明化学致癌物会改变这些终端，而炎症负荷也会影响这些过程的结局。为了解析这一过程，过去数十年里具有高敏感度和高精确度的技术获得了极大的突破。这些技术与快速发展的生物信息学相结合，使我们开始能够将终身暴露（暴露组学）与终身代谢组、蛋白组、微生物组、转录组、表观基因组和其他组学整合分析。我们乐观地预测，经过下一个十年的努力，新的系统工具将会被开发出来，这些工具不仅能协助我们确定可作为癌症风险分子标志物的个体权重化的风险标签，还能够开发出用于癌症的化学预防和个体化治疗的精准方法。

化学物质致癌是一个多阶段过程，通常是由环境、生活和饮食中以复合物形式存在的化合物致癌原引发（表 23-1，表 23-2）。典型的例子是烟草烟雾，它可诱发多部位肿瘤，其中以肺癌的发生风险最高。大多数致癌原不能直接与细胞内成分相互作用，但它们可被机体的代谢系统（其在进化过程中的功能原本是清除机体内毒素和修饰内源性物质）激活为具有致癌性和致突变性的亲电子产物，亲电子化合物能够天然地被亲核物质（如 DNA 和蛋白质）所吸引，进而通过共价键与 DNA 结合，从而导致基因损伤。一旦进入体内，虽然一些化合物可直接发挥致癌作用，但大多数致癌物要经过代谢激活（获得致癌能力）或代谢解毒的竞争过程。在人群中，这些竞争性代谢过程以及机体修复 DNA 损伤的能力和控制细胞生长的能力存在极大的变异，这是人群中患癌风险个体差异的发生基础，也反映出基因—环境相互作用，这种相互作用体现了遗传特征影响着化学致癌物暴露后的致癌效应[55,56]。这种基本代谢、DNA 修复和细胞生长控制等的差异性导致人群中个体对化学物质暴露的敏感性的差异。例如，尽管吸烟与心血管疾病、肺气肿、慢性阻塞性肺疾病（chronic obstructive pulmonary disorder，COPD）等有关，但只有大约 10%的吸烟者会发生肺癌。在肿瘤发生的这一多阶段过程中，化学物质-DNA 相互作用引起的主要基因改变被称为肿瘤起始[13,14,57]。因此，起始细胞发生了不可逆的改变，比正常细胞具有更高的发生恶性转化的风险。肿瘤启动子区的表观遗传学改变加速了起始细胞的克隆扩增[58,59]。选择性克隆增殖优势会导致癌前病变细胞的形成。这些细胞数量更多、增殖更迅速，是化学致癌物、致癌病毒和其他因子进一步作用的目标群体，因而也更易形成肿瘤。这一过程中，基因和表观遗传学的改变进一步累积[58,59]。癌基因的激活、抑癌基因和 DNA 修复基因的失活导致基因组的不稳定性或突变体表型，加速了基因改变的发生[29,60,61]。这一过程之后，将会相继发生恶性转化、肿瘤进展和转移。调控化学物质致癌效应的分子机制正逐渐被阐明，这些理论也正在帮助研究人员建立更好的研究人类癌症风险和易感性的方法。这些研究成果将逐渐用于开发有效的预防和干预策略。而且，针对抑癌基因 *TP53* 等这类“管家基因”的研究将为开发新的、靶向性治疗方法提供机遇。

表 23-1　人类化学物致癌示例

器官系统（特定病理）	化学致癌物	共致癌物
肺（小细胞和非小细胞）	吸烟	石棉
	金属：As，Be，Cd，Cr，Ni	
	BCME	
	汽车尾气	
胸膜间皮	石棉	吸烟
口腔	吸烟	
	槟榔	熟石灰 [$Ca(OH)_2$]
食管	吸烟	酒精
鼻腔鼻窦	鼻烟	玻璃粉
	异丙醇	
皮肤（阴囊）	切削油	
	煤烟尘[a]	
肝脏（血管肉瘤）	黄曲霉毒素 B_1	HBV，HCV
	氯乙烯	酒精
膀胱	芳香胺（如 4-ABP 和联苯胺）	
	烟草来源的芳香胺[b]	
ALL	苯	
淋巴和造血系统恶性肿瘤	环氧乙烷	

4-ABP，4-氨基联苯；ALL，急性淋巴细胞白血病；BCME，二氯甲醚；HBV，乙肝病毒；HCV，丙肝病毒。

[a] 早在 225 年前就有关于职业化学致癌的报道。

[b] 有详细的证据[1]。可在 1971 年启动的国际癌症研究机构专题研究计划中，发现一篇关于全面评估化学品对人类致癌风险的论文。

表 23-2 化学物致癌的一些里程碑事件

年份	事件/发现	参考文献
公元前 3000	埃德温·史密斯纸草文稿首次书面描述癌症(乳腺)	2
公元前 1500	埃及人用砷治疗肿瘤	2
1620	托马斯·温纳警告人们不要过度使用烟草	3, 4
1742	Hermann Boerhaave 和 Jean Astruc 认为炎症与癌症有关	3, 5, 6
1775	Percival Pott 描述了烟灰暴露与烟囱清洁工阴囊癌之间的关系	7
1863	Rudolf Virchow:癌症往往发生在慢性炎症部位	8
1879	Harting 和 Hesse:肺癌是矿工的一种职业病	9
1909	第一个治疗梅毒的化疗药物[砷苯类似物,化合物 606,或 salvarsan(撒尔佛散)]	10
1910	病毒被发现能致癌	11
1932	雌性激素(雌激素)会导致小鼠乳腺癌	12
1941	提出了化学致癌物致癌的两阶段:启动和促进作用	13, 14
1950	吸烟与肺癌有关	15, 16
1956	亚硝胺类致癌	17
1956	证明酶能被化学致癌物激活	18
1962, 1963	发现化学致癌物能使 DNA 和蛋白质甲基化的证据	19, 20
1964—1968	黄曲霉毒素 B_1 是一种真菌毒素,在大鼠中致癌;与 DNA 结合,对人类也是致癌的	21~23
1968	DNA 修复缺陷与癌症有关	24
1971	发现 Rb 基因致癌的“二次打击”理论,发现抑癌基因	25
1971	提出致癌的表观遗传学机制	26
1973	艾姆斯法用于测定化学致癌物的致突变性	27
1974	有证据表明化学致癌物质在人体组织中被激活形成 DNA 加合物	28
1974	突变体表型概念确定	29
1976	化学致癌物与 DNA 结合和基因-环境相互作用的个体间变异	30
1973	发现癌基因	31, 32
1977	发现肿瘤干细胞	33
1979	发现人类肿瘤中最常改变的基因-p53	34, 35
1981	首次定量评估环境和遗传学对癌症发生的影响	36
1982	介绍了分子流行病学的一般结构/模型	37
1983	单核苷酸多态性能导致肿瘤发生	38
1988	化学致癌物引起位点特异性突变	39
1990	发现结肠癌的序列突变	40
1991	P53 被确定为抑癌基因	41
1991	确定与特定环境和化学致癌物相关的 *p53* 选择性突变(突变热点)	42, 43
2001	人类基因组草图	44, 45
2002	肿瘤中的 MicroRNA 改变	46

续表

年份	事件/发现	参考文献
2002	基因表达标签预测预后	47
2005	介绍了暴露组的概念(个体从受孕到死亡所受的全部暴露)	48
2006	定义的两种人类癌症类型(结肠癌和乳腺癌)的遗传图谱	49
2006	MicroRNA 标签预测预后和生存	50
2006	FDA 批准 HPV 疫苗[重组人乳头瘤病毒四价(6、11、16、18 型)疫苗]	51
2011	美国国家研究委员会提出的开发疾病新分类的框架中介绍了精准医学	52
2012	Victor Velculescu:检测癌症患者血液循环中的染色体变化	53
2012	使用整合个人组学资料在个体水平上区分健康和疾病状态	54

癌症发生的多个阶段

癌症发生在概念上可被分为四个阶段:肿瘤起始、肿瘤促进、恶性转化和肿瘤进展(图 23-1,框 23-1)。起始和促进阶段的区别是通过对病毒和化学致癌物的研究发现的[13,14,57],并在小鼠皮肤癌模型中被正式确认。在这一模型中,小鼠局部皮肤被单次涂抹多环芳烃(polycyclic aromatic hydrocarbon,PAH 即诱发剂)继而重复涂抹巴豆油(即促进因素)[13]。在多种啮齿类动物的组织(包括膀胱、结肠、食管、肝脏、肺、乳腺、胃和气管)的癌症发生过程中也确定了肿瘤起始和促进阶段[59]。在过去的 65 年里,化学物质致癌的过程已被系统解析,相应的模式被逐渐明确,啮齿类动物和人类癌症发生过程中的相同和不同之处也逐渐被发现[63]。癌症发生需要良性过度增生细胞向恶性细胞的转化,而侵袭和转移则是基因和表观遗传学进一步改变的表现[64]。在人类研究这一过程只能通过间接的方式,分析生活方式或职业暴露于化学致癌物的相关信息。但是,对年龄依赖的癌症发生率的分析表明,肿瘤发展速率与时间的 6 次方成正比,这说明肿瘤发生至少需要 4 到 6 个相互独立的步骤[65]。在一些肿瘤中,现已部分明确这一过程中特异性的遗传学事件的时序安排。例如,在肺癌[66]和结肠癌[67]发生过程中已经发现了高概率出现的序列性遗传学和表观遗传学改变。测序技术的进展使得我们能够确定许多肿瘤标志性的基因组学特征。在常见的实体肿瘤,如起源于结肠、乳腺、脑或胰腺等的肿瘤中,平均有 33~66 个基因出现可影响蛋白产物的细微的体细胞突变[68]。特定类型的肿瘤可能含有远高于或远低于这一平均水平的突变。例如,在黑色素瘤和肺癌中,通常每个肿瘤含有大约 200 个非同义突变,反映出这些类型肿瘤的发生过程中存在强大的致突变原(分别是紫外线(ultraviolet,UV)和吸烟)[68]。

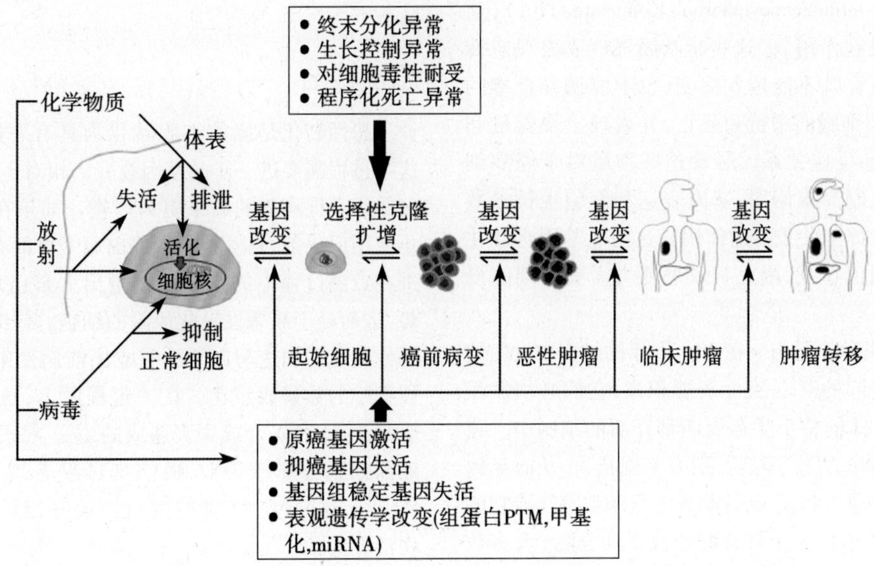

图 23-1 化学物致癌的多个步骤可以从概念上分为四个阶段:肿瘤发生、肿瘤促进、恶性转化和肿瘤进展。原癌基因的激活和抑癌基因的失活是由化学暴露引起的 DNA 共价损伤引起的突变事件。突变的积累,而不一定是它们发生的顺序,构成了癌变的多个阶段。在这些阶段,由于化学物质的暴露,也会发生表观遗传的变化

框 23-1 癌症发生的多个阶段

癌症发生包括四个阶段：

1. 肿瘤起始：正常细胞的最初变化，发生在化学致癌的早期，包括不可逆的基因突变（基因毒性起始）或表观遗传的变化（非基因毒性启动），使这些细胞能够形成肿瘤。

2. 肿瘤促进：起始细胞群的选择性克隆扩增，引起额外遗传变化而具备生长优势，从而有恶性转化的危险。肿瘤促进因子一般是非基因毒性的，不能单独驱动肿瘤发生，并且需要长时间重复暴露。

3. 恶性转化：指癌前细胞转化为表达恶性表型的细胞。额外的基因改变、癌前细胞持续暴露于 DNA 破坏因子会增加恶性转化的可能性，并可能是通过原癌基因的激活和抑癌基因的失活来介导。

4. 肿瘤进展：随着时间的推移，恶性细胞有表达恶性表型、获得更多侵袭性特征的趋势。恶性表型的一个显著特征是基因组不稳定和生长失控的倾向。在这一过程中，还会发生进一步的遗传和表观遗传变化，包括原癌基因的激活和抑癌基因的功能丧失。

肿瘤起始

关于肿瘤起始的早期概念认为，化学物质致癌的最初变化是不可逆的基因损伤。但近年来有关人类肺和结肠癌前病变组织的分子研究表明，表观遗传学的改变是癌症发生的一个早期事件。基因启动子区域的 DNA 甲基化会在转录水平引起抑癌基因的沉默[69]。因此从广义上讲，化学致癌物可被分为两类——基因毒性物质［例如苯并(a)芘或 B(a)P，通常被认为在起始阶段发挥作用］和非基因毒性物质［例如 2,3,7,8-四氯二苯并二噁英(3,7,8-tetrachlorodibenzo-p-dioxin，TCDD)或佛波酯(12-O-tetradecanoylphorbol-13-acetate，TPA)，通常被认为在促进阶段起作用］。这些非基因毒性或表观遗传性物质在作用的靶器官既不能诱发突变，也不能诱导直接的 DNA 损伤。它们调控细胞的增殖和死亡，并表现出暴露量和肿瘤形成之间的剂量-反应关系。尽管这些物质对于癌症细胞形成的具体作用机制尚未阐明，基因表达和细胞生长参数的改变可能在其中发挥至关重要的作用。这些非基因毒性化合物具有时间性和阈值特征，因此其致癌能力需要长期的慢性接触。

总之，大多数人类肿瘤是由于在 20~30 年的过程中发生的 2~8 个序列性改变引起的[68]。突变若要积累，它们必须发生于能够增殖并且在机体的整个生存周期都存活的细胞中。化学致癌物通过改变 DNA 的分子结构，引发基因错误，从而导致 DNA 合成中的突变。通常状况下，这是由于化学致癌物或它的某个功能基团与 DNA 中的一个核苷酸形成了加合物（大多数种类的化学致癌物均会引发这一过程，详见“致癌原代谢”部分）。大体而言，在动物模型中，致癌原-DNA 加合物的数量和发生的肿瘤数目之间存在正相关性[70,71]。因此，无法形成致癌原-DNA 加合物的组织几乎不能形成肿瘤。致癌原-DNA 加合物的形成是化学物质致癌理论的核心，它对于肿瘤起始（非基因毒性致癌物的描述参见“致癌原代谢”）是必需的，但不是充分的。DNA 加合物形成会导致癌基因的激活或抑癌基因的失活。因此，DNA 加合物形成被归类为肿瘤起始事件（参见下文“肿瘤进展”和“癌基因和抑癌基因”）。

肿瘤促进

肿瘤促进包括了起始细胞的选择性克隆扩增。由于突变的累积速率和细胞分裂的速率成正比，或至少是与干细胞更新速率成正比，起始细胞的克隆扩增会产生大量有进一步发生基因改变和恶性转化风险的细胞群[64,68]。促癌剂一般不具有基因毒性，也不单独致癌，并且经常（而非总是）不需要代谢激活即可产生生物学效应。这些促癌剂的特征是，可缩短组织暴露于肿瘤启动因子后肿瘤形成的潜伏期，或增加组织中肿瘤的形成数量。此外，它还可与低剂量的肿瘤启动因子（该剂量本身不足以单独致癌）协同作用诱发肿瘤的形成。巴豆油（从巴豆种子中分离获得）作为促癌剂在小鼠皮肤致癌中被广泛应用。在促癌剂中，巴豆油中作用最强的组 TPA 的作用机制被了解得最为透彻，它通过激活蛋白激酶 C 发挥作用[72]。同时具有肿瘤起始和肿瘤促进作用的化合物或制剂被称为完全致癌物（如苯并芘和 4-氨基联苯）。随着用于促癌分析的模型系统的成熟发展，在动物模型中鉴定新的促癌剂的能力获得极大提升。此外，在培养的细胞内表达的重组蛋白激酶 C 的同工酶，可用于测定配体的结合能力[73]。具有促癌特性的化合物、复杂化合物混合物或其他制剂包括二噁英、佛波酯、2,3,7,8-四氯二苯并-对-二噁英、过氧化苯甲酰、大环内酯、溴甲基苯蒽、蒽啉、苯酚、糖精、色氨酸、二氯二苯三氯乙烷(dichlorodiphenyltrichloroethane，DDT)、苯巴比妥、香烟凝集物、多氯联苯(polychlorinated biphenyls，PCB)、杀鱼菌素、环磺酸盐、雌激素和其他激素类、胆汁酸、紫外线、创伤、擦伤和其他慢性刺激（如盐水灌洗等）[74]。

恶性转化

恶性转化是癌前细胞转化为具有恶性表型细胞的过程。这个过程需要进一步的基因改变。相对于总剂量而言，频繁反复暴露于促癌剂的后果更为严重。如果在发生恶性转化前停止使用促癌剂，良性肿瘤或癌前病变可能会自行消退。肿瘤促进在致癌过程中的作用是扩增出大量已启动的、具有生长优势、进而处于高恶性转化风险的细胞。该细胞群中的部分细胞恶性转化的加速与良性肿瘤或癌前病变中细胞分裂速率和分裂细胞的数量成正比。在一定程度上，这些进一步的基因改变是由于 DNA 合成失真造成的[75]。将恶性转化概率较低的癌前细胞暴露于 DNA 损伤剂可显著增加恶性转化的发生率[76]。这一过程可能是通过原癌基因的激活和抑癌基因的失活介导的。

肿瘤进展

肿瘤进展包括恶性表型的出现和随时间推移细胞获得更多的侵袭性特征。此外，转移也包括了肿瘤细胞分泌蛋白酶的能力,从而使肿瘤细胞向原发部位以外的部位侵袭。恶性表型的显著特征之一是基因组的不稳定性倾向和细胞生长失控[77]。在这一过程中,会发生更多的基因和表观遗传学改变,其中仍然包括原癌基因的激活和抑癌基因的失活。原癌基因主要通过两种方式激活:对于 *ras* 基因家族来说,点突变经常发生在基因高度特异区域(如第 12、13、59 或 61 位密码子),而 *myc*、*raf*、*HER2* 和 *jun* 等多个基因家族成员则可因包含这些基因的染色体节段的扩增等引起表达升高。如果一些癌基因易位到强大的启动子的附近,这些基因也会过表达,例如 B 细胞恶性肿瘤中 *bcl-2* 基因易位到免疫球蛋白重链基因的启动子区。抑癌基因功能缺失通常是双重原因造成的,最常见的情况是一个等位基因发生点突变(由 DNA 加合物、DNA 复制错误或 DNA 修复错误引发),另一个等位基因因重组事件、染色体不分离或高甲基化等原因而缺失。这些改变赋予细胞生长优势和局部侵袭的能力,并最终导致向远隔部位转移扩散。虽然有证据表明特定突变事件的发生有明显的时间顺序,但是决定因素是突变的累积,而不是突变的顺序或是突变发生时所处的肿瘤发生阶段[68]。目前来自基因表达芯片的证据表明,人类肿瘤进展的模式是可替代型的,而非相互排斥型。原发肿瘤和其转移灶的基因表达谱是相近的,提示原发肿瘤的分子进展一般都在其转移灶中得以保留[78]。

过去十年间,基因测序技术发现了在常见的人类肿瘤中存在的基因组标志性改变。Vogelstein 及其同事最近将这些基因特征定义为包括一小部分“高山”(在大部分肿瘤中发生改变的基因)和绝大多数的“丘陵”(很少发生改变的基因)[68]。大约有 140 个基因当发生基因内改变时会驱动肿瘤形成。典型的肿瘤通常包括 2 到 8 个这种控制细胞命运、细胞生存和基因组稳定性的“驱动基因”的突变。其他“伴随突变”不具备选择性生长优势。总而言之,在原发肿瘤和转移灶中明确这些特殊基因及其功能对于原发肿瘤的分子诊断和个体化治疗中靶向治疗策略的选择具有重要临床价值。

表观遗传学和化学物质致癌

表观遗传学研究的是不伴有 DNA 序列变化的基因活性的改变[79]。表观遗传学研究的较为清楚的机制包括 DNA 甲基化和组蛋白修饰,它们均在不影响 DNA 序列的情况下改变基因的表达水平。另一种可归类为“表观遗传”的机制是微小 RNA(microRNA,miRNA;图 23-2,框 23-2)对于癌症的影响(详见后述)。非基因毒性和基因毒性化学致癌原均会影响这些表观学过程。在细胞水平,暴露于环境因素会留下表观遗传学标记,这些标记可用于开发新的风险评估和肿瘤预防的分子标志物[80,81]。

DNA 的甲基化被 DNA 甲基转移酶(DNA methyltransferases,DNMT)家族催化。在哺乳动物体细胞中,DNA 甲基化发生于 CpG 二核苷酸的胞嘧啶残基;在胚胎干细胞中,CpG 和非 CpG 序列均可发生 DNA 甲基化。DNMT 的表达及对 DNA 甲基化的间接作用受 DNMT3L、淋巴特异性螺旋酶、miRNA 和 piRNA(Piwi-interacting RNA)等的调控[82]。越来越多研究表明,许多化学致癌原影响了 DNA 甲基化。例如,在小鼠和肺癌患者中,烟草特异性致癌原 4-(N-甲基亚硝胺基)-1-(3-吡啶基)-1-丁酮[4-(methylnitrosoamino)-1-(3-pyridyl)-1-butanone,NNK]可诱导 DNMT 表达升高和抑癌基因的高甲基化[83]。苯并(a)芘和许多其他的非基因毒性和基因毒性化学致癌原均被发现可导致异常的甲基化模式[82,84]。化学致癌原通过多种机制导致异常甲基化模式。例如,烟草的烟雾可通过以下机制改变 DNA 甲基化:①诱导 DNA 损伤,刺激 DNMT1 募集;②尼古丁具有下调 DNMT1 mRNA 和蛋白表达的能力;③影响 DNA 结合因子,

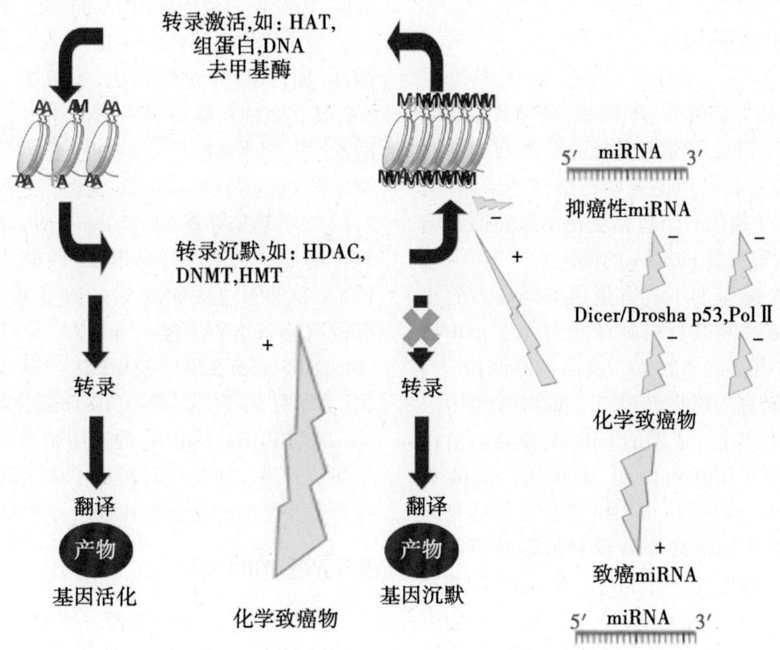

图 23-2 化学致癌物的表观遗传影响。化学致癌物可以影响表观基因组学中不同酶的活性。A,乙酰基;M,甲基;DNMT,DNA 甲基转移酶;HAT,组蛋白乙酰转移酶;HDAC,组蛋白脱乙酰酶;HMT,组蛋白甲基转移酶

框 23-2 表观遗传学

表观遗传学描述的是基因活性的变化而不是 DNA 序列的变化。它包括 *DNA* 甲基化的变化[致癌物质修饰甲基化酶(如 DNMT)引起的低甲基化/高甲基化],组蛋白尾部修饰[致癌物引起乙酰化、甲基化、瓜氨酸化、泛素化、SUMO 化和磷酸化过程相关酶类的变化(如 HDAC)]、小非编码 RNA(如基因异常、生物合成机器和/或表观遗传学机制引起的 miRNA 的改变)所引发]。

如 Sp1 的表达和活性;④导致缺氧,上调 HIF1 氧表达,进而引起甲硫氨酸腺苷转移酶 2A 表达升高[85](图 23-2)。

染色质是 DNA 缠绕于组蛋白八聚体形成的复合物,主要由组蛋白 H2A、H2B、H3 和 H4 组成。组蛋白 N 末端尾部区域内的转录后修饰(如:乙酰化、磷酸化和甲基化)可影响基因表达水平。调控组蛋白修饰的酶类包括:组蛋白去乙酰化酶(histone deacetylases,HDAC),组蛋白乙酰转移(histoneacetyltransferases,HAT)和组蛋白甲基转移酶(histonemethyltransferases,HMT)。化学致癌原可改变这些酶类的活性。例如,苯并(a)芘处理细胞会导致转录活跃的染色质标志物—组蛋白 H3 上第 4 位赖氨酸的三甲基化(H3 trimethylated at lysine 4,H3K4Me3)和 H3 上第 9 位赖氨酸的乙酰化(H3 acetylated at lysine 9,H3K9Ac)的早期富集,降低 DNMT1 和长散在重复序列-1(L1)启动子的结合。接下来,会引发细胞内 DNMT1 依赖于蛋白酶体途径的降解和 L1 启动子 CpG 岛区域持续的胞嘧啶甲基化减少[86]。与之相似的是,长期暴露于低剂量的烟草相关致癌原会导致永生化的支气管上皮细胞(HBEC-3KT)恶性转化,HDAC 表达增加,细胞周期非依赖的 DNMT1 稳定性增加和 DNA 高甲基化[87]。

化学物质致癌中的 miRNA

miRNA 的表达受到包括炎症因子、自由基和化学致癌原等在内的一系列因素的调控[88~91]。化学致癌原在体外和体内对每一个 miRNA 的特殊效应已在其他论著中详细阐述,读者可参考[91]。本章节的目的在于提供一个包括受化学致癌原影响的关键 miRNA 和调控机制等有关 miRNA 的概述。

miRNA 是长度约 22 个碱基的不具有蛋白编码能力的小 RNA,可调控 mRNA 的稳定性和其蛋白翻译能力[92]。miRNA 的表达受到转录因子及抑癌基因产物 p53 蛋白等的调控[93],且参与了包括肿瘤侵袭和转移等癌症进程[94]。miRNA 是由一个发卡前体经 Dicer 酶加工产生。成熟的 miRNA 整合到被称为 RNA 诱导沉默复合体(RNA-induced silencing complex,RISC)的蛋白复合物中,此复合物引导 miRNA 结合互补的靶向 RNA。RISC 与靶 RNA 的结合导致靶 RNA 降解或阻断后者翻译,从而阻止了相应的蛋白的生成。由于每一种 miRNA 调控着大量基因,化学暴露或炎症导致的 miRNA 表达的改变会引起一系列后果。每一种生物均编码数以百计的 miRNA,它们影响着包括细胞增殖、分化、存活和代谢等在内的关键生物学过程。自从 miRNA 被发现以来[95~97],miRNA 对基因的转录后调控已成为基因调控的重要且广泛存在的方式。在人类中,大约有 60%的蛋白编码基因受到 miRNA 调控[98,99]。由于 miRNA 的高度特异性和对基因表达的强大抑制能力,miRNA 表达调控的异常与包括肿瘤在内的许多疾病有关。这些 miRNA 在治疗领域中潜在的应用价值也逐渐引起人们关注[100~104]。不足为奇的是,miRNA 也已成为肿瘤诊断、预后和治疗预后判断的临床分子标志物[105,106]。由于暴露于环境或内生化学物质会引起 miRNA 水平发生改变,miRNA 也可能用于生物监测。由于 miRNAs 能够从靶向组织中释放入血流,因此,通过无创取样(尿液、粪便等)开展 miRNA 的分析也成为可能[107~109]。

致癌 miRNA(OncomiR)

2002 年,Croce 研究小组首次将 miRNA 和肿瘤的发生联系起来,他们发现 miR-15a 和 miR-16-1 在 B 细胞慢性淋巴细胞白血病(chronic lymphocytic leukemia,CLL)患者中表达降低[46]。自此以后,许多已知的 miRNA 基因被发现存在于通常与肿瘤相关的基因组区域[110]。因此,miRNA 本身也被认为发挥抑癌基因或癌基因的功能。而环境致癌原可通过下调抑癌功能的 miRNA 和上调致癌 miRNA 的表达而改变 miRNA 的表达。

致癌 miRNA 是在驱动癌症表型中具有决定作用的 miRNA。正如本章所探讨的那样,肿瘤是一系列生物途径中所参与基因的大量的遗传学和表观学异常的累积所致。尽管存在这种复杂性,某些特定肿瘤可能依赖于单个的、强大的癌基因,消除这个癌基因能够逆转恶性表型。支持这一理论的经典成功例证是,在慢性髓细胞性白血病中,使用 BCR-ABL 激酶的抑制剂靶向 Philadelphia 染色体可发挥良好治疗效果[111,112]。另一个例证是 Herceptin 和其在治疗 $Her2^+$ 乳腺癌中的成功[113,114]。单个癌基因也能影响 miRNA 的表达。例如,Myc 能够诱导致癌 miRNA17/92 簇表达,抑制抑癌 miRNA(如 let-7,miRNA-29)的表达[115,116]。致癌 miRNA 控制着许多癌症相关通路,因此靶向致癌 miRNA 的潜能非常具有吸引力。方法之一是确定能够引起致癌 miRNA 表达升高或失衡的外源性和内源性(如自由基)化学物质。miR-21 是一种关键的致癌 miRNA,其在多种人类肿瘤中上调[90,117]。暴露于诱癌剂(如亚砷酸盐[118]、活性氧[118]、过氧化氢[119]、UV 辐射[120]、TPA[121] 和 NO 等[122])会上调 miR-21 表达。此外,miRNA-21 缺失可抑制 7,12-二甲基苯并蒽(7,12-dimethylbenz[a]anthracene,DMBA)/TPA 诱导的皮肤癌。miR-21 的靶点包括多个抑癌基因如 PTEN 和 TPM1,及 DNA 错配修复基因如 MSH2 和 MSH6[117]。其他致癌 miRNA(包括 miRNA's-17/92,-20,-106,-107,-141,-146,-155,-181,-200,-221/222,-373 等)也被发现是化学致癌物[如苯并芘-7,8-二醇-9,10-环氧化物(B[a]P-7,8-diol 9,10-epoxide,BPDE),DMBA]的作用靶点[92,123],这些致癌物会引起其表达升高。这让我们初步了解了防治这些化学物质相关癌症所需要靶向的化合物和致癌 miRNA 的分子靶标特征。

抑癌性 miRNA

多种肿瘤与 miRNA 表达异常相关,miRNA 表达谱已成为肿瘤分型的一种方式[105,124~126]。通常,肿瘤细胞中具有抑癌基因功能的 miRNA 表达水平降低[100,127~130]。每一种抑癌性 miRNA 可调控在不同肿瘤相关通路中发挥作用的一系列基因的表达。尽管每一种抑癌性 miRNA 只有部分直接靶点被阐明，可以确定的是一种抑癌性 miRNAs 缺失的整体影响会促进癌症进程的一个或多个方面。在一些情况下，动物模型的实验结果表明缺失某一特定的抑癌性 miRNA 会导致肿瘤发生，而重新表达该抑癌性 miRNA 又可以抑制肿瘤[129,131~133]。对 miRNA-34a 的研究是例证之一。miRNA-34a 是 p53 转录网络的组分之一[134]，可调控肿瘤干细胞的存活[135,136]，它可能是目前临床试验中最具有应用前景的 miRNA 之一[127,136]。miRNA-34a 在肿瘤中表达降低，在不同类型肿瘤的动物模型中被重新表达后可阻断肿瘤起始和/或抑制肿瘤生长[137~142]。因此，miRNA 替代疗法在肿瘤治疗中可能具有相当大的应用前景。但是，与其他基于小 RNA 的治疗方法类似，目前最大的瓶颈是如何将 RNA 输送到靶向位点[130,133,143,144]。针对这一挑战，研究人员已开发出了一系列给药系统。许多方法使用的是商业化合成的分子，这种分子通过新的化学修饰以提高稳定性[144~146]。此外，合成的 RNA 通常不是以成熟单链 miRNA 的形式，而是以双链形式生产出来。因为双链形式不仅能增强稳定性，还可以激发哺乳动物防御系统识别双链 RNA。为了克服细胞 RNA 摄取的屏障，化学修饰的 RNA 通常情况下与另一种分子（如胆固醇）等耦联或被包裹入纳米颗粒[123,141]。这其中的负面影响包括：①修饰后的分子的特异性和功能可能会与天然 miRNA 不同，导致疗效降低；②产生诸如免疫应答、包装成分的毒性、激活补体系统等不良反应；③成本增加。通过腺病毒或慢病毒载体输送小 RNA 前体的策略在动物模型中经常使用，但在人体中的安全性尚未明确。因此，尽管研究者在系统递送治疗性小 RNA 方面取得了一定的成功，但仍面临着诸如安全性、效率和经济成本等一系列的挑战。

化学致癌物引起抑癌性 miRNA 表达改变（通常是降低）的例子很多，已在相关综述中详细论述[91]。需要强调的是暴露于烟草烟雾的小鼠的肺中抑癌性 miRNA let-7 家族和 miR-34b 的表达的降低。有趣的是，停止抽烟 1 周后，let-7 家族的表达水平得到恢复。但是，有一部分 miRNA（miR-34b、miR-345、miR-421、miR-450b、miR-466 和 miR-469）的表达只得到部分恢复。因此，miRNA 可作为效应的生物标志物。只有暴露于高剂量，并且持续足够长的时间才能引发与 miRNA 改变相关的吸烟相关癌症进程[147]。

化学致癌原诱导的 miRNA 表达改变的机制

在低剂量和短期暴露下，环境致癌原诱发的 miRNA 水平的改变是可逆的；而在更高剂量和长时间暴露下，则会出现不可逆的改变。这些不可逆的 miRNA 改变对于未来的肿瘤表型的出现具有预测价值[91,147]。化学致癌原导致 miRNA 表达失衡和改变的机制主要包括基因异常、生物合成机制的改变，和/或表观遗传学机制[92,115,116]（框 23-2）。基因异常包括染色体重排、基因扩增、缺失和突变[92]。第一篇在肿瘤发生中明确 miRNA 作用的研究论文中阐述了这一过程。miRNA-15/16-1 簇被发现在慢性淋巴细胞白血病中表达缺失，进而累积减少[46]。生殖细胞突变也被发现与该簇 miRNA 的累积减少有关[148]。多种机制会导致 miRNA 生物合成机制改变，从而影响 miRNA 水平。例如，关键生物合成酶 Dicer 和 Drosha 和或它们复合物的突变会导致 miRNA 产生的异常[149]。实际上，已发现一系列化学致癌原（如 PAH，杂环化合物，亚硝胺，吗啉，乙基亚硝基脲，苯衍生物，羟胺和烯烃等）通过与 Dicer 结合影响 miRNA 成熟[91,149]。近年来环境化学致癌原对于 miRNA 机器的影响已研究的较为清楚[91]，概括起来主要通过三种机制。第一，出于对 DNA 损伤的反应，p53 与 miRNA 相互联系会调节胞核中 miRNA 基因的表达。第二，环境致癌原的亲电子代谢物会与 miRNA 前体的亲核位点结合，形成 miRNA 加合物，导致其在细胞质中不能接近 Dicer 的催化口袋。第三，环境致癌原的代谢物会在 miRNA 催化位点近端与 Dicer 结合，抑制 miRNA 前体的成熟[91]（图 23-2）。但是，致癌性 miRNA 上调的机制仍不清楚。这一机制对于更好地理解化学物质致癌和化学预防具有重要的意义。因此，多项正在进行的研究力图发现能够抑制致癌性 miRNA 生物合成的特异性小分子抑制剂[150]。

由于非基因毒性致癌原也可以影响 miRNA 的表达[91]，因此存在 DNA 损伤反应途径之外的调控 miRNA 表达的机制。如表观遗传学机制（如抑癌性 miRNA 的高甲基化），对于转录机器的直接影响和转录后修饰均可调控 miRNA 表达。例如，结肠癌中 miRNA-124a 的高甲基化导致癌基因 Cdk6 激酶的表达上调和抑癌基因 Rb 的磷酸化[151]。后续已有越来越多的其他抑癌性 miRNA 被发现存在 CpG 岛的高甲基化[152~155]。miRNA 也被发现可以靶向和改变 DNMT 和其他表观修饰酶类（HDAC 和组蛋白乙酰转移酶）的活性[156~159]（图 23-2）。在这一过程中，致癌原反过来又可以发挥不可或缺的作用。例如，硫化镍尽管只是一种弱的致突变剂，但却是一种强力致癌原，能够通过启动子-DNA 高甲基化下调 miRNA-152 表达[157]。与之类似的是，ROS 通过作用于 DNMT1 增加 miR-199a 和 miR-125b 启动子的甲基化，从而抑制 miR-199a 和 miR-125b 表达[160]。

miRNA 由 RNA 聚合酶Ⅱ（Pol Ⅱ）及相关因子转录[92,161,162]。因此，环境致癌原对 Pol Ⅱ和相关因子的影响显然会导致 miRNA 转录调控异常，进而改变 miRNA 水平。例如，作为 p53 的直接的和保守性靶基因，miR-34a 和 miR-34b/c 介导了 p53 诱导凋亡、细胞周期阻滞和衰老[163]。当 p53 发生突变时（通常由环境致癌原诱导[164]），miR-34a 和 miR-34b/c 的转录活性也受到影响[165]。与之相似的是，环境致癌原也可影响 Pol Ⅱ的活性[166]。

总之，现已明确化学致癌原能够改变 miRNA 的表达。如同许多生物实体一样，这些改变是对暴露于化学刺激的适应性反应。miRNA 发挥作用的机制包括激活 p53、细胞周期阻滞、诱导凋亡（通过抑癌性 miR-34 家族）。原癌基因突变（“起始”，例如 k-ras）能诱导 let-7 家族等其他抑癌性 miRNA 的表达[167]。长期、持续的暴露会导致 miRNA 表达出现不可逆的改变。例如 miR-34 和 let-7 家族成员的失活会导致 p53 的抑制和 k-ras 的激活[91,168]。如果 miRNA 替代治疗成为主流，这将成为改变甚至是逆转化学致癌原诱导的癌症进程的强有力的工具。有趣的是，近期研究发现，哺乳动物摄取的植物来源的 miRNA 能够在哺乳动物（包括人类）体内被检测到，并且在哺乳动物体内具有活性，可发挥抑制肿瘤的作用[169~171]。

基因-环境交互作用和个体差异

人类化学物致癌的奠基石是基因-环境交互作用（图 23-3，

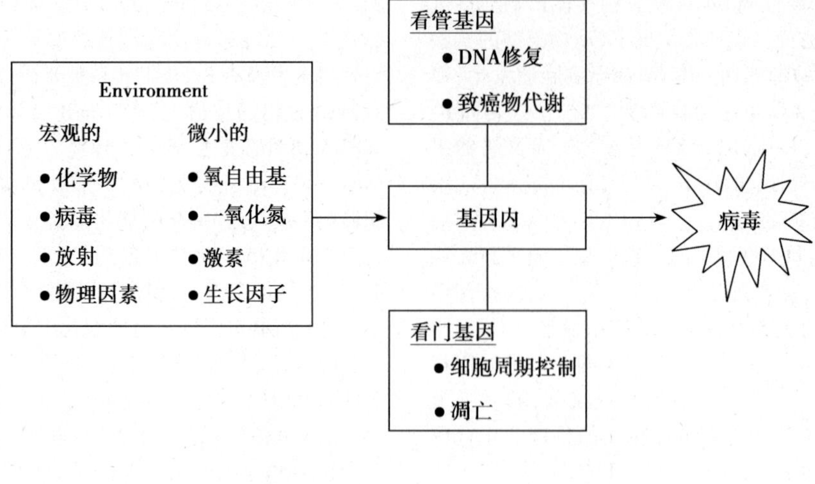

图 23-3 基因-环境相互作用的概念是多方面的：①环境化学物质被代谢基因的产物所改变；②环境化学物质破坏致癌物质代谢基因的表达（诱导或抑制）；③环境暴露导致癌症相关基因的变化（突变）。癌症相关基因分为看门基因（如 APC）和看管基因（如 MSH1 和 MLH1）基因。这些基因与外部和内部环境因子的相互作用可能导致维持基因稳定性和细胞增殖的调控通路紊乱

框 23-3）[56,172]。这一复杂系统中宿主元素的遗传变异决定了潜在的个体间对化学物致癌易感性的差异。在化学物致癌中起作用或可能起作用的蛋白质的功能多态性包括代谢外源物质的酶（激活或解毒）、DNA 损伤修复酶、激活磷酸化级联信号系统的细胞表面受体和细胞周期控制基因（如作为信号转导级联组分的癌基因和抑癌基因）。

> 框 23-3 基因-环境交互作用
>
> 已确定的修饰对化学致癌物反应的基因包括那些参与致癌物代谢（如 p450）、DNA 修复（如 NER）、细胞信号、细胞周期和激素调节的基因。

化学物质或外源物质遇到生物系统就会因机体的代谢而发生改变，这是基因-环境交互作用的第一层面。大概 40 年前人们就已知道致癌物代谢的能力及在这些代谢过程中形成大分子加合物的能力存在个体间差异[30]。细胞色素 P450（CYP）多基因家族很大程度负责对人类环境中大量不同的化学致癌物的代谢激活和解毒[173]。细胞色素 P450 是 Ⅰ 相代谢酶，其作用是把一个氧原子加到底物上。这类酶可被多环芳烃和氯化烃诱导[173]。Ⅱ 相代谢酶则作用于已被氧化的底物，也参与外源物质的代谢。一些 Ⅱ 相代谢酶是甲基转移酶、乙酰转移酶、谷胱甘肽转移酶、尿苷 5 基转二磷酸葡糖醛酰转移酶、磺基转移酶、烟酰胺腺嘌呤二核苷酸（nicotinamide adenine dinucleotide，NAD）-和烟酰胺腺嘌呤一核苷酸磷酸酯（nicotinamide adenine dinucleotide phosphate，NADP）-依赖的醇脱氢酶、醛和类固醇脱氢酶、醌还原酶、NADPH 硫辛酰胺脱氢酶、偶氮还原酶、醛酮还原酶、转氨酶、酯酶和水解酶。激活和解毒的途径通常是竞争性的，这为致癌物代谢致 DNA 损伤因子的倾向性的个体差异提供了进一步可能。当基因-环境交互作用的第二个层面即出现酶被诱导或被抑制时，情况就更为复杂。此时，环境暴露改变了基因表达，暴露于特定化合物会引起负责致癌物代谢的基因的上调或抑制。

基因-环境交互作用的第三个层面发生于化合物改变基因结构（环境诱发的异常 DNA）。前致癌物一旦经过代谢激活成为最终的致癌物，即可共价结合到包括 DNA 在内的细胞大分子上。这种 DNA 损伤可通过几种不同机制修复[174]。DNA 修复速率和精确度差异可影响致癌原加合物的形成量（如生物有效剂量），以及最后的遗传损伤数量。细胞周期控制基因（丝氨酸/苏氨酸激酶、转录因子、细胞周期蛋白、细胞周期依赖蛋白激酶抑制剂和细胞表面受体）多态性的影响效果还很不清楚。然而，分子流行病学证据表明，这类基因的一些常见变异在化学致癌易感性方面发挥一定作用[175]。多态性作为人群潜在的易感标志的评价参见其他著作[176]。

致癌物代谢

肿瘤易感性的个体间差异和有效的人类肿瘤风险评价包括确定可遗传的宿主因素和进行暴露评估。历史上曾通过使用特定的药物（如咖啡因，异喹胍、右美沙芬、氨苯砜和异烟肼等）来测定代谢多态性。如今，这些方法已被更直接的基因检测所取代。基因检测使对无法获得指示药物的众多宿主因素的研究成为可能，并已被广泛用于多种肿瘤[177~181]。这些研究对药物基因组学、致癌物质活化和解毒倾向的遗传指标等领域均产生了重要影响[182,183]。

CYP P450 多态性（参与了致癌原激活），以及谷胱甘肽-S-转移酶、尿苷二磷酸（uridine diphosphate，UDP）、葡萄糖醛酸转移酶、磺基转移酶和 N-酰基转移酶（均参与了致癌原的激活和解毒）等可以解释人群肿瘤易感性的差异。有证据表明，功能完整的 *GSTM1* 基因的缺失与烟草相关肺癌的风险增加有关[184]。同样，*GSTM1* 和 *GSTT1* 基因的缺失增加了氡暴露引起

的肺癌的风险[185]。CYP2A13 是最活跃的参与烟草特异性致癌物 NNK 代谢激活的 CYP P450 成员，CYP2A13 基因的多态性与肺腺癌风险显著降低相关[186]。研究发现，XRCC1、GSTM1 和 COMT 多态性与吸烟女性的肺癌风险密切相关，这支持了该疾病中修复、烟草代谢和雌激素代谢之间存在相互作用，也使得关于女性肺癌风险增加的争论延续下去[187]。此外，UDP 葡萄糖醛酸转移酶（如 *UGT1A1*、*UGT1A9* 和 *UGT2B7*）也与头颈部肿瘤有关。*NAT1* 和 *NAT2* 基因活性降低的变异体可导致慢乙酰基化表型，遗传了这种变异体的人更容易发生芳香胺诱导的膀胱癌。这种情况可能也发生于因吸入烟草烟雾而暴露的人群中[188,189]。在过去的 25 年间，对致癌原代谢、个体间变异和肿瘤风险的认识已取得了长足的进步，相关进展可参见综述[190]。

多环芳香烃（PAH）如苯并芘［B（a）P］是第一类被化学分离的致癌物[191]。它们是由数量不等的融合苯环组成的化合物，由矿物燃料和植物材料不完全燃烧所产生，也是常见环境污染物。PAH 本身是惰性物质，需要代谢才发挥其生物学作用[191]。这一代谢过程包括多个步骤，包括起始的环氧化（细胞色素 P450）、环氧化物的水合作用（环氧化物水合酶）和随后的烯键间的环氧化[173,192]，从而形成了最终的致癌代谢物。以苯并芘为例，形成的是苯并芘-7，8-二醇-9，10-环氧化物（BPDE）[193]。细胞色素 P450（如 CYP1A1）代谢的生物学已被阐明，这为细胞色素在人群中可诱导性及其个体间差异提供了分子基础，而 CYP 的含量在人群也被发现存在变异[194]。BPDE 芳烃环的第 10 位可自发打开形成一个可与包括 DNA 在内的细胞大分子共价结合（加合物）的正碳离子。在所形成的若干种加合物中，含量最丰富的是与脱氧鸟苷环外氨基加合的产物（［7R］-N2-［10-7β，8a，9a-三羟基-7，8，9，10-四氢化苯并芘基］-脱氧鸟苷；［7R］-*N2*-［10-（7β，8a，9a-trihydroxy-7，8，9，10-tetrahydro-benz［a］pyrene）yl］-deoxyguanosine，BPdG）。单电子氧化是 PAH 激活的另一条通路，即在中间位置（L 区）形成一个自由基阳离子。在鸟嘌呤 C8 位形成的 DNA 加合物（BP-6-C8Gua 和 BP-6-C8dGua）和在鸟嘌呤和腺嘌呤的 N7 位形成的（BP-6-N7Gua 和 BP-6-N7Ade）可发生自发脱嘌呤。有确切证据证明，这些加合物可通过尿液排出[195]。

在香烟烟雾、汽车尾气、工业环境和某些煮熟的食物中均含有芳香胺。4-氨基联苯被认为是引起吸烟者和橡胶业工人膀胱癌的元凶[196]。此外，硝基多环芳烃是芳香胺经硝基还原作用生成的环境污染物。芳香胺还可通过依赖乙酰辅酶 A 的乙酰化作用转变为芳香酰胺[197]。乙酰化表型在人群中存在差异。具有快速乙酰化表型的人患结肠癌风险增高（尤其是吸烟者）[198]，而具有慢乙酰化表型的人患膀胱癌风险增高[198]。后一个相关性可能源于芳香胺通过 *N*-氧化激活是芳香胺代谢的竞争途径。*N*-羟基化产物一旦质子化（如在膀胱中）则性质活泼，可致 DNA 损伤。

芳香胺和芳香酰胺的最初激活步骤都是由 CYP1A2 催化的 *N*-氧化。*N*-羟基芳胺与 DNA 的反应可被酸催化，进而被乙酰辅酶 A 依赖的 *O*-乙酰化酶或 3′-磷酸腺苷-5′磷酰硫酸依赖的 *O*-磺基转移酶激活。*N*-芳基羟肟酸由 *N*-羟基芳胺乙酰化或芳香酰胺的 *N*-羟基化形成，它们无亲电子性而需要进一步激活。这其中主导的途径是通过乙酰转移酶催化的重排反应形成有活性的 *N*-乙酰氧基芳香胺。磺基转移酶将其催化形成 *N*-磺酰氧基芳香胺。这个复杂的通路最终形成两种主要类型的加合物，即酰胺（乙酰化）和胺（未乙酰化）。

在烹饪过程中，氨基酸、肌酐和葡萄糖的热分解（>150℃）可产生杂环胺。杂环胺被认为是食品致突变剂，它们可形成 DNA 加合物，诱发灵长类的肝脏肿瘤[199]。这些化合物可被 CYP1A2 激活，其代谢物可在人体内形成 DNA 加合物。杂环胺的 N-羟基代谢物如 2-氨基-3-甲基咪唑-［4，5-f］喹啉（IQ）可直接与 DNA 反应。*N*-羟基代谢物的酶促 *O*-酯化在食物致突变剂激活中起关键作用。由于 N-羟基代谢物是乙酰转移酶的良好底物，因此这些化合物可能与结直肠癌相关。

黄曲霉（*aspergillus flavus*）的代谢物黄曲霉毒素（B1、B2、G1 和 G2）可污染麦子、谷物和坚果。在发展中国家，饮食摄入的黄曲霉毒素和肝癌发病率成正相关，而这些地方的粮食霉变率很高。在黄曲霉毒素 B1 和 G1 的第 8、9 位存在一个烯烃双键，可被几种细胞色素 P450 氧化[173,192]，提示 8、9 位的双烯键是激活位点。进一步支持该机制的证据来自对肝癌中 DNA 加合物和 TP53 突变率的研究。在食物霉变很常见的中国和非洲，肝癌患者 *TP53* 第 249 位密码子 G∶C 颠换为 T∶A 的频率很高[42,43,200]。这一现象与黄曲霉素 B1 的代谢激活和致癌物-脱氧鸟苷加合物的脱嘌呤形成一致。

致癌性 *N*-亚硝胺是环境中普遍存在的污染物。在食物、酒精性饮料、化妆品、切削油、液压油、橡胶制品和烟草中均可检出 N-亚硝胺[201]。烟草特有的 *N*-亚硝胺（tobacco-specific *N*-nitrosamines，TSN）如 NNK 并非由热分解形成，它是鼻烟和嚼烟具有高致癌性的原因[202]。TSN 的非对称性使得其既可形成小的烷基加合物，也可形成大的加合物：如 NNK 代谢物可产生带正电荷的吡啶-氧代丁基离子或带正电荷的甲基离子，二者均可使 DNA 烷基化[70,203]。内源性亚硝胺可由胺单独与硝酸盐或胺与亚硝酸盐在酸存在下反应形成。因此，在乙醛（来自乙醇）存在时，亚硝酸盐（常被用来腌制肉类）和 L-半胱氨酸可形成 N-亚硝基噻唑-4-羧基酸。*N*-二甲基亚硝胺可被乙醇诱导的 CYP2E1 催化发生进行羟基化，形成不稳定的 a-羟基亚硝胺。后者可被分解成甲醛和甲基重氮氢氧化物。甲基重氮氢氧化物及其相关化合物是强烷化剂，可在 DNA 多个部位添加小的功能基团。

非遗传毒性致癌物可在微环境中通过影响激素和生长因子而起作用，或通过自由基的作用间接导致 DNA 损伤和突变。这些化学物质没有活性或活性极低，不能通过代谢激活。它们的另一个特征是在生物系统中持久存在，导致在食物链中不断蓄积。它们可通过至少三种机制激活氧自由基形成：有机氯和 Ah 受体相互作用诱导细胞色素 P450 及相关的氧自由基形成；与其他受体如 IFN-γ 受体相互作用，刺激初级免疫应答元件，也会产生氧自由基；一些物质如石棉可与二价铁反应促进氧自由基形成。产生的氧自由基可导致 DNA 损伤。一些所谓的“非遗传毒性”致癌物更应当被看作“氧自由基的激发物”。确实,涉及氧自由基形成的慢性炎症状态也是癌变的风险因素[204~208]。

DNA 损伤和修复

化学致癌物诱发肿瘤风险的个体差异的另一方面体现在机体对化学致癌物所致 DNA 损伤的修复能力的差异。DNA 损伤可启动复杂的信号传递网络[209]。致癌物可通过形成大的芳香族加合物、小的烷基加合物、氧化作用、二聚作用及脱氨作用改变 DNA 的化学结构。此外,致癌物还可引起 DNA 的双链或单链断裂。化学致癌物还可引起 DNA 表观遗传学改变,如改变 DNA 甲基化状态,从而引起特定基因的表达沉默[69]。在环境中存在的化学致癌物为是混合存在的,因此各种环境暴露所形成的致癌物-DNA 加合物种类繁杂。

近来发现了许多 DNA 修复基因,也发现了越来越多的多态性。分子流行病学研究表明这些属性中的遗传学变异可能成为人类肿瘤的危险因素,并可用于定制肿瘤化疗方案[210,211]。通常,该类型分子流行病学研究最初关注的是如工人、服用治疗性药物或吸烟者等高暴露人群。已在吸烟相关的肿瘤中发现了一系列 DNA 修复基因的多态性[212]。最近,出现了一种称为“hide-then-hit”假说的理论,这种理论强调了 DNA 修复相关的变异体在逃避检查点监测中的重要作用。只有那些由低外显率的 DNA 修复基因的变异体引起的修复能力轻微受损的细胞才能够在不触发细胞周期检查点监测的情况下获得生长机会,并积累起肿瘤形成所需的遗传学改变[213]。

BPDE 可与脱氧鸟苷的环外氨基(N2)反应,并占据 DNA 双螺旋小沟,这是多环芳烃所特有的特征。BPDG 这个加合物可能是苯并芘在哺乳动物体内形成的最常见和持续存在的加合物,而其他形式则只是可能存在。加合物如 BPDG 被认为可引发 ras 基因突变,该基因突变在吸烟相关性肺癌中很常见[214,215]。芳香胺加合物比较复杂,因为芳香胺有乙酰化和非乙酰化中间产物,可与脱氧鸟苷和脱氧腺苷的 C8、N2 甚至还有 O6 结合。但大多数加合物还是 C8 脱氧鸟苷加合物,主要占据 DNA 双螺旋大沟[216]。

黄曲霉毒素 B1 和 G1 通过 8、9 位烯烃键的羟基化激活,在脱氧鸟苷 N7 位形成加合物。它们相对不稳定,在中性 pH 下的半衰期约为 50h;其脱嘌呤产物可在尿液中检测到[217]。黄曲霉毒素 B1-N7-脱氧鸟苷加合物也可以通过开环产生两个嘧啶加合物。此外,另一种情况是如果原加合物发生水解,可形成黄曲霉毒素 B1-8,9-二氢二醇,从而恢复原来的 DNA 分子结构[218]。

DNA 烷基化可以发生在许多位点,或者是在某些 N-亚硝胺的代谢激活之后,或者是直接通过 *N*-烷基脲(*N*-甲基-*N*-亚硝基脲)或 *N*-亚硝基胍的作用。在 DNA 中形成损伤的质子化烷基官能团通常攻击以下亲核中心:腺嘌呤(N1、N3 和 N7)、胞嘧啶(N3)、鸟嘌呤(N2、O6 和 N7)和胸腺嘧啶(O2、N3 和 O4)。其中一些病变已知是可以修复的(*O*6-甲基脱氧鸟苷),而另一些则不能修复(*N*7-甲基脱氧鸟苷)。这就解释了为什么 *O*6-甲基脱氧鸟苷是一种促突变性病变,而 *N*7-甲基脱氧鸟苷则不是[219,220]。

DNA 损伤的另一个潜在致突变原因是 DNA 甲基化胞嘧啶残基的脱氨作用。5-甲基胞嘧啶约占脱氧核苷酸的 3%。在这种情况下,CpG 二核苷酸的脱氨导致了 TpG 错配。这种病变修复后通常会恢复 CpG;然而,修复可能导致突变(TpA)[221]。如果尿嘧啶糖基化和 G-T 错配修复不充分,胞嘧啶脱氨也能产生 C→T 转变。

氧自由基损伤可形成胸腺嘧啶乙二醇或 8-羟基脱氧鸟苷加合物。暴露于有机过氧化物(儿茶酚、对苯二酚、4-硝基喹啉-N-氧化物)可导致氧自由基损伤。然而,在脂质过氧化和某些酶的催化循环过程中以及环境(如烟草烟雾)也会产生氧自由基和过氧化氢[204,222]。某些药物和塑化剂可以刺激细胞产生过氧化物酶体。当炎症细胞暴露于像佛波酯这类的肿瘤促进剂时,蛋白激酶 C 可介导氧自由基的下形成[223]。氧自由基可通过诱导 NO 合成酶参与脱氨反应[224]。

维持基因组完整性需要减少 DNA 损伤。因此,DNA 修复能力下降与癌症发生、出生缺陷、过早衰老和寿命缩短有关。DNA 修复酶作用于化学致癌物引起的 DNA 损伤部位,已知的作用机制主要有 6 种:直接 DNA 修复、核苷酸切除修复、碱基切除(direct DNA repair, nucleotide excision repair, base excision, BER)修复、非同源末端连接(双链断裂修复)、错配修复和同源重组(homologous recombination, HR)(复制后修复)[225,226]。

在非致命性 DNA 损伤存在的情况下,细胞周期进展被推迟以进行修复。这个高度协调的过程涉及多个基因。DNA 损伤识别传感器触发信号转导级联反应,下游因子与负责 DNA 修复的蛋白协同作用,将细胞周期阻滞于 G1 和 G2 期。虽然至少有六种不同的修复机制,但其中五种即含有完成 DNA 修复所必需的用以逐步完成修复功能的大量蛋白复合物。

一般来说,DNA 修复需要损伤识别、损伤清除或切除、再合成或小片段合成以及连接。至今已克隆出 130 余个参与了其中 5 种 DNA 修复途径的人类基因。这些基因及其特殊功能的列表可以参见其他著作[227]。这些基因负责 DNA 修复的保真度;当它们有缺陷时,突变率增加,表现出突变体表型[29,60,61]。发生于至少 30 个 DNA 修复相关基因的突变与癌症易感性增加或过早衰老有关(表 23-3)[227]。此外,部分基因中的常见多态性的作用与基因-环境相互作用场景中易感性的增加有关(这经 Weston 和 Harris 讨论过[176])。事实上,分子流行病学证据表明,与吸烟有关的肺癌与核苷酸切除修复基因 XPC(ERCC2)的多态性有关[228]。

直接 DNA 修复受 DNA 烷基转移酶的影响。在没有 DNA 链断裂的情况下,这些酶催化烷基基团从烷基化的碱基(例如,*O*6-甲基脱氧鸟苷)转移到其自身活性位点的半胱氨酸残基。因此,该酶的一个分子只能够修复一个 DNA 烷基化损伤,这是一种自杀机制。启动子高甲基化导致的这一机制失活与结肠癌中 Kras 基因 G→A 突变有关[229]。

表 23-3　与 DNA 修复基因突变相关的疾病易感性和疾病综合征的例证

基因	功能	疾病或肿瘤
肿瘤易感性		
MMRa		
MLH1	损伤识别	遗传性非息肉病性大肠癌 2b，胶质瘤
MLH2	DNA 结合	遗传性非息肉病性大肠癌 1，卵巢癌
MSH3	—	子宫内膜癌
MSH6	滑动夹	子宫内膜癌，遗传性非息肉病性大肠癌 1
PMS1	损伤识别	遗传性非息肉病性大肠癌 3
PMS2	修复启动	遗传性非息肉病性大肠癌 4，胶质母细胞瘤
NER		
BRCA-1	将 *p53* 转录导向 DNA 修复通路	乳腺癌，卵巢癌
RB1	细胞周期限制	视网膜母细胞瘤、乳腺癌和进展性骨肉瘤
DSB		
BRCA-2	调节 RAD51	乳腺癌，胰腺癌
HR		
RAD54	解旋酶	结肠癌，乳腺癌，非霍奇金淋巴瘤
其他		
TP53（DSB，NER，HR）	细胞周期控制；核酸外切酶；凋亡；DNA 结合	结肠癌，在人类癌症中普遍存在的躯体缺陷；遗传于利-弗劳梅尼综合征和部分乳腺癌
hOgg1（多种）	糖基化酶	肿瘤易感性
着色性干皮病（XP）		
NER		
XPD	DNA 解旋酶	皮肤和神经系统，但发病晚于 XPA
XPB	DNA 解旋酶	皮肤病变
XPG	核酸内切酶	急性阳光过敏，症状轻微；晚期皮肤癌
XPC（和 BER）	核酸外切酶	精神发育迟滞；皮肤敏感性；头小畸型
DDB1 和 *DDB2*	与特异性 DNA 损伤结合	XPE——轻微的皮肤敏感
XPA	损坏传感器	XPA——皮肤和神经问题：最严重的 XP
XPC	损坏传感器	XPC——皮肤、舌头和嘴唇癌症
XPE	损坏传感器	XPE——神经正常
PRR		
POLH	聚合酶	XPV——轻微至严重皮肤敏感；神经正常
其他综合征		
NER		
Cockaynes		
CSB	ATP 酶	皮肤、眼睛、神经和躯体异常；身材矮小；进行性耳聋、智力低下、神经退行性变、早逝；有时与 XPB 一起出现
Juberg-Marsidi		

续表

基因	功能	疾病或肿瘤
ATRX	假定的解旋酶	地中海贫血/精神发育迟滞
SB		
Nijmegen		
NBS1	Nibrin,细胞周期控制	小头症;精神发育迟滞;免疫缺陷;生长迟缓;辐射敏感性;倾向恶性肿瘤
共济失调毛细血管扩张症(Ataxia-telangiectasia)		
ATM	磷酸化	神经系统缺陷,表现为不能协调肌肉动作;皮肤和角膜毛细血管扩张; 白血病、淋巴瘤和其他恶性肿瘤(乳腺癌?)
MRE11(共济失调样)	核酸外切酶	DNA 损伤的敏感性;基因组不稳定性;端粒缩短;异常减数分裂; 重度联合免疫缺陷症
PRKDC	丝/苏氨酸激酶	严重联合免疫缺陷(SCID)
Bloom 综合征		
BLM	DNA 解旋酶	自发性淋巴及其他恶性肿瘤发生率高;高发 SCE
范可尼贫血(Fanconi anemia)		
FANCA-G	蛋白控制	多个先天畸形;染色体的断裂;全血细胞减少症。端粒缩短
Werner 综合征		
WRN	DNA 解旋酶/核酸外切酶	早衰、身材矮小、核酸外切酶快速进展的白内障; 结缔组织和肌肉的丧失、过早动脉硬化、增加恶性肿瘤的风险
RecQ4	DNA 解旋酶	骨肉瘤;早衰

BER,修复机制;DSB,双链断链;HR,同源重组;MMR,错配;NER,核酸剪切;PRR,复制后;SB,链断裂。

DNA 核苷酸切除修复需要损伤识别、预切除、切除、间隙填补和连接。所谓的切补核酸酶复合物包括 16 种或更多的不同蛋白。由大体积 DNA 加合物(如 BPDE-dG 和 4ABP-dC)引起的大的 DNA 变形可被着色性干皮病(xeroderma pigmentosum, XPA)识别,被内切酶 XPF、XPG 和 FEN 去除。接下来,小片段由聚合酶(pol 和 pol e)合成,最后进行游离末端连接。

碱基切除修复也可移除含有加合物的 DNA 片段,但其靶点通常是小加合物(如 3-甲基腺嘌呤),因此碱基切除修复与直接修复有重叠。加合物通过糖基化酶(hOgg1 和 UDG)移除,一种脱嘌呤核酸内切酶(APE1 或 HAP1)降解受损链的一些碱基,接下来合成补丁(pol β)和连接(DNA 连接酶:Ⅰ、Ⅱ、Ⅲα、Ⅲβ 和Ⅳ)。

DNA 错配时有发生,因为切除修复过程掺入了未经修饰的或传统的但不互补的 Watson-Crick 碱基,在 DNA 螺旋中彼此相对。通过错配修复过程,修复转换错配(G-T 或 A-C)的效率要高于颠换错配(G-G、A-A、G-A、C-C、C-T 和 T-T)。纠正错配的机制类似于前面描述的核苷酸切除、修复和再合成,但它通常涉及包含错配的 DNA 大片段的切除。由于错配识别蛋白需要在 GATC 识别序列中同时与错配和未甲基化腺嘌呤结合,因此它会去除整个插入的 DNA 序列。然后,聚合酶使用亲本模板链来填补空白。

暴露在电离辐射和氧化作用可致双链 DNA 断裂。双链 DNA 断裂会导致复制和转录的抑制以及杂合性丢失。双链 DNA 断裂修复是通过 HR 完成的。在 HR 中,DNA-蛋白激酶介导了游离端连接,同时 DNA-蛋白激酶也保护游离端免受核水解攻击。然后 DNA 的游离端通过 DNA 连接酶Ⅳ进行连接。已知编码 DNA 修复酶的基因包括 XRCC4、XRCC5、XRCC6、XRCC7、HRAD51B、HRAD52、RPA 和 ATM。

复制后修复是一种损伤耐受机制,发生于受损模板上的 DNA 复制过程中。当在模板链上检测到 DNA 损伤时,DNA 聚合酶在复制叉处停止。另一种可能是聚合酶跨过损伤位点,在新合成的链上留下一个缺口。填补这一缺口的方法有两种:一种是通过螺旋状核蛋白(RAD51)介导的过程,将同源母链与子链重组;另一种是当一个核苷酸缺口存在时,哺乳动物 DNA 聚合酶插入一个腺嘌呤残基。因此，这种机制可能导致重组事件以及碱基错配。

持续存在而无法修复的 DNA 损伤可阻断 DNA 复制。细胞已经进化出翻译跨损伤合成（translesion synthesis，TLS）DNA 聚合酶来绕过这些障碍[230]。这些 TLS 聚合酶大多数属于最近发现的 Y 家族，比复制型聚合酶的严谨度低得多，因此容易出错。突变频率的增加是细胞生存的进化交换。

突变体表型

与正常细胞相比，肿瘤细胞有大量的基因异常。这些异常包括大的改变，如染色体非二倍数（即异倍体）、染色体易位或重排，也包括很小的 DNA 序列改变，如缺失、插入和单个核苷酸替换。因此，癌变涉及三个层面的错误：①染色体分离；②内源性自由基或环境致癌物引发的 DNA 损伤修复；③DNA 复制。Loeb 在 1974 年率先提出突变体表型的概念[29,60]，以解释癌细胞相对于正常细胞而言具有的大量突变。在人类细胞和动物模型致癌过程中分子分析的最新进展完善了对突变体表型的认识[61,231]，突变体表型也与 Nowell 提出的克隆选择理论相联系（图 23-4）[232]。一般来说，突变体表型假说认为正常细胞的突变率不足以解释在癌细胞中发现的大量突变。因此，人类肿瘤表现出较高的突变率，增加了肿瘤获得有利突变的可能性。该假说预测肿瘤是由含有数十万种突变而不是少数特异的驱动突变的细胞组成的。因此，肿瘤内的恶性细胞构成了一个高度异质性的群体[231]。

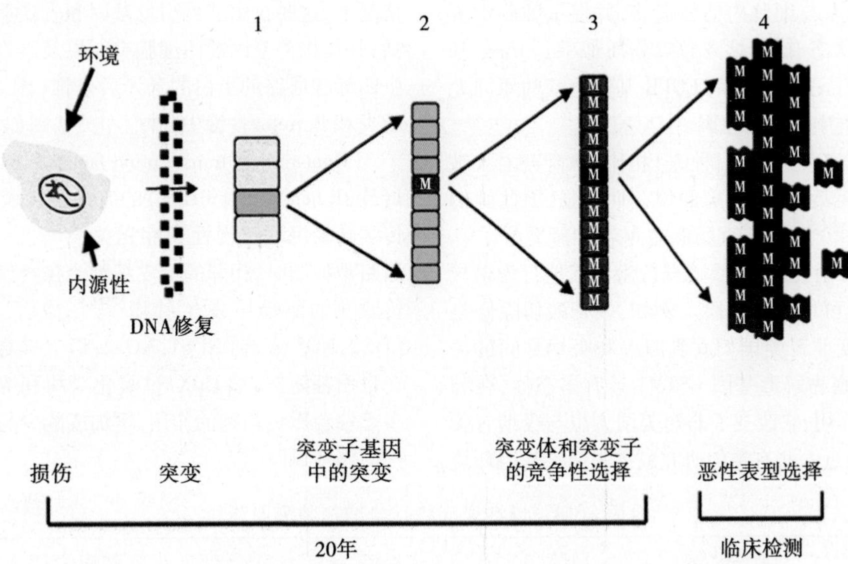

图 23-4　肿瘤进展过程中的突变积累。①当 DNA 损伤超过细胞无错误修复 DNA 的能力时，就会产生随机突变。②这些随机突变可导致克隆扩增和突变体基因突变（M）。③突变体的重复选择在增变基因中产生共选突变体。④从突变癌细胞群中，可以选择脱离宿主调控细胞复制、侵袭和转移机制的细胞

化学物致癌的种族、性别和社会经济差异

基因多态性也可能部分解释了不同性别、种族和民族之间与癌症相关化学致癌物风险的增加。围绕这个问题最大的争议之一是女性吸烟者患肺癌的风险。最初的研究发现，吸烟的女性比吸烟的男性患肺癌的风险更高，这在生物学上可以用多种方式加以解释[233]。一些证据（尽管不完全一致）表明雌激素可能在肺癌中发挥作用。男女之间风险因素和肿瘤特征的差异已有报道，女性患者具有以下特征：更易于罹患肺腺癌，从不吸烟者风险更高，多环芳烃 DNA 加合物水平更高，编码 CYP P450（CYP）1A1 的基因表达水平更高，p53 基因中 G：C→T：A 颠换更常见，表皮生长因子受体（epidermal growth factor receptor，EGFR）突变更频繁[187]。影响激活酶和解毒酶的遗传性基因多态性也可以解释不同性别对烟草致癌物易感性的不同[234]。此外，与吸烟习惯或环境和职业接触有关的一些生活方式和行为因素也可以解释一些性别差异[235]。然而，近年来，吸烟的男性和女性对肺癌易感性的差异受到了质疑[236,237]。

一个一致的结论是，与不吸烟的男性相比，不吸烟的女性患肺癌的风险更高[237,238]；与未暴露于环境性吸烟（environmental tobacco smoke，ETS）的不吸烟的女性相比，暴露于 ETS 导致不吸烟女性患肺癌的风险更高[239~244]。这种风险可能与多态性有关。例如，在女性人群中，一个常见的基因多态性将不吸烟者分为两个大致相等的群体，一个群体（GSTM1 无效等位基因的纯合携带者）对于 ETS 诱发的肺癌的风险显著高于另一个群体（野生型 GSTM1 等位基因的杂合或纯合携带者）[240]。在类似的背景下，*13q31.3* 的基因变异改变了磷脂酰肌醇聚糖-5（glypican-5，GPC5）基因的表达，而 GPC5 的下调可能会导致从不吸烟者肺癌的发生[245,246]。在从不吸烟的人群中发现的与肺癌风险相关的其他基因是：LEM 域结合蛋白 3（LEM domain-containing protein 3，LEMD3），跨膜 Bax 抑制剂结合基序｛含基

序的跨膜 Bax 抑制剂(transmembrane Bax inhibitor containing motif,TMBIM),阿托品样 7-2(ataxin 7-like 2,ATXN7L2),包含 E 的 Src 同源 2 结构域(Src homology 2 domain containing E,SHE),α-胰蛋白酶抑制剂重链 H2(inter-α-trypsin inhibitor heavy chain H2,ITIH2),Nudix(核苷二磷酸连接部分 X)型基序 5 [Nudix(nucleoside diphosphate linked moiety X) type motif 5,NUDT5],EGFR 和棘皮微管相关蛋白样 4-间变性淋巴瘤激酶(echinoderm microtubule-associated protein like 4-anaplastic lymphoma kinase,EML4-ALK5)}融合基因[243,247,248]。同样,α(1)ATD 携带者发生肺癌的风险会增加 70%~100%[249]。最后,就像 p53 的情况一样,k-ras 的突变谱似乎随着吸烟情况的不同而有很大的不同:G→T 的颠换在吸烟者中更常见,而 G→A 的转换在从不吸烟者中更常见。K-ras 和 EGFR 突变通常是相互排斥的,说明它们有序地参与细胞内信号通路,并提示肺癌中不同的致癌机制与吸烟状态有关:烟草致癌物质似乎是 k-ras 基因突变的直接原因,而目前还不清楚 EGFR 基因突变的原因尤其是在从不吸烟的人群中突变的原因。

就种族而言,与高加索人种(白种人)相比,非裔美国人被诊断出患有乳腺癌的年龄更小,肿瘤的侵袭性更强,因此她们的乳腺癌生存率更低[250,251]。结直肠癌也存在种族差异[252]。虽然这些差异可以用社会经济差异、筛查行为和其他行为差异来解释,但生物学差异可以影响风险。例如,核苷酸切除修复基因的多态性可能改变非裔美国妇女乳腺癌和吸烟之间的关系[253]。此外,化学致癌物解毒基因 GSTM1 具有多态性,在肺癌的发展过程中发挥作用,它改变了非裔美国人患与吸烟有关的肺癌的风险[254]。最近一些有趣的研究成果强调了基因环境的交互作用。这些发现表明,家庭收入与乳腺癌(尤其是 ER 阴性)患者 p53 突变频率有关。此外,高收入患者 p53 突变可能比其他患者更少,这表明与社会经济地位相关的终生暴露可能会影响乳腺癌生物学[255,256]。

慢性炎症和肿瘤

一个多世纪前,德国病理学家 Virchow 就推测炎症与肿瘤相关[8]。在世界范围内,感染和炎症导致的肿瘤占全部肿瘤的 25%(表 23-4)[204]。炎性反应会释放化内源性化学物质和自由基。这些活性氧(ROS)和活性氮(RNS)是机体对病原微生物和有毒物质的生理保护反应时产生的。在慢性炎症(如慢性病毒性肝炎)和氧自由基超负荷(如血色沉着病,炎症性肠炎)的情况下,这些自由基可引发基因和表观遗传改变。这些改变包括:肿瘤相关基因的体细胞突变以及涉及 DNA 修复、凋亡和花生四烯酸通路的蛋白的翻译后修饰(图 23-5)[8]。在溃疡性结肠炎和 Barretts 食管中,肿瘤相关基因如 p16、Runt 相关转录因子 3(Runt-related transcription factor 3,RUNX3)和 MutL 同源物 1(MutL homolog 1,MLH1)的启动子区域甲基化引起的表观遗传学转录沉默与慢性炎症相关[257,258]。基质细胞 TGF-β 信号通路被抑制时,相邻的上皮细胞会在炎症介导的基因和表观遗传改变的驱动下发生肿瘤[259]。最后,与产生自由基[例如 COX2,NOS 家族(NOS1,NOS2;但大多数是 NOS3)]或对已存在自由基防护(如 GpX、过氧化氢酶和 MnSOD)有关的基因的多态性会影响药物的作用,增加或减少与外源性化学致癌物相关的癌症风险[260]。

表 23-4 慢性炎症和感染增加肿瘤风险

疾病	肿瘤位置	风险	疾病	肿瘤位置	风险
遗传性			盆腔炎症性疾病(PID)	卵巢	3
血色沉着病	肝	219	寄生虫		
克罗恩病	结肠	3	埃及血吸虫	膀胱	2~14
溃疡性结肠炎	结肠	6	日本血吸虫	结肠	2~6
获得性			肝吸虫	肝	14
病毒			化学/物理/代谢		
乙型肝炎	肝	88	胃酸倒流	食道	50~100
丙型肝炎	肝	30	石棉	肺胸膜	>10
细菌性			肥胖	多器官	1.3~6.5
幽门螺杆菌	胃	11			

"18%的人类癌症,也就是每年 160 万例,与感染有关。"——B. Stewart and P. Kleihues, World Cancer, Report, IARC Press, Lyon 2003, p57.

类风湿关节炎是一种慢性炎症性疾病,但不会明显增加癌症(例如关节肉瘤)风险。致癌性人乳头状瘤病毒是不伴有炎症的慢性感染致癌的例子。

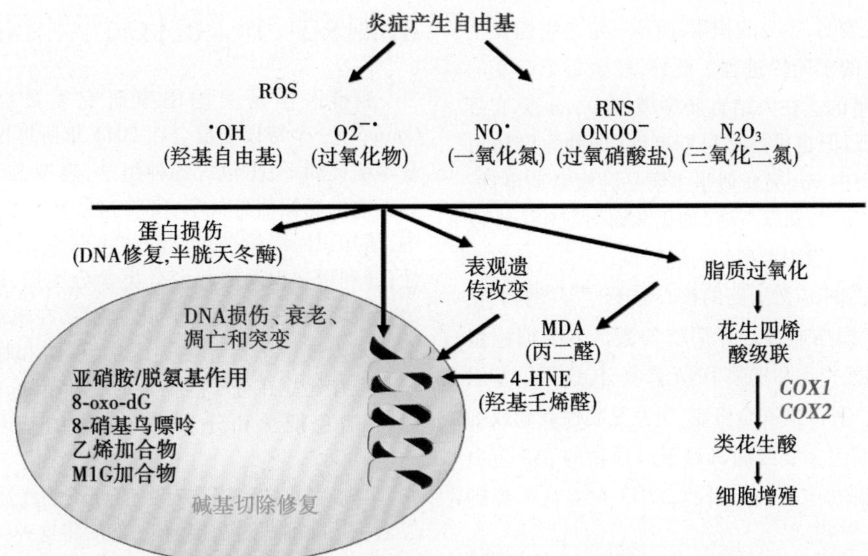

图 23-5 慢性炎症过程中产生多种活性氧(ROS)和活性氮(RNS)。活性物质可以引起 DNA 损伤(包括癌症相关基因的点突变),和参与 DNA 修复,细胞凋亡,细胞周期的关键蛋白的修饰。这种作用是直接或间接通过脂质过氧化反应的激活和产生活性醛[如丙二醛(MDA)和羟基壬烯醛(4-HNE)]完成的

癌基因和抑癌基因

长期接触致癌物、突变累积、突变体表型发展和数十年的克隆选择导致肿瘤。虽然每个肿瘤的表型性状有显著差异,但通常都获得了无限复制、生长信号自给自足、对抑生长信号不敏感、逃避凋亡、组织侵袭、持续的血管生成和转移的能力[64]。这些表型性状体现肿瘤细胞中存在复杂的生化通路分子环路和蛋白质机器[269]。

编码肿瘤发生相关分子环路的基因分属于许多功能类别,并且在历史上被从概念上分为癌基因和抑癌基因两类[269,270](框 23-4)。癌基因和抑癌基因的描述详见本书第4~7章。我们以癌基因 ras 和抑癌基因 TP53 为例论述化学致癌物的分子靶点。

> 框 23-4 肿瘤基因中的突变热点
>
> 致癌基因和抑癌基因是化学致癌物的作用靶点。包括 *K-ras* 和 *p53* 在内的许多基因都含有化学致癌物靶向的特定序列,从而导致成为突变"热点"。这些突变会导致它们编码的 RNA 和蛋白质的表达和活性发生变化。

在实验动物中发现的经化学物质诱导的癌基因中,激活的 *ras* 基因家族占据绝大多数。*ras* 基因家族成员编码分子量为 21kD 的蛋白质(p21);这些蛋白是膜结合蛋白,具有 GTP 水解酶活性,可与其他蛋白形成复合物。*ras* 基因编码的小 G 蛋白(结合鸟嘌呤核苷酸)可通过信号转导级联反应介导强烈的增殖反应。化学致癌物激活原癌基因的第一个直接证据是通过体外研究得到的[271]。用苯并芘二醇环氧化物(BPDE)处理野生型人 *Ha-ras* 基因重组克隆(pEC),接下来将其转染到小鼠 NIH-3T3 细胞,发现该转化细胞出现了与从人体肿瘤包括膀胱肿瘤(pEJ)中分离出的激活的 *ras* 基因相同的点突变(位于第 12 或 61 密码子)。在化学物致癌的动物模型和各种环境暴露产生的人类肿瘤中,均发现 *ras* 突变[272~275]。例如,在人类肺腺癌的分子致病过程中,吸烟可致 K-ras 突变[276]。在啮齿动物中反复使用多环芳烃(3-甲基胆蒽、DMBA 和苯并芘)可诱导良性和恶性肿瘤。大部分这些良性及恶性病变中的 *ras* 基因都发生了位于第 12 位或第 61 位密码子的突变。与之相似,用 DMBA 或 *N*-甲基-*N*-亚硝基脲处理大鼠产生的乳腺癌也出现了 *ras* 第 12 位或第 61 位密码子的突变。在 DMBA(肿瘤启动)和 TPA(肿瘤促进)诱导的小鼠皮肤癌模型中也检测到了上述突变。用乙烯基氨基甲酸酯、羟基脱氧草蒿脑或 *N*-羟基-2-乙酰氨基芴处理的小鼠肝脏也出现了 ras 突变。相同位点的点突变也被发现存在于用 *N*-甲基-*N*-亚硝基脲或 γ-射线处理的小鼠胸腺淋巴瘤,用甲基甲磺酸酯、α-丙内酯、二甲基氨基甲酰氯或 *N*-甲基-*N9*-硝基-*N* 亚硝基胍处理引起的其他啮齿动物皮肤癌中。

这些数据提示,化学致癌物可产生位点特异性突变,部分原因是基于最终致癌物的核苷选择性。有趣的是,最近在 K-ras 基因的 12 和 13 个密码子上发现了(+)-抗 BPDE 的非共价结合位点[277]。然而,特定突变的持续存在还取决于氨基酸的替代,因为突变蛋白的功能改变赋予细胞选择性克隆生长优势。在化学激活的 *ras* 基因中发现的突变类型会引起构象变化,改变蛋白结合(GTPase 激活蛋白)能力,从而导致 *ras*-MAP 激酶通路持续激活。现有证据支持 *ras* 激活与恶性转化及肿瘤起始相关的学说。将激活的 *ras* 基因转染到没有组成性 *ras* 基因激活的良性乳头瘤中会引发恶性进展[275,278]。这些以及其他结果提示,在化学致癌过程中存在 *ras* 突变。同样,将激活的 *ras* 基因转染到永生化的人支气管上皮细胞也会导致恶性转

化[279,280]。*Ki-ras* 基因突变也是结直肠癌发生的早期或晚期变化之一[281]。这些发现表明，突变的积累，而不一定是它们发生的顺序，影响肿瘤发生的多阶段进程。此外，发生每个突变的癌变阶段不一定是固定的。在人结直肠癌模型中，ras 突变最常在恶性转化阶段出现，但也可能是早期事件（即肿瘤启动）；而在啮齿动物皮肤模型中，*ras* 突变似乎主要是肿瘤启动事件。这些差异可能反映了不同的暴露类型（如化学物类型和慢性或急性暴露类型），或是不同组织类型的功能所致。

抑癌基因 *TP53* 是细胞应激通路的核心分子[282]。例如，化学致癌物引起的 DNA 损伤通过翻译后修饰激活 p53 抑癌蛋白，通过参与细胞周期检查点和增强 DNA 修复，传递保护基因组的信号[283]，并作为一种故障安全机制，引发复制性衰老或细胞凋亡[284,285]。*TP53* 基因突变或病毒癌蛋白导致的 p53 蛋白失活会使这些细胞防御功能丧失。因此，*TP53* 突变在人类肿瘤中很常见并不意外[286,287]。

TP53 的分子分析可为癌症的环境病因学提供线索（表 23-5）。前文（见“DNA 损伤和修复”）已经提示激活的致癌物与 DNA 共价结合是非随机的。因此，特定的 DNA 损伤的形成在某种程度上可由所产生的突变推断出来。一个明显的例子是前述的 *TP53* 基因的 249 位密码子突变，它几乎可在所有黄曲霉毒素相关肝细胞癌中检测到[41,289,290]。这种关联性可能由两种不同的机制引起。第一，密码子 249（AGG）的第三个碱基可能对激活的黄曲霉毒素 B1 突变异常敏感。如前所述，黄曲霉毒素 B1-8，9-氧化物与脱氧鸟苷的 N7 共价结合形成突变前损伤。第二，携带 249 密码子损伤的细胞可能具有重要的选择性生长优势。也有证据表明这两种因素存在联合作用[291]。另一个间接证据指向特定分子事件的典型例子是 *TP53* 突变可指示紫外线相关皮肤癌中的嘧啶二聚体形成[292]。在吸烟与肺癌的病例中，G：C 到 T：A 颠换则提示激活的大分子致癌物（如多环芳烃）形成了加合物[41,293]。

表 23-5 人类肿瘤中 TP53 的突变谱[288]

致癌物类型	肿瘤	突变
黄曲霉毒素 B1	肝癌	密码子 249（AGG 6 AGT）
日光	皮肤癌	未翻译的 DNA 链上双嘧啶突变（CC 6 TT）
烟草烟雾	肺癌	未翻译的 DNA 链上 G：C 6 T：A 突变（常见于密码子：157，248，和 273）
烟草和酒精	头颈部肿瘤	p53 突变频率增加（尤其是密码子 157 和 248）
氡	肺癌	密码子 249（AGG 6 ATG）
氯乙烯	肝血管瘤	A：T 6 T：A 颠换
马兜铃酸	尿路上皮癌	A→T 颠换

精准医学、分子流行病学和预防

精准医学是美国国家研究委员会（National Research Council）一个特设委员会在 2011 年所提出的一个概念[52]，其基本前提如下：①包含各种组学、表型、临床和流行病学数据等在内的癌症信息共享；②将这些数据集成到一个知识网络中，该知识网络检查来自信息共享的每一层数据之间的互联性；③利用知识网络开发分类学分类器，以提高患者的诊断、治疗策略的决策和健康产出；最后，在机制和观察性研究中，这些知识被用于指导生物医学、预防和临床研究（图 23-6）。精准医疗建立在分子生物学的组学革命、生物信息学、肿瘤代谢、肿瘤免疫学和分子流行病学的基因-环境概念的进展之上。

与接触化学致癌物有关的分子癌症流行病学中最大的挑战之一是准确地测定接触量，然后将这种接触与癌症风险联系起来。从这个意义上说，到目前为止，结果令人失望。传统上，由 Perera 和 Weinstein 在 1982 年首次定义的算法[37]涉及对暴露的评估[什么化学物质和有多少化学物质，例如，有多少烟草烟雾，或更具体地说，有多少 B（a）P；BPDE；TSN]、体内剂量（体液和组织中有多少这种化学物质，例如，尼古丁/可替宁的量）、生物有效剂量（化学物质与生物实体的相互作用；如 BPDE 加合物）、早期生物学反应（如 TP53 突变和 k-ras 突变）、结构功能改变（如 TP53 下游功能和 k-ras 过表达）以及临床疾病（癌症）。与此算式交织在一起的是遗传因素和个体的易感性（例如，代谢酶如前面讨论的 p450 的多态性）。因此，分子癌症流行病学的一个目标是确定准确预测疾病风险的生物标志物（暴露、影响和易感性）。不幸的是，到目前为止，除了易感性标记物[例如，BRCA1/2 用于乳腺癌风险，结肠腺瘤样息肉（adenomatous polyposis coli，APC）用于家族性结肠癌等]，很少有真正准确的生物标志物存在。部分原因是识别生物标志物需大量资金、人力和时间，然后才能根据这些标志物提前（大部分可以提前几十年）准确评估癌症风险。

为此目的，在过去十年中，随着新的、高敏感性的和复杂的技术的出现，这一概念正在演变。例如，“组学”领域发展迅速，在化学致癌物暴露和暴露引起的癌症风险领域得到了应用。利用遗传信息（基因组学），已确定易感性的生物标志物。除了 BRCA1 或 APC 等例子外，代谢酶的多态性和 DNA 修复途径也得到了论证。基因组学与其他“组学”（加合物组学、表观基因组学、转录组学、蛋白质组学、微生物组学、代谢组学和细胞分裂组学）结合在一起，如果能与环境化学物质暴露适当地联系起来，将可以成为一个强大的工具。一个不断发展的概念就是“暴露组”[48,294]。一般来说，环境暴露组包括个体从受孕到死亡所经历的每一次暴露。暴露分为三大类：①内部暴露（代谢、内源性循环激素、身体形态、身体活动、肠道菌群、炎症和衰老）；②特定的外部暴露（辐射、感染、化学污染物、饮食、烟草、酒精、职业和医疗干预）；③更广泛的社会/经济影响（教育、经济状况、心理压力和气候）。虽然这一概念在流行病学研究中有明显的用途，用于在人群水平上确定危险因素；但将数字与暴露组（暴露组学）联系起来并进行量化将是设计化学预防策略的必要步骤（图 23-6 和图 23-7）。

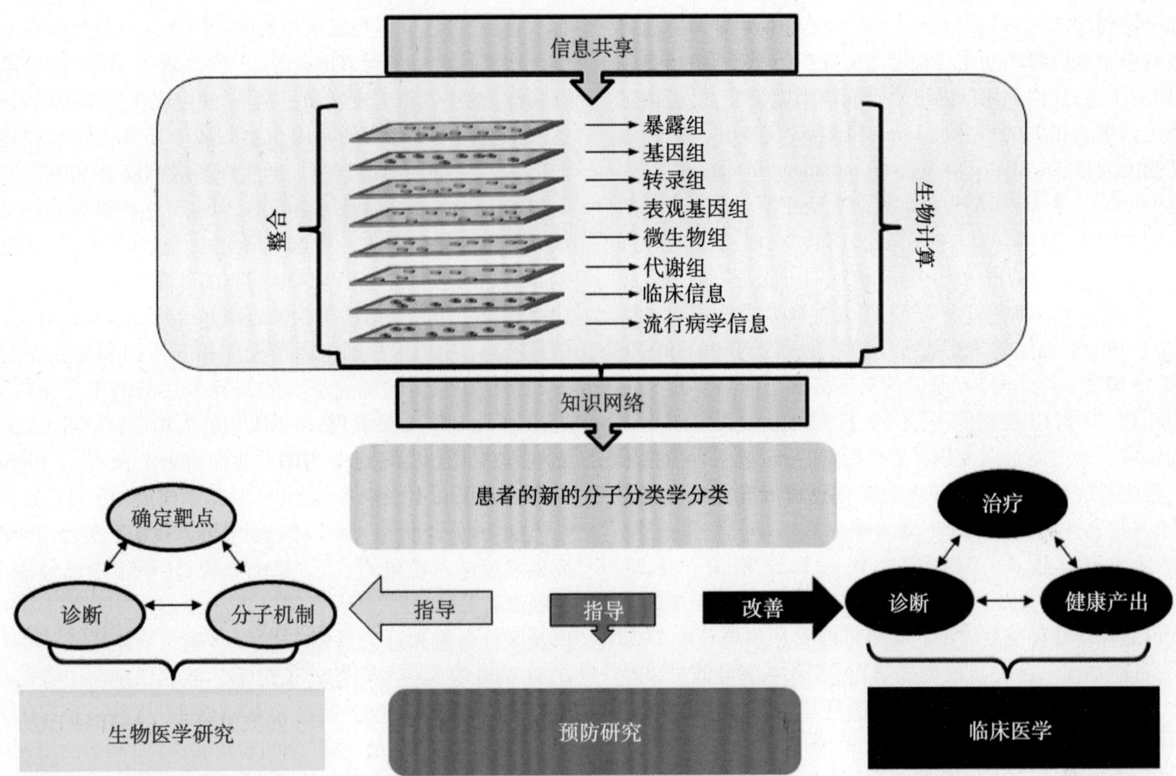

图 23-6　精准医学。2011 年 3 月,应美国国立卫生研究院(National Institutes of Health)院长的要求,美国国家研究委员会(National Research Council)成立了一个特设委员会,讨论基于分子生物学定义人类疾病"新分类"的可行性、必要性、范围、影响和后果。精准医学的概念包括四个基本前提[52]。首先,包含各种各样的组学、表型、临床和流行病学数据的每一种疾病的信息共享。其次,这些数据被集成到一个知识网络中,该网络检查来自信息共享的每一层数据的互连性。再次,利用知识网络开发新的分类学分类器,以提高患者诊断、治疗策略的决策和健康产出。最后,这些知识被用于指导生物医学和临床医学机制性和观察性研究中。如果实现了这一点,精准医疗的优势可被用于包括癌症在内的大多数(如果不是全部)疾病类型

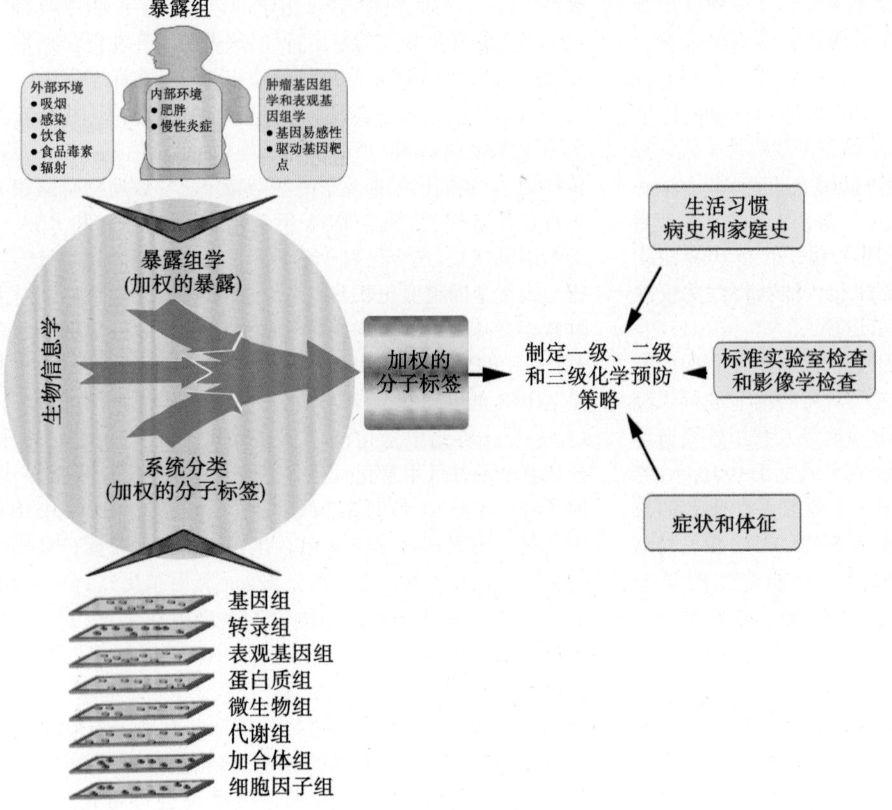

图 23-7　将暴露组学与分类学相结合,制定一级预防和化学预防策略的加权风险标签。在过去的十年里,随着技术的爆炸式发展、广泛而庞大的数据集的生成,我们可以利用生物信息学将暴露组与收集到的各种"组学"结合起来,生成一个加权的、精确的风险标签。量化个体或人群的内在的、特定的和一般的外部暴露(暴露组学),然后将其与个体或人群的分子特征联系起来,就可以生成个体或人群的风险标签。进一步、持续性考虑体征/症状、标准实验室检查和家族史等信息,将会汇聚出一项有针对性的一级预防和化学预防策略,可降低个体或高危人群的致癌风险

如今需要重新考虑这一理论。因为极其困难的一个任务是直接将单个基因组的变化与特定类型癌症的风险联系起来。例如,如前所述,我们利用基因组学研究体细胞突变,已经确定了与特定致癌物相关的特异性 k-ras 和 *TP53* 突变热点。肿瘤的体细胞突变目录(catalog of somatic mutations in cancer,COSMIC)表明,k-ras 是 ras 亚型中最常见的突变亚型。在所有分析的肿瘤中,22%的肿瘤含有 k-ras 突变,而含 N-ras 突变的肿瘤占 8%,含 H-ras 突变的占 3%。k-ras 被证明可能是一种预后指标,或可指导治疗。抑癌基因 *TP53* 在大多数人类癌症中发生突变,是已知的最常见的突变基因(例如,在大约 50%的肺癌中发现 *TP53* 突变)[41]。与 *ras* 基因的突变多发生于高度特异的区域(12、13、59 和 61 位密码子)不同,*TP53* 的突变发生于更为广泛的区域。这可能是因为只有某些特定的 ras 突变会为细胞带来正性生长优势,而 *TP53* 抑癌功能丧失的特异性较低。然而,对于一些恶性肿瘤,TP53 突变为癌症病因学提供了线索,其特异性标记(热点)与特定的致癌暴露相关(表 23-5)[41~43,55,286,295,296]。*TP53* 突变与其他基因损伤的进一步区别在于其可能存在几种突变表型。突变可能只是单纯导致 *TP53* 的缺失,可能存在一种失活的突变蛋白;或者突变可能带来生长优势。已有几项研究对 *TP53* 的表达进行了探索,虽然其在预后中的作用尚未明确,但它可能指导治疗方案的选择。为此,最近的进展促进了对"癌症景观"的解读[68],确定了驱动基因,分属于调控细胞命运、细胞存活和基因组维护等不同的信号通路。对这些驱动基因突变的理解,将有助于合成在特定个体的特定癌症内针对这些分子通路的新药,从而为个性化医疗提供特定的治疗方案。

随着微阵列和其他 RNA 检测技术的出现[如实时定量 PCR(polymerase chain reaction)],转录组学也得到了发展,特定的癌症亚型以及特定的化学致癌物暴露有关的转录特征已被确定。例如,乳头瘤病毒感染与细胞周期相关基因的失调有关,这些基因大多为 E2F 基因和 E2F 调控基因[297]。丙型肝炎病毒(hepatitis C virus,HCV)相关的肝细胞癌(Hepatocellular Carcinomas,HCC)样本中表达上调的基因多可被归类于代谢通路,其中最具代表性的是芳基烃类受体(aryl hydrocarbon receptor,AHR)信号通路和蛋白泛素化通路。这些通路此前曾被报道与癌症尤其与 HCC 进展相关。在 HCV 相关的非 HCC 组织样本中,上调的基因已被证明属于炎症和天然获得性免疫途径,且大多数过表达基因属于抗原递呈途径[298]。

迄今为止,大多数研究环境暴露引起的转录组变化的研究都依赖于外周血。Wild 等人已经对这些研究的细节进行了综述分析[294],此处概括了一些亮点。Thomas 等人利用外周血单核细胞进行研究,发现低浓度苯(浓度等于或低于 0.1ppm)与 AML 通路基因及 CYP2E1 表达改变有关。这是一个重要的发现,因为它表明苯以剂量依赖的方式改变疾病(AML)相关通路和基因,在空气中低至 100ppb 的浓度下即能产生明显效果[299]。另一项研究表明,接触苯的工人的造血祖细胞中与白血病有关的染色体发生了变化[300]。其他研究人员发现,与对照组相比,接触苯浓度超过 31ppm 的工人端粒长度略长,但差异显著($P=0.03$)[301]。最后,CYP2E1 基因的多态性已被证明与苯诱导微核有关,并可能与暴露在工作环境中的工人罹患癌症的风险增高相关[302]。

有趣的是,许多与吸烟相关的基因表达变化与炎症和氧化应激通路有关。最近,Tilley 等人[303]发现了一种"慢性阻塞性肺病样"的小气道上皮转录组特征,并发现在健康吸烟者中,表达水平变化幅度最大的基因主要归属于外来物质和氧化相关的类别。Beane 等研究表明,虽然许多吸烟应答基因在大气道上皮的表达在戒烟后是可逆转的,但也有一些吸烟应答基因在戒烟后持续异常表达。在这一研究中,他们还发现,在吸烟者差异表达的基因中,CYP P450 参与的外来物质代谢、维生素 A 代谢和氧化还原酶活性等相关通路都得到了富集;而趋化因子信号通路、细胞因子-细胞因子受体相互作用和细胞黏附分子等通路则在吸烟的肺癌患者的差异表达基因中富集[304]。最近,同一组研究人员发现,与不吸烟的人相比,吸烟的人的正常支气管气道上皮细胞中 SIRT1 活性显著上调[305]。Pierrou 等人[306]发现,在不吸烟者、健康吸烟者和 COPD 吸烟者的大气道上皮细胞中,氧化相关基因的表达发生了显著变化,其他的研究也发现这一现象[307,308]。总的来说,转录组学已经表明,区分吸烟有关的通路、区分暴露于和未暴露于烟草烟雾的个体,以及区分当前和过去暴露于烟草烟雾的个体均已成为可能。正如 Wild 等人[294]所述,转录组学还能够识别与二噁英(细胞生长增殖、葡萄糖代谢、凋亡和 DNA 复制、修复)、金属烟雾(炎症、氧化应激、磷酸盐代谢、细胞增殖和凋亡)和柴油尾气(炎症和氧化应激)相关的特定特征。在人类肺组织中,599 个转录本的基因表达特征能够将从不吸烟者与当前吸烟者区分开来。CYP1 家族成员(包括 CYP1A1、CYP1A2 和 CYP1B1)是吸烟上调最多的基因之一。吸烟引起的基因上调最明显的是芳香烃受体阻遏物(aryl hydrocarbon receptor repressor,AHRR)。有趣的是,在戒烟 10 年后,吸烟者仍然有 6 个基因(SERPIND1、AHRR、FASN、PI4K2A、ACSL5 和 GANC)的表达显著高于从不吸烟者[309]。与此同时,转录组学的研究已经证明了与特定的化学致癌物暴露相关的特定特征,这表明了存在促进癌症的潜在机制,并有助于确定与癌症风险相关的生物标志物。

表观基因组描述表观基因组变化的总体情况[在特定细胞类型中伴随 DNA 和 DNA 相关结构(如组蛋白)存在的表观遗传标记]。我们已经描述了一些与特定化学致癌物暴露相关的表观遗传事件(主要是 DNA 甲基化、组蛋白修饰和 RNA 介导的基因沉默)。迄今已有一些研究试图将特定的化学致癌物暴露与表观基因组变化联系起来。总的来说,化学致癌物对人类群体表观基因组的影响仅限于吸烟(MTHFR 和 CDKN2A 高甲基化;GPR15、MSH3、NISCH 及 CYP1A1;RPS6KA3、ARAF,尤其是 AHRR 低甲基化)、苯(alu、长穿插核苷酸原件、PTEN、ERCC3、p15、p16 高甲基化;STAT3、MAGE-1 低甲基化)、镉(长穿插核苷酸原件低甲基化)、空气污染(长穿插核苷酸原件、组织因子、F3、ICAM-1 和 TLR-2 低甲基化,以及 alu、IFN-γ 和 IL-6 高甲基化)、烟煤排放(p16 高甲基化)、工作场所暴露(iNOS 高甲基化;SATα 和 NBL2 低甲基化,mgmt 高甲基化),砷(alu、长穿插核苷酸原件、RHBDF1、p16 及 p53 高甲基化)[310~345]。需要指出的是,在最近的多项研究中,AHRR 低甲基化已被发现是吸烟的一种常见的生物标志物[313,316~321,323,346]。此外,重要的是,最近的研究表明,表观遗传学被证明对确定当前和过去的吸烟史都很有用。过去的暴露可以被检测到,甚至可能根据它们在特定基因上留下的表观遗传足迹进行量化。Zhang 等人[347]发现凝血因子Ⅱ(凝血酶)受体样(factor Ⅱ (thrombin) receptor-like,F2RL3)甲基化强度与吸烟状态有很强的相关性;在控制潜在混杂因素后,这种相关性仍然存在。无论是当前的吸烟强度还是终生吸烟的包×年数,F2RL3 甲基化强度与剂量-反应呈明显的负相关。在戒烟者中,F2RL3 的甲基化强度从接近于最近戒烟者的水平逐渐增加到接近于长期戒烟者(>20 年)的水平。EPIC 和 NOWAC 等机构最近的一项研究发现,与从不吸烟的人相比,在以前和现在的吸烟者中分别有 8 个和 897 个 CpG 位点的甲基化程度不同。戒烟者的 8 个候选标记物显示,它们的甲基化水平从典型的现吸烟者水平逐渐恢复到从不吸烟者水平。使用累积(涵盖不同时间窗)吸烟强度的进一步分析,明确了三类生物标志物:短期和长期生物标志物(分别测量过去 10 年和过去 10~30 年吸烟的影响),以及戒烟后 30 多年检测到的终生生物标志物[348]。这些研究表明,通过表观遗传学,有希望检测烟草烟雾暴露的短期至终身生物标记物,更广泛地说,有可能识别暴露的时变性生物标记物。

人类的组蛋白标记(翻译后修饰)最近也被评估与化学致癌物暴露有关。吸烟可使 HDAC2 蛋白表达降低 54%,活性降低 47%,同时可增强 Akt1 和 HDAC2 的磷酸化;工作场所接触镍与 H3K4me3 的增加和 H3K9me2 的减少有关;暴露于苯与组蛋白 H4 和 H3 乙酰化、H3K4 甲基化降低有关,并增加 Topo Ⅱα 启动子的 H3K9 甲基化;接触砷与 H3K4me2 的增加以及整体 H3K9ac 和 H3K9me2 水平的变化有关[349~352]。

在人类群体中,miRNA 的变化与暴露于香烟烟雾(吸烟者中有 40 个 miRNA 上调,包括 miR-21、-16、-17、-29a、-221 和 -223;miR-15a、-199b、-125b、-218、-487 和-4423 等表达抑制)、工作场所暴露(电炉钢厂工人暴露后 miR-21 和-222 较暴露前增加)、苯(上调 miR-34a、-205、-10b、let-7d、miR-185 和 423-5p-2;下调 miR-133a、-543、hsa-miR-130a、-27b、-223、-142-5p、-320b)、空气污染(上调 miR-132、-143、-145、-199a*、-199b-5p、-222、-223、-25、-424、-582-5p)、砷(上调 miR-190、-29a、-9、-181b);下调 mir -200 b)有关[349,353~361]。有趣的是,miRNA 水平已经被证明在戒烟后可以回到基线水平[355]。总的来说,越来越明显的是,表观基因组学为化学致癌物质的暴露提供了有用的、特异的生物标志物,而且这些变化可以在人类身上检测到。此外,观察到一些变化是可逆的,而一些变化是不可逆转的;因此可以仔细监测当前和过去的暴露及其对临床后果的影响。

与炎症负荷细胞因子组学、蛋白质组学、代谢组学和微生物组学相关的环境致癌物的影响仍在不断出现。Moore 等人已详细回顾了"基因组"技术在人群砷暴露研究中的应用[362]。读者可以参阅这篇文献了解详细内容。简言之,基因组分析显示长期砷暴露可能增加暴露膀胱组织中染色体改变的风险,而染色体 17p 丢失是砷暴露膀胱癌患者独有的,其与 p53 失活或异常蛋白表达无关。此外,在人体组织或外周细胞中,砷在很多研究中已被证明能改变基因表达(经常包括参与细胞周期调节、细胞凋亡、DNA 损伤反应的基因)、表观遗传事件(例如,p16 和 p53 启动子区域的高甲基化)、蛋白质组学特征(例如,人 b-defensin-1 和 ADAM28 的水平降低),以及代谢组学特征[362]。在一些与 HCV 和肝硬化相关的例子中,最近发现与健康对照组相比,血清中 IL-1α、IL-1β、IL-2R、IL-6、IL-8、CXCL1、CXCL9、CXCL10、CXCL12、MIF 和 β-NGF 有显著上调[363]。

尽管个体化医疗的概念已经存在了几十年(可能会有人争论,几个世纪以来医疗一直是针对个体化的症状施治),但直到最近,我们才达到一个临界点,技术使我们能够更精确地使用个体化医疗(精准医疗)[52]。从最广泛的意义上说,精准医疗是针对个体患者的特征进行医学治疗,它超越了目前基于表型性生物标志物将患者划分为不同治疗组的方法。现在,有了灵敏的仪器和收集大量化学致癌物数据的能力,我们准备开始打包、集成和量化大型数据集,以精确测量化学致癌物暴露。我们已经讨论了暴露组学,这是实现此目标的关键第一步。将这种暴露量化仍然是一个挑战,但是迎接这个挑战将带来真实和精确的数字,这些数字可以与通过不同的"组学"端点获得的大量数据集汇集而成的量化分类资料相关联[52]。在这种情况下,我们将有可能绘制出精准的风险标签用于精准医学和化学预防(框 23-5 和图 23-7)。

框 23-5　暴露组

暴露组包括个体从受孕到死亡所经历的每一次暴露。包括:①内部暴露(代谢、内源性循环激素、身体形态、身体活动、肠道菌群、炎症、衰老);②特定的外部暴露(辐射、感染、化学污染物、饮食、烟草、酒精、职业和医疗干预);③更广泛的社会经济影响(教育、经济状况、心理压力和气候)。将暴露组与代谢组学、蛋白质组学、微生物组学、转录组学和表观基因组学联系起来,会使我们识别出能作为肿瘤风险评估的个体风险标签,并开发出精准医学方法用于肿瘤预防和治疗。

致谢

我们感谢 Glory Johnson 和 Karen Yarrick 在编辑方面提供的帮助。本研究(部分)得到了美国国立卫生研究院校内研究项目、国家癌症研究所和癌症研究中心项目的支持。

(杨文　向威　宗倩妮 译　于乐兴　李亮 校)

部分参考文献

2 Hajdu SI. A note from history: landmarks in history of cancer, part 1. *Cancer*. 2011;**117**:1097-1102.

3 Hajdu SI. A note from history: landmarks in history of cancer, part 2. *Cancer*. 2011;**117**:2811-2820.

5 Astruc J. *Traite de Tumeurs et des Ulceres*. Paris: P. Guillaume Cavelier; 1759.

6 Boerhaave H. *Opera Omnia Medica*. Holland: Neapoli: S. Abbate; 1742.

7 Pott P. *Cancer Scroti in Chirurgical Observations Relative to the Cataract, the Polypus of the Nose, the Cancer of the Scrotum, the Different Kinds of Ruptures, and the Mortification of the Toes and Feet*. London: Hawes, Clarke and Collins; 1775:63-65.

9 Hajdu SI. A note from history: landmarks in history of cancer, part 3. *Cancer*. 2012;**118**:1155-1168.

11 Rous P. A transmissible avian neoplasm. (sarcoma of the common fowl.). *J Exp Med*. 1910;**12**:696-705.

13 Berenblum I, Shubik P. A new, quantitative, approach to the study of the stages of chemical cartinogenesis in the mouse's skin. *Br J Cancer*. 1947;**1**:383-391.

15 Doll R, Hill AB. Smoking and carcinoma of the lung; preliminary report. *Br Med J*. 1950;**2**:739-748.

18 Conney AH, Miller EC, Miller JA. The metabolism of methylated aminoazo dyes. V. Evidence for induction of enzyme synthesis in the rat by 3-methylcholanthrene. *Cancer Res*. 1956;**16**:450-459.

21 Barnes J, Butler WH. Carcinogenic activity of aflatoxin to rats. *Nature*. 1964;**202**:1016.

22 Sporn MB, Dingman CW, Phelps HL, et al. Aflatoxin B1: binding to DNA in vitro and alteration of RNA metabolism in vivo. *Science*. 1966;**151**:1539 - 1541.

25 Knudson AG Jr. Mutation and cancer: statistical study of retinoblastoma. *Proc Natl Acad Sci U S A*. 1971;**68**:820 - 823.

27 Ames BN, Durston WE, Yamasaki E. Carcinogens are mutagens: a simple test system combining liver homogenates for activation and bacteria for detection. *Proc Natl Acad Sci U S A*. 1973;**70**:2281 - 2285.

28 Harris CC, Genta VM, Frank AL, et al. Carcinogenic polynuclear hydrocarbons bind to macromolecules in cultured human bronchi. *Nature*. 1974;**252**:68 - 69.

29 Loeb LA, Springgate CF, Battula N. Errors in DNA replication as a basis of malignant changes. *Cancer Res*. 1974;**34**:2311 - 2321.

30 Harris CC, Autrup H, Connor R, et al. Interindividual variation in binding of benzo[a]pyrene to DNA in cultured human bronchi. *Science*. 1976;**194**:1067 - 1069. 2013;582 - 768.

31 Stehelin D, Varmus HE, Bishop JM, et al. DNA related to the transforming gene(s) of avian sarcoma viruses is present in normal avian DNA. *Nature*. 1976;**260**:170 - 173.

32 Varmus HE, Vogt PK, Bishop JM. Integration of deoxyribonucleic acid specific for Rous sarcoma virus after infection of permissive and nonpermissive hosts. *Proc Natl Acad Sci U S A*. 1973;**70**:3067 - 3071.

34 Lane DP, Crawford LV. T antigen is bound to a host protein in SV40-transformed cells. *Nature*. 1979;**278**:261 - 263.

35 Linzer DI, Levine AJ. Characterization of a 54K dalton cellular SV40 tumor antigen present in SV40-transformed cells and uninfected embryonal carcinoma cells. *Cell*. 1979;**17**:43 - 52.

36 Doll R, Peto R. The causes of cancer: quantitative estimates of avoidable risks of cancer in the United States today. *J Natl Cancer Inst*. 1981;**66**:1191 - 1308.

37 Perera FP, Weinstein IB. Molecular epidemiology and carcinogen-DNA adduct detection: new approaches to studies of human cancer causation. *J Chronic Dis*. 1982;**35**:581 - 600.

41 Hollstein M, Sidransky D, Vogelstein B, et al. p53 mutations in human cancers. *Science*. 1991;**253**:49 - 53.

42 Hsu IC, Metcalf RA, Sun T, et al. Mutational hotspot in the p53 gene in human hepatocellular carcinomas. *Nature*. 1991;**350**:427 - 428.

43 Bressac B, Kew M, Wands J, et al. Selective G to T mutations of p53 gene in hepatocellular carcinoma from southern Africa. *Nature*. 1991;**350**:429 - 431.

44 Lander ES, Linton LM, Birren B, et al. Initial sequencing and analysis of the human genome. *Nature*. 2001;**409**:860 - 921.

45 Venter JC, Adams MD, Myers EW, et al. The sequence of the human genome. *Science*. 2001;**291**:1304 - 1351.

46 Calin GA, Dumitru CD, Shimizu M, et al. Frequent deletions and down-regulation of micro- RNA genes miR15 and miR16 at 13q14 in chronic lymphocytic leukemia. *Proc Natl Acad Sci U S A*. 2002;**99**:15524 - 15529.

48 Wild CP. Complementing the genome with an "exposome": the outstanding challenge of environmental exposure measurement in molecular epidemiology. *Cancer Epidemiol Biomarkers Prev*. 2005;**14**:1847 - 1850.

51 Group FIS. Quadrivalent vaccine against human papillomavirus to prevent high-grade cervical lesions. *N Engl J Med*. 2007;**356**:1915 - 1927.

52 National Research Council Committee on AFfDaNToD. The National Academies Collection: Reports funded by National Institutes of Health. *Toward Precision Medicine: Building a Knowledge Network for Biomedical Research and a New Taxonomy of Disease*. Washington (DC): National Academies Press (US) National Academy of Sciences; 2011.

54 Chen R, Mias GI, Li-Pook J, et al. Personal omics profiling reveals dynamic molecular and medical phenotypes. *Cell*. 2012;**148**:1293 - 1307.

55 Loeb LA, Harris CC. Advances in chemical carcinogenesis: a historical review and prospective. *Cancer Res*. 2008;**68**:6863 - 6872.

57 Friedewald WF, Rous P. The initiating and promoting elements in tumor production: an analysis of the effects of tar, benzpyrene, and methylcholanthrene on rabbit skin. *J Exp Med*. 1944;**80**:101 - 126.

64 Hanahan D, Weinberg RA. Hallmarks of cancer: the next generation. *Cell*. 2011;**144**:646 - 674.

68 Vogelstein B, Papadopoulos N, Velculescu VE, et al. Cancer genome landscapes. *Science*. 2013;**339**:1546 - 1558.

91 Izzotti A, Pulliero A. The effects of environmental chemical carcinogens on the microRNA machinery. *Int J Hyg Environ Health*. 2014;**217**:601 - 627.

95 Lagos-Quintana M, Rauhut R, Lendeckel W, et al. Identification of novel genes coding for small expressed RNAs. *Science*. 2001;**294**:853 - 858.

190 Rendic S, Guengerich FP. Contributions of human enzymes in carcinogen metabolism. *Chem Res Toxicol*. 2012;**25**:1316 - 1383.

191 Herenblum I. 3:4-benzpyrene from coal tar. *Nature*. 1945;**156**:601.

232 Nowell PC. The clonal evolution of tumor cell populations. *Science*. 1976; **194**:23 - 28.

239 Fontham ET, Correa P, Reynolds P, et al. Environmental tobacco smoke and lung cancer in nonsmoking women. A multicenter study. *JAMA*. 1994;**271**:1752 - 1759.

240 Bennett WP, Alavanja MC, Blomeke B, et al. Environmental tobacco smoke, genetic susceptibility, and risk of lung cancer in never-smoking women. *J Natl Cancer Inst*. 1999;**91**:2009 - 2014.

283 Lane DP. Cancer. p53, guardian of the genome. *Nature*. 1992;**358**:15 - 16.

292 Brash DE, Rudolph JA, Simon JA, et al. A role for sunlight in skin cancer: UV-induced p53 mutations in squamous cell carcinoma. *Proc Natl Acad Sci U S A*. 1991;**88**:10124 - 10128.

第24章　激素相关癌症的内分泌和遗传学基础

Leslie Bernstein, PhD ■ Xia Pu, PhD ■ Jian Gu, PhD

概述

目前在美国，激素反应性组织发生的癌症占所有新诊断出的男性癌症的30%以上，占所有新诊断出的女性癌症的近40%。鉴于内源性激素明显影响这些癌症的罹患风险和总体发病率，如果患者因其他缘由使用激素类药物(例如避孕、更年期激素调整或预防流产)，就会存在影响患癌风险。根据激素类药物使用的时机和组织特异性效应，一些化合物会降低癌症的风险，而另一些会增加"激素依赖性"癌症的风险。本章集中介绍女性的乳腺癌、子宫内膜癌和卵巢癌，以及男性的前列腺癌，综述激素在癌症发生发展中的作用，包括流行病学和内分泌学的证据。本文还将综述外源性激素与乳腺癌、子宫内膜癌和卵巢癌风险之间的关系。此外，本文汇总了人们对乳腺癌、子宫内膜癌、卵巢癌和前列腺癌的遗传易感性的当前认识。虽然其他癌症(如宫颈癌、透明细胞阴道腺癌、甲状腺癌、睾丸癌和骨肉瘤)也可能与激素相关，但不在本章阐述之列。

来自实验室、临床和流行病学的大量证据表明，激素在人类多种癌症发生中起重要作用。Bittner基于小鼠雌激素和乳腺癌的研究结果，最先提出了激素可以增加肿瘤发生率的理论[1]。该理论已被提炼成与乳腺癌、子宫内膜癌、前列腺癌、卵巢癌、甲状腺癌、骨恶性肿瘤和睾丸癌相关的流行病学假说[2,3]。这些癌症的潜在机制认为肿瘤是靶器官受到激素长期刺激的结果，而这些靶器官的正常生长和功能本身也由一种或多种类固醇或多肽激素所控制。越来越多的证据表明：组织在内环境中接触到的激素的有效含量受到遗传学上的严格调控[4]。因此，运动或使用外源性激素等外部因素可以直接改变激素在体内的分布模式，目前研究还是认为激素相关癌症的易感性是由多个基因乃至多种因素共同决定[5,6]。

激素作用于靶器官诱导癌症，主要通过促进细胞增殖，其他潜在机制还包括诱导细胞的代谢活化或直接结合DNA(脱氧核糖核酸)。癌细胞的恶性表型取决于细胞分裂过程中发生的一系列基因变异，但在正常细胞向表现特定表型癌细胞的转化过程中，发生变异的基因及其变异次序尚不清楚(图24-1)。候选的癌症相关基因包括内分泌和生长因子信号通路的成员[4,7,8]、DNA修复基因、肿瘤抑制基因和癌基因[9,10]。除了体细胞突变，生殖细胞中也有报道发生肿瘤抑制基因*BRCA1*和*BRCA2*的突变，其与乳腺癌和卵巢癌的易感性相关[11~14]。生殖细胞系中的*TP53*的突变与家族性乳腺癌风险增加有关[15]。然而，这些基因的突变在大多数散发性乳腺癌中似乎并不存在。最近的全基因组关联分析(GWAS)的研究发现了许多常见的、低外显率的散发性癌症的易感位点[16]。

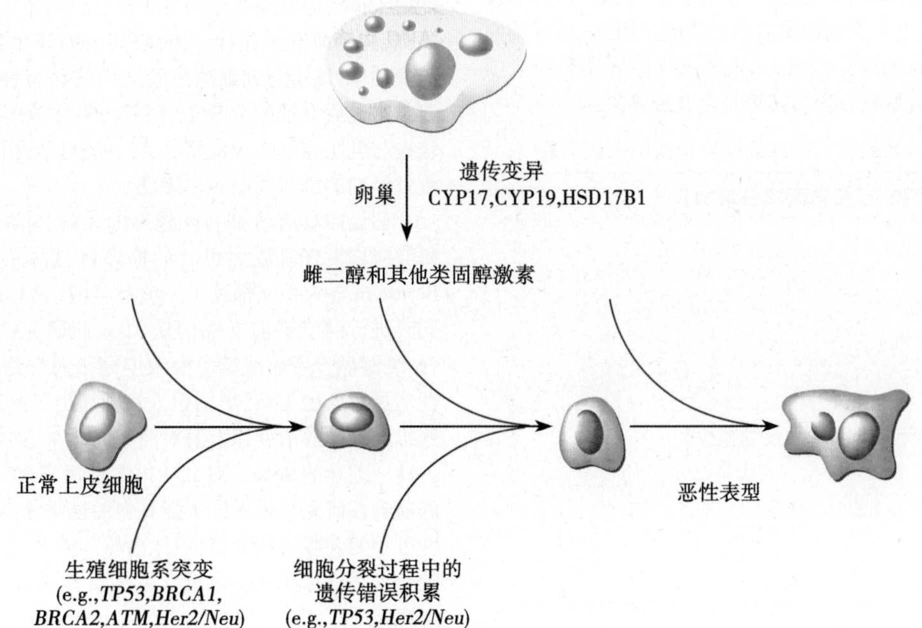

图24-1　雌二醇和其他类固醇激素(如孕酮)促进乳腺细胞增殖，促进关键信号通路成员基因的DNA随机复制错误的积累，导致肿瘤恶性表型。在生殖细胞中发生的肿瘤抑制相关基因突变加速了肿瘤恶性表型的发生

目前在美国，激素相关癌症占所有新诊断的男性癌症的30%以上，占所有新诊断的女性癌症的近40%。鉴于内源性激素明显影响这些癌症的风险和总体发病率，如果患者出于其他治疗目的接受激素类药物（例如用于避孕、更年期激素调整或预防流产），就会存在影响癌症风险的可能[17]。本章集中介绍女性的乳腺癌、子宫内膜癌和卵巢癌、以及男性的前列腺癌，综述激素在癌症发生发展中的功能和角色，包括流行病学和内分泌学的证据。本章还将综述外源性激素与乳腺癌、子宫内膜癌和卵巢癌风险之间的关系。虽然其他不太常见的癌症（如宫颈癌、透明细胞阴道腺癌、甲状腺癌、睾丸癌和骨肉瘤）也可能与激素相关，但在本章不做阐述。

乳腺癌

乳腺癌是女性最为常见的癌症；预计 2014 年美国将新诊断出 232 670 例侵袭性乳腺癌病例和 62 570 例原位乳腺癌病例，同时有 40 430 名美国女性将死于乳腺癌[18]。由于乳腺 X 光造影筛查、激素治疗和靶向 *HER2/neu* 药物治疗的广泛应用，乳腺癌的死亡率自 1990 年以来一直持续下降[19~21]。已有的证据表明雌激素是刺激乳腺细胞增殖的主要激素因子[2,3]。此外，黄体酮可以进一步增加乳腺细胞的增殖率[22]。后一个结论主要基于一个观察，即乳腺细胞的有丝分裂活动在月经的黄体期达到高峰，此外有越来越多的文献表明，同时接受孕激素类药物可显著增加雌激素替代治疗（ERT）诱导乳腺癌的风险[23~28]。

乳腺癌最常见的激素相关危险因素是初潮年龄提早、绝经年龄推迟、第一次足月妊娠年龄过大和体重超重（表 24-1）。从乳腺癌的年龄-发病率曲线上可以看出排卵是风险评判的重要因素[17]。乳腺癌病例首先发生在青年期，发病率的增加率随着年龄的增长而急剧上升，直到绝经期后显著降低。乳腺癌发病率在绝经后的增长率约为绝经前的六分之一。这个年龄-发病率曲线在很大程度上受到卵巢活动的影响。因此，理解排卵的发生、规律和终止的决定因素，无论是遗传因素还是环境因素，对研发有效的乳腺癌预防方式都是至关重要的。

表 24-1 已确定的乳腺癌激素风险和保护因素列表

危险因素（雌激素和/或黄体酮接触增加）
初潮过早
更年期过晚
肥胖（绝经后女性）
激素替代治疗
保护因素（雌激素和/或黄体酮接触减少）
哺乳期
早期足月妊娠
体力活动（运动）

生育因素

月经初潮年龄过早是乳腺癌的一个既定危险因素[3]。一般来说，月经初潮每推迟一年，乳腺癌的风险降低 5%～6%，这种关系可以根据排卵月经周期正常化后的年龄进一步修正。在一项针对年轻女性的研究中，Henderson 等人报告称，12 岁或 12 岁以下就开始正常月经周期的女性罹患乳腺癌的风险比那些初潮较晚且经历了长期不规则周期的女性高几乎四倍[29]。还有研究进一步表明，罹患乳腺癌女性的女儿体内的雌激素和黄体酮水平高于未患乳腺癌女性的同龄女儿[30]。

尽管初潮和排卵在某种程度上是由遗传学决定的，通过一些措施干预女性在生育期内经历的排卵月经周期数也很重要[31]。大量的体育活动可能会推迟初潮的到来[32]。例如，研究表明芭蕾舞演员的平均初潮年龄为 15.4 岁，而对照组为 12.5 岁。青春期适度的体育活动可导致不排卵的月经周期。经常进行中度体力活动（每学年每周平均消耗至少 600 千卡的能量）的女孩发生无排卵月经周期的可能性几乎是不太进行体育运动女孩的三倍[33]。Bernstein 等人报道，利用休闲时间锻炼身体的生活方式显著影响年轻女性（<40 岁）、老年女性、绝经后女性（55~64 岁）的乳腺癌风险，包括非洲裔美国人和亚裔美国人[34~37]。在病例-对照研究和队列研究中，越来越多的证据表明体育锻炼可降低乳腺癌风险，尽管这些研究在分组及收益最多的组别上会有差异[38~40]。

较晚进入更年期和绝经前较长时间处于排卵周期也会增加患乳腺癌的风险。自然绝经期发生在 45 岁之前女性的风险是 55 岁之后才绝经女性的一半[41]。双侧卵巢切除术或盆腔照射诱导的人工绝经也会显著降低乳腺癌的风险，且比 50 岁之前的绝经带来的保护作用更为显著[41~43]。自然绝经后，卵巢产生雌激素的水平逐渐下降，但其产生少量睾酮的功能则得以延续。

此外，体重与乳腺癌风险之间的相关性取决于绝经状态。在绝经后的女性中，体重每增加 10kg 会导致乳腺癌风险增加 80%[44]。这种相关性效应的一个解释是，体重较重的绝经后女性由于体内脂肪组织中的芳香化酶会将肾上腺雄激素（雄烯二酮）转化为雌激素，因而具有较高的循环雌激素水平。在绝经前女性中，体重与乳腺癌风险之间的相关性还没有那么明确，或与绝经后女性的情况正好相反；对于绝经前女性来说，体重较重与乳腺癌风险较低相关[45]。这可能是由于体重较重会导致月经期的排卵周期频率降低。

假设卵巢活动影响乳腺癌的风险，病例-对照研究和队列研究应该发现乳腺癌患者的循环雌二醇水平高于健康女性。Bernstein 等人撰文描述了一项在美国（洛杉矶）和中国（上海）同时进行的绝经前女性的病例-对照研究的结果[46]。总体而言，乳腺癌患者血清雌二醇浓度高出对照组 14%，其中中国女性超过对照组 17%，美国白人女性超出对照组 11%。洛杉矶对照组的雌二醇浓度比上海对照组高 21%，而体重因素的影响仅占这一差异的 25%。对九项内源性激素和绝经后乳腺癌风险的前瞻性研究结果提供了强有力的证据表明：较高的雌二醇浓度可预测乳腺癌风险，其中体内雌二醇含量最高的前五分之一的女性相比那些处于最低含量的女性承受了高达两倍的乳腺癌风险[47]。

初次生产年龄

与未产妇相比，首次足月妊娠年龄较小（例如 20 岁之前）

的女性患乳腺癌的风险低至约 50%。足月妊娠年龄较晚的女性所受到的保护作用会变弱[48]。首次足月妊娠年龄较大(例如 30 多岁)的女性比未产妇罹患乳腺癌的风险更大。这种首次足月妊娠年龄不同带来的看似矛盾的翻转效应已被流行病学研究反复证实。

足月妊娠对乳腺癌风险的即刻影响是短期增加的。在三年内生育过的女性罹患乳腺癌的风险几乎是那些至少在 10 年前生育女性的三倍,尽管两者具有相似的年龄、产次和初次生育年龄[49]。根据这些结果,似乎首次怀孕对乳腺癌风险有两个相互矛盾的影响:短期风险增加,长期风险则大幅降低[49]。

这一明显的悖论有一个涉及雌激素分布模式及孕期催乳素分泌和代谢生理学的解释。在怀孕的前三个月中,体内雌二醇活性水平迅速上升,其对初次怀孕的影响比对随后的怀孕更为显著[50]。因此,就乳腺组织而言,雌激素在怀孕早期施加的效应所增加的风险等同于将乳腺组织在相对较短的时间内经历了数个排卵周期[51]。在分子水平上,怀孕期间的激素变化可能会在一些已经积累了相关突变的体细胞中诱导不可逆的分化和凋亡,而这些是乳腺癌发生发展的必要条件。然而从长远来看,怀孕早期对乳腺癌风险的不良影响可以被完成妊娠后的两个有益的激素作用所抵消。据报道与未产妇相比,经产妇的催乳素水平明显较低[52~54]。催乳素是一种多肽激素,调节泌乳,并增强雌激素对乳腺组织的作用。此外据报道,经产妇体内的活性雌二醇水平低于未产妇[51]。

有切实证据表明,泌乳可降低绝经前女性罹患乳腺癌的风险,但对绝经后女性的作用则不明确[55~58]。在两份文献中,Enger 等人的研究显示,母乳喂养超过 15 个月的美国产妇的乳腺癌风险显著降低,其中绝经前降低 35%,绝经后降低 30%(与情况相似的、但从未哺乳过的女性相比)[55,58]。在美国,母乳喂养率随着时间的推移而变化;一些研究可能没有发现母乳喂养的女性具有较低的乳腺癌风险,那是因为具有足够长的哺乳期的女性所占人口比例很小。在上海市的绝经前和绝经后的女性中,常有母乳喂养延长至每名儿童 1 年以上的情况,因此可以观察到随着母乳喂养时间的延长,乳腺癌风险的降低呈现显著的剂量依赖效应[59]。婴儿接受辅食的时间以及母乳喂养的频率和单次持续时间也可能会导致观察上的不一致。此外,哺乳可以通过减少女性经历的总月经周期的数量来降低乳腺癌风险,因为母乳喂养会导致完成妊娠后恢复排卵的时间大大延迟。

膳食

许多研究关注的焦点是各国之间的饮食差异,特别是摄食脂类的方式,来解释从低风险国家迁移到高风险国家后乳腺癌发生率的高低和变化[60]。乳腺癌的死亡率和发病率与饮食中的人均脂肪消耗量高度相关(相关系数分别为 r=0. 93 和 r=0. 84)[60]。如前所述,营养可能通过改变初潮年龄和体重来影响乳腺癌的发生率,但即使在对这些因素进行统计学修正后,脂肪摄入与乳腺癌死亡率的相关性仍然非常显著。

尽管理论上认为饮食中的脂肪摄入可能是乳腺癌风险的一个重要因素,但也有许多关于脂肪摄入和乳腺癌的病例-对照研究发现疾病组和对照组之间的差异很小。同样,大多数使用进食量-进食频率问卷开展的总体脂肪、饱和脂肪或植物脂肪与乳腺癌关系的队列研究发现:各类脂肪的摄入对乳腺癌风险几乎没有影响。根据总脂肪摄入量和乳腺癌风险的统合研究分析,最高脂肪摄入量组与最低脂肪摄入量组相比,病例-对照研究中的乳腺癌风险增加的程度为 14%[总比值比(OR)= 1. 14;95%置信区间(CI) 0. 99~1. 32]。队列研究中的风险增加程度为 11%(OR=1. 11;95% CI 0. 99~1. 25)[61]。一项在超过 48 000 名女性中开展的"女性健康倡议"(The Wonmen's Health Initiative)的随机试验检验了如下假设:将总脂肪摄入量减少到能量摄入的 20%,并每天摄入至少 5 份蔬菜水果和 6 份谷物,可以显著降低癌症尤其乳腺癌的风险[62]。在随机分组后开展的为期平均 8. 1 年随访中,坚持规定膳食的女性罹患乳腺癌的相对风险度(RR)比没受干预的对照组低,尽管结果在统计学上并不十分显著(RR=0. 91;95%CI=0. 83~1. 01),但依然提示饮食对乳腺癌风险的影响。

高纤维膳食有助于预防乳腺癌,可能是因为纤维减少了肠道对雌激素的再吸收,这些雌激素来源于胆道系统的排出[63]。由于缺乏有关特定食物纤维含量的数据,加上没有可靠的生化技术用于定量食物中各类型纤维的比例,通过流行病学研究评估纤维摄入量一直问题很多。但通过病例-对照研究,而非队列研究,可以发现膳食纤维的摄入量与乳腺癌风险之间存在明确的反比关系[64]。

有一些研究表明在接受了低脂高纤维的膳食干预后,血清中的雌激素水平降低[65,66]。统合研究分析表明,在膳食脂肪摄入减少之后,绝经前女性的雌二醇水平平均降低 7. 4%,绝经后女性的雌二醇水平平均降低 23%[66]。上述分析无法区分这种作用是膳食结构改变本身造成的直接作用,还是由于绝经前女性的排卵周期受到干预造成的间接作用;但是不论是哪种作用机制,降低雌二醇水平对于预防乳腺癌来说都是非常重要的。

外源性激素

激素疗法和口服避孕药是女性可能接触到的外源性激素,其同内源性激素功能相似,因此被视为潜在的乳腺癌风险因素。

口服避孕药

口服避孕药与乳腺癌风险之间的关系一直是许多综述的主题。近期有一篇文献对涉及超过 15 万女性的 54 项有关联合口服避孕药(COC,联合口服避孕药将雌激素和黄体酮结合在同一片剂中)对乳腺癌风险影响的研究进行综合分析[67]。分析的结果表明,联合口服避孕药的使用对罹患乳腺癌的风险具有轻微增加的作用,其中当前使用者和近期使用者的相对风险分别为 1. 24 和 1. 16。首次使用联合口服避孕药的年龄与近期使用所带来的风险具有相关性。20 岁之前开始使用联合口服避孕药的女性近期使用后罹患乳腺癌的风险最高。然而,在近期使用者中,使用联合口服避孕药的总时间与乳腺癌风险的增加无关。

汇总统计分析研究目前主要集中于年轻女性,因为大多数联合口服避孕药的使用者尚未达到围绝经期和绝经期[67]。一项基于人群的病例-对照研究,"女性避孕和生殖经验(女性保健)研究"(The Wonmen's Contraceptive and Reproductive Experiences,Women's CARE),在美国的五个地区进行,涵盖了 4 500 多名 35~64 岁的新诊断的乳腺癌患者和 4 500 多名同龄对照受试者[68]。本研究旨在评估口服避孕药对已不再服用的女性罹患乳腺癌风险的影响。在该研究中,目前仍然在服用口服避孕药的受试者相对较少;许多女性在至少 20 年前就已经停止使用避孕药。结果发现使用口服避孕药的时间长短、配方中的雌激素剂量、首次使用的年龄、上次使用后的时间间隔、使用药物相对怀孕的时间等因素和乳腺癌风险之间并无显著关联。此外,年轻女性(35~44 岁)的结果与老年女性(45~64 岁)相似,而后者更可能使用过早期配方,而近期不再使用避孕药。

国际癌症研究机构对所有关于联合口服避孕药和乳腺癌风险的现有文献进行回顾,得出结论:口服避孕药的当前使用者和近期使用者的乳腺癌风险增加,尤其是 35 岁以下、首次口服避孕药在 20 岁之前的女性[69]。这些风险的增加会随着年龄增加而消失,在停止口服避孕药后,风险的增加将在 10 年内彻底消失。

激素治疗

激素治疗最初是为减少更年期症状而设计的,但因其在降低骨质疏松症风险方面的功效以及据称在降低心脏病风险方面的益处而广受欢迎。最初的配方是雌激素替代治疗(ERT)。使用激素疗法的女性人数在 20 世纪 70 年代中期增加,直到人们对 ERT 增加子宫内膜癌的风险提出担忧。在 20 世纪 80 年代,周期性使用雌激素-黄体酮的激素治疗方案被广泛推荐和使用,以消除与雌激素单独治疗相关的子宫内膜癌风险的增加。最初,治疗方案是一个持续的疗程,在 28 天周期的前 15~20 天内给予雌激素,然后在 5~10 天内同时给予雌激素和孕激素。最近,持续的联合疗法因为减少了月经样出血的发作和易于给药而受到欢迎。

基于女性长期(如超过 10 年)使用 ERT 的研究表明,接触激素治疗的女性患乳腺癌风险约每年增加了 3%[70]。在美国,通常使用马源性结合雌激素进行治疗。据估计,标准剂量方案的使用(0.625mg/d)导致乳腺癌风险每年增加约 2.2%。

一组汇集了 51 项流行病学研究和 16 万名女性的乳腺癌激素作用研究,评估了激素治疗对乳腺癌风险的影响[55]。数据分析显示,80%的女性采用雌激素单一疗法,12%的女性采用激素联合疗法。该研究显示,激素治疗(主要是 ERT)增加了乳腺癌风险,在队列研究、基于人群的病例-对照研究和基于医院的病例-对照研究中,接受治疗的女性相对于未接受治疗的女性,其相对风险分别为 1.09、1.15 和 1.14。在使用激素治疗至少十五年的女性中,风险进一步显著增加(RR = 1.58)。在五年或同等参考时间内使用激素治疗的女性中,使用激素治疗的风险每年增加 2.3%(P = 0.000 2)(图 24-2)。然而,不管曾经使用激素治疗时间的长短,停止治疗五年或五年以上的女性罹患乳腺癌的风险就只有不显著的轻微增加。

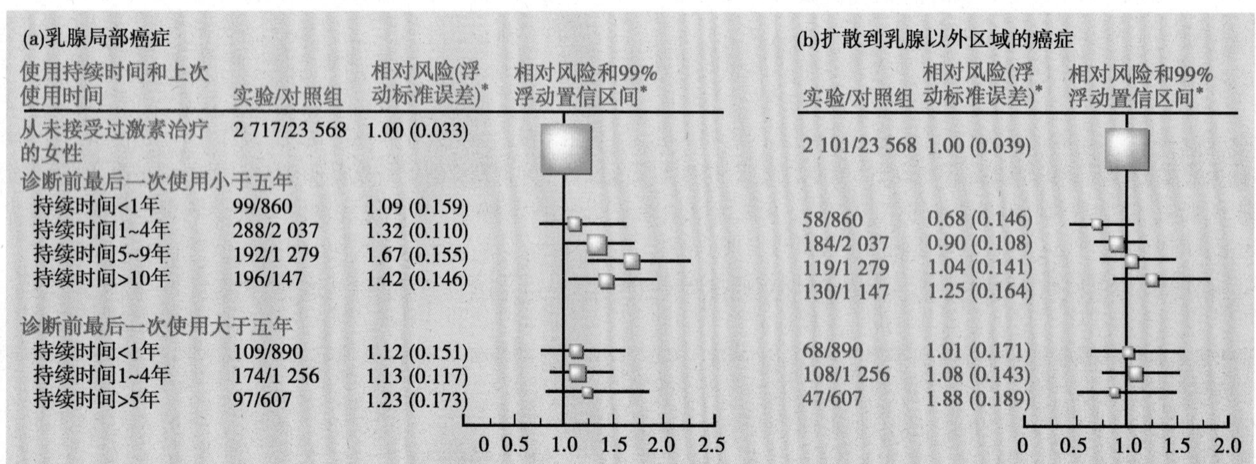

图 24-2 (a,b)近期激素治疗持续的时间和次数影响乳腺癌的相对风险,根据相对于非使用者的肿瘤扩散程度,按项目、诊断年龄、绝经时间、体重指数、产次和首胎出生时女性的年龄分层研究。"诊断前五年内最后使用"的标准包括当前用户。* 浮动标准误差(FSE)和浮动置信区间(FCI),根据每个类别的浮动方差计算得出

在英国进行的"百万女性研究"(Million Women Study)也获得了一致的结果,该研究招募了年龄在 50~64 岁、接受过常规乳腺造影筛查的女性队列[61]。在这项研究中,当前接受 ERT 治疗女性的乳腺癌发病率显著高于从未接受激素治疗的女性(RR=1.30;95% CI 1.22~1.38)。乳腺癌风险随着当前用户接受激素治疗的时间延长而增加,其中激素治疗 5~9 年的相对风险为 1.32,10 年或 10 年以上的相对风险为 1.37。

"女性健康倡议"的随机试验,比较了单独使用雌激素与安慰剂的 50~79 岁的进行过子宫切除术的女性的乳腺癌发病率,并评估了雌激素联合孕激素方案与安慰剂的子宫完整的同龄女性的乳腺癌发病率。雌激素单用方案包括 0.625mg/d 的马源性结合雌激素,而联合方案包括 0.625mg/d 的马源性结合雌激素和 2.5mg/d 的甲羟黄体酮醋酸酯[27,71]。"女性健康倡议"的随机试验中关于 ERT 治疗的研究结果有些出乎意料,平均随访 7.1 年后,乳腺癌的相对风险并没有提高(RR=0.80;95% CI 0.62~1.04)[72]。研究发现 ERT 似乎可显著降低导管癌风险,尽管在该试验中由于样本数量太少无法从肿瘤组织学上看出较大的风险差异。与导管肿瘤相比,小叶癌的风险升高,导管癌与小叶癌的比较近乎具有统计学意义(P=0.054)。此外,局部癌症的风险有一定程度降低(P=0.09),但区域性癌症的风险未受影响。

"女性健康倡议"只研究了持续联合治疗方案(CHT)。1999—2000 年的三项观察性研究表明,与单用雌激素方案相比,CHT 具有更大的乳腺癌罹患风险[24,25,73]。例如:Ross 等人

发现,每五年的 CHT 治疗相比,单独 ERT 治疗增加了近四倍的乳腺癌罹患风险[25]。"女性健康倡议"比较了持续 CHT 治疗和安慰剂试验,获得了类似先前研究的风险评估(RR = 1.24; 95% CI 1.01~1.54)[27]。

Lee 等人统合分析了 CHT 激素治疗方案对乳腺癌风险影响,区分开了顺序(循环)联合方案与持续联合方案的疗效,整合了乳腺癌激素作用研究和"女性健康倡议"的结果[27,55,74]。总体而言,使用 CHT 方案的女性罹患乳腺癌的风险显著增加,每年递增 7.6%[74]。但是,并非所有的研究都提供了黄体酮水平时间表。此外,研究确实呈现了顺序和持续的 CHT 方案在诱导乳腺癌风险上的微小差异,两者导致的乳腺癌年增长风险分别为 8.9%和 10.3%。值得注意的是,斯堪的纳维亚的研究结果表明,持续治疗比顺序治疗方案对乳腺癌风险的影响更大。这一差异在美国的"百万女性研究"中并不明显。在美国,持续联合方案的孕激素总剂量与顺序方案相似,而在斯堪的纳维亚半岛,持续联合方案的孕激素剂量要比顺序治疗方案高得多。因此,大量数据表明,联合治疗中的孕激素成分大大增加了单纯雌激素导致的乳腺癌风险。因此,美国和斯堪的纳维亚之间的研究结果差异可能是由于孕激素剂量的不同造成的。

最近,"女性健康倡议"调查了激素治疗停止后的乳腺癌风险,发布了关于 CHT 的健康风险和益处的报告[75]。激素治疗后近 2.4 年的随访显示,被随机分配到雌激素加孕激素联合治疗组的女性罹患侵袭性乳腺癌的风险仍然较高(RR = 1.27; 95% CI 0.91~1.78),尽管其置信区间涵盖了 1.0[75]。

CHT 的激素治疗可能会增加小叶癌和导管-小叶乳腺癌的风险,特别是那些被判定为小叶组织成分超过 50% 的乳腺癌[76]。55~74 岁的老年女性,目前使用 CHT 罹患小叶癌和导管-小叶癌的风险相比没有接受治疗的女性分别增加了 2.7 倍和 3.3 倍。

在美国和德国,减少联合治疗并不显著影响乳腺癌发病率[77~79]。值得注意的是,在 2002 年"女性健康倡议"公布联合治疗结果前,美国的乳腺癌发病率就开始下降了[26]。一份对 1975—2003 年监测、流行病学和最终结果(SEER)登记处的数据显示,从 1999 年起 45 岁或以上的所有女性的侵袭性乳腺癌发病率均下降;2002 年和 2003 年,旧金山的 59~69 岁女性中,雌激素受体阳性的乳腺癌发病率急剧下降[78]。来自美国乳腺造影筛查登记处的 78 份数据表明,激素治疗在 1999 年达到高峰,然后开始减少,"女性健康倡议"发表调查结果后减少得更为明显[80]。Robbins 和 Clarke 分析了加利福尼亚州 58 个郡的乳腺癌发病率后证实了这一点,乳腺癌发病率在 2001~2004 年间下降,因为加利福尼亚州医疗中心记录在案的联合治疗减少[81]。老年女性乳腺癌发病率下降的部分原因可能是乳腺造影筛查的减少,但是基于乳腺造影诊断技术发现,原位乳腺癌的发病率并没有像侵袭性乳腺癌的发病率一样下降[78]。"加州健康访谈调查"(California Health Interview Survey)显示,过去两年内,参加乳腺造影筛查的女性人口比例并无显著变化[81]。

子宫内膜癌

在与激素有关的癌症中,病因学最为清楚的是子宫内膜癌。子宫内膜癌主要的人口统计学特征和非人口学的危险因素都可以根据子宫内膜接触雌激素的剂量累积效应来解释的,且不受黄体酮的影响[2,3]。

子宫内膜的有丝分裂活性

Key 和 Pike 对正常月经周期中子宫内膜有丝分裂活性的现有数据进行了总结[82]。有丝分裂率在月经周期的第 1~4 天很低,然后迅速增加,直到第 19 天保持稳定,之后有丝分裂率在月经周期的其余时间基本上降至零。子宫内膜有丝分裂活动受到雌激素刺激或黄体酮的明显调控,在此之前一般有 4 天左右的延迟期。

孕激素在子宫内膜拮抗雌激素活性的细胞学基础已经很清楚了[2]。孕激素降低雌二醇受体的浓度,增加了 17-β-羟甾类脱氢酶Ⅱ型酶的活性,后者可将雌二醇转化为雌激素酮,而雌激素酮是一种生物学功能较弱、与雌激素受体结合较弱的雌激素[83,84]。黄体期的黄体酮可使子宫内膜细胞分化为分泌状态,而黄体酮水平减弱则导致子宫内膜组织的周期性脱落。

细胞有丝分裂的频率是子宫内膜癌风险的主要决定因素,而细胞分裂活性是由累积接触的非拮抗的雌激素含量所控制的,基于这个概念,我们可以很容易地预测子宫内膜癌最重要的危险因素(表 24-2)。怀孕和口服避孕药使子宫内膜同时接触到持续高水平的雌激素和孕激素,可以防止子宫内膜癌的发展。ERT 治疗和肥胖则会增加风险。所有这些可以影响子宫内膜癌风险的预测因素都在流行病学的研究中得到反复证实[2]。

表 24-2 已确定的子宫内膜癌的激素风险和保护因素的列表

危险因素(增加接触无孕激素拮抗的单纯雌激素)
雌激素替代治疗
肥胖
口服避孕药
绝经较晚
保护因素(减少接触无孕激素拮抗单纯的雌激素)
妊娠
联合口服避孕药

雌激素治疗

在 20 世纪的 60~70 年代,激素疗法以无孕激素拮抗的单纯雌激素替代治疗(ERT)的模式在美国获得了广泛的普及[85]。与此同时,绝经后女性子宫内膜癌的发病率也迅速增加,特别是在使用 ERT 更为普遍的美国西部各州[86]。到 1975 年,流行病学的病例-对照研究发表结果显示:ERT 治疗与子宫内膜癌风险之间有很强的相关性[87,88]。目前已有数十项研究进一步证明,ERT 治疗后子宫内膜癌的风险相对较高。其风险与激素使用的剂量和时间都有密切相关,但即使只是接受中等持续时间的中等剂量治疗,子宫内膜癌的风险也会有较高地相对增加。使用 ERT 达五年或更长时间的女性,相比从未使用过这种疗法的女性,其患病风险大约增加了 3.5 倍(图 24-3a)[17]。

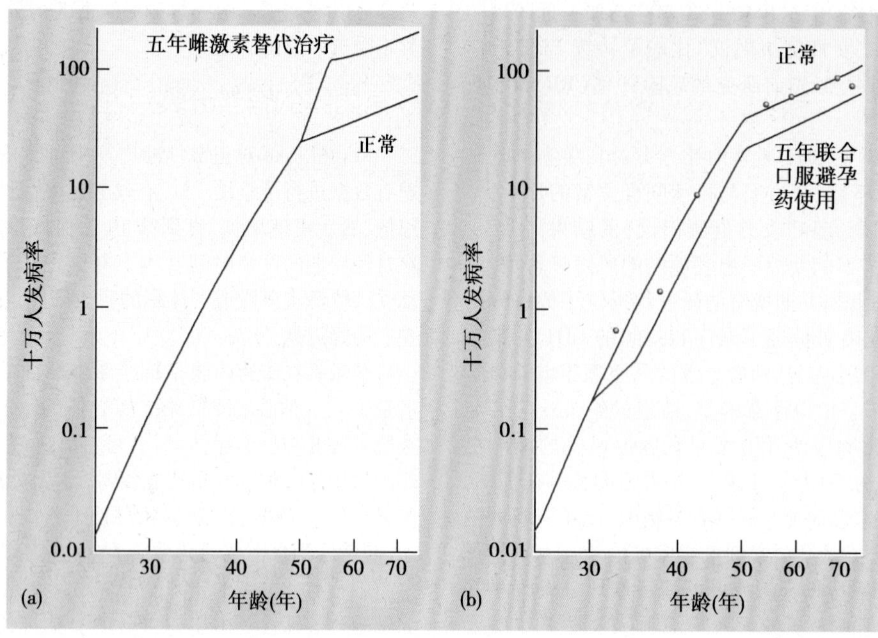

图 24-3 五年内使用雌激素治疗(ERT)(a)和联合口服避孕药(COC)(b)的女性子宫内膜癌发病率-年龄对应图。数据来自英国伯明翰癌症登记处 1968—1972 年的数据。这些数据在很大程度上避免了由于美国较高的子宫切除术和卵巢切除术率对年龄-发病率曲线的干扰。点表示实际发病率数据;实线标记"正常",数学模型根据癌症的主要已知危险因素预测发病率。资料来源:Henderson et al. 1993[17]。经美国科学促进会许可转载

虽然雌激素的使用明显增加了侵袭性子宫内膜癌的发病率,但看似矛盾的是,接受过激素治疗的子宫内膜癌患者的总体死亡率却要比未接受激素治疗的子宫内膜癌患者低得多[89]。事实上,与同龄的健康女性相比,接受过激素治疗的子宫内膜癌患者的寿命几乎没有缩短。其原因尚不完全清楚,但这一现象可能是因为雌激素使用者通常接受更多的医学保健和监测。使用 ERT 治疗的女性往往会受到更严密的检查,因为药物经常会导致阴道出血。良好的生存率也部分由于一些雌激素诱导的良性增生患者被误诊为子宫内膜癌的原因。曾经接受过 ERT 治疗的女性罹患子宫内膜癌的风险介于当前接受和从未接受过 ERT 治疗女性之间,但是曾经接受过治疗的女性,即使在多年不再接受治疗,其罹患子宫内膜癌的风险仍明显高于基线水平[90]。

基于上述原因,新的激素治疗方案通常遵循以下两种方案之一:顺序或联合采用雌激素和黄体酮。顺序治疗试图重现正常月经周期的激素模式,尽管所使用的雌激素和孕激素水平都较低。因此,有人可能预测这种激素治疗方案的实施只能部分抵消单纯使用非拮抗 ERT 治疗造成的子宫内膜癌风险的增加。Pike 等人的研究表明,如果激素治疗中每月添加黄体酮不足 10 天,则子宫内膜癌的风险仅能被微弱降低[91]。而每月使用孕激素超过 10 天或采用孕激素与雌激素持续使用的治疗方案并不会增加子宫内膜癌的风险[91]。

在英国进行的"百万女性研究"也支持了这方面的观察,该研究包括在 1996—2001 年招募的 716 738 名未患癌症或未行子宫切除术的绝经后女性[74]。与从未接受任何激素治疗的女性相比,曾经使用持续 CHT 作为最近一次激素治疗方案的女性罹患子宫内膜癌风险明显较低,相对风险为 0.71(95% CI 0.56~0.90)。然而,对于使用环支睾酮的女性,其风险与未使用环支睾酮的女性无差异(RR=1.05;95% CI 0.92~1.22)。单独使用雌激素治疗的女性病例很少,因为自 20 世纪 70 年代中后期以来,这种疗法已很少用于子宫完好的女性患者。在接受雌激素单独治疗的女性中,子宫内膜癌的相对风险显著低于以往研究观察到的风险(RR=1.45;95% CI 1.02~2.06)。正如所料,肥胖通过雌激素途径导致子宫内膜增生,并增加了子宫内膜癌的风险,在肥胖女性中使用 CHT 治疗,其子宫内膜癌的风险的降低程度最大,而在非肥胖女性中使用雌激素单独治疗,其子宫内膜癌的风险的增加程度最大[82,92]。

"百万女性研究"的作者还对已发表的关于 CHT 对子宫内膜癌风险影响的研究进行了广泛的评估,包括他们自己的研究[74]。总的来说,在所有研究中,接受持续 CHT 治疗的女性对比从未接受过治疗的女性,其子宫内膜癌的相对风险为 0.88(95% CI 0.75~1.03)。然而,该结果是基于相对较少的病例——共 6 个包括"女性健康倡议"的研究项目,总共只有 265 例患者的数据可用于此项分析[93]。循环 CHT 治疗导致的子宫内膜癌的相对风险是 1.14(95% CI 1.01~1.28),该结果也是基于 6 个项目共 456 例病例的基础上,其中有四个项目与对持续 CHT 治疗的调查采用的项目是相同的[74]。总体看来,相对从未接受任何激素疗法的女性,采用雌激素和黄体酮每天一起使用的激素治疗方案(连续 CHT 方案)可以轻微地预防子宫内膜癌的风险,而循环使用黄体酮的治疗方案则略微提高子宫内膜癌的风险。

他莫昔芬,一种作用于乳腺的雌激素拮抗剂,可作为子宫内膜雌激素受体激动剂,同 ERT 治疗相似,其可以提高子宫内膜癌的风险[94]。此外,他莫昔芬在之前接受过 ERT 治疗和体重较高的女性中会导致更大的子宫内膜癌风险[94]。他莫昔芬在子宫内膜和乳腺中分别发挥激动剂和拮抗剂的相反作用,其

分子机制尚不完全清楚。

体重

在年轻女性中，体重越高患乳腺癌的风险越低，而在老年女性中，体重越高患乳腺癌的风险越高。与乳腺癌不同的是，在任何年龄段的女性中，体重越高，其患子宫内膜癌的风险越大。对绝经后女性的研究表明，体重较重的女性相对体重较轻的女性罹患子宫内膜癌的风险增至两倍[95,96]。脂肪组织富含芳香化酶系统，可以将雄烯二酮转化为雌酮。反过来，雌酮则可以直接转化为雌二醇。此外，肥胖女性血液中的雌激素与蛋白的结合程度较低，因此绝经后的肥胖女性体内具有生物活性的雌二醇的含量高于单纯从外周雄激素二酮转化为雌二醇的含量。

绝经前的肥胖女性罹患子宫内膜癌风险升高的机制并不明确[96]。虽然肥胖确实与绝经前女性体内具有生物活性的雌二醇水平的轻微升高有关，但仅凭这一点似乎不足以解释如此显著的影响。更可能的解释是，绝经前女性的肥胖与闭经和黄体期黄体酮水平低下有关，从而导致子宫内膜长期接触没有被拮抗的雌激素[97]。

"女性健康倡议"的研究结果发表之后，CHT 治疗逐渐减少，肥胖已成为决定绝经后女性罹患子宫内膜癌风险更重要的因素之一。"美国癌症协会癌症预防研究Ⅱ营养队列"的研究显示，肥胖引起的子宫内膜癌风险显著受到女性是否接受过 CHT 治疗的影响[98]。体型和身体质量指数（kg/m^2）的增加与绝经后女性的子宫内膜癌风险之间的相关性取决于患者是否接受过 CHT 治疗，从未接受过 CHT 治疗的女性风险升高，但是接受过 CHT 治疗的女性风险则不受影响[98]。

口服避孕药

雌激素在诱导子宫内膜癌的主要作用得到了进一步实验证据支持，在相对较短时间内顺序使用口服避孕药，可在月经周期的大部分时间内为机体提供无孕激素拮抗的单纯的雌激素[96,99]。这种强效作用可通过同时给予孕激素而减轻。一系列的病例-对照研究和队列研究共同表明，每日同时使用雌激素和孕激素的联合口服避孕药，可将子宫内膜癌的风险每年降低 11.7%（图 24-3b）[17]。停用口服避孕药后的至少 3 年内使用无孕激素拮抗的单纯的 ERT 治疗则会抵消口服避孕药带来的降低风险的益处[100]。

产次

子宫内膜癌的另一个主要的已确定的危险因素是低产次，可以很容易地用非拮抗雌激素的假说解释[95]。子宫内膜癌的最高风险发生在没有生育过的女性中，而且风险随着女性产次的增加而降低。没有生育过的女性患子宫内膜癌的风险是产次大于三次的女性的 3~5 倍。由于黄体酮水平在妊娠期间持续升高，抑制了子宫内膜的有丝分裂活动，因此预期会出现这种效果。

卵巢癌

现有的流行病学数据显示，在上皮性卵巢癌的四种主要组织病理学亚型（浆液性、子宫内膜型、透明细胞型和黏液性肿瘤）中，激素接触是一致的风险因素（可能黏液性肿瘤除外）。传统认为，上皮性卵巢癌（以下简称卵巢癌）的细胞来源被描述为卵巢表面的单层细胞；因为这些细胞在每次排卵中或排卵后都会进行复制增殖，所以暂停排卵可以预防卵巢癌的发生[101]。这个被称为"不间断排卵"的假说得到了流行病学数据的支持。流行病学数据表明，随着产次和 COC 使用的增加，女性罹患卵巢癌的风险降低，而两者均可导致排卵停止（表 24-3）[102~109]。然而越来越多的证据表明，输卵管和腹膜的浆液性肿瘤与浆液性卵巢癌具有相同的流行病学数据，这使人们开始质疑这种疾病的流行病学基础不是排卵行为和随后的伤口愈合；相反，其基础可能是生育和口服避孕药的使用导致的激素环境变化[110]。此外，更年期激素治疗与卵巢癌风险之间存在明显的相关性，这表明激素环境而不是排卵行为本身影响卵巢癌的风险。

表 24-3　已确定的与卵巢癌相关的激素风险和保护因素的列表

危险因素（排卵次数增加）
绝经年龄推迟
保护因素（排卵次数减少）
妊娠
口服避孕药

与乳腺癌和子宫内膜癌一样，卵巢癌的年龄-发病率曲线表明更年期在决定风险中的重要性。如果将卵巢的年龄从月经初潮起算起，并在停止排卵和绝经时期的卵巢年龄增长速率矫正为正常卵巢的 30%，则卵巢癌的年龄-发病率曲线符合线性重对数坐标图（Linear Log-Log Plot），与其他熟悉的非激素依赖性的上皮肿瘤类似[17]。

产次

产次一直被认为是卵巢癌风险的一个保护因素[102~104]。在女性第一次生产后，卵巢癌的风险降低大约 40%，而再次生产则降低 10%[103~105,111~113]。尽管首次生产带来的风险降低的部分原因可能是一种人为因素，如未产妇对照组中包括了卵巢癌高危的不孕女性在内，但是这种因素并不足以解释首次生育降低卵巢癌风险的显著性[114]。年龄较大（35 岁或以上）女性相比年轻女性的（25 岁以下）从生育中获得保护益处更大，但这个结果并没有在所有的研究中被观察到，因此需要进一步的跟进研究的验证[103~105,112,115]。

口服避孕药

流行病学的研究表明，口服避孕药的使用可降低卵巢癌的风险，其效果与观察到的子宫内膜癌的保护作用类似，且与持续用药的时间有关[104~109]。一项对 45 项流行病学研究的联合分析表明，使用任何口服避孕药都能降低 27% 的卵巢癌风险（95% CI 0.70~0.76），每使用五年可降低 20% 的风险[109]。这项分析还表明随着时间的推移，风险降低的程度有所减弱；最后一次使用口服避孕药在 10 年内的女性的五年发病风险降低

29%，而最后一次使用口服避孕药在20~29年前的女性的五年发病风险仅降低15%。然而，风险的降低可以持续了几十年。在本研究中，在不同的组织病理学亚型中观察到了统计学上显著性的异质性，其中黏液性肿瘤的风险降低在统计上并不显著。

假说认为，停止排卵是通过生育和口服避孕药来预防卵巢癌的机制；然而，另一种解释可能是机体通过口服避孕药和怀孕获得高水平的黄体酮。在正常月经周期内，每天平均接触的黄体酮浓度约为3.5ng/ml，而口服避孕药的女性则为9.2ng/ml[116,117]。同样，怀孕与高黄体酮水平有关。一项对雌性猕猴的研究表明，口服避孕药中使用的孕激素可诱导卵巢上皮细胞凋亡，从而起到预防卵巢癌的作用[118]。此外，体外实验证明雌激素能促进卵巢肿瘤细胞的生长，而这种作用可被黄体酮阻断[119,120]。

激素治疗

近年来，有关激素治疗和卵巢癌风险的流行病学证据已经越来越清楚。对2007年发表的基于人群的病例-对照研究[105,121~127]和队列研究[128~132]的文献进行了详细的统合分析，结果表明，每接受五年的更年期ERT治疗，会增加22%的卵巢癌风险（$P<0.0001$）。这种相关性在所有文献中基本上一致，只有一篇报道两者没有相关性[121]。在显示相关性的13份文献中，两者相关性的剂量效应关系是明确的。

对接受更年期雌激素-孕激素治疗的结果进行分析也得出清楚的相关性，但一致性较差。基于人群的病例对照研究[105,121,123~126,129]、队列研究[130~132]和“女性健康倡议”实验[93]的统和分析结果显示，每接受五年的CHT治疗，卵巢癌的风险增加10%（$P=0.001$）。单纯雌激素治疗与CHT治疗的风险差异具有统计学意义（$P=0.004$），提示在ERT治疗中添加黄体酮可改善雌激素的作用。这些分析为黄体酮对卵巢癌风险的保护作用提供了进一步的支持。

目前尚不清楚CHT的疗效是否因顺序或持续联合用药方案而异。四项研究阐明了这个问题。“百万女性研究”没有发现用药与否对卵巢癌风险影响的差异[131]，但是缺乏用药使用时间的资料。美国国立卫生研究院退休人员协会的队列研究报告，顺序联合治疗的卵巢癌风险高于持续联合治疗，但两种方案都会增加卵巢癌的风险[130]。美国的一项病例-对照研究报告显示，两种联合治疗方案均降低了患卵巢癌的风险，而瑞典的一项病例-对照研究发现，顺序联合治疗增加了卵巢癌风险，但是连续联合治疗没有增加风险[125,126]。但是在瑞典，持续联合治疗与顺序联合治疗相比，所用黄体酮的剂量更高，这可能解释了瑞典研究中该方案与卵巢癌缺乏相关性[28]，在这方面需要进一步的后续研究。

考虑到更年期激素治疗的这些发现，我们可以从一个新的角度来看待生育和口服避孕药降低卵巢癌风险的观察结果，特别是这两个保护因素的作用机制可能通过增加黄体酮的水平来发挥作用。这与一种新近提出的学术观点具有一致性，即卵巢表面的单层细胞可能不是卵巢癌的起源。

前列腺癌

前列腺癌是美国男性最常被诊断的癌症，预计2014年将有233 000例前列腺癌病例。前列腺癌是男性癌症死亡的第二大原因，仅次于肺癌，每年约有29 480人死于前列腺癌[18]。前列腺是雄激素的靶器官，雄激素被认为是前列腺上皮细胞分裂的主要刺激因子。因此，雄激素是前列腺癌发生的主要原因之一。直到最近，只有间接证据支持雄激素在前列腺癌发展中的因果作用[7,133]。“前列腺癌预防试验”（Prostate Cancer Prevention Trial，PCPT）使用一种降低前列腺雄激素作用的药物开展研究，其结果首次直接证实雄激素在前列腺癌发生过程中发挥重要的调控作用[134]。评估雄激素在前列腺癌发生发展中的功能是困难的，部分原因是男性缺乏像女性一样容易测量的激素相关表型（例如初潮、更年期、生育经验）。此外，使用外源性雄激素治疗疾病的男性患者相对较少。

前列腺癌的流行病学主要由三个观察结果构成：①发病率和死亡率在不同国家和种族-民族间存在显著差异，前列腺癌在高风险（非洲裔美国人）和低风险（日本和中国土著）人群之间的历史报道差异可高达80倍[135]；②隐匿性亚临床前列腺癌的发生率在人群中相对比较普遍[136]；③前列腺癌发病率与年龄显著相关性[7]。前列腺癌在50岁之前极其罕见，但它仍然是美国男性最常见的癌症，很大程度上是因为随着年龄的增长，前列腺癌发病率的增长速度比其他任何癌症都要快。

男性激素在前列腺癌发展中发挥作用的一些间接证据来自对有高、中、低前列腺癌风险的健康男性的激素含量的比较。尽管研究没有显示白人和非裔美国男性在睾丸激素水平上的差异[12,137,138]，最近的证据表明，非裔美国人的雌二醇水平高于白人和拉丁裔[139]。亚洲男性的循环睾酮水平在任何年龄段相对于白人和非洲裔美国人都没有更低，却有着较低的雄烷二醇葡萄糖醛酸苷水平[140,141]。这种激素反映的是5α-还原酶的活性（5α-还原酶是一种前列腺酶，能将睾酮生物活性化为二氢睾酮，后者是最具生物活性的人类雄激素）。基于这些结果和假定的雄激素在前列腺细胞增殖中的作用，Ross等人提出5α-还原酶抑制剂可能是前列腺癌的有效化学预防剂[140]。

另外一些间接证据表明雄激素在前列腺癌发病机制中起作用。在大多数前列腺腺癌的动物模型中，雄激素是前列腺癌发生发展所必需的[142]。在阉人、遗传导致的5α-还原酶活性降低、雄激素活性极低和前列腺高度发育不良的男性中[7]从未报道过前列腺癌的发生。前列腺癌，至少在发病初期，几乎都是雄激素依赖性的，雄激素剥夺治疗在过去几十年来一直是治疗早期转移性前列腺癌的主要方法。

循环雄激素与前列腺癌风险之间的关系已被多项研究调查，但具体结果并不一致。“内源性激素和前列腺癌合作团队”（Endogenous Hormones and Prostate Cancer Collaborative Group）对18项前瞻性研究的大型汇总分析发现，前列腺癌的风险与睾酮、双氢睾酮、硫酸脱氢表雄酮、雄烯二酮、雄烯二醇葡醛内酯或雌二醇的循环水平均没有相关性[143]。循环性激素结合球蛋白与前列腺癌的风险降低有关联，其含量处于最高五分位的男性与处于最低五分位的男性相比，相对风险降低了14%。性激素结合球蛋白调节循环系统中游离睾酮和雌二醇的水平，也可能在类固醇信号中发挥作用[144]。虽然大多数循环雄激素似乎不影响前列腺癌的风险，但这些研究的一个重要考量因素是，单次激素的测量是否能准确反映个体的平均激素水平的全貌。

有关雄激素在前列腺癌中作用的最令人信服的证据来源于 PCPT 项目[134]。在 PCPT 项目中，18 882 名 55 岁或以上的前列腺特异性抗原(PSA)正常的健康男性，被随机分配接受 5 毫克每日的 5α-还原酶抑制剂-非那雄胺或安慰剂。七年后，所有男性都被指定接受试验结束时的前列腺活检。药物组的前列腺癌发病率降低了约 25%。然而，矛盾的是，在药物组中，高恶性等级的前列腺癌发病率在统计上显著增加了 25%。这种奇怪的结果引起了关于 5α-还原酶抑制剂是否预防前列腺癌的激烈争议。例如，有人认为，这一发现表示非那雄胺可在前列腺中引起人为的破坏性形态变化，或者高恶性等级的前列腺癌风险的增加是由于非那雄胺诱导前列腺体积减小而导致的检测偏差[145]。另外，有人认为这些结果预示着明确的生物学基础；例如，Ross 等认为高级别的前列腺癌前体细胞可能携带雄激素受体基因的遗传学变异(拷贝数倍增、基因突变)，在缺乏雄激素的环境中可增殖[146]。因此，具有 5α-还原酶Ⅱ型基因突变的前列腺癌细胞对抑制剂的反应不同于没有这种基因突变的细胞，而非那雄胺由于前列腺内睾酮水平的增加，选择性地刺激前列腺癌前体细胞发生高恶性级别的病变。彻底解读这些结果的潜在机制可对前列腺癌的公共卫生领域的发展产生深远的影响。

遗传学的决定因素

家族性风险

乳腺癌家族史与疾病风险增加有关[4]。当家族中有一名女性早年患病或患有双侧乳腺癌疾病时，这一点尤其明显。总体而言，患有乳腺癌女性的一级亲属患病风险增加了两到三倍，而在绝经前患有双侧乳腺癌的女性的一级亲属患病风险增加了九倍。有一个以上的一级亲属罹患乳腺癌的女性也具有非常高的风险(五倍及以上)。

类似的，基于人群的病例-对照研究表明，卵巢癌患者的一级亲属患卵巢癌的风险增加了两到三倍[147,148]。根据一项经典的双胞胎研究，乳腺癌和卵巢癌的遗传率约为 25%[149]。家族史对子宫内膜癌风险的影响仍然存在争议[150~155]。与乳腺癌和卵巢癌不同的是，双胞胎的遗传研究显示子宫内膜癌并没有很强的遗传因素[149]。

前列腺癌也是一种高度家族性疾病。与没有前列腺癌家族史的男性相比，一级亲属患前列腺癌的男性风险大约增加了两到三倍，而且这种增加在不同种族群体中都明显存在[156]。与乳腺癌一样，当一个男性有多个一级亲属患前列腺癌或患前列腺癌的亲属在相对较年轻的时候被诊断出疾病时，其患病风险会进一步升高[157]。双胞胎研究表明前列腺癌的遗传性约为 42%，是所有散发性癌症中最高的[149]。

基因和变异

过去的二十年间，我们在确定癌症的易感等位基因方面取得了非凡的成就。等位基因的遗传易感性可大致分为高、中、低外显率[5]。高外显率等位基因通常具有≥10 的相对风险和>50%的终生风险；中外显率等位基因的相对风险为 2~9(大部分为 5 或更低)，终身风险为 20%~50%；而低外显率等位基因的相对风险<2(大多为 1~1.5)，终生风险为 10%~19%。高外显率和中外显率基因的有害突变很少见(一般为 1%或更低)，而低外显率等位基因的有害突变在一般人群中很常见(主要为>5%)。高外显率等位基因，如乳腺癌的 *BRCA1* 和 *BRCA2*，是通过家系连锁分析和定位克隆鉴定而来[11,12]。生殖细胞的 *BRCA1* 突变携带者终生罹患乳腺癌和卵巢癌的风险分别为 60%~80%和 30%~40%。而生殖细胞 *BRCA2* 突变的携带者罹患腺癌和卵巢癌的风险估计分别为 40%~50%和 10%~15%[158]。

从家族性癌症综合征中发现了更多的高外显率的等位基因，包括 Li-Fraumeni 综合征中的 *TP53* 突变、Peutz-Jeghers 综合征中的 *STK11/LKB1* 突变和 PTEN hamartoma 肿瘤综合征中的 *PTEN* 突变[15,159,160]。遗传性非息肉性结直肠癌(HNPCC 或 Lynch 综合征)患者罹患子宫内膜癌的终身风险达到 40%~60%，且 Lynch 综合征相关的错配修复基因(如 *MLH1*、*MSH2*、*MSH6*)的突变被认为是子宫内膜癌的高外显率等位基因[161,162]。尽管经过 20 年的努力，仍然没有发现前列腺癌具有一致的高外显率等位基因[6]。

乳腺癌和卵巢癌的中外显性的等位基因主要存在于 DNA 修复基因中，最显著的是那些与 Fanconi 贫血(FA)-BRCA 通路相关的基因[163,164]。这些等位基因是通过对 DNA 修复缺陷综合征的连锁分析、候选基因的重新测序以及最近的全外显子组测序发现的。Fanconi 贫血(FA)是一种罕见的隐性染色体不稳定综合征，以儿童期再生障碍性贫血、骨髓衰竭和细胞对 DNA 交联剂敏感为特征[165]。到目前为止，已在 FA 患者中鉴定出 15 个基因的突变。这些基因的产物与熟知的 DNA 损伤反应蛋白相互作用，包括 BRCA1、ATM 和 NBS1 在内，并参与多种细胞 DNA 修复途径，特别是双链断裂后的同源重组(HR)修复[165,166]。FA 相关基因的纯合突变导致 FA 综合征，而其杂合突变则使携带者罹患乳腺癌和卵巢癌的风险增加。*BRCA2*(*FANCD1*)是 FA 相关基因之一。有趣的是，除了易患乳腺癌和卵巢癌，*BRCA2* 也是前列腺癌的一种中等外显率基因：与没有发生 *BRCA2* 突变的男性相比，具有生殖系 *BRCA2* 突变的男性患前列腺癌的风险几乎高出五倍[167,168]。另外两个 FA 相关基因，*FANCJ/BRIP1*(BRCA1 相互作用蛋白)和 *FANCN/PALB2*(BRCA2 相互作用蛋白)，也被证明是乳腺癌和卵巢癌的中等外显率等位基因[164,166,169~171]。除了 FA 相关基因外，许多其他的与 DNA 修复和细胞周期控制相关的基因被确定为乳腺癌和卵巢癌的中度外显等位基因。例如，细胞周期检查点激酶 *CHEK2* 中的一种截短变异(1100delC)导致女性乳腺癌风险增加约两倍和男性乳腺癌风险增加 10 倍[172]。*ATM* 突变在双等位基因的情况下会导致共济失调毛细血管扩张，而单等位基因突变携带者则乳腺癌易感，估计相对风险为 2.4[173]；两种同源重组基因 *RAD51C* 和 *RAD51D* 的有害突变是卵巢癌的中等外显率等位基因，而不是乳腺癌的[174,175]。在 DNA 聚合酶 delta 基因(*POLD1*)的校对区发生生殖细胞系突变会带来很高的子宫内膜癌风险[176]。参与前列腺的正常发育和雄激素反应的一个关键决定基因同源框转录因子 *HOXB13* 的一个错义突变 Gly84Glu 是前列腺癌的风险因子。该突变是从超过 200 个前列腺癌家系中测序鉴定出的，且最近的一项统合分析研究了 24 213 例病例和 73 631 例对照，发现这种突变增加了四倍的前列腺癌的风险(OR=4.07;95% CI 3.05~5.45)[177,178]。

所有高外显率和中等外显率的等位基因加起来决定乳腺癌家族风险的20%~25%[179]。普通癌症的家族风险被认为较大部分是由常见的低外显率的等位基因造成的(在一般人群中次要等位基因频率>5%)。直接对不相关病例和对照病例之间的等位基因频率进行比较的关联研究是识别低外显率等位基因最有效的方法。从20世纪90年代中期开始的早期癌症关联研究采用的是一种候选基因方法,即在与特定癌症的生物学和病因相关的基因中选择潜在的功能变异,主要是单核苷酸多态性(SNP)。候选基因通常编码参与激素生物合成、DNA修复、细胞周期控制、细胞生长、凋亡和其他重要细胞功能的蛋白,这些功能的异常会导致癌症的发生。然而,尽管最初有数百个SNP被候选基因关联研究报告为潜在的癌症易感性位点,但很少有在后续更大规模的验证研究中获得令人信服的证据[180]。从候选基因关联研究中发现的唯一令人信服的乳腺癌低外显率等位基因是caspase-8(*CASP8*)基因中的功能性SNP(Asp302His):次要等位基因(His等位基因的频率为13%)以剂量依赖的方式对乳腺癌具有保护作用(每个等位基因OR=0.88;95% CI 0.84~0.92)。这一结果是基于对16 423例乳腺癌患者和17 109名对照者的分析得出的[181]。此外,候选基因的关联研究并没有从卵巢癌、子宫内膜癌或前列腺癌中找到令人信服的易感SNP。

2005年GWAS技术的出现开创了一个基因关联研究的新时代[182]。利用高通量的基因分型平台,可以同时检验数十万到数百万个SNP,GWAS允许一种不可知论的研究方法,不需要事先知道基因功能或单核苷酸多态性的先验知识。GWAS通过一组SNP标记基因组中所有已知的常见变异,揭示了特定等位基因与疾病风险之间的关系。截至2014年12月,超过250篇关于癌症风险的GWAS文献确定了数百种常见的、低外显率的大约35种癌症类型的SNP[16]。到目前为止,已在不同种族群体的乳腺癌和前列腺癌中鉴定出最多的易感性SNP:包括分布在28个染色体区域的70多个乳腺癌易感性SNP和分布在47个染色体区域的80个前列腺癌易感性SNP。相比之下,卵巢癌的研究在9个染色体区域中鉴定出20个易感性SNPs,而子宫内膜癌只鉴定出一个位于染色体17q12的位点[16]。不同癌症通过GWAS识别到的易感性SNPs数量的差异可归因于不同的样本大小(乳腺癌和前列腺癌更常见,其GWAS样本量大于卵巢癌和子宫内膜癌)和不同的遗传性(子宫内膜癌遗传性远低于其他三个癌症)。几乎所有这些SNP都具有一定的风险,等位基因的OR值小于1.5。大多数SNP都具有癌症位点的特异性;然而,有几个区域对多种癌症和其他病症也显示出多效性的影响,例如,位于染色体5p15.33的*TERT-CLPTM1L*位点有一些常见的特异性SNP,决定至少10种癌症(包括乳腺癌、卵巢癌和前列腺癌)的易感性[183~185]。

此外,在癌基因*MYC*附近的染色体8q24区域与包括乳腺癌、卵巢癌和前列腺癌在内的至少7种恶性肿瘤有关[186]。这些SNP中的绝大多数位于基因间或内含子区,有些位于完全的“基因沙漠”区域,因此,在大多数易感区域的致病变异和致病基因是未知的。然而,新出现的对已鉴定的DNA区域进行精细的定位和对候选基因的功能研究已经为研究特定癌症的病因提供了重要的生物学理解。

对于乳腺癌,10q26位点的*FGFR2*是一种酪氨酸激酶受体,在5%~10%的乳腺肿瘤中过表达,是最强的乳腺癌风险相关基因。*FGFR2*的第二个内含子中至少存在三个可能的致病SNP,经被确定可以与*FGFR2*的启动子相互作用,并且有证据表明这些致病SNP具有等位基因特异性的转录因子结合[187,188]。乳腺癌的另一个强易感基因是位于11q13的*CCND1*,有一项精细的基因图谱研究发现三个独立的SNP与ER阳性的乳腺癌相关[189]。染色质构象研究表明所有三个SNP都与转录增强子或沉默子及它们的靶基因*CCND1*相互作用[189]。在与激素相关的乳腺癌病因中,有两个乳腺癌易感性SNP靠近雌激素受体ER通路相关基因,其中6q25.1的SNP rs3757318位于ERα基因*ESR1*上游约200kb处,21q21的SNP rs2823093与*NRIP1/RIP140*相近,后者与ERα相互作用的,抑制ER信号传导并抑制其促有丝分裂的作用[190,191]。这两个基因是否是这两个区域的主效致癌因素尚值得进一步研究。其他可能的乳腺癌易感基因包括生长因子、癌基因、肿瘤抑制因子,以及参与DNA修复、细胞周期调控、乳腺发育、端粒维持、凋亡和肿瘤侵袭性的基因[5]。总的来说,目前发现的常见低外显率的等位基因可以解释了大约14%的乳腺癌家族风险[192]。而据估计,现有GWAS平台可通过测序更大的样本库鉴定出1 000多个新的乳腺癌易感性SNP;但是,单独的SNP发挥的作用非常小,OR主要在1.02~1.05。所有这些已确定和尚未确定的常见低外显率SNP估计约占乳腺癌家族风险的28%[192]。

在卵巢癌中,GWAS在9个染色体区域鉴定出20个易感性SNP:2q31,3q25,8q21,8q24,9p22.2,10p12,17q12,17q21和19p13区域出现在白人群体,两个独立的区域出现在中国汉族群体[193,194]。这些区域的主效致病基因包括两个同源框基因*HOXD1*和*HOXD3*(均在2q31处)、一个多聚二磷酸腺苷酸(ADP)核糖聚合酶(PARP)基因*TiPARP*(3q25)、在8q21处的染色质修饰蛋白4c(*CHMP4C*))、癌基因*MYC*(8q24),9p22.2的DNA结合锌指基因*BNC2*,17q12的同源域包含转录因子*HNF1B*和19p13的BRCA1相互作用基因*BABAM1/MERIT40*。总之,这些SNP只能解释卵巢癌家族风险的5%。

在子宫内膜癌中,GWAS迄今为止只鉴定出一个位点,即17q12处的*HNF1B*[195,196]。该区域的SNP也与浆液性和透明细胞性卵巢癌、前列腺癌和2型糖尿病相关[193,197,198~200]。*HNF1B*编码包含同源域的转录因子超家族的一个成员,是一个转录激活因子[201]。*HNF1B*的表达在许多癌症中发生改变,根据不同的组织环境可能分别发挥抑癌基因或致癌基因的作用。最近的一项精细映射研究将子宫内膜癌与*HNF1B*的第一个内含子中的单个信号关联并表明:其关键的SNP位于*HNF1B*的扩展启动子,该启动子包含负调控元件,并与*HNF1B*在子宫内膜肿瘤中的表达有关[202]。

前列腺癌是最具有遗传性的癌症之一,与其他癌症相比,前列腺癌的GWAS研究发现了最多的易感性变异。所有已鉴定的易感性SNP可解释约30%的前列腺癌家族风险。与乳腺癌相似,47个从前列腺易感位点中鉴定出的潜在致病基因与许多细胞功能相关，如 DNA 修复、细胞周期控制、端粒维持、细胞生长、细胞黏附和雄激素受体信号传导[6]。有几个区域的具有显著的重要性，如多效性的 8q24 位点位于 *MYC* 癌基因附近，其涵括独立与前列腺癌风险相关的 SNP 数量最多[6]。功能研究表明，这个区域的 SNP 位于转录增强子，可以通过与 *MYC* 基因远程互作来调控其表达[203,204]。另外一个多效性的区域 5p15 至少有四个独立的位点位于 *TERT* 基因的启动子或内含子区域，且最新的精细基因图谱定位研究表明其与前列腺癌的风险相关[205]。此外，对正常前列腺组织的基因表达分析表明，其中一个位点与 *TERT* 的表达有关，为疾病的易感性提供了一种可能的机制[205]。19q13 位点包含了编码丝氨酸蛋白酶的激肽释放酶（KLK）家族蛋白的基因，其中以 PSA（由 *KLK3* 基因编码）最为熟知。一项精细图谱研究发现，*KLK3* 基因中有一个常见的 SNP 错误编码（rs17632542，Ile179Thr），该 SNP 与前列腺癌风险关系最为显著[206]。这个 SNP 也与血清 PSA 水平显著相关[207]。如前所述，17q21 位点上的 *HOXB13* 基因中有一个罕见的错码突变 Gly84Glu 是前列腺癌的一个中等外显等位基因。有趣的是，*HOXB13* 基因中常见的 SNP 也与前列腺癌风险有关[208]。该位点的精细映射研究发现一群位于 *HOXB13* 内部或上游的 SNP 簇与前列腺癌的风险高度相关。此外，这些常见的 SNP 频率较低、部分与 Gly84Glu 突变相关。这是第一个通过常见 SNP 检测到的适度的 GWAS 关联，由具有较高相对风险的罕见主效变异所驱动，为基因调控的合成关联导致癌症易感性的现象提供了证据[209]。最后，Xq12 位点的 SNP rs5919432 位于距离 AR 基因的 77kb 处，提示 AR 变异在前列腺癌病因学中的作用[210]。

尽管目前在鉴定高、中、低外显率等位基因方面取得了巨大的进展，但各种类型的散发性癌症中仍有超过 50% 的家族风险无法解释。通过国际合作，分析超大样本量（大于 10 万病例），找寻剩余常见的、低外显率和影响力非常小的等位基因，全面揭示癌症遗传性。癌症研究中越来越多地应用了全外显子组测序和全基因组测序，通过大样本分析鉴定罕见的、未知的高、中外显率等位基因。此外，其他形式的易感性变异，如基因结构变化（如拷贝数变化）和遗传相互作用（基因-基因和基因-环境相互作用）可能会解释一些当前尚未发现的遗传性[211]。

结论

随着我们对流行病学的危险因素与激素水平间关系的理解不断加深，对激素相关肿瘤的一级预防途径也越来越清晰。控制肥胖对子宫内膜癌和绝经后的乳腺癌都有明显的影响。获取更多儿童饮食和运动、青春期发育及与青春期/青年期的激素生理学相关的信息，为女性乳腺癌、卵巢癌和子宫内膜癌的预防提供更多依据。化学预防试验显示：他莫昔芬可以有效降低高危妇女罹患乳腺癌的风险，而雌激素受体调节剂雷洛昔芬和芳香化酶抑制剂阿那曲唑可以降低绝经后高危妇女患乳腺癌的风险。因 COC 和 CHT 处方的推广，卵巢癌和子宫内膜癌的激素化学预防成为现实。目前已完成一项全国范围内的使用 5α-还原酶抑制剂非那雄胺预防前列腺癌的试验，为评估雄激素在前列腺癌中的作用提供了坚实可靠的证据。随着我们对增加癌症风险的基因突变和多态性的深入了解，将能更好的个性化预测激素相关肿瘤的易感性，以为高风险人口亚群提供干预策略。

（王旭　雷群英　译　王义平　雷群英　校）

部分参考文献

4 Henderson BE, Feigelson HS. Hormonal carcinogenesis. *Carcinogenesis*. 2000;**21**(**3**):427–433.

5 Ghoussaini M, Pharoah PD, Easton DF. Inherited genetic susceptibility to breast cancer: the beginning of the end or the end of the beginning? *Am J Pathol*. 2013;**183**(**4**):1038–1051.

6 Eeles R, Goh C, Castro E, et al. The genetic epidemiology of prostate cancer and its clinical implications. *Nat Rev Urol*. 2014;**11**(**1**):18–31.

8 Chan JM, Stampfer MJ, Giovannucci E, et al. Plasma insulin-like growth factor-I and prostate cancer risk: a prospective study. *Science*. 1998;**279**(**5350**):563–566.

11 Miki Y, Swensen J, Shattuck-Eidens D, et al. A strong candidate for the breast and ovarian cancer susceptibility gene BRCA1. *Science*. 1994;**266**(**5182**):66–71.

12 Wooster R, Bignell G, Lancaster J, et al. Identification of the breast cancer susceptibility gene BRCA2. *Nature*. 1995;**378**(**6559**):789–792.

13 Søgaard M, Kjaer SK, Gayther S. Ovarian cancer and genetic susceptibility in relation to the BRCA1 and BRCA2 genes. Occurrence, clinical importance and intervention. *Acta Obstet Gynecol Scand*. 2006;**85**(**1**):93–105.

17 Henderson BE, Ross RK, Pike MC. Hormonal chemoprevention of cancer in women. *Science*. 1993;**259**(**5095**):633–638.

22 Key TJ, Pike MC. The role of oestrogens and progestagens in the epidemiology and prevention of breast cancer. *Eur J Cancer Clin Oncol*. 1988;**24**(**1**):29–43.

25 Ross RK, Paganini-Hill A, Wan PC, et al. Effect of hormone replacement therapy on breast cancer risk: estrogen versus estrogen plus progestin. *J Natl Cancer Inst*. 2000;**92**(**4**):328–332.

27 Chlebowski RT, Hendrix SL, Langer RD, et al. Influence of estrogen plus progestin on breast cancer and mammography in healthy postmenopausal women: the Women's Health Initiative Randomized Trial. *JAMA*. 2003;**289**:3243–3253.

28 Lee SA, Ross RK, Pike MC. An overview of menopausal oestrogen-progestin hormone therapy and breast cancer risk. *Br J Cancer*. 2005;**92**(**11**):2049–2058.

29 Henderson BE, Pike MC, Casagrande JT. Breast cancer and the oestrogen window hypothesis. *Lancet*. 1981;**2**(**8242**):363–364.

34 Bernstein L, Henderson BE, Hanisch R, et al. Physical exercise and reduced risk of breast cancer in young women. *J Natl Cancer Inst*. 1994;**86**(**18**):1403–1408.

38 McTiernan A, Kooperberg C, White E, et al. Recreational physical activity and the risk of breast cancer in postmenopausal women: the Women's Health Initiative Cohort Study. *JAMA*. 2003;**290**:1331–1336.

56 Newcomb PA, Storer BE, Longnecker MP, et al. Lactation and a reduced risk of premenopausal breast cancer. *New Engl J Med*. 1994;**330**:81–86.

62 Prentice RL, Caan B, Chlebowski RT, et al. Low-fat dietary pattern and risk of invasive breast cancer: the Women's Health Initiative Randomized Controlled Dietary Modification Trial. *JAMA*. 2006;**295**(**6**):629–642.

67 Collaborative Group on Hormonal Factors in Breast Cancer. Breast cancer and hormonal contraceptives: collaborative reanalysis of individual data on 53,297 women with breast cancer and 100,239 women without breast cancer from 54 epidemiological studies. *Lancet*. 1996;**347**(**9017**):1713–1727.

68 Marchbanks PA, McDonald JA, Wilson HG, et al. Oral contraceptives and the risk of breast cancer. *N Engl J Med*. 2002;**346**:2025–2032.

71 Committee TW'sHIS. Effects of conjugated equine estrogen in postmenopausal women with hysterectomy. *JAMA*. 2004;**291**:1701–1712.

72 Stefanick ML, Anderson GL, Margolis KL, et al. Effects of conjugated equine estrogens on breast cancer and mammography screening in postmenopausal women with hysterectomy. *JAMA*. 2006;**295**(**14**):1647–1657.

73 Schairer C, Lubin JH, Triosi R, et al. Menopausal estrogen and estrogen-progestin replacement therapy and breast cancer risk. *JAMA*. 2000;**283**:485–491.

75 Heiss G, Wallace R, Anderson GL, et al. Health risks and benefits 3 years after stopping randomized treatment with estrogen and progestin. *JAMA*. 2008;**299**(**9**):1036–1045.

91 Pike MC, Peters RK, Cozen W, et al. Estrogen-progestin replacement therapy and endometrial cancer. *J Natl Cancer Inst*. 1997;**89**(**15**):1110–1116.

93 Anderson GL, Judd HL, Kaunitz AM, et al. Effect of estrogen plus progestin on gynecologic cancers and associated diagnostic procedures: the Women's Health Initiative randomized trial. *JAMA*. 2003;**290**:1739–1748.

94 Bernstein L, Deapen D, Cerhan JR, et al. Tamoxifen therapy for breast cancer and endometrial cancer risk. *J Natl Cancer Inst*. 1999;**91**(**19**):1654–1662.

102 Adami HO, Hsieh CC, Lambe M, et al. Parity, age at first childbirth, and risk of ovarian cancer. *Lancet*. 1994;**344**(**8932**):1250–1254.

109 Collaborative Group on Epidemiological Studies of Ovarian Cancer. Ovarian Can-

cer and oral contraceptives: collaborative reanalysis of data from 45 epidemiological studies including 23,257 women with ovarian cancer and 87,303 controls. *The Lancet*. 2008;**371**:303-314.

114 Ness RB, Cramer DW, Goodman MT, et al. Infertility, fertility drugs, and ovarian cancer: a pooled analysis of case-control studies. *Am J Epidemiol*. 2002;**155(3)**:217-224.

119 Risch HA. Hormonal etiology of epithelial ovarian cancer, with a hypothesis concerning the role of androgens and progesterone. *J Natl Cancer Inst*. 1998;**90(23)**:1774-1786.

129 Lacey JV Jr, Mink PJ, Lubin JH, et al. Menopausal hormone replacement therapy and risk of ovarian cancer. *JAMA*. 2002;**288**:334-341.

130 Lacey JV Jr, Brinton LA, Leitzmann MF, et al. Menopausal hormone therapy and ovarian cancer risk in the National Institutes of Health-AARP Diet and Health Study Cohort. *J Natl Cancer Inst*. 2006;**98(19)**:1397-1405.

131 Beral V, Bull D, Green J, et al. Ovarian cancer and hormone replacement therapy in the Million Women Study. *Lancet*. 2007;**369(9574)**:1703-1710.

134 Thompson IM, Goodman PJ, Tangen CM, et al. The influence of finasteride on the development of prostate cancer. *New Engl J Med*. 2003;**349**:215-224.

143 Roddam AW, Allen NE, Appleby P, et al. Endogenous sex hormones and prostate cancer: a collaborative analysis of 18 prospective studies. *J Natl Cancer Inst*. 2008;**100(3)**:170-183.

149 Lichtenstein P, Holm NV, Verkasalo PK, et al. Environmental and heritable factors in the causation of cancer—analyses of cohorts of twins from Sweden, Denmark, and Finland. *N Engl J Med*. 2000;**343(2)**:78-85.

158 Antoniou A, Pharoah PD, Narod S, et al. Average risks of breast and ovarian cancer associated with BRCA1 or BRCA2 mutations detected in case Series unselected for family history: a combined analysis of 22 studies. *Am J Hum Genet*. 2003;**72(5)**:1117-1130.

163 D'Andrea AD. Susceptibility pathways in Fanconi's anemia and breast cancer. *N Engl J Med*. 2010;**362(20)**:1909-1919.

192 Michailidou K, Hall P, Gonzalez-Neira A, et al. Large-scale genotyping identifies 41 new loci associated with breast cancer risk. *Nat Genet*. 2013;**45(4)**:353-361, 361e1-2.

208 Eeles RA, Olama AA, Benlloch S, et al. Identification of 23 new prostate cancer susceptibility loci using the iCOGS custom genotyping array. *Nat Genet*. 2013;**45(4)**:385-391, 391e1-e2.

第 25 章 电离辐射

David J. Grdina, PhD

概述

许多实验性和流行病研究已证实电离辐射具有致癌作用。本章简要总结了电离辐射对于生物系统的影响、适应性和旁观者效应、辐射致癌的细胞及分子机制以及控制恶性进展的药物治疗手段。

辐射损伤理论的发展

1895 年伦琴发现 X 射线。此后不久,人们就认识到了暴露于电离辐射的危害。在老式 X 射线发生器的操作人员中可观察到急性皮肤反应。1902 年报道了第一例辐射诱导的癌症,该癌症发生在皮肤溃疡处。几年之内,类似的皮肤癌大量涌现,并于 1911 年首次出现了五名射线工人罹患白血病的报道[1]。图 25-1 描述了电离辐射与生物组织的相互作用,以及辐射损伤如何产生。电离是分子的一个电子从轨道逃逸,产生带正电荷或"离子化"分子的过程。这些分子极度不稳定,能迅速发生化学变化,产生自由基。这一过程最常见的产物就是水分解产生的超氧阴离子自由基(O_2^-)、过氧化氢(H_2O_2)和高反应性羟自由基。这种羟自由基寿命极短,仅能与周围 4nm 半径范围内的其他分子相互作用[2]。活跃线粒体使活性氧(ROS)大量增加,级联放大 ROS 损伤信号[3]。"ROS 介导的 ROS 释放"(ROS-induced ROS release, RIRR)过程是其潜在机制之一。在强大的氧化应激负荷下,ROS 在线粒体内增加达到阈值,触发线粒体通透性转换孔(mitochondrial permeability transition, MPT)或内膜阴离子通道(inner membrane anion channel, IMAC)开放,继而导致线粒体膜电位同步下降,以及暂时性的电子传递链生成 ROS 增加。大量 ROS 释放到胞质,作为第二信使激活邻近线粒体内的 RIRR[4,5]。辐射能在数分钟内生成短寿命的活性氧或氮,同时伴有可逆性线粒体膜电位去极化[3]。单个线粒体的辐射损伤能够通过可逆性钙离子依赖的 MPT 传递到相邻线粒体,导致 ROS 生成的增加。这种由级联反应导致的 ROS 增加和传递会靶向损伤重要的生物分子,导致细胞死亡,这些重要生物分子包括 DNA、核骨架、胞质转运系统、线粒体膜和细胞膜。ROS 可被内源性抗氧化剂如超氧化物歧化酶(SOD)或外源性加入的抗氧化剂清除。

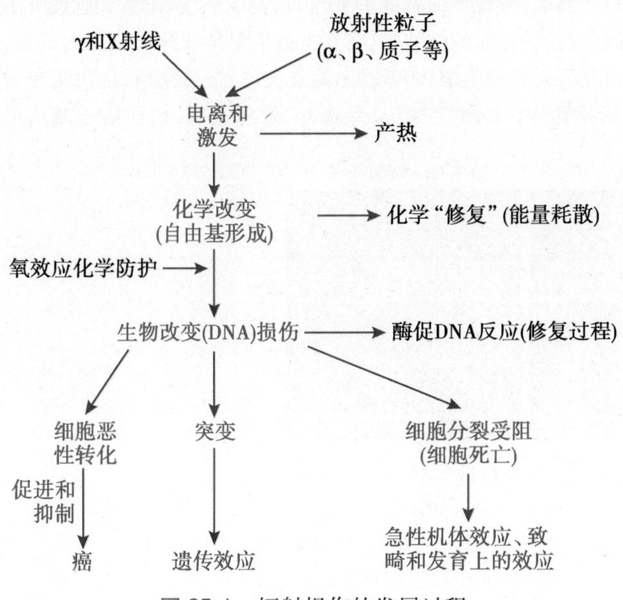

图 25-1 辐射损伤的发展过程

辐射对细胞和组织的主要作用效应

细胞杀伤

辐射能够通过凋亡和间期死亡杀死细胞[6~8]。在受到辐射几小时内,细胞进入凋亡程序,并通常于分裂间期死亡。相对低剂量的辐射暴露能诱导细胞凋亡性死亡[6],这也是造成造血细胞或淋巴细胞高剂量辐射暴露后死亡的重要方式之一。

辐射诱导的凋亡依赖 *p53* 基因及 *p53* 非依赖性信号通路的功能活性[9],其作用核心都是激活名为"含半胱氨酸的天冬氨酸蛋白水解酶(caspase)"的蛋白酶[10]。有研究提出 *p53* 依赖的凋亡可能涉及诱导氧化还原相关基因的转录,导致 ROS 形成,细胞因氧化应激而死亡[11]。

辐射诱导细胞死亡的第二个机制是细胞增殖异常。辐射通过抑制细胞增殖杀伤哺乳动物细胞。人类通常仅在受到 100cGy 以上的全身性辐射后,才出现急性辐射暴露相关症状。

诱发突变

在人类细胞中诱导单基因突变的研究可缩小到几个基因座,其中位于 X 染色体可编码次黄嘌呤-鸟嘌呤磷酸转移酶的基因(HPRT)尤其引人关注[12,13]。辐射剂量低至 10cGy 甚至 1cGy 时,人类细胞中的辐射诱变与辐射剂量成线性关系,且剂量率效应不显著[14,15]。DNA 结构分析显示,多数辐射诱导的人类细胞突变是大规模遗传事件(包括整个激活基因的缺失)的结果,常会影响同一染色体的其他位点[16]。

对人类而言,辐射诱变的主要威胁是诱导生殖细胞突变,使突变基因的效应得以遗传。对于高剂量率暴露而言,单个生殖细胞的诱变率大体在 10^{-5}~10^{-4}/cGy。单个位点的诱变率在

10^{-8}～10^{-7}/cGy。减少暴露时间至少能将啮齿动物模型中的突变率降低一半以上。结合不同遗传终点事件数据，低剂量辐射暴露的遗传突变倍增剂量（使自发突变率增加2倍所需的辐射剂量）在100cGy以内。

染色体畸变

辐射能诱导两种类型的哺乳动物细胞染色体畸变。第一类被称为“不稳定”畸变，对于分裂细胞而言是致命的。这类畸变包括双着丝粒、环形染色体、染色体大段缺失和断裂。每种畸变的发生频率与辐射的细胞毒性大小密切相关。

第二种类型称为“稳定”畸变，包括染色体小段缺失、易位和一些不影响细胞分裂和增殖的异倍体改变。辐射诱导的异位染色体通过细胞复制代代相传，并最终出现在整个细胞克隆中[17,18]。

染色体片段缺失和易位会导致基因突变。特定染色体异常与特定肿瘤类型相关，例如Burkitt淋巴瘤中的8∶14染色体易位。染色体异常还会导致某些癌基因激活，例如视网膜母细胞瘤（RB）中染色体13q14缺失。

辐射诱导的基因组不稳定性

辐射暴露能在单个细胞中诱导一类可遗传的不稳定基因组，复制多代后，子代的遗传改变频率持续性增加。这是辐射的非靶效应，最终结局包括恶性转化、特定基因突变和染色体畸变。

早期证据来自对辐射体外诱导细胞恶性转化的动力学研究[19,20]。辐射产生的恶性转化灶并非起源于单个损伤细胞。相反，辐射能诱导细胞群中20%～30%的细胞产生一种不稳定性，从而提高继发恶性转化的可能性，而继发恶性转化发生的频率极低，约为10^{-6}。每一代的各个细胞发生继发转化的频率相同，并且都可发生突变[21]。

随后，一系列针对不同的遗传终点事件的实验研究证实了该现象[22～25]。就突变而言，在辐射后存活细胞形成的细胞克隆群中，约10%的克隆群的自发突变频率显著高于正常细胞来源的克隆群[26,27]。在辐射后，突变频率的升高能维持约30～50代。那些胸苷激酶基因座突变的辐照细胞的子代出现小卫星[28]和微卫星[29]不稳定性的增加。

研究发现，染色体不稳定性的传递一般发生在体内[30,31]，但辐射诱导下，不同小鼠染色体的敏感性截然不同[32,33]。研究表明，在受辐射之后的许多代子细胞群中，细胞死亡率持续增加[34～36]。染色体不稳定性和恶性转化常与迟发性增殖障碍相关[38,39]，有证据提示，DNA是导致迟发性增殖障碍的重要靶点之一[40]。

近期一项新研究提出并证实了“迟发性抗辐射效应”的存在。这种效应表现为：用含硫醇的药物例如N-乙酰半胱氨酸和卡托普利处理细胞，细胞内的抗氧化酶如锰超氧化物歧化酶（MnSOD）水平升高。此后持续几小时至几天内，细胞对电离辐射的抵抗能力增强[41,42]。其背后的机制是硫醇还原剂激活了氧化还原敏感的核转录因子κB（NFκB），从而使得MnSOD的转录增强。胞内MnSOD水平升高10～20倍能防止甚至消除辐射诱导的氧化损伤，使细胞的存活率提高10%～30%。

受辐射细胞群中的旁观者效应

细胞核一直被认为是辐射所致生物效应的重要靶点。然而，近来的研究表明，靶向细胞质的辐射也具有显著的致突变效应。损伤信号能从受辐射的细胞传递到临近细胞群，诱导其他未受辐射的细胞产生生物学效应[43]，例如“旁观者”效应。

低通量的α粒子辐照细胞单层培养物后，仅有1/1 000～1/100的细胞被α粒子穿透，但细胞中出现姐妹染色单体互换（sister chromatid exchanges，SCE）的频率升高至20%～40%[44]。受辐射细胞可分泌细胞因子或其他因子，这是“旁观”细胞中氧化代谢上调的主要机制[45,46]。图25-2是一个“旁观者”效应的例子。用来自受辐射细胞的条件培养液孵育未受辐射的细胞，可观察到细胞毒效应，说明与受辐射细胞释放到培养基中的因子有关[47]。当某个细胞群受到低通量的α粒子辐射后，旁观者细胞中出现特定基因突变[48,49]以及染色体畸变[50,51]的频率升高。

然而，旁观者细胞的DNA损伤与直接受辐射细胞有所不同：直接受辐射的细胞中，突变类型主要是部分或全基因缺失；而在旁观者细胞中，90%以上是点突变[52]，提示氧化代谢在旁观者细胞中上调[45,46]。“旁观者”效应表明，损伤信号能从受

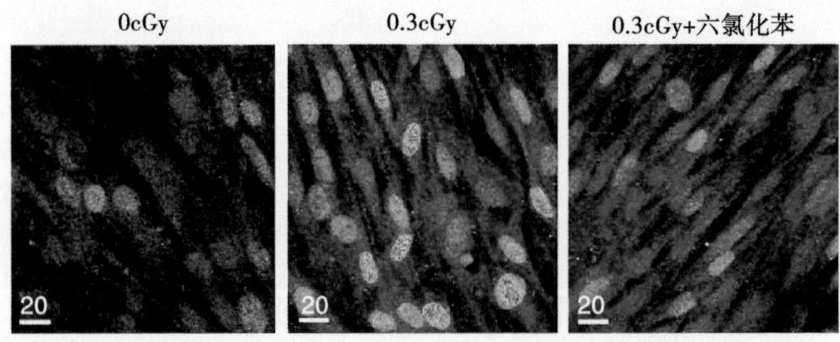

图25-2 辐射的旁观者效应。原位免疫荧光呈现的是单层培养的人二倍体成纤维细胞中$p21^{Waf1}$基因表达。在受到0.3 cGy的辐射后（小于1%～2%的细胞核被α粒子穿透），细胞群中未受辐射的细胞出现了$p21^{Waf1}$基因表达升高（中图）。经六氯化苯处理后，这一效应被抑制。六氯化苯能抑制缝隙连接介导的细胞间交流（右图）

辐射细胞传递到未受辐射细胞。

适应性反应

最初,研究人类淋巴细胞的学者提出“适应性反应”,他们观察到人淋巴细胞在受到 1~10cGy 的低剂量电离辐射之后,对辐射抵抗性变强,能够抵抗随后至少 2Gy 的高剂量辐射[53]。适应性反应的产生与蛋白从头合成相关,因为蛋白合成抑制剂(例如放线菌酮)可以阻断这一效应[54]。适应性反应可视为细胞间应激反应的结果。最被广泛研究的是 MnSOD(一种在细胞线粒体中的抗氧化酶)介导的适应性反应,在正常细胞和癌细胞中均能发生。例如,小鼠皮肤 JB6P+上皮细胞受到 10cGy 辐射之后,表现出了对 2Gy 辐射抵抗能力的增强。在此过程中,一系列 NFκB 调控基因上调,包括 MnSOD、p65、磷酸化胞外信号相关激酶、cyclin B1 和 14-3-3Z[55]。细胞中 MnSOD 合成增加促进适应性反应,不仅体现在细胞受到低剂量电离辐射时[55],也表现在细胞暴露于细胞因子 TNFα[56]以及多种还原剂时,如氨磷汀和 *N*-乙酰半胱氨酸[42,57]。用 NFκB 抑制剂和/或 MnSOD 反义寡聚核苷酸或 MnSOD 的 siRNA 能完全抑制上述还原剂诱导的适应性反应[55,56]。辐射和细胞因子诱导的适应性反应都是氧化损伤的结果,然而与硫醇诱导的还原反应不同,前者 NFκB 是通过还原 p50 和 p65 亚基的半胱氨酸残基激活的[58,59],并且该机制在慢性硫醇暴露中持续存在[60]。

目前已发现,细胞是否恶性以及受辐射的方式是介导适应性反应的影响因素。在每次高剂量辐射前给予低剂量辐射预暴露,肿瘤细胞中出现 survivin 基因介导的适应性反应[61]。survivin 是细胞凋亡抑制蛋白(IAP)家族的成员之一,最初发现于肿瘤细胞中,是肿瘤细胞发挥抵抗力的重要因素[62,63],高表达的 Survivin 能升高肿瘤细胞对辐射及化疗药物所致细胞杀伤作用的抵抗,减少细胞凋亡[64~66]。1/3 的适应性反应在正常细胞中出现,在缺氧诱导因子 HIF-1α 诱导下[67],小剂量辐射使这些细胞代谢方式从氧化磷酸化转变为有氧糖酵解。

DNA 损伤

用 X 射线对 DNA 相互作用进行示踪分析,发现 DNA 中损伤的聚集,这导致复杂性 DNA 双链断裂(double-strand break, DSB)[68]。特定类型的 DNA 碱基损伤(例如 8-羟基脱氧鸟苷和胸腺嘧啶乙二醇形成)具有极为重要的潜在生物效应,但目前的实验结果提示,单一或数个碱基对于辐射的致突变效应作用或许很小。成簇 DNA 损伤包括无碱基位点、嘌呤或嘧啶氧化[69]。高线性能量传递(high-LET)辐射造成 DNA 的复杂性损伤,最终诱导 DNA 断裂增加[70]。

细胞通过一系列复杂的信号通路来识别并修复 DNA 损伤。ATM 基因是 DNA 损伤的探测器,可通过磷酸化激活多种参与细胞周期调控和 DNA 修复的多种蛋白。DNA 双链断裂(DNA double-strand break, DSB)修复中,两种不同机制发挥互补的作用:一是非同源末端连接(non-homologous end-joining, NHEJ),这种方式几乎不需要 DNA 末端同源序列,修复过程易发生错误;二是同源重组(homologous recombination, HR),这种方式需要严格的同源性,修复错误极少[71]。一种包含了 Ku70、Ku80、DNA-PK 催化亚基 DNA-PKcs、XRCC4 和连接酶Ⅳ的蛋白复合体参与 NHEJ。NBS1/MRE11/RAD50 复合体[72]参与 NHEJ 中的核水解过程,并在 HR 过程中也发挥作用。HR 过程也涉及一种蛋白复合体,其中包括了 RAD51 和 RAD50 上位蛋白基团的其他因子[73]。已有研究报道了乳腺癌易感基因 BRCA1 和 BRCA2[74~76],以及 Fanconi 贫血家族蛋白[77]与重组修复的密切关系。多数未修复或错误修复的 DSB 会造成大范围的基因改变,表现为染色体异常。然而,在辐射诱发的肿瘤中,尚未发现特异性的基因改变。

辐射诱发肿瘤的一般特征

电离辐射在不同物种的各个年龄段(包括胎儿)的多数组织中诱发癌症。对人类而言,电离辐射也具有致癌性。然而,电离辐射是一个相对较弱的致癌物和致突变原。辐射所致的恶性肿瘤的组织学类型与自然发生的肿瘤一致,但分布类型可能不同。从辐射暴露到临床上肿瘤出现之间存在明确的潜伏期。

辐射致癌是一个随机的过程,发生率随辐射剂量的增加而升高,且无阈值剂量。但致癌效应的强度不受辐射剂量的影响。辐射导致的癌症似乎是一个“全或无”现象。致癌的剂量-效应关系在小型动物不同部位、性别和品种间存在差异[78~80]。对于低线性能量传递的辐射而言,诱发癌症的频率在辐射剂量 0~300cGy 范围内大致随剂量的增加而升高。在一些病例中,高辐射剂量下,肿瘤发生率趋于平缓,甚至降低。这一现象反映了细胞杀伤效应。在辐射剂量达到 200~300cGy 时,剂量-效应曲线根据肿瘤类型有所不同,但大体上呈线性二次型或近似线性关系。对于高线性能量传递的辐射而言,肿瘤发生率随剂量的增加升高而更显著。0~20cGy 辐射剂量间,剂量-效应曲线近乎线性[78,81]。

在实验动物中,辐射诱癌能被某些药物抑制,这些药物在体外被用作抑制辐射介导的恶性转化效应,例如氨磷汀是目前唯一获得食品药品监督管理局(FDA)批准用作临床辐射防护的药物[82]。图 25-3 的 Kaplan-Meier 生存曲线中显示,在对 B6CF1 杂交鼠进行 2Gy 低线性能量传递射线全身辐照 30 分钟之后,使用 400mg/kg 的氨磷汀,能显著抑制雄性和雌性动物的肿瘤发生。Kaplan-Meier 生存曲线反映出氨磷汀可使淋巴网状细胞肉瘤死亡率降低,即经药物处理的受辐射动物的生存曲线向未受辐射的对照组动物的生存曲线偏移[83~85]。每只患淋巴网状细胞肉瘤实验动物的死因[83]由资深病理学家通过大体及镜下病理观察判定(包括白血病和淋巴瘤)。同样地,还发现某些蛋白酶抑制剂能够抑制多种系统肿瘤[86]。众所周知,激素环境对于辐射诱发的某些浸润性癌十分重要,尤其是卵巢癌和乳腺癌。

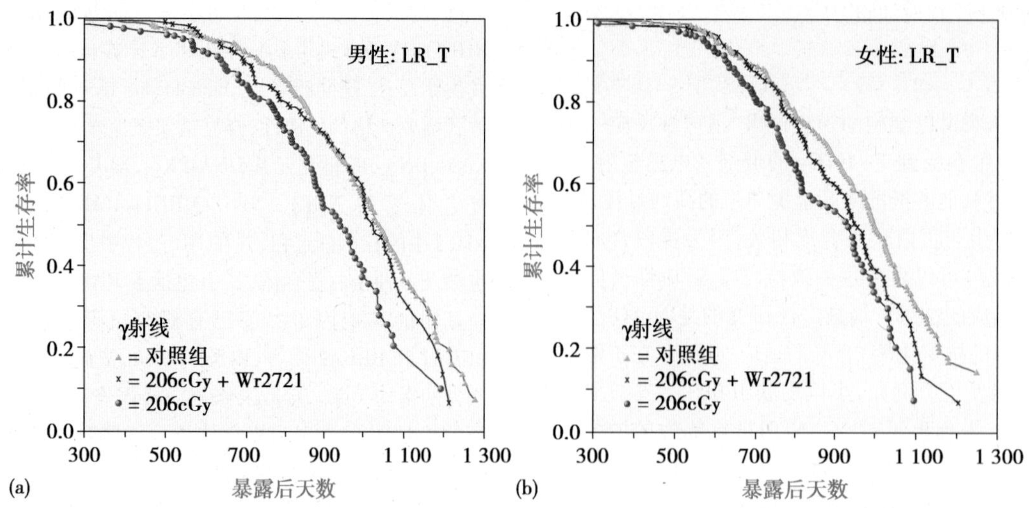

图 25-3　(a,b)淋巴网状细胞肉瘤(LR-T)的生存曲线。肉瘤取自受辐射(206cGy)后使用或未使用氨磷汀的死亡动物,并由组织病理分析确定。LR-T 包括组织细胞白血病和淋巴瘤、淋巴细胞-淋巴母细胞白血病和淋巴瘤、髓系白血病、未分化白血病和淋巴瘤以及混合组织细胞性白血病和淋巴瘤

辐射诱癌中的基因易感性

鲜有证据表明基因与多数人类癌症相关,但基因的确与一些罕见的遗传病有关,这些遗传病可以作为理解辐射-基因相互作用的基础。例如,患有遗传性视网膜母细胞瘤(RB)的患者的体细胞中带有杂合的 RB 基因,辐射诱导发生骨肉瘤的风险显著增加[87],而痣样基底细胞癌综合征患者在受辐射的部位发生基底细胞癌的风险也较高。辐射还与早发乳腺癌高发生率相关。*p53*[88]或 *ATM*[89]抑癌基因杂合突变的转基因小鼠对辐射高度敏感,容易诱发癌症。而 *ATM* 和 *p53* 的杂合突变分别与共济失调性毛细血管扩张症和 Li-Fraumeni 综合征(家族性癌症综合征)有关,均属于人类癌症前驱疾病。

人群流行病学研究

目前大量关于辐射诱癌的研究数据来源于针对受辐射人群的流行病学研究。这些人群主要来自:①长期随访的广岛和长崎核弹爆炸幸存者[90,91];②暴露于医疗 X 射线的人群[92,93]。这些研究收集了大量辐射剂量-效应的数据,这些数据来自辐射诱发的至少 5 个组织部位的恶性肿瘤中。可惜的是,这些流行病学研究中可用的剂量-效应的数据大部分是剂量相对较高的辐射暴露(大于 10cGy)。因此,只能通过高剂量辐射的剂量-效应关系推断低剂量辐射的风险,其中剂量-效应关系的类型是关键。

在人流行病学研究中观察到的剂量-效应为线性或线性二次型关系(例如,在低剂量范围内为线性,高剂量范围内为二次线性),尽管在极低剂量范围内,未必如此(低于阈值则无效应存在)[94,95]。线性关系说明在各个辐射剂量下,每厘戈瑞(cGy)辐射产生的风险比例恒定;而线性二次型说明在低剂量辐射范围内,每厘戈瑞的辐射产生的风险较小。线性模型假设简化了由高剂量效应推断低剂量效应的过程和相应风险评估。决定辐射剂量危险性的关键因素是风险模型的确定。风险的评估多年来都基于一个绝对风险模型。这个模型假设一定的辐射剂量能诱导一定数目的癌症发生。除了自然的癌症发生外,还发生了辐射诱导的癌症。罹癌风险的增加表示为每百万辐射暴露的人每年每 cGy(年平均率)超过自然水平的癌症发生率(或癌症死亡),或每百万辐射暴露的人每年每 cGy 超过自然水平的癌症事件总数(给定辐射剂量预期的总风险或自然寿命内发生癌症的事件总数)。绝对风险模型假设剂量-效应间总体为线性关系,尽管经特定的修正后为线性二次型。因为在广岛的辐射中包含了少部分的中子,所以在当地原子弹爆炸幸存者的研究中,辐射剂量以西弗(Sv)而非 Gy 为单位。该单位能将中子的相对生物效应(relative biological effectiveness,RBE)计算在内。

一项新的有关核弹爆炸幸存者的数据分析显示,某些癌症的辐射诱发风险更接近于相对风险模型[90]。相对风险模型表示辐射以剂量依赖的模式增加全年龄段癌症的自然发生率。由于额外癌症风险与癌症自然发病率正相关,辐射诱发的癌症主要发生于自然癌症发生时,不受辐射暴露时年龄的影响。因此,辐射诱发癌症的病例在老年人中最多。尽管在白血病、骨癌和肺癌例外,多种实体癌的相对风险模型与流行病学的研究结果相符。这些涉及医疗辐射暴露的研究中的风险评估与原子弹爆炸幸存者的研究相似[93,96,97],高剂量放射治疗病例中的差异可以归因于辐射的细胞杀伤效应和分段放疗[92]。在肺癌的分段高剂量放疗中可见辐射诱发的肿瘤相对减少[98]。但在乳腺癌中并非如此,尽管乳腺癌中低剂量-效应的持久辐射与损伤效应的减少有关[97]。

辐射诱导的继发性癌

单纯的用于传统治疗的射线可能并非继发性癌的重要诱因。这种设想的理论基础是:临床放疗中的辐照是局限性的,对正常组织的辐射剂量已调至最小。并且,电离辐射更倾向于产生细胞毒性而非致突变性。在临床治疗中,使用高剂量的辐射能够杀伤潜在的向癌细胞转化的细胞。但霍奇金病的治疗和强度调制放射治疗(intensity-modulated radiation therapy,IMRT)可能是一个例外。霍奇金病的治疗采用低剂量的射线辐

照相对较大的组织，因而较多正常组织受到了低剂量的辐照[99]。评估显示，IMRT 会使继发性肿瘤发生率升高至传统放疗的近两倍，对于生存期 10 年的患者而言，从 1% 升高至 1.75%[100]。儿童患者的风险可能更高。

低剂量辐射暴露

利用充足的原子弹爆炸幸存者的数据，研究者已经可以对受到小于 0.5Sv 辐射的幸存者进行分析。这些数据可用于 5~10cGy 的低剂量辐射进行初步风险评估[95]。这些数据表明在该剂量范围内具有显著的风险，与剂量-效应线性关系一致，其任何可能阈值的置信上限为 6cGy。

一项几乎覆盖所有低剂量辐射相关研究的系统分析显示，癌症全发病率及特定癌症发病率均无显著增加。对来自英国[101]和加拿大[102]的大量辐射工作人员的分析表明，白血病和所有癌症的风险估计均与根据原子弹爆炸幸存者的数据推断出的结果一致，无证据显示低剂量辐射会导致敏感性的意外增加，表明现存辐射防护标准可能存在明显误差。

（危晏平 译　曹琦琪　李亮 校）

部分参考文献

1 Upton AC. Historical perspectives on radiation carcinogenesis. In: Upton AC, Albert RE, Burns FJ, Shore RE, eds. *Radiation Carcinogenesis*. New York: Elsevier; 1986:1-10.

2 Roots R, Okada S. Protection of DNA molecules of cultured mammalian cells from radiation-induced single strand scissions by various alcohols and SH compounds. *Int J Radiat Biol*. 1972;**21**:329-342.

6 Little JB. Cellular effects of ionizing radiation. I & II. *N Engl J Med*. 1968;**278**:308-315, 369-376.

12 Albertini RJ. Validated biomarker responses influence medical surveillance of individuals exposed to genotoxic agents. *Radiat Prot Dosimetry*. 2001;**97**:47-54.

23 Little JB. Radiation-induced genomic instability. *Int J Radiat Biol*. 1998;**74**:663-671.

27 Little JB, Nagasawa H, Pfenning T, Vetrovs H. Radiation-induced genomic instability: delayed mutagenic and cytogenetic effects of X rays and alpha particles. *Radiat Res*. 1997;**148**:299-307.

33 Ponnaiya B, Cornforth MN, Ullrich RL. Radiation-induced chromosomal instability in BALB/c and C57BL/6 mice: the difference is as clear as black and white. *Radiat Res*. 1997;**147**:121-125.

34 Seymour CB, Mothersill C, Alper T. High yields of lethal mutations in somatic mammalian cells that survive ionizing radiation. *Int J Radiat Biol Relat Stud Phys Chem Med*. 1986;**50**:167-179.

35 Chang WP, Little JB. Delayed reproductive death in X-irradiated Chinese hamster ovary cells. *Int J Radiat Biol*. 1991;**60**:483-496.

39 Redpath JL, Gutierrez M. Kinetics of induction of reactive oxygen species during the post-irradiation expression of neoplastic transformation in vitro. *Int J Radiat Biol*. 2001;**77**:1081-1085.

41 Murley JS, Kataoka Y, Weydert CJ, Oberley LW, Grdina DJ. Delayed cytoprotection after enhancement of *Sod2* (*MnSOD*) gene expression in SA-NH mouse sarcoma cells exposed to WR-1065, the active metabolite of amifostine. *Radiat Res*. 2002;**158**:101-109.

42 Murley JS, Kataoka Y, Cao D, Li JJ, Oberley LW, Grdina DJ. Delayed radioprotection by NFκB-mediated induction of Sod2 (MnSOD) in SA-NH tumor cells after exposure to clinically used thiol-containing drugs. *Radiat Res*. 2004;**162**:536-546.

43 Little JB. Genomic instability and bystander effects: a historical perspective. *Oncogene*. 2003;**22**:6978-6987.

47 Mothersill C, Seymour CB. Cell-cell contact during gamma irradiation is not required to induce a bystander effect in normal human keratinocytes: evidence for release during irradiation of a signal controlling survival into the medium. *Radiat Res*. 1998;**149**:256-262.

50 Little JB, Nagasawa H, Li GC, Chen DJ. Involvement of the nonhomologous end joining DNA repair pathway in the bystander effect for chromosomal aberrations. *Radiat Res*. 2003;**59**:262-267.

51 Azzam EI, de Toledo SM, Gooding T, Little JB. Intercellular communication is involved in the bystander regulation of gene expression in human cells exposed to very low fluences of alpha particles. *Radiat Res*. 1998;**150**:497-504.

53 Olivieri G, Bodycote J, Wolff S. Adaptive response of human lymphocytes to low concentrations of radioactive thymidine. *Science*. 1984;**223**:594-597.

55 Fan M, Ahmed KM, Coleman MC, Spitz DR, Li JJ. Nuclear factor-kB and manganese superoxide dismutase mediate adaptive resistance in low-dose irradiated mouse skin epithelial cells. *Cancer Res*. 2007;**67**:3220-3228.

56 Murley JS, Kataoka Y, Baker LL, Diamond AL, Morgan WF, Grdina DJ. Manganese superoxide dismutase (SOD2)-mediated delayed radioprotection induced by the free thiol form of amifostine and tumor necrosis factor κB. *Radiat Res*. 2007;**167**:465-474.

57 Murley JS, Kataoka Y, Weydert CJ, Oberley LW, Grdina DJ. Delayed radioprotection by nuclear transcription factor κB-mediated induction of manganese superoxide dismutase in human microvascular endothelial cells after exposure to the free radical scavenger WR1065. *Free Radic Biol Med*. 2006;**40**:1004-1016.

58 Matthews JR, Wakasugi N, Virelizier JL, Yodoi Y, Hay RT. Thioredoxin regulates the binding activity of NF-κB by reduction of a disulphide bond involving cysteine 62. *Nucleic Acids Res*. 1992;**20**:3821-3830.

59 Murley JS, Kataoka Y, Hallahan DE, Roberts JC, Grdina DJ. Activation of NFκB and *MnSOD* gene expression by free radical scavengers in human microvascular endothelial cells. *Free Radic Biol Med*. 2001;**30**:1426-1439.

61 Grdina DJ, Murley JS, Miller RC, et al. A survivin-associated adaptive response in radiation therapy. *Cancer Res*. 2013;**73**(**14**):4418-4428.

63 Marivin A, Berthelet J, Plenchette S, Dubrez L. The inhibitor of apoptosis (IAPs) in adaptive response to cellular stress. *Cells*. 2012;**1**:711-737.

64 Lu B, Mu Y, Cao C, et al. Survivin as a therapeutic target for radiation sensitization in lung cancer. *Cancer Res*. 2004;**64**:2840-2845.

67 Lall R, Ganapathy S, Yang M, et al. Low-dose radiation exposure induces a HIF-1-mediated adaptive and protective metabolic response. *Cell Death Diff*. 2014;**21**:836-844.

68 Goodhead DT. Initial events in the cellular effects of ionizing radiations: clustered damage in DNA. *Int J Radiat Biol*. 1994;**65**:7-17.

71 Jackson SP. Sensing and repairing DNA double-strand breaks. *Carcinogenesis*. 2002;**23**:687-696.

81 Ullrich RL. Tumor induction in BALB/c mice after fractionated or protracted exposures to fission-spectrum neutrons. *Radiat Res*. 1984;**97**:587-597.

82 Grdina DJ, Murley JS, Kataoka Y. Radioprotectants: current status and new directions. *Oncology*. 2002;**63**:2-10.

83 Grdina DJ, Carnes BA, Grahn D, Sigdestad CP. Protection against late effects of radiation by *S*-2-(3-aminopropylamino)-ethylphosphorothioic acid. *Cancer Res*. 1991;**51**:4125-4130.

84 Carnes BA, Grdina DJ. *In vivo* protection by the aminothiol WR-2721 against neutron-induced carcinogenesis. *Int J Radiat Biol*. 1992;**61**:567-576.

85 Grdina DJ, Carnes BA, Nagy B. Protection by WR-2721 and WR-151327 against late effects of gamma rays and neutrons. *Adv Space Res*. 1992;**12**:257-263.

88 Kemp CJ, Wheldon T, Balmain A. p53-deficient mice are extremely susceptible to radiation-induced tumorigenesis. *Nat Genet*. 1994;**8**:66-69.

93 Little MP, Weiss HA, Boice JD Jr, et al. Risks of leukemia in Japanese atomic bomb survivors, in women treated for cervical cancer, and in patients treated for ankylosing spondylitis. *Radiat Res*. 1999;**152**:280-292.

99 Goffman TE, Glatstein E. Intensity-modulated radiation therapy. *Radiat Res*. 2002;**158**:115-117.

第 26 章　紫外线辐射致癌

James E. Cleaver, PhD ■ Susana Ortiz-Urda, MD, PhD, MBA ■ Radhika Gulhar, BA ■
Sarah T. Arron, MD, PhD ■ Lionel Brookes, 3rd, PhD ■ David L. Mitchell, PhD

概述

细胞 DNA 暴露于太阳紫外线(UV)所形成的 UV 光产物是皮肤癌变的第一步,后进一步产生鳞状细胞癌、基底细胞癌和黑色素瘤。光产物由相邻嘧啶之间形成的二聚体组成,并通过核苷酸切除修复(nucleotide excision repair, NER)机制修复。两类 NER 在损伤识别机制上有所不同:在全基因组切除修复(global genome repair, GGR)中,非转录区 DNA 损伤由 DDB2 和 XPC 蛋白识别;而在转录偶联修复(transcription-coupled repair, TCR)中,通过转录 RNA 聚合酶停滞点来识别损伤部位。T=C 光产物是主要诱变产物,未修复的 DNA 损伤易通过低保真聚合酶 Pol H 产生 C 至 T 或 CC 至 TT 突变。相对 GGR 针对全基因组修复而言,TCR 能有效降低转录区突变频率。着色性干皮病中 GGR 缺陷会导致皮肤癌发病提前和发病率增加,且通常包含普通人群鲜有的 UV 型基因突变。Cockayne 综合征中 TCR 缺陷与光过敏、发育和神经系统紊乱有关,但尚未发现与癌症的相关性。

皮肤癌的流行病学

皮肤癌发病率和发病年龄

非黑色素瘤皮肤癌(nonmelanoma skin cancers, NMSC)是美国每年新发癌症中最常见的[1,2],占癌症总数的 30%~40%,且近百年来发病率稳定增加[3,4]。皮肤癌发病风险与地理位置、皮肤类型、各种光过敏、光照增强和光防护应用以及维生素 D 有关[4~10]。在儿童和青少年时期暴露于易感因素,其发生皮肤癌的风险将更大[5,11]。因此,NMSC 是为数不多已明确致病原因的恶性肿瘤之一。黑色素瘤与日光的关系以及作用机制尚不清楚[12,13],但可能与急性晒伤有关而非日光暴露的累积剂量[5,14]。

常染色体隐性遗传病着色性干皮病(xeroderma pigmentosum, XP)的研究强调 DNA 是紫外线辐射(ultraviolet radiation, UVR)的重要损伤靶点。在该疾病中,DNA 修复缺陷导致 NMSC 和黑色素瘤风险增加[12,13]。美国普通人群首次诊断 NMSC 的中位年龄是 60 岁以后,而 XP 患者癌变加速,中位发病年龄在 10 岁之前(图 26-1)[12,13],XP 患者黑素瘤风险也有所增加,但增幅较低。因此,XP 患者 NMSC 发病早于黑色素瘤,而非 XP 患者黑素瘤通常早于 NMSC 发生。

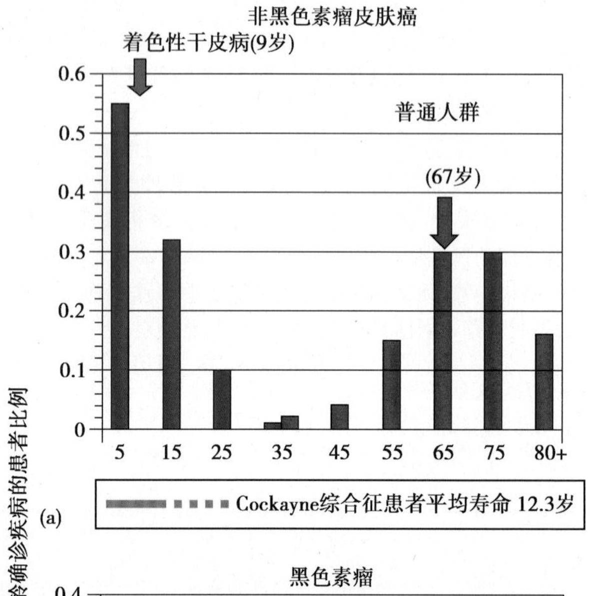

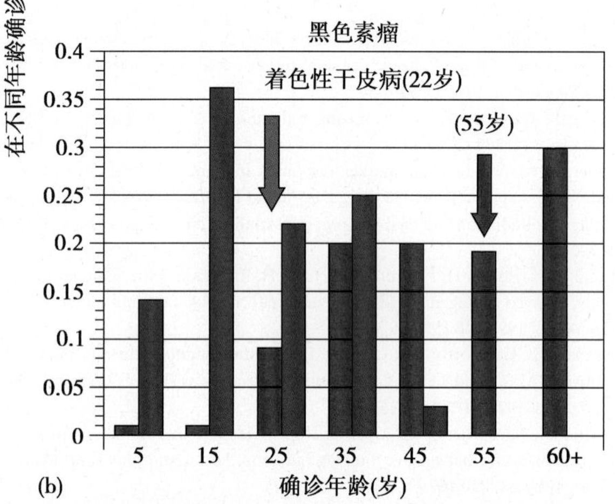

图 26-1　与美国普通人群相比,着色性干皮病(XP)患者首次诊断癌症的年龄和类型。(a)非黑色素瘤皮肤癌(NMSC)患者的确诊年龄分布。(b)黑素瘤患者的确诊年龄分布。同时患有 NMSC 和黑素瘤的患者纳入两组统计。图示年龄是每个十年的中值。XP 人群:蓝色;普通人群:红色。箭头表示确诊中位年龄。橙色线条显示 Cockayne 综合征患者的年龄分布:实心线止于平均死亡年龄(12.25 岁),虚线延伸至最大报告年龄。XP 和普通人群数据来源[27]

导致皮肤癌的日光光谱和波长

紫外线辐射可分为三个波长范围:UVA、UVB 和 UVC。UVA(320~400nm)有光致癌作用并参与光老化,但只能被 DNA 和蛋白质微弱吸收,其损伤机制可能涉及活性氧(reactive oxygen species, ROS),ROS 可继发性损伤 DNA[15]。然而最新证据表明 UVA 也可直接诱导人类细胞 DNA 损伤[19]。UVB(290~

320nm)波长与 DNA 和蛋白质在吸收光谱的上段重叠,主要通过使 DNA 发生直接光化学损伤而导致皮肤癌。UVC(240~290nm)不存在于外界日光中,但可由低压汞消毒灯(254nm)产生。UVC 与 DNA 吸收峰(260nm)十分接近,被广泛用于实验研究。大气平流层中臭氧可吸收 UVR,所以波长小于 300nm 的辐射到达地球表面的量极少。虽然 UVA 和 UVB 只占太阳发射波长的极小部分(10^{-9}),但它们是日光致病作用的主要原因。

日光诱导的 DNA 光产物

DNA 的吸收光谱与紫外线引起的细胞死亡、突变和光产物形成密切相关[20~24]。被 DNA 吸收的能量可产生分子改变,涉及单个碱基、相邻与非相邻碱基以及 DNA 与蛋白质的相互作用。不同波长紫外线产生的 DNA 光产物相对比例不一样。

相邻嘧啶二聚体是最常见的 DNA 光产物,主要有两种分别是环丁烷嘧啶二聚体(cyclobutane pyrimidine dimer,CPD)和[6-4]嘧啶二聚体([6-4] pyrimidine dimer,[6-4] PD),后者约占光产物总量 25%。[6-4] PD 可引起 DNA 螺旋弯曲 47°,而 CPD 则使 DNA 弯曲 7°。[6-4] PD 可在 UVB 作用下进一步转变为其光学异构体,即 Dewar 嘧啶酮[25]。

光产物在染色质中的分布取决于碱基序列、DNA 二级结构以及 DNA-蛋白质相互作用[24,26,27]。由于胞嘧啶比胸腺嘧啶更有效地吸收较长波段的紫外线辐射,因此经 UVB 辐照后更容易形成含胞嘧啶的 CPD[28]。在胸腺嘧啶-胞嘧啶二聚体处更易诱导产生胞嘧啶 CPD 和[6-4] PD,它们可能在 UVB(日光)致突变中起重要作用[29]。通过 UVB 而非 UVC,甲基化胞嘧啶生成 CPDs 的能力可增加 1.7 倍[30]。p53 基因中 PyrCG 序列甲基化可增加热点突变位点上 CPD 和[6-4] PD 的形成[31,32]。其他较少见的损伤包括嘌呤-嘌呤光加合物、嘌呤-嘧啶光加合物、光水化反应和光氧化反应[33]。虽然这些光产物仅占 CPD 总量的 3%~4%,但不能排除其可造成一些特定位点的突变前损伤。

皮肤癌变中的遗传因素

识别 DNA 中 UV 光产物

DNA 中 UV 光产物的修复(核苷酸切除修复,NER)包括识别光产物、组装切除复合物、置换切除片段和置换片段的聚合等连续步骤[34]。着色性干皮病(XP)患者的细胞缺乏 NER 使人们意识到 NER 的重要性[35,36]。NER 有两种主要途径(图 26-2):转录偶联修复(TCR)和全基因组切除修复(GGR),但识别 DNA 损伤的机制不尽相同[34,37-39]。TCR 能够更快地从转录活跃基因的转录链中去除损伤,而 GGR 作用于非转录区域且速度较慢[40,41]。[6-4] PD 的半衰期为 2~6 小时,CPD 是 12~24 小时,在啮齿动物细胞中切除 CPD 需要更长时间[42,43]。

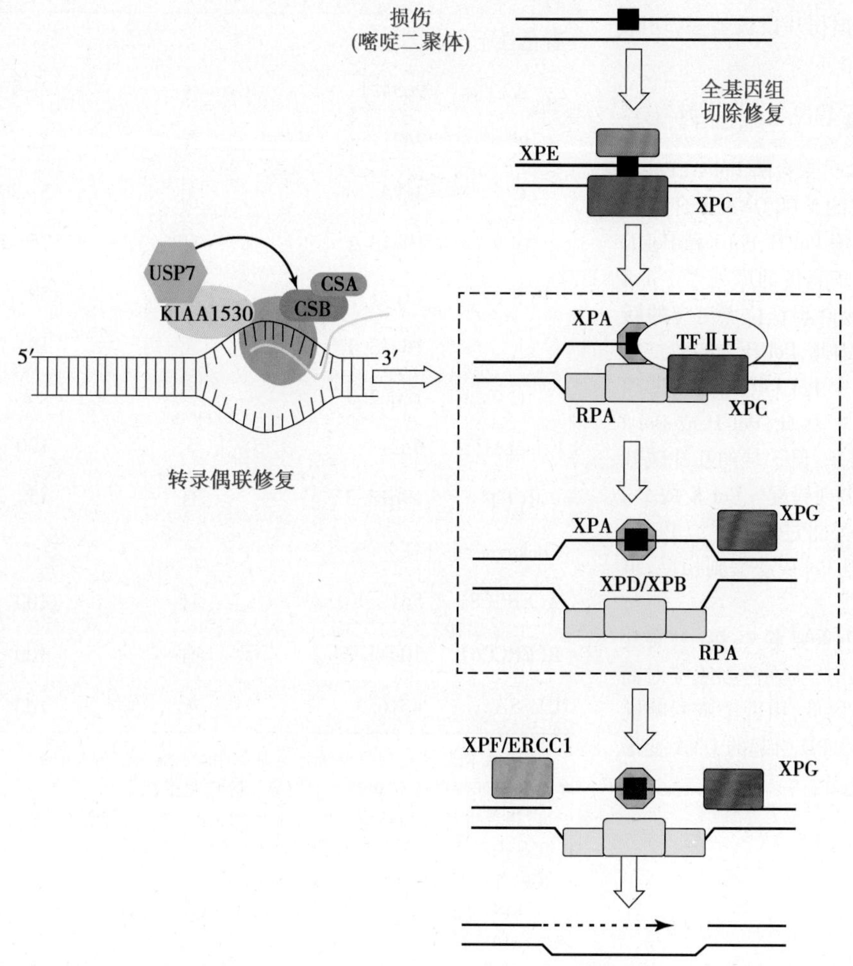

图 26-2　[6-4] PD 和 CPD 核苷酸切除修复(全基因组切除修复和转录偶联修复)的生物化学步骤。首先,全基因组切除修复起始于 DDB2 和 XPC 基因产物,转录偶联修复起始于 RNA 聚合酶Ⅱ停滞和 CSA、CSB 和 UVSSA 使转录复合物在损伤 DNA 处松脱,随后 XPA 和 RPA 结合到光产物上,募集解旋酶 XPB 和 XPD 进行局部解链。接着,由 UV 特异性内切核酸酶(XPF/ERCC1 和 XPG)进行 5′和 3′端内切。剪切和随后的聚合释放出一含 CPD 的 29 个碱基的寡核苷酸,并激活隐性核酸内切酶 XPG 进行最后的剪切

全基因组切除修复(GGR)包括三个阶段:先是 DDB1/DDB2(XPE)复合物结合[44,45];随后 DDB1/DDB2 利用 E3 连接酶活性,通过泛素化招募 XPC/HR23B/centrin[46~49];最后 XPC 蛋白结合嘧啶二聚体对侧的非损伤链,在 DNA 双螺旋之间插入肽链将二聚体置于双螺旋外[50,51]。

转录偶联修复(TCR)起始于 RNA 聚合酶Ⅱ在受损碱基的转录停滞处,随后特异性 TCR 因子 CSA、CSB、UVSSA 以及 XABP(XPA 的结合配体)协助移除或降解停滞的 RNA 聚合酶Ⅱ,使 NER 蛋白能够进入受损位点[52,53]。CSB 是 SWI2/SNF2 染色质重塑蛋白家族成员之一,TCR 与 CSB 的染色质重塑功能密切相关[54,55]。RNA 聚合酶Ⅱ在 DNA 链上的延伸与组蛋白 H2B(H2Bub)的泛素化与去泛素化相关,紫外线损伤引起的染色质失衡使组蛋白 H3[56] 倾向于去泛素化和乙酰化。切除阻碍转录的光产物后,H2Bub 恢复平衡,转录继续进行。

核苷酸切除修复的机制

在识别 DNA 损伤后,XPA/RPA 稳定开放螺旋,XPA/RPA 对[6-4] PD 的亲和力高于 CPD,它可与具有解旋活性的 10 亚基转录因子 TFIIH,以及 3′-5′(XPB)和 5′-3′(XPD)核酸酶相互作用[57,58]。开放的螺旋首先被 ERCC1/XPF 核酸酶剪切,暴露出 3′OH 末端,由 DNA 聚合酶 D、增殖细胞核抗原(PCNA)和单链结合蛋白共同作用延伸碳链[59,60]。XPG 是一种隐性核酸酶,它从 3′端切割到损伤位点,而 ERCC1/XPF 从 5′端剪切到 CPD[60]。一段长达 27~29 个核苷酸的损伤片段被剪去,切除产生的缺口由连接酶 I 连接[61]。

UV 光产物的致突变性和低保真 DNA 聚合酶

许多光产物可以阻碍参与复制的 B 类聚合酶 Pol A、Pol D 和 Pol E,但这些光产物能被损伤特异性的 Y 类 DNA 聚合酶绕过[62~64]。由于活性位点扩大,Y 类聚合酶 Pol H、Pol I 和 Pol K 保真性较低,这使得聚合酶能够读取非信息性的序列[65]。Pol H 复制各种 DNA 损伤的能力最强[66],易在损伤位点对应的新生链中插入腺嘌呤(称“A 规则”)[67]。因此,Pol H 忠实地复制含胸腺嘧啶的 CPD[68~71]。在复制过程中 Pol I 优先插入鸟嘌呤,其能够复制含胞嘧啶的光产物[72,73]。因此,Pol H 或 Pol I 在二嘧啶光产物对应的新生链中插入碱基,但 3′端的互补碱基将因错误插入或光产物引起的失真而出现错配。Pol K 或 Pol Z 可通过错配的 3′端延伸来完成复制旁路过程[74~76]。Pol H 的缺失可导致 XPV 组突变增加[77,78],但 Pol Z 缺失则相反,可降低突变率[79]。

复制旁路机制对 UV 致突变有两个重要意义:第一,突变最常发生在胞嘧啶是光产物组分的地方,因为在胸腺嘧啶对面插入腺嘌呤是正确的,不会发生突变。因此,由两个胸腺嘧啶形成的 CPD 是不致突变的。第二,[6-4] PD 引起的 DNA 变形比 CPD 严重,所以更可能致死而非致突变。

DNA 修复相关的疾病

着色性干皮病

着色性干皮病(XP)是一种罕见的常染色体隐性遗传病,在美国的发病率为 1/250 000[12]。患者(纯合型)对阳光敏感,皮肤、眼睛等器官暴露于阳光中会发生退行性变化,经常导致癌变。另外一些着色性干皮病患者还伴有进行性神经病变。杂合型(双亲)没有任何临床症状。XP 发病的中位年龄为 1~2 岁,而 NMSC 首诊的中位年龄为 9 岁(图 26-1)[12,13]。患者皮肤呈现出似经过多年日晒的性状,皮肤萎缩、色素沉着、毛细血管扩张并可能进展为 NMSC 和黑色素瘤。在年龄小于 20 岁的人群中,XP 患者出现 NMSC 的概率为正常人的 2 000 倍,且寿命大约减少 30 年。有些患者会在日后出现骨髓增生异常和白血病。

在 NER 异常的患者中,有 8 个互补组相当于 NER 各个组分,通过 XPG 和非常罕见的 ERCC1 来弥补 XPA 异常[80]。另一组 XP 患者是低保真聚合酶 Pol H 突变(表 26-1)。由于 CPD 和非二聚体光产物的修复缺陷,XP 患者的细胞复制时 UV 损伤突变增加[81]。着色性干皮病患者中 UV 诱发癌变主要原因是细胞丧失 NER 能力或者 Pol H 失活,两者均会导致持续性基因损伤增加(突变、基因重排、缺失和基因组不稳定)。

表 26-1 人类 UV 损伤修复相关基因[d]

组别(基因)	染色体定位	中枢神经系统和发育异常	DNA 相对修复率(%)[a]
着色性干皮病			
A	9q34. 1	有	2~5
B[b]	2q21	有	3~7
C	3q25	无	5~20
D[b]	19q13. 2	有	25~50
E	11p11~12	无	50
F	16q13. 1	无	18
G	13q32. 3	有	<2
V(pol H)	6p21	无	100
ERCC1[c]	19q13. 32	有	15
Cockayne 综合征			
A(ERCC8)	5q12. 1	有	100[a]
B(ERCC6)	10q11. 23	有	100[a]
UVSSA	4p16. 3	无	100[a]

[a]DNA 相对修复率主要统计全基因组切除修复,Cockayne 综合征主要是转录偶联修复异常而全基因组切除修复正常。

[b]患者也具有 Cockayne 综合征症状:侏儒症、皮肤苍老、精神迟滞。B 组被认定为 ERCC3、D 组为 ERCC2、F 组为 ERCC4、G 组为 ERCC5。一些患者也有毛发硫营养不良的症状。

[c]ERCC1 突变非常罕见,会导致脑眼面骨骼综合征——一种新生儿致死性功能异常。

[d]更多信息请登录 http://www. photobiology. info/和 http://www. cgal. icnet. uk/DNA_Repair_Genes. html

Cockayne 综合征

Cockayne 综合征(CS)是一种常染色体隐性遗传疾病,出生后有光过敏、侏儒症、视网膜变性、小头畸形、失聪、神经系统缺陷、身体发育迟滞等症状[82,83]。主要症状是小脑萎缩伴有浦肯野(Purkinje)细胞缺失引起的行走和平衡困难[84]。尽管 CS 患者寿命处于 XP 患者皮肤癌的发病年龄,但未在 Cockayne 综合征患者中发现光致癌,使之与 XP 相区别(图 26-1)[82]。Cockayne 综合征患者涉及 CS 基因突变,包括 *CSA* 和 *CSB*[83,85],症状与着色性干皮病 B、D 和 G 组类似[86]。CS 蛋白促进 RNA 聚合酶Ⅱ从 DNA 受损部位移除,从而允许 NER 机制进入(图 26-2)。另一种基因产物 UVSSA 也有助于 TCR,但 *UVSSA* 基因突变只产生轻微的光过敏[87,88]。

CSA 和 CSB 蛋白还可与线粒体和自噬中的氧化磷酸化相互作用,协助维持细胞氧化还原平衡[89],不难想象,它们在线粒体的作用使其在中枢神经发育和神经病理学中发挥着比核内转录偶联修复更重要的作用[90]。

毛发硫营养不良症

毛发硫营养不良症(trichothiodystrophy,TTD)是一种罕见的常染色体隐性遗传病,患者具有缺硫的脆性毛发和鱼鳞癣,毛发呈小的纤维状且易碎。患者头发蛋白中半胱氨酸/胱氨酸的含量只有正常个体的 15%~50%。患者身体和智力发育迟滞的严重程度不同,通常有面容异常如双耳突出和下巴萎缩,智力呈低下到严重迟钝,表现不等[91]。根据对 UV 的敏感性和 DNA 修复缺陷可将此病分为几种类型[92,93],最严重的患者有 *XPB* 和 *XPD* 突变[92],其他几种已知 TTD 相关基因不涉及 DNA 修复。

引起着色性干皮病的 *XPD* 突变位于 DNA 解旋酶功能域,而引起 TTD 的则是 RNA 解旋酶功能域和蛋白 C 末端的错义突变[94]。有些 TTD 患者并无 *XPB* 或 *XPD* 突变,而是由一个调节 TFIIH 活性的 8-kDa 亚基发生突变所致[95]。

致癌作用

突变和皮肤癌的类型

勒布(Loeb)是第一个认识到癌细胞高频突变的人,并引入突变体表型的概念[96]。例如,三阴性乳腺癌的突变率是一般细胞的 13.3 倍,而正常细胞每次分裂只有 0.6 个突变[97]。NMSC 和黑色素瘤的突变率最高,其中大部分是日光暴露引起的 C 至 T 或 CC 至 TT 置换[98,99]。与全基因组的其他区域相比,正常细胞和癌细胞在转录区的突变减少,这提示细胞倾向于转录偶联修复[97,98,100]。转录偶联修复减少的患者,即 Cockayne 综合征患者,理论上基因转录区突变率更高因此癌症发生率更高。然而事实上,CS 患者并不像 Cs-a 或 Cs-b 小鼠那样因致癌物暴露而患皮肤癌[101],因此,必须预防或延迟 CS 的突变细胞进展为癌症。

非黑色素瘤皮肤癌

鳞状细胞癌(squamous cell carcinoma,SCC)和基底细胞癌(basal cell carcinoma,BCC)都有 UV 型基因突变驱动肿瘤发展。光化性角化病作为 SCC 的癌前病变,有许多相同的突变谱和全基因表达谱[102~104]。SCC 的初始分子变化是 *p53* 的 UV 型突变,它导致日光暴露区域的皮肤克隆扩增,这些扩增的克隆原先只局限在增殖单位内[105]。在正常皮肤中,50% 的 SCC 具有 *p53* 突变,而在着色性干皮病患者中,突变频率为 90%[106~110]。UV 照射时,p53 功能丧失会造成 DNA 复制中基因组不稳定[111~113]。大多数基因组不稳定是不具有生长优势的"乘客突变",突变的 *p53* 才是 SCC 有力驱动因素。

鳞状细胞癌的基因突变涉及 Notch、*KNSTRN*、着丝粒基因、*EGF*、*RAS*、*NFkb*、*JNK2* 和 *MMP9*[114~118]。日光 UV 照射,可导致原癌基因 *H-RAS* 和 *N-RAS* 的第 61 位密码子发生 TT 位点的激活突变[119~122]。

Sonic Hedgehog 信号通路参与基底细胞癌和基底细胞母斑综合征(basal cell nevus syndrome,BCNS),其中跨膜受体(PTC)和膜蛋白(SMO)通过与 PTC 结合的细胞外蛋白 Hedgehog(HH)调节信号转导[123]。在一般人群中大多数 UV 型基底细胞癌突变位于 PTC 基因,少数发生在 *SMO* 基因,极少有 *HH* 突变[109,124~126]。然而,在着色性干皮病患者中,突变集中于 *SMO* 和 *HH* 基因[127,128]。

黑色素瘤

黑色素瘤涉及 MAPK 通路一系列的基因突变、缺失和扩增(拷贝数变化),MAPK 通路是调节细胞增殖和分化的磷酸化级联反应(图 26-3)[129~135]。BRAF(V600E)是一种常见突变,但

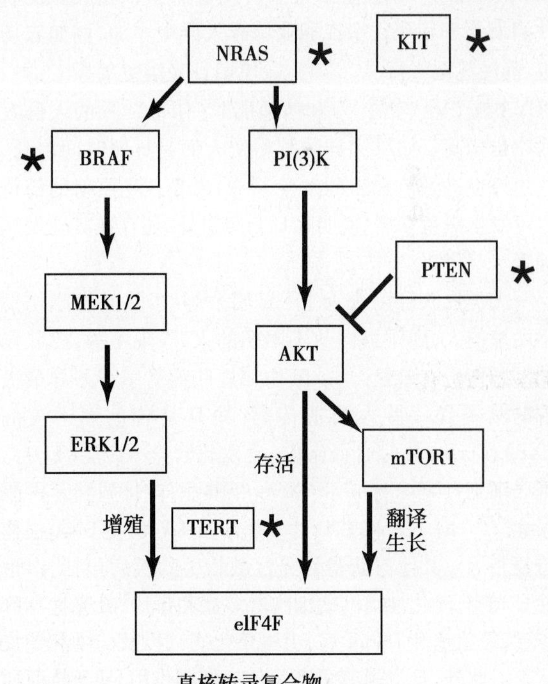

图 26-3　黑色素瘤相关的信号转导通路。着色性干皮病患者和一般人群中由于 UV 照射而引发的突变基因标注星号。TERT 突变是 UV 型,但未在着色性干皮病患者中发现。注意黑色素瘤常见基因突变 *BRAF*(V600E)并非 UV 诱导型,但 UV 可导致 *BRAF* 的其他突变体[136]。着色性干皮病最常见的基因突变是 *PTEN*,而普通人群黑色素瘤最常见的是 MAPK 通路

这种突变不属于 UV 型[137,136]。相比之下，XP 来源的黑色素瘤 *BRAF* 基因中 11 个突变有 10 个是 UV 型且与 V600E 不同[136]。已在 hTERT 的启动子区发现导致基因活化的 UV 型突变[138,139]。除点突变外，黑色素瘤还有显著的蛋白激酶基因易位[140]。着色性干皮病患者的色素痣和黑色素瘤一般呈雀斑样，且有高频(53%~61%) UV 型 *PTEN* 基因失活突变[136]。不同于一般黑色素瘤中 *PTEN* 突变频率较低，XP 来源的黑色素瘤 *PTEN* 基因突变频率远高于 *BRAF*、*NRAS* 和 *KIT*。

致谢

本工作得到了来自加州大学旧金山分校(JEC)及其西蒙纪念基金会的学术评议会(JEC)的 E. A. Dickson 名誉教授的支持。

结论

皮肤肿瘤发病人数占每年新增癌症病例数的 30%[141]。流行病学和实验室研究证实，日光暴露是皮肤癌的直接原因[142]，高剂量紫外线成分是皮肤癌高发病率的主要原因。非黑色素瘤皮肤癌(NMSC，包括基底细胞癌和鳞状细胞癌)和黑色素瘤易发生于被日光照射的身体部位(如男性的面部和躯干，女性的面部和腿部)，其发病率与急性日光照射或日照累积相关。皮肤肿瘤发病率和死亡率在职业暴露人群中增加，例如农场主、渔民甚至飞行员[6,143~145]。使用日光浴室美黑[145,146]、PUVA 或 UVA 疗法[147]和西地那非(伟哥)[148]的人群发病率也增高。如果涂抹防晒霜使人们受日照时间增长，这也可促进黑色素瘤的发生[149]。未受日光照射的部位也可发生黑色素瘤，说明除日光照射外，还存在其他发病因素[12,150,151]。

人类皮肤可以分为 Ⅰ~Ⅳ 四个等级，从经常晒伤但不晒黑的人，到晒黑但从不晒伤的人，表现不等，皮肤癌的易感性也有差异[152]。晒伤和皮肤癌易感性差异最极端的例子是一些人类遗传病，尤其是着色性干皮病(XP)、Cockayne 综合征(CS)、毛发硫营养不良症(TTD)、基底细胞母斑综合征(BCNS)、卟啉症、白化病和苯丙酮尿症[12]。XP、CS 和 TTD 的发病涉及 UV 相关 DNA 损伤修复基因。其他与获得性光过敏相关的疾病包括，多形性日光疹、光化性类网状细胞增多症和痒疹、日光性荨麻疹、红斑狼疮和 Darier 病(毛囊角化病)，以及药物和免疫状态。此外，日光暴露可产生免疫抑制作用，导致抗原递呈的 Langerhans 细胞消失，上表皮出现不良角化的角质细胞(凋亡的日光灼伤细胞)，前列腺素释放引起的血管舒张可导致红斑反应[153]，器官移植和艾滋病患者的免疫抑制也使皮肤癌发病率增加[154]。

(曹琦琪 译　董亚萍　文文 校)

部分参考文献

12 Kraemer KH, Lee MM, Andrews AD, Lambert WC. The role of sunlight and DNA repair in melanoma and nonmelanoma skin cancer. The xeroderma pigmentosum paradigm. *Arch Dermatol*. 1994;**130**:1018-1021.

13 Bradford PT, Goldstein AM, Tamura DT, et al. Cancer and neurologic degeneration in xeroderma pigmentosum: long term follow-up characterises the role of DNA repair. *J Med Genet*. 2011;**48**:168-176.

25 Taylor JS, Cohrs MP. DNA, light. and Dewar pyrimidinones: the structure and significance of TpT3. *J Am Chem Soc*. 1987;**109**:2834-2835.

26 Mitchell DL, Jen J, Cleaver JE. Relative induction of cyclobutane dimers and cytosine photohydrates in DNA irradiated in vitro and in vivo with ultraviolet C and ultraviolet B light. *Photochem Photobiol*. 1991;**54**:741-746.

27 Mitchell DL, Jen J, Cleaver JE. Sequence specificity of cyclobutane pyrimidine dimers in DNA treated with solar (ultraviolet B) radiation. *Nucleic Acids Res*. 1992;**20**:225-229.

29 Mitchell DL, Cleaver JE. Photochemical alterations of cytosine account for most biological effects after ultraviolet irradiation. *Trends Photochem Photobiol*. 1990;**1**:107-119.

34 Hoeijmakers JH. Genome maintenance mechanisms for preventing cancer. *Nature*. 2001;**411**:366-374.

35 Cleaver JE. Defective repair replication in xeroderma pigmentosum. *Nature*. 1968;**218**:652-656.

36 Cleaver JE. Xeroderma pigmentosum: a human disease in which an initial stage of DNA repair is defective. *Proc Natl Acad Sci U S A*. 1969;**63**:428-435.

37 Cleaver JE, Lam ET, Revet I. Disorders of nucleotide excision repair: the genetic and molecular basis of heterogeneity. *Nat Rev Genet*. 2009;**10**: 756-768.

38 Sancar A, Lindsey-Boltz LA, Unsal-Kacmaz K, Linn S. Molecular mechanisms of mammalian DNA repair and the DNA damage checkpoints. *Annu Rev Biochem*. 2004;**73**:39-85.

40 Hanawalt PC. Transcription-coupled repair and human disease. *Science*. 1994;**266**:1957-1958.

46 Fitch ME, Nakajima S, Yasui A, Ford JM. In vivo recruitment of XPC to UV-induced cyclobutane pyrimidine dimers by the DDB2 gene product. *J Biol Chem*. 2003;**276**:46909-46910.

49 Groisman R, Polanowska J, Kuraoka I, et al. The ubiquitin ligase activity in the DDB2 and CSA complexes is differentially regulated by the COP9 signalosome in response to DNA damage. *Cell*. 2003;**113**:357-367.

50 Min JH, Pavletich NP. Recognition of DNA damage by the Rad4 nucleotide excision repair protein. *Nature*. 2007;**449**:570-575.

51 Maillard O, Solyom S, Naegeli H. An aromatic sensor with aversion to damaged strands confers versatility to DNA repair. *PLoS Biol*. 2007;**5**:e79.

52 Lindsey-Boltz LA, Sancar A. RNA poymerase: the most specific damage recognition protein in cellular responses to DNA damage. *Proc Natl Acad Sci U S A*. 2007;**104**:13213-13214.

53 Schwertman P, Lagarou A, Dekkers DHW, et al. UV-sensitive syndrome protein UVSSA recruits USP7 to regulate transcription-coupled repair. *Nat Genet*. 2012;**44**:598-602.

55 Newman JC, Bailey AD, Weiner AM. Cockayne syndrome group B protein (CSB) plays a general role in chromatin maintenance and remodeling. *Proc Natl Acad Sci U S A*. 2006;**103**:9613-9618.

56 Mao P, Meas R, Dorgan KM, Smerdon MJ. UV damage-induced RNA polymerase II stalling stimulates H2B deubiquitylation. *Proc Natl Acad Sci U S A*. 2014;**111**:12811-12816.

58 Wood RD. DNA damage recognition during nucleotide excision repair in mammalian cells. *Biochimie*. 1999;**81**:39-44.

59 Sancar A. Mechanisms of DNA excision repair. *Science*. 1994;**266**:1954-1956.

60 Fagbemi AF, Orelli B, Scharer OD. Regulation of endonuclease activity in human nucleotide excision repair. *DNA Repair*. 2011;**10**:722-729.

64 Ohmori H, Friedberg EC, Fuchs RPP, et al. The Y-family of DNA polymerases. *Mol Cell*. 2001;**8**:7-8.

65 Trincao J, Johnson RE, Escalante CR, et al. Structure of the catalytic core of S. cerevisiae DNA polymerase h: implications for translesion synthesis. *Mol Cell*. 2001;**8**:417-426.

68 Johnson RE, Prakash S, Prakash L. Efficient bypass of a thymine-thymine dimer by yeast DNA polymerase eta. *Science*. 1999;**283**:1001-1004.

82 Nance MA, Berry SA. Cockayne syndrome:review of 140 cases. *Am J Med Genet*. 1992;**42**:68-84.

87 Nakazawa Y, Sasaki K, Mitsutake N, et al. KIAA1530/UVSSA is responsible for UV-sensitive syndrome that facilitates damage-dependent processing of stalled RNA polymerase IIo in TC-NER. *Nat Genet*. 2012;**44**:586-592.

88 Zhang X, Horibata K, Saijo M, et al. Mutations in KIAA1530/UVSSA cause UV-sensitive syndrome destabilizing ERCC6 in transcription-coupled DNA

repair. *Nat Genet*. 2012;**44**:593–597.

89 Scheibye-Knudsen M, Croteau DL, Bohr VA. Mitochondrial deficiency in Cockayne syndrome. *Mech Aging Dev*. 2013;**134**:275–283.

90 Cleaver JE, Brennan-Minnella AM, Swanson RA, et al. Mitochondrial reactive oxygen species are scavenged by Cockayne Syndrome B protein in human fibroblasts without nuclear DNA damage. *Proc Natl Acad Sci U S A*. 2014;**111**:13487–13492.

96 Loeb L. Mutator phenotype may be required for multistage carcinogenesis. *Cancer Res*. 1991;**51**:3075–3079.

97 Wang Y, Waters J, Leung ML, et al. Clonal evolution in breast cancer revealed by single nucleus genome sequencing. *Nature*. 2014;**512**:155–160.

98 Lawrence MS, Stojanov P, Polak P, et al. Mutational heterogeneity in cancer and the search for new cancer-associated genes. *Nature*. 2013;**499**:214–218.

99 Pleasance ED, Cheetham RK, Stephens PJ, et al. A comprehensive catalogue of somatic mutations from a human cancer genome. *Nature*. 2010;**463**:191–196.

113 Laposa RR, Huang EJ, Cleaver JE. Increased apoptosis, p53 up-regulation, and cerebellar neuronal degeneration in repair-deficient Cockayne syndrome mice. *Proc Natl Acad Sci U S A*. 2007;**104**:1389–1394.

124 Epstein EH. Basal cell carcinomas:attack of the hedgehog. *Nat Rev Cancer*. 2008;**8**:743–754.

136 Masaki T, Wang Y, DiGiovanna JJ, et al. High frequency of PTEN mutations in nevi and melanomas from xeroderma pigmentosum patients. *Pigment Cell Melanoma Res*. 2014;**27**:454–464.

137 Davies H, Bignell GR, Cox C, et al. Mutations of the BRAF gene in human cancer. *Nature*. 2002;**417**:949–954.

141 Scotto J, Fears TR, Fraumeni JF. *Incidence of Nonmelanoma Skin Cancer in the United States*. Bethesda, MD: U.S. Department of Health and Human Services, NIH Publication No. 83–2433; 1983.

151 Noonan FP, Recio JA, Takayama H, et al. Neonatal sunburn and melanoma in mice. *Nature*. 2001;**413**:271–272.

153 Kripke ML. Immunological effects of ultraviolet radiation. *J Dermatol*. 1991;**18**:429–433.

第 27 章　炎症与肿瘤

Jelena Todoric, MD, PhD ■ Atsushi Umemura, MD, PhD ■ Koji Taniguchi, MD, PhD ■ Michael Karin, PhD

概述

流行病学和实验研究有力支持了慢性炎症促进恶性肿瘤发生发展这一长期以来的观点，持续性病毒和细菌感染、自身免疫性疾病、环境刺激物甚至肥胖都会引发炎症，这种预先存在的炎症会促进肿瘤发展，而且是近 20%癌症所致死亡的罪魁祸首。炎症也可继发于癌症发展，这种“肿瘤诱发性炎症”在许多癌症的恶性进展和播散转移中发挥重要作用。尽管使用常用抗炎药物如阿司匹林可降低癌症风险，但是目前针对癌症相关炎症的临床治疗远未满足人们的需求。

慢性炎症与癌症

炎症与肿瘤相关的观点由德国病理学家 Rudolf Virchow 于 19 世纪首次提出。他发现实体肿瘤中存在免疫细胞浸润，从而提出炎症可能是肿瘤发生的原因。但直到一个多世纪后，流行病学研究表明慢性炎症与近 20%的癌症死亡有关，这才重新激起人们探索炎症与癌症之间关系的兴趣。最近，确凿的证据表明炎症是癌症的一个关键标志，一些潜在的关键分子机制也被阐明[1]。此外，炎性微环境是包括一些造血系统恶性肿瘤在内的许多癌症的重要组成部分，甚至在尚未与炎症建立直接因果关系的肿瘤中亦是如此[2]。值得注意的是，只有 10%的癌症与生殖细胞突变有关，而绝大多数(90%)是由体细胞获得性突变引起的，其中很多可能与慢性炎症的微环境有关。然而，在大多数情况下，由持续感染和自身免疫性疾病引发的慢性炎症(表 27-1)扮演着肿瘤促进者角色[3]。最典型的例子之一是炎症性肠病(inflammatory bowel disease, IBD)，例如溃疡性结肠炎大大增加了结直肠癌(colorectal cancer, CRC)患病风险[3]。同样，幽门螺杆菌持续感染引发慢性胃炎并可导致胃癌。乙型肝炎病毒(hepatitis B virus, HBV)或丙型肝炎病毒(hepatitis C virus, HCV)感染引起慢性肝炎，最终导致肝细胞癌(HCC)。HCC 是全球癌症相关死亡的主要原因之一，目前大约 85%的 HCC 起源于 HBV 或 HCV 感染引起的慢性肝损伤。

在过去的一代中，肥胖已成为许多发达国家的主要公共健康问题，肥胖能够增加包括癌症在内的各类疾病风险。肥胖诱导低水平的可影响多器官系统的持续炎症，是目前几乎所有类型癌症的常见风险因素之一。另外，长期使用抗炎药物如阿司匹林或选择性环氧合酶-2(cyclooxygenase-2, COX-2)抑制剂可以大大降低癌症风险。这些现象进一步证实了炎症是癌症的主要原因之一，也是癌症恶性进展和播散转移的重要驱动因素。

表 27-1　与感染因素相关的主要癌症部位和类型

感染因素	癌症部位和类型
幽门螺旋杆菌	胃癌
乙型或丙型肝炎病毒	肝癌
人类乳头瘤病毒	宫颈癌；生殖器癌；口咽癌
EB 病毒	鼻咽癌
埃及血吸虫	膀胱癌
人类免疫缺陷病毒	非霍奇金淋巴瘤；Kaposi 肉瘤；宫颈癌

截至 2008 年，全球 16%左右的癌症可归因于各类感染因素。其中最突出的是幽门螺旋杆菌、HBV、HCV 和 HPV。

值得注意的是，仅在某些癌症起始或恶性转化之前就已存在慢性炎症。在多数癌症中，癌症发生发展诱导的局部炎性微环境，进一步促进肿瘤进展。了解炎症与癌症之间的联系对于制定更好的预防和治疗策略至关重要。

炎细胞、微环境与癌症

巨噬细胞

巨噬细胞是肿瘤微环境中数量最多的免疫细胞。肿瘤相关巨噬细胞(tumor-associated macrophages, TAM)在原发和转移部位均具有促肿瘤特性[4]，并在癌症发展中发挥支持作用。TAM 的促肿瘤功能能够影响癌细胞增殖和存活、血管生成、癌细胞侵袭、运动、内外渗透以及抑制细胞毒性 T 细胞反应[5,6]。在肿瘤起始和早期促成时期，TAM 分泌细胞因子和生长因子刺激具有致癌突变的起始上皮细胞增殖存活[7]。目前尚不清楚，肿瘤发展的早期阶段的巨噬细胞在通过极化获得促肿瘤特性之前能否消除异常细胞。巨噬细胞大致可分为两个亚群：经典激活的 M1 巨噬细胞和替代激活的 M2 巨噬细胞[8]。M1 型巨噬细胞表达和分泌多种促炎细胞因子、趋化因子和效应分子，包括 IL-12、IL-23、肿瘤坏死因子(tumor necrosis factor, TNF)和 iNOS，而 M2 型巨噬细胞释放抗炎因子，如 IL-10、TGF-β 和精氨酸酶-1。在肿瘤早期进展期间，某些因素导致 TAM 表型向 MS 转换，从而提供允许肿瘤生长的免疫抑制微环境。巨噬细胞暴露于由 $CD4^+$ T 细胞和/或癌细胞产生的 IL-4[5,9]、生长因子例如集落刺激因子-1(colony-stimulating factor-1, CSF1)[10]、GM-CSF[11]以及癌症分泌的 TGF-β 可转化为促肿瘤的 M2 表型，但 TAM 的确切起源仍具争论。大多数 TAM 可能来源于循环 $Ly6C^+$ 单核细胞[12~14]，但是骨髓(bone marrow, BM)是单核细胞的主要产生部位这一经典观点受到最近研究结果的挑战——这些研究表明髓外造血才是肿瘤浸润单核细胞的储存库。然而，谱系追踪实验证明，脾脏在这过程中的贡献很小，至少在一些肿瘤模型中 BM 仍然是产生 TAM 的单核细胞的主要来源[16]。CSF1 除了能够促进 TAM 增殖和激活，还是主要的谱系调节因子和巨噬细胞的趋化因子[17]。在恶性转化期间，多数肿瘤中提供营养和氧合作用的血管急剧增加，这一过程被称为"血管生成转换"。表达 TIE2 的 TAMs 主要通过血管内皮生长因子（vascular endothelial growth factor，VEGF）调节这一过程[18]。$TIE2^+$巨噬细胞还能促进癌细胞转移和向血管迁移[19]。此外，巨噬细胞介导肿瘤床的部分免疫抑制，抑制细胞毒性 $CD8^+$细胞，这将在下文进一步讨论（表 27-1）。

T 和 B 淋巴细胞

许多肿瘤表达可被 T 淋巴细胞识别的抗原，对实体肿瘤微环境的分析揭示存在 T 细胞浸润。然而，尽管部分患者仍存在主动免疫应答，包括细胞毒性 $CD8^+$ T 细胞的浸润，但这并未阻断肿瘤的进展。这表明存在一种抵抗肿瘤免疫的免疫抑制机制。这种机制依赖 $CD4^+Foxp3^+$调节性 T 细胞（Treg）的聚集，Treg 细胞在维持免疫自身耐受中起关键作用[21]。此外，Treg 细胞还可产生多种细胞因子，例如促进肿瘤进展的 RANK 配体（RANKL），最初是在乳腺癌中阐明了 RANKL 的作用[22]。应激相关或损伤相关分子模式（damage-associated molecular pattern，DAMP）参与了肿瘤 $CD8^+$T 细胞反应，损伤组织或死亡癌细胞通过 DAMP 可以促进免疫应答。$CD8\alpha^+$ 组树突状细胞（DC）产生的 I 型干扰素也有利于激活抗癌免疫[23]。DC 和巨噬细胞表达主要组织相容性复合物（major histocompatibility complex，MHC）I 类分子，并向细胞毒性 $CD8^+$ T 细胞呈递抗原。然而，表达膜结合或可溶形式的组织相容性白细胞抗原（histocompatibility leukocyte antigen，HLA）分子的巨噬细胞可以直接抑制自然杀伤（nature killer，NK）细胞和其他 T 细胞亚群的激活[24]。此外，HLA-G 和 HLA-E 可以抑制 NK 细胞分泌干扰素 IFN-γ，IFN-γ 是 $CD8^+$T 细胞活化的重要介质[25]。癌细胞或免疫细胞上可表达抑制性受体程序性细胞死亡蛋白 1（programmed cell death protein 1，PD-1）和细胞毒性 T 淋巴细胞抗原 4（cytotoxic T lymphocyte antigen 4，CTLA-4），在配体的激活下，会控制免疫应答的强度并抑制 T 细胞受体（T-cell receptor，TCR）和 B 细胞受体（B-cell receptor，BCR）信号传导[26]。已证明 TAMs 可上调 PD-1 配体表达应对肿瘤缺氧区域的缺氧诱导因子 1 体（hypoxia inducible factor 1α，HIF-1α），从而抑制 T 细胞[27]。此外，TAMs 还分泌多种细胞因子和趋化因子直接抑制 T 细胞活化并募集免疫抑制性 Treg 细胞。Th17 细胞产生炎性细胞因子 IL-17A 和 IL-17F，早期结肠癌募集 Th17 细胞，加速肿瘤进展[28]。B 淋巴细胞也存在于肿瘤微环境中，皮肤癌或鳞状细胞癌的小鼠模型中，B 细胞通过激活髓系细胞促进肿瘤进展[29,30]。在前列腺癌中，新募集的 B 细胞通过促炎细胞因子淋巴毒素促进侵袭性去势抵抗型肿瘤的进展[31]。浸润肿瘤的 B 细胞也可在某些肿瘤局部高浓度 TGF-β 在作用下，呈现出免疫抑制表型，抑制细胞毒性 T 细胞的活化。

癌症相关成纤维细胞

癌症相关成纤维细胞（cancer-associated fibroblasts，CAF）是位于肿瘤微环境内的成纤维细胞，CAF 通过刺激癌细胞增殖、促进血管生成和改变细胞外基质（extracellular matrix，ECM）的结构来促进肿瘤发生[32~37]。在正常组织中，成纤维细胞通过 TGF-β 介导的信号负调控上皮细胞增殖，防止肿瘤生长起始。相反的，CAF 表现出促炎和促肿瘤特性[38]，并产生多种趋化因子和细胞因子，包括骨桥蛋白（osteopontin，OPN）、CXCL1、CXCL2、IL-6、IL1-2、CCL-5、基质衍生因子（stromal-derived factor，SDF-1α）和 TNF[39,40]。在肿瘤发生的早期阶段，成纤维细胞"感知"邻近上皮细胞增殖增加引起的组织结构变化，激活成纤维细胞中促炎信号[41~43]。此外，定植免疫细胞分泌的介质会增强 CAF 的促炎特性[40]。例如，由于少量血液从有漏隙血管中渗出，B 细胞的抗体可沉积在肿瘤床中，并诱导定植的免疫细胞分泌 IL-1；这又反过来促进成纤维细胞转化为促炎症表型[44,45]。肿瘤缺氧也会影响 CAF，上调 CAF 产生 TGF-β 也和某些趋化因子的能力[46]。CAF 促进肿瘤的主要机制是分泌细胞因子和趋化因子，将免疫细胞募集到肿瘤微环境中并改变其功能。例如，CAF 分泌 CCL2 在肿瘤中募集巨噬细胞，分泌免疫抑制细胞因子 TGF-β 抑制 NK 和 $CD8^+$T 细胞的功能[47]，同时诱导 Treg 细胞分化[48]。CAF 来源的 CXCL13 介导 B 细胞在雄激素剥夺前列腺癌的募集，导致去势抵抗[46]。

癌症中的促炎和抗炎细胞因子

细胞因子是由许多类型的细胞，特别是免疫细胞产生和释放的小分子蛋白质，通过特定膜受体起到细胞—细胞间通讯的介质作用[7]。细胞因子通常在炎症反应中被诱导，通过癌症内在效应（癌细胞增殖、存活和侵袭性质）和癌症外在效应（肿瘤微环境），提供炎症和癌症之间的重要联系（图 27-1）[49]。TNF 和 IL-6 是研究最深入的致癌细胞因子，它们在大多数癌症中过度表达（表 27-2），从而将炎症与癌症联系起来[50]。转录因子像是 NF-κB、信号转导和转录激活因子 3（signal transducer and activator of transcription 3，STAT3）和 AP-1 是细胞因子信号转导通路的主要下游效应物，在许多癌症中被激活，它们协作调节许多癌症相关的病理生理过程，包括细胞增殖和存活、分化、免疫、代谢和转移[51]。

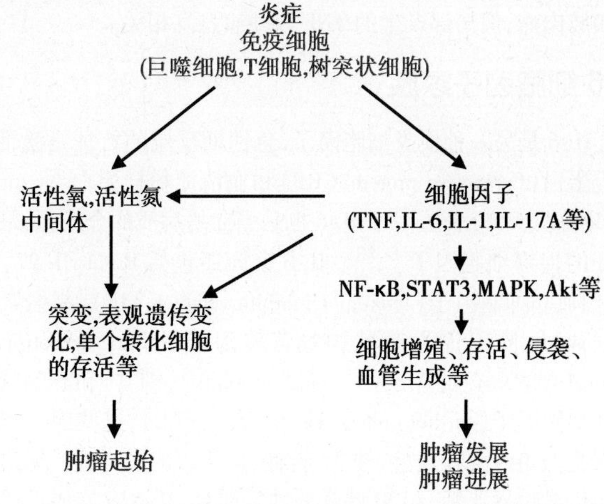

图 27-1　炎症在肿瘤起始、发展和进展中的作用

表 27-2 炎症和癌症的炎性介质

炎性介质	对肿瘤和免疫细胞的作用	转导通路
TNF	促炎、细胞存活或死亡	NF-κB,MAPK
IL-6	促炎、细胞增殖或存活	JAK/STAT3,ERK,Akt
IL-11	保护组织、细胞增殖或存活	JAK/STAT3,ERK,Akt
IL-1	促炎、激活免疫细胞	NF-κB,MAPK
IL-17A	促炎、增加炎症	NF-κB,MAPK
IL-12	促炎、Th1 分化	JAK/STAT4
IL-23	促炎、Th17 分化	JAK/STAT3,STAT4
IL-10	抗炎、抑制 NF-κB	JAK/STAT3
IL-22	保护组织、细胞增殖或存活	JAK/STAT3
TGF-β	抗炎、肿瘤发生的双重作用	Smad,MAPK

肿瘤坏死因子

肿瘤坏死因子(tumor necrosis factor,TNF)是细胞因子大家族的奠基成员,是应对各种病原体产生炎症和免疫反应的主要激活因子[52,53]。TNF 是恶病质和数种急性和慢性炎症性疾病的重要介质,如败血症、类风湿性关节炎(rheumatoid arthritis,RA)和 IBD。TNF 主要由巨噬细胞产生,巨噬细胞在病原体相关分子模式(pathogen-associated molecular pattern,PAMP)如脂多糖(lipopolysaccharide,LPS)的作用下通过 Toll 样受体(toll-like receptor,TLR)激活。TNF 与 TNF 受体(TNFR)1 和/或 TNFR2 结合激活几种信号转导通路。根据细胞环境,通路被激活并诱导产生其他炎性细胞因子,例如 IL-6 和 IL-1,调控细胞存活和死亡。升高的 TNF 表达在多个环节促进肿瘤发生和转移,包括细胞转化、存活、增殖、侵袭和血管生成[52,53]。TNF 诱导 NF-κB 活化,进一步激活 β-catenin,导致非干细胞去分化,使结肠直肠癌小鼠模型的细胞获得肿瘤起始能力[54]。临床上已有 TNF 抑制剂用于治疗 RA 和 IBD。尽管高剂量 TNF 已被用于治疗四肢肉瘤,但局部产生的 TNF 与肿瘤息息相关。

IL-6 细胞因子家族

IL-6 是另一种促炎细胞因子,急性期反应的特征是激活 C 反应蛋白(C-reactive protein,CRP)和血清淀粉样蛋白 A(serum amyloid A,SAA)表达[55]。IL-6 也是癌症恶病质的介质,是最具特征的促癌细胞因子[56,57]。IL-6 家族还包括 IL-11、IL-27、IL-31、白血病抑制因子(leukemia inhibitory factor,LIF)、制瘤素 M(oncostatin M,OSM)、睫状神经营养因子(ciliary neurotrophic factor,CNTF)、心肌营养素-1(cardiotrophin-1,CT-1)和心肌营养素样细胞因子(cardiotrophin-like cytokine,CLC),这些因子控制着细胞增殖、存活、迁移、侵袭、转移、血管生成和炎症。通过与共同信号传导亚基 gp130 偶联的独特受体,IL-6 家族成员激活 JAK-STAT3 通路、SH2-SHP-2-Ras-Raf-MEK-ERK 通路和 PI3K-Akt-mTOR 通路。STAT3 在效应物中被认为是致癌基因,是癌症中 gp130 信号传导的主要下游介质[58,59]。IL-6 和 IL-11 由许多不同类型的细胞产生,包括免疫细胞、成纤维细胞和上皮细胞。IL-6、IL-11 和 STAT3 在许多实体瘤中高表达。最新研究认为 IL-11(IL-6 家族成员)在小鼠胃肠道(gastrointestinal,GI)肿瘤发生过程中起重要作用[60]。IL-6 拮抗剂已被批准用于治疗 RA 和相关疾病,但在癌症中尚需进一步评估。

白细胞介素 1

IL-1 是另一种由多种细胞类型产生的主要促炎和促癌细胞因子[61]。IL-1 诱导发热并在败血症中扮演重要角色。IL-1 有两型:IL-1α 和 IL-1β,都通过 IL-1 受体(IL-1R)激活 NF-κB、JNK、p38 和 ERK,并诱导表达其他细胞因子。尽管在蛋白质水平上 IL-1α 和 IL-1β 仅有 26%的相似性,但它们功能类似。已开发出数种 IL-1 拮抗剂用于治疗炎性疾病,但在癌症中的功效需要进一步测试。

白细胞介素 17A

IL-17A 是 IL-17 家族成员,主要由可产生 IL-17 的 T 辅助细胞(Th17)、γδT 细胞和先天淋巴细胞(innate lymphoid cells,ILC)产生[62,63]。IL-17A 保护细胞免受细菌和真菌侵害,并且与自身免疫疾病如牛皮癣有关。IL-17A 通过 IL-17 受体 A(IL-17RA)激活 NF-κB、JNK、p38 和 ERK,并促进肿瘤发生、转移、血管生成和化疗耐药[64]。IL-17A 诱导产生包括 TNF、IL-6 和 IL-17 在内的多种促炎细胞因子,表明 IL-17A 在炎症级联扩大中起重要作用。IL-17A 还在异型小肠细胞发挥作用,促进结直肠癌小鼠模型中异常隐窝的生长和进展[64]。

IL-12 和 IL-23

IL-12 和 IL-23 是异二聚体促炎因子,有相同的 p40 亚基和 IL-12 受体(IL-12R)β1 亚基[65]。它们由抗原呈递细胞产生,是 T 细胞反应的调节的关键参与者。IL-12 刺激产生 IFN-γ 的 Th1 细胞(一般是抗肿瘤)的生成,而 IL-23 与 IL-6、TGF-β 一起促进 Th17 细胞(一般是促肿瘤)的发育。

IL-10 和 IL-22

IL-10 是 IL-10 家族的典型抗炎细胞因子,通过主要在免疫细胞中表达的 IL-10 受体 1(IL-10R1)激活 JAK-STAT3 通路[66]。IL-10 的抗炎活性是通过抑制 NF-κB 活性发挥的。IL-10 敲除小鼠自发产生类似人 IBD 的慢性结肠炎。IL-22 是 IL-10 细胞因子家族的另一成员,作用和 IL-10 相反,是促炎因子,由可产生 IL-17 和 IL-22 的 T 辅助细胞(Th22)和 ILC 细胞产生。IL-22 还通过 IL-22 受体 1(IL-22R1)激活 JAK-STAT3 途径,IL-22 受体 1 仅在上皮细胞而不在免疫细胞上表达。IL-22 调节与宿主防御和自身免疫疾病相关的天然反应,与 IL-6 细胞因子家族的作用方式类似,促进细胞增殖、存活、组织再生、转移和血管生成[67]。

转化生长因子

转化生长因子(transforming growth factor-beta,TGF-β)是抗炎细胞因子 TGF-β 超家族的典型成员[68]。TGF-β 结合异二聚

体Ⅰ型和Ⅱ型 TGF-β受体(TGF-RⅠ和 TGF-RⅡ)通过 JNK、p38 和 MAPK,激活 Smad 通路和非 Smad 通路。TGF-β 还抑制细胞增殖并调节 Treg 细胞和 Th17 细胞分化。TGF-β 在癌症进展中起双重作用[69],在正常细胞和早期癌中发挥抑制作用,在肿瘤晚期则促进恶性进展、侵袭和转移。

炎症和肿瘤发生

肿瘤发生由起始、发展和转移这几步组成,伴随着肿瘤血管和淋巴管新生,为生长中的肿瘤提供必要营养和氧气,也为转移播散提供了途径。通过释放炎症介质,慢性活化的 TAM 和 CAF 控制肿瘤微环境的恶性进展和肿瘤血管新生。

肿瘤起始

起始阶段涉及诱导致癌基因突变,导致癌基因激活和/或抑癌基因缺失。通过为正常细胞提供优于临近细胞的生长和存活优势,这些突变使正常细胞转变为异常细胞。炎症细胞产生的活性氧(ROS)和活性氮中间体(RNI)等介质可导致细胞 DNA 损伤并获得致癌突变。这些反应性中间体也会引起基因组不稳定并可加速细胞增殖,但过量产生会导致细胞死亡。炎症促进肿瘤起始的另一种机制是产生生长因子和细胞因子,赋予肿瘤祖细胞干细胞样表型或刺激干细胞扩增,从而扩大环境诱变剂可以作用的细胞群。然而,这种机制更类似于早期肿瘤产生,这将在下文讨论。

在大多数情况下,至少需要 4~5 个突变才可以诱发癌症,单个突变不足以引起癌变[70,71]。因此,肿瘤起始需要持续暴露于 ROS 和 RNI,产生不可逆、持久的 DNA 损伤和累积突变的可分裂细胞。慢性炎症还导致表观遗传改变,例如 DNA 甲基化和组蛋白修饰,进一步促进肿瘤起始。

肿瘤发展

肿瘤发展是从单个肿瘤起始细胞生长到克隆群体,最后产生原发性肿瘤的过程,免疫或炎细胞产生的促肿瘤细胞因子和生长因子是肿瘤发展的核心。例如,TNF 和 IL-6 激活 AP-1、NF-κB 和 STAT3 以诱导维持细胞增殖存活的基因。促进血管新生的细胞因子为原发性肿瘤提供供应氧气和营养的血管,从而令肿瘤生长。

炎症和血管新生

如前所述,肿瘤生长过程对血液的需求增加。炎细胞是血管生成细胞因子(例如 VEGF)的重要来源。肿瘤缺氧可导致 CAF 活化,增加趋化因子的产生,从而将更多的炎细胞和免疫细胞招募到缺氧的肿瘤中[46]。

肿瘤转移

转移是肿瘤进展的最后阶段,最终导致超过 90%的癌症死亡。转移是一个复杂的过程,需要癌细胞、免疫/炎细胞和基质成分的密切合作。起初,癌细胞通过丧失细胞极性和细胞-细胞黏附获得间充质特征,导致移动性和侵入上皮基底膜并进入血管或淋巴管的能力增加[72],这个过程称为上皮-间质转换(epithelial-mesenchymal transition,EMT),EMT 的特征是 E-钙粘蛋白表达缺失。接下来,癌细胞浸润到血管和淋巴管中。炎症通过产生分别激活癌细胞中 NF-κB 和增加血管通透性的介质来促进 EMT 和血管内渗透。接下来转移的起始细胞存活并在循环系统播散。据估计,进入循环的癌细胞中只有约 0.01%最终存活以及产生微转移[73]。中性粒细胞上调可黏附分子,通过整合素介导的附着,允许循环中癌细胞从血管外渗到组织液[74],最后,单个转移祖细胞与免疫、炎症和基质细胞相互作用并开始增殖[75],全身性炎症可以加强循环癌细胞与靶器官的附着并动员中性粒细胞,癌症患者循环中的几种促炎细胞因子上调表达内皮细胞或靶器官的黏附分子,促进转移细胞的附着。

炎症相关癌症:疾病举例和治疗

结直肠癌

炎症性肠病和结直肠癌

炎症性肠病(inflammatory bowel disease,IBD)患者患结直肠癌(colorectal cancer,CRC)的风险升高,这被称为结肠炎相关癌症(colitis-associated cancer,CAC)。虽然 IBD 仅占所有 CRC 病例的 2%~3%[76,77],但 20%IBD 患者在疾病发生 30 年内发生 CAC。小鼠的 CAC 样疾病可以由促癌化合物氧化偶氮甲烷(azoxymethane,AOM)与黏膜刺激剂葡聚糖硫酸钠盐(dextran sulfate sodium salt,DSS)诱发,病理类型类似结肠炎[78]。该模型说明,IL-6/IL-11-STAT3 轴和 NF-κB 是癌前期肠上皮细胞增殖存活和 CAC 发育所必需的[7,79]。

散发性结直肠癌和炎症

散发性 CRC 不由明显的结肠炎症发展而来,但同样表现出广泛炎症浸润,被称为"肿瘤引起的炎症",在其肿瘤微环境高表达许多细胞因子[7]。长期摄入非甾体抗体-COX-2 酶抑制剂的药物(nonsteroidal anti-inflammatory drugs,NSAID)如阿司匹林可降低散发性 CRC 和遗传性 CRC 的相对风险,提示炎症在自发性 CRC 发展过程扮演重要作用[76]。腺瘤性息肉病(*adenomatous polyposis coli*,*APC*)肿瘤抑制基因,编码负调节 Wnt-n 信号通路,是散发性 CRC 中最常见的突变基因(60%),胚系 *APC* 突变引起家族性腺瘤性息肉病(familial adenomatous polyposis,FAP)。因此,*Apc*^{min} 突变小鼠和特异性敲除肠上皮细胞 *Apc* 基因小鼠是研究散发性 CRC 和 FAP 良好模型。这些小鼠的结直肠腺瘤在失去正常 *Apc* 等位基因后上皮屏障蛋白缺失,导致微生物产物进入肿瘤而不是邻近组织[28],这些微生物产物激活巨噬细胞产生 IL-23 并扩增释放 IL-17 的细胞群,激活 IL-17RA 促进肿瘤进展[64]。

肠道微生物群和结肠直肠癌

胃肠道是人体内最大的共生细菌库[82],共生细菌通过宿主-微生物相互作用影响肠道的各种生理功能,微生物群生态失调可导致各种胃肠道疾病,包括 IBD 和 CRC。在动物实验模型和临床流行病学研究发现了肠道微生物群构成组成和胃肠道癌症的相关性。然而,尽管众所周知幽门螺杆菌可诱发胃炎和胃癌,CRC 的肠道细菌仍有待鉴定[76]。病原微生物可能通过激活慢性炎症、改变肿瘤微环境、诱导基因毒反应和代谢促进肠道肿瘤发生,保护性或有益微生物缺失也可引起这种病理改变。

癌症预防、治疗和副作用

CRC 的常规疗法包括手术、化疗和放疗。鉴于越来越多的证据表明炎症会引发并促进 CAC 和散发性 CRC，为研发通过药物减少炎症来预防或治疗 CRC 和其他胃肠道癌症提供理论依据。如前所述，已证明 NSAID 和选择性 COX-2 抑制剂可有效预防 CRC。促炎细胞因子的抑制剂，如 TNF、IL-6、IL-1、IL-17A 和 IL-23 的中和抗体或诱饵受体，或者 JAK、STAT3、IKK 和 NF-κB 细胞因子抑制剂，有希望用于治疗 CAC 和自发性 CRC。但是，这类药物不太可能作为单一疗法发挥作用，因此应与化疗或放疗联合进行验证。值得注意的是，JAK 抑制剂可有效治疗 IBD，但会产生黏膜炎症、贫血、血小板减少症、肝功能障碍和感染等副作用。黏膜炎症是细胞毒性化疗剂量的主要限制因素，因此，细胞因子活性抑制剂（IL-6，IL-17A 和 IL-23 可促进黏膜愈合）与化疗药物联合使用时，应谨慎用药。某些化疗药物更适合联合用药，如最近在 *Apc* 突变小鼠中发现 5-FU 与 IL-17A 中和抗体联用效价更高[64]。

另一种控制胃肠炎症的方法是使用益生元或益生菌，使宿主微生物组趋于稳定从而抑阻止癌症发展[83]。研究发现膳食中的碳水化合物、纤维、不饱和 n-3 脂肪酸、维生素、矿物质和植物化学物质（白藜芦醇和姜黄素）可以减少炎症和 CRC 风险，但潜在分子机制尚不清楚[76]。

胰腺癌

炎症和胰腺导管腺癌

胰腺导管腺癌（pancreatic ductal adenocarcinoma，PDAC）是一种侵袭性恶性肿瘤，5 年总体生存率不足 5%[84]。PDAC 的主要特征是由 ECM、成纤维细胞、血管和免疫细胞组成的显著结缔组织病变[85]，细胞环境中富含炎症因子、生长因子和蛋白酶，刺激恶性细胞增殖存活[86,87]。促炎细胞因子 IL-6、IL-8 和 TNF 以及抗炎细胞因子 IL-10 和 TGF-β 的水平增加，与 PDAC 患者的恶病质和不良预后有关[88-91]。研究证实，胰腺 *KRAS* 突变小鼠中早期 PanIN 病变向 PDAC 进展依赖于 IL-6 激活的 JAK-STAT3 通路[92]。此外，IL-6 诱导胰腺癌细胞表达 VEGF 从而促进血管新生[93]。虽然高剂量 TNF 对癌细胞有毒性作用，但在 PDAC 微环境中，TNF-TNFR2 结合导致 EGF 受体及其配体 TGF-β 的上调，促进癌细胞增殖[94]。IL-10 和 TGF-β 则能促进免疫表型从 Th1（抗肿瘤活性）向 Th2（肿瘤活性）转变[95]。

PDAC 治疗的抗炎策略

在高度免疫原性癌症（如皮肤黑色素瘤和膀胱癌）中发现，激活抗肿瘤免疫反应的治疗策略有效，例如过继癌症反应性 T 细胞和免疫检查点抑制剂[96]。用特异性单克隆抗体阻断抑制性受体 CTLA-4 和 PD-1 或用 CD25 单抗中和 Treg 细胞可激活抗肿瘤免疫[97,98]。然而，这种策略迄今为止对 PDAC 疗效并不显著，可能原因是存在额外的尚未发现的免疫抑制机制。能与可溶性 IL-6 受体结合的 IL-6 单克隆抗体 Siltuximab 和 Tocilizumab，目前正在卵巢癌（clinicaltrials. gov）和 PDAC 患者中进行评估。Ruxolitinib 是一种选择性 JAK1/JAK2 抑制剂，于 2011 年被 FDA 批准用于治疗骨髓纤维化。Ruxolitinib 可以阻断 IL-6 对 STAT3 的激活，显著提高复发或治疗难治性 PDAC（clinicaltrial. gov）患者组的存活率。IL-6 中和抗体或 JAK 抑制剂是否可以增强靶向 PDAC 的细胞毒性 T 细胞活化将是令人感兴趣的课题。

肝癌

病因和发病机制

HCC 是第五大常见癌症和第三大癌症死亡的原因。超过 90% 的 HCC 有慢性肝病和 HBV 或 HCV 持续性感染的背景。HCC 其他风险因素包括脂肪肝病、黄曲霉毒素、酒精和遗传性疾病（如血色素沉着症）。HCC 表型和分子异质性反映了病理起源不同。因此，尽管 hTERT、β-catenin 和 *p53* 基因改变常见于 HCC，也无法证实它们就是 HCC 的驱动基因。鉴于 HCC 一般发展于广泛炎症和纤维化的肝脏中，炎症在 HCC 中的作用尤为重要。

治疗

早期 HCC 可进行手术切除（全或部分肝切除术）、肝移植或局部消融治疗，然而，70% 的 HCC 在治疗 5 年后复发。如果肿瘤在诊断时已经处于晚期或复发，则除化学栓塞外还考虑全身使用分子靶向药物。尽管如此，HCC 的 5 年生存率仍然很低（<8%）。

蛋白激酶抑制剂索拉非尼是目前唯一被批准用于晚期 HCC 的全身性药物，索拉非尼治疗组患者的中位生存期仅比对照组长 2. 8 个月（分别为 10. 7 个月和 7. 9 个月）。虽然在索拉非尼批准后，人们应用许多靶向 HCC 相关信号通路的药物进行了临床试验，但是一线药物（Brivanib、Sunitinib、Erlotinib 和 Linifanib）或二线药物（Brivanib 和 Everolimus）均未呈现阳性结果。目前，正在 RAS（+）HCC 患者中进行 MET 抑制剂 Tivantinib 和 MEK 抑制剂 Refametinib 的临床试验。然而，因为 *RAS* 突变患者不足不超过 5%，这些药物仅能使部分 HCC 患者获益[99]。

对 HCC，人们依旧知之甚少，其异质性和复杂的分子特征是临床试验失败的原因。药物的肝脏毒性也是临床试验失败的主要原因。值得注意的是，肝硬化常常限制 HCC 患者的治疗选择。与安慰剂相比，Rapalog Everolimus 不仅不能延长总生存期，并且会导致肝损伤率增加。有趣的是，雷帕霉素处理或肝细胞特异性敲除 mTORC1 的 raptor 亚基（Rapalog 的分子靶点）可增加 IL-6 生成并激活小鼠原癌基因转录因子 STAT3。此外，mTORC1 活性丧失导致低程度肝脏炎症，促进 HCC 进展[100]。

肥胖、炎症和潜在治疗选择

西方国家的部分 HCC 患者并无病毒感染[101]，这些患者多数患有肥胖症，表现为代谢综合征和非酒精性脂肪性肝炎（nonalcoholic steatohepatitis，NASH）——严重形式的非酒精性脂肪性肝病（nonalcoholic fatty liver disease，NAFLD）[102]。肥胖使男性 HCC 风险增加 4. 5 倍[103]。由于肥胖率在世界范围内迅速增加，人们开始广泛关注肥胖与肝脏肿瘤发生的关联。从肥胖促进小鼠 HCC 发展的现象出发，科学家进行机制研究，发现肥胖通过升高 TNF 和 IL-6[104] 促进肝脏低程度炎症，进一步增加 HCC 风险。IL-6 信号转导对非肥胖人群的 HCC 进展也很重要，HCC 祖细胞或干细胞扩增和肿瘤恶性进展依赖自分泌 IL-6 信号[105,106]。此外，肥胖[107,108] 和 HBV/HCV 感染[109] 可诱导肝细胞内质网（endoplasmic reticulum，ER）应激，促进人类肝细胞增多症[110]。ER 应激会促进 NASH 样疾病和小鼠 HCC 的进展[111]。有趣的是，通过缓解 ER 应激或抑制肝细胞 TNF 信号，可以减缓小鼠 HCC 进展。这些研究结果表明抗 TNF 药物和缓解 ER 应激的“化学伴侣”可能能够预防或改善 NASH 和进展而成的 HCC。

（曹琦琪 宋玉婷 译 于晗 于乐兴 校 陈瑶 审）

部分参考文献

1 Karin M. Nuclear factor-kappaB in cancer development and progression. *Nature.* 2006;**441(7092)**:431-436.

2 Mantovani A, Allavena P, Sica A, Balkwill F. Cancer-related inflammation. *Nature.* 2008;**454(7203)**:436-444.

4 Biswas SK, Allavena P, Mantovani A. Tumor-associated macrophages: functional diversity, clinical significance, and open questions. *Semin Immunopathol.* 2013;**35(5)**:585-600.

5 Coussens LM, Zitvogel L, Palucka AK. Neutralizing tumor-promoting chronic inflammation: a magic bullet? *Science.* 2013;**339(6117)**:286-291.

6 Qian BZ, Pollard JW. Macrophage diversity enhances tumor progression and metastasis. *Cell.* 2010;**141(1)**:39-51.

7 Grivennikov SI, Greten FR, Karin M. Immunity, inflammation, and cancer. *Cell.* 2010;**140(6)**:883-899.

11 Su S, Liu Q, Chen J, et al. A positive feedback loop between mesenchymal-like cancer cells and macrophages is essential to breast cancer metastasis. *Cancer Cell.* 2014;**25(5)**:605-620.

13 Franklin RA, Liao W, Sarkar A, et al. The cellular and molecular origin of tumor-associated macrophages. *Science.* 2014;**344(6186)**:921-925.

14 Qian BZ, Li J, Zhang H, et al. CCL2 recruits inflammatory monocytes to facilitate breast-tumour metastasis. *Nature.* 2011;**475(7355)**:222-225.

18 Lin EY, Pollard JW. Tumor-associated macrophages press the angiogenic switch in breast cancer. *Cancer Res.* 2007;**67(11)**:5064-5066.

21 Spranger S, Spaapen RM, Zha Y, et al. Up-regulation of PD-L1, IDO, and T(regs) in the melanoma tumor microenvironment is driven by CD8(+) T cells. *Sci Transl Med.* 2013;**5(200)**:200ra116.

22 Tan W, Zhang W, Strasner A, et al. Tumour-infiltrating regulatory T cells stimulate mammary cancer metastasis through RANKL-RANK signalling. *Nature.* 2011;**470(7335)**:548-553.

27 Noman MZ, Desantis G, Janji B, et al. PD-L1 is a novel direct target of HIF-1alpha, and its blockade under hypoxia enhanced MDSC-mediated T cell activation. *J Exp Med.* 2014;**211(5)**:781-790.

28 Grivennikov SI, Wang K, Mucida D, et al. Adenoma-linked barrier defects and microbial products drive IL-23/IL-17-mediated tumour growth. *Nature.* 2012;**491(7423)**:254-258.

30 Affara NI, Ruffell B, Medler TR, et al. B cells regulate macrophage phenotype and response to chemotherapy in squamous carcinomas. *Cancer Cell.* 2014;**25(6)**:809-821.

31 Ammirante M, Luo JL, Grivennikov S, Nedospasov S, Karin M. B-cell-derived lymphotoxin promotes castration-resistant prostate cancer. *Nature.* 2010;**464(7286)**:302-305.

34 Bhowmick NA, Neilson EG, Moses HL. Stromal fibroblasts in cancer initiation and progression. *Nature.* 2004;**432(7015)**:332-337.

37 Levental KR, Yu H, Kass L, et al. Matrix crosslinking forces tumor progression by enhancing integrin signaling. *Cell.* 2009;**139(5)**:891-906.

40 Erez N, Truitt M, Olson P, Arron ST, Hanahan D. Cancer-associated fibroblasts are activated in incipient neoplasia to orchestrate tumor-promoting inflammation in an NF-kappaB-dependent manner. *Cancer Cell.* 2010;**17(2)**:135-147.

45 Mantovani A. La mala educación of tumor-associated macrophages: diverse pathways and new players. *Cancer Cell.* 2010;**17(2)**:111-112.

46 Ammirante M, Shalapour S, Kang Y, Jamieson CA, Karin M. Tissue injury and hypoxia promote malignant progression of prostate cancer by inducing CXCL13 expression in tumor myofibroblasts. *Proc Natl Acad Sci U S A.* 2014;**111(41)**:14776-14781.

48 Yang L, Pang Y, Moses HL. TGF-beta and immune cells: an important regulatory axis in the tumor microenvironment and progression. *Trends Immunol.* 2010;**31(6)**:220-227.

49 Hanahan D, Weinberg RA. Hallmarks of cancer: the next generation. *Cell.* 2011;**144(5)**:646-674.

53 Balkwill F. Tumour necrosis factor and cancer. *Nat Rev Cancer.* 2009;**9(5)**:361-371.

56 Taniguchi K, Karin M. IL-6 and related cytokines as the critical lynchpins between inflammation and cancer. *Semin Immunol.* 2014;**26(1)**:54-74.

58 Yu H, Pardoll D, Jove R. STATs in cancer inflammation and immunity: a leading role for STAT3. *Nat Rev Cancer.* 2009;**9(11)**:798-809.

64 Wang K, Kim MK, Di Caro G, et al. Interleukin-17 receptor a signaling in transformed enterocytes promotes early colorectal tumorigenesis. *Immunity.* 2014;**41**:1052-1063.

68 Pickup M, Novitskiy S, Moses HL. The roles of TGFbeta in the tumour microenvironment. *Nat Rev Cancer.* 2013;**13(11)**:788-799.

76 Terzic J, Grivennikov S, Karin E, Karin M. Inflammation and colon cancer. *Gastroenterology.* 2010;**138(6)**:2101.e5-2114.e5.

79 Greten FR, Eckmann L, Greten TF, et al. IKKbeta links inflammation and tumorigenesis in a mouse model of colitis-associated cancer. *Cell.* 2004;**118(3)**:285-296.

85 Gukovsky I, Li N, Todoric J, Gukovskaya A, Karin M. Inflammation, autophagy, and obesity: common features in the pathogenesis of pancreatitis and pancreatic cancer. *Gastroenterology.* 2013;**144(6)**:1199.e4-1209.e4.

86 Feig C, Gopinathan A, Neesse A, Chan DS, Cook N, Tuveson DA. The pancreas cancer microenvironment. *Clin Cancer Res.* 2012;**18(16)**:4266-4276.

92 Lesina M, Kurkowski MU, Ludes K, et al. Stat3/Socs3 activation by IL-6 transsignaling promotes progression of pancreatic intraepithelial neoplasia and development of pancreatic cancer. *Cancer Cell.* 2011;**19(4)**:456-469.

96 Dougan M, Dranoff G. Immune therapy for cancer. *Annu Rev Immunol.* 2009;**27**:83-117.

100 Umemura A, Park EJ, Taniguchi K, et al. Liver damage, inflammation, and enhanced tumorigenesis after persistent mTORC1 inhibition. *Cell Metab.* 2014;**20(1)**:133-144.

101 El-Serag HB. Hepatocellular carcinoma. *N Engl J Med.* 2011;**365(12)**:1118-1127.

103 Calle EE, Teras LR, Thun MJ. Obesity and mortality. *N Engl J Med.* 2005;**353(20)**:2197-2199.

104 Park EJ, Lee JH, Yu GY, et al. Dietary and genetic obesity promote liver inflammation and tumorigenesis by enhancing IL-6 and TNF expression. *Cell.* 2010;**140(2)**:197-208.

111 Nakagawa H, Umemura A, Taniguchi K, et al. ER stress cooperates with hypernutrition to trigger TNF-dependent spontaneous HCC development. *Cancer Cell.* 2014;**26(3)**:331-343.

第 28 章 RNA 肿瘤病毒

Robert C. Gallo, MD ■ Marvin S. Reitz, PhD

概述

反转录病毒是一类基因组为二倍体 RNA 的包膜病毒,因其含有反转录酶而被定义为反转录病毒。反转录酶是一种 DNA 聚合酶,能将 RNA 反转录成 DNA 后再整合至宿主细胞的染色体中,此过程通常会导致遗传物质的捕获和/或改变,从而在细胞之间进行信息传递。这种信息传递过程可导致被感染的细胞发生癌变,但为偶然事件。反转录病毒也与免疫缺陷和神经系统疾病有关,尽管感染过程通常没有症状。反转录病毒也能够进入生殖系统,成为物种遗传互补的一部分,而这些病毒被称为内源性反转录病毒。虽然大多数反转录病毒仅能在非人物种中引起白血病/淋巴瘤,但人类 T 淋巴细胞病毒-1 型(HTLV-1)可在少数被感染的患者中引起成人 T 细胞性白血病/淋巴瘤,以及神经系统疾病和其他病理变化。尽管科学家不认为人类免疫缺陷病毒-1 型(HIV-1)是一种肿瘤病毒,但其与几种类型肿瘤的发病率的增加有关,特别是那些由人乳头瘤病毒和 EB 病毒引起的肿瘤。

反转录病毒发现于 20 世纪初期,Ellerman 和 Bang[1] 通过无细胞滤液在鸡的体内传播了白血病,Rous[2] 同样在鸡的体内成功传播了肉瘤。Bittern 对小鼠乳腺肿瘤的研究[3] 和 Gross 对小鼠白血病的研究[4] 将这些发现扩展到了哺乳动物。Gross 意识到病毒接种新生小鼠对白血病研究的重要性,他的发现在多方面标志着现代反转录病毒研究的开端。Jarrett 证明了猫的白血病是由一种类似的病毒引起的,这是首次证实白血病在远交系物种中存在自然传播[5,6],Kawakami 和 Theilen 及其同事首次证明了反转录病毒能够在灵长类动物尤其是长臂猿和新世界猴[7~9] 中引发白血病。

这些病毒的生物学检测方法可以追溯到 20 世纪 50 年代,但是直到 70 年代早期发现病毒含有反转录酶(RT),人们才对它们的生命周期有了深入的理解[10,11]。这些知识为反转录病毒的检测提供了一种更简便、更快捷、更灵敏的方法。20 世纪 70 年代的另一个重要发现是一些反转录病毒[如罗斯肉瘤病毒(RSV)]含有导致细胞转化和肿瘤发生的基因(癌基因),这些基因是反转录病毒捕获的细胞内基因(原癌基因)。这些工作使得很多相似的基因得以确认,并使人们认识到反转录病毒在细胞生长和肿瘤转化中的作用。

尽管反转录病毒的研究工作在 20 世纪 70 年代引起了人们的关注,但当时人们仍普遍认为反转录病毒不会引起人类疾病,甚至可能不存在于人类中。但一些研究结果表明事实并非如此。人类 T 细胞白血病病毒-1 型(HTLV-1)是迄今发现的第一个具有传染性的人类反转录病毒,Gallo 和他的同事发现它是一种特殊的病毒[13~16],并且很快证实是成人 T 细胞白血病(ATL)的病原体。ATL 是一种在多个地区流行的白血病,包括日本南部和加勒比海地区[17~21]。随后很快 HTLV-Ⅱ[22] 被发现,尽管 HTLV-Ⅱ普遍存在,但并未发现其与任何疾病有确切的关联。另有研究证明 HTLV-1 能够引起脐带血 T 细胞的恶性转化[23]。

几年后,免疫缺陷和恶性肿瘤在同性恋群体中开始流行,尤其在美国的同性恋群体中。人类反转录病毒的第一个成员是从患有获得性免疫缺陷综合征(AIDS)的人群中分离出来的[24]。当能够对这种病毒进行大规模培养时[25],研究人员证明了它就是艾滋病的病原体[26~27]。这种现在被称为人类免疫缺陷病毒Ⅰ型(HIV-1)的病毒已在全球范围内流行,并造成了当前全球医疗和经济的灾难。此外,人们还发现了一种与之相关的 HIV-2 病毒[28],但其致病性似乎远低于 HIV-1[29]。

分类

反转录病毒科作为病毒中的一个大家族,研究人员最初根据其生物学效应用多重标准对其进行了分类[30]。其亚科包括在宿主中引起白血病或其他恶性肿瘤的癌病毒;导致慢性退行性疾病的"慢"病毒;以及在受感染的培养物中产生"泡沫"细胞病变效应的泡沫病毒。根据它们的基因组结构亚科可进一步对其划分(表 28-1)。历史上研究人员是根据电子显微镜照片中病毒初期和成熟时的形态对它们进行分类的(表 28-2)。依据反转录病毒是通过感染传播还是在物种种系内传播,可以将之分为外源性或内源性反转录病毒。

表 28-1 反转录病毒分组

致癌病毒
• 禽类白血病-肉瘤病毒(ALSV)
• 禽网状内皮细胞增生病毒
• 哺乳动物细胞白血病和肉瘤病毒(小鼠/猫 C 型病毒)
小鼠乳腺肿瘤病毒
• 灵长类 D 型病毒(Mason-Pfizer 猴病毒/猿类 AIDS 病毒)
• 人类 T 细胞白血病病毒/牛白血病病毒/猿 T 细胞白血病病毒
慢病毒(包括免疫缺陷病毒)
泡沫病毒

表 28-2 反转录病毒形态

A 型颗粒	• 有或无突出尖峰
• 胞内核心的形成和出芽	D 型颗粒
• 脑池内 A 型颗粒(IAP)是内源性的原病毒产物	• Mason-Pfizer 猴病毒,猿类 AIDS 病毒
• 非感染型	• 胞内核衣壳形成,在质膜出芽
B 型颗粒(MMTV)	• 偏心核
• 核心形成发生在胞质中	• 尖刺样突出少
• 在胞膜出芽后,成熟为偏位核心	慢病毒
• 表面尖刺样突出	• Visna-maedi,EIAV,CAEV,SIV,HIV,FIV,BIV
C 型颗粒	• 同 C 型颗粒一样形成核心和出芽
• 大多数致癌 RNA 病毒	• 成熟核心凝聚成锥体型
• 最初在质膜上形成电子致密斑	泡沫病毒
• 质膜出芽	• IAP 样核心
• 核心成熟产生位于中心的核心	

结构

反转录病毒颗粒由核结构或衣壳组成,包含两条相同的单链 RNA,被脂质双分子层的包膜包围。整个病毒颗粒,或细胞外病毒颗粒的直径为 100nm。基因组 RNA 通常由 8 000~9 500 个核苷酸组成,最简单的反转录病毒包含三个主要的基因(*gag*、*pol* 和 *env*)。所有这些基因都包含在病毒颗粒中(图 28-1)。基因组 RNA 在其两端含有重复区域,称为 R 区。整合在宿主细胞基因组中的 DNA(脱氧核糖核酸)结构中包含 R 区和其他调控序列即长末端重复序列(LTP)(图 28-1)。反转录病毒通常由于其基因组的大面积缺失而造成复制缺陷,这些缺失的基因组有时可由来自宿主细胞的癌基因取代。接下来将介绍的是具有复制能力的反转录病毒的基因组和蛋白质。

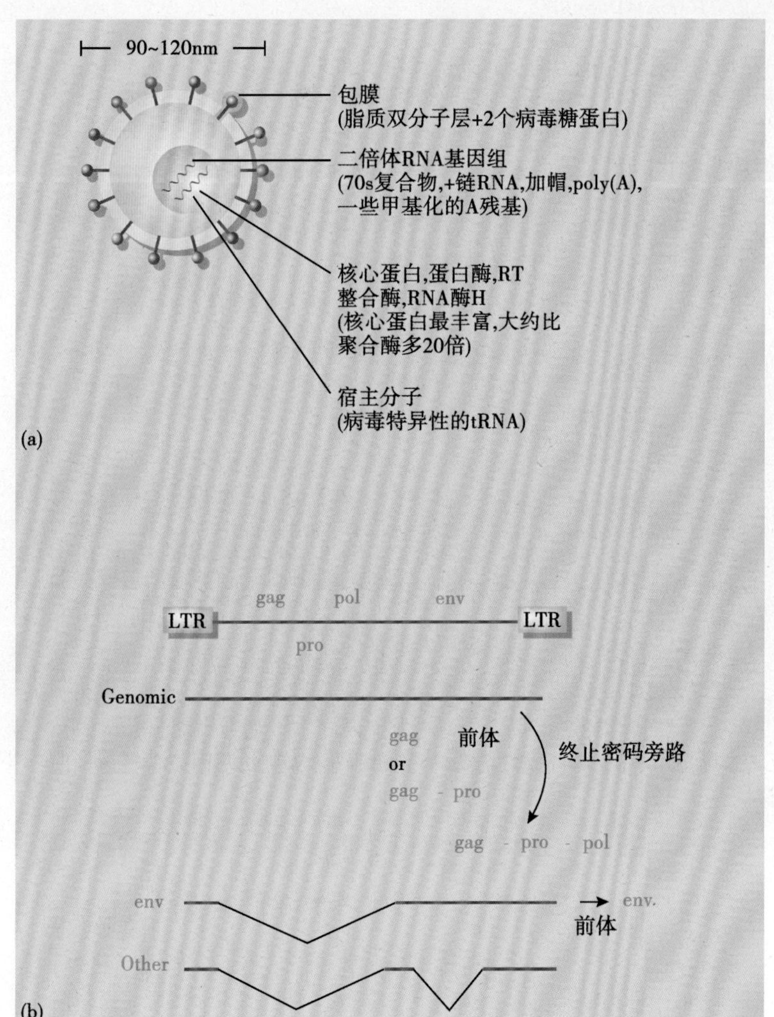

图 28-1 (a)典型反转录病毒的颗粒结构。(b)典型反转录病毒的基因组结构。有完全复制能力的反转录病毒会产生一条编码 gag 和 pol 产物的全长核糖核苷酸(RNA)和一条编码 env 的单链剪切 RNA。一些反转录病毒也会产生较小的多重拼接信息。env,包膜;gag,核心蛋白;pol,聚合酶;pro,蛋白酶

病毒基因组和基因产物

鉴于篇幅原因,不再对反转录病毒的基因组结构和病毒蛋白进行详细介绍,感兴趣的读者可以参考 Teich 等的文章[30]了解详情。相关示意图见图 28-2 和图 28-3。

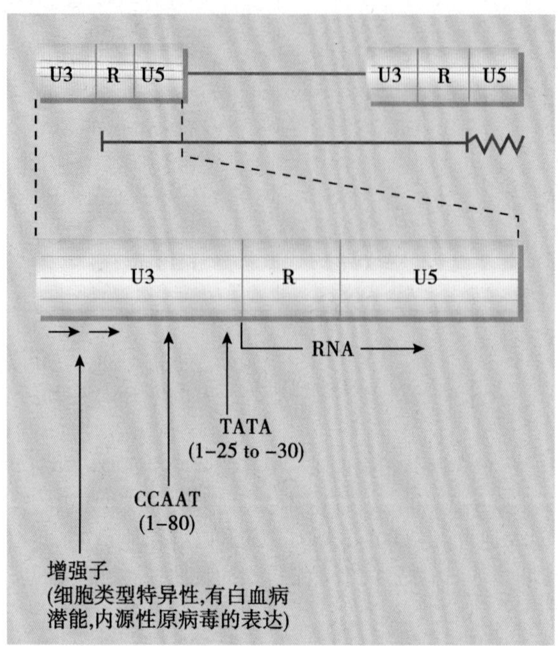

图 28-2 长末端重复(LTR)结构。具有复制能力的反转录病毒在 5′和 3′末端含有相同的 LTR。5′LTR 的 U3 部分包含所有病毒或细胞基因启动转录所必需的增强子和启动子元件。CA,衣壳;FeLV,猫白血病病毒;IN,整合酶;MA,基质蛋白;MMTV,Moloney 乳腺肿瘤病毒;MuLV,鼠白血病病毒;NC,核衣壳;PR,蛋白酶;RT,反转录酶

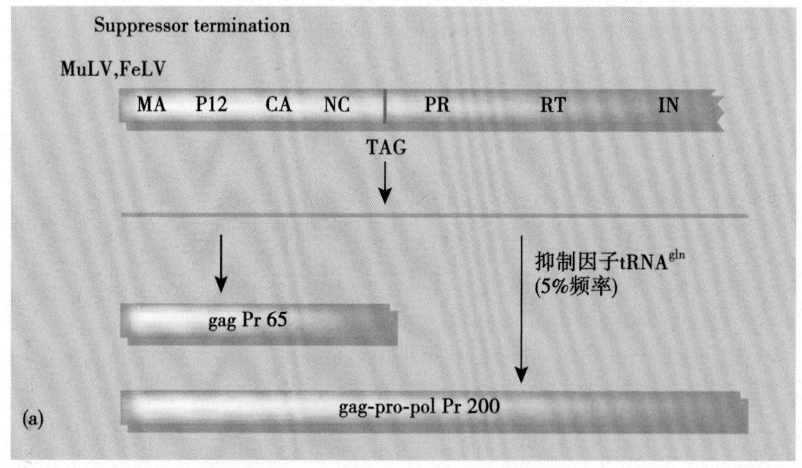

图 28-3 不同的反转录病毒用不同的方法绕过 *gag* 终止密码子,从全长基因组转录生成前 *pol* 产物

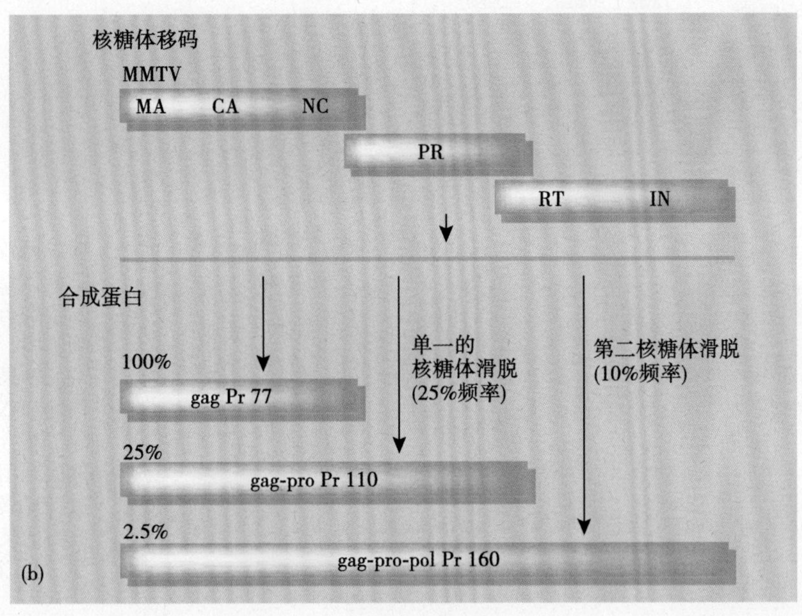

图 28-3(续)

基因组变异

上文描述的基因组结构代表了最简单的反转录病毒;其他反转录病毒,特别是慢病毒和 HTLV 组的成员(包括相关的牛白血病病毒,BLV),则含有额外的基因并具有更复杂的基因组结构。HIV-1 共编码 6 种调节蛋白,包括激活病毒 RNA 表达的蛋白,调节病毒 RNA 剪接方式的蛋白,以及干扰宿主免疫功能的蛋白。额外的基因也可导致更复杂的 RNA 剪接方式,其中包括许多调控基因的多重剪接。与此类似,HTLV-1 编码至少 5 个额外的蛋白质,包括(如 HIV)一种激活病毒 RNA 表达的蛋白质和另一种调节病毒 RNA 剪接模式的蛋白质。最近的证据表明[31~33],一种分子量为 31kDa,名为 HTLV-1 bZIP 的蛋白(HBZ)从 3′LTR 进行转录,由负链 RNA 翻译而来,在感染的 T 细胞和未培养的 ATL 细胞中表达。HBZ 蛋白与包括 CREB 和 Jun 家族成员[34,35]的细胞 bZIP 转录因子结合,抑制 Tax 介导的病毒转录并促进 ATL 细胞的增殖。目前,这是 HTLV-1 一种新的遗传学特征。小鼠乳腺肿瘤病毒(MMTV)和泡沫病毒也编码了包括激活病毒 RNA 表达的蛋白质在内的其他蛋白质。其他反转录病毒,特别是那些急性转化的病毒(如禽类和哺乳动物肉瘤病毒)通常具有复制缺陷,其基因组的一部分缺失并由具有转化能力的细胞内基因取代。这些病毒需要有复制能力的辅助病毒才能进行传播和复制。

复制周期

由于篇幅原因,这里不再对病毒的复制周期进行详细描述,相关步骤详见参考文献[36~39],图 28-4~图 28-6 以缩略图的形式介绍了其中的一些步骤。应注意一些反转录病毒复制周期的关键点:首先,通过整合反应形成原病毒,并获得从被感染的细胞中不能移除的病毒稳定遗传副本。受感染的细胞可以并持续存在于宿主体内,每当细胞分裂时,原病毒就会传递给两个子代细胞。此外,当生殖细胞被感染时,它们就会成为子代基因组的一部分。因此,5%或更多的人类基因组是由既往反转录病毒感染的原病毒组成的。然而,整合并不总是很准确,可能会发生基因的缺失和重排。被整合的原病毒偶尔也会被删除或重排。由于这些原因,尽管某些内源性原病毒的确能够表达,但大多数会存在缺陷并且通常不表达。并且,这种大规模外来 DNA 的插入可能会对进化过程产生深远的影响。其次,在原病毒形成后,病毒基因产物的转录和翻译完全依赖于细胞内的因子。因此,反转录病毒通常在静止期细胞中保持沉默。感染细胞的活化,例如当免疫系统细胞被抗原刺激或细胞被激素激活时,可以激活病毒的表达,该表达由病毒 LTR 中的一系列转录因子结合位点来调节。此外,复杂的反转录病毒(如 HTLV 和 HIV)编码的转录激活因子可以显著影响病毒 RNA 聚合酶启动子的活性[40~45]。

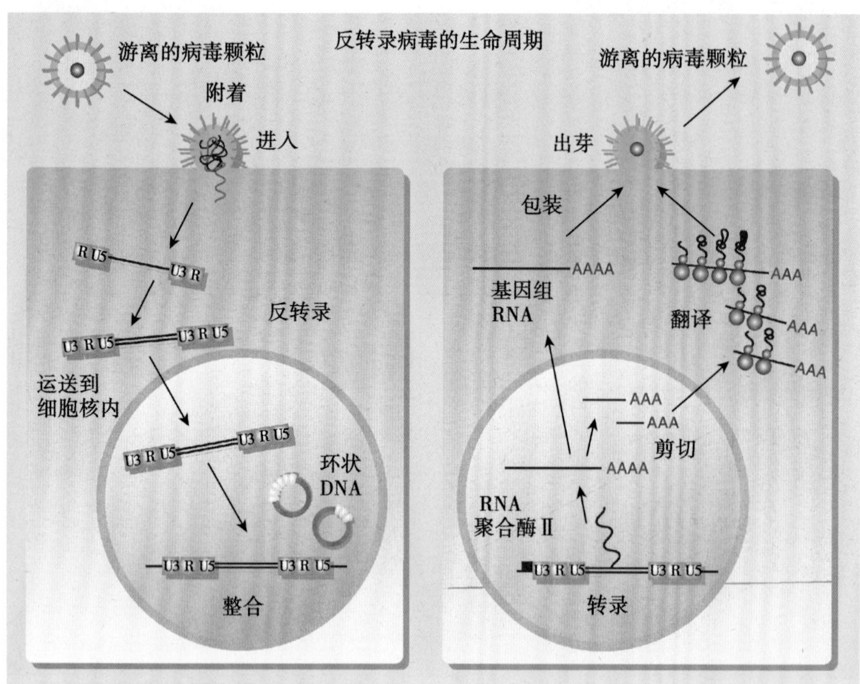

图 28-4 反转录病毒的生命周期。反转录病毒与特异性细胞膜受体结合后，病毒和细胞膜发生融合，核心病毒颗粒进到细胞中。反转录酶指导生成双链反转录病毒基因组脱氧核糖核酸（DNA），在整合酶定向指导下整合到宿主细胞 DNA 中。然后利用宿主细胞的转录机制进行反转录病毒转录，最终形成新的反转录病毒从细胞膜出芽，进行新一轮的感染

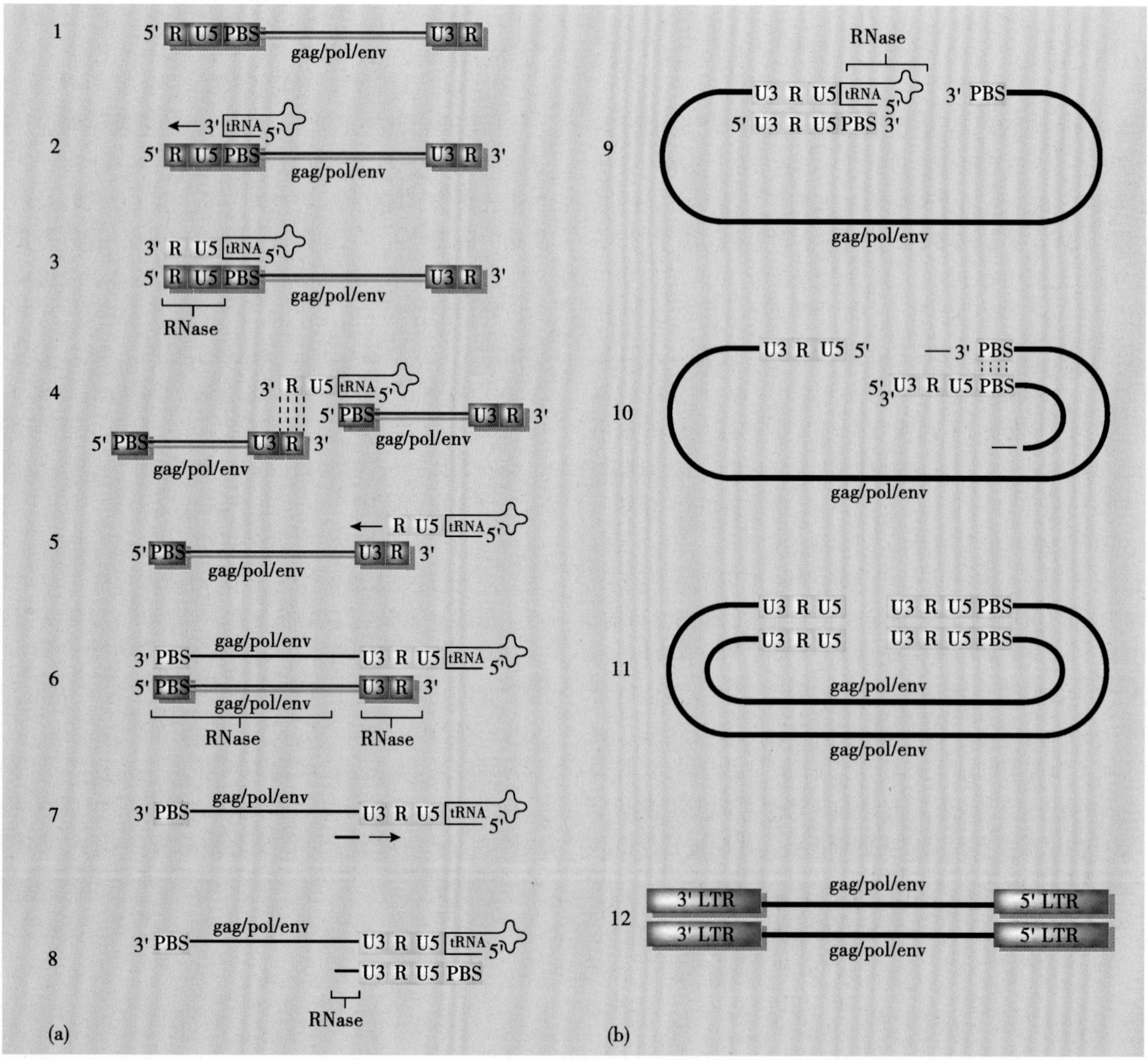

1 5' R U5 PBS gag/pol/env U3 R

2 3' tRNA 5' ; 5' R U5 PBS gag/pol/env U3 R 3'

3 3' R U5 tRNA 5' ; 5' R U5 PBS gag/pol/env U3 R 3' ; RNase

4 3' R U5 tRNA 5' ; 5' PBS gag/pol/env U3 R 3' ; 5' PBS gag/pol/env U3 R 3'

5 R U5 tRNA 5' ; 5' PBS gag/pol/env U3 R 3'

6 3' PBS gag/pol/env U3 R U5 tRNA 5' ; 5' PBS gag/pol/env U3 R 3' ; RNase RNase

7 3' PBS gag/pol/env U3 R U5 tRNA 5'

8 3' PBS gag/pol/env U3 R U5 tRNA 5' ; U3 R U5 PBS ; RNase

(a)

9 RNase ; U3 R U5 tRNA 5' 3' PBS ; 5' U3 R U5 PBS 3' ; gag/pol/env

10 U3 R U5 5' 3' PBS ; 5' 3' U3 R U5 PBS ; gag/pol/env

11 U3 R U5 U3 R U5 PBS ; U3 R U5 U3 R U5 PBS ; gag/pol/env ; gag/pol/env

12 3' LTR gag/pol/env 5' LTR ; 3' LTR gag/pol/env 5' LTR

(b)

图 28-5 反转录。从单链核糖核苷酸基因组前体（a）反转录合成并整合到宿主细胞 DNA 的双链脱氧核糖核苷酸（DNA）（b）

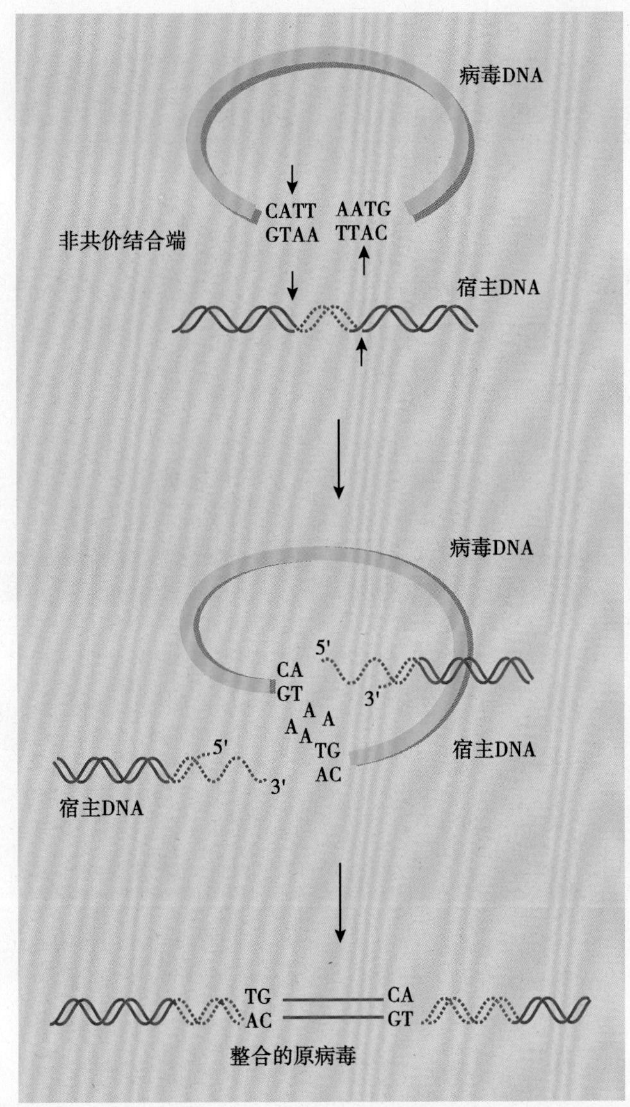

图 28-6　整合。新反转录合成的双链反转录病毒脱氧核糖核酸（DNA）基因组和一段染色体 DNA 被反转录病毒整合酶蛋白特异性剪切。伴随着反转录基因组中两个碱基对的缺失和宿主 DNA 中的 4～6 个碱基对的重复。反转录病毒基因组插入到被剪切的宿主 DNA 后，DNA 重新连接

肿瘤的发生机制

一些反转录病毒具有急性转化的能力，它们能够直接转化细胞。反转录病毒诱导被感染宿主体内肿瘤的形成，除了通过急性转化病毒引起的细胞转化外，还涉及多种机制，如图 28-7 所示。

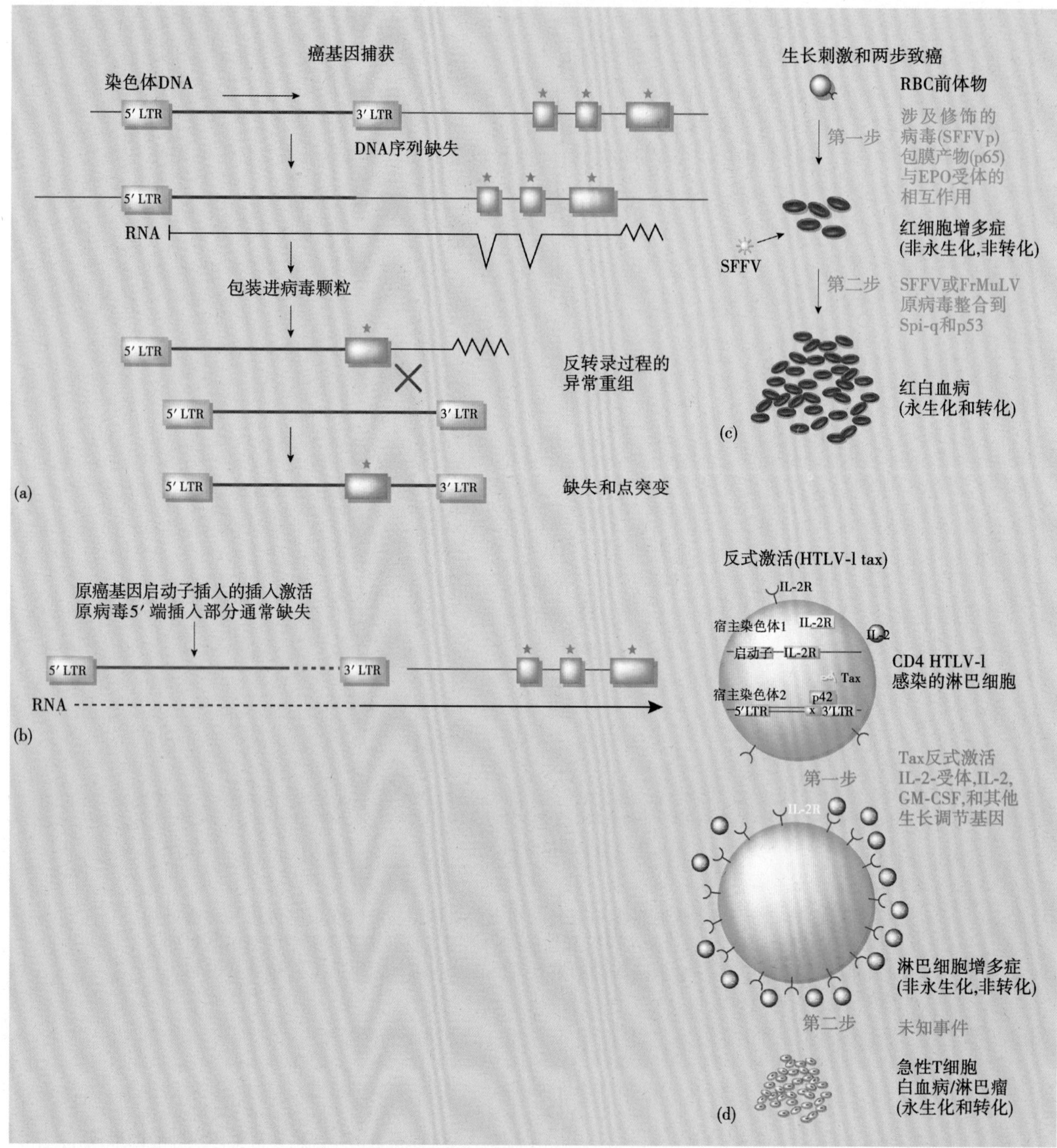

图 28-7 反转录病毒诱导肿瘤发生的四种机制。(a)癌基因捕获。细胞原癌基因(*v-onc*)的突变形式被转移(转导)至正常细胞,从而诱导转化(* c-癌基因)。(b)插入激活。LTR 定向转录增强(* c-癌基因)后,原癌基因表达率显著增加。(c)生长刺激和两步致癌。来自脾脏病灶形成病毒(SFFV)的变异 env 蛋白与促红细胞生成素(EPO)受体结合,导致红细胞增生。这增加了对实际转化事件敏感的目标人群,即 *SPi-1* 或 *TP53* 基因的反转录病毒插入中断。FrMuLV,Friend 鼠白血病病毒。(d)反式激活。病毒反式激活蛋白(在人类 T 细胞白血病病毒 I 型的 Tax)通过反式激活生长调节基因导致潜在目标群体的扩大。然后,未知的第二事件诱导这些细胞克隆体的实际转化

癌基因的捕获

当细胞原癌基因在病毒复制过程中，通过插入病毒基因组而被病毒捕获，通常会产生急性转化病毒。这个过程通常会引起原癌基因的遗传改变，从而产生癌基因或显性转化基因。同样，此过程通常也会引起病毒的复制缺陷，导致其需要辅助病毒协助才能进行复制。辅助病毒提供蛋白来帮助缺陷病毒 RNA 包装成病毒颗粒，这些颗粒称为假性病毒。

最早发现的致癌病毒是 RSV，它是导致鸡肉瘤的传播源[2]，它也是最早发现的急性转化病毒之一，通过捕获细胞基因 *src* 而产生致癌性[12]。RSV 病毒中的 *src* 基因直接独立地插入其他病毒基因的 3′端[46,47]。因为转化缺陷的 RSV 病毒在 *src* 基因上有突变，而含有 *src* 基因的重组病毒有转化能力[48~50]，所以认为 RSV 的转化能力完全来源于病毒的 *src* 基因（*v-src*）。这些发现使人们认识到正常细胞的基因在被修饰后，在适当的环境下能够发生恶性转化。

易感宿主在急性转化反转录病毒感染后的数天至数周内会产生肿瘤。因为急性转化反转录病毒的转化能力非常强，大部分被感染的细胞都会发生转化，产生的肿瘤往往是多克隆的。雏鸡经 RSV 感染可诱导多种相关类型的肿瘤发生，特别是纤维肉瘤和组织细胞肉瘤。动物越年轻，越容易形成肿瘤。1 月龄以下的雏鸡可在数天内形成多发性、进展迅速的肿瘤并可导致动物死亡。在有免疫反应的情况下，如在成年鸡体内肿瘤往往会退化和消失。向幼鸟体内注射 *v-src* DNA 也可诱导肿瘤，进一步证实了 *v-src* 可诱发肿瘤[51]。与反转录病毒感染相比，用 DNA 形成肿瘤的效率较低，说明了细胞对功能性 DNA 的摄取效率较低。

尽管效率低，RSV 也能够在幼龄啮齿类动物中引发肿瘤，但这种肿瘤仅局限于接种部位。随着动物年龄的增长，肿瘤可能会随着免疫能力的增强而趋于退化。较低的致瘤潜能可能反映了 RSV 在啮齿类动物细胞中的复制能力降低或逐步下降[52,53]。

Abelson 鼠白血病病毒（A-MuLV）是包含癌基因的急性转化反转录病毒的另一个典型代表。用复制能力强的 *MuLV*[54,55] 感染裸鼠，使得大多数 *MuLV* 基因被原癌基因 *c-abl*[56]（一种作为抗癌药物伊马替尼靶点的酪氨酸激酶）的修饰拷贝所替换。与大多数病毒癌基因及其细胞对应物一样（如表 28-3 所示），*v-abl* 的 *abl* 部分在遗传上与 *c-abl* 不同。重组的 A-MuLV 不能合成任何病毒基因，仅编码含有部分 *Gag* 和 *Abl*（*v-Abl*）的融合蛋白。在 *v-Abl* 上存在的 Gag 氨基末端部分使其被酰胺化并转运至细胞膜，这对于 A-MuLV 的转化功能至关重要。缺乏功能性病毒基因意味着 A-MuLV 有复制缺陷，只有在辅助病毒的协助下才能感染和转化靶细胞。A-MuLV 可在幼鼠体内诱导 B 细胞淋巴瘤，但成年动物通常会抵抗 A-MuLV 的致瘤作用[57]。

表 28-3　病毒癌基因（*v-onc*）和细胞癌基因（*c-onc*）的区别

通常只有部分细胞癌基因存在于 v-onc 中
v-onc 衍生自加工过的 mRNA，无内含子和侧翼序列
某些癌基因（*myc* 和 *mos*）丧失细胞控制元件（启动子/抑制子以及 RNA 去稳定子），其自身表达水平可能会发生改变
缺失/重排可能影响蛋白质本身的结构：
• 含 Tyr 区域的 c-src 的 C 端缺失可导致宿主细胞激酶介导的磷酸化失控
• 由于细胞外结构域的缺失，v-erb B 与 EGF 受体的不同
v-onc 基因通常与对转化功能重要的病毒序列融合：
• gag-abl 获得对转化活性重要的膜定位的肉豆蔻酰化信号
• *v-fms* 是 CSF-1 受体和 *gag* 基因融合的产物，后者提供了嵌入细胞膜中的信号序列

如图 28-7 所示，关于反转录病毒基因组如何获得细胞基因序列，研究人员已经提出了几种模型。在一种情况下（图 28-7a），反转录病毒整合到宿主细胞基因组中的原癌基因上游[58]。随后的缺失将原病毒的 3′部分和原癌基因的 5′部分移除，将病毒基因组与细胞序列融合，形成了包括部分 *gag* 基因的融合蛋白阅读框。该基因在病毒 LTR 的调控下转录、加工并与辅助病毒基因组共同包装形成假型反转录病毒颗粒。当假型病毒感染靶细胞时，反转录酶介导两个病毒 RNA 的 3′末端会进行重组，将一个 3′LTR 放在被转导的细胞基因的末端，从而使合成的双链 DNA 整合到宿主细胞 DNA 中。在第二个模型中（图 28-7b），复制能力强的病毒再次整合到原癌基因的上游。在个别情况下，3′LTR 中的终止信号不能被识别，转录通过其下游基因进行。然后，较大的组合转录本经过剪接或重组，移除病毒区域的 3′部分和细胞区域的 5′部分，形成一个病毒-原癌基因融合的开放的阅读框，这个阅读框随后被假型化，用于感染细胞和生成整合型 DNA。该过程需要病毒和细胞基因之间的同源区域，来促进重组或合适区域的剪接信号以形成融合的开放阅读框。虽然在融合区域中的禽类反转录病毒 MC29 的 *pol* 基因和鸡 *c-myc* 中发现了这种同源性的例子[58~59]，但这种同源性在大多数反转录病毒中并不显著，说明上述第一种情况可能更常见。

插入诱变

大多数引起宿主肿瘤的反转录病毒不会诱导急性转化，这些病毒含有极少的 *gag*、*pol* 和 *env* 基因的互补体，并且具有复制能力。由于这些病毒中的许多种类都可诱导白血病发生并在遗传上有一定的相关性，因此统称其为白血病病毒。这些病毒的代表包括禽类、鼠类、猫科类和长臂猿白血病病毒。反转录病毒诱导的白血病种类随病毒株而异，一些 GaLV 株与淋巴细胞性白血病有关[7,60]，而另一株与髓性白血病有关[61]。这些病毒缺乏急性转化癌基因意味着它们不能直接转化，更不能在体外转化靶细胞。由于特定肿瘤的所有肿瘤细胞的原病毒的插入位点是相同的，所以从这一特征可明显看出宿主感染引起的白血病及其他肿瘤起源于相同的克隆。这表明导致恶性转化的感染极为罕见,提示反转录病毒的感染在转化之前(并暗示导致其转化)。同时这说明了特殊插入位点的重要性,并由此产生了插入诱变的概念。在这类病毒性肿瘤中,原病毒常常整合在已知的细胞原癌基因附近。病毒LTR的插入(或原病毒插入原癌基因的调节区)会导致其表达失调,进而导致细胞生长或分化失控。另外一种情况,病毒的插入可能会干扰阻止转化的基因的表达。这种插入突变的机制显然需要病毒具有高复制的能力,因为整合在一定程度上是随机发生的,因此白血病可能只发生在少数受感染的动物当中,且潜伏期(从感染到白血病发病的时间)可能相当长。

禽类白血病病毒(ALV)是典型的简单白血病病毒。ALV在鸟类中呈水平和垂直传播。在感染后数月内,B细胞淋巴母细胞开始在法氏囊内聚集[62]。随着法氏囊的退化,许多增大的滤泡消退,但一些肿瘤结节仍持续存在并生长,最终导致转移性淋巴瘤。这些肿瘤通常在*c-myc*(一种细胞原癌基因)附近有显著的原病毒整合[63~65],这些肿瘤中的*c-myc* RNA的表达明显高于正常对照的细胞。转录通常从3′LTR开始[66],产生病毒-细胞的嵌合转录本,但不再需要病毒基因的持续表达和病毒的复制。

插入诱变可能在MMTV和小鼠乳腺肿瘤中也起着关键作用。MMTV与ALV一样,可以进行水平或垂直传播,并且在乳腺肿瘤细胞中通常也存在类似的主要的原病毒。MMTV的整合发生在含*Int-1*原癌基因约30kbp序列的周围(不在30kbp序列内)[67~69],*Int-1*的表达通常仅发生在妊娠中期胚胎的神经管和睾丸减数分裂后期的细胞中,这提示其在乳腺细胞中的异常表达可促进MMTV导致的肿瘤发生。在小鼠中转入MMTV LTR调控的*int-1*基因会导致小鼠发生乳腺肿瘤,而用其他几种基因(包括*c-myc*)中的任何一个取代*int-1*时,也会导致肿瘤的发生[70~73],该结果表明肿瘤的发生可由乳腺特异性启动子来调控任何一个原癌基因而引起。

生长刺激和两阶段致癌

引起红细胞增多的Friend鼠白血病病毒(F-MuLV)代表了另一种类型的转化复制缺陷型反转录病毒。与这些类型中的其他病毒不同,F-Mulv不编码细胞来源的癌基因。含TM和SU蛋白部分的*env*基因内部缺失会产生无功能的env蛋白,该缺陷的env可作为促红细胞生成素(Epo)的类似物,并通过与Epo受体的相互作用激活红细胞前体细胞的生长[74]。这会导致感染小鼠出现红白血病及明显的脾肿大[75]。在裸鼠体内产生的红细胞不会形成肿瘤,也没有永生化。所以F-MuLV引起的脾肿大和红细胞增多更准确地说是增生。然而,红细胞增生经过一段较长时间的潜伏期,之后的遗传改变将有偶发的可能使一个复制中的细胞转化,导致单克隆红系白血病。如图28-7c总结。

反式激活

病毒LTR近距离插入突变引起的原癌基因表达激活,或由整合事件导致的对负调控序列的干扰,称为顺式激活。一些白血病病毒的基因组比简单的白血病病毒(如AlV和MuLV)更复杂,并含有执行调节功能的额外基因。HTLV和BLV是两个典型的例子。这些病毒(像简单的白血病病毒)具有复制能力,在其基因组中不含已转换的原癌基因,仅能在少数感染宿主中诱导单克隆造血系统恶性肿瘤。然而,它们与急性转化病毒相似,被其转化培养的细胞并不需要肿瘤发生所需的特定整合位点(图28-7d)。HTLV是ATL的病原,ATL是一种单克隆T细胞淋巴瘤/白血病,具有常见的皮肤症状,在日本南部和加勒比等多个地区流行[17~19,21,76],也是类似多发性硬化症的神经系统疾病的病因,称为热带痉挛性下肢瘫痪或HTLV相关脊髓病[77]。

HTLV和BLV所编码的蛋白质分别称为Tax[41~44]和p34 Tax[78],其通过与转录因子的协同作用结合到病毒LTR来激活自身的表达。这种由蛋白质产物而非DNA调控区激活的方式被称为反式激活,这些病毒蛋白被称为反式激活因子。HTLV-1也编码其他几种蛋白质,包括调节HTLV-1 mRNA复杂剪接模式的蛋白质Rex[79~80],HTLV-1编码三种功能未知的蛋白质:p30(Ⅱ),另一种结合转录因子CREB结合蛋白/p300(CBP/p300)的反式激活蛋白[81];p12(Ⅰ),激活转录因子NFAT并结合到IL-2受体的胞质结构域[82~83];p13(Ⅱ),定位于线粒体并与法尼基焦磷酸合成酶(一种参与原癌基因*ras*活化的酶)相互作用[84~85]。Tax是许多人关注的焦点,因为它在病毒LTR反式激活病毒复制周期中发挥重要的作用,其激活还可以扩展到细胞基因,包括IL-2受体、淋巴毒素和粒细胞-巨噬细胞刺激因子的基因[86~90]。因此有观点认为,细胞基因间的交叉反式激活表明因TAX导致的生长调控异常在其引起的细胞转化中发挥了重要的作用。

一系列实验证据表明,Tax确实可以在白血病的发生过程中发挥作用。在感染HTLV-I的转化T细胞或白血病ATL细胞中,HTLV-I原病毒通常带有大范围的缺失,但Tax的开放阅读框几乎总能被保留下来。转入受病毒LTR或T细胞特异性启动子调控的Tax基因,可使转基因小鼠发生淋巴细胞白血病等肿瘤[91~94]。然而,T细胞淋巴瘤与ATL细胞的表型是不同的[91~92]。TAX可在体外与*ras*协同作用,直接转化大鼠的成纤维细胞系或转化大鼠原代胚胎细胞[95,96],表明Tax确实具有致癌性。当*Tax*基因被插入到复制能力强但存在转化缺陷的松鼠猴疱疹病毒突变株的基因组中时,人造血细胞可在体外被嵌合病毒感染并转化,且转化细胞在形态学和细胞表面表型上与ATL细胞相似[97],表明Tax在ATL的发病机制中确实很重要。与F-MuLV白血病的发生相似,ATL的发生可能需要后续的步骤。HTLV-1感染后只有极小部分发展成ATL,表明单纯的感染是不够的,缺乏共同的整合位点,说明插入性突变在ATL发生中不起作用。更有可能的是,白血病细胞只有在培养后才表达病毒正链RNA[98],这说明,当细胞成为白血病细胞时,它们不再需要病毒的表达,并且在ATL白血病发生过程中一定存在后续的遗传步骤。

目前研究人员对Tax反式激活和转化的信号转导通路已经有了更好的认识。Tax与ATF/CREB转录因子的家族成员有关[99~103],而HTLV-I LTR中有三个ATF/CREB结合位点。一些细胞基因如血清应答因子(SRF)和NF-κB/Rel,可通过相同的通路被Tax反式激活。Tax还可通过NF-κB反式激活其

LTR 以及一些细胞基因的启动子如 IL-2 和 IL-2 受体启动子[62,104~105]。这取决于 Tax 和 MEKK1 相互作用引起的 NF-κB 抑制剂 IkB 的磷酸化。磷酸化的 IkB 通过泛素化和蛋白酶体降解，使 NF-κB 的核定位信号暴露，从而可以被转运到细胞核中，通过与病毒 LTR 中存在的 NF-κB 增强子结合而激活基因的表达。Tax 也可直接影响细胞周期：Tax 能与细胞周期抑制剂 p16/INK4a 结合，干扰其抑制 CDK4 激酶活性的能力，CDK4 是一种在 G1/S 进展期重要的细胞周期蛋白激酶[106,107]。Tax 也能介导细胞周期蛋白 D3[108] 的磷酸化，并通过 ATF/CREB 信号上调 E2F 的表达[107,109]。这两者都可能导致细胞周期的失调，而细胞周期失调常常导致 p53 介导的细胞凋亡[110]。Tax 导致 p53 失调[111~113]，引起细胞的过度增殖和永生化。Tax 可通过 NF-κB 依赖的以及与 p53 竞争结合 CBP/p300 的机制来抑制 p53 的功能。Tax 还可抑制参与 G2/M 期转换的蛋白质 MAD1[114]。令人感兴趣的是 Tax 可干扰 p16/INK4a 和 p53 通路，而这些基因或其活性的改变在自然发生的癌症中十分普遍。

从病毒 RNA 负链翻译的 HBZ 蛋白也可能是 HTLV-1 导致白血病发生的决定因素。HBZ 是唯一能在 ATL 细胞中持续表达的病毒基因产物[115]。HBZ 与 CREB 和 Jun 家族成员组成异源二聚体[31]，支持 ATL 细胞的增殖[115]。*HBZ* 转基因小鼠出现类似于 ATL 的皮肤病变和 T 细胞淋巴瘤[116]。*Tax/HBZ* 双转基因小鼠与 *HBZ* 单转基因小鼠的表型无明显差异[117]。HBZ 蛋白及其转录产物似乎具有不重叠的功能。HBZ mRNA 在没有 HBZ 蛋白的情况下可支持 ATL 细胞的增殖[115]。HBZ 的转录物中含有剪接变异体，二者中较短的称做 SP1，另一个为 SP2。SP1 亚型负调节依赖 Tax 和 c-Jun 的转录。因此，HBZ 蛋白的一个功能似乎是抑制病毒蛋白的表达。相反，HBZ 蛋白可以与 JunD 蛋白协同作用上调端粒酶（hTERT）的表达[118]。Tax 蛋白还可以通过上调 HBZ 的表达来增加病毒基因表达调控的复杂性[119]。

人类免疫缺陷病毒

HIV 虽然不被认为是肿瘤病毒，但其感染会导致一些类型肿瘤的发病率显著增加，其中大多数肿瘤是与其他病毒如人乳头瘤病毒（HPV）或 Epstein-Barr 病毒（EBV）的共同感染有关[120,121]。反转录病毒也与被感染动物的免疫缺陷有关，如 FeLV。最著名的免疫致病性病毒是可引起 AIDS 的 HIV-1。由于在肿瘤细胞中没有发现 HIV-1，因而其机制一定是间接的。其中最明显的例子是它对人类疱疹病毒 8（HHV-8）[也被称为卡波西肉瘤（KS）疱疹病毒（KSHV）] 发病机制的影响[122]。HHV-8 是导致 KS 和 B 细胞淋巴瘤即外周积液淋巴瘤（PEL）的明确病因[123]。HHV-8 很少会在缺乏 HIV-1 或没有免疫抑制性的条件下引发这些疾病。HIV-1 的感染大幅增加了这些疾病的患病风险[120,121]，但并未在肿瘤细胞中发现 HIV-1。自有效的病毒抑制疗法出现以来，KS 的发病率急剧下降，这进一步证实了 HIV 感染作为辅助因素的作用。在 HIV 感染的情况下，非霍奇金淋巴瘤（NHL）的发病率也显著升高，其中大部分 AIDS-NHL 病例与 EBV 感染有关。HIV-1 的感染也会增加儿童平滑肌肉瘤[121]（与 EBV 相关）、宫颈癌、肝癌（分别与 HPV 和乙型、丙型肝炎病毒感染相关）的风险。感染 HIV 病毒的人往往更容易感染这些病毒，同时感染 HIV 和其中一种病毒的人群患癌症的风险似乎也会更高。这些肿瘤细胞和 KS 一样并未感染 HIV-1，表明 HIV-1 起间接的作用。

免疫缺陷可能在 HIV 感染引发的癌症发病率升高中发挥重要的作用，尤其是病毒性的癌症。然而，HIV 也可能在肿瘤发生中产生更直接的作用。Tat（与 HTLV-I Tax 功能同源的 HIV 反式激活蛋白）转基因小鼠，可引发类似 KS 的病变[124]。Tat 以旁分泌的方式加速 KS 小鼠异种移植模型中肿瘤的发生[125]。一部分 AIDS-NHL 与 EBV 无关，其发病率增加的原因尚不清楚。一些证据表明了 HIV 病毒蛋白，特别是 p17 基质蛋白的作用。即使没有检测到病毒 RNA 或复制，病毒蛋白在感染者的淋巴结中持续存在的时间也会延长[126]。HIV 转基因小鼠的 B 细胞淋巴瘤的发病率显著升高[127]。尽管删除了部分 *gag* 和 *pol* 基因，病毒的转基因仍可以表达多种病毒蛋白，包括 p17。最近，p17 被报道在体外能通过结合和激活趋化因子受体 CXCR1 和 2[128] 促进淋巴管的生成。

内源性反转录病毒

内源性反转录病毒是物种正常遗传互补的一部分，构成了各种哺乳动物基因组的很大一部分（高达 5%）。基于它们类型和数量的差异，许多内源性反转录病毒都是在物种形成之后出现的。由于反转录病毒插入的随机性，以及存在数目之多，使得它们对进化过程产生了深远的影响。目前尚不清楚内源性反转录病毒是否在人类癌症或其他疾病中发挥作用。首先，大部分内源性反转录病毒由于出现缺失而存在缺陷，尽管有些只有少数点突变且极少数内源反转录病毒仍具有复制能力。

其次，内源性反转录病毒即使在 RNA 水平也不表达。这可能是由于它们的 LTR 调控区发生了突变，或者位于染色质的转录失活区，或者是因为 LTR 中启动子序列的甲基化。在正常胎盘或畸胎瘤中，内源性病毒通常表达为 RNA、蛋白质或病毒体，这可能是因为很多内源性反转录病毒的 LTR 中存在激素反应元件。内源性反转录病毒的整合可能导致隐性突变。小鼠的 Hr（无毛）和 D（淡棕色）隐性表型与受影响位点的内源性反转录病毒的存在有关[129~131]，突变的逆转与原病毒的缺失有关。这些现象说明了人群中存在类似现象的可能性。

事实上，在复制的胰淀粉酶基因上游插入 GaLV 相关原病毒会促使该酶在唾液中表达[132~134]，并可能使人类增加对富含淀粉食物的摄入。

一种特异性内源性反转录病毒 RNA 在胎盘中高度表达，其产物为合胞素。合胞素可能在人类胎盘形态发生中起重要的作用，其表达失调与先兆子痫的发生有关[135,136]。研究发现 AKR 小鼠通过内源性 MuLV 表达和重组的复杂过程而引发白血病，但一般来说，目前内源性反转录病毒基因的表达或其表达缺失与人类疾病是无关的[137~139]。

最近，发现于 1988 年的考拉反转录病毒（KoRV）引起了人们的关注[140,141]。考拉反转录病毒已经在考拉种群中存在了几个世纪[142]，在澳大利亚北部变成内源性反转录病毒，而在南部主要是外源性反转录病毒。KoRV 可造成感染考拉[143~145] 发生免疫缺陷和淋巴瘤（危及考拉种群），并且可以迅速侵入考拉的生殖细胞系[144,146]。考拉反转录病毒与 GaLV 的关系最为密切[141],该病毒起源于亚洲鼠种的跨种传播[147]。

同一物种成员之间内源性反转录病毒的整合模式和数量不尽相同,这表明它们不是完全稳定的,许多这类病毒目前对其宿主来说并非是必要的。但既然它们能够作为固定的遗传元件存在,就表明它们曾发挥了重要的作用。相同受体的反转录病毒之间会相互干扰,这是因为感染会阻断或下调细胞表面受体的表达,以避免细胞被重复感染。内源性反转录病毒不再重要的原因可能是内源性反转录病毒干扰或阻止的致病性反转录病毒已不存在。

反转录病毒载体和基因治疗

随着对特定基因在不同疾病中作用的认识的进一步加深,通过基因疗法治疗疾病,或导入所需基因已经成为可能。目前基因治疗的主要障碍之一是无法有效且特异地将目的基因运输到合适的组织和细胞中。通过 DNA 转染运送或导入细胞(用化学物质或电荷使细胞膜部分通透性增加)的方法效率相对较低,特异性不高,一般不适用于体内运送。用基因枪运送,将金微粒表面的 DNA 直接射入皮肤和肌肉中,直接注射的 DNA 可在体内表达,但这些方法的特异性不是很强,可能更适合 DNA 疫苗的运送。

另一种方法是用重组病毒将目的基因运载到合适的组织中,这种基因运送的方法叫做转导。病毒具有高度的组织特异性,原则上,转导可能是基因运送的最佳途径。不同的病毒包括腺病毒已被用于基因的输送,但腺病毒的缺点是缺乏持久性,重复使用后有可能引起宿主对病毒蛋白产生免疫反应。反转录病毒载体可能是研究最透彻,最具发展前景的转导载体[148~151]。它们具有整合的能力,所以理论上只需导入一次。此外,就像在急性转化复制缺陷型反转录病毒中那样,载体基因组不需要编码任何病毒蛋白就能进行整合。转导目的基因唯一的要求是载体 RNA 包含合适的包装信号,并且两端都有 LTR。它们的组织和细胞趋向性可通过不同细胞包膜的假型化而改变[152]。形成病毒颗粒所需的蛋白由某些表达所有病毒蛋白的细胞系提供,而表达这些蛋白的基因本身并不能被包装。当含有目的基因的 RNA 被转染到有包装能力的细胞系中,只有载体 RNA 会被包装成病毒颗粒。由于假型化 RNA 不编码病毒蛋白,病毒颗粒只能进行单次的感染和整合。这使得在没有任何反转录病毒蛋白的情况下,目的基因能够稳定的表达,这可能会诱发免疫应答,从而清除遗传改变的细胞。迄今为止,大多数反转录病毒载体都是以 MuLV 的 Moloney 株(Mo-MuLV)为基础制作的[148~151]。Mo-MuLV 载体能有效地感染包括人类细胞在内的多种细胞类型。而今,现有的研究表明慢病毒反转录病毒载体有一定的发展前景。其优点是能够利用与天然慢病毒感染休眠细胞相同的机制来转导不分裂的细胞[153,154]。

反转录病毒载体存在一些潜在的问题。第一个问题是:在载体的包装过程中可能通过同源重组而产生具有复制能力的辅助病毒。目前已有两种方法可以将这种可能性降到最小。第一种方法是将病毒的结构基因放置在不同的遗传单元上,这样多同源重组必然发生在产生有复制能力的辅助病毒之前。第二种方法与第一种方法并不排斥,例如,通过使用异源启动子进行辅助病毒 RNA 的转录使表达辅助病毒蛋白单元之间的同源区域最小化。第二个潜在的问题是:发生在原癌基因附近的整合有导致肿瘤发生的风险。虽然风险似乎很小,但并非没有。在一项基因治疗研究中,这个原因导致了 7 只猴子中有 3 只罹患淋巴瘤[155]。Mo-MuLV 在人类细胞中的复制能力较差,但其他潜在的反转录病毒载体并非如此。通过严格排除具有复制能力的辅助病毒来最大限度地减少整合事件,在一定程度上可避免但仍不能完全消除该问题。事实上,应用不含可复制辅助病毒的慢病毒载体来治疗患重症联合免疫缺陷 X1 的年轻患者时,似乎已经导致 LMO2 原癌基因启动子附近发生了插入,随后在其中几个患者中发生了白血病样克隆性 T 细胞生长[156]。第三个问题是表达并非无限期持续;反转录病毒的启动子会随时间的推移而失活。另一个局限性是反转录病毒的遗传容量仅有 8~9kb,这限制了它们只能递送一两个基因。

结论

对反转录病毒的研究产生了当今很多的分子生物学技术并拓展了分子生物学的知识。这在细胞转化和肿瘤发生方面尤其明显,这是因为许多反转录病毒既能致癌,又可以(急性转化病毒)捕获有潜在致癌能力的细胞基因。反转录病毒是第一个显示遗传信息可以从 RNA 到 DNA 逆向转录的例子。反转录的发现和阐明为克隆和鉴定 mRNA 提供了方法。极大促进了对基因表达及功能的理解。此外,对病毒转录的调控、反转录 RNA 的加工、病毒进入的机制、病毒蛋白的加工以及病毒装配的研究,丰富了我们关于转录调控、RNA 剪切、翻译调控、膜的生物化学及融合、以及蛋白质加工和蛋白质间相互作用的知识。了解反转录病毒是如何包装和传递遗传物质是今后将这些病毒成功应用到临床的基础——将治疗性基因成功运送到适合的细胞和组织来治疗人类疾病。正在进行的新一代载体研究使我们更加接近这一目标。

反转录病毒研究对人类健康最重要的贡献可能是发现了 HTLV-I 和 HIV-1 这两种致病的人类反转录病毒。20 世纪 70 年代,作为尼克松总统抗癌大战的一部分,许多反转录病毒的研究都得到病毒-癌症计划(VCP)的资助。由于没能找到人类癌症相关的病毒以及人们对反转录病毒的存在日渐增长的怀疑导致了 VCP 的终止。然而,不久之后,就发现了 HTLV-I 与 ATL 的关联。尽管这一发现未能优化 ATL 的治疗,但有益于其预防,例如通过血液样本的筛查和避免通过母乳喂养传播来预防 HTLV-I 的感染,因为母乳喂养是婴儿常见的感染途径。有趣的是,VCP 和反转录病毒研究最重要的成果是较快发现并鉴定了一种与癌症没有直接联系但具有免疫缺陷的病毒,即 HIV-1。HIV-1 被发现并被证明是 AIDS 的病因,研究人员在短时间内建立了血液检测的方法,开发出基于其反转录酶和蛋白酶结构测定的疗法并成功进行了应用。反转录病毒的分离、培养和鉴定技术的合理应用,促进了这些研究的快速发展。

(刘康栋 赵四敏 译 路静 陈新焕 孙文 校)

部分参考文献

4 Gross L. Neck tumors, or leukemia, developing in adult C3H mice following inoculation, in early infancy, with filtered (Berkefeld N), or centrifugated (144,000 X g). *Ak-leukemic Extracts Cancer*. 1953;**6(5)**:948–958.

6 Jarrett WF, Martin WB, Crighton GW, Dalton RG, Stewart MF. Transmission experiments with leukemia (lymphosarcoma). *Nature*. 1964;**202**:566–567.

13 Kalyanaraman VS, Sarngadharan MG, Poiesz B, Ruscetti FW, Gallo RC. Immunological properties of a type C retrovirus isolated from cultured human T-lymphoma cells and comparison to other mammalian retroviruses. *J Virol*. 1981;**38(3)**:906–915.

14 Poiesz BJ, Ruscetti FW, Gazdar AF, Bunn PA, Minna JD, Gallo RC. Detection and isolation of type C retrovirus particles from fresh and cultured lymphocytes of a patient with cutaneous T-cell lymphoma. *Proc Natl Acad Sci U S A*. 1980;**77(12)**:7415–7419.

15 Poiesz BJ, Ruscetti FW, Reitz MS, Kalyanaraman VS, Gallo RC. Isolation of a new type C retrovirus (HTLV) in primary uncultured cells of a patient with Sezary T-cell leukaemia. *Nature*. 1981;**294(5838)**:268–271.

16 Reitz MS, Poiesz BJ, Ruscetti FW, Gallo RC. Characterization and distribution of nucleic acid sequences of a novel type C retrovirus isolated from neoplastic human T lymphocytes. *Proc Natl Acad Sci U S A*. 1981;**78(3)**:1887–1891.

17 Catovsky D, Greaves MF, Rose M, et al. Adult T-cell lymphoma-leukaemia in Blacks from the West Indies. *Lancet*. 1982;**1(8273)**:639–643.

18 Hinuma Y, Nagata K, Hanaoka M, et al. Adult T-cell leukemia: antigen in an ATL cell line and detection of antibodies to the antigen in human sera. *Proc Natl Acad Sci U S A*. 1981;**78(10)**:6476–6480.

19 Kalyanaraman VS, Sarngadharan MG, Nakao Y, Ito Y, Aoki T, Gallo RC. Natural antibodies to the structural core protein (p24) of the human T-cell leukemia (lymphoma) retrovirus found in sera of leukemia patients in Japan. *Proc Natl Acad Sci U S A*. 1982;**79(5)**:1653–1657.

20 Robert-Guroff M, Ruscetti FW, Posner LE, Poiesz BJ, Gallo RC. Detection of the human T cell lymphoma virus p19 in cells of some patients with cutaneous T cell lymphoma and leukemia using a monoclonal antibody. *J Exp Med*. 1981;**154(6)**:1957–1964.

21 Yoshida M, Miyoshi I, Hinuma Y. Isolation and characterization of retrovirus from cell lines of human adult T-cell leukemia and its implication in the disease. *Proc Natl Acad Sci U S A*. 1982;**79(6)**:2031–2035.

22 Kalyanaraman VS, Sarngadharan MG, Robert-Guroff M, Miyoshi I, Golde D, Gallo RC. A new subtype of human T-cell leukemia virus (HTLV-II) associated with a T-cell variant of hairy cell leukemia. *Science*. 1982;**218(4572)**:571–573.

24 Barre-Sinoussi F, Chermann JC, Rey F, et al. Isolation of a T-lymphotropic retrovirus from a patient at risk for acquired immune deficiency syndrome (AIDS). *Science*. 1983;**220(4599)**:868–871.

25 Popovic M, Sarngadharan MG, Read E, Gallo RC. Detection, isolation, and continuous production of cytopathic retroviruses (HTLV-III) from patients with AIDS and pre-AIDS. *Science*. 1984;**224(4648)**:497–500.

26 Gallo RC, Salahuddin SZ, Popovic M, et al. Frequent detection and isolation of cytopathic retroviruses (HTLV-III) from patients with AIDS and at risk for AIDS. *Science*. 1984;**224**:500–503.

27 Sarngadharan MG, Popovic M, Bruch L, Schupbach J, Gallo RC. Antibodies reactive with human T-lymphotropic retroviruses (HTLV-III) in the serum of patients with AIDS. *Science*. 1984;**224(4648)**:506–508.

31 Mesnard JM, Barbeau B, Devaux C. HBZ, a new important player in the mystery of adult T-cell leukemia. *Blood*. 2006;**108(13)**:3979–3982.

32 Cavanagh MH, Landry S, Audet B, et al. HTLV-I antisense transcripts initiating in the 3′LTR are alternatively spliced and polyadenylated. *Retrovirology*. 2006;3:15.

33 Ludwig LB, Ambrus JL Jr, Krawczyk KA, et al. Human immunodeficiency virus-type 1 LTR DNA contains an intrinsic gene producing antisense RNA and protein products. *Retrovirology*. 2006;3:80.

34 Gaudray G, Gachon F, Basbous J, Biard-Piechaczyk M, Devaux C, Mesnard JM. The complementary strand of the human T-cell leukemia virus type 1 RNA genome encodes a bZIP transcription factor that down-regulates viral transcription. *J Virol*. 2002;**76(24)**:12813–12822.

35 Lemasson I, Lewis MR, Polakowski N, et al. Human T-cell leukemia virus type 1 (HTLV-1) bZIP protein interacts with the cellular transcription factor CREB to inhibit HTLV-1 transcription. *J Virol*. 2007;**81(4)**:1543–1553.

41 Felber BK, Paskalis H, Kleinman-Ewing C, Wong-Staal F, Pavlakis GN. The pX protein of HTLV-I is a transcriptional activator of its long terminal repeats. *Science*. 1985;**229(4714)**:675–679.

42 Fujisawa J, Seiki M, Kiyokawa T, Yoshida M. Functional activation of the long terminal repeat of human T-cell leukemia virus type I by a trans-acting factor. *Proc Natl Acad Sci U S A*. 1985;**82(8)**:2277–2281.

44 Sodroski J, Rosen C, Goh WC, Haseltine W. A transcriptional activator protein encoded by the x-lor region of the human T-cell leukemia virus. *Science*. 1985;**228(4706)**:1430–1434.

61 Kawakami TG, Kollias GV Jr, Holmberg C. Oncogenicity of gibbon type-C myelogenous leukemia virus. *Int J Cancer*. 1980;**25(5)**:641–646.

62 Leung K, Nabel GJ. HTLV-1 transactivator induces interleukin-2 receptor expression through an NF-kappa B-like factor. *Nature*. 1988;**333(6175)**:776–778.

64 Hayward WS, Neel BG, Astrin SM. Activation of a cellular onc gene by promoter insertion in ALV-induced lymphoid leukosis. *Nature*. 1981;**290(5806)**:475–480.

65 Neel BG, Hayward WS, Robinson HL, Fang J, Astrin SM. Avian leukosis virus-induced tumors have common proviral integration sites and synthesize discrete new RNAs: oncogenesis by promoter insertion. *Cell*. 1981;**23(2)**:323–334.

66 Payne GS, Bishop JM, Varmus HE. Multiple arrangements of viral DNA and an activated host oncogene in bursal lymphomas. *Nature*. 1982;**295(5846)**:209–214.

67 Nusse R, Varmus HE. Many tumors induced by the mouse mammary tumor virus contain a provirus integrated in the same region of the host genome. *Cell*. 1982;**31(1)**:99–109.

76 Robert-Guroff M, Nakao Y, Notake K, Ito Y, Sliski A, Gallo RC. Natural antibodies to human retrovirus HTLV in a cluster of Japanese patients with adult T cell leukemia. *Science*. 1982;**215(4535)**:975–978.

89 Tschachler E, Bohnlein E, Felzmann S, Reitz MS Jr. Human T-lymphotropic virus type I tax regulates the expression of the human lymphotoxin gene. *Blood*. 1993;**81(1)**:95–100.

91 Grossman WJ, Kimata JT, Wong FH, Zutter M, Ley TJ, Ratner L. Development of leukemia in mice transgenic for the tax gene of human T-cell leukemia virus type I. *Proc Natl Acad Sci U S A*. 1995;**92(4)**:1057–1061.

92 Hall AP, Irvine J, Blyth K, Cameron ER, Onions DE, Campbell ME. Tumours derived from HTLV-I tax transgenic mice are characterized by enhanced levels of apoptosis and oncogene expression. *J Pathol*. 1998;**186(2)**:209–214.

101 Suzuki T, Fujisawa JI, Toita M, Yoshida M. The trans-activator tax of human T-cell leukemia virus type 1 (HTLV-1) interacts with cAMP-responsive element (CRE) binding and CRE modulator proteins that bind to the 21-base-pair enhancer of HTLV-1. *Proc Natl Acad Sci U S A*. 1993;**90(2)**:610–614.

120 Goedert JJ. The epidemiology of acquired immunodeficiency syndrome malignancies. *Semin Oncol*. 2000;**27(4)**:390–401.

121 Rabkin CS. Epidemiology of AIDS-related malignancies. *Curr Opin Oncol*. 1994;**6(5)**:492–496.

125 Guo HG, Pati S, Sadowska M, Charurat M, Reitz M. Tumorigenesis by human herpesvirus 8 vGPCR is accelerated by human immunodeficiency virus type 1 Tat. *J Virol*. 2004;**78(17)**:9336–9342.

156 Hacein-Bey-Abina S, Von KC, Schmidt M, et al. LMO2-associated clonal T cell proliferation in two patients after gene therapy for SCID-X1. *Science*. 2003;**302(5644)**:415–419.

第 29 章　疱疹病毒

Jeffrey I. Cohen, MD

概述

目前已从人体中分离出 8 种疱疹病毒:其中两种 Epstein-Barr 病毒(EBV)和卡波西肉瘤(Kaposi sarcoma, KS)相关疱疹病毒(KSHV)与人类肿瘤相关。已在移植后淋巴组织增生性疾病、鼻咽癌和某些类型的胃癌、伯基特淋巴瘤(Burkitt lymphoma)、霍奇金淋巴瘤(Hodgkin lymphoma)和某些其他淋巴肿瘤患者的病变中检测到 EBV 的存在,而 KSHV 与卡波西肉瘤、原发性积液性淋巴瘤和卡斯尔门病有关。这些病毒编码的蛋白质对于潜伏期的建立、细胞的转化和免疫逃逸有着重要作用。

疱疹病毒的特性

疱疹病毒是有包膜的 DNA 病毒,具有潜伏性感染和裂解性感染的能力。疱疹病毒能在人体内建立潜伏性感染并具有从潜伏期重新激活的能力,确保了病毒源能够感染先前未经感染的个体。大多数成年人携带有潜伏期的单纯疱疹病毒 1 型,水痘-带状疱疹病毒,人疱疹病毒 6 型和 7 型,以及 EBV。疱疹病毒复制的几个特征对于维持潜伏期和致癌性非常重要,下面将以 EBV 为例来说明疱疹病毒感染与癌症的相关性。

首先,病毒 DNA 只能在细胞中存在。EBV 基因组通常以多拷贝环状游离体的形式存在于潜伏感染的 B 细胞中。其次,由于病毒转化的细胞必须逃避免疫清除,EBV 的复制需要 100 多种病毒蛋白;然而,EBV 潜伏感染 B 细胞只需要表达 12 个或更少的基因[1~3]。这些有限的基因产物可防止病毒的频繁复制,避免被感染细胞的死亡,并限制免疫系统识别和破坏病毒潜伏感染细胞。再次,特定的病毒蛋白可与宿主细胞蛋白相互作用或直接反式激活其他细胞基因,促进细胞的增殖和永生化。几种 EBV 蛋白可与细胞蛋白相互作用,激活病毒和细胞基因的转录或参与细胞内的信号转导通路。

EBV:一种致癌的人类疱疹病毒

EBV 基因在转化淋巴细胞中的表达

原代 B 细胞被 EB 病毒感染后可发生细胞转化,导致细胞无限增殖。体外培养的被 EBV 生长转化并潜伏感染的 B 淋巴细胞可表达八种 EBV 蛋白和数种非翻译的 RNA(表 29-1)。EBV 核蛋白 EBNA-1、EBNA-2、EBNA-LP、EBNA-3A、EBNA-3B 和 EBNA-3C 组成 EBV 核抗原复合物。EBNA-1 与 EBV DNA 上的 oriP 序列(病毒 DNA 复制的起始部)结合,并使病毒基因

表 29-1　筛选的 EBV 基因及其细胞同源物和活性

基因	表达方式	细胞同系物	活性
EBNA-1	潜伏,裂解	无	保持游离基因,反式激活病毒基因,抑制细胞凋亡
EBNA-2	潜伏	Notch	反式激活病毒和细胞基因,抑制细胞凋亡
EBNA-3A,B,C	潜伏	无	调节 EBNA-2 活性,反式激活细胞基因
EBNA-LP	潜伏	无	增加 EBNA-2 活性
LMP1	潜伏,裂解	CD40	反式激活细胞基因,抑制细胞凋亡
LMP2	潜伏	无	防止 EBV 重新激活,反式激活 Akt
EBER	潜伏	无	上调细胞基因
BARF-1	裂解	CSF-1R	抑制 IFN-α
BCFR1	裂解	IL-10	抑制 IFN-γ 和 IL-12
BNLF2a	裂解	无	阻断抗原特异性 CD8 T 细胞识别
BHRF1	裂解	Bcl-2	抑制细胞凋亡
BALF1	裂解	Bcl-2	调节 BHRF1 活性
BGFL5	裂解	无	阻断 MHC Ⅰ类和Ⅱ类的合成
BILF1	裂解	GPCR	从细胞表面移除 MHC Ⅰ类
BLLF3	裂解	无	上调 IL-10,TNF-α,IL-1β
BPLF1	裂解	无	抑制 Toll 样受体信号转导
BZLF1	裂解	无	抑制 IFN-γ 作用,抑制 p53 功能,抑制 TNF-α,引发裂解性感染

组以游离的形式存在于转化的 B 细胞中[4]。EBNA-1 也可反式激活其自身的表达。四个不同启动子中的任何一个均可启动 EBNA-1 转录本的表达。Cp 和 Wp 启动子可在体外的类淋巴母细胞系中表达 EBNA-1；Qp 启动子可在伯基特淋巴瘤、鼻咽癌和霍奇金淋巴瘤的组织中表达 EBNA-1；Fp 启动子被用于在病毒裂解复制过程中表达 EBNA-1[5]。EBNA-1 通过蛋白酶体[6]抑制其自身的蛋白质降解并限制自身的翻译[7]，这两者均可能降低细胞对 $CD8^+$ 细胞毒性 T 细胞的呈递。然而，EBNA-1 仍然是 $CD4^+$ 细胞攻击的对象[8~11]。EBNA-1 还可抑制 p53[12] 表达引起的细胞凋亡。

EBNA-2 反式激活 EBV LMP1[13] 和 LMP2[14]，以及细胞基因 *CD21*、*CD23*、*c-myc* 和 *c-fgr* 的表达[15,16]。EBNA-2 通过 GTGGGAA 片段靶向结合蛋白 Jκ 与 LMP1、LMP2、Cp EBNA 和 CD23 启动子结合，并激活这些启动子[17]。EBNA-2 与 Notch 受体在功能上同源，在发育过程中利用 Jκ 调节基因的表达[18]。EBNA-2 也可与 DNA 结合蛋白 PU 相互作用来反式激活 LMP1 启动子[19] 并与 AUF 相互作用来反式激活 EBNA Cp 启动子[20]。EBNA-2 的反式激活结构域对 B 淋巴细胞的转化至关重要[21]。该结构域可与转录因子 TFⅡB 和 TATA 结合蛋白相关因子 TAF40[22] 相互作用。EBNA-2 还可抑制 Nur77 介导的细胞凋亡[23]。

EBNA-LP 作用于 EBNA-2 并增强其反式激活 LMP1 和 LMP2[24] 的能力。尽管 EBNA-LP 在体外与 Rb 和 p53 结合[25]，但这些相互作用的重要性尚不确定。去除 EBNA-LP 的羧基末端可以显著降低病毒转化 B 淋巴细胞的能力[26]。

EBNA-3A、EBNA-3B 和 EBNA-3C 之间无明显的相关性。EBNA-3 蛋白与 Jκ 结合，阻止其结合 DNA，从而抑制 EBNA-2 的反式激活作用[27]。EBNA-3C 可以上调 LMP1 和 CD21 的表达。EBNA-3C 与人肿瘤转移蛋白 Nm23-HI 结合，抑制其活性从而促进伯基特淋巴瘤细胞的转移[28]。EBNA-3C 通过破坏 p27 来降解 Rb 并增强其激酶活性[29,30]。EBNA-3A 和 EBNA-3C 对于体外 B 淋巴细胞的转化至关重要，而 EBNA-3B 则并不是必要的[31,32]。

LMP1 在裸鼠体内发挥转化癌基因的作用[33]。EBV 阴性的伯基特淋巴瘤细胞因 LMP1 的表达而导致 B 细胞的聚集并增加绒毛状突起。LMP1 上调 bcl-2、bfl-1 和 A20 并抑制 Bax，以保护 B 细胞免于凋亡[34,35]。上皮细胞中 LMP1 的表达可抑制细胞的分化[36]。

LMP1 是 CD40 的功能性同源物，CD40 是肿瘤坏死因子受体（TNFR）家族的成员[37]。LMP1 的羧基末端可在体外与 TNFR 相关因子（TRAFs）1、2、3 和 5，TRADD、RIP 和 JAK3 相互作用[38]。LMP1 作为 CD40 的结构型活性形式，可激活 NF-κB、应激活化蛋白激酶、STAT、黏附分子、B7 共刺激分子、JNK 以及 B 细胞的增殖[39]。LMP1 可在 B 细胞中上调黏附分子、Fas、CD40 和 MMP-9 的表达[40]，并上调上皮细胞中 EGF 的表达[41]。LMP1 抑制 Tyk2 的磷酸化，导致干扰素（IFN）-α 的信号转导被抑制[42]。LMP1 对于 EBV 转化 B 淋巴细胞十分重要[43]。对包含有 EBV 的人淋巴瘤的分析表明 LMP1 与 TRAF-1、TRAF-3 共定位并激活 NF-κB[44]。

LMP2 对于 B 细胞的转化不是必需的[45]，但可以诱导上皮细胞表型的转化并增强其运动性[46,47]。LMP2 可通过交联细胞表面的免疫球蛋白，阻止因应答 B 细胞受体复合物激活而导致的 EBV 感染原代 B 细胞的裂解重激活。LMP2 与 B 细胞受体复合物偶联的 *syk* 蛋白酪氨酸激酶及 *src* 家族有关[48]。LMP2 与这些蛋白质的结合会导致其结构型磷酸化，这抑制了它们介导病毒再激活信号的能力[48,49]。表达 LMP2 的转基因小鼠的 B 细胞即使在没有正常 B 细胞受体信号转导活性的情况下也能存活[50]。LMP2 可以激活上皮细胞中 β-catenin 和 Ras/PI3K/Akt 信号通路并引起细胞转化[51,52]。LMP2 还能激活 mTOR 并增加 c-myc 的表达[53]。

两种 EBV 编码的 RNA，EBER-1 和 EBER-2，是潜伏感染的 B 细胞中最多的 EBV RNA；然而，它们并不是潜伏或溶解性 EBV 感染所必需的，但可能有助于 B 细胞转化[54,55]。EBER 上调了 bcl-2 和 IL-10[56] 的表达，并与双链 RNA 激活的蛋白激酶和 IFN 诱导的寡腺苷酸合成酶相互作用[57,58]。

EBV 基因组的 BART 和 BHRF1 结构域至少编码了 44 种 miRNA；BART 和 BHRF1 microRNA 都可以下调细胞基因表达，抑制细胞凋亡，增强 B 细胞的增殖[59]。EBV 还可编码增强转化的细胞 rRNA[60]。EBV microRNA 和 LMP1 均由感染细胞的外泌体分泌，可能促进肿瘤的发生[61,62]。

EBV 基因在生产性感染中的表达

EBV 感染上皮细胞可以导致生产性感染，伴随病毒复制和被感染细胞的裂解。即早期基因编码病毒基因表达的调节因子，包括 BZLF1 和 BRLF1 蛋白，作为引发裂解性感染的开关。BZLF1 蛋白抑制 TNF-α 的信号转导[63] 并帮助病毒逃避 T 细胞反应[64]。BZLF1 蛋白抑制 IFN-γ 受体的表达[65]，并抑制 p53[66] 的功能。早期基因编码参与病毒 DNA 合成的蛋白质，而晚期基因编码结构蛋白质。

在生产性感染中表达的三种病毒基因是细胞基因的功能性同源物，对于 EBV 感染的 B 细胞的存活至关重要[67~68]。EBV BCRF-1 蛋白与 IL-10 同源并具有 IL-10 的活性[69]。BCRF-1 是 B 细胞的一种生长因子并可抑制活化的外周血单核细胞释放 IFN-γ，还可以抑制巨噬细胞分泌 IL-12。

EBV BARF-1 蛋白可以作为 CSF-1[70] 的可溶性受体发挥作用，抑制人单核细胞分泌 IFN-α。EBV BNLF2a 蛋白与 TAP 复合物相互作用以阻断抗原特异性 CD8 T 细胞的识别[71]。EBV BHRF1 蛋白与 bcl-2 同源并保护细胞免于凋亡[72]。EBV BALF1 也与 bcl-2 同源并拮抗 BHRF1[73] 的抗细胞凋亡作用。

临床方面

EBV 感染通常通过唾液传播。该病毒直接感染 B 细胞或口咽上皮细胞，然后扩散到上皮下的 B 细胞[74]。在初次感染期间，有若干百分比的外周血 B 淋巴细胞感染 EBV 并获得在体外无限增殖的能力。自然杀伤（NK）细胞、CD4 T 细胞以及 HLA 和 EBNA 或 LMP 限制性细胞毒性 T 细胞可以控制潜伏感染的 B 淋巴细胞。T 和 B 细胞相互作用释放淋巴因子和细胞因子，使患者产生多种急性传染性单核细胞增多症的临床表现。恢复后，外周血中潜伏感染 EBV 的 B 细胞比例保持在 $1/10^6 \sim 1/10^5$。这些淋巴细胞是 EBV 持续存在的主要部位，并且是上皮表面持续感染的病毒来源。

EBV 感染后早期发生的 B 细胞肿瘤通常是淋巴组织的增生过程引起的，其中 B 细胞潜伏病毒感染是增殖的主要原因。相反，鼻咽癌在原发性 EBV 感染后很久才发生，而病毒基因表达对恶性细胞的生长影响较小。

淋巴组织增生性疾病

EBV 与先天性或后天性免疫缺陷患者的 B 细胞淋巴组织增生性疾病有关。X 染色体连锁淋巴组织增生综合征是男性遗传性免疫缺陷疾病；大多数患者死于致命的淋巴组织增生性疾病或急性重症肝炎，但有些患者则会患低丙种球蛋白血症或 EBV 阳性淋巴瘤并存活下来。已鉴定了在 X 连锁淋巴组织增生综合征中突变的基因 *SAP*[75]，其编码含有 SH2 的蛋白质，可以与 B 细胞和 T 细胞上的 SLAM 相互作用，并且与 NK 细胞和 T 细胞上的 2B4 相互作用。抗 CD20 抗体(利妥昔单抗)可有效治疗一些 X 连锁淋巴组织增生疾病和急性 EBV 感染的患者[76]。其他易导致严重 EBV 感染的细胞蛋白突变包括 XIAP、ITK、CD27、MagT1、CTP 合成酶 1 和 PI3K110δ 的突变。

EBV 淋巴组织增生性疾病可发生在因器官移植或 AIDS 而发生免疫抑制的患者中[77~79]。淋巴组织增生性疾病发展的危险因素包括患者在移植前血清 EBV 呈阴性，并接受了 T 细胞耗竭骨髓的移植或输入了抗淋巴细胞抗体。淋巴组织增生性疾病变最常见于淋巴结，肝，肺，肾，骨髓或小肠内。移植患者的肿瘤通常为淋巴瘤；一些患者有增生性病变。这些肿瘤中增殖的淋巴细胞通常没有染色体易位。

AIDS 相关性淋巴瘤可以是全身性(淋巴结或结外淋巴)淋巴瘤或原发性中枢神经系统淋巴瘤。大多数移植接受者的 B 细胞肿瘤和 AIDS 患者的中枢神经系统淋巴瘤都包含 EBV，AIDS 患者中约 50%的其他类型淋巴瘤也含有 EBV。艾滋病患者的淋巴瘤通常是免疫母细胞淋巴瘤或伯基特淋巴瘤；后者大多数都有 *c-myc* 易位。

来自受移植者或患有 EBV 淋巴组织增生性疾病的 AIDS 患者的组织中可见 EBER 表达，包括 EBNA-1、EBNA-2 和 LMP1 的表达(表 29-2)。外周血中的 EBV 病毒负荷可以用于预测疾病的发展与患者治疗后的随访。EBV 基因的表达是细胞毒性 T 细胞的攻击对象，它的表达对治疗具有重要的意义。EBV 特异的细胞毒性 T 细胞，非辐射的供体白细胞或 HLA 配型的异源细胞毒性 T 细胞都对一些 EBV 淋巴细胞增生病患者有治疗效果[80~86]。抗 CD20 抗体(利妥昔单抗)可使一部分患者的病情得到缓解，并且在一些研究中，当具有淋巴增生性疾病[87]风险的受移植者血液中的 EBV 病毒 DNA 升高时，抗 CD20 抗体可用作预防性治疗，但仍有其他一些研究显示预防性治疗可能是不必要的[88]。

表 29-2 与 EBV 潜在基因表达相关的疾病

疾病	RARTS	EBERS	EBNA-1	EBNA-2	LMP1	LMO2
伯基特淋巴瘤	+	+	+	−	−	−
鼻咽癌	+	+	+	−	+	+
霍奇金淋巴瘤	+	+	+	−	+	+
外周 T 细胞淋巴瘤	+	+	+	−	+	+
淋巴组织增生性疾病	+	+	+	+	+	+

伯基特淋巴瘤

血清流行病学的研究显示，伯基特淋巴瘤与非洲 EBV 之间存在密切关联[89,90]。非洲有超过 90%的伯基特淋巴瘤与 EBV 有关，然而美国只有约 20%的伯基特淋巴瘤与该病毒有关。非洲伯基特淋巴瘤患者通常具有高水平的抗 EBV 抗原的抗体，并且可以从其组织中分离出病毒。

伯基特淋巴瘤含有导致 *c-myc* 基因表达失调的染色体易位。最常见的染色体易位 t(8;14)是将一部分 *c-myc* 癌基因易位到免疫球蛋白重链基因的附近。不太常见的易位包括 *c-myc* 分别易位 κ 或 λ 免疫球蛋白轻链基因的附近，即 t(2;8)和 t(8;22)。这些易位导致 *c-myc* 基因的组成性高表达。目前通过抑制 *c-myc* 基因来治疗伯基特淋巴瘤的新方法正在研究中[91]。

EBV 相关的地方性伯基特淋巴瘤的发生是分阶段进行的。首先，EBV 感染可能扩大了可分化和可增殖的 B 细胞池。其次，慢性地方性疟疾可引起 T 细胞抑制和 B 细胞增殖。最后，增强分化 B 细胞的增殖可提高 *c-myc* 基因发生相互易位[t(8;14)和 t(8;22)]的可能性，使 *c-myc* 部分被免疫球蛋白相关转录增强子所调控，进而形成单克隆肿瘤。

鼻咽癌

非角化性鼻咽癌均与 EBV 有关。鼻咽癌患者具有高水平的针对 EBV 抗原的抗体。关于中国台湾男性的一项前瞻性研究表明，携带 EBV 病毒衣壳抗原(VCA)的 IgA 抗体和抗 EBV 脱氧核糖核酸酶抗体的人，比不含这些抗体的人患鼻咽癌的风险更高[92]。这些抗体可用于鼻咽癌患者的早期筛查及治疗预后的预测。另一项研究表明，定时检测晚期鼻咽癌患者血浆中 EBV DNA 的水平可监测患者的病情并判断预后[93]。鼻咽癌组织中每个细胞都含有 EBV 的基因组。这些 EBV 感染相关的肿瘤是单克隆的，表明 EBV 感染发生于癌细胞生长之前。与伯基特淋巴瘤不同，EBV 与鼻咽癌的关联是一致且普遍的。输注 EBV 特异性细胞毒性 T 细胞可使部分难治性鼻咽癌患者得到缓解[94]。

霍奇金淋巴瘤

具有传染性单核细胞增多症病史的人发生霍奇金淋巴瘤的风险较高[95]。霍奇金淋巴瘤患者通常比一般人群具有更高水平的 EBV VCA 抗体滴度。40%~60%的霍奇金淋巴瘤患者的组织中含有 EBV 基因组。HIV 感染者或发展中国家的霍奇金淋巴瘤患者比 HIV 未感染或发达国家的霍奇金淋巴瘤患者更易携带 EBV 基因组[96]。EBV 基因组是单克隆的，位于 Reed-Sternberg 细胞中。EBV 更常与侵袭性霍奇金淋巴瘤亚型(特别是混合细胞型)有关。EBV 阳性霍奇金淋巴瘤患者和淋巴组织增生性疾病患者的肿瘤源于后生发中心的细胞[97]。11 例具有可测量病灶的复发性霍奇金淋巴瘤患者在接受输注细胞毒性 T 细胞治疗后，2 例患者获得完全缓解，1 例患者部分缓解，5 例患者病情稳定，3 例患者无反应[98]。输注丁酸精氨酸和更昔洛韦可诱导 EBV 胸苷激酶表达和更昔洛韦磷酸化以及诱导细胞凋亡，可使部分 EBV B 细胞恶性肿瘤患者产生抗肿瘤应答[99]。

其他与 EBV 相关的肿瘤

在非霍奇金淋巴瘤中也可以检测到 EBV。EBV 阳性弥漫性大 B 细胞淋巴瘤患者的预后较 EBV 阴性淋巴瘤患者差[100]。用 LMP2 转导的自身抗原呈递细胞治疗 EBV 阳性非霍奇金淋巴瘤，可增加一些复发患者中 LMP2 特异性细胞毒性 T 细胞出现的频率以及肿瘤应答。在外周 T 细胞淋巴瘤患者的组织中可检测到 EBV DNA[101] 和潜伏蛋白[102]。在无潜在免疫缺陷的中枢神经系统淋巴瘤、病毒相关噬血细胞综合征患者的 T 细胞、鼻腔 T 细胞淋巴瘤、腭扁桃体癌、喉癌和血管免疫母细胞性 T 细胞淋巴瘤患者中均可检测到 EBV DNA。在胸腺癌和淋巴瘤样肉芽肿病患者的 B 细胞中可检测到 EBV DNA 和核抗原。

目前已在 AIDS 患者的平滑肌肉瘤中发现了 EBV DNA[103]，并且在器官受移植者的平滑肌肿瘤中检测到病毒 RNA 和 EBNA-2[104]。约 7%的原发性胃癌，特别是在未分化的淋巴上皮瘤样癌中也检测到 EBV 呈阳性。

KSHV 和恶性肿瘤

1994 年，Chang 等人[105] 在 AIDS 患者的卡波西肉瘤组织中检测到一种新的人疱疹病毒即卡波西肉瘤相关疱疹病毒（KSHV）的序列。KSHV 存在于无临床症状人群的 B 细胞中。源自原发性渗出性淋巴瘤患者的 B 细胞系可维持 KSHV 于潜伏状态，并且可以通过添加佛波醇酯或丁酸盐诱导裂解病毒复制。KSHV 体外感染真皮微血管内皮细胞会导致细胞转化并维持长期感染。细胞变成纺锤形，失去接触抑制特性并获得锚定非依赖性生长的能力[106]。虽然 KSHV 可转化骨髓来源的内皮细胞，但病毒只存在于小部分细胞中[107]。

病毒蛋白

一些 KSHV 蛋白对于转化，建立潜伏期和调节对病毒的免疫应答非常重要[108~110]。KSHV 编码大量的细胞同源物（表 29-3），可以根据这些同源物在原发性渗出性淋巴瘤中表达的时间，将它们分为不同的类别[111]。*KSHV K1* 基因在啮齿动物成纤维细胞中的表达可导致细胞转化[112]。K1 蛋白诱导细胞中的酪氨酸磷酸化[113] 并激活 Akt 信号通路[114]。K1 蛋白可以抑制细胞凋亡[115] 并促使 B 细胞中的组成型钙依赖性信号激活[116]。

表 29-3　筛选的 KSHV 基因及其细胞同源物和活性

基因	表达类别	细胞同源物	活性
K1	Ⅱ	ITAM 结构域	转化，激活信号通路
K2	Ⅰ	IL-6	B 细胞生长因子，血管生成，造血功能
K3	Ⅲ	无	减少表面 MHC Ⅰ类
K4	Ⅱ	MIP-1α	趋化因子受体拮抗剂；血管生成；趋化作用
K4.1	Ⅱ	MIP-1α	趋化因子受体激动剂；血管生成；趋化作用
K5	Ⅱ	无	抑制 NK 细胞活性；减少表面 MHC Ⅰ类；促进单核细胞增殖
K6	Ⅱ	MIP-1α	趋化因子受体激动剂；血管生成；趋化作用
K8	Ⅲ	无	抑制 P53
K9	Ⅱ	IRF	抑制 IFN 活性，转化，抑制 p53
K10.5（LANA-2）	Ⅱ	IRF	抑制 IFN 活性，抑制细胞凋亡；抑制 p53
K11.1	Ⅰ	IRF	抑制 IFN 活性
K12（Kaposin A）	Ⅱ	无	转化
K12（Kaposin B）	Ⅱ	无	增加细胞因子 mRNA 的稳定性
K14	Ⅱ	OX-2	诱导促炎细胞因子
K15（LAMP）	Ⅲ	无	结合 TRAF，抑制 B 细胞受体信号转导
ORF4	Ⅱ	CR2	补体结合蛋白
ORF16	Ⅱ/Ⅲ	Bcl-2	抑制细胞凋亡
ORF45	Ⅲ	无	抑制 IFR7
ORF50	Ⅲ	无	增加 CD21 和 CD23 表达，降低 IRF7
ORF63	Ⅲ	NLR proteins	抑制 NLRP1
ORF71	Ⅰ	FLIP	抑制细胞凋亡；激活 NF-κB
ORF72	Ⅰ	Cyclin D	细胞周期进展，抑制 Rb
ORF73（LANA-1）	Ⅰ	无	保持游离基因，抑制 p53 和 Rb
ORF74	Ⅱ	GPCR	血管生成，转化和增殖

表达类别Ⅰ类＝潜伏基因，在非诱导的原发性渗出性淋巴瘤细胞中表达，不由佛波酯诱导；Ⅱ类＝在 TPA 诱导的非诱导细胞中表达；Ⅲ类＝裂解基因，仅在 TPA 诱导后表达（包括许多结构蛋白和 DNA 复制酶）。FLIP，FLICE 抑制蛋白；GPCR，G 蛋白偶联受体；IRF，干扰素调节因子；ITAM，基于免疫受体酪氨酸的活化基序；MHC，主要组织相容性复合物；MIP，炎症蛋白中的巨噬细胞；NK，自然杀伤细胞；Rb，视网膜母细胞瘤蛋白；TRAF，TNFR 相关因子

KSHV K2 基因编码 IL-6 的同源物(vIL-6)。IL-6 是一种 B 细胞生长因子,可作为淋巴肿瘤的自分泌生长因子,促进细胞增殖[117]。vIL-6 可防止体外 IL-6 依赖性的 B9 细胞死亡[118],促进血细胞生成,诱导 VEGF 并促进血管生成[119]。K3[免疫识别调节因子 1(MIR1)]和 K5(MIR2)蛋白通过泛素化,诱导 MHC(主要组织相容性复合物)I 类分子和 IFN-γ 受体 1 从细胞表面快速胞吞[120~122]。K5 蛋白还可下调 ICAM-1 和 B7.2,从而抑制 NK 细胞介导的细胞毒性作用[123],并移除内皮细胞表面的 CD31[124]。

KSHV K4、*K4.1* 和 *K6* 基因分别编码三种趋化因子:病毒巨噬细胞炎性蛋白(MIP)-Ⅱ,-Ⅲ 和-Ⅰ。vMIP-1 抑制依赖于 CCR5[118] 的 HIV 病毒株的复制。vMIP-1 和 vMIP-Ⅲ 分别是 CCR8[125] 和 CCR4[126] 的趋化因子的受体激动剂,而 vMIP-Ⅱ 是一种广谱的趋化因子受体拮抗剂[127]。vMIP-Ⅱ 是嗜酸性粒细胞的化学引诱物,可与 CC 和 CXC 趋化因子结合,阻断趋化因子诱导的钙流通[128]。

KSHV K9、K11.1 和 K10.5 蛋白分别称为病毒 IFN 调节因子(vIRF)-1、-2 和-3。这些蛋白均能抑制病毒介导的 IFN-α 启动子的激活[129]。vIRF1 可以抑制 MHC-1 的转录和表面表达[130]。vIRF1 和 vIRF3 可以抑制 p53 介导的细胞凋亡[131,132] 并转化 NIH 3T3 细胞[133]。vIRF3(也称为 LANA2)保护细胞免受 p53 诱导的细胞凋亡[134~135]。KSHV ORF45 可以阻断 IRF7 的活性并抑制 IFN-α 和 β 的活化[136]。

KSHV K12 基因座编码几种称作 Kaposin 的蛋白。Kaposin A 可以诱导细胞转化[137]。Kaposin B 通过激活 MAP 激酶相关蛋白激酶 2 和抑制细胞因子 mRNA 的降解来促进细胞因子的表达[138,139]。KSHV K14 蛋白,一种细胞 OX2 蛋白的同源物,可以刺激单核细胞产生促炎因子如 TNFα、IL-1β 和 IL-6[140]。KSHV ORF4 蛋白可以抑制补体系统[141]。*KSHV ORF16* 编码 bcl-2 的同源物并抑制 bax 诱导的细胞凋亡[142]。*ORF71* 编码与细胞 FLIP 同源的蛋白,可阻止细胞凋亡。ORF71 与 Atg3 结合并保护细胞免于自噬。KSHV ORF71 可以激活 NF-κB,促进肿瘤的生长,是 KSHV 感染的淋巴瘤细胞存活所必需的[143~147]。*KSHV ORF72* 编码了一种细胞周期蛋白 D 的同源物,其可以结合并激活 cdk6,磷酸化 p27,刺激正常静止期的成纤维细胞周期进展[148~149],导致病毒细胞周期蛋白磷酸化从而使 Rb 失活[150]。

KSHV ORF73 编码 LANA1,它是定位于病毒 DNA 的游离基因,可以在细胞分裂期间将游离基因连接到染色体上[151]。KSHV LANA1 是分裂细胞中维持游离基因所必需的,并可反式激活其自身的启动子。此外,LANA1 可以抑制 p53 和 Rb 的活性[152,153],上调 β-catenin 的表达并使其稳定[154],还可以上调和激活凋亡抑制蛋白[155],诱导 HIF 的细胞核聚集[156],并激活 c-myc[157]。转基因小鼠中 LANA 的表达可导致淋巴瘤[158]。LANA 还可抑制 TGF-β 的信号转导[159]。*KSHV ORF74* 编码与细胞 IL-8 受体同源的 G 蛋白偶联受体;然而,与后者蛋白不同,KSHV 受体具有组成型活性并可诱导细胞增殖[160]。ORF74 蛋白可以诱导血管生成[161],激活 Akt 信号通路[162],并诱导内皮细胞的增殖、增加血管通透性[163~165]。ORF74 可以激活 NF-κB 和 JNK,上调 IL-1,IL-8,TNF-α 和 FGF,并抑制病毒裂解基因的表达[166]。

KSHV K15 编码潜伏相关膜蛋白(LAMP)并与 TRAF 1,2 和 3[167] 相互作用。K15 抑制酪氨酸磷酸化和细胞内钙流动,从而抑制 B 细胞受体的信号[168]。KSHV 编码的几个 microRNA 位于 K12 和 ORF71 之间或 K12 内部,这几个 microRNA 在潜伏期间表达并可以在患者血浆中检测到[169]。这些 microRNA 对 NF-κB 活化和阻断潜伏感染细胞的细胞周期阻滞非常重要[109,170]。KSHV microRNA 也可靶向细胞基因[171]。

临床方面

KSHV 的血清阳性率从小于美国正常献血者的 5% 到英国 HIV 阳性的男同性恋群体的 30%~35% 不等[172]。KSHV 抗体在非洲和地中海人群中更为常见。至少 85% 的卡波西肉瘤患者有 KSHV 抗体[173]。女性卡波西肉瘤的患病率低于男性,血清 HIV 阳性女性的 KSHV 抗体阳性率也低于血清 HIV 阳性的男性。HIV 阳性同性恋男子的 KSHV 血清阳性对卡波西肉瘤的后续发展有预测价值[174]。活动期卡波西肉瘤或多中心 Castleman 病患者的 KSHV DNA 水平要高于缓解期患者,并且原发性渗出性淋巴瘤患者的 KSHV DNA 的水平也会升高[175]。该病毒对大多数健康个体并不致病,并可以终生处于潜伏期;然而,在免疫功能低下者中,它与卡波西肉瘤有着密切的关联。因此,尽管感染 KSHV 似乎是卡波西肉瘤发展所必需的,但仅有这一个因素可能还不够,还需要其他辅助因子的参与,如 HIV 和细胞免疫功能受损。KSHV 可在同性恋男性中通过性传播,也可在女性中通过性和静脉注射药物传播。在某些地区的人群(如非洲)中,KSHV 可能是从母婴垂直传播以及同胞之间进行传播的[176]。另外 KSHV 已被发现可以通过肾移植进行传播[177,178]。

卡波西肉瘤

几乎所有经典型的卡波西肉瘤、非洲地方性卡波西肉瘤、HIV 阴性受移植者和同性恋男性的卡波西肉瘤以及 AIDS 患者的卡波西肉瘤的活检中均可以检出 KSHV[179,180]。KSHV 存在于肿瘤的内皮细胞和梭形细胞中,但不存在于正常的内皮细胞中[181]。大多数肿瘤细胞处于病毒潜伏感染,但 HIV 阳性卡波西肉瘤中 1%~5% 的梭形细胞显示裂解性 KSHV 感染。卡波西肉瘤可以是多克隆,寡克隆或单克隆。大约 50% 的卡波西肉瘤患者的外周血单核细胞中存在 KSHV,其存在可预测恶性肿瘤的发生[172]。在卡波西肉瘤患者的唾液中也可检测到 KSHV,但很少在精液中检测到。一些 KSHV 蛋白在卡波西肉瘤组织中表达(表 29-4)。一些报道显示,膦甲酸和更昔洛韦降低了卡波西肉瘤病变的发生率,但并非所有研究都显示如此[182,183]。西多福韦对已形成的病变无效[184]。相比之下,HIV 蛋白酶抑制剂被报道可诱导卡波西肉瘤病变的消退[185]。IL-12 与多柔比星脂质体联合,可在接受 HAART 治疗的患有卡波西肉瘤的 AIDS 患者中引起肿瘤应答,这种应答将随 IL-12 的治疗而持续[186]。据报道,西罗莫司[187]、伊马替尼[188]、贝伐单抗[189] 和紫杉醇[190] 都具有抗卡波西肉瘤的活性。

表 29-4 与 KSHV 基因表达相关的疾病

基因	卡波西肉瘤	原发性渗出性淋巴瘤	Castleman 病
LANA(ORF73)	+	+	+
K12(Kaposin)	+	+	–
ORF72(v-cyclin)	+	+	–
ORF71(v-FLIP)	+	+	+
ORF74(GPCR)	+	–	–
K10.5(vIRF3)	–	+	+
K9(vIRF1)	–	–	+
K2(vIL-6)	–	±	+

原发性渗出性淋巴瘤

在 AIDS 患者的原发性渗出性淋巴瘤中也发现了 KSHV[180,181,191]。这些体腔的 B 细胞系淋巴瘤位于胸膜，腹膜或心包腔，通常含有 EBV 和 KHSV 基因组。在非 AIDS 患者中也发现了一些 KSHV 阳性的淋巴瘤。

多中心 Castleman 病

KSHV 可以在一些多中心 Castleman 病患者的活检样本中发现，尤其是浆细胞型患者[180,181,192~194]。这种疾病通常是多克隆的，表现为全身的淋巴结受累，发热和高球蛋白血症。这些症状的出现归因于 IL-6 和 vIL-6[195]水平的升高。在 HIV 阳性患者的组织活检中，KSHV 的检出率高于 HIV 阴性的患者。KSHV 存在于病变的外套层免疫母细胞的 B 细胞中。在一些 KSHV 相关 Castleman 病患者中，齐多夫定联合缬更昔洛韦表现出了一定的活性[196]。

总结

- 两种疱疹病毒，爱泼斯坦-巴尔病毒(EBV)和卡波西肉瘤相关疱疹病毒(KSHV)，与人类肿瘤有关。
- EBV 与伯基特淋巴瘤，霍奇金和非霍奇金淋巴瘤，移植后淋巴组织增生性疾病，T 细胞淋巴瘤，鼻咽癌和某些类型的胃癌有关。
- EBV 转化的 B 细胞和 EBV 移植后淋巴组织增生病变可表达 EBNA-1、-2、-3s、-LP、LMP1、LMP2 和包括 EBER、BART 在内的 RNAs。伯基特淋巴瘤仅表达 EBNA-1、EBER、BARTs。霍奇金淋巴瘤和鼻咽癌表达 EBNA-1、LMP1、LMP2、EBER 和 BART。
- EBV EBNA-1 对于在细胞复制期间维持病毒游离体是十分重要的。EBNA-2 可以反式激活几种病毒和细胞启动子，并且是 Notch 受体的功能性同源物。EBNA-3′s 可以调节 EBNA-2 的活性，并反式激活病毒基因。LMP1 是 CD40 的功能性同源物，并与 TNFR 相关因子结合以上调 NF-κB，STAT，JNK 和应激活化蛋白激酶。
- KSHV 与原发性渗出性淋巴瘤、卡波西肉瘤和卡斯尔门病有关。
- 三种 KSHV 相关肿瘤中均表达 LANA(ORF73)和 v-FLIP(ORF71)。其他 KSHV 蛋白，包括：Kaposin(K12)，v-cyclin(ORF72)，G 蛋白偶联受体(GPCR，ORF74)，v-IRF3(K10.5)，v-IRF1(K9)和 v-IL-6(K2)并非在所有与病毒相关的恶性肿瘤中都表达。
- LANA 可以在复制过程中维持病毒的游离体并抑制 Rb 和 p53 的活性。KSHV v-FLIP 是细胞 FLIP 的同源物，可以抑制细胞凋亡并激活 NF-κB。卡波西肉瘤会增强细胞因子的活性，v-cyclin 抑制 Rb 并促进病毒感染的细胞周期的进展，病毒 GPCR 有助于 KSHV 感染细胞的增殖。v-IRF1 和 v-IRF3 可以抑制干扰素和 p53 的活性，而 v-IL-6 可以作为 B 细胞生长因子起作用。

(刘康栋 路静 译 赵继敏 李鑫 孙文 校)

部分参考文献

1 Longnecker R, Kieff E, Cohen JI. Epstein-Barr virus. In: Knipe DM, Howley PM, Cohen JI, Griffith DE, Lamb RA, Martin MA, Racaniello V, Roizman B, eds. *Fields Virology*. Philadelphia: Lippincott Williams & Wilkins; 2013:1898–1959.

2 Thorley-Lawson DA, Gross A. Persistence of the Epstein-Barr virus and the origins of associated lymphomas. *N Engl J Med*. 2004;**350**:1328–1337.

3 Price AM, Luftig MA. Dynamic Epstein-Barr virus gene expression on the path to B-cell transformation. *Adv Virus Res*. 2014;**88**:279–313.

8 Hislop AD, Taylor GS, Sauce D, Rickinson AB. Cellular responses to viral infection in humans: lessons from Epstein-Barr virus. *Annu Rev Immunol*. 2007;**25**:587–617.

37 Uchida J, Yasui T, Takaoka-Shichijo Y, et al. Mimicry of CD40 signals by Epstein-Barr virus LMP-1 in B lymphocyte responses. *Science*. 1999;**286**:300–303.

59 Klinke O, Feederle R, Delecluse HJ. Genetics of Epstein-Barr virus microRNAs. *Semin Cancer Biol*. 2014;**26**:52–59.

62 Meckes DG Jr, Gunawardena HP, Dekroon RM, et al. Modulation of B-cell exosome proteins by gamma herpesvirus infection. *Proc Natl Acad Sci U S A*. 2013;**110**:E2925–E2933.

67 Horst D, Verweij MC, Davison AJ, Ressing ME, Wiertz EJ. Viral evasion of T cell immunity: ancient mechanisms offering new applications. *Curr Opin Immunol*. 2011;**23**:96–103.

74 Cohen JI. Epstein-Barr virus infection. *N Engl J Med*. 2000;**343**:481–492.

76 Milone MC, Tsai DE, Hodinka RL. Treatment of primary Epstein-Barr virus infection in patients with X-linked lymphoproliferative disease using B-cell-directed therapy. *Blood*. 2005;**105**:994–996.

85 Leen AM, Bollard CM, Mendizabal AM, et al. Multicenter study of banked third-party virus-specific T cells to treat severe viral infections after hematopoietic stem cell transplantation. *Blood*. 2013;**121**:5113–5123.

86 Bollard CM, Rooney CM, Heslop HE. T-cell therapy in the treatment of post-transplant lymphoproliferative disease. *Nat Rev Clin Oncol*. 2012;**9**:510–519.

89 Grömminger S, Mautner J, Bornkamm GW. Burkitt lymphoma: the role of Epstein-Barr virus revisited. *Br J Haematol*. 2012;**156**:719–729.

91 Schmitz R, Young RM, Ceribelli M, et al. Burkitt lymphoma pathogenesis and therapeutic targets from structural and functional genomics. *Nature*. 2012;**490**:116–120.

92 Chien Y-C, Chen J-Y, Liu M-Y, et al. Serological markers of Epstein-Barr virus infection and nasopharyngeal carcinoma in Taiwanese men. *N Engl J Med*. 2001;**345**:1877–1882.

93 Lin JC, Wang WY, Chen KY, et al. Quantification of plasma Epstein-Barr virus DNA in patients with advanced nasopharyngeal carcinoma. *N Engl J Med*. 2004;**350**:2461–2470.

94 Louis CU, Straathof K, Bollard CM, et al. Adoptive transfer of EBV-specific T cells results in sustained clinical responses in patients with locoregional nasopharyngeal carcinoma. *J Immunother*. 2010;**33**:983–990.

95 Hjalgrim H, Askling J, Rostgaard K, et al. Characteristics of Hodgkin's lymphoma after infectious mononucleosis. *N Engl J Med*. 2003;**349**:1324–1332.

98 Bollard CM, Gottschalk S, Torrano V, et al. Sustained complete responses in patients with lymphoma receiving autologous cytotoxic T lymphocytes targeting

Epstein-Barr virus latent membrane proteins. *J Clin Oncol*. 2014;**32**:798–808.

99 Perrine SP, Hermine O, Small T, et al. A phase 1/2 trial of arginine butyrate and ganciclovir in patients with Epstein-Barr virus-associated lymphoid malignancies. *Blood*. 2007;**109**:2571–2578.

101 Bollard CM, Gottschalk S, Torrano V, et al. Sustained complete responses in patients with lymphoma receiving autologous cytotoxic T lymphocytes targeting Epstein-Barr virus latent membrane proteins. *J Clin Oncol*. 2014;**32**:798–808.

105 Chang Y, Cesarman E, Pessin MS, et al. Identification of herpesvirus-like DNA sequences in AIDS-associated Kaposi's sarcoma. *Science*. 1994;**266**:1865–1869.

108 Damania B, Cesarman E. Kaposi's sarcoma-associated herpesvirus. In: Knipe DM, Howley PM, Cohen JI, Griffith DE, Lamb RA, Martin MA, Racaniello V, Roizman B, eds. *Fields Virology*. Philadelphia: Lippincott Williams & Wilkins; 2013:2080–2128.

109 Giffin L, Damania B. KSHV: pathways to tumorigenesis and persistent infection. *Adv Virus Res*. 2014;**88**:111–159.

110 Cesarman E. How do viruses trick B cells into becoming lymphomas? *Curr Opin Hematol*. 2014;**21**:358–368.

117 Chatterjee M, Osborne J, Bestetti G, et al. Viral IL-6-induced cell proliferation and immune evasion of interferon activity. *Science*. 2002;**298**:1432–1435.

118 Moore PS, Bashoff C, Weiss RA, Chang Y. Molecular mimicry of human cytokine and cytokine response path-way genes by KSHV. *Science*. 1996;**274**:1739–1744.

127 Bashoff C, Endo Y, Collins PD, et al. Angiogenic and HIV-inhibitory functions of KSHV-encoded chemokines. *Science*. 1997;**278**:290–294.

150 Chang Y, Moore PS, Talbot SJ, et al. Cyclin encoded by KS herpesvirus. *Nature*. 1996;**382**:410.

152 Friborg J, Kong W, Hottiger MO, et al. p53 inhibition by the LANA protein of KSHV protects against cell death. *Nature*. 1999;**402**:889–894.

155 Lu J, Jha HC, Verma SC, Sun Z, et al. Kaposi's sarcoma-associated herpesvirus-encoded LANA contributes to viral latent replication by activating phosphorylation of survivin. *J Virol*. 2014;**88**:4204–4217.

160 Arvanitakis L, Geras-Raaka E, Varma A, et al. Human herpesvirus KSHV encodes a constitutively active G-protein–coupled receptor linked to cell proliferation. *Nature*. 1997;**385**:347–350.

169 Chugh PE, Sin SH, Ozgur S, et al. Systemically circulating viral and tumor-derived microRNAs in KSHV-associated malignancies. *PLoS Pathog*. 2013;**9**:e1003484.

172 Martin JN, Ganem DE, Osmond DH, et al. Sexual transmission and the natural history of human herpesvirus 8 infection. *N Engl J Med*. 1998;**338**:948–954.

174 Gao SJ, Kingsley L, Hoover DR, et al. Seroconversion of antibodies to Kaposi's sarcoma-associated herpesvirus related latent nuclear antigens prior to onset of Kaposi's sarcoma. *N Engl J Med*. 1996;**335**:233–241.

180 Sullivan RJ, Pantanowitz L, Casper C, Stebbing J, Dezube BJ. HIV/AIDS: epidemiology, pathophysiology, and treatment of Kaposi sarcoma-associated herpesvirus disease: Kaposi sarcoma, primary effusion lymphoma, and multicentric Castleman disease. *Clin Infect Dis*. 2008;**47**:1209–1215.

186 Little RF, Aleman K, Kumar P. Phase 2 study of pegylated liposomal doxorubicin in combination with interleukin-12 for AIDS-related Kaposi sarcoma. *Blood*. 2007;**110**:4165–4171.

187 Stallone G, Schena A, Infante B, et al. Sirolimus for Kaposi's sarcoma in renal-transplant recipients. *N Engl J Med*. 2005;**352**:1317–1323.

194 Uldrick TS, Polizzotto MN, Yarchoan R. Recent advances in Kaposi sarcoma herpesvirus-associated multicentric Castleman disease. *Curr Opin Oncol*. 2012 Sep;**24(5)**:495–505.

195 Polizzotto MN, Uldrick TS, Wang V, et al. Human and viral interleukin-6 and other cytokines in Kaposi sarcoma herpesvirus-associated multicentric Castleman disease. *Blood*. 2013;**122**:4189–4198.

196 Uldrick TS, Polizzotto MN, Aleman K, et al. High-dose zidovudine plus valganciclovir for Kaposi sarcoma herpesvirus-associated multicentric Castleman disease: a pilot study of virus-activated cytotoxic therapy. *Blood*. 2011;**117**:6977–6986.

第30章　乳头瘤病毒与宫颈肿瘤

Michael F. Herfs, PhD ■ Martin C. Chang, MD, PhD, FCAP, FRCPC ■ Christopher P. Crum, MD, FRCP

概述

HPV 相关领域的研究正在不断发展中，人们对其发病机制有了新的认识，使用 HPV 检测的筛查方法也得到了改进，研制出了针对更广泛 HPV 类型的疫苗。人们更精确地描述了鳞柱状上皮交界处的特征，并且正在讨论其是否有潜力成为针对年龄超过疫苗接种最佳时间的女性的预防靶点。HPV 检测在对 30 岁以上女性的筛查中发挥了主要作用，而阴道涂片检测主要对 20 岁到 30 岁之间的女性有意义，同时减少或取消了对 20 岁以下女性的宫颈癌筛查。为了预防宫颈癌变，随着新型更广谱疫苗（如 9 价疫苗）的出现，靶向更广泛的 HPV 类型已经成为现实。

人类乳头状病毒（HPV）与宫颈肿瘤的因果关系是一个公认的事实。研究该病毒不仅可以阐明病毒的致癌机制，改进宫颈癌的诊断和筛查方法，还可探讨宿主对病毒的免疫应答机制。从最初的描述性形态学研究，到分子生物学研究，再到分子免疫学研究，技术的进步对揭示病毒致癌机制、宿主免疫应答和疫苗研究防治均起到了推动作用。

定义、HPV 靶细胞，以及感染和转化的机制

定义

生殖"感染"最佳的定义是临床上或者阴道镜镜检观察到含有乳头状瘤脱氧核糖核酸（DNA）的扁平或隆起的湿疣。在这种情况下，感染性病毒很有可能在上皮内被识别（图 30-1）。目前，感染的定义范围已经扩大，只要携带了 HPV DNA，或有与 HPV 相关的癌前病变以及癌均可称为 HPV 感染。然而，在晚期病变中更有可能发现整合的病毒 DNA 而不是病毒颗粒（图 30-2）[1]。正如之后详述的（见题为"危险因素"的章节），HPV DNA 可能与无明显异常改变，临床上或者形态上显著的活动性感染以及晚期肿瘤有关（表 30-1、表 30-2）。显著的 HPV 感染的标志是受累组织的形态学发生改变，这不是传统意义上的 HPV 核酸导入培养细胞后所产生的变化，而是指与 HPV 核酸存在始终相关的形态学改变。根据宿主因素和感染的 HPV 类型，可将其定义为低级别或高级别的生殖系统癌前病变，两者均不同于正常的上皮（图 30-1、图 30-2）。

HPV 靶细胞和感染机制

传统上认为 HPV 感染起源于外宫颈鳞状上皮基底层，以及宫颈中柱状上皮被鳞状上皮所取代的区域（转化区）。以此推测，宫颈复层黏膜中的微小创伤或擦伤使基底细胞暴露于病毒颗粒，从而使病毒进入增殖的基底上皮细胞[5]。有一些证据支持这一假说，如基底细胞中存在 HPV DNA 和核糖核酸，在假病毒暴露前破坏上皮表面（从而暴露基底细胞）可增强假病毒对鳞状上皮的实验性感染[6]。尽管基底角质细胞感染可能导致产毒性感染以及随后在子宫颈外部和其他黏膜部位（阴道、外阴）发生癌变（或癌前病变），但是这一假说与长期观察结果并不一致——经长期观察大约 90% 的宫颈癌（或癌前病变）特

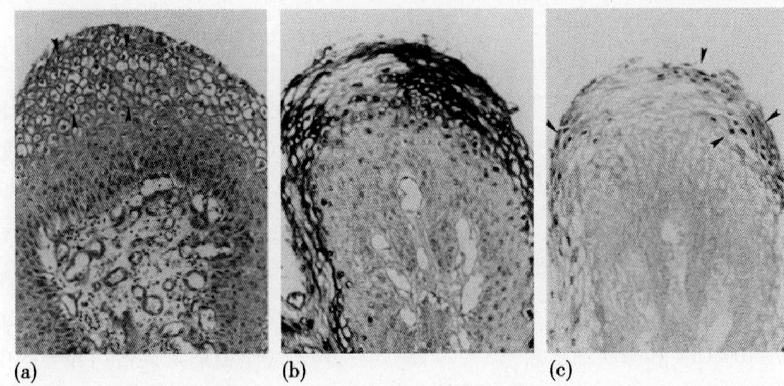

图 30-1　典型的低危型子宫颈人乳头瘤病毒（HPV）（HPV 6 型或 11 型）感染（湿疣）的病理组织学。（a）HPV 感染的形态学特征包括浅表上皮细胞核异型，并伴有明显的胞质晕（箭头）。底层细胞含有最低限度的核异型。（b）与生物素标记的 HPV 6 型和 HPV 11 型（VIRATYPE, Life Technologies, Gaithersburg, MD）脱氧核糖核酸（DNA）探针进行原位杂交图像。在浅表细胞的核和胞质中深染的物质为 HPV DNA 以及病毒复制过程中产生的核酸。（c）HPV 衣壳蛋白的免疫过氧化物酶染色，显示在浅表上皮中有若干细胞核深染（箭头）

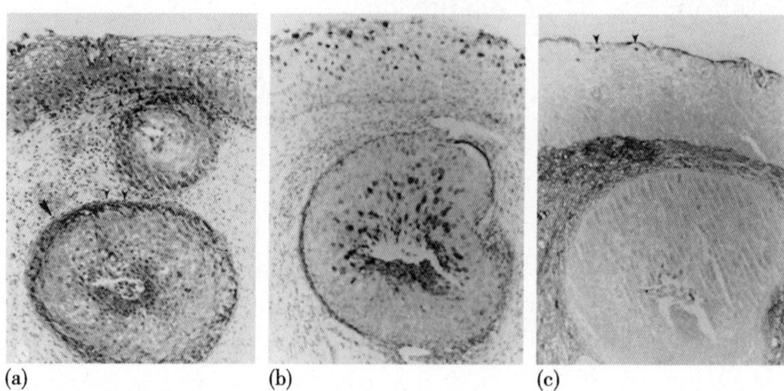

图 30-2 高危型人乳头瘤病毒(HPV)(即 16、31、33 和 35)相关子宫颈上皮内瘤变的组织病理学。(a)病变累及浅表及腺窝(腺体)上皮(大箭头)。显示凹陷细胞异型性(右上方),此外在底层细胞有显著的核异型(小箭头)。(b)与 31、33 和 35 型 HPV DNA 混合探针进行原位杂交图像。染色分布与图 30-1b 相似。(c)与图 30-1c 不同,免疫染色显示的衣壳蛋白很少,染色阳性的细胞核也少

表 30-1 定义

HPV,人类乳头瘤病毒。
CIN,宫颈上皮内瘤变,乳头瘤病毒相关的鳞状上皮病变。低级别 CIN(CIN Ⅰ)指上层上皮细胞核异型性、扁平或外生的湿疣。高级别 CIN(CIN Ⅱ或Ⅲ)指累及上皮全层的异型性。HPV 相关病变包括 HPV 感染如湿疣,高级别 CIN 和各种浸润性癌等 HPV 相关病变。
隐匿性或潜伏性 HPV,感染 HPV 但无明显形态学改变。
高危型 HPV,已证明与癌症有关联的 HPV 亚型(不是对癌症风险的评估,其在高危型 HPV 之间不尽相同)。
低危型 HPV,不引起肿瘤的 HPV 亚型。
VLP,病毒样颗粒,体外产生的类似乳头瘤病毒的病毒颗粒。

表 30-2 生殖系统 HPV 及其相关疾病[2~4]

HPV	相关疾病
16	50%以上高级别 CIN 和癌(鳞状细胞癌和腺癌)
18	10%鳞状细胞癌,50%腺癌和原位腺癌以及 90%神经内分泌癌
31,45	5%~10%CIN 和鳞状细胞癌
33,39,52,52,55,56,8,59,68	少于 3%CIN 和鳞状细胞癌
6,11,40,42,53,54,57,66,84	低危型 HPV,在癌中基本检测不到
61,62,64,67,69~72,81,cp6108,iso39	没有足够的证据证明其风险

异性发生于在鳞柱状上皮交界处(SCJ)[7]。多年来,人们猜测这种特定的微环境含有多能细胞,这些细胞由于其生物学特性或所处的位置易于被 HPV 感染。最近在宫颈 SCJ 处发现了残留胚胎(Müllerian)细胞的离散群体[8]。这些 SCJ 细胞除了参与成人宫颈重塑(化生、增生)外[9],还有望作为 HPV 的靶标,并因此被认为是宫颈癌的前体细胞。在该模型中,基底角质细胞仍然易受 HPV 影响,但敏感度相对于 SCJ 细胞较低。

无论 HPV 最初感染何种细胞,HPV 首先均通过成熟病毒衣壳与基底膜上硫酸乙酰肝素蛋白多糖的结合进入宿主细胞。然后,在 HPV 次要衣壳蛋白 L2 弗林(转化酶)共识别位点的剪切诱导衣壳构象改变,从而使 HPV 衣壳被内吞[10]。但是内吞途径和 HPV 细胞受体仍然存在争议,可能的 HPV 受体包括 α6 整合素等[11]。

肿瘤转化机制

HPV 感染导致肿瘤转化的机制已逐渐被阐明,至少由四个部分组成(图 30-3)[12]。第一种是病毒癌蛋白直接作用于细胞周期,这是分别由致癌性 HPV(高风险)的 E6 或 E7 蛋白与 TP53 或 Rb 蛋白相互作用介导的(图 30-3)。这些癌蛋白还可直接影响其他细胞周期调节因子如细胞周期蛋白 E[13],这会导致细胞周期蛋白依赖性激酶抑制剂 p16 表达代偿性升高[14,15]。第二种效应是由病毒癌蛋白介导的中心体复制异常,导致基因组不稳定,最后造成等位基因失衡[2,16],后者包括染色体 3p 的改变和 3q25-27 的特异性扩增[17,18]。第三种是由 E6 介导的端粒酶表达上调和扰乱正常的复制性衰老[19]。这些事件的发生根本上都是由于病毒癌蛋白(E6 和 E7)的表达所造成的。第四种是甲基化导致的抑癌基因失活[20]。例如 E7 蛋白对 E-钙黏蛋白的表观遗传抑制作用增强了 HPV 感染细胞的迁移性[21]。

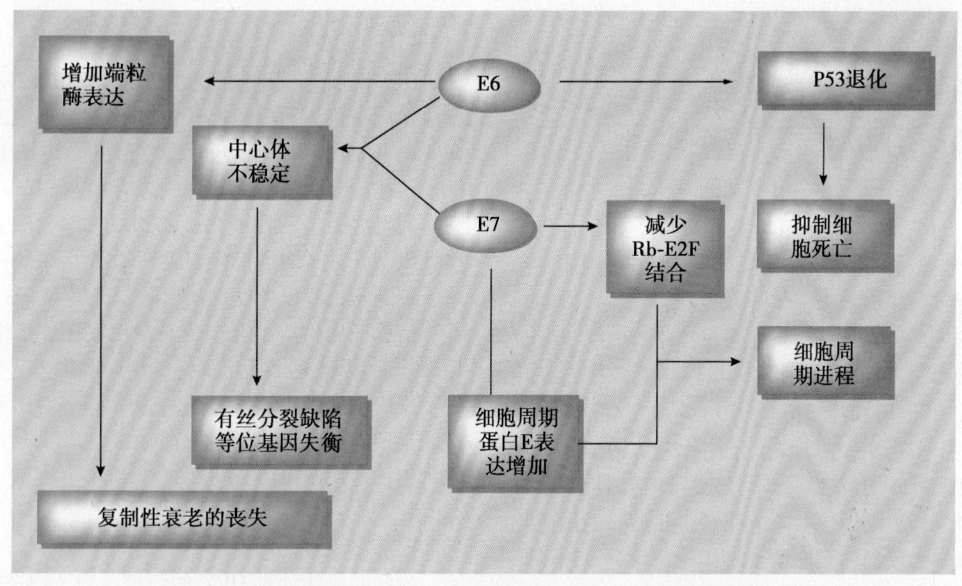

图 30-3 人乳头瘤病毒相关肿瘤转化的可能机制示意图

HPV 和人生殖系统肿瘤

危险因素

HPV 感染在年轻、性活跃的人群中普遍存在,感染率在生育早期达到高峰。HPV 感染通常是短暂的,并且随着年龄的增长而逐渐减少[22,23]。然而,持续感染同一类型的 HPV 与当前或之后罹患宫颈癌的风险密切相关[24]。至少有 30 种 HPV 亚型与宫颈癌有关,这些病毒亚型的危险性有显著的梯度差异。HPV 6 型和 11 型是典型的低危型,与生殖器疣(湿疣)相关[25,26]。相比之下,HPV 16 型是典型的高危型,出现在 50%以上的宫颈癌中[27]。HPV 18 主要与腺癌和神经内分泌癌相关[28,29]。然而,所有这些 HPV 均可存在于细胞学检查正常的女性中。还有许多其他类型的 HPV 与癌症相关,但其发生率较低。目前,已将中危和高危的 HPV 亚型合并为同一类别。无论感染高危型或低危型 HPV,都不能排除另一种不同危险型的 HPV 感染,这意味着感染一种病毒可能作为随后感染高危 HPV 的替代标记。在风险预测方面,正常巴氏宫颈涂片检查发现的大多数 HPV 都与患宫颈癌风险有一定关联[3],尽管相关程度低。

如果在一位女性生殖道内发现高危型 HPV,那么她患上高级别鳞状上皮内病变(HSIL)的风险如何?一般情况下,大约 15%的育龄女性携带高危型 HPV。HSIL 的风险从低于 5%到超过 80%不等,这取决于巴氏涂片是否正常、是否含有少量或非诊断性异型细胞(意义不明的异型鳞状上皮细胞[ASCUS]),或是否发生 HSIL。若重复检出感染同一类型的 HPV,那么即使巴氏涂片正常,风险也会增高近 20%[30]。据有力的理论推测,型内序列变异影响 HPV 16 感染后的结果[31]。然而,若要在治疗中应用这个信息需要进一步统一研究设计和结果,并需要更清楚地了解型内序列变异影响高级别宫颈上皮内瘤变(CIN)或癌症发生风险的机制。

年轻、性活跃的女性感染 HPV 和发生浸润前宫颈癌变的风险最高,此风险随着年龄的增长而显著下降。高达 39%的青少年可能首次检查就是阳性[22]。HPV 检出指数随着更年期的临近而进一步下降,这可能表明了从早期性行为开始和暴露于 HPV 以来产生了长期有效的免疫反应[23,24]。

免疫抑制的人尤其是器官移植患者患肛门-生殖器肿瘤或 HPV 感染已被充分报道[32]。人体免疫缺陷病毒(HIV)感染一直是研究的热点,HIV 阳性的女性中 HPV 阳性和持续性阳性的风险会增高[33]。此外,有研究发现 CD4 细胞计数<200 个/μL 的人持续性感染 HPV 的风险是 CD4 细胞计数正常者(>500 个/μL)的 1.9 倍(95%可信区间 CI 1.5~2.3)[33]。HIV 阳性的女性感染 HPV 后继发鳞状上皮内病变的风险也显著增加[34],虽然进展期癌前病变的比例增加不明显,但病变持续的风险增加[34,35]。感染 HIV 的女性患浸润性癌的风险不尽相同,但可能受免疫抑制的水平和持续时间的影响[36]。这与男同性恋者形成了鲜明对比,男同性恋者患肛门癌的风险在 HIV 感染人群中最高,尤其是应用抗反转录病毒治疗以后[37]。

总之,病毒和宿主相关的多种因素在病毒暴露之前、之中和之后以及病变进展过程中共同影响乳头瘤病毒相关性肛门生殖器肿瘤风险。

临床医学应用

宫颈癌的预防以巴氏涂片为基础,因为大多数宫颈癌由宫颈癌前病变(CIN)进展而来,而且通常需要很多年,所以检测这些癌前病变对预防宫颈癌至关重要。最近对巴氏试验指南进行了修订,以与在筛查中使用 HPV 检测的指南相一致。下一节将一并讨论这些问题。癌前病变可在医院用阴道镜识别,然后用醋酸鉴定[38]。可充分利用阴道镜对病变部位进行活检,常用方法是门诊去除病灶,包括冷冻治疗、激光和最近发展的宫颈环形电切术[39]。宫颈环形电切术针对整个转化区,切除病灶并用表皮再植的快速修复方法取代慢性修复过程。切除或消融后复发的原因可能是切除不当,也可能是治疗后又感染了其他 HPV。如果是切除,切缘阳性者复发的概率明显更高。再感染其他型 HPV 似乎能够解释为什么许多高级别癌前病变经消融后，复发的却是低级别癌前病变。除了免疫抑制的女性外，再次感染同一类型 HPV 的情况并不常见，在本章最后讨论了这些发现在癌症预防中的潜在意义。

巴氏涂片异常者管理过程和初筛中的 HPV 检测

宫颈细胞学检查异常的女性，HPV 检测是一种可行的管理方法。因为 HPV 与宫颈癌密切相关，而且在宫颈中高危型 HPV 感染占主导地位，因此大部分细胞学检查为低级别或高级别癌前病变的女性都有高危型 HPV 感染。因此，HPV 检测对这部分人群价值有限。然而，对那些具有非诊断性鳞状上皮异型（ASCUS）的女性，管理则陷入困境，临床医生必须决定是用阴道镜治疗还是进行巴氏涂片随访。

HPV 检测为给予阴道镜治疗或巴氏涂片随访的选择提供了又一种方法，可通过新的液基细胞学技术立即检测细胞学样本来实现。新一代 HPV 检测技术如杂交捕获Ⅱ试验的敏感性很高，在组织学证实为浸润前病变的女性中检出率达 95%[40]。如果 HPV 阴性，患有 ASCUS 的女性发生高级别 CIN 的风险<1%；但若 HPV 阳性，其发生高级别 CIN 的风险为 20%[40]。在有异常腺体细胞的涂片中也有类似的结果[41]。最近，该检测已被批准作为巴氏涂片的辅助检查，用于 30 岁以上女性的筛查。HPV 检测的依据是正常涂片和 HPV 检测均为阴性时的高阴性预测价值，如果双阴性则可延长筛查间隔。最近，美国癌症协会和美国预防工作组提出了如下筛查建议：首先，除非有宫颈癌病史，否则不建议对 21 岁以下和 65 岁以上的女性进行首次筛查。第二，将 21~65 岁女性的筛查间隔延长至 3 年。第三，如果伴有 HPV 检测，30 岁以上女性的筛查可延长至 5 年（见 http://www.uspreventiveservicestaskforce.org/uspstf/uspscerv.htm，http://www.cancer.org/Cancer/news/News/new-screening-guidelines-for-cervical-cancer）[42]。这些新的筛查建议可能会影响到筛查费用的保险支付。

诊断 HPV 感染的替代标志

早期宫颈癌的实验室管理基于既往研究制订的高危型 HPV（如 HPV 16）与 HSIL（CIN Ⅱ级和Ⅲ级）关联的标准。但是区分浸润前病变与良性炎症过程有一定困难，并且可能影响管理的决策。

提高诊断方法的准确性是那些旨在寻找生物标志物以简化鉴别 HPV 相关肿瘤与相似病变的研究的重点所在。由于 HPV 会干扰细胞功能，所以宿主基因的改变可能是 HPV 感染的"替代标记"。已报道在宫颈癌中表达上调的宿主基因包括端粒酶、p16ink4、细胞周期蛋白 E、Ki-67、MN 等[14]，其中一些基因如 Ki-67、细胞周期蛋白 E 和 p16ink4 在区分组织异常方面具有实用价值[14,15]。下肛门-生殖道专业课题组最近建议将 p16 染色作为组织学评价的辅助手段，阳性结果表现为连续水平线性（或块状）染色[43]。这种生物标记物最合适的用途是通过推断是否存在致癌 HPV 来印证组织学检查中 CIN2 或 CIN3 的诊断。多达 70% 以上的 CIN1 病变中此标记物可呈阳性染色，但仅 p16 免疫染色不能用于 CIN2 或 CIN3 的诊断[44]。此外，p16 强染色并不一定代表病变进展，经组织学证实 CIN2 病变中高达 67% 的病变会在 3 年内消退[45]。

临床管理

HPV 相关宫颈肿瘤的临床管理正不断调整，与切除病灶的方法保持一致。大多数巴氏涂片检测为低级别或高级别 CIN 或非典型涂片 HPV 阳性的女性需要行阴道镜检查。在检查阴性或活检诊断为低级别 CIN 的患者中，有 10%~13% 的人将在两年内发展为经活检确认的高级别 CIN。许多医生会随访那些低级别异常和阴道镜检查阴性的患者，在 6~12 个月内进行重复细胞学检查以关注发病风险。

活检证实的高级别 CIN 通常用宫颈环形电切术或锥形活检来处理，因此一个给定病例的结局取决于区分高级别和低级别上皮内病变的组织学标准的应用[44]。对所有子宫颈异常女性的长期随访（不论是否治疗）通常包括巴氏涂片评估，但最终也将包括定期的 HPV 检测。

预防

为阐明机体针对 HPV 的免疫反应，人们已经从研究融合蛋白和线性表位进展到体外生产病毒样颗粒（VLP）（图 30-4）[45~48]。VLP 是通过在真核表达系统中表达完整的乳头瘤病毒晚期区而产生的。VLP 含有可产生宿主免疫的构象表位，并可用于研究（或产生）宿主免疫[49,50]。这种研究方法是最具前景的，因为它提供了具有高度免疫原性的完整的病毒颗粒。最近大规模的试验已经证实了 VLP 疫苗接种的优点，证明疫苗可高度有效预防它所针对的 HPV 的感染及病变[51,52]。目前正在进行的测试多价疫苗的试验不仅包含 HPV 16，还包含 HPV 18、6 和 11 亚型（后两种针对生殖器疣）。实验结果显示，对未感染 HPV 的女性，该疫苗可有效预防 HPV 导致的宫颈和生殖器感染（有效率 95% 或以上）[53]。对已感染 HPV 的女性，其预防效果较低，HPV 相关疾病的发生仅降低不足 20%[54]。然而，对无特定疫苗的 HPV 类型，疫苗的有效率是 27%，对特定类型如 31、45 和 52 有交叉保护作用。因此接种 HPV 16 和 18 疫苗人群获益巨大[55]。此外，目前更多针对 HPV L2 的广谱疫苗正在研究中[56]。这些新的、更广谱的疫苗有望解决某些 HPV 类型流行的地区差异。鳞柱状上皮交界处与宫颈癌之间的紧密联系以及该部位起源细胞的发现，提高了预防性切除这个区域，进而显著降低宫颈癌风险的可能性。全世界宫颈癌的年发病率比阴道/外阴癌高出近 20 倍，这进一步证明了鳞柱状上皮交界处对癌症风险的潜在影响[57]。有趣的是，对冷冻消融后的 HPV 感染，以及鳞柱状上皮交界切除或消融后的局部复发模式和 CIN 分级差异的研究都表明，切除鳞柱状上皮

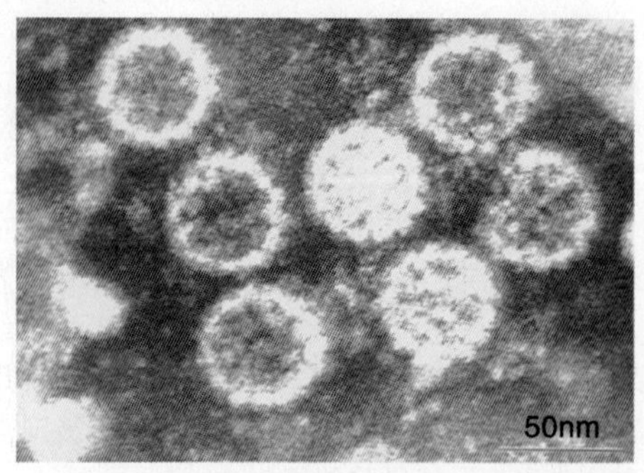

图 30-4 体外产生的乳头瘤病毒颗粒电子显微镜扫描图

交界处可能会对癌前病变风险产生深远的影响。这些信息能否转化为可行的癌症预防策略尚不清楚，还有待进一步的研究[58]。

（赵继敏 李鑫 译 陈新焕 赵继敏 陈瑶 校）

部分参考文献

1 Cullen AP, Reid R, Campion M, Lorincz AT. Analysis of the physical state of different human papillomavirus DNAs in intraepithelial and invasive cervical neoplasm. *J Virol*. 1991;**65**:606–612.

3 Koutsky LA, Holmes KK, Critchlow CW, et al. A cohort study of the risk of cervical intraepithelial neoplasia grade 2 or 3 in relation to papillomavirus infection. *N Engl J Med*. 1992;**327**:1272–1278.

4 FUTURE II Study Group. Quadrivalent vaccine against human papillomavirus to prevent high-grade cervical lesions. *N Engl J Med*. 2007;**356**:1925–1927.

7 (a) Marsh M. Original site of cervical carcinoma; topographical relationship of carcinoma of the cervix to the external os and to the squamocolumnar junction. *Obstet Gynecol*. 1956;7:444–452; (b) Richart RM. Cervical intraepithelial neoplasia. *Pathol Annu*. 1973;**8**:301–328.

8 Herfs M, Yamamoto Y, Laury A, et al. A discrete population of squamocolumnar junction cells implicated in the pathogenesis of cervical cancer. *Proc Natl Acad Sci U S A*. 2012;**109**:10516–10521.

9 Herfs M, Vargas SO, Yamamoto Y, et al. A novel blueprint for 'top down' differentiation defines the cervical squamocolumnar junction during development, reproductive life, and neoplasia. *J Pathol*. 2013;**229**:460–468.

10 Kines RC, Thompson CD, Lowy DR, Schiller JT, Day PM. The initial steps leading to papillomavirus infection occur on the basement membrane prior to cell surface binding. *Proc Natl Acad Sci U S A*. 2009;**106**:20458–20463.

13 Kreider JW, Howett MK, Wolfe SA, et al. Morphologic transformation in vivo of human uterine cervix with papillomavirus from condylomata acuminata. *Nature*. 1985;**317**:639.

14 Keating JT, Cviko A, Riethdorf S, et al. Ki-67, cyclin E, and p16INK4 are complementary surrogate biomarkers for human papilloma virus-related cervical neoplasia. *Am J Surg Pathol*. 2001;**25**:884–891.

15 Sano T, Masuda N, Oyama T, Nakajima T. Overexpression of p16 and p14ARF is associated with human papillomavirus infection in cervical squamous cell carcinoma and dysplasia. *Pathol Int*. 2002;**52**:375–383.

18 Rader JS, Gerhard DS, OíSullivan MJ, et al. Cervical intraepithelial neoplasia III shows frequent allelic loss in 3p and 6p. *Genes Chromosomes Cancer*. 1998;**22**:57–65.

19 Klingelhutz AJ, Foster SA, McDougall JK. Telomerase activation by the E6 gene product of human papillomavirus type 16. *Nature*. 1996;**380**:79–82.

22 Rosenfeld WD, Rose E, Vermund SH, et al. Follow-up evaluation of cervicovaginal human papillomavirus infection in adolescents. *J Pediatr*. 1992;**121**:307–311.

24 Bory JP, Cucherousset J, Lorenzato M, et al. Recurrent human papillomavirus infection detected with the hybrid capture II assay selects women with normal cervical smears at risk for developing high grade cervical lesions: a longitudinal study of 3091 women. *Int J Cancer*. 2002;**102**:519–525.

25 de Villiers EM, Gissmann L, zur Hausen H. Molecular cloning of viral DNA from human genital warts. *J Virol*. 1981;**40**:932–935.

26 Gissmann L, Wolnik L, Ikenberg H, et al. Human papillomavirus types 6 and 11 DNA sequences in genital and laryngeal papillomas and in some cervical cancers. *Proc Natl Acad Sci U S A*. 1983;**80**:560–563.

27 Durst M, Gissman L, Ikenberg H, zur Hausen H. A papillomavirus DNA from a cervical carcinoma and its prevalence in cancer biopsy samples from different geographic regions. *Proc Natl Acad Sci U S A*. 1983;**80**:3812.

29 Stoler MH, Walker AN, Mills SE. Small cell neuroendocrine carcinoma of the cervix: a human papillomavirus type 18 associated cervix cancer. *Lab Invest*. 1989;**60**:92A.

32 Fairley CK, Sheil AG, McNeil JJ, et al. The risk of ano-genital malignancies in dialysis and transplant patients. *Clin Nephrol*. 1994;**41**:101–105.

33 Ahdieh L, Klein RS, Burk R, et al. Prevalence, incidence, and type-specific persistence of human papillomavirus in human immunodeficiency virus (HIV)-positive and HIV-negative women. *J Infect Dis*. 2001;**184**:682–690.

35 La Ruche G, Leroy V, Mensah-Ado I, et al. Short-term follow up of cervical squamous intraepithelial lesions associated with HIV and human papillomavirus infections in Africa. *Int J STD AIDS*. 1999;**10**:363–368.

36 Parkin DM, Wabinga H, Nambooze S, Wabwire-Mangen F. AIDS-related cancers in Africa: maturation of the epidemic in Uganda. *AIDS*. 1999;**13**:2563–2570.

38 Richart RM. Current concepts in obstetrics and gynecology: the patient with an abnormal Pap smearóscreening techniques and management [review]. *N Engl J Med*. 1980;**302**:332–334.

40 Solomon D, Schifman M, Tarone R. Comparison of three management strategies for patients with atypical squamous cells of undetermined significance: baseline results from a randomized trial. *J Natl Cancer Inst*. 2001;**93**:293–299.

42 Hoyer H, Scheungraber C, Kuehne-Heid R, et al. Cumulative 5-year diagnoses of CIN2, CIN3 or cervical cancer after concurrent high-risk HPV and cytology testing in a primary screening setting. *Int J Cancer*. 2005;**116(1)**:136–143.

44 Crum CP. Our wages of CIN. *Obstet Gynecol*. 2012;**120**:1261–1262.

45 Moscicki AB, Ma Y, Wibbelsman C, et al. Rate of and risks for regression of cervical intraepithelial neoplasia 2 in adolescents and young women. *Obstet Gynecol*. 2010;**116**:1373–1380.

47 Zhou J, Sun XY, Stenzel DJ, Frazer IH. Expression of vaccinia recombinant HPV 16 L1 and L2 ORF proteins in epithelial cells is sufficient for assembly of HPV virionlike particles. *Virology*. 1991;**185**:251–257.

50 Rose RC, Bonnez W, Reichman RC, Garcea RL. Expression of human papillomavirus type 11 L1 protein in insect cells: in vivo and in vitro assembly of viruslike particles. *J Virol*. 1993;**67**:1936–1944.

51 Kirnbauer R, Booy F, Cheng N, et al. Papillomavirus L1 major capsid protein self-assembles into virus-like particles that are highly immunogenic. *Proc Natl Acad Sci U S A*. 1992;**89(24)**:12180–12184.

52 Ghim SJ, Jenson AB, Schlegel R. HPV-1 L1 protein expressed in cos cells displays conformational epitopes found on intact virions. *Virology*. 1992;**190(1)**: 548–552.

53 Koutsky LA, Ault KA, Wheeler CM, et al. Proof of Principle Study Investigators. A controlled trial of a human papillomavirus type 16 vaccine. *N Engl J Med*. 2002;**347**:1645–1651.

54 Harper DM, Franco EL, Wheeler C, et al. GlaxoSmithKline HPV Vaccine Study Group. Efficacy of a bivalent L1 virus-like particle vaccine in prevention of infection with human papillomavirus types 16 and 18 in young women: a randomised controlled trial. *Lancet*. 2004;**364**:1757–1765.

57 Chaturvedi AK. Beyond cervical cancer: burden of other HPV-related cancers among men and women. *J Adolesc Health*. 2010;**46(4 Suppl)**:S20–S26.

58 Herfs M, Somja J, Howitt BE, et al. Unique recurrence patterns of cervical intraepithelial neoplasia after excision of the squamocolumnar junction. *Int J Cancer*. 2015;**136**:1043–1052.

第 31 章 肝炎病毒与肝脏肿瘤

Hongyang Wang, MD ■ Guangwen Cao, MD, PhD ■ Jing Fu, MD, PhD ■ Guishuai Lv, MD

概述

肝炎是肝脏的一种炎症，由病毒感染或肝脏暴露于有毒物质如酒精或黄曲霉毒素 B 所引起。肝炎病毒是世界范围内最常见的肝炎病因，其中乙型肝炎病毒（HBV）和丙型肝炎病毒（HCV）可引起持续性的肝脏感染，并进一步发展为慢性肝炎、肝硬化，最终形成肝细胞癌（hepatocellular Carcinoma，HCC）。HBV 属于肝病毒科正肝病毒属，具有不完整的环形双链 DNA 基因组，包含四个重叠的开放阅读框（ORFs），分别编码外壳蛋白（HBsAg）、核心蛋白（HBcAg 和 HBeAg）、聚合酶和多功能非结构蛋白 X（HBx）。HBV 基因型和亚基因型具有明显的地理分布特征。在东亚，HBV 基因型以 B 型和 C 型较为流行。病毒性肝炎全球发病率的差异可能在于 HCV 和 HBV 流行情况的差异。据估计，57%的肝硬化可归因于 HBV（30%）或 HCV（27%）感染，78%的 HCC 可归因于 HBV（53%）或 HCV（25%）感染。在中国，高达 80%的 HCC 可归因于 HBV 感染，约 20%的 HCC 患者 HCV-RNA 检测呈阳性。除了 HBV 编码蛋白的致癌作用，HBV 感染诱导的病毒或宿主 DNA 突变也参与了 HCC 的发生。与 HBV 不同，HCV 属于黄病毒科肝病毒属，其基因组为单链正义 RNA。HCV 不在宿主基因组整合，也不包含任何已知的癌基因。HCV 诱发 HCC 的主要机制包括 HCV 病毒蛋白的致癌作用、脂肪变性和胰岛素抵抗、慢性炎症和纤维化、氧化应激和染色体不稳定。本章重点介绍肝炎以及 HBV 和 HCV 感染相关 HCC，包括流行病学、结构和基因型、病毒在 HCC 形成中的作用，以及早期诊断和预防。肝炎病毒选择性地感染特定宿主，增加其恶性肝脏肿瘤风险，这给全球医疗带来了负担。因此，肝炎和肝脏肿瘤发病率的上升对于公共卫生非常重要。

肝炎和肝脏肿瘤

肝脏疾病是世界范围内的主要疾病和死亡原因，包括乙型肝炎病毒（HBV）和丙型肝炎病毒（HCV）感染，酒精性肝病（ALD），非酒精脂肪性肝病（NAFLD）及肝硬化和 HCC[1]。因其在世界范围内的高发病率和不良的长期临床结局（包括肝功能失代偿引起的过早死亡、肝硬化和 HCC），肝脏疾病导致了严重的公共健康问题。在这些肝脏疾病中，由于疾病易感性、隐匿性和难治性，肝炎和 HCC 严重危害人类健康[1]。

人类肝炎病毒

选择性感染人肝细胞并导致肝脏疾病的病毒被称为人类肝炎病毒，包括甲型肝炎病毒（HAV）、HBV、HCV、丁型肝炎病毒（HDV）和戊型肝炎病毒（HEV）。HAV 或 HEV 通过粪-口传播途径，引起暂时性肝脏感染，可出现无症状感染或暴发性疾病。HAV 作为一种单链 RNA 病毒，是全球急性病毒性肝炎的主要病因，偶尔可引起急性肝衰竭。HEV 是一种单链无包膜 RNA 病毒，在一些亚洲和非洲国家流行。孕妇和慢性肝病患者在感染 HEV 后是暴发性肝衰竭的高危人群[2]。HBV（单独或合并感染 HDV 或重叠感染 HDV）和 HCV 可引起持续性肝脏感染，常导致慢性肝炎、肝硬化，最终形成 HCC。

HBV

HBV 属于肝病毒科正肝病毒属，具有长度约为 3.2kb 的环形不完整双链 DNA 基因组。HBV 基因组包含四个重叠的开放阅读框（ORF），分别编码外壳蛋白（HBsAg）、核心蛋白（HBcAg 和 HBeAg）、聚合酶和多功能非结构蛋白 X（HBx）。前 S（PreS）区包含前 S1（核苷酸 2848-3204）和前 S2（核苷酸 3205-154）两部分，与编码聚合酶基因（P 基因）的区域重叠。增强子Ⅱ（EnhⅡ；核苷酸 1636-1744）和基础核心启动子（BCP；核苷酸 1751-1769）区域与 X 基因重叠（核苷酸 1374-1835）。HBV 基因组包含两个调节 HBV 启动子转录的增强子，其中 BCP 控制前核心和核心区域的转录。入肝细胞后，HBV 进入肝细胞核。HBV 基因组在细胞核内形成一个松散的环状 DNA，随后转变为双链共价闭合环形 DNA（cccDNA）。HBV cccDNA 转录所有的病毒 RNA，包括作为复制 RNA 中间体的前基因组（pg）RNA。pgRNA、病毒核心蛋白和聚合酶蛋白在细胞浆中组装进入核壳体，随 pgRNA 在病毒聚合酶的作用下转变为 HBV DNA。在慢性 HBV 感染者体内，每日约有 10^{11} 个病毒颗粒被释放入循环系统，这些病毒颗粒在血浆中被清除的半衰期约为 1.2 天。在病毒复制过程中，部分双链 HBV DNA 是在病毒聚合酶的逆转录活性作用下由 RNA 中间体生成的。由于 HBV 逆转录酶缺乏校对功能，HBV 感染者在 HBeAg 阳性阶段其突变率为 $1.5\times10^{-5}-5\times10^{-5}$ 核苷酸替换/位点/年[3,4]。然而，极为重叠的 ORFs 限制了 HBV 基因组的演变，维持了病毒复制所需的重要蛋白质功能[5]。在免疫选择压力的作用下，具有可塑性的 HBV 基因组可行成多种病毒突变体。

目前已鉴定出八种 HBV 基因型（基因型 A-H），这些基因型在整个 HBV 基因组的序列差异大于 8%，或在 S 区的序列差异大于 4%。若全部核苷酸序列的差异为 4%～8%，这些基因型可进一步分为不同的亚基因型。基因型 A 的亚基因型 1～5，基因型 B 的亚基因型 1～8，基因型 C 的亚基因型 1～8 和基因型 D 的亚基因型 1～7 最近已被命名。HBV 基因型和亚基因型有独特的地理分布[3,6,7]。HBV 基因型 A1、A3、A4 和 A5 在非洲，尤其是西非流行，而基因型 A2 在欧洲流行。基因型 B 和 C 在亚洲流行。在 B 和 C 基因型中，亚基因型 B2 和 C2 在亚洲大部分地区流行。亚基因型 C4 偶见于澳大利亚的土著居民，常被称为澳大利亚土著亚型。亚基因型 B3～B8、C1、C3 和 C5～C8 出现在印度尼西亚和菲律宾。基因型 D 在北非、北亚、南亚、地中海地区和大多数欧洲国家流行。穆斯林种族中亚基因型 D1 最常见。亚基因型 D2 在俄罗斯和波罗的海地区流行。亚基因型 D4 和 D6 分别在大洋洲和印度尼西亚流行。HBV 基因型 E 在西非和中非流行。HBV 基因型 F、G 和 H 在中美洲和南美洲流行。HBV 基因型和亚基因型不仅与临床结局相关，还与对干扰素-α 治疗的反应性有关[7,8]。在 HBV 基因型 B 和 C 流行的东亚，基因型 B 更容易引起年轻人的急性感染，且比基因型 C 更容易被清除，而基因型 C 在急性感染后可引起更高的持续感染率，也更易引起肝硬化和 HCC[8～11]。因此，HBV 基因分型不仅对于重构人类和 HBV 进化史非常重要，而且也有助于揭示 HBV 感染的临床转归及对抗病毒治疗的反应。

发生在免疫系统不成熟的围生期或童年早期的感染常导致慢性 HBV 感染。成人 HBV 感染大多无症状或经历过一个急性期。侵入性医疗程序、家庭接触 HBV 携带者、身体护理和美容治疗，以及缺乏 HBV 疫苗接种是成人急性乙型肝炎的主要危险因素。在中国大陆，约有 8.5%的成人急性乙型肝炎患者将发展成慢性感染[9]。HBV 基因型 C 型（与 B 型相比）和 D 型（与其他 HBV 基因型相比）更容易在急性病程后引起持续感染[9,11]。人类白细胞抗原（HLA）在 *HLA-DP* 和 *HLA-DQ* 区域的基因多态性参与了 HBV 感染后的免疫失衡（如 Th1/Th2 细胞，Th17/Treg 细胞，中性粒细胞/淋巴细胞，中性粒细胞/$CD8^+$T 细胞以及 Th1/Th2 细胞因子平衡），这种免疫失衡可导致 HBV 持续感染并可能引起慢性肝脏炎症[12～14]。*HLA-DP* 等位基因多态性的发生率在不同种族间差异显著。根据 NCBI 数据库（http://www.ncbi.nlm.nih.gov/projects/snp/），可促进慢性 HBV 感染的 *HLA-DP*（或 *HLA-DQ*）等位基因是亚洲人群中的主要等位基因[13,14]，但在欧洲人群中却是变异等位基因。这可能是 HBV 持续感染更常发生在亚洲而非欧洲的原因之一。这些 *HLA-Ⅱ* 基因多态性可能使宿主更易维持慢性 HBV 感染，促进疾病相关 HBV 突变的免疫选择，并影响 HBV 突变引起肝硬化和 HCC 的风险。

HBV 与 HCC

通常情况下，如果缺乏有效治疗，所有的慢性肝炎最终都将发展成终末期肝病（end-stage liver diseases，ESLD），例如肝硬化和 HCC。大多数 ESLD 的临床结局较差。HCC 是全球范围内肿瘤致死的主要原因，其全球发病率的差异主要是由于 HCV 和 HBV 流行的差异[1]。2013 年，世界卫生组织报道原发性肝脏肿瘤在全球引起 745 517 例死亡，其中 HCC 是主要的组织类型[15]。另一有关全球死亡率的述评指出 2010 年 HCV 相关 HCC 的死亡人数约为 195 700。在中国，HCC 是第二大肿瘤致死原因，2009 年其致死率是 24.15/100 000[16]。中国每年约有 383 203 人死于肝脏肿瘤，占全球肝脏肿瘤死亡人数的 51%[16]。在中国，高达 80%的 HCC 病例可归因于 HBV 感染，约有 20%的 HCC 患者 HCV-RNA 检测阳性[17]。

流行病学

全球约有 20 亿人曾暴露于 HBV，其中 3.5 亿人是慢性 HBV 感染者。据估计 57%的肝硬化可归因于 HBV（30%）或 HCV（27%）感染，78%的 HCC 可归因于 HBV（53%）或 HCV（25%）感染[18]。台湾的一项前瞻性研究表明，对于 HBsAg 和 HCV 抗体双阳性的人群，累积寿命（30～75 岁）男性和女性的 HCC 发病率分别为 38.35%和 27.40%；对于仅有 HBsAg 阳性的人群，HCC 发病率分别为 27.38%和 7.99%；对于 HBsAg 和 HCV 抗体均为阴性的人群，HCC 发病率分别为 1.55%和 1.03%[19]。前瞻性流行病学研究已证实男性、年龄增长、肝硬化、高病毒载量、HBeAg 阳性、HBV 基因型 C（与基因型 B 相比）、低白蛋白、丙氨酸氨基转移酶（ALT）升高，以及病毒 A1762T/G1764A 突变均可独立增加 HBV 慢性感染患者的 HCC 风险[11,19～23]。HBV 的“突变-选择-适应”，即一种病毒进化过程，参与了 HCC 的发生。在这个过程中，特别是在 HBeAg 血清转换过程中，HBV 累积 HCC 风险相关突变，这些突变主要发生在 HBV 基因组的核心启动子区和前 S 区[24～26]。A1762T/G1764A 突变可预测 HCC 的发生，可能是因为这种突变发生在进化过程的早期[27]。在 HCC 发生前收集得到的有关人群、临床和病毒因素的信息可评估患者预后，并能在 HBV 感染者中预测肝癌发生。

HBV 突变在肝癌发生中的作用

在长期进化过程中，HBV 抗原诱导的免疫应答不足会选择 HCC 相关的 HBV 基因突变。只有最适应免疫系统的 HBV 株/变异体才能在肝脏中生存和发展。HLA-Ⅱ抗原和其他炎症因子，如 NF-κB 和 STAT3 的遗传倾向性可能参与了 HBV 感染时免疫失衡，导致了持续感染和肝脏慢性炎症，最终促进了 HCC 风险相关 HBV 突变的产生[13,28,29]。炎症因子至少部分通过激活胞苷脱氨酶促进 HBV 突变。

宿主体细胞突变

胞苷脱氨酶及其类似物不仅可以促进 HBV 突变的形成，还可以促进体细胞的突变，它们的表达和活性可被炎症过程中的促炎细胞因子激活[5]。已发现，在一些关键基因中存在许多重要的 HCC 相关体细胞突变，如 RNA 编辑基因（*ADAR1*、*ADAR2*、*KHDRBS2* 和 *RTL1*）、染色质重塑基因（*ARID1A*、*ARID1B* 和 *ARID2*）、DNA 结合基因（*HOXA1*）、生长因子信号通路基因（*CDH8*、*CDK14*、*CNTN2*、*ERRFI1*、*RPS6KA3*、*P62* 和 *PROKR2*）、转录调节基因（*AXIN1*、*CCNG1*、*CTNNB1*、*IRF2*、*NFE2L2*、*PARP4*、*PAX5*、*ST18*、*TP53*、*TRRAP* 和 *ZNF717*）、细胞结构修饰基因（*FLNA* 和 *VCAM1*）、表观遗传修饰基因（*MLL3*）和 JAK/STAT 通路基因（*JAK1* 和 *JAK2*）[30]。这些体细胞突变会影响到可作为肝癌侵袭治疗靶点的重要信号通路。

HBV 编码蛋白的功能

①HBV 衣壳蛋白、中等（前 S2/S）或大衣壳蛋白（前 S1/前 S2/S）截短体的过量生成可以激活细胞信号转导通路或内质网（ER）应激通路，通过上调细胞周期蛋白 A 的表达、激活 c-Raf-1 和细胞外调节激酶（ERK）信号通路来刺激细胞增殖。S 蛋白在 ER 中的累积可激活未折叠蛋白反应并引起氧化应激。表皮生长因子受体（EGFR）过度表达发生在 40%～70%的人类 HCC 中，与肿瘤发生密切有关[31]。EGFR 介导的 Raf-MEK-ERK 和 PI3K-Akt 通路的异常活化在许多人类肿瘤，包括 HCC 中均很常见，并与肿瘤的生长和进展密切相关[32]。此外，同源配体或 EGFR 高表达引起的 EGFR 通路活化与肝癌预后不良密切相

关。②HBx可作为多个细胞信号通路的反式激活子,包括参与HBV相关HCC发生的Wnt通路,还可通过与肿瘤抑制子APC相互作用来激活Wnt/β-catenin通路。HBx能够增强HCC的侵袭和转移能力。例如,近期有研究利用HBx转基因小鼠和人HBV相关HCC样本,证实HBx的表达可促进肝脏祖细胞(hepatic progenitor cells,HPCs)的扩增和致瘤性,进而在乙基二硫代氨基甲酸酯(DDC)诱导的小鼠模型中介导肿瘤形成。这些研究为HBx在慢性肝炎感染和肝脏肿瘤中的作用提供了新的解释[33]。羧酸末端截短型HBx蛋白(Ct-HBx)是HBV DNA整合到宿主基因组后的一种常见形式,与全长型HBx相比,Ct-HBx可以更有效地增强HCC细胞的侵袭和转移能力。HBV基因组整合至人端粒酶逆转录酶(TERT)基因启动子区常以高克隆比例出现,这种整合可增加TERT的表达[5]。整合到特定宿主基因组位点的倾向和插入片段的特征能否赋予HBV整合更大的致癌潜能有待进一步阐明。

肝癌的早期诊断和预防

HCC在世界各国的5年总生存率约为10%。这种令人沮丧的临床转归部分是由于缺乏及时诊断的有效方法,仅有30%~40%的HCC患者在诊断后适于接受有效的治疗。甲胎蛋白(AFP)是临床应用的肝癌诊断生物标志物,但在常规使用20ng/ml作为临界值时,其敏感性较低(25%~65%),尤其是早期肝癌的检测[34]。此外,许多非恶性慢性肝脏疾病患者的血清AFP浓度亦升高,包括15%~58%的急性-慢性肝炎患者和11%~47%肝硬化患者[34]。因此,目前急需新的、可靠的诊断标志物来改善HCC患者的临床结局。

Glypican-3(GPC3)是一种硫酸乙酰肝素糖蛋白,在约70%的肝癌病例中高表达[35],但在癌前病变和正常肝组织中表达较低[36]。GPC3被认为是肝癌诊断的生物标志物,多项研究证实GPC3是一种有吸引力的肝脏肿瘤特异性靶点[37]。此外,临床前探索性研究亦表明GPC3是最有希望的HCC标记物之一[38]。目前,GPC3病理检测试剂盒已用于HCC的诊断和分型,尤其是肝脏良恶性肿瘤的鉴别诊断,因此为GPC3阳性HCC的治疗提供了一个有效的干预策略[37]。因GPC3对患者个体化治疗具有诊断价值且可避免对良性病变的过度治疗,GPC3试剂盒已被中国食品药品监督管理局(CFDA)批准在临床推广应用。Dickkopf-1(DKK1)是一种经典Wnt信号通路的分泌型拮抗剂,在HCC组织中过表达,但在相应的非癌组织中检测不到。一项大规模多中心研究表明DKK1在肝癌诊断中可代偿AFP的作用,增加AFP阴性HCC患者的检出率,并可鉴别诊断HCC与非恶性慢性肝脏疾病[38]。一项涵盖正常人、慢性乙型肝炎、肝硬化和HCC的大规模人群研究表明一种血浆microRNA组合(血浆miR-122、miR-192、miR-21、miR-223、miR-26a、miR-27a和miR-801)是潜在的高准确性的肝癌诊断循环标志物。此microRNA组合含有七个通过多元logistic回归模型筛选出的microRNA,在肝癌诊断中具有高准确性,尤其是对于可在治疗中获益的BCLC早期(0和A)HCC患者[39]。

重要的是,近零距离光交联和串联亲和纯化证实前S1的受体结合区可以与主要在肝脏表达的多次跨膜转运体牛磺胆酸钠协同转运多肽(NTCP)特异性相互作用。这表明NTCP是HBV和HDV的功能性受体,因此,它对于HBV感染及HBV相关HCC的治疗具有重要意义[40]。

乙肝疫苗接种对HBV未感染者有效。然而,针对全球3.5亿HBV携带者,抗病毒药物治疗对慢性HBV感染者有效。活动性炎症刺激的HBV复制对于HBV诱导的肝癌发生是必不可少的。与非活动性HBV携带者相比,HCC更易发生于活动性慢性乙型肝炎患者,即使这些患者口服了核苷类似物进行治疗[41]。IFN-α和/或核苷类似物的标准抗病毒治疗可明显减轻肝脏炎症,改善肝功能,进而显著降低HBV感染者的HCC发生并提高HCC患者手术治疗后的生存率[41~43]。此外,现有的研究表明肝癌患者miR-26的表达水平与其存活率及对IFN-α辅助治疗的反应相关,microRNA在肝组织中的表达模式在男性和女性HCC患者间存在差异[44]。值得注意的是,这些结果包含了HBV阳性率高的中国患者。HBV复制是炎性环境中HCC进化的驱动因素。因为大约30%的男性和10%的女性HBV携带者在其一生中可能会发展成HCC,所以确定哪些HBV感染者更易发展为HCC非常重要,并需要具有成本效益的抗病毒治疗和对早期肝癌的定期筛查。抗病毒治疗有助于肝功能的正常化,可降低HBV相关HCC的复发,提高术后生存率。中国东方肝胆外科医院开展的随机对照试验(RCT)表明核苷酸/核苷类似物(NA)可显著减少肝癌复发和肝癌相关死亡。与对照组相比,HCC患者接受抗病毒治疗可显著降低早期复发率,改善术后6个月的肝功能($P<0.001$)。这些肝功能恢复的HCC患者较未恢复者具有更高的2年无复发生存(RFS)率。此外,在接受抗病毒治疗组,Ct-HBx在肝癌邻近肝脏组织的表达可显著预测更差的RFS[43]。

在世界范围内手术切除仍是具备良好肝功能HCC患者的一线治疗手段,但术后5年的复发率高达70%。在切除的肿瘤组织、癌旁组织和外周血中能检测到一些预示HCC术后复发的预后因素。在肿瘤中,中性粒细胞/CD8$^+$ T细胞和Treg/CD8$^+$ T细胞比值升高,促血管生成因子如缺氧诱导因子-1-α(HNF-1-α)和细胞生长/存活相关因子如CD24的高表达,以及炎症信号通路如Wnt、NF-κB和STAT3等通路的激活可预测肝癌的早期复发。在癌旁组织中,高水平HBV DNA、HBV突变、高密度的巨噬细胞、激活的星状细胞和肥大细胞、高水平的巨噬细胞集落刺激因子/受体及胎盘生长因子、Th1/Th2样细胞因子转换、炎症相关标志和肿瘤发生相关通路的激活可预测HCC晚期复发。术前外周血中高水平HBV DNA、HBV突变和基因型、中性粒细胞/淋巴细胞高比值、高浓度的巨噬细胞迁移抑制因子和骨桥蛋白预示着HCC预后不良[45]。作为一种化学治疗药物,索拉非尼部分通过靶向抑制过度激活的、与术后肝再生相关的ERK通路发挥作用。目前,索拉非尼是第一个可显著延长晚期肝癌患者生存的系统性药物。最近,研究证实早期肝癌患者手术切除后使用索拉非尼可抑制术后复发并改善预后。因此,尽管缺乏特异性,索拉非尼目前仍是肝癌患者的标准治疗药物[46]。

随着HBV感染人数的增多,早期诊断和及时治疗对于炎症驱动的肝癌更为重要。即使靶向激酶依赖是肿瘤治疗的有效策略,EGFR抑制剂在肝癌患者中显示出令人失望的临床结果。有关研究报道了在炎症驱动的肝癌形成过程中，Kuffer 细胞或巨噬细胞中的 EGFR 信号通路发挥了重要作用[40]。EGFR 为肝脏巨噬细胞转录生成 IL-6 所必需，后者启动肝细胞增殖和肝癌发生。重要的是，EGFR 阳性肝脏巨噬细胞的出现与 HCC 病人较短的生存期相关[47]。此研究表明非肿瘤细胞中的 EGFR 具有肿瘤促进作用，这可能带来更有效的精准治疗策略。EGFR 阳性 Kupffer 细胞可能成为一种预后标志物和潜在的 HCC 治疗靶点。

丙肝病毒

HCV 属于黄病毒科的肝炎病毒属。它是一个小包膜病毒，带有单链正义 RNA 基因组，长度 9.6kb。它以高度脂化的病毒颗粒形式循环。目前有六种已知的主要基因型和许多亚基因型。这种遗传变异性促进了病毒的持久性，产生了免疫逃逸的病毒突变体，并对抗病毒治疗形成耐受。

HCV 病毒一旦进入细胞，病毒 RNA 基因组暴露并在细胞质内转录为单个含有 3 011 个氨基酸的长链多肽[48]。在宿主和病毒蛋白酶作用下，HCV 多肽剪切生成 10 种病毒蛋白。这些蛋白质进一步分类为结构蛋白（C、E1 和 E2）和 NS 蛋白（p7、NS2、NS3、NS4A、NS4B、NS5A 和 NS5B）。结构蛋白参与子代病毒的组装，形成两种衣壳糖蛋白（E1 和 E2）和一种核衣壳蛋白（核心蛋白）[49,50]。核心蛋白不仅对病毒颗粒的组装至关重要，并且具有多种调节功能，包括胞内转录、病毒诱导的转化和信号转导[51]。NS 蛋白负责病毒的复制和传播[52,53]。HCV 基因组在编码衣壳蛋白的高变区出现快速突变，以逃避免疫监视。大多数的 HCV 感染者发展为慢性感染，并最终转为肝硬化。

2005 年，预计有超过 1.85 亿人 HCV 抗体阳性，占世界人口的 2.8%。但是，HCV 流行率在不同国家、地域、年龄和风险群体间存在明显差异，从 0.1%到 5%不等。受灾最严重的地区是亚洲中东部和北非。在美国，估计有 390 万人（占总人口的 1.8%）感染 HCV。中国过去被认为是 HCV 感染相对高发地区。根据 1992 年在中国大部分地区进行的一次全国流行病学调查，总人口中 HCV 感染率预计平均为 3.2%，输血或血液制品是主要的感染途径。自 1993 年以来，对 HCV 抗体的强制性筛查和其他防止血源性疾病传播的预防措施广泛实施，HCV 感染新发率已急剧下降。2006 年的全国性调查表明中国 HCV 感染率仅为 0.43%[54]。

HCV 基因型在世界各地也呈现出显著差异[1]。HCV 变异体可分为六种基因型。HCV-1b 是世界范围内最常见的基因型，与肝硬化和慢性肝炎患者相比，HCV-1b 在 HCC 患者中更常见。美国以基因型 1a 为主，欧洲和中国以基因型 1b 型为主。在中国，1b 基因型占 68.4%，2a 基因型占 19.5%[55]。有趣的是，基因型 1b 病毒更易通过输血和医疗程序传播，而基因型 6a 病毒更易通过静脉药物使用（IDU）和性传播[56]。在一定程度上，西方国家和中国 HCV 基因型的差异可能与每个国家人群对 Peg-IFN-α 和利巴韦林（RBV）治疗的反应性有关[57]。此外，在白细胞介素（IL）-28B 基因区域附近的单核苷酸多态性也被发现与 HCV 感染者接受 Peg-IFN-α/RBV 治疗的有效性有关[58]。中国 HCV 患者的 rs12979860 C 等位基因的频率高于白种人患者。一项大规模队列研究表明中国 HCV 感染者的主要病毒基因型为 1b（占 60%～70%），宿主 IL28b rs12979860 基因型主要为 CC（占 84%）[59]。这些数据表明，IL28B 等位基因频率和 HCV 基因型的全球差异可能解释了为何中国患者对 Peg-IFN-α/RBV 治疗的反应更好。

HCV 与 HCC

全球有 1.3 亿～1.5 亿人慢性感染 HCV[60]。只有少数感染者能自行清除病毒，大多数 HCV 感染者，55%～85%，发展为慢性 HCV 感染，并具有较高的患肝硬化和 HCC 的风险[61~63]。慢性 HCV 感染者在 20 年内发展为肝硬化的风险为 15%～30%。升高的 HCV 载量显著增加 HCC 风险。据估计，HCV 感染使 HCC 的发生风险上升至 17 倍[64]。HCV 感染至肝硬化发病的平均时间为 13～25 年，至 HCC 发病的时间为 17～32 年[65]。在 HCV 感染的肝硬化患者中，HCC 的年发病率为 3%～5%[66]。此外，有效清除 HCV 感染可降低肝病相关的总体死亡率和 HCC 发生率，这表明了 HCV 的重要作用[67]。

HCV 是一种 RNA 病毒，具有独特的细胞质内生命周期。与 HBV 感染不同，HCV 不存在宿主基因组整合，也不包含任何已知的致癌基因。HCV 诱导肝癌发生的机制错综复杂，已知的一些机制包括 HCV 病毒蛋白的致癌作用、脂肪变性和胰岛素抵抗、慢性炎症和纤维化、氧化应激和染色体不稳定性[68~71]。有报道称在实验动物模型中，HCV 编码的蛋白-核心蛋白、E2、NS3 和 NS5A-通过与许多影响细胞存活、增殖、迁移和转化的宿主因子和信号通路相互作用，直接参与致瘤过程[72~74]。HCV 核心蛋白还可以影响或结合脂肪酸转运和分解代谢中起重要作用的一些分子[72~74]。HCV 相关的肝脂肪变性、胰岛素抵抗和氧化应激可导致慢性肝脏炎症、凋亡和纤维化。这些机制对慢性 HCV 患者肝硬化和 HCC 的发生至关重要。

预防和治疗

由于缺乏疫苗，HCV 感染的一级预防主要是降低高危人群的病毒暴露。在 HCV 感染者中，有 15%～45%的人可在 6 个月内不经任何治疗而自行清除病毒。当需要治疗时，目前 HCV 的标准治疗是以干扰素和 RBV 联合抗病毒治疗，这对所有的 HCV 基因型都有效。以干扰素为基础的有效治疗方案已应用许多年，实现对抗病毒治疗的持续病毒学应答（SVR）与发病率和死亡率的改善有关[75,76]。此外，随着直接口服抗病毒药物（DAA）的快速发展，无干扰素治疗方案治疗 HCV 感染正在成为现实，它们比干扰素治疗更有效、更安全、耐受性更好。DAA 方案也可以显著降低检测要求，增加治愈率，进而简化 HCV 治疗。

12 周疗程的无干扰素治疗方案的 SVR 率为 90%或更高。人们期待这种治疗方案可以尽早应用于大多数无肝硬化的 HCV 患者[77,78]。无干扰素 DAA 方案在肝硬化患者中的应用经验有限，现有数据表明一些方案的 SVR 率较低[79]。因此，HCV 的早期诊断和及时治疗是很重要的。

（付静　译　吕桂帅　于乐兴　校）

部分参考文献

1 Wang FS, Fan JG, Zhang Z, Gao B, Wang HY. The global burden of liver disease: the major impact of China. *Hepatology*. 2014;**60(6)**:2099–2108.

2 Wedemeyer H, Pischke S, Manns MP. Pathogenesis and treatment of hepatitis e virus infection. *Gastroenterology*. 2012;**142(6)**:1388–1397.e1.

4 Orito E, Mizokami M, Ina Y, et al. Host-independent evolution and a genetic classification of the hepadnavirus family based on nucleotide sequences. *Proc Natl Acad Sci U S A*. 1989;**86(18)**:7059–7062.

6 Yin J, Zhang H, He Y, et al. Distribution and hepatocellular carcinoma-related viral properties of hepatitis B virus genotypes in Mainland China: a community-based study. *Cancer Epidemiol Biomarkers Prev*. 2010;**19(3)**:777–786.

8 Wai CT, Chu CJ, Hussain M, Lok AS. HBV genotype B is associated with better response to interferon therapy in HBeAg(+) chronic hepatitis than genotype C. *Hepatology*. 2002;**36**:1425–1430.

9 Zhang HW, Yin JH, Li YT et al. Risk factors for acute hepatitis B and its progression to chronic hepatitis in Shanghai, China. *Gut*. 2008;**57(12)**:1713–1720.

11 Chan HL, Tse CH, Mo F, et al. High viral load and hepatitis B virus subgenotype ce are associated with increased risk of hepatocellular carcinoma. *J Clin Oncol*. 2008;**26(2)**:177–182.

12 Kamatani Y, Wattanapokayakit S, Ochi H et al. A genome-wide association study identifies variants in the HLA-DP locus associated with chronic hepatitis B in Asians. *Nat Genet*. 2009;**41(5)**:591–595.

15 Globocan. *Estimated Incidence, Mortality and Prevalence Worldwide in 2012* (2012), http://globocan.iarc.fr/Pages/fact_sheets_cancer.aspx (accessed 12 October 2015).

18 Perz JF, Armstrong GL, Farrington LA, Hutin YJ, Bell BP The contributions of hepatitis B virus and hepatitis C virus infections to cirrhosis and primary liver cancer worldwide. *J Hepatol*. 2006;**45(4)**:529–538.

19 Huang YT, Jen CL, Yang HI, et al. Lifetime risk and sex difference of hepatocellular carcinoma among patients with chronic hepatitis B and C. *J Clin Oncol*. 2011;**29(27)**:3643–3650.

20 Wong VW, Chan SL, Mo F, et al. Clinical scoring system to predict hepatocellular carcinoma in chronic hepatitis B carriers. *J Clin Oncol*. 2010;**28**:1660–1665.

21 Lee MH, Yang HI, Liu J, et al. Prediction models of long-term cirrhosis and hepatocellular carcinoma risk in chronic hepatitis B patients: risk scores integrating host and virus profiles. *Hepatology*. 2013;**58**:546–554.

22 Yuen MF, Tanaka Y, Fong DY, et al. Independent risk factors and predictive score for the development of hepatocellular carcinoma in chronic hepatitis B. *J Hepatol*. 2009;**50**:80–88.

27 Li Z, Xie Z, Ni H, et al. Mother-to-child transmission of hepatitis B virus: evolution of hepatocellular carcinoma-related viral mutations in the post-immunization era. *J Clin Virol*. 2014;**61(1)**:47–54.

29 Zhang Q, Ji XW, Hou XM, et al. Effect of functional nuclear factor-kappaB genetic polymorphisms on hepatitis B virus persistence and their interactions with viral mutations on the risk of hepatocellular carcinoma. *Ann Oncol*. 2014;**25(12)**:2413–2419.

30 Ji X, Zhang Q, Du Y, et al. Somatic mutations, viral integration and epigenetic modification in the evolution of hepatitis B virus-induced hepatocellular carcinoma. *Curr Genomics*. 2014;**15(6)**:1–12.

31 Buckley AF, Burgart LJ, Sahai V, Kakar S. Epidermal growth factor receptor expression and gene copy number in conventional hepatocellular carcinoma. *Am J Clin Pathol*. 2008;**129**:245–251.

33 Wang C, Yang W, Yan HX, et al. Hepatitis B virus X (HBx) induces tumorigenicity of hepatic progenitor cells in 3,5-diethoxycarbonyl-1,4-dihydrocollidine-treated HBx transgenic mice. *Hepatology*. 2012;**55(1)**:108–120.

34 Gao H, Li K, Tu H, et al. Development of T cells redirected to glypican-3 for the treatment of hepatocellular carcinoma. *Clin Cancer Res*. 2014;**20**:6418–6428.

35 Marrero JA, Lok ASF. Newer markers for hepatocellular carcinoma. *Gastroenterology*. 2004;**127**:S113–S119.

36 Shen Q, Fan J, Yang XR, et al. Serum DKK1 as a protein biomarker for the diagnosis of hepatocellular carcinoma: a large-scale, multicentre study. *Lancet Oncol*. 2012;**13(8)**:817–826.

37 Zhao J, Yu L, Gao X, et al. Plasma microRNA panel to diagnose hepatitis B virus–related hepatocellular carcinoma. *J Clin Oncol*. 2011;**29(36)**:4781–4788.

38 Nakatsura T, Yoshitake Y, Senju S, et al. Glypican-3, overexpressed specifically in human hepatocellular carcinoma, is a novel tumor marker. *Biochem Biophys Res Commun*. 2003;**306(1)**:16–25.

40 Yan H, Zhong G, Xu G, Li W, et al. Sodium taurocholate cotransporting polypeptide is a functional receptor for human hepatitis B and D virus. *Elife*. 2012;**1**:e00049.

41 Cho JY, Paik YH, Sohn W, et al. Patients with chronic hepatitis B treated with oral antiviral therapy retain a higher risk for HCC compared with patients with inactive stage disease. *Gut*. 2014;**63(12)**:1943–1950.

42 Papatheodoridis GV, Lampertico P, Manolakopoulos S, Lok A. Incidence of hepatocellular carcinoma in chronic hepatitis B patients receiving nucleos(t)ide therapy: a systematic review. *J Hepatol*. 2010;**53**:348–356.

43 Yin J, Li N, Han Y, et al. Effect of antiviral treatment with nucleotide/nucleoside analogs on postoperative prognosis of hepatitis B virus-related hepatocellular carcinoma: a two-stage longitudinal clinical study. *J Clin Oncol*. 2013;**31**:3647–3655.

44 Ji J, Shi J, Budhu A, et al. MicroRNA expression, survival, and response to interferon in liver cancer. *N Engl J Med*. 2009;**361(15)**:1437–1447.

45 Chen L, Zhang Q, Chang W, Du Y, Zhang H, Cao G. Viral and host inflammation-related factors that can predict the prognosis of hepatocellular carcinoma. *Eur J Cancer*. 2012;**48(13)**:1977–1987.

47 Lanaya H, Natarajan A, Komposch K, et al. EGFR has a tumour-promoting role in liver macrophages during hepatocellular carcinoma formation. *Nat Cell Biol*. 2014;**16(10)**:972–981, 1–7.

49 Fusco DN, Chung RT. Novel therapies for hepatitis C: insights from the structure of the virus. *Annu Rev Med*. 2012;**63**:373–387.

54 Chen YS, Li L, Cui FQ, et al. A seroepidemiological study on hepatitis C in China. *Zhonghua Liu Xing Bing Xue Za Zhi*. 2011;**32**:888–891.

57 Ghany MG, Liang TJ. Current and future therapies for hepatitis C virus infection. *N Engl J Med*. 2013;**368**:1907–1917.

60 WHO (World Health Organization). *Hepatitis C*. Rep. 164. Geneva: WHO; 2014. http://www.who.int/mediacentre/factsheets/fs164/en/.

67 Hino K, Okita K. Interferon therapy as chemoprevention of hepatocarcinogenesis in patients with chronic hepatitis C. *J Antimicrob Chemother*. 2004;**53**: 19–22.

77 Zeuzem S, Jacobson IM, Baykal T, et al. Retreatment of HCV with ABT-450/r-ombitasvir and dasabuvir with ribavirin. *N Engl J Med*. 2014;**370(17)**:1604–1614.

78 Feld JJ, Kowdley KV, Coakley E, et al. Treatment of HCV with ABT-450/rombitasvir and dasabuvir with ribavirin. *N Engl J Med*. 2014;**370(17)**:1594–1603.

79 Afdhal N, Reddy KR, Nelson DR, et al. Ledipasvir and sofosbuvir for previously treated HCV genotype 1 infection. *N Engl J Med*. 2014;**370(16)**:1483–1493.

第 32 章　寄生虫

Mervat Z. El Azzouni, MD, PhD ■ Radwa G. Diab, MD, MBBCH, PhD

概述

研究发现寄生虫可能在肿瘤的发生中发挥一定的作用。埃及血吸虫已被证实在膀胱癌(BC)的发生发展中扮演着重要的角色。其他种类的血吸虫如日本血吸虫被认为是结直肠癌的致癌物,特别在远东地区。华支睾吸虫和后睾吸虫被证实可诱发肝胆管癌。在非洲,Epstein-Barr 病毒(EBV)感染和伯基特淋巴瘤(BL)之间具有很强的相关性,而恶性疟原虫在其中发挥了明显的促进作用。慢性炎症被认为是寄生虫诱发癌症最常见的机制;然而某些致癌物质、癌基因、DNA 突变和其他因素也都被认为在寄生虫感染过程中发挥了增强致癌的作用。值得注意的是,尽管有上述数据,但是某些寄生虫似乎可以调节宿主的免疫反应,从而对癌症起到抑制或预防的作用。重新评估传染性病原体的临床重要性有广阔的前景,也是一个未来需要关注的问题。

寄生虫感染的严重程度与其流行程度密切相关[1]。因此,如果相对罕见的某些肿瘤在一个寄生虫病流行地区过度频发的话,就需要考虑寄生虫在肿瘤发生中所起的作用。在这方面,两个最有趣的例子是血吸虫病与膀胱癌以及疟疾与伯基特淋巴瘤的关系。既往经典的参考文献已进行过相关的报道[2]。

血吸虫病和膀胱癌

1911 年,Fergusson 首次在埃及发现血吸虫可能在诱导膀胱癌中具有潜在作用[3];1994 年,国际癌症研究机构(IARC)最终确认了这一问题,认为寄生虫是一种致癌物质[4]。如果在全国大范围筛查并实施包括控制钉螺数量和大规模治疗运动在内的预防措施,血吸虫膀胱癌(BBC)理论上是可以预防的[5]。

流行病学方面

欧洲、北美洲和非洲北部是膀胱癌发病率最高的地区[6]。在西方国家,吸烟和职业暴露是主要危险因素;然而由于吸烟习惯的改变,膀胱癌的发病率和死亡率在过去的十年中有所下降[7]。在发展中国家特别是非洲和中东地区,埃及血吸虫慢性感染约占膀胱癌病因的 50%[8],其中埃及男子的死亡率最高(16.3/100 000)[9]。埃及血吸虫感染和膀胱癌之间的相关性比其他任何一种寄生虫感染都密切的多[10],并且被划分为一类致癌物[11]。埃及血吸虫与膀胱癌之间的关系最初是通过病例对照研究和膀胱癌发生与寄生虫流行的密切关系而建立的。在临床上,这基于寄生虫卵的存在和血吸虫诱发的 BC 病理组织学的改变进一步明确了血吸虫与膀胱癌发生间的密切联系[12]。

膀胱癌在形态学上具有异质性。超过 90% 的癌症是移行细胞癌(TCC)[13],例如与吸烟和职业危害有关的膀胱癌[14]。在非洲,膀胱鳞状细胞癌(SCC)在血吸虫流行的埃及费拉欣和莫桑比克、津巴布韦和赞比亚(前罗德西亚)中发病率非常高[15~17]。然而,随着发展中国家城市化和工业化的进展,风险因素的变化导致膀胱癌类型向 TCC 转变[7]。在埃及,20 世纪 60 年代修建的高坝导致水流的变化,这直接影响到钉螺的中间宿主,埃及血吸虫逐渐被曼氏血吸虫所取代,而曼氏血吸虫引起的是肠道疾病,不是泌尿系统疾病[18]。此外,自 1977 年以来,埃及开展了有效的口服药物治疗运动,明显减少了泌尿系统血吸虫病的发生[19]。值得注意的是,尽管埃及的埃及血吸虫感染率大幅下降,膀胱癌仍然是男性中最常见的癌症。这是因为血吸虫相关性膀胱癌发病率的下降逐渐被吸烟相关性膀胱癌发病率的增长所抵消[20]。这一点可由埃及鳞状细胞癌的发病率从 20 世纪 80 年代的 78% 下降到 2005 的 27% 并向移行细胞癌转化的现象中得到证实[21]。2001—2010 年在埃及进行了另一项回顾性研究,研究对象分为两组:第一组为 2001 年至 2005 年的 1 002 例患者,第二组为 2006 年至 2010 年的 930 例患者。作者发现,BBC 的发病率从第一组的 80% 下降到第二组的 50%。此外,对两组的比较发现,移行细胞癌的发病率从 20% 显著上升至 66%,鳞状细胞癌从 73% 显著降低至 25%[22]。Hamed 等人[23]提出了血吸虫性膀胱癌发生率在埃及各省普遍下降的另一个原因,即气候变暖的趋势,最高温度超过 45℃ 和全年高温天数的增加影响了钉螺宿主的生存以及血吸虫病的传播。

随着感染时间的延长和感染程度的加重,膀胱癌与血吸虫感染的相关性逐渐增强[24]。在埃及,运河的长年灌溉导致的再感染风险与膀胱癌直接相关,并与控制措施和安全有效的治疗呈负相关[25]。由于每天在农村地区接触被感染的水源,学龄儿童尤其危险[26]。此外,值得注意的是,在伊拉克、肯尼亚沿海、加纳、马拉维、莫桑比克、赞比亚和津巴布韦的血吸虫流行地区,埃及血吸虫与膀胱癌之间存在高度相关性,而在尼日利亚、非洲南部和沙特阿拉伯地区这些埃及血吸虫中度到高度流行的区域,埃及血吸虫与膀胱癌之间缺乏相关性[27]。通常,血吸虫病影响农业地区,尤其是那些依赖灌溉农业的地区。19 世纪问题变得更加严重,新的灌溉工程和人口的增加共同增加了暴露于寄生虫的可能性[28]。

埃及血吸虫的地理分布不同也导致了易感人群的年龄和性别分布上的不同。血吸虫非流行地区膀胱癌的发病年龄高峰在60~70岁[29]。在埃及、苏丹、伊拉克、赞比亚、马拉维和津巴布韦，膀胱癌发病年龄高峰在40~49岁[10]。在血吸虫流行国家，血吸虫性膀胱癌的男女发病比例平均为5∶1[30]，这可以解释为，农村地区的农业劳动需要长期接触受感染的水域，这些活动通常是由男性而不是女性进行的[5]。最近的观察表明，1995年至2005年在埃及女性中由血吸虫引起的膀胱癌的发病率呈上升趋势。这是由于越来越多的男性农民从尼罗河谷和三角洲迁移到城市和边境省份寻找工作。因此，女性需要代替她们丈夫从事农业工作，继而增加了她们被感染的风险[23]。而另一项研究发现，与2000年至2010年维多利亚湖沿岸坦桑尼亚西部的男性相比，女性更容易受到血吸虫性膀胱癌的影响(51.4%)[31]。

泌尿系统血吸虫病诊断标准的差异影响血吸虫性膀胱癌的流行率。因离心尿标本中没有血吸虫卵而排除血吸虫病在许多因血吸虫纤维化而导致膀胱收缩的病例中是与事实不符的，因为致密的瘢痕组织会阻止血吸虫卵从黏膜下层脱落[25]。因此，通过扩大诊断血吸虫膀胱病的标准，包括应用最新的高灵敏度和特异性的影像学和分子生物学技术，血吸虫性膀胱癌的流行率有望得到更准确地统计。

血吸虫性膀胱癌的发展

膀胱癌细胞在能够快速生长、侵袭和转移之前，需要获得某些特性。慢性感染可导致血吸虫卵留在膀胱壁中。膀胱黏膜细胞的增殖是由持续的刺激和炎症引起的。这种黏膜的损害会增加尿路感染的概率[32]。此外，炎症部位诱导活化的巨噬细胞与产生致癌的N-亚硝胺和活性氧自由基有关[33]。黏膜纤维化和由慢性炎症及细菌感染引起的排尿困难，会导致尿路梗阻，从而延长了尿道上皮与这些致癌物质接触的时间[34]。

硝酸盐还原菌和泌尿系统血吸虫可以通过释放N-亚硝基化合物介导胺的N-亚硝基化[35]。在分子水平上，这些化合物与特定碱基和DNA序列的致瘤烷基化有关[36~38]，导致癌基因、抑癌基因和细胞周期控制基因的突变[5]。与血吸虫性膀胱癌相关的分子事件包括*H-ras*基因[39]的激活、*p53*[40]的失活和视网膜母细胞瘤(*Rb*)基因的失活[41]。2010年，Botelho等人[42]提出寄生虫提取物通过*K-ras*基因的致癌突变而具有致癌能力。不同级别的血吸虫性膀胱癌其*p53*的突变频率也不相同[43]。据报道，对于埃及的血吸虫性膀胱癌[44]大约86%含有*p53*外显子5、6、8和10的突变，并且在疾病早期，突变型*p53*激活程度的范围是0~38%，而在肿瘤晚期为33%~86%[43]。另一方面，在一组日本膀胱癌患者中，长期的吸烟史并没有增加*p53*突变的频率，而是导致了异常的AT∶GC的突变模式[44]。*p53*基因的突变主要与CpG二核苷酸的转变有关，而在血吸虫性膀胱癌中这种转变较多。这些转变可以用血吸虫卵引起的宿主免疫反应产生的一氧化氮的作用进行解释。炎症反应释放的一氧化氮可以通过5-甲基胞嘧啶的脱氨基作用直接导致这种突变，或者间接通过其形成内源性N-亚硝基化合物的能力导致DNA烷基化而形成突变[45]。在大多数研究病例中发现：血吸虫性膀胱癌中*p53*基因频繁失活可能是由*MDM2*基因编码的蛋白质过表达造成的，从而导致DNA损伤的积累和侵袭性的临床病程[46]。

癌症的发展与失控的细胞周期密切相关[47]。在53%的血吸虫性膀胱癌中发现了细胞周期依赖的蛋白激酶(CDK)抑制剂$p16^{Ink4}$基因的缺失和突变[48]。此外，在埃及92%的鳞状细胞癌中发现了*CDKN2*基因所在的9号染色体的缺失[49]。

人乳头状瘤病毒

人乳头状瘤病毒和血吸虫性膀胱癌之间是否存在关联尚未明确[50]。Khaled等人[51]进行的一项研究表明，在40例BBC病例中，有23例感染了HPV。最近，一项使用质谱技术的研究显示，所有血吸虫性膀胱癌血液检测样本都与HPV-16 DNA有关[52]。

血吸虫病过程中的代谢观测值

在关于血吸虫性膀胱癌的研究中，色氨酸通过甲酰犬尿氨酸途径代谢生成烟酸引起了人们很大的兴趣[53]。这种关注最初来自工业肿瘤学；而且，曾经在埃及高发的经典糙皮病在流行病学方面也支持这一观点，此类疾病在非洲其他血吸虫病流行但膀胱鳞状细胞癌报道不多的地区并不高发。在糙皮病中，从色氨酸到烟酸的甲酰犬尿氨酸途径代谢非常活跃，经此代谢途径产生大量的色氨酸中间产物[25]。

由于饮食习惯的地域差异，我们对血吸虫感染在色氨酸代谢紊乱中所起作用的理解变得复杂。事实上，5-羟色胺代谢物如5-羟基吲哚乙酸，在以芭蕉为食的非洲人排出量大，在其他饮食习惯的非洲人中排出量低[54]。在莫桑比克和南非的血吸虫病患者之间也发现了类似的饮食习惯差异。埃及农民不吃芭蕉，主要以豆类、扁豆和大米为生。那些患有血吸虫性癌症患者可将色氨酸转化为3-羟基烟酸、邻氨基苯甲酸、5-羟基吲哚乙酸和犬鸟氨酸。摄入一定量的色氨酸可增加这些代谢产物的排泄。因此，血吸虫病不应该被认为是色氨酸代谢产物异常排泄的唯一原因，无论有无癌症，泌尿系统血吸虫病几乎普遍伴有尿路感染。因此，菌群可能导致一些色氨酸代谢物的假性蓄积[25]。

潜在致癌的色氨酸代谢物可能是存在于血吸虫膀胱炎症的真正致癌物，它主要由肝脏代谢模式决定。与此相关的因素是同时发生的肝脏曼氏杆菌感染，吡哆醛缺乏症和长期蛋白质饥饿。如果这些因素中有任何一项出现严重异常，就会导致肝酶或辅酶因子缺乏，进而形成一定数量的潜在致癌代谢物[55,56]。感染曼氏杆菌的小鼠肝脏药物代谢能力明显下降[57]。感染日本血吸虫的小鼠肝脏的诱变剂失活能力也相应降低[58]，导致诱变剂在宿主体内的存留时间延长[59]。致癌物质的剂量似乎是膀胱肿瘤侵袭性的决定因素，如果持续暴露在低剂量的N-亚硝基化合物下，低级别的肿瘤也可以转化为高级别的肿瘤。这至少部分解释了血吸虫性膀胱癌大多表现为高度侵袭的鳞状细胞癌的原因[60]。

血吸虫性膀胱癌的细胞凋亡

慢性血吸虫病发生的几种细胞遗传学变化导致的一项负面影响是，细胞凋亡的减少可以促进肿瘤的发生[12]。2009 年，Botelho 等人[61]的研究表明，暴露于埃及血吸虫的总抗原（蠕虫提取物）细胞分裂速度比未暴露于该抗原的细胞更快，而且死亡数也更少。这是由于 *bcl-2* 水平的增加，*bcl-2* 是一种可以通过抑制细胞凋亡促进肿瘤发生的基因。血吸虫性膀胱癌患者中的 *Bcl-2* 基因过表达在 SCC 中发生上调，而在 TCC 中未发现上调[62]。

良性和血吸虫性膀胱癌前病变的病理学

活血吸虫卵堵塞膀胱静脉诱导剧烈的迟发型超敏反应，导致瘤状突起，小结节或息肉。在血吸虫膀胱炎中，乳头状瘤表面覆盖着一层或两层扁平细胞，这些细胞与基底部的移行上皮细胞融合，本质上是肉芽肿，而不是癌前病变。随着炎症和纤维化反复发生，一些移行上皮细胞被隔离在膀胱黏膜下层，并在中央腔周围形成球状排列。当它们进入膀胱腔时，囊性结构变成假腺结构。这些结构作为腺性膀胱炎的一部分，有时是癌前病变；腺瘤可能起源于柱状上皮细胞，其内层细胞已经分化。在血吸虫病患者中，经常发生鳞状上皮化生，它是一种常见的慢性炎症的伴生疾病。这种类型的化生是一种膀胱癌的癌前病变，因此，黏膜白斑作为一种癌前病变具有重要的临床意义[25]。

发病部位

在西方国家患者中，膀胱癌常发生在膀胱三角区；在埃及患者中，该疾病通常发生在远离输尿管的区域，主要发生在膀胱前壁和后壁。这一特性强化了其与血吸虫感染的关联，因为膀胱三角区黏膜下组织的稀少或完全缺失阻碍了血吸虫卵大量沉积[25]。

组织学分类

在过去的几十年中，血吸虫病相关膀胱肿瘤的病理类型发生了显著的变化[10]。1962—1967 年和 1987—1992 年相比，结节性肿瘤（83.4%～58.7%）和鳞状细胞癌（65.8%～54.0%）的发病率有所下降，但乳头状肿瘤（4.3%～34.8%）和移行细胞癌（31.0%～42.0%）的发病率有所上升。通过比较 2001—2005 年和 2006—2010 年两个时期，也得到了类似的结果[22]。血吸虫的感染程度在不同类型癌症的发生中起着重要作用；鳞状细胞癌通常与体内中度和/或高度蠕虫负荷有关，而移行细胞癌更常见于感染程度较低的区域[63~65]（图 32-1）。血吸虫性膀胱腺癌由于容易引发明显的染色体变异和细胞高度增殖而更具有侵袭性[66]。另一种罕见而独特的鳞状细胞癌变异体是血吸虫性膀胱疣状癌（图 32-2）。尽管有观点不同的报道，但大多数疣状癌可发展为浸润性鳞状细胞癌，所以与鳞状细胞癌一样预后不良[67]。

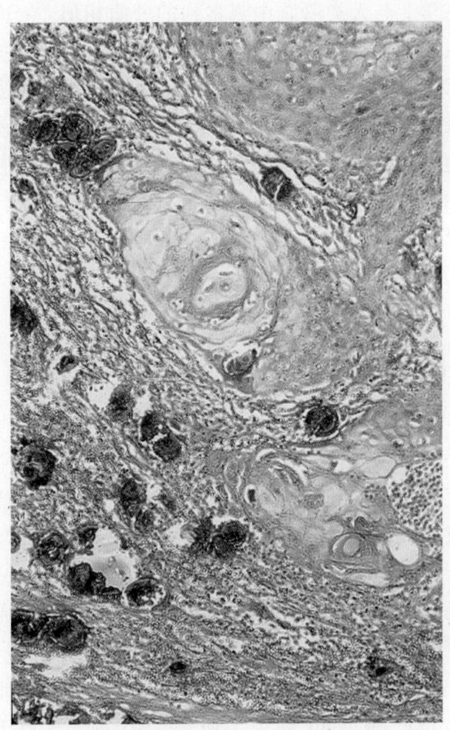

图 32-1　血吸虫性膀胱癌。浸润性，分化良好的鳞状细胞癌，伴有邻近埃及血吸虫卵的钙化（H&E×100）

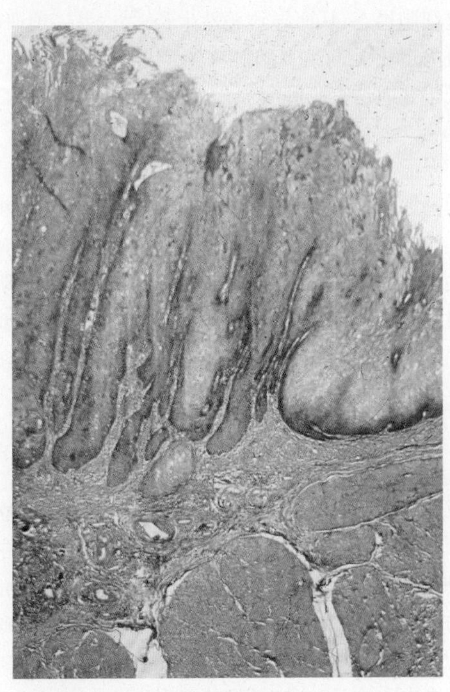

图 32-2　膀胱疣状肿瘤（无侵袭性）表面呈细长的丝状突起（H&E×40）

血吸虫性膀胱癌实验数据

在一些非人灵长类动物中，埃及血吸虫感染可导致上皮细胞增殖、鳞状上皮化生和膀胱移行细胞癌[68]。这种类型的肿瘤在形态学上与人类膀胱中观察到的肿瘤相似[69]，这说明埃及血吸虫和膀胱癌之间是有联系的。这些早期的实验观察很重要，因为还没有发现埃及血吸虫卵、冻干蠕虫和血吸虫病患者的尿液对小鼠有致癌作用[70,71]。然而，2-2-乙酰-氨基氟似乎比单独使用药物更能促进感染血吸虫的小鼠良恶性肿瘤的生长[72]。由于血吸虫感染对尿路上皮细胞具有直接增殖效应，因此血吸虫感染可能作为晚期共致癌剂，加速膀胱癌的进程[73]。

血吸虫病和其他部位的癌症

大肠

在亚洲，日本血吸虫的肠道感染被认为是导致结直肠癌(CRC)发生的重要因素。雌性日本血吸虫产卵量非常大(每对蠕虫每天产卵 2 000 只)，而曼氏血吸虫产卵量要少得多，因此引起的病理问题也就少得多[74]。在上海，患有肠道血吸虫病和大肠癌的患者要比患有自发性肠癌的患者平均年轻 6 岁。此外，血吸虫性结直肠癌中男女比例始终高于非血吸虫性癌[75,76]。最近，Madouly 等人[76]研究了曼氏血吸虫相关的结直肠癌，研究显示其具有独特的病理特征，通常类似于结肠炎诱导的癌症。寄生状态与微卫星不稳定性密切相关，微卫星不稳定是 DNA 修复缺陷的标志[77]，而 DNA 修复缺陷又影响正常的结肠上皮细胞稳态，从而导致恶性生长[78]。另一项研究表明，与曼氏血吸虫相关的结直肠肿瘤的特点是 *bcl-2* 过表达，且凋亡活性低于普通结直肠肿瘤[79]。

肝脏

在中国四川农村进行了一项关于肝癌和先前诊断为血吸虫病相关性的研究。人们发现既往的血吸虫感染与肝癌有显著的相关性，其中一小部分疾病(27%)可归因于肝炎阴性人群中的血吸虫病[80]。实验数据显示，在乙型肝炎和丙型肝炎阴性的大猩猩的高分化肝细胞癌内存在残留的血吸虫卵引起的严重肉芽肿反应[81]。

淋巴瘤

血吸虫病和淋巴瘤之间的关系鲜有报道[82]。孤立的原发性膀胱 T 细胞淋巴瘤的发生是对血吸虫病异常的免疫反应[83]。偶有一些关于淋巴瘤患者的肝脾型血吸虫病和慢性肠道感染的曼氏杆菌和日本血吸虫的病例报道。检测到的淋巴瘤类型为组织细胞性淋巴瘤[84]和大 B 细胞淋巴瘤[82,85,86]；淋巴瘤细胞在虫卵栓子和成虫周围增殖[86]。

其他器官

免疫组织化学研究证实了有三名前列腺血吸虫病患者发生侵袭性前列腺鳞状细胞癌，这些患者来自前列腺癌低发病率人群[87]。Mazigo 等人[88]报道了坦桑尼亚三例前列腺腺癌与埃及血吸虫感染相关。

一名 34 岁白人女性的病例报道中怀疑存在子宫颈血吸虫病。子宫颈涂片显示细胞学改变，提示子宫颈不典型增生和绒毛膜内存在埃及血吸虫卵，周围有肉芽肿性炎。患者对吡喹酮反应良好，并且所有临床和病理学表现均缓解。因此，子宫颈血吸虫病被认为是一种不典型增生可治愈的病因。子宫颈血吸虫病可能在 HPV 诱导的子宫颈不典型增生和宫颈癌中发挥辅助作用[89]。

血吸虫病致癌性评价

根据公认的国际标准，感染埃及血吸虫是人类致癌的因素(第 1 组)；感染曼氏血吸虫对人类致癌作用无法归类(第 2 组)；感染日本血吸虫可能是人类致癌的因素(第 2B 组)[90]。

东亚肝吸虫病

肝脏和胰腺

华支睾吸虫病和后睾吸虫病是由胆道系统内人类肝吸虫引起慢性感染所导致的。华支睾吸虫、泰国肝吸虫和猫肝吸虫是三种亲缘关系密切的吸虫，它们的生命周期相似，对胆道的病理生理作用也相同[91]。全球有近 3 500 万人感染华支睾吸虫，其中中国有约 1 500 万感染者[92]。华支睾吸虫病在中国、韩国、越南和俄罗斯部分地区最为流行[93]。类似的泰国肝吸虫在泰国也导致了肝吸虫病。胆管癌(CCA)是一种发生于胆管的癌症，是肝吸虫感染最严重的并发症。泰国和韩国异常高的 CCA 发病率与高流行性的后睾吸虫病和华支睾吸虫病密切相关[91]；因此，2009 年华支睾吸虫和泰国肝吸虫已经被国际癌症研究机构(IARC)列为“人类致癌物”(第一组)[94,95]。然而，猫肝吸虫感染不能归类于人类致癌物(第三组)[94~96]。世界上有记录的最高 CCA 发病率出现在泰国东北部，那里 70%～90%的人口感染了泰国肝吸虫。在华支睾吸虫广泛流行的韩国，CCA 占肝癌的 20%以上。

胆管导管内乳头状瘤是一种癌前病变，常与黏蛋白分泌过多有关。最近的几篇文章表明该疾病与华支睾吸虫感染有关。Suh 等人[97]报道 16 例胆管导管内乳头状瘤中有 5 例与华支睾吸虫感染有关(31%)。Jang 等人[98]报道，当 CCA 与华支睾吸虫感染相关时，导管内乳头状瘤比普通腺瘤更为常见。

人类感染华支睾吸虫是由于食用了被肝吸虫感染的生的或未煮熟的淡水鱼。进入人体后，寄生虫在十二指肠中脱囊，上升到胆管和胆小管并在那里成熟，导致胆管上皮细胞增生和纤维化。亚硝基化合物是致癌作用的催化剂。在远东地区，传统的中国腌制食品如咸鱼、干虾米和香肠等普遍存在亚硝胺[99]。感染泰国肝吸虫的男性体液内已被证实含有亚硝基化合物的前体[100]。胰腺导管也可能感染华支睾吸虫；这通常导致鳞状上皮化生和黏液腺增生。

疟疾

伯基特淋巴瘤(BL)在典型疟疾带的地理分布表明节肢动物媒介可能在肿瘤发生中发挥作用[101,102]。BL 是一种高度侵袭性的 B 细胞非霍奇金淋巴瘤且是人类生长最快的肿瘤[103]。提示 BL 发病机制的两大主要流行病学线索是 EBV 的早期感染和与疟疾的地理联系。这两种情况会导致 B 细胞增生,这几乎可以肯定是诱发 BL 淋巴瘤的主要病因。最近的数据显示,赤道区非洲儿童的发病率与高收入国家急性淋巴母细胞淋巴瘤(ALL)类似,每年每 100 000 名 0～14 岁儿童中,就有 3～6 名儿童发病,占该地区所有儿童癌症的 30%～50%。这与儿童中疟疾发病的高频率和高强度有关[104]。世界其他地区的发病率情况虽然了解有限,但比非洲赤道区要低得多[105]。根据非洲的这些数据,这种病被命名为地方性 Burkitt 淋巴瘤(eBL)。

马达加斯加共和国[108]和西非 Imesi 地区[109]进行了大力度抗疟疾预防行动,研究人员在这两个地区没有观察到 eBL 的增加(实际上是减少),因此认为不太可能是防御疟疾服用的药物促进了 BL[106,107]的发生。有趣的是,最近的研究表明氯喹可以在癌症流行地区的癌症预防中发挥作用[110,111]。在地方病流行区,BL 的最高发病率紧随严重恶性疟原虫疟疾之后,而疟疾的预防可以降低淋巴瘤的发病率[108,109]。

研究 eBL 患者和对照组患者的镰刀状细胞的频率具有重要意义。有镰刀状细胞的人在儿童早期就能免于恶性疟原虫的致命影响以及强烈的网状内皮细胞刺激,这种刺激有时会发展为高反应性疟疾性脾肿大[112]。暴露在低氧状态下的镰刀状细胞不能支持寄生虫在体外生长。另一个类似的现象是在血红蛋白 AS 基因型的个体中,疟疾的死亡率较低、IgM 水平和淋巴增殖也较少(以脾脏大小衡量)。这也许可以解释为什么具有镰刀状细胞的儿童患恶性疟原虫寄生虫血症可能性比较低。然而,大多数试图将 eBL 与 AS 基因型血红蛋白联系起来的研究都未发现统计学意义[113,114]。其他血红蛋白病,如遗传性球形红细胞增多症,也可抵抗疟疾。如果 eBL 在两种球形红细胞增多症都存在的人群中(如巴布亚新几内亚[115])数量很少,这也可以为疟疾作为 eBL 形成的辅助因素提供强有力的支持证据[113]。

携带大量寄生虫抗原的疟疾患者易发生 eBL 的其中一种解释是疟疾患者产生很多非特异性和“无用”的抗体,而它们无法识别和应对小克隆性恶性淋巴细胞所带来的威胁[116]。

疟疾和 EBV

流行病学观察提供了更有力的证据将 eBL 的发生与疟疾对 EBV 感染的增强作用联系起来[117]。eBL 只发生在疟疾普遍且高发的地区;而在无疟疾地区,如城市中心,eBL 是不存在的。活性较强的细胞和血清学反应发生在疟疾感染期间[118]。这就提出了一个可能的论点,即在疟疾人群中持续的网状内皮组织刺激使感染 EBV 的非洲患者发展成为一种肿瘤性疾病,而不是如传染性单核细胞增多症那样的自限性疾病[119]。疟疾诱导 BL 的增强作用是 B 细胞的增殖。恶性疟原虫红细胞膜蛋白 1(PfEMP1)的半胱氨酸丰富的区域 1α(CIDR1α)表达于感染的红细胞表面。在急性疟疾中,这种蛋白会导致携带 EBV 的循环 B 细胞数量增加[120,121]。这可以用两种机制来解释:首先,这种蛋白质刺激记忆 B 细胞的复制,包括 EBV 感染的 B 细胞[122]。其次,CIDR1α 可以诱导受感染的 B 细胞产生病毒,从而导致其他 B 细胞被感染[122～124]。急性疟疾促进了 B 细胞的增殖,也降低了 EB 病毒的特异性 T 细胞反应[101,113,125]。这导致更多的 EB 病毒感染细胞,促进了染色体易位和淋巴瘤的生成[126]。Chattopadhyay 等人[127]发现了一种仅存在于 EBV 特异性 CD8+T 细胞的疟疾相关性异常改变。

非洲 eBL 患儿出现自身抗体,其自身抗体的滴度升高与 EBV 病毒衣壳抗原(VCA)或 EBNA[128]滴度无线性相关,提示与 EBV 无关的因素导致了免疫失衡和自身抗体的产生。上述结论得到了另一些观察性研究结果的支持,即患有急性恶性疟原虫的白种人会产生自身抗体[129,130],而体外实验表明,作为对疟疾抗原的反应[131],正常人的淋巴细胞可以产生自身抗体。

染色体畸变和淋巴瘤的生成

c-myc 过表达似乎是典型和非典型 BL 发病机制的核心。尽管 *c-myc* 易位发生在所有 BL 病例中,但在该疾病的地方性和散发性类型存在易位模式上的差异。通常散发性 BL 发生染色体易位,涉及 8 号染色体上 *myc* 基因 5′端序列,以及 14 号染色体上免疫球蛋白重链 S 区域或附近的序列。相比之下,eBL 的特征是染色体易位涉及 8 号染色体上 *myc* 上游的序列,以及 14 号染色体 JH 区域内或附近的序列易位[131]。疟疾可直接产生与 BL 相关的染色体易位,其机制之一是与 toll 样受体(TLR)[104]的相互作用,TLR 在疟疾感染中受到某些激动剂(如疟原虫色素和 CpG 富集 DNA)的刺激,进而激活适应性免疫系统。这是因为它们能够在 B 细胞中诱导活化诱导胞苷脱氨酶(AID),这种酶可以诱导高变区突变和类别转换重组,并激活 B 淋巴细胞[132～134]。

近期证据

一些研究证实了几种寄生虫与肿瘤发生的关系,如隐孢子虫与肠癌的关系[135,136]。Certad 等人[135]的研究首次记录了人类起源的微小隐孢子虫能在小鼠中诱发癌症。另一种阴道毛滴虫可能在宫颈癌的发生中起作用,但在前列腺癌中的作用仍存在争议[137]。神经囊虫病也与血液恶性肿瘤有关系[138]。其机制是寄生虫引起的免疫调节、DNA 损伤和慢性炎症导致的一氧化氮的释放[139]。人们还研究了粪类圆线虫与肝胆管癌[140]和卡波西肉瘤[141]的关系,以及弓形虫在脑肿瘤[142,143]和淋巴瘤[144]中的作用。这些寄生虫可能都与癌症的发展有关。然而,目前的证据尚不足以将它们列在 IARC 名单内[137]。

鉴于最近对寄生虫作用的重新评估，人们发现，感染原及其产物可以调节多种宿主免疫反应，通过这些反应，它们可以正向或负向地调节癌症的发生和/或进展。有趣的是，某些类型的病原体，包括寄生虫，可以降低肿瘤发生的风险或导致癌症消退[145]。人们发现克氏锥虫可以降低啮齿动物结肠癌的发生率[146]，并且在临床和实验室研究了线虫减轻疾病的能力，如炎症性肠炎（溃疡性结肠炎，克罗恩病），多发性硬化症和过敏性反应[147,148]。其对癌症病理学特别是胃肠道肿瘤的适用性，是一个有待研究的问题[145]。

总结

在寄生虫病高度流行的国家，当罕见的肿瘤以异常频率出现时，寄生虫就会引起人们的高度重视。研究发现许多寄生虫在肿瘤发生中可能发挥作用。然而，并不是其所有都被 IARC 定义为真正的致癌物。慢性炎症、免疫调节、某些致癌物质的过表达、DNA 突变和细胞凋亡抑制是寄生虫诱发肿瘤发生的常见机制。此外，在许多情况下，其他感染因子的协同存在也被证明是肿瘤发生的一个增强因素。可以应用流行病学、细胞遗传学和动物研究来证明寄生虫与癌症之间的关系。通过对黏膜下虫卵沉积、N-亚硝基化合物的持续高水平导致 DNA 的突变、细胞凋亡的抑制以及泌尿系统上皮组织的组织病理学改变等机制的研究，埃及血吸虫被证明在膀胱癌的形成中发挥着重要的作用。人类乳头状瘤病毒也被怀疑在这一过程中起辅助作用。日本血吸虫的其他种类被列为结直肠癌的致癌物质，尤其在远东地区。其他蠕虫如华支睾吸虫病和后睾吸虫病已被证实可诱发肝癌。在非洲，BL 和 EBV 感染之间存在很强的相关性，并有证据表明恶性疟原虫的确在其中有明显的促进作用。由于几种寄生虫感染与慢性炎症相关，因此更多种类的寄生虫被认为可能是人类的致癌物质。然而，这一结论尚需强有力的证据，特别是细胞遗传学证据。值得注意的是，尽管多种寄生虫对肿瘤存在促进作用，但某些寄生虫似乎可以调节宿主的免疫反应，从而引起癌症的消退或起预防作用。因此重新评估传染性病原体的临床重要性有广阔的前景，也是一个未来需要关注的问题。

（路静 陈新焕 译 李鑫 赵四敏 校 孙文 审）

部分参考文献

7 Ploeg M, Aben KK, Kiemeney LA. The present and future burden of urinary bladder cancer in the world. *World J Urol*. 2009;**27**:289–293.

11 International Agency of Research on Cancer. Infection with schistosomes (*Schistosoma haematobium*, *Schistosoma mansoni* and *Schistosoma japonicum*). *IARC Monogr Eval Carcinog Risks Hum*. 1994;**61**:45–119.

12 Zaghloul MS. Bladder cancer and schistosomiasis. *J Egypt Natl Canc Inst*. 2012;**24**:151–159.

21 Felix AS, Soliman AS, Khaled H, et al. The changing patterns of bladder cancer in Egypt over the past 26 years. *Cancer Causes Control*. 2008;**19**(**4**):421–429.

22 Salem HK, Mahfouz S. Changing patterns (age, incidence, and pathologic types) of Schistosoma-associated bladder cancer in Egypt in the past decade. *Urology*. 2012;**79**(**2**):379–383.

23 Hamed MA, Ahmed SA, Hussein AS, El Feel A. Time series trend of bilharzial bladder cancer in Egypt and its relation to climate change: a study from 1995–2005. *IJPCR*. 2014;**6**(**1**):46–53.

27 Bustinduy AL, King CH. Helminthic infections: schistosomiasis. In: Farrar J, Hotez P, Junghanss T, Kang G, Lalloo D, White N, eds. *Manson's Tropical Diseases*, 23rd ed. Philadelphia, PA: Elsevier/Saunders; 2014:698–725.

29 La Vecchia C, Nagri B, D'Avanzo B, Savoldelli R, Franceshi S. Genital and urinary tract diseases and bladder cancer. *Cancer Res*. 1991;**51**:629–631.

34 Zaghloul MS, Gouda I. Bladder cancer and schistosomiasis: is there a difference for the association. In: Canda AE, ed. Bladder Cancer from Basic Science to Robotic Surgery. Croatia: In Tech open publisher, Rajeko; 2012:195–218.

36 O'Brien PJ. Radical formation during the peroxidase-catalised metabolism of carcinogens and xenobiotics. The reactivity of these radicals with GSH, DNA and unsaturated fatty lipid. *Free Radical Biol. Med*. 1988;**4**:216–226.

42 Botelho MC, Machado JC, de Costa JM. Schistosoma hematobium and bladder cancer. *Virulence*. 2010;**1**(**2**):84–87.

45 Lozano JC, Nakazawa H, Cros MP, Cabral R, Yamasaki H. G:T mutations in p53 and H-ras genes in esophageal papillomas induced by N-nitroso methyl benzyamine in two strains of rats. *Mol Carcinog*. 1994;**9**:33–39.

46 Osman I, Scher HI, Zhang ZF, et al. Alterations affecting the p53 control pathway in bilharzial-related bladder cancer. *Clin Cancer Res*. 1997;**3**:531–536.

50 Chung KT. The etiology of bladder cancer and its prevention. *J Cancer Sci Ther*. 2013;**5**(**10**):346–361.

52 Yang H, Yang K, Khafagi A, et al. Sensitive detection of human papilloma virus in cervical, head/neck, and schistosomiasis-associated bladder malignancies. *Proc Natl Acad Sci*. 2005;**102**(**21**):7683–7688.

59 Aji T, Matsuoka H, Ishii A, et al. Retention of a mutagen, 3 amino-1-methyl-5 H-pyrido[4,3,6] indole (Trp P2) in the liver of mice infected with S. japonicum. *Mutat Res*. 1994;**305**:265.

62 Chaudhary KS, Lu KS, Abel PD, et al. Expression of Bcl-2 and p53 oncoproteins in schistosomiasis-associated transitional and squamous cell carcinoma of the urinary bladder. *Br J Urol*. 1997;**79**:78–84.

66 Shabaan AA, Elbaz AE, Tribukait B. Primary nonurachal adenocarcinoma in the bilharzial urinary bladder: deoxyribonucleic acid flow cytometric and morphologic characterization in 93 cases. *Urology*. 1998;**51**:469.

76 Madbouly KM, Senagore AJ, Mukerjee A, et al. Colorectal cancer in a population with endemic *Schistosoma mansoni*: is this an at-risk population? *Int J Colorectal Dis*. 2007;**22**(**2**):175–181.

77 Soliman AS, Bondy ML, El-Badawy SA, et al. Contrasting molecular pathology of colorectal carcinoma in Egyptian and Western patients. *Br J Cancer*. 2001;**85**(**7**):1037–1046.

78 Itzkowitz SH, Yio X. Inflammation and cancer IV. Colorectal cancer in inflammatory bowel disease: the role of inflammation. *Am J Physiol Gastrointest Liver Physiol*. 2004;**287**(**1**):G7–17.

79 Zalata KR, Nasif WA, Ming SC, et al. p53,Bcl-2 and C-Myc expressions in colorectal carcinoma associated with schistosomiasis in Egypt. *Cell Oncol*. 2005;**27**(**4**):245–253.

80 Qiu DC, Hubbard AE, Zhong B, Zhang Y, Spear RC. A matched, case–control study of the association between Schistosoma japonicum and liver and colon cancers, in rural China. *Ann Trop Med Parasitol*. 2005;**99**(**1**):47–52.

88 Mazigo HD, Zinga M, Heukelbach J, Rambau P. Case series of adenocarcinoma of the prostate associated with Schistosoma haematobium infection in Tanzania. *J Global Infect Dis*. 2010;**2**(**3**):307–309.

89 Dzeing-Ella A, Mechaï F, Consigny PH, Zerat L, et al. Case report: cervical Schistosomiasis as a risk factor of cervical uterine dysplasia in a traveler. *Am J Trop Med Hyg*. 2009;**81**(**4**):549–550.

91 Lim JH. Liver Flukes: the Malady Neglected. *Korean J Radiol*. 2011;**12**(**3**):269–279.

93 Qian MB, Chen YD, Liang S, Yang GJ, Zhou XN. The global epidemiology of clonorchiasis and its relation with cholangiocarcinoma. *Infect Dis Poverty*. 2012;**1**:4. http://www.idpjournal.com/content/1/1/4.

94 Bouvard V, Baan R, Straif K, et al. WHO international agency for research on cancer monograph working group: a review of human carcinogens—part B: biological agents. *Lancet Oncol*. 2009;**10**:321–322.

99 Schwartz DA. Cholangiocarcinoma associated with liver fluke infection: a preventable source of morbidity in Asian immigrants. *Am J Gastroenterol*. 1986;**81**(**1**):76–79.

103 De Leval L, Hasserjan RP. Diffuse large B-cell lymphomas and Burkitt lymphoma. *Hematol Oncol Clin North Am*. 2009;**23**:791–827.

110 Maclean KH, Dorsey FC, Cleveland JL, Kastan MB. Targeting lysosomal degradation induces p53-dependent cell death and prevents cancer in mouse models of lymphogenesis. *J Clin Invest*. 2008;**118**:79–88.

111 Dang CV. Antimalarial therapy prevents Myc-induced lymphoma. *J Clin Invest*. 2008;**118**(**1**):15–17.

112 Morrow RH, Sever JL, Henderson BE. Antibody levels to infectious agents other than Epstein-Barr virus in Burkitt's lymphoma patients. *Cancer Res*. 1974;**34**:1212.

113 Whittle HC, Brown J, Marsh K, et al. T-cell control of Epstein-Barr virus-infected B-cells is lost during P falciparum malaria. *Nature*. 1984;**312**:449.

119 O'Conor GT. Persistent immunologic stimulation as a factor in oncogenesis with special reference to Burkitt's tumor. *Am J Med*. 1970;**48**:279.

120 Moormann AM, Chelimo K, Sumba OP, Cynthia JB, Chelimo K. Exposure to holoendemic malaria results in elevated Epstein–Barr virus loads in children. *J Infect Dis*. 2005;**19**:1233–1238.

125 Mulama D, Chelimo K, Collins O, Jura W, Otieno J, et al. EBNA-1 specific effector T cell deletion associated with holoendemic malaria exposure in the etiology of endemic Burkitt's lymphoma (P3063). *J Immunol*. 2013;**190**:187.7.

135 Certad G, Benamrouz S, Guyot K, et al. Fulminant cryptosporidiosis after near-drowning: a human Cryptosporidium parvum strain implicated in invasive gastrointestinal adenocarcinoma and cholangiocarcinoma in an experimental model. *Appl Environ Microbiol*. 2012;**78**(**6**):1746–1751.

141 Lin CJ, Katongole-Mbidde E, Byekwaso T, Orem J, Rabkin CS, Mbulaiteye SM. Intestinal parasites in Kaposi Sarcoma patients in Uganda: indication of shared risk factors or etiologic association. *Am J Trop Med Hyg*. 2008;**78**(**3**): 409–412.

143 Thomas F, Lafferty KD, Brodeur J, et al. Incidence of adult brain cancers is higher in countries where the protozoan parasite Toxoplasma gondii is common. *Biol Lett*. 2012;**8**(**1**):101–103.

第五篇

流行病学、预防及检测

第 33 章　全球的癌症负担：当前和未来的观点

Jacques Ferlay, MSc, ME ■ Christopher P. Wild, PhD ■ Freddie Bray, PhD

概述

癌症曾被认为是多发生于高收入国家的一种疾病，但目前，在全球非感染性疾病引起的死亡中仅癌症就占三分之一，癌症已成为导致人类死亡的主要原因。在未来几十年，由于人口数量和生活方式的改变，同时基于不断发展的人类统计学和流行病学的转变，全球癌症仍将保持高发趋势。据统计 2012 年全球新增 1 400 万新发癌症病例和 800 万癌症死亡病例，预计到 2030 年将增加 55%。本章从以下三点进行叙述。第一，介绍世界不同地区癌症的规模和常见癌症形式的显著差异。第二，指出癌症发病率的转变特点，明确了常见癌症发病率的上升和特征的变化与社会和经济变革有关。第三，处于转型状态的国家癌症的不均衡状态。在这些国家中，有关癌症发病率和死亡率的上升数据有限，且缺乏国家癌症管理计划。最后讨论通过规划和发展以人口为基础的癌症登记来改善在资源有限的情况下如何控制癌症。

引言

癌症曾被视为是工业化国家和高收入国家的一种疾病，如今却成为世界上大多数国家的发病率和死亡率的主要原因之一。世界卫生组织(WHO)2011 年的死亡率数据统计结果显示：从死亡原因方面来看，癌症的死亡率高于缺血性心脏病、中风、慢性阻塞性肺病合并下呼吸道感染等几种疾病的死亡率总和。目前，癌症致死数占 NCD(非传染性疾病)相关死亡总数的四分之一。在 70 岁以下的人群中，癌症致死数占 NCD 相关死亡总数的三分之一。在未来的二三十年中，随着人口数量和生活方式的转变，以及人口统计学和流行病学转变，癌症的全球发病趋势将会持续上升。据统计，2012 年全世界增加 1 400 万癌症新发病例和 800 万癌症死亡病例，2030 年这些数据将增加 55%。

癌症快速发展的趋势将极大地影响发展中国家和正在经历快速社会和经济变革的国家。因此，在非洲、亚洲和拉丁美洲，癌症负担将会持续不成比例地增加，这将会给这些医疗资源较差的国家带来更大的医疗负担，使这些国家难以满足日益增加的癌症患者对癌症治疗服务的需求。

本章有三个主要的目的。首先，通过全球癌症统计数据分析，强调了世界不同地区癌症的规模和常见癌症形式的显著差异。从国家层面来看，在按性别划分的癌症发病率或死亡率统计中，有 20 种不同类型的癌症居于发病率或死亡率的前五名。在此，我们简要地回顾和阐述癌症特定的模式。其次，我们从时间角度指出癌症负担的转变特性，表明癌症发病率的上升和模式转变与国家内部的社会和经济变化有关，并利用人类发展指数(HDI)的变化趋势作为这些变化的国家指标。最后，我们将评估现状说明与这些描述性结果的特定目的联系起来，以倡导和支持癌症控制行动的实施。我们强调处于转型中国家目前存在的不均衡现象，不断增加的癌症负担往往是由于缺乏准确的癌症控制数据以及相应的国家癌症管理计划造成的。资源有限的国家可以通过开发基于人口的癌症登记(PBCR)来统计相关癌症数据，进而完善癌症控制的规划。最后，我们强调需要在给予癌症治疗、管理和保守治疗的同时实施预防策略，并将这些策略纳入非传染性疾病计划。

在此介绍之后，下一节将回顾癌症关键指标的定义、可用的数据来源，用于在国家层面得出癌症发病率、死亡率和流行率的估计方法以及 GLOBOCAN 内的全球估计。第三节按发展水平和世界上最常见的八种癌症的分布情况分析了癌症负担的主要方面，并简要指出所观察到变化的主要原因。第四部分着重讨论了人类发展和社会经济转型如何改变世界范围内的癌症规模和进程。最后一节将这些发现与均衡实施国家癌症控制政策合理联系起来，以避免日益增加的负担。我们讨论了在资源有限的环境中，迫切需要更完善的癌症数据作为全球癌症控制战略的组成部分。本章所包含的描述性流行病学为确定一级和二级预防的优先次序提供了强有力的支持，这是未来降低不断增加的癌症负担的基本手段。

定义、数据来源与研究方法

众所周知，国际癌症研究机构(IARC)是全球癌症信息的权威参考来源；此外，在过去 40 年中，该机构不断更新全球癌症的预测数据。自 1975 年开始，对世界不同地区 12 种常见癌症的新发例数进行广泛评估[1]，IARC 现在可通过 GLOBOCAN 系列按性别和年龄提供 27 种癌症的国家整体发病率、死亡率和患病率的具体国家详细预估[2]。我们一直强调使用本国可获得的信息来直接预估癌症的严重程度，无论是来自 PBCR(新的癌症病例)还是来自生命登记系统(癌症死亡)。随着数据质量的提高和数据可用性的增多，GLOBOCAN 的每次数据更新都会改进估算方法。最新版本载有 2012 年的评估情况[2]，包括按性别分类的 184 个国家和 30 个世界区域的全部数据集的表格和图形描述的在线工具(http://globocan.iarc.fr)。在接下来的讨论中，我们定义了本章中使用的发病率、死亡率和患病率的核心指标，以及构建全球癌症概况的基础数据资源。

发病率即新增病例数，可以表示为在每单位时间(通常以年为单位)的绝对病例数、每 100 000 人次的比率，或者在没有相互竞争的死因的情况下，表示为发展到一定年龄(通常高达 75 岁)的癌症的累积风险(以百分比表示)。发病率数据是由 PBCR 通过定期和系统地收集特定人群中所有新发癌症病例的信息所得出的。PBCR 可能覆盖整个国家人口，但更多的是覆盖较小的地区，特别是在发展中国家，只覆盖主要地区（城市）。目前，以人口为基础的癌症登记仅覆盖了不到四分之一的世界人口，亚洲（占总人口的8%）和非洲（占总人口的11%）登记人数更少[3]。如果仅考虑高质量数据[例如《五大洲癌症发病率》（CI5）系列最新卷（X）中包含的数据集[4,5]]，癌症登记比例更低，只有14%的世界人口被符合CI5纳入标准的癌症登记机构所覆盖。目前，大约每三个国家（主要是高收入国家）中就有一个拥有高质量的PBCR。目前虽然资源匮乏地区注册中心的信息很多不符合CI5的质量标准，但这些客观的数据对癌症控制仍具有独特的重要性（参见“整合基于人口的癌症登记”一节）。PBCR还可以通过追踪癌症患者的生存状态产生生存统计数据。生存率表示癌症患者不因癌症死亡的概率，可在缺乏死亡率数据的情况下根据发病率估计死亡率，反之亦然。

死亡率是死亡的发生率，与发病率一样，可用死亡人数、比率或累计风险来表示。死亡率是发病率和病死率（与生存相反）的产物。世界卫生组织收集并提供死亡率统计数据。这些数据的优势是具有全国覆盖性和长期可获得性，但对一些国家来说，人口覆盖并不完善，因此而产生令人难以置信的低死亡率，而在另一些国家，死因信息的可信度受到质疑。截至2003年，提供数据的国家中只有不到一半向世卫组织报告高质量的统计数字，但死亡率统计数据却已覆盖了约三分之一的世界人口[6]。虽然几乎所有欧美国家都有全面的死亡登记系统，但大多数非洲和亚洲国家（包括人口众多的尼日利亚、印度、印度尼西亚和巴基斯坦）并没有该系统。用于估计中国癌症负担的死亡率数据可以从“疾病监测点”项目的抽样调查中获得。该项目虽然仅覆盖了中国人口总数的6%左右，但由于其样本包括城市和农村地区，这些统计数据被认为具有全国代表性。

患病率是指在某一特定时间点，受疾病影响的人口中存活的个体的绝对数量（或相对比例）。虽然发病率和死亡率被认为是衡量癌症负担的关键指标，但患病率是提供医疗服务发展策略的重要补充指标。然而，与发病率和死亡率不同，癌症患病率没有明确的定义。总（或完全）患病率是某一特定人群患病后在特定时间内存活的概率，一般是指在过去的某段时间被诊断为癌症的人，即使该人在多年前癌症已被治愈。除了记录生存癌症患者的数量外，患病率的应用通常体现在癌症服务规划的过程中，可根据患病率划分为癌症医治的不同阶段，即只考虑那些需要某种形式的癌症服务的人。因此，癌症患病率通常指被诊断为癌症的患者在给定年数后，仍存活的人数[7]。我们在本章中使用了5年患病率，并且在本章中，5年患病率是指在2012年以前的5年中被诊断为癌症的存活人数，以区分治疗之前的医疗需求（诊断、初步治疗和随访）。对于需要某种形式的医疗服务超过5年的癌症幸存者来说，这些数据可能不太具有参考价值，例如对于患乳腺癌的女性来说，在确诊后的几十年中，它仍然是一种影响平均预后的慢性疾病[8]。

GLOBOCAN中癌症的全球发病率、死亡率和患病率估计值由所在国家的最新和最可靠的国内数据源构建而成。在估算过程中使用的方法已在各种报告中进行了详细描述，并在表33-1中进行了总结[2,7,9]。

表33-1 2012年数据质量和估算方法：在GLOBOCAN上提交的184个国家的状况

		状态	国家数量
死亡率			
	数据质量		
	1	人口动态登记	95
	2	不完整的人口动态登记	2
	3	其他来源（癌症登记，口头尸检调查等）	7
	4	无数据	80
	方法		
	1	预测比率/适用于2012年的比率	95
	2	根据区域比率的加权平均数进行估算	1
	3	根据国家发病率估计和模拟存活率进行估算	85
	4	邻近国家或同一地区登记的比率	3
			184
发病率			
	数据质量		
	1	高质量的国家数据或高质量的区域数据	67
	2	国家数据（比率）	24
	3	区域数据（比率）	18
	4	频率数据	13
	5	无数据	62

续表

状态			国家数量
	方法		
	1	预测比率/适用于 2012 年的比率	58
	2	使用模拟发病率与死亡率从国家死亡率估计中估计	22
	3	使用模型生存从国家死亡率估计中估计	32
	4	估计为本地比率的加权平均值	27
	5	使用不同癌症的相对频率数据对“所有癌症”的年龄/性别特定比率进行划分	12
	6	邻近国家或同一地区登记的比率	33
			184
患病率			
	方法		
	1	根据国家发病率估计和特定国家的生存情况估算	32
	2	根据国家发病率估算和汇总区域存活率估算	152
			184

全球癌症的多样性

世界范围内的癌症负担

表 33-2 列出了 2012 年 27 种主要癌症和所有癌症（不包括非黑色素瘤皮肤癌）按性别分类的预计新增病例和死亡病例，以及在 75 岁之前患癌的风险。图 33-1 显示了按洲和地区/国家划分的癌症发病率和死亡率以及 5 年患病率的分布情况。2012 年有 1 400 多万新增癌症病例，820 万癌症死亡病例，3 200 多万癌症患者（确诊后 5 年内）。约二分之一的癌症发生在亚洲，其中近四分之一（22%）发生在中国，另有 7%发生在印度。另外四分之一的癌症发生在欧洲，其余的在美洲和非洲，1%在大洋洲。在亚洲和非洲中，癌症相关的死亡率较高，在欧洲和北美则较低，这一现象反映了预后较差的癌症类型出现的频率，以及某些可在早期治疗的常见癌症的低生存率。

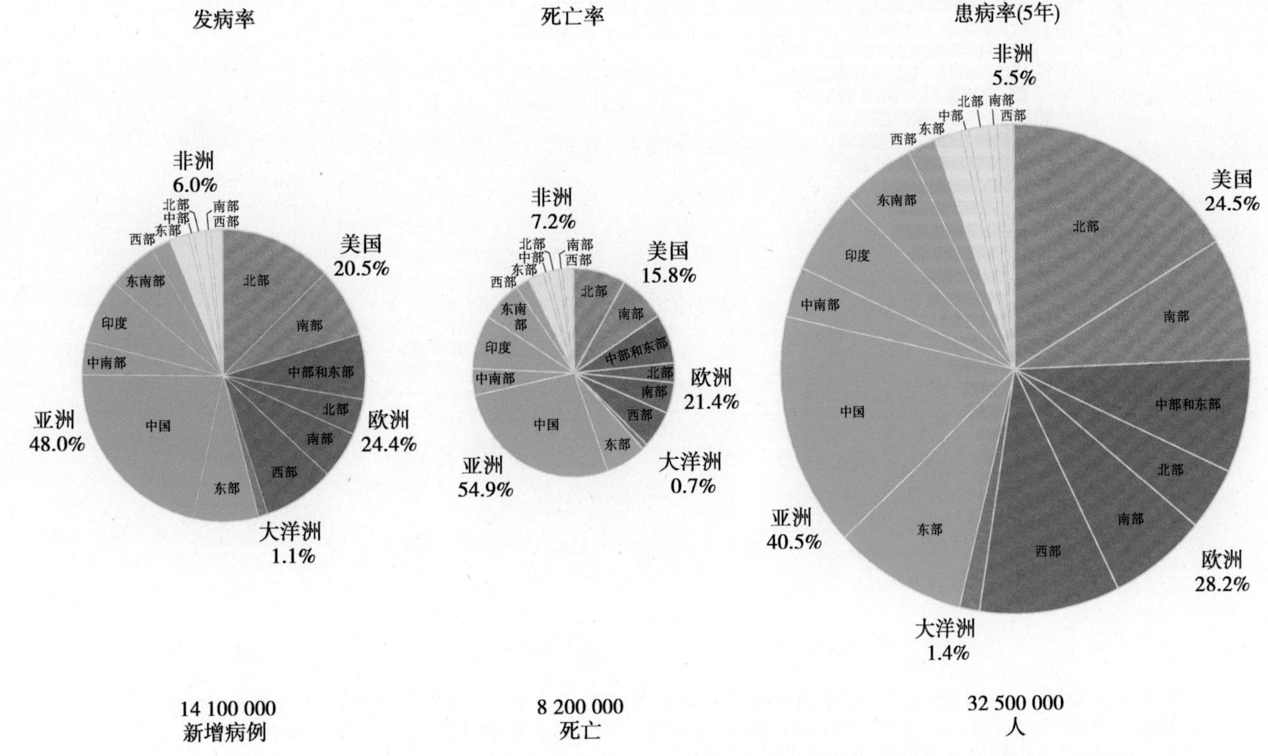

图 33-1 2012 年全球癌症负担：按大陆分列的估计发病率、死亡率和 5 年患病率

从新增病例数(180 万例)和死亡病例数(160 万例)这两个方面来看,肺癌仍然是全世界最常见的癌症。从整体水平来看,乳腺癌是第二常见的癌症(170 万例),但其在癌症致死方面排名第五(52.2 万人死亡),说明其预后相对较好。在发病率方面,紧随其后的依次为结直肠癌(140 万例,69.4 万例死亡)、前列腺癌(110 万例,30.7 万例死亡)和胃癌(95.2 万例,72.3 万例死亡)。这五种癌症几乎占到 2012 年全球癌症发病率负担的一半。

截至 2012 年底的前 5 年内,约有 3 250 万人诊断出癌症并存活(表 33-2)。截至目前,患病率最高(男性和女性)的癌症是女性乳腺癌(图 33-2),约有 630 万女性患有这种疾病。患病率位于第二的癌症是前列腺癌(男性,390 万例),紧随其后的是结直肠癌(350 万例)。患病率综合反映了发病率和预后情况,肺癌是全球最常见的癌症,但其预后较差,5 年患病率(190 万)与年度死亡率相当接近,排名第四。

按发展水平分类的癌症类型

在下面的讨论中,我们使用人类发展指数(HDI)的四个级别(低、中、高和极高)代表社会和经济的发展程度[10](http://hdr.undp.org/en)。HDI 是出生时预期寿命、受教育机会和收入[国内生产总值(GDP)]的综合衡量标准。虽然 HDI 与国民总收入(GNI)高度相关,但 HDI 也可作为一个国家在卫生和教育领域的支出情况的指标(图 33-3a)。图 33-3b~33-3e 根据广泛的 HDI 水平描述了全球不同的癌症发病率和死亡率概况。不同癌症的发病情况取决于生殖和生活方式这些关键的决定因素,以及早期发现和临床干预措施等卫生服务。人群能否得到这些卫生服务取决于个别国家的资源水平和发展的均衡程度,即取决于社会和经济转型的程度。在 HDI 水平高或非常高的地区(图 33-3c),乳腺癌、肺癌、结直肠癌和前列腺癌占总体癌症发病率的一半,而胃癌位居第五。这是许多高收入国家常见的癌症"前五位"分布情况,这些地区的癌症发病率占全球癌症负担的 56%,与世界癌症发病率分布水平相当(图 33-3b)。同样值得注意的是,预后情况极差的胰腺癌目前在高 HDI 和极高 HDI 国家中的患病率排名第五位,是癌症死亡的原因之一。在低 HDI(图 33-3e)和中等 HDI(图 33-3d)区域,常见癌症依然是食管癌、胃癌、肝癌和宫颈癌。中等 HDI 地区的癌症发病概况与中国相同,因中国人口规模达 13.5 亿,中国的癌症负担占中等 HDI 负担的五分之二。在低 HDI 的地区包括许多东非和其他撒哈拉以南非洲国家,与 HIV/AIDS(人类免疫缺陷病毒感染与获得性免疫缺陷综合征)相关的癌症负担依然存在,比如卡波西肉瘤,是由人类疱疹病毒-8 引起的与艾滋病毒相关的癌症。然而,由于 HIV 患病率的下降和高活性抗反转录病毒疗法的广泛应用,与艾滋病毒相关癌症的发生率正在下降[11~13]。

在男性群体中,欧洲和美洲的男性具有较高癌症死亡率的风险,包括哈萨克斯坦和中国在内的一些中亚和东亚国家的男性癌症死亡率也在升高,在这些国家,肺癌是男性癌症发病率和死亡率最常见的原因。在女性群体中,非洲东部和南部的女性面临着很大的死亡风险,在这些地区的许多国家,宫颈癌和乳腺癌的负担都很高。

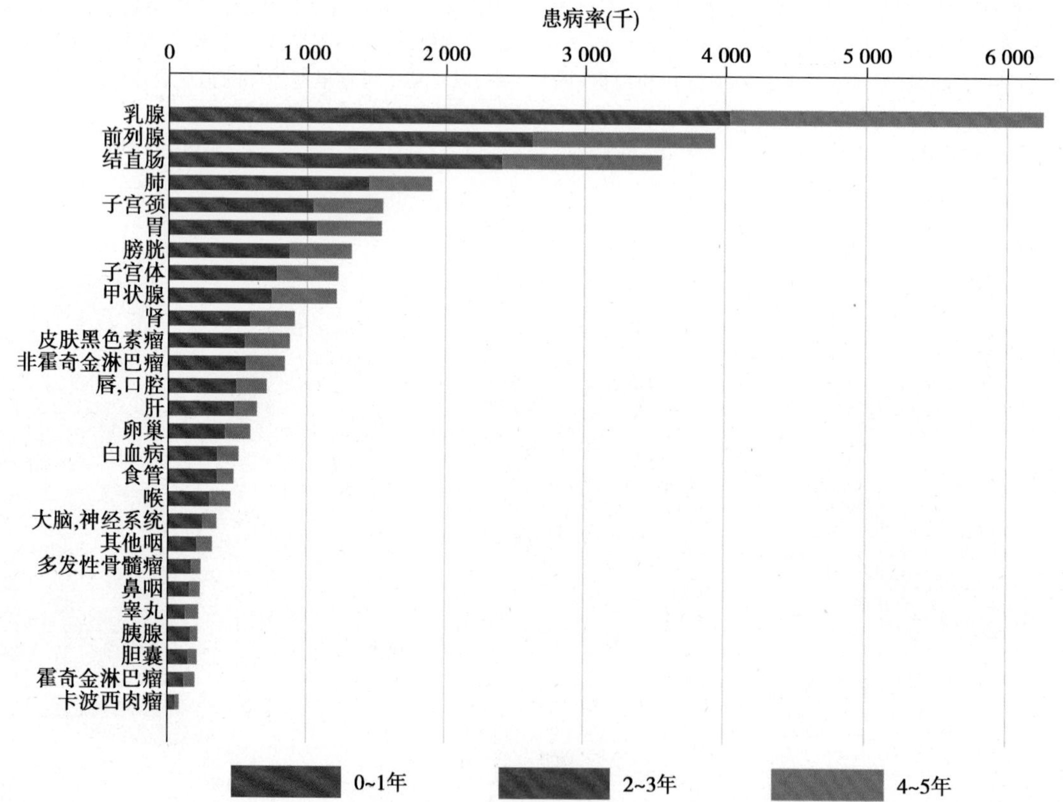

图 33-2 全球 5 年癌症患病率(百万)的柱状图;堆积条形表示分别在 2012 年、2010—2011 年和 2008—2009 年诊断的 2012 年底存活患者中的患病率;例如,诊断后<1 年、2~3 年和 4~5 年。性别和年龄均为 15 岁及以上,按患病率大小排序。数据来源:GLOBOCAN 2012

表 33-2　2012 年全球按癌症部位和性别划分的癌症发病率、死亡率和患病率估计

癌症位点	发病率						死亡率						患病率		
	两性		男性		女性		两性		男性		女性		两性	男性	女性
	病例数（×1 000）	累计风险（0~74）	病例数（×1 000）	累计风险（0~74）	病例数（×1 000）	累计风险（0~74）	死亡数（×1 000）	累计风险（0~74）	死亡数（×1 000）	累计风险（0~74）	死亡数（×1 000）	累计风险（0~74）	数量（×1 000）		
唇，口腔	300	0.5	199	0.6	101	0.3	145	0.2	98	0.3	47	0.1	702	467	235
鼻咽	87	0.1	61	0.2	26	0.1	51	0.1	36	0.1	15	0.0	229	162	67
其他咽部	142	0.2	115	0.4	27	0.1	96	0.2	78	0.3	19	0.1	310	251	59
食管	456	0.7	323	1.1	133	0.4	400	0.6	281	0.9	119	0.3	465	337	128
胃	952	1.4	631	2.0	320	0.8	723	1.0	469	1.4	254	0.6	1 538	1 031	507
结肠和直肠	1 361	2.0	746	2.4	614	1.6	694	0.9	374	1.0	320	0.7	3 543	1 953	1 590
肝	782	1.1	554	1.7	228	0.6	746	1.0	521	1.6	224	0.6	633	453	180
胆囊	178	0.2	77	0.2	101	0.3	143	0.2	60	0.2	82	0.2	205	90	115
胰腺	338	0.5	178	0.6	160	0.4	330	0.4	174	0.5	157	0.4	211	114	97
喉	157	0.3	138	0.5	19	0.1	83	0.1	73	0.2	10	0.0	442	389	53
肺	1 825	2.7	1 242	3.9	583	1.6	1 590	2.2	1 099	3.3	491	1.2	1 893	1 267	626
皮肤黑色素瘤	232	0.3	121	0.4	111	0.3	55	0.1	31	0.1	24	0.1	870	453	417
卡波西肉瘤	44	0.1	29	0.1	15	0.0	27	0.0	17	0.1	10	0.0	80	55	25
乳腺	1 677	4.6	—	—	1 677	4.6	522	1.4	—	—	522	1.4	6 255	—	6 255
子宫颈	528	1.4	—	—	528	1.4	266	0.8	—	—	266	0.8	1 547	—	1 547
子宫体	320	1.0	—	—	320	1.0	76	0.2	—	—	76	0.2	1 217	—	1 217
卵巢	239	0.7	—	—	239	0.7	152	0.4	—	—	152	0.4	587	—	587
前列腺	1 112	3.8	1 112	3.8	—	—	307	0.6	307	0.6	—	—	3 924	3 924	—
睾丸	55	0.1	55	0.1	—	—	10	0.0	10	0.0	—	—	215	215	—
肾	338	0.5	214	0.7	124	0.3	143	0.2	91	0.3	53	0.1	907	581	326
膀胱	430	0.6	330	1.0	99	0.2	165	0.2	123	0.3	42	0.1	1 319	1 018	301
大脑，神经系统	256	0.3	140	0.4	117	0.3	189	0.3	106	0.3	83	0.2	343	190	153
甲状腺	298	0.4	68	0.2	230	0.6	40	0.1	13	0.0	27	0.1	1 206	271	935
霍奇金淋巴瘤	66	0.1	39	0.1	27	0.1	25	0.0	15	0.0	10	0.0	188	108	80
非霍奇金淋巴瘤	386	0.5	218	0.6	168	0.4	200	0.3	115	0.3	84	0.2	832	463	369
多发性骨髓瘤	114	0.2	62	0.2	52	0.2	80	0.1	43	0.1	37	0.1	229	125	104
白血病	352	0.4	201	0.5	151	0.4	265	0.3	151	0.4	114	0.3	501	285	216
除非黑色素瘤皮肤癌除外的所有癌症	14 090	18.5	7 427	21	6 663	16.4	8 201	10.5	4 653	12.7	3 548	8.4	32 544	15 362	17 182

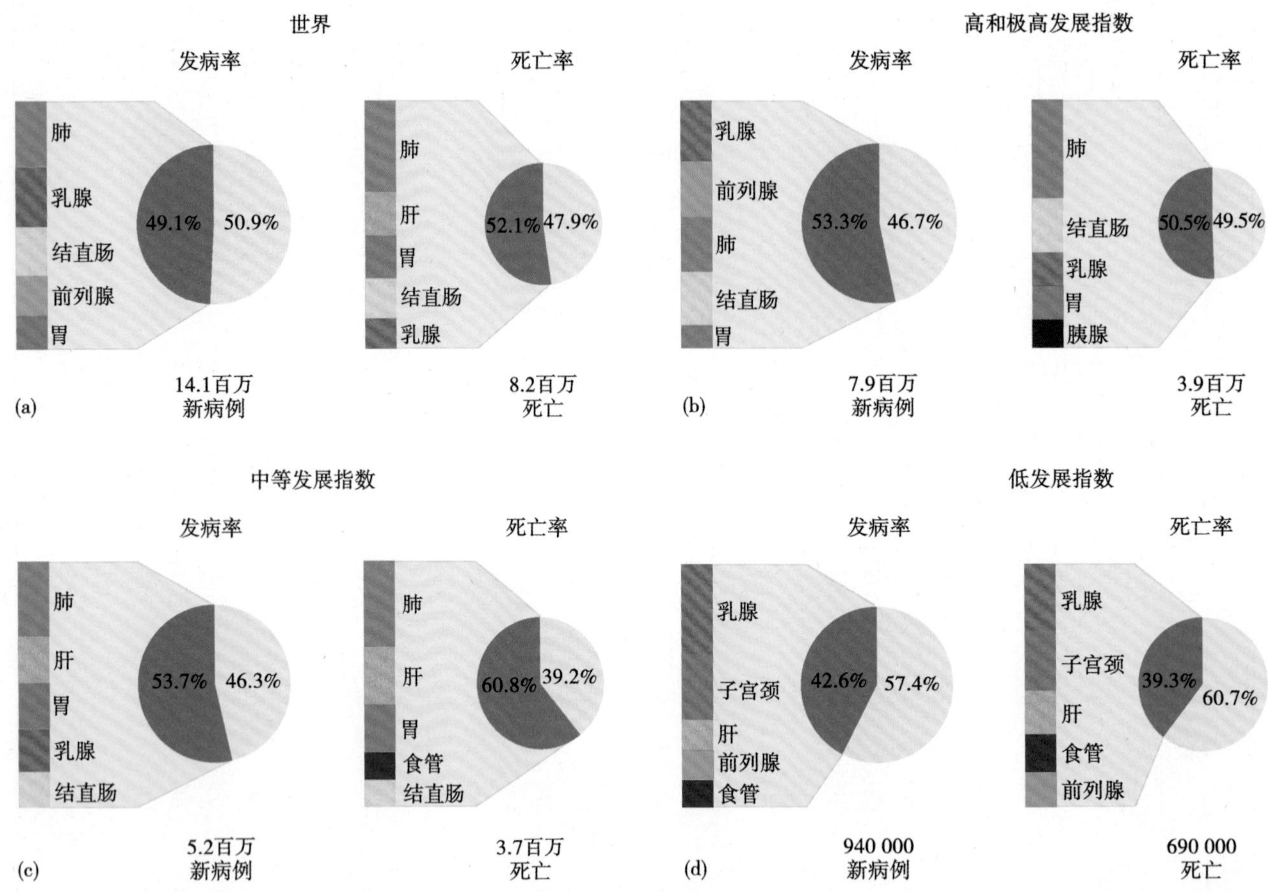

图 33-3 (a)2012 年全球发病率和死亡率以及人类发展水平最常见的五种癌症;(b)高和极高 HDI;(c)中 HDI;(d)低 HDI

八种主要癌症类型的模式

以下是对全球八种最常见癌症的全球模式的简要描述。

肺癌

肺癌仍然是全世界最常见的癌症。新增病例超过 180 万例(占癌症总发病率的 13%),死亡人数近 160 万人(占癌症总死亡率的 20%)。三分之一以上的新确诊病例发生在中国。在 38 个国家中,肺癌是男性癌症发病率的首要原因;在 89 个国家中,它是男性癌症死亡率的首要原因,在 26 个国家中是最常见的女性癌症死亡原因。无论一个国家的经济水平如何,肺癌的死亡率均较高并且相当稳定,其死亡率的模式和趋势与发病率相似。肺癌最近的趋势反映了因吸烟而导致的流行病学的转变[14],在男性中,处于吸烟流行后期的高度发达国家肺癌发病率已经达到顶峰并开始呈现下降趋势,但肺癌在女性中发病率继续上升。只有少数几个国家和地区(北欧、澳大利亚和美国)几十年来吸烟率一直在下降,其女性肺癌发病率最近达到了峰值,且部分出现下降趋势。然而,在包括中国和印度尼西亚在内的许多中等收入国家,男性吸烟的普遍程度急剧上升[15]。在未来,肺癌以及其他与吸烟相关的癌症负担取决于未来具有性别特异性的吸烟模式,包括吸烟持续的时间、戒烟程度和吸入烟草的类型[16]。

乳腺癌

乳腺癌是迄今为止最常见的癌症,也是女性因患癌症死亡的主要原因。据估计有 170 万新发乳腺癌病例(占女性所患癌症的 25%)和 50 万因乳腺癌死亡病例(占女性所有癌症死亡的 15%)。在 140 个国家中,乳腺癌是女性最常见的癌症诊断类型,在 101 个国家中,乳腺癌是引起癌症死亡的最常见原因之一。在欧洲和北美洲,预计有约 42% 的乳腺癌新确诊病例和 34% 的癌症死亡患者。乳腺癌的全球死亡率相差约 2.5 倍,在欠发达国家乳腺癌的病死率更高。虽然在世界大多数地区乳腺癌的发病率普遍上升(图 33-4a),但在一些高度发达的国家,乳腺癌的发病率在过去十年左右达到峰值并有所下降,这可能与癌症的全国筛查以及在一些国家全人群 HRT(激素替代疗法)使用率的降低有关。自 20 世纪 80 年代末和 90 年代初以来,一些高度发达国家的乳腺癌死亡率一直在下降,这是由于癌症的早期诊断和治疗包括有效疗法等方面取得的突破。

前列腺癌

在全球范围内,前列腺癌位居男性最常见癌症的第二位,也位居男性癌症死亡原因第五位,每年预计新增前列腺癌病例 110 万例(占男性所有癌症的 15%),30 万例死亡病例(占男性所有癌症死亡的 7%)。据估计,2012 年有 60%的新增前列腺癌病例发生在欧洲和北美洲,但该地区因前列腺癌死亡患者只占全球前列腺癌死亡总人数的 41%。在以黑色人种为主的国家和地区(在加勒比地区和撒哈拉以南非洲的部分地区)前列腺癌患者的死亡率最高,但在某些北欧国家前列腺癌的死亡率也很高。前列腺癌的发病率在全球范围内的差异超过 25 倍。发病率最高的地区是澳大利亚、新西兰、北欧、西欧以及北美。据 2012 年统计数据,全球 87 个国家男性中最常见的癌症类型是前列腺癌,主要发生在人类发展水平较高或非常高的国家,但也出现在中部和非洲南部的几个国家。20 世纪 80 年代末,随着前列腺特异性抗原(PSA)检测的普及,北美和北欧国家的前列腺癌发病率急剧上升;在 20 世纪 90 年代,许多资源最丰富的国家也出现了类似的情况(图 33-4b)。虽然目前一些发达国家的前列腺癌发病率趋于平稳,但在向更高社会和经济水平转变的国家中其发病率持续上升。

结直肠癌

结直肠癌发病率占全球癌症发病率的近 10%,是男性第三常见的癌症(约 74.6 万例),女性第二常见的癌症(61.4 万例)。该疾病导致约 69.4 万人死亡,是全球癌症死亡原因中位居第四。几乎三分之二的新增病例发生在人类发展水平高或极高的国家,其中一半发生在欧洲和美洲。结直肠癌在发展水平较高的国家中是一种常见的癌症,其发病率随着发展水平而增加,在东欧(斯洛伐克、匈牙利和捷克共和国)和韩国的男性结直肠癌发病率较高。在宫颈癌历史发病率较低的国家,如东地中海地区,女性的结直肠癌发病率往往仅次于乳腺癌。世界各国结直肠癌总的发病率相差 10 倍,在大多数非洲国家发病率往往相对较低。与发病率一致的是,除加勒比地区外,女性的结直肠癌死亡率低于男性。结直肠癌发生规模及其发展时间是特定国家人类发展转变的关键标志。在许多向更高发展水平过渡的国家中,结直肠癌的发病率逐步上升;而在已经达到人类发展最高水平的国家,结直肠癌发病率增加的趋势似乎正趋于稳定或下降(图 33-4c)。

胃癌

胃癌位居全球最常见癌症的第五位,预计新增病例 95.2 万例(占癌症总发病率的 7%)和死亡病例 72.3 万(占总死亡率的 9%)。几乎四分之三的胃癌新增病例发生在亚洲,其中超过五分之二的胃癌新增病例发生在中国。世界各国的胃癌发病率相差近 10 倍;男性的胃癌发病率大约是女性的两倍。以年龄为标准来划分发病率,则东亚、中欧和东欧的胃癌发病率最高。非洲和北美洲的胃癌发病率仍然相对较低。在过去的 50 年里,几乎所有国家的胃癌发病率和死亡率都在下降(图 33-4d)。这可能与幽门螺杆菌感染的患病率变化有关,幽门螺杆菌感染是胃癌发生的主要危险因素,目前正在探索预防幽门螺杆菌感染的方法,以获得最佳的公共卫生预防方法[17]。胃癌的总体发病率的下降主要是由于非贲门型胃癌发病率下降,相比之下贲门癌在同一人群中近二三十年内的发病率一直保持稳定甚至上升。

肝癌

肝癌在全球癌症发病率和死亡率负担中分别占 6% 和 9%。肝癌是全球第二大癌症死亡原因,预计死亡人数约为 74.6 万人。肝癌在最常见的男性癌症中位居第五位(55.4 万新发病例,占总数的 8%),在最常见的女性癌症中排第九位(22.8 万例,占总数的 3%)。几乎四分之三的新增肝癌病例发生在人类发展水平较低和中等的地区;中国的肝癌发病率和死亡率占全球的一半以上。鉴于肝癌的高死亡率(总死亡率与发病率之比,0.95),我们发现肝癌死亡率与发病率的地理模式和发展趋势非常相似。截至目前,按年龄标准划分的肝癌发病率以蒙古最高。东亚、东南亚、非洲和美拉尼西亚的肝癌发病率升高。肝癌发病率在大多数高度发达的地区往往较低。不发达国家肝癌发病率高的原因是乙型肝炎病毒慢性感染和饮食广泛暴露于黄曲霉毒素。在已引进乙肝疫苗(从 20 世纪 80 年代初开始)并实现人口完全覆盖的国家,未来几十年的肝癌发病率有望降低。由于经济发展,一些国家(例如中国的部分地区)减少了黄曲霉毒素的暴露,并且发展中国家正在将重点转移到干预农民的生活习惯上[18]。随着丙型肝炎病毒感染的增加以及肥胖率的上升和酗酒,肝癌的发病率可能会相应增加[19]。

子宫颈癌

宫颈癌是全球第七大常见的癌症,从发病率(52.8 万新发病例)和死亡率(26.6 万例死亡)来看,宫颈癌在女性癌症中排名第四。约 70%的全球宫颈癌发生在人类发展水平低或中等的地区,印度发病人数超过全球新发病例的五分之一。各国宫颈癌的发病率差别很大。全球 184 个国家中,宫颈癌依然是 39 个国家中女性最常见的癌症,在 45 个国家当中,宫颈癌是女性癌症死亡的首要原因。宫颈癌患病率风险升高主要存在于撒哈拉以南的非洲、亚洲部分地区以及中美洲和南美洲的一些国家。发病率最低的地区是西欧、北美、澳大利亚、新西兰和地中海东部。除极少数地区外,许多国家过去 30 年宫颈癌发病率都有所下降(图 33-4e)。这一趋势反映了随着国家经济的转型等社会因素的变化,在资源丰富的国家,实施有效的筛查方案能够显著降低宫颈癌发病率。相比之下,近年来乌干达宫颈癌发病率下降相关的证据很少,几个东欧和中亚国家的宫颈癌发病率也在上升。最近发现,性行为的变化会增加感染高危人乳头瘤病毒的风险,在缺乏有效筛查计划的情况下,会导致宫颈癌发病率上升[20]。

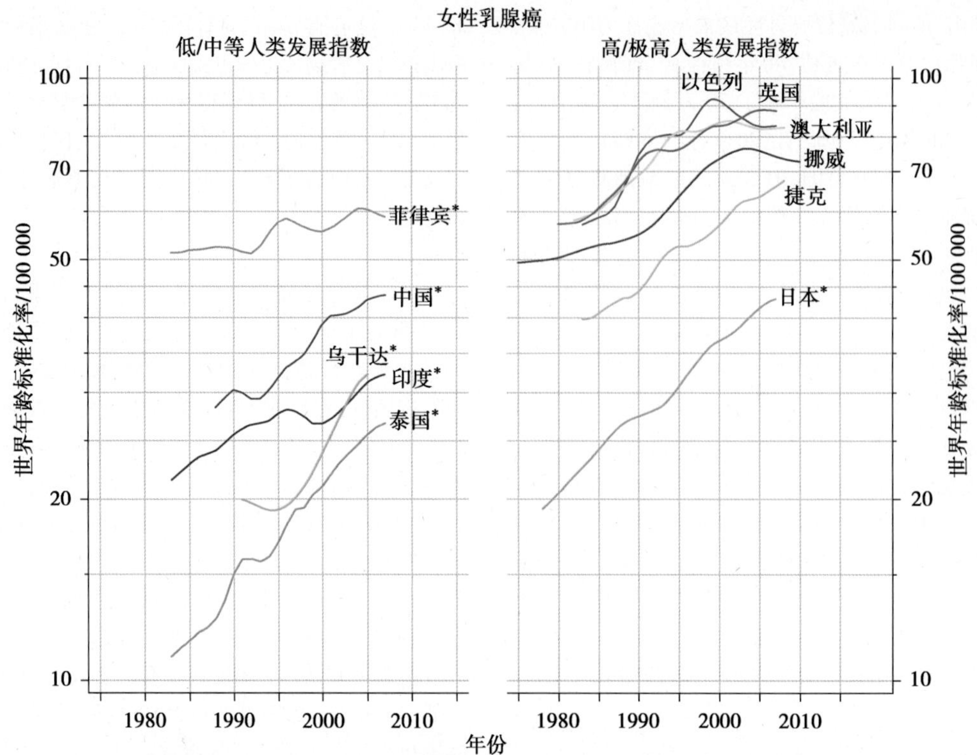

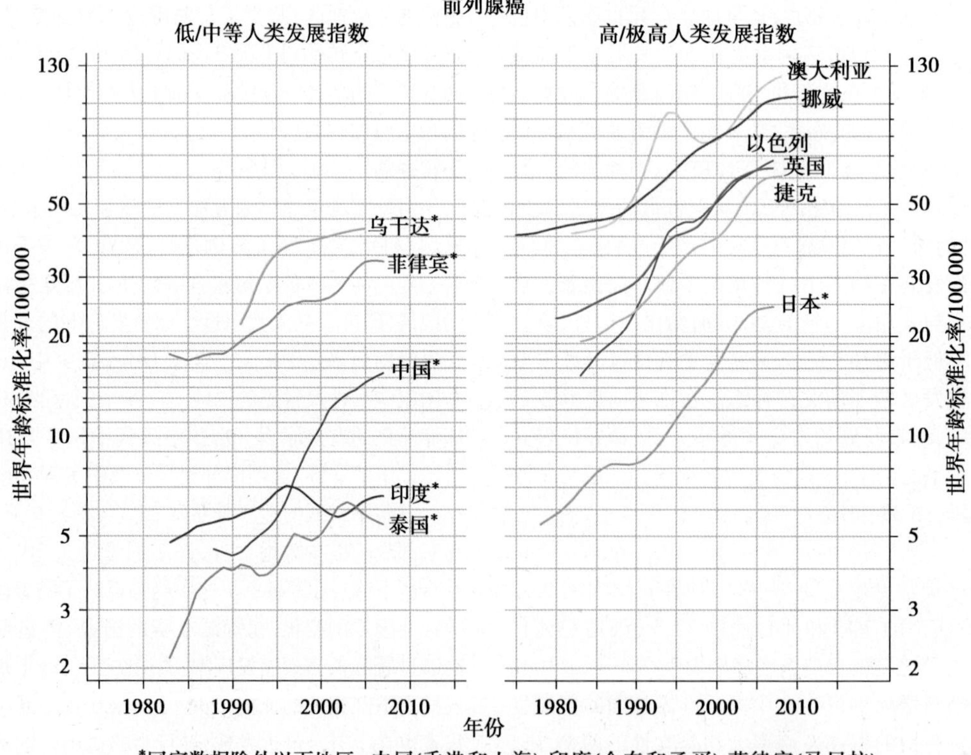

图 33-4 使用低度回归处理的(a)女性乳腺癌,(b)前列腺癌,(c)结肠直肠癌(男性),(d)胃癌(男性)和(e)子宫颈癌发病率的时间趋势。资料来源:五大洲的癌症发病率

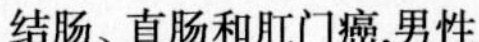

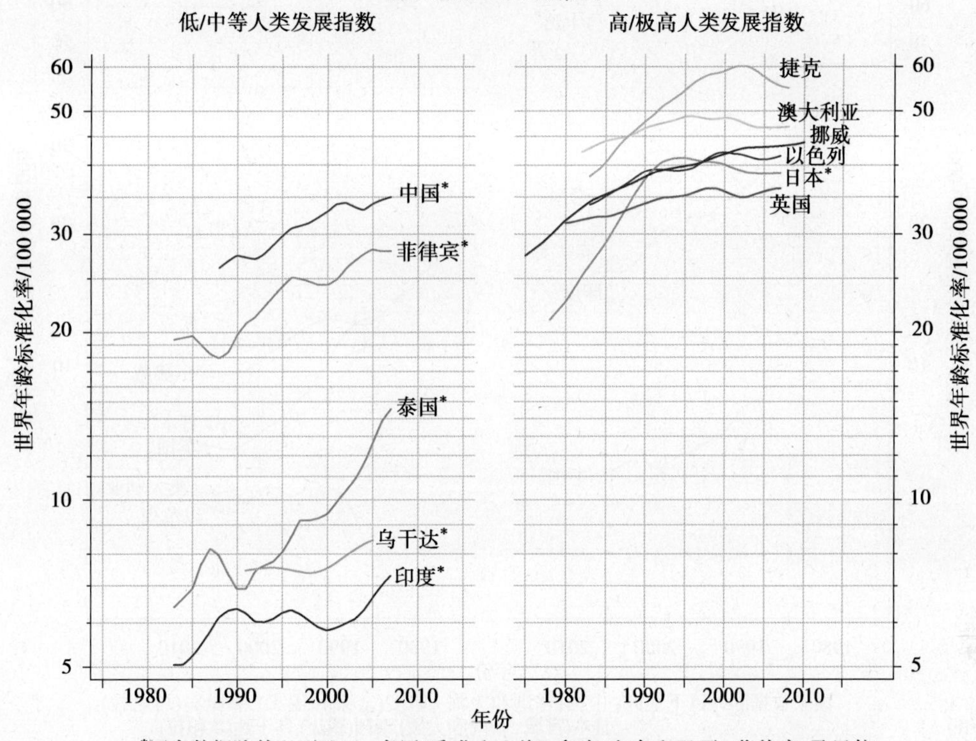
结肠、直肠和肛门癌,男性
低/中等人类发展指数
高/极高人类发展指数
世界年龄标准化率/100 000
中国*
菲律宾*
泰国*
乌干达*
印度*
捷克
澳大利亚
挪威
以色列
日本*
英国
年份
*国家数据除外以下地区:中国(香港和上海),印度(金奈和孟买),菲律宾(马尼拉),
日本(宫城、长崎和大阪),泰国(钱迈),乌干达(坎帕拉)

(c)

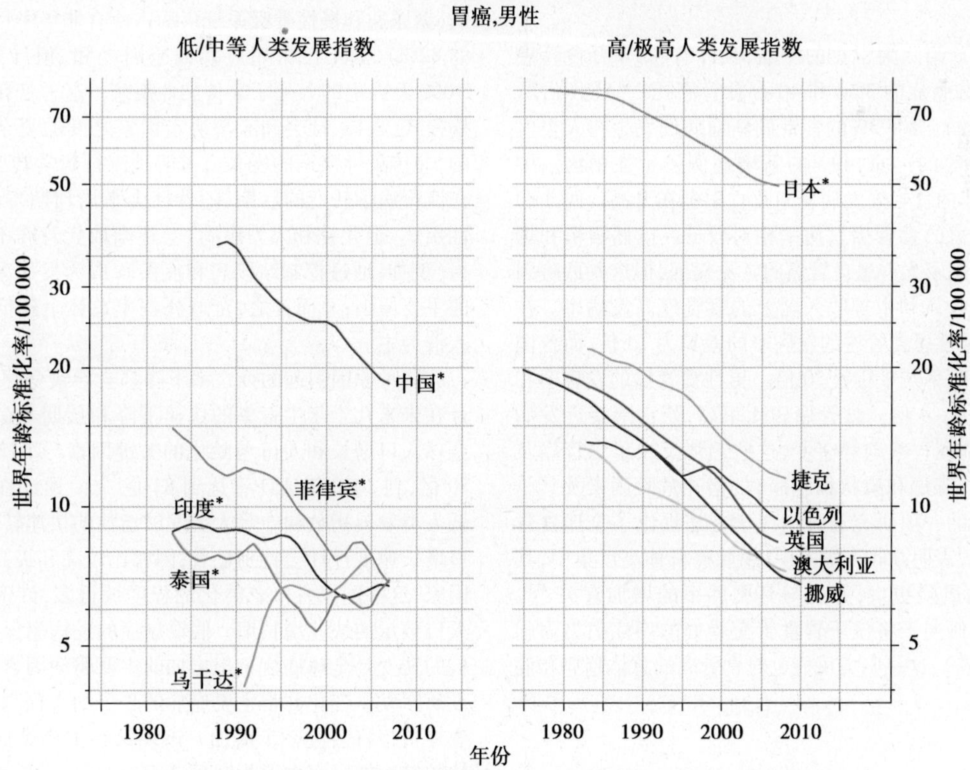
胃癌,男性
低/中等人类发展指数
高/极高人类发展指数
世界年龄标准化率/100 000
中国*
菲律宾*
印度*
泰国*
乌干达*
日本*
捷克
以色列
英国
澳大利亚
挪威
年份
*国家数据除外以下地区:中国(香港和上海),印度(金奈和孟买),菲律宾(马尼拉),
日本(宫城、长崎和大阪),泰国(钱迈),乌干达(坎帕拉)

(d)

图 33-4(续)

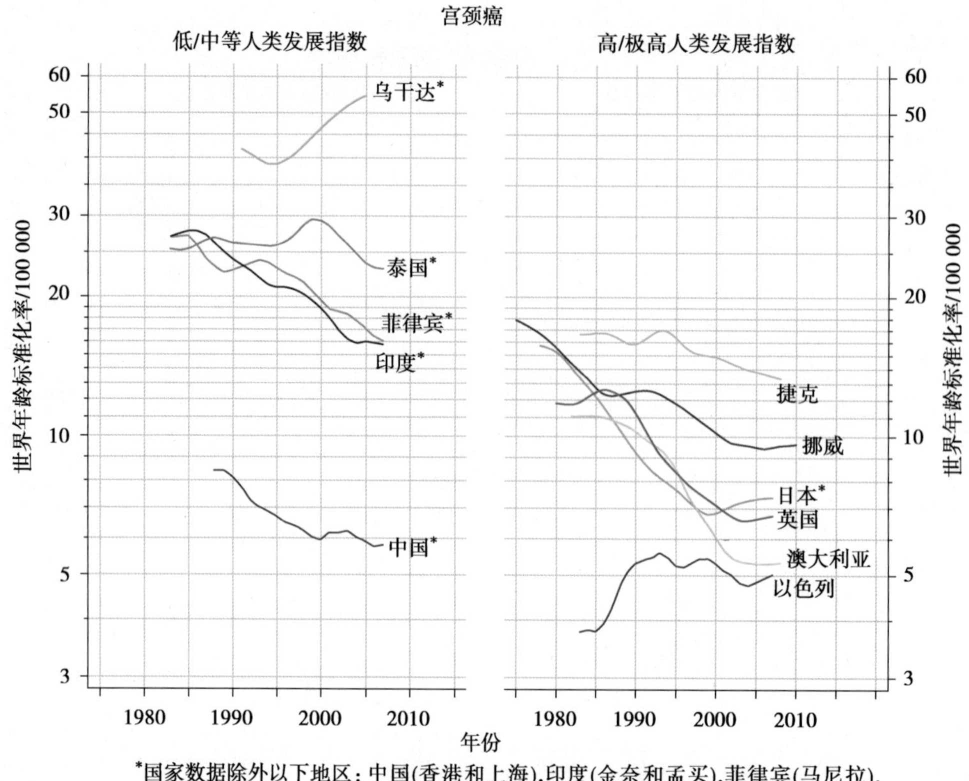

图 33-4(续)

食管癌

食管癌是全球第八大常见的癌症，预计有 45.6 万食管癌新发病例(占所有癌症的 3%)和 40 万食管癌死亡病例(占所有癌症死亡的 5%)。约 73%的食管癌新增病例发生在人类发展水平较低或中等的国家，49%的新增病例发生在中国。中亚、东亚以及东非的食管癌发病率和死亡率都在升高。西非和一些拉丁美洲国家的食管癌发病率相对较低。虽然酒精和烟草是导致高收入国家人群患食管癌的常见病因，但这些危险因素并不能解释低收入和中等收入国家的食管癌高发病率。在世界各国之间，男性患食管癌的发病率的差异为 15 倍，而各国女性食管癌的发病率几乎相差 20 倍。男性食管癌的发病率和死亡率是女性的 2~4 倍。食管癌病死率高，死亡率接近发病率，而且发病率和死亡率趋势多变，这些趋势反映了食管癌及其主要组织亚型(腺癌和鳞状细胞癌)的潜在危险因素及其分布的变化。最近的一项研究通过组织学方法提供了全球食管癌发病率的预估，表明高收入国家中，患腺癌群体高度集中，其中男性患腺癌的风险更大，并且与其肥胖率的增加有关[21]。目前我们越来越倾向于将位于胃食管交界处的癌症归类为腺癌(而不是贲门癌)，这一归类可能也对食管癌的总体趋势和癌症负担产生影响。

全球癌症转变

癌症规模的变化

2011 年，有 3 600 万人死于非传染性疾病(癌症、心血管疾病、糖尿病和慢性呼吸系统疾病占所有非传染性疾病死亡人数的 82%)，其死亡率超过其他原因之和，预计到 2030 年将有 5 000 万以上的人死于非传染性疾病。这种变化是由健康与疾病模式、人口、社会和经济决定因素之间的复杂相互作用造成的，非传染性疾病的增多也可能是流行病学转变的一部分[22]。在流行病学转变的后期，随着社会平均预期寿命增加，非传染性疾病(退化性和人为疾病)会逐渐取代营养不良和感染大流行(例如：通过控制结核病和疟疾)，成为发病率和死亡率上升的主要原因；总而言之，全球死亡率总体上较低但死亡以老年人群为主。

各种原因引起的死亡率下降都会导致全球生育率下降，预计在未来几十年生育率的快速下降和预期寿命的增加会成为全球人口增长和人口老龄化的关键因素。2012 年全球人口为 70 亿，到 2030 年预计将达到 83 亿[23]。预计在目前被归类为低人类发展指数和中等人类发展指数的快速转型国家中，其人口增长速度预计会特别显著；因相比较高和极高人类发展指数国家，这些国家人口老龄化的程度低得多，许多国家将会进入人口数量的快速增长期。假设癌症的发病率保持不变，人口结构的转变是全球癌症负担增加的主要驱动因素：如果允许癌症发病率发生变化并将主要癌症的趋势纳入预测体系时，未来的癌症负担将会进一步增加。该现象在主要癌症发病率增长最快的转型期国家中尤为明显。无论如何，人口结构的变化和基本比率的变化都会使得 4∶1 这一比例上升[9]；在人口构成方面，预计 2025 年全球新增癌症病例近 1 900 万例，到 2030 年增加到 2 160 万例，而 2012 年预计为 1 410 万例(图 33-5)。人口的增长比例和未来癌症新增病例与目前的发展水平成反比，因此在低 HDI 地区人口及新增癌症病例的数量相对增长最大。中等 HDI 国家将经历最大的绝对人口增长，因此其癌症负担将会在 2025 年出现最大的绝对增长。预计到 2030 年，拉丁美洲、亚洲和非洲的癌症发病率将增加 60%~70%。

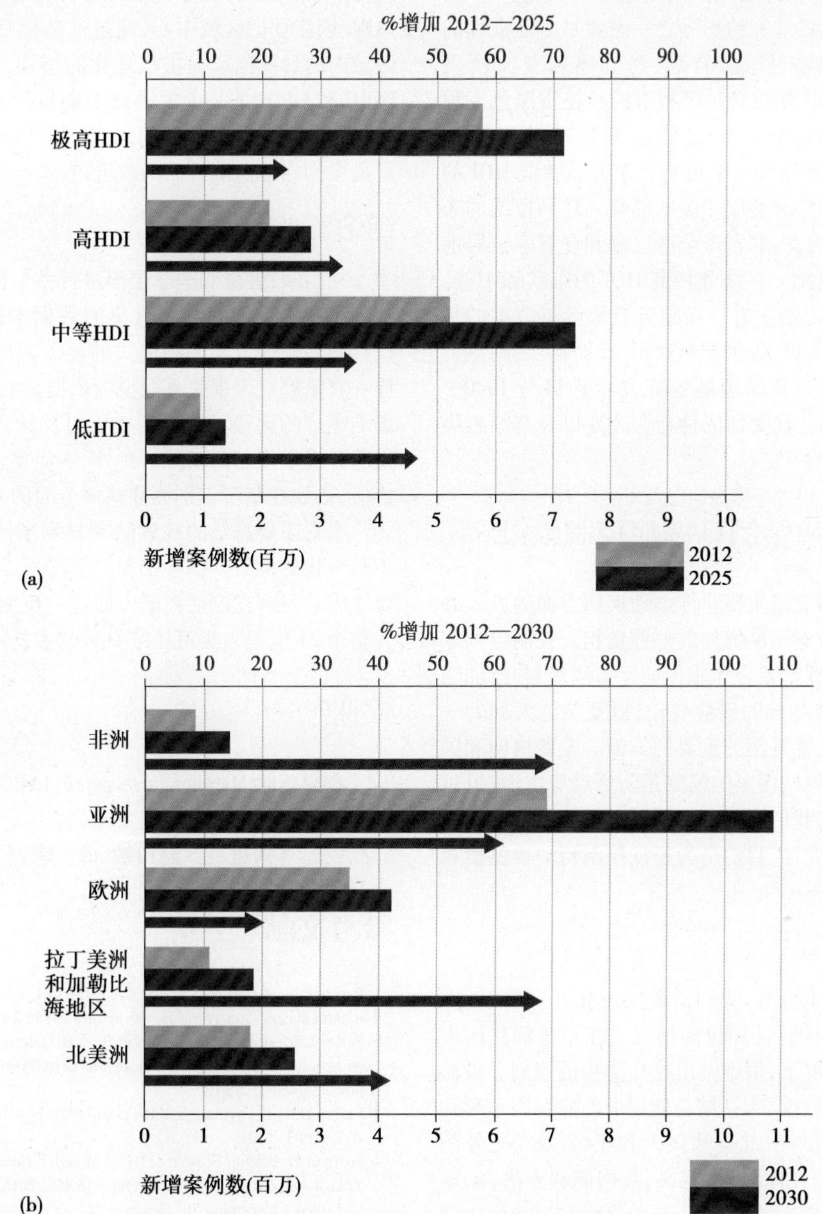

图 33-5　(a)通过 HDI 描述 2012—2025 年癌症发病率增长百分比(b)世界五个区域 2012—2030 年癌症发病率增长百分比的条形图

癌症谱的变化

癌症已成为人类死亡的主要原因之一，老年人退行性疾病(如脑血管病和中风)死亡率的降低也意味着癌症是延长平均预期寿命的主要障碍之一。随着国家向更高的人类发展水平过渡，癌症负担在癌症谱和规模上都在发生变化，并具有过渡性特征：从全球角度来看，与良好生活条件相关的癌症(例如：乳腺癌、结直肠癌和前列腺癌)的发病率已经超过了感染相关性癌症(例如：宫颈癌和胃癌)的发病率。结直肠癌在 HDI 达到中等或更高水平的国家中发病率迅速上升，进一步体现了西方化生活方式的影响：一些生殖、饮食、代谢和激素风险因素导致人口患病率不断变化(与西方观察到的水平相近)以及相应的疾病风险增加[24]。

科威特是一个资源丰富的国家，其 HDI 在所有阿拉伯国家中得分最高。科威特目前的癌症概况与许多西方国家相似(与 Amani Elbasmy 博士的个人交流)，如乳腺癌、前列腺癌和结直肠癌(与澳大利亚登记的数据相似，但科威特的总体发病率比澳大利亚低三倍)，某些类型的癌症(如白血病和非霍奇金淋巴瘤)的相对重要性不断上升。但人们对在男性中排名第 10 位睾丸肿瘤的致病因素的了解仍然有限[25]。

人们已经注意到，Omran 的流行病学转变的基本模型未能把握全面性质，因此不能把握死亡率转变的非同步性，并且流行病学转变的模型可能和社会类型同样存在多样性[26]。对于癌症来说，在没有解决感染对癌症的影响的情况下，将“癌症转变”简单地描述为癌症是非传染性疾病是过于片面化[27]。据统计，发生在撒哈拉以南的非洲约三分之一癌症是由传染性病原体引起的，包括宫颈癌、肝癌、胃癌、膀胱癌和卡波西肉瘤[28]。虽然在乌干达的坎帕拉和津巴布韦的哈拉雷黑色人种中观察到乳腺癌、前列腺癌和结直肠癌发病率的快速上升[12-13]，但其相应的宫颈癌发病率也有所上升。在低 HDI 的东非地区，常见的是与感染和贫困相关的癌症。在马拉维的布兰太尔，宫颈癌、卡波西肉瘤、非霍奇金淋巴瘤和食管癌位居前五位，排在女性乳腺癌之前。在高和极高 HDI 的东欧和中亚，年轻女性宫颈癌死亡率不断上升。在缺乏有效筛查方案的情况下，白俄罗斯、塔吉克斯坦、吉尔吉斯斯坦、亚美尼亚、阿塞拜疆、乌克兰、俄罗斯和哈萨克斯坦的癌症发生趋势与 1940—1950 年前后出生的连续几代女性的性行为改变以及持续感染 HPV 的风险增加有关[29]。

利用描述性流行病学制订癌症控制政策

显然，在控制癌症和其他主要非传染性疾病方面的投入必须进行阶段性改变，以应对不断增加的癌症负担。在制定国家癌症控制战略并将这些战略整合到非传染性疾病规划时，加强系统监测，包括以人口为基础的癌症登记，以及实施人群的一级预防和早期发现政策，都是至关重要的方面。发展机构和国际合作伙伴在支持资源短缺国家的癌症预防活动等方面，可以发挥独特的作用。最后，我们讨论了在资源有限的条件下加强癌症监测系统建设的必要性，目的是为癌症控制行动提供信息参考。

整合基于人口的癌症登记

为了规划和评估卫生服务，我们需要知道在人口层面（在国家、一个省或一个重要部门层面）的情况。在不了解社区中癌症的规模和概况的情况下，很难做出癌症防控的规划。虽然使用高质量的癌症监测数据（包括结合使用的癌症发病率和死亡率）最为理想，但对除欧洲、北美和澳大利亚/新西兰之外的许多发展中国家来说（如在标题为“定义，数据源和方法”的章节中讨论的），各自的数据来源、基于人口的癌症登记和生命登记系统在可用性、数据质量以及人口覆盖面等方面十分有限。值得注意的是，PBCR 即使在资源有限的情况下也是可行的，并且用于规划和开发登记系统也有相应的参考材料[30]。目前实际情况是只有 67 个国家（主要是高收入国家）配备了高质量的 PBCR 系统，而在 62 个国家（主要是低收入国家）中没有可靠的数据。许多发展中国家存在着其他卫生服务面临的同样障碍，例如缺乏财政资源和专业知识。

然而，近年来对非传染性疾病的政治认识发生了变化，世界各国领导人在 2011 年商定了解决全球 NCD 的政策，包括承诺在 2013 年之前制定预防和控制非传染性疾病政策，以及通过了 2025 年的 9 个全球目标（包括将非传染性疾病过早死亡率降低 25%）。其中重要的是，所有国家都同意收集癌症发病率数据，并将这些数据作为监测癌症负担进展的 25 个指标之一，国际癌症研究中心领导的全球癌症登记发展倡议（GICR）伙伴关系（http://gicr.iarc.fr）旨在通过提供 PBCR 来帮助和加快不同国家癌症控制目的的实现。实现这些目标的关键方法是在非洲、亚洲、拉丁美洲、加勒比和太平洋群岛建立 6 个 IARC 癌症登记区域中心，通过这些癌症登记区域中心向一定区域内的目标国家提供本地化的培训、专业支持和宣传方案。IARC 和 GICR 的一个关键的中期目标是通过规划和开发 PBCR 支持 50 个资源有限的国家，为 2018 年癌症控制行动提供可衡量的癌症监测方面的改进措施。

结论

在国家、区域和全球层面进行基于证据的癌症控制的重要基础是癌症登记和利用收集的数据来描述癌症的流行病学。世界各地癌症发病率和模式的显著差异及其随时间的变化趋势一直是癌症因果关系假说的依据，也是衡量预防性干预措施影响癌症的途径。关于疾病负担及其变化模式的信息也是卫生服务提供规划的基础。此外，癌症登记对于研究也有很好的价值，例如在基于识别癌症病例方面的人群研究。

本章简要总结的观察结果显示了国际癌症控制的差异和不断变化的挑战。癌症已是中低收入国家人口过早死亡的重要原因。只有在癌症控制方面进一步加大投入，癌症才不会成为整个 21 世纪人类可持续发展的主要障碍。

致谢

我们感谢 Mathieu Laversanne，IARC 对本章部分图片所进行的工作。

（刘康栋 赵四敏 译 李鑫 陈新焕 于乐兴 审）

参考文献

1 Parkin DM, Stjernsward J, Muir CS. Estimates of the worldwide frequency of twelve major cancers. *Bull World Health Organ*. 1984;**62**:163–182.

2 Ferlay J, Soerjomataram I, Dikshit R, et al. Cancer incidence and mortality worldwide: sources, methods and major patterns in GLOBOCAN 2012. *Int J Cancer*. 2014. doi: 10.1002/ijc.29210.

3 Parkin DM. The evolution of the population-based cancer registry. *Nat Rev Cancer*. 2006;**6**:603–612.

4 Forman D, Bray F, Brewster DH, et al. (eds). *Cancer Incidence in Five Continents*. Vol. X (electronic version). Lyon: IARC; 2013. Available at: http://ci5.iarc.fr (accessed 2 December 2013).

5 Bray F, Ferlay J, Laversanne M, et al. Cancer incidence in five continents: inclusion criteria, highlights from volume X and the global status of cancer registration. *Int J Cancer*. 2015;**137**(**9**):2060–2071.

6 Ferlay J, Steliarova-Foucher E, Lortet-Tieulent J, et al. Cancer incidence and mortality patterns in Europe: estimates for 40 countries in 2012. *Eur J Cancer*. 2013;**49**:1374–1403.

7 Mathers C, Ma Fat D, Inoue M, et al. Counting the dead and what they died from: an assessment of the global status of cause of death data. *Bull World Health Organ*. 2005;**83**:171–177.

8 Bray F, Ren JS, Masuyer E, Ferlay J. Estimates of global cancer prevalence for 27 sites in the adult population in 2008. *Int J Cancer*. 2013;**132**:1133–1145.

9 Bray F, Jemal A, Grey N, Ferlay J, Forman D. Global cancer transitions according to the human development index (2008-2030): a population-based study. *Lancet Oncol*. 2012;**13**:790–801.

10 United Nations Development Programme. *Human Development Report*. 2013, http://hdr.undp.org/en (accessed 12 February 2013).

11 Chaabna K, Bray F, Wabinga HR, et al. Kaposi sarcoma trends in Uganda and Zimbabwe: a sustained decline in incidence? *Int J Cancer*. 2013;**133**(**5**):1197–1203.

12 Chokunonga E, Borok MZ, Chirenje ZM, Nyakabau AM, Parkin DM. Trends in the incidence of cancer in the black population of Harare, Zimbabwe 1991–2010. *Int J Cancer*. 2013;**133**:721–729.

13 Wabinga HR, Nambooze S, Amulen PM, Okello C, Mbus L, Parkin DM. Trends in the incidence of cancer in Kampala, Uganda 1991–2010. *Int J Cancer*. 2014;**135(2)**:432–439. doi: 10.1002/ijc.28661

14 Lopez A. Changes in tobacco consumption and lung cancer risk: evidence from national statistics. In: Hakama M, Beral V, Cullen V, Parkin DM, eds. *Evaluating Effectiveness of Primary Prevention of Cancer*. Lyon: IARC Scientific Publications No. 103; 1990:133–149.

15 Jha P. Avoidable global cancer deaths and total deaths from smoking. *Nat Rev Cancer*. 2009;**9(9)**:655–664. doi: 10.1038/nrc2703. Epub 2009 Aug 20. Review. PubMed PMID: 19693096.

16 Thun M, Peto R, Boreham J, Lopez AD. Stages of the cigarette epidemic on entering its second century. *Tob Control*. 2012;**21(2)**:96–101.

17 Herrero R, Parsonnet J, Greenberg ER. Prevention of gastric cancer. *JAMA*. 2014;**312(12)**:1197–1198. doi: 10.1001/jama.2014.10498. PubMed PMID: 25247512.

18 International Agency for Research on Cancer. Pitt JI, Wild CP, Baan RA, Gelderblom WCA, Miller JD, Riley RT, Wu F, eds. *Improving Public Health through Mycotoxin Control*. Lyon, France: IARC Scientific Publication, No 158.; 2012.

19 McGlynn KA, London WT. The global epidemiology of hepatocellular carcinoma: present and future. *Clin Liver Dis*. 2011;**15**:223–243, vii–x.

20 Vaccarella S, Lortet-Tieulent J, Plummer M, Franceschi S, Bray F. Worldwide trends in cervical cancer incidence: impact of screening against changes in disease risk factors. *Eur J Cancer*. 2013;**49(15)**:3262–3273.

21 Arnold M, Soerjomataram I, Ferlay J, Forman D. Global incidence of esophageal cancer by histological subtype in 2012. *Gut*. 2014;**64**:381–387.

22 Omran AR. The epidemiologic transition. A theory of the epidemiology of population change. *Milbank Mem Fund Q*. 1971;**49**:509–538.

23 United Nations Population Division. *World Population Prospects, the 2010 Revision*. 2010, New York: United Nations, http://esa.un.org/wpp/index.htm (accessed 12 October 2015).

24 Bray F. Transitions in human development and the global cancer burden. In: Wild CP, Stewart B, eds. *World Cancer Report 2014*. Lyon, France: International Agency for Research on Cancer; 2014.

25 Maule M, Merletti F. Cancer transition and priorities for cancer control. *Lancet Oncol*. 2012;**13(8)**:745–746. doi: 10.1016/S1470-2045(12)70268-1. PubMed PMID: 22846827.

26 Caldwell JC. Population health in transition. *Bull World Health Organ*. 2001;**79(2)**:159–160.

27 Gersten O, Wilmoth JR. The cancer transition in Japan since 1951. *Demogr Res*. 2002;7:271–306.

28 De Martel C, Ferlay J, Franceschi S, et al. Global burden of cancers attributable to infections in 2008: a review and synthetic analysis. *Lancet Oncol*. 2012;**13**:607–615.

29 Bray F, Lortet-Tieulent J, Znaor A, Brotons M, Poljak M, Arbyn M. Patterns and trends in human papillomavirus-related diseases in Central and Eastern Europe and Central Asia. *Vaccine*. 2013;**31(Suppl 7)**:H32–H45.

30 Bray F, Znaor A, Cueva P, et al. *Planning and Developing Population-Based Cancer Registration in Low- and Middle-Income Settings*. Lyon, France: International Agency for Research on Cancer; 2014. IARC Technical Publication No. 43.

第34章 癌症的流行病学

Xifeng Wu, MD, PhD ■ Xia Pu, PhD ■ Stephanie C. Melkonian, PhD ■ Margaret R. Spitz, MD, MPH

概述

根据世界卫生组织(WHO)的数据,全世界每年有超过1 400万新增的癌症病例。随着流行病学的不断发展,发展中国家的癌症发病率有所上升,甚至超过一半的新发病例在中低收入国家。本章将回顾癌症在发达国家和发展中国家之间的差距、传统的致癌因素以及最近出现的致癌因素,尤其是吸烟和与均衡能量摄入有关的因素。本文还将通过对现有的以及新兴的基因组学、流行病学、代谢组学和转录组学相关信息的总结,预测癌症的风险和预后。

癌症统计学数据

全球癌症统计数据

根据世界卫生组织(WHO)的统计,每年有超过1 400万新确诊的癌症病人,并有800万死亡病例与癌症相关[1]。全球范围内发病率排名前10的癌症有肺癌(13%)、乳腺癌(11.9%)、结肠直肠癌(9.7%)、前列腺癌(8%)、胃癌(6.8%)、肝癌(5.5%)、宫颈癌(3.7%)、食管癌(3.2%)、膀胱癌(3%)和非霍奇金淋巴瘤(2.7%)[1]。癌症在男性和女性之间的发病率也有所不同;在男性中,最常见的是肺癌(16.7%)、前列腺癌(15%)、结直肠癌(10%)、胃癌(8.5%)和肝癌(7.5%),在女性中最为常见的是乳腺癌(22.5%)、结直肠癌(9.2%)、肺癌(8.8%)、宫颈癌(8%)和子宫内膜癌(5%)(不包括皮肤非黑色素瘤)[1]。据统计,如果未来几年癌症发病率按照目前的趋势继续下去,截至2030年,每年的癌症新发病例将达2 360万例。2013年,全球范围约820万人死于癌症,其中包括男性470万人(57%)和女性350万人(48%),男性与女性的比例为10:8[1]。

美国癌症统计学数据

2014年,美国有超过160万新增癌症病例,并有将近60万人死于癌症[2]。根据美国国立癌症研究所监测、流行病学和最终结果数据库(SEER)的数据,除了非黑色素瘤,在美国,男性群体中,发生率最高的癌症包括前列腺癌(27%)、肺癌(14%)、结肠直肠癌(8%)、膀胱癌(6.6%)、皮肤黑色素瘤(5.1%)、肾癌(4.6%)、非霍奇金淋巴瘤(4.5%)、口腔癌(3.5%)、白血病(3.5%)和胰腺癌(2.8%)。女性中最常见的癌症包括乳腺癌(29%)、肺癌(13%)、结肠直肠癌(8%)、子宫内膜癌(6.5%)、甲状腺癌(5.9%)、黑色素瘤(4%)、非霍奇金淋巴瘤(4%)、肾癌(3.1%)、胰腺癌(2.8%)和卵巢癌(2.7%)[3]。从总发生率来看,每10万名男性中就有529.4名男性患有癌症,每10万名女性中有411.3名女性患有癌症。近年来,随着初级预防和筛查方式的进步使得结直肠癌、前列腺癌和肺癌的发生迅速减少,癌症的总发病率也相应出现下降[3]。然而,皮肤黑色素瘤、食管腺癌、甲状腺癌、肝癌、肾癌、肛门癌、胰腺癌以及人类乳头瘤病毒阳性的口咽癌的发病率呈现上升趋势[4]。尽管癌症的总死亡率在20世纪的一段时期中呈上升趋势,但在过去的二十年中,癌症的死亡率一直在稳步下降(从1991年的215.1/10万人的死亡率下降为2010年的171.8/10万人)[2,3]。

癌症发病率和死亡率在不同种族和不同社会经济地位(SES)的群体之间有很大不同。无论是在全球范围内还是在美国,这些不同都引起了人们对于癌症健康差异的关注。

癌症健康差异

癌症健康差异是指不同人群之间癌症发病率、患病率和死亡率的差异,这些差异基于以下因素:种族、民族、贫困、社会经济地位、教育程度、医疗服务以及各种不同的行为、环境、生活方式和职业暴露[5~7]。消除癌症负担的差异是当今世界的首要关注点。

癌症发病率和死亡率在美国不同种族间存在差异

癌症发病率和死亡率在不同种族之间中有相当大的差异(广义上定义的非西班牙裔白人,黑色人种,亚裔美国人/太平洋岛民,美洲印第安人/阿拉斯加原住民和西班牙裔美国人)。癌症发病率在非裔美国人(AA)男性中所占比率最高(554.5/10万人),其次是白人(499.7/10万人),西班牙裔美国人(393.5/10万人),亚洲/太平洋岛民(310.1/10万人)和美洲印第安人/阿拉斯加原住民(293.5/10万人)(图34-1a)[4]。非洲裔美国人男性的癌症死亡率最高(253.9/10万人),几乎是亚裔美国人的两倍(131.1/10万人),亚裔美国人癌症的发病率和死亡率在这五个种族或民族中处于最低水平(图34-2a)[2,4]。除肾癌之外,黑色人种在其他部位癌症中的发病率和死亡率都要高于白人[4,8]。

在女性中,白人的癌症发病率最高(414.8/10万人),其次依次为非裔美国人(393.8/10万人),西班牙裔美国人(324.2/10万人),亚裔美国人/太平洋岛民(279.8/10万)和美洲印第安人/阿拉斯加原住民(261.0/10万人)(图34-1b)。黑色人种中女性的癌症死亡率最高(166.2/10万人),相对而言,亚洲/太平洋岛民的癌症死亡率最低(91.1/10万人)(图34-2b)。总的来说,亚裔美国人/太平洋岛民、美洲印第安人/阿拉斯加原住民和西班牙裔美国人在四个最常见癌症发病部位中的癌症发病率和死亡率均低于白人[3]。然而,与感染相关的癌症(子宫颈癌、胃癌和肝癌)在非白种人中更常见。胃癌和肝癌在亚裔美国人/太平洋岛民中的发病率最高,西班牙裔美国人的宫颈癌发病率最高[9]。

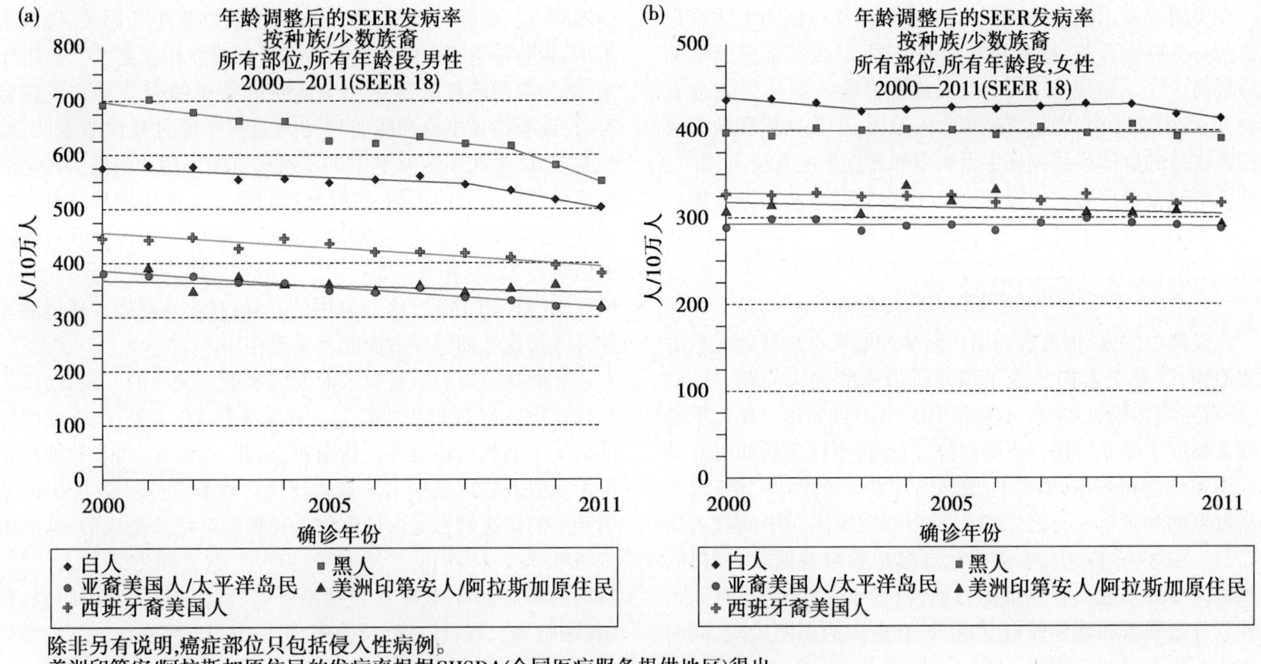

除非另有说明,癌症部位只包括侵入性病例。
美洲印第安/阿拉斯加原住民的发病率根据CHSDA(合同医疗服务提供地区)得出。
西班牙裔和非西班牙裔与白人、黑人、亚裔/太平洋岛民和美洲印第安/阿拉斯加原住民并不相互排斥。
西班牙裔美国人和非西班牙裔美国人的发病率数据由北美癌症登记协会(NAACCR)提供。
西班牙裔识别算法排除阿拉斯加本地注册的病例。
发病率为每10万人,年龄根据2000美国标准人口(19个年龄组——人口普查P25~1130)调整。
回归线计算使用 Joinpoint Regression Program 4.1.0版计算,2014年4月,美国国家癌症研究所。
发病数据来源:SEER 18区(旧金山、康涅狄格、底特律、夏威夷、爱荷华、新墨西哥、西雅图、犹他、亚特兰大、圣若泽蒙特雷、洛杉矶、阿拉斯加本地登记、佐治亚州农村、加利福尼亚不包括SF/SJM/LA、肯塔基州、路易斯安那州、新泽西州和佐治亚州不包括ATL/RG)。

图 34-1 (a,b)1999—2011 年,美国,按种族/民族和性别合并一起的所有癌症发病率。资料来源:http://seer.cancer.gov/faststats/selections.php?series=race

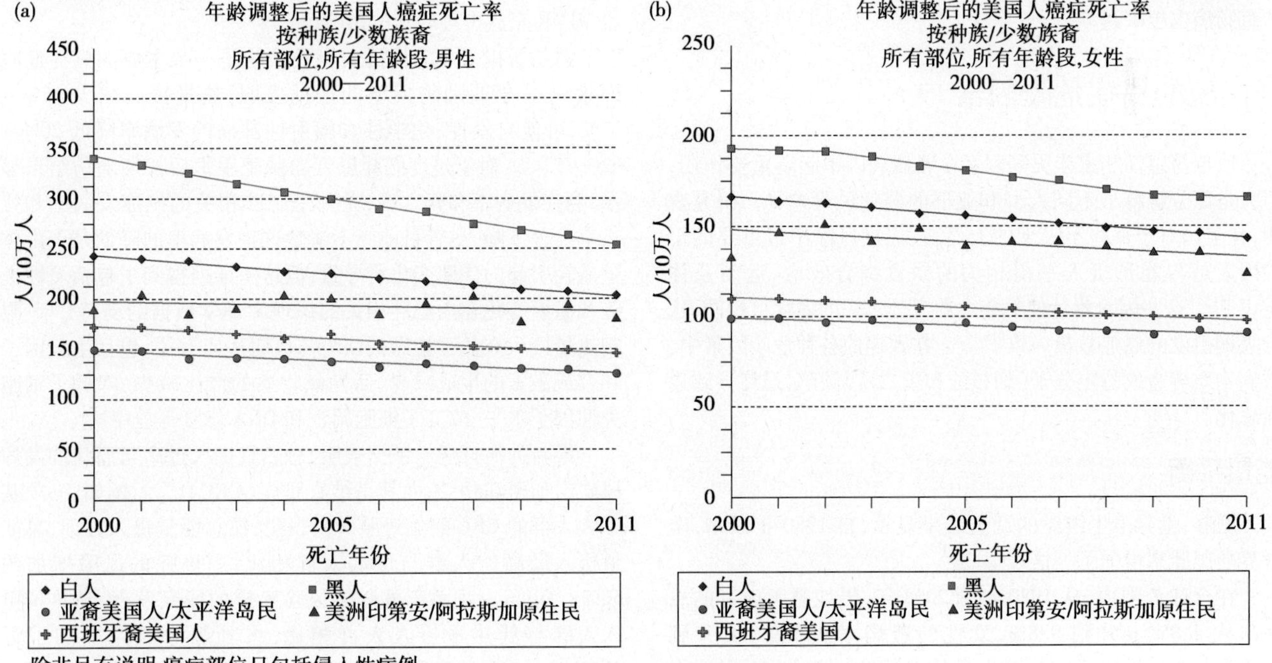

除非另有说明,癌症部位只包括侵入性病例。
美洲印第安/阿拉斯加原住民的发病率根据CHSDA(合同医疗服务提供地区)得出。
西班牙裔和非西班牙裔与白人、黑人、亚裔/太平洋岛民和美洲印第安/阿拉斯加原住民并不相互排斥。
死亡率数据来源:美国疾病控制与预防中心,国家卫生统计中心,美国死亡率档案。
死亡率为每10万人,年龄根据2000美国标准人口(19个年龄组——人口普查P25~1130)调整。
回归线计算使用 Joinpoint Regression Program 4.1.0版计算,2014年4月,美国国家癌症研究所。

图 34-2 (a,b)1999-2011 年,美国,按种族/民族和性别合并一起的所有癌症死亡率。资料来源:http://seer.cancer.gov/faststats/selections.php?series=race

在美国等发达国家，低收入的社会群体往往因为无法获得充足的有关癌症预防、检测和治疗的资源，导致其罹患癌症的风险较高[5,7,9]。通常来说，少数民族和低收入群体之间会有重叠，但我们注意到，即使有经济收入原因，少数民族和缺乏医疗服务支持的群体往往在癌症发病率和死亡率上有所不同[9]。这些人群通常在疾病进入晚期阶段才选择就医，从而导致癌症的发病率和死亡率上升[7,9]。

癌症在发展中国家的差异

在发展中国家，传染病和围产期孕产妇死亡是导致死亡的主要原因，以至于人们忽视了癌症所造成的健康问题[6]。然而，所有主要传染性疾病（不包括 HIV/AIDS）导致的死亡率已出现大幅度下降并将保持下降趋势，但非传染性疾病如癌症的死亡率预计会在未来 30 年内增加[6,7,10,11]。全世界 50%以上的新发癌症和每年三分之二癌症死亡病例发生在中低收入国家[1,11]。在这些国家中，癌症问题更多地影响着低收入群体，这些群体中大多数人有抽烟的习惯，营养水平较差，长时间的户外紫外线暴露和其他职业暴露，具有更高的患癌风险，同时还无法获得充足的医疗服务[12]。

尽管癌症的长期生存率在高收入国家的人群中已超过 60%，而在发展中国家却仅为 20%。可能是由于基础设施较差和可用于早期检测方法的匮乏，在发展中国家中大约 70%的癌症在诊断时都处于晚期[1,12]。感染诱发的癌症（如宫颈癌和肝细胞癌）的发病率，在中低收入国家一直处于较高的水平[1,7]。然而，随着这些国家工业化发展以及可变风险因素（如久坐的生活方式和西方化饮食等）的增加，这些因素在癌症的发病过程中变得越来越突出。在西方国家癌症更为普遍，如乳腺癌和结直肠癌也越来越多[7]。

新出现的癌症危险因素

遗传易感性和家族史等因素在癌症病因中起着重要作用，但只是部分解释了不同人群和亚群的癌症风险差异。研究表明，在美国对于那些不吸烟的人而言，癌症风险中最重要的可控因素是与能量摄入平衡相关的饮食综合效应、运动及体重[13,14]。这些因素累计使每年大约三分之一的癌症可预防，这与吸烟引发的癌症数量一致[15,16]。在致癌的各种危险因素中，致癌物质可造成特定分子（如核酸和蛋白质）缺陷，最终导致癌症恶化。

能量平衡

肥胖：世界卫生组织的调查结果显示，自 1980 年以来，全世界的肥胖率增加了一倍[17]。

在全球范围内，从 1980 年到 2008 年，男性肥胖患者的患病率从 4.8%上升到 9.8%，女性的患病率从 7.9%上升到 13.8%[17,18]。世界卫生组织估算，截至 2008 年，在 20 岁以上的成年人中有超过 14 亿人体重超标，在这些超重的人群中，将近 5 亿人患有肥胖[17]。美国是肥胖率最高的国家。超过三分之一（34.9%）的成年人被认为肥胖，其中不同种族和社会经济亚群的肥胖率有很大差异[19]。例如，非西班牙裔黑色人种肥胖的年龄调整率最高（47.8%），其次是西班牙裔美国人（42.5%）。肥胖可能通过胰岛素和类胰岛素生长因子、性激素水平、脂肪细胞衍生因子或脂肪因子和癌症相联系[20-22]。近年来，脂肪组织已被公认是一个活跃的重要的内分泌和代谢器官，在调节能量平衡和脂肪代谢的过程中通过释放激素肽，如瘦素、脂联素和细胞因子 TNF-α 发挥重要作用。根据所讨论的癌症部位和人群的不同，肥胖导致的癌症人群比例从结直肠癌（CRC）的 14%到子宫内膜癌的 50%不等[23]。遗传因素对体重的影响较大，为 40%～70%[24-26]。研究表明，遗传变异，尤其是 FTO、MC4R 和 TMEM18 等基因的变异，在个体对致胖环境的易感性或抵抗性的差异方面起着重要作用[27]。

肥胖这一曾经被高收入西方国家重点关注的问题，已成为全球疾病负担的主要因素[18]。在未来的 20 年里，超重或肥胖的成年人的数量将会在包括南亚、东非、东南亚、西非和加勒比等中低收入的国家中出现最大比例的增长[18,28]。发展中国家肥胖率的快速增长是由城市化进程和经济增长造成的，这些因素将继续改变人们的生活和劳动环境、饮食和生活方式[18,28]。目前的研究表明，肥胖在包括结肠癌、乳腺癌、子宫内膜癌、肾（肾细胞）癌、胃贲门癌、胰腺癌、胆囊癌和肝癌在内的几种癌症中均发挥作用[20]。

体力活动和能量摄入

大量观察性研究显示癌症发生随体力活动水平增加而降低[29]。流行病学证据表明，体力活动与结直肠癌的发病风险之间存在关联[30]。研究表明，与活动水平最低的个体相比，活动水平最高个体患癌风险降低约 30%[30]。体力活动与其他癌症（如前列腺癌、子宫内膜癌、乳腺癌、肺癌和肾癌）之间相关性的证据并不一致，这表明这些相关性可能还受到体重指数（BMI）和家族史等因素的影响[31]。

总热量摄入或能量摄入也被认为是一个主要的癌症危险因素[32]。早期动物模型的证据表明，热量摄入减少 15%～53%，可使自发性、化学性和辐射性肿瘤的发病率降低 20%～62%[32-34]。对于过度肥胖患者的减肥手术后长期随访结果显示，癌症发病率和死亡率，尤其是肥胖相关的癌症发病率和死亡率显著下降，尽管目前尚不清楚这种发病率的降低是否由体重减轻引起的代谢变化所导致，但这一证据得到了包括慢性炎症和激素变化在内肥胖相关的病理生理学数据的支持[35]。限制热量摄入有益于控癌被认为与代谢适应有关，包括生长因子和合成激素的生成减少、活性氧物质的产生减少、降低了细胞炎性因子水平、改变了细胞凋亡和 DNA 修复等程序[32]。

最新的流行病学证据表明，总热量摄入过高与癌症的发病风险增加密切相关，尤其是结直肠癌（CRC）[36]。例如，一项基于大人群的 CRC 病例对照研究表明，在总能量摄入方面，总能量摄入最高的人群与最低人群相比，患癌症的风险增加约 56%。同样，一项关于乳腺癌风险家族的研究发现，高热量摄入人群与低热量摄入人群相比，患乳腺癌风险增加了近 60%[37]。前列腺癌和肾癌的病例对照研究也表明，高热量摄入与癌症风险增加有关[38,39]。然而，流行病学研究中对总热量摄入的测量往往容易因使用自我报告的数据而产生偏倚和错误分类，导致关于能量摄入和体力活动的研究结果不一致[38,39]。

代谢、激素和生长因子的改变会影响参与 DNA 修复、细胞增殖和凋亡的基因的调控和表达，这些改变与多食和少动有关[40]。规律的锻炼和热量限制能显著降低胰岛素和类胰岛素生长因子水平[41]。锻炼可能改变内源性的性激素、激素和生长因子的水平，影响机体免疫应答，减少肥胖和中心性肥胖症，起到一定的防癌作用[40]。

饮食

在西方国家，将近三分之一的癌症发病被认为与饮食因素有关[42]。早期将饮食与癌症病因学联系起来发现，世界各地的人群饮食摄入模式不同，癌症发病率也各不相同，这表明饮食模式可能与癌症病因学有关。为了进一步研究这种关联性，研究人员开展了数百项病例队列的前瞻性研究，评估饮食习惯在癌症风险中所起的作用。几篇综述总结了饮食摄入与癌症风险之间的关系[42~45]。

简单地说，患癌风险有关饮食因素，如肉类摄入量，摄入脂肪的消耗，水果和蔬菜的摄入量等方面，都已被广泛研究。一项 meta 分析表明，较高红肉摄入量可使 CRC 的患病风险增加 28%~35%，而加工肉类的摄入可使 CRC 的患病风险增加 20%~40%[46,47]。吃肉与患胃癌的风险关系相比 CRC 较小，与膀胱癌、乳腺癌、子宫内膜癌、胶质瘤、胰腺癌、前列腺癌和肾癌的关系的一致性也较低[46]。病例对照研究表明，过高的脂肪摄入可使患乳腺癌风险最高增加 35%；然而，由于前瞻性研究不太容易产生病例研究中常见的偏倚（即回忆偏差），所以前瞻性研究并没有发现脂肪摄入与癌症风险之间的关联，这表明方法上的偏差可能是造成一些病例对照研究结果出现误差的原因[48]。研究还表明，大量摄入水果和蔬菜可预防 5%~12% 的癌症[49]。水果和蔬菜中存在的物质可能具有抗癌作用，这些物质包括二硫硫醇、异硫氰酸盐、吲哚-3-甲醇、大蒜化合物、异黄酮、蛋白酶抑制剂、皂苷、植物甾醇、肌醇六磷酸、维生素 C、D-柠檬烯、叶黄素、叶酸、β-胡萝卜素、番茄红素、硒、维生素 E、类黄酮和膳食纤维[50]。这些物质已被证明在雌激素代谢、保护 DNA 免受氧化损伤、DNA 甲基化和细胞增殖中发挥作用[51]。

电子烟

电子烟，也被称为“电子蒸气烟（vaping）”，它采用电池供电，提供含有尼古丁的蒸气，而不是传统香烟的吸入烟雾[52]。电子烟市场在不断增长，据估计 2014 年一年电子烟的销售额约为 22 亿美元[53]。电子烟作为传统香烟的替代品，在帮助戒烟和减少烟草危害方面仍存在争议。有证据表明，电子烟因使用便捷比传统香烟更难戒掉[52]。美国食品药品监督管理局（FDA）的报告指出，电子烟含有许多致癌的化学物质[54]。2014 年 4 月，FDA 宣布将对电子烟设备进行监管，使其符合烟草产品的既定监管条款的相关规定。长期使用电子烟的危害还有待观察。

遗传易感性

虽然癌症主要是由环境暴露引起的，但遗传易感性在癌症的发病中也起着重要作用[55]。易感基因分为罕见的高外显变异[优势比（OR）]>10、中外显变异（OR 2~5）、或常见的低外显变异（OR 1.2~1.5）。已知的遗传性癌症并不常见，其通常与高外显基因有关。例如，BRAC1 和 BRCA2 基因的胚系突变是导致大多数遗传性乳腺癌/卵巢癌综合征的原因，其他几种癌症的患病风险也会因此而相应的增加，如前列腺癌和胰腺癌[56]。MLH1 和 MLH2 基因可导致大多数遗传性非息肉性大肠癌（HNPCC）的发生[57]。有两个 RB1 基因突变副本的儿童发展成儿童视网膜母细胞瘤的风险高达 90%[58]。

虽然这些遗传性癌症综合征的外显率很高，但它们只占所有癌症病例的很小一部分。大多数癌症是偶发性的，归因于大量常见的低外显率基因。历史上看，候选基因方法只是确定了少数几个真正的癌症易感性位点，如膀胱癌的 GSTM1 和 NAT2，乳腺癌的 CASP[59~61]。造成问题的主要原因在于平台的低通量、有限的研究规模和能力、基因-环境相互作用的不可重复性等，最重要的是未能选择功能型突变变体来进行功能评估。近年来，全基因组关联分析研究（GWAS）的井喷式发展彻底改变了遗传易感性的研究。迄今为止，有超过 250 篇关于 GWAS 的癌症风险的报道，已经将数以百计的单核苷酸多态性（SNP）确定为 35 个癌症部位的遗传易感性变体，包括 48 个区域前列腺癌的 95 个 SNP，28 个区域乳腺癌的 81 个 SNP，12 个区域肺癌的 17 个 SNP（已出版的 GWAS 目录可在 http://www.genome.gov/gwastudies 查阅），这些基因变异多位于基因沙漠和基因间区。然而，一些已确定的易感性基因为癌症的病因学提供了重要的生物学线索，如含有烟碱乙酰胆碱受体基因的 15q25.1 号染色体的肺癌易感性位点[62~64]，含有雌激素受体 1 的 6q25.1 号染色体的乳腺癌易感性位点[65,66]，和含有雄激素受体结合区的多个前列腺癌易感性位点[67]。除了这些特定的癌症易感性区域之外，许多“热点”区域也被发现具有多种癌症易感性位点。例如，癌基因 MYC 两侧的 8q24 染色体区域含有 5 种癌症的易感性位点，包括乳腺癌、结直肠癌、膀胱癌、前列腺癌和卵巢癌。5p15.33 号染色体位于 TERT-CLPTM1L 区域，存在至少 6 种癌症的易感性位点，包括黑色素瘤、基底细胞癌、胶质瘤、肺癌、膀胱癌、乳腺癌、前列腺癌、胰腺癌和睾丸癌。染色体 11q13 的第三区含有至少 4 种癌症的易感性位点，包括前列腺癌、肾脏癌、结直肠癌和乳腺癌。该区域的主要信号是 TPCN2 和 MYEOV 附近的基因区间[68,69]。

尽管 GWAS 方法在确定癌症易感性位点方面取得了成功，但每个区域只提供一个小的癌症风险优势比，并且这些低外显率的基因位点的临床应用尚不明确。这些 GWAS 研究提示易感基因的生物学机制在很大程度上是未知的，下一步的研究需要解释基因与环境的相互作用关系，探索已确定热点基因的功能相关性，并确定这些位点的生物学机制。

新兴方法和技术

在过去的十年里，科技的飞速发展对癌症流行病学产生了巨大的推动作用。尤其是各种“组学”技术正在以前所未有的速度改变着流行病学研究的格局。除了基因组学外，表观基因组学、转录组学、蛋白质组学和代谢组学都被应用于癌症的流行病学研究。然而，由于研究设计和一些干扰因素，到目前为止这些技术尚未在癌症流行病学的研究中被充分使用。与作为稳定性状的遗传变异不同，表观遗传、RNA、蛋白质和代谢物水平的分子特征受环境暴露、病理状态、样品采集和处理以及技术可重复性的影响。加以合适的研究设计（前瞻研究，纵向研究)，标准化数据收集，控制良好的样本收集及操作步骤，成熟的技术，这些"组学"方法将有可能发现新的癌症风险生物标记并明确癌症流行病学研究结果。

下一代测序(NGS)

GWAS 在识别遗传易感性位点方面的成功要得益于基因组技术的进步，以及人类基因组单体型图计划。GWAS 在识别新的基因易感性位点方面卓有成效；但 GWAS 仅检测了普通等位基因，并且 GWAS 的检测结果仅一小部分地解释了癌症遗传可能性[70]。下一代测序(NGS)(例如外显子或全基因组测序)有助于识别癌症缺失的遗传能力。使用 NGS 案例研究癌症的关联性已经取得很多成功。PALB2 的一个种系突变被鉴定为家族性胰腺癌的易感基因，是将 NGS 应用于癌症基因发现的早期成果之一[71]。NGS 的研究发现能引起蛋白质缺陷的 POLE 和 POLD1 胚系变异是结直肠腺瘤和腺癌的高外显率易感基因，这进一步增加了我们对该疾病病因的理解[72]。年初，NGS 在颅内生殖细胞肿瘤(IGCT)患者中发现，JMJD1C 中有大量新的和罕见的种系变异，这表明 JMJD1C 是这种罕见脑肿瘤的易感基因。JMJD1C 编码组蛋白去甲基化酶，是雄激素受体的共激活因子[73]。最近，NGS 发现编码端粒蛋白复合物一个成员的 POT1 的种系突变可导致家族性黑色素瘤和胶质瘤[74,75]。

表观基因组关联研究(EWAS)

表观遗传变化是指在不影响 DNA 序列的情况下调控基因表达的变化。表观基因组是位于动态外部环境和静态人类基因组之间的结合点。表观基因组具有广泛的个体间差异。表观遗传学关联研究(EWAS)一般是指对全基因组表观遗传学谱的研究，是一种探究疾病病因、预测治疗反应和临床结果的新工具[76]。例如，一项前瞻性的乳腺癌 EWAS 研究认为血液甲基化标记在乳腺癌风险预测方面比 8 个 GWAS 识别的单核苷酸多态性位点具有更好的预测能力[77]。同样，全基因组甲基化分析发现，对于雌激素受体亚型和患者临床预后来说甲基化标记是其可靠预测因子[78]。尽管表观基因组具有动态优势，即可捕获由遗传因素和环境因素相互作用导致的癌症过程，但在进行 EWAS 研究方面仍然存在着挑战，包括样本选择和处理、表型暴露，样本大小和人口选择。因此，相关研究结果也应持谨慎态度，因为表观遗传的变化既可能是特定表型的原因，也可能是该表型的结果。MicroRNA(miRNA)是另一种重要的表观遗传修饰因子，其在转录后可调控人类三分之一的基因[79]。有证据表明 miRNA 在细胞增殖、分化和细胞死亡等许多导致癌症的过程中发挥作用。MiRNA 组是指基因组中全部 RNA 谱。由于 MiRNA 和靶基因之间存在复杂的调控网络，全面分析 MiRNA 组将进一步阐明癌症病因、治疗效果和潜在的治疗分子[79,80]。

微生物组

慢性感染有致癌作用，全球癌症发病率中，约 16% 由感染性疾病导致。这种通过病原体，如病毒来促进癌症的机制，也有较为详尽的描述。例如，幽门螺杆菌和丙型肝炎病毒(HCV)通过损伤上皮和炎症来促进癌症的发展。然而，最新的证据也表明，癌症的发生和发展可能不仅是因为一种病原体，还可能是与我们微生物组的整体变化有关[81]。

微生物只占健康人体质量的 1%~2%，但据估计，微生物细胞的数量是人体细胞的 10 倍，微生物基因(即微生物组)的数量估计是人类基因数量的 100 倍[82,83]。因为人类基因组编码的代谢过程与相关微生物群的代谢过程相关，NGS 技术使研究人员能够探索细菌微生物群及其在代谢和炎症中的作用，这两个因素与癌症的发生有关。16S rRNA 基因存在于所有微生物中，是描述微生物群落结构的重要工具[83]。早期的动物模型将微生物群落的变化与致癌作用，特别是结直肠癌的发生联系起来。在肿瘤中，微生物群的促癌作用主要是由于机体稳态的失衡，而不是特定病原体的感染。不同个体间的微生物群差异性受多种因素的影响，包括宿主生理学、病理学、环境、生活方式(饮食)和行为因素，而微生物群落的结构是影响癌症的重要危险因素，包括肥胖[83~85]。人们对这一领域的研究才刚刚起步，微生物群和宿主之间在致癌方面的复杂关系目前被揭示出的只是冰山一角[86~88]。未来这一领域的工作对于癌症的诊断、预防和治疗具有重大意义[81]。

其他组学和数字流行病学

癌症是一种复杂的疾病，由多种环境和宿主因素相互作用引起。因此，从整体上研究这些因素之间的相互作用，而非割裂地来看每一部分，对于找到癌症发生的因果关系至关重要。"相互作用组"是一个新的术语，它指的是一个细胞或有机体在不同因素(通常是生物分子)作用下导致某一状态或疾病时的相互作用整体网络[89]。这种网络通常用相互连接的线路图来描述。例如，*Notch2* 的相互作用组发现了一种新的肿瘤抑制基因 *WWP2*，它是 *Notch2* 的负调控因子[90]，用传统的候选基因方法是无法发现这一基因的。此外，全基因组-环境相互作用研究(GEWIS)可以解决遗传和环境因素之间的联合效应和相互作用问题[91]。一项针对 CRC 的探索性 GEWIS 发现，SNP 与超重之间存在显著的相互作用，两者之间的相互作用增加了 CRC 的患病风险[92]。

基于通信技术设备、成像、先进统计方法和生物信息学工具开发的"数字流行病学"的进展促进了癌症流行病学的发展[93]。传统流行病学数据是通过个人随访来收集的，这既费时又费力。随着数字技术的进步，这些数据现在可以通过手机和互联网收集。数字革命及时地为基于计算机的数据挖掘提供了资源。与此同时，复杂的统计和生物信息学工具是分析大数据以得出有意义结论的基础。但是，许多流行病学专家没有受过专业的设计培训，无法分析这些大数据和进行复杂且昂贵的高通量研究。所以，当前迫切需要专业的研究团队和新的培训方法。

未来方向与展望

过去，癌症流行病学家过于专注病因的研究，现在研究人员迫切地需要拓宽他们在整个转化谱中的视野[94]。Khoury 等人[95]总结了转化流行病学的路线图，这对转化研究的每一步都有影响。Spitz[96,97]等人提出了"整合流行病学"的概念，整合流行病学扩大了流行病学的范畴，它将传统的流行病学研究设计与先进的分析和数据挖掘工具紧密结合，整合并分析来自多个信息源的资料，分析对风险评估，预后及治疗效果等多个节点的影响。癌症流行病学的分析方法是多层次的整合。Taplin 等人[98]构建了一个跨癌症连续体的多层次分析模型，该模型是基于多层次背景的影响，通过相互依赖及相互作用来影响行为这一假设而进行构建的。Lynch 和 Rebbeck 将这种方法扩展到“多层次生物和社会整合构建”（MBASIC）框架中，将宏观环境、个体因素与生物学相结合，以探索多因素之间关系，并以此来指导研究设计和统计或机制模型，从而进一步研究这些关系[99]。

癌症流行病学的核心含义是知识整合，即整合信息的过程，加速研究成果的转化和应用。该过程包括三个关键过程：知识管理、综合和转化。

采用这种数据整合和知识集成方法验证过的风险预测模型可以提高筛选效果，具有重大的公共卫生意义。而且，风险预测工具可以被纳入更小、更强大和“更智能”的预防试验设计中。开发风险预测模型，需基于严格的统计学方法，综合各种风险因素。通过量化个体层面的风险，该模型为癌症监测、干预设计及受试者招募提供了参考[100]。多变量统计 GAIL 模型是乳腺癌预测的一个范例，它可以根据女性当前的年龄、初潮时的年龄、初产时的年龄、乳腺癌的家族史和以往的乳腺活检次数来评估女性患乳腺癌的风险。目前该模型已经扩展包含了暴露、遗传和表型变异等综合因素[101~103]。研究人员还增加了其他的乳腺癌危险因素，如体重指数、乳腺密度和营养，以适度改善鉴别效果[104~107]。Tammemagi 等人[108]收集了前列腺癌、肺癌、结直肠癌、卵巢癌（PLCO）筛查试验的大量数据，建立了一个曲线下阴影面积（AUC）为 0.8 的肺癌风险预测模型，其风险预测模型在对肺癌检测方面比国家肺癌筛查试验（NLST）标准更为敏感。Wen[109]等人开发了一系列肝细胞癌模型，变量包括乙型肝炎病毒（HBV）和丙型肝炎病毒（HCV）感染以及一组血清生物学标志物。

风险模型对于癌症流行病学研究成果的实施非常重要。已公布的模型，预测识别能力普遍较低，AUC 大多在 0.55~0.70 之间，因此面临巨大的挑战[100]。研究人员一直在致力于提高模型的预测能力，例如，DNA 的甲基化谱使乳腺癌风险模型的 AUC 增加了 9.8%[77]，并且 DNA 修复分析可以将膀胱癌风险模型的 AUC 提高 10%[110]。对于风险模型来说，主要问题在于模型验证，尤其是使用高通量数据和中间生物标志物数据时的模型验证。通过协作提供外部验证来评估开发模型的实用性和通用性至关重要。

结论

Lam 等人[94]总结了 21 世纪影响转化癌症流行病学的四大驱动力：规模日益壮大的科学团队合作、新兴的基因组技术及其在大规模流行病学研究中的应用、多层次数据分析和干预，以及越来越复杂的分析技术，这使得有效整合大型多层次数据成为可能。这些特征使得癌症流行病学迅速发展，成为一门综合性研究的“工具科学”，整合了癌症各个方面的信息，最终架起了发现和转化之间的桥梁。

（刘康栋　路静 译　陈新焕　赵四敏　于乐兴 校）

部分参考文献

3 Siegel R, Ma J, Zou Z, et al. Cancer statistics, 2014. *CA Cancer J Clin.* 2014;**64(1)**:9–29.

7 Jones LA, Chilton JA, Hajek RA, et al. Between and within: international perspectives on cancer and health disparities. *J Clin Oncol.* 2006;**24(14)**:2204–2208.

9 Ward E, Jemal A, Cokkinides V, et al. Cancer disparities by race/ethnicity and socioeconomic status. *CA Cancer J Clin.* 2004;**54(2)**:78–93.

10 Kamangar F, Dores GM, Anderson WF. Patterns of cancer incidence, mortality, and prevalence across five continents: defining priorities to reduce cancer disparities in different geographic regions of the world. *J Clin Oncol.* 2006;**24(14)**:2137–2150.

18 Malik VS, Willett WC, Hu FB. Global obesity: trends, risk factors and policy implications. *Nat Rev Endocrinol.* 2013;**9(1)**:13–27.

22 Park J, Morley TS, Kim M, et al. Obesity and cancer—mechanisms underlying tumour progression and recurrence. *Nat Rev Endocrinol.* 2014;**10(8)**:455–465.

23 Calle EE, Kaaks R. Overweight, obesity and cancer: epidemiological evidence and proposed mechanisms. *Nat Rev Cancer.* 2004;**4(8)**:579–591.

24 Stunkard AJ, Foch TT, Hrubec Z. A twin study of human obesity. *JAMA.* 1986;**256(1)**:51–54.

29 Kushi LH, Doyle C, McCullough M, et al. American Cancer Society Guidelines on nutrition and physical activity for cancer prevention: reducing the risk of cancer with healthy food choices and physical activity. *CA Cancer J Clin.* 2012;**62(1)**:30–67.

31 McTiernan A. Mechanisms linking physical activity with cancer. *Nat Rev Cancer.* 2008;**8(3)**:205–211.

33 Tannenbaum A, Silverstone H. The influence of the degree of caloric restriction on the formation of skin tumors and hepatomas in mice. *Cancer Res.* 1949;**9(12)**:724–727.

45 Key TJ, Allen NE, Spencer EA, et al. The effect of diet on risk of cancer. *Lancet.* 2002;**360(9336)**:861–868.

52 Electronic cigarettes (e-cigarettes). *CA: Cancer J Clin.* 2014;**64(3)**:169–170.

53 Cobb NK, Abrams DB. The FDA, e-cigarettes, and the demise of combusted tobacco. *N Engl J Med.* 2014;**371(16)**:1469–1471.

55 Lichtenstein P, Holm NV, Verkasalo PK, et al. Environmental and heritable factors in the causation of cancer—analyses of cohorts of twins from Sweden, Denmark, and Finland. *N Engl J Med.* 2000;**343(2)**:78–85.

56 Lindor NM, McMaster ML, Lindor CJ, et al. Concise handbook of familial cancer susceptibility syndromes—second edition. *J Natl Cancer Inst Monogr.* 2008;**(38)**:1–93. doi: 10.1093/jncimonographs/lgn001.

58 Gallie BL. Retinoblastoma gene mutations in human cancer. *N Engl J Med.* 1994;**330(11)**:786–787.

59 Dong LM, Potter JD, White E, et al. Genetic susceptibility to cancer: the role of polymorphisms in candidate genes. *JAMA.* 2008;**299(20)**:2423–2436.

62 Amos CI, Wu X, Broderick P, et al. Genome-wide association scan of tag SNPs identifies a susceptibility locus for lung cancer at 15q25.1. *Nat Genet.* 2008;**40(5)**:616–622.

65 Zheng W, Long J, Gao YT, et al. Genome-wide association study identifies a new breast cancer susceptibility locus at 6q25.1. *Nat Genet.* 2009;**41(3)**:324–328.

66 Garcia-Closas M, Couch FJ, Lindstrom S, et al. Genome-wide association studies identify four ER negative-specific breast cancer risk loci. *Nat Genet.* 2013;**45(4)**:392–398, 398e1-2.

68 Chung CC, Chanock SJ. Current status of genome-wide association studies in cancer. *Hum Genet.* 2011. doi: 10.1007/s00439-011-1030-9.

71 Jones S, Hruban RH, Kamiyama M, et al. Exomic sequencing identifies PALB2 as a pancreatic cancer susceptibility gene. *Science.* 2009;**324(5924)**:217.

76 Rakyan VK, Down TA, Balding DJ, et al. Epigenome-wide association studies for common human diseases. *Nat Rev Genet.* 2011;**12(8)**:529–541.

79 Berindan-Neagoe I, Monroig PC, Pasculli B, et al. MicroRNAome genome: a treasure for cancer diagnosis and therapy. *CA: Cancer J Clin.* 2014. doi: 10.3322/caac.21244:n/a-n/a.

81 Schwabe RF, Jobin C. The microbiome and cancer. *Nat Rev Cancer.* 2013;**13(11)**: 800–812.

84 Ley RE, Turnbaugh PJ, Klein S, et al. Microbial ecology: human gut microbes associated with obesity. *Nature.* 2006;**444(7122)**:1022–1023.

85 Tilg H, Kaser A. Gut microbiome, obesity, and metabolic dysfunction. *J Clin Invest.* 2011;**121(6)**:2126–2132.

86 Ahn J, Sinha R, Pei Z, et al. Human gut microbiome and risk for colorectal cancer. *J Natl Cancer Inst.* 2013;**105(24)**:1907–1911.

89 Vidal M, Cusick ME, Barabasi AL. Interactome networks and human disease. *Cell.* 2011;**144(6)**:986–998.

91 Thomas D. Gene–environment-wide association studies: emerging approaches.

Nat Rev Genet. 2010;**11**(**4**):259–272.

94 Lam TK, Spitz M, Schully SD, et al. "Drivers" of translational cancer epidemiology in the 21st century: needs and opportunities. *Cancer Epidemiol Biomarkers Prev*. 2013;**22**(**2**):181–188.

95 Khoury MJ, Gwinn M, Ioannidis JPA. The emergence of translational epidemiology: from scientific discovery to population health impact. *Am J Epidemiol*. 2010;**172**(**5**):517–524.

96 Spitz MR, Caporaso NE, Sellers TA. Integrative cancer epidemiology—the next generation. *Cancer Discov*. 2012;**2**(**12**):1087–1090.

97 Spitz MR, Wu X, Mills G. Integrative epidemiology: from risk assessment to outcome prediction. *J Clin Oncol*. 2005;**23**(**2**):267–275.

100 Pu X, Ye Y, Wu X. Development and validation of risk models and molecular diagnostics to permit personalized management of cancer. *Cancer*. 2014;**120**(**1**):11–19.

103 Gail MH. Value of adding single-nucleotide polymorphism genotypes to a breast cancer risk model. *J Natl Cancer Inst*. 2009;**101**(**13**):959–963.

109 Wen CP, Lin J, Yang YC, et al. Hepatocellular carcinoma risk prediction model for the general population: the predictive power of transaminases. *J Natl Cancer Inst*. 2012;**104**(**20**):1599–1611.

110 Wu X, Lin J, Grossman HB, et al. Projecting individualized probabilities of developing bladder cancer in white individuals. *J Clin Oncol*. 2007;**25**(**31**):4974–4981.

第 35 章 癌症预防的行为学方法

Errol J. Philip, PhD ■ Jamie S. Ostroff, PhD

概述

某些健康行为增加了癌症发生的风险。据估计，全世界 35%的癌症相关死亡可通过健康的生活方式来避免。本章综述了癌症发病的行为学危险因素以及癌症预防的行为学干预方法。吸烟、不健康饮食、肥胖、久坐不动的生活方式、阳光和紫外线暴露等行为危险因素均与癌症的病因有关。我们倡导健康行为，并倡议医务人员开展健康咨询，有效普及癌症预防。

吸烟

吸烟仍然是癌症发病率和死亡率的首要可预防性病因。在美国，每年因使用烟草导致近五分之一或约 48 万人过早死亡(*US Surgeon General Report 2014*)。吸烟所导致的癌症死亡至少占总癌症死亡人数的 30%，占男性肺癌死亡人数的 87%和女性肺癌死亡人数的 70%(*Cancer Facts & Figures 2014*)。除肺癌外，吸烟还会增加患口腔癌、喉癌、咽喉癌、食管癌、胃癌、肝癌、胰腺癌、肾脏癌、膀胱癌、子宫颈癌、结/直肠癌以及急性髓系白血病的风险(资料来源：*Cancer Facts & Figures 2014*)。二手烟暴露也是肺癌发生的危险因素，每年约有 3 400 名不吸烟的成年人因吸入二手烟而死于肺癌(*Cancer Facts & Figures 2014*；*SGR*，*2014*)。抽雪茄会导致肺癌、口腔癌、咽喉癌、喉癌和食管癌的发生(资料来源：*CDC*，*Consumption of Cigarettes and Combustible Tobacco-United States*，*2000-2011*，*2012*)。无烟烟草产品增加了患口腔癌、喉癌、食管癌和胰腺癌的风险。

自 1964 年第一份美国外科医生关于吸烟与健康的报告发布以来，吸烟者的数量急剧下降。但目前仍然有 18.1%或者超过 4 200 万的美国成年人吸烟(资料来源：*CDC*，*Current cigarette smoking among adults-United States*，*2005-2012*，*2014*)。2012 年，约有 20.5%的男性和 15.8%的女性吸烟。非裔美国人、美洲原住民、低收入群体、受教育程度较低者、同性恋群体以及滥用药物者和患有精神疾病者更有可能吸烟成瘾。幸运的是，香烟的日消费量已有所下降，而且大约 22%的吸烟者并非每日吸烟(资料来源：*CDC*，*Current cigarette smoking among adults—United States*，*2005-2012*，*2014*)。

另一个好消息是，青年吸烟人数也显著下降。据报道，1997 年将近一半(48%)的男性高中生和超过三分之一(36%)的女性高中生在过去的一个月里使用了某种形式的烟草-香烟、雪茄或无烟烟草产品。2012 年，男学生吸烟率降至 23%，女学生降为 18%。(资料来源：*Cancer Facts & Figures 2010*；*CDC*，*Tobacco Product Use Among Middle and High School Students-United States*，*2011 and 2012*，*2013.*)。另一方面，越来越多的人担心电子烟、水烟袋和其他无烟烟草产品的使用也有潜在风险[1,2]。

医疗环境中全面禁烟

美国公共卫生服务机构提出了烟草使用和依赖临床指南(PHS 指南)[3]，该指南在 2008 年更新并代表了当前最佳方案，提供有效的循证烟草治疗的信息。

简短建议

PHS 指南建议使用简短建议。如表 35-1 所示，医生：询问、评估、建议、协助和安排。鼓励医疗人员每次问诊病人吸烟状况。一旦确定了病人为吸烟者，临床医生应该评估其戒烟的意愿，并制订烟草依赖治疗计划。临床医生应该强烈建议患者戒烟，告知患者持续吸烟的患癌风险及其他危害，戒烟有益疾病治疗。另一个策略，教育并协助吸烟者消除戒烟障碍，如制订戒烟计划和实施方案，如有需要可使用临床药物治疗，帮助他们克服顾虑和障碍。对于不愿戒烟的患者，临床医生应该提供鼓励性咨询，鼓励他们戒烟或减少日常吸烟量。最后，倡导临床医生提供后续支持，例如向吸烟者推荐其他渠道，如戒烟热线或临床烟草依赖治疗专家。

表 35-1 治疗烟草依赖的“5A”模型

询问烟草使用情况	了解和记录来访者的烟草使用状态(策略 A1)
建议戒烟	以清晰、有力、个性化的方式敦促戒烟(策略 A2)
评估戒烟意愿	吸烟者是否愿意在这个时候尝试戒烟？(战略 A3)
协助戒烟	对于有戒烟意愿的吸烟者提供药物治疗，并提供咨询服务或额外治疗以帮助患者戒烟(策略 A4) 对于目前没有戒烟意愿的吸烟者，提供旨在增加未来戒烟意愿的干预措施(策略 B1 和 B2)
安排随访	对于有戒烟意愿的吸烟者，应安排随访联系人，在戒烟后的第一周安排随访(策略 A5) 对于目前没有戒烟意愿的吸烟者，请在下次随诊时建议其解决烟草依赖和戒烟相关问题。

药物疗法

指南强烈建议在咨询的同时配合药物治疗，以达到最佳的戒烟效果。几种安全有效的戒烟药物：尼古丁替代疗法(NRT)(贴片、口香糖、口服液、鼻喷雾器和吸入器)、安非他酮(Wellbutrin)和伐尼克兰(Chantix)。戒烟药物、剂量、持续时间、潜在禁忌证和副作用列表参见表35-2。联合与延长使用药物治疗可提高烟草依赖治疗的有效性。个性化治疗的方法需要更多的研究,根据吸烟者的戒烟意愿、社会文化因素、性别、年龄和健康状况来调整干预措施。关于尼古丁成瘾的遗传基础的神经学研究,可为高危人群制定精确的干预措施。

表35-2 烟草治疗药物治疗指南

药品名称	用量	用法	是否处方药	预防措施/禁忌	不良反应	病人教育
• 尼古丁贴片 NicoDermCQ® Habitr®	吸烟11支/d及以上: • 21mg/24h • 14mg/24h • 7mg/24h 吸烟小于10支/d: • 14mg/24h • 7mg/24h	 • 6周 • 2周 • 2周 • 6周 • 2周	• 非处方药 • 医疗补助只能凭处方报销	• 无法控制的高血压	• 皮肤刺激 ○ 发红 ○ 肿胀 ○ 瘙痒 • 睡眠中断 ○ 噩梦 ○ 多梦	• 指导患者每天更换贴片部位 • 如果睡眠受到干扰,病人应在就寝前取下补片
• 戒烟口香糖 Gum®	• 2mg,每天吸烟24支或更少者 • 4mg,每天吸烟25支或更多者 • 不要超过24片口香糖/24h	• 最多12周	• 非处方药 • 医疗补助只能凭处方报销	• 牙齿松动 • 口腔干燥	• 呃逆 • 胃不适 • 颌骨疼痛	• 定时嚼口香糖 • 每片口香糖咀嚼30分钟 • 咀嚼前15分钟和咀嚼时,除了水,不要吃/喝任何东西
• 尼古丁含片 Commit®	• 2mg,在醒来后30分钟以后抽第一支香烟者 • 4mg,在醒来后30分钟内抽第一支香烟者 不要超过20粒/24h	• 最多12周	• 非处方药 • 医疗补助只能凭处方报销	• 口腔干燥	• 口喉局部刺激 • 胃部不适	• 使用含片前15分钟及使用期间,除水外,避免进食/饮用任何东西 • 每片含片需要20~30分钟溶解
• 尼古丁吸入系统 Nicotrol Inhaler®	• 6~16次/d	• 最多6个月	• 处方药		• 口喉局部刺激 • 胃部不适	• 每个药筒吸80~100次,每次20分钟以上 • 指导病人像抽雪茄一样使用吸入器,使颊黏膜吸收
• 尼古丁鼻喷雾剂 Nicotrol NS®	• 0.5mg/吸入/鼻孔,1~2次/h或注射长期备用医嘱	• 最多12周	• 处方药	• 鼻窦感染	• 鼻子/眼睛/上呼吸道刺激	
• 安非拉酮 Zyban® Wellbutrin SR®	• 150mg/d,3天,然后 • 150mg每日两次	• 12周	• 处方药	• 癫痫发作史 • 进食障碍史 • 贪食症 • 厌食症	• 失眠 • 口干 • 烦躁 • 头晕	• 与吸烟重叠1~2周 • 不需要缓慢停药
• 伐伦克林 Chantix®	• 1~3天:0.5mg,然后 • 4~7天:0.5mg一日两次,然后 • 第8天~治疗结束:1mg每日两次	• 12周 • 如果病人已戒烟,可再接受12周的治疗,以防止复发	• 处方药	• 肾脏问题或透析 • 怀孕或计划怀孕 • 母乳喂养	• 轻度恶心 • 睡眠问题 • 头痛	• 饭后服用药物时要喝一满杯水 • 每次给药间隔8小时 • 睡前几小时服用此药,以避免烦躁不安

目前,关于电子香烟究竟会促进或阻碍戒烟,以及电子香烟是否能减少传统香烟和其他可燃烟草产品的危害,争论甚多,数据较少[4]。美国临床肿瘤学协会和美国癌症研究协会最近发表了一篇关于电子香烟的文献综述和政策声明[5]。肿瘤学家应建议吸烟者停止吸入传统香烟,鼓励使用 FDA(食品和药物管理局)批准的戒烟药物并提供戒烟咨询。并向患者说明长期使用电子烟戒烟并不能获益,且仍有潜在风险。

预防吸烟

预防与烟草有关的癌症需要制定和实施有效的烟草预防方案[6]。在最新版的全面烟草控制计划实践过程中,疾病控制和预防中心(CDC)建议:基于社区干预的全国计划聚焦于:①通过烟草管制政策(即税收、无烟法)防止青少年开始吸烟;②鼓励成年人和青少年戒烟;③避免接触二手烟;④查明烟草对不同群体引起影响的差别并且消除其影响。烟草的预防方案也应将具有高生物易感性和受社会文化因素影响的儿童纳入目标人群,因为这些因素可能会增加其开始规律吸烟的风险。

癌症二级和三级预防

一批新的证据表明,对于癌症患者来说吸烟也可导致一些不良后果,如手术并发症增加、治疗相关毒性增加、治疗有效性降低、生活质量较差、复发风险增加、二次原发肿瘤风险增加、非癌症相关并发症和死亡率增加,并降低其存活率[7~9]。尽管存在这些风险,但报告显示至少有 15.1%的成年癌症幸存者仍然吸烟[10]。诊断后继续吸烟和初次戒烟后再次吸烟应被视为一个可干预的临床问题。事实上,肿瘤学领导组织逐渐达成共识,认为烟草使用评估和治疗应被视为一种护理质量的衡量标准[11~14]。不幸的是,最近一项关于执业肿瘤学医生的调查显示,肿瘤专业的医生只向 25%的病人提供戒烟建议[15]。只有一半的国家癌症研究所指定的综合癌症中心向吸烟患者提供一些类型的戒烟方案[16]。这些调查结果凸显了在癌症治疗中查明并解决烟草治疗方案实施障碍的必要性。

有必要查明和解决癌症护理中戒烟方面的障碍。患者戒烟可能因患者自身因素(羞耻、无助、成瘾),医生因素(缺乏培训和转诊选择,缺乏对患者戒烟能力和兴趣的信心),以及系统因素(对吸烟者的识别不足、费用问题)[17]等妨碍了控烟方案有效实施。需要对患者、医者以及系统等级策略进行进一步研究,来使吸烟者持续参与基于循证的烟草治疗。

能量平衡:饮食、运动和体重

能量平衡与饮食、运动和体重之间密切联系,能量平衡问题已经被证明是导致全球癌症负担的一个重要因素。能量平衡与癌症的发生发展之间密切相关,目前关于这些因素与癌症的发生和预后相关的机制尚在研究中。

据估计,肥胖和饮食因素所致癌症在美国癌症病例中占近 35%。强有力的证据表明,超重与许多常见癌症的发病率以及较差的预后有关。饮食与癌症密切相关,以蔬菜为基础,限制肉类和奶制品的摄入,通常会降低癌症发病风险。参与体育活动也有助于防癌。

倡导所有患者和存活者依据健康的生活方式开展癌症防控。防控指南包括健康饮食,达到并保持正常体重,进行有规律的体育活动,这些是癌症防控和延长癌症患者长期生存的关键因素。

在美国,超重仍然是防癌的一个重要的可控危险因素[18,19],缺乏运动和饮食因素进一步增加了患癌风险。这三个因素相互关联,统称为能量平衡,是癌症防控的主要目标。目前有大量研究表明,原发和继发性癌症风险的增加、相关并发症的出现、生活质量受损、疾病预后更差都与能量平衡相关[20]。

国家癌症预防和控制组织已经发布了生活方式行为指南。美国癌症协会强调了保持健康体重、采用健康饮食和定期锻炼的重要性[21,22]。这些建议总结见表 35-3。重要的是,这些建议与非癌的疾病预防指南在大方向上相一致,遵循这些建议还将有助于降低其他慢性病的风险,如心血管疾病、糖尿病和高血压。然而,尽管国家努力提高人们对于健康生活方式的理解与采纳,但普通人群和癌症存活者的依从性仍然较低[23,24]。最近,“能量平衡”一词被强调用于临床实践和肿瘤学中[25],加强饮食、锻炼和体重之间的联系,使患者不再仅单独关注某一因素。

表 35-3　ACS 成人癌症预防和控制能量平衡指南

达到并保持健康的体重	• 通过控制摄入和消耗的能量,强调以植物为基础的饮食,限制高热量的食物和饮料,来平衡能量的摄入和消耗
定期参加体育活动	• 每周进行 150 分钟的适度运动(如快步走)或 75 分钟的剧烈运动(如慢跑),并避免久坐不动
保持健康饮食	• 强调以植物为基础的饮食,包括全谷物和每天 2.5 杯水果和蔬菜,同时限制加工食品和红肉的摄入量 • 饮酒应限制在男性每天 1 标准杯和女性每天 1 标准杯(1 标准杯约 30ml)

最近一项针对近 11.2 万名非吸烟者的研究,通过 14 年的随访,调查了遵守 ACS 健康指南与疾病结局之间的关系。作者报告说,严格地遵守健康建议能够降低患癌和所有病因导致的死亡风险[26]。下一节将概述有关能量平衡与癌症之间关系的最新研究发现。认识了饮食、体重和运动间的协同和关联后,后续将就这些因素在美国四种最常见癌症中分别重点讨论。

饮食与癌症

乳腺癌

过去三十年里,饮食和乳腺癌之间的潜在联系受到了广泛关注。世界癌症研究基金会(WCRF)报告说,基于观察性研究,某些饮食模式,包括大量水果和蔬菜的摄入,以及家禽、鱼类和低脂乳制品的消费,能够降低患乳腺癌的风险[27]。Brennan 等人在 2010 年的关于多种饮食模式的研究中,对 39 个病例的对照和队列研究的系统回顾和 meta 分析中报告了类似的发现[28]。尽管水果和蔬菜的摄入在严格的饮食方案中起主要作用,但几乎没有证据支持只摄入蔬菜和水果具有保护作用[29]。"妇女健康倡议"(Women's Health Initiative)的一项随机临床试验涉及近5万名绝经后女性,该试验旨在研究减少脂肪摄入量是否会影响癌症风险。在8年的随访期间,脂肪摄入量的减少仅与疾病风险的轻微降低相关,而在浸润性乳腺癌中则未见差异[30]。最后,有证据表明,对于绝经前和绝经后的女性来说[27,29],饮酒可能会以剂量反应的方式增加患乳腺癌的风险,然而,最近的一项数据荟萃(meta)分析表明,目前还没有证据表明食用红肉会增加患乳腺癌的风险[31]。

前列腺癌

研究饮食与前列腺癌关系的文献已经十分成熟,最近的研究表明,其相关性可能因前列腺癌的侵袭性而有所不同。Ma和Chapman进行了系统性回顾[32],他们认为需要进一步的研究来解释这一潜在的影响,还没有可靠的证据来对饮食在前列腺癌中的作用提出明确的建议。尽管如此,仍有证据表明食用蔬菜和大豆具有保护作用,乳制品会增加患前列腺癌相关疾病的风险。Kirsh等人的研究表明[33],摄入大量十字花科蔬菜(如卷心菜、西蓝花)的男性患前列腺癌的风险较低。通过对PLCO试验的进一步分析,乳制品的摄入可能会增加患前列腺癌的风险[27]。有报告显示,乳制品摄入量较高的人群中,近3万名男性患非侵袭性癌症的风险略有增加[34]。而乳制品摄入量与侵袭性更强的类型的癌症之间没有联系。

结直肠癌

科学家研究了营养对结直肠癌发生发展的潜在影响。最近的一些国际报告和meta分析指出,有充足的证据表明,食用红肉和加工肉制品会增加患结肠癌、结直肠癌和直肠癌的风险[27,35]。最近的meta分析发现[36],肉类摄入与癌症风险之间存在剂量效应关系,每天摄入50g,风险增加21%,每天摄入100g,风险增加29%[35]。相比之下,推荐的瘦肉摄入量大约为85g。

纤维与疾病风险之间的关系也受到极大关注,尽管已有可信的生物学机制,但早期的报告并没有发现纤维摄入与结直肠癌之间明显有关[37~39]。然而,最近研究指出了两者之间的关系[40,41]。一个基于25项前瞻性研究的系统综述,报告了谷物纤维和全谷物与降低结直肠癌风险之间的剂量-反应关系[42]。研究人员报告说,每天摄入10克纤维可以显著降低10%的患癌风险,并建议成年人每天摄入25克纤维。

饮酒也与结直肠癌的风险增加有关[35]。Huxley通过回顾103项队列研究发现,与不饮酒者或轻度饮酒者相比,大量饮酒的人患结直肠癌的风险增加了60%。在男性参与者中,这种关系尤为突出[43]。Chung等人对钙和维生素D与结直肠癌的关系进行了系统性的综述[44],并报道了不一致的结果。重要的是,虽然有证据表明增加钙的摄入量可以降低患结肠癌的风险,但这一益处必须与前列腺癌风险的潜在增加进行权衡。目前,还没有关于增加钙摄入量作为降低癌症风险的方法的建议。

肺癌

WRCF/AICR(美国癌症研究所)的报告表明,在吸烟者和非吸烟者中,水果和蔬菜的摄入量越高,患肺癌的风险越低[27]。但是,报告指出,尽管存在这种相关性,但其与吸烟导致肺癌的风险相比,健康饮食的保护作用微乎其微。

肥胖与癌症

过去的30年里,肥胖率急剧上升,超过35%的美国成年人被认为是肥胖者[45]。2003年的一份报告估计,在所有癌症死亡病例中,由体重超标引起的死亡占14%~20%[46],再加上饮食摄入问题所导致的癌症,总共约占三分之一。肥胖可能很快就会超过烟草,成为癌症的主要可预防风险因素[27,47]。普通人群体重的空前增加,加上超重导致的癌症风险增加,意味着1 400万癌症幸存者中估计有1 000万人超重或肥胖[48~50]。WCRF/AICR发表的一份报告,以及Renehan在2008年更新的一份综述,都指出了超重和许多常见癌症之间存在联系[27,51]。这些癌症包括结肠癌、肾癌、胰腺癌和食管癌,男性的甲状腺癌和胆囊癌、女性的子宫内膜癌、卵巢癌和绝经后乳腺癌。

乳腺癌和前列腺癌

成年后体重超标和体重增加都与患乳腺癌的风险有关[52,53]。Vrieling等人的meta分析进一步指出[54],体重增加与雌激素/黄体酮阳性乳腺癌之间关联更强。肥胖对前列腺癌的影响取决于疾病的严重程度,这一关系有待更详细的研究。肥胖状态与被诊断为晚期疾病的风险更大[55],与复发风险更高[56]和预后较差有关[57]。相比之下,Wright等人在美国国立卫生研究院饮食与健康研究的报告称,大量男性受试者BMI(体重指数)与早期疾病风险之间呈负相关[58]。由于遗传性肥胖男性的筛查和诊断的困难,这种复杂关系还需深入研究。

结直肠癌和其他值得注意的发现

大多数研究以及最近一项包含超过56项观察性研究的meta分析都表明体重与患结直肠癌风险之间存在正相关[59],其中男性中的相关性最强[35,46]。Norat等人指出[35],这种关联在研究BMI之外的体脂分布指标时更为一致,腹部脂肪超重与癌症风险增加的相关性更强。

子宫内膜癌仍然是与超重联系最紧密的癌症,约有60%的新发病例与肥胖有关[60]。肥胖女性子宫内膜癌的发病率是正常女性的2~3.5倍[61]。在欧洲,一项关于肥胖与子宫内膜癌的大规模研究,对100万名女性进行了近40年的跟踪调查,报告称,与正常体重的女性相比,肥胖女性患子宫体癌的可能性要高出2.5倍[62]。

体育锻炼与癌症

参与体育活动仍然是健康指南的一个重要组成部分,能降低患许多常见癌症的风险[22]。

乳腺癌和前列腺癌

运动和患乳腺癌的风险之间的关系已被广泛研究并得到证实[63]。研究人员对70多份观察性报告进行了回顾,将经常运动的人与不常运动的人进行比较,发现经常运动的人患乳腺癌的绝对风险降低了20%~30%[61,64]。Liu等人对40多份报告进行了系统的回顾和meta分析[65],其中包括200多万人和近9万例癌症病例,他们得出结论,参与体育活动可使患前列腺癌总体风险降低10%。

结直肠癌和肺癌

运动与结直肠癌之间的关系也得到了相当多的实证关注。2009年,Wolin等人完成了一项包含50多项研究的meta分析[66],报告了运动使患结直肠癌的总体风险降低24%,在病例对照研究中其下降更为显著。Harris 和 Thune 报道了与结肠癌相关的类似发现，报道了运动与癌症风险之间的剂量-反应关系的证据[67,68]。然而，在 7 项直肠癌研究中，没有证据表明两者之间存在关联。

在一项 Emaus 和 Thune 报告的以队列研究为主的综述中[69]，从事体育运动的人群患肺癌的风险降低了 23%，在病例对照研究中从事体育运动的人群患肺癌的风险降低了 38%。进一步的 meta 分析报告了类似的结果，风险降低取决于运动强度，适度运动使肺癌相关风险降低 13%，有规律的运动使肺癌相关风险降低 30%[70]。最近的一项系统性综述指出，需要进一步研究运动与肺癌尤其是女性肺癌之间的关系，有 10 项研究报告表明，体育运动与肺癌之间存在负相关，但有几乎同样多的研究报告表明两者之间没有关联[71]。

能量平衡与癌症存活率

随着许多常见癌症存活率的提高，一些新出现的研究开始关注生活方式在癌症预后和生存率中的作用。这一领域的相关研究与临床项目都在试图将癌症的诊断作为一个患者教育的机会[72]，并且抓住这个时期能够激励患者和幸存者改变生活方式[73-75]。在一项关于体育锻炼与癌症存活率的系统综述中，作者对 27 项已发表的研究进行总结，证明体育锻炼能降低所有原因引起的死亡率包括乳腺癌和结肠特异性癌症死亡率[76]。Davies 等人的综述指出[77]，低脂肪、高纤维的健康或严格的饮食方案可能与降低癌症复发和进展的风险有广泛的联系，这种联系依然需要进一步的研究。还应明确健康的饮食习惯与体育锻炼是否能够维持满意的体重。最后，Parekh 等人在对乳腺癌、结肠癌和前列腺癌相关文献的系统回顾中报告说[78]，大多数研究表明超重与癌症存活率呈负相关。然而，作者指出，乳腺癌在这一文献中所占比例过高，许多研究肥胖和癌症存活率的研究最初并不是为了研究这些结果。鉴于这些新发现，美国临床肿瘤学会（American Society of Clinical Oncology）创建了一个方案，鼓励肿瘤学家向癌症存活者提供体重管理的重要性相关咨询[79]。

促进饮食和体育运动的行为改变

医务工作者的建议对于促进能量平衡和生活方式改变方面具有重要作用，虽然一些人可能需要更加深入的干预。对于那些需要更多帮助的人可以提供循证的行为生活方式计划。为期 6~12 个月的方案中，通常采用小组的形式，包括了饮食咨询，控制热量摄入，参与体育锻炼。这类计划通常能使体重减轻 5%~10%[80]，并提供许多疾病标志物的临床相关改善情况，以及可信的因降低癌症风险而带来的下游获益[81,82]。坚持减肥仍然是一个挑战，医务工作者应该持续支持那些寻求改变的患者[83]。行为改变影响癌症结局的证据越来越多，有证据表明，减肥手术可以降低癌症风险[84]，合理饮食和运动可以改善癌症存活者的生物学指标[85]。

皮肤癌的致癌风险行为

皮肤癌通常分为黑色素瘤和非黑色素瘤皮肤癌。黑色素瘤不太常见，但比其他类型的皮肤癌更具侵袭性，每年约有 6.8 万美国人患病[86]。暴露于太阳或室内晒黑设备的紫外线辐射（UVR）是患皮肤癌的一个重要风险因素，目前已有完善的预防皮肤癌的行为策略[87]。不使用人工日光浴床[88]，尽可能避免无保护的暴露在阳光下——尤其是正午强烈的阳光下。当不可避免地暴露在阳光下时，应建议个人尽量使用广谱防晒霜［即对 UVA（紫外线 A）和 UVB（紫外线 B）辐射均有效，防晒系数（SPF）须达 30 或以上］，出门前约 30 分钟涂抹，然后每隔 2 小时或接触水后再涂一次。最重要的是，防晒霜只提供部分的紫外线防护，应尽量避免暴露于强烈阳光，穿防晒衣物（即帽子、长袖衣物）。

不幸的是，只有 30% 的美国成年人经常使用防晒霜和/或防晒服[89]。值得注意的是，调查显示，即使癌症存活者也不能始终保护自己免受紫外线的伤害，尤其是那些最可能暴露在紫外线下的年轻存活者[50,90,91]。

结论

降低行为风险对癌症预防的重要性已得到充分证实[92]。2020 年健康人类目标强调促进健康行为[93]，如不吸烟、保持健康的体重、低脂肪高纤维的饮食、体育运动，以及限制紫外线的暴露。

（路静　赵继敏　译　李鑫　陈新焕　孙文　校）

部分参考文献

3 Fiore M, Jaén C, Baker T, et al. Treating tobacco use and dependence: 2008 update U.S. Public Health Service Clinical Practice Guideline executive summary. *Respir Care*. 2008;**53**(**9**):1217-1222.

5 Brandon TH, Goniewicz ML, Hanna NH, et al. Electronic nicotine delivery systems: a policy statement from the American Association for Cancer Research and the American Society of Clinical Oncology. *J Clin Oncol*. 2015;**33**(**8**):952-963.

6 Centers for Disease Control and Prevention. Best Practices for Comprehensive Tobacco Control Programs-2014. Atlanta: U.S. Department of Health and Human Services, Centers for Disease Control and Precention, National Center for Chronic Disease Prevention and Health Promotion, Office on Smoking and Health, 2014.

10 Underwood JM, Townsend JS, Stewart SL, et al. Surveillance of demographic characteristics and health behaviors among adult cancer survivors—behavioral risk factor surveillance system, United States, 2009. *Morb Mortal Wkly Rep Surveill Summ*. 2012;**61**(**Suppl 1**):1-23.

18 Danaei G, Vander Hoorn S, Lopez AD, Murray CJ, Ezzati M. Causes of cancer in the world: comparative risk assessment of nine behavioural and environmental risk factors. *Lancet*. 2005;**366**(**9499**):1784-1793.

21 Rock CL, Doyle C, Demark-Wahnefried W, et al. Nutrition and physical activity guidelines for cancer survivors. *CA J Clin*. 2012;**62**(**4**):243-274.

22 Kushi LH, Doyle C, McCullough M, et al. American Cancer Society Guidelines on nutrition and physical activity for cancer prevention: reducing the risk of cancer with healthy food choices and physical activity. *CA Cancer J Clin*. 2012;**62**(**1**):30-67.

23 Blanchard CM, Courneya KS, Stein K. Cancer survivors' adherence to lifestyle behavior recommendations and associations with health-related quality of life: results from the American Cancer Society's SCS-II. *J Clin Oncol*. 2008;**26**(**13**):2198-2204.

26 McCullough ML, Patel AV, Kushi LH, et al. Following cancer prevention guidelines reduces risk of cancer, cardiovascular disease, and all-cause mortality. *Cancer Epidemiol Biomarkers Prev*. 2011;**20**(**6**):1089-1097.

28 Brennan SF, Cantwell MM, Cardwell CR, Velentzis LS, Woodside JV. Dietary patterns and breast cancer risk: a systematic review and meta-analysis. *Am J Clin Nutr*. 2010;**91**(**5**):1294-1302.

30 Prentice RL, Caan B, Chlebowski RT, et al. Low-fat dietary pattern and risk of invasive breast cancer: the Women's Health Initiative Randomized Controlled Dietary Modification Trial. *JAMA*. 2006;**295**(**6**):629-642.

31 Alexander DD, Morimoto LM, Mink PJ, Cushing CA. A review and meta-analysis of red and processed meat consumption and breast cancer. *Nutr Res Rev*. 2010;**23(2)**:349–365.

32 Ma RW, Chapman K. A systematic review of the effect of diet in prostate cancer prevention and treatment. *J Hum Nutr Diet*. 2009;**22(3)**:187–199; quiz 200–2.

33 Kirsh VA, Peters U, Mayne ST, et al. Prospective study of fruit and vegetable intake and risk of prostate cancer. *J Natl Cancer Inst*. 2007;**99(15)**:1200–1209.

36 Chan DS, Lau R, Aune D, Vieira R, Greenwood DC, Kampman E, et al. Red and processed meat and colorectal cancer incidence: meta-analysis of prospective studies. *PLoS One*. 2011;**6(6)**:e20456.

37 Schatzkin A, Lanza E, Corle D, et al. Lack of effect of a low-fat, high-fiber diet on the recurrence of colorectal adenomas. Polyp prevention trial study group. *N Engl J Med*. 2000;**342(16)**:1149–1155.

38 Park Y, Hunter DJ, Spiegelman D, et al. Dietary fiber intake and risk of colorectal cancer: a pooled analysis of prospective cohort studies. *JAMA*. 2005;**294(22)**:2849–2857.

41 Bingham SA, Day NE, Luben R, et al. Dietary fibre in food and protection against colorectal cancer in the European Prospective Investigation into Cancer and Nutrition (EPIC): an observational study. *Lancet*. 2003;**361(9368)**:1496–1501.

42 Aune D, Chan DS, Lau R, et al. Dietary fibre, whole grains, and risk of colorectal cancer: systematic review and dose–response meta-analysis of prospective studies. *BMJ*. 2011;**343**:d6617.

43 Huxley RR, Ansary-Moghaddam A, Clifton P, Czernichow S, Parr CL, Woodward M. The impact of dietary and lifestyle risk factors on risk of colorectal cancer: a quantitative overview of the epidemiological evidence. *Int J Cancer*. 2009;**125(1)**:171–180.

46 Calle EE, Rodriguez C, Walker-Thurmond K, Thun MJ. Overweight, obesity, and mortality from cancer in a prospectively studied cohort of U.S. adults. *N Engl J Med*. 2003;**348(17)**:1625–1638.

48 Howlader N, Noone AM, Krapcho M, et al. *SEER Cancer Statistics Review, 1975–2008*. Bethesda, MD: National Cancer Institute; 2011.

50 Coups EJ, Ostroff JS. A population-based estimate of the prevalence of behavioral risk factors among adult cancer survivors and noncancer controls. *Prev Med*. 2005;**40(6)**:702–711.

51 Renehan AG, Tyson M, Egger M, Heller RF, Zwahlen M. Body-mass index and incidence of cancer: a systematic review and meta-analysis of prospective observational studies. *Lancet*. 2008;**371(9612)**:569–578.

52 Michels KB, Mohllajee AP, Roset-Bahmanyar E, Beehler GP, Moysich KB. Diet and breast cancer: a review of the prospective observational studies. *Cancer*. 2007;**109(Suppl 12)**:2712–2749.

54 Vrieling A, Buck K, Kaaks R, Chang-Claude J. Adult weight gain in relation to breast cancer risk by estrogen and progesterone receptor status: a meta-analysis. *Breast Cancer Res Treat*. 2010;**123(3)**:641–649.

55 Cao Y, Ma J. Body mass index, prostate cancer-specific mortality, and biochemical recurrence: a systematic review and meta-analysis. *Cancer Prev Res*. 2011;**4(4)**:486–501.

58 Wright ME, Chang SC, Schatzkin A, et al. Prospective study of adiposity and weight change in relation to prostate cancer incidence and mortality. *Cancer*. 2007;**109(4)**:675–684.

59 Ning Y, Wang L, Giovannucci EL. A quantitative analysis of body mass index and colorectal cancer: findings from 56 observational studies. *Obes Rev*. 2010;**11(1)**:19–30.

60 Calle EE, Kaaks R. Overweight, obesity and cancer: epidemiological evidence and proposed mechanisms. *Nat Rev Cancer*. 2004;**4(8)**:579–591.

64 Friedenreich CM. Physical activity and breast cancer: review of the epidemiologic evidence and biologic mechanisms. *Recent Results Cancer Res*. 2011;**188**: 125–139.

65 Liu Y, Hu F, Li D, et al. Does physical activity reduce the risk of prostate cancer? A systematic review and meta-analysis. *Eur Urol*. 2011;**60(5)**:1029–1044.

66 Wolin KY, Yan Y, Colditz GA, Lee IM. Physical activity and colon cancer prevention: a meta-analysis. *Br J Cancer*. 2009;**100(4)**:611–616.

67 Harriss DJ, Atkinson G, Batterham A, et al. Lifestyle factors and colorectal cancer risk (2): a systematic review and meta-analysis of associations with leisure-time physical activity. *Colorectal Dis*. 2009;**11(7)**:689–701.

70 Tardon A, Lee WJ, Delgado-Rodriguez M, et al. Leisure-time physical activity and lung cancer: a meta-analysis. *Cancer Cause Contr*. 2005;**16(4)**:389–397.

72 Demark-Wahnefried W, Aziz NM, Rowland JH, Pinto BM. Riding the crest of the teachable moment: promoting long-term health after the diagnosis of cancer. *J Clin Oncol*. 2005;**23(24)**:5814–5830.

76 Ballard-Barbash R, Friedenreich CM, Courneya KS, Siddiqi SM, McTiernan A, Alfano CM. Physical activity, biomarkers, and disease outcomes in cancer survivors: a systematic review. *J Natl Cancer Inst*. 2012;**104(11)**:815–840.

79 American Society for Clinical Oncology. Obesity and Cancer Toolkit Alexandria, VA: American Society for Clinical Oncology; 2015 [3/1/2015]. Available from: http://www.asco.org/practice-research/obesity-and-cancer.

85 Rock CL, Byers TE, Colditz GA, et al. Reducing breast cancer recurrence with weight loss, a vanguard trial: the Exercise and Nutrition to Enhance Recovery and Good Health for You (ENERGY) Trial. *Contemp Clin Trials*. 2013;**34(2)**: 282–295.

91 Tercyak KP, Donze JR, Prahlad S, Mosher RB, Shad AT. Multiple behavioral risk factors among adolescent survivors of childhood cancer in the Survivor Health and Resilience Education (SHARE) program. *Pediatr Blood Cancer*. 2006;**47(6)**:825–830.

第 36 章　膳食和营养在癌症病因研究与预防中的作用

Steven K. Clinton, MD, PhD ■ Elizabeth Grainger, PhD, RD ■ Edward L. Giovannucci, MD, ScD

概论

由于评估全球不同人群膳食暴露和癌症结局的工具日益完善，越来越多的科学研究开始关注营养素、食物、膳食模式和癌症风险之间的关联，包括了观察性研究、流行病学队列研究以及一些基于机制研究的人体干预试验。这些研究工作都强有力地显示膳食模式是全球癌症负担的主要风险因素，若干公共卫生组织也由此制定了预防癌症的膳食指南。这些指南包括保持健康体重和定期参加体育活动等一系列相关建议，通过调整膳食安排和运动行为模式来降低癌症风险。接受了多种治疗的癌症患者通过个性化咨询营养领域的专业人员（如注册营养师），可在保持最佳健康状态的同时降低药物毒性并巩固治疗效果。如今，膳食和体育活动在癌症生存中的作用得到了越来越广泛的认可，未来可能会出现更具体的个性化生存指南，用以降低癌症复发的风险，缓解癌症治疗的长期并发症，改善健康和生活质量。

在上两个世纪中，随着食品生产、加工、储存方式的改进及运输能力的提高，膳食结构在全世界发生了重大变化。在此期间，由于公共卫生措施的实施、职业安全性的提高和营养缺乏综合征发病率的降低等一系列综合因素，发达国家的预期寿命有了显著提高。随着人口老龄化，癌症及心血管疾病等慢性病逐渐成为人群发病和死亡的主要原因。在美国，久坐不动的人群中患有肥胖症的人越来越多，已成为近几十年的一大特点，而且呈全球蔓延趋势。虽然发达国家的部分群体仍然面临营养缺乏，如穷人、老年人、酗酒者和慢性病患者，但人们逐渐意识到，营养过剩才是许多慢性疾病（包括癌症）的病因，困扰着绝大部分人口。基于实验室、临床和流行病学的研究显示，癌症的复杂病因与特定营养素和某些膳食模式息息相关。

建立一个整合了膳食、营养及癌症相关信息的概念体系非常重要，有助于明确膳食在癌症预防和治疗中的作用，为公众和患者提供指导。我们将从预防、治疗和生存三个方面展开探讨。美国国立癌症研究所（National Cancer Institute）、美国癌症协会（American Cancer Society，ACS）、世界卫生组织（World Health Organization，WHO）和美国癌症研究中心/世界癌症研究基金会（American Institute for Cancer Research/Word Cancer Research Fund）等组织已经发布了在全体人群中均具有可行性的膳食和营养目标建议，这可能有助于通过一级预防降低总体癌症负担（表 36-1）。这些建议通常是基于循证医学和系统性回顾的研究证据所制定的。部分人群，特别是那些因环境暴露、

表 36-1　营养和癌症预防指南

	美国癌症研究中心[1]	美国心脏协会和美国心脏病学会[2,3]	美国人膳食指南[4]a	美国癌症协会[5]
体重	确保儿童和少年期的体重在 21 岁之前朝着正常 BMI 范围的偏低端发展。从 21 岁开始，将体重保持在正常范围内避免体重增加	对于超重的人，建议参加附带专业指导的促进低热量膳食的生活方式项目（持续时间大于 6 个月） 医疗团队应使用 NHLBI 体重指数（BMI）表将风险分级并确定干预措施	通过改善膳食和体育活动来预防和/或减少超重和肥胖 控制卡路里摄入量 对于超重的人，摄入更少来自食物和饮料的热量 在生命周期的每个阶段保持适当的卡路里平衡	在整个生命中实现并保持健康的体重 在整个生命周期中尽可能瘦，但体重不要过低；在所有年龄段都避免体重增加过多 定期进行体育锻炼，同时限制摄入高热量食物和饮料
体育活动	每天至少进行 30 分钟中等强度活动 随着健康状况的改善，每天至少进行 60 分钟的中等强度活动或 30 分钟的高强度活动 限制久坐的习惯	每周参加 2 小时 30 分钟的中等强度活动或 75 分钟的高强度有氧运动 若想减轻体重，每周进行 150 分钟的有氧运动。建议更高强度（每周 200~300 分钟）以保持体重减轻并防止复重	增加体育活动，减少久坐时间	采取积极运动的生活方式 成人：每周至少进行 150 分钟的中等强度或 75 分钟的高强度活动 限制久坐行为，如坐、躺、看电视或其他基于屏幕的娱乐活动

续表

	美国癌症研究中心[1]	美国心脏协会和美国心脏病学会[2,3]	美国人膳食指南[4]a	美国癌症协会[5]
植物性膳食	每天至少吃五份（至少400g）各种非淀粉类蔬菜和水果 每顿饭都要吃相对未加工的谷物和豆类 限制精制淀粉类食物	强调摄入蔬菜、水果和全谷物的膳食模式，包括低脂乳制品、家禽、鱼类、豆类、非热带植物油和坚果		
蔬菜和水果	每天至少吃五份（至少400g）各种非淀粉类蔬菜和水果	强调蔬菜和水果摄入的膳食模式	增加水果和蔬菜的摄入量 吃各种蔬菜，尤其是深绿色、红色和橙色蔬菜，以及豆类和豌豆	每天至少吃2.5杯[b]蔬菜和水果
面包、谷物和谷类	每顿饭都要吃相对未加工的谷物和豆类 限制精制淀粉类食物	植物性膳食模式，包括全谷物	保证谷物摄入至少有一半是全谷物 通过用全谷物代替精制谷物来增加全谷物摄入量	选择全谷物而不是精制谷物产品
动物产品	选择吃红肉的人每周摄入量应少于500g，摄入极少量加工肉类	包括低脂乳制品、家禽和鱼类的膳食模式；限制摄入红肉	选择各种蛋白质食物，包括海鲜、瘦肉、家禽、和鸡蛋 增加无脂或低脂牛奶和奶制品的摄入量	限制加工肉类和红肉的消费
膳食脂肪	少量食用能量密集的食物 谨慎食用“快餐”（如有）	减少来自饱和脂肪的热量比 目标定为从饱和脂肪中获得5%~6%热量的膳食模式 减少来自反式脂肪的热量比	保证来自饱和脂肪的热量占比不到10% 每天摄入的胆固醇少于300mg 保持尽可能少的反式脂肪酸摄入	
加工食品和精制糖	避免含糖饮料	限制甜食和含糖饮料的摄入	减少摄入来自添加糖的热量	
盐和钠	避免用盐腌制、盐渍或含盐的食物；保存食物时不使用盐 限制添加盐的加工食品的摄入量，以确保每天摄入量少于6g（2.4g钠）	每天摄入不超过2 400mg的钠 进一步将钠摄入量减少至每天1 500mg，可使血压进一步降低	将每日钠摄入量减少至少于2 300mg。某些人群，包括非洲裔美国人，糖尿病或慢性肾病患者，以及所有51岁及以上的成年人，应将钠摄入量减少至每天1 500mg	
酒精	如果饮酒，限制男性每天饮酒不超过两杯，女性每天饮酒不超过1杯[c]		如果饮酒，应该适量饮用 女性每天最多饮用1杯[c]，男性每天最多饮用2杯[c]	如果喝酒精饮料，应限制饮酒量 女性每天饮酒不超过1杯[c]，男性每天饮酒不超过2杯[c]
其他	不推荐将膳食补充剂用于预防癌症 除非另有建议，否则癌症生存者应该努力遵循膳食、健康体重和体育活动方面的建议		选择符合长期营养需求的膳食模式，摄入适当水平的热量	增加社区、工作场所和学校平价健康食品的供应

BMI，体重指数；NHLBI，美国国家心肺血液研究所。

[a]更新版美国膳食指南计划于2016年发布并可通过以下网址查看 http://health.gov/dietaryguidelines/

[b]1杯≈240ml。

[c]1杯≈30ml。

家族史或有癌变前病症而具有较高罹患特定类型癌症风险的人,更容易接受为其定制的膳食和生活方式干预措施,以降低他们罹患特定类型癌症的机会。另一类对此极为关注的是积极接受癌症治疗的患者,他们希望了解膳食和营养干预对巩固治疗效果、减少副作用的频率和严重程度所起到的作用。这些问题是多种多样的,并且最好通过有注册营养师(Registered Dietitian,RD)参与的治疗团队在医疗诊所中解决。最后,由于癌症的早期发现以及治疗干预措施的发展,癌症生存者的数量正在迅速增加。完成癌症治疗的患者正在寻求关于膳食和生活方式干预的指导来降低癌症复发风险(二级预防),减轻癌症治疗过程中长期存在的一些并发症,包括治疗相关的次生肿瘤及持续性的器官功能失调。因此,参与癌症治疗和长期健康管理的人员越来越多地被要求在这个科学研究极少的领域提供循证指导。但是,目前相关科学研究很少,且供应商推出的替代性膳食和营养干预的产品缺乏与疗效和安全性相关的可靠数据。这样的情况下,本就脆弱的癌症生存者经常成为盲目膳食调整的牺牲品。虽然本章侧重于预防,但我们也将简要回顾治疗和生存阶段,并为关注膳食和营养干预的个人和团体提供咨询信息。

在膳食、营养和癌症领域开展的研究绝大部分都侧重于病因学和预防。因此,本章着重介绍公共卫生模型,并集中介绍了可减轻大批人群总体癌症负担的干预措施。然后,我们讨论了特定器官常见癌症预防方法的证据。本章不会详细介绍有关膳食成分在特定癌症病因中作用的文献(这些文献很复杂,通常是不完整的,有时还相互矛盾),只是提供了一个通用指南,主要强调了该领域的新兴概念。最后,我们简要概述了膳食和营养在提高疗效和生存方面所起的作用。

膳食、营养和癌症研究中的方法问题

简要探讨一下膳食指南制定的原则是有意义的。理想情况下,可以通过随机和前瞻性试验,针对膳食和营养摄入量差异实现无偏检测和风险量化。遗憾的是,长期的营养研究成本过高,控制或测量膳食模式和营养摄入在科学上过于困难,限制了其可行性。所以,目前的疾病预防营养指南是以各种不同流行病学方法和实验室调研的整合信息为基础。而正因为此,大多数指南是由美国国立癌症研究所(National Cancer Institute)、美国癌症协会(ACS)、美国癌症研究中心(American Institute of Cancer Research, AICR)/世界癌症研究基金会(World Cancer Research Fund, WCRF)和世界卫生组织等[1,2,5,6]召集的专家委员会制定的。根据因果关系的标准,对流行病学研究、临床调查和实验室研究中获得的证据进行审核和讨论,其中因果关系定义为伴随着一系列已知情况或条件而出现的特定事件或结局。在营养学中,单一营养素缺乏综合征和补充维生素后症状的完全逆转就是因果关系的充分体现。例如,膳食中缺乏水果和蔬菜会导致维生素 C 缺乏症,而这很容易通过补充维生素 C 迅速逆转。然而,膳食和癌症之间的关系比单一营养缺乏综合征要复杂得多。为了确定因果关系,某一时间肿瘤的发生与其致病因素的相关性结论是以多个既定标准为基础的。这些标准经过多年发展,包括一致性、关联强度、生物梯度、时序性、特异性、生物学合理性、生物学机制、一致性和实验证据[7]。由于大多数癌症的病因涉及多种因素,并且人们对这些因素的相互作用知之甚少,因此很难准确地定量饮食因素引起的风险。根据年龄、性别、种族、社会经济地位、宿主遗传因素,以及许多环境、职业和生活方式变量等因素,人类癌症表现出惊人的差异。这些因素与膳食之间极有可能进行复杂的相互作用。这里需要强调的一点是,与证明高风险环境暴露对癌症的影响(例如吸烟对肺癌的影响)相比,同样清晰地证明膳食与癌症的关联要复杂得多。

人类膳食评估

营养流行病学研究面临的特殊难题在于食物暴露的广泛性,这与许多致癌的环境暴露如香烟烟雾完全不同。表 36-2 详述了营养学研究中使用的各类研究设计的优势和局限性。营养流行病学的研究重点包括营养素、非营养素生物活性成分和膳食模式。营养素包括供应能量的大量营养素,涵盖脂类、碳水化合物和蛋白质,以及各种构成要素,如必需脂肪酸和氨基酸、微量营养素维生素和矿物质。营养素的缺乏会导致相应的综合征。非营养素成分包括数千种潜在的生物活性物质,特别是水果和蔬菜中富含的物质,例如纤维、多酚和类胡萝卜素。目前,制定膳食模式的策略可以帮助更好地理解多变量的综合效应,例如地中海饮食、全素饮食或营养过剩饮食,然而,目前仍缺乏评估膳食模式的标准化定义和统计方法。

表 36-2 用于评估膳食和疾病关系的研究类型

研究类型	方法	优势	限制
生态/相关研究	观察单位是由鉴别者位置(日本与美国,北纬与南纬)决定的全体人口 将群体的死亡率或发病率与营养素或食物摄入量的估计值进行比较	经常会发现癌症发病率和膳食模式方面的巨大差异,并且可以由此进行假设	不同人口之间经常存在许多膳食和生活方式上的差异;因此,疾病发病率和膳食因素之间的相关性会被已知或未知的变量所混淆 癌症发病率数据和膳食模式在国家之间可能无法进行类似的定量
病例对照研究	找出患有疾病的个体,以及没有该疾病的一组相似的匹配受试者 从病例和对照中获得关于过去膳食和营养素的信息以进行比较	研究可以在相对较短的时间内进行	如果选择的对照组不具有代表性,则可能发生选择偏差 当患有疾病的受试者的感知和对过去膳食习惯的回忆发生改变时,可能会发生回忆偏倚。当参与者熟悉特定的膳食/疾病假设时,通常会发生这种情况

续表

研究类型	方法	优势	限制
前瞻性/队列研究	确定研究人群并评估膳食模式。在一段时期内随访该人群，关注其疾病结局和对膳食风险因素的接触情况的变化	可以定期监测膳食摄入量；膳食评估不依赖于长期记忆，并且受回忆偏倚的影响较小；可以定期进行生化检测	确诊疾病可能需要很长一段时间，因此队列研究通常需要多年的随访 需要大量受试者来补偿退出的受试者、在随访过程中丢失的受试者，和/或出现目标结局的频率过低的可能性 长期、大型前瞻性研究费用昂贵
随机对照试验	对个人根据具体特征进行筛选；确定适当的目标人群并将其随机分配到对照组（标准操作）或干预组。跟踪受试者的疾病结局或其他生物标记	尤其适用于测试可以掺入药丸或胶囊中的化合物（维生素和矿物质），可在数年内以双盲的方式提供给受试者	很难针对许多营养和癌症假设（减肥、运动、膳食脂肪、纤维、水果和蔬菜）进行实施，因为膳食改变的试验无法双盲 在大规模的干预研究中操作单一膳食成分很困难，因为食物很复杂，且含有许多化合物 对食物变化的依从性可能难以界定 随机对照试验可能需要很长时间才能完成并且可能非常昂贵

大多数人群研究的主要局限性特征是无法精确量化膳食摄入量。估算食物或营养素的日常摄入量，以及考虑随时间而改变的个体差异，是一个关键的研究领域[8~10]。人体营养素摄入量的估算基于两个步骤。第一步，必须通过采访、调查问卷或膳食记录来确定食物的摄入量及食物种类[11]。第二步，利用这些信息来计算营养素摄入量，前提是已经建立了一个可对被调查人群摄入的各种食物中含有的每一种营养素进行精确定量的数据库。在此过程中，每个步骤的差错都会给研究营养素和癌症的联系带来挑战。人类膳食包含了一系列复杂的食物，具有显著的日常和季节差异。膳食的复杂性在不同种族、文化和地理区域之间也存在显著差异。因此通常需要为不同的人群或亚人群制定不同的评估方法。未来的进展将部分取决于对营养素暴露生物标志物的识别上。开发有效且可靠的营养素摄入量生物标志物将有望提高流行病研究的精确度，因为根据摄入量估计减少了参与者在分类时犯错的情况[12]。最后，对于食物中许多可能影响癌症风险的生物活性化合物（包括来自植物的各种非营养素植物化学物质），由于缺乏食物成分数据库，评价营养素摄入水平对我们仍然是一个挑战[13]。

实验室模型

营养素或食物的成分及其相互作用对癌症发生的影响可以在越来越多的动物模型中进行严格测试。尽管从动物模型中获得的信息外推到人类时必须谨慎，但它们确实为流行病学研究提出的二者关系在生物学合理性方面提供了重要证据。大多数实验动物的营养需求已经得以精准确认，并且可以使用纯化的成分来配制用于癌症研究的膳食。基于转基因和敲除技术的新动物模型的迅速出现为检测特定遗传基因和膳食变量之间的相互作用提供了新的机遇[14]。

预防癌症的公共卫生指南

在本章的开始，我们汇总了美国癌症研究所/世界癌症研究基金会（AICR/WCRF）、美国癌症协会（ACS）和美国心脏协会（American Heart Association，AHA）等组织机构[1,2,3,5]发布的关于癌症预防和健康领域的公共卫生膳食指南。公共卫生方法是一种预防性策略，通过减少整个人群的不良膳食习惯，降低整体疾病发病率。实行膳食指导需要媒体、食品工业、公共卫生工作人员、医疗从业者、教育工作者和政府机构之间通力合作[1]。要取得成功，膳食指导必须明确可行、风险极小、社会成本低并且对人类有益[1]。此外，与粮食和农业相关的经济问题也可能影响确定营养指南的决策，尤其是政府机构的决策。在营养方面，过去的工作已取得了成功。例如，虽然对少数患有血黄素沉着症的个体存在一定风险，但通过对谷物进行铁强化来预防贫血已经使许多儿童和成年女性受益。目前提供的循证膳食建议的合理程度已有一定的确定性，且将风险降至最低，并有极大造福公共卫生的潜力[1,6,15,16,17]。表 36-1 总结了目前基于人群的膳食建议，这些建议可以共同降低慢性病风险，包括癌症[1,4,5]。2016 年初，美国国立卫生研究院将发布《美国膳食指南》的修订版，并建议由关注疾病预防策略的人士进行审核。

营养和癌症预防的公共卫生指南

保持健康的体重

越来越多的研究证明，久坐行为、体重增加、超重和肥胖是人类癌症的主要风险因素[1~3,5,18~23]。体重指数（body mass index，BMI）大于 25kg/m² 的女性和 BMI 大于 27kg/m² 的男性应尽快减肥。体重仅减轻 5%～10%，就能改善健康状况并降低多种癌症的发病率及严重性[20~23]。减轻体重的最佳方式是降低总热量摄入并增加热量消耗，来实现负能量平衡，从而让体重在一段时期内适度但持续地减轻。对于大多数人来说，每周最多减重 1～2 磅是适宜的。通过流行的减重膳食实现快速减肥并不会促使个人建立起健康的膳食和体育活动模式，并且这些方法不能持续减轻体重[3]。人们日益清楚地认识到，在一生中保持健康的体重可能是预防许多常见恶性肿瘤最关键的方法之一[1,2,5,18]。

每天参加体育活动和每周数天进行中到高强度运动

通过体育活动来消耗能量是保持健康体重和预防成人体重增加的关键组成部分，而成人体重增加与多种癌症风险相关[1,5,24]。此外，许多研究都表明，每天进行体育活动与定期规律性中等至高强度运动相结合，可以降低癌症风险，且不受体重和膳食的影响[25~27]。体育活动应纳入日常生活中，并在每周超过一半天数定期进行中到高强度运动。一般公认的建议是每周至少进行 150 分钟的中等强度活动或 75 分钟的高强度运动[1,5,28]。

摄入富含水果、蔬菜和各种全麦和谷物的植物性膳食

数百项研究已经证实了水果和蔬菜摄入量与癌症风险之间的关系[1]。绝大多数研究表明，植物性膳食对多个部位的癌症风险具有明显的预防作用。水果和蔬菜不仅含有多种维生素、矿物质、纤维和植物化学物质，而且其能量密度低于其他大多数食物。每餐都应有各种非淀粉类水果和蔬菜，目标是每天至少食用五份（或至少 400～600g）水果和蔬菜。此外，豆类也是重点摄入对象，豆类提供蛋白质、纤维、维生素 B 和铁，还应重点摄入可提供膳食纤维、维生素 B 和大量植物化学物质的全麦面包、谷物和意大利面。由于植物性膳食可与适度食用瘦肉搭配，因此不应将这种膳食模式认为是素食膳食模式。

尽量减少食用高能量密度食物和含糖饮料

这项建议对于全面预防体重增加和肥胖至关重要。富含加工食品的饮食通常富含精制糖和/或脂肪，这些糖和/或脂肪会给饮食带来过多的热量且无法提供维生素、矿物质和具有生物活性的植物化学物质。近几十年来，含糖加工食品的消费量显著增加，目前占总摄入热量的 15%以上[29,30]。这主要是由于含糖饮料，特别是苏打水的消费日益增加[1]。含糖饮料与儿童、青少年和成人的超重和肥胖风险增加有关，因此应尽可能少摄入碳酸饮料。

对于喜欢红肉的人，建议食用中等份量并减少高度加工红肉的摄入量

人们常常发现，素食为主的人群患各种疾病的风险较低，包括某些类型的癌症；然而，在排除其他变量的情况下，肉类是否在促进癌症中起到的特定作用仍未明确。此外，肉类是许多营养素的重要来源，如蛋白质、铁和维生素 B_{12}。因此，每周适当食用不超过 510g 的红肉（牛肉、羊肉和猪肉）不会显著增加癌症风险，特别是在肉类没有完全取代水果、蔬菜和全谷类的情况下。不同的烹饪方法会产生致癌物质，其对癌症的影响仍在研究中[31]。谨慎做法是适度摄入长时间用火煮熟的肉类[32]。历史上，食用各种加工肉类（包括烟熏、腌制或腌制肉类）的人群患各种癌症的风险更高。因此，建议限制这些肉类产品的摄入[1,33]。对于选择肉类的人来说，明智的做法是选择多种来源的肉，包括新鲜的鸡肉、鱼肉和火鸡肉[1]。

如果饮酒，应该限制饮酒量

适度饮酒的风险和潜在好处仍然是一个争论性话题。虽然酒精或特定类型的酒精饮料对健康的影响方面仍是一个活跃的研究领域，但长期饮酒与口咽癌、喉癌、食道癌和乳腺癌（包括绝经前和绝经后）密切相关这一结论已经得到证实[1,5]。吸烟在口腔癌和上呼吸消化道癌症的发病机制中会与酒精协同作用。大量摄入酒精饮料也会引发肝癌和结肠癌[1]。即使每日适量饮酒，也可能轻微增加患乳腺癌的风险[1,34]。鉴于有证据表明适度饮酒可能降低患心脏病的风险，因此个人应根据自己的健康情况来决定是否饮酒。如果饮酒，女性每天不超过 1 杯，男性不超过 2 杯[1,2,5]。

食品保鲜、加工和准备的最佳方式

盐对人类健康至关重要，但其正常需求量远低于美国膳食中常见的水平[35]。盐腌食品与胃癌有关，而胃癌是全球最主要的恶性肿瘤之一，特别是在发展中国家。尽管盐与肿瘤的关系尚不确定，但富含盐的加工肉类饮食与多种癌症的风险相关，因此应适量食用[1,36]。在高温下烹饪、烤制和炭烧的肉类容易含有某些化学致癌物质，应适量食用[1]。食品供应中的微生物污染是全球的一个主要问题。最关键的是，食用被真菌黄曲霉毒素污染过的谷物和豆类会大幅增加患肝癌的风险，政府机构须采取公共卫生措施来进行限制。

膳食补充剂并非健康膳食的必需组成成分

越来越多的美国民众定期服用自选的营养素或营养补充剂。公众认为营养补充剂和替代药物是一种预防和治疗包括癌症在内的多种疾病的自我疗法的重要方式[1,24]。多种维生素及矿物质补充剂通常价格低廉、易于摄入，在摄入剂量与推荐膳食供给量（recommended dietary allowance，RDA）一致时，基本无副作用且无需处方即可获得。鲜有证据表明，日常膳食补充剂可以在整体人群水平起到预防癌症的效果[5,37]。虽然美国人按照上述膳食建议均可达到足够的营养素摄入量，但提供推荐膳食供给量为基础的标准多维生素/矿物质补充剂可能对部分人有益而无害。含有高浓度特定营养素和其他成分的补充剂正在大量上市，如草药、提取物和浓缩物。消费者应该意识到，目前几乎没有与膳食补充剂相关的健康声明及补充剂成分安全性和有效性的规定，因此，购买时应保持怀疑和谨慎的态度。美国国立卫生研究院膳食补充剂办公室通过网络为关注补充剂的消费者提供相关信息。

专注于特定癌症的研究工作的总结

任何食物、营养元素或饮食习惯不可能对所有癌症都产生相同作用[1,5,24]。因此，在研究营养与癌症风险之间的关系时，要重点区开每个组织或器官的检查数据。基于遗传学检测、家族史、致癌因素暴露和恶化前病症的研究，将提高我们对特定癌症高风险人群的识别能力，为高危个体提供量身定制的膳食建议和化学预防策略，特异性地预防各类癌症。以下简要总结了膳食、营养与特发或常见癌症风险之间关系的研究进展。有关其他信息请参阅表 36-3。

表 36-3 世界癌症研究基金(WCRF)/美国癌症研究所(AICR)指南

美国癌症研究所/世界癌症研究基金总结的有关膳食、营养、体育活动和预防癌症的有力证据

↓↓	确认风险降低
↓	很可能降低风险
↑↑	确认风险增加
↑	很可能增加风险
•	不太可能对风险产生重大影响

	口腔癌,舌咽癌,喉癌(2007)	鼻咽癌(2007)	食道癌(2007)	肺癌(2007)	胃癌(2007)	胰腺癌(2007)	胆囊癌(2007)	肝癌(2007)	结肠直肠癌(2011)	乳腺癌(绝经前)(2010)	乳腺癌(绝经后)(2010)	卵巢癌(2014)	子宫内膜癌(2013)	前列腺癌(2014)	肾癌(2007)	皮肤癌(2007)
含有膳食纤维的食物									↓↓							
黄曲霉毒素								↑↑								
非淀粉类蔬菜[1]	↓		↓		↓											
葱属蔬菜					↓											
大蒜									↓							
水果[2]	↓		↓	↓	↓											
红肉									↑↑							
加工肉制品									↑↑							
广式咸鱼		↑														
高钙膳食[3]									↓							
盐,含盐和咸的食物					↑											
血糖负荷													↑			
饮用水中的砷				↑↑												↑
马黛茶			↑													
酒精饮料[4]	↑↑		↑↑					↑	↑[4] / ↑↑[4]	↑↑	↑↑				•	
咖啡					•								↓		•	
β-胡萝卜素[5]				↑↑										•		•
体育活动[6]									↓↓		↓		↓			
肥胖[7]			↑↑			↑↑	↑		↑↑	↓	↑↑	↑	↑↑	↑	↑↑	
成年时身高						↑			↑↑	↑	↑↑	↑↑		↑		
出生时超重										↑						
哺乳										↓↓	↓↓					

[1]证据包括含有类胡萝卜素的食物对口腔癌、舌咽癌、喉癌的影响;含有β-胡萝卜素的食物对食道癌的影响;含有维生素C的食物对食道癌的影响。

[2]证据包括含有类胡萝卜素的食物对口腔癌、舌咽癌、喉癌和肺癌的影响;含有β-胡萝卜素的食物对食道癌的影响;含有维生素C的食物对食道癌的影响。

[3]证据来自牛奶和针对结肠直肠癌使用补充剂的研究。

[4]确认对男性患结肠直肠癌风险增加,女性患结肠直肠的风险很可能增加。证据显示对肾癌有副作用。

[5]证据来自针对肺癌使用补充剂的研究。

[6]确认结肠癌的风险增加,不包括直肠癌。

[7]晚期前列腺癌的风险很可能增加,不包括非晚期前列腺癌。

结肠和直肠

结直肠癌是世界上第三位最常见的癌症,在美国癌症死因中位居第三[1,38]。通过对遗传因素及癌前病变特征的描述,有助于确定化学预防的高危人群,开展临床前试验的饮食干预研究。结直肠癌的死亡率国际间差异巨大(图 36-1)。虽然诊断方法的不同可能是造成这种差异的部分原因,但在不同国家间观察到的超过十倍的差异尚无法解释[1]。亚洲国家死亡率较低,可能在于文化和生活方式而非工业化的差异[1,40,41]。日本和中国移民到美国后发病率急剧增加[42],这清楚地表明,国家间的差异主要来自环境影响而非遗传背景[43,44]。对结直肠癌发病率的时间趋势研究,特别是自 20 世纪 40 年代以来在日本的研究,有力地表明了患病的主要因素是西方文化相关的膳食和生活方式(图 36-2)。

能量平衡、体质和体育活动

能量摄入、体育活动、身体各种测量数据或肥胖都与结肠癌风险密切相关。如果不将它们作为一个整体来看待,很难对每个因素在结肠癌中的作用进行定量或确认。有报道,持续的体育活动与结肠癌风险之间反向关联[1,45~47]。数项研究发现,身体质量指数(BMI)或肥胖与结肠癌风险升高之间存在关联[1,44,48~50]。研究发现,一些国家(美国、中国、瑞典和日本)中,无论男性或女性,肥胖和不运动往往伴有结肠癌风险,不管此类运动是职业运动还是娱乐活动[1]。同时,肥胖与结肠腺瘤风险有关[51]。一些证据表明,身高(可能代表儿童期和青春期的净能量摄入量)也与结肠癌的高风险有关[52~54]。对啮齿动物的结肠癌模型研究发现,自由饮食组动物[55]癌症发生率升高,而限制摄入组[56]癌症发生率降低。整体而言,有足够的证据表明体育活动、适当的能量平衡以及维持理想的 BMI 可降低患结肠癌的风险[1,47]。

膳食模式

一般来说,富含红肉和加工肉类、高脂肪,而水果、蔬菜和纤维含量较低的西方膳食模式与结肠癌风险增加有关[1,57,58]。总脂肪摄入、脂肪饱和度或不同来源的脂肪与结肠癌的危险性之间的关系仍是一个活跃的研究领域,但至今尚无确定结论[1,5,42,59~62]。例如,图 36-3 展示的是一个基于人群的病例对照研究,该研究表明美国的华人移民中 60%的结直肠癌风险是由膳食脂肪引起的。其他队列研究报告显示,来自红肉的脂肪而非总脂肪可能会增加结肠癌风险[50,61,63~65]。饮食中的加工肉类中不仅含有脂肪,还可能有可疑致癌物质,已确认为结肠癌的风险因素[1,47,66,67]。因此,结肠癌高危个体应考虑减少红

肉和加工肉类的摄入。目前正在进行的研究针对的是复杂的膳食模式(例如地中海式膳食),而不是单一变量因素,研究中的新数据也证明了健康膳食模式的益处[68,69]。

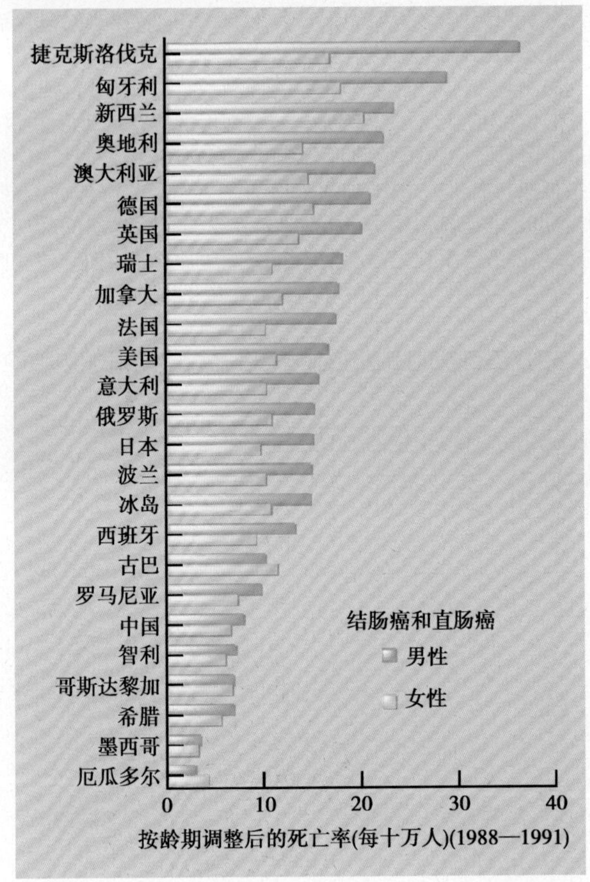

图 36-1　选定国家结肠癌和直肠癌患者按年龄调整后的死亡率(每 10 万人)[39]

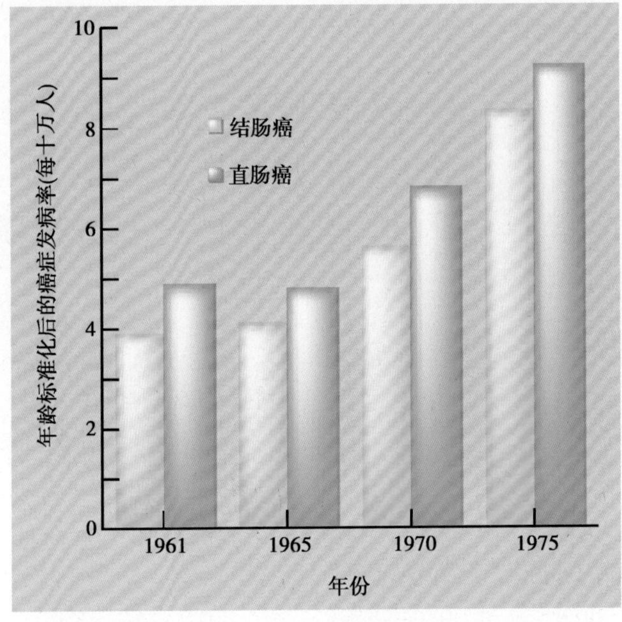

图 36-2　1960—1977 年日本年龄标准化后的结肠癌和直肠癌发病率(每 10 万人)

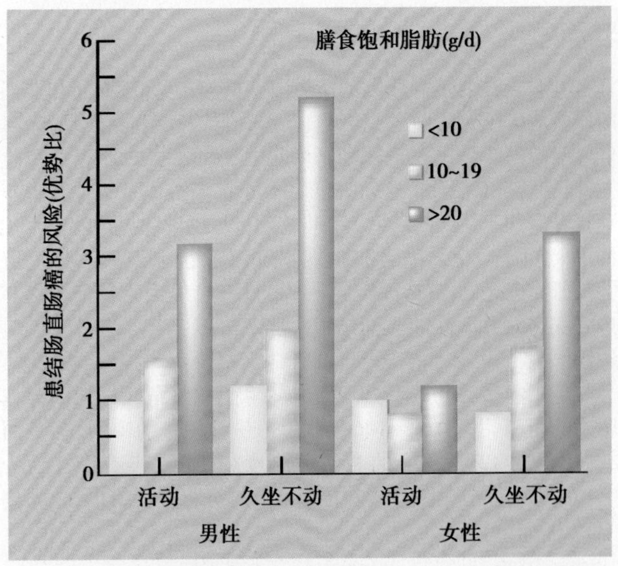

图 36-3　根据膳食脂肪摄入量和体育活动水平划分的中国移民到美国人群的结直肠癌风险[42]

水果,蔬菜和纤维

富含植物的产品,特别是富含谷物和蔬菜的膳食模式通常与结肠癌风险降低相关,许多研究者推测纤维含量是一个主要的介导因素[1,15,26,59,61,70~73]。膳食纤维的化学成分特别复杂,非常遗憾的是,人类流行病学研究中纤维摄入量的定量和定性评估非常困难。然而,大多数研究表明,富含多种含纤维食物的膳食对健康可能是有益的。欧洲大型前瞻性癌症调查(European Prospective Investigation into Cancer, EPIC)研究结果发现,在所调查的超过 50 万的男性和女性中,每日膳食中谷物、水果或蔬菜中膳食纤维每增加 10g,结肠癌风险降低 13%[74,75]。一些干预试验评估了特定类型的膳食纤维对结肠癌风险的影响,迄今为止尚未取得明确结果[76~80]。尚未确定任何一种类型或类别的水果、蔬菜或谷物的特定作用。不过,多样化植物性膳食模式是一种可取的策略。

酒精

生态学、队列和基于人群的病例对照研究表明,酒精摄入量与结肠癌风险之间存在正相关关系[1,5,47,81~83]。酒精也与结直肠腺瘤的高风险有关[1,5,47]。总体而言,这些影响更多与酒精摄入量有关,而不是酒精来源[1,5]。研究表明,与酒精相关的癌症危险性升高主要发生在直肠或远端结肠[65]。最近的研究表明摄入大量叶酸或甲硫氨酸,似乎可以减轻酒精的影响,这两种酸对于正常的甲基代谢特别是脱氧核糖核酸(DNA)甲基化都至关重要[81]。众所周知酒精对甲基代谢有不良影响,这说明酒精会通过这种机制增加结直肠癌的风险。然而,叶酸在癌变各个阶段的作用仍有待确定[84]。

总之,结直肠癌风险的增加与缺乏体育活动的生活方式,高 BMI,富含单糖、高脂肪食物(尤其是红肉和加工肉类)的富人或西方膳食模式,水果、全谷物和蔬菜的低摄入以及饮酒相关[1,5,47]。叶酸、甲硫氨酸、肉类和特定纤维成分的各自作用有待进一步研究[1,5]。这些成分与其他导致风险的因素(例如早期膳食暴露、运动、结肠微生物和遗传学等)之间会产生许多潜在的相互影响。目前,在提出结肠癌预防建议时,应考虑整体膳食模式和体育活动的综合影响,而不是只关注单一因素。

乳腺癌

乳腺癌在北美和西欧的富裕国家最为常见,在亚洲和非洲的许多地区较少见[1,5,38],与结直肠癌一样,我们观察发现,来自低风险国家的移民在迁移到高风险国家[1,5,38,43]之后患病风险上升,特别是其后代。这一观察结果表明,营养以及其他在青年和青春期处于活跃的环境因素可能对随后的乳腺癌风险产生长期重大影响[1,5,38]。早孕和哺乳能降低乳腺癌的风险[1,23,85]。有数项研究也提出,富裕国家的一些膳食和营养因素特征会提高患乳腺癌的风险,并简要总结了这些特点[1,5]。

饮酒

越来越多的证据表明,酒精摄入和乳腺癌危险性之间存在明确的正相关性[1,5,23]。每天饮用一份常规量的啤酒、葡萄酒或白酒(约 12g 乙醇)的相对危险度(relative risk,RR)约为 1.4,而每天三份则危险度加倍。最近有分析报告指出,乳腺癌风险与每日饮酒量增加 10g 之间存在线性关系,即使在不同的雌激素/孕激素亚型中也是如此[34,86]。

能量平衡,体重和肥胖

越来越多的证据表明,肥胖、成年人体重增加和缺乏体育活动是乳腺癌的重要风险因素[1,5,23,87,88]。能量摄入对乳腺癌的促进作用已经通过对啮齿动物研究得到了充分证实,研究方式为限制膳食或能量摄入[89,90],以及对自由采食进行回归分析[55,91]。总的来说,成年人坚持较高强度的体育活动可在一定程度上降低乳腺癌的危险性(降低约 25% 风险),并且该保护效果可能与成年人 BMI 或体重增加无关[88,92~94]。然而,要明确能量摄入、能量消耗、人体测量和乳腺癌风险之间的确切关系,必须要考虑女性生命周期中各个关键时期的不同。这些因素可能在青春期、生育年龄和绝经后产生不同的影响。

膳食脂肪

关于膳食脂肪对乳腺癌危险性影响的争论可通研究图 36-4

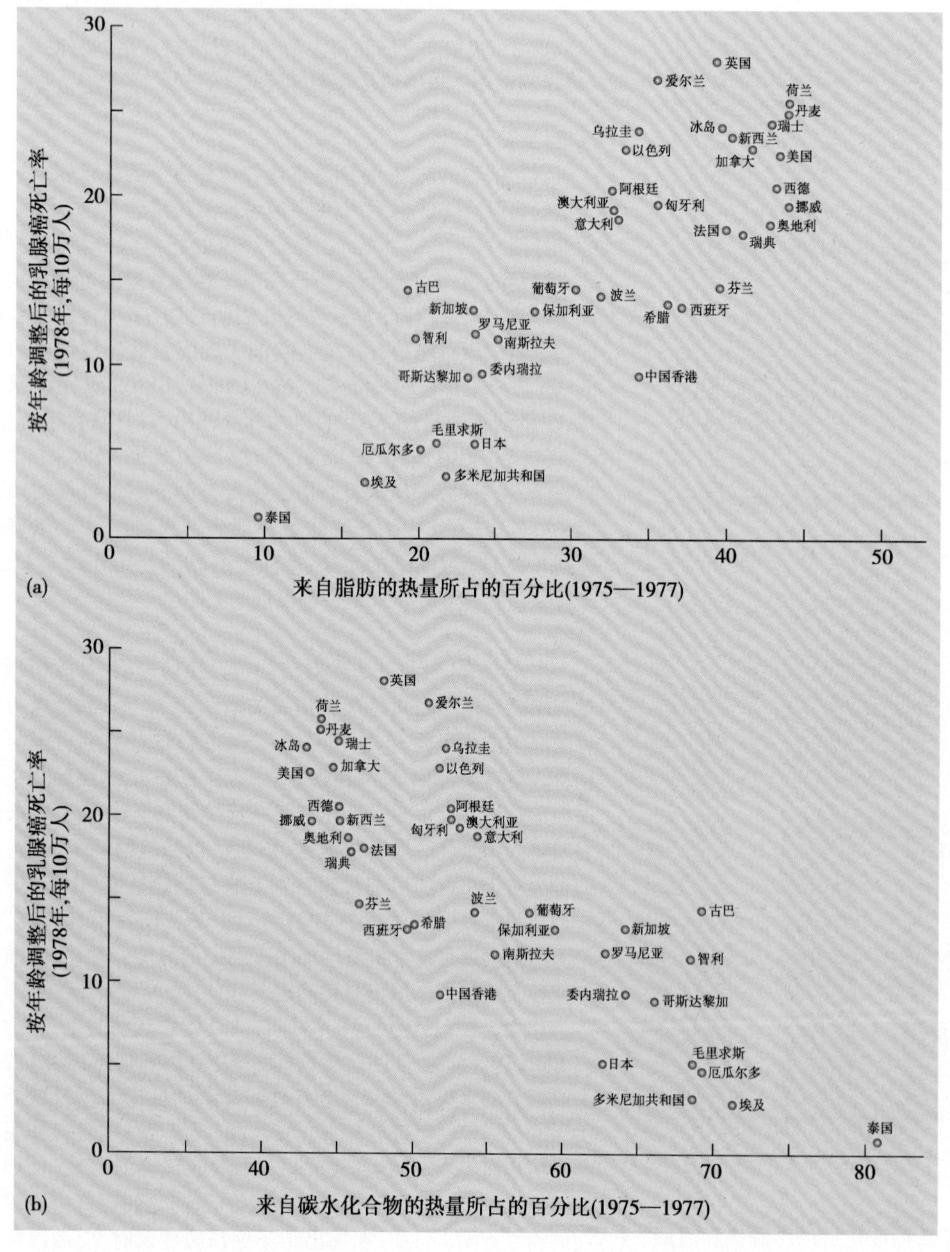

图 36-4 (a)膳食脂肪预估摄入量(来自脂肪的热量所占的百分比)和(b)碳水化合物预估摄入量(来自碳水化合物的热量所占的百分比)和按年龄标准化的乳腺癌死亡率的相关性

展示的具有代表性的数据得到理想的解答。地域研究显示，各国家和地区的乳腺癌发病率与人均脂肪预估摄入量之间存在很强的相关性[60,96]。乳腺癌发病率、人均脂肪占能量供给百分比在国家之间差别很大。从膳食中脂肪含量较低的低风险地区(例如日本)迁移到膳食中脂肪含量高的高风险地区(例如美国)的人群，乳腺癌发病率显著增加[43,97]。时间趋势研究也证实了膳食脂肪与乳腺癌相关联。在第二次世界大战后的几十年里，日本的人均每日脂肪预估摄入量有所上升。而在此期间，日本的乳腺癌死亡率也上升了超过 30%。相关性并不能证明因果关系，许多研究者认为，脂肪摄入也许只是一些仍未发现的，与膳食和环境相关的危险因素的一个指标，而这些因素才是真正的关键风险因素。许多病例对照和队列研究已经探讨了脂肪摄入与乳腺癌风险之间的关系，然而得出的结论却不一致[98~101]。虽然流行病学数据未提供关于膳食脂肪和乳腺癌的确切结果，但是来自 100 多项使用化学致癌物质、激素、辐射或病毒诱导乳腺癌的动物研究表明，脂肪是乳腺癌发生率增加的独立危险因素(图 36-5)[1,55,91,102]。一项针对乳腺癌治疗女性的随机干预研究表明，能够将膳食脂肪摄入降低到约 33g/d 的女性，乳腺癌复发风险降低 24%(对照组为 51g/d)[103]。尽管两组之间的差异没有统计学意义，但在妇女健康倡议的大型随机化研究中也出现了类似的趋势[98]。一项大规模 EPIC 研究随访了超过 33 000 名女性共 11.5 年，发现总脂肪和饱和脂肪含量高的膳食与 ER(+)PR(+)疾病风险显著增加有关，但与 ER(-)PR(-)的乳腺癌无关[104]。总体而言，成年期脂肪摄入量的减少与乳腺癌风险的降低之间的关系仍未得到确定，青春期和生育年龄的膳食模式可能对未来的乳腺癌风险更为关键[1]。

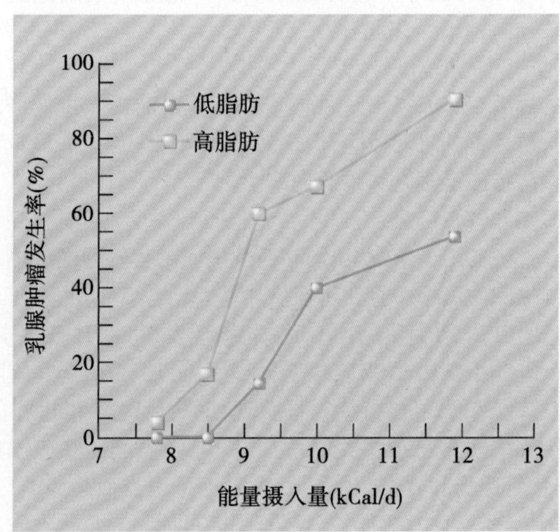

图 36-5　低热量和高脂肪膳食在不同热量摄入水平对 C3H 雌性小鼠自发性乳腺肿瘤发生的影响[90]

其他膳食因素

总体而言，富含蔬菜、水果和谷物的植物性膳食模式可能在降低乳腺癌风险方面发挥了一定作用，但特定植物成分对乳腺癌风险的决定性和具体作用尚未得到证实[1,5,23,101,105]。摄入特定维生素或矿物质与乳腺癌风险之间不存在一致的相关性，因此，使用膳食补充剂预防乳腺癌的建议仍有待确定[1,5]。膳食中包含的其他生物活性化合物(如大豆异黄酮、木脂素和纤维)可能对乳腺癌有一定作用，但证据的强度仍不足以进行推荐[1,5,101]。总之，预防乳腺癌最行之有效的方法是定期进行高强度体育活动，避免或限制摄入酒精饮料，以及通过体育活动和能量限制来控制体重增加或肥胖。

前列腺癌

前列腺癌是美国男性中最常见的恶性肿瘤之一，在非裔美国人群中尤为常见[1,38]。前列腺癌是一种老年男性疾病，它的国际分布类似于结肠癌和乳腺癌；因此，认为它与富人膳食模式相关[1,106]。膳食与前列腺癌之间的关系尚未明确界定，预防该疾病的具体建议仍然是推测性的。由过多的能量摄入和缺乏体育活动导致的体重增加和肥胖对前列腺癌起到的作用在人体研究中已获得了相关的证据，并且在啮齿动物研究中已经得到了明确证实[1,18,106~109]。有证据表明，这些因素对晚期前列腺癌风险上升的影响是最明显的[22]。国际和国内相关性研究表明，前列腺癌死亡率与人均总脂肪摄入量之间存在关联[1,106]。同样，一些分析性流行病学研究和病例对照研究显示，前列腺癌与总脂肪或者高脂肪食物(特别是动物性食物中的饱和脂肪)摄入之间存在关联[1,106~108,110,111]。

多项研究表明，维生素 E 和硒等特定营养素可能会影响患前列腺癌的风险[112]。在随机接受维生素 E 补充的男性中观察到患前列腺癌的风险显著降低[112]。目前，通过各种间接证据，已经对硒在预防前列腺癌中可能起到的作用有了一定的假设[1,113~116]。迄今为止规模最大的前列腺癌化学预防试验，即硒和维生素 E 化学预防试验(Selenium and Vitamin E Chemoprevention Trial，SELECT)，于 2001 年秋季在随机选取的 33 000 名男性中开始。研究设计成由维生素 E、硒和安慰剂组成的 2×2 析因设计。中位随访 5.4 年后，未发现硒、维生素 E 或两者的组合对前列腺癌有保护作用[117]。现在正在研究钙和维生素 D 作为通过复杂膳食和内分泌因子网络发挥相互作用来调节前列腺癌风险的有效因子的可能性[118]。几项大型队列研究表明，高钙膳食会增加前列腺癌风险[1,22,118~122]。高钙摄入和日晒不足会抑制维生素 D[$1,25(OH)_2$]的内源性产生。前列腺细胞表达维生素 D 受体，与配体结合后会诱导分化途径。这些复杂的关系推动了许多细胞培养、动物和队列研究，其中一些研究表明维生素 D 与前列腺癌风险之间存在负相关关系，除了补充不足和少量摄入以外，尚不确定其他的益处[123~126]。

水果和蔬菜的总摄入量并未显示出与前列腺癌风险持续降低的关联性[1,22,106]。然而，在前瞻性健康专业人员随访研究中，曾反复出现患前列腺癌风险降低与食用番茄和加工番茄制品相关的现象[127~131]。基于这些研究结果推测：类胡萝卜素番茄红素可能是番茄产品具有抗癌特性的原因，尽管在番茄食品中发现的其他化合物也可能起到重要作用[131~137]。然而，现在断定番茄红素针对前列腺癌具有保护作用，或者番茄红素是番茄产品中唯一可能造成这种关联的成分，还为时过早[138]。有趣的是，有几组对食用番茄产品或番茄红素补充剂的受试者进行的干预发现，血液和前列腺组织的癌症生物标记得到了调节[135,139~141]。

总之，流行病学研究和有限数量的实验室研究表明，富人膳食模式对前列腺癌风险有一定影响。尽管特定成分的作用尚未明确且正在积极研究中，但在普遍存在富人膳食模式、肥胖和久坐生活方式的国家中，前列腺癌的发病率确实较高。

肺癌

肺癌是目前世界上最常见的恶性肿瘤，也是癌症相关死亡的主要原因[1]。吸烟是大多数肺癌病例的诱因，并且肺癌发生率随着香烟生产、销售及广告的全球化同步增长[1]。某些职业性接触(如石棉或辐射)可能与吸烟协同增加肺癌风险[1]。与烟草的作用相比，膳食和营养的潜在影响相对较小。然而，人类营养流行病学中经常发现，水果和蔬菜摄入量与肺癌风险之间存在反比关系[1,142~144]。许多人假设，水果和蔬菜中的β-胡萝卜素或来自β-胡萝卜素转化成的维生素A可能是这些食物中的关键活性剂[1,145]。然而，两组在高危人群中进行的随机对照干预试验发现，在每天补充20mg或30mg β-胡萝卜素数年后，男性吸烟者的肺癌发病率没有降低，甚至还有所上升[146]。最近一项针对72 000多名中国女性的研究报告指出，在接触侧流烟的女性中，膳食中摄入富含生育酚的食物与肺癌发病呈负相关。相反，补充维生素E会显著增加整体肺癌风险，尤其是肺腺癌[147]。这些报告强调，富含水果和蔬菜的膳食的保护作用可能涉及许多相互作用的成分，无法通过补充单一因素[1,148]来实现。总体而言，消除吸烟和职业风险因素是降低肺癌发病率最有效的方式。对于高风险个体而言，经常食用各种水果、蔬菜和其他植物性食物，可以起到一定程度的预防肺癌作用。

口腔癌，喉癌和口咽癌

与肺癌一样，口腔癌和喉癌与烟草制品的使用密切相关[1,2,24]。几十年来的病例对照研究证明，酒精饮料的摄入与这些组织的癌症之间存在关联。许多研究发现，酒精和口腔癌存在剂量反应关系，并且与烟草使用无关(图36-6)[150,151]。其他证据来源于对更高风险的人群(例如酗酒者)研究。美国的

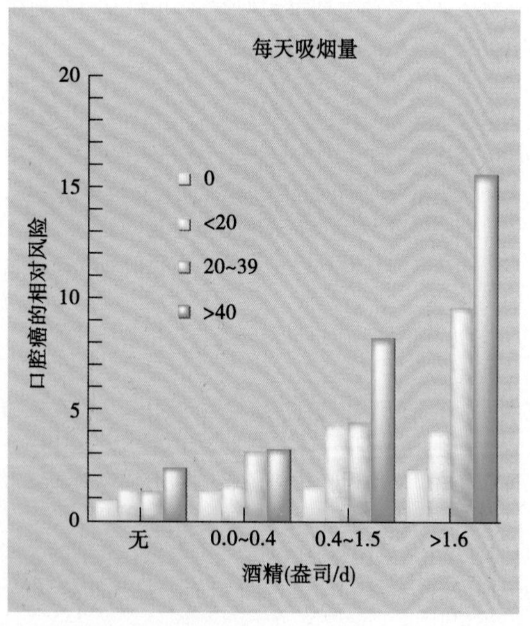

图36-6 酒精摄入量和吸烟之间的相互作用对口腔癌相对风险的影响[149]。1盎司≈30ml

基督复临安息日会成员和摩门教徒等不饮酒人群的风险很低[152,153]。值得注意的是，在动物实验中将纯酒精加入营养充足的健康膳食来喂食，不会产生口腔癌。因此，需要对相关问题进一步评价，例如人类与啮齿类动物的生化学差异、酒精直接致癌作用的证据不足、人类消费的酒精饮料中存在的致癌物、饮酒场所存在的被动吸烟情况、或其他重要致癌物的相互作用及营养缺乏等。流行病学和实验室研究都表明，富含水果和蔬菜的膳食具有保护作用[1,49,154]。此外，临床和实验室研究表明，维生素A和类似物或代谢物以及某些类胡萝卜素可能对口腔癌和呼吸道上皮癌起到抑制作用[155]。总之，烟草制品是口腔和咽喉癌的主要致癌原因，特别是与饮用含酒精饮料结合的情况下[1]。有必要进一步研究维生素A及衍生物、其他植物化学物质和多样化植物性膳食在高危群体预防中起到的作用。

食管癌

食管鳞状细胞癌是全球第八大常见癌症，在不同国家之间和一个国家不同的地理区域之间的差异可达数百倍[1,154]。大多数发达国家的相关性分析和病例对照研究表明，食管鳞状细胞癌的主要风险因素是乙醇和吸烟[1]，其风险与饮酒量成比例上升[1,156,157]。许多研究显示，虽然饮酒与吸烟会产生显著的相加作用，但控制吸烟后，癌症危险性与酒精摄入量存在剂量反应关系[1]。酒精摄入量的增加通常伴随许多营养素摄入的不足，这被认为会使个体患病风险更高。例如，酒精可能与叶酸、维生素B_{12}和甲基代谢相互作用以调节食管癌的风险[158]。一些研究表明，食管癌风险与食用新鲜水果和蔬菜之间存在负相关[1,143,159]。在亚洲的某些地区，高食管癌风险的原因不一定是饮酒，而可能与当地缺乏新鲜水果、蔬菜和动物产品的膳食有关，同时当地人维生素A、维生素C、核黄素、锌和一些微量元素(如钼)的摄入量也偏低[1,160,161]。总之，吸烟和饮酒是最主要的病因。有人提出一种或多种营养素的摄入过低可能提高了富裕人群的患病风险，但这尚未得到完全确定。最重要的膳食预防措施是多吃水果及蔬菜[1]。

食管腺癌和胃贲门癌

在过去的二十年中，美国和西欧国家的食管远端腺癌和胃贲门腺癌的发病率一直在迅速增加[162]。自20世纪70年代中期以来，白人男性的食管远端腺癌发病率上升了超过350%[163]。正在吸烟或曾经吸过烟可能是其中一个危险因素[163,164]。然而，经过持续观察发现，患病风险与BMI和(或)腹部肥胖之间存在正相关关系[165~168]。随着肥胖在美国广泛出现，食管腺癌和胃贲门癌的发病率也呈现类似趋势[169]。患病机制仍在调查中；然而，据推测，肥胖可能易导致胃食管反流病。其他与腺癌风险上升相关的营养因素包括富含动物脂肪但纤维、水果和蔬菜含量低的膳食模式[170,171]。除肥胖之外，须进一步进行研究来阐明其他导致食管腺癌发病率急剧增加的风险因素，并制定有效的干预策略。

胃癌

胃癌是全球第四大常见癌症[39]。各国的发病率差异很大，亚洲部分地区(如日本)和南美洲的发病率最高。据记载，在过去的一个世纪，许多富裕国家胃癌发病率显著下降。美国

目前的发病率全球最低，而在 1930 年，胃癌是美国人中最常见的恶性肿瘤。近年来，研究人员已经确定了胃贲门癌和远端胃癌的发病模式存在差异，说明二者病因不同。在病因学上，贲门腺癌通常与从远端食管化生引起的癌症分为一组，二者组织类似，且可能包含相同的风险因素。目前尚无令人信服的特定食物和营养素与胃癌有关的证据。然而，正处于研究中的几个变量被认为可能与其有一定关联，其中包括：①富含水果和蔬菜的膳食保护作用[172,173]；②现代食品加工和储存的保护作用，以此减少食品的腐烂变质；③用盐腌制、浸渍和硝酸盐保存食品而导致风险上升[174]；④幽门螺杆菌感染及与膳食因素的相互作用[175,176,177]；⑤食物中发现的天然致癌物质或前体物质，如硝酸盐类[178]；⑥食品储存和制备过程中产生的致癌物质；⑦在胃的酸性环境中从膳食中的前体物质（如硝酸盐）合成的致癌物质[1,164,175,176]。

肝癌

原发性肝细胞癌在美国和北欧较少见。相比之下，它是撒哈拉以南非洲和亚洲的发展中国家最常见的癌症类型之一，目前是全球第六大常见癌症[1]。在许多高风险地区，乙型肝炎和丙型肝炎感染似乎是主要的致病因素，这些地区病原携带者的相对危险度高达 200 倍[179]。涉及致癌真菌产品（如某些黄曲霉毒素）的食品污染也可能在某些人群中导致风险上升[1]。黄曲霉毒素污染常见于没有采取适当食品加工和储存方式的地区。高黄曲霉毒素暴露人群通常存在乙型肝炎感染率和寄生虫感染率高，营养缺乏较为严重，患病风险可能取决于三个因素的相互作用。在低风险国家，肝癌发病机制中的相关饮食因素包括肥胖、超重、非酒精性脂肪性肝炎（nonalcoholic steatohepatitis，NASH）综合征和饮酒[1,59,72,180,181]。数据还表明，这些风险因素之间可能存在累加效应或协同作用[182]。据推测，肝癌主要发生在持续接触酒精、病毒性肝炎和毒素而导致肝硬化的人群中。越来越多的研究认为咖啡摄入与肝癌风险降低相关，并且有限的证据表明，食用鱼类和定期进行体育活动也可能降低患肝癌的风险[183~186]。

胰腺癌

胰腺癌经常在晚期才被发现，所以死亡率极高。吸烟已被确定为致病因素之一[24,187]，每天至少吸一包烟的人群患胰腺癌的风险约为不吸烟人群的四倍[1]。有限的证据表明，富含红肉和加工肉类、酒精、含果糖的食物和饱和脂肪的膳食可能会提高患胰腺癌的风险[188]。肥胖和过多能量摄入与胰腺癌风险呈正相关[1,188,189]，并获得动物模型研究的支持[190]。

子宫内膜癌

总体而言，子宫内膜癌显示出与其他富人癌症（例如乳腺癌、结肠癌和前列腺癌）类似的国际分布。子宫内膜癌与能量摄入过多、缺乏体育活动、肥胖和高血糖负荷之间关联的证据也日益增多[1,18,20,97,108,187]。咖啡被发现对子宫内膜癌有保护作用，一些研究表明，每日饮用一杯咖啡，患病风险降低 7%~8%[20,191]。还有一些研究表明，水果和蔬菜在降低子宫内膜癌风险方面有一定作用[1,192]。目前，最合适的建议是通过减少能量摄入，定期体育锻炼以及采取富含水果、蔬菜和谷物的膳食模式来避免肥胖。

卵巢癌

卵巢癌的发病率和死亡率存在相当大的国际和地理差异。这种疾病在西方文化的国家中更为常见，特别是在社会经济地位较高的群体[1,187]。虽然目前有越来越多的证据显示肥胖会增加患病风险，但膳食成分以及哺乳在卵巢癌发病机制中的作用仍有待进一步研究[21]，特别是其与低生育率和特定遗传性基因异常等已知风险因素之间的关系[1]。

膀胱癌

膀胱癌在工业化国家更为常见，特别是在吸烟人群、城市地区人群以及社会经济地位较低的人群中[1,59,143,193,194]。大多数流行病学和病例对照研究支持频繁食用水果和蔬菜会降低膀胱癌风险的假设[1,143,193,195]。富含十字花科蔬菜（如西蓝花）的膳食与吸烟人群和不吸烟人群的膀胱癌风险降低有关，但这不包括其他类别的水果和蔬菜[195]。液体摄入可能影响膀胱癌的风险[1,196]。对液体摄入的前瞻性评估发现，每日总液体摄入量与膀胱癌风险之间存在明显的负相关，但没有证据显示特定液体来源的益处或风险[196]。最近的一些研究据指出，富含红肉和加工肉类的膳食可能是膀胱癌的重要致癌原因[197~199]。实验室研究发现，高剂量的非营养性甜味剂（如甜蜜素和糖精）可能是啮齿类动物膀胱癌发生的弱诱发剂或促进剂，但它们对人类癌症的影响可能非常小[1]。

研究进展

与癌症预防相关的特定食物、营养素和膳食成分

许多癌症高危人群将注意力集中在特定的食物或营养素上，部分原因是大众媒体进行了广泛营销和宣传。当学术杂志报道的某一单项实验或预实验结果与以前的结果矛盾或不一致而使读者感到疑惑时，新闻媒体会促进这种趋势。以下部分简要总结了所选食物成分或营养素的相关数据，可能有助于医生回答来自不同患者的具体询问。

维生素

维生素 A

维生素 A 对上皮组织的正常生长和发育至关重要。维生素 A 缺乏在发展中国家的许多地方很常见，但在美国很少发生。维生素 A 来自牛奶和内脏肉类中的视黄醇及其酯类，以及黄色和绿叶蔬菜中的 β-胡萝卜素和一些其他维生素原 A 类胡萝卜素。研究认为，食用富含维生素 A 的食物对于多种类型的癌症具有保护作用[1,5,143]。然而，没有明确证据表明补充维生素 A 可以降低健康膳食的人群或个人患癌症的风险。尽管许多实验室模型研究表明缺乏维生素 A 增加了组织对化学致癌作用的易感性，但对于在摄入充足维生素 A 的人群中过量补充维生素 A 可以降低风险这一观点，并未得到证据支持。在化学预防试验中使用维生素 A 和合成类维生素 A 作为药理学试剂来确定其在特定高危人群中的疗效是转化研究的一个重要领域[200]。

维生素 D

维生素 D 是一种通过膳食获得的激素类营养素,它是通过阳光照射内源性产生的。众多证据表明,维生素 D 在结肠癌、前列腺癌、乳腺癌等多种癌症亚型中都起到重要作用,不过,目前尚不清楚维生素 D 与剂量反应的明确关系,以及维生素 D 在每日推荐摄入量之外的益处[1,119]。最近的研究表明,维生素 D 缺乏可能比过去认识到的情况更常见,并且可能带来癌症风险[201]。许多人类肿瘤的癌细胞表达 1,25-二羟基维生素 D3 的受体,并在体外对该药物有反应,但这在人类癌症中的病理生理学意义仍有待确定,特别是在剂量远超最低风险剂量的情况下[5,202]。

维生素 E

维生素 E 家族包含八个化合物,统称为生育酚。植物油、鸡蛋和全谷物是膳食中维生素 E 的主要来源。维生素 E 的抗氧化和可清除自由基剂的特性可能在抑制癌症发生中发挥作用[202,203]。然而,很少有啮齿动物、流行病学或干预措施研究为支持摄入维生素 E 补充剂提供有力的证据,特别是使用超出预防癌症要求剂量的情况[1,204]。

维生素 C

维生素 C 包括抗坏血酸和脱氢抗坏血酸,它不仅是水溶性抗氧化剂,也是中间代谢过程中几种酶促反应的组成部分之一。柑橘类水果、叶类蔬菜、番茄和马铃薯能提供丰富的维生素 C。尽管有大量的相关文献,但很少有证据显示膳食中的维生素 C 对大多数人类癌症的发生起关键作用,而且只有少数研究表明富含维生素 C 的膳食可能对癌症有保护作用[5]。补充剂方面的研究尽管数量很少,但未能证明可降低患癌症的风险[205]。一些证据认为,维生素 C 能通过抑制致癌物亚硝胺的生成,来降低与亚硝胺相关的癌症如胃癌的发生率[206]。目前,没有证据表明在富含新鲜水果和蔬菜的均衡膳食的基础上额外摄入维生素 C 补充剂对人类癌症有预防或治疗作用[1,5]。

叶酸

叶酸是氨基酸、甲基和核苷酸的正常代谢所必需的水溶性 B 族维生素。它存在于许多蔬菜、水果、豆类和全谷物中,在美国的强化谷物产品中也含有叶酸[207]。叶酸在 DNA 甲基化中发挥重要作用,这可能对基因表达和组织分化的正常调节至关重要。目前,流行病学和实验室研究已经开始有众多证据表明,叶酸不足可能与多种恶性肿瘤的风险有关,特别是结肠癌和乳腺癌[208]。经常饮酒且膳食中叶酸含量低的人患癌症的风险也可能更高[5,16,111,209]。然而,由于叶酸对 DNA 代谢和细胞增殖至关重要,高含量叶酸有促进癌变的可能,我们对此应该更加谨慎[84,210]。

矿物质

钙

钙被认为可以降低患结肠癌的风险,但会增加患前列腺癌的风险[1,5]。例如,一些前瞻性队列研究发现,结肠癌患者的钙和维生素 D 摄入量显著降低[1,5,211]。对结肠癌高风险患者而言,每天补充 1.2g 钙能降低结肠细胞增殖率[47,212]。目前有多项确定补钙对息肉形成影响的临床试验正在进行,初期报告发现有一定的好处。与此相反,多项前瞻性研究已经证明,来自膳食和补充剂的钙与前列腺癌风险上升有关[118,121,213],特别是具有更具浸润性的癌症。如今,适当的做法是从各种食物摄入 RDA 水平的钙。对于年龄在 19 岁至 50 岁之间的人,RDA 为 1 000mg/d,50 岁以上则为 1 200mg/d。

硒

硒是饮食中所需浓度非常低的矿物质,男性和女性的 RDA 均为 55μg/d。谷物、燕麦、海鲜和肉类都是硒的良好来源。硒是谷胱甘肽过氧化物酶的重要成分,利用谷胱甘肽的还原当量参与体内过氧化氢和有机氢过氧化物的清除。因此,硒对细胞和组织抵抗氧化损伤有帮助。由于食物中的硒含量对土壤浓度非常敏感,因此流行病学研究面临的一个主要难题就是膳食中硒摄入量的准确估算,特别是在食品深加工和长途运输的发达国家。来自不同地理区域的饲料作物中的硒含量或组织硒含量与某些癌症的死亡率之间存在负相关关系[1,5,113]。一项具有里程碑意义的人体干预试验报告称,硒补充剂可降低患肺癌、结肠癌和前列腺癌的风险[113]。然而,以上结果需要更大规模的随机对照试验来验证。由于硒的安全和潜在毒性剂量之间的范围很窄,当个体选择使用硒补充剂时,推荐个人每日摄入量为 55μg,且不超过 200μg[1,5]。

食品和食品成分

豆制品

生活在日本和中国等经常食用大豆食品的国家的人患乳腺癌、结肠癌和前列腺癌的风险,要低于美国等不常食用大豆食品的人群。然而,除了大豆之外,还有许多其他原因可能与这种地理差异有关。大豆食品含有多种成分,包括大豆蛋白、异黄酮、木脂素和皂苷等,这些成分的抗癌作用已在实验室模型中进行了研究[214,215]。尽管目前正在进行许多研究,但没有令人信服的证据证明使用大豆补充剂、大豆提取物、纯大豆浓缩物或目前市面上其他大豆成分将显著影响人类癌症风险。有人对大豆对于乳腺癌或子宫内膜癌的风险和益处提出了一些担忧。几种大豆异黄酮具有与雌激素类似的化学结构,并且可以与雌激素受体结合并发挥弱雌激素的功能。尽管这仍然存在争议,但我们可以认为大量植物雌激素确实可以促进细胞增殖。目前,乳腺癌高风险女性最好避免使用浓缩的异黄酮补充剂,但作为植物性膳食的一部分,适量的摄入大豆食品不会增加癌症风险[37,216~220]。

β-胡萝卜素

富含 β-胡萝卜素的食物与低癌症危险性相关,包括许多水果和蔬菜。然而,最近包含药物剂量 β-胡萝卜素的干预试验明确针对可以通过 β-胡萝卜素补充剂来产生植物性膳食的益处产生提出了质疑。两项大型 β-胡萝卜素干预研究表明,摄入超过饮食来源剂量的 β-胡萝卜素会提高吸烟人群患肺癌的风险[146,221]。虽然 β-胡萝卜素是一种潜在的抗氧化剂和维生素 A 的来源,但不应该提倡使用补充剂来预防癌症,而应该提倡富含类胡萝卜素的膳食。

番茄红素

番茄制品的鲜红色是由非维生素原类胡萝卜素的番茄红素产生的。对番茄红素的兴趣源自许多研究表明,摄入番茄制品可以降低多种癌症的风险,特别是前列腺癌[129,130,133]。最近的 WCRF/AICR 持续更新项目报告得出结论,番茄红素和前列腺癌之间的关系非常有限，无法得出结论[1,22]。因此，目前明智的做法是将番茄和番茄制品加入基于水果和蔬菜的富含类胡萝卜素的膳食模式中。

Omega-3 脂肪酸、鱼油和橄榄油

富含总脂肪的膳食能量密度高，可能导致能量过剩和肥胖。因此，大多数健康膳食模式的总脂肪摄入量略低于目前的美国膳食模式。然而，脂质的种类也可能对癌症产生影响。鱼肉富含的 Omega-3 脂肪酸可通过多种机制影响细胞，包括调节生物活性脂质（如前列腺素和白三烯）的生成。动物模型显示 Omega-3 脂肪酸对前列腺和乳腺癌等癌症有一定的抑制作用[222]。研究显示总脂质、饱和脂肪和其他脂质摄入量指标与癌症呈正相关性，而橄榄油与癌症缺乏关联，因此引起了人们对橄榄油的关注。与其他脂类一样，橄榄油也会造成能量过剩并诱发肥胖，但可在某些食谱中用于取代那些可能与癌症和心血管疾病有更大关联的其他脂质。总之，目前尚没有关于脂质来源或脂肪酸谱和人类癌症风险之间相关性的确切数据，因此无法给予具体建议[1,5]。

有机和天然食品

政府监管机构将继续评估相关信息，并在食品标签中使用“有机”一词向怀有期望的消费者提供最新标准和建议。一般而言，该术语是指在不使用合成杀虫剂或除草剂的情况下种植的食物，并且已经扩展到包括非转基因食物。目前，很少有研究表明，与标准农业生产的相同食品相比，食用有机食品将大大降低癌症风险[1,5]。一项通过在 9.3 年里随访 60 多万名女性来评估有机食品摄入量和癌症风险相关性的著名的前瞻性研究发现，除了非霍奇金淋巴瘤（non-Hodgkin lymphoma）外，有机食品的摄入与癌症总发病率或癌症亚型发病率无关[223]。

食品中的杀虫剂、除草剂和环境污染物

水果和蔬菜中存在低浓度的杀虫剂和除草剂的残留物。总体而言，研究尚未明确确定与接触低浓度现代药物相关的癌症风险，大部分数据支持多吃水果和蔬菜的建议。其他问题涉及肉类（包括鱼肉）中某些环境毒素的蓄积，但缺乏明确的癌症风险证据。当然，通过工业或农业暴露大剂量接触此类化合物则具有明显毒性并有可能增加癌症危险性。最重要的是，监管机构必须对这些化合物进行持续的监测，并确保食品供应中其含量符合预期的安全水平[1,5]。

人造甜味剂（阿斯巴甜和糖精）

人造甜味剂是目前市场上许多低能量食品的基础。目前，阿斯巴甜与癌症之间没有明确关系。当给予剂量远超人类摄入量时，糖精会略微提高膀胱癌的风险。人类流行病学研究尚未确定摄入糖精或阿斯巴甜是人类癌症的风险因素[1,5]。

糖

高度精制的单糖可以提供热量，但不提供任何天然食品中含有的营养素。含有大量单糖的膳食往往缺乏营养素，也可能导致肥胖和激素变化，从而可能提高癌症风险。然而，糖本身并不是致癌物质，在健康膳食模式的前提下，膳食中含有适量的甜食无须担忧[1,5]。

茶

目前正在对绿茶和红茶进行临床研究，以确定这些产品是否对人体具有抗癌特性，从而支持实验室研究得出的数据。到目前为止，尚未有研究证明茶可以降低任何人类癌症的风险，但重要的研究正在进行中[1,5]。

癌症生存：癌症治疗期间和之后的膳食和营养指南

虽然本章的重点是膳食和营养在癌症病因研究和预防中的作用，但我们还是简要介绍了癌症生存期间膳食和营养的新兴领域。现在认为，“癌症生存”是在癌症诊断时开始并且延续至癌症患者的整个生命过程。膳食和营养可能在癌症生存者的几个组成部分中发挥作用，包括：

（1）巩固治疗的收益并降低急性治疗相关毒性的发生频率或严重程度；

（2）一个治疗阶段结束后促进恢复；

（3）为患有癌症恶病质以及无法治愈或晚期癌症的终末期的患者提供支持；

（4）通过降低疾病复发、癌症二级预防和减少晚期并发症的发生频率和严重程度，提高整体存活率和健康程度，来促进患者长期存活。

按目前的速度，美国每年有超过 120 万人被诊断患有癌症，超过 1 000 万人为癌症生存者。癌症患者或癌症生存者获取膳食和营养的科学建议的愿望非常强烈，而当前的研究无法满足他们的要求。美国癌症协会（ACS）最近发表的一篇综述总结了营养和体育活动研究的状况，并提供了与癌症生存者沟通的指南（表 36-4）[37]。

表 36-4　癌症生存者的公共卫生指南

	美国癌症协会[37]	国家综合癌症网络[224]
体重	达到并保持健康的体重（BMI 在 $18.5 \sim 25kg/m^2$）。在癌症治疗后，应通过膳食、体育活动和行为策略结合起来控制体重增加或减重	保持健康的体重。在癌症治疗和幸存期间体重增加和超重可能增加复发风险并降低幸存概率
体育活动	定期参加体育活动。避免不活动，并在诊断后尽快恢复正常的日常活动。目标是每周锻炼至少 150 分钟，包括每周至少 2 天力量训练	每周至少 5 天进行至少 30 分钟的中等强度活动，或在至少 3 天进行 20 分钟以上的高强度活动。此外，每周至少进行 2 天力量训练

续表

	美国癌症协会[37]	国家综合癌症网络[224]
植物性膳食	采取富含蔬菜、水果和全谷物的膳食模式	以丰富食物种类为目标。保持均衡膳食,包括一半熟的或生的蔬菜,四分之一瘦肉蛋白(鸡肉、鱼肉、瘦肉或奶制品)和四分之一的全谷物
蔬菜和水果	很少有研究评估水果、蔬菜和癌症 复发或幸存的关联性。与2010年美国膳食指南一致,癌症生存者每天至少应摄入2~3杯[a]蔬菜和1.5~2杯[a]水果来保持健康	每天至少吃五份水果和蔬菜。使用植物调味料,如草药和香料
面包、谷物和谷类	选择全谷物产品,而非精制谷物产品。多吃高纤维食物	选择全谷物。选择高纤维面包和谷物。避免精制食物和高糖食物
动物产品	限制加工肉类和红肉的摄入量。避免在高温下烹饪这两种肉和其他高脂肪蛋白质	选择鱼肉、家禽和豆腐等瘦肉蛋白。限制红肉和加工肉类 每周至少吃两次富含脂肪的鱼肉。选择低脂乳制品。选择脱脂牛奶、低脂酸奶和低脂奶酪
膳食脂肪	限制摄入高脂肪和添加糖的食品和饮料,以促进健康的体重控制	每周至少吃两次富含脂肪的鱼,如鲑鱼、沙丁鱼和金枪鱼罐头。核桃,菜籽油和亚麻籽是对心脏健康有益的ω-3脂肪的额外来源
加工食品和精制糖盐和钠	限制摄入高脂肪和添加糖的食品和饮料,以促进健康的体重控制	避免精制食物和高糖食物
酒精	酒精饮料(分别为女性每天最多1杯[b],男性每天最多2杯[b])可以降低患心脏病的风险,但过量饮酒可能会提高特定癌症的风险。对于医疗保健提供者来说,为个体生存者量身定制饮酒建议非常重要	限制饮酒量。酒精与癌症风险有关。男性每天饮酒不应超过2杯[b],女性每天饮酒不超过1杯[b]
补充剂	在开具或服用补充剂之前,应尽一切努力通过膳食来源获得所需的营养素。只有在生物化学或临床证明营养素缺乏时才应考虑补充剂	健康的膳食模式是摄入足够维生素和矿物质的理想策略,而不是补充剂。没有证据表明膳食补充剂能独立提供与健康膳食模式相同的抗癌益处。一些高剂量补充剂实际上可能会提高癌症风险

[a] 1杯≈240ml。

[b] 1杯≈30ml。

对于许多癌症患者而言,膳食和营养给了他们一个对抗由于应对癌症治疗过程中出现的严重失控感的机会。当患者感觉自己能积极参与治疗过程中时,他们的生活质量将得到提高。然而,大多数情况下,没有足够的科学证据来帮助患者选择最佳膳食和营养信息。癌症生存者面对着令人眼花缭乱的膳食信息来源,包括出于善意的家人和朋友、医务工作者,以及营销产品或宣传膳食方法的付费出版物。再加上许多医务工作者(包括医师和护士)缺乏营养学相关培训和知识,癌症生存者因此经常感到困惑或容易被误导。尽管目前没有明确和详细的指导方针,但以下提供了与患者沟通和指导进行进一步癌症生存者研究的框架。

积极治疗阶段

由于针对更多临床情景建立了多模态干预,因而癌症治疗通常包括手术、放射、化学疗法或生物治疗,以及这几种方法联合应用进行综合干预。指导正在接受治疗的患者的关键在于提供个人化的营养支持。护理团队应通过评估体重、胖瘦体质以及是否存在进食或消化障碍来监测个人营养需求。某些癌症的治疗可能会通过癌症患者的进食、消化、吸收和营养代谢受损而危害患者的营养状况。例如,可能短期出现食欲不振、恶心、呕吐、味觉和嗅觉改变、便秘和腹泻。在此期间,通过个人化定制干预措施来为患者提供营养支持,可提高他们的生活质量。对一些无法维持正常能量摄入的患者而言，可以在膳食中使用商业化配制和测试的营养产品。为高营养并发症风险的患者在早期介绍注册营养师可以预防更严重的营养不良的情况出现，而这种营养不良可能会给医疗团队提供最佳治疗强度带来困难[37]。

在癌症治疗期间使用营养补充剂是有争议的，并且缺乏相关研究提供详细的指导。例如，一些临床医生认为在化疗或放疗期间给予高剂量抗氧化剂（维生素 C 或维生素 E，硒等）的补充剂可能会降低将癌细胞中氧化应激作为作用机制的治疗效果。然而，也有人认为抗氧化补充剂可通过限制对正常组织（例如骨髓）的损害给患者带来好处。一般而言，临床医生应告知正在接受化疗或放射治疗的患者将抗氧化剂量限制在不超过 RDA 的水平，并避免摄入其他富含抗氧化成分的草药或提取物的其他产品。例如，当叶酸剂量超过 RDA 水平时，会影响甲氨蝶呤（methotrexate）或 5-氟尿嘧啶（5-fluorouracil，5-FU）等涉及叶酸代谢途径的抗代谢药剂化疗的效果。对于这些患者，不提倡每天摄入超过 RDA 水平的叶酸补充剂[37]。

治疗后恢复

在癌症治疗的连续过程中，许多患者都会在完成强化治疗后的几天或几周内探索膳食和营养干预，来提高生存率。在此期间，患者与医疗护理提供者的联系频率降低，并开始担心治疗效果和治疗恢复的情况。应在治疗计划中加入膳食和体育活动以恢复患者肌肉组织和功能状态。医务工作者必须继续向患者提供有关补充剂和替代医学治疗的情况，并根据需要提供指导。连续的个人营养状况评估会确认那些因治疗引起的长期严重营养缺乏症的患者，例如在口咽癌、食道癌、胃癌、胰腺癌、肠癌等癌症治疗中常见吞咽困难、吸收障碍和肠道变化。注重能量平衡并确保充分摄入必需营养素至关重要。例如，胃手术或回肠末端切除可能导致维生素 B_{12} 缺乏，必须通过肠外方式给予补充[37]。注册营养师可以为每个人提供风险评估和个人化咨询。

晚期癌症

一般而言，癌症的恶化往往伴随食欲不振，并且即便不迅速出现并发症或共病状态，也会出现显持续的体重减轻和其他营养不良的症状。然而，许多家庭和看护人员认为缓解营养不足将显著延长患者的生命。实际上，问题的关键是未能控制癌症的发展而非营养不良。通常，患者和护理人员会因患者食欲不振和食物选择而产生冲突。医疗团队应该保持警惕，时刻留意并解决因食物引发的冲突，促进相互理解，并为家庭成员提供健康指导。在癌症晚期，膳食和营养干预可以提高患者的健康状况和生活质量。营养师和医疗团队可以帮助患者选择合适的食物和膳食模式，在癌症晚期帮助患者维持营养状况时，患者常常会伴有疼痛控制问题以及由麻醉镇痛药引起的便秘。可以将一些药物与有限的体育活动相结合，以增强患者的食欲并改善肠功能。在某些情况下还需要额外的营养支持[37]。

癌症复发和长期治疗并发症的预防

从癌症中完全康复的患者会担心原发性癌症的复发。此外，某些癌症的生存者是次生肿瘤的高发人群。实际上，口腔癌或肺癌生存者每年可能有约 10% 的高概率患上与吸烟有关的继发性肿瘤。许多癌症生存者也面临发生与治疗有关的其他部位癌症的风险。例如，通过基于依托泊苷（etoposide）的化学疗法治愈睾丸癌的患者患继发性白血病的风险更高；用纵隔放射治疗的青少年淋巴瘤的生存者患继发性乳腺癌的风险更高。很少有研究来确立最佳膳食模式以预防疾病复发或在相同或不同部位的继发性肿瘤。一般而言，大多数专家着重于本章前部分以及各种预防癌症的群体的膳食建议[1,5,37]。

随着癌症生存者人数的不断增加以及医疗人员在监测的时间加长，膳食干预的潜在目标的长期治疗并发症也越来越明确。例如，接受乳腺癌化疗治疗的女性过早绝经可能导致加速骨质疏松症[225]，这可能需要调整膳食中的钙含量和体育活动。年轻人和儿童的纵隔放射可能导致早发冠状动脉粥样硬化。医疗护理人员应强调在早期干预膳食和运动模式，以保持血液中健康的胆固醇和甘油三酯水平。虽然目前几乎没有关于膳食和营养的研究为癌症生存者提供明确的指导，但我们预计，随着患者需求的增加和美国国立卫生研究院（NIH）对癌症生存者问题的重视，未来这一领域的研究将得到迅速发展。

（葛阳 译　陈瑶　于乐兴 校）

部分参考文献

1 World Cancer Research Fund. *Food, Nutrition and the Prevention of Cancer: A Global Perspective.* Washington, DC: American Institute for Cancer Research; 2007.

2 Eckel RH, Jakicic JM, Ard JD, et al. AHA/ACC guideline on lifestyle management to reduce cardiovascular risk: a report of the American College of Cardiology/American Heart Association Task Force on Practice Guidelines. *J Am Coll Cardiol.* 2013;**63(25 Pt B)**:2960–2984.

3 American College of Cardiology/American Heart Association Task Force on Practice Guidelines. Based on a systematic review from the The Obesity Expert Panel. Executive summary: Guidelines (2013) for the management of overweight and obesity in adults: a report of the American College of Cardiology/American Heart Association Task Force on Practice Guidelines and the Obesity Society published by the Obesity Society and American College of Cardiology/American Heart Association Task Force on Practice Guidelines. Based on a systematic review from the The Obesity Expert Panel, 2013. *Obesity (Silver Spring).* 2013;**22(Suppl 2)**:S5–S39.

4 U.S. Department of Agriculture and U.S. Department of Health and Human Services. *Dietary Guidelines for Americans, 2010.* Washington, DC: US Government Printing Office; 2010.

5 Kushi LH, Doyle C, McCullough M, et al. American Cancer Society Guidelines on nutrition and physical activity for cancer prevention: reducing the risk of cancer with healthy food choices and physical activity. *CA Cancer J Clin.* 2012;**62(1)**:30–67.

7 Weed DL, Greenwald P, Kramer BS (eds). *In Cancer Prevention and Control.* New York: Marcel Dekker, Inc; 1995:385–402.

10 Willett W. *Nutritional Epidemiology*, 3rd. ed. New York: Oxford University Press; 2012.

12 Colditz GA, Willet WC. Epidemiologic approaches to the study of diet and cancer. In: Alfin-Slater RB, Kritchevsky D, eds. *Human Nutrition: A Comprehensive Treatise.* New York: Plenum; 1991:1–51.

15 National Academy of Sciences Committee on Diet and Health Food and Nutrition Board N.R.C. Commission on Life Sciences, ed. *Diet and Health: Implications for Reducing Risk of Chronic Disease.* Rockville, MD: Academy Press; 1989.

18 Calle EE, Rodriguez C, Walker-Thurmond K, Thun MJ. Overweight, obesity, and mortality from cancer in a prospectively studies cohort of U.S. adults. *N Engl J Med.* 2003;**348(17)**:1625–1638.

20 World Cancer Research Fund/American Institute for Cancer Research, *Continuous Update Project Report. Food, Nutrition, Physical Activity, and the Prevention of Endometrial Cancer.* 2013.

21 World Cancer Research Fund / American Institute for Cancer Research, *Continuous Update Project Report. Food, Nutrition, Physical Activity, and the Prevention*

of Ovarian Cancer. 2014.

22 World Cancer Research Fund / American Institute for Cancer Research, *Continuous Update Project Report. Food, Nutrition, Physical Activity, and the Prevention of Prostate Cancer.* 2014.

23 World Cancer Research Fund / American Institute for Cancer Research, *Continuous Update Project Report. Food, Nutrition, Physical Activity, and the Prevention of Breast Cancer.* 2010.

24 Eyre H, Kahn R, Robertson RM. Preventing cancer, cardiovascular disease, and diabetes. A common agenda for the American Cancer Society, the American Diabetes Association, and the American Heart Association. *Stroke.* 2004;**35**:1999–2010.

28 United States Department of Health and Human Services. *Physical Activity Guidelines for Americans.* Rockville, MD: United States Department of Health and Human Services; 2008.

34 Smith-Warner SA, Spiegelman D, Yaun SS, et al. Alcohol and breast cancer in women: a pooled analysis of cohort studies. *JAMA.* 1998;**279(7)**: 535–540.

37 Rock CL, Doyle C, Demark-Wahnefried W, et al. Nutrition and physical activity guidelines for cancer survivors. *CA Cancer J Clin.* 2012;**62(4)**:243–274.

43 Haenszel W. Cancer mortality among the foreign-born in the United States. *J Natl Cancer Inst.* 1961;**26**:37.

47 World Cancer Research Fund/American Institute for Cancer Research, *Continuous Update Project Report. Food, Nutrition, Physical Activity, and the Prevention of Colorectal Cancer.* 2011.

59 Armstrong B, Doll R. Environmental factors and cancer incidence and mortality in different countries, with special reference to dietary practices. *Int J Cancer.* 1975;**15(4)**:617–631.

62 Willett WC, Hunter DJ, Stampfer MJ, et al. Dietary fat and fiber in relation to risk of breast cancer. An 8-year follow-up. *JAMA.* 1992;**268(15)**:2037–2044.

69 Romaguera D, Vergnaud AC, Peeters PH, et al. Is concordance with World Cancer Research Fund/American Institute for Cancer Research guidelines for cancer prevention related to subsequent risk of cancer? Results from the EPIC study. *Am J Clin Nutr.* 2012;**96(1)**:150–163.

85 Colditz GA, Bohlke K. Priorities for the primary prevention of breast cancer. *CA Cancer J Clin.* 2014;**64(3)**:186–194.

90 Tannenbaum A. The dependence of tumor formation on the composition of the calorie-restricted diet as well as on the degree of restriction. *Cancer Res.* 1945;5:616.

100 Holmes MD, Hunter DJ, Colditz GA, et al. Association of dietary intake of fat and fatty acids with risk of breast cancer. *JAMA.* 1999;**281**:914–920.

103 Chlebowski RT, Blackburn GL, Elashoff C, et al. Dietary fat reduction in postmenopausal women with primary breast cancer: phase III Women's Intervention Nutrition Study (WINS). *J Clin Oncol.* 2005;**23(16S)**:3S (ASCO conference proceedings abstract).

131 Zu K, Mucci L, Rosner BA, et al. Dietary lycopene, angiogenesis, and prostate cancer: a prospective study in the prostate-specific antigen era. *J Natl Cancer Inst.* 2014;**106(2)**:djt430.

146 Omenn GS, Goodman GE, Thornquist MD, et al. Risk factors for lung cancer and for intervention effects in CARET, the Beta-Carotene and Retinol Efficacy Trial. *J Natl Cancer Inst.* 1996;**88(21)**:1550–1559.

168 Steffen A, Huerta JM, Weiderpass E, et al. General and abdominal obesity and risk of esophageal and gastric adenocarcinoma in the European Prospective Investigation into Cancer and Nutrition (EPIC). *Int J Cancer.* 2015;**137(3)**:646–657.

183 Arem H, Moore SC, Park Y, et al. Physical activity and cancer-specific mortality in the NIH-AARP Diet and Health Study cohort. *Int J Cancer.* 2014;**135(2)**:423–431.

188 World Cancer Research Fund/American Institute for Cancer Research, *Continuous Update Project Report. Food, Nutrition, Physical Activity, and the Prevention of Pancreatic Cancer.* 2012.

195 Michaud DS, Spiegelman D, Clinton SK, Rimm EB, Willett WC, Giovannucci EL. Fruit and vegetable intake and incidence of bladder cancer in a male prospective cohort. *J Natl Cancer Inst.* 1999;**91(7)**:605–613.

208 de Batlle J, Ferrari P, Chajes V, et al. Dietary folate intake and breast cancer risk: European prospective investigation into cancer and nutrition. *J Natl Cancer Inst.* 2015;**107(1)**:367.

210 Mason JB. Folate consumption and cancer risk: a confirmation and some reassurance, but we're not out of the woods quite yet. *Am J Clin Nutr.* 2011;**94(4)**:965–966.

219 Shu XO, Zheng Y, Cai H, et al. Soy food intake and breast cancer survival. *JAMA.* 2009;**302(22)**:
2437–2443.

220 Guha N, Kwan ML, Quesenberry CP Jr, Weltzien EK, Castillo AL, Caan BJ. Soy isoflavones and risk of cancer recurrence in a cohort of breast cancer survivors: the Life After Cancer Epidemiology study. *Breast Cancer Res Treat.* 2009;**118(2)**:395–405.

221 The Alpha-Tocopherol Beta-Carotene Cancer Prevention Study Group. The effect of vitamin E and beta carotene on the incidence of lung cancer and other cancers in male smokers. *N Engl J Med.* 1994;**330(15)**:1029–1035.

223 Bradbury KE, Balkwill A, Spencer EA, et al. Organic food consumption and the incidence of cancer in a large prospective study of women in the United Kingdom. *Br J Cancer.* 2014;**110(9)**:2321–2326.

224 National Comprehensive Cancer Network. Nutrition for Cancer Survivors. 2015. Available from: http://www.nccn.org/patients/resources/life_after_cancer/nutrition.aspx

第 37 章 癌症的化学预防

William N. William, Jr., MD ■ Waun Ki Hong, MD ■ Scott M. Lippman, MD

概论

癌症化学预防领域的基础是肿瘤形成的两种现象：区域性癌变和多步骤癌变。准确的癌症风险模型对于化学预防至关重要，并可加速化学预防中的药物开发。美国食品药品监督管理局（the Food and Drug Administration, FDA）已经批准了多种化学预防策略。本章简述了已完成的以西方人群中四种主要癌症（肺癌、结直肠癌、前列腺癌和乳腺癌）为主的化学预防临床试验，以及发病部位不确定的肿瘤化学预防研究，并探讨了癌症的疫苗预防。

化学预防的生物学原理

癌症化学预防领域主要基于肿瘤形成的两种现象：①区域性癌变，即上皮内瘤变（intraepithelial neoplasia, IEN，或称癌前病变）的多灶性发展或一种或多种 IEN 的克隆扩散；②多步骤癌变，由遗传不稳定性驱动并积累导致遗传和表观遗传变化[1~4]。这些过程会刺激癌变细胞逃逸细胞凋亡，进而具备强大的复制潜能和持续的血管生成能力，导致 IEN 和癌症进展。针对多步骤致癌的癌症化学预防是在浸润性癌变之前进行化学预防干预。由于一些重要共性，包括遗传和表观遗传异常、细胞失控和某些表型特性，故可将用于癌症治疗的药物用于癌症化学预防研究[5]。区域性癌变过程使得诸如系统性给药方法控制整个上皮区域中扩散接触致癌物的致癌结果变得具有吸引力。FDA 已经批准了几种 IEN 治疗方法。

癌症风险性模型

精确的癌症风险性模型对于化学预防至关重要。现已建立基于临床/人口统计学因素的乳腺癌风险模型（Gail 模型）和肺癌风险性模型（Spitz 模型），并确定了风险性增加的标志物，包括前期临床/组织病变[6,7]。这些风险模型和病变辨识在整个人群的基础上是有效的，但是对于鉴别个体风险帮助不大。近期有研究表明，整合了基因组学（体细胞基因表达阵列和宿主 DNA 修复能力）和代谢组学的临床肺癌风险模型比单独的临床模型能更准确地评估风险[8~10]。巴雷特食管（Barrett's esophagus）是已确立的但只能在一定程度上预测完全食管癌风险的模型，然而相比之下，整合了特定杂合子丢失（loss of heterozygosity, LOH）和 DNA 含量谱（DNA-content profile）的显著巴雷特食管模型却能区分高食管癌风险性（6 年内患病率达 79%）和低食管癌风险性（超过 6 年患病率为 0%）的人群[11]。在口腔黏膜白斑病中，染色体 3p 和/或 9p 特定位点的杂合性丢失使得患口腔癌的风险性大大提高（与不具备这种杂合性丢失的口腔黏膜白斑病相比）[12~14]，特别对于之前接受过口腔癌治疗的患者而言[15]，这个标记是迄今为止第一个也是唯一一个已经完成的个体化的、基于分子的随机口腔癌化学预防试验的选择标准，该试验称为厄洛替尼（erlotinib）预防口腔癌研究[16,17]。对于患有口腔黏膜不典型增生或具有喉部癌前损伤的患者而言，高癌症风险与 CYCLIN D1 基因型相关（第 4 外显子的 870 位点 A/G 单核苷酸多态性）[18]。最近的研究表明，CYCLIN D1 的高表达表型结合高风险 CYCLIN D1 基因型可提高喉部不典型增生患者的癌症风险[19]。因此，根据癌症风险模型选择高危人群进行化学预防可提高干预措施的治疗指数，有助于该领域的药物研发。

化学预防试验

本节列举了已完成的以西方世界人群中的四个主要患癌部位（肺、结直肠、前列腺和乳腺）为主的化学预防临床试验，以及部位不确定的化学预防研究。还讨论了疫苗对癌症预防的作用。

肺部

癌前病变

临床和转化化学预防试验，包括 5 项阴性结果的临床随机试验，这些试验证实在已发生组织化生的吸烟人群中，维生素 A 类药物在逆转肺部癌前病变方面无效或效果很小[20]。尽管总体上是阴性数据，但鼓舞人心的Ⅱb 期临床数据出现在了以下四项研究中，分别是：9-顺式-维 A 酸（9-cis-retinoic acid）对 RAR-β 和 Ki-6 的调控[21,22]，肌醇对 PI3 激酶基因表达途径的调控[23]，布地奈德（budesonide）对 CT 检测到的外周结节的调控[24]，以及茴香脑二硫醇硫酮（anethole dithiolthione）[25]和伊洛前列素（iloprost）[26]对支气管发育异常的调控。

原发性肺癌的预防

美国国家癌症研究所发起的 α-生育酚（alpha-tocopherol）和 β-胡萝卜素（beta-carotene）（alpha-tocopherol, beta-carotene, ATBC）癌症预防研究是 α-生育酚和 β-胡萝卜素预防原发性肺癌的Ⅲ期临床试验。ATBC 研究中包含 29 133 名 50~69 岁的男性吸烟者，这些吸烟者平均每天吸一包香烟并持续大约 36 年[27]。这项试验是 2×2 析因设计，以随机、双盲和安慰剂对照的方式给予受试者提供 α-生育酚（50mg/d）和 β-胡萝卜素（20mg/d）。析因设计允许该项研究的科学家能够分别评价每个药物的个体效应。经过中位随访时间为 6.1 年的随访后发现，β-胡萝卜素治疗的受试者出现了肺癌发生率（上升 18%，$P=0.01$）和总死亡率（上升 8%，$P=0.02$）都显著上升。α-生育酚对肺癌死亡率没有显著影响,也没有证据表明 α-生育酚和 β-胡萝卜素之间存在相互作用[28]。

β-胡萝卜素和维生素 A 功效试验(Beta-Carotene and Retinol Efficacy Trial,CARET)在 17 000 名吸烟者和石棉工人中测试了 β-胡萝卜素(30mg/d)与棕榈酸视黄酯(plus retinyl palmitate)(25 000IU/d)合用的效果[29]。其初步结果证实了 ATBC 研究的主要发现,即在高危人群中合用 β-胡萝卜素增加了肺癌发生风险。ATBC 研究和 CARET 测试中均无证据显示 β-胡萝卜素能增加非吸烟者、曾经吸烟者或轻度(<1 包/d)吸烟者的肺癌发病率。

SPT 预防

第二原发性肿瘤(second primary tumor,SPT)预防方面,已经完成了两项大规模的Ⅲ期视黄酸临床试验:一项在欧洲[研究棕榈酸视黄酯和/或 N-乙酰-半胱氨酸(N-acetyl-L-cysteine)][31],另一项在美国(研究低剂量 13cRA)[32]。两者均未显示出在整体人群中 SPT 发生率降低。1 151 位已切除Ⅰ期非小细胞的肺癌患者的随机对照试验也表明,与安慰剂相比,硒并不能预防 SPT[33]。

结直肠

结直肠临床试验设计主要采用的替代终点为腺瘤性息肉的发生、反应以及过度增生标志。

舒林酸(sulindac)和塞来昔布(celecoxib)可有效治疗(但不能预防)家族性腺瘤性息肉病(familial adenomatous polyposis,FAP)患者的腺瘤[34,35]。大剂量塞来昔布(800mg/d)可使大肠息肉发生率降低 28%,更难得的是,还可让很难切除的十二指肠息肉发生率降低 14%(与安慰剂相比)[36]。这些研究促使 FDA 临时批准将塞来昔布用作 FAP 患者内镜和外科治疗的辅助手段。然而,由于在这种高风险环境中(大剂量塞来昔布具有心肌毒性)进行确证试验存在很大困难,FDA 随后又将塞来昔布从 FAP 患者息肉治疗的可用药名录中删除。钙剂(1 200mg/d)在总体上能使散发性腺瘤的风险降低 15%[37],对晚期疾病作用甚至更大(与安慰剂组对照)。CAPP-1 和 CAPP-2 试验研究了阿司匹林(aspirin,600mg,每日 1 次)分别对患有 FAP 遗传性结直肠癌(colorectal cancer,CRC)综合征和林奇综合征(Lynch syndrome)患者的影响。CAPP-1 发现在进行中位数为 17 个月的治疗后,阿司匹林治疗组中息肉数量有所降低(23%),并且最大息肉体积变小。CAPP-2 发现在平均 55.7 个月的随访后,完成至少 2 年治疗的受试者中,CRC 风险显著降低(59%)[38,39]。

4 项随机对照试验测试了阿司匹林预防散发性腺瘤的疗效,结果表明接受阿司匹林治疗 1 年或以上的患者复发性腺瘤显著减少[40~43]。在医师健康研究和妇女健康研究(Women's Health Study,WHS)中,阿司匹林对男性和女性的结直肠癌发生风险没有保护作用。然而,经过 18 年的整体随访后,WHS 最近的结果表明阿司匹林可以显著降低健康女性患 CRC 的风险[44]。最近对英国医师阿司匹林试验和英国短暂缺血性卒中阿司匹林试验的汇总分析发现,阿司匹林能使结直肠癌的发生风险明显降低 26%。该效应在治疗至少 5 年后最为明显并且至少 10 年内都不会消失[45]。后者研究结果与近期一项大规模队列研究结果一致,该队列研究包括 47 000 名来自卫生职业随访研究的受试者,结果表明结直肠癌风险的降低有明显的剂量和时间依赖性[46]。

三项随机对照临床试验评估了选择性环氧合酶抑制剂(coxibs)(与安慰剂对照)在具有结直肠息肉史的患者中预防散发性腺瘤的效果。万络(Vioxx)预防腺瘤性息肉试验(the Adenomatous Polyp Prevention on Vioxx,APPROVe)测试了罗非昔布(rofecoxib),并且在 APC 和预防结肠直肠腺瘤性息肉(Prevention of Colorectal Sporadic Adenomatous Polyps,PreSAP)试验中测试了不同剂量的塞来昔布。临时心血管事件的发生率在 APPROVe 和 APC 试验中较预期高,而在 PreSAP 试验中并未出现[47~49]。尽管罗非昔布对结直肠腺瘤有显著抑制作用,但因为这些安全性事件,相关数据和安全性监视委员会很早就终止了所有三项随机对照临床试验,且该药的制造商已将其从世界市场撤市。在 APPROVe 试验(2 587 名随机受试者)中,罗非昔布使腺瘤减少了 24%[50]。在 APC 试验(2 035 名随机患者)中,不同药物组的腺瘤发生率差异明显,分别为 37.5%(400mg 塞来昔布,每日两次),43%(200mg 塞来昔布,每日两次)和 60%(安慰剂)($P<0.001$)[51];严重的心血管不良事件发生率以剂量依赖的方式显著升高。在 1 561 名随机患者中进行的的 PreSAP 试验发现,腺瘤的发生率为 33.6%(400mg 塞来昔布,每日 1 次)和 49.3%(安慰剂)($P<0.001$)[47]。PreSAP 试验中心血管事件的风险并未上升。在最近对 APC 患者进行的延伸性分析表明:严重的心血管事件发生率在停药 2 年后消退,而抑制腺瘤的效果仍持续存在(尽管效果降低),尤其是对晚期腺瘤。最近一项塞来昔布安慰剂对照试验的汇总分析(双盲且计划对非关节炎疾病患者至少进行 3 年随访)结果表明,在心血管疾病风险性较低的人群(占试验总人数的 15%~20%)中,任何剂量(最高 400mg,一天 2 次)都不会增加严重心血管事件的发生率。这些结果有力地表明,低基线心血管疾病风险能够改善风险-收益,并有助于选择患者进行未来的 COX-2 特异性 NSAID(nonsteroidal anti-inflammatory drug,非甾体抗炎药)的试验[52]。

以降低结直肠腺瘤的风险性为目的的维生素和饮食(低脂肪,富含水果蔬菜和纤维)的临床试验结果大多数为阴性[53,54]。钙剂能够降低 19%(有一定统计学意义)的腺瘤风险[37],并能在长期随访中维持该水平[55]。叶酸的两项随机对照试验表明,0.5 或 1mg/d 的剂量不能降低腺瘤风险;一项研究的亚组分析表明,叶酸(1mg/d)甚至可能增加晚期或多发性腺瘤的风险[43,56]。

针对低剂量二氟甲基鸟氨酸(DFMO)和舒林酸的临床前研究支持了一项随机对照临床试验的结果,该临床试验让 375 位有腺瘤切除(不小于 3mm)病史的患者同时服用 DFMO(500mg)和舒林酸(150mg;与安慰剂对照),持续 36 个月[根据入组时是否服用低剂量阿司匹林(81mg)以及不同的临床中心来分层][57]。结直肠腺瘤复发率如下:一个或多个腺瘤复发率为 41.1%(安慰剂)对比 12.3%[联用;相对风险(RR)= 0.30;95%置信区间(CI)0.18~0.49;$P<0.001$];一个或多个晚期腺瘤复发率为 8.5%(安慰剂)对比 0.7%(联用;RR=0.085;95% CI 0.011~0.65;$P<0.001$);多发性腺瘤为 13.2%(安慰剂)对比 0.7%(联用;RR=0.055;95%CI 0.007 4~0.41;$P<0.001$)。长期以来,组合化学预防策略一直被认为具有增强单药活性和

降低毒性的巨大潜力，这一联合用药试验里程碑性的进展进一步巩固了这种观点。

乳腺

由于乳腺癌预防试验（breast cancer prevention trial，BCPT）的结果得到了非常重要的阳性结果，因此选择性雌激素受体调节剂（the selective estrogen-receptormodulator，SERM）他莫昔芬（tamoxifen）成为第一个获得 FDA 批准的化学预防剂。由国家外科辅助乳腺及肠道项目（the National Surgical Adjuvant Breast and Bowel Project，NSABP）进行的 BCPT 在 13 388 例乳腺癌高危女性患者中比较了他莫昔芬与安慰剂对乳腺癌的效果[58]。主要的高风险入组标准是年龄大于 60 岁且有小叶原位癌（lobular carcinoma in situ，LCIS）病史，或者是根据 Gail 模型 5 年内患乳腺癌风险为 1.66%的 35~59 岁妇女。实际上按总体均值，5 年内患乳腺癌的风险为 3.2%。在中位 55 个月的随访中，在他莫昔芬组和安慰剂组发现的原发侵袭性乳腺癌分别为 89 例和 175 例，他莫昔芬组相对安慰剂组降低了 49%（$P<0.000\,01$）。他莫昔芬仅在雌激素受体（estrogen-receptor，ER）阳性亚组中观察到的乳腺癌相对风险性的降低，而在其他年龄组和风险性组中没有明显差别。他莫昔芬非显著性地降低了总体乳腺癌的死亡率。有益的次级结果发现，他莫昔芬组骨折发生率下降了 19%。与他莫昔芬相关的次级不良反应包括子宫内膜癌、血管疾病和白内障概率的增加。

虽然 BCPT 成功地验证了其最初的假设，但也提出了几项关键的未解决问题，例如他莫昔芬对致死率的影响，最适的持续时间，结果的普遍化以及预防与治疗相比较的问题。FDA 随后批准将他莫昔芬用于降低高风险女性患乳腺癌的风险。对于高危女性，FDA 建议服用他莫昔芬 20mg/d，持续 5 年，并对莫昔芬相关风险进行警示。FDA 基于一致的次级辅助性数据，也批准了他莫昔芬用于降低对侧乳腺癌的发病率[59]。

NSABP B-24 研究在 1 804 例患原位导管癌（ductal carcinoma in situ，DCIS）的患者接受切除和放射治疗后的 5 年中测试了他莫昔芬（20mg/d）与安慰剂相对照的作用[60]。中位随访 74 个月后，在他莫昔芬组和安慰剂组中，所有乳腺癌（浸润性和非浸润性）在 5 年内的发生率分别为 8.2%和 13.4%，相对风险降低 43%（$P=0.000\,9$）。他莫昔芬组在所有浸润性乳腺癌 5 年的累积发病率为 4.1%，而安慰剂组为 7.2%（$P=0.004$）。FDA 批准将他莫昔芬用于降低局部治疗（切除和放射）乳腺 DCIS 的风险。

国际乳腺癌干预研究（the International Breast Cancer Intervention Study，IBIS-I）将 7 410 名妇女随机分组，发现他莫昔芬使乳腺癌风险降低了 32%[60]。该试验和 BCPT（该领域两项较强的随机对照试验）的阳性结果仅限于 ER 阳性的癌症。IBIS-I 长期随访报告显示，他莫昔芬降低乳腺癌风险的效应可以至少持续 10 年，且大多数副作用在 5 年治疗期后消失，包括所有严重不良反应（例如血栓和子宫内膜癌）[61]。这些长期发现对将他莫昔芬用于预防乳腺癌的风险/收益具有重要意义。

他莫昔芬和雷洛昔芬（raloxifene）的研究（the Study of Tamoxifen and Raloxifene，STAR）测试了 SERM 雷洛昔芬对比 SERM 他莫昔芬在乳腺癌预防方面是否具有更高的疗效和更低的毒性[62]。为期 5 年，共有 19 747 名患乳腺癌风险较高的绝经后妇女被随机分配到他莫昔芬组（20mg/d）或雷洛昔芬组（60mg/d）。在长期随访中，雷洛昔芬组的浸润性乳腺癌发病率略高（RR = 1.24；95%CI 1.05~1.47），但子宫癌的发病率低于他莫昔芬（RR = 0.55；95%CI 0.36~0.83）此外，雷洛昔芬组的血栓栓塞和白内障发病率在数据上显著低于他莫昔芬组。他莫昔芬和雷洛昔芬在减少非浸润性乳腺癌方面作用类似[63]。雷洛昔芬被 FDA 批准用于降低高风险或患有骨质疏松症的绝经后妇女的浸润性乳腺癌风险。

这些开创性试验之后进行的是针对第三代 SERM 的化学预防效果的研究。拉索昔芬（lasofoxifene）的绝经后评估和风险降低试验研究了拉索昔芬对骨密度（bone mineral density，BMD）较低的绝经后女性的影响[64,65]。研究显示，浸润性乳腺癌减少 79%，ER 为阳性的乳腺癌减少 83%。在一项名为 Generations Trial 的类似的Ⅲ期预防试验中，接受阿佐昔芬（arzoxifene）治疗的低 BMD 绝经后妇女的浸润性乳腺癌减少了 56%[66,67]。这些试验发现，拉索昔芬和阿咗昔芬均可降低非椎骨和椎骨骨折的风险；然而，诸如雷洛昔芬和他莫昔芬的第三代 SERM 仍会提高静脉血栓栓塞的风险。

最近一项纳入所有 9 项大规模的Ⅲ期 SERM 预防试验[68]的荟萃分析发现，所有 SERM 降低了整体和 ER 阳性的乳腺癌的发病率。并且除雷洛昔芬外，所有 SERM 均能降低 DCIS 发病率。

主要基于阿那曲唑、单独的他莫昔芬或联合（the Anastrozole，Tamoxifen Alone or in Combination，ATAC）试验[69]的结果，芳香化酶抑制剂在绝经后妇女中对乳腺癌的预防作用吸引了很多关注。乳腺预防 3（Mammary Prevention 3）号试验将 4 560 名绝经后高危妇女随机分组，服用 25mg 依西美坦（exemestane）或安慰剂，持续 5 年。浸润性乳腺癌的年发病率降低了 65%，体现了依西美坦的作用[风险比（hazard ratio，HR）= 0.35；95%CI 0.18~0.70]。各组在骨折、心血管发病率或其他癌症方面没有差异[70]。IBIS-Ⅱ试验在 3 864 名高危绝经后妇女中评估每日服用 1mg 阿那曲唑或安慰剂对照，持续 5 年，也证实芳香酶抑制剂能降低浸润性乳腺癌的发病率（HR = 0.47；95%CI 0.32~0.68）。阿那曲唑还可降低皮肤癌、妇科癌、胃肠道癌和其他癌症的发病率。阿那曲唑组疼痛、关节僵硬、血管舒缩症、眼睛干涩和高血压的发生率更高，但两组间骨折的发生率在数据上不存在显著差异[71]。用于预防雌激素受体阴性乳腺癌的药物正在开发中，但迄今为止，尚未发现有效药物。

前列腺

前列腺癌的发生过程受雄激素驱动，一项持续 7 年的前列腺癌预防试验（the Prostate Cancer Prevention Trial，PCPT）的大型随机对照试验在 18 882 名 55 岁及以上且直肠指检（digital rectal exam，DRE）和前列腺特异性抗原（prostate-specific antigen，PSA）水平均为正常的男性中测试了非那雄胺（finasteride，5mg/d）的作用，与安慰剂对照。非那雄胺能抑制 5-α-还原酶（5-α-reductase）将睾酮转化为二氢睾酮（dihydrotestosterone）这种功能更强大的雄激素。它虽然在 7 年内使前列腺癌患病率降低了 24.8%[72]，却增加了高级别疾病的发生率——非那雄胺组为 6.4%，而安慰剂组为 5.1%。非那雄胺还降低了高级别前列腺 IEN 风险[73]。PCPT 分析也显示良性前列腺肥大症状减少和性功能副作用增加，尽管最近的详细分析发现非那雄胺对性功能的影响很小[74]。PCPT 次要发现显示，PSA 水平正常的男性患前列腺癌的风险较高，包括高级别疾病[75]，且服用和未服用非那雄胺的男性 PSA 筛查结果存在差异[76,77]。高级别疾病发生率上升的负面结果极大地降低了公众对用非那雄胺预防前列腺癌的关注。另一个主要问题是在前列腺癌预防试验中密集的 PSA/DRE 筛查及早期前列腺癌检测，可能意味着非那雄胺的预防作用可能更多是针对临床表现为惰性的前列腺癌，而非恶性程度较高的前列腺癌。

然而，一些分析对此类问题提出了质疑[77~83]。最近一份长期（18 年）随访报告试图解释发现高级别病变的重要性（例如，非那雄胺驱动的假象与新的非那雄胺引起的高级别癌症对比），该研究发现总体生存率或确诊前列腺癌后患者的生存率在不同组之间没有显著差异[84]。

度他雄胺（dutasteride）降低前列腺癌发生率的研究在 8 231 名 50~75 岁、PSA 水平介于 2.5 和 10ng/mL 之间且 6 个月内前列腺活检阴性的男性中比较了服用度他雄胺 0.5mg/d 与安慰剂对照的情况。参与者在治疗的第 2 年和第 4 年接受超声引导的活检。度他雄胺组的前列腺癌相对风险降低了 22.8%（95%CI 15.2~29.8；$P<0.001$）。在第 1 年到第 4 年之间，度他雄胺组和安慰剂组分别出现 29 和 19 例 Gleason 分数为 8~10 的癌症（$P=0.15$）；然而，在第 3 到第 4 年之间，度他雄胺组有 12 例 Gleason 分数为 8~10 的肿瘤。而安慰剂组仅有 1 个（$P=0.003$）。度他雄胺组中急性尿潴留更少见，但是心力衰竭以及勃起功能障碍和性欲减退的复合式终点更常见[85]。

另一项硒和维生素 E 癌症预防试验（the Selenium and Vitamin E Cancer Prevention Trial，SELECT）的大规模随机对照试验已于近期终止。报告结果显示，在由 35 533 名相对健康男性组成的异质群体中，单独或联合使用试验中剂量和剂型的硒和维生素 E，对前列腺癌没有预防作用。维生素 E 组中前列腺癌风险上升的趋势（$P=0.06$；RR＝1.13；99%CI 0.195~1.35）[86]在进一步随访中出现了统计学差异[87]。最近的一项 SELECT 后续分析研究了硒或维生素 E 是否对硒含量低于平均水平的男性有益。结果恰恰相反，没有证据表明干预对硒含量低于平均水平的男性有益；而且，对于趾甲中硒含量低于平均水平的男性，补充维生素 E 会使前列腺癌的风险提高 63%，这种效果对于高级别前列腺癌更为明显[88]。

疫苗

在中国台湾，通过为儿童接种乙肝疫苗，大大降低了肝癌的发病率和死亡率，这为使用疫苗预防感染相关性癌症提供了概念验证[89]。

人乳头瘤病毒（HPV）感染已确认为宫颈癌的主要风险因素，通过免疫接种预防病变相关感染的分子靶向治疗，是一种非常有效的途径，能够预防宿主细胞的早期损伤，以防止其进一步发生肿瘤。癌症化学预防的一个里程碑式进展是最近 HPV 疫苗预防女孩和年轻女性 HPV 感染的随机对照试验，以及随后 FDA 对 HPV 疫苗接种的上市批准。

一项名为女性联合单方面降低子宫颈内/子宫颈阴道部疾病（Females United to Unilaterally Reduce Endo/Ectocervical Disease，FUTURE）发生率Ⅰ号的安慰剂对照（Ⅲ期）试验评估了涵盖 HPV6、11、16 和 18 型的四价疫苗在 16~24 岁女性中对肛门生殖器疾病的预防作用。主要复合终点为在没有 HPV 感染的病毒性证据且根据协议属于易感群体的妇女中出现生殖器疣、外阴或阴道 IEN 或癌症，以及宫颈 IEN，原位腺癌或与 HPV6、11、16 或 18 型相关的癌症。该疫苗能够 100%有效地预防每一个共同主要终点事件的发生[90]。同样地，FUTURE Ⅱ 研究发现，四价疫苗在年龄分布为 15 到 26 岁之间且没有 HPV 感染的病毒性证据的女性中使主要复合终点［宫颈 IEN（2 级和 3 级）、原位腺癌或与 HPV16 或 18 型相关的癌症］风险降低了 98%[91]。

另一项Ⅲ期试验在 18 644 名年龄在 15 至 25 岁之间女性中测试了二价（HPV16 和 18 型）疫苗的作用。在没有 HPV 感染证据的女性中，与 HPV16 或 18 型相关的 2 级宫颈 IEN 作为主要终点下降了 90%[92]。在 18~25 岁的年轻女性中进行的群体随机对照试验中，二价疫苗已被证明针对 HPV16 或 18 型持续感染具有高效保护作用，并且对 HPV31、33 和 45 型有部分交叉保护作用[93]。

在男性中，四价 HPV 疫苗也被证明可以减少 HPV 感染和相关外生殖器病变[94]以及肛门 IEN[95]。女性接种 HPV 疫苗（二价疫苗）也能减少口腔 HPV 感染。但目前尚不清楚这最终是否能预防与 HPV 相关的头颈部鳞状细胞癌[96]。目前尚未发现 HPV 疫苗具有加速 HPV 清除的作用，因此不太可能对已感染患者起到预防癌症的作用[97]。

全部肿瘤

在美国进行的两项大型试验，研究了 β-胡萝卜素降低总体癌症发病率的作用。医师健康研究（the Physicians' Health Study，PHS）进行了为期 12 年的 β-胡萝卜素对总体癌症发病率影响的测试[98]。β-胡萝卜素在总体癌症（包括肺癌）发病率方面没有显著性差异。这一群体中只有 11%是现时吸烟者。女性健康研究对 β-胡萝卜素也得出了相似的结果[99]。PHS Ⅱ 的结果已于最近揭晓。这项大规模（N＝14 641 名男性）随机安慰剂对照研究表明，与安慰剂相比，每日低剂量服用多复合维生素使总体癌症发病率降低［分别为每 1 000 人・年中 17.0 和 18.3 例；风险比（HR）＝0.92；95%CI 0.86~0.998；$P=0.04$］，主要体现在具有既往癌症史的个体中。具体部位癌症的发生率没有降低[100]。这种并不显著的抗肿瘤作用的临床意义尚未确定。

结论

临床癌症化学预防业已成熟，FDA 批准了几种预防癌症或预防/治疗上皮内瘤样病变的药物。最近的例子是雷洛昔芬用于在高风险女性中预防浸润性乳腺癌，HPV 疫苗用于预防肛门生殖器癌。FDA 目前已批准的癌症预防药物包括双氯芬酸（diclofenac）、卟吩姆钠（photofrin）［与光动力疗法（photodynamic therapy，PDT）联合］、他莫昔芬、乙型肝炎疫苗（hepatitis B vaccine）、卡介苗（bacillus Calmette-Guerin）、戊柔比星（valrubicin）、马索罗酚（masoprocol）、5-氟尿嘧啶（5-FU）、氨基乙酰丙酸（aminolevulinic acid）（与 PDT 联合）和 HPV 疫苗。在阿司匹林和塞来昔布防治结直肠肿瘤的研究中，通过特定干预措施使患者获益最大化、伤害最小化的个体化治疗方法正不断进步。当前，组合制剂是癌症化学预防最有希望的方向之一。前文讨论过的 DFMO-舒林酸用于结直肠腺瘤的试验结果，有力支持了制剂组合可增加有效单一药物的获益（活性）/风险（毒性）比这一概念。基于该试验，化学预防性制剂组合可成为标准的临床治疗措施，同时应将其他活性组合制剂纳入临床试验[101]。

总结

癌症化学预防水平的不断提高推动着癌症治疗进程。临床化学预防领域已经取得诸多成效，十分鼓舞人心，例如，20 世纪 90 年代后期，FDA 批准将他莫昔芬用于降低浸润前和浸润性乳腺癌的风险，之后又批准将雷洛昔芬和 HPV 疫苗分别用于降低浸润性乳腺癌和宫颈癌风险。新近发现，芳香化酶抑制剂在绝经后妇女中有预防乳腺癌的作用，且副作用更低。一项结合了舒林酸和二氟甲基鸟氨酸（DFMO）的随机对照试验（RCT）显示，结直肠腺瘤发生率显著降低了 70%（晚期腺瘤中超过 90%），突显了组合制剂对化学预防的重要性，同时也预示着该方法可成为临床治疗的标准。

（程宁涛 译　葛阳　陈瑶 校）

参考文献

The complete reference list can be found on the Wiley Companion Digital Edition of this title (see inside front cover for login instructions).

6 Gail MH, Brinton LA, Byar DP, et al. Projecting individualized probabilities of developing breast cancer for white females who are being examined annually. *J Natl Cancer Inst*. 1989;**81**:1879–1886.

27 The Alpha-Tocopherol, Beta Carotene Cancer Prevention Study Group. The effect of vitamin E and beta carotene on the incidence of lung cancer and other cancers in male smokers. *N Engl J Med*. 1994;**330**:1029–1035.

29 Omenn GS, Goodman GE, Thornquist MD, et al. Effects of a combination of beta carotene and vitamin A on lung cancer and cardiovascular disease. *N Engl J Med*. 1996;**334**:1150–1155.

35 Steinbach G, Lynch PM, Phillips RK, et al. The effect of celecoxib, a cyclooxygenase-2 inhibitor, in familial adenomatous polyposis. *N Engl J Med*. 2000;**342**:1946–1952.

41 Baron JA, Cole BF, Sandler RS, et al. A randomized trial of aspirin to prevent colorectal adenomas. *N Engl J Med*. 2003;**348**:891–899.

45 Flossmann E, Rothwell PM, British Doctors Aspirin Trial, et al. Effect of aspirin on long-term risk of colorectal cancer: consistent evidence from randomised and observational studies. *Lancet*. 2007;**369**:1603–1613.

47 Arber N, Eagle CJ, Spicak J, et al. Celecoxib for the prevention of colorectal adenomatous polyps. *N Engl J Med*. 2006;**355**:885–895.

48 Bresalier RS, Sandler RS, Quan H, et al. Cardiovascular events associated with rofecoxib in a colorectal adenoma chemoprevention trial. *N Engl J Med*. 2005;**352**:1092–1102.

49 Solomon SD, McMurray JJ, Pfeffer MA, et al. Cardiovascular risk associated with celecoxib in a clinical trial for colorectal adenoma prevention. *N Engl J Med*. 2005;**352**:1071–1080.

50 Baron JA, Sandler RS, Bresalier RS, et al. A randomized trial of rofecoxib for the chemoprevention of colorectal adenomas. *Gastroenterology*. 2006;**131**:1674–1682.

51 Bertagnolli MM, Eagle CJ, Zauber AG, et al. Celecoxib for the prevention of sporadic colorectal adenomas. *N Engl J Med*. 2006;**355**:873–884.

57 Meyskens FL Jr, McLaren CE, Pelot D, et al. Difluoromethylornithine plus sulindac for the prevention of sporadic colorectal adenomas: a randomized placebo-controlled, double-blind trial. *Cancer Prev Res (Phila)*. 2008;**1**:32–38.

58 Fisher B, Costantino JP, Wickerham DL, et al. Tamoxifen for prevention of breast cancer: report of the National Surgical Adjuvant Breast and Bowel Project P-1 Study. *J Natl Cancer Inst*. 1998;**90**:1371–1388.

60 Cuzick J, Forbes J, Edwards R, et al. First results from the International Breast Cancer Intervention Study (IBIS-I): a randomised prevention trial. *Lancet*. 2002;**360**:817–824.

62 Vogel VG, Costantino JP, Wickerham DL, et al. Effects of tamoxifen vs raloxifene on the risk of developing invasive breast cancer and other disease outcomes: the NSABP Study of Tamoxifen and Raloxifene (STAR) P-2 trial. *JAMA*. 2006;**295**:2727–2741.

70 Goss PE, Ingle JN, Ales-Martinez JE, et al. Exemestane for breast-cancer prevention in postmenopausal women. *N Engl J Med*. 2011;**364**:2381–2391.

71 Cuzick J, Sestak I, Forbes JF, et al. Anastrozole for prevention of breast cancer in high-risk postmenopausal women (IBIS-II): an international, double-blind, randomised placebo-controlled trial. *Lancet*. 2014;**383**:1041–1048.

72 Thompson IM, Goodman PJ, Tangen CM, et al. The influence of finasteride on the development of prostate cancer. *N Engl J Med*. 2003;**349**:215–224.

84 Thompson IM Jr, Goodman PJ, Tangen CM, et al. Long-term survival of participants in the prostate cancer prevention trial. *N Engl J Med*. 2013;**369**:603–610.

85 Andriole GL, Bostwick DG, Brawley OW, et al. Effect of dutasteride on the risk of prostate cancer. *N Engl J Med*. 2010;**362**:1192–1202.

89 Chiang CJ, Yang YW, You SL, et al. Thirty-year outcomes of the national hepatitis B immunization program in Taiwan. *JAMA*. 2013;**310**:974–976.

90 Garland SM, Hernandez-Avila M, Wheeler CM, et al. Quadrivalent vaccine against human papillomavirus to prevent anogenital diseases. *N Engl J Med*. 2007;**356**:1928–1943.

91 Group FIS. Quadrivalent vaccine against human papillomavirus to prevent high-grade cervical lesions. *N Engl J Med*. 2007;**356**:1915–1927.

92 Paavonen J, Jenkins D, Bosch FX, et al. Efficacy of a prophylactic adjuvanted bivalent L1 virus-like-particle vaccine against infection with human papillomavirus types 16 and 18 in young women: an interim analysis of a phase III double-blind, randomised controlled trial. *Lancet*. 2007;**369**:2161–2170.

94 Giuliano AR, Palefsky JM, Goldstone S, et al. Efficacy of quadrivalent HPV vaccine against HPV Infection and disease in males. *N Engl J Med*. 2011;**364**:401–411.

95 Palefsky JM, Giuliano AR, Goldstone S, et al. HPV vaccine against anal HPV infection and anal intraepithelial neoplasia. *N Engl J Med*. 2011;**365**:1576–1585.

100 Gaziano JM, Sesso HD, Christen WG, et al. Multivitamins in the prevention of cancer in men: the Physicians' Health Study II randomized controlled trial. *JAMA*. 2012;**308**:1871–1880.

第 38 章　癌症的筛查及早期诊断

Otis W. Brawley, MD, MACP

概述

癌症筛查是早期发现癌症的一种有效的干预手段。筛查的首要目的是降低疾病的死亡率，其次是在降低发病率的前提下成功治愈疾病。为了保证筛查的有效性，需在疾病处于局部，并可通过干预成功阻止其进展的阶段进行。然而，某些癌症的病程并无以上所述阶段，因此筛查是无效的。我们可以通过前瞻性的随机化研究来评估某种癌症是否具有可筛查性：将入组的具有癌症风险的人群随机纳入筛选干预组或对照组，定期进行或不进行干预；试验中两组确诊为癌症的患者都应给予适当的治疗；通过长期随访比较两组患者的死亡率。需要注意的是，对研究进行评估需按照疾病筛查的目的进行，成功的筛查试验可以降低死亡率。用前瞻性随机试验来评估某项筛查是很有必要的，因为一些筛查试验会提高患者的总体生存率和 5 年生存率，却不会降低其死亡率或死亡风险。总而言之，筛查试验的益处和风险对决定是否推荐或使用某项筛查是非常重要的。

癌症筛查是一种在癌症高危人群中早期发现无症状恶性肿瘤的方法。筛查阳性表明患者可能已经罹患癌症，需要进行必要的额外“诊断”检测来确诊或排除疾病。对于有症状的人，同样的筛查通常被认为是“可确诊的”而不是筛查性的[1]。

筛查的目的不仅是为了发现疾病，更是为了减少晚期疾病的发病率，并在疾病进程中找到可以通过治疗来预防死亡的节点。在临床研究中，癌症死亡率的降低表明达到了对疾病导致的死亡进行预防的目的[2]。一些筛查试验可降低与治疗相关的发病率并/或改善患者的生活质量；也有些筛查主要致力于识别并治疗癌前病变以防微杜渐。

筛查的主要标准

对于高发疾病和对社会有重要影响的癌症，筛查是最有效和最高效的方式。临床前期是指隐匿性肿瘤在转移或出现症状前可通过筛查被发现的时期。成功的癌症筛查需具备以下几个要素：癌症在个体内要有一定的临床前期，以确保在扩散之前可以通过定期筛查在目标人群中检出；与出现症状后的治疗相比，患者接受提前治疗的获益更大；筛选试验的准确度和成本应在患者可接受的范围内[1]。

早期筛查项目的评估

对筛查试验的评估应主要看其是否发现了癌症，是否真正延长了患者的生存时间，以及筛查是否降低了受试者死于该疾病的风险。如果没有严格的研究设计，筛查试验的评估就容易受到很多偏倚的影响，使结论无效。

评估筛查试验的偏倚类型

领先时间偏倚：从筛查发现隐匿性症状到疾病进展再到症状出现的时间被称为领先时间。接受筛查的人群总是有生存率更好的倾向，因为筛查使诊断的时间提前了。领先时间偏倚存在时，早期筛查只提前患者的诊断时间，却并没有延长患者的生存期（图 38-1）。由于领先时间偏倚的存在，生存率的提高或 5 年生存率的改善不能单独用来评估筛查试验。

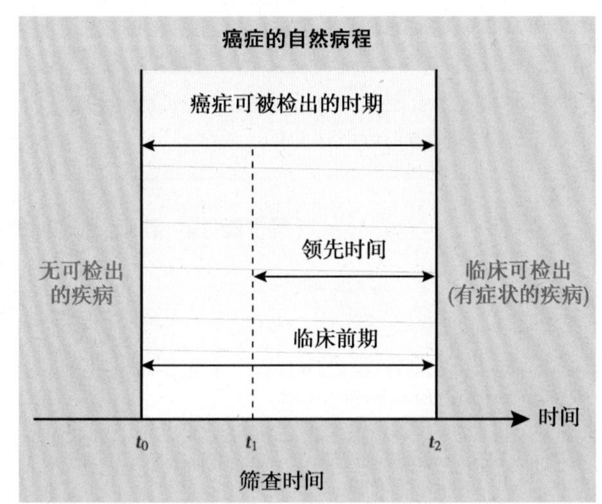

图 38-1　癌症的自然病程。在图中，$t_2 \sim t_0$ 是临床前筛查的可检测期，称为“临床前期”；$t_2 \sim t_1$ 是通过筛选诊断可提前的时间，称为“领先时间”。假设临床前期呈指数分布，个体通过筛查可检出疾病的预期领先时间等于临床前期阶段分布的平均值

病程偏倚：是指发现对人群造成较小威胁的癌症的偏倚（图 38-2）。生长较慢且临床前期较长的癌症更有可能在筛查中被发现。生长速度更快、更具侵袭性、临床前期较短的癌症更容易逃避检测，可能在两次定期筛查之间出现症状而被诊断。与未接受筛查的人群相比，筛查发现肿瘤的癌症患者中，生长缓慢肿瘤的比例更高，因此其生存率看上去会比未筛查组更好。

过度诊断：是指一些肿瘤符合所有恶性肿瘤的组织学标准，但并不一定会导致死亡，而且如果没有筛查，患者也不会知晓（图 38-3）[3]。过度诊断是病程偏倚的一个极端的例子。过度诊断分两种：第一种：虽然疾病在组织学上与癌前病变或癌症难以区分，但其在生物学上没有进展的倾向[4]。这种情况常见于筛检出的子宫颈癌前病变和前列腺癌及甲状腺癌[5]。第二种：疾病虽为致命的肿瘤，但对特定的患者来说却不是致命

的原因，她/他可能在临床前期就死于其他原因[4]。在某个人群中持续较高的发病率可能是由于领先时间，或将未筛查的队列纳入筛查项目以及过度诊断。

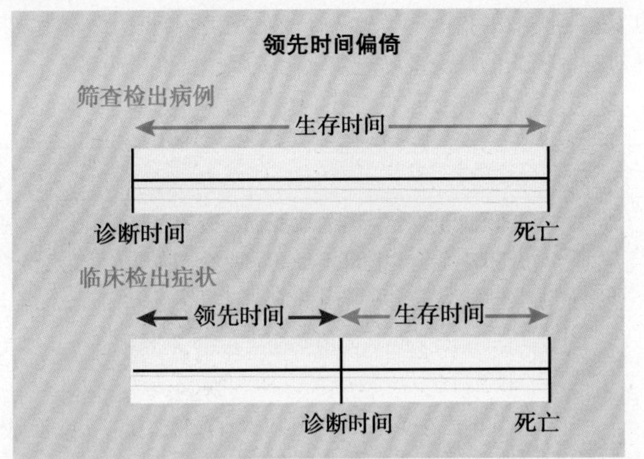

图 38-2　领先时间偏倚。需要注意的是，筛查发现病例和诊断发现病例均在同时死亡，但由于领先时间偏倚，筛查发现病例的生存时间显得更长

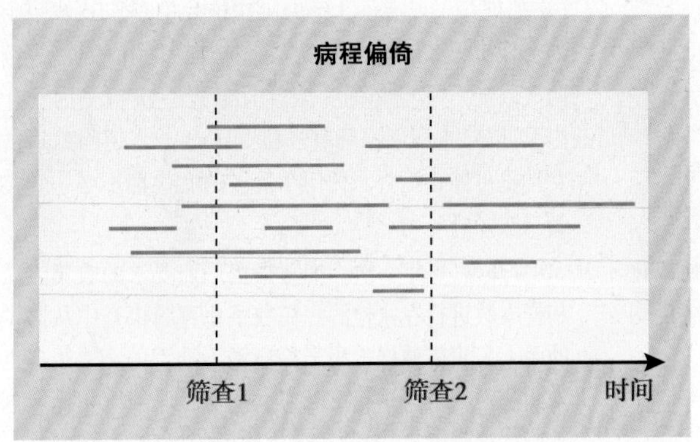

图 38-3　病程偏倚。该图中横线代表了在筛查中能检测到肿瘤的临床前期。在 8 例临床前期长的肿瘤中，这两种筛查可检出 6 例，而在 6 例临床前期短的病例中只能检出其中的 2 例

选择偏差：是指参与筛查的个体可能与不参与筛查的个体存在明显的差异，例如，他们可能更有健康意识，更注重控制风险因素，更有疾病意识，依从性更好，其总体的生活习惯也更健康[6]。选择偏倚可以产生比预期更好的筛查结果，甚至可能影响旨在克服该偏倚的研究结果的普适性。例如，与一般美国人群相比，参加国家肺筛查试验（NLST）的吸烟者和戒烟者，肺气肿、心脏病和糖尿病的发病率明显更低。

在随机试验中，当研究者征得了干预组受试者的同意，而对照组的受试者没有意识到自己在研究中，就有可能发生特有的选择偏差。在这种情况下，干预组健康状况不佳的人可以拒绝参与试验，而对照组的人则没有这种机会[7]。

筛查的特点

灵敏性和特异性：敏感性或阳性率是指当某项试验应用于真正患有该病的人群时，检出阳性结果的概率。特异性或真阴性率是指没有患病的人群检出阴性结果的概率（表 38-1）。在筛查试验中，高敏感性和高特异性都是可取的，然而，二者往往是负相关的。虽然高灵敏度的检测可以成功地筛查出大多数的隐匿性疾病，但低特异性的检测会导致很多假阳性和额外的检查。

表 38-1　筛查试验评估

	患病	状态
筛查试验结果	是	否
阳性	a	b
阴性	c	d

敏感性 = a/（a+c）；特异性 = d/（b+d）；阳性预测值（PPV）= a/（a+b）；阴性预测值（NPV）= c/（c+d）。

阳性预测值和阴性预测值：阳性预测值（PPV）是指筛查阳性的患者罹患目标疾病的概率（表 38-1），阴性预测值（NPV）是指筛查阴性的患者不患目标疾病的可能性，是筛查试验阴性结果再次确认值的量化。可以说，筛查中较高的 NPV 更重要，因为这意味着很少有患者会漏诊或延误诊疗。

效能和效力：筛查研究通常要评估干预措施的有效性，即该试验是否能拯救参与试验人群的生命。另一个因素是当干预被广泛使用时的效力。一些大型临床试验会评估其筛查的效力，尽管这些研究可能会受到知情同意的健康志愿者的影响[1]。最终，筛查干预的效力评估应该结合现实情况进行，而不是通过实验性研究来确定，诸如试验者的经验、与时俱进的筛查技术的进步、人群可接受性和成本效益等因素均需要考虑在内。

评估筛查干预的研究设计

描述性研究：是最容易进行的筛查性研究，为疾病控制提供了一手的证据。该研究是不受控制的观察性研究，并且基于医生、诊所或癌症登记处的经验。描述性研究可以产生有用的信息，但由于观察者固有的偏倚，该证据较为薄弱；并且该研究没有对照组，无法评估其试验效能。

病例对照研究：是典型的回顾性研究，通过比较一组会出现预期结果（疾病、死亡、间期癌等）的患者（病例组）与不会出现预期结果的患者（对照组），以评估可能导致该结果的因素[8]。病例组和对照组的关键特征必须进行匹配，如年龄、性别和社会经济地位。病例对照研究的成本通常较低，而且能比前瞻性研究更快地提供证据[8]。该研究面临着如何避免偏倚的问题，其结果也很容易被不可控因素混淆。

前瞻性随机临床试验（prospective randomized clinical trial，RCT）：是评估最为严格的筛查试验，通常用来比较随机接受筛查邀请的试验组与接受常规护理的对照组之间疾病的特异性死亡率。该设计通过随机化使设计者选择偏差和其他偏差的混淆效应最小化。死亡率终点不受领先时间偏倚、病程偏倚或过度诊断的影响。RCT 应该通过治疗意向（intention-to-treat，ITT）进行分析，这意味着最终结果是基于入组和未入组患者之间的比较，而不是筛查组和未筛查组间的比较。如果分析时只包括筛查人的信息将会导致偏倚。

庞大的样本量、过高的费用以及较长的研究持续时间，都限制了前瞻性随机对照试验的开展数量。一些人认为，全因死

亡率比疾病特异性死亡率更适合作为研究的主要终点,因为它避免了死因判断方面的潜在偏见,也避免了由于诊断和治疗干预导致的其他死因无法衡量的缺点。RCT 需要更大研究规模和更高的花费来衡量全因死亡率,因此经济上并不划算[9]。

一些医学机构和专业机构通过调研科学文献来制定筛查建议或指南[5]。美国预防服务工作组(The US Preventive Services Task Force,USPSTF)以设计非常严格的筛查指导流程而闻名,该流程旨在将利益冲突、经济、智力和情感的影响最小化[10]。这些建议可以在 www. uspreventiveservicestforce. org 网站上找到。美国癌症协会(The American Cancer Society,ACS)也发布了类似的指南(表 38-2)。很多医学专业协会也发布了针对特定疾病的指南或筛查建议。

表 38-2 美国癌症协会在一般风险无症状人群中早期检测癌症的筛查指南

肿瘤部位	受试人群	筛查方法	筛查频率等推荐
乳腺	女性 年龄:40~44 岁	乳腺 X 线造影	参加筛查的女性需理解乳腺癌筛查的益处、局限性及可能的危害。女性应该在 40~44 岁之间开始每年一次的乳腺 X 线造影筛查
	女性 年龄:45~54 岁	乳腺 X 线造影	具有一般乳腺癌风险的女性应在 45 岁开始进行年度乳腺癌筛查
	女性 年龄:55 岁以上	乳腺 X 线造影	年龄在 55 岁或以上的女性应该每两年接受一次筛查,但她们可能会选择接收年度筛查
宫颈	女性 年龄:21~65 岁	子宫颈抹片检查和 HPV DNA 检测	宫颈癌筛查应在 21 岁开始。对于 21~29 岁的女性,每 3 年需接收一次常规的或者液相子宫颈抹片检查。对于 30~65 岁的女性,每 5 年需接受 HPV 检测和抹片检查(更加推荐),或者每 3 年做一次抹片检查。65 岁以上的女性 10 年以内连续 3 次以上抹片检查阴性或者连续两次以上两种检查均为阴性且最近一次检查为 5 年内,可以停止宫颈癌筛查。接受了全子宫切除术后的女性也可停止筛查。任何年龄段的女性都不必一年接受一次筛查
结直肠	50 岁以上的人群	粪便潜血试验(FOBT)或粪便组化检测(FIT)检出癌症的敏感度均大于 50%	从 50 岁开始,每年一次。推荐根据厂商要求的收集方法和样本数进行在家检测。在数字化直肠检查中从医生的手上采集粪便样本用于检测是不推荐的。使用愈创木脂法马桶取样进行 FOBT 也是不可取的。相比愈创木脂法检测隐血,人群对组化检测的接受度更高,且二者的灵敏度和特异性相当。无需重复 FOBT 以验证检测呈阳性的样本
		粪便 DNA 检测	从 50 岁开始,每 3 年一次
		可屈乙状结肠镜检(FSIG)	从 50 岁开始,每 5 年一次。可单做此项检查或每 5 年 1 次 FSIG 配合每年 1 次高敏感度的 FOBT 或 FIT
		双对比的钡灌肠检查(DCBE)	从 50 岁开始,每 5 年一次
		结肠镜检	从 50 岁开始,每 10 年一次
		结肠 CT	从 50 岁开始,每 5 年一次
子宫内膜	绝经后的女性		绝经期处于一般风险的女性应该熟知子宫内膜癌的风险及症状。当发现不明原因的出血时应及时告知医生
肺	年龄在 55~74 岁之间健康状况良好,每年吸烟量大于 30 包的吸烟者及戒烟者	低剂量螺旋 CT(LDCT)	在高水平的肺癌筛查和治疗中心工作的临床医生应该就年龄在 55~74 岁之间,目前健康状况良好,在过去 15 年内每年至少吸烟 30 包的吸烟者和戒烟者是否接受筛查进行讨论。在决定是否开始肺癌筛查之前,临床医生应对筛查者进行知情介绍,对于 LDCT 筛查肺癌的潜在益处、局限性和危害要有充分的了解,共同协商达成决议。在与吸烟者的讨论中,戒烟咨询仍然是临床优先关注的重点,吸烟者需被告知存在罹患肺癌的高风险。筛查不应被视为戒烟的替代选择

续表

肿瘤部位	受试人群	筛查方法	筛查频率等推荐
前列腺	50 岁以上的男性	直肠指检(DRE)和前列腺特异性抗原检测(PSA)	寿命预期达 10 年以上的男性应与相应的医疗机构协商是否接受前列腺癌筛查,在做出决定前需充分了解筛查的潜在受益、风险以及不确定性等。如果受检者未充分知情而做出决策,就不能实施前列腺癌筛查
癌症相关检查	20 岁以上的人群		在定期的体检中,检查项目应包含对于甲状腺、睾丸、卵巢、淋巴结、口腔、皮肤等癌症的排查,同时还需要进行烟草、日晒、饮食及营养、高危因素、性习惯、环境及职业暴露因素等方面的健康咨询

计划性筛查与机会性筛查　在有组织的筛查项目中,受试者对于筛查推荐项目的依从性将被追踪记录,筛查质量也会通过系统审查记录。很多欧洲国家都是这样进行筛查的。而在美国,大多数筛查是机会性筛查,对依从性或筛查质量的跟踪很有限。美国的一些乳房 X 光检查确实达到了世界级的高标准。然而,在美国和欧洲,对其他疾病的筛查仍缺乏普适性的标准。

乳腺癌筛查

乳腺癌是全球范围内最常见的女性肿瘤性疾病,排在肿瘤致死的第一位。美国女性诊断为乳腺癌的中位年龄为 61 岁,乳腺癌致死的中位年龄为 68 岁[11]。

乳腺癌筛查方法

乳腺 X 线造影:是一种对乳房进行 X 线检查的方法,它能以最小的 X 线剂量为乳房生成高质量的前后视图(CC)和中间斜向视图(MLO)图像。有证据表明,数字成像可使结果得到更准确的解读,并提高对乳腺高密度女性的诊断准确率,而其对绝经后女性的诊断则与传统胶片的成像效果相似[12]。

首次筛查出现异常解读的概率比之后做乳腺 X 线造影要高出 5%~10%。大多数异常可通过附加不同角度的乳腺 X 线造影或超声检查进行确认。仍无法确定的异常可通过超声或 X 线引导的细针穿刺、芯针活检或手术切除进行活检。

迄今为止,已有 9 项乳腺癌筛查的随机对照试验发表(表 38-3)。这些试验在纳入女性的年龄范围、使用的筛查方式[单独使用乳腺 X 线造影(mammography,MMG)或与临床乳腺检查(clinical breast examination,CBE)联用]、筛查间隔、随访时间等方面均存在差异。这几项随机对照试验都开始于现代辅助化疗之前,其中大部分在现代辅助化疗开展之前已完成,还有一些在激素疗法出现之前就已结束。筛查和诊断设备也有所改进[13]。专家们试图通过非随机研究和数学模型来分析这些研究的局限性和缺陷[14,15]。好的筛查项目有可能降低乳腺癌死亡的风险目前已成为共识[8]。

表 38-3　乳腺癌筛查随机试验

研究	随机性	样本数量	干预	随访	研究发现
健康保险计划,美国,1963	个体	60 565~60 857	持续 3 年 MMG 和 CBE	18 年	RR=0.77(95%CI 0.61~0.97)
马尔摩,瑞典,1976	个体	42 283	每 18~24 个月做 2 个视野的 MMG,共 5 次	12 年	RR=0.81(95%CI 0.62~1.07)
科帕尔贝里,瑞典,1977	地理集群	试验组:38 405~39 034;对照组:37 145~37 936	50 岁以下每两年做 3 次单视野的 MMG;50 岁以上女性每 33 个月做 3 次单视野的 MMG	12 年	RR = 0.82(95% CI,0.64~1.05)东约特兰
科帕尔贝里,瑞典,1977	地理集群	干预组:38 562~39 051 对照组:18 478~18 846	50 岁以下每两年做 3 次单视野的 MMG;50 岁以上女性每 33 个月做 3 次单视野的 MMG	12 年	RR = 0.68(95% CI 0.52~0.89)
爱丁堡,英国	根据诊所分群	试验组:23 266 对照组:21 904	首次做双视野 MMG 和 CBE,之后每年做 CBE,在第 3、5、7 年做单视野 MMG	10 年	RR = 0.84(95% CI 0.63~1.12)
NBSS-1,加拿大,1980	个体	试验组:25 214(进入 CBE 后 100%筛查)对照组:25 216	持续 4~5 年的年度双视野 MMG 和 CBE	13 年	RR = 0.97(95% CI 0.74~1.27)

续表

研究	随机性	样本数量	干预	随访	研究发现
NBSS-2, Canada, 1980	个体	试验组:19 711(进入CBE后100%筛查) 对照组:19 694	年度双视野MMG和CBE	11~16年(平均13年)	RR = 1.02(95% CI 0.78~1.33)
斯德哥尔摩,瑞典,1981	根据生日集群	干预组:从40 318减少到38 525 对照组:从19 943增加到20 978	每28个月1次单视野MMG,共2次	8年	RR = 0.80(95% CI 0.53~1.22)
哥德堡,瑞典,1982	复杂	干预组:21 650 对照组:29 961	首次双视野MMG,之后每18个月做1次单视野MMG,共4次;前3次单次读取,第4次做2次读取	12~14年	RR = 0.79(95% CI 0.58~1.08)
AGE Trial	个体	160 921*(53 884入组;106 956未入组)	试验组小于等于48周岁每年1次MMG(首次双视野,之后中外侧斜位单视野),68%在首次筛查时同意入组,70%后期同意入组(81%接受了1次以上的筛查)	10.7年	RR = 0.83(95% CI 0.66~1.04)

* 译注:疑似原书数据有误,应为160 840例。

关于是否应该在其40岁或50岁时对正常风险的女性开展筛查,一直存在着巨大的争论。争论的核心是缺乏来自随机对照试验的证据以明确40~49岁女性的乳腺X线造影筛查是否有效。有些研究数据表明,对40多岁的女性进行筛查有显著的益处,而其他研究则未证实这一点[16]。最新的随机对照试验为AGE研究,这个研究中的一些患者可能接受了现代辅助治疗[17]。该研究总共纳入了53 884名年龄在39~41岁之间的女性,对照组并不知道自己已入组研究并接受"常规医疗护理"。在10.7年的随访中,筛查组与对照组相比,乳腺癌死亡的相对风险降低了17%,但该差异并无统计学意义(RR = 0.83,95%CI 0.66~1.04)[17]。USPSTF对包括AGE在内的大型随机对照试验进行了荟萃分析(表38-4),该分析认为在随访11~20年后,40~49岁入组的女性在接受了2~9轮的筛查后,死亡率相对危险度降低了15%(RR = 0.85,95% CI,0.75~0.96)[18]。换句话说,1 904名女性参加筛查就可以预防或延缓1名乳腺癌患者的死亡[19]。据估计,在10年的筛查中有一半以上的女性曾出现过假阳性。将筛查间隔改为每两年进行一次虽然略微降低了检出率,但可将假阳性率降低近一半[20]。

表38-4 所有年龄段乳腺癌筛查试验中乳腺癌死亡率的合并RR

年龄(岁)	试验数	乳腺癌死亡率的RR(95% CI)	预防1例乳腺癌死亡的NNI(95% CI)
39~49	8	0.85(0.75~0.96)	1 904(929~6 378)
50~59	6	0.86(0.75~0.99)	1 339(322~7 455)
60~69	2	0.68(0.54~0.87)	377(230~1 050)
70~74	1	1.12(0.73~1.72)	未统计

CI,可信区间;NNI,需接受筛查的人数;RR,相对风险度。

与50多岁的女性相比,40多岁女性的乳腺密度(X线检查参数)更高,这使得解读40岁组女性乳腺的X线造影结果更加复杂。研究表明,不同影像科医生解读乳腺X线结果的准确性、灵敏度和特异性各异,但总体上该检查的有效性随着患者年龄的增长而提高[21,22]。在定期筛查的女性中,间期癌在40~49岁的女性中更为普遍[23]。

临床乳腺检查(CBE)和乳房自检(BSE):合格的CBE应由受过专业训练的健康机构从业者对乳房进行小范围的物理触诊,触诊范围包括乳头、乳房周围和腋窝[24]。在某些情况下,特别在发展中国家,这种方法可能是唯一可行的乳腺癌筛查方法[18]。

CBE作为单一的筛查方式还未进行前瞻性随机对照试验评估。由于X线造影无法识别一小部分可触及的肿块乳房,因此指南中乳腺癌的筛查包括了常规CBE,并且推荐在乳腺X线造影之前进行。也有一些数据表明,在坚持定期使用高质量乳房X线造影进行筛查的情况下,CBE对于乳腺癌检出的贡献较小[18]。

BSE作为乳腺癌的筛查方法具有简单、方便、无创的优点。每月乳房自检一度被广泛提倡[25]。然而,两项前瞻性随机对照试验则表明BSE作为筛查方法缺乏有效性,甚至还可能有害,但这两项研究都存在一些方法学上的问题[26,27]。每月乳房自检的推广使人们忽略了乳腺X线检查的重要性,并给一些乳腺癌患者提供了错误的提示;同时增加了未患病人群罹患乳腺癌的焦虑,可能会产生假阳性。目前美国和欧洲没有任何的专业机构鼓励每月乳房自检,而是提倡"乳房意识",鼓励乳腺可能异常的人群尽早咨询医疗人员[25,28]。

筛查有效性的评估

虽然乳腺癌筛查的随机对照试验提示筛查利大于弊,但评估社区常规筛查项目的有效性并非易事。1989—2011 年,美国人口中年龄调整后的死亡率下降了 35%。数学模型评估显示,乳腺癌筛查和治疗方法的改进(特别是激素治疗)各占死亡率下降原因的一半[29]。

乳腺癌筛查的危害

任何一种筛查试验都有其相应的危害。在 10 年的筛查中,略超半数的女性会出现假阳性,至少需要再次影像学检查来确认是否患病[30,31]。调查显示,即使癌症通过进一步检查被排除的 3 个月后,仍有约四分之一的人处于痛苦和焦虑中[32]。假阴性则会带来错误的安全感。在借助乳腺 X 线造影诊断的乳腺癌筛查中,过度诊断的概率估计从 0 到 54%不等,大多数的评估认为过度诊断概率为 10%~30%[14,33]。

乳腺 X 线造影也使乳腺导管原位癌(ductal carcinoma in situ,DCIS)的诊断率大幅上升。在此之前,DCIS 的诊断率极低,其常在乳腺癌切除术后意外被发现,但现在美国每年有超过 7 万例病例经筛查后确诊 DCIS,但这尚不能表明早期发现和治疗能够降低 DCIS 的死亡率。一般认为多数 DCIS 病变不会发展为侵袭性癌[15,34],因此目前有过度治疗的趋势。如果重新命名 DCIS,将"癌"字去掉可能会更加准确[36]。未来医学基因组学或许能帮助我们区分哪些是需要积极治疗的肿瘤(原位癌和真正的癌症),以及哪些是可以观察而暂时不需要处理的肿瘤。

新的技术

数字乳腺断层摄影(digital breast tomosynthesis,DBT)和三维乳腺 X 线造影是较新的技术,或可提高检测的敏感度并减低重检率[37]。

磁共振成像(MRI)检测乳腺癌比乳腺 X 线造影更灵敏,但特异性更低[38]。首检使用 MRI 会产生大量的假阳性结果,而联用其他方法复查之后假阳性率会逐渐下降。但对于乳腺密度显著升高和因乳腺癌易感基因突变而患病风险升高的女性,MRI 为癌症提供了一个可检出的时间窗。

超声成像多年来一直被用作诊断。乳腺 X 线造影筛查高密度型乳腺有一定的局限性,因而引起了使用超声成像进行乳腺癌初筛或将其作为乳腺 X 线造影辅助手段的热潮[39,40]。

2003 年,美国放射学会影像网络(ACRIN)启动了一项多中心试验,研究了由于家族史和高乳腺密度而导致乳腺癌高风险的女性[41,42]。研究表明联用乳腺 X 线造影和超声的检出率比单用乳腺 X 线造影更高,每 1 000 名女性中可多检出 4.2 个乳腺癌(11.8 vs 7.6/1 000)。然而,假阳性和活检阴性率也很高。虽然这一研究能显著提高高危人群中直径较小、淋巴结阴性的乳腺癌的诊断率,但尚不清楚是否能降患者的低死亡率,同时未来超声波筛查的潜力也受质疑[40]。因此,目前并不提倡使用超声检查作为常规的筛查手段。

三维自动乳腺超声也在逐步进入临床应用。与传统超声相比,它提供了更标准化的成像,并且可以由技术人员完成,而不一定需要放射科医生进行操作。目前这一技术仅用于诊断,未来是否可以联合乳腺 X 线造影和 CBE 进行乳腺癌初筛是值得关注的。

筛查建议

从 2015 年开始,ACS 指南建议女性需了解乳腺癌筛查的潜在益处、局限性和危害。乳腺癌平均风险的女性应该从 45 岁开始定期接受乳腺 X 线造影。年龄在 45~54 岁之间的女性应每年接受检查。55 岁及以上的女性应每 2 年筛查一次,也可选择继续进行每年一次的检查。女性也可在 40~44 岁之间开始年度筛查。只要是整体健康状况良好,预期寿命在 10 年及以上的女性均应继续接受筛查。从 2015 年开始,美国癌症协会建议不使用临床乳腺检查对平均乳腺癌风险的女性进行乳腺癌筛查。ACS 指南适用于接受乳腺 X 线造影进行筛查的女性。

2009 年 USPSTF 建议 50~75 岁的女性每 1~2 年做一次乳腺 X 线造影[43],但是不推荐 CBE 用于常规筛查,认为其缺乏有益的证据。工作小组建议不要对 40~49 岁的女性进行"常规"的乳腺 X 线造影,但可在医生与患者充分讨论明确风险解除疑虑后再做决定。

2014 年 12 月,USPSTF、美国医师学会和加拿大定期健康体检任务小组建议从 50 岁开始常规筛查[44]。欧盟的癌症预防咨询委员会建议通过有组织的筛查项目对 50~69 岁的女性进行筛查[45]。

即使缺少随机对照研究数据的支持,根据以往的数据,美国癌症协会建议高乳腺癌风险的女性可以在 30 岁时开始进行每年一次的乳腺 X 线造影和磁共振成像(MRI);如果受检者和医生进行了充分的沟通,认为提前开始筛查很有必要,那么在 30 岁之前也可开始筛查[38]。然而,在高风险人群中进行前瞻性 RCT 几乎是不可行的。以下群体被定义为高风险人群:携带 *BRCA1* 或 *BRCA2* 突变;基于家族史终生患乳腺癌的概率升高 20%~25%或更高的人群;患高风险的遗传综合征,如 Li-Fraumeni 综合征或 Cowden 病;或曾接受过高剂量的胸部放射治疗的女性[22]。

结直肠癌

在世界范围内,结直肠癌是男性第三高发、女性第二高发的癌症,其致死人群占所有癌症致死人数的 8%。在美国,结直肠癌是第三高发的癌症,也位居男性和女性癌症死因的第三位。虽然大多数病例是在 60~80 岁时确诊,但是在 40~50 岁的人群中,其发病情况呈上升趋势,也越来越受到关注[11]。

考虑到腺瘤性息肉是癌前病变的重要证据,结直肠癌筛查的主要任务一方面是检测早期腺癌,另一方面是检测并切除腺瘤性息肉。结直肠息肉高发年龄为 50 岁以上的人群。1/2 到 2/3 的结直肠息肉是腺瘤性的,少数可能会发展为癌症。据估计,小于 1cm 的腺瘤性息肉进展为侵袭性病变大概需要 10 年[46]。其他息肉,包括偶发性增生性息肉和炎性息肉,在结直肠癌的发展过程中无显著作用[47]。

结直肠癌的筛查方法

研究表明,定期监测项目中的一些检查有可能会降低结直肠癌的死亡率。这些检查包括:

1. 粪便潜血试验(FOBT)的目的是发现由息肉(尤其是>2cm 的息肉)等造成的出血。常规的 FOBT 包括愈创木脂法粪便潜血试验(gFOBT)和粪便免疫化学检测(FIT)。

gFOBT 通过血红素的假过氧化物酶活性检测粪便中的潜血。由于红肉、十字花科蔬菜和某些水果中的过氧化物酶能在该试验中产生阳性反应,因此检测前需要进行饮食调整。gFOBT 复水后(rehydration of gFOBT)可提高检测的敏感性,但同时也增加了假阳性率[48]。gFOBT 可以在医师处进行，但患者最好在家中采集标本送至实验室进行处理。粪便血检呈阳性需后续进行结肠镜检查。

gFOBT 的局限性导致了其应用量下降，但一些高灵敏度的测试仍然在使用。目前不推荐在直肠指检（DRE）中收集粪便进行 gFOBT。

FIT 对人的球蛋白有反应。FIT 不会像 gFOBT 那样受饮食影响，也不会与上消化道出血后被消化的血产生反应。粪便血红蛋白阈值可根据个人风险或项目要求设置，以平衡敏感性和特异性。FIT 通常在实验室里进行操作，检测的灵敏度随样品处理的延迟而下降，即使是 5 天的延迟灵敏度也会大幅度下降[49]。

在 1 000 例有或无结直肠癌症状的门诊患者中，当血红蛋白阈值为 75ng/ml 时，通过 FIT 检测 3 个样本对结直肠癌诊断的敏感度为 94. 1%，特异性为 87. 5%。另一项在 FIT 后进行结肠镜检查的筛查发现与未服用阿司匹林的患者相比，服用低剂量阿司匹林的患者晚期肿瘤的检出率更高，而特异性略微下降[50]。

对 gFOBT 和 FIT 的系统回顾表明，这两种检测不相伯仲[51]。癌症或大息肉引起的出血可能是间歇性的。一般来说，FIT 需要约一周两次的检测，而 gFOBT 需要一周 3 次。一定程度上，FIT 正在取代 gFOBT。

2. 粪便 DNA（sDNA）检测可以在结肠息肉脱落的细胞和结肠腔内的恶性肿瘤中检测与结直肠肿瘤相关性较好的 DNA 标记物。现有的 sDNA 检测侧重于 K-RAS 癌基因中大于 21 个的单独点突变、BAT-26 探针（微卫星不稳定性的标志物）和 DNA 完整性分析（DIA）标志物，而三者联用可以提高灵敏度[52]。与粪便血检一样，任何呈阳性的粪便血检或 DNA 检测都必须进行结肠镜检查，以排除息肉或癌症的存在。

3. 软性乙状结肠镜检查（FSIG）的范围为 60cm，是一种相对简单的检查方法，准备工作较少，可以检查一半左右的结肠[53]。一般情况下，该检查不需要麻醉患者。远端的肠息肉提示近端肠息肉或癌症的风险升高。如果 FSIG 呈阳性，则推荐患者进行结肠镜检查。

FSIG 已有发布的质控参数，强调操作者需进行适当的培训，操作者需达到以下要求：能够检查的范围需大于 40cm，能达到基于年龄和性别预期的腺瘤检出率以及具备对可疑腺瘤进行活检的能力。

4. 钡剂灌肠是通过钡剂（单对比研究）或钡剂与注入空气的对比[双对比钡剂灌肠研究（DCBE）]对肠道进行的 X 线检查。DCBE 对恶性肿瘤和息肉的敏感性高于单对比研究。如果患者的检查呈阳性，下一步应通过结肠镜检查确认[54]。

DCBE 可检出小的恶性病变和息肉，目前早期发现并切除息肉可降低死亡率，这可作为证明 DCBE 有效性的间接证据。通过结肠镜检和 DCBE 均能检出的腺瘤性息肉的比例受到病变大小的显著影响。在所有目前推荐的筛查试验中，钡灌肠的使用率最低。

5. 结肠镜检查在结肠直肠癌筛查中有一个独特的优势，即可以直接观察整个肠道，90% 的检查在盲肠结束，在检查过程中可以发现并切除有临床指征的腺瘤[24,55]。肠镜检查主要在门诊进行，虽然清醒镇静是标准的操作，也有一些患者会接受全身麻醉。适当的肠道准备对确保肠道清洁至关重要。

乙状结肠镜检查更为复杂，由于镇静、活检或息肉切除而引起并发症的风险更高。任何大小的息肉都可导致出血，但切除大的息肉或结肠近端息肉时更容易出血。肠穿孔的风险随着年龄增长而增加，在患有憩室疾病的个体中其风险更高。500 名医疗保险人群中约 1 人会发生肠穿孔，而在总体人群中其发生率约为 1/1 000。

1 256 名结肠镜检查阴性的成人 5 年后接受再次筛查仍未发现癌症，其中 201 名（16%）受检者检出 1 个或多个腺瘤，其中 16 人处于进展期[56]。这一研究结果表明结肠镜检结果正常的人群中结直肠癌的 5 年风险极低。

另一项研究对马尼托巴省 35 000 名无症状且结肠镜检阴性的患者随访了 10 年，观察到预期的 5 年结直肠癌发病率降低了 45%，10 年发病率降低了 72%[57]。这提示最初的结肠镜检结果存在错误。

结肠镜检查后结肠直肠癌风险降低的持续时间取决于检查的质量和息肉是否被完全切除。质控强调培训和经验的重要性，质控需注意以下方面：建议适当的风险评估和记录；在肠道准备和黏膜显示良好的情况下检查至盲肠；具备发现息肉并安全切除的能力；息肉样病变的记录和切除；及时并妥善处理不良事件；对后续组织病理学结果的随访；合理的筛查推荐或根据指南的推荐进行再次筛查；持续的绩效评估并在必要时采取纠正措施。

6. CT 结肠镜或虚拟结肠镜是一种成像过程，通过结合多个螺旋 CT 扫描并进行计算来创建结肠内部的二维或三维图像。这些图像可以进行不同视图的旋转，组合成一个完整的“虚拟”视图[54]。

对 CT 结肠镜检查的评估通常包括 CT 检查和之后的光学结肠镜检查，结肠镜检人员对 CT 结果并不知情。虽然 2D 成像的早期结果令人失望，但最近对 CT 结肠镜检查进行了连续的评估，当使用更快的扫描仪、更新 3D 管腔显示、以及使用数字减影法进行粪便标记时，CT 结肠镜检出大腺瘤的敏感性与结肠镜检等同。借助以上进展，一项研究利用连续 CT 和结肠镜检对无症状人群进行了筛查，该研究发现该筛检方法检出大腺瘤的敏感性达到了 94%，单个患者检出大于等于 6mm 腺瘤的敏感性为 89%[58]。

在 ACRIN/NCI 合作试验中[59]，CT 结肠镜检查检出 90% 的大（≥10mm）腺瘤和癌症的特异性达 86%，检出息肉的敏感性为 84%。CT 结肠镜检查发现了 30 个大的病变，而光学结肠镜检查并未检出。在 18 个≥10mm 的病变中，5 个经结肠镜检查确认为真阳性。虽然 CT 结肠镜检查对于≤6mm 的病变的敏感性较低，但这种病变一般没有临床意义。对于≥1cm 的病变，CT 结肠镜检查结果与光学结肠镜检查非常相似[58]。

CT 结肠镜检查与光学结肠镜检查一样，同样需要肠道准备和严格的饮食。由于 CT 结肠镜检查完全依赖于影像学，无法对息肉进行进一步的处理，因此推荐息肉≥6mm 的患者后续进行治疗性结肠镜检查和息肉切除术[59]。

结直肠筛查试验

在未出现症状时，gFOBT 可在早期发现结直肠癌病变，这是最早的结直肠筛查可挽救生命的证据。继这一发现后，欧洲和美国都开展了评估 FOBT 有效性的前瞻性试验。在明尼苏达试验中，46 551 名 50~80 岁之间的无症状参与者被随机邀请参加年度筛查、两年筛查或常规检查[60]。gFOBT 阳性的患者将接受结肠镜检查。年度筛查组、两年筛查组和常规对照组的 13 年累积死亡率分别为每 1 000 人中 5. 33、8. 33 和 8. 83。经过 18 年的随访，年度 gFOBT 和两年 gFOBT 都与死亡率降低相关，且有统计学意义;癌症发病率分别降低了 20%和 18%[48]。结直肠癌的成功预防归因于腺瘤性息肉的发现和切除。在另外两个试验中,两年一次的 gFOBT 筛查也发现了类似的结果[61]。

乙状结肠镜检查:在 20 世纪 90 年代早期,两项病例对照研究评估了乙状结肠镜筛查的准确性,研究表明筛查可使结直肠癌的死亡风险降低 70%或更多[62,63]。另有 5 项随机对照试验报道了乙状结肠镜筛查试验的发病率和死亡率。通过对上述 5 项试验结果的荟萃分析,研究人员发现结直肠癌的死亡率降低了 28%(RR=0.72,95%CI 0.65~0.80),发病率降低了 18%(RR=0.82,95%CI 0.73~0.91),左侧结肠癌的发病率降低了 33%(RR=0.67,95%CI 0.59~0.76)[64,65]。

每 5 年一次的粪便血检联合 FSIG 的检出率优于单用 FOBT 或 FSIG。FOBT 可检测近端结肠的病变(近端结肠已超出 FSIG 的检测范围),对于远端结肠病变,FSIG 比 FOBT 具有更高的敏感性和特异性。一项 RCT 筛查试验针对年龄≥40 岁的无症状个体进行了 5~11 年的随访,结果表明接受年度 FOBT 和乙状结肠镜检查的患者的结直肠癌死亡率低于仅接受乙状结肠镜检查的患者(0.36 vs 0.63/1 000;$P=0.53$)[64]。USPSTF 根据建模得出以下结论,每 5 年进行 1 次 FSIG 并结合每 3 年 1 次高灵敏度的 FOBT 与每 10 年 1 次结肠镜筛查的效果等同[65]。

结肠镜检查:目前还没有设置死亡终点的前瞻性随机对照试验来评估结肠镜检查是否能预防结直肠癌死亡。在明尼苏达的试验中,每年接受 FOBT 筛查的患者中 40%以上最终至少接受了一次结肠镜检查,这或许是评估其效能最有力的证据。此外,另有病例对照研究表明,结肠镜检查和息肉切除对结肠直肠癌的发病率和死亡率有显著的影响[66,67]。

结直肠癌筛查建议

如表 38-2 所示,ACS 对平均风险人群推荐了 7 个结直肠癌的常规筛查项目,筛查可从 50 岁开始[68,69],包括一年一次的高敏感性 FOBT(gFOBT 或 FIT);sDNA(间隔未知);每 5 年 1 次的 FSIG,年度高灵敏度的 gFOBT 或首次筛查后每 5 年 1 次的 FIT 和 FSIG 检查;每 5 年进行一次 DCBE 结肠全检;或每 10 年进行一次结肠镜检查。事实上,大多数接受筛查的成年人都会进行 gFOBT 或 FIT 或结肠镜检查。如果内镜医师经验丰富,并对准备充分的患者进行>40cm 的镜检,那么间隔 10 年进行一次 FSIG 筛查也是合理的。由于敏感性低,因此不再推荐进行年度 DRE 筛查,但 DRE 应在 FSIG 或结肠镜检查前进行。虽然美国的机构对≥50 岁成人的结直肠癌筛查的价值有强烈的共识,但 USPSTF 指出,目前尚没有足够的证据支持或反对利用 CT 结肠镜或 sDNA 检查进行筛查。

针对高危人群的指南建议尽早开始筛查并对结肠进行更彻底的检查(表 38-5)。高危人群包括有腺瘤性息肉或结直肠癌家族史、家族性腺瘤样息肉病(FAP)、遗传性非息肉病性结肠直肠癌(HNPCC)或有炎性病史的人[70]。

表 38-5　高于平均风险人群结直肠息肉及结直肠癌早筛监测指南

风险分类及描述	筛查方式	筛查起始年龄	筛查间隔及建议
中度风险			
单发小腺瘤性息肉(<1cm)	结肠镜检查	息肉诊断时	最早的息肉切除后 3 年内进行 TCE 检查;如结果为阴性则按照平均风险人群筛查指南进行筛查
单发大腺瘤性息肉(≥1cm),或多发腺瘤性息肉	结肠镜检查	最早的息肉诊断时	最早的息肉切除后 3 年内进行 TCE 检查;如正常每 5 年进行 1 次 TCE
结直肠癌根治性切除史	TCE[a]	切除后 1 年内	如正常,每 3 年进行 1 次 TCE;如第二次 TCE 结果正常,则每 5 年 1 次
年龄小于 60 岁一级亲属或两个以上一级亲属(不限年龄)患结直肠癌或腺瘤性息肉	TCE[a]	40 岁或者在家族最早发病年龄的 10 年前,选择二者中更早的时间开始筛查	每 5 年进行 1 次 TCE
非一级亲属患结直肠癌	与平均风险人群相同		
高风险			
家族 FAP 病史	用内镜进行早期检测,咨询基因检测,转专科护理	青春期	如果基因检测为阳性或确定有息肉,考虑结肠切除术;如均为阴性则每 1~2 年做 1 次内镜
家族 HNPCC 病史	结肠镜检查,咨询基因检测	21 岁	如未经过检测或者基因检测为阳性,每 2 年进行 1 次结肠镜检直到 40 岁;40 岁之后,每年 1 次结肠镜检
炎症性肠病	结肠镜检查并做不典型增生活检	全肠炎开始 8 年后;左侧结肠炎发病 12~15 年后	每 1~2 年进行 1 次结肠镜检

FAP,家族性腺瘤样息肉病;HNPCC,遗传性非息肉病性结直肠癌;TCE,全套结肠检查。

[a] TCE 包括结肠镜检查、DCBE 或 CT 结肠镜检查。当结肠镜检查不能显示整个结肠时,应在结肠镜检查中增加 CT 结肠镜检查或 DCBE 检查。

宫颈癌

宫颈癌是全球女性第三大最常见的癌症，在癌症导致的死亡中排名第4[11]，在非洲和亚洲的一些地区，宫颈癌仍然是女性癌症死亡的主要原因。治疗和早期诊断的进步使宫颈癌的死亡率急剧下降，特别是美国和西欧，1980年宫颈癌的死亡率比1930年降低了70%以上[71]。

早期检测的改善归功于20世纪20年代George Papanicolaou博士开发的巴氏试验或涂片。在很多西方国家，20世纪40年代末到50年代，这一方法得到了广泛的应用[72]。巴氏试验可用以诊断早期癌症和癌前病变[不典型增生或宫颈上皮内瘤变(CIN)]，诊断后有多种治疗方法可供选择。通过巴氏试验，可治疗的癌前病变的检出率要比癌症高很多，因此筛查导致的宫颈癌发病率的下降远比其死亡率的下降更为显著[73]。

筛查和诊断方法

总体来说，巴氏试验的技术含量极低[69]。它通常采集来自宫颈鳞状柱状上皮交界处或转化区的脱落的上皮细胞，子宫颈外和宫颈内的样本都需要采集。两个样品分别涂在玻璃载玻片的一侧，快速固定以防止其在空气中干燥。切片染色后由细胞学分析人员在显微镜下镜检。巴氏试验虽然操作简单，但其准确性高度依赖于高质量的标本获取、良好的玻片制备、专业的显微镜检查及结果分析解读[69]。

巴氏涂片有很高的错误率。据估计取样错误约占假阴性试验的三分之二，其余三分之一为涂片的分析错误。巴氏涂片筛查的特异性为98%，敏感性为51%[74]。美国国立癌症研究院于1988年发布了Bethesda系统(表38-6)，"为细胞病理学报告规定了统一的格式。目的在于使用标准化的术语来交流相关的临床信息"[75]。

表38-6 Bethesda系统(2001)

样本类型	传统涂片(巴氏涂片)与液基细胞学检测等方法的对比
样本量是否充足	
充足可评估	描述了宫颈内或移形区内基本情况和其他指标，如局部模糊出血和炎症等
不充足	样本不合格/未处理(注明原因)，或者样本经过处理和检测但对上皮细胞异常的描述不充分(注明原因)
总体分类(可选)	无上皮内瘤变或恶性病变 上皮细胞异常；见描述或结果(在适当的位置注明"鳞状细胞"或"腺细胞") 其他：见描述或结果(例如：大于40岁的女性观察到子宫内膜细胞)
自动阅片	如果病例是由自动化方法检测，注明方法和结果
辅助检查	提供简要的关于检测方法和报告结果的表述，以便临床医生更易理解
无上皮内病变及恶性病变的描述	当没有瘤变细胞证据时，在上面的总分类中或者在报告的描述/结果部分予以说明，是否发现有机物或其他非瘤组织
有机物	阴道毛滴虫 形态与念珠菌一致的真菌 提示细菌性阴道炎的菌群变化 形态与放线菌一致的细菌 与单纯疱疹病毒感染一致的细胞改变
其他非瘤发现	与炎症有关的细胞活性改变(包括典型的修复变化)以及宫内辐射性避孕器
(选择性报告：不限于表格内列举的情况)	子宫切除后腺细胞的状态 细胞萎缩
其他上皮细胞异常	子宫内膜细胞(在≥40岁样本中，需注明是否鳞状上皮内病变阴性)
鳞状细胞	意义不明的非典型鳞状细胞(ASCUS)，无法排除高度鳞状上皮内病变(HSIL) 低度的鳞状上皮病变(ISIL)，包含HPV/轻度不典型增生/CIN1 高度鳞状上皮内病变，包含中到重度不典型增生，CIS/CIN2和CIN3有浸润可疑特征 鳞状细胞癌

续表

样本类型	传统涂片(巴氏涂片)与液基细胞学检测等方法的对比
腺细胞	非典型 　宫颈细胞(NOS 或者描述中注明) 　子宫内膜细胞(NOS 或者描述中注明) 　腺细胞(NOS 或者描述中注明) 　宫颈内细胞,瘤状物 原位宫颈内腺癌 腺癌 　宫颈内 　子宫内 　子宫外的 　无具体说明的
其他恶性瘤状物	标注
专业意见及建议(可选)	建议应当简明,且与专业机构发布的临床随访指南一致(可引用相关刊物)

筛查有效性的临床研究

巴氏涂片筛查相对便宜,接受度也很高,但尚未开展评估其有效性的随机对照试验。自从美国开始巴氏涂片检测,其宫颈癌的死亡率出现了长期的下降,这可能是巴氏涂片筛查降低死亡率最令人信服的证据[25]。由于子宫切除率的增加和宫颈癌治疗的进步等因素,在广泛使用该检查之前,死亡率已经开始下降。然而,发病率和死亡率的下降如此之大,不能完全归功于治疗方法的改进。此外,从 20 世纪 50 年代到 70 年代,挪威较晚才开始使用宫颈癌筛查,其宫颈癌死亡率却相对保持不变,而对于较早采用该方法筛查的冰岛,死亡率则下降了 70% 以上[71]。大量的病例对照研究也显示了宫颈癌筛查的益处。目前大多数被诊断为宫颈癌的美国女性在确诊前 5 年内都没有接受过宫颈癌筛查,这也是筛查可降低发病率的有力证据[76,77]。

癌前病变通常需要数年才能发展为癌症,因此正常风险女性每 3 年进行一次筛查既可[78]。过度诊断和过度治疗也是一个值得关注的问题,观察性研究表明,未经治疗的病变如不明意义的不典型鳞状细胞通常会自行消退[79]。目前常采用分诊、观察病情以及重复检查等策略避免过度治疗[80]。

新的筛查技术

液基细胞学使用与常规巴氏涂片相似的标本采集技术。它同样依赖于收集足够的样品,但样品悬浮在固定液中,经过分散、过滤后使单层细胞分布在载玻片上。经计算机辅助的液基细胞学诊断为异常的玻片,须再由细胞学专家对其进行阅片诊断[81]。

由于伪影(血液、黏液等)的减少以及细胞不重叠,液基细胞学诊断的准确性得以提高。研究表明,液基细胞学在细胞学异常发生率较低的人群中具有更高的敏感性[81]。应用严格循证标准分析发现,与传统的巴氏试验相比,液基细胞学检测在敏感性或特异性方面并没有显著的优势。然而,液基细胞学大大减少了样本不足的问题。

某些人类乳头状瘤病毒(HPV)亚型的持续感染与宫颈癌有很强的相关性[82]。通过检测 HPV DNA 或 HPV RNA 可以更好地诊断宫颈不典型增生。HPV 检测越来越多地被当作一种辅助检测手段,用于对细胞学检测不正常的女性进行分类,例如检出了意义不明的非典型鳞状细胞(ASCUS)或意义不明的非典型腺上皮细胞(AGUS)。此外,在年龄≥30 岁的女性中,HPV 筛查试验也有替代巴氏涂片的趋势[83]。印度的一项前瞻性随机试验表明,HPV 检测可检测到高度不典型增生和早期宫颈癌,通过治疗可降低其死亡率[84]。美国食品药品监督管理局(FDA)已批准了一项 HPV DNA 检测,该检测可单独用于初级筛查。该筛查不适用于 20 多岁的女性,因为 30 岁以下的女性普遍存在活动性和暂时性的 HPV 感染。HPV 作为筛查方式或许消耗的资源更少,可行性更强[85]。

筛查建议

2012 年,美国癌症协会(ACS)、美国阴道镜与宫颈病理学会(ASCCP)和美国临床病理学会(ASCP)对 25 个专业机构提供的数据进行了系统的联合分析,共同发布了宫颈癌的筛查指南[86]。2012 年 USPSTF 也发布了类似的指南[85]。与很多欧洲国家的指南相比,虽然这些新指南支持进行更积极的筛查,但新指南也规定了比以前更合理、更经济的筛查方法。然而,尽管有充分的证据表明,过度筛查会浪费资源,并可能造成潜在的危害,很多美国临床医生仍不愿减少宫颈癌筛查的频次[78]。

筛选的指南的特别建议:

- 21 岁以下的女性无论何时开始性活动都不应接受筛查。
- 21~29 岁之间的女性每 3 年进行 1 次细胞学筛查(常规涂片或液基细胞学检查)。此年龄段女性不进行常规 HPV 检测,但是当诊断出 ASCUS 时,可作为备选检查。30~65 岁之间的女性,推荐每 5 年进行一次 HPV 和细胞学联合筛查。大于 65 岁的女性也可继续进行每 3 年 1 次的细胞学检查。
- 大于 65 岁的女性如果 3 次连续的细胞学检查都呈阴性或者在 10 年内 2 次连续的联合检查呈阴性,且最近一次检查为 5 年内,则无需继续筛查。

- 任何年龄的女性都无需做年度筛查。

这些建议是为具有平均风险的女性制定的,并不适用于高风险人群,例如有宫颈癌病史的女性;出生之前接触过己烯雌酚的人群;以及因药物治疗或感染人类免疫缺陷病毒(HIV)而免疫功能受损的人群。已摘除宫颈的女性不再接受筛查,除非她们有CIN2病史或其他更严重的宫颈疾病。上述人群在治疗后应遵循:30~65岁女性至少进行20年的筛查,即使在筛查期内年龄已超过65岁也应继续筛查。筛查方法不随是否接种过HPV疫苗而改变。

前列腺癌

前列腺癌是世界范围内第二常见的癌症,也是男性癌症死亡的第六大常见原因[11],其发病率和死亡率在不同地区的变化较大。在美国男性中,前列腺癌是最常见的非皮肤癌,也是癌症导致死亡的第二大原因;非洲裔男性、美洲高加索男性和斯堪的纳维亚男性的死亡率更高,而亚洲则最低。

一部分前列腺癌是侵袭性的,死亡风险很高。不幸的是,这些患者直到局部进展或转移时才会出现症状。老年男性的前列腺癌通常生长缓慢或无痛。可通过病理分级和基因组检测来区分有临床指征和无临床指征的局限性前列腺癌。

筛查和诊断方法

直肠指检(DRE)的目的是发现硬结节区,并提示前列腺癌发生风险。DRE有三个主要的局限性:该检测高度依赖于操作者;大多数可触及的癌症已不是早期癌症;很多临床上重要的前列腺癌位于触诊难以触及的区域。DRE常被推荐作为筛查的一部分,因为它可以检测到其他检测遗漏的前列腺癌;可预测分级较高的疾病;成本低;并能检测其他异常,如良性前列腺增生。即便如此,在早期的欧洲前列腺癌随机研究中,尽管在PSA值处于正常范围(<4.0ng/ml)的患者中,有四分之一到三分之一的前列腺癌是由DRE检测到的,该研究认为DRE作为一种独立的检测手段,其价值仍然有限[88]。

前列腺特异抗原(PSA)是一种由前列腺上皮成分分泌的糖蛋白。前列腺癌的进展与血清PSA升高相关。20世纪80年代早期,血清PSA测定首次被用于监测转移性疾病。截至1992年,该检查在患者中已有很高的接受度,并成为美国广泛使用的筛查方法。然而,很久以后才将其反应特征研究清楚[89]。现在我们已经知道血清PSA在除癌症外的多种情况下也会升高,如良性前列腺增生、炎症、腺体损伤等。PSA筛查法既能筛查出前列腺癌,也会漏掉很多患者。PSA筛查是否能降低死亡率是当今癌症医学最紧迫的问题之一[90]。

越来越多的证据支持PSA检测单独或与DRE联用可以有效地发现局部疾病[88,91]。约有四分之一年龄≥50岁的男性的PSA>4ng/dl,他们最终会通过活检被诊断罹患前列腺癌。降低截断值可使检测更加敏感,但同时也降低了其特异性。

前列腺癌预防试验(PCPT)随机选取了19 000多名年龄≥55岁、初始PSA为3.0ng/ml的男性,并将其随机分为服用非那雄胺或安慰剂组[92]。受试者每年接受一次血清PSA和DRE筛查,该筛查持续了7年(共8次),试验中14%的受试者被诊断罹患前列腺癌。在PSA和DRE正常的男性中,另有14%在研究终点时通过前列腺活检被诊断罹患前列腺癌[92]。而在PCPT中超过25%的男性被诊断罹患前列腺癌,这一比例显著偏高,表明该研究存在过度诊断。PCPT还显示,将4ng/ml作为PSA值的正常上限,或将PSA在一年内增加1ng/ml作为标准而漏诊的患者与诊断出的患者的数量相似。PSA筛查没有自然的界值。事实上,有些前列腺癌患者诊断时血清PSA<0.6ng/ml[89]。

经直肠超声(TRUS)将小的直肠探头放置在前列腺上部,可以使整个腺体成像。然而,前列腺癌并没有特定的可供评估的超声特征。单一采用TRUS进行筛查,其敏感性和特异性均较差。但它可用来准确测量腺体的大小和体积,并指导前列腺穿刺活检。

直肠内MRI不用于筛查,但其正逐步在前列腺诊断评估和确诊患者的随访中发挥作用。

前列腺癌治疗的临床试验

在PSA检测时代开始之前,一项研究对767名局限性前列腺癌患者进行了随访,发现其中仅少部分人死于前列腺癌,这意味着出现了很高比例的过度诊断。经过20年的随访,Gleason评分2~4分,5分和6分的患者比例分别为4%~7%、6%~11%、18%~30%,只有这些患者死于前列腺癌[87]。该研究提出了一个问题,对局部或局部晚期前列腺癌进行治疗是否有益,是否可以挽救生命。20世纪90年代末发表的前瞻性随机对照试验首次证明了对局部晚期患者进行治疗是有积极效果的。这些研究表明,放疗和激素治疗比单纯放疗更有优势[94,95]。

2002年,斯堪的那维亚前列腺癌小组-4研究(SPCG-4)首次证明局部疾病治疗可以挽救生命。他们随机选择了695名患有临床局限性前列腺癌的男性进行根治性前列腺切除术或观察等待,如有必要则进行激素治疗。随访发现(中位随访时间12.8年),前列腺切除术组有14.6%的患者死亡,而观察等待组有20.7%的患者死亡($RR=0.75, P=0.007$)。预防一例死亡所需的治疗人数为15人。该研究中只有不到15%的参与者的PSA检测呈阳性[96]。我们可以预测,在经过筛选的人群中,预防癌症死亡所需要的治疗人数会更高。

前列腺干预与观察试验(PIVOT)随机选择了731名PSA筛查为阳性的前列腺癌患者进行根治性前列腺切除术或观察等待[97]。随访发现(中位随访时间12年),前列腺切除术可导致患者的死亡率绝对值降低2.9%,同时可使前列腺癌的特异性死亡率降低2.6%,但均无统计学意义。亚组分析表明,PSA>10ng/ml的男性和中度及高危患者的死亡率有一定程度的降低,虽然这一比例较小,但具有统计学意义[97]。

总的来说,SPCG-4和PIVOT研究表明,治疗性干预在确诊的患者中仅拯救了少部分人的生命,还有相当一部分确诊为前列腺癌的男性被过度诊断和过度治疗,研究者也正在努力区分这部分患者。

前列腺癌的筛查效果

自从1989年FDA批准PSA用于前列腺癌的随诊后,前列腺癌的筛查率急剧上升。之后FDA批准了PSA用于疑似疾病的诊断，但不用于筛查。血液检测操作的简便性使得在健康展会和社区活动中进行大规模的 PSA 筛查成为可能，由于检出率的提高，美国的前列腺癌发病率也随之上升。

在 PSA 检测被批准之前的 20 年里，前列腺癌的死亡率也一直在上升。1993 年其发病率达到顶峰，自那以后，美国经年龄调整的前列腺癌死亡率下降了 40%[98]。尚不清楚这种下降在多大程度上是由于筛查造成的。Etzioni 和 Feuer[99]认为，考虑到前列腺癌的自然病程是长期的，在广泛开展 PSA 检测的头十年中其死亡率的下降不太可能完全归因于 PSA 检测。前列腺癌死亡率在 21 个国家有所下降[100]。在美国和少数的其他国家 PSA 筛查是很常见的。

前列腺癌死亡率下降的可能原因有：①将前列腺癌归类为潜在死亡原因的趋势发生了改变，②不同阶段前列腺癌治疗水平的显著提高[101]。20 世纪 70 年代末随着死亡率开始上升，世界卫生组织（WHO）改变了用于判定死因的算法，并在 1991 年恢复使用较老的算法，几乎与此同时前列腺癌的死亡率开始下降，这可以作为支持原因一的证据[102]。以下证据支持原因二：前列腺癌在老年男性中高发，通过有效的治疗，即使中位生存期增加 2~3 个月，也可能导致前列腺癌的死亡率下降，因为其他死因的权重也在增加。也有人推测，过度使用新的激素疗法可能会增加心血管疾病相关的死亡，从而减少了前列腺疾病的死亡[103]。综上所述，除了筛查可能有积极的预防作用外，以上三种方法都可能导致了美国前列腺癌死亡率的下降。

流行病学研究表明，截至 2000 年，前列腺癌远端转移的诊断率出现了显著的下降。假设筛查会导致疾病诊断由远端转移转换到局部疾病，NCI 的癌症干预预警模型网络（CISNET）估计美国前列腺癌死亡率下降的 45%~70%归因于筛查所致的疾病诊断阶段的转化[99]。

总之，评估筛查效果最有效的方法是长期的、设置死亡率终点的大型前瞻性随机对照试验。目前已有 5 项此类试验，但都有一定的局限性。美国 NCI 多中心前列腺、肺、结肠直肠和卵巢试验（PLCO）和欧洲多中心随机前列腺癌研究（ERSPC）的质量更高[88,91]。

PLCO 于 1992 年启动[91]，近 77 000 名年龄在 55~74 岁之间的男性被随机分配进行年度 PSA 检查或常规检查，观察期为 6 年。在 13 年的随访中，随机分配接受年度筛查的男性前列腺癌死亡率出现了增加，且具有统计学意义（RR = 1.09，95% CI，0.87~1.36）[91]。本试验有一个局限性，即对照组的 PSA 检测率高，并降低了数据的权重。相比筛查与不接受筛查，PLCO 是常规筛查与机会性筛查的最佳对比方式。

ERSPC 于 1991 年启动[88]，7 个国家最终报告了结果。对 182 160 名年龄在 50~74 岁之间的男性进行的初步分析发现，前列腺癌特异性死亡率并没有降低，但 55~69 岁男性的前列腺癌特异性死亡率显著下降。该研究的中位随访时间为 11 年，并在第 13 年进行数据校正，前列腺癌死亡率相对降低了 21%（RR=0.79，95% CI 0.68~0.91）。随访 11 年统计发现，预防一例前列腺癌死亡需要诊断和治疗的男性为 37 例，在 13 年时，数据经校正后为 27 例[104~106]。

将 ERSPC 的发现应用到美国人口中，意味着每 200 名筛查确诊的男性中，约有 8 人在 13 年后存活；而每 200 名接受根治性前列腺切除术的男性中，就有 1 人死于手术。剩下的 191 名男性将经历诊断和治疗的不良影响，但他们罹患前列腺癌的命运却不会改变。13 年后，其中 32 名男性会死于前列腺癌，目前还不清楚剩下的 159 名幸存者中有多少人将来会死于前列腺癌。

如果除去这部分瑞典的参与者，ERSPC 试验的结果是阴性的。瑞典的筛查效果非常好，荷兰的筛查效果也略有成效，整体而言四个国家的筛查在统计学上患者并没有受益的趋势。ERSPC 中芬兰接受筛查的人群占比最高，但在随访 12 年后并没有表现出受益的证据[107]。瑞典的筛查结果更好有可能是由以下原因造成的：一、前列腺癌死亡的风险更高；二、瑞典的随机方案可能在筛查组中产生了一种“健康志愿者”的选择偏倚，而在对照组中并没有这种偏倚。筛查组患者是知情的，而对照组并不知道他们处于临床试验中[101]。

筛查建议

美国、欧洲和加拿大的一些专业机构已经发布了前列腺癌的筛查指南，这些机构也都担心筛查的风险收益比。目前普遍认同，只有在被筛查者完全知情同意的情况下才能进行筛查，且需要由本人和医生共同做出决定[108~110]。指南不支持在公共场所进行大规模的筛查。ERSPC 的研究者也认为数据不支持广泛的筛查[106]。

ACS 2010 指南指出，前列腺癌早期检测的利害关系尚不明确，现有的证据也不足以支持推荐或反对常规的 PSA 筛查[109]。美国癌症协会呼吁是否接受筛查应由医患进行充分讨论后共同决定。

USPSTF 2012 指南认为有足够的证据支持 PSA 检测弊大于利，因此建议不要常规使用 PSA 进行筛查[10]。工作组也表示，一些男性将继续要求筛查，他们的医生也将继续提供筛查。与 ACS 和 AUA 类似，他们认为在这种情况下的筛查应该尊重知情患者的选择[10]。

2013 年，AUA 对 300 多项研究进行了系统回顾并更新了指南[110]。该研究得出结论，55~69 岁的男性从筛查中获益最大，尽管“仅有中等强度的证据表明筛查有益，而筛查危害的证据却很强。”即使是 55~69 岁的男性，AUA 也将医患共同判断利弊平衡并决策放在首位[111]。委员会建议每两年进行一次筛查，不必每年一次；建议以下人群不必接受筛查：40 岁以下的男性、40~54 岁的平均风险男性、大部分超过 70 岁的男性和预期寿命小于 10~15 年的男性。他们建议对 40~54 岁的高危男性和大于 70 岁健康状况良好的男性进行个体化筛查。

笔者认为，男性应该被告知筛查的潜在好处和相关的危害，尤其是过度诊断的风险。对于大多数人来说，观察是合理的选择。做出筛查决定时还应保证一旦诊断为癌症，不要即刻采取激进的治疗方法。

肺癌

无论是在美国还是在世界范围内，肺癌都是最常见的非皮肤类癌症，也是男性癌症死亡的主要原因和女性癌症死亡的第二大原因[11,19]。

筛查和诊断方法

20 世纪 50 年代初首次提倡使用胸部 X 光检查用于筛查，

到1960年,已开展了多项肺癌筛查运动。始于1971年的“梅奥肺项目”(Mayo Lung Project,MLP)招募了9 200多名男性吸烟者,每4个月或每年随机对他们进行一次胸透和痰细胞学检查,为期6年,该项目一直随访到现在[112,113]。经过13年和20年的随访,经过严格筛查被诊断出的肺癌的数量大量增加,疾病特异性生存率也显著提高[113,114]。但肺癌导致的死亡率并未降低,表明筛查可在不降低死亡率的情况下提高患者的生存率。在另一项研究中,筛查组约有18%的癌症被判断为过度诊断[115]。另外三项大型随机试验采用不同的筛查计划进行胸透和痰细胞学研究,也同样证实了MLP的发现[116,117]。

这些胸透研究非常有局限性,没有随机选择未筛查的对照组,并且这些研究中使用的是20世纪60年代到70年代的X光检查和治疗技术。美国PLCO重新评估了肺癌筛查的有效性[118]。参与者被随机分配进行为期4年的年度前后视图胸片筛查或常规检查(不筛查),中位随访时间为12年,PLCO没有发现X线胸片筛查对降低死亡率有优势[119]。

螺旋计算机断层扫描(CT)对小结节的诊断比胸透更敏感。低剂量计算机断层扫描(LDCT)使用平均1.5mSv的辐射在15秒内进行肺部扫描,这一技术促进了2002年NLST的启动[120]。大约53 000名肺癌高危人群被随机分配到2组,分别接受3次年度LDCT或单次前后胸部的X光检查。该研究的中位随访时间为6.5年,与接受胸部X光检查组相比,LDCT扫描组肺癌的死亡率相对降低了20%(95% CI 6.8~26.7;P=0.004)[120]。这相当于肺癌死亡率分别为247人和309人每10万人每年。LDCT组中患者的全因死亡率降低了6.7%(95%CI 1.2~13.6;P=0.02),这在前瞻性随机对照试验中较为少见。肺癌筛查避免了大量的高风险参与者的死亡,而在风险很低的参与者中几乎没有预防作用。这些发现为基于风险的筛查提供了实证支持[121]。

LDCT筛查显然是有前景的,但也有局限性。在全国肺筛查试验(NLST)中,96.4%的阳性结果是不真实的[120]。阳性结果需要额外的检查证实,主要是常规的CT扫描,但在某些情况下,需要进行穿刺活检、支气管镜、纵隔镜或开胸,这些额外的检查必然会造成患者的焦虑情绪、额外的花费和并发症(如肺活检后的气胸或血胸)。NLST报告显示接受侵入性诊断手术后的60天内有16例患者死亡;这一操作是否是死因尚不明确。在这些参与者中,6人未患癌症。因此,评估算法以减少侵入性的诊断程序也越来越引起关注[122,123]。

筛查的其他危害包括理论上由LDCT和过度诊断导致的辐射可能会诱发癌症。据估算NLST中过度诊断率约为18.5%(95% CI 5.4~30.6%)[124]。有趣的是,这与MLP中得出的结论非常相似[112]。虽然过度诊断无法在在世的人身上证明,但一项尸检研究发现有六分之一的肺癌在死亡前并没有得到诊断[125]。也有人认为NLST需要更长时间的随访才能准确地对过度诊断进行估算。

筛查建议

ACS,美国胸科医师学会(AACP)和美国临床肿瘤学会(ASCO)建议临床医生与符合以下NLST筛查标准的患者讨论是否接受筛查:年龄为55~74岁、有吸烟史,每年吸烟量≥30包,目前吸烟或在过去的15年里戒烟,健康状况相对良好。

讨论应包括与LDCT筛查肺癌相关的益处、不确定性和危害。选择接受肺癌筛查的人应在具备LDCT检查的专业机构加入相应的筛查项目,该机构还应具备擅长评估、诊断和治疗异常肺部病变的多学科团队。如果没有高质量的筛查项目,筛查导致危害的风险可能大于受益[70,126]。指南还建议只要受试者一经确诊为肺癌可通过治疗延长生命,就应接受每年进行一次的LDCT。所有筛查指南均强调应帮助吸烟者戒烟。

睾丸癌

睾丸癌相对来说并不高发[11],而且治疗通常很成功。超过70%的转移性睾丸癌的患者可获得长期完全缓解。

筛查和诊断方法

睾丸癌的诊断通常是由于患者或医生发现了阴囊异常而被诊断。可疑肿块需通过超声和活检进一步评估。

虽然睾丸的自我触诊很简单,但现有的数据表明,它的特异性和预测价值都很低,即使提倡这种检查,频率也不会太高[127]。自我检查会导致错误的预警,给医疗系统带来负担并增加医疗成本。健康教育可能是较为实用的干预措施,应鼓励男性在发现肿块或结节或睾丸的大小、形状与以往相比发生变化时及时就医。患者在意识到睾丸异常后的延迟就诊与生存率不佳显著相关。

筛查建议

对平均风险的男性不建议进行睾丸癌的常规筛查。美国家庭医师学会建议,对于13~39岁,有隐睾症、睾丸固定术或睾丸萎缩病史的高危男性应进行睾丸触诊[127]。

肝细胞癌

肝细胞癌(HCC)是全球第四大常见癌症[128]。中国的年龄标准化发病率是北美的40倍。美国的发病率也在升高[11]。

慢性乙型和丙型肝炎是主要的风险因素。其他风险因素包括酒精性肝硬化、血色素沉着、抗胰蛋白酶缺乏症、糖原储积病、迟发性皮肤卟啉症、酪氨酸血症和肝豆状核变性[128]。在非洲部分地区,HCC的高发病率可能与摄入受黄曲霉毒素污染的食物有关。

目前,有四种类型的肿瘤标志物被用于或适用于筛查试验:癌胚抗原和糖蛋白抗原、酶和同工酶、基因和细胞因子[129]。血清AFP是一种胎儿特异性糖蛋白抗原,在筛查中应用最为广泛。在高危人群中,其检测敏感性为39%~97%,特异性为76%~95%,阳性预测值(PPV)为9%~32%。AFP不是HCC的特异性指标,在肝炎、怀孕和生殖细胞肿瘤中也会升高[128]。

已有研究将超声和CT成像作为AFP的辅助筛查手段[130]。这些试验的敏感性和特异性有限。在中国开展的一项前瞻性随机研究使用了AFP和肝脏超声检查(US)作为筛查方法,该研究发现筛查组中HCC的死亡率较低[83.2 vs 131.5/100 000,死亡率比为0.63(95% CI 0.41~0.98)]。这项研究的结果在不同的报道中有所不同,目前还不清楚这是否是有意进行的筛选分析[131,132]。

筛查建议

一般人群中不提倡进行筛查，而在高危人群中筛查的优势仍受到质疑。

子宫内膜癌

子宫内膜癌是最常见的妇科恶性肿瘤，在美国和西欧，大约有四分之一的子宫内膜癌在诊断时已处于晚期。

筛查和诊断方法

子宫内膜癌筛查的有效性从未在前瞻性 RCT 中评估过。Pap 检查偶尔可显示子宫内膜异常，但该检测对于鉴别子宫内膜癌并不敏感，不应用来进行子宫内膜癌的筛查。筛查的金标准是子宫内膜活检。近来，经阴道超声（TVU）筛查也引起了关注[133]。两项设计严谨的研究采用了 TVU 和活检进行筛查，筛查结果令人失望，并且出现了明显的伤害，例如子宫穿孔。

筛查建议

目前，不建议对一般风险的女性进行子宫内膜癌的常规筛查。美国癌症学会建议绝经期女性了解子宫内膜癌的风险和症状，并强烈建议向医生报告不明原因的出血或点状出血[134]。

美国癌症学会建议对子宫内膜癌高危的女性采取基于风险的筛查方法[69]。高风险女性包括携带 HNPCC 相关突变（Lynch 综合征）、已知亲属携带突变而有携带突变风险、家庭成员中疑似有结肠癌常染色体显性遗传倾向但未经基因检测证实的女性[269]。在充分讨论筛查受益、风险和局限性的基础上，罹患或怀疑患有 Lynch 综合征的女性应在 35 岁开始接受子宫内膜检查[84]。

卵巢癌

卵巢癌是所有妇科癌症中死亡率最高的，死亡人数占美国所有癌症死亡人数的 6%[11]。最近的研究表明，很多所谓的卵巢癌实际上是原发性输卵管癌，还有少数表现为原发性腹壁肿瘤。大多数女性在出现症状后被诊断为“卵巢癌”，但只有 19%的患者病变部位在卵巢[19]。

筛查和诊断方法

盆腔检查：对卵巢癌检测的敏感性和特异性都很低，因此不能单独用来筛查。然而，最近的研究表明如果对早期症状进行评估，可能会得到更准确的诊断。

CA-125 是研究最广泛的卵巢癌血清标志物。它是一种肿瘤相关抗原，主要用于上皮性卵巢癌手术切除后的监测。目前使用的检测方法——CA-125 Ⅱ同时使用了 OC125 和 MC11 两种抗体[135]。CA-125 水平>30~35U/ml 即为异常。虽然大多数晚期卵巢癌患者的 CA-125 水平升高，但只有一半的早期卵巢癌患者的检测结果呈阳性。此外，非癌性卵巢疾病患者的 CA-125 水平也可升高[136]，存在其他癌症、有既往激素使用史以及吸烟均可影响 CA-125 的水平。

超声检查：腹部超声检查的特异性低，因此在卵巢癌筛查中的应用效果不佳[137]。经阴道超声检查（TVU）能发现小肿块，但对恶性肿瘤的诊断能力较差。彩色多普勒超声用于区分良恶性肿块被寄予了厚望，但研究显示它并没有提高诊断的准确性。目前的数据不能支持独立的 TVU 或其他影像方法用于筛查平均风险的无症状女性[138]。

CA-125 和超声联合：一般和高危女性的非随机队列研究表明，单独使用 CA-125 或超声（腹部或阴道）的特异性水平尚可接受，但敏感性有限，阳性试验的预测价值较低。筛查的高特异性尤其重要，因为当筛查呈阳性时，需要腹腔镜和/或开腹手术来排除卵巢癌。前瞻性随机对照试验中已经评估了联合使用 CA-125、ROC CA-125 算法和成像的多模式方法。PLCO 是前瞻性的 RCT，它招募了 78 237 名年龄在 55~74 岁之间的女性，共有 39 115 名患者被随机分配接受卵巢癌筛查，接受基线 CA-125 和 TVU 检测，然后再进行 3 次年度 TVU 和 5 次 CA-125 检查。研究发现 1 万名女性中每年有 2.1 人死于卵巢癌，而对照组为 2.6 人（RR=1.18，95% CI 0.82~1.71）。

同时也开展了一些针对卵巢癌高危女性的筛查研究[138]。英国卵巢癌筛查联合试验（UKCTOCS）[139,140]将 20 万年龄 50~74 岁平均风险的绝经后女性随机分配到常规检查组（n=10 万）；CA-125 及超声检测后进行包含了血清 CA-125 检测的年度多模式筛查（n=50 000）；或持续 7 年的年度超声筛查，6~8 周后重复检查（n=50 000）。该研究发现多模式筛查将总体平均死亡率降低了 20%（RR=0.80，95% CI 0.60~0.98）。

血清蛋白组学：模式识别算法正在开发中，用来识别关键的肽段集合以区分卵巢癌病例和对照。将单独或辅助蛋白质组检测用以卵巢癌筛查的前景广阔，但目前仍未实现。

筛查建议

大型组织机构不建议对中等风险的女性进行卵巢癌筛查，USPSTF 尤其不建议进行筛查[141]。1994 年 NIH 共识委员会得出结论，所有女性都应进行详细的家族病史采集，应该为两名或两名以上一级亲属有卵巢癌患病史的女性提供妇科肿瘤医生（或其他专科医生）咨询，因为这些女性有 3%的机会患遗传性卵巢癌综合征[142]。对于已知患有遗传性卵巢癌综合征的女性，如 BRCA1 和 BRCA2 基因存在突变，包括乳腺-卵巢癌综合征，特定位点的卵巢癌综合征以及 HNPCC，应进行年度直肠阴道盆腔检查、CA-125 检查以及 TVU 直到生育或 35 岁，之后建议进行预防性双侧卵巢切除术。据估算，患有这些遗传综合征的女性仅为 0.05%，而她们一生中患卵巢癌的风险约为 40%。

黑色素瘤和其他皮肤癌

皮肤癌在世界范围内以及在美国都很常见，几乎占所有恶性肿瘤的一半[11]。最常见的是基底细胞癌和鳞状细胞癌，被称为非黑色素瘤皮肤癌（NMSC）。虽然延迟诊断和治疗可能会导致高发病率，但 NMSC 是可以治愈的。但黑色素瘤却是癌症死亡的重要原因之一。在美国，虽然黑色素瘤占所有皮肤癌病例的 2%，但绝大多数皮肤癌的死亡病例是由黑色素瘤引起的。

筛查和诊断方法

近年来，由于死亡率不断上升，人们对黑色素瘤筛查的兴趣日益增长。其筛查主要由临床医生视诊或自行视诊完成，最好对皮肤进行2~3分钟的全面检查，因为皮肤癌通常发生在没有直接暴露在阳光下的部位。在美国，医疗保健人员通常不进行皮肤检查，皮肤科医生检查比初级保健医生更常见。皮肤基底细胞癌可能表现为扁平生长或小的隆起的粉红色或红色半透明发亮区域，在轻微损伤后可能会出血。皮肤鳞状细胞癌可以表现为一个逐渐变大的肿块，通常表面粗糙，也可以表现为一个扁平、略带红色、生长缓慢的斑块。黑色素瘤表现为大小、形状或颜色随时间变化的痣或其他皮肤病变，被总结为一种ABCD算法，该算法描述了病变的不对称性[A]、边界的不均匀[B]、颜色的变化[C]和直径的变化[D]。Cochrane综述支持增加"E"类，即"进化"，以强调病变随时间变化的重要性。然而，大多数皮肤科医生似乎更倾向于通过整体的外观（难看程度）进行诊断，而不会对特征进行逐步评估。

病例对照研究表明，提高对黑色素瘤及其症状的认识可以早日发现病变，或在病变厚度较薄时及时发现[143]。与有病史者或对照的人群相比，经皮肤科医生常规筛查诊断的高危患者在诊断时的病灶往往较薄。

自1985年以来，美国皮肤病学会皮肤癌筛查项目已经筛查了超过60万不同风险类别的人[144]。除了检测到超过35 000个NMSC外，通过筛查诊断的黑色素瘤与以往的对照相比更有可能小于1.5mm。皮肤癌在高危人群中的筛查效能更高，例如年龄为>20岁的非典型痣综合征、先天性黑素细胞痣的白人患者、具有特殊表型特征的患者或有NMSC病史的患者[144]。

目前尚无RCT评估皮肤癌筛查是否能降低死亡率。一些大型的观察性研究认为它是有效的。苏格兰发起了一项筛查活动，旨在提高人们对黑色素瘤的认识并早期发现黑色素瘤，此次活动的结果发现筛查可能与患者的死亡率下降有关。在德国某地区开展了一项为筛查有效性提供证据的皮肤癌研究项目，该项目共有36万名参与者[145,146]。尽管筛查中出现了很多假阳性，但在2年的时间内，男性黑色素瘤的发病率提高16%，女性提高38%，并在干预期结束后恢复到基线水平。干预期结束的五年后，该地区黑色素瘤的死亡率仅为德国其他地区的一半[147,148]。澳大利亚也正在开展一项基于社区的自查与临床皮肤检查相互对比的随机试验，该研究在随访15年后将得出黑色素瘤死亡率的统计[69,149]。

筛查建议

美国癌症协会建议在定期的体检中进行皮肤检查[69]。美国预防医学学会建议对高危人群进行定期的皮肤全面检查，包括白种人、白皮肤的人、存在色素沉着病变（发育不良或非典型痣）、若干大的非瘤性的色素痣、数量较多的小痣、中度雀斑或家族性发育不良痣综合征等。

USPSTF建议大家警惕皮肤异常，尤其是高危人群[149]。任务小组（The Taskforce）则认为还不能确定将全身皮肤检查作为常规筛查项目是否能够早期发现皮肤黑色素瘤、基底细胞癌或鳞状细胞皮肤癌。

口腔癌

男性口腔癌比女性高发[11]，大约三分之一的口腔癌被诊断时处于局部阶段[150]。

筛查和诊断方法

口腔癌一般可由患者及医护人员（尤其是牙科医生）进行检查时发现。为提高筛查的效率，可着重检查90%的鳞状细胞癌发生的高危部位，如口腔底、舌腹侧方和软腭复合体。白斑和红斑病变是鳞状细胞癌最早和最严重的症状[151]。虽然新的筛检技术还在评估中，例如甲苯胺蓝检查、细胞刷检、组织反射率和自体荧光技术，但尚无确凿的证据表明任何一种新的技术优于传统的口腔检查。

印度喀拉拉邦开展了一项聚类随机对照试验，将年龄≥35岁的高危男性和女性随机分为三组，每隔3年由专业的卫生工作者进行3轮口腔视诊[152]。与对照组相比，干预组的96 517名参与者的口腔癌死亡人数减少了21%（RR=0.79，95%CI 0.51~1.22），相比吸烟者和饮酒者群体，干预组死亡人数减少高达34%。

虽然有些人主张把口腔检查作为牙科和内科诊所体检的一部分，但这一建议未被广泛接受，因此口腔体检并未得到推广。实际上，口腔癌风险最高的人（吸烟者和酗酒者）接受牙科和内科检查的可能性比风险较低的人还要小。需要警惕的常见症状包括唇或口腔溃疡、口腔出血、口腔或牙龈持续出现白色或红色斑块、口腔肿胀和/或疼痛、喉咙痛和吞咽困难。

结论

在短期内，减少癌症死亡最有效的方法还是早期发现和合理治疗。由于可行性的限制、资源的不足、质量的参差不齐以及合理系统的缺乏，早期筛查的益处并没有在全球范围内普及。无论是个体水平还是群体，机会性筛查都不如系统性筛查高效。我们需要建立一个早期发现和干预的综合系统，提高参与度，并更好地应用任何能够改善疾病控制的早期筛查新技术，确保项目中所有的要素高效运行并相互关联和依赖。系统的方法不仅有可能提高质量，还有可能减少小错误的数量，避免筛查效率逐渐下降，同时还可以避免导致不必要死亡的大错误。虽然要建立真正的以人群为基础的筛查项目必须克服许多实际障碍，但有组织的筛查系统最有可能实现降低晚期癌症发病率的目标，从而避免过早死亡。

（陈淑桢 译 孙文 何慧斯 校）

部分参考文献

1 Croswell JM, Ransohoff DF, Kramer BS. Principles of cancer screening: lessons from history and study design issues. *Semin Oncol*. 2010;**37**:202–215.

3 Welch HG, Black WC. Overdiagnosis in cancer. *J Natl Cancer Inst*. 2010;**102**:605–613.

4 Baker SG, Prorok PC, Kramer BS. Lead time and overdiagnosis. *J Natl Cancer Inst*. 2014;**106**:109.

8 Marmot MG, Altman DG, Cameron DA, Dewar JA, Thompson SG, Wilcox M. The benefits and harms of breast cancer screening: an independent review. *Br J Cancer*. 2013;**108**:2205–2240.

10 Moyer VA. Screening for prostate cancer: U.S. preventive services task force recommendation statement. *Ann Intern Med*. 2012;**157**:120–134.

16 Nelson HD, Zakher B, Cantor A, et al. Risk factors for breast cancer for women aged 40 to 49 years: a systematic review and meta-analysis. *Ann Intern Med*. 2012;**156**:635–648. doi: 10.7326/0003-4819-156-9-201205010-00006.

18 U.S. Preventive Services Task Force. Screening for breast cancer: U.S. Preventive Services Task Force recommendation statement. *Ann Intern Med*. 2009;**151**:716–726, W-236.

20 Mandelblatt J, van Ravesteyn N, Schechter C, et al. Which strategies reduce breast cancer mortality most? Collaborative modeling of optimal screening, treatment, and obesity prevention. *Cancer*. 2013;**119**:2541–2548.

21 Harris R, Yeatts J, Kinsinger L. Breast cancer screening for women ages 50 to 69 years a systematic review of observational evidence. *Prev Med*. 2011;**53**:108–114.

25 Smith RA, Manassaram-Baptiste D, Brooks D, et al. Cancer screening in the United States, 2014: a review of current American Cancer Society guidelines and current issues in cancer screening. *CA Cancer J Clin*. 2014;**64**:30–51.

29 Berry DA, Cronin KA, Plevritis SK, et al. Effect of screening and adjuvant therapy on mortality from breast cancer. *N Engl J Med*. 2005;**353**:1784–1792.

36 Esserman LJ, Thompson IM Jr, Reid B. Overdiagnosis and overtreatment in cancer: an opportunity for improvement. *JAMA*. 2013;**310**:797–798.

38 Saslow D, Boates C, Burke W, et al. American Cancer Society guidelines for breast screening with MRI as an adjunct to mammography. *CA Cancer J Clin*. 2007;**57**:90–104. Available on line at http://caonline.amcancersoc.org.

47 Shaukat A, Mongin SJ, Geisser MS, et al. Long-term mortality after screening for colorectal cancer. *N Engl J Med*. 2013;**369**:1106–1114.

48 Mandel JS, Church TR, Bond JH, et al. The effect of fecal occult-blood screening on the incidence of colorectal cancer. *N Engl J Med*. 2000;**343**:1603–1607.

51 Burch JA, Soares-Weiser K, St John DJ, et al. Diagnostic accuracy of faecal occult blood tests used in screening for colorectal cancer: a systematic review. *J Med Screen*. 2007;**14**:132–137.

52 Imperiale TF, Ransohoff DF, Itzkowitz SH, et al. Multitarget stool DNA testing for colorectal-cancer screening. *N Engl J Med*. 2014;**370**:1287–1297.

60 Mandel JS, Bond JH, Church TR, et al. Reducing mortality from colorectal cancer by screening for fecal occult blood. Minnesota Colon Cancer Control Study [published erratum appears in N Engl J Med 1993 26;329(9):672]. *N Engl J Med*. 1993;**328**:1365–1371.

68 Levin B, Lieberman DA, McFarland B, et al. Screening and surveillance for the early detection of colorectal cancer and adenomatous polyps, 2008: a joint guideline from the American Cancer Society, the US Multi-Society Task Force on Colorectal Cancer, and the American College of Radiology. *CA Cancer J Clin*. 2008;**58**:130–160.

73 Janerich DT, Hadjimichael O, Schwartz PE, et al. The screening histories of women with invasive cervical cancer, Connecticut. *Am J Public Health*. 1995;**85**:791–794.

74 Kulasingam SL, Havrilesky L, Ghebre R, Myers ER. *U.S. Preventive Services Task Force Evidence Syntheses, Formerly Systematic Evidence Reviews. Screening for Cervical Cancer: A Decision Analysis for the US Preventive Services Task Force*. Rockville, MD: Agency for Healthcare Research and Quality (US); 2011.

75 Solomon D, Davey D, Kurman R, et al. The 2001 Bethesda System: terminology for reporting results of cervical cytology. *JAMA*. 2002;**287**:2114–2119.

84 Sankaranarayanan R, Nene BM, Shastri SS, et al. HPV screening for cervical cancer in rural India. *N Engl J Med*. 2009;**360**:1385–1394.

85 Moyer VA. Screening for cervical cancer: U.S. Preventive Services Task Force recommendation statement. *Ann Intern Med*. 2012;**156**:880–891, W312.

86 Saslow D, Solomon D, Lawson HW, et al. American Cancer Society, American Society for Colposcopy and Cervical Pathology, and American Society for Clinical Pathology screening guidelines for the prevention and early detection of cervical cancer. *CA Cancer J Clin*. 2012;**62**:147–172.

87 Albertsen PC, Hanley JA, Fine J. 20-year outcomes following conservative management of clinically localized prostate cancer. *JAMA*. 2005;**293**:2095–2101.

88 Schroder FH, Hugosson J, Roobol MJ, et al. Screening and prostate-cancer mortality in a randomized European study. *N Engl J Med*. 2009;**360**:1320–1328.

89 Thompson IM, Ankerst DP, Chi C, et al. Operating characteristics of prostate-specific antigen in men with an initial PSA level of 3.0 ng/ml or lower. *JAMA*. 2005;**294**:66–70.

91 Andriole GL, Crawford ED, Grubb RL 3rd, et al. Mortality results from a randomized prostate-cancer screening trial. *N Engl J Med*. 2009;**360**:1310–1319.

97 Wilt TJ, Brawer MK, Jones KM, et al. Radical prostatectomy versus observation for localized prostate cancer. *N Engl J Med*. 2012;**367**:203–213.

106 Schroder FH, Hugosson J, Roobol MJ, et al. Screening and prostate cancer mortality: results of the European Randomised Study of Screening for Prostate Cancer (ERSPC) at 13 years of follow-up. *Lancet*. 2014;**384**:2027–2035.

107 Kilpelainen TP, Tammela TL, Malila N, et al. Prostate cancer mortality in the Finnish randomized screening trial. *J Natl Cancer Inst*. 2013;**105**:719–725.

110 Carter HB, Albertsen PC, Barry MJ, et al. Early detection of prostate cancer: AUA guideline. *J Urol*. 2013;**190**:419–426.

115 Marcus PM. Estimating overdiagnosis in lung cancer screening. *JAMA Intern Med*. 2014;**174**:1198.

120 Aberle DR, Berg CD, Black WC, et al. The National Lung Screening Trial: overview and study design. *Radiology*. 2011;**258**:243–253.

126 Bach PB, Mirkin JN, Oliver TK, et al. Benefits and harms of CT screening for lung cancer: a systematic review. *JAMA*. 2012;**307**:2418–2429.

131 Zhang BH, Yang BH, Tang ZY. Randomized controlled trial of screening for hepatocellular carcinoma. *J Cancer Res Clin Oncol*. 2004;**130**:417–422.

140 Goff BA, Mandel LS, Drescher CW, et al. Development of an ovarian cancer symptom index: possibilities for earlier detection. *Cancer*. 2007;**109**:221–227.

141 Moyer VA. Screening for ovarian cancer: U.S. Preventive Services Task Force reaffirmation recommendation statement. *Ann Intern Med*. 2012;**157**:900–904. doi: 10.7326/0003-4819-157-11-201212040-00539.

144 Geller AC, Zhang Z, Sober AJ, et al. The first 15 years of the American Academy of Dermatology skin cancer screening programs: 1985–1999. *J Am Acad Dermatol*. 2003;**48**:34–41.

第六篇

临床基本原则

第 39 章　病理新视角：预测临床疾病进程，精准靶定疾病病因

Carlos Cordon-Cardo，MD，PhD ■ Adolfo Firpo-Betancourt，MD，MPA

概述

病理学是基础医学与临床医学的桥梁学科，本章节通过阐述及机制论述，来了解疾病发展过程的病理变化和潜在分子事件。肿瘤性疾病因研究发展迅速而作为本章重点内容。病理学主要包括两个目标——解释疾病病因[来自"Pathos"（希腊语）"疾病"]及疾病分类，从而为临床提供诊断服务。现代病理学系还涉及教育内容，包括医学生培养、住院医师及从业人员培训；基于医院的临床服务则通常可以分为三个部门，包括解剖病理学（外科病理学、细胞学和尸检）、临床病理学（包括从血库和凝血到化学和微生物学等各种实验室服务），以及分子病理学（通常包含体细胞遗传学、细胞遗传学和流式细胞术）。过去的二十年，我们见证了从对疾病整体分析所做的组织学诊断到更客观及准确地针对个体化特征的研究转变过程。传统分类正转变为个体化分类，从而针对分类制定个性化治疗方案，以优化疗效与更精准预测预后（表 39-1）。这种综合诊疗模式推动了循证治疗方案的选择，产生高性价比和个体化的治疗方案。将重点以患者为中心进行疾病分类和辅助治疗选择，拓展至对治疗进行监测（如通过肿瘤基因型评估治疗指数和突变负荷），并能通过早期诊断来管理高危患者（图 39-1）。最终达到发现病因、针对病因进行有效治疗，并从医疗服务转向以人群为基础的健康医疗管理的目的。

表 39-1　从疾病常规诊断到综合预测平台的病理学演变

	经典病理学	分子和系统病理学
诊断和分期	对临床变量、组织病理学和生物标志物进行描述性分析，从而将患者分为不同疾病阶段；对治疗选择价值有限	对临床变量、组织形态学和肿瘤分子特征进行客观、定量多维度分析，以确定患者个体化肿瘤表型和基因型
预后评估	传统人群和队列分类用于推断疾病进展和治疗反应，通常是非特指	患者的疾病特征和分子肿瘤特征可用于预测药物敏感性和放疗反应，从而优化疗效
治疗选择	分组管理方法是将患者按照疾病类别进行分组，采用预先确定的基于人群的方案治疗，而不是患者特异性方案	个体化综合护理模式推动循证治疗方案的选择，以优化临床治疗效果为终点；患者个体化治疗能够提高生存率和生活质量
	将患者以疾病类别"分组"的诊断和预后方法	精准、预测性和高性价比；个体化患者管理

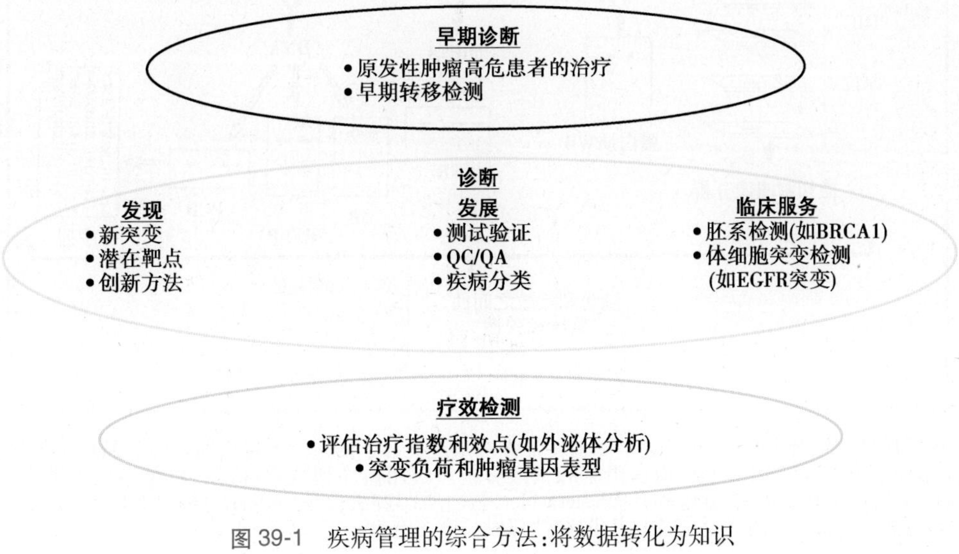

图 39-1　疾病管理的综合方法：将数据转化为知识

从解剖和临床病理到分子和预测性综合诊断

病理学的学术起源可以追溯到16世纪至17世纪的意大利。当时医生进行系统性尸检,以进一步了解疾病。正是在Benivieni(1443—1502年)和Morgagni(1682—1771年)所著的文字记载中,以详细尸检研究为基础,首次发现了临床病理相关性。这种描述性的大体解剖方法被以Bichat(1771—1802年)为代表的法国和英国的"组织病理学"学派所取代,最终定义以德国Muller(1801—1858年)和Virchow(1821—1902年)为代表的"细胞病理学"[1]。细胞被定义为生命的基本单元以及大多数疾病的发病基础,并通过所起源组织的病理学变化表现出来(图39-2)[2]。生物化学、免疫学和遗传学的发展被引进到临床医学领域中,并在20世纪中后期促进产生新的医疗技术设备。分子病理学即从这些研究中发展而来,将组织学与免疫组织化学(IHC)和遗传技术相结合,以检测相关的表型/基因型,从而建立患者个体化评估(图39-3)[3,4]。

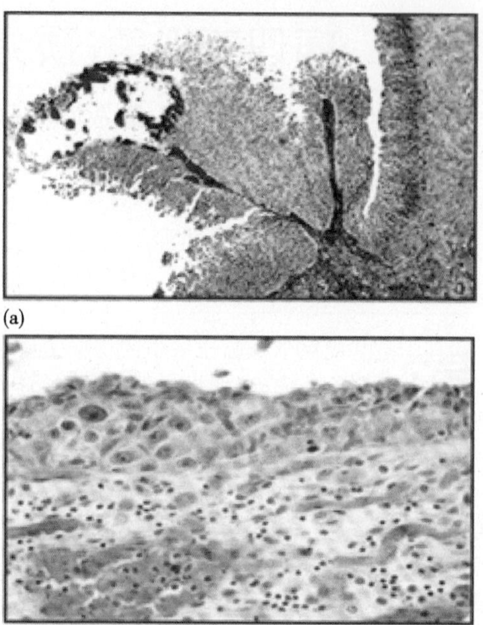

图39-2 (a,b)细胞分析。显微镜作为一种新型装置,能够让Dr. Rudolf Virchow(1821—1902年)实现将细胞描述为生命单元并探索病因。根据组织发生进行疾病分类。图显示为苏木精-伊红(HE)染色的肿瘤组织切片,高倍镜显示非浸润性乳头状移行细胞癌;低倍镜显示膀胱原位移行细胞癌

多年来病理学家的角色已经发生改变。传统病理学家的主要任务是通过人体组织的形态学分析和体液中某些化学物质和生物分子的分析来诊断患者。肿瘤的诊断包括对组织样本和体液进行分析,发现与恶性转化和肿瘤进展相关的特征。获取组织标本、细胞和液体(如血液、尿液和渗出液)途径包括手术活检、内窥镜活检、细针穿刺活检、静脉穿刺、骨髓穿刺、组织表面刮片以及从尿液或痰中收集脱落细胞。获取的组织或细胞标本经过一系列分析进行诊断。通过光镜评估标本的形态学特征,几乎是多年来唯一的诊断方法,并且与所有新型方法相比,目前仍然是标准诊断方法。酶组织化学和电子显微镜的应用,包括生物化学与亚细胞结构分析拓展了微观解剖结构的内涵。近代在肿瘤诊断中,细胞遗传学、DNA含量分析、分子遗传学分析和IHC研究已经作为光学显微镜的重要辅助手段,并扩展到深度基因型-表型特征。这些方法尤其是免疫组织化学方法,显著提高我们确定人类肿瘤分化方向的能力。新一代DNA测序平台和RNA表达阵列等新一代高通量技术的加入,

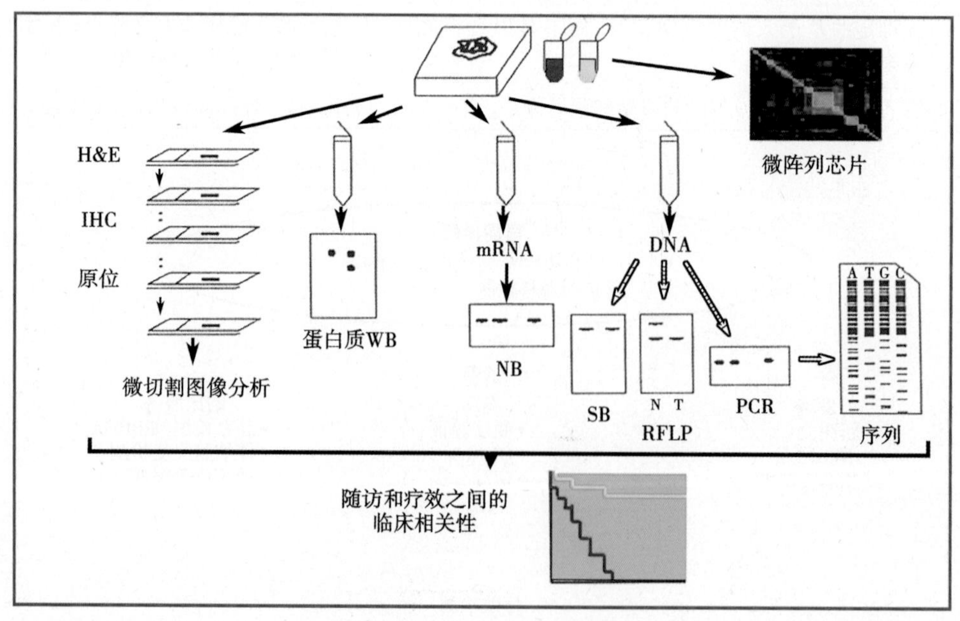

图39-3 分子病理。结合组织学、免疫化学和遗传学方法来定义分子谱系。运用低通量和高通量技术将表型和基因型进行整合,这些技术包括组织学、蛋白组学和核酸分析。应用微序列技术可以在单个序列中进行多个分析。HE,苏木精-伊红染色;IHC,免疫组化;WB,Western blot,蛋白质印迹法;NB,northern blot,RNA印迹法;SB,southern blot,DNA印迹法;PCR,聚合酶链反应;RFLP,限制性片段长度多态性

构成了分子病理学的基础，同时为当前的分类提供了有价值的信息和依据[5]。现代病理学的主要目标是整合来自诸多技术库的数据，并将其转化为知识，充分运用这些知识以便更好地管理患者以及发展为某些特定疾病的高危人群。

分子病理

分子病理学即在生化、免疫和遗传水平上研究疾病的起源和发病机制。肿瘤是一种主要由遗传突变和表观遗传紊乱引起的克隆性疾病[6,7]，这意味着任何特定的肿瘤都起源于一个单细胞（克隆性），这个细胞经特定分子改变触发启动肿瘤发生，受基因控制而缺乏激活细胞死亡或免疫监视的途径，因此向侵袭和转移扩散途径发展，最终形成恶性表型。尽管有许多肿瘤起源于病毒感染（肿瘤病毒），其中某些病毒蛋白（肿瘤蛋白）可增强增殖能力并消除凋亡反应，例如某些人类乳头状瘤病毒亚型，但大多数肿瘤可定义为由遗传或体细胞突变驱动的疾病。对此病理学不同于医学遗传学，医学遗传学的主要目的是确定与遗传性疾病相关的异常携带胚系突变，而肿瘤分子病理学旨在识别和了解肿瘤疾病发生和进展过程中的异常机制。相关研究目标包括：①根据对特定肿瘤类型中出现的复杂表型（指纹）或独特分子变化的识别，确定肿瘤的最终诊断和分类；②利用敏感分子检测技术进行早期肿瘤检测，从而进行治疗干预；③通过评估相关分子预测标志，提供临床相关预后信息；④协助选择个体化治疗方案，从而获得针对性治疗并避免不必要的药物毒性。设计配套的诊断方法以指导针对性的临床试验和个体化的肿瘤治疗。临床诊断还包括对小的残留病灶进行分析并提供早期复发的证据，这些证据通常来自肿瘤细胞新的耐药克隆。已经有大量循证医学证据表明基于分子标记所制定的针对性的治疗方案能够提高治愈机会并提高肿瘤患者的生活质量。

分子病理学是临床和基础生物医学学科之间的桥梁。分子病理学转化研究包括两个方面：临床病理对肿瘤的研究结果延伸至基础研究，以及将实验室研究结果有效地转化到临床实践中。因此，分子病理学有助于将生物学研究发现转化并运用到临床诊断、预后和治疗应用中。

分子技术的应用使我们在和肿瘤发生发展密切相关的细胞生长、分化、基因组完整性及程序性细胞死亡等知识的理解认识方面取得了长足进步[3-5]。某些生物学标记物如 *TP53* 肿瘤抑癌基因的改变，在特定肿瘤类型中与肿瘤生物学行为相关[8]。同样，利用一定特征的患者队列和经过适当筛选的正常和肿瘤配对样本进行前瞻性临床分析，可以更好地解释这些基因发生突变对肿瘤所造成的影响。对肿瘤基因突变和基因表达谱改变的研究结果之间差异性的出现，可能源自所使用的探针或研究方法不同所致。研究时应注意观察存活的肿瘤、肿瘤坏死程度、正常细胞与肿瘤细胞比率以及病变的分期和分级。不同的方法在特异性、敏感性、检测时间和成本上各不相同，通常针对特定病种，用特定方法检测特定的标志物。应用全谱系分子方法评估组织标本，以及针对靶向治疗特定靶点检测，已导致组织标本使用处理以及组织库的原有模式发生了变化。应不断更新方案以达到保证样品满足临床分子检测最佳需求。在日常工作中这意味着应尽可能预留部分样本，以进行下一步分子诊断。在诊断时添加预测分析环节将增强临床制定有效治疗方案的能力。

膀胱癌分子病理分类模型

膀胱癌是第五大常见的非皮肤性实体恶性肿瘤，也是继前列腺癌之后第二大常见的泌尿生殖系肿瘤[9-11]。发达国家膀胱癌的患病率是发展中国家的 6 倍。由于膀胱癌具有反复复发的特点，因此膀胱镜检查和尿细胞学检查，以及麻醉下反复的肿瘤切除，导致膀胱癌成为医疗保健系统花费高昂的恶性肿瘤之一[9-11]。大多数膀胱癌患者临床表现为排尿困难和血尿[12]。膀胱镜检查和活检评估发现两种不同的浅表（非浸润性）型病变：低级别肿瘤通常是乳头状（Ta 低级别尿路上皮癌）和高级别原位癌（Tis 或 CIS）病变。CIS 是一种扁平的高级别肿瘤，5 年内 60%~80%的病例发展为浸润性膀胱癌，40%的患者死亡[13-15]。这两种不同临床病理的实体肿瘤揭示了新的基于分子遗传学研究的膀胱癌发生发展模型[16-22]。两种不同的基因通路描述了早期膀胱肿瘤的演变以及晚期膀胱癌的进展[23,24]。浅表乳头状膀胱肿瘤的特征是原癌基因如 *H-RAS*、*FGFR3* 和/或 *PI3K* 发生获得性突变，以及 9 号染色体长臂的缺失（*9q*）。CIS 病变的特征是肿瘤抑制基因 *p53*、*RB* 和/或 *PTEN* 发生缺失突变[25-40]。这些突变是侵袭性膀胱癌的主要遗传性前期病变。基于这些数据提出膀胱肿瘤进展模型，其中两个独立的基因通路揭示早期膀胱肿瘤的演变（图 39-4）。

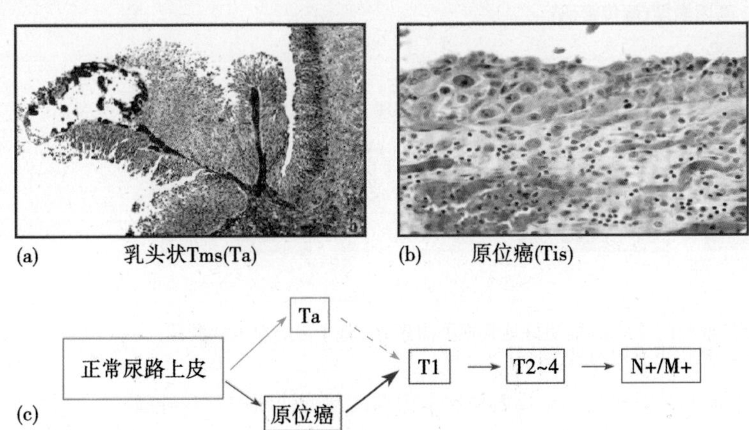

图 39-4　疾病分类的分子模式：以膀胱癌为例。膀胱肿瘤作为实体肿瘤，其临床表现为非浸润性乳头状（Ta）肿瘤，倾向于复发但不进展为浸润性肿瘤，或非浸润性异常增生的原位癌（Tis），病变倾向于浸润并进展为临床侵袭性疾病，最终转移扩散。多种技术包括表达谱分析，也揭示了这两个阶段的分子分类，即浅表性和浸润性膀胱癌。浅表乳头状膀胱肿瘤的特征是癌基因（如 *H-RAS*、*FGFR3* 和 *PI3K*）和/或 9 号染色体（9q）缺失突变；而原位癌的特征是肿瘤抑癌基因（如 *p53*、*RB* 和 *PTEN*）的突变

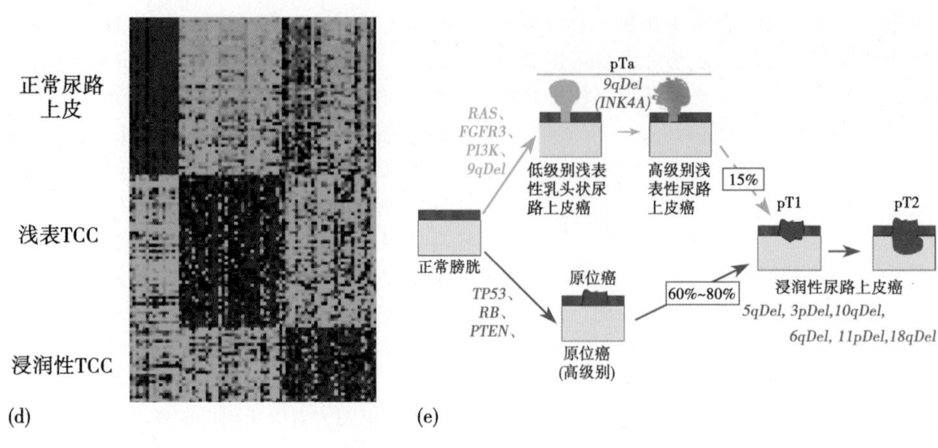

图 39-4(续)

系统病理学和预测肿瘤学

大多数诊断平台基于单纯的检测工具，通常应用一种特定的技术来提取形态或生物标志信息。系统病理学代表一种全新的、全面的个体化医学概念。“系统病理学”通过应用新技术如图像分析、模式识别和定量多重生物标志物，整合临床变量、组织学和细胞特征以及分子特征(图 39-5)[41-46]。通过苏木素-伊红染色的甲醛溶液固定、石蜡包埋组织切片和抗体/探针荧光标记分析物，使细胞水平定量原位成像研究成为可能。通过对组织学研究，分析包括信号通路在内的肿瘤表型特征，并利用患者临床数据和组织标本来构建临床风险状态的基线特征[42,44]，生成的数据可以转化为具有可供临床操作、用于机器学习和生成人工智能的实施工具。为提高治疗效果，还可以生成高精度的患者管理预测性算法，最终提供给用户方便使用的报告，为患者预后概率提供个体化的预测。例如，可以预测前列腺癌复发时间和根治性前列腺切除术后临床治疗失败时间[45,46]。以前列腺癌为模型可以进一步说明系统病理学概念。近年来前列腺癌诊断和临床分期方面的问题日益突出，早期筛查的广泛应用导致晚期疾病的发病率急剧下降。此外早期诊断导致了临床评估的权重，约 85%的诊断患者被归类为低或中等风险，而当前风险分层工具(如 Gleason 评分)与临床转归的相关性较低[47-51]。鉴于目前传统诊断方法给出的分层预测信息的局限性，临床难以明确患者为高危或惰性人群。前列腺特异性抗原(prostate-specific antigen, PSA)既不是前列腺癌的敏感指标，也不是前列腺癌的特异指标，对大多数患者来说 PSA 在预测临床意义方面也不尽人意。随着早期检测的开展，当前的 Gleason 分级系统应用出现了明显问题，因该分级主观性强，缺乏可重复性，尤其是诊断以 Gleason 4 为主的高级别病变。当多个预后指标在一起分析时，会出现结果的不一致性，例如患者可能具有高 PSA 但“低风险”的 Gleason 评分(例如 6 分或 6 分以下)。此外在判断手术切缘情况时存在很大的主观因素。因此临床急切需要另外一种定量、客观的方法，这些方法源自对单个患者组织样本的分析，以提供个体化的风险预测(图 39-6)。

第一版精准病理分析平台旨在对前列腺癌患者切除前列腺后进行风险评估[45,46,52]。这项“前列腺切除术后”评估使用切除后组织预测疾病侵袭性及患者可能的疾病进展，或术后 5 年内复发的生化指标(通过检测 PSA 和 PSA 的升高)。这些评估指标作为疾病的客观基线特征，有助于医生预测肿瘤进展风

(i) 临床数据和预后数据 } **注明记录**
(ii) 数字形态学和形态学统计
(iii) 分子病理学特征
(iv) 临床实验参数 } **表型(表达基因)**
(v) 基因组变量和基因突变 } **基因表型(遗传密码)**

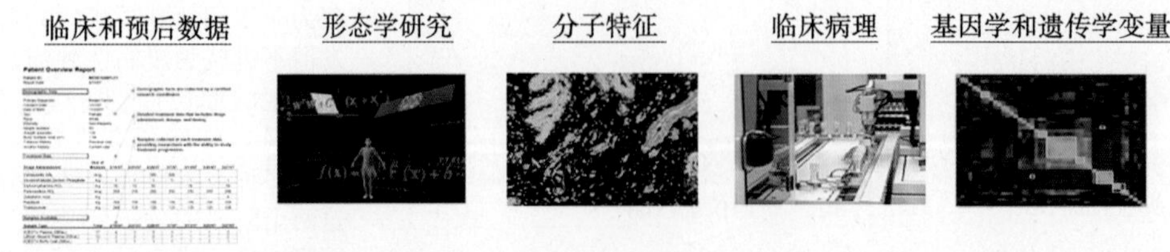

基于计算机程序的平台可以提供更加准确的诊断，并能更好地管理肿瘤患者。基于更高精度的测试，提供更有效的患者诊疗

图 39-5 系统病理学。利用人工智能和计算机程序集成表型和基因型的新型诊断和预测肿瘤学平台

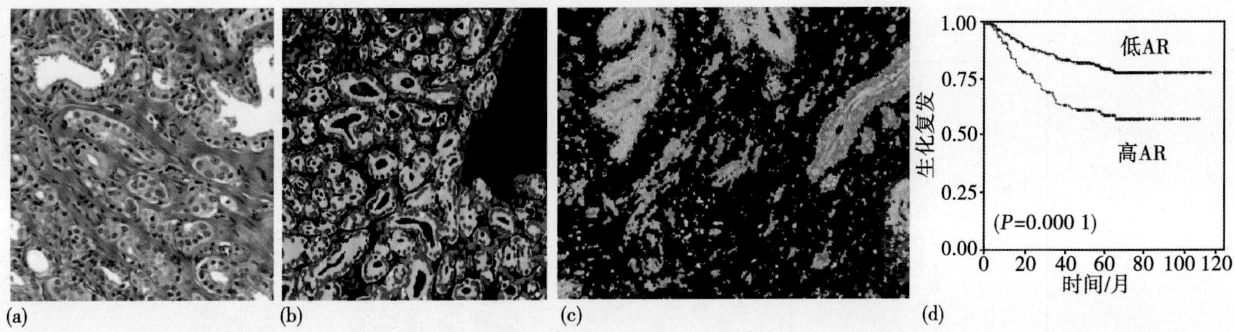

图 39-6　结果预测的综合方法:以前列腺癌为模型。运用数字化技术将苏木精-伊红染色组织切片(a)转换成形态测量图像,从而可以量化微观解剖特征(如腺体数量)(b)。利用对临床相关生物标志物(如雄激素受体或 AR,通过 Ki67 标记增殖指数)(c)的抗体蛋白分析,可以量化生物标志,并对临床患者进行针对性分层,如低和高水平 AR 的前列腺癌患者

险及指导治疗。这项研究来自 Memorial Sloan-Kettering Cancer Center,New York 的 758 名患者,该研究预测模型优于独立的临床因素和其他常见的术后风险因素,如手术切缘阳性、包膜外侵犯,同样也优于预测患者术后进展的整合因素。术后分析为诊治提供重要生物特征信息,并提高风险分层的准确性[风险比(HR)11.4,一致性指数(CI)0.84,$P<0.000\ 1$]。通过根治性前列腺切除术,该平台能够给出一份个体化风险评估报告:①为具有复发性生化指标的患者提供更多风险评估信息;②预测手术时疾病严重进展程度和复发的 PSA 水平;③协助给出正确辅助治疗决策[45,46,52]。

接下来的第二项则集中在对前列腺穿刺活检的研究[53],即基于诊断时的活检组织来预测疾病进展,并进行早期病理分期(可能处在潜在惰性疾病阶段)。它能够帮助医生正确评估该男性患者疾病严重程度,并作出更明智的治疗决策。这项研究是针对 1 027 名来自国际多机构队列的患者进行,该模型在患者风险预估方面优于独立的临床因素和其他综合工具,如列线图。这一版活检评估将重要的生物识别信息整合到诊疗特征中,具有显著的风险分层准确性(HR 3.47,CI 0.73,$P<0.001$),帮助医生对患者采取个体化治疗模式。在诊断时即为临床提供风险评估信息,帮助泌尿科医生:①预测治疗后(如前列腺切除术)的疾病进展;②作出客观、明智的治疗决策;③辨认看似低危的高危患者;④将临床上不明确的中危患者重新分类为高风险或低风险;⑤帮助患者缓解对于一些未知情况的焦虑心情。对于仅行放疗的患者,最初的活检样本和相关的 Gleason 评分将是研究疾病的唯一"组织资源"。对于不能切除的前列腺癌评估,这项研究为前列腺相关肿瘤提供了仅有的机会。值得一提的是该模型在一个小型放射治疗队列探索性研究中得以验证。此外,对于正处于监测或观察中的低风险患者,活检结果评估可以帮助临床决定是否应避免保守方案而选择积极治疗方案。特别是对于初次监测人群应用前景尤为看好。简而言之,采用针吸活检法对一组组织特征良好的男性队列(n=181)监测研究发现,综合分析能够成功预测该组患者需要进行治疗的时间(如退出监测时机),其 CI 为 0.65,HR 为 3.6($P<0.000\ 1$)。

将上述研究结果延伸至药理学分析,结果表明前列腺切除术后评估与临床实践相比,其性价比为 2 100 美元/QALY(质量调整寿命年)。同样,临床重要的中间风险人群活检评估的初步性价比分析显示节省了 2 300 美元的成本。一项基于来自 23 名全国泌尿科医师诊治的 233 名前列腺癌患者的精准分析显示,在关键性的中危和高危患者群体中,成本节约了 1 889 美元[54-56]。

从对症治疗到病因学治疗

细胞内环境平衡状态受 4 个关键程序调控:增殖(细胞周期分裂)、分化、衰老和细胞死亡(细胞凋亡)[4,7]。推测组织更新由组织特异性干细胞通过程序调节来完成[57-62]。许多特性都归因于干细胞,其应具备两个基本特征:①干细胞能够自我更新,通过细胞分裂产生新的干细胞;②干细胞是多能祖细胞,通过不对称细胞分裂产生具有分化特点的瞬时扩增细胞。当然,这些细胞也显示出未分化表型(图 39-7)。

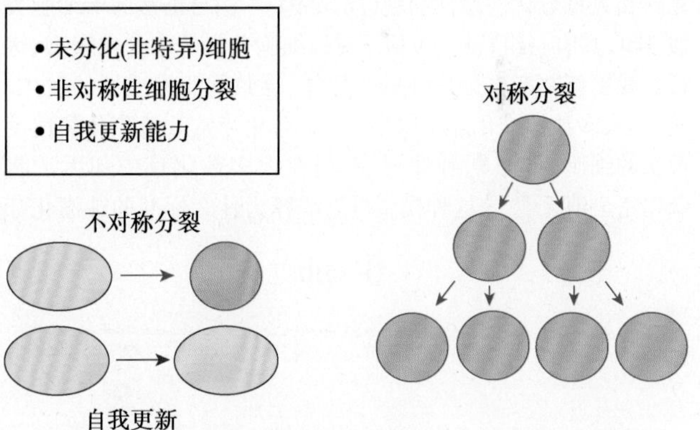

图 39-7　干细胞与分化细胞的特性。干细胞的基本特征包括未分化表型、不对称细胞分裂和自我更新能力,分化细胞特征为对称分裂也被称为有丝分裂。非对称性细胞分裂或自我更新完成后的原始细胞持续发挥其生理功能,而有丝分裂中的原始细胞在经过核分裂和细胞分裂后消失,产生两个相同的子细胞

肿瘤是用于定义一组疾病的术语,其特征是不受调节的细胞增殖、异常分化和缺陷性凋亡。关于肿瘤发生有两个主要假说:"随机模型",推测每个肿瘤细胞都能产生一个全新的肿瘤;"肿瘤干细胞(cancer stem cell,CSC)模型",它提出肿瘤细胞处于分级状态,只有少数几个干细胞具有启动肿瘤的潜能(图 39-8)[58-62]。对于后一种模型,所有肿瘤可能具有相同的初始转化

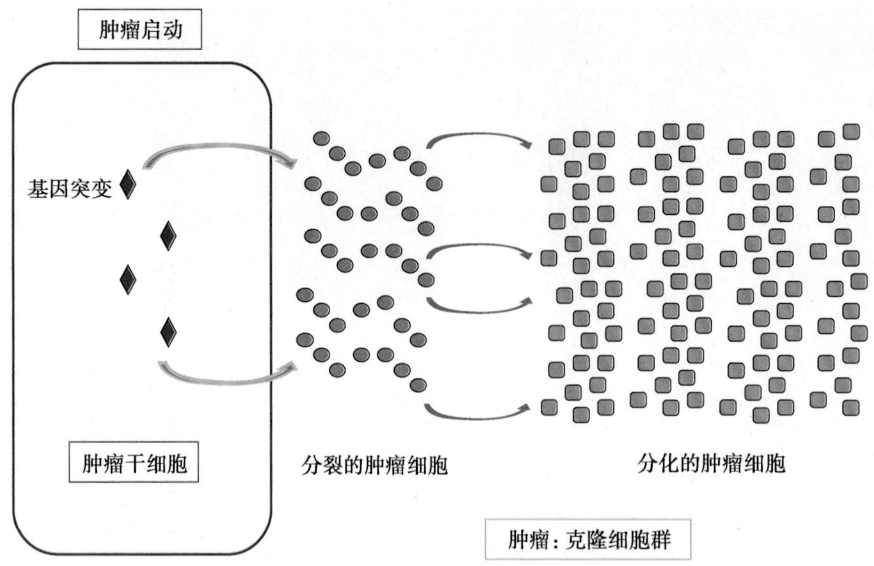

图 39-8　肿瘤发生和进展的干细胞模型。研究假设肿瘤转化起源于能够维持基因调控的组织干细胞、基于下调的凋亡程序和有利于逃避免疫监测的 HLA 阴性表型。这种转化的肿瘤干细胞进行自我更新和不对称的细胞分裂，产生快速增殖的分化克隆，形成具有分化特征的肿瘤异质群体

事件。影响这种独特的体细胞（即所谓的成人干细胞）转化的原因是多方面的（例如病毒感染、化学致癌物和自发突变）。转化事件产生一个 CSC 来完成肿瘤启动和肿瘤分级。支持这一假设的事实就是肿瘤是一种克隆性疾病，即从单个细胞进化而来并发展后代。

CSC 假说认为，除了 CSC 外肿瘤还包括一小部分转化扩增克隆和大量分化性恶性细胞（图 39-9）[62]。与正常的干细胞类似，CSC 具有一组特性，包括不对称细胞分裂的未分化表型，进行自我更新并产生分化性的克隆体，导致肿瘤异质性的发生。此外，大多数标准化疗难以根除 CSCs，化疗常常清除分裂速度最快的细胞，即早期肿瘤反应，但在大多数化疗中却无法将 CSC 完全消灭[62]。这种模型可以解释为什么标准的肿瘤化疗开始可以造成肿瘤缩小，最终由于存活的 CSC 导致肿瘤复发。

对“耐药”与“无应答”表型进行识别至关重要。化疗耐药是克服敏感性状态后获得的一种现象，而无应答是一种新现象，并不意味着先前存在应答表型。CSC 高表达多药耐药蛋白（multidrug resistance protein，MRP），包括多药耐药 1（multidrug resistance 1，MDR1）或 P-糖蛋白。此外，尽管不对称分裂的发生机制尚不清楚，但是体外试验研究证据表明，即使在使用某些传统有丝分裂抑制剂如紫杉醇的情况下，不对称分裂仍然可以发生。综上所述，尽管某些化疗药物能够作用于 CSC，但仍然可以赋予 CSC 持续存活的无应答表型能力。随后这些存活的 CSC 产生耐药性克隆，最终成功导致治疗耐受（图 39-9）。本实验室首次报道了前列腺癌模型 CSC 亚群[63]。研究揭示了

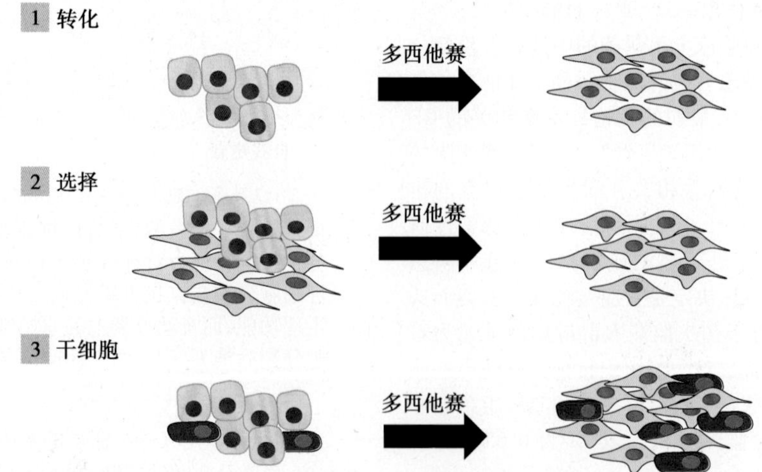

图 39-9　肿瘤干细胞与化疗耐药。用于解决化疗耐药性的不同模型：转化模型是指敏感性肿瘤转变为耐药克隆性肿瘤；选择模型遵循 Darwinian 假设，即原发未治疗肿瘤存在异质性亚群，当敏感性克隆死亡时，耐药克隆存活并增殖；干细胞模型则认为肿瘤干细胞代表肿瘤一个小亚群，且对大多数传统药物无反应，当敏感细胞死亡时，肿瘤干细胞通过自我更新和不对称细胞分裂产生新的耐药克隆增殖

这种 CSC 在化疗耐药过程中所做的“贡献”。这些耐药 CSC 表现为一种未分化表型，其特征为上皮分化标记物（如细胞角蛋白18）缺失与细胞膜 HLA Ⅰ型表达缺失，以及由 *Notch* 和 *Hedgehog* 基因编程发育途径的激活[63,64]。更加重要的是，实验室开发的模型能够首次分离和识别临床前列腺癌组织中的 CSC，并阐明了一种新的治疗策略，即在免疫缺陷小鼠模型中使用患者源性肿瘤移植物抑制 *Notch* 和 *Hedgehog* 信号通路可消除前列腺癌术后复发。最近，通过收集化疗耐药 CSC 模型基因表达谱的患者数据集，发现转录因子 *GATA2* 调节一个由 *IGF2* 驱动的多激酶程序，该程序有助于在致死性前列腺癌中发生化疗耐药和肿瘤形成[65]。值得注意的是，该研究首次从循环肿瘤细胞中提取来自患者的异种移植物，这有助于临床试验对前列腺癌富有应用前景的新型治疗组合（多西他赛或卡巴齐他赛联合双 *IGF1R/INSR* 抑制剂）的验证。最初的前列腺癌转化模型已拓展到其他肿瘤包括乳腺癌、结肠癌以及胶质瘤和肉瘤。

与既往报道相似，这些 CSC 一般表现出组织相容性负向特征，即缺乏单个或簇状瘤细胞 HLA Ⅰ型表达，并与局部侵袭性行为和转移能力相关[64]。此外，胚胎干细胞也具有 HLA 阴性表型。据报道人类植入前胚胎为 HLA Ⅰ型和Ⅱ型阴性，这种现象排除了由于父系抗原的表达而产生的排斥反应，直到出现胎盘产生血-组织屏障。对于 CSC 来说组织相容性阴性表型具有重要临床意义，由于 CSC 具有免疫逃逸特点，可以解释宿主突变的相容性，以及肿瘤扩散和转移能力。此外，它还可能与新型肿瘤免疫靶向治疗中观察到的临床治疗失败有关，例如当使用活化的 T 淋巴细胞时，靶细胞表达 MHC 至关重要。

总之，我们已经能够在人类肿瘤细胞系和组织样本中识别一种新定义的前列腺 CSC，利用 HLA Ⅰ型表面标记物分离出这一群体细胞，并证明其肿瘤驱动能力。并且还发现在人类乳腺癌、结肠癌、肺癌和膀胱癌以及肉瘤和胶质母细胞瘤中都存在类似的 CSC 群，这一事实进一步证明 CSC 具有普遍性。这种人类 CSC 的发现在临床诊断和实验室分析以及针对 CSC 和分化性克隆的治疗新策略研发具有重要临床意义（图 39-10）。

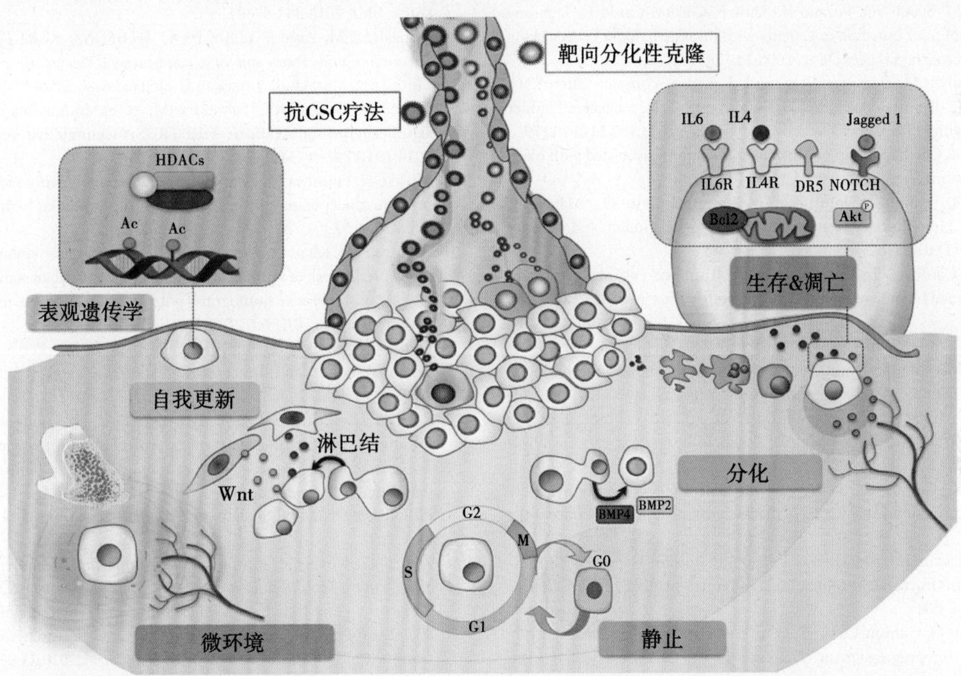

图 39-10 针对症状学和病因的治疗模式。该模型假设需要针对两种不同的细胞亚群根治肿瘤：分化性肿瘤克隆和肿瘤干细胞。这幅图展示了抗肿瘤干细胞（anti-CSC）疗法与抗分化肿瘤克隆的疗法相结合的各种不同途径方法，包括将未分化克隆转化为分化克隆的表观遗传因子，以及针对微环境的新型指标

（王海月 译，林冬梅 审校）

参考文献

1 Virchow R. *Cellular Pathology*. London: John Churchill; 1860.

2 Rosai J. *Guiding the Surgeon's Hand, The History of American Surgical Pathology*. Washington, D.C.: American Registry of Pathology; 1997.

3 Cordon-Cardo C. Applications of molecular diagnostics: solid tumor genetics can determine clinical treatment protocols. *Mod Pathol*. 2001;**14**:254–257.

4 Cordon-Cardo C. Mutation of cell cycle regulators: biological and clinical implications for human neoplasias. *Am J Pathol*. 1995;**147**:545–560.

5 Donovan MJ, Cordon-Cardo C. Predicting high-risk disease using tissue biomarkers. *Curr Opin Urol*. 2013;**23**:245–251.

6 Clark WH. Tumour progression and the nature of cancer. *Br J Cancer*. 1991;**64**:631–644.

7 Hanahan D, Weinberg RA. The hallmarks of cancer. *Cell*. 2000;**100**:57–70.

8 Vousden KH, Prives C. Blinded by the light: the growing complexity of p53. *Cell*. 2009;**137**:413–431.

9 Ferlay J, Soerjomataram I, Ervik M, et al. *Cancer Incidence and Mortality Worldwide: IARC CancerBase No. 11*. International Agency for Research on Cancer: Lyon, France; 2013.

10 Siegel R, Ma J, Zou Z, Jemal A. Cancer statistics, 2014. *CA Cancer J Clin*. 2014;**64**:9–29.

11 Ye F, Wang L, Castillo-Martin M, et al. Biomarkers for bladder cancer management: present and future. *Am J Clin Exp Urol*. 2014;**2**:1–14.

12 Holmang S, Hedelin H, Anderstrom C, Johansson SL. The relationship among multiple recurrences, progression and prognosis of patients with stages Ta and T1 transitional cell cancer of the bladder followed for at least 20 years. *J Urol*. 1995;**153**:1823–1826.

13 Botteman MF, Pashos CL, Redaelli A, Laskin B, Hauser R. The health economics of bladder cancer: a comprehensive review of the published literature. *Pharmacoeconomics*. 2003;**21**:1315–1330.

14 Cordon-Cardo C, Cote RJ, Sauter G. Genetic and molecular markers of urothelial premalignancy and malignancy. *Scand J Urol Nephrol*. 2000;**34(Suppl. 205)**:82–93.

15 Eble JN, Sauter G, Epstein JI, Sesterhenn IA. *WHO Classification of Tumors: Pathology and Genetics of Tumours of the Urinary System and Male Genital Organs*. Lyon: IARC Press; 2004.

16 Presti JC, Reuter VE, Galan T, Fair WR, Cordon-Cardo C. Molecular genetic alterations in superficial and locally advanced human bladder cancer. *Cancer Res*. 1991;**51**:5405–5409.

17 Dalbagni G, Presti J, Reuter V, Fair WR, Cordon-Cardo C. Genetic alterations in bladder cancer. *Lancet*. 1993;**324**:469–471.

18 Dalbagni G, Cordon-Cardo C, Reuter V, Fair WR. Tumor suppressor gene alterations in bladder carcinoma: translational correlates to clinical practice. *Surg Oncol Clin N Am*. 1995;**4**:231–240.

19 Sanchez-Carbayo M, Socci N, Charytonowicz E, Prystowski M, Childs G, Cordon-Cardo C. Molecular profiling of bladder cancer using cDNA microarrays: defining histogenesis and biological phenotypes. *Cancer Res*. 2002;**62**:6973–6980.

20 Sanchez-Carbayo M, Socci ND, Lozano JJ, Haab BB, Cordon-Cardo C. Profiling bladder cancer using targeted antibody arrays. *Am J Pathol*. 2006;**168**:93–103.

21 Sanchez-Carbayo M, Socci ND, Lozano JJ, Saint F, Cordon-Cardo C. Defining molecular profiles of poor outcome in patients with invasive bladder cancer using oligonucleotide microarrays. *J Clin Oncol*. 2006;**24**:778–789.

22 Jia AY, Castillo-Martin M, Domingo-Domenech J, et al. A common MicroRNA signature consisting of miR-133a, miR-139-3p, and miR-142-3p clusters bladder carcinoma in situ with normal umbrella cells. *Am J Pathol*. 2013;**182**:1171–1179.

23 Sanchez-Carbayo M, Cordon-Cardo C. Molecular alterations associated with bladder cancer progression. *Semin Oncol*. 2007;**34**:75–84.

24 Castillo-Martin M, Domingo-Domenech J, Karni-Schmidt O, Matos T, Cordon-Cardo C. Molecular pathways of urothelial development and bladder tumorigenesis. *Urol Oncol*. 2010;**28**:401–408.

25 Fradet Y, Cordon-Cardo C, Thomson T, et al. Cell surface antigens of human bladder cancer defined by mouse monoclonal antibodies. *Proc Natl Acad Sci USA*. 1984;**81**:224–228.

26 Fradet Y, Cordon-Cardo C, Whitmore WF, Melamed MR, Old LJ. Cell surface antigens of human bladder tumors: definition of tumor subsets by monoclonal antibodies and correlation with growth characteristics. *Cancer Res*. 1986;**46**:5183–5188.

27 Cordon-Cardo C, Wartinger D, Petrylak D, et al. Altered expression of the retinoblastoma gene product as predictor of outcome in bladder cancer. *J Natl Cancer Inst*. 1992;**84**:1251–1256.

28 Sarkis A, Dalbagni G, Cordon-Cardo C, et al. Detection of p53 mutations in superficial (T1) bladder carcinomas as a marker of disease progression. *J Natl Cancer Inst*. 1993;**85**:53–59.

29 Orlow I, Lianes P, Lacombe L, Dalbagni G, Reuter VE, Cordon-Cardo C. Chromosome 9 deletions and microsatellite alterations in human bladder tumors. *Cancer Res*. 1994;**54**:2848–2851.

30 Sarkis AS, Dalbagni G, Cordon-Cardo C, et al. Association of p53 nuclear overexpression and tumor progression in carcinoma in situ of the bladder. *J Urol*. 1994;**152**:388–392.

31 Lianes P, Orlow I, Zhang ZZ, et al. Altered patterns of MDM2 and TP53 expression in human bladder cancer. *J Natl Cancer Inst*. 1994;**86**:1325–1330.

32 Gruis NA, Weaver-Feldhaus J, Liu Q, et al. Genetic evidence in melanoma and bladder cancers that p16 and p53 function in separate pathways of tumor suppression. *Am J Pathol*. 1995;**146**:1199–1206.

33 Orlow I, Lacombe L, Hannon GJ, et al. Deletion of the p16 and p15 genes in human bladder tumors. *J Natl Cancer Inst*. 1995;**87**:1524–1529.

34 Cordon-Cardo C, Zhang ZF, Dalbagni G, et al. Cooperative effects of p53 and pRB alterations in primary superficial bladder tumors. *Cancer Res*. 1997;**57**:1217–1221.

35 Orlow I, LaRue H, Osman I, et al. Deletions of the INK4A gene in superficial bladder tumors: association with recurrence. *Am J Pathol*. 1999;**155**:105–113.

36 Mo L, Zheng X, Huang HY, et al. Hyperactivation of Ha-ras oncogene, but not Ink4a/Arf deficiency, triggers bladder tumorigenesis. *J Clin Invest*. 2007;**117**:314–325.

37 Puzio-Kuter SA, Castillo-Martin M, Shen TH, et al. Inactivation of p53 and Pten promotes invasive bladder cancer. *Genes Dev*. 2009;**23**:675–680.

38 Karni-Schmidt O, Castillo-Martin M, HuaiShen T, et al. Distinct expression profiles of p63 variants during urothelial development and bladder cancer progression. *Am J Pathol*. 2011;**178**:1350–1360.

39 Jia AY, Castillo-Martin M, Bonal DM, Sánchez-Carbayo M, Silva JM, Cordon-Cardo C. MicroRNA-126 inhibits invasion in bladder cancer via regulation of ADAM9. *Br J Cancer*. 2014;**110**:2945–2954.

40 Gaya JM, López-Martínez JM, Karni-Schmidt O, et al. ΔNp63 expression is a protective factor of progression in clinical high grade T1 bladder cancer. *J Urol*. 2015;**193**:1144–1150.

41 Donovan MJ, Costa J, Cordon-Cardo C. Systems pathology: a paradigm shift in the practice of diagnostic and predictive pathology. *Cancer*. 2009;**115**:3078–3084.

42 Capodieci P, Donovan M, Buchinsky H, et al. Gene expression profiling in single cells within tissues. *Nat Methods*. 2005;**2**:663–665.

43 Saidi O, Cordon-Cardo C, Costa J. Technology insights: will systems pathology replace the pathologist? *Nat Clin Pract Urol*. 2007;**4**:39–45.

44 Donovan MJ, Cordon-Cardo C. Genomic analysis in active surveillance: predicting high-risk disease using tissue biomarkers. *Curr Opin Urol*. 2014;**24**:303–310.

45 Cordon-Cardo C, Kotsianti A, Verbel D, et al. Improved prediction of prostate cancer recurrence through systems pathology. *J Clin Invest*. 2007;**117**:1876–1883.

46 Donovan MJ, Hamann S, Clayton M, et al. A systems pathology approach for the prediction of prostate cancer progression after radical prostatectomy. *J Clin Oncol*. 2008;**26**:3923–3929.

47 Shariat S, Roehrborn C. Using biopsy to detect prostate cancer. *Rev Urol*. 2008;**10**:262–280.

48 Rosario D, Lane JA, Metcalfe C. Short term outcomes of prostate biopsy in men tested for cancer by prostate specific antigen: prospective evaluation within ProtecT study. *BMJ*. 2012;**344**:d7894.

49 Gonzalez CM, Averch T, Boyd LA. *AUA/SUNA White Paper on the Incidence, Prevention and Treatment of Complications Related to Prostate Needle Biopsy*. Linthicum, Maryland: American Urological Association; 2012.

50 Yaskiv O, George AK, Fakhoury M, et al. Improving detection of clinically significant prostate cancer: MRI/TRUS fusion-guided prostate biopsy. *J Urol*. 2014;**191**:1749–1754.

51 Miyake H, Fujisawa M. Prognostic prediction following radical prostatectomy for prostate cancer using conventional as well as molecular biological approaches. *Int J Urol*. 2013;**20**:301–311.

52 Donovan MJ, Khan FM, Powell D, et al. Postoperative systems models more accurately predict risk of significant disease progression than standard risk groups and a 10-year postoperative nomogram: potential impact on the receipt of adjuvant therapy after surgery. *BJU Int*. 2012;**109**:40–45.

53 Donovan MJ, Khan FM, Fernandez G, et al. Personalized prediction of tumor response and cancer progression on prostate needle biopsy. *J Urol*. 2009;**182**:125–132.

54 Zubek VB, Konski A. Cost effectiveness of risk-prediction tools in selecting patients for immediate post-prostatectomy treatment. *Mol Diagn Ther*. 2009;**13(1)**:31–47.

55 Zubek VB, Khan FM. *Cost-Minimization Analysis of Biopsy-based Risk Stratification Tools in Intermediate-risk Prostate Cancer Patients*. 15th Annual Meeting of ISPOR (International Society for Pharmacoeconomics and Outcomes Research). May, 2010.

56 Zubek VB, Khan FM, Karvir H. *Cost-Minimization Analysis of Biopsy-Based Risk Stratification Tools in Intermediate and High Risk Prostate Cancer Patients Based on Results from Physician Case Studies*. 16th Annual Meeting of ISPOR (International Society for Pharmacoeconomics and Outcomes Research). May, 2011.

57 Cordon-Cardo C. Cancer Stem Cells. *Ann Oncol*. 2010;**21**:93–94.

58 Dick JE. Stem cell concepts renew cancer research. *Blood*. 2008;**112**:4793–4807.

59 Magee JA, Piskounova E, Morrison SJ. Cancer stem cells: impact, heterogeneity, and uncertainty. *Cancer Cell*. 2012;**21**:283–296.

60 Valent P, Bonnet D, De Maria R, et al. Cancer stem cell definitions and terminology: the devil is in the details. *Nat Rev Cancer*. 2012;**12**:767–775.

61 Visvader JE, Lindeman GJ. Cancer stem cells: current status and evolving complexities. *Cell Stem Cell*. 2012;**10**:717–728.

62 Vidal SJ, Rodriguez-Bravo V, Galsky M, Cordon-Cardo C, Domingo-Domenech J. Targeting cancer stem cells to suppress acquired chemotherapy resistance. *Oncogene*. 2014;**33**:4451–4463.

63 Domingo-Domenech J, Vidal SJ, Rodriguez-Bravo V, et al. Suppression of acquired Docetaxel resistance in prostate cancer through depletion of Notch and Hedgehog dependent tumor initiating cells. *Cancer Cell*. 2012;**22**:373–388.

64 Cordon-Cardo C, Fuks Z, Eisenbach L, Feldman M. Expression of HLA-A,B,C antigens on primary and metastatic tumor cell populations of human carcinomas. *Cancer Res*. 1991;**51**:6372–6380.

65 Vidal SJ, Rodriguez-Bravo V, Quinn SA, et al. A targetable GATA2-IGF2 axis confers aggressiveness in lethal prostate cancer. *Cancer Cell*. 2015;**27**:223–239.

第40章 癌症的分子诊断学

Roshni D. Kalachand, MBBCh, MD ■ Bryan T. Hennessy, MD ■ Robert C. Bast Jr., MD ■
Gordon B. Mills, MD, PhD

概述

分子诊断学是指利用与癌症有关的分子变化以促进检测、诊断、监测和/或治疗。分子生物标志物常用于癌症组织研究，但也可用于分析易于获得的患者样本（如唾液、痰、血液、尿液和粪便），从而可以最大限度地减少对侵入性活检的需求。传统的血液生物标志物-癌胚抗原（carcinoembryonic antigen, CEA）、前列腺特异性抗原（prostate specific antigen, PSA）、人绒毛膜促性腺激素（human chorionic gonadotropin, hCG）、甲胎蛋白（alpha-fetoprotein, AFP）、CA125 和 CA15-3 已被用于监测对治疗的反应以及检测疾病的复发，其临床效用往往取决于对残留病变或复发疾病的有效治疗。早期检测不仅需要具有高灵敏度的生物标志物来检测临床前疾病以及理想情况下的转移前疾病，而且还需具有高度特异性来进行有效而经济的筛查。两阶段策略通常是最有希望的，即升高的生物标志物导致影像学检查或将影像学结果与生物标志物联合以提高阳性预测值。癌症特异性基因组畸变已被确定，可用于指导治疗以及预测患者亚群的预后。曲妥珠单抗显著改变了 HER2 扩增乳腺癌患者的预后，表皮生长因子受体（epidermal growth factor receptor, EGFR）抑制剂在治疗转移性 EGFR 突变阳性非小细胞肺癌中的作用也是如此。由于单个驱动基因畸变往往不足以预测治疗反应，因此基因特征以及包含 DNA、RNA 和/或蛋白质畸变在内的多标志物系列作为有效生物标志物的可能性正在被评估。一个由多种生物标志物组成的系列（Onco-Type Dx®）已被证明在预测激素受体阳性乳腺癌患者除激素治疗外是否需要化疗方面非常有用。随着靶向治疗逐渐成为现实，对这些治疗方法的耐药性的出现也是可以预测的，这些耐药性通常通过基因扩增、继发性突变或靶向分子畸变下游信号机制的重新激活发生。寻找分子生物标志物，即所谓的伴随诊断，对一线治疗耐药性和二线治疗反应进行预测，目前是靶向药物开发的内在要求。然而，这些新兴的综合技术尚未惠及大多数癌症患者。对通过高通量技术鉴定的大量畸变的解读、充足而高质量组织样本的获取、成本以及临床验证仍然是开发和实施有效生物标志物的重大挑战。战略性的利用生物信息学、国际合作、开发前瞻性收集含有新鲜冷冻组织的临床注释生物数据库，以及在大量前瞻性数据中进行临床验证，这些都是将有用的分子生物标志物引入临床实践的关键。

引言

分子诊断学包括应用分子生物标志物（框 40-1）来检测、诊断或监测癌症，以及评估患者预后或预测可能使患者受益的治疗干预措施。最终，分子诊断学的发展有望促进癌症治疗的个体化，其目标在于将单个癌症患者的治疗效益最大化，同时将毒性降到最低。分子诊断学在临床管理中的发展和应用已取得重要进展。本章概述了癌症分子诊断学的现状，此外还对将生物标志物驱动的方法纳入未来个性化癌症治疗发展的可能途径，以及新技术和可能需要解决和克服的问题和障碍进行回顾。

框 40-1 癌症生物标志物

癌症生物标志物包括肿瘤细胞、基质、正常组织或体液的任何特征，这些特征有助于检测、诊断、监测、确定预后或预测治疗的反应或毒性。因此，生物标志物包括 DNA、RNA、蛋白质、碳水化合物、脂质或代谢物的改变，以及肿瘤细胞、肿瘤微环境或宿主基因组的生物物理特征和反应。病理检查和影像学技术提供了传统的肿瘤组织学和分期信息，迄今为止指导着患者管理。然而，这些方法并没有考虑到癌症在分子水平上肿瘤间和肿瘤内的全部异质性。通过考虑不同平台交叉的多个分子生物标志物的概况，个体化的筛查、预防和治疗应该可以得到充分改善。

用于癌症筛查和早期检测的分子生物标志物

早期发现意味着在早期发展阶段诊断癌症。至关重要的是早期诊断发生在以目前可用的疗法可实现治愈的肿瘤发展阶段。筛查策略通常要求较高的灵敏度和特异性。通过识别发生特定癌症的高风险个体以及降低评估高风险个体的特异性障碍，可促进早期诊断[1-4]。筛查是一个术语，用于在早期可治愈阶段促进发现肿瘤的方法。有效的癌症筛查策略必须具有成本效益，可被患者接受，并与干预和假阳性结果的有限发病率相关。由于对整个人群的筛查很少是可行的，因此通常需要患者风险评估指南来确定以预防和早期诊断癌症为目标的适当方法。随着我们对癌症分子异质性认识的深入，可以将新标准添加到描述理想的筛查生物标志物的常规标准中（框 40-2）。因此，由于大多数癌症治疗仅对少数癌症患者有效，未来有用的筛查生物标志物也可指导个体患者的适当治疗。

框 40-2 最佳筛查试验

五个关键术语描述筛查试验的标准：灵敏度、特异性、选择性以及阳性和阴性预测值。灵敏度是通过测试检测到的疾病病例的部分（真阳性数/真阳性数加上假阴性数）。特异性是没有癌症的病例通过测试检测为阴性的部分（真阴性数/真阴性数加假阳性）。选择性表示的是筛查试验区分不同类型癌症的能力。当测试结果是连续变量时，灵敏度和特异性呈反向相关，并且以一种任意的方式对疾病的存在设置临界，这意味着结果错误的临床后果。在大多数有效的筛查方法中，两阶段策略已被证明是最佳的，该策略包括初次诊断测试以及随后进行的二次测试，二次测试可优化灵敏度和/或特异性并超出仅进行一次单独的初步测试所能达到的水平（例如，巴氏宫颈涂片后的阴道镜检查）。这种方法有助于控制假阳性结果的后果、侵入性方法和成本。人群中该疾病的流行率也影响筛查测试表现：在低流行率环境中，即使是非常好的测试也具有较差的阳性预测值（检测结果阳性的患者中正确诊断的比例，即真阳性数/真阳性数加上假阳性数）。因此，了解该病的流行情况是解释筛查检测结果的一个关键先决条件。筛查相对不常见的癌症（如卵巢癌和胰腺癌）比筛查更常见的癌症（如乳腺癌或前列腺癌）需要更强的特异性。

新兴的放射学和内窥镜技术为小肿瘤的早期发现提供了越来越灵敏的非侵入性方法。尽管存在一些争议，但与常规胸片相比，低剂量计算机断层扫描似乎能在吸烟高危人群中发现早期肺癌，并降低肺癌相关死亡率[5]。同样，作为 *BRCA1/2* 基因突变携带者的早期乳腺癌检测策略，将每年一次的双侧乳房磁共振成像加入年度乳腺 X 线检查中，可以减少使用双侧预防性乳房切除术来降低这些患者患乳腺癌的风险[6,7]。在结肠癌中，结肠镜检查使整个结肠中小病灶可视化的能力使其成为比双对比钡灌肠更为理想的筛查方法。然而，这些工具依赖于肿瘤的解剖学特点进行检测，而分子标记可以在解剖学检测之前的早期以及或许癌变前期识别癌症。此外，可以检测体液（尿液、粪便和血液）中的生物标志物，从而避免患者因准备内窥镜检查而可能产生的不适，以及放射性成像中潜在的有害电离辐射。

筛查通常适用于那些有确凿证据表明存在相关生存益处的人群，以及为确保成本效益，癌症是常见死亡原因的人群。例如，尽管存在争议，美国大多数监管机构都建议对 40 岁及以上的女性进行每年一次的乳房 X 线检查[8]。或者，可使用风险评估将选择的患者分层进行筛查，如果风险足够高，则进行预防。这样，在有风险的患者中保持较高的癌症检出率的同时，避免了大量个体接触假阳性筛查试验和不必要的活检。目前，与肺癌筛查一样，风险评估主要基于患者的特定因素，包括年龄、家族史和社会因素（如吸烟）。然而，一些分子标记，如癌症易感性基因（如 *BRCA1*、*BRCA2* 和 *p53*）的突变，已经证明可用于有风险人群的识别。

目前临床实践中用于筛查、预防和早期检测的分子生物学标志物

前列腺癌

前列腺特异性抗原（prostate-specific antigen，PSA）通常以非常低的水平存在于血液中，浓度在 0~4.0ng/ml 之间。PSA 水平升高与潜在的前列腺癌有关。尽管血清 PSA 测定在前列腺癌筛查中广泛应用，但仍存在争议[9]。高达 15%的前列腺癌可以在无 PSA 升高的情况下发生。PSA 水平可因前列腺感染、刺激、良性前列腺肥大或近期射精而升高。因此，PSA 并非前列腺癌筛查足够敏感或特异的标志物。PSA 筛查可引起不必要的活检、过度诊断和过度治疗的高发生率，从而导致发病。前列腺切除术和放射治疗都可能与阳痿和尿失禁有关。被诊断为侵袭性较弱（Gleason 评分<7）的前列腺癌患者可以在患癌症的情况下存活数十年，通常死于共患疾病。根据大型多中心试验判断，50 岁以上男性的 PSA 筛查可使前列腺癌特异性死亡率降低 20%，尽管这可能会或不会转化为总体死亡率的降低[10,11]。在过去，在与患者讨论筛查相关风险后，PSA 筛查被推荐用于年龄超过 50 岁、预期寿命为 10 年或更长时间的男性[12]。美国预防卫生工作组现在建议不要使用 PSA 进行筛查[13]。美国泌尿学协会（American Urological Association，AUA）则有更具细微差别的年龄相关指南[14]。AUA 建议不要对 40 岁以下的男性进行 PSA 筛查。在 40 岁到 54 岁之间，PSA 筛查仅被推荐给非洲裔美国男性或具有阳性家族史而患病风险增加的男性。对于年龄在 55~69 岁之间的男性而言，在过去十多年里，每 1 000 名筛查的男性中可预防一人因前列腺癌而死亡，这一益处必须与筛查和治疗相关的已知危害进行权衡。70 岁以上的男性不推荐 PSA 筛查。

血液中的 PSA 大多与血清蛋白结合。少量 PSA 不与血清蛋白结合，被称为游离 PSA，其中的一种同种型[-2]proPSA（前 2 肽前列腺特异性抗原），与前列腺癌高度相关。PSA、游离 PSA 和[-2]proPSA 组合的单一评分，即前列腺健康指数（PSA Health Index，PHI），在 PSA 水平在 4~10ng/ml 之间的男性中 PHI 显示比单独 PSA 筛查的灵敏度增加，但尚未被广泛地用作前列腺癌的筛查工具[15]。

卵巢癌

卵巢癌的患病率相对较低——在美国为 1/2 500——这意味着早期卵巢癌检测策略必须对临床前疾病具有相对较高的灵敏度（>75%）以及非常高的特异性（99.6%）以获得至少 10%的阳性预测值，即对发现的每例卵巢癌进行 10 次操作。血清 CA125 受到最多关注，但其作为独立筛查试验缺乏灵敏度或特异性。两阶段的筛查策略有望更为有效。随着时间的推移，血清生物标志物水平的增高会提示经阴道超声（transvaginal sonography，TVS）以检测需要进行剖腹手术的病变。随着每年对卵巢癌平均风险女性 CA125 的测定，研究者已经开发了一种计算机算法以确定每个女性自身基线的偏差。如果 CA125 显著升高，则进行 TVS 检查；如果成像异常，则行剖腹手术。如果 CA125 无变化，则女性在 1 年内复查；如果

CA125轻度升高，则在3个月内获取生物标志物水平。基于此策略，一项由MD Anderson协调的对5 000多名健康绝经后妇女的研究，进行了18次操作以发现2例临界癌症和10例75%在Ⅰ期或Ⅱ期的侵袭性癌症[16]。检测每例癌症所需的操作不超过三次。在英国进行了一项更大规模的随机试验，涉及20万人，旨在测试这种策略对生存率和死亡率的影响。应计项目前两年的数据表明，两阶段策略可以增加早期发现的疾病比例[17]。利用每位妇女基线的偏差，而不是仅使用CA125的单一界定，使检测到的卵巢癌病例数量增加了一倍[18]。这项研究的结果将在不久的将来进行报道，如果结果令人满意，它将改变实践。由于只有80%的卵巢癌表达CA125，因此需要其他标志物对所有卵巢癌进行早期检测。可同时检测多种血清标志物技术的发展，与提高灵敏度而不牺牲特异性的统计学方法的创建相关联，蕴含着巨大的希望。

子宫颈癌

通过宫颈巴氏涂片细胞学检查发现和治疗宫颈上皮内瘤变（cervical intra-epithelial neoplasia，CIN）癌前阶段的国家宫颈癌筛查项目的建立，使宫颈癌的发病率和死亡率降低了80%。单独巴氏涂片的假阴性率为20%~40%，通过定期筛查（每3年一次）可以部分克服这一问题。人乳头瘤病毒（human papilloma virus，HPV），尤其是16型和18型，对宫颈癌的发生至关重要。宫颈涂片检测HPV DNA可使子宫颈癌的检出率比细胞学筛查提高30%，并可将筛查间隔延长至5年[19]。目前正在考虑将基于HPV的筛查纳入指南。然而，重要的是，巴氏涂片和HPV DNA作为初步筛查，随后通过阴道镜进行可视化和病理学评估作为二次筛查。

高危个体

对于有较强癌症家族史的患者，特别是具有癌症高风险基因组生物标志物的携带者，存在特定的指南。当与特定（通常是遗传）生物标志物相关的癌症风险足够高时，建议将重点放在预防上，而不是早期发现。由于预防策略通常比筛查对生活质量的影响更大，因此，识别与极高癌症风险相关的遗传突变，需要对患者进行教育以及谨慎的共同决策。此外，遗传性生物标志物测试对家庭成员具有重要意义。预防性手术和化学预防是特别有效的降低风险的技术，专门留给风险最高的人。预防性卵巢切除术和/或乳房切除术对*BRCA1*/*BRCA2*突变携带者具有最好的保护作用，可将卵巢癌和乳腺癌的风险降低90%以上[20,21]。然而，一些患者更愿意进行乳房X线检查、磁共振成像或其他筛查方法来推迟手术干预，要么出于个人偏好，要么为了允许生育。在与极高风险患者讨论早期发现和预防的选择时，需要考虑许多因素（例如，伦理和成本），该医学领域是一个快速发展的专业[22-24]。

乳腺癌和卵巢癌

在有显著乳腺癌和/或卵巢癌病史的家庭中，利用临床预测模型（如BRCAPRO模型），现在可以在少数病例中确定关键的癌症风险生物标志物（通常是遗传突变）[25]。这些模型可用于指导特定的分子测试，以进一步风险分层并指导随后的筛查或预防。*BRCA1*和*BRCA2*的遗传突变分别占所有乳腺癌和卵巢癌的5%~10%和10%~15%[26,27]。此外，在没有显著家族史的情况下，大约15%的患有三阴性乳腺癌或高级别浆液性卵巢癌的患者会携带有害的*BRCA1/2*种系突变。此外，*BRCA1/2*突变指导卵巢癌的治疗，如下节所述。大约12%的高风险女性不携带*BRCA1/2*突变，估计这些人群有另一种诱发癌症的基因组改变[28]，这表明需要改进检测方法以识别额外的风险生物标志物。研究较少的乳腺癌易感基因包括*CHEK2*、*ATM*、*RAD51C*、*BRIP1*、*PALB2*、*NBS1*、*LKB1*、*PTEN*、*p53*、*XRCC1*和*STK11*，但由于遗传突变的罕见性，这些基因通常未被评估[29-32]。最近，上述基因已被整合到多重测序分析中，这些与较低的癌症发展频率有关的基因，为患者决策提供了更多的信息和更大的挑战。

结肠癌

家族性腺瘤性息肉病（familial adenomatous polyposis，FAP）和遗传性非息肉病性结肠癌（hereditary nonpolyposis colon cancer，HNPCC）易患早发型家族性/遗传性结肠癌。它们的特征分别是结肠腺瘤性息肉病（adenomatous polyposis coli，APC）基因和DNA错配修复基因中的种系突变。在HNPCC中，使用针对错配修复蛋白的抗体筛查常规肿瘤分子已取代临床风险模型以指导筛查（如修订的Bethesda指南）。然而，肿瘤分子筛查导致对HNPCC基因检测过度，因为10%~15%的病例表现为散发病[33]。将临床风险预测模型与肿瘤分子筛查相结合，或检测散发病的分子标志物（*MLH1*启动子甲基化和/或*BRAF* V600E基因突变）来检测肿瘤，可以在保持高检出率的同时，提高HNPCC的筛查水平[34]。管理指南要求对FAP进行外科癌症预防（结肠切除术）以及对HNPCC进行密集的结肠镜筛查。

在最近的一项研究中，粪便血红蛋白检测结合粪便DNA检测突变的K-Ras、异常的*NDRG4*和*BMP3*甲基化以及B-肌动蛋白[35]。与9 989名可评估的具有平均风险参与者的标准粪便免疫组化检测（fecal immmunohistochemical test，FIT）相比，复合Cologuard®检测显示检测结直肠癌的灵敏度更高（92.3% vs 73.8%，$P=0.002$），检测晚期癌前病变的灵敏度更高（42.4% vs 23.8%，$P<0.001$），高级别发育异常息肉检出率较高（69.2% vs 46.2%，$P=0.004$），检测1cm或以上无蒂锯齿状息肉的检出率更高（42.4%和5.1%，$P<0.001$）。然而，DNA检测的特异性略低于FIT（86.6%比94.9%）。基于这些结果，美国FDA于2014年批准该测试用于50岁以上的个体。

未来的早期检测和筛查方法

虽然目前的早期检测方法已经对某些恶性肿瘤如宫颈癌的死亡率产生了影响，然而低灵敏度、由于假阳性而使用不必要的侵入性诊断程序以及过度诊断/治疗仍然是重要的问题。此外，许多肿瘤类型，如卵巢癌和胰腺癌，无法从这些方法中获益。患者仍呈现晚期疾病，因此预后较差。循环肿瘤生物标志物的升高可能需要相当大的肿瘤体积。小体积的癌症可以在较早的时段诱发自身抗体。新的分子筛查技术，包括循环DNA，RNA和外泌体，有可能补充现有的基于蛋白质的筛查标记并彻底改变早期癌症检测，同时促进准确的风险评估和个体治疗计划。

目前用于预测效果和治疗反应性的分子生物标志物

尽管预测癌症患者预后的分子生物标志物是有用的，但更大的临床应用在于可预测从特定癌症治疗中获益的生物标志物。这两种类型之间有相当大的重叠，因为那些预测特定癌症治疗对特定患者有益的生物标志物将预测改善的预后。

乳腺癌

激素受体

激素受体（hormone receptor，HR）阳性乳腺癌约占所有乳腺癌的 70%，并以雌激素受体（estrogen receptor，ER）alpha 和/或黄体酮受体（progesterone receptor，PR）的表达为标志。HR 生物标志物可识别那些通过抗激素治疗对生长抑制敏感的乳腺肿瘤，这些治疗包括 ER 部分激动剂/拮抗剂（如他莫昔芬），ER 下调剂（如氟维司群）和芳香酶抑制剂（如来曲唑）[36,37]。在临床实践中，使用免疫组织化学对所有乳腺癌的 HR 蛋白表达进行常规评估。然而，尽管进行了 5 年的辅助抗激素治疗，仍有相当一部分早期 HR 阳性的妇女乳腺癌复发，并且大多数患有转移性 HR 阳性乳腺癌的女性对抗激素治疗产生耐药。因此，在美国，每年有超过 25 000 名患有 HR 阳性乳腺肿瘤的女性死亡，这一数字超过了每年其他所有类型乳腺癌的总和。

多参数基因表达谱

我们预测 HR 阳性乳腺癌患者接受抗激素药物治疗后治愈可能性的能力已经显著提高。*Oncotype Dx*（表 40-1）基于 21 个基因的表达，可预测辅助药物他莫西芬对单个淋巴结阴性 HR 阳性乳腺肿瘤患者的益处，并根据与他莫西芬耐药性相关的特征选择患者进行细胞毒性化疗[38]。然而，尽管这一方法具有临床应用价值，但除了已知的肿瘤分级、HER2 和 HR 水平的作用外，这一方法和类似的检测方法，如 PAM50 和 Mammoprint，并没有增加我们对 HR 阳性乳腺癌中抗激素耐药机制的了解[36,38,39]。磷脂酰肌醇-3 激酶（phosphatidylinositol-3-kinase，PI3K）/AKT/mTOR 和丝裂原活化蛋白激酶（mitogen-activated protein kinase，MAPK）通路是 HER2 等膜受体酪氨酸激酶（receptor tyrosine kinases，RTKs）作用的主要介质，并介导抗激素治疗的耐药性[40]。mTOR 抑制剂依维莫司将对抗激素治疗有耐药性的 HR 阳性乳腺癌妇女的无进展生存期提高了大约 60%[41]。然而，缺乏对该药物反应的预测性分子生物标志物。

表 40-1 *Oncotype Dx* 的 21 个基因系列及基于功能进行细分

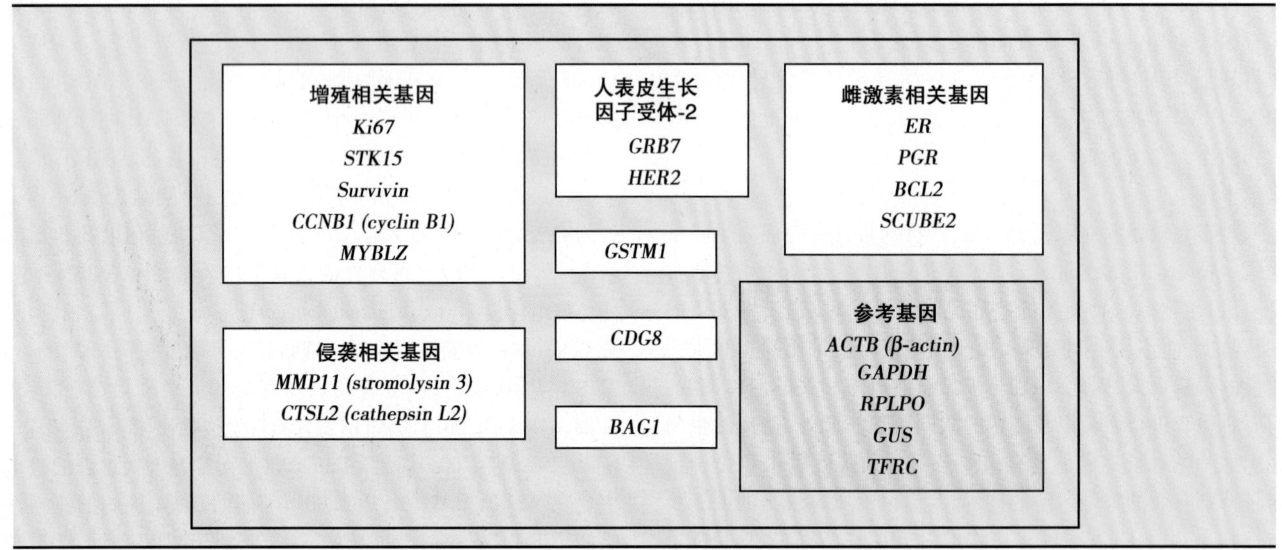

人表皮生长因子受体-2（HER2）

在 15%～20%的侵袭性乳腺癌中，有编码 HER2 的癌基因扩增并伴有蛋白过表达。HER2 过表达决定了侵袭性乳腺肿瘤表型和预后不良[42]。将靶向 HER2 的重组人源化单克隆抗体曲妥珠单抗（Herceptin）和细胞毒性化疗联合治疗转移性和早期 HER2 癌基因扩增的乳腺癌患者，提高了应答率和生存率[43]。因此，HER2 是乳腺肿瘤对曲妥珠单抗和其他 HER2 靶向疗法（例如帕妥珠单抗、拉帕替尼和 TDM1）反应性的生物标志物[44]。最近，HER2 还被证实可预测 15%～20%由 HER2 驱动肿瘤发生的晚期胃癌患者对基于曲妥珠单抗化疗的反应[45]。

HER2 过表达的乳腺癌和胃癌中有相当一部分最初对曲妥珠单抗没有反应，或对曲妥珠单抗产生耐药性。这可能是通过一种不结合曲妥珠单抗（p95-HER2）的切割形式的 HER2，通过上调其他膜 RTKs，如 IGF1R 或 MET，或上调 PI3K/AKT 通路介导的[46-49]。后者可以通过 PTEN（一种负性 PI3K/AKT 调节剂）的突变失活、PTEN 缺失或 PIK3CA 突变（编码 PI3K 的 p110α 亚基的癌基因）发生[50]。事实上，在以抗 HER2 靶向治疗 HER2 阳性乳腺癌时，PI3K 通路的激活以及 PIK3CA 和 PTEN 的突变是负面预后标志物[51]。

因此，美国临床肿瘤学会（American Society of Clinical Oncology，ASCO）的一个小组建议，应该确定所有侵袭性乳腺癌的 HER2 状态[52]。该小组提出了一种依赖于准确且可重复分析性能的检测算法，包括新近可用的明场原位杂交（in situ hybridization,ISH)类型,并详细说明了可靠地减少检测变异的元素(如样本处理、分析排除和报告标准)。这强调了在可靠性和临床实用性方面都需要对所有预测性的标志物进行质量控制和方法验证。

卵巢癌:BRCA1/2

大约 20%的高级别浆液性卵巢癌具有潜在的遗传性或体细胞 *BRCA1/2* 突变,导致其同源重组缺陷,而同源重组是修复双链 DNA 断裂的必要途径[53]。这些肿瘤依赖于替代性的 DNA 修复机制,如碱基切除修复,其中 PARP 酶是关键。PARP 的抑制剂利用 *BRCA1/2* 突变的卵巢癌易受 DNA 损伤。在一项随机Ⅱ期试验中,与安慰剂相比,PARP 抑制剂奥拉帕尼用于铂敏感复发性 *BRCA1/2* 突变卵巢肿瘤的维持治疗时,其无进展生存期提高了 82%[54]。奥拉帕尼现在已经被批准用于该适应证,其他 PARP 抑制剂和其他用途的批准迫在眉睫。耐药机制包括 *BRCA1/2* 突变的功能恢复、53BP1(一种参与替代性 DNA 修复机制的蛋白)缺失以及 PI3K/AKT/mTOR 通路的上调[55]。奥拉帕尼与 PI3K 抑制剂 BKM120 的联合应用,在高级别浆液性卵巢癌和三阴性乳腺癌的早期临床研究中显示出活性[56]。

肺癌

表皮生长因子受体

可逆的表皮生长因子受体(epidermal growth factor receptor,EGFR)酪氨酸激酶抑制剂(tyrosine kinase inhibitors,TKIs)吉非替尼和厄罗替尼以及不可逆的 pan-HER TKI 阿法替尼和达克替尼为大约 10%~30%的非小细胞肺癌患者提供了有效的治疗。这些患者的肿瘤带有激活的 EGFR 突变,常见的突变位于外显子 19 和 21[57-60]。尽管在男性和从前吸烟者中也观察到 EGFR 突变,但亚裔女性非吸烟者合并腺癌是典型的表型。虽然在 EGFR 突变型肺癌中使用达可替尼进行一线治疗与令人印象深刻的无进展生存期(18.2 个月)相关,而且阿法替尼在外显子 19 突变中表现出最大的功效,但一种 TKI 优于另一种 TKI 的益处尚未确定。

EGFR 抑制剂的多重获得性耐药机制,包括 *EGFR* 的二次突变(T790M)和 MET 扩增[61],限制了 EGFR 靶向治疗的疗效。新的 EGFR TKIs 在Ⅰ/Ⅱ期研究中显示出治疗或预防耐药的前景,目前正在更大规模的临床试验中进行评估[62],有望转化为肺癌患者的有效治疗方法。

间变性淋巴瘤激酶和 ROS-1

导致致癌基因融合的两种可靶向的染色体基因重排,指导了晚期肺腺癌的新疗法[63,64]。间变性淋巴瘤激酶(anaplastic lymphoma kinas,ALK)和 ROS-1 基因易位分别存在于 4%~6% 和 1%~2%的晚期肺腺癌患者中,使其对 ALK、ROS-1 和 MET 抑制剂克唑替尼显著敏感。从确定这些靶标到克唑替尼获得批准之间的短周期,使人们对不再需要从药物发现和实施应用的传统较长时间的演变感到兴奋。克唑替尼对 ALK 和 ROS-1 重排肿瘤的应答率超过 70%,中位无进展生存期分别为 11 个月和 19 个月。基因过表达、旁路机制和继发性突变通常导致获得性耐药,尽管与 EGFR 突变的非小细胞肺癌不同,在疾病进展过程中可在单个肿瘤观察到多种突变类型。在早期临床试验中,涉及第二代 ALK 抑制剂如色瑞替尼以克服获得性耐药的策略显示出前景[65]。

基于这些结果,对所有晚期肺腺癌(或具有腺癌成分的肺肿瘤),无论其临床特征如何,都建议常规分子检测 EGFR 和 ALK。可能由于抽样错误而不含腺癌成分,但由于临床特征(年轻,从不吸烟)而怀疑含有腺癌成分的肿瘤也可以进行检测[66]。

结肠癌

微卫星不稳定性

目前的指南建议在Ⅱ期结肠癌的"高风险"患者中使用基于 5-氟尿嘧啶的辅助化疗,这些患者定义为存在高级别肿瘤,伴有淋巴管空间侵犯及肿瘤穿孔的证据,和/或少于 12 个淋巴结摘除手术。大约 11%的Ⅱ期结肠癌具有错配 DNA 修复缺陷,表现为微卫星不稳定性[67]。这些肿瘤在没有辅助化疗的情况下具有良好的预后。因此,指南建议对Ⅱ期结肠癌进行错配修复蛋白的常规免疫组织化学检测,如其不存在则无需辅助化疗。

KRAS、BRAF 和 NRAS

KRAS 是 EGFR 下游的原癌基因,通过 Ras-Raf-MAPK 通路启动信号传递。大约 60%的转移性结直肠癌具有良好的野生型 *KRAS* 谱,预测其对抗 EGFR 单抗、西妥昔单抗和帕尼单抗敏感。*KRAS* 突变主要存在于外显子 2 的第 12 和第 13 个密码子上,预测对这些疗法耐药,如同更罕见的 *NRAS* 突变一样[68-71]。下游 *BRAF* 突变发生在约 5%~9%的病例中,并与不良预后相关,尽管未从 EGFR 抑制剂获益的报道尚不确定。

胃肠道间质瘤:KIT 和 PDGFRA

胃肠道间质瘤(gastrointestinal stromal tumors,GIST)与 *KIT*(80%的 GIST)或血小板衍生生长因子受体 A(platelet-derived growth factor receptor A,*PDGFRA*;5%~10%的 *GISTs*)基因的初级活化突变有关,该突变导致组成型 RTK 活化[72]。抑制 KIT 和 PDGFRA 的伊马替尼(Gleevec)在大约 85%无法切除或转移性疾病的患者中获得临床益处,中位无进展生存期为 20~24 个月,尽管外显子 11 突变患者的结果优于外显子 9 突变。更高剂量的伊马替尼可为外显子 9 突变的病例带来更大的益处。对伊马替尼的获得性耐药机制是多种多样的,主要涉及 *KIT* 外显子 13、14 或 17 二次突变的出现。在伊马替尼耐药的 *GIST* 患者中,新型激酶抑制剂如舒尼替尼、尼洛替尼、达沙替尼和瑞格非尼,可以抑制突变蛋白的功能并恢复抗肿瘤活性。

黑素瘤

BRAF

所有黑色素瘤中大约有一半携带 *BRAF* V600E 基因突变,导致 MAPK 通路的组成型下游激活,从而产生对 BRAF 抑制剂(如维罗非尼和达拉非尼)的敏感性[73,74]。临床上,对这些药物的反应持续时间很短,中位进展时间为 6~7 个月。克服 MAPK 通路代偿性过度激活引起耐药性的新方法包括预先联合 BRAF 和 MEK 抑制剂(如曲美替尼),从而提高效力并降低治疗的毒性[75]。

NRAS

MEK 抑制剂可能在治疗 *NRAS* 突变型黑色素瘤中发挥重

要作用,这种黑色素瘤约占所有黑色素瘤的15%~20%,其在生物学上特别具有侵袭性。有趣的是,MEK抑制剂与免疫疗法结合可以显示出活性[76]。

KIT

少数(3%)*BRAF/NRAS*阴性的黑色素瘤携带*KIT*原癌基因突变,尤其是在黏膜和肢端黑色素瘤中。使用伊马替尼或舒尼替尼进行靶向治疗是可行的治疗选择,能够提供持久的反应,有证据表明在伊马替尼治疗后肿瘤进展时尼洛替尼具有活性[77,78]。

慢性粒细胞白血病

Bcr-Abl 染色体异位

大多数慢性粒细胞白血病(chronic myeloid leukemia,CML)病例是由Abl激酶的组成性激活驱动的,这是断裂点簇集区(breakpoint cluster region,Bcr)与Abl激酶易位的结果(费城染色体)。伊马替尼靶向治疗抑制Abl激酶活性,显著改善了CML患者的预后。然而,尽管最初对患者有益,伊马替尼可能会出现耐药性。此外,伊马替尼治疗晚期"原始细胞危象"CML的疗效有限[79]。耐药性主要是由于Abl激酶域的新突变干扰药物结合。因此,研究者开发了新的Abl激酶抑制剂(AKIs),其中尼洛替尼、达沙替尼和博舒替尼获得了监管批准。不幸的是,所有可用的AKIs对某些激酶域的突变都表现为无活性,最常见的是*Bcr-Abl*(*T315I*)突变的交叉耐药。第三代AKI帕纳替尼在*Bcr-Abl*(*T315l*)突变CML和其他一些多重耐药突变中表现出临床益处。然而,在临床开发期间,可能与选择药物高剂量相关的心血管毒性问题,阻碍了监管部门的批准。对帕纳替尼剂量优化的试验正在进行中[80]。

淋巴瘤

CD20 和其他生物标志物

生物标志物靶向治疗对非霍奇金淋巴瘤(non-Hodgkin lymphoma,NHL)的治疗有显著效果[81,82]。嵌合的抗CD20抗体利妥昔单抗的开发,预示着NHL治疗方法进入了一个新时代。利妥昔单抗目前是滤泡性淋巴瘤一线治疗的标准单药疗法,并可与其他CD20阳性B细胞淋巴瘤的化疗联合使用。随后,利妥昔单抗的放射免疫偶联物(^{90}Y-替伊莫单抗和^{131}I-托西莫单抗)的开发和批准进一步改善了预后。

抗体的临床评价在很大程度上基于对淋巴瘤细胞表面抗原表达的认识,这导致了抗CD22(如未偶联的依帕珠单抗)、CD80(galiximab)、CD52(阿仑单抗)、CD2(西普珠单抗)、CD40(SGN-40)和CD30抗体的开发[83]。抗CD30抗体本妥昔单抗与一种名为vedotin的药物结合,可将细胞毒性药物靶向传递给CD30阳性的霍奇金淋巴瘤或间变性大细胞淋巴瘤,产生了毒性可接受的显著临床效益。它最近被批准用于自体干细胞移植后复发的霍奇金淋巴瘤和复发的间变性大细胞淋巴瘤。目前,正在研究将其用于化疗之前。

口咽癌

人乳头瘤病毒

在过去的二十年,口咽癌(oropharyngeal cancer,OPC)的流行病学发生了变化,有研究报告在西方国家所有OPC中有60%~70%存在HPV p16亚型。使用p16免疫组织化学很容易进行分子肿瘤检测,其与HPV FISH具有高度一致性。大型临床试验的回顾性分析表明,与HPV阴性的OPCS相比,在HPV相关的OPCS中放化疗具有更高的反应率和生存率[84]。因此,HPV是未来OPCs治疗研究的重要分层工具,并可能决定着不同的治疗方法。关于HPV相关性OPCs可能受益于较低强度放化疗的建议需要进一步的评估。

用于癌症监测的分子生物标志物

许多循环生物标志物用于监测癌症对治疗的反应和/或早期发现癌症患者的复发性疾病。

甲胎蛋白和人绒毛膜促性腺激素

许多生殖细胞肿瘤[大多数男性睾丸癌,妊娠滋养细胞疾病(绒毛膜癌)和罕见卵巢癌]产生循环肿瘤标志物[甲胎蛋白(Alpha-fetoprotein,AFP),人绒毛膜促性腺激素(human chorionic gonadotropin,hCG),乳酸脱氢酶(lactate dehydrogenase,LDH)][67]。这些生物标志物可用于诊断、分期、监测治疗反应以及检测早期肿瘤复发。由于复发性生殖细胞肿瘤可以通过细胞毒性化疗治愈,特别是在早期发现复发时,因此即使没有明显的疾病,在患者随访期间肿瘤标志物水平的提高是开始挽救治疗的一个指标。评价治疗反应时必须考虑标志物的半衰期。

AFP是一种糖蛋白,通常由胎儿卵黄囊,肝脏和胃肠道产生,但不由正常成人组织产生。AFP在生殖细胞肿瘤中重新表达,包括卵黄囊肿瘤和胚胎癌。hCG是由合体滋养细胞产生的一种糖蛋白,由两个亚基α和β组成。α亚基为三种垂体营养激素所共有:FSH,LH和TSH;β-亚基组成hCG的酶促和免疫独特区。分析仅检测β亚基(β-hCG)。在男性中,它对睾丸癌具有高度特异性,特别是绒毛膜癌细胞和5%~10%的纯精原细胞瘤。LDH反映"肿瘤负荷"、生长速度和细胞增殖,具有独立的预后意义。在约80%的晚期精原细胞瘤和约60%的晚期非精原细胞生殖细胞肿瘤中,LDH升高。LDH同工酶1对生殖细胞肿瘤的特异性和敏感性似乎高于同工酶2~5[85]。

CA125

CA125是MUC16基因的黏液性跨膜糖蛋白产物,分子量最高可达5mD。CA125最为人所知的是作为卵巢癌标志物,尽管观察到其在子宫内膜癌、输卵管癌、肺癌、乳腺癌和胃肠道癌以及包括子宫内膜异位症在内的相对良性疾病中也可升高。单独使用一次CA125对卵巢癌的筛查不够敏感或特异[86]。此外,20%的卵巢癌的CA125水平不会升高。然而,血清CA125对于跟踪治疗反应、预测治疗预后以及检测卵巢癌患者的复发非常有用。在卵巢癌一线铂类化疗期间,应定期随访CA125水平(如每3周)。CA125水平在最低点、3个月正常化的CA125和CA125半衰期是无进展和总生存期的强预测因子[87-89]。手术和铂类化疗初始治疗后血清CA125正常化的失败,是卵巢癌患者预后不良的一个特别不祥的指征。

国家综合癌症网络(National Comprehensive Cancer Network,NCCN)(www.nccn.org)建议,在先前治疗卵巢癌之后临床缓解的女性中,如果在最初诊断时血清CA125水平升高,则在每次随访时评估血清CA125水平。在记录CA125升高后,临床疾病复发的中位时间超过 4 个月，尽管在正常范围内的增高可以产生更长的提前期。在英国进行的一项大型随机研究得出结论，疾病复发的女性在 CA125 升高接受治疗时总体生存获益不足，尽管只有 25% 的对照组和实验组的女性及时接受了最佳联合化疗[90]。考虑到症状复发与死亡之间的间隔相对较短，以 CA125 检测早期复发至少可以为接受已知药物和新型药物提供时间。然而存在这样的争议，即应该与每位患者讨论使用 CA125 来监测复发。

CA15-3 and CA27.29

CA15-3 和 CA27.29 是检测外周血中循环 MUC1 抗原的特异性方法[91]。一些研究支持这种循环标志物在早期乳腺癌中的预后相关性，尽管监测基于 MUC1 的血清标志物已经证明在制定治疗决策中具有实用性[92,93]。ASCO 认为现有数据不足以推荐使用 CA15-3 或 CA27.29 进行乳腺癌筛查、诊断、分期或监测患者复发，因为缺乏早期发现复发可提高生存率的确凿证据[91]。虽然目前的数据不能推荐单独使用 CA15-3 或 CA27.29 来监测治疗反应，但 CA15-3 或 CA27.29 的上升可用于指示无易测指标疾病的治疗失败。但是，在新疗法的前 4~6 周解释 CA27.29 或 CA15-3 水平升高时应谨慎，因为可能会出现虚假的早期升高。这些建议也适用于使用 CEA（carcinoembryonic antigen，癌胚抗原）监测转移性结肠癌。

CA19-9

糖类抗原 19-9 主要在胃肠道癌患者的血清中升高。血清 CA19-9 最大的作用是监测胰腺癌的治疗反应。对于接受积极治疗的局部晚期或转移性胰腺癌患者，ASCO 建议每 1~3 个月测量一次血清 CA19-9 水平[94]。CA19-9 连续升高提示在治疗过程中出现进展性疾病，但在治疗改变开始前应寻求确定性研究（如 CT 扫描）。

癌胚抗原

癌胚抗原（carcinoembryonic antigen，CEA）是细胞黏附糖蛋白[95]，其产生于胎儿发育期间，通常不存在于健康成人的血液中，尽管在重度吸烟者中水平升高。结直肠癌、胃癌、胰腺癌、肺癌、乳腺癌和甲状腺髓样癌患者的血清 CEA 可能升高。ASCO 制定了临床实践指南用于监测结直肠癌患者的血清 CEA 水平，如果血清 CEA 有助于分期和手术计划，则要求其在术前检测血清 CEA。对于Ⅱ期和Ⅲ期结直肠癌患者，术后 CEA 水平应每 3 个月进行一次，如果该患者是手术（如肝切除）或转移性疾病进行化疗的潜在人选，则应至少进行 3 年。CEA 也是监测转移性结直肠癌全身治疗反应的首选标志物。

前列腺特异性抗原

检测血清 PSA 对确诊前列腺癌的男性很重要。PSA 升高的速度可以预测前列腺癌的预后。在前列腺癌诊断前一年内 PSA 水平升高超过 2.0ng/ml 的前列腺癌患者，在根治性前列腺切除术后死于前列腺癌的风险更高。PSA 水平、临床分期和 Gleason 肿瘤分级是大多数用于前列腺癌风险评估的列线图和预测模型的组成部分[96]。此外，血清 PSA 可作为疾病治疗反应的指标。

对于最初治疗有治愈目的的前列腺癌患者，应每 6~12 个月评估血清 PSA 水平，为期 5 年，此后每年评估一次。PSA 水平升高表明生化功能衰竭，通常发生在临床可检测到的复发前数年。由于生化衰竭可能代表一个单独的局部复发，因此识别这些患者很重要，因为他们可能是挽救治疗的候选者。

新型分子生物标志物及其检测平台

恶性肿瘤的特征在于导致个体癌症特性的多个分子异常。驱动畸变可以发生在生殖细胞系基因组中，也可以在癌症基因组和/或蛋白质组中以体细胞或获得的方式发生。无论是以循环肿瘤细胞（circulating tumor cells，CTCs），还是以循环核苷酸、蛋白质或代谢物的形式，新的癌症生物标志物不仅可以在肿瘤或其微环境中检测到，还可以在循环中检测到。

综合癌症基因组和蛋白质组特征的新型高通量分子技术为生物标志物的鉴定创造了许多新的可能性，特别是集成了许多标志物交叉信息的多标志物（如多基因）系列的开发。许多早期的高通量手段，如基因甲基化分析、基因芯片、比较基因组杂交、质谱/光谱和基于微珠的分析方法正在被下一代测序所取代。基因表达谱已被广泛开发以确定各种人类肿瘤的良好和不良预后亚组[97]。目前，甲基化分析检测早期癌细胞 DNA 甲基化异常的能力正在研究中。高通量反相裂解蛋白阵列（reverse phase protein lysate array，RPPA）蛋白质组学技术允许同时分析多种特定激酶和其他蛋白的表达和激活[98-102]。该平台特别适合研究癌症中的激酶信号传导，以及治疗期间和化学预防期间的高风险组织中新型药物（如 TKIs）的分子效应（图 40-1）。新兴的质谱分析方法，如多重反应监测（multiple reaction monitoring，MRM）和 SWATH，可以在没有高质量抗体的情况下提供候选基因的额外信息，而且质谱分析对生物标志物的发现尤其有用。基因组和蛋白质组学平台一起提供可以合并的信息，以开发反映全球 DNA、RNA 和蛋白质异常的特征变化。这些可能能够胜过仅从其中一个平台的单一技术检查中获得的数据[103]。例如，蛋白质组学研究可以通过提供翻译后修饰和蛋白质相对水平和激活的信息来增强基因组系列检测。同样地，数据集、有效数据管理系统、通路综合分析以及“荟萃分析”是成功开发分子标记的关键组成部分[104-106]。

新的生殖细胞系生物标志物

生殖细胞系基因组可能含有尚未开发的有价值的新型癌症风险生物标志物，以及特定抗癌治疗的毒性和有效性的生物标志物。例如，生殖细胞系多态性与 *EGFR* 抑制剂厄洛替尼在肺癌中的毒性和功效有关[107]。最近对生殖细胞系基因组的大规模研究也开始发现大量的癌症易感性标志物，其中许多具有低外显率，从而提高了我们利用新的生殖细胞系生物标志物预测癌症高风险以及对治疗反应的能力[108-110]。

高风险和早期发现癌症的组织特异性生物标志物

早期的恶性变化可能是特定组织癌症高风险的一个指标。随着可采用微创方法获得可能有风险或有患癌风险的组织（例如痰液、支气管灌洗液、血液、粪便、尿液或乳头抽出物）中带有早期瘤变的细胞，研究用于筛查具有致癌风险和早期恶变的组织标志物变得更加可行。迄今为止，由于成本、侵入性、缺乏大型前瞻性结果验证研究以及缺乏标准化指南，这些潜在有用的方法大多局限于小型临床研究。

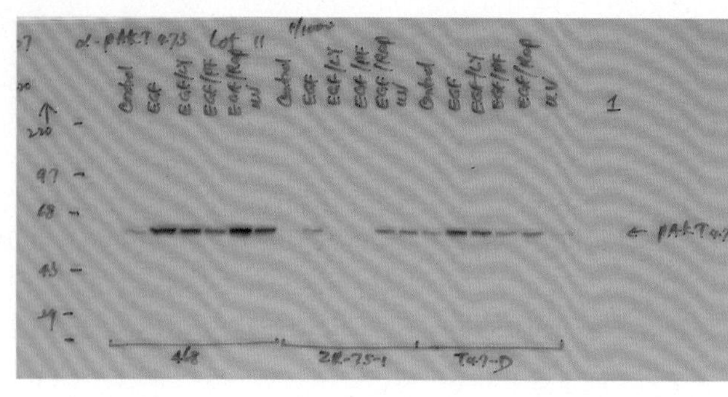

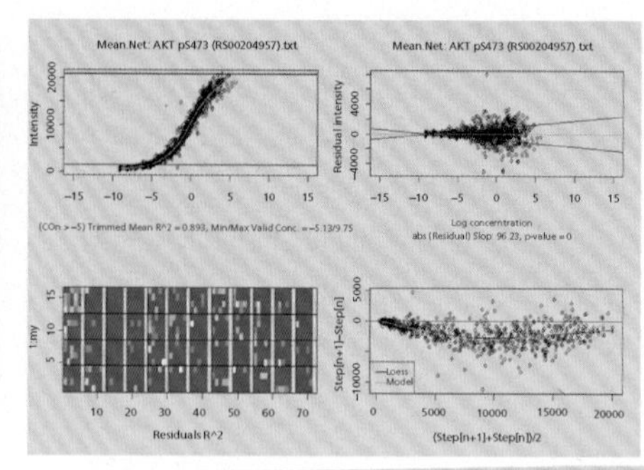

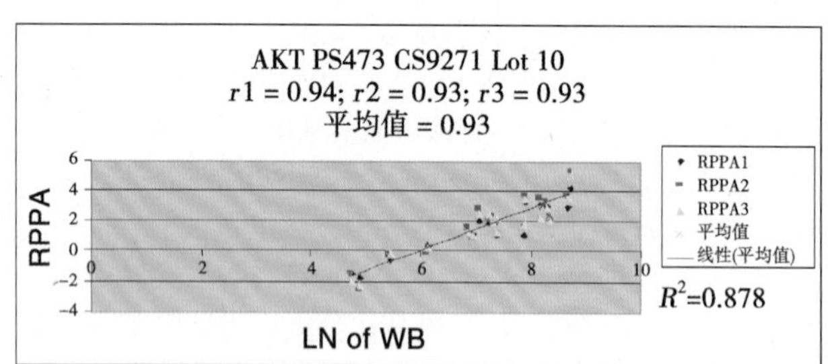

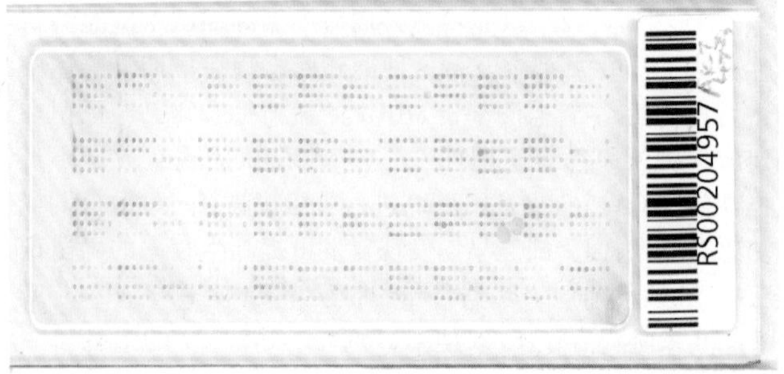

图 40-1 反相裂解蛋白阵列(RPPA)抗体的验证。将来自细胞系的蛋白质裂解物在硝酸纤维素包被的载玻片上连续稀释,然后用抗磷酸化 Akt 的单特异性抗体进行信号检测和扩增。连续稀释曲线用于定量。与蛋白质印迹结果进行比较证实 r 值为 0.878。右上图为染色定量和质量控制

尽管使用常规细胞学检查痰液在早期筛查肺癌并未降低癌症特异性死亡率,但目前正在研究将分子检测方法应用于痰液和支气管灌洗液,以尝试检测与癌变前期和早期恶性支气管上皮细胞相关的分子变化[111]。例如,用特异位点探针对染色体区 5p15、7p12(EGFR)、8q24(C-Myc)和 6 号染色体的着丝粒进行 FISH 检测,可显著提高痰和支气管冲洗样本中恶性肿瘤检测的敏感性[112]。

癌症特异性生物标志物

如前所述,在确定单一生物标志物和多标志物系列(如 *Oncotype Dx*)以预测对靶向治疗的反应和克服耐药性方面已取得进展。然而,在其他癌症类型中这方面的进展更为有限。新兴的篮子临床试验可能部分解决了这一不足。篮子试验是基于对不同癌症类型中发生的常见分子畸变的观察,其在同一试验中评估了靶向治疗对特定分子畸变的作用,而不论其癌症类型[113]。

将来,早期药物活性的药效学生物标志物也必须在临床前肿瘤模型中加以定义,然后在患者样本中进行确认,以确保患者正在接受生物相关的药物剂量。在这方面,药物对肿瘤的最佳靶标抑制作用可能比药物的最大耐受剂量更为重要。然而,大多数药物的最佳药物活性是否依赖于最大靶标抑制、曲线下面积或波谷值尚不清楚。来自系统生物学如敏感性分析的规则可能提供有关所需的最佳抑制模式的指南。该方法可优化药物疗效,降低毒性,特别是脱靶毒性,并有助于早期识别无应答者,以便向替代疗法进行分流。例如,哌立福辛诱导肿瘤中 AKT 的抑制与使用多种哌立福辛给药方案的肿瘤生长抑制作用显著相关。此外,在开始治疗后不久使用蛋白质组学测定如 RPPA 对肿瘤中多个 PI3K/AKT 通路成员的激活状态进行综合评估,在预测肿瘤对 PI3K 通路抑制剂的反应方面可能优于单一标志物。

血清和尿液生物标志物

新的血清生物标志物在癌症筛查、预测肿瘤对特定治疗的反应性以及监测肿瘤对治疗的反应方面具有潜在的应用价值。如前所述,虽然传统的血清癌症生物标志物常规用于癌症监测,但其在筛查中因无法达到最佳灵敏度和特异性而应用受限[114-116]。通过监测个体标志物水平随时间的增加可以改善特异性,但几乎肯定需要标志物系列来增加筛查的灵敏度。关于血清生物标志物的筛查实用性的常规概念是其检测应当在适当情况下通过影像学、活检或增加监测来引发临床评估。或者,新的血清标志物可以在通过其他方法筛查后使用以增加后者的特异性。因此,一种新的生物标志物可能允许定义一个可疑的乳房 X 线病变,视情况采取连续监测或立即活检。

基于质谱的无偏倚方法,可从血液或尿液中存在的蛋白质组或代谢组中确定新的血清生物标志物,具有鉴定能从早期发展阶段发现肿瘤的生物标志物系列的潜力。由于卵巢癌的诊断处于晚期,患者预后不佳,以及缺乏一种完善的筛查方法,卵巢癌已经成为几项此类研究的主题。两种通用方法已被使用:识别独特的特征以及发现那些可以组装成系列的离散标记。然而,没有一种基于质谱的方法在大规模的前瞻性样本组中得到验证[117]。

在尿液中,FISH 或使用 IHC 或反转录酶(reverse transcriptase,RT)-聚合酶链反应(polymerase chain reaction,PCR)检测细胞角蛋白(例如角蛋白 19、20)的灵敏度可能高于膀胱和尿路上皮癌筛查的常规细胞学检测[118]。一个包含染色体 3、7、9p21 和 17 杂交探针的商用试剂盒(UroVysion)被用于尿液的 FISH 分析。该 FISH 分析检测膀胱癌的灵敏度和特异性分别为 60%和 82.6%。相反,与尿液细胞学相关的灵敏度和特异性分别为 24.1%和 90.5%。因此,对于染色体 3、7、9 和 17 的 FISH 测定可能比细胞学具有更高的灵敏度,并且在检测尿路

上皮癌方面具有相似的特异性。表 40-2 总结了已被研究作为促进膀胱癌筛查的潜在工具的各种方法[119]。

表 40-2　尿细胞学、膀胱肿瘤抗原(bladder tumor antigen, BTA)免疫检测、核基质蛋白 22(nuclear matrix protein-22, NMP22)检测、免疫细胞、尿 FISH 对早期发现膀胱癌的灵敏度、特异性及阳性预测值

	灵敏度(%)	特异性(%)	PPV(%)
PSA	72	93	25
尿液细胞学	48~73	48~100	48~69
BTA	53	77	63
NMP22	71	66	21
ImmunoCyt	78~81	74~100	26
FISH	69~71	78~95	68

注:血清前列腺特异性抗原(prostate-specific antigen, PSA)在前列腺癌筛查中仅作为参考。ImmunoCyt 目前被美国食品和药物管理局批准用于监测复发性膀胱癌。ImmunoCyt 使用三种单克隆抗体混合物检测尿液中的膀胱癌细胞。其中一种抗体针对的是一种高分子量形式的糖基化癌胚抗原 19A211。另外两种抗体, LDQ10 和 M344, 是抗膀胱癌的特异性黏蛋白,并用荧光素标记。

来源:*Hu 2007. Reproduced with permission of Oxford University Press.*

循环肿瘤细胞

循环肿瘤细胞(circulating tumor cells, CTCs)在癌症筛查、靶标识别、反应预测以及监测对治疗的反应方面具有潜在的应用价值。事实上, CTCs 和最近的循环肿瘤 DNA 的预测和预后功效已经在转移性乳腺癌中得到证实[120,121]。CTCs 在乳腺癌筛查中实用性的初步研究正在进行中[122]。在卵巢癌中,一些 FIGO Ⅲ/Ⅳ期卵巢癌患者可以检测到外周血 CTC-特异性 *p53* 序列,表明该方法可用作早期检测的基本构件[123]。

由于需要扩增底物,使用 CTCs 研究分子生物标志物目前限于基因表达特征。然而, CTCs 具有用"液体"活组织检查替代侵入性肿瘤活检的潜力,并且有助于早期进入肿瘤基因组和蛋白质组获取预测治疗反应和耐药性的分子生物标志物,如在肺癌和前列腺癌中所证实[124,125]。一个主要的挑战是难以在有限数量的细胞中收获 CTCs 和探索分子标记。目前正在探索 CTCs 富集的方法,包括增强密度梯度体系[126]。目前,我们正在研究新的 DNA 和蛋白质提取方法,以检测 CTCs 中的突变和蛋白质表达/激活变化,后者利用 RPPA 技术[127,128]。

循环核苷酸

DNA、RNA、microRNA 和蛋白质从肿瘤细胞中释放出来并且可在循环中找到。循环生物标志物具有反映体内所有肿瘤部位发生过程的潜力,这些过程无法通过对原发肿瘤和/或转移部位的分析检测到。因此,"液体"活组织检查可提供肿瘤活组织检查无法获得的信息的潜力令人振奋。此外,它们将避免对肿瘤活组织检查的需要,特别是重复肿瘤活检以确定治疗后的肿瘤反应和分子演化。肿瘤可以将大量核苷酸释放入循环,高达 20%的循环 DNA 来源于患者肿瘤。因此,如同 *KRAS* 和 *p53* 突变一样,诸如突变、重排、拷贝数增加、microRNA 或 RNA 水平增加的任何异常,都可以在循环中检测到。然而,循环中的 DNA 数量和检测肿瘤相关异常的能力在不同的肿瘤类型中差异显著。尽管如此,基于循环 DNA 的商业测试正在变为可能。

验证新的分子生物标志物所面临的挑战

用于描述癌症基因组或蛋白质组以定义新的生物标志物系列的新型无偏倚技术易受可重复性的挑战,这可归因于用有限数量的癌症样本同时测定许多基因或蛋白质标志物。大量潜在的生物标志物组合引入了一个重要的可能性,即未发现的关联只是偶然的结果。对新的生物标志物研究严格的训练、测试和验证方法对有意义地影响患者管理至关重要。迄今为止,大多数新的生物标志物系列的研究并未对患者管理产生影响,这些研究不是因为没有解决这个多参数问题,就是因为其未采用足够强大的统计方法进行验证。不可过分强调生物信息学和生物统计学支持新的分子诊断学发展的重要性。

在将分子标记系列常规用于患者管理之前,需要在大量记录良好的病例中对其进行严格的验证,以测试其临床效用。数个预试系列的适用性仍在验证中[129,130]。设计用于发现和验证生物标志物的新型分子研究的一个主要障碍是,经常缺乏可用的大量充分保存和注释的组织或血液样品可与使用新兴技术的结果相关联。特别是,新的高通量方法通常限制用于新鲜冷冻样本(而石蜡包埋的样品更丰富)。因此,一种流行的生物标志物开发模型包括在冷冻组织中使用新的高通量分析技术(如转录谱)进行发现,然后使用应用于石蜡包埋组织的中等通量技术(如 RT-PCR)进行验证。分子标志物在何种特定组织类型中进行临床使用验证,这种界定至关重要[131,132]。利用蛋白质组或全基因组表达谱发现生物标志物的新型综合方法现在重新定义了肿瘤库收集和存储肿瘤样本的方法,主要重点放在新鲜冷冻样本上[133,134]。

目前,不可能将所有可用的调查技术应用于每个人,甚至无法应用于每个具有癌症发展高风险的患者。抛开成本问题,一个挑战是从活检、细胞或血清样本中获取足够的材料。实际上,对基因组 DNA 或 RNA 进行全面分析需要几百纳克,但是从细针穿刺中获得的 DNA 和 RNA 的数量是以皮克为单位。此外,活组织检查通常肿瘤含量相对较低,从而使分析复杂化。至于 CTCs 和循环核苷酸, DNA 和 RNA 的产量甚至更小。PCR 扩增可以提高 mRNA 的产量,但 PCR 产生的错误并不罕见。应对蛋白质含量低的方法最少。如前所述, MRM 和其他质谱方法可以补充基于抗体的方法。目前,我们正在探索具有 DNA 序列的"条形码"抗体,以便允许使用已经应用于 DNA 检测的扩增方法。这些主要困难需要解决以促进新型分子技术在癌症诊断中的常规应用。

建议

新型癌症生物标志物的有效发现需要整合多个关键因素,

包括合作研究、获得合适的人体组织样本组、用于分析的标准化试剂和技术、识别和量化组织和液体中的候选生物标志物、疾病的小鼠模型、综合的生物信息学平台和实现自动化,所有这些因素都是实现诸如人类基因组计划的关键。关于肿瘤标本生物库、标本处理和质量控制、验证、性能和化验分析解释的标准操作程序(standard operating procedures,SOPs)应在国家或理想情况下在国际层面制定,以减少对可能不可靠的研究结果的担忧,并允许准确汇总和比较交叉研究结果。美国癌症研究协会(American Association for Cancer Research,AACR)、美国食品药品管理局(Food and Drug Administration,FDA)、美国国家癌症研究所(National Cancer Institute,NCI)癌症生物标志物合作组织以及欧洲肿瘤标志物组织已经确定了开发有效生物标志物的关键程序。这些策略可以通过创建国家生物样本资源库来促进,例如人类癌症生物数据库(Cancer Human Biobank),其检索美国各中心的高度临床注释的肿瘤样本,并在可用于分析之前根据 SOPs 进行处理。

由于生物标志物发现程序使用高通量基因组、转录组和蛋白质组学方法描述组织特征,因此开发适当且集中的计算基础设施对于允许存储、利用和整合源自新型"组学"技术的大量异构数据至关重要。这样的计算资源应该便于所有调查人员访问,保护机密性,并避免重复工作。这些资源应该有助于数据挖掘、检索和自动化分析,从而促进跨分子平台和数据集之间的数据整合,并促进特定畸变与临床终点的关联。随着引入和升级新的"组学"技术,应保持数据流通。数据库访问应该促进新的生物统计方法,从而进一步提升我们选择临床有用的癌症生物标志物的能力。考虑到可用的数据量远远超过任何群体充分挖掘和解释数据的能力,目前正在实施一些方法以促进整个社区的样本和数据共享。NCI 的 Biospecimen 和 Biorepositories 研究分部为建立高质量的生物库提供了有效的工具和资源。大量的在线数据存储库,如癌症基因组图谱门户网站和临床蛋白质组肿瘤分析联盟,现已公开可用,便于不同研究小组对生物标志物的查询。

从使用新型高通量技术获得的数据中选择新的生物标志物需要仔细考虑,以便从真正的生物关系中识别出偶然的关联。错误的生物标志物发现可能来自选择偏倚、过度拟合、患者间相关性、多样性和多个临床终点,必须将这些因素排除,并使用准确的统计方法和研究设计,其中包括样本量,以使符合为明确临床应用而预先确定的性能特征的标志物能够被识别。在将新的生物标志物可能引入临床管理之前,应在前瞻性随机研究中测量生物标志物对成本的影响,并仔细选择临床结果,以便进行验证[135]。然而,研究成本以及监管和医疗市场的限制常常使此类临床试验不切实际。改进的研究设计涉及回顾性样本,如 ProBE 法,已被开发成为替代方案。或者,对已存档的前瞻性采集样本进行回顾性分析,或对已发表和未发表的队列进行系统回顾的合并分析,也可以提供高水平的证据,只要这些研究设计中确保高质量的特定要求得到满足即可。此外,研究人员和政策制定者转向模拟建模以预测新的生物标志物对结果的影响。模拟建模可以优化灵敏度、特异性和成本,此外还可以确定可能需要更明确的生物标志物的杠杆点。这种方法已用于评估可屈性乙状结肠镜检查对结直肠癌筛查的成本效益。

美国国家科学院医学研究所(Institute of Medicine of the National Academies)的一个开发基于生物标志物的癌症筛查、诊断和治疗工具的委员会,为癌症开发基于生物标志物的工具提出了一套正式的建议(框 40-3)。

框 40-3　为癌症开发基于生物标志物的工具的建议摘要

发现和开发生物标志物所需的方法、工具和资源

1. 联邦机构应该开发一种有组织的、发现生物标志物的综合方案,并促进新技术的发展。
2. 行业和其他资助者应建立国际联盟以生成和分享竞争前期的生物标志物数据。
3. 资助者应重点关注开发通路生物标志物,以扩大适用性。
4. 资助者应赞助示范项目,以开发能够预测已经上市的药物对患者疗效和安全性的生物标志物。
5. 政府机构和其他资助者应持续支持前瞻性收集样本的高质量生物库。
6. 生物标志物的开发和验证应该具有较高的阴性预测值,以预测对靶向治疗的反应,特别是那些高成本的靶向治疗。

生物标志物开发所需的指南、标准、监督和激励措施

7. 政府机构和其他利益相关者应该制定一个透明的流程,为生物标志物的开发、鉴定、验证和使用制定明确的共识标准和指南。
8. FDA 和行业应共同努力促进诊断-治疗联合的共同开发和批准。
9. FDA 应明确界定并规范其对临床决策中使用的生物标志物检测的监督。
10. 医疗保险和医疗补助服务中心应该在 CLIA 下开发一个分子诊断学的专业领域

临床评估和 sdoption 所需的方法和流程

11. 医疗保险和医疗补助服务中心应该修订和更新诊断测试的编码和定价系统。
12. 医疗保险和医疗补助服务中心以及其他支付者应该为新的生物标志物检测的保险范围条件制定标准。

作为保险范围条件的一个组成部分,应该建立高质量的基于人群的程序,以评价生物标志物检测的效力和成本效益。

来源:来自美国国家科学院医学研究所

结论

总之,在某些形式的癌症(如乳腺癌)中分子诊断学的发展已经取得了重大进展。最近的分子研究已经揭示了癌症的生物学异质性和复杂性,这就需要应用更多的癌症基因组和蛋白质组的全球性研究来鉴定新的生物标志物,从而促进对癌症认识、治疗和早期检测的进一步进展。实际上,高通量技术的应用已经显著提高了预测特定癌症治疗反应性的能力。对癌症分子异质性认识的提高，以及能够描述这种异质性的分子技术的迅速改进已经揭示了癌症分子诊断学发展的可能性。最终，这些方法不仅可以提高我们在早期阶段诊断癌症的能力，还可以同时分析能够促进患者护理个性化的分子靶点。实现这些目标就必须克服目前阻碍将传统和新型分子技术成功应用于癌症诊断的许多挑战。随着高通量技术在新型分子癌症诊断学的发展中获得越来越多的立足点，建立强大的协作和生物信息学方法以实现高通量数据存储、整合、分析和验证将至关重要。

（曾瑄　译）

参考文献

The complete reference list can be found on the Wiley Companion Digital Edition of this title (see inside front cover for login instructions).

1 Fisher B, Costantino JP, Wickerham DL, et al. Tamoxifen for the prevention of breast cancer: current status of the National Surgical Adjuvant Breast and Bowel Project P-1 study. *J Natl Cancer Inst*. 2005;**97**:1652–1662.

2 Barrett-Connor EL, Mosca L, Collins P, et al. Effects of raloxifene on cardiovascular evenets and breast cancer in postmenopausal women. *N Engl J Med*. 2006;**355**:125–137.

5 The National Lung Screening Trial Team. Reduced lung-cancer mortality with low-dose computed tomographic screening. *N Engl J Med*. 2011;**365**:395–409.

6 Kriege M, Brekelmans CT, Boetes C, et al. Efficacy of MRI and mammography for breast cancer screening in women with a familial or genetic predisposition. *N Engl J Med*. 2004;**351**:427–437.

10 Schroder FH, Hugosson J, Roobol MJ, et al. Screening and prostate-cancer mortality in a randomized European study. *N Engl J Med*. 2009;**360(13)**:1320–1328.

11 Andriole GL, Crawford ED, Grubb RL 3rd, et al. Mortality results from a randomized prostate-cancer screening trial. *N Engl J Med*. 2009;**360**:1310–1319.

12 Basch E, Oliver TK, Vickers A, et al. Screening for prostate cancer with prostate-specific antigen testing: American Society of Clinical Oncology Provisional Clinical Opinion. *J Clin Oncol*. 2012;**30(24)**:3020–3025.

13 Moyer VA, on behalf of the U.S. Preventive Services Task Force. Screening for prostate cancer: U.S. Preventive Services Task Force recommendation statement. *Ann Int Med*. 2012;**157**:120–134.

14 Carter HB, Albertsen PC, Barry MJ, et al. *Early Detection of Prostate Cancer: AUA Guideline*. Linthicum, MD: American Urological Association Education and Research, Inc.; 2013.

16 Lu KH, Skates S, Hernandez MA, et al. A 2-stage ovarian cancer screening strategy using the Risk of Ovarian Cancer Algorithm (ROCA) identifies early-stage incident cancers and demonstrates high positive predictive value. *Cancer*. 2013;**119(19)**:3454–3461.

17 Menon U, Gentry-Maharaj A, Hallet R. Sensitivity and specificity of multimodal and ultrasound screening for ovarian cancer, and stage distribution of detected cancers: results of the prevalence screen of the UK Collaborative Trial of Ovarian Cancer Screening (UKCTOCS). *Lancet Oncol*. 2009;**10(4)**:327–340.

18 Menon U, Ryan A, Kalsi J, Gentry-Maharaj A, et al. Risk algorithm using serial biomarker measurements doubles the number of screen-detected cancers compared with a single-threshold rule in the United Kingdom Collaborative Trial of Ovarian Cancer Screening. *J Clin Oncol*. 2015;**33(18)**:2062–2071.

19 Ronco G, Dillner J, Elfström KM. Efficacy of HPV-based screening for prevention of invasive cervical cancer: follow-up of four European randomised controlled trials. *Lancet*. 2014;**383(9916)**:524–532.

27 Bolton KL, Chenevix-Trench G, Goh C. Association between BRCA1 and BRCA2 mutations and survival in women with invasive epithelial ovariancancer. *JAMA*. 2012;**307(4)**:382–390.

32 Couch FJ, Hart SN, Sharma P, et al. Inherited mutations in 17 breast cancer susceptibility genes among a large triple-negative breast cancercohort unselected for family history of breast cancer. *J Clin Oncol*. 2015;**33(4)**:304–311.

33 Pérez-Carbonell L, Ruiz-Ponte C, Guarinos C. Comparison between universal molecular screening for Lynch syndrome and revised Bethesda guidelines in a large population-based cohort of patients with colorectal cancer. *Gut*. 2012;**61(6)**:865–872.

38 Paik S, Shak S, Tang G, et al. A multigene assay to predict recurrence of tamoxifen-treated, node-negative breast cancer. *N Engl J Med*. 2004;**351**:2817–2826.

42 Slamon DJ, Clark GM, Wong SG, et al. Human breast cancer: correlation of relapse and survival with amplification of the HER-2/neu oncogene. *Science*. 1987;**235**:177–182.

51 Majewski IJ, Nuciforo P, Mittempergher L, et al. PIK3CA mutations are associated with decreased benefit to neoadjuvant human epidermal growth factor receptor 2-targeted therapies in breast cancer. *J Clin Oncol*. 2015;**33(12)**:1334–1339.

52 Wolff AC, Hammond EH, Hicks DG. Recommendations for human epidermal growth factor receptor 2 testing in breast cancer: American Society of Clinical Oncology/College of American Pathologists Clinical Practice Guideline Update. *J Clin Oncol*. 2013;**31(31)**:3997–4013.

53 Hennessy BT, Timms KM, Carey MS. Somatic mutations in BRCA1 and BRCA2 could expand the number of patients that benefit from poly (ADP ribose) polymerase inhibitors in ovarian cancer. *J Clin Oncol*. 2010;**28(22)**:3570–3576.

56 Matulonis UA, Wolff G, Barry W, et al. *Phase I of Oral BKM120 or BYL719 and Olaparib for High-Grade Serous Ovarian Cancer or Triple-Negative Breast Cancer: Final Results of the BKM120 Plus Olaparib Cohort*. Proceedings of the 106th Annual Meeting of the American Association for Cancer Research; 2015 April 18–22; Philadelphia, PA. Philadelphia (PA): AACR; 2015. Abstract nr CT324.

57 Rosell R, Carcereny E, Gervais R. Erlotinib versus standard chemotherapy as first-line treatment for European patients with advanced EGFR mutation-positive non-small-cell lung cancer (EURTAC): a multicentre, open-label, randomised phase 3 trial. *Lancet Oncol*. 2012;**13(3)**:239–246.

58 Fukuoka M, Wu YL, Thongprasert S. Biomarker analyses and final overall survival results from a phase III, randomized, open-label, first-line study of gefitinib versus carboplatin/paclitaxel in clinically selected patients with advanced non-small-cell lung cancer in Asia (IPASS). *J Clin Oncol*. 2011;**29(21)**:2866–2874.

59 Yang JC, Wu YL, Schuler M. Afatinib versus cisplatin-based chemotherapy for EGFR mutation-positive lung adenocarcinoma (LUX-Lung 3 and LUX-Lung 6): analysis of overall survival data from two randomised, phase 3 trials. *Lancet Oncol*. 2015;**16(2)**:141–151.

60 Jänne PA, Ou S-HI, Kim D-W, et al. Dacomitinib as first-line treatment in patients with clinically or molecularly selected advanced non-small-cell lung cancer: a multicentre, open-label, phase 2 trial. *Lancet Oncol*. 2014;**15(13)**:1433–1441.

63 Shaw AT, Kim DW, Nakagawa K. Crizotinib versus chemotherapy in advanced ALK-positive lung cancer. *N Engl J Med*. 2013;**368(25)**:2385–2394.

64 Shaw AT, Ou SH, Bang YJ. Crizotinib in ROS-1 rearranged non-small cell lung cancer. *N Engl J Med*. 2014;**371(21)**:1963–1971.

65 Shaw AT, Kim DW, Mehra R. Cetirinib in ALK-rearranged non-small cell lung cancer. *N Engl J Med*. 2014;**370(13)**:1189–1197.

66 Leighl NB, Rekhtman N, Biermann WA. Molecular testing for selection of patients with lung cancer for epidermal growth factor receptor and anaplastic lymphoma kinase tyrosine kinase inhibitors: American Society of Clinical Oncology endorsement of the College of American Pathologists/International Society for the Study of Lung Cancer/Association of Molecular Pathologists guideline. *J Clin Oncol*. 2014;**32(32)**:3673–3679. doi: 10.1200/JCO.2014.57.3055.

68 Douillard JY, Oliner KS, Siena S, et al. Panitumumab-FOLFOX4 treatment and RAS mutations in colorectal cancer. *N Engl J Med*. 2013;**369**:1023–1034.

70 Van Cutsem E, Köhne CH, Láng I, et al. Cetuximab plus irinotecan, fluorouracil, and leucovorin as first-line treatment for metastatic colorectal cancer: updated analysis of overall survival according to tumor KRAS and BRAF mutation status. *J Clin Oncol*. 2011;**29(15)**:2011–2019.

72 Cioffi A, Maki RG. GI stromal tumors: 15 years of lessons from a rare cancer. *J Clin Oncol*. 2015;**33(16)**:1849–1854. doi: JCO.2014.59.7344.

73 Chapman PB, Hauschild A, Robert C, et al. Improved survival with vemurafenib in melanoma with BRAF V600E mutation. *N Engl J Med*. 2011;**364**:2507–2516.

74 Hauschild A, Grob JJ, Demidov LV, et al. Dabrafenib in BRAF-mutated metastatic melanoma: a multicentre, open-label, phase 3 randomised controlled trial. *Lancet*. 2012;**380**:358–365.

75 Long GV, Stroyakovskiy D, Gogas H, et al. Combined BRAF and MEK inhibition versus BRAF inhibition alone in melanoma. *N Engl J Med*. 2013;**371**:1877–1888.

76 Johnson DB, Puzanov I. Treatment of NRAS-mutant melanoma. *Curr Treat Options Oncol*. 2015;**16(4)**:15.

77 Hodi FS, Corless CL, Giobbie-Hurder A, et al. Imatinib for melanomas harboring mutationally activated or amplified KIT arising on mucosal, acral, and chronically sun-damaged skin. *J Clin Oncol*. 2013;**31(26)**:3182–3190.

90 Rustin G, van der Burg M, Griffin C. Early versus delayed treatment of relapsed ovarian cancer (MRC OV05/EORTC55955): a randomised trial. *Lancet*. 2010;**376(9747)**:1155–1163.

91 Harris L, Fritsche H, Mennel R, et al. American Society of Clinical Oncology. American Society of Clinical Oncology 2007 update of recommendations for the use of tumor markers in breast cancer. *J Clin Oncol*. 2007;**25(33)**:5287–5312.

94 Locker GY, Hamilton S, Harris J, et al. American Society of Clinical Oncology 2006 update of recommendations for the use of tumor markers in gastrointestinal cancer. *J Clin Oncol*. 2006;**24**:5313–5327.

100 Stemke-Hale K, Gonzalez-Angulo AM, Lluch A, et al. An integrative genomic and proteomic analysis of PIK3CA, PTEN, and AKT mutations in breast cancer. *Cancer Res*. 2008;**68**:6084–6091.

102 Hennessy BT, Lu Y, Poradosu E, et al. Quantified pathway inhibition as a pharmacodynamic marker facilitating optimal targeted therapy dosing: proof of principle

with the AKT inhibitor perifosine. *Clin Cancer Res*. 2007;**13**:7421–7431.
113 Sleijfer S, Bogaerts J, Siu LL. Designing transformative clinical trials in the cancer genome era. *J Clin Oncol*. 2013;**31(15)**:1834–1841.
120 Cristofanilli M, Budd GT, Ellis MJ, et al. Circulating tumor cells, disease progression, and survival in metastatic breast cancer. *N Engl J Med*. 2004;**351**:781–791.
121 Dawson SJ, Tsui DW, Murtaza M, et al. Analysis of circulating tumor DNA to monitor metastatic breast cancer. *N Engl J Med*. 2013;**368**:1199–1209.
127 Becker FF, Wang XB, Huang Y, et al. Separation of human breast cancer cells from blood by differential dielectric affinity. *Proc Natl Acad Sci U S A*. 1995;**92**:60–864.
132 Segal E, Friedman N, Kaminski N, Regev A, Koller D. From signatures to models: understanding cancer using microarrays. *Nat Genetics*. 2005;**37(suppl)**:S38–S45.
135 Hartwell L, Mankoff D, Paulovich A, Ramsey S, Swisher E. Cancer biomarkers: a systems approach. *Nat Biotechnol*. 2006;**24**:905–908.

第 41 章 影像学检查使用原则

Lawrence H. Schwartz, MD

概述

影像学检查是临床肿瘤学不可分割的一部分。较之于 X 线平片,计算机断层扫描(computed tomography,CT)可以提供更多的诊疗信息。采用[18]F-氟代脱氧葡萄糖的代谢成像通过与 CT 提供的解剖学相结合可以达到最佳诊断效能。新一代磁共振与 CT 功能关联成像是精准评估的又一大进步。采用标记药物的特殊分子靶向成像也逐渐兴起。在影像监控下进行的介入操作在很大程度上取代了部分开放性手术,提高了患者舒适度,为其节约了时间成本和医疗费用。

影像学检查在肿瘤学的方方面面均扮演了重要而基础的角色。放射学检查在肿瘤检测、表征、分期和疗效监测方面均提供了非常重要的信息。随着技术进步,肿瘤相关影像学检查逐渐发展成为预后和预测生物标志物,在临床中可独立应用或与其他组织及血清生物标志物联合应用。其他肿瘤相关影像学检查的应用还包括肿瘤筛查,如乳腺 X 线摄片、肺癌低剂量 CT 筛查、仿真结肠镜。此外,影像学检查引导的介入治疗近年来得到了长足的发展,大大减少了侵入性肿瘤治疗的数量。

断层影像学检查,包括利用电离辐射的 CT 和正电子发射断层扫描(positron emission tomography,PET)以及非电离辐射的磁共振(magnetic resonance,MR)成像,在肿瘤患者诊疗中发挥主要作用,极大改善了传统影像学检查的不足。传统影像学检查如 X 线平片尽管操作简便、辐射剂量低且费用低廉,但在肿瘤患者的诊疗中作用非常有限。

肿瘤患者的影像学评估取决于肿瘤类型、疾病分期以及检查的特殊临床指征。肿瘤相关影像学检查的临床指征范围很广,包括筛查、有症状患者的诊断、其他影像学检查异常发现的进一步评估、治疗或干预后疾病反应或进展的评估以及治疗并发症的评价。在每项影像学检查申请前必须熟知临床场景,包括需要提供哪些临床信息、影像学检查能否提供所需证据,尤其重要的是根据检查结果下一步应采取怎样的措施以改变治疗方案及患者预后。

融合影像学检查与包括基因组学和蛋白质组学检测在内的其他诊断方法相结合,可以获得肿瘤患者更多信息。事实上,临床越来越需要影像学检查在简单的解剖可视化和肿瘤定位以外提供更多有用的信息。当代肿瘤学要求影像学检查可以将基础分子改变可视化,以更好理解肿瘤发生发展过程并最终影响临床实践。

分子影像学产生于 20 世纪 90 年代初,最早以 PET 显像和葡萄糖类似物探针[^{18}F]-2-氟代-2-脱氧-D-葡萄糖(fluoro-2-deoxy-D-glucose,FDG)的使用为标志。近年来 FDG-PET 已经成为肿瘤患者评估最重要的检查之一,可以同时评估原发肿瘤及其转移灶,并监测疗效。PET 显像本身对解剖学细节显示欠佳,需要联合 CT 扫描提供的更精细形态解剖学信息。PET/CT 以及 PET/MRI 联合双模态扫描可以提供综合信息,在多种肿瘤和临床适应证中优于单一 PET、CT 或 MRI 的诊断价值。随着分子影像学的进步,新型靶点、技术以及肿瘤特异性显像探针的发展将为精准诊断提供更多信息。PET 显像及其他分子影像学技术与 MRI 相结合在评估细胞代谢、细胞增殖、组织缺氧、细胞凋亡、受体表达、基因表达、血管生成和信号转导中应用越来越广泛。未来分子影像学检查有望解决当前肿瘤学诊断中存在的诸多问题。尽管技术发展日新月异,影像学检查工作者有责任对新型分子成像技术谨慎研究以明确其是否真正有效和具备成本效益。图像引人入胜并不代表可以改善患者治疗方案及预后。

非侵入性解剖学和分子影像学检查意欲在患者诊疗中发挥作用,需要进行基于假说和循证医学的研究。鉴于影像学检查是诊断评估的基础,更好地理解不同检查的应用指征可以进行更有效的患者评估。该部分的系列章节聚焦于肿瘤患者,概述了影像学检查使用原则。影像学检查在临床处理中占据核心地位,本书所提供的信息实为日常临床实践中的通用指南。

(彭攀 译,吴宁 审校)

延伸阅读

Apolo AB, Pandit-Taskar N, Morris MJ. Novel tracers and their development for the imaging of metastatic prostate cancer. *J Nucl Med*. 2008;**49**:2031–2041.

Boss DS, Olmos RV, Sinaasappel M, Beijnen JH, Schellens JH. Application of PET/CT in the development of novel anticancer drugs. *Oncologist*. 2008;**13(1)**:25–38.

Czernin J, Ta L, Herrmann K. Does PET/MR imaging improve cancer assessments? Literature evidence from more than 900 patients. *J Nucl Med*. 2014;**55(Supplement 2)**:59S–62S.

Farwell MD, Pryma DA, Mankoff DA. PET/CT imaging in cancer: current applications and future directions. *Cancer*. 2014;**120(22)**:3433–45.

Fleming IN, Manavaki R, Blower PJ, et al. Imaging tumour hypoxia with positron emission tomography. *Br J Cancer*. 2015;**112(2)**:238–250.

Gerstner ER, Sorensen AG, Jain RK, Batchelor TT. Advances in neuroimaging techniques for the evaluation of tumor growth, vascular permeability, and angiogenesis in gliomas. *Curr Opin Neurol*. 2008;**21(6)**:728–735.

Heron DE, Andrade RS, Beriwal S, Smith RP, et al. PET-CT in radiation oncology: the impact on diagnosis, treatment planning, and assessment of treatment response. *Am J Clin Oncol*. 2008;**31(4)**:352–362.

Iagaru A, Mittra E, Minamimoto R, et al. Simultaneous whole-body time-of-flight 18F-FDG PET/MRI: a pilot study comparing SUVmax with PET/CT and assessment of MR image quality. *Clin Nucl Med*. 2015 Jan;**40(1)**:1–8.

Kim JH, Choi SH, Ryoo I, et al. Prognosis prediction of measurable enhancing lesion after completion of standard concomitant chemoradiotherapy and adjuvant temozolomide in glioblastoma patients: application of dynamic susceptibility contrast perfusion and diffusion-weighted imaging. *PLoS One*. 2014;**9(11)**:e113587.

Kuehl H, Veit P, Rosenbaum SJ, Bockisch A, Antoch G. Can PET/CT replace separate diagnostic CT for cancer imaging? Optimizing CT protocols for imaging cancers of the chest and abdomen. *J Nucl Med*. 2007;**48(suppl 1)**:45S–57S.

Kundra V, Silverman PM, Matin SF, Choi H. Imaging in oncology from the University of Texas M. D. Anderson Cancer Center: diagnosis, staging, and surveillance of prostate cancer. *AJR Am J Roentgenol*. 2007;**189**(**4**):830–844.

Malviya G, Nayak TK. PET imaging to monitor cancer therapy. *Curr Pharm Biotechnol*. 2013;**14**(**7**):669–682.

Schaefer JF, Schlemmer HP. Total-body MR-imaging in oncology. *Eur Radiol*. 2006;**16**(**9**):2000–2015.

Tanvetyanon T, Eikman EA, Sommers E, Robinson L, Boulware D, Bepler G. Response by PET scan versus CT scan to predict survival after neoadjuvant chemotherapy for resectable non-small cell lung cancer. *JCO*. 2008;**26**:4610–4616.

Veit P, Ruehm S, Kuehl H, et al. Lymph node staging with dual-modality PET/CT: enhancing the diagnostic accuracy in oncology. *Eur J Radiol*. 2006;**58**(**3**):383–389.

Wirth A, Foo M, Seymour JF, Macmanus MP, Hicks RJ. Impact of [18f] fluorodeoxyglucose positron emission tomography on staging and management of early-stage follicular non-hodgkin lymphoma. *Int J Radiat Oncol Biol Phys*. 2008;**71**(**1**):213–219.

Wong TZ, Paulson EK, Nelson RC, Patz EF Jr, Coleman RE. Practical approach to diagnostic CT combined with PET. *AJR Am J Roentgenol*. 2007;**188**(**3**):622–629.

Zhao B, Schwartz LH, Larson SM. Imaging surrogates of tumor response to therapy: anatomic and functional biomarkers. *J Nucl Med*. 2009;**50**(**2**):239–249.

第 42 章　肿瘤患者的介入治疗

Judy U. Ahrar, MD ■ Michael J. Wallace, MD ■ Rony Avritscher, MD

概述

近几十年来，影像引导下的各种介入技术在肿瘤诊治方面蓬勃发展。经皮穿刺活检是诊断的第一步，且能推动和不断改进疾病治疗方案。影像引导下的介入治疗，如肝动脉栓塞术，肝肿瘤消融术，及门静脉栓塞术，在原发性肝癌或肝转移癌患者中已得到广泛应用。姑息性介入治疗使许多患者获益，例如下腔静脉滤器置入术、胆汁引流及胆道支架置入术、肾动脉栓塞术等；甚至可以获得根治性的治疗，比如消融术。因此，微创介入治疗将成为肿瘤诊治过程中不可缺少的重要组成部分。

在过去的几十年里，肿瘤诊断技术的进步、新型抗癌药物的研发和外科治疗水平的提高，极大地改善了肿瘤患者的生存预后，也带动了影像引导下的各种介入技术在肿瘤诊治方面的蓬勃发展。得益于影像医学的发展，更多肿瘤患者表现为原发或单个器官的转移，相应地，他们能从局部治疗中获得比全身治疗更好的疗效。标准的影像诊断方法可用于发现肿瘤，微创经皮穿刺技术可以确立诊断，并且可以局部根治或姑息性地治疗肿瘤患者。目前，已有研究发现导管/器械、栓塞剂、化疗药物及输送系统的改良与肿瘤患者预后的提高有关，因此，这些方面的研究兴趣被重新激发出来。本文中，我们讨论肝脏血管介入、泌尿生殖系统介入、胸部介入，几种姑息性治疗方法及其他影像引导的介入治疗方案（静脉滤器置入、穿刺活检、瘤内基因治疗）。

肝血管介入

在针对肿瘤患者的介入放射诊疗，也就是肿瘤介入领域中，肝脏长期占据了重要地位。肝脏的介入诊断与治疗之所以应用广泛，原因很多，主要是因为肝脏是各种肿瘤最常见的远处转移器官，且容易经皮穿刺操作。而因为肿瘤独特的血供特点，肝脏肿瘤特别适宜经导管给药治疗。肝脏肿瘤主要由肝动脉供血，而正常肝脏组织由门静脉系统供血。这种特性使得肿瘤介入医师在治疗肝脏病灶时，不伤及肿瘤周围的正常组织。

动脉灌注治疗

动脉灌注的目的是通过将化疗药直接递送到肿瘤的供血动脉，以获得更好的肿瘤反应。动脉灌注治疗的基本原理是基于首过效应：当药物直接进入会对其进行代谢的组织中时，会发生首过效应。因此，相较于全身化疗，动脉灌注治疗能够使化疗药物在局部肿瘤内的浓度成倍增加，而体循环中浓度低，减少了化疗药物全身毒副作用和药量。动脉灌注治疗也被视作克服药物最大耐受剂量的方法之一[1]。

动脉灌注治疗最早被报道用于结直肠癌肝转移患者的治疗。在 Mocellin 等[2]的荟萃分析中，共纳入了 10 项随机对照试验，对比了肝动脉灌注化疗（hepatic arterial infusion，HAI）与系统化疗治疗结直肠癌肝转移的疗效。虽然研究结果提示以氟尿嘧啶为基础的 HAI 组，肿瘤的治疗反应率优于系统化疗组，但对比 HAI 和氟尿嘧啶联合奥沙利铂或伊立替康的化疗方案时，两组的肿瘤治疗反应率类似，甚至系统化疗组的治疗反应率优于 HAI 组。此外，该研究还认为，基于氟尿嘧啶的 HAI 治疗并未改善结直肠肝转移患者的生存预后。因此，仍有必要对基于新型抗癌药物的 HAI 进行深入研究，以明确动脉灌注治疗在肿瘤局部治疗中的确切作用与地位。

动脉栓塞治疗

经导管肝动脉栓塞的目的是完全或部分阻塞肿瘤滋养血管，从而使肿瘤缺血，生长停滞，最终发生坏死。当肝动脉主干被栓塞后，栓塞点附近的侧支循环会迅速建立。因此，还应追踪新建立的侧支循环血管的供血情况，明确其是否为肿瘤供血，否则应当同时栓塞侧支循环。中央大血管栓塞程度越严重，侧支循环血流就越丰富。因此，为了尽可能使肿瘤发生最大程度地缺血坏死，应同时栓塞远端终末血管。周围血管（肝段或肝亚段）可以同轴置入微导管，采用小粒径颗粒进行栓塞。

多种栓塞剂被成功用于肝动脉的栓塞治疗。最常用的栓塞剂包括可吸收性明胶海绵颗粒和粉末、聚乙烯醇颗粒、纤维蛋白胶、氰基丙烯酸正丁酯（n-butyl cyanoacrylate，NBCA）、乙碘油、微球和无水乙醇。吸收性明胶海绵条或者不锈钢弹簧圈多用于中央性血管栓塞，较少用于肿瘤的栓塞治疗。

栓塞后综合征是肝动脉栓塞术后最常见并发症，主要表现为发热、恶心、乏力、白细胞计数升高和肝功能损害等，症状多具有自限性。误栓非靶血管所致的并发症包括胆囊炎、胰腺炎和胃十二指肠溃疡等。其他严重并发症如肝坏死、肝衰竭、肝脓肿，但并不常见。在肝动脉栓塞时，如果没有识别出肝内动静脉瘘，栓塞剂可进入肝静脉系统，并异位栓塞至肺循环，进而导致呼吸衰竭。Hemingway 和 Allison 等[3]报道了 10 年内 284 名患者共行 410 次肝动脉栓塞治疗的情况，其结果显示：肝动脉栓塞术后轻度并发症发生率为 16%，严重并发症发生率为 6.6%，死亡率为 2%。

动脉化疗栓塞术

动脉化疗栓塞是联合使用化疗药与栓塞剂，经动脉注入肝脏肿瘤组织内。其原理为肿瘤的主要供血动脉被栓塞后，引起肿瘤缺血，并和注入的化疗药物起到协同作用。该技术由 Yamada[4]在 1977 年首次提出，现已成为肿瘤介入治疗中的主要方法。而一种来自罂粟籽油的碘化酯——碘化油的出现，又进一步推动了动脉化疗栓塞术的发展。碘化油非常适用于化疗栓塞,它对肝细胞性肝癌和某些肝转移癌具有极高的亲和性和趋向性,可以被优先摄取;碘化油还可与化疗药物和栓塞剂可逆性结合与释放,而不改变药物特性,起到药物载体的作用[5,6]。Maeda 等[7]认为这可能同肿瘤血管高渗透性及阻滞性增强有关:新生成的肿瘤血管渗透性较高,且肿瘤内缺乏淋巴系统,使高分子量药物滞留在肿瘤细胞间质的时间延长,从而发挥了药物缓释作用。阻滞性增强也部分解释了肿瘤内碘油蓄积或与化疗药物共轭聚合后药物浓度增加的原因。

目前化疗栓塞的诸多方案中,最常用的药物是多柔比星,其常与顺铂及丝裂霉素联用。化疗药物与碘化油混合后,缓慢注入肿瘤滋养血管以发挥抗癌作用。近年来,载药(多柔比星和伊立替康)洗脱微球(drug-eluting beads,DEB)作为一种新的药物递送系统开始逐渐应用于肝动脉化疗栓塞中。其他栓塞剂,如吸收性明胶海绵颗粒,也可增加化疗栓塞效果,进一步促进肿瘤缺血。操作中,应保留肿瘤供血动脉的近端,以在重复治疗时增加肿瘤缓解。

经导管动脉化疗栓塞术可用于无法外科根治的肝细胞癌、胆管癌及肝转移癌、联合外科切除或消融射频、肝移植前的桥接治疗。两项临床随机试验[8,9]的结果表明,化疗栓塞治疗可使无法外科根治的肝细胞癌(hepatocellular carcinoma,HCC)患者获益。随着化疗药物和栓塞材料的不断研发及改良,化疗栓塞治疗肝癌显出了巨大潜力,如利用化疗栓塞联合抗血管生成药物治疗肿瘤并抑制肿瘤复发和转移[10,11]。而 C 形臂锥形束 CT 的使用,也使化疗栓塞术中横断面成像成为可能(图 42-1):

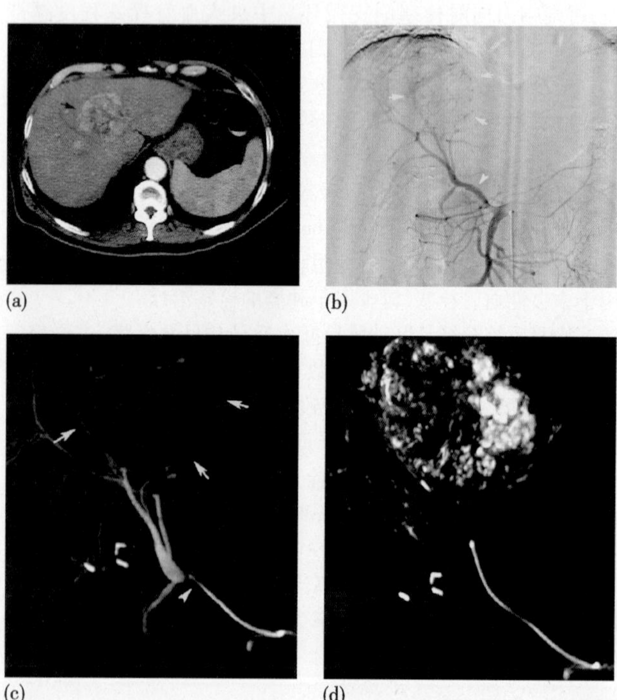

图 42-1 71 岁老年男性,患者无法手术根治肝细胞癌,行经导管动脉化疗栓塞术。(a)经导管动脉化疗栓塞前 CT 扫描:第Ⅳ肝段有一较大的、孤立的、富血供肿块(箭头所指);(b)DSA 显示右侧肝动脉起源于肠系膜上动脉近端(箭头所指)。该血管也供应位于左肝Ⅳ段的肿瘤(箭头所指);(c)C 臂 CT 影像显示,操作过程中 3F 导管尖端在远端异位右侧肝动脉,确定供应肝细胞癌的血管来源(箭头所指);(d)C 臂 CT 影像显示,在化疗栓塞后碘化油在整个病灶中沉积

锥形束 CT 使选择性栓塞的水平更高,通过多平面和三维图像获得动脉血管解剖图,并更加准确地评估栓塞程度[12]。

肝动脉内近距离放疗

放疗栓塞术是指经动脉导管注入载有放射性核素钇 90(^{90}Y)的栓塞剂。与化疗栓塞原理类似,都是将栓塞剂选择性的注入肿瘤的供养动脉内引起肿瘤缺血坏死。^{90}Y 是一种纯 β 辐射的短半衰期放射性物质。由于肿瘤内部血流是周围肝实质血流的数倍,因此相对于外照射而言,放疗栓塞术增加了局部病灶的放射剂量,同时又降低放射性肝炎等并发症的发生。

TheraSphere bead(MDS Nordion,Ottawa,Canada)1999 年获 FDA 批准上市,用于伴有门脉癌栓的肝癌患者的辅助治疗或肝移植前桥接治 SIR-Spheres(Sirtex Medical,Lane Cove,Australia)联合氟尿苷用于治疗结肠癌肝转移瘤。为了保证该操作的安全性,需要明确腹腔动脉及肠系膜上动脉的变异情况,以避免带有放射活性的微粒误栓非靶血管。多项研究已证实^{90}Y 放疗栓塞术可安全地治疗无手术切除指征的肝细胞癌和结肠癌肝转移瘤患者[13-15]。

局部消融

影像引导下肿瘤消融治疗主要包括温度消融和化学消融。化学消融术包括经皮瘤内无水乙醇注射(percutaneous ethanol injection,PEI),以及用热水、高渗盐水、醋酸或者化学药物导致肿瘤细胞死亡。温度消融是通过将光、声、电等导入局部肿瘤内,产生低温(冷冻消融)或高温(射频消融、微波消融、激光消融、高强度聚焦超声),从而使局部肿瘤发生凝固型坏死或促使细胞发生脱水、结晶而死亡。这些消融手术可以在手术室由介入医生或者外科医生在影像引导下完成。无水乙醇是化学消融中最常用的药物[16]。无水乙醇被注入到肿瘤细胞中,可以引起肿瘤细胞及其血管内皮细胞迅速脱水,蛋白质变性和小血管栓塞[17]。对原发性肝癌,PEI 治疗效果良好;但对肝转移癌,PEI 治疗效果则不如热消融治疗。其原因主要是由于无水乙醇在肝转移癌中非均质分布所致。在原发性肝癌患者中,由于大多数患者有肝硬化病史,肿瘤组织周围的肝组织较硬,使无水酒精能够在肿瘤内弥散分布;而肝转移瘤患者多数无肝硬化病史,肿瘤比周围的肝脏组织硬,影响了无水酒精的弥散分布,进而导致 PEI 治疗后疗效降低。Ebara 等[18]报道了 20 年内,以 PEI 治疗直径≤3cm 的 HCC 患者 270 例,结果显示:术后 3 年局部复发率为 10%,3 年和 5 年生存率分别为 81%和 60%。

Livraghi 等[19]对比了 PEI 和射频(radiofrequency,RF)消融治疗 HCC(直径≤3cm)的疗效差异:RF 消融组,52 例肿瘤病灶有 47 例(90%)达到完全坏死,每个肿瘤平均行 1.2 次 RF 消融治疗;PEI 治疗组,60 例肿瘤病灶有 48 例(80%)达完全坏死,每个肿瘤平均行 4.8 次 PEI 治疗。RF 消融组严重并发症 1 例(血胸),轻度并发症 4 例(出血、胆道出血、胸膜渗出、胆囊炎),而 PEI 组无并发症发生。Lencioni 等[20]报道了随机应用 RF 或 PEI 治疗肝硬化患者 102 例。虽然两组患者的 1 年和 2 年生存率无显著差异,但其 1 年和 2 年局部无复发生存率却有显著不同(1 年局部无复发生存率:RF 组 98%,PEI 组 83%;2 年局部无复发生存率:RF 组 96%,PEI 组 62%)。但该研究纳入患者局限,仅纳入了小于等于 5cm 的单个 HCC 病灶,或至多

3 个 HCC 病灶且单个病灶最大长径 ≤3cm 的患者。Ebara 等[18]的研究结果尽管更支持 RF 消融，但其研究中有高达 25%的病例因解剖结构而无法行 RF 消融治疗，这强调了 PEI 在小肿瘤治疗中仍有一定作用。热消融不仅能够根治小肝癌，也能使结肠癌肝转移患者获益。Gillams 和 Lees 等[21]报道热消融治疗结肠癌肝转移，患者术后平均生存时间从 21~25 个月增加至 39 个月。

门静脉栓塞术

成功的肝切除依赖于剩余肝脏实质的功能。当门静脉被阻塞，来自肠道的促肝细胞生长因子（肝细胞生成素 A、胰岛素、胰高血糖素）就会分流到血管没有被栓塞的肝段[22]。结果导致那些门静脉被阻塞的肝段发生萎缩，而肝脏其他区域出现增生。这样，门静脉栓塞术（portal vein embolization，PVE）作为外科术前准备，被用于预期剩余肝脏（future liver remnant，FLR）体积处于临界状态的拟做肝切除的患者，诱导其肝脏增生（图 42-2）。

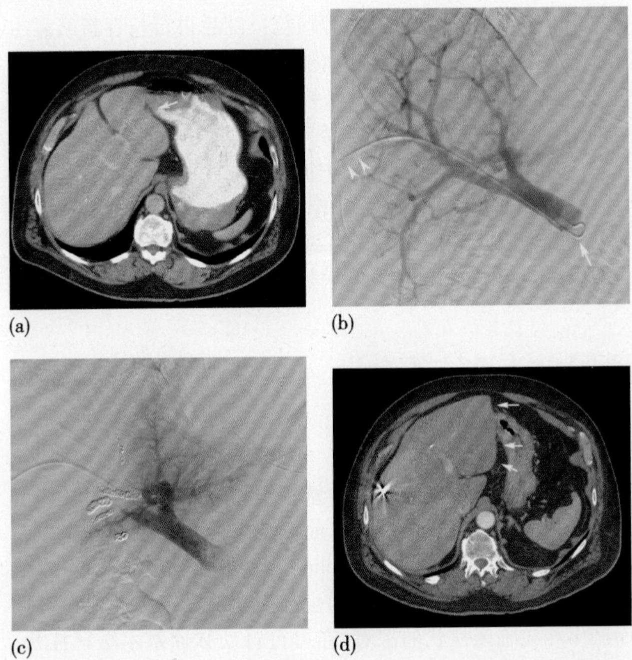

图 42-2　直肠癌肝转移患者，52 岁，男性，采用三基丙烯（Tris-acryl）颗粒和弹簧圈，经同侧右肝扩展至第Ⅳ肝段的门静脉栓塞术（PVE）。(a) PVE 前 CT 扫描显示残余肝脏剩余体积（FLR）比值［FLR/TELV（total estimated liver volume，TELV）= 17%］（箭头所指）；(b) 门静脉造影 DSA 显示在门静脉右支有一 6F 血管鞘，在门静脉主干有一 5F 导管（箭头所指）；(c) 最后的 DSA 造影显示，从第Ⅳ段到第Ⅷ段的门静脉分支被栓塞，而保留了通畅的门静脉血流供应剩余左侧肝；(d) 右肝扩展至第Ⅳ肝段 PVE 术后 1 个月 CT 扫描显示，FLR 升高（FLR/TELV = 27%）（箭头所指）。FLR 升高程度为 10%

PVE 的适应证：无基础肝病、肝功能正常者 FLR<20%；伴有严重肝损伤者 FLR<30%；肝硬化代偿期 FLR<40%[23]。扩大右半肝切除术，包括Ⅳ段在内的改良的术前门脉栓塞可以获得理想的肝脏增生。应用不同的栓塞剂，门脉栓塞术后 FLR 平均增加 46%~70%。PVE 安全性高，主要引起栓塞侧门静脉分支周围肝细胞凋亡，因此并不发生栓塞后综合征及肝脏坏死。而 Madoff 等[24]报道了肝切除术前行 PVE 的患者 44 例，所有患者在外科术后均未出现肝衰竭。

PVE 术中常用的栓塞剂包括纤维蛋白胶、吸收性明胶海绵、凝血酶、栓塞颗粒、弹簧圈、无水乙醇等。在美国，最常用栓塞剂为栓塞微粒与弹簧圈。

最近，有回顾性研究和荟萃分析结果提示，肝切除术前门静脉栓塞术可提高外科手术效果[23,25]。因此，门静脉栓塞术在很多肝病治疗中心已被视作外科术前常规治疗。

关于肝细胞癌的思考

肝细胞癌发病率为世界第五，死亡率为世界第三[26]。肝癌在世界范围内广泛流行，其中原因和肝硬化和肝炎发病率上升有关。外科切除肿瘤仍是根治肝细胞癌的首选治疗之一。然而，仅 20%~30%的患者可行根治性肝癌切除[27]。肝部分切除术后五年生存率约为 50%[28]。但由于原发灶的播散、未发现的肝内微小转移灶和异质性病变等原因，外科切除术后复发率极高。肝移植能够根治肝细胞癌及潜在肝病，其适应证包括肝硬化患者和其他不能手术切除的患者。对不适合肝癌切除术和肝移植的患者，则可选择消融术和动脉内介入治疗（栓塞术、化疗栓塞、放疗栓塞）。消融治疗，尤其是射频消融，不仅能够根治小肝癌，还能对中期及晚期患者进行姑息性治疗。对晚期肝癌患者而言，传统肝癌全身化疗因治疗反应率低，效果不佳。近几年发现一种具有抗血管生成、促细胞凋亡和 Raf 激酶抑制活性的多激酶抑制剂—索拉非尼。该药的患者耐受度高，是第一种经统计学证实可以显著提高晚期肝细胞癌患者总体生存率的有效药物[29]。

西方国家的肝细胞癌患者与包括日本在内的亚洲国家的肝细胞癌患者的肿瘤特点不同[30]，因此在介入治疗前，还需进行病因学评估。西方国家的结节型肝细胞癌发病率低于 25%，而在日本则接近 75%。对于中期以前的肝细胞癌患者，消融技术对周围肝实质损伤小，保留了患者接受二次治疗的条件，此外又可以作为肝移植前的桥接治疗，为等待供肝期间的患者或无法肝移植的患者提供肝移植机会。目前，推荐单个病灶最大长径小于 5cm 或 3 个病灶直径之和小于 3cm，且不适合外科根治性切除和肝移植的患者，可行经皮射频消融术[31]。

化疗栓塞主要适用于无法外科根治，且无肝外转移的大肝癌或多发结节型肝细胞癌。有研究提出化疗栓塞的效果优于单纯栓塞、保守治疗或两者联合应用。Llovet 等[9]报道：37 例接受单纯栓塞治疗的患者，1 年生存率为 75%，2 年生存率为 50%；40 例接受化疗栓塞的患者，1 年生存率为 82%，2 年生存率为 63%；35 例接受保守治疗的患者，1 年生存率为 63%，2 年生存率为 27%。由于该研究生存率差异显著，故在研究早期便终止实验。另一项由 Lo 等[8]进行的研究证实了在无法手术切除的肝细胞癌患者中，化疗栓塞（碘化油、顺铂、吸收性明胶海绵）组患者的生存率显著优于对照组（仅接受对症治疗）。化疗栓塞组患者的 1、2 和 3 年生存率分别为 57%、31%和 26%；对照组患者的 1、2 和 3 年生存率分别为 32%、11%和 3%。无法手术切除且伴有门脉栓塞的患者，钇-90 放射性栓塞的应用已获 FDA 批准,可作为新辅助治疗,或作为肝移植术前的桥接治疗,但仍需大量随机对照试验证实其作用。

关于肝转移癌的思考

结肠癌肝转移

肝脏是结肠癌的首站转移器官也是唯一转移器官,这些患者多死于肝脏病变。因此,局部病变的有效控制对改善患者预后具有积极作用。尽管外科切除是治疗肝转移癌的首选治疗,但许多患者因伴发疾病而不适合手术。目前新型全身化疗药的应用能够延长肝转移癌患者生存期[32]。局部消融或外科手术联合消融治疗则可使有伴发病或者两叶受累而不适合手术的患者获益。有研究证实,肝内≤5 个转移灶,且单个病灶直径小于 5cm 的患者行局部消融联合外科手术治疗后,术后五年生存率为 24%~44%[33,34]。PVE 也可使无法手术切除的肝转移患者获得手术机会[23]。动脉灌注和放疗栓塞治疗肝转移癌可达到姑息治疗目的。新型化疗药物联合动脉灌注治疗以替代传统姑息治疗的研究也正在进行中。SIR 微球(树脂微球)放疗栓塞联合氟尿苷治疗结肠癌肝转移目前已获批准在临床上使用。

神经内分泌瘤肝转移

肝动脉栓塞或肝动脉化疗栓塞的适应证之一还包括具有内分泌活性的不可切除的神经内分泌瘤肝脏多发转移。其治疗目的是缩小肿瘤体积并减少激素分泌。肝动脉栓塞或化疗栓塞、对症治疗、生物化疗后的五年生存率分别为 50%~60%、40%~80%和 50%~60%[35]。Motertel 等[36]报道了他们在 10 年中对 111 例神经内分泌瘤肝转移患者行血管栓塞治疗的经验。这些肿瘤多为富血供肿瘤,其中 71 名患者接受了序贯交替栓塞化疗方案(达卡巴嗪联合多柔比星序贯治疗,链佐星联合 5-氟尿嘧啶交替化疗)。研究显示,单独血管栓塞的治疗反应率为 60%,血管栓塞与化疗栓塞联合应用的治疗反应率为 80%。血管栓塞术后,胰岛细胞癌与类癌肝转移患者的中位生存期分别为 37 个月和 49 个月。此外,二次栓塞对具有内分泌活性的神经内分泌瘤肝转移也能有效缓解临床症状。

肝动脉化疗栓塞治疗神经内分泌瘤肝转移疗效最佳,序贯周期性化疗栓塞方案则可达到有效姑息治疗的目的。Gupta 等[37]报道了 81 名类癌肝转移患者分别行单纯肝动脉栓塞和肝动脉化疗栓塞,通过影像学评估其中 69 例患者的治疗反应,部分反应(partial response,PR)者占 67%,病情稳定(stable disease,SD)者占 16%,肿瘤进展者占 8.7%。在 PR 患者中,平均反应持续时间为 17 个月。63%的患者的肿瘤相关综合征得到缓解,无进展中位生存期为 19 个月,中位生存期为 31 个月。随后,Gupta 等[38]又对比了上述 69 名类癌肝转移患者与 54 名胰岛细胞癌肝转移患者接受单纯栓塞或化疗栓塞后的治疗效果:类癌肝转移患者的治疗反应率及无进展生存时间均显著长于胰岛细胞癌肝转移患者(67% vs 35%;23 个月 vs 16 个月)。尽管在对比化疗栓塞与单纯栓塞时,未能证实类癌患者的生存差异,但化疗栓塞在一定程度上确实提高了胰岛细胞癌患者的总体生存期(32 个月 vs 18 个月)和治疗反应率(50% vs 25%)。

射频消融术可用于缓解神经内分泌瘤转移瘤的相关症状。Berber[39]进行的一系列研究表明,RFA 治疗 222 名神经内分泌性转移瘤患者,其症状完全缓解率为 63%,症状部分缓解率为 95%。放疗栓塞术是另一种可选择的能够减轻神经内分泌瘤肝转移肿瘤负荷的微创疗法。

其他肝转移瘤

其他肿瘤肝转移常常由于受侵范围广而不适合局部介入治疗。但是,某些特殊类型的原发肿瘤肝转移瘤可通过介入治疗获益。这些原发肿瘤包括眼黑色素细胞瘤、平滑肌肉瘤、乳腺癌以及肾细胞癌,发生肝转移后可行化疗栓塞治疗。在 30 名患有眼黑色素细胞瘤肝转移的患者中,应用化疗栓塞联合顺铂治疗后的反应率为 46%,平均生存期为 11 个月[40]。首次化疗栓塞后,最长生存期为 5 年。而在过去,此类患者一旦出现肝转移仅能生存 2~6 个月。另一研究结果显示,对比卡铂和福莫司汀灌注化疗,治疗反应率分别为 38%和 40%[40]。肝动脉免疫栓塞术治疗此类患者的也显示了不同的治疗反应率。14 名平滑肌肉瘤肝转移患者,首先接受了 4 周一次的化疗栓塞(顺铂、150~250μm 的聚乙烯醇颗粒),随后再行长春新碱灌注化疗[41],治疗反应率可达 70%,反应持续时间 4~19 个月(中位持续时间:9 个月)。与之相比,异环磷酰胺和多柔比星全身化疗的治疗反应率仅为 15%。需要注意的是,这些肿瘤并不常见,大多数病例是在临床研究中进行治疗。在 MD Anderson,肝转移癌化疗栓塞操作方法与肝细胞癌类似,这也提示了富血供转移瘤比乏血供肿瘤获益更多。但不论是缓解症状还是延长生存期,对这些转移瘤的介入治疗都应权衡利弊后决定。

泌尿生殖系统的介入

肾动脉栓塞

肾癌根治术前的肾动脉栓塞主要用以减少术中出血。尽管早期的研究成果并未证实术前肾动脉栓塞对改善肾癌患者生存预后具有积极作用,但 Zielinski 等[42]研究结果显示,术前肾动脉栓塞可延长肾癌患者的生存期。因局部肿瘤体积过大而产生相应临床症状的患者,亦可行肾动脉栓塞术缓解症状;或对不能手术的肾细胞癌患者进行减瘤治疗[43]。肾动脉栓塞还可用于动静脉分流所致充血性心衰的治疗。有肾功能不全或孤立肾的患者,为尽可能保留多的肾功能,可行部分肾动脉栓塞。

肾消融术

热消融术在肾细胞癌的治疗中地位愈发重要。尽管选择性部分肾切除仍然是肾癌治疗的金标准,但射频消融术已具备取代之势(图 42-3)。射频消融创伤小、并发症发生率低[44],适用于有较高手术并发症风险者、孤立肾或双侧肿瘤不适合手术切除者以及拒绝手术者。例如,有遗传性疾病者,如 von Hippel-Lindau 病,其肾脏多发肿瘤发生率高,可通过多次射频消融进行治疗,并保护肿瘤周围正常的肾实质。

Gervais 等[45,46]证实了射频消融的疗效同肿瘤的大小、位置直接相关,外生型肿瘤较中央型治疗效果更佳。这是因为肿

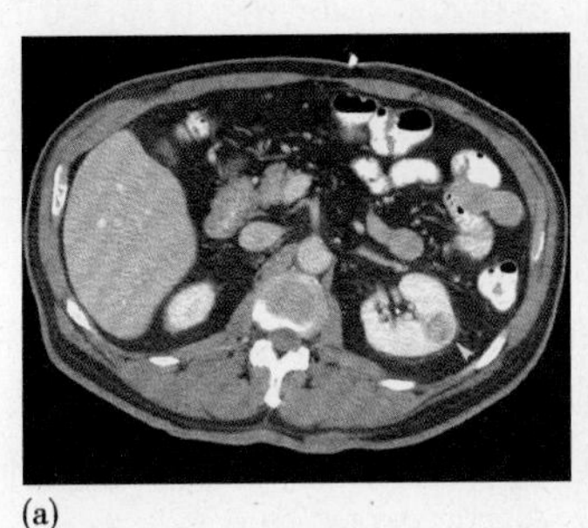
(a)

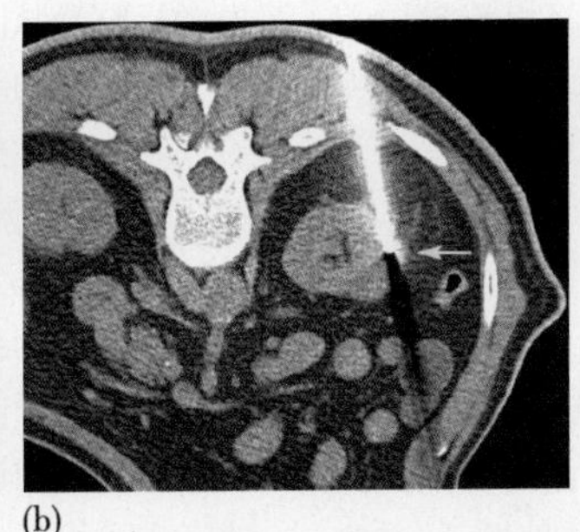
(b)

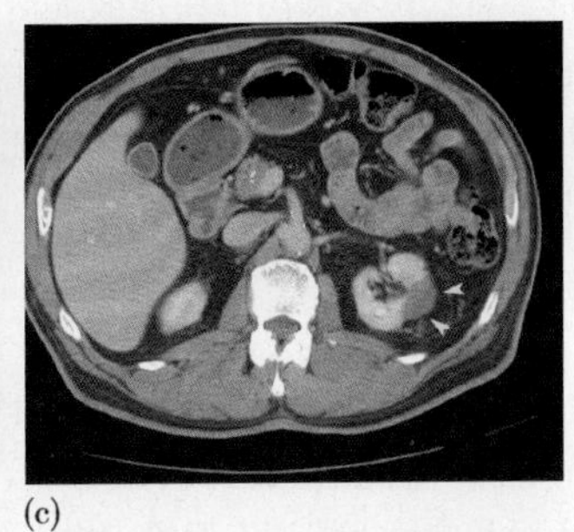
(c)

图 42-3 对一名 62 岁经活检确诊为肾细胞癌的老年患者进行经皮射频消融。(a)RF 消融前的增强 CT 显示左肾有增强团块(箭头);(b)俯卧位 RF 消融时的 CT 显示肿瘤部位的单针电极(箭头);(c)RF 消融后的增强 CT 显示肾脏治疗部位无残留的增强影

瘤周围的脂肪组织有助于手术定位,同时在消融过程中能起到绝缘作用。肿瘤的大小也会影响消融效果:肿瘤小于 4.0cm 时,完全坏死率可达 90%。而直径较大或者中央型的病灶,单次治疗不能彻底消融,还需两次或多次消融。中央型癌灶由于距离血管近,血流产生的“热沉效应”降低了肿瘤内部温度,影响消融疗效。而髓质肿瘤消融术后并发症的发生风险也相应增加。肾癌射频消融术后最常见的并发症为出血。Gervais 等[45,46]观察了 100 例肾细胞癌患者,射频消融术后出血的发生率为 5%。术后出血可发生在肾集合系统或局限在肾包膜下,若出血发生在肾脏集合系统造成尿路梗阻,则需行输尿管支架置入术以解除梗阻。

Ahrar 等[44]报道了经皮 RF 消融术治疗 29 例肾癌患者(瘤体 30 个)。瘤体平均最大直径为(3.5±0.24)cm。原发肿瘤完全消融率为 96%。平均和中位随访时间分别为 10 个月和 7 个月。RF 消融后严重并发症发生率为 12%;3 名患者出现大量血尿和尿路梗阻。术后出血均已成功治愈。1 名患者出现了持续的前腹壁薄弱。未见消融后明显的肾功减退报道。

胸部介入治疗

肺的消融

热消融可用于原发性肺癌及肺转移癌患者的治疗。早期肺癌的患者可通过消融获得根治,是早期肺癌的理想治疗选择之一。对瘤荷较大的肿瘤,消融也能够缓解、减轻肿瘤的相关症状[47]。肺的消融术主要用于不能手术的原发性肺癌和肺转移癌。

Simon 等[48]报道了肺 RF 消融治疗 153 例(瘤体 189 例)无法手术的原发性或转移性肺癌患者。研究结果显示,射频消融术后 1 年、2 年、3 年、4 年和 5 年生存率:在Ⅰ期非小细胞肺癌患者中分别为 78%、57%、36%、27%和 27%;在直肠癌肺转移患者中分别为 87%、78%、57%、57%和 57%。RF 消融术后气胸发生率为 28.4%。若患者消融术后出现气胸而无临床表现可行保守治疗;若症状明显,或气胸量持续进展,则需行胸腔置管引流。在 Simon 等[48]的报道中,操作相关的 30 天内死亡率为 2.6%。

胸腔积液是肺消融术后另一常见并发症。Baere 等[49]报道在 60 例接受 RF 消融的肺肿瘤患者中,9%的患者在治疗后立即出现少量胸腔积液,60%的患者在术后 24~48 小时通过 CT 扫描发现胸腔积液。10%的患者消融后出现咯血。咯血一般在消融术后第 1~9 天出现,持续 2~13 天。这些并发症一般具有自限性,不需要治疗即可痊愈。

肺的化疗栓塞

肺的化疗栓塞可以用于多种肺部肿瘤治疗。肺的化疗栓塞目的是将化疗药物注入肿瘤内,同时阻断肿瘤的血液供应。为此,通过将化疗药物与栓塞剂同时注入到供血给肿瘤的支气管动脉内。栓塞延缓了化疗药物的洗脱速度,从而延长了化疗药物在肿瘤内的停留时间。

2005 年,Vogl 等[50]验证了 23 例不可切除肺转移癌患者接受丝裂霉素-碘油支气管动脉化疗栓塞的疗效。研究结果显示,支气管动脉化疗栓塞安全可行,患者耐受度高。研究中未观察到严重并发症;35%的患者对治疗表现为局部反应,26%的患者治疗后肿瘤大小不变,39%的患者出现肿瘤进展速度减缓。(译者注:这篇文献发表年代相对早,目前临床实践中,碘化油一般不用于支气管动脉栓塞,取而代之,是采用颗粒进行栓塞,会获得更高的安全性。)

姑息治疗

经皮胆汁引流

胆管腔内梗阻多由胰腺癌、胆管癌和壶腹癌等引起;胆管外压性梗阻则多由淋巴瘤、肝细胞癌和肝转移癌等压迫所致。不能手术的恶性胆道梗阻患者,可以通过胆汁引流解除胆道梗阻,包括内镜下和经皮两种方式。经皮胆汁引流术包括了内引流、外引流或内-外引流。

经皮胆汁引流可缓解因胆道梗阻所致的恶性梗阻性黄疸、瘙痒、胆管炎等症状,或为抗肿瘤治疗提供准备。但无论内镜下引流还是经皮引流治疗,目前都无法提高患者的生存期。一般情况下,治疗技术的选择多由治疗团队根据当地的诊疗经验及技术条件决定。

相较于外引流,内引流后患者穿刺点疼痛轻、导管周围胆汁漏发生率较低、因细菌逆流入血所致的败血症较少,在临床中应用更有优势。而经皮穿刺的方法能够迅速将引流导管置入胆道内,将胆汁引出,迅速解除梗阻,降低胆道压力。无论哪种引流方法,引流治疗后的黄疸部分缓解率或完全缓解率可达到 73%~100%[51]。

经皮胆道支架

Speer 等[52]对比了经皮胆道支架置入和内镜下胆道支架置入的疗效差异:将 70 例恶性胆道梗阻的患者,随机分配到经皮胆道支架置入组和内镜下胆道支架置入组。结果提示:黄疸缓解成功率:内镜支架置入为 81%,经皮支架置入为 61%。内镜支架置入组的并发症发生率为 19%,而经皮支架置入组为 67%。另外,内镜支架和经皮支架置入术后的 30 天死亡率分别为 15%和 33%。

支架置入术的最常见并发症包括胆管炎、出血和胆汁漏。塑料支架比金属支架更易引起胆管炎[53]。塑料支架易移位,通畅性平均维持 3~4 个月[53]。自膨式金属支架术后通畅率维持时间更长,但价格相较于其他支架昂贵。金属支架在球囊扩张时有可能发生移位,但是远期自发移位率低,甚至可忽略不计。非覆膜金属支架不能取出。尽管支架技术有很多优点,但是支架内肿瘤生长或者支架两端内膜增生引起的再狭窄仍然是一个复杂的问题。

肌肉、骨的消融

多数前列腺癌、乳腺癌和肺癌患者在死亡时已存在骨转移。这部分患者常常合并疼痛、病理性骨折等,生活质量受到了极大的影响[54]。外照射是治疗骨转移癌性疼痛的金标准。大多数患者的疼痛症状能在外照射后得到缓解。但仍有少部分患者对放疗不敏感,使得治疗反应率和持续缓解率不理想[55]。

当患者主诉中度或者重度肌肉骨骼疼痛,疼痛是局部病灶所致且经影像学资料证实,并且能通过经皮路径治疗者,可选择消融治疗[56]。

适宜消融的病灶包括典型的溶骨性或者溶骨和成骨混合性病灶,或者混有软组织的病灶。射频消融与冷冻消融对缓解那些经标准治疗困难的转移病灶的疼痛安全、有效。重要的是,患者术后生存质量可以得到显著提高。Goetz 等[57]报道了 43 例骨转移癌性疼痛病例接受 RF 消融治疗:95%的患者疼痛症状缓解,阿片类药物的使用剂量得到明显降低。单次消融治疗对绝大多数患者有效,并且能够较长时间缓解疼痛。

综合应用

下腔静脉滤器置入

癌症患者血栓形成率高,肺栓塞风险大。有抗凝治疗禁忌证或充分抗凝后再次发生肺栓塞的患者可首选经皮穿刺腔静脉内滤器置入。腔静脉滤器种类很多,例如可回收滤器以及磁共振成像(MRI)兼容滤器。

Wallace 等[58]报道了 308 例患有血栓栓塞疾病的恶性肿瘤患者行腔静脉滤器置入术。267 例实体瘤患者的中位生存时间为 145 天,41 例囊性肿瘤患者的中位生存时间为 207 天。转移瘤或者弥漫性疾病的患者的死亡风险是局部病灶的患者的 3.7 倍,而有深静脉血栓形成和出血史的患者的死亡率是无深静脉血栓和出血史的患者的 2 倍。腔静脉滤器置入术后的严重并发症包括肺动脉栓塞、腔静脉阻塞、腹膜后出血和滤器移位等。

围术期预防性的可回收下腔静脉滤器置入术是常见的操作技术之一,其适应证为有血栓栓塞病史且需行外科手术者,或者在手术后有栓子形成风险的高危患者。一旦患者可以接受系统的抗凝治疗,那么应该计划置入下腔静脉可回收滤器。

静脉狭窄支架置入

腔内或腔外的恶性肿瘤常常引起腔静脉综合征[59]。腔静脉综合征中,肿瘤通过侵犯和占位,或者通过纵隔、腹膜后以及盆腔的淋巴结转移,对腔静脉产生外压性改变,进而导致腔静脉狭窄或者梗阻。放疗和化疗治疗腔静脉综合征的并发症包括纵隔纤维化和血栓性静脉炎[59]。

上腔静脉综合征的典型表现分为以下 4 种:①中枢神经系统症状,包括头痛、视力模糊和认知功能异常;②咽喉水肿及其产生的呼吸困难和声音嘶哑;③鼻部或者面部水肿;④静脉充血和扩张的其他征象[60]。另外,腔静脉狭窄或者阻塞时常伴有肿瘤压迫纵隔或者侵入血管内部。Parish 等[61]报道确诊恶性上腔静脉栓塞的患者,平均生存期为 7 个月。而血管支架对恶性肿瘤引起的腔静脉栓塞的症状缓解率达到 68%~80%[59]。

活检

经皮穿刺活检是诊断癌症的有效方法之一,包括心肌在内的所有组织都可以经皮穿刺活检。各种各样的穿刺针(11~25G)和活检钳均可获得有效的病理标本。目前,活检枪已能自动化完成活检操作。然而,即便活检结果阴性仍不能排除恶性肿瘤的可能,阴性的活检结果只能反映抽样误差。大多数成人的病灶活检可在门诊选择性地完成。

纵隔和肺的活检主要在 CT 引导下完成[62]。肺癌或者肺转移癌的经胸针吸活检的准确率达到 90%~98%[63],免疫缺陷患者的局部肺感染的诊断率为 73%[64]。肺和纵隔穿刺活检的严重并发症有:体循环的空气栓塞、出血、心包填塞、穿刺路径恶性细胞的播散和脓胸。气胸是最常见并发症,CT 引导下活检的气胸发生率为 22%~45%[65,66]。而 Cox 等[67]在其研究中表示,CT 引导下进行穿刺活检,气胸发生的概率与小病灶(<2cm)和肺气肿的存在密切相关。

84%~95%的患者可以通过 CT、超声和 MRI 引导的腹部穿刺活检获得到足够的诊断组织以用于细胞学检查。对肝脏、胰腺、肾、肾上腺、脾脏、卵巢和其他器官进行活检时,使用 20~23G(gauge)的穿刺针的活检敏感性为 86%,特异性为 98%,准确性为 90%。在一项纳入 63 180 例患者的研究中,活检后并发症发生率为 0.16%。穿刺路径恶性细胞种植的发生率为 0.05%[68-70]。

经皮骨髓穿刺活检的平均准确性是 80%。有报道在 178 例原发性骨肿瘤的患者中,经皮穿刺活检的诊断准确率为

78%[71]。这一活检手段检出恶性肿瘤的准确率(83%)高于良性肿瘤(64%)。

经颈静脉肝内门体分流术

经颈静脉肝内门体分流术(transjugular intrahepatic portosystemic shunt,TIPS)通过在肝脏和门脉系统之间架桥并置入金属支架,形成肝内门体分流通道,是一种公认的能够有效降低门脉高压的治疗方法。其适应证主要包括:食管胃静脉曲张破裂出血、顽固性腹水、门静脉高压性胃病、肝性胸腔积液和布加综合征等。伴有肝病的肿瘤患者同样也可以接受 TIPS 治疗。Wallace 等[72]报道了 38 例患有恶性肿瘤和肝脏疾病的患者接受 TIPS 治疗,97%的患者达到技术成功。19 例患者中只有一例发生再出血(5%)。12 例患者中 9 例胸、腹水消失或者明显好转(75%)。TIPS 支架内膜增生引起的分流道再狭窄或闭塞是令人担忧的术后并发症,近年来覆膜支架与 TIPS 专用支架的应用使分流道通畅率大大提高,使得 TIPS 在肝癌门静脉高压合并症治疗方面具有广阔发展前景。

(袁筑慧　龚涛 译,李肖 审校)

参考文献

The complete reference list can be found on the Wiley Companion Digital Edition of this title (see inside front cover for login instructions).

1 Collins JM. Pharmacologic rationale for regional drug delivery. *J Clin Oncol*. 1984;**2**(**5**):498–504.

2 Mocellin S, Pilati P, Lise M, Nitti D. Meta-analysis of hepatic arterial infusion for unresectable liver metastases from colorectal cancer: the end of an era? *J Clin Oncol*. 2007;**25**(**35**):5649–5654.

3 Hemingway AP, Allison DJ. Complications of embolization: analysis of 410 procedures. *Radiology*. 1988;**166**(**3**):669–672.

4 Yamada R, Nakatsuka H, Nakamura K, et al. Hepatic artery embolization in 32 patients with unresectable hepatoma. *Osaka City Med J*. 1980;**26**(**2**):81–96.

5 Nakakuma K, Tashiro S, Hiraoka T, et al. Studies on anticancer treatment with an oily anticancer drug injected into the ligated feeding hepatic artery for liver cancer. *Cancer*. 1983;**52**(**12**):2193–2200.

8 Lo CM, Ngan H, Tso WK, et al. Randomized controlled trial of transarterial lipiodol chemoembolization for unresectable hepatocellular carcinoma. *Hepatology*. 2002;**35**(**5**):1164–1171.

9 Llovet JM, Real MI, Montana X, et al. Arterial embolisation or chemoembolisation versus symptomatic treatment in patients with unresectable hepatocellular carcinoma: a randomised controlled trial. *Lancet*. 2002;**359**(**9319**):1734–1739.

10 Liapi E, Georgiades CC, Hong K, Geschwind JF. Transcatheter arterial chemoembolization: current technique and future promise. *Tech Vasc Interv Radiol*. 2007;**10**(**1**):2–11.

11 Yoshizawa H, Nishino S, Shiomori K, Natsugoe S, Aiko T, Kitamura Y. Surface morphology control of polylactide microspheres enclosing irinotecan hydrochloride. *Int J Pharm*. 2005;**296**(**1–2**):112–116.

12 Wallace MJ, Murthy R, Kamat PP, et al. Impact of C-arm CT on hepatic arterial interventions for hepatic malignancies. *J Vasc Interv Radiol*. 2007;**18**(**12**):1500–1507.

13 Geschwind JF, Salem R, Carr BI, et al. Yttrium-90 microspheres for the treatment of hepatocellular carcinoma. *Gastroenterology*. 2004;**127**(**5 Suppl**):S194–S205.

14 Salem R, Lewandowski RJ, Atassi B, et al. Treatment of unresectable hepatocellular carcinoma with use of ^{90}Y microspheres (TheraSphere): safety, tumor response, and survival. *J Vasc Interv Radiol*. 2005;**16**(**12**):1627–1639.

15 Stubbs RS, Cannan RJ, Mitchell AW. Selective internal radiation therapy (SIRT) with ^{90}Yttrium microspheres for extensive colorectal liver metastases. *Hepatogastroenterology*. 2001;**48**(**38**):333–337.

16 Livraghi T, Giorgio A, Marin G, et al. Hepatocellular carcinoma and cirrhosis in 746 patients: long-term results of percutaneous ethanol injection. *Radiology*. 1995;**197**(**1**):101–108.

18 Ebara M, Okabe S, Kita K, et al. Percutaneous ethanol injection for small hepatocellular carcinoma: therapeutic efficacy based on 20-year observation. *J Hepatol*. 2005;**43**(**3**):458–464.

19 Livraghi T, Goldberg SN, Lazzaroni S, Meloni F, Solbiati L, Gazelle GS. Small hepatocellular carcinoma: treatment with radio-frequency ablation versus ethanol injection. *Radiology*. 1999;**210**(**3**):655–661.

20 Lencioni RA, Allgaier HP, Cioni D, et al. Small hepatocellular carcinoma in cirrhosis: randomized comparison of radio-frequency thermal ablation versus percutaneous ethanol injection. *Radiology*. 2003;**228**(**1**):235–240.

21 Gillams AR, Lees WR. Survival after percutaneous, image-guided, thermal ablation of hepatic metastases from colorectal cancer. *Dis Colon Rectum*. 2000;**43**(**5**):656–661.

22 Yokoyama Y, Nagino M, Nimura Y. Mechanisms of hepatic regeneration following portal vein embolization and partial hepatectomy: a review. *World J Surg*. 2007;**31**(**2**):367–374.

24 Madoff DC, Abdalla EK, Gupta S, et al. Transhepatic ipsilateral right portal vein embolization extended to segment IV: improving hypertrophy and resection outcomes with spherical particles and coils. *J Vasc Interv Radiol*. 2005;**16**(**2 Pt 1**):215–225.

25 Abulkhir A, Limongelli P, Healey AJ, et al. Preoperative portal vein embolization for major liver resection: a meta-analysis. *Ann Surg*. 2008;**247**(**1**):49–57.

27 Yamada R, Kishi K, Sato M, et al. Transcatheter arterial chemoembolization (TACE) in the treatment of unresectable liver cancer. *World J Surg*. 1995;**19**(**6**):795–800.

28 Bruix J, Sherman M. Management of hepatocellular carcinoma. *Hepatology*. 2005;**42**(**5**):1208–1236.

31 Chen MS, Li JQ, Zheng Y, et al. A prospective randomized trial comparing percutaneous local ablative therapy and partial hepatectomy for small hepatocellular carcinoma. *Ann Surg*. 2006;**243**(**3**):321–328.

32 Goldberg RM, Sargent DJ, Morton RF, et al. A randomized controlled trial of fluorouracil plus leucovorin, irinotecan, and oxaliplatin combinations in patients with previously untreated metastatic colorectal cancer. *J Clin Oncol*. 2004;**22**(**1**):23–30.

33 Lencioni R, Crocetti L, Cioni D, Della Pina C, Bartolozzi C. Percutaneous radiofrequency ablation of hepatic colorectal metastases: technique, indications, results, and new promises. *Invest Radiol*. 2004;**39**(**11**):689–697.

34 Gillams AR, Lees WR. Radio-frequency ablation of colorectal liver metastases in 167 patients. *Eur Radiol*. 2004;**14**(**12**):2261–2267.

35 Ramage JK, Davies AH, Ardill J, et al. Guidelines for the management of gastroenteropancreatic neuroendocrine (including carcinoid) tumours. *Gut*. 2005;**54**(**Suppl 4**):iv1–iv16.

36 Moertel CG, Johnson CM, McKusick MA, et al. The management of patients with advanced carcinoid tumors and islet cell carcinomas. *Ann Intern Med*. 1994;**120**(**4**):302–309.

37 Gupta S, Yao JC, Ahrar K, et al. Hepatic artery embolization and chemoembolization for treatment of patients with metastatic carcinoid tumors: the M.D. Anderson experience. *Cancer J*. 2003;**9**(**4**):261–267.

38 Gupta S, Johnson MM, Murthy R, et al. Hepatic arterial embolization and chemoembolization for the treatment of patients with metastatic neuroendocrine tumors: variables affecting response rates and survival. *Cancer*. 2005;**104**(**8**):1590–1602.

44 Ahrar K, Matin S, Wood CG, et al. Percutaneous radiofrequency ablation of renal tumors: technique, complications, and outcomes. *J Vasc Interv Radiol*. 2005;**16**(**5**):679–688.

45 Gervais DA, McGovern FJ, Arellano RS, McDougal WS, Mueller PR. Radiofrequency ablation of renal cell carcinoma: part 1, Indications, results, and role in patient management over a 6-year period and ablation of 100 tumors. *Am J Roentgenol*. 2005;**185**(**1**):64–71.

46 Gervais DA, Arellano RS, McGovern FJ, McDougal WS, Mueller PR. Radiofrequency ablation of renal cell carcinoma: part 2, lessons learned with ablation of 100 tumors. *Am J Roentgenol*. 2005;**185**(**1**):72–80.

48 Simon CJ, Dupuy DE, DiPetrillo TA, et al. Pulmonary radiofrequency ablation: long-term safety and efficacy in 153 patients. *Radiology*. 2007;**243**(**1**):268–275.

49 de Baere T, Palussiere J, Auperin A, et al. Midterm local efficacy and survival after radiofrequency ablation of lung tumors with minimum follow-up of 1 year: prospective evaluation. *Radiology*. 2006;**240**(**2**):587–596.

50 Vogl TJ, Wetter A, Lindemayr S, Zangos S. Treatment of unresectable lung metastases with transpulmonary chemoembolization: preliminary experience. *Radiology*. 2005;**234**(**3**):917–922.

52 Speer AG, Cotton PB, Russell RC, et al. Randomised trial of endoscopic versus percutaneous stent insertion in malignant obstructive jaundice. *Lancet*. 1987;**2**(**8550**):57–62.

56 Callstrom MR, Charboneau JW. Image-guided palliation of painful metastases using percutaneous ablation. *Tech Vasc Interv Radiol*. 2007;**10**(**2**):120–131.

57 Goetz MP, Callstrom MR, Charboneau JW, et al. Percutaneous image-guided radiofrequency ablation of painful metastases involving bone: a multicenter study. *J Clin Oncol*. 2004;**22**(**2**):300–306.

58 Wallace MJ, Jean JL, Gupta S, et al. Use of inferior vena caval filters and survival in patients with malignancy. *Cancer*. 2004;**101**(**8**):1902–1907.

59 Carrasco CH, Charnsangavej C, Wright KC, Wallace S, Gianturco C. Use of the Gianturco self-expanding stent in stenoses of the superior and inferior venae cavae. *J Vasc Interv Radiol*. 1992;**3**(**2**):409–419.

60 Kee ST, Kinoshita L, Razavi MK, Nyman UR, Semba CP, Dake MD. Superior vena cava syndrome: treatment with catheter-directed thrombolysis and endovascular stent placement. *Radiology*. 1998;**206**(**1**):187–193.

62 Gupta S, Seaberg K, Wallace MJ, et al. Imaging-guided percutaneous biopsy of mediastinal lesions: different approaches and anatomic considerations. *Radiographics*. 2005;**25**(**3**):763–786; discussion 86–88.

63 Westcott J. Lung biopsy. In: Dondelinger RF, Rossi P, Kurdziel JC, Wallace S, eds. *Interventional Radiology*. Stuttgart: Thieme; 1990:9–17.

66 Kazerooni EA, Lim FT, Mikhail A, Martinez FJ. Risk of pneumothorax in CT-guided transthoracic needle aspiration biopsy of the lung. *Radiology*. 1996;**198**(**2**):371–375.

67 Cox JE, Chiles C, McManus CM, Aquino SL, Choplin RH. Transthoracic needle aspiration biopsy: variables that affect risk of pneumothorax. *Radiology*. 1999;**212**(**1**):165–168.

69 Stewart CJ, Coldewey J, Stewart IS. Comparison of fine needle aspiration cytology and needle core biopsy in the diagnosis of radiologically detected abdominal lesions. *J Clin Pathol*. 2002;**55**(**2**):93–97.

71 Ayala AG, Zornosa J. Primary bone tumors: percutaneous needle biopsy. Radiologic-pathologic study of 222 biopsies. *Radiology*. 1983;**149**(**3**):675–679.

72 Wallace MJ, Madoff DC, Ahrar K, Warneke CL. Transjugular intrahepatic portosystemic shunts: experience in the oncology setting. *Cancer*. 2004;**101**(**2**):337–345.

第 43 章　肿瘤外科学原则

Mark Bloomston, MD, FACS ■ Kenneth K. Tanabe, MD, FACS ■ Raphael E. Pollock, MD, PhD, FACS ■ Donald L. Morton, MD, FACS(deceased)

概述

肿瘤外科学是外科的一个顶级专业学科，目前在美国针对该专科有一个专业认证程序。肿瘤外科医生是一类针对肿瘤问题以外科手术为主要治疗方式的肿瘤学专家，他们聚焦于外科认知与外科技术。因此，肿瘤外科医生对实体恶性肿瘤的自然史有着透彻的理解，在肿瘤活检和分期方法方面有着丰富的经验，这些知识可用于制定实体肿瘤多学科治疗方案，并可通过积极的个人参与来执行。通过此类相关的研究机会，我们将提升对癌症患者的综合诊治能力。

尽管癌症患者的多种全身性治疗方法取得了显著进展，但手术治疗仍然是大多数实体恶性肿瘤的主要治疗方法，并且在癌症从预防到诊断，再到治愈性治疗、延长生存和姑息性治疗等全程治疗的各个阶段中发挥重要作用。为了最大限度地提高疗效，肿瘤外科医生必须成为肿瘤治疗团队中的一员，并时常成为患者咨询的首位肿瘤专科医生。肿瘤外科医生通常负责为可疑病变建立组织学诊断，这可能涉及某种手术操作、影像学引导或其他病理活组织检查方法。肿瘤外科医生通常负责将活检结果传达给患者，完成肿瘤分期所需的程序，并启动患者与多学科肿瘤学团队其他成员之间的后续互动。基于这些责任，大多数情况下是肿瘤外科医生首次向患者解释将用于治疗特定恶性肿瘤的各种治疗方法的顺序和基本原理。因此，为了获得最大的效果，肿瘤外科医生必须掌握不同的治疗方案、特定恶性肿瘤的自然病史，以及如何将这些知识整合到精心设计的、合理的多学科治疗过程中。肿瘤外科医生通常也有责任提供关于预后的最新进展，并决定后续治疗和监测，以及早发现肿瘤复发。在这些方面，肿瘤外科医生几乎完全不同于其他外科医生，因为他们对特定患者的责任既包含对疾病的急性处理也包含长期治疗。

多年来，肿瘤外科的发展实践形成了一个完整的循环。最初，外科医生试图通过只切除大体病变来保守的治疗癌症。不幸的是，这导致了极高的局部复发率和后续的高死亡率。19 世纪末，外科医生开始实施根治性整块切除术和截肢术用以治疗恶性疾病。这些技术虽产生了积极的结果但方式却常常是不规范的。随着其他可替代的、有效的治疗方式出现，特别是 20 世纪 20 年代的放射治疗和 20 世纪 40 年代的化疗出现，外科切除的方向再次变得保守，其重点变成器官保存和尽可能的功能恢复。

对于手术切除后但合并肿瘤的微转移，仍有很高复发可能性的患者，辅助化疗（单独或联合放射治疗）提高了其无瘤生存率，提升了生活质量。随机临床试验研究证实了辅助化疗对多种肿瘤的积极作用，包括乳腺癌、结直肠癌、胰腺癌、骨肉瘤、睾丸癌、卵巢癌和某些肺癌等。

外科手术是治疗局限的、原发性疾病最有效的方法。手术切除的原则是对原发肿瘤实施整块切除，即试图切除所有相连续和相邻的解剖部位上的大体和微观肿瘤。对于某些肿瘤类型，局部淋巴结的清扫是外科初始治疗的重要组成部分。在许多情况下，当疾病被早期诊断和切除时，手术切除是唯一的治愈性手段，并常常因此获得较高的长期生存率。直观地说，一旦肿瘤从主要部位扩散到远处，手术切除在疾病治疗中的作用就变得很小，这似乎是合乎逻辑的。事实上，手术治疗也正在广泛应用于转移性肿瘤。在切除各种转移部位（包括肝、肺或脑）后，可以在某些特定的患者中观察到生存期的延长。尤其是众多当前的研究显示，结直肠癌肝转移完整切除的 5 年生存率超过 50%。随着更有效的全身细胞毒性和靶向治疗不断地延长各类肿瘤患者的生存期，残留转移部位的切除或消融术的应用也越来越广泛。

手术遵循零级动力学原理（非线性动力学），其中 100% 的切除细胞被破坏。相比之下，化疗和放疗则遵循一级动力学原理（线性动力学，即浓度/剂量与杀伤效果成正比），其中每次治疗仅能杀灭一小部分肿瘤细胞。正基于这个原因，这些疗法仅作为补充性治疗手段。手术切除可减轻肿瘤负荷，提高旨在消除微残余病灶的非手术辅助治疗的功效，从而降低复发风险并延长生存期。

在过去几十年中，许多复杂的癌症手术相关的发病率和死亡率均显著降低。这些结果在一定程度上可归因于手术技术的进步、患者的筛选以及大型临床中心的区域化。例如医院的规模显著影响胰十二指肠切除术后的围术期风险和长期存活率[1]。此外，肿瘤切除更局限的趋势正带来良好的肿瘤学预后。具体而言，保乳手术已经成为乳腺癌患者乳房切除术的替代方案，骨和软组织肉瘤患者进行肢体保留成为可能，并且直肠癌患者保留括约肌功能和性功能亦常常能够实现。由于外科手术越来越多地与其他治疗方式相结合，因此大多数实体肿瘤患者的治疗方案必须由一个多学科团队来制定，该团队包括放射科、肿瘤内科以及肿瘤外科医生等。为了在癌症患者的诊治过程中能发挥主要作用，成功的肿瘤外科医生必须能够协调和整合整个肿瘤学团队的工作，同时重视患者的尊严和生活质量。

肿瘤外科学发展史

肿瘤学（oncology，希腊语中的 onkos 意思是肿块或肿瘤，而 logos 意思是研究）是一门研究肿瘤疾病的科学。早期作者认为，某些家庭、种族和工人阶层更容易发生肿瘤性转化。1862年美国埃及古物学家 Edwin Smith 发现了最早的癌症手术治疗记录[2]。这篇记录写于大约公元前1600年的埃及，其依据的教义可能要追溯到公元前3000年。这位埃及作者建议外科医生应积极处理可能通过手术治愈的肿瘤，而非治疗那些可能致命的肿瘤。

Hippocrates（公元前460—375年）是第一个描述肿瘤相关临床症状的人。他建议不要治疗那些晚期肿瘤患者，因为他们若接受非外科治疗反而能享受更好的生活质量[3]。他还创造了术语"癌"（蟹腿样肿瘤）和"肉瘤"（肉性肿块）。在公元2世纪，Galen 发表了他的肿瘤分类，并将癌症描述为由过量黑胆汁引起的全身性疾病[4]。Galen 警告说癌症是一种全身性疾病，它并不能通过手术获得治愈，相反手术加速了患者的死亡。这一强烈反对癌症手术的告诫持续了1 500多年，直到18世纪病理学家发现癌症在扩散到其他解剖部位之前通常会先在局部生长。在安全可靠的全身麻醉药出现之前，外科手术主要用于处理创伤或严重的感染问题，诸如脓肿引流等。在那个时代，癌症手术主要包括截肢或烧灼躯干、四肢的表面肿瘤。患者通常不愿意接受肿瘤手术带来的痛苦，因为这种治疗方式几乎不可能提高生存率。

在18世纪和19世纪，解剖病理学的进步导致了尸体解剖的增加，这反过来又推动和加深了对人体解剖和生理学更好的理解。Morgagni、Le Dran 和 Da Salva 的早期研究证实，在肿瘤远处传播之前存在一个局部生长的初始阶段。这使人们认识到并非所有肿瘤都是全身性扩散的，某些恶性肿瘤仅通过局部侵袭性生长便可导致死亡。Percival Pott（1714—1788）是第一个描述与癌症发展相关的特定病因的人。1775年 Pott 发现在已进入青春期的烟囱清洁工的阴囊癌的发病率很高，并建议实施广泛的局部切除治疗。1829年法国外科医生 Joseph Recamier（1774—1852）第一次描述了肿瘤播散的复杂过程。1809年美国外科医生 Ephraim McDowell 实施了第一次有记录的选择性肿瘤切除手术，他成功地从一名患者身上切除了一个22磅重的卵巢肿瘤，这名患者后来活了30年。McDowell 的工作还包括12例卵巢肿瘤切除手术，这大大激发了人们对癌症患者选择性手术的兴趣。

外科医生最初感到挫败，因患者在手术过程中所经历的极度不适以及缺乏可有效降低感染发生的药物。1842年 Crawford Long（1815—1878）是第一个在全身麻醉中使用乙醚的人，然而是 John Collins Warren（1778—1856）和 William T. G. Morton（1819—1868）的报告才让麻醉的潜力引发了公众关注。Warren 发表的第一篇关于乙醚麻醉的文章（1846年）中提到的手术是选择性舌癌切除术，手术切除了颌下腺和部分舌骨。Warren 还负责编写了第一本美国本土作者的肿瘤外科教科书《肿瘤手术观察》，并于1838年出版。Joseph Lister（1827—1912）是第一个报道在选择性手术中成功应用灭菌的人。1867年，Lister 依据 Pasteur 关于细菌引起感染的观点引入了石炭酸作为一种灭菌剂与外科器械的热消毒一起使用。此外，Lister 还引入了可吸收线以及留置引流管来消除手术伤口的分泌物和无效腔。

即便出现了灭菌和全身麻醉，肿瘤外科手术在19世纪下半叶和20世纪初仍然有很高的死亡率。癌症很少能在早期阶段被诊断出来，因此很少有患者能够实施根治性手术。那些尝试手术切除恶性病变的外科医生受限于基础麻醉的条件，这也是与患者高死亡率密切相关的独立危险因素。当时还没有抗生素，手术器械也很简陋。当时显微镜评估手术切缘冷冻组织的重要性尚未得到重视，外科医生对肿瘤边缘的评估仅相信自己的肉眼。然而那个时代的一些重要进步也导致了肿瘤外科学的快速发展。随着对精细手术技术、温和组织处理的不断重视和抗菌理念的应用，Albert Teodore Billroth（第一次胃切除术，喉切除术和食管切除术）、William Stewart Halsted（整块切除术，根治性乳房切除术）等外科先驱以及许多其他当时的外科医生定义并拓展了肿瘤外科学的领域（表43-1）[3]。

表43-1 肿瘤外科学发展的里程碑事件

时间	事件	术者
1775年	癌症的病因学基础	Percival Pott
1809年	选择性卵巢切除术	Ephraim McDowell
1829年	肿瘤转移过程	Joseph Recamier
1846年	乙醚麻醉	John Collins Warren
1867年	石炭酸灭菌	Joseph Lister
1873年	喉头切除术	Albert Theodore Billroth
1878年	直肠肿瘤切除术	Richard von Volkman
1880年	食管切除术	Albert Theodore Billroth
1881年	胃切除术	Albert Theodore Billroth
1890年	根治性乳房切除术	William Stewart Halsted
1896年	卵巢切除术治疗乳腺癌	G. T. Beatson
1904年	根治性前列腺切除术	Hugh H. Young
1906年	根治性子宫切除术	Ernest Wertheim
1908年	腹会阴联合切除术	W. Ernest Miles
1909年	甲状腺手术（诺贝尔奖）	Theodore Emil Kocher
1910年	颅骨切开术	Harvey Cushing
1912年	脊髓切断术治疗疼痛	E. Martin
1913年	胸段食管切除术	Franz Torek
1927年	肺转移瘤切除术	George Divis
1933年	肺切除术	Evarts Graham
1935年	胰十二指肠切除术	Allen O. Whipple
1945年	肾上腺切除术治疗前列腺癌	Charles B. Huggins
1957年	肢体隔离热灌注	Oliver Creech
1958年	国家辅助性乳腺和肠道工程组织（NSABP）开展前瞻性随机试验	Bernard Fisher
1965年	癌症激素疗法	Charles Huggins
1971年	微血管吻合游离组织移植	Harry Buncke

为有效控制原发肿瘤而持续进行的创新已经大大改善了手术预后和生存质量。伴随微血管外科的进展，现已实现复杂的游离自体组织移植，如游离空肠移植来重建消化系统或骨肌皮瓣来重建四肢和其他活动的身体部位（如下颌等）。自动吻合器、腹腔镜/机器人器械以及高分辨率的光学设备的应用已极大促进了微创肿瘤外科的发展，减少了患者的不适和恢复时间（图 43-1）。

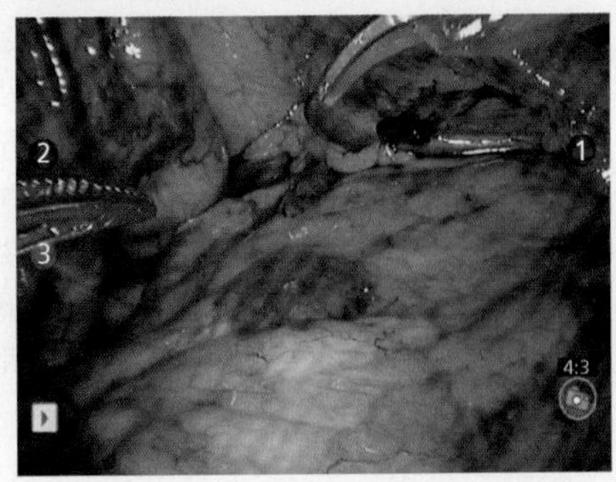

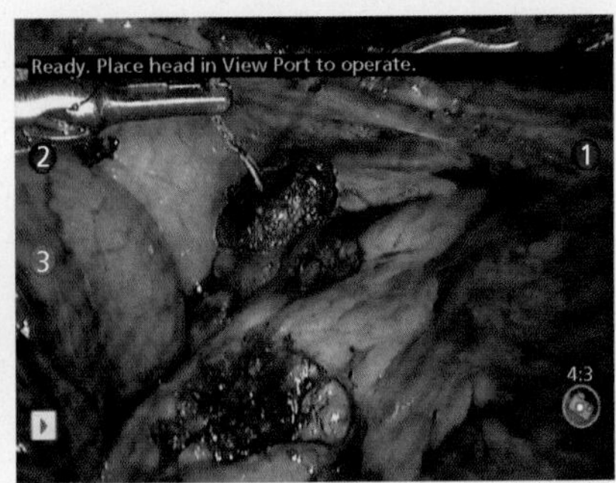

图 43-1　胰岛素瘤机器人摘除术

机器人技术的迅速发展正在改变传统的外科干预方式。其潜在的优势在于机器人手术操作者可通过充满了多维关节的机器人"手腕"实现可伸缩手的直接延伸，从而避免了腹腔镜手术操作中刚性器械交叉的障碍。将光电可视化系统集成到机器人显示器中，使其具有超常视觉敏锐度的三维立体术野。接通显示的图像可配合放大或缩小手术游离动作（例如缝线放置和置管等），减弱可移动解剖结构操作的震颤效应，尤其在微观水平上。分子放射探针可用于显像具有众多不良遗传特征的肿瘤细胞成分，其不断的发展预示着未来介入放射科和微创肿瘤外科专家将在手术室中一起合作，应用激光或者结合术中导航系统、各种视觉界面如直接视网膜显示系统等以获取那些恶性肿瘤的显微解剖信息。

随着术前合并症处理和围术期重症治疗的不断进步，现在已可以安全地实施越来越复杂的外科手术。对肿瘤扩散模式更加成熟的认识也为微创手术提供了更多的机会，其中一个例子便是在早期黑色素瘤和乳腺癌中使用淋巴结标记和前哨淋巴结活检以替代常规的淋巴结清扫术。另外，对复发风险的更深入认识导致了更多而非更少的扩大手术切除，这方面的一个例子是选择性应用全肝切除及原位肝移植术治疗早期的肝细胞癌。

现代肿瘤外科学

肿瘤外科医生是一类将大部分时间用于研究和治疗恶性肿瘤疾病的外科专家。他们必须具备必要的知识、技能和临床经验以便能为癌症患者实施标准的和超常规的手术方式。肿瘤外科医生必须能够准确诊断肿瘤并鉴别侵袭性肿瘤病变与良性反应过程。另外，肿瘤外科医生应该对放射肿瘤学、肿瘤内科学、诊断与介入放射学有深入地理解。他们还必须有能力组织跨学科的癌症研究。肿瘤外科医生也应接受病理学方面的培训，因为他们要为病理医生切除恰当的肿瘤标本并决定手术切缘是否充足。肿瘤外科医生应与肿瘤内科医生共同承担癌症治疗的"初级保健医生"角色。几乎所有癌症患者最初都将由这两类专家中的一个进行管理，因此他们将承担协调个体化患者进行恰当多模式治疗的最终责任。

鉴于目前多学科治疗模式对癌症患者而言极为复杂，众多癌症中心已开发出相应的设备以提供必要的专业诊疗规划、临床治疗、患者支持服务和临床试验入组信息。综合性癌症中心通常附属于医疗学术机构并能提供完整的肿瘤治疗、临床试验、康复和社会服务以及基础和转化研究项目，以便将新知识从实验室转移到临床应用。目前，肿瘤外科医生在理解癌症患者序贯治疗方面所发挥的作用越来越大。

肿瘤外科学不仅仅是一门外科专业技术，更多的是一门认知科学。除了一小部分代表性手术如胰十二指肠切除术、保肢手术、腹膜后肉瘤手术、肢体隔离热灌注和复杂的肝切除术等，肿瘤外科医生进行的大部分外科手术与没有受过肿瘤学训练的外科医生进行的外科手术类似。区分这两种类型外科医生的依据不仅仅是如何做一个特定手术所需的知识，而更多的是对如何和何时做手术的理念，即对当代多模式癌症治疗的认知。对癌症的表现形式和复发形式的深入理解以及对推动肿瘤增殖和扩散的机制的认识是肿瘤外科医生特殊认知体系的重要组成部分。

随着癌症治疗在基因组学、蛋白质组学和代谢组学时代继续向前迈进，人们对研究人类肿瘤组织的需求不断增加。至少，肿瘤外科医生可以协助确保获取这些重要的组织，从而为癌症研究做出贡献。实际上，肿瘤外科医生可以做的不仅仅是被动地提供肿瘤组织。对实体肿瘤病理生理学的透彻理解，加上对手术室、病理科的解剖知识和工作流程的深入了解，使得肿瘤外科医生在组织、维护、优化和监督有效的组织获取和肿瘤入库中扮演着关键角色。因而，肿瘤外科医生已成为转化科学团队的重要成员。此外，肿瘤外科医生与病理医生、研究人员合作，将有机会为之提供有意义的临床信息，这些信息可用于标注归档的存储库组织并协助创建组织芯片。这些都是有价值的工具，其应用可从探索性的、产生假说的回顾性研究延伸到特定实验室发现的确认。

作为外科团体的一大分支，肿瘤外科医生是向普通外科和其他外科专业同事传播癌症信息的重要渠道。他们在大型外科会议上做学术报告、主导医院肿瘤委员会并为癌症患者提供咨询服务。由于肿瘤外科医生在癌症的初次诊断中发挥着主导作用，因此他们在癌症预防和筛查项目中也经常发挥领导作用。全国性的多模式临床试验小组也依赖于肿瘤外科专业知识来辅助进行试验设计、建立手术质量控制标准、就外科治疗标准(包括手术适应证)对培训试验参与者进行培训、确保研究级别肿瘤和自体正常组织的安全获取以用于相关研究,以及协助准确的收集、分析数据和展示试验结果。

多学科管理

实体肿瘤的多学科管理要求肿瘤外科医生在有关治疗方式排序的决策中发挥关键作用,例如直肠癌合并可切除的肝转移患者最终治疗可能包括肝切除、直肠切除、直肠放疗和全身化疗。一般情况下,这些治疗的顺序是先术前放化疗,然后是直肠切除(如腹会阴联合切除或低位前切除术),随后是肝脏切除,最后是辅助化疗——这是一种激进的方法,但能让一部分患者获得长期生存。然而,由于认识到这些患者死亡的最大风险来自全身复发,最近出现了一种趋势即从化疗开始而不是以化疗结束。这种方法还有另外一个优势,即对新辅助治疗的反应性可作为一项重要的预后评估指标。此外,肿瘤缩小可能会降低肝切除或直肠切除的难度。以前肝和肠的手术很少同时进行,但现在更常见的是同时进行,因为有数据显示这种方式对特定的患者是安全的。现在,更常见的情况是在这两种手术分别进行时通常先进行肝脏切除。这种方法基于这样的事实,虽然术前化疗很少对结肠或直肠手术有任何不良影响,但是已知化疗的累积会增加化疗引起肝脏病变的风险,从而导致肝脏手术并发症发生。采用短疗程辅助放疗如分 5 次,剂量 25Gy,术后 1 周进行而不是传统的 5 周放疗疗程,这种方法缩短了 3 种模式治疗所需的时间,也缩短了化疗的休息时间。选择多模式治疗顺序的基本原则也同样适用于其他大多数实体肿瘤,这是肿瘤外科医生不可或缺的知识。

儿童肿瘤医生率先使用联合治疗模式(放射疗法结合化疗和手术)来有效治疗儿童肿瘤。多模式治疗已实现了对儿童局限性视网膜母细胞瘤的有效控制。儿童 Wilms 瘤患者的治愈率为 75%,如果手术治疗后进行化疗,在某些情况下再进行放疗,则治愈率比单纯手术提高 40%。胚胎性横纹肌肉瘤对放疗、化疗和手术的联合治疗效果最好。直到最近,多模式治疗的有效性也只是偶尔在成人肿瘤中被证实,其中一个显著的例子是骨肉瘤和软组织肉瘤的治疗方法。外科手术是大多数四肢骨骼和软组织肉瘤的一种公认的局部治疗方法,但如果单独使用常常会导致治疗失败。在过去,即便是在切除了原发肿瘤的肢体之后仍有大约 50% 的软组织肉瘤患者和 80% 的骨肉瘤患者最终死于远处转移。因此,需要发展多模式的治疗方案以改善这些预后。术前经动脉阿霉素化疗再加放疗可导致多达 75% 的患者出现肿瘤细胞广泛坏死,这种有效的术前治疗使得局部切除肉瘤和尽可能保留功能性肢体成为现实。而且,此方案的局部复发率与截肢患者一样低,长期效果来看,在功能和心理上均优于截肢患者。此外,其总体生存率和无瘤生存率均没有下降。多模式综合治疗对包括结直肠癌在内的其他实体恶性肿瘤也有效。具体地说,临床试验已证实对Ⅱ期或Ⅲ期直肠癌使用新辅助放化疗可提高疗效和保肛率。多模式治疗还被证实可以提高结直肠癌肝转移的可切除率和长期生存率[5]。

与外科手术和放疗不同,全身治疗如化疗、免疫疗法和激素疗法可以杀灭已经转移到远处的肿瘤细胞。与那些有明显临床病变的患者相比,这些全身性疗法对肿瘤负荷较小(甚至亚临床)的患者有更大的治愈机会。因此,手术和放射治疗可能有助于减轻特定患者的肿瘤负荷,从而最大限度地发挥随后的全身治疗的作用。治疗的目标是治愈还是姑息取决于特定肿瘤的分期。如果癌症局限且没有扩散的证据,则很有可能根除癌症并获得治愈。当癌症扩散到无法治愈的程度时,我们的目标是改善症状以及尽可能长时间地提高活动能力和生活质量。如果患者出现远处转移或肿瘤附近重要结构广泛浸润的证据,通常认为是无法治愈的。然而,有些患者即便有远处转移,仍有治愈的可能。具体而言,孤立性肝或肺转移瘤患者通过切除治疗,抑或播散性生殖细胞或胃肠道间质瘤患者仅用全身治疗都仍可能获得治愈。在判断患者无法治愈之前应获得远处转移的组织学证据。偶尔,探查手术可能是必要的,目的是确定肺部或肝脏可疑病变的组织学类型。在极少数情况下,临床实际情况可能毫无疑问的指向远处转移,此时患者可能在没有病理活组织检查的情况下就确定是无法治愈的。对于各个解剖部位的肿瘤都有一定的局部标准来确定患者是否是无法治愈的,然而其他一些解剖因素可能仅提示预后不良,并非是判断不可治愈的绝对指标。在模棱两可时,众多的研究若不能证实转移或无法治愈的局部浸润,患者应因此获益并实施治愈性治疗。

治疗方式的选择不仅取决于癌症的类型和进展程度,还取决于患者的一般状况和是否有合并症存在,例如患有严重肺气肿或肝功能衰竭可能是手术禁忌;有糖尿病基础病的患者更容易出现糖皮质激素治疗的毒性反应;肾脏疾病可能增加一些化疗药物如顺铂或异环磷酰胺的毒性。扩大的分期手术可能表明肿瘤局限于原发部位和/或区域淋巴结,因此有可能通过局部治疗获得治愈。然而,大约 60% 的局部恶性肿瘤最终复发,这表明许多此类患者在初次诊断时就已出现亚临床的转移。如果全身治疗与局部治疗相结合,治愈的可能性可能会提高。化疗药物必须在肿瘤细胞数量低到足以被破坏及患者可耐受剂量时才能使用。治愈的机会很可能是在疾病的早期或手术后,因为这时肿瘤负荷已减至最低。辅助化疗显著改善了一些恶性肿瘤的手术效果,主要是因为其杀灭了手术区外临床检测不到的恶性细胞。新辅助化疗开始于局部和区域治疗之前,也可以减少远隔肿瘤的微转移,同时显著降低原发肿瘤的细胞数量。

传统意义上,手术切除在可切除实体恶性肿瘤的治疗顺序中一直处于第一位,但越来越多的证据表明,在治疗计划的后期尤其在肿瘤晚期,手术切除可能更有效。化疗和放疗都是遵循一级动力学原理发挥作用,但因肿瘤细胞具有异质性特征,可以预期在这些治疗后,残存肿瘤细胞的耐药性复制可能会在原发肿瘤中持续存在。这种耐药异质性更可能发生在化疗药灌注不良且相对缺氧的大肿瘤中,因此对放射疗法也不敏感。由于手术是遵循零级动力学原理进行的,它能有效地切除对其他治疗方式不敏感的局部残留的原发肿瘤细胞。

从实际应用的角度来看,在术前应用化疗可以提供关于治疗反应性的重要预后信息,有效的新辅助治疗有助于规划额外的术后辅助化疗。此外,早期的全身治疗还可以杀灭潜在的隐匿性微转移病灶。在某些情况下,术前治疗(或"转化"治疗)可用于将肿瘤从不可切除状态缩小到可切除状态(图 43-2)。

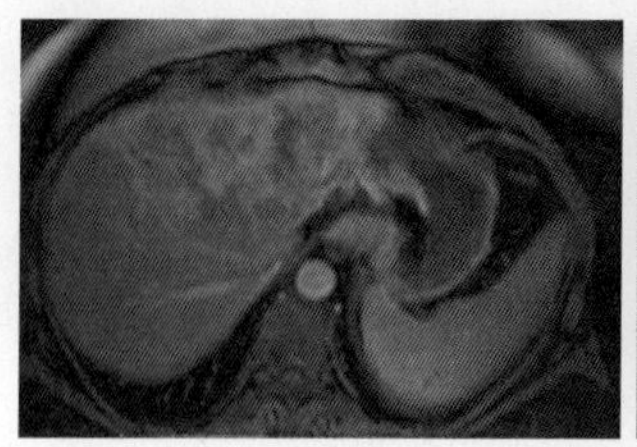
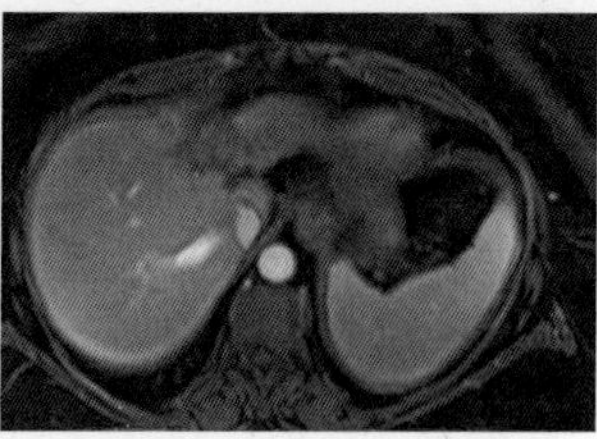

图 43-2 无法切除的肝内胆管癌(全部 3 条肝静脉受累)新辅助化疗药吉西他滨和顺铂实现降期

肿瘤外科治疗的组成成分

预防外科

随着对易癌基因突变作用的认识不断扩大,可以预见预防性手术将扩大到其中的一些患者。在这种情况下,肿瘤外科医生必须对遗传咨询的适应证、局限性和伦理问题有深入的认识,因为外科医生有责任提醒其他有风险的家庭成员并安排做相应的检测。新出现的预防性手术适应证不断增多,诸如溃疡性结肠炎伴发育异常、家族性腺瘤性息肉病、多发性内分泌肿瘤综合征和遗传性乳腺癌等,进一步强化了其在已经确定的恶性肿瘤的预防作用。评估预防性手术的风险-获益比是至关重要的,但往往是不准确的。未来更廉价和可靠的遗传筛选技术将会出现,加上来自分子流行病学新领域的见解不断成熟,我们对风险人群的预防性手术获益的认识会更加准确。

病理活检和诊断

实体瘤的诊断取决于对病灶的定位和活检。活检的结果将用于确定肿瘤的组织学分型和/或分级,这是制定最佳治疗的先决条件。若在治疗前未确认活检病理为恶性,就会造成明显的治疗错误。即使有来自其他医院的活检报告也必须在治疗前获取并重新检查之前的活检玻片。这是至关重要的,因为在最初病理诊断时往往会出现错误。

外科医生在许多实体肿瘤的初次诊断中发挥关键作用,包括决定是否以及如何对肿块进行病理活组织检查。在临床可疑乳房肿块合并异常乳房 X 线照片的病例中,作为一种限制手术数量、倡导多学科治疗和可能的新辅助治疗的策略,对肿块行针芯穿刺活检而并非切除活检通常是合适的。相反,对于合并慢性病毒性肝炎以及具有肝细胞癌特征性动脉增强肿块的患者,如果切除是最合适的治疗方式,则通常不建议进行针刺活检。对于可疑黑色素瘤的皮肤色素沉着病变,要选择正确的活检方式就需要了解正确的术中组织操作,以避免深部阳性切缘残留所造成的肿瘤厚度测量错误,并要认识到临床上仅有部分非典型痣行活检这一窘境。对此,完全切除活检在多数情况下是合适的。对于可疑软组织肉瘤的肿块,其活检策略包括周密的规划以获取足够的组织进行组织学研究、最大限度地减少组织平面的破坏和潜在的播种,以及设置穿刺活检针道位于辅助或新辅助放射治疗的区域内。对于引发胆总管梗阻的非常小的病变,其活检假阴性结果的可能性相对较高,而且越是可能治愈的病变,其体积就越小且越难获得真阳性的结果。所以,即使是没有活检阳性结果,通常也会在这种情况下实施外科切除。由于远处转移的诊断常常会改变整个治疗计划,外科医生通常会决定如何在创伤最小、敏感最高的转移部位实现组织学诊断。活检方式选择的基本原则是肿瘤外科医生必备的知识。

当肿瘤接近体表或累及可以用相应的可视仪器(如支气管镜、结肠镜或膀胱镜)检查的腔道时,活检是最容易的。乳腺癌、舌癌、直肠癌均可见或可触诊,其中一部分也可切除以明确诊断。相反,一些深部的病灶可能会生长到相当大才会引起症状,超声、计算机断层扫描(CT)和磁共振成像(MRI)都可用于在侵入性病理活检时定位这些病灶。尽管影像学引导的针刺活检对某些患者可能是适合的,但探查性手术偶尔也是必要的,以便获取明确的活检组织并确定组织学诊断。在某些情况下,可能需要比经皮穿刺活检更大的组织样本才能明确肿瘤性质,如淋巴瘤等,因此常需要手术活检。幸运的是,现在已经可以在门诊应用腹腔镜等微创技术常规实施这类手术了。

活检可疑病变常用 3 种方法:针刺活检(细针穿刺抽吸或针芯穿刺)、切取活检及切除活检。无论采取何种方法,只有获得具有代表性的肿瘤切片,才能建立正确的病理诊断。肿瘤外科医生必须意识到,在只有一小部分肿瘤组织提交病理检查的情况下,针刺活检和切取活检可能会出现假阴性。为诊断提供足够的组织是外科医生的责任,必要时肿瘤定位也是其责任之一。充足的组织可以为合格的病理医生提供诊断依据,而不充足的组织则不能,这是很显然的。

细针穿刺抽吸(fine needle aspiration,FNA)活检是一种用针和注射器从肿瘤中抽取细胞的细胞学技术。该技术可以在影像学引导下进行,特别适合相对难以接近的病变,例如深部的内脏肿瘤。由于吸入物是分散的细胞而不是完整的组织,恶性肿瘤的诊断通常依赖于检测细胞内的异常特征如核多形性等,因此与其他活检技术相比,FNA 假阴性率更高。此外,由于缺乏完整的肿瘤结构,FNA 无法鉴别侵袭性和非侵袭性恶性肿瘤,阴性结果并不能排除恶性肿瘤。因此,应根据不同的临床情况,例如鉴别原位癌和浸润性恶性肿瘤时,选择其他类型的活检方法可能更为合适。

针芯穿刺活检是最简单的组织学诊断方法(相对于细胞学诊断),可用于皮下和肌肉肿块以及一些内部脏器(如肝、肾和胰腺)的活组织检查。其他的优势是该方法便宜,并且对周围组织造成的干扰最小。切割针芯穿刺活检采用大口径针头进行,如 Vim Silverman 或 truo-cut 器械,该技术能获取一小块完整的肿瘤组织,这为病理医生研究癌细胞与周围微环境之间的浸润关系提供了条件。在针刺活检时,虽然肿瘤细胞针道种植的风险很小,但如果能准确定位针道以便在最后手术时整块切除,则完全可以避免这类风险。如果组织标本体积较小,则针刺活检可能不太合适,因其增加了穿刺失败或活检组织不能代表整个肿瘤的可能性。因此,对于恶性肿瘤阴性的针刺活检报告,如果与临床表现不一致,应持怀疑态度并再行切取或切除活检以确认。

切取病理活检包括切除一小部分肿瘤。切取活检最好在活检切口能被完全切除的情况下进行,因为在活检时若出现任何肿瘤细胞溢出,则可以实施确切的手术切除。对于较深的皮下或肌肉内的肿块,若最初的针刺活检不能确定诊断时就适合选择切开活检。当肿瘤太大以至于完整的局部切除会破坏广泛的组织平面,并将对随后根治性的广泛局部切除产生不良影响时，切取活检也是合适的。如果可能的话，切取活检应该尽量切除肿瘤的深部和正常组织的边缘。切取活检与针刺活检有同样的缺点，即切除的部分或许不能代表整个肿瘤，因此，活检阴性也不能排除残余肿块癌变的可能性。

切除活检即完整切除了目标肿块，适用于直径小于3cm的小且散在的肿块，因为在这种情况下，肿块的完整切除并不会影响后续更广泛的切除，而广泛切除可能是达到局部根治所必要的条件。切除活检使得病理医生能够检查整个病变，然而这种方法对大体积肿瘤是有禁忌的。这是因为活检过程可能会把肿瘤细胞散布到整个大的手术区域，导致必须实施再次根治性手术才能广泛且完整地切除这一区域。因此对于骨骼和软组织肿块，当怀疑肉瘤的诊断时，切除活检通常是禁忌的。切除活检也适用于结肠息肉样病变、甲状腺和乳腺结节、淋巴结、小的皮肤病变，以及病理医生无法通过切取活检明确诊断时。当病变的性质可疑、有切除的必要（无论诊断是什么）而且具有非毁伤性手术可行性时，也可直接通过手术切除未活检的肿块。这类手术的例子包括对FNA后诊断不明确的甲状腺结节行甲状腺次全切除术，以及对可能是炎症性或肿瘤性的盲肠肿块行右半结肠切除术，对于后一个例子，结肠镜活检只有在肿瘤呈阳性时才具有诊断价值。外科医生应该用缝合线或金属夹标记切除的活检组织边缘，以便在切除不完全且需要进一步切除时可以在原位准确地识别出阳性切缘。

活检切口的设计也非常重要。不合理的切口可能会不必要地切开额外的组织平面，从而造成随后的放疗区域或根治手术切除范围扩大，例如四肢的肿瘤最好取平行于肢体长轴的活检切口，这有利于对包含活检路径在内的组织实施确定性的整块切除（图43-3）。由于血肿可导致组织平面受到污染引发肿瘤细胞扩散，因此应在闭合活检切口时谨慎止血。如果在活检后立即进行最终的手术切除，则应丢弃器械、手套、长袍和窗帘，并用未使用的替代品替换。

活检时应仔细筛选淋巴结，若因术后感染而致区域淋巴结

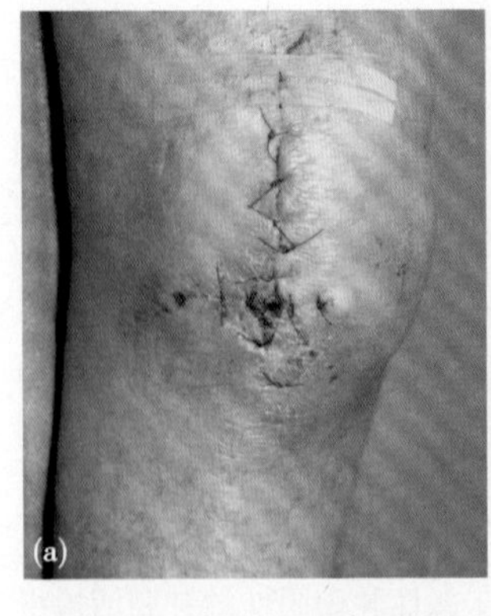

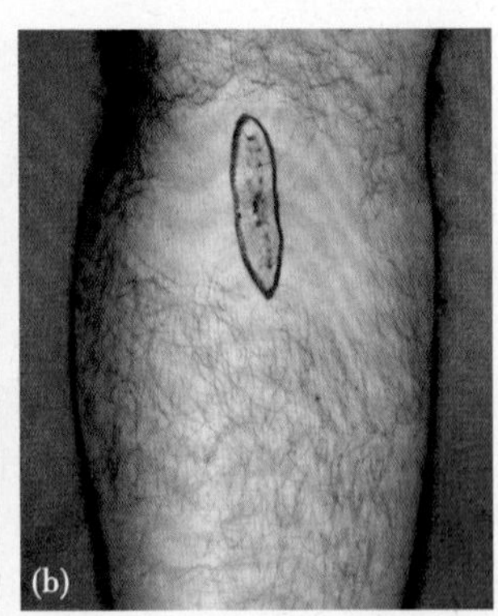

图43-3 合理和不合理的活检切口。（a）一位在髌腱上有十字形活检瘢痕的滑膜肉瘤患者。注意感染切口的红斑。设计不合理的活检瘢痕需要一个大范围的软组织和骨联合切除才能涵盖所有受侵犯的组织平面。不幸的是，肿瘤在活检时侵入了关节间隙，这位患者最终需要膝以上截肢来治疗这个本可以保全肢体的小肉瘤；（b）一个方向合理的下肢切开活检瘢痕。注意与肢体长轴平行的瘢痕对齐，并细密缝合小的活检创面。整个瘢痕都可以被手术切除（蓝色椭圆），同时最大程度保留了正常组织

反应性增大时，选择腋窝淋巴结活检可能要优于腹股沟淋巴结。其他一些注意事项也值得关注，例如保存在甲醛中的淋巴结标本不能用于细胞遗传学或流式细胞免疫表型分析，以及淋巴瘤的实验室检查通常需要未固定的无菌组织。在未使用鼻咽镜、食管镜和支气管镜仔细检查原发肿瘤之前，不应对颈部淋巴结进行活检，因为颈上增大的淋巴结通常是由喉部、口咽或鼻咽部的原发性肿瘤转移而来。与此不同，锁骨上增大的淋巴结更常是由原发性胸、腹腔或乳腺肿瘤转移而来。

可以通过冰冻或石蜡切片来制备用于病理检查的肿瘤标本。若活检时取冰冻切片，一般在10分钟内即可获得病理诊断。冰冻切片常应用在大手术中评估其可切除性或术中检查肿瘤切缘。若被活检冰冻切片证实为恶性，则可能是放弃根治性手术而采用姑息治疗的指征。有时需要行纵隔镜、腹腔镜、胸腔镜、开胸探查，甚至开腹探查来获取足够的代表性的组织标本进行显微镜检查，以明确诊断或肿瘤分期。

肿瘤分期

肿瘤分期是用于描述个体特定肿瘤恶性进展的解剖学范围的系统。分期系统汇集了原发肿瘤的相关预后因素，例如大小、分级和部位等，以及向区域部位（例如淋巴结或远处转移部位）播散的信息。准确地肿瘤分期对于规划合适的治疗方案和判断预后都至关重要。如果没有准确的分期，就不能有效地比较不同研究中心的治疗结果，新的治疗方法只有通过对比当前同期肿瘤的治疗效果才能实现恰当的评估。

肿瘤分期的重要性已得到公认，因此国际上和各国都试图把肿瘤患者的分期进行标准化。但到目前为止，还没有一个单一的系统被普遍接受。美国癌症联合委员会（AJCC）推荐了一个从Ⅰ期（局部小恶性肿瘤）到Ⅳ期（远处转移扩散）的分期系统[6]。AJCC和国际抗癌联盟（Union Internationale Contre Cancer，UICC）都采用了一种共享的TNM系统，其根据原发肿瘤（T）、有无淋巴结转移（N）以及有无远处转移（M）来定义癌症。随着T后数字的逐渐升高，如T_1、T_2、T_3或T_4，表明病变的大小或穿透深度逐渐增加，这通常与预后较差密切相关。无淋巴结转移者被定义为N_0，有淋巴结转移者为N_1，若淋巴结受累范围更广可采用附加数字。最后，远处转移是通过在M后面加上数字1表示转移，或者数字0表示未转移。因此，一个既没有扩散到区域淋巴结，也没有转移到远处部位的小病灶将被定义为$T_1N_0M_0$，一个累及区域淋巴结但没有远处转移的较大病灶可被定义为$T_2N_1M_0$，一个既累及区域淋巴结又有远处转移的大病灶将被定义为$T_3N_1M_1$。对于某些肿瘤类型，例如软组织肉瘤，增加了G用于恶性程度分级，高级别肿瘤的分化程度较低，并且更易发生转移。

TNM系统有4种按时间顺序的分类方法：临床分类（cTNM或TNM）代表首次明确治疗前疾病进展的程度，它是由体格检查、影像学检查、内镜检查、活检、手术探查和其他任何相关的发现来确定的；病理分类（pTNM）包含了手术时或从完全切除的标本病理检查中获得的附加信息，这一分类对计划辅助治疗是尤其有用的；也可以添加y前缀来表示初始全身或放疗后的病理分期（ypTNM）；再治疗分类（rTNM）用于分期在无瘤生存期后复发的肿瘤，包括临床和/或病理的复发证据；最后，尸检分类（aTNM）是基于死后的尸体检查。

肿瘤的扩散模式

一般来说，恶性肿瘤有 4 种扩散模式：①直接向周围组织扩散；②通过淋巴管扩散；③通过血行扩散；④通过浆膜腔种植扩散。然而，许多癌症通过上述一种以上的途径传播，并且转移过程的顺序仍不可预知，例如乳腺癌或黑色素瘤患者可能在肺、肝或骨骼中出现远处转移而并无淋巴结转移的迹象。表 43-2 总结了人类不同肿瘤的扩散模式。

表 43-2　人类常见恶性肿瘤的扩散模式

肿瘤	血行扩散	淋巴转移	局部浸润（局部复发）
腺癌			
乳腺	++++	+++	++
子宫内膜	+	++	+
卵巢	++	+++	++++
胃	++++	++++	+++
胰腺	++++	++++	+++
结肠	+++	+++	+
肾	++	++	++
前列腺	+++	+++	+++
肝脏	+	+	++++
表皮细胞癌			
肺	++++	+++	++
口咽	++	+++	+++
喉	+	+++	++
子宫颈	+	++++	+++
移行细胞癌			
膀胱	++	+++	++++
皮肤肿瘤			
鳞状细胞癌	+	++	+
黑色素瘤	+++	+++	++
基底细胞癌	0	0	+
肉瘤			
骨	++++	+	+
软组织	++++	+	+++
脑肿瘤	0	0	++++

注：未发生；0，<1%；+，1%～<5%；++，5%～<15%；+++，15%～<30%；++++，30%～50%。

癌细胞也可以通过组织间隙和组织平面直接浸润扩散。有些肿瘤如软组织肉瘤和胃或食管的腺癌可沿着可触及肿块的组织平面向外浸润相当长的一段距离（10～15cm）。其他一些肿瘤如皮肤基底细胞癌则很少能向肿瘤边缘外浸润超过几毫米。尽管大多数中枢神经系统（central nervous system，CNS）肿瘤很少发生转移，但它们可能会穿透附近的脑组织，而且某些部位的 CNS 肿瘤可能通过干扰 CNS 的重要功能而导致死亡。

肿瘤细胞可轻易进入淋巴管并通过这些管道向局部淋巴结渗透或形成栓塞。渗透是一群肿瘤细胞沿着淋巴管生长的过程，这一过程通常发生在乳腺癌的皮肤淋巴管和前列腺癌的神经周围淋巴管中。淋巴浸润在所有类型的上皮恶性肿瘤中都很常见，但皮肤基底细胞癌（<0.1%的病例转移到局部淋巴结）和间叶瘤（如肉瘤，仅 2%～5%的病例转移到淋巴结）除外。

肿瘤细胞可沿淋巴管扩展至局部或远处的淋巴结，这具有重要的临床意义。肿瘤细胞可在局部淋巴管内移动并能通过侧支淋巴管道扩散至附近的淋巴结。淋巴结转移开始局限于包膜下间隙，在这个阶段淋巴结并未增大，可能看起来与正常无异。随后肿瘤细胞逐渐向淋巴窦浸润，逐步取代淋巴结实质并改变其形态和结构。淋巴结之间很少有直接浸润扩散，因为淋巴结的包膜直到肿瘤晚期才能被穿透。然而，当受累的淋巴结直径超过 3cm 时，肿瘤通常会浸润到包膜外，进入周围的脂肪组织。

淋巴液自腹内脏器和下肢引流入乳糜池，然后进入胸导管，最后进入左颈内静脉，通过这条路径，肿瘤细胞可以从淋巴系统自由地进入血液系统。肿瘤学者最初认为，实体肿瘤是首先累及局部淋巴结，然后通过胸腔导管进入血液，最后经血液播散到身体的其他部位。目前，大多数肿瘤学家支持的另一种解释是区域淋巴结中癌细胞的存在表明宿主-肿瘤关系是不和谐的，同时这也造成远处转移的风险很高。

癌细胞可以通过胸导管或直接侵犯血管进入血液。毛细血管并不能抵御肿瘤细胞的侵袭，小静脉也经常受侵犯，但厚壁动脉却很少被累及。静脉壁内经常会形成一条延伸至内皮下区域的神经丛，这为肿瘤通过薄静脉壁提供了一个入口。当血管内皮受破坏时就会形成血栓并很快被肿瘤侵入，这种血栓和肿瘤的结合可能会分离形成大的肿瘤栓子。血管侵犯在癌和肉瘤中都很常见，并且预后不良。某些类型的肿瘤有明显的沿静脉成柱状生长的趋势，例如肾细胞癌可以侵入到肾静脉并可沿下腔静脉延伸至右心房。在这种情况下，若进行工程浩大的体外循环下的整块移除，仍有可能会获得长期生存甚至治愈。

肿瘤细胞偶尔会透过器官壁侵入浆膜腔，许多肿瘤细胞可以在无基质的悬浮液中生长并在腹膜腔内广泛传播或附着于浆膜表面。因此，广泛的腹膜种植在胃肠道和卵巢癌中很常见。与之类似，恶性神经胶质瘤也可通过脑脊液在 CNS 内广泛传播。

虽然我们对肿瘤的传播途径已经有了很多了解，但这一过程背后的机制仍知之甚少。有些癌症在临床发现时就已发生转移，而另一些类型相同、位于同一组织器官的癌症却可能会停留局部数年。尽管原发肿瘤可能是隐匿且无症状的，甚至是无法检测到的，但转移灶的临床表现却可能是十分明显的，例如来自支气管或乳腺隐匿癌的脑转移通常会被误认为是原发性的良性 CNS 肿瘤。

术前准备

外科治疗前肿瘤患者的准备是十分重要的，目的是减少围术期并发症、加速健康状态恢复到疾病前，以及避免可能的术后辅助治疗延迟。在实施外科大手术之前应尽一切努力纠正营养不良、恢复缺失的血容量、纠正电解质失衡。极度营养不良的患者准备大手术时可使用全胃肠外营养（total parenteral nutrition，TPN），尽管纠正过程缓慢，但 TPN 可以通过恢复正氮平衡来阻止营养状况进一步恶化。如果不提前纠正严重的生理、生化缺陷，可以预见癌症大型手术后的并发症率和死亡率可能会很高。

择期手术内在风险的评估是复杂且不准确的，因为其影响因素众多。患者的身体状况包括心肺储备、合并症、某些手术固有的功能失调、肝肾功能、手术的目的（根治性/姑息性）都与此评估相关。手术的技术复杂性、麻醉的方式以及相关医护人员的经验都会对手术的并发症产生影响。对此有不同的风险评估模式，如美国麻醉医师学会的五级体质状况分类（表43-3）和东部肿瘤协作组的五步体力状态评分（表43-4），都可能有助于评估某些患者对择期手术的耐受性。

表43-3 美国麻醉医师学会：体质状况分级

等级	描述
P-1	正常健康人
P-2	有轻微系统性疾病
P-3	有严重系统性疾病
P-4	有严重系统性疾病，并持续威胁生命
P-5	不手术难以存活的濒死患者
P-6	确证为脑死亡，其器官拟用于器官移植手术

来源：Saklad 1941[7]，经 *Wolters Kluwer* 许可转载。

表43-4 东部肿瘤协作组：体力状况分级及相应的 Karnofsky 评分

等级	描述
0	完全正常，能够无限制地进行所有患病前活动（Karnofsky 100）
1	体力活动受限，但可以走动并能从事较轻或久坐性质的工作，例如轻家务/办公室工作（Karnofsky 80~90）
2	能走动，能自理，但不能从事任何工作活动，日间不少于50%时间可以起床活动（Karnofsky 60~70）
3	生活仅能部分自理，日间50%或以上时间卧床或坐轮椅。
4	完全不能活动，不能自理，完全被限制在床上或轮椅上（Karnofsky 30 或以下）

来源：改编自 Etzioni 2003[15]，经 *Springer* 许可转载。

美国外科医师学会外科手术风险评估系统（www.riskcalculator.facs.org）可用于术前评估相关风险。该评估系统纳入了21项患者特征，这些特征可以在线输入并用于预测九种可能与手术相关的结果，包括死亡、任何并发症、严重并发症和手术部位感染等。该计算器是基于2009年至2012年参与美国外科医师协会/国家外科质量改进项目（ACS/NSQIP）的393家医院里的140多万例手术数据开发而成[8]。

手术死亡率是指手术后30天内发生的死亡率。在癌症患者中，潜在的疾病是手术死亡率的主要决定性因素。虽然与其他成年人相比，众多手术在老年患者中的并发症发生率更高，但高龄本身不应成为患者获得潜在治愈性手术机会的禁忌。由于高龄患者的手术本身就是高风险的，因此要判断姑息性手术的指征是相当困难的，例如对于癌症引起的广泛转移性病变或症状性肠梗阻，姑息性手术的围手术期死亡率可达20%~30%，在这种情况下，风险-获益比和最终手术目标必须尽可能明确并且被患者、家属和外科医生所接受。

癌症手术患者术前应用化疗和/或放疗的频率越来越高。在部分病例中，这些治疗可能与围术期并发症的增加有关，例如在术前几周内使用抗血管内皮生长因子抗体贝伐单抗可能会增加切口愈合相关并发症的风险[9]，由于这种靶向治疗的半衰期有21天，因此建议在择期手术前至少6~8周停用贝伐单抗。

术中注意事项

一旦决定进行手术治疗就必须为特定的外科患者仔细规划手术方式。必须认识到，最好的（通常也是唯一的）治愈机会在于首次切除，因为当组织平面、淋巴管和血管潜在暴露于肿瘤细胞时，肿瘤细胞就可能会在手术区域内移位，而且随后的复发可能很难与正常的术后炎症反应和瘢痕相鉴别。

"非接触技术"的原则是肿瘤外科必须坚持的，这一观点是基于切除过程中直接接触和处理肿瘤会增加肿瘤细胞局部种植和栓塞的风险。尽管较少的临床证据支持这一原则，但对于直接侵犯到血管的肿瘤如侵犯到大静脉或腔静脉的肝细胞癌或肾肿瘤，这一原则可能有一定的有效性。虽然没有确证证实违反该原则是有害的，但是避免粗暴处理肿瘤以及术中小心避免肿瘤破裂的一般原则是十分合理的。同样的，每一次切除肿瘤的尝试都应该非常注重细节，同时要避免过多的失血或过长的手术时间。尽管相邻的多脏器切除其本质上可能导致手术时间延长和失血增多，但对此类复杂手术如肝大部分切除术、胰腺切除术和腹膜后肿瘤切除等的熟练程度和经验可能会降低手术并发症发生率并增加其肿瘤学获益。

肿瘤手术的分类

对于低级别肿瘤，确保瘤周正常组织有足够边缘的局部切除可能就是合适的治疗手段，因为这类肿瘤很少转移到区域淋巴结或广泛浸润邻近组织，基底细胞癌和腮腺混合性肿瘤就属于这一类。相反，通过浸润邻近组织而广泛传播的肿瘤如软组织肉瘤、食管癌和胃癌，则必须切除更大范围的正常组织。在切缘和肿瘤之间的这一较宽的组织边界也可作为一种保护屏障，防止术中肿瘤细胞穿透过离断的淋巴管和血管。若之前曾单独行切开活检，则切口可能已有肿瘤细胞种植，为了要囊括可能受侵犯的组织，超出原始切口范围的广泛皮肤、皮下肌肉、脂肪和筋膜的切除是非常必要的。

恶性肿瘤通常没有真正的包膜却常有假包膜包绕，假包膜是由正常的组织和散在其中的肿瘤细胞压缩形成的。这种假包膜的存在看似可能很容易被原位剜除，适合单纯的肿瘤摘除术，然而这种方式必须予以避免，因为单纯摘除术将会遗留穿透过假包膜的微侵犯，注定会导致患者局部复发。理想状况下，外科医生应始终在正常组织中操作，在切除肿瘤的过程中不要碰到或甚至直接看到肿瘤，切除过程应谨小慎微以免肿瘤细胞溢出。因许多肿瘤是通过淋巴转移，手术的目的就是将原发肿瘤和相应引流区的淋巴结连同所有相关的组织一并切除，这种手术方式适用于引流肿瘤的淋巴结位于肿瘤床附近或者仅有一条淋巴引流通道且其可以在不牺牲重要结构的情况下被切除时。此外，应尽量避免切断所累及的淋巴管道以降低局部复发的风险。

目前，人们普遍认为整块的区域淋巴结清扫适用于临床证实淋巴结受累的转移瘤。然而，在许多情况下肿瘤已经扩散超过区域淋巴结。虽然在这种情况下手术切除的治愈率可能很低(20%～50%)，但过度的悲观情绪不应该成为这类患者接受适当手术治疗的阻碍。整块切除受累的淋巴结可能提供唯一的治愈机会或至少可以提供有效的局部姑息性控制。因此，不应将局部淋巴结受累视为手术禁忌，而应将其视为辅助治疗如放疗或化疗的可能适应证。

对于大多数类型的癌症，建议常规地切除靠近原发恶性肿瘤的区域淋巴结，即使是肿瘤并未临床累及这些结构。这一建议是基于多个淋巴结出现镜下微侵犯时手术切除后的局部复发率很高，以及仅用触诊评估可能的淋巴结受累有很高的错误率。在临床淋巴结阴性的癌和黑色素瘤中，有 20%～40%可以检测到其区域淋巴结有肿瘤微转移。

淋巴结清扫的范围仍然存在争议。前哨淋巴结切除术现在已是一种成熟的技术，用于在特定肿瘤类型中发现早期的淋巴结病变。这种方法首先由 Morton 等[10]引入用于黑色素瘤，现在也被应用于乳腺癌[11]和其他一些肿瘤[12]的治疗。最初，该技术是依靠在肿瘤部位注射蓝色的生物染料，再肉眼追踪这种染料沿淋巴管流向淋巴结。然而，现在已经实现向染料中添加放射性标记的同位素并使用手持式伽马探测仪监测淋巴引流路径以定位前哨淋巴结。前哨淋巴结切除术是一种低并发症的手术，它可以准确地实现局部淋巴结的分期，并识别出 60%～80%不需要根治性淋巴结清扫的黑色素瘤和乳腺癌患者。

手术技术、麻醉和支持治疗(输血、抗生素、液体和电解质治疗)的进步，使得更彻底、更广泛和时间更长的手术操作能够更加安全的实施。如果没有远处转移的证据，这类手术提供了一个其他方法所无法实现的治愈可能，并且这已在无远处转移证据的一些特定肿瘤中得到证实，例如一些生长缓慢、可能达到巨大体积且局部浸润广泛但无远处转移的原发肿瘤。对于一些分布广泛且几乎无法手术的肿瘤应考虑扩大根治性手术，因为偶尔也有患者被治愈。然而，这类手术应该仅限经验丰富的外科医生进行，因为只有他们能够选择那些最有可能获益的患者。盆腔脏器切除术就是一个精心设计的根治性手术的例子，它能够治愈经放射治疗的复发性宫颈癌和某些分化良好的局部进展直肠腺癌患者。该手术切除了骨盆内的所有脏器(膀胱、子宫和直肠)和软组织，然后通过结肠造口来恢复肠功能，再通过输尿管-肠段(回肠或乙状结肠)吻合来建立尿道引流。采用盆腔脏器切除术治疗的 5 年无复发生存率为 25%。在实施大范围切除术(如半侧骨盆切除术、上肢截肢术、头颈部癌切除手术或全骨盆脏器切除术)之前，肿瘤外科医生也有责任促成患者术后情绪和心理的康复。

虽然从理论上讲，肿瘤一旦转移到远处就不能再通过手术切除治愈，但经验证明并非如此，有时切除肝脏、肺部或其他部位内的转移性病灶也可获得长期生存。另外，通常对具有良好生物学特性和全身化疗反应的肿瘤实施转移瘤切除术较单独的化疗可以显著延长生存时间，并将此类晚期疾病转化为慢性病也并不罕见。在实施这类手术前应完善大量的检查以排除拟手术区域外的其他身体部位的扩散转移。

一些仅有肝转移的患者实施手术切除仍可能受益，尤其是结直肠肿瘤来源时。术前评估、手术技术和全身治疗方面的不断进步均促成对此类患者采取越来越积极的治疗方法。虽然过去肝转移可切除性判断是由其数量、大小和分布决定的，但最近则是由能否实现全部切除并切缘阴性(R_0)以及保留足够的功能性肝体积决定而非肿瘤数量。即便是对合并局限、可切除的肝外肿瘤及肝转移瘤的晚期患者，只要所有病灶都能实现安全切除，也可能会通过外科治疗获益。此外，当最初不具备手术切除指征时，可通过以下方法处理：①通过术前化疗缩小肿瘤；②通过术前门静脉栓塞或分期肝切除扩大残余肝脏体积；③应用热消融方法联合切除。上述方法均可增加适合行肝转移瘤手术切除的患者数量。随着越来越激进的方法不断应用，目前的研究报道这类肿瘤完全切除后的 5 年生存率已超过 50%[13]。

外科手术有时只用于缓解症状而非治愈肿瘤，从而延长患者舒适而有意义的生命。姑息性手术可能有助于缓解疼痛、出血、梗阻或感染，当然手术应该在对患者无不良风险的前提下进行。当没有更好的非手术的姑息治疗能改善生活质量时，即便不能延长生存期姑息性手术也是适用的。相反，不能改善生存质量的手术对患者无益。有姑息性手术指征的实例包括：①结肠造口、肠-肠吻合或胃-空肠吻合术以缓解肠梗阻；②脊髓切断或腹腔神经阻滞术以控制疼痛；③肝管-空肠吻合术以缓解胆道梗阻和瘙痒；④截肢术治疗四肢肿瘤的顽固性疼痛；⑤单纯乳房切除术治疗合并肿瘤感染、巨大溃疡且局部可切除的乳腺癌(即使存在远处转移)；⑥梗阻性结肠癌切除术，即使存在播散转移。减瘤手术是姑息性手术的一种特殊应用。在一些患者中，分布广但孤立的局部播散的恶性肿瘤不能实现所有病灶的全部切除，此时应用减瘤术可能是有效的，这类肿瘤包括生物惰性肿瘤或那些产生局部/激素症状的转移性神经内分泌肿瘤。肿瘤导致的出血、内脏穿孔、脓肿形成或空腔脏器梗阻(如胃肠道、重要血管或呼吸道)有时需要急诊外科手术干预。急诊手术也适用于侵入 CNS 或在颅内密闭空间施加压力而破坏关键神经元的肿瘤减压。正在接受急诊手术评估的癌症患者可能由于近期的骨髓抑制而出现中性粒细胞或血小板减少。有时，在预期过了最近一次化疗的骨髓抑制低谷期后再对这类患者实施手术可以避免可能的不良后果。由于急诊手术相关的风险很高，必须让每位患者及其家属充分了解拟行手术的风险和获益，如果患者能在该急诊手术中活下来，还要让他们了解其他可用的有效治疗方法。

肿瘤切除后的重建手术显著改善了许多癌症患者的生活质量。微血管吻合技术的常规应用使得含有皮肤、肌肉和/或骨骼的复合移植物能够自由移植到手术所造成的身体缺陷部位。乳房切除后的乳房重建、作为肢体肉瘤或下颌骨切除重建手术一部分的组织移植，以及使用游离空肠移植进行的呼吸、消化道重建等，这些都是复杂的癌症问题在联合手术治疗方面取得显著进展的例子。在未来，组织工程这门新兴学科的应用将极大地拓展组织重建的应用领域。将来组织工程学有可能定制培养出神经、脂肪、肌肉、骨软骨或其他身体组成部分，用于替代癌症综合治疗中需要切除的组织[14]。

肿瘤/肿瘤外科质量控制

对个人和机构数据持续不断的评估提供了改进质量体系的机会,这一体系可以促成更安全的手术实施,以及对改善肿瘤预后的新标记物或疗法的识别。肿瘤科特别是肿瘤外科医生已经准备建立相应的数据库用于明确癌症发展的始动因素、手术并发症的预测因子、肿瘤预后的标志物和治疗计划的可能变动。通过跨机构联合这些综合的数据集用于深入研究罕见的肿瘤和/或治疗手段。各机构联合创建的肿瘤标记库将成为非常强大的研究工具,除了可用于改进治疗流程之外还可以用来识别潜在的药物靶点。美国外科医师学会肿瘤专业委员会成立了一个超过 1 500 个相关研究机构参与的论坛,目的是监督肿瘤治疗的质量。通过这种准入机制,要求各机构必须拥有顶尖的临床肿瘤服务、肿瘤委员会领导力、制定治疗计划和提供教育培训的肿瘤讨论会、质量改进计划(部分是通过遵守公认的治疗指南,例如 NCCN 指南),以及一个综合的肿瘤登记处,以保证肿瘤治疗的质量。肿瘤外科医生应该为此做出表率。

肿瘤外科的未来

预计在未来 10 年内,癌症将取代心血管疾病成为美国人的第一大死因。人口老龄化将导致对肿瘤手术的需求暴增,到 2020 年,接受肿瘤手术的患者数量预计将增加 24%~51%(表 43-5)[15]。如果实施这些手术的外科医生一旦出现短缺,其结果将不可避免地降低肿瘤患者获得治疗的机会。为了防止这种情况发生,需要严格评估和改进外科医生应对工作负担增加的能力。鉴于美国每年培养的肿瘤外科医生不超过 50 名,显然传统的肿瘤外科学教育在学术医疗中心和大型的医疗保健社区中的作用将继续发挥下去,而且其可能面临的扩张压力也越来越大。

表 43-5 预计肿瘤手术量:2010—2020 年

手术	2000 年[a]	2010 年[b]	2020 年[b]	增加(2000—2020 年)
乳腺(诊断)	364 800	416 100(14.1%)	464 100(27.2%)	99 300
乳腺(切除)	392 700	440 200(12.1%)	485 600(23.7%)	92 900
门诊总量	757 500	856 300(13.0%)	949 700(25.4%)	192 200
乳腺(乳房切除)	90 400	106 000(17.3%)	123 700(36.8%)	33 300
结肠切除	96 300	113 700(18.1%)	141 100(46.5%)	44 800
直肠切除	27 800	33 300(19.7%)	40 900(47.0%)	13 100
胃切除	9 400	11 100(17.6%)	13 700(45.1%)	4 300
胰腺切除	3 900	4 700(19.7%)	5 800(47.4%)	1 900
食管切除	1 400	1 700(24.0%)	2 100(51.2%)	700
住院总量	229 200	270 500(18.0%)	327 100(42.7%)	97 900

[a] 列出的住院患者手术量是 2000 年实施的手术总量,基于 2000 年的全国住院患者抽样数据(NIS);列出的门诊手术量(乳腺诊断和乳腺切除术)是基于 1996 年全国门诊手术调查数据(NSAS)。
[b] 列出的 2010 年和 2020 年的数字均为预测;列出的百分比显示为相对于 2000 年的增长率。
来源:改编自 Etzioni 2003[15],经 *Springer* 许可转载。

随着多学科模式治疗的复杂性日益增加,放化疗在新辅助治疗的地位更加凸显,肿瘤外科医生将不得不越来越多地参与到临床试验设计中。要想在这个领域有所作为,就必须要掌握特定恶性肿瘤的自然病史,这便需要拓展突变基因及其同源蛋白相关的知识体系,因为这些突变基因及其同源蛋白可驱动实体肿瘤增殖和转移。无论是在接受培训还是在投入毕生的自我学习期间,肿瘤外科医生都必须对这些知识有更多的了解。

自 2014 年开始,医学界已设立肿瘤外科学委员会的认证,这是增强肿瘤外科学地位的一项重要举措。在过去的半个世纪,外科专业经历了前所未有的变革,如今已成为一门独立的学科,拥有专业知识、技术、解剖学挑战和重点关注的疾病。肿瘤外科学亦尤如此,它融合了技术和认知,具备强大的吸引力。逐渐出现了一种新的认识,即肿瘤外科医生具有普通外科训练无法获得的专业知识:恶性疾病自然病史知识、癌症多学科治疗知识,当然还包括如何实施一些罕见且技术要求高的肿瘤手术的知识。这些因素再加上对快速增长的人力需求的认识,促成了一个肿瘤外科学专业委员会认证机构的建立。认证委员会命名为"综合普通外科肿瘤学委员会",认证过程包括笔试和口试两部分。有资格参加这些考试的仅限于美国研究生医学教育委员会(American Council of Graduate medical Education, ACGME)认可的肿瘤外科学奖学金项目的毕业生,这意味着此类奖学金项目的毕业生若不能获得 ACGME 认可,在其毕业时将没有资格参加综合普通外科肿瘤学委员会的认证。这一规定有效地限制了该委员会年度合格候选人的总数,使得在过去几年中全美的奖学金申请人数量增长了一倍。该委员会的认证将提升并增强肿瘤外科医生的地位和影响,亦可有助于其他国家类似认证机构的发展,从而提升全球癌症诊疗水平。

(顾宗廷 译,王成锋 审校)

参考文献

1 Birkmeyer JD, Warshaw AL, Finlayson SR, et al. Relationship between hospital volume and late survival after pancreaticoduodenectomy. *Surgery*. 1999;**126**:178–183.

2 Breasted JH. *The Edwin Smith Surgical Papyrus*. Chicago: University of Chicago Press; 1930.

3 Hill GJ II., Historic milestones in cancer surgery. *Semin Oncol*. 1979;**6**:409–427.

4 Antman KA, Eilber FR, Shiu MH. Soft tissue sarcomas: current trends in diagnosis and management. *Curr Prob Cancer*. 1989;**13**:339–367.

5 Choti MA, Sitzmann JV, Tiburi MF, et al. Trends in long-term survival following liver resection for hepatic colorectal metastases. *Ann Surg*. 2002;**235**:759–766.

6 Edge SB, Byrd DR, Compton CC, et al. (eds). *American Joint Committee on Cancer (AJCC) Cancer Staging Manual*, 7th ed. New York: Springer-Verlag; 2010.

7 Saklad M. Grading of patients for surgical procedures. *Anesthesiology*. 1941;**2**:281.

8 Bilimoria KY, Liu Y, Paruch JL, et al. Development and evaluation of the universal ACS NSQIP surgical risk calculator: a decision aid and informed consent tool for patients and surgeons. *J Am Chem Soc*. 2012;**217**:833–842.

9 Scappaticci FA, Fehrenbacher L, Cartwright T, et al. Surgical wound healing complications in metastatic colorectal cancer patients treated with bevacizumab. *J Surg Oncol*. 2005;**91**:173–180.

10 Morton DL, Wen D-R, Wong JH, et al. Technical details of intraoperative lymphatic mapping for melanoma. *Arch Surg*. 1992;**127**:392–399.

11 Giuliano AE, Kirgan DM, Guenther JM, Morton DL. Lymphatic mapping and sentinel lymphadenectomy for breast cancer. *Ann Surg*. 1994;**220**:391–398.

12 Koch WM, Choti MA, Civelek AC, Eisele DW, Saunders JR. Gamma probe-directed biopsy of the sentinel node in oral squamous cell carcinoma. *Arch Otolaryngol Head Neck Surg*. 1998;**124**:455–459.

13 Pawlik TM, Scoggins CR, Zorzi D, et al. Effect of surgical margin status on survival and site of recurrence after hepatic resection for colorectal metastases. *Ann Surg*. 2005;**241**:715–722.

14 Patrick CW Jr, Mikos AG, McIntire LV. *Frontiers in Tissue Engineering*. New York: Pergamon Press; 1998.

15 Etzioni DA, Liu JH, Maggard MA, O'Connell JB, Ko CY. Workload projections for surgical oncology: will we need more surgeons? *Ann Surg Oncol*. 2003;**10**:1112–1117.

第 44 章　肿瘤放射治疗学原则

Philip P. Connell, MD ■ Ralph R. Weichselbaum, MD

概述

近十余年来，科技的重大进步和发展促进了肿瘤放射治疗技术的突破和创新。同时，在辐射如何作用于人体组织和细胞的基础生物学方面，我们也有了快速而深入的了解。这里我们总结了有关肿瘤治疗的一些开创性的关键进展。本章生物学内容主要涉及电离辐射对细胞 DNA 损伤的分子反应，包括 DNA 损伤修复、细胞周期阻滞和死亡、细胞信号传导以及原始肿瘤细胞（肿瘤干细胞）对治疗结果的影响。当辐射在肿瘤中产生炎性微环境时，调节免疫功能的药物也提供了潜在的治疗机会。有关准确预测细胞对辐射内在敏感性的较前沿的生物学技术，以及能够调节这种辐射敏感性的药物，本章也进行了详细介绍。最后，本章回顾了提高临床放射治疗准确性和实用性的主要基础物理技术的创新。尽管取得了这些进展，尚有一些挑战悬而未决从而限制了放射治疗的发展，如何克服这些剩余的问题将成为这一领域未来创新的热点。

引言

自 1895 年人类发现 X 射线，以及开展其对组织影响的研究之后不久，就开展了肿瘤放射治疗这一医学领域的应用[1]。第一种放疗设备就是使用低能阴极射线管或镭填充的玻璃管对邻近肿瘤进行单次大野照射。1920 年至 1950 年间，技术发展改善了光束输出和可传输的能量水平。这一进步非常重要，因为早期使用的低能量（200~500kV）X 射线对组织的渗透性较差，导致皮肤灼伤。20 世纪 50 年代，钴 60 设备和直线加速器的发展，可以传递“超电压”辐射能量（≥1MeV），是一个重大进展，因为这些高能量的光子可以更深入地渗透到组织中。另一个重要进展是使用分割治疗，即将大剂量治疗分为多个小剂量。这使得正常组织对辐射的耐受性更好。在随后的几十年中，在治疗传送技术、成像和肿瘤生物学方面的进一步改进，使肿瘤放射治疗学更接近理想目标——最大化肿瘤局部控制的同时，最小化正常组织的毒性。

肿瘤放射治疗学的一般原则

肿瘤在局部生长，并通过淋巴或血液途径全身播散。因此，成功的治疗通常需要针对所有受累部位进行治疗。肿瘤治疗的 3 种主要方式（手术、放射治疗和化疗）可以单独使用，也可以联合应用。手术和放射治疗通常用以治疗局部区域的肿瘤。手术既可以是治疗性的，也可以是诊断性的，因为肿瘤切除为组织病理检测提供了组织。放射治疗有时可作为一种替代手术非侵入性的方式，具有保存器官的可能性。用作辅助治疗时，术前放疗可使肿瘤更易于切除，也可用于手术后微小残留病灶的治疗。与这些局部疗法不同，化疗可用于治疗转移性疾病或降低潜在的微转移风险。化疗也可以作为放射增敏剂，增加放疗的局部肿瘤控制。这 3 种模式的最佳联合是根据肿瘤类型、解剖位置、肿瘤分期和其他患者因素而个体化定制的。每一种模式都有不同的风险，需要相互平衡，以便为每个患者提供最佳风险-受益比的治疗。大多数临床放射治疗方案采用分割治疗，单次治疗为小剂量（剂量单位为 Gy），而不是一次大剂量治疗。现代放射治疗的常见疗程一般是平均治疗 6~8 周，每周治疗 5~6 次。分割放疗的概念建立在早期临床观察的经验基础上，即每天小剂量的照射可以导致癌细胞死亡，同时正常的组织可以恢复。放射性生物学家对此提出了各种机制解释，但我们对这一过程的理解仍在不断深入。例如，正常组织健康细胞的自我修复能力是正常组织耐受性的一个重要组成部分。

放射治疗在组织层面的影响通常用 S 形曲线来表示，x 轴表示辐射剂量（图 44-1）。理想情况下，肿瘤控制概率的 S 形

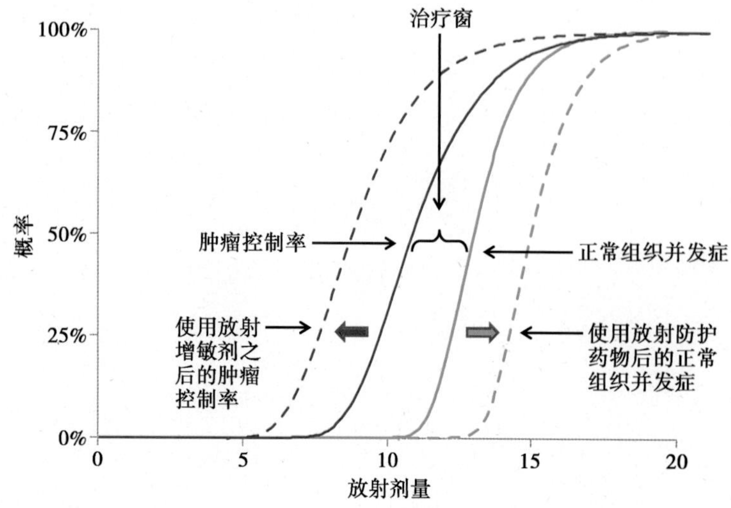

图 44-1　组织水平的放射治疗影响。实线 S 形曲线表示肿瘤控制的理想化概率和正常组织并发症的风险。虚线曲线表示加入了调节辐射敏感性的药物之后的预期效应

曲线位于正常组织毒性的曲线左侧。这两条曲线之间的间隔为治疗窗，其表示可以成功消除肿瘤同时保持正常组织耐受性的剂量范围。这些曲线表明，对于任何组织，存在一个放疗剂量的区间，在此区间外，剂量变化产生的影响很小。然而，在曲线的陡峭部分内，剂量的微小变化就能在临床疗效方面产生很大的差异。代表肿瘤杀伤和周围正常组织毒性的剂量-效应曲线之间存在着独特的关系，这在不同临床情况下差异很大。图 44-1 中的曲线描述了一个理想化的情况，而在现实中，实际肿瘤与邻近正常组织的敏感性之间的关系通常要复杂得多。

放射治疗的生物效应

细胞和组织的放射反应

细胞对放射治疗的分子反应

1Gy 的剂量照射导致每个细胞产生约 10^5 个电离事件，每个细胞核产生大约 1 000~2 000 条单链 DNA 断裂（SSBs）和大约 40 条双链 DNA 断裂（DSBs）。这种 DNA 损伤引起了越来越多的非 DNA 修复/检查点相关机制的激活，这些机制介导了重要的细胞应答[2]。辐射诱导的 DSBs 通常被认为是与临床放射治疗相关的主要致死事件。这种损伤引起许多细胞反应，包括 DNA 损伤识别、导致细胞周期检查点激活的信号转导、应激反应基因的诱导和协调、DNA 修复和/或凋亡级联的激活（图 44-2）。MRN 蛋白复合物（Mre 11、Rad 50 和 NBS 1）和变性共济失调（ATM）蛋白是 DNA 损伤的中枢传感器，这些蛋白在 DSBs 上迅速积累。ATM、相关蛋白共济失调、毛细血管扩张症和 Rad3 相关蛋白（ATR）是 PI-3 激酶家族的成员，在识别 DNA 损伤和启动应答方面起着重要作用。ATM 和 ATR 可能具有部分重叠的功能；然而，ATM 优先识别 DSBs，而 ATR 优先感知复制-阻断 DNA 的作用，它们都可以磷酸化下游的靶点，从而调节细胞周期检查点、凋亡、衰老、自噬和 DNA 修复的途径。染色质蛋白组蛋白 H2AX 是这类磷酸化靶点之一，它的激活导致染色质结构变得不那么浓缩和易于接受修复蛋白的出现，因此 H2AX 磷酸化是一种很容易被荧光显微镜观察到的 DSB 形成和修复的标记物。磷酸化的 H2AX 对辐射反应至关重要，因为它促进其他传感器/效应蛋白的合成，包括 53BP 1、MDC1 和 BRCA 1。

DSBs 的修复

细胞同源重组（HR）和非同源端连接（NHEJ）是 DSBs 修复的主要途径。这两条通路均在传感器/效应蛋白的出现后起作用[2]。在 HR 中，细胞识别出一段同源 DNA，并从这个同源 DNA 模板中复制缺失的遗传信息[3]。与之相比，NHEJ 通路处理断裂的 DNA 末端并使其重新出现，有时使用一个微同源区[4]。NHEJ 通路被认为是在 G_0/G_1 期间修复辐射诱导的 DSBs 的主要途径。普遍接受的模型包括 Ku 70/80、Artemis 和 DNA-PKcs 复合物与 DNA 末端的结合和处理。DSB 随后被 Ligase Ⅳ/XRCC 4 复合物 5 所重排[5]。由于 NHEJ 有时需要在解除之前处理 DSB 结束，通过这一途径进行修复可能容易出错。相比之下，HR 是 DSB 修复的一种普遍无错误的模式，因为修复模板是未损坏的姐妹染色单体。HR 需要包括关键重组酶 RAD 51 在内的许多蛋白质的作用，以及促进其在 DNA 上组装的其他因素，包括 BRCA 2、RAD 52 和 RAD 51[3]。除了这种 DSB 修复功能外，HR 蛋白还能促进对复制阻断性损伤（如链间 DNA 交联剂的损伤）和折叠复制叉的耐受性。一些常见的化疗药物作为放射增敏剂的原理可能是因为它们干扰了这些通路。

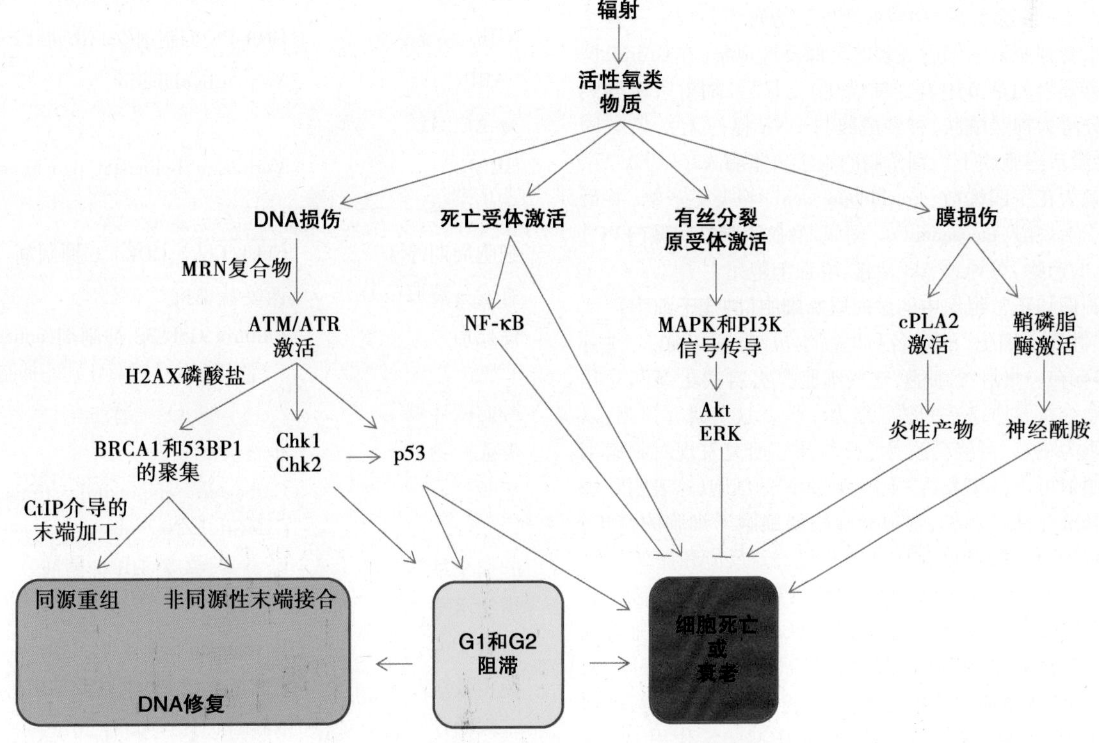

图 44-2　辐射暴露后发生的分子反应概览

放疗诱导的细胞周期阻滞和死亡

哈特维尔、乐仕和亨特[2]等早期报道了细胞周期在辐射暴露后阻滞在 G_1 和 G_2 期。激活的 ATM 和 ATR 会导致关键下游效应激酶如 Chk 1 和 Chk 2 的磷酸化。活化后，Chk 1 和 Chk 2 磷酸化磷酸酶 CDC25A，进而降解。因此，CDC25A 不能去磷酸化激活 CDK 2，最终导致细胞周期阻滞。重要的是，Chk 2 也使 p53 磷酸化，导致 p21 介导的细胞周期阻滞，这些受损细胞随后面临一个关键时期，尤其在辐射损伤没有完全修复的情况下[6]。受损细胞可能因损伤未修复而发生有丝分裂障碍，也有可能只是通过衰老而失去增殖能力。放射诱导的衰老与 p16/Rb 和 p53/p21 肿瘤抑制因子的激活有关。细胞也可能经历凋亡而死亡，经典的途径包括依赖 p53 的细胞凋亡蛋白酶级联的激活。此外，辐射诱导的细胞表面"死亡受体"（TNF、Fas 或 TRAIL 的受体）的激活，可导致凋亡性死亡。但自相矛盾的是，这些死亡受体在某些情况下也能通过激活转录因子核因子 κB（NFκB）来抑制细胞凋亡而产生细胞保护作用。

放疗后细胞信号传导的主要途径

组织被射线照射后导致活性氧类物质（radical oxygen species，ROS）的形成，并与包括 DNA 在内的多种细胞内物质相互作用。这些 ROS，包括超氧化物和羟自由基，通过耗尽细胞中的抗氧化剂，如谷胱甘肽[7]的通路被激活，从而促进存活、抗凋亡反应和转录改变。净效应是可变的和细胞类型依赖的，但这通常包括激活细胞表面受体，如含有表皮生长因子受体（EGFR）的 ErbB 家族，从而激活其他下游通路，如级联的丝裂原活化蛋白激酶（MAPK）超家族（ERK、JNK 和 p38）和磷脂酰肌醇 3 激酶（PI3K）通路[2]。这些途径倾向于通过 Akt 和 Erk 信号途径促进抗凋亡信号[8]。辐射也能触发自分泌机制，包括转化生长因子 α（TGFα）的释放，转化生长因子 α 结合并激活 EGFR 8，另外的促炎症细胞因子如肿瘤坏死因子-α（TNF-α）和白细胞介素-6[9]也会释放，这些都会导致旁观者效应——这是一种邻近未受到照射的细胞表现的类似反应现象（在 Grdina 博士关于电离辐射的章节中有详细描述）。最后，辐射可诱导膜基鞘磷脂分解为神经酰胺，神经酰胺与 DNA 损伤无关[10]。同样，辐射能激活细胞膜上识别磷脂的胞浆磷脂酶 A2（CPLA 2），并将其降解为花生四烯酸（arachidonic acid）等炎症产物，并最终降解成二十烷酸（eicosanoid）。例如，溶血磷脂酰胆碱（LPC）是 cPLA 2 的产物，可导致 Akt 活化，增强细胞死亡[11]。

在受照射肿瘤和正常组织中的肿瘤原始细胞（肿瘤干细胞）

尽管"肿瘤干细胞"的命名和生物学机制方面存在一些分歧，但显然存在一批肿瘤细胞，这些细胞具有自我更新和分化为促进肿瘤维持异质谱系的独特能力[12-14]。这些研究预测，以肿瘤干细胞为靶点，可能会改善治疗结果。研究发现对肿瘤细胞群体的照射可以富集表达"干细胞"标记的细胞，这表明肿瘤干细胞具有抗药性。例如，辐射导致胶质细胞干细胞的富集，这些干细胞表现出优先激活 DNA 损伤检查点反应和提高 DNA 修复能力[15]。介导这种辐射耐受性的潜在机制尚不清楚，醛脱氢酶 1（ALDH 1）可能是部分原因。ALDH 1 蛋白在肿瘤细胞中的高表达可能是由于醛分解代谢活性所致。众所周知，ALDH 1 还与范可尼贫血相关的 DNA 修复基因协同作用，提示 ALDH 1 的活性可能在修复 DNA 加合物中起一定作用[16]，从而促进了干细胞克隆的辐射抗性。肿瘤干细胞的另一个有趣的特点是他们倾向于用 HR 修复来修复 DSBs[17]，这表明 HR 抑制剂可能代表着一种耗尽肿瘤干细胞库的治疗策略。另外，盐霉素和噻嗪是针对肿瘤干细胞研发的化合物[18,19]，但临床上还没有它们与放射治疗联合的试验。

放射增敏药物的发展

肿瘤往往与放射敏感的正常组织相邻，这限制了可以安全使用的放疗剂量。因此，能优先作用于肿瘤的放射增敏药物将是非常有利的。例如，恶性胶质瘤治疗后的局部复发是致命的，肿瘤特异性增敏药物可能会增加肿瘤的可治愈性。相比之下，一些肿瘤，如前列腺癌，已经可以通过放射治疗治愈，但需要非常高的剂量，毒性很大。在这种情况下，肿瘤特异性放射增敏剂可在保持疗效的基础上，降低放疗剂量并减少副作用。标准化疗药物仍然是提高放疗局部疗效的常用药物。我们最近发表了一篇综述，详细介绍了特定靶点放射增敏剂的研究进展[2]。本章不可能对这些新药物进行详尽的讨论，表 44-1 列举了多种此类药物。其中许多药物的目标蛋白是感知辐射损伤和协调细胞反应的蛋白质，而另一些药物则是利用肿瘤中存在的缺氧或异常氧化还原的环境。这些药物最终能否成功，将取决于它们是否有能力提高放射治疗指数（见图 44-1 中关于这一概念的说明）。然而真正有效的肿瘤特异性放射增敏剂的研发是非常困难的。

表 44-1 可调节辐射效应的药物

作用水平（靶点）	辐射增敏剂或保护剂
活性氧自由基	阿米福汀，吡多胺，UROD RNAi
DNA 损伤反应 DSB 识别	Mirin，atm/atr 抑制剂（例如 KU-55933），DT 01
HR 修复	RS-1，RI-1，RAD51 表达调节剂
NHEJ 修复	DNA-PK 抑制剂（如 NU7441，Salvicine）
PARP	Veliparib，olaparib
染色质组织	
HDAC	Vorinostat，belinostat，panobinostat
细胞应答	
细胞周期停滞	Chk1/Chk2，CDK4/6 抑制剂
有丝分裂原信号	西妥昔单抗
促死信号	Pifithrin，GSK-3β 抑制剂，anticeramide，细胞色素 C 过氧化物酶抑制剂
肿瘤微环境	
炎症产物	他汀类
乏氧	Carbogen，efaproxiral，tirapazamine，MGd，EZN-2968
肿瘤干细胞	盐霉素、噻嗪、HR 抑制剂
组织水平	
血管生成	Bevizumab
免疫效应	CTLA-4、抗 PD-1、IL-2 SBRT
基因治疗	NFerade、HSV-tk、G 207
细胞重组	Palifermin

放射治疗联合基因治疗

广泛的临床前研究和少数临床试验已经将基因治疗与放射治疗联合，利用复制缺陷病毒传递放射增敏药物、细胞因子、抑癌基因和免疫激活化合物。例如，TNFerade（Ad.Egr-TNF11D）是一种复制缺陷的腺病毒载体，由编码肿瘤坏死因子-α的启动子上游的放射和化学诱导元件组成，是一种直接的放射增敏剂和免疫激活剂。这利用了辐射诱导的Egr-1启动子，使肿瘤坏死因子-α在放射治疗靶区内特异性分泌[20]。早期临床试验表明TNFerade在软组织肉瘤、食道癌、头颈部和直肠癌患者的治疗反应率相当高[21]。然而，胰腺癌的随机Ⅲ期研究中，尽管早期肿瘤有生存改善的趋势，生存期却未能提高[22]。

其他试验采用了酶/前药的方案，例如单纯疱疹病毒胸苷激酶（HSV-tk）的直接表达，将前药更昔洛韦磷酸化成一种干扰DNA复制的有毒代谢物。虽然这一概念很有说服力，但Ⅲ期随机研究未能显示改善多形性胶质母细胞瘤的生存[23]。类似的方案将HSV-tk与另一种"自杀基因"（如胞嘧啶脱氨酶）结合起来，将前药5-氟胞嘧啶转化为5-FU[24]。这种方案与前列腺放射治疗的联合，尚未在Ⅱ～Ⅲ期试验中显示有效性。最后，有方案将肿瘤病毒与放射治疗联合，提出了一些病毒可以通过优先感染和裂解癌细胞来与放射治疗协同的概念。例如，一种复制型单纯疱疹病毒Ⅰ型（HSV-1）已用于治疗恶性胶质瘤和局部晚期头颈部肿瘤的放射治疗[25]。同样，近期一项Ⅰ期试验中，将一种呼肠孤病毒与姑息性放射治疗联合使用[26]。

免疫调节药物联合放射治疗

辐射在肿瘤中产生炎症微环境，通过损伤的细胞增加抗原表达和免疫识别。这些效应包括主要组织相容性复合体Ⅰ类（MHC-I）表达的增加，抗原肽库的改变，调节性T细胞的减少，以及细胞因子和黏附分子的上调，这些细胞因子和黏附分子可以招募和激活CD8细胞毒性T淋巴细胞和树突状细胞[2]。辐射也会损伤免疫抑制过程[27,28]。这种免疫调节的能力使放射治疗和免疫治疗的联合成为可能[29]。在前列腺癌中的治疗中已经进行了相关研究，例如将标准放射治疗和编码PSA的基因治疗性疫苗相联合[30]。其他类似的方案包括：不同的疫苗、未成熟树突状细胞的瘤内注射或输注肿瘤浸润淋巴细胞的过继免疫治疗。这些试验通常显示出很好的免疫应答。例如，高剂量IL-2和立体定向体放疗治疗转移性黑色素瘤或肾癌，与单用高剂量IL-2治疗的历史对照组相比，疗效显著提高[31]。类似的方案包括：将放射治疗与细胞毒性T淋巴细胞相关抗原4（CTLA-4）或程序性死亡因子1（PD-1）的拮抗剂联合，肿瘤细胞可借用这些抗原来逃避免疫系统[32]。

热疗联合放射治疗

体外设备产生的微波、超声波或射频（RF）能量，可对病灶进行局部加热。实验表明，高于41℃的温度可杀伤细胞，高于42.5℃的温度可使细胞的死亡率剧增[33]。当细胞处于S期时，高热导致的死亡最为明显，这与蛋白质变性的机制一致[34]。高温和辐射组合产生的致死效应具有协同作用[35]，可能是因为辐射引起的DNA损伤修复所需的蛋白质变性。然而临床上这种明显的协同作用并不常见，两种治疗的疗效似乎只是独立的。几个随机临床试验测试了放疗±热疗的组合，结果并不一致。此外，临床上热疗的一个难点是如何将热量均匀地输送到较深的解剖部位。因此，临床上使用热疗最多的仍是浅表的皮肤癌和乳腺癌。

保护正常组织免受放射损伤

放疗导致的正常组织的早期副作用，主要是因为损伤了快速增殖的细胞更新系统，而晚期副作用一般与血管损伤、纤维化和健康细胞针对正常组织的再群体化不良有关。辐射还会产生突变，导致继发性肿瘤，尤其是在儿童患者中更为常见。因此，大量辐射防护药物的研发以期尽量减少这一问题。"辐射保护剂"定义为在辐射暴露前预防性给予的药物，而辐射"缓解剂"则是在辐射照射期间或之后使用。第三类药物为"治疗性药物"，可增加辐射照射后正常组织的修复。研发这类药物的主要挑战是它们不能保护肿瘤细胞也免受辐射引起的死亡[2]。由于篇幅限制，不可能对这些新药进行详尽的讨论；表44-1中列举了其中一些药物。含有巯基的化合物，例如阿米福汀，具有清除活性氧的作用，从而吸收辐射产生的活性氧[36]。阿米福汀是这类药物中唯一获得FDA批准的，也是这类药物中研究最多的药物[37]。由于担心对肿瘤的保护，阿米福汀的广泛使用受到限制；然而临床上几乎没有证据表明这种情况的存在[38]。近期研究侧重于非硫醇类药物，例如影响细胞周期分布或辐射诱导凋亡的药物[39-43]。治疗性药物，是那些减少内皮细胞损伤、炎症级联和组织缺血的药物[44,45]。放疗后可使用多种生长因子来促进正常细胞增殖。例如角质形成细胞生长因子（Palifermin）可在局部晚期头颈癌的放化疗期间减少黏膜炎的发生率[46]。

可预测放射治疗效果的分子指标

根据肿瘤的遗传和表观遗传特征，基因组分析方法越来越多地用于恶性肿瘤的分类和临床结果的预测。这有助于推动个体化医疗的实现，其中个体化的治疗方案是根据患者特定的分子分型和肿瘤特征量身定制的。我们在此只讨论预测放射治疗疗效的系统。放射敏感性指数（RSI）就是这样一种方法，它利用10个基因的mRNA水平来预测一系列人类癌细胞系的放射敏感性[47]。它在五个独立的临床数据集中得到了临床验证，包括直肠、食管、头颈部和乳腺癌的放化疗或单纯放疗[48]。我们研发了一种类似的干扰素相关损伤特征法（IRDS），成功地预测了辅助化疗的疗效和放疗后的局部区域控制[49]。此外，我们最近报道了一种新的方法来量化癌症治疗中DNA修复通路的效率[50]。重组能力评分（recombination proficiency score，RPS）是根据参与DNA修复通路的四个基因（Rif1、PARI、RAD51和Ku80）的表达水平计算出来的，这些基因的高表达会产生低的RPS。我们在临床上验证了RPS系统在乳腺癌和非小细胞肺癌（NSCLCs）中的应用。RPS低的肿瘤预后不良，这表明HR抑制导致基因组不稳定，从而加速恶性进展。如果NSCLC患者接受以铂类为基础的辅助化疗，这种与低RPS相关的不良预后会减少，这表明HR抑制和以铂类药物为基础的相关敏感性抵消了与低RPS相关的不良预后。我们目前正在测试该系统是否能同样地预测肿瘤的放射敏感性。另一种预测放射敏感性的方法是通过比较基因组杂交阵列或第二代测序结果来寻找基因改变[51,52]，这些方法正在迅速发展，未来几年可能会发生彻底的改变。

现代放射治疗的物理和临床进展

放射治疗大多为使用直线加速器产生高能（6～20mV）光子的体外放疗（XRT）。还有少数 XRT 通过其他粒子束完成，可以为电子、质子、碳离子或中子。患者通常每天在固定的治疗台上完成治疗，光束从多个角度照射至患者的肿瘤区域。每个直线加速器都连接在一个"机架"上，它可以绕着治疗台旋转。作为 XRT 的一种替代方法，也可以将放射源放置在肿瘤附近进行治疗（即近距离治疗）。通过这些模式的多种组合，放射治疗得以广泛地应用（见表 44-2）。某些情况下，这些模式的高级组合可以提供更好的治疗比。特定模式的确定取决于以下几个因素，包括可预测的肿瘤放疗疗效、邻近正常组织对辐射损伤的敏感性以及特定癌种的非放疗替代方案。

表 44-2　不同类型放射治疗的临床应用实例

	光子分割外照射 三维适形放疗；调强放射治疗	外照射消融治疗 立体定向放射治疗 立体定向放射外科	粒子束外照射治疗 质子或碳离子束治疗	腔内或插植近距离治疗
常用适应证	许多	脑转移 早期肺癌 寡转移病灶	小儿恶性肿瘤 葡萄膜黑色素瘤脊索瘤	前列腺癌 宫颈癌
插图	一例肛管癌采用不同类型的 X 线外照射治疗，黄色阴影区表示靶体积，包括肛门/直肠和引流淋巴结区域。盆骨和膀胱代表邻近的正常组织 基于 IMRT 的计划更加符合目标的形状，从而减少正常组织的照射 3D-CRT：45Gy，1.8Gy/fx IMRT：45Gy，1.8Gy/fx	这些治疗方法包括：能够给予消融剂量的放疗方法，使用单次照射或少量的 1～5 次大分割放疗 采用多个相交光束，生成高适形度的计划，显著降低正常组织受照射量 脑转移的 SRS：18Gy 单次放疗 SBRT 治疗肺癌：12Gy/次，5 次	质子束可在组织中产生特定的剂量分布 XRT 用于治疗儿童髓母细胞瘤的全脑全脊髓区域 以质子为基础的治疗减少了脊柱前部的正常组织的受量 光子　质子 全脑全脊髓照射：36Gy，1.8Gy/次	放射源位于靶区内或附近。减少了对周围组织的照射。这是一种常用且有效的治疗前列腺癌的方法，通过直肠超声实时成像指导会阴路径放置永久性粒子 X 线平片显示整个前列腺的小粒子（造影剂充满膀胱） 插植体放疗剂量：145Gy
区别特点	这些治疗是最广泛使用的放射治疗形式	先进的靶向性能够实现陡峭的剂量梯度，允许大剂量的分割照射 必须以精确的摆位和图像引导技术为基础	需要专门而昂贵的回旋加速器设备。对于某些疾病，质子治疗可以降低 XRT 的毒性	邻近的正常组织受照射量很低。解剖屏障限制近距离放疗仅适用于小部分癌症类型

XRT，体外照射；3D-CRT，三维适形放疗；IMRT，调强放射治疗；SBRT，立体定向放射治疗；SRS，立体定向放射外科。

三维适形放射治疗、调强放射治疗和影像引导放射治疗

近年来 CT 影像和三维（3D）治疗计划软件的结合显著地提高了放射治疗的质量。此外，通过加速器自动形成各种放疗野的能力使许多技术得以实现。射线束的形状现在通常是利用多叶准直器（MLCS）产生，其是位于直线加速器末端的小型金属自动控制模块。这种基于硬件的创新与治疗优化软件相结合，创造了三维适形放射治疗（3D-CRT）的技术。剂量师、物理师和医师联合制定最优的 3D-CRT 治疗计划，使计划既符合

标准(即高剂量"包裹"在靶体积周围),又具有同质性(即在靶体积内的剂量差异很小)。与以往的方法相比,3D-CRT 能更有效地覆盖肿瘤,同时更好地保护邻近的正常器官。

调强放射治疗(IMRT)是另一种常用的 XRT 方法。如同 3D-CRT 一样,IMRT 利用多个交叉的 X 射线束对靶区进行治疗。在 IMRT 计划中,光束的强度被调制成网格模式以提供更适合的剂量分布。IMRT 计划软件是基于用户定义的肿瘤覆盖和正常组织保护的目标,利用迭代算法进行治疗优化。这种高度的适形性对于治疗邻近不规则正常组织的肿瘤优势显著[53]。近年来 IMRT 的广泛使用增加了肿瘤剂量并降低了毒性。例如,IMRT 已作为头颈部肿瘤保留器官的标准治疗,可以保护唾液腺,从而减少口干[54]。IMRT 还可以采用同步加量的方法,对不同部位的肿瘤进行不同剂量的治疗[55]。

虽然这些技术进展提供了更好的放疗计划,但实际上患者治疗很大程度上取决于每天重复执行该计划的能力。患者的日常摆位和体内器官运动(如呼吸运动)的多变性都会破坏这种治疗实施的准确性。图像引导放射治疗(IGRT)解决了这个问题。现在的直线加速器通常配备"机载"成像设备,提供千伏级 X 线或锥形束 CT 扫描的实时(或几乎实时)诊断成像。某些情况下,可在特定组织中植入射线不能透射的标记用于病人位置的微调[56]。此外,有一些软件可以解决生理运动,例如呼吸运动对放疗的影响。因为 IGRT 能减少摆位误差的大小,治疗靶区的体积也会相应减少[2]。

使用大分割方式的放疗消融方法

近年来由于治疗精度的改进,放疗的方式发生了转变,使得采用较高单日放疗剂量和较短疗程的放疗(即大分割 RT)成为可能。总治疗时间的减少,一定程度上抵消了在较长体外放疗期间发生的肿瘤细胞群的增殖(加速再增殖),进而产生治疗获益[57]。单次立体定向放射外科技术(SRS)是大分割放疗的极端版本,用于颅内肿瘤的消融治疗[58]。分次立体定向放射治疗(SBRT)是一种类似的治疗颅外病灶的方法,分割次数少而单次剂量较大[59]。SRS 和 SBRT 的使用必须依赖于之前提及的采用了提高放疗计划和实施准确性的方法,才能使治疗更小体积的病灶成为可能。这些模式的安全性和有效性已被证明。例如,对较小脑转移瘤进行单次 20Gy 照射之后可以取得很高的局部控制率,或对肝转移灶进行 20Gy/3 次治疗后可以取得>80%~85%的局部控制率。早期 NSCLC 通过短疗程的 SBRT 治疗(3~5 次分割,每次 12~20Gy)也能取得很好的疗效[60]。但 SBRT 的最佳分割模式尚未完全明确。需要考虑包括肿瘤体积和邻近正常组织特点在内的多个因素,才能决定在特定临床情况下,是采用 SBRT 还是采用多次分割的体外照射模式更合适[61,62]。

近距离治疗

近距离治疗是一种将放射源放置在肿瘤附近的放疗方法。对于某些肿瘤其疗效可能优于外照射。通过改变放射源的强度、位置和暴露时间,可以实现肿瘤内高度适形的辐射剂量分布。同时能保护邻近的正常器官,受到相对较低的剂量照射。放射源可通过插植放置,即将其直接放置到目标组织中。或者,将放射源放置在与目标组织相邻的管腔内(例如,体腔或肠腔内,称为腔内近距离治疗)。在某些情况下,近距离治疗提供了更优的剂量分布。然而,近距离治疗并没有 XRT 的应用那么广泛,因为只有少数临床情况下,才可以分清靶区的解剖结构,进而安全使用放射源。因此宫颈癌、前列腺癌、乳腺癌和皮肤癌是最常使用近距离治疗的瘤种。例如,前列腺癌的近距离治疗可能优于增加剂量的 XRT[63]。但许多解剖部位不适合采用近距离治疗,因为 XRT 的治疗比超过了近距离治疗。此外,如果放射源错位或在放置后移位,近距离治疗有增加副作用的潜在风险[64]。

粒子束治疗

粒子治疗是体外放疗的一种形式,其射线束是由电子、质子、碳离子或中子组成的粒子束,而不是光子[65]。近年来,质子束治疗的应用有所增加,尤其值得关注。当质子束穿过组织时,大部分能量会在粒子静止之前迅速沉积。这种沉积发生在组织的特定深度(称为布拉格峰),可通过改变质子束的能量进行控制。其临床意义是,质子束可以减少靶区附近正常组织的辐射损伤,特别是比肿瘤更深的组织。这一特点可以减少治疗并发症,因此质子在儿童疾病中的使用迅速增长—尤其对于儿童颅内肿瘤,正常脑组织受照剂量的减少可以减少 XRT 的神经认知后遗症。此外,位于脊柱附近的肿瘤,如脊索瘤或椎旁软骨肉瘤,是质子束治疗的明确适应证,因为其可使这些相对放疗抵抗的肿瘤得到更高剂量的治疗,同时减少周围正常组织的辐射损伤[66]。

某些类型粒子束每单位能量沉积也能产生更高的相对生物效率(RBE)。例如,质子的 RBE 是光子的 1~1.2 倍,而中子或碳离子,RBE 可以是光子的 4~10 倍。需要进一步的研究来明确,相对于以光子为基础的治疗,这些 RBE 的差异是否有更好的,或者是更差的治疗比。例如,质子或碳离子束加速器的建造成本很高,需要更大的空间和更多训练有素的工作人员。

结论,放疗的发展方向

近年来科技的巨大进步,影响了肿瘤患者的放射治疗模式。同时,我们对控制人体细胞和组织辐射效应的基本生物机制的理解也有了很大的提高。然而,一些尚未解决的问题仍然限制了放射治疗的应用,在未来的几十年里,这些剩余的问题或许是指导我们在该领域取得进展的重要因素[2]。其中一个问题是细胞内在的辐射抵抗降低了许多肿瘤的局部控制率。例如,在胶质母细胞瘤等肿瘤中,尽管使用了先进的放疗技术和非常高的放疗剂量,但肿瘤局部控制率仍然很低。我们需继续加深对潜在生物问题的探索来解决这一问题。我们还需要研制更多的药物,可使肿瘤细胞对辐射更为敏感,或者用以保护正常组织。在未来的放射治疗中还需要更多的个体化治疗。目前,是否放疗以及放疗的关键参数(例如剂量和体积),是基于疾病分期进行选择。当放疗敏感性的分子预测指标在实际应用中变得更加准确和方便时,基于患者生物学的个体化的信息将更准确地指导治疗。

(邓垒　译,周宗玫　审校)

参考文献

The complete reference list can be found on the Wiley Companion Digital Edition of this title (see inside front cover for login instructions).

1 Connell PP, Hellman S. Advances in radiotherapy and implications for the next century: a historical perspective. *Cancer Res*. 2009;**69**(**2**):383–392.

2 Liauw SL, Connell PP, Weichselbaum RR. New paradigms and future challenges in radiation oncology: an update of biological targets and technology. *Sci Transl Med*. 2013;**5**(**173**):173sr2.

4 Thompson LH, Schild D. Recombinational DNA repair and human disease. *Mutat Res*. 2002;**509**(**1–2**):49–78.

6 Eriksson D, Stigbrand T. Radiation-induced cell death mechanisms. *Tumour Biol*. 2010;**31**(**4**):363–372.

8 Dent P, Yacoub A, Contessa J, et al. Stress and radiation-induced activation of multiple intracellular signaling pathways. *Radiat Res*. 2003;**159**(**3**):283–300.

10 Kolesnick R, Fuks Z. Radiation and ceramide-induced apoptosis. *Oncogene*. 2003;**22**(**37**):5897–5906.

15 Bao S, Wu Q, McLendon RE, et al. Glioma stem cells promote radioresistance by preferential activation of the DNA damage response. *Nature*. 2006;**444**(**7120**):756–760.

17 Al-Assar O, Mantoni T, Lunardi S, Kingham G, Helleday T, Brunner TB. Breast cancer stem-like cells show dominant homologous recombination due to a larger S-G2 fraction. *Cancer Biol Ther*. 2011;**11**(**12**):1028–1035.

20 Hallahan DE, Mauceri HJ, Seung LP, et al. Spatial and temporal control of gene therapy using ionizing radiation. *Nat Med*. 1995;**1**(**8**):786–791.

21 Weichselbaum RR, Kufe D. Translation of the radio- and chemo-inducible TNFerade vector to the treatment of human cancers. *Cancer Gene Ther*. 2009;**16**(**8**):609–619.

22 Herman JM, Wild AT, Wang H, et al. Randomized phase III multi-institutional study of TNFerade biologic with fluorouracil and radiotherapy for locally advanced pancreatic cancer: final results. *J Clin Oncol*. 2013;**31**(**7**):886–894.

29 Kamrava M, Bernstein MB, Camphausen K, Hodge JW. Combining radiation, immunotherapy, and antiangiogenesis agents in the management of cancer: the Three Musketeers or just another quixotic combination? *Mol Biosyst*. 2009;**5**(**11**):1262–1270.

31 Seung SK, Curti BD, Crittenden M, et al. Phase 1 study of stereotactic body radiotherapy and interleukin-2—tumor and immunological responses. *Sci Transl Med*. 2012;**4**(**137**):137ra74.

33 Dewey WC, Hopwood LE, Sapareto SA, Gerweck LE. Cellular responses to combinations of hyperthermia and radiation. *Radiology*. 1977;**123**(**2**):463–474.

35 Sapareto SA, Hopwood LE, Dewey WC. Combined effects of X irradiation and hyperthermia on CHO cells for various temperatures and orders of application. *Radiat Res*. 1978;**73**(**2**):221–233.

36 Yuhas JM, Yurconic M, Kligerman MM, West G, Peterson DF. Combined use of radioprotective and radiosensitizing drugs in experimental radiotherapy. *Radiat Res*. 1977;**70**(**2**):433–443.

37 Brizel DM, Wasserman TH, Henke M, et al. Phase III randomized trial of amifostine as a radioprotector in head and neck cancer. *J Clin Oncol*. 2000;**18**(**19**):3339–3345.

46 Le QT, Kim HE, Schneider CJ, et al. Palifermin reduces severe mucositis in definitive chemoradiotherapy of locally advanced head and neck cancer: a randomized, placebo-controlled study. *J Clin Oncol*. 2011;**29**(**20**):2808–2814.

49 Weichselbaum RR, Ishwaran H, Yoon T, et al. An interferon-related gene signature for DNA damage resistance is a predictive marker for chemotherapy and radiation for breast cancer. *Proc Natl Acad Sci U S A*. 2008;**105**(**47**):18490–18495.

50 Pitroda SP, Pashtan IM, Logan HL, et al. DNA repair pathway gene expression score correlates with repair proficiency and tumor sensitivity to chemotherapy. *Sci Transl Med*. 2014;**6**(**229**):229ra42.

53 Bortfeld T. IMRT: a review and preview. *Phys Med Biol*. 2006;**51**(**13**):R363–R379.

54 Lin A, Kim HM, Terrell JE, Dawson LA, Ship JA, Eisbruch A. Quality of life after parotid-sparing IMRT for head-and-neck cancer: a prospective longitudinal study. *Int J Radiat Oncol Biol Phys*. 2003;**57**(**1**):61–70.

55 de Arruda FF, Puri DR, Zhung J, et al. Intensity-modulated radiation therapy for the treatment of oropharyngeal carcinoma: the Memorial Sloan-Kettering Cancer Center experience. *Int J Radiat Oncol Biol Phys*. 2006;**64**(**2**):363–373.

56 Shirato H, Harada T, Harabayashi T, et al. Feasibility of insertion/implantation of 2.0-mm-diameter gold internal fiducial markers for precise setup and real-time tumor tracking in radiotherapy. *Int J Radiat Oncol Biol Phys*. 2003;**56**(**1**):240–247.

57 Schmidt-Ullrich RK, Contessa JN, Dent P, et al. Molecular mechanisms of radiation-induced accelerated repopulation. *Radiat Oncol Investig*. 1999;**7**(**6**):321–330.

58 Leksell L. The stereotaxic method and radiosurgery of the brain. *Acta Chir Scand*. 1951;**102**(**4**):316–319.

59 Potters L, Kavanagh B, Galvin JM, et al. American Society for Therapeutic Radiology and Oncology (ASTRO) and American College of Radiology (ACR) practice guideline for the performance of stereotactic body radiation therapy. *Int J Radiat Oncol Biol Phys*. 2010;**76**(**2**):326–332.

60 Grills IS, Mangona VS, Welsh R, et al. Outcomes after stereotactic lung radiotherapy or wedge resection for stage I non-small-cell lung cancer. *J Clin Oncol*. 2010;**28**(**6**):928–935.

61 Hoyer M, Roed H, Sengelov L, et al. Phase-II study on stereotactic radiotherapy of locally advanced pancreatic carcinoma. *Radiother Oncol*. 2005;**76**(**1**):48–53.

62 Timmerman R, McGarry R, Yiannoutsos C, et al. Excessive toxicity when treating central tumors in a phase II study of stereotactic body radiation therapy for medically inoperable early-stage lung cancer. *J Clin Oncol*. 2006;**24**(**30**):4833–4839.

63 Jabbari S, Weinberg VK, Shinohara K, et al. Equivalent biochemical control and improved prostate-specific antigen nadir after permanent prostate seed implant brachytherapy versus high-dose three-dimensional conformal radiotherapy and high-dose conformal proton beam radiotherapy boost. *Int J Radiat Oncol Biol Phys*. 2010;**76**(**1**):36–42.

64 Bogdanich W. *At V.A. Hospital, a Rogue Cancer Unit*. 2009, New York City: The New York Times; June 20 [cited 2012 September 29], http://www.nytimes.com/2009/06/21/health/21radiation.html?_r=0. (accessed 12 October 2015)

65 Durante M, Loeffler JS. Charged particles in radiation oncology. *Nat Rev Clin Oncol*. 2010;**7**(**1**):37–43.

66 Schulz-Ertner D, Tsujii H. Particle radiation therapy using proton and heavier ion beams. *J Clin Oncol*. 2007;**25**(**8**):953–964.

第 45 章　肿瘤内科学原则

WilliamN. Hait, MD, PhD ■ JamesF. Holland, MD, ScD(hc) ■ EmilFreiIII, MD(deceased) ■ DonaldW. Kufe, MD ■ RobertC. BastJr. , MD ■ WaunKiHong, MD, DMSc(Hon)

概述

肿瘤内科学临床实践的发展速度快于其他任何医学领域。众多恶性肿瘤的分子基础及其分子亚型的发现，使得临床医生面临着一系列令人眼花缭乱的新信息。由于这个专业的基本原则应该保持不变，因此它们需要为这些新增加的信息提供框架。为此，本章试图定义那些适用于肿瘤患者治疗的不变领域，并通过对它们的理解来组织文中提出的大量新内容。

肿瘤内科学是由内科学分出的一个亚学科，这一医学分支的标志是能从事癌症的诊疗，安全地使用对患者具有风险的主要是和现代分子生物学相关的药物。今天，正在进入个体化医学。肿瘤内科学家应当懂得恶性转化的分子生物学基础，并能将这些知识用于癌症患者的预防、早期发现和治疗。对于肿瘤患者，应当从癌变过程中的病因学、病理发生学、病理学、遗传学、免疫学和生物化学角度考虑，并从人文主义角度将患者视作一位和这种可怕疾病抗争的战友。

肿瘤内科学家的培训最初是在癌症研究所、血液科和药理学系开展。美国内科学委员会在 1971 年将肿瘤内科学确定为一个独立的学科[1]。肿瘤内科学家和血液学家对造血组织的肿瘤疾病具有重叠的兴趣，并且在培养上述两个领域的亚专科医生方面具有共同的历史兴趣。但是，由于每个学科变得更加复杂，个体化的培训计划已成为首选方法。

本章我们将介绍肿瘤内科学并定义这一亚专业临床实践中的重要原则。

原则

某些原则蕴含在肿瘤内科学实施过程中，如表 45-1 所示。尽管这些原则虽然不是数学上推导出的或经过严格的验证，但仍然可供那些没有经验的年轻医生和经验丰富的老专家参考。

表 45-1　肿瘤内科学的原则

癌症治疗应当是多学科的，需要其他相关同行共同讨论
对癌症需要敏锐的临床思考和组织学检查证实
预防优于治疗
癌症内科治疗的基础是对药物作用机制、可能发生的不良反应，药物耐药机制的明确知识和对治疗原则的充分了解
早期癌症患者比晚期更能达到根治。初次治疗比二线治疗效果更好
最好的治疗多数是通过临床试验发现的
癌症的监测必须根据一定设想
癌症患者需要终身获得肿瘤学照顾

癌症的治疗是多学科的，需要和有关亚专业同道协商

肿瘤内科学的成功取决于能否与其他学科特别是肿瘤外科学、肿瘤放射治疗学、泌尿学、骨外科学、放射学和病理学的高效合作。另外，与肿瘤护理学、肿瘤精神病学、肿瘤神经病学、妇科肿瘤学、康复医学的合作也十分重要，对于低龄的患者还需要和儿童肿瘤专家合作。癌症治疗中最常见的并发症是感染疾病和近年来出现的自身免疫疾病，这需要联合感染科和风湿免疫科专家共同处理。目前，由于很多患者可以长期存活，肿瘤内科学家需要与基层医师合作以随访患者，有时还需要与心理学家和精神病学家配合。有时还需要处理这些长期存活患者的复杂问题和治疗后遗症。

肿瘤内科学家常常需要参与患者治疗的最后决策，例如手术和放疗的时机，是否进行根治性或姑息性处理？是否观察等待，还是进行积极治疗？都需要征询肿瘤内科学家的意见。多数患者在确诊为癌症以前都经过其他医师看过，包括家庭医师和实习医师，他们将患者转给肿瘤内科学家或其他专家。肿瘤内科学家必须认识到他们对多系统疾病患者管理的兴趣和持续作用，并与他们进行有效沟通。如果缺少他们，肿瘤内科学家就必须处理所有的内科问题。本书包括各种疾病的详细描述、治疗方法、药理学、免疫学、神经病学、精神病学、生物化学、流行病学以及分子生物学和癌症导致的并发症等。同时还包括癌症急症、康复和肿瘤学专家和医学信息科学及政府的关系等。熟悉以上问题就构成了肿瘤内科学的原则。

考虑到癌症是基于临床智慧，而诊断则依据组织检查

肿瘤内科学家首先必须是一个能够胜任癌症诊断、排除和治疗的内科医师。很多疾病的症状和体征可以很像癌症，因此肿瘤内科学家就必须熟悉癌症以外的其他疾病。相反，内科学家和肿瘤内科学家也必须知道癌症像过去的梅毒一样是“最大的伪装者”，因此在各种情况下都应当在鉴别诊断中考虑癌症的可能性[2]。肿瘤内科学家必须认识到，癌症的病理生理学、遗传易感性、分子亚型和基础药理学是癌症有效治疗的基石。所有癌症患者并不完全相同，诊断相同而生物行为各异。越来越多的资料表明，癌症可以分为许多不同的分子亚型，各种分子亚型的预后和对治疗都有微妙的差异。正如白血病和淋巴瘤那样，更精细的分型能改善治疗的疗效。高效诊断检测的临床应用可以识别对治疗反应不同的实体肿瘤亚组，促进了导致当今治疗的改善。

对于过去患过癌症的患者，有时会新出现一些复杂的综合征，例如肺功能不全、脑膜脑病或难于定性的疼痛等，必须有客

观的标准能说明是癌症引起的,否则不能简单都归咎为癌症。因为癌症患者也可以患其他疾病,例如肺纤维化、中枢神经系统疾病或疼痛性疾病,如椎间盘突出。若没有确凿的证据,任何症状不可归因于癌症,但每次都必须怀疑是否由癌症引起。

为了确定这些发现是由癌症引起的,需要病理学检查证实。现代肿瘤内科学家需要了解癌症和癌前病变的组织病理学表现,还要有复杂的核酸序列(DNA 和 RNA)谱、基因转录、蛋白质翻译和染色体异常等方面的知识,才能适当地诊断和处理患者。这些进展将有可能让我们知道哪些是容易发生癌症的高危人群,还有哪些患者或被认为已经治愈的患者由于肿瘤微小残留容易复发。也有例外,那就是肿瘤内科学家可以在没有病理学诊断时开始治疗,这就是肿瘤学急症,例如脊髓压迫、上腔静脉压迫综合征。但这些情况通过现代的影像和活检技术常可以很快安全获得组织学诊断。细胞学诊断在具有明确临床综合征的患者提供足够的依据。但是,支气管、胃、子宫颈和体液的细胞学可以有一定假阳性,所以确诊十分重要。循环肿瘤细胞和游离肿瘤 DNA 的使用可以帮助诊断和监测患者,但是这些替代方法还没有得到充分验证。在特殊情况,例如颅内、胸内或腹腔等体腔肿瘤,活检有时会导致一定风险,具有高度特异性的生化和分子标记物很有帮助。但是,如有可能最好取得组织学证据。

癌症患者的处理需要了解肿瘤的遗传学、生物学和药理学以及社会心理学在癌症的发生或诊断过程中对患者和医师的影响

肿瘤内科学的实施需要医师的智慧、敏感和足智多谋。最好是在当患者相对来说无症状的时候发现癌症。这样,可以让患者知道在发现癌症以前已经患有癌症,能鼓舞患者证明癌症并不意味着即将或一定导致死亡。肿瘤内科学家可以强调癌症需要长期的演变,从有致癌物刺激,遗传突变,具有生存优势的细胞选择和发生癌症的几个阶段。由于这样的过程很长需要几年或几十年,认识这样的过程很有价值。平均来说一个恶性细胞需要 5 年以上,倍增 30 次才能达到 1cm(10 亿细胞)大小的肿块。特别是对于需要患者及时做出决定手术、放疗或后来时有这样的知识很重要,因为等待 1~2 周获得足够的数据和建议,对患者很可能并没有负面影响。相反,某些恶性肿瘤如急性髓性白血病,需要立即采取治疗,因为诊断时即存在近乎致命的 10^{12} 恶性细胞。

越来越多的证据表明,由于微妙的基因组学和表观基因组学改变,个体被认为具有癌症的遗传易感性。肿瘤学家应当综合考虑癌症诊断、采取的干预对患者和家属的影响。有的患者和家属可能很敏感因此情绪很不稳定。有些癌症和癌症预防可能是慢性过程,正如糖尿病或高血压的处理一样。同样,肿瘤学家必须认识环境暴露可以增加患癌的风险,应当采取措施降低这样的影响。

肿瘤内科学家应当区分哪些癌症是可以治愈的,哪些是目前尚不能治愈的("将可治愈的")。如果早期发现,大多数癌症都是可以治愈的;如果发现较晚,大多数癌症都是无法治愈的。前者可能由少数基因组改变驱动并且局限于一个或两个关键途径,而后者可能在若干途径中存在多个变化,这使得治疗成功的可能性降低。因此,肿瘤内科学家必须认识到预防、筛查和早期发现的重要性,并且必须积极地教育同行和患者。

正是由于我们对肿瘤生物学的了解越来越深入,鼓舞我们相信未来总会有一天所有癌症都将预防或根治。过去多数人认为癌症一旦有了转移就意味着不能根治,但从高剂量甲氨蝶呤治愈转移性绒毛膜上皮癌后[3,4],这种观念首次被打破。目前能够通过内科治疗获得根治的癌症已经很多(表 45-2)。还有一些虽然单独内科治疗不能治愈但和手术、放疗适当结合也能达到根治(表 45-3)。

表 45-2 可以通过化疗根治的肿瘤

绒毛膜癌
儿童急性淋巴细胞白血病
Burkitt 淋巴瘤
霍奇金病
急性早幼粒细胞白血病
大滤泡中心细胞淋巴瘤
睾丸胚胎癌
毛细胞白血病

表 45-3 通过与手术、放疗联合可以治愈的肿瘤[a]

加区域性治疗
肾母细胞瘤(Wilms 瘤)
骨肉瘤
尤文(Ewing)瘤
胚胎性横纹肌肉瘤
乳腺癌
小细胞肺癌
上气道和上消化道鳞状细胞癌[b]
卵巢腺癌
没有区域治疗的胸腺瘤
成人急性淋巴细胞白血病
急性粒细胞白血病
淋巴瘤某些亚型

[a] 定义是单独化疗的治愈率<50%,化疗加区域性治疗疗效明显优于单独区域性治疗(即化疗只能消灭微小转移病灶)。

[b] 多数的治愈率<50%。

患者的疗效常常受到就诊时一般状况的影响。肿瘤学家有责任识别癌症可能复发和转移的征象。因此,肿瘤内科学家必须了解患者、家属和病历、X 线片、病理片和其他重要的原始资料。很重要的一点是了解患者如何无偏见地做出最后决定。此外,还需要知道患者和家属在评估肿瘤情况时可能会有哪些行为方面的改变。例如,当发现肺部结节有可能是恶性,患者和家属都很"恐慌"的时候,就是规劝他们戒烟的最好时机[5]。癌症的诊断会导致超乎寻常的情绪负担。第一次将诊断、侵犯范围告知患者时,根据患者的态度和表现出的弱点等,肿瘤内科学家应该向患者提出建议,并且将这些情况告知其他可能接触该患者的医师。

向患者解释病情、可能的治疗和其他有关处理,必须根据

该患者的知识和情感状况个体化对待。永远不要对患者说谎，对于不能一下子接受全部诊断和处理的患者，可以逐步向患者说明全部病情。“你的患者无权知道你所知道的全部事实，正像你不必告诉他你葫芦里都有什么药一样”是一百多年前福尔摩斯人道、合乎伦理的原则[6]。扭曲事实或否认一些事实，例如有没有转移都是不诚实的。同样，否认事实告诉患者是良性或能治愈，以致患者没有机会做出最好决定，也是违背患者自己、家属、宗教信仰和法律的。家属坚持说患者不能承受往往造成双重错误：常常患者早已知道或已经察觉你们不让他知道病情，这样患者会把自己的预后和从其他患者来获得的信息不加分析地联系在一起。大家应当读一下托尔斯泰的著作《伊凡・伊里奇之死》，就可以让任一对此存在怀疑的肿瘤学家了解不确定所带来的恐惧和患者直接、诚实但人道、亲切的交流价值。当患者问到“我还有希望吗？”肿瘤学家应当永远给予正面回答。希望是人类特有的性格，支撑继续努力，毋庸置疑所有肿瘤学家和患者都希望有较好的结局。

治疗致命性疾病对医护人员也能造成损伤。在完成重要任务时遭遇障碍会有失落感，特别是在知识型任务和隐形障碍。如果肿瘤学家面对的是一种致命性疾病而自己又缺少有效办法。特别是在短期内有年轻或与自己熟悉的患者由于复发或对治疗抗拒而连续死亡时，对肿瘤学家的影响更强烈。会导致一种无能为力的挫折感，甚至抑郁。经常遭遇这种挫折可能使医师崩溃。

我们知道目前很多癌症还不能治愈。明确肿瘤内科学家能在实践和概念方面可能解决这一复杂问题，就可以减轻自己的困惑。我们的公民们对癌症研究，无论是基础研究还是临床研究，都很尊敬。综合治疗的概念“我是团队的一个成员”可能减轻已经竭尽全力但以悲剧结局告终导致的自责。共同战斗的其他同志之间的友情也会让我们克服失败的情绪，因为我们的武器过于原始。其他肿瘤学家会理解内科医师的伤痛，因为大家可能都会遭遇相同的困境。

应当从长远角度来看我们目前遇到的挫折，我们正在为克服目前的困境而努力。参与系统的学术研究，无论是学院式的或是医学教育的延续，肿瘤学会、地方协作组织等都可以提供在学术方面的安全感。肿瘤内科学家应当具有健全的理念和健全的身体，意味着休息、锻炼、营养和乐趣。要达到乐趣，前面三项是先决条件。业余爱好和休假，包括短期休息和锻炼，是良好心理健康的组成部分。

最后，广大肿瘤学家还可以从很多继续教育课程受益，包括医学中心组织的、通过网络以及全国性会议，例如美国临床肿瘤学会、美国血液学会和像《肿瘤医学》这一类的教科书等。

预防胜于治疗

John Hopkins 医学院的 Bert Vogelstein 医师创新性的工作表明：从正常上皮细胞通过化生、间变转化为肿瘤的渐进过程，遗传变异也同时逐渐增加，这一过程可以长达数年[7]。同样，慢性粒细胞白血病从慢性期通过加速期而变成急性期，需要更多的染色体和遗传基因的异常。对于环境致癌物的暴露，例如最常见的因为尼古丁成瘾导致的吸烟，可以显著加速支气管黏膜癌变的过程。这些突变活化复杂的信号通路，打破细胞活化和抑制之间的正常平衡，使细胞增殖失控。而且毋庸置疑，很多这样的分子变异也会使癌症对治疗抗拒。正是如此，癌症诊断、治疗越早，效果越好。此外，这样的癌变过程为干预提供了大量时间，可以预防易感个体的癌症形成，即所谓的疾病拦截。

非甾体抗炎药抑制肠上皮内的环氧化酶，能够预防大肠癌的发生[8,9]。乙肝疫苗已经降低过去在东方最常见的肝炎病毒导致的慢性炎性反应和细胞损伤造成的肝癌的发病率[10]。丙型肝炎的新治疗方法也降低肝癌的发生[11]。维 A 酸能降低重度吸烟患者第二个原发癌的发病率[12]；他莫昔芬和雷洛昔芬能预防高危患者乳腺癌的发病[13]。小的外科手术干预，例如结肠多发性息肉切除[14]和原位子宫颈癌环状电切手术[15]能分别预防结肠癌和子宫颈癌的发生。

不但如此，肿瘤内科学家还要决定高危人群是否应当进行内科或外科预防治疗。最终将延伸至细微的遗传学变异，例如单核苷酸多态性和循环生物标记物等。此外，对于预防性药物需要长期监视，因为一般需要每日服用数年。目前，肿瘤内科学家需要决定哪些人群需要应用他莫昔芬预防乳腺癌、维 A 酸预防头颈部癌、口服避孕药预防卵巢癌。肿瘤内科学家时常建议患者，关于具有 BRCA1 和 BRCA2 突变妇女双侧卵巢切除和乳腺切除的获益。同样，肿瘤学家应当明确乙肝疫苗预防肝癌，人乳头瘤病毒疫苗预防子宫颈癌的效果[16]。肿瘤学家也必须对治疗尼古丁成瘾的各种临床症状起到主导作用，并且教育医师和公众通过适当的筛查做到早期发现的重要性。

肿瘤内科学家应当向患者和家属说明好的营养和健康性行为以及对某些癌症现有的筛查检测方法。本书有几章是关于预防和早期发现的，美国国立癌症研究所（NCI）和美国癌症协会（ACS）有很多关于这些问题的出版物可以提供给患者和他们的家属。NCI 癌症信息服务部（800-4-CANCER）和 ACS 全国癌症信息中心（800-ACS-2345）可以免费提供这些资料，也可以在他们的网站获得。

发展中的癌症治疗

癌症化疗的起源始于观察到芥子气衍生物，如氮芥，可以治疗淋巴瘤患者，随后发现靶向 DNA 合成（抗代谢物）和微管功能（长春花生物碱和紫杉醇）的生化途径，然后发展到联合化疗及靶向治疗的时代。这些新药可能比传统的靶向 DNA 或微管的癌症化疗药物毒性低。

适当地应用这些新靶向治疗就需要对于一般恶变的分子通路以及每个患者肿瘤细胞的具体通路有一定的了解。最近这样的范例很多，包括伊马替尼通过慢性粒细胞白血病慢性期的致癌转化蛋白（Bcr-Abl）[17]；吉非替尼治疗非小细胞肺癌的靶点是患者表皮生长因子受体的突变[18]；资料表明，厄罗替尼对表皮生长因子受体突变的非小细胞肺癌具有生存获益[19]；曲妥珠单抗对 HER-2/neu 癌基因有过度表达的转移性乳腺癌有效[20]；西妥昔单抗治疗大肠癌的靶点是表皮生长因子受体[21]；贝伐单抗治疗大肠癌的靶点是血管上皮生长因子受体和阻断新生血管生成[22]；维罗非尼能够抑制黑色素瘤患者突变的 BRAF 基因[23]。

今天，我们正处于免疫肿瘤学的现代时代。这一时代始于 Dr. Steve Rosenberg 在 NCI 的开创性工作，发现某些 T 细胞亚群可用于治疗难治性黑色素瘤和肾细胞癌[24]。今天，随着免疫检查点抑制剂(例如 ipilimumab)的出现,肿瘤内科学家面临一系列新的治疗挑战,因为需要额外的技能来管理自身免疫副作用。

此外,必须认识到耐药性的重要性,并在发生时识别它。对于复发患者在选药时则需要考虑可能的交叉耐药问题。有些天然产物由于和三磷酸腺苷(p-糖蛋白,MRPs)介导的转运系统而发生多药耐药表型。相同类型的药物(例如紫杉类)或序贯应用相同作用机制的内分泌治疗(例如芳香化酶抑制剂)疗效会有所下降。此外,肿瘤内科学家需要熟悉药物靶点敏感和耐药的突变,例如 EGFR 抑制剂,BRAF 抑制剂,abl 抑制剂和 BTK 抑制剂(Bruton's tyrosine kinase)等。

癌症患者的治疗包括应用对宿主的支持。对于肿瘤的作用,药物的产物对患者的正常组织以及对精神和情绪的影响,以及对疾病过程和患者本人的了解都具有重要意义。同样,也必须注意给患者合适的剂量和给药方法。医师应当对用药可能发生的不良反应,药物对正常组织的作用有充分的了解。此外,我们还需要了解药物对正常组织靶分子的作用以及药物和药物的相互作用以避免不必要的毒性。

正是有了有效的抗生素和血小板输注使我们很早就能治愈急性白血病;集落刺激因子(如 G-CSF 和 GM-CSF)对于药物引起的粒细胞减少,重组促红细胞生成素对药物引起的贫血都具有明显的效用。目前已经有改善血小板减少症的方法,而不再全靠血小板输注。

应用细胞因子收集循环中的原始造血(CD34)细胞,方便得到骨髓造血的前体细胞。因此,造血干细胞输注正在代替自体骨髓输注。新抗生素使粒细胞减少比过去安全,而预防性应用口服的抗生素和抗真菌药物能减少患者必须住院的需要。这些支持措施的进展使得我们应用设计剂量和方法进行化疗更为安全或不必降低剂量。

有效的抗呕吐药物使化疗患者比过去不那么痛苦。目前受到广泛欢迎的心理肿瘤学专业的出现,可以促进患者比较平静地接受根治性治疗或姑息性治疗。

静脉给药可能刺激静脉壁或外渗导致静脉周围炎,如果患者静脉解剖异常或肥胖反复穿刺或需要长期滴注,最好放置中心静脉管。这样可以减少多次周围静脉穿刺的困难和浪费的时间。惧怕穿刺是很多患者不愿接受治疗的原因之一,如果永久性置管就可以避免这一问题。

60 岁的老人多数会有其他疾病的治疗,因此开药时必须注意是否和其他药物有矛盾。因此,必须明确所开药物之间没有导致严重不良反应的相互作用。目前,医师都可以访问互联网查到药物的相互作用、药物说明书和如何监视疗效和毒性。肿瘤内科学家应用电子病历能够节约时间,通过网络计算剂量和医嘱,可以避免差错。这样的系统同时还能建立数据库,进一步了解发展趋向和未能预期的结果。

有的患者可以通过适当的手术、放疗和(或)化疗获得治愈。但对于已经有了广泛转移的患者可能就完全不能治愈。有的根治性治疗可能相对来说会导致短期毒性。在另一方面,有的保守措施目的是保存生成但不避免毒性;姑息治疗的目的通常是采取一定措施而不降低患者的生活质量,哪怕是短期的。同样,对于预防性治疗由于对象是无症状的人而且是长期用药,同样需要不影响生活质量。最近两个癌症预防的研究说明高剂量的环氧化酶Ⅱ抑制剂长期应用可以导致心血管疾病发生率增高,给制药企业带来严重麻烦[25]。

半个世纪以前哥伦比亚医学院教授 RobertF. Loeb 提出的一些应用于各种疾病的简单原则,似乎已经被广泛接受和应用。但是由于对癌变的深入了解,对于这些原则需要重新考虑。

例如第一个原则是"效不更方",如果好就继续下去。这意味着医师必须衡量任何干预措施对肿瘤和宿主两方面的影响。从治疗儿童急性淋巴细胞白血病的例子,长春新碱加泼尼松是特别好的诱导方案,但到了 1968 年人们提出一个问题,是否改用抗代谢物诱导疗效会更好?通过一组儿童患者在应用长春新碱加泼尼松诱导缓解以后随机分成两组:一组继续长春新碱加泼尼松,另一组改用抗代谢物。第一组患者很快耐药并复发,而第二组换用抗代谢物的患者则有的持续缓解和有些患者获得治愈(癌症和白血病研究组 B,未发布资料)。所以,Robert F. Loeb 的第一个原则对癌症并不一定永远正确,对这些患者序贯治疗方案可能特别重要。肿瘤学的根治多数和临床上潜在的肿瘤(微小残存肿瘤)生物学相关。而现实的临床表现并不能使我们看到。RobertF. Loeb 的第一原则可能对临床上可见的肿瘤比较合适。

治疗的第二原则是疗效不好应当停止。多数治疗方案成功的机会都不大,如果治疗 8 周还没有出现疗效就应停药;但有的患者治疗不到 8 周肿瘤就有缩小。尽管如此,在大多数情况下进行第二个月的治疗还是有利的,因为在影像学检查中,有据可查的肿瘤直径的早期增大或疼痛增加确实可以导致肿瘤消退,特别是对于某些形式的激素治疗以及免疫治疗。在停止治疗之前,应通过直接测量来寻找证据,包括循环肿瘤细胞和 ctDNA 的生物标志物,这些证据有助于决定停止无效治疗。放射性核素的骨吸收增加可能是骨骼愈合的迹象,甚至是先前未曾怀疑的病变,这不是终止治疗的合适终点。尽管进行了治疗,但出现新的转移性沉积物或先前发现的肿瘤持续生长,不宜继续该方案。

希波克拉底誓言中 Primum non nocere(首先是不要带来伤害)对在肿瘤学中应当重新评价[26]。因此,治疗的第二个原则不能延伸到毒性反应,除非是致命或严重致残的。现有的治疗药物很多都具有一定毒性,如果要求完全避免不良反应,那就意味着让很多患者等待着被肿瘤夺去生命。虽然有些高剂量药物治疗在杀灭肿瘤细胞的同时对正常细胞也有杀伤,但可以治愈一些肿瘤,还有一些可得到有意义的缓解。这样,患者都能恢复,有些肿瘤细胞可能就不能再生长。而为了避免毒性(有致命风险)而采用低剂量治疗,比为了最大限度获益而应用合适剂量患者所付出的代价反而更高。据我们所知,目前根治性和亚根治性化疗以及免疫治疗具有一定毒副反应,但导致患者死亡的很罕见。为了避免毒性而降低标准剂量,多数患者都不能获益[27,28]。对个别患者可以调整剂量但必须慎重,应当考虑采用其他能降低毒性而不降低剂量的方法。

第三个治疗的原则是"如果你不知道该做什么,就不要做"是避免不规范的治疗。有些情况下,匆忙决策或更糟糕地匆忙去做什么,会导致灾难性的后果。除了肿瘤学急症和某些白血病,由于时间紧迫,很少有机会观察症状和体征的演变或征询其他专家从新的角度考虑。但是如果患者有疼痛应当及时镇痛，其他治疗可以慢慢按规范制订。需要和其他疾病特别是炎症进行鉴别诊断的时候，医师应当明确延迟不会影响疾病死亡率或其他可能存在疾病的发病。不要把投入观察和会诊的时间看作浪费。在现有治疗的疗效较差或未知的情况下，应首先考虑进行临床试验。

治疗的第四个原则是"治疗永远不要带给患者比疾病更大的痛苦"这要用总的风险来衡量。肿瘤学专家知道，为了取得将来真正的疗效，患者需要忍受一定不良反应。患者可能看不到这点，因为有时药物的毒性症状可能比原来由癌症引起的症状还要重。肿瘤内科学家必须说服患者为了争取长期生存，需要忍受目前短时的生活质量方面的损失。说明这一重要问题是我们的责任。随着通过临床试验新抗肿瘤药物和无数新治疗方法的迅速涌现，越来越难评价哪些可能具有根治效果，哪些是姑息性的。当然在特定的情况，例如新确诊的早期和低度恶性病变和只能进行姑息治疗的终末期患者，决定就比较容易。对所有患者合适的目标是最大限度地争取最长的存活时间和最好的生活质量。有些患者治疗导致的毒性超过了可能延长寿命的价值，这常常直接和患者的年龄相关。由癌症导致的疼痛和行动不便有时会对治疗有利，只要有短暂和部分减轻患者就会觉得有效。但只是减轻将死患者的痛苦延缓死亡不是我们的目的，我们努力的方向是有意义的疗效。

肿瘤内科学家必须重视现实，并告诉患者哪些是可能的哪些是不大可能达到的目的。这样做的时候，往往符合治疗原则和人道，包括希望。

最后，肿瘤内科学家必须记住，不是患者对治疗失败，而是治疗对患者无效。粗心的使用前者表述在不经意间意味着对患者的不尊重，而对治疗无效患者的极其脆弱状态缺乏了解。

早期治疗治愈率高于晚期，首次治疗的效果优于二线治疗

由于目前还没有完全有效的预防方法，肿瘤内科学家必须推荐能早期发现最早可能存在的癌症的检测方法。包括乳腺X线摄影、结肠镜、粪便潜血试验、肛门和前列腺指诊、子宫颈巴氏涂片以及皮肤和口腔等看有无癌前病变如白斑和化生的痣。很快我们将有一系列生物标记物鉴定是否有早期癌症或癌前病变。例如原位导管癌、前列腺上皮肿瘤、结肠息肉和子宫颈上皮化生。前已述及，癌症进展过程会伴有基因突变或基因表达异常，导致细胞生存超过死亡。很多这样的改变可以使肿瘤细胞在恶劣环境特别是乏氧和低 pH 状态下生存。有些这样的改变也使更多的肿瘤细胞多治疗耐药。

以下情况说明，通常有些细胞株具有原发耐药或具有耐药机制。例如，对 EGFR 抑制剂初始有效后进展的肺腺癌患者可能会获得某些基因突变，这些突变使可能会导致这些激酶抑制剂无效[29]。这种现实使首次治疗显得非常重要。因此，肿瘤内科学家及其团队必须确保他们掌握了所有必要的信息，以便为初始治疗提供最佳选择。例如，对乳腺癌患者必须了解雌激素和孕激素受体的状态以及正确测量的 HER2/neu 癌基因，对非小细胞肺癌必须根据 EGFR，ALK 和其他基因组改变对其进行亚型分型。否则可能会影响初始治疗。同样，对急性粒细胞白血病首次治疗也必须具有全基因表型和风险基因表型的资料才不至于犯错误。而且，对伊马替尼的耐药和 P-糖蛋白和 BCR：ABL 基因的特异性突变相关。明确了这些变化，可以使用新药来克服这些形式的耐药性。最后，对肺癌和黑色素瘤患者的正确治疗方法需要根据分子分型来选择正确的治疗方法。

对于早期肿瘤负荷很低的患者的优势，使得医师和患者都能充分接受手术后或称辅助化疗的概念，当然我们也知道有些患者，即使不是多数，他们复发的风险和肿瘤负荷已经是 0。但术后辅助治疗已经说明在一些肿瘤，尤其是单手术治愈率较低的，能够提供治愈率，而单化疗不能治愈转移性病灶。乳腺癌、肾母细胞瘤（Wilms 瘤）和骨肉瘤都是这方面主要的范例。还有很多肿瘤辅助化疗能够延长无病生存时间和生存时间，例如Ⅱ、Ⅲ期乳腺癌[30,31]，Ⅲ期卵巢癌[32]和Ⅲ期结肠癌[33]。最近的资料表明对乳腺癌切除标本的转录谱检测可以帮助识别哪些患者需要辅助治疗[34]。

因为辅助治疗的目标是针对原发肿瘤的远处微小转移灶，术前"新辅助化疗"的结果已经在一些类型的肿瘤开展。这一治疗对早期微小转移灶可以起到作用以外，新辅助化疗还有两种意义：一是如果原发肿瘤缩小可以预测微小转移灶也会敏感，如果原发肿瘤没有无效，则意味着微小转移灶应当改用其他方案[35]；二是如果原发肿瘤缩小可以不必手术，而进行根治性放射治疗。在头颈部癌有些已经获得成功，大量乳腺癌患者也可以如此[36]。还有时候化疗后同样也能根治，手术技术可以比较容易。由于手术对于边缘细胞很难确定一定切净。诱导化疗或同步放化疗在其他肿瘤例如肛门癌，可以显著增加放疗的疗效，而减少手术的必要性。

过去，复发癌的治疗常取决于医师的经验而定。而相关治疗的疗效预测则随时代而定。例如，ER/PR 强阳性的乳腺癌一线内分泌治疗的疗效有效的几率大于 50%。而且缓解期也相对较长，可达 18 个月[37]。但在复发患者二线治疗的有效率减半，缓解期也较短[38]。如今，动态监测循环肿瘤细胞、ctDNA 以及二次活检标本的基因组分析有望帮助复发患者最佳治疗方法的选择。

最好的治疗常常是通过临床试验发现的

最常见和最致命的癌症，例如转移性肺癌、结肠癌、乳腺癌，现有的治疗通常不能达到治愈的效果。复发晚期的患者几乎很难治愈，甚至也不能看到疗效。而且，多种现有的治疗都有不良反应，只能有限地延长生存时间。虽然如此，多数患者还是接受标准治疗而不接受实验性治疗。很多时候，最好的治疗可能是能通过临床试验。

目前，越来越多的患者参与治疗选择的决策。他们通过网络获得广泛的信息。患者通常忧虑他们接受的不是最好的治疗，在开始治疗前可能恰当地提出一些具有挑战性的问题。肿瘤内科学家可以请教更有权威的专家，讨论这些试验是否能够改善标准治疗的效果，而不是仅仅相等。

必须确定患者现在是否能够治愈，不然会有很多伦理问题。对于不能治愈的转移性患者，参加系统设计的临床试验，接受研究性新药治疗不但合乎伦理而且重要，可以尽早参加。这样可以评价疗效，而不受传统治疗的毒性限制剂量。传统的治疗还可以导致耐药或免疫抑制。这些都可能对研究药物的活性有负面影响。

对于预后特别不佳，而且没有成熟治疗的患者，拖延应用毒性很小或风险很少的研究性治疗无论从资源投入和时间来说都是一种不智之举。这样剥夺了患者获得短期生存和得到裨益的机会。不成功的治疗比参加临床研究更具风险。

我们应当在开始和患者讨论治疗的时候就告诉患者临床试验的可能性。太多的患者未能从医师那里，而是从朋友或网络那里知道临床试验。对于转移性乳腺癌患者未经传统化疗就直接参加Ⅱ期临床试验和已知方案的疗效并没有限制差别[39]。目前，对于已经证明对细胞株有效并且在动物模型证明安全的分子靶向药物可以直接进入临床试验。人和小鼠的药代动力学有很大差异，所以即使是设计良好的临床试验也需要十分谨慎。如何确定新的靶向治疗药物应该和我们早期抗癌药物临床试验不同。例如，伊马替尼的Ⅰ期临床试验并未达到最大耐受剂量（MTD），而是根据“最大生物学剂量”即能最高抑制靶酶的剂量[40]。同样，应用动态影像技术如 PET（正电子发射断层摄影）可以在肿瘤体积变化以前预测伊马替尼对胃肠间质瘤（GIST）的疗效[41]。最后，一些新的药物在早期的临床研究中显示出令人鼓舞的疗效，将进一步促进患者及其医生参加经过恰当设计的临床研究。

因此，在所有癌症都可以预防或治愈以前，最好的肿瘤内科学家的标志就是让患者参加临床试验。目前还没有一定可以改善癌症预后或真正能预测的疗效的措施，所以开展研究是必要的。

临床医师不能像大学、研究所或医院的研究人员有那么多的时间和精力从事临床研究。但即使是全科医师也能通过协作组或与癌症中心合作参加临床试验，这样的机会不能错过。每个肿瘤学家应当在培训期间就参加临床试验。肿瘤内科学家的责任是和患者探讨参加临床试验而对最后的决定没有偏见。我们有很多理由期望临床研究进展能够更快，就像儿科肿瘤学那样，将研究作为治疗的一部分整合到肿瘤内科学临床实践中去。对于社区肿瘤学家同样可以像其他同行或学术中心一样通过电脑、电子邮件和电传很方便地获得信息参与诊断、预防及治疗的临床试验。有些肿瘤学家工作量太大，以致他们没有足够的时间参加临床研究，这样他们的患者就有可能无法及时获得研究新进展带来的好处。临床研究应当成为通往基础科学的桥梁，以及理解新的癌症分子生物学所带来的振奋人心[42]。

癌症的监测必须根据经过验证的设想

在完成根治治疗及获得完全缓解或辅助治疗以后，监测复发的早期征象是基于我们逻辑性概念，就是越早发现治疗的结果越好。虽然原则上是如此，但在临床上很罕见。有几种可能导致这样不合逻辑的结果，包括监测的实验不敏感或缺乏特异性，以及进一步的治疗无效，等等。对于复发率低的患者，有可能由于伴随的心理或身体的疾病，由于急着做出肯定的诊断而导致假阳性结果。但是对于有些类型的肿瘤可进行有效的挽救治疗，如生殖细胞瘤、大细胞淋巴瘤、霍奇金病、骨肉瘤、乳腺癌、前列腺癌等。如果这部分患者没有检测是否复发则是不可宽恕的错误。肿瘤学家必须明确检测实验，如肿瘤标记物、影像研究等的预测价值，并在相应的特异肿瘤应用。

多数国家，除了美国，都应用标准的定量诊断实验[系统国际单位（SI）]。如果不熟悉 SI 单位就很难读国际医学杂志。我们将具有代表性的列举在表 45-4 中，以便读者可以方便地对贯穿于论文中的单位（特别是美国）进行换算。

表 45-4 肿瘤学重要实验室检查的国际单位

项目	参考值	现用单位	转换系数	参考值	单位符号
白蛋白	4.0~6.0	g/dl	10.0	40~60	g/L
甲胎蛋白放射免疫测定	0~20	ng/ml	1.00	0~20	g/L
胆红素					
总胆红素	0.1~1.0	mg/dl	17.10	2~18	μmol/L
结合胆红素	0~0.2	mg/dl	17.10	0~4	mol/L
钙	8.8~10.3	mg/dl	0.249 5	2.20~2.58	μmmol/L
胆固醇	<200+	mg/dl	0.025 86	<5.20	μmmol/L
皮质醇	4~19	g/dl	27.59	110~520	nmol/L
肌酐	0.6~1.2	mg/dl	88.40	50~110	mol/L
纤维蛋白原	200~400	mg/dl	0.01	2.0~4.0	g/L
葡萄糖	70~110	mg/dl	0.055 51	3.9 * 6.1	μmmol/L
血红蛋白					
男性	14.0~18.0	g/dl	10.0	140~180	g/L
女性	11.5~15.5	g/dl	10.0	115~155	g/L

续表

项目	参考值	现用单位	转换系数	参考值	单位符号
免疫球蛋白					
IgG	500~1 200	mg/dl	0.01	5.00~12.00	g/L
IgA	50~350	mg/dl	0.01	0.50~3.50	g/L
IgM	30~230	mg/dl	0.01	0.30~2.30	g/L
IgD	<6	mg/dl	10	<360	mg/L
IgE	20~1 000	ng/ml	1.00	20~1 000	g/L
铁	80~180	g/dl	0.179 1	14~32	μmol/L
铁结合力	250~460	g/dl	0.179 1	45~82	μmol/L
低密度脂蛋白(LDL)	50~190	mg/dl	0.025 86	1.30~490	mmol/L
高密度脂蛋白(HDL)	30~70	mg/dl	0.025 86	0.80~1.80	mmol/L
镁	1.8~3.0	mg/dl	0.411 4	0.80~1.20	mmol/L
	1.6~2.4	mEq/L	0.500		
肾上腺素(去甲肾上腺素)	0~2.0	mg/24h	5.458	0~11.0	μmol/d
渗透压	280~300	mOsm/kg	1.00	280~300	nmol/kg
磷(无机磷)	2.5~5.0	mg/dl	0.322 9	0.80~1.60	mmol/L
钾	3.5~5.0	mEQ/L	1.00	3.5~5.0	mmol/L
总蛋白	6~8	g/dl	10.0	60~80	g/L
5 羟色胺	8~21	g/dl	0.056 75	0.45~1.20	mol/L
游离甲状腺素(T_4)	0.8~2.8	ng/dl	12.87	10~36	pmol/L
三碘甲腺原氨酸(T_3)	75~220	ng/dl	0.015 36	1.2~3.4	nmol/L
尿酸盐(尿酸)	2.0~6.0	mg/dl	59.48	120~360	μmol/L
尿素氮	8~18	mg/dl	0.357 0	3.0~6.5	mmol/L
香草扁桃酸	<6.8	mg/24h	5.046	<35	μmol/d

肿瘤学的终身照顾

良好的医患关系不应当在控制癌症播散失败时就终结。肿瘤内科学家必须熟悉姑息治疗的原则和方法，并与其他能控制症状的专家合作，例如神经病学家、精神病学家和临终关怀的同事们。如果能认识我们的责任是对患者终身照顾，这样在患者突然复发的时候就不会有被遗弃的失落感。

当然，我们也有责任和患者及家属共同解决临终计划。甚至我们对患者的遗嘱、律师的能力和其他事务也可以提出建议。这种责任在有些州尤为重要，因为美国这些州规定需要将 DNR(Do Not Resuscitate，放弃抢救)写在患者死前的医嘱单上。在这些州，如果没有这样的医嘱，护士发现患者显然已经死亡，由于法律规定，她必须作为急诊呼叫医师来抢救。

但多数时候，如果患者由于癌症逐渐进展生命力衰竭，我们已经无力使患者起死回生，抢救治疗无效而死亡的时候，这种过程就没必要了。抢救的努力应当针对那些并未预期会死亡还有恢复希望的患者，正如其他住院或门诊的患者，例如肺栓塞、心律失常、误吸和类似的可导致肿瘤患者意外死亡的情况。很多患者特别是老年和肿瘤进展的情况，可以和家属平静地讨论是否需要抢救，避免患者无谓的痛苦，也免得活着的家属遭受折腾。如果可能，多数患者会签署生前遗嘱或委托代理人办理。

由于涉及法律方面的影响，在获得特定宗教顾虑的地方或有些不能控制感情的家属不能接受他爱的人逝去，肿瘤内科学家就应当花费一定时间向他们解释这种意料中的死亡。DNR 表格是一些技术文件，也是医学进入新平台的组成部分。

肿瘤内科学家应当对每一个患者预先了解他们的意见，避免给患者、家属和医务人员带来不必要的伤痛和麻烦。也可以进一步避免任何患者和家属之间的严重纠纷。如果出现僵局，为了解决这样患者临终期难于解决的问题，有时可以请其他医师代替。

但是，DNR 医嘱并不意味不需要给患者死前的姑息治疗。如果能够清楚的判断对患者继续治疗只能给患者带来痛苦而不会有疗效，签署 DNR 医嘱后，则应停止积极的治疗。

总结

肿瘤内科学家正站在现代分子生物学和医学实践的交叉点，并通常是决定是否将癌症研究用于临床的最后途径。目前，有关的信息迅速涌现使我们对癌症发生过程了解越来越深入，并正在转化为有效的治疗、预防或支持治疗方法。

越来越多的研究说明：癌基因和抑癌基因通过正常自分泌和旁分泌信号通路而起作用；癌症不仅是癌细胞本身的疾病，而且依赖新生血管、成纤维细胞、平滑肌细胞、巨噬细胞、淋巴细胞等的支持。这样，也提供了很多不同的治疗新靶点。恶性转化实际是由于基因异常长期积累而成的多步骤疾病。这种认识可以指导我们制订合理的预防策略和对高危患者开展靶向治疗。针对这些通路的靶向治疗不但有效而且毒性反应比传统的化疗要低。这种对于基础研究的发现澄清了一些过去的无知。尽管今天我们很多肿瘤的内在本质还未十分清楚，但已经能治愈某些癌症。无疑，前途是光明的。

60 年前我们首次应用药物治愈癌症，目前临床成就也会同样获得突出成果。目前药物的数目越来越多，大批新的遗传工程类药物能提高机体的抗病能力，还有一些药物正在早期发展中。影像技术的发展将继续对癌症的早期发现、分期、治疗和监测做出革命性贡献。肿瘤生化标志物将提高癌症诊断和监测能力，并可能为治疗提供新的靶点。

近十年来，几乎所有的癌症在诊断或治疗方面都有一定进展。同样，癌症预防也有相当成果。肿瘤学家对维护人民健康必须承担更多的责任。我们应当重视推进生活方式、膳食和锻炼身体等大家都知道的措施。医学也需要政治支持才能迅速改善，例如提高烟草税等。多数州之间已经开始协调共同努力。但联邦政府在解决吸烟这一瘟疫的力度还不够。

我们离胜利还很遥远，但我们现在有着许多充满希望的前进方向，其中必定会有一条路能给我们带来超乎预期的成果。作为肿瘤内科学的基础信息表明肿瘤学进展得越来越快，具有启示意义的是将科学成就转化为临床实践。这些无疑都会给肿瘤内科学和癌症患者带来鼓舞。

（张宁宁 陶丹 译，石远凯 审校）

参考文献

1 Kennedy BJ, Calabresi P, Carbone PP, et al. Training program in medical oncology. *Ann Intern Med*. 1973;**78**:127–130.

2 Holland J. The diseases that cancer causes. *J Chron Dis*. 1963;**16**:635.

3 Hertz R, Li MC, Spencer DB. Effect of methotrexate therapy upon choriocarcinoma and chorioadenoma. *Proc Soc Exp Biol Med*. 1956;**93**:361–366.

4 Holland JF. Methotrexate therapy of metastatic choriocarcinoma. *Am J Obstet Gynecol*. 1958;**75**:195–199.

5 Mitka M. "Teachable moments" provide a means for physicians to lower alcohol abuse. *JAMA*. 1998;**279**:1767–1768.

6 Holmes O. Medical Essays, 1842–1882. New York, NY: Houghton, Mifflin and Company; 1891.

7 Vogelstein B, Fearon ER, Hamilton SR, et al. Genetic alterations during colorectal-tumor development. *N Engl J Med*. 1988;**319**:525–532.

8 Thun MJ, Namboodiri MM, Heath CW Jr. Aspirin use and reduced risk of fatal colon cancer. *N Engl J Med*. 1991;**325**:1593–1596.

9 Koehne CH, Dubois RN. COX-2 inhibition and colorectal cancer. *Semin Oncol*. 2004;**31**:12–21.

10 O'Brien TR, Kirk G, Zhang M. Hepatocellular carcinoma: paradigm of preventive oncology. *Cancer J*. 2004;**10**:67–73.

11 Lawitz E, Lawitz MS, Lawitz R, et al. Simeprevir plus sofosbuvir, with or without ribavirin, to treat chronic infection with hepatitis C virus genotype 1 in non-responders to pegylated interferon and ribavirin and treatment-naive patients: the COSMOS randomised study. *Lancet*. 2014;**384**(9956):1756–1765.

12 Hong WK, Lippman SM, Itri LM, et al. Prevention of second primary tumors with isotretinoin in squamous-cell carcinoma of the head and neck. *N Engl J Med*. 1990;**323**:795–801.

13 Vogel VG, Costantino JP, Wickerham DL, et al. Effects of tamoxifen vs raloxifene on the risk of developing invasive breast cancer and other disease outcomes: the NSABP Study of Tamoxifen and Raloxifene (STAR) P-2 trial. *JAMA*. 2006;**295**:2727–2741.

14 Thiis-Evensen E, Hoff GS, Sauar J, et al. Population-based surveillance by colonos-copy: effect on the incidence of colorectal cancer. Telemark Polyp Study I. *Scand J Gastroenterol*. 1999;**34**:414–420.

15 Boardman LA, Steinhoff MM, Shackelton R, et al. A randomized trial of the Fischer cone biopsy excisor and loop electrosurgical excision procedure. *Obstet Gynecol*. 2004;**104**:745–750.

16 Koutsky LA, Ault KA, Wheeler CM, et al. A controlled trial of a human papillomavirus type 16 vaccine. *N Engl J Med*. 2002;**347**:1645–1651.

17 Druker BJ, Talpaz M, Resta DJ, et al. Efficacy and safety of a specific inhibitor of the BCR-ABL tyrosine kinase in chronic myeloid leukemia. *N Engl J Med*. 2001;**344**:1031–1037.

18 Lynch TJ, Bell DW, Sordella R, et al. Activating mutations in the epidermal growth factor receptor underlying responsiveness of non-small-cell lung cancer to gefitinib. *N Engl J Med*. 2004;**350**:2129–2139.

19 US Food and Drug Administration, 2004. Available at: www.fda.gov division.

20 Slamon DJ, Leyland-Jones B, Shak S, et al. Use of chemotherapy plus a monoclonal antibody against HER2 for metastatic breast cancer that overexpresses HER2. *N Engl J Med*. 2001;**344**:783–792.

21 Cunningham D, Humblet Y, Siena S, et al. Cetuximab monotherapy and cetuximab plus irinotecan in irinotecanrefractory metastatic colorectal cancer. *N Engl J Med*. 2004;**351**:337–345.

22 Hurwitz H, Fehrenbacher L, Novotny W, et al. Bevacizumab plus irinotecan, fluorouracil, and leucovorin for metastatic colorectal cancer. *N Engl J Med*. 2004;**350**:2335–2342.

23 Sosman JA, Kim KB, Schuchter L, et al. Survival in BRAF V600-mutant advanced melanoma treated with vemurafenib. *N Engl J Med*. 2012;**366**:707–714.

24 Rosenberg SA, Yang JC, Restifo NP. Cancer immunotherapy: moving beyond current vaccines. *Nat Med*. 2004;**10**(9):909–915.

25 Masters BA, Kaufman M. Painful withdrawal for makers of Vioxx: pulling of arthritis drug raises questions on marketing, safety risks. *Washington Post*. 2004; Sect. A:1, 8.

26 Holland JF. Ethics for a clinical investigator. Non primum non nocere. *Am J Med*. 1979;**66**:554–555.

27 Frei E III. Combination cancer therapy: presidential address. *Cancer Res*. 1972;**32**:2593–2607.

28 Frei E III, Canellos GP. Dose: a critical factor in cancer chemotherapy. *Am J Med*. 1980;**69**:585–594.

29 Kobayashi S, Boggon TJ, Dayaram T, et al. EGFR mutation and resistance of non-small-cell lung cancer to gefitinib. *N Engl J Med*. 2005;**352**:786–792.

30 Early Breast Cancer Trialists' Collaborative Group. Systemic treatment of early breast cancer by hormonal, cytotoxic, or immune therapy. 133 randomised trials involving 31,000 recurrences and 24,000 deaths among 75,000 women. *Lancet*. 1992;**339**:71–85.

31 Perloff M, Norton L, Korzun AH, et al. Postsurgical adjuvant chemotherapy of stage II breast carcinoma with or without crossover to a non-cross-resistant regimen: a Cancer and Leukemia Group B study. *J Clin Oncol*. 1996;**14**:1589–1598.

32 McGuire WP, Hoskins WJ, Brady MF, et al. Cyclophosphamide and cisplatin compared with paclitaxel and cisplatin in patients with stage III and stage IV ovarian cancer. *N Engl J Med*. 1996;**334**:1–6.

33 Moertel CG, Fleming TR, Macdonald JS, et al. Levamisole and fluorouracil for adjuvant therapy of resected colon carcinoma. *N Engl J Med*. 1990;**322**:352–358.

34 Paik S, Shak S, Tang G, et al. A multigene assay to predict recurrence of tamoxifen treated, node-negative breast cancer. *N Engl J Med*. 2004;**351**:2817–2826.

35 Rosen G, Caparros B, Huvos AG, et al. Preoperative chemotherapy for osteogenic sarcoma: selection of postoperative adjuvant chemotherapy based on the response of the primary tumor to preoperative chemotherapy. *Cancer*. 1982;**49**:1221–1230.

36 Jacquillat C, Weil M, Baillet F, et al. Results of neoadjuvant chemotherapy and radi-

ation therapy in the breast-conserving treatment of 250 patients with all stages of infiltrative breast cancer. *Cancer*. 1990;**66**:119–129.

37 Sawka CA, Pritchard KI, Shelley W, et al. A randomized crossover trial of tamoxifen versus ovarian ablation for metastatic breast cancer in premenopausal women: a report of the National Cancer Institute of Canada Clinical Trials Group (NCIC CTG) trial MA.1. *Breast Cancer Res Treat*. 1997;**44**:211–215.

38 Robertson JF, Osborne CK, Howell A, et al. Fulvestrant versus anastrozole for the treatment of advanced breast carcinoma in postmenopausal women: a prospective combined analysis of two multicenter trials. *Cancer*. 2003;**98**:229–238.

39 Costanza ME, Weiss RB, Henderson IC, et al. Safety and efficacy of using a single agent or a phase II agent before instituting standard combination chemotherapy in previously untreated metastatic breast cancer patients: report of a randomized study—Cancer and Leukemia Group B 8642. *J Clin Oncol*. 1999;**17**:1397–1406.

40 Druker BJ, Sawyers CL, Kantarjian H, et al. Activity of a specific inhibitor of the BCR-ABL tyrosine kinase in the blast crisis of chronic myeloid leukemia and acute lymphoblastic leukemia with the Philadelphia chromosome. *N Engl J Med*. 2001;**344**:1038–1042.

41 Demetri GD, von Mehren M, Blanke CD, et al. Efficacy and safety of imatinib mesylate in advanced gastrointestinal stromal tumors. *N Engl J Med*. 2002;**347**:472–480.

42 Weinberg RA. The biology of cancer. In: *Garland Science*. New York, NY: Taylor and Francis Group, LLC; 2007.

第 46 章 姑息治疗和疼痛管理

Cardinale B. Smith, MD, MSCR

概述

姑息治疗是癌症综合治疗的重要组成部分。姑息治疗与缓解病症、延长生存和根治性治疗同步进行。姑息医学专家侧重给予多种照护帮助患者及其家属,包括控制症状、心理社会支持、医患交流。其照护目标涉及患者的病情、预后、价值观和偏好以及照护的转变。癌症患者常常经受着由疾病本身或相关治疗所带来的明显的症状困扰。姑息治疗的有益作用早已被证明。当姑息治疗整合到早期肿瘤治疗中,其与生活质量、抑郁、生存期的显著改善相关。正因如此,应将姑息治疗贯穿到整个癌症的治疗过程,无论是目的在于治愈的早期疾病,还是侧重于获得最佳生活质量的更晚期疾病中。目前,国内和国际组织的临床指南均推荐姑息治疗应常规整合到肿瘤的综合治疗中。

姑息治疗

姑息治疗是侧重于缓解痛苦和帮助那些患有严重威胁生命疾病的患者及家庭获得最佳生活质量一种医疗照护[1]。姑息治疗的目的是确认和设法解决生理、心理社会及疾病的实际负担,并作为额外层面的支持提供给重病患者。姑息治疗与所有适当的有效治疗和延长生命的干预措施同时进行。姑息治疗专家提供疼痛及其他症状的评估和治疗;应用沟通技巧与患者、家属和同事进行交流;帮助进行复杂的医疗决策,在确认和尊重患者意愿和目标的基础上设定治疗目标;促进医疗知情治疗的协调性和持续性;在医疗机构内和贯穿整个疾病过程中为患者、家庭陪护者及同事提供实际支持。癌症患者的姑息治疗应该始于疾病确诊之时。治疗的重心应该随着疾病病程演变而改变,支持治疗和症状管理应伴随着抗肿瘤治疗同时进行。

数个随机研究已证明,早期姑息治疗联合标准肿瘤治疗能够获益[2,3]。在这些研究中,姑息治疗显示能够改善晚期患者的情绪、生活质量和潜在的生存。因此,肿瘤学指南目前推荐将常规的姑息治疗整合到常规的肿瘤治疗中。2012 年美国临床肿瘤学协会(American Society for Clinical Oncology, ASCO)发表了临时意见,推荐对任何转移性癌症和/或高症状负荷的患者联用姑息治疗[4]。2013 年医学研究所的报告《提供高质量癌症照护》推荐,癌症治疗团队应重视姑息治疗、心理社会支持和适时转换到终末期的临终关怀[5]。

在为癌症患者提供有质量的姑息治疗时,应该包含一些核心内容。其中包括:

- 对患者的全面评估
- 有效的沟通
- 先进的治疗方案
- 症状管理
- 终末期照护
- 悲伤和居丧期的支持

患者的全面评估

患者的全面评估由美国国立综合癌症网络(National Comprehensive Cancer Network, NCCN)指南和国家质量论坛上所详述的姑息治疗核心要素来进行指导,涉及全面评估癌症和癌症治疗对患者及家庭的影响[6]。除了常规的病史,患者的评估包括评估患者的社会团体支持及癌症的诊断和治疗对患者生活质量、精神和社交状态的影响,还要评估患者的治疗预期和治疗目标。通过对患者的全面评估可以增强医患交流,帮助医师了解患者对治疗方案依从性的潜在障碍。这种评估因多学科团队参与而得到完善,致力于所有医学、心理社会学方面的诊断治疗,帮助缓解患者及家属的痛苦。

沟通

有效的沟通是肿瘤医师与患者关系的重要组成部分,并有助于提供最高质量的癌症治疗。1998 年 ASCO 的一项调查研究显示,近 60%的被调查者每个月会有 5~20 次向患者告诉坏消息。尽管面对这么多挑战,仅有不到 10%的被调查者接受过正规的告知坏消息的培训[7]。在 2004 年 ASCO 年会发表的类似调查中,肿瘤医师报道,与讨论治疗目标相比,在骨髓穿刺活检时更容易观察、也更容易获得反馈[8]。缺乏培训对癌症患者和服务者产生负面影响。不良的沟通技巧会使患者减少参与决策[9]、错失用心回应患者关切的时机、患者讨论有关健康生活质量问题的意愿被忽视,并且增加了在生命终末期接受抗肿瘤治疗的概率[10]。反之,有效的沟通显示能影响到所期望的结果,如患者的满意度、治疗的依从性、减少患者痛苦和降低医生过度劳累[11,12]。

这里有关于如何传达坏消息与设立治疗目标的现行方案(表 46-1)[13,14]。这些方案适用于大多数情况,包括新诊断的癌症、癌症复发、疾病进展和过渡到临终关怀。沟通过程试图达到 4 个主要目标:收集患者信息以了解他们愿意听到的消息;提供符合患者需要和意愿的信息;减少情绪影响和坏消息接收者所经历的孤独感;制订与患者偏好相匹配的治疗方案。当与患者及家属交流时,最好采用开放式问题。例如,"你的希望和恐惧是什么?"以及"在你的生命中什么是重要的?"[14]。

尽量避免用可能发生意想不到后果的语言，如“我们没有什么能为您做到了”以及“您想让我们尝试一切可能吗？”[14]。相反，尝试如下语言，如“我们将尽所能给予您最佳的生活质量”或“我们将非常积极地处理您的症状。”此外，最好避免使用术语和委婉用语，取而代之是使用朴实、简单的语言。一旦确立了治疗目标，那么确立以目标偏好为中心的治疗方案比较容易。这里有一些现行的培训项目，用以对肿瘤学医师的特定技能进行培训，在表 46-2 中列出了可利用的资源。

表 46-1 告知坏消息和确立治疗目标的方案

推荐	备注
构建恰当的谈话设置	• 在谈话前确定最合适的参与者（家庭成员和提供医疗服务的人员）
	• 预留充足的时间
	• 在谈话前确定说哪些话
知晓患者和家属已经了解的信息	• “迄今为止，关于您的病情您知道哪些信息？”
	• 这些可以纠正任何错误信息，并主导谈话在他们已知的病情的基础上进行
深入了解患者和家属的希望和期待	• 帮助区分可实现和不可实现的目标
设定可实现的目标	• 基于现有临床病情的基础上建议可实现的目标和达到目标的最佳方式
	• 综合评定疾病缓解治疗的恰当性
	• 尽量用通俗易懂的言语解释为什么不能达到那些不可实现的目标
带有感情的回应	• 允许沉默和主动倾听非常重要
	• 让患者和家属表达他们的感情
	• 一旦他们表达了感情，及时使用一些回应话语，如“我能明白这对你来说有多么难过”
制订方案并执行	• 总结治疗方案以确保在谈话中你的解释和决定是与患者和家属一致的，以及通过这个治疗方案将如何达到既定目标
	• 制订一个继续随访的计划
	• 告知患者和家属你的联系方式，并告知他们如果有更多的问题或担忧可与你联系
	• 如有必要，再次评估并修订方案

来源：参考文献 13 和 14。

表 46-2 姑息治疗的网络资源

• www. capc. org：Center to Advance Palliative Care：学习基本姑息治疗技术的基础教育内容。向在建立或加强姑息治疗过程中寻求帮助的临床工作人员或医疗机构提供技术上的支持
• www. vitaltalk. org：帮助服务人员学习沟通技能的网站
• www. epeconline. net：Education on Palliative and End of Life Care（EPEC）：综合课程涵盖姑息治疗基础；免费下载的链接点及教学指南
• www. palliativedrugs. com：症状控制用药的详尽信息
• www. aahpm. org：American Academy of Hospice and Palliative Medicine：医师会员组织及其内部教育资料和公开出版物
• www. hms. harvard. edu/cdi/pallcare：Center for Palliative Care at Harvard Medical School：面向专业人员的教育课程及其他继续教育项目
• www. nationalconsensusproject. org：National Consensus Project for Quality Palliative Care：临床实践指南
• http://endoflife. stanford. edu/：Joint project of the US Veterans Administration and SUMMIT，Stanford University Medical School. 涵盖姑息医学的基础课程

预立医疗自主计划

一旦患者的治疗目标被确立，其应以预立遗嘱的形式来记录。预立遗嘱由两个重要部分组成：医疗护理委托书或医疗护理预立代理人和治疗指示[15]。通常所用的综合的预立遗嘱是生命维持治疗的医嘱（MOLST）或生命维持治疗的医师医嘱（POLST），其目前在超过 40 多个州正在使用或开展[16]。POLST 适用于癌症患者且预后评估为 1~2 年者。其特别提到了医疗的决策和选择，这些在不远的将来可能会涉及，包括心肺复苏、抗感染的抗生素、人工营养和补液，以及患者是否愿意再次入院治疗。此外，它可在医疗机构内通用。与传统的做法相比，POLST 似乎关系到更好地接受体现患者治疗偏好的医疗护理（减少住院和生命维持治疗），增进代理人理解患者目标和偏好，提高了记录偏好的普及性、清晰度和特异性[17-19]。重要的是每个癌症患者要有预立遗嘱，以利于避免困惑和矛盾，有备于将来的医疗，并保证患者的意愿得以遵循。

症状管理

癌症患者经历很多由治疗或疾病本身所引起的生理和心理的症状。症状管理的基本内容包括：①定期、反复规范化评估；②正确开具处方用药，包括安全使用阿片类止痛药、止痛治疗的辅助方法以及处理其他常见不适症状和综合征；③熟练地处理治疗相关的不良反应。目前在姑息治疗中还没有症状评估的金标准。虽然有几种评估工具，但是最常用评估工具是埃德蒙顿症状评估量表，它由9种视觉模拟评估量表或数字化评分量表构成，可联合评估大多数常见机体和心理的症状[20]。疼痛是癌症患者最常见的症状[21]。最常见的非疼痛症状是便秘、恶心和呕吐、厌食/恶病质、呼吸困难、谵妄和焦虑[21]。这些症状的处理将在以下章节讨论。

疼痛

国际癌痛研究学会将疼痛定义为：与实际或潜在的组织损伤或类似损伤相关联一种不愉快的感觉和情绪体验[22]。虽然疼痛的原因和损伤的类型多种多样，但疼痛的一系列复杂神经生理学现象可归纳为两大类：伤害感受性疼痛（包括躯体痛和内脏痛）和神经病理性疼痛[23]。躯体痛的特点是定位明确、间断性或持续性疼痛，常被描述为隐痛、虫咬痛、搏动样痛或痉挛样痛（如，骨转移）。内脏痛是由分散在心血管、呼吸道、胃肠道和泌尿生殖系统的伤害感受器所介导的。其往往被描述为深部疼痛、挤压痛和绞痛，常放射到某一表皮部位，这种皮肤放射痛程度轻微。神经病理性疼痛在临床上常被描述为烧灼样痛、刺痛或伴有放电痛发作的麻木感。癌症病史采集应包括疼痛主诉的描述，其包含患者对疼痛和强度的描述、性质、加重或减轻的因素、是否放射到其他部位、确切的发作和爆发痛情况。疼痛对日常生活、睡眠、情绪和情感的影响也应评估。

癌痛治疗策略的指导原则应包括：①详细评估患者的疼痛；②做出疼痛诊断；③理解治疗目标和患者的偏好；④制订和执行最佳的治疗和诊断策略；⑤不断地重新评估疼痛程度和镇痛情况；⑥专门提供另外的治疗策略。至关重要的是，不要因为患者感到“太多的疼痛”而使患者未得到充分的评估。已经制定了癌痛治疗的一系列规则[24,25]。世界卫生组织癌痛和姑息治疗大纲提倡三阶梯止痛治疗原则，其提倡首先用非阿片类镇痛［如非甾体抗炎药物（NSAIDs）］，然后滴定到弱阿片类药物以至强阿片类药物[23]。同样，NCCN疼痛管理指南提供了轻度、中度和重度癌痛的阶梯式治疗原则以及快速安全的阿片类药物滴定止痛策略[26]。癌痛治疗总则列在表46-3。癌痛处理分为药物治疗、介入治疗和心理治疗。

表46-3 癌症疼痛镇痛药物使用指南

根据特定的疼痛类型选择特定的药物
1. 阐明患者的疼痛：疼痛性质、部位、持续时间、强度和之前使用非阿片类或阿片类药物后疼痛缓解程度
2. 详细完成医学和神经学病史采集和体格检查。评估放疗、手术和/或化疗在疼痛治疗中可能发挥的作用
3. 评估疼痛的心理因素，了解疼痛对患者的影响
4. 根据患者具体情况选择合适的给药途径
（1）口服给药是最简单的给药方法
（2）不能口服或拒绝胃肠外给药的患者，考虑颊黏膜或直肠给药。对需要迅速提高阿片用量来控制癌痛的患者开始静脉间断推注或持续输注
（3）不能建立静脉通道或居家患者采用间断推注或持续皮下输注
（4）全身使用阿片类药物出现限制性副作用的患者选择硬膜外或鞘内给药
（5）住院或居家特定选择的患者使用PCA泵
5. 掌握现有阿片类药物的药理作用。根据患者个体化需求进行剂量滴定
（1）起始剂量至少是先前所用镇痛药物的等效剂量或略高于等效剂量，开始滴定
（2）规律给药（根据需要口服给药每次间隔3~4小时，静脉给药每次间隔15~60分钟）
（3）如果患者没有使用过阿片类药物，告知患者根据情况需要可使用阿片类药物
（4）根据按需给药原则，初始给予“解救药物”的剂量相当于常规24小时总剂量10%
（5）告知患者使用的是何种止痛药物，并要求患者报告过度镇静或意识模糊等不良反应。密切监测不良反应
6. 联合用药产生累加的止痛作用以降低副作用或控制其他症状
（1）掌握多种能增加镇痛作用辅助用药，如抗惊厥药、皮质类固醇
（2）使用神经兴奋剂降低镇静作用，如咖啡因、右旋安非他命、哌甲酯、莫达非尼
（3）使用抗抑郁药、抗惊厥药和其他镇痛药处理神经病理性疼痛
7. 预防并治疗副作用
（1）密切注意呼吸抑制，必要时应用纳洛酮（稀释剂量以避免急性戒断）
（2）使用神经兴奋剂对抗镇静作用
（3）使用止吐药抑制阿片药物的催吐作用
（4）采用个体化方案预防和治疗便秘
（5）通过更换镇痛药物治疗肌阵挛或使用抗焦虑药控制肌阵挛
8. 密切注意药物耐受的发展
（1）辨别药物耐受与肿瘤进展
（2）认识到无耐受极限
（3）如果目前使用的阿片药物剂量无法提高，可转换成其他阿片类药物
（4）如果出现一种或多种难治的副作用，可考虑阿片类药物转换

PCA，患者自控镇痛。

药物治疗是最常用的癌痛治疗方法。药物治疗的概要详细地列在表 46-4。选择正确镇痛治疗以达到最大限度缓解疼痛和最低限度的不良反应,轻度疼痛可从使用非阿片类药物开始。对于使用非阿片类药物,如对乙酰氨基酚、NSAIDs 和辅助药物(WHO 第一阶梯药物)不能控制的中度疼痛患者,可以单独或联用所谓的弱阿片类激动剂(可待因、氢可酮和曲马多),即第二阶梯止痛治疗。重度疼痛的患者应选择强阿片类药物(吗啡、氢吗啡酮、芬太尼、美沙酮、羟考酮、羟吗啡酮或左啡诺),即第三阶梯止痛治疗。在所有不同级别的癌痛中,针对特定的适应证可以使用一些 NSAIDs 和辅助药物。多种阿片类止痛药物应用于临床,见表 46-4。

表 46-4 治疗中重度疼痛的常用阿片类镇痛药物

	胃肠外/mg	口服/mg	转换系数(静脉:口服)	备注
吗啡	10	30	1∶3	阿片类镇痛药对比的标准用药;老年人用药剂量要降低
氢吗啡酮	1.5	7.5	1∶5	短效药物
芬太尼	25μg = 1mg 静脉吗啡	—	—	半衰期短,有经皮给药和经黏膜给药剂型
可待因	130	200	1∶1.5	常与非阿片类镇痛药联用,部分生物转化为吗啡
羟考酮	—	20	—	也可与非阿片类镇痛药联用,但后者有剂量限制性
羟吗啡酮	1	10	1∶10	无口服剂型
美沙酮[a]	—	—	—	—

[a] 美沙酮具有复杂的药代动力学和药效学特征,这使得确定等效镇痛剂量特别困难。在美沙酮剂量滴定和调整前应咨询有经验的临床医师。

阿片类药物的选择应基于患者止痛药物用药史、肝肾功能(见表 46-5)、副作用和疼痛严重程度来做出。短效阿片类药物通常用于阿片类药物的滴定或爆发痛时按需给药(必要时)。在有效、稳定的阿片类药物治疗 24 小时后,应考虑转换为长效剂型治疗。长效阿片类药物可以使患者血药水平更稳定,减少疼痛再发生,提高依从性,减少医源性依赖。给予患者的解救药物剂量应相当于常规 24 小时总剂量的 10%[27,28]。总之,阿片类药物剂量、用药途径和滴定应根据患者的医疗需要、治疗目标和不良反应情况进行专门制订。阿片类药物没有最小和最大剂量限定。阿片类药物剂量需要滴定至能维持患者的疼痛缓解和阿片类药物相关的副作用间的理想平衡状态。

表 46-5 肝肾疾病患者的阿片类药物使用指南

	肾脏疾病[a]		肝脏疾病	
	肾衰竭	透析	稳定的肝硬化	重症肝病
吗啡	勿用	勿用	慎用↓剂量↓频率[b]	勿用
		不被透析		
羟考酮	慎用↓剂量↓频率[b]	慎用	慎用↓剂量↓频率[b]	慎用↓剂量↓频率[b]
氢吗啡酮	首选↓剂量↓频率[b]	首选	慎用↓剂量↓频率[b]	慎用↓剂量↓频率[b]
		不被透析,毒性最小		
芬太尼	首选	首选	首选	首选
		不被透析,毒性最小		
可待因	勿用	勿用	勿用	勿用
美沙酮[c]	首选,但需咨询	首选,但需咨询	首选,但需咨询	首选,但需咨询
		不被透析,毒性最小		

[a] 避免肾脏疾病患者使用缓释口服阿片类药物和芬太尼贴剂。注意即使"最安全的"阿片类药物也是不可透析的。

[b] ↓剂量意思是剂量降低 25%~50%。↓频率意思是减少短效阿片类药物的常规使用次数,从每 4 小时 1 次延长至每 6 小时 1 次。

[c] 在开始用或调整美沙酮剂量之前,应向有经验的临床医师咨询。

介入治疗可分为 6 种主要类型:①痛点注射;②外周神经阻滞;③自主神经阻滞;④硬膜外和鞘内注射;⑤外科方法;⑥神经刺激方法。这些操作技术不在此章节中介绍,已在别处详细描述[29]。

癌痛的心理治疗包括精神疗法、认知-行为疗法和精神类药物干预。这些技术在以下 3 种临床情况最为有用:①间断性、可预测的疼痛处理（如操作相关性疼痛）；②活动诱发的疼痛处理（如运动时疼痛）；③慢性癌痛的处理[30,31]。

便秘

便秘被定义为干结的大便次数减少及排便困难。便秘是姑息治疗领域是一种常见疾病，并且超过95%的接受阿片类药物治疗癌症相关性疼痛的患者受便秘困扰[15]。便秘最常见的两个病因是阿片类药物不良反应和疾病进展。严重便秘能引起肠梗阻、肠穿孔，并能导致严重的并发症。对于中性粒细胞减少的患者，严重便秘可促进细菌穿过结肠入血，导致菌血症并可能诱发败血症。罗马标准对便秘的定义为出现2种或2种以上伴随症状[32]：

- 排便时至少25%的时间在使劲
- 至少25%的时间大便干结
- 至少25%的时间排便不完全
- 每周排便≤2次

便秘的评估应该包括患者既往的排便习惯、液体摄入、近期饮食变化、目前服药情况及全面体格检查，包括直肠指检，但中性粒细胞减少的患者需谨慎。此外，如果不能明确诊断，可以进行腹部影像学检查以证实大便的存在。

便秘可通过非药物方法和药物干预进行治疗。非药物的措施包括尽可能增加液体摄入及在结肠蠕动活跃的清晨、步行后和饭后30分钟常规如厕。药物治疗便秘可以通过口服或直肠给药，具体总结见表46-6。目前没有单一合理的泻药使用办法。最初的方案通常包括刺激剂，如番泻叶，每日1次或2次，并根据治疗反应调整给药。大便软化剂，如多库酯钠，常被开具处方，但在这种情况下并不有效[33]。无论开始使用哪种肠道治疗方案，都应个体化并根据治疗反应进行调整。需要重视的是，预防是治疗便秘的最好方法。在开始使用阿片类药物时就应开始使用预防性肠道治疗方案，并应持续至患者使用阿片类药物的整个过程。

表46-6 治疗便秘常用的缓泻剂

药物类型	制剂	起始剂量	作用机制	备注
口服				
润滑剂	矿物油	5~10ml/d	润滑大便表面，使其更容易通过肠道	不良反应包括类脂性肺炎和油性大便漏，255石蜡和氢氧化镁被认为最安全
膨胀成形剂	甲基纤维素、糠麸、洋车前子	糠麸每日8g 其他每日3~4g	增加大便体积，刺激蠕动	对轻度便秘疗效好。注意须至少摄入200~300ml水。虚弱的患者可能形成粘滞团块而引起肠梗阻 可引起胃肠胀气和腹胀
渗透剂（不被吸收的糖）	乳果糖	每日15~30ml	通过渗透作用在肠腔内保留水分	甜味可能不能被忍受。腹胀、腹部绞痛和胀气较常见
盐	氢氧化镁 双膦酸盐钠	每日2.4~4.8g	高渗透压化合物引起整个肠腔水分潴留，直接刺激肠蠕动	强泻药，大多用于内镜操作的肠道准备。可能导致液体和电解质紊乱。心力衰竭和肾功能不全的患者慎用
蒽醌类药物	番泻叶	最大量100mg/d	直接刺激肌间神经从而诱导肠蠕动	常与多库酯钠合用。可能引起腹部绞痛。疑为肠梗阻时禁用
多酚类药物	比沙可啶	每日10mg	刺激小肠、结肠分泌和运动	可能导致腹部绞痛
直肠给药				
润滑剂	矿物油灌肠	灌肠1次	用于保留灌肠以排空或人为去除嵌顿的大便	疗效取决于肠道保留油剂的能力
渗透剂	甘油	栓剂纳肛1次	通过渗透作用软化大便	
盐	磷酸钠	灌肠或栓剂纳肛1次	从粪便中释放结合水。可刺激直肠或远端结肠蠕动	可能改变液体和电解质平衡。心力衰竭和肾功能不全的患者慎用
多酚类药物	比沙可啶	10mg栓剂纳肛	促进结肠蠕动	活性取决于比沙可啶是否触及直肠壁
皮下给药				
外周阿片类受体拮抗剂	甲基纳曲酮	<38kg：0.15mg/kg 38~<62kg：8mg 62~114kg：12mg >114kg：0.15mg/kg （四舍五入）	在胃肠道选择性阻断阿片类物质与μ受体的结合	仅用于阿片类药物引起的便秘

恶心呕吐

报道显示 40%~70%癌症患者受到恶心呕吐的影响[34]。恶心呕吐能极大地导致患者和家属的心理困扰，并影响其整体的生活质量[35]。恶心是一种主观感受，其定义为想呕吐的不愉快感觉，并可能与自主神经症状相关，包括面色苍白、冷汗、心动过速和腹泻。呕吐是由于膈肌和腹部肌肉收缩导致胃内容物通过口腔强制性排出。恶心和呕吐的病理生理机制比较复杂，涉及四个通路（化学感受器触发区、大脑皮层、胃肠道的外周通路和前庭系统）。当这些通路受到刺激时，就能引发恶心和呕吐[36,37]。

恶心和呕吐的病因多种多样，但重要的是要明确原因从而选择针对性的有效治疗。癌症患者最常见的病因是化疗引起恶心和呕吐（chemotherapy-induced nausea and vomiting, CINV）和阿片类药物引起的恶心后呕吐、肠梗阻和便秘。一旦明确了恶心呕吐可能的病因，就应开始针对性的治疗。有一些指南用于指导抗肿瘤治疗患者的 CINV 的预防和治疗[38]。最常用方法是在明确病因的基础上，应用针对相关受体的最有效拮抗药物。这种治疗策略在高达 80%~90%的患者中是有效的。一些医生建议，不管推测的病因是什么，都可开始经验用止吐药物，如具有代表性的多巴胺受体拮抗剂[39-41]。目前没有基于发病机制的治疗和经验治疗之间直接比较结果。

治疗应包括针对缓解症状病因的非药物和药物措施。非药物措施包括避免强烈气味或其他诱发恶心的因素、少食多餐、剧烈呕吐时限制食物摄入[42]、采用放松技巧[43]、针灸和穴位按摩[44]。在化疗期间渐进性肌肉放松和心理意象引导也是能获益的[45]。全世界最常用的止吐药有甲氧氯普胺、地塞米松、氟哌啶醇、丁溴东莨菪碱和赛克力嗪。止吐药有片剂、口腔溶解片、静脉注射剂、直肠栓剂和皮下注射剂。应考虑选择合适的止吐药的给药方式以达到最大止吐功效。在表 46-7 中列出了止吐药物、给药途径及其性质。

表 46-7　治疗恶心呕吐的常用止吐药

受体作用部位	药物名称	剂量/用法	不良反应
多巴胺拮抗剂(D_2)	氯丙嗪	10~25mg PO q4~6h, 25~50mg IM q3~4h	肌张力失调，静坐不能，镇静和体位性低血压
	氟哌啶醇	10~20mg PO, IV/SQ 饭前和睡前或 q6h	肌张力失调和静坐不能
	甲氧氯普胺	10~20mg PO q6h, 5~10mg IV q6h 或 25mg 纳肛 q6h	肌张力失调，静坐不能，梗阻者出现腹部绞痛
	普鲁氯嗪	5~10mg PO q6~8h 或 25mg 纳肛 q12h	肌张力失调，静坐不能和镇静
	奥氮平	5~10mg PO 每日 1 次持续 5 天	
组胺拮抗剂(H_1)	赛克力嗪	25~50mg PO/SQ 或纳肛 q8h	口干，镇静，皮下注射部位可能出现皮肤刺激
	苯海拉明	25~50mg PO/IV/SQ q4~8h	镇静，口干和尿潴留
	异丙嗪（亦作用于 D2 和 ACH）	12.5~25mg PO, IV/IM 纳肛 q4~6h	口干，肌张力失调，静坐不能和镇静
乙酰胆碱拮抗剂（ACH）	格隆溴铵	0.2mg IV/SQ q4~6h	口干，视力模糊，意识模糊，尿潴留，肠梗阻
	Hycosamine	0.125~0.25mg PO/SL q4h 或 0.25~0.5mg IV/SQ q4h	口干，视力模糊，意识模糊，尿潴留，肠梗阻
	东莨菪碱	0.1~0.4mg IV/SQ q4h 或 1.5mg 透皮贴剂 q72h	口干，视力模糊，意识模糊，尿潴留，肠梗阻
5-羟色胺拮抗剂（$5HT_3$）	多拉司琼	100mg PO qd	头痛，腹泻
	格拉司琼	2mg PO qd	头痛，便秘，虚弱
	昂丹司琼	4~8mg PO/IV 或溶解片 IV q4~8h（最大量 32mg/d）	头痛，便秘，虚弱
	帕洛诺司琼	0.25mg IV 开始化疗前[a]	头痛，便秘
P 物质拮抗剂	阿瑞匹坦	125mg PO 化疗第一天，80mg PO 化疗第二天、第三天[a]	头痛
	福沙吡坦	150mg IV 化疗第一天	头痛，注射部位疼痛
其他			

续表

受体作用部位	药物名称	剂量/用法	不良反应
皮质类固醇	地塞米松	10~20mg PO/IV 每个治疗日	高血糖,胃肠道出血,失眠,精神错乱
大麻类	屈大麻酚	2~20mg PO 每日分次给药	眩晕,年轻者出现欣快感而年老者出现烦躁不安,偏执狂反应,嗜睡
苯二氮䓬类药物	劳拉西泮[b]	0.5~2mg PO/IV q4~6h	镇静,呼吸抑制
生长抑素类似物	奥曲肽	100mcg IV/SQ q8~12h 或 100mcg/h CIV	心动过缓,头痛,萎靡,高血糖

[a] 不能有效终止已经发生的恶心或呕吐,此种情况不推荐使用。

[b] 最适用于预期性恶心和呕吐。

厌食症/恶病质综合征

厌食症/恶病质综合征(anorexia/cachexia syndrome,ACS)的特征是瘦体重异常或过度的丢失。晚期癌症患者 ACS 发生率高达 80%[46]。ACS 通常是疾病进展的标志。一项由美国东部肿瘤协作组对参加临床试验的 3 047 名癌症患者进行的多中心回顾分析显示,患者化疗后体重比化疗前体重下降超过 5%,预示早期死亡[47]。体重下降具有独立预测价值,不依赖于疾病分期、肿瘤组织学和患者体力状态[47]。

ACS 治疗首先应关注控制其诱发因素。因为厌食是困扰大多数癌症患者的常见症状,所以药物治疗的根本就集中在缓解症状上。在Ⅲ期临床试验中显示,皮质类固醇和孕激素这两类药物是有效的[48,49]。尽管这些药物并不能延长患者生存期,但有助于提高患者生活质量。皮质类固醇,常用地塞米松 4mg/d(尽管可使用 2~20mg/d),可短期减轻癌症相关的厌食。这项研究结果也被其他的研究复制出来,并且泼尼松龙和甲强龙也同样被证实是有效的[50]。因为皮质类固醇食欲刺激作用的维持时间较短,并且副作用随着使用时间的延长而逐渐增加,因此皮质类固醇最常用于预期生存期不超过 6 周的患者。醋酸甲地孕酮同样能够以剂量依赖的方式改善食欲,起效时间通常在用药 1 周以后。以醋酸甲地孕酮的起始剂量 160mg/d 治疗,超过 60% 患者的整体状态得到改善。以增加体重为目的,醋酸甲地孕酮的最佳用药剂量为 480~800mg/d。仅有 25% 的患者在用药数周后见效[51]。醋酸甲地孕酮的不良反应呈剂量相关性,因此从低剂量开始服用并进行剂量滴定是非常重要的。不良反应包括深静脉血栓(尤其在与化疗同时进行的患者中)、水肿、高血糖和肝酶升高。大麻素(屈大麻酚的合成形式)也能改善患者的食欲,但作用有限,并且不能显著增加体重。一项屈大麻酚和醋酸甲地孕酮对照的随机试验显示,醋酸甲地孕酮组患者的食欲和体重增加得到明显改善[52]。联合使用屈大麻酚和醋酸甲地孕酮的疗效并不优于单用醋酸甲地孕酮。屈大麻酚不良反应包括镇静、意识模糊和感知障碍。

呼吸困难

呼吸困难是呼吸过程中出现的不舒适或不愉快的感觉。根据原发病灶部位、疾病分期和转移部位的不同,呼吸困难的发病率差别很大,范围为 21%~79%[53]。感觉呼吸困难是一种由多种病因引起的主观体验。呼吸急促和缺氧并不足以反映患者症状的严重程度[54]。许多中重度呼吸急促的患者并没有呼吸困难的主诉。相反,患者虽没有呼吸急促,却主诉重度呼吸困难。因此基于患者的主诉进行评估非常重要。治疗目标是缓解患者自觉呼吸困难的症状,而非纠正客观变量(呼吸急促和低血氧饱和度)。

治疗呼吸困难最常用的方法包括氧疗和阿片类药物。3 项随机对照交叉研究评价了使用氧气(4 或 5L/min)对比空气治疗呼吸困难的晚期癌症患者。其中两项研究评价了呼吸室内空气的低氧血症的患者,发现氧疗是更获益的[55,56]。第三项研究评价了非低氧血症的癌症患者,发现氧疗和吸入空气在降低呼吸困难程度方面无差别[57]。阿片类药物是治疗呼吸困难的可选药物。在呼吸困难的癌症患者中进行的几项随机对照研究证实阿片类药物有益。对于非阿片类药物耐受的患者,每 4 小时口服起始剂量为 2.5~5mg 的硫酸吗啡或其等效剂量静脉注射就能有效。对于已经正在使用阿片类药物的患者,在其基础剂量上再增加 25% 才能达到缓解呼吸困难的作用[58]。

终末期

死亡是每个患者都要面对的一个自然过程。大约 10% 的人是突然意外死亡的,而另外 90% 则是因为疾病逐渐恶化直至生命终结[5]。"两条路通向死亡"[59]。一条平常的路常见于大多数患者中,表现为意识逐渐减弱而导致昏迷直至死亡。另一条是困难之路,特征是表现为无睡眠、精神恍惚及躁动的终末期谵妄。这给患者本人、家庭及亲人带来极大的痛苦[59]。患者家属报告的在生命最后一周最常见的症状有乏力、呼吸困难和口干,而最痛苦的症状是乏力、呼吸困难和疼痛[60]。高质量姑息治疗临床实践指南强调,患者家属应该接受一些关于濒临死亡症状和体征的教育,而教育的方式应与其发育程度、年龄及文化程度相适应[6]。患者和家属可能仍然关注血糖或血压控制,这样的预防措施应该纳入预期寿命中。停用药物治疗常常需要对风险和副作用超过可能缺乏获益进行详细地讨论。最初应该尝试用最小有创的药物治疗;只有不得已时,才启用最有创的方法。在生命终止前的最后几小时会出现多种生理变化,以下总结了一些最常见的变化[61,62]。

1. 虚弱和乏力　当患者临近死亡时,虚弱和乏力通常会加重。患者会全天卧床,对包括与他人见面在内的日常活动缺乏兴趣。

2. 经口进食减少　大多数濒临死亡的患者缺乏食欲、停止饮水。很多照顾患者的人认为是患者"放弃"或者"饿死"。有必要向患者及其家属说明,在患者濒死阶段对食物和水的需要量是减少的。一些证据表明,长时间厌食并不会让患者感觉不适。一项研究发现,97% 的停止进食的濒死患者并不感到饥饿或仅在刚开始时有饥饿感[63]。有人提出,终末期的厌食症诱发了酮症,而酮症使患者感到安适愉快、减少了不适,这实际上可能对临终的患者是有益的[61,64]。两项关于晚期癌症患者肠外[65]和肠内营养[66]的荟萃分析研究发现,这两种治疗均不能改善患病率和死亡率,而实际上增加了并发症的比率。关于濒死患者是否需要补液治疗还缺乏直接的证据,并且专家的意见也不一致[61,67-69]。一些研究显示,胃肠外补液治疗可预防和治疗某些病例的终末期谵妄[67,68,70]。另一些研究认为,脱水与口渴这些不良症状有关[69,71,72]。仍有专家认为,这些数据并不支持脱水与症状相关,而且补液治疗并不能改善患者的舒适度[63,70]。晚期癌症患者死亡前数周的随机对照研究显示,与安慰剂组相比,症状、生活质量或生存无改善[73]。对每个患者进行评估确定治疗风险获益比是很重要的。即使进行补液,也要注意减轻口渴感并维持患者的舒适度,同时注意口腔卫生。口腔清洁可以用棉签蘸取冷的液体(如水、柠檬水或柠檬汁)来进行。

3. 谵妄　在高达半数的病例中可能找到谵妄的可逆性因素,终末期谵妄的治疗通常集中于以药物控制症状上[72]。要针对谵妄的症状进行治疗,同时应该尝试处理可逆的病因。尽管谵妄大多发生于生命结束前的最后几个小时至几天,但某些情况下经过治疗干预谵妄可以被逆转[72,74]。安定类药物是主要的治疗药物,无论对活动减少型还是对过度活跃型谵妄均有效。在这些药物中,氟哌啶醇是可选的药物,它具有镇静作用弱、抗胆碱能及心血管副作用较少的优点。谵妄治疗的常用药物见表 46-8。

表 46-8　谵妄的药物治疗

药物名称	剂量/用法	备注
氟哌啶醇	0.5~5mg PO/IV/IM/SC q6~12h	最常用的药物。可能会延长 QT 间期
氯丙嗪	12.5 ~ 50mg PO/IV/IM q8~12h	与氟哌啶醇作用类似,但镇静作用、抗胆碱作用和降低血压的作用更明显
劳拉西泮	0.5~2mg PO/SL/IV q4~8h,必要时滴定	最常与氟哌啶醇联用的二线药物。也可通过连续输注的方式用于需要高度镇静的难治性病例。可能会加重老年患者的谵妄。肝衰竭的患者慎用
利培酮	从 0.5~1mg/d 开始口服,滴定至 4~6mg/d	一项研究显示与氟哌啶醇相比,两者的副作用没有明显差别。由于只能口服,临床应用受到限制
奥氮平	5mg PO qhs 并滴定至起作用(最大剂量 20mg/d)	癌症患者对奥氮平反应不佳的危险因素包括:年龄大于 70 岁、有痴呆病史、中枢神经系统转移、缺氧、活动减退的谵妄
咪达唑仑	1mg/h IV 并滴定至起作用	最常用于需要镇静的难治性病例

悲伤和居丧

居丧是指由死亡所致的一种失落的状态[75]。悲伤被定义为面对失落和哀痛的一种情感反应,并常指与失落相关的社交措辞[75]。悲伤的类型有以下几种:预期悲伤、简单悲伤和复杂悲伤。预期悲伤是指在死亡之前患者和家属心中的哀痛,它有助于居丧期的调整。简单悲伤是悲伤反应的最常见类型,并在社会上被认为是正常的。复杂悲伤是指长时间持续存在的悲伤反应,它以不能恢复到丧失亲人之前的功能水平为特征[76]。姑息治疗在死亡之前、死亡期间和死亡后为患者和其照顾者提供悲伤和居丧服务,以帮助促进顺利地度过悲伤期。

临终关怀和姑息治疗两者都可以在丧亲前为预防复杂悲伤提供有效的干预措施。这些干预措施可以降低照顾者患重度抑郁症的风险[77]。由包括内科医师、社会工作者、护士、心理学家和牧师在内的姑息治疗多学科团队对患者和照顾者进行心理社会评估,从而鉴别出那些易患复杂悲伤的高风险人群。姑息治疗团队能够在患者死亡之前提供基本的实际帮助,如协助预立遗嘱、经济援助、鼓励看护者个体化医疗照顾,还有在患者过世后通过提供咨询服务或推荐其他的支持服务的方式来给予帮助。

临终关怀

临终关怀是一种关怀照顾理念。临终关怀的目的在于维持最好的生活质量,而不是延长那些预期生存期少于 6 个月的患者的生存时间。它与姑息治疗的区别在于,姑息治疗是与其他根治性及延长生存时间的治疗同时进行的。美国从 1974 年开始有临终关怀服务,并从 1982 年起作为 Medicare 临终关怀福利的一部分由 Medicare 提供资金[78]。

临终关怀是唯一的 Medicare 福利,其包括药物治疗、耐用的医疗设备和持续的全天候获得服务和支持。在患者过世后也可为患者家庭成员提供居丧服务。Medicare 临终关怀福利覆盖所有与癌症诊断相关的服务。患者仍能获得治疗其他疾病的 Medicare 福利。

大多数的临终关怀是在家中进行的。在其他地点也可以提供临终关怀,如住院临终关怀机构、养老院、疗养院和医院。据估计,2011 年美国所有死亡者中接近 45% 的人接受了一个临终关怀项目的服务,而参与临终关怀项目的所有患者中 38% 被诊断为癌症[79]。在一项对比接受临终关怀者与未接受临终关怀者生存的研究中,临终关怀能延长某些终末期重症癌症患者的生存[80]。接受临终关怀的患者平均生存时间明显延长:肺癌患者延长 39 天,胰腺癌患者延长 21 天,而结肠癌患者至少延长 33 天[80]。

总结

姑息治疗是一种以患者及其家庭为中心的多学科治疗,它关注为患者缓解痛苦和提供最佳的生活质量。这些患者不仅包括接受根治性和延长生命治疗的患者,也包括不再接受癌症特定治疗的患者。据估计,35% 的癌症患者将死于所患的疾病[81]。在肿瘤领域中,改善患者的生活质量受到越来越多的关注。这些患者不仅包括正在接受化疗的患者、生命即将终结的患者，还包括癌症幸存者。癌症治疗过程中可能会出现大量的症状。姑息治疗是癌症综合治疗不可或缺的一部分。确诊时就开始的姑息治疗是最有效的，使患者在整个病程中都得到关注。从诊断开始，肿瘤科医师就在讨论根治性治疗或姑息性治疗选择上起着关键作用。评估患者的目标是同样的重要。要让患者意识到，接受抗肿瘤治疗并不妨碍他们获得姑息治疗的帮助。越来越强调姑息治疗在肿瘤学中的重要性将改善疾病预后并减少一些肿瘤科医师治疗危重症患者的压力。

为了应对越来越多的重症患者、高质量症状控制的需求增加、渴望提高医疗协作和预立医疗自主计划的需求增多，在最近 20 年姑息治疗经历着快速的发展。自 2000 年以来医院的姑息治疗项目的数量已经增加了 138%[82]。姑息治疗教育的发展得到医学教育联络委员会（Liaison Committee on Medical Education，LCME）和毕业生医学教育评审委员会（Accreditation Council for Graduate Medical Education，ACGME）的支持。LCME 授权医学院校行姑息医学教育。ACGME 要求肿瘤专业的学生进行姑息医学的培训。大量的以互联网为基础的资源可供医师在实践中使用，帮助他们获取更深入的关于姑息治疗的信息和教育（表 46-2）。

（于晶琳 译，吴世凯 审校）

参考文献

The complete reference list can be found on the Wiley Companion Digital Edition of this title (see inside front cover for login instructions).

1 Morrison RS, Meier DE. Clinical practice. Palliative care. *N Engl J Med.* 2004;**350**(**25**):2582–2590.

2 Temel JS, Greer JA, Muzikansky A, et al. Early palliative care for patients with metastatic non-small-cell lung cancer. *N Engl J Med.* 2010;**363**(**8**):733–742.

3 Bakitas M, Lyons KD, Hegel MT, et al. Effects of a palliative care intervention on clinical outcomes in patients with advanced cancer: the Project ENABLE II randomized controlled trial. *JAMA.* 2009;**302**(**7**):741–749.

4 Shih YC, Ganz PA, Aberle D, et al. Delivering high-quality and affordable care throughout the cancer care continuum. *J Clin Oncol.* 2013;**31**(**32**):4151–4157.

5 Field MJ, Cassel CK. *Approching Death: Improving Care at the End of Life.* Institute of Medicine: Washington, DC; 1997.

6 National Consensus Project for Quality Palliative Care. Clinical Practice Guidelines for quality palliative care, executive summary. *J Palliat Med.* 2004;**7**(**5**):611–627.

8 Buss MK, Lessen DS, Sullivan AM, Von Roenn J, Arnold RM, Block SD. A study of oncology fellows' training in end-of-life care. *J Support Oncol.* 2007;**5**(**5**):237–242.

9 Beach WA, Easter DW, Good JS, Pigeron E. Disclosing and responding to cancer "fears" during oncology interviews. *Soc Sci Med.* 2005;**60**(**4**):893–910.

10 Detmar SB, Muller MJ, Wever LD, Schornagel JH, Aaronson NK. The patient-physician relationship. Patient-physician communication during outpatient palliative treatment visits: an observational study. *JAMA.* 2001;**285**(**10**):1351–1357.

11 Baile WF, Aaron J. Patient-physician communication in oncology: past, present, and future. *Curr Opin Oncol.* 2005;**17**(**4**):331–335.

12 Zachariae R, Pedersen CG, Jensen AB, Ehrnrooth E, Rossen PB, von der Maase H. Association of perceived physician communication style with patient satisfaction, distress, cancer-related self-efficacy, and perceived control over the disease. *Br J Cancer.* 2003;**88**(**5**):658–665.

13 Baile WF, Buckman R, Lenzi R, Glober G, Beale EA, Kudelka AP. SPIKES-A six-step protocol for delivering bad news: application to the patient with cancer. *Oncologist.* 2000;**5**(**4**):302–311.

19 Hammes BJ, Rooney BL, Gundrum JD. A comparative, retrospective, observational study of the prevalence, availability, and specificity of advance care plans in a county that implemented an advance care planning microsystem. *J Am Geriatr Soc.* 2010;**58**(**7**):1249–1255.

20 Bruera E, Kuehn N, Miller MJ, Selmser P, Macmillan K. The Edmonton Symptom Assessment System (ESAS): a simple method for the assessment of palliative care patients. *J Palliat Care.* 1991;**7**(**2**):6–9.

22 International Association for the Study of Pain. http://www.iasp-pain.org/AM/Template.cfm?Section=Pain_Defi… isplay.cfm&ContentID=1728, accessed 23 November, 2010.

24 Du Pen SL, Du Pen AR, Polissar N, et al. Implementing guidelines for cancer pain management: results of a randomized controlled clinical trial. *J Clin Oncol.* 1999;**17**(**1**):361–370.

25 Moulin DE, Clark AJ, Gilron I, et al. Pharmacological management of chronic neuropathic pain—consensus statement and guidelines from the Canadian Pain Society. *Pain Res Manag.* 2007;**127**(**1**):13–21.

26 Levy MH, Adolph MD, Back A, et al. Palliative care. *J Natl Compr Cancer Netw.* 2012;**10**(**10**):1284–1309.

28 Davies AN, Dickman A, Reid C, Stevens A-M, Zeppetella G. The management of cancer-related breakthrough pain: recommendations of a task group of the Science Committee of the Association for Palliative Medicine of Great Britain and Ireland. *Eur J Pain.* 2009;**13**(**4**):331–338.

29 Miguel R. Interventional treatment of cancer pain: the fourth step in the World Health Organization analgesic ladder? *Cancer Control.* 2000;**7**(**2**):149–156.

33 Hawley PH, Byeon JJ. A comparison of sennosides-based bowel protocols with and without docusate in hospitalized patients with cancer. *J Palliat Med.* 2008;**11**(**4**):575–581.

36 Wood GJ, Shega JW, Lynch B, Von Roenn JH. Management of intractable nausea and vomiting in patients at the end of life: "I was feeling nauseous all of the time…nothing was working". *JAMA.* 2007;**298**(**10**):1196–1207.

38 (NCCN) NCCN. Antiemesis. NCCN Clinical Practice Guidelines in Oncology. Version 1.2013; http://www.nccn.org/professionals/physician_gls/pdf/antiemesis.pdf (accessed 28 January 2013).

39 Stephenson J, Davies A. An assessment of aetiology-based guidelines for the management of nausea and vomiting in patients with advanced cancer. *Support Care Cancer.* 2006;**14**(**4**):348–353.

41 Bruera E, Belzile M, Neumann C, Harsanyi Z, Babul N, Darke A. A double-blind, crossover study of controlled-release metoclopramide and placebo for the chronic nausea and dyspepsia of advanced cancer. *J Pain Symptom Manage.* 2000;**19**(**6**):427–435.

49 Servaes P, Verhagen C, Bleijenberg G. Fatigue in cancer patients during and after treatment: prevalence, correlates and interventions. *Eur J Cancer.* 2002;**38**(**1**):27–43.

51 Loprinzi CL, Michalak JC, Schaid DJ, et al. Phase III evaluation of four doses of megestrol acetate as therapy for patients with cancer anorexia and/or cachexia. *J Clin Oncol.* 1993;**11**(**4**):762–767.

57 Bruera E, Sweeney C, Willey J, et al. A randomized controlled trial of supplemental oxygen versus air in cancer patients with dyspnea. *Palliat Med.* 2003;**17**(**8**):659–663.

63 McCann RM, Hall WJ, Groth-Juncker A. Comfort care for terminally ill patients. The appropriate use of nutrition and hydration. *JAMA.* 1994;**272**(**16**):1263–1266.

64 Musgrave CF, Bartal N, Opstad J. The sensation of thirst in dying patients receiving i.v. hydration. *J Palliat Care.* 1995;**11**(**4**):17–21.

65 Koretz RL, Lipman TO, Klein S, American Gastroenterological Association. AGA technical review on parenteral nutrition. *Gastroenterology.* 2001;**121**(**4**):970–1001.

66 Koretz RL, Avenell A, Lipman TO, Braunschweig CL, Milne AC. Does enteral nutrition affect clinical outcome? A systematic review of the randomized trials. *Am J Gastroenterol.* 2007;**102**(**2**):412–429; quiz 468.

73 Bruera E, Hui D, Dalal S, et al. Parenteral hydration in patients with advanced cancer: a multicenter, double-blind, placebo-controlled randomized trial. *J Clin Oncol.* 2013;**31**(**1**):111–118.

79 National Hospice and Palliative Care Organization. NHPCO's Facts and Figures Hospice Care in America. http://www.nhpco.org/sites/default/files/public/Statistics_Research/2012_Facts_Figures.pdf, accessed January 2015; 2012.

80 Connor SR, Pyenson B, Fitch K, Spence C, Iwasaki K. Comparing hospice and non-hospice patient survival among patients who die within a three-year window. *J Pain Symptom Manage.* 2007;**33**(**3**):238–246.

81 Siegel RL, Miller KD, Jemal A. Cancer statistics, 2015. *CA Cancer J Clin.* 2015;**65**(**1**):5–29.

82 Center to Advance Pallaitive Care. *Public Opinion Research on Palliative Care: A Report Based on Reseach by Public Opinion Strategies*; 2011.

第 47 章　心理社会肿瘤学

Jimmie C. Holland, MD ■ Talia W. Wiesel, PhD

概述

本章向肿瘤科医生介绍心理社会肿瘤学的现状，这是一个在过去 30 年里发展起来的亚学科。主要是对焦虑、抑郁和谵妄的基本治疗，包括药理学，以及基于证据的心理治疗干预。自 2008 年获得美国医学研究所（Institute of Medicine）的批准以来，这一领域已经成熟起来。该机构表示，高质量的癌症医疗服务必须将心理社会功能领域评估纳入常规。美国外科医生学会癌症委员会（American College of Surgeons Commission on Cancer）大力推动了这项进程。在 2015 年，该委员会将心理痛苦筛查列入标准质量鉴定，要求所有癌症中心都应该建立并推广此项目，以识别并分诊心理痛苦的患者。这极大地推动了所有新进患者常规心理筛查的发展，以确保心理问题得到早期识别和适当处理。在美国心理社会肿瘤学会（American Psychosocial Oncology Society，APOS）的帮助下，这些项目正在全美范围内推广实施。APOS 为癌症工作者组织了培训、咨询和持续督导。事实上，正是由于国家对于癌症相关政策的变化，现今的癌症患者在处理疾病时有了不同的感受。我们已经将重点转向以患者为中心的照护模式，包括对患者的整体照护。

精神病学术语似乎不能很好地描述癌症患者的情绪反应，他们正在寻找方法来面对一个压倒性的但却“真实”的现实。诸如勇气和力量之类的词语会显得更为恰当。

J. C. Holland，Cancer Medicine，1973，P992

简介

上面这句话出现在 1973 年的《癌症医学》上。在过去的 40 多年里，癌症治疗的人性化方面并没有改变患者的情绪。然而，现在有一系列的干预措施可以让患者坚持走完疾病治疗之路。造成这一显著变化的部分原因与心理社会肿瘤学的贡献有关。这些变化发生的原因可能如下：首先，评估量表工具的发展，这些量表作为工具定量地测量了患者的主观症状，而这些症状以前被认为是无法测量的。其次，利用这些量表进行临床试验，从而发展了有循证依据的干预措施。在 20 世纪 90 年代末，上述这些都被整合到第一版关于痛苦管理的《NCCN 肿瘤临床实践指南》（NCCN 指南®）中[1]。第三部分是美国医学研究所在其 2008 年的报告中第一次出现的声明，即全人管理，其中指出，心理社会领域必须纳入日常照护路径[2]。这个项目被美国外科医生学会癌症委员会提升到一个更高的层面，在 2015 年，该组织要求那些获得认证的癌症中心制定一项计划，来识别和转诊心理痛苦的患者以获得适当的治疗[3]。这使得心理肿瘤学家努力帮助癌症中心的多学科团队实施这项新政策[4,5]。在未来，患者会通过常规筛查程序更早得到识别。然而，新的流程给肿瘤学工作者繁忙的临床工作带来了更大的负担，但是这可以确保真正有心理痛苦的患者得到专业团队的治疗或转诊寻求更专业的心理社会照护。图 47-1 列出用于评估和治疗疾病的 NCCN 指南®，该指南建议对所有新患者进行心理痛苦筛查[6]。NCCN 指南推荐在繁忙的临床工作中用单条目筛查心理痛苦的患者（图 47-2）。临床工作中发现在提问“在 0 到 10 分的范围内你的痛苦程度有几分”这个问题时，对于患者来说这个问题是可接受的、简洁的以及没有病耻感的。这种提问就是“心理痛苦温度计”，它在国际上得到广泛应用，包括一个量表与问题清单，找出痛苦的常见原因。验证性研究发现，分数大于等于 4 分时应让工作人员进行二次评估来确定痛苦的性质，以及是否需要将患者转诊到精神卫生专科、社会工作者或神职人员那里。

本章主要概述了肿瘤科医生快速评估和管理最常见的精神科并发症所需要的基本信息[7]。

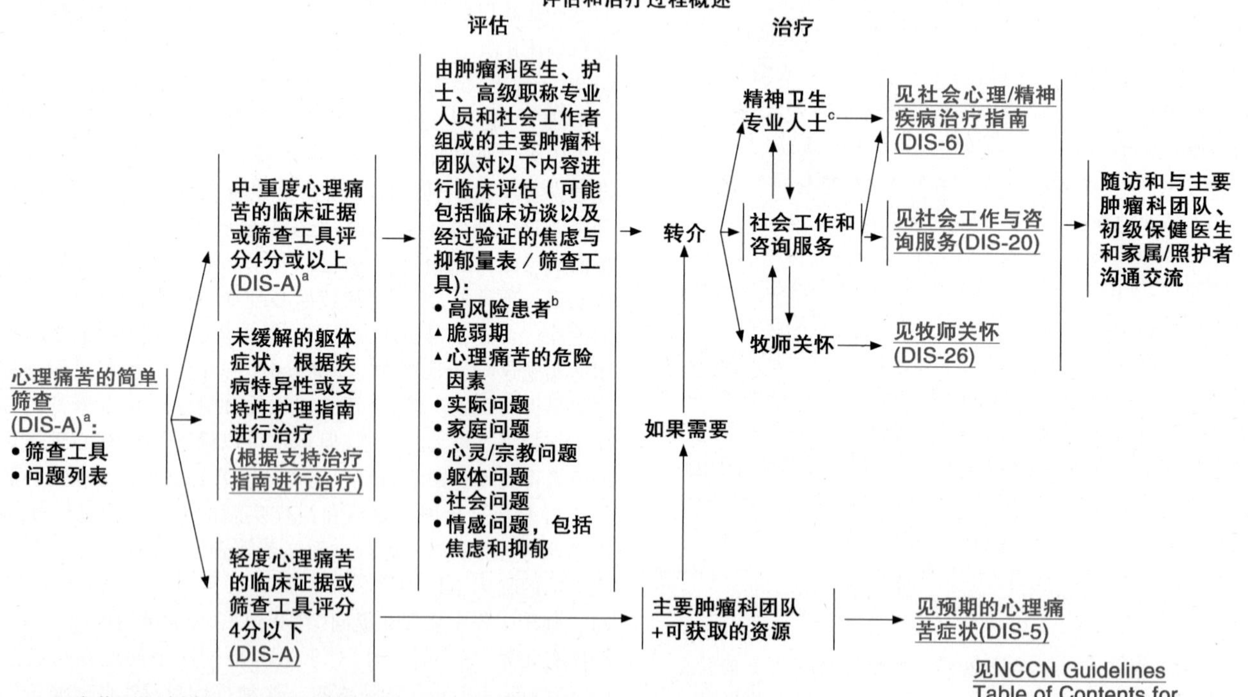

图 47-1 NCCN 指南®。来源：Reproduced with permission from the NCCN Clinical Practice Guidelines in Oncology (NCCN Guidelines®) for Distress Management V. 2. 2014. © 2014 National Comprehensive Cancer Network, Inc. All rights reserved. The NCCN Guidelines and illustrations herein may not be reproduced in any form for any purpose without the express written permission of the NCCN. To view the most recent and complete version of the NCCN Guidelines, go online to NCCN. org. NATIONAL COMPREHENSIVE CANCER NETWORK®, NCCN®, NCCN GUIDELINES®, and all other NCCN Content are trademarks owned by the National Comprehensive Cancer Network, Inc.

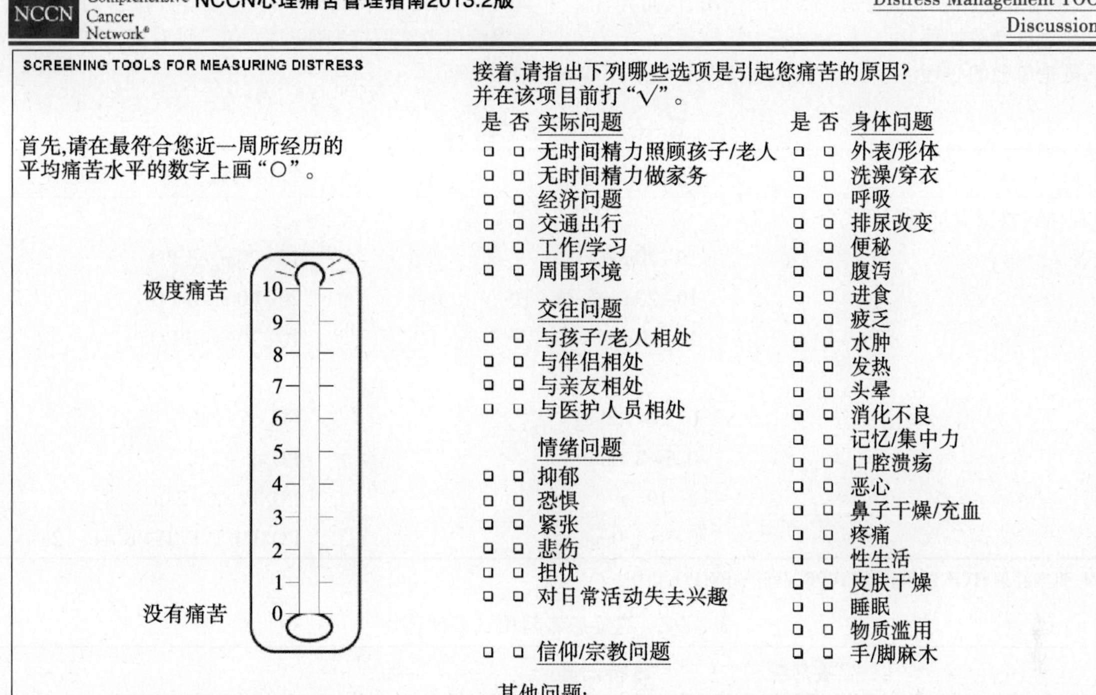

NCCN National Comprehensive Cancer Network® NCCN心理痛苦管理指南2013.2版

NCCN Guidelines Index
Distress Management TOC
Discussion

SCREENING TOOLS FOR MEASURING DISTRESS

首先,请在最符合您近一周所经历的平均痛苦水平的数字上画"○"。

极度痛苦 10 9 8 7 6 5 4 3 2 1 0 没有痛苦

接着,请指出下列哪些选项是引起您痛苦的原因?并在该项目前打"√"。

是	否	实际问题	是	否	身体问题
□	□	无时间精力照顾孩子/老人	□	□	外表/形体
□	□	无时间精力做家务	□	□	洗澡/穿衣
□	□	经济问题	□	□	呼吸
□	□	交通出行	□	□	排尿改变
□	□	工作/学习	□	□	便秘
□	□	周围环境	□	□	腹泻
			□	□	进食
		交往问题	□	□	疲乏
□	□	与孩子/老人相处	□	□	水肿
□	□	与伴侣相处	□	□	发热
□	□	与亲友相处	□	□	头晕
□	□	与医护人员相处	□	□	消化不良
		情绪问题	□	□	记忆/集中力
□	□	抑郁	□	□	口腔溃疡
□	□	恐惧	□	□	恶心
□	□	紧张	□	□	鼻子干燥/充血
□	□	悲伤	□	□	疼痛
□	□	担忧	□	□	性生活
□	□	对日常活动失去兴趣	□	□	皮肤干燥
			□	□	睡眠
			□	□	物质滥用
□	□	信仰/宗教问题	□	□	手/脚麻木

其他问题:________________

DIS-A

图 47-2　NCCN 心理痛苦温度计。来源:Reproduced with permission from the NCCN Clinical Practice Guidelines in Oncology(NCCN Guidelines®) for DistressManagement V. 2. 2014. © 2014 National Comprehensive Cancer Network, Inc. All rights reserved. The NCCN Guidelines and illustrations herein may not be reproduced in any form for any purpose without the express written permission of the NCCN. To view the most recent and complete version of the NCCN Guidelines, go online to NCCN. org. NATIONAL COMPREHENSIVE CANCER NETWORK®, NCCN®, NCCN GUIDELINES®, and all other NCCN Content are trademarks owned by the National Comprehensive Cancer Network, Inc.

临床管理

易感人群

具有下列特点的患者更容易存在心理痛苦的问题[8]

- 以前有过精神系统疾病(抑郁和物质依赖)
- 认知问题
- 语言或沟通障碍
- 存在共患病
- 社会问题(家庭、经济以及独居)
- 灵性或宗教方面的考虑

癌症患者易感心理痛苦的不同时间点[8]

- 发现疑似癌症的症状
- 被告知诊断癌症
- 等待肿瘤组织的活检和基因组检测,确定突变并指导靶向治疗
- 等待首次治疗
- 治疗间的过渡
- 治疗结束
- 从积极治疗转向安宁缓和医疗
- 进展期肿瘤与终末期
- 生存期间恐惧癌症复发。

在这些患者中,大多数肿瘤科工作人员可以较好管理。情境性焦虑、悲伤、失眠、疲劳、恐惧和担忧这些症状都是常见的,安抚和药物都会有效果。然而,一些患者经历了更多的困难,并有明显的痛苦,这需要更积极的干预。症状管理中最常见的精神障碍概述如下:焦虑、抑郁、自杀风险、谵妄和人格障碍。

焦虑障碍

焦虑是对疾病威胁的一种反应,但这也是一系列代谢状态的变化和药物作用的结果,需要对这些问题进行仔细地临床检查。它可能伴随着恐慌发作(心动过速和过度通气)和抑郁症状。治疗包括心理治疗,尤其是认知行为疗法;放松和冥想以及线上干预都很有用。如果焦虑症状一直持续或加重,一些药物是有帮助的。表 47-1 列出了最常用的药物。然而,奥氮平,一种抗精神病性药物,也常常超适应证用于治疗严重的焦虑症,并取得了良好的效果。

抑郁障碍和自杀风险

抑郁障碍

悲伤是癌症正常反应的一部分,然而更为重要的症状是乐趣的缺乏(快感缺失)、无助和绝望。它们常常导致治疗延后甚

至停止，影响治疗结果。与之相伴的症状还可有失眠、疲劳和厌食，但应注意与癌症相关症状鉴别。药物副作用、代谢异常、副肿瘤综合征也可导致抑郁。

治疗既可是单独的心理治疗手段，包括支持性心理治疗和认知治疗，也包含放松和冥想等行为干预手段。症状持续或加重时，为获得良好疗效，可联合心理疗法和药物手段。表 47-2 是癌症患者常用抗抑郁药物，包含针对疲乏和注意力减退的精神兴奋药。

表 47-1 焦虑的药物治疗

药物	起始剂量	维持剂量
选择性 5-羟色胺再摄取抑制剂		
艾司西酞普兰	10~20mg	10~20mg/d PO
氟西汀	10~20mg 每早一次	20~60mg/d PO
西酞普兰	10~20mg	10~20mg/d PO
苯二氮䓬类		
阿普唑仑	0.25~1.0mg	PO q6~24h
氯硝西泮	0.5~2.0mg	PO q6~24h
地西泮	2~10mg	PO/IV q6~24h
劳拉西泮	0.5~2.0mg	PO/IM/IVP/IVPB q4~12h

缩写：IM，肌肉注射；IVP，静脉注射；IVPB，静脉输液；PO，口服。

表 47-2 癌症患者常用抗抑郁药物

药物	起始剂量	维持剂量	评价
选择性 5-HT 再摄取抑制剂			
西酞普兰	10mg/d	20~40mg/d	
艾司西酞普兰	5~10mg/d	10~20mg/d	恶心、性功能障碍
氟西汀	10~20mg/d	20~60mg/d	半衰期长；恶心、性功能障碍；强 CYP2D6 抑制剂
帕罗西汀	20mg/d	20~60mg/d	恶心、镇静；强 CYP2D6 抑制剂
舍曲林	25~50mg/d	50~150mg/d	恶心
三环类抗抑郁药			
阿米替林	25~50mg/d，睡前	50~200mg/d	高度镇静，抗胆碱能不良反应，对神经病理性疼痛有效
地西帕明	25~50mg/d	50~200mg/d	中度镇静，抗胆碱能不良反应
去甲替林	25~50mg/d，睡前	50~200mg/d	中度镇静，对神经病理性疼痛有效 增加活力；改善性功能障碍；癫痫患者慎用
其他药物			
安非他酮	100mg/d	100~400mg/d 450mg/d 缓释(XL)； 400mg/d 缓释(SR)	恶心、唾液减少；对神经病理性疼痛可能有效 镇静、促进食欲、止吐
度洛西汀	20~40mg/d	60mg/d	恶心
米氮平	15mg，每日睡前	15~45mg，每日睡前 50~100mg，每日	恶心；可用于治疗神经病理性疼痛、潮热
去甲文拉法辛	50mg，每日	75~225mg/d；	心血管不良反应
文拉法辛	18.75~37.5mg/d	缓释(XR)，每日一次	恶心、焦虑、激越
精神兴奋药			
右旋苯丙胺	2.5mg，每日两次	5~20mg	激活、恶心、心脏不良反应；通常耐受较好
哌甲酯	5mg，每日两次	10~60mg	
莫达非尼	50mg，每日两次	50~200mg	头痛、恶心、眩晕、唾液减少；仅在早晨给药
阿莫达非尼	50mg	50~200mg	

来源：引用自文献 7。

自杀风险

有许多患者这样说，"事情恶化到无法忍受之时，我就会结束自己的生命"。不过很少会走到这一步。这似乎代表了一种在疾病面前控制情绪的方式。然而，任何自杀倾向都必须严肃对待，小心评估。关于自杀想法，也必须去探究。可以这样开始对话，"最近是否有感到不想再继续活下去了？"若患者已有大致想法，要更加注意。高自杀风险患者有以下特点：

- 既往精神问题史或自杀企图
- 控制不良的严重疼痛
- 晚期疾病
- 轻度谵妄（干扰正常理性判断）
- 酒精和药物滥用

识别有高度自杀风险的患者[8]：

- 初诊即为晚期疾病
- 自杀风险在第 1 个月内最高，但此后 6 个月内仍保持在高水平
- 肺部癌症患者有最高的自杀率，其次是头颈癌、胃癌、胰腺癌和结肠癌
- 大手术或重建手术
- 情绪低落、绝望或因为成为负担而导致的自责
- 癌痛严重且控制不佳

评估患者的自杀风险时理应想到可能归属于精神科急救的范畴。在完全评定自杀风险之前，患者都应该有人看护。若有较大自杀可能，有必要将患者置于安全环境中。对于晚期癌症患者则尽量不要变换环境，及时处理躯体症状，尤其是疼痛。必要时可咨询精神科专业人士，并让家人在家中小心看护。

谵妄

谵妄常见于住院患者和老年人，前者尤见于术后，后者可能是由不易察觉的轻度认知失调所引起。谵妄通常可有多种原因，包括发热、药物、代谢紊乱、中枢神经系统癌转移、副癌综合征（paraneoplastic disorders）等，因而常常得不到有效识别和及时治疗。其典型症状是急性发作的意识波动、意识错乱、精神运动性迟滞或激越。对于环境的知觉障碍（错觉）和幻视或幻听较为常见，通常是偏执的。控制谵妄症状的药物包括抗精神病药物、苯二氮䓬类和主要用于重症监护室的短效麻醉药。患者必须置于安全环境中，为防止患者拔除引流管或静脉输液管而伤害到自己，可使用躯体约束。发病初期即应紧密观察，最好是安置在重症监护室或是有熟悉人物在场的安静房间。陪护的家属可以安抚患者，并使其重新定向。表 47-3 是癌症患者常用抗谵妄药物。

表 47-3　癌症患者常用抗谵妄药物

药物	用量及用法	评价
抗精神病药		
氟哌啶醇	0.5~5mg，PO/IM/IV，q30min~12h	
氯丙嗪[a]	25~100mg，PO/IM/IV，q4~12h	
利培酮	2.5~5mg，PO，q12h	
奥氮平	2.5~5mg，PO/IM，q12~24h	
喹硫平	12.5~50mg，PO，q12h	
苯二氮䓬类		
劳拉西泮	0.5~2mg，PO/IM/IV，q1~4h	仅用于酒精戒断性谵妄
米达唑仑[a]	0.003mg/（kg·h），IV，滴定至起效（每位麻醉医师）	
麻醉药		
丙泊酚[a]	0.5mg/（kg·h），Ⅳ，滴定至起效	快速起效，作用时间短
α2-肾上腺素受体激动剂		
右美托咪定	1mcg/kg 缓慢输注超过 10 分钟，之后维持在 0.2~0.7mcg/（kg·h）	快速起效，作用时间短；对认知功能无影响
重症监护室用法：丙泊酚和右美托咪定快速起效，作用时间短		

[a] 通常用于 ICU 静脉持续泵入。
缩写：IM，肌肉注射；IV，静脉注射；PO，口服。
来源：引用自文献 7。

人格障碍

人格障碍的患者较为棘手，因为这本身并非某种特定的精神障碍，因此肿瘤医生须关注患者可能影响治疗的异常想法和行为。以下是癌症治疗中较为棘手的几种人格障碍。

偏执型人格障碍。此类患者多疑，易激惹，可能会争辩不停并且迁怒于肿瘤治疗团队成员。

边缘型人格障碍。此类患者情绪易外露，可能有自杀企图，情绪波动大，常对治疗团队提出不可能的任务。因此有必要划定界限并将治疗计划告知团队成员。

表演型人格障碍。患者好夸大症状，所表现的情绪强烈时甚至难以控制。易受他人影响，表现出性暗示。了解患者这些

特点很重要。

自恋型人格障碍。患者以自我为中心,自负,希望得到"特殊"对待,不关心他人需求。

强迫型人格障碍。患者在意疾病和治疗的任何一个小细节,对自己、他人要求甚高。不够灵活,可能有强迫性仪式动作。

依赖型人格障碍。此类患者缺乏自信,需要经常性的保证和安慰,优柔寡断。这些特质可能会干扰到治疗,因而经常需要很多时间来进行情绪支持。

患者的这些特征是人格模式的一部分,对肿瘤科医生而言,主要任务是知晓并能够识别,避免对患者的异常行为做出不专业的反应。一个肿瘤治疗团队最好重点关注有严重人格障碍的患者,理解其所承受的压力。但是精神科诊治常会使患者生气,甚至拒绝访谈。

心理社会干预

许多临床试验为非药物性的心理社会干预提供了循证基础[5,9]。

癌症照护中的心理治疗

认知治疗

虽然目前仍以支持性心理治疗为主,但基于认知的疗法已经展现出了效果。认知行为治疗广泛应用于焦虑、抑郁症状[10]及创伤后应激障碍的治疗。它是一种短期疗法,旨在解决当下应对疾病的问题,协助患者以更为建设性的方式直面恐惧和担忧。此种问题聚焦的疗法鼓励患者以积极的态度看待疾病,同家属一起解决挑战。人际心理疗法聚焦于受疾病影响的人际关系,尝试将被改变的角色联系起来。肿瘤心理治疗医生可以迅速学会以上疗法。对于哀伤等特殊问题,目前也有专门疗法。其他还有针对不同疾病分期或年龄阶段的疗法,主要是少年、青年和老年患者。尊严疗法和正念疗法致力于生命晚期的问题,旨在提供一种安慰性的态度。

行为干预

行为干预对于肿瘤患者的价值已经证实。人声或磁带引导的渐进式肌肉放松疗法有助于治疗失眠和焦虑,患者一旦掌握,便可在需要时使用。正念减压疗法/冥想是来自于东方的佛教传统方法,已进行了大量研究,并广泛应用。冥想对于焦虑有镇静功效,可以个人或团体为单位进行练习,最好是每天坚持。引导式想象同样有舒缓心情之功效。锻炼身体于身心都有益处,若病情允许,患者最好养成每日锻炼身体的习惯。

团体治疗和在线治疗

时间证明了心理社会支持团体的价值。成员们仅仅是分享经验和互帮互助就能让团体发挥很好的作用。今天,通过电话和网络所联系起来的虚拟团体同样常见,事实证明,同样有效。虽然相关研究还较少,但是这种新的方法因其成本远低于传统方法,使用者日益增多,以后会更加常见。诸如 Cancer Care 和 Cancer Support Community 之类的倡导组织提供了求助热线和咨询网站一类的服务,后者有可靠的信息和精神科医生的指导。通过电话,咨询者甚至能够识别患有某些特定肿瘤的患者的心理处境。寻求心理支持可咨询以下优质信息源:Cancer Care(www.cancercare.org)和 Cancer Support Community(www.cancersupportcommunity.org)。

从免费的电话在线咨询到付费一对一访谈,患者如今已能接触到许多不同种类的心理支持服务。虽然保险尚未完全覆盖精神科门诊和心理门诊的费用,但是在可见的将来此种不足可能会改善。另外,肿瘤心理医生仍难以满足目前的临床需求,其中一个原因是工作薪酬太低。

补充治疗

今天已有许多种的干预方法,肿瘤患者可以选择适合自己生活方式的治疗技术。艺术疗法是一种非常好的情绪表达方式;音乐和舞蹈疗法也能提供心理支持;写作和引导性写作同样有效。大部分肿瘤治疗中心都提供了一体化的治疗方案,患者可选择包括针灸、营养建议,以及心理和行为干预在内的辅助治疗。

职业倦怠

照护癌症患者不仅需要治疗团队的时间,还会耗费情感。当压力在程度上增长或在时间上延长时,即可导致倦怠综合征(burnout syndrome)。调查显示,约三分之一的肿瘤科医生会受到影响[11-17],在放射肿瘤科医生中这一比例更高[18-20]。职业倦怠综合征最初由 Freudenberger[21] 在 1974 年描述,包含 3 个维度:情感耗竭、人格解体(共情能力下降)和低成就感[22]。职业倦怠对医生有着双重影响——专业表现方面,干扰临床判断[23,24];个人生活上,导致医生更高的自杀率。

根据一份覆盖 7 000 名医生的全国性调查问卷,肿瘤科医生的职业倦怠率为 37.9%,稍低于其他内科医生(48.8%)[25]。他们经常情绪低落,不过,哪怕是重新选择,依然愿意选择肿瘤科医生这个职业。

职业倦怠成因多为长期的高难度工作、日益提高的要求和工作-生活冲突。医生的工作时长中位数为 50 小时/周,而肿瘤科医生每周工作时长中位数长达为 63 小时[26]。与各科医生相比,肿瘤科医生产生职业倦怠的风险最高[27]。而医疗纠纷又增加了发生职业倦怠的风险。

只要有预警和早期干预的意识,职业倦怠就可防可治。前瞻性研究显示,使用自我觉察技巧和正念冥想培训过的医师会有更强的共情能力和更少的沮丧情绪[28,29]。锻炼于身心都有益处,医护人员应适当锻炼。研究人员们也在调查医学院校关于"坚韧"的课程[30,31]。积极评价职业价值、平衡工作与生活和职业规划,都能使医生较少产生职业倦怠[32,33]。鼓励肿瘤科医生向家人寻求心理支持同样也可减少职业倦怠。在家庭和婚姻中出了难以意识到的问题时,许多医生总是把压力怪罪到工作上。

总结

就对癌症患者的心理支持而言,今日的大环境已大大好过 40 年前。得益于宣传教育,社会公众对癌症了解得更多,而这也相应减少了人们对于癌症的恐惧和病耻感。医疗的进步延长了 1 400 万癌症患者的生命。今天,临床上的肿瘤治疗团队更能与患者共情，与患者相识，成为患者的依靠。此外，癌症患者还能获得社会服务和健康资源，以及营养师、康复医疗和辅助治疗等方面的帮助。通过定期访谈，压力较大的患者在疗程早期就能被发现，并会得到心理咨询师的帮助。与 1973 年的第 1 版《癌症医学》所描述的情形相比，治疗过程中对患者生活质量的关切，这 40 年来取得了长足发展。心理社会肿瘤学作为一门独立的学科，积极参与了这一进程，并产生了一系列成果，包括循证的心理、行为和药物干预方法。如今的挑战在于将心理社会领域的知识融入癌症患者的日常照护中，充分确保承受压力的患者病有所医。

（唐丽丽　韩鑫坤　周城城 译，唐丽丽 审校）

参考文献

1 Holland JC, Benedeti C, Breitbart W, et al. Update: NCCN practice Guidelines for the management of psychosocial distress Version 1.2000. *Oncology*. 1999;**11(11A)**:459-507 © 1999 National Comprehensive Cancer Network.

2 Institute of Medicine. *Cancer Care for the Whole Patient: Meeting Psychosocial Health Needs*. Washington, DC: The National Academies Press; 2008.

3 Jacobsen PB, Wagner L. A new quality standard: the integration of psychosocial care into routine cancer care. *J Clin Onc*. 2012;**30**:1154-1159.

4 Pirl WF, Fann JR, Greer JA, et al. Recommendations for the implementation of distress screening programs in cancer centers: Report from the American Psychosocial Oncology Society (APOS), Association of Oncology Social Work (AOSW), and Oncology Nursing Society (ONS) joint task force. *Cancer*. 2014;**120**:2946-2954.

5 Holland JC, Breitbart WS, Jacobsen PB, Loscalzo MJ, McCorkle R, Butow PN. *Psycho-Oncology*, 3rd ed. New York, NY: Oxford University Press; 2015.

6 Holland JC, et al., NCCN Clinical Practice Guidelines in Oncology (NCCN Guidelines®) Distress Management Version 2. © 2014 National Comprehensive Cancer Network, Inc. Available at NCCN.org (accessed 1 February 2015); 2014.

7 Holland JC, Golant M, Greenberg DB, et al. *Psycho-Oncology: A Quick Reference on the Psychosocial Dimensions of Cancer Symptom Management*; New York, NY: Oxford University Press; 2015.

8 Holland JC, Weiss Wiesel T, Nelson CJ, Roth AJ, Alici Y. *Geriatric Psycho-Oncology: A Quick Reference on the Psychosocial Dimensions of Cancer Symptom Management*. New York, NY: Oxford University Press; 2015.

9 Golant M, Loscalzo M, Walsh M. *Psychological Non-pharmacological Interventions. Psycho-Oncology: A Quick Reference on the Psychosocial Dimensions of Cancer Symptom Management*, 2nd ed. New York, NY: Oxford University Press; 2015.

10 Watson M, Kissane D. *Handbook of Psychotherapy in Cancer Care*. Wiley; 2011.

11 Ramirez AJ, Graham J, Richards MA, et al. Burnout and psychiatric disorder among cancer clinicians. *Br J Cancer*. 1995;**71**:1263-1269.

12 Shanafelt T, Dyrbye L. Oncologist burnout: causes, consequences, and responses. *J Clin Oncol*. 2012;**30**:1235-1241.

13 Allegra CJ, Hall R, Yothers G. Prevalence of burnout in the U.S. Oncology community: results of a 2003 survey. *J Oncol Pract*. 2005;**1**:140-147.

14 Whippen DA, Canellos GP. Burnout syndrome in the practice of oncology: results of a random survey of 1,000 oncologists. *J Clin Oncol*. 1991;**9**:1916-1920.

15 Arigoni F, Bovier PA, Mermillod B, Waltz P, Sappino AP. Prevalence of burnout among Swiss cancer clinicians, paediatricians and general practitioners: who are most at risk? *Support Care Cancer*. 2009;**17**:75-81.

16 Grunfeld E, Whelan TJ, Zitzelsberger L, Willan AR, Montesanto B, Evans WK. Cancer care workers in Ontario: prevalence of burnout, job stress and job satisfaction. *CMAJ*. 2000;**163**:166-169.

17 Grunfeld E, Zitzelsberger L, Coristine M, Whelan TJ, Aspelund F, Evans WK. Job stress and job satisfaction of cancer care workers. *Psychooncology*. 2005;**14**:61-69.

18 Dyrbye LN, Shanafelt TD. Physician burnout: a potential threat to successful health care reform. *JAMA*. 2011;**305**:2009-2010.

19 Kuerer HM, Eberlein TJ, Pollock RE, et al. Career satisfaction, practice patterns and burnout among surgical oncologists: report on the quality of life of members of the Society of Surgical Oncology. *Ann Surg Oncol*. 2007;**14**:3043-3053.

20 Balch CM, Shanafelt TD, Sloan J, Satele DV, Kuerer HM. Burnout and career satisfaction among surgical oncologists compared with other surgical specialties. *Ann Surg Oncol*. 2011;**18**:16-25.

21 Freudenberger HJ. Staff burnout. *J Soc Issues*. 1974;**30**:159-165.

22 Cherniss C. *Staff Burnout: Job Stress in Human Services*. Beverly Hill: Sage Publications; 1980.

23 Shanafelt TD, Balch CM, Dyrbye L, et al. Special report: suicidal ideation among American surgeons. *Arch Surg*. 2011;**146**:54-62.

24 Dyrbye LN, Thomas MR, Massie FS, et al. Burnout and suicidal ideation among U.S. medical students. *Ann Intern Med*. 2008;**149**:334-341.

25 Shanafelt TD, Boone S, Tan L, et al. Burnout and satisfaction with work-life balance among US physicians relative to the general US population. *Arch Intern Med*. 2012;**172**:1377-1385.

26 Wetterneck TB, Linzer M, McMurray JE, et al. Worklife and satisfaction of general internists. *Arch Intern Med*. 2002;**162**:649-656.

27 Jena AB, Seabury S, Lakdawalla D, Chandra A. Malpractice risk according to physician specialty. *N Engl J Med*. 2011;**365**:629-636.

28 Krasner MS, Epstein RM, Beckman H, et al. Association of an educational program in mindful communication with burnout, empathy, and attitudes among primary care physicians. *JAMA*. 2009;**302**:1284-1293.

29 Epstein RM. Mindful practice. *JAMA*. 1999;**282**:833-839.

30 Epstein RM, Krasner MS. Physician resilience: what it means, why it matters, and how to promote it. *Acad Med J Assoc Am Med Coll*. 2013;**88**:301-303.

31 Dyrbye LN, Power DV, Massie FS, et al. Factors associated with resilience to and recovery from burnout: a prospective, multi-institutional study of US medical students. *Med Educ*. 2010;**44**:1016-1026.

32 Shanafelt T, Chung H, White H, Lyckholm LJ. Shaping your career to maximize personal satisfaction in the practice of oncology. *J Clin Oncol Off J Am Soc Clin Oncol*. 2006;**24**:4020-4026.

33 Shanafelt TD, Novotny P, Johnson ME, et al. The well-being and personal wellness promotion strategies of medical oncologists in the North Central Cancer Treatment Group. *Oncology*. 2005;**68**:23-32.

第 48 章　癌症康复医学原则

Michael D. Stubblefield, MD ■ David C. Thomas, MD, MHPE David C. Thomas, MD, MHPE ■ Kristjan T. Ragnarsson, MD

概述

目前,美国有 1 400 多万的癌症生存者,其中许多癌症生存者忍受着由于疾病本身及各种治疗(例如手术、化疗、放疗)的相关并发症所带来痛苦。恢复和维持癌症生存者的身体功能和生活质量往往需要比较专业的康复支持和服务。癌症康复专家致力于与癌症及其治疗相关的神经肌肉、肌肉骨骼、疼痛和功能障碍等方面识别、评估和康复。本文聚焦于这一富有挑战性的群体康复领域,具体阐述其原则与相关实践。

引言

癌症康复专家聚焦在与癌症相关的神经肌肉、肌肉骨骼、疼痛和功能障碍的识别、评估和康复,强调对于躯体功能恢复和维持以及保持良好的生活质量。目前美国有超过 1 400 万癌症生存者[1]。预计到 2020 年这一数字将增加至 1 800 万[2]。大多数癌症生存者忍受着疾病本身及治疗相关并发症所带来的痛苦,其中常常混杂很多医学上的合并症,需要接受专门的康复服务。本章节讨论康复医学专家在恢复和维持癌症生存者身体功能和保证生活质量方面的作用,所选择的癌症生存者群体包括患有颅脑肿瘤、头颈部肿瘤、乳腺癌及那些脊髓功能障碍(spinal cord dysfunction, SCD)的患者。

康复团队

有组织性、计划性的康复项目可以显著改善患者的身体功能和社区融合[3-6]。这一项目的主要部分就是跨学科的癌症康复与相关调适团队。团队的构成人员是根据康复项目的理念和规模、机构类型以及患者失能的严重程度来组织建立的。在理想情况下,团队应由理疗医师来主导。团队的成员及其角色如表 48-1 所示。

表 48-1　跨学科癌症康复小组

团队成员	职能分工
照顾者	作为患者的延伸,给予患者的支持以及与治疗团队建立关系
牧师	评估以及协助患者和护理人员提供相关精神需求
营养治疗师	评估患者的营养状况,评估癌症对身体的额外代谢需求,建议最佳饮食的条件,如热量摄入,选择的最佳食物成分,容易吞咽,以及适合患者个人的口味等
职业治疗师	评估和制订康复计划,重点关注上肢运动和力量范围以及自我护理培训活动
患者	作为团队的成员积极参与治疗的各个方面的决策
物理治疗师	评估并制订康复计划,以改善关节活动范围,加强肌肉强度和耐力,重点是改善相关功能性技能,如床上活动,移动,轮椅运动以及有或没有辅助设备的行走
医师	引导康复团队制订切合实际的目标,并制订适当的康复计划,包括预防计划,恢复,支持和姑息治疗
假肢矫形师	根据患者的需要评估和制造假肢或特殊牙套(矫形器)
心理治疗师	评估患者的认知和行为,包括智力、性格、个人历史、意志和对疾病的反应,并协助患者和护理人员制订应对医疗疾病的计划
娱乐治疗师	为每位患者提供满足他们的个人需求的活动,如艺术和/或音乐疗法,组织对患者重要的社交活动
康复护师	评估患者的特定护理需求,并确定包括患者和护理人员的相关教育的计划
语言矫正师	评估并为口腔沟通障碍患者提供治疗,并与职业治疗师和营养师密切合作,评估吞咽障碍的相关病情并进行护理
社会工作者	评估患者心理社会方面需求并设定相关计划,特别是出院计划,促进顺利过渡到社区,确保护理的连续性以及确保在出院后获得适当的后续服务
职业咨询师	评估可能重返工作岗位患者的需求,并设立计划,协助其重新重返工作角色

颅脑恶性肿瘤

脑损伤可能是由颅脑原发肿瘤、脑转移或手术、放疗和化疗等引起的。所表现出的症状和与此导致的功能缺陷差异很大,而和中风后观察到的症状相似(表 48-2)。脑肿瘤患者的功能恢复与急性脑卒中患者相似[7]。所出现的功能缺陷与脑内病灶的位置和大小有关,这些功能缺陷的差异需要个体化评估和制订个体化治疗计划。所有患有脑肿瘤和运动功能及日常生活活动(activity of daily living,ADL)受损的患者均应接受康复治疗,希望能帮助此类患者恢复上述两方面的功能,更好地帮助患者,使其可以独立生活。脑肿瘤患者在康复机构的住院时间通常比创伤性脑损伤和中风患者要短一些[8,9]。通过简单的指导,治疗师的培训和提供辅助设备可以帮助此类患者迅速恢复更好的功能甚至完全独立生活。对于预期生存期长而失能较为严重的患者,住院进行"综合性康复计划"可能是最佳的选择。通过功能训练来增加萎缩肌肉的强度和舒展挛缩关节及肌肉,可以有效地恢复患者的运动功能和自理能力。通过反复舒展拉伸所有关节,配合适当的药物治疗,以及有针对性地注射肉毒杆菌毒素可以有效缓解痉挛。某些患者的平衡障碍和步态异常可能与肌肉无力、疲乏、痉挛、本体感觉丧失以及视力和认知能力下降有关。上述功能的缺损都会增加跌倒的风险。通过增加肌肉强度的训练和有氧运动,使用适当的助行器(手杖、拐杖、助行器)进行平衡和步态训练,穿合适的鞋和矫形器,改善家庭和工作的环境,减少镇静剂的使用等均可以降低此类风险。疼痛控制和解决关节挛缩同等重要。各种视觉上的缺陷,包括复视和视野缺陷,需要经常通过使用交替的眼罩或特殊的眼镜来解决。语言障碍,如构音障碍和失语症,沟通技能受损,需要评估和妥善管理,往往可以通过引入替代的沟通方法,如写作、打字、手语和图片来解决。

表 48-2 与脑肿瘤相关的康复问题

- 瘫痪
- 痉挛
- 关节挛缩
- 疼痛
- 感觉障碍
- 视野缺损
- 复视
- 失语症
- 构音障碍
- 吞咽困难
- 共济失调
- 认知和行为缺陷
- 视知觉缺陷
- 心理社会职业缺陷

不同程度的神经心理变化与影响大脑半球的癌症相关,包括记忆力,判断力,视觉感知等能力的下降。仔细评估这些功能缺陷后,对患者和家属进行相关宣教是至关重要的。通过神经心理修复和补偿策略,例如提供一本"记忆簿"可能也会有所帮助。

脊髓功能障碍

脊柱的原发性肿瘤并不常见,最常见的是多发性骨髓瘤。骨转移更为常见,有 5% 的癌症患者尸检发现有骨转移[10]。脊髓功能障碍(spinal cord dysfunction,SCD)最常见的病因是转移性硬膜外压迫[11],此外也可能是由放疗、化疗或外科手术引起的医源性损伤。脊柱肿瘤最常见的初始症状是疼痛。不同程度的神经功能障碍可能是突然发生的,也可能是逐渐发生的,这取决于肿瘤的生长速度和部位。神经学水平是指双侧感觉和运动功能正常脊髓节段水平。低于这一水平的神经系统缺陷,可使用美国脊髓损伤协会(亚洲)损伤量表[American spine Injury Association(ASIA) impairment scale]进行分类[12]。病变引起的神经病变水平和并发症程度有助于预测功能预后。生命的预后因癌症类型而异。脊柱转移瘤的中位生存期为 7.7 个月,结肠癌和肺癌患者预期生存期较差,而肉瘤、前列腺癌、肾癌和乳腺癌患者预期生存期更长一些[13]。

大多数脊柱转移采用非手术治疗。当神经功能缺损迅速发生时,通常需要采用手术减压和/或放疗。脊柱转移和原发肿瘤可能导致脊柱不稳定,应该采用手术方法使其稳定[14]。患有 SCD 肿瘤患者的康复取决于他们的神经科,肿瘤科,内科,疼痛和社会支持状态的评估[11]。SCD 合并严重瘫痪和感觉缺失,伴有膀胱和肠道功能异常,需要特殊的医疗和护理照顾,以及后续各个相关功能情况的综合康复(表 48-3)。泌尿道并发

表 48-3 脊髓功能障碍相关情况

- 运动障碍
- 失去知觉
- 压疮
- 泌尿功能障碍
- 肠道功能障碍
- 性功能障碍
- 疼痛
- 痉挛
- 自主反射障碍
- 关节挛缩
- 循环障碍
- 直立性低血压
- 水肿
- 深静脉血栓性静脉炎
- 呼吸衰竭
- 代谢紊乱
- 内分泌激素失调
- 心理问题
- 社会问题
- 职业问题

症、压疮、深静脉血栓/肺栓塞、关节挛缩和其他并发症的预防必须强调相关的医疗及护理措施，例如及时实施间歇膀胱导管置入，预防性抗凝，合适的床位放置和至少每2小时变换体位，一定的运动和锻炼，日常肠排空以及关注情感支持。物理和职业治疗师旨在恢复患者身体活动度和自理能力技能。伴有辅助设备的行动装置可能适用许多低平面不完全性SCD的患者，但是对于那些神经功能完全的胸椎或颈椎平面SCD的患者，将需要手动或电动轮椅。不完全SCD患者可能从步行训练中获益，包括体重支持，如悬吊。那些完全胸椎平面SCD的患者需要矫形器来稳定他们的膝关节或脚踝。许多低腰椎平面SCD可能从踝-足矫形器中获益，以此补偿踝部肌肉无力，如足下垂需要额外使用拐杖或步行器来步行。最近开发的外骨骼机器人电动设备，具有多种控制机制，有望使完全截瘫的人重新获得一定程度的独立和功能的行走[15]。一旦在医学上和功能上被认为是合适的，患有SCD的患者就可以出院，并获得必要的辅助设备、护理用品、个人帮助以及后续医疗护理的指导。

头颈部恶性肿瘤

当前头颈部肿瘤(head and neck cancer,HNC)多模式治疗包括手术和/或调强放射治疗(intensity-modulated radiation therapy,IMRT)联合或不联合铂类为基础的化疗。手术通常包括切除原发肿瘤，以及颈部淋巴结清除，分为根治性[切除所有淋巴结，副神经(spinal accessory nerve,SAN)，胸锁乳突肌(sternocleidomastoid,SCM)，颈内静脉(internal jugular vein,IJV)]，改良根治性(切除所有淋巴结，但是备选一个或多个SAN,SCM,IJV)，或选择性(保留通常在根治性颈部淋巴结清扫中切除的一个或多个淋巴结区)[16]。通常颈部淋巴结清扫范围越大，造成肩部功能异常，疼痛和生活质量下降越严重[17]。尽管SAN的切除或损伤是主要原因，但是损伤其他重要结构，包括颈根分支和颈神经丛，对相关功能损伤也起到重要作用[18-20]。斜方肌无力(SAN受损)和肩回旋肌群(rotator cuff,RTC)无力(神经根分支受损)影响肩胛胸的运动，进而可以导致肩部肌肉骨骼不适，如RTC肌腱炎和粘连性关节囊炎[21]。颈丛及其分支以及颈部神经根分支损伤，可以导致神经病理性疼痛[20]。

放疗可以损伤放射野内的任何结构，包括神经、肌肉、肌腱、韧带、血管、淋巴管和骨骼[22]。HNC放疗的晚期效应包括神经根病变，颈椎和/或臂丛神经病变，以及位于放射野内脑神经或其他神经的单一神经病变。放疗的晚期效应还包括吞咽困难、构音障碍、口腔干燥、牙关紧闭、头颅下垂综合征、颈部肌张力障碍、肩关节功能障碍、颈和/或肩部疼痛和其他多个不良后遗症[23-26]。手术和放疗的联合可能会累加相关功能损伤的发病率。HNC生存者晚期效应的治疗方式多样，取决于具体问题。物理疗法是大部分功能障碍治疗的主要方式。在两项前瞻随机研究中，HNC患者伴有SAN功能性麻痹/神经切除术和肩部功能障碍，渐进式阻力训练(progression resistance training,PRT)在缓解肩部疼痛，提高一定的运动锻炼和改善失能状态上比标准的物理治疗显示更有效[27,28]。对物理治疗无效的伤害性疼痛(RTC肌腱炎，粘连性关节囊炎)可能需要非甾体抗炎药(nonsteroidal anti-inflammatory drugs,NSAIDs)或阿片类镇痛药。肩部注射可能在某些患者中有效，但是在慢性神经肌肉功能障碍时通常只能产生短暂效果。神经病理性疼痛和肌肉痉挛初始治疗应该采用神经稳定类药物(加巴喷丁，普瑞巴林、度洛西汀、三环类抗抑郁药)[22]。HNC如果影响到口腔，咽喉，和/或食管的结构和功能，可以导致吞咽困难。吞咽困难可以导致相关并发症，如吸入性肺炎和营养不良。康复首先需要综合的评估，开始于采用液体或不同类型食物的床旁吞咽测试，之后根据需要进行咽，喉，食管的视频荧光照相术和内窥镜检查。改善吞咽的训练包括加强无力肌肉的运动，确定吞咽时头和颈部恰当的体位，对液体和不同黏度食物的仔细喂养，提供口内设备和合适的瓶子，杯子，盘子和餐具，和有时采用特定的手术治疗。

乳腺癌

乳腺癌的治疗包括乳腺肿瘤切除术，乳房切除术，前哨淋巴结活检和腋窝淋巴结清扫术，以及联合(或不联合)放疗和化疗[29]。乳腺癌及其治疗存在多种潜在的并发症，主要是由于疾病和手术、放疗、化疗及治疗中使用的其他药物的影响而产生，这些并发症均可以从康复干预中获益。

淋巴水肿发生率为6%~28%[30]。乳房切除术，腋窝淋巴结扩大清扫，放疗，和阳性的淋巴结均增加发生淋巴水肿的风险[31]。淋巴水肿的治疗选择包括综合物理疗法，弱激光疗法(low-level laser therapy,LLLT)，药物治疗和手术[32]。综合物理疗法(包括综合性抗淋巴瘀滞疗法)可能包括人工淋巴引流(manual lymphatic drainage,MLD)，渐进式运动，低拉伸压缩绷带，穿着合适的梯度压缩服装，淋巴水肿区的皮肤护理和其他方面的教育。

乳腺癌生存者的上肢疼痛和功能障碍由多种因素引起(表48-4)[33]。这些障碍的康复治疗具有很大的差异性，但是通常包括物理疗法和药物治疗，如NSAIDs，阿片类药物，治疗神经稳定类药物，不定期注射药物(例如对RTC肌腱炎进行关节内糖皮质激素注射)[33]。选择乳房切除术的女性常常需要乳房重建手术，植入的填充物可以由生理盐水、硅胶或复合材料等制成。其他人优先选择使用外部乳腺假体，由硅胶或轻质量泡沫或纤维填充制成。这些内衣的尺寸和一致性各不相同，但都要求穿着定制的文胸和服装才能达到最佳的美容效果。

表48-4 乳腺癌生存者的上半身疼痛障碍

肌肉骨骼
术后疼痛
肩袖疾病
二头肌肌腱炎
粘连性关节囊炎
骨转移瘤
上髁炎
De Quervain病(桡骨茎突狭窄性腱鞘炎)
关节痛
关节炎
神经肌肉
颈神经根病

续表

软脑膜疾病
臂丛病
多发性神经病
化疗诱导的周围神经病变
糖尿病周围神经病变
单神经病
肩胛背侧神经(菱形肌 C5)
肩胛上神经(冈上肌和冈下肌 C5-C6)
胸长神经(前锯肌 C5-C6-C7)
胸外侧神经(胸大肌和胸小肌 C5-T1)
胸内神经(胸大肌和胸小肌 C5-T1)
胸背神经(背阔肌 C6-C7-C8)
正中神经
腕管综合征
尺神经
肘管神经
尺管神经
桡神经
桡神经沟
乳癌术后疼痛综合征
肋间臂神经痛
复杂局部疼痛综合征
淋巴血管
淋巴水肿
腋网综合征
深静脉血栓
血栓后综合征
体壁
蜂窝织炎
放射性皮炎

来源:Stubblefield and Keole 2014[33]. Reproduced with permission from Elsevier.

四肢恶性肿瘤

原发性肢体恶性肿瘤需要手术治疗。确切的手术类型取决于肿瘤的部位、大小、类型、分级、分期以及患者的年龄和一般健康状况。其主要目的是通过切除肿瘤边缘较宽的部位,清除所有恶性肿瘤,或根治性切除整个骨骼或受肿瘤影响的部位来切除肿瘤。随后的手术目标是对所致缺陷进行重建达到最佳功能和美观。虽然肢体截肢已经有几百年的历史,但近年来,通过扩大局部或局部切除和重建来挽救肢体已成为主要目标,目前约 90%的病例选择手术干预。这两种手术方式的生存和无疾病生存期类似,并且近几年随着化疗,放疗或两者序贯应用明显提高。

骨转移比原发性骨肿瘤更常见,但多倾向于转移至脊柱而不是四肢。骨肿瘤通常最初表现多为局部疼痛或病理性骨折。病理性骨折需要内固定,同时使用甲基丙烯酸甲酯(骨水泥),这样可以减轻疼痛,早期恢复活动能力,减轻护理压力,并使患者心理得以安慰。无论是计划截肢或保肢手术,术前康复在确诊患肢肿瘤后便应立即开始。这包括讨论手术和预期的术后康复过程,建立切实可行的预期目标,并由成功康复的截肢者提供咨询服务。同时,适当的体育锻炼计划应该从四肢和躯干的强化训练开始,同时应该对受影响的下肢进行不负重的步行训练。

局部切除肿瘤,保留肢体重建,可获得与截肢相同的无病生存期。但更重要的是患者将保留更好的功能,形象和情绪的适应。我们的目的是切除有活性的肿瘤,同时保留邻近的神经、肌腱和血管。患癌的骨骼可以通过移植新鲜冷冻的同种异体骨骼,自体骨移植或安装人造金属假体来替代。另一种选择是,在骨肿瘤切除后,可以将肢体放置在一个外固定装置中,通过定期调整固定针和固定架来保持骨端之间的牵张,有利于新骨生长。这种方法通常是儿童和青少年的首选。这将最终填补骨端之间的间隙,使得骨长度合适并愈合坚固。下肢保留手术后的康复治疗是漫长的、高强度的,是手术成功的关键。其中包括术后第一天对未受累肢体的强化训练,但受累肢体的强化训练的强度和负重程度取决于具体的肢体重建和术后过程。对大多数人来说,长期效果很好,可以做到完全自理,能够在没有辅助设备的情况下行走。

对于侵及神经和血管的较大的肿瘤,截肢可能是首选的手术方式,所以无法保留患肢。然而在保证肿瘤根治术的基础上最大限度地保留肢体长度是可取的,这样使得假肢更容易安装到残肢上。因此,最好避免在后足、胫骨远端或股骨髁上区域进行截肢。膝下截肢最好保留 12~18cm 的胫骨,膝上截肢也应保留相似长度的股骨。术后 2 天即应开始进行物理和职业治疗,使用助行器、拐杖,最终使用假肢和拐杖来改善肌肉力量、关节活动和步行训练。所有的下肢假体都需要一个定制的塑料套座来固定残肢,内置硅胶衬垫以保持舒适,通常还需要几层袜子来固定萎缩的残肢。附着于膝关节下假体关节窝的有一种小腿和脚踝机械装置,而膝关节上假体也有一种膝关节机械装置。从最基本的到微处理器控制和电池电源,膝关节假体和脚踝关节假体的机械装置在设计上均存在很大的差异。因此,功能和经济成本差别也很大。

上肢癌症可以进行保肢手术治疗,然而肢体近端肿瘤可能会侵及神经和血管,需要进行肩关节切断术,甚至肩胛胸廓截断术。根据个人的情况、能力和需求,可以选择多种假体用于整形或功能应用。

结论

癌症管理的重点集中在预防、早期诊断和治疗,但在有效的治疗之后,许多癌症患者会经历神经肌肉、肌肉骨骼、疼痛以及导致身体残疾的功能障碍。随着癌症预后的改善,为了确保患者可以重返以前的社会角色,最大程度上恢复功能就显得尤为重要。因此,多学科协作的康复治疗是癌症患者整体管理的重要组成部分。需要对每位患者进行充分的评估,确定精准明确的功能缺陷,适当的康复干预应立即与其他治疗同时开始。

(韩颖　韩瑜　寇芙蓉　王龙 译,刘巍 审校)

参考文献

1 Siegel R, Ma J, Zou Z, Jemal A. Cancer statistics, 2014. *CA Cancer J Clin.* 2014;**64(1)**:9-29.

2 Mariotto AB, Yabroff KR, Shao Y, Feuer EJ, Brown ML. Projections of the cost of cancer care in the United States: 2010-2020. *J Natl Cancer Inst.* 2011;**103(2)**:117-128.

3 Cole RP, Scialla SJ, Bednarz L. Functional recovery in cancer rehabilitation. *Arch Phys Med Rehabil.* 2000;**81(5)**:623-627.

4 Franklin DJ. Cancer rehabilitation: challenges, approaches, and new directions. *Phys Med Rehabil Clin N Am.* 2007;**18(4)**:899-924, viii.

5 Hinterbuchner C. Rehabilitation of physical disability in cancer. *N Y State J Med.* 1978;**78(7)**:1066-1069.

6 Harvey RF, Jellinek HM, Habeck RV. Cancer rehabilitation. An analysis of 36 program approaches. *JAMA.* 1982;**247(15)**:2127-2131.

7 Geler-Kulcu D, Gulsen G, Buyukbaba E, Ozkan D. Functional recovery of patients with brain tumor or acute stroke after rehabilitation: a comparative study. *J Clin Neurosci.* 2009;**16(1)**:74-78.

8 Greenberg E, Treger I, Ring H. Rehabilitation outcomes in patients with brain tumors and acute stroke - Comparative study of inpatient rehabilitation. *Am J Phys Med Rehab.* 2006;**85(7)**:568-573.

9 O'Dell MW, Barr K, Spanier D, Warnick RE. Functional outcome of inpatient rehabilitation in persons with brain tumors. *Arch Phys Med Rehab.* 1998;**79(12)**:1530-1534.

10 Parsch D, Mikut R, Abel R. Postacute management of patients with spinal cord injury due to metastatic tumour disease: survival and efficacy of rehabilitation. *Spinal Cord.* 2003;**41(4)**:205-210.

11 Stubblefield MD, Bilsky MH. Barriers to rehabilitation of the neurosurgical spine cancer patient. *J Surg Oncol.* 2007;**95(5)**:419-426.

12 International standards for neurological classification of spinal cord injury, revised 2002. Chicago, IL: American Spinal Injury Association; 2002.

13 Wang JC, Boland P, Mitra N, et al. Single-stage posterolateral transpedicular approach for resection of epidural metastatic spine tumors involving the vertebral body with circumferential reconstruction: results in 140 patients. Invited submission from the Joint Section Meeting on Disorders of the Spine and Peripheral Nerves, March 2004. *J Neurosurg Spine.* 2004;**1(3)**:287-298.

14 Fourney DR, Frangou EM, Ryken TC, et al. Spinal instability neoplastic score: an analysis of reliability and validity from the spine oncology study group. *J Clin Oncol.* 2011;**29(22)**:3072-3077.

15 Chen G, Chan CK, Guo Z, Yu H. A review of lower extremity assistive robotic exoskeletons in rehabilitation therapy. *Crit Rev Biomed Eng.* 2013;**41(4-5)**: 343-363.

16 Inoue H, Nibu K, Saito M, et al. Quality of life after neck dissection. Archives of otolaryngology—head & neck surgery. 2006;**132(6)**:662-666.

17 Kuntz AL, Weymuller EA Jr. Impact of neck dissection on quality of life. *Laryngoscope.* 1999;**109(8)**:1334-1338.

18 Umeda M, Shigeta T, Takahashi H, et al. Shoulder mobility after spinal accessory nerve-sparing modified radical neck dissection in oral cancer patients. *Oral Surg Oral Med Oral Pathol Oral Radiol Endod.* 2010;**109(6)**:820-824.

19 Roh JL, Yoon YH, Kim SY, Park CI. Cervical sensory preservation during neck dissection. *Oral Oncol.* 2007;**43(5)**:491-498.

20 Dilber M, Kasapoglu F, Erisen L, Basut O, Tezel I. The relationship between shoulder pain and damage to the cervical plexus following neck dissection. *Eur Arc Otorhinolaryngol.* 2007;**264(11)**:1333-1338.

21 Stubblefield MD. Cancer rehabilitation. *Semin Oncol.* 2011;**38(3)**:386-393.

22 Stubblefield MD. Radiation fibrosis syndrome: neuromuscular and musculoskeletal complications in cancer survivors. *PM R.* 2011;**3(11)**:1041-1054.

23 Rong X, Tang Y, Chen M, Lu K, Peng Y. Radiation-induced cranial neuropathy in patients with nasopharyngeal carcinoma. A follow-up study. *Strahlenther Onkol.* 2012;**188(3)**:282-286.

24 Tuan JK, Ha TC, Ong WS, et al. Late toxicities after conventional radiation therapy alone for nasopharyngeal carcinoma. *Radiother Oncol.* 2012;**104(3)**:305-311.

25 Chen AM, Hall WH, Li J, et al. Brachial plexus-associated neuropathy after high-dose radiation therapy for head-and-neck cancer. *Int J Radiat Oncol Biol Phys.* 2012;**84(1)**:165-169.

26 Smillie I, Ellul D, Townsley R, et al. Head drop syndrome secondary to multimodality treatments for head and neck cancer. *Laryngoscope.* 2013;**123(4)**:938-941.

27 McNeely ML, Parliament M, Courneya KS, et al. A pilot study of a randomized controlled trial to evaluate the effects of progressive resistance exercise training on shoulder dysfunction caused by spinal accessory neurapraxia/neurectomy in head and neck cancer survivors. *Head Neck.* 2004;**26(6)**:518-530.

28 McNeely ML, Parliament MB, Seikaly H, et al. Effect of exercise on upper extremity pain and dysfunction in head and neck cancer survivors—a randomized controlled trial. *Cancer.* 2008;**113(1)**:214-222.

29 NCCN Clinical Practice Guidelines in Oncology (NCCN Guidelines) Breast Cancer. Available from: http://www.nccn.org/professionals/physician_gls/pdf/breast.pdf, accessed 9 May 2014.

30 DiSipio T, Rye S, Newman B, Hayes S. Incidence of unilateral arm lymphoedema after breast cancer: a systematic review and meta-analysis. *Lancet Oncol.* 2013;**14(6)**:500-515.

31 Tsai RJ, Dennis LK, Lynch CF, Snetselaar LG, Zamba GK, Scott-Conner C. The risk of developing arm lymphedema among breast cancer survivors: a meta-analysis of treatment factors. *Ann Surg Oncol.* 2009;**16(7)**:1959-1972.

32 Paskett ED, Dean JA, Oliveri JM, Harrop JP. Cancer-related lymphedema risk factors, diagnosis, treatment, and impact: a review. *J Clin Oncol.* 2012;**30(30)**: 3726-3733.

33 Stubblefield MD, Keole N. Upper body pain and functional disorders in patients with breast cancer. *PM&R.* 2014;**6(2)**:170-183.

第 49 章　整合肿瘤学在癌症治疗中的作用

Gabriel Lopez, MD ■ Richard T. Lee, MD ■ Alejandro Chaoul, PhD ■ M. Kay Garcia, DrPH, MSN, LAc ■ Lorenzo Cohen, PhD

概述

整合医学(integrative medicine)一直寻求以一种综合、个体化、循证且安全的方式将传统医学和补充治疗相融合。整合肿瘤学(integrative oncology)则用以描述整合医学在癌症治疗中的应用。整合肿瘤学是一个不断发展的多学科领域。本章主要回顾整合医学在肿瘤治疗中的作用,重点阐述有效的沟通,全面回顾循证的证据,指导医护工作者以及患者如何将整合医学有效融合到癌症治疗中。现有的研究发现大部分癌症患者渴望与他们的医生探讨整合医学相关的话题。主动询问患者关于补充医学的使用,提供循证的建议,指导患者在这个不断变化的领域中科学应用,是医护专业人员的职责。正文详细介绍了身心治疗、按摩以及针灸的主要研究成果。身心治疗可以帮助改善患者的情绪、睡眠质量、身体功能以及整体健康。按摩对于缓解疼痛、焦虑以及帮助放松有益。有大量证据支持针灸在症状管理中的应用,例如化疗导致的恶心、呕吐以及疼痛;另有初步研究发现针灸有可能对放疗引发的口腔干燥以及其他症状有缓解作用。目前,有许多权威资源可以帮助患者更合理地使用补充治疗,同时也让医护人员有循证指南可遵循。

引言

整合医学是指联合传统医学和最安全、最有效的补充医学的一种治疗方法。尽管整合医学这样一个治疗理念在肿瘤治疗中的应用尚不成熟,但许多美国的癌症综合治疗中心仍不断尝试对整合医学的概念进行实践,并称其为“整合肿瘤学”。随着整合肿瘤学被广泛关注,国立①癌症研究所(National Cancer Institute, NCI)成立了一个癌症补充与替代医学办公室(Office of Cancer Complementary and Alternative Medicine),美国癌症协会(American Cancer Society)致力于利用网站评估补充治疗方法,整合医学学术健康中心联合会(Consortium of Academic Health Centers for Integrative Medicine, CAHCIM)成立了一个肿瘤治疗工作组,随之整合肿瘤学协会(Society for Integrative Oncology, SIO)也成功建立。本章主要是回顾整合医学在肿瘤治疗中的作用,重点阐述有效的沟通,全面回顾循证的证据,用具体实例指导医护工作者及患者如何将整合医疗有效融合到癌症治疗中。

① 如无特殊说明,本文中“国立”都是指美国国立机构。

定义

补充与整合医学国立中心(National Center for Complementary and Integrative Health, NCCIH)[前身为“补充与替代医学国立中心(National Center for Complementary and Alternative Medicine, NCCAM)”]和大多数美国调查将补充与替代医学(complementary and alternative medicine, CAM)定义为:非常规的多种药物和健康护理为基础的体系、操作及产品[1]。尽管有证据表明一些 CAM 方法有效,但是仍不足以将其纳入传统医学范畴,另一些 CAM 在应用时还缺乏相关的证据。替代医学是应用非传统治疗模式代替传统治疗,且无论是否有证据表明其有效的一种治疗模式。与此对应,补充医学被定义为应用 CAM 联合传统医学的一种治疗模式,同样无论是否有证据证明其有效。具有资质或在认证机构工作的医疗保健专家,均可在行业规范内为患者提供 CAM 治疗。治疗团队包括医生、护士、物理治疗师、心理学家、针灸医生以及按摩师。各个学科的临床工作者应该具有高度专业知识,了解所有的治疗选择,且各学科之间应公开地交流和探讨。

整合医学一直寻求以一种综合、个体化、循证且安全的方式将传统医学和补充治疗相融合。CAHCIM 对整合医学的定义为:“关注治疗者与患者之间的关系,强调治疗关乎整个人,且具有循证的支持,利用各种适合的治疗途径、医疗专家以及学科,以达到理想健康状态和最佳治疗目的一种医学实践。”[2]。整合医学在肿瘤治疗中的应用被称之为“整合肿瘤学”。CAM 和补充与整合医学(complementary and integrative medicine, CIM)经常互换使用。但值得注意的是,当使用 CAM 时,它包括可被视为替代的治疗方法,并且可替代传统治疗;但是 CIM 并不包括替代治疗途径。

应用

根据世界卫生组织(World Health Organization, WHO)的评估,超过 80% 发展中国家的患者,在他们治疗初期主要依赖非传统治疗方式[3];在发达国家的患者,同样也会寻求补充治疗的应用。2007 年,美国疾病控制中心(US Centers for Disease Control)的一项调查显示在过去的 12 个月里,38% 的成年人曾经使用过 CAM 治疗[4];2012 年的数据即将发布。

在肿瘤患者以及肿瘤家庭中,CAM 的使用率要高于普通人群。预计 48%~69% 的美国肿瘤患者正在使用 CAM 治疗,若将精神修行包括在内,则此比例更高[5]。因此,超过 69% 的肿瘤患者采用过 CAM 治疗,且在晚期患者中的使用率更高[5,6]。

多数情况下,选择 CAM 治疗的患者并非不满足于单纯的传统治疗,他们只是希望尽一切可能接受所有治疗,而重获新生和提高生活质量。他们采用 CAM 来降低不良反应、提高生活质量、刺激免疫反应、防止肿瘤复发和其他原发肿瘤[5,7]。这些患者还可以通过 CAM 治疗其他慢性病如关节炎、心脏病、糖尿病以及慢性疼痛等。

沟通

研究表明无论是成年或是儿童肿瘤患者均没有从医生、药剂师、护士或是 CAM 临床工作者那里获取到充足的 CAM 治疗信息或是与之谈论过 CAM 治疗的应用[8]。预估大约 38%~60%接受 CAM 治疗的肿瘤患者并没有有效告知其治疗团队[6,7]。大部分患者不会提及 CAM 治疗,因为没有医护人员主动询问过,因此患者可能认为这并不是什么重要的事情。这种交流的缺乏可能引发相当严重的后果,例如一些草本植物或是营养补充剂可能具有一定毒性,或者对抗肿瘤治疗有干扰作用。患者普遍没有意识到药品和营养补充剂的区别。美国食品药品监督管理局(United States Food and Drug Administration, FDA)批准的药品,是需要充足的临床证据证明其有效性、安全性和生产质量控制,然而营养补充剂则是由 1994 年颁布的《膳食补充剂健康与教育法》(Dietary Supplement Health and Education Act,DSHEA)管理,而不是 FDA。因此由 DSHEA 管理的营养补充剂并没有像 FDA 批准的药品那样具有严格的审查标准。此外,营养补充剂并不能用于治疗、预防或是治愈疾病。然而,患者普遍认为“天然的”就是安全的,但其实不然,很多草本植物和营养补充剂可能影响多种药物相互作用,同时可能增加患癌风险和器官毒性,因此对患者教育非常重要[9,10]。

现有的研究发现大部分癌症患者渴望与他们的医生探讨 CAM 相关的话题。为提供最佳的医护服务,肿瘤学家不仅应熟知 CAM 的应用,并且还要愿意与患者沟通交流各种治疗方法,这在肿瘤界已达成共识。主动询问患者接受补充治疗情况是医疗专家的责任;最理想的情况是在患者开始接受补充治疗之前,就开始进行此类讨论,无论是营养治疗、身心治疗或其他治疗。

在交流沟通时,一些策略可使对话变得更有意义。其中一种方法就是把 CAM 的话题作为患者入院评估的一部分[11]。例如,当问及用药史时,医生应该询问患者摄入的任何保健品及药品,包括非处方药、维生素、矿物质、草本植物,甚至是患者的饮食摄入也应有所了解。医生也可以考虑让患者把服用的草本植物和营养补充剂带到医院进行评估。医生也可以通过询问治疗团队的其他成员,来获得患者既往病史的情况,以此来了解患者是否曾经拜访过 CAM 治疗师,如理疗师或按摩师。如果发现 CAM 相关的问题,临床医生需要根据患者的需求与他们做融入感情的交流,同时专家应当了解当前的学科现状[12]。换句话说,这种谈话策略需要平衡临床客观性和与患者的感情连接,保证医患双方均能从中受益。善于倾听患者需求的临床医生,较容易营造出一种舒适的氛围,使患者更愿意谈论关于 CAM 治疗的话题。此外,医生还需要具有开放的态度,愿意回顾循证的参考文献,并且乐于向其他医疗专家进行咨询。只有这样,临床医生才能确保患者能从值得信赖的资源,获取关于 CAM 的可靠信息,同时肿瘤医生应该保证充足时间与患者讨论这些信息[13]。

证据

整合肿瘤学是一个不断发展的多学科领域。近年来,关于整合肿瘤学的研究呈急速增长的态势。在接下来的小节里,我们将列举出一些迄今为止整合肿瘤学的主要研究成果,其中以下是 CAM 主要研究领域,且有充足证据为患者建议此类治疗:身心治疗、按摩以及针灸。虽然不断有新的其他领域的研究,如触摸治疗、顺势疗法、天然产品以及特殊饮食,但由于缺乏证据还尚不能为患者推荐。

身心治疗

有这样一种观点,认为我们的所思所感可以影响我们的健康和治疗,这一观点可以向上追溯几千年。在传统中医治疗、藏医治疗、古希腊医学、印度阿育吠陀医学以及世界其他国家的传统治疗中都非常重视患者的思想、情绪、行为对健康的影响。

大量证据表明慢性应激对健康具有损害作用,前者几乎影响着机体所有的生物系统[14]。不受控制的慢性应激可通过端粒缩短来加速衰老[15],也可能增加罹患心脏疾病的风险[16]、导致睡眠障碍[17],引发消化障碍[18],甚至诱发抑郁[19]。另有研究发现应激也可能降低患者对健康筛查和治疗的依从性[20]。此外,应激还有可能导致患者放弃健康饮食和锻炼习惯,这些良好的生活方式可以帮助预防肿瘤和其他疾病的发生。

关于慢性应激影响肿瘤发生的证据较少;然而,确有大量证据表明慢性应激可促进肿瘤的生长和进展[21,22]。这其中潜在的机制非常复杂,但与交感神经和下丘脑-垂体轴-肾上腺轴的长期活化有关[23]。这些通路的持续激活(如去甲肾上腺素和皮质醇)可产生不同的作用,包括刺激肿瘤入侵,肿瘤血管再生,炎症反应,免疫系统紊乱,降低失巢凋亡,甚至干扰化疗效果[24]。潜在的信号通路可为临床研究者提供机会,探索如何破坏应激对肿瘤的影响,从而研发出包括行为和药理学(如β阻断剂)的治疗方法。

应激相关的生理变化与肿瘤微环境变化的临床意义还尚未被广泛研究。但这些变化足以影响患者的短期健康,甚至改变疾病进展,危害患者的长期健康。因此,建议患者参与一些降低应激的治疗是明智的。

身心治疗被定义为:为改善心理功能从而影响身体功能以及症状的各种治疗手段。身心治疗包括放松训练、催眠治疗、视觉表象、冥想、生物反馈疗法、瑜伽、太极拳、气功、其他基于运动的治疗、认知行为疗法(cognitive behavioral therapy, CBT)、团体支持、自生训练、灵性及艺术表达治疗如美术、音乐或舞蹈。随着研究的深入,那些被发现有益的治疗有希望融入传统治疗的行列。

研究发现一旦疾病确诊,患者总是积极尝试改变他们的生活方式,希望可以掌控他们的治疗过程[25]。被证明有效的应激管理方法有渐进式肌肉放松、腹式呼吸、引导性想象法以及社会支持。在抗肿瘤治疗之前参与应激管理治疗可以帮助患者提高治疗耐受性,降低副作用的发生率。支持性表达小组治疗也被发现对肿瘤患者是有帮助的。即使一些数据支持使用艺术表达治疗如音乐治疗[26]、美术治疗[27]、表达写作[28]以及日记可以提高患者的生活质量，但是缺乏大量的试验证明其有效性，且已有的试验样本量较小，并常缺乏对照组。另有研究表明心理社会干预可降低肿瘤患者的焦虑、抑郁以及情绪障碍，并可以帮助提高他们的应对技能[29]。

Newell 等[30]通过回顾肿瘤患者的心理治疗，建议使用自我实践和催眠相关的治疗来控制患者的恶心呕吐的症状，并提出放松训练和引导性想象法还需要进一步的研究证明其潜在的作用。Ernst 等人[31]分析了 2000—2005 年间有关身心治疗的证据，发现目前有充分的证据表明放松治疗可以缓解由化疗所引发的焦虑、高血压、失眠以及恶心。另外，近期的研究发现催眠治疗，尤其是自我催眠，可减轻患者在治疗期间的痛苦和不适[32]。此外，NIH 技术评估小组发现有力证据证明催眠可以缓解癌性疼痛[33]。另有研究发现，催眠可以有效治疗成人和儿童肿瘤患者的预期性恶心，降低术后恶心呕吐的发生率，并改善患者对侵入性医疗操作的适应能力。若与 CBT 相结合，催眠还可以降低乳腺癌患者在放疗结束以及结束后 1 至 6 个月后的疲劳状况[34]。

对于瑜伽、太极和冥想包括正念减压疗法（mindfulness-based stress reduction，MBSR）融合癌症护理的研究表明：这些身心疗法可以改善治疗期间的肿瘤患者以及癌症生存者的生活质量，包括改善情绪、睡眠质量、身体功能以及整体健康[35]。

冥想练习中被研究最广泛的是 MBSR。在过去几年发表的有关冥想的大型随机对照试验发现，在乳腺癌女性肿瘤患者中，MBSR 可以降低自我评价的焦虑和抑郁症状，并改善睡眠质量；对于长期用药（如激素治疗）所导致的身心副作用也有缓解作用，其中包括明显降低情绪紊乱和应激症状。针对癌症患者设计的特别版本 MBSR 被称为正念癌症康复（mindfulness-based cancer recovery，MBCR）；有研究发现，在心理痛苦温度计得分大于等于 4 分的乳腺癌患者中，MBCR 可以降低患者的应激症状并提高生活质量[36]。除此之外，与对照组相比，MBCR 和支持性表达治疗组均表现出更正常的日间皮质醇水平。

越来越多的基于运动的身心治疗，如印度瑜伽、西藏瑜伽以及中国太极拳、气功，都是通过结合身体动作或运动，呼吸技巧以及冥想来加强健康和幸福感。印度瑜伽（“yoga”是梵文，意为“结合”）是西方文化中最广泛应用的东方传统；强调精神和肉体的结合，或身体、呼吸以及心灵的和谐同步。瑜伽在肿瘤领域越来越受到欢迎。实际上，一些系统综述和荟萃分析显示练习瑜伽可改善肿瘤患者和癌症生存者的生活质量[37,38]。另有研究表明瑜伽可以治疗睡眠障碍[39]以及疲劳[40]。瑜伽还可通过降低炎症信号和调节应激激素[41]，来改善由乳腺癌治疗所引起的行为症状，如疲劳[42]。因此，瑜伽实际上可能会影响患者对生活质量的感知以及症状之外的生物通路。虽然大部分关于瑜伽的研究都是在早期乳腺癌女性患者中进行的，但有更多的研究正努力将这些发现拓展到晚期乳腺癌患者和肺癌生存者以及看护人员中[43]。

虽然太极拳和气功在肿瘤领域的研究甚少[44]；但研究成果却令人鼓舞，发现太极拳和气功可以降低患者的疲劳和痛苦，改善外周循环系统和功能有氧代谢能力，从而降低术后体液和细胞免疫的紊乱。

按摩

按摩已展现出对肿瘤和肿瘤相关症状的缓解作用。作为操作性接触治疗，一个懂得肿瘤患者需求的按摩治疗师可以为患者带来最大的益处[45]。接受过肿瘤按摩相关训练的按摩师，才是最安全的按摩操作者。在一些选定的患者中，应谨慎施加压力，避免按压入深层组织或骨头，这样可以有效减轻挫伤、出血、或受伤的风险。近期进行过手术或接受过辐射的部位，应该避免按压。在患有四肢淋巴水肿的患者中，按摩治疗师应该调整手法，最大限度保证患者安全。正规淋巴水肿治疗作为物理治疗项目的一部分，可以帮助患者改善症状[46]。

目前的证据显示，按摩可以帮助患者缓解疼痛、焦虑、疲劳、痛苦以及增加放松感[47,48]。按摩缓解情绪和疼痛的作用只被证实具有短期效果，目前尚没有证据表明其可长期改善情绪和疼痛[49,50]。轶事记录和个案报曾表明按摩可以缓解化疗引发的周围神经病变。按摩脚部、手部和头部可以带来较好的治疗效果，这是因为这些部位对触觉刺激极为敏感，从而可以使人放松，增进健康。另有研究发现，按摩为治疗师和患者提供了特殊的交流机会，这对双方的健康都有益处[51]。除了症状缓解，研究还发现按摩也具有全身效应，可通过按摩降低皮质醇水平[52]。未来需要更多的研究用以了解按摩的机制以及确立治疗方案（最佳按摩类型、按摩量），进而可以更好地确定按摩在肿瘤症状管理中的。

针灸

针灸是传统中医中常见的理疗方法，在中国已有几千年的历史；在世界范围内，被至少 78 个国家使用。根据传统中医的理论，针灸的针、热量或压力实施在特殊的穴位上可以帮助身体调理气血运行。针灸最常见的形式是使用实心、无菌、不锈钢针刺入身体的不同部位，旨在减少生物电阻力并增加电传导。刺入的针灸针可手动操作或利用轻微电流刺激穴位。无菌不锈钢、金（半永久的）针或者“钉”有时也会被刺入耳上，并会保留 3~5 天。

在癌症治疗领域，针灸对症状管理的相关证据最为有力。研究发现针灸有利于控制多种原因引起的恶心呕吐（如化疗所致恶心呕吐、术后恶心呕吐以及孕吐）[53,54]；另外虽然有较多证据表示针灸可以控制疼痛，但在肿瘤领域的证据较为有限。一个纳入 29 项试验的大型个体患者水平数据荟萃分析发现，在患有慢性疼痛的非肿瘤患者中（$N=14\ 597$），真针灸组的疼痛控制明显优于不实施针灸的小组（50% vs 30%，$P<0.001$）和假针灸组（40% vs 42.5%，$P<0.001$）。

与疼痛和恶心相比，针灸对其他症状管理的证据等级较弱；然而，一些初步研究发现针灸可能有助于持续减轻放射性口腔干燥的严重程度[55,56]。另有证据指出针灸有可能治疗或者帮助控制一些症状，如便秘、食欲不振、周围神经病变、热潮红、疲乏、失眠症、睡眠障碍、呼吸困难、焦虑、抑郁及白细胞减少症；然而研究质量较差，需要进一步地研究[57]。只要操作正确规范，针灸是一种安全，侵入性小，副作用极小的一种治疗手段。最常见的副作用有昏厥、挫伤以及轻度疼痛。尽管少见，针灸也具有潜在的感染风险，因此只有具有执业证书和丰富经验的健康保健专业人员才能进行针灸治疗。

针灸治疗的作用机制还尚未完全明确，但有充足的证据支持使用针灸对化疗性恶心呕吐和疼痛进行管理。尽管目前对于控制其他癌症相关症状和癌症治疗相关症状方面证据不充分，作为一种低风险和低成本的治疗选择，当治疗副作用无法控制或传统治疗方法无效时，针灸可能对肿瘤治疗有额外价值。

教育资源

由于资源的快速更新，一个综述会很快过时，并随着网络发表的简便，越来越多的科学审查机构通过网络提供电子综述。我们列举了一些提供可靠信息的机构网站（表 49-1）。

表 49-1 有关循证资源的网站推荐

机构/网站	网址/URL
Cochrane 回顾组织	www. cochrane. org
纪念斯隆-凯特琳癌症中心	www. mskcc. org/cancer-care/integrative-medicine/about-herbs
天然药物数据库	www. naturaldatabase. com/
天然标准	www. naturalstandard. com/
NCI 癌症补充与替代医学办公室	www. cancer. gov/cam
得克萨斯大学安德森癌症中心整合医学项目	www. mdanderson. org/integrativemed

美国癌症协会（American Cancer Society，ACS）以及 NCI 癌症补充与替代医学办公室（Office of Cancer Complementary and Alternative Medicine，OCCAM）均向患者和公众提供有关补充治疗的教育资源。天然药物数据库（Natural Medicines Comprehensive Database）提供关于补充治疗的循证综述。Cochrane 回顾组织始建于 1993 年，是一个国际非营利独立组织，也提供补充治疗相关的系统综述。

天然标准由多学科、多机构发起，致力于研究补充与替代治疗。它遵循一个类似的过程，在历史和民俗的观点之外，建立了深入的证据和基于共识的科学数据分析。纪念斯隆凯特琳癌症治疗中心的整合医学服务提供循证综述，作为"关于草本植物、植物性治疗药物 & 其他药物"网络资源的一部分。得克萨斯大学安德森癌症中心整合医学项目也为患者和医护人员提供网络资源，使他们有机会学习更多有关整合医学在癌症看护中的循证作用。

整合肿瘤学的临床实践

整合肿瘤学有能力提高癌症护理的质量，通过额外的治疗选项帮助患者改善健康，症状管理以及生活质量。目前，大多数的大型医学中心都会在传统治疗的基础上，提供一些补充医学治疗手段[58]。为了创造全面的癌症整合医疗，这些类型的治疗方法不仅要避免潜在的相互作用，还要与进行中的治疗形成协同作用。若要达到这种效果，整合肿瘤学方法需要是循证的、个体化的且是安全的。

得克萨斯大学安德森癌症中心整合医学中心就是一个很好的例子。此中心利用一个基于卫生保健的生物心理社会模式（图 49-1）作为临床框架，指导整个癌症患者的服务实施，从预防到治疗，再到院外生存；并且对医护人员也提供一些服务。他们的临床服务针对具体的医疗情况提供解决方法，例如疼痛、焦虑或如何适当使用草本植物和营养补充剂，并且作为 spa 服务的一部分不向患者开放。此中心同时提供个体和团体的医护服务，患者可以接受住院和门诊的医生咨询、针灸、按摩、身心治疗如冥想、音乐治疗等。另外，物理治疗可提供运动咨询，营养师可提供营养咨询，心理医生也可为所有患者提供情绪管理和行为咨询。患者也可免费参加集体课程，如冥想、瑜伽、太极拳、气功、音乐治疗、运动及烹饪课程。所有的工作人员每周举行一次会议，讨论对新患者的挑战以及如何帮助配合患者治疗。临床记录在电子健康档案中可以查询。作为常规治疗的一部分，患者需要完成症状和生活质量的量表调查，这些信息也是临床研究的重要资料，可帮助医护人员了解这些医

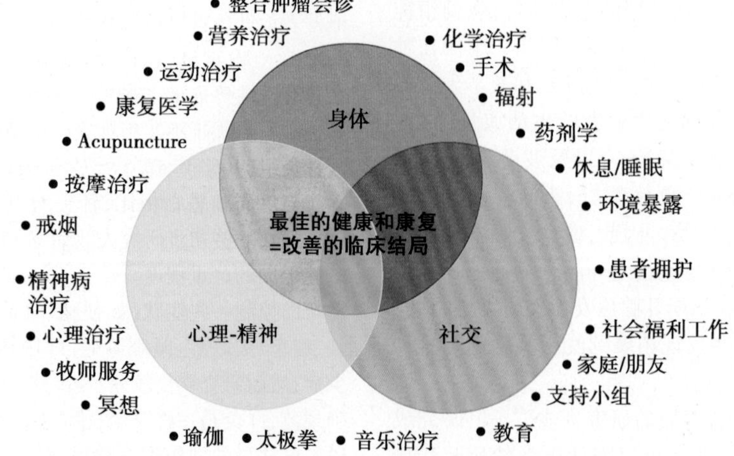

图 49-1 整合医学中心模式。基于卫生保健的生物心理社会模式，我们中心为癌症护理框架发挥作用

疗服务对患者临床治疗的影响。整合医学中心也会与类似的支持服务机构共同合作，如缓和医疗、精神病治疗、疼痛中心以及康复服务。大部分的转诊都来自这些服务领域以及主治肿瘤医师。

结论

整合肿瘤学是一个快速发展的学科，具有附加治疗选择和有效症状控制方面的巨大潜力。一个整合方法也给患者提供了一个更加个性化的治疗体系以满足他们的需求。大部分的患者或是正在使用补充治疗，或是想要了解补充治疗，传统医学系统有责任提供给患者合适的教育和医疗服务。整合治疗的医学模型要求一种以患者为中心的方式，关注患者的需求并促进交流能力。另外，传统和非传统医学从业者一并致力于研发整合模式也是非常重要的。这样，通过使用所有合适的治疗模式，癌症患者将会接受最好的医学治疗。

（邹宝华　瞿慧敏　译，丛明华　审校）

参考文献

The complete reference list can be found on the Wiley Companion Digital Edition of this title (see inside front cover for login instructions).

1 NCCAM. National Center for Complementary/Alternative Medicine of the National Institutes of Health. What is complementary and alternative medicine? (2015) http://nccam.nih.gov/health/whatiscam/ (accessed January 15, 2015).

4 Barnes PM, Bloom B, Nahin R. CDC National Health Statistics Report #12. Complementary and Alternative Medicine Use Among Adults and Children: United States, 2007. December 10, 2008.

5 Richardson MA, Sanders T, Palmer JL, Greisinger A, Singletary SE. Complementary/alternative medicine use in a comprehensive cancer center and the implications for oncology. *J Clin Oncol*. 2000;**18**(**13**):2505–2514.

6 Navo MA, Phan J, Vaughan C, et al. An assessment of the utilization of complementary and alternative medication in women with gynecologic or breast malignancies. *J Clin Oncol*. 2004;**22**(**4**):671–677.

9 Ulbricht C, Chao W, Costa D, Rusie-Seamon E, Weissner W, Woods J. Clinical evidence of herb-drug interactions: a systematic review by the natural standard research collaboration. *Curr Drug Metab*. 2008;**9**(**10**):1063–1120.

11 Verhoef MJ, White MA, Doll R. Cancer patients' expectations of the role of family physicians in communication about complementary therapies. *Cancer Prev Control*. 1999;**3**(**3**):181–187.

14 Chrousos GP, Gold PW. The concepts of stress and stress system disorders. Overview of physical and behavioral homeostasis. *JAMA*. 1992;**267**(**9**):1244–1252.

15 Epel ES, Blackburn EH, Lin J, et al. Accelerated telomere shortening in response to life stress. *Proc Natl Acad Sci U S A*. 2004;**101**(**49**):17312–17315.

19 Hammen C. Stress and depression. *Annu Rev Clin Psychol*. 2005;**1**:293–319.

20 Prasad SM, Eggener SE, Lipsitz SR, Irwin MR, Ganz PA, Hu JC. Effect of depression on diagnosis, treatment, and mortality of men with clinically localized prostate cancer. *J Clin Oncol*. 2014;**32**(**23**):2471–2478.

21 Lutgendorf SK, Sood AK, Antoni MH. Host factors and cancer progression: biobehavioral signaling pathways and interventions. *J Clin Oncol*. 2010;**28**(**26**):4094–4099.

22 Lutgendorf SK, Sood AK, Anderson B, et al. Social support, psychological distress, and natural killer cell activity in ovarian cancer. *J Clin Oncol*. 2005;**23**(**28**):7105–7113.

23 Lutgendorf SK, Sood AK. Biobehavioral factors and cancer progression: physiological pathways and mechanisms. *Psychosom Med*. 2011;**73**(**9**):724–730.

24 Thaker PH, Han LY, Kamat AA, et al. Chronic stress promotes tumor growth and angiogenesis in a mouse model of ovarian carcinoma. *Nat Med*. 2006;**12**(**8**):939–944.

26 Archie P, Bruera E, Cohen L. Music-based interventions in palliative cancer care: a review of quantitative studies and neurobiological literature. *Support Care Cancer*. 2013;**21**(**9**):2609–2624.

29 Devine EC, Westlake SK. The effects of psychoeducational care provided to adults with cancer: meta-analysis of 116 studies. *Oncol Nurs Forum*. 1995;**22**(**9**):1369–1381.

30 Newell SA, Sanson-Fisher W, Savolainen NJ. Systematic review of psychological therapies for cancer patients: Overview and recommendations for future research. *J Natl Cancer Inst*. 2002;**94**(**8**):558–584.

31 Ernst E, Pittler MH, Wider B, Boddy K. Mind-body therapies: are the trial data getting stronger? *Altern Ther Health Med*. 2007;**13**(**5**):62–64.

33 NIH Technology Assessment Panel. Integration of behavioral and relaxation approaches into the treatment of chronic pain and insomnia. NIH Technology Assessment Panel on Integration of Behavioral and Relaxation Approaches into the Treatment of Chronic Pain and Insomnia. *JAMA*. 1996;**276**:313–318.

34 Montgomery GH, David D, Kangas M, et al. Randomized controlled trial of a cognitive-behavioral therapy plus hypnosis intervention to control fatigue in patients undergoing radiotherapy for breast cancer. *J Clin Oncol*. 2014;**32**(**6**):557–563.

35 Chaoul A, Milbury K, Sood AK, Prinsloo S, Cohen L, et al. Mind-body practices in cancer care. *Curr Oncol Rep*. 2014;**16**:417.

36 Carlson LE, Doll R, Stephen J, et al. Randomized controlled trial of mindfulness-based cancer recovery versus supportive expressive group therapy for distressed survivors of breast cancer. *J Clin Oncol*. 2013;**31**(**25**):3119–3126.

37 Cramer H, Lange S, Klose P, Paul A, Dobos G. Yoga for breast cancer patients and survivors: a systematic review and meta-analysis. *BMC Cancer*. 2012;**12**:412.

38 Bower JE, Garet D, Sternlieb B, et al. Yoga for persistent fatigue in breast cancer survivors: a randomized controlled trial. *Cancer*. 2012;**118**(**15**):3766–3775.

39 Mustian KM, Sprod LK, Janelsins M, et al. Multicenter, randomized controlled trial of yoga for sleep quality among cancer survivors. *J Clin Oncol*. 2013;**31**(**26**):3233–3241.

40 Bower JE, Greendale G, Crosswell AD, et al. Yoga reduces inflammatory signaling in fatigued breast cancer survivors: a randomized controlled trial. *Psychoneuroendocrinology*. 2014;**43**:20–29.

41 Chandwani KD, Perkins G, Nagendra HR, Raghuram NV, et al. Randomized, controlled trial of yoga in women with breast cancer undergoing radiotherapy. *J Clin Oncol*. 2014;**32**(**10**):1058–1065.

42 Kiecolt-Glaser JK, Bennett JM, Andridge R, et al. Yoga's impact on inflammation, mood, and fatigue in breast cancer survivors: a randomized controlled trial. *J Clin Oncol*. 2014;**32**(**10**):1040–1049.

43 Milbury K, Chaoul A, Engle R, et al. Couple-based Tibetan yoga program for lung cancer patients and their caregivers. *Psychooncology*. 2015;**24**:117–120.

45 Collinge W, MacDonald G, Walton T. Massage in supportive cancer care. *Semin Oncol Nurs*. 2012;**28**(**1**):45–54.

46 Torres Lacomba M, Yuste Sanchez MJ, Zapico Goni A, et al. Effectiveness of early physiotherapy to prevent lymphoedema after surgery for breast cancer: randomised single blinded, clinical trial. *BMJ*. 2010;**340**:b5396.

48 Russell NC, Sumler S-S, Beinhorn CM, Frenkel M. Role of massage therapy in cancer care. *J Altern Complement Med*. 2008;**14**(**2**):209–214.

49 Wilkinson SM, Love SB, Westcombe AM, et al. Effectiveness of aromatherapy massage in the management of anxiety and depression in patients with cancer: a multicenter randomized controlled trial. *J Clin Oncol*. 2007;**25**(**5**):532–539.

51 Collinge W, Kahn J, Walton T, et al. Touch, Caring, and Cancer: randomized controlled trial of a multimedia caregiver education program. *Support Care Cancer*. 2013;**21**(**5**):1405–1414.

52 Listing M, Krohn M, Liezmann C, et al. The efficacy of classical massage on stress perception and cortisol following primary treatment of breast cancer. *Arch Womens Ment Health*. 2010;**13**:165–173.

53 NIH. Acupuncture. NIH Consensus Statement. 1997;**15**(**5**):1–34.

54 Ezzo J, Vickers A, Richardson MA, et al. Acupuncture-point stimulation for chemotherapy-induced nausea and vomiting. *J Clin Oncol*. 2005;**23**(**28**):7188–7198.

55 Meng Z, Garcia MK, Hu C, et al. Randomized controlled trial of acupuncture for prevention of radiation-induced xerostomia among patients with nasopharyngeal carcinoma. *Cancer*. 2012;**118**:3337–3344.

56 Simcock R, Fallowfield L, Monson K, et al. ARIX: a randomised trial of acupuncture v oral care sessions in patients with chronic xerostomia following treatment of head and neck cancer. *Ann Oncol*. 2013;**24**:776–783.

57 Garcia MK, McQuade J, Haddad R, et al. Systematic review of acupuncture in cancer care: a synthesis of the evidence. *J Clin Oncol*. 2013;**31**(**7**):952–960.

第 50 章　卫生服务研究

Michaela A. Dinan, PhD ■ Bradford R. Hirsch, MD, MBA ■ Amy Abernethy, MD, PhD

概述

卫生服务研究（health services research, HSR）涵盖多领域内容，自提出至今已有 100 多年历史。HSR 旨在评估医疗卫生服务对患者和人群的影响，从而进一步了解医疗保健在癌症领域的作用、效果和成本。目前，临床工作者和科研人员较推崇“从科研到临床应用”为创新型生物医学研究的目标。然而，在临床实施干预措施前、中、后各阶段，患者、医生和医疗体系可能会受到诸多因素影响，从而影响医疗保健效果。虽然卫生服务研究是一个与时俱进、深奥难懂的复杂概念，但是为了准确地量化、评估、优化现在及未来的癌症研究，基本理解其内容是必要的。

引言：什么是卫生服务研究？

卫生服务研究（health services research, HSR）涵盖多学科内容，旨在评估医疗保健对患者和人群的影响。虽然各学科侧重点不同，但具有相似之处，使其均可以纳入 HSR 研究范围。不同卫生服务研究的基础研究方法相同，即针对目标结局，实施治疗或干预措施，以便更好地理解和指导临床实践。

为了帮助医疗保健消费者选择最佳治疗或干预方案，基于 Institute of Medicine（IOM）定义，HSR 侧重医疗保健以下 3 个方面：①医疗保健获得方式：②医疗保健质量；③医疗保健费用（针对需方患者来说，cost 翻译成费用，针对供方翻译成“成本”），以便患者了解到最优的治疗方案和预防措施[1]。此外，IOM 还汇总了当下 HSR 热点研究方向（表 50-1）。

表 50-1　卫生服务研究热点

序号	研究热点
1	医疗机构组织与融资
2	医疗卫生服务的获取方式
3	医务人员、患者和医疗服务消费者的行为学研究
4	医疗卫生服务质量
5	临床预后研究
6	医疗决策和医学信息学
7	医疗相关职业人员研究

HSR 涉及多学科领域，生物统计学家、经济学家、临床医生和卫生服务研究人员等都是其重要参与者。在癌症领域，内科学、外科学和放射治疗学等临床、病理和影像专家的专业知识是研究临床相关问题、提高医疗保健质量所必需的。其中，科研人员和临床医生的密切合作对于确保 HSR 研究的科学性、有效性和临床意义至关重要。

HSR 在癌症领域应用广泛。例如，侧重于诊疗以延长生存时间、提高生活质量（quality of life, QOL）、为医疗决策提供证据、为获得医疗卫生服务提供便利、确保医疗卫生服务与指南的一致性或探究医疗保健带给癌症患者的经济影响。除了上述研究内容和其他潜在结果外，为推动癌症研究进展，还应从患者及其家属、临床医生和其他医务人员、医疗服务提供方、医疗服务支付方、其他相关行业人员和政策制定者等在内的多个利益相关者角度开展研究。

卫生服务研究在癌症领域的意义

在癌症领域开展卫生服务研究是我们确定癌症范围、提高癌症护理水平的主要手段。但是，基础研究和临床试验等在可控条件下获得的结果，在外推到大样本人群或真实世界研究时不一定适用。这是因为，临床试验侧重于特定干预方式的疗效或特定干预方式在特定条件下发挥效用的能力；而 HSR 仅侧重于干预措施在真实世界中发挥效用的能力即有效性，其目的在于将干预措施推广到更广泛、更多样化的人群中以提高其有效性从而促进人群健康。

目前，用于确定癌症范围并预测其发展风向的癌症卫生服务研究已在全国范围内开展。例如，一项基于人群的监测、流行病学和预后（Surveillance, Epidemiology, and End Results, SEER）登记系统研究显示，2014 年美国癌症新发病例 1 665 540 例，死亡病例 585 720 例。随着人口老龄化加剧，癌症新发病例和死亡病例数可能还会不断增加。2010 年美国癌症直接治疗成本为 1 245 亿美元，在调整人口结构后，到 2020 年，预计将增加到 1 578 亿美元[2]。而由于采用昂贵的创新型疗法、推广无证据支撑的先进技术、现有治疗方法不恰当使用（过高或过低）以及患者实际需求和过高期望之间的矛盾，实际癌症治疗成本可能会更高。针对当前医疗资源和基础设施需求激增的问题，卫生服务研究为此提供了新思路。

卫生服务研究的多学科领域

实践过程中，卫生服务研究涵盖多学科领域——卫生经济学、流行病学、定性研究和实施性研究。为更好地解决科学问题，基于数据、方法学和专业知识的实际需求，各学科应运而生并逐渐发展。虽然学科间存在差异，但“异”中有“同”，各学科的共同目标都是实现因果关系推断。例如，预后研究关注治疗方式或暴露因素与结局的关系（例如新型治疗方式对生存状态的影响）；卫生经济学关注医疗成本和资源利用度；流行病学关注暴露因素和暴露方式;卫生服务研究关注医疗系统内直接或间接的暴露或治疗问题。

卫生服务研究的研究设计概述

卫生服务研究可采用多种研究设计方案,可分析数据类型包括一手数据(作为临床试验的一部分,经前瞻性收集获得)和二手数据(最初为其他目的收集)。其中,随机对照试验(randomized clinical trials,RCTs)可将研究者感兴趣的干预措施随机施加给受试者,被认为是临床试验的金标准。RCTs 通常采用单盲法,即医生不知道受试者的分组情况;也可以采用双盲法,即医生和受试者均不知道分组情况。RCTs 确保干预措施随机施加给受试者,有助于避免偏倚。

观察性研究对研究对象不施加任何干预措施,主要用于探索暴露与结局的关系,且多是回顾性研究。观察性研究分为描述性和分析性两种:描述性研究包括病例报告(系列)、生态学研究和横断面研究,用于提出假设;分析性研究包括纵向队列研究和病例对照研究,用于验证暴露与结局间关系的相关假设。

癌症卫生服务研究的相关二级数据库

众所周知,研究效果和数据质量密切相关。由于各数据库适用条件不同,卫生服务研究人员需联合使用多个数据库才能解决研究问题。一手数据的质量在很大程度上取决于仪器设定和数据收集过程中遇到的问题;二手数据的质量通常受到收集目的的影响。例如,账单数据(又名医保数据)通过医疗服务申请单和收款单获得,利用该数据的研究在统计分析时应考虑其固有局限性。

可用于分析的常见癌症二级数据库包括临床登记系统、管理数据库、临床试验数据库以及数据量日益增加的电子病例系统(electronic medical record,EMR)(本章其他部分将详细描述)。深入了解各数据库的优劣势对于有效开展统计分析至关重要(表 50-2)。临床登记系统可以收集特定人群、特定地区、医疗系统或互联网内癌症患者的数据,不仅包含高质量的短期暴露和结局数据、目标研究疾病的临床数据,还可以收集潜在混在因素,从而开展大样本研究;其缺点是随机性差,缺少中长期随访以及非目标研究疾病的数据(如心血管疾病)。

表 50-2　常见大型二级数据库的主要优势和局限性

数据来源	二级数据库	优势	局限性
疾病登记系统	SEER NCDB EMR	• 短时间内、高质量的暴露和结局数据 • 临床数据丰富 • 可收集潜在的混杂因素 • 覆盖人群广	• 不能对关键因素进行随机化控制 • 长期随访效果差 • 缺少非研究疾病的数据资料
管理数据	CMS(Medicare) VA(Veterans Affairs) Kaiser Permanente	• 覆盖人群广 • 数据收集高效 • 通过患者特定标识可实现长期随访 • 可与其他数据来源的数据库链接	• 不能对关键因素进行随机化控制 • 数据准确度低 • 临床资料不全面
临床试验研究	协作组研究 行业研究 机构研究	• 随机化 • 临床数据丰富	• 预选研究对象 • 多为小样本研究 • 失访偏倚

管理数据库由医疗保险机构(例如 Medicare)、综合医疗保健系统(例如 Veterans Affairs Hospitals)或大型医疗保健组织(例如 Kaiser Permanente)定期收集,具有覆盖人群广、数据可用性高以及可长期随访的优势。此外,不同于临床资料丰富但由于研究成本和科学性而局限于小样本的临床试验,管理数据库有更好的人群代表性。但是该数据库也存在局限性,其收集目的是追踪医疗保健资源使用及支付情况,从而影响数据粒度即数据统计的粗细程度。以医保数据为例,索赔日期和医疗服务项目等数据信息的可信度很高,然而,癌症分期等非关键信息不一定会记录。

链接不同类型的数据库有助于抵消单一数据库的局限性。例如,临床登记数据和临床试验数据存在数据不完整、缺乏长期随访的问题,可通过链接医保数据库(如 Medicare)增加随访和生存数据。

数据,在任何设计方案中都是极其重要的,但是数据类型与研究设计间存在高度特异性。接下来,我们会针对不同研究背景及方法讨论各数据库的用法。鉴于 SEER 数据库和 National Cancer Data Base(NCDB)在癌症卫生服务研究中发挥着核心作用,本节将详细介绍。

SEER 数据库

通过汇总具有高度代表性的癌症登记数据,SEER 数据库收集了美国 28%癌症患者详细的临床和病理信息,但是缺乏治疗方案、成本费用和卫生服务提供方的数据资料。上述局限性,可通过链接其他数据库,生成宽数据而得到解决。例如通过 National Cancer Institute(NCI)与 Centers for Medicare and Medicaid Services(CMS)合作,链接 Medicare 管理数据和医保数据从而建立 SEER-Medicare 数据库。CMS 的医疗保险服务覆盖超过 97%的 65 岁及以上的美国人，为评估 SEER 数据库所含对象的卫生服务利用率和成本提供了有利条件。目前，SEER-Medicare 数据库已用于种族差异、临床医生或医院机构特征、癌症筛查、癌症治疗方式选择（即手术、化疗和放疗）、相关并发症、死亡率和医疗成本等方面的癌症医疗质量研究[3]。值得注意的是，虽然 SEER-Medicare 数据库功能强大，但仅包含 65 岁及以上人群的相关数据。

美国国家癌症数据库（NCDB）

另一个被广泛使用的癌症专用数据库是美国国家癌症数据库（National Cancer Data Base，NCDB），由美国癌症协会（American Cancer Society）和美国外科医师协会癌症委员会（American College of Surgeons' Commission on Cancer，COC）联合建立。NCDB 成立于 1989 年，是一个全国性的、全面的、以医院为基础的临床监测数据库。数据来源于 1 500 多家经 COC 认证的机构，包括 3 000 万例现患者和 70%新发癌症患者的信息[4]。该数据库优势在于规模大，包含全美大多数癌症病例，因此可用于研究国家医疗模式，新型外科手术以及罕见癌症的治疗方法。作为一个外科数据库，NCDB 包括患者手术和生存状况等详细信息。然而，该数据库也存在如下问题：部分数据的编码信息不可靠；化疗、放疗或非癌症相关健康问题的数据不详细；无复发、再发或后续治疗的信息。

卫生服务研究的统计分析

本节将重点介绍适用于绝大多数卫生服务研究的常用统计分析方法。HSR 通过分析目标人群的数据资料从而描述或推断该人群的一般情况。统计描述指通过均数、频数、频率、统计图或其他方式来描述、概括数据的一般情况；统计推断和统计分析是通过较为专业且复杂的统计学方法做出统计推论，例如判断两组数据之间的差异是否具有统计学意义。

多因素分析和单因素分析的异同点

实际分析过程中，选择单因素分析还是多因素分析是常见问题之一。单因素分析用于描述、总结单个变量的情况，例如有吸烟史者占总研究人群的百分比。多因素分析用于解释因变量和其他多个自变量之间的关系，较为复杂。

由于多因素分析通过控制变量来调整潜在混杂因素，单因素分析与多因素分析又被称为“未调整性分析”和“调整性分析”。需要控制的变量是指与研究结局相关的临床变量，例如年龄、疾病分期、疾病等级以及与暴露（结局）相关的任何变量，以便控制潜在混杂因素对结果的影响。同单因素分析相比，多因素分析对可能会影响结果推论的潜在混杂因素进行了调整，其结果更能反映暴露和结局的真实关系。此外，如果忽略变量间的交互作用则可能得出错误结论。HSR 主要是在控制混杂因素的基础上探讨特定治疗、条件或暴露如何影响特定结局。

多因素分析

多元回归分析是卫生服务研究中使用最广泛的多因素分析方法之一。19 世纪末，Francis Galton 提出“回归”这一概念，用于预测异常豌豆植株（高大或矮小）的后代植株高度，这些后代植株的高度更接近或者说又“回归”到了总体豌豆植株的高度[5]。最简单的回归是通过在双变量散点图上绘制一条直线，得到一个变量的平均值与另一个变量的关系函数。随着数学和计算机领域的迅猛发展，更为复杂的数学模型加入预测行列中来，通过多个“自变量”的值，可以对“因变量”作出更为合理的统计预测。模型有多种类型，经过不断改进和发展，可对各种类型的变量进行描述、预测及建模。例如，线性回归模型用于对连续型数据建模；Logistic 回归模型（将结局定义为 0 或者 1）用于对二分类数据建模；Cox 比例风险模型（生存变量包括结局事件，如死亡、复发或发生该事件的时间）用于对生存数据建模。不同模型的统计指标不同：线性回归模型构建因变量均值与各自变量的函数（例如，用性别和身高来预测平均体重）；Logistic 回归模型估计暴露因素相关的优势比（OR）；Cox 比例风险模型得到风险比（HR）。其他常用多因素分析方法还有 χ^2 检验，例如 Cochran-Mantel-Haenszel 检验[6,7]，其实质是在控制混杂因素的前提下，通过计算 χ^2 来判断两变量之间的关联程度。

多元回归分析的另一优势是可以观测到两独立变量之间的交互作用。当变量仅影响某组研究对象的治疗效果时，该变量与分组变量之间即存在交互作用。例如，一项纳入 3 项随机对照试验的非小细胞肺癌（NSCLC）meta 分析结果显示：鳞状细胞癌、接受培美曲塞治疗和治疗效果不佳 3 个变量间存在显著的交互作用，因此证实，培美曲塞可改善非鳞状细胞癌患者预后状况，是非鳞状 NSCLC 的首选药物[8]。

偏倚和混杂

偏倚和混杂是卫生服务研究中的重要概念。混杂因素是指任何混淆、模糊或以其他方式影响研究变量的因素。“confound”来自拉丁语，意为“倾倒在一起”[9]，表示变量间关联被混杂因素混淆、歪曲的情况。以一项关于转移性疾病的回顾性研究为例，该研究表明患有轻度侵袭性疾病并因其转移而接受手术的患者的生存时间更长。在此例中，我们所观测到的，接受手术与生存期延长之间的关联被非侵袭性疾病与手术和生存之间的关联所混淆。

偏倚一词源于古法语“biais”，意思是“倾斜”[9]，也是描述混杂影响的一种方式，表示所观察到的关联有所偏重或偏向，从而使两变量之间的关联出现假阳性（正偏移、负偏移）或假阴性（结果偏向于零假设）。

癌症卫生服务研究中关于偏倚的典型例子是 NSCLC 患者的生存分析。多项研究显示，是否接受 PET 扫描与患者生存率相关，并得出接受 PET 扫描可以提高患者生存率这一结论。然而，深入研究发现，PET 扫描更适用于需要手术和根治治疗的早期患者，不适用于晚期或发生转移的患者。由此可见，PET 扫描与提高生存率的关系受到选择偏倚的影响，即仅轻度患者才进行 PET 扫描，从而错误地估计了 PET 扫描与生存率提高之间的关系[10,11]。

观察性卫生服务研究存在常见偏倚。其中，遗漏变量偏倚是其主要偏倚之一，几乎存在于所有卫生服务研究中。此偏倚常发生在以下两种情况：①某变量与研究结局和暴露因素均相关；②作为对照而被遗漏。例如，在 PET-NSCLC 方案中，疾病分期与是否接受 PET 扫描和生存状态均相关，但不包括在模型中。

当干预或暴露措施非随机地施加给研究对象时，会产生选择偏倚。正如上述PET-NSCLC方案中，PET扫描选择性地应用于早期患者。回忆偏倚指某群体比其他群体更易回忆起某事件。例如，患有某种罕见癌症的患者，对既往环境暴露因子及自身暴露情况，印象更为深刻，而这些环境暴露因素常被非癌症患者忽视或遗忘。失访偏倚是由于研究对象患病状况及对某些因素的暴露情况与失访者可能会不尽相同，从而导致的系统误差。无应答偏倚发生在自评调查中，参与自评者要比目标全体人群有更强的表达欲。错分偏倚是指暴露或结局被错误分类。另外，如果研究者事先了解研究对象的暴露或治疗情况，可能会对其采取与对照组不可比的方法探寻可能与某病或某结局相关的因素，从而导致错误的结论，产生访谈者偏倚。

偏倚和混杂的最小化

减小混杂的方法有多种，但个别方法仅适用于研究设计阶段。因此，在研究设计阶段初期，要由统计学和HSR专家对研究方法和研究方案等问题进行把控。例如，RCTs通常根据关键变量分层以确保得到均衡可比的干预组和对照组；多元回归分析通常会调整或控制潜在混杂因素。然而，上述方法均无法对那些无法观测到的变量加以控制，而此类变量几乎存在于所有观察性HSR研究中并发挥着不同程度的干扰作用。因此，在这些变量的混杂作用未得到证实之前，不应将任何观察到的关联结果报告为因果关系。

减小偏倚的常用方法包括匹配、分层、亚组分析和工具变量分析。

匹配，即要求对照组与干预组在某些因素或特征上保持一致，以构建各方面均相似的两组研究群体。通过间接法评估匹配效果，确保非匹配变量在组间更为接近。

当组间存在多个不同因素时，对所有因素精确匹配较困难，可用倾向性评分预测个体接受治疗或暴露于某因素的可能性（或倾向性）[12]，再根据评分对研究对象直接进行匹配或分层分析，以减小组间差异，更好地评估暴露因素或治疗方式。

分层法或亚组分析的思想与匹配法相似，将研究对象按照某一特征或可疑的混杂因素分为不同组（例如疾病分期、患者年龄、体力状态等）再展开分析。

上述方法均能识别混杂因素并对其进行控制和校正。与之相比，工具变量法是通过避免所有混杂因素来控制、消除偏倚。若某变量与模型中随机解释变量高度相关，但与随机误差项不相关，这个变量就称为工具变量。例如，研究对象与可提供PET扫描的场所的最近距离，与疾病阶段或生存状态（结局）无直接关系，但可以预测研究对象进行PET扫描的可能性（暴露）。然而，功能性越强的工具变量越难被识别，而且通常是不可用的。值得注意的是，上述任何一种方法都不能完全消除真实世界卫生服务研究的偏倚。因此，识别、减小偏倚对于准确地解释观察性卫生服务研究结果至关重要。

内部效度和外部效度

内部效度指研究结果能否反映研究对象的情况，换句话说，内部效度用来反映研究结果在研究对象中的可信程度。任何研究必须具有内部效度以便进行临床层面的解释。其影响因素包括选择偏倚、随访偏倚、回忆偏倚、错分偏倚、访谈者偏倚、混杂因素影响以及任何与暴露相关的系统误差。

外部效度指在研究对象内观察到的结果是否可以推广到研究样本之外。各研究的外部效度并非完全相同。例如，许多RCTs仅限于有较少合并症的年轻患者，其研究结果不适合外推到高龄、病情严重或已经过预处理的患者。

卫生服务研究的研究类型

Meta分析与系统综述

系统综述，作为Meta分析的第一步，指对特定问题的相关文献进行彻底的、系统的概括和总结。Meta分析是全面收集所有相关研究并逐个进行严格评价和分析，再用定量合成的方法对资料进行统计学处理得出综合结论的过程。为保证有效性，Meta分析通过高质量、系统化地概括现有文献，纳入所有相关数据，利用异质性分析评估是否存在发表偏倚，利用敏感性分析验证研究结果以确保效应估计值更为可信。Meta分析和系统综述作为循证医学的主要组成部分，在验证普适性和了解临床意义方面尤其重要。

随机对照试验

长期以来，随机对照试验（RCTs）一直被认为是个体试验中具有最高证据效力的研究方法。通过将患者随机分配到对照组（安慰剂或金标准）或试验组，RCTs可用于药效评估、行为干预、化学预防和筛查。尽管RCTs具有较好的验证假设的能力并具有诸多优势，但对于医疗保健提供者和研究人员来说，彻底了解其优劣势对于准确合并、解释研究结果至关重要，从而更好地指导临床实践和卫生服务研究。

RCTs的显著优势是“随机化”，这是消除潜在偏倚的唯一的、最可靠的方法，也是进行“反事实推断”的重要研究方法。“反事实推断”指对现实情况进行否定而重新表征，以构建一种新可能性假设的过程。例如，假设同一个患者分别接受治疗A和治疗B会有怎样不同？如果时间可以倒退，那么对同一个患者进行不同的治疗，结局会改变吗？虽然此种假设是不现实的，但是在实践过程中，我们通过RCTs随机分配研究对象可以实现间接推断——患者分别接受治疗A或治疗B会有怎样的影响。混杂导致的潜在偏倚是观察性研究的主要局限性，而RCTs的最根本优势就是能避免混杂因素的影响。

随机对照试验的潜在局限性

RCTs无法解决卫生服务研究的所有问题，最重要的原因是由于伦理道德问题难以在各组之间达到均衡，难以避免对照组与试验组的沾染。以局限性前列腺癌的两种最终治疗方式——根治性前列腺切除术与放疗为例，医生和患者通常都不愿意被随机地分配到某一治疗方案之中。因此，针对此两种治疗方式展开的RCTs也因样本量或外部效度问题受到限制[13]。在英国，此类研究招募的研究对象同意随机化的比例仅为二十分之一[14]。

即便满足了伦理学要求，样本量适当，RCTs仍存在其他局限性。因此,在解释"阴性结果"时,应确保 RCTs 有足够说服力来应对所出现问题。

RCTs 的另一个局限性是外部效度低。RCTs 的研究对象通常需要符合严格纳入标准且具有高度代表性,因此研究结果往往优于基于社区人群的研究。例如一项关于局部乳腺癌化疗效果的经典 Meta 分析显示,在纳入的 194 项研究中,由于 69 岁以上研究对象较少,因而无法得知 70 岁以上妇女化疗的效果[15]。

RCTs 的设计、招募、随访和分析过程往往需要数十年或更长时间才能完成进而得到研究结果。而这些研究在完成前可能已经过时,特别是自然史长、进展速度快的癌症(如乳腺癌)。RCTs 无法评估某种治疗手段在一般人群中的效果,无法确定试验条件下和实际实践中风险或效益的一致程度,无法描述在真实世界中干预措施的接受度、利用度、成本费用或其他特征。虽然 RCTs 是验证治疗方式是否有效的最佳研究证据之一,但是为了对治疗方案的真实影响和有效性进行全面的评估,仍需要将观察性研究作为补充研究。

观察性研究

观察性研究不区分暴露组和对照组,也不对任何感兴趣因素加以控制。顾名思义,观察性研究是利用医保数据、疾病登记数据、大型医疗机构数据库(例如 Veterans Affairs)以及临床试验数据等多种数据库的资料进行二次分析。基于人口登记系统的 SEER 数据库覆盖了 28% 的美国人口;NCDB 是一个基于医院的注册数据库,拥有超过 1 500 个 COC 认证机构,收集了全美 70% 的新诊断癌症病例[4];Nationwide Inpatient Sample (NIS)包含自 2012 年以来美国共 44 个州的出院数据,占所有社区医院的 20%[16];大型医保数据库,例如 Medicare 数据库和大型私立保险公司数据库,可通过与基线库、治疗库、死因库等其他数据库合并连接,获取更为全面、详细的医疗数据信息。

偏倚或混杂是观察性研究的主要局限性。上节已讨论一系列减小偏倚或混杂的方法以避免得出无效结论。虽然存在局限性,但观察性研究仍然在卫生服务研究的多领域发挥重要作用,而这些是 RCTs 无法解决的。例如,吸烟是癌症最重要的危险因素,许多观察性研究已证实吸烟与多种癌症的发生相关,而 RCTs 无法对其关系进行验证。

观察性研究的优点如下:①不同于研究机构或癌症中心的研究,观察性研究是基于社区的真实世界研究,可提供干预措施的实际实施情况与真实效果;②与试验研究相比,观察性研究成本低、样本量大、易随访且具有足够统计学效力探索罕见疾病的治疗方式和危险因素。

观察性研究的常见类型

观察性研究通常分为描述性研究和分析性研究两种。分析性研究类似于随机试验,目的在于评估暴露因素或治疗方式与结局的因果关系。此外分析性研究还可用于验证某特定假设,例如,对于要接受手术治疗的患者来说,大医院的治疗效果是否优于小医院。描述性研究指总结某特定群体的一般特征或结局变量,以及生成假设以便在下一步的研究中验证假设。

病例对照研究和队列研究是分析性研究的两种常见类型。在癌症卫生服务研究中,病例对照研究常用于评估环境暴露因素(如吸烟、遗传、地理、药物、饮食等)与癌症发生可能性(结局)的关联。以现在确诊的患有某特定疾病的患者作为病例,以不患有该病但具有可比性的个体作为对照,通过询问、实验室检查或复查病史,搜集两组研究对象既往各种可能的危险因素的暴露史,继而做出统计推断。其优势在于可分析罕见癌种的危险因素;难点在于对照组和病例组除暴露因素以外,其他各方面应保持一致,以确保在获取既往信息时,两组之间回忆偏倚不会相差太大。

队列研究根据某一特定人群是否暴露于某可疑因素或暴露程度分为不同的亚组,追踪观察两组或多组成员结局(如疾病)发生的情况,其分组在结果出现前就已经确定好。卫生服务研究中有许多研究属于队列研究范畴,包括临床试验、疾病登记和其他回顾性或前瞻性研究。这些研究常被用来探索新兴医疗技术如高级成像、PET 扫描[17],以及前列腺癌强调放射治疗(IMRT)技术[18]等新兴医疗技术的使用情况和成本费用。

前瞻性队列研究是为了特定目的而收集数据并对其进行分析。而回顾性队列研究是利用已经收集的数据进行分析。虽然两者存在差异,但统计分析方法相似。前瞻性研究,特别是收集、分析数据前已制定详细计划的前瞻性研究,较少采用可识别虚假关联的亚组分析或其他统计方法。观察性队列研究的优势在于能在长时间随访过程中发现罕见暴露因素,例如原子弹辐射暴露对若干年后发生白血病或其他癌症的影响。卫生服务研究中,队列研究是最常用的观察性研究方法,用于比较特定治疗方式对患者预后的影响。例如,考虑到在前列腺癌患者中开展关于前列腺切除术与放射治疗的大规模 RCTs 的困难性,最终采用队列研究比较两种治疗方式的预后效果(Sun 2014)。

描述性研究包括生态学研究、横断面研究和病例报告(系列)。不同于分析性研究,此类研究的目的在于产生假设而不是验证假设。生态学研究是在群体水平上研究某种暴露因素与结局之间的关系[19]。例如,多项癌症生态学研究已证实,由于文化、环境、饮食或生活方式等不同,美国与其他国家在某些癌症如乳腺癌或前列腺癌的发病风险上存在差异[20]。生态学研究虽然能提供病因线索,产生病因假设,但不能确定个体水平上暴露与结局的关系。

横断面研究是通过收集、描述特定时间和(或)特定范围内人群中的疾病或健康状况和有关因素的分布状况,从而为进一步的研究提供病因线索。然而,此类研究存在一个严重局限性,即难以判断暴露与结局的时间先后顺序,因而论证因果关系的能力较差。

病例报告(系列)是指通过描述小样本量研究对象的暴露和结局关系进而评估新型治疗方式的效果。以一项关于联合使用免疫检查点抑制剂和放疗的病例报告研究为例,该研究表明,放疗可以诱导机体免疫反应,因而对转移性黑色素瘤患者进行局部放射治疗即可治疗所有病变部位[21]。

大多数回顾性研究缺乏个体危险因素和病情的详细资料。此外,若我们在研究开始前就已经知晓某因素与结局或暴露有较强关联,那我们可能会采取与收集其他因素不可比的方法去收集此因素的相关资料。数据质量的好坏决定最终分析结果的准确性。数据中关键暴露因素、结局变量和潜在混杂因素等数据资料的可靠性决定其内部效度。再次以医保数据为例,由于索赔日期和类型编码等与支付相关的数据资料，需要经过严格审计核实，因而真实可靠。然而，不影响索赔的轻微并发症（例如便秘）等数据资料，其完整性和可靠性相对较低。因此，熟悉待分析数据的基本情况对于研究至关重要。

建模研究

建模研究指通过算法描述暴露因素、研究结局和混杂因素间的复杂关系[22]。在指导政策、指南、治疗方法或医疗费用报销等方面，建模研究发挥着重要作用，避免了运用干预性研究或传统观察性研究高耗时、高成本和相对复杂的局限性。建模研究还可用于探索无法在实践中直接观察或获得的数据，例如成本费用或治疗的远期影响。就卫生服务研究来说，建模研究主要用于探索各种决策算法、新型干预措施、政策及患者个人因素与成本、效益的关系。研究中常采用质量调整寿命年（QUALYs）作为评价癌症患者疾病负担的客观指标。成本效果分析通过报告增量成本效益比（ICER）描述替代性治疗或其他暴露因素的相对成本和效益。

例如，乳腺癌癌型检测（Oncotype DX 检测）可以预测接受化疗的相关益处，且已有研究证明该检测能够帮助医生制定更优的化疗方案，节省化疗成本费用[23]。建模研究的优点在于能发现多种因素对结局的影响，例如，可以根据干预措施、受检者年龄和化疗费用调整乳腺癌癌型检测节省成本估计值。建模的主要缺点是必须做出多种假设，而这可能影响研究结果。

医疗质量

IOM 将医疗质量定义为“向个人和人群提供的医疗卫生服务在提高预期健康水平方面的可能性，以及医疗卫生服务与现有专业知识水平的一致程度”，广义定义是“尊重患者自身价值和偏好的医疗卫生服务”[24,25]。尽管现有治疗手段和医疗技术已得到实质性提高，但是影响患者健康状态、医疗质量和成本费用的主要决定因素仍然未得到正确认识，这可能与临床多样性[26,27]和患者未能获得基本医疗保健有关[28]。

一项基于高容量医院、长达 30 余年的研究发现，病例容量大或就诊人数多的医疗机构的患者预后效果更好[29]。20 年后，上述结果被一项 Meta 分析证实。该 Meta 分析纳入了 128 项研究，发现在 40 个不同的高容量医疗机构实施外科手术的住院死亡率较低[30]。另一项研究发现，在低容量医疗机构接受食管切除术或胰切除术等复杂手术的风险较高，其术后 30 天内死亡率比高容量医疗机构高 5%～10%[31]。然而，这些研究本质上都是观察性研究，对于“高容量”的定义各不相同，且患者对于高容量医疗机构的倾向性可能导致选择偏倚。医疗质量也可能受到地理因素、患者数量、癌症专家人数或其他因素影响。例如，腹腔镜结肠切除术[32]和临终关怀[33]的占比在各区域间存在较大差异。

Donabedian 在 1950 年提出一系列描述医疗结构、过程和结果的度量指标，并一直沿用至今[1]。结构指医疗环境及相关的人力、财力资源，例如人力资源配置、资格认证和规模等机构特征；过程指在疾病诊疗过程中医患双方的行为，该过程通常由国家综合癌症网络（National Comprehensive Cancer Network，NCCN）或美国临床肿瘤学会（American Society of Clinical Oncology，ASCO）等国家级机构发布的指南定义；结果指患者的预后情况，通常由总体生存率、疾病特异性生存率、客观缓解率、疾病进展时间和治疗副作用等指标来反映。而由于病例复杂、疾病严重程度不同和存在超出可控范围的混杂因素等原因，在癌症领域采用“结果”相关指标常引起争论，不过该问题已引起关注并逐渐得到解决。

尽管影响医疗质量的潜在因素有很多，但是最根本的挑战在于如何使用基于“结果”和“结构”的结局指标来定义医疗质量，从而激励医务人员和改善医疗系统。例如，基于“结果”的结局指标可能受到病例复杂性的影响；“择优挑选”或采用其他纳入方式可能会增加收益但不会改善医疗质量。而基于“结构”的结局指标取决于医院容量、医院位置、病例复杂性和医院多方面资源配置情况，无法适用于所有研究。因此，无论是研究还是实践，评估医疗质量均应以“过程”为主。例如，目前 Healthcare Effectiveness Data and Information Set（HEDIS）评估医疗质量的大部分主流指标都基于“过程”，如癌症筛查、免疫接种或疾病的特殊治疗[34]。但是“过程”可能存在未得到充分利用、滥用或误用的情况。未得到充分利用常发生于即使有推荐指南但未考虑患者能否接受、参与研究的情况。由于指南很少考虑不适用条件，滥用和误用两种情况较难被发现。例如，虽然 PET 扫描不适用于所有乳腺癌或结直肠癌患者，但交界性 CT 扫描或其他经验性研究认为 PET 扫描属于合理指征。若治疗记录缺失，误用同样难以识别，而治疗记录在回顾性研究中通常无法获得。

卫生服务研究 2.0

卫生服务研究在过去 20 年中迅速发展，很大部分原因在于计算、生成、储存、链接、分析和解释大型数据库的能力得到大幅提升。但是直到 1970 年，运用当时最先进的机电台式计算机进行单因素回归分析仍需 24 小时[35]。近年来，个人计算机、互联网和现代移动设备的出现为卫生服务研究提供了前所未有的发展机遇，即从患者、医疗服务提供者、医疗系统的角度全面捕获和分析医疗卫生服务。IOM 提出“学习型医疗体系（learning health system，LHS）”，即结合自然科学、信息学、激励机制和文化内涵实现医疗体系的不断提高和创新，收集更多数据信息，制定最佳医疗服务支付方案[36]。LHS 更深层的意义在于通过快速学习患者反馈信息，实现个性化医疗服务从而为医疗决策提供建议[37]。虽然 LHS 的理念已经逐渐普及，但评估疗效和引导未来研究领域的“实例”才刚刚兴起。例如，LHS 方法正被用于评估生物制剂在儿童克罗恩病中的作用[38]。

EMR 记录了每位患者完整的医疗服务电子信息，是 LHS 的基础。EMR 数据，在编码标准化后近似于登记数据，其数据类型不同，编码标准化方式不同。结构化数据（例如实验室数据）需要经过数据清洗转换为单一、通用的数据类型；非结构化数据（例如 PDF 格式的临床记录、病理报告）需要先转换为可编码的电子格式。

致力于 LHS 的研究人员众多，涉及传统卫生组织、政府机构和基因组公司等。通过链接 EMR 与外部数据库，可实时获得真实世界数据。而进一步实现将决策支持纳入常规医疗程序，不仅需要患者基因组学、疾病治疗史和预测结果等具体数据,还需要了解如何从科学技术、法医学、道德伦理和临床实践的角度进行数据管理。面对日益上涨的医疗成本和不对等的医疗效果,癌症学研讨会更侧重于负担得起的医疗保健,提出通过 LHS 寻找解决方案以节约医疗保健和临床研究成本[39]。

结局和终点

卫生服务研究可以采用任何与医疗保健相关的结局或终点指标,此外,多种结局和终点已构成当前卫生服务研究的研究主体,QOL、成本、质量、获得途径、医疗模式和疗效比较研究(cost-effectiveness ratio,CER)等多种结局指标也已成为当前卫生服务研究的研究主体。

患者报告结局

患者报告结局(patient reported outcome,PRO)是基于患者临床症状和其他患者关心问题而得,并非由临床医生或医疗保健人员记录生成。

随着互联网的普及和计算机领域的飞速发展,获得和收集纵向 PRO 信息愈发便利。当下,PRO 的收集和利用已成为一个独特的研究领域,大量计算机与 QOL 研究人员通力合作,以期更有效率地实现研究目标。QOL 是 PRO 重要组成部分,我们将在下一章节对其具体内容做更为详细的讲解与讨论。

PRO 具有下列优点:①数据收集效率高;②与医生报告相比,准确性高;③可预测客观临床结果,如生存状态、患者满意度和一般健康信息[40]。PRO 可分为通用型和特异型(针对各类疾病),各有利弊[41]。通用型 PRO 的优势主要包括其适用疾病的类型比较广泛以及证明其有效性和与传统客观指标关联度的文献数量较多[41]。

虽然已有大量研究使用了 PRO 方法,但在癌症领域,仅有少数进行了评估,包括 EORTC QOL Questionnaire(EORTC QLQ-C30)、Functional Assessment of Cancer Therapy(FACT)、MD Anderson Symptom Inventory(MDASI)、PRO version of the Common Terminology Criteria for Adverse Events(PRO-CTCAE)和 PRO Measurement Information System(PROMIS)[40]。经过验证、标准化和比较,PRO 方法的可靠性已得到大幅提高,并运用于临床试验设计以及向 FDA 提交的新药申请书。

目前,已实现在 LHS 中通过 PRO 收集患者的音频资料已成为现实。与传统 PRO 相比,电子型患者报告结局(electronic PROs,EPRO)的优点更多,包括成本低、医患双方参与度高以及可以使用计算机自适应测试(computer adaptive testing,CAT)有效利用个性化数据。基于上述优点,EPRO 数据可用于通知医护人员,提供决策支持以及在护理时间内向医患双方实时提供帮助。

生活质量

生活质量(quality of life,QOL)的测量方法复杂多样,每一种都适用于特定领域(例如疲劳,尿路症状,医疗事件),各领域又包括多个研究项目。衡量特定测量方法利用度的关键指标包括可靠性、内部一致性、可重复性和效度(内容和结构)。以简表-36 项(short form-36 item,SF-36)为例,该调查问卷已用于数百项研究和多种疾病类型,并有大量文献验证了其可靠性和适用性。而特定疾病的生活质量测量方法能针对性地、更好地评估对应患者群体的关键影响因素。例如,对于前列腺癌患者,泌尿功能和性生活质量应直接通过特定疾病测量工具进行评估,如国际勃起功能指数(International Index of Erectile Function,IIEF)和美国泌尿系统协会(American Urologic Association,AUA)。因此,选择最佳生活质量指标需要全面了解该疾病相关症状和结局[40]。此外,生活质量研究还可用于实际应用或 QOL 量化,例如用于调整生存分析以描述存活人数和生活质量。

合理评估生活质量存在如下局限性:①涵盖众多领域和项目,多种评估方式以及功能障碍和症状的不同排序方式都会阻碍其标准化和验证;②不具有普适性,例如,老年患者对性功能关注度低,残疾患者基线水平与非残疾患者不同;③疲劳、冷漠、心智功能下降或整体健康状态不佳可能会影响问卷完成度或导致数据缺失,该情况常见于姑息治疗。同时,患者整体表现不良与参与不积极密切相关并可能导致报告偏倚。

医疗成本

正如本章前面所述,由于人口老龄化和新兴医疗技术的兴起,美国的癌症医疗成本迅速增加。准确量化成本、了解成本驱动因素以及对备选治疗方案建模是癌症卫生服务研究的重要组成部分。通过此类分析,有助于了解研究的总体成本、成本效益、成本效用以及成本效果,为其提供一个统一的框架并设置通用阈值,从而客观地、合理地告知政策制定者、报销方、付款方、医疗人员和患者相关决策。

但是,即使是最基本的成本分析也比预期要复杂。例如,在同一机构接受相同治疗方案的不同患者可能会为相同的服务支付截然不同的费用(例如保险费用差异)。由于医疗服务的本质以及"权利"这种法律资格(例如急救),"客户"不能被拒之门外。因此,医疗机构用来平衡有无能力支付者的方法并不能为一个模糊、复杂的定价系统奠定基础,在该系统中,临床医生往往无法得知治疗成本。而在其他服务中,收费是事先告知消费者的,并由服务提供方提出商议与讨论。

综上,需综合考虑医疗成本的估测方法和支付角度,包括保险费用(付款人视角)、患者自费费用(患者视角)、总实际支付费用、总费用、由于生产力下降而损失的工资以及家庭成员和其他陪护人员的额外经济负担(社会视角)。在所有医疗成本指标中,由于保险公司的介入,医疗收费清单和实际需支付医疗成本差异最大,即多数患者实际支付费用较少。另外,一些干预措施可能会改变后续医疗保健策略和效果,此类"间接成本"也会影响总成本。而治疗策略改变以及额外服务引起的成本变化,即边际成本,通常用于反映治疗策略改变带来的增量影响。因此,考虑到医疗成本的计算复杂性以及既定医疗保健成本的潜在变化,相关研究应密切关注医疗成本估测的各细节和假设。

捆绑式医疗支付

目前,许多医疗机构已不再使用"点选收费系统",即各项医疗服务、医疗用品或药物都与支付相关联,而是将患者在住院期间的所有医疗费用"捆绑"到一起,按照疾病诊断相关分类(DRG)编码制定的报销率一次性支付给医院。DRG 编码是基于入院诊断和其他因素对住院费用的合理估计而制定。此外，外科手术的相关费用也可以“捆绑”支付，包括整个手术过程、术后护理以及并发症的治疗等费用。上述捆绑式医疗支付系统旨在激励医务人员和医疗机构提供更为有效的医疗服务，并将并发症发病率降至最低。

成本效果分析

除了简单汇总外，还有几种成本分析方法可以提供客观数据以辅助患者、医务人员、支付方和政策制定者进行医疗决策。常规分析方法包括成本效果分析和建模研究（本章前面已介绍）。据国立卫生与临床研究所（National Institute for Health and Clinical Excellence，NICE）的定义，成本效果分析是一项经济研究，通过单一指标（即获得寿命年、减少的死亡病例数或新发病例数）衡量不同干预措施的效果，然后与替代干预措施比较[42]。其中，最关键的衡量指标是增量成本效益（ICER），干预措施是否“划算”取决于资源可用度和目标人群的支付意愿。一项关于能挽救 500 多条生命的干预措施的研究发现每生命年可节省成本的中位数约为 42 000 美元[43]（1995 年美元），该结果为美国公民的支付意愿提供了参考值；全球卫生倡议、疫苗接种和疟疾治疗均具有很高的成本效益，每生命年节省至少 100 美元；从 50 岁开始，每 10 年进行一次结肠镜检查，每生命年可节省约 11 000 美元[44]。世界卫生组织建议根据人均国内生产总值（GDP）衡量成本效益[45]。因此，可将干预措施分为以下 3 个等级：高成本效益（低于人均 GDP）、低成本效益（人均 GDP 的 1 到 3 倍）和不具有成本效益（高于人均 GDP 的 3 倍以上）。以 2012 年美元为例，上述 3 个等级依次为低于 50 000 美元，50 000~15 0000 美元和高于 150 000 美元。成本效益分析通常用 ICER 描述研究结果。例如，若某干预措施支付费用为 60 000 美元每质量调整生命年，那么 ICER 低于 60 000 美元的新干预措施就是具有成本效益的。在美国当前所采取的干预措施中，ICER 低于 50 000 美元通常被认为是具有成本效益的。成本效果分析为患者、医务人员和政策制定者在成本、医疗保健和治疗疗效等方面做出合理权衡提供了一个详细、客观的研究框架。

疗效比较研究

根据 Agency for Healthcare Research and Quality（AHRQ）定义，疗效比较研究旨在通过研究各治疗方案的效果、益处和副作用从而辅助医疗决策[46]。大约 25 年前，“相对有效性”这一概念被提出，最初用于“帮助患者、患者家属或医务人员与决策者一起做出更明智的决定”的研究[47]。在实践中，疗效比较研究主要指对两种干预措施效果进行比较的研究（通常是观察性的）。2010 年，Patient Protection and Affordable Care Act（PPACA）建立了 Patient-Centered Outcomes Research Institute（PCORI），旨在资助项目、开展研究或评估医疗效果，并且强调将成本和成本效益均纳入研究范围[48]。因此，近年来，成本和成本效益问题是疗效比较研究的热点。

疗效比较研究不是一种特定的分析技术或方法，而是对现有观察性研究的重新构架，将重点放在治疗策略的比较上。大多数疗效比较研究基于队列研究，如本章前面所述，通过模拟 RCTs 比较两个治疗组从而进行因果推断。值得注意的是，同其他观察性研究一样，疗效比较研究也存在偏倚和混杂。

（李敏娟 译，魏文强 审校）

参考文献

The complete reference list can be found on the Wiley Companion Digital Edition of this title (see inside front cover for login instructions).

1 Donabedian A. Evaluating the quality of medical care. 1966. *Milbank Q.* 2005;**83(4)**:691-729.

2 Mariotto AB, Yabroff KR, Shao Y, Feuer EJ, Brown ML. Projections of the cost of cancer care in the United States: 2010-2020. *J Natl Cancer Inst.* 2011;**103(2)**:117-128. Epub 2011 Jan 2012.

3 Warren JL, Klabunde CN, Schrag D, Bach PB, Riley GF. Overview of the SEER-Medicare data: content, research applications, and generalizability to the United States elderly population. *Med Care.* Aug 2002;**40(8 Suppl)**:IV-3-IV-18.

5 Pearson K. *The Life, Letters and Labors of Francis Galton.* London: Cambridge University Press; 1930.

7 Mantel N, Haenszel W. Statistical aspects of the analysis of data from retrospective studies of disease. *J Natl Cancer Inst.* Apr 1959;**22(4)**:719-748.

8 Scagliotti G, Brodowicz T, Shepherd FA, et al. Treatment-by-histology interaction analyses in three phase III trials show superiority of pemetrexed in nonsquamous non-small cell lung cancer. *J Thorac Oncol: official publication of the International Association for the Study of Lung Cancer.* Jan 2011;**6(1)**:64-70.

10 Dinan MA, Curtis LH, Carpenter WR, et al. Stage migration, selection bias, and survival associated with the adoption of positron emission tomography among medicare beneficiaries with non-small-cell lung cancer, 1998-2003. *J Clin Oncol.* Aug 1 2012;**30(22)**:2725-2730.

11 Chee KG, Nguyen DV, Brown M, Gandara DR, Wun T, Lara PN Jr. Positron emission tomography and improved survival in patients with lung cancer: the Will Rogers phenomenon revisited. *Arch Intern Med.* Jul 28 2008;**168(14)**:1541-1549.

12 D'Agostino RB Jr. Propensity score methods for bias reduction in the comparison of a treatment to a non-randomized control group. *Stat Med.* 1998;**17(19)**:2265-2281.

13 Penson DF. An update on randomized clinical trials in localized and locoregional prostate cancer. *Urol Oncol.* Jul-Aug 2005;**23(4)**:280-288.

14 O'Reilly P, Martin L, Collins G. Few patients with prostate cancer are willing to be randomised to treatment. *BMJ.* Jun 5 1999;**318(7197)**:1556.

15 Early Breast Cancer Trialists Group. Effects of chemotherapy and hormonal therapy for early breast cancer on recurrence and 15-year survival: an overview of the randomised trials. *Lancet.* May 14-20 2005;**365(9472)**:1687-1717.

16 AHRQ. Health Care Utilization Project: Overview of the National (Nationwide) Inpatient Sample (NIS). 2015; http://www.hcup-us.ahrq.gov/nisoverview.jsp.

17 Dinan MA, Curtis LH, Hammill BG, et al. Changes in the use and costs of diagnostic imaging among Medicare beneficiaries with cancer, 1999-2006. *JAMA.* Apr 28 2010;**303(16)**:1625-1631.

18 Dinan MA, Robinson TJ, Zagar TM, et al. Changes in initial treatment for prostate cancer among Medicare beneficiaries, 1999-2007. *Int J Radiat Oncol Biol Phys.* Apr 1 2012;**82(5)**:e781-e786.

20 Buell P. Changing incidence of breast cancer in Japanese-American women. *J Natl Cancer Inst.* Nov 1973;**51(5)**:1479-1483.

21 Postow MA, Callahan MK, Barker CA, et al. Immunologic correlates of the abscopal effect in a patient with melanoma. *N Engl J Med.* Mar 8 2012;**366(10)**:925-931.

22 Ringel JS, Eibner C, Girosi F, Cordova A, McGlynn EA. Modeling health care policy alternatives. *Health Serv Res.* Oct 2010;**45(5 Pt 2)**:1541-1558.

23 Vanderlaan BF, Broder MS, Chang EY, Oratz R, Bentley TG. Cost-effectiveness of 21-gene assay in node-positive, early-stage breast cancer. *Am J Manag Care.* 2011;**17(7)**:455-464.

25 IOM. *Crossing the Quality Chasm: A New Health System for the 21st Century.* Washington, DC: National Academy Press; 2001.

27 Fisher ES, Wennberg DE, Stukel TA, Gottlieb DJ, Lucas FL, Pinder EL. The implications of regional variations in Medicare spending. Part 1: the content, quality, and accessibility of care. *Ann Intern Med.* Feb 18 2003;**138(4)**:273-287.

28 McGlynn EA, Asch SM, Adams J, et al. The quality of health care delivered to adults in the United States. *N Engl J Med.* Jun 26 2003;**348(26)**:2635-2645.

29 Luft HS, Bunker JP, Enthoven AC. Should operations be regionalized? The empirical relation between surgical volume and mortality. *N Engl J Med.* Dec 20 1979;**301(25)**:1364-1369.

30 Dudley RA, Johansen KL, Brand R, Rennie DJ, Milstein A. Selective referral to high-volume hospitals: estimating potentially avoidable deaths. *JAMA.* Mar 1 2000;**283(9)**:1159-1166.

31 Begg CB, Cramer LD, Hoskins WJ, Brennan MF. Impact of hospital volume on operative mortality for major cancer surgery. *JAMA.* Nov 25 1998;**280(20)**:

1747–1751.

32 Reames BN, Sheetz KH, Waits SA, Dimick JB, Regenbogen SE. Geographic variation in use of laparoscopic colectomy for colon cancer. *J Clin Oncol*. Nov 10 2014;**32**(**32**):3667–3672.

33 Morden NE, Chang CH, Jacobson JO, et al. End-of-life care for Medicare beneficiaries with cancer is highly intensive overall and varies widely. *Health Aff (Millwood)*. Apr 2012;**31**(**4**):786–796.

34 Havrilesky LJ, Moorman PG, Lowery WJ, et al. Oral contraceptive pills as primary prevention for ovarian cancer: a systematic review and meta-analysis. *Obstet Gynecol*. Jul 2013;**122**(**1**):139–147.

35 Ramcharan R. Regressions: Why Are Economists Obsessed with Them? *Finance & Development*. 2006;**43**(**1**). http://www.imf.org/external/pubs/ft/fandd/2006/03/basics.htm

36 IOM. *Roundtable on value & science-driven health care*. 2014.

37 Abernethy AP, Etheredge LM, Ganz PA, et al. Rapid-learning system for cancer care. *J Clin Oncol*. Sep 20 2010;**28**(**27**):4268–4274.

38 Abernethy AP. Demonstrating the learning health system through practical use cases. *Pediatrics*. Jul 2014;**134**(**1**):171–172.

39 Shih YC, Ganz PA, Aberle D, et al. Delivering high-quality and affordable care throughout the cancer care continuum. *J Clin Oncol*. Nov 10 2013; **31**(**32**):4151–4157.

40 Basch E, Abernethy AP, Mullins CD, et al. Recommendations for incorporating patient-reported outcomes into clinical comparative effectiveness research in adult oncology. *J Clin Oncol*. Dec 1 2012;**30**(**34**):4249–4255.

41 Dinan MA, Compton KL, Dhillon JK, et al. Use of patient-reported outcomes in randomized, double-blind, placebo-controlled clinical trials. *Med Care*. Apr 2011;**49**(**4**):415–419.

43 Tengs TO, Adams ME, Pliskin JS, et al. Five-hundred life-saving interventions and their cost-effectiveness. *Risk Anal: an official publication of the Society for Risk Analysis*. Jun 1995;**15**(**3**):369–390.

44 Sonnenberg A, Delco F. Cost-effectiveness of a single colonoscopy in screening for colorectal cancer. *Arch Intern Med*. Jan 28 2002;**162**(**2**):163–168.

45 WHO. World Health Organization. Cost effectiveness and strategic planning (WHO-CHOICE) 2015; http://www.who.int/choice/costs/CER_thresholds/en/.

47 Comparative effectiveness: its origin, evolution, and influence on health care. *J Oncol Pract*. Mar 2009;**5**(**2**):80–82.

48 Kinney ED. Comparative effectiveness research under the Patient Protection and Affordable Care Act: can new bottles accommodate old wine? *Am J Law Med*. 2011;**37**(**4**):522–566.

第七篇

个体化治疗

第 51 章　个体化医学在抗肿瘤药物研发中的发展

Nicholas C. Dracopoli, PhD ■ Lqbal Grewal PhD, DSc, FRCPath ■ Chris H. Takimoto, MD, PhD, FACP ■ Peter F. Lebowitz, MD, PhD

概述

随着抗肿瘤药物研发的不断发展,个性化医学的概念已不再是一个可望而不可即的概念,并逐渐成为抗肿瘤药物研发的典范。确定伴有哪些分子特征的肿瘤最有可能从药物中获益成为现代抗肿瘤药物研发中的重要组成部分。此外,针对患者个体的个体化医学方法也正在出现。例如自体免疫细胞的工程,就是针对患者个体或单一瘤种的肿瘤疫苗。

越来越多的研究成果表明,通过生物标志物选择个体化医学的方法可以为患者提供更多的帮助,并能使抗肿瘤药物获得更快地批准。个体化医学策略在抗肿瘤药物研发中的益处是多方面的,包括增加药物研发总体成功的可能性,缩小 3 期注册性临床试验规模,以及提高患者临床获益的可能性。近期,Falconi 及其同事回顾性统计分析了自 1998 年至 2012 年针对 676 例非小细胞肺癌患者所进行的 1、2 和 3 期临床试验的结果[1]。未经选择的患者有效率仅为 11%。然而,应用生物标志物进行人群筛查后的患者,其有效率提高了近 6 倍,达到 62%。客观证据已经显示出通过预测性生物标志物进行筛选可以提高抗肿瘤药物研发的成功率。利用特异的遗传和/或蛋白质标志物,许多重要的抗肿瘤药物得以研发成功并获批,这种方法体现了抗肿瘤药物研发的模式的转变。

引言

越来越多的生物标志物被纳入个体化药物研发中,这将增加药物研发过程的复杂性,为抗肿瘤药物的发展带来挑战。由于伴随诊断与药物研发靶点的一致性使得精准医疗得以逐步实现。随着科学的发展,需要在一些个体化医学领域进行拓展,以寻求更大的发展。一些示例包括:

1. 诊断性多生物标志物组　除了少数例外,多数成功的个体化医学项目都是检测单个基因或蛋白质。随着对数千个数据点的多通路复合分析方法成为主流,全基因组检测开始出现。生物标志物诊断技术的发展源于临床策略的发展,这其中包含早期临床试验中生物标志物的发现以及后续注册性临床研究中的确认。

转录谱就是多基因诊断技术的成功案例之一。通过这一技术,可以辨别应答者与非应答者的基因表达谱。在试验中转录谱可作为样本的验证集来检测其预测价值、敏感性和特异性。这一技术在临床上已开始应用,如 Oncotype Dx(Genomic Health, Redwood City, California), MammaPrint(Agendia BV, Amsterdam, the Netherlands)和 H/I(AvariaDX, Carlsbad, California)。与潜在应答者相比,这些检测技术可以更好地鉴别出那些不能从治疗中获益的患者。

2. 肿瘤免疫个体化医学　虽然肿瘤细胞的分析已成为个性化医学的支柱,但现在也可以通过调节肿瘤的其他成分(如免疫细胞和基质细胞)在临床获益。

随着针对细胞微环境新疗法的出现,相关的新分析技术也正在研发中。但多种细胞类型、多标志物检测的复杂性对新型免疫治疗的发展提出了挑战。

3. 个性化治疗　包括自体细胞工程和个体化肿瘤抗原技术,将在下文详细介绍。

虽然个体化医学在肿瘤药物的研发中得以实现,但随着对肿瘤学机制和生物学的深入研究,其正在成为一个更加复杂的命题。本章中,我们试图涵盖一些关键的问题,这些关键问题对于理解本章内容将提供帮助。

生物标志物及伴随诊断在个体化医学中的作用

生物标志物类型

在大多数个体化药物研发中,生物标志物及其伴随诊断是重要的组成部分。如表 51-1 所示,生物标志物可分为预测、预后和终点替代指标三大类。所有这些生物标志物不仅在药物研发中起到了至关重要的作用,而且是个体化医学发展的驱动力。与整体人群相比,通过生物标志物识别出来的人群更有可能从治疗中获益。随着分子诊断技术和人类基因组序列完成的共同发展,为发现预测药物疗效或降低药物毒性的生物标志物创造了新的机会。

现阶段,大量的生物标志物被发现,但多数生物标志物并未应用于临床。2014 年 10 月,GOBIOM 数据库(www.gvkbio.com)列出了超过 45 000 个生物标志物。相当于人类基因组中每一个基因存在两个生物标志物！这表明,生物标志物一词被过度使用,大部分生物标志物都无法在研究中应用。绝大多数的生物标志物均缺乏特异性,如果不应用有效的分析方法和相关数据以确认其作为生物标志物的作用,将无法在研究或临床应用中得到有效应用。

生物标志物在整个药物开发过程中有不同的用途,如作用机制(mechanism of action, MOA)、药效学(pharmacodynamic, PD)、预后、预测疗效、耐药性和替代指标(表 51-1)。生物标志物最常见的用途是作为 MOA 标志物,通过评估下游信号通路成员的蛋白磷酸化来确认药物是否达到预期的目标及下游的生物学效应。PD 标志物被广泛应用于药物动力学(pharmacokinetic,PK)分析,以确定生物有效剂量,并为 2 期疗效研究确定药物剂量。预后标记物是指在无特定药物干预的情况下疾病可能的发展过程,并在某些肿瘤中被广泛应用于预测原发肿瘤切除术后复发的可能性(如 Mammaprint 和 Oncotype Dx)。预测标志物测试用于预测特定治疗的反应,将在下文中进行详细讨论。越来越多的生物标记被用于检测疗效和监测耐药性,生物标志物在预测酪氨酸激酶抑制剂治疗耐药性上已经取得了相当大的成就。

表 51-1 生物标志物类型和诊断

标记物	功能	检测方法
药物动力学/作用机制	• 确定药物对靶标有无影响,并对生物途径产生的影响 • 评估作用机制 • PK/PD 相关性和确定剂量和时间表 • 确定生物有效剂量	• 药物开发过程中使用的研究测试 • 尚未发展成熟的伴随诊断
预测	• 确定药物治疗时最可能有反应或最不可能发生不良事件的患者	• 伴随诊断试验(如:赫赛汀、表皮生长因子受体)
药物耐药	• 确定导致获得性耐药的机制	• 突变分析(例如伊马替尼治疗的 CML 中 BCR-ABL 突变)
预后	• 预测疾病进程而不依赖任何治疗方式	• 已批准的检测
替代品	• 批准的注册终点	• 商业化诊断检测

伴随诊断的成就与挑战

作为个体化抗肿瘤药物发展的成功典范,截至 2015 年 1 月,FDA 批准 20 项伴随诊断,并广泛应用于肿瘤患者的治疗中[2]。这 20 项伴随诊断详见表 51-2。许多重要因素均体现在本表中。首先,所有伴随诊断操作简单,均用于检测药物靶点状态,或药物耐药通路下游的靶点状态,如 KRAS 基因[3,4]。每项伴随诊断均为单一靶点检测,用于检测激活药物靶点的体细胞遗传变化,包括基因扩增(HER2,KIT)、突变[KRAS、表皮生长因子受体(epidermal growth factor receptor,EGFR)、BRAF]或易位(ALK)。其次,所有获批的信号传导抑制剂的伴随诊断均针对检测靶向通路或其下游通路上存在的驱动突变。相反,如细胞毒性药物、表观遗传调节剂、免疫疗法等药物机制目前尚无 FDA 批准的伴随诊断。为何信号传导抑制剂的伴随诊断可以成功研发而针对其他药物机制的伴随诊断未获成功呢?主要是由于信号传导抑制剂研发将驱动基因的突变作为药物研发的靶点。这种快速检测技术假设驱动基因突变导致肿瘤的增殖与转移是药物的靶点,只有携带驱动基因突变的患者才可以从抑制剂治疗中获益。这种假设可以在确定有效药物剂量的 1 期临床试验中便得以证实。相反,如果在 2 期临床试验中通过收集样本进行分子图谱分析形成假设,将使得预测标记的开发变得十分困难。在这种情况下,伴随诊断的研发是一个循序渐进的过程,包括生物标记物假设的产生、假设的测试与验证,以及最终形成伴随诊断。

表 51-2 2014 年 10 月批准的 FDA 伴随诊断列表

检测手段	公司名称	药物	分子学手段	作用靶点
therascreen KRAS RGQ PCR Kit	Qiagen	Erbitux(cetuximab) 艾比妥(西妥昔单抗)	PCR 聚合酶链式反应	KRAS
—	—	Vectibix(panitumumab) 维克替比(帕尼单抗)	—	—
EGFR PharmDx Kit	DAKO	Erbitux(cetuximab) 艾比妥(西妥昔单抗)	IHC 免疫组化	EGFR
—	—	Vectibix(panitumumab) 维克替比(帕尼单抗)	—	—
therascreen EGFR RGQ PCR Kit	Qiagen	Gilotrif(afatanib) 阿法替尼(阿法坦尼)	PCR 聚合酶链式反应	EGFR
C-KIT PharmDx	DAKO	Gleevec(imatinib mesylate) 格列卫(甲磺酸伊马丁尼)	IHC 免疫组化	KIT

续表

检测手段	公司名称	药物	分子学手段	作用靶点
INFORM HER-2/NEU	Ventana Medical Systems	Herceptin(trastuzumab) 赫赛汀(曲妥珠单抗)	FISH 荧光原位杂交技术	HER2
PATHVISION HER-2 DNA Probe kit	Abbott Molecular	Herceptin(trastuzumab) 赫赛汀(曲妥珠单抗)	FISH 荧光原位杂交技术	HER2
PATHWAY ANTI-HER-2/NEU(4B5)	Ventana Medical Systems	Herceptin(trastuzumab) 赫赛汀(曲妥珠单抗)	IHC 免疫组化	HER2
INSITE HER-2/NEU Kit	Biogenex Laboratories	Herceptin(trastuzumab) 赫赛汀(曲妥珠单抗)	IHC 免疫组化	HER2
SPOT-Light HER2 CISH Kit	Life Technologies	Herceptin(trastuzumab) 赫赛汀(曲妥珠单抗)	CISH 色素原位杂交	HER2
Bond Oracle HER2 IHC System	Leica Biosystems	Herceptin(trastuzumab) 赫赛汀(曲妥珠单抗)	IHC 免疫组化	HER2
HER2 CISH PharmDx Kit	Dako Denmark A/S	Herceptin(trastuzumab) 赫赛汀(曲妥珠单抗)	CISH 色素原位杂交	HER2
INFORM HER2 DUAL ISH DNA Probe Cocktail	Ventana Medical Systems	Herceptin(trastuzumab) 赫赛汀(曲妥珠单抗)	CISH 色素原位杂交	HER2
HERCEPTEST	Dako Denmark A/S	Herceptin(trastuzumab) 赫赛汀(曲妥珠单抗)	IHC 免疫组化	HER2
—	—	Perjeta(pertuzumab) 帕妥珠单抗	—	—
—	—	Kadcyla(ado-trastuzumab emtansine) 曲妥珠单抗-美坦新偶联物	—	—
HER2 FISH PharmDx Kit	Dako Denmark A/S	Herceptin(trastuzumab) 赫赛汀(曲妥珠单抗)	FISH 荧光原位杂交技术	HER2
—	—	Perjeta(pertuzumab) 帕妥珠单抗	—	—
—	—	Kadcyla(ado-trastuzumab emtansine) 曲妥珠单抗-美坦新偶联物	—	—
THxID BRAF Kit	bioMerieux	Mekinist(trametinib) 曲美替尼	PCR 聚合酶链式反应	BRAF
—	—	Tafinlar(dabrafenib) 达拉非尼	—	—
cobas EGFR mutation test	Roche Molecular Systems	Tarceva(erlotinib) 厄洛替尼(特罗凯)	PCR 聚合酶链式反应	EGFR
VYSISALK Break Apart FISH Probe Kit	Abbott Molecular	Xalkori(crizotinib) 克唑替尼	FISH 荧光原位杂交技术	ALK
COBAS 4800 BRAF V600 mutation test	Roche Molecular Systems	Zelboraf(vemurafenib) 威罗菲尼	PCR 聚合酶链式反应	BRAF
BRACAnalysis CDx™	Myriad Genetic Laboratories, Inc.	Lynparza™(olaparib) 奥拉帕尼	PCR 聚合酶链式反应	BRCA1/2
Ferriscan	Resonance Health Analysis Services Pty Ltd	Exjade(deferasirox) 恩瑞格(地拉罗司)	MRI 磁共振	肝铁

来源:Data from http://www.fda.gov/MedicalDevices/ProductsandMedicalProcedures/InVitroDiagnostics/ucm301431.htm.

免疫治疗的发展就是伴随诊断研发中的一个典型的例子。抗 PD-1 抗体作为免疫检查点抑制剂已经显示出了显著的生存获益并成为免疫调节剂的新先锋[5]。此类药物通过抑制免疫检查点和防止肿瘤逃避宿主免疫系统发挥作用。然而,早期的临床数据显示,将免疫检查点的表达作为预测性生物标志物来进行检测十分复杂。对于 PDL1 高表达的肿瘤,PD1 抑制剂的有效率可提高 3~4 倍,但对于无表达者也可能对 PD1 抑制剂有反应。因此,仅检测检查点的表达可能不足以作为这种新型药物的预测指标,可能需要研发新型的分子图谱来预测对此类免疫调节药物的反应。

除了 FDA 批准的抗肿瘤药物伴随诊断外,还有许多检测在美国临床实验室改进修正案(Clinical Laboratory Improvement Amendment,CLIA)和美国病理学会(College of American Pathology,CAP)认证的实验室中进行研究与临床应用。这些检测包含了从单一的基因检测到复杂的分子谱分析。其中一些检测表现出较强的验证分析性能和临床实用性,而另一些则没有较好的特征。最近,许多实验室研发了包含 30~300 个常见肿瘤突变基因的测序模板。这些测序模板越来越多应用于筛选肿瘤患者入组合适的临床研究。其中代表性的测序模板是由基金会医学公司提供的 FoundationOne。该测序模板针对福尔马林固定石蜡包埋组织(formalin-fixed paraffin-emmbedded tissue,FFPET)进行 230 个肿瘤基因测序以检测突变。这些检测结果可用来指导患者进入恰当的临床试验,或超适应证用药。

伴随诊断发展策略

伴随诊断的发展——临床前

伴随诊断(companion diagnostic,CDx)发展的第一步是形成预测性生物标志物假说。理想情况下,在新的治疗药物或靶点确定之时即形成预测性生物标志物假说。预测性生物标志物假说概括了预测药物敏感性或耐药性的确定与检测的方法。在药物研发的早期阶段,该假说应当包含对生物靶点和药物 MOA 的全面理解。由此将产生一系列候选预测性生物标志物,这些生物标记物将经过严格地临床前及临床中的检测来评估其作为 CDx 检测的意义。候选生物标志物可以预测药物敏感性或耐药性,但无论何种情况,CDx 协同发展的策略是相似的。

如上所述,在一些临床研究中将预测性生物标志物定义为药物的靶点。例如,以肿瘤耐药突变为靶点的临床研究,有可能使用该突变作为预测性生物标志物,选择患者在早期临床试验中进行评估来验证其有效性。

该方法已用于针对伴有 T790M 耐药突变的 NSCLC 患者二代 EGFR 抑制剂的研发[6]。在其他情况下,预测性生物标记物可能仅为靶点的高表达,如伴有 HER2/Neu 高表达的乳腺癌患者可以从曲妥珠单抗治疗中获益[7]。目前已获批准的抗肿瘤药物 CDx 检测主要是检测与药物分子靶点直接相关的单个基因或蛋白。

预测性生物标志物本身的特性可能会影响其临床结果。例如,以二进制判断是否存在突变的生物标志物,因其阳性结果易于判定是临床试验中最简单的评估方法。而以连续性变量作为生物标志物则较为复杂,如免疫组织化学染色强度或基因扩增程度或拷贝数,这类生物标志物需要在实际临床研究中建立判断阳性的临界值。而以微阵列标志物或由多种不同检测产生的复合性参数为例的多元性检测则更为复杂。综上所述,随着预测性生物标志物越来越复杂,临床试验验证的负担也在增加。

如果药物 MOA 缺乏明显的特征,那么预测性生物标志物假设便难形成,可能需要进一步探索性研究。例如,一种新的治疗方法在一组具有分子特征的肿瘤细胞株中探索与明确其分子特征,甚至进一步明确与药物敏感性或耐药性密切相关的基因变化情况。迄今为止,与药物敏感性相关的复杂的基因信号尚未有助于伴随诊断;然而,该方法仍可能是发现生物标志物的有效工具。可以在储存的肿瘤组织中确定任何新发现的候选预测性生物标志物的普遍性,从而探索潜在的临床相关性。最终,探索预测性生物标志物假说将为临床进一步评估产生一系列有希望的候选试验。

一旦确定了一系列潜在候选的预测性生物标志物,就应评估预测性生物标志物假设的强度。可以在相关的体外细胞系和体内肿瘤模型中进行临床前试验以探索相关候选生物标志物的预测潜力。预测性生物标志物的存在应该与一系列肿瘤模型中的药物敏感性强烈相关。来自患者的异种移植物的确认发现将进一步支持候选预测性生物标志物的临床相关性。预测生物标志物假设的强度可以显著影响所研究的患者群体的选择。如果预测性生物标志物的预测潜力非常强,那么作为快速概念验证策略,早期试验中的治疗可能仅限于生物标志物阳性的患者。然而,如果生物标志物相关性较弱,则可在临床开发早期对生物标志物阳性和生物标志物阴性患者均进行治疗。

CDx 开发的最后临床前步骤是准备适用于临床试验的合格实验室分析。如果用于患者筛查,理想的检测方法应该是简单、可靠、敏感并且具有快速周转性。分析循环肿瘤细胞、血浆蛋白或检测甲醛溶液固定、石蜡包埋的肿瘤储存组织比需要新鲜肿瘤组织活检的检测更具优势。几种不同预测性生物标志物候选物的原型分析可用于临床前试验中的探索性评估和早期临床研究中非筛选研究患者入组[8]。然而,完整的 CDx 检测需要完整的分析验证,理想情况下应在关键后期试验开始之前进行。临床研究团队和处理预测性生物标志物物流的相关研究人员之间的仔细协调对于确保一致的样品处理、运输和试验结果的转变至关重要。

早期临床试验中 CDx 的开发

开发药物治疗所需的程序已颇具特征,但验证 CDx 所需的步骤往往不太受重视。过去,预测性生物标志物通过对临床试验数据进行事后分析进行回顾性研究,以产生假说[9]。然而,这种缓慢、线性的思维方式已经过时,并且不符合新疗法与 CDx 检测快速发展的要求。在现代,积极的共同发展计划至关重要。

CDx 的开发可以强烈影响传统的首次应用于人类的 1 期肿瘤研究的设计。这些试验传统上是在癌症患者中进行的,其经典的研究终点包括剂量选择、药代动力学、毒性谱和最大耐受剂量的确定。1 期试验也常常包含药效学生物标志物研究终点,例如受体占有率或靶点抑制,以评估靶点参与和下游通路调节。这些药效学试验可有助于选择推荐的 2 期试验剂量;然而,它们通常不用作伴随诊断,并且它们的使用仅限于早期开发试验。一项传统的实体肿瘤 1 期肿瘤学研究将入组各种晚期肿瘤类型的患者，与其生物标志物状态无关，以确保快速确定毒性谱，收集药代动力学数据，并建立可靠的剂量建议。

越来越多的 1 期肿瘤试验将药物活性的早期评估纳入剂量选择后立即开放的扩展队列中。这种在特定人群中建立快速概念验证的尝试削弱了独立的 2a 期疗效试验在许多当前药物研发项目中的作用[10,11]。然而，它也相应地增加了 1 期试验的规模和复杂性。一个重要的早期决定在于是否在这些扩展队列中限制性入组生物标志物阳性的患者，或者采取全部纳入、包含所有生物标志物未知患者的方法。如果生物标志物假说是有说服力的，并且预计生物标志物阴性的患者不会从治疗中受益，那么就有充分的理由限制性纳入生物标志物阳性的患者。一种流行的 1 期研究策略是在剂量递增阶段纳入非选择性患者，但是在扩展队列中限制性纳入生物标志物阳性患者。这种改进方法为在被认为最有可能对试验性治疗作出反应的概念验证人群中观察疗效信号提供了早期机会。其缺点是如果预测生物标志物的普遍性低，则必须筛选许多患者，而这将进一步增加研究的复杂性。或者，如果在 1 期扩展研究中使用全部纳入或生物标记分层方法，则应强制性地回顾性确定所有患者中的预测性生物标志物状态。

即使采用生物标志物富集策略，这些早期试验的探索性质也应该强制实施临床均衡措施。在收集到足够的支持性临床数据之前，必须避免对候选预测性生物标志物的效用进行过于严格的假设。在 CDx 开发中，生物标志物的错误设定并不罕见，并且初始的候选预测性生物标志物可能被这些探索性临床试验中鉴定的新标志物所取代。例如，激酶抑制剂克唑替尼的首个 1 期试验最初主要针对有 cMET 变异的肿瘤患者，因为这是该药物主要发现的靶点。然而，克唑替尼也是一种有效的 ALK 酪氨酸激酶抑制剂；在 1 期试验中，EML4/ALK 易位被确定为进一步肺癌发展的最终伴随诊断[12]。

后期临床试验中 CDx 的开发

在关键注册试验开始之前，预测性生物标志物试验应经过全面的分析验证。理想情况下，只有一个在中心实验室进行分析的验证版本应该用于 2b 期或 3 期试验[8]。如果在临床验证中使用两个版本的 CDx 分析，则需要进行桥接诊断研究。由于后期试验将需要大量的患者和研究中心，在广阔的地理区域内统一实施 CDx 将带来额外的后勤挑战。当项目过渡到后期开发阶段时，必须仔细考虑这些因素，因为重点已从生物标志物探索转向验证完整的伴随诊断。

后期 CDx 开发临床试验的设计将在很大程度上取决于迄今为止收集的关于拟议 CDx 的临床数据。如果预测性生物标志物检测是明确的，并且在生物标志物阴性的患者中仍然预期很少或没有活性，那么可以采用纯富集策略（图 51-1）。该方法仅关注生物标志物阳性患者，可以考虑相对传统的 2b 期和 3 期研究设计。然而，如果在生物标志物阴性患者中仍然可能存在有意义的药物活性，则应考虑包括生物标志物阳性和生物标志物阴性患者的生物标志物分层研究设计（图 51-2）。生物标志物分层随机试验的研究设计选择非常大，这是一个快速发展的临床研究领域。以下部分讨论了富集和生物标志物分层临床试验设计的一些一般说明性实例。

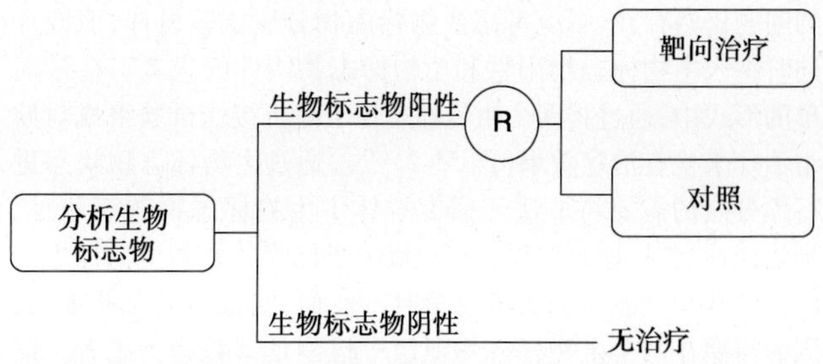

图 51-1　靶向富集设计。R，随机

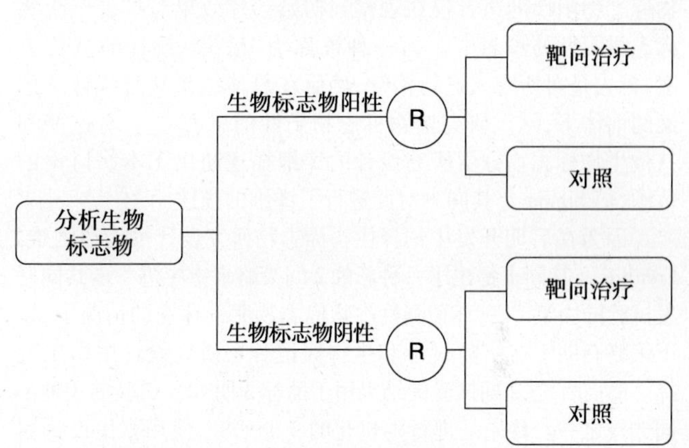

图 51-2　生物标志物分层设计。R，随机

富集研究设计

在纯粹的富集策略中，随机研究仅在生物标志物阳性患者中进行，并且研究设计保持相对传统（图 51-1）[13]。由于在减少分子异质性的肿瘤患者中预期的临床获益更大，如果生物标志物强烈预测治疗效果，则所得的随机试验将小于相应的未选择患者的试验。相对于全部纳入治疗的研究设计方法，富集设计的效能取决于预测性生物标志物的普遍性和在生物标志物阴性患者中治疗的有效性。当生物标志物存在于不到一半的潜在患者中且在标志物阴性患者中治疗效果最小时，富集设计将比未选择的试验中随机化的患者数少得多[9,13]。然而，取决于预测性生物标志物的普遍性，可能需要筛选许多患者以确定足够的生物标志物阳性的患者。

CDx 开发的纯富集策略的缺点是生物标志物的阴性预测值是未知的，因为这些患者被排除在研究之外。至少有一个 CDx 被批准用于新治疗药物的例子后来未能证明其具有医学或临床效用。对于转移性结直肠癌患者，抗 EGFR 抗体西妥昔单抗的最初批准包括使用免疫组织化学记录 EGFR 表达情况的 CDx 检测。然而，后来的试验证明，西妥昔单抗在 EGFR 阴性和 EGFR 阳性患者中同样有效[14]，这意味着 CDx 缺乏医学效用。因此，成功的富集策略注册项目可能需要在生物标志物阴性患者中进行额外测试，作为批准后的保证。尽管如此，富集临床试验设计仍然很受欢迎，并且有许多成功的肿瘤学 CDx 共同开发项目已经使用了这种方法。最近突出的例子包括批准 vemurafenib 在 BRAF V600E 突变的恶性黑色素瘤患者[15]和克唑替尼在 EML4/ALK 易位的 NSCLC 患者中的注册[12]。

生物标志物分层设计

如果预测性生物标志物检测的特征是明确的，但临床验证的问题仍然存在，则应考虑生物标志物分层试验设计，该设计同时纳入生物标志物阳性和生物标志物阴性的患者。在最简单的形式中，通过将两个生物标志物组随机接受试验组或对照组治疗来检查治疗效果(图 51-2)[9]。通过生物标志物状态进行预分层的需要将取决于研究群体中生物标志物的普遍性。当效能适当时，该研究设计可提供关于治疗效果和生物标志物的预测和预后能力的大部分信息。然而，这也是相对低效的，因为需要在两个生物标志物亚组中检测足够数量的患者。已对该方法提出了大量的修改，即通过使用不同的统计分析计划来提高效率[9,13]。一些实例包括顺序累加设计，其开始纳入生物标志物阳性的患者仅在观察到初始治疗效果后扩展至生物标志物阴性的患者[9]。另一种被称为“后退”设计的替代方案，首先是对所有人进行治疗，然后在总体结果缺乏统计学意义的前体下，侧重研究生物标志物阳性的患者[16]。对这些和其他生物标志物分层研究设计的详细描述超出了本次讨论的范围，但 Simon 及其同事对此进行了详细的描述[9,13,16]。

因为在后期开发中选择生物标志物研究设计可能很困难，Freidlin 及其同事提出了一种新的 2 期策略来指导进一步共同开发试验的决策[17]。在预测性生物标志物明确存在的情况下，以下策略有助于在富集设计和生物标记分层研究设计中做出选择。简而言之，2 期试验的结果用于推荐 3 期 CDx 试验的 4 种不同选择之一。首先是进行随机化的 3 期研究，使用富集设计仅纳入生物标志物阳性的患者，因为该药物是有效的并且诊断确定了专有的治疗人群。其次是实施随机生物标志物分层设计，因为在标志物阳性和标志物阴性患者中治疗均有效，但生物标志物具有一定预测临床结局的能力。再次是无论生物标志物状态而纳入所有患者，因为该药物是广泛有效的，而生物标志物缺乏临床效用。最后，第四种选择是不进入 3 期研究并停止所有进一步的开发，因为该药物在任何人群中都缺乏疗效。

使用 Freidlin 的 2 期研究策略，患者被随机分配到试验组和对照治疗组，并确定预测性生物标志物状态[17]。首先在生物标志物阳性人群中评估治疗效果，然后根据结果评估总体人群或生物标志物阴性亚组。Freidlin 概述了该方法的决策算法，其结果输出是推荐的 3 期研究策略。在本例中，无进展生存的风险比被用于评估治疗效果，尽管它可以适应各种 2 期研究终点。这种方法很好地突出了药物研发科学家在设计一项 CDx 开发项目时所面临的决策。然而，该生物标志物 2 期试验的一个潜在缺点是它可能是庞大而复杂的，并且它可能推荐更加庞大而复杂的 CDx 3 期试验。

如果在 2 期研究结束时对预测性生物标志物持续存在问题，那么在 3 期试验阶段仍有可能发现或改进现有的诊断。为了探索和调整新的预测性生物标志物，同时评估治疗效果，已经提出了一些创新的适应性 3 期研究设计。例如，生物标志物适应的阈值设计可以为 3 期试验中连续性或分级的预测性生物标志物的检测阳性选择最佳分割点[18]。如果在关键性试验开始时尚未确定生物标志物阳性阈值，则这是有效的，它保留检测整体广泛治疗效果的统计效能。这种方法的一种更广泛的变化，称为适应性生物标志物设计，可以同时分析几种不同的预定义的二元生物标志物的预测能力，允许选择与临床结果最相关的一种[13,18]。

如果在 2 期研究结束时仍无候选的预测性生物标志物，则可以在 3 期患者中进行基因表达谱分析，Freidlin 及其同事提出了一种新的适应性特征设计，该设计前瞻性地定义了预测性生物标志物特征并在同一项关键 3 期试验中验证了其与治疗效果的相关性[19]。在该研究设计中，预测性生物标志物特征是在训练子集中开发的，并在独立的、互斥的患者亚组中进行验证，同时保留评估整体治疗效果的统计效能。在模拟试验中，当敏感患者的比例较低时，适应性特征设计减少了拒绝积极治疗的机会；然而，当治疗广泛有效时，它仍然可检测到与传统试验相似的整体治疗效果。Freidlin 等最近发表了该方法的一种更具统计学稳健性的版本，称为交叉验证的适应性特征设计，其利用完整的患者群体进行特征开发和验证。[20]适应性特征设计的既定目标之一是允许制药公司投资药物基因组学用于患者筛选的生物标志物，同时不影响 3 期研究数据支持的更广泛适应证的机会[19]。在单次试验中进行生物标志物的发现和验证是一个有吸引力的概念，但目前没有已获批的 CDx 使用这种方法。因此，这对于未来的 CDx 开发仍然是一个很有希望的，但目前仅是理论上的选择。

CDx 开发中的监管考虑因素

在一项双重药物诊断共同开发项目中，目标是将预测性生物标志物验证为 CDx，同时在一系列统一的临床试验中证明新疗法的安全性和有效性(图 51-3)。批准一种新治疗药物的监

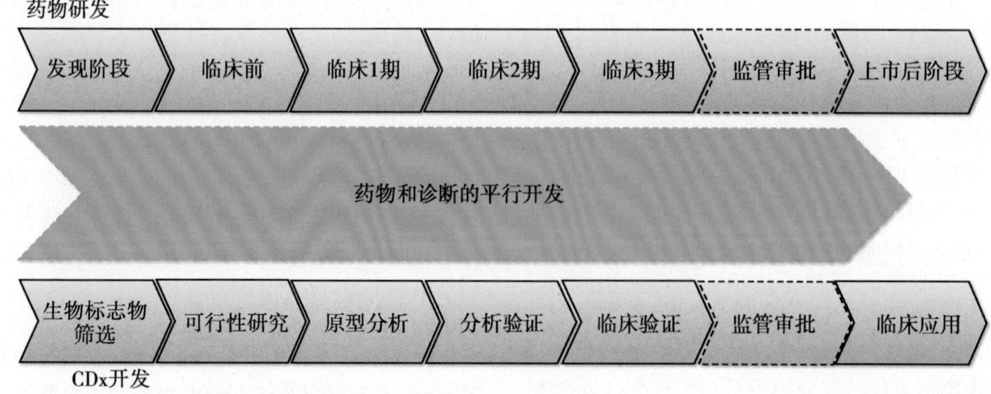

图 51-3 药物-诊断共同开发模型显示了药物研发过程和平行伙伴(CDx)开发过程，争取在 3 期研究结束时获得一致的监管机构共同批准。资料来源：Olsen 2014. 8 Used under CC BY(http://creativecommons.org/licenses/by/3.0/)

管标准已明确界定,但 CDx 的监管期望在随着科学的发展而变化。

由于认识到滥用辅助诊断检测可能会对患者造成潜在伤害,因此,辅助诊断检测一直受到越来越多的监管审查。例如,假阳性诊断结果可能使癌症患者暴露于毒性治疗而且获益的机会最小,而假阴性测试可能使患者失去可能有效的治疗。为了被标记为伴随诊断,预测性生物标志物必须显示出分析有效性、临床有效性和医学效用。分析有效性要求在相关实验室条件下进行稳健性和可重复性的技术证明[13,21,22]。如果存在金标准参考检测,则还应确定正式的准确性参数,例如特异性和灵敏度。分析验证主要是一种基于实验室的练习,可以在储存的组织库中的临床标本上进行;然而,临床有效性和医疗效用的证明则需要适当设计的临床试验。临床有效性通过预测性生物标志物与特定临床终点或治疗效果的相关性来定义[13,21,22]。例如,特定基因易位可预测对新疗法的客观反应。最后,也是最重要的,通过显示生物标志物的使用可改善临床结局,从而实现医学或临床效用[13,21,22]。

2004 年,FDA 发布了一份题为“药物-诊断共同开发概念文件”的文件,该文件解决了治疗药物和诊断产品协调发展的挑战[21]。此外,FDA 已就此及相关主题发布了指南[23];但是,正如 Fridyland 等所描述的那样,在设计和实施 CDx 共同开发项目时仍存在许多战略困境[22]。

个体化免疫治疗

肿瘤免疫学的最新进展为推进个体化免疫治疗提供了强有力的科学依据。这是一个快速发展的药物开发领域,其中基于免疫的治疗可以针对单个患者定制,或者新的基于免疫的预测性生物标志物可以用于选择最有可能受益于特定治疗的患者。后面的方法与前面讨论的个体化医疗方法相似。前文提到的个体化免疫治疗方法指的是针对每一个特定的患者采取特定的治疗方法。虽然个体化免疫治疗的技术和逻辑方面还存在很显著的问题,但是个体化免疫治疗可能显著影响疾病的疗效,这点具有很大的吸引力。

肿瘤的免疫治疗能够蓬勃发展得益于很多令人激动的发现。这些研究揭示了肿瘤是如何影响机体的免疫系统的。新药临床试验探索了肿瘤的免疫动力学[24]。新的免疫疗法如治疗前列腺癌的肿瘤疫苗,靶向作用于免疫检查点治疗恶性黑色素瘤的单克隆抗体等已经获批,并证实免疫系统可以成功消除肿瘤[24-26]。宿主对肿瘤免疫应答和肿瘤侵犯免疫系统机制间复杂关系的探索成为了目前广泛研究的领域。但是肿瘤本质上具有多样性,在不同患者身上具有不同的特点,并通过多种方法破坏免疫系统。肿瘤细胞与机体免疫系统间的作用机制复杂,每个患者都具有独特的特点,因此建议采取个体化的方法利用机体的免疫系统提供最合适的治疗。

近期,肿瘤免疫治疗领域发展迅速,在很多方面都有创新性的治疗进展。最流行的免疫治疗策略是特异性的 T 细胞激活,这种治疗策略在前期的实验中取得了成功。其他治疗的结果如肿瘤疫苗仍存在争议,这些治疗在一些肿瘤中看到了疗效但并不是对所有肿瘤都有疗效[27]。目前受到人们关注的一项新技术为 T 细胞重新编码,这项技术针对肿瘤应用基因修改的方法重新编码了机体自身的免疫细胞。这项技术在体外改变了自体 T 细胞后再回输至患者体内。此外,如免疫表型等分子分析的新方法通过收集患者的信息用于制定个体化的免疫治疗方案。在这方面,大量的研究对患者特异性的基因和分子进行分析,应用这些信息针对肿瘤制定个体化的免疫治疗。

识别基因改变,发现独特的抗原

肿瘤细胞经过大量的突变和其他表观遗传改变在理论上是可以被免疫系统识别的。理解这些改变的本质并将之转化为有用的信息可以用于制定个体化的免疫治疗。多种技术可以用全 DNA/RNA 基因测序以破译表观遗传学调控来确定可以用来描述特定患者肿瘤特征的肿瘤细胞内的转录变异。发现患者活检或其他组织样本中特定 T 细胞抗原表位和免疫表型可以用来确定肿瘤细胞的蛋白突变。通过确定具有可以被免疫系统识别的表型的独特的蛋白序列,研究者可能研发个体化的疫苗治疗复发的肿瘤患者。这样,确定对患者特异性的表型可以帮助制定个体化治疗,这种基于患者的生物学特征的个体化治疗可以使患者的疗效最大化。

描述肿瘤的基因特征同样可以用于 T 细胞的再编码,因为它可以帮助发现独特的 T 细胞结合抗原,研发个体化的 T 细胞免疫治疗。可以通过两种基因方法来编码 T 细胞。第一,肿瘤细胞的基因序列可以揭示发生在细胞表面受体的突变,这有助于选择靶抗原,进而针对这种靶抗原重新编码 T 细胞。考虑到肿瘤内部的异质性,可能有必要选择多种突变抗原。第二,肿瘤细胞可能随着时间而发生改变,他们可能丢失最初的抗原或者增加新的细胞表面突变。因此,必须仔细监控选择的肿瘤抗原的任何变化。整个过程必须在一段时间后进行重复来发现未来的突变并选择新的靶抗原,因此也无法通过这种治疗清除所有的肿瘤细胞。监测肿瘤细胞以及抗肿瘤免疫应答是针对特异性抗原进行 T 细胞编码成功的关键。

为了确定独特的肿瘤特异性抗原以及建立监测特异性抗肿瘤 T 细胞应答的方法,动物实验为我们提供了有用的信息,这些信息可以用来建立人类的治疗方法[29]。一种联合应用全外显子、转录组测序分析和质谱技术的方法用来鉴定包含新表位多肽的鼠肿瘤模型。鼠疫苗联合这些多肽可以产生强烈的抗肿瘤 T 细胞应答,这种方法具有潜在的疗效。这些研究打开了在肿瘤患者中建立个体化疫苗和抗肿瘤 T 细胞应答的 PD 监控的大门。

应用个体化肿瘤特异性抗原的个体化疫苗

激活人免疫系统的肿瘤疫苗在鼠模型中显示出潜在的疗效,但在人的试验中并没有取得成功[30]。肿瘤疫苗理论上可以激活宿主依赖的针对包含在疫苗中肿瘤相关抗原的免疫应答。为了使其发生,给予的抗原必须被抗原呈递细胞如树突状细胞(dendritic cell,DC)吞噬。DC 必须处理抗原,抗原与人白细胞抗原(human leukocyte antigen,HLA)分子形成复合物,被处理的抗原在复合物表面,之后迁移至淋巴结,淋巴结可以将抗原/HLA 复合物呈递给 T 细胞。这一过程激活了可能进入血液中并迁移至肿瘤的 T 细胞,通过免疫应答来杀死肿瘤细胞。一个成功疫苗的一个重要特征就是这个抗原可以被肽段处理,这样才可以与 HLA 分子合理的结合。

目前正在研究新方法用以发现哪些肿瘤来源的抗原可以作为可以被免疫系统有效识别的好的肿瘤抗原。可以预测多肽和不同HLA等位基因比如NetMHC结合能力的复杂的工具可以用来决定免疫系统识别肿瘤变化的强度[31]。在这种方法中,每一种多肽都被分配一个基于与HLA结合强度的评分。这种方法可以用来判断宿主免疫系统是否有识别肿瘤变化的潜力。然而,高的识别能力并不一定与好的疫苗疗效有关。为了进一步改善产生强大免疫应答的机会。可以进行实验来判断哪一种表型参与了抗肿瘤应答。通过比较NetMHC评分和其他多肽以确定哪些具有最强免疫原性。具有最强免疫原性的患者可以被选出来,这个方法可以用于选择多肽和患者信息以研发个体化疫苗[31]。

个体基因型为基础的疫苗

血液系统恶性肿瘤患者独特的抗原决定簇可以诱导肿瘤特异性免疫。例如,B细胞恶性肿瘤通常起源于表达免疫球蛋白分子的单克隆。免疫球蛋白的可变区独特的氨基酸序列叫作个体基因型(idiotype,Id)。因此对于一个患者,Id为肿瘤相关抗原,这种抗原可以作为疫苗的特异性靶向抗原[32]。B细胞淋巴瘤免疫球蛋白的肿瘤特异性Id已经被成功用于研制分泌肿瘤来源免疫球蛋白的细胞系。可以提纯这些免疫球蛋白用于研制疫苗[33]。

尽管Id为基础的疫苗在临床中获得成功,但在这个领域的进展是很有限的[34]。最大的问题是每位患者的肿瘤细胞表达独特的Id,疫苗需要具有患者特异性,需考虑到每一个个体。此外,对每位患者进行测序并针对每位患者的Id研发疫苗存在逻辑问题。然而,针对肿瘤相关Id专门制作的单克隆抗体的临床试验正在进行并显示出显著的疗效,许多患者获得长期缓解[34]。一些通过这种方法治疗的患者因为Id发生了突变阻碍了抗Id抗体的结合对治疗耐药。

因为Id来源于自身蛋白,很多Id为基础的疫苗并不能产生很好的免疫应答。因为这个原因,临床试验力图通过将这些抗原与DC结合改善免疫系统对抗原的吞噬和呈递进而改善疫苗的免疫原性。这种方法无论是在人体中还是细胞中都看到了一定的疗效。例如,一项临床试验应用Id诱导的DC用于治疗B细胞淋巴瘤患者。通过T细胞增殖抗Id检测结果显示8/10患者显示出疗效。

患者特异性肿瘤浸润淋巴细胞的应用

就像之前讨论的一样,肿瘤细胞具有很多基因突变和其他重排,这些会产生新的抗原决定基,抗原决定基可以作为新抗原诱导抗肿瘤T细胞获得疗效[36]。目前已经发现很多具有免疫原性的肿瘤具有大量的突变,具有识别肿瘤细胞表达抗原能力的T淋巴细胞经常出现肿瘤浸润[37]。肿瘤浸润淋巴细胞(tumor infiltrating lymphocyte,TIL)的出现认为在判断细胞免疫治疗和其他形式治疗恶性黑色素瘤患者的疗效中发挥重要作用[38-40]。基于这种观点,已经尝试应用患者自身的TIL进行细胞免疫治疗恶性黑色素瘤。在这种治疗方法中,对患者TIL进行收集,实验室进行扩增,产生大量TIL后回输体内。尽管这种个体化治疗在恶性黑色素瘤患者中获得了成功,在上皮肿瘤中能否获得成功仍不明确[41]。上皮肿瘤与恶性黑色素瘤相比包含的突变更少,这使得他们免疫原性更少[42]。在此领域已经有了一些进展,比如绘制上皮肿瘤突变抗原图谱。尽管一些个案报道证实TIL在上皮肿瘤中看到了令人期待的疗效,但是探索这些新信息进而研发有效的治疗策略仍然是一个未解决的问题[43]。

应用肿瘤细胞作为抗原进行以DC为基础个体化免疫治疗

尽管可以对独特的肿瘤相关突变肽进行鉴定,但是因为他们可能不会被DC细胞呈递,只有一小部分关键的突变可以被免疫系统识别。为了被DC呈递,特异性的抗原决定基必须与HLA结合,但是并不是所有肽都会与HLA结合。这限制了很多肿瘤特异性T细胞克隆的诱导,进而导致肿瘤逃逸。因此可以克服这一问题的个体化肿瘤来源的基因令人期待。就这点来说,包含大量已知或未知的全死亡肿瘤制剂可以用来帮助诱导针对肿瘤细胞的多克隆性T细胞应答[44,45]。因此,DC装载全部肿瘤肽链与只装载一部分肽链相比,在呈递肿瘤抗原成分给T细胞方面会有明显的优势。此外,这种方法可以真正提供个体化治疗因为对患者自身的肿瘤具有特异性。很显然这种免疫治疗的方法具有吸引力,但是很多问题仍需解答。例如,以凋亡细胞、坏死细胞、全溶解产物形式存在的死亡肿瘤细胞是否是诱导DC更好的抗原目前尚不明确[46-48]。另一种方法是应用扩增的肿瘤来源RNA产生肿瘤抗原[49]。应用全肿瘤细胞制剂促进DC的临床试验可以促进有效的抗肿瘤免疫并获得临床疗效。目前已经有报道经过自体肿瘤细胞介导的DC疫苗治疗后出现持续完全缓解的晚期恶性黑色素瘤患者[45]。通过肿瘤细胞裂解物介导的DC疫苗治疗肾细胞癌以及在临床试验中通过DC为基础的治疗前列腺癌都可以看到临床获益[50]。

总结

肿瘤具有高度的异质性,每位患者的情况都不相同,这就使得个体化治疗引起高度的重视。可以预料到个体化的免疫治疗在利用免疫系统的力量和精确性提高抗肿瘤免疫疗效方面发挥重要作用。然而,这种方法要求新技术和大量的研究。尽管在这一领域已经取得了很大进展,但是很多问题仍然没有得到解答。如何鉴定抗原以及如何确定抗原的优先顺序?我们如何选择性地激活免疫应答并且避免毒性?最佳的免疫分析方法是什么?要求对每位患者处理细胞和抗原自体治疗的可行性?毫无疑问,对个体化治疗进行研究来解答这些问题并通过个体化免疫治疗提高肿瘤患者的疗效将是未来几年发展的中心。

(史幼梧 韩颖 郑博 译,石远凯 审校)

参考文献

The complete reference list can be found on the Wiley Companion Digital Edition of this title (see inside front cover for login instructions).

1 Falconi A, Lopes G, Parker JL. Biomarkers and receptor targeted therapies reduce clinical trial risk in non-small-cell lung cancer. *J Thorac Oncol*. 2014;**9**(**2**):163–169.

2 Food and Drug Administration (2014), *List of Cleared or Approved Companion Diagnostic Devices*, http://www.fda.gov/MedicalDevices/ProductsandMedicalProcedures/InVitroDiagnostics/ucm301431.htm (accessed 23 December 2014).

3 Lièvre A, Bachet JB, Le Corre D, et al. KRAS mutation status is predictive of response

to cetuximab therapy in colorectal cancer. *Cancer Res.* 2006;**66**(**8**):3992-3995. doi: 10.1158/0008-5472.CAN-06-0191 DOI:10.1158%2F0008-5472.CAN-06-0191. PMID 16618717.

4 Pao W, Wang TY, Riely GJ, et al. KRAS mutations and primary resistance of lung adenocarcinomas to gefitinib or erlotinib. *PLoS Med.* 2005;**2**(**1**):e17.

5 Herbst RS. A study of MPDL3280A, an engineered PD-L1 antibody in patients with locally advanced or metastatic tumors. *J Clin Oncol.* 2013. (suppl; abstr 3000).

6 Yu HA, Riely GJ, Lovly CM. Therapeutic strategies utilized in the setting of acquired resistance to EGFR tyrosine kinase inhibitors. *Clin Cancer Res.* 2014;**20**:5898-5907.

7 Fornier M, Risio M, Van Poznak C, Seidman A. HER2 testing and correlation with efficacy of trastuzumab therapy. *Oncology* (Williston Park). 2002;**16**(**10**):1340-8-1351-2; discussion 1352, 1355-8.

8 Olsen D, Jorgensen JT. Companion diagnostics for targeted cancer drugs - clinical and regulatory aspects. *Front Oncol.* 2014;**4**:105.

9 Simon R. Drug-diagnostics co-development in oncology. *Front Oncol.* 2013;**3**:315.

10 Dahlberg SE, Shapiro GI, Clark JW, Johnson BE. Evaluation of statistical designs in phase I expansion cohorts: the Dana-Farber/Harvard Cancer Center experience. *J Natl Cancer Inst.* 2014;**106**(**7**).

11 Manji A, Brana I, Amir E, et al. Evolution of clinical trial design in early drug development: systematic review of expansion cohort use in single-agent phase I cancer trials. *J Clin Oncol.* 2013;**31**(**33**):4260-4267.

12 Kwak EL, Bang YJ, Camidge DR, et al. Anaplastic lymphoma kinase inhibition in non-small-cell lung cancer. *N Engl J Med.* 2010;**363**(**18**):1693-1703.

13 Simon R. Clinical trial designs for evaluating the medical utility of prognostic and predictive biomarkers in oncology. *Per Med.* 2010;**7**(**1**):33-47.

14 Chung CH, Mirakhur B, Chan E, et al. Cetuximab-induced anaphylaxis and IgE specific for galactose-alpha-1,3-galactose. *N Engl J Med.* 2008;**358**(**11**):1109-1117.

15 Chapman PB, Hauschild A, Robert C, et al. Improved survival with vemurafenib in melanoma with BRAF V600E mutation. *N Engl J Med.* 2011;**364**(**26**):2507-2516.

16 Simon R, Wang SJ. Use of genomic signatures in therapeutics development in oncology and other diseases. *Pharmacogenomics J.* 2006;**6**(**3**):166-173.

17 Freidlin B, McShane LM, Polley MY, Korn EL. Randomized phase II trial designs with biomarkers. *J Clin Oncol.* 2012;**30**(**26**):3304-3309.

18 Jiang W, Freidlin B, Simon R. Biomarker-adaptive threshold design: a procedure for evaluating treatment with possible biomarker-defined subset effect. *J Natl Cancer Inst.* 2007;**99**(**13**):1036-1043.

19 Freidlin B, Simon R. Adaptive signature design: an adaptive clinical trial design for generating and prospectively testing a gene expression signature for sensitive patients. *Clin Cancer Res.* 2005;**11**(**21**):7872-7878.

20 Freidlin B, Jiang W, Simon R. The cross-validated adaptive signature design. *Clin Cancer Res.* 2010;**16**(**2**):691-698.

22 Fridlyand J, Simon RM, Walrath JC, et al. Considerations for the successful co-development of targeted cancer therapies and companion diagnostics. *Nat Rev Drug Discov.* 2013;**12**(**10**):743-755.

25 Kantoff PW, Higano CS, Shore ND, et al. Sipuleucel-T immunotherapy for castration-resistant prostate cancer. *N Engl J Med.* 2010;**363**:411-422.

26 Hodi FS, O'Day SJ, McDermott DF, et al. Improved survival with ipilimumab in patients with metastatic melanoma. *N Engl J Med.* 2010;**363**:711-723.

27 Melero I, Gaudernack G, Gerritsen W, et al. Therapeutic vaccines for cancer: an overview of clinical trials. *Nat Rev Clin Oncol.* 2014;**11**:509-524.

28 Noguchi M, Sasada T, Itoh K. Personalized peptide vaccination: a new approach for advanced cancer as therapeutic cancer vaccine. *Cancer Immunol Immunother.* 2013;**62**:919-929.

29 Yadav M, Jhunjhunwala S, Phung QT, et al. Predicting immunogenic tumour mutations by combining mass spectrometry and exome sequencing. *Nature.* 2014;**515**:572-576.

30 Palena C, Abrams SI, Schlom J, Hodge JW. Cancer vaccines: preclinical studies and novel strategies. *Adv Cancer Res.* 2006;**95**:115-145.

31 Duan F, Duitama J, Seesi SA, et al. Genomic and bioinformatic profiling of mutational neoepitopes reveals new rules to predict anticancer immunogenicity. *J Exp Med.* 2014;**211**:2231-2248.

32 Muraro E, Martorelli D, Dolcetti R. Successes, failures and new perspectives of idiotypic vaccination for B-cell non-Hodgkin lymphomas. *Hum Vaccin Immunother.* 2013;**9**:1078-1083.

34 Meeker T, Lowder J, Cleary ML, et al. Emergence of idiotype variants during treatment of B-cell lymphoma with anti-idiotype antibodies. *N Engl J Med.* 1985;**312**:1658-1665.

35 Timmerman JM, Czerwinski DK, Davis TA, et al. Idiotype-pulsed dendritic cell vaccination for B cell lymphoma: clinical and immune responses in 35 patients. *Blood.* 2002;**99**:1517-1526.

36 Vogelstein B, Papadopoulos N, Velculescu VE, Zhou S, Diaz LA, Kinzler KW. Cancer genome landscapes. *Science.* 2013;**339**:1546-1558.

37 Robbins RF, Lu YC, El-Gamil M, et al. Mining exomic sequencing data to identify mutated antigens recognized by adoptively transferred tumor-reactive T cells. *Nat Med.* 2013;**19**:747-752.

38 van Rooij N, van Buuren MM, Philips D, et al. Tumor exome analysis reveals neoantigen-specific T-cell reactivity in an ipilimumab-responsive melanoma. *J Clin Oncol.* 2013;**31**:e439-e442.

41 Wedén S, Klemp M, Gladhaug IP, et al. Long-term follow-up of patients with resected pancreatic cancer following vaccination against mutant K-ras. *Int J Cancer.* 2011;**128**:1120-1128.

42 Tran E, Turcotte S, Gros A, et al. Cancer immunotherapy based on mutation-specific CD4+ T cells in a patient with epithelial cancer. *Science.* 2014;**344**:641-645.

43 Turcotte S, Gros A, Hogan K, et al. Phenotype and function of T cells infiltrating visceral metastases from gastrointestinal cancers and melanoma: implications for adoptive cell transfer therapy. *J Immunol.* 2013;**191**:2217-2225.

44 de Gruijl TD, van den Eertwegh AJM, Pinedo HM, Scheper RJ. Whole-cell cancer vaccination: from autologous to allogeneic tumor- and dendritic cell-based vaccines. *Cancer Immunol Immunother.* 2008;**57**:1569-1577.

45 O'Rourke MG, Johnson M, Lanagan C, et al. Durable complete clinical responses in a Phase I/II trial using an autologous melanoma cell/dendritic cell vaccine. *Cancer Immunol Immunother.* 2003;**52**:387-395.

46 Sauter B, Albert ML, Francisco L, Larsson M, Somersan S, Bhardwaj N. Consequences of cell death: exposure to necrotic tumor cells, but not primary tissue cells or apoptotic cells, induces the maturation of immunostimulatory dendritic cells. *J Exp Med.* 2000;**191**:423-434.

47 Jarnjak-Jankovic S, Pettersen RD, Saeboe-Larssen S, Wesenberg F, Olafsen MRK, Gaudernack G. Preclinical evaluation of autologous dendritic cells transfected with mRNA or loaded with apoptotic cells for immunotherapy of high-risk neuroblastoma. *Cancer Gene Ther.* 2005;**12**:699-707.

49 Muller MR, Grunebach F, Nencioni A, Brossart P. Transfection of dendritic cells with RNA induces CD4- and CD8-mediated T cell immunity against breast carcinomas and reveals the immunodominance of presented T cell epitopes. *J Immunol.* 2003;**170**:5892-5896.

50 Holtl L, Zelle-Rieser C, Gander H, et al. Immunotherapy of metastatic renal cell carcinoma with tumor lysate-pulsed autologous dendritic cells. *Clin Cancer Res.* 2008;**8**:3369-3376.

第八篇

化　疗

第 52 章　化疗药物、基于机制的药物和生物制剂的临床前和早期临床开发

Axel-R. Hanauske, MD, PhD, MBA ■ Daniel D. Von Hoff, MD, FACP

概述

在过去 10 年中，药物开发的方法发生了巨大变化。由于对癌细胞分子生物学的深入了解，大部分经验方法已基本被抛弃，取而代之的是生物学促进的、基于假设的转化方法。尽管有这种明显进展，但是临床药物开发试验的分层序列基本保持不变，分为 3 个阶段。本章概述了早期临床开发的各个步骤，包括药物开发过程的里程碑、国家癌症研究所的作用以及转向基于机制的药物开发。其中概述了这些新型药剂临床开发中的挑战，并提供了对早期临床药物开发所涉及的复杂性的基本理解。

在过去十年中，虽然大多数国家的整体年龄校正癌症死亡率一直在下降，但仍极需开发治疗晚期癌症患者的新型药剂。人们认为还需要开发用于治疗"早期癌症"患者的新型药剂（在转移性疾病证据之前或上皮内瘤形成的状态下）[1,2]。后一种治疗早期癌症的方法，过去被称为化学预防，代表了一种可能对疾病产生巨大影响的新概念。

在本章中，我们描述了从发现到初始安全性（Ⅰ期）临床试验的新型药剂开发的基本原理。在此过程中，我们讨论了一些研究，这些研究说明了近年来引入药物开发的新方法。本章主要关注新化学实体的开发，而不是生物制剂的开发，尽管本文概述的一些原则也适用于这些药剂的开发。

作为概述，图 52-1 描述了新型药剂开发的经典阶段。使用该基本过程，已经开发了超过 150 种用于治疗患有各种恶性肿瘤的患者以及治疗早期癌症的新型药剂。虽然这是一个令人印象深刻的可用于治疗各种癌症患者的药剂列表，但鉴于各种类型癌症的生物多样性，我们仍需对我们的医疗设备进行重大补充。随着为新型药剂的适当检测开发新策略，必须了解已获批用于特定适应证的药物。人们还需意识到是否应该在"前线"环境中或在抢救或姑息治疗环境中开发新单药或联合用药。在了解所有抗癌药物及其官方批准的适应证的基础上，再结合图 52-1 和图 52-2，有助于理解如何设计将获得监管机构批准的关键临床试验，最重要的是为患者提供有效且安全的新药。

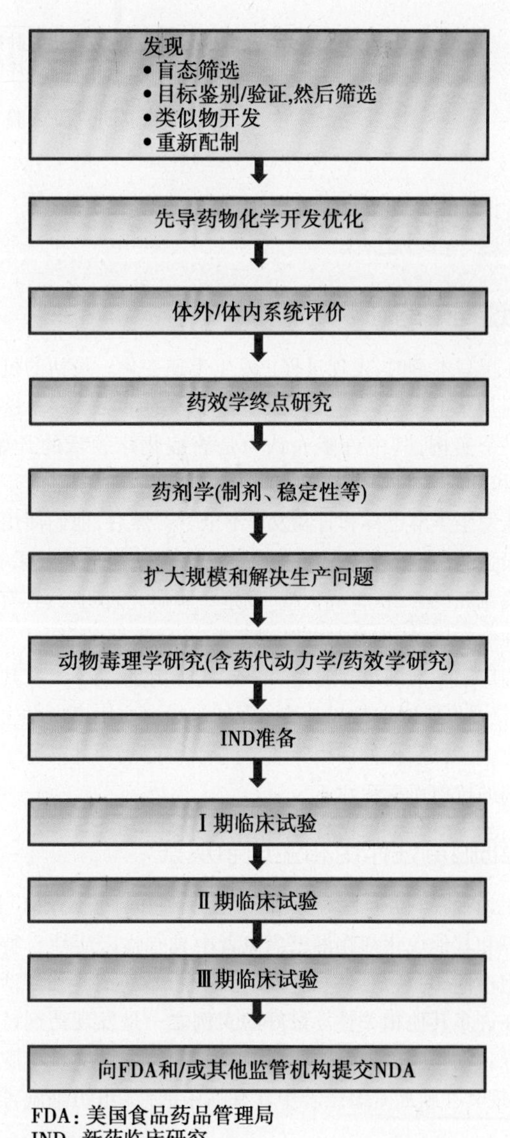

图 52-1　新型抗癌药剂的开发阶段

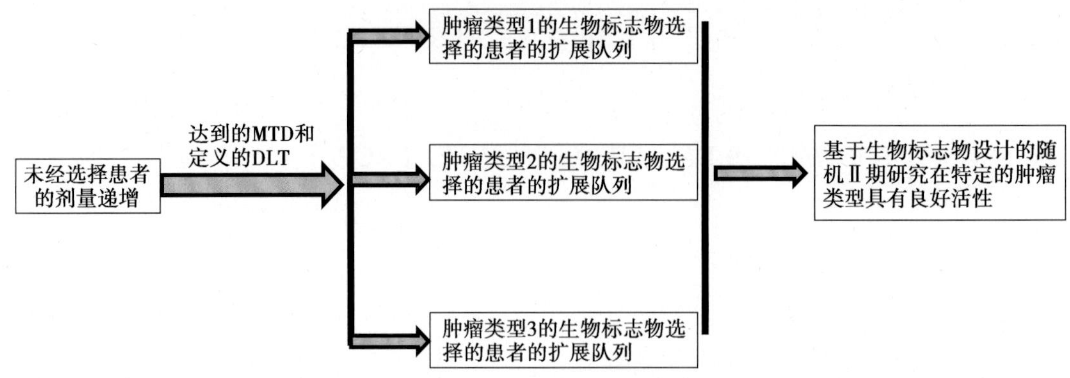

图 52-2 早期阶段试验设计的例子，具有靶向药物和患者富集

发现过程的进展

发现过程中的临床观察

在撰写本章时，发现过程正发生迅速变化。最初的抗癌药物发现是基于临床医生和临床前科学家的重要观察。这种观察的一个实例，其中许多人认为是癌症化疗领域的开始，是 Adair 和 Bogg 在 1931 年观察到第一次世界大战中暴露于硫芥的军队发生了淋巴样和骨髓发育不全[3]。然后，他们使用这种毒性很强的药剂硫芥治疗许多癌症患者。该药剂的效果有限。对相关氮芥（第二次世界大战）的进一步研究表明，其具有更强的抗肿瘤作用，特别是对淋巴瘤患者[4,5]。

临床医生准确观察的另一个典型实例是，Farber 及其同事发现，接受肝脏提取物或叶酸治疗的年轻白血病患者发生白血病恶化[6]。然后他们使用叶酸拮抗剂治疗患者，并描述了这些拮抗剂的抗白血病活性。

组织细胞毒性作用和生理学观察

正如观察到芥子气导致淋巴结、脾脏和骨髓发育不全（随后氮芥和其他烷化剂在淋巴瘤患者中具有临床活性），特定组织细胞毒性（对特定组织类型具有毒性）与药剂的临床活性之间存在许多其他相关性。最好的实例之一是发现药剂链脲佐菌素导致动物胰岛细胞破坏（导致糖尿病）[7]。尝试链脲佐菌素，发现其在胰岛素瘤患者中具有临床活性（组织细胞毒性作用）[8]。

在早期动物毒理学研究中，顺铂引起动物睾丸和卵巢发育不全，随后发现其在睾丸或卵巢癌患者中具有显著活性[9-11]。

通过一系列新型抗癌剂开发研究，Heidelberger 合成了 5-氟嘧啶[12,13]。Elion 和 Hitchings 的观察结果（基于核酸控制细胞生长的假设）推测嘌呤和嘧啶类似物可用于癌症治疗，这肯定导致产生 6-巯基嘌呤、6-硫鸟嘌呤和许多其他有用的抗癌剂[14-16]。虽然仍有明显的重要临床、毒理学和生理学观察空间，但这些观察结果可能不会成为未来药物发现的主导。

国家癌症研究所药物发现计划在药物发现过程中的早期和持续作用

在 20 世纪 60 年代早期，美国国家癌症研究所（National Cancer Institute，NCI）开始在发现和开发新型抗癌剂方面发挥重要的领导作用。这在当时是关键性的，因为业界认为在该领域的投资在经济上不可行且风险很高。NCI 通过建立国家服务中心（National Service Center，NSC）开始其领导，该中心为所有化学家、生物学家和其他感兴趣的研究者提供所有化合物的交换所（以及一系列化合物）。将化合物提交至 NSC，指定 NSC 编号（例如，用于米托蒽醌的 NSC 3101139），并在一系列体外和体内临床前模型中进行检测。通过体外和体内抗肿瘤活性的某些障碍的药剂被 NCI 机构认为是“决策网络”，用于将它们纳入毒理学研究并最终进入临床试验。

NCI 早期尝试使用最初从口腔癌患者获得的 KB 鳞状细胞癌细胞系对大量化合物进行筛选。在称为 P388 和 L1210 的两种白血病小鼠中进一步评估对该细胞系有活性的化合物[17,18]。这些体外和体内筛选确实产生了具有抗白血病和淋巴瘤临床活性的化合物（例如，长春花生物碱和亚硝基脲）。寻找具有针对实体瘤的抗肿瘤活性的药剂不太成功[18]。1975 年，NCI 对其评估过程进行回顾，包括抗实体瘤化合物的体内评价（自体动物肿瘤和在裸鼠中作为异种移植物生长的人肿瘤）。Staquet 及其同事对这项重大实验进行了非常重要的回顾性分析[19]。他们的分析结果详见表 52-1。

表 52-1 最具预测性的动物模型：1978—1982 年国家癌症研究所经验

合理预测[a]	完全无法预测
P388 白血病（小鼠）	Lewis 肺
L1210 白血病（小鼠）	CD8（乳腺）
Bl6 黑色素瘤（小鼠）	Co38（结肠）
MX-1 乳腺[b]	LXI[b]（肺）
	CXI[b]（结肠）

[a] 特别是既存肿瘤的消退。
[b] 异种移植物。
来源：改编自 Staquet 1983。

如表所示，P388 和 L1210 白血病小鼠持续用于预测临床中新型药剂的活性，在免疫活性小鼠中生长的 B16 小鼠黑素瘤实体瘤自体模型也是如此。唯一可预测临床抗肿瘤活性的人肿瘤异种移植物是在裸鼠中生长的 MX Ⅰ乳腺肿瘤异种移植物。这些模型的预测性不具有肿瘤特异性，而是通常预测临床活性的那些系统中的体内活性[18]。在 Staquet 及其同事的报告中，同样重要的是发现在这些模型中既存在肿瘤的实际消退以及存活≥45 天的动物的百分比，甚至是这些药物最终临床疗效的更强预测因子[19]。

2001 年，Johnson 等[20]报道了 NCI 临床前体外和体内模型中药物活性与新型药剂临床活性之间的关系。令人感兴趣的是，对于可获得异种移植物和Ⅱ期临床数据的 39 种药剂，如果在至少三分之一的检测异种移植物模型中存在活性，则至少观察一些Ⅱ期试验中的临床活性。特别值得注意的是，如果在检测的异种移植物的三分之一或更多中存在临床前活性，则该化合物有 45%的可能具有临床活性。在该相同研究中，仅非小细胞肺癌（nonsmall-cell lung cancer，NSCLC）异种移植物预测具有针对相同组织学（例如，非小细胞肺癌）的临床活性。因此，尽管这些体内评估系统经常受到诽谤，但当对其进行系统的大规模评价时，一些模型似乎是临床活性的合理预测因子（尽管不是肿瘤特异性预测因子）。

表 52-1 中另外注意到的结果是，几个模型被判断为完全无法预测临床活性。一些模型，如 Lewis 肺模型，继续用于证明许多新型药剂进入临床试验（特别是新型药剂，如血管生成抑制剂）。重要的是，正在考虑基于仅在 Lewis 肺癌、CD8、Co38、LXI 或 CX1 模型中的临床前活性使新型药剂进入临床的研究者注意到大量既往经验，证明它们不能预测临床活性。

然而，想要取得最大成功，重要的是记住 Staquet 及其同事用于临床活性证据的参数（与临床前模型相关）：肿瘤缩小。因此，他们的发现可能不适用于新一代更多的细胞抑制剂（而不是在 20 世纪 60 年代至 80 年代评估的细胞毒性剂）。

NCI 于 1985 年对其评价策略进行了进一步的修订，当时他们原位植入大量 60 种人肿瘤细胞系用于筛选目的[18,21-25]。他并尝试更多原发肿瘤类型，纳入乳腺癌、肺癌、结肠癌、肾癌、脑癌、卵巢癌、前列腺癌和黑色素瘤人肿瘤细胞系[18,22,23]。在将这一概念引入药物评价过程时，研究界对如何选择这些细胞系进行了大量讨论。许多研究者认为选择具有过快倍增时间的细胞系，不代表分裂更慢的实体瘤。然而，这种 60 种细胞系筛选系统是目前已有的系统。通过访问 NCI 的网站 http://dtp.nci.nih.gov/branches/btb/ivclsp.html，可以了解更多有关 60 种细胞系成功的信息。然后在传统的体内模型中评价在细胞系筛选中被认为具有活性的药剂（基于参考文献 18 和 23 中概述的标准并基于其他标准，如疾病特异性活性）以确定它们的治疗指数。如果发现它们具有活性，它们将进入临床前毒理学研究（见下文）[24,25]。

NCI-60 细胞系系列的真实预测性尚不清楚，因为尚无已发表的关于该方法对临床抗肿瘤活性的真实预测性的分析。然而，对 NCI-60 细胞系结果的许多极好的分析已产生了一些非常极具挑战性和有用性的研究工具。

作为唯一使用 60 种细胞系筛选结果的初始实例，Paull 及其同事描述了一种方法（他们称之为 COMPARE 程序），其中使用在 60 种细胞系筛选中评价的化合物作为种子，COMPARE 程序用于检测具有与 60 种细胞系相似活性模式（或指纹）的化合物[26]。然后，计算相关系数以描述其他药剂与种子化合物活性模式的接近程度。如 Weinstein 及其同事所述，似乎如果两种化合物具有相似的相关系数，这将预测化合物具有相似作用机制或相似的细胞内靶标[27]。如果新型活性化合物的相关系数与在 NCI 筛选中评价的化合物相比较低，则可能显著增加对新型化合物的关注，因为它很可能具有新的（独特的）作用机制。

癌症研究界的附加重要性和重大关注是 NCI-60 细胞系是否存在特定靶标（激酶、端粒酶、错配修复蛋白和受体）[28-30]。最近，对该细胞系系列进行完整的全外显子组测序，并在所有基因的 6%中鉴定出可能影响蛋白质功能的遗传变化[31]。这些品系的精确分子表征肯定不仅有助于评价新化合物，而且还报道了鉴定指示辐射响应性的基因特征[32]。

历史上，NCI 探索的其他临床前模型用于评价值得关注的化合物，这些模型用于评价直接从患者体内取得肿瘤的药剂。有两种系统，包括体外人肿瘤克隆测定（human tumor cloning assay，HTCA）和体内肾下囊系统（subrenal capsule system，SRC）。但是这些测定被认为在逻辑上太难以用作评价大量化合物的前期筛选[33-36]。

最近，已确定生长肿瘤组织的方法，该肿瘤组织直接取自患者或直接从糖尿病和严重免疫受损的小鼠中取得适当储存的肿瘤库。这导致患者来源的异种移植物更准确地反映原始患者肿瘤的病理和分子特征[37-41]。虽然这些模型对于个性化医疗中的常规临床用途可能仍不可行，但它们确实在早期药物开发过程中提供了另一进展，并且可助于识别敏感的肿瘤类型和耐药性的分子模式。它们特别适用于基于机制的治疗方法的开发[42]。随着免疫治疗疗法（例如，抗-CTLA-4、抗-PD1 和抗-PD-L1 单克隆抗体）的出现，使用同种异体移植物植入免疫活性小鼠的临床前小鼠模型将更常使用[43]。

随着患者肿瘤的完整外显子组测序变得可负担，已经发表了尝试产生类似于在个体患者中检测到的相同异常组合的小鼠模型。然后，使用抗癌剂治疗这些“替身”模型，患者将接受在模型中表现出活性的药物[44]。

基于机制的（“靶向”）药物发现和评价

随着分子技术和细胞生物学知识的爆炸式增长，现在有一系列令人难以置信的新方法可用于发现肿瘤细胞与正常细胞中存在的潜在靶标。

基于机制的治疗方法的惊人实例是伊马替尼的开发，其具有抗慢性髓性白血病和抗胃肠道间质肉瘤的显著活性。为了展望伊马替尼的发展时间表，伊马替尼的发现和开发的基础生物学背景工作实际上始于 1960 年在慢性髓性白血病（CML）中发现费城染色体[45]。这实际上是在任何类型的癌症中发现的首个一致的染色体异常。异常涉及 9 号和 22 号染色体的易位[46]。在 1990—1993 年中完成的工作记录了易位使得 9 号染色体上的 ABL 基因（非受体酪氨酸激酶）移至邻近 22 号上的 BCR（断点簇区域）基因。这种易位编码 BCR-ABL 蛋白，其是组成型表达的 210kDa 转化酪氨酸激酶，负责约 95%的 CML 患者[47,48]。这种异常的酪氨酸激酶不存在于患者的正常细胞中;因此,它是开发具有抗 CML 活性的药剂的极好靶标。

进行筛选以发现具有抗 BCR-ABL 酪氨酸激酶特异活性的化合物,并通过靶向作用于三磷酸腺苷结合位点(ATP 袋)。发现该药剂(CGP57148,又称 STI 571,伊马替尼)是该激酶最具选择性的抑制剂[49]。在体外和体内对该药剂进行检查,发现其对 BCR-ABL 阳性细胞具有选择毒性[49-51]。1999 年和 2000 年的Ⅰ期和Ⅱ期试验记录了伊马替尼对 CML 具有显著活性,特别是在疾病的慢性期[52,53]。如上所述,这个令人印象深刻的药物开发实例从确定目标到记录化合物对疾病的临床活动确实跨越了近 40 年(如果从发现目标开始计算,仅需 10 年,p210 BCR-ABL 酪氨酸激酶)。值得注意的是,其他工作表明,伊马替尼还具有抗其他几种肿瘤性疾病的显著活性,例如,胃肠道间质肉瘤,这些疾病具有 KIT 致癌基因异常,已获得总共 9 种不同适应证的监管部门批准。

尽管不在本章的范围内,但各种其他靶向治疗剂也显示出显著的临床抗肿瘤活性(抗雌激素、抗雄激素、芳香酶抑制剂和 CD20、CD52、HER-2/neu 等单克隆抗体)。然而,在撰写本章时,靶向范围也有一些令人失望的情况。例如,已开发用于靶向具有 ras 突变的肿瘤的法尼基转移酶抑制剂未显示出抗胰腺癌活性,即使它们具有抗乳腺癌和急性白血病的明显临床活性[54-56]。靶向难点的另一实例是发现尽管表皮生长因子受体(EGFR)在许多恶性肿瘤中上调,但 EGFR 激酶的小分子抑制剂或 EGFR 的单克隆抗体的活性未表现出与 EGFR 表达增加相关(至少通过目前可用的测量受体或其激酶的方法)[57]。最近的研究表明法尼基转移酶抑制剂在 Hutchinson-Gilford 早衰中具有有益作用[58,59]。

显然,如果靶向治疗欲在主要肿瘤类型中取得成功,还有很多工作要做。在最近的一项工作中,Druker 和 Lydon[60]概述了从伊马替尼开发所学到的经验教训。这些经验教训为思考改进基于机制的方法提供了指导,包括以下内容:

1. 确定适合药物开发的靶向分子。鉴别 BCR-ABL 酪氨酸激酶作为引起 CML 的激酶(即,作为靶向的单一分子缺陷)是重要的。激酶是一种“疾病基因”。为了成功,人们可能应该有一个对病程至关重要的靶标。
2. 可以在患者中轻易测量经验证的替代终点的可用性,以确保新药剂确实干扰期望靶标并具有期望效应。
3. 改进对于药物设计(例如,结晶学和分子建模)而言很重要的技术,以优化化合物的选择性(特异性)。

随着我们对细胞联系的理解的提高,无疑我们将继续努力开发基于机制的药剂[60-65]。然而,鉴于临床开发新药剂所需的大量工作和大量资源,明智地选择目标非常关键[66]。此外,已经清楚的是,已鉴别靶标的生物学作用在整个患者的临床过程中可能不是静态的。因此,早期药物开发已经使人们认识到重复活检是理解灵敏度和耐药性机制所必需的。进行治疗前和治疗后活检仍是临床上的挑战,并且在所有肿瘤类型中可能均不可能。

除了靶向肿瘤细胞外,现在很明显,靶向肿瘤细胞的环境正在发挥全新的重要性。鉴于发现直接抗 VEGF-A 的单克隆抗体贝伐珠单抗基本上改善了结直肠癌、非小细胞肺癌以及可能还有乳腺癌患者的生存期(与化疗联合使用时),令人兴奋的血管生成领域让所有临床医生都感到乐观[67-69]。很明显,该药剂还具有抗肾细胞和卵巢癌的单药活性[70,71]。虽然贝伐珠单抗可中和 VEGF 受体 2,但最近雷莫芦单抗(另一种单克隆抗体)引起了人们很大的兴趣,因为它与细胞外结构域结合并直接阻断 VEGF 受体 2。从概念上讲,这会阻碍所有配体的结合,而不仅仅是 VEGF-A 与受体的结合[72,73]。靶向 VEGF 和 PDGF 途径(改变血管生成过程)的小分子,例如,舒尼替尼(SU1248)或瑞格非尼(BAY73-4506),也显示出显著的临床抗肿瘤活性。由抗血管生成化合物的成功开发所启发的研究也产生了非常重要的见解,即不仅通过信号通路网络诱导和维持肿瘤血管生成,而且血管生成因子的自分泌和旁分泌环也可能对肿瘤干细胞发挥关键作用[74]。尽管获得了这些令人印象深刻的进展和新作用机制,但影响肿瘤环境的新药物仍需要本章所述的药物开发步骤。抗血管生成化合物的最大挑战之一是鉴别预测性生物标志物,其足以选择患者进行治疗决策。

随着早期临床试验设计向分子特征性肿瘤发展,生物标志物的开发仍存在挑战,原因如下[75]:

- 缺少对肿瘤生物学或候选药物作用机制的全面了解;
- 缺少可靠、可重复、足够灵敏或特异的方法用于测量候选生物标志物分子;
- 缺少在早期阶段研究中观察到的统计学把握度可以转移到更大规模的研究中(Ⅱ期或Ⅲ期)。

有关实例,见相关参考文献[76,77]。

由于这些复杂性,进入Ⅰ期的药物通常缺乏相关的,具有临床意义的药效标记物。Ⅰ期生物标志物的验证需要在剂量递增阶段或至少在需要足够大样本特别是在表达候选生物标志物或生物标志谱的患者人群进行合理的生物统计学的后续扩张队列中,对Ⅰ期试验进行概念重新设计,允许在正在进行的研究中进行学习的自适应研究设计,以及随机剂量确定的Ⅱ期试验(图 52-2)[78,79]。即使存在稳健和预测 PD 标记物,继续剂量递增直至达到最大耐受剂量(maximally tolerated dose, MTD)可能是明智的,从而在考虑急性和延迟毒性设计剂量范围。在统计模拟的基础上,Hoering 及其同事提出了Ⅰ/Ⅱ期杂交研究设计,其中包括最初的传统剂量递增,随后是改良的单臂Ⅱ期部分,包括剂量和时间表优化和疗效测试。这将有助于确定进入大型随机研究的最佳剂量[80]。

开发蛋白质工程化合物的特殊方面

蛋白质工程化合物如单克隆抗体、肽、肽体或融合蛋白是针对可溶性肽配体或膜结合受体而开发的。在Ⅰ期研究期间,这些化合物可能无法提供剂量限制性毒性(dose-limiting toxicitie, DLT)或 MTD。当长期给予治疗时,超过 20mg/kg 的绝对剂量也可能引起对非特异性蛋白质相关毒性的担忧。由于单克隆抗体的产生可能发生在病毒转化的细胞中,尽管努力去除病毒,残留的病毒载量——如果长时间施用非常高剂量的蛋白质也可能是一个问题。出于这些原因,选择剂量和时间表以便以后的Ⅱ期或Ⅲ期研究开发,通常是依赖于“生物有效剂量(biologically effective dose, BED)”或“生物活性剂量(biologically active dose, BAD)”。该剂量方案可源自动物模型中的 PK 观察。例如,可使用在小鼠中导致异种移植物反应的单克隆抗体的最小血浆浓度，并且在Ⅰ期研究中导致相应或更高血浆浓度的剂量可进行到后期Ⅱ期或Ⅲ期试验中。然而，这种方法对患者的剂量和时间表具有显著风险，其具有次优效力并且在完成和分析Ⅲ期试验后需要随后的改进。然而，动物模型可能不具有预测性，可能需要物种特异性抗体/工程蛋白，这与人体试验中使用的不同。因此，蛋白质工程药物如单克隆抗体的开发将极大地受益于稳健和预测性 PK/PD 建模以及尽可能早期在临床前和临床研究过程中应用可靠的生物标志物。如果没有 PK/PD 模型，生物标志物，MTD 和明确药物相关的 DLT，随后试验的剂量和时间表的选择意味着即使化合物具有令人鼓舞的早期临床活性，也会盲目选择。它存在丢失潜在活性化合物的风险以及影响生命周期管理的非常晚期的剂量/进度优化研究。肿瘤类型的 Encore 研究在完成的Ⅲ期研究中显示出阴性或阳性结果，可能在伦理上存在争议。这就产生了使用Ⅰ期研究设置和添加扩展队列以优化剂量和调度以实现最大靶点阻断作用，并在人类中提供概念的早期证据的挑战。这种方法还可能包括患者内剂量递增，尽管这些应在个别情况下并在适当的护理下考虑。

免疫治疗抗体的开发很有前景。通常，临床使用和开发中的化合物对细胞具有负面影响，例如，通过关闭代谢或生殖途径或阻断受体或下游磷酸化事件。相反，免疫治疗性抗体对免疫检查点受体/配体的阻断使免疫系统重新激活。因此，这些新化合物的活性不是直接在肿瘤上，而是在免疫系统上。这类药物的早期试验需要涉及检测以确定细胞免疫应答，延迟肿瘤缩小的意识，包括肿瘤病变初始增加的可能性，以及对新的毒性的认识（例如，垂体、甲状腺炎和由于免疫系统过度活化导致的自身免疫状态，这可能需要免疫抑制治疗[81-83]。

用于评估靶点的化合物来源

毫无疑问，针对靶点开发新药物的最合理方法是了解该靶点的晶体结构（至少对于非生物制剂而言）并合理设计药物与该靶点的相互作用[60,61,66]。但是对于绝大多数靶点，并无晶体结构。幸运的是，通常可采用分子筛选来帮助识别靶点抑制[84]。因此，药物开发团队有必要获得主要的化合物库，以便用于高通量系统识别药物靶点。NCI 一直是包括自然产品在内的化合物库的重要资源[85]。NCI 已经为研究者建立了 NCI 多样性化合库（http://dtp.nci.nih.gov/branches/dscb/diversity_explanation.html）。此外，还有一些额外的化合库供研究者使用（例如，http://htbc.stanford.edu/compounds.html；http://www.chemdiv.com 等）。

临床研究药物准备

配方

用于临床前药理学、毒理学和临床研究的药物或化合物的制剂是药物开发中经常被忽视但非常重要的方面。在进行动物药理学和毒理学之前，非常希望有一个计划用于临床研究的最佳配方[86]。

困难的配方往往导致长期的开发计划，偶尔会导致化合物的开发几乎停止。紫杉醇肯定是这种情况，紫杉醇需要溶解一种难以溶解的含有 cremaphor 的组合，这可能会导致一些患者发生特异性反应[87]。多种其他抗癌药物（紫杉醇除外）都有明显的配方问题，包括依托泊苷［最终配方使用 20mg 依托泊苷、2mg 柠檬酸、30mg 苯甲醇、80mg 改良聚山梨醇酯 80/吐温 80、650mg 聚乙二醇 300 和 30.5%（V/V）乙醇］、CPT-11（拓扑异构酶Ⅰ抑制剂）（使用在患者血清和肿瘤中被羧酸酯酶分解的前药方法解决）、多西紫杉醇（使用聚山梨醇酯 80 的制剂溶解）和其他几种。如果需要一种外来配方用于静脉注射，那么临床研究的开始可能会有很大的延迟。通常，只有已经用于患者的制剂可用于配制新药。最近，在配方领域取得了一些重要进展。例如，将紫杉醇包装成特制的白蛋白颗粒（称为“nab-技术”）已经改变了紫杉醇的特性，并导致了 nab-paclitaxel 在乳腺癌、非小细胞肺癌和胰腺中令人印象深刻的活性[88-90]。

在配制过程中经常出现的另一个主要问题是口服给药途径是否优于静脉给药途径。通常，对于细胞毒药物，担心药物在胃肠道吸收存在更大的可变性。这种可变性可能导致某些患者的不可预测和潜在的严重副作用，但某些患者又不会出现。此外，患者对口服药物摄入的依从性受到质疑，特别是如果这些药物可引起恶心或呕吐。因此，一般而言，如果可配制用于静脉和口服的药物，则优选开发静脉内给药制剂。保证在吸收不是问题的情况下完全确定化合物的药理学。例外情况是该化合物在其临床前活性检测中具有很大的时间表依赖性。在这种情况下，口服制剂可能更令人满意[91]。此外，如果预计药物会反复（例如每天）长时间服用，口服应用的开发可能是有利的。

开发药效学终点（替代标记物）的检测法

抗癌药物的开发在很大程度上是经验性的。更具体地说，之前并没有强调确保新药物实际上作用于它的设计靶点。对于更多基于机制的药物设计，已经建议尝试进行一些测定方法以确定该药物是否对靶点具有期望的作用（即药效学终点）。由于可假设任何化合物都会发挥各种生物效应，因此这种检测方法可能无法反映药物生化或临床效果的全部。

该领域变得至关重要。例如，Hidalgo 及其同事测量了接受 EGFR 拮抗剂的患者皮肤活检中 EGFR 的磷酸化[92]。此外，对培美曲塞有应答可能是与胸苷酸合成酶和 mrp-4 的表达水平以及抗肿瘤活性有关。丝氨酸-苏氨酸激酶抑制剂 enzastaurin 的表达与 GSK-3 的表达有关[93,94]。这些替代标志物伴随基于机制的药物开发是非常重要的。如果没有这些标记物，它们的开发将会很迷茫，而且如果化合物失败，则不清楚它是否是不适当的靶点或新药物是否不作用于靶点（药代动力学和各种其他可能的原因）。

动物药理学

动物药理学研究很少是开发新抗癌药物的主要部分［至少在准备研究新药（investigational new drug，IND）申请中］。当然，例外的是口服抗癌药物，它们需要进行生物利用度研究。动物药理学研究中其他的重要信息包括①药物的器官分布，包括在肿瘤中的渗透和停留时间（特别适用于在脂质体中配制的化合物，或者是白蛋白包裹的纳米颗粒配制的新化合物）；②渗透到中枢神经系统中或其他区域[95,96]。

Collins 及其同事描述了另一种可从动物药理学中收集的非常有力的信息[97]。这项经常被遗忘的工作表明在小鼠 LD_{10} 的浓度×时间(C×T)之间以及和患者 MTD 的 C×T 之间存在直接关系。基本上,小鼠的 C×T 等同于人类的 C×T。这种重要的关系似乎在大多数动物物种通用,可作为患者新药Ⅰ期研究剂量递增的目标(见下文)。其他人的工作证实了这种关系,并记录了如何利用这种关系来确定患者血清中的药物浓度(因此应该用于体外模型系统)[98,99]。

动物毒理学

动物毒理学研究是任何药物开发项目关键的部分。一般而言,迄今为止用于毒理学研究的模型(小鼠、大鼠或比格犬,因为这些动物模型的胆道系统更接近人类)已为开发新的抗癌药物提供了极好的安全数据(例如,在患者的初始Ⅰ期临床研究中并未发生灾难性事件)。一个必须更加谨慎的领域是核苷和抗代谢物。例如,氟达拉滨磷酸盐的起始剂量过高,第一剂量水平在患者观察到大量骨髓毒性,这可能是因为氟达拉滨需要通过脱氧胞苷激酶活化,而且这种酶的水平在人类癌细胞中比在小鼠和犬骨髓细胞中高得多[100,101]。培美曲塞(MTA,LY231514)是一种多靶点酶抑制剂,被批准用于治疗患有间皮瘤和非小细胞肺癌患者,也有类似的问题,但动物毒性比患者毒性更严重[102]。因此,研究者在检查核苷类似物或其他抗代谢物的动物毒性研究结果时,应警惕动物与人之间不一致的可能性。特别是当在创新的配方如纳米颗粒中研究抗癌药物时,显得尤为重要[103]。

如上所述,正式毒理学研究所需的常用动物物种是小鼠或大鼠以及比格犬[104]。对于单克隆抗体和其他生物制剂而言,经常需要灵长类动物模型。DeGeorge 等发表了美国食品药品管理局(Food and Drug Administration,FDA)对毒性要求的精彩评论[104]。在欧洲,在患者中进行Ⅰ期研究前,只需使用两种鼠类(小鼠和大鼠)作为必需的毒理学研究[105]。但是,如果这些物种的耐受剂量(mg/m^2)广泛存在差异,那么在开始患者的Ⅰ期临床研究之前,必须进行额外的狗毒理学研究。

一般而言,所使用的动物模型在预测某些器官类型的毒性(如骨髓抑制)方面是可靠的[106,107]。但是,发现狗对肾、肝和胃肠道毒性有些过度预测[108]。鼠和犬模型通常不能很好地预测神经系统、胰腺、皮肤和肺部毒性。这些模型在预测其他器官毒性方面是不完美的,并且偶尔在一个物种(例如鼠类物种)中发现毒性,但在另一物种(例如狗)中不存在毒性。这通常可归因于物种之间药物代谢的差异。如果在小鼠中发现不可接受的毒性,仍然应该考虑犬或灵长类动物研究,因为它们可能不会表现出小鼠模型中所报道的毒性。已经发现有些化合物在小鼠毒理学研究中有心脏毒性,但犬模型正确预测患者不会发现严重的心脏毒性[109]。

如下所述,动物毒理学研究对于帮助确定患者开始药物Ⅰ期研究的起始剂量是最关键的。

IND(研究新药)申请准备

在美国和大多数其他国家开始临床试验之前,有必要准备 IND 申请并将该文件分发给监管机构(例如 FDA)。IND 的必要组成部分列于表 52-2 中。

表 52-2 研究新药(IND)申请

1. 封面——表格 1571
(a) 申办者的姓名、地址和电话号码等
(b) 临床研究
(c) 承诺在 IND 生效之前不开展临床研究
(d) IRB 承诺
(e) 承诺遵守所有监管要求
(f) 负责监测人姓名和头衔
(g) 安全责任人姓名和头衔
(h) 任何转移义务,例如临床研究组织
(i) 申办者签名
2. 目录
3. 介绍性陈述和一般研究计划
4. FDA 留档
5. 研究者小册子
6. 协议
7. CMC 信息
8. 药理学和毒理学资料
9. 既往人类对研究药物的经验
10. 补充资料

CMC,化学、制造和控制;FDA,美国食品药品管理局;IND,研究新药。

更详细的信息参见 FDA 网站:http://www.fda.gov/drugs/developmentapprovalprocess/howdrugsaredevelopedandapproved/approvalapplications/investigationalnewdrugindapplication/default.htm.

如果在提交 IND 文件包后 30 天内未获得 FDA 的任何评论,可开始新药的临床研究。当然,如果 FDA 在 30 天等待期内需要额外信息,则必须在Ⅰ期研究开始之前提供该信息并获批准。

早期临床研究

0 期临床研究

0 期研究设计在常规Ⅰ期研究之前进行。从概念上讲,它们为后期Ⅰ期研究的药代动力学/药效学关系,起始剂量和其他参数提供参考信息。0 期研究的持续时间很短(通常只有一个疗程),并且使用剂量远远低于随后Ⅰ期研究的起始剂量。监管要求已在 FDA 指导文件缩略版 IND 公布,该指南于 2006 年 1 月发布的并且比完整 IND 文档的要求容易。鉴于伦理考虑(无治疗获益),未能加速药物开发和增加资源消耗,这种研究设计已经基本被淘汰[110-115]。

Ⅰ期临床研究

这是新药在患者(或正常志愿者)的首次研究。几篇优秀的综述是关于Ⅰ期研究方法[116-118]。第一次在人类进行的Ⅰ期研究的目的是该药物是首先在患者进行还是首先在正常志愿者进行而定。

正常志愿者与患者的Ⅰ期研究

通常在正常志愿者而不是患者中进行新抗癌药物的Ⅰ期临床研究。引用该方法的首要原因是正常志愿者有正常的器官功能,不像患者会受恶性肿瘤,恶性肿瘤之前的治疗影响。此外,正常志愿者通常不会使用其他合并药物(通常Ⅰ期研究中平均为 10 人),这可能使新药的药代动力学和副作用特征复杂化[119]。但是,照顾癌症患者的临床医生经常认为在正常志愿者进行的Ⅰ期研究是浪费宝贵时间,并且是延迟了向有需要的人:晚期癌症的患者给予有效药物的操作。但是,随着许多新细胞抑制剂而非细胞毒性剂的开发,这些药物是非致癌剂,首先在正常志愿者中尝试新药的兴趣越来越大——正如在其他药物开发领域如心脏病学中所做的那样。

对于给予正常志愿者的新药物,当然,必须证明它在适当的临床前系统中是非致癌的和非致突变的。然后可开始在正常志愿者中进行初步研究。

在正常志愿者中进行的新抗癌药物的初始临床研究的目标比在晚期癌症患者中进行初始临床研究更受限制。目标包括以下内容:

1. 以起始剂量给药时确定单剂量药物的临床药理学(并且可能在其他剂量水平下,以确保药物的线性动力学)。该临床药理学信息将包括峰值血浆水平,药物的半衰期和药物的曲线下面积(area under the curve,AUC)。此外,可收集一些药效学数据,例如药物是否在特定的正常组织(例如白细胞)中靶向靶标。

2. 确定新药在开始剂量(并且可能在其他剂量水平下)多日给药(通常不超过 5~7 天)的临床药理学,以确保不发生药物的累积。该药物的临床药学内容将包括峰值血浆水平、谷值水平、药物的半衰期、药物的 AUC 和稳态血浆水平。此外,还可收集一些药效学数据,例如,药物是否在特定正常组织(例如白细胞、颊黏膜细胞、唾液、毛发和指甲)中靶向靶标。

3. 确定这些志愿者是否存在针对这些低剂量药物的任何副作用。这通常通过安慰剂对照来完成。这可通过平衡随机化(为每一名接受新药的正常志愿者匹配一名接受安慰剂的正常志愿者)或不平衡随机化(每两名或更多名接受新药物的正常志愿者匹配一名接受安慰剂正常志愿者)。

使用正常志愿者进行新药的初始研究的想法是,获得药代动力学数据将提供清晰重要的可变性较小(相对比晚期癌症患者的变异性)的信息。据认为,这些可靠信息实际上可能会缩短患者新药Ⅰ期临床研究的时间,并且能让晚期癌症患者接受更有效的给药物量和新药物的时间表,这将使他们有更好治疗获益的机会。但是,即使在低剂量下将新细胞抑制剂给予正常志愿者人群也存在问题。最近,将细胞抑制剂服给予正常志愿者,并且在每日低剂量的给药时引起非常严重的皮肤反应(单次剂量未见)。虽然没有生命危险,但它表观上很严重,实际推迟了患者的给药时间。总之,在肿瘤学药物开发界,给予正常志愿者新的抗癌药物仍然存在争议。

高级恶性肿瘤患者的Ⅰ期研究目标包括:

1. 确定药物的 MTD。MTD 是推荐用于随后新药物Ⅱ期研究的剂量。

2. 确定新药的定性和定量毒性。在传统的Ⅰ期研究中,根据国际公认的表格和观察 DLT 对毒性进行分级描述。这些表格定期更新,并在 http://ctep.cancer.gov/protocolDevelopment/electronic_applications/ctc.htm 下发布。最近 DLT 的剂量被称为"NTD"或非耐受剂量。

3. 获得有关新药物临床药理学的可靠信息。最近再次强调了对这一重要方面的需求[120]。

4. 获得关于新药物的药效学信息(例如,新药物的特定血浆浓度是否与特定靶点相互作用/调节特定靶点)。这些研究可使用组织样品(正常和肿瘤)、外周血细胞、皮肤活组织检查、渗出液、血清蛋白、颊黏膜细胞或新成像技术来完成。

5. 记录抗肿瘤活性的早期证据(例如,客观应答、肿瘤标志物下降和临床获益)。

选择Ⅰ期研究的时间表和给药途径

Ⅰ期研究中最常探讨的时间表包括①单次剂量,每 3 周或 4 周重复一次;②每天一次,5 次,每 3 周或每 4 周重复一次;③每周一次,4 次,每 6 周重复一次;④每周一次,3 次,每 4 周重复一次;⑤连续输注 120 小时;⑥每天一次,21 次,每 28 天重复一次。当然,新药物有更多信息(例如,药代动力学/药效学信息),可能有必要探索其他时间表。选择使用哪种时间表(例如,推注与更频繁给药例如每日一次×5 次或每日一次×21 次时间表的选择)最常基于①临床前模型中抗肿瘤活性的时间依赖性;②药物在临床前模型中的药代动力学(最终来自患者数据);③非常重要的关于作用机制和临床前数据(例如,药物在"靶点"的停留时间发挥作用)。请读者注意,根据临床前动物模型中最活跃的时间表制定时间的决定,需要考虑到动物肿瘤比大多数类型人类癌症(除了白血病或侵袭性淋巴瘤之外)具有更快的倍增时间和更高的生长分数这一事实。

就给药途径而言,用于开发新药物的经过验证的方法(即使新药物使用口服途径)是通过静脉内给药途径进行Ⅰ期研究。静脉内给药研究随后可进行口服Ⅰ期研究。这通常是因为:①确定了静脉注射途径的药物(许多癌症患者可能有胃肠道异常,他们可能有其他药物的低度恶心(如镇痛药物),或吞咽困难,并且依从性可能是一个问题);②在静脉注射途径中,毫无疑问药物可能达到最大血药浓度峰值;③首先具有正确的静脉内给药物量,然后进行该药物的口服Ⅰ期研究,可评估药物口服剂型的生物利用度。

随着新的细胞抑制剂的引入,其更具有时间表依赖性,仅开发口服形式的药物(例如他莫昔芬、卡培他滨、伊马替尼和维罗非尼)变得越来越普遍。使用药物的口服制剂,在时间表中有更多的调整空间(例如,每天一次×5 天,休息 2 天;每天一次×5 天;以及每天一次×42 天)。但是,必须记住,用于Ⅰ期研究的时间表不能与动物毒理学中使用的时间表差别太大,并且应该在新药批准后在更不受控制的临床中进行管理。有了更好的诊断工具,对患者的药物遗传学变异性认识逐渐提高。药物遗传学变异可能对临床活性和毒性的差异很重要，因此在选择基于机制的药物的剂量和时间表时可能需要考虑[121]。

计算Ⅰ期试验的起始剂量

计算起始剂量的标准包括使用小鼠或大鼠 LD10（或 MTD）的十分之一或狗的最低毒性剂量（toxic dose low，TDL）的三分之一或六分之一。TDL 被定义为产生毒性效应的最低剂量，通常是指剂量如果加倍，不会导致致死亡。使用小鼠或狗的剂量来指导起始剂量的决定是考虑了剂量将计划用于使用的较低或更保守的起始剂量[122]。

因为动物毒理学研究经常以 mg/kg 为单位，所以以 mg/m^2 计算动物和人之间的所有剂量是至关重要的[123,124]。表 52-3 详述了 Freireich 等[123]提出的换算系数，将动物的 mg/kg 换算为至 mg/m^2。

表 52-3　对于人类起始剂量，将毫克每千克（mg/kg）改为毫克每平方米（mg/m^2）的换算系数

动物模型	mg/kg 换算为 mg/m^2 的换算系数
小鼠	3
大鼠	6
猴子	12
狗	20
人	37

来源：改编自 Freireich 1966。

为了证明如何计算新药的起始剂量，我们使用拓扑异构酶Ⅰ抑制剂 CPT-11[125]的开发实例，在 CPT-11 的动物毒理学研究中，最敏感的动物物种是小鼠使用每周计划。对于 CPT-11，小鼠每周给予 CPT-11 的 MTD 是 70mg/kg。使用转换因子 3（表 52-3），以 mg/m^2 水平表示的小鼠 MTD 为 70mg/kg×3 = $210mg/m^2$。然后，使用小鼠信息的人体起始剂量将是小鼠 MTD 的十分之一或 210 的十分之一或每周给予 $21mg/m^2$。如果狗是 CPT-1 最敏感的动物物种，我们会使用该犬的毒理学信息来确定我们 CPT-11 的起始剂量。

剂量递增的方法

剂量递增方法用于确定 DLT，DLT 又定义 MTD。副作用用于滴定进一步的剂量增加，并假设剂量、毒性和活性之间存在单一关系。

在Ⅰ期研究中用于剂量递增的方法通常是改良的 Fibonacci 研究方案[118,126]。但是，如表 52-4 所示，现在Ⅰ期研究中有几种剂量递增的方法，大多数其他剂量递增方法都是为了尽量减少接受极低剂量和无效剂量新药物的患者数量，并试图改善伦理规范[134,136,137]。改良的 Fibonacci 研究方案是最常用的剂量递增方法。但是，它可能出现最多的接受无效剂量的患者数量，主要是因为虽然初始剂量递增很大，但最终逐渐减少剂量递增百分比至后续每个剂量水平仅增加 33%。表 52-5 详述了经典的改良 Fibonacci 剂量递增方案。使用改良的 Fibonacci 方案开始新药Ⅰ期临床研究的真正好处是具有极好的安全性记录。特别当新药的动物毒理学研究中具有陡峭的剂量-毒性曲线时，优选该方法。

表 52-4　Ⅰ期研究中剂量递增的方法

方法	提倡者
Fibonacci 改良法	Hansen[126]
双倍递增法	Gottlieb[127]
	Freireich（个人通讯）
药理学指导法	Collins[97]
2 倍 AUC 法	Evans[128]
几何平均数+扩展因子 2	Erlichmann[129]
持续重新评估法	O'Quigley[130,131]
（和改良的持续重新评估法）	Faries[132]
加倍滴定设计	Simon[133]
患者选择法	Freedman[134,135]

表 52-5　Ⅰ期研究中改良的 Fibonacci 剂量递增方案

剂量水平	剂量	较上一个剂量的提高量/%
1	N	开始剂量
2	2 N	100
3	3,3 N	67
4	5 N	50
5	7 N	40
6	12 N	33
7	16 N	33
以上	—	—

随同改良的 Fibonacci 法，对于每个剂量水平，通常按照 3+3 设计每个剂量水平。必须小心操作。通常，将新剂量水平的第一位患者（患者 1）纳入研究并观察 3 周。如果在患者 1 中没有注意到毒性，则患者 2 入组相同剂量水平并观察至少 2 周（注意，此时患者 1 将进入他/她的第二疗程）。如果在患者 2 中没有注意到毒性，则可在患者 2 观察 2 周后入组患者 3。尽管让患者更快地进入Ⅰ期研究面临着多方面的压力，但遵循这种方法可提供最高程度的安全性，并在新药（或其代谢产物）具有特别长半衰期或具有非线性动力学的情况下提供额外的保护。当人们正在处理作为前药的药物（如 CPT-11）时，也必须小心并且可能使用改良的斐波纳契方法，并且提供有限的活性代谢物的信息。

如果剂量水平没有达到 DLT（参见下面的定义），则对于下一队列患者，剂量逐步增加。如果特定剂量水平的 3 名患者中只有一名达到 DLT，那么最多可有 3 名患者入组该剂量水平。如果 3 个或 6 名患者中的两名或更多患者达到 DLT，则剂量水平已经超过药物的 MTD。然后，在前一个剂量水平中入组其他的患者，以确保剂量水平是正确的 MTD-新药物进入Ⅱ期研究的剂量。值得注意的是，标准Ⅰ期研究中每个剂量水平需要 3 名患者没有真正的科学依据[138]。每剂量水平 3+3 队列大小

设计的主要理由是，到目前为止，它为Ⅰ期研究提供了良好的安全记录，允许在较低剂量水平下进行更彻底的药代动力学和可能的药效学评估，使用简单，机构审查委员会通常也能接受，并且没有与模型相关的额外费用。在最近的文献综述中，回顾性地分析了 1 235 个Ⅰ期研究，尽管人们担心 3+3 队列大小可能比更复杂的基于模型的队列大小更差，但 3+3 队列大小方法是目前未知最常使用的方法[139,140]。

表 52-4 中列出的下一个剂量递增方法是倍增法。该方法是为了尽量减少无效剂量水平的患者数量。该方法提供更快速的剂量递增。从理论上讲，它可能会导致剂量过高而伴随着严重的毒性（尽管在文献中找不到任何问题的例子）。这种剂量递增的倍增法（n，2n，4n，8n，16n……）现在可能是Ⅰ期研究中至少在药物不会引起毒性的低剂量水平下最常用的剂量递增方法之一。

Simon 等[133]介绍的剂量递增的另一种方法是，每剂量水平使用一名患者即加速滴定设计。他们介绍了两种设计（设计Ⅰ和Ⅱ）。对于设计Ⅰ，每剂量水平的一名患者队列在剂量水平之间以 40%的递增进行治疗。第一个 DLT，队列总共扩大到 3 名新患者。对于设计Ⅱ，每剂量水平仅有一名患者，但是在不同水平之间剂量递增 100%，第一次 DLT，该水平也扩展至 3 名新患者。然后，递增以 40%的增量进行。在设计Ⅰ和Ⅱ，如果患者在之前的疗程中具有 0 级或 1 级毒性，则允许患者增加剂量。

现在很少使用的另一种Ⅰ期剂量递增方法是 1990 年 Collins 等提出的方法。该方法也称为药理学指导的剂量递增方法。该方法基于一项重要的工作，显示小鼠的 LD 10（或 MTD）下 C×T 血浆消除曲线（AUC）下面积等于人体中 MTD 的 AUC。基本上，该发现为研究者提供了目标 AUC。在实践中，在每个剂量水平，AUC 是经过患者接受该剂量新药物确定的。然后使用该水平的 AUC 来确定下一剂量递增将是什么（如果药物的动力学是线性的）。使用该方法进行药理学指导的剂量递增需要实时药代动力学，这在临床有时难以实现。但是，它可能导致更强烈的剂量递增。已有一些建议改进该方法，一些Ⅰ期临床研究组已经实施[141,142]。

为了尽量减少接受无效剂量新药的患者数量而引入的最激进的概念是 O'Quigley 及其同事在 1990 年提出的持续重新评估方法。该模型已被反复评论并被其他作者改进[130-132,143-145]。在这种改进的连续重新评估方法（modified continual reassessment method，MCRM）中，一组临床医生估计临床可能发生毒性的剂量下限和上限（基于动物毒理学数据）。然后使用贝叶斯方法构建剂量-毒性曲线。Ⅰ期研究以小鼠 LD 10 或 MTD 的十分之一或狗的 TDL 的三分之一或六分之一开始。但是，不同之处在于只有一名患者进入第一剂量水平。在适当的随访量（通常 2~3 周）后，判断患者是否有毒性（≥1 级）。如果无毒性，则参考剂量-毒性曲线以确定下一次剂量递增。只要剂量低于估计的 MTD（剂量-毒性曲线上），剂量递增通常可通过加倍剂量来进行。CRM/MCRM 方法已经使用一段时间。有几篇综述评论了连续重新评估改进法进行的研究结果[141,146,147]。一般来说，MCRM 似乎没有减少完成Ⅰ期研究所需的时间，实际上也没有大量减少进入Ⅰ期研究的患者人数。在下一位患者接受治疗之前，它确实需要快速和完整地提供毒性信息。它确实缩短了达到接近研究 MTD 的剂量所需的时间，并且 MCRM 有助于减少一个Ⅰ期研究可能接受无效（<80%的 MTD）剂量的患者的数量（参见下面的应答率信息），但因此也可能增加中毒剂量治疗的患者数量。CRM 方法的一个潜在问题是当毒性发生较晚时，那么在剂量确定过程中无法捕获。这一点很重要，因为最近的一篇综述发现，在基于机制的化合物早期研究中，57%的≥3 级毒性在第一疗程完成后发生[148]。这一观察结果与基于机制的药物治疗后的长期低级别毒性的观察结果也可能定义了“DLT”，这已被国际回顾性分析证实[149,150]。CRM 的改进可能有助于考虑这些重要方面，但尚不清楚它们是否具有一般实用性[151]。Iasonos 和 O'Quigley 最近分析了公布的改进剂量探索研究的情况，包括对最初提出的持续重新评估方法的各种修改[152]。作者得出结论，Ⅰ期研究中的改进设计至少是安全的，并且可适应各种Ⅰ期临床情况。

贝叶斯Ⅰ期研究设计已经开发用于基于机制的新化合物的联合Ⅰ期研究，但尚未在临床上广泛使用。这些数学方法也关注毒性的起始时间[153,154]。

在Ⅰ期试验中选择患者的另一个常见问题是是否应该只有患有某种疾病的患者进入该研究（例如，仅患有前列腺癌的患者）。有趣的是，这种情况并不常见，但当更多针对特定疾病的药物被纳入Ⅰ期临床研究时可能会更频繁地提出。在此之前，大多数Ⅰ期研究，特别是细胞毒性试验，可能会继续允许患有各种恶性肿瘤的患者入组。

MTD 和 DLT 定义

MTD 的经典定义是导致 6 名患者中的一名或更少患者患有 DLT 的最高剂量。该 MTD 是通常推荐的剂量，用于在Ⅱ期临床研究单药使用的剂量。但是，欧洲研究小组使用的 MTD 有不同的定义，在新药研究前，必须仔细审查 MTD 定义。

DLT 的定义是根据 NCI 不良事件（NCI Common Toxicity Criteria for Adverse Events，NCI CTCAE）常见毒性标准≥3 级非血液学或 4 级血液学（例如，绝对中性粒细胞计数<500/μl）毒性。在以下网站上查找：http://ctep. cancer. gov/protocolDevelopment/electronic_applications/CTC。HTM。

关于Ⅰ期研究是否总应该定义 MTD 和 DLT 的问题经常被讨论。在临床研究中，这个问题越来越多地在基于机制的药物（例如，单克隆抗体和激酶抑制剂）的临床研究中提到。与定义 MTD 不同，越来越强调定义 BED（使用药效学测量）。值得注意的是，BED 和 MTD 通常彼此非常接近。此外，Ⅰ期研究止于 BED 时要非常谨慎。如果仅使用 BED，伊马替尼的Ⅰ期研究可能已经过早停止。新的证据表明，CML 细胞对伊马替尼耐药的一种机制可能归因于低剂量暴露。如果使用更高剂量的伊马替尼来杀死这些肿瘤细胞克隆，这将是有益的。

Ⅰ期研究患者的选择标准

表 52-6 详述了包含在Ⅰ期研究中的传统选择标准。这些仅作为指南提供。由于Ⅰ期临床研究理论上可能对患者构成风险，因此已经努力形成额外的评分系统或检测方法，这些评分系统或检测方法比传统的资格标准更准确预测Ⅰ期研究入选候选患者的预后[155-158]。这些系统更新了关于癌症生物学的新信息，例如，Olmos 及其同事的一项研究得出结论，循环肿瘤细胞的数量-以及白蛋白、乳酸脱氢酶和转移部位的数量-可用于更好地预测Ⅰ期患者的预后[159]。已采取类似措施预测哪些

表 52-6 患者进入Ⅰ期试验的常用选择标准

1. 年龄≥18 岁
2. 病理证实诊断为任何恶性实体瘤
3. 不需要可测量的疾病
4. 预期寿命≥12 周
5. 卡诺夫斯基的表现状态≥70%(ECOG≤2)
6. 充足的器官功能:
(a) 中性粒细胞≥1 500/μl,血红蛋白≥9g/dl
(b) 血小板≥100 000/μl
(c) 具有正常限度的血清胆红素
(d) SGOT≤3×ULN(除非由于疾病,否则≤5×ULN 是可接受的)
(e) 血清肌酐在正常范围内,计算肌酐清除率≥60ml/min
(f) 无需药物控制的心房或室性心律失常;在过去的 6 个月内没有发生缺血事件
(g) 没有需要积极治疗的癫痫病史;没有中枢神经系统恶性肿瘤的临床证据
7. 必须用尽所有治疗,这种治疗更可能为患者提供机会(包括研究性治疗)或必须处于没有标准治疗的情况
8. 在进入前 4 周内(丝裂霉素 C 或亚硝基脲 6 周)不得接受任何化疗,并从该疗法的毒性作用中完全恢复
9. 患者不得接受任何伴随的放射治疗
10. 患者必须从先前治疗的可逆毒性中恢复
11. 女性患者必须无生育需求或非哺乳期,并且在研究开始时和每个疗程前使用充分的避孕措施并且妊娠试验结果阴性
12. 男性患者也必须使用充分的避孕措施
13. 不应出现其他严重的并发疾病或活动性感染,这将危及患者接受(合理安全)方案中概述的化疗的能力
14. 必须努力将伴随药物减少到必需药物,是为了控制疼痛,患者舒适或危及生命所需的药物
15. 患者必须签署知情同意书。患者必须了解他/她的疾病的肿瘤性质,并在被告知要遵循的程序,治疗的实验性质,替代方案,潜在的益处,副作用,风险和不适之后自愿同意

SGOT,血清谷氨酸-草酰乙酸转氨酶;ULN,正常上限。

患者可能出现严重的药物相关毒性,这些患者可能被排除在Ⅰ期临床研究之外[160,161]。这些努力旨在检测哪个患者可能从研究参与中受益,但也确保药物足够的生命周期在患者人群中得到充分的评估。另一方面,讨论了Ⅰ期研究是否有偏差,入组人群在药物上市后不具有代表性。事实上,即使最终推荐的Ⅱ期剂量用于随后的Ⅲ期研究并在随后的Ⅲ期研究中得到证实,批准后"真实世界"的使用表明剂量和时间表的修改很频繁[162]。这些修改通常是由对毒性的担忧导致的,但是必须记住,剂量减少也可能导致临床受益减少。

传统排除标准也值得讨论几点。首先,一个重要的问题是老年患者是否应参加Ⅰ期临床研究。值得注意的是 Bowen 等的研究[163]表明患者的实际年龄对新药的Ⅰ期研究遇到的毒性没有影响。与这些研究结果相反,Schwandt 等[164]在他们的回顾性分析中发现,超过 500 名 70 岁以上的患者实际上发生毒性的可能性略有增加,但作者得出结论,这种风险在Ⅰ期研究的可接受范围内。两项研究都得出结论,单独的年龄因素并不是Ⅰ期研究的患者排除标准。

其次,在Ⅰ期研究中出现的最有趣的新问题之一(由于更多靶向药物的开发)是仅有肿瘤表现特定靶点的患者可以进入Ⅰ期研究。这似乎是有道理的,因为如果患者肿瘤具有靶点(例如,雌激素受体或 HER2/neu,CD20 或 CD52 阳性,或 BCR-ABL 重排或突变的 c-kit),患者更有可能对新药物做出应答。已经强烈要求在Ⅱ期研究仅包括携带靶点的患者[165]。相当清楚的是,如果药物确定仅对具有靶点的肿瘤起作用,并且明确新药物的作用机制仅针对特点靶点。那么非常清楚靶点在患者肿瘤中的存在应该是进入研究的标准。此外,必须确定用于测量该特定靶点的检测方法是准确且可重复的。在这种情况下,随着肿瘤在临床过程中改变其分子特征,留样组织或血液样本不可能在肿瘤进化的后期产生相关信息[166]。当满足这些标准时,限定表达靶点的患者人群效果非常好,如在携带 EML-ALK 易位的非小细胞肺癌患者中使用 ceritinib 进行的Ⅰ期研究所示[167]。选择存在肿瘤靶点的患者进入新药物研究策略将会成为标准。因为我们可以更好地确定新药物的确切作用机制。至此,基于在外周组织或肿瘤活组织检查中存在特定靶点来选择患者,对于Ⅰ期研究领域中的许多化合物来说仍然是不确定。

最后,在Ⅰ期研究中选择患者的常见问题是是否应该仅将具有某种疾病的患者纳入研究(例如,仅患有前列腺癌的患者)。有趣的是,这种情况并不常见,但当更多针对特定疾病的药物被纳入Ⅰ期临床研究时可能会更频繁地提出。

虽然传统的Ⅰ期研究仅作为大型随机研究的引入期,但最近在基于机制研究的药物开发的进展已经允许一种新的但仍然是实验性的监管方法来批准药物。2012 年，FDA 发布了一项新指南，即可基于有限数据获得基于机制的化合物的“突破性指定”（http://www.fda.gov/downloads/drugs/guidancecomplianceregulatoryinformation/guidances/ucm358301.pdf）[168,169]。这是一种很有前景的药物开发新模型，2013 年已经用于两种抗癌药物（obinutuzumab 和 ibrutinib）和一种非癌症药物，在本章撰写时，2014 年已经用于 5 种抗癌化合物（ofatumumab，ceritinib，idelalisib，ibrutinib 和 pembrolizumab）和一种非癌症药物。Ceritinib 仅根据Ⅰ期数据通过此流程获得批准。但是，基于突破性指定的批准是初步批准，FDA 将强制要求后续研究以确定患者的利益-风险比。

Ⅰ期研究中的药物联合

在Ⅰ期研究中，道德规范更为直接，研究中将新药物与已经批准的药物相联合。在这种情况下，患者将至少接受一种已证实具有临床活性的药物（通常是批准的小分子）。在Ⅰ期临床研究中，新型抗癌药物也可与传统放射治疗相结合[170]。该领域的临床研究活动数量日益增多，至少有单克隆抗体（如曲妥珠单抗、利妥昔单抗和西妥昔单抗）的初步经验证明当与标准化疗药联合使用时临床活性增加。另一方面，也有小分子的例子，其中联合策略至少在未经选择的患者人群中尚未得到验证[171]。尽管如此，这仍然是一个积极探索的领域，最近增加了基于机制的药物诸如信号转导抑制剂与标准化疗药组联合使用。一般指导原则包括标准药物通常应以日常使用的剂量和时间表给药（如果可能的话，以其批准的剂量和时间表使用）。这提高了研究者和患者对研究设计的接受度。尽管这些模型的预测价值尚未确定，但应在临床前模型中（如果可能的话）制定药物给药顺序。通过从标准药物的推荐/可接受剂量开始，然后在固定剂量的标准药物中加入新药物。一般而言，新药的起始剂量为单独新药 MTD（或适用的 BED）的 25%（如果与标准药物没有重叠毒性）。根据初始水平情况，新药物的下一剂量水平将是其 MTD 的 50%，其 MTD 的 75%，然后是其 MTD 的 100%（如果可能的话）。还有一些复杂的模型报道为Ⅰ期联合研究中使用的剂量递增提供了额外的依据[172]。

特别关注涉及基于机制的药物早期研究，Yap 等[173]最近完善地总结了许多基于耐药性逆转、药物给药顺序、向基础治疗添加新药物、交替药物和脉冲时间表的基本概念的试验设计。因此，有许多联合机会可以通过替代途径解决垂直耐药或水平耐药，并在药物开发中联合用药的决定必须基于肿瘤生物学的熟悉掌握[174]。无论最终应用哪种方法，我们应该始终谨记，基于机制的药物在联合使用时可能会产生意想不到的毒性，但是不应该允许在剂量方面做出妥协，使两种药物都以次优剂量或次优的靶点抑制作用给药[177,176]。最近，NCI 研究药物指导委员会的临床试验设计工作组发布了以下一系列建议：如何合理地选择Ⅰ期研究的联合应用[177]：

- 新联合应在方案中解释明确的药理学或生物学基础以及假设。
- 在方案中应描述该联合如何转化为临床获益以及该联合开发在Ⅰ期研究后的后续发展步骤。
- 研究的设计应解决 DLT，PK 相互作用可能导致毒性的可能性，以及这种相互作用的机制基础的假设。

Ⅰ期临床试验是治疗性的吗？

Ⅰ期试验有时被认为是非治疗性的，即没有治疗意图或对患者无益。这一含义需要加以纠正，因为有几项研究已经证明，实际上，在参与新药的单药Ⅰ期试验的晚期恶性肿瘤患者中可看到常规反应（完全和部分缓解）[178-182]。报道的缓解率范围为 5%至 7%（完全缓解率约为 1%）。但是，也有更高缓解率的例子，特别是在Ⅰ期联合试验中[52,183-186]。注意到大多数缓解率是药物 MTD 缓解率的 80%~120%。Roberts 及其同事回顾了在同行评审期刊上发表的 213 项研究（6 474 名癌症患者）[187]。他们指出总体缓解率为 3.8%。值得注意的是，他们发现在 12 年的研究期内，缓解率有所下降（1991—1994 年为 6.2% vs 1999—2002 年为 2.5%）。在观察期间，毒性死亡率也从 1.1%（1991—1994 年）下降到 0.06%（1999—2002 年）。根据这些数据，作者得出结论，风险与获益比可能已经提高。在对 24 项Ⅰ期研究分析中，Jain 等人发现基于 RECIST 的应答与患者的总体生存之间存在相关性[188]。这一发现也支持在Ⅰ期试验中使用应答作为结局指标的价值。对于头颈癌，Garrido-Laguna 的一项研究表明，进入Ⅰ期研究的患者无进展生存期与最后一次使用 FDA 批准药物治疗的无进展生存期相似[157]。感兴趣的是是否稳定疾病的类别将成为越来越多的利益衡量标准（特别是持续≥4 个月的稳定疾病）。对这类非进展型患者感兴趣，并且可能越来越多地将其用作确定新药在Ⅰ期研究中是否具有某些抗肿瘤作用的标准[189]。但是，使用 WHO 或 RECIST 标准实际上对患者的应答（无应答与应答）进行二分法，是基于或多或少的任意阈值。使用肿瘤缩小作为连续变量反而提供关于抗肿瘤活性的更精确的信息，因此越来越多地单独使用这个指标或与功能成像程序组合使用以评估在早期临床试验中研究的新化合物的生物活性[165,186,188,190]。许多已经发表了其他检测抗癌活性早期迹象的尝试。它们包括肿瘤反应的免疫因素，测量肿瘤代谢或灌注的功能成像程序，以及肿瘤生长率计算[167,191-195]。一种实验方法是测量肿瘤生长时间作为相对快速的终点确定临床活性。该终点是基于 Claret 及其同事对结直肠癌的两项大型随机Ⅲ期研究的模型提出的，虽然它仍然是实验性的，未在Ⅰ期研究中验证，但它是在早期临床开发阶段鉴定药物活性的潜在有价值的其他工具[196,197]。

确定新药物是否具有某些抗肿瘤活性的另一种方法是使用患者作为自己的对照的概念[198]。在这种方法中，从患者即将进入新药物Ⅰ期试验的时间开始，将他们先前的治疗方案作为比较，直到患者在没有进行性疾病的情况下进行试验。如果患者在新的Ⅰ期研究中的时间周期（B 期）比他/她在之前的治疗时间长，则该药物被判断为对患者肿瘤的自然病史有一些影响。如果Ⅰ期试验中 30%的患者（在 MTD 或其附近）的 B 期比 A 期长，则该药物可能是有希望的。临床医生在Ⅰ期试验舞台上越来越多地使用这种方法。

关于Ⅰ期研究的一般问题

有关患者参与Ⅰ期临床试验的伦理学的内容越来越多[134,199-203]。在最近的出版物中,人们注意到,经常引用的观点认为患者是出于利他主义的动机,患者参加Ⅰ期试验的动机包括以下[186,203-206]:

1. 希望改善他们的状况(高动机)
2. 亲戚和朋友施加的压力(高动机)
3. 亲戚和朋友施加的压力(高动机)
4. 医生的建议或信任(低动机)
5. 利他主义(低动机)

这些发现再次强调了患者从临床开发团队获得所有事实的重要性,以便他们能够就是否参加Ⅰ期临床试验做出明智的决定[207]。但是,有几项研究发现,早期临床研究的预后,支持治疗和实验性质的重要信息往往被临床医生忽略或被患者误解,因此"治疗误解"是医患关系的真正风险[208-210]。有兴趣的是,在此背景下,据 Berger 等人的一项研究报道,挪威肿瘤学试验中的知情同意文件的长度在 1987 年至 2007 年期间翻了一番[211]。对于美国来说,这种观察当然也是正确的。它不一定是生物复杂性的反映,而是日益复杂的法律和行政政府环境的结果。对于包括额外活组织检查或生物标记物的研究,通常需要由患者签署几个单独的知情同意书。尽管有这些手续复杂,但一些研究表明,患者参与Ⅰ期试验可提高患者的希望和食欲水平,这两者都是衡量生活质量的指标[212,213]。特别是年轻患者可能也有兴趣了解参与临床试验的医生/机构是否可能存在潜在的利益冲突[214]。

从失败中吸取教训是早期药物开发的重要组成部分。本章编写的一个突出例子是开发破坏胰岛素样生长因子途径(IGF-受体抑制剂)药物的巨大努力。以下这些方面可能导致靶向 IGF 受体的单克隆抗体的临床失败:次优的 PK 和 PD 行为,患者选择,缺乏预测性和稳健性的生物标志物,基于非预测性细胞系数据的肿瘤选择,缺乏明确的癌症驱动突变,从生物基因数据中检索到的 IGF 拷贝数,以及对 IGF 血清浓度升高的错误解释,其可能解释是与肿瘤缺氧相关的旁观者效应。在此背景下,Camaccho 及其同事进行的一项有趣的分析发现,在美国临床肿瘤学会年会上提出的Ⅰ期临床试验中,只有约三分之二实际上是全文发表了[215]。这是不幸的,因为患者为这些试验投入时间、健康和希望,并预期治疗结果将以适当详细的方式与医学界分享。

正如本章开头所述,早期研究中化合物类型的变化是显著的。确定的几种类型化合物:①没有"脱靶"作用的化疗药物;②基于机制的药物(高剂量)可能具有显著且通常有毒性的"脱靶"效应;③基于机制的生物化合物,超过最大值没有进一步影响;④免疫治疗化合物不仅有毒性,而且早期研究中的传统疗效终点可能不充分。在今天的Ⅰ期研究时代,根据化合物的类型和其他误导性风险结果定制早期临床评估方法变得非常重要。

未来的技术可能会对Ⅰ期试验产生影响

在过去的 10 年中,新药的研发已经从经典的细胞毒性药物转变为基于分子机制的化合物。但是,最初希望的更快和更有效的药物开发过程并没有得到满足,开发的早期阶段和后期阶段往往是缓慢、复杂和昂贵的。需要包含预测性和稳健性生物标志物、药代动力学和药效学的新试验设计。在某些多靶点药物研究中,生物标志物标签是必需的[216]。

此外,功能成像(例如动态磁共振成像、正电子发射断层扫描和单光子发射计算机断层扫描)的快速发展可能通过帮助研究人员评估药效学终点和可能评估抗肿瘤作用的早期证据而对Ⅰ期临床试验产生巨大影响。

最近关于血清蛋白质组学的报道(具有预测疾病存在的不同蛋白质模式)代表了肿瘤标志物的新模式,这些标志物肯定会对检测新药物的早期效应有用[217,218]。

上述和其他新技术应该有助于Ⅰ期研究者尽早确定一个特定的新药是否有助于特定患者,并改善愿意参与新药Ⅰ期试验的患者的获益前景。

结论

自 20 世纪 30 年代早期开始系统性抗癌治疗以来,已发现超过 150 种药物具有抗癌活性,并已获得美国食品和药物管理局的批准。尽管付出巨大的努力,癌症仍然是最大的医疗保健负担之一,只有少数转移性癌症可以治愈。随着抗癌药物的开发,已经建立了开发过程标准化方法并且提供新药可能带来的益处的客观评估方法。过去 10 年中,我们对癌细胞的分子生物学和癌症细胞组的理解获得特别显著的加速,这对于如何开发针对特定分子过程的新药的理解产生了很大的影响。在本章的撰写中,开发这种基于机制的药物的努力已经在很大程度上取代了针对细胞生长的一般特征的更传统的化疗药物的开发。但是,不可忘怀的是初始的基于偶然性的观察有多重要,并且这些观察结果使得国家癌症研究所为确定临床药物发现的潜在先导物和预测临床活性的临床前试验做出了广泛的努力。这是现在所谓的"个性化"医学的开始——彼时还未有对突变事件复杂性的基本理解。确定伊马替尼作为慢性粒细胞白血病的活性药物为药物开发的新时代的一个里程碑,并激发了对成药靶标和随后药物开发的深入研究。尽管在基于机制的药物早期开发方面取得了巨大进步,但临床方法基本上没有改变,并且基于不同的终点分为 3 期(Ⅰ期、Ⅱ期和Ⅲ期)。随着对如何最好地开发基于机制的药物的逐渐理解,正在修补一些临床开发阶段,基于贝叶斯方法的新的Ⅰ期设计变得越来越流行。基于机制的药物也可能具有不同于传统化疗药物毒性的毒性,这需要加以考虑。只有当肿瘤表达靶点分子异常时,它们的使用才有意义。考虑到起始治疗时肿瘤可能发生生物漂移,将患者纳入特定试验的治疗决定,重复活检可能是必要的。当我们进入这个新的令人兴奋的抗癌治疗时代时,成像技术、蛋白质组学和代谢组学等新技术将增加我们对如何开发更具活性和耐受性的药物的理解。

(李志铭 译,姜文奇 审校)

参考文献

The complete reference list can be found on the Wiley Companion Digital Edition of this title (see inside front cover for login instructions).

4 Goodman LS, Wintrobe MM, Damashek W, Goodman MJ, Gilman A. Nitrogen Mustard Therapy – Use of methyl-bis (β-chlorethyl)amine hydrochloride and tris (β-chloroethyl)amine hydrochloride for Hodgkin's disease, lymphosarcoma, leukemia and certain allied and miscellaneous disorders. *JAMA*. 1946;**132**:126–132.

6 Farber S, Diamond LK, Mercer RD, Sylvester RF Jr, Wolff JA. Temporary remissions in acute leukemia in children produced by folic acid antagonist 4-aminopteroyl-glutamaic acid (aminopterin). *N Engl J Med*. 1948;**238**:787–793.

15 Elion GB, Hitchings GH, Vanderwerff H. Antagonists of nucleic acid derivatives. VI. Purines. *J Biol Chem*. 1951;**192**:505–518.

16 Elion GB. Nobel Lecture. The purine path to chemotherapy. *Biosci Rep*. 1989;**9**:509–529.

19 Staquet MJ, Byar DP, Green SB, Rozencweig M. Clinical predictivity of transplantable tumor systems in the selection of new drugs for solid tumors: rationale for a three-stage strategy. *Cancer Treat Rep*. 1983;**67**:753–765.

23 Grever MR, Schepartz SA, Chabner BA. The National Cancer Institute: cancer drug discovery and development program. *Semin Oncol*. 1992;**19**:622–638.

37 Seol HS, Kang H, Lee SI, et al. Development and characterization of a colon PDX model that reproduces drug responsiveness and the mutation profiles of its original tumor. *Cancer Lett*. 2014;**345**:56–64.

38 Julien S, Merino-Trigo A, Lacroix L, et al. Characterization of a large panel of patient-derived tumor xenografts representing the clinical heterogeneity of human colorectal cancer. *Clin Cancer Res*. 2012;**18**:5314–5328.

43 Das TM, Pryer NK, Singh M. Mouse tumour models to guide drug development and identify resistance mechanisms. *J Pathol*. 2014;**232**:103–111.

45 Nowell PS, Hungerford DA. A minute chromosome in human granulocytic leukemia. *Science*. 1960;**132**:1497.

52 Druker BJ, Talpaz M, Resta DJ, et al. Efficacy and safety of a specific inhibitor of the BCR-ABL tyrosine kinase in chronic myeloid leukemia. *N Engl J Med*. 2001;**344**:1031–1037.

63 Hanahan D, Weinberg RA. The hallmarks of cancer. *Cell*. 2000;**100**:57–70.

65 Hanahan D, Weinberg RA. Hallmarks of cancer: the next generation. *Cell*. 2011;**144**:646–674.

74 Goel HL, Mercurio AM. VEGF targets the tumour cell. *Nat Rev Cancer*. 2013;**13**:871–882.

78 Hollebecque A, Postel-Vinay S, Verweij J, et al. Modifying phase I methodology to facilitate enrolment of molecularly selected patients. *Eur J Cancer*. 2013;**49**:1515–1520.

81 Hoos A, Eggermont AM, Janetzki S, et al. Improved endpoints for cancer immunotherapy trials. *J Natl Cancer Inst*. 2010;**102**:1388–1397.

82 Wolchok JD, Hoos A, O'Day S, et al. Guidelines for the evaluation of immune therapy activity in solid tumors: immune-related response criteria. *Clin Cancer Res*. 2009;**15**:7412–7420.

104 DeGeorge JJ, Ahn CH, Andrews PA, et al. Regulatory considerations for preclinical development of anticancer drugs. *Cancer Chemother Pharmacol*. 1998;**41**:173–185.

116 Eisenhauer EA, O'Dwyer PJ, Christian M, Humphrey JS. Phase I clinical trial design in cancer drug development. *J Clin Oncol*. 2000;**18**:684–692.

118 Von Hoff DD, Kuhn J, Clark GM. Design and conduct of Phase I trials. In: Staquet M, Sylvester R, Buyse M, eds. *EORTC*. Oxford: Oxford University Press; 1984:210–220.

121 Deenen MJ, Cats A, Beijnen JH, Schellens JH. Part 2: pharmacogenetic variability in drug transport and phase I anticancer drug metabolism. *Oncologist*. 2011;**16**:820–834.

130 O'Quigley J, Pepe M, Fisher L. Continual reassessment method: a practical design for Phase I clinical trials in cancer. *Biometrics*. 1990;**46**:33–48.

132 Faries D. Practical modifications of the continual reassessment method for phase I cancer clinical trials. *J Biopharm Stat*. 1994;**4**:147–164.

136 Ratain MJ, Mick R, Schilsky RL, Siegler M. Statistical and ethical issues in the design and conduct of Phase I and II clinical trials of new anticancer agents [see comments]. *J Natl Cancer Inst*. 1993;**85**:1637–1643.

139 Rogatko A, Schoeneck D, Jonas W, Tighiouart M, Khuri FR, Porter A. Translation of innovative designs into phase I trials. *J Clin Oncol*. 2007;**25**:4982–4986.

143 Piantadosi S, Fisher JD, Grossman S. Practical implementation of a modified continual reassessment method for dose-finding trials. *Cancer Chemother Pharmacol*. 1998;**41**:429–436.

148 Postel-Vinay S, Gomez-Roca C, Molife LR, et al. Phase I trials of molecularly targeted agents: should we pay more attention to late toxicities? *J Clin Oncol*. 2011;**29**:1728–1735.

149 Postel-Vinay S, Collette L, Paoletti X, et al. Towards new methods for the determination of dose limiting toxicities and the assessment of the recommended dose for further studies of molecularly targeted agents – Dose-Limiting Toxicity and Toxicity Assessment Recommendation Group for Early Trials of Targeted therapies, an European Organisation for Research and Treatment of Cancer-led study. *Eur J Cancer*. 2014;**50**:2040–2049.

150 Paoletti X, Le TC, Verweij J, et al. Defining dose-limiting toxicity for phase 1 trials of molecularly targeted agents: results of a DLT-TARGETT international survey. *Eur J Cancer*. 2014;**50**:2050–2056.

151 Liu S, Yin G, Yuan Y. Bayesian data augmentation dose finding with continual reassessment method and delayed toxicitiy. *Ann Appl Stat*. 2013;**7**:1837–2457.

153 Tighiouart M, Liu Y, Rogatko A. Escalation with overdose control using time to toxicity for cancer phase I clinical trials. *PLoS One*. 2014;**9**:e93070.

160 Hyman DM, Eaton AA, Gounder MM, et al. Nomogram to predict cycle-one serious drug-related toxicity in phase I oncology trials. *J Clin Oncol*. 2014;**32**:519–526.

168 Darrow JJ, Avorn J, Kesselheim AS. New FDA breakthrough-drug category – implications for patients. *N Engl J Med*. 2014;**371**:89–90.

169 Darrow JJ, Avorn J, Kesselheim AS. New FDA breakthrough-drug category – implications for patients. *N Engl J Med*. 2014;**370**:1252–1258.

173 Yap TA, Omlin A, de Bono JS. Development of therapeutic combinations targeting major cancer signaling pathways. *J Clin Oncol*. 2013;**31**:1592–1605.

176 Hu-Lieskovan S, Robert L, Homet MB, Ribas A. Combining targeted therapy with immunotherapy in BRAF-mutant melanoma: promise and challenges. *J Clin Oncol*. 2014;**32**:2248–2254.

177 Paller CJ, Bradbury PA, Ivy SP, et al. Design of Phase I combination trials: recommendations of the Clinical Trial Design Task Force of the NCI Investigational Drug Steering Committee. *Clin Cancer Res*. 2014;**20**:4210–4217.

178 Von Hoff DD, Turner J. Response rates, duration of response, and dose response effects in phase I studies of antineoplastics. *Invest New Drugs*. 1991;**9**:115–122.

181 Jones RL, Olmos D, Thway K, et al. Clinical benefit of early phase clinical trial participation for advanced sarcoma patients. *Cancer Chemother Pharmacol*. 2011;**68**:423–429.

184 Thödtmann R, Depenbrock H, Dumez H, et al. Clinical and pharmacokinetic Phase I study of Multitargeted antifolate (LY231514) in combination with cisplatin. *J Clin Oncol*. 1999;**17**:3009–3016.

第 53 章 肿瘤生长动力学

Elizabeth Comen, MD ■ Teresa A. Gilewski, MD ■ Larry Norton, MD

概述

动力学是研究作用于物体的力大小与物体运动随时间变化的一门科学。动力学是肿瘤学的核心概念,肿瘤进展反映了肿瘤细胞数量、肿瘤团块大小以及侵犯部位随时间的变化过程。本章的目的是阐明动力学在肿瘤生长过程中的理论意义和实际应用。正如时间和空间密切相关,肿瘤生长动力学和肿瘤微环境也是如此。在本章我们将讨论肿瘤细胞增殖、生长的动力学,为改善肿瘤化疗提供一定的理论基础。

引言

动力学是对运动的研究,或者通俗地讲是对大小、形状、距离、速度或其他任何可定量的物质随时间变化的研究。因此,动力学应被视为肿瘤学的核心内容。肿瘤发生发展的全部内容,都是围绕肿瘤细胞数量、肿瘤团块大小以及侵犯部位随时间变化的函数。肿瘤发病率和死亡率是这些变化的结果,用无复发生存期、无进展生存期和总生存期来衡量。不仅如此,肿瘤在分子水平上,并非一个停滞的过程,而是涉及基因完整性、拷贝数和表达、翻译后修饰,以及 RNA 和蛋白质产生、降解等一系列过程的异常,这些都是与时间相关的。不能从时间变化的角度分析和解释肿瘤生物学行为,可能忽略现象的本质,而导致概念上和临床上的谬误。

本章的目的是根据最新的肿瘤研究成果阐明肿瘤生长动力学在肿瘤学中的理论意义和实际应用。了解以时间依赖方式评估肿瘤发生发展时,肿瘤细胞在空间上随时间变化的重要性。比如肿瘤细胞与基质之间的相互作用很大程度上影响肿瘤生长。肿瘤生长动力学与肿瘤微环境就像时间和空间一样,密不可分。在本章,我们将通过评估肿瘤动力学行为以及基质介导肿瘤生长的作用,为更好地理解肿瘤发生发展过程提供新的见解。

肿瘤医学中的疑惑

肿瘤研究提示了众多疑惑,即在一组现象中,各个现象都确实存在,但似乎看起来不能共存。这些疑惑提示理论存在缺陷,在这里我们将从动力学角度解释、阐明部分疑惑。

肿瘤病因的多样性

首先,我们需要考虑肿瘤细胞在基因形态和拷贝数方面表现出多种多样的变化,这与恶性肿瘤形成的理论基础是一致的。恶性肿瘤是各种异常累积的结果,有一些因素独立于基因组学变化,这也正是肿瘤病因多样性的体现。这些变化涉及生长过程的自给自足、对抗生长和促凋亡信号的不敏感,以及获得侵袭、转移、诱导血管生成和无限增值的能力等。然而,这一理论如何与原位癌形成的理论相一致?原位癌临床表现为良性——无转移并很少出现大肿块,但却与它们演变形成的恶性肿瘤一样具有异常的遗传学基因。

恶性肿瘤病因多样性呈现的另一个疑惑,涉及组织学分级、肿瘤大小、邻近区域(主要是淋巴结)以及远隔部位侵犯之间的显著关联。这些特征组合在一起,我们可能会忽略它们是不同生物过程的表现,包括形态形成、有丝分裂、细胞凋亡以及转移。事实上,"转移"行为呈现出许多令人深省的疑惑。19 世纪末期,Halsted 利用当时盛行的力学假设原发性乳腺癌的恶性传播可通过切除含有该乳腺癌的整个乳房以及相邻的同侧腋窝内容物而得到控制。根治性乳房切除术的理念是肿瘤细胞通过侵入乳房中的淋巴管进入身体的其他部分,而淋巴管与体循环连接前须经过腋窝。许多研究似乎都支持 Halsted 的论点。根治性乳房切除术确实治愈了一些患者,如果保留乳房的话,他们中的大多数患者都将死于转移性乳腺癌,这在 19 世纪的观察性研究中得到验证。因此,是否发生淋巴侵犯是一个强有力的预后因素。最值得注意的是近期研究发现,前哨淋巴结活检证实了乳腺中淋巴管和肿瘤细胞的共流动模型。然而,人们如何引用 Halsted 的理论解释那些接受根治性切除术时未出现腋窝淋巴结侵犯的患者仍然发生远处转移?

分子分型与肿瘤干细胞概念

肿瘤的另一个疑惑是根据基因表达谱进行肿瘤分子分型。毫无疑问,肿瘤的基因表达不同,与临床上有意义的观察终点如无病生存、总生存以及化疗获益相关[1]。检测肿块的一小部分样本就可以提供关于整个肿瘤生物学行为有用的信息,似乎肿瘤中的所有细胞都携带着关键的信息。然而,这一现象如何与大家普遍认为的、实验得知的肿瘤干细胞学说相一致,即只有极少数的肿瘤细胞具有形成新肿瘤的能力?这些细胞被称为肿瘤干细胞或肿瘤起始细胞。

肿瘤:局部 vs 全身性疾病

众所周知,乳腺癌在早期通常是一种全身性疾病,系统性辅助治疗如激素和化疗可改善患者无病生存和总生存。但这如何解释良好的局部控制也可以提高生存?如放射治疗保乳术后残余的乳房组织可以改善预后。事实上,似乎每 4 例通过放射治疗预防局部复发的患者中,可以挽救 1 例患者避免发生远处转移。如果疾病是早期转移,为什么局部控制没有起作用?实践中或许可以找到部分答案。组织病理学分析显示,在原发肿瘤切除部位边缘外几厘米处通常可以发现乳腺癌细胞。这引发了新的问题：这些细胞如何到达那里，这些细胞和远处转移之间的关系是什么？

Gompertzian 生长曲线

肿瘤的另一个疑惑涉及肿瘤的生长曲线。例如乳腺癌的生长曲线不能简单地通过指数或线性动力学解释，而是遵循 S 形曲线，其介于以上两种曲线之间（图 53-1）[2]。该生长曲线不仅在临床上可直接观察到，还符合逻辑推断。例如，回顾性分析临床确诊的乳腺癌患者 X 线片，预估肿瘤从一个细胞增长到 10^9 或 10^{10} 个细胞平均需要 2 年。如果所有细胞紧密地包在一起，这个细胞数相当于 1～10cm^3 的肿瘤体积，在诊断原发肿物时这是一个合理的大小范围。

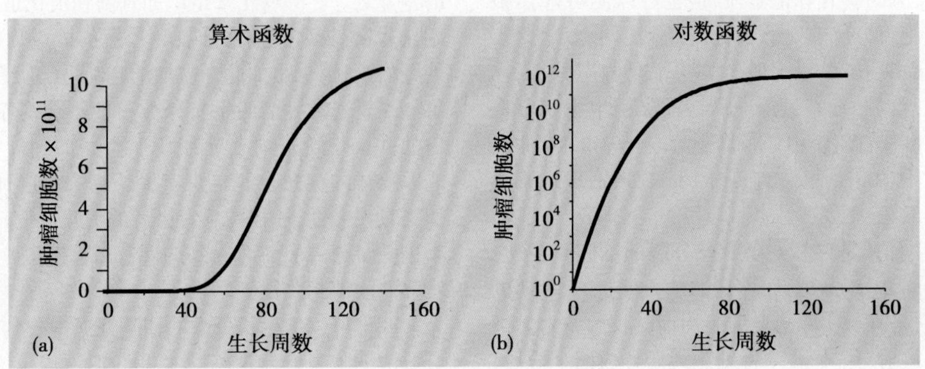

图 53-1　（a，b）两种函数下 Gompertzian 生长曲线

现在让我们想象一下如果肿瘤呈线性生长会发生什么？这意味着肿瘤将从 1 个细胞生长到两个细胞，然后是 3 个细胞、4 个细胞，以此类推。按照这种曲线，肿瘤从 1 个细胞增长到 10^9 或 10^{10} 个细胞（1～10cm^3）需要 2 年时间，那么增长到 2～20cm^3 需要再过 2 年，生长到 3 倍尺寸 3～30cm^3 仍需要再过 2 年。对于未经治疗的原发肿瘤，这种缓慢增长显然是不切实际的。因此，肿瘤不可能呈线性增长。

指数动力学也不符合肿瘤的生长曲线。指数生长涉及连续的倍增时间，也就是说，如果一个细胞分裂成两个细胞需要一周时间；按照指数动力学，两个细胞分裂成四个也需要一周；四个分裂成八个也需要一周；以此类推。几十年前，Howard Skipper 及其同事用指数动力学解释小鼠白血病生长及对治疗的反应，为大部分实验和临床化疗奠定了理论基础。但指数动力学是否适用于人类疾病？让我们再看一下原发性乳腺癌 2 年内从一个细胞增长到 10^9 或 10^{10} 个细胞的情况。如果它以指数方式生长到这么大并继续以指数方式生长，此后肿块将每 22～24 天增加一倍，这意味着肿瘤在诊断后 7 周内即可达到 4～40cm^3 大小。这是一种爆炸性生长速率，与一般医学经验不符。因此，指数动力学也不适用于肿瘤生长曲线。然而，有丝分裂确实是从一个细胞产生两个细胞，因此在细胞数很少的早期阶段，肿瘤必定是近似指数生长。这确实是一个疑惑。

解决这个疑惑的唯一方法是假设肿瘤开始以指数方式生长，随着肿瘤变大，逐渐趋向于缓慢生长。随时间推移呈指数下降的生长方式，确实符合肿瘤实际的生长曲线[3]。1825 年 Benjamin Gompertz 提出这一生长曲线，自那以后一直是所有生物数学中最常用的曲线之一。图 53-1 显示了两种函数下肿瘤的生长曲线：算术函数和对数函数。"S"形状在算术函数中很明显，但在对数函数中，随着肿块变大，相对生长速率似乎持续减小。事实证明，Gompertzian 动力学在优化改进抗肿瘤化疗方案中非常有用，不仅在乳腺癌（首次发现），还包括淋巴瘤、儿童肉瘤和其他恶性肿瘤。如果 Gompertzian 生长曲线普遍存在，那它普遍存在的原因是什么？

在本章中，我们将利用动力学提供的框架探讨致癌机制、肿瘤起始细胞行为、病理组织学分级和转移扩散曲线等问题。我们将利用细胞增殖的基本原理探索肿瘤生长和细胞异质性的原因，在现代分子学中寻求 Gompertzian 生长曲线的病因学；阐述生长动力学在肿瘤医学中的实际应用，认识 Gompertzian 生长曲线对抗肿瘤药物剂量调整的指导意义；进一步探索动力学研究新领域，包括预测预后、治疗选择、治疗靶点以及预防等方面。

细胞增殖动力学

关于肿瘤细胞如何分裂的研究为肿瘤疑惑提供了一些答案，但它自己本身也存在未解之谜。肿瘤由肿瘤细胞和支持它的基质构成，因此首先通过肿瘤细胞增殖动力学讨论肿瘤动力学是合理的。

生长分数评估

有丝分裂或细胞分裂是体细胞数量随时间增加的基本生物学过程。术语"生长"适用于描述一个细胞群体积的增加，以体积（cm^3）或重量（mg）为单位进行测量评估。生长主要是细胞数量增加的结果，但也受个体细胞大小、水肿、细胞外基质变化、出血和宿主细胞（如白细胞）浸润等影响。相反，术语"增殖"仅指细胞数量的增加，以细胞数量作为时间的函数来测量评估。细胞经过一系列步骤进行分裂，这些步骤统称为有丝分裂或"细胞"循环。

对细胞动力学的研究者来说，理解评估细胞周期阶段的方法是非常重要的，因为在所有科学领域，概念与其量化指标密不可分[4]。最简单的方法，可以在显微镜载玻片上计数处于分裂期的细胞。该方法计算出的有丝分裂指数可用于粗略评估

M 期细胞百分比。评估有丝分裂指数还可以通过 stathmokinetic 技术方法来改善，该技术是在特定时间应用药物阻断有丝分裂过程后再进行计数，目前只限于实验。通过免疫组织化学染色检测 Ki-67 蛋白表达也可以评估细胞增殖活性，Ki-67 蛋白存在于所有增殖细胞中而在非增殖细胞中不存在。现在大多使用 Ki-67 染色，但历史上最有效的技术是胸苷标记指数（thymidine labeling index，TLI）。该方法是用带放射性标记的胸苷培养液培养细胞，最常见的胸苷标记是氚，但也可以使用^{14}C。被放射标记的肿瘤细胞百分比即处于 S 期的细胞比例。

除了 stathmokinetic 技术，以上所有方法都是静态分析，体现的是某一个时间点而非动态过程[5]。因此又引申出一个概念，即生长分数，指肿瘤细胞群中处于复制阶段（S+G2 期）的细胞比例。人们曾应用 TLI 评估人白血病的生长分数，现在不再使用。

TLI 的一个应用延伸是计算处于有丝分裂的细胞百分比。该技术根据暴露时间计算被放射性标记的从 S 期进入 M 期的细胞数量。因此，它是唯一实际测量细胞周期时长的技术。数十年前使用该动态放射自显影技术将细胞周期分成四个阶段：G_1 期（DNA 合成前期），合成核糖体和蛋白质，为 DNA 合成的准备阶段；S 期（DNA 合成期），此期主要是合成 DNA；G_2 期（DNA 合成后期），此期细胞 DNA 合成停止，主要是 RNA 和蛋白质的大量合成，为有丝分裂做准备；M 期（有丝分裂期），母细胞分裂成两个子细胞。术语“有丝分裂”通常指 M 期，而形容词“有丝分裂”指细胞参与自我复制的全过程，包括 G_1、S、G_2 和 M 期。而特定观察期内不分裂的细胞，称为 G_0 期细胞。M 期的时间变化最小，在大多数哺乳动物细胞中持续约 1 小时；G_2 期通常为 3 小时。但总细胞周期变异很大，人类肿瘤细胞周期平均为 2~4 天，这种变异大多是由 G_1 期变化导致的。成人有丝分裂周期很长，而果蝇仅需几分钟，哺乳动物胚胎也只需数小时。

在 G_1 期，正常哺乳动物体细胞含有二倍体，因此 DNA 含量也是两倍（2N）。在 S 期，细胞 DNA 含量从 2N 增加到 4N（少数所谓的 S_0 细胞在 S 期可能会停止 DNA 合成，极少数细胞可能停滞在 G_2 期而不进入 M 期）。在细胞大小上 G_0 期细胞往往小于 G_1 期细胞，且 RNA 和蛋白质含量较少。细胞增殖过程中 DNA 含量变化可通过流式细胞术的一系列方法进行分析。荧光激活的细胞分选中，流式细胞仪根据 S 期 DNA 含量、RNA 含量、细胞大小、抗体（例如 Ki-67）标记、溴脱氧尿苷和/或氚标记脱氧胸苷摄取等标记或这些标记的不同组合自动计数。新鲜组织也可以检测，如白血病、胸水或腹水中的肿瘤细胞、酶促分解的实体瘤，或从石蜡包埋标本中收集的细胞。通过检测每个细胞的 DNA 含量，流式细胞仪还可以鉴定 G_0-G_1 峰中异常 DNA 含量，称为非整倍体。存在明显非整倍体的情况下可能无法检测 S 期细胞比例，这是该方法的一个局限。

生长分数、死亡分数、肿瘤大小和治疗反应

采用先前的检测技术，已检测到 2%~20%细胞在肿瘤的任何时间段都处于 S 期。因为 S 期占细胞周期的 1/4 到 1/2，生长分数通常为 4%~80%，平均<20%。对于特定的组织，无论恶性或良性，尽管该组织中处于不同周期的细胞数不断变化，但细胞周期是相当稳定的。通过动物实验，已观察到肿瘤增殖动力学的细微变化。当细胞在体外培养时，细胞可以变大，细胞分裂周期时长也可以发生显著变化。肿瘤生长过程中生长分数变化的重大发现之一是生长分数随着肿瘤增大而降低。这是 Gompertzian 生长的原因还是结果？稍后我们进行讨论。

随着肿块增大，恶性组织较良性组织其生长分数降低的速率更慢。这是在细胞动力学中，恶性和良性组织之间为数不多的差异之一。一些正常组织如骨髓和消化道黏膜，与许多肿瘤相比，具有较高的生长分数和较短的分裂周期，甚至与同部位的肿瘤相比，也是如此。这是细胞动力学研究展现的另一个疑惑。尽管恶性肿瘤的生长分数可能不会高于其起源的正常组织的生长分数，但在特定组织学类型的肿瘤中，高 S 期比例和非整倍体的存在通常与快速生长相关。这种快速生长提示肿瘤更具侵袭性，往往预示着患者的治疗反应较差。这些观察结果进一步放大了前面提到的疑惑，即组织学分级、肿瘤大小和转移之间的相关性。

或许可以从生长分数的伴随概念中找到部分答案，即死亡分数或细胞丢失分数，它是指单位时间内由细胞死亡造成细胞团块丢失的比例。细胞丢失分数很难实际测量，因为凋亡作为细胞死亡的常见途径，可能很少留下解剖学痕迹。通常根据预期生长速率（根据测量的生长分数计算）与实际生长速率比较来推断。细胞丢失分数高的影响是显著的。例如，尽管大量细胞处于有丝分裂期，皮肤基底细胞上皮瘤生长仍然很缓慢。这是因为细胞丢失速率超过细胞增长速率。每次有丝分裂都存在一定的突变频率。与较低细胞丢失率的肿瘤相比，较高细胞丢失率的肿瘤需要进行更多次有丝分裂使其增大。因此，细胞丢失率直接与突变率相关。

实际上，细胞更新速率与肿瘤发生有关。甲状腺刺激激素水平升高易发生甲状腺癌。慢性热损伤伴代偿性增生及继发于太阳损伤的增生可以导致皮肤癌。造血障碍及慢性粒细胞白血病时骨髓的过度增殖很可能与急性白血病的发生发展相关。良性结肠上皮细胞和乳腺上皮细胞过度增殖与肿瘤转化明显相关。化学致癌需要生长促进因子。基于对霍奇金淋巴瘤和胃肠道肿瘤的研究发现，抗肿瘤药物治疗后大量肿瘤细胞死亡，残存肿瘤细胞会发生代偿性地过度增殖，这种增殖更易形成耐药。

但“细胞丢失分数”这个概念本身也存在疑惑。化疗通过破坏肿瘤细胞、诱导凋亡而使肿瘤缩小。已经有大量实验证明有丝分裂细胞，特别是处于 S 期的细胞，非常容易受化疗影响。如果肿瘤生长分数<20%，意味着处于 S 期的细胞比例为 5%~10%，假设自发性细胞丢失分数大于零，化疗是如何进一步增加细胞丢失分数使细胞减少超过 90%？此外，有尝试使用雌二醇促进乳腺癌细胞进入 S 期以增加化疗效果，但并未产生预期的治疗获益。

另一个疑惑是关于化疗对正常宿主组织的影响。化疗对快速增殖的骨髓、消化道黏膜和毛囊等有明显损伤，但这些组织通常可以从化疗的影响中恢复。然而，有些增长速度并不比这些正常组织快的肿瘤，化疗后肿瘤细胞减少且并不能恢复，如急性白血病、恶性淋巴瘤、绒毛膜癌和生殖细胞癌，因此可以通过化疗治愈而不摧毁那些具有强生长动力的正常组织。

这又引出系列问题，为什么肿瘤生长分数随着肿瘤增大而

减小,但比正常组织低?生长和细胞丢失分数与组织学分级、肿瘤大小和转移有何潜在关系?处于有丝分裂期的细胞如此少,化疗又是如何起作用的?即使是恶性度极高的肿瘤,治疗时细胞都处于有丝分裂状态吗?要寻求这些疑惑的答案,我们的重点需从单个细胞动力学扩展到整个细胞群的动力学。

化疗反应的动力学

通过一系列分析研究,我们发现肿瘤生长呈 Gompertzian 曲线或非常接近 Gompertzian 曲线是唯一可信的生长曲线。然而,一些非 Gompertzian 生长曲线理念也是有用的,值得进一步讨论。其中,最主要的是美国南方研究所 Howard Skipper 及其同事的研究[6],他们发现白血病呈指数生长,通过有效治疗后又呈指数下降。这意味着无论治疗时肿瘤多大,杀死的细胞百分比总是相同的。当绘制对数细胞数与时间的函数时发现,似乎治疗引起的细胞对数死亡总是相同的:1 个对数级意味着 90%的细胞被杀死,2 个对数级意味着 99%的细胞被杀死,以此类推。如果特定药物的特定剂量可以将 10^6 个细胞减少至 10^5 个细胞,则相同的处理下,10^4 个细胞可以减少至 10^3 个。

与之相关的第二个重大发现是,很多药物对细胞的对数杀伤随剂量的增加而增加。因此,消除大的肿瘤需要更高的药物剂量。此外,如果使用两种及以上药物时,引起的细胞对数杀伤效应是相乘的,即如果某一剂量的药物 A 可以引起 1 个对数级细胞死亡,某一剂量的药物 B 也可以引起 1 个对数级细胞死亡,则 A 与 B 联合(剂量与单药应用时相同),可以引起 2 个对数级细胞死亡。

第三个发现是诺贝尔奖获得者 Max Delbrück 和 Salvador Luria 关于基因突变对干扰产生耐药的研究[7]。尽管 Delbrück 和 Luria 研究的是细菌对病毒感染的抵抗,但是 Skipper 及其同事基于 Lloyd Law 应用采用 Delbrück-Luria 模型,评估了化疗的耐药性[8]。这种耐药是在没有选择压力的情况下,出现遗传学变异进而影响长期生存,而不是对选择压力的反应。事实上,这个概念类似于达尔文自然选择进化理论,只是应用于细胞层面而非生物体层面。可以用一种新的方法阐述这一概念:假设在一次有丝分裂中细菌或哺乳动物细胞发生特定突变的概率为 x,则不发生突变的概率为 1-x。在 y 次有丝分裂中,不发生突变的概率是 $(1-x)^y$。如果每次有丝分裂产生两个活细胞(没有细胞丢失),则 1 个细胞生长为 N 个细胞需要 N-1 次有丝分裂。因此,在 N 个细胞中不发生任何突变的概率是 exp[(N-1)*ln(1-x)],这是一个非常小的概率。如果在模型中考虑细胞丢失的因素,则需要更多次有丝分裂以至生长到 N 个细胞,那么不发生突变的概率更小。临床上肿瘤发生耐药突变是很常见的,几十年的实验研究也证明了这一点。这也可以解释为什么非整倍体,作为一种常见的遗传学变异,与细胞更新速率密切相关;也可以解释原发肿瘤大小与转移扩散之间的正相关性,因为肿瘤越大,发生突变的概率越高,而突变的细胞更易发生转移扩散。

基于这种进化模型,一些理论家建议,当两种同样有效的化疗方案应用时,如果它们不能以全剂量同时给药,则应该改成严格地交替给药以便在产生耐药突变之前尽快地杀死细胞[9]。另外一些学者则认为基因突变更可能发生在诊断前,因此尽可能杀死在诊断时已存在的各个细胞亚群更为重要[10-12]。前一种观点认为在肿瘤治疗中应尽早开始辅助治疗以提高疗效,但许多试验并未发现原发性乳腺癌术前化疗的优势,这与后一种观点更为一致。事实上,虽然这两种观点都有理论依据,但实验证据,包括大型的前瞻性临床试验更支持第二种观点。后一种观点也可以解释以下现象:一些肿瘤特别是恶性淋巴瘤、急性白血病和乳腺癌,首次化疗未达到治愈,之后再应用同一化疗时细胞仍具有敏感性[13]。因此,所有化疗失败不能归因于永久耐药性的产生,而是由于未清除细胞的持续存在。一些残存的细胞可能导致肿瘤复发,这些细胞只是相对(而非绝对)对所用的药物不敏感,只是未与足量药物或足够时间接触以致于未被清除[14]。这类似于抗生素剂量不足导致细菌感染复发,即使如此,这些细菌在体外对药物还是敏感的。然而,无论是感染还是肿瘤,长期或反复低剂量治疗可通过耐药细胞的选择而产生绝对耐药。

是否可以通过调整剂量或给药时间克服这种问题?如前所述,严格的药物交叉或联合应用并未证明是有效的。中等程度的剂量增加可以提高疗效,包括原发性和转移性乳腺癌、儿童急性淋巴细胞白血病和成人生殖细胞肿瘤。然而,也没有证据证明剂量与疗效之间有严格的相关性。例如,环磷酰胺剂量超过 600mg/m^2、阿霉素剂量超过 60mg/m^2 并不会改善乳腺癌辅助化疗的疗效。需要进行自体移植的患者,移植前的大剂量化疗也未证明是一种有利的策略。

然而,调整给药时间是可行的,一定程度上可以提高疗效。Skipper 及其同事根据呈指数生长的小鼠白血病模型提出"对数杀伤"理论,后来转化成 Gompertzian 生长曲线[15]。图 53-2 和图 53-3 是 Gompertzian 生长曲线的计算机模拟。图 53-2a 显示的是对化疗敏感的肿瘤:箭头表示给药时间,在前三个治疗周期,由于化疗诱导的对数杀伤,每次给药后肿瘤体积缩小,下一次给药前体积又增大。第四周期后停止给药,最终达到 10^{10} 个肿瘤细胞(虚线所示)并继续生长,这个细胞数量已经达到临床可评估的数量。图 53-2b 显示了相同的四周期化疗,但给药时间间隔缩短(剂量密集化疗)的情况下,肿瘤生长的变化。由于化疗周期间隔缩短,肿瘤细胞没有足够的时间再生,每次给药后肿瘤细胞数越来越少。在 Gompertzian 生长曲线中,细胞杀伤速率与生长速率成正比,因为处于 S 期的细胞更易被杀伤。肿瘤体积越小,生长指数越高,被杀伤的细胞指数也越高。在图 53-2b 中第四周期化疗结束后,尽管肿瘤生长不再受治疗影响,但达到 10^{10} 个肿瘤细胞所需时间更长(以较小体积开始再生),转化到临床上就是改善患者预后。事实上,原发性乳腺癌、恶性淋巴瘤、儿童尤文氏肉瘤的前瞻性随机临床试验已证实,剂量密集化疗可以改善总生存[16-19]。目前治疗淋巴瘤的 14 天 CHOP 方案化疗已被广泛使用(使用粒细胞集落刺激因子支持),旧标准是 21 天方案化疗[18]。

图 53-3 显示的是在初始治疗前就存在化疗耐药的肿瘤 Gompertzian 生长曲线。图中用两条生长曲线说明,一条黑色和一条红色,黑色表示对治疗敏感的细胞(黑色箭头所示),红色表示对治疗不敏感的细胞(红色箭头所示),但是总肿瘤体积是两者之和。采用平行的方式,红色箭头所指的"红色"细胞对治疗敏感,黑色箭头所指的"黑色"细胞对治疗不敏感。图 53-3a 中"黑色"治疗和"红色"治疗交叉给药,图 53-3b 中序贯给药。

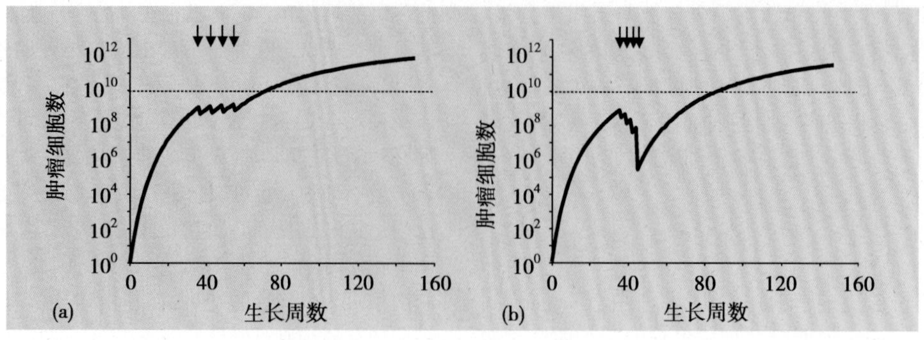

图 53-2 (a,b)剂量强度对肿瘤生长的影响

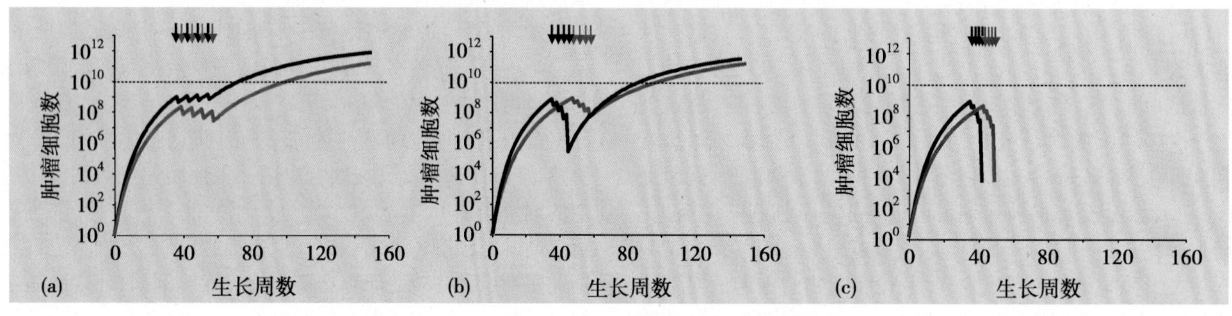

图 53-3 (a~c)序贯剂量强度对肿瘤生长的影响

显然,序贯给药对"黑色"细胞的杀伤作用更强,但对"红色"细胞的作用相差不大,细胞杀伤越多,增加到 10^{10} 个细胞所需的时间越长,患者预后越好。图 53-2b 显示的细胞杀伤作用更强是因为"黑色"治疗更密集(时间间隔短)。在乳腺癌的辅助化疗中,阿霉素初次使用就是这样序贯进行的,现已成为标准治疗[20]。意大利米兰国家癌症研究所进行的一项前瞻性随机辅助化疗试验证实了这一方案的有效性[21]。阿霉素 4 周期,随后三药 CMF 联合(环磷酰胺、甲氨蝶呤和 5-氟尿嘧啶)8 周期的序贯给药方式与交叉给药相比,在无病生存和总生存方面都有优势。同样,乳腺国际组织(02-98 研究)已经公布,紫杉醇仅在序贯给药时才会增加阿霉素的疗效,而不是在减低剂量的情况下同时使用[22](两组 CMF 疗程均相同,因此不会影响序贯治疗优于联合治疗的结论)。

图 53-3c 通过缩短"黑色"和"红色"治疗间隔进一步验证了序贯治疗的有效性。由于化疗引起的对数杀伤很强,可以排除肿瘤细胞再生长。北美乳腺组织 CALGB9741 大规模随机临床试验验证了剂量密集方案的有效性。在 G-CSF 支持下应用阿霉素加环磷酰胺 4 周期,每周期 14 天,然后序贯 4 周期紫杉醇,每周期 14 天。与每周期 21 天化疗方案相比,剂量密集方案不仅改善了患者无病生存和总生存,而且由于粒细胞保留(使用 G-CSF)和其他可能因素而毒性较低[16]。最近,对 10 项随机对照试验的系统评价和荟萃分析显示,剂量密集方案可提高患者总生存和无病生存,特别是在激素受体阴性的乳腺癌中[17]。在其中 3 项试验(共 3 337 例患者)中,剂量密集方案与标准化疗方案相比(化疗药物相同),可提高总生存[死亡风险比(hazard ratio,HR)= 0.84,95%置信区间(confidence interval,CI)= 0.72~0.98,P = 0.03]以及无病生存(复发或死亡 HR = 0.83,95%CI = 0.73~0.94,P = 0.005)。在其他 7 项试验中(共 8 652 例患者),剂量密集方案与标准化疗方案相比(化疗药物及剂量不同),仍可提高总生存及无病生存(死亡 HR = 0.85,95%CI = 0.75~0.96,P = 0.01;复发或死亡 HR = 0.81,95%CI = 0.73~0.88,P<0.001)[17]。图 53-4 比较了接受剂量密集方案与常规化疗方案患者的风险比[17]。

图 53-3b 体现的治疗曲线与现在化疗和生物制剂联合治疗的理念相关。长期、持续用药可以抑制肿瘤生长,但不适合图 53-5 所模拟的化疗杀死肿瘤细胞的能力。图 53-5a 中,化疗结束后开始接受生长抑制剂治疗(斜线阴影框所示);图 53-5b 中,同时给予"红色"治疗与生长抑制剂治疗。显然,图 53-5b 中达到 10^{10} 个细胞所需时间更长。原因是,"黑色"细胞在早期被抑制(对"红色"治疗不敏感);而"红色"细胞被"红色"治疗抑制的同时还被生长抑制剂抑制,因此每个治疗周期之间存活的细胞非常少,意味着对数杀伤也越强(如图 53-3c 所示)。这或许可以解释 HER2 抑制剂曲妥珠单抗在 HER2 过表达的原发性乳腺癌中的治疗作用。NCCTGN9831 试验中,患者先接受阿霉素联合环磷酰胺化疗 4 周期,然后每周使用紫杉醇;在紫杉醇治疗期间,同时或序贯使用曲妥珠单抗(曲妥珠单抗连续使用 1 年),结果表明同时接受紫杉醇和曲妥珠单抗治疗的患者乳腺癌复发的概率更小[23]。美国 Memorial Sloan-Kettering 癌症中心的研究人员完成了一项Ⅱ期研究,证明了剂量密集化疗以及同时用药具有良好的有效性,进一步验证了上述研究结果。

然而,生长抑制剂也不是必须总与化疗同时使用。图 53-6 显示了生长抑制剂对化疗的影响(斜线阴影框所示)。在图 53-6a 中,化疗结束后再给予生长抑制剂(不抑制化疗),对细胞生长的影响与图 53-5a 相同。然而在图 53-6b 中,生长抑制剂对"红色"细胞生长影响较为复杂。因为生长抑制剂比图 53-5a 中更早使用,对细胞生长抑制作用更大;但同时生长抑制剂减弱了化疗的作用(红色箭头所示),这又有利于细胞生长。通过计算生长到 10^{10} 个细胞所需的时间得出,该曲线下其净效应是中性的。如果生长抑制剂对细胞的杀伤作用更强或对化疗药物的影响更弱一点,那么其净效应是对患者有益的。但是,如

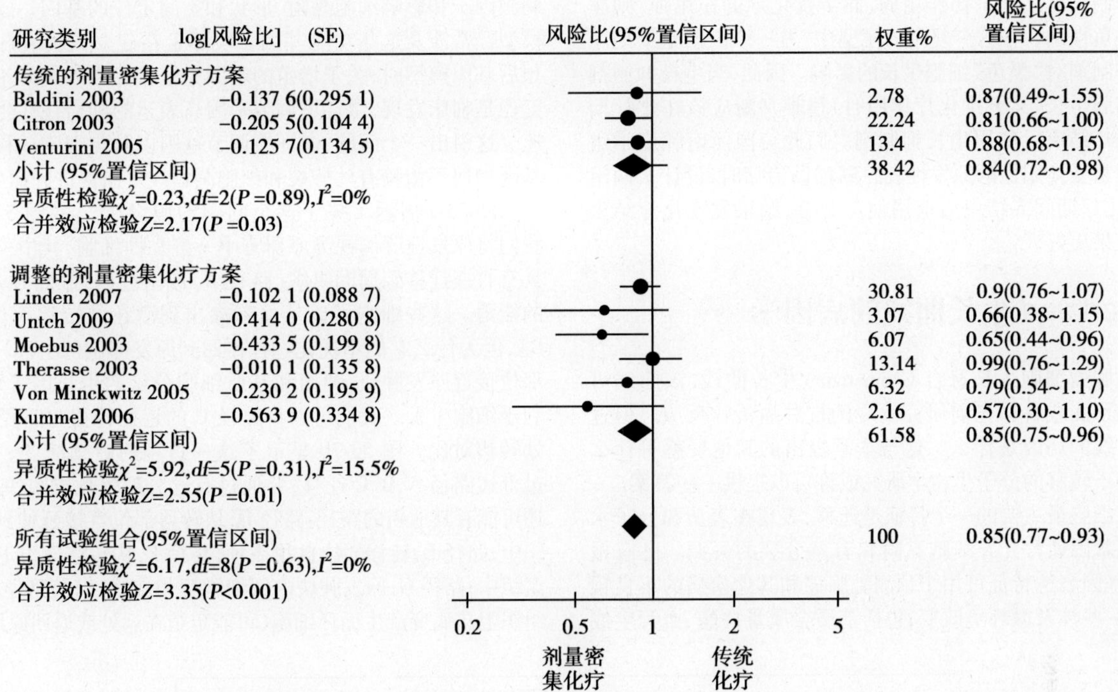

图 53-4 比较接受剂量密集化疗与常规化疗患者总生存的风险比森林图。来源:Bonilla et al. 2010[17]

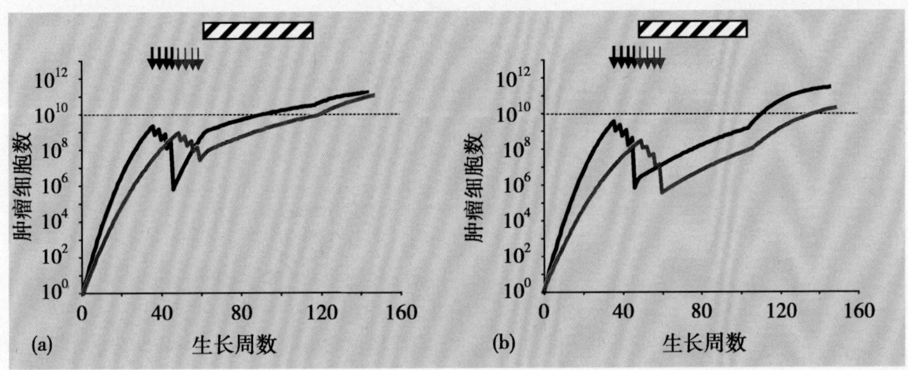

图 53-5 (a,b)生长抑制剂对肿瘤生长的影响(不抑制化疗)

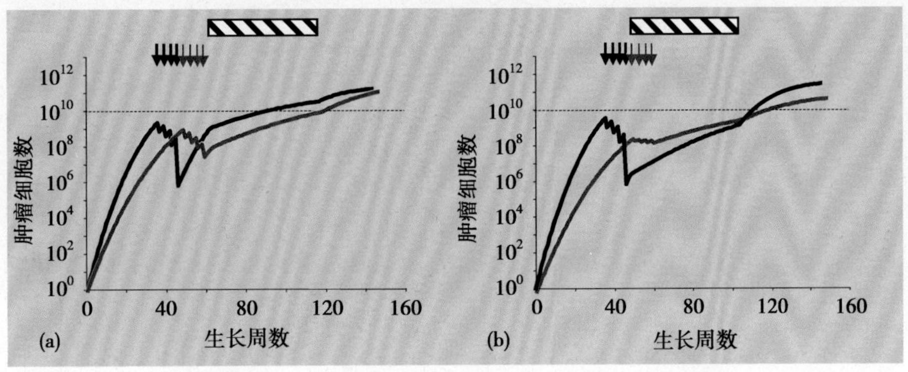

图 53-6 (a,b)生长抑制剂对肿瘤生长的影响(抑制化疗)

果生长抑制剂对细胞杀伤作用弱，而干扰化疗的作用强，则净效应将是负性的。在这个复杂的模型中，另一个因素是早期应用生长抑制剂对“黑色”细胞生长的影响。因此，当生长抑制剂既抑制细胞生长，又干扰化疗作用时，很难判断应该在化疗期间还是化疗结束后使用生长抑制剂。因此美国西南肿瘤学组在研究激素受体阳性的原发性乳腺癌辅助治疗时，设计了两组试验，即化疗期间或结束后应用他莫昔芬，结果发现化疗结束后给药效果更好[24]。

Gompertzian 生长曲线的病因学

恶性肿瘤细胞生长符合 Gompertzian 生长曲线，该曲线可以很好地预测或解释先前研究发现的抗肿瘤治疗反应。但这种生长曲线的病因是什么？这与本章提出的其他疑惑有什么关系？关于转移的分子生物学研究或许可以提供一些答案。

肿瘤细胞最主要的一个特征是迁移，表现在表型和分子水平上。癌基因通常介导细胞黏附和有丝分裂的失调。已有报道，多个基因表达特征可用于预测乳腺癌和其他疾病的不良预后，其中一些涉及微环境改变，包括基质金属蛋白酶、血管生成刺激因子和影响细胞黏附、形状和空间定位的基因。迁移实验模型经常涉及这些功能基因。实际上在建立人类乳腺癌不良预后基因模型时，关于增殖的基因完全排除在外。无论实验研究还是临床发现，微环境调节基因高表达的肿瘤往往生长更迅速。这引出一个问题：微环境调节基因以及与细胞迁移相关的基因如何不依赖有丝分裂和细胞凋亡改变而促进肿瘤生长？

图 53-7 展示了关于这个问题的假设[25]。在图 53-7a 中，我们将原发性肿瘤视为原器官中一群黏性细胞，其中一些细胞具有直接迁移到周围组织（路径 A）或附近血管（路径 B 和 C）的能力。这些细胞可以从血管渗出到潜在的转移部位（路径 B），但为什么它们不优先选择再回到原发部位（路径 C）？这些部位接近原发肿块，肿瘤和基质细胞分泌的生长因子更多，更利于细胞生长。我们可以将路径 C 的近处转移与路径 B 的远处转移对比。图 53-7b 显示了这一过程的后续演变。细胞通过上述路径 A、B、C 迁移，并通过有丝分裂生长成团块。此外，还可能有其他新的路径：路径 D，从转移部位直接延伸到周围组织中；路径 E，转移部位自我播种；路径 F，从转移部位返回到原组织中；路径 G，原发肿块内部细胞互相交换；以及路径 H，原发组织卫星病变产生循环细胞（可能定植在远处或返回原组织）。

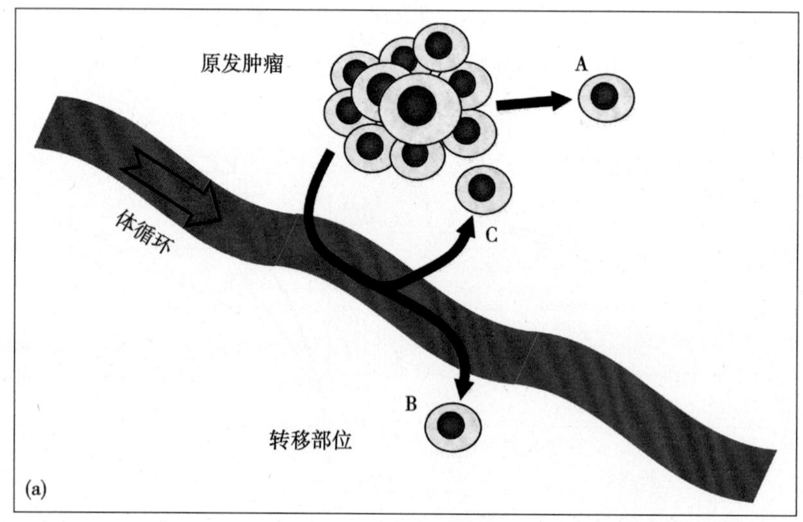

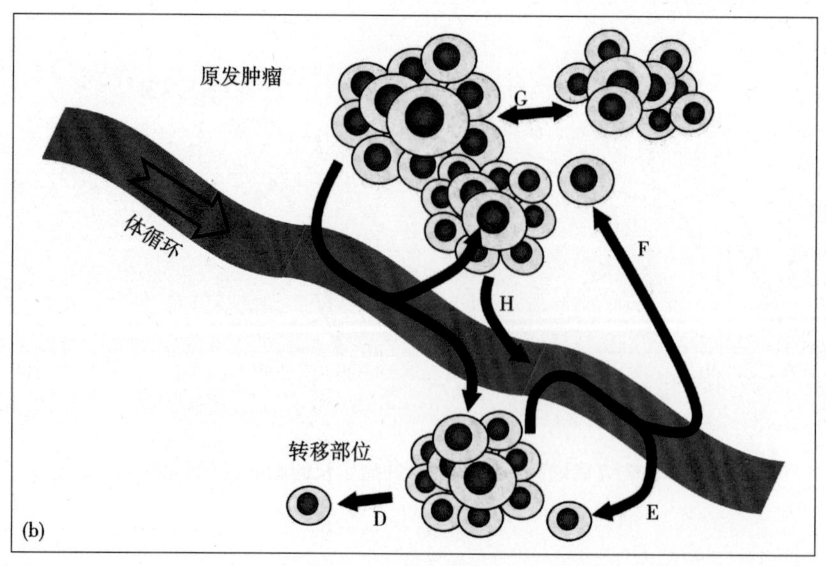

图 53-7 （a）早期迁移曲线和（b）晚期转移曲线

尽管这些路径还有待进一步证实，但它们对肿瘤生长动力学的影响是显然的。图 53-7b 中，肿块不是一个个离散的、有组织的实体，而是多个小团块的组合或聚集。每个团块都是独立的，可能通过吸引髓源性内皮细胞前体及富含细胞因子的白细胞诱导自身的血液供应。这不仅可以解释为什么肿瘤血管丰富，还可以解释恶性间变时组织结构的显著异型性。此外，由于每个团块很小，细胞生长速率相对较快，尽管肿瘤生长分数与原组织相比并不特别大，肿瘤依旧可以迅速增大。

原肿瘤器官中存在自我播种的细胞群（图 53-7a 路径 C），这些细胞可以重新进入血液循环（图 53-7b 路径 H），这可以解释为什么原发病灶清除后仍需要放射治疗残存的“正常”组织。原发病灶内部（路径 G）细胞互相交换可以解释肿瘤起始细胞或干细胞在整个肿块中播散，使得检测基因表达谱时临床取样变得切实可行。

原发肿块从外向内生长（自我播种）以及从内向外生长（有丝分裂）为 Gompertzian 生长曲线提供了一些诠释。举一个最简单的例子，一个球体，表面积与直径的平方成正比，体积与直径的立方成正比；随着质量变大，相对应的直径（d）变大，表面积与体积的比率下降，与 1/d 成正比。由于从外向内生长发生在表面，生长分数可能降至 1/d 的倍数。也就是说，随着质量增加，相对生长速率下降，这正是 Gompertzian 生长曲线体现的。由于肿块不是完美的球体，所以表面积不是与直径的平方成正比，而是介于直径的平方和立方之间。细胞生长的过程越具侵袭性，肿块的表面越不规则，越接近直径的立方。例如，如果自我播种非常明显，表面积可能与 $d^{2.9}$ 成正比，生长分数将降至 $d^{2.9}/d^3$ 的倍数，与 1/d 相比这是非常缓慢的。这可以解释前面提到的疑惑，正常组织表面积与 d^2 成比例，因此随着体积增加肿瘤组织生长分数下降更缓慢。

这个曲线可以解释间变、生长速率、肿瘤大小和转移之间潜在的关系。那些涉及细胞血管渗出形成自我播种的功能基因，也会参与远处转移过程。因此，区域淋巴结容易受累的肿瘤更可能发生远处转移，因为这两种过程涉及的基因调控是相似的，尽管不是完全相同，这也是造成差异的原因。实际上，癌变前的基因谱与侵袭性肿瘤相比可能仅有略微不同，这可以解释虽然是两种类型病变，但涉及的基因异常却类似。例如，乳腺原位导管细胞癌可能自我播种的能力并不高，如缺乏进入或离开血液循环的能力；不能适时改变种植部位微环境；或者不能吸引髓源性基质细胞。这种推理也可以解释肿瘤与正常组织细胞增殖周期是相似的。在原发部位形成团块的那些细胞可能是非常正常的，除非由于异常播种重新定居。从这方面讲，原发性乳腺癌可以看作是数十到数千个胚胎乳房细胞的集合，而其中每个细胞都接近正常。

播种细胞的生长很大程度上依赖于基质，特别是骨髓来源的细胞，这些细胞有助于血管生成和基质形成。当它们受到攻击时，也会影响肿瘤。这就是为什么当只有 5% 或更少细胞处于 S 期时，由于化疗对骨髓的显著影响，化疗仍可以有效地对抗肿瘤。自我播种模型与肿瘤休眠有何相关性，以及手术切除对这种休眠的影响是值得大家进一步关注的话题[26]。

肿瘤自我播种与肿瘤微环境之间的相互关系

如前所述，自我播种模型不仅依赖于肿瘤细胞固有的迁移性，还依赖于非肿瘤细胞，它可以支持循环肿瘤细胞迁移到远处并在远处存活。最终，肿瘤微环境或“土壤”也影响肿瘤细胞生长和增殖能力。肿瘤微环境是基质细胞、细胞外基质、血管系统和其他支持细胞的复杂组合。每一个因素都可能影响肿瘤的生长和迁移。对这些非肿瘤细胞尤其免疫系统的认识，引起越来越多的人对癌症免疫疗法的兴趣。自 19 世纪末 Rudolf Virchow 首次认识到肿瘤内存在白细胞以来，免疫疗法仍具有很多挑战。最近，越来越多证据表明，实体瘤和免疫调节细胞之间存在着一种重要的相互作用。实验模型表明固有免疫系统对原发性肿瘤的生长和转移至关重要，协同抑制或促进肿瘤生长、侵袭和转移[27]。的确，肿瘤浸润淋巴细胞、肿瘤周围淋巴结及相关分子特征可能与预后有关。最近 3 项研究发现，肿瘤浸润淋巴细胞与乳腺癌预后存在潜在相关[28-30]。此外肿瘤浸润基质细胞和免疫细胞的功能可能与其在血液循环或非肿瘤组织中的功能截然不同[31,32]。例如，新诊断的乳腺癌患者骨髓中发现散在肿瘤细胞预示患者总体预后不良，但并非所有骨髓中发现肿瘤细胞的患者都会发展成多发性骨转移[33]。最近，两项独立研究表明白细胞在介导肿瘤生长和转移过程中可能发挥新的作用。这些研究表明改善肿瘤患者的预后，不仅需要治疗肿瘤细胞，还需要治疗基质内和血液循环中关键的免疫调节因子。

第一，随着肿瘤浸润白细胞影响肿瘤生物学行为的证据越来越多，在乳腺癌中人们开始应用基因组学分析技术识别肿瘤浸润白细胞中的突变，而该技术通常用于识别肿瘤细胞内的突变。人们将肿瘤浸润白细胞中发生的突变与循环白细胞、上皮细胞（口腔拭子）以及乳腺癌细胞本身发生的突变进行比较。共检测了 20 例乳腺癌样本的肿瘤浸润白细胞及 20 例相匹配的外周血/口腔拭子白细胞，其中 8 例鉴定出的基因突变只发生在肿瘤浸润白细胞中，而肿瘤细胞本身或外周血/口腔拭子样本中均未发现这些突变。重要的是，肿瘤浸润白细胞发生的突变包含在白血病基因中，包括 *BCOR*、*TET2* 和 *EZH2*[34]。这是首次发现体细胞致癌突变仅发生在肿瘤浸润白细胞，而不是上皮细胞或外周循环血中。值得注意的是，这些肿瘤浸润白细胞在形态学上完全“正常”。目前正在研究这些突变的肿瘤浸润白细胞在肿瘤发生、发展中的作用。

第二，中性粒细胞，通常与抗感染有关，似乎对癌症有极化作用。具体来说，中性粒细胞可根据细胞因子的相对浓度以促肿瘤形成[35]或抗转移[36]方式发挥作用。例如，在小鼠乳腺癌模型中已证明中性粒细胞可被原发肿瘤激活，而这些激活的中性粒细胞可抑制肿瘤细胞转移到肺部[36]。在转移部位，不同细胞因子水平似乎介导中性粒细胞不同功能，进而抑制或促进生长。在这方面，肿瘤微环境似乎可以适时地调节免疫功能。在新诊断的无转移的乳腺癌患者中，进一步研究中性粒细胞功能。入组患者在进行肿块或乳房切除术时提取外周血中性粒细胞。将这些中性粒细胞与健康受试者中性粒细胞比较。体外实验表明，乳腺癌患者的中性粒细胞对某些乳腺癌细胞系有细胞毒性作用，而健康受试者没有[36]。说明原发性乳腺癌患者激活的中性粒细胞能够杀死癌细胞，而健康受试者的中性粒细胞没有这种能力。目前正在进行研究以评估刺激乳腺癌患者中性粒细胞是否可以改善预后。越来越多研究指出肿瘤细胞和造血细胞（微环境和外周血）之间的相互作用对肿瘤发病机制和治疗反应有影响。模拟肿瘤生长曲线无疑需要将肿瘤微环境的作用纳入其中。

结论

在这一章中，我们回顾了细胞和细胞群生长动力学，为改进肿瘤化疗方案提供了一定的理论基础。此外，我们从动力学角度研究、解释了各种临床和实验现象，从宏观上认识肿瘤分子学与恶性行为之间的联系。最后，肿瘤生长动力学与肿瘤微环境也密切相关，这种微环境作用既可以在原发肿瘤部位，也可以在转移部位。随之新兴的免疫肿瘤学，虽然仍有许多挑战，但为肿瘤患者治疗带来新的希望。

（王先火　张婷婷　译，张会来　审校）

参考文献

1 van't Veer LJ, Paik S, Hayes DF. Gene expression profiling of breast cancer: a new tumor marker. *J Clin Oncol*. 2005;**8**:1631–1635.

2 Norton LA. Gompertzian model of human breast cancer growth. *Cancer Res*. 1988;**48**:7067.

3 Laird AK. Dynamics of growth in tumors and normal organisms. *Monogr Natl Cancer Inst*. 1969;**30**:15.

4 Steel GG. Autoradiographic analysis of the cell cycle. Howard and Pelc to the present day. *Int J Radiat Biol*. 1986;**49**:227.

5 Frei E III, Whang J, Scoggins RB, et al. The stathmokinetic effect of vincristine. *Cancer Res*. 1964:18–25.

6 Skipper HE, Schabel FM Jr, Wilcox WS. Experimental evaluation of potential anticancer agents XIII. On the criteria and kinetics associated with "curability" of experimental leukemia. *Cancer Chemother Rep*. 1964;**35**:1.

7 Luria SE, Delbruck M. Mutations of bacteria from virus sensitivity to virus resistance. *Genetics*. 1943;**28**:491.

8 Law LW. Origin of resistance of leukaemic cells to folic acid antagonists. *Nature*. 1952;**169**:628.

9 Goldie JH, Coldman AJ. A mathematic model for relating the drug sensitivity of tumors to their spontaneous mutation rate. *Cancer Treat Rep*. 1979;**63**:1727.

10 Shapiro DM, Fugmann RA. A role for chemotherapy as an adjunct to surgery. *Cancer Res*. 1957;**17**:1098.

11 Schabel FM. Concepts for the systemic treatment of micrometastases. *Cancer*. 1975;**35**:15.

12 Norton L. Implications of kinetic heterogeneity in clinical oncology. *Semin Oncol*. 1985;**12**:231.

13 DeVita VT. The relationship between tumor mass and resistance to treatment of cancer. *Cancer*. 1983;**51**:1209.

14 Holland JF. Clinical studies of unmaintained remissions in acute lymphocytic leukemia. In: *The Proliferation and Spread of Neoplastic Cells. 21st Annual Symposium on Fundamental Cancer Research* 1967. Baltimore, MD: Williams & Wilkins; **1968**:453–462.

15 Norton L, Simon R. Tumor size, sensitivity to therapy, and the design of treatment schedules. *Cancer Treat Rep*. 1977;**61**:1307.

16 Citron ML, Berry DA, Cirrincione C, et al. Randomized trial of dose-dense versus conventionally scheduled and sequential versus concurrent combination chemotherapy as postoperative adjuvant treatment of node-positive primary breast cancer: first report of Intergroup Trial C9741/Cancer and Leukemia Group B Trial 9741. *J Clin Oncol*. 2003;**21**:1431–1439.

17 Bonilla L, Ben-Aharon I, Vidal L, Gafter-Gvili A, Leibovici L, Stemmer SM. Dose-dense chemotherapy in nonmetastatic breast cancer: a systematic review and meta-analysis of randomized controlled trials. *J Natl Cancer Inst*. 2010;**102(24)**:1845–1854.

18 Held G, Schubert J, Reiser M, et al. Dose-intensified treatment of advanced-stage diffuse large B-cell lymphomas. *Semin Hematol*. 2006;**43(4)**:221–229.

19 Womer RB, West DC, Krailo MD, et al. Randomized comparison of every-two-week vs every-three-week chemotherapy in Ewing sarcoma family tumors. *J Clin Oncol*. 2008;**26(Suppl. 15)**:10504.

20 Perloff M, Norton L, Korzun AH, et al. Postsurgical adjuvant chemotherapy of stage II breast carcinoma with or without crossover to a non-cross-resistant regimen: a Cancer and Leukemia Group B study. *J Clin Oncol*. 1996;**14(5)**:1589–1598.

21 Bonadonna G, Zambetti M, Moliterni A, et al. Clinical relevance of different sequencing of doxorubicin and cyclophosphamide, methotrexate, and Fluorouracil in operable breast cancer. *J Clin Oncol*. 2004;**22(9)**:1614–1620.

22 Francis P, Crown J, Di Leo A, et al. Adjuvant chemotherapy with sequential or concurrent anthracycline and docetaxel: Breast International Group 02–98 randomized trial. *J Natl Cancer Inst*. 2008;**100(2)**:121–133.

23 Baselga J, Perez EA, Pienkowski T, Bell R. Adjuvant trastuzumab: a milestone in the treatment of HER2-positive early breast cancer. *Oncologist*. 2006;**11(Suppl. 1)**:4–12.

24 Albain KS, Green SJ, Ravdin PM, et al. Adjuvant chemohormonal therapy for primary breast cancer should be sequential instead of concurrent: initial results from Intergroup trial 0100 (SWOG-8814). *Proc Am Soc Clin Oncol*. 2002;**21**; abstr 143.

25 Norton L, Massagué J. Is cancer a disease of self-seeding? *Nat Med*. 2006;**12**:875–878.

26 Demicheli R, Miceli R, Moliterni A, et al. Breast cancer recurrence dynamics following adjuvant CMF is consistent with tumor dormancy and mastectomy-driven acceleration of the metastatic process. *Ann Oncol*. 2005;**16(9)**:1449–1457.

27 Grivennikov SI, Greten FR, Karin M. Immunity, inflammation, and cancer. *Cell*. 2010;**140(6)**:883–99.

28 Mohammed ZM, et al. The relationship between lymphocyte subsets and clinico-pathological determinants of survival in patients with primary operable invasive ductal breast cancer. *Br J Cancer*. 2013;**109(6)**:1676–84.

29 Loi S, et al. Prognostic and predictive value of tumor-infiltrating lymphocytes in a phase III randomized adjuvant breast cancer trial in node-positive breast cancer comparing the addition of docetaxel to doxorubicin with doxorubicin-based chemotherapy: BIG 02–98. *J Clin Oncol*. 2013;**31(7)**:860–7.

30 Adams S, et al. Prognostic value of tumor-infiltrating lymphocytes in triple-negative breast cancers from two phase III randomized adjuvant breast cancer trials: ECOG 2197 and ECOG 1199. *J Clin Oncol*. 2014;**32(27)**:2959–2966.

31 Orimo A, Weinberg RA. Stromal fibroblasts in cancer: a novel tumor-promoting cell type. *Cell Cycle*. 2006;**5(15)**:1597–601.

32 Li HJ, et al. Cancer-stimulated mesenchymal stem cells create a carcinoma stem cell niche via prostaglandin E2 signaling. *Cancer Discov*. 2012;**2(9)**:840–855.

33 Braun S, Vogl FD, Naume B, et al. A pooled analysis of bone marrow micrometastasis in breast cancer. *N Engl J Med*. 2005;**353(8)**:793–802.

34 Comen E, Kleppe M, Wen H, et al. Somatic leukemogenic mutations associated with infiltrating white blood cells in breast cancer patients. San Antonio Breast Cancer Symposium. PD1-4; 2014.

35 Fridlender ZG, Sun J, Kim S, et al. Polarization of tumor-associated neutrophil phenotype by TGF-beta: "N1" versus "N2" TAN. *Cancer Cell*. 2009;**16(3)**:183–194.

36 Granot Z, Henke E, Comen EA, et al. Tumor entrained neutrophils inhibit seeding in the premetastatic lung. *Cancer Cell*. 2011;**20(3)**:300–314.

第 54 章　用药剂量、时序及联合治疗的原则

William N. Hait, MD, PhD ■ Joseph P. Eder, MD

概述

抗肿瘤药物的研发是非常复杂的，并且成功率很低。进入临床试验的新药大约只有 10%的机会被监管部门批准并最终可供患者使用。监管部门将根据药物的安全性和有效性决定是否批准进入临床，而合适的药物剂量和用药时序则是药物安全性和有效性的重要决定因素。对于研发领域的研究人员而言，了解如何最佳评估目前可用的或正在研发中的多种治疗药物的合适剂量和用药时序是一项关键技能。在激素类和小分子药物的平台上，随着单克隆抗体、可替代蛋白支架以及肿瘤疫苗的加入，这个专业领域变得更为复杂。在本章中，我们以细胞毒药物为例，阐述了制定合适用药剂量和用药时序的基本原则；此外，讨论了许多能影响量效关系的变量，包括肿瘤的特征、肿瘤微环境、宿主特点如药物代谢酶和药物清除机制；最后对选择合适剂量和时序而成功的抗肿瘤药物临床试验设计进行了总结。

背景

确证新型的具有临床活性的药物在肿瘤化疗的发展过程中至关重要。表 54-1 列举了一些新药和正在探索的细胞通路和靶点的新型靶向药。对于经典的细胞毒性化疗药物，剂量是决定其抗肿瘤活性及毒副反应的一个重要因素[1]。这些药物可直接或间接地损伤 DNA 或抑制细胞分裂，但是药靶相互作用与细胞的致死率之间的定量关系并不明确。高剂量化疗（基础剂量的 4~10 倍）序贯造血干细胞移植，已证实可治愈特定的血液肿瘤。不论对于任何药物或任何治疗目的，FDA 非常明确地指出药物的剂量-反应关系是中心。“暴露-反应信息是确定药物安全性和有效性的核心。也就是说，只有了解了疗效和不良反应的确定暴露剂量时，才能确定该药物是安全有效的[2]。”

生物治疗制剂（如干扰素、白细胞介素、单克隆抗体、激素）和酪氨酸激酶抑制剂的剂量对其疗效的影响很复杂；对于这些药物的剂量-反应效应，还没有统一的明确的证据。而目前靶

表 54-1　肿瘤治疗的分子靶点

靶点分类	举例
细胞周期	细胞周期蛋白依赖性激酶，细胞周期蛋白，细胞周期蛋白依赖性激酶抑制剂和有丝分裂小管相关蛋白
细胞分化	维 A 酸和维生素 D 核内类固醇受体
细胞凋亡	*BCL2*，*NF-kB*，*TP53*，*TNFSF10* 和 *FAS*
血管生成	*KDR*，内皮整合素和 *PDGFRB*
细胞表面信号受体	胰岛素样生长因子受体（*IGF*），*ERBB* 受体家族和 *KIT*
肿瘤转移	基质金属蛋白酶和趋化因子受体
细胞内信号元件	*BCR-ABL1*，*ras*，*raf*，*MADD*，PI3 激酶，mTOR，*src*，蛋白激酶 C，局部黏着斑激酶（*PTK2*：蛋白酪氨酸激酶 2），间变性淋巴瘤激酶（*ALK*），*STAT* 家族蛋白，以及蛋白激酶中的 *MAP* 家族
核转录因子	例如，4 号类固醇激素
潜在靶点	端粒酶
	DNA 甲基化［人类 DNA 甲基转移酶（MeTase）］，蛋白酶体 20S，法尼基转移酶，组蛋白去乙酰化酶和 hsp90（伴侣蛋白）
细胞表面抗原	例如，CD20

向药物的疗效与药靶相互作用的程度有更为明确的关系，例如单克隆抗体的受体占有率（receptor occupancy，RO）或激酶抑制剂的磷酸化抑制程度（机制方面的证据）及可测量的药效学效应（原理方面的证据）。在进行靶标筛选的患者中，靶点磷酸化抑制比单纯的药物剂量强度与临床疗效的关系更为密切（概念方面的证据）。这在临床药物中已经在替代使用中。

除药物剂量以外，用药时序对于治疗指数也很重要。与用药时序相关的细胞动力学研究促进了诸如阿糖胞苷（cytarabine，ara-C）等药物在白血病基础研究及临床应用中的进展（参

见标题为“骨髓细胞动力学”部分)[3,4]。大部分分子靶向药物,无论是小分子抑制剂还是单克隆抗体,在临床上均进行持续给药,这将会显著改变其临床毒性特征。

联合化疗在血液系统恶性肿瘤、小儿实体瘤、睾丸癌、卵巢癌的治愈性治疗以及乳腺癌、肺癌、肠癌和骨肉瘤的辅助治疗中至关重要[5,6]。在下面各小节中都会讨论联合化疗的基本原理,其主要包括:①经验:几乎所有在临床上已证实有治愈效果的治疗都涉及联合用药(表54-2);②遗传不稳定会导致肿瘤细胞异质性,最终表现为肿瘤治疗中的耐药[6-8];③靶向特定的肿瘤驱动突变的信号转导抑制剂,除了在一些慢性粒细胞白血病(chronic myelogenous leukemia,CML)患者中使用的伊马替尼外[9],总是会诱导耐药,可以通过联合第二种药物(如在黑色素瘤中使用达拉非尼和曲美替尼)[10]或使用具有更广谱靶标尤其针对耐药突变的第二代药物(如在*EML4/ALK*突变的NSCLC中使用色瑞替尼)[11,12]进行耐药逆转。尽管研究人员通常对药物剂量的选择和联合化疗方案的选择进行单独考虑,但这二者之间具有重要且复杂的关系[13,14]。近年来,在研发中的用于肿瘤治疗的分子靶标的数量显著增加(见表54-1)。临床研究的主要挑战不仅是要最大限度地提高单药的有效性,还需要将药物整合到最佳的联合治疗策略中。

表54-2 治疗儿童急性淋巴细胞白血病(ALL)的药物数量及治愈方案

	化疗药物的数量							
	1	2	3	4	5	6	7	8
年份	1948	1954	1956	1960	1965	1974	1985	1988
药物	甲氨蝶呤	MP	泼尼松	长春新碱	甲氨蝶呤[a]	阿霉素	天冬酰胺	ara-C
CR/%	20~40	40~92	80~95	>95	>95	>95	>95	>95
治愈/%	0	0	0	15	5~35	55	75	80

[a] 鞘内甲氨蝶呤。

CR,完全缓解;MP,6-巯基嘌呤;ara-C,阿糖胞苷。

用药剂量

在基础实验体系如在培养的肿瘤细胞系中,药物剂量和毒性之间的关系可能接近线性对数(即指数)[15]。例如,化疗药物剂量的线性增加将导致培养的人乳腺癌细胞MCF7的数量呈对数级别减少[16]。当药物剂量为IC_{90}的倍数(即肿瘤细胞数量减少90%时的药物剂量或浓度)时,肿瘤消退的反应非常好。在临床上可明显观察到的肿瘤,其总负荷估计为$5\times10^{11}\pm10^{1}$(11±1 logs)。因此,要产生良好的肿瘤部分缓解(例如,50%~90%肿瘤消退)的药物剂量最多只能使肿瘤细胞减少1-log,这也只是“指数冰山”的10%。影响剂量效应的因素很多,将在以下小节中一一列出[17,18]。

影响剂量效应的因素

抗肿瘤药物的分类

理想的抗肿瘤药物可以通过引起多个对数级别的肿瘤细胞死亡来维持药物剂量和肿瘤细胞对数减少(log tumor cell reduction,log-TCR)之间的线性关系。电离辐射是最接近这一理想模式的治疗方案。在化疗药物中,烷化剂可诱导DNA损伤,其在维持剂量/log-TCR的关系上要优于其他类别的化疗药。烷化剂主要在细胞周期的S期和M期表现出抗肿瘤活性,但与其他化疗药物不同的是,它们也可在整个细胞周期中保持抗肿瘤活性。对照研究表明烷化剂在化疗敏感的肿瘤如白血病和淋巴瘤中具有明显的剂量效应,但在实体肿瘤特别是那些上皮来源的肿瘤中,剂量效应并不明显[19,20]。靶向嘌呤和嘧啶的抗代谢类药物主要在细胞增殖期中发挥作用,因此当发生药代动力学耐药时,需要通过增加暴露持续时间使更多的细胞进入增殖期而非通过增加药物剂量来克服。这也适用于诱导DNA损伤的拓扑异构酶Ⅰ/Ⅱ抑制剂和抗微管药物,这两类药物也只在DNA合成或有丝分裂纺锤体装配时具有抗肿瘤活性[21,22]。

针对激素受体、生长因子受体和细胞内激酶信号等靶标的药物具有不同的剂量效应关系。一旦此类药物与受体/激酶的相互作用进入饱和状态,药物剂量进一步增加,疗效将不会进一步提高[23]。因此,这些药物类似于抗代谢药物,一旦达到药物的饱和水平,剂量递增将不会产生进一步的临床获益。在慢性期或加速期CML患者中应用比标准剂量稍高的伊马替尼虽然可使一部分患者获益,但获益百分率较低且反应的持续时间也较短[24,25]。

肿瘤因素

肿瘤细胞内在敏感性

肿瘤对所给药物越敏感,其剂量效应越陡峭。因此,如果单位剂量药物能产生0.5log-TCR,那么将该剂量加倍则可产生高达1.0 log的肿瘤细胞死亡,这在临床上仅代表肿瘤的部分缓解。在化疗敏感的肿瘤中,单位剂量药物产生3 log-TCR,剂量加倍则可产生高达6 log-TCR,当然这个过程会受到肿瘤细胞异质性和耐药性(参见“耐药性”一节)的影响。6 log-TCR将达到肿瘤完全缓解,临床可明显获益,最重要的是,达到肿瘤治愈或根治。对于患有常见上皮来源的转移性肿瘤(如乳腺癌)的患者,使用标准单药化疗仅可在最多30%的患者中诱导肿瘤部分缓解(<1 log-TCR),联合化疗则会诱导出现更高的部分缓解率和较低的(10%~20%)完全缓解率。而在化疗敏感的肿瘤患者(例如,非霍奇金淋巴瘤、霍奇金病和生殖细胞肿瘤)中应用联合化疗则可以实现多个级别的log-TCR[26]。

肿瘤负荷

肿瘤负荷一直是化疗应答的负性预测因子。这一发现首次在小鼠移植瘤模型中得到证实。在小鼠模型中，肉眼可见的(即可触知的)肿瘤通常对化疗的反应最小；而相同类型的肿瘤如果其负荷只在微观水平，对化疗反应更好并且有治愈可能[26,27]。

对患者的平行观察试验得到与动物实验一致的结果，如辅助治疗可以治愈早期乳腺癌患者，但并不能治愈发生明显转移的乳腺癌患者。细胞丢失(即细胞凋亡)和细胞生长相平衡，以及无肿瘤新生血管形成均会延迟微观转移灶的生长。大多数可长期存活的肿瘤患者体内可能存在具有耐药性的微观肿瘤，这也会对治疗策略产生影响(参见“肿瘤的细胞动力学-生长分数”一节)。

使用分子技术对微小残留肿瘤进行检测和分类使得对患者的微观转移灶进行研究成为可能[26]。可以从辅助化疗研究中推断微观病灶的动力学特征(参见“辅助化疗”一节)。

耐药性

基础研究中通常通过“压力选择”的方法来诱导耐药性的产生，即将靶细胞暴露于药物浓度逐渐增加的环境中进行诱导。药物抗性通常表示为导致耐药细胞系产生 50% 抑制所需的药物浓度(IC_{50})除以亲本敏感细胞系所需的浓度(IC_{50})。有关耐药性的详细介绍，请参阅“联合化疗”一节和第 62 章。

肿瘤的细胞动力学-生长分数

影响肿瘤细胞 log-TCR 的主要因素为肿瘤的生长分数(growth fraction，GF)及细胞周期特异性药物的剂量。周期循环中细胞(即具有有丝分裂活性的细胞)的代增时间比肿瘤体积倍增时间短得多[28-32]。因此，肿瘤内许多细胞是濒死细胞，或处于“非循环”状态即 G_0/G_1 期中。肿瘤的 GF 是指循环中细胞与肿瘤细胞总数的比率。

对于常见的上皮来源的实体瘤，GF 通常小于 5%[33,34]。GF 为 5% 的实体瘤对细胞周期特异性药物的敏感性最差，而对其他化疗药物的敏感性各异。但是通过重复化疗可以使休眠的非循环细胞进入必要的生长期而成为循环细胞，并因此使化疗增效。对于低 GF 的肿瘤，延长暴露于细胞周期特异性药物的时间可能会使化疗增效。相比之下，对于高 GF 的肿瘤如 Burkitt 淋巴瘤，在较短的时间内接受相同的治疗甚至相同剂量的治疗即可产生多个 log-TCR[1]。最近对肿瘤长期克隆进化模型的研究发现了负责肿瘤持续增殖的特定的肿瘤祖细胞(cancer progenitor cell，CPC)。在这个模型中，具有自我更新能力的 CPC 可产生肿瘤内所有的祖细胞和分化细胞，但 CPC 只占所有肿瘤细胞的一小部分[35]。与正常组织干细胞一样，CPC 对化疗和放疗具有极强的抵抗力[36]。治愈性治疗方案与姑息性治疗方案之间的差别可能归因于 CPC 的相对敏感性以及不具备自我更新能力的祖细胞和分化癌细胞的敏感性。明确 CPC 中的治疗靶点有助于研发更有效的抗肿瘤治疗方案。

肿瘤缺氧

肿瘤实验及临床实体肿瘤中都会发生缺氧，这种情况可能是由于血管生成不足和肿瘤代谢活性高(氧消耗高)引起的。肿瘤内的氧分布是异质的，甚至一小部分缺氧细胞都可以明显影响化疗疗效。距离血管越远的肿瘤细胞，接触到的化疗药物的浓度就越低。并且，随着距血管的距离变远，肿瘤细胞的增殖能力也降低，其中就会包含一部分对细胞周期特异性药物耐药的非增殖细胞。某些化疗药物需要氧气作为毒性或代谢反应的中间体[37]。除此之外，缺氧会引起肿瘤的某些基因表达水平发生改变。缺氧诱导因子 1(hypoxia-inducible factor 1，HIF1)通过增加血管生成来阻止缺氧的细胞进入增殖周期并抑制其凋亡。缺氧会促进肝细胞生长因子(hepatocytes growth factor，HGF)的分泌及其受体 MET 的表达，进一步促进血管生成，增加转移和耐药的发生率[38,39]。三磷酸腺苷结合盒(adenosine triphosphate-binding cassette，ABC)蛋白如 p-糖蛋白(p-glycoprotein，PgP)的表达可能增加，从而引起对化疗药物的耐药。缺氧还会影响 *TP53* 突变细胞，降低对 DNA 损伤或靶向细胞周期的药物的凋亡反应[40]。对于缺氧是否可作为抗肿瘤治疗的靶点，研究人员在许多临床试验中利用生物还原烷化剂如丝裂霉素 C 和硝基咪唑(在氧环境中可作为电子受体)进行尝试，遗憾的是没有或只有很少的临床获益[41,42]。化疗敏感性下降的现象并不具有普遍性，在选定的细胞系(如肾脏)中，某些药物在常氧条件下的效果甚至低于缺氧条件[43]。放射治疗尤其需要氧分子来产生细胞毒性[44]。

癌基因依赖-生长因子信号

维持癌细胞转化状态导致明显的代谢和遗传压力。在这种条件下维持肿瘤细胞生存需要强的抗凋亡信号因子，干扰此信号通道将导致肿瘤细胞死亡。特别的是，突变的癌基因(如 CML 中的 *BCR-ABL*)或突变的生长因子受体[如肺癌中的 *EGFR*、黑素瘤中的 *BRAF* 和胃肠道间质瘤(gastrointestinal stromal tumors，GIST)中的 *CKIT*]也为肿瘤细胞提供了必要的生存信号，阻断这些途径会在这部分患者中产生显著的临床获益。诊断性分子检测的出现，能够识别这部分患者并选择适当的治疗方案。

宿主因素

骨髓细胞动力学

由于骨髓的增殖活性高且 DNA 修复能力相对缺乏，骨髓抑制是许多化疗药物的剂量限制性毒副反应。因此探索骨髓和肿瘤之间的细胞动力学差异已成为建立选择性的临床策略的基础[4,28]。

正常骨髓可在阿糖胞苷治疗后 1~2 周内恢复，几乎没有累积性骨髓抑制。对于许多患者而言，与阿糖胞苷治疗周期间的正常骨髓细胞相比，急性髓性白血病(acute myelogenous leukemia，AML)细胞的恢复是不完善的。体外的 AML 细胞对生长因子如 G-CSF 和 GM-CSF 的敏感性要低于正常的骨髓细胞[45]。因此，在阿糖胞苷诱导的骨髓抑制出现后，骨髓内 CSF 会反应性增加，由于正常骨髓的恢复可能比 AML 细胞更快，所以此时连续给药即可产生累积的治疗效应。

类似的变化也会发生在其他增殖组织中，如在胃肠道中，化疗药物会引起细胞有丝分裂停滞，从而导致肠道上皮细胞(如参与吸收液体的细胞)的丢失。这像骨髓一样也需要一个恢复期[46]。

药代动力学

药代动力学因素通常会影响剂量-反应曲线。如果药物的灭活酶变得饱和，则毒性和抗肿瘤作用可能会不成比例地增加，例如用 5-氟尿嘧啶(5-fluorouracil，5-FU)的某些剂量方案时就会观察到此现象[47,48]。

如果药物激活系统饱和，则可能发生相反的效果。异环磷酰胺是一种药物前体，在肝脏中被氧依赖性药物代谢酶细胞色素 P450 激活为具有生物活性的 4-羟基衍生物。异环磷酰胺的 3 天常规剂量（每天 1 200～2 400mg/m^2）比环磷酰胺（600mg/m^2）更高，是因为异环磷酰胺的 P450 活化速率相对较慢。随着环磷酰胺剂量的增加，会以恒定比例向活性 4-羟基环磷酰胺转化。但是，对于异环磷酰胺，一旦 P450 酶系统变得饱和，转化为活性形式的异环磷酰胺的比例就会降低，从而使其在较高剂量下失去有效的抗肿瘤作用[37]。

临床试验和剂量效应

患者的剂量选择

药物的清除率将决定总药物暴露[浓度曲线下面积（AUC）乘以时间]，药物在小鼠体内的 AUC 与其毒性相关。这种 AUC 与药物暴露及毒性的关系也适用于人类，并且可以通过小鼠模型的数据进行预测[49]。Ⅰ期临床试验中初始剂量的选择过程详见第 44 章。在大多数情况下，药物剂量是在Ⅰ期临床试验中确定的，后期会再根据患者的体表面积（body surface area，BSA）、体重或药物暴露（AUC）进行个体化剂量选择。

利用 Dubois BSA 公式可在不同物种之间类比地选择药物剂量。研究人员期望通过此公式进行类似的剂量调整后可以减少患者之间药物清除率的差异，并且也可用来确定首次人类（first time in human，FTIH）试验中的药物初始剂量。BSA 有助于儿童白血病中细胞毒药物的剂量选择，并且随后被纳入药物的标准用法中[50,51]。但最近的文献综述和机构经验发现 BSA 与正在研发的或常用的抗癌药物（除紫杉醇、口服白消安和替莫唑胺外）的清除率之间并无显著相关性[52,53]。

BSA 可能与肾小球滤过率、血容量和基础代谢率相关[52]。然而，与肝脏代谢酶诱导的药物清除变异相比，这些因素引起的药物清除变异很小（<25%），并且 BSA 和代谢活动之间也无相关性[52]。

细胞色素 P450 3A4（家族 3，亚家族 A 和多肽 4）是人类中最普遍的代谢酶，负责 55% 以上药物的代谢清除[54]。最近的研究利用非癌症药物的清除率（例如咪达唑仑的清除率[55]）来预测 CYP3A4 的代谢活动，表明通过该途径代谢的药物可能具有潜在的临床效用，例如多西紫杉醇[56]。酶促途径负责清除 5-FU 和 6-巯基嘌呤（6-mercaptopurine，6-MP），并通过 UGT1A1 进行葡糖醛酸化作用以清除伊立替康的活性成分 SN-38（见个别章节）。编码这些代谢酶的基因都可能出现多态性，这将影响药物的代谢过程并且与药物毒性相关。具有 *UGT1A1* *28 7/7 纯合基因型的人葡糖醛酸化能力降低，SN-38 的代谢受阻，导致出现更高的药物暴露（AUC）。一些研究也证实了 *1A1* *28 基因型确实与 SN-38 暴露及严重中性粒细胞减少、腹泻之间存在明显的相关性[57]。药物遗传学分析可指导未来个体化的剂量选择，并且在药物研发早期发挥重要作用。基于 DNA 的检测尚未商业化，故目前尚无临床角色。

由血清肌酐估算的肾小球滤过率确实与拓扑替康、依托泊苷和卡铂的毒性相关。事实上，由血清肌酐计算出的 AUC（Calvert 公式）现已用于卡铂的剂量选择[51]。目前，这些用于计算药物剂量的方法（利用 AUC 计算卡铂剂量除外）仍在研究中，临床实践中经典的化疗药物依然基于 BSA 进行剂量选择。

批准用于临床的及正在研发的所有酪氨酸激酶抑制剂采用平台剂量给药，并不根据体重或 BSA 进行调整。抗肿瘤单克隆抗体的剂量选择也不遵循经典的剂量递增直至出现毒副反应，但可根据细胞表面糖蛋白的受体占有率估算以细胞表面蛋白为靶点的药物的剂量（如抗 PD1 免疫检查点剂）或耗尽循环蛋白所需的药物的剂量[血管内皮生长因子（vascular endothelial growth factor，VEGF）和贝伐单抗]。

实时药代动力学和患者的安全

药代动力学研究提供了关于剂量效应的重要信息。这些研究表明血清药物水平与给定剂量药物的 AUC 有显著差异。对于用于急性白血病患者的甲氨蝶呤和 6-MP 以及移植前采用的高剂量白消安和卡莫司汀，药物或其活性代谢物（或两者均有）的 AUC 水平与毒性及治疗效果密切相关[58-61]。

在筛选后的 ALL 或 DLBCL 患者中给予高剂量[>1mg/m^2（译者注）]甲氨蝶呤后，检测其血浆药物水平，可用来确定这些患者中甲酰四氢叶酸拯救所需的剂量及持续时间[62]。实体瘤患者中给予相同剂量的紫杉醇，其 AUC 也有显著差异；但随后几天根据 AUC 进行的剂量的实时调整显著减少了需要吗啡治疗的黏膜炎的发生，并可缩短住院时间[63]。

敏感肿瘤的剂量效应

很少有临床研究将剂量强度作为一个独立的随机变量。在一项由癌症和白血病协作组 B（cancer and Leukemia Group B，CALGB）发起的研究中，596 名 AML 患者接受 4 个周期为期 5 天的阿糖胞苷治疗，随机分为 3 个剂量强度组：①每日 100mg/m^2（标准组）；②连续输注 400mg/m^2；③在第 1、3 和 5 天进行每天 2 次的输注（3g/m^2，3 小时内输注完成，每 12 小时输注一次）[3]。对于 60 岁及以下的患者，100mg/m^2 组 4 年后持续完全缓解率为 24%，400mg/m^2 组为 29%，3g/m^2 组为 44%（$P=0.002$），表明药物剂量增加时临床反应更好。但是老年患者反应欠佳。在急性淋巴细胞白血病（acute lymphocytic leukemia，ALL）中，维持化疗的剂量对疾病缓解的持续时间也有重要影响[64]。同样地，在小细胞肺癌研究中，尽管采用的是过时的治疗方案，联合化疗依然具有明显的剂量效应[65]。

在 AML 患者的初始治疗中，采用高剂量的蒽环类药物联合标准剂量的阿糖胞苷可提高年轻患者和老年患者的完全缓解（complete response，CR）率，并延长无进展生存期（progression free survival，PFS）[66]。

针对新型的激酶抑制剂的剂量-反应效应的研究较少，倾向于每日给予最大耐受剂量，故几乎没有机会再增量。在慢性期或加速期 CML 患者和 GIST 患者中增加伊马替尼的剂量可提高部分患者的缓解率。若是由于药物代谢清除增加、PgP 活性增加或 *BCR-ABL* 基因扩增引起的伊马替尼耐药，或是 BCR-ABL 激酶本身发生突变的情况下，增加伊马替尼的剂量也可使部分患者获益[24,25,67,68]。

在治疗个体患者时，如果可以治愈，药物剂量是关键的影响因素。因此，对于白血病、淋巴瘤、睾丸癌、儿童实体瘤及乳腺癌的常规剂量辅助治疗，即使存在明显的毒副反应风险，也不应减少剂量。而对于有耐药性的肿瘤，当以姑息治疗为目标时，应主要根据毒副反应来调整药物剂量。

外周血干细胞和骨髓移植

急性和慢性白血病及淋巴瘤患者接受同种异体骨髓移植可获得较长时间的无病生存期(即治愈),但由于存在移植物抗白血病的效应,并不能独立评估由药物剂量所贡献的效应。

在复发性淋巴瘤患者中应用高剂量化疗联合后续的挽救性自体干细胞移植,这类研究是关于剂量反应的最有说服力的证据[69,70]。通常使用烷化剂和基于全身放疗的方案进行移植前的预处理,因为它们的剂量限制性毒性是骨髓抑制。而对于不同的化疗药物,在非骨髓抑制的毒性变为剂量限制性毒副反应之前,药物剂量可达到基线水平的 3~20 倍。鉴于在药物剂量递增至基线的 2~4 倍时,AUC 与血清药物水平均有明显的重叠,故高剂量化疗联合干细胞移植时能更好地对药物的剂量效应进行对比。在非霍奇金淋巴瘤及睾丸癌患者中应用高剂量化疗联合挽救性自体干细胞移植可以提高完全缓解率,并获得治愈效果[70,71]。但是,由于毒副反应可能是致命的,所以高剂量化疗只能在专科中心中进行[72]。

辅助化疗

随机研究

细胞动力学研究为许多治疗方案的设计提供了实验基础。以下对相关的历史进行简要回顾。

Skipper 等[15]发现了药物治疗与肿瘤存活分数之间的基本指数关系。对于给定的药物和给定的剂量,TCR 分数是恒定的。尽管这种指数关系可能被其他因素所改变,例如耐药性和微环境,但它仍然是细胞动力学和化疗的基本原则。Norton 和 Simon[73]利用 Gompertzian 理论对化疗缓解间期的治疗进行分析,证明了后期强化治疗的潜在巨大获益。Goldie 和 Coldman[74]提出了突变导致耐药的理论,将肿瘤负荷及固有突变率同治愈潜力联系起来。Hryniuk 及其同事不仅在白血病和淋巴瘤中发现了显著的剂量反应效应,而且在相对不敏感的肿瘤如乳腺癌中也发现了明显的剂量反应效应[75-77]。

进行辅助治疗时,肿瘤负荷是微观级别的,所以此阶段是证明剂量效应的理想模式。在微观级别的肿瘤环境中,许多可以减少肿瘤杀伤的因素(肿瘤大小、血管分布异常且减少、GF 低、缺氧和肿瘤异质性增加)和促进化疗耐药的因素并不明显。例如,在转移性乳腺癌患者中应用环磷酰胺、甲氨蝶呤与 5-FU 联合化疗(CMF)或环磷酰胺、阿霉素和 5-FU 联合化疗(CAF),仅可产生短暂的部分缓解和少量的完全缓解,但在乳腺癌辅助治疗中,应用此联合化疗可使疾病复发率和死亡率降低 20%~30%[78]。在结肠癌中也可以看到类似的现象[79]。

在乳腺癌治疗中,研究人员期望通过增加辅助化疗的剂量来改善患者的无病生存期,但得到了混杂的结果。由 CALGB 发起的研究首次得到了强有力的阳性证据[19]。此研究将伴有淋巴结转移的乳腺癌患者随机分到不同剂量强度的 CAF 方案组(4 个周期)中:高剂量组,600mg/m^2 环磷酰胺,60mg/m^2 阿霉素和 600mg/m^2 5-FU,每 3~4 周一次;低剂量组的药物剂量分别为 300mg/m^2,30mg/m^2 和 300mg/m^2。2 年无复发曲线相差 10%,且此差异维持了 10 年。相比于低剂量组,高剂量组的死亡率也降低了约 20%。在占 20%的 *ERBB2*(*HER2/neu*)过表达的肿瘤中,剂量效应最为显著。对于没有 *ERBB2* 过表达的肿瘤,则没有观察到明显的剂量效应[20,80,81]。但是,假如没有分子标志物的存在,就不会发现这种亚群效应。

然而,由国家外科辅助乳腺和肠道项目(National Surgical Adjuvant Breast and Bowel Project,NSABP)实施的另外两项研究却未能证实在乳腺癌辅助治疗时,环磷酰胺剂量增加 2 倍或 4 倍会影响患者的复发或生存[80,81]。因此,研究人员猜测在 CAF 方案的对照研究中,阿霉素的剂量可能更重要。但是,另一项乳腺癌的辅助治疗研究也给出了阴性结果,患者随机分到三个剂量强度的阿霉素组中[82](60mg/m^2、75mg/m^2 和 90mg/m^2,均给予标准剂量的环磷酰胺),此时患者的无病生存期或总生存期(overall survival,OS)也并无差异。所以,对于阿霉素而言,60mg/m^2 可能是一个阈值剂量,超过该阈值剂量也不会产生更多的获益。

有关药物剂量的主要临床试验看似得到了不一致的结果,其原因已经成为临床前研究和作用机制研究的热点,但结果依然未明。可以推测,在大型对照研究的分析中,极有可能忽略掉了一个未被明确的重要的影响因素,这可能就是解释阴性结果的重要阻碍。

剂量密集化疗

剂量密集化疗是通过缩短治疗之间的间隔来增加药物强度,但并不增加药物的总剂量。这种药物强度的增加是通过在给定的时间内逐步增加剂量或周期数来实现的。使用中性粒细胞集落刺激因子是剂量密集疗法的基本要求。CALGB 9741 研究的中期结果显示,在乳腺癌的辅助治疗中应用剂量密集的环磷酰胺、阿霉素和紫杉醇的双周方案(同时给药或序贯给药),与标准的 3 周方案相比,可降低每年的复发风险或死亡风险。剂量密集组中,DFS[风险比(risk ratio,RR)= 0.74,P = 0.10]和 OS(RR = 0.69,P = 0.013)明显延长。序贯给药和同时给药组的 DFS 或 OS 没有差异,故剂量强度和用药时序之间没有相关性。此初步报告支持剂量密集方案可以提高化疗的疗效,但是也会增加毒副反应[82]。虽然所有的研究并未全部完成,但最终的随机试验结果并没有证实这些初步结论[83]。

小结

在临床中,剂量效应通常与肿瘤基本的化疗敏感性相关。因此,对化疗高度敏感的 Burkitt 淋巴瘤、ALL 和睾丸癌,对剂量强度的反应也很敏感,可达到治愈的效果。而对化疗相对不敏感的肿瘤如胃肠道肿瘤和肺癌,其对化疗反应差,也不受剂量强度的影响。在肿瘤患者身上依然有许多未知的尚无法解释的因素发挥作用,其中包括促进肿瘤发生的来源于特定肿瘤类型或特定肿瘤患者的固有遗传背景、体细胞和非转化间质细胞的影响、肿瘤干细胞及其他未被认知的因素的新功能。对于这些影响因素的作用,研究人员尚未从经典的体外和体内模型中得到明确的研究结果。

给药时序

药物的给药时序及效果

阿糖胞苷

Skipper 及其同事使用细胞周期特异性药物阿糖胞苷对

L1210 小鼠白血病进行了详细的定量研究[4,15]。当阿糖胞苷在适当的时间持续给药，且给予正常骨髓恢复的时间间隔时，可产生最佳的治疗效果。研究人员将他们的研究结果外推至 AML 患者，给予患者 5~7 天的连续输注，间隔 2~3 周后再进行重复治疗。在 AML 患者中，该方案可诱导 30%~40%的完全缓解率，而其他方案(例如每日静脉内给药)仅为 10%[4,84,85]。利用柔红霉素和阿糖胞苷联合化疗可进一步提高完全缓解率，并且此方案成为 40 多年来成人 AML 诱导治疗的支柱(详见"骨髓细胞动力学"一节)。

吉西他滨

吉西他滨(一种与阿糖胞苷结构相似的核苷类似物)的剂量限制性毒性是骨髓抑制[86,87]。与阿糖胞苷不同，吉西他滨在实体瘤特别是胰腺癌、乳腺癌和非小细胞肺癌中也具有抗肿瘤活性。每周一次或每两周一次的吉西他滨推注治疗耐受性良好，毒性主要为骨髓抑制。在临床试验和动物实验中，考虑到骨髓抑制、胃肠道毒性和低血压等毒副反应，若通过连续输注的方式给予吉西他滨，则需要降低药物剂量[87]。

甲氨蝶呤

由 Li 及其同事提出的间歇性甲氨蝶呤疗法(连续推注 5 天，每 3~4 周一个周期)可治愈妊娠性绒毛膜癌[88]。Goldin 等[89]也证实间歇性甲氨蝶呤疗法治疗 L1210 小鼠白血病的疗效要优于连续性甲氨蝶呤化疗(每日)。一项随机对照研究结果显示，间歇性甲氨蝶呤方案治疗 ALL 患者的完全缓解率显著优于每日治疗[90]。这一观察结果与 Schimke 等随后的发现一致[91]，相比于间歇性接触甲氨蝶呤，在体外持续接触甲氨蝶呤会产生更多的耐药性。此外，间歇性甲氨蝶呤给药后发生耐药的机制为药物转运缺陷，而连续给药后的耐药则是由基因扩增引起[91,92]。骨髓恢复和黏膜细胞更替相关的动力学因素，在制定阿糖胞苷给药方案中很重要，同时也是甲氨蝶呤给药方案的重要决定因素。

氟尿嘧啶

在临床研究中，通常以静脉推注的形式给予每日 350~450mg/m^2 的 5-FU，持续 5 天。使用该方案时，骨髓抑制是剂量限制性毒性。也可以将此剂量加倍后，进行超过 5 天的连续静脉滴注，在这种情况下，黏膜炎和腹泻成为剂量限制性毒性[93]。

当通过连续滴注而不是间歇推注给药时，氟脱氧尿苷(fluorodeoxyuridine，FUDR)的毒性更大。例如，每日剂量在 30~50mg/m^2 范围时即可产生毒性。从生化角度推测，连续滴注 FUDR 时可能对 DNA 合成有更大的影响，而其他用药方案则对宿主组织的核糖核酸(RNA)及 RNA 合成具有相对较大的影响[93]。关于不同用药时间影响治疗指数的数据很少(亚叶酸的调节将在本章后面进行讨论)。目前正在研究更长时间的全身给药方案[94]。

卡培他滨是 5-FU 的口服前体药物。它使给药效率更高且更简便，便于长期管理。卡培他滨可以在治疗结直肠癌和胃癌的 FOLFOX 方案中替代 5-FU[95]，但它并不能在所有适应证中都取代 5-FU 的静脉注射。

因此，5-FU 的作用机制、耐药性和交叉耐药性根据所选的药物和给药方案等因素而有所不同[96]。

烷化剂

烷化剂包括一类异质性的可与 DNA 相互作用的化合物。这种相互作用可导致培养的哺乳动物细胞发生恶性转化以及促进患者肿瘤的发生。这些药物的细胞毒性作用是通过添加烷基(CH3)和/或链内和链间交联产生的，如果没有通过 DNA 损伤修复机制进行完全修复，则会直接损害或阻止 DNA 复制或产生致死的双链断裂。而转化细胞中的 DNA 损伤修复机制通常都是缺陷的。这种相互作用也解释了烷化剂的致畸和致癌潜力。

就抗肿瘤作用而言，不同的烷化剂具有相同的效力，差异主要在于毒副反应。对于二氯铂类化合物，其毒性的变异很大，但其抗肿瘤作用与 X 线辐射非常相似。由于反式加合物的性质不同，它们的毒性基本不同。关于烷化剂的大多数实验数据表明，烷化剂的抗肿瘤效应和毒副反应与药物剂量相关，与用药时间无关[97](关于环磷酰胺和异环磷酰胺的具体讨论，参见"药代动力学"和"辅助化疗"章节)。

蒽环类药物

心脏毒性是蒽环类药物的重要的迟发性毒副反应。在实验中发现，连续输注蒽环类药物时，可维持较低的血药浓度，而推注相同剂量的蒽环类药物所产生的峰值浓度会造成更强的心脏毒性。Weiss 和 Manthel[98]首次证明每周一次的阿霉素化疗比总剂量相同的标准三周方案产生的心脏毒性更低。Legha 及其同事发现，阿霉素连续滴注 4 天的三周方案所产生的心脏毒性要低于静脉推注方案，后续的随机研究也证实了这一观察结果[99-101]。阿霉素持续静脉滴注方案可在心脏毒性出现之前使总累积剂量增加 30%~50%。在基础实验和初步的临床研究中，脂质体多柔比星可能比阿霉素的心脏毒性要低[102,103]。在目前临床实践中，可在部分患者中使用心脏保护剂右丙亚胺预防心脏毒性[104]。

依托泊苷

依托泊苷是拓扑异构酶Ⅱ抑制剂，可诱导 DNA 双链断裂，只对循环周期中的细胞有作用。依托泊苷通常用于实体瘤的联合化疗，特别是与顺铂进行联合。临床前研究表明依托泊苷的输注必须在顺铂输注期间和之后立即进行，以达到最佳的治疗效果；这是因为依托泊苷和顺铂具有协同作用，如抑制 DNA 修复。在小细胞肺癌中，依托泊苷的最佳剂量方案为每日一次，连用 5 天，每 3~4 周一个周期，这与本章前面关于骨髓和肿瘤细胞动力学的讨论以及对细胞周期特异性药物反应的讨论一致[105]。

微管蛋白结合药物

虽然长春新碱和长春碱是细胞周期特异性药物，但没有其他方案优于标准的每周给药方案[106]。从目前有限的数据来看，长春瑞滨也是如此。在紫杉醇化疗中主要考虑的是急性组胺样毒性，这可能与溶剂(聚氧乙烯蓖麻油)相关；抗组胺药和皮质类固醇可以缓解这种毒性。尽管一些随机试验表明紫杉类药物更长时间输注具有优势[107]，但从实际操作和经济学因素考虑，门诊患者一般采用 1 至 3 小时的静脉输注。

在乳腺癌和卵巢癌患者中，紫杉醇每周输注方案的疗效要优于间歇给药方案[108,109]。血浆中紫杉醇浓度高于 0.1mol/L 的持续时间与骨髓抑制的发生相关[107]。尽管神经病变是与剂量相关的副作用，中性粒细胞减少似乎与用药计划相关，而非剂量[110]。

间歇给药的用法

对于大多数直接或间接靶向 DNA 或有丝分裂纺锤体的化疗药，不论是单药化疗还是联合化疗，间歇性给药方案的疗效(例如，每隔 3~4 周连续用药 5 天，共 4 个疗程)通常优于其他方案(例如，连续用药即每日用药)。Burkitt 淋巴瘤中环磷酰胺和甲氨蝶呤的使用、绒毛膜癌中的甲氨蝶呤和放线菌素 D 的使用、骨髓瘤中美法仑的使用、AML 中阿糖胞苷的使用及 ALL 中甲氨蝶呤的使用都是如此[111]。应用于霍奇金病、ALL 和儿童实体肿瘤的联合化疗也是如此[106,111,112]。基础实验和临床研究发现在快速增殖的肿瘤中给予间歇性强化治疗是更优效的，其原因可能是间歇化疗将静息的 G_0/G_1 细胞募集到活跃的细胞周期中。而对于更惰性的、低 GF 的肿瘤，持续用药疗效可能更好，但这需要更多的研究进一步证实[113]。

支持治疗的进展推动了间歇性强化疗法的发展。在乳腺癌的剂量密集辅助治疗中应用中性粒细胞集落刺激因子[114]，或在化疗完成骨髓恢复后进行白细胞分离和使用 G-CSF 治疗，均可以收获足够的外周血循环干细胞，用以解救四个疗程的中等强度化疗[115]。

持续给药

直肠癌的辅助治疗使用 5-FU 持续输注(6 周)联合局部放疗，局部复发和远处转移的发生率均降低[116]。卡培他滨是一种口服药物，在体内经过生物转化成 5-FU。卡培他滨单药连续给药 14 天，以 21 天为一个周期，有效率要优于静脉注射 5-FU 和甲酰四氢叶酸，但没有生存获益[117,118]。卡培他滨单药或联合化疗在难治性乳腺癌中也具有抗肿瘤活性。目前研究人员正在探索在联合化疗和联合放疗中同时应用连续静脉滴注氟尿嘧啶与口服卡培他滨的效果。卡培他滨三周方案可显著降低其剂量限制性毒性(手足综合征)的发生。

靶向激酶抑制剂

由于与作用机制相关的原因，许多新的靶向药物均采用连续口服给药，如伊马替尼在 CML 和 GIST 中的临床应用[113,119]。在临床和临床前模型中发现，持续抑制肿瘤细胞或肿瘤血管网络中的增殖性生长信号，或持续阻断肿瘤细胞的生存通路信号是十分必要的。在疾病稳定的肾细胞癌患者中随机停用多靶点酪氨酸激酶抑制剂索拉非尼，结果显示，对于继续接受索拉非尼治疗的患者，6 个月时 PFS 优势明显优于安慰剂组，这与临床前模型的结论相吻合[120]。而对于其他药物，如多靶点激酶抑制剂舒尼替尼，它类似于 DNA 损伤剂和有丝分裂纺锤体抑制剂，使用间歇性给药方案时患者的耐受性会更好[121]。

联合化疗

原因

联合化疗的根本原因：①肿瘤细胞异质性及其对耐药性的影响；②临床中联合化疗的成功。在临床实践中，特定类型肿瘤中联合化疗方案的药物选择取决于药物在该瘤种中的活性及不同的毒性谱。优选具有最高单药活性的药物，特别是可以诱导完全缓解的药物(如果存在这样的药物)，同时考虑纳入不同作用机制的药物以解决肿瘤异质性问题。

临床中的联合化疗

联合化疗存在着大量的临床先例，如在儿童 ALL 的治疗中联合使用多种活性药物，使用的药物数量与治愈率之间存在直接的相关性(见表 54-2)。事实上，基本上所有的治愈性化疗方案都涉及两种药物的联合，常常是 3 种或更多的药物(表 54-3)。但在联合化疗的每次用药时，并不需要包含所有药物。例如，在乳腺癌或儿童软组织肿瘤的总治疗过程中，多柔比星和环磷酰胺后序贯使用紫杉醇化疗。正常组织的耐受性通常会限制可单次给予的化疗药物的数量。

表 54-3　肿瘤化疗-治愈不同肿瘤所需药物的数量

肿瘤	治愈所需的药物数量	辅助或新辅助	治愈所需的药物数量
急性淋巴细胞白血病(儿童)	4~7	肾母细胞瘤	2~3
妊娠绒毛膜癌[a]		胚胎性横纹肌肉瘤	2~3
早期	1~3	成骨肉瘤	3
进展期	2~4	软组织肉瘤	3
急性髓系白血病	3+	卵巢癌	3~4
睾丸癌	3	乳腺癌	2~4
Burkitt 淋巴瘤[b]	1~4	结直肠癌	2
霍奇金病	4~5	ⅢA 期非小细胞肺癌	2
弥漫性组织细胞性淋巴瘤	4~5	局限期小细胞肺癌	2~4

[a] 一种药物是有治愈性的，但是使用两种或更多药物可以获得更高的治愈率。

[b] 一种药物可治愈非洲 Burkitt 淋巴瘤，但两种或更多种药物联合使用更好。

目前的研究已经证实针对DNA或有丝分裂纺锤体的化疗药物与其他作用机制的药物联合使用时可具有协同作用或相加效应。分子靶向药物，无论是单克隆抗体还是小分子抑制剂，均可以与细胞毒药物或其他靶向药物联合使用。曲妥珠单抗是靶向*ERBB2*的单克隆抗体，与多柔比星和紫杉醇具有协同作用。25%的乳腺癌患者肿瘤表面存在*ERBB2*，但是只有*ERBB2*基因扩增的患者可以从曲妥珠单抗治疗中获益[122]。需要注意的是，在选择联合用药时要慎重考虑毒副反应。曲妥珠单抗联合阿霉素会增加心脏毒性，但与紫杉醇联合使用时，心脏毒性较小。非霍奇金淋巴瘤的化疗方案（环磷酰胺、羟基甲砜霉素/多柔比星、硫酸长春新碱和泼尼松）联合单克隆抗体利妥昔单抗，可以提高疾病缓解率但不增加毒性。在雌激素受体（estrogen receptor，ER）阳性的转移性乳腺癌患者的治疗中，芳香化酶抑制剂（aromatase inhibitor，AI）和*mTOR*抑制剂依维莫司的联合使用显著延长了患者的PFS[123]。并且，在ER受体阳性的乳腺癌患者中联合使用AI和CDK 4/6抑制剂palbociclib（哌柏西利）进行治疗，也可延长患者的PFS[124]。但是新药和老药联合使用的效果并不能随意推测，比如细胞毒药物化疗联合厄洛替尼和吉非替尼的治疗方案却并不能使肺癌患者获益[125]。

目前新型的靶向药物可以靶向多个靶标。理论上，靶向血管生成途径中多个靶标（如VEGFR和PDGFR）的小分子药物，会比单独靶向一个靶标的药物产生更大的临床获益。比如，多靶点抑制剂索拉非尼和舒尼替尼在部分临床试验中获得了成功，但是贝伐单抗以及部分仅靶向*VEGFR2*的小分子药物却失败了[12]。

联用的抗肿瘤药物可以针对同一靶蛋白或针对肿瘤生长过程一条必需信号通路中的不同蛋白。曲妥珠单抗和帕妥珠单抗可以与ERBB2受体的不同表位相结合，这两种单克隆抗体的联合使用可以显著延长ERBB2阳性的转移性乳腺癌患者的OS[126]。在BRAF^{V600E}黑色素瘤患者中联合使用BRAF和MEK抑制剂也可以提高疾病缓解率，延长患者的PFS和OS[10]。全反式维A酸和三氧化二砷可以与急性早幼粒白血病细胞中的PML蛋白相互作用，诱导疾病的持久缓解[127]。

单克隆抗体与小分子抑制剂相结合的技术已经成熟，如乳腺癌中使用的T-DM1是曲妥珠单抗和奥瑞他汀相结合的药物，或在霍奇金淋巴瘤的治疗中可以将放射性钇加入抗CD30的抗体中[128,129]。

肿瘤细胞异质性和耐药性

肿瘤起源于克隆，但伴随着肿瘤形成，DNA不稳定性会增加，从而导致子细胞的突变增加，这称为“克隆进化”，最终导致肿瘤细胞异质性的产生。这种进化会筛选出具有更高存活能力的后代细胞，表现为更高的增殖能力、对细胞凋亡的抵抗、更强的转移或侵袭潜力、对正常细胞生长因子的依赖性降低和诱导血管生成的能力增强[130]。肿瘤细胞的异质性将增加潜在治疗靶点的数量及多样性，所以更为需要进行联合治疗。

最初，肿瘤耐药被认为只是对单个药物有抗性。但多药耐药的发现则需要我们重新思考联合化疗的原因[131]。ABC家族转运蛋白（如ABCB1、PgP）、多药耐药蛋白（如ABCC1）和乳腺癌相关蛋白（如ABCG2）的表达与多药耐药相关，并且此耐药几乎只发生在天然药物中。延长底物药物如阿霉素低剂量暴露，可能会克服这些转运蛋白介导的耐药性[132]。然而，谷胱甘肽转移酶、DNA修复和拓扑异构酶Ⅱ的改变也可能与多药耐药性相关[133]。

最近对多细胞耐药的研究结果表明是这群细胞的凋亡设定点发生了改变[134]。体外耐药和体内耐药之间的差异正在改变着联合化疗的策略[135]。尽管长期的药物暴露会诱导稳定的耐药细胞系，但急性的药物暴露可能导致短期的可逆转的耐药性。目前研究人员正在探索短期耐药与长期耐药在机制上的相关性，推测可能是遗传因素从中发挥作用。

根据肿瘤的分子分型可以选择相应的治疗方案，但是同一时间点的同一肿瘤中存在着异质性，同一肿瘤在不同的时间点也存在着异质性，同一患者的不同肿瘤转移灶也会存在异质性。针对这一复杂问题，研究人员正在开发新的治疗策略（更详细的讨论参见第41章）。

细胞动力学

由于肿瘤缺氧和GF较低，实体瘤中存在很多处于G_1期或G_0期的潜在的克隆形成细胞，这一发现可能为联合化疗的应用提供了理论基础[27,28,33]。因此，使用细胞周期特异性药物可以杀死具有有丝分裂活性的细胞，而添加非细胞周期特异性药物（例如烷化剂）可以杀伤处于非增殖期的肿瘤细胞。重复周期化疗让正常组织得以恢复，且不需降低药物剂量，同时通过增加营养物质、氧气和血管供应使G_0/G_1期肿瘤细胞进入增殖期。

同步化

抑制DNA合成或阻止细胞有丝分裂的药物可在体外和体内使肿瘤细胞或正常细胞实现同步化。而利用激素类药物可以使肿瘤细胞实现同步化，但并不影响基本的正常细胞。

但是在肿瘤患者体内，由于肿瘤异质性的存在，只有一部分肿瘤细胞可以在激素类药物的干预下实现同步化。所以如何利用激素类药物实现全部肿瘤细胞的同步化仍然需要继续探索[136,137]。

调节剂

一些无细胞毒性的药物可以通过降低化疗对正常组织的毒性（例如甲酰四氢叶酸和甲氨蝶呤的联用）或通过增强抗肿瘤效果（如5-FU和甲酰四氢叶酸在结肠癌辅助治疗和晚期治疗中的联合使用）来改善已有化疗药物的治疗指数[138-144]。

从生化角度讲，5-FU的代谢产物氟脱氧尿苷一磷酸（fluorodeoxyuridine monophosphate，FdUMP）可以与胸苷酸合成酶（thymidylate synthase，TS）的底物位点相结合，从而抑制DNA合成及细胞复制。这种抑制的稳定性及持续时间受甲酰四氢叶酸的代谢产物5,10-亚甲基四氢叶酸的影响，此产物也可以与TS结合，产生所谓的三元复合物（FdUMP-TS-5,10-亚甲基四氢叶酸）。在临床前研究中，不论是体外实验还是体内实验，甲酰四氢叶酸均可以增加5-FU的治疗指数。许多临床试验将5-FU治疗与5-FU和甲酰四氢叶酸联合治疗的效果进行比较，结果发现在转移性结直肠癌患者中应用5-FU/亚叶酸钙联合治疗后疗效更佳，且只轻度增加了黏膜炎和腹泻的发生率。并且在结肠癌的辅助治疗和晚期治疗中，5-FU与甲酰四氢叶酸的组合均可以提高患者的存活率[143,144]。

贝伐珠单抗（Avastin）可以与VEGF结合并阻断其生物活

性。VEGF 是作用于内皮细胞的一种重要的促有丝分裂和抗细胞凋亡因子（见第 11 章）。VEGF 通过与内皮细胞表面的 VEGF 受体 2（即 KDR）和血小板衍生的生长因子受体 β（platelet-derived growth factor receptor beta，PDGFRB）相结合，增加内皮细胞的通透性，从而导致肿瘤内的组织间压（interstitial fluid pressure，IFP）增加。结肠癌、乳腺癌、肺癌、头颈部肿瘤、宫颈癌和皮肤肿瘤中的 IFP 均明显高于正常组织[145-148]。肿瘤 IFP 增加将阻碍各种物质在肿瘤血管中的转运；降低肿瘤 IFP 或调节微血管压力可以增加靶向药物或低分子量示踪化合物在肿瘤血管中的转运[149,150]。越来越多的证据表明 PDGFRB 和 KDR 酪氨酸激酶在肿瘤 IFP 增加过程中发挥着至关重要的作用，这使得它们成为干预肿瘤组织高液压的候选靶标[151-154]，并且可以联合化疗药物来使化疗增效。贝伐珠单抗可降低晚期结直肠癌患者肿瘤组织中的 IFP，并增加肿瘤中钆的摄取。伊立替康、5-FU 和甲酰四氢叶酸联合贝伐珠单抗的方案可以显著延长转移性结直肠癌患者的生存期[155]。正如这两项研究结果所示，调节肿瘤内的 IFP 可以在不增加患者毒副反应的情况下选择性地增加肿瘤内的药物水平，这为所有类型的实体瘤提供了一个具有广谱意义的治疗策略。

贝伐珠单抗（和类似药）与细胞毒性化疗联合治疗在许多肿瘤但非全部肿瘤中，显示了 PFS 和 OS 的获益。鉴于 VEGF 的作用机制很复杂，尚不能确定到底是哪种机制介导这种作用。在大多数情况下，VEGF 靶向治疗不管是用于同时性联合治疗还是序贯性联合治疗都比其单药治疗更有效，说明 VEGF 靶向治疗更倾向于作为调节剂发挥作用。

耐药性的影响

化疗药物具有细胞毒性和抗增殖作用，但是肿瘤细胞对化疗药物的反应是有异质性的，所以联合化疗显得更为重要。联合化疗的最初原因就是避免治疗的耐药。

关于耐药性的初步研究证实耐药性与药物外排增加、靶点突变或扩增、细胞内药物失活等引起的作用部位药物水平下降相关。最近的研究更关注药物与其靶受体相互作用后引起药物敏感、耐药或者细胞凋亡（程序性细胞死亡）的机制。化疗药引起的细胞损伤具有触发细胞凋亡级联反应的共同特性，此过程需要能量、酶和细胞结构才能完成[156]。除细胞凋亡外，在某些情况下，由药物诱导的 ATP 耗竭，会引起坏死性细胞死亡[157]。最后，在用细胞毒药物、激素类药物或放射治疗后，营养和/或氧气的缺乏会引起自噬，这是一种高度保守的细胞存活过程，也会导致耐药的发生[158]。必须在药物治疗指数的背景下去观察耐药性，因为从根本上，耐药性意味着在携带肿瘤的宿主中，并不存在与毒性相关的选择性细胞毒性。此现象可能在治疗开始时即存在或在治疗过程中变得更为明显。大多数抗肿瘤药物都会出现这种治疗指数低下的情况。

逆转耐药性

另一种对化疗的改进方法即逆转耐药性，其中研究最多的是由 PgP 介导的多药耐药性。维拉帕米和其他几种脂溶性杂环药物，包括环孢菌素类似物，可以抑制 PgP 的功能，从而减少许多天然抗肿瘤药物（多柔比星、长春新碱、紫杉烷等）从细胞中流出，进而增加药物毒性。B 细胞肿瘤、AML 及肉瘤中 PgP 的表达上调。某些药物会引起多药耐药，在使用这些药物治疗后，肿瘤中 PgP 的表达也会增加[159]。但通过抑制 PgP 的功能来逆转耐药的策略尚未在临床试验或临床实践中获得成功。

分子生物学/靶向治疗

剂量和时序的影响

最近关于靶向治疗的临床有效性的概念，让研究人员对靶向治疗重获希望。在肿瘤治疗中，研究人员已经合成针对癌细胞及其表面的独特分子靶标（例如，融合基因、突变和重组基因）的小分子药物和单克隆抗体，但其靶向的特异性却依然缺乏[160-162]。

表 54-1 列出的是目前正在研发的抗肿瘤靶标，可针对这些分子和生化通路选择联合治疗。许多药物在临床前研究中显示出良好的抗肿瘤活性，为临床上的联合治疗提供了基础。这些药物在分子水平上的累积效应表明，可能多样化的靶点相互作用和序贯或同时攻击关键细胞行为导致了相互作用。

另一个重要关注点是预期毒性的多样性。传统的化疗药物出现的与药物剂量相关的毒性通常存在于增殖明显的组织中，并且此毒性在不同药物之间具有相对的一致性；而分子靶向药物不同药物的毒性谱差异很大，这与经典的抗肿瘤药物明显不同。研究人员正在对分子靶向药的抗肿瘤特性、不同靶向药之间的相互作用以及靶向药与其他抗肿瘤药物之间的相互作用进行广泛研究。

联合治疗的实验模型

经典的抗肿瘤药物主要限于那些可以直接或间接引起 DNA 损伤的药物；而分子生物学时代的药物具有更多的不同的抗肿瘤机制。实际上，许多有趣的临床前研究利用实验模型已经证实了联合治疗具有相加或协同效应。Rideout 和 Chou 对临床前模型和计算机分析的相关文献进行了综述[163]。

未来的联合化疗将受到药物数量及其相互作用的显著影响。在血液系统、儿童和胚胎肿瘤的治愈性治疗中，利用作用机制不同的药物进行联合治疗获得了成功。

临床上经常使用的术语“相加性”和“协同性”目前还没有明确的定义。在考虑这些术语时，相比于药物在患者身上的治疗指数，药物对肿瘤的选择性是关键。如果两种具有相加性治疗效果的药物具有不同的剂量限制性毒性，毒性是不加成的，则应将总体抗肿瘤效果描述为相加性效应。当抗肿瘤效果大于“相加性”时，术语“协同作用”可能是更合适的。

表 54-4 比较了联合化疗和联合治疗的各种特点。若要纳入不同种类的药物，则需要更有效的临床试验设计，例如Ⅱ期/Ⅲ期联合研究设计。未来临床研究会整合越来越多的定量分子标志物和“实时”药理学参数。这些有效的方法将会提高临床试验的效率和有效性。

癌基因和抑癌基因可以通过干扰生长信号、血管生成或 DNA 修复过程来阻碍细胞周期的正常推进。通过肿瘤分型可以鉴定出个体患者中的特定基因或信号通路异常，有助于精确选择可能在该患者中最有效的药物，这就是个体化肿瘤治疗的目的。

表 54-4 联合化疗与联合治疗的对比

组合	联合化疗	联合治疗
药物种类	一类药物,抗增殖药物	从所有种类[a]中选择
药物数量	2~5	4~12+
毒性	毒性主要发生在骨髓及胃肠道(大剂量)、心脏、神经系统和肺	毒性谱多样,包括与剂量相关的毒性;毒性通常无加性效应;毒性有限,药物选择性更多
临床试验设计	已建立好的、固定的设计	灵活、创新、半贝叶斯;患者参与
终点	经典;R、dR、DFS、OS	MRT
与基础科学的结合	受限	广泛、可操作;PK、PD;靶点

[a] 化疗、免疫疗法、内分泌药物、抗血管生成、抗基质药物、基因疗法和细胞周期控制药物[抗细胞周期蛋白(CDK 家族)、转录控制和反义 RNA]。

DFS,无病生存期;dR,缓解持续时间;MRT,微束放射治疗;OS,总生存期;PD,药效学;PK,药代动力学;R,缓解(部分缓解或完全缓解)。

肿瘤化疗的综合方法

肿瘤化疗于半个多世纪前就已经开始。现在使用的化疗药物多起源于生物靶向治疗。例如,Hitchings 和 Elion 研发了抑制嘌呤合成的特异性药物,如 6-MP 和 6-TG;Heidelberger 利用 5-FU 靶向 RNA 合成;Farber 利用氨基蝶呤靶向叶酸还原途径。这些创新不仅为肿瘤治疗奠定了基础,也成为研究转化肿瘤细胞的工具。

天然药物如长春花生物碱、蒽环霉素和紫杉类药物可选择性杀伤具有增殖活性的肿瘤细胞。这些药物可以与其他对增殖细胞具有活性的药物进行组合(例如,激素、烷化剂和辐射)。新研发的药物的最佳使用方案就是将它们整合到越来越复杂的联合治疗中,以便得到更大的治疗指数。对于目前经典的主要抑制增殖的化学药物也是如此。

分子生物学的快速发展增加了抗肿瘤药物的种类。除了经典的抗增殖和诱发 DNA 损伤的化合物之外,还有激素、免疫毒素以及侵袭和转移抑制剂。之后发现的还有具有独特结构和数量的能够靶向特定分子的受体和激酶,且其在肿瘤中激活的途径需要进一步阐明。

显而易见的是,绝大多数肿瘤只有用针对特定类型肿瘤的最高活性的药物进行联合治疗才能获得成功。理想的情况是,这些药物具有不同的剂量限制性毒性。经验主义是当代肿瘤治疗发展的重要组成部分,而合理的药物发现、类似物开发、临床前建模、精确的病理诊断、精准的疾病分期和临床试验设计都是当今肿瘤治疗获得成功的基础。

分子生物学的突破为肿瘤治疗带来了巨大的机遇和挑战。在这些突破的基础上,一个完美的分子诊断不仅要明确肿瘤的起源和方式,还要明确其生存所必需的信号。肿瘤发生和转移的具体过程已成为抗肿瘤治疗的靶点(见表 54-1)。制药技术的发展不仅为临床提供了小分子药物,还提供了单克隆抗体、免疫交联物、核酶、反义 RNA 和重组病毒等。

抗肿瘤治疗现在会联合很多不同作用机制的药物,以更广泛的治疗方法来对抗肿瘤的异质性。这些组合中有一些药物是现在的标准治疗,因为已经证实它们可以提高缓解率并延长生存(见表 54-4)。未来肿瘤治疗领域需要克服的挑战包括:①开发不伴有预期的显著的急性毒性的细胞抑制剂;②不同类别的靶向药物(表 54-5)联合使用时的用药剂量和时序问题;③为适当类型的肿瘤和个体患者选择特定的治疗方案。

表 54-5 不同种类药物的联合治疗

药物	作用的肿瘤
化疗+其他全身性治疗	
化疗+免疫治疗	
顺铂+赫赛汀	乳腺癌
紫杉醇+赫赛汀	乳腺癌
CHOP+利妥昔单抗	淋巴瘤
化疗→MRT→免疫恢复→疫苗	
化疗联合同种异体淋巴细胞移植	
化疗+内分泌治疗	
长春新碱+泼尼松	急性淋巴细胞白血病
化疗+他莫昔芬	乳腺癌
化疗+分化剂	
柔红霉素+ATRA	急性早幼粒细胞白血病
化疗+抗血管生成治疗	
IFL+贝伐珠单抗	结直肠癌

ATRA,全反式维 A 酸;IFL,伊立替康/ 5-氟尿嘧啶/亚叶酸;MRT,微束放射治疗。

随着分子生物学发挥着越来越重要的作用,肿瘤治疗相关的临床和基础研究将继续推动肿瘤治疗的加速发展。

(段晶晶 邓婷 译,巴一 审校)

参考文献

The complete reference list can be found on the Wiley Companion Digital Edition of this title (see inside front cover for login instructions).

1 Frei E 3rd, Canellos GP. Dose: a critical factor in cancer chemotherapy. *Am J Med.* 1980;**69(4)**:585–594.

4 Skipper HE, Schabel FM Jr, Wilcox WS. Experimental evaluation of potential anticancer agents. XXI. Scheduling of arabinosylcytosine to take advantage of its S-phase specificity against leukemia cells. *Cancer Chemother Rep.* 1967;**51(3)**:125–165.

10 Robert C, Karaszewska B, Schachter J, et al. Improved overall survival in melanoma with combined dabrafenib and trametinib. *N Engl J Med.* 2015;**372(1)**:30–39.

14 Hryniuk W, Frei E 3rd, Wright FA. A single scale for comparing dose-intensity of all chemotherapy regimens in breast cancer: summation dose-intensity. *J Clin Oncol.* 1998;**16(9)**:3137–3147.

16 Frei E 3rd, Cucchi CA, Rosowsky A, et al. Alkylating agent resistance: in vitro studies with human cell lines. *Proc Natl Acad Sci U S A.* 1985;**82(7)**:2158–2162.

19 Wood WC, Budman DR, Korzun AH, et al. Dose and dose intensity of adjuvant chemotherapy for stage II, node-positive breast carcinoma. *N Engl J Med.* 1994;**330(18)**:1253–1259.

23 Dowsett M. Clinical development of aromatase inhibitors for the treatment of breast and prostate cancer. *J Steroid Biochem Mol Biol.* 1990;**37(6)**:1037–1041.

24 Zonder JA, Pemberton P, Brandt H, Mohamed AN, Schiffer CA. The effect of dose increase of imatinib mesylate in patients with chronic or accelerated phase chronic myelogenous leukemia with inadequate hematologic or cytogenetic response to initial treatment. *Clin Cancer Res.* 2003;**9(6)**:2092–2097.

27 Norton L, Simon R, Brereton HD, Bogden AE. Predicting the course of Gompertzian growth. *Nature.* 1976;**264(5586)**:542–545.

32 Tannock I. Cell kinetics and chemotherapy: a critical review. *Cancer Treat Rep.* 1978;**62(8)**:1117–1133.

36 Visvader JE, Lindeman GJ. Cancer stem cells in solid tumours: accumulating evidence and unresolved questions. *Nat Rev Cancer.* 2008;**8(10)**:755–768.

39 Engelman JA, Janne PA. Mechanisms of acquired resistance to epidermal growth factor receptor tyrosine kinase inhibitors in non-small cell lung cancer. *Clin Cancer Res.* 2008;**14(10)**:2895–2899.

40 Achison M, Hupp TR. Hypoxia attenuates the p53 response to cellular damage. *Oncogene.* 2003;**22(22)**:3431–3440.

49 Baker SD, Verweij J, Rowinsky EK, et al. Role of body surface area in dosing of investigational anticancer agents in adults, 1991–2001. *J Natl Cancer Inst.* 2002;**94(24)**:1883–1888.

51 Jodrell DI, Egorin MJ, Canetta RM, et al. Relationships between carboplatin exposure and tumor response and toxicity in patients with ovarian cancer. *J Clin Oncol.* 1992;**10(4)**:520–528.

55 Dresser GK, Spence JD, Bailey DG. Pharmacokinetic-pharmacodynamic consequences and clinical relevance of cytochrome P450 3A4 inhibition. *Clin Pharmacokinet.* 2000;**38(1)**:41–57.

58 Evans WE, Crom WR, Abromowitch M, et al. Clinical pharmacodynamics of high-dose methotrexate in acute lymphocytic leukemia. Identification of a relation between concentration and effect. *N Engl J Med.* 1986;**314(8)**:471–477.

64 Pinkel D, Hernandez K, Borella L, et al. Drug dosage and remission duration in childhood lymphocytic leukemia. *Cancer.* 1971;**27(2)**:247–256.

73 Norton L, Simon R. The Norton-Simon hypothesis revisited. *Cancer Treat Rep.* 1986;**70(1)**:163–169.

78 Early Breast Cancer Trialists' Collaborative Group. Polychemotherapy for early breast cancer: an overview of the randomised trials. *Lancet.* 1998;**352(9132)**:930–942.

82 Citron ML, Berry DA, Cirrincione C, et al. Randomized trial of dose-dense versus conventionally scheduled and sequential versus concurrent combination chemotherapy as postoperative adjuvant treatment of node-positive primary breast cancer: first report of Intergroup Trial C9741/Cancer and Leukemia Group B Trial 9741. *J Clin Oncol.* 2003;**21(8)**:1431–1439.

83 Swain SM, Tang G, Geyer CE Jr, et al. Definitive results of a phase III adjuvant trial comparing three chemotherapy regimens in women with operable, node-positive breast cancer: the NSABP B-38 trial. *J Clin Oncol.* 2013;**31(26)**:3197–3204.

90 Frei E 3rd, Karon M, Levin RH, et al. The effectiveness of combinations of antileukemic agents in inducing and maintaining remission in children with acute leukemia. *Blood.* 1965;**26(5)**:642–656.

97 Teicher BA, Holden SA, Eder JP, Brann TW, Jones SM, Frei E 3rd. Influence of schedule on alkylating agent cytotoxicity in vitro and in vivo. *Cancer Res.* 1989;**49(21)**:5994–5998.

100 Smith LA, Cornelius VR, Plummer CJ, et al. Cardiotoxicity of anthracycline agents for the treatment of cancer: systematic review and meta-analysis of randomised controlled trials. *BMC Cancer.* 2010;**10**:337.

109 Pignata S, Scambia G, Katsaros D, et al. Carboplatin plus paclitaxel once a week versus every 3 weeks in patients with advanced ovarian cancer (MITO-7): a randomised, multicentre, open-label, phase 3 trial. *Lancet Oncol.* 2014;**15(4)**:396–405.

112 Devita VT Jr, Serpick AA, Carbone PP. Combination chemotherapy in the treatment of advanced Hodgkin's disease. *Ann Intern Med.* 1970;**73(6)**:881–895.

113 Heinrich MC, Corless CL, Demetri GD, et al. Kinase mutations and imatinib response in patients with metastatic gastrointestinal stromal tumor. *J Clin Oncol.* 2003;**21(23)**:4342–4349.

121 Motzer RJ, Hutson TE, Olsen MR, et al. Randomized phase II trial of sunitinib on an intermittent versus continuous dosing schedule as first-line therapy for advanced renal cell carcinoma. *J Clin Oncol.* 2012;**30(12)**:1371–1377.

122 Slamon D, Eiermann W, Robert N, et al. Adjuvant trastuzumab in HER2-positive breast cancer. *N Engl J Med.* 2011;**365(14)**:1273–1283.

129 Francisco JA, Cerveny CG, Meyer DL, et al. cAC10-vcMMAE, an anti-CD30-monomethyl auristatin E conjugate with potent and selective antitumor activity. *Blood.* 2003;**102(4)**:1458–1465.

131 Gottesman MM, Ling V. The molecular basis of multidrug resistance in cancer: the early years of P-glycoprotein research. *FEBS Lett.* 2006;**580(4)**:998–1009.

147 Less JR, Posner MC, Boucher Y, Borochovitz D, Wolmark N, Jain RK. Interstitial hypertension in human breast and colorectal tumors. *Cancer Res.* 1992;**52(22)**:6371–6374.

151 Ferrara N, Gerber HP, LeCouter J. The biology of VEGF and its receptors. *Nat Med.* 2003;**9(6)**:669–676.

154 Willett CG, Boucher Y, di Tomaso E, et al. Direct evidence that the VEGF-specific antibody bevacizumab has antivascular effects in human rectal cancer. *Nat Med.* 2004;**10(2)**:145–147.

158 Hait WN, Jin S, Yang JM. A matter of life or death (or both): understanding autophagy in cancer. *Clin Cancer Res.* 2006;**12(7 Pt 1)**:1961–1965.

160 Druker BJ, Lydon NB. Lessons learned from the development of an abl tyrosine kinase inhibitor for chronic myelogenous leukemia. *J Clin Invest.* 2000;**105(1)**:3–7.

第 55 章 肿瘤药物药理学

Manish R. Sharma, MD ■ Mark J. Ratain, MD

概述

本书中的其他章节已经详细讲述了肿瘤系统治疗中所涉及的生物学及临床指征。本章节主要涉及临床药理学的相关准则及其在肿瘤系统性治疗中的应用。同时，阐述如何应用药代动力学及药效学理论来提升肿瘤药物的治疗指数。美国食品药品管理局(Food and Drug Administration, FDA)对每种上市药品都会进行临床药理学及生物药代动力学的相关审核(http://www.fda.gov/downloads/AboutFDA/ReportsManualsForms/Staff PoliciesandProcedures/ucm073007.pdf)。FDA 的审核结果可以在其官网上通过检索药品名称获得，(http://www.accessdata.fda.gov/scripts/cder/drugsatfda/)审核报告中时常会有药品说明书中所没有的内容。本章节将借助 FDA 对药品审核标准提问模式来介绍肿瘤药物的临床药理，并以实例阐述。

药物一般特性

药物分子的理化性质及其制剂处方在临床药理学和生物药物审核中的关键考虑因素

FDA 在 2000 年引入生物药物分类系统(biopharmaceutics classification system, BCS)以制定新化学分子实体得到临床研究豁免体内生物等效性研究的标准。体外渗透性及溶解度研究可预测体内生物等效性表现这一概念，最早由 Amidon 等[1]提出。BCS 1 级药物(高渗透性/高溶解度)可申请豁免体内生物等效性研究。之后，Wu and Benet[2]基于高渗透率化合物易于从排泄途径(尿液和胆汁)重吸收，所以主要依赖代谢途径清出体外的假设，提出了生物药物表观分布系统(Biopharmaceutics Drug Disposition Classification System, BDDCS)。很多口服的激酶抑制剂抗肿瘤药均为高渗透性/低溶解度化合物，属于 BCS 2 级及 BDDCS 2 级药物。此类药物易受到食物对药物吸收的影响；肠道外排转运体相关的药物-药物相互作用；肝脏摄取/外排转运体或代谢[3]。

有哪些抗肿瘤机制及治疗指征？

抗肿瘤三大类治疗药物包括细胞毒类药物、生物类药物和小分子非细胞毒类药物。在本章节表 55-1 中列举了每一类药物的代表药物以及它们的作用机制。值得说明的是，酪氨酸激酶抑制剂的作用机制可能还不明确，甚至在某一药物已经明确表现出对某个适应证的治疗作用后依然如此。例如，瑞戈非尼有效抑制多种酪氨酸激酶，但是究竟是哪种机制延长化疗失败的结直肠癌转移患者的生存期仍然尚不明确[4]。

究竟有哪些给药途径及剂量？

治疗癌症可能的给药途径包括静脉给药、口服、血管内、脏器内、皮下或肌肉注射给药。很多方面的因素决定何种给药途径为最佳选择。不言自明，静脉给药的方式可使 100% 的药物进入血液。对于口服用药，最终进入血液循环系统的药物占所有给药剂量的比例称之为生物有效利用度。换言之，生物有效利用度是口服药物后血药浓度曲线下面积(area under the curve, AUC)占据同等药物剂量静脉给药后血药浓度(AUC)的比值。生物有效利用度同时受到吸收及首过效应两方面影响。首过效应为口服药物吸收后在进入全身血液循环系统前在消化道和肝脏代谢中损失的部分。口服药物给药方便且理论上价格相对低廉，但却有在不同患者个体间及同一患者内生物有效利用度不均一的劣势[5]。影响口服生物利用度的因素包括患者依从性，药物从剂型中释放的情况，药物在胃肠道内的稳定性，影响药物溶解及吸收的因素(包括食物的影响)，药物进入血液循环系统前代谢的部分，以及同时服用的其他药物(影响吸收及代谢)[6]。血管内及脏器内给药可以在肿瘤附近达到更高的血药浓度[7-9]。最后，曲妥珠单抗治疗乳腺癌的使用经验表明，通过皮下给药的方式可以达到与静脉给药相近的给药效果[10]。

表 55-1 抗肿瘤药物及其作用机制

(a) 细胞毒类药物	药物举例	作用机制
烷化剂	环磷酰胺	与 DNA 交联
铂类药物	顺铂，卡铂，奥沙利铂	与 DNA 交联
抗生素类抗肿瘤药物	多柔比星	抑制拓扑异构酶Ⅱ；稳定拓扑异构酶Ⅱ-DNA 复合物
抗代谢类抗肿瘤药物	抗叶酸类药物：甲氨蝶呤 嘧啶类似物：5-氟尿嘧啶 嘌呤类似物：6-巯基嘌呤	抑制核苷酸整合入 DNA

续表

微管蛋白结合药物	长春花生物碱类:长春新碱、艾立布林、伊沙匹隆	加速或抑制微管蛋白聚合
喜树碱类	伊立替康	抑制拓扑异构酶Ⅰ,诱导 DNA 链断裂
(b) 生物类药物	**药物举例**	**作用机制**
单克隆抗体	拮抗 CD20:利妥昔单抗 拮抗 HER2:曲妥珠单抗 拮抗 EGFR:西妥昔单抗,帕尼单抗 拮抗 PD-1:帕博利珠单抗,纳武利尤单抗 拮抗 VEGF:贝伐珠单抗	与细胞表面受体或信号转导介质结合以阻断信号传递,以及增强抗体依赖型细胞毒性
抗体-药物聚合体	恩美曲妥珠单抗	与 HER2 受体结合以呈递微管蛋白结合剂入细胞
基于蛋白质类药物	阿柏西普	与 VEGF-A,-B,-C 结合
白细胞介素	IL-2,干扰素	增强免疫系统活性
自体细胞免疫治疗	恩扎卢胺	激活免疫系统对前列腺癌抗原产生反应
(c) 小分子非细胞毒类靶向药物/作用机制	**药物举例**	
EGFR 抑制剂	厄洛替尼,阿法替尼	
HER2 抑制剂	拉帕替尼	
ALK 抑制剂	克唑替尼,塞瑞替尼	
VEGFR2 抑制剂	索拉非尼,舒尼替尼,帕唑帕尼	
BRAF 抑制剂	维莫非尼,达拉非尼	
MEK 抑制剂	曲美替尼	
mTOR 抑制剂	依维莫司,替西罗莫司	
BCR-ABL 抑制剂	伊马替尼,尼洛替尼	
KIT 抑制剂	伊马替尼,舒尼替尼,瑞戈非尼	
PARP 抑制剂	奥拉帕利	
ER 拮抗剂	他莫昔芬,氟维司群	
芳香化酶抑制剂	阿那曲唑,来曲唑,依西美坦	
芳香化酶受体拮抗剂	氟他胺,比卡鲁胺,恩扎卢胺	
CYP171 抑制剂	阿比特龙	
蛋白酶体抑制剂	硼替佐米,卡非佐米	
布鲁顿酪氨酸激酶抑制剂	伊布替尼	

肿瘤临床药理总论

临床药理及临床研究中如何确定给药剂量?

抗肿瘤药物的最佳给药剂量为最大抗肿瘤效果,最小化严重不良反应,同时将不同患者间药代动力学差异降到最低。除个别药物外,由于历史原因细胞毒类药物通常依据体表面积确定给药剂量,尽管身高体重仅为影响药代动力学差异性众多因素中的两个[11]。生物大分子类药物通常依据患者体重制定给药剂量,而小分子非细胞毒类药物通常所有患者使用统一剂量。由于传统观点认为剂量越大疗效越强,Ⅰ期临床试验还要确定最大耐受剂量(maximum tolerated dose,MTD),定义为严重不良反应达到一定比例之前的最大剂量[12]。

人们越来越认识到，传统的抗癌药物治疗模式还不尽完善的两个原因。首先，它无法评估患者个体间治疗反应和/或毒性变异的来源，因此也不便于个体化给药。其次，由于对靶向信号途径的饱和生物利用度或饱和效应，许多生物制剂和小分子非细胞毒性药物在低于 MTD 下也可能获得最大的疗效[13,14]。一些最近批准的抗癌新药在上市后被要求进行上市后临床试验以确定替代剂量，而理想的方法是在上市前就进行随机剂量比较研究、药代动力学取样和暴露-药效反应分析[15]。

选择药效反应终点（即临床或替代终点）或生物标记物（统称为药效学）的依据是什么？在临床药理学和临床研究中如何衡量它们？

抗癌治疗的传统药效反应终点是总生存期（overall survival，OS）、无进展生存期（progression-free survival，PFS；定义为死亡或疾病进展-以先发生者为准）或客观反应率，定义为肿瘤最大直径之和缩小至少 30%［借用实体瘤疗效评价（response evaluation criteria in solid tumors，RECIST）标准］[16]。虽然 RECIST 作为评价药物疗效的指标还有许多局限性，但它仍然是最常用的方法[17]。国家癌症研究所药物指导委员会（Investigational Drug Steering Committee，IDSC）提出了关于选择抗癌疗法二期试验终点和在新抗癌治疗早期临床试验中使用生物标记物的建议[18,19]。

血浆（或其他生物液体）中的活性部分是否得到适当的鉴定和测量，以评估药代动力学参数和暴露-反应关系？

许多抗癌疗法需要激活后才能发挥其抗癌效果，活化过程涉及正常组织或肿瘤组织中的化学或酶反应。在大多数情况下，药物激活过程发生在细胞内，因此在血浆中无法测量到药物的活性成分。例如，顺铂在细胞内与水分子发生化学反应，产生一种带正电荷的水化物，攻击 DNA 上的亲核位点[20]。抗代谢类抗肿瘤药物，如吉西他滨、5-氟尿嘧啶和甲氨蝶呤，分别在细胞内发生磷酸化，磷酸核糖化和多聚糖反应，以发挥它们的最大作用[21-23]；另一些抗癌药物主要在肝脏被激活，因此其活性成分可以而且应该在血浆中测量，以探索有效的暴露-响应关系。一个例子是拓扑异构酶交联剂伊立替康，它被肝羧酸酯酶转化为活性部分 SN-38，后者释放到全身血液循环，可用来预测伊立替康发生严重不良反应的概率[24]。

药物暴露-药效反应关系

反映药物有效性的暴露-反应关系有哪些特点？

抗癌治疗的结果取决于药代动力学和药效学。药代动力学指的是用药剂量和血药浓度之间的关系，而药效学指的是浓度（或暴露）和"反应"之间的关系，药物反应广义定义为药物的任何可测量的效应，包括药物的疗效、毒性或者以上两者之外的其他作用。暴露-反应关系有助于确定药物在不引起严重毒性的情况下有效的目标暴露范围（通常称为治疗指数）。很多抗癌药物的治疗指数都很窄。

一般来说，任何药物都可以被视为具有最大效应和中位剂量（最大效应 50% 所需的剂量）。基于所有药物效应都需要与受体的初始相互作用的假设，Wagner 提出了一个广义的 S 曲线药物效应模型（图 55-1）[25]。只在细胞周期的某些阶段（阶段特异性）起作用的药物，通常与在细胞周期的任何阶段都起作用的药物（非阶段特异性药物）相比，具有不同的药效学曲线。对于细胞周期非相特异型药物，例如环磷酰胺和其他烷化剂，可以使用简单的对数线性模型来表示其药效曲线。如下所示：

$$\text{存活率} = \text{治疗细胞数}/\text{对照细胞数} = e^{-KC} \qquad (1)$$

该模型具有陡峭的暴露-反应曲线，因为随着药物浓度（C）的增加，药效继续成比例增加。对于任何 K（在等式 1 中），药物浓度 C 每增加 $2.3/K$，将导致抗肿瘤作用增加 1-log（图 55-2a）[26,27]。

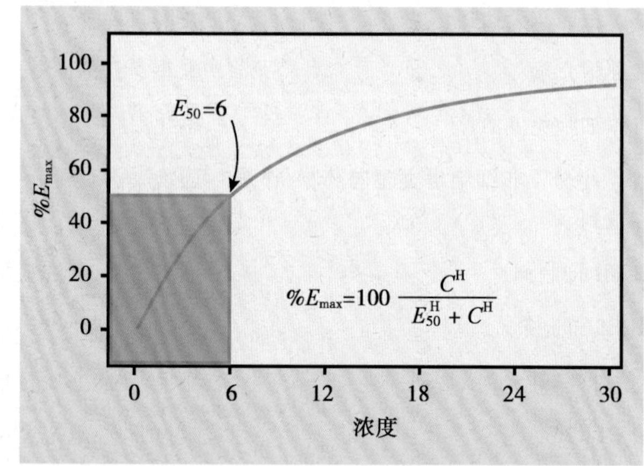

图 55-1 Wagner 提出的 E_{max} 模型示例。最大效应为 100%，药物浓度为 6 时，药效达到 50%。幂数 H，也称为 Hill 常数，决定曲线的形状，通常在 1 到 2 之间

对于细胞周期特异性药物，如抗代谢药物，暴露-反应关系要复杂得多。根据定义，有些细胞并不处于特定的细胞周期之中，因此细胞在药物暴露期间对药物的影响不敏感（或相对不敏感）。这一点不能通过增加剂量来克服，但却可以通过增加药物暴露的持续时间来解决[28]。结果是暴露反应曲线出现平台（图 55-2b）。更为复杂的是，血浆浓度可能不足以预测那些进行细胞内合成代谢以产生活性代谢物的药物的临床效果，例如阿糖胞苷和许多其他抗代谢类肿瘤药。

恩美曲妥珠单抗（trastuzumab emtansine，T-DM1）是一种抗体-药物偶联剂，由一种针对 HER2 胞外结构域的重组人源化单克隆抗体与一种微管蛋白稳定剂结合而成。T-DM1 是一种新药，已经对其暴露-反应关系进行了充分研究。T-DM1 用于治疗 HER2 阳性转移性乳腺癌的病例中，在调整基线风险因素后，第 1 个治疗周期第 21 天较高的谷浓度的患者，其 OS、PFS 均更好。事实上，暴露于中位浓度水平以下的患者的 OS 和 PFS 与拉帕替尼联合卡培他滨的有效对照组相当，提示剂量增加可能改善这部分患者的有效性。其他抗癌治疗药物暴露-反应关系总结见表 55-2。尽管仍有争议，基于药物暴露-反应关系，已经建议对许多酪氨酸激酶抑制剂进行治疗药物监测[43]。

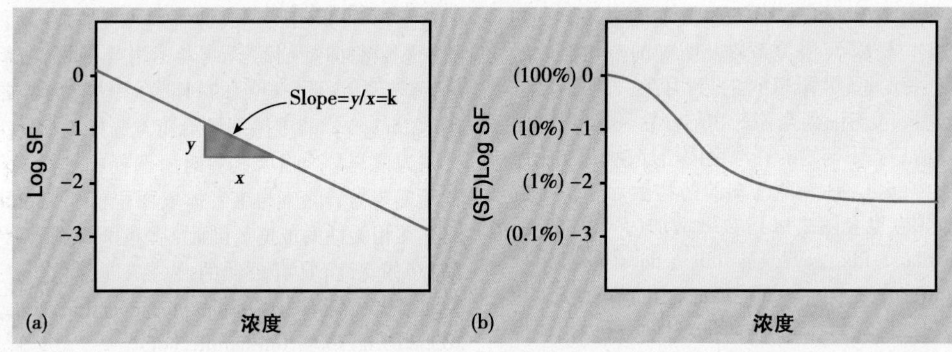

图 55-2　(a)药效不会饱和药物的药效学曲线及(b)药效会饱和药物的药效学曲线。在图中最简单的药效学模型(a)中,药物浓度与肿瘤细胞残存对数间存在线性关系。在药效学模型(b)中,药物疗效有最大极限,在达到一定浓度之后,药物剂量与药效曲线达到阈值不再变化。缩写:SF,肿瘤细胞残存比例

表 55-2　目前已经确定药物暴露量与疗效关系的抗肿瘤药物举例

药物	疾病	参考文献
阿昔替尼	肾细胞癌	Rini *et al.* [31]
白消安	异体干细胞移植	Bleyzac *et al.* [32]
卡铂	卵巢癌	Jodrell *et al.* [33]
达沙替尼	慢性粒细胞白血病	Wang *et al.* [34]
厄洛替尼	非小细胞肺癌	Tiseo *et al.* [35]
5-氟尿嘧啶	头颈部肿瘤	Milano *et al.* [36]
伊马替尼	慢性粒细胞白血病,胃肠道间质瘤	Larson *et al.* [37] Demetri *et al.* [38]
甲氨蝶呤	急性淋巴细胞白血病	Evans *et al.* [39]
高三尖杉酯	慢性粒细胞白血病	FDA review[a]
培唑帕尼	肾细胞癌	Suttle *et al.* [40]
舒尼替尼	肾细胞癌,胃肠道间质瘤	Houk *et al.* [41]
曲妥珠单抗	胃癌,胃食管癌	Cosson *et al.* [42]
恩美曲妥珠单抗	HER2 阳性乳腺癌	Wang *et al.* [30]
维莫非尼	黑色素瘤	FDA review[b]

这只是一个说明性的列表,而不是一个全面的列表。
[a] http://www.accessdata.fda.gov/drugsatfda_docs/nda/2012/203585Orig1s000ClinPharmR.pdf
[b] http://www.accessdata.fda.gov/drugsatfda_docs/nda/2011/202429Orig1s000ClinPharmR.pdf

出于用药安全考虑的药物暴露-反应关系有哪些特征?

用药安全性的药物暴露-反应关系与疗效的药物暴露-反应关系很类似,区别在于研究方向是药物潜在的严重毒性,而不是疗效测量。许多细胞毒性药物的历史经验已经体现出阐明这种药物暴露-反应关系的价值。大剂量甲氨蝶呤后的毒性与延迟清除甲氨蝶呤的毒性之间的关系导致常规使用治疗药物监测血浆甲氨蝶呤浓度以指导四氢叶酸给药[44]。紫杉醇用药量与中性粒细胞减少(可推广至其他细胞毒性治疗)的关系最好使用非线性模型进行描述,该模型考虑了血药浓度对骨髓抑制的间接影响,并且此类模型为许多药物的剂量和间隔提供了优化参考[45,46]。另一个具有明显药物暴露-反应安全性关系特征的药物是卡铂,它是顺铂的类似物。与顺铂不同,卡铂的用药剂量限制毒性是血小板减少,该不良反应与药物剂量、患者肾功能、治疗前血小板计数和先前治疗均有关[47]。卡铂产生的血小板最低值与卡铂的清除率有关,卡铂的清除率与患者肌酐清除率成正比关系。因此,卡铂治疗后有严重血小板减少的高危患者可在用药前就提前确定,并且可以通过监测肌酐清除率来调整药物剂量。尽管已经有很多在治疗过程中通过监测血药浓度来避免严重药物不良反应的尝试,但这些尝试通常都无法产生有临床意义的结果。

维莫非尼是一种口服小分子 BRAF 激酶抑制剂，作用于转移性黑色素瘤患者中具有 V600E 或 V600K 突变的个体。它同时具有明确的用药安全暴露-反应关系以及明确的药物疗效暴露-反应关系（值得注意的是，尽管 FDA 的药物标签表明该药物可能与或者不与食物一起服用，但当该药物与食物一起服用时，吸收量会增加）。随着稳态下药物的谷浓度的增加，鳞状细胞癌的发生率（鳞状细胞癌，SCC，是一种已知的药物治疗相关的癌症，治疗相关不良反应）也会随之以指数级增加（$P<0.0001$）（http://www.accessdata.fda.gov/drugsatfda_docs/nda/2011/202429Orig1s000ClinPharmR.pdf）。即便如此，由于生存获益超过了药物安全风险，依然不建议降低用药量以预防药物相关性鳞状细胞癌。

抗肿瘤药是否延长 QT 或 QTc 间期？

许多药物由于延迟心室的去极化和复极导致延长 QT 间期。QT 间期由两个公认的公式中的一个来计算由心率校正后的 QT 间期（QTc）。QT 间期延长可导致室性心动过速（特别是尖端扭转型室性心动过速，Tdp），甚至可能进一步导致心搏骤停。由于心源性猝死风险的增加是一个重大的用药安全问题，FDA 和其他监管机构要求药物生产厂家在新药临床开发过程中充分评估该项风险。2005 年，FDA 制定了国际指南来全面规范 QT 研究的设计和数据解读，这些指导规范经 FDA 整合为一个针对药品生产行业颁布的指南文件（Guidance for Industry: E14 Clinical Evaluation of QT/QTc Interval Prolongation and Proarrhythmic Potential for Non-Antiarrhythmic Drugs. FDA, October 2005）。在该指南中，FDA 建议将 ΔΔQTc（与基线 QTc 相比的变化值，经安慰剂效应校正后）作为药物对 QT 影响的全面研究终点指标，并且使用 95% 单侧置信区间的上限（等同于 90% 双侧置信区间的上限）衡量药物对 QTc 延长作用的最大平均值应小于 10ms，方可得出该药物没有明显延长 QTc，进而产生安全风险的结论。

尼洛替尼是一种口服小分子 BCR-ABL 及其他激酶抑制剂，用于慢性髓系白血病的治疗。依据 E14 指南，对健康志愿者进行了一项全面的 QT 研究，尽管该研究中健康志愿者体内的药物浓度低于癌症患者在批准治疗剂量下预期可达到的血药浓度，仍然明确证明了药物稳态浓度与 ΔΔQTc 之间的关系。（http://www.accessdata.fda.gov/drugsatfda_docs/nda/2007/022068s000_ClinPharmR.pdf）。基于此，不建议低钾血症、低镁血症或长 QT 综合征患者这类对 QTc 延长类药物敏感患者使用该药物。更进一步，FDA 要求药物生产厂家发起一项风险评估及控制计划（REMS）以将“QT 间期延长及其心脏风险降至最低”。（https://www.accessdata.fda.gov/drugsatfda_docs/label/2010/022068s001rems.pdf）。作为 REMS 的一部分，在药品说明书上的黑框警告中，处方医生和患者应注意避免同时使用已知延长 QT 间期的药物以及 CYP3A4 酶抑制剂和食物，这两类药物相互作用都会大大增加患者体内的药物浓度。建议在药物治疗前的基线检查时、开始治疗后 1 周以及之后定期进行心电图监测，包括药物剂量调整后也要重新进行心电图检查（Tasigna 处方信息 http://www.accessdata.fda.gov/drugsatfda_docs/label/2007/022068lbl.pdf）。

药品生产厂家选择的给药剂量和方案是否与剂量、浓度和反应之间的已知关系一致，是否存在任何未解决的用药剂量或给药问题？

虽然大多数抗癌治疗的剂量和方案都是根据剂量-浓度-反应关系来选择的，但仍有一些尚未解决的剂量问题，例如高三尖杉酯，一种蛋白质合成抑制剂，批准用于对两种或两种以上酪氨酸激酶抑制剂耐药或者不耐受的慢性髓系白血病患者。尽管该药物说明书建议的剂量为在诱导剂量之后，按照体表面积 1.25mg/m² 的维持剂量给药。选择 1.25mg/m² 的维持剂量是因为该剂量为临床试验时所选择的剂量。药品审查人员没有发现药物清除率与患者体表面积（body surface area，BSA）之间存在相关性的证据。因此，基于 BSA 给药会导致较小体型的患者（如女性）具有更低的血药浓度，而这与疗效下降直接相关。（http://www.accessdata.fda.gov/drugsatfda_docs/nda/2012/203585Orig1s000ClinPharmR.pdf）。

另一个例子是卡巴他赛，一种微管稳定剂，该药被批准用于在多西他赛治疗后激素治疗抵抗的转移性前列腺癌患者。在该药用于晚期前列腺癌的Ⅱ期临床试验中，初始剂量为每 3 周给药 20mg/m²，如果在第 1 个化疗周期中未观察到 2 级以上毒性，则允许将计量增加至 25mg/m²。尽管在 71 名患者中只有 21 名在第 2 个周期内可以升级，但生产厂家在Ⅲ期临床试验中选择了 25mg/m² 每 3 周给药一次的化疗剂量方案治疗前列腺癌。根据现有的数据，治疗效果与用药剂量之间没有明确的关系，但药物 AUC 与 3 级及以上中性粒细胞减少的发生率呈正相关。由此推断，部分患者可以通过从低的剂量开始用药，避免调整用药剂量，以及额外使用生长因子支持的需要（http://www.accessdata.tda.gov/drugsatfdadocs/nda/2010/2010235000clinpharmr.pdf）。最后，当一种药物在一种新的药物中被研究并被批准用于新的适应证时，通常都会遇到如何确定给药剂量的问题。以曲妥珠单抗为例，在曲妥珠单抗联合化疗治疗转移性 HER2 阳性胃/胃食管交界（gastroesophageal junction，GEJ）癌疗效的Ⅲ期临床中，使用了曲妥珠单抗用于治疗乳腺癌的批准用药剂量[48]。随后，一篇病例报告和生产厂家的药代动力学回顾表明，该药用于转移性胃/GEJ 癌时的清除率比用于乳腺癌时要高约 70%[49]。一种可能的解释是转移性胃癌患者有更高的肿瘤负荷和更多的循环 HER2 胞外结构域水平，从而导致药物更快的从患者体内清除。另一种可能性是胃癌患者可能具有较低的白蛋白浓度，导致药物清除率较高，标准剂量与较高剂量曲妥珠单抗目前正在 HER2 阳性转移胃/GEJ 患者的随机Ⅲ期试验中进行研究（Heloise 研究；NCT 01450696）。

药物及其主要代谢物的药代动力学特征是什么？

单剂量和多剂量给药的药代动力学参数有哪些？

药代动力学是一门研究药物的吸收、分布、代谢和排泄的学科。药代动力学中的一个基本概念是药物清除，即从体内清除药物，类似于肌酐清除的概念。在临床实践中，药物的清除率很少是直接测量的，而是按以下方法之一计算的

$$\text{药物清除率}=\text{剂量}/\text{AUC} \tag{2}$$

$$\text{药物清除率}=\text{输注速率}/C_{ss} \tag{3}$$

AUC 代表随时间累积的总药物暴露量，是药代动力学和药效学分析的重要参数。如公式 2 所示，清除率仅仅是剂量与 AUC 的比率，因此在相等的给药剂量下，AUC 越高，清除率就越低。如果通过持续输注方式给药并达到稳定状态，则可通过单次测量血浆药物浓度（C）来估计清除率，如公式 3 所示。

药物清除率在概念上可以被认为是分布和消除的函数。在最简单的药代动力学模型中,

$$药物清除率=VK \quad (4)$$

其中 V 是表观分布容积,K 是清除常数。V 是药物最初分布的液体体积,因此 V 越高,初始浓度越低。K 是清除常数,它与半衰期成反比,半衰期是血浆浓度下降 50%所消耗的时间。当半衰期较短时,K 值较高,血浆浓度迅速下降。因此,高 V 和高 K 都会导致高清除率和相对较低的血浆浓度。

在大多数抗肿瘤治疗的Ⅰ期临床试验中,药代动力学取样在首次给药后的多个时间点进行,并且在多次给药后再次进行,后者可能达到,也可能达不到稳态浓度。对于单剂量采样,所给出的参数通常包括观察到的最大浓度(C_{max})、最大浓度时的时间(T_{max})、AUC、V、清除率和半衰期。对于多剂量采样,除了在给药前可能添加最低浓度(C_{min})外,参数通常与单剂量给药时相同。

药代动力学参数可以用以下两种方法之一来描述。第一种方法为非隔室模型,经两个步骤得出药代动力学参数。在这个过程中,首先估算出每个患者的 C_{max} 和 AUC 等参数,然后汇总计算出群体的药代动力学参数。非隔室模型分析可快速完成,并且不需要特殊的分析软件。第二种方法为是群体药代动力学模型,为一步过程,通过构建一个非线性的包含一个或多个隔室的混合效应模型,估计患者群体的药物代谢动力学参数。群体药代动力学模型有几个优点:①它可以用稀疏的(较少的时间点)采样数据来完成;②它不易丢失数据;③它可以很容易地包含使患者间变异性最小化的协变量。群体药代动力学模型的缺点是它需要使用特殊的软件,并且需要经过相应训练方可掌握软件的使用方法[50]。感兴趣的读者可以从实际操作这些软件中受益。对普通读者来说,有几点需要强调。药代动力学模型的有效性在很大程度上取决于用于建立模型的数据的质量,因此,药物输注必须精确定时,必须提取足够数量的血样,血样必须按时抽取,并且分析方法必须敏感且特异。此外,必须对数据进行适当加权,以避免由于药物浓度接近分析检出限时分析误差概率增加而产生结果偏差,使用特定模型获得的结果应与使用非隔室模型分析的结果进行比较。在已知时间点以外的模型外推必须非常小心。

药物吸收的特点有哪些?

对药物吸收的差异是药代动力学中患者间变异性的主要来源。药物吸收的速度和程度取决于它在肠黏膜的溶解度和渗透性。在药代动力学模型中,吸收通常由一阶速率常数 K_a 估计。吸收是可以饱和的,这意味着当给药剂量超过某一阈值剂量后,继续增加剂量不会导致的更高的血药浓度。BCS 1 类药物具有高渗透性和高溶解度,吸收速度快且完全,而 BCS 2~4 类中药物的吸收可变,并受多种因素的影响。例如,许多小分子酪氨酸激酶抑制剂的吸收受限于细胞膜外转运蛋白,如 P-糖蛋白(也称为 ABCB 1)、乳腺癌耐药蛋白(ABCG 2)和多药耐药蛋白家族(ABCC 家族)的成员。作为一种耐药机制,同样的细胞膜外转运蛋白可能在癌细胞中过度表达[51]。饮食因素对于药物吸收也非常重要,因为许多口服抗癌药物与餐同服时吸收增强,导致与食物一起服用时血药浓度增加(并可能增加不良反应),特别是高脂肪食物更为明显。例如厄洛替尼、拉帕替尼、尼洛替尼、培唑帕尼、维莫非尼和阿比特龙,阿比特龙与高脂肪食物同服时的 AUC(与隔夜禁食相比)增加 10 倍[52-54]。这些口服抗癌药通常建议空腹服用,尽管事实上食物增加了药物的吸收率,这一点与非癌症药物相反(与餐同服以增加药物吸收);理论上,如果患者未能严格遵照说明书建议空腹服药,那么发生药物不良反应风险就会增加[53,55]。许多口服抗癌药都是弱碱性的,它们的溶解度受到 pH 影响,如果患者同时使用质子泵抑制剂或其他抗胃酸药物则可能减少口服抗癌药物的吸收。如果患者同时使用质子泵抑制剂或其他抗胃酸药物既可能由医生处方,也可能由患者自行购买的非处方药。例如与抗胃酸药合用时达沙替尼、厄洛替尼、吉非替尼和尼洛替尼时可显著降低血药浓度[56]。当医生开出这些激酶抑制剂处方时,应指示患者避免使用可能会影响这些药物的复杂性的抑酸剂。

药物表观分布的特点是什么?

在药代动力学模型中,模型中每个室的体积分布受到许多因素的影响。最显著的是药物的水溶性和蛋白结合。亲水性化合物,如甲氨蝶呤,可以溶解到液体集合中(如胸膜积液或腹水),并显著延迟药物从中央(血浆)室的清除[57]。另一方面,聚乙二醇化脂质体多柔比星是被设计成疏水药物的一个例子。与普通多柔比星相比,它的表观分布容积非常小,主要是局限于血管之内,因为血管内皮细胞紧密连接的脂质体的防止外渗,这可能也就解释了其心脏毒性较小的原因[58]。蛋白结合率对于药物起效是非常重要的,因为只有游离的药物才能达到其作用靶点,也只有游离的药物可以被清除。维莫德吉是一种与-1-酸糖蛋白(AAG)和白蛋白具有高度可逆性结合的药物,导致血浆中未结合药物浓度低于总药物浓度的 1%,因此药物的清除率较低。AAG 水平约占患者间药动学差异的 70%,这表明这是影响药物"伴随药物或疾病状态"的药动学的最重要因素[59]。低蛋白血症可能会增加未结合药物的比例,但这一现象对维莫德吉和大多数其他药物的临床意义仍不清楚[60]。

质量平衡研究是否表明肾脏或肝脏是主要的消除途径?

质量平衡研究涉及给人类使用放射性标记药物,通过测量血液、尿液和粪便中不同时间点的放射性,以了解肝代谢、胆道排泄和尿排泄在多大程度上起到了药物清除的作用。生物样本也被用来鉴定和量化母体药物及其代谢物[61]。FDA 指南建议,任何代谢产物在稳定状态下的浓度超过母体 AUC 的 10%时,都应该在临床前动物模型中进行毒理学评估(https://www.fda.gov/OHRMS/DOCKETS/98fr/FDA-2008-D-0065-GDL.pdf)。

有许多抗癌药物主要通过肾或肝途径来清除的。如卡铂和甲氨蝶呤主要以原型经肾脏清除。由此,基于患者肾功能可计算卡铂的剂量。其计算简单,如公式 5 所示[62]。

$$卡铂剂量(mg)=(目标\ AUC)\times(GFR+25) \quad (5)$$

甲氨蝶呤经尿液途径清除,可引起肾小管的沉淀,引起肾毒性。研究表明,因为甲氨蝶呤在 pH 较高时更容易溶解,碱化尿液可预防高剂量甲氨蝶呤肾毒性和其他毒性[63,64]。另一方面,所有的紫杉醇类药物(包括紫杉醇、白蛋白紫杉醇、多西他赛和卡巴他赛)都经历了广泛的肝代谢和胆道排泄,需对肝功能不全患者重新调整剂量[65]。进行良好的器官功能障碍研究有助于指

导肾和/或肝功能受损患者选择最合适的抗癌治疗剂量/方案。理想情况下,这些研究应在药物上市前完成,但也有在上市后阶段完成此类研究的例子,如伊马替尼和索拉非尼[66,67]。

药物代谢的特点是什么?

如果通过质量平衡方法研究经历显著代谢的药物,那么需要解决一些后续问题。肝脏摄取率在 0 到 1 之间变化,大致上是一种衡量血液单次通过肝脏时从系统循环中清除药物的效率的指标。肝脏低摄取率(<0.3)药物,不受肝脏血流的影响。但其清除率与血浆蛋白结合有关。与之相反,高摄取率(>0.7)的药物清除率与肝血流量相关,但不受血浆蛋白结合的影响。肝动脉灌注去氧氟尿苷而非 5-FU 治疗肝转移瘤的概念是基于去氧氟尿苷具有较高的肝摄取率,高剂量可局部给药而不引起全身毒性[68]。负责新陈代谢的酶可分为 3 个代谢阶段:修饰(第一阶段)、结合(第二阶段)或排泄(第三阶段)。第一阶段反应包括氧化、还原和水解,通常由肝微粒体中丰富的细胞色素 p450 酶催化。在第二阶段反应中,第一阶段反应的活性代谢物与带电粒子结合,使它们更亲水。最后,在第三阶段反应中,ATP 结合(abc)转运蛋白家族的成员将第二阶段产物转移到细胞外介质中。例如,伊立替康首先被羧酸酯酶(第一阶段)活化为其活性代谢物 SN-38,然后被 CYP3A4 代谢为非活性代谢物氨基戊烷羧酸(APC)。然后,SN-38 通过 UDP 葡萄糖醛酸合成酶 1 多肽 A1(UGT1A1;第二阶段)被葡萄糖醛酸化为 SN-38 葡萄糖醛酸(SN-38-G)。SN-38-G 通过 ABCC2 转运体(第三阶段)排泄到胆汁中[69]。对于伊立替康,部分药物和这三种代谢物(APC、SN-38 和 SN-38-G)占质量平衡研究中平均放射化学 AUC 的 93%,表明这些是起关键作用的药物代谢酶[70]。通常首先在人肝微粒体或人肝细胞中进行体外研究,然后在动物体内进行研究,最后在人体内进行研究以确定起关键作用的药物代谢酶。液相色谱-质谱(LC-MS)技术现在广泛用于药物代谢研究中进行鉴定和测定药物代谢产物[71]。

药物排泄的特点是什么?

药物排泄的特征不仅包括药物是主要通过胆汁还是肾脏途径排出,还包括被排出的特定代谢物和参与其排泄的转运体。某些药物的排泄过程可能是直接的,而其他的药物可能相当复杂。继续以伊立替康举例。当 SN-38-G 从胆汁中排出后,大肠埃希菌等肠道细菌可以通过产生 b-葡萄糖醛酸酶将化合物转换回活性代谢物 SN-38,并且这种 SN-38 可以被重新吸收并返回到肝脏,这种现象被称为肠肝循环。事实上,伊立替康给药后 SN-38 的药代动力学模型要求包含肝肠循环以准确地描述观察到的数据[72]。顺铂同样经历了复杂的排泄过程,其在肾小管中既有主动分泌又有再吸收[73,74]。

根据药代动力学参数,剂量-浓度关系的线性或非线性程度如何?

线性药代动力学模型的主要特点是

$$dC/dt = -KC \tag{6}$$

这表明药物浓度的瞬时变化率仅取决于当前的药物浓度。无论药物浓度有多高,清除率和半衰期都将保持不变,这一原则的一个应用是 AUC 不受药物给药间隔方案变化的影响。例如,60mg/m^2 剂量的多柔比星单次给药的 AUC,等于分 3 次每天(或每周)20mg/m^2 剂量的 AUC 总和,也等于 96 小时输注相同剂量的 AUC。第二个应用是,AUC 与剂量成比例。因此,如果已经测量了 60mg/m^2 剂量的 AUC,则可以估计同一患者 90mg/m^2 剂量的 AUC 为前者的 1.5 倍。通过绘制药物在不同给药剂量下所得到的 AUC 这一简单图表,即可判断该药物是否具有线性药代动力学。

最简单的线性药代动力学模型如图 55-3 所示:

$$C(t) = \frac{剂量}{V}(e^{-kt}) \tag{7}$$

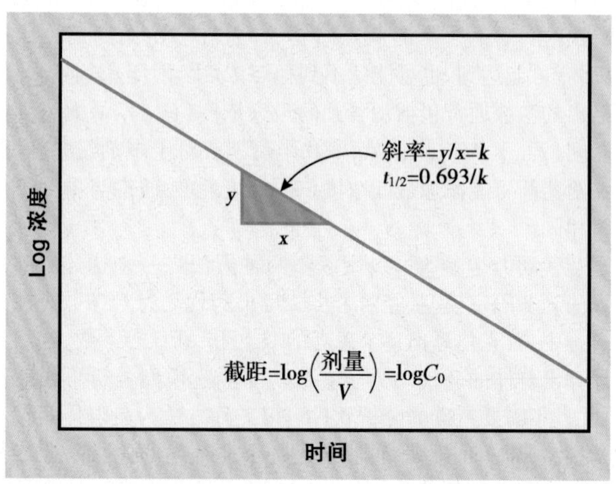

图 55-3 一室线性药物浓度-时间曲线图。C_0 表示初始浓度,假设瞬时给药和分配。半衰期为 $\log_e(2)/k$。V,表观分布容积

这个模型假设药物瞬时完成给药,并且完全的分布也是瞬时的。这些假设通常是无效的。如果药物是在时间(t)内持续注射给药。在给药的过程中,由于药物的浓度在增加,必须对模型进行校正。

$$C(t) = \frac{剂量}{VKT}(1 - e^{-kt}) \tag{8}$$

输注结束后,药物浓度的衰减速度与瞬间完成给药情况下的速度相同。因此,如果 T 表示输液时间,那么输液后的药物浓度可以表示为

$$C'(t) = C(T)e^{-k(t-T)} \tag{9}$$

通常,药代动力学数据要比图 55-3 所示更加复杂,并且可能更加适合使用多室模型上,通常为两个或三个隔室(图 55-4)。必须强调的是,这些隔室仅是理论性的,不一定与任何解剖空间或生理过程相关。

非线性药代动力学的存在意味着药物的药代动力学行为方面是可饱和的。非线性模型的数学运算超出了本章的范围,但是这些原理与几种抗癌药物非常相关[75,76]。药物的变化和药物的作用机制相反,改变非线性动力学的药物的给药方案可能显著影响 AUC,并可能改变临床效果。

非线性药代动力学通常发生于主要代谢产物或运输途径饱和的时候。这种非线性药代动力学行为通常在高剂量时导致清除率降低,使得 AUC 以超过比例的速度大幅增加。如果缩短药物输注时间,在较高的峰值血浆浓度下,清除速度相对

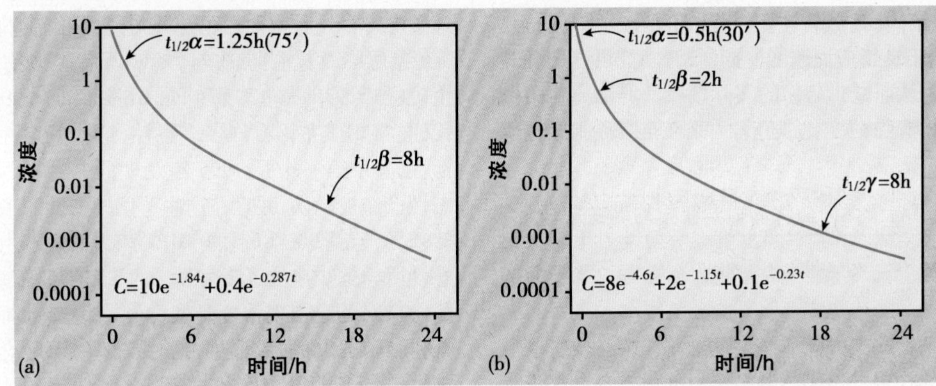

图 55-4　典型 2 室(a)和 3 室(b)线性药代动力学模型的浓度-时间曲线。这两条曲线非常相似,假定两条曲线的初始药物浓度均为 10。注意,对于每个隔室均有一个项,相应的半衰期等于 $t_{1/2}=\log(2)/k^n$,其中 k^n 是第 n 项

较慢。5-FU 就是这种情况,可能是因为将 5-FU 转化为二氢氟尿嘧啶的二氢嘧啶脱氢酶发生饱和[77-79]。5-FU 可使用多种给药方案,其非线性药代动力学行为可能是其严格要求遵照方案给药的原因。因为其配方的原因,紫杉醇也被证明具有非线性药代动力学[80-82]。因此,在固定剂量下,通过较短的(3 小时 vs 24 小时)输注时常给予紫杉醇时,AUC 较高,尽管这并不会导致毒性增强[83]。

相反的情况是当药物从胃肠道的吸收(或肾小管的再吸收)是饱和的。在这种情况下,剂量的增加导致 AUC 的增加低于比例。具有饱和吸收的药物的例子包括类似天然化合物的药物在胃肠道的吸收通常是由显示饱和动力学的叶酸类似物(如甲氨蝶呤或亮氨酸)和氨基酸类似物(如美法仑)的主动转运过程介导的[84-86]。顺铂由于其肾小管再吸收饱和而呈现非线性药物动力学特性[74,87]。与 20 分钟输注相比,24 小时持续输注的血浆中游离铂增加 42%。

缓慢给药后药动学参数是否随时间变化?

当给药速率等于药物消除速率时,即为稳态。累积比率与稳态下的暴露(由 C_{max}、AUC 或 C_{min} 测量)与单次剂量后的暴露相关,并且与剂量间隔成反比。虽然这个比率可以用单剂量药代动力学参数来预测,但直接用观测数据来测量这个比率更为准确。对于单室药动学药物,稳态时间与半衰期成正比,且与剂量和给药间隔无关。在实践中,通常认为在 4~5 个半衰期内达到稳态。稳态时的血浆浓度(C_p^{ss})可以估计为

$$C_p^{ss}=S\times F\times D/\mathrm{CL}\times\tau \qquad (10)$$

其中 S 是盐因子(译者注:表示盐类药物电离为游离的离子形态比例),F 是生物利用度,D 是剂量,CL 是清除率,τ 是给药间隔。不遵医嘱服用药物可以随时间降低 C_p^{ss},而药物-药物相互作用和饮食情况可以随时间增加或减少 C_p^{ss}。有一些特定的抗癌药物,很容易随着时间的推移,C_p^{ss} 产生变化。例如,环磷酰胺对参与其代谢的 CYP450 酶的自我诱导作用导致其在 96 小时输注结束时的 CL 大约加倍[88]。尽管其机制尚不清楚,但一项针对胃肠道肿瘤患者的前瞻性研究表明,伊马替尼在稳定之前的治疗前 90 天,其血药浓度减少了大约 30%[89]。对于伊马替尼等具有明确暴露-反应关系的药物,由于随着时间推移血药浓度发生缓慢的变化,可以考虑对患者进行治疗性药物监测。

志愿者和患者的药代动力学参数在受试者间和受试者内的变异性是什么?变异性的主要原因是什么?

药代动力学参数的患者间变异性对优化抗癌治疗具有潜在的重要意义。参数的变异程度通常表示为变异系数(标准差与平均值之比),可通过非隔室模型或群体药代动力学模型进行估计。由于生物利用度的变异性,口服制剂的药动学变异性高于静脉制剂。

例如,在一项依托泊苷的研究中,口服与静脉注射药物的 AUC 的变异系数分别为 58% 和 28%[90]。

表 55-3 列出了癌症患者的患者间药代动力学变异的潜在来源,其中许多也是群体药代动力学模型中患者间药代动力学变异的潜在来源,表 55-3 中的变量可以作为药代动力学模型协变量进行研究,可检验加入这些变量进入模型后,是否显著降低了患者间的变异性,或者并提高了整体模型与观察数据的拟合度。联合用药可以通过影响吸收、消除和蛋白质结合来解释变异性。与志愿者相比,患者更常见的不良反应,如恶心/呕吐和体重减轻,可导致治疗情境发生变化。低白蛋白血症更常见于癌症患者,可能导致更高的生物制剂清除率。例如,在进展期胃癌或胃癌患者中,曲妥珠单抗的群体药动学模型发现,降低血清白蛋白水平与增加药物清除率有关[42]。类似地,使用先前建立的群体药代动力学模型(使用来自其他癌症患者的数据开发)对进展期胃癌患者接受贝伐单抗治疗的清除率进行估计,证明低白蛋白患者的药物清除率更快[91]。餐前状态对患者间和患者体内的药代动力学变异性都有显著影响。阿比特龙的群体药代动力学模型表明,食物中脂肪含量较高与阿比特龙合用降低其生物利用度。另一方面,去势耐药的转移性前列腺癌患者(与健康受试者相比)清除率较低[92]。

由于需要在以后的时间点对同一受试者进行重复的药代动力学抽血取样,因此很难估计患者个体内的药代动力学变异性。例如,肿瘤医生常常面临对同一患者反复给药后脊髓抑制增加的临床情况。这通常被认为是由于化疗的累积效应,使患者对随后的剂量更加敏感。然而,也有可能患者对药物的清除率降低,从而导致药物浓度增加,进而诱发更严重的骨髓抑制。

器官功能的变化是个体内药代动力学变异性的主要来源，肾功能可能因为进行性疾病（输尿管梗阻并发症的治疗量耗竭）或由于治疗（顺铂）的不良反应而改变。同样，肾功能可能会随着时间的推移而改善，从而减少药物的实际接触。肝功能也可能发生变化，产生药物清除的变化，随着时间的推移可能导致毒性增加。

表 55-3 癌症患者个体间药代动力学变异的潜在来源

影响吸收性的因素
恶心/呕吐[a]
手术、放疗和/或化疗史[a]
影响肠道运动的止吐药（如甲氧氯普胺）[a]
患者依从性[a]
肠内药物代谢和/或药物转运酶的遗传差异[a]
膳食状态（对于具有显著食物影响因素的药物）[a]
影响药物分布
减肥[a]
肥胖
体脂减少（亲脂性药物）[a]
胸腔积液或腹水（甲氨蝶呤）[a]
影响消除的因素（代谢和/或排泄）
肝功能不全
肾功能不全
药物代谢和/或药物转运酶的遗传差异
低蛋白血症（生物类药物）
联合用药
影响蛋白质结合的因素
低蛋白血症[a]
同时使用的其他药物[a]

[a] 患者体内药代动力学变化的潜在来源。

内在因素

哪些内在因素（年龄、性别、种族、体重、身高、疾病、遗传多态性、妊娠和器官功能障碍）影响药物浓度和/或反应，药物浓度的任何差异对疗效或安全反应有何影响？根据已知的浓度-反应关系及其变异性以及所研究的组、健康志愿者与患者与特定人群的对比，建议对这些组中的每一组进行哪些剂量方案调整（如果有的话）？

由于患者内在因素会影响抗肿瘤药物的浓度，如果对浓度的影响足够大，也会影响药物疗效或安全性，那么在某些人群中避免使用该药物，或进行剂量调整可能是必要的。例如，6-巯基嘌呤是一种常用于治疗儿童急性淋巴细胞白血病的药物。6-巯基嘌呤及其前药硫唑嘌呤和嘌呤类似物 6-硫鸟嘌呤主要由硫嘌呤 S-甲基转移酶（thiopurine S-methyltransferase，TMPT）代谢。TMPT 基因有许多多态性，这些多态性降低了 TMPT 的活性，其中第一个是 1995 年发现的[93]。自那以后，其他的多态性已经被确认，并且在这些罕见的变异的频率上有明显的种族差异，但是 90%以上的 TMPT 酶失活病例由 3 个等位基因多态性所导致。遗传了 2 个失活的 TMPT 等位基因的个体（<1%的人口），均会出现重度骨髓抑制。相当比例的遗传一个失活等位基因的个体（人群中占比约 3%~14%）会经历中重度骨髓抑制；临床药物遗传学实施联合会已经发表指南，建议对该患者群体减少用药剂量[94]。类似地，接受伊立替康治疗的 UGT1A1＊28 纯合子患者会有更高的 SN-38 活性代谢产物血液浓度，进而严重中性粒细胞减少的风险也更高。这表明在这些患者中减少剂量是有必要的[24]。

在其他情况下，即使调整药物剂量或避免使用的建议已纳入药品说明书，也可能不需要调整剂量和/或避免使用该药物。这一点可以通过推荐肾损伤患者降低卡培他滨剂量来说明（Xeloda prescribing information，http://www.accessdata.fda.gov/drugsatfda_docs/label/2005/020896s016lbl.pdf）。在一篇关于该建议的评论文章中[95]，Ratain 指出，推荐 Cockcroft-Gault 公式估算肌酐清除率 31~50ml/min 的患者推荐降低剂量 25%的建议，是建立在 Cockcroft-Gault 这一被诟病不够准确的公式基础之上[96]。这个公式会低估妇女和高血清肌酐个体，低体重，老年患者的肌酐清除率。此外，这种肾损害的定义并没有针对 BSA 进行相应调整。结果就是，一个小个女人可能会降低给药剂量，而一个大个男人可能就不会，即使他们在进行 BSA 调整过后的血清肌酐清除率是相同的。

外在因素

哪些外部因素（药物、草药制品、饮食、吸烟和饮酒）会影响给药剂量-药物浓度和/或反应关系，以及药物浓度差异会影响治疗反应吗？根据已知的暴露-反应关系及其变异性，如果需要的话，你会建议如何调整给药方案？

药物与药物的相互作用可以通过减少或增加药物浓度而降低治疗疗效或安全性，并对药物治疗反应产生影响。患者常常将处方药、非处方药与抗癌药同时使用，有时肿瘤医生并不知道这种常见药物相互作用的机制是诱导或抑制 CYP450 酶和抑制 P-糖蛋白转运体。例如，具有潜在治疗意义的药物-药物相互作用是他莫昔芬和抗抑郁药选择性 5-羟色胺再摄取抑制剂（selective serotonin reuptake inhibitor，SSRI）。帕罗西汀是一种 SSRI，通常用于治疗抑郁症或与他莫昔芬治疗相关的潮热，也是他莫昔芬活化为代谢产物内皮氧芬时所需的 CYP2D6 酶的强抑制剂[97]。在一项前瞻性临床试验中，12 名服用他莫昔芬的乳腺癌患者在帕罗西汀联合用药 4 周前后接受药代动力学取样。野生型 CYP2D6 等位基因同源的受试者的内皮氧芬浓度下降了 64%，但 CYP2D6 基因变异的女性仅下降了 21%[98]。在一项对 80 名服用他莫昔芬的妇女进行的前瞻性研究中报告了类似的结果，其中大约 30%的妇女在服用了 4 个月后服用了各种 SSRI[99]，尽管降低内源性氧芬浓度的确切临床意义仍在研究中[100]，但这些数据结果已足以建议在他莫昔芬治疗的患者中避免使用强 CYP2D6 酶抑制剂（如帕罗西汀和氟西汀）的 SSRI，以免在控制他莫昔芬副作用的同时影响其正常疗效的发挥[101]（Brisdelle 处方信息，http://www.accessdata.fda.gov/drugsatfda_docs/label/2013/204516s000lbl.pdf）。

尽管抗肿瘤药物通常是联合用药，但研究药物之间潜在的药代动力学和/或药效学相互作用的研究相对较少。例如，紫杉醇和顺铂（卵巢癌的一种重要化疗方案）联合使用，如果先使用顺铂的话，就会降低紫杉醇的清除率[102]。另一方面，紫杉醇和卡铂没有类似的药动学相互作用，但紫杉醇可以减轻卡铂引起的血小板减少[103]，已经在巨核细胞水平上提出解释这一现象的机制[104]。联合治疗的另一个问题是药物可能联合用药，但并不考虑它们是否与饮食条件相匹配。例如，卡培他滨和拉帕替尼联合用于转移性乳腺癌的治疗。卡培他滨被标记为每天两次与食物一起服用，而拉帕替尼（与食物接触显著增加）则被标记为在可能的情况下每天空腹服药一次[105]。为了使患者最大限度地遵守两种药物的规定剂量和给药方案，将同时服用药物的膳食条件进行匹配是有意义的。

除了药物，许多其他外在因素亦可影响药物浓度和对抗癌药物的反应。例如，吸烟诱导的 CYP1A1 及其对肺癌患者厄洛替尼药物浓度的影响。目前吸烟者中厄洛替尼的剂量递增研究表明，维持剂量每天 300mg，在接受该剂量治疗的患者中，稳定的谷底血浆浓度和皮疹和腹泻的发生率与已经戒烟者或从未吸烟者每天维持剂量 150mg 的情况相似[106]。圣约翰草（贯叶连翘）是一种癌症患者常用的抗抑郁草药，是一种已知的孕烷 x 受体配体（pregnane X receptor，PXR），可诱导转录 PXR 调节基因，如 CYP3A 和 UGT[107-110]，已经证实与圣约翰草同时服用，可显著减少伊立替康、伊马替尼和多西他赛的药物浓度[111-113]。葡萄柚汁则刚好相反，葡萄柚汁是一种有效的 CYP3A4 抑制剂，已被证明能增加西罗莫司的药物浓度，这意味着它可能对其他作为 CYP3A4 底物的抗癌药物也有同样的作用[114]。

普通生物类药品

根据生物制药分类系统（BCS）的原则，这种药物和制剂属于哪一类？溶解度、渗透性和溶解性数据如何支持这种分类？

正如本章开头所讨论的，BCS 根据体外渗透性和溶解度的测量来预测药物在体内的性能，而 BDDC 预测药物在体内的分布和药物在肠和肝中的相互作用。BCS 1 类药物具有高溶解性。溶出度高，渗透性好，因此没有必要进行体内生物等效性研究。因为 BCS 2 类药物具有溶解度低、渗透性强的特点，许多激酶抑制剂都属于这一类。BCS 3 类药物具有高溶解度和低渗透性，而 BCS 4 类药物具有低溶解度和低渗透性。BDDCS 1 类药物具有很高的溶解度，在肠道和肝脏中的转运体作用很小，这意味着它们主要通过代谢消除。由于 p-糖蛋白外排不是 BDDCS 1 类药物的主要清除方法，这些药物往往能透过血脑屏障，并在脑内有良好的分布。BDDCS 2 类药物溶解度低，外排转运体效应在肠道占主导地位，吸收和转运均在肠道内，肝脏的外排和摄取均对药物的药代动力学产生影响。BDDCS 3 类药物具有高溶解度，以吸收转运作用为主。

食品对剂型中药物的生物利用度有什么影响？应提出哪些对于与膳食或膳食类型有关的用药剂量建议（如有）？

一般来说，高脂膳食对 BDDCS 1 类药物的吸收程度几乎没有影响，增加 BDDCS 2 类药物（如许多激酶抑制剂）的浓度，降低 BDDCS 3 类药物的暴露率。食物可能会影响人体药代动力学，包括延缓胃排空，刺激胆汁流动，改变胃肠道 pH 值，增加内脏血流量，改变药物的肠道代谢，以及与药物或剂型的物理/化学相互作用[90]。在食物效应研究中，FDA 建议报告药物浓度参数（如 C_{max} 和 AUC）组间几何平均值的比率，以及 90%的置信区间范围。如果进食后服药 90%的置信区间在 80%~125%范围内，则认为进食与否不影响生物等效性，而超出该范围则认为食物对药品的作用将产生显著影响（FDA《食物效应生物利用度和联邦生物等效性研究》行业指南，2002 年）。

小分子非细胞毒性药物已被证实与食物同服会增加血药浓度，包括厄洛替尼、拉帕替尼、尼洛替尼、帕唑帕尼、维莫非尼和阿比特龙。最近的一个例子是二代 ALK 抑制剂塞瑞替尼在 ALK 重排的非小细胞肺癌中显示了疗效，塞瑞替尼是 BCS 4 类化合物，是 p-糖蛋白顶端外排转运体的底物。生产厂家基于对健康受试者在空腹、低脂或高脂饮食条件下单次服用 500mg 的药代动力学数据，获得了 FDA 的新药加速批准。

FDA 使用药代动力学模型来预测在稳定状态下每日 750mg 和 600mg 的多剂量塞瑞替尼后食物的影响，该模型预测食物增加塞瑞替尼的 C_{max} 和 AUC 分别为 68%和 67%。与食物同服药物时的每日 600mg 与空腹服药每日 750mg 效果相当。（http://www.accessdata.fda.gov/drugsatfda_docs/nda/2014/205755Orig1s000ClinPharmR.pdf）。该药物说明书推荐为每日空腹服用 750mg，因为这是关键临床试验中使用的剂量。FDA 发布了一项上市后的要求，对患者与食物同服药物时每日 450mg 与空腹服药每日 750mg 进行对比评估，可以推测，低剂量的非劣化证据将使生产厂家更新药品说明书。

结论

如前所述，在各类抗癌药物中，都能找到理解临床药理学可以提高这些药物临床应用的实例。因为其目的是在保持耐受性的同时最大限度地提高疗效。肿瘤医生需要理解用药剂量与药物浓度（药代动力学）之间的基本关系，如整体人群的药物浓度和治疗反应（药效学）。肿瘤医生还需要了解某个患者的反应与一般患者不同的方式和原因，以及药物效应随时间变化的原因（患者个体间和患者个体内的变异性）。当出现问题时，药品说明书是一个合理的研究起点，但是基于问题的 FDA 临床药理学和生物药剂学综述提供了说明书上可能遗漏的更详细的答案。由于许多关于抗癌疗法的临床药理学的新观察是在药物上市后进行的，因此也推荐随时对新发表文献进行阅读整理。

（郑凯 译，张艳华 审校）

参考文献

The complete reference list can be found on the Wiley Companion Digital Edition of this title (see inside front cover for login instructions).

3 Benet LZ. The role of BCS (biopharmaceutics classification system) and BDDCS (biopharmaceutics drug disposition classification system) in drug development. *J Pharm Sci*. 2013;**102**(**1**):34–42.

6 Stuurman FE, Nuijen B, Beijnen JH, Schellens JH. Oral anticancer drugs: mechanisms of low bioavailability and strategies for improvement. *Clin Pharmacokinet*. 2013;**52**(**6**):399–414.

11 Bins S, Ratain MJ, Mathijssen RH. Conventional dosing of anticancer agents: precisely wrong or just inaccurate? *Clin Pharmacol Ther*. 2014;**95**(**4**):361–364.

18 Seymour L, Ivy SP, Sargent D, et al. The design of phase II clinical trials testing cancer therapeutics: consensus recommendations from the clinical trial design task force of the national cancer institute investigational drug steering committee. *Clin Cancer Res Off J Am Assoc Cancer Res*. 2010;**16**(**6**):1764–1769.

19 Dancey JE, Dobbin KK, Groshen S, et al. Guidelines for the development and incorporation of biomarker studies in early clinical trials of novel agents. *Clin Cancer Res Off J Am Assoc Cancer Res*. 2010;**16**(**6**):1745–1755.

24 Ramchandani RP, Wang Y, Booth BP, et al. The role of SN-38 exposure, UGT1A1*28 polymorphism, and baseline bilirubin level in predicting severe irinotecan toxicity. *J Clin Pharmacol*. 2007;**47**(**1**):78–86.

25 Wagner JG. Kinetics of pharmacologic response. I. Proposed relationships between response and drug concentration in the intact animal and man. *J Theor Biol*. 1968;**20**(**2**):173–201.

26 Jusko WJ. A pharmacodynamic model for cell-cycle specific chemotherapeutic agents. *J Pharmacokinet Biopharm*. 1973;**1**:175–200.

28 Skipper HE, Schabel FM Jr, Mellett LB, et al. Implications of biochemical, cytokinetic, pharmacologic, and toxicologic relationships in the design of optimal therapeutic schedules. *Cancer Chemother Reports Part 1*. 1970;**54**(**6**):431–450.

30 Wang J, Song P, Schrieber S, et al. Exposure-response relationship of T-DM1: insight into dose optimization for patients with HER2-positive metastatic breast cancer. *Clin Pharmacol Ther*. 2014;**95**(**5**):558–564.

31 Rini BI, Garrett M, Poland B, et al. Axitinib in metastatic renal cell carcinoma: results of a pharmacokinetic and pharmacodynamic analysis. *J Clin Pharmacol*. 2013;**53**(**5**):491–504.

33 Jodrell DI, Egorin MJ, Canetta RM, et al. Relationships between carboplatin exposure and tumor response and toxicity in patients with ovarian cancer. *J Clin Oncol Off J Am Soc Clin Oncol*. 1992;**10**(**4**):520–528.

34 Wang X, Roy A, Hochhaus A, Kantarjian HM, Chen TT, Shah NP. Differential effects of dosing regimen on the safety and efficacy of dasatinib: retrospective exposure-response analysis of a phase III study. *Clin Pharmacol Adv Appl*. 2013;**5**:85–97.

35 Tiseo M, Andreoli R, Gelsomino F, et al. Correlation between erlotinib pharmacokinetics, cutaneous toxicity and clinical outcomes in patients with advanced non-small cell lung cancer (NSCLC). *Lung Cancer*. 2014;**83**(**2**):265–271.

38 Demetri GD, Wang Y, Wehrle E, et al. Imatinib plasma levels are correlated with clinical benefit in patients with unresectable/metastatic gastrointestinal stromal tumors. *J Clin Oncol Off J Am Soc Clin Oncol*. 2009;**27**(**19**):3141–3147.

39 Evans WE, Relling MV, Rodman JH, Crom WR, Boyett JM, Pui CH. Conventional compared with individualized chemotherapy for childhood acute lymphoblastic leukemia. *N Engl J Med*. 1998;**338**(**8**):499–505.

40 Suttle AB, Ball HA, Molimard M, et al. Relationships between pazopanib exposure and clinical safety and efficacy in patients with advanced renal cell carcinoma. *Br J Cancer*. 2014;**111**(**12**):2383.

42 Cosson VF, Ng VW, Lehle M, Lum BL. Population pharmacokinetics and exposure-response analyses of trastuzumab in patients with advanced gastric or gastroesophageal junction cancer. *Cancer Chemother Pharmacol*. 2014;**73**(4):737–747.

43 Yu H, Steeghs N, Nijenhuis CM, Schellens JH, Beijnen JH, Huitema AD. Practical guidelines for therapeutic drug monitoring of anticancer tyrosine kinase inhibitors: focus on the pharmacokinetic targets. *Clin Pharmacokinet*. 2014;**53**(**4**):305–325.

45 Karlsson MO, Molnar V, Bergh J, Freijs A, Larsson R. A general model for time-dissociated pharmacokinetic-pharmacodynamic relationship exemplified by paclitaxel myelosuppression. *Clin Pharmacol Ther*. 1998;**63**(**1**):11–25.

46 Minami H, Sasaki Y, Saijo N, et al. Indirect-response model for the time course of leukopenia with anticancer drugs. *Clin Pharmacol Ther*. 1998;**64**(**5**):511–521.

47 Egorin MJ, Van Echo DA, Tipping SJ, et al. Pharmacokinetics and dosage reduction of cis-diammine(1,1-cyclobutanedicarboxylato)platinum in patients with impaired renal function. *Cancer Res*. 1984;**44**(**11**):5432–5438.

50 Mould DR, Upton RN. Basic concepts in population modeling, simulation, and model-based drug development-part 2: introduction to pharmacokinetic modeling methods. *CPT: Pharmacometr Syst Pharmacol*. 2013;**2**:e38.

51 Deng J, Shao J, Markowitz JS, An G. ABC transporters in multi-drug resistance and ADME-Tox of small molecule tyrosine kinase inhibitors. *Pharm Res*. 2014;**31**(**9**):2237–2255.

53 Szmulewitz RZ, Ratain MJ. Playing Russian roulette with tyrosine kinase inhibitors. *Clin Pharmacol Ther*. 2013;**93**(**3**):242–244.

56 Budha NR, Frymoyer A, Smelick GS, et al. Drug absorption interactions between oral targeted anticancer agents and PPIs: is pH-dependent solubility the Achilles heel of targeted therapy? *Clin Pharmacol Ther*. 2012;**92**(**2**):203–213.

57 Evans WE, Pratt CB. Effect of pleural effusion on high-dose methotrexate kinetics. *Clin Pharmacol Ther*. 1978;**23**(**1**):68–72.

60 Benet LZ, Hoener BA. Changes in plasma protein binding have little clinical relevance. *Clin Pharmacol Ther*. 2002;**71**(**3**):115–121.

61 Penner N, Klunk LJ, Prakash C. Human radiolabeled mass balance studies: objectives, utilities and limitations. *Biopharm Drug Dispos*. 2009;**30**(**4**):185–203.

62 Calvert AH, Newell DR, Gumbrell LA, et al. Carboplatin dosage: prospective evaluation of a simple formula based on renal function. *J Clin Oncol Off J Am Soc Clin Oncol*. 1989;**7**(**11**):1748–1756.

64 Relling MV, Fairclough D, Ayers D, et al. Patient characteristics associated with high-risk methotrexate concentrations and toxicity. *J Clin Oncol Off J Am Soc Clin Oncol*. 1994;**12**(**8**):1667–1672.

66 Miller AA, Murry DJ, Owzar K, et al. Phase I and pharmacokinetic study of sorafenib in patients with hepatic or renal dysfunction: CALGB 60301. *J Clin Oncol Off J Am Soc Clin Oncol*. 2009;**27**(**11**):1800–1805.

72 Rosner GL, Panetta JC, Innocenti F, Ratain MJ. Pharmacogenetic pathway analysis of irinotecan. *Clin Pharmacol Ther*. 2008;**84**(**3**):393–402.

73 Reece PA, Stafford I, Davy M, Freeman S. Disposition of unchanged cisplatin in patients with ovarian cancer. *Clin Pharmacol Ther*. 1987;**42**(**3**):320–325.

75 Wagner JG, Szpunar GJ, Ferry JJ. A nonlinear physiologic pharmacokinetic model: I. Steady-state. *J Pharmacokinet Biopharm*. 1985;**13**(**1**):73–92.

77 Collins JM, Dedrick RL, King FG, Speyer JL, Myers CE. Nonlinear pharmacokinetic models for 5-fluorouracil in man: intravenous and intraperitoneal routes. *Clin Pharmacol Ther*. 1980;**28**(**2**):235–246.

80 Gianni L, Kearns CM, Giani A, et al. Nonlinear pharmacokinetics and metabolism of paclitaxel and its pharmacokinetic/pharmacodynamic relationships in humans. *J Clin Oncol Off J Am Soc Clin Oncol*. 1995;**13**(**1**):180–190.

90 Singh BN, Malhotra BK. Effects of food on the clinical pharmacokinetics of anticancer agents: underlying mechanisms and implications for oral chemotherapy. *Clin Pharmacokinet*. 2004;**43**(**15**):1127–1156.

91 Han K, Jin J, Maia M, Lowe J, Sersch MA, Allison DE. Lower exposure and faster clearance of bevacizumab in gastric cancer and the impact of patient variables: analysis of individual data from AVAGAST phase III trial. *AAPS J*. 2014;**16**(**5**):1056–1063.

94 Relling MV, Gardner EE, Sandborn WJ, et al. Clinical Pharmacogenetics Implementation Consortium guidelines for thiopurine methyltransferase genotype and thiopurine dosing. *Clin Pharmacol Ther*. 2011;**89**(**3**):387–391.

98 Stearns V, Johnson MD, Rae JM, et al. Active tamoxifen metabolite plasma concentrations after coadministration of tamoxifen and the selective serotonin reuptake inhibitor paroxetine. *J Natl Cancer Inst*. 2003;**95**(**23**):1758–1764.

103 Calvert AH. A review of the pharmacokinetics and pharmacodynamics of combination carboplatin/paclitaxel. *Semin Oncol*. 1997;**24**(**1 Suppl 2**):S2-85–S2-90.

106 Hughes AN, O'Brien ME, Petty WJ, et al. Overcoming CYP1A1/1A2 mediated induction of metabolism by escalating erlotinib dose in current smokers. *J Clin Oncol Off J Am Soc Clin Oncol*. 2009;**27**(**8**):1220–1226.

107 Moore LB, Goodwin B, Jones SA, et al. St John's wort induces hepatic drug metabolism through activation of the pregnane X receptor. *Proc Natl Acad Sci U S A*. 2000;**97**(**13**):7500–7502.

114 Cohen EE, Wu K, Hartford C, et al. Phase I studies of sirolimus alone or in combination with pharmacokinetic modulators in advanced cancer patients. *Clin Cancer Res Off J Am Assoc Cancer Res*. 2012;**18**(**17**):4785–4793.

第 56 章　叶酸拮抗剂

Peter D. Cole, MD ■ Lisa Figueiredo, MD ■ Joseph R. Bertino, MD

概述

叶酸拮抗剂(antifols)是一类细胞毒药物,可用于抗肿瘤,抗微生物,抗炎和免疫抑制治疗。虽然已开发出多种叶酸拮抗剂,但甲氨蝶呤(4-氨基-4-脱氧-10-N-甲基-蝶酰谷氨酸;MTX)是历史最久,也是应用最广的叶酸拮抗剂。MTX 仍然是用于治疗急性淋巴细胞白血病、骨肉瘤和绒毛膜癌患者化疗方案中的必需药物,并且是治疗淋巴瘤、乳腺癌、膀胱癌和头颈癌的重要药物。此外,它还用于非恶性疾病患者,如类风湿性关节炎、牛皮癣、自身免疫性疾病和移植物抗宿主病。本章节将回顾 MTX 的临床应用和代谢,并从结构上讨论那些已被开发用于克服耐药性或作用于细胞内其他靶点的叶酸拮抗剂。

历史概述

在 20 世纪 40 年代初期,联合观察结果显示,患有急性白血病患者常伴随有叶酸缺乏症,而叶酸缺乏症患者的骨髓巨幼细胞在形态学上与白血病细胞相似,这使得一些研究人员认为白血病可能与 B 族维生素缺乏有关。然而,研究很快发现给白血病患者补充叶酸不仅无效,而且还加速了疾病的进程[1]。因此,治疗这些白血病患者的努力方向转为使用叶酸类似物在药理学上模拟叶酸缺乏,这些类似物具有拮抗维生素的作用。氨蝶呤(4-氨基-4-脱氧 PGA;AMT;图 56-1)是这类制剂中第一个能够使 16 例急性白血病患者中 5 例达到临时缓解的药物[2]。该报告是肿瘤化学治疗的一个里程碑,是第一个通过合理药物设计成功得到有效抗肿瘤药物的例子。

由于最初的研究表明 AMT 在治疗儿童急性白血病中有效,因此叶酸拮抗剂引起了人们持久的关注。虽然效力较 AMT 低,但在 20 世纪 50 年代早期,4-氨基-4-脱氧-10-N-甲基-蝶酰谷氨酸(MTX)仍取代了 AMT,因为由 AMT 引起的毒性更大且更不可预测[3-5]。为了克服肿瘤细胞对 MTX 的耐药性或找到叶酸相关途径新的作用靶点,新的叶酸拮抗剂——经过合理设计的叶酸或 MTX 类似物——已经合成。本章将讨论最近获得 FDA 批准用于肿瘤治疗的两种药物——普拉曲沙和培美曲塞。

MTX 的作用机制

叶酸拮抗剂通过以下几种方式发挥作用:与叶酸竞争阻止其被摄入细胞;抑制叶酸辅酶的形成;抑制一种或多种由叶酸酶介导的反应。到目前为止,临床重要的抗肿瘤叶酸类似物似乎主要通过抑制二氢叶酸还原酶(dihydrofolate reductase,DHFR)或胸苷酸合成酶(thymidylate synthase,TS)起作用。DHFR 抑制剂的原型是 4-氨基取代的蝶呤化合物,例如 MTX 或 AMT(图 56-1)。用氨基取代 4-羟基部分使叶酸类似物对 DHFR 的亲和力增加数千倍。MTX 对于 DHFR 的 K_i 低于 10^{-10}M,远低于天然底物二氢叶酸的微摩尔水平 K_m。通过在弱酸性 pH 环境下,按化学计量抑制 DHFR,MTX 阻断了细胞的叶酸供应,而这些叶酸是细胞从头合成胸苷酸所必需消耗的(图 56-2)[6]。在快速分裂的细胞中,胸苷酸生物合成的抑制使胸苷三磷酸池减少,从而 DNA 合成减少,最终导致细胞死亡。

经典叶酸拮抗剂如 MTX 在细胞内代谢成多聚谷氨酸类物质,后者可显著影响其功能发挥和细胞毒性机制[8]。叶酸多聚谷氨酸合成酶(folylpolyglutamate synthetase,FPGS)将底物 γ-羧基键中的谷氨酸残基添加到叶酸辅酶和经典叶酸拮抗剂分子上的谷氨酸残基的上。这使得在原来的分子增加了 7~8 谷氨酸残基,增加了其分子质量和负电荷,从而显著减少其外流,进而在稳态下胞内积聚增多[9]。FPGS 的表达量和功能在肿瘤和非肿瘤组织之间存在差异[10],这就解释了为什么叶酸拮抗剂对肿瘤细胞存在一定的选择性[11]。在暴露于相同浓度 MTX 的情况下,大量处于 G_0 期的细胞群比分裂活跃的细胞群更易受到 MTX 的影响,这也许是因为前者往往缺乏 FPGS。

MTX 聚谷氨酸盐比 MTX 本身更能有效地抑制 DHFR,因为它们虽然能够像 MTX 一样与 DHFR 紧密结合,但解离速度却很慢[12]。此外,MTX 聚谷氨酸盐还是其他叶酸复合酶的有效抑制剂,包括 TS[13] 和两种嘌呤从头合成的限速酶:甘氨酰胺

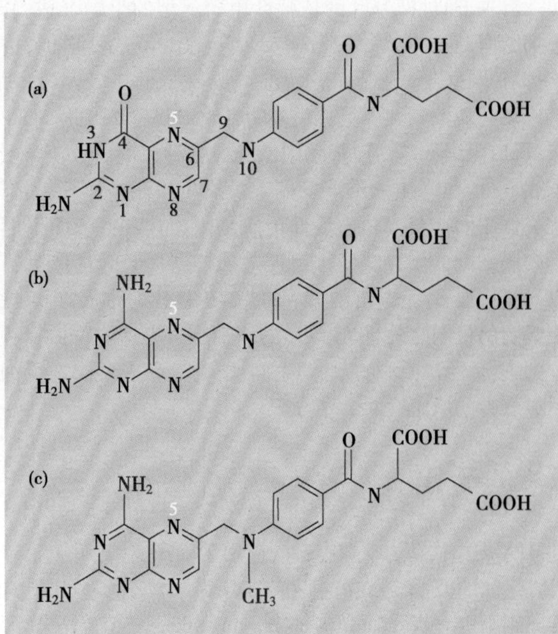

图 56-1　叶酸的化学结构以及结构上相关的叶酸拮抗剂,AMT 和 MTX。(a)叶酸(碟酰谷氨酸)。(b)氨蝶呤(4-氨基-PGA)。(c)甲氨蝶呤(4-氨基-N-10-甲基 PGA)

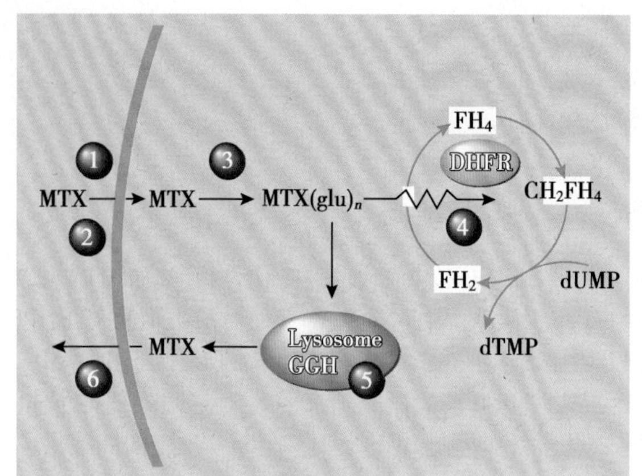

图 56-2 MTX 和 MTX(glu)$_n$ 主要作用部位。MTX 通过减少的叶酸载体(1)或膜叶酸结合蛋白(2)进入细胞。MTX 被胞质中的叶酸多聚谷氨酸合成酶(3)代谢成 MTX(glu)$_n$,二氢叶酸还原酶(4)的有效抑制剂。MTX(glu)$_n$ 可被溶酶体中的 γ-谷酰基水解酶(GGH)(5)水解为 MTX。略缩语:CH_2FH_4,N_5,N_{10}-亚甲基四氢叶酸;dTMP,脱氧一磷酸胸腺嘧啶核苷;dUMP,脱氧一磷酸尿嘧啶核苷;FH_2,二氢叶酸;FH_4,四氢叶酸;MTX,甲氨蝶呤;MTX(glu)$_n$,MTX 多聚谷氨酸盐

核糖核苷酸(glycinamide ribonucleotide,GAR)转移酶和氨基咪唑甲酰胺核糖核苷酸(aminoimidazole carboxamide ribonucleotide,AICAR)转移酶[14]。DHF-聚谷氨酸盐和 10-甲酰基-DHF-聚谷氨酸盐是这两种酶的有效抑制剂,在 MTX 抑制 DHFR 后水平升高[15]。因此,对于 MTX,无论是在抑制癌细胞过程中发挥细胞毒作用[16],还是在风湿病患者中发挥抗炎作用[17,18],都或多或少与其抑制 DHFR 后进而抑制嘌呤从头合成有关。

MTX 发挥抗肿瘤或抗炎作用的其他可能作用机制也值得关注。首先,通过抑制叶酸依赖性甲硫氨酸的生物合成,MTX 导致细胞内同型半胱氨酸(homocysteine,Hcy)浓度增加,进而使 S-腺苷-同型半胱氨酸(S-adenosyl-homocysteine,SAH)增加,这是许多叶酸依赖性甲基化反应的有效抑制剂。因此,MTX 的暴露,可以阻断 ras 在胞膜上定位,这是一种关键信号转导蛋白的家族成员,在许多人类癌症发生发展中被激活。其次,MTX 的抗炎作用和部分抗肿瘤活性可能是因为其在低浓度下能够抑制内皮细胞的增殖[20]。临床前数据证明,低剂量甲氨蝶呤可以通过抗血管生成作用抑制肿瘤微转移灶的进展[21]。除了前面提到的机制之外,快速增殖的癌细胞过表达线粒体和甘氨酸-丝氨酸途径相关的酶,近期人们认为,这种表型决定了细胞对甲氨蝶呤的敏感性。

MTX 的药代动力学

MTX 的药代动力学数据常规应用于临床实践,平衡了疗效和毒性之间的关系,这在抗癌药物当中是为数不多的[23]。对急性淋巴细胞白血病(acute lymphoblastic leukemia,ALL)患儿的回顾性分析显示,较低的 MTX 清除率[24]和较高的 MTX 浓度[25]与降低复发风险有关。关于 ALL 患者的前瞻性随机对照试验数据更令人振奋:比较按体表面积给药和基于药代动力学数据的个体化给药的结果显示,个体化治疗组的完全连续缓解率显著提高[26]。然而,有可能这些结果是方案特异性的,正如其他人发现,在某些亚群中,药理学指导的强化治疗效果较差[27]。

吸收

按 15~30mg/m^2 的剂量口服给药后,1~5 小时后出现血药浓度高峰。食物、不可吸收的抗生素、胆汁酸盐和肠道通过时间缩短都会影响 MTX 的吸收,在这些情况下,药物的吸收可能相对较差且不可预测[28,29]。因此,建议用空腹清水送服。尽管如此,按照 25mg/m^2 的给药剂量,每日间隔 6 小时口服 4 次,超过 85%的 ALL 儿童患者血浆 MTX 浓度>0.5μM,表明了该口服方案的可行性[30]。

分布

静脉给予 MTX 后,初始分布容积(V_d)约为 0.18L/kg 体重。初始分配阶段的 $t_{1/2}$ 为 30~45min;$t_{1/2}$β 是 3~4 小时。稳态 V_d 介于 0.4L/kg 和 0.8L/kg 之间[31]。

使用高剂量 MTX(>3g/m^2)后,将在 10^{-4}~10^{-3}mol/L 范围内达到血药浓度高峰[32]。在这样的浓度下,跨膜转运达到饱和状态,使得 MTX 的进一步流入局限于被动扩散。包括亚叶酸(leucovorin,LV)在内的还原叶酸的摄取也会受到抑制。关于淋巴母细胞中 MTX 代谢的体外研究也表明,过高的胞外药物浓度会阻碍 MTX 代谢成多聚谷氨酸盐[33]。

约 50%的 MTX 与血浆蛋白(尤其是白蛋白)结合[34,35]。MTX 的 7-羟基代谢物与血浆蛋白的结合率为 90%,但在临床观察到的浓度下,不会干扰 MTX 与血浆蛋白的结合。人体中从各组织到血浆,浓度最高的部位是肝脏和肾脏,其次是胃肠道。人体高剂量输注 MTX 后,其血浆水平延长,是由于胃肠道梗阻导致的转运率下降造成的。

由于血脑屏障和主动从中枢神经系统中清除 MTX 的外排机制[36],脑脊液(cerebrospinal fluid,CSF)MTX 浓度约为血浆中的 1%;因此,常规剂量 CSF 无法达到有效的杀伤细胞的浓度,只有在剂量为 500mg/m^2 或更高时才可达到目的[37]。高剂量全身 MTX 给药后,腰椎 CSF 和脑室脑脊液浓度相似。高剂量甲氨蝶呤(HDMTX)可能能够在治疗非白血病软脑膜病患者中替代鞘内药物注射[38]。然而,最近关于中枢神经系统定向治疗 ALL 患儿的 Meta 分析得出结论:使用 HDMTX 增加脑脊液穿透的努力,并没有达到降低这类人群中枢神经系统复发率的预期效果[39]。

由于 MTX 在 CSF 中累积量很少,即使给予小剂量口服 LV 也可显著增加 CSF 叶酸浓度。这种系统性挽救,特别是如果在 MTX 后过早给予,可以拯救脑脊液中的白血病细胞[40]。

当通过留置脑室导管注入 MTX 时,至少需要 48 小时才能达到有效的治疗浓度(>10^{-6}M)[41]。相反,当 MTX 通过腰椎注入脑脊液时,它却不能很好地分布到脑室。有学者提出改良方案,即建议多次小剂量鞘内注射 MTX[42]。鞘内注射后,MTX 缓慢进入体循环,$t_{1/2}$ 为 8~10h[36]。没有 LV 拯救的情况下多次施用鞘内注射 MTX 可观察到其全身毒性。鞘内注射 MTX 的药理学特征和脑室内 MTX 的含量可能会受到脑膜白血病的影响,亦可因腰椎穿刺时患者的体位而改变[43]。临床观察到 MTX 治疗后予放疗,患者也许会出现神经毒性症状,可能是由

于放疗对血脑屏障产生了影响[44]。

由于 MTX 积聚"第三次间隔"或注射部位，使其缓慢持续释放入血，导致血清中 MTX 浓度持续存在，增加了胸腔或腹腔积液患者 HD-MTX 中毒的风险[45]。在这些情况下，使用更高剂量的 LV 并延长 LV 抢救的时程可能是必要的，直到血清 MTX 水平降低至 0.05×10^{-6}M 以下。

代谢

MTX 的主要代谢产物是由肝醛氧化酶作用产生的 7-羟基 MTX（7-OH MTX）（图 56-3），其对 DHFR 的抑制作用仅为 MTX 的 1%[46]。其水溶性也较 MTX 小，而且高剂量后可能导致肾毒性[47]。

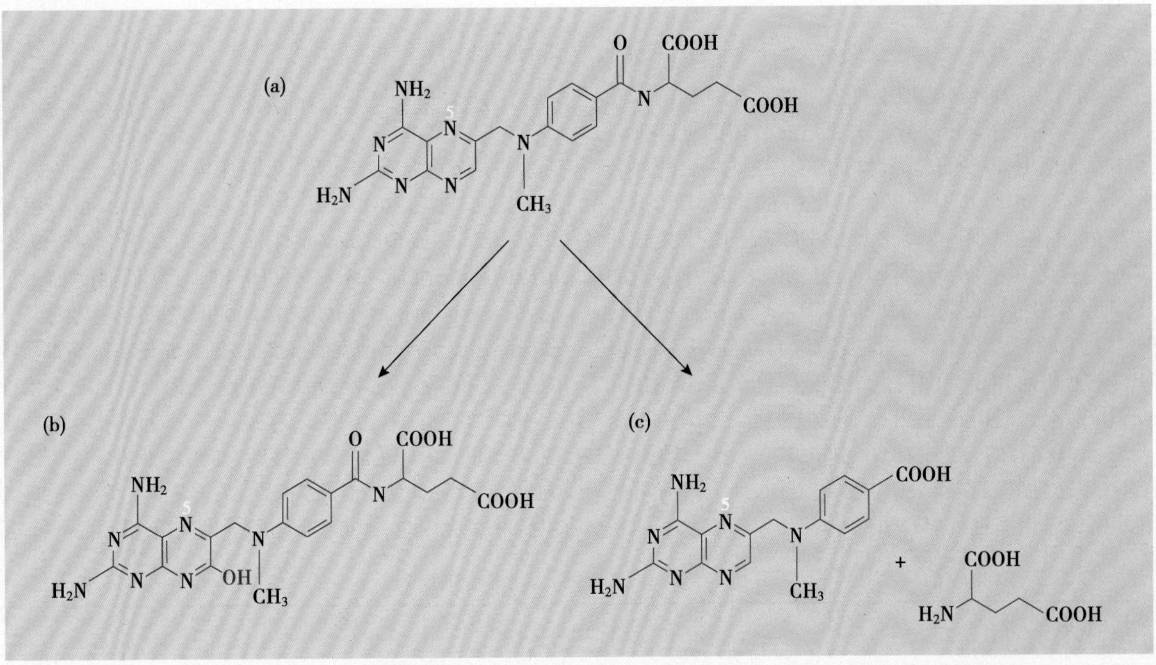

图 56-3　MTX 分解代谢。MTX（a）在肝脏中转化成 7-羟 MTX（b）。此外，肠杆菌可将 MTX 分子切割成 dAMPA 和谷氨酸盐（c）

第二种不太主要的 MTX 代谢途径发生在肠道中。MTX 被细菌水解为蝶呤（4-脱氧-4-氨基-N10-甲基蝶酸；dAMPA）和谷氨酸（图 56-3）[48]。dAMPA，如 7-OH MTX，也是一种相对无活性的代谢产物，其对 DHFR 的亲和力仅为 MTX 的 1/200。尿中 dAMPA 排泄量不到给药剂量的 5%。

MTX 的第三种谢产物是 MTX 聚谷氨酸。如前所述，MTX 聚谷氨酸是至少与 MTX 一样有效的 DHFR 抑制剂，并且与 DHFR 的解离速率比 MTX 慢[12]。由于 γ-谷氨酰水解酶（GGH）在血浆中具有将叶酰-和 MTX-聚谷氨酸转化为单谷氨酸的活性，因此在血浆或尿液中未发现 MTX 聚谷氨酸盐。与 MTX 类似，7-OH MTX 也在细胞内聚谷氨酰胺化，这些聚谷氨酸类物质在胞内的积聚可能使 MTX 发挥细胞毒性作用[49]。

可以通过测量循环红细胞（red blood cell，RBC）中的 MTX-聚谷氨酸浓度来监测对口服 MTX 方案的依从性[50-52]。骨髓内的有核 RBC 前体细胞将累积并代谢循环 MTX。代谢后的 MTX 聚谷氨酸将在成熟 RBC 的整个生命周期中停留于胞内[53]，而未代谢的 MTX 将逐渐被外排出[54]。

排泄

大多数 MTX（及其代谢产物 7-OHMTX 和 DAMPA）直接从尿液中排泄[55,56]。由于近端小管中的活跃分泌，MTX 的肾清除率可超过肌酐清除率[57]。MTX 清除率在患者间广泛存在差异，而这与肾功能无关[58]。据报道，MTX 排泄与年龄成反比，因为经肾脏排泄药物的血浆清除率与肾功能的成熟密切相关。研究发现儿童往往能比成人更快地清除 MTX，并且随着年龄的增长清除率降低[59]。MTX 通过有机酸转运蛋白排泄，可被丙磺舒或其他弱有机酸竞争抑制如阿司匹林或青霉素 G。一些药物如头孢菌素、磺胺甲噁唑，会抑制远端小管的重吸收，MTX 的清除会因此而增加。

通常不到 10% 的 MTX 会通过粪便排泄[60]。按 30~80mg/m^2 每日 4 次静脉给药后，0.4%~20% 通过微管多重有机酸转运蛋白（cMOAT；ABCC2；MRP2）排出进入胆汁。在基因敲除小鼠模型（$ABCC2^{-/-}$；$ABCG2^{-/-}$）中显示：两种转运蛋白在清除 MTX 和 7-OH-MTX 中起重叠作用。已经鉴定出这些转运蛋白具有多态性，存在突变，导致其表达和活性的差异，影响全身 MTX 暴露浓度。因此，具有 ABCC2 和/或 ABCG2 突变或杂合多态性的患者可能会有更高的 MTX 中毒风险[61]。

药物相互作用

癌症患者使用的一些药物，包括抗生素，可能会改变 MTX 的肾排泄，增加毒性或降低疗效。据报道，MTX 与非甾体抗炎药之间存在有害甚至致命的不良反应，尤其是萘普生和酮洛芬[62,63]。这种毒性增加可能是由于肾脏分泌的竞争导致的肾脏消除减少[57]。其他常用的有机药物也可能增强 MTX 的毒性，如保泰松，水杨酸盐和丙磺舒[64,65]。丙磺舒增加 MTX 在荷瘤小鼠体内的疗效，但在临床上并没有以此为目的的应用[66]。

甲氧苄啶(抗菌剂)与 MTX 一起使用导致毒性增加亦有报道。据推测,这种叶酸拮抗剂对哺乳动物 DHFR 只有很弱的亲和力,可以降低叶酸储存量,尤其是对于亚临床叶酸缺乏症患者,这使得骨髓细胞更容易受到 MTX 毒性的影响[67]。接受 MTX 治疗的患者亦应避免饮酒,因为会增加肝纤维化和肝硬化的风险。

药物基因组学

越来越多的数据表明,之所以不同患者间对叶酸拮抗剂的疗效反应和毒性存在差异,是因为人群中负责叶酸代谢的酶在基因上存在与生俱来的遗传变异。关于这些数据的更详细讨论超出了本章的范围,但一直是综合评论的主题[68-71]。简而言之,功能多态性已在 DHFR、亚甲基四氢叶酸还原酶(MTHFR)、氨基咪唑甲酰胺核糖核苷酸转化酶(ATIC)、还原叶酸载体(RFC)、GGH、蛋氨酸合成酶(MTR)、蛋氨酸合成酶还原酶(MTRR)、亚甲基四氢叶酸脱氢酶(MTHFD)、丝氨酸羟甲基转移酶(SHMT)、TS 和溶质载体有机阴离子转运蛋白基因 1B1(SLCO1B1)的基因启动子或编码区中描述。许多多态性在人群中存在频率较高,并且与急性淋巴细胞白血病[72-77]或类风湿性关节炎患者中较高的复发率或毒性相关[78]。这些数据表明,如果这些多态性基因在较大的群体中复制,那么将有可能基于每位患者的基因型进行 MTX 的个体化治疗。

基因-环境相互作用可以调节基因型变异对毒性的影响。例如,人们观察到一些血清同型半胱氨酸(功能性叶酸缺乏的标志物)的变异可以通过 MTHFR 基因中的两种常见功能多态性来解释,即 C677T 和 A1298C,但仅限于饮食叶酸摄入减少的情况[79,80]。在强制性服用叶酸补充剂的国家,充足的膳食叶酸可以消除遗传多态性的影响。

临床应用

临床用量表

自从 60 多年前 MTX 引入临床以来,MTX 已经按照各种剂量方案实施(表 56-1)。在头颈癌患者的 MTX 试验中,剂量为 50 500mg/m² 或 5 000mg/m²,同时用 LV“救援”治疗,观察到剂量反应的趋势分别:5/24、5/16 和 9/18。于较低剂量下缺乏反应的患者,在 5 000mg/m² 剂量方案下可呈现一定反应性[81]。一项实验研究强调了剂量调度的重要性,该研究显示对高剂量 MTX 的耐药性,可能不会影响持续低剂量方案[82]。在联合治疗中,确定 MTX 的最佳剂量方案是复杂的(表 56-2)。当 MTX 与 5-氟尿嘧啶(5-FU),L-天冬酰胺酶,以及与阿糖胞苷和 6-巯基嘌呤或 6-硫鸟嘌呤一起使用时,测序成为很重要的步骤。表 56-2 总结了包括 MTX 在内的一些常见药物组合的使用,以及序列特异性。

表 56-1 甲氨蝶呤(MTX)常用剂量表

剂量时间表	应用及评价
口服	
每周或每 2 周(15~25mg,顿服或分次服用)	主要用于银屑病、类风湿性关节炎等良性疾病
每周或每 2 周(20~30mg/m²)	ALL 的维持治疗
肠外给药	
每周脉冲式用药(30~60mg/m²)	绒毛膜癌,ALL
间隔用药(150~500mg/m²,每周)	ALL,NHL;需要 LV 解救,10~15mg/m²,q6h×6~8 剂
高剂量用药(500~12 000mg/m² 每周或隔周)	骨肉瘤,ALL,肿瘤性脑膜炎;需要 LV 解救

略缩语:ALL,急性淋巴细胞白血病;LV,亚叶酸;NHL,非霍奇金淋巴瘤。

表 56-2 甲氨蝶呤(MTX)联合化疗

联合用药	使用要点	联合效果	评价
5-氟尿嘧啶	MTX 用药需早于 5-FU 24 小时	协同	
蒽环类药物		增效	
博来霉素		增效	黏膜毒性增加
糖皮质激素	同时使用	协同	用于 ALL
环磷酰胺	同时使用	增效	
阿糖胞苷	同时使用	增效或协同	
门冬酰胺酶	如果 MTX 早于门冬酰胺酶 24 小时用药	协同	用于 ALL,AML
	如果两者同时用药	拮抗	
长春碱类		增效	

略缩语:ALL,急性淋巴细胞白血病;AML,急性髓细胞白血病;5-FU,5-氟尿嘧啶。

MTX 治疗肿瘤现况

急性淋巴细胞白血病

在急性淋巴细胞白血病患者的治疗中，MTX 几乎是所有多药治疗方案的组成部分之一，并且一些诱导缓解方案也包括 MTX。除全身用药外，MTX 还可用于治疗脑膜白血病和预防 CNS 复发。

在缓解后早期的强化治疗治疗阶段，MTX 可以口服或肠外给药。一些肠外给药的方案中已纳入中等剂量（100~500mg/m²/剂量）或高剂量（≥1 000mg/m²）的 MTX，增加了早期骨髓细胞中 MTX-聚谷氨酸的积累[83]，以克服其抗药性，并改善了包括 CNS 和睾丸在内等受保护部位的渗透性[84]。虽然 HD-MTX 预防 CNS 复发的效果尚未得到明确证实[39]，但随着中等剂量或高剂量 MTX 的使用，单纯的睾丸复发率似乎有所下降[85]。随机试验表明，逐步提高剂量的静脉给药与口服 MTX 相比，随机分配到静脉给药组进行间歇维持治疗的患者 5 年无事件生存率（EFS）显著改善[86-89]。然而，在一些研究中，EFS 的增加是以增加血液学和神经毒性为代价的[90-93]。

在后续维持治疗阶段，目前大多数治疗方案有赖于每周使用低剂量（20~50mg/m²）MTX 与每日巯嘌呤结合，并且需要延长使用周期。早期研究表明，在缓解治疗阶段，每周两次治疗（20mg/m²）优于连续每日口服用药[94]。还显示了口服分剂量的有效性（每 6 小时给予 25~30mg/m²，每周 4~6 次）[30]。

急性髓性白血病

目前 MTX 在治疗急性非淋巴细胞白血病患者中的价值还比较有限。在使用含 MTX 的治疗方案：泼尼松、长春新碱、甲氨蝶呤和巯基嘌呤（POMP）[95]或含 L-天冬酰胺酶的 MTX（“Capizzi 方案”）的成人 AML 患者中，大约四分之一能达到完全缓解[96,97]。在多数人群中，使用 LV 解救的大剂量方案对外周血细胞计数具有短暂而快速的影响，但却没有产生骨髓缓解[98]。MTX 之所以在治疗这种疾病中疗效不佳，是由于 MTX 在胞内聚谷氨酰胺化不足以及治疗后靶酶 DHFR 的增加进而导致药物在细胞内难以保留造成的[99]。

淋巴瘤

Ⅱ期临床研究表明中至高剂量的 MTX（200mg/m² 至 3g/m²）联合 LV 解救可以使大细胞淋巴瘤患者产生短暂消退，基于此，一些中、高级淋巴瘤的联合用药方案中已将 MTX 联合 LV 解救纳入其中。在一些方案（例如，M-BACOD）中，MTX 在药物治疗后的白细胞减少期间与 LV 一起使用，因为 MTX/LV 组合几乎没有骨髓毒性[100]。一些实验研究表明 MTX 和阿糖胞苷产生了叠加和协同的作用，基于此[101]，该组合也被用于治疗这种疾病的方案中（例如，COMLA 方案：环磷酰胺、长春新碱、MTX、阿糖胞苷和 LV）。同样，部分文献记载了一些 Burkitt 淋巴瘤患者对应用 MTX[102,103]在内的治疗方案呈现一定反应性。对于 Burkitt 淋巴瘤患者，高剂量 MTX 联合 LV 解救治疗已被加入 CVAD，阿糖胞苷和鞘内治疗以及其他联合化疗方案中。

原发性中枢神经系统淋巴瘤患者的大多数治疗方案包括高剂量 MTX，因为常规放射剂量可能导致神经毒性。在 226 例原发性中枢神经系统淋巴瘤患者的回顾性研究中，那些接受 HDMTX 方案后进行放疗的患者存活率提高，同时没有增加晚期神经毒性风险[107]。

绒毛膜癌

绒毛膜癌的独特之处在于，使用甲氨蝶呤或放线菌素 D 单药治疗可获得相当好的治疗效果[108]。这种肿瘤对甲氨蝶呤异常敏感的机制尚不完全清楚，但绒毛膜癌细胞可能通过合成长链聚合谷氨酸有效地积累和保留这种药物。JAR（人绒毛膜癌）细胞系对叶酸和叶酸拮抗剂具有活化受体偶联摄取作用（胞吞作用）[109]。目前治疗这种恶性肿瘤的方案是 MTX 与其他药物联合使用，特别是对“低风险”或复发患者[110]。

乳腺癌

单药应用甲氨蝶呤导致大约 30% 的乳腺癌患者复发。当与氟尿嘧啶联合使用时，连续使用甲氨蝶呤和 5-FU 可将反应率提高到 50%，并可提高辅助治疗时的无病生存率[111]。研究者使用环磷酰胺、甲氨蝶呤及 CMF 方案（甲氨蝶呤氟尿嘧啶）辅助治疗也显著减少复发风险[112]；对于更多应用保守手术治疗的局部病变的乳腺癌女性患者，亦可作为新辅助治疗方案[113]；同时也可以在晚期、进展的患者中发挥作用[114]。甲氨蝶呤、5-FU 和长春瑞滨（VMF）联合使用代替环磷酰胺，同样能够在进展患者中发挥作用[115]。与含烷基化剂的方案相比，这种组合的另一个优点是减少了长期毒性（不孕、致癌）。最后，值得注意的是，每日口服环磷酰胺联合低剂量口服 MTX（2.5mg，每日 2 次×2 天/周）在重度经预处理的晚期转移性乳腺癌患者中显示出活性[116]。

胃肠道恶性肿瘤

抗叶酸药物对胃肠道恶性肿瘤的治疗效果有限。甲氨蝶呤在这些疾病治疗中的作用主要是调节并有可能提高 5-FU 的疗效。通过抑制嘌呤的合成，使用甲氨蝶呤预处理增加了磷酸核糖焦磷酸盐含量，这是 5-FU 核苷酸形成所必需的前提[117]。最近在结肠癌患者中使用高剂量 MTX 和 LV/5-FU 的试验数据强调了，甲氨蝶呤和 5-FU 之间需要 7~24 小时的间隔[118]。然而，在一项随Ⅲ期研究中，5-FU 联合甲氨蝶呤与标准持续输注 5-FU 相比毒性增加，但总生存率却无明显差异。基于这些发现，5-FU 仍然是晚期胃癌的治疗标准药物[119-121]。

泌尿生殖器系统恶性肿瘤

单独甲氨蝶呤（100mg/m²）或高剂量（≥500mg/m²）联合 LV 解救，在晚期膀胱癌治疗中具有积极作用。报告的反应率（约 30%）与另一种最有效的单药顺铂相似。包括甲氨蝶呤与顺铂、长春碱和阿霉素（M-VAC）的联合用药已获得可观的长期临床缓解[122]。随机试验的荟萃分析发现，使用含甲氨蝶呤方案的新辅助治疗具有一定生存优势[123]。

头颈癌

甲氨蝶呤是一种治疗晚期头颈部肿瘤的有效药物。大剂量甲氨蝶呤联合 LV 抢救方案的反应率从 30% 提高到 50%，但缓解时间和生存率没有提高[124]。甲氨蝶呤亦可与 5-FU 联合治疗这种疾病，有效率高达 60%[125,126]。虽然观察到不同的毒性，但给药顺序和给药时间尚未显示影响反应率。

肺癌

甲氨蝶呤作为常规剂量单用或高剂量联合 LV 解救，在非小细胞肺癌(NSCLC)中仅具有微弱的活性。这种药物在小细胞肺癌中确实活性有限，并已与他药联合治疗该疾病。普拉曲沙是一种非经典的抗叶酸药物，已被证明对接受过其他治疗方案的 NSCLC 患者有效，稍后将对此进行详细讨论[127]。

骨肉瘤

骨肉瘤对传统剂量的甲氨蝶呤反应较差。然而，高剂量甲氧蝶呤自 20 世纪 70 年代问世以来一直是治疗的主要药物之一[128]。随机试验的前后结果显示了化疗的优势，包括高剂量甲氨蝶呤与 LV 挽救[129]。不同的研究探讨甲氨蝶呤峰值浓度和浓度-时间曲线下面积(AUC)是否是骨肉瘤的重要预后因素[130]。关于甲氨蝶呤暴露与结果之间是否存在相关性仍存在争议[131]。最近的一项研究分析了甲氨蝶呤药代动力学、毒性与骨肉瘤患儿生存的关系。虽然生存结果与峰值浓度或 AUC 无关，但 48 小时内甲氨蝶呤浓度与生存有显著相关性，证实系统 MTX 暴露是影响治疗结果的重要预后因素[132]。

肿瘤性脑膜炎

鞘内注射甲氨蝶呤通常是治疗实体瘤癌性脑膜炎的一个组成部分。高剂量静脉注射甲氨蝶呤($8g/m^2$)联合 LV 挽救是唯一的治疗方法[38]，这可能是一个合理的选择，因为在肿瘤性脑膜炎存在的情况下，甲氨蝶呤的抗肿瘤浓度更容易达到治疗目的[133]。

副作用

血液毒性

MTX 靶向作用于叶酸依赖酶的表达，这种靶向具有细胞周期特异性，这与它们在 DNA 合成中的作用一致。自我更新快的组织，具有较高比例的 S 期细胞，因此更有可能被叶酸拮抗剂所破坏。所有骨髓祖细胞都受到甲氨蝶呤的影响，但通常以中性粒细胞减少为主，在给药后 10 天中性粒细胞数目达到最低点，一般在第 14~21 天开始恢复。MTX 对骨髓的影响与剂量有关，但在患者之间存在相当大的差异。遗传变异[71 134 135]、亚临床叶酸缺乏症、肾功能不全、放射治疗、化疗或感染造成的骨髓损伤，以及曾使用复方新诺明预防卡氏肺孢子菌病均可能使患者更易出现血液(和胃肠道)毒性。年轻患者通常比老年人更能耐受甲氨蝶呤，这可能与该药物在肾脏的清除率有关。LV 的应用可以预防或减少甲氨蝶呤毒性，并允许更大剂量叶酸拮抗剂的使用。

胃肠道毒性

即使是高剂量的甲氨蝶呤，恶心和呕吐的症状通常也是轻到中度的。相反，黏膜炎是甲氨蝶呤治疗的常见副作用。黏膜炎通常在接触药物后 3~5 天出现。这是甲氨蝶呤毒性的早期毒性，发生时应停止用药。更严重的胃肠道毒性表现为腹泻，可进展为严重的血性腹泻。当这种情况合并中性粒细胞减少时，患者就有很高的盲肠炎、败血症甚至死亡的风险。这些严重的副作用通常发生在肾功能不全的情况下，通常由高剂量甲氨蝶呤(≥$500mg/m^2$/剂量)导致，但也可能发生在接受常规剂量治疗的患者中。用药过程中应监测甲氨蝶呤血药浓度和血肌酐水平，并给予适当剂量的 LV，并辅以对症支持治疗(详见下文讨论)。

肾毒性

肾毒性有时发生在高剂量甲氨蝶呤治疗后，在低剂量治疗期间很少发生。当发生肾毒性时，甲氨蝶呤清除延迟，随后导致严重的骨髓和胃肠道毒性，这可能是致命的，尤其是在成年人[136]。这种毒性的产生是由于甲氨蝶呤及其不溶性代谢物 7-OH 甲氨蝶呤在肾小管沉积造成的(图 56-3)，同时该药物亦有可能对肾小管造成直接损害[47]。通过充分的水化、碱化尿液以及渗透性利尿剂的使用，甲氨蝶呤和 7-OH 甲氨蝶呤的溶解度增加，使这一问题得到明显的改善。部分患者，即使采用这种方案(表 56-3)，也会出现肾功能损害；因此，密切监测甲氨蝶呤和血肌酐水平是必要的[137]。对于那些因急性肾功能不全继发甲氨蝶呤清除延迟的患者，增加 LV 剂量，已成为抵消高甲氨蝶呤不良反应的常规治疗策略[137]。

甲基黄嘌呤，如咖啡因或氨茶碱，可能在改善 MTX 延迟清除中发挥作用。MTX 可以增加血清腺苷浓度，从而降低肾小球滤过率[17]。因此，腺苷受体竞争性拮抗剂，如甲基黄嘌呤，可能作为一种特殊的利尿剂，以增加 MTX 的消除[138]。

极高水平的 MTX($>10^{-3}$M)很难解救，即使是使用大剂量的 LV[139]。通过腹膜透析或血液透析去除 MTX 也是无效的，因为该药物具有广泛的蛋白结合性。炭柱吸附型人工肾已经成功地应用于少数患者，但在治疗后 MTX 水平会发生反弹，因此疗效受到限制[140]。甲氨蝶呤体外清除方法，如高通量血液透析和血液透析过滤，其效果各不相同，但均为有创方法，其 MTX 水平仅出现短暂而轻微的下降，并且需要联合或每日重复使用才能有效降低 MTX 浓度[141,142]。口服木炭和消胆胺也可以结合肠道中的 MTX，从而限制了其肠肝循环和毒性[143]。胸腺嘧啶[$1\sim3g/(m^2\cdot d)$]也能够解救 MTX 毒性，但这种代谢产物一般不存在[144]。重组细菌羧肽酶——谷卡匹酶[羧肽酶-G2($CPDG_2$)]，是一种通过水解的方法切断 MTX 的肽键形成谷氨酸盐和 dAMPA 的酶(图 56-3)。有报道称，在给药后 1 小时内，全身 MTX 浓度可迅速降低>95%[145,146]。对于发生危及生命毒性的高危患者，静脉或鞘内给予 MTX 后，在 96 小时内给予羧肽酶 G2 并联合 LV 效果明显[146-148]。上述大多数研究是在成人中进行的，但最近对儿科患者的回顾性研究也得出了类似的得出结论[150]。

肝毒性

长期每周低剂量服用 MTX 治疗银屑病、类风湿关节炎或者 ALL 患者与门脉纤维化有关，而且在一些患者中，出现了明显的肝硬化[151]。在癌症患者中，肝酶的急性升高通常发生在 MTX 治疗后的几天内，但很快恢复正常，但即使升高到正常上限的 10~20 倍，似乎也不能预测慢性肝毒性[152,153]。同时使用地塞米松可能增加 MTX 诱导的肝毒性[154]。在这些患者中应避免使用酒精和其他肝毒性药物。

表 56-3　高剂量甲氨蝶呤(MTX)支持治疗

水化、碱化预处理
治疗前 8~12 小时,患者应接受 1.5L/m^2 生理盐水或 5%葡萄糖注射液,同时使用 100mEq HCO_3 和 20mEq KCl/L 持续水化直至尿液 pH 达到 7.0 及以上
检测
用药 24 小时后应监测 MTX 血药浓度;分别在用药前、用药后 24 小时、用药后 48 小时检测血肌酐水平
额外的 LV 解救
用药后 24 小时 MTX 水平>10^{-6}M 时使用 LV 解救。MTX 血药浓度达到 10^{-6}M 时,提高 LV 剂量至 100mg/m^2 q 6h;MTX 血药浓度达到 5×10^{-6}M 时,提高 LV 浓度至 200mg/m^2 q 6h
在 MTX 血药浓度<10^{-8}M 之前,需要每日监测 MTX 水平并持续使用 LV 解救

略缩语:LV,亚叶酸。

中枢神经系统毒性

鞘内及静脉给予高剂量 MTX 会带来轻到重度的急性神经系统毒性。已有部分报道指出意外过量的情况下(鞘内>100mg)可导致死亡。随着对由 MTX 引起的神经毒性的病理生理学的更深入了解,现已开始出现治疗性干预措施来预防或治疗这种并发症。

鞘内注射 MTX 最常见的直接副作用表现为严重头痛、发热、脑膜炎、呕吐和脑脊液细胞增多。这些表现认为是由化学性蛛网膜炎引起的,亦可能是由腺苷释放引起的,腺苷在中枢神经系统是一种强效的内分泌物质[155]。腺苷的这种作用通过低剂量系统地应用茶碱类药物得到改善,如氨茶碱和茶碱,它们是腺苷受体的竞争性拮抗剂[138]。如果这些症状持续,可能需要调整剂量或改用阿糖胞苷。大剂量 MTX 全身治疗后几天即可发生急性毒性反应,表现为头痛、麻痹、失语症或癫痫发作。它通常是短暂的,在 2~3 天内就会消散[156]。

亚急性神经毒性(给药后 7~14 天)在 5%~18%接受鞘内 MTX 和/或静脉高剂量 MTX 的患者中被观察到。最严重的表现为四肢运动瘫痪、脑神经麻痹、癫痫甚至昏迷。虽然亚急性抗叶酸诱导的神经毒性的发病机制可能是多因素的,但同型半胱氨酸稳态的破坏可能发挥关键作用。MTX 通过抑制甲硫氨酸的再甲基化,导致患者血浆和脑脊液中同型半胱氨酸含量增加[157]。同型半胱氨酸可通过诱导神经组织和血管内皮的氧化损伤而引起神经毒性[158,159]。此外,同型半胱氨酸及其代谢产物是具有兴奋毒性的氨基酸(谷氨酸类似物),可激活 n-甲基-d-天冬氨酸(NMDA)类谷氨酸受体。MTX 的亚急性神经毒性可以通过天冬氨酸受体的拮抗剂来改善,如右美沙芬或美金刚[160-162]。

MTX 诱发的迟发性神经毒性可能与多达 80%的急性淋巴细胞白血病患儿的慢性脱髓鞘性脑病有关,影像学改变的大小似乎与静脉 MTX 的剂量和给药次数多少有关[92,93]。计算机体层成像扫描显示皮质萎缩,脑室扩大,颅内弥漫钙化。虽然最常见的原因是归咎于鞘内注射 MTX 联合颅脑放疗,但也有报道称,仅接受高剂 IV MTX 治疗也可引起脑病。迟发性神经毒性的发病机制可能是髓鞘相关成分叶酸依赖性甲基化过程障碍造成的[163]。

对于在接受鞘内注射 MTX 过量(>100mg)的患者,建议立即用脑室灌注清除脑脊液[164]。在鞘内给予致命剂量 MTX 的动物模型中,同样通过鞘内使用羧肽酶 G2 被证明可以降低动物的死亡率,这被认为是治疗鞘内 MTX 并发症的首选方法[165]。在这些病例中没有提到鞘内或全身应用 LV,因为这种毒性不太可能是由抑制 DHFR 引起的。

肺毒性

虽然肺毒性并不常见,但在长期接受低剂量口服 MTX 治疗的患者中,MTX 引起的肺毒性已引起关注[166]。临床表现通常包括咳嗽、呼吸困难、发烧和低氧血症。胸片表现不具备特异性,可表现为片状间质浸润影。同时接受类固醇治疗的患者必须排除卡氏肺孢子菌感染。组织学检查显示弥漫性间质淋巴细胞浸润,并可见巨细胞和非干酪样肉芽肿。在一些患者中,可观察到外周血嗜酸性粒细胞增多,这增加了过敏性肺炎的可能性。这一过程可能进展为肺纤维化,在肺毒性尚且可逆的情况下及时停用 MTX 是很重要的。一些患者出院后,没有复发。

皮肤毒性

MTX 导致的皮肤毒性通常发生在 5%~10%的患者中。表现为红斑性皮疹,特征性见于颈部和上躯干。皮疹伴瘙痒通常可持续几天亦可相对不易察觉。应用中等剂量 MTX 后出现皮肤血管炎的亦有报道[167]。在大剂量或过量使用甲氨蝶呤后发生严重全身 MTX 毒性时,皮肤可形成严重的大疱和脱屑[168]。

致畸及突变效应

叶酸缺乏通过使 DNA 低甲基化改变基因表达,使 DNA 双联中的胸腺嘧啶为尿嘧啶所取代,进而促进 DNA 双链断裂。因此,叶酸缺乏能够直接促进促进肿瘤的形成[169]。众所周知,MTX 是强效堕胎药,尤其在早期妊娠阶段。尽管如此,对于 MTX 的致畸及致癌效应,却缺乏直接的证据。

其他毒性

有报道称,长期低剂量 MTX 用药会导致骨质疏松[170],这也许是因为 MTX 能够直接抑制成骨细胞的分化[171]。亦有报道称,高剂量 MTX 可导致发热、癫痫、再放射反应、光毒性、过敏反应。较高剂量用药方案还会引起脾脏的炎症,从而出现肋膜炎和左上腹疼痛的表现。另有研究表明,在使用 MTX 的情况下,机体会产生红细胞 IgG-3 抗体,从而诱发急性溶血性贫血[172]。

叶酸拮抗剂耐药性

尽管含 MTX 化疗方案的疗效已经在很多不同恶性肿瘤的治疗中取得了很大的进步,但即便是在化疗敏感恶性肿瘤中,无疾病进展期依然难以得到显著延长。和许多其他抗肿瘤药物一样,MTX 疗效的发挥同样受到固有耐药和获得性耐药的限制。MTX 耐药机制可分为以下几种类型:①细胞转运机制受损使药物胞内累计含量下降;②聚谷氨酸化降低或去谷氨酸化过程增强使 MTX 多聚谷氨酸盐形式积累下降;③DHFR 含量或活性增加;④DHFR 基因突变,使其与 MTX 亲和力较正常减低。除了上述机制,DHFR 和 FPGS 的活性受到细胞周期的影响,细胞周期相关基因失调将对抗代谢药物的耐药性产生深刻影响。

MTX 固有耐药

叶酸拮抗剂固有敏感性与线粒体酶表达有关[22]。在许多种肿瘤细胞中,由于受到 myc 基因的驱动,参与代谢丝氨酸、叶酸、甘氨酸的酶表达上调。这种表达的异质性,使不同正常组织对叶酸拮抗剂的敏感性出现差异。

通过 RFC 转运 MTX 的功能出现障碍,使得很多肿瘤出现了固有耐药。叶酸拮抗剂转运功能受损大部分是由于 RFC 出现量或质的改变。这其中可能涉及 RFC 基因本身的突变直接影响其转运活性;启动子甲基化及 3′非翻译区改变使 RFC 基因沉默;转录因子功能失活使 RFC 基因沉默;而且在叶酸拮抗剂耐药细胞中,RFC 基因复制也出现了异常[173]。通过骨肉瘤组织活检获取标本并进行反转录-聚合酶联反应发现,RFC 表达过程中,mRNA 含量下降[174]。在其他肿瘤中,RFC 表达下降可由启动子区甲基化异常导致[175,176]。

有研究报道称,与转运功能改变相关的 RFC 基因突变在耐药细胞[177]及白血病细胞[178]中出现。RFC 基因的单核苷酸多态(SNPs)会使蛋白质对叶酸拮抗剂的亲和力减低,然而却对叶酸具有持久而充分地亲和力,从而使细胞持续生长。其他已知的 SNPs 选择性的提高叶酸亲和力并增加胞内叶酸储备。然而一项研究分析了来自 246 例白血病患儿的样本,结果只有 3 例出现了有效的 RFC 多态性,这表明至少在这个群体中,SNPs 并不是产生 MTX 固有耐药性的主要原因[179]。

多聚谷氨酸盐使经典叶酸拮抗剂更易在胞内停留。因此,缺乏 FPGS 活性的细胞,耐药性相对增加。也许就是形成长链 MTX 多聚谷氨酸盐能力的差异能够解释为什么 AML 比 ALL 的 MTX 耐药性强[180,181]。类似的,来自对 MTX 耐药的软组织肉瘤组织的肿瘤细胞往往形成长链 MTX 多聚谷氨酸盐的能力较低[182,183]。和 T 细胞来源的 ALL 细胞相比,B 细胞来源的 ALL 细胞具有更高的 FPGS 活性,因此后者胞内积聚了更多的长链 MTX 多聚谷氨酸盐[184,185]。研究发现,AML、ALL 细胞系和原始细胞之间[186],耐药和敏感肉瘤细胞之间[187]的 FPGS 对 MTX 的亲和性是不同的;而且,从 L1210 细胞和小鼠肝细胞分离出来的 FPGS 被长链多聚谷氨酸盐抑制的程度也是不同的。上述这些事实都说明了不同组织表达不同的 FPGS 亚型(剪接变异体)[10]。

众所周知,目标酶 DHFR 表达的增加是 MTX 获得性耐药的机制,但同样能够导致固有耐药的发生。在 3′非翻译区出现的核苷酸多态降低了抑制性微小 RNA 片段(miR-24)的结合,这使得 DHFR 表达增加,即便是在没有暴露于 MTX 的情况下[188]。尽管起初人们认为这种 SNP 存在于 11%~16%的日本人群中[189],但在其他人群众,这种 SNP 出现的概率更低[190]。

视网膜母细胞瘤蛋白的缺失在很多种类型的肿瘤细胞中出现,在 MTX 固有耐药过程中亦发挥了重要的作用。在视网膜母细胞瘤蛋白缺失的情况下,转录因子 E2F 的表达增加,进而使一些 DNA 复制相关基因,包括 DHFR,表达增加[191]。

p-糖蛋白过表达不会导致 MTX 耐药。然而,MTX 确是一些蛋白的作用底物,如多药耐药蛋白 1-5(ABCC1-5)[192,193]以及乳腺癌耐药蛋白(ABCG2)[194]。ABCC5[193]和 ABCG2[195]能够转运 MTX 和 MTX 多聚谷氨酸盐。一些体外研究表明这些蛋白过度表达会产生 MTX 耐药性[193,196,197],并且会影响白血病患者对治疗的反应[198,199]。但是,在其他疾病中,这些蛋白在何种程度上引起 MTX 固有耐药尚不明确。

MTX 获得性耐药

目前通过对实验室和临床样本的研究已经阐明了 4 种 MTX 获得性耐药机制:基于 DHFR 基因扩增的 DHFR 活性增强;DHFR 基因突变改变了 DHFR 对 MTX 的亲和力;通过 RFC 转入胞内的 MTX 减少;长链多聚谷氨酸盐形成减少。在药物转入细胞内的关键环节,无论是 RFC 基因突变还是缺失,都会使 MTX 摄取减少并进而导致 MTX 耐药。尽管在白血病患者中,RFC 基因多态性似乎并不是固有耐药的常见机制,但是对于 ALL 复发的患者来说,由于 RFC 基因异常使 MTX 转运减少却是白血病细胞耐药的主要机制[200]。

暴露于 MTX 使 DHFR 蛋白含量快速升高,因为 MTX 与 DHFR 结合后将阻止其与自身 mRNA 结合进而解除对其转录的抑制作用[201]。研究表明,基于基因扩增的不稳定且可逆的耐药性往往与含 DHFR 扩增的"双微染色体"有关[202]。而高水平且稳定的耐药性与 MTX 结合区域异常有关,通常指那些单一染色区[203-207]。在包含人类细胞在内的多种细胞系中,DHFR 都存在点突变,人们发现这些点突变会使 MTX 与 DHFR 结合发生改变,并且这些突变还会使 DHFR 结合 MTX 部位的氨基酸残基产生疏水作用[208]。

尽管在多种 MTX 耐药细胞系中发现了多聚谷氨酸盐减少[209],但这些细胞的耐药性确是多种耐药机制发挥作用的。耐药细胞中 MTX 多聚谷氨酸盐的水解往往是由于转入溶酶体增多[210]及 GGH 活性增强[183,211]所致。最近一些研究充分证明了,GGH 基因启动子及编码区的表观遗传学异常和 SNPs 可影响 GGH 表达,最终影响叶酸拮抗剂的治疗效果[212-214]。然而亦有研究表明,短暂使用 MTX 处理的 GGH 过表达的肿瘤细胞,并不会产生耐药性[215]。

克服 MTX 耐药性的新策略

随着人们不断加深对叶酸生理学、MTX 毒性、耐药性的理解,并且掌握了 MTX 靶酶的晶体学数据,合理的设计出新的叶酸拮抗剂已是大势所趋[208]。新设计出的叶酸拮抗剂至少具备如下至少一点特性：具备更强的 RFC 结合力以更多地转入胞内，或者能够独立于 RFC 入胞；能够不依赖聚谷氨酸化过程发挥作用，或者具备更高的 FPGS 亲和力以增强多聚谷氨酸化过程；能够更强的抑制 DHFR 或 TS；具备更强的嘌呤合成关键酶抑制作用。

氨蝶呤（AMT）——古老的叶酸拮抗剂

临床试验和临床前试验数据都支持我们重新评价 MTX 的“前辈”，4-氨基-蝶酰-谷氨酸（AMT；图 56-1），这可是第一个在白血病患者中达到临床缓解的叶酸拮抗剂[2]。和 MTX 相比，AMT 具备一些优势：AMT 具有 20~40 倍于 MTX 的临床疗效[216]；白血病患者的体外实验表明，AMT 能够更有效地被 FPGS 转化成多聚谷氨酸类物质（更高的 V_{max}/K_m 比）[217]，从而增加胞内的蓄积[218]；完全的口服生物利用度[219]。一项Ⅱ期临床试验表明，27%难治 ALL 患儿口服 AMT 后临床上达到明显的缓解[220]。另一项Ⅱb 期临床试验表明，在使用多药治疗的具有高复发风险的新诊断的 ALL 患儿中，AMT 能够很安全的替代 MTX 而不会具备更多的毒副作用[134]。最新的临床前数据表明 AMT 能够使过敏性皮炎的患者获益[221]。

普拉曲沙——二代 DHFR 抑制剂

与 MTX 相似，普拉曲沙（10-炔丙基-10-去氮甲氨蝶呤；PDX；图 56-4），能够完全阻断 DHFR，限制胸腺嘧啶的合成和细胞分裂。PDX 对 RFC 和 FPGS 具有很高的亲和力，这使得其能够更好且更具选择性的进入并停留在肿瘤细胞内[222]。最终，和 MTX 相比，PDX 展现了 14 倍于 MTX 的胞内流入率[223]，并且能够更有效地抑制肿瘤的生长[224]。

通常普拉曲沙通过静脉给药。全身暴露总量（AUC）和最高血药浓度（C_{max}）呈剂量依赖性。清除 PDX 的 $t_{1/2}$ 是 12~18 小时。大约占给药剂量 1/3 的药物会以原型的形式随尿液排出体外，该药物的清除率随肌酐清除率下降而减低。PDX 的药物动力学特性在多周期药物治疗后并不会发生明显的改变[225]。

PDX 与吉西他滨[226]和硼替佐米[227]联合用药的临床前研究结果，促使人们将这种药物组合用在淋巴瘤患者身上，相关的临床试验正在开展。T 细胞淋巴瘤患者的总反应率明显高于 B 细胞淋巴瘤，表明含 PDX 的药物方案对 T 细胞恶性肿瘤具有较高的选择性[228]。PROPEL 研究是一项关于普拉曲沙治疗复发难治外周 T 细胞淋巴瘤的回顾性研究。该研究总共纳入了 115 例患者，大部分都进行过长期多周期治疗。总的反应率是 29%，基于此研究结果，FDA 已经批准 PDX 用于治疗复发难治 T 细胞淋巴瘤[229]。此外，在治疗 NSCLC 和复发难治皮肤 T 细胞淋巴瘤患者中，PDX 同样显示出了较高的活性及可接受的毒副反应[230]。一项最近的研究表明，LV 在体内外具有保护性作用，可解救 PDX 的毒性[231]。

培美曲塞——以作用于 TS 为主的多种叶酸依赖酶抑制剂

培美曲塞｛N-[4-[2-(2-氨基-3，4-二氢-4-氧-7H-吡咯并[2，3-d]嘧啶-5-烷基)乙基]苯甲酰基]-左旋谷氨酸；图 56-4｝能够抑制 TS、DHFR 及甘氨酸核糖核苷甲酰基转移酶。最初该药被视为一种多靶点叶酸拮抗剂，然而其主要作用于 TS，因为研究表明其与 TS 的亲和力更强，这一点可以通过终产物抑制试验证明[232,233]。培美曲塞通过 RFC 和质子耦联叶酸转运体转入胞内。培美曲塞在胞内能够快速地被 FPGS 多聚谷氨酸化，其 K_m 值比 MTX 低两个计量等级。和普拉曲沙一样，培美曲塞一般通过静脉给药。其 AUC 及 C_{max} 呈剂量依赖性。对于肾功能正常的患者，培美曲塞半衰期为 3.5 小时。培美曲塞的 PK 在多周期药物治疗后并不会发生明显的改变[234]。临床上发现，血中 Hcy 浓度升高会增加培美曲塞的毒性。Hcy 浓度升高与营养性叶酸缺乏及 5-甲基四氢叶酸减少有关，后者为甲硫氨酸合成所必需，其缺乏往往是继发于亚甲基四氢叶酸还原酶变异。在后续药物方案中补充这些维生素，不但能够减轻毒性而且还能够使患者耐受更多周期的治疗，进而提高治疗的反应性[235]。

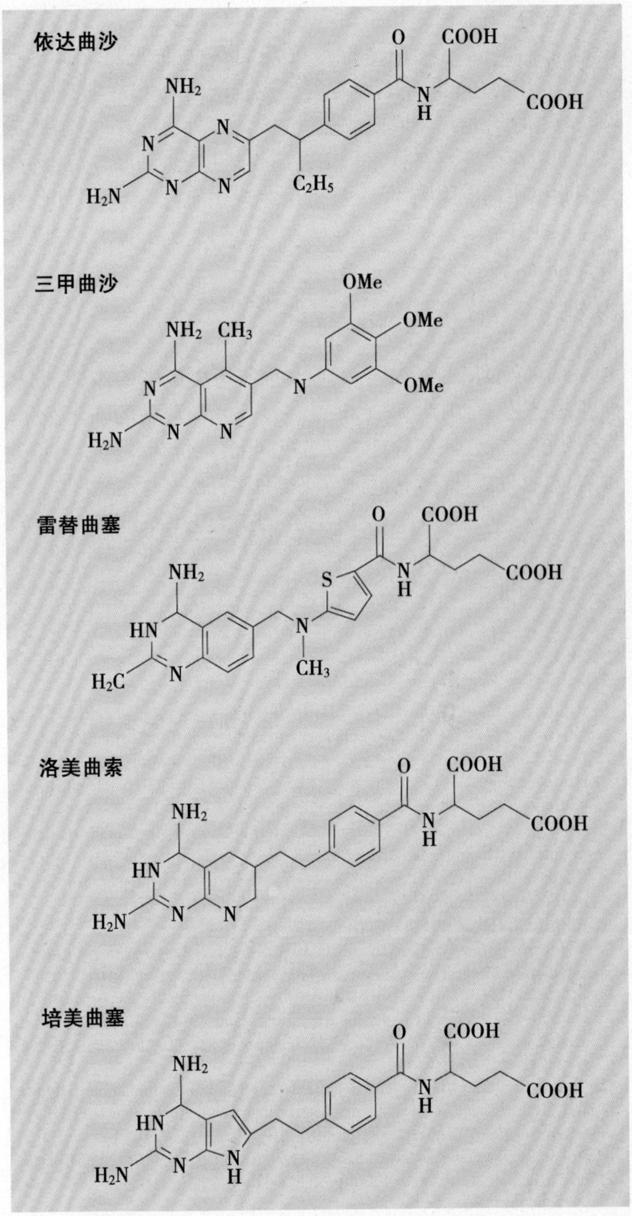

培美曲塞在多种肿瘤类型中具有光谱的活性[236]。基于一项Ⅲ期临床试验的研究结果，培美曲塞和顺铂联合可作为晚期 NSCLC 治疗的一线方案[237]。一项名为 PARAMOUNT 的Ⅲ期

图 56-4　临床上热门的叶酸拮抗剂新星

临床试验评估了使用培美曲塞在NSCLC维持治疗中的效果。该研究证明了，培美曲塞能够提高无疾病进展期及总生存期[238]。该药还能够单药治疗复发或难治的NSCLC，此外还能够与顺铂联合治疗胸膜间皮瘤[235,239]。此外，尚有一些前临床及Ⅰ期临床研究旨在探索培美曲塞在乳腺癌、结肠癌、成神经管细胞瘤中的应用[240-242]。针对上述这些研究，多项Ⅱ期临床试验正在开展。

致谢

Barton A. Kamen，MD，PhD，本章节历史版本的作者，因恶性肿瘤已故于2012年。Bart是一位令我们尊敬的临床医生、临床研究者、教师、基础科学家，曾在叶酸拮抗剂领域做出重要贡献，包括发现叶酸结合蛋白并阐明其特征。

（毛宇　陈馨蕊　译，王华庆　审校）

参考文献

The complete reference list can be found on the Wiley Companion Digital Edition of this title (see inside front cover for login instructions).

1 Farber S, Cutler EC, Hawkins JW, Hartwell Harrison J, Converse Peirce E, Lenz GG. Action of pteroylglutamic conjugates on man. *Science*. 1947;**106**:619–621.

2 Farber S, Diamond L, Mercer RD, Sylvester RF Jr, Wolff JA. Temporary remissions in acute leukemia in children produced by folic acid antagonist, 4-aminopteroyl-glutamic acid (aminopterin). *N Engl J Med*. 1948;**238**:787.

6 Osborne MJ, Freeman MB, Huennekens FM. Inhibition of dihydrofolic reductase by aminopterin and amethopterin. *Proc Soc Exp Biol Med*. 1958;**97**:429–431.

8 Chabner BA, Allegra CJ, Curt GA, et al. Polyglutamation of methotrexate. Is methotrexate a prodrug? *J Clin Invest*. 1985;**76**(**3**):907–912.

16 Allegra CJ, Hoang K, Yeh GC, Drake JC, Baram J. Evidence for direct inhibition of de novo purine synthesis in human MCF-7 breast cells as a principal mode of metabolic inhibition by methotrexate. *J Biol Chem*. 1987;**262**(**28**):13520–13526.

17 Cronstein BN, Naime D, Ostad E. The antiinflammatory mechanism of methotrexate. Increased adenosine release at inflamed sites diminishes leukocyte accumulation in an in vivo model of inflammation. *J Clin Invest*. 1993;**92**(**6**):2675–2682.

22 Vazquez A, Tedeschi PM, Bertino JR. Overexpression of the mitochondrial folate and glycine-serine pathway: a new determinant of methotrexate selectivity in tumors. *Cancer Res*. 2013;**73**(**2**):478–482.

23 Stoller RG, Hande KR, Jacobs SA, Rosenberg SA, Chabner BA. Use of plasma pharmacokinetics to predict and prevent methotrexate toxicity. *N Engl J Med*. 1977;**297**(**12**):630–634.

26 Evans WE, Relling MV, Rodman JH, Crom WR, Boyett JM, Pui CH. Conventional compared with individualized chemotherapy for childhood acute lymphoblastic leukemia. *N Engl J Med*. 1998;**338**(**8**):499–505.

30 Winick N, Shuster JJ, Bowman WP, et al. Intensive oral methotrexate protects against lymphoid marrow relapse in childhood B-precursor acute lymphoblastic leukemia. *J Clin Oncol*. 1996;**14**(**10**):2803–2811.

31 Huffman DH, Wan SH, Azarnoff DL, Hogstraten B. Pharmacokinetics of methotrexate. *Clin Pharmacol Ther*. 1973;**14**(**4**):572–579.

40 Thyss A, Milano G, Etienne MC, et al. Evidence for CSF accumulation of 5-methyltetrahydrofolate during repeated courses of methotrexate plus folinic acid rescue. *Br J Cancer*. 1989;**59**(**4**):627–630.

81 Woods RL, Fox RM, Tattersall MH. Methotrexate treatment of squamous-cell head and neck cancers: dose–response evaluation. *Br Med J (Clin Res Ed)*. 1981;**282**(**6264**):600–602.

82 Pizzorno G, Mini E, Coronnello M, et al. Impaired polyglutamylation of methotrexate as a cause of resistance in CCRF-CEM cells after short-term, high-dose treatment with this drug. *Cancer Res*. 1988;**48**(**8**):2149–2155.

89 Matloub Y, Bostrom BC, Hunger SP, et al. Escalating intravenous methotrexate improves event-free survival in children with standard-risk acute lymphoblastic leukemia: a report from the Children's Oncology Group. *Blood*. 2011;**118**(**2**):243–251.

90 Mahoney DH Jr, Shuster JJ, Nitschke R, et al. Acute neurotoxicity in children with B-precursor acute lymphoid leukemia: an association with intermediate-dose intravenous methotrexate and intrathecal triple therapy—a Pediatric Oncology Group study. *J Clin Oncol*. 1998;**16**(**5**):1712–1722.

101 Edelstein M, Vietti T, Valeriote F. The enhanced cytotoxicity of combinations of 1-beta-D-arabinofuranosylcytosine and methotrexate. *Cancer Res*. 1975;**35**(**6**):1555–1558.

107 Blay JY, Conroy T, Chevreau C, et al. High-dose methotrexate for the treatment of primary cerebral lymphomas: analysis of survival and late neurologic toxicity in a retrospective series. *J Clin Oncol*. 1998;**16**(**3**):864–871.

108 Hammond CB, Hertz R, Ross GT, Lipsett MB, Odell WD. Primary chemotherapy for nonmetastatic gestational trophoblastic neoplasms. *Am J Obstet Gynecol*. 1967;**98**(**1**):71–78.

112 Bonadonna G, Moliterni A, Zambetti M, et al. 30 years' follow up of randomised studies of adjuvant CMF in operable breast cancer: cohort study. *BMJ*. 2005;**330**(**7485**):217.

125 Coates AS, Tattersall MH, Swanson C, Hedley D, Fox RM, Raghavan D. Combination therapy with methotrexate and 5-fluorouracil: a prospective randomized clinical trial of order of administration. *J Clin Oncol*. 1984;**2**(**7**):756–761.

128 Jaffe N, Frei E 3rd, Traggis D, Bishop Y. Adjuvant methotrexate and citrovorum-factor treatment of osteogenic sarcoma. *N Engl J Med*. 1974;**291**(**19**):994–997.

134 Cole PD, Drachtman RA, Masterson M, et al. Phase 2B trial of aminopterin in multiagent therapy for children with newly diagnosed acute lymphoblastic leukemia. *Cancer Chemother Pharmacol*. 2008;**62**(**1**):65–75.

138 Bernini JC, Fort DW, Griener JC, Kane BJ, Chappell WB, Kamen BA. Aminophylline for methotrexate-induced neurotoxicity. *Lancet*. 1995;**345**(**8949**):544–547.

146 Buchen S, Ngampolo D, Melton RG, et al. Carboxypeptidase G2 rescue in patients with methotrexate intoxication and renal failure. *Br J Cancer*. 2005;**92**(**3**):480–487.

157 Cole PD, Beckwith KA, Vijayanathan V, Roychowdhury S, Smith A, Kamen BA. CSF folate homeostasis during therapy for acute lymphoblastic leukemia. *Pediatr Neurol*. 2009;**40**(**1**):35–42.

160 Drachtman RA, Cole PD, Golden CB, et al. Dextromethorphan is effective in the treatment of subacute methotrexate neurotoxicity. *Pediatr Hematol Oncol*. 2002;**19**(**5**):319–327.

165 Adamson PC, Balis FM, McCully CL, et al. Rescue of experimental intrathecal methotrexate overdose with carboxypeptidase-G2. *J Clin Oncol*. 1991;**9**(**4**):670–674.

177 Zhao R, Assaraf YG, Goldman ID. A mutated murine reduced folate carrier (RFC1) with increased affinity for folic acid, decreased affinity for methotrexate, and an obligatory anion requirement for transport function. *J Biol Chem*. 1998;**273**(**30**):19065–19071.

178 Jansen G, Mauritz R, Drori S, et al. A structurally altered human reduced folate carrier with increased folic acid transport mediates a novel mechanism of antifolate resistance. *J Biol Chem*. 1998;**273**(**46**):30189–30198.

188 Mishra PJ, Humeniuk R, Longo-Sorbello GS, et al. A miR-24 microRNA binding-site polymorphism in dihydrofolate reductase gene leads to methotrexate resistance. *Proc Natl Acad Sci U S A*. 2007;**104**(**33**):13513–13518.

200 Gorlick R, Goker E, Trippett T, Waltham M, Banerjee D, and Bertino JR. Intrinsic and acquired resistance to methotrexate in acute leukemia. *N Engl J Med*. 1996;**335**(**14**):1041–1048.

201 Ercikan-Abali EA, Banerjee D, Waltham MC, Skacel N, Scotto KW, and Bertino JR. Dihydrofolate reductase protein inhibits its own translation by binding to dihydrofolate reductase mRNA sequences within the coding region. *Biochemistry*. 1997;**36**(**40**):12317–12322.

202 Alt FW, Kellems RE, Bertino JR, and Schimke RT. Selective multiplication of dihydrofolate reductase genes in methotrexate-resistant variants of cultured murine cells. *J Biol Chem*. 1978;**253**(**5**):1357–1370.

208 Schweitzer BI, Dicker AP, Bertino JR. Dihydrofolate reductase as a therapeutic target. *FASEB J*. 1990;**4**(**8**):2441–2452.

209 Pizzorno G, Chang YM, McGuire JJ, Bertino JR. Inherent resistance of human squamous carcinoma cell lines to methotrexate as a result of decreased polyglutamylation of this drug. *Cancer Res*. 1989;**49**(**19**):5275–5280.

222 Marchi E, Mangone M, Zullo K, O'Connor OA. Pralatrexate pharmacology and clinical development. *Clin Cancer Res*. 2013;**19**(**24**):6657–6661.

229 O'Connor OA, Pro B, Pinter-Brown L, et al. Pralatrexate in patients with relapsed or refractory peripheral T-cell lymphoma: results from the pivotal PROPEL study. *J Clin Oncol*. 2011;**29**(**9**):1182–1189.

232 Chattopadhyay S, Moran RG, Goldman ID. Pemetrexed: biochemical and cellular pharmacology, mechanisms, and clinical applications. *Mol Cancer Ther*. 2007;**6**(**2**):404–417.

238 Paz-Ares LG, de Marinis F, Dediu M, et al. PARAMOUNT: final overall survival results of the phase III study of maintenance pemetrexed versus placebo immediately after induction treatment with pemetrexed plus cisplatin for advanced nonsquamous non-small-cell lung cancer. *J Clin Oncol*. 2013;**31**(**23**):2895–2902.

239 Vogelzang NJ, Rusthoven JJ, Symanowski J, et al. Phase III study of pemetrexed in combination with cisplatin versus cisplatin alone in patients with malignant pleural mesothelioma. *J Clin Oncol*. 2003;**21**(**14**):2636–2644.

242 Morfouace M, Shelat A, Jacus M, et al. Pemetrexed and gemcitabine as combination therapy for the treatment of Group3 medulloblastoma. *Cancer Cell*. 2014;**25**(**4**):516–529.

第 57 章　嘧啶和嘌呤类抗代谢药

Robert B. Diasio, MD

概述

基于核酸对细胞复制至关重要的基本原理，开发出了嘧啶和嘌呤类抗代谢药物。不论在细菌、病毒还是肿瘤细胞中，嘧啶和嘌呤碱（及其核苷）是合成核酸所必需的“构建单元”，针对这些潜在的位点来设计药物可以有效地抑制核酸的合成。本章提出了目前用于治疗癌症的各种尿嘧啶/胸腺嘧啶、胞苷/脱氧胞苷、次黄嘌呤/鸟嘌呤和腺苷抗代谢物或类似物，并回顾了药物代谢、作用机制、临床药理学、临床有效性和毒性。

基于核酸对细胞复制至关重要的基本原理，开发出了嘧啶和嘌呤类抗代谢药物。不论是在细菌、病毒，还是肿瘤细胞，嘧啶和嘌呤碱（及其核苷）是合成核酸所必需的“构建单元”，针对这些潜在的位点来设计药物可以有效地抑制核酸的形成。考虑到肿瘤细胞（例如白血病细胞）相较正常细胞（例如淋巴细胞或粒细胞）增殖快速，设计类似嘧啶或嘌呤碱或核苷前体结构的药物的进一步逻辑是希望它们可以破坏核酸的合成。所谓“抗代谢”是指这些药物可以模拟嘧啶和嘌呤碱（及其核苷）天然结构，进入与自然状态下效应底物相似的细胞生物化学途径去合成嘧啶和嘌呤。然而，这些抗代谢物细微的分子结构差异可以干扰 DNA 和 RNA 合成。自然状态下的核酸合成破坏以数种方式进行。嘧啶或嘌呤类抗代谢物可与天然存在的效应物竞争性的结合核酸合成途径中的关键酶，从而扰乱 DNA 或 RNA 合成所需的天然嘧啶和嘌呤核苷酸库；嘌呤或嘧啶还可以直接掺入 DNA 或 RNA 中，导致功能失调的核酸合成；亦或因为 DNA 或 RNA 试图修复异常而导致核酸断裂[1]。

嘧啶类抗代谢物

潜在的嘧啶类抗代谢抗肿瘤药物可能包括自然状态下的嘧啶碱基，尿嘧啶，胞嘧啶或胸腺嘧啶或其核糖/脱氧核糖核苷的结构修饰的类似物（图 57-1a）。胸腺嘧啶类抗代谢物，如齐多夫定（azidothymidine，AZT），虽然其治疗病毒感染很有效，但在治疗肿瘤时并不如尿嘧啶和胞嘧啶类抗代谢物。

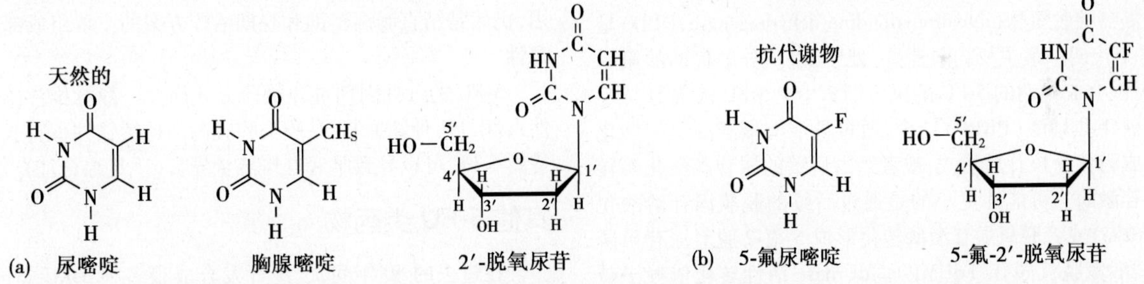

图 57-1　尿嘧啶/胸腺嘧啶类抗代谢物。(a) 天然的尿嘧啶和胸腺嘧啶结构，尿嘧啶脱氧核糖核苷（2′-脱氧尿苷）。(b) 在尿嘧啶和 2′-脱氧尿苷结构基础上修饰而成的抗代谢物：5-氟尿嘧啶和 5-氟-2′-脱氧尿苷

尿嘧啶抗代谢物

多年来，已有数种尿嘧啶类抗代谢物在多种恶性肿瘤治疗中显示出潜在的活性。目前在美国仍然活跃使用的尿嘧啶类抗代谢物仅为 5-氟尿嘧啶（5-fluorouracil，5-FU）类药物（图 57-1），包括母体药物 5-FU，其脱氧核糖核苷即 5-氟脱氧尿嘧啶（氟尿苷，FUdR 或 FdUrd），5-FU 的前体药物卡培他滨。直到今天，5-氟脱氧尿嘧啶偶尔用于肝动脉输注。在世界其他地区，特别是亚洲，其他的 5-FU 前体药（例如，UFT，S-1）已经广泛使用，但在美国，卡培他滨是唯一获批的[2]。

5-FU

5-FU 是最先合理合成的抗肿瘤药物之一[3]。开发这种抗代谢药的灵感源于观察到快速生长的肿瘤细胞需要外源性尿嘧啶来支撑（超过乳清酸的天然合成途径形成的内源性尿嘧啶）。外源性形成的尿嘧啶可转化为脱氧尿苷酸（dUMP），其在 5，10 亚甲基四氢叶酸的存在下，通过甲基基团转移至尿嘧啶的第五位，合成 DNA 所需的胸苷酸（图 57-1 和图 57-2）。5-FU 是尿嘧啶的近似类似物，由于相似的构象，包括类似的范德华半径，氟在尿嘧啶的第五位置有效地取代氢。从图 57-2 中可以看出，这允许 5-FU 进入尿嘧啶天然参与的生化途径。

代谢

5-FU 给药后进入循环，可作为小分子经肾小球滤过后直接排到尿液，或取决于不同组织而进入合成代谢和分解代谢途径，从而有效地代替尿嘧啶和尿嘧啶衍生代谢物并作为基质参与酶促步骤。进入循环中的 5-FU 将近 85% 会被直接分解代

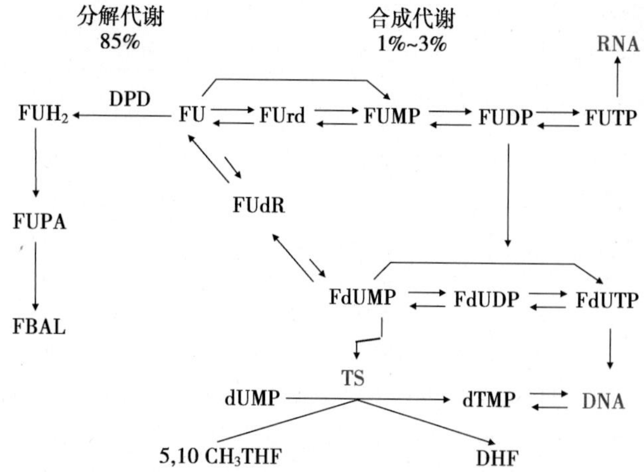

图 57-2 5-FU 的代谢及作用位点。5-FU 可以进入左侧的分解代谢或右侧的合成代谢途径。5-FU 给药后大约 85%会通过二氢尿嘧啶脱氢酶(DPD)限速酶分解代谢为二氢氟尿嘧啶(FUH_2),然后代谢为氟尿丙酸(FUPA),最终代谢为氟-β-丙氨酸(FBAL),从尿液中排出;仅仅 1%~3%的被用于合成代谢。5-FU 首先被合成代谢为核苷类,进而核苷酸(这些代谢产物和酶促步骤在参考文献 2,3 中有详细阐述)。3 个主要的作用位点为:①在 5,10-甲基四氢叶酸(5,10CH_3THF)存在下,单磷酸氟脱氧尿苷(FdUMP)抑制胸苷酸合成酶(TS);②三磷酸氟尿苷(FUTP)掺入至 RNA 中;③三磷酸脱氧5 氟尿苷(FdUTP)掺入 DNA 中,尿嘧啶转葡萄糖基酶将其移除后导致 DNA 的破碎

谢,10%~15%的通过尿液排出体外,1%~3%的被用于合成代谢。二氢嘧啶脱氢酶(dihydropyrimidine dehydrogenase,DPD)是 5-FU 整个代谢中最主要的限速酶,处于 5-FU 分解代谢的第一步,是可供合成代谢的 5-FU 的决定因素[4]。5-FU 大部分与 5-磷酸核糖-1-焦磷酸(PRPP)结合,通过乳清酸核苷酸焦磷酸化酶转化成为核糖核苷酸形式,或者经由后续的尿苷磷酸化酶转换为尿苷激酶。可能性更小的是通过后续的脱氧尿苷磷酸化酶(dUrdase)或者脱氧尿苷激酶转化形成 5-氟-2 脱氧尿苷单磷酸(单磷酸氟脱氧尿苷,FdUMP)。dUrdase 活性转化依赖于碱基位置而不是逆反应。5-FU 核苷酸类(尤其是 FdUMP,FUTP,FdUTP)的形成对 5-FU 发挥活性至关重要(详见后述)。关于个体化代谢步骤的详细信息在其他地方提供[2,3]。

理论上讲,5-FU 形成核苷酸进而发挥潜在关键作用中的任何受阻均可导致 5-FU 的耐药[5]。因此,这包括抑制 5-FU 吸收到细胞中,5-FU 转化为核苷,然后再到核苷酸的过程中任何酶活性限制。此外,减少尿苷磷酸化酶/激酶或乳清酸磷酸核糖基转移酶可能导致 5-FU 核苷酸的水平降低。

5-FU 的代谢和药理学不同于其他药物之处在于"生化调制",即 5-FU 的重要酶促活性或关键位点作用可以受添加一个重要的化学品或前体到关键代谢步骤的影响[6]。最好的例子是使用甲酰四氢叶酸(亚叶酸),它通常与 5-FU 一起给药,从而增加足够量的 5,10-甲基四氢叶酸,这样可确保后者与 FdUMP 的和胸苷酸合成酶(thymidylate synthase,TS)组合形成三元复合物,进而抑制 DNA 合成。

作用机制

5-FU 通过其核苷酸代谢物在 3 个不同位点发挥作用来展现抗癌活性(图 57-2)。在 5,10-甲基四氢叶酸存在下,FdUMP 抑制 TS(FdUMP 实际上对 TS 的亲和力大于天然底物 dUMP),抑制胸苷酸(TMP)的形成,而 TMP 对 DNA 的合成至关重要。这一直被认为是氟尿嘧啶类药物的主要作用机制[5]。第二种可能的机制是 5-FU 核苷酸氟尿酸三磷酸酯(fluoro uridylate triphosphate,FUTP)掺入 RNA 代替天然的尿嘧啶核糖核苷酸 UTP。考虑到它对小 RNAs 的影响,这种 RNA 的掺入可能也很重要[2]。第三个机制与第二个机制有些类似,是将 5-FU 脱氧核苷酸 FdUTP 掺入 DNA 代替天然胸苷酸核苷酸 TTP。在这种情况下,包含 FdUTP 的 DNA 在尿嘧啶转葡萄糖基酶诱导下进行剪切修复时会导致 DNA 断裂,这被认为是细胞毒性的原因[3]。

临床药理学

5-FU 通常以静脉推注或静脉输注的形式给药。静脉注射后 5-FU 在肝脏首过后迅速清除,超过 85%的 5-FU 迅速经过初始的分解代谢为失活的二氢氟尿嘧啶(dihydrofluorouracil,FUH_2)[3]。在这种情况下,5-FU 的半衰期约为 13±7 分钟,清除率约为 600±200ml/(min · m^2)[4]。通过连续输注超过 5 天或选用长时间的动态泵输注,预期可以保持相对稳定且低水平的 5-FU 浓度[2]。分解代谢效率存在变异性,主要决定因素是 DPD,即 5-FU 分解代谢的限速步骤。在一小部分但很显著的人群中(5%)存在 DPD 编码基因(*DPYD*)的编码变异,导致 DPD 活性降低,使得更多的 5-FU 从分解代谢移转至合成代谢途径,进而导致毒性增加[7,8]。

临床用途及适应证

5-FU 继续被广泛用于治疗几种常见的恶性肿瘤,包括结直肠癌,特定的皮肤肿瘤和乳腺癌。它通常与其他药物一起使用,仍然是结直肠癌辅助和晚期治疗方案的主要组成部分[2]。

毒性

5-FU 的毒性因剂量和给药方式而异。静脉推注给药的急性毒性包括骨髓抑制、黏膜炎和腹泻。持续输注保持长时间的暴露 5-FU 可以导致掌底红斑感觉异常(手足综合征)[2,3]。

其他 5-FU 类药物

在过去的 60 年间,已经开发合成很多种 5-FU 类的药物,其中很大部分都是 5-FU 的前体药物。

5-氟脱氧尿苷

背景

5-氟脱氧尿苷(FdUrd,FUDR)是 20 世纪 50 年代末与 5-FU 同时合成的 5-FU 的脱氧尿苷,目前用途相对有限。其结构如图 57-1 所示。

代谢

FdUrd 可以作为 5-FU 的前体药物,经脱氧尿苷或胸苷磷酸化酶转化为 5-FU。然而,因为它是脱氧尿苷或胸苷激酶的良好底物,所以很可能直接快速地转化为 FdUMP,而 FdUMP 是 5-FU 的主要活性代谢物之一。

作用机制

在 5,10 亚甲基四氢叶酸存在下,FdUMP 与 TS 可形成不可逆的三元络合物,进而阻断 DNA 合成。由于大多数给药的 FdUrd 将直接代谢为 FdUMP,因此 FdUrd 是一种相对纯的 S 相抑制剂[9]。

临床药理学

如今，当使用 FdUrd 时，它主要是通过植入式泵持续进行肝动脉灌注[10]。

临床活性

FdUrd 主要用于肝细胞癌和结直肠癌肝脏转移的治疗。

毒性

随着肝动脉输注时间的延长，主要毒性是肝毒性，包括胆道硬化和转氨酶的偶尔升高[2,3]。

卡培他滨

背景

开发 5-FU 口服制剂进行了很多尝试，这种药物不仅要提供更方便的服法，还需要模仿 5-FU 输注的理想效果[11]。在美国，卡培他滨是食品药品管理局(Food and Drug Administration, FDA)批准的唯一一种口服制剂，而在亚洲和欧洲还有其他的 5-FU 口服制剂。

代谢

卡培他滨通过三种酶的连续作用转化为 5-FU：①肝脏羧酸酯酶，首先将药物水解为 5′-脱氧-5-氟胞苷；②胞嘧啶脱氨酶，进而将该衍生物脱氨基为 5′-脱氧-5-氟尿苷(5′-dFUrd)；③胸苷酸磷酸化酶，最终将 5′-dFUrd 水解为 5-FU(图 57-3)。与大多数正常组织相比，肿瘤组织中胸苷酸磷酸化酶活性更高，因此卡培他滨具有潜在的选择性益处，可提高治疗指数。

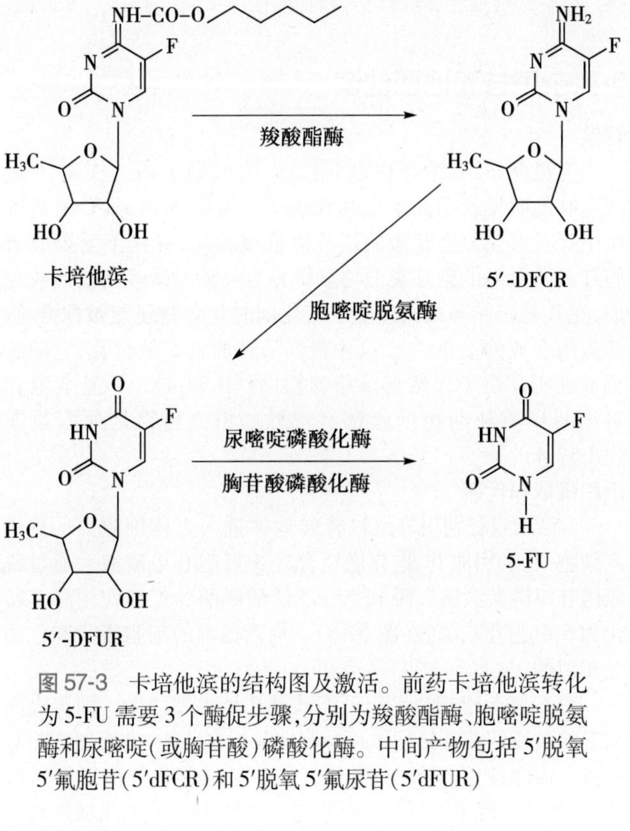

图 57-3　卡培他滨的结构图及激活。前药卡培他滨转化为 5-FU 需要 3 个酶促步骤，分别为羧酸酯酶、胞嘧啶脱氨酶和尿嘧啶(或胸苷酸)磷酸化酶。中间产物包括 5′脱氧 5′氟胞苷(5′dFCR)和 5′脱氧 5′氟尿苷(5′dFUR)

作用机制

转化为 5-FU 后，作用机制与 5-FU 相同(见上文)。

临床药理学

卡培他滨是更友好的 5-FU 替代给药方法且可提供类似 5-FU 长期输注的效果。

临床活性

卡培他滨与 5-FU 具有相似的活性，通常用于治疗结直肠癌和乳腺癌。

毒性

卡培他滨的毒性与 5-FU 相似，手足综合征是主要的毒性，见于卡培他滨持续使用后。有趣的是，欧洲和美国人群对卡培他滨的剂量耐受性存在差异。尽管叶酸水平等外部因素可能会起作用，但仍不清楚其基础是什么[12]。

胞嘧啶抗代谢产物

具有临床抗癌活性的胞嘧啶抗代谢产物主要是核苷，其中主要的结构修饰是在分子的糖基而不是碱基。目前，临床上常用 4 种胞嘧啶抗代谢物。这些药物包括阿糖胞苷(ara-C)、5-氮胞苷(和相关的地西他滨)和吉西他滨(图 57-4)。

阿糖胞苷

背景

从海洋生物海绵 *Cryptotethya crypta* 分离得到的 ara-C 是一种天然物质。阿拉伯糖苷糖将这种化合物与胞嘧啶脱氧核糖核苷区别开来，脱氧核糖核苷通常是 DNA 的一个组成部分，2′-OH 基团是相对于胞嘧啶和糖基间的 N-糖基键的顺式构象(图 57-4)[13]。如今，ara-c 合成被用于商业使用。其在癌症化疗中的有效性促进了其他阿拉伯糖苷化合物的合成，如嘌呤抗代谢物 2-氟-ara-单磷酸腺苷和奈拉滨(见下文讨论)。

代谢

在通过核苷转运体进入细胞后，ara-C 必须首先通过脱氧胞苷激酶的作用转化单磷酸阿糖胞苷(ara-CMP)，然后进一步磷酸化为二磷酸阿糖胞苷(ara-CDP)和三磷酸阿糖胞苷(ara-CTP)，后者对静止细胞活性至关重要(图 57-5)[14]。

Ara-C 的分解代谢或降解可通过胞苷脱氨酶的作用发生，将 ara-C 转化为失活的 ara-U，或经脱氧胞苷酸脱氨酶，将 ara-CMP 转化为失活的 ara-UMP。脱氨作用增强会减少 ara-C 向细胞内的转运，是耐药增加的基础；其他任何潜在导致活性代谢物 ara-CTP 的减少的机制也会导致药物耐药。

作用机制

一般认为，ara-C 的作用机制发生在几个可能的部位。Ara-CTP 是一种有效的 DNA 多聚体 α、β、γ 的抑制剂，可抑制 DNA 合成、延伸、修复。另一种作用机制为 ara-CTP 掺入 DNA 后，它可以作为 DNA 终止子终止 DNA 的延伸[15]。

临床药理学

胃肠道存在广泛着脱氨基作用，故 ara-C 的口服生物利用度较差。这就需要静脉内给药，通常是通过持续输注。Ara-C 在血浆、肝脏和各种外周组织中代谢为 ara-U，80% 的 ara-U 排泄到尿液中。Ara-C 还可以穿过血脑屏障进入脑脊液。

临床活性

Ara-C 是一种有效的抗白血病药物，常被用作急性髓细胞白血病(acute myelogenous leukemia, AML)的标准诱导方案。在急性淋巴细胞白血病(acute lymphocytic leukemia, ALL)和慢性髓源性白血病以及其他血液学恶性肿瘤(如非霍奇金淋巴瘤)中也有活性。有趣的是，该药在非血液系统的实体瘤中基本上没有活性。

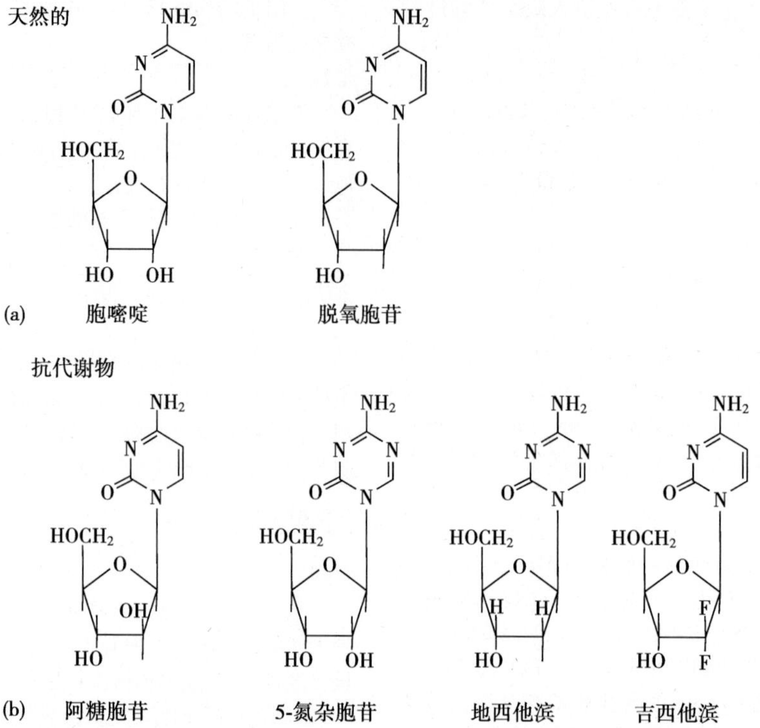

天然的

(a) 胞嘧啶 脱氧胞苷

抗代谢物

(b) 阿糖胞苷 5-氮杂胞苷 地西他滨 吉西他滨

图 57-4 胞嘧啶/脱氧胞苷类抗代谢物。(a)天然的胞嘧啶和脱氧胞苷结构图;(b)胞嘧啶核苷糖基部位修饰后而合成的抗代谢物,阿糖胞苷、5-氮杂胞苷、地西他滨和吉西他滨

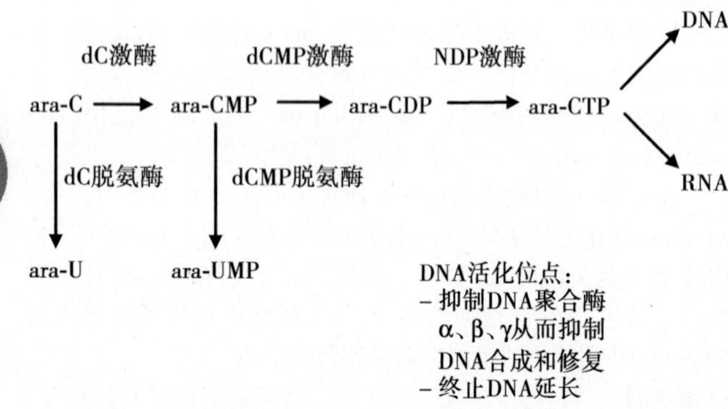

图 57-5 阿糖胞苷(ara-C)的代谢及作用位点。阿糖胞苷依次通过脱氧胞苷激酶(dC 激酶),脱氧胞苷酸激酶(dCMP 激酶)和二磷酸核苷激酶(NDP 激酶)转化为三磷酸阿糖胞苷(ara-CTP)。通过胞嘧啶脱氨酶(CdR 脱氨酶)和脱氧胞苷酸脱氨酶(dCMP 脱氨酶)转化为失活产物。图中显示了 ara-C 的作用位点。Ara-CMP,单磷酸阿糖胞苷;ara-CDP,二磷酸阿糖胞苷;ara-U,阿糖尿苷;ara-UMP,阿糖尿苷酸

毒性

毒性因剂量和给药方式而异。正如人们所预测的,最突出的毒性之一是骨髓抑制。在标准的 7 天方案中可以看到,骨髓抑制峰值为 7~14 天,特别是在使用高剂量($2\sim3g/m^2$)的情况下。伴随骨髓抑制的还有其他血液毒性,特别是血小板减少。其他毒性包括胃肠道症状,如恶心、厌食和呕吐,以及腹泻、黏膜炎和胰腺炎时的腹痛,大剂量时有小脑毒性。

5-氮杂胞苷和地西他滨

背景

为提高 ara-C 治疗白血病疗效,人们做了新的探索,5-氮杂胞苷的研发就是其中成功代表。因为很多对 ara-C 耐药肿瘤中存在着脱氧胞苷激酶活性降低或缺失,寻找不需要脱氧胞苷激酶激活的胞苷类似物显得尤为关键。许多类似物被合成,尤其是嘧啶环结构发生了变化同时化合物还能被尿苷-胞苷激酶合成的核苷[13]。其中最具活性的是 5-氮胞苷,它随后也被证实存在于天然真菌培养物中(图 57-4)。5-氮杂胞苷对细菌和哺乳动物细胞都有毒性。相关药物是地西他滨(图 57-4)。

细胞摄取和代谢

5-氮杂胞苷利用等位核苷转运体进入人体细胞。一旦进入细胞内,利用尿苷-胞苷途径合成 5-氮胞苷单磷酸。通过脱氧胞苷单磷酸激酶和脱氧胞苷二磷酸激酶的连续作用将其转化为 5-氮胞苷三磷酸(图 57-6)。地西他滨的细胞吸收和代谢是相似的。

对 5-氮杂胞苷的耐药可能通过几种机制产生。细胞表面缺乏或改变的核苷转运体可抑制细胞摄取药物,进而导致相对抵抗。内源性尿苷和/或胞苷可与 5-氮胞苷竞争性进行磷酸化,导致活性降低。同样,尿苷-胞苷激酶表达减少或缺失也可能产生耐药性。分解代谢酶(如胞苷脱氨酶)活性的增加可能导致 5-氮杂尿苷的产生增加,后者缺乏细胞毒性[13]。

作用机制

5-氮胞苷三磷酸是关键的代谢产物。有几个关键的作用位点。5-氮胞苷三磷酸首先与天然的 CTP 竞争进入 RNA。5-

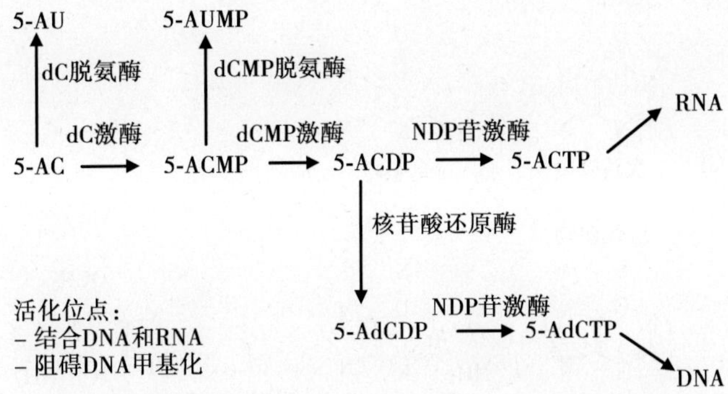

图 57-6　5-氮杂胞苷的结构及作用位点。5-氮杂胞苷(5-AC)的代谢途径如图。5-氮杂胞苷经过脱氧胞苷激酶(dC 激酶)和脱氧胞苷酸激酶(dCMP 激酶)作用后转化为二磷酸 5 氮杂胞苷酸(5-ACDP)。5-ACDP 经过二磷酸核苷激酶(NDP 激酶)可转化为三磷酸 5 氮杂胞苷酸(5-ACTP),或者通过核苷酸还原酶(Rib Red)转化为二磷酸 5 氮杂脱氧胞苷酸(5-AdCDP)。5-AdCDP 通过 NDP 激酶转化为三磷酸 5 氮杂脱氧胞苷酸(5-AdCTP)。5-AC 通过胞嘧啶脱氨酶(dC 脱氨酶)和脱氧胞苷酸脱氨酶(dCMP 脱氨酶)转化为失活产物。图中显示了 5-AC 的作用位点。5-AU = 5 氮杂尿苷;5-ACMP,5 氮杂胞苷酸;5-AUMP,5 氮杂尿苷酸

氮杂胞苷三磷酸与 RNA 结合,对 RNA 的加工和功能产生多种不利影响,包括抑制核糖体 328S 和 18S 的形成,改变转运 RNA 的受体功能,破坏多核糖体的组装,从而抑制蛋白质合成[9]。此外,5-氮杂胞苷三磷酸可以掺入 DNA,在 DNA 复制后抑制 DNA 甲基化[13]。正是这种效应引发了大家的特别兴趣,去研究它对甲基化后的表观遗传的效应。地西他滨有类似的作用机制,包括去甲基化或干扰 DNA 的甲基化。结果,肿瘤抑制基因的正常功能恢复,细胞生长得到控制。作为一种典型的抗代谢物,地西他滨也可掺入核酸中,与许多潜在靶点相互作用,产生直接的细胞毒性效应,导致癌细胞快速分裂死亡。

临床药理学

5-氮杂胞苷通过静脉输注给药,然后迅速脱氨基为 5-氮杂尿苷。妇女和老年人的血浆清除率通常较低,因此在这些人群中应谨慎使用。

临床活性

对于 5-氮杂胞苷和地西他滨,在 AML 和骨髓发育不良中都观察到了临床活性[16]。如前所述,5-氮杂胞苷对 DNA 甲基化的抑制作用特别重要,因为它能够在临床和实验上上调表观抑制基因的表达。

毒性

与抗代谢物组的其他成员相似,5-氮胞苷和地西他滨的主要剂量限制性毒性是骨髓抑制,特别是中性粒细胞减少和血小板减少。在推注给药时,恶心和呕吐尤其常见。其他毒性,尤其在高剂量 5-氮胞苷给药时,还观察到肝功能异常、高胆红素血症、肌肉压痛和无力、中枢神经系统毒性伴有嗜睡、精神错乱,甚至昏迷[17]。鉴于此,在出现肝功能衰竭或精神状态异常的情况下使用这些药物时应谨慎。

吉西他滨

背景

吉西他滨是一种合成的核苷类似物,其中脱氧胞苷中的氢被两个氟取代[13]。它的结构如图 57-4 所示。

细胞摄取和代谢

与其他抗代谢物相似,吉西他滨利用细胞的核苷转运体进入人体细胞。一旦进入细胞内,它必须利用细胞的天然脱氧胞苷途径进行合成代谢,形成吉西他滨三磷酸以获得活性;而作为母体药物它是没有活性的(图 57-7)[18]。

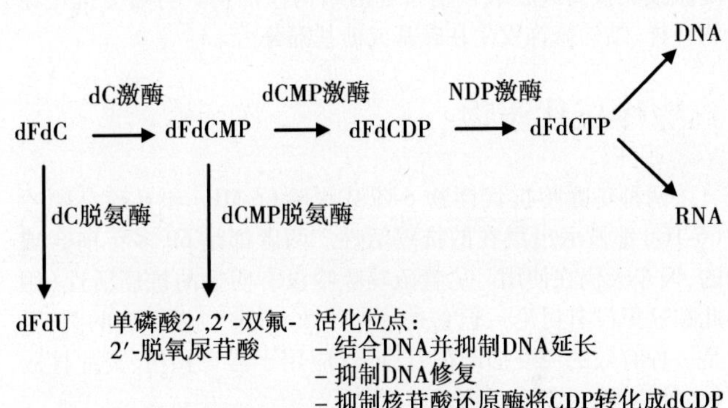

图 57-7　吉西他滨(dFdC)的代谢及作用位点。吉西他滨的代谢途径如图所示。最初吉西他滨必须经过脱氧胞苷激酶(dC 激酶),脱氧胞苷酸激酶(dCMP 激酶),二磷酸核苷激酶(NDP 激酶)转化为 dFdCTP。和阿糖胞苷一样,dFdC 也是通过胞嘧啶脱氨酶(dC 脱氨酶)和脱氧胞苷酸脱氨酶(dCMP 脱氨酶)转化为失活产物。图示了 dFdC 的作用位点。dFdU = 2′,2′-双氟-2′-脱氧尿苷;dFdCMP,单磷酸 2′,2′-双氟-2′-脱氧胞苷酸;dFdCDP,二磷酸 2′,2′-双氟-2′-脱氧胞苷酸;dFdCTP,三磷酸 2′,2′-双氟-2′-脱氧胞苷酸

吉西他滨有几个理论上的耐药位点。核苷转运体的缺陷或改变可抑制吉西他滨的细胞摄取并导致相对抗性[13]。代谢上,耐药性可通过关键的合成代谢酶(如脱氧胞苷激酶)活性降低或分解代谢酶(如胞苷脱氨酶或脱氧胞苷脱氨酶)活性增加而获得。

作用机制

吉西他滨三磷酸是一种重要的代谢产物。提示的作用位点有数个。其中大家认为最重要的是终止 DNA 链或掺入 DNA 后进一步抑制 DNA 的合成[19]。吉西他滨三磷酸也被认为能直接抑制 DNA 聚合酶 α、β、γ,并能导致链终止和 DNA 合成的抑制以及 DNA 修复。最后,吉西他滨三磷酸还能够抑制核苷还原酶,通过消耗急需的脱氧核苷库进一步抑制 DNA 合成。

临床药理学

考虑到 2′,2′-二氟-2′-脱氧尿苷(dFdU)的快速脱氨基作用,吉西他滨通常经静脉输注给药。妇女和老年人的血浆清除率通常较低,因此在这些人群中应谨慎使用。

临床活性

尽管吉西他滨与 ara-C 具有结构相似性和相同的作用部位,但它的临床应用范围更广,包括多个实体瘤,如胰腺癌、肺癌(小细胞和非小细胞)、卵巢癌、膀胱癌和乳腺癌,以及血液系

统恶性肿瘤，包括霍奇金淋巴瘤和非霍奇金淋巴瘤。

毒性

主要的剂量限制性毒性是骨髓抑制，表现为中性粒细胞减少和较小程度的血小板减少。当输注超过 30 分钟时，血液毒性倾向于更严重。其他常见的毒性包括流感样症状，包括发烧、头痛、肌痛和关节痛。

嘌呤抗代谢物

抗肿瘤的嘌呤抗代谢物包括针对鸟嘌呤和腺嘌呤天然嘌呤碱或其核糖或脱氧核糖核苷的结构修饰物。与嘧啶抗代谢物一样，结构修饰发生在碱基或糖基部分[20]。

鸟嘌呤抗代谢物

两种鸟嘌呤抗代谢物 6-巯基嘌呤(6-MP)和 6-硫鸟嘌呤(6-TG)都显示出潜在的抗癌活性。两者都是 60 多年前合成的，但今天仍在使用。尽管硫唑嘌呤没有明显的抗癌活性(因此在这里没有讨论)，但它是一种导致 6-MP 缓慢释放的前药，是一种有效的免疫抑制剂，已广泛应用于器官移植、炎症性肠病(如克罗恩病)和风湿病。

天然的

(a) 次黄嘌呤 鸟嘌呤

抗代谢物

(b) 6-巯基嘌呤 6-硫鸟嘌呤 奈达滨

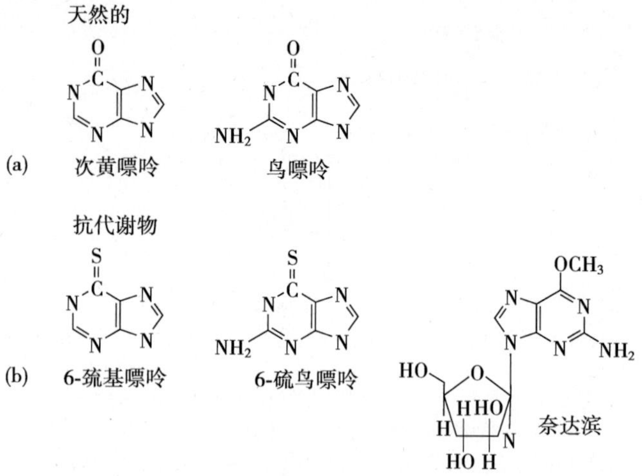

图 57-8 次黄嘌呤和鸟嘌呤类抗代谢物。(a)天然存在的次黄嘌呤和鸟嘌呤。(b)在次黄嘌呤和鸟嘌呤结构上进行不同修饰而合成的抗代谢物，分别为 6-巯基嘌呤(6-MP)，6-硫鸟嘌呤(6-TG)和奈达滨，即脱氧鸟苷抗代谢物 9-β-D-阿拉比诺呋喃基鸟嘌呤(ara-G)的前药

6-巯基嘌呤

背景

6-MP 的结构与天然存在的嘌呤碱次黄嘌呤(图 57-8a)密切相关；在第六位，硫醇取代羟基。和其他抗代谢物一样的特征，6-MP 可以进入天然代谢物所使用的合成代谢和分解代谢途径，是经次黄嘌呤而实现。

代谢

摄入细胞后，6-MP 可立即被次黄嘌呤鸟嘌呤焦磷酸化酶(hypoxanthine guanine phosphoribosyltransferase，HGPRT)合成为单磷酸硫代肌苷(6-thioinosine monophosphate，TIMP)。TIMP 可以进一步被重组为三磷酸酯，然后被整合到 DNA 中。6-MP 的代谢如图 57-9 所示。

减少合成代谢或增加分解代谢(主要由磷酸酶介导)致 TIMP 减少可导致耐药。

作用机制

TIMP 被认为是通过抑制了嘌呤从头合成而发挥抗代谢作用，这使得核酸合成所需的天然嘌呤核苷酸池的大小受到干扰(图 57-9)。

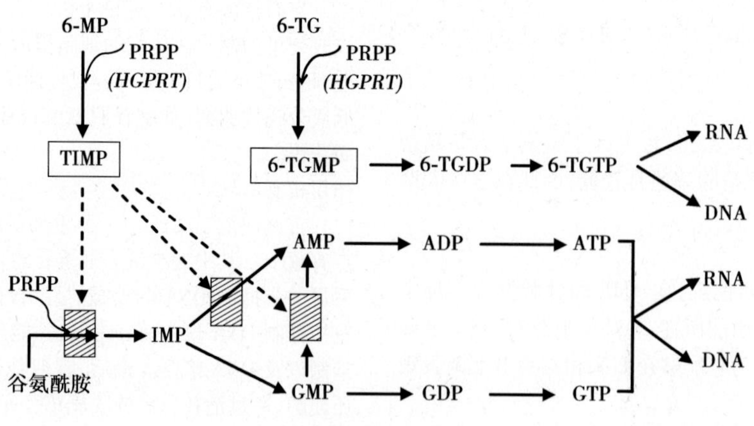

图 57-9 6-巯基嘌呤(6-MP)和 6-硫鸟嘌呤(6-TG)的代谢及作用位点。在 5-磷酸核糖-1-焦磷酸(PRPP)存在情况下，通过次黄嘌呤鸟嘌呤焦磷酸化酶(HGPRT)作用，6-MP 代谢为单磷酸硫代肌苷(TIMP)，6-TG 代谢为单磷酸硫鸟苷酸(6-TGMP)。TIMP 通过抑制嘌呤从头合成的 3 个关键步骤来发挥活性：①抑制谷氨酰胺在 PRPP 存在下生成肌苷单磷酸(IMP)；②抑制 IMP 向 AMP 的转化；③抑制 GMP 向 AMP 的转化。而通过后续核苷酸激酶的激活，6-TGMP 最终可转化为二磷酸硫鸟嘌呤核苷酸(6-TGDP)，之后为三磷酸硫鸟嘌呤核苷酸(6-TGTP)。6-TGTP 掺入至 DNA 和 RNA 中发挥活动，导致正常核酸功能受阻。AMP，单磷酸腺苷；ADP，二磷酸腺苷；ATP，三磷酸腺苷；GMP，单磷酸鸟苷；GDP，二磷酸鸟苷；GTP，三磷酸鸟苷

临床药理学

6-MP 是口服的（通常为 90mg/m^2），尽管其吸收可能随峰值浓度和峰值时间的变化而不稳定。6-MP 与血清蛋白的结合很小，游离药物的半衰期在 20～45 分钟[21]。

6-MP 经黄嘌呤氧化酶代谢。因为在肿瘤环境中使用的其他药物，如别嘌呤醇，在其代谢过程中也使用相同的酶，这可能导致潜在的严重药物相互作用，并伴随毒性增加（会导致更多的 6-MP 有活性代谢物产生）。因此，在合并用药情况下，6-MP 的剂量通常减少 50%～75%[22]。

另一个重要的 6-MP 临床药理学发现是药物遗传学。由于 TPMT 基因存在变异，硫嘌呤甲基转移酶（thiopurine methyltransferase，TPMT）在人群中的表达存在变异，因此代谢和活性药物的可获得性可能会有所不同。现在可以在 6-MP 给药前筛选这些 TPMT 变异体，从而避免毒性[23]。

临床活性

尽管已经被引入临床超过 50 年，目前 6-MP 在急性淋巴细胞白血病，尤其是儿童患者中仍然具有临床作用。6-MP 在实体瘤中缺乏疗效。由于其免疫抑制作用，它也被用于非肿瘤性疾病（如克罗恩病）。

毒性

6-MP 的主要毒性是骨髓抑制。其他毒性包括胃肠道，特别是厌食、恶心、呕吐和腹泻。也可见到肝毒性。因此，应避免经常使用肝毒性药物。最后，6-MP 和它的前药硫唑嘌呤一样，可以产生免疫抑制，基于此会增加感染的风险。

6-硫鸟嘌呤

背景

6-TG 和 6-MP 一样，是最早于 20 世纪 50 年代合成的嘌呤类抗代谢产物之一，也是鸟嘌呤类抗代谢产物家族的成员。其结构如图 57-8 所示。

代谢

摄入细胞后，6-TG 利用鸟嘌呤途径中的内源性酶合成代谢，如图 57-9 所示。6-TG 与 6-MP 的区别在于它直接转化为 6-TG 核苷酸单磷酸，然后再到核苷酸二磷酸和核苷酸三磷酸，然后可以掺入到 RNA 和 DNA 中。与其他抗代谢物类似，合成代谢酶活性降低或分解代谢酶活性增加都可能产生耐药性[20]。

作用机制

6-TG 的作用机制被认为是它掺入 RNA 和 DNA 后干扰核酸的合成和功能[24]。

临床药理学

6-TG 通常口服。其口服生物利用度变异，在给药后 2～4 小时出现峰值。它的代谢不同于 6-MP，不经黄嘌呤氧化酶代谢。因此，与 6-MP 不同，与别嘌呤醇合并用药时无需减少 6-TG 的剂量来避免毒性作用。

然而，6-TG 与 6-MP 一样，都是 TPMT 的底物，在 TPMT 基因遗传变异而导致其表达下降的情况下，必须调整受影响的个体的剂量。TPMT 缺乏症很常见（约占所有患者的 10%），因此建议在给药前进行 TPMT 筛查[23]。

临床活性

6-TG 在 AML 中有活性，有时用于缓解诱导和维持治疗。6-TG 也用于 ALL。

毒性

骨髓抑制是主要的毒性。其他毒性包括口炎和胃肠道毒性，特别是厌食、恶心/呕吐和腹泻。肝毒性也见于很大比例的患者，特别是胆汁淤积性黄疸和偶尔的转氨酶升高。因此，应避免同时使用肝毒性药物。最后，与 6-MP 一样，6-TG 也可致免疫抑制，增加感染风险。

奈达滨

背景

奈达滨是脱氧鸟苷抗代谢物 9-β-D-阿拉比诺呋喃基鸟嘌呤（ara-G）的前药，具有细胞毒性。它是一种新的嘌呤抗代谢物，被开发用于对氟达拉滨耐药的患者（见下文讨论）。其结构如图 57-8 所示。

代谢

作为前药，奈达滨必须首先通过腺苷脱氨酶（adenosine deaminase，ADA）介导去甲基化而转化为 ara-G[25]。一旦被核苷转运体转运到肿瘤细胞中，ara-G 被合成为核苷三磷酸（ara-GTP），这是活性代谢物。它利用与天然嘌呤合成代谢途径中的相同的酶（图 57-10）。与其他抗代谢物相似，分解代谢酶的活性可能影响相应的耐药性。

作用机制

Ara-GTP 掺入 DNA 后显示出活性，可导致 DNA 碎裂和凋亡。与其他抗代谢物类似，ara-GTP 与天然存在的脱氧鸟苷三磷酸（deoxyguanosine triphosphate，dGTP）竞争性掺入 DNA。在与长链 DNA 的 3′端结合后，进一步结合到 DNA 就被抑制，导致细胞凋亡和细胞死亡。其他作用机制尚不能排除，但目前仍不清楚[26]。

临床药理学

奈达滨是一种可溶性前体药物，通常通过 2～3 小时的静脉滴注给药。奈达滨和 ara-G 都不会被血浆蛋白显著结合，而是通过肾脏被清除[27]。

临床活性

奈达滨于 2005 年被 FDA 批准用于 T 细胞急性白血病或 T 细胞淋巴母细胞性淋巴瘤患者，这些患者包括既往化疗无效或至少两线化疗方案后复发的[28]。

毒性

常见的毒性反应包括不适、发热、恶心和骨髓抑制。严重的（3 级和 4 级）神经系统毒性发生在 10%～15%的患者中，可能包括中枢神经系统的副作用，例如昏迷、癫痫发作、脑病和周围神经病变。

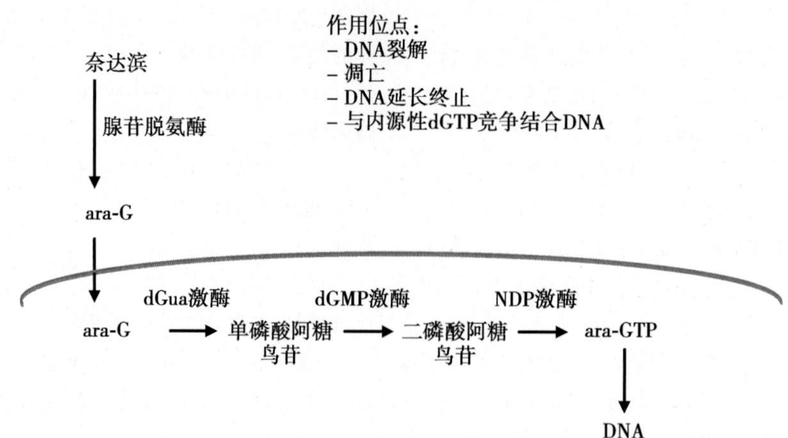

图 57-10 奈达滨的代谢及作用位点。作为前体药物，静脉给药后首先通过腺苷脱氨酶(ADA)去甲基化而转化为 ara-G。9-β-D-阿拉比诺呋喃基鸟嘌呤(ara-G)通过核苷转运体进入细胞中后，在脱氧鸟苷激酶(dGua 激酶)作用下单磷酸化为 ara-GMP，然后通过后续核苷酸激酶，脱氧鸟苷酸激酶(dGMP 激酶)和二磷酸核苷激酶(NDP 激酶)，转化成活性代谢物核苷三磷酸(ara-GTP)。图显示了 ara-GTP 的作用位点

腺苷抗代谢物

腺苷类似物代表了另一大类的嘌呤抗代谢物。与依赖于嘌呤碱基内结构修饰的鸟嘌呤抗代谢物不同，腺苷抗代谢物依赖于分子中糖基结构的变化。这一结构变化导致腺苷脱氨酶 ADA 的有效性下降。脱氧腺苷第二位的卤素被氟达拉滨中的氟取代，被克拉屈滨中的氯取代，取得了预设的效果。目前，有几种腺苷抗代谢药被批准用于临床(图 57-11)。这些药物包括氟达拉滨、克拉屈滨和氯法拉滨。第四种腺苷样类似物，戊他汀(脱氧可福霉素)，是一种天然存在的嘌呤类似物，首次发现于抗生素链霉菌的发酵液中。其结构类似腺苷酸在 ADA 反应中的过渡形式。它是 ADA 最有效的抑制剂之一，更多细节将在其他地方介绍[20]。

氟达拉滨

背景

氟达拉滨，又称 9-β-D-阿糖腺苷-2-氟磷酸或 F-ara-AMP，其结构如图 57-11 所示。

代谢作用

静脉给药后，它迅速脱磷至 F-ara A(图 57-12)。然后通过核苷转运体进入细胞。在细胞内，在三磷酸腺苷(ATP)和脱氧胞苷激酶的存在下，它被转化为核苷酸单磷酸，然后依次转化为 F-ara-ATP[29]。

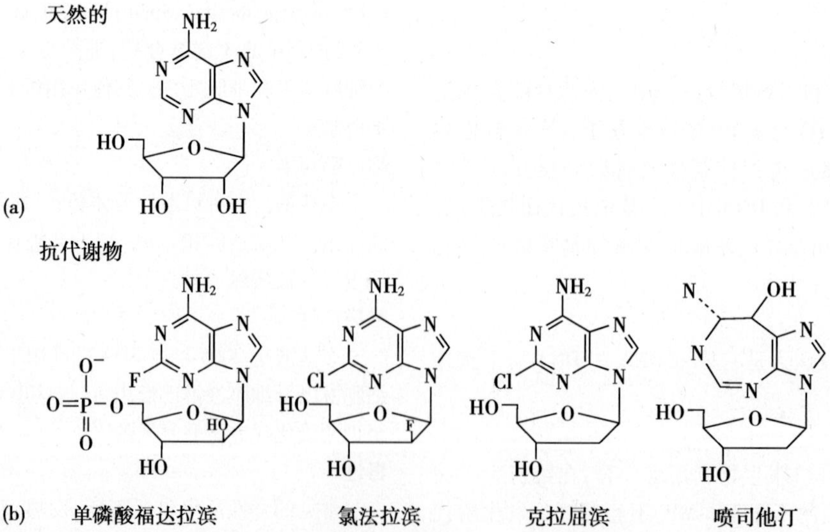

天然的

(a)

抗代谢物

(b) 单磷酸福达拉滨 氯法拉滨 克拉屈滨 喷司他汀

图 57-11 腺苷抗代谢物。(a)天然的嘌呤碱腺苷。(b)在腺苷结构上修饰而成的抗代谢物单磷酸福达拉滨，氯法拉滨和克拉屈滨。第四种腺苷酸类似物为喷司他汀(本章节中未讨论)，是从抗生素链霉菌的发酵液中首先提取的天然存在的嘌呤类似物。其结构类似于 ADA 反应中腺苷的过渡形式

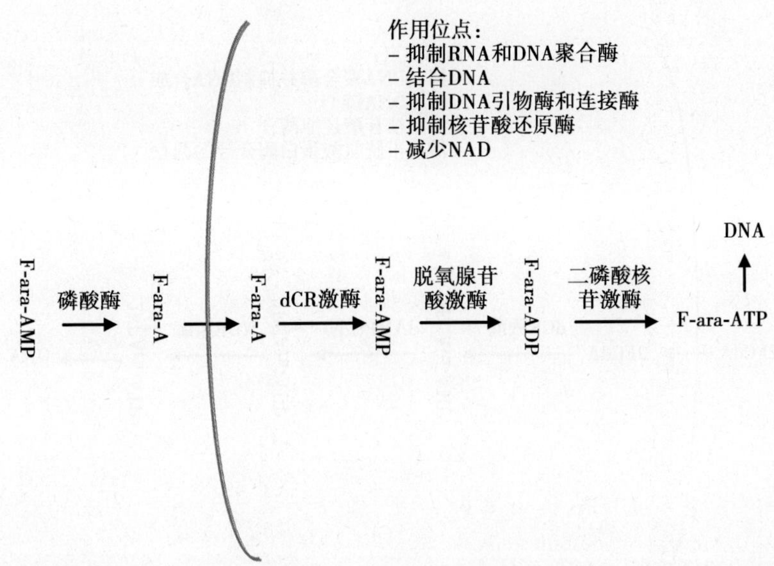

图 57-12　福达拉滨（F-ara-AMP）的代谢及作用位点。静脉注射后，F-ara-AMP 迅速脱磷至 2-氟阿糖腺苷（F-ara-A）。然后通过核苷转运体进入细胞。在细胞内的脱氧胞苷激酶（dCR 激酶）的作用下转化为核苷酸单磷酸 F-ara-AMP，然后通过核苷酸激酶［脱氧腺苷酸激酶（dAMP 激酶）和二磷酸核苷激酶（NDP 激酶）］转化为活性代谢产物 F-ara-ATP。图显示了 F-ara-ATP 的作用位点。F-ara-ADP，2-氟二磷酸阿糖腺苷；F-ara-ATP，2-氟三磷酸阿糖腺苷

作用机制

F-ara-ATP 作为一种活性代谢产物来发挥药物作用。它与天然代谢产物三磷酸脱氧腺苷（dATP）可进行竞争。

临床药理学

F-ara-AMP 必须通过静脉给药。峰浓度在 3～4 小时后观察到。几乎 25%的药物以原形经尿液排出。

临床活性

这种嘌呤抗代谢物首次批准用于慢性淋巴细胞性白血病中并显示活性。在其他几种血液系统恶性肿瘤中也有疗效，包括早幼粒细胞白血病、惰性非霍奇金淋巴瘤、皮肤 T 细胞淋巴瘤、套细胞淋巴瘤和华氏巨球蛋白血症，而其在非血液系统实体瘤中基本上没有活性[30]。

毒性

限制 F-ara-AMP 临床应用的两个主要副作用是骨髓抑制和免疫抑制。骨髓抑制通常表现为淋巴细胞减少和血小板减少。发热常见于骨髓抑制。免疫抑制主要是 T 细胞介导的，对 B 细胞的影响要小得多。淋巴细胞计数，特别是 CD4 细胞，经常在 F-ara-AMP 后降低，可能需要一年以上才能恢复。骨髓抑制和免疫抑制的联合效应可能导致机会性感染风险增加，如白色念珠菌感染、卡氏肺胞菌或水痘带状疱疹病毒感染。推荐预防性使用覆盖卡氏肺胞菌的抗生素，在给予 F-ara-AMP 治疗时推荐同时予以甲氧苄啶、磺胺甲噁唑，后者是联合治疗的首选药物。其他不太常见的毒性包括厌食、恶心、呕吐、腹泻和腹痛，有时唾液增多，味觉异常（金属味），皮疹和口腔炎[20]。实验室异常包括一过性肝酶升高和肾功能不全。

克拉屈滨

背景

克拉屈滨是一种嘌呤脱氧腺苷类似物。其结构如图 57-11 所示。

代谢作用

在使用细胞的核苷转运体进入细胞后，它通过脱氧胞苷激酶（dC 激酶）合成代谢为克拉屈滨单磷酸酯，最终转化为克拉屈滨三磷酸酯，即活性代谢物[31,32]（图 57-13）。克拉屈滨的代谢改变可导致耐药，尤其是 dC 激酶活性的降低，因为这是该药合成代谢的关键步骤。同理，分解代谢酶特别是 5′-核苷酸酶的表达增加可能有助于耐药。

作用机制

活性代谢物克拉屈滨三磷酸酯与天然存在的 dATP 竞争性结合至 DNA 中，在 DNA 中它可以导致 DNA 链延长的终止。另外，由于关键的脱氧核糖核酸池的不平衡和核糖核苷酸还原酶的抑制，还会造成 DNA 的合成和修复障碍。

临床药理学

克拉屈滨可以口服。该药物主要通过肾脏排泄，约 50%进入尿液，25%以原形排出。这种药物可以通过血脑屏障进入脑脊液。

临床活性

克拉屈滨最初被 FDA 批准用于治疗毛细胞白血病，现在仍然是治疗这种疾病的药物选择。对初发或复发的毛细胞白血病的其有效率为 60%或更高。该药对低级别淋巴组织增殖性疾病也有疗效。对 CLL 和非霍奇金淋巴瘤患者具有潜在活性[33,34]。

毒性

标准剂量下的主要剂量限制性毒性是骨髓抑制，为血小板减少和中性粒细胞减少。其他毒性包括恶心、呕吐、腹泻和神经毒性。克拉屈滨还可引起免疫抑制，淋巴细胞数量减少，特别是 CD4 阳性细胞。这些降低的计数可能需要结束治疗数年后才能恢复。CD4 计数的减少使患者易患机会性感染。

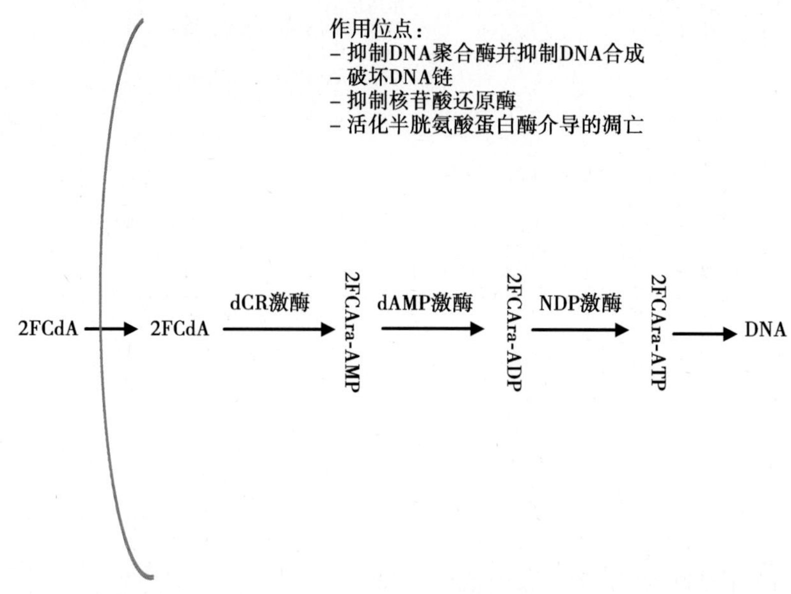

图 57-13 克拉屈滨(2FCdA)的代谢及作用位点。静脉注射后，克拉屈滨使用核苷转运体进入细胞后，通过脱氧胞苷激酶(dCR 激酶)合成代谢为克拉屈滨单磷酸酯，2FCAra-AMP，然后通过核苷酸激酶[脱氧腺苷酸激酶(dAMP 激酶)和二磷酸核苷激酶(NDP 激酶)]最终转化为活性代谢物克拉屈滨三磷酸酯，即 2FCAra-ATP。该图同时显示了 ara-2FCAra-ATP 的作用位点。2FCAra-AMP，克拉屈滨单磷酸酯；2FCAra-ADP，克拉屈滨双磷酸酯；2FCAra-ATP，克拉屈滨三磷酸酯

氯法拉滨

背景

为研发比氟达拉滨和克拉屈滨潜在更有效的腺嘌呤类似物，合成了氯法拉滨(图 57-11)。这种 2-卤-2′-脱氧阿拉伯糖氟腺嘌呤类似物具有 2-氯腺嘌呤苷元，不受 ADA 失活影响。与氟达拉滨和克拉屈滨相比，其结构中氟在 2′位的糖基的配置，可能有助于抑制嘌呤核苷磷酸化酶的磷酸化作用[20]。

代谢作用

进入肿瘤细胞后，氯法拉滨必须被合成代谢为三磷酸酯，这是一种活性代谢产物。氯法拉滨的化学性质可能有助于减少分解代谢，进而提高疗效。实际上，氯法拉滨相较氟达拉滨或克拉屈滨，是更好的脱氧胞苷激酶底物[35]。

合成代谢减少或分解代谢增加而引起的代谢紊乱可导致耐药。

作用机制

几个可能的作用位点包括：掺入 DNA 后导致链终止，从而抑制 DNA 合成；通过抑制 DNA 聚合酶 α、β 和 γ 来抑制 DNA 的合成，进而干扰 DNA 链的延长以及 DNA 的合成与修复。通过抑制核糖核苷酸还原酶使细胞内脱氧核糖核苷酸池耗竭，进一步抑制了 DNA 的合成[36,37]。

临床药理学

氯法拉滨通常作为静脉注射给药，剂量为 2～40mg/m^2，持续 5 天。半衰期约为 5 小时，血浆峰浓度可高达 2. 5μmol/L，但患者之间存在差异。据估计，50%～60%的给药可能会以原形排泄到尿液中。目前，肾功能不全或肝功能不全患者药物使用尚缺乏数据指导。

临床活性

FDA 于 2004 年批准氯法拉滨用于儿童难治性 ALL。它也被用于成人急性髓细胞白血病和骨髓增生异常综合征。临床上特别值得注意的是氯法拉滨与阿糖胞苷的联合应用，据报道疗效增强而毒性不增加。这被认为是 ara-C 浓度增强的结果[38-40]。

毒性

主要的毒性表现是骨髓抑制，这会增加感染的风险。多达 25%的患者会出现肝脏转氨酶升高。其他副作用包括厌食，恶心，另外皮疹在儿童中很常见。

(郭曦　刘天舒 译)

参考文献

1 Chabner BA. General principles of cancer chemotherapy. In: Brunton LL, Chabner BA, Knollmann BC, eds. *Goodman & Gilman's the Pharmacological Basis of Therapeutics*, 12th ed. New York: McGraw-Hill; 2011.
2 Grem JL, Chabner BA, Ryan DR. 5-Fluoropyrimidines. In: Chabner BA, Longo DL, eds. *Cancer Chemotherapy and Biotherapy; Principles and Practice*, 5th ed. Philadelphia, PA: Walters Kluwer Lippincott Williams & Wilkins; 2011.
3 Diasio RB, Harris BE. Clinical pharmacology of 5-fluorouracil. *Clin Pharmacokinet*. 1989;**4**:215–237.
4 Heggie GD, Sommadossi JP, Cross DS, Huster WJ, Diasio RB. Clinical pharmacokinetics of 5-fluorouracil and its metabolites in plasma, urine, and bile. *Cancer Res*. 1987;**478**:2203–2206.
5 Wilson PM, Danenberg PV, Johnston PG, Lenz HJ, Ladner RD. Standing the test of time: targeting thymidylate biosynthesis in cancer therapy. *Nat Rev Clin Oncol*. 2014;**11**:282–298.
6 Anderson N, Lokich J, Bern M, Wallach S, Moore C, Williams D. A phase I clinical trial of combined fluoropyrimidines with leucovorin in a 14-day infusion. Demonstration of biochemical modulation. *Cancer*. 1989;**63**:233–237.
7 Diasio RB, Beavers TI, Carpenter JT. Familial deficiency of dihydropyrimidine dehydrogenase. Biochemical basis for familial pyrimidemia and severe 5-fluorouracilinduced toxicity. *J Clin Invest*. 1988;**81**:47–51.

8 Chong CR, Zirkelbach JF, Diasio RB, Chabner BA. Pharmacogenetics. In: Chabner BA, Longo DL, eds. *Cancer Chemotherapy and Biotherapy; Principles and Practice*, 5th ed. Philadelphia, PA: Walters Kluwer Lippincott Williams & Wilkins; 2011.

9 Veselý J. Mode of action and effects of 5-azacytidine and of its derivatives in eukaryotic cells. *Pharmacol Ther*. 1985;**28**:227–235.

10 Kemeny NE, Schwartz L, Gönen M, et al. Treating primary liver cancer with hepatic arterial infusion of floxuridine and dexamethasone: does the addition of systemic bevacizumab improve results? *Oncology*. 2011;**80**:153–159.

11 de Bono JS, Twelves CJ. The oral fluorinated pyrimidines. *Invest New Drugs*. 2001;**19**:41–59.

12 Midgley R, Kerr DJ. Capecitabine: have we got the dose right? *Nat Clin Pract Oncol*. 2009;**6**:17–24.

13 Chabner BA, Glass J. Cytidine analogues. In: Chabner BA, Longo DL, eds. *Cancer Chemotherapy and Biotherapy; Principles and Practice*, 5th ed. Philadelphia, PA: Walters Kluwer Lippincott Williams & Wilkins; 2011.

14 Chou TC, Arlin Z, Clarkson BD, Phillips FS. Metabolism of 1-D-arabinofuranosylcytosine in human leukemic cells. *Cancer Res*. 1977;**37**:3561–3570.

15 Ohno Y, Spriggs D, Matsukage A, Kufe D. Effects of 1-d-arabinofuranosylcytosine incorporation on elongation of specific DNA sequences by DNA polymerase. *Cancer Res*. 1988;**48**:1494–1498.

16 Kantarjian H, Oki Y, Garcia-Manero G, et al. Results of a randomized study of 3 schedules of low-dose decitabine in higher-risk myelodysplastic syndrome and chronic myelomonocytic leukemia. *Blood*. 2007;**109**:52–57.

17 Glover AB, Leyland-Jones BR, Chun HG, Davies B, Hoth DF. Azacitidine: 10 years later. *Cancer Treat Rep*. 1987;**71**:737–746.

18 Shewach DS, Hahn TM, Chang E, Hertel LW, Lawrence TS. Metabolism of 2′,2′-difluoro-2-deoxycytidine and radiation sensitization of human colon carcinoma cells. *Cancer Res*. 1994;**54**:3218–3223.

19 Ruiz van Haperen VW, Veerman G, Vermorken JB, Peters GJ. 2′,2′-Difluorodeoxycytidine (gemcitabine) incorporation into RNA and DNA of tumour cell lines. *Biochem Pharmacol*. 1993;**46**:762–766.

20 Hande KR. Purine antimetabolites. In: Chabner BA, Longo DL, eds. *Cancer Chemotherapy and Biotherapy; Principles and Practice*, 5th ed. Philadelphia, PA: Walters Kluwer Lippincott Williams & Wilkins; 2011.

21 Zimm S, Collins JM, Riccardi R, et al. Variable bioavailability of oral mercaptopurine: is maintenance chemotherapy in acute lymphoblastic leukemia being optimally delivered? *N Engl J Med*. 1983;**308**:1005–1009.

22 Zimm S, Collins JM, O'Neill D, Chabner BA, Poplack DG. Inhibition of first-pass metabolism in cancer chemotherapy: interaction of 6-mercaptopurine and allopurinol. *Clin Pharmacol Ther*. 1983;**34**:810–817.

23 Lennard L. Implementation of TPMT testing. *Br J Clin Pharmacol*. 2014;**77**: 704–714.

24 Karran P, Attard N. Thiopurines in current medical practice: molecular mechanisms and contributions to therapy-related cancer. *Nat Rev Cancer*. 2008;**8**:24–36.

25 Nelson JA, Carpenter JW, Rose LM, Adamson DJ. Mechanisms of action of 6-thioguanine, 6-mercaptopurine and 8-azaguanine. *Cancer Res*. 1975;**35**: 2872–2878.

26 Gandhi V, Keating MJ, Bate G, Kirkpatrick P. Nelarabine. *Nat Rev Drug Discov*. 2006;**5**:17–18.

27 Sanford M, Lyseng-Williamson KA. Nelarabine. *Drugs*. 2008;**68**:439–447.

28 Cohen MH, Johnson JR, Justice R, Pazdur R. FDA drug approval summary: nelarabine (Arranon) for the treatment of T-cell lymphoblastic leukemia/lymphoma. *Oncologist*. 2008;**13**:709–714.

29 Gandhi V, Plunkett W. Cellular and clinical pharmacology of fludarabine. *Clin Pharmacokinet*. 2002;**41**:93–103.

30 Montillo M, Ricci F, Tedeschi A. Role of fludarabine in hematological malignancies. *Expert Rev Anticancer Ther*. 2006;**6**:1141–1161.

31 Griffig J, Koob R, Blakley RL. Mechanisms of inhibition of DNA synthesis by 2-chlorodeoxyadenosine in human lymphoblastic cells. *Cancer Res*. 1989;**49**:6923–6928.

32 Fukuda Y, Schuetz JD. ABC transporters and their role in nucleoside and nucleotide drug resistance. *Biochem Pharmacol*. 2012;**83**:1073–1083.

33 Grever MR, Lozanski G. Modern strategies for hairy cell leukemia. *J Clin Oncol*. 2011;**29**:583–590.

34 Sigal DS, Miller HJ, Schram ED, Saven A. Beyond hairy cell: the activity of cladribine in other hematologic malignancies. *Blood*. 2010;**116**:2884–2896.

35 Zhenchuk A, Lotfi K, Juliusson G, Albertioni F. Mechanisms of anti-cancer action and pharmacology of clofarabine. *Biochem Pharmacol*. 2009;**78**:1351–1359.

36 Nagai S, Takenaka K, Nachagari D, et al. Deoxycytidine kinase modulates the impact of the ABC transporter ABCG2 on clofarabine cytotoxicity. *Cancer Res*. 2011;**71**:1781–1791. PMID: 21245102.

37 Aye Y, Stubbe J. Clofarabine 5'-di and -triphosphates inhibit human ribonucleotide reductase by altering the quaternary structure of its large subunit. *Proc Natl Acad Sci U S A*. 2011;**108**:9815–9820.

38 Ghanem H, Kantarjian H, Ohanian M, Jabbour E. The role of clofarabine in acute myeloid leukemia. *Leuk Lymphoma*. 2013;**54**:688–698.

39 Bryan J, Kantarjian H, Prescott H, Jabbour E. Clofarabine in the treatment of myelodysplastic syndromes. *Expert Opin Investig Drugs*. 2014;**23**:255–263.

40 Wiernik PH. Optimal therapy for adult patients with acute myeloid leukemia in first complete remission. *Curr Treat Options Oncol*. 2014;**15**:171–186.

第 58 章 烷化剂和铂类抗肿瘤化合物

Zahid H. Siddik, PhD

概述

烷化剂和铂类化合物是治疗多种癌症的高效抗肿瘤药物。这些药物能靶向 DNA(脱氧核糖核酸),但需要通过自发或代谢途径转化激活,以诱导单功能 DNA 加合物的形成以及链间和链内的交联。这种损害使得 DNA 解旋和/或弯曲,由此带来的畸变被特异的 DNA 损伤识别蛋白识别后激活检查点,进而阻滞细胞周期的运行,使细胞有时间修复损伤并存活。如果细胞 DNA 受到广泛损伤且无法完成修复,则激活 p53 依赖性或非依赖性细胞凋亡途径(程序性细胞死亡)来影响抗肿瘤药物疗效。由于烷化剂和铂类化合物的活化产物不具有对肿瘤细胞选择性,它们还会与正常细胞的 DNA 和其他内源性大分子相作用,从而引起严重的副作用;其中某些毒性可能是不可逆的和累积性的,因此表现为剂量限制的障碍。另一个缺点是,肿瘤细胞本身内源性或者获得性的遗传学改变能抑制细胞凋亡并且诱导细胞对烷化剂和铂类化合物产生耐药性。耐药的机制主要表现为药物累积的减少、药物失活的增加、DNA 修复的增加、DNA 损伤识别系统对损伤的识别障碍及凋亡信号转导途径的异常。因此,我们亟须采取合理的策略来应对这些耐药机制,以使患者获得更佳的疗效。

引言

癌症的标志包括持续活化的增殖信号和无限复制的能力,这些生物学特征导致肿瘤体积不可控制地增长[1,2]。这与肿瘤细胞缺乏对 DNA(脱氧核糖核酸)复制和细胞周期反馈性或抑制性调控的特点相符合。因此,靶向 DNA 或者与 DNA 共价作用以抑制 DNA 复制,进而抑制细胞增殖的治疗药物已成为临床上癌症患者治疗的基石。这些药物被广泛地称为 DNA 烷化剂,其中包括以铂类为基础的抗肿瘤化合物。这些药物能形成单功能和/或双功能加合物,其中双功能加合物能以链间和链内 DNA 交联等多种形式存在。

烷化剂作为治疗药物的发现要追溯到 1914—1918 年间的第一次世界大战,当时氯气或硫磺芥子气等毒气在化学战中被广泛地用于抵抗敌军士兵。1917 年德军在比利时伊普尔镇附近对英国、加拿大和法国士兵首次使用硫磺芥子气(图 58-1)。在对死亡士兵进行尸检时发现,芥子气具有重度骨髓抑制作用,并且可导致淋巴组织再生不良[3]。于是,有关此类药物可能用于治疗癌症的想法被概念化,但是芥子气的严重毒性与不良反应禁止了它在临床上的应用。在 20 世纪 40 年代初,耶鲁大学 Goodman 和 Gilman 的工作最终发现了反应轻且毒性更低的氮芥(图 58-2)[4,5]。氮芥是第一个在淋巴瘤的抗肿瘤临床试验中进行测试的药物,它所表现出的疗效为现代癌症化疗奠定了坚实的基础,同时也催生了更多有效低毒的烷化剂的开发,其中有些药物至今仍然是临床抗癌配备中的组成部分。除氮芥以外,几种其他结构类型的烷化剂也相当引人注目,包括氮丙啶、己糖醇环氧化物、烷基磺酸盐、亚硝基脲和三嗪/肼。这些药物和含铂抗肿瘤药物是本章论述的主体。

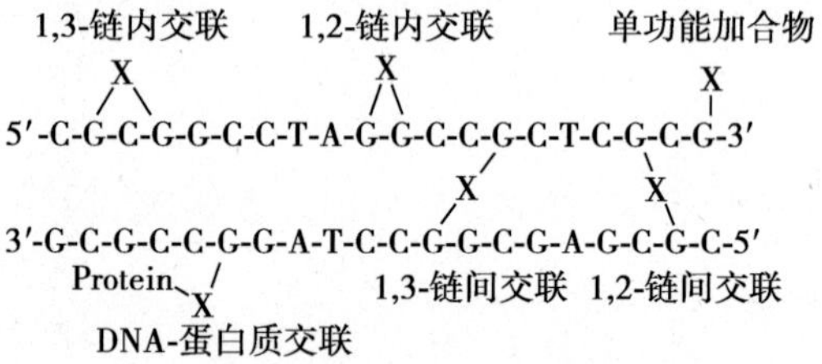

1,3-链内交联　1,2-链内交联　单功能加合物

5′-C-G-C-G-G-C-C-T-A-G-G-C-C-G-C-T-C-G-C-G-3′

3′-G-C-G-C-C-G-G-A-T-C-C-G-G-C-G-A-G-C-G-C-5′

Protein　1,3-链间交联　1,2-链间交联

DNA-蛋白质交联

图 58-1　DNA 损伤药物诱导的单功能 DNA 加合物和链间和链内交联(X 为烷基或者铂类化合物)

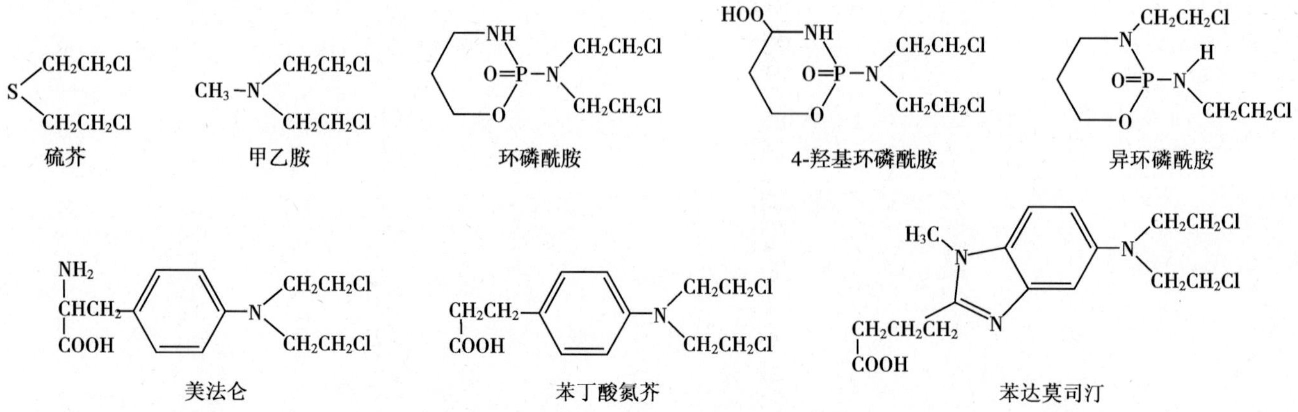

硫芥　甲乙胺　环磷酰胺　4-羟基环磷酰胺　异环磷酰胺

美法仑　苯丁酸氮芥　苯达莫司汀

图 58-2　硫磺芥子气与氮芥类化合物的结构

细胞毒性的主要机制

烷化剂和铂类化合物可以转化为高活性产物，并广泛地与含有富电子（亲核）中心（如氮和硫原子）的内源性大分子结合形成有力的化学键。这种大分子可以是多肽、蛋白质或核酸，但是与 DNA 的相互作用是其发挥细胞毒效应的基础。如果仅发生单一的烷基化或铂化反应时，这些高活性产物与 DNA 的相互作用是单功能性的，而当它们与 DNA 上两个不同碱基的亲核中心形成共价键，并诱导交联或形成加合物时则为双功能性。此外，这些交联的形成主要是通过鸟嘌呤的 N7 位点，可以发生于 DNA 链间（在相对应的 DNA 链之间；主要由烷化剂诱导）或者链内（在同一条 DNA 链上；主要由铂类药物诱导）（图 58-1）。

尽管烷化剂与 DNA 的偶然性作用可能受到许多因素的影响，如活性烷基化部位的形成、解毒和核获取等，但是其与 DNA 的实际作用则具有位点的特异性。例如，富电子的鸟嘌呤的 N7 位点能优先促进与带正电荷的烷基化产物共价结合。当鸟嘌呤在 5′-GC-3′或 5′-GXC-3′序列（其中 X 为任意核苷酸）时，氮芥更有利于与其形成链间 GG 交联，也就是说，核苷酸序列可进一步促进它们的交互作用[6,7]。另一方面，丝裂霉素 C 具有 DNA 小沟区的趋向性，所以更优先与 5′-CG-3′序列中的 N2-鸟嘌呤（胞嘧啶位于鸟嘌呤之前）相交联。O6-鸟嘌呤和 N3-胞嘧啶的烷基化亦可发生。

在 20 世纪 60 年代早期，N7-二胍基交联在烷化剂的细胞毒性中所起关键作用被确定[6,9]。尽管可以设想 DNA 的链间交联能阻止双链在基因组复制过程中的分离，并导致细胞毒作用，但是这并不肯定。单功能的链间和链内加合物显然都具有细胞学效应，包括抑制 DNA 合成、诱导细胞周期停滞和细胞凋亡。然而，双功能药物比单功能加合物具有更强的效力。这种细胞学效应是由烷化剂或铂类药物所诱导的 DNA 特异性扭曲和解旋的最终结果，通过在 DNA 损伤处的不同蛋白质协调组装并激活许多信号通路来进一步诱导。最终的细胞学效应取决于药物浓度，进而是 DNA 受损的程度。DNA 轻度损伤可诱导细胞周期停滞，通过 DNA 修复可促进细胞存活，而广泛的 DNA 损伤且超过其修复能力时会激活细胞凋亡。这些情况在肿瘤细胞和正常细胞中均可发生，且肿瘤细胞和正常细胞对 DNA 损伤的相对耐受性差异较小，因此不可避免带来的副作用限制了药物的更大剂量使用。

烷化剂

双功能烷化剂

氮芥

自 1946 年有关氮芥的临床有效性初步报告发表后不久，相关研究进一步通过结构-活性关系评估许多氮芥类化合物的抗肿瘤能力。在少数进入临床试验的化合物中，有个别被 FDA 批准并且至今仍在使用。如图 58-2 所示，除了氮芥之外，还包括环磷酰胺、异环磷酰胺、美法仑、苯丁酸氮芥和苯达莫司汀。该图中也列出 4-过氧氢环磷酰胺，它是活性 4-羟基环磷酰胺的前体药物。

Colvin 等已经较好描述了氮芥与 DNA 之间作用反应的事件顺序和特异性[10]。这类药物的双氯乙烷基团在 DNA 中 N7-鸟嘌呤的主要烷基化中起着至关重要的作用，但是烷基化亦可发生但是少见于 O6-鸟嘌呤和 N3-和 N7-腺嘌呤位点处。烷基化具有位点特异性且需要 5′-GXC-3′序列中的鸟嘌呤（其中 X 为任意核苷酸）。为了交互作用，氯乙烷基团环化形成高反应性氮杂环丙烷离子中间体，其更容易作用于富电子位点，如图 58-3 中的 N7-鸟嘌呤位点所示。为了烷基化反应，氮杂环丙烷离子可能首先重排为反应性正碳离子中间体。由于存在双氯乙烷基团，这使得在交联 DNA 的过程中出现连续的双功能烷基化。如上所述，氮芥类化合物更倾向于与 DNA 产生链间交联，其中 1,3-交联为常见的相互作用方式。然而，DNA-DNA 链内，DNA-蛋白和 DNA-谷胱甘肽亦可形成交联，但并没有产生细胞毒性的可能性。DNA 的链间交联为关键损伤，根据 Roberts 等的研究结果显示，双功能 DNA 的链间交联对细胞的杀伤效应是单功能 DNA 加合物所产生效应的 100 倍[11]。

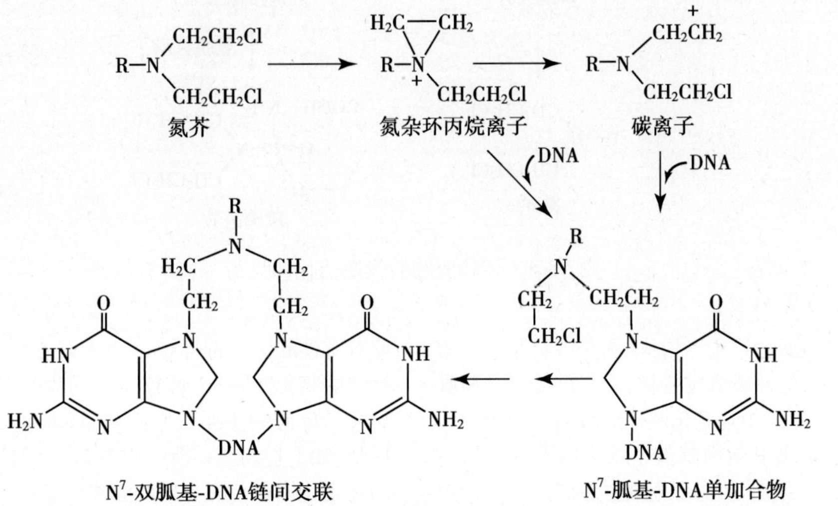

图 58-3　氮芥通过 DNA 烷基化形成的链间交联

所有氮芥类药物都是中性，它们必须被激活后才能与DNA的靶位点相互作用。例如，氮芥在生理pH条件下能自发激活，但是这种快速激活正是氮芥带来许多不良反应的主要原因。分子化学修饰不仅在稳定氮芥同源物方面发挥至关重要的作用，而且能影响调节输送、分布和反应活性的理化特点，以提高其临床实用性[12]。带有一个氧氮磷杂环已烯环的环磷酰胺，选自1 000多种氧氮磷杂环己烯候选物，它的化学惰性和对代谢活化的依赖性是一种理想的特征[13,14]。它激活的主要部位在肝脏，其中由P450介导的混合功能氧化酶反应引发了一系列复杂的化学转化事件，部分如图58-4所示[15-18]。4-羟基环磷酰胺是最重要的代谢物，它相对非极性且可以很容易分布全身，包括肿瘤组织。这种代谢物可直接由前体药物4-氢过氧环磷酰胺形成(图58-2)，能有效清除接受自体骨髓移植患者的骨髓抽取液中的肿瘤细胞[19]。在生理pH条件下，少量的4-羟基环磷酰胺与醛磷酰胺平衡存在，醛磷酰胺相对不稳定并自发先后分解为高活性的磷酰胺氮芥和氮芥。

丙烯醛是环磷酰胺代谢生成的重要副产物，在醛磷酰胺转化为磷酰胺氮芥的过程中产生(图58-4)[18]。丙烯醛可导致出血性膀胱炎这一严重的副作用[20]，但它潜在的抗肿瘤活性还是令人感兴趣的。虽然在使用模型化合物二氯-4-氢过氧环磷酰胺进行的研究发现，自发释放的丙烯醛缺乏细胞毒性[21]，但其他研究均表明，丙烯醛确实具有抗肿瘤和致癌活性，而它能被O6-烷基鸟嘌呤-烷基转移酶灭活[22-24]。乙醛脱氢酶在调节活性中也起着重要作用，它通过将醛磷酰胺转化为无活性的羧基磷酰胺代谢物，最终有80%的环磷酰胺剂量经尿液排泄。当肿瘤细胞异常过表达这种酶时，无疑会导致对环磷酰胺的耐药性[25]。因此，肝脏、造血祖细胞、肠道干细胞和黏膜吸收细胞的高水平乙醛脱氢酶与环磷酰胺相比其他烷化剂更低的肝脏、胃肠道和血液学毒性降低有关。由于钠丢失和肾小管对水重吸收导致的抗利尿作用，大剂量环磷酰胺可导致代谢物经尿液排泄功能障碍并导致水肿[26]。电解质失衡也可能导致研究报道的大剂量化疗所导致的剂量限制性和致命的心脏毒性[27]。临床上需要充分认识这一缺陷，监测给药剂量以防发生严重的不良反应。

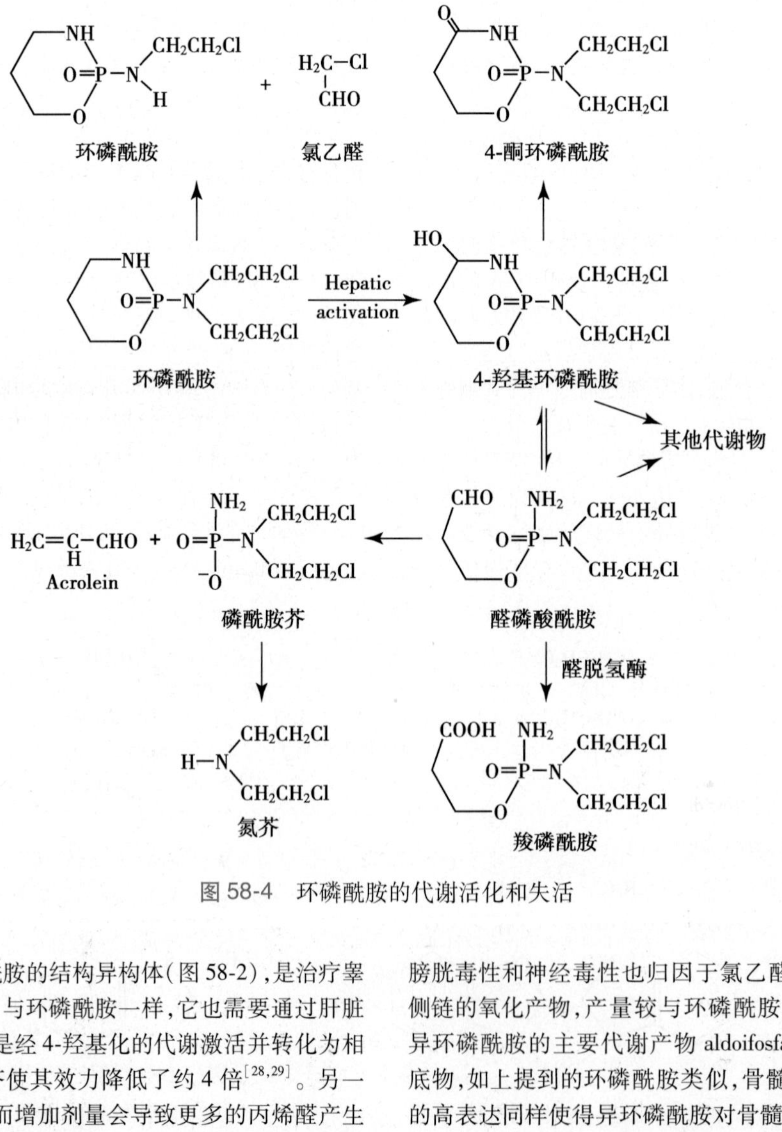

图58-4 环磷酰胺的代谢活化和失活

异环磷酰胺是环磷酰胺的结构异构体(图58-2)，是治疗睾丸癌和肉瘤的重要药物。与环磷酰胺一样，它也需要通过肝脏混合功能氧化酶激活，但是经4-羟基化的代谢激活并转化为相应的活性异环磷酰胺氮芥使其效力降低了约4倍[28,29]。另一方面，为补偿较低的效力而增加剂量会导致更多的丙烯醛产生和累积，这会增加尿路上皮毒性的发生概率，因此需要使用基于硫醇的美司钠来灭活这种有毒副产物。异环磷酰胺的肾脏、膀胱毒性和神经毒性也归因于氯乙醛的形成[30]，它是氯乙烷侧链的氧化产物，产量较与环磷酰胺多(约50% vs 约10%)。异环磷酰胺的主要代谢产物aldoifosfamide也属乙醛脱氢酶的底物，如上提到的环磷酰胺类似，骨髓和胃肠道中乙醛脱氢酶的高表达同样使得异环磷酰胺对骨髓和胃肠道的低毒性。

美法仑、苯丁酸氮芥和苯达莫司汀在结构上没有环磷酰胺和异环磷酰胺具有的氧氮磷杂环，因此它们不需要代谢活化。

但是药物的代谢仍在肝脏中进行。相反，这些药物具有不饱和的吸电子芳环（图 58-2），能缓和双氯乙烷基团的活化和氮杂环丙烷离子的形成从而尽可能降低不良反应。由于带有苯丙氨酸的结构特征，美法仑能更主动进入细胞和突破血脑屏障[31-33]。这些氮芥类化合物已是多种恶性肿瘤的重要治疗手段，如美法仑用于治疗多发性骨髓瘤、乳腺癌和卵巢癌[34]，苯丁酸氮芥用于治疗卵巢癌、慢性淋巴细胞白血病、霍奇金和非霍奇金淋巴瘤[35-37]，苯达莫司汀用于治疗慢性淋巴细胞白血病和淋巴瘤[38]。据报道苯达莫司汀的耐受性高于结构类似的苯丁酸氮芥，因此是一种更具成本效益的治疗药物[39]。

氮丙啶

氮丙啶，也称为乙烯亚胺，通过三元杂环氮丙啶环烷基化。如图 58-5 所示，氮丙啶类药物包括噻替派（N，N'，N"-三亚乙基硫代磷酰胺）和丝裂霉素 C 和三亚乙基三聚氰胺。另外还有六甲基三聚氰胺，其类似于三亚乙基三聚氰胺，但缺乏经典的氮丙啶环。噻替派和丝裂霉素 C 在包括难治性骨肉瘤和膀胱癌在内的多种疾病的治疗中具有重要的临床意义[40,41]。含有大剂量的噻替派的联合用药方案加[42]/不加[43]自体干细胞支持已被用于乳腺癌的治疗。另外，六甲基三聚氰胺已被用于复发性卵巢癌的挽救治疗[44]。

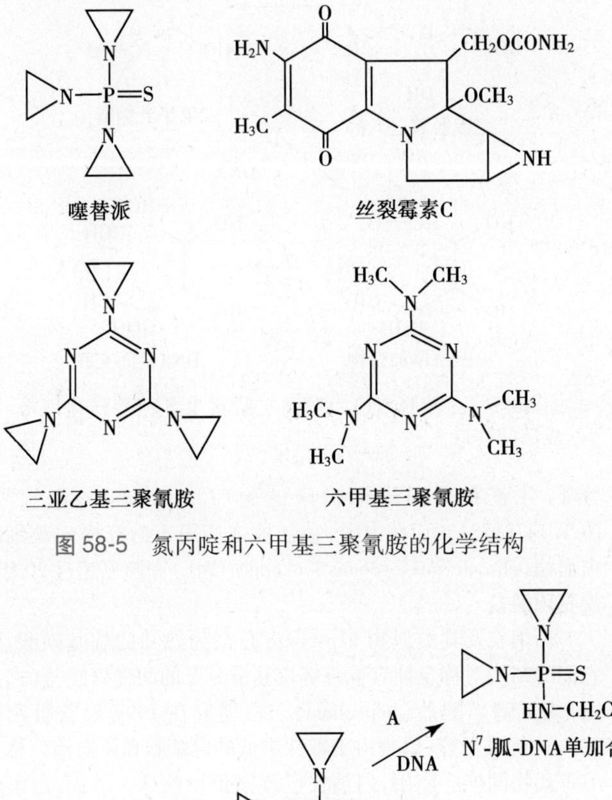

图 58-5　氮丙啶和六甲基三聚氰胺的化学结构

噻替派化学结构中的氮丙啶环不带电荷，这使得它与 RNA（核糖核酸）、DNA、蛋白质和硫醇（如谷胱甘肽）中富电子中心的反应性弱于其他由结构类似氮丙啶环形成的氮芥化合物。在 DNA 中，噻替派的烷基化位点位于全部 4 个核苷酸中，尤其是 O2-胞嘧啶，N1-胸腺嘧啶，N1-、N2-和 N7 腺嘌呤，以及 N1-、N7-和 O6-鸟嘌呤[45]。然而，与其他烷化剂一样，N7-鸟嘌呤仍然是首选位点，能形成鸟嘌呤-鸟嘌呤（GG）和腺嘌呤-鸟嘌呤（AG）链间交联，主要是 1，2-交联[46]。这些交联按顺序形成，在 N7-鸟嘌呤处通过第一反应形成单功能加合物，接着与附近鸟嘌呤产生第二反应并形成交联，如图 58-6 中的途径 A 所示。交联也可通过将噻替派代谢为替派（硫被氧取代），然后打开氮丙啶环并转化为含氯乙基的交联化合物，正如氮芥类药物中所见[47]。另外，氮丙啶环可被切割以介导 N7-鸟嘌呤烷基化，形成单功能 DNA 加合物（图 58-6，途径 B）进而诱导 DNA 单链断裂并促进细胞死亡[48,49]。

与噻替派不同，丝裂霉素 C 与 DNA 相互作用时需要还原代谢形成白三叠氮基亚油基以促进单功能加合物的形成[50]。丝裂霉素 C 的 C10 处自发分子内重排并清除氨基甲酸酯基团，导致与 DNA 相反链的二级烷基化反应，进而诱导细胞毒性 1，2-GG 链间交联损伤（图 58-7）。有趣的是，丝裂霉素 C 更多地导致 DNA 的 N2-鸟嘌呤位点烷基化，尤其当鸟嘌呤存在于螺旋 DNA 双链的 5'-嘌呤-CG-吡啶-3'序列中时[8]。

基于三亚乙基三聚氰胺结构中氮丙啶环的存在，该药物进行烷基化的方式可能与如上对噻替派所描述的方式相同。然而，对于六甲基三聚氰胺，需要在肝脏中进行代谢激活[51,52]。代谢中产生的羧基胺中间体：N-羟甲基五甲基三聚氰胺，重排为反应性亚胺离子，是负责 DNA 中鸟嘌呤烷基化的主要物质（图 58-8）。六甲基三聚氰胺代谢或可产生双羧基胺产物——N，N'-二羟甲基-四甲基三聚氰胺[53]，并可能导致 DNA 的双功能链间交联。基于三羧基胺的六甲基三聚氰胺前体药物——三甲基三聚氰胺，尤其容易形成这种交联[54]。值得注意的是，已有临床试验关注三甲基三聚氰胺[55]，但由于其有限的临床效果[56]和/或药物配方/稳定性问题[57]，此药物的开发并未继续。

己糖醇环氧化物

二环氧化物 1，2∶5，6-二脱水半乳糖醇（DAG）及其前体药

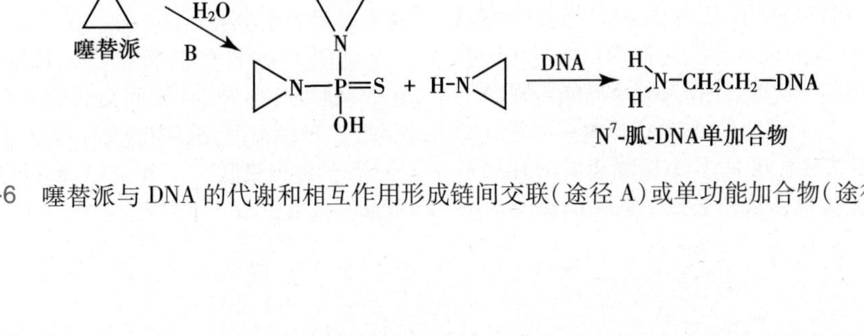

图 58-6　噻替派与 DNA 的代谢和相互作用形成链间交联（途径 A）或单功能加合物（途径 B）

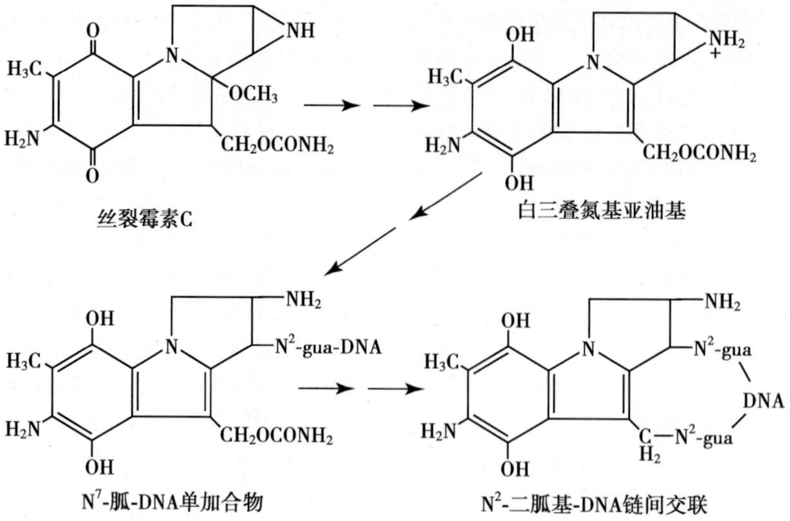

丝裂霉素C　白三叠氮基亚油基　N^7-胍-DNA单加合物　N^2-二胍基-DNA链间交联

图 58-7 丝裂霉素 C 诱导的 DNA 链间交联

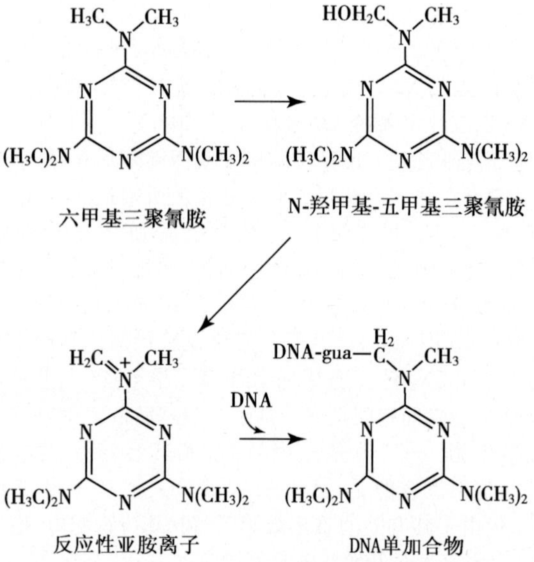

六甲基三聚氰胺　N-羟甲基-五甲基三聚氰胺　反应性亚胺离子　DNA单加合物

图 58-8 六甲基三聚氰胺的激活以形成 DNA 加合物

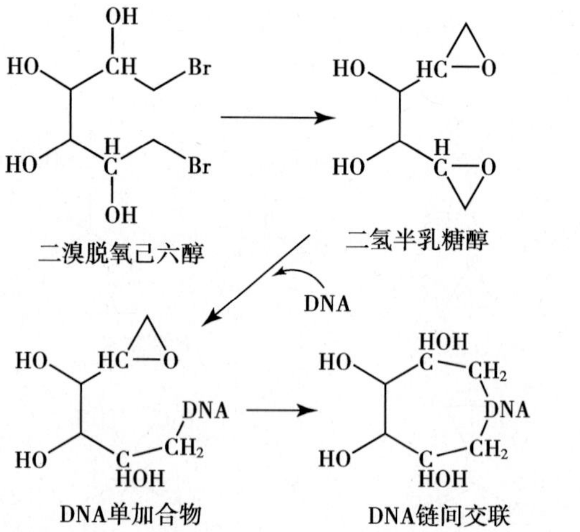

二溴脱氧己六醇　二氢半乳糖醇　DNA单加合物　DNA链间交联

图 58-9 二溴脱氧己六醇向二脱水半乳糖醇转化以形成链间交联

物 1,2 二溴脱氧己六醇(DBD),如氮丙啶类,也通过一个张力三环进行烷基化(图 58-9)。DAG 和 DNA 之间的化学相互作用导致 N7-鸟嘌呤的烷基化[58],这是其他几种烷化剂通常的优选位点。据检测,在无细胞、细胞的和龄齿动物体内系统中,N7-单胍基和 N7-二胍基衍生物是分别代表单功能和链间交联的 DNA 加合物的两种主要产物[58-61]。

在一些抗肿瘤实验模型中,DBD 和 DAG 均显示出与烷化剂类似的抗肿瘤活性,而在其他实验中则不同。例如,在亚硝基脲(BCNU)抗性的 L1210 白血病模型中观察到,DAG 与其缺乏交叉耐药性[62]。在这两种己糖醇中,DAG 具有更高的化学稳定性和更好的临床前抗肿瘤活性[63,64]。然而,DBD 和 DAG 都在 20 世纪 70 年代开展临床研究,并在胃肠道癌症和肺癌中表现出一些治疗活性[65,66]。有趣的是,这些己糖醇类能穿过血脑屏障[67-69],后续的临床试验发现 DAG 在脑癌患者的有效率达 44%[66]。最近 DAG 在美国和欧洲被授予脑癌的孤儿药的称呼,并正在美国进行临床试验(ClinicalTrials. gov 编号:NCT01478178)。而在中国,它已被推广用于治疗慢性粒细胞白血病(chronic myelogenous leukemia,CML)和肺癌超过 20 年。

烷基磺酸盐

白消安及其类似物 hepsulfam 是最为熟知的烷基磺酸盐,它们的结构对称且拥有被直链烷基链分开的两种磺酸盐(白消安)或氨基磺酸盐(hepsulfam)。白消安在 1999 年获批用于 CML 的标准治疗,但是由于毒性更低的羟基脲和靶向治疗格列卫等药物的推广使用,白消安已逐渐退出临床。然而,白消安仍用于同种异体干细胞或骨髓移植的治疗中[70,71]。尽管在人肿瘤模型中,hepsulfam 比白消安更有效[72,73],但在临床试验中并未显示治疗作用。

如图 58-10 中的白消安所示,磺酸盐或氨基磺酸盐是负责在 N7-鸟嘌呤形成 GG 链间交联烷基化反应的关键基团[74,75]。然而,这种由白消安形成的交联存在争议[76],并且提出另外一种 GA 的链内交联[77]。很显然,已报道任何交联都与药物的细胞毒性相关。

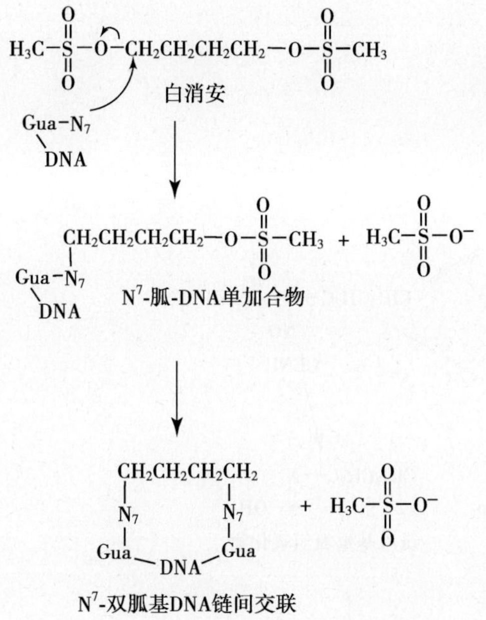

图 58-10　白消安诱导的 DNA 链间交联

亚硝基脲

Montgomery 与其同事就 2-氯乙基亚硝基脲(CENU)作为尿素衍生物在结构-活性关系和临床开发基础等方面开展大部分工作[78-80]。如图 58-11 所致,有 4 种能穿透血脑屏障的类似物进入临床[81,82]。BCNU(Carmustine)和 CCNU(Lomustine)对多种癌症均有效,包括胶质瘤、胶质母细胞瘤、多形细胞瘤、胃肠道肿瘤、乳腺癌和多发性骨髓瘤。链脲佐菌素(Zanosar)对胰岛细胞癌有效,主要是因为它通过葡萄糖转运蛋白 GLUT2 摄取,而该蛋白在胰岛细胞中高表达[83]。由于缺乏任何优于其他亚硝基脲的优势而停止使用甲基-CCNU(Semustine)。亚硝基脲临床应用的局限性主要在于它们的严重副作用,包括造血和肾毒性,链脲佐菌素由于依靠 GLUT2 转运蛋白而主要表现为对正常胰岛 β 细胞的实质性毒性[84]。因此,新的亚硝基脲药物的开发工作仍在继续。如图 58-11 所示,第三代类似物,Fotemustine(Muphoran),已在脑癌和伴有/不伴脑转移的转移性黑色素瘤中显示出活性,并已在澳大利亚、巴西、中国和欧洲获得批准,而在美国未获批[85,86]。

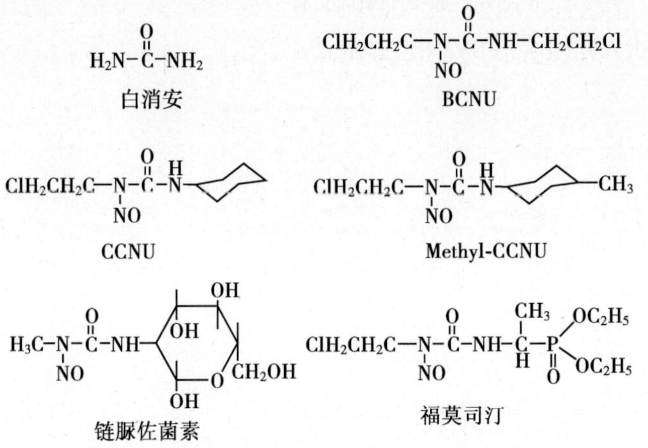

图 58-11　尿素和选择的氯乙基亚硝基脲衍生物的化学结构

众所周知,作为双功能 DNA 链间交联剂的 CENU 是不稳定的,例如 BCNU 的半衰期短,约 50 分钟[82];几种分解产物如图 58-12 所示。某些 CENU 有一个不寻常的特点,就是它们可以产生异氰酸酯,进而螯合包括组蛋白和其他核蛋白质中赖氨酸的 ε-氨基,然而对于螯合蛋白是否促进细胞毒性的意见仍存有分歧[79,87,88]。另一个不寻常的特点就是 CENU 可以烷基化 DNA 中的 O6-鸟嘌呤,可能是借助形成的 2-氯乙基二氮烯羟化物及其类似物 2-羟乙基二氮烯羟化物(图 58-12)[81,82]。这些化合物重排成正碳离子导致在 O6-鸟嘌呤的烷基化并形成单加合物[89]。O6 烷基化反应在上调表达 O6-烷基鸟嘌呤-DNA 烷基转移酶起着重要作用,其能修复 O6-加合物,增加抗性,而反过来使用 O6-苄基鸟嘌呤抑制这个酶的活性能增加肿瘤细胞对亚硝基脲的敏感性[89-91]。然而,来自 N7-鸟嘌呤烷基化的加合物通常是其中最主要的化合物,特别是当这个嘌呤位于 GGG 序列的中间时[92]。这些 DNA 单加合物迅速形成(通常在 1 小时内),但随后缓慢转化为具有细胞毒性的 N7-二胍基链间交联,该过程可能长达 8 小时。值得注意的是,N3-胞嘧啶-N1-脒基交联也是通过 O6-氯乙基-鸟嘌呤单加合物环化成 O6,N1-乙醇鸟嘌呤五环中间体而形成的,其作用于胞嘧啶的 N3 位点并与鸟嘌呤的 N1 位点交联后,促进乙醇鸟嘌呤环的开放和重排[82,93,94]。从空间角度考虑还有一个提议,CENU 中只有 CG 交联是链间的,具有同样细胞毒性的 GG 加合物则是链内的。

单功能烷化剂

下文讨论的一些单功能烷化剂的结构如图 58-13 所示。

肼

在临床前共测试了 400 多种肼类化合物,但只有丙卡巴肼获得临床批准并用于治疗多种恶性肿瘤,特别是霍奇金淋巴瘤、肺癌和黑色素瘤。对于它的活化知之甚少,但是氧化偶氮基-丙卡巴肼的代谢氧化是其中重要的一步。该代谢物重排成活性甲基重氮中间体,进一步形成 O6-和主要的 N7-甲基-鸟嘌呤加合物,然后自发地脱嘌呤诱导单链断裂[95-97]。DNA-DNA 或者 DNA-蛋白质交联尚未见报道。自 20 世纪 70 年代初以来研究的另一种肼类化合物为硫酸肼,但是它的临床有效性不确定,在美国亦未获得批准。

三嗪

最容易辨别的三嗪类化合物是六甲基三聚氰胺(Altretamine)、达卡巴嗪(DTIC-Dome)和替莫唑胺(Temodar)。其中,六甲基三聚氰胺也可能是一种双功能烷基化药物,因此,在"氮丙啶"下,它与上文提到的三甲基三聚氰胺非常相似并归于一类。达卡巴嗪已被用于治疗多种恶性肿瘤,包括霍奇金淋巴瘤、肉瘤、恶性黑色素瘤和胰岛细胞瘤。替莫唑胺是达卡巴嗪的咪唑四嗪衍生物,它对星形细胞瘤、黑色素瘤具有特别的活性。三嗪甲基化 O6-和 N7-鸟嘌呤[98],但是与肼一样,需要代谢活化以进行细胞毒性烷基化反应并促进 DNA 单链断裂[99]。对于达卡巴嗪,肝内活化为[甲基-三嗪基]-咪唑-甲酰胺(MTIC)并产生活性 DNA 甲基化甲基重氮离子。相反,替莫唑胺作为 MTIC 的前体药物起作用,并自发产生活性物质[100]。

异喹啉生物碱

两种天然存在并引起关注的四氢异喹啉生物碱分别是曲贝替定(ecteinascidin-743, Yondelis)和 Zalypsis。曲贝替定是第

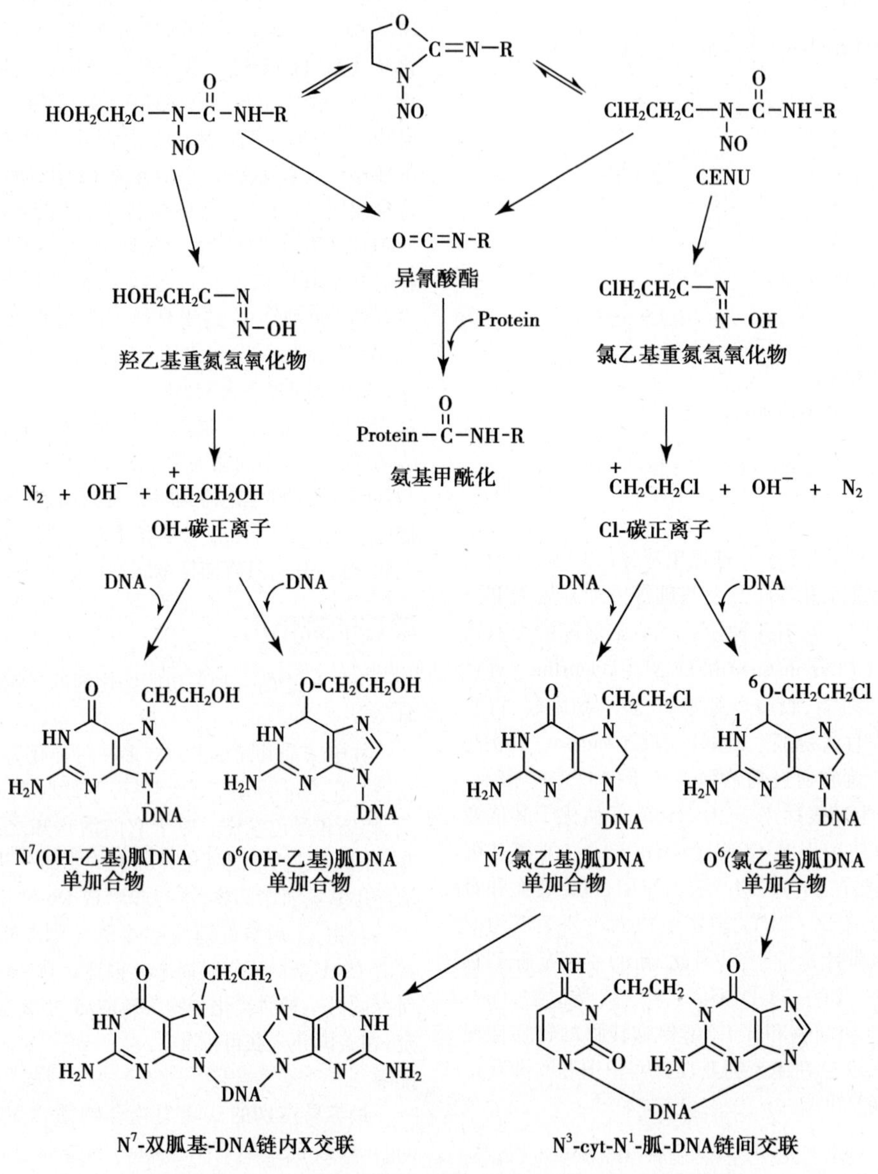

图 58-12 氯乙基亚硝基脲(CENU)的活化并与 DNA 相互作用

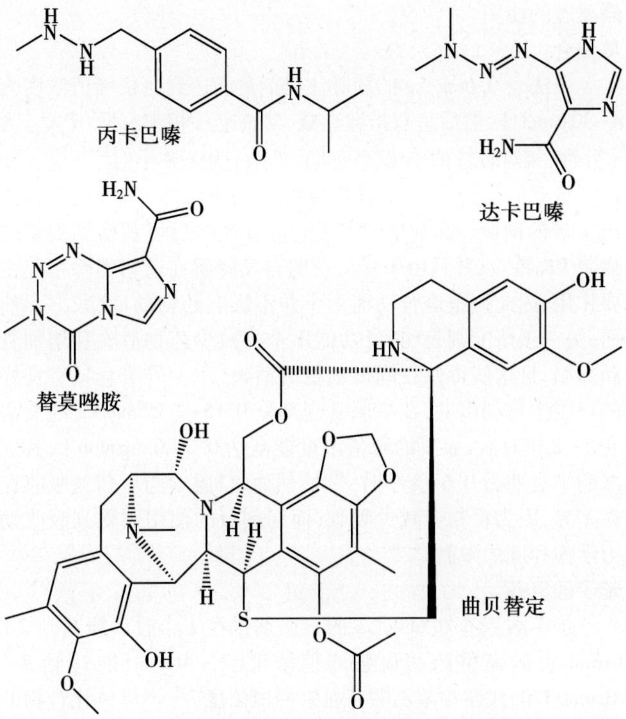

图 58-13　单功能烷化剂的结构

一种海洋衍生的抗肿瘤药物，在欧洲、俄罗斯和韩国已获批用于治疗癌症，特别是晚期软组织肉瘤和铂类耐药卵巢癌[101]。而在美国的则尚待批准。该药物最初以非共价的方式结合到DNA小沟中单一链的TCG、CGG、AGC或GGC序列，随后羧基胺基团脱水产生亚胺离子中间体，继而烷基化相反链中鸟嘌呤的非常见N2位点。曲贝替定诱导的单功能加合物转录偶联的核切除修复（transcriptionally coupled nuclear excision repair，TC-NER）蛋白Rad13/ERCC5募集到DNA损伤位点并诱导链断裂和细胞死亡。曲贝替定的另一个在几种双功能烷化剂中并未发现的不寻常的特征是，p53肿瘤抑制活性的缺乏使其抗肿瘤活性增加3倍[103]。Zalypsise基本上是曲贝替定的合成衍生物，具有与母体分子相同的作用模式[104,105]，目前正在进行临床试验。

分解与代谢

在治疗配方和医学处理方面，烷化剂最初必须处于非活性状态以保持最大的分子效力，直至给予患者使用。如上所述，对于烷化剂，例如替莫唑胺和环磷酰胺，这种效力分别通过生物环境中的自发分解或通过代谢活化来实现。所产生的具有强亲电子特点的活性物质是其抑制肿瘤生长的关键，但它们本身也易于通过与水的水解反应，或通过与细胞中丰富的亲核靶标直接失活交互作用后分解。硫醇，如三肽谷胱甘肽或富含半胱氨酸的金属硫蛋白是交互作用的主要靶点。在某些情况下，谷胱甘肽S-转移酶可促进谷胱甘肽的失活。因此，通过抑制其合成来消耗谷胱甘肽能增强这些药物的抗肿瘤活性[106]。相比而言，谷胱甘肽的存在对于丝裂霉素C的双功能活化是重要的[107]。在药物处置方面，烷化剂在肝脏和肝外组织的代谢也起着重要作用。除了羟基化之外，其他反应包括在亚硝基脲中所观察到的脱氯和脱氮也很重要[87]。如前所述，胃肠道和造血细胞中高水平的醛脱氢酶可以通过对环磷酰胺代谢产物进行解毒来保护细胞。此外，代谢可能受到其他药物的影响，如苯巴比妥可以增加微粒体酶活性和无活性代谢产物的生成和处置的速率[108,109]。

烷化剂耐药

烷化剂的主要临床限制是肿瘤细胞的耐药性。这种耐药性可能是在肿瘤发展过程中固有产生的，也可能是肿瘤细胞通过药物选择压力所获得的。在许多肿瘤中，单一的耐药机制较为罕见，而多种机制则比比皆是，正如已报道的美法仑[110]和替莫唑胺[111]。因此，为了在难治性癌症中获得抗肿瘤效果的任何尝试，都需要克服其多种耐药的机制，而这项工作更具有挑战性。然而，对各个机制的认识能让我们识别肿瘤细胞内信号网络的弱点，并以此开发合成致死的方法[112]。另外，明确一种耐药机制，如果克服这一机制能作为细胞凋亡的主要触发因素。

一般而言，肿瘤细胞的耐药性可归因于：①细胞内药物浓度降低；②细胞失活增加；③DNA修复增强；④凋亡信号的下调。由于L型氨基酸转运蛋白的下调，在耐药细胞中观察到其对美法仑摄取的减少[110,113]。然而，绝大多数烷化剂通过扩散进入细胞，且不受转运蛋白的影响。由于含硫醇化合物或巯基相关酶，如谷胱甘肽、金属硫蛋白、γ-谷氨酰半胱氨酸合成酶（参与谷胱甘肽合成）和谷胱甘肽S-转移酶（增加药物与谷胱甘肽的结合）的水平升高，烷化剂的失活增加可导致耐药[114-118]。醛脱氢酶的水平升高也会导致失活增加，因为这很容易促进环磷酰胺和其他相关的烷化剂的解毒作用[119,120]。

烷化剂靶向结合DNA，持续存在的DNA加合物与细胞毒性有关。在耐药肿瘤细胞中，这些加合物得到有效的修复。如上所述，其中一种修复机制涉及O6-烷基鸟嘌呤-烷基转移酶，其逆转DNA中O6-鸟嘌呤的初始烷基化并防止链间交联的形成。因此，这种烷基转移酶的上调表达能增加癌症耐药性，正如人神经胶质瘤细胞对BCNU所表现出的耐药性[121]。相比而言，错配修复（mismatch repair，MMR）通路能增强O6-烷基鸟嘌呤加合物（O6-甲基≫O6-乙基）的细胞毒性反应[122]，而当MMR通路的缺陷时则相反会促进甲基-烷基化剂替莫唑胺的耐药性[123]。交联的修复可通过核苷酸切除修复（nucleotide excision repair，NER）和替代的非同源末端连接（nonhomologous end-joining，NHEJ）通路来进行。因此人肿瘤细胞中NER和NHEJ系统的修复增强会导致对环磷酰胺、美法仑和苯丁酸氮芥的耐药性[124-127]。而如上所述，单功能烷化剂曲贝替定则相反，NER蛋白Rad13/ERCC5能参与增强其活性[102]。

加合物形成和链间交联通过细胞凋亡杀死细胞，这在许多烷化剂，包括环磷酰胺和替莫唑胺中均已得到证实[128,129]。DNA损伤会激活一系列复杂的信号转导通路，这些通路汇聚于凋亡机制中并诱导细胞死亡。具体而言，核苷酸碱基的烷基化会诱导DNA的解旋和折叠，由此产生的构象变化被专门的识别蛋白感测，进而转导DNA的损伤信号。由此导致特异性基因的转录激活，最终激活半胱天冬酶，并执行细胞凋亡的死亡程序。由于其中涉及大量蛋白质，例如ATR、Chk1、Chk2、p53、Bak和Bax，细胞凋亡程序中的任何关键步骤遭受破坏，均可以抑制凋亡并导致烷化剂耐药。例如，通过突变或其他方法使

p53 功能丧失会导致替莫唑胺耐药[111,130]。干细胞样胶质母细胞瘤细胞对替莫唑胺耐药则表现为 Mdm2 蛋白的过表达，其能增加蛋白酶体的降解进而抑制 p53 的功能[131]。另一方面，在某些癌症中过表达的 Bcl-2 蛋白能与 BAX 结合，进而阻断 caspase-9/caspase-3 级联反应，抑制环磷酰胺所诱导的细胞凋亡[128]。另外，在 BAX 低表达的人 B 细胞 CLL 和 U87MG 胶质母细胞瘤细胞中可观察到对环磷酰胺、苯丁酸氮芥和替莫唑胺的耐药性[132,133]。

尽管在组织培养和龄齿动物模型中均可观察到肿瘤细胞中对烷化剂药物的耐药性，但情况并非总是如此。举一个经典的例子，使用药物直接注射 EMT-6 乳腺肿瘤小鼠将产生对环磷酰胺的耐药性，而在体外当这种癌细胞暴露于环磷酰胺时并没表现出耐药性[134]。这表明，某些机制可导致烷化剂药物的耐药，如 TGF-β(转化生长因子-β)的影响、肿瘤低灌注状态、细胞内 pH 变化和肿瘤微环境，它们只能在体内发挥作用[135-137]。

临床药理学

药物的药代动力学(pharmacokinetics，PK)决定其药效学(pharmacodynamics，PD)，这种 PK-PD 关系对于我们进一步理解药物活性和毒性的基础，以及设计最大化抗癌活性和最小化毒副作用的方案都是不可或缺的。对烷化剂的药理学已经研究了 60 多年，但早在 1952 年就很明确，理想的烷化剂应该以非活性的形式给药并在患者肿瘤中转化为活性状态[12,138]。现将这些我们关注的药物在临床药理学的基本知识总结如下。

环磷酰胺

全身剂量 50～75mg/kg 的环磷酰胺能达到 400μmol/L 的血浆完整药物浓度，随后药物衰减的半衰期为 3～10 小时[139-141]。血浆峰值浓度达 50～100μmol/L 的磷酰胺芥代谢物约在 3 小时出现。有趣的是，它的曲线下面积(area under the curve，AUC)和 4-羟基-环磷酰胺代谢物在静脉和口服给药时相似，这提示两种给药途径均能达到治疗效果。但是不同患者在药物 PK 方面存在较大的差异，这可能是由于环磷酰胺给药后通过自发诱导的代谢，或者是同时使用其他诱导代谢的药物，如苯巴比妥[109,142,143]。然而，在常规剂量范围内，PK 的变化并不会显著影响其毒性或疗效[144]。对此的一个解释就是，活性代谢物的最终 AUC 未受影响，表现为静滴 90 分钟的环磷酰胺所产生 4-羟基环磷酰胺的 AUC 达 105～110μmol/L，这与静注 4 天的环磷酰胺所能达到的 AUC 相似[145]。虽然在骨髓移植中大剂量环磷酰胺是一个引人关注的方案，但是药代动力学的饱和性限制了它的疗效[146]。环磷酰胺的主要排泄途径是经尿液，占总剂量的 60%～70%，排泄物主要为无活性的代谢产物[147,148]。肾脏功能似乎与环磷酰胺的毒性没有相关性，这表明活性的代谢产物主要通过自发分解，而不是经肾脏排泄。

异环磷酰胺

有关异环磷酰胺临床 PK 的数据有限的，它的 PK 特点似乎与环磷酰胺相似。然而，来自异环磷酰胺的活性 4-羟基代谢物的水平低于环磷酰胺[149-151]。与环磷酰胺一样，异环磷酰胺具有口服的生物利用度并能自发诱导其自身代谢[141,152]。这两种药物的相似性可能导致临床使用上的难以选择，但是与环磷酰胺相比，由于侧链代谢在不同患者间可能存在着更大差异，以及合并用药对代谢途径的影响，均可能更多地影响异环磷酰胺的使用[153-155]。

美法仑

美法仑 0.6mg/kg 的静脉注射剂量能达到血浆峰值浓度为 4～13μmol/L，然后呈双指数衰减，其快速 α 相半衰期($T_{1/2\alpha}$)为 8 分钟，相对较慢的 β 相半衰期($T_{1/2\beta}$)为 1.8 小时[156,157]。在该剂量下能达到的平均 AUC 为 8μmol · h/L，且 24 小时能排泄约 13%的剂量。高剂量的美法仑静脉注射后可观察到类似的血浆 PK 特点，并且由于美法仑的自发降解在药物消除中起主要作用，因此据报道肾功能不全并不影响药物的清除[158]。然而，另一项研究则表明，肾功能不全将减少药物清除和增加骨髓抑制，且这些毒性在降低剂量后消失[159]。美法仑具有良好的口服生物利用度，在口服常规剂量 0.15～0.25mg/kg 的美法仑 1～2 小时后，血浆的峰值浓度能高达 0.2～0.6μmol/L，其衰减的半衰期为 0.6～3 小时[160]。然而，口服给药后药物吸收存在差异，因为食物会减少吸收，而高剂量的使用则受到吸收动力学饱和度的限制[161-163]。

苯丁酸氮芥

苯丁酸氮芥 0.6mg/kg 的口服剂量在 1 小时后能达到 2～6μmol/L 的完整药物血浆峰值浓度，2～4 小时能达到 2～4μmol/L 的代谢物苯乙酸芥血浆峰值浓度[157]。母体化合物的 β 相半衰期为 92 分钟，代谢物的半衰期为 145 分钟。在另一项研究中，4 天内口服每天剂量为 0.8～0.9mg/kg 的 PK 分析表明，第一天约 10μmol · h/L 的苯丁酸氮芥的 AUC 在第 4 天下降了 17%，后续在每 4 周的治疗周期中仍逐步下降[164]。这表明，与环磷酰胺和异环磷酰胺一样，苯丁酸氮芥也可能会自发诱导自身的代谢和排泄，但是另一种可能性是，重复给药会减少肠道的吸收。据报道，口服苯丁酸氮芥的 PK 有 2 倍到 4 倍的个体间和个体内变异[165]。有趣的是，该药物或其代谢产物苯乙酸芥的血浆 AUC 并不受食物摄入的影响[166]。

苯达莫司汀

苯达莫司汀 5mg/kg 静脉推注的剂量在血浆中能被快速清除，$T_{1/2\alpha}$ 为 10 分钟，而 $T_{1/2\beta}$ 为 36 分钟，最终得到的 AUC 约 28μmol · h/L[167]。它的口服生物利用度良好(0.25～0.94，均值为 0.57)。该药物经肝脏混合功能氧化酶代谢，主要的代谢产物为 N-去甲基和 γ-羟基-苯达莫司汀[168]。已知谷胱甘肽能结合这些代谢物，且在静推剂量的患者血浆中能观察到另一种代谢物二羟基-苯达莫司汀[169]。药物的总排泄量占静推剂量的 76%，通过尿液和粪便排泄的药量类似。仅约 5%的剂量作为未改变的母体药物被回收，这表明苯达莫司汀被广泛代谢。

噻替派

噻替派 12mg/m^2 静脉注射的剂量能使母体药物的血浆峰值浓度达到 5μmol/L，然后以 $T_{1/2\alpha}$ 8 分钟的和 $T_{1/2\beta}$ 2 小时的半衰期双相衰减，最终得到约 9μmol · h/L 的 AUC[170]。给药 2 小时后，代谢物替派的峰值浓度为 1μmol/L，它在血浆中的持续时间长于噻替派。在 24 小时内尿液排泄约 30%的剂量，其中 1.5%为未改变的药物，大多数为(约 24%的剂量)作用不明确的反应性代谢物。因此，噻替派的生物转化是广泛的。在一项使用高剂量(高达 900mg/m^2)持续灌注 4 天的研究中，第一天就达到噻替派的血浆峰值浓度，但是接下来 3 天逐渐下降约 30%[171]。高剂量的噻替派也带来相应的高血浆 AUC 值(高达 600μmol · h/L)。噻替派也可经腹腔注射给药，腹腔吸收迅速并且能达到与静脉注射使用相似的血浆浓度[172]。但是腹膜中药物 AUC 比血浆高 4 倍以上，这为局限于腹膜的癌症采取腹腔给药的方式提供了强大的理论支持。

亚硝基脲

BCNU 60~170mg/m² 静脉滴注后的 PK 特点已被研究，它能达到 5μmol/L 的血浆峰值浓度，然后它以 $T_{1/2\alpha}$ 6 分钟的和 $T_{1/2\beta}$ 68 分钟的半衰期双相衰减[173]。高剂量（300~750mg/m²）BCNU 在标准化为 1g/m² 的恒定剂量时，其 PK 表明血浆的峰值浓度为超滤 BCNU 7.8μmol/L，平均 AUC 为 9μmol·h/L[174]。这代表仅约 23%的血浆 BCNU 具有烷基化的生物可利用性。CCNU 130mg/m² 口服使用的 PK 研究发现，血浆中未能检测到母体药物，可能是由于 CCNU 快速转化为反式-4-羟基 CCNU 和顺式-4-羟基 CCNU[175]。在给药 2~4 小时后，这两种代谢物达到 3μmol/L 的峰值浓度。羟基-CCNU 代谢物的血浆清除半衰期约为 1~3 小时。

白消安

白消安不能溶解于水溶液的特点使得该药主要用作口服制剂。口服 1mg/kg 的白消安后药物的吸收率差异大，血浆峰值浓度波动于 1~10μmol/L，AUC 波动于 10~85μmol/L，血浆清除半衰期波动于 1~7 小时[176]。但是幼儿患者（2 个月至 3.6 岁）的血浆峰值浓度偏低（1~5μmol/L），平均清除时间比成人提高 34%，而 AUC 始终保持低于成人 3 倍[177]。2002 年以来，白消安的静脉剂型 Busulfex 已可获及，现已被广泛使用，特别是因为它的良好的耐受性并能带来更稳定的剂量依赖性线性 PK[178]。因此，将 0.8mg/kg 的白消安以 Busulfex 剂型静脉推注后，血浆峰值浓度能达到 15μmol/L，然后以约 3 小时的半衰期开始下降，最终得到的平均 AUC 为 80μmol/L。

替莫唑胺

替莫唑胺 150mg/m² 口服后迅速吸收，1 小时后达到血浆峰值浓度 40μmol/L，并得到 116μmol·h/L 的 AUC[179,180]。该药物在血浆中快速被清除，半衰期为约 1.8 小时。食物摄入能减少吸收，使峰值浓度降低 32%，AUC 降低 9%，并能使达到峰值浓度的时间延迟至 2.3 小时。替莫唑胺静脉滴注 90 分钟能达到 38μmol/L 的药物峰值浓度和 127μmol·h/L 的 AUC，这与口服给药的 PK 相似，证明该药物能在肠道快速完全地被吸收。约 38%~39%剂量的替莫唑胺在 7 天内被清除，其中大部分（37.7%）以尿液排泄，其余（0.8%）部分以粪便排出。

曲贝替定

当曲贝替定采用每周静脉输注 1 或 3 小时连用 3 周停 1 周的方案时，它的最大耐受剂量（maximum tolerated dose，MTD）约为 0.6mg/m²[181]，这表明该药物具有高效力。曲贝替定的血浆浓度和 AUC 随着剂量线性增加。在 MTD 时，1 小时输注能达到 15nmol/L 的平均峰浓度，43nmolh/L 的平均 AUC，末端相血浆半衰期约为 4 天。相比之下，3 小时输注所得到的相应数据分别是 8nmol/L、31nmol/L 和 2 天。采用每 21 天输注 24 小时的方案，MTD 为 1.5mg/m²，但是在第一个和第五个疗程之间总体清除率显著升高[182]。第一个疗程采用这个 MTD 给药后所得到的血浆峰浓度为 2.4nmol/L，AUC 为 74nmolh/L，末端相血浆半衰期约为 4 天。根据剂量调整后这个 AUC 值与采用较短时间（1 小时或 3 小时）输注所得到的 AUC 值相一致。曲贝替定的生物转化发生于肝脏，几种代谢物均通过患者的尿液和粪便排出[183]。

不良反应

鉴于烷化剂能靶向 DNA，正常组织有可能受到这些药物的影响，特别是那些具有高增殖比率的组织器官。然而，任何器官均可出现治疗毒性，其中的原因包括组织器官能特异性增加活性药物和/或毒性代谢物的累积。因为治疗指数狭窄，每种烷化剂均会产生一些副作用，其中一些副作用是轻微的，而另一些则成为剂量限制性毒性并影响临床应用。

造血系统毒性，尤其是对粒细胞和血小板的影响，是烷化剂相关的最常见剂量限制性毒性。但是正如替莫唑胺所表现的一样，这种血液学毒性是可逆的。有趣的是，环磷酰胺和异环磷酰胺的骨髓抑制作用较小，这可能与醛脱氢酶的存在相关，因为它能灭活造血干细胞和幼稚粒细胞的醛磷酰胺代谢物。在其他烷化剂导致严重的造血系统毒性时，具体的应对措施包括采用粒-巨噬细胞集落刺激因子（GM-CSF）和粒细胞集落刺激因子（G-CSF）。采取这些保护措施可以允许我们为了增加抗肿瘤疗效而提高剂量。然而，使用这些保护性药物并非没有额外的并发症[184]。高剂量治疗中正常造血细胞的 DNA 烷基化相应增加，因此继发白血病可发生于 10%以上的患者中，是一个严重的副作用。同样的，因为 DNA 是其靶点，烷化剂是高风险的致畸药，特别是在孕期的前三个月[185]。

胃肠道表达的醛脱氢酶可保护自身免受环磷酰胺和异环磷酰胺的毒性作用。然而，其他烷化剂能靶向胃肠道中快速增殖的细胞并导致副作用，尤其是在高剂量的方案中。例如，高剂量的美法仑和噻替派能诱发口腔炎、食道炎和腹泻。涉及胃肠道的恶心呕吐反应部分由中枢神经系统效应所介导，这可能是因为药物的高亲脂性和它们穿过血脑屏障的能力。幸运的是，恶心呕吐可以使用止吐药加以控制，包括多巴胺和 5-羟色胺拮抗剂[186]以及更新指南的相关推荐[187,188]。

白消安、一定程度的美法仑、环磷酰胺和苯丁酸氮芥等药物的使用均与肺损伤有关[189]，可表现为干咳、呼吸困难，可能发展为肺功能不全甚至死亡。Busulfan 诱发的肺毒性可发生于开始治疗 6 周以，病情可迅速发展，根据不同的治疗方案（包括大剂量化疗），这种肺毒性可影响 3%~34%的患者。高剂量治疗也可诱发肝脏毒性，骨髓移植后可发生致命的静脉闭塞性疾病综合征，这种综合征部分以肝脏肿大为表现，在接受环磷酰胺和白消安治疗的患者中，该综合征有高达 25%的发生概率[190,191]。标准剂量的美法仑、白消安、苯丁酸氮芥和曲贝替定治疗后可发生轻度和短暂的肝脏毒性，这与更严重的肝硬化、纤维化和胆汁淤积也有关系。亚硝基脲也有肝毒性，其中 BCNU 与高达 26%比例的患者肝功能异常有关，通常这个毒性是可逆的，但在少数病例中则是致命的。

性腺损害是烷化剂的一种严重副作用，在使用环磷酰胺、苯丁酸氮芥、美法仑、白消安、氮芥、CCNU 和 BCNU 后可出现，但是多数情况下停药后在数年内可以逆转[192]。而含丙卡巴肼的方案，会给大多数接受治疗的淋巴瘤男性患者带来永久性不育症。在女性患者中，丙卡巴肼和环磷酰胺可诱导卵巢功能衰竭和短暂性闭经[193]。25 岁以上的女性患者罹患卵巢功能衰竭的风险显著增高，而 30 岁以上的女性出现月经不规则的风险则高出 12 倍。

尽管环磷酰胺和异环磷酰胺对造血系统和胃肠道的毒性反

应轻微,但是他们导致的出血性膀胱炎却很严重[194]。白消安、噻替派和替莫唑胺也有这种副作用。然后,使用硫醇如美司钠来灭活它们的代谢物,充分水化以强迫尿液对代谢物的排泄可对膀胱黏膜带来保护作用。肾毒性也是烷化剂治疗的一个严重的副作用,特别是使用亚硝基脲类治疗。在一项使用 200mg/m^2 的 BCNU 或甲基-CCNU 治疗 6 个疗程的研究中,肾功能损害很常见,主要表现为血尿素氮和肌酐的升高[195]。在一些患者中,肾损害表现为肾小管萎缩、间质纤维化和肾小球硬化。

心脏毒性也可能是由环磷酰胺、异环磷酰胺和白消安所导致的严重副作用,且已知大剂量环磷酰胺所导致的心脏毒性是致死性的[196-198]。病理学依据表明内皮损伤和出血性心肌炎是特异性的药物诱导心脏毒性反应。神经毒性则相反,作为一种严重的并发症,在标准剂量的白消安或 BCNU 使用后它并不常见,但是在大剂量输注或者通过颈动脉以标准剂量给药后,神经毒性会变严重[199-201]。

烷化剂可以导致严重的脱发,特别是环磷酰胺、异环磷酰胺和白消安[202]。联合用药方案中加入长春新碱或多柔比星可以进一步加重该副作用。该毒性可能是因为亲脂性代谢物渗透至毛囊所致[203],但它通常是可逆转的。烷化剂的其他罕见毒性则包括过敏反应和一过性的抗利尿作用。

铂类抗肿瘤化合物

最常见的铂类抗肿瘤化合物是顺铂[顺-二氨二氯铂(Ⅱ)],它是一种中性的方形平面无机复合物,具有两个不稳定的氯基和两个稳定的氨基配体,呈顺式配位。这种化学几何学特点很重要,因为具有类似反式几何结构的反铂(图 58-14)使得该分子的细胞毒性降低约 20 倍。然而,对于反式几何结构的低效力也存在例外的情况[204]。顺铂在 1844 年的时候被称为 Peyrone 盐,而它的细胞毒性直到 1969 年才被发现。这是 Rosenberg 研究组的偶然观察到的现象,他们将铂电极浸入大肠埃希菌培养基中来传递直流电以阻止细胞分裂,但是细胞仍继续以细丝状生长。深入研究发现铂电极与培养基中的营养物质起反应并形成数个化合物,其中包括顺铂,其有效地阻止大肠埃希菌中的细胞分裂。顺铂最终作为抗肿瘤药物而被开发,并在 1978 年获得美国食品药品管理局(Food and Drug Administration,FDA)批准用于临床[205]。

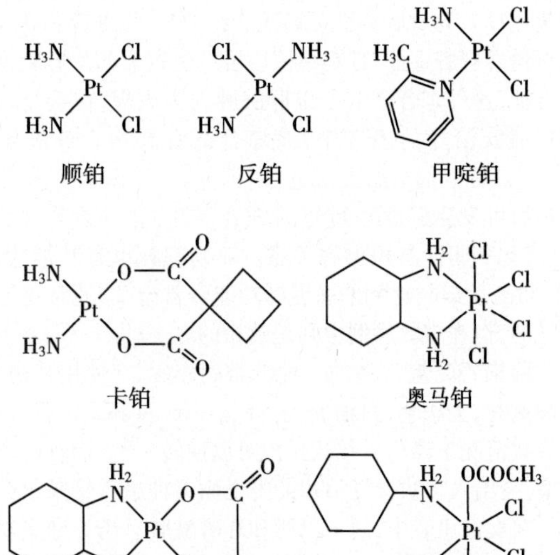

顺铂 反铂 甲啶铂

卡铂 奥马铂

奥沙利铂 沙铂

图 58-14 顺铂及其选择性类似物的结构

顺铂类似物的研发基础

自 FDA 批准以来,顺铂已被广泛用于多种癌症的治疗,包括睾丸癌、卵巢癌、头颈癌、膀胱癌和宫颈癌[206]。其中由于顺铂在化疗方案中的引入,使用睾丸癌的治愈率从 10% 增加到 85%。虽然顺铂稳定且方便使用,但是它也表现出一些主要的临床局限性。基于此原因,研究者合成了数百个铂分子以选出具有更广谱的抗癌活性和更少的毒性反应的铂类同源替代化合物。在 1979 年至 1999 年的 20 年间,23 种铂类药物进入临床试验,其中大部分未能证明其临床有效性,往后也未再有新的铂类药物[207]。部分药物的分子结构如图 58-14 所示,其中只有卡铂、奥沙利铂是获得 FDA 批准的其他铂类化合物。顺铂与其他具有方形平面的类似物都含有二价状态的铂(Ⅱ)中心结构,但是其他的如八面体奥马铂则含有四价铂(Ⅳ)原子。

顺铂的主要缺点在早年即明显表现出来,其对肾脏和外周神经有着不可逆并且累积的毒性。这种剂量限制性的肾毒性促使研究者寻找更安全的铂类似物。在 20 世纪 80 年代早期,Harrap 研究组对大约 300 种铂类似物进行筛查,最终选用卡铂开展的下步的临床试验[208]。这个类似物含有双齿环丁二羧酸配体,取代了两个氯原子(图 58-14),这个结构改变足以减轻肾毒性和外周神经毒性。然而,在临床有效性方面,卡铂与顺铂是类似的。因此,顺铂难治的癌症对卡铂完全交叉耐药[209,210]。寻求缺少交叉耐药性类似物的兴趣被重新点燃,而这需要对氨基配体进行修饰。数种这样的类似物进入临床试验,包括含有双齿 1,2-二氨基环己烷组分的奥马铂和奥沙利铂,以及一个氨基被甲基吡啶替换的吡铂(图 58-14)。最终只有奥沙利铂在特定的难治性癌种中显示出有效性[208]。与其他化合物相比,沙铂结构中的一个氨基被环己烷基团取代,在临床上作为口服药进行试验。尽管已经显示出一些活性[211],但是就如吡铂一样,沙铂未来的临床应用仍不明确[207]。

铂类化合物的作用基础

尽管顺铂、卡铂和奥沙利铂都被认为是化学惰性的,但是它们具有临床活性。为了表现出活性,中性铂分子在水中或生物环境中自发转化为活性化合物。这需要将顺铂中的氯或卡铂和奥沙利铂中的二羧酸配体替换为水分子,如图 58-15 中顺铂所示[212,213]。得到的物质在水溶液中能平衡存在,但是在生物环境中,因为氯-单水合物可立即与生物分子中的亲核位点发生反应,所以无法建立平衡。卡铂中的双齿环丁烷-二羧酸(CBDCA)配体减缓了水化反应,这能反过来降低药物的效力,因此临床上需要使用卡铂剂量比顺铂高 4 倍[214]。另外,奥沙利铂的双齿草酸结构相对来说更不稳定,而它的效力能与顺铂相当。铂(Ⅳ)化合物,如沙铂,在水性环境中是稳定的,并且它们还原为铂(Ⅱ)化合物是水合反应的先决条件。令人惊讶的是,奥马铂具有高度反应性,能与血浆蛋白迅速结合[215],这表明 Pt(Ⅳ)化合物中平面配体的性质决定分子的还原和活化速度(氯≫乙酸盐)。

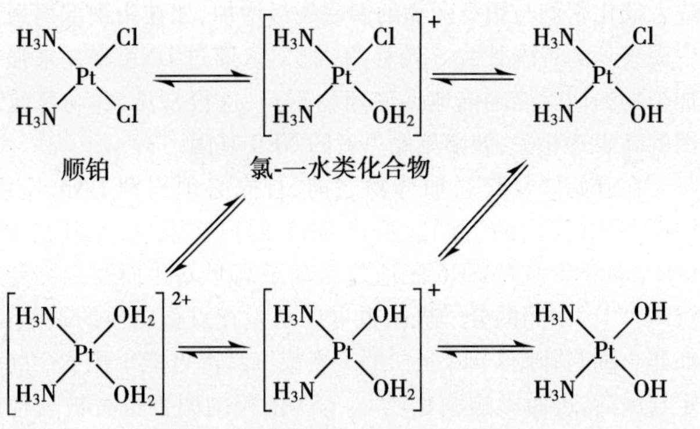

图 58-15 顺铂发生水合作用并成为活化的铂类化合物

铂类药物与 *DNA* 的相互作用

有几项研究的结果表明 DNA 是铂类药物的主要细胞毒性靶点[216]。铂类药物在激活后立即与内源性大分子发生反应，它们很可能以完整的中性状态进入细胞核，进行原位水合并与 DNA 相互作用，主要的结合位点是鸟嘌呤的 N7。铂类药物可以通过不同构型形成链间和链内交联（见图 58-1）。与氮芥化合物一样，当鸟嘌呤位于 5′-GC-3′序列时，很容易形成链间交联[217]。

顺铂诱导的链间交联具有生物学效应，包括细胞毒性和抑制 DNA 依赖性 RNA 聚合酶的转录活性[218,219]，但是现有的证据表明链内加合物的形成是更有力的细胞毒性损伤。这与低活性的反铂无法形成链内加合物相符合[219]。此外，85%~90%由顺铂形成的加合物是 1,2-链内 AG 和 GG 交联，其他的加合物是 1,3-链内 GXG 交联（其中 X 为任意核苷酸）、链间 GG 交联和单官能加合物，各占 2%~6%的比例。链间交联的比例低可能与它们不稳定的性质有关，容易缓慢地转化为稳定的链内加合物[217,220]。DNA-蛋白质交联和单官能加合物虽可形成，但它们并不具有细胞毒性。基于反铂可大量形成这类加合物[221]，或它们无法抑制 DNA 依赖的 RNA 聚合酶这两个事实得出了这一推断[222,223]。

含有 DACH 的铂类化合物（如奥沙利铂）能克服顺铂的耐药性的能力引起了极大的关注[224]。有趣的是，由类似的模型药 DACH-硫酸根-铂（Ⅱ）所形成的单加合物、链间和链内加成物谱与顺铂形成的基本相似[225]。因此，克服顺铂耐药性的原因得归因于奥沙利铂与顺铂所形成的 DNA 加合物之间微妙的化学差异（图 58-16）。因为顺铂和卡铂能形成相同的双功能加合物，所以它们能发挥类似细胞毒作用。

DNA 损伤信号和细胞死亡

顺铂形成的交联只需要少量即足以抑制 DNA 复制，这表

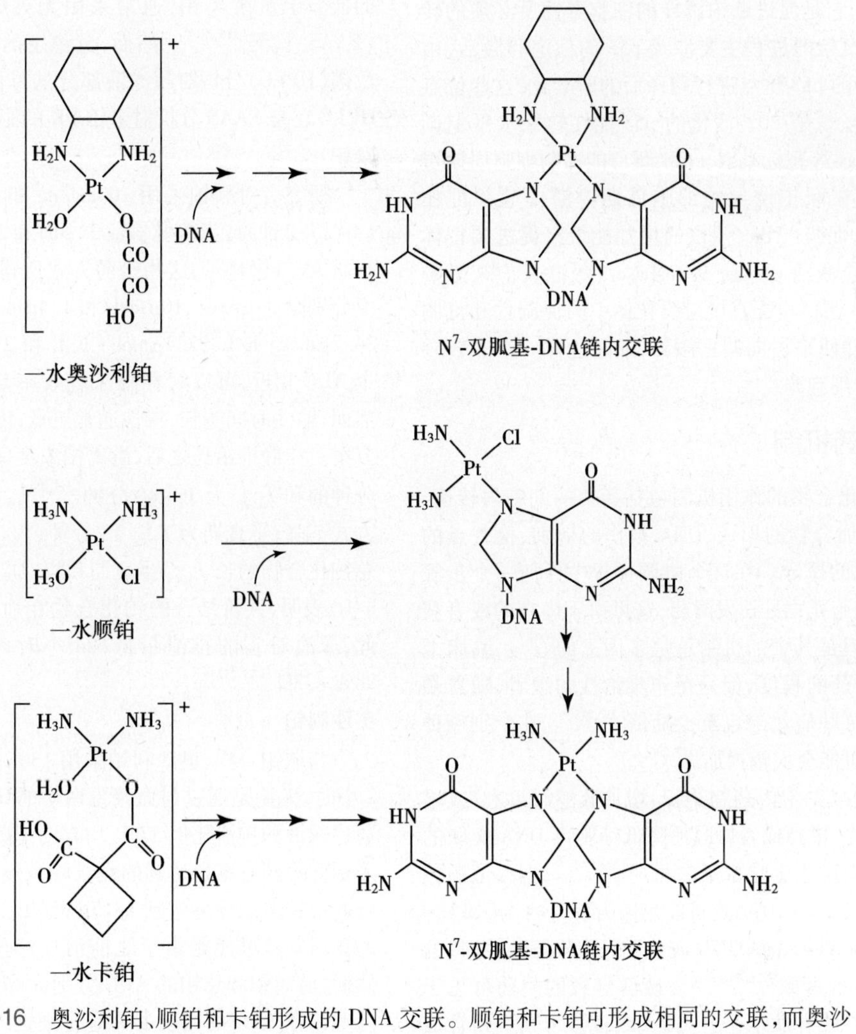

图 58-16 奥沙利铂、顺铂和卡铂形成的 DNA 交联。顺铂和卡铂可形成相同的交联，而奥沙利铂形成的交联则是通过二氨基环己烷配体与铂原子相连，而在结构上有别于顺铂和卡铂

明该药物的高效力[226]。因此,交联形成是理解铂类药物诱导细胞死亡的基本点。然而,在顺铂耐药的细胞中,顺铂与奥沙利铂之间活性的差异值得进一步讨论。链内和链间加合物均能诱导 DNA 在损伤部位的解旋和弯曲。例如,顺铂链内交联能将 DNA 解旋 13°~23°并使其弯曲 32°~34°[227],而链间交联能将双螺旋展开 79°,并弯曲 45°[217,228]。而奥沙利铂形成的链间交联则可诱导 DNA 解旋 82°并弯曲 61°。这种由不同的铂类药物所导致的 DNA 构象差异可被 DNA 损伤传感器蛋白质所识别。例如,非组蛋白染色体蛋白 HMGB1 和 MMR 蛋白 hMLH1、hMSH2 和 hMSH6 能识别顺铂的 GG 交联,而不能识别沙铂和临床有效的奥沙利铂所形成的交联[228-230]。正因如此,MMR 蛋白缺失将导致顺铂耐药,而非奥沙利铂耐药[230,231]。同样的,HMGB1 不能识别有效性低的反铂所形成的链间交联[232]。因此,特定蛋白质对奥沙利铂诱导的 DNA 局部扭曲的进行识别后,绕过被顺铂阻滞的信号通路而促进了其他不同信号通路的传导,使得奥沙利铂得以激活 DNA 损伤检查点而克服顺铂的耐药性。然而,特异性地识别奥沙利铂加合物的蛋白质尚有待明确。

DNA 损伤检查点激活几种激酶,如 ATR、Chk1 和 Chk2,他们能相互协调起作用并激活靶蛋白。这其中关键的靶蛋白是肿瘤抑制因子 p53,它是促进顺铂诱导的细胞毒性所必须的转录因子[233]。这个复杂的过程主要涉及 p53 的稳定和激活,由检查点激酶在关键的 p53 位点进行翻译后的磷酸化,这些位点包括丝氨酸-15 和丝氨酸-20。活化的 p53 能在转录水平上调表达包括 p21 和 Bax 等靶标基因。p21 蛋白能抑制细胞周期蛋白依赖性激酶,并在顺铂诱导的细胞周期停滞中起关键作用[234]。另一方面,促凋亡 Bax 蛋白的增加能最终促进凋亡体复合物的形成,其能激活 caspase-9/caspase-3 级联反应来影响细胞凋亡[235]。p53 蛋白也能直接与线粒体中的促凋亡和抗凋亡蛋白相互作用,并使平衡向凋亡倾斜,通过这样一个非转录依赖的方式来激活细胞凋亡[233]。

铂类药物的耐药机制

如前所述,铂化合物的作用机制包括药物的细胞内转运、药物的激活、DNA 加合物的形成、DNA 损伤的识别、检查点的激活以及细胞凋亡的诱导。在这个协调过程中任何一个步骤的中断都将抑制细胞死亡并诱发耐药,这可由于内在的或者获得性的因素所致,但是其中的机制总是多因素的[236]。临床上很难去定义铂类耐药的程度,但是在非难治性的患者,随着顺铂的剂量翻倍,其抗肿瘤效果也至少翻倍[237,238]。在个别癌种里面,耐药的概率可能会大幅增加[233,236]。

肿瘤细胞通过减少胞内药物累积、增加硫醇浓度和/或增加 DNA 加合物修复,单独或者协同地降低细胞毒 DNA 交联的水平或持久性,进而发生生化水平的耐药[239,240]。据报道顺铂的胞内累积可减少 20%~70%,这可能是因为参与内流(如 Ctrl 低表达)和外排(如 ATP7A、ATP7B 或 ATP11B 的表达增加)的转运蛋白水平的改变所致[236,241,242]。硫醇导致的耐药可见于金属硫蛋白和/或谷胱甘肽水平升高后,或者参与其生物合成的酶表达增加,如谷胱甘肽相关的 γ-谷氨酰半胱氨酸合成酶,或者催化它们与铂类药物的偶联失活增加,如在头颈部癌患者中观察到的谷胱甘肽 S-转移酶[236,243]。通过 DNA 修复来强化加合物的清除能翻倍地促使药物耐药,这很常见,并与修复基因的高表达相关,如卵巢癌患者的 NER 基因[244]。

在开始修复交联加合物之前,首先必须识别 DNA 损伤。因而 MMR 蛋白的下调能阻止 DNA 的损伤识别,尤其是 hMLH1、hMSH2 和 hMSH6 能通过启动子高甲基化而发生突变或沉默[236]。耐药的分子机制也可以是检查点蛋白质的缺陷,例如非小细胞肺癌 Chk2 蛋白的突变或沉默都可能干扰 p53 的稳定与激活,进而影响凋亡[245]。p53 依赖的凋亡也可被其他因素抑制,包括 Bcl-2 蛋白、凋亡蛋白抑制剂和 Her-2/neu,PI3K/Akt 以及 Ras/MAPK 通路的表达上调[236]。p53 本身也可突变,这可能是顺铂耐药的最大影响因素[233,246]。

临床药理学

顺铂或奥沙利铂作为完整分子的 PK 很复杂,因为它们能快速和自发转化为活性物质,活性物质能进而与蛋白质发生不可逆结合而失活。因此,对铂"总量"的分析并不能反映未与失活蛋白质结合的"游离"部分(生物可利用的母体药物和活性物质)。于是,血浆中的 PK 包括估计的总铂和血浆超滤液中的低分子量游离铂,通常采用无火焰原子吸收分光光度法(FAAS)检测[215,247]。然而,更稳定的卡铂适合采用高效液相色谱(HPLC)分析对超滤液部分的母体药物进行分析,但采用 HPLC 还是 FAAS 分析对卡铂 PK 的影响较小[248,249]。

顺铂

研究者对顺铂采用 100mg/m^2 的标准剂量通过静脉推注(4~15 分钟)或者静脉输注 3 小时和 24 小时的血浆 PK 分别进行研究,结果显示,这些给药方式所得到的游离铂物质的峰浓度分别是 44μmol/、10μmol/和 1. 4μmol/L,对应的 AUC 分别是 24. 7μmol · h/L、27. 4μmol · h/L 和 27. 8μmol · h/L[250]。这 3 个 AUC 相近,可以解释临床有效率与给药方案无关的原因。然而,输注时间越长,毒性通常更低,因此可以作为优选的用药方案。在静推给药之后,游离铂浓度呈双相下降,$T_{1/2\alpha}$ 为 6~10 分钟的和 $T_{1/2\beta}$ 为 36~40 分钟[215,251]。总血浆铂浓度则呈三相方式下降,半衰期为 $T_{1/2\alpha}$ 13 分钟,$T_{1/2\beta}$ 43 分钟和 $T_{1/2\gamma}$ 5. 4 天。总铂化合物的长 $T_{1/2\gamma}$ 半衰期和相对应的较高 AUC(908μmol · h/L)表明,共价结合的铂化合物在血浆停留时间的延长。因此,尿液对它的排泄量低,24 小时内的排泄率仅为剂量的 28%~33%[215,252]。

奥沙利铂

与顺铂一样,奥沙利铂采用 130mg/m^2 标准剂量静脉输注 2 小时,无论是通过与血浆蛋白质的共价结合,还是 24 小时内通过尿液的排泄比例 37%,均有助于奥沙利铂的快速清除[215]。采用此用药方案所达到的血浆峰浓度为 6. 2μmol/L,在第 5 疗程时总铂的浓度可达到 18. 5μmol/L。游离铂与总铂峰浓度间的 3 倍差异可能是由于之前治疗疗程中蛋白结合铂的累积。然而,游离铂和总铂的 AUC 分别为 61μmol/L 和 1 062μmol/L,与顺铂在 AUC 的比较上具有合理性[215,247]。血浆游离铂呈三倍指数衰减,半衰期为 $T_{1/2\alpha}$ 17 分钟,$T_{1/2\beta}$ 16 小时和 $T_{1/2\gamma}$ 约 270

小时。

卡铂

卡铂的低反应活性使其 24 小时内尿液排泄比例约为 77%，其中绝大部分是卡铂原型药物[215,249]。卡铂采用 550mg/m^2 的剂量能达到 251μmol/L 的总铂峰浓度，这反映的也可能是完整的卡铂药物浓度，主要是因为卡铂与血浆蛋白质的缓慢反应动力学，以及总铂、游离铂和完整药物相似的 $T_{1/2\alpha}$ 和/或 $T_{1/2\beta}$ 值[215,247]。游离铂呈双相衰减，$T_{1/2\alpha}$ 为 23 分钟，$T_{1/2\beta}$ 为 2 小时；而总铂则呈三相衰减，$T_{1/2\alpha}$ 和 $T_{1/2\beta}$ 与游离铂接近，分别是 22 分钟和 1.9 小时，$T_{1/2\gamma}$ 延长至 5.8 天。总铂、游离铂和完整卡铂所得到的的 AUC 分别是 1 385μmol/L、506μmol/L 和 456μmol/L，这也支持完整的卡铂正是血浆游离铂的主要构成部分。

不良反应

顺铂的剂量限制性毒性是累积且不可逆的肾毒性，表现为肾小球滤过率降低，并以急性局灶性肾小管坏死、肾小管扩张和管型形成为主要特征[253,254]。血清电解质紊乱包括低镁血症可在超过 50%的患者中发生[255]。这可能是由于肾小管对顺铂的主动运输导致肾小管中的药物浓度的增加[256]。然而，水化和强迫利尿可能减低肾脏损伤的严重程度和/或发生率。奥沙利铂和卡铂的肾毒性较少，它们仅通过肾小球滤过清除[215,257]。基于这个药物清除的特点，Calvert 公式以肾功能水平来个体化计算卡铂剂量，现在的标准用法正是如此[257]。

累积性的耳毒性也是顺铂的一个重要的并发症，通常表现为耳鸣和听力损失，在幼儿患者更容易出现[258]。高频听力损失是第一个征象，当剂量超过 100mg/m^2 时中频听力逐渐累及，最后当累积剂量超过 400mg/m^2 时约有一半的患者听力完全丧失[259]。与放射治疗的联合会加重耳毒性。而卡铂和奥沙利铂耳毒性的发生率较低，可能是因为它们在耳蜗的药物积累浓度较顺铂低[260-262]。

3 种铂类药物均可出现外周神经病变[261]。顺铂导致外周神经病变的发生率更高，具有累积性和不可逆性，主要表现为感觉神经病变，当累积剂量超过 300mg/m^2 时发生率高达 50%。通常表现为刺痛性感觉异常、虚弱、震颤和味觉丧失，甚至可见癫痫发作。对头颈癌患者经动脉注射顺铂治疗后可发生严重的神经毒性。奥沙利铂的外周神经病变是剂量限制性的，可表现急性或者慢性病程，其中慢性外周神经毒性的症状可在停药后缓解，40%的患者在 6~8 个月后症状消失。卡铂的神经毒性最低，发生率仅为 4%~6%。针对外周神经毒性的化学防护已有数种策略，其中包括使用硫醇化合物和维生素 E[261]。

顺铂是最具致吐性的抗肿瘤药物之一。剂量大于 50mg/m^2 时，呕吐的发生率达 90%，采用更低的剂量能降低呕吐的发生率（30%~90%）[263]。相比之下，治疗剂量的卡铂和奥沙利铂具有中度的致吐风险。止吐药能缓解这个不良反应，包括多巴胺拮抗剂甲氧氯普胺和羟色胺受体拮抗剂，如昂丹司琼、格雷司琼和多拉司琼。

骨髓抑制与铂类药物的使用有关，但是其通常是可逆的。顺铂导致的血液学毒性主要表现为白细胞减少症，而卡铂诱导的血小板减少症正是其剂量限制性毒性，严重时甚至可导致内出血。奥沙利铂导致的中性粒细胞减少症和血小板减少症均有报道。这三种铂类药物可能观察到的其他几种副作用包括肺毒性、肝毒性、脱发和/或过敏反应。

（林泽晓　黄慧强 译）

参考文献

The complete reference list can be found on the Wiley Companion Digital Edition of this title (see inside front cover for login instructions).

2 Hanahan D, Weinberg RA. Hallmarks of cancer: the next generation. *Cell*. 2011;**144**:646–674.

12 Brock N. Oxazaphosphorine cytostatics: past-present-future. Seventh Cain Memorial Award lecture. *Cancer Res*. 1989;**49**:1–7.

14 Brock N. The history of the oxazaphosphorine cytostatics. *Cancer*. 1996; **78**:542–547.

20 Emadi A, Jones RJ, Brodsky RA. Cyclophosphamide and cancer: golden anniversary. *Nat Rev Clin Oncol*. 2009;**6**:638–647.

21 Flowers JL, Ludeman SM, Gamcsik MP, et al. Evidence for a role of chloroethylaziridine in the cytotoxicity of cyclophosphamide. *Cancer Chemother Pharmacol*. 2000;**45**:335–344.

25 Magni M, Shammah S, Schiro R, et al. Induction of cyclophosphamide-resistance by aldehyde-dehydrogenase gene transfer. *Blood*. 1996;**87**:1097–1103.

28 Colvin M. The comparative pharmacology of cyclophosphamide and ifosfamide. *Semin Oncol*. 1982;**9**:2–7.

38 Tageja N, Nagi J. Bendamustine: something old, something new. *Cancer Chemother Pharmacol*. 2010;**66**:413–423.

49 Musser SM, Pan SS, Egorin MJ, et al. Alkylation of DNA with aziridine produced during the hydrolysis of N,N',N''-triethylenethiophosphoramide. *Chem Res Toxicol*. 1992;**5**:95–99.

51 Ames MM, Sanders ME, Tiede WS. Role of N-methylolpentamethylmelamine in the metabolic activation of hexamethylmelamine. *Cancer Res*. 1983;**43**:500–504.

56 Judson IR, Calvert AH, Gore ME, et al. Phase II trial of trimelamol in refractory ovarian cancer. *Br J Cancer*. 1991;**63**:311–313.

59 Institoris E. In vivo study on alkylation site in DNA by the bifunctional dianhydrogalactitol. *Chem Biol Interact*. 1981;**35**:207–216.

71 Hassan M. The role of busulfan in bone marrow transplantation. *Med Oncol*. 1999;**16**:166–176.

74 Bedford P, Fox BW. DNA-DNA interstrand crosslinking by dimethyanesulphonic acid esters. Correlation with cytotoxicity and antitumour activity in the Yoshida lymphosarcoma model and relationship to chain length. *Biochem Pharmacol*. 1983;**32**:2297–2301.

78 Schabel FM Jr. Nitrosoureas: a review of experimental antitumor activity. *Cancer Treat Rep*. 1976;**60**:665–698.

82 Gnewuch CT, Sosnovsky G. A critical appraisal of the evolution of N-nitrosoureas as anticancer drugs. *Chem Rev*. 1997;**97**:829–1014.

87 Lemoine A, Lucas C, Ings RM. Metabolism of the chloroethylnitrosoureas. *Xenobiotica*. 1991;**21**:775–791.

92 Hartley JA, Gibson NW, Kohn KW, Mattes WB. DNA sequence selectivity of guanine-N7 alkylation by three antitumor chloroethylating agents. *Cancer Res*. 1986;**46**:1943–1947.

96 Tweedie DJ, Erikson JM, Prough RA. Metabolism of hydrazine anti-cancer agents. *Pharmacol Ther*. 1987;**34**:111–127.

101 D'Incalci M, Badri N, Galmarini CM, Allavena P. Trabectedin, a drug acting on both cancer cells and the tumour microenvironment. *Br J Cancer*. 2014;**111**:646–650.

106 Hamilton TC, Winker MA, Louie KG, et al. Augmentation of adriamycin, melphalan, and cisplatin cytotoxicity in drug-resistant and -sensitive human ovarian carcinoma cell lines by buthionine sulfoximine mediated glutathione depletion. *Biochem Pharmacol*. 1985;**34**:2583–2586.

108 Cohen JL, Jao JY. Enzymatic basis of cyclophosphamide activation by hepatic microsomes of the rat. *J Pharmacol Exp Ther*. 1970;**174**:206–210.

122 Hickman MJ, Samson LD. Role of DNA mismatch repair and p53 in signaling induction of apoptosis by alkylating agents. *Proc Natl Acad Sci U S A*. 1999;**96**:10764–10769.

125 Torres-Garcia SJ, Cousineau L, Caplan S, Panasci L. Correlation of resistance to nitrogen mustards in chronic lymphocytic leukemia with enhanced removal of melphalan-induced DNA cross-links. *Biochem Pharmacol*. 1989;**38**: 3122–3123.

132 Bosanquet AG, Sturm I, Wieder T, et al. Bax expression correlates with cellular drug sensitivity to doxorubicin, cyclophosphamide and chlorambucil but not fludarabine, cladribine or corticosteroids in B cell chronic lymphocytic leukemia.

Leukemia. 2002;**16**:1035–1044.
135 Teicher BA, Holden SA, Ara G, Chen G. Transforming growth factor-beta in in vivo resistance. *Cancer Chemother Pharmacol*. 1996;**37**:601–609.
148 Wagner T, Heydrich D, Jork T, et al. Comparative study on human pharmacokinetics of activated ifosfamide and cyclophosphamide by a modified fluorometric test. *J Cancer Res Clin Oncol*. 1981;**100**:95–104.
157 Alberts DS, Chang SY, Chen HS, et al. Comparative pharmacokinetics of chlorambucil and melphalan in man. *Recent Results Cancer Res*. 1980;**74**:124–131.
180 Agarwala SS, Kirkwood JM. Temozolomide, a novel alkylating agent with activity in the central nervous system, may improve the treatment of advanced metastatic melanoma. *Oncologist*. 2000;**5**:144–151.
182 van Kesteren C, Cvitkovic E, Taamma A, et al. Pharmacokinetics and pharmacodynamics of the novel marine-derived anticancer agent ecteinascidin 743 in a phase I dose-finding study. *Clin Cancer Res*. 2000;**6**:4725–4732.
195 Schacht RG, Feiner HD, Gallo GR, et al. Nephrotoxicity of nitrosoureas. *Cancer*. 1981;**48**:1328–1334.
206 Prestayko AW, D'Aoust JC, Issell BF, Crooke ST. Cisplatin (cis-diamminedichloroplatinum II). *Cancer Treat Rev*. 1979;**6**:17–39.
207 Wheate NJ, Walker S, Craig GE, Oun R. The status of platinum anticancer drugs in the clinic and in clinical trials. *Dalton Trans*. 2010;**39**:8113–8127.
215 Graham MA, Lockwood GF, Greenslade D, et al. Clinical pharmacokinetics of oxaliplatin: a critical review. *Clin Cancer Res*. 2000;**6**:1205–1218.
217 Malinge JM, Giraud-Panis MJ, Leng M. Interstrand cross-links of cisplatin induce striking distortions in DNA. *J Inorg Biochem*. 1999;**77**:23–29.
227 Bellon SF, Coleman JH, Lippard SJ. DNA unwinding produced by site-specific intrastrand cross-links of the antitumor drug cis-diamminedichloroplatinum(II). *Biochemistry*. 1991;**30**:8026–8035.
232 Kasparkova J, Brabec V. Recognition of DNA interstrand cross-links of cis-diamminedichloroplatinum(II) and its trans isomer by DNA-binding proteins. *Biochemistry*. 1995;**34**:12379–12387.
233 Martinez-Rivera M, Siddik ZH. Resistance and gain-of-resistance phenotypes in cancers harboring wild-type p53. *Biochem Pharmacol*. 2012;**83**:1049–1062.
257 Calvert AH, Newell DR, Gumbrell LA, et al. Carboplatin dosage: prospective evaluation of a simple formula based on renal function. *J Clin Oncol*. 1989;**7**:1748–1756.
262 Hellberg V, Wallin I, Eriksson S, et al. Cisplatin and oxaliplatin toxicity: importance of cochlear kinetics as a determinant for ototoxicity. *J Natl Cancer Inst*. 2009;**101**:37–47.

第 59 章　DNA 拓扑异构酶靶向药

Anish Thomas, MBBS, MD ■ Susan Bates, MD ■ William D. FiggSr, Pharm D ■ Yves Pommier, MD, PhD

概述

DNA 拓扑异构酶靶向药广泛用于多种癌症的治疗。这类药物通过引起拓扑异构酶连接的 DNA 断裂并阻断裂解复合物的再连接而起作用。尽管拓扑异构酶靶向药具有广谱活性,但其结构、药代动力学和药效学特征在一定程度上限制了其疗效和安全性。为了规避其限制性并进一步发挥其活性,一些新型抑制剂正在研发之中,包括新的剂型和实现靶向运输的药物。最近有关细胞对拓扑异构酶靶向药物敏感性的机制研究使我们能够预测该类药物的活性,并能精准地选择最有可能的患者。了解药物代谢酶、转运蛋白和影响药物药理作用的其他蛋白质的遗传变异,有助于进一步个性化使用此类药物。

引言

人类基因组由长链双螺旋 DNA 聚合物(参与构成 46 条染色体)组成,该 DNA 聚合物长约 1.8 米,密集蜷缩在直径仅其长度百万分之一的细胞核中。当两条基因链分离进行转录和复制时,使用拓扑异构酶松弛 DNA 超螺旋是必需的,因为染色质的核小体结构限制并产生 DNA 超螺旋。此外,Ⅱ型拓扑异构酶在有丝分裂中是必需的,其用于复制后基因组在子细胞之间均匀分布。由此可见,拓扑异构酶是普遍存在并对所有生物体是必需的,因为其可防止并松弛 DNA 和 RNA 的缠绕,且在转录和复制过程中松弛 DNA 超螺旋。

拓扑异构酶在历史上命名为第一拓扑异构酶,即大肠埃希菌拓扑异构酶Ⅰ[1]和小鼠拓扑异构酶Ⅰ[2]。值得注意的是,大多数抗癌剂和抗菌剂是抗癌化疗药物的组成部分,在术语"拓扑异构酶"出现之前就已经被独立发现,其拓扑异构酶靶标具有高度特异性。

拓扑异构酶生物学

人体细胞包含 6 个拓扑异构酶基因,其中 3 个基因编码的拓扑异构酶是抗癌药物靶标,即拓扑异构酶Ⅰ、拓扑异构酶Ⅱα 和拓扑异构酶Ⅱβ(表 59-1)[3-5]。

表 59-1　拓扑异构酶的特征

基因	染色体	蛋白质	药物	药物机制	极性[a]	主要功能
TOP1	20q12-q13.1	Top1	喜树碱类	旋转	3′-Y	核超螺旋松弛
		100kDa 单体	英德诺斯	旋转		
TOP1MT	8q24.3	Top1mt	无			线粒体超螺旋松弛
		70kDa 单体				
TOP2A	17q21-q22	Top2α	蒽环类	ATP 酶链通路	5′-PY	解链/复制
		170kDa 二聚体	蒽醌类 鬼臼毒素类			
TOP2B	3p24	Top2β				转录
		180kDa 二聚体				
TOP3A	17p12-p11.2	Top3α	无	酶链通路	5′-PY	使用 BLM 进行 DNA 复制[b]
		100kDa 单体				
TOP3B	22q11.22	Top3β				RNA 拓扑异构酶
		100kDa 单体				

[a] 催化酪氨酸和断裂 DNA 末端之间的共价连接。

[b] 布鲁姆综合征,RecQ 螺旋酶。

拓扑异构酶介导的 DNA 断裂类型是每个拓扑异构酶特异性的(图 59-1、表 59-1)。这些催化中间体称为裂解复合物(图 59-1b、图 59-1c)。逆向降解反应通过核糖羟基末端向酪氨酰-DNA 键的攻击进行。拓扑异构酶Ⅰ和拓扑异构酶Ⅰmt 共价连接到断裂的 3′端,而其他拓扑异构酶Ⅱα、拓扑异构酶Ⅱβ、拓扑异构酶Ⅲα 和拓扑异构酶Ⅲβ 连接到断裂的 5′端,通过切割和重排 DNA 骨架,无需核酸酶和连接酶的协助。拓扑异构酶Ⅰ和拓扑异构酶Ⅰmt 切割并重排一条 DNA 链,而拓扑异构酶Ⅱα 和 β 切割并重排两条 DNA 双链,四碱基对交错切割(图 59-1)。DNA 切割再连接机制是所有拓扑异构酶的共同机制,其利用酶催化酪氨酸残基作为亲核剂而与破坏的 DNA 末端共价连接。DNA 拓扑异构酶Ⅲα 和Ⅲβ 所连接的 DNA 3′末端与 5′末端极性相反,拓扑异构酶Ⅲα 和Ⅲβ 与 DNA 断端的 5′末端形成共价键(表 59-1,图 59-1b,1c)。拓扑异构酶在生化上是有区别的。拓扑异构酶Ⅰ和拓扑异构酶Ⅰmt 在没有核苷酸或金属辅助因子的情况下以单体形式发挥作用,而拓扑异构酶Ⅱα 和Ⅱβ 以二聚体的形式发挥作用,需要 ATP 和 Mg^{2+} 催化。拓扑异构酶Ⅲα 和Ⅲβ 也需要 Mg^{2+},但以单体形式发挥作用,不需要 ATP 催化。值得注意的是,拓扑异构酶Ⅲ的底物有所不同。拓扑异构酶Ⅰ和拓扑异构酶Ⅱ均处理双链 DNA,而拓扑异构酶Ⅲ的底物则需要单链核酸(拓扑异构酶Ⅲα 需要 DNA,拓扑异构酶Ⅲβ 需要 RNA)。

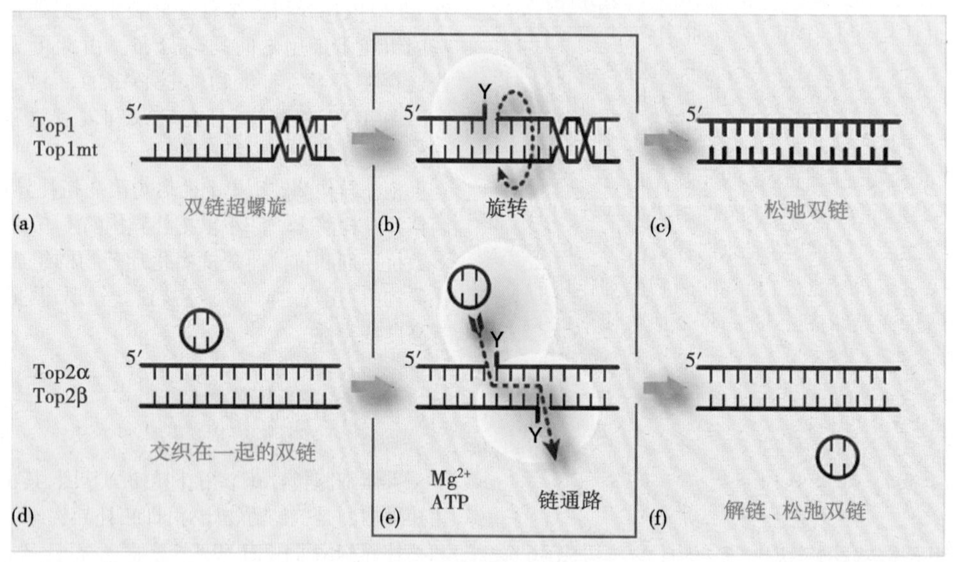

图 59-1 拓扑异构酶的分子机制。(a~c)拓扑异构酶Ⅰ(核 DNA 的 top1 和线粒体 DNA 的 Top1mt)通过可逆地切割一条 DNA 链来松弛超螺旋 DNA(a),在酶催化酪氨酸和切口 DNA 的 3′端(Top1 裂解复合物:Top1cc;b)之间形成共价键。这种反应允许断裂的链绕完整的链旋转。快速重排可使 Top1 解离(c)。(d-f)拓扑异构酶Ⅱ作用于两个 DNA 双链。它们作为同源二聚体,通过在催化酪氨酸和 DNA 断裂的 5′端(Top2cc;e)之间形成共价键来切割两条链。这种反应允许完整的双链通过 Top2 同型二聚体(红点箭头;e)。Top2 抑制剂会捕获 Top2CC 并阻止正常释放(f)。拓扑异构酶裂解复合物(b 和 d)是拓扑异构酶抑制剂的靶点

作用机制

拓扑异构酶抑制剂的常见作用机制和分子药理学:通过界面抑制捕获拓扑异构酶裂解复合物

拓扑异构酶裂解复合物通常是高度可逆,因此在没有拓扑异构酶抑制剂的情况下存在时间短暂,很难检测到。这是因为裂解复合物的重新连接是由断裂末端的重排驱动的,断裂端本身是由双链 DNA 的两个基本结构特征决定的,即:①相邻碱基在每条链内通过 π-π 相互作用堆叠;②碱基对。双链 DNA 可被视为“强大的分子拉链”,其通过氢键相互作用在相对的链上配对。

临床拓扑异构酶抑制剂通过产生拓扑异构酶连接的 DNA 断裂而起作用,当药物分子在拓扑异构酶-DNA 裂解复合物的界面处紧密结合时,药物阻断了裂解复合物的再连接。药物结合的选择性和强度通过以下方式确定:①药物与切割位点的碱基堆积;②拓扑异构酶的氢键网络(图 59-2)。由于药物在切割位点结合,通过错配 DNA 末端来阻止 DNA 的再连接,而 DNA 末端通常是攻击磷酸酪氨酰键所必需的。这种结合模式即“界面抑制”概念的由来,它不仅适用于蛋白质-DNA 界面,而且适用于蛋白质-蛋白质界面,如微管蛋白及 mTOR 抑制剂[6]。药物结合的裂解复合物晶体结构已经牢固确立了拓扑异构酶Ⅰ和拓扑异构酶Ⅱ靶向药物的机制[6]。每种药物的结构特征(化学支架、氢键供体及受体的差异)(图 59-3)说明了药物对拓扑异构酶Ⅰ、拓扑异构酶Ⅱ裂解复合物的选择性及不同拓扑异构酶抑制剂在不同类别中的 DNA 序列选择性和基因组靶向[5,7]。

了解拓扑异构酶抑制剂的细胞毒性非常关键,这是由于拓扑异构酶裂解复合物与相关的拓扑异构酶催化抑制分开。除了在定义的分子环境中,正是拓扑异构酶裂解复合物(DNA 断裂和相关的拓扑异构酶-DNA 共价复合物)杀死了癌细胞。这将拓扑异构酶抑制剂从经典酶抑制剂,如抗溶剂中分离出来。

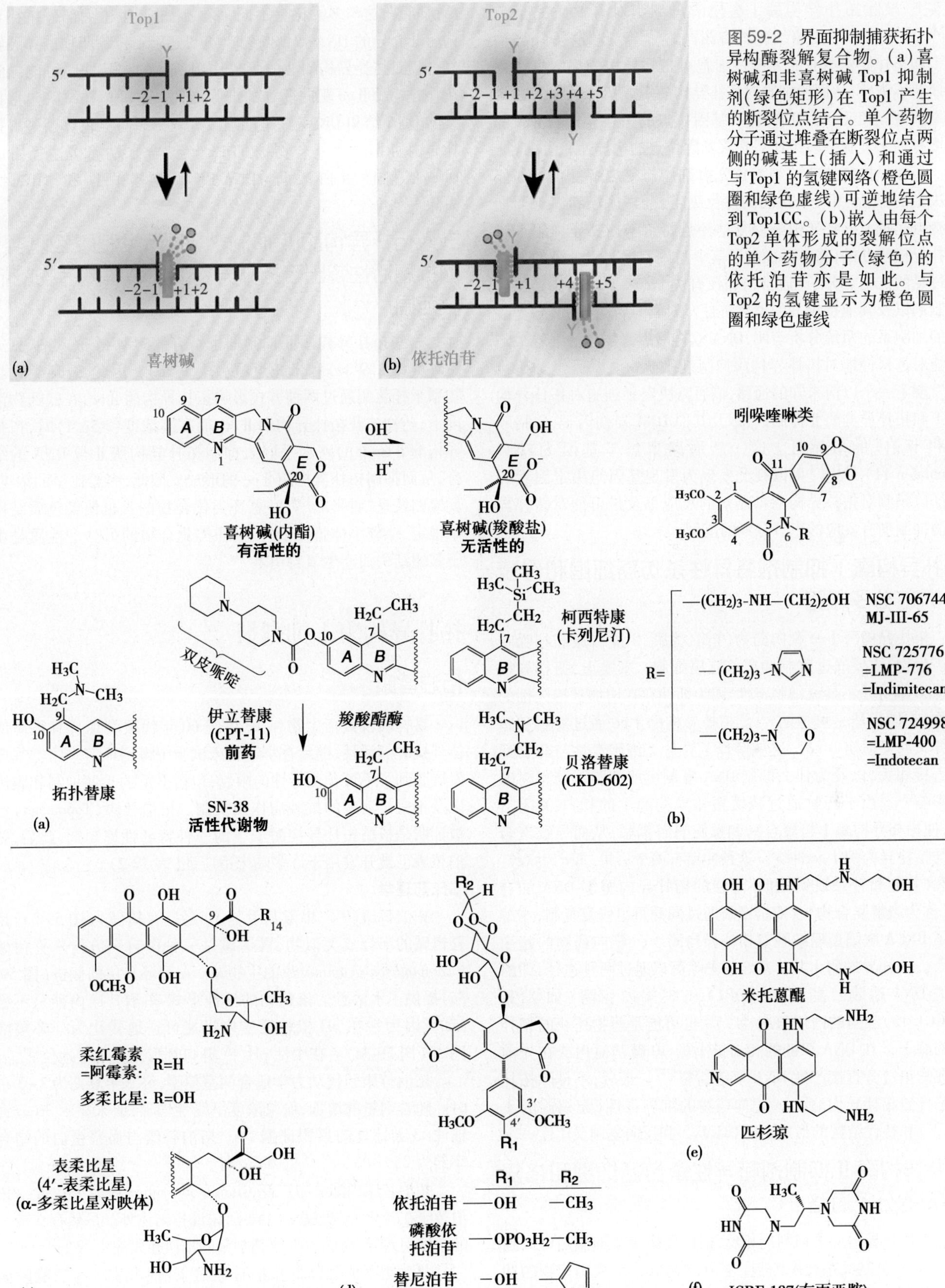

图 59-2 界面抑制捕获拓扑异构酶裂解复合物。(a)喜树碱和非喜树碱 Top1 抑制剂(绿色矩形)在 Top1 产生的断裂位点结合。单个药物分子通过堆叠在断裂位点两侧的碱基上(插入)和通过与 Top1 的氢键网络(橙色圆圈和绿色虚线)可逆地结合到 Top1CC。(b)嵌入由每个 Top2 单体形成的裂解位点的单个药物分子(绿色)的依托泊苷亦是如此。与 Top2 的氢键显示为橙色圆圈和绿色虚线

图 59-3 临床拓扑异构酶抑制剂。(a)喜树碱衍生物在生理 pH 下不稳定,在几分钟内形成羧酸衍生物。伊立替康是一种前药,需要将其转化为 SN-38 以捕获 Top1CC。(b)非喜树碱吲哚喹啉衍生物的临床试验。(c)蒽环类衍生物。(d)去甲基表鬼臼毒素衍生物。(e)米托蒽醌。(f)右丙亚胺,Top2 催化抑制剂

事实上,敲除拓扑异构酶Ⅰ会使酵母细胞对喜树碱完全免疫[8],降低酶水平使癌细胞具有耐药性[3,5]。此外,拓扑异构酶Ⅰ和拓扑异构酶Ⅱ的突变使细胞对拓扑异构酶裂解复合物的捕获不敏感,从而使细胞对拓扑异构酶Ⅰ或拓扑异构酶Ⅱ具有高抗性。相反,与HER2同一基因位点的拓扑异构酶ⅡA的扩增有助于乳腺癌多柔比星在该基因位点的选择性和活性。

拓扑异构酶捕获的结果首先由细胞修复裂解复合物的能力决定的,然后由两个共同的途径决定:凋亡途径和细胞周期检查点途径。拓扑异构酶修复途径是特定于拓扑异构酶Ⅰ或拓扑异构酶Ⅱ的,将在后面的段落中讨论。促凋亡分子的缺陷和过量的抗凋亡分子(通常与癌症有关)赋予了对拓扑异构酶抑制剂以及其他抗癌剂的整体抗性。对具有特定DNA修复改变的细胞系的系统分析表明,DNA双链断裂修复中的细胞缺陷可能对选择性地对拓扑异构酶抑制剂敏感[9]。基因组分析最近发现了一个以前未知的通路,该通路决定了细胞对拓扑异构酶Ⅰ和拓扑异构酶Ⅱ抑制剂(以及其他DNA损伤因子,包括顺铂和卡铂)的敏感性。这一新通路聚焦于基因SLFN11(Schlafen 11)[10,11]。可以视此发现为发现基因组决定因素和特征以预测对拓扑异构酶抑制剂的反应以及最可能对拓扑异构酶抑制剂有反应的患者分期的范例。

拓扑异构酶Ⅰ抑制剂特异性杀伤癌细胞和修复DNA的分子通路

拓扑异构酶Ⅰcc靶向药物(拓泊替康、伊立替康和吲哚喹啉衍生物)主要通过复制冲突杀死癌细胞。事实上,拓扑异构酶Ⅰcc本身并不具有细胞毒性,因为即使存在增加其持久性的药物,它们仍然是可逆的[12]。拓扑异构酶Ⅰcc通过复制和转录分叉冲突损伤DNA。这就解释了为什么细胞毒性与药物暴露直接相关,以及为什么抑制DNA复制可使细胞不受喜树碱的影响[4]。由于药物通过减缓拓扑异构酶Ⅰ的切口-关闭活性,使拓扑异构酶Ⅰ与聚合酶和螺旋酶解耦联,从而导致聚合酶与拓扑异构酶Ⅰcc冲突。这种冲突有两个后果,即产生双链断裂(复制和转录缺失)和不可逆的拓扑异构酶Ⅰ-DNA加合物(称为裂解复合物)。双链断裂通过同源重组修复复制,这解释了BRCA缺陷型癌细胞对拓扑异构酶Ⅰcc靶向药物的超敏性[9]。拓扑异构酶Ⅰ共价复合物去除可以通过两种途径,即酪氨酰-DNA-磷酸二酯酶1(TDP1)和3′端内切酶(如XPF-ERCC1.13)参与的内切酶途径[13]。也可能是药物捕获的拓扑异构酶Ⅰcc在DNA双链的相对链上的10碱基对内或在先前存在的单链旁直接产生DNA双链断裂[14]。最后,不排除拓扑缺陷导致拓扑异构酶Ⅰcc靶向药物的细胞毒性(超螺旋的累积[15])和替代结构的形成,如R环1[16]和反向复制叉[17]。

拓扑异构酶Ⅱ抑制剂特异性杀伤癌细胞和修复DNA的分子通路

与拓扑异构酶Ⅰ抑制剂相反,拓扑异构酶Ⅱ抑制剂可以独立于DNA复制叉杀死癌细胞。拓扑异构酶Ⅱcc靶向药物的冲突机制涉及拓扑异构酶Ⅱ和RNA聚合酶Ⅱ的转录及蛋白水解,通过破坏拓扑异构酶Ⅱ二聚体导致DNA双链断裂。或拓扑异构酶Ⅱ同型二聚体界面通过机械张力分离。值得注意的是,90%被依托泊苷捕获的拓扑异构酶Ⅱcc不协调,因此存在单链断裂,这与多柔比星不同,多柔比星产生了大部分拓扑异构酶Ⅱ介导的DNA双链断裂[4,5]。最后,不排除药物诱导裂解复合物对拓扑异构酶Ⅱ的隔离作用所致的拓扑缺陷可能导致拓扑异构酶Ⅱcc靶向药物的细胞毒性。这种拓扑缺陷包括持续的DNA结和DNA链,可能导致有丝分裂时染色体断裂。拓扑异构酶Ⅱ共价复合物被TDP2[13]结合末端连接途径[ku、DNA依赖性蛋白激酶(DNA-PK)、连接酶Ⅳ和XRCC4]去除[9,18]。

嵌入拓扑异构酶Ⅱ抑制剂(蒽环类和蒽二酮类)的抗癌活性超出了拓扑异构酶Ⅱ裂解复合物的捕获范围

一些拓扑异构酶Ⅱ抑制剂也是有效的DNA嵌入剂,见于蒽环类(图59-3c)和米托蒽醌(图59-3e)。因此,蒽环类化合物和米托蒽醌通过两种方式影响拓扑异构酶Ⅱcc:在低药物浓度下,药物捕获拓扑异构酶Ⅱcc,而在高浓度(>5μM)时,拓扑异构酶Ⅱcc外的高水平嵌入抑制拓扑异构酶Ⅱ与DNA的结合,从而抑制拓扑异构酶Ⅱcc的形成。因此,多柔比星的浓度-反应曲线呈"钟形"[4,19]。蒽环类化合物嵌入也使染色质结构不稳定,伴核小体排出[20]。蒽环类化合物的另一个性质是由于其醌结构而产生氧自由基[21]。

拓扑异构酶Ⅰ抑制剂

拓泊替康

喜树碱及其衍生物在20世纪60年代被发现具有很高的体外抗肿瘤活性,随后在早期临床试验中得到证实[22-24]。临床发展受到了不可预测毒性的限制,包括严重的骨髓抑制和腹泻以及不完全清楚的抗肿瘤作用机制。拓泊替康(Topotecan)已被证明是核酶拓扑异构酶1[25]的一种特异性抑制剂,此后,拓泊替康已被开发用于许多临床适应证(表59-2)。

临床药理学

拓泊替康(9-二甲氨基甲基-10-羟基喜树碱)(图59-3a)是喜树碱的半合成类似物,喜树碱是一种源自东方树木喜树碱(*Camptotheca acuminata*)的生物碱。A型环9位的侧链(图59-3a)提供了水溶性。该药物的活性形式-拓泊替康内酯是不稳定的,因为它在pH依赖反应中迅速可逆地转化为开环羧酸酯[12](图59-3a)。在中性pH下,开口环形式占主导地位[26]。

拓泊替康药代动力学适合两室模型,终末半衰期为2~3小时。随着剂量的增加,血浆浓度呈线性增加,但未显示30分钟输注×5天计划的累积证据[27]。拓泊替康与血浆蛋白的结合率约为35%[27]。

拓泊替康内酯分布广泛,稳态平均分布容积为75L/m^2。拓泊替康在转化为羧酸盐后主要随尿液排出体外。虽然存在较大的个体间差异,但约30%给药剂量的排泄在尿液中不变[27]。

肾功能不全会降低拓泊替康血浆清除率,轻度功能障碍(肌酐清除率40~60ml/min)和中度功能障碍(肌酐清除率20~39ml/min)分别降低至正常值的67%和34%[28]。因此,肾功能受损时,建议调整药物剂量。肝功能损害不影响拓泊替康清除率,肝功能不全患者无需调整剂量[29]。

表 59-2　DNA 拓扑异构酶靶向药

药物类型	药名	FDA 批准年份	批准指示
喜树碱	伊立替康	1996	结直肠癌
	拓扑替康	1996	宫颈癌、卵巢癌、小细胞肺癌
蒽环类	多柔比星	1974	乳腺癌、急性淋巴细胞白血病、急性髓系白血病、Wilms 瘤、神经母细胞瘤、软组织和骨肉瘤、卵巢症、膀胱移行细胞癌、甲状腺癌、胃癌、霍奇金淋巴瘤、非霍奇金淋巴瘤、支气管肺癌
	聚乙二醇化脂质体多柔比星	1999	艾滋病相关卡波西肉瘤、多发性骨髓瘤、卵巢癌
	柔红霉素	1979	急性淋巴细胞白血病、急性髓系白血病
	伊达比星	1990	急性髓系白血病
蒽醌类	米托蒽醌	1987	急性非淋巴细胞白血病、晚期激素难治性前列腺癌
鬼臼霉素	依托泊苷	1984	小细胞肺癌、睾丸癌
	替尼泊苷	1992	急性淋巴细胞白血病

FDA,美国食品药品管理局。

虽然经典的给药途径是静脉注射,但也可口服。拓泊替康口服制剂的目的是维持足够长的药物暴露时间,众所周知该药物在体内外均有最高抗肿瘤功效[12],而无需输液泵[30]。批准的口服剂量为 2.3mg/m²,每天一次,连续 5 天重复使用。每 21 天重复一个疗程。拓泊替康的口服生物利用度约为 35%[27],生物利用度低可能是由于拓泊替康内酯在肠道内水解所致,产生吸收不良的开环形式。口服拓泊替康显示出与小细胞肺癌静脉注射剂量相当的临床活性[31]。

临床应用

拓泊替康单药疗法在美国和欧洲被批准用于初始或后续化疗失败后的转移性卵巢癌患者以及复发小细胞肺癌患者。它还被批准与顺铂联合治疗复发或耐药的宫颈癌(ⅣB 期)[32]。

拓泊替康在其他类型肿瘤中也有临床活性,包括儿童髓母细胞瘤[33]、非小细胞肺癌[34]、骨髓增生综合征、慢性粒细胞白血病[35]、尤文氏肉瘤[36]、横纹肌肉瘤[37]、多发性骨髓瘤[38]。除了宫颈癌中批准的顺铂联合治疗外,还开展了 Top1 抑制剂与其他抗肿瘤药物的联合治疗。在临床前期研究中进行了协同和添加剂组合的观察,如组蛋白脱乙酰基酶抑制剂、PARP 抑制剂,并对患者的一些药物组合策略进行了研究[39,40]。拓泊替康可扩散到脑脊液,可用于脑转移的治疗[41]。

用药时间管理

在Ⅰ期临床试验中,已经评估了拓泊替康的各种方案。美国食品药品管理局(Food and Drug Administration,FDA)推荐复发性卵巢癌和小细胞肺癌中拓泊替康的剂量为 1.5mg/m²,静脉输注 30 分钟以上,在 21 天周期的第 1 天至第 5 天。

尽管与拓泊替康用药剂量和时间相关的 3 级或 4 级骨髓抑制的发生率很高,但拓泊替康仍然是治疗的标准。为了减轻这种毒性反应,在Ⅰ期和Ⅱ期临床试验中,评估了多种用药剂量和时间的变化[42,43]。据报告,卵巢癌患者每周服用拓泊替康(第 1、8 和 15 天服用 4mg/m²)的疗效与标准疗程相当,但毒性更小[43]。在小细胞肺癌中,周疗程尚未与 5 天疗程进行比较[31]。在宫颈癌患者中,拓泊替康与顺铂联合应用已被批准,即在第 1 天、第 2 天和第 3 天,拓泊替康的推荐剂量为 0.75mg/m² 静脉注射 30 分钟以上,第 1 天联合顺铂 50mg/m² 静脉注射,每 21 天重复一次[44]。

毒性

拓泊替康的剂量限制性毒性是骨髓抑制,主要是中性粒细胞减少,也可发生血小板减少和贫血。在剂量为 1.5mg/(m²·d)持续 5 天的情况下,拓泊替康在第一个治疗周期后白细胞计数最低下降 80%~90%。中性粒细胞减少的程度与完整内酯曲线下面积(area under the curve,AUC)或总药物浓度有关[45]。对于基线中性粒细胞计数<1 500/mm³ 或血小板技术<100 000/mm³ 的患者,不应给予拓泊替康治疗[47]。

如上所述,肾功能不全会降低拓泊替康清除率并增加毒性。与血液毒性相关的其他因素包括高龄和既往治疗,如铂类给药(尤其是卡铂)、放射治疗[46]。在接受拓泊替康连续 5 天治疗的高危患者中,拓泊替康剂量降低到 1.0mg/(m²·d)或 1.25mg/(m²·d),可降低严重骨髓抑制的发生率。造血生长因子、输血和疗程调整有助于管理骨髓抑制。3 天、每周或口服给药的替代方案与低骨髓抑制有关。

比骨髓移植相对少见的拓泊替康的其他毒性包括皮疹、发热、疲劳、恶心、呕吐、黏膜炎和血清转氨酶升高[48]。大多数非血液学副作用通常是可控的。静脉注射给药引起腹泻并不常见,但口服拓泊替康有报道。危及生命的罕见非血液学毒性包括间质性肺病和中性粒细胞减少性结肠炎。

伊立替康

伊立替康(Irinotecan)是一种强效的水溶性喜树碱衍生物。

临床药理学

伊立替康(CPT-11)是喜树碱(SN-38)的强效 7-乙基-10-羟基类似物的前药(图 59-3a)[45],在 C-10 处含有一个双哌啶取代基,为肠外给药提供水溶性。伊立替康通过酯酶进行广泛的代谢转化,转化为其活性代谢物 SN-38(图 59-3a)。伊立替康前药被羧酸酯酶活化为生物活性化合物 SN-38。这就解释了伊立替康比 SN-38 体外细胞毒性测定的活性低几个数量级的原因。

伊立替康的血浆峰浓度和 AUC 随着给药剂量的增加而相应增加，提示存着线性药物动力学。SN-38 的血浆 AUC 仅为伊立替康的 2%～8%，表明仅有一小部分伊立替康转化为其活性形式 SN-38。伊立替康和 SN-38 均以活性内酯形式和无活性羧酸盐形式存在。与拓泊替康相似，两种形式均处于 pH 依赖的平衡状态。

静脉输注伊立替康后血浆浓度呈多指数下降。伊立替康的平均终末消除半衰期为 6～12 小时，SN-38 的平均终末消除半衰期为 10～20 小时，均比拓泊替康长得多。伊立替康和 SN-38 的内酯形式在给药后血浆中的比例相对较大，这是由于内酯形式与白蛋白的优先结合[26]。SN-38 的血浆蛋白结合率为 95%，而伊立替康约为 50%[45]。

与拓泊替康不同，伊立替康主要通过胆汁排出体外[45]。SN-38 和伊立替康的肾排泄仅占给药剂量的小部分。尿苷 5′-二磷酸葡萄糖醛酸基转移酶（UGT1A1；由 *UGT1A1* 基因编码）的 1A1 等位形式介导 SN-38 的葡萄糖醛酸化为非活性代谢物 SN-38G（参见“药物基因组学”的章节）。与 *UGT1A1* 基因多态性相关的 UGT1A1 酶活性存在广泛的个体差异[51,52]。此外，酶的多态性与引起家族性高胆红素血症的疾病有关，如 Crigler-Najjar 胆红素血症和 Gilbert 综合征[53]。*UGT1A1* 多态性可显著改变伊立替康的代谢，从而影响其在个别患者的毒性，建议对携带 *UGT1A1* 特定变体的患者减少剂量。伊立替康也被 CYP3A4 介导的氧化代谢灭活[54]。多态性变异体的影响将在随后的章节中更详细地讨论。

临床应用

伊立替康在美国和欧洲被批准与 5-氟尿嘧啶和四氢叶酸联合治疗转移性结直肠癌。同时也被批准用于 5-氟尿嘧啶治疗后复发或进展的转移性直肠癌患者[49,50]。

伊立替康单药或与其他药物联合治疗已在多种类型肿瘤显示出临床活性，包括广泛期小细胞肺癌[56]、宫颈鳞状细胞癌[57]、复发性胶质母细胞瘤[58]、胃癌、食管癌[59]、非小细胞肺癌[60]、胰腺癌[61]、横纹肌肉瘤[62]和卵巢癌[63]。

用药时间管理

伊立替康单药治疗通常在第 1 天、第 8 天、第 15 天和第 22 天静脉滴注 125mg/m^2 超过 90 分钟，然后休息 2 周（6 周治疗周期）。另一种给药方案是 350mg/m^2，每 3 周静脉输注 60 分钟。对于 5-氟尿嘧啶难治性转移性结直肠癌患者，每周和每 3 周一次用药显示出了相似的疗效和生活质量。每 3 周一次的治疗方案与严重腹泻的低发生率显著相关[64]。

与 5-氟尿嘧啶和四氢叶酸联合用药时，伊立替康的给药方案为第 1 天、第 8 天、第 15 天和第 22 天（6 周治疗周期），125mg/m^2 静脉输注超过 90 分钟。替代给药方案为第 1 天、第 15 天和第 29 天（6 周治疗周期），180mg/m^2，超过 90 分钟。

毒性

腹泻和骨髓抑制是伊立替康最常见的毒性。迟发性腹泻在伊立替康治疗超过 24 小时后发生。如不及时处理，会导致危及生命的脱水和电解质失衡[65]。约三分之一接受每周剂量治疗的患者出现 3 级或 4 级迟发性腹泻。晚期腹泻的发病时间中位数为 5 天（3 周给药）和 11 天（每周给药）[49,55]。游离肠腔 SN-38（胆汁或 SN-38G 去结合）是迟发性腹泻的原因。SN-38 引起直接的黏膜损伤，导致水、电解质吸收不良和黏液过度分泌过多[66]。晚期腹泻应及时用洛哌胺、补充必要的水和电解质。若患者出现肠梗阻、发热或严重的中性粒细胞减少，抗生素治疗是必要的。迟发性腹泻的易感因素包括高龄、状态不佳和既往的腹壁手术放射治疗[67]。有危险因素的患者应考虑降低起始剂量。在开始下一疗程前，治疗相关腹泻应已完全解决。建议减少 3 级和 4 级腹泻患者的用药剂量。已经研究了各种降低其严重性的措施，但没有一种措施在实践中起到既定的作用[68]。2005 年，FDA 批准了对 *UGT1A1* 变异等位基因 *28 的诊断试验，该等位基因表达减少导致清除率降低和毒性增加[69]。然而，还已知其他影响酶表达的等位基因变异，并影响葡萄糖醛酸化的药物清除率（下文将详细讨论）。

伊立替康在输液期间或 24 小时内所致的早期腹泻不太常见。伊立替康所致的早期腹泻一般时间短，严重病例少。这是由于伊立替康抗胆碱能酶活性介导的胆碱能综合征[70]。这种胆碱能综合征往往发生在高剂量伊立替康的血浆峰值。其他胆碱能症状包括腹部绞痛、鼻炎、流泪和流涎。症状的平均持续时间为 30 分钟，通常对阿托品反应迅速。

可观察到的伊立替康的其他常见毒性包括恶心、呕吐、腹痛、便秘、厌食、乏力、发烧、体重下降和脱发。罕见但危及生命的非血液毒性包括间质性肺病和过敏反应。肺毒性的危险因素包括先前存在的肺病、使用肺毒性药物、辐射和使用集落刺激因子。在伊立替康治疗期间和治疗后数周内，应监测有危险因素患者的呼吸症状[71]。

喜树碱类似物和非喜树碱拓扑异构酶 I 抑制剂

如上所述，喜树碱衍生物有几个公认的局限性。其在生理 pH 下于数分钟内通过内酯 E 开环失活（图 59-3a）。由于内酯形式是抗肿瘤活性所必需的，故这会引起药物抗肿瘤活性丧失。其他局限性包括药物去除后被捕获的 DNA-拓扑异构酶 I 裂解复合物快速逆转以及由 ATP 结合盒（ABC）转运介导的耐药性[12]。

目前正在临床研发的几种新型喜树碱衍生物旨在弥补喜树碱及其衍生物的一些缺点（表 59-3）。来源于对母体药物修饰的喜树碱类似物一直是一个活跃的研究领域[72]。盐酸贝洛特肯（Belotecan）是一种水溶性喜树碱类似物，目前正在临床研发治疗小细胞肺癌和卵巢癌[73]。Costecan（Karenitecin）（图 59-3a）是一种口服活性高亲脂性半合成喜树碱，正在研发用于卵巢癌。由于其亲脂性，与水溶性喜树碱相比，Costecan 表现出增强的组织渗透性和生物利用度，对药物耐药性不太敏感。

在不影响喜树碱抗肿瘤活性的前提下，已采取了几种方法来稳定喜树碱内酯环[19]。吲哚类喹啉是一类非喜树碱类的拓扑异构酶 I 抑制剂，具有较好的化学稳定性，能产生稳定的 DNA-拓扑异构酶 I 裂解复合物。与喜树碱相比，此类药物有独特的 DNA 切割位点，已证明对喜树碱抗性细胞株具有活性，并产生抗逆转的 DNA 蛋白质交联。此类药物对过表达 ATP 结合盒转运体、ATP 结合盒亚家族 G 成员 2（ABCG2）和多药耐药（MDR-1）[74]的细胞也显示出较少或无耐药性。解决 E 环不稳定性的其他方法包括将 E 环转化为五元环，这将使药物完全稳定[75]。

表 59-3　处于临床研究的拓扑异构酶Ⅰ型抑制剂

	药物/药物类	评论
喜树碱类似物	贝洛替康	水溶性喜树碱类似物
	柯西特康	亲脂半合成喜树碱
	Lipotecan	内酯环修饰以增加抗肿瘤效力
	希明替康	吉咪替康的酯前体药物
靶向运输拓扑异构酶Ⅰ抑制剂	脂质体/纳米颗粒/聚乙二醇化制剂	
	MM-398 安能得	伊立替康的纳米脂质体制剂
	CPX-1	伊立替康-氟尿嘧啶脂质体复方
	Firtecan pegol	SN-38 的聚乙二醇制剂
	CRLX101	基于环糊精的喜树碱聚合物缀合物
	抗体-药物偶联物 Sacituzumab govitecan	靶向拓扑异构酶Ⅱ抑制剂抗原的人源化 IgG1 抗体与伊立替康的代谢活性产物 SN-38 偶联而成
	喜树碱结合物 HA-伊立替康	伊立替康-透明质酸复合
	Etirinotecan pegol(NKTR-102)	伊立替康通过可生物降解的连接体与聚乙二醇核偶联而成
非喜树碱拓扑异构酶Ⅰ型抑制剂	吲哚喹啉类衍生物	较好的化学稳定性,能产生稳定的 DNA-拓扑异构酶Ⅰ裂解复合物,不受药物流泵的影响

靶向运输拓扑异构酶Ⅰ抑制剂

目前正在探索几种改善喜树碱靶向运输和肿瘤定位的方法。这些方法涉及广泛,包括:①脂质体或纳米颗粒制剂,以增加血浆半衰期和肿瘤定位;②抗体结合靶向运输;③改善药代动力学特性和暴露的结合剂。

脂质体/纳米颗粒制剂

脂质体是具有水核心的微小磷脂球[76]。由于其双相性,脂质体可以作为亲脂性药物和亲水性药物的载体;亲水性药物倾向于包埋在核心中,而疏水性药物包埋于脂质双层中。喜树碱的稳定脂质体包封通过减少药物在生理 pH 的暴露和延长内酯活性药物的存在时间使其向无活性羧酸盐形式的转化最小化。聚乙二醇化增加了共轭生物分子的大小和分子量[77]。与非聚乙二醇化分子相比,聚乙二醇化分子显示出半衰期延长、血浆清除率降低及不同的生物分布。脂质体的聚乙二醇化进一步改善了稳定性和循环时间。聚合物纳米粒是药物载体,其设计具有特定的尺寸和表面特性,有利于药物在肿瘤中沉积[78]。这些制剂通过一个被称为增强渗透保持效应的过程来改善肿瘤的"被动"靶向性,其中,由于肿瘤血管系统的异常渗漏,大分子渗透并滞留于肿瘤组织中。

MM-398(NAL-IRI)是一种伊立替康蔗糖酯的纳米脂质体包封装。在临床前研究中,与药物的自由形式相比,MM-398 改善了伊立替康和 SN-38 的药物动力学和肿瘤生物分布,在剂量限制毒性的器官中蓄积较少[80]。在先前接受过吉西他滨治疗的转移性胰腺癌患者中,MM-398 联合 5-氟尿嘧啶和四氢叶酸显示出临床活性[81]。

CRLX101 是一种由喜树碱组成的纳米颗粒治疗剂,与线性环糊精-聚乙二醇共聚物共价结合组成[72]。CRLX101 在溶液中自组装成纳米颗粒,与母体药物喜树碱相比,溶解度增加了 1 000 倍以上。CRLX101 目前正在肾癌、卵巢癌和直肠癌患者中进行评估。

抗体-药物偶联物

喜树碱与单克隆抗体结合产生的抗体-药物偶联物(ADC)正在研制中,旨在促进靶向药物向肿瘤的输送。Sacituzumab govitecan 是针对滋养层细胞表面抗原的人源化抗体(TROP-2)与 SN-38 通过 PH 敏感性接头偶联而成[82]。TROP-2 是一种Ⅰ型跨膜钙转导蛋白,在多种上皮癌表达,而正常组织表达有限。抗体与 *TACSTD2* 基因编码的 TROP-2 结合后选择性地进入癌细胞。Sacituzumab govitecan 对三阴性乳腺癌和小细胞肺癌疗效正在研究之中。

喜树碱偶联物

依替诺替康聚乙二醇是一种长效的拓扑异构酶Ⅰ抑制剂,由伊立替康通过可生物降解的连接体与聚乙二醇核偶联而成。连接体在体内缓慢水解形成活性形式 SN-38。该药物旨在提供长期持续暴露于 SN-38,同时降低与过高的伊立替康和 SN-38 血浆浓度相关的毒性。在晚期乳腺癌患者的三期临床试验中,依替诺替康聚乙二醇的用药方案为每 21 天以 145mg/m^2 剂量静脉注射一次[83]。透明质酸伊立替康是伊立替康与透明质酸结合的静脉制剂[84]。透明质酸通过 CD44 选择性地与癌细胞结合,从而增强膜的流动性并可能减少副作用。

拓扑异构酶Ⅱ抑制剂

临床上使用的拓扑异构酶Ⅱ靶向药物可分为嵌入式和非嵌入式拓扑异构酶Ⅱ抑制剂。嵌入式拓扑异构酶Ⅱ抑制剂具有化学多样性，包括多柔比星、蒽环类以及蒽醌类药物（图 59-3c，3e）。非嵌入式的拓扑异构酶Ⅱ抑制剂包括表鬼臼毒素、依托泊苷和替尼泊苷（图 59-3d；表 59-2）。

蒽环类（Anthracyclines）

蒽环类抗生素，最初是从链霉菌发酵产物中分离出来的，数十年前，在鉴定拓扑异构酶之前，就已被证明具有抗肿瘤活性。直到 1984 年才发现蒽环类药物可抑制拓扑异构酶 2[85]。多柔比星（Doxorubicin），又称阿霉素，是第一代蒽环类药物的代表；表柔比星和伊达比星属第二代蒽环类药物，旨在降低 ABC 转运体的心脏毒性和药物外排。蒽环类药物具有广泛的抗人类癌症活性，广泛用于治疗、辅助和姑息治疗，既作为单一药物，也作为联合治疗方案。

多柔比星是最常用的蒽环素（图 59-3c）。蒽环是亲脂性的，但在氨基糖附近存在大量的羟基产生两性分子。多柔比星与细胞膜结合，包括心磷脂和血浆蛋白。柔红霉素与多柔比星的区别在于 C14 上有一个单独的羟基（图 59-3c），具有独特的抗肿瘤活性谱。伊达比星是柔红霉素（4-去甲氧基柔红霉素）的半合成衍生物，不含 4-甲氧基（图 59-3c）。表柔比星是多柔比星的一种表聚物，氨基糖上的 C4′羟基位于赤道位置，而不是轴向位置，这增加了其亲脂性。这些类似物的抗肿瘤活性均不如两种原来的蒽环类药物，但限制多柔比星和柔红霉素的毒性[86]。

临床药理学

多柔比星的药动学呈线性，静脉注射后呈三相分布。最初的半衰期很短，大约 5 分钟，这表明组织摄取快；第二阶段大约 10 小时，代表其代谢；最后阶段缓慢，24~48 小时，多柔比星从包括 DNA 在内的多个结合位点逐渐释放[87]。多柔比星及其主要代谢产物多柔比星醇的血浆蛋白结合率约为 50%~90%[88]。多柔比星不能透过血脑屏障。

多柔比星的血浆清除主要是通过代谢和胆汁。该药物在肝脏中被醛酸酮还原酶广泛代谢，产生具有抗肿瘤活性的二氢二醇衍生物多柔比星，还可被 NADPH 依赖性细胞色素 P450 还原酶分解糖苷键并释放苷代谢物[89]。肝功能受损患者多柔比星和多柔比星醇的清除率降低[90]。肾清除率对药物清除并不重要，故肾衰竭患者不需要进行剂量调整。

多柔比星脂质体包封已成功地作为一种不丧失药效并降低药物毒性的策略[91]。聚乙二醇化多柔比星脂质体是多柔比星的一种脂质体制剂，与未包封多柔比星相比，其具有较长的半衰期及网状内皮系统的摄取延迟（这是由于聚乙二醇聚合物黏附在脂质锚上），同时有稳定的药物保留（这是由于脂质体通过硫酸铵化学梯度包封）[92]。这种药物的药代动力学特征是循环时间延长和分布体积减小，从而促进肿瘤吸收。

临床应用

多柔比星被用于多种类型的癌症。FDA 批准其用于原发性乳腺癌切除术后腋窝淋巴结浸润的辅助化疗。多柔比星还用于急性淋巴细胞白血病和髓性细胞白血病的治疗，以及非霍奇金淋巴瘤和霍奇金淋巴瘤的联合治疗。多柔比星对多种实体瘤有活性，包括乳腺癌、卵巢癌、膀胱癌、甲状腺癌、胃癌、肺癌、软组织癌和骨肉瘤。聚乙二醇化脂质体多柔比星用于治疗既往系统治疗失败或不耐受的艾滋病相关卡波西肉瘤，还可作为联合治疗的一部分用于多发性骨髓瘤[93,94]。另外，还可用于在铂基治疗后的进展性或复发性卵巢癌[95]。

表柔比星的活性谱与多柔比星非常相似，但毒性较低[96]。表柔比星被用于原发性乳腺癌、食管癌、胃癌、软组织和子宫肉瘤的辅助治疗[97]。

柔红霉素（图 59-3c）主要用于急性淋巴细胞白血病和急性髓性白血病的诱导方案。在儿童实体瘤中也有活性，但对成人实体瘤的活性很小。伊达比星主要用于治疗急性髓性白血病和急性淋巴白血病[98]。

用药时间管理

单剂多柔比星的治疗方案为每 21 天静脉注射 60~75mg/m^2。在联合治疗方案为每 21~28 天静脉注射 40~75mg/m^2。柔红霉素为每日 30~60mg/m^2 静脉注射，连续 3 天。伊达比星为每日 12mg/m^2 静脉注射，连续 3 天。表柔比星为每 3 周注射 100~120mg/m^2。聚乙二醇化脂质体多柔比星治疗艾滋病相关的卡波西肉瘤的用法为每 21 天静脉注射 20mg/m^2，治疗卵巢癌的用法为每 28 天静脉注射 50mg/m^2。

毒性

所有的蒽环类药物都会造成心脏损伤，导致严重甚至危及生命的并发症[99,100]。心脏损伤是多柔比星长期治疗的主要剂量限制性毒性。多柔比星和柔红霉素的心脏毒性比表柔比星和伊达比星更常见[96]。心脏毒性的急性表现为心电图异常，包括 ST-T 升高和心律失常，从治疗开始到治疗后的数周内均可发生。心脏毒性的慢性表现是心肌病，可以早在治疗结束后 1 年内发生，也可在治疗后 1 年后发生。

多柔比星相关的心肌病和充血性心力衰竭是剂量依赖性的。风险以非线性方式与总累积剂量成比例增加（550mg/m^2 时高达 1%~5%，600mg/m^2 时为 30%，1g/m^2 或更高时为 50%），具有明显的个体差异[101]。当药物的累积剂量超过 550mg/m^2 体表面积时，这些并发症的发生率高的令人无法接受[102]。给药方式在累积性心脏毒性中起着重要作用，且可能与推注有关[103]。为了减少心脏毒性，研究了连续输注方案。已经研究了超过 48 小时或 96 小时的输注方案，表现出副作用的变化，对具有较少的恶心、呕吐和心脏毒性[104]，但允许剂量超过常规限值。尽管有明显的优势，但连续输注方案难以实施意味着其在社区中没有显著的应用。

多柔比星的心脏毒性可归因于氧化还原反应和活性氧（reactive oxygen species，ROS）生成；然而，ROS 清除剂不能阻止这种毒性[102,105]。最近的数据表明，拓扑异构酶Ⅱβ[106]拓扑异构酶Ⅱα在肿瘤中的高表达，这是多柔比星抗肿瘤活性的分子基础，而拓扑异构酶Ⅱβ则在心肌细胞和非复制细胞中表达[13,107]。多种证据表明，拓扑异构酶Ⅱβ在多柔比星诱导的心肌病发展中的作用。拓扑异构酶Ⅱβ-多柔比星-DNA 三元分裂复合物可诱导心肌细胞 DNA 双链断裂，导致心肌细胞死亡。经证实，拓扑异构酶 2β 缺失的小鼠胚胎成纤维细胞对多柔比星诱导的细胞死亡具有抵抗力[108]。最近的研究还表明，线粒体拓扑异构酶(拓扑异构酶Ⅰmt)通过促进线粒体 DNA 复制和维持功能性氧化磷酸化来对抗多柔比星的细胞毒性。

一些因素增加了蒽环类药物心脏毒性的风险。最强的预测因子是累积药物剂量[109]。其他危险因素包括药物暴露时的年龄、同时服用其他心脏毒性药物、胸部辐射和先前存在的心血管疾病。在保持疗效的同时,已经采取了许多方法来降低心脏毒性的风险。这些包括交替的给药时间表、蒽环类分子的修饰以及 β-肾上腺素能阻滞剂或右丙亚胺(dexrazoxane)的辅助治疗[108]。最近的证据表明,存在正常单核苷酸多态性的拓扑异构酶Ⅰmt 突变是多柔比星心脏毒性的潜在决定因素[107]。

右丙亚胺(图 59-3f)是一种乙二胺四乙酸(EDTA)类螯合剂,通过结合脂质过氧化后细胞内储存释放的铁来防止蒽环类药物的损害[110]。与仅用蒽环类药物治疗的乳腺癌患者相比,用右丙亚胺治疗的患者发生心脏事件的次数更少[111]。右丙亚胺在美国和欧洲被批准用于已接受 300mg/m^2 多柔比星或 540mg/m^2 表柔比星治疗的晚期或转移性乳腺癌患者。然而,人们对使用右丙亚胺降低化疗反应和更多骨髓抑制的可能性存在担忧[112]。因此,多柔比星为基础的化疗中,不推荐常规使用右丙亚胺。建议接受多柔比星治疗的患者继续进行心脏监测[113]。

蒽环类药物的其他毒性包括骨髓抑制、黏膜炎、脱发、恶心、呕吐、腹泻和皮肤色素沉着。骨髓抑制是急性剂量限制性毒性。白细胞计数在给药 7 天内开始下降,10~14 天达到最低点,1~2 周后恢复。血小板减少和贫血相对较轻。注射部位的红斑(反应性红斑)是良性的,与外渗不同,后者可导致严重的局部并发症,如周围组织严重坏死。先前放射部位的炎症可导致难以预料的并发症,包括心包炎、胸腔积液和皮疹。表柔比星组的恶心、呕吐和脱发的发生率低于多柔比星组[96]。

与多柔比星相比,聚乙二醇化脂质体多柔比星的毒性特征是黏膜和皮肤毒性、轻度骨髓抑制、降低的心脏毒性降低及轻微脱发。掌跖红斑感觉障碍是观察到的最常见的 3 级或 4 级毒性,常发生于第二或第三个周期,发生频率高于接受传统多柔比星的患者[114]。黏膜皮肤毒性是剂量限制性的。掌跖红斑感觉异常的病理生理机制尚不清楚。据推测,在局部创伤后,聚乙二醇化脂质体多柔比星可能通过手足深层的微毛细血管排泄腺渗出,此处脂质体的亲水层促进其积聚[115]。聚乙二醇化脂质体多柔比星的心脏毒性降低使得其累积剂量比多柔比星大。急性超敏反应通常发生在第一次输注时[116]。

新型蒽环类药物

虽然蒽环类药物具有广谱的活性、结构、药动学和药效学特征,但其疗效和安全性受到了一定限制。为了规避这些限制性并进一步开发其活性,开发了新型的蒽环类和蒽环类结合物。

氨柔比星(amrubicin)是一种完全合成的蒽环类药物,其结构类似于多柔比星,具有有效的拓扑异构酶 2 抑制活性,仅在日本被批准用于非小细胞肺癌和小细胞肺癌[117]。氨柔比星本身抗肿瘤作用较弱,需要转化为其活性形式 amrubicinol 才能发挥作用[118]。在临床前的研究中,氨柔比星几乎没有引起心脏毒性。氨柔比星的心脏毒性较低,是因为比多柔比星相比,其低水平累积和代谢优势[119]。在小细胞肺癌的二线治疗中,尽管其有较好的回应率,但与托泊替康相比,氨柔比星并不能提高生存率[120]。在小细胞肺癌的一线治疗中,氨柔比星联合顺铂优于伊立替康联合氨柔比星[121]。

蒽醌类药物(anthracenediones)

米托蒽醌(mitoxantrone)(图 59-3e)是一种有效的拓扑异构酶Ⅱ抑制剂,部分来源于早期的假设,即蒽环类药物的心脏毒性可能取决于氨基糖的存在[122]。由于强心苷类的苷元具有比母体化合物更低的心脏毒性,人们认为一种插入 DNA 但不含氨基糖的多环芳香分子可能是一种无心脏毒性的有效抗肿瘤剂。与多柔比星相比,米托蒽醌的抗肿瘤谱是有限的。米托蒽醌用于急性非淋巴细胞白血病的初步治疗,其对晚期去势抵抗前列腺癌和乳腺癌有活性。米托蒽醌的剂量限制毒性在实体瘤患者中为白细胞减少,而在白血病患者中剂量限制性毒性可能是口炎。其他不良反应通常是轻度或中度的。心脏影响,特别是充血性心力衰竭,可能是值得关注的,尤其是以前接受过蒽环类药物治疗、纵隔放疗或心血管疾病患者。

匹杉琼(pixantrone)(图 59-3e)是一种结构类似于米托蒽醌的氮杂蒽醌。在临床前模型中,与多柔比星相比,匹杉琼活性增强,心脏毒性降低,自由基形成减少[123]。匹杉琼单剂挽救疗法已获得了欧盟的有条件上市许可,用于治疗多重复发或难治性侵袭性非霍奇金 B 细胞淋巴瘤[124]。匹杉琼的推荐方案为第 1 天、第 8 天和第 15 天给药 50mg/m^2,每周期 28 天,最多 6 个周期。最常见的副作用是骨髓抑制(特别是中性粒细胞)、恶心、呕吐和虚弱。该药物在美国不允许使用。

鬼臼毒素类(epipodophyllotoxins)

鬼臼毒素(podophyllotoxin)是从盾叶鬼臼和桃儿七中分离出来的天然产物[125]。虽然鬼臼毒素及其衍生物的抗癌活性在 20 世纪 40 年代就已为人所知,但鬼臼毒素的抑制性毒性阻碍了其进一步的发展。去甲基鬼臼毒素拓扑异构酶Ⅱ抑制剂是鬼臼毒素的衍生物,这是保留抗肿瘤活性的结果,其毒性较低。

依托泊苷(etoposide)

依托泊苷(VP-16)(图 59-3d)是第一个公认的拓扑异构酶Ⅱ抑制剂抗癌药物[126]。与许多其他拓扑异构酶抑制剂一样,在了解其作用机制和药理学之前,对其临床活性和批准的评价。

临床药理学

依托泊苷不溶于水,这给作为增溶剂的载体的快速给药和药物过敏反应带来困难。磷酸依托泊苷是依托泊苷的水溶性酯,浓度高达 20mg/ml,是努力克服此问题的结果,已被 FDA 批准用于静脉注射[127]。磷酸依托泊苷的水溶性也减轻了静脉注射时药物沉淀的风险。体内磷酸依托泊苷通过去磷酸化迅速转化为活性部分,即依托泊苷。磷酸依托泊苷的药代动力学、毒性和临床活性与依托泊苷相似。

依托泊苷具有双相药代动力学特征,分布半衰期约为 1.5 小时,终末消除半衰期为 4~11 小时。静脉注射后 AUC 与血浆峰值浓度呈线性关系[128]。尽管脑脊液中依托泊苷的含量低于脑室外肿瘤和血浆中的含量,但可能超过最低细胞毒性水平,可能对中枢神经系统定向治疗有用[129]。

依托泊苷与血浆蛋白高度结合,平均游离血浆分数为 6%。

由于游离药物具有生物活性,降低蛋白质结合的条件会增强药物的药理作用[130]。肾衰竭患者依托泊苷清除率有所下降,中度肾功能损害患者建议调整剂量。胆汁排泄是一种次要的清除途径,肝梗阻患者的清除率不受影响[131]。

虽然依托泊苷典型的给药途径是静脉注射,但也可以口服[132]。与静脉注射相比,口服依托泊苷的生物利用度在患者体内及患者间均有很大的变化,范围从40%~75%。口服生物利用度也随药物剂量的不同而变化,在低剂量时效果更好[133]。尽管口服依托泊苷的药效有限,但它允许长期给药,并得到了FDA的批准。

临床应用

依托泊苷可与其他药物联合用于难治性睾丸肿瘤和小细胞肺癌的一线治疗。依托泊苷在其他肿瘤类型中也表现出临床活性,包括非霍奇金淋巴瘤、白血病、卡波西肉瘤、神经母细胞瘤和软组织肉瘤。它也是骨髓和外周干细胞抢救前准备方案的重要组成部分。

用药时间管理

对于小细胞肺癌的治疗,依托泊苷与其他药物联合使用,静脉注射剂量为80~120mg/m^2,治疗第1~3天使用,每疗程为21~28天。睾丸癌经典剂量为50~100mg/(m^2·d),第1~5天或100mg/(m^2/d),第1天、第3天和第5天使用,每21~28天重复一次。

暴露的持续时间是依托泊苷活性的一个重要决定因素,许多研究表明长期服用可使活性最大化[134,135]。在小细胞肺癌中,3~5天给药比单天给药有更好的疗效[135,136]。为了确定给药时间比标准的3~5天治疗时间长,可能进一步提高依托泊苷的治疗指数,开发了延长的口服剂量方案。然而,在第三阶段的试验中,接受21天口服依托泊苷治疗的小细胞肺癌患者与3~5天给药患者相比,其应答率或生存率没有任何改善[137]。

毒性

骨髓抑制是依托泊苷静脉注射、口服的主要剂量限制性毒性。给药后7~14天和9~16天分别出现粒细胞和血小板最低值。骨髓恢复通常在第20天完成。其他可能的毒性包括过敏或其他输液反应,表现为发热、支气管痉挛和低血压。与口服依托泊苷相关的毒性包括恶心、呕吐和黏膜炎。

替尼泊苷(teniposide)

替尼泊苷(VM-16)(图59-3d),依托泊苷类似物,是鬼臼毒素的半合成衍生物。替尼泊苷的糖环不同于依托泊苷。尽管在依托泊苷之前对患者进行了分离和评估,但早期对超敏反应的关注和低剂量使用导致了该药物的发展缓慢[132]。在体外,替尼泊苷比依托泊苷更有效地杀死癌细胞,这可能与其更好的细胞摄取有关[138-140]。

与依托泊苷相比,更大比例的替尼泊苷是与蛋白质结合的[141],而肾功能与替尼泊苷清除率的相关性较小[142]。骨髓抑制是替尼泊苷的剂量限制性毒性。它也能产生超敏反应。替尼泊苷被批准用于治疗难治性儿童急性淋巴细胞白血病。很少有研究能接研究这两种药剂的活性。

治疗相关的继发性急性白血病(t-AML)

拓扑异构酶2抑制剂的主要并发症之一,尤其是依托泊苷和米托蒽醌,是急性继发性白血病,约5%的患者发生。治疗相关的急性髓细胞性白血病(t-AML)的特点是发病相对较快(治疗后仅几个月发生),并且在11q23和50多个伴侣基因上存在涉及混合性白血病(MLL)基因座的反复平衡易位[143]。所提出的分子机制是通过在不同的染色体上分离两个药物捕获的拓扑异构酶2裂解复合物,这与转录冲突和不合法的重排有关[144]。拓扑异构酶2β与这些分离的裂解复合物的产生有关[144,145]。

药物基因组学

已证明药物代谢酶、转运体和其他蛋白质的遗传变异影响包括伊立替康和多柔比星在内的拓扑异构酶抑制剂的药理学,对这些基因变异的理解将允许对每种药物进行个体化给药,目的是提高疗效和减少毒性。

伊立替康(irinotecan)

葡萄糖醛酸基转移酶ⅠA

几种酶和药物转运体参与了伊立替康的清除。伊立替康剂量变化受*UGT1A*、*CYP3A*和*ABC*基因家族遗传多态性的影响。这些基因的等位基因变体改变了功能活性,从而导致伊立替康代谢的个体差异,并使患者易受可变毒性的影响。

已描述的*UGT1A1*基因的启动子和编码区的单核苷酸多态性显著影响伊立替康的代谢和毒性[146,147]。变异被描述为等位基因,由符号“*”和数字表示。虽然有超过113个基因变体,但仅描述了几个变体影响伊立替康的药效学(*6、*27、*28、*36、*37、*60、*93)。本章重点介绍*28和*6变种,这些变种在临床上与支持性研究相关。通过该途径清除SN-38有助于伊立替康诱导的毒性的个体间变异,该毒性与*UGT1A1*(*UGT1A1*28*)近端启动子区的变异等位基因相关。*UGT1A1*28*(rs8175347,也称为UGT1A1 7/7基因型)等位基因在启动子区的TATA盒中有七个二核苷酸重复,而野生型*UGT1A1*1*等位基因有六个重复,导致转录、蛋白表达和酶活性降低。在白种人和非裔美国人中,*UGT1A1*28*的频率分别为0.26~0.31和0.42~0.56[148,149]。与*1/*1患者相比,*UGT1A1*28*纯合子变异体患者对SN-38的全身暴露增加,血浆SN-38G/SN-38比率降低,并且通常出现剂量限制性的严重腹泻或中性粒细胞减少[52,150-153]。*UGT1A1*6*多态性的特点是*UGT1A1*外显子1的单核苷酸替换,导致表达减少,毒性增加,与*UGT1A1*28*类似。*UGT1A1*6*(rs4148323)变异在亚洲人中出现频率较高(频率为0.13~0.25)[154],并且与亚洲人伊立替康相关腹泻和中性粒细胞减少有关[150,155,156]。

在每2周[157]或每3周[158]接受伊立替康单剂治疗或伊立替康与氟尿嘧啶[159,160]、卡培他滨[161]、或卡培他滨和奥沙利铂[162]联合治疗的患者中,评估了以*UGT1A1*基因型为导向的伊立替康给药的概念。尽管患者群体和治疗方案存在差异,但这些研究的普遍共识是,具有*28/*28基因型的患者具有最高的伊立替康相关毒性风险,需要将剂量减少40%。自2005年以来,美国食品和药物管理局建议,对于*UGT1A1*28*纯合子变种的个体,减少伊立替康的初始剂量(至少一个水平),因为其有更高的中性粒细胞减少风险。

许多 meta 分析评估了 *28/ *28 基因型与毒性风险的关系为伊立替康剂量函数。Hoskins 等[51](n=821)表明，*28/ *28 患者在高/中剂量下的严重血液毒性明显较高。Hu 等[163](n=1 998)表明，*28/ *28 患者 3~4 级中性粒细胞减少症的风险显著增加，高剂量组高于中、低剂量组。最近对 16 项结直肠癌研究(n=2 328)的 meta 分析显示，与 *1/ *1(OR=4.79,95% CI=3.28~7.01,P<0.000 01)或 *1/ *28(OR=3.44,95% CI=2.45~4.82,P<0.000 01)相比，无论伊立替康剂量多少，*28/ *28 患者中性粒细胞减少症 3~4 级的发生率更高[164]。

伊立替康药物遗传学的研究主要集中在 *UGT1A1* *28 等位基因与伊立替康相关毒性的关系。*UGT1A1 *28* 基因分型对事先减少剂量的临床效用取决于 *UGT1A1 *28* 是否也影响治疗效果，迄今为止的研究一直存在矛盾。最近的一项 meta 分析发现，*UGT1A1 *28* 基因型(纯合子、杂合子或野生型)与伊立替康治疗相关的生存率没有差异，包括总体数据(n=1 524 例患者)和无进展生存率(n=1 494 例患者)[165]。因此，虽然已证明 *28 基因分型经济有效，但临床实用性尚不清楚[166,167]。迄今为止，有关 *28 是否影响治疗效果的研究一直是矛盾的，而且由于大多数严重毒性(中性粒细胞减少或腹泻)的发生是通过在随后的周期中减少剂量来管理的，因此临床实施仍有待确定。

除 UGT1A1 外，*UGT1A7* 和 *UGT1A9* 基因的变体也参与了患者间伊立替康相关毒性的差异。*UGT1A7* 主要参与肝外代谢(位于肠内)，并负责解毒 SN-38，而 *UGT1A9* 对于肝内 SN-38 与 SN-38G 的结合是必要的[168]。*UGT1A7 *2*、*UGT1A7 *3* 或 *UGT1A7 *4* 多态性可能导致伊立替康代谢和相关毒性改变[169-172]。据报道，*UGTA9 *1* 纯合子患者的腹泻严重程度高于 *UGTA9 *9* 或 *UGTA9 *22* 携带者[172,173]。

总之，这些研究表明，临床结果可能是单倍型复杂组合的结果，涉及 UGT 代谢解毒(*UGT1A1*、*UGT1A7* 和 *UGT1A9*)途径的关键基因组变异[168,171]。

CYP3A 和药物转运体

CYP3A4 和 *CYP3A5* 基因对伊立替康氧化代谢为非活性代谢产物 APC 和 NPC 至关重要。体外研究表明，变种(*CYP3A4 *16* 或 *CYP3A4 *18* 或 *CYP3A5 *3*)活性降低，导致氧化代谢率降低，从而减少 APC 和 NPC 代谢产物的产生[173,174]。然而，这些基因变异与伊立替康治疗结果的相关性仍有待阐明。

伊立替康的清除也依赖于 ABC 药物转运体，该转运体存在于胆小管膜上，促进伊立替康及其代谢物的分泌[175]。ABCB1 和 ABCC2 的特异性多态性可影响伊立替康的药物配置和肿瘤反应[176]。虽然 ABCC2 *2 单倍体与伊立替康诱导的低腹泻发生率相关[177]，但 ABCC2(rs374066)和 ABCG2(rs2231137)变异的患者 3 级腹泻发生率较高[173,178,179]。用新型药物代谢酶和转运体(DMET)微阵列基因分型平台对伊立替康诱导的胃肠道毒性药物基因组学研究，确定了 3 个附加的单核苷酸多态性，这些单核苷酸多态性分别对应 *ABCG1*、*ABCC5* 和 *OATP1B1/SLCO1B1* 转运体基因[180]。此外，最近的一项研究表明，*OATP1B1* 和肿瘤 *OATP1B3* 可调节以伊立替康为基础的化疗后暴露、毒性和生存率[181]。

多柔比星(doxorubicin)

基因多态性存在于介导多柔比星代谢、转运和药理作用的基因中，但这些变异的临床意义及其对多柔比星疗效和毒性的影响近年来才得到评价。多柔比星的药代动力学参数有明显的个体差异[182]，累积剂量是多柔比星引起心脏毒性的最重要的危险因素。

多柔比星的主要代谢产物是 13-C 醇、多柔比星二辛醇，由羰基还原酶 1(CBR1)、CBR3 和醛酮还原酶 1C3(AKR1C3)代谢。功能性单核苷酸多态性在 CBR1、CBR3 和 AKR1C3 中具有特征。已描述了 *CBR1* 中两个对 CBR1 活性或表达有功能影响的单核苷酸多态性(rs1143663 和 rs9024)[183,184]。迄今为止，*CBR1* 基因多态性影响的研究有限，在乳腺癌患者中未发现任何关联[185]。然而，rs9024 杂合子和另一个 CBR1 变异体(与之连锁不平衡)的患者多柔比星清除率较低[186]。

与野生型相比，*CBR3* G730A(rs1056892)和 G11A(rs8133052)中两个常见的单核苷酸多态性呈连锁不平衡状态，其体外催化效率降低[187]。有研究认为野生型 *CBR3* G730A 等位基因表现出较高的活性和表达增加，与儿童癌症幸存者中蒽环相关充血性心力衰竭的风险相关[188]。亚洲乳腺癌患者肿瘤组织中 CBR3 表达较高，其变异与多柔比星高 AUC 有关[185]。在同一队列中，G11A 次要等位基因除影响多柔比星药代动力学和 CBR 表达外，还与更大的血液毒性和疗效相关[185]。Voon 等[189]研究也显示，G11A 次要等位基因与多柔比星低 AUC 及长总生存期相关。然而，对乳腺癌患者的其他研究显示，这些变异对多柔比星药代动力学[186]或生存率[190]没有影响。

一项体外研究表明，与野生型相比，醛酮还原酶 1C3(AKR1C3)基因外显子 5 中 508 C>T(rs3575889)和 538 C>T(rs34186955)的两个非同义单核苷酸多态性编码的酶显著降低多柔比星代谢[191]。在一项亚洲乳腺癌患者的临床研究中，上述 2 个单核苷酸多态性没有被确定；然而，检测到了两个内含子变异体 IVS4-212 C>G(rs1937840)和 IVS4+218G>A(rs1937841)。在多柔比星为基础的治疗后，AKR1C3 IVS4-212 GG 等位基因与更严重的血液毒性和更长的总体、无进展生存期相关[189]。

已证实一些转运体参与了多柔比星的转运，包括 ABCB1、ABCC1、ABCC2、ABCG2、RALBP1 和 SLC22A16。多柔比星是 ABCB1 的底物，ABCB1 介导的多柔比星外流可导致实验室和动物模型的疗效下降。抑制 ABCB1 可能导致多柔比星毒性增加。3 种高频 *ABCB1* 多态性，即 1236C>T(rs1128503)、2677G>A/T(rs2032582)和 3435C>T(rs1045642)被提出可改变底物药物的药代动力学，但在文献中存在一些争议，既有阳性研究，也有阴性研究。这可能是由于不同的患者群体、其他协变量和个体底物药物所致。一项针对亚洲患者的小型研究发现，多柔比星药代动力学受损，导致暴露水平显著增加，清除率降低；然而，该研究仅涉及少数患者[192]。此外，尽管 2677A 等位基因与多柔比星和环磷酰胺治疗乳腺癌患者的总生存期较短和无进展生存期相关，但 C1236T、G2677T 和 C3435T 单核苷酸多态性对生存率无影响[193]。在多柔比星为基础的亚洲乳腺癌患者中，*ABCB1* G2677T/A 与药物清除率和血小板毒性相关，*ABCB1* IVS26+59 T>G 与总生存率相关[189]。3435T 等位基因与多柔比星和硼替佐米治疗的多发性骨髓瘤患者无进展生存期延长显著相关，与假设的功能或表达丧失一致[194]。其他研究发现

ABCB1 基因型对多柔比星的反应没有影响[195]。在欧洲人群中发现的一个额外的 *ABCB1* G1199T/A(rs2229109)变异体,与其他三个连锁不平衡变异体不同,在临床上研究较少,但已被证明对多柔比星的外流和毒性具有功能性影响[196]。考虑到不同人群的研究不一致,*ABCB1* 单核苷酸多态性对多柔比星配置的功能意义仍然存在争议。

ABCG2 介导的多柔比星耐药性取决于获得性突变(R482T/G)[197]。在一项乳腺癌患者的临床研究中,没有观察到与 *ABCG2* 421C>a 多态性相关的多柔比星药动学显著性差异[192],该多态性曾被证明比野生型具有更低的 ATP 酶活性[198]。其他 ABC 家族成员的表达,包括 ABCB5、ABCB8、ABCC5 和 RALBP1,也会对多柔比星产生耐药性;然而,临床意义仍不清楚。

有机阳离子输出器 SLC22A16 运输多柔比星到细胞。*SLC22A16* A146G(rs714368)的纯合子可能有较高的多柔比星 AUC[199],同一次要等位基因及连锁不平衡的其他 *SLC22A16* 单核苷酸多态性(T312C 和 T755C 变异体)在多柔比星和环磷酰胺辅助治疗乳腺癌期间不太可能有剂量延迟[193]。在 SLC22A16 T1226C(rs12210538)携带者中,剂量延迟的发生率较高,表明毒性增加[193]。

在一项涉及 1 697 名患者(其中 3.2%的患者存在急性或慢性毒性)82 个基因单核苷酸多态性的蒽环素诱导心脏毒性的药物基因组预测因子研究中,发现了 5 个显著的相关性,多态性位于 NAD(P)H 氧化酶复合物(CYBA rs4673、NCF4 rs1883112 和 RAC2 rs13058338)和多柔比星转运体(ABCC1 rs45511401、ABCC2 rs8187694 和 RS8187710)[200]。Rossi 等[201]同时显示 CYBA rs4673 和 NCF4 rs1883112 与含多柔比星化疗的淋巴瘤患者毒性相关。降低 ROS 的基因多态性可能导致多柔比星治疗后的疗效或毒性增加,可能包括超氧化物歧化酶Ⅱ(SOD2)、谷胱甘肽 S-转移酶(GSTS)或 NAD(P)H:醌氧化还原酶 1(NQO1)的变体。此外,药物遗传学研究还评估了 *ERBB2* 和 *TOP2A* 基因拷贝数作为多柔比星应答的预测因子,结果相互矛盾[202-204]。

柔红霉素、表柔比星及依托泊苷

关于柔红霉素、表柔比星及依托泊苷的药物基因组学的数据有限。使用 DMET 平台对儿童柔红霉素进行的药物基因组学研究发现,FMO3 和 GSTP1 单倍型与柔红霉素药代动力学的相关性可能影响疗效和毒性[205]。表柔比星和多柔比星醇的主要失活途径是尿苷二磷酸葡萄糖醛酸转移酶 2B7(UGT2B7)催化的葡萄糖醛酸化。具有 UGT2B7 802 C>T 纯合子次要等位基因的乳腺癌患者可能从辅助性表柔比星化疗中获益最多[206]。在用环磷酰胺、表柔比星和 5-氟尿嘧啶辅助治疗乳腺癌的药理学研究中,与表柔比星相比,NQO2 外显子单核苷酸多态性与较高的表柔比星暴露有关。NQO1、CBR、UGT 酶和转运体的多态性变体对表柔比星或其代谢产物没有影响[207]。最后,通过一项全基因组关联研究,利用 HapMap 细胞系上产生的数据,鉴定出 63 种导致依托泊苷诱导细胞毒性的遗传变异[208]。

展望

拓扑异构酶抑制剂是抗癌药物的基本成分。以下 4 点与它们的未来用途有关:①新的制剂和靶向给药方法(例如脂质体和抗体偶联物)可以在限制剂量限制毒性的同时实现肿瘤的靶向性选择性。②详细了解药物的化学局限性(喜树碱的化学不稳定性和蒽环类的氧化还原反应)和毒性分子机制,设计出新的拓扑异构酶抑制剂,如非喜树碱拓扑异构酶Ⅰ抑制剂(吲哚喹啉 LMP 衍生物)、避免与拓扑异构酶Ⅱβ抑制相关的严重毒性(蒽环类药物的心脏毒性和由表鬼臼毒素引起的继发性白血病)的拓扑异构酶Ⅱα特异性抑制剂。③更好地理解敏感性的分子基础将能更好地选择抗肿瘤药物的组合[10,11]。到目前为止,抗肿瘤药物组合是由经验发展而来,但未来进一步深入了解基因组学和表观基因组学将有助于开发合理的抗肿瘤药物组合疗法。④最后,预测拓扑异构酶抑制剂的活性,并根据肿瘤基因组特征等现代技术精准选择患者仍然是至关重要的[10,11,209]。虽然这些药物在个体化医学时代之前就已被确认,但确实有特定的细胞靶点,因此了解它们是很重要的。识别药物敏感性和抵抗力的分子基础是很重要的,以便在未来制定策略做出最佳的治疗选择。

(李志铭 译,姜文奇 审校)

参考文献

1 Wang JC. Interaction between DNA and an *Escherichia coli* protein omega. *J Mol Biol*. 1971;**55(3)**:523-533.

2 Champoux JJ, Dulbecco R. An activity from mammalian cells that untwists superhelical DNA—a possible swivel for DNA replication (polyoma-ethidium bromide-mouse-embryo cells-dye binding assay). *Proc Natl Acad Sci U S A*. 1972;**69**:143-146.

3 Pommier Y. *DNA Topoisomerases and Cancer*. New York, Dordrecht, Heidelberg, London: Springer & Humana Press; 2012.

4 Pommier Y. Drugging topoisomerases: lessons and challenges. *ACS Chem Biol*. 2013;**8(1)**:82-95.

5 Gheeya J, Johansson P, Chen QR, et al. Expression profiling identifies epoxy anthraquinone derivative as a DNA topoisomerase inhibitor. *Cancer Lett*. 2010;**293(1)**:124-131.

6 Pommier Y, Marchand C. Interfacial inhibitors: targeting macromolecular complexes. *Nat Rev Drug Discov*. 2012;**11(1)**:25-36.

7 Capranico G, Binaschi M. DNA sequence selectivity of topoisomerases and topoisomerase poisons. *Biochim Biophys Acta*. 1998;**1400**:185-194.

8 Nitiss J, Wang JC. DNA topoisomerase-targeting antitumor drugs can be studied in yeast. *Proc Natl Acad Sci U S A*. 1988;**85**:7501-7505.

9 Maede Y, Shimizu H, Fukushima T, et al. Differential and common DNA repair pathways for topoisomerase I- and II-targeted drugs in a genetic DT40 repair cell screen panel. *Mol Cancer Ther*. 2014;**13(1)**:214-220.

10 Zoppoli G, Regairaz M, Leo E, et al. Putative DNA/RNA helicase Schlafen-11 (SLFN11) sensitizes cancer cells to DNA-damaging agents. *Proc Natl Acad Sci U S A*. 2012;**109(37)**:15030-15035.

11 Barretina J, Caponigro G, Stransky N, et al. The Cancer Cell Line Encyclopedia enables predictive modelling of anticancer drug sensitivity. *Nature*. 2012;**483(7391)**:603-607.

12 Pommier Y. Topoisomerase I inhibitors: camptothecins and beyond. *Nat Rev Cancer*. 2006;**6(10)**:789-802.

13 Zhang H, Zhang YW, Yasukawa T, Dalla Rosa I, Khiati S, Pommier Y. Increased negative supercoiling of mtDNA in TOP1mt knockout mice and presence of topoisomerases IIalpha and IIbeta in vertebrate mitochondria. *Nucleic Acids Res*. 2014;**42(11)**:7259-7267.

14 Pommier Y, Jenkins J, Kohlhagen G, Leteurtre F. DNA recombinase activity of eukaryotic DNA topoisomerase I; effects of camptothecin and other inhibitors. *Mutat Res*. 1995;**337(2)**:135-145.

15 Koster DA, Palle K, Bot ES, Bjornsti MA, Dekker NH. Antitumour drugs impede DNA uncoiling by topoisomerase I. *Nature*. 2007;**448(7150)**:213-217.

16 Sordet O, Redon CE, Guirouilh-Barbat J, et al. Ataxia telangiectasia mutated activation by transcription- and topoisomerase I-induced DNA double-strand breaks. *EMBO Rep*. 2009;**10(8)**:887-893.

17 Ray Chaudhuri A, Hashimoto Y, Herrador R, et al. Topoisomerase I poisoning results in PARP-mediated replication fork reversal. *Nat Struct Mol Biol*. 2012;**19**:417-423.

18 Gomez-Herreros F, Romero-Granados R, Zeng Z, et al. TDP2-dependent

non-homologous end-joining protects against topoisomerase II-induced DNA breaks and genome instability in cells and in vivo. *PLoS Genet*. 2013;**9**(**3**):e1003226.

19 Pommier Y, Leo E, Zhang H, Marchand C. DNA topoisomerases and their poisoning by anticancer and antibacterial drugs. *Chem Biol*. 2010;**17**(**5**):421–433.

20 Pang B, Qiao X, Janssen L, et al. Drug-induced histone eviction from open chromatin contributes to the chemotherapeutic effects of doxorubicin. *Nat Commun*. 2013;**4**:1908.

21 Doroshow JH. Effect of anthracycline antibiotics on oxygen radical formation in rat heart. *Cancer Res*. 1983;**43**(**2**):460–472.

22 Gottlieb JA, Guarino AM, Call JB, Oliverio VT, Block JB. Preliminary pharmacologic and clinical evaluation of camptothecin sodium (NSC-100880). *Cancer Chemother Rep*. 1970;**54**(**6**):461–470.

23 Moertel CG, Schutt AJ, Reitemeier RJ, Hahn RG. Phase II study of camptothecin (NSC-100880) in the treatment of advanced gastrointestinal cancer. *Cancer Chemother Rep*. 1972;**56**(**1**):95–101.

24 Muggia FM, Creaven PJ, Hansen HH, Cohen MH, Selawry OS. Phase I clinical trial of weekly and daily treatment with camptothecin (NSC-100880): correlation with preclinical studies. *Cancer Chemother Rep*. 1972;**56**(**4**):515–521.

25 Hsiang YH, Liu LF. Identification of mammalian DNA topoisomerase-I as an intracellular target of the anticancer drug camptothecin. *Cancer Res*. 1988;**48**(**7**):1722–1726.

26 Burke TG, Munshi CB, Mi Z, Jiang Y. The important role of albumin in determining the relative human blood stabilities of the camptothecin anticancer drugs. *J Pharm Sci*. 1995;**84**(**4**):518–519.

27 Herben VMM, Huinink WWTB, Beijnen JH. Clinical pharmacokinetics of topotecan. *Clin Pharmacokinet*. 1996;**31**(**2**):85–102.

28 O'Reilly S, Rowinsky EK, Slichenmyer W, et al. Phase I and pharmacologic study of topotecan in patients with impaired renal function. *J Clin Oncol*. 1996;**14**(**12**):3062–3073.

29 O'Reilly S, Rowinsky E, Slichenmyer W, et al. Phase I and pharmacologic studies of topotecan in patients with impaired hepatic function. *J Natl Cancer Inst*. 1996;**88**(**12**):817–824.

30 Gerrits CJH, Schellens JHM, Burris H, et al. A comparison of clinical pharmacodynamics of different administration schedules of oral topotecan (hycamtin). *Clin Cancer Res*. 1999;**5**(**1**):69–75.

31 Eckardt JR, von Pawel J, Pujol JL, et al. Phase III study of oral compared with intravenous topotecan as second-line therapy in small-cell lung cancer. *J Clin Oncol*. 2007;**25**(**15**):2086–2092.

32 GlaxoSmithKline. *HYCAMTIN- Topotecan Hydrochloride for Injection Package Insert*. Research Triangle Park, NC: GlaxoSmithKline; 2015.

33 Stewart CF, Iacono LC, Chintagumpala M, et al. Results of a phase II upfront window of pharmacokinetically guided topotecan in high-risk medulloblastoma and supratentorial primitive neuroectodermal tumor. *J Clin Oncol*. 2004;**22**(**16**):3357–3365.

34 Joppert MG, Garfield DH, Gregurich MA, et al. A phase II multicenter study of combined topotecan and gemcitabine as first line chemotherapy for advanced non-small cell lung cancer. *Lung Cancer*. 2003;**39**(**2**):215–219.

35 Beran M, Estey E, O'Brien S, et al. Topotecan and cytarabine is an active combination regimen in myelodysplastic syndromes and chronic myelomonocytic leukemia. *J Clin Oncol*. 1999;**17**(**9**):2819–2830.

36 Hunold A, Weddeling N, Paulussen M, Ranft A, Liebscher C, Jurgens H. Topotecan and cyclophosphamide in patients with refractory or relapsed Ewing tumors. *Pediatr Blood Cancer*. 2006;**47**(**6**):795–800.

37 Walterhouse DO, Lyden ER, Breitfeld PP, Qualman SJ, Wharam MD, Meyer WH. Efficacy of topotecan and cyclophosphamide given in a phase II window trial in children with newly diagnosed metastatic rhabdomyosarcoma: a children's oncology group study. *J Clin Oncol*. 2004;**22**(**8**):1398–1403.

38 Kraut EH, Crowley JJ, Wade JL, et al. Evaluation of topotecan in resistant and relapsing multiple myeloma: a Southwest Oncology Group Study. *J Clin Oncol*. 1998;**16**(**2**):589–592.

39 Bruzzese F, Rocco M, Castelli S, Di Gennaro E, Desideri A, Budillon A. Synergistic antitumor effect between vorinostat and topotecan in small cell lung cancer cells is mediated by generation of reactive oxygen species and DNA damage-induced apoptosis. *Mol Cancer Ther*. 2009;**8**(**11**):3075–3087.

40 Kummar S, Chen A, Ji JP, et al. Phase I Study of PARP Inhibitor ABT-888 in Combination with Topotecan in Adults with Refractory Solid Tumors and Lymphomas. *Cancer Res*. 2011;**71**(**17**):5626–5634.

第 60 章　靶向微管和有丝分裂过程的药物

Eric K. Rowinsky, MD

概述

许多疾病的治疗在很大程度上归功于天然来源的药物,恶性疾病也不例外。数十亿年的进化压力使得植物、真菌和微生物能够产生高效且特异的毒素。在 20 世纪 50 年代和 60 年代,许多以有丝分裂过程为靶标的植物类衍生物和其他天然产物表现出了显著的抗癌活性,从那时开始,微管就被认为是具有重要研究意义的亚细胞靶点。

第一类广泛使用的靶向微管的药物是来源于植物的长春碱类化合物,几十年来一直是姑息疗法和治疗恶性肿瘤的主要药物。而具有独特作用机制和抗癌谱的植物类衍生物紫杉烷的发现,使人们重新对微管和有丝分裂过程产生兴趣,不仅将其作为开发癌症治疗药物的靶点,同时作为验证其他治疗癌症药物的靶标。最近,一些植物和海洋衍生化合物以及其他合成制剂,被发现对微管和其他有丝分裂成分具有更独特的破坏作用,包括从土壤黏菌和海绵动物中分别分离出的环氧酮类和海绵素 B 类化合物。这其中还包括强力的抗菌药物,如美坦辛和多拉司他丁的类似物,它们是抗体-药物偶联物的组成部分。本章内容集中于微管作为治疗靶点的确立以及抗微管药物作为治疗方案如何应用。

引言

许多疾病的治疗需要依赖于天然来源的药物,恶性疾病的治疗也不例外。事实上,数十亿年的进化压力已经导致植物、真菌和微生物通过自然选择,能够产生高效而特异的毒素。在 20 世纪 50 年代和 60 年代,一些植物来源的化合物和其他天然产物被发现能通过影响有丝分裂纺锤体来终止有丝分裂,进而在晚期恶性肿瘤患者中显示出显著的抗癌活性。自那以后,微管就被认为是具有重要研究意义的亚细胞靶点。

第一类广泛使用的靶向微管的药物是来源于植物的长春碱类化合物,过去几十年来一直是治疗恶性肿瘤的主要药物。具有独特作用机制和抗癌谱的植物衍生紫杉烷的发现,使人们重新对微管和有丝分裂过程产生兴趣,不仅将其作为开发癌症治疗药物的靶点,同时作为验证其他治疗癌症药物的靶标。最近,一些植物和海洋衍生化合物以及其他对微管和其他有丝分裂成分(例如有丝分裂激酶)具有更独特破坏作用的合成剂已经被发现,并被加入我们的治疗决策中,包括从土栖黏杆菌中分离的 epothilones 类似物(如 ixabepilone)和从海绵动物中分离的软海绵素 B(如艾日布林)。它们还包括强效的抗微管药物,例如美坦辛和多拉司他丁的类似物,它们是抗体-药物偶联物(antibody-drug conjugate, ADC)的成分,利用单克隆抗体(monoclonal antibodie, mAb)将其选择性地传送到表达相应抗原的癌细胞。本章重点介绍微管作为靶点进行治疗的发展历程,以及作为治疗方案的抗微管药物,尤其是长春碱类化合物和紫杉烷类和正在进行临床评估的几类有前景的抗微管药物。

微管作为抗癌治疗的靶点

微管是细胞骨架高度协调和统一的组成部分,可被各种天然产物(如长春碱类化合物、紫杉烷、埃博霉素、软海绵素等)以及越来越多的合成化合物破坏[1-6]。微管与微丝和中间丝共同构成细胞骨架,维持细胞结构。微管在细胞增殖过程中最重要的功能是其作为细胞骨架和有丝分裂纺锤体的组成部分来实现染色体分离,对细胞分裂至关重要。微管同时在整个细胞周期中参与许多其他关键功能的实现,包括囊泡和细胞器的胞内运输,使许多蛋白包括癌蛋白在胞内转移、运动、黏附以及亚细胞器和受体的锚定等[1-8]。细胞骨架,特别是微管,也会影响基因表达和信号转导,反之亦然;然而,这些相互作用的机制尚不清楚。转录因子的特异性表达与药物介导的微管解聚反应之间的关系已经被广泛报道,对相关机制的深入研究为理解特异性基因的差异表达提供了参考。最终,细胞骨架可以通过各种生长因子来介导细胞反应[9],而抗微管药物可以破坏这些功能。

微管结构与动力学

微管是由两种球状亚基 α-微管蛋白单体和 β-微管蛋白单体组成的二聚体结构,每个微管蛋白单体由约 450 个氨基酸组成,分子量为 50kD[10]。α/β-微管蛋白二聚体通过形成线状的原纤维组装成微管。通常,微管是由 13 条原纤维平行组合而成,但在体外也观察到由更少或更多的原纤维组成的微管。由于原纤维独特的排列特点,微管具有明显的极性。原纤维的形状是一个中空的管状,微管蛋白头尾相接,一个二聚体的 α-微管蛋白亚基与另一个二聚体的 β-微管蛋白亚基接触,如图 60-1 所示。因此,原纤维的一端将暴露 α-微管蛋白亚基,而另一端将暴露 β-微管蛋白亚基。这些末端分别被称为正端和负端。原纤维以相同的极性平行排列,因此,在微管中的正端,只有 β-微管亚基暴露,而另一端负端,只有 α-微管蛋白亚基暴露。在正端,有三磷酸鸟苷(guanosine triphosphate, GTP)结合、快速组装和网状延伸,而负端由于组装速度慢出现缩短。微管的独特功能与它们的聚合动力学有关,包括细胞内 α/β 微管蛋白二聚体和微管聚合物之间,以及 α/β 微管蛋白二聚体持续地释放到可溶性微管蛋白池之间的平衡。微管蛋白聚合是通过成核-伸长机制,短小的微管的"核"缓慢形成之后,α/β 微管蛋白二聚

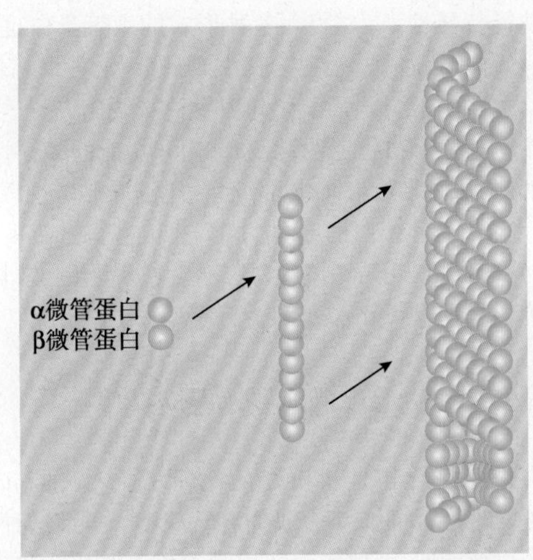

图 60-1　α/β-微管蛋白二聚体的原理图模型，以蓝色和黄色的阴影代表其单体。二聚体线性地结合形成原丝，然后再横向相连形成微管的空心圆柱形壁。原丝可以在微管轴上慢慢地扭曲，尽管这里显示的是平行的，就像在包含 13 个原丝的微管中一样。在大多数微管中，横向接触涉及 α-α 和 β-β 单体相互作用。因此，每种类型的单体都沿微管周围的浅螺旋路径接触

体在其末端可逆的、非共价的连接导致微管快速伸长。在微管的两端，游离的 α/β 微管蛋白二聚体和微管之间保持动态平衡[1-7]。每个微管蛋白分子与两分子 GTP 相连。N 端与 α 微管蛋白结合的 GTP 不可替换，而在 E 端与 β 微管蛋白结合的核苷可以与游离的鸟苷二磷酸（guanosine diphosphate，GDP）交换。微管的组装过程利用 GTP 的水解提供能量。

微管蛋白以高亲和力结合 GTP，并且随着 GTP 连接到延伸着的微管末端，GTP 也被逐渐水解为 GDP 和 Pi[11]。Pi 最终分解，留下由微管连接 GDP 组成的微管骨架。直到微管蛋白亚基与微管分离，GDP 核苷酸一直保持不可替换状态。尽管在微管的每一端同时发生微管蛋白的聚合和解离，导致微管的伸长和缩短，但是在更活跃的正端处的总长度变化比在负端处的长度变化更为明显。如果在体外观察聚合反应，会发现初始存在延迟期，之后微管会快速合成直到达到平台期。在完整的细胞中，微管的负端锚定在两个微管组织中心（microtubule-organizing center，MTOC），而正端则游离在细胞质中自由地向细胞边缘辐射。中心体作为大多数细胞的主要 MTOC，是有丝分裂纺锤体的起源点；同时，高尔基体也可以作为微管成核的平台[12]。中心体的成核是对称的，而高尔基相关的微管成核可以形成一个不对称的微管网络。在间期，MTOC 组织微管向细胞质提供极性，并参与蛋白质的运输，其中包括多种癌蛋白。

踏板运动和动态不稳定性

在活细胞中有两个主要过程控制着微管的动力学[1-15]。第一种称为“踏板”，是微管一端的净生长和另一端的净缩短[8]。在有丝分裂后期纺锤体的形成和染色体的分离以及其他微管相关活动都是通过踏板运动发生的。第二种动态过程称为动态不稳定，是指在微管的正端在缓慢持续生长和快速缩短的状态之间的自由转换状态[11,13-15]，动态不稳定依赖于 GTP 的水解和交换循环。从机制上看，位于微管末端的 GTP 帽模型，由 GTP 或 GDP 与相关的非交换性 Pi 组成，其可以保持微管稳定，从而使微管在正端生长，这很可能解释了动态不稳定的过程。从本质上讲，微管生长和缩短之间的转换取决于微管的末端构象，其中生长的末端由一层 GTP-微管亚基（GTP 帽）稳定，而缩短端则失去了 GTP，允许最终的 GDP-微管二聚体与微管点阵分离[16]。

微管与有丝分裂

在有丝分裂开始的时候，连接在 MTOC 上的间期排列的微管会分解，取而代之的是更活泼的纺锤体微管[2,13,17,18]。此时在 MTOC 中的是另一种微管蛋白 γ-微管蛋白，它与其他蛋白质结合形成一个称为 γ-微管环状复合体的锁垫圈状结构。这种复合物是 α/β-微管蛋白二聚体开始聚合的模板；它将负端盖住，使微管的生长发生在游离的正端[19]。最近发现的一种叫做 augmin 的蛋白质复合物，其与 γ-微管环复合体相互作用，增加有丝分裂纺锤体起源处周围的微管密度，因此它对于 MTOC 依赖的纺锤形微管的形成至关重要[20]。当新组装的微管的纺锤形阵列组织起来时，核膜破裂并释放致密的染色体和有丝分裂前复制的中心体，分列在有丝分裂纺锤体的两极。有丝分裂过程中动态不稳定的速度加快，从而使有丝分裂纺锤体形成并附着在染色体上。在大多数细胞中，有丝分裂进展迅速，构成有丝分裂纺锤体的高度动态的微管使它们对破坏聚合运动的抗菌药物敏感[3,13]。

有丝分裂纺锤体的装配和功能离不开微管的动态不稳定性和踏板运动，而构成有丝分裂纺锤体的微管的高度动态性是中期染色体的精确定位和其附着在有丝分裂纺锤体上以及后期染色体分离所必需的。动态不稳定性和踏板运动使有丝分裂纺锤体的微管能够进行大范围的生长和缩短，这通常被称为搜索和捕捉，本质上是探测细胞质，直到运动中它们的正端连接到染色体上。即使是单个染色体也不能达到双极附着在纺锤体上，也许是由于药物诱导的微管动力学抑制，细胞不会度过前中期/中期阶段，而是会因为一系列纺锤体组装检查点的复杂过程而发生凋亡[21,22]。虽然在低浓度的微管抑制剂存在下，有丝分裂纺锤体也能形成，但细胞无法通过有丝分裂检查点进入有丝分裂在中期/后期[13,17,22]。这种有丝分裂纺锤体动力学的干扰在关键的有丝分裂检查点可能延缓细胞周期的进展，最终通过检查点和有丝分裂激酶复杂的相互作用触发细胞凋亡[7,13,17,22]。在未受干扰的正常状态下，染色体倍数的波动、动态不稳定和踏板运动，包括在着丝点处的纺锤体中加入微管蛋白，在纺锤体极处丢失微管蛋白，在中期对染色体产生强大的张力，促进细胞加速进入有丝分裂后期。在后期，附着在染色体上的微管经历缩短，而另一个微管亚群，称为极间微管，变长，导致染色体的极性运动。抗菌药物抑制纺锤体-微管的踏板运动和动态不稳定性，降低纺锤体张力，阻碍从中期到后期的进程，从而触发细胞死亡[3-5,13,17,18,23,24]。在间期微管曾被报道过存在相似的阳性端帽活性，是由腺瘤性息肉病大肠埃希菌蛋白 Forins 和 EB1 介导的。

微管动力学与功能多样性的调控

微管蛋白胞内池与微管聚合物之间动态平衡的方向受多种因素的影响，这些因素调节聚合所需微管蛋白的临界浓度，包括 GTP/GDP 比值、离子微环境、细胞周期调节剂以及各种微管相关蛋白（microtubule-associated protein，MAP）和调节蛋白[1,4,5,25,26]。MAP 在不同组织中参与微管的多种功能，可作为直接和间接靶点用于肿瘤治疗[26]。大多数的 MAP 有利于微管聚合，包括低分子量的 tau 蛋白（分子量 40～60kD）和高分子量（200～300kD）的 MAP1、MAPc（腺苷三磷酸酶）、MAP2、MAP4 和 XMAP215 等[4,25-27]。其他调节蛋白包括 stathmin、XKCM1、XKIF2 和剑蛋白，它们负责微管的解聚[27]。MAP 通常有两个结合域，一个与微管结合，促进微管聚合的初始成核步骤，另一个负责微管与其他细胞成分的连接。当然还有其他的 MAP，例如动力蛋白（GTPases）和驱动蛋白（ATPases），发挥微管运动蛋白的作用，将化学能转化为动能，使各种溶质和亚细胞器沿微管移动[1,4,5,25-27]。运动蛋白在有丝分裂、减数分裂前期活动和细胞器转运中起着关键作用，是抗肿瘤治疗的潜在靶点之一（见“靶向有丝分裂的运动蛋白和激酶”部分）[28,29]。

除 MAP 外，同型异构体的存在和翻译后修饰的差异也是微管在不同组织中的功能多样性的原因之一。在人类细胞中，α-微管蛋白和 β-微管蛋白至少有 6 种亚型，它们的 C 端氨基酸序列存在多样性，并由一个多基因家族编码，该家族在进化过程中一直高度保守[4,30-33]。微管蛋白亚型在不同组织中的表达分析显示了一种尽管高度保守但复杂的同型分布模式，提示了它们的功能特异性[1,4,5,25-27]。各种形式的微管蛋白也经历了各种翻译后修饰，通过微管结合酶实现磷酸化、去甲基化、聚糖苷化、δ2 微管蛋白形成、乙酰化和多聚谷氨酸化[34,35]。翻译后修饰赋予微管聚合物稳定性，以及结构和功能的多样性[34,35]。当微管解聚时，大多数修饰被可溶性酶迅速逆转。翻译后修饰一般发生在 α-微管蛋白的 C 端，这个区域富含带负电的谷氨酸，使微管伸出相对不规则的尾端，并接触运动蛋白。因此，翻译后修饰似乎可以调节运动蛋白与微管的相互作用。

长春碱类化合物：简介及适应证

长春碱类化合物是从粉红色长春花（*catharanthus roseus* G. Don）中自然提取的或半合成的含氮碱类。早期这种植物由于具有降血糖活性，因此作为药用筛选出这些化合物，但是最终相比之下发现，它的细胞毒作用的重要性更大。许多长春碱类化合物经历了广泛研究，但只有长春新碱（vincristine，VCR）、长春碱（vinblastine，VBL）和长春瑞滨（vinorelbine，VRL）被批准在美国和其他地方使用，而长春氟宁（vinflunine，VFL）和去乙酰长春酰胺（vindesine，VDS）只在某些地区被批准使用。硫酸长春新碱脂质体注射剂也被美国和某些地方批准使用。

长春碱类化合物是由两个基本的多环单元组成的二聚体结构（图 60-2），一个吲哚核（catharanthine）和一个二氢吲哚核（文朵灵）与其他复杂成分连接在一起[36-38]。从结构上看，除了在文朵灵核上有一个取代物外，VCR 和 VBL 在结构上是相同的，VCR 和 VBL 分别具有甲酰基和甲基。虽然这种微小的差异并没有从根本上改变这些药物的机制和与微管蛋白的结

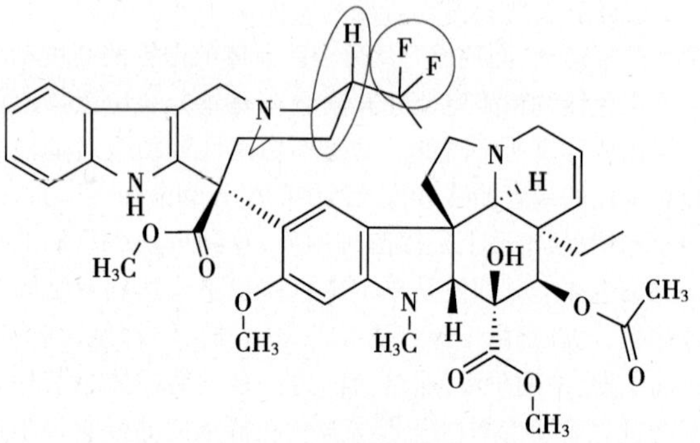

长春氟宁

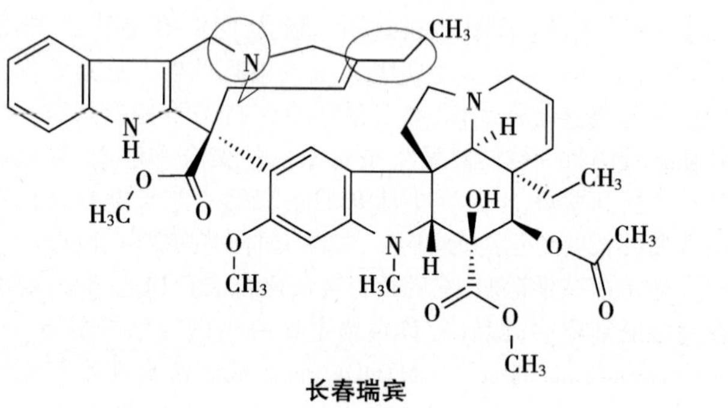

长春瑞宾

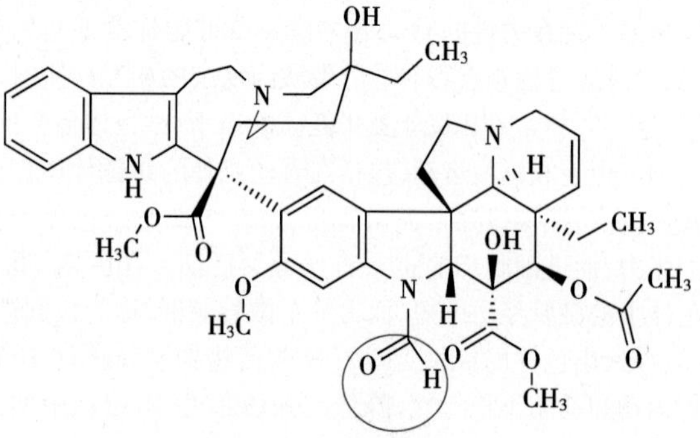

长春新碱

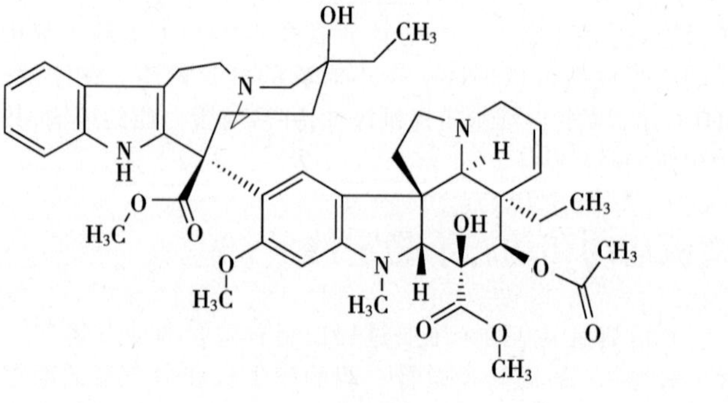

长春碱

图 60-2 长春碱类化合物的化学结构，以长春碱为参照物进行结构修改

合特性，但是 VCR 和 VBL 的抗癌谱和毒理学作用却有很大的不同[4,36-41]。

VCR 更常用于治疗儿童恶性肿瘤，部分原因是儿童恶性肿瘤对 VCR 的内在敏感性普遍较高，并且儿童对 VCR 的治疗剂量具有更好的耐受性。然而，无论是儿童还是成年人，VCR 都是治疗急性淋巴细胞白血病（acute lymphocytic leukemia，ALL）、慢性髓系白血病（chronic myeloid leukemia，CML）急淋变以及霍奇金淋巴瘤和非霍奇金淋巴瘤的化疗方案的重要组成部分。VCR 在肾母细胞瘤、尤因肉瘤、神经母细胞瘤和横纹肌肉瘤的联合治疗中也发挥了一定的作用，并可用于治疗多发性骨髓瘤（VAD 方案：VCR、阿霉素和地塞米松），以及复发性小细胞肺癌、软组织肉瘤和骨肉瘤等。该试剂还被用作联合方案的组成部分，如 PCV（丙哌嗪，洛莫司汀和 VCR）方案，用于早期和晚期间变性星形细胞瘤和少突胶质细胞瘤[42]。更重要的是，在其他疾病的治疗中也有广泛的用途，如 VCR 联合血小板输注在治疗难治性自身免疫性血小板减少方面是有效的；VCR 在治疗非恶性和免疫介导的疾病如自身免疫性溶血性贫血、溶血性尿毒症综合征、血栓性血小板减少性紫癜和类固醇依赖性肾病综合征方面也被证实有一定治疗作用[38-40,43]。

VBL 一直是生殖细胞恶性肿瘤和某些晚期淋巴瘤化疗的主要药物之一[38]。多年来，由顺铂、VBL 和博来霉素组成的 PVB 方案是生殖细胞癌的标准治疗方案；然而，由于顺铂-依托泊苷方案具有更少的毒副作用，这种情况下大多数 VBL 已被依托泊苷所取代。对于霍奇金淋巴瘤，VBL 常与阿霉素、博来霉素、长春新碱和达卡巴嗪（doxorubicin，bleomycin，vinblastine，and dacarbazine，ABVD）联合使用[38]。这种方案要么单独使用，要么与氮芥、VCR、普罗嗪和泼尼松（nitrogen mustard，VCR，procarbazine，and prednisone，MOPP）交替使用，这些药与 ABVD 无交叉耐药，或者混合使用（MOPP/ABV），即同时包括 VCR 和 VBL。已观察到 VBL 作为单一药物或与其他抗癌药物联合应用于晚期和/或复发性乳腺癌、膀胱癌和肺癌，以及卡波西肉瘤、绒毛膜癌、慢性粒细胞白血病终末期、皮肤 T 细胞淋巴瘤和组织细胞增生症 X 的抗癌活性[38]。由于其对血小板的亲和力，输注 VBL 或 VBL 联合血小板对某些难治性自身免疫性血小板减少症患者是有效的[38,43]。VBL 也单独或与其他药物联合治疗卡波西肉瘤和膀胱癌、乳腺癌和某些类型的中枢神经系统恶性肿瘤[38,44-48]。

半合成的 VBL 衍生物长春瑞滨（5′-norhydro-VBL，VRL），它在长春碱核上进行了结构修饰，使得与其他长春碱类化合物相比，其亲脂性大大提高，在美国被批准单药或与顺铂联合使用治疗非小细胞肺癌，并在其他地方批准用于治疗晚期乳腺癌患者。该药物在晚期卵巢癌和淋巴瘤中也显示了临床活性，但尚未明确其在治疗这些癌症中的独特机制。VRL 还被证明可以为老年和/或工作能力降低的晚期乳腺癌和肺癌患者提供良好的治疗效果[4,38,44-48]。

其他的一些长春碱类化合物或经典长春碱类化合物的新衍生物可用于治疗恶性肿瘤。一种研究广泛的长春碱类化合物去乙酰长春酰胺（desacetyl-VBL caroxyamide），它是 VBL 的半合成衍生物以及人类代谢产物，20 世纪 70 年代在美国以外的几个地区进行过研究。一些报告中显示，非小细胞肺癌患者对于 VDS 联合顺铂或丝裂霉素的应答率似乎优于标准方案或单一使用这些药物[38,40,41]。此外，在 ALL、CML 急变期、恶性黑色素瘤、各种儿科实体瘤和晚期肾癌、乳腺癌和食管癌中已经观察到了抗癌活性。此外，双氟化长春碱类化合物 VFL 在膀胱、乳腺、肺和其他部位癌症中显示出显著的临床活性[4,38,44-52]。在欧洲，VFL 被批准作为既往含铂方案失败的晚期尿路上皮癌患者的治疗方案[52]。

最后，VCR 的基于鞘磷脂和胆固醇的脂质体纳米粒制剂在美国注册，用于治疗至少两种治疗方案后疾病进展的费城染色体阴性的成人 ALL 患者[53,54]。尽管脂质体制剂允许递送更高的 VCR 剂量，在循环系统停留的时间更长，并且与标准 VCR 相比，将更多的 VCR 递送至靶组织，但是新形式的 VCR 的获益优于标准 VCR 的程度仍然未知。

作用机制

长春碱类化合物主要通过破坏微管功能来诱导细胞毒性，特别是组成有丝分裂纺锤体的微管，导致分裂停滞于中期导致细胞死亡[2-7,36-38,55-59]。然而，它们有许多与微管有关或无关的其他活性，包括抑制蛋白质和核酸的合成、升高氧化的谷胱甘肽水平、改变膜脂和脂质代谢、升高环腺苷酸（cyclic adenosine monophosphate，cAMP）水平和通过钙-钙调蛋白阻断 cAMP 磷酸二酯酶的作用[38]。只有在高浓度条件下微管破坏效应才会发生，然而在体内不易达到这一条件，以下药物在临床实践应用中已经实现的纳摩尔浓度可以诱导典型的抗微管作用。长春碱类化合物还破坏血小板和其他富含微管蛋白的细胞的结构完整性。除阻断有丝分裂外，长春碱类化合物和其他抗微管药物扰乱非有丝分裂细胞周期阶段的细胞，由于微管参与了许多非有丝分裂功能，所以这并不难理解[38,57-59]。长春碱类化合物与微管蛋白上的位点（vinca 结构域）迅速并可逆地结合，与紫杉烷类、秋水仙碱、鬼臼毒素和 GTP 不同，但类似于美登素和其他几种植物生物碱。

长春碱类化合物似乎有两个不同亲和力的结合位点[2,4,6,7,10,37,38,51,55-57,60-65]。长春碱类化合物与位于微管末端的高亲和力位点（Kd，1～2μmol）结合导致低浓度条件下（<1μmol）微管蛋白交换的有效抑制。在低长春碱类化合物浓度下，依赖于微管动力学的过程（踏板运动和动态不稳定性）被破坏，但微管总量不受影响。总体导致的结果是中期/后期交界处的有丝分裂阻滞。长春碱类化合物与位于微管两侧的低亲和力位点（Kd，0.25～3.0mmol）结合后，因微管蛋白解聚或微管螺旋成聚合体或原纤维时伸展而形成不完全晶体，而导致微管总量降低，最终导致微管解体。这些作用发生在高药物浓度（>1～2μmol）的情况下，通过一种自传播机制，最初仅涉及药物结合的几个位点，逐渐削弱原纤维之间的横向相互作用，从而暴露新的位点并加强的解聚作用。

长春碱类化合物在中期/后期过渡阶段可诱导有丝分裂的有效阻滞[2,4,66]。核膜破裂后，长春碱类化合物阻止有丝分裂纺锤体的形成，降低染色体着丝点处的张力。虽然染色体可能浓缩，但它们仍然分散在细胞中。染色体沿长轴分离，但仍在着丝粒处附着[2,4,9,13,18,24,58,59,67]。有丝分裂进程停滞在有丝分裂中期，染色体“粘”在纺锤体两极，无法移动到赤道面。后期促进复合物的细胞周期信号被阻断，导致细胞无法从中期向后期过渡，使细胞凋亡随之死亡。在没有分裂后期或胞质分裂的情况下可能会出现细胞周期进展，导致染色质解凝和形成多裂核[2,4,13,24]。构成有丝分裂纺锤体的微管动力学破坏而不解聚，最终诱导细胞凋亡，这其中涉及促凋亡基因的表达以及促凋亡蛋白的激活和抗凋亡蛋白的失活（见“长春碱类化合物的作用机制”和“长春碱类化合物的耐药机制”和“紫杉烷类化合物的作用机制和耐药性”）[2,4,9,13,18,21,23,51,67-72]。然而，诱导凋亡并不取决于是否存在完整的TP53检查点。P21是G_2/M期检查点，控制细胞进入有丝分裂的蛋白质，它的丢失可能通过加速药物损伤的细胞进入细胞分裂期而使肿瘤细胞对长春碱类化合物和紫杉烷敏感[23,68-70]。

长春碱类化合物引起的微管解聚及其对细胞增殖、有丝分裂阻滞和有丝分裂纺锤体断裂的影响出现在一系列研究中，其结果表明，细胞生长抑制与中期阻滞直接相关[18]。在最低有效药物浓度下，中期细胞的增殖和阻断被抑制，而有丝分裂纺锤体很少甚至没有微管的解聚或破坏。随着药物浓度的增加，停止有丝分裂的纺锤体中，无论潜在的机制是什么，微管和染色体以类似于大多数抗菌药物作用的方式分解[2-4,13,14]。

除了它们对肿瘤细胞的直接毒性外，长春碱类化合物以及美登木素生物碱、紫杉醇和各种其他抗微管药物通过抑制与新生血管生成相关的过程而产生出乎意料的抗癌作用[73]。这些抗血管生成效应最可能是由于药物诱导的血管内皮细胞的微管不稳定引起的；然而，这些作用对临床抗癌活性的相对贡献尚不清楚。

不同组织和肿瘤对长春碱类化合物敏感性不同的原因是多因素的。一种可能的解释是组织微管蛋白亚型不同导致的差异敏感性，这可能影响细胞内药物的积累和药物与微管蛋白的结合[4,33,74-75]。另一种可能是微管相关蛋白和微管蛋白转录后修饰的类型和浓度的差异可能影响药物与微管蛋白的相互作用，以及细胞通透性和滞留性的差异，可能会影响长春碱类化合物和微管蛋白形成的复合物的形成和稳定性[76]。其他可能的因素包括微管蛋白亚型的差异（见“长春碱类化合物的耐药机制”和“紫杉醇的耐药机制”）、GTP含量、GTP水解速率和细胞渗透率[74,77-81]。

耐药机制

大量临床前模型显示，肿瘤细胞对长春花生物碱类药物会迅速产生耐药性，这可能与药物积累和存储减少有关。长春花生物碱的耐药性主要涉及两种机制。第一种是“经典”多效性或叫多药耐药（multidrug-resistant，MDR），可以分为原发性耐药和继发性耐药。尽管许多介导MDR的蛋白已经被鉴定出来，但最广为人知的是ATP结合盒（ATP-bingding cassette，ABC）转运蛋白，它属于已知最大的转运蛋白基因家族，可在细胞间转运多种底物[82,83]。这些细胞内和细胞外的跨膜蛋白运输内源性和外源性物质，形成了细胞对长春花生物碱类和其他高分子天然产物的耐药性。ABC转运蛋白包括一种具有通透性的糖蛋白（permeability glycoproteins，Pgp）、由MDR1基因编码蛋白MDR1（ABC亚家族B1）和多药耐药蛋白（MRP；ABC亚家族C2）[82]。

MDR1为分子量为170kDa的Pgp，属于一种能量依赖跨膜泵，主要调控大量疏水底物由细胞内向细胞外转运[82]。该蛋白在多种正常组织中组成性过表达，其中包括肾小管上皮细胞、结肠黏膜、肾上腺髓质，以及源自组成性过表达Pgp的组织的肿瘤组织。Pgp是一种ATP酶，可与长春花生物碱类药物结合，并将该类药物泵出细胞外，这一过程需要ATP形式的能量。MDR表型也赋予细胞对其他天然高分子化合物的交叉耐药，如紫杉类、蒽环类、鬼臼乙叉苷和秋水仙碱。与长春花生物碱耐药性相关的特异性Pgp和秋水仙碱或紫杉烷耐药性细胞的Pgp相比，在消化后显示出轻微的抗原和氨基酸序列差异以及不同的氨基酸图谱[84-87]。事实上，在VCR耐药的细胞单克隆中产生的两种蛋白，主要发生了翻译后N-糖基化和磷酸化修饰，进而导致结构多样性，这解释了与赋予MDR的其他药物相比，所使用的特定药物的耐药程度更大，也可能解释MDR细胞间耐药的变化模式。药物敏感肿瘤细胞与长春花生物碱耐药细胞株中细胞膜上的神经节苷脂在组成上存在差异，这些耐药机制产生的临床结果尚不清楚。然而一项儿童急性淋巴细胞白血病的研究显示，体外测定的VCR耐药性与P-糖蛋白的过表达并无相关性[88]。

MRP1蛋白是一种与MDR1具有15%氨基酸同源的跨膜蛋白，其分子量为190kDa，体外研究显示，它参与细胞对长春花生物碱类药物的耐药[39,82,83,89-92]。MRP1表达于多种肿瘤组织，包括肺癌、结肠癌、乳腺癌、膀胱癌、前列腺癌以及白血病，并且MRP1表达与细胞多药耐药表型相关联。MRP1转运谷胱甘肽修饰的烷化剂和外源性化合物如依托泊苷、阿霉素等，但MRP1只导致外源性化合物产生耐药。MRP1的耐药谱还包括长春花生物碱和甲氨蝶呤[39,82,83,89-92]。尽管科学家已鉴定了几种在体外与长春花生物碱细胞耐药相关的ABC转运体，与MDR1和MRP1的耐药机制比较，临床中这些ABC转运体的原发或继发性的耐药机制尚不清楚。

体外经不同结构和功能特点的药物处理后，由MDR1和MRP介导的药物耐药具有可逆性，如钙通道阻滞剂、钙调素抑制剂、洗涤剂、孕激素、抗雌激素制剂、抗生素、抗高血压药、抗心律失常药、抗疟药和免疫抑制剂，可以逆转耐药，这一直是临床研究的热点[39,82,93,94]。这些耐药逆转剂可直接与P-糖蛋白结合，阻断细胞毒类药物的外排作用，增加了药物在细胞内的浓度。然而，MDR调节剂，尤其是MDR1逆转剂的存在，使耐药调节的临床研究陷入混乱，它可以增加正常细胞对药物的摄取，减少胆汁和药物清除，并导致细胞毒性增强[39,82,93,94]。总而言之，由于MDR1的表达与大量耐药蛋白的过表达相关，因此，针对MDR1和MRP药理调节剂的临床策略未能有效逆转对长春花生物碱的耐药性[82]。

在对长春花生物碱和紫杉类具有耐药的肿瘤细胞中，临床前研究和临床研究中均显示，由于α和β微管蛋白存在基因突变、翻译后修饰、微管蛋白同型异构体的表达，特别是β-Ⅲ微管蛋白同型异构体表达，α和β微管蛋白结构和功能发生改变[95-106]。此外，这些研究表明，β-Ⅲ微管蛋白同型异构体可作为有益的临床预后和预警的标志物。β-Ⅱ微管蛋白的表达似乎依赖于TP53的抑制功能，这也可能与长春花生物碱的耐药性有关[107]。

MAP蛋白，特别是MAP4的过表达也与长春花生物碱耐药性具有相关性[75]。MAP蛋白的过表达和α、β微管蛋白改变，促进了细胞对微管形成抑制剂的耐药性，主要通过增加微管的稳定性、促进纵向二聚体内和纵向二聚体间相互作用和/或原纤维两侧的相互作用等机制抑制微管组装。此外，这些“超稳定"微管两侧对紫杉类药物敏感(参见"紫杉类,耐药机制")。体外经长春花生物碱药物持续作用的肿瘤细胞显示这种微管蛋白的修饰,但是由微管蛋白或 MAP 变异导致的"超稳定"微管分子机制尚不清楚。

细胞对药物的通透性和滞留能力的改变也可影响长春花生物碱-微管蛋白复合物的形成和稳定[51,79,108-114]。细胞可迅速摄取长春花生物碱并在细胞内滞留,依据细胞类型差异,长春花生物碱在细胞内外的浓度比可高达 5~500 倍[80,81]。小鼠白血病细胞中,VCR 的细胞内浓度比细胞外浓度高 5~20 倍,对其他长春花生物碱类药物,其胞内的药物浓度为胞外浓度的 150~500 倍[81,108,115]。细胞对于长春花生物碱的摄入和滞留也存在显著差异,而细胞对长春花生物碱的滞留与药物作用的持续时间和效能相关。如在人离体肝细胞中,VRL 与其他长春花生物碱类药物相比,具有更迅速摄入和代谢的能力[116];在另一个动物模型中进行的研究显示,对于短时间接受药物暴露的细胞,VCR 比 VBL 具有更高的药物效应,其主要依赖 VCR 在细胞内显著的滞留能力。一种药物在细胞内滞留性的主要决定因素是药物的亲脂性。与轴突微管比较,VRL 对有丝分裂纺锤体微管具有更强的破坏作用,这是由于 VRL 长春碱环的差异使 VRL 具有更高的亲脂性,增加了 VRL 在组织内的滞留[114]。相对其他长春花生物碱而言,VRL 治疗具有较低的神经毒性,这主要由于药物滞留和亲脂性差异导致长春花生物碱对轴突微管的不同治疗效果。关于长春花生物碱在细胞内滞留的反应机制尚不完全清楚,但可能与微管蛋白结合特性和其他几个因素相关。不同肿瘤对于药物的摄入能力主要与微管蛋白同型体、吸收和排出的差异性及细胞内药物滞留相关。最后,与制剂载体相关的药代动力学差异似乎影响组织摄取。在临床前研究中,对于 VSLI,脂质体包埋似乎与循环时间和肿瘤细胞通透性增加有关[53]。在施用 VSLI 后,肿瘤摄取 VCR 增加一部分可能是由于脂质体制剂增强了细胞的通透性和滞留能力所致。

药理学

细胞药理学

大部分长春花生物碱的转运主要是与温度无关的非饱和机制,类似于简单扩散,而温度依赖性可饱和过程则不太重要[117]。虽然药物浓度和治疗持续时间是药物蓄积和细胞毒作用的决定因素,但是高于临界阈值浓度的药物暴露持续时间可能是细胞毒作用最重要的药理学决定因素[80]。当治疗持续时间保持不变时,细胞毒作用直接取决于药物的细胞外浓度。对于长时间暴露于 VCR 而言,其浓度在 1~5nmol/L 范围内,可产生 50%的抑制作用[118]。

临床药理学

长春花生物碱的临床药理学在几十年前进行了深入研究,主要反映了这样一个事实,即没有灵敏、特异和可靠的分析方法能够测定毫克级剂量给药后所产生的微小血药浓度。早期研究因为使用放射性标记药物和分析方法,结果可能受到干扰。长春花生物碱类药物,尤其是 VCR 和 VBL,可能发生自发降解,其降解产物可用高压液相色谱(high-pressure liquid chromatography,HPLC)加以分离。放射性标记化合物与 HPLC 结合,改进了各种化学基团的分离方法。放射免疫分析(radioimmunoassay,RIA)和酶联免疫吸附分析(enzyme-linked immunosorbent assay,ELISA)方法可以测量 pmol 级的药物浓度;然而,这些方法不能区分母体化合物和其衍生物,因此可能无法提供足够关于降解产物和代谢物的定量信息。为了解决这一问题,具有更高敏感性和特异性的 mAb 已被应用于改良的 RIA 和 ELISA 方法。此外,近来提取方法的进步和检测方法学的新技术发展提高了色谱方法的灵敏度和特异性,尤其是串联质谱和高效液相质谱的联用。表 60-1 总结了长春花生物碱类药物的药代动力学特征,其全面展示了静脉给药短暂注射后的人血浆三相清除情况。除 VSLI 外,这些药物的药代动力学行为典型表现为分布广泛(volumes of distribution,Vd),早期清除率高,终末半衰期长,主要在肝脏代谢,通过胆汁/粪便排出。所有的长春花生物碱类药物都很类似,有相对较短的 α 和 β 相,这可能是由于药物在外周组织中快速分布和吸收,与微管蛋白结合并形成血液成分。然而,终末(γ)相相对持续时间较长,是由于组织隔离并且缓慢释放药物,记录显示变化可达 4 倍之多。

长春新碱

长春新碱(vincristine,VCR)在给药后迅速从中央室分配到外周室。可广泛与血浆蛋白和成形的血液成分结合,特别是含有大量微管蛋白的血小板,负荷 VCR 的血小板被巨噬细胞吞噬后可直接损伤巨噬细胞的功能,减少血小板的破坏,这是使用 VCR 治疗血小板消耗异常疾病,如难治性血小板减少症的主要原因[38,43]。相比之下,VCR 和所有其他长春花生物碱类药物很难穿过血脑屏障,可能是因为分子量大,并且是 ABC 转运泵的有高亲和力的底物,而 ABC 转运泵能保持血脑屏障完整性。给予常规剂量($1.4mg/m^2$)治疗时,通过快速静脉输注,血药浓度峰值可达 0.4μmol/L[38,117,119-124]。总 VCR 的清除比较缓慢,这反映出其与组织有效结合并可缓慢释放。已有报道显示其半衰期($T_{1/2}$)可达 23~85 小时[38,117,119-124]。VCR 主要由肝胆系统代谢和排泄。放射性标记的 VCR 给药 72 小时后,尿中可检测到接近 12%的放射性活性产物(其中 50%是代谢产物),粪便中可检测到接近 70%的放射性活性产物(其中 40%是代谢产物)[38,117,119-126]。在人类和动物实验中都可检测到多达 11 种代谢物[113]。目前从鉴定的 VCR 代谢物的性质来看,该药物主要由肝细胞色素 P450 CYP3A 代谢,无论从人类胆汁中分离出的 4-去乙酰 VCR 和 N-去甲酸 VCR,还是从经 VCR 培养的胆汁中发现的 4′-脱氧-3′羟基-VCR 和 3′,4′-环氧 VCR 的含氮氧化物都提示这一点[38,117,119-127]。尽管证据很少,但是有研究显示血药浓度峰值和全身暴露是 VCR 导致的神经毒性的决定因素,这一观点目前仍存在争议[127]。

长春碱

长春碱(vinblastine,VBL)的药理学表现与 VCR 类似。VBL 以标准剂量快速静脉注射后,血药浓度的峰值接近 0.4μmol/L[38,117,128]。药物的组织分布也很广泛。与 VCR 相似,VBL 与血浆蛋白和成形血液成分结合的量也相当大。不仅如此,VBL 分布很迅速,α 相和 β 相半衰期只有 4 分钟和 1.6 小时。有报道显示,终末相半衰期为 20~24 小时。与 VCR 一样,VBL 也是主要通过肝胆系统进行代谢。VBL 的主要代谢模式是肝脏代谢,胆汁排泄。通过粪便排泄的母体化合物很少,这表明代谢是相当主要的。细胞色素 P450 CYP3A 的亚型主要用于其生物转化[116]。至少有一种代谢产物,4-去乙酰基-VBL 或 VDS,和母体化合物的活性是一样的,可从人体中检出,也可从尿液和粪便中少量检出。

表 60-1 长春花生物碱类药物的药代动力学及毒理学特征

	长春新碱	长春碱	长春地辛	长春瑞滨	长春氟宁	硫酸长春新碱脂质体注射液
标准成人剂量/($mg \cdot m^{-2}$)	1~2(每周)	6~8(每周)	3~4(每周)	15~30(每周)	320(每3周)	2.25(每周)
药代动力学特征	三相	三相	三相	三相	多相	二相
血浆半衰期						
α/min	<5	<5	<5	<5	—	—
β/min	50~155	53~99	55~99	49~168	—	—
γ/min	23~85	20~64	20~24	18~49	40	7.66[a]
清除率/($L \cdot h^{-1} \cdot kg^{-1}$)	0.16	0.74	0.25	0.4~1.29	0.64	0.35(L/h)
主要途径	肝脏代谢,胆汁清除	肝脏代谢,胆汁清除	肝脏代谢,胆汁清除	肝脏代谢,胆汁清除	肝脏代谢,胆汁清除(≈66%);肾脏(≈33%)	肝脏代谢,胆汁清除
主要毒性	神经毒性	中性粒细胞减少症	中性粒细胞减少症	中性粒细胞减少症	中性粒细胞减少症	中性粒细胞减少症
其他毒性	便秘,SIADH	脱发,神经毒性,黏膜炎	脱发,神经毒	神经毒性呕吐,便秘,黏膜炎	神经毒性,肌痛,疲劳,厌食,便秘,恶心/呕吐,贫血,注射部位,血小板减少,低钠血症	神经毒性,血小板减少症,贫血

[a] 表示非隔室半衰期。
SIADH,抗利尿激素分泌失调症。

长春瑞滨

长春瑞滨(vinorelbine,VRL)的药理学行为和其他长春花生物碱类药物相似,血药浓度下降呈双指数模型或三指数模型方式。静脉给药后,血药浓度迅速下降,然后进入相当缓慢的清除相($T_{1/2}$,18~49 小时)[38,46,47,129,130]。据报道,血浆蛋白结合率为 80%~91%,主要与 α_1-酸糖蛋白、白蛋白和脂蛋白结合。VRL 在体内广泛分布,并大量储存在体内除脑和睾丸之外的所有组织中。该药物还与血小板大量结合。VRL 在体内广泛分布反映出药物具有亲脂性,在长春花生物碱类药物中是最高的。虽然报道显示 VRL 在人肺组织中的浓度比在血浆中的浓度高 300 倍,分别是 VDS 和 VCR 在肺内浓度的 3.4 倍和 13.8 倍,但是组织与血浆分布的比例仅为 20∶80。经肝脏代谢和胆汁排泄的代谢物和 VRL 是药物代谢的主要方式[8,46,47,129-132]。接近 33%~80% 的 VRL 以原药形式通过粪便排泄,而通过尿液排泄的仅占 16%~30%的药物总代谢量,且大多数都是 VRL 代谢产物。细胞色素 P450 亚型 CYP3A 主要参与人体的生物转化过程[46-48,132-137]。主要代谢产物为 4-O-去乙酰-VRL、3,6-环氧-VRL 和几种羟基-VRL 异构体。大多数代谢产物没有生物活性。虽然 4-O-去乙酰-VRL 的活性可能与 VRL 一样,但是由于其浓度较小,因此无关紧要。

一项研究发现,在肝功能正常的老年患者和年轻患者中,VRL 的全身清除率[1.2L/(h·kg)]和平均 $T_{1/2}$(大约为 26 小时)是相似的。如果患者的肝转移病灶累计超过脏器的 75%,对药物清除率具有不利影响;在这些患者中,药物清除率可以通过单乙基甘油二甲基苯胺的清除实验加以预测,该实验可以评价 CYP3A4 的功能[137]。在评估 VRL 药代动力学时,可以选择地塞米松作为检验 CYP3A4 代谢的探针[131]。虽然血清中胆红素的浓度无法准确预测 VRL 清除率,但是在少数患者中的确发现胆红素水平明显升高与清除率显著降低相关。VRL 在口服时具有生物活性。在动物实验中,服用氚标记的 VRL 后,可以检测到 100%的放射活性,而在人体实验中,经过粉末填充和液体填充的胶囊形式给药后,母体化合物的生物利用度分别为 43%和 27%,食物对凝胶填充胶囊的生物利用度产生的影响可忽略不计[129,138,139]。给药后 1~2 小时达到峰浓度(C_{max}),个体间差异适中。

长春氟宁

已证实长春氟宁(vinflunine,VFL)的药代动力学在临床相关剂量(30~400mg/m^2)下是线性的[49,50]。VFL 在静脉内给药后先经过多指数衰减,处于快速初始分布阶段。VFL 与其他长春花生物碱类似,其末相的 Vd 很大(2.42L/kg 或 35L/kg),表明 VFL 广泛分布到富含微管蛋白的大组织隔室[49,50]。VFL 的总清除率很大[43.9L/h,0.640L/(h·kg)],反映了其最初的快速分布并与富含微管蛋白的组织结合。VFL 清除相 $T_{1/2}$ 约为 40 小时,这反映了它从外周室中清除缓慢。VFL 与人血浆蛋白中度结合(67.2%)。在临床可达到的 VFL 浓度范围内,蛋白质结合是不饱和的,主要涉及高密度脂蛋白和血清白蛋白;与 α_1-酸性糖蛋白和血小板的结合可忽略不计(<5%)。三分之二的 VFL 通过肝脏代谢和胆汁排泄处理,肾脏排泄占三分之一[140,141]。除主要代谢物,由多种酯酶形成的 4-O-脱乙酰-VFL(DVFL)外,肝脏代谢由 CYP3A4 介导。DVFL 与母体化合物活性相当,清除相 $T_{1/2}$ 约 120 天。在体外研究中,尚未证实 VFL 抑制或诱导 CYP3A4 和其他 CYP 代谢酶;然而,VFL 与酮康唑共同给药,分别导致 VFL 和 DVFL 暴露增加 30%和 50%。尽管 VFL 具有广泛的肝脏代谢和排泄,但在一项研究中,25 名患有不同程度肝功能不全的患者,他们的 VFL 和 DVFL 药代动力学相似。尽管如此,还是建议对肝功能不全患者进行 VFL 剂量调整(见"给药方法、剂量和方案")[142]。与年龄<70 岁的对照组相比,≥80 岁患者的 VFL 清除率显著降低,建议老年患者(≥75 岁)减少剂量(见"给药方法、剂量和方案")。

硫酸长春新碱脂质体注射液

与传统的非脂质体给药相比,硫酸长春新碱脂质体注射液(vincristine sulfate liposome injection,VSLI)给药后 VCR 的药代动力学表现为 VCR 中心腔室的清除率要低得多[53]。VSLI 脂质体的脂质组成和大约 100ηm 的平均粒径有助于低蛋白质结合，导致纳米颗粒的循环时间延长[53]。体外蛋白质结合试验表明，VSLI 吸收的人血浆蛋白量可忽略不计。在体外人血浆试验中，24 小时释放大约 18%～39%的被脂质体包裹的 VCR。这些特征可能是在肿瘤和巨噬细胞吞噬系统（例如，淋巴结、骨髓、脾和肝）的组织中 VSLI 优先积累的原因，可能是由于这些组织中微血管孔更大，以及通透性和滞留能力较强[143]。在人肿瘤异种移植物的小鼠研究中，使用单剂量 VSLI 后，VSLI 在肿瘤中的累积速度明显快于非肿瘤组织[144]。与非肿瘤组织相比，肿瘤组织中药物的间质含量在 1 小时时约高出 70 倍，48 小时时仍保持较高水平。结合起来看，这些分布数据与 VSLI 从循环中清除、在肿瘤部位积聚的过程一致，VSLI 在肿瘤组织中充当一个储库，在局部释放 VCR 以增强抗癌活性。

人类受试者接受 VSLI（剂量为 2.25mg/m^2）治疗后，平均血浆清除率为 345ml/h [53]。峰值血浆浓度（C_{max}）值平均为 1 220ng/ml，而消除半衰期（$T_{1/2}$）平均为 7.66 小时，总 Vd 和稳态 Vd 的平均值分别为 3.57L 和 2.91L。在静脉内给 VSLI 后，96 小时后粪便排泄占给药药物的 69%，尿液排泄不足 8%。

药物相互作用

长春花生物碱类药物，尤其是 VCR 和 VBL，在体外实验中均显示能增加甲氨蝶呤在肿瘤细胞内聚集，这个调节作用是由长春花生物碱类药物的药物外排阻滞效应介导的。但是，体内研究发现，要实现这个效应的 VCR 的最小浓度（0.1μmol/L）是瞬间达到的[145-147]。体外研究还发现，长春花生物碱类药物可以抑制鬼臼素向细胞内流入，降低细胞毒性，但是这一效应的临床结果仍然未知[148]。左旋天冬酰胺酶可以降低长春花生物碱类药物，特别是 VCR 的肝脏清除率，因此合用可能会导致毒性增加。为了尽可能减少这种相互作用，推荐 VCR 在左旋天冬酰胺酶给药前 12～24 小时给药。在 VFL 和聚乙二醇化脂质体多柔比星之间可以观察到药代动力学相互作用，分别导致 15%～30%的增加以及 VFL 和阿霉素暴露降低 2～3 倍，但对于阿霉素和代谢物的浓度没有影响。在体外研究中，这种变化可能与脂质体上吸附 VFL 和两种化合物的血液分布改变有关。因此，联合用药时应谨慎。基于体外研究的结果，VFL 与紫杉烷、紫杉醇和多西紫杉醇（CYP3A 底物）之间可能存在相互作用。

长春花生物碱类药物治疗导致的癫痫发作与苯妥英钠浓度未达到治疗剂量有关，很可能是由于该药物诱导了 CYP3A 介导的苯妥英钠清除[149-152]。在 VCR 和 VBL 治疗后 1～10 天，都会显示苯妥英钠水平降低。任何长春花生物碱类药物与红霉素、伊曲康唑、酮康唑、利托那韦、酮康唑、葡萄柚汁和其他 CYP3A 抑制剂一起使用时，都可能由于肝脏代谢减少而导致严重毒性反应[41,152,153]。应避免使用诱导 CYP3A4 的药物，如利福平和贯叶连翘（圣约翰草），因为它们可能加速长春花生物碱的清除并增加药物暴露[50]。与戊巴比妥和 H_2 组胺拮抗剂同时给药时，也会通过调节肝细胞色素 P450 的代谢过程而影响 VCR 的清除[152,154]。另一种可能存在潜在的药物相互发生作用的情况出现在同时有卡波西肉瘤（Kaposi's sarcoma）和获得性免疫缺陷综合征的患者身上，需要同时接受 3′-叠氮-3′脱氧胸腺嘧啶（AZT）和长春花生物碱类药物的治疗，长春花生物碱类药物会抑制醛糖酸化 AZT 为 5′-O 醛糖酸[155]。另有一系列严重的毒性反应见诸报道，包括抗利尿激素分泌异常综合征（syndrome of inappropriate antidiuretic hormone secretion，SIADH）、双侧脑神经麻痹、周围神经病变、脑神经麻痹、心力衰竭，以及同时接受硝苯地平和伊曲康唑治疗的儿童 ALL 患者在 VCR 治疗后出现的心血管副作用，提示这些药物可能增加长春花生物碱类药物的神经毒性和心血管毒性[154]。最后，由于同时使用 P450 诱导皮质类固醇类药物，使 P450 的代谢发生变化，导致儿童体内 VCR 药动学出现明显的个体之间和个体内的差异[150,151]。联合使用丝裂霉素 C 和长春花生物碱类药物与肺毒性有关（参见“毒性，杂项”部分）。

毒性

尽管长春花生物碱类药物的结构和药理学特点相似，但是其主要毒性反应不同。VCR 的主要毒性是神经毒性，而 VBL、VDS、VRL、VFL 和 VSLI 的主要毒性是骨髓抑制。但是，如果重复使用 VBL、VDS、VRL、VFL 和 VSL，或在先天敏感的患者中使用这些药物，也会发生外周神经毒性。

神经毒性

尽管长春花生物碱类药物结构相似，但是毒性反应明显不同。所有长春花生物碱类药物都有典型外周神经毒性反应，其中 VCR 的毒性尤其明显。典型的神经毒性反应是外周对称混合性感觉-运动和自主神经的多神经病变[37,38,41,48,156-160]。主要的病理改变为轴突变性和轴突传导减慢，这主要由药物导致微管功能紊乱所致。在开始时，通常仅仅是对称的感觉神经异常以及距离依赖性麻木（首先发生在肢体远端）。随着连续给药，会出现神经性疼痛和深部腱反射缺失，其后可能出现足下垂，腕下垂，运动功能障碍，共济失调和瘫痪。可能发生背痛、骨痛和肢体痛。电生理研究可以明确提示正常神经传导的速度；但是，可以发现感觉和运动神经动作电位的幅度减小以及远端潜伏延迟，与轴突变性相似[156-160]。脑神经毒性反应非常罕见，可能发生声嘶、复视、颌关节疼痛、面神经麻痹以及喉麻痹[38,161,162]。VCR 很少进入颅脑，因此中枢神经系统反应发生极其少见，如混乱、精神状态改变、抑郁、幻觉、焦虑、失眠、惊厥、昏迷、SIADH 以及视觉障碍[38,48,163-165]。也有可能继发于内侧橄榄耳蜗束破坏导致听力受损的相关报道。急性严重的自主神经毒性并不常见，但是在高剂量化疗中（剂量大于 2mg/m^2）或由于肝功能异常导致药物清除下降的患者中可能发生这种毒性[38,158-160,164-169]。自主神经毒性反应表现包括便秘、腹部痉挛、麻痹性肠梗阻、尿潴留、站立性低血压和高血压[38,156-159,166-169]。类似 Guillain-Barré 综合征表现的急性神经毒性反应也有发生[160]。成人接受 VCR 治疗时，当剂量累积到 5～6mg 时就可能开始出现神经毒性反应，当剂量累积到 15～20mg 时症状可能变得严重。神经毒性通常存在蓄积性，结束治疗后通常需要几年时间才可以缓慢恢复。治疗后偶尔也可能发生短时间症状加重[170]。尽管既往认为儿童发生神经毒性的风险低于成人，老年人尤其易感，但是事实上，这些明显的年龄差异可能是源于早年剂量计算不精确，因为在婴儿中选择体表面积计算剂量而在儿童和成人中选择体重计算剂量。在婴儿中，现在根据体重计算 VCR 剂量，由于广泛的组织内分布，从药理学角度看，这样计算可能会更精确。既往存在神经病变，如 Charcot-Marie-Tooth 病，1 型遗传性感觉神经病变，Guillain-Barré 综合征和儿童脊髓灰质炎的患者，更易发生神经毒性[171-173]。在合并肝功能不全或梗阻性肝脏疾病的患者中使用 VCR 会导致发生神经毒性的风险增高，这是由于药物代谢异常，胆汁排泄延迟所致[174,175]。由于 CEP72 启动子区域的遗传多态性，其编码参与微管形成的中心体蛋白，与 VCR 相关的周围神经病变风险和严重程度增加有关[176]。如果这一发现在其他人群中普遍存在，就可为这种广泛使用的抗癌药物的安全剂量提供依据。

目前知道预防长春花生物碱类药物神经毒性的唯一有效方法是间断给药、降低给药剂量以及降低给药频率[166,176,177]。尽管使用了几种解毒剂，包括维生素 B_1、维生素 B_{12}、亚叶酸、维生素 B_6 以及神经活性药物（如镇静剂、安定药、抗惊厥药），但是这些治疗的疗效并不确定[38,127,178-180]。亚叶酸对于接受致死剂量长春花生物碱类药物的老鼠模型具有保护作用，在人类中也有关于其成功挽救过量长春花生物碱类药物治疗的相关报道；但是缺乏前瞻性试验验证。亚叶酸治疗过量 VCR 化疗的推荐剂量为每次 15mg，24 小时内每 3 小时 1 次，然后为每 6 小时 1 次，最少持续 48 小时[38]。另外还有其他具备神经保护作用的药物已取得令人满意的效果。在一项随机双盲试验中，使用 VCR 治疗的同时给予谷氨酸可以降低神经毒性[180]。在动物模型中，促肾上腺皮质激素类似物（ORG2766）对 VCR 引起的神经病变有保护作用，在一项双盲、安慰剂对照的试验中该结果也得到验证[38]。其他几种药物，包括神经生长因子、胰岛素生长因子-1 以及氨磷汀，在试验模型中都证实可以改变神经毒性的自然进程，但是在临床上，这些药物还没有确切证据证明其疗效。与 VCR 相比，VBL、VDS、VRL 和 VFL 导致严重神经毒性的发生率较低[114,181]。与 VCR 或 VBL 相比，VRL 与轴突微管的亲和力低，在临床观察中也已经得到证实[36,38,48,114,181]。VSLI 给药后会发生典型的长春花生物碱类神经毒性，但该药物已经在先前接受 VCR 的患者中进行了大量评估，并且尚未研究 VCR 和 VSLI 的相对神经毒性作用。

骨髓抑制

中性粒细胞减少症是 VBL、VDS、VRL 和 VFL 的主要剂量限制性毒性，在 VSLI 中也很常见。血小板减少和贫血通常并不常见也不严重。中性粒细胞减少通常发生在给药后的 7~11 天，14~21 天基本恢复。骨髓抑制没有明显的蓄积性。尽管 VCR 很少与血液学毒性相关，但是某些情况如无意中过量用药和肝功能不全时会发生骨髓抑制，导致药物暴露增加。

胃肠道反应

除了自主神经功能紊乱所致的胃肠道反应，其他的胃肠道毒性也会发生[37,38,41,48,127,182,183]。胃肠道自主神经功能紊乱，表现为腹胀、便秘和腹痛，最常由 VCR 引起，其他长春花生物碱类药物在高剂量治疗时或提高药物暴露量时（如肝功能异常，给药过量）也可以引起这些毒性反应。自主神经异常的早期表现为由小肠转运减慢引起粪便堆积在结肠上段。数字化检查可以观察到直肠排空，腹部 X 线检查也可以用于诊断该情况，证明高剂量灌肠剂和泻药治疗有效。因此建议所有接受 VCR 治疗的患者服用常规预防性药物以防止发生便秘。严重自主神经毒性反应可能导致麻痹性肠梗阻、肠坏死，甚至肠穿孔。肠梗阻可能类似"急腹症"，通常在治疗结束后采取保守措施可缓解。接受大剂量 VCR 治疗或合并肝功能异常的患者，特别容易出现自主神经毒性引起的严重胃肠道并发症。尽管预防性使用一些药物可以降低毒性反应的报道不时见诸笔端，包括乳果糖、雨蛙素、甲氧氯普胺以及胆囊收缩素类似物（sincalide，辛卡利特），但是这些药物也可能通过影响胆汁排泄和/或肠肝循环来改变长春花生物碱的药代动力学行为，最终导致药物清除率增加[38]。VBL 引起黏膜炎、口腔炎和咽炎的比例高于 VCR，但在 VFL、VRL 和 VDS 中并不少见。恶心、呕吐和腹泻的发生率也很低。可以发生短时无症状的血清转氨酶和碱性磷酸酶水平升高。在 VRL 中偶有发生胰腺炎的报道[182]。

其他毒性反应

所有长春花生物碱类药物是有效的糜烂性毒剂，如果发生药物外渗，可能导致严重的组织损伤。此警告应该适用于 VSLI，因为没有证据表明如果出现外渗，该药物可防止组织损伤。如果发现可疑药物外渗，需要立即停止使用化疗药并尽量吸出任何残留在组织中的药物[38,184-189]。在试验中发现，冷敷会加重毒性反应，而热敷可以限制损伤。为了减轻痛苦和潜在蜂窝织炎的发生，可以选择以下治疗：立即进行局部加热，每日 4 次，每次 1 小时，连续 3~5 天；使用 25 号规格的注射针沿顺时针方向选择 6 个注射点在周围组织中皮下注射透明质酸酶 150~1 500U（15U/ml 溶于 6ml 0.9% 盐水中），一点一针[187-189]。在动物模型中使用亚叶酸、苯海拉明、氢化可的松、异丙肾上腺素、碳酸氢钠以及维生素 A 膏进行治疗均无效[185]。推荐立即与外科协商进行早期清创术。沿输液静脉走行可能发生局部不适以及静脉炎，伴有血管硬化，但是治疗后进行充分血管冲洗会尽可能减少静脉炎的发生。

接受 VRL 和 VCR 治疗的患者发生轻度可逆性脱发的比例分别为 10% 和 20%。使用长春花生物碱类药物也可以发生急性心肌缺血、无缺血证据的胸痛、无明确病因的发热、雷诺现象和手足综合征[190-192]。大约 5% 的患者出现以呼吸困难为主要表现的呼吸道症状，当长春花生物碱与丝裂霉素 C 合用时尤为多见[193,194]。肺毒性的发作可以是急性的，典型表现是支气管痉挛和呼吸困难，与过敏反应类似。另一种类型的毒性表现亚急性可逆反应，包括咳嗽和呼吸困难，偶尔可见间质性浸润。这种反应基本在给药 1 小时之内发生。在严重病例中使用皮质类固醇可以获益，严重病例可以恢复并且不会出现并发症。没有明确的证据表明 VRL 是导致慢性肺毒性的原因。

所有长春花生物碱都可引起 SIADH，接受密集水化的患者特别容易发生继发于 SIADH 的严重低钠血症[36-38,48,127]。此外，研究人员还注意到，SIADH 也与血浆抗利尿激素水平升高有关，通常在治疗后 3 天内恢复。低钠血症通常可以通过限制液体摄入量加以纠正。VBL 可引起光敏反应，可能由角膜刺激和肌肉反应引发[195]。如果不小心将长春花生物碱类药物进行了鞘内注射，将导致上行性脑脊髓病，并且通常是致命的。有报道指出立即进行脑脊液回抽，同时采用乳酸林格液配以新鲜冷冻血浆(15ml/L)以 55ml/h 速度灌注 24 小时能够达到很好疗效,有两例患者经过这种治疗后得以存活,虽伴有明显截瘫表现,但是大脑功能得以完整保留[196]。为了防止这种错误的发生,建议不要同时进行甲氨蝶呤鞘内注射和 VCR 静脉注射治疗,并且避免将这两种药物同时应用[197]。药物所致肝转氨酶升高也有报道,尤其是使用 VSLI 时。

给药方法、剂量与方案

临床建议应用长春花生物碱类药物时采取快速静脉滴注的方式。静脉滴注速度过慢会增加静脉炎以及注射部位局部反应的发生率,因此在静脉完全冲洗干净之前不能拔出导管。在体重超过 10kg 的患儿中,VCR 推荐剂量为静脉滴注每周 1.5~2.0mg/m^2,在更小的患儿中,推荐剂量为每周 0.05~0.65mg/m^2。对于成人,传统的推荐剂量为每周 1.4~2.0mg/m^2。在患儿中 VCR 实际用量不超过 2.0~2.5mg,在成人中不超过 2.0mg,这是 VCR 的封顶剂量,是基于在少部分接受高剂量化疗患者中发生严重胃肠道毒性反应报道基础上规定的。但是,支持这个结论的药理学和毒理学证据非常有限,而且有证据显示这个结论应当重新验证,特别是患者的药代动力学表现和耐受性存在非常大的差异。VCR 的清除在不同患者中存在明显差别(最高可达 11 倍),一些患者可以耐受非常高的药物剂量治疗却几乎没有毒性反应。不仅如此,成人接受 2.0mg 药物治疗时,安全性问题和治疗疗效两方面都没有达到封顶效应[198]。在任何情况下,特别是当 VCR 用于可能治愈的病例时,不要因为轻微的周围神经毒性反应而减量。相反的,如果发生严重的神经毒性反应时,如严重的伴有症状的感觉变化,运动神经及脑神经缺陷,以及肠梗阻等,需要调整剂量,直至毒性反应缓解。在明确为姑息治疗的情况下,如果发生中度神经毒性时也可以选择减量,延长周期给药时间或换药治疗。为防止严重自主神经毒性导致严重后果,特别是重度便秘情况的发生,也建议常规采取预防措施。

静脉注射 VSLI 的推荐剂量为每周 2.25mg/m^2。VSLI 是通过混合制造商提供的试剂盒中的 3 种成分来制备的,包括 VCR 硫酸盐,磷酸钠和鞘磷脂/胆固醇脂质体注射液。按照步骤,VSLI 应该呈现为白色到灰白色的半透明悬浮液,基本上不含可见的异物和聚集物,由鞘磷脂/胆固醇脂质体组成,其中脂质体的平均直径约为 100 纳米。超过 95%的药物被包裹在脂质体中。将该方法得到的溶液用 5%葡萄糖注射液或 0.9%氯化钠注射液稀释至终体积为 100ml,静脉注射 1 小时。

含 VBL 的化疗方案大都采用 VBL 每周 6mg/m^2 快速静脉给药的方式。儿童和成人的推荐剂量分别为每周 2.5mg/m^2 和 3.7mg/m^2,根据血液学耐受情况剂量可以按每周 1.8mg/m^2 和 2.5mg/m^2 逐渐增加,儿童可达到每周 12.5mg/m^2。单药 VLB 治疗时,推荐每周给药总量在成人可达到 18.5mg/m^2;但是事实上由于骨髓抑制,这些剂量远高于大多数患者可以耐受的剂量,即使降低给药频率也不可行。由于剂量相同的 VBL 导致的白细胞减少症严重程度存在很大差异,不建议给药频率短于每周一次。曾有 5 天连续给药的使用方法,VBL 剂量为每天 1.5~2.0mg/m^2,生物相关血浆浓度大约为 2.0nmol/L,但是由于延长给药时间会导致药物分布广泛的同时与周围组织紧密结合,这种给药方法的获益可能很少。

针对 VRL,通常选择每周 30mg/m^2 或每两周一次的给药方案,通过侧臂进行 6~10 分钟快速静脉给药(或者缓慢静推后选择 5%葡萄糖或 0.9%氯化钠冲管)或者进行超过 20 分钟的短时静滴。给药速度越快,局部静脉毒性越低。口服给药,每周一次,每次 80~100mg/m^2 的方案一般耐受良好,但是目前口服剂型未获得上市许可。其他的给药方式包括小剂量长期口服治疗,间歇性高剂量给药以及延时静脉给药。

VLF 的推荐剂量为 320mg/m^2,每 3 周静脉输注 20 分钟。依据世界卫生组织或美国东部肿瘤协作组,ECOG 评分为 1 或 0,并有盆腔放疗史的患者,建议将剂量减低至 280mg/m^2。若第一个周期未发生血液学毒性导致治疗延迟或剂量减少的情况,后续周期应将剂量增加到 320mg/m^2。

由于具有明显的局部腐蚀能力,长春花生物碱类药物不可进行肌内注射、皮下、膀胱内或腹腔内注射。在临床意外事故中,将 VCR 和其他长春花生物碱类药物直接进行鞘内注射会导致严重的脑脊髓病,其特征性表现为上行性运动和感觉神经病变,脑病以及死亡(见毒性反应:神经毒性)。

尽管指南对肝功能异常患者的特殊计量没有详细规定,但是由于肝脏在处理长春花生物碱类药物中起到重要作用,因此对于那些伴有肝功能异常,特别是肝脏分泌功能异常的患者,应当考虑调整给药剂量[181]。对于 VCR、VRL、VDS 和 VBL,当总胆红素水平在 1.5~3.0mg/dl 之间时,建议减量 50%,(对于 VRL,当总胆红素水平在 2.0~3.0mg/dl 之间时,建议减量 50%),血浆总胆红素水平超过 3.0mg/dl 的患者,至少减量 75%。针对肝功能不全患者的给药指南尚未制定,应采取保守的给药方式,可能与之前提到的无包膜的长春花生物碱指南类似,因为肝脏代谢和胆道排泄是 VSLI 代谢的主要过程。然而,在中度肝功能不全患者(Child-Pugh B)中评估了 VSLI 的药代动力学,剂量调整后的最大血浆浓度和暴露与具有正常肝功能的患者相当[49]。对于轻度(Child-Pugh A 级)和中度(Child-Pugh B 级)肝损害患者,VFL 的推荐剂量分别为 250mg/m^2 和 200mg/m^2,详见处方信息。

肾功能损害的剂量减少不适用于任何一种除 VFL 外的长春花生物碱类,对于中度(肌酐清除率在 40~60ml/min)和严重(肌酐清除率在 20~40ml/min)的患者,推荐的起始剂量分别为每 3 周 280mg/m^2 和 250mg/m^2[53]。

因为药物清除与年龄相关,也建议将老年患者的 VFL 剂量减少。在年龄介于 75~80 岁之间的患者和年龄超过 80 岁的患者中,推荐剂量分别为每 3 周 280mg/m^2 和 250mg/m^2。

紫杉烷类药物:引言和适应证

作用于微管的紫杉烷类药物,其主要的作用机制、药理学、临床适应证和毒性反应与长春花生物碱有很大不同。人们对紫杉烷类的兴趣始于 1963 年,发现太平洋紫杉(短叶红豆杉)树皮的粗提取物在临床前研究中显示出了显著的抗癌活性。1971 年,Wall 和其同事确定紫杉醇为树皮提取物的活性成分。然而,太平洋紫杉原材料的匮乏阻止了大量紫杉醇化合物的提取和制备,此外,其水溶性差的特点进一步阻碍了紫杉醇化合物的发展[199]。科学家们确定了紫杉烷类新的作用机制,并为必要的临床前研究和有限的临床研究提供了充足供应后,人们对紫杉烷类的研究得以维持。早期,对来源丰富并多为可再生资源的紫杉烷类进行研究,促成了多西紫杉醇的半合成方法,方法是在 10-脱乙酰基巴卡丁Ⅲ上添加一条侧链,10-脱乙酰基巴卡丁Ⅲ

是一种非活性紫杉烷前体，来源于针叶及其他数量丰富的杉树[200]。这种可行的半合成方法，解决了紫杉醇的供应问题。最近，一种紫杉醇与白蛋白的结合配方[蛋白紫杉醇注射粒子(protein-bound paclitaxel particles for injection，PBPPI)]，又名 nab-紫杉醇或纳米白蛋白紫杉醇，在多个地区广泛获批上市[201]。

图 60-3 显示了紫杉醇、多西紫杉醇和卡巴他赛的结构，是由一个 15-mer 的紫杉烷环与一个罕见的 4-mer 环氧内酯组成的复杂酯类。在紫杉醇和多西紫杉醇的紫杉烷环的 C13 位连接一个脂性侧链，而非 10-脱乙酰基巴卡丁Ⅲ，对抗微管活性极其重要[202]。紫杉醇和多西紫杉醇的结构差异位于紫杉醇的 C10 位点乙酰基置换和 C-13 侧链上，这使多西紫杉醇比紫杉醇具有稍强的水溶性和效力，然而这些结构和水溶性差异的临床意义尚未完全清楚。最近加入治疗方案的另一种药物是卡巴他赛，是多西紫杉醇的二甲氧基衍生物，是由 10-脱乙酰基巴卡丁Ⅲ半合成所形成的单一非对映异构体[203]。与多西紫杉醇相比，卡巴他赛更有效，对 Pgp 和药物跨膜射流泵具有更低的亲和力，这在一定程度上解释了其在多西紫杉醇耐药性癌症中的活性显著的原因[204]。

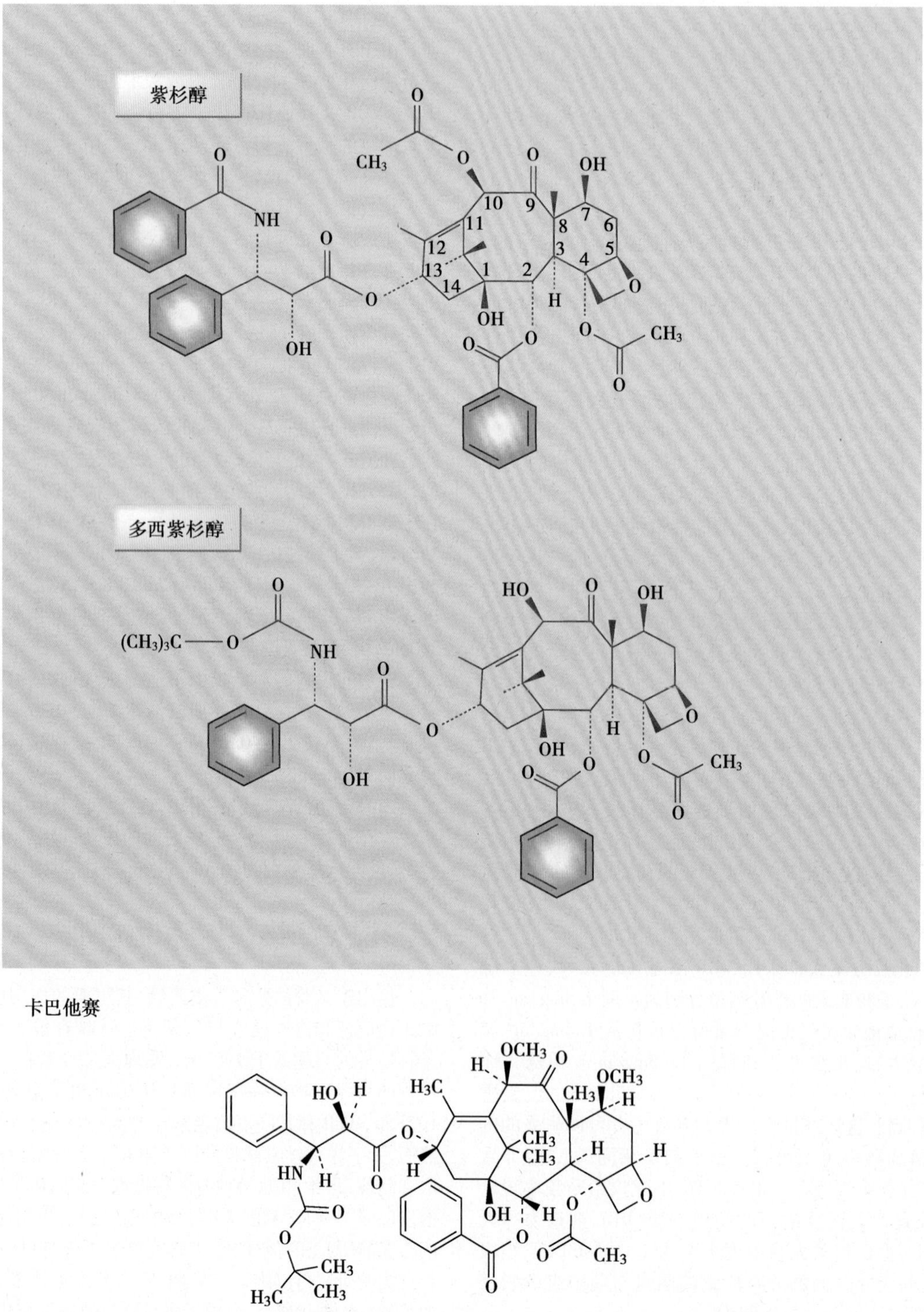

紫杉醇

多西紫杉醇

卡巴他赛

图 60-3　紫杉烷的化学结构：紫杉醇、多西紫杉醇和卡巴他赛

临床适应证

紫杉醇最早在美国和其他国家获批准上市，用于卵巢癌的一线治疗或后续化疗失败的卵巢癌患者。在Ⅲ期随机临床研究中发现，在姑息性手术切除的Ⅲ期或Ⅳ期卵巢癌患者中使用紫杉醇联合铂类药物作为初始化疗使用，可以获得生存受益[205]。在美国，紫杉醇还用于治疗联合化疗失败的转移性乳腺癌以及辅助化疗后 6 个月内复发的乳腺癌患者，包括既往使用过蒽环类药物的患者[206]。紫杉醇还可用于淋巴结阳性乳腺癌的辅助治疗，并按标准的阿霉素联合化疗顺序进行。在临床试验中，激素受体阳性和激素受体阴性肿瘤患者的总体无病生存率和总体生存率均有较好的改善，但这种改善仅在激素受体阴性肿瘤患者中得到了无可辩驳的证实[207-209]。研究还证明，在转移性乳腺癌和早期高危乳腺癌患者中选择含有紫杉醇药物的序贯方案，尤其是剂量密集方案和每周方案后，已取得了引人注目的结果。然而，这些疗效结果尚不能推广到其他情况和/或其他紫杉烷类药物[210,211]。紫杉醇或其他紫杉烷类药物的每周方案与较低频率给药方案相比，不良反应发生率较低，特别是骨髓抑制的发生率低。

其他的以紫杉醇为基础的联合方案治疗的特殊适应证也获得批准。在转移性乳腺癌患者的一线化疗中，吉西他滨联合紫杉醇方案的生存期优于单药紫杉醇，因此，吉西他滨联合紫杉醇方案获得批准。与此类似，曲妥珠单抗联合紫杉醇被用于转移性 HER-2 阳性乳腺癌的一线治疗[212]。紫杉醇也可用于淋巴结阳性或阴性的 HER-2 阳性乳腺癌（激素受体阴性或至少有一个高危特征）的辅助治疗，作为阿霉素、环磷酰胺和曲妥珠单抗方案的一部分[213,214]。在美国，紫杉醇还被批准用于与 AIDS 有关的 Kaposi 肉瘤的二线治疗，以及联合顺铂作为无法放疗或失去根治性手术机会的ⅢB 期和Ⅳ期非小细胞肺癌患者的一线治疗[215,216]。贝伐单抗、紫杉醇、卡铂三药联合用于治疗ⅢB 和Ⅳ期非鳞癌的非小细胞肺癌也获得批准[217]。

在美国，多西紫杉醇最早被批准用于治疗蒽环类药物化疗失败的转移性或局部晚期乳腺癌患者，后来适应证范围扩大到所有化疗失败后的治疗[200]。后续研究证明，在蒽环类药物化疗失败的局部晚期或转移性乳腺癌患者中，卡培他滨联合多西紫杉醇方案的疗效优于多西紫杉醇单药，因此含卡培他滨的联合方案获得批准[218]。多西紫杉醇的适应证还包括联合环磷酰胺及阿霉素用于局限性乳腺癌标准局部治疗后的辅助化疗[219]。在非小细胞肺癌中，多西紫杉醇最早被批准用于治疗含铂方案化疗失败的无法切除的局部晚期或转移性肺癌，随后，多西紫杉醇联合顺铂被批准作为这部分患者的一线化疗方案[220]。多西紫杉醇联合泼尼松治疗激素抵抗型前列腺癌的生存期优于米托蒽醌联合强的松的方案，因此被批准用于前列腺癌的治疗[221]。不仅如此，紫杉烷类药物在治疗头颈部鳞癌中也取得了很好的疗效。因此，在美国，多西紫杉醇联合顺铂和 5-FU 被批准用于局部晚期患者的新辅助治疗[222]。多西紫杉醇联合顺铂和 5-FU 被批准用于初治、晚期胃癌和食管交界处的腺癌，而紫杉醇联合雷莫芦单抗用于复发或难治性患者[223,224]。针对曾使用含有多西紫杉醇的治疗方案，并发展为去势抵抗性的转移性前列腺癌，卡巴他赛联合强的松的疗效优于米托蒽醌联合泼尼松，因此被批准用于治疗此类患者[225]。

PBPPI 是在美国和其他地区获得批准最新上市的紫杉烷类药物，是将紫杉醇溶于 3%～4% 的人血白蛋白所得到的药物，与人血液中白蛋白浓度相似[201]。PBPPI 最初被批准用于联合化疗失败或辅助化疗 6 个月内复发的转移性乳腺癌患者[226]。一项随机试验表明，局部晚期或转移性非小细胞肺癌患者使用 PBPPI 联合卡铂治疗的客观缓解率高于紫杉醇联合卡铂治疗；但总生存期相近[227]。此外，PBPPI 联合吉西他滨用于转移性胰腺癌的一线治疗，因为该方案的总生存期高于单独使用吉西他滨[201]。

必须指出的是，紫杉醇、多西紫杉醇、卡巴他赛及 PBPPI 的抗瘤谱是相同的，在多种肿瘤中均有抗癌活性，包括子宫内膜癌、膀胱癌、小细胞肺癌、生殖细胞肿瘤、淋巴瘤和黑色素瘤。不同紫杉烷类药物在临床疗效和适应证上的差别，可能是由于调整策略、研究设计以及剂量制订的不同所导致，而并非是某种紫杉烷类药物的固有优势。与长春花生物碱相比，紫杉烷类药物在儿童恶性肿瘤中似乎没有相应的活性。

作用机制

紫杉醇与微管结合位点不同于其他抗微管抑制剂的结合位点，其中包括交换 GTP 位点、秋水仙碱、鬼臼毒素和长春碱的结合位点。紫杉醇与 β-微管蛋白亚单位 N 端 31 个氨基酸结合，亦可能涉及其他位点[199,228-234]。紫杉醇可以与微管壁网眼侧面由几个疏水氨基酸组成的空腔结合，大约位于原纤维单体的中段[3-7,199,234,235]。多西紫杉醇与微管的结合位点与紫杉醇相同，多西紫杉醇对于该位点有更高的亲和力，是紫杉醇的 1.9 倍，多西紫杉醇诱导微管蛋白组装所需的一种关键性蛋白的浓度比紫杉醇低 2.1 倍[233,236-240]。多西紫杉醇在一定药物浓度下具有更高效能，可以产生更强的细胞毒作用，然而人们尚不清楚能否将其转化为更高的临床治疗效果。临床前和临床研究结果表明，紫杉烷类药物可能存在不完全交叉耐药，提示临床工作者给药物剂量和联合方案应有所差别。虽然如此，紫杉醇、多西紫杉醇和其他紫杉烷类药物的抗癌谱几乎相同。虽然长春花生物碱和紫杉烷类药物对有丝分裂纺锤体结构破坏的影响相似，但它们的作用机制各不相同。紫杉烷类药物结合 β-微管蛋白亚基后，通过静电相互作用稳定微管原纤维之间的侧向接触[7]。实际上，这种相互作用通过影响微管两端的微管蛋白解离速率，降低了细胞质中游离微管蛋白的浓度，并促进聚合反应的成核和延伸，从而稳定微管，防止解聚和增强聚合[2-7,55,239-245]。

紫杉烷类与聚合微管蛋白的结合增强了微管的稳定性。在亚化学计量浓度下，紫杉烷类抑制微管的活动，并且没有显著提高微管蛋白聚合的速率[2-7,55,239-245]。在临床所能达到的高浓度下，紫杉烷类药物可诱导微管蛋白聚合并加快微管团块的形成。经过紫杉烷类处理的细胞，其微管非常稳定，可有效抵抗由低温、钙离子、GTP 以及长春花生物碱和秋水仙碱等解聚剂导致的解聚作用。这些作用抑制了微管的踏板运动和动态不稳定性，对在有丝分裂和无丝分裂的细胞周期中维持正常的微管动力学至关重要[2,3,13,17,20]。紫杉烷类的化学计量和亚化学计量结合抑制细胞的增殖,主要是在有丝分裂的中期和晚期诱导持续的有丝分裂阻滞;形态学上的变化,如细胞间期微管束的形成,表明间期微管也会受到影响。由于紫杉烷类对微管的动态干扰与有丝分裂纺锤体的形成密切相关,因此细胞在有丝分裂期对紫杉烷类药物最敏感。

紫杉烷类干扰有丝分裂过程和诱导有丝分裂阻滞,触发细胞凋亡。目前,介导细胞死亡的作用机制尚不完全清楚。紫杉烷类药物对负责染色体分离的功能性有丝分裂纺锤体的形成具有破坏作用,并最终激活有丝分裂检查点,有丝分裂检查点是有丝分裂的主要细胞周期控制机制,其作用是防止染色体的错误分离。有丝分裂检查点导致染色体分离的延迟,这些染色体经复制后成为姐妹染色单体进入有丝分裂,直到每对染色体都与有丝分裂纺锤体的两极建立连接。紫杉烷类药物阻止纺锤体与着丝点的连接,因此特定的信号转导通路被激活,通过抑制后期具有促进作用的复合物来延迟有丝分裂过程[22,246-248]。经紫杉烷类药物处理的细胞最终进入后期并经历有丝分裂,但未附着的着丝点将导致染色体向多个方向分裂;染色体分离是随机的,多极分裂后部分细胞分裂失败。由此产生的子细胞是非整倍体,可能由于一个或多个基本染色体的丢失,部分细胞将死亡。

紫杉烷类药物引起的微管扰动会引起有丝分裂检查点的延迟,最终通过细胞凋亡的内在途径介导细胞死亡[22,75,244-262]。这一过程涉及多种调控成分,如肿瘤抑制基因 TP53、细胞周期蛋白依赖性激酶抑制剂(如 p21/waf1)以及其他蛋白激酶的调控因子[244,245,262]。细胞被阻滞在 G2/M 期,随后细胞执行细胞凋亡或通过 G2/M 进入细胞分裂[248,259]。凋亡的启动包括促凋亡分子 Bax 和 Bad 的活化和抗凋亡调节分子 Bcl-2 和 BclxL 的失活[248,259-261]。紫杉烷类和其他微管抑制剂诱导激酶活化 Bcl-2 磷酸化,所涉及的激酶包括 Jun 氨基末端激酶(JNK)和其促凋亡的效应因子 BIM 和 C-Raf、细胞外信号调节诱导磷酸化激酶 1 和 2(ERK1 和 ERK2)、细胞凋亡信号调节激酶(ASK)、周期蛋白依赖性激酶 1(CDK1)、cAMP 依赖蛋白激酶 A 和 BCL-2 家族成员蛋白激酶[69,250,260-264]。Bcl-2 家族蛋白的磷酸化(失活)和促凋亡分子的磷酸化(激活)促进细胞凋亡内源性途径和下游效应因子半胱天冬酶活化[257,259]。紫杉烷类药物也可诱导细胞死亡,而与半胱天冬酶的活化无关[241,265]。

研究显示,紫杉烷类药物也会干扰非增殖细胞的间期微管,表现为微管束形成[248]。紫杉烷类药物亦可诱导转录因子和介导细胞增殖的酶的产生,触发细胞凋亡和炎症反应[252,262,266,267]。紫杉烷类药物在体内和体外都能增强电离辐射,最有可能是通过抑制细胞周期中对辐射最敏感的 G2/M 期的进展来实现的[268-272]。此外,紫杉烷类药物抑制血管生成的浓度低于诱导细胞毒性的浓度,但抗血管生成作用对紫杉烷类药物抗癌作用的贡献尚未完全清楚[258,273,274]。

与长春花生物碱类似,紫杉烷类药物也能诱导许多其他细胞效应,这些效应可能与它们对微管动力学的破坏作用有关,也可能无关。虽然紫杉烷类药物主要阻断有丝分裂相的细胞周期变化,但它们阻止了 G0 期向 S 期的转变[260,275]。紫杉烷类对有丝分裂间期细胞的干扰主要包括对细胞膜微管蛋白的破坏、间期细胞骨架的破坏、涉及生长因子信号转导的微管损伤及通过活性氧诱导血管内皮生长因子的表达下降[38,276,277]。

紫杉烷类药物可扰乱正常组织以及恶性肿瘤组织,这些影响在一定程度上是通过破坏微管动力学来介导的。紫杉醇抑制人类中性粒细胞相关的形态和生化过程,包括趋化、迁移、扩散、极化、过氧化氢的生成及对微生物的吞噬功能[38]。紫杉醇能够拮抗淋巴细胞的功能、cAMP 的代谢、抑制淋巴细胞增殖。同时,紫杉醇模拟细菌脂多糖内毒素对巨噬细胞的影响,导致细胞迅速消耗肿瘤坏死因子(TNF-α)受体,并释放 TNF-α[261,266,267]。这类药物还能诱导 TNF-α 基因表达,这些作用机制不涉及紫杉醇对微管组装的破坏作用,提示其抗肿瘤作用涉及多种细胞因子的活化[266]。此外,研究显示,紫杉醇抑制增生性视网膜病变模型的脉管上皮成纤维细胞增殖和收缩,以及心脏和周围血管成形术后内膜平滑肌细胞的增殖[278,279]。由紫杉醇涂层的心脏动脉支架有效降低了成纤维细胞增殖和内膜增生的发病率,并获得美国和其他国家的药物监管机构的批准使用[280,281]。紫杉醇抑制一些特殊细胞的分泌功能,如大鼠离体胰岛的分泌、大鼠肝细胞的蛋白质分泌、肾上腺嗜铬细胞经烟碱受体刺激儿茶酚胺的分泌功能[38]。

尽管 PBPPI 对于恶性或非恶性组织的作用与传统配方的紫杉醇和多西紫杉醇相似,但 PBPPI 中紫杉醇与白蛋白的结合增加了肿瘤组织中紫杉醇分子的积累。白蛋白有几个特点,使其成为一个有吸引力的肿瘤药物载体。它是内源性疏水分子的天然载体,以可逆的非共价方式结合,主要通过与 60-kDa 糖蛋白(gp60)细胞表面受体结合,促进内皮细胞对与蛋白结合或未与蛋白结合的血浆成分的转运。在白蛋白与 gp60 结合后,复合物与细胞内蛋白质小窝蛋白-1 相互作用,随后形成内吞囊泡(细胞膜穴样内陷),将复合物转运至细胞内。骨粘连蛋白也被称为酸性分泌蛋白,富含半胱氨酸(SPARC),由于与 gp60 具有序列同源性,因此也能结合白蛋白[201,282-284]。与小窝蛋白-1 类似,SPARC 在多种恶性肿瘤中表达,包括乳腺癌、肺癌和前列腺癌,以及这些肿瘤和其他肿瘤的基质中表达,这可能是肿瘤内白蛋白积累以及 PBPPI 等白蛋白结合药物积累的原因。然而,SPARC 在肿瘤和/或间质中的表达尚不能够准确预测 PBPPI 的抗癌活性[201,282-286]。

PBPPI 是作为紫杉醇/聚氧乙烯蓖麻油制剂的替代药品而开发的,是平均粒径 130μm 与白蛋白结合的紫杉醇颗粒制剂,不需使用任何溶剂。它是由紫杉醇和人血清白蛋白的冻干配方制成的胶体悬浮液。人血清白蛋白使药物颗粒稳定在 130μm 的平均大小,可防止毛细血管阻塞,并且因为不含溶剂而不需要特殊的预先给药或输注[201,282-284]。此外,以接受人类肿瘤异种移植的无胸腺小鼠为实验对象的研究表明,PBPPI 可向肿瘤细胞递送更高的紫杉醇浓度,从而比同等剂量的紫杉醇在聚氧乙烯蓖麻油制剂中的抗癌活性高。与聚氧乙烯基蓖麻油制剂相比,SPARC-白蛋白的相互作用也可能导致紫杉醇在全身的分布和清除更快。

耐药机制

研究显示,紫杉烷类药物的低剂量长时间给药导致的细胞耐药存在两种常见机制。最具特征的机制是由 ABC 多药转运子家族成员介导的 MDR 型。与紫杉烷类耐药相关的最重要的 ABC 转运子是 170kDa Pgp 流出泵或 MDR1 编码基因产物 MDR1

(ABC 亚家族 B1,ABCB1)和 MDR2(ABC 亚家族成员 ABCB4)(见长春花碱:耐药简介、适应证和机制)[83,86,87,233,287,288]。此外,低剂量紫杉烷类继发的耐药似乎是由胆汁酸盐输出蛋白(BSEP,别名 ABCC11)引起的[293,294]。与长春新碱不同,ABCC1(MRP1)和 ABCC2(MRP2)并不参与紫杉醇的转运[289-292]。就鼠类而言,在紫杉醇耐药细胞中发现的 Pgp 特殊种类与亲代细胞衍生的长春新碱和秋水仙素耐药细胞中 Pgp 相似,但不雷同[92,287,288]。这些细胞与许多其他天然产物具有交叉耐药性,由 MDR 导致的紫杉醇和多西紫杉醇的耐药能被多种膜激活药物所逆转,包括钙通道阻滞剂、他莫昔芬、环孢素 A 和抗心律失常药[287,291-294]。甚至参与紫杉醇和多西紫杉醇溶解的载体聚乙烯蓖麻油和聚山梨酯-80 的主要成分都能逆转紫杉烷类的耐药,但是即使聚氧乙酰蓖麻油的胞质浓度对于逆转 MDR 是足够的,在临床使用时,充分调节浓度后的聚山梨酯-80 也不足以克服多西紫杉醇耐药[291,292]。直至今日,克服由紫杉烷类和其他 MDR 药物导致的耐药在临床上进展甚微。但是已经开展许多有关 MDR 调节子的研究,这些调节子可以减少紫杉烷类清除,增加毒性(如维拉帕米、环孢素 A),以上内容综合解释了药物对 MDR 调节的固有作用。然而,MDR 调节子并不影响紫杉烷类的清除和毒性,似乎也并不增强药物的抗肿瘤活性[293,294]。

尽管卡巴他赛的效力类似于多西紫杉醇在癌细胞系和对多西紫杉醇敏感的人肿瘤异种移植物中的效力,但卡巴他赛在多西紫杉醇耐药的癌细胞系和具有 MDR 表型的人肿瘤异种移植物中保留相关活性,这是由于对 Pgp 的底物亲和力较低所导致的。与多西紫杉醇 4.8~59 的耐药率相比,卡巴他赛的耐药率从 1.8 到 10 不等[203,204]。在多西紫杉醇治疗去势抵抗性前列腺癌失败后,Pgp 底物亲和力的差异能在多大程度上解释卡巴他赛的活性,但目前尚未明确。

与长春花生物碱类药物类似,几株由高浓度药物引起的紫杉烷类耐药的人类细胞株在延长治疗期发生 α 和 β 微管结构性的改变和微管单体结合,致微管受损(见长春花生物碱:耐药简介、适应证和机制)[106,107,295-307]。这些细胞有丝分裂纺锤体两极缺乏正常的微管,当缺乏药物时,微管的组装变慢。微管组装过程需要紫杉烷类持续存在。而且,这些变化对长春花生物碱类药物也敏感。在一些实验体系中,紫杉醇耐药的细胞具有 β-微管等位基因突变,其突变涉及紫杉烷类的潜在结合位点的突变,特别是 215、217 和 228 位亮氨酸突变成组氨酸、精氨酸或苯丙氨酸[297,299,300,306]。低水平表达导致药物耐受,然而,高水平的突变位点的表达导致微管组装损害、细胞周期停滞和增殖的失败,所有这些情况都能通过加入紫杉醇共培养而逆转。尽管在紫杉烷类耐药细胞系中已经报道了微管蛋白同型基因突变、基因扩增和同型转换,但几乎没有迹象表明其机制与临床相关,即使发生,也可能只是罕见的事件[306]。在一项检查来自非小细胞肺癌、卵巢癌、卵巢癌异种移植物和卵巢癌细胞系的紫杉醇天然和紫杉醇耐药样品的研究中,未发现 βⅠ-微管蛋白突变[306]。然而,βⅠ-微管蛋白外显子 1 中的沉默多态性以非常低的频率被检测到,表明与多态性不相关[306]。

在临床前研究中,微管蛋白含量、微管蛋白亚型谱和微管蛋白聚合动力学的改变导致对紫杉烷类药物产生耐药性,现有的证据表明,这些机制可能解释了临床上对紫杉烷类药物反应的多样性[306]。如前所述,存在多种 α-和 β-微管蛋白同种型,其由位于不同染色体上并具有组织和细胞特异性表达模式的不同基因编码。这些微管蛋白同种型可以进行翻译后修饰,从而改变微管与 MAP 的相互作用并改变它们的功能。预测分子模型,用于检查微管蛋白结合剂对不同 β-微管蛋白同种型的亲和力如何变化,可以用来解释敏感性的差异。例如,紫杉醇被认为是通过微管内的纳米孔扩散到微管内面向内腔的结合位点。有研究者预测,这种运动是通过氢键形成来介导的,所述氢键涉及所有 β-微管蛋白同种型中的丝氨酸 275,除了 βⅡ-和 βⅥ-微管蛋白[306]。已显示紫杉醇抗性肿瘤具有高水平的 β-微管蛋白Ⅰ、Ⅲ和Ⅳa 同种型[20,100-107,295-306,308,309]。高水平瘤内 βⅢ-微管蛋白是细胞 β-微管蛋白的最小元件,βⅢ-微管蛋白的动态不稳定性增加,阻碍微管组装,并导致紫杉烷类耐药,这些已在产生获得性紫杉烷类耐药的细胞系和紫杉烷类耐药的肿瘤活检组织中得到了证实[100-106,298-307,310-322]。βⅢ-微管蛋白的缺乏与体外微管组装速度增快相关,而过表达与微管组装速率降低有关。

各种微管蛋白同种型的功能差异尚未完全阐明,而微管蛋白经历的翻译后修饰又增加了另一层复杂性。促凋亡蛋白和抗凋亡蛋白,包括 TP53 和 Bcl2,通过微管连接或运输。抗微管药物通过内在的凋亡途径诱导细胞凋亡,主要是由 Bcl2 家族成员介导[23,306,317,318]。凋亡原蛋白 Bim 被拴在微管上,经紫杉醇治疗后,Bim 从微管转移到线粒体[306,319]。Bim 高表达的癌细胞比低表达的癌细胞更容易受到紫杉烷类药物的细胞毒性作用的影响。β-微管蛋白同种型或翻译后修饰的差异表达如何影响抗微管药物结合,转运和释放诱导细胞凋亡的因子的能力尚不完全清楚;然而,特定 β-微管蛋白同种型和 MAP 的表达与一系列癌症(包括肺癌、卵巢癌、乳腺癌和前列腺癌)中的耐药性有关[20,100-107,295-306,308,309]。

异常增生的信号可能提高紫杉烷类引起凋亡的阈值而导致紫杉烷类耐药。例如,胰岛素样生长因子-Ⅰ可以保护蒽环类和紫杉烷类药物对乳腺癌细胞的细胞毒作用,这可能是通过激活磷脂酰肌醇 3-激酶(PI3K)途径而诱导抗凋亡诱导因子磷酸化(失活)实现的[320]。其他可能影响药物诱导细胞凋亡门槛的因子包括:TP53、HER-2、auora2 激酶、survivin 和 BRAC1。着丝粒相关丝氨酸/苏氨酸激酶和 aurora2-激酶参与中心体分离,两极纺锤体的形成和染色体动粒在有丝分裂纺锤体的附着,似乎覆盖有丝分裂组装检查点,并诱导紫杉烷类药物耐药[21,22,306]。另外,凋亡抑制蛋白家族成员之一的 survivin 的过表达能够抑制 caspase 活性和抗微管药物诱导的细胞凋亡。BRAC1 通过 DNA 修复保持基因组稳定,是一种肿瘤抑制因子,似乎与遗传性乳腺癌和卵巢癌有关。阻断 BRAC1 似乎在紫杉烷类药物耐药中发挥了作用。诱导 BRAC1 表达可增强紫杉烷类诱导的细胞凋亡[306,321]。与 DNA 阻断剂不同,TP53 肿瘤抑制因子突变的丢失并不影响微管聚集药物的耐药[306]。

MAP 涉及紫杉烷类药物和其他抗微管药物引起的凋亡抵抗机制。例如,主要在神经元组织中表达的 Tau 和 MAP2,以及主要的非神经元 MAP,MAP4,它们与微管结合并稳定微管以防止解聚[28-28]。乳腺癌中的 Tau 表达与紫杉醇耐药性有关,其表现为通过微管壁阻断紫杉醇,并限制紫杉醇进入微管内腔表面[316,322]。MAP4 赋予了微管稳定性,TP53 的诱导导致 MAP4

减少而导致对 VBL 的敏感性增加，但对紫杉醇的敏感性降低[323,324]。

微管-多价螯合蛋白 stathmin 在许多血液和实体恶性肿瘤过表达，是一种主要的细胞溶质磷蛋白，通过与微管蛋白异二聚体结合并诱导微管不稳定来调节有丝分裂纺锤体。stathmin 的过度表达降低了乳腺癌细胞对紫杉醇和 VBL 的敏感性[306]。stathmin 的高度表达也与紫杉醇和顺铂治疗上皮性卵巢癌患者的不良预后有关[295,306]。最后，其他细胞骨架成分的改变，特别是 γ-肌动蛋白的降低和 γ-肌动蛋白的调节因子，与抗微生物药物的耐药性有关[306]。

HER-2 是表皮生长因子受体家族成员之一，大约 30%的乳腺癌患者存在 HER-2 扩增或过表达，或扩增伴随过表达，HER-2 转染的细胞增加紫杉醇耐药；体外高表达 HER-2 也涉及紫杉醇耐药[325,326]。HER-2 过度表达也可能通过诱导参与 G2/M 检查点的 P21 而抑制 CDK1，参与抗微管药物诱导的凋亡抵抗；或直接磷酸化（失活）CDK1，可能会阻止紫杉醇介导的有丝分裂和凋亡的启动。与这种关系一致，用抗 HER-2 抗体曲妥珠单抗使 HER-2 表达下调可以增加乳腺癌细胞对紫杉烷类药物的敏感性，与单独的紫杉烷相比，曲妥珠单抗与紫杉醇或多西紫杉醇的组合与存活率增加有关[325,226]。然而，存在扩增 HER-2 不会对一线紫杉醇化疗的反应产生不利影响[212]。在一项研究中发现，伴有 HER-2 表达或扩增，或既表达又扩增的淋巴结阳性乳腺癌患者在阿霉素联合环磷酰胺辅助治疗后继续紫杉醇治疗都有获益，而且不受雌激素受体状态影响；而在 HER-2 阴性的患者中则没有获益[287]。

临床药理学

概况

紫杉类通常是静脉给药，紫杉醇给药剂量在 175~225mg/m^2 之间，用药 3 小时，多西紫杉醇给药剂量在 75~100mg/m^2 之间，用药 1 小时，PBPPI 260mg/m^2，30~40 分钟给药，或 25mg/m^2（卡巴他赛），也有其他给药方法，特别是每周给药方案在实际给药时普遍使用（见给药方法、剂量和方案）。对于非小细胞肺癌（卡铂）或胰腺癌患者，对于在一线转移性环境中非小细胞肺癌（用卡铂）或胰腺癌（用吉西他滨）患者，PBPPI 分别在每 21 天或 28 天的第 1、8 和 15 天以 100mg/m^2 或 125mg/m^2 的剂量注入。在大多数情况下，紫杉醇和多西紫杉醇口服给药的生物利用度很低且不稳定，这可能部分由于 Pgp 过表达以及肠上皮细胞的 P450 代谢能力和/或肝脏和/或肠的首过效应的综合作用所致。正如表 60-2 所示，紫杉类药物有如下药理学特点：广泛分布，迅速并有效的与除中枢神经系统之外的所有组织结合，半衰期长，主要在肝脏代谢，胆汁分泌和粪便排泄。卡巴他赛在某些方面有所不同，特别是其穿透血脑屏障的能力，这可以通过其降低 Pgp 的底物亲和力来解释。

表 60-2 紫杉烷：比较药代动力学和毒理学特征

参数	紫杉醇	PBPPI	多西他赛	卡巴他赛
成人标准剂量/（mg·m^{-2}·3 周$^{-1}$）	175~225（3 小时输注）	260（30 分钟输注）	75~100（1 小时输注）	25（1 小时输注）
成人标准剂量/（mg·m^{-2}·周$^{-1}$）	80	100~125（每 4 周×3 周）[b]	30~36	
药代动力学行为（临床相关剂量）	三相	双相	三相	三相
剂量比例药代动力学	紫杉醇可消除和分配的可饱和；由媒介物引起的伪非线性	剂量与 360mg/m^2 成比例	剂量与 360mg/m^2 成比例	剂量与 115mg/m^2 成比例，剂量与 30mg/m^2 成比例
血浆半衰期（终末期）	10~20 小时	27 小时	10~20 小时	95 小时
清除率	20~25L/h[a]	15L/（h·m^2）	36L/h	48.5L/h
主要路线	肝脏代谢和胆汁消除	肝脏代谢和胆汁消除	肝脏代谢和胆汁消除	肝脏代谢和胆汁消除
主要毒性	中性粒细胞减少	中性粒细胞减少	中性粒细胞减少	中性粒细胞减少
其他毒性	脱发，神经毒性，肌痛，关节痛，过敏反应，虚弱	脱发，神经毒性，关节痛，过敏反应，恶心，呕吐，腹泻，皮肤毒性	脱发，皮肤和指甲毒性，虚弱，肌痛，关节痛，流体潴留，神经毒性，过敏反应	腹泻，疲劳，虚弱，恶心，呕吐，神经毒性，便秘，脱发，皮肤和指甲毒性，过敏反应，关节痛

[a] 175mg/m^2，超过 3 小时（剂量方案）。
[b] 联合吉西他滨（胰腺癌）或卡铂（非小细胞肺癌）治疗，每 4 周 100~125mg/（m^2·周）×3 周。
PBPPI，蛋白紫杉醇注射粒子。

紫杉醇

紫杉醇的药代动力学行为是非线性或假非线性的[292,327-329]。非线性表现在给药时间较短时会更明显，使紫杉醇血浆浓度更高，药物排泄和组织分布过程的饱和更有效。饱和的分布和排泄过程有可能部分由于紫杉醇的非线性表现，组织分布在低血药浓度下就可以达到饱和（在 3 小时给药方案中紫杉剂量可以低于 175mg/m²），而同时排泄过程却需要高浓度时才会饱和（在 3 小时给药方案中紫杉剂量要高于 175mg/m²）。非线性表现的潜在后果是药物剂量增加时可能导致药物接触和毒性不成比例的增加而药物剂量降低时会导致药物接触不成比例的降低。然而，有效剂量范围相对较宽。但是，使用短时间注射方法也会导致血浆中助溶剂聚氧乙烯酰胺蓖麻油浓度过高，而这样可能会通过结合紫杉醇并抑制药物分散模拟非线性表现（假-非线性）[330,331]。

紫杉醇在血浆中的药理学行为已被模拟为三相或双相。最初的快速下降代表向外周隔室的分布和药物的消除。后期阶段部分是由于紫杉醇从外周隔室流出相对缓慢。它的 Vd 比体内水的体积大得多，表明大量药物与血浆蛋白或其他组织成分结合，有可能是微管蛋白。血浆蛋白的结合率非常高并且可逆，范围从 89%~98%[292]。白蛋白和 α1-酸糖蛋白与药物结合同等重要而脂蛋白与药物结合较少[332-334]。通常没有药物与紫杉醇同时给药，包括雷尼替丁、地塞米松、苯海拉明、多柔比星、5-氟尿嘧啶、顺铂都会明显地改变蛋白结合[334]。富含微管蛋白的血小板的药物结合广泛且可饱和，并且用放射性标记的紫杉醇进行动物分布研究表明由于异常的大脑和睾丸等部位，可能由于异生素外排泵所引起的大量摄取和保留[335,336]。

清除率与身体表面积密切相关，基于这个参数可以提供合理的剂量。在 3~96 小时给药方案中，人体的血药浓度峰值高于 0.05~10μmol/L，而在三腔体液如腹水中的药物浓度高于 0.1μmol/L。在体外，这种浓度能诱导相应的生物效应，但是药物渗透到中枢神经系统是可以忽略的[292,337,338]。紫杉醇分布的主要模式是肝脏代谢、胆汁排泄。肝脏代谢紫杉醇，然后紫杉醇及紫杉醇的代谢产物被分泌到胆汁[292,336,339-344]。在老鼠实验中，给予放射性标记的紫杉醇，6 天内回收的粪便中发现 98%的放射活性物；在人类，5 天内排泄的粪便中发现接近 71%给药剂量的紫杉醇以母药化合物或代谢产物的形式排出，6α-羟基紫杉醇是最主要的组成成分，占总量的 26%；未代谢的紫杉醇只占 5%。紫杉醇的肾脏清除和代谢占给药剂量的 14%[292]。人体中，细胞色素 P450 多功能氧化酶影响药物的分散，尤其是同工酶 CYP2C8 和 CYP3A4，它们将紫杉醇代谢为 6α-羟基紫杉醇（主要）和另一种羟基化的代谢产物，两种代谢产物在体内的活性都比紫杉醇低得多，可能是由于其极性比较大阻止了细胞内吸收[92,336,339-342]。紫杉醇代谢的个体差异相当大，可能是由于 P450 代谢的遗传药理学不同以及同时给药影响代谢[292,341-344]。

药效学研究揭示一些药动学参数可以代表与紫杉醇主要毒性相关的药物暴露，其中最重要且不变的关系是中性粒细胞减少症的程度与血药浓度持续维持在 0.05~0.1μmol/L 之上的药物暴露时间之间的关系[292,345]。一项前瞻性药动学决定因素的预测分析研究涉及数百名晚期 NSCLC 患者，结果发现当采用顺铂联合紫杉醇治疗时，紫杉醇剂量无论是 135mg/m² 还是 250mg/m²，只要给药时间超过 24 小时，那么紫杉醇稳态血浆浓度的高低与抗肿瘤活性，无病生存期和总生存期就没有多少关系[345]。

多西紫杉醇

多西紫杉醇（1 小时方案）在血浆中的药代动力学类似于紫杉醇。在剂量低于或等于 115mg/m² 时其血浆中药动学为三相，并且呈线性表现[200,346-351]。多西他赛分布阶段迅速（α-和 β 相 $T_{1/2}$ 值分别为 4 分钟和 36 分钟）和终末半衰期长（$T_{1/2\gamma}$ 范围，在一项研究中为 11.1~18.5h），与前面讨论的紫杉醇的原因相同。一项群体研究发现，药物血浆浓度数据显示出三相药动学分布，其他药动学参数如下：终末相半衰期为 12.4 小时，清除率为 1L/(h·m²)，稳态分布体积为 74L/m²[200,346-351]。决定多西紫杉醇清除率最重要的因素是体表面积，肝功能和血浆 α1-酸糖蛋白浓度，而年龄和血浆白蛋白水平对于清除率也有明显影响，虽然作用较小。和紫杉醇相似，血浆蛋白结合率很高（>80%~90%），并且主要与 α1-酸糖蛋白、白蛋白和脂蛋白结合[352,353]。与紫杉醇一样，多西他赛广泛分布于外周组织并缓慢释放，但药剂不会进入带有 Pgp 外排泵屏障的“庇护场所”，例如未受干扰的中枢神经系统。狗和老鼠的放射性标记药物的实验中，70%~80%的总放射活性物由粪便排泄，而尿液排泄仅为 10%以下。在有限的人体研究中，给肿瘤患者给予放射性标记的多西紫杉醇，大约 6%和 75%的给药放射性分别在 7 天内排出。并且在第一个 48 小时中有大约 80%的放射性物质在 1 种主要和 3 种次要代谢物中排出，非常少量（<8%）由未转化的多西紫杉醇组成。肝细胞色素 P450 多功能氧化酶，尤其是 CYP3A，其活性是 CYP3A4、CYP3A5、CYP3A7 和 CYP3A43 活性的总和，负责大部分多西紫杉醇的代谢[354-356]。与紫杉醇的紫杉环被代谢不同，多西紫杉醇中 C-13 侧链会被代谢[354-357]。这些代谢产物的活性似乎比多西紫杉醇低。

毒性反应，尤其是中性粒细胞减少症发生的主要药动学决定因素是药物暴露以及血浆药物浓度超过生物有效浓度的时间[351]。一项Ⅱ期多西紫杉醇群体药动学决定因素分析实验发现，预处理后的血浆 α1-酸糖蛋白浓度是转移性乳腺癌患者至疾病进展时间的决定因素；而在晚期肺癌患者中，药物暴露和预处理后血浆 α1-酸糖蛋白浓度都是致疾病进展时间的决定因素。相反，预处理后血浆 α-酸糖蛋白浓度和严重中性粒细胞减少症和中性粒细胞减少性发热的发生存在明显负相关。多西紫杉醇的清除率还与 CYP3A4 的活性有关，可以通过红霉素呼吸实验进行测定。

PBPPI

在临床研究中，评估 PBPPI 给药剂量为 80~360mg/m² 时，紫杉醇药代动力学与给药剂量成比例，在 30~180 分钟范围内与输注时间无关[285,286,358,359]。与聚氧乙烯化蓖麻油中配制的紫杉醇相比，PBPPI 的清除率高出 43%，Vd 高出 53%，且在末端 $T_{1/2}$ 中没有明显的差异。对于晚期乳腺癌患者，推荐剂量为 260mg/m²，总清除率平均为 15L/(h·m²)，Vd 平均为 632L/m²，这表明在使用 PBPPI 后紫杉醇具有广泛的血管外分布和/或组织结合。在体外，紫杉醇约有 89%~98%为蛋白结合。在一项患者自身对照试验中，血浆中 PBPPI 形式(6.2%)的未结合紫杉醇的比例明显高于溶剂型紫杉醇(2.3%)，这可能导致与基于溶剂的 PBBPI 相比，未结合的紫杉醇暴露更高[358-359]，如预期的那样，PBBPI 和溶剂型紫杉醇具有相似的代谢特征。粪便和尿液排泄占 PBBPI 给药总量的约 20%和 4%。在尾静脉注射 20mg/kg 紫杉醇后 24 小时，将放射性标记的紫杉醇从 PBBPI 和聚氧乙烯化紫杉醇制剂分配到红细胞和肿瘤组织中，研究药物动力学和分配放射性标记的紫杉醇。在 MX-1 人乳腺癌异种移植物中尾静脉注射 20mg/kg 紫杉醇后，检测血浆药代动力学并将放射性标记的紫杉醇从 PBBPI 和聚氧乙烯化紫杉醇制剂分配到红细胞和肿瘤组织 24 小时的研究中，分布 PBPPI 快速而广泛，表现为与聚氧乙烯化蓖麻油配方相比，浓度-时间曲线下面积(area under the curve，AUC)值下的 *Vd* 大 5 倍，C_{max} 和面积低得多[285,358,359]。此外，PBBPI 显示血浆紫杉醇在所有时间点的浓度显著下降，并更有效地分布到 MX-1 肿瘤中。紫杉醇的肿瘤 AUC 值平均为 PBBPI 的 1.6 倍，PBBPI 的终末半衰期值显著长于聚氧乙烯化蓖麻油制剂(17.1 小时 vs 4.0 小时)。PBPPI 半衰期的延长可归因于红细胞渗透和随着血浆水平 PBPPI 释放紫杉醇而导致暂时储存。

卡巴他赛

在以 10～30mg/m² 剂量给予卡巴他赛的临床研究中，血浆的配置是三相且与剂量成比例的[203,360,361]。类似于紫杉醇和多西紫杉醇，药剂从中央隔室的分布是快速的，而从外周隔室消除缓慢，这很可能是由于广泛的组织分布和与微管蛋白的亲密结合；在群体药代动力学研究中 α-、β-和 γ-相 $T_{1/2}$ 值分别平均为 4.4 分钟、1.6 小时和 95 小时；卡巴他赛的血浆清除率为 48.5L/h[203,360,361]。卡巴他赛在血液和血浆之间均匀分布，其 Vd 很大，稳态时平均为 2.64L/m²。卡巴他赛与人血清蛋白(主要是 almumin 和脂蛋白)的结合在体外为 89%～92%。

卡巴他赛在肝脏中广泛代谢(>95%)，主要由 CYP3A4 和 CYP3A5 同工酶(80%～90%)代谢，在较小程度上由 CYP2C8 代谢[361]。卡巴他赛是人血浆中的主要循环部分，但也检测到 7 种代谢物，其中 3 种是活性的并且由去氧甲基化形成，其中主要的一个占卡巴他赛总量的 5%。大约 20 种卡巴他赛的代谢物被排泄到人尿和粪便中。给予放射性标记的卡巴他赛后，大约 80%的给药剂量在 2 周内消除，其中 76%和 3.7%的代谢物分别通过粪便和尿液排出。

药物相互作用

紫杉类药物和其他化疗药物由给药次序决定的药动学和毒理学相互作用众所周知[362]。最突出的顺序依赖效应发生在铂类化合物和紫杉类药物之间，尤其在延迟紫杉类药物给药方案中。关于给药次序问题的报道主要集中在紫杉醇上，这可能与多西紫杉醇给药时间较短(1 小时)有关。顺铂给药后继以紫杉醇(24 小时方案)治疗方案较相反的顺序治疗方案，会导致更严重的中性粒细胞减少症，因为紫杉醇在顺铂后给药会导致紫杉醇清除率降低 33%[363,364]。最少毒性的给药顺序是先紫杉醇后顺铂，在体外实验中发现这样做细胞毒作用强，因此成为临床用药方式[364]。与卡铂单药治疗相比，当紫杉醇给药后继以卡铂联合化疗，无论 3 小时给药或 24 小时给药方案，联合化疗导致的中性粒细胞减少症相同而血小板减少症更少，通过药代动力学的相互作用无法解释[365,366]。在采用紫杉醇 24 小时给药方案时，紫杉醇在多柔比星前使用和在多柔比星后使用相比，会引起更严重的中性粒细胞减少症和黏膜炎，这极可能是在紫杉醇后给药时，多柔比星和阿霉素的清除率会下降接近 32%所致[367-369]。在采用紫杉醇 3 小时给药方案时，没有发现明显的多柔比星和紫杉醇用药顺序引起的药理学和毒理学相互作用；但是在两种顺序中，多柔比星的清除率都会降低，与不含紫杉醇方案的相同多柔比星累积剂量相比，紫杉醇(3 小时给药方案)和多柔比星(快速滴注)联合方案都会导致更高的充血性心脏毒性发生率(见毒性部分)[367,368]。尽管在紫杉醇联合表柔比星的方案中报道过表柔比星和它的代谢产物的清除率相似，但是没有观察到增加心脏毒性的趋势[370]。这些药物相互作用的确切原因还不清楚。药动学相互作用不足以解释联合方案增加心脏毒性的原因，而且有实验数据显示在心肌细胞内，紫杉醇可以增加多柔比星代谢为具有心脏毒性代谢产物的能力。多西紫杉醇似乎并不影响多柔比星的药动学过程，但是和紫杉醇相同，在人类心脏中多西紫杉醇能增强多柔比星代谢为毒性代谢物的能力[371]。肝脏或胆汁 P-糖蛋白竞争性运输蒽环类药物和紫杉醇或其聚氧乙烯化蓖麻油介质(或两者兼有)是另一种可能[291,362,367]。在多西紫杉醇中没有发现相似的作用，多西紫杉醇中不含聚氧乙烯化的蓖麻油。在紫杉醇(24 小时方案)前使用环磷酰胺较相反顺序会导致更严重的血液学毒性[372]。在体外实验中发现与紫杉类药物存在用药顺序相关细胞毒作用的药物包括 5-氟尿嘧啶、依托泊苷、阿糖胞苷、氟达拉滨、黄酮吡多和其他抗肿瘤药物[362]。在人肿瘤异种移植模型中发现，紫杉醇和多西紫杉醇都会诱导胸苷磷酸化酶的活性，导致口服嘧啶药物前体药卡培他滨的代谢活化作用增强[373,374]。

紫杉类药物与其他种类药物之间，尤其是那些依赖于细胞色素 P450 酶代谢的药物之间的相互作用都有报道[374]。一些细胞色素 P450 混合功能氧化酶诱导剂，如抗惊厥药苯妥英钠和苯巴比妥，在体外实验中发现会加快紫杉醇和多西紫杉醇在微粒体中的代谢，在同时接受这些抗惊厥药物治疗的儿童和成人中，药物清除迅速，可耐受更高剂量的药物[292,336,340,342,362,367,368,375-378]。临床前研究证明多西紫杉醇可以明显降低可能需要肝脏 CYP3A4 诱导产生药物相互作用的倾向[344]。相反的，体外研究发现，许多抑制细胞色素 P450 混合功能氧化酶的药物，如苯海拉明、红霉素、西咪替丁、睾丸素、酮康唑、氟康唑、咪达唑仑、聚氧乙烯蓖麻油和皮质类固醇，会干扰紫杉醇和多西紫杉醇在微粒体的代谢。除了之前提到的强大的 CYP3A 抑制剂和诱导剂，包括柚子汁和药草产物(如圣约翰草和菊科植物)，也可能对紫杉类药物的药代动力学相互作用产生潜在影响。虽然已经意识到使用不同 H2 受体拮抗剂对于细胞色素 P450 抑制活性不同，其作为预处理方案重要成分可能不同程度影响药物清除率，带来相应毒性，但是在随机临床试验中并未发现药物之间毒理学和药理学存在差异[379]。早期关于多西紫杉醇的临床试验综述未发现皮质类固醇会明显改变多西紫杉醇的清除率。另外，华法林和紫杉类药物的相互作用确有报道，可能是蛋白结合移位效应所致[380]。用曲妥珠单抗和紫杉醇联合治疗乳腺癌患者会增加充血性心力衰竭的发生率,但这种观察结果的解释尚未阐明[381-383]。

临床前研究表明,PBPPI 与聚氧乙烯化蓖麻油紫杉醇相比具有相似的药物相互作用[286,359]。在体外,西咪替丁、雷尼替丁、地塞米松不会影响白蛋白与 PBPPI 中的紫杉醇结合。尽管紫杉醇代谢被许多药物抑制,如酮康唑、维拉帕米、地西泮、奎尼丁、地塞米松、环孢素、替尼泊苷、依托泊苷以及长春新碱,但是在体内正常给药情况下,无法达到体外实验需要的药物浓度。在体外,睾酮、17α-乙炔基雌二醇、视黄酸和一种特殊的 CYP2C8 抑制剂——栎精,也会抑制主要代谢产物 6α-羟基紫杉醇的形成。与聚氧乙烯化蓖麻油紫杉醇类似,PBPPI 给药后,其中紫杉醇的药动学可能会发生改变,这是与底物、诱导剂或 CYP2C8 和/或)CYP3A4 抑制剂相互作用的结果。

毒性

概况

紫杉类药物的主要毒性反应为骨髓抑制。但是,尽管结构相似,不同药物之间的毒性反应谱还是存在明显不同。

紫杉醇

紫杉醇的主要毒性是中性粒细胞减少[384]。通常在给药后 8~10 天出现,基本在 15~21 天恢复。对于严重的中性粒细胞减少,主要的临床治疗策略基于目前可以提供的最佳治疗骨髓抑制的方法。但是,中性粒细胞减少基本上没有蓄积性,严重中性粒细胞减少的持续时间即使在既往接受过很多治疗的患者中也是短暂的。血浆紫杉醇的药代动力学参数反映药物暴露情况,特别是血浆浓度持续高于生理相关水平(0.05~0.10μmol/L;见临床药理学)的时间长短与中性粒细胞减少的严重程度相关,这可能解释了为什么在长时间滴注方案中中性粒细胞减少更加严重[385,386]。由于紫杉醇即使在快速给药方案中也体现了分布广泛而且亲和力好的特点,因此延时给药可能也并不意味着带来更高的抗肿瘤活性。采用紫杉醇 175mg/m^2 以上剂量持续 24 小时给药方案或 225mg/m^2,3 小时给药方案,即使在初治患者中,在许多周期中也会出现化疗后 5 天内发生中性粒细胞绝对值低于 500/μl 的情况。即使既往接受过大量化疗的患者通常也可以耐受紫杉醇 175~200mg/m^2 3 小时或 24 小时方案的化疗。高频率给药方案,特别是紫杉醇 80~100mg/m^2 每周治疗方案,较单次给药方案中性粒细胞减少的严重程度更轻(见给药方法、剂量和方案)。严重血小板减少性和贫血性患者除了预处理造成严重造血能力减少的患者外,其他近期患者的急性期反应发生率为 30%,但随着有效预防的出现和广泛采用,其发生率约为 1%~3%[377-393]。

大多数严重反应的特点是伴有支气管痉挛、荨麻疹和低血压的呼吸困难,尤其在第一次治疗后的前 10 分钟,并且在第二次治疗后较少发生。大多数过敏性反应(hypersensitivity reactions,HSR)通常在停止治疗后完全消退,偶尔用抗组胺药,补液和血管加压剂治疗后也会完全消退。在经过大剂量皮质类固醇治疗后,有些发生过敏反应的患者再次接受了紫杉醇治疗,但是这种情况不适用于所有患者[384,387-390],经历过紫杉醇相关 HSR 的患者仍然可以顺利接受多西紫杉醇的治疗[351]。轻微的过敏反应,如面部潮红和皮疹,发生率为 40%,而且特别重要的是这些轻度 HSR 不会发展为严重反应。HSR 的发生似乎主要与聚氧乙烯化蓖麻油溶剂中非免疫介导的组胺或组胺样物质释放有关,但是紫杉醇本身可能也有部分原因[384,393]。在一些病例中,补体激活也是原因之一[394]。尽管减慢输液速度,延长输液时间降低了严重 HSR 的发生率,但是如果患者在给药前接受皮质类固醇和 H_1 组胺及 H_2 组胺拮抗剂预处理的话,那么无论是 3 小时方案还是 24 小时方案,严重反应的发生率都很低(见给药方法、剂量和方案)。当评价紫杉醇两种不同给药方式的相对安全性时(24 小时∶3小时),如果给予预处理,那么接受紫杉醇 3 小时或 24 小时治疗的患者发生严重反应的概率相似,都很低(2.1%∶1.0%)[384,395]。

外周神经毒性主要体现在感觉神经表现,如麻木和感觉异常。紫杉醇的主要神经毒性表现呈现为手套-袜子样分布[384,396,397]。通常伴有对称性远端粗纤维(本体感觉、振动觉)和细纤维(温度觉、针刺觉)介导的感觉缺失。症状最快可以在高剂量(≥250mg/m^2)给药后 24~72 小时发生,但是更多时候发生在经过 135~250mg/m^2 每 3 周给药或 80~100mg/m^2 每周给药方案治疗多个周期以后,因此存在蓄积性。严重神经毒性反应要求避免长期采用紫杉醇 250mg/m^2 以上剂量 3 小时或 24 小时化疗,但是如果选择紫杉醇单药常规剂量(<200mg/m^2)化疗,即使在既往接受过具有神经毒性药物,如顺铂治疗的患者中也很少发生严重神经毒性。接受紫杉醇短时治疗方案(如 3 小时)的患者较接受紫杉醇缓慢滴注(如 24 小时或 96 小时)方案治疗的患者可能更容易发生神经毒性,提示峰浓度可能是决定神经毒性的主要药理学基础。神经毒性的发生率在 3 小时紫杉醇滴注联合顺铂化疗方案治疗的患者中特别高。远端、对称的距离依赖性神经缺陷表明紫杉醇引起的感觉和运动神经轴突缺失与逆死性神经病变相似,这种病变可能源于细胞内或轴突转运,但是仅有部分患者在胳膊和腿部同时出现症状,包括面部(口周麻木),粗纤维为主合并广泛的反射消失提示神经病变发生。两种类型的神经病变都依赖于紫杉醇剂量或联合顺铂化疗[364,398]。运动神经和自主神经功能异常也可能发生,在大剂量化疗和伴有糖尿病、酒精中毒导致神经毒性的患者中尤其多见。尽管在一些试验模型中,报道中或缺乏充分可信度的随机研究中提出,使用氨磷汀、谷氨酸、吡哆醇、含巯基净化剂药物和抗惊厥药可以减轻紫杉醇引起的神经毒性,但是目前没有确切证据显示任何特别方法可以有效改善发生的症状或预防神经毒性的发生或恶化[398-400]。

紫杉醇也可以发生视神经受损,其典型表现为出现一些暗点[401]。急性脑病见于高剂量化疗后(>600mg/m^2),可以发展为昏迷、死亡[402]。既往接受过脑放疗的患者进行紫杉醇治疗后出现短暂的急性脑病非常少见[403]。

紫杉醇可以产生短暂肌痛,但是缺乏发生肌炎的生理或生化证据。肌痛主要发生在经过 170mg/m^2 以上剂量治疗后的 2~5 天[384,404]。肌肉和神经病变的组合症状通常发生在紫杉醇每周方案持续治疗的过程中,需要延长休息时间。总的看来,非甾体抗炎药物对于缓解和预防症状作用很小,有症状的患者在给药后 2~5 天预防性给予麻醉药可能有效。有报道称抗组胺类药物可以预防肌痛的发生。皮质类固醇治疗,特别是化疗后 24 小时开始给予泼尼松 10mg 每天 2 次连续 5 天治疗，可能会减轻肌痛和关节痛，另外加巴喷丁、谷氨酸和抗组胺药也对治疗或预防反应有益。

在早期研究中，由于发生严重 HSR 的概率很高，因此要常规给予心电监护，从而发现紫杉醇可以引发心律不齐，通常没有症状或后果；因而这些反应在临床上的相关性也并不清楚[384,405]。最常见的心律不齐表现为短暂的心动过缓。积累的经验告诉我们，没有血流动力学影响的单纯性无症状心动过缓不需要停用紫杉醇。严重心动过缓，包括 Mobitz 1 型（Wenckebach 综合征）、Mobitz 2 型和Ⅲ度房室传导阻滞都有发生，但是在大宗 NCI 的资料中显示，发生率仅为 0.1%[406]。大多数报道显示为无症状发作。因为这些事件是在早期注册临床试验中接受持续心电监护的患者中发生的，因此当心电监护不再作为常规使用时，Ⅱ～Ⅲ度房室阻滞可能漏报了。有趣的是，有报道指出，无论是动物还是人类，进食紫杉属植物和与紫杉醇有关的食物后都会影响心脏自主节律和传导性，证明是紫杉醇导致了心动过缓。心肌梗死、心肌缺血、房性心律失常和室性心动过速都可以发生，但是在紫杉醇和这些事件之间是否存在必然联系还未确定。没有证据显示紫杉醇长期治疗会导致进行性心衰加重。紫杉醇治疗期间不需要进行常规心电监护，但是，建议对那些不能耐受心动过缓的患者施行心电监护，如合并房室传导阻滞或室性心衰的患者。尽管大量合并心脏功能异常和心脏病病史的患者在早期临床试验中受到入组限制，但是后来的报道证实在一些伴有心脏高危因素的妇科肿瘤患者中进行紫杉醇治疗来看，耐受性良好[357]。另一方面，反复接受紫杉醇 3 小时滴注联合阿霉素快速滴注方案治疗的患者，发生充血性心脏毒性的频率高于同等剂量阿霉素但不伴有紫杉醇化疗的频率（见药物相互作用）。一项研究结果表明，初治晚期乳腺癌患者接受单药阿霉素 60mg/m^2 化疗，当阿霉素累积剂量达到 480mg/m^2 时，发生心脏毒性的患者不超过 5%，而在此基础上联合紫杉醇 3 小时滴注治疗的患者中，发生充血性心脏毒性的比例高达 25%[367]。但是当类似的患者接受同样的化疗方案治疗，只要阿霉素的累积用量不超过 360mg/m^2，那么发生心脏毒性的比例不超过 5%。实验室研究和早期临床试验都证明，去铁胺可能会减轻阿霉素和紫杉醇联合方案的心脏毒性[407,408]。在Ⅲ期临床试验中发现，当乳腺癌患者接受曲妥珠单抗联合紫杉醇治疗时，发生充血性心衰的可能性远高于紫杉醇单药治疗的患者；因此，建议联合用药的患者需接受严格的心电监护[212-214]。

胃肠道毒性很少发生，包括恶心、呕吐和腹泻。高剂量紫杉醇可能引起黏膜炎，尤其在伴有白细胞减少的患者中经常发生，因为这些患者的黏膜保护屏障更易受损，另外在接受长时间滴注治疗的患者中发生率较高。罕见的中性粒细胞减少性小肠结肠炎和胃肠道坏死也见于一些报道，尤其在接受高剂量紫杉醇联合阿霉素或环磷酰胺治疗的患者中有相关报道[409,410]。也有关于发生严重肝功能受损和胰腺炎的报道，但是都很罕见。在接受 3 小时方案化疗的一组患者中，报道称急性双侧肺炎的发生率低于 1%，而且可以发现间质性肺毒性和实质性肺毒性两种表现，但是发生临床上明显肺毒性症状的却很少[391,411]。

紫杉醇可以导致可逆性脱发，而且随着连续给药，可以发生所有体毛的脱落。脱发似乎与剂量相关，而且这种关系仅发生在每周给药方案中。尽管紫杉醇并非糜烂性毒剂，但是如果发生大量液体渗漏于血管外，还是会导致中度软组织损伤。注射部位和沿注射静脉走行可以发生炎性反应[412]。指甲改变也有发生，特别多见于接受每周方案治疗的患者中[370]。既往接受过放疗的部位可以发生回忆反应。紫杉醇引起的味觉改变也很普遍。

多西他赛

与紫杉醇相似，多西紫杉醇的主要毒性反应也是中性粒细胞减少[200,413,414]。当接受剂量 75～100mg/m^2 静滴 1 小时治疗时，中性粒细胞数量通常低于 500/μl。中性粒细胞减少通常发生在给药后 8 天，到 15～21 天方能完全缓解。当采用低剂量高频率治疗，如每周方案治疗时，中性粒细胞减少的发生率明显降低（见给药方法、剂量和方案）。导致中性粒细胞减少最重要的决定因素是既往治疗的程度，α1-酸性糖蛋白和药物暴露在高于生物学相对浓度的持续时间似乎也是重要的决定因素（见临床药理学）。血小板和红细胞数目不会经常受到明显影响。

尽管多西紫杉醇的配方中并不含有聚氧乙烯化的蓖麻油，但是未经过预处理的患者中，大约 31% 会发生 HSR，只是通常反应轻微[200,413,414]。不仅如此，严重的反应，如呼吸困难、支气管痉挛、低血压，经常发生在头两个周期的给药后数分钟内。这些症状一般在停止化疗后 15 分钟内缓解，而且再次给药后通常不会再次发生，偶尔需要使用 H_1 组胺拮抗剂。使用皮质类固醇和 H_1 和 H_2 组胺拮抗剂进行预处理治疗可以明显降低 HSR 的发生率和严重程度（见给药方法、剂量和方案）。与紫杉醇相似，发生过严重 HSR 的患者在症状缓解并经过皮质类固醇和 H_1 组胺拮抗剂治疗后，可以再次使用多西紫杉醇。尽管在紫杉醇治疗中发生 HSR 的患者还可以接受多西紫杉醇的治疗，但是这种方案并没有经过严格的研究加以证实。

在早期研究中发现，当患者接受多程多西紫杉醇治疗后会发生特异性的液体潴留综合征，特点为水肿、体重增加和浆膜腔积液增加（心包、胸腔、腹水）[200,413-416]。体液潴留看起来与低蛋白血症或心脏、肾脏、肝脏功能异常无关，但是与肾小球通透性增加有关。肾小球滤过试验揭示了包含 2 个阶段的过程，即蛋白质和水进行性蓄积在间质空隙中，以及从第二到第四周期中发生的进行性淋巴回流不良。在缺乏预防性药物治疗的早期研究中，当多西紫杉醇的累积用量低于 400mg/m^2 时，体液潴留现象通常并不明显；但是，当累积剂量达到或超过 400mg/m^2 时，体液潴留的发生率和严重程度明显升高，经常导致给药延迟或终止给药。预防性使用皮质类固醇包括或不包括 H_1、H_2 组胺拮抗剂可以降低体液潴留的发生率，在发生毒性反应前增加给药周期数，提高多西紫杉醇的累积用量（见给药方法、剂量和方案）[415]。事实上，当广泛采用皮质类固醇进行预处理治疗后，药物相关性体液潴留已经很少发生了。结束多西紫杉醇治疗后，体液潴留现象可以缓慢缓解，发生严重毒性的患者在结束治疗后的几个月后也可以完全恢复。尽早积极选择温和的利尿剂缓慢加量进行治疗，从保钾利尿剂开始，可以有效地改善体液潴留。接受低剂量（60～75mg/m^2）化疗的研究发现，在每个周期中体液潴留的发生率较低，但是这可能是总的给药累积剂量较低的结果，而且低剂量治疗的抗肿瘤疗效也无法确定。

尽管由多西紫杉醇导致的神经感觉和神经肌肉反应与紫杉醇相似，但是与紫杉醇相比，这些症状的发生率较低，严重程度较轻[200,397,413,414,417]。在一项Ⅲ期临床研究中发现，接受多西紫杉醇联合卡铂一线方案化疗的晚期卵巢癌患者发生神经毒性的可能性和严重程度较接受紫杉醇联合卡铂方案化疗的患者更轻[417,418]。在初治患者中发生轻度至中度周围神经毒性的大约为 40%。既往接受过顺铂治疗的患者发生神经毒性的可能性增加。神经毒性的性质与紫杉醇引起的神经毒性相似，主要为感觉神经异常[364,396-400]。患者经常主诉麻痹和麻木，周围运动神经异常也可以发生。接受多西紫杉醇小于 100mg/m^2 多次治疗的患者很少发生严重神经毒性，除非患者既往合并某些其他的异常或疾病，如酒精滥用。

尽管心血管反应，包括心绞痛、心律失常、心脏传导异常、充血性心衰、高血压和低血压，在早期治疗研究中都被偶尔提及，但是没有确切证据证实多西紫杉醇与这些事件有关联。与紫杉醇相比，多西紫杉醇引起口腔炎更为多见，尤其是在延时给药的过程中，虽然这种情况已经很少出现。恶心、呕吐、腹泻很少发生，偶尔可见严重反应。

沿输液静脉走行发生静脉炎和注射部位发生炎症反应偶尔可见；但是，通常不会发生静脉外渗液导致的严重组织损伤。在治疗后数天，偶尔会发生短暂的没有发炎征象的关节痛和肌肉痛。在接受较大蓄积量治疗，特别是接受多西紫杉醇每周方案连续治疗的患者中，最多见的主诉是身体不适，即无力[419]。

50%~75%的患者会出现皮肤毒性反应[364,420]，但是，通过预处理可以减少这个副作用的发生。典型表现为前臂、手部和/或足部出现一种红斑样瘙痒的斑丘红疹。手足脱皮作为常见手-足综合征的一种表现，使用维生素 B_6 或冷敷可能会有效果，另外，以色素沉着、起皱、甲脱离、溃疡、易碎和指甲缺失为特点的指甲营养不良也有报道[318,420]。在接受低剂量高频率（如每周方案）治疗的患者中，皮肤和指甲改变似乎更为常见。偶尔会因为泪管狭窄而导致过度流泪[421]。其他少见的事件可能与多西紫杉醇有关，也可能无关，包括意识混乱、多态性红斑、中性粒细胞减少性小肠结肠炎、肝炎、肠梗阻、间质性肺炎、癫痫发作、肺纤维化、放疗后回忆反应以及视力损害。

PBPPI

PBPPI 的毒性反应与紫杉醇相似，中性粒细胞减少是主要剂量限制性毒性反应[201,283-286,358,359]。其他大多数因紫杉醇引起的毒性反应也发生在 PBPPI 中。与配方中含有聚氧乙烯酰胺蓖麻油的紫杉醇相比，PBPPI 引起的过敏反应，特别是严重的过敏反应明显减少。不需要进行预处理来预防过敏反应。在以 PBPPI 或紫杉醇为基础的方案治疗晚期乳腺癌或非小细胞肺癌的随机研究中，毒性情况相似。中性粒细胞减少和神经毒性是 PBPPI 的主要毒性。其他相对常见的副作用包括关节痛、肌痛、乏力、疲劳、黏膜炎和腹泻。在其他紫杉醇配方中更为常见的其他毒性也有发生，包括过度流泪、结膜炎、化疗后回忆反应、Stevens-Johnson 综合征、中毒性表皮坏死溶解、光敏反应以及先前接受过卡培他滨治疗的患者可患有手足综合征。

卡巴他赛

卡巴他赛的不良反应在定性和定量上与多西紫杉醇非常相似[203,225,359,360]。最常见的毒性是中性粒细胞减少症。与前面讨论的其他紫杉烷类药物一样，中性粒细胞减少是一种非累积性的、短暂的毒性。在卡巴他赛联合泼尼松与米托蒽醌联合强的松的Ⅲ期关键随机试验中，先前接受多西他赛治疗的去势抵抗的前列腺癌患者中，82%的患者出现 3~4 级中性粒细胞减少症，8%出现中性粒细胞减少性发热，还有几名患者出现了致命的不良感染事件。严重贫血（11%）和血小板减少症（4%）远不常见[225]。常见的非血液学毒性主要为胃肠道毒性：腹泻（47%，所有级别）、恶心（34%）、呕吐（22%）和便秘（20%）。重要的是，在这群先前接受多西他赛治疗的患者中，只有<1%的患者存在严重的（3~4 级）周围神经病变。其他与疾病和药物无关的常见的不良反应包括疲劳（37%）、乏力（20%）和血尿（17%）。最常见的非血液学 3~4 级不良反应是腹泻（6%）、疲劳（5%）和乏力（5%）。<4%的患者可能发生过敏反应和严重的 HSR（呼吸困难需要支气管扩张剂，低血压需要治疗，晕厥，或心动过缓）。常规的预处理，包括组胺 H_1 和 H_2 受体拮抗剂和皮质类固醇（见给药方法、剂量和方案），建议在 30 分钟前进一步减少。肌痛、关节痛、口腔炎、黏膜炎、周围水肿少见，且程度较轻（1~2 级）。33%的患者发生脱发。有时可能会出现恶心、呕吐和严重腹泻。随机临床试验中出现了腹泻和电解质失衡导致的死亡[225]。在接受卡巴他赛治疗的患者也被报道出现了其他的胃肠道毒性，包括出血、穿孔、肠梗阻、小肠结肠炎、胃炎、肠梗阻和持续便秘。腹痛和压痛、发热、持续便秘、腹泻以及伴或不伴有中性粒细胞减少可能是严重胃肠道毒性的早期表现，应及时给予评估和治疗。在这时延迟或停止卡巴他赛的治疗可能是必要的。转移酶升高很少被观察到。

给药方法、剂量和方案

紫杉醇

确定紫杉烷类药物（主要是紫杉醇）的最佳剂量和给药方案是过去十年来许多评估的重点。这些研究的综合结果表明在不同的方案中，紫杉醇都具有显著的抗癌活性。虽然没有一个特定的方案对所有类型的肿瘤都具有极佳疗效，但在乳腺癌的辅助治疗中，每周方案被证明比每 3 周方案的疗效更好[422,423]。然而一般来说，毒性效应取决于方案。紫杉醇的早期临床研究都被限定为 24 小时方案，这主要是由于在短时间给药方案中，严重 HSR 的发生率明显增加，但是随着有效的预处理方案的发展，进行了大量关于剂量范围的研究。

虽然最初紫杉醇 135mg/m^2，24 小时给药方案批准用于治疗难治和复发的卵巢癌患者，但是后来调整为 175mg/m^2，3 小时给药方案用于治疗这类患者以及其他适应证患者。对于晚期乳腺癌和卵巢癌患者，随机临床研究综合结果显示，延长注射时间的方案（24~96 小时）偶尔会提高有效率，但是其他疗效指标似乎并不依赖给药持续时间。紫杉类药物在外周组织广泛分布，同时组织与药物紧密地长时间结合，这似乎可以解释为什么在体内短时给药方案和延时给药方案的抗肿瘤活性没有实质性差别，而在体外实验中却有本质的不同[385,424,425]。间歇给药方案引起相当大的兴趣，尤其是紫杉醇每周 1 小时给药方法，与每 3 周给药一次的方案相比，骨髓抑制相当轻微[422-424,426,427]。不仅如此，报道显示对于某些疾病情况，与每3周给药一次方案相比，周疗方案疗效更佳，尤其是治疗早期（辅助治疗）和晚期乳腺癌患者时（见临床适应证）十分明显[210,422,423]。但是，没有确切证据证明对紫杉类药物3周方案治疗耐药的肿瘤，周疗会产生确实的疗效。尽管如此，对那些容易出现严重骨髓抑制的患者，周疗方案可能有优势，但是也似乎会导致神经肌肉毒性反应发生率升高。

紫杉醇推荐剂量为175mg/m²，3小时以上给药，或135～175mg/m²，24小时以上给药（少见），每3周一次。在晚期肺癌、头颈部癌和卵巢癌患者中进行的几个随机临床试验显示，紫杉醇剂量超过135～175mg/m²的24小时给药方案与常规剂量相比，并没有表现出更突出的疗效[385,424,428]。在转移性乳腺癌患者中进行的一项Ⅲ期临床试验也得到了几乎同样的结论，紫杉醇超过175mg/m²的3小时治疗方案并没有获得更好的疗效[429]。以下的推荐剂量并非常规方案：200mg/m²，1小时以上单次给药或者分为3次给药，每3周一疗程；140mg/m²，96小时以上，每3周一次；以及4周内80～100mg/m²周疗持续3或4周。在获得性免疫缺陷综合征引起的卡波西肉瘤患者中进行评价的最常见方案为紫杉醇135mg/m²，3小时或24小时，每3周重复和100mg/m²每两周重复[215]。紫杉醇也可以进行胸腔和腹腔给药。腹腔内给药获得了生物学相关的血浆浓度，而且腹膜腔内的药物浓度比血浆浓度高几倍。推荐以下的预处理方案防止发生主要的HSR：地塞米松20mg口服或静脉注射，化疗前12小时和6小时各一次；H_1组胺拮抗剂（如苯海拉明，50mg静脉注射），化疗前30分钟；以及H_2组胺拮抗剂（如西咪替丁，300mg；法莫替丁，20mg；或雷尼替丁，150mg静脉注射），化疗前30分钟。化疗前30分钟给予单剂量皮质类固醇（地塞米松20mg静脉注射）似乎也可以有效预防主要的HSR。

药物分布的主要模式为肝脏代谢和胆汁分泌，因此肝功能不全患者使用紫杉醇时需要调整剂量。前瞻性研究显示，与未合并肝功能不全的患者相比，存在中度或重度血清肝细胞酶和/或胆红素水平升高的患者，更容易发生严重毒性反应。因此，推荐合并中度肝功能障碍患者将紫杉醇剂量至少减少50%[430]。当肝脏转氨酶升高到正常上限（upper limit of normal，ULN）的10倍，并将胆红素提高到ULN的1.26～2.0倍时，建议将3小时给药方案下的紫杉醇剂量从175mg/m²降低到135mg/m²。如果胆红素进一步升高到5.0倍，并伴转氨酶升高到ULN的10倍，那么紫杉醇的使用剂量建议降低到90mg/m²。对于更多的转氨酶和/或肝排泄功能障碍的情况，尚未制定相应的建议剂量。由于肾脏对总体药物清除的贡献最小（5%～10%），所以合并严重肾功能不全的患者似乎不需要调整药物剂量[292,431]。基于药物的药理学表现，特别是紫杉烷类药物在体内广泛分布的特点，仅发生周围性水肿和浆膜腔积液时，不需要调整剂量。

聚氧乙烯化蓖麻油紫杉醇要避免与可塑化聚氯乙烯（polyvinyl chloride，PVC）装置或设备接触，因为这样可能会增加患者暴露于从PVC注射袋或注射套浸出的可塑剂的风险。紫杉醇溶液需要稀释并储存在玻璃或聚丙烯瓶子中或适合的塑料袋中（聚丙烯或聚烯烃），并且通过非PVC的给药装置给药，如聚乙烯内衬。装置包括一个带有多微孔膜的线型过滤器，孔径不超过0.22μm。

多西紫杉醇

多西紫杉醇用于晚期乳腺癌的剂量范围为60～100mg/m²（静脉注射1小时），在所有其他适应证中作为单一药物或与其他药物联合使用的剂量范围为75mg/m²。值得注意的是，大多数临床评估集中在这一范围的上限剂量（75～100mg/m²），而使用多西紫杉醇（60mg/m²）治疗的患者数据相对较少[200]。虽然一些未经治疗或最低限度预处理的患者可以耐受多西紫杉醇100mg/m²治疗，而且这也是许多地区在选择适应证时唯一批准的剂量，但从毒理学角度来看，75mg/m²似乎更合理，适用于较重治疗的患者[432]。与紫杉醇相同，多西紫杉醇也可以采用每周1小时的输液给药方法，尽管与传统的每3周一次的频率相比，周疗方案在抗肿瘤活性方面并没有明确的获益[210,418]，但周疗方案的血液毒性更低。多西紫杉醇周疗方法的主要毒性反应是蓄积性乏力和神经毒性，避免给药剂量超过每周36mg/m²。尽管使用聚山梨醇酯-80取代聚氧乙烯基蓖麻油（紫杉醇助溶剂）合成紫杉醇，但是如果患者不进行预处理治疗，仍然会导致HSR和严重的液体潴留发生率相对较高，有几种有效的预处理方案可以采用，最常用的方案是地塞米松8mg，每天口服两次连续3天，在多西紫杉醇给药前1天开始，多西紫杉醇给药前30分钟可以给予H_1和H_2组胺拮抗剂，也可以不用[413,414]。对于前列腺癌转移的患者，考虑同时使用泼尼松，建议在使用多西他赛前8小时、3小时和1小时口服8mg地塞米松。即使是在没有出现HSR的患者中也不推荐在不使用皮质类固醇的情况下使用多西紫杉醇，因为药物相关性液体潴留是一种慢性毒性反应，可以导致停药[414,415]。

一项以多西紫杉醇药物动力学为研究目的的回顾性研究发现，没有合并高胆红素血症的患者中，如果肝脏转氨酶水平升高（1.5倍或以上）同时碱性磷酸酶水平升高（2.5倍或以上），无论这种升高是否是肝转移的结果，多西紫杉醇清除都下降了大约25%[346-349,433]。因此，对于这样的患者，建议减量至少25%。虽然合并中度或重度肝脏排泄功能不全（高胆红素血症）的患者可能需要更大幅度的药物减量，但肝脏在药物处理中的几乎排他作用导致制造商不建议将多西他赛用于转氨酶升高超过ULN 1.5倍，同时碱性磷酸酶升高超过2.5倍，或胆红素值升高的受试者。与紫杉醇类似（见紫杉醇方法、剂量和方案），仅合并肾功能不全和/或浆膜腔积液不是调整剂量的合理理由。与紫杉醇的情况类似（见紫杉醇方法、剂量和方案），多西紫杉醇不建议与塑化PVC设备接触。为了尽量减少患者与可浸出的增塑剂DEHP的接触，应使用瓶子（玻璃或聚丙烯）或塑料袋（聚丙烯或聚烯烃）对多西紫杉醇进行制备和储存，并通过内衬聚乙烯的给药装置进行给药。

PBPPI

PBPPI最初在美国获得监管批准，用于治疗联合化疗失败的晚期乳腺癌或辅助化疗后6个月内复发的转移性乳腺癌患者[226]。这一适应证的推荐剂量为260mg/m²，30分钟静脉注射给药；然而，在其他不同的给药方案中也观察到了明显的抗癌活性，在100～150mg/m²的剂量范围内尤为明显，具体用法与紫杉醇和多西他赛类似，30分钟静滴，每周一次，连续3周，4周重复。PBPPI之后很快就在美国和其他地方注册作为局部晚期或转移性胰腺癌患者或非小细胞肺癌的一线治疗，125mg/ m^2 或 100mg/ m^2，30~40 分钟静脉注射，每周一次，连续 3 周，28 天重复，可与卡铂或吉西他滨分别合用[200,227]。化疗前不推荐预处理以预防 HSR 或水肿。不必要一定使用专门的非 DEHP（即非 PVC）容器和给药装置，也不建议使用嵌入过滤器。伴有肝功能不全（胆红素 1.5>mg/dl）和肾功能不全患者的最佳剂量尚不清楚；但是，与其他紫杉烷类药物类似，肾脏排泄是可以忽略的。制造商建议：当伴有中度或重度肝功能缺陷（定义为胆红素升高不超过 ULN 的 5 倍），伴或不伴转氨酶 ULN 升高不超过 ULN 的 10 倍时，晚期或转移性乳腺癌患者或非小细胞肺癌患者的剂量应分别从 260mg/ m^2 减少到 200mg/ m^2 或从 100mg/ m^2 减少到 80mg/ m^2。PBPPI 不推荐用于胆红素超过 ULN 1.5 倍的胰腺癌患者。只要胆红素值不超过 1.5 倍，转氨酶升高低于 ULN 10 倍的患者无需减少剂量。对于胆红素超过 ULN 5 倍的患者，制造商不推荐使用 PBPPI。在 PBPPI 治疗期间出现严重中性粒细胞减少症和/或血小板减少的患者建议停止治疗，直到充分恢复才能重新使用 PBPPI，此外在随后的治疗中需要减少剂量。对于严重感觉神经病变的患者，建议停止治疗，直到症状恢复到轻度或中度表现时，开始减量的后续疗程。对于接受 PBPPI 加吉西他滨治疗的胰腺癌患者，PBPPI 治疗在发生 3 级黏膜炎或腹泻时暂停，在毒性消退至 1 级或更低水平后恢复低剂量。最后，如果使用 PBPPI 加吉西他滨治疗的患者出现 2 级或 3 级皮肤毒性，建议减少 PBPPI 的剂量，如果毒性持续，建议停止治疗。

卡巴他赛

卡巴他赛用于先前使用含有多西紫杉醇的治疗方案的去势抵抗的转移前列腺癌患者的治疗[203,225,360,361]。该药物的具体剂量为 25mg/ m^2，60 分钟静脉注射，每 3 周一次，并在整个治疗过程中每日口服泼尼松 10mg。其他方案尚未得到充分评估。以下预处理方案建议在每次卡巴他赛给药前至少 30 分钟静脉注射以降低 HSR 的风险和/或严重性：苯海拉明 25mg 或等价的 H_1 组胺拮抗剂，地塞米松 8mg 或等价的类固醇，以及 H2-组胺拮抗剂如雷尼替丁 50mg 或等价的其他药物。建议进行止吐预防，并可根据需要口服或静脉注射。与多西紫杉醇一样，卡巴他赛也是在聚山梨醇-80 中配制的，用乙醇稀释，然后在 0.9%氯化钠溶液或 5%葡萄糖溶液中稀释。由于聚山梨醇酯-80 有潜在的过滤增塑剂的能力，所以无论是 PVC 输液容器或聚氨酯输液器都不能用于制备或管理卡巴他赛。卡巴他赛的管理应该使用名义上孔径为 0.22μm 的管路过滤器（也指 0.2μm）。

目前还没有对卡巴他赛进行专门的肝损害试验，因此合并肝功能不全或肾功能损害的患者也没有相应的剂量推荐。虽然多西紫杉醇和卡巴他赛有相似的清除模式，像多西紫杉醇一样调整卡巴他赛的剂量似乎是合理的，但制造商并没有正式推荐卡巴他赛用于肝功能不全的患者。根据人群药代动力学数据，轻度至中度（30ml/min≤肌酐清除率）患者的清除率无显著差异，不确定需要减少此类受试者的药物剂量。然而，严重肾功能损害（肌酐清除率<30ml/min）和终末期肾病患者应谨慎使用。与紫杉醇、多西紫杉醇和 PBPPI 类似，当有相关的各程度的中性粒细胞减少症、腹泻和/或周围神经病变时，卡巴他赛的剂量应进行调整和/或进行相应治疗。例如，如果患者在 30mg/ m^2 剂量水平治疗后，尽管使用了包括生长因子在内的适当药物，仍出现了中性粒细胞减少程度≥3 级，且持续至少 7 天的情况，则需要将剂量减少到 20mg/ m^2。对于出现≥3 级腹泻或持续性腹泻的患者，尽管有适当的药物、液体和电解质替代或 2 级周围神经病变，仍应坚持卡巴他赛治疗，直到症状改善或消退，然后将剂量减少到 20mg/ m^2。卡巴他赛不应用于已发展为 3 级严重周围神经病变的患者。

其他加强微管聚合的天然化合物

紫杉烷类化合物的成功经验引发了人们寻找其他可以加强微管聚合药物的兴趣，从而在过去 20 年里发现了几种效果较好的化合物，其中与此关联最密切的是埃博霉素。埃博霉素是最初从土壤中的溶纤维素黏细菌中分离提取到的大环内酯类化合物。其他促进微管蛋白聚合的天然产品包括圆皮海绵内酯（从 Caribbean 海绵 *Discodermia dissoluta* 中分离提取）、eleutherobin（从软珊瑚 *Eleutherobia* sp. 中提取），莱利霉素（从海生海绵 *Cacospongia mycofijiensis* 中提取）、peloruside A（从新西兰海洋海绵 *Mycale hentscheli* 中提取）、箭根酮内酯（植物源性的自然类固醇）和 sarcodictyins（从地中海 stoloniferan 珊瑚 *Sarcodictyon roseum* 中提取）。其中一些化合物与紫杉醇竞争性与微管结合，而且与紫杉类药物结合位点一致或邻近（埃博霉素、圆皮海绵内酯、eleutherobins 和 sarcodictyins）；但其他的一些化合物，如莱利霉素和 peloruside A，似乎只与微管的特定部位结合[2-7,237,316]。因为 eleutherobin、epothilones A 和 B 和圆皮海绵内酯竞争性地抑制紫杉醇与微管的结合，因此可以发现并确认一个共同的药效基团，这可能有助于开发出具有更理想生物学特性的杂交结构[237,240,316]。有趣的是，圆皮海绵内酯和紫杉醇在体外表现出协同的细胞毒性，这表明它们的微管结合位点和微管效应不相同[433]。然而，在一种完全合成的圆皮海绵内酯 XAA296 的早期临床试验中发现了意想不到的肺毒性[434]。大多数上述化合物，特别是 epothilone B，圆皮海绵内酯和箭根酮内酯在体外研究中都表现出与 ABC 转运或低或无的亲和性，对紫杉烷类耐药细胞具有不同程度的活性，包括表达 βⅢ微管的恶性肿瘤细胞（epothilone B，箭根酮内酯）。尽管这些特性的临床意义还不完全清楚，但在临床上已经证明埃博霉素在既往接受过紫杉烷类药物治疗，并且其中一部分还明确为紫杉类耐药的患者具有相当疗效。在所有促进微管聚合的非紫杉醇类微管聚合剂中，埃博霉素的研发进展最快，而埃博霉素 B 类似物伊沙匹隆已被注册用于治疗不再受益于紫杉醇的晚期乳腺癌患者。

伊沙匹隆和埃博霉素

埃博霉素 A 和埃博霉素 B（帕妥匹隆）是由 16 元大环内酯类聚酮化合物，埃博霉素 B 除了在 C12 的位置上增加了一个甲基集团外，二者的结构几乎完全相同。体外对肿瘤细胞系的研究表明，埃博霉素 B 比埃博霉素 A 活性更高。埃博霉素 A 和埃博霉素 B 在体外均比紫杉醇或多西紫杉醇药效强，平均半抑制浓度（IC_{50}）值在低纳摩尔范围[435,436]。将埃博霉素 B 的内酯转化为内酰胺,就合成了埃博霉素 B 的半合成衍生物伊沙匹隆(氮杂埃坡霉素 B)(图 60-4)。这种结构修饰提高了溶解度,降低了血浆蛋白的结合,比其前体具有更高的代谢稳定性。埃博霉素,特别是埃博霉素 B 类似物与 β 微管蛋白结合的独特机制,至少在一定程度上,可能促使它们拥有相对于紫杉烷类而言更强的效力和更广泛的功能,以及稳定酵母微管的能力[437]。埃博霉素 A 和埃博霉素 B 良好的抗癌活性使人振奋,在大环内酯环上进行进一步改进,产生了 deoxyepothilone B(埃博霉素 D),它拥有和埃博霉素 A 和埃博霉素 B 相似的抗肿瘤活性。

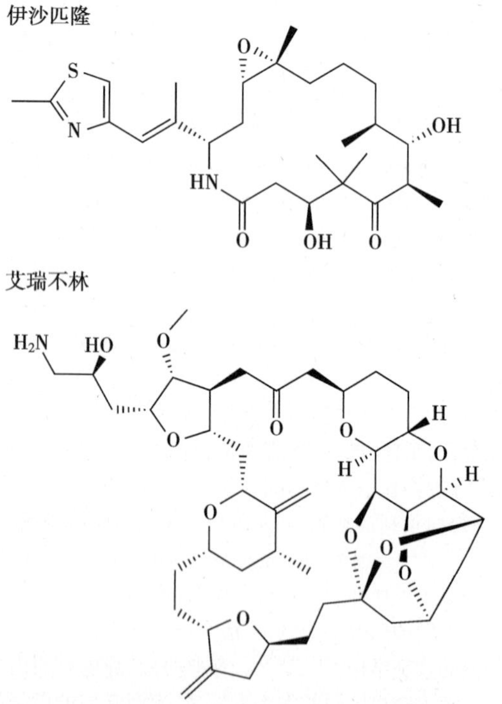

伊沙匹隆

艾瑞不林

图 60-4 伊沙匹隆和艾瑞不林的化学结构

临床适应证

伊沙匹隆被注册为在紫杉烷、蒽环类药物和卡培他滨失败后,治疗转移性或局部晚期乳腺癌的单一用药药物,与卡培他滨联合用于治疗蒽环和紫杉烷类药物治疗失败的患者[438]。伊沙匹隆和其他埃博霉素,尤其是埃博霉素 B,在其他各种恶性肿瘤中也显示出抗癌活性。主要对那些对紫杉烷类药物敏感的肿瘤效果好,例如非小细胞肺癌、前列腺癌和卵巢癌[439,440]。

作用机制

与天然的埃博霉素 A 和埃博霉素 B 一样,伊沙匹隆能稳定微管并诱导细胞凋亡[433,436,440,441]。伊沙匹隆对人类和小鼠肿瘤异种移植瘤有显著的抗肿瘤活性,并且对紫杉醇耐药的细胞系和肿瘤反应活跃,包括那些 Pgp 和/或 βⅢ-或者 βⅣ-微管同形像表达升高的肿瘤细胞[433,435,436,440,441]。埃博霉素 A 和埃博霉素 B 及其相关类似物在体外竞争性地抑制紫杉醇与微管蛋白聚合物的结合,推测埃博霉素与紫杉烷的结合位点可能重叠[435-437]。它们也有类似的结合亲和力。事实上,埃博霉素和紫杉烷具有相同的药效基团用于微管结合[237,240]。体外环境下,埃博霉素 A 和埃博霉素 B 促进微管聚合,其动力学与紫杉醇相似,但埃博霉素 B 似乎比埃博霉素 A 和紫杉醇诱导作用更强。与紫杉烷药物类似,埃博霉素在缺少 GTP 和/或 MAP 的情况下依然可以诱导微管聚合,导致微管变长、变硬,对低温、钙离子的稳定性增强,从而提高微管稳定性,保证微管集合成束[237,435-437,439-446]。此外,埃博霉素诱导有丝分裂纺锤体形成异常,导致细胞周期阻滞在 G2/M 期。在低浓度条件下,埃博霉素 B 不会诱导有丝分裂停滞,但是可以改变增殖细胞形成大的异倍体细胞,使细胞在 G_1 期发生细胞凋亡。因此,延迟有丝分裂可能不是这些药物凋亡细胞凋亡的主要原因[446]。

尽管埃博霉素和紫杉烷在机械构造上具有相似性,但利用电子晶体学进行研究的结果表明埃博霉素与 β 微管通过独特独立的分子间相互作用发挥药物作用,这可能是这些药物破坏各种 βⅢ、βⅣ微管蛋白以及其他微管同分体更不易受紫杉烷类药物影响的原因[446]。此外,使细胞对紫杉烷类产生耐药性的 β 微管蛋白的各种突变不会显著改变埃博霉素 A 和 B 的细胞毒性,但微管蛋白突变的临床意义还不清楚[296]。

埃博霉素的一个重要特点似乎是微管扰动导致细胞死亡的机制。而在埃博霉素中,对伊沙匹隆的研究最多。紫杉烷类诱导的细胞凋亡是通过线粒体介导的途径传递信号的,涉及了细胞色素 C 的释放和 Apaf-1 和 caspase-9 的活化,而伊沙匹隆诱导的细胞凋亡涉及了 caspase-3 和 caspase-8 的活化[447-450]。在紫杉醇难治性卵巢癌细胞中,伊沙匹隆能够诱导 p53 依赖的 p53 上调凋亡调节剂(PUMA),从而激活 caspase-2、死亡效应因子 Bax 和细胞凋亡[451,452]。

耐药机制

与紫杉烷类和长春花生物碱相比,转运蛋白 Pgp 和 MRP1 的过表达对埃博霉素的细胞毒性影响最小,因为它们是这些转运蛋白的弱底物[2,3,240,433,437,440,441,446]。埃博霉素 A 和 B 在对紫杉醇耐药的 P-糖蛋白(ABCB1)高表达的人类肿瘤细胞中具有很强的抗增殖活动,并且,从伊沙匹隆治疗有效患者体内获取的肿瘤样本表明 MDR1 和 MRP1 显著表达,这些蛋白质在埃博霉素的临床应用时可能不会导致相关的耐药性[453,454]。在体外,埃博霉素 B 类似物伊沙匹隆不是乳腺癌抵抗蛋白(breast cancer resistance protein,BCRP)的底物。

在临床前系统观察中,肿瘤细胞具有各种各样的 β 微管蛋白突变,例如对微管稳定至关重要的 βⅠ微管蛋白突变,而这些似乎导致了细胞对埃博霉素耐药,然而这些观察的临床意义仍是未知的[296]。临床前研究还提示存在其他耐药机制,例如 α 微管蛋白突变,微管蛋白同分体表达改变,以及 MAP 结构和功能改变等[433,435,440,443,454]。

临床药理学

伊沙匹隆在采用 15~57mg/m² 剂量给药时,表现为剂量-比例药代动力学模式(表 60-3)[435,440,454]。40mg/m² 单次给药后,平均 C_{max} 为 252ng/ml(变异系数 56%),终末期 $T_{1/2}$ 平均为

表 60-3　伊沙匹隆和 Eribulin：药物动力学和毒理学特性的比较

参数	伊沙匹隆	Eribulin
标准成人剂量[mg/(m^2·3 周)]	40(3h 静脉注射)；若身体表面积超过该值，应以 2.2 为上限	—
标准成人剂量(mg/m^2/周)	16(每 4 周三次)	1.4(每 3 周两次)或 1.4(每 4 周三次)，2~5min 静脉注射
药代动力学行为(临床相关剂量)	多指数	双指数
剂量比例效应的范围(mg/m^2)	15~57	0.25~4.0
血浆半衰期(终末期)	52h	40h
清除速度	36~40L/h	1.15~2.42L/h
主要排泄方式	肝脏新陈代谢和胆道排泄	肝脏新陈代谢和胆道排泄
主要的毒性效应	神经毒性，中性粒细胞减少	中性粒细胞减少
其他毒性	超敏反应，贫血，血小板减少	神经毒性，疲劳，血小板减少，贫血

52 小时。因此，如果每 3 周给药一次，预计不会有药物积累。与紫杉烷类和长春花生物碱类药物相似，伊沙匹隆的稳态分布容积很大，平均值超过 1 000L。在体外，其与人血清蛋白的结合率在 67%~77%之间，而在人类血液中血液-血浆浓度比在 0.65~0.85 之间。伊沙匹隆全身消除的主要方式是肝脏代谢。静脉注射放射性标记的伊沙匹隆后，约 86%的剂量在 7 天内消除；主要是不活跃的代谢物通过粪便和尿液排泄，粪便和尿液的排泄量分别占药物剂量的 65%和 21%，排出的母体化合物分别约占总剂量的 1.6%和 5.6%。体外主要代谢途径为 CYP3A4 氧化代谢。超过 30 种无活性代谢产物通过尿液和粪便排出，但没有一种代谢产物的量超过给药剂量的 6%。

药物相互作用

体外使用人类肝微粒体研究发现，伊沙匹隆的临床相关浓度不会影响 CYP3A4、CYP1A2、CYP2A6、CYP2B6、CYP2C8、CYP2C9、CYP2C19 或者 CYP2D6 的活性，因此可能不会影响作为这些酶的底物药物的药物动力学表现和代谢情况[435,440,454]。然而，与单独使用伊沙匹隆相比，与强效 CYP3A4 抑制剂酮康唑联合使用伊沙匹隆可使伊沙匹隆的 AUC 值平均增加 79%。考虑到和酮康唑及类似的 CYP3A4 强效抑制剂联合使用时的影响，如果不能改换其他治疗方案，那么应考虑调整剂量，并应监测患者的毒性。由于轻度或中度 CYP3A4 抑制剂(如红霉素、氟康唑或维拉帕米)对伊沙匹隆药物暴露的影响还缺少临床研究，所以如果在伊沙匹隆治疗期间必须使用此类药物，应十分谨慎。与单用伊沙匹隆相比，共同服用有效的 CYP3A4 代谢诱导物利福平使伊沙匹隆 AUC 减少了 43%，并且可以预计其他强有力的 CYP3A4 诱导物，如地塞米松、苯妥英、卡马西平、利福平、苯巴比妥也可能起到同样的作用，从而可能降低伊沙匹隆的浓度；因此，在与伊沙匹隆合用时应考虑无或低 CYP3A4 诱导效应的药物。圣约翰草可能会不可预测地降低伊沙匹隆的血浆浓度，应避免使用。如果患者必须与强 CYP3A4 诱导剂联合用药，可以考虑逐步调整剂量。研究表明，在接受伊沙匹隆(40mg/m^2)联合卡培他滨(1 000mg/m^2)治疗的癌症患者中，伊沙匹隆对卡培他滨和 5-氟尿嘧啶的 C_{max} 和 AUC 值的影响适度，且无临床相关性，特别是联合治疗的合理性已经得到确切有效的数据支持。

伊沙匹隆在相关的临床浓度下不抑制 CYP 酶，预计不会改变其他药物的血浆浓度。关于这一点，接受伊沙匹隆(40mg/m^2)联合卡培他滨(1 000mg/m^2)治疗的患者与其分别接受的伊沙匹隆和卡培他滨相比，伊沙匹隆的 C_{max} 值下降 19%，卡培他滨的 C_{max} 值下降 27%，5-氟尿嘧啶 AUC 增加 14%。基于支持联合治疗具有独特作用的临床疗效数据，这种相互作用与临床无关。

毒性效应

在伊沙匹隆单药或联合卡培他滨治疗时，最常见的严重毒性是外周神经毒性，总结见表 60-3[435,439,440,454,455]。最常见的症状包括烧灼感、感觉过敏、感觉迟钝、感觉异常和神经性疼痛。既往接受过含紫杉醇药物化疗的乳腺癌患者，在伊沙匹隆单药化疗后，大约 63%的患者会发生周围神经病变，在联合卡培他滨治疗后的患者中发生率大约为 67%；但是，严重毒性(Ⅲ度和Ⅳ度)反应的发生率分别为 14%和 23%。既往接受过大量化疗的患者发生神经毒性的时间较早，在头 3 个周期中，大约 75%的患者会发生神经毒性或神经病变加重，而且在四周期化疗后症状最重。尽管根据对临床试验数据的大量回顾性分析，先前接触过神经毒性药物似乎不容易发生神经病变，但值得注意的是，神经病变程度至少为中度神经病变的患者被排除在早期研究之外。合并肝功能不全和糖尿病的患者发生严重神经病变的风险增加(见给药方法、剂量和方案)。在临床试验中发现，减少药物用量、推迟给药时间和终止给药可以缓解周围神经病变(见给药方法、剂量和方案)。经过终止给药和/或减量给药处理后，由紫杉烷类、长春花生物碱和艾日布林引起的症状可以迅速缓解，中位时间为4~6周，严重毒性可以恢复至Ⅰ度毒性，几乎所有3~4级事件在发病后12周内都能消退到这个水平。

剂量依赖性的骨髓抑制，特别是中性粒细胞减少，在伊沙匹隆化疗中经常发生。而血小板减少和红细胞减少并不常见。在伊沙匹隆联合卡培他滨化疗的患者中，36%患者会发生Ⅳ度中性粒细胞减少(<500个/μl)，而单药化疗组中的Ⅳ度中性粒细胞减少发生率为23%；但是，伊沙匹隆联合卡培他滨化疗中，中性粒细胞减少性发热和中性粒细胞减少性感染的发生率分别为5%和6%，而单药化疗组中，两者分别为3%和5%。连续化疗不会加重骨髓抑制，提示造血干细胞没有受到明显影响。发生严重中性粒细胞减少的患者建议减量治疗，伴有中度肝功能受损的患者建议调整剂量(见"给药方法、剂量和方案"部分)。由于伊沙匹隆溶于聚氧乙烯酰胺蓖麻油，需要注意由溶剂导致的严重过敏反应。过敏反应表现包括脸红、皮疹、呼吸困难和支气管痉挛。基于这个原因，建议所有患者在化疗前1小时左右接受 H_1 和 H_2 组胺拮抗剂预处理(见"给药方法、剂量和方案部分")。如果发生严重过敏反应，应当停止化疗并积极给予支持治疗(如肾上腺素、皮质类固醇)。在临床研究中，尽管给予了各种预处理方案，仍然有1%左右的患者会发生严重过敏反应。有报道指出，发生过敏反应的患者，在加入皮质类固醇(例如化疗前30分钟地塞米松20mg静脉注射或化疗前60分钟口服)、H_1 和 H_2 组胺拮抗剂和延长给药时间后，仍然可以再次接受这种药物化疗。

接受伊沙匹隆化疗的患者在围化疗期可以出现认知功能障碍、嗜睡和不协调运动，这可能是因为溶剂中含有乙醇。围化疗期还可以发生肌肉痛和关节痛，也可以发生一系列心脏异常，包括心肌梗死、室上性心律失常、左心室功能不全、心绞痛、心房扑动、心肌病和心肌缺血，但是这些症状的发生不一定与伊沙匹隆直接相关。罕见的毒性反应偶有发生，包括肠梗阻、结肠炎、胃排空不全、食管炎、吞咽困难、胃炎、胃肠道出血、肝功能损害、多形性红斑、肌肉痉挛、牙关紧闭和肾衰竭。

给药方法、剂量和方案

伊沙匹隆推荐剂量为40mg/m²，每次静脉注射3小时以上，每3周给药一次[436,440,454,455]。因为缺乏人体表面积超过2.2m²的患者的药物剂量数据，所以，这些患者的药物剂量应以体表面积2.2m²来计算。虽然评估过间断给药方案的范围，特别是4周为一周期，连续3周给药，每周给药16mg/m²。目前最有疗效的剂量方案是每3周给药一次，每次3小时，但是迄今为止，间歇性给药方案中还没有显示出更好的疗效。伊沙匹隆仅与配套的稀释液稀释后才能用于静脉注射。稀释液是非热解溶液，含52.8%(w/v)纯化的聚氧乙烯蓖麻油和39.8%(w/v)无水乙醇，而且需要乳酸套环注射剂进一步稀释，或0.9%氯化钠注射液(在加入所组成的伊沙匹隆溶液之前，使用碳酸氢钠将pH调整在6.0至9.0之间)。为了降低严重超敏反应的发生机会，给药前大约1小时，所以患者都要接受预处理治疗，包括 H_1 组胺拮抗剂(例如苯海拉明50mg口服或相当的药物)和 H_2 组胺拮抗剂(例如口服雷尼替丁150~300mg或相当的药物)。对于有超敏反应病史的患者，除了使用的 H_1 组胺和 H_2 组胺拮抗剂进行预处理，还建议给予皮质类固醇进行预处理(例如，地塞米松20mg化疗前30分钟静脉给药，或化疗前60分钟口服给药)。

发生临床相应级别神经病变和/或骨髓抑制的患者推荐调整剂量和/或治疗延迟。对于发生Ⅱ度神经病变并持续至少7天或Ⅲ度病变持续不足7天的患者，建议给药剂量减少20%。对于出现长时间Ⅲ度神经病变或任何Ⅳ度毒性的患者，建议停止治疗。出现中性粒细胞计数<500/μl持续至少7天和/或伴发热，血小板计数<25 000/μl，或血小板计数<50 000/μl伴出血的患者也建议给药剂量减少20%。除外疲乏，肢端红肿症和/或关节痛/肌痛，发生其他类型的Ⅲ度(严重)毒性反应的患者也建议给药剂量减少20%。任何类型的Ⅳ度(禁止)非血液学毒性都建议终止用药。研究显示，在伴有轻度到严重肝损伤患者中使用伊沙匹隆时，当患者的胆红素水平波动在ULN的1~1.5倍范围，或AST水平超过ULN并伴有胆红素升高低于ULN 1.5倍时，伊沙匹隆的AUC值增长22%；而且，无论AST水平如何，只要患者的胆红素水平超过ULN的1.5~3倍，伊沙匹隆的AUC值增长30%；只要患者的胆红素水平超过ULN的3倍，伊沙匹隆的AUC值增长81%。少部分伴有严重肝功能不全(胆红素超过ULN3倍)的患者可以耐受10mg/m²和20mg/m²单药治疗。伴有AST或ALT升高至ULN 10倍以内和胆红素水平升高至ULN 1.5倍以内的患者，推荐伊沙匹隆单药治疗减量至32mg/m²。伴有AST或ALT升高至ULN 10倍以内和胆红素水平升高至ULN 1.5~3.0倍的患者，推荐伊沙匹隆单药治疗减量至20mg/m²。如果患者耐受，在后续化疗周期中，伊沙匹隆剂量可以增加，但是不能超过30mg/m²。伴有重度肝功能不全，即AST或ALT升高超过ULN 10倍或胆红素水平升高超过ULN 3.0倍的患者，不推荐使用伊沙匹隆。伴有AST、ALT和/或胆红素水平超过ULN的患者，不推荐伊沙匹隆和卡培他滨的联合方案。伴有AST和ALT低于ULN 2.5倍且胆红素水平正常的患者，推荐伊沙匹隆标准剂量(40mg/m²)。

伊沙匹隆很少通过肾脏排泄，但是，在肌酐水平升高超过ULN 1.5倍患者中没有进行伊沙匹隆单药治疗的相关评估。伊沙匹隆单药治疗的群体药代动力学分析显示，轻度至中度肾功能不全(肌酐清除率>30ml/min)对于伊沙匹隆药代动力学没有产生影响。尚未在肌酐清除率<50ml/min患者中进行伊沙匹隆联合卡培他滨化疗方案的评估。应当避免合并使用强效CYP3A4抑制剂(例如酮康唑、伊曲康唑、克拉仙霉素、阿扎那韦、奈法唑酮、沙奎那韦、泰利霉素、利托那韦、氨普那韦、茚地那韦、奈非那韦、地拉韦啶或伏立康唑)(见"药物相互作用")。葡萄柚汁可能会影响药物代谢的清除，要避免饮用。基于药代动力学研究，如果必须与强效CYP3A4抑制剂合并使用，那么伊沙匹隆剂量必须要减为20mg/m²，这时应将伊沙匹隆的AUC与未用抑制剂的AUC校正。如果停用强效抑制剂，那么在采用伊沙匹隆推荐剂量给药之前，建议给予1周的洗脱期。

甲磺酸艾日布林和其他促进微管蛋白解聚的天然产品

其他几种天然或半合成药剂能与微管蛋白的长春花或秋

水仙碱结合域结合，这些药物已经得到批准或正在被评估。甲磺酸艾日布林（eribulin mesylate）是海洋天然产品软海绵素 B（halichondrin B）的一种大环酮类似物，该药物最初从海生海绵 *Halichondria okadai* 中分离出（图 60-4），自在世界范围内被登记后，已经成为继蒽环类抗生素和紫衫烷类治疗女性晚期乳腺癌无效后最有效的药物。甲磺酸艾日布林和其他软海绵素 B 类似物能与微管蛋白结合并抑制其聚合，干扰有丝分裂纺锤体的形成和着丝粒动力，诱导有丝分裂停止进而引起细胞凋亡，并在亚纳米范围内具有生长抑制特性，在临床前研究中具有显著的抗癌活性[456-458]。Hemiasterlin（HTI-286 和 E7974）是一种从海生海绵中分离出的天然产品，其合成也处于临床开发阶段[459]。Hemiasterlin 及其类似物与微管蛋白上的长春花结合域结合，干扰正常的微管动力学，在化学计量浓度下使微管解聚。它们作为 Pgp 的底物，活性比长春花生物碱和紫杉烷类弱得多，而在人类肿瘤异种移植物中具有显著的抗癌活性，这包括那些表达 Pgp 的肿瘤[460,461]。Hemiasterlin 也与长春花生物碱以及能与微管蛋白上长春花结合位点结合的其他药物存在交叉耐药性，但与紫杉烷类，伊沙匹隆和秋水仙碱类交叉耐药性较弱。在临床前研究中，这种耐药性至少部分由 α-微管蛋白的突变和/或不同于 Pgp，ABCG2，MRP1 或 MRP3 的 ABC 药物泵介导[460,461]。

其他的促进微管蛋白聚合的强效天然产品是多拉司他汀（dolastatins），是从海兔 *Dolabella auricularia* 中提取的一系列寡肽。多拉司他汀能非竞争性地抑制长春花生物碱与微管蛋白的结合，微管蛋白聚合以及微管蛋白依赖性 GTP 的水解[462]。多拉司他汀也能保持微管蛋白上秋水仙素结合活性的稳定，同时在皮摩尔到低钠摩尔范围内具有细胞毒活性[462]。奥利斯他汀（auristatin）是一种强效的多拉司他汀-10 类似物，已经被整合入几种 ADC 中，包括靶向 CD30 的本妥昔单抗（brentuximab vedotin）（参见"携带抗微管药物有效载荷的抗体-药物偶联物"一节）。

大多数针对肿瘤血管系统的研究是抑制恶性血管生成的发展，但有几种抗微管的药物能通过抑制血管内皮细胞中微管蛋白的功能迅速关闭现有的肿瘤血管系统的功能[463,464]。自从 20 世纪 90 年代末以来，combretastatins 和 N-乙酰秋水仙碱-O-磷酸（N-acetylcolchicinol-O-phosphate）已作为多种癌症的抗血管药物得到广泛的临床发展，它们与秋水仙碱相似并结合在微管蛋白的秋水仙碱结构域；然而，它们还没有显示出良好的治疗指标。

甲磺酸艾日布林

1986 年，Hirata 和 Uemura 从稀有的日本海生海绵 *H. okadai* 中提取出一种大聚醚大环内酯物 halichondrin B。基于它在临床前模型中强效的抗癌活性，并根据其他已知的抗微管和细胞毒性药物对其进行了进一步的评价[458]。虽然 halichondrin B 的抗增殖作用与其他抗微管药物相似，它们的作用机制确是不同的[458]。然而，尽管它在临床前研究中表现出显著的抗癌活性，却没有足够数量的天然来源。但是十多年后，结构活性研究表明大环内酯 C1-C38 部分赋予了 halichondrin B 的抗微管活性，同时一种完全合成、结构简化的甲磺酸艾日布林衍生物也得到开发，并保留了其母体化合物甲磺酸艾日布林的高效能。

临床适应证

甲磺酸艾日布林已在许多恶性实体瘤中显示出临床活性，但它在世界范围内被登记用于治疗转移性乳腺癌患者，这些患者之前接受过至少两种化疗方案来治疗转移性疾病。与其他相关抗癌药物相比［紫杉烷类，卡培他滨（capecitabine），吉西他滨（gemcitabine）和 VRL］，该药物提高了总生存率，但是该研究不能充分衡量甲磺酸艾日布林与该组任一特定单一药物相比的优越性[465]。除此之外，最近研究表明相比于利用达卡巴嗪（dacarbazine）治疗接受过至少两种化疗方案无效的软组织肉瘤患者，甲磺酸艾日布林治疗方案具有更高的总生存率；甲磺酸艾日布林也被批准用于治疗不可手术切除的脂肪肉瘤的患者，这些患者曾接受过含蒽环类药物的治疗。甲磺酸艾日布林在晚期头颈癌、膀胱癌、前列腺癌、卵巢癌、胰腺癌和肺癌患者中有显著的活性[458]。

作用机制

艾日布林发挥其作用的机制不同于其他微管解聚剂。甲磺酸艾日布林与微管正极末端高亲和力结合，每个微管最多 15 个结合位点，并抑制了微管的动态不稳定性。艾日布林的结合位点与紫杉烷类和长春花生物碱不同，艾日布林被认为对一些伴有 MDR 或 β-微管蛋白突变的癌细胞具有活性[456-458]。它是 VBL 结合位点的非竞争性抑制剂，它与 β-微管蛋白的结合位点同长春花生物碱位点稍微有所不同。与长春花生物碱相似的是艾日布林抑制微管蛋白的聚合和微管的生长阶段；与长春花生物碱不同的是艾日布林并没有影响微管的缩短[456-458,466,467]。甲磺酸艾日布林被认为具有"末端中毒"机制，它要么与微管蛋白末端直接结合，要么诱导出微管蛋白聚集物与可溶性微管蛋白竞争添加到微管的生长末端。通过这些步骤，eribulin 阻碍了有丝分裂纺锤体的形成，使细胞周期停留在 G_2/M 期。长时间停滞在 G_2/M 期和有丝分裂检查点相关干扰的不完全修复可导致细胞凋亡，这可以通过 Bcl-2 的磷酸化，caspase-3 和 caspase-9 的线粒体活化释放细胞色素 C 以及 PARP 的裂解得到证明[466]。甲磺酸艾日布林可以在微管蛋白表面或其附近保持相对稳定，这使其比其他 halichondrin B 类似物在肿瘤细胞内保留更长时间。虽然艾日布林和长春花生物碱都能抑制 β-微管蛋白上核苷酸的交换和 β-微管蛋白残基的交联，但是这两种药物形成的聚合物结构是不同的。长春花生物碱形成大而稳定的结构抑制微管，而 halichondrin B 和艾日布林都形成更小且不稳定的微管蛋白聚合物。除了抑制微管的生长，艾日布林将微管隔离成球形聚集体，这与长春花生物碱形成的环状或螺旋状的聚集体不同。另外，与长春花生物碱不同的是，艾日布林没有导致微管末端的外展以及 α/β 微管蛋白异二聚体的连接。艾日布林独特的机制对于之前给予其他类型抗微管药物的患者的临床治疗十分重要的。

耐药机制

艾日布林的细胞耐药机制并未完全为人所知；然而，因为eribulin能干扰微管动力学使细胞周期停留在 G_2/M 期，所以循环细胞最易受艾日布林活动影响[458-462,466,467]。虽然如此，参与有丝分裂纺锤体动力学和间期功能的微管的相对药物敏感性尚不清楚。与长春花生物碱和紫杉烷类相似，艾日布林的耐药性似乎是MDR1赋予的；然而，这一现象的临床意义尚不清楚。在临床前研究中艾日布林对于多种人类肿瘤有强大的疗效，这疗效强于紫杉烷类和长春花生物碱。在含有β-微管蛋白突变的耐紫杉醇的人类卵巢癌细胞与表达相对高浓度βⅢ-微管蛋白同型的肿瘤细胞中，艾日布林也能引起相关程度的抑制[458-462,467]。

临床药理学

甲磺酸艾日布林在0.25~4.0mg/m² 的剂量范围内呈剂量-比例的药代动力学(表60-3)。静脉给药时，血浆分布是双相的，具有快速的初始分布相和缓慢的消除相。Eribulin消除半衰期平均为40h；估计其表观分布容积范围为43~114L/m²，在上述剂量范围系统清除率为1.15~2.42L/(h·m²)。在浓度为100~1 000ng/ml时，甲磺酸eribulin的血浆蛋白结合率为49%~65%[458,467]。多次给药与单次给药的药物暴露量相当。每周给药均未见药物积聚。

对癌症患者使用甲磺酸放射标记的艾日布林后，未代谢的艾日布林是其主要循环物质。Eribulin在粪便中的排泄量不变，同时其代谢物浓度占比不足母体化合物浓度的<0.6%，这证实艾日布林代谢是微不足道的。母体化合物和4种CYP3A4生成的单氧代谢产物由肝脏进行代谢。少量的艾日布林(约9%)以母体化合物形式经肾脏排出。

药物相互作用

在原发性人类肝病中，甲磺酸艾日布林对CYP1A、CYP2C9、CYP2C19和CYP3A没有诱导作用[458,467]。它能抑制肝脏微粒体中CYP3A4的活性，但不足以大量增加CYP3A4底物的血浆浓度。人微粒体中艾日布林浓度高达5μmol/L时，未检测到艾日布林显著抑制CYP1A2、CYP2C9、CYP2C19、CYP2D6和CYP2E1。体外药物相互作用的研究表明，艾日布林对可充当CYP酶底物的药物的代谢和血浆浓度没有显著影响。艾日布林是一种低亲和力的底物且作为药物外排转运体Pgp的弱抑制剂。

正如体外试验预测的那样，目前临床研究的结果表明即使艾日布林与CYP3A4抑制剂和诱导剂存在的药物-药物相互作用也是微不足道的[467]。当艾日布林与酮康唑(ketoconazole)(CYP3A4强效抑制剂和Pgp抑制剂)联合给药或者与利福平(rifampin)(CYP3A4强效诱导剂)联合给药时，并没有观察到相关药物代谢动力学的相互作用。

毒性反应

接受艾日布林治疗的患者中，最常见的不良反应是中性粒细胞减少症。在一项关键试验中，503名进行乳腺癌重度治疗的患者中，57%的患者在21天周期的第1天和第8天接受剂量为1.4mg/m² 的艾日布林治疗，他们的中性粒细胞计数最低点为1 000/μl甚至更低[458,465,467]。5%的患者出现发热性中性粒细胞减少。12%的患者因中性粒细胞减少而需要减少剂量和小于1%的患者因中性粒细胞减少而需要停药；19%的患者需要使用粒细胞集落刺激因子。中性粒细胞计数到达最低点的时间平均为13天，而从重度中性粒细胞减少(<500/μl)恢复正常的时间平均要8天。分别有小于1%和2%的患者出现3级或以上血小板减少症和贫血。艾日布林治疗组中其他常见的不良反应包括疲劳(54%)、秃顶(45%)和外周神经病变(35%，其中8%达3级或4级)。神经病变以感觉病变为主，但运动病变也存在。大约5%的患者主要因外周神经病变而停药，其发生率与使用紫杉烷类的亚组相似。在以往存在或不存在轻中度神经病变的患者中，严重(3级或4级)神经病变的发生率相似。最近的一项随机Ⅱ期研究显示，艾日布林和伊沙匹隆在神经病变的发生率和严重程度方面没有显著差异；然而，伊沙匹隆引起的神经病变逆转得更快[467]。在21天周期的第1天和第8天短暂静脉输注剂量为1.4mg/m² 的艾日布林时，日本患者出现严重毒性反应的发生率更高[467]。在一项涉及26例患者的无对照开放式心电图研究中，不论艾日布林浓度如何，第8天可出现QT延长，而第1天无QT延长。因此，建议对可能易受心电图扰动影响的患者进行心电图监测和限制(见"甲磺酸艾日布林和其他促进微管蛋白解聚的天然产品"和"方法、剂量和方案")。

在0级或1级肝转氨酶升高的预处理患者中，约18%的艾日布林治疗患者经历了至少2级转氨酶升高。经艾日布林治疗的患者中很少发生严重的不良事件，包括口腔炎、腹泻、便秘，恶心、呕吐、厌食、肌痛、关节痛、泪液增多、体重减轻、发热、贫血和头痛。

方法、剂量和方案

对于转移性乳腺癌患者，在21天周期的第1天和第8天给药，静脉注射甲磺酸艾日布林的剂量为1.4mg/m²，持续2~5分钟。还可以在28天周期的第1天，第8天和第15天给药，给药剂量为1.4mg/m²。对转移性乳腺癌患者的两种给药方案进行直接比较，结果表明21天的治疗方案有稍高的反应率，尽管这个结果不显著[458,467]。每瓶含有1mg甲磺酸艾日布林，被5∶95的乙醇和水配比为0.50mg/ml无色无菌溶液用于注射。从小瓶中取出所需的艾日布林，与100ml 0.9%的氯化钠注射液混合。不能用葡萄糖稀释或给药。不需要使用皮质类固醇或抗组胺药物进行预处理，因为它的水溶性不需要亲脂性载体，如聚山梨酯-80或聚氧乙烯基蓖麻油(可导致超敏反应)。

对轻度(Child-Pugh A)和中度(Child-Pugh B)肝损害的患

者，推荐使用较低起始剂量的甲磺酸艾日布林，分别为 1.1mg/m² 和 0.7mg/m²[458,467]。这种药物还没有在患有严重肝功能不全的患者中进行评估。对中度或重度肾损伤的患者（肌酐清除率为 15~49ml/min），推荐起始剂量为 1.1mg/m²。如果中性粒细胞<1 000/μl 和/或血小板计数<75 000/μl 和/或其处在非血液学毒性的 3~4 级，艾日布林不应该在每 21 天疗程中 1~8 天的第 8 天使用。第 8 天的药量最多可延迟 1 周。如果在 15 天内毒性没有消退或改善到至少二级严重程度，应该停止给药。如果在 15 天内毒性消退或改善到至少二级严重程度，艾日布林的给药剂量为 1.1mg/m²，下一个周期给药不应迟于 2 周。如果毒性相似，建议第二次剂量减少到 0.7mg/m²。艾日布林的剂量减少后不应再加量。

建议对患有充血性心力衰竭、慢性心律失常、电解质紊乱以及使用延长 QT 间期药物治疗的患者进行心电图监测。治疗前应纠正低钾血症和低镁血症，治疗期间应定期检测电解质水平。对患有先天性长 QT 综合征的患者不应使用艾日布林。

作用于有丝分裂的运动蛋白和激酶

尽管微管是有丝分裂纺锤体器官中最主要的蛋白质成分，但是还有许多其他蛋白质，如有丝分裂驱动蛋白，中心体蛋白和有丝分裂激酶，在有丝分裂机制和有丝分裂前细胞周期检查点的进程中扮演关键角色。在过去的十年里，许多亚细胞成分已经被认为是治疗癌症的靶点。

有丝分裂驱动蛋白

驱动蛋白（kinesins）是运动蛋白，将 ATP 水解释放的能量转化为机械力，用于运输物质（如细胞器、相关成分）沿微管的运动，参与形成有丝分裂纺锤体细胞内的组织以及微管的结构[28,29,468,469]。

有丝分裂驱动蛋白作用于增殖细胞的有丝分裂[28,29,468-470]。在有丝分裂过程中，不同的、具有高度特异性的有丝分裂驱动蛋白在有丝分裂纺锤体形成的各个方面起着关键作用，包括纺锤体两极的建立、纺锤体极的组织、染色体排列和分离，以及微管动力学的调节。有丝分裂纺锤体两极的建立是纺锤体形成中发生最早的事件之一，它需要一种特殊的驱动蛋白即运动蛋白 KSP（也称作 Eg5）的参与，KSP 除了参与有丝分裂外，没有其他用途。在正常组织中 KSP mRNA 的表达与增殖细胞 KSP 的优先表达一致，优先是相对于正常邻近组织和有丝分裂后的神经元而言。作为有丝分裂纺锤体形成并发挥作用的基本要素，KSP 和有丝分裂驱动蛋白提供了干扰细胞周期的有效靶点。

在过去的十年里，几种 KSP 抑制剂被用作抗癌治疗的药物。Ispinesib 是一种多环、含氮的杂环，是 KSP 运动区 ATP 酶的变构抑制剂，包含一个 12nM 的 Ki，是一种潜在的 KSP 抑制剂，在临床前研究中，实体瘤和血液恶性肿瘤中都能有效地诱导有丝分裂停滞[28,29,468-470]。与许多其他已经纳入临床评估的 KSP 抑制剂相似，ispinesib 对 KSP 的选择性比其他驱动蛋白超家族的成员高 10 000 倍，并且阻断了功能性有丝分裂纺锤体的形成，因而导致细胞周期有丝分裂的停止，进而导致细胞死亡。在荷瘤小鼠体内，ispinesib 和一些其他 KSP 抑制剂具有抗肿瘤活性，与紫杉烷类活性相当，甚至更高，从而形成了单极有丝分裂的特征，这与培养细胞时观察的现象一致。KSP 抑制剂在对紫杉烷敏感和紫杉烷抗性的细胞中都有效，这些细胞或过表达多药耐药性产物 Pgp，或产生 β-微管蛋白突变。有趣的是，KSP 抑制剂与紫杉烷类的结合对有丝分裂阻滞和细胞死亡产生一种拮抗效应，这表明 KSP 抑制剂与紫杉烷类的结合使用可能不起作用。尽管高度特异性的 KSP 抑制剂在实体瘤和恶性白血病肿瘤（如乳腺癌、淋巴瘤和多发性骨髓瘤）中均显示出抗肿瘤活性，在临床相关剂量下，高增殖率组织的毒性（即中性粒细胞减少症）是显著的，因此需要使用粒细胞集落刺激因子。KSP 抑制剂独特的临床作用至今还没有被阐明。

有丝分裂着丝粒相关驱动蛋白（mitotic centromere-associated kinesin，MCAK）是驱动蛋白 13 家族的成员，通过从聚合物端除去微管蛋白亚单位调节微管动力学，是肿瘤治疗发展中另一潜在靶点[471]。MCAK 的解聚活性在纺锤体形成，纠正微管-动粒的错误连接和染色体运动过程中发挥着关键作用。因此，有丝分裂激酶、Aurora-A 和 Aurora-B、polo-like 激酶 1 以及 CDK1 对 MCAK 的精准调节对于保证有丝分裂时染色体的准确分离和染色体的稳定性具有重要作用。有越来越多的数据表明 MCAK 在癌细胞中异常调控，因而导致了肿瘤发生、侵袭、转移和耐药，最可能的原因是由于染色体不稳定性增加和癌细胞中微管细胞骨架的重构。更有趣的是，最新观察表明 MCAK 作为一种新的癌抗原或者有丝分裂调节剂，这可能成为一种治疗癌症的新型分子靶点。

着丝粒相关蛋白 E（centromere-associated protein E，CENP-E）是另一种有丝分裂驱动蛋白。CENP-E 与着丝粒相关，在有丝分裂早期染色体运动过程中发挥重要作用，并将有丝分裂纺锤体机制与有丝分裂检查点的调节因子相结合，实现细胞周期由中期向后期的转变[472]。抑制 CENP-E 可诱导细胞复制过程中细胞周期的停滞，进而出现细胞凋亡或细胞死亡。在临床前研究中发现，GSK-923295 在一系列人肿瘤异种移植裸鼠模型中具有广泛的抗瘤谱，包括结肠癌、乳腺癌、卵巢癌、肺癌和其他肿瘤[469]。

有丝分裂激酶

有丝分裂激酶（mitotic kinases），特别是 Aurora 激酶和 polo-like 激酶，正在被评估用于抗肿瘤治疗的开发[473]。Aurora 激酶包括 3 个重要的家族成员（Aurora-A、Aurora-B 和 Aurora-C）。aurora 激酶调控有丝分裂过程中的染色体分离和胞质分裂。这些激酶的异常表达和异常的活性可能导致非整倍体形成和肿瘤发生，从而形成多种类型的人类癌症中。Aurora-A 和 Aurora-B 激酶在有丝分裂过程中发挥不同的作用。Aurora-A 激酶，主要分布于中心体周围区域，当子中心体形成有丝分裂中的纺锤体时，该酶为纺锤体招募重要的成分，如 γ-微管蛋白。Aurora-B 激酶分布于分裂间期染色体靠近着丝粒的位置上，当有丝分裂起始染色体浓缩时，Aurora-A 和 Aurora-B 激酶共同负责组蛋白 H3 的磷酸化。在细胞分裂形成两个子细胞的过程中需要收缩环的参与，两种激酶在收缩环发挥功能的过程中也起着不同的作用。Aurora-C 激酶具有高度特异性，然而它在有丝分裂过程中发挥的作用尚不明确，但它似乎补充了 Aurora-B 激酶的作用。在多种类型的癌症中，这 3 种激酶的表达量都增加。高效的、高选择性或非选择性的 Aurora-A 和 Aurora-B 激酶的小分子抑制剂正用于临床研究，这些小分子抑制剂在人类肿瘤实验模型中都表现出阻断细胞周期进程并诱导细胞凋亡的作用。它们主要的毒性是导致中性粒细胞减少，虽然已观察到其抗癌活性，尤其是抗白血病恶性肿瘤的作用，但这些抑制剂独特的临床作用尚未阐明，很可能是由于潜在的易感恶性肿瘤和造血细胞的治疗指数范围过窄[473]。

与 Aurora 激酶家族类似，polo-like 激酶、NIMA 相关激酶以及其他有丝分裂激酶家族都参与了中心体周期并调节纺锤体的功能，而 Bub1、BubR1 和 Mps1 激酶参与调控纺锤体形成的检查点[474,475]。在细胞分裂、DNA 损伤修复路径、细胞凋亡以及细胞周期进程中，一些家族成员，如 polo-like 激酶 1，也参与关键步骤的调控。polo-like 激酶 3 是一种多功能的应激反应蛋白，能对 DNA 损伤和/或有丝分裂纺锤体破坏释放的信号作出反应。polo-like 激酶的小分子抑制剂正用于临床研究，其在临床前研究中已证明对实体瘤和血液病恶性肿瘤有广谱的抗癌活性[474,475]。与有丝分裂驱动蛋白和 Aurora 激酶在临床开发相似，其在癌症治疗中的独特作用尚未发现，可能是在相关剂量水平出现血液毒性，主要是中性粒细胞的减少。

携带抗微管药物有效载荷的抗体-药物偶联物

抗体疗法具有许多优于细胞毒剂的优点，主要是每种 mAb 对其靶抗原的特异性[476,477]。自从 20 世纪 70 年代初它们被发现以来，mAb 就已经作为一种治疗剂，近年来已取得相当大的成效。但是 mAb 也有其缺点，包括固有细胞毒性差以及对恶性肿瘤的穿透性不佳。然而，mAb 与有效的细胞毒性剂结合能优势互补——即 mAb 对肿瘤的特异性和细胞毒剂的有效性。ADC 利用 mAb 对抗原的高度特异性这一特点，有选择地向癌细胞输送一种高毒性的药物，从而增加了作为 ADC 有效载荷的细胞毒性剂的选择性和治疗窗。ADC 的设计依赖于肿瘤特异性抗原的正确选择，这些抗原可用于抗体的结合并向其靶点的传递。ADC 的基本原理在于癌细胞抗原表达的特异性，这使得药物能被输送到靶组织，而相对较少地进入很少或不表达抗原的正常组织中。同样地，肿瘤细胞中靶抗原的表达水平决定了药物的输送以及对正常组织的影响。如果一种靶抗原没有在肿瘤细胞中表达，那 ADC 的摄取就会减少，这将减弱对细胞的毒性，导致毒性药物在细胞外的积聚，引起对正常细胞非特异性的毒性作用。由于抗微管药物在细胞内起作用，故靶抗原将 ADC 输送至细胞内部是至关重要的。如果靶抗原没有介导 ADC 的内化，药物就无法达到足够的浓度以发挥毒性作用，而 ADC 最终也会使正常细胞受到毒性影响。靶抗原在形成肿瘤的癌细胞中表达的同一性也很关键。除此之外，靶抗原必须容易从血液中获取。最后，由于只有极少量的药物能发挥作用，所以有效载荷必须高度有效。微管合成的高效抑制剂，美登木素生物碱衍生物（maytansinoids）和多拉司他汀（dolastatins）是加入 ADC 中的主要药物，这些 ADC 是在美国或其他地方注册的[476-479]。

在 20 世纪 70 年代初，科学家首次从埃塞俄比亚的一种灌木中分离出了苯甲安山克罗内酯（benzoansamacrolide）和美登木素（maytansine）类似物，maytansine 的有效性是长春花生物碱和其他抗微管药物的 100~1 000 倍，其发现引起了人们极大的兴趣。然而，全身用药导致的胃肠道不良反应，周围神经病变以及血液毒性的高发生率令人难以接受[480,481]。maytansine 与微管蛋白的结合位点与长春花生物碱的结合位点有重叠，而与秋水仙素的结合位点不同。长春花生物碱和 maytansinoids 都能与 β-微管蛋白亚基结合。maytansinoids 类药物对微管蛋白结合的构效关系与其体外活性密切相关，缺乏其他主要影响因素，这表明抑制有丝分裂是 maytansinoids 抗肿瘤效应的主要机制。现已表明 maytansine 通过与微管蛋白中的关键巯基结合而起作用[480]。maytansinoids 对位于微管末端的微管蛋白有很高的亲和力，而对遍及整个微管上的位点亲和力较低。微管动力学的抑制导致细胞周期停滞在 G_2/M 期，最终导致细胞凋亡。maytansinoids 的高效性使其成为与抗体结合的理想药物。两种 maytansine 的衍生物——emtansine[也被称作 DM1（图 60-5a）]和 ravtansine[也被称作 DM4（图 60-5b）]——已经广泛用于与不可逆性子（linkers）的结合。曲妥珠单抗-emtansine 是第一个被研发的 ADC，它适用于使用曲妥珠单抗的转移性乳腺癌的女性患者（见第 108 章）。曲妥珠单抗-emtansine 的细胞毒性效应可能因癌细胞募集到胞内的 DM1 的浓度不同而变化，胞内高浓度导致细胞的快速凋亡，较低浓度导致细胞运输受阻和有丝分裂障碍，最低浓度导致对 T-DM1 反应不佳[481]。HER-2 扩增晚期乳腺癌对曲妥珠单抗-emtansin 的原发耐药性似乎相对较弱，但多数经曲妥珠单抗-emtansin 治疗的患者表现出获得性耐药性。耐药性的机制尚不能完全解释，但可能与限制曲妥珠单抗和癌细胞结合有关。低效的内化作用，癌细胞中 HER-2-ADC 复合物回收的加强，曲妥珠单抗溶酶体降解受损以及 HER-2 在细胞内的转运都可能导致曲妥珠单抗-emtansine 的细胞毒性效应减弱。其毒性效应也会受到 MDR 蛋白的影响而削弱，MDR 蛋白负责将 DM1 泵出癌细胞。

多拉司他汀及许多由其合成的衍生物被广泛用于临床试验，但这些药物并没有表现出明显的抗肿瘤活性及/或良好的治疗指标（见"甲磺酸 eribulin 和其他促进微管蛋白解聚的天然产品"）。然而，ADC 类药物本妥昔单抗（brentuximab vedotin）针对患有复发难治性霍奇金淋巴瘤和间变性大细胞淋巴瘤的患者已经获得监管批准（见第 64 章），这种药物由多拉司他汀的类似物单甲基澳瑞他汀 E（monomethyl auristatin E，MMAE）共价连接 CD30 组成（来源于 TNF 家族的Ⅱ型跨膜蛋白质）。本妥昔单抗的毒性载荷 MMAE 可以稳定地连接在抗体上，只有 2%MMAE 在人血浆中停留 10 天后释放，但在 CD30 受体介导内化作用之后可选择性地被溶酶体酶或组织蛋白酶 B 切割[480]。除了要求 CD30 表达之外，多种因素如内化作用，细胞内运输，酶切作用以及与 MMAE 有关的确切因素也决定了体外肿瘤细胞的敏感性。

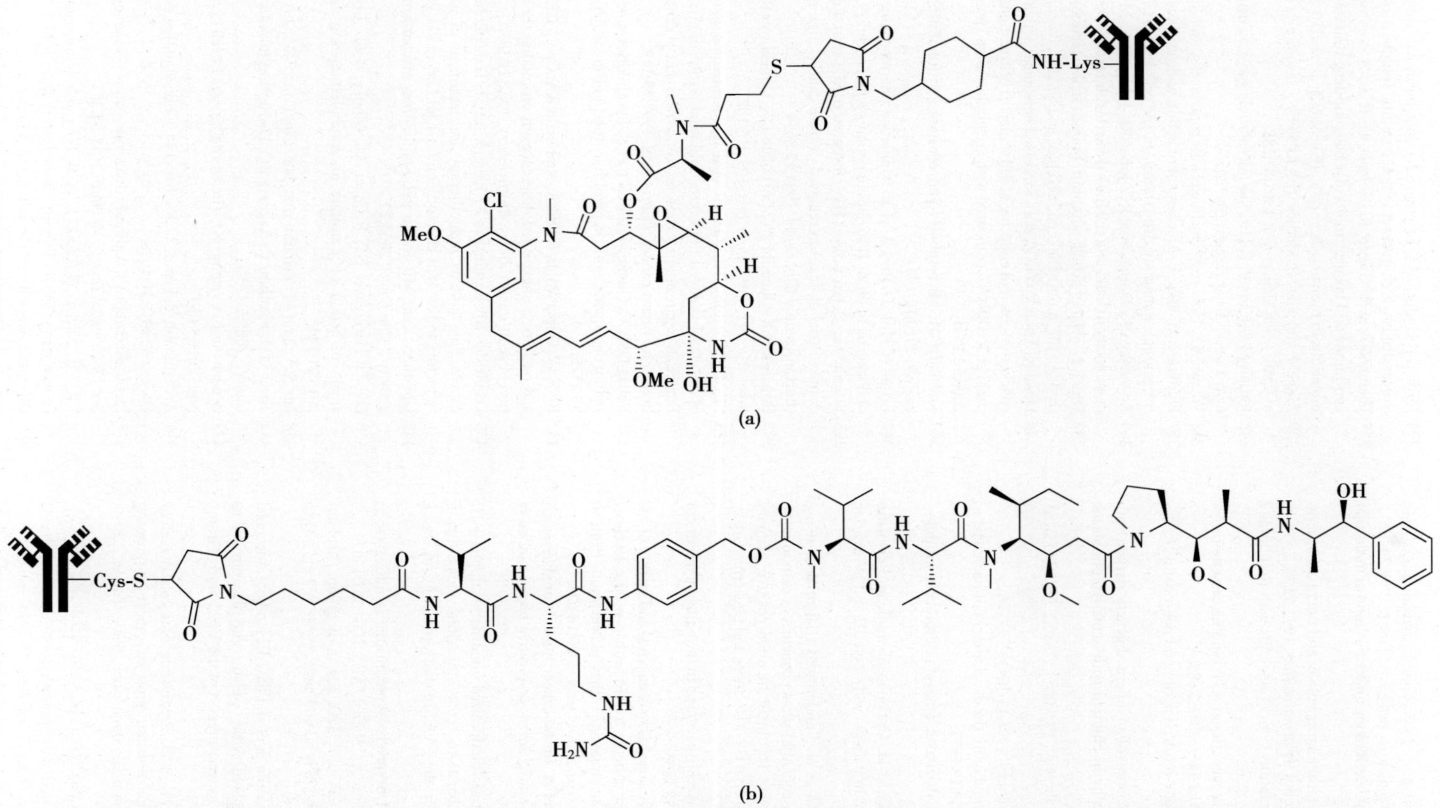

(a)

(b)

图 60-5　ADC 曲妥珠单抗-emtansin(a)和本妥昔单抗(b)及其各自的细胞毒性有效载荷 emtansin(DM1)和一甲基澳瑞他汀 E 的化学结构

(陈耐飞　吕铮　译,崔久嵬　审校)

参考文献

The complete reference list can be found on the Wiley Companion Digital Edition of this title (see inside front cover for login instructions).

2 Jordan MA, Wilson L. Microtubules as a target for anticancer drugs. *Nat Rev Cancer*. 2004;**4**:253.

13 Wilson L, Panda D, Jordan MA. Modulation of microtubule dynamics by drugs: a paradigm for the actions of cellular regulators. *Cell Struct Funct*. 1999;**24**:329.

29 Vale RD, Milligan RA. The way things move: looking under the hood of molecular motor proteins. *Science*. 2000;**288**:88.

38 Rowinsky EK, Donehower RC. The clinical pharmacology and use of antimicrotubule agents in cancer chemotherapeutics. *Pharmacol Ther*. 1992;**52**:35.

61 Himes RH. Interactions of the Catharanthus (vinca) alkaloids with tubulin and microtubules. *Pharmacol Ther*. 1991;**51**:256.

82 Lockhart A, Tirona G, Kim B. Pharmacogenetics of ATP binding cassette transporters in cancer and chemotherapy. *Mol Ther*. 2003;**2**:685.

158 Quasthoff S, Hartung HP. Chemotherapy-induced peripheral neuropathy. *J Neurol*. 2002;**249**:9.

175 Diouf B, Crews KR, Lew G, et al. Association of an inherited genetic variant with vincristine-related peripheral neuropathy in children with acute lymphoblastic leukemia. *JAMA*. 2015;**313**:815.

199 Rowinsky EK, Donehower RC. Drug therapy: paclitaxel (Taxol). *N Engl J Med*. 1995;**332**:1004.

200 Cortes JE, Pazdur R. Docetaxel. *J Clin Oncol*. 1995;**13**:2643.

201 Ma WW, Hidalgo M. The winning formulation: the development of paclitaxel in pancreatic cancer. *Clin Cancer Res*. 2013;**19**:5572.

203 Villanueva C, Bazan F, Kim S, et al. Cabazitaxel: a novel microtubule inhibitor. *Drugs*. 2011;**71**:125.

205 McGuire WP, Hoskins WJ, Brady MF, et al. Cyclophosphamide and cisplatin compared with paclitaxel and cisplatin in patients with stage III and IV ovarian cancer. *N Engl J Med*. 1996;**334**:1.

207 Citron ML, Berry DA, Cirrincione C, et al. Randomized trial of dose-dense versus conventionally scheduled and sequential versus concurrent combination chemotherapy as postoperative adjuvant treatment of node-positive primary breast cancer: first report of Intergroup Trial C9741/Cancer and Leukemia Group B Trial 9741. *J Clin Oncol*. 2003;**21**:1432.

210 Sparano JA, Wang M, Martino S, et al. Weekly paclitaxel in the adjuvant treatment of breast cancer. *N Engl J Med*. 2008;**358**:1663.

216 Bonomi P, Kim K, Fariclough D, et al. Comparison of survival and quality of life in advanced nonsmall cell lung cancer patients treated with two dose levels of paclitaxel combined with cisplatin versus etoposide with cisplatin: results from an Eastern Cooperative Oncology Group trial. *J Clin Oncol*. 2000;**18**:623.

219 Martin M, Pienkowski T, Mackey J, et al. Breast cancer international research group 001 investigators. Adjuvant docetaxel for node-positive breast cancer. *N Engl J Med*. 2005;**352**:2302.

220 Fossella F, Pereira JR, von Pawel J, et al. Randomized, multinational, phase III study of docetaxel plus platinum combinations versus vinorelbine plus cisplatin for advanced nonsmall-cell lung cancer: the TAX 326 study group. *J Clin Oncol*. 2003;**21**:3016.

221 Tannock IF, de Wit R, Berry WR, et al. Docetaxel plus prednisone or mitoxantrone plus prednisone for advanced prostate cancer. *N Engl J Med*. 2004;**351**:1502.

222 Posner MR, Hershock DM, Blajman CR, et al. TAX 324 study group. Cisplatin and fluorouracil alone or with docetaxel in head and neck cancer. *N Engl J Med*. 2007;**357**:1705.

224 Van Cutsem E, Moiseyenko VM, Tjulandin S, et al. Phase III study of docetaxel and cisplatin plus fluorouracil compared with cisplatin and fluorouracil as first-line therapy for advanced gastric cancer: a report of the V325 Study Group. *J Clin Oncol*. 2006;**24**:4991.

225 de Bono JS, Oudard S, Ozguroglu M, et al. Prednisone plus cabazitaxel or mitoxantrone for metastatic castration-resistant prostate cancer progressing after docetaxel treatment: a randomised open-label trial. *Lancet*. 2010; **376**:1147.

226 Gradishar WJ, Tjulandin S, Davidson N, et al. Phase III trial of nanoparticle albumin-bound paclitaxel compared with polyethylated castor oil-based paclitaxel in women with breast cancer. *J Clin Oncol*. 2005;**23**:7794.

227 Socinski MA, Bondarenko I, Karaseva NA, et al. Weekly nab-paclitaxel in combination with carboplatin versus solvent-based paclitaxel plus carboplatin as first-line therapy in patients with advanced nonsmall-cell lung cancer: final results of a phase III trial. *J Clin Oncol*. 2012;**30**:2055.

228 Manfredi JJ, Parness J, Horwitz SB. Taxol binds to cellular microtubules. *J Cell Biol*. 1982;**94**:688.

229 Schiff PB, Fant J, Horwitz SB. Promotion of microtubule assembly in vitro by taxol. *Nature*. 1979;**22**:665.

230 Horwitz SB, Cohen D, Rao S, et al. Taxol: mechanisms of action and resistance. *J Natl Cancer Inst Monogr*. 1993;**15**:55.

235 Jordan A, Hadfield JA, Lawrence NJ, McGowan AT. Tubulin as a target for anticancer drugs which interact with the mitotic spindle. *Med Res Rev*. 1998;**18**:259.

237 Giannakakou P, Gussio R, Nogales E, et al. A common pharmacophore for epothilone and taxanes: molecular basis for drug resistance conferred by tubulin mutations in human cancer cells. *Proc Natl Acad Sci U S A*. 2000;**97**:2904.

239 Ringel I, Horwitz SB. Studies with RP56976 (Taxotere): a semisynthetic analogue of taxol. *J Natl Cancer Inst*. 1991;**83**:288.

243 Jordan MA. Kamath K How do microtubule-targeted drugs work? An overview. *Curr Cancer Drug Targets*. 2007;**7**:730.

248 Weaver BA. How taxol/paclitaxel kills cancer cells. *Mol Biol Cell*. 2014;**25**:2677.

252 Dumontet C, Sikic B. Mechanism of action and resistance to antitubulin agents: microtubule dynamics, drug transport, and cell death. *J Clin Oncol*. 1999;**17**:1061.

265 Rowinsky EK, Donehower RC, Jones RJ, Tucker RW. Microtubule changes and cytotoxicity in leukemic cell lines treated with taxol. *Cancer Res*. 1988;**48**:4093.

282 Desei N. Nanoparticle albumin bound (nab) technology: targeting tumors through the endothelial gp60 receptor and SPARC. *Nanomedicine*. 2007;**3**:339.

286 Desai N, Trieu V, Yao Z, et al. Increased anticancer activity, intratumor paclitaxel concentrations, and endothelial cell transport of cremophor-free, albumin-bound paclitaxel, ABI-007, compared with cremophor-based paclitaxel. *Clin Cancer Res*. 2006;**12**:1317.

306 Kavallaris M. Microtubules and resistance to tubulin-binding agents. *Nat Rev Cancer*. 2010;**10**:194.

347 Bruno R, Hille D, Riva A, et al. Population pharmacokinetic/pharmacodynamics of docetaxel in phase II studies in patients with cancer. *J Clin Oncol*. 1998;**16**:186.

395 Eisenhower E, ten Bokkel HW, Swenerton KD, et al. European-Canadian randomized trial of Taxol in relapsed ovarian cancer: high vs low dose and long vs short infusion. *J Clin Oncol*. 1994;**12**:2654.

396 Rowinsky EK, Chaudhry V, Cornblath DR, Donehower RC. The neurotoxicity of taxol. *Monogr Natl Cancer Inst*. 1993;**15**:107.

415 Piccart MJ, Klijn J, Paridaens R, et al. Corticosteroids significantly delay the onset of docetaxel-induced fluid retention: final results of a randomized study of the European organization for research and treatment of cancer, investigational drug branch for breast cancer. *J Clin Oncol*. 1997;**15**:149.

435 Bollag DM, McQueney PA, Zhu J, et al. Epothilones, a new class of microtubule-stabilizing agents with a taxol-like mechanism of action. *Cancer Res*. 1995; **55**:2325.

437 Bode CJ, Gupta ML Jr, Reiff EA, Suprenant KA, Georg GI, Himes RH. Epothilone and paclitaxel: unexpected differences in promoting the assembly and stabilization of yeast microtubules. *Biochemistry*. 2002;**41**:3870.

438 Lechleider RJ, Kaminskas E, Jiang X, et al. Ixabepilone in combination with capecitabine and as monotherapy for treatment of advanced breast cancer refractory to previous chemotherapies. *Clin Cancer Res*. 2008;**14**:4378.

443 Goodin S, Kane MP, Rubin EH. Epothilones: mechanism of action and biologic activity. *J Clin Oncol*. 2004;**22**:2015.

456 Dybdal-Hargreaves NF, Risinger AL, Mooberry SL. Eribulin mesylate: mechanism of action of a unique microtubule-targeting agent. *Clin Cancer Res*. 2015;**21**:2445.

458 Jain S, Vahdat LT. Eribulin mesylate. *Clin Cancer Res*. 2011;**17**:6615.

463 Tozer GM, Kanthou C, Baguley BC. Disrupting tumour blood vessels. *Nat Rev Cancer*. 2005;**5**:423.

473 Goldenson B, Crispino JD. The aurora kinases in cell cycle and leukemia. *Oncogene*. 2015;**34**:537.

474 Archambault V, Lépine G, Kachaner D. Understanding the polo kinase machine. *Oncogene*. 2015;**10**:1038.

477 Iyer U, Kadambi VJ. Antibody drug conjugates—Trojan horses in the war on cancer. *J Pharmacol Toxicol Methods*. 2011;**64**:207.

478 Klute K, Nackos E, Tasaki S, et al. Microtubule inhibitor-based antibody-drug conjugates for cancer therapy. *Onco Targets Ther*. 2014;**7**:2227.

480 Chari RV, Martell BA, Gross JL, et al. Immunoconjugates containing novel maytansinoids: promising anticancer drugs. *Cancer Res*. 1992;**52**:127.

第 61 章 激素受体阳性乳腺癌患者的内分泌治疗

Aman U. Buzdar, MD, FACP ■ Shaheenah Dawood, MD, MBBch, FACP, FRCP, MPH, CPH ■
Harold A. Harvey, MD ■ Virgil Craig Jordan, OBE, PhD, DSc, FMedSci

概述

19 世纪初，生殖内分泌系统在乳腺癌治疗中的重要性开始得到体现。大约在这个时候，人们意识到卵巢切除可以对大约三分之一的绝经前晚期乳腺癌女性有一定的治疗价值。然而，只有当雌激素受体(estrogen receptor, ER)被发现时，人们才有可能充分了解卵巢切除和其他相关治疗方法如卵巢放疗、肾上腺切除和垂体切除术治疗乳腺癌的机制。对雌激素和孕激素相关通路的研究不仅有助于更深入地了解乳腺癌发生过程中致癌途径的相关机制，而且还可以确定潜在的治疗干预靶点。本章讨论了雌激素和孕激素受体(progesterone receptor, PR)通路的最新研究进展，以及其潜在的干预靶点。此外，还阐述和比较了不同内分泌药物在早期和晚期乳腺癌治疗中的药理学及疗效。

孕激素产生和作用的生物学

孕激素参与了多种组织的发育、分化、增殖、凋亡和代谢的调控行为，在肿瘤的发生发展中具有重要的意义。此外，孕激素也是雌激素、雄激素和肾上腺皮质类固醇的前体。靶组织上的一些孕激素效应是通过转录介导的，而一些其他的作用迅速的效应并不涉及直接的转录介导。孕激素(图 61-1)包括天然存在的激素孕酮，孕烷中的 17α-乙酰氧基孕酮衍生物系列，19-去甲睾酮衍生物(雌烷)和在甾烷系列中的诺地孕酮及其相关化合物。在人体中孕酮是最重要的孕激素。

合成和产生地点

孕酮产生于合成途径的早期，包括胆固醇转化为雄激素、孕激素和雌激素。绝经后，在没有激素替代的情况下，肾上腺成为孕激素(通过孕烯醇酮的转化)以及其他性激素的主要来源。在绝经前的女性中，孕酮主要来源于卵巢的黄体，但在妊娠第 8 周后，胎盘孕酮的产生量大大超过卵巢来源的孕酮。胎盘滋养细胞是胎盘分泌孕酮的优势细胞。为了囊胚植入，分泌型子宫内膜的发育过程需要孕酮的参与。孕酮的水平在月经周期的黄体期通常为 25ng/ml，但在妊娠晚期可高达 150ng/ml。

作用机制

孕酮在 RNA 转录调控中的作用机制是通过一系列复杂的相互作用来实现的，这些相互作用是通过激素与其同源受体的

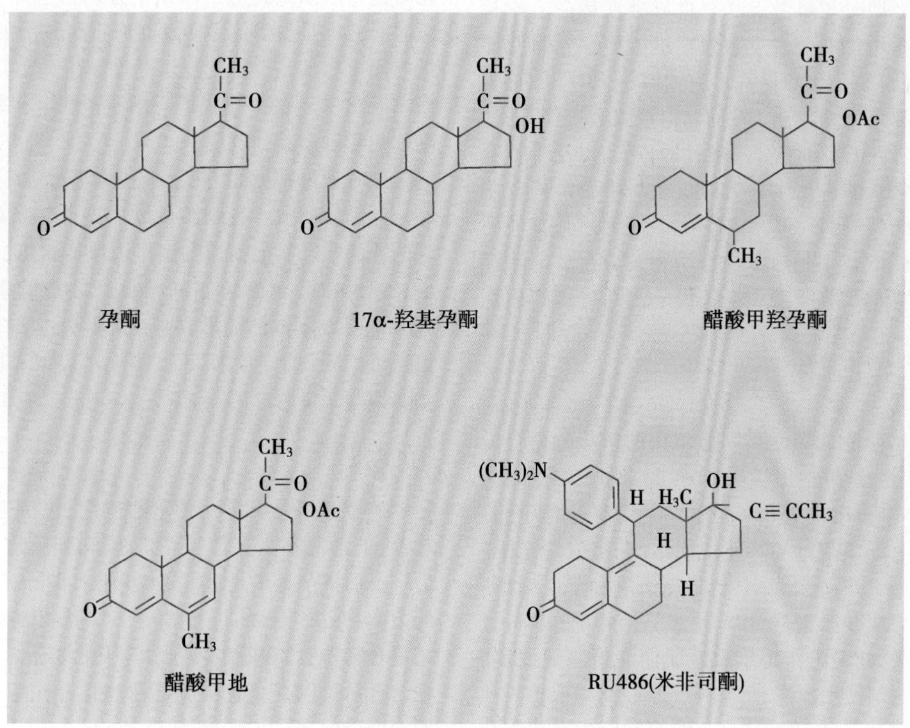

图 61-1 孕酮、17α-羟基孕酮和合成孕酮的结构

结合而启动的。PR 有两种亚型,称为 PR-A 和 PR-B,它们具有不同的生物学活性。PR-B 介导孕酮的刺激活性,而 PR-A 的作用是抑制 PR-B 和其他类固醇受体的活性[1-3]。这两种亚型的作用是由单个基因编码的,其表达比例在生殖组织中因发育状态、激素水平和组织类型而有所不同。PR 的两个亚型都含有 AF-1 和 AF-2 的转录激活结构域,PR-B 也含有一个额外的 AF-3 结构域,其功能是促进其细胞和启动子的特异性活性。PR 两种异构体的配体是完全相同的。

在缺乏激素的情况下,细胞核内的 PR 是与热休克蛋白(HSP-90、70、60 和 40)复合物(HSP-90、70、60 和 40)相关的一种不活跃的单体状态,且是转录失活的[4,5]。孕酮与 PR 的结合导致热休克蛋白的解离,受体配体二聚体的形成,这些受体配体二聚体仍定位于核内,并与位于靶基因上的高度选择性孕酮反应元件(progesterone response element,PRE)结合[6]。需要注意的是,靶细胞不仅必须区分从其他类固醇激素中区分出孕酮,而且还需要从其他的疏水分子中区分出孕酮。这种高度的鉴别仅限于在基因组序列存在 PR 和 PRE 的细胞[6,7]。下一步是 PR 的转录激活,这是与许多辅助激活因子(包括类固醇受体辅激活因子 1(SRC-I)、转录介导因子 2 和维 A 酸辅激活因子 3)相互作用的结果[6-9]。SRC-1 与 PR 的 N-末端 AF-1 和 C-末端 AF-2 相互作用。这有助于增强 SRC-1 与 PR 的配体反应性羧基端 AF-2 协同配体无关的氨基末端 AF-1 的功能。PR-共激活物复合物然后进一步与具有组蛋白乙酰化酶活性的其他蛋白质相互作用,从而导致染色质重塑,增加转录蛋白对启动子的识别[8]。

生理作用

孕激素涉及了一系列良性生理变化,从分泌活性到乳腺间质组织的水肿变化。其对肿瘤发生的影响主要与子宫内膜肿瘤的风险降低和绝经期时与雌激素联合进行激素替代治疗时乳腺肿瘤的风险略微增加有关。孕激素在维持受孕方面发挥着关键作用:子宫内膜的分化和促进子宫内膜进入分泌期;阴道黏膜上皮的成熟和角化;抑制排卵;抑制促性腺激素释放;乳腺上皮的增殖和在乳腺上皮细胞分泌活性的诱导;以及肾脏利钠和利尿作用。孕激素的一些生理效应仅在与雌激素具有协同作用的靶组织中能观察到,而其他的一些效应似乎与其他类固醇激素、肽类激素和/或生长因子的作用相关。在制定治疗策略时,必须考虑孕激素、雌激素和生长因子之间可能的相互作用。

孕激素的合成

合成的孕激素是孕酮或睾酮类固醇结构的衍生物。合成孕激素最常见的 17-羟基孕酮、甲氧基孕酮(Provera)、甲孕酮乙酸甲酯(medroxyprogesterone acetate,MPA)、甲地孕酮(medroxyprogesterone acetate,MA)(Megace)、炔诺酮、庚酸炔诺酮、醋酸炔诺酮、异炔诺酮、甲基炔诺酮、地索高诺酮和孕二烯酮。两种应用最广泛的合成孕激素是 MPA 和 MA,结构上在 C6-C7 只有一个键的差异。MPA 可作为口服或肌内注射制剂使用,而 MA 可作为口服制剂使用。

合成孕激素在避孕、与雌激素联合作为绝经后激素替代疗法(hormone replacement therapy,HRT)和在子宫癌和乳腺癌中内分泌治疗的应用最为广泛。在绝经后 HRT 中,孕激素被添加到雌激素替代物中,主要是为了减少雌激素单独治疗时相关的子宫癌风险,尽管将孕激素添加到雌激素中对乳腺癌风险的影响已变得越来越令人担忧[10]。在绝经前女性中,孕激素和抗孕激素主要用于避孕[11]。孕激素还经常单独用于某些具有更年期症状但不被建议服用雌激素的妇女。

转移性乳腺癌

孕激素和 PR 在人乳腺癌中得到了广泛的研究。PR 阳性的肿瘤患者对内分泌治疗(不一定是孕激素)有更高的缓解概率,并且在大多数情况下,在生存期和无疾病间隔方面,预后都要好一些[12]。在转移性乳腺癌患者中,MPA 和 MA 均能产生类似的使血清雌激素水平下降的作用,30% 的患者能对治疗产生缓解[13]。用于转移性乳腺癌的治疗的孕激素主要是 MA。转移性乳腺癌对 MA 的反应不仅是通过 ER 和/或 PR 的存在,而且还要通过患者对以前的激素治疗是否能产生缓解来预测的。随机临床研究表明孕激素与他莫昔芬、氨鲁米特和芳香化酶抑制剂在治疗转移性乳腺癌的二线和后线治疗中疗效类似[13,14]。目前,孕激素对激素受体阳性转移性乳腺癌的治疗主要是在选择性 ER 调节剂(例如他莫昔芬)和芳香化酶抑制剂后疾病进展的患者中使用。因此,孕激素通常被用作激素受体阳性转移性乳腺癌患者的第三线或更后线的治疗(图 61-2)。

子宫癌的治疗

孕激素也被用于治疗子宫内膜癌[15]。在子宫腺癌中,80% 的患者可以通过局部治疗得到治愈。在复发的情况下,外源性孕激素对于部分患者而言是一种有效的治疗方法:30% 以上的复发患者对外源性孕激素可以产生客观缓解。ER 和 PR 的状态在这些肿瘤中可以被测定,这些受体的存在与肿瘤的分化、患者的预后以及其对孕激素治疗的应答相关。治疗缓解的持续时间并不是由受体是否存在来进行预测的,而且这一缓解持续时间可以从几个月到几年不等。在不到 10% 的患者中,缺乏 ER 和 PR 表达的肿瘤仍能对孕激素产生客观缓解。

副作用和孕激素的剂量

孕激素最常见的不良反应是体重增加,这是由于食欲增加和液体潴留所致。其刺激食欲的副作用常被用于治疗癌症引起的恶病质。其他报道的副作用包括潮热、出汗、阴道出血、恶心、呼吸困难、血栓栓塞和罕见的心血管事件,如心力衰竭。MA 和 MPA 不同的剂量方案在剂量-反应效应的研究中已经被报道过。MA 的推荐剂量为 160mg/d,MPA 的推荐剂量至少为 400~500mg/d[16]。

抗孕激素

抗孕激素具有广泛的治疗应用,包括避孕、引产或治疗乳腺癌、子宫内膜异位症、子宫肌瘤和脑膜瘤[17]。最古老和应用最广泛的抗孕激素是 RU 38486 或米非司酮,它是 19-去甲孕酮的衍生物,在 11β 的位置含有二甲基氨基酚取代基[11,18]。这一复合物口服能够有效吸收,与 PR 结合具有高度的亲和力并在结合后可以改变共调节蛋白的相互作用。它既具有拮抗作用,又具有一定的激动剂活性,因此被认为是一种 PR 调节剂。它与前列腺素一起用于终止早孕[18]。

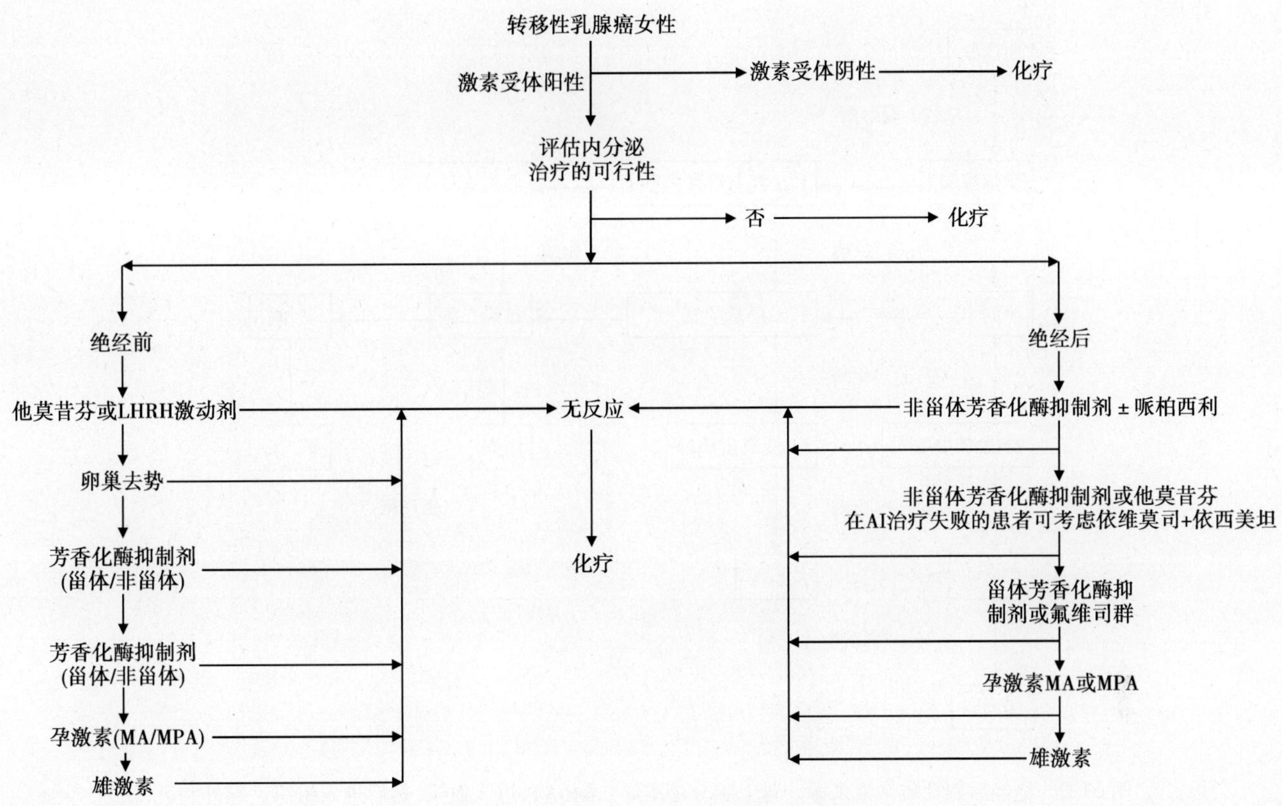

图 61-2　转移性乳腺癌内分泌治疗策略

雌激素产生和作用的生物学

许多天然产生的内源性雌激素在女性体内产生，ER-α 和 β 介导的作用最强的是雌二醇，其次是雌酮和雌三醇。3 种化合物均含有碳 3 羟基的酚类 A 环和 D 环第 17 位的 β-OH 或酮，酚醛 A 环是它们与 ER 选择性高度结合的主要结构特征。天然产生的雌激素的主要作用是通过刺激生长因子的增加［如转化生长因子-α（TGF-α）］和抑制性生长因子（如转化生长因子-β）的降低来调节细胞的生长[19]。这些生长因子被认为是通过与其各自的膜受体相互作用而启动或阻止细胞周期的，其调节机制是一个自分泌环。生长因子（如胰岛素样生长因子-1（IGF-1）的旁分泌（细胞-细胞）也可在调节上皮细胞的复制中发挥作用。

生物合成途径

芳香化酶复合物位于内质网，由细胞色素 P450 血红素蛋白（P450 芳香族，芳香化酶）和大多数细胞共有的烟酰胺腺嘌呤二核苷酸磷酸组成，其主要功能是向细胞色素 P450 传递电子[20]。在雌激素生物合成途径中，参与雄烯二酮转化为雌酮的主要酶是芳香化酶。芳香化酶是 CYP 19 基因的产物，编码 503 个氨基酸的多肽，分子量为 55kDa。芳香化酶在雄烯二酮转化为雌酮的过程中催化了 3 种不同的甾体羟基化。前两种反应产生 19-羟基和 19-醛结构，第三种，尽管仍有争议，可能涉及含有甲酸释放的 C-19 甲基基团酸[21]。

产生部位

许多组织能表达芳香化酶，从而合成雌激素，这些组织包括卵巢、胎盘、下丘脑、肝脏、肌肉、脂肪组织和恶性乳腺肿瘤组织[22]（图 61-3）。在绝经前女性中，卵巢是芳香化酶和雌激素产生的最重要部位。黄体生成素（luteinizing hormone，LH）通过膜细胞室控制雄烯二酮的产生，而卵泡刺激素（follicle stimulating hormone，FSH）则促进颗粒细胞芳香化酶的表达。通过协同作用，LH 促进芳香化酶底物的产生，而 FSH 则增加芳香化酶的数量，使雌二醇的产量在排卵时增加 8~10 倍。

绝经后妇女，雌激素的产生几乎完全发生在腺外组织。雄烯二酮主要由肾上腺产生，少部分由卵巢产生，由脂肪组织[23]等外周组织中表达的芳香化酶转化为雌酮，然后由 17-羟基类固醇脱氢酶转化为雌二醇。通过这一途径，绝经后妇女每天产生大约 100mg 的雌酮，在肥胖妇女中可观察到更高雌酮水平[24]。部分雌酮也被转化为雌二醇，以产生循环血浆浓度约为 10~20pg/ml 的游离雌二醇。据估计，人乳腺肿瘤组织中雌二醇的水平约是血浆中的 4~6 倍[25]。维持这种高浓度的机制尚未完全确定；然而，通过芳香化酶途径产生的局部物质很可能与类固醇硫酸盐酶的其他途径有关，这种酶可将硫酸雌酮水解为雌酮[26]。

作用机制

循环的雌激素与性激素结合球蛋白（sex hormone binding globulin，SHBG）结合，结合解离后雌激素进入细胞与主要位于细胞核内的 ER 结合，并与热休克蛋白（主要是 Hsp 90）结合，使其稳定下来。ERα-和 β 均为雌激素依赖的核转录因子，分别由位于不同染色体上的 ESR 1 和 ESR 2 编码[27]，具有不同的组织分布和转录调节活性。ERα 主要表达于女性生殖道，包括子宫、阴道和卵巢，以及乳腺、下丘脑、内皮细胞和血管平滑肌。ERβ 主要在前列腺和卵巢中表达，在肺、脑、骨和血管中表

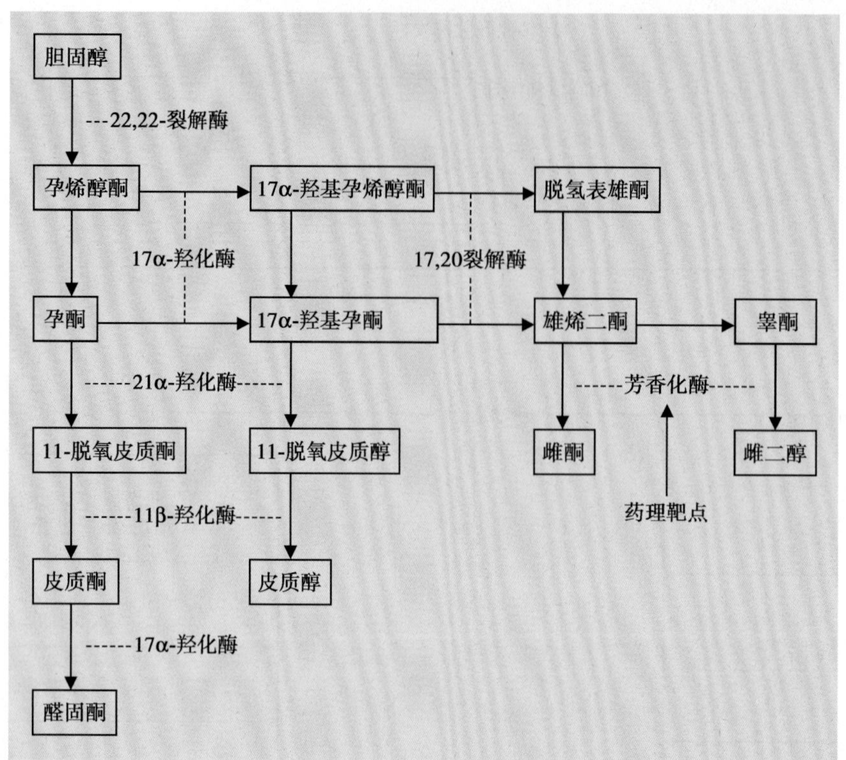

图 61-3 绝经后妇女雌激素来源。肾上腺分泌雄烯二酮(A),进入血浆,然后进入组织。腺外和乳腺肿瘤组织含有将 A 转化为雌酮(E_1)和雌二醇(E_2)或雌酮硫酸盐(E_1)转化所必需的酶。这些类固醇在血浆中循环,并以 pg/ml 表示

达较低。ERα 和 β 受体在多个组织中共同表达,其中最显著的是乳腺组织,它们在此可形成同源或异二聚体。

雌激素与 ER 的结合导致受体构象的改变,ER 从而从稳定蛋白中释放出来。雌激素-ER 同型二聚体复合物之后结合到位于启动子区域的被称为雌激素反应元件(estrogen response element,ERE)特定的核苷酸序列上。这种结合的相互作用还涉及许多核蛋白,共调节因子,以及转录过程中的其他组成部分。雌激素的基因组效应主要是通过调节应答基因的转录而合成的蛋白质。已经成熟的两种对于雌激素敏感乳腺癌主要的治疗方法,要么是通过阻止雌激素的产生,要么是抑制其与雌激素受体的相互作用。

致癌效应

对于单独使用合成雌激素或作为口服避孕药的一部分使用对于癌症发展的影响这一问题令人担忧。研究报道妊娠前 3 个月内雌二乙烯雌激素(合成雌激素)的摄入与暴露在子宫内的子代晚期的阴道透明细胞癌和宫颈腺癌的发生率相关,这是首次发现雌激素的发育暴露与人类癌症的增加有关[28,29]。研究还表明,作为绝经女性的 HRT 的一部分,无拮抗的雌激素增加子宫内膜癌的风险 5~15 倍[30],这一增加的风险可以通过孕酮的加入得到干预[31]。在绝经后女性中,乳腺癌风险与 HRT 的关系在两项大型试验中被报道。妇女健康倡议(Women's Health Initiative,WHI)是一项大型前瞻性试验,将女性随机分为安慰剂组或 HRT 组。研究结果显示,服用雌激素-孕激素联合治疗的女性患乳腺癌的总风险增加了 24%,但没有子宫的女性服用雌激素的风险比服用安慰剂的妇女减少了 23%[10,32]。在 WHI 试验的延长扩展阶段,研究结果进一步显示在累积随访期内,乳腺癌风险仍有一定程度的提高[HR 1.28,95%CI(可信区间)1.11~1.48][33]。百万女性研究(Million Women Study,MWS)是一项大型队列研究,研究结果显示了进行或未进行 HRT 治疗的女性患侵袭性乳腺癌的相对风险(relative risk,RR)[34]。在雌激素-孕激素联合治疗的妇女中,侵袭性乳腺癌的 RR 增加了 2,单用雌激素的女性的 RR 增加了 1.3。

流行病学研究还发现高水平的天然雌激素与癌症的发展有一定的相关性。在超重的女性中可以观察到高水平的天然雌激素。WHI 试验中,在从未接受过 HRT 的绝经后女性中,超重的女性(体重指数>31.1)患乳腺癌的风险高于身材相对苗条的女性(体重指数<22.6)(RR=2.52)[32];一项涉及从未接受过外源性雌激素治疗的女性的病例队列研究中,发现高水平的天然雌激素也与乳腺癌风险有关[35]。研究结果显示,与循环雌二醇水平较低的妇女相比,血清雌二醇水平较高的妇女(≥6.83pmol/L 或 1.9pg/ml)的 RR 为 3.6(95% CI,1.3~10.0)。

骨矿物质密度也被证明是一种雌激素暴露的标志。据报道,高内源性雌激素浓度与老年妇女的骨密度增高有关[36]。绝经后骨密度增高的妇女患乳腺癌的概率也较高[37]。这些研究表明循环雌激素作为乳腺癌风险的标记的潜在益处。然而,由于绝经后妇女的循环雌激素的基线水平较低,而且绝经前妇女循环雌激素水平与月经周期的重要相关性导致检测时间点的选择具有重要性,因此将其作为标记的可靠性存在争议。无论如何,已经有足够的证据表明雌激素与激素敏感的乳腺癌的发展有关,这就催生了许多干预性的试验,这些试验通过药物

的靶点阻止雌激素的产生或阻断其与受体的相互作用。

选择性雌激素受体调节剂与抗雌激素

早在一个多世纪前，激素在乳腺癌发展过程中所起的作用就已被发现，1896 年，Beatson 观察到，切除一部分乳腺癌患者的卵巢可以使疾病缓解[38]。虽然最初还不清楚这一效应是由于消除了绝经前妇女雌激素的主要来源而引起的。临床前的研究证实了雌激素可以促进 ER 阳性乳腺癌细胞的增殖[39]，许多流行病学研究也发现雌激素与乳腺癌风险的相关性[32-37]。随着雌激素在乳腺癌发生和进展中的重要作用被发现，两组药物被开发用于来拮抗雌激素的作用。第一组药物主要阻止雌激素与其受体的相互作用，包括选择性雌激素受体调节剂（selective estrogen receptor modulator，SERM）和抗雌激素。SERM 包括他莫昔芬、雷洛昔芬和托瑞米芬，它们在某些组织（骨、肝和心血管系统）具有雌激素激动剂的特性，在其他组织（脑和乳腺）具有雌激素拮抗剂的特性，在子宫中具有混合激动剂/拮抗剂的雌激素特性。包括氟维司群在内的抗雌激素与 SERM 的区别在于它们都是雌激素的拮抗剂。第二组药物则通过阻断芳香化酶的作用而阻断雌激素的产生，被称为芳香化酶抑制剂。在本节中，我们将回顾各种 SERMs 和抗雌激素在临床实践中用于治疗和预防激素受体阳性乳腺癌（图 61-4）。

他莫昔芬

作用方式

他莫昔芬是一种非甾体三苯乙炔化合物，它通过竞争性地抑制雌二醇与 ER 的结合而发挥其作用，从而消除了雌激素的刺激效应，使细胞处于复制周期的 G_1 期[40]。他莫昔芬是乳腺中的雌激素拮抗剂，是子宫内膜和骨中的雌激素激动剂，这种生物学特性的平衡正是目前他莫昔芬治疗策略的关键。

他莫昔芬的高治疗指数允许其在剂量上可以有较大的差异，不同的治疗时间表和剂量取决于不同的国家及其评估这种药物有效性的临床试验。在美国，他莫昔芬的推荐剂量为 10mg 每日两次或 20mg 每日 1 次。在其他国家则是 10mg 每日 3 次或 20mg 每日 2 次。

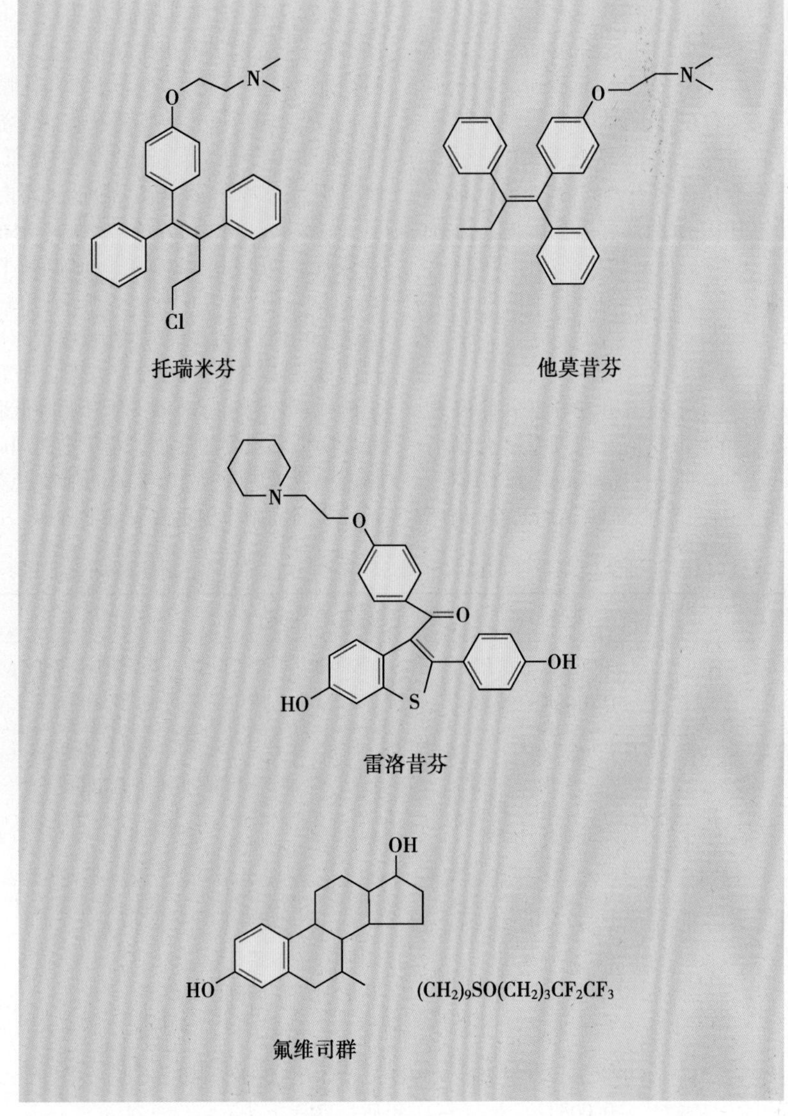

图 61-4　选择性雌激素受体调节剂（SERM）和抗雌激素的结构

他莫昔芬口服给药并迅速吸收，在4~6周内达到稳定的血清水平。细胞色素P450亚型CYP2D6和CYP3A4在肝脏中将他莫昔芬代谢为N-脱甲基他莫昔芬（主要代谢物）和4-羟基他莫昔芬（次级代谢物），这两种物质都有可能进一步代谢为4-羟基-N-去甲基他莫昔芬（次级代谢物去甲基他莫昔芬），后者对ER的亲和力比他莫昔芬高30~100倍[41]。他莫昔芬具有长达7天的血清半衰期，次级代谢产物N-去甲基他莫昔芬具有更长的半衰期14天[42]。长时间的血清半衰期可能是为什么当他莫昔芬治疗停止时，未常规的记录到戒断反应的发生。目前还没有发现用他莫昔芬治疗致畸的临床病例。但由于致畸性的可能性尚不清楚，因此不推荐用于妊娠妇女。此外，已知他莫昔芬会对有排卵周期的绝经前妇女产生卵巢刺激，因此，服用他莫昔芬的有怀孕概率的妇女应接受各种避孕方法的建议[43]。

他莫昔芬在晚期乳腺癌

他莫昔芬是晚期绝经后女性内分泌治疗的选择之一，ER阳性的患者更有可能从中获益[44]。最近的数据表明，芳香化酶抑制剂在一线治疗中是更优的选择，我们将在“芳香化酶抑制剂”一节中更详细地讨论这一问题。

他莫昔芬是绝经前晚期乳腺癌患者一线内分泌治疗的选择之一。四项研究的Meta分析表明，他莫昔芬产生的缓解率和总生存率（overall survival，OS）类似于卵巢切除术后[45]。但是，有了高效促黄体生成素释放激素（luteinizing hormone-releasing hormone，LHRH）激动剂如戈舍瑞林（Zoladex）的研制，其可以通过阻止LH从垂体释放而减少类固醇类激素的产生，LHRH激动剂和他莫昔芬的组合已成为有效的治疗选择，meta分析显示联合治疗相比单用LHRH激动剂可以显著提高无进展生存时间和总生存时间[46]。因此，最新的指南表明，单独或联合使用LHRH激动剂和他莫昔芬是治疗绝经后前晚期激素受体阳性疾病的合适选择[47]（图61-3）。

他莫昔芬在辅助治疗

许多随机临床试验已经解决了他莫昔芬在早期乳腺癌患者辅助治疗中的有效性问题。最近由早期乳腺癌专家合作小组（Early Breast Cancer Trialists' Collaborative Group，EBCTCG）更新了含有145 000个早期乳腺癌患者的94项辅助治疗（化疗和/或激素疗法）试验进行的概述和Meta分析的结果[48]。EBCTCG报告显示，在ER阳性的患者中使用5年辅助他莫昔芬后，不管年龄、PR状况、绝经状态或化疗的使用情况如何，乳腺癌的年死亡率会降低31%，这一获益在持续15年的随访后仍然存在。在这一报告中，他莫昔芬治疗1年疗效不大，5年的他莫昔芬疗效明显高于2年，尚需长期随访以评估5年以上他莫昔芬治疗的疗效。一些前瞻性临床试验探讨了他莫昔芬辅助治疗大于5年的疗效（表61-1）[49-53]。B-14试验，一个美国乳腺与肠道外科辅助治疗研究组（National Surgical Adjuvant Breast and Bowel Project，NSABP）的临床试验，淋巴结阴性ER阳性的女性患者接受他莫昔芬治疗5年后，随机接受安慰剂或继续他莫昔芬的治疗。但对于延长他莫昔芬治疗，7年的随访结果没有显示出额外的优势。与5年后停止他莫昔芬治疗的患者相比，他莫昔芬治疗延长的患者无病生存期（disease-free survival，DFS）缩短（78% vs 82%，$P=0.03$）。最近两项大型Ⅲ期临床试验的长期随访数据也公布了，这些试验将完成了5年他莫昔芬辅助治疗的早期乳腺癌患者随机分为停止内分泌治疗和延长内分泌治疗5年组[50,51]。辅助他莫昔芬：长vs短（Adjuvant Tamoxifen：Longer Against Shorter，ATLAS）试验中，纳入了12 894名早期乳腺癌女性。在ER阳性的6 846名女性中，研究人员报告了相比5年的他莫昔芬治疗，10年的他莫昔芬治疗后乳腺癌复发（$P=0.002$）、乳腺癌死亡（$P=0.002$）和总死亡（$P=0.01$）风险的显著下降。研究结果显示，在随访的5~14年间，10年他莫昔芬治疗绝对降低乳腺癌复发风险和死亡率分别为3.7%和2.8%。然而，子宫内膜癌的累积风险也增加了（3.1% vs 1.6%），其绝对死亡率增加了0.2%。在辅助他莫昔芬提供更多（Adjuvant Tamoxifen Treatment Offer More，aTTom）试验中，纳入6 953名早期乳腺癌女性[51]。与ATLAS试验结果相似，乳腺癌复发、乳腺癌特异性死亡和总死亡下降，支持了他莫昔芬10年的治疗方案。研究结果显示，持续5年以上的他莫昔芬治疗从第7年开始降低乳腺癌的复发风险，在10年后降低乳腺癌的死亡。鉴于这两项临床试验的证据，目前的指南建议考虑使用10年辅助他莫昔芬治疗[47]。但他莫昔芬治疗带来的副作用也需要仔细考虑。

表61-1 持续5年以上辅助他莫昔芬与5年他莫昔芬治疗对比的随机对照临床试验的疗效数据

试验	治疗	复发风险	乳腺癌特异性死亡	无病生存	总生存
ECOG[53]（1996）	继续vs停止	15% vs 25%（$P=0.014$，ER+患者）	8% vs 8.6%	85% vs 73%（$P=0.10$）	86% vs 89%（$P=0.81$，ER阳性）
NSABP-14[49]（2001）	继续vs停止	NR	NR	78% vs 82%（$P=0.03$）	91% vs 94%（$P=0.07$）
Scottish cancer trials breast group[52]（2001）	继续vs停止	5.2% vs 7.1%	23% vs 15%	54% vs 61%（$P=0.15$）	59.5% vs 68%（$P=0.12$）
ATLAS[50]（2012）	继续vs停止	RR=0.81（绝经前） RR=0.85（绝经后）	12.2% vs 15%（$P=0.01$）5~14年 RR=0.75（$P=0.002$）10年后	NR	NR
aTTom[51]（2013）	继续vs停止	28% vs 32%（$P=0.003$）	RR=0.75（$P=0.007$）10年后	NR	24.5% vs 26.1%（$P=0.1$）

他莫昔芬和化疗

最新的EBCTCG更新显示,以蒽环为基础的化疗方案的加入,每年可降低<50岁和50~69岁乳腺癌女性的死亡率38%和20%[48]。然而,内分泌治疗的加入,例如他莫昔芬,是否能进一步降低ER阳性的乳腺癌的死亡率？在3 330例ER阳性或ER状态未知的乳腺癌女性,单纯化疗的患者中28.1%发生复发,而在接受化疗和5年他莫昔芬治疗有17.5%复发,P值具有统计学意义[48]。同样,在ER阳性或ER状态未知的乳腺癌女性,与单用他莫昔芬相比,50岁以下接受化疗和他莫昔芬治疗的妇女中,EBCTCG报告的复发率为0.64(SE=0.08),年乳腺癌死亡率为0.65(SE=0.10)。此外,在50~69岁年龄组的妇女中也出现了类似的趋势。在ER阳性乳腺癌患者中,单纯辅助化疗是不够的,他莫昔芬的加入是非常重要的。EBCTCG还探讨了化疗和他莫昔芬的次序问题。在50~69岁妇女中,与单独使用他莫昔芬的妇女相比,接受化疗和他莫昔芬联合治疗妇女的复发率和年乳腺癌死亡率分别为0.80(SE=0.03)和0.90(SE=0.03)。与单用他莫昔芬相比,接受化疗后再使用他莫昔芬治疗的妇女复发率和年乳腺癌死亡率分别为0.77(SE=0.08)和0.80(SE=0.10)[48]。西南肿瘤学研究组(SWOG)8814的研究也探讨了治疗顺序的问题。该研究报告称,在CAF(环磷酰胺、阿霉素和5-氟尿嘧啶)后给予他莫昔芬,DFS和OS优于同时使用或他莫昔芬单独治疗[54]。这些研究表明,化疗序贯激素的治疗可能是一个更好的选择。

乳腺癌的预防

观察发现,长期他莫昔芬治疗可降低早期乳腺癌患者对侧乳腺癌的发生率和风险,这一现象激发了人们对于他莫昔芬预防乳腺癌发生的研究兴趣。囊括了5个主要的乳腺癌预防临床试验,纳入了28 000名乳腺癌患者的研究结果概述显示他莫昔芬将乳腺癌的发病率降低了38%(P<0.000 1)[55]。对于ER阴性的患者无影响,但ER阳性患者发病率降低了48%(P<0.000 1)。

然而,接受预防性他莫昔芬治疗的患者子宫内膜癌发生率增加(RR 2.4;P=0.000 5),静脉血栓栓塞事件也增加(相对危险度为1.9;P<0.000 1)。因此,在考虑使用他莫昔芬作为预防时,应平衡利弊,对于他莫昔芬在育龄年轻女性中不加限制的使用应谨慎。这方面的例外是,他莫昔芬被用于降低高危妇女患乳腺癌的风险,这是美国食品药品管理局(Food and Drug Administration,FDA)批准的第一种药物。因此,预防性使用他莫昔芬应评估个体患乳腺癌的风险。有导管原位癌、小叶原位癌、不典型增生或有BRCA 1/2有害突变女性被认为是乳腺癌发生的高危人群,对于他莫昔芬治疗的理想人群,其治疗目标是他莫昔芬的获益大于相关不良事件的风险[56-58]。他莫昔芬相关的不良事件意味着评价芳香化酶抑制剂的预防作用也是重要的。评价芳香化酶抑制剂作为预防治疗的研究结果将在题为“芳香化酶抑制剂”的章节中讨论。

雷洛昔芬

雷洛昔芬是一种苯并噻吩二代SERM,被FDA批准用于治疗和预防骨质疏松症和降低患骨质疏松症或浸润性乳腺癌高风险的绝经后女性患浸润性乳腺癌的风险[59-62]。但其在转移性乳腺癌中没有显著的抗肿瘤活性,因此未被批准用于治疗晚期乳腺癌。4项大型前瞻性临床试验报道了雷洛昔芬作为乳腺癌化学预防的有效性。雷洛昔芬评估的多重结果试验(Multiple Outcomes of Raloxifene Evaluation,MORE)纳入了7 705名绝经后骨质疏松症女性,随机接受雷洛昔芬或安慰剂,其主要终点是骨折的发生,这也是第一个表明雷洛昔芬可以作为乳腺癌化学预防的潜在药物的主要临床试验[59]。在这项试验中,经过4年的治疗,雷洛昔芬降低了ER阳性浸润性乳腺癌的发生风险84%(RR 0.16,95%CI 0.09,0.30)。雷洛昔芬相关连续结果(Continuing Outcomes Relevant to Evista,CORE)试验是MORE试验的延伸,该试验对同意继续参加的实验的MORE参与者额外进行了4年的随访研究,旨在进一步研究雷洛昔芬治疗对浸润性乳腺癌发病率的影响[60]。在为期8年的MORE和CORE中,研究者报告的在雷洛昔芬组和安慰剂组相比总浸润性乳腺癌和ER阳性浸润性乳腺癌的减少率分别为66%(HR,0.34;95%CI,0.22~0.50)和76%(HR,0.24;95%CI,0.15~0.40)。雷洛昔芬用于心脏(Raloxifene Use for the Heart,RUTH)试验的目的是研究雷洛昔芬对10 101例绝经后女性冠状动脉事件和乳腺癌发生率的影响[61]。研究人员发现,乳腺癌的减少程度与其他研究中他莫昔芬相似。NSABP P-2试验是一项前瞻性、双盲、随机的临床试验,比较他莫昔芬和雷洛昔芬对19 747名绝经后女性预防浸润性乳腺癌的疗效和安全性[62]。研究人员报告了他莫昔芬与雷洛昔芬在降低浸润性乳腺癌风险方面的疗效显示(RR=1.02;95%CI 0.82~1.28)。在副作用方面,与他莫昔芬相比,雷洛昔芬有着更少的妇科和血栓栓塞事件。有趣的是,雷洛昔芬降低了浸润性乳腺癌的风险,但对导管原位癌的发生率没有影响。

拉索昔芬

拉索昔芬是一种第三代非甾体SERM,与ER α-和β都可以高亲和力地选择性结合,并且中位抑制浓度比雷洛昔芬和他莫昔芬比报道的高出10倍。此外,与其他SERM相比,它还表现出更好的口服生物利用度,因为增加了对肠壁葡萄糖醛酸苷的抵抗力[63]。在绝经后妇女中,拉索昔芬被证明可以减少骨丢失、骨吸收和低密度脂蛋白胆固醇。在一项前瞻性临床试验中,8 556位骨密度T值-2.5或更低的绝经后女性随机接受5年的拉索昔芬或安慰剂治疗[64]。研究人员报告说,与安慰剂相比,在绝经后骨质疏松女性中使用拉索昔芬会降低ER阳性的乳腺癌、冠心病、中风以及非脊椎和脊椎骨折的风险。然而,据报道,它也与静脉血栓栓塞事件的风险增加有关。

托瑞米芬

托瑞米芬(Fareston)是他莫昔芬的结构衍生物,在实验动物中显示了相似的抗雌激素和雌激素特性。一般而言,托瑞米芬具有高度蛋白结合特性,因此具有长的血清半衰期。托瑞米芬的效应不如他莫昔芬,因此,临床研究评估的托瑞米芬的剂量高达240mg/d。托瑞米芬与他莫昔芬存在交叉耐药,但临床试验表明,它与他莫昔芬具有相似的疗效和副作用,因此可作为治疗晚期乳腺癌的一种替代方法[65,66]。但在辅助治疗中,还没有充分的数据推荐其使用。

曲洛司坦

曲洛司坦(Modrenal)是一种抗肾上腺药物,其常用于治疗库欣综合征。然而,曲洛司坦调节雌激素对ER的结合能力引起了人们对其阻止乳腺肿瘤细胞增殖的兴趣。对几项小型研究进行的Meta分析,评估了绝经后晚期乳腺癌患者曲洛司坦的使用情况和临床获益。需要进一步的试验来评估其作为晚期乳腺癌内分泌治疗的价值[67]。

氟维司群

氟维司群(Faslodex)是一种无激动剂性质的抗雌激素药物,与他莫昔芬不同的是,它具有以下作用机制:它可以结合、阻断和增加ER蛋白的降解,通过与ER的相互作用和下调细胞中ER蛋白的表达导致ER信号通路的抑制,还与PR表达的显著下调有关[68,69]。两个Ⅲ期的前瞻性临床试验的联合分析对比了氟维司群(250mg,肌内注射,每月1次)组和阿那曲唑对既往他莫昔芬治疗后疾病进展的晚期乳腺癌患者的疗效,经过15.1个月的中位随访时间,结果提示氟维司群与阿那曲唑的疗效[中位至疾病进展时间(times to progression,TTP)为5.5个月vs 4.1个月],两组的耐受性均良好,不良事件的发生率相似[70]。随后,另一项随机临床研究对比了氟维司群(250mg,肌内注射)与他莫昔芬一线治疗绝经后晚期乳腺癌(其肿瘤为HR阳性或HR状态未知)[71]。中位随访14.5个月后,结果显示氟维司群不劣于他莫昔芬未能得到证明,但在亚组分析中HR+患者氟维司群与他莫昔芬疗效相似。一项Ⅲ期的随机对照临床试验对比了氟维司群(250mg肌内注射)与依西美坦治疗非甾体芳香化酶抑制剂治疗失败的绝经后晚期乳腺癌患者的疗效[72]。结果显示,总客观缓解率(7.4% vs 6.7%;$P=0.736$)和至疾病进展时间(两组均为3.7个月)在氟维司群和依西美坦组中相似,提示对于非甾体芳香化酶抑制剂治疗失败的患者氟维司群并不优于甾体芳香化酶抑制剂依西美坦。由于氟维司群在每月250mg(之前批准的用药方案)的治疗剂量中需要3~6个月才能达到稳定的血浆水平,临床试验评估了标准给药方案与负荷剂量方案。在一项Ⅲ期双盲多中心临床试验中,之前内分泌治疗进展的绝经后ER阳性晚期乳腺癌患者随机接受氟维司群500mg或250mg,每月一次肌内注射的治疗[73]。结果显示500mg的负荷剂量在未明显增加毒性的同时能显著延长PFS(HR 0.8,95% CI 0.68~0.94,$P=0.006$)。基于以上结果,氟维司群500mg被批准用于内分泌治疗进展的绝经后HR+晚期乳腺癌患者。由于500mg的剂量方案优于250mg的剂量方案,是否500m的氟维司群在一线治疗HR+晚期乳腺癌患者优于芳香化酶抑制剂?一项Ⅱ期开放随机临床试验种,绝经后晚期乳腺癌患者随机接受一线的氟维司群或阿那曲唑治疗[74]。结果显示,氟维司群相比阿那曲唑能显著延长患者的至疾病进展时间。这项研究最新的结果显示氟维司群500mg相比阿那曲唑能显著提高OS[75]。试验正在研究新批准剂量的富夫罗特剂是否比芳香化酶抑制剂更好地治疗激素受体阳性的晚期乳腺癌。确认这一结果的Ⅲ期的临床试验(FALCON试验)正在进行中。

SERM和抗雌激素的副作用

SERM和抗雌激素相关的副作用主要是由于阻断雌激素对各种组织的刺激作用而产生的。最常见的副作用是潮热、夜汗和阴道干燥,这与更年期女性相似。其他不常见但比较重要的副作用与骨、血管和致癌相关。

骨质疏松症

雌激素对维持绝经前女性的骨健康具有重要意义,常被推荐用于预防绝经后女性骨质疏松症的发生。长期服用抗雌激素有可能导致绝经前女性过早的发生骨质疏松症。然而,由于SERM的部分雌激素激动剂作用,临床研究表明他莫昔芬治疗与骨密度降低无关[76],而雷洛昔芬被批准用于治疗骨质疏松症。

冠心病

雌激素可以降低低密度脂蛋白胆固醇水平,并提高高密度脂蛋白胆固醇水平,因此长期使用抗雌激素可能会提高冠心病的发生风险。然而,他莫昔芬的雌激素作用已被证明能降低女性患者的循环胆固醇水平[77,78]。临床研究结果提示他莫昔芬可以显著降低或有趋势地降低冠心病的风险[79]。雷洛昔芬也被证明能降低血清胆固醇水平[80];然而,在一项大型随机临床试验未能证明其可以降低冠心病的风险[61]。

血栓栓塞

许多研究结果提示他莫昔芬的预防性或治疗性使用与血栓栓塞事件的发生相关[55,81]。这与HRT或雷洛昔芬治疗中的报道类似。已知有血栓栓塞性疾病史的患者在决定长期使用他莫昔芬治疗之前应该仔细评估。

子宫内膜癌

研究表明,他莫昔芬治疗可能导致子宫内膜增厚、增生和子宫肌瘤[82]。子宫内膜增厚与子宫基质成分有关,而非上皮成分[83]。评估他莫昔芬治疗和预防乳腺癌疗效的临床试验表明,他莫昔芬的治疗导致子宫内膜肿瘤包括子宫内膜癌和小部分肉瘤的发生风险增加[84,85]。他莫昔芬治疗下发展的子宫内膜癌不是高级别子宫内膜癌,因此预后一般不会太差,而子宫内膜肉瘤一般与预后较差有关,因为其更差的组织学和更高的分期[86]。因此,在接受他莫昔芬治疗的患者中,所有发生持续阴道出血的患者都应进行妇科检查和子宫内膜活检。值得注意的是,这种增加的风险仅限于绝经后女性,绝经前的女性不存在子宫内膜癌增加的风险。在直接比较雷洛昔芬与他莫昔芬预防乳腺癌的实验(STAR试验)中,他莫昔芬组发生了36例子宫内膜癌,而雷洛昔芬组发生了23例(RR,0.62;95%CI,0.35~1.08)[62]。在评估5年辅助他莫昔芬治疗延长到10年的ATLAS和aTTom试验中,研究结果显示,长时间的他莫昔芬治疗增加了子宫内膜癌的发生率和因子宫内膜癌导致的死亡率。使用三苯氧胺的风险似乎仅限于治疗时间内[50,51]。在随机国际乳腺癌干预研究(International Breast Cancer Intervention Study,IBIS-I)(一项预防性研究,患者随机接受他莫昔芬或安慰剂),他莫昔芬组与安慰剂组相比,他莫昔芬治疗过程中的不良事件(包括深静脉血栓、肺栓塞和子宫内膜癌)发生率较安慰剂组增加,但在他莫昔芬治疗停止后的随访中并没有观察到[87]。

其他副作用

抗雌激素和SERM也与白内障和视网膜病变等眼部副作用有关[88,89]。临床前的研究提示他莫昔芬能引起肝脏中的致癌作用;然而,并未在人体中观察到肝癌的发生率升高[70]。

芳香化酶抑制剂

与SERM和抗雌激素相比,芳香化酶抑制剂的作用是阻断负责雌激素生物合成途径最后一步的酶复合物,从而从根本上阻止ER底物的产生。此外,与他莫昔芬不同,芳香化酶抑制剂没有部分雌激素激动剂作用。尽管卵巢是芳香化酶的主要来源,芳香化酶抑制剂不能有效抑制卵巢雌激素产生到绝经后的水平,可能是由于促性腺激素的代偿性升高以维持足够的雌激素产生。相反,芳香酶抑制剂可以充分地抑制绝经后女性雌激素的产生。

根据其抑制芳香化酶的特异性和能力，芳香化酶抑制剂被分为第一、第二和第三代芳香酶抑制剂（表 61-2）。它们根据其作用机制进一步细分为甾体（不可逆、Ⅰ型）和非甾体（可逆，Ⅱ型）抑制剂。Ⅰ型抑制剂，包括福美坦和依西美坦，通过共价结合芳香化酶不可逆抑制其功能从而导致其永久失活，即使在停药后仍持续存在，直到周围组织合成新的酶为止。Ⅱ型抑制剂，包括阿那曲唑、来曲唑和法德罗唑，只有抑制剂占据催化中心，才能可逆地与芳香化酶的活性部位结合，阻止底物的形成。在这一节中，我们将集中在新的第三代芳香化酶抑制剂来曲唑，阿那曲唑和依西美坦，这些在今天的临床实践中经常被使用的药物。这些芳香化酶抑制剂已经挑战了他莫昔芬作为黄金标准的内分泌治疗地位，现在是绝经后激素敏感乳腺癌患者的首选治疗，无论是在早期或晚期的治疗中，只要患者有中度或高度复发风险。

第一代

氨鲁米特是镇静剂格鲁米特的衍生物，最初作为细胞色素 P450 N-介导的类固醇羟基化的抑制剂而被引入。然而，这种化合物的作用是相当非特异性，因为这种药物在胆固醇代谢转化为活性甾体产物的过程中影响了许多羟基化步骤，总体来说，在乳腺癌女性中使用氨鲁米特加糖皮质激素会产生与其他内分泌治疗相似的疗效。氨鲁米特标准剂量（1 000mg/d）的副作用包括药物性皮疹、发热和嗜睡[91]。选择性更强的第二代和第三代芳香酶抑制剂的开发后，氨鲁米特现在很少用于乳腺癌的治疗。

表 61-2　典型芳香化酶抑制剂的结构和分类

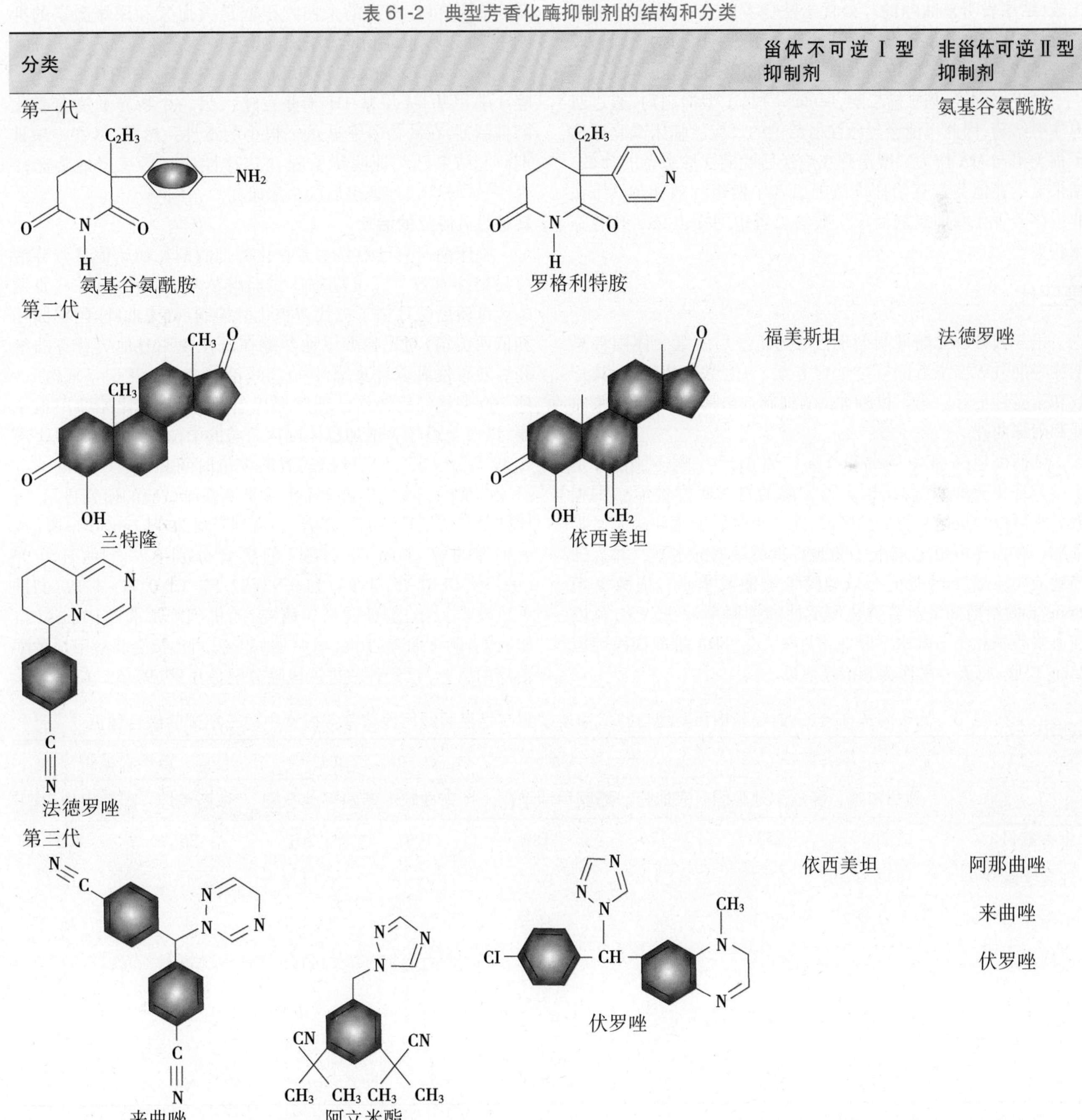

分类	甾体不可逆Ⅰ型抑制剂	非甾体可逆Ⅱ型抑制剂
第一代		氨基谷氨酰胺
第二代	福美斯坦	法德罗唑
第三代	依西美坦	阿那曲唑 来曲唑 伏罗唑

化合物以增加芳香化酶抑制的特异性和效力的近似顺序显示。

第二代

市场上的两种第二代芳香化酶抑制剂是法德罗唑和福美坦。法德罗唑(4-[5,6,7,8-四氢咪唑-(1,5-a)-吡啶-5基]苯甲腈)是一种高效的Ⅱ型芳香化酶抑制剂。两个大型多中心Ⅲ期临床试验比较了法德罗唑和MA在他莫昔芬内分泌经治的患者的疗效。两组在至疾病进展时间、总缓解率、缓解持续时间和OS方面均无显著差异[92]。当法德罗唑和他莫昔芬作为绝经后晚期乳腺癌一线治疗,研究结果显示两组疗效相似但法德罗唑的耐受性更好[93]。随机双盲临床试验也对比了法德罗唑和来曲唑在晚期乳腺癌的疗效,研究结果显示来曲唑疗效优于法德罗唑在晚期乳腺癌的随机双盲试验中也与来曲唑进行了比较,结果表明来曲唑的疗效优于法德罗唑[94]。法德罗唑毒性反应轻微,主要是恶心、厌食、疲劳和潮热。因为法德罗唑较氨鲁米特有重大提高,因此在日本被批准用于治疗乳腺癌。

福美坦(4-羟基雄烯二酮,Lentaron)是Ⅰ型抑制剂,通过肌内注射给药,因此可能会导致注射部位的反应。临床试验评估了福美坦与MA作为二线治疗在绝经后晚期女性患者的疗效,结果显示在他莫昔芬治疗失败的患者中两组疗效相似[95],在非甾体芳香化酶抑制剂治疗失败的患者中同样也显示其有临床获益[96]。

第三代

第三代芳香化酶抑制剂现已成为绝经后激素受体阳性早期或晚期乳腺癌患者的标准治疗方案,与他莫昔芬相比,其疗效和耐受性更好。第三代芳香化酶抑制剂包括依西美坦、来曲唑和阿那曲唑。

依西美坦(6-亚甲基-雄甾-1,4-二烯-3,17-二酮,阿诺新)是Ⅰ型芳香化酶抑制剂,结构上与该酶的自然底物雄烯二酮相似。它可以很快地从胃肠道吸收,在2小时后可达到最大血浆浓度。和福美坦相比,能更有效地降低雌激素的水平。并且已经被证明比福美坦能更有效地降低雌激素水平。依西美坦25mg/d的给药剂量对芳香化酶活性的抑制率为97.9%,可以使血浆雌酮和雌二醇水平降低约90%[97]。FDA批准依西美坦25mg口服,每天一次作为其治疗剂量。

阿那曲唑(阿立米酯),Ⅱ型抑制剂,是一个强大而有选择性的口服后快速吸收的苯并三唑衍生物,2小时后达到峰值浓度,7天后达到稳定状态,人体半衰期约为32.2小时[98]。阿那曲唑1mg或10mg,每天一次,持续28天,显示分别能降低整个身体芳构化达96.7%和98.1%[98]。FDA批准的给药方案是阿那曲唑每日口服1mg。

来曲唑{4,4-[(1H-1,2,4-三唑-1-基)亚甲基]双苯甲腈,弗隆},一种Ⅱ型抑制剂,体内外研究证明是一种高效的芳香化酶抑制剂。对比其他芳香化酶抑制剂,有更强抑制雌激素血浆水平作用。当给成年雌鼠口服,以1mg/(L·d),持续14天,观察到手术切除卵巢后来曲唑降低了子宫重量[99]。健康志愿者的临床研究以及进展的绝经后乳腺癌患者Ⅰ期临床也显示口服0.25mg/d小剂量的来曲唑引起最大血浆和尿雌激素的抑制[100]。FDA批准和推荐来曲唑给药方案是口服,每天2.5mg。

伏罗唑{R83842;R76713;6-[(s)4-氯苯基)-1H-1,2,4-三唑-1-基甲基]-1-甲基-1H-苯并三唑},另一个特异Ⅱ型芳香化酶抑制剂,在动物研究显示了很小的毒性。然后,尽管一项Ⅲ期研究结果已经证明伏罗唑在转移性绝经后患者的临床疗效[101]。该药已经退出后续临床研究。

转移性乳腺癌的治疗

临床前研究已经显示芳香化酶抑制剂在初始他莫昔芬治疗后继续有效[102],Ⅱ期临床试验继续验证其疗效,一些Ⅲ期临床试验已经评估了三代芳香化酶抑制剂(来曲唑、阿那曲唑和依西美坦)对比醋酸甲地孕酮在既往使用过他莫昔芬的绝经后转移性乳腺癌患者中的二线治疗疗效(表61-3)。在一项769例绝经后转移性乳腺癌患者研究中,对比醋酸甲地孕酮,依西美坦显著增加总体临床获益的中位持续时间(60.1周 vs 49周,$P=0.025$),肿瘤进展的中位时间和中位生存期[103]。一项相似的764例来自2个关键Ⅲ期临床试验的研究显示,对比接受醋酸甲地孕酮的患者,随机到阿那曲唑(1mg/d口服)或者阿那曲唑(10mg/d口服)的患者分别有一个估计0.97(97.5% CI 0.75~1.24)和0.92(97.5% CI,0.71~1.19)的进展风险[104]。关键Ⅲ期临床研究,随机到阿那曲唑(1mg/d口服)或者阿那曲唑(10mg/d口服)患者,对比接受醋酸甲地孕酮治疗的患者,已经评估进展风险分别是0.97(97.5% CI 0.75~

表61-3 比较阿那曲唑、来曲唑和依西美坦与醋酸甲地孕酮在绝经后服用他莫昔芬妇女中的三期试验综合数据

	联合数据		第一次试验		第二次试验		第一次试验	
	阿那曲唑	醋酸甲地孕酮	来曲唑	醋酸甲地孕酮	来曲唑	醋酸甲地孕酮	依西美坦	醋酸甲地孕酮
患者数目	263	253	174	189	199	201	366	403
客观缓解[a]/%	12.6	12.2	23.6	16.4	16.1	14.9	15	12
临床获益[b]/%	42.2	40.3	34.5	31.7	26.7	23.4	37	35
进展/%	57.4	59.3	53.4	56.1	51.3	50.7	48	53
中位TTP/月	5	5	5.6	5.5	3	3	5	5
中位获益间期/月	18.3	15.7	33	18	17.5	15.4	15	12
中位生存期/月	28.7	21.5	25.3	21.5	28.6	26.2	NA	28

[a] 客观缓解=完全缓解+部分缓解。
[b] 临床获益=完全缓解+部分缓解+超过6个月的疾病稳定。
缩略语:NA,没有可用的;TTP,疾病进展时间。

1.24）和 0.92（97.5% CI，0.71～1.19）[104]。在 1mg/d 和 10mg/d 计量间，没有观察到有统计差异的计量-反应差异。接下来的 2 年生存随访，接受阿那曲唑（1mg/d）组的 2 年生存率是 56.1%，接受醋酸甲地孕酮组是 46.3%[105]。一项 555 例他莫昔芬进展后的绝经后转移性乳腺癌女性也评估到相似的来曲唑疗效[106]。来曲唑（2.5mg/d）的总反应率是 36% 和 35%，而来曲唑（0.5mg/d）的总反应率是 27% 和 33%，醋酸甲地孕酮的总反应率是 32%。来曲唑（2.5mg/d）的中位缓解持续时间是 33 个月，醋酸甲地孕酮和来曲唑（0.5mg/d）的中位缓解持续时间都是 18 个月。也观察到支持来曲唑 2.5mg/d 的延长肿瘤进展时间和生存趋势优势[106]。

随着第三代芳香化酶抑制剂在绝经后转移性乳腺癌患者二线治疗上的成功，直接对比他莫昔芬，集中转到一线治疗（表 61-4）。在一项Ⅱ期研究中，对比依西美坦（25mg/d）和他莫昔芬（20mg/d）用于转移患者的一线治疗，发现较他莫昔芬，接受依西美坦组获得更好的客观缓解率（完全缓解+部分缓解）和中位缓解持续时间[107]。该研究随后扩展到三期临床，结果报道对比他莫昔芬，依西美坦组耐受性好，获得显著延长的无进展生存（10.9 月 vs 6.7 月）[108]。两项关键的Ⅳ期研究联合分析显示纳入的 1 021 例转移性绝经后乳腺癌女性，一线阿那曲唑（1mg/d）对比他莫昔芬[109]。中位随访激素受体阳性肿瘤患者（占患者比例 59.8%）18.5 个月，接受阿那曲唑治疗组中位进展时间显著优于接受他莫昔芬组（10.7 月 vs 6.4 月，$P=0.022$）。同样的，在一项多中心双盲一线Ⅲ期临床研究中，入组 907 例局部进展或转移的绝经后乳腺癌患者，给予来曲唑（2.5mg/d）对比他莫昔芬（20mg/d）[110]。中位随访 32 个月，报道显示接受来曲唑治疗组患者的疾病进展时间（中位 9.4 个月 vs 6.0 个月；$P<0.0001$），治疗失败时间（中位 9.0 个月 vs 5.7 个月；$P<0.0001$）和总体客观缓解率（32% vs 21%；$P=0.0002$）上都显著优于接受他莫昔芬组患者。来曲唑组和他莫昔芬组中位 OS 分别是 34 个月和 30 个月。已发表数据清晰显示芳香化酶抑制剂，特别是三代抑制剂，已经证明在进展期乳腺癌患者中疗效显著优于他莫昔芬。尽管如此，目前背景下还没有证据证明一种芳香化酶抑制剂优于另一种。

表 61-4　比较阿那曲唑、来曲唑和依西美坦与他莫昔芬一线治疗绝经后转移性乳腺癌妇女的疗效数据

	Ⅱ期研究				Ⅲ期研究			
	来曲唑	他莫昔芬	依西美坦	他莫昔芬	阿那曲唑[a]	他莫昔芬[a]	阿那曲唑[b]	他莫昔芬[b]
患者数目	453	454	61	59	170	182	340	453
客观缓解/%	30	20[c]	41	14	21	17	33	30
临床获益/%	49	38[c]	56	42	59	46[c]	56	56
TTP/月	9	6[c]	9	5	11	6[c]	8	8
TTF/月	6	6[c]	NR	NR	8	5	6	6

[a] 北美研究。
[b] 欧洲研究。
[c] 差异有统计学意义。
缩略语：NR，没有达到；TTF，治疗失败时间；TTP，疾病进展时间。

随着第三代芳香化酶抑制剂在转移性乳腺癌患者一线治疗被证明有效，研究集中转向于调查提高疗效的方法上。一种方法是芳香化酶抑制剂联合抗雌激素氟维司群。芳香化酶抑制剂的机制是最终导致低雌激素环境，临床前模型显示氟维司群在如此环境下依然发挥很好作用[111]。此外，临床前模型显示氟维司群和一种芳香化酶抑制剂的联合，可以通过下调几个已知与耐药发展相关的信号分子来实现延迟耐药的发展[112]。3 项随机临床研究已经在转移性激素受体阳性绝经后乳腺癌女性中对比了氟维司群和一种芳香化酶抑制剂的联合与单用芳香化酶抑制剂的疗效[113-115]。这些研究中氟维司群每月给药剂量 250mg。在一项Ⅲ期开放标签随机研究中［氟维司群和阿那曲唑联合治疗（Fulvestrant and Anastrozole Combination Therapy，FACT）］，原发疾病后首次复发的患者随机接受氟维司群联合阿那曲唑或者阿那曲唑单药[113]。研究者观察到加用氟维司群后，对于进展时间（10.8 个月 vs 10.2 个月，$P=0.91$）和中位 OS 均没有临床获益（37.8 个月 vs 38.2 个月，$P=1.00$）。在一组非甾体芳香化酶抑制剂进展后患者，作者观察到氟维司群联合阿那曲唑的疗效与单药氟维司群或者依西美坦相似。一项命名为 SWOG 的Ⅲ期研究中，既往未经治疗的乳腺癌患者被随机分为接受氟维司群联合阿那曲唑或者单药阿那曲唑[114]。作者报道联合组显著提高无进展生存（15 个月 vs 13.5 个月，$P=0.007$）。一项多中心随机安慰剂对照的Ⅲ期试验［一项非甾体芳香化酶抑制剂进展后芙仕得联合或不联合瑞宁得对比依西美坦的研究（Study of Faslodex with or without concomitant Arimidex vs exemestane following progression on nonsteroidal Aromatase inhibitors，SoFEA）］，转移性乳腺癌女性在接受非甾体芳香化酶抑制剂复发或进展后，随机分到接受氟维司群联合阿那曲唑组或者氟维司群联合安慰剂组或者单药氟维司群组[115]。毫无疑问，这 3 个试验由于入组患者类型不同导致观察到不同结果。例如，在 FACT 试验中，3/4 患者已经接受前线芳香化酶抑制剂治疗，在 SoFEA 试验中，患者必须是非甾体芳香化酶抑制剂进展后才符合入组标准。这与参与 SWOG 试验中大部分患者没有接受之前的芳香化酶抑制剂队列形成对比。然而，由于观察到的结果不尽相同，而且事实上，目前认为氟维司群的使用剂量是次优的，因此，在这个时候不能得出有关氟维司特和芳香化酶抑制剂联合治疗的确切结论。目前的指南对于激素受体阳性的绝经后转移性乳腺癌女性，芳香化酶抑制剂依然是首选的一线治疗方法，推荐多种可用的内分泌药物序贯治疗策略[47](图 61-2)。

辅助研究

随着第三代芳香化酶抑制剂证明在 HR+转移性乳腺癌绝经后女性的治疗疗效,研究转而集中于证明它们在早期乳腺癌的辅助治疗疗效。随着公然的子宫内膜癌风险增加和他莫昔芬使用相关的血栓栓塞事件发生,另一种选择是使用芳香化酶抑制剂。评估第三代芳香化酶抑制剂的辅助研究已经探索它们在前期辅助治疗和辅助他莫昔芬治疗之后使用的疗效(表 61-5;图 61-5)。接下来的篇章将回顾主要辅助试验的结果。

表 61-5 芳香化酶抑制剂辅助治疗绝经后早期乳腺癌妇女的疗效数据

试验	药物	中位随访(月)	无病生存(95%CI 或 P 值)
首次治疗			
ATAC	5 年阿那曲唑 vs 5 年他莫昔芬	120	0.86(0.78~0.95)
BIG 1-98	5 年来曲唑 vs 5 年他莫昔芬	8.7 年	0.86(0.78~0.96)
他莫昔芬之后			
MA17	5 年他莫昔芬后继续 5 年来曲唑或者安慰剂	30	0.58(0.45~0.76)
IES	2~3 年他莫昔芬后继续依西美坦或他莫昔芬累计 5 年	55.7	0.76(0.66~0.88)
NSABP B-33	5 年他莫昔芬后继续 5 年依西美坦或者安慰剂	30	0.68(P=0.07)
ITA	2~3 年他莫昔芬后继续阿那曲唑或他莫昔芬累计 5 年	64	0.56(0.35~0.89)
ABCSG 试验 6a	5 年他莫昔芬后继续 3 年阿那曲唑或安慰剂	62.3	0.62[a](0.40~0.96)

[a] 复发风险。

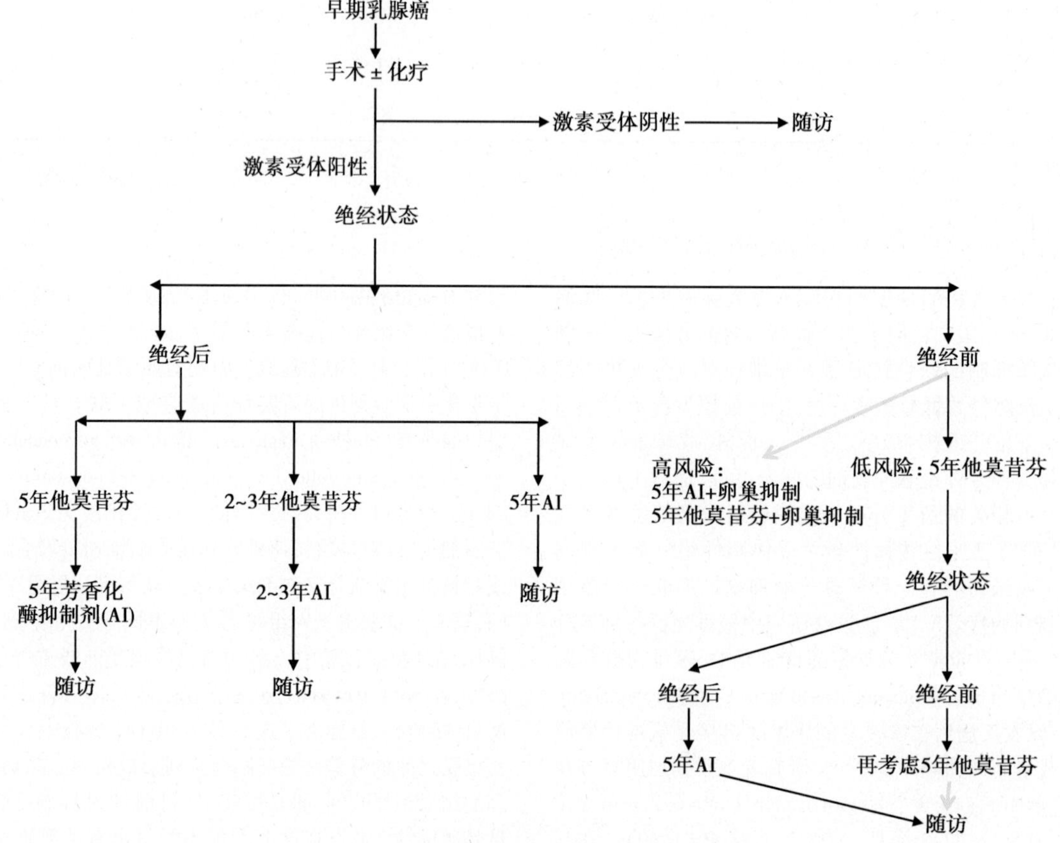

图 61-5 非转移性乳腺癌女性内分泌治疗的程序

绝经后女性早期疾病的前期治疗

瑞宁得、他莫昔芬单用或者联合（Arimidex, Tamoxifen, Alone or in Combination, ATAC）试验，是一项 9 366 例早期绝经后乳腺癌患者的随机双盲试验，目的在于与阿那曲唑联合他莫昔芬相比，比较 5 年他莫昔芬或者阿那曲唑治疗的疗效与耐受性[116]。中位随访 33 个月的计划分析，因为他莫昔芬单用组缺乏优良的疗效和耐受性导致联合组终止。该研究的主要研究终点是 DFS，次要研究终点是复发时间（time to recurrence, TTR）、新对侧乳癌发生率、距远处复发时间（time to distant recurrence, TTDR）和 OS。中位随访激素受体阳性患者 120 个月，阿那曲唑组 DFS 显著优于他莫昔芬组（HR = 0.86, 95% CI 0.78 ~ 0.95, P = 0.003），同样 TTR, TTDR 和对侧乳癌发生率也是阿那曲唑组获益。两组的总体死亡率没有显著差异（HR = 0.95, 95% CI 0.84 ~ 1.06, P = 0.7）[117]。

国际乳腺组织（Breast International Group, BIG）1-98 试验随机了 8 028 例激素受体阳性的绝经后乳腺癌患者。BIG 1-98 包含了 2 个主要辅助组，对比 5 年来曲唑和 5 年他莫昔芬，以及 2 个序贯治疗组：包含 2 年来曲唑、后续 3 年他莫昔芬组和 2 年他莫昔芬、后续 3 年来曲唑组[118]。主要研究终点是无病间期（disease-free interval, DFI）。随机后中位随访 8.7 年，对比接受他莫昔芬治疗组的患者，接受来曲唑治疗组显著提到 DFI（HR 0.86, 95% CI 0.78 ~ 0.96）和 OS（HR 0.87, 95% CI 0.77 ~ 0.999）[119]。

绝经后妇女他莫昔芬治疗后（转换策略）

第二个需要探索的问题是早期绝经后乳腺癌患者，在辅助他莫昔芬治疗后，序贯使用第三代芳香化酶抑制剂，这是转换策略的常用方法。MA17 研究是一项随机、双盲、延长的辅助阶段安慰剂对照的试验，入组的 5 187 例绝经后女性既往接受过 5 年的辅助他莫昔芬治疗[120]。由于在第一次中期分析观察到来曲唑比对照组疗效更优，该研究最终终止了。在更新的分析中，中位随访 30 个月，来曲唑组对比安慰剂组显著延长 DFS（HR = 0.58, 95% CI 0.45 ~ 0.76; P < 0.001）[121]。对比安慰剂，来曲唑耐受性很好，降低阴道出血，增加低度潮热、关节炎、关节痛和肌痛。研究提前终止后，对照组患者给予来曲唑治疗。在接受他莫昔芬治疗中位 2.8 年后，最新更新报道显示选择来曲唑的女性对比没有接受的女性 DFS 改善[122]。在统计调整后的探索性分析中，对于交叉效应，研究者报道中位随访 64 个月，延长的辅助来曲唑治疗在 DFS 和 OS 上均优于安慰剂组[123]。研究者进一步指出，尽管在初始诊断绝经前或绝经后女性中，在 5 年他莫昔芬后继续延长辅助来曲唑治疗是获益的，但看来对初始绝经后女性的预后影响更大[124]。

组间依西美坦研究（Intergroup Exemestane Study, IES）调查了在 2 ~ 3 年辅助他莫昔芬治疗后序贯依西美坦治疗的疗效和安全性。试验入组了 4 742 例患者，他们随机分配到继续他莫昔芬，或者在 5 年治疗的剩余时间转换到依西美坦治疗。中位随访 30.6 个月，数据显示转换到依西美坦治疗比继续他莫昔芬治疗获得显著改善的 DFS（HR = 0.68, 95% CI 0.56 ~ 0.82; P < 0.001）[125]。中位随访 55.7 个月，对比继续他莫昔芬组，转换到依西美坦组获得 DFS 24% 的改善（HR = 0.76, 95% CI 0.66 ~ 0.88, P = 0.000 1）和 OS 15%（HR = 0.85, 95% CI 0.71 ~ 1.02, P = 0.08）的提高[126]。NSABP B-33 试验，类似于 IES 试验，是一项继 5 年他莫昔芬后评估 5 年依西美坦对比 5 年安慰剂的随机试验[127]。由于 MA17 研究结果，NASBP B-33 研究被提前终止和破盲。尽管提前关闭和患者交叉，对比安慰剂组，接受依西美坦的原队列组观察到有统计差异的 4 年 DFS 获益（91% vs 89%; HR = 0.68; P = 0.07）[127]。

早期乳腺癌辅助他莫昔芬对比依西美坦试验（TEAM）是一项Ⅲ期研究，目的在于比较前期依西美坦单用对比完成 5 年他莫昔芬后序贯依西美坦治疗的疗效[128]。超过 9 000 例患者被招募到该试验。研究者指出 2 组治疗策略的 5 年 DFS 没有显著差异（风险比 0.97, 95% CI 0.88 ~ 1.08; P = 0.60），并且得出结论：对于早期绝经后乳腺癌患者，依西美坦在他莫昔芬之前或之后使用都是合适选择。

几个更小的试验也注意到芳香化酶抑制剂的治疗顺序问题。意大利他莫昔芬阿那曲唑（Italian Tamoxifen Anastrozole, ITA）和阿立米酯他莫昔芬 95/澳大利亚乳腺癌研究组 8（Arimidex Nolvadex 95/Austrian Breast Cancer Study Group 8, ARNO 95/ABCSG 8）已经证明在 2 ~ 3 年他莫昔芬后转换到阿那曲唑显著降低复发风险[129,130]。在 ABCSG 试验 6a，绝经后女性在接受辅助他莫昔芬治疗后随机分组到阿那曲唑或者安慰剂组[131]。中位随访 62.3 个月后，对比安慰剂组，接受阿那曲唑组女性获得 38% 的复发风险降低（HR = 0.62; 95% CI = 0.40 ~ 0.96, P = 0.031）。把前面提到的试验总结起来，很清楚对于激素受体阳性的绝经后乳腺癌女性，辅助使用芳香化酶抑制剂不论先于他莫昔芬还是序贯其后，均优于单用他莫昔芬。两种策略都是推荐并纳入国际指南的。

芳香化酶抑制剂在绝经前女性的使用

从早期总结的数据来看，在辅助阶段芳香化酶抑制剂是优于他莫昔芬的。由于他们不同的作用机制，芳香化酶抑制剂仅被使用于绝经后女性。他莫昔芬是唯一推荐用于激素受体阳性的绝经前乳腺癌患者辅助使用。抑制卵巢雌激素产生在接受他莫昔芬绝经前女性中的治疗价值尚不确定[132]。挑战数据已经发表，提示化疗继发性卵巢抑制（即发展为闭经状态）是与降低复发风险相关的，指导年轻乳腺癌女性推荐基于个体讨论使用他莫昔芬联合促性腺激素释放激素类似物[133,134]。我们知道卵巢剥除的实际应用并没有导致结果改善，尽管从小于 40 岁绝经前女性复发和 DFS 的角度观察到获益趋势。然而，记住这些研究的绝大部分没有在两组进行卵巢剥除和他莫昔芬对比，所以是否卵巢剥除优于他莫昔芬单用是不确定的。

国际乳腺癌研究组（International Breast Cancer Study Group, IBCSG）在 2003 年发起了 2 个Ⅲ期随机临床试验，集中于早期激素受体阳性的绝经前乳腺癌患者[卵巢功能抑制试验（Suppression of Ovarian Function Trial, SOFT），他莫昔芬和依西美坦试验（Tamoxifen and Exemestane Trial, TEXT）]，为了确定辅助芳香化酶抑制剂是否比三苯氧胺改善 DFS，并确定卵巢抑制的价值[135,136]。TEXT 研究随机分组早期绝经前乳腺癌患者进入 5 年的依西美坦联合卵巢抑制治疗组或者 5 年的他莫昔芬联合卵巢抑制治疗组。SOFT 研究随机分组早期绝经前乳腺癌患者进入 5 年的他莫昔芬单用组，他莫昔芬联合卵巢抑制组，或者依西美坦联合卵巢抑制治疗组。来自 TEXT 和 SOFT 的联合分析，研究者观察到中位随访 68 个月，接受依西美坦联合卵巢抑制治疗的患者比接受他莫昔芬联合卵巢抑制治疗的患者显著改善 5 年 DFS（91.1% vs 87.3%，HR 0.72，95% CI 0.60～0.85，P<0.001）[133]。接受依西美坦治疗的女性 3 或 4 级 AE 发生率更高（30.6% vs 29.4%）[135]。SOFT 随机了超过 3 000 例激素受体阳性的早期绝经前乳腺癌患者，分为接受他莫昔芬单药组，他莫昔芬联合卵巢抑制组，或者依西美坦联合卵巢抑制组，基本目标是确定卵巢抑制的价值[136]。研究者报告中位随访总人群 67 个月后，单变量分析中对比单药他莫昔芬，联合卵巢抑制没有显著改善 5 年 DFS（86.6% vs 84.7%，P=0.10）。在调整协变量的多变量模型中，对比他莫昔芬单药，他莫昔芬联合卵巢抑制导致乳腺癌复发、第二种侵袭性癌症或者死亡的相对危险度降低 22%（P=0.03）。作者进一步观察到，在有足够高复发风险接受化疗的绝经前妇女中，接受他莫昔芬单药女性 5 年无乳腺癌发生率是 78%，接受他莫昔芬联合卵巢抑制的女性 5 年无乳腺癌发生率是 82.5%（当对比他莫昔芬单药 HR 0.78；95% CI 0.60～1.02），接受依西美坦联合卵巢抑制的女性 5 年无乳腺癌发生率是 85.7%（当对比他莫昔芬单药 HR 0.65；95% CI 0.49～0.87）。研究者报告随着治疗开始年份的增加，卵巢抑制的不依从性增加。报道显示卵巢抑制引起更频繁的副作用包括潮热、失眠、抑郁、阴道干燥、肌肉骨骼症状、高血压，以及葡萄糖不耐受。接受卵巢抑制的女性骨质疏松发生率更高。在第三个随机Ⅲ期试验［澳大利亚乳腺癌和结直肠癌研究组（Austrian Breast and Colorectal Cancer Study Group，ABCSG）-12］，1 803 例接受Ⅰ期或者Ⅱ手术的激素受体阳性的绝经前女性患者随机分到阿那曲唑联合卵巢抑制治疗组或者他莫昔芬联合卵巢抑制治疗组，使用或者不使用唑来膦酸[137]。该研究的主要研究终点是 DFS，次要终点是 RFS 和 OS。中位随访 94.4 个月后，研究者报告他莫昔芬和阿那曲唑组 DFS 没有显著差异，尽管接受阿那曲唑联合卵巢抑制组患者死亡风险比接受他莫昔芬联合卵巢抑制组更高（HR=1.63；95% CI，1.05～1.45；P=0.030）。有趣的是，观察到唑来膦酸的增加与 DFS 改善相关。已经假设多种原因来解释 ABCSG-12 和 TEXT 及 SOFT 的不一致结果；最重要的一点是 TEXT/SOFT 有更高的统计效力来回答卵巢抑制和芳香化酶抑制剂在绝经前女性中的地位。长期随访 TEXT 和 SOFT 对于年轻患者确定长期疗效和相关的毒性是至关重要的。

基于之前提供的证据，作者推荐在激素受体阳性的早期绝经后乳腺癌患者辅助治疗中提前使用芳香化酶抑制剂。目前绝经后女性的辅助内分泌治疗指南基于患者个体风险获益推荐芳香化酶抑制剂作为初始治疗或者他莫昔芬初始治疗后使用[138]。使用芳香化酶抑制剂超过 5 年目前不推荐，正在进行的临床试验将回答这种方法临床效用的问题。绝经前女性的故事有点更复杂。使用他莫昔芬 10 年或者使用卵巢抑制联合芳香化酶抑制剂在更新的指南都被列入其中，具体选择需要基于个体风险评估和副作用的讨论[47]。对前面描述的辅助试验的长期随访，有望更好的定义芳香化酶抑制剂用于辅助治疗的长期疗效结果、副作用和描述所需治疗的持续时间。

新辅助治疗

新辅助治疗用于在外科局部治疗之前降低肿瘤分期，允许更多患者进行保乳手术，或者使不能手术的病例可能手术。第三代芳香化酶抑制剂已经证明了在进展期和早期疾病的疗效，研究它们带来的术前获益是重要的。

对比新辅助化疗试验，探索乳腺癌治疗内心分泌疗效的新辅助研究是小很多的。几个试验已经在激素受体阳性的绝经后乳腺癌患者中比较了新辅助他莫昔芬对比新辅助第三代芳香化酶抑制剂[139-143]。临近术前的瑞宁得、他莫昔芬或者两者联用试验（Immediate Preoperative Arimidex，Tamoxifen，or Combined with Tamoxifen，IMPACT），在 330 例激素受体阳性的绝经后乳腺癌患者中对比了术前 3 个月的阿那曲唑和他莫昔芬或者二者联合的疗效[139]。观察到 3 组总体反应无差异（37% vs 36% vs 39%）。然而，124 例基线需要乳房切除的女性，外科医生考虑 46%用了阿那曲唑的患者可以做保乳手术，对比之下，考虑有 22% 接受他莫昔芬的患者可以做保乳手术（P=0.03）[139]。相似的，术前瑞宁得对比术前他莫昔芬（PROACT）试验，随机将 451 例绝经后女性分为 3 个月新辅助阿那曲唑或者他莫昔芬，联用或者不联用化疗，报告显示单用内分泌治疗组患者，基线时接受阿那曲唑治疗的患者的可行手术率提高了 43.0%，而接受他莫昔芬治疗的患者为 30.8%（P=0.04）[140]。

在 P024 研究，337 例绝经后女性随机分配到接受 4 个月新辅助来曲唑或者他莫昔芬，发现来曲唑组的总体反应率（55% vs 36%，P<0.001）和保乳手术率显著提高（45% vs 35%，P=0.022）[138]。另外，在 P024 研究，来曲唑组和他莫昔芬组的反应率差异在 ErbB-1 阳性和/或 ErbB-2 阳性的亚组最显著（88% vs 21%，P = 0.000 4）；然而，研究的这部分基本上证据不足[142]。在 151 例患者的小样本随机研究中，依西美坦也被报道在新辅助治疗中比他莫昔芬获得更有效的临床总体反应（76.3% vs 40%；P=0.05）和保乳手术率（依西美坦 36.8% vs 他莫昔芬 20%；P=0.05）[140]。

在 ACOSOG Z1031 Ⅱ期试验中，3 种芳香化酶抑制剂被用于术前比较。超过 300 例临床分期Ⅱ到Ⅲ的绝经后乳腺癌女性入组了这项主要终点是临床反应的研究[144]。接受依西美坦、来曲唑和阿那曲唑患者的临床反应分别是 62.9%、74.8% 和 69.1%。手术结果、术前内分泌预后指数（Preoperative Endocrine Prognostic Index，PEPI）评分或者被检查的 Ki67 抑制率（次要研究终点）都没有差异。

目前，临床试验之外，芳香化酶抑制剂新辅助内分泌治疗被推荐用于因不适合术前化疗相关并发症的绝经后女性[145]。几个包括新辅助内分泌治疗合适时间的问题仍有待于以后的临床试验来解决。

乳腺癌的化学预防

如前讨论，他莫昔芬的副作用限制了其在乳腺癌的预防使用。进一步试验观察到他莫昔芬和雷洛昔芬预防性使用降低了 ER+乳腺癌 50%发生率，因此，寻找一种能进一步降低乳腺癌发生率的药物是很重要的。芳香化酶抑制剂，鉴于它们已经证明的对于 HR+乳腺癌的疗效，是可行选择。ATAC 试验[117]中位随访 100 个月，对比他莫昔芬组，阿那曲唑可以显著降低 HR+对侧乳腺癌的发生率（HR 0.60，95% CI 0.42～0.85，P=0.004）。同样在 BIG-98 试验[118,119]，来曲唑组比他莫昔芬组有更少的对侧乳腺癌例子（16 例 vs 27 例）。IES 研究[126]中位随访 55.7 个月，随着进展为 ER+对侧乳腺癌，观察到依西美坦组有 17 例对侧乳腺癌，对比他莫昔芬组的 35 例对侧乳腺癌，依西美坦显著降低了对侧乳腺癌发生率（HR=0.56，95% CI 0.33～0.98，P=0.04）。

这些试验说明第三代芳香化酶抑制剂对比他莫昔芬降低了大约超过40%~50%的对侧乳腺癌发生率。通过外推,这意味着这些芳香化酶抑制剂可能降低大约70%~80%的ER+对侧乳腺癌发生率[142]。随着如此印象深刻的结果,大型随机临床试验被设计来观察芳香化酶抑制剂在初始预防使用的作用[147,148]。一项Ⅲ期试验,4 560例中等患乳腺癌风险的绝经后女性随机分到接受依西美坦或安慰剂[147]。作者报道说中位随访35个月后,依西美坦组检测到11例侵袭性乳腺癌,安慰剂组检测到32例侵袭性乳腺癌。对比安慰剂,使用依西美坦转变为侵袭性乳腺癌年发生率65%的相对降低(HR 0.35,95%CI 0.18~0.70,P=0.002)。观察到两组微小的生活质量差异,两组的骨骼骨折、其他癌症、治疗相关的死亡和心血管事件没有显著差异。一项第二阶段的Ⅲ期试验(IBIS-Ⅱ),1 920例高风险患乳腺癌的绝经后女性随机分为接受阿那曲唑或者安慰剂5年[148]。中位随访5年后,阿那曲唑组检测到40例乳腺癌,安慰剂组检测到85例(HR 0.47,95% CI 0.32~0.68,P<0.000 1)。随访7年的累计发病率:阿那曲唑是2.8%,安慰剂组是5.6%。鉴于对比他莫昔芬描述的数据和更好的副作用数据,目前指南推荐中到高风险患乳腺癌的绝经后女性使用芳香化酶抑制剂[47]。

副作用

骨骼疾病

如前所讨论,雌激素缺乏与骨质疏松症风险增加相关,特别是对于乳腺癌女性[149]。然而他莫昔芬,通过雌激素激动剂作用于骨骼,显示对骨健康有益处[76],所有3个三代芳香化酶抑制剂显示增加骨丢失。在120个月的ATAC试验分析中,对比他莫昔芬,阿那曲唑组骨折率显著增加(451例骨折 vs 351例骨骼,HR 1.33,95% CI 1.15~1.55;P<0.000 1);尽管如此,在接受5年治疗后,阿那曲唑和他莫昔芬组的骨折率差异不显著(110 vs 112,OR 0.98,95% CI 0.74~1.30,P=0.9)[117]。

在BIG1-98试验,中位随访60.3个月,9.3%的来曲唑组患者发生骨折,他莫昔芬组骨折发生率6.5%,手腕是最常见骨折部位[150]。相似的观察也出现在IES试验中位随访55.7个月时,对比他莫昔芬组5%的骨折率,依西美坦组骨折率显著增加到7%(比值比=1.45,95% CI 1.13~1.87;P=0.003)[151]预防或者逆转芳香化酶抑制剂相关的骨丢失的一个方法是使用双膦酸盐。在两个随机择泰-弗隆辅助协调试验(Z-FAST和ZO-FAST)综合分析中,1 667例患者接受辅助来曲唑,提前接受唑来膦酸或者当骨密度降到-2时结束[152]。随访12个月,提前使用唑来膦酸组相比延迟使用的腰椎骨密度增加了5.2%。需要长期随访来证实这些结果。

心血管疾病

绝经后乳腺癌女性可能因为她们的年龄、绝经状态、相关的共病状态以及暴露于乳腺癌治疗的化疗药物,有一个更高的心血管事件风险。如前描述,他莫昔芬,通过它的雌激素激动剂功能,已经显示有降脂功能从而轻度降低心血管事件[79]。阿那曲唑没有显示出明显改变脂肪分布[153,154],在辅助阶段,服用阿那曲唑与服用他莫昔芬女性经历的心肌梗死相似[117]。在BIG1-98实验,中位随访51个月,对比他莫昔芬组女性,来曲唑组女性经历了显著增高的低级别胆固醇升高和心血管事件(除缺血性心脏病和心力衰竭外)[119]。对比他莫昔芬组患者,来曲唑组的低级别胆固醇升高,或许是如前提高的他莫昔芬降脂效果反应。研究显示依西美坦除了对高密度脂蛋白胆固醇略有下降外[155],依西美坦对脂质水平没有明显影响。IES研究,中位随访55.7个月,所有患者心血管事件(排除血栓栓塞事件)在依西美坦和他莫昔芬组没有看出不同,对比0.8%的他莫昔芬治疗组患者出现心肌梗死,约1.3%的依西美坦治疗组患者出现心肌梗死(P=0.08)。尽管将需要更长的随访来评估临床使用第三代芳香化酶抑制剂的心血管效应,乳腺癌女性一般来说由于多种因素有更高的风险发展心血管事件,因此应适当监测和管理。

其他副作用

芳香化酶抑制剂一个重要的副作用是关节痛的发展,它能显著影响生活质量。例如,BIG1-198实验中,来曲唑相关的关节痛事件是20.3%,对比观察到的服用他莫昔芬女性是12.3%(P<0.001)[119]。临床治疗的依从性和关节痛试验(COMPliance and Arthralgia in Clinical Therapy,COMPACT)是一项开放标签试验,主要研究终点是观察关节痛依从性[156]。将近2 000个绝经后女性接受了提前的阿那曲唑。研究者注意到随着时间推移,阿那曲唑的依从性逐渐降低。伴随关节痛平均分和不依从性之间的显著相关性。芳香化酶抑制剂相关的其他副作用包括阴道干燥和性交困难。尽管芳香化酶抑制剂的治疗增加了血管舒缩症状和阴道出血/分泌物的风险,大规模临床试验已经显示这些事件的发生率比他莫昔芬治疗经历的要低[116-130]。另外,这些试验也报道了接受芳香化酶抑制剂组女性的血栓栓塞事件和子宫内膜癌发生率比接受他莫昔芬患者要低很多。

内分泌耐药

我们很确定在激素受体阳性的乳腺癌患者辅助和转移阶段治疗管理方面走了很长的路。尽管内分泌治疗在转移性患者是有效的,只有30%HR+乳腺癌患者有客观缓解,伴随几乎只有内分泌治疗的50%临床获益增加[157]。在临床实践中,内分泌药物的顺序使用能够产生对激素依赖性转移性乳腺癌的长期缓解。事实上,尽管如此,内分泌耐药问题也是遇到的。辅助阶段临床试验已经证明接近50%激素受体阳性乳腺癌患者可以从内分泌治疗获益,剩下的发展为原发或者获得性内分泌耐药。几种耐药模式是临床试验中一般遇到的。原发耐药描述了尽管ER表达的肿瘤对ER靶向治疗内在抵抗的情形。获得性耐药描述了ER+肿瘤对如内分泌治疗起始有反应然后进展。药物选择性耐药描述了ER+肿瘤对特定内分泌药物耐药的情形。

肿瘤对内分泌耐药的机制,总体来说,只有部分被理解[158]。芳香化酶抑制剂耐药不仅仅因为这些药物抑制雌二醇水平的失败,也是因为细胞成分发生了改变,如生长因子受体通路[159]。部分内分泌耐药机制包括细胞表面生长因子受体激活[包括表皮生长因子受体,人表皮生长因子受体2(human epidermal growth factor receptor 2,HER2)和IGF-1受体]和受体酪氨酸激酶下游元素的激活[包括磷脂酰肌醇3激酶(phosphatidylinositol 3-kinase,PI3K)、AKT和哺乳动物雷帕霉素靶蛋白(mammalian target of rapamycin,mTOR)]。这些通路的激活或者失调很大程度上导致 ER 信号通路的配体独立激活，从而导致这些通路变成对临床应用的内分泌药物耐药。随着对耐药机制的理解加深，已被介绍的选择性靶向药物当与内分泌治疗结合可以克服耐药。

靶向 HER2 通路

已知大约 1/5 的新诊断乳腺癌患者有 HER2 过表达或者扩增，并且通常与预后不良有关。一系列抗 HER2 药物(例如，曲妥珠单抗、拉帕提尼、帕托株单抗和 TDM-1)的引进，很大程度上改变了这类乳腺癌亚型的自然史。临床前证据显示 HER2 和 ER 通路的交联导致已有内分泌治疗的耐药[160-162]。基于该证据，在联合优于内分泌单用的假说下，一系列临床试验研究抗 HER2 药物和内分泌治疗的联合作用。TANDEM 试验是一个Ⅲ期研究，随机了绝经后 HR+/HER2-转移性乳腺癌患者到曲妥珠单抗联合阿那曲唑或者阿那曲唑单药组[163]。研究者注意到联合组有统计学意义，尽管临床 PFS 获益不显著(HR 0.63；95% CI，0.47~0.84；中位 PFS，4.8 个月 vs 2.4 个月；P=0.001 6)，并且两组 OS 没有差异。第二项试验中，HR+/HER2-绝经后乳腺癌患者被随机分到接受拉帕提尼联合来曲唑或者来曲唑单药组，研究者观察到加入拉帕提尼可以显著降低疾病进展风险(HR 0.71；95% CI 0.53~0.96；P=0.019，中位 PFS 8.2 个月 vs 3.0 个月)[164]。

靶向 PI3K 激酶通路

PI3K 通路已知和 mTOR 一起作为信号转导激酶通路来调节细胞成长、增殖和生存。mTOR 存在于两个多蛋白复合物中，mTORC1 由 mTOR 组成，与 mTOR(raptor)的调节蛋白有关，是 AKT 的下游，而 mTORC2 与 mTOR(rictor)雷帕霉素不敏感伴侣相关，mTORC2 磷酸化 AKT。PI3K 通路激活导致 AKT 磷酸化，AKT 的磷酸化反过来导致 mTORC1 及其效应物的磷酸化[4E 结合蛋白 1(4E-BP-1)增加细胞增殖、存活和血管生成；S6 激酶 1(S6K1)调节细胞生长]。临床前证据显示 PI3K 通路激活与内分泌治疗耐药相关，S6K1 负责磷酸化 ERS 的激活域[165,166]。一系列研究也证明 mTOR 抑制逆转内分泌抵抗，特别当 mTOR 抑制剂与内分泌治疗结合时候[167,168]。这样的证据导致一系列 mTOR 抑制剂的发展，很多结合内分泌治疗的研究在临床试验开展。Ⅲ期试验(HORIZON)检测 mTOR 抑制剂西罗莫司的临床疗效，1 112 个既往没有接受过芳香化酶抑制剂的 HR+转移性乳腺癌患者，随机分到接受来曲唑或者来曲唑联合西罗莫司组。这个研究当观察到来曲唑联合西罗莫司极不可能证明比来曲唑单用 PFS 获益后，关闭了试验[169]。Ⅲ期临床口服依维莫司乳腺癌试验 2(BOLERO-2)试验检测了依维莫司(抑制 mTORC1 激酶的雷帕霉素类似物)，入组既往非甾体芳香化酶抑制剂进展后的 HR+转移性乳腺癌患者，随机分到接受依维莫司联合依西美坦或者依西美坦单用组[170]。入组患者必须是前线来曲唑或者阿那曲唑耐药后患者，也就是辅助治疗期间或完成后 12 个月内复发；对于转移性患者，要求治疗期间或者治疗结束后 1 个月内疾病进展。在这些对非甾体芳香化酶抑制剂耐药患者人群，研究者证明联合组获得显著差异的 4.6 个月中位 PFS 改善(P<0.000 1)。尽管这种获益没有延续到次要终点 OS 的显著提高(31 个月 vs 26.6 个月，P=0.14)。依维莫司加入依西美坦后，增加了毒性，包括口腔炎(3 级，8% vs 1%)、肺炎(3 级，3% vs 0%)、肝功能不全和高血糖。第三个试验[他莫昔芬联合依维莫司(TAMRAD)]是一个随机的Ⅱ期试验，在 111 例既往使用过芳香化酶抑制剂的女性中，评估依维莫司和他莫昔芬的联合对比他莫昔芬单用[171]。TAMRAD 研究的主要研究终点是 6 个月的临床获益率，显示在接受他莫昔芬联合依维莫司组比单药他莫昔芬显著提高 6 个月的临床获益率(61% vs 42%)。通过限制前线芳香化酶抑制剂进展的患者入组，BOLERO-2 和 TAMRAD 试验很大程度上选择肿瘤通过 PI3K/AKT/mTOR 通路驱动的患者入组，这也能够解释与 HORIZON 研究不一致性的结果。目前依维莫司和依西美坦联合已经被推荐用于前线芳香化酶抑制剂进展后的患者使用[47]。因为依维莫司的加入具有显著而独特的毒性，在治疗之前与患者的讨论沟通很重要。

靶向 CDK4/6 通路

细胞周期依赖性激酶(cyclin-dependent kinase，CDK)与调控蛋白质细胞周期蛋白在控制进展中起着关键作用。控制细胞周期的基因改变是最具吸引力的 CDK 靶向药物治疗的潜在靶点[172]。CDK4/6 和细胞周期 D 调节 pRb 的磷酸化(视网膜瘤)，过磷酸化的结果导致转录因子释放，允许细胞从周期的 G1 到 S 期的[173]。帕博西利(PD-0332991)是一个选择性的，可逆的小分子 CDK4/6 抑制剂，在人乳腺癌细胞系的临床前研究已经显示在 ER+和 HER2-扩增亚型中有潜在活性[174]。在这些亚型中，导致 pRb 高磷酸化的阻滞很大程度上导致细胞周期阻滞在 G1 期。一项单臂的Ⅱ期 36 个严重乳腺癌患者是 RB 蛋白阳性表达，单药帕博西利在一些 HR+乳腺癌患者中显示出活性[175]。相关的 3/4 级毒性包括暂时性中性粒细胞和血小板减少。一项随机开放标签的Ⅱ期 PALOMA 试验，165 例既往没有因为疾病进展接受过治疗的 HR+HER2-转移性绝经后乳腺癌患者，随机接受来曲唑或者来曲唑联合帕博西利[176]。注意到来曲唑基础上加上帕博西利，提高 PFS 从 10.2 个月到 20.2 个月(HR 0.488，95% CI 0.319~0.718，P=0.000 4)。相对于单药来曲唑组，3/4 级的中性粒细胞减少(54% vs 1%)和疲乏(4% vs 1%)被报道在帕博西利/来曲唑组有更高的发生率。基于这些结果，FDA 加速获批了帕博西利联合来曲唑在激素受体阳性转移性乳腺癌患者的一线治疗。最近 PALOMA-3 试验结果发表，随机了超过 500 例内分泌治疗治疗复发或者进展的 HR+HER2-转移性乳腺癌患者，接受氟维司群单药或者联合帕博西利[177]。这个Ⅲ期试验纳入了接受戈舍瑞林的绝经前和围绝经期患者。研究者报道了帕博西利加入氟维司群后 PFS 显著增加(9.2 个月 vs 3.8 个月，P<0.001)。

促性腺激素释放激素类似物与卵巢功能

随着早期年轻绝经前乳腺癌患者辅助化疗预后的改善，过早绝经问题和与化疗相关的不孕不育已经成为重要问题。在小于 35 岁接受化疗的女性，长期闭经率接近 10%，在 35~40 岁间女性化疗后闭经率接近 50%，40 岁以上化疗后闭经率上升到 85%[178]。卵巢早衰相关的不孕不育能够影响近 30%年轻乳腺癌女性的治疗决定[179]。目前没有接受化疗的绝经前女性生育保护标准。2013 版美国临床肿瘤学会(American Society of Clinical Oncology,ASCO)生育保护指南推荐对在开始试图保护生育问题之前,对化疗和/或放疗引起的不孕不育风险尽早预先讨论[180]。推荐生育年龄妇女的保育手段包括胚胎、卵母细胞冷冻保存和卵巢盆腔放射治疗中的换位术。促性腺激素释放激素类似物同时联合化疗的使用已经被探索作为卵巢功能保护的一个方法。促性腺激素释放激素类似物的卵巢功能保护已经被假定通过几个机制发生,包括 FSH 中断分泌,子宫卵巢灌注减少,和没有分化的生殖干细胞的保护[181]。一系列动物和人体模型数据已经显示促性腺激素释放激素类似物的使用与短暂卵巢抑制相关,或许可以保护卵巢功能[181-185]。尽管临床数据推荐使用促性腺激素释放激素类似物作为卵巢功能保护已经有冲突。在诺雷德拯救卵巢功能试验(ZORO)中,随机了 60 例 ER-乳腺癌患者,她们计划接受蒽环紫杉类化疗或者化疗联合戈舍瑞林,研究者发现两组恢复卵巢功能没有统计差异[185]。相似的,绝经前乳腺癌患者的卵巢保护试验(Ovarian Protection Trial in Premenopausal Breast Cancer Patients, OPTION)随机了 227 例患者到单用化疗组或者联合戈舍瑞林,两组的卵巢保护没有发现差异[186]。对比一系列研究,已经发现使用促性腺激素释放激素类似物的获益。Ⅲ期 PROMISE-GIM6 试验,随机了 281 例早期绝经前乳腺癌患者,接受单用化疗或者化疗联合促性腺激素释放激素类似物曲普瑞林,研究者观察到早期更年期发生率有一个 17%的完全下降[187]。最近这项研究的长期随访结果被报道[188]。研究者注意到中位随访 7.3 年,两组的 5 年 DFS 没有差异(单用化疗组 83.7% vs 化疗联合曲普瑞林组 80.5%,$P=0.519$)。化疗单用组有 4 位怀孕,化疗联合曲普瑞林组有 8 位怀孕(OR 1.84;95% CI 0.54~6.27,$P=0.39$)。在 IBCSG-/SWOG-Ⅲ期试验(POEMS),HR-绝经前乳腺癌患者被随机到接受化疗或者化疗联合格式瑞林[189]。主要研究终点是 2 年原发性卵巢衰竭。化疗单用组 2 年卵巢衰竭率是 22%,化疗联合戈舍瑞林组是 8%(OR=0.30,95% CI 0.10~0.87,$P=0.03$)。化疗单用组有 13 位怀孕,化疗联合戈舍瑞林组有 22 位怀孕(OR=2.22,95% CI 1.00~4.92,$P=0.05$)。该研究的局限性包括没有达到目标收益(416 个目标收益,214 个随机报告),38%的患者缺少终点数据,数据没有根据疾病危险因素进行分层(HER2,淋巴结状态,疾病分期)。2013ASCO 指南目前没有推荐促性腺激素释放激素类似物作为一个生育保护手段,注意到在卵巢功能保护方面它的疗效还证据不足[180]。这一章的作者推荐生育保护尽早被讨论,并且包括所有方法的优缺点都要讨论。

结论

总之,目前对于不论早期还是进展期 HR+乳腺癌患者管理的一些内分泌药物都是可及的,他们靶向 ER 和 PR 通路不同位点的机制各不相同。他莫昔芬已经广泛应用于各阶段乳腺癌的前线治疗,仍然是绝经前患者治疗的中心选择。新的数据显示对高复发风险的早期绝经前患者使用有卵巢功能抑制作用的芳香化酶抑制剂与改善预后相关。绝经后女性非交叉抵抗芳香化酶抑制剂的引入已经改变了治疗建议,目前处于早期和晚期乳腺癌治疗的前沿。然后,关于芳香化酶抑制剂使用的几个问题仍然包括辅助阶段的使用时间和与他莫昔芬的使用顺序。另外在三个第三代芳香化酶抑制剂中,没有头对头的比较来支持一种抑制剂显著优于另一种。此外,使用芳香化酶抑制剂也并非没有副作用,可用不同的方法(例如,唑来膦酸,地诺单抗的使用)来预防骨丢失,骨丢失对于生活质量有显著影响。我们也已经在内分泌药物耐药发展的理解机制上取得了长足进展,如依维莫司目前获批与芳香化酶抑制剂联用。包括 MA 和醋酸甲孕酮的孕激素已经发展,是尝试用于他莫昔芬和芳香化酶抑制剂耐药的有用药物。

最后,随着更多抗激素疗法的出现,我们对加强耐药的分子通路理解增加,建立治疗乳腺癌内分泌药物的最佳顺序是至关重要的。这可能会延长内分泌疗法的使用时间,因此,推迟细胞毒性化疗成为必要的选择。

(李懿　叶慧 译,胡夕春 审校)

参考文献

The complete reference list can be found on the Wiley Companion Digital Edition of this title (see inside front cover for login instructions).

45 Crump M, Sawka CA, DeBoer G, et al. An individual patient-based meta-analysis of tamoxifen versus ovarian ablation as first line endocrine therapy for premenopausal women with metastatic breast cancer. *Breast Cancer Res Treat.* 1997;**44(3)**:201–210.

46 Klijn JG, Blamey RW, Boccardo F, et al. Combined tamoxifen and luteinizing hormone-releasing hormone (LHRH) agonist versus LHRH agonist alone in premenopausal advanced breast cancer: a meta-analysis of four randomized trials. *J Clin Oncol.* 2001;**19(2)**:343–353.

48 Early Breast Cancer Trialists' Collaborative Group (EBCTCG). Effects of chemotherapy and hormonal therapy for early breast cancer on recurrence and 15-year survival: an overview of the randomised trials. *Lancet.* 2005;**365(9472)**:1687–1717.

49 Fisher B, Dignam J, Bryant J, Wolmark N. Five versus more than five years of tamoxifen for lymph node-negative breast cancer: updated findings from the National Surgical Adjuvant Breast and Bowel Project B-14 randomized trial. *J Natl Cancer Inst.* 2001;**93(9)**:684–690.

50 Davies C, Pan H, Godwin J, Gray R, Arriagada R, et al. Long-term effects of continuing adjuvant tamoxifen to 10 years versus stopping at 5 years after diagnosis of oestrogen receptor-positive breast cancer: ATLAS, a randomised trial. *Lancet.* 2013;**381(9869)**:805–816.

51 Gray RG, Rea D, Handley D, Bowden SJ, Perry P. aTTom: long-term effects of continuing adjuvant tamoxifen to 10 years versus stopping at 5 years in 6,953 women with early breast cancer. *J Clin Oncol.* 2013;**31** (suppl; abstr 5):2013.

54 Albain KS, Barlow WE, Ravdin PM, et al. Adjuvant chemotherapy and timing of tamoxifen in postmenopausal patients with endocrine-responsive, node-positive breast cancer: a phase 3, open-label, randomised controlled trial. *Lancet.* 2009;**374(9707)**:2055–2063.

56 Fisher B, Costantino JP, Wickerham DL, et al. Tamoxifen for prevention of breast cancer: Report of the National Surgical Adjuvant Breast and Bowel Project P-1 Study. *J Natl Cancer Inst.* 1998;**90**:1371–1388.

62 Vogel VG, Costantino JP, Wickerham DL, et al. Effects of tamoxifen vs raloxifene on the risk of developing invasive breast cancer and other disease outcomes: The NSABP Study of Tamoxifen and Raloxifene (STAR) P-2 trial. *JAMA.* 2006;**295**:2727–2741.

72 Chia S, Gradishar W, Mauriac L, et al. Double-blind, randomized placebo controlled trial of fulvestrant compared with exemestane after prior nonsteroidal aromatase inhibitor therapy in postmenopausal women with hormone receptor-positive, advanced breast cancer: results from EFECT. *J Clin Oncol.* 2008;**26(10)**:1664–1670.

73 Di Leo A, Jerusalem G, Petruzelka L, et al. Results of the CONFIRM phase III trial comparing fulvestrant 250 mg with fulvestrant 500 mg in postmenopausal women with estrogen receptor-positive advanced breast cancer. *J Clin Oncol.* 2010;**28(30)**:4594–4600.

75 Ellis MJ, Llombart-Cussac A, Feltl D, et al. Fulvestrant 500 mg versus anastrozole 1 mg for the first-line treatment of advanced breast cancer: overall survival analysis from the phase II first study. *J Clin Oncol.* 2015;**33(32)**:3781–7. doi: 10.1200/JCO.2015.61.5831

87 Cuzick J, Forbes JF, Sestak I, et al. Long-term results of tamoxifen prophylaxis for

breast cancer – 96-month follow-up of the randomized IBIS-I trial. *J Natl Cancer Inst*. 2007;**99(4)**:272–282.

113 Bergh J, Jönsson PE, Lidbrink EK, et al. J FACT: an open-label randomized phase III study of fulvestrant and anastrozole in combination compared with anastrozole alone as first-line therapy for patients with receptor-positive postmenopausal breast cancer. *Clin Oncol*. 2012;**30(16)**:1919–1925.

114 Mehta RS, Barlow WE, Albain KS, et al. Combination anastrozole and fulvestrant in metastatic breast cancer. *N Engl J Med*. 2012;**367(5)**:435–444.

115 Johnston SR, Kilburn LS, Ellis P, et al. Fulvestrant plus anastrozole or placebo versus exemestane alone after progression on non-steroidal aromatase inhibitors in postmenopausal patients with hormone-receptor-positive locally advanced or metastatic breast cancer (SoFEA): a composite, multicentre, phase 3 randomised trial. *Lancet Oncol*. 2013;**14(10)**:989–998.

117 Cuzick J, Sestak I, Baum M, et al. Effect of anastrozole and tamoxifen as adjuvant treatment for early-stage breast cancer: 10-year analysis of the ATAC trial. *Lancet Oncol*. 2010;**11(12)**:1135–1141.

119 Regan MM, Neven P, Giobbie-Hurder A, et al. Assessment of letrozole and tamoxifen alone and in sequence for postmenopausal women with steroid hormone receptor-positive breast cancer: the BIG 1-98 randomised clinical trial at 8 · 1 years median follow-up. *Lancet Oncol*. 2011;**12(12)**:1101–1108.

120 Goss PE, Ingle JN, Martino S, et al. A randomized trial of letrozole in postmenopausal women after five years of tamoxifen therapy for early-stage breast cancer. *N Engl J Med*. 2003;**349(19)**:1793–1802.

125 Coombes RC, Hall E, Gibson LJ, et al. A randomized trial of exemestane after two to three years of tamoxifen therapy in postmenopausal women with primary breast cancer. *N Engl J Med*. 2004;**350(11)**:1081–1092.

127 Mamounas EP, Jeong JH, Wickerham DL, et al. Benefit from exemestane as extended adjuvant therapy after 5 years of adjuvant tamoxifen: intention-to-treat analysis of the National Surgical Adjuvant Breast and Bowel Project B-33 trial. *J Clin Oncol*. 2008;**26(12)**:1965–1971.

128 van de Velde CJ, Rea D, Seynaeve C, et al. Adjuvant tamoxifen and exemestane in early breast cancer (TEAM): a randomised phase 3 trial. *Lancet*. 2011;**377(9762)**:321–331. doi: 10.1016/S0140-6736(10)62312-4.

135 Pagani O, Regan MM, Walley BA, et al. Adjuvant exemestane with ovarian suppression in premenopausal breast cancer. *N Engl J Med*. 2014;**371(2)**:107–118.

136 Francis PA, Regan MM, Fleming GF, et al. Adjuvant Ovarian Suppression in Premenopausal Breast Cancer. *N Engl J Med*. 2014;**372(5)**:436–446.

137 Gnant M, Mlineritsch B, Stoeger H, et al. Zoledronic acid combined with adjuvant endocrine therapy of tamoxifen versus anastrozol plus ovarian function suppression in premenopausal early breast cancer: final analysis of the Austrian Breast and Colorectal Cancer Study Group Trial 12. *Ann Oncol*. 2015;**26(2)**:313–320.

148 Cuzick J, Sestak I, Forbes JF, et al. Anastrozole for prevention of breast cancer in high-risk postmenopausal women (IBIS-II): an international, double-blind, randomised placebo-controlled trial. *Lancet*. 2014;**383(9922)**:1041–1048.

156 Hadji P, Jackisch C, Bolten W, et al. COMPliance and Arthralgia in Clinical Therapy: the COMPACT trial, assessing the incidence of arthralgia, and compliance within the first year of adjuvant anastrozole therapy. *Ann Oncol*. 2014;**25(2)**:372–377.

176 Finn RS, Crown JP, Lang I, et al. The cyclin-dependent kinase 4/6 inhibitor palbociclib in combination with letrozole versus letrozole alone as first-line treatment of oestrogen receptor-positive, HER2-negative, advanced breast cancer (PALOMA-1/TRIO-18): a randomised phase 2 study. *Lancet Oncol*. 2015;**16(1)**:25–35. pii: S1470-2045(14)71159-3.

177 Turner NC, Ro J, André F, et al. Palbociclib in Hormone-Receptor-Positive Advanced Breast Cancer. *N Engl J Med*. 2015;**373(3)**:209–219. doi: 10.1056/NEJMoa1505270.

185 Gerber B, von Minckwitz G, Stehle H, et al. Effect of luteinizing hormone- releasing hormone agonist on ovarian function after modern adjuvant breast cancer chemotherapy. The GBG 37 ZORO study. *J Clin Oncol*. 2011;**29**:2334–2341.

186 Leonard RC, Adamson D, Anderson R, et al. The OPTION trial of adjuvant ovarian protection by goserelin in adjuvant chemotherapy for early breast cancer. *J Clin Oncol*. 2010;**28(suppl)**:15S.

188 Lambertini M, Boni L, Michelotti A, et al. Long-term outcome results of the phase III PROMISE-GIM6 study evaluating the role of LHRH analog (LHRHa) during chemotherapy (CT) as a strategy to reduce ovarian failure in early breast cancer (BC) patients. *J Clin Oncol*. 2014;**32(suppl 26**: abstr 105).

189 Moore HCF, Unger JM, Phillips K-A, et al. Phase III trial (Prevention of Early Menopause Study [POEMS]-SWOG S0230) of LHRH analog during chemotherapy (CT) to reduce ovarian failure in early-stage, hormone receptor-negative breast cancer: an international Intergroup trial of SWOG, IBCSG, ECOG, and CALGB (Alliance). *J Clin Oncol*. 2014;**32**:5s (suppl; abstr LBA505).

第 62 章　药物耐药性及其临床规避

Jeffrey A. Moscow, MD ■ Kenneth H. Cowan, MD, PhD ■ Branimir I. Sikic, MD

概述

初始治疗时对化疗药物敏感的肿瘤通常会发生耐药，常见的临床现象是开始治疗有效，复发后治疗不再有效。实验室和临床研究已经认证了一系列的耐药发生机制，有些机制是某些药物所特有的，另一些是各种类型药物所共有的机制。这些机制包括药物在细胞中积聚和解毒的改变；药物靶点的突变；药物作用靶点表达的变化；以及替代信号转导通路的激活。耐药机制明确后，已经研究出一些克服耐药和改善临床结局的措施。

播散性肿瘤绝大多数有效治疗是以细胞毒性药物或靶向药物的系统性治疗为基础的。另外，局限性肿瘤在手术或放疗后给予的辅助化疗，通过清除无法检测的微小病灶或镜下残留肿瘤，对部分患者可以提供显著的生存获益。然而，肿瘤对化疗方案的反应千差万别，因耐药导致的治疗失败却经常可见。

药物耐药的临床现象促进了对抗肿瘤药物作用机制及其耐药机制的研究。可以预期的是，依据这些重要研究信息，通过合理设计新的非交叉耐药的药物、对已知药物研发新的药物输送剂型或已知药物联合治疗、或研发对已知药物可能增加活性或逆转耐药的治疗方法，药物的耐药有可能被规避。早年通过对耐药细胞系传代的实验研究已经明确了药物的耐药机制，近年基因组技术的进展使临床耐药肿瘤的耐药机制可以被直接确认。

单种药物的通用耐药机制

重复暴露于单种抗肿瘤药物的实验选择出的耐药，通常会导致部分同类药物的交叉耐药。这种现象可以用以下的机制解释：结构和生物化学类似的化合物具有相同的药物转运载体，相似的药物代谢通路，以及同样的胞内细胞毒性靶标。

通常，耐药细胞仍然保持了对不同作用机制的其他类型的细胞毒性药物的敏感性。因此，对烷化剂或抗叶酸类药物耐药的细胞，通常对其他类型药物敏感，如蒽环类药物。例外的是存在交叉性多药耐药，即患者或肿瘤细胞对既往从未治疗过的结构和功能不同的药物产生了耐药。尽管这些药物在细胞内作用的位点不同，但产生多药耐药（multidrug-resistance，MDR）现象的药物具有共同的代谢通路或药物外排系统。

本章节将阐述药物的耐药机制。某些特殊类型药物的耐药机制将在后续章节中进行更详细讨论。

降低药物的蓄积

降低细胞内细胞毒药物的水平是一种最常见的耐药机制。因极性、水溶性药物不能透过细胞膜的双脂质层，需要特殊的机制以进入细胞。肿瘤细胞可以通过下调药物摄取机制对这类药物产生耐药。例如，抗叶酸药物甲氨蝶呤需要特殊的运输载体才能进入细胞内。高亲和力的叶酸受体、叶酸携带体（SLC19A1）和质子偶联叶酸转运体（SLC46A1）的减少，以及这些药物摄取机制的下调，已经被认为是甲氨蝶呤产生耐药的原因[1]。对于可轻易透过细胞膜的疏水的非极性药物，通过提高药物外排泵的活性可以降低细胞内药物的浓度。例如，P-糖蛋白（*MDR1/ABCB1*）药物外排泵的过度表达是这类耐药机制的典型[2]。

改变药物的代谢

降低药物活性、增强药物的失活、改变必需的协同因子也会导致某些抗肿瘤药物的耐药。例如通过改变特异性激酶和磷酸核糖基转移酶挽救酶来降低核苷类似物转化成细胞毒性的核苷及核苷酸，可能导致对这些抗癌药物的耐药[3]。另外一个耐药的例子是，降低羧基酯酶的水平-而其活性是将 TOPO 异构酶 I 抑制剂 CPT-11 转化成活性代谢产物 SN-38 所必需的[4]。

另一方面，通过增强脱氨酶的表达而增加嘧啶和嘌呤类似物的失活，与这些药物的耐药有关[5]。最后，辅助因子水平的变化也会改变药物的毒性。例如，5-氟脱氧尿嘧啶核苷单磷酸酯（5-fluorodeoxyuridine monophosphate，FdUMP）与其靶酶胸苷酸合成酶形成理想的抑制复合物时，需要 5，10-亚甲基四氢叶酸辅助因子的共同参与[6]。细胞内辅助因子水平的变化，将导致对氟尿嘧啶的耐药。

增强修复或提高细胞对药物性损伤的耐受性

细胞对细胞膜和 DNA 损伤具有复杂的修复系统，而改变修复程序会影响药物的敏感性。例如顺铂，其细胞毒作用涉及链内 DAN 交联，通过增强 DNA 的修复产生耐药。相反，错配修复机制（mismatch repair，MMR）的缺失使细胞对顺铂-诱导的 DNA 损伤产生耐受。在这种形式的铂类耐药中，修复系统无法识别铂类药物-DNA 加合物，因而无法激活正常的程序性细胞死亡反应。

增强解毒率

细胞对抗癌药物和其他外源性物质的代谢过程，通常经过以下 3 个解毒步骤。尽管并不是每个步骤对任何药物代谢都是必需的，这个概念是展示细胞解毒机制的一个有用的框架。3 个步骤中任何一步的改变将影响药物或毒素的敏感性或耐药性。第一步药物代谢是由细胞色素 P-450 复合功能氧化酶所介导的。通常，药物或外源性物质转变成更亲电子的活化的中间体，这个过程可能增加了毒性。在第二步反应中，药物/外源物质通过与谷胱甘肽（GSH）、葡糖醛酸形成偶联物，使代谢产物转化成低活性的，也可能是低毒性的形式-这些反应被多种同工酶所催化，分别包括谷胱甘肽 S 转移酶（glutathione S-transferase，GST）、尿苷二磷酸（UDP）、葡萄糖醛基转移酶和硫酸酯酶。第三步解毒机制是通过能量依赖的跨膜外排泵，包括前面描述过的 MRP（ABCC）家族成员，将原型药物/外源性物质或其代谢产物外排。

改变药物的靶标

抗肿瘤药物的酶作用靶标性质的改变会降低药物的疗效和产生耐药，常见于酪氨酸激酶抑制剂（tyrosine kinase inhibitor，TKI）。这些突变通常发生在 TKI 结合位点，是在选择性压力下发生的获得性耐药突变。同样，其他酶抑制剂的直接靶标产生的突变会导致细胞毒化疗药物的耐药，包括二氢叶酸还原酶（dihydrofolate reductase，DHFR）与甲氨蝶呤、胸苷酸合成酶与氟尿嘧啶，以及拓扑异构酶Ⅰ和Ⅱ抑制剂与喜树碱类药物耐药的关系。

改变基因表达

提高或降低靶酶的表达也会导致耐药。这种变化可发生于基因表达和调控通路的任何位点，包括 DNA 缺失或扩增、转录或转录后 RNA 水平控制的变化及蛋白质转录后修饰的改变。另外，通过改变药物靶标的表达，与致癌相同的分子机制也会导致耐药。增强 DHFR 的表达是对甲氨蝶呤耐药的机制；而降低拓扑异构酶Ⅰ的表达与喜树碱类药物耐药相关。

替代信号通路的激活

靶向药物如 TKI 的耐药可以通过激活替代信号通路而产生，即使主要的致癌因素已经被成功抑制，替代信号的激活仍然会提供持续的生长刺激信号。在接受 EGFR 和 ALK 抑制剂治疗的肺癌患者中发现了一些旁路信号通路的激活[7]。这些替代通路包括 MET 扩增、HGF 高表达、*PIK3CA* 突变、*BRAF* 突变和 *HER2* 扩增。替代耐药通路被确定后，患者可接受相应的抑制剂治疗。接受 BRAFV600 突变抑制剂治疗的恶性黑素瘤患者的耐药机制包括：*BRAF* 扩增、A-RAF 和 C-RAF 活性增强、*NRAS* 和 *MEK1* 突变以及 *NF1* 缺失[8]。克服 BRAF 抑制剂耐药的一个策略是同步抑制 RAF-MEK-ERK 通路中一个以上激酶。这个策略已经在一项随机临床试验中被验证是成功的，即 BRAF 突变的转移性恶性黑素瘤患者接受 BRAF 抑制剂维罗非尼（vemurafenib）单药对比维罗非尼联合 MEK 抑制剂 cobimetinib[9]。联合治疗组患者的中位无进展生存时间为 9.9 个月，缓解率 68%，而维罗非尼单药仅 6.2 个月和 45%。

要点

单药耐药的机制

- 降低药物蓄积
- 改变药物代谢
- 增强 DNA 修复
- 加强解毒
- 药物靶标突变
- 改变药物靶标的表达

对多种药物耐药的通用机制

药物转运介导的多药耐药（MDR）

通过增强多种药物外排泵，即 ATP 结合盒（ABC）蛋白的表达，可对多种抗肿瘤药物产生原发性及获得性的交叉耐药（表 62-1）。ABC 蛋白大家族由 48 种转运蛋白所构成，并组合成 ABCA-ABCG 7 个亚家族。这些亚家族中至少有 3 个直接与 MDR 有关，称为 MDR1/P-糖蛋白（ABCB1），多药耐药相关蛋白 1（MRP1），（ABCC1）和 BCRP/MXR/ABC-P（ABCG2）。由 P-糖蛋白（MDR1 或 ABCB1）介导的典型的 MDR 相关耐药的药物罗列于表 62-2。相似但不完全相同的另外一种 MDR 现象是由能量依赖的多药耐药蛋白（MRP）家族成员药物外排活性造成的，包括 MRP1 或 ABCC1[10]。

表 62-1 ABC 转运体相关的多药耐药（MDR）

- P-糖蛋白/MDR1/ABCB1-介导的经典 MDR
- MRP 家族成员介导的 MDR（目前至少有 3 个成员，与 MDR 药物外排和解毒有关的 ABCC 1、ABCC 2 和 ABCC 3 中的 MRP 1、2 和 3）
- BCRP（ABCG2）-介导的 MDR（被认为与米托蒽醌和蒽环类药物耐药有关的 ABC 半转运体）

表 62-2 经典（P-糖蛋白介导）MDR 的交叉耐药模式

分类	药物
蒽环类	多柔比星
	柔红霉素
	米托蒽醌
抗生素	放线菌素 D
	普卡霉素
抗微管药物	长春新碱
	长春碱
	秋水仙碱
鬼臼毒素	依托泊苷
	替尼泊苷

通过高级别晚期卵巢癌肿瘤样本的全基因测序已经研究了获得性耐药的遗传基础。基因测序结果发现，约 8%化疗后复发患者因获得性突变导致 ABCB1 多药转运基因表达增强[11]。这些患者均接受过紫杉类和/或多柔比星治疗，而上述药物都是 P-糖蛋白转运体的底物。突变包括位于 ABCB1 启动子的融合及基因 5′区域的易位。

在肿瘤细胞暴露于紫杉类药物如卡巴他赛的同时抑制 P-糖蛋白，发现了紫杉类药物替代的耐药机制[12]。这些替代耐药机制包括诱导上皮细胞向间充质转变（EMT）；通过过度表达 β 微管的 TUBB3 亚型，增加微管代谢的不稳定性。

另外一种重叠但有所不同的 MDR 现象与最近发现的一种可能的外排转运体，乳腺癌耐药蛋白（BCRP 或 ABCG2）的增强表达相关[13]。MDR 也被发现与肺癌耐药蛋白（lung resistance protein，LRP）的过度表达有关。LRP 相关耐药机制尚不明确，LRP 单独作用是否能够导致耐药也不清楚。据推测，作为一种穹窿体主蛋白，LRP 涉及核浆转运并可能阻止药物进入细胞核[14]。

细胞死亡通路抑制相关的多药耐药

尽管化疗药物引起的细胞毒是其与多种分子靶点的相互作用产生的，抗癌药物导致的细胞死亡至少部分是通过下游事件，最终依赖于 1 型（凋亡）或 2 型（自噬）程序性细胞死亡或凋亡通路实现的。凋亡是一种有序的细胞死亡程序，具有可预测的分子和形态学变化，包括细胞核固缩和破碎，间核小体内切裂解使 DNA 片段化，胞浆凋亡小体形成，及浆膜改变，如磷脂酰丝氨酸移位到细胞表面[15,16]。自噬是一种亚细胞成分大量降解的途径，是细胞对多种应激的反应，如营养剥夺[17]。自噬涉及了自噬体/自溶酶的形成，可以被 PI3 激酶抑制剂所抑制，如 3-甲基腺苷和渥曼青霉素（wortmannin）。

尽管凋亡可能既有 TP53 依赖性的又有非依赖性的，细胞对 DNA 损伤反应通常都由 TP53 所调控[18]。如简化程序图所示（图 62-1），抗癌治疗引起的 DNA 损伤与 TP53 相关，其机制尚不完全清楚。根据特定的细胞类型和损伤，TP53 的表达可能启动以下两条可能的通路之一：凋亡或细胞周期阻滞和修复过程。对于凋亡通路占优势的细胞，TP53 失去功能或缺乏将减弱因 DNA 损伤引起的凋亡，导致相应的耐药和受损伤细胞的存活。

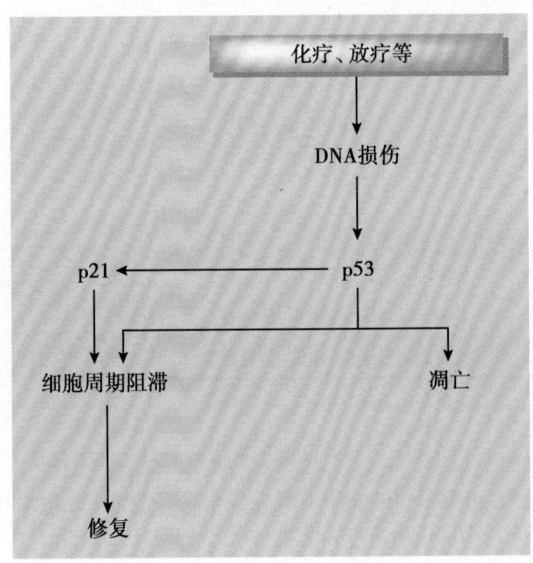

图 62-1　抗肿瘤治疗应激下细胞应答的替代途径

其他细胞死亡信号通路组成包括：丝裂原活化蛋白激酶（mitogen-activated protein kinase，MAPK）信号级联反应，涉及细胞对外源性因素反应的调控，如对基因治疗或细胞毒化疗的反应；细胞外刺激调节激酶（ERK1/2）通路，与细胞对生长因子的增殖反应相关联；p38 和应激激活/c-Jun N 端蛋白激酶（SAPK/JNK）通路。这些相互作用的通路的调控使肿瘤细胞对细胞毒性药物治疗产生不同的反应，即激活凋亡，或激活细胞周期阻滞和修复并导致对治疗的耐药[19]。

尽管其机制尚不完全清楚，抗凋亡家族成员（Bcl-2 和 Bcl-XL）和促凋亡家族成员（Bax、Bak、Bad 和 Bid）表达的平衡会影响细胞对毒性药物的相对敏感性[20]。实际上，BCL-2 及其抗凋亡同类物的上调会增强淋巴细胞对糖皮质激素和放疗的细胞毒作用以及化疗药物所致 DNA 损伤的抵抗[21,22]。抗凋亡蛋白 BCL-2 和 Bcl-XL 水平的上调将导致肿瘤细胞对 DNA 损伤性抗癌药敏感性降低—这种耐药现象表现为肿瘤细胞存活，对 DNA 损伤耐受性提高以及遗传不稳定性。这种遗传不稳定性可能导致进一步的突变并激活其他耐药机制及转变为侵袭性更强的肿瘤行为[20]。尽管 BCL-2 家族蛋白及该家族的多域促凋亡成员在形成 1 型（凋亡）程序性细胞死亡中的作用已经被广泛论证，但最近的研究发现这些蛋白也调控 2 型（自噬）和非凋亡程序性细胞死亡[23]。

BCL-2 家族成员在靶向治疗的耐药中也发挥了重要作用[24]。BIM 和 PUMA 是两个促凋亡 BCL2 家族成员，它们的表达可以由癌基因靶向激酶抑制剂所诱导，如突变的 EGFR 和 BRAF、BCR-ABL 融合基因及扩增的 HER2 抑制剂。BIM 表达缺失已显示可抑制凋亡和对这些癌基因抑制剂的耐药。这样，突变型和野生型 TP53、BCL2 家族成员、MAPK 家族成员，及其他与调控凋亡和/或自噬相关的蛋白表达对肿瘤细胞的临床敏感性有明显的影响。这些蛋白的任何一种都是研究药物的靶点[20,25]。

宿主-肿瘤相互作用引起的耐药因素

在体外实验中敏感的化疗药物，在体内实验中无法清除肿瘤细胞的现象，可能是由于解剖学或药理学原因所致。例如，在尚未建立额外的 CNS 直接给药的治疗方案前，因许多药物无法透过血-脑和血-睾屏障而达到足够的药物浓度，急性淋巴细胞性白血病经常发生这些部位的复发[26]。在巨大实体肿瘤中，因过度生长而血供不足，使到达肿瘤的药物减少。另外，在大肿块血供差的区域发生了酸中毒和乏氧会干扰某些药物的细胞毒性。肝脏或其他正常组织对前体药物激活的改变也可能影响药物的疗效，如环磷酰胺。

Teicher 和 Herman 的研究[27]显示，肿瘤-宿主相互作用可能通过非预期的途径影响药物的药代动力学及产生肿瘤耐药。该研究发现，在体内实验中筛选出对环磷酰胺和顺铂耐药的肿瘤细胞，在体外实验中通常对药物敏感。当肿瘤细胞再植入裸鼠，体内耐药重新出现。这些研究结果提示，耐药肿瘤可能拥有细胞耐药因子，这些因子仅与宿主因素协同发挥作用，因此，仅在体内通过改变药物的药代动力学而产生耐药。如果这种新的宿主依赖的肿瘤耐药机制被证明是常见的，这些结果就可以解释为何传统的体外测试无法在全部病例中预测临床疗效。

肿瘤干细胞与耐药

肿瘤干细胞的概念来源于研究观察到的一种现象，即在同一个肿瘤中不同的恶性细胞形成肿瘤的能力不同。这些肿瘤干细胞，或“肿瘤形成细胞”，在肿瘤细胞中仅占小于 1%，但具有可塑性或有能力在致瘤性与非致瘤性状态之间转变，并且是引起抗肿瘤耐药的重要因素[28]。复发的肿瘤富含肿瘤干细胞，并且这些细胞亚群已知高表达多药耐药转运体和其他耐药基因。同时，肿瘤干细胞也提供了新的抗肿瘤靶点，包括抑制Notch、Wnt及Hedgehog通路。

获得性耐药的遗传基础和肿瘤异质性

对各个肿瘤基因进行高通量深度测序发现多种肿瘤存在瘤内的异质性[29]。这些数据支持了肿瘤分支进化的模式，许多相互竞争的克隆在生长速度、转移潜能和对各种药物的敏感性方面存在差异。抗肿瘤药物耐药的许多依据来源于这个模型。耐药正常组织如结肠和肾来源的肿瘤优势克隆，其耐药通常与肿瘤起源的正常细胞的耐药相同。在优势克隆对特定药物敏感的肿瘤中，肿瘤初次诊断时同时存在耐药弱势克隆的概率较高。导致癌症的致癌性突变可影响药物敏感性，通过驱动细胞复制，提高了肿瘤细胞对增殖细胞具有杀伤作用的化疗药物的敏感性。然而，在抗肿瘤治疗完全缓解后，获得性耐药的产生来自耐药克隆，部分耐药克隆可能治疗前已经存在，而另一些则可能在治疗中产生。耐药的出现表现为药物敏感克隆的消失，且耐药克隆过度生长。这种现象是达尔文"适者生存"理论在肿瘤细胞中的例证[30]。通过比较患者个体顺序样本的DNA序列以及不同患者间耐药的演变，已经有越来越多证据表明了耐药机制的异质性以及这些机制的本质[31]。

深度测序同样揭示了不同肿瘤间遗传不稳定性和突变率存在差别。导致遗传不稳定性差异的影响因素尚不清楚，除了已经了解到部分肿瘤存在MMR缺陷。MMR缺陷与高频率的点突变有关，并且可能对免疫治疗有较好疗效，可通过免疫检查点抑制剂（如CTLA4，PD-1和PDL-1）增强抗肿瘤免疫[30]。除了肿瘤突变负荷，对恶性黑素瘤标本的测序已经发现了一种新抗原，其与CTLA-4抑制剂伊匹木单抗（ipilumumab）或者tremelimumab疗效良好有明确的关系[32]。

全基因测序和靶向基因测序可发现"可操作突变"，如BRAFV600E或HER2扩增，由此可指导选择特殊的靶向药物。这种概念已经在一些临床试验中被测试，如NCI-MATCH（NCT02465060）、TRACERx（NCT01888601）、DARWIN（NCT02183883）和BATTLE-2（NCT01248247）。甚至，有些亚克隆的检测可以预测对某个治疗的无效，由此可选择性应用非交叉耐药的药物对抗这种亚克隆[30]。所谓的"液体活检"分析了循环血液中游离的肿瘤DNA，也能够在肿瘤患者中检测到可以靶向的突变和耐药性突变。

总之，基于肿瘤性包块及其转移灶是由遗传学相同的克隆所组成的理念，可以将肿瘤设想为树状结构，中心是肿瘤干细胞，从树干发出的树枝是多种进化的克隆。因此，肿瘤成为了具有异质性，既相似又不完全相同的细胞集合，在原发肿瘤灶和远处转移灶均存在这种情况。选择性压力，如既往接受过的治疗，会塑造患者肿瘤细胞特征，空间分离的克隆会发展出不同的耐药机制。原发肿瘤灶和转移灶的多次活检标本的深度测序研究揭示了具有有机体样性质的肿瘤图像。肿瘤的异质性倾向于既有遗传学又有表观遗传学的多面性。因此，克服耐药的策略必须考虑任何一种药物耐药机制的多面性，因为在同一患者体内不同的细胞群可能具有不同的耐药机制。

要点

获得性多药耐药机制

- 增强药物外排泵的作用
- 抑制细胞死亡通路
- 宿主-肿瘤相互作用
- 休眠的肿瘤干细胞
- 肿瘤异质性

避免或克服耐药的潜在临床策略

克服化疗失败的方法包括防止耐药发生的各种方法（表62-3）。对引起耐药机制的各种因素的了解，使我们能够选择更有效的治疗方案。典型的例子是，已经创建的包含非交叉耐药的强烈联合化疗能足够快速地清除肿瘤细胞以防止选择出具有多重耐药的肿瘤细胞克隆。另一种办法是开发能够逆转或避免临床耐药的治疗方法。

表62-3 克服或规避耐药的途径

预防	强烈的多药联合治疗
	关注与耐药机制相关的各种因素
	同时阻断耐药通路
规避	药物筛选程序和合理的药物设计
	规避药物摄取缺陷
	剂量递增
	运用其他转运机制的药物
	能够逆转外排增加的药物
	增强药物活性或疗效的联合因素
	药物失活的抑制
	新治疗方法
	免疫治疗
	抑制替代信号通路
	增强凋亡通路
	拮抗相同靶点的非交叉耐药类似物

逆转ABC转运体介导的耐药

尽管小鼠模型的临床前研究显示了P-糖蛋白抑制剂的疗效，逆转MDR药物治疗人类实体肿瘤的临床试验绝大多数是令人失望的。尽管大量的逆转MDR药物在数百个临床前实验中被研发，但没有任何一个开发成为临床有用的药物。逆转MDR药物的临床试验存在明显的障碍，包括：①逆转MDR药物通过影响MDR相关的细胞毒药物的药代动力学和药效动力学，增加了化疗药物的毒性；②某些早期MDR1逆转药物本身的毒性使其无法使用足够剂量，如维拉帕米；③缺乏对患者肿瘤MDR1/ABCB1表达的筛查；④肿瘤复发时，耐药涉及了其他转运体和其他耐药机制；⑤对MDR1多样性如何影响MDR1抑制剂的易感性缺乏了解[2]。因为 P-糖蛋白和其他 ABC 转运体在肿瘤生物学和耐药方面起着重要的作用，一旦临床耐药被确诊，运用非药理学的措施通过抑制这些转运体的活性有可能改善临床结局。

核酸类似物耐药的逆转

作为 ABC 转运体底物的亲脂性细胞毒性药物，在细胞内药物的积聚会因上调这些转运体而受到限制，而依赖于特殊转运体而摄入细胞的亲水性的核酸类似物，就不存在这个问题。因此，与 MDR 相反，这个问题的关键是逆转排出泵的活性，通过增加细胞摄取克服对核酸类似物的耐药。这些方法包括合成亲脂性更强的核酸类似物的前体药，使其比较容易透过细胞膜；使用纳米传递系统以避开核苷转运体；甚至运用基因治疗以增强核苷转运体在肿瘤中的表达[33,34]。

靶向药物的耐药

BCR/ABL

伊马替尼是第一个被批准的酪氨酸激酶抑制剂，对 *BCR/ABL* 融合基因突变驱动的慢性髓性白血病（chronic myeloid leukemia，CML）具有显著的疗效。伊马替尼和 BCR/ABL 已经成为了一类激酶抑制剂耐药机制的重要范例，包括发生点突变直接影响药物结合，或改变 BCR/ABL 蛋白构象降低药物结合[35,36]。在耐药的 CML 标本中已经发现了超过 100 个点突变。对 CML 样本的 *BCR/ABL* 融合基因的深度测序已经能够确定耐药克隆，甚至在接受伊马替尼治疗的早期就可以检测到这些克隆。*BCR/ABL* 相关的一些 DNA 修复通路的异常活化增强了遗传不稳定性，与伊马替尼耐药性点突变高发生率有关[36]。值得关注的是，FDA 批准了数个新的对伊马替尼耐药有效的 BCR/ABL 激酶抑制剂，包括达沙替尼、尼洛替尼、博舒替尼（bosutinib）和泊那替尼（ponatinib）。

EGFR

针对表皮生长因子受体 EGFR 的药物包括两类。EGFR 单克隆抗体被批准用于结肠癌和头颈部癌，以及肿瘤细胞生长依赖于野生型 EGFR 的恶性肿瘤；小分子 EGFR TKI 被批准用于治疗 EGFR 活性突变的非小细胞肺癌（nonsmall-cell lung cancer，NSCLC）。抗 EGFR 单抗和 TKI 均发生了耐药，其机制具有可预测的相似性和不同点。EGFR 突变可导致耐药，但耐药性突变发生的位点在不同的药物间存在差异：第一代 EGFR TKI 如厄洛替尼和吉非替尼的主要突变是 T790M，影响了这类药物所靶向的 ATP 结合区；而抗 EGFR 单抗西妥昔单抗的耐药发生于多个位点，改变了单抗的结合表位，包括 S492R、S464L、G465R 和 I491M[11]。

同时对两种 EGFR-抑制剂耐药的情况也可能发生，通过激活旁路信号通路使相同的下游信号效应持续活化，如激活了同属 EGFR 家族的酪氨酸激酶受体 HER2 以及 MET。甚至，因肿瘤组织学转变而出现同时对抗 EGFR TKI 和单抗耐药的情况，通常被描述为 EMT，这种现象以丢失泛表皮标记 E-钙黏蛋白、增强了间叶相关抗原波形蛋白和纤维连接蛋白的表达为特征，失去了对 EGFR 靶向药物的敏感性。在肺癌中，有一种非预期的对突变 EGFR 抑制剂的耐药机制是，14% 的病例从非小细胞肺癌转变成了小细胞肺癌[37]。

目前尚不清楚为何单个肿瘤会发生不同的耐药机制，为何在一种肿瘤中发生的旁路激活而不会在另外一种肿瘤中发生。然而，NSCLC 与结肠癌之间的差别之一是，NSCLC 中 EGFR 的活性突变是其驱动基因，所以 EGFR 耐药突变起了非常重要的作用；而 EGFR 信号仅仅是结肠癌多种上调的信号通路之一，因此旁路信号激活在这种情况下更常见。

逆转 EGFR 靶向药物耐药的策略包括 4 个方面。第一，对于 NSCLC，正在研发针对突变 EGFR 的活性更强的新药，可同时靶向活性突变和 T790M 耐药突变，这样可以确保提高这些药物的治疗指数，并且消除发生耐药性突变的可能性。两种第三代 EGFR 抑制剂已经显示对常见的 T790M 耐药突变有效。这两个药物是罗西替尼（CO-1686）[38] 和 AZD9291[39]。第二，联合应用抗 EGFR TKI 和抗 EGFR 单抗对 EGFR 双重抑制，正在开展临床研究以验证这种方法能够更完全地抑制 EGFR 信号的假设。第三，抗 EGFR 药物联合应用一些旁路信号抑制剂，如 MET 和 MEK 抑制剂。第四，可能抑制 EMT 的药物，如组蛋白去乙酰化酶抑制剂联合 EGFR 抑制剂，可能起到预防和逆转耐药的作用。

ALK

间变性淋巴瘤激酶（anaplastic lymphoma kinase，*ALK*）基因的重排是肺腺癌第二个最常见的癌基因突变（仅次于 *EGFR*）。克唑替尼是首个被 FDA 批准的 ALK 激酶抑制剂，但不可避免地发生了对克唑替尼耐药，机制包括 ALK 点突变和旁路信号通路的激活[40]。FDA 已经批准了色瑞替尼作为第二代 ALK 抑制剂，可以部分克服克唑替尼的耐药[41,42]对克唑替尼耐药的患者，色瑞替尼治疗可获得 56% 的缓解率，中位无进展生存时间 7 个月[42]。

BRAF

大约 50% 的恶性黑素瘤是由 *BRAF* 基因活性突变所引起的，最常见的是 V600E 突变。FDA 已经批准了两种激酶抑制剂，维罗非尼（vemurafenib）和达拉菲尼（dabrafenib），抑制 V600E 突变的 BRAF。然而，几乎所有的病例均发生了对这些激酶抑制剂的耐药，包括 *NRAS* 和 *MEK1* 突变，*BRAF* 扩增，NF1 丢失和其他 MAPK 通路的改变[8]。正如前文所述，同时抑制突变的 BRAF 和 MEK 已经成为一种成功的延迟恶性黑素瘤对 BRAF 抑制剂耐药的策略[9]。

活性 *BRAF* 突变在其他肿瘤类型中也有较低比例的发生，包括在 10% 的结肠癌中。结肠癌对 BRAF 抑制剂耐药的机制主要是因 MAPK 通路基因的改变，导致了 MAPK 通路的持续活化，包括 *KRAS* 和 *BRAF* 扩增，以及 *MEK1* 突变[43]。

布鲁顿酪氨酸激酶

伊布替尼是一种不可逆的布鲁顿酪氨酸激酶（Bruton's tyrosine kinase，BTK）结合剂，BTK 是一种 B 细胞发育和生存的关键酶。伊布替尼抑制 BTK 在多种 B 细胞恶性肿瘤中有临床疗效，包括套细胞淋巴瘤和慢性淋巴细胞白血病。伊布替尼的耐药机制包括位于药物结合半胱氨酸残基的 BTK 基因中 *C481S* 突变，以及 *PLCγ2* 突变导致了 B 细胞受体的自我激活[44]。

总结和展望

抗肿瘤药物耐药机制的多样性，以及肿瘤生物学的异质性，使抗肿瘤治疗充满挑战。然而，明确耐药机制后，可以采取有效措施克服临床耐药并改善治疗疗效。这些措施包括设计可能非相同耐药机制的新药；研发靶向耐药通路的联合治疗方案。即使尽了各种努力，很多肿瘤仍然将对传统化疗和靶向治疗产生耐药。

（曹军宁 译）

参考文献

1 Matherly LH, Wilson MR, Hou Z. The major facilitative folate transporters solute carrier 19A1 and solute carrier 46A1: biology and role in antifolate chemotherapy of cancer. *Drug Metab Dispos*. 2014;**42**(**4**):632–649.

2 Amiri-Kordestani L, Basseville A, Kurdziel K, Fojo AT, Bates SE. Targeting MDR in breast and lung cancer: discriminating its potential importance from the failure of drug resistance reversal studies. *Drug Resist Updat*. 2012;**15**(**1-2**):50–61.

3 Drahovsky D, Kreis W. Studies on drug resistance. II. Kinase patterns in P815 neoplasms sensitive and resistant to 1-beta-D-arabinofuranosylcytosine. *Biochem Pharmacol*. 1970;**19**(**3**):940–944.

4 Haaz MC, Rivory LP, Riche C, Robert J. The transformation of irinotecan (CPT-11) to its active metabolite SN-38 by human liver microsomes. Differential hydrolysis for the lactone and carboxylate forms. *Naunyn Schmiedeberg's Arch Pharmacol*. 1997;**356**(**2**):257–262.

5 Hunt SW 3rd, Hoffee PA. Amplification of adenosine deaminase gene sequences in deoxycoformycin-resistant rat hepatoma cells. *J Biol Chem*. 1983;**258**(**21**): 13185–13192.

6 Houghton JA, Maroda SJ Jr, Phillips JO, Houghton PJ. Biochemical determinants of responsiveness to 5-fluorouracil and its derivatives in xenografts of human colorectal adenocarcinomas in mice. *Cancer Res*. 1981;**41**(**1**):144–149.

7 Camidge DR, Pao W, Sequist LV. Acquired resistance to TKIs in solid tumours: learning from lung cancer. *Nat Rev Clin Oncol*. 2014;**11**(**8**):473–481.

8 Van Allen EM, Wagle N, Sucker A, et al. The genetic landscape of clinical resistance to RAF inhibition in metastatic melanoma. *Cancer Discov*. 2014;**4**(**1**):94–109.

9 Larkin J, Ascierto PA, Dreno B, et al. Combined vemurafenib and cobimetinib in BRAF-mutated melanoma. *N Engl J Med*. 2014;**371**(**20**):1867–1876.

10 Cole SP. Multidrug resistance protein 1 (MRP1, ABCC1), a "multitasking" ATP-binding cassette (ABC) transporter. *J Biol Chem*. 2014;**289**(**45**):30880–30888.

11 Arena S, Bellosillo B, Siravegna G, et al. Emergence of Multiple EGFR Extracellular Mutations during Cetuximab Treatment in Colorectal Cancer. *Clin Cancer Res*. 2015;**21**(**9**):2157–2166.

12 Duran GE, Wang YC, Francisco EB, et al. Mechanisms of resistance to cabazitaxel. *Mol Cancer Ther*. 2015;**14**(**1**):193–201.

13 Ishikawa T, Nakagawa H. Human ABC transporter ABCG2 in cancer chemotherapy and pharmacogenomics. *J Exp Ther Oncol*. 2009;**8**(**1**):5–24.

14 Slovak ML, Ho JP, Cole SP, et al. The LRP gene encoding a major vault protein associated with drug resistance maps proximal to MRP on chromosome 16: evidence that chromosome breakage plays a key role in MRP or LRP gene amplification. *Cancer Res*. 1995;**55**(**19**):4214–4219.

15 Adams JM, Cory S. Bcl-2-regulated apoptosis: mechanism and therapeutic potential. *Curr Opin Immunol*. 2007;**19**(**5**):488–496.

16 Hanahan D, Weinberg RA. Hallmarks of cancer: the next generation. *Cell*. 2011;**144**(**5**):646–674.

17 Levine B, Kroemer G. Autophagy in the pathogenesis of disease. *Cell*. 2008;**132**(**1**): 27–42.

18 Vousden KH, Lu X. Live or let die: the cell's response to p53. *Nat Rev Cancer*. 2002;**2**(**8**):594–604.

19 Abrams SL, Steelman LS, Shelton JG, et al. The Raf/MEK/ERK pathway can govern drug resistance, apoptosis and sensitivity to targeted therapy. *Cell Cycle*. 2010;**9**(**9**):1781–1791.

20 Thomas S, Quinn BA, Das SK, et al. Targeting the Bcl-2 family for cancer therapy. *Expert Opin Ther Targets*. 2013;**17**(**1**):61–75.

21 Herr I, Debatin KM. Cellular stress response and apoptosis in cancer therapy. *Blood*. 2001;**98**(**9**):2603–2614.

22 Stahnke K, Fulda S, Friesen C, Strauss G, Debatin KM. Activation of apoptosis pathways in peripheral blood lymphocytes by in vivo chemotherapy. *Blood*. 2001;**98**(**10**):3066–3073.

23 Levine B, Sinha S, Kroemer G. Bcl-2 family members: dual regulators of apoptosis and autophagy. *Autophagy*. 2008;**4**(**5**):600–606.

24 Hata AN, Engelman JA, Faber AC. The BCL2 family: key mediators of the apoptotic response to targeted anticancer therapeutics. *Cancer Discov*. 2015;**5**(**5**):475–487.

25 Mohell N, Alfredsson J, Fransson A, et al. APR-246 overcomes resistance to cisplatin and doxorubicin in ovarian cancer cells. *Cell Death Dis*. 2015;**6**:e1794.

26 Poplack DG, Reaman G. Acute lymphoblastic leukemia in childhood. *Pediatr Clin N Am*. 1988;**35**(**4**):903–932.

27 Teicher BA, Herman TS, Holden SA, et al. Tumor resistance to alkylating agents conferred by mechanisms operative only in vivo. *Science*. 1990;**247**(**4949 Pt 1**):1457–1461.

28 Mertins SD. Cancer stem cells: a systems biology view of their role in prognosis and therapy. *Anti-Cancer Drugs*. 2014;**25**(**4**):353–367.

29 Swanton C. Intratumor heterogeneity: evolution through space and time. *Cancer Res*. 2012;**72**(**19**):4875–4882.

30 Jamal-Hanjani M, Quezada SA, Larkin J, Swanton C. Translational implications of tumor heterogeneity. *Clin Cancer Res*. 2015;**21**(**6**):1258–1266.

31 Patch AM, Christie EL, Etemadmoghadam D, et al. Whole-genome characterization of chemoresistant ovarian cancer. *Nature*. 2015;**521**(**7553**):489–494.

32 Snyder A, Makarov V, Merghoub T, et al. Genetic basis for clinical response to CTLA-4 blockade in melanoma. *N Engl J Med*. 2014;**371**(**23**):2189–2199.

33 Adema AD, Bijnsdorp IV, Sandvold ML, Verheul HM, Peters GJ. Innovations and opportunities to improve conventional (deoxy)nucleoside and fluoropyrimidine analogs in cancer. *Curr Med Chem*. 2009;**16**(**35**):4632–4643.

34 Hung SW, Mody HR, Govindarajan R. Overcoming nucleoside analog chemoresistance of pancreatic cancer: a therapeutic challenge. *Cancer Lett*. 2012;**320**(**2**):138–149.

35 Jabbour EJ, Cortes JE, Kantarjian HM. Resistance to tyrosine kinase inhibition therapy for chronic myelogenous leukemia: a clinical perspective and emerging treatment options. *Clin Lymphoma Myeloma Leuk*. 2013;**13**(**5**):515–529.

36 Lamontanara AJ, Gencer EB, Kuzyk O, Hantschel O. Mechanisms of resistance to BCR-ABL and other kinase inhibitors. *Biochim Biophys Acta*. 2013;**1834**(**7**): 1449–1459.

37 Sequist LV, Waltman BA, Dias-Santagata D, et al. Genotypic and histological evolution of lung cancers acquiring resistance to EGFR inhibitors. *Sci Transl Med*. 2011;**3**(**75**):75ra26.

38 Sequist LV, Soria JC, Goldman JW, et al. Rociletinib in EGFR-mutated non-small-cell lung cancer. *N Engl J Med*. 2015;**372**(**18**):1700–1709.

39 Janne PA, Yang JC, Kim DW, et al. AZD9291 in EGFR inhibitor-resistant non-small-cell lung cancer. *N Engl J Med*. 2015;**372**(**18**):1689–1699.

40 Wilson FH, Johannessen CM, Piccioni F, et al. A functional landscape of resistance to ALK inhibition in lung cancer. *Cancer Cell*. 2015;**27**(**3**):397–408.

41 Friboulet L, Li N, Katayama R, et al. The ALK inhibitor ceritinib overcomes crizotinib resistance in non-small cell lung cancer. *Cancer Discov*. 2014;**4**(**6**):662–673.

42 Shaw AT, Kim DW, Mehra R, et al. Ceritinib in ALK-rearranged non-small-cell lung cancer. *N Engl J Med*. 2014;**370**(**13**):1189–1197.

43 Ahronian LG, Sennott EM, Van Allen EM, et al. Clinical acquired resistance to RAF inhibitor combinations in BRAF-mutant colorectal cancer through MAPK pathway alterations. *Cancer Discov*. 2015;**5**(**4**):358–367.

44 Woyach JA, Furman RR, Liu TM, et al. Resistance mechanisms for the Bruton's tyrosine kinase inhibitor ibrutinib. *N Engl J Med*. 2014;**370**(**24**):2286–2294.

第九篇

生物治疗与基因治疗

第 63 章　细胞因子、干扰素和造血生长因子

Suhendan Ekmekcioglu, PhD ■ Elizabeth A. Grimm, PhD

概述

细胞因子是免疫反应的重要介质，机体内几乎每个细胞均可产生。生长促进因子或抑制因子可细分为白细胞介素（interleukin，IL）、淋巴因子、单核因子、趋化因子和造血生长因子。在肿瘤中，某些细胞因子直接作用于内皮细胞的生长、分化或存活，而另一些细胞因子则通过吸引影响血管生成的炎症细胞或诱导次生细胞因子或其他调节血管生成的介质发挥作用。促炎细胞因子和趋化细胞因子影响肿瘤环境，控制浸润造血效应细胞的数量和性质，抑制或促进肿瘤生长。细胞因子在调节免疫反应中的重要作用可能使肿瘤产生有效的免疫反应或抑制抗原呈递细胞（antigen-presenting cell，APC）的功能。

对于细胞因子的理解现在认为是刺激因子和抑制因子相互作用的复杂过程。许多控制这一过程的分子已经被克隆并进入临床试验。现在很清楚的是，调控细胞因子具有多效性的特点，同时，表现出明显的功能冗余。

本章的主题包括已知的临床相关 IL、干扰素和选定的生长因子的生物学特性、它们用于癌症患者治疗的理论基础以及所积累的临床经验。

细胞因子，是由包括各种恶性肿瘤细胞在内的机体内几乎每个细胞均可产生的多种多样的信号分子家族，是免疫反应的重要介质。总体上，一些细胞因子起刺激生长的作用，另外一些起抑制作用。与恶性肿瘤临床相关的细胞因子可进一步分类为 IL、单核因子、趋化因子和造血生长因子。在恶性肿瘤中，一些细胞因子直接作用于内皮细胞的生长、分化或生存，而另外一些细胞因子通过吸引炎性细胞影响血管生成，或诱导间接细胞因子或其他介质调节血管生成。促炎症细胞因子和趋化细胞因子影响肿瘤环境并控制浸润性造血效应细胞的数量和性质，从而抑制或者加快肿瘤生长。细胞因子在调节免疫反应中起重要作用，可能针对肿瘤产生有效的免疫应答，或抑制抗原呈递细胞的功能。使用免疫刺激性 IL 引发恶性肿瘤患者免疫激活，最常用的是 IL-2，在一些恶性肿瘤的治疗中取得了成功。可推测抗原存在于肿瘤细胞，各种免疫刺激性细胞因子，尤其是 IL，现在已用于患者试图引发、增强或刺激微弱的或以前不存在抗肿瘤免疫反应。除了刺激免疫反应的作用，一些 IL 已被用于在化疗或骨髓移植（bone marrow transplantation，BMT）后刺激各种类型的血细胞的生长和分化，起到加快恢复的作用。

IL 决定白细胞的可溶性蛋白质或糖蛋白产物的产生，这些产物又调节其他白细胞的反应。IL 主要通过旁分泌相互作用产生影响。病原体暴露和抗原特异性相互作用启动的 IL 级联反应最初是局限的，IL 的功能由旁分泌相互作用所介导，相关的特异受体有区别地表达于不同的细胞类型，包括造血和免疫细胞，但也包括内皮细胞和其他细胞。现已明确许多细胞因子多效性的本质使得它们可以影响几乎所有的器官系统（图 63-1）。细胞因子可能具有自己独特的受体，但也可以与其他细胞因子共享一个“公共”受体（表 63-1，表 63-2）。

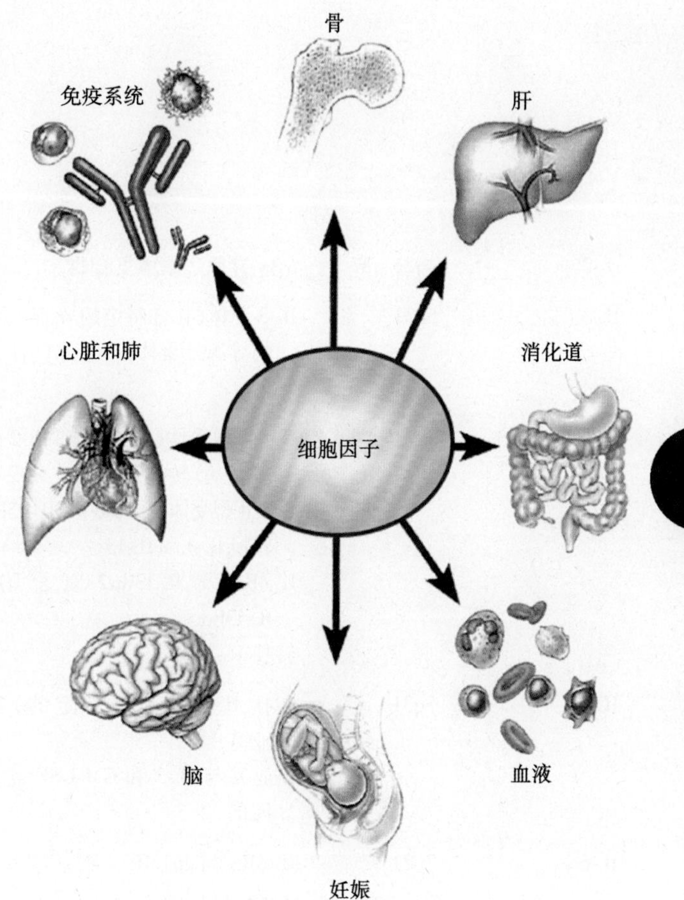

图 63-1　除了本身在造血和免疫方面的作用，“造血”生长因子能影响多个器官系统包括（但非仅限于）：骨骼重塑、呼吸循环功能、肝脏功能和胃肠道

表 63-1 造血生长因子受体的类型

类型	特点	受体举例
Ⅰ型细胞因子受体	不具有内在的激酶活性。受体作为衔接分子的结合位点，导致细胞底物的磷酸化	IL-1，IL-2，IL-3，IL-4，IL-5，IL-6，IL-7，IL-9，IL-13，IL-18，IL-21，GM-CSF，G-CSF，EPO，TPO，白血病抑制因子
Ⅱ型细胞因子受体	包含细胞外纤连蛋白类Ⅲ型结构域	干扰素及 IL-10
具有与络氨酸激酶结构域的受体（Ⅲ型）	大细胞外免疫球蛋白样结构域，单次跨膜纺丝区域，和胞质络氨酸激酶结构域	FMS（M-CSF 受体），FLT-3，c-kit（SCF 受体），PDGFR
趋化因子受体	七个跨膜纺丝 G 蛋白连锁区域	IL-8
肿瘤坏死因子家族	胞外结构域富含半胱氨酸重复序列，胞质的 80 个氨基酸“死亡区域”	肿瘤坏死因子和 Fas

缩略语：EPO，促红细胞生成素；G-CSF，粒细胞集落刺激因子；GM-CSF，粒细胞巨噬细胞集落刺激因子；IL，白细胞介素；M-CSF，巨噬细胞集落刺激因子；SCF，干细胞因子；TPO，血小板生成素。

表 63-2 白细胞介素（IL）

	染色体定位	受体	选择性生物学活性
IL-1	2q13	IL-1RⅠ和 IL-1RⅡ	IL-1 作用于几乎每一个器官系统，促进急性期反应诱导多种细胞因子产生 上调细胞表面因子的表达 与其他细胞因子具有协同作用，刺激造血祖细胞的增殖 影响免疫调节 调节内分泌功能 影响骨骼的形成 IL-1R 在神经传递中作为辅助因子
IL-2	4q26-q27	αβγ 异源三聚体复合物	诱导 T 细胞、B 细胞和 NK 细胞的增殖和活化
IL-3	5q31	IL-3 受体（IL-3 特定的 α 亚基和 β 亚基的异源二聚体）	刺激多向造血祖细胞，特别是当与其他细胞因子联合使用时（SCF、IL-1、IL-6、G-CSF、GM-CSF、EPO 和 TPO）
IL-4 和 IL-13	5q31	IL-4Ⅰ型受体（IL-4Rα 和 IL-2 受体的 γc 链亚基）转换 IL-4 IL-4Ⅱ型受体（IL-4Rα 及 IL-13Rα1 亚基）转换 IL-4 和 IL-13 IL-4Rα 及 IL-13Rα2 复合物或两个 IL-13Rα 转换 IL-13	IL-4 和 IL-13 均参与过敏反应（诱导 IgE 转变）
IL-5	5q31	包括 IL-5Rα（IL-5 特定的）和一个 β 亚基 β 亚基与 IL-3 和 GM-CSF 复合物是共同的	调节嗜酸性细胞的产生、功能、生存和迁移 增强嗜碱性粒细胞的数量和功能
IL-6	7p21	IL-6Rα 与 gp130	B-和 T-细胞发育和功能 血栓形成 急性期蛋白的合成 抑制肝脏白蛋白排泄 破骨细胞骨吸收 神经分化

续表

	染色体定位	受体	选择性生物学活性
IL-7	8q12-q13	由 IL-7Rα(CD127)和共同 γc 链亚基组成	对 T-和 B-细胞的发育至关重要
IL-8	4q12-q13	存在 IL-8Rα 和 IL-8Rβ	各种白细胞,尤其是中性粒细胞的强效趋化剂 抑制不成熟的髓系祖细胞的集落形成 提高角质化细胞和内皮细胞的增殖
IL-9	5q31. 1	IL-9 受体	支持红细胞祖细胞的无性克隆成熟 作为一种肥大细胞分化因子 阻止淋巴瘤凋亡 在 B-细胞反应中与 IL-4 协同作用 增强神经元分化
IL-10	1q31-q32	IL-10 受体,IFN 受体	抑制 Th1 细胞和单核/巨噬细胞的细胞因子合成 刺激 B 细胞增殖 参与由 EB 病毒和 TNF 受体诱导的 B 细胞转化
IL-11	19q13. 3-q13. 4	IL-11Rα 和 gp130 亚基 gp130=位于 5q11 的 CD130 IL-6,制瘤素 M 和白血病抑制因子也使用 gp130 亚基	血栓形成因子 刺激多系祖细胞、红细胞生成、髓细胞生成、淋巴细胞生成 在动物模型中使黏膜炎减退 刺激破骨细胞发育 抑制脂肪细胞 刺激神经细胞增殖
IL-12	IL-12A:3p12-q13. 2	IL-12Rβ1 和 IL-12Rβ2 链与 gp130 有关	在抗感染中重要的前炎症细胞因子
	IL-12B:5q31. 1-q33. 1		Th1 的发育 刺激和抑制造血功能
IL-15	4q31	高亲和力受体需要 IL-2Rβ 和 γ 链以及 IL-15Rα 链	触发的预活化的 B 细胞的增殖和免疫球蛋白的产生 $CD8^+$记忆性 T 细胞的数量可能由 IL-15(刺激性)与 IL-12(抑制性)间的平衡所控制 刺激 NK 细胞的增殖,活化 $CD4^+$或 $CD8^+$T 细胞 促进诱导 LAK 细胞和 CTL 刺激肥大细胞增殖 促进多毛细胞白血病和慢性淋巴细胞白血病细胞的增殖
IL-16	15q26. 1	发挥生物活性需要 四次跨膜蛋白 CD9	$CD4^+$细胞(T 细胞,单核细胞,嗜酸性粒细胞的趋化因子) 可能与哮喘和炎性肉芽肿有关 对 HIV-1 具有抗病毒作用
IL-17	2q31	IL-17 受体	可能部分介导 T 细胞在感染中的作用 刺激上皮细胞、内皮细胞、成纤维细胞和巨噬细胞表达多种炎性细胞因子 促进成纤维细胞维持造血祖细胞增长的能力 促进树突状细胞祖细胞的分化 可能参与类风湿关节炎和移植物排斥的发病机制
IL-18	11q22. 2-q22. 3	IL-18R	促进 IFN-γ 和 TNF 的产生 靶向于 T 细胞,NK 细胞及巨噬细胞 促进 Th1 对病毒的免疫反应

续表

	染色体定位	受体	选择性生物学活性
IL-19	1q32	IL-20R1 及 IL-20R2	诱导的 IL-6 和 TNF-α
IL-20	1q32	IL-20R1 和 IL-20R2	诱导炎症相关的基因,例如 TNF-α,MRP1 和 MCP-1
IL-21	4q26-27	IL-21R	主要调控 T 细胞的增殖和分化 调节细胞介导的免疫,清除肿瘤
IL-22	12q14	IL-22R1 和 IL-10R2	上调急性期反应物的产生 诱导静息 B 细胞产生 ROS
IL-23	12q13	IL-12Rb1 和 IL-23R	IL-2 的一个独特的功能是优先诱导记忆 T 细胞增殖
IL-24	1q32	IL-20R1 和 IL-20R2	诱导 IL-6、TNF-a、IL-1b、IL-12 和 GM-CSF 功能上,它与 IL-10 作用相反
		IL-22R1 和 IL-20R2	感染 Ad-IL24 导致肿瘤细胞 Bcl-2 和 Bcl-XL(抗凋亡蛋白)下调,Bax 和 Bak(前凋亡蛋白)上调
IL-25	14q11	IL-17BR	IL-25 诱导 IL-4,IL-5 和 IL-13 的基因表达和蛋白质产生
IL-26	12q14	IL-20R1 和 IL-10R2	抗病毒感染的免疫保护作用
IL-27	12q13	TCCR/WSX-1 和 GP130	引发早期的 Th1 细胞 与 IL-12 协同诱导 T 细胞和 NK 细胞产生 IFN-γ
IL-28A、28B 和 29	19q13	IL-28R1 和 IL-10R2	抗病毒活性
IL-31	12q24	IL-31RA 和抑瘤素 M 受体	促进皮炎及过敏性和非过敏性疾病中上皮细胞所特有的反应
IL-32	16p13. 3	蛋白酶 3	诱导其他促炎细胞因子和趋化因子,如 TNF-α,IL-1β,IL-6 和 IL-8 诱导 IκB 下调 磷酸化 p38 MAPK 信号通路
IL-33	9p24. 1	ST2	激活 NF-κB 和 MAP 激酶 驱动体外极化的 Th2 细胞产生 Th2 相关细胞因子 诱导 IL-4、IL-5、IL-13 的表达 导致黏膜器官的严重病理改变
IL-35	19p13. 3	IL-12Rβ2 和 gp130	促进调节性 T 细胞的抑制活性 诱导血清 IL-10 和 IFN-g 水平 降低 IL-17 的诱导
IL-36	IL-36A:2q12-q14. 1	IL-1Rrp2 和 IL-1RAcP	激活 NF-κB 和 MAP 激酶
	IL-36B:2q14		在皮肤生物学中起重要作用
	IL-36G:2q12-q21		参与免疫反应的启动和调节
	IL-36RN:2q14		
IL-37	2q12-q14. 1	IL-18R	调节炎性反应
IL-38	2q13	IL36R	减少 IL-36g 诱导的 IL-8 的产生

本章的主要内容包括已知与临床相关的 IL 和经选择的一些细胞因子的生物学特点、用于治疗癌症患者的原理以及积累的临床经验。

白细胞介素

白细胞介素-1(IL-1)

IL-1(IL-1α 和 IL-1β)是一种原型的多效细胞因子,这种分子几乎影响所有的细胞类型[1,2]。因为 IL-1 是一种强效的炎症性细胞因子,所以发挥对人体有益的影响和产生严重毒性之间的治疗窗非常狭窄。因此,减少 IL-1 产生和/或降低其活性的化合物也正在临床试验中探索。

IL-1 的生物学活性

IL-1 具有调节多种基因和表面受体的表达的能力,因此作用广泛。事实上,IL-1 可以增加自身的表达,以及许多其他细胞因子(包括 IL-1RA)、细胞因子受体(包括 IL-2、IL-3、IL-5、GM-CSF 和 c-kit)、炎性递质(如环氧合酶和诱导型一氧化氮合酶)、肝急性期反应物、生长因子(包括但不限于成纤维细胞生长因子、角质形成细胞生长因子、肝细胞生长因子、神经生长因子、胰岛素样生长因子、阿替普酶)、凝血因子、神经肽、脂质相关基因、细胞外基质分子及癌基因(如 c-jun,cabl,c-fms,c-myc,c-fos)的表达[1]。最近关于炎症-癌症联系的数据表明,炎性成分存在于大多数肿瘤组织的微环境中,包括那些与明显的炎症过程的无因果联系的成分。因此,作为一个促炎症细胞因子,IL-1 也可能是生理和病理血管生成的主要的促血管生成刺激因子。

IL-1 家族几乎与每一个人体器官系统的功能和功能障碍有关。事实上,据报道,感染(病毒,细菌,真菌和寄生虫),血管内凝血,癌症(实体肿瘤和恶性血液病),阿尔茨海默氏病,自身免疫性疾病,外伤,缺血性疾病,胰腺炎,移植物抗宿主病,移植排斥以及运动后的健康受试者中 IL-1 产生均增加[1]。

曾有人建议,IL-1 与其天然拮抗剂之间的平衡实际上最与疾病相关[3]。这种平衡可因不同的疾病以不同的方式改变。例如,在心肌梗死或手术后患者以及人类免疫缺陷病毒(HIV)-1 的无症状感染者中,循环中 IL-1RA 的水平显著升高,而 IL-1β 水平无升高。一方面,在传染性,炎症或自身免疫性疾病患者的体液中,内源性 IL-1RA,与 IL-1β 的摩尔"比率"通常是 10~100,与 IL-1β 水平相比,IL-1RA 的水平可能是疾病严重程度的更好的指标。另一方面,在急性髓细胞白血病(acute myelogenous leukemia,AML)中 IL-10 自发表达,但是即使在 GM-CSF 刺激下,IL-1RA 的基因表达仍受到抑制[4,5]。在晚期的及生存期差的慢性粒细胞白血病(chronic myeloid leukemia,CML)患者中,IL-1RA 受到抑制,而 IL-1β 升高[6]。在 AML 和 CML 患者中,IL-1β 作为一种自分泌生长因子,暴露于降低 IL-1 活性的分子中,IL-1 可抑制白血病增殖[7,8]。已有报道,在实体肿瘤中(黑色素瘤,肝母细胞瘤,肉瘤,鳞状细胞癌,移行细胞癌和卵巢癌)中 IL-1α,IL-1β,和/或 IL-1RA 成组产生,并且在某些情况下与转移潜能相关。但是,IL-1 和肿瘤生长之间的关系是复杂的。

IL-1 的临床应用

IL-1α 和 IL-1β 都进行了治疗癌症的临床试验[65]。在一般情况下,每一种亚型的 IL-1 均是静脉注射的急性毒性较皮下注射大。皮下注射会引起显著的局部疼痛,红斑和肿胀。在几乎所有的患者都观察到剂量相关的寒战和发热,甚至应用 1ng/kg 的剂量也出现发热。几乎所有接受 100ng/kg 及以上剂量静脉注射给药的 IL-1 患者均会出现显著的低血压,可能是因为诱导产生一氧化氮的缘故。

即使是在剂量低至 1 或 2ng/kg 的情况下,IL-1 输入人体后显著增加循环 IL-6 水平,并导致白细胞计数上升。在骨髓储备正常的患者中也观察到了血小板增加。此外,外周血单核细胞计数和佛波醇诱导的过氧化产物显著增加。与骨髓良好功能的患者相反,再生障碍性贫血的患者接受每日剂量为 30~100ng/kg 的 IL-1α 连续 5 天治疗并未增加外周血细胞计数或骨髓细胞构成[9]。然而,在化疗后给予两次 IL-10 显著地缩短了中性粒细胞减少的持续时间[10],并且 IL-1α(5 天)显著地减少了血小板减少的持续时间[11]。总体而言,IL-1 的毒性显著,影响到其治疗获益。

IL-1RA 也已经对人体给药。当在健康志愿者中进行静脉注射时,它在生化、血液学、内分泌指标方面没有副作用或变化。这些研究 IL-1 在健康人中没有调节体温、血压或造血的功能。

白细胞介素-2(IL-2)

IL-2 最初被描述为一个 T 细胞生长因子,但其功能超出了淋巴细胞活化及增殖,虽然 T 细胞似乎仍然是其主要的靶点[12]。

IL-2 的生物学活性

IL-2,主要作为一个 T 细胞生长因子,但是也对 B 细胞、NK 细胞和淋巴因子活化的杀伤细胞产生影响。IL-2 与其三聚体受体复合物结合后,发生内在化,并诱导细胞周期进程,其与一系列明确的基因表达相关联[13]。第二能性反应通过二聚体受体 IL-2β,也被称为中间亲和力二聚体复合物(kDa,10^{-9}),涉及几个亚型的淋巴细胞的分化成淋巴因子活化的 LAK 杀伤细胞[14]。该反应发生在接受 IL-2 的癌症患者中[15,16],原先被认为是 IL-2 的抗肿瘤作用的一个重要组成部分。

IL-2 的临床应用

IL-2 对肿瘤免疫治疗的发展有着深远的影响。应用 IL-2 及其抗肿瘤 T 细胞过继免疫治疗是首个有效治疗人类肿瘤的免疫疗法[17]。自 1992 年以来,大量使用高剂量 IL-2(HD IL-2)的临床试验显示,两种晚期癌症(肾细胞癌和恶性黑色素瘤)的完全缓解率达到了 7%[18-22]。其中许多完全缓解持续了 10 年以上。HD IL-2 可能增强对癌细胞的免疫反应。它的抗癌活性与它作为 T 淋巴细胞生长因子的能力、刺激抗原非依赖性 NK 细胞和 LAK 细胞的能力以及它在恶性肿瘤部位增加淋巴细胞的能力密切相关。HD IL-2 的显著不良反应主要是由于严重的血管舒张和毛细血管渗漏综合征,包括低血压、心律失常、肝肾毒性。它的管理需要住院患者的重症护理类设置,因此它被推荐出现极少的并发症和状态良好的患者使用。IL-2 有 1%~2% 的致死风险,这也强调了选择适合这种治疗方式的患者的重要性[23]。

历史上，HD IL-2 首次是被用于联合生物化学治疗疗法，这种疗法通常包括顺铂、长春碱、达卡巴嗪或顺铂、长春碱和替莫唑胺，同时联合生物制剂 IFN-α 和 IL-2。然而，生存率的轻度提高却伴随着毒性的显著增加[24]。最近，随着 ipilimumab 等药物显示出持久的效应，HD IL-2 作为单一药物的作用变得越来越具有争议性。一种合理的方法是将两种经批准的治疗Ⅳ期黑色素瘤的免疫疗法——ipilimumab 和 IL-2 结合起来。目前还没有关于免疫疗法的准确测序的数据。一些黑色素瘤专家认为，IL-2 在早期治疗中使用效果最好，此时患者的病情较有限（M1a 疾病），且有良好表现。一项小型研究表明，NRAS 突变型黑色素瘤患者的反应率可能更高（47%），但这一发现还需要进一步验证[25]。2005 年的一项研究中，36 名晚期黑色素瘤患者接受了 ipilimumab（每 3 周 0.1～3mg/kg）和 IL-2 的联合治疗，总缓解率为 22%[26]。评估 ipilimumab 在过继细胞治疗中的作用的研究正在进行中。延长或提高 HD IL-2 或 ipilimumab 治疗效果的另一种方法是将免疫疗法与 BRAF 抑制剂联合治疗 BRAFV600 突变的晚期黑色素瘤患者[27]。临床前研究显示，BRAF 抑制剂治疗后，肿瘤活检组织中黑色素瘤抗原表达和肿瘤浸润淋巴细胞数量增加，这与肿瘤体积缩小和坏死增加有关[28,29]。目前的工作是检查接受 vemurafenib 的患者的肿瘤活检，以评估肿瘤内 T 细胞积聚的机制和动力学，并描述免疫浸润细胞的特异性和功能，以设计更成功的 BRAF 抑制剂和免疫治疗的联合治疗方案。

白细胞介素-3（IL-3）

Lee 和 Ihle 首先将 IL-3 描述为 Moloney 白血病病毒诱导的 T 细胞淋巴瘤发病机制相关的 T 细胞产物[30]。这种分子备受关注，因为它在体内外都具有刺激多系造血祖细胞的能力[30-37]。

IL-3 的生物学特性

已证实在体外及体内多系正常的造血祖细胞的均对 IL-3 具有反应。在体外，在半固体培养基中 IL-3 联合其他细胞因子，例如 SCF、IL-6、IL-1、G-CSF、GM-CSF、EPO 或 TPO，可诱导 CFU-GM、CFU-EO、CFU-Baso、BFU-E 和 CFU-GEMM 的增殖，并可刺激悬浮培养的纯化的 $CD34^+$ 细胞的增殖[31]。事实上，与其他细胞因子联合，特别是 SCF、IL-6、IL-1、FL、G-CSF 和/或 EPO，IL-3 被包括在几乎所有体外扩增造血干细胞和祖细胞的方案中。

IL-3 的临床应用

IL-3 已被用于各种临床试验，包括外周血干细胞动员，化疗后和移植以及骨髓衰竭状态。大多数的研究表明，IL-3 本身的影响有限。然而，与其他生长因子联合，试验结果证明了显著的益处。例如，在动员研究中，IL-3 本身无动员作用，但是它可显著增加 G-CSF 诱导的所有类型祖细胞的产生以进行高剂量化疗后的造血重建。移植后，已证实联合应用 IL-3 和 GM-CSF 较单独应用 IL-3 或 GM-CSF 可更有效地促进骨髓移植物的植入。联合应用 IL-3 和 GM-CSF 较 G-CSF 可更有效地促进血小板的恢复，但对于髓细胞生成的益处相仿。在部分但并非所有的临床试验中，发现化疗后 IL-3 可降低中性粒细胞减少和/或血小板减少的程度。

白细胞介素-4（IL-4）及白细胞介素-13（IL-13）

IL-4 和 IL-13 是密切相关的[38-40]。它们对 B 细胞、单核细胞、树突状细胞及成纤维细胞的生物学和免疫调节功相仿。IL-4 和 IL-13 的基因位于 5 号染色体上相同的区域。IL-4 和 IL-13 启动子的主要调节序列是相同的，从而可解释它们在活化的 T 细胞和肥大细胞的有限的表达模式。此外，IL-4 和 IL-13 受体为复合受体，至少有一条链——IL-4RA 相同。这一点，以及 IL-4 和 IL-13 信号转导的相似之处，可解释这两种细胞因子之间的生物学特性的显著的重叠。然而，由于 T 淋巴细胞缺乏 IL-13 受体，IL-13 不能调节 T 细胞的分化，这是这两种细胞因子的一个主要区别。因此，尽管这两种分子的功能存在很多重叠之处，但是存在调节机制以保证其独特的功能。

IL-4 及 IL-13 的生物学活性

IL-13 的可发挥很多但不是所有 IL-4 的生物学作用。但是，IL-4 具有 T-细胞生长因子活性以及驱动 Th0 前体细胞向 Th2 细胞谱系分化的能力，这些有别于 IL-13。Th2 细胞分泌 IL-4 及 IL-5 并优先刺激体液免疫。与此相反，产生 IL-2 和 IFN-γ 的 Th1 细胞，优先刺激细胞免疫。

IL-4 和 IL-13 在小鼠体内的具有强抗肿瘤活性[41]。它在体外以及在裸鼠体内可以抑制某些人类肿瘤细胞株的增殖。IL-13 对人乳腺癌细胞的具有类似的抗增殖效应。此外，由 IL-13 和截短形式的假单胞菌外毒素 A 组成的嵌合蛋白对人类肾细胞癌具有特定的细胞毒活性，但对正常的造血细胞不具毒性[42]。

IL-4 的临床试验

尽管临床前研究显示 IL-4 非常有希望，然而迄今为止，这种分子应用于人类的临床试验表明，虽然这种分子是安全无毒的，但是在包括黑色素瘤、肺癌及艾滋病相关的卡波西肉瘤的许多种癌症中仅观察到个别的抗肿瘤活性[43-45]。

白细胞介素-6

IL-6 于 1986 年被首次克隆[46]。这是一个典型的细胞因子，具有功能的多效性和重复性。IL-6 参与免疫反应、炎症和造血。IL-6 是一个由 212 个氨基酸组成的 21～30kDa 的糖蛋白，IL-6 与特定受体结合，该受体需要相同的 130kDa 的膜糖蛋白以介导信号转导，像已经描述过的包括 IL-2 在内的多种细胞因那样[47,48]。

IL-6 的生物学活性

IL-6 影响下丘脑-垂体轴、骨吸收以及免疫系统的体液和细胞免疫[49-53]，是保证 B 和 T 淋巴细胞的正常发育和功能的一个强有力的和必不可少的因素[54]。这种分子也参与了其他生物的活动，如髓系白血病细胞株分化为巨噬细胞、巨核细胞的成熟、神经分化、破骨细胞发育。作为一个急性期反应的主要的诱导因子[55]，这种细胞因子可能在败血症的发病机制中发挥作用。

IL-6 作为骨髓瘤/浆细胞瘤、角质形成细胞、肾小球系膜细胞、肾细胞癌和卡波西肉瘤的生长因子，并促进造血干细胞的生长。另一方面，IL-6 也抑制髓性白血病细胞系和某些肿瘤细胞株的生长。已证明在许多种炎症状态下血清 IL-6 的活性和血清急性期蛋白水平显著相关。IL-6 是与淋巴瘤的 B 症状有关的一种递质[56]。血清 IL-6 水平升高也与霍奇金淋巴瘤和非霍奇金淋巴瘤的预后不良相关[57-60]。在弥漫性大细胞淋巴瘤中,多因素分析显示 IL-6 水平是完全缓解率和无复发生存的一个最重要的独立预后因素[58]。IL-6 水平也可作为肾细胞癌和多发性骨髓瘤的一项预后因素,也观察到前列腺癌和卵巢癌患者 IL-6 水平升高。IL-6 可能也是淋巴组织增生性疾病 Castleman 病全身表现的病因[61]。IL-6 水平升高也是胰腺癌的不良预后因素[62]。

IL-6 的临床应用

在接受化疗或自体移植的患者中,在可耐受剂量下,IL-6 仅有微弱或无增强血小板活性的作用。毒性包括发热和贫血[63-65]。IL-6 也被作为抗肿瘤药物试用于治疗黑色素瘤和肾细胞癌。有效率一直较低(<15%)[55]。因为高水平的 IL-6 与在许多种癌症的不良预后相关并且在某些肿瘤中作为自分泌/旁分泌生长因子,所以就 IL-6 抑制剂进行临床研究可能是有价值的。

综上所述,IL-6 是癌症中最无所不在的并且不受调节的细胞因子,在几乎每一项肿瘤研究中均发现 IL-6 水平增高。如第 14 篇参考文献所述,IL-6 的作用与包括乳腺癌、肺癌、大肠癌、卵巢癌、前列腺癌、胰腺癌、多发性骨髓瘤、神经胶质瘤、黑色素瘤、肾细胞癌、白血病、淋巴瘤及 Castleman 病的几乎每一种肿瘤均相关。临床前和转化性研究支持 IL-6 在不同的恶性肿瘤中均发挥作用,为靶向治疗研究提供了生物学基本原理。多种化合物可拮抗 IL-6 的生成,包括皮质类固醇、非甾体抗炎药物、雌激素和细胞因子。靶向生物疗法包括 IL-6 偶联毒素和针对 IL-6 及其受体的单克隆抗体。例如,一种嵌合型鼠抗人 IL-6 抗体,CNTO328,已在一项 1 期试验中用于 B 细胞非霍奇金淋巴瘤、多发性骨髓瘤及 Castleman 病受试者[66]。此治疗获得了肿瘤缓解和疾病控制,尤其是在 Castleman 病中观察到了显著的治疗反应[67]。

白细胞介素-7(IL-7)

IL-7 能够在缺乏基质细胞的情况下诱导 B 细胞祖细胞增殖,基于上述特点,IL-7 被确定和克隆[68-76]。目前已经明确,这种细胞因子是由骨髓和胸腺的基质干细胞所分泌,并且对于 B 和 T 细胞的发育是不可替代的[69-71]。事实上,在基因敲除小鼠观察到除去 IL-7 或部分 IL-7 受体将不可避免地导致淋巴细胞发育的重要缺陷,因此 IL-7 必不可少。

IL-7/IL-7 受体的生物学活性

产生 T 细胞和 B 细胞的主要部位分别是胸腺和骨髓。胸腺 T 细胞是骨髓祖细胞生成的子代。大量的细胞因子在 B-和 T-细胞的发育中发挥作用。然而,多数单一细胞因子基因敲除的小鼠表现出相对正常的 B-和 T-细胞系列,这表明许多细胞因子的功能是多余的。相反,IL-7 缺乏的小鼠存在胸腺和骨髓显著的淋巴细胞缺失。总体来说,基因实验所确定的各种淋巴因子在体内的作用明显不同。IL-2 和 IL-4 的功能为在免疫反应中影响淋巴细胞群的成熟,而 IL-7 在淋巴细胞的产生和扩增中起显著的主导作用。所有的淋巴细胞来自造血干细胞。在克隆共同淋巴祖细胞阶段 IL-7R 上调,可引起在单细胞水平上的所有淋巴谱系的发生[74]。在淋巴细胞发育中 IL-7R-介导的信号发挥作用至少通过以下 3 个主要的途径:提高增殖,触发谱系特异的发育程序,并维持适当的经选择细胞的活性。

发现在 T 细胞耗竭状态下 IL-7 水平升高,因此 IL-7 在促进 T 细胞扩增中发挥作用[75]。还发现在慢性淋巴细胞性白血病和 Burkitt 淋巴瘤中 IL-7 水平升高,并且过量表达 IL-7 基因的转基因小鼠的淋巴细胞发育显示出了巨大变化,在某些情况下,可能会导致形成淋巴肿瘤[76]。

白细胞介素-8(IL-8)

IL-8 最早发现于 1987 年,是强效的前炎症趋化因子,诱导中性粒细胞穿过血管壁(趋化性)[77]。这种分子属于一个趋化因子超家族,其成员包括中性粒细胞活化肽-2、血小板因子-4、生长相关细胞因子(也称为黑色素瘤生长刺激活性)和 IFN-诱导蛋白-10,所有这些趋化因子都是负责各种细胞的定向迁移。IL-8 受体与人疱疹病毒-8 所编码的基因显示出高度的同源性 HHV-8[79,80]。

IL-8 的生物学活性

炎症刺激聚集循环中的白细胞,尤其是中性粒细胞,产生趋化因子,以起到防御作用,并引导它们到达损伤部位。在中性粒细胞作用的趋化因子中,IL-8 是最有效的之一[81]。暴露于趋化因子后,中性粒细胞被活化,并在几秒钟内形状发生改变。中性粒细胞形状变化的过程至关重要。它是由细胞整合素类的和肌动蛋白细胞骨架所调节。整合素类的活化和上调也使中性粒细胞黏附于血管壁内皮细胞,继而迁移进入组织。

IL-8 可诱发肿瘤生长,是因为 IL-8 具有促血管生成活性,一种促进血管形成的特性。一方面,将抗 IL-8 抗体给予表达 IL-8 的人肺癌移植瘤的 SCID 小鼠,已显示出获益[82]。另一方面,IL-8 的抗肿瘤作用也有报道。在这方面一个有趣的事实是已发现肺癌和黑色素瘤患者 IL-8 水平升高。IL-8 可能是胰腺癌和黑色素瘤的一种生长因子[78]。在黑色素瘤中,IL-8 水平与肿瘤细胞生长和转移的可能性相关,将肿瘤细胞暴露于 IFN(已明确对于黑色素瘤具有抗肿瘤活性)可降低 IL-8 的水平并且抑制肿瘤细胞的增殖[83]。已建议将阻断 IL-8 或 IL-8R 作为一个治疗策略[78]。

白细胞介素-9(IL-9)

人 IL-9 最初是作为人巨核细胞白血病的促有丝分裂因子被确定和克隆的。接着,发现 IL-9 的靶细胞包括广泛的细胞[84,85]。

IL-9 的生物学活性

对 IL-9 有反应的细胞成分包括红细胞祖细胞、人 T 细胞和 B 细胞、胎儿胸腺细胞、胸腺淋巴瘤和未成熟的神经元细胞系[84]。

在 EPO 的作用下 IL-9 可支持红系祖细胞克隆性成熟。相反,粒细胞或巨噬细胞集落形成(CFU-GM,CFU-G,或 CFU-M)通常是不受 IL-9 影响。比较 IL-9 对胎儿和成人祖细胞影响的实验已经表明,IL-9 对胎儿细胞更有效。活化的细胞也更可能对于该细胞因子的反应更显著。除了其促增殖活性,IL-9 也似乎是一种有效的调节肥大细胞的效应分子。

IL-9 对正常 T 细胞对无作用,而对淋巴瘤细胞具有显著活性,这是一个有趣的自相矛盾的现象。这种差别可由以下观察到的现象解释,成熟的 T 细胞经过长时间的体外培养后获得对IL-9发生反应的能力，而他们同时也获得了肿瘤细胞系的特性。对转基因小鼠进行的观察也证明失调IL-9的产生失调具有致癌潜能，因为5%～10%的过表达这种细胞因子的小鼠发生了淋巴母细胞淋巴瘤[85]。与这些资料相一致，目前已有数据明确显示人霍奇金淋巴瘤和间变性大细胞淋巴瘤产生IL-9[84]。即便如此，IL-9的病理生理作用仍然难以明确。

白细胞介素-10(IL-10)

IL-10是一种多效的细胞因子，是在1989年发现的由鼠Th2细胞所产生的一种活性物质[86,87]。它最初被指定为细胞因子合成抑制因子，因为它能够抑制某些细胞因子的产生[88]。有趣的是，IL-10显示与Epstein-Barr病毒基因组中的开放阅读框架-BCRF1具有显著的DNA和氨基酸序列的同源性[88]。事实上，BCRF1蛋白质产物显示了许多细胞IL-10的生物学特性，因此，被称为病毒IL-10。

IL-10的生物学活性

IL-10抑制Th1细胞产生的细胞因子的合成，包括IL-2、IFN-γ、GM-CSF、淋巴毒素、单核细胞衍生的IL-1α和β、IL-6、IL-8、TNF-α、GM-CSF和G-CSF。外源性IL-10也可以抑制IL-10的表达[87]。同时，IL-10诱导IL-1受体的合成，IL-1受体可为巨噬细胞所拮抗。IL-10也抑制CD28共刺激途径，因此，IL-10作为一个决定性的机制以确定T细胞将有助于免疫反应或无变应性。

从分子角度来看，IL-10在转录水平并在转录后水平抑制细胞因子的表达[89]。这两种机制似乎需要新的蛋白质的合成。在细胞水平，Th1细胞因子合成的抑制间接通过IL-10对抗原呈递细胞(APC)的影响所介导，因为抑制发生时，是由巨噬细胞而不是B细胞作为APC[90]。单核细胞/巨噬细胞存在时，IL-10抑制静止T细胞的增殖，包括Th0、Th1、Th2细胞的$CD4^+$ T细胞克隆。高浓度的IL-2仅可部分逆转这种抑制作用，提示增殖降低仅可部分反应IL-2产生的减少。IL-10也可以提高$CD8^+$T细胞的细胞毒活性。所有这些影响都支持IL-10在调节炎症反应中具有重要作用。与对其他谱系细胞的抑制效应相反，IL-10对B细胞和肥大细胞具有刺激作用[91]。例如，IL-10可强烈刺激活化B细胞的增殖和分化。

IL-10在癌症中的作用，应在一个高度复杂的生物难题的框架内考虑。已知IL-10对适应性和先天免疫细胞介质具有多效性。虽然一些研究表明，IL-10能够积极介导免疫抑制，但是一些实验模型描述了相对截然相反的结论。关于IL-10和抗肿瘤免疫之间关系的最新数据支持IL-10对恶性细胞具有有效的免疫攻击，这对IL-10作为免疫抑制因子促进肿瘤免疫逃逸的传统的观念进行了挑战。

白细胞介素-11(IL-11)

IL-11最初以血小板生成因子为特征，现在已知IL-11在众多的其他系统中表达并具有活性，包括肠道、睾丸和中枢神经系统[92,93]。临床上，这种细胞因子已被美国FDA批准用于改善化疗引起的血小板减少症。

IL-11的生物学活性

IL-11最初是从造血微环境中的细胞中分离而来，并可能在这样的环境中作为旁分泌或自分泌生长因子。IL-11与其他早期和后期作用的生长因子产生协同作用，刺激不同阶段和不同谱系的造血作用。与IL-3、IL-4、IL-7、IL-12、IL-13、SCF、FLT-3配体和GM-CSF发生协同作用，IL-11刺激原始干细胞的增殖、定型为多向祖细胞及其的分化[92]。IL-11和TPO对多系细胞的协同效应可能部分由SCF/c-kit的相互作用所介导。

IL-11与IL-3、TPO或SCF对巨核细胞和血小板生成的各个阶段具有协同刺激作用[94,95]。IL-11单独或与其他细胞因子(IL-3、SCF或EPO)联合，可刺激红细胞生成的多个阶段。IL-11还调节髓系祖细胞的分化和成熟。IL-11与SCF联合刺激髓系细胞的集落形成。IL-11与IL-13或IL-14的联合，可减少粒细胞和髓系集落爆炸的比例，同时增加巨噬细胞数量。IL-11与SCF或IL-4联合可有效地支持在原代培养的B细胞的产生。IL-11和IL-4也可以逆转IL-3对早期B-淋巴细胞的发展的抑制作用。对B细胞分化的促进作用可能由T细胞介导。

IL-11与IL-3、GM-CSF和SCF共同刺激人类原代白血病细胞、髓细胞性白血病细胞系、巨核母细胞性细胞系和红白血病细胞株的增殖，并刺激白血病鼓风集落的形成。

白血病细胞表达IL-11mRNA和IL-11反义寡核苷酸抑制白血病细胞的生长表明，IL-11在白血病细胞株中可能作为自分泌生长因子[96]。虽然IL-11刺激鼠浆细胞瘤细胞和鼠杂交瘤细胞的增殖，但是IL-11对人骨髓瘤/浆细胞瘤细胞生长的影响是有争议的[92]。

IL-11的临床应用

IL-11是获得FDA批准的第二种IL。它用于化疗引起的血小板减少症的二级预防和减少非髓系恶性疾病患者的血小板输注的需要。

白细胞介素-12(IL-12)

IL-12最初被确定为NK细胞刺激因子[97]。随后的研究表明，IL-12对Th1细胞的发展至关重要[98]。事实上，似乎从先天免疫反应到获得性免疫有一个共同的途径；细胞内病原体刺激巨噬细胞产生IL-12，促进幼稚细胞群Th1细胞的发展。可以利用这种途径设计新型免疫疗法和疫苗。

IL-12的生物学活性及其在人类疾病的作用

IL-12是一种强力前炎症分子，其在抵抗细菌、真菌和寄生虫的感染中必不可少。它在感染的几个小时内产生，激活NK细胞，并通过NK细胞诱导产生IFN-γ，增强吞噬细胞吞噬和杀菌活性及释放前炎症细胞因子的能力，其中包括IL-12本身。IL-12也是一种重要的免疫调节分子，尤其是Th1免疫反应。它在感染和炎症的早期阶段产生，随后发生抗原特异的免疫反应，有利于Th1 T细胞的分化和功能，同时抑制Th2细胞的分化。IL-12并不会引起外周血静止T细胞和NK细胞的增殖；它可能促进各种有丝分裂原诱导的T细胞增殖，并且对预活化的T细胞和NK细胞有直接的促增殖效应。

IL-12与其他造血因子的协同促进早期多能造血祖细胞和各谱系前体细胞的存活和增殖[99]。虽然在体外IL-12多表现为造血刺激作用，但是在体内IL-12的治疗效果表现为降低骨髓造血以及短暂的贫血和中性粒细胞减少，这是通过IFN-γ介导的效应。

IL-12 的临床应用

IL-12 具有开发为治疗过敏症和感染性疾病辅助治疗药物的潜力[100]。此外，IL-12 恢复现有耐受性或无反应性状态的能力，使得它称为应对传染性病原体或肿瘤的疫苗成分的候选。在过去几年中，在肿瘤以及人类免疫缺陷病毒感染者和慢性乙型肝炎和丙型肝炎患者中已经开始进行 1 期临床试验。迄今为止，给予慢性丙型肝炎患者 IL-12 治疗未显示出获益[101]。在高剂量的 IL-12 治疗癌症患者方面更令人担忧的是，观察到急性造血、肝脏、胃肠道毒性，并且有几例受试者死亡的报道。在长期治疗中，主要是肺毒性。曾有人建议，如果在开始每天给药之前 1～2 周单次注射给药，IL-12 的一些严重的毒性反应可以得到减轻[102]。

白细胞介素-15（IL-15）

IL-15 与 IL-2 的部分生物学活性相仿[103]。

IL-15 的生物学活性

与 IL-2 相似，IL-15 能够触发正常 B 淋巴细胞的增殖和免疫球蛋白的产生。但是，只有当 B 细胞已在体外被多克隆有丝分裂原预活化，或当它们与其他刺激物共同培养时，才可以获取这些生物学功能，IL-15 也刺激 NK 细胞和活化的 $CD4^+$ 和 $CD8^+$T 细胞的增殖，并促进溶细胞的效应细胞的诱导（例如淋巴因子激活的杀伤细胞）。最后，动物 $CD8^+$ 记忆性 T 细胞的数目在 IL-15 的刺激作用和 IL-12 的抑制作用下保持平衡[104]。

对 IL-15 的应答性可区分恶性 B 细胞和正常 B 淋巴细胞。与正常 B 淋巴细胞不同，正常 B 淋巴细胞需要预活化以在 IL-15 的作用下增殖，慢性 B 细胞恶性肿瘤患者的白血病细胞在 IL-15 作用下的增殖与体外预活化无关，这主要与恶性 B 淋巴细胞的 IL-2R 系统的 β 和 γ 链相关[103]。即便如此，这些白血病中 IL-15 不能被视为自分泌因子，因为它不是由白血病细胞本身产生的。相反，这些患者中的 IL-15 主要来源于单核细胞/巨噬细胞谱系的细胞[103]。

白细胞介素-17（IL-17）

人 IL-17 与毒松鼠猴疱疹病开放阅读框 63-13 在氨基酸水平与有 72% 的整体序列同源性[105]。

IL-17 的生物学活性

虽然在数量上不多，研究表明，IL-17 可能是一种 T 细胞诱导或促进炎症的可溶性因子[106]。IL-17 也可以刺激上皮细胞，内皮细胞和成纤维细胞以及巨噬细胞表达多种细胞因子[99]。暴露于 IL-17 的细胞因子释放显示是细胞特异性的。例如，在 IL-17 作用下，成纤维细胞产生 IL-1、G-CSF、IFN-γ、IL-6 和 IL-8，巨噬细胞产生 TNF-α、IL-1β、IL-1Rα、IL-6、IL-10 和 IL-12[107]。IL-17 还具有间接的造血活性，IL-17 可增强成纤维细胞的容量以支持 $CD34^+$ 造血祖细胞的增殖以及向中性粒细胞的分化[108,106]。IL-17 也能促进树突状细胞祖细胞的成熟[109]。由于 IL-17 能够分化早期的干细胞，因此它与宿主 T 细胞同种异体刺激和移植排斥反应有关。

白细胞介素-18（IL-18）

IL-18（IFN-γ 诱导因子）首先被描述为诱导小鼠脾脏细胞产生 IFN-γ 的一种血清活性物质[110]。IL-18 的分子量为 18～19kDa，与 IL-1 具有同源性[111,112]。与 IL-1β 相仿，IL-18 最初被合成为缺乏信号肽的无活性前体分子（前-IL-18），经 ICE 裂解为活性分子[113,114]。

IL-18 的生物学活性

T 淋巴细胞、NK 细胞和巨噬细胞是 IL-18 的主要靶细胞。例如，IL-18 直接刺激人体血液中的 $CD4^+$T 淋巴细胞和 NK 细胞产生 TNF，并且在促进 Th1 淋巴细胞对病毒抗原的长期持久的反应中发挥重要作用。IL-18 似乎不是内源性致热原，但是仍然可能有助于炎症和发热，因为它是一种 TNF、趋化因子和 IFN 的有效的诱导剂[115]。在 IFN-γ 诱导的情况下，IL-18 作为有丝分裂原或 IL-2 的共同刺激物。事实上，缺乏切割前-IL-18 为期活性形式的 ICE 的小鼠，在内毒素的作用下不产生 IFN-γ。

白细胞介素-21（IL-21）

IL-21，是与 IL-2 和 IL-15 最密切相关的细胞因子，与骨髓中 NK 细胞群增殖和成熟相关，并与成熟的 B 细胞群和 T 细胞群的增殖相关[116]。IL-21 与先天免疫反应的激活和 Th1 反应相关。IL-21 在调节的 B 细胞免疫球蛋白的产生中也起着关键作用[117]。

白细胞介素-24（IL-24）

在 1995 年被发现时，IL-24 最初被命名为黑色素瘤分化相关基因 7（mda-7）。它是通过消减杂交技术在 IFN-β 和瑞香素治疗后的黑色素瘤细胞中确定的，IFN-β 和瑞香素可导致终末分化和生长停滞[118]。在 2001 年，人们发现 mda-7 编码一种分泌蛋白，其与 IL-10 表现出显著的同源性，是 IL-10 家族的另一个成员。这种分子被正式指定为 IL-24[119]。人 IL-24 是由活化的外周血单核细胞分泌的，是两种异源二聚体受体 IL-22 R1/IL-20 R2 和 IL-20 R1/IL-20 R2 的配体[120]。IL-24 也作为一种肿瘤抑制癌基因，其蛋白产物在黑色素细胞、痣细胞以及一些初期黑色素瘤组成性表达，但不在黑色素瘤的转移性病灶中表达[121,122]。这可能是肿瘤抑制基因具有免疫刺激特性的第一个例子[123]。

IL-24 的生物学活性

IL-24 有许多有趣而独特的性能，包括直接杀死癌细胞的活性，较高的旁观者抗肿瘤活性，免疫调节活性和抗血管生成的特性。作为抗肿瘤制剂，mda-7/il-24 是真正独一无二的显示出对肿瘤细胞选择性抗肿瘤活性，并有能力利用不同的信号转导途径介导肿瘤细胞死亡的制剂。

IL-24 的临床应用

基于其卓越的属性和在动物模型中有效的抗肿瘤治疗作用，这种细胞因子已经迈出了进入临床的重要一步。在一项 1 期临床试验中，瘤内注射以腺病毒作为载体的 MDA-7/IL-24（INGN241）是安全的，引起肿瘤调控及免疫活化的过程，并显示出显著的临床活性[124,125]。

白细胞介素-26（IL-26）

减法杂交联合代表性差异分析确认，IL-26/AK155 是一种在感染水疱性口炎病毒、人巨细胞病毒和单纯疱疹病毒 1 型后在人 T 细胞中上调的基因[126]。它具有抗肿瘤的能力。它有能力转变这些培养中的细胞。IL-26 蛋白与人 IL-10 有 24.7%的氨基酸同源和 47%的氨基酸相似。结构分析表明，IL-26 包含 6 个单环，具有 4 个高度保守的半胱氨酸残基，它被假定为与二聚体的形成有关，这与 IL-10 相类似。据测定，IL-26 在 HVS 转化后的 T 细胞中特异性高表达。

白细胞介素-27(IL-27)

在 2002 年，Pflanz 及其同事[127]描述了一种新的异二聚体细胞因子，与 IL-12 相关。这种细胞因子被命名为 IL-27。其与 IL-12 共同作用触发幼稚 $CD4^+$T 细胞产生 IFN-γ。他们还确定 IL-27 是 TCCR/WSX-1 的配体，Ⅰ类细胞因子受体家族的一个新成员，对于 Th1 的发展很重要[128]。最近的研究表明 IL-27 具有能够诱导肿瘤特定的抗肿瘤活性和免疫，抗肿瘤活性主要是通过 $CD8^+$T 细胞和 IFN-γ 介导的[129]。

白细胞介素-28(IL-28)及白细胞介素-29(IL-29)

IL-28 家族在人基因组序列中被确定，命名为 IL-28 A、IL-28 B 和 IL-29。这些分子与Ⅰ型干扰素和 IL-10 家族有较远的相关。IL-28 和 IL-29 是由病毒感染引起，并显示出抗病毒活性。此外，IL-28 和 IL-29 与异二聚体的Ⅱ型细胞因子受体相互作用，这种受体包括 IL-10 Rβ 和一个单独的Ⅱ型受体链，命名为 IL-28Rα。现在，它们被分类为Ⅲ型干扰素，并且由它们的有效抗病毒和抗肿瘤特性所决定它可以替代Ⅰ型干扰素。鉴于 IL-28/29 主要影响上皮细胞、黑色素细胞及其衍生的肿瘤细胞以及肝细胞，这些细胞因子有可以应用，包括作为癌症和黑色素瘤的抗肿瘤治疗等几个潜在领域的治疗当中[130]。

白细胞介素-31(IL-31)

IL-31 是 Th2 细胞优先产生的四螺旋束细胞因子。IL-31 信号通过 IL-31 受体 A 和抑瘤素 M 受体组成的受体传导。活化的单核细胞表达 IL-31 受体 A 和抑瘤素 M 受体 mRNA，而上皮细胞组成表达两种基因。需要特别说明的，数据表明 IL-31 可能参与促进皮炎和上皮细胞的反应，其表现为过敏性和非过敏性疾病的特点[131]。

白细胞介素-35(IL-35)

IL-35 是异源二聚体 IL-12 细胞因子家族的一个新成员。IL-35 是 Treg 细胞所产生的一种新颖的抑制性细胞因子，有助于其的抑制性活性。此外，异位表达的 IL-35 调节幼稚 T 细胞的活性，而重组 IL-35 抑制 T 细胞的增殖。由于 IL-35 可能完全由 Treg 细胞及其他具有调节潜能的细胞群体所分泌，它代表了一种新的潜在的治疗性靶点，通过调节 Treg 细胞活性治疗癌症和自身免疫性疾病[132]。

白细胞介素-37(IL-37)

自 1977 年发现 IL-1 以来，IL-1 家族的细胞因子列表不断扩展[133]。IL-37 最初被定义为 IL-1 家族成员 7(IL-1F7)，在淋巴结、胸腺、骨髓、肺、睾丸、子宫和胎盘中检测到转录物[134]。TGF-β 和一些 Toll 样受体(TLR)配体通过诱导 PBMCS 产生高水平的 IL-37；促炎细胞因子，如 IL-18、IFN-γ、IL-1β 和 TNF 适度增加 IL-37 的水平[135]。此外，单核细胞中 IL-37 的表达已被证明可减少对转导促炎信号很重要的几种细胞内激酶，例如黏着斑激酶、STAT1、p38MAPK 和 c-jun。因此，IL-37 被认为是炎症的许多关键调节剂之一。

干扰素

IFN 是涉及抗病毒防御，细胞生长调节和免疫激活的大型多功能分泌蛋白家族。IFN 有 3 种类型：Ⅰ型(IFN-α，IFN-β)、Ⅱ型(IFN-γ)和Ⅲ型(IFN-λ)。每种 IFN 类型都具有序列相似性，通过特定的细胞表面受体复合物(表 63-3)发送信号，并通过激活多种信号途径(包括 JAK-STAT 途径等)来调节其作用。JAK-STAT 信号事件导致转录因子复合物和同或异二聚体 STAT 分子的激活，以及随后与 IFN 刺激应答元件、γ 激活序列和 IFN 调节基因启动子中的 STAT 结合位点的结合，从而导致转录因子复合物和同种或异二聚体 STAT 分子的激活。诱导这些 IRG 的转录激活[136]。

表 63-3 干扰素(IFN)

分类		刺激因素	受体	信号分子
Ⅰ类干扰素	IFN-α IFN-β	病毒 其他微生物	IFNAR：IFNAR1-IFNAR2	• JAK1 和 TYK2 • STAT1-STAT2-IRF9 复合物 • STAT1-STAT1 复合物
Ⅱ类干扰素	IFN-γ	抗原-MHC 复合物 激活 NK 细胞配体 IL-12 加 IL-18 TLRs	IFNGR：IFNGR1-IFNGR2	• JAK1 和 JAK2 • STAT1-STAT1 复合物
Ⅲ类干扰素	IFN-λ	病毒 其他微生物	IL10R2 和 IFNLR1	• JAK1 和 TYK2 • STAT1-STAT2-IRF9 复合物 • STAT2-STAT2 复合物

编码Ⅰ、Ⅱ和Ⅲ型 IFN 的基因分别聚集在人类的 9、12 和 19 号染色体上。在与相对少量的高亲和力受体结合后发生细胞作用。干扰素与其为数不多的高亲和力受体结合，从而启动细胞的反应。这一效应可调控蛋白转录，从而调控基因表达而

产生相应蛋白，此类蛋白在相应部位通常是不表达或低表达的。这些干扰素刺激基因的产物构成多种生物学效应的基础，包括：病毒抑制、免疫调节、抗细胞增殖、促进凋亡及抗血管生成。然而，仍不能确定究竟是哪种特异的干扰素刺激基因产物发挥了多种生物学效应和治疗作用；同样，抗肿瘤效应的特异性细胞机制也是不清楚的。抗肿瘤效应可能源于对细胞活性和增殖能力或对肿瘤细胞抗原表达的直接影响，也可能源于对免疫效应因子或内皮细胞群的调节。IFN 调节基因表达，调节细胞表面蛋白质的表达及促进新酶类的合成。基因表达的改变导致了其他细胞因子受体的调整、免疫效应细胞表面的调节蛋白的聚集以及调节细胞生长和功能的酶类的活化。在细胞水平，这些效应转化为分化状态、增殖和死亡率及多种细胞类型的功能活动的改变。诱导的蛋白质及其产物能够在细胞及治疗患者的血清中检测出来。对这些物质的测量或者免疫效应细胞的数量可用于确定生物活性分子、剂量、方案及给药途径。

在人体中的抗肿瘤效应

天然的和重组的干扰素在各种恶性肿瘤患者中都显示出一定的抗肿瘤活性。在超过十余个恶性肿瘤中单独应用 IFN-α2 被证明有临床获益。IFN 独特的分子学及细胞学效应是其他治疗机制的补充。大部分基因及生物反应调节效应在 24~48 小时达高峰，这与静脉注射或皮下注射后数分钟至数小时血清中浓度达最大值不相符[137-139]。静脉推注后，IFN-α2 的 α 相半衰期很短（小于 60 分钟），总的平均半衰期是 4~5 小时，血清中可检测浓度的时间是 12 小时。肌内注射或皮下注射，达峰时间为 3~8 小时[137]。IFN-β 的药理学特点是肌内注射或皮下注射时无法在血清中检测到药物浓度，但是确实发生了生物学反应调节作用及治疗效应[139]。脂质体 IFN 与未改进的 IFN 在动力学上有明显的差异[140-142]。每周一次给药即可使 7 天内 IFN-α2 的可测血清浓度超过体外基因诱导及细胞学效应所需的浓度。聚乙二醇化 IFN-α2 可有效用于治疗转移性肾癌、CML 及黑色素瘤[142,143]。

血液肿瘤

IFN-α2 用于 CML 新诊断患者可达到大于 75% 治疗缓解率[144,145]。少数患者出现完全的细胞遗传学缓解，年轻患者的缓解率更高。然而，由于干扰素有相当大的副作用，如果在大约 1 年的治疗后没有发现细胞遗传学改善，许多临床医生选择停止治疗。在研发出酪氨酸激酶抑制剂之前，干扰素是大多数 CML 患者的首选治疗方法。随着甲磺酸伊马替尼的研发而且干扰素的毒性比酪氨酸激酶抑制剂更强，干扰素越来越少应用于慢性粒细胞白血病中的治疗之中。近年来，联合治疗，如干扰素加伊马替尼，在临床试验中已使慢性粒细胞白血病患者得到长期缓解，并已成为新诊断慢性粒细胞白血病患者的标准治疗。法国 Spirit 试验显示，使用伊马替尼和 peg-IFN 联合使用单独与 IFN 相比，分子应答率更高[146]。但另一项研究未能证明其对无进展生存率有所改善[147]。因此，在推荐这组组合之前，我们仍需要额外的临床数据。

IFN-γ 已被用作 CML 的治疗方法，并且表现出不同程度的细胞遗传学改善[148]，但未能在随后的研究中显示任何效果，因此，不建议用于治疗 CML。

实体瘤

相对于单独应用细胞毒药，IFN-α2 单药治疗转移性黑色素瘤可获得大约 15% 的有效率[149-152]。因为反应的持久性通常建议将 IFN 与 DTIC 分开作为治疗转移性黑色素瘤的治疗方案。与化疗及 IL-2 联合，有效率可高达 45%，但是毒性也随之增加，而无进展生存期或总生存期未见明显延长[24,152-156]。一些临床试验中 IFN-α2 用于具有高复发风险患者（Ⅱb 期或Ⅲ期）的术后辅助治疗，可获得无病生存期及总生存期的延长[143,157-160]。对辅助治疗中生活质量调整的生存期进行分析，IFN-α2 仍然占优势[161]。因此，IFN-α2 在美国已成为Ⅱb 期或Ⅲ期黑色素瘤患者的标准治疗方法，该应用得到了荟萃分析的支持[161,162]。欧洲一项长期应用脂质体 IFN-α2 的大型临床试验已明确 IFN-α2 可提高高风险患者的无病生存期[163]。

脂质体 IFN 治疗转移性黑色素瘤的疗效使得人们进行了创新的试验设计：根据疲乏及厌食调整的剂量进行长期给药，试验结果表明可延长无病生存期[143,160,164]。

IFN 已广泛应用于肾细胞癌的治疗当中。有临床试验表明 IFN-α2 用于转移性肾癌可获得 4%~26% 的有效率，几个临床试验的平均有效率为 15%[165]。随后的工作是评价干扰素和其他生物反应调节剂，包括 IL-2 或与化疗药物，特别是 5-氟尿嘧啶（5-Fu）的联合使用。IFN-α 和 IL-2 联合应用已广泛应用于转移性肾细胞癌患者的治疗当中。第一阶段和第二阶段的试验表明，其有效率约为 20%，CR 率为 5%[166]。在两个比较 IFN-α 单独或联合其他治疗的随机试验中，生存率有统计学意义的显著增加[167,168]。其他随机临床试验表明那些即使存在远处转移灶仍切除肾脏，然后接受 IFN-α 治疗的患者有最大的生存期获益[169,170]。总之，由于许多研究未能显示接受联合细胞因子治疗的转移性肾细胞癌患者的生存优势，因此不能推荐其作为标准治疗。其他实体瘤例如卵巢癌、膀胱癌及基底细胞癌也有部分病例对 IFN-α 有效，尤其是那些肿瘤负荷比较小的患者[171-173]。

由于Ⅰ型和Ⅲ型干扰素的共享基因诱导谱导致了对Ⅲ型干扰素在癌症治疗中潜在作用的研究。Ⅲ型干扰素能有效地对抗反应性癌细胞，同时由于受体分布的限制，其副作用比Ⅰ型干扰素少[174]。最近在一项关于Ⅲ型干扰素对丙型肝炎病毒作用的第一阶段研究中，最近证实了Ⅲ型干扰素相比Ⅰ型干扰素的副作用较少。一些接受Ⅰ型干扰素治疗的患者出现中性粒细胞减少或贫血，但接受Ⅲ型干扰素治疗的患者仍然没有症状[175]。数据表明，Ⅲ型干扰素在癌症治疗中起到积极作用，副作用很少或没有，但仍处于起步阶段。

造血生长因子的作用

通过一系的精密的分裂过程，造血干细胞分化产生所有的血细胞。从功能上看，这些早期祖细胞具有自我更新、增殖和分化能力。造血系统的发展、动态平衡性、运输及反应能力均由一个复杂的、由细胞间信号介导的通信网络进行严格调控。这些信号是由直接的细胞与细胞、细胞与基质的接触或可溶性细胞因子介质的释放所触发。

造血生长因子的识别和克隆为血液学实践带来了革命性的变化。在粒细胞 G-CSF 和粒细胞巨噬细胞 GM-CSF 出现前，提高中性粒细胞减少症患者的白血细胞计数是不可想象的。今天,生长因子常规用于治疗化疗后中性粒细胞减少症,相对较少地,用于治疗化疗后血小板减少和贫血。它们也可以用于移植前干细胞的动员,扭转各种非恶性疾病中的血细胞减少,并且有可能调动免疫系统对抗感染和癌症。

促红细胞生成素

促红细胞生成素(erythropoietin,EPO)是调节红细胞生成的主要激素。它在治疗各种疾病相关的贫血中具有明确的作用(表 63-4)。

表 63-4 造血生长因子

染色体定位	受体	选定的生物活性
EPO7q21 GM-CSF 5q31. 1	EPO 受体 Ⅰ型受体 α(CD116)和(CDw131)β 亚基	促进红细胞前体的增殖、分化和存活 刺激多向祖细胞,BFU-E,粒细胞,巨噬细胞以及嗜酸性粒细胞克隆生长 诱导血管内皮细胞的迁移和增殖 激活成熟的吞噬细胞(中性粒细胞,巨噬细胞,嗜酸性粒细胞)
G-CSF17q11. 2-q12	G-CS 受体(CD114)	调节中性粒细胞的产生和功能
M-CSF1p21-p13	Fms(CD115)	影响单核细胞/巨噬细胞发育和功能的多个方面 刺激造血 诱导破骨细胞的生成 有利于维持妊娠 降低胆固醇水平 影响小神经胶质细胞的功能
SCF12q22-12q24	c-kit(CD117)	在多个水平促进造血 在胚胎期影响原始生殖细胞和黑色素细胞的迁移 影响免疫调节细胞(B 和 T 细胞,肥大细胞,NK 细胞,树突状细胞) 影响造血细胞的黏附特性
TPO3q27-q28	Mpl(CD110)	血小板生成的主要调节者 与 EPO 协同刺激红系祖细胞经济的生长 与 IL-3 和 SCF 协同刺激造血干细胞的增殖并延长其生存期

EPO 的生物学活性

EPO 向早期红系祖细胞[红系爆发集落形成单位(BFU-E)]提供增殖信号,并向后期的红系前体细胞[红系集落形成单位(CFU-E)]提供分化信号。EPO 也能促进巨核细胞分化、B 细胞增殖和内皮细胞趋化。

EPO 与恶性肿瘤

一方面,在因恶性肿瘤导致的贫血患者中,尤其是血液恶性肿瘤患者中,常发现高水平的内源性 EPO 在另一方面,在许多肿瘤患者中,甚至是在因恶性肿瘤导致的贫血患者中,存在内源性 EPO 的相对缺乏。换而言之,虽然这种分子的浓度提高了,但是仍然达不到与贫血程度相适应的水平。某些家族性红细胞增多症的病例归于 EPO-高敏细胞的出现。增高的 EPO 反应是由于患者体内形成了截短的 EPO 受体,其负性调节区域缺失[176]。

EPO 的临床应用

EPO 用于治疗存在绝对或相对的内源性 EPO 水平缺乏的贫血最有效。EPO 首先成功地用于纠正慢性肾衰竭相关贫血的替代治疗,EPO 也可有效地增加实体肿瘤和恶性血液疾病以及许多其他疾病患者的血红蛋白[177]。

EPO 通常用于血红蛋白<10g/dl 的显著贫血的患者。美国 FDA 建议适当使用 EPO 以避免输血,而不是使血红蛋白水平正常化。然而,在癌症患者中,不是所有的患者均出现治疗反应,那些内源性 EPO 水平最高的患者获益的可能性较小。

粒细胞-巨噬细胞集落刺激因子

粒细胞-巨噬细胞集落刺激因子(granulocyte macrophage colony-stimulating factor,GM-CSF)是第一个进入临床试验的 CSF。如今,它已在许多国家被批准用于治疗化疗或移植后中性粒细胞减少症,治疗移植物植入失败以及外周血干细胞动员。

GM-CSF 的主要生物学活性

GM-CSF 刺激多能干细胞的增殖,刺激 BFU-E、粒细胞、巨噬细胞和嗜酸性粒细胞克隆的生长。GM-CSF 也增强了大多数吞噬细胞,包括中性粒细胞、巨噬细胞和嗜酸性粒细胞的功能活性。

GM-CSF 与恶性肿瘤

髓样白血病细胞和细胞系中的自分泌表达的 GM-CSF 被认为在肿瘤形成中发挥作用[178]。肿瘤自主产生的 GM-CSF(或 G-CSF)也被认为是癌症患者类白血病反应的一个可能的病理生理机制[179]。此外,在类风湿性关节炎患者的滑液存在 GM-CSF 的生物学活性,表明它可能增强与这种疾病相关的组织破坏。

已证明 GM-CSF 治疗接受诱导治疗的 AML 患者是安全和有效的。这种分子可缩短中性粒细胞减少持续时间,并降低老年患者的严重感染率。GM-CSF 还用于加速异基因 BMT 后的骨髓重建。这种分子也提高了异体或自体移植后的移植物植入失败或延迟患者的生存。最后，应用 GM-CSF 进行外周血造血干细胞动员产生的集落数目显著多于未应用 GM-CSF，并且移植后接受 GM-CSF 动员的祖细胞的患者中性粒细胞、血小板和红细胞恢复更快，住院时间更短。

粒细胞集落刺激因子

粒细胞集落刺激因子为中性粒细胞减少及其后遗症（感染）的治疗带来了革命性的变化。它在全世界被广泛应用，被认为是显著有效并且几乎没有副作用[180,181]。

CSF 的生物学活性

G-CSF 是一个造血祖细胞向中性粒细胞谱系生长和分化的相对特异的刺激因子。它还能保护中性粒细胞免于凋亡，并增强其功能（趋化，吞噬，氧化反应，杀菌活性）。最后，G-CSF 使成熟的中性粒细胞从骨髓释放进入血液循环。

G-CSF 与人类疾病

在健康人，G-CSF 平均值±标准差水平为 25±19.7pg/ml。G-CSF 水平在感染时增加 30 倍，感染性休克时增加 10 000 倍[182]。一些实体肿瘤患者出现白细胞计数显著增加。其中一些患者血清 G-CSF（或 GM-CSF）水平升高，可能是白细胞计数上升的原因[179]。据推测，G-CSF（或 GM-CSF）是由肿瘤本身所产生。

AML 患者存在 G-CSF 受体基因的点突变，导致严重的先天性中粒细胞减少症。这些突变截断了 G-CSF 受体胞质区的 C-末端，因此被推测中断了受体的成熟信号[183]。

将 G-CSF 作为实体瘤和淋巴瘤标准剂量化疗的辅助治疗的研究证实，在应用 G-CSF 周期中，中性粒细胞减少的持续时间、住院天数以及抗生素治疗天数显著降低。在小细胞肺癌患者中进行的安慰剂对照的研究显示，G-CSF 对发热性中性粒细胞减少具有临床显著意义的保护作用[184]。高剂量化疗后，当患者接受 G-CSF 治疗时，中性粒细胞减少及其相关并发症的恢复更快速。这些研究表明，G-CSF 支持可以增加非清髓性化疗的剂量强度。在移植中，G-CSF 可减少中性粒细胞减少症和感染[185]。G-CSF 也用于动员自体外周血造血干细胞，这些细胞被用于接受清髓性或骨髓抑制化疗的患者以加速造血恢复[186]。

已研发了一种新型的 G-CSF，G-CSF 单甲氧基乙二醇的共轭体。聚乙二醇化的 G-CSF 肾脏清除率降低，因此半衰期延长。血清清除率与中性粒细胞数直接相关。因此，化疗后仅需皮下应用一次聚乙二醇化的 G-CSF（Neulasta）。基于随机双盲临床试验的结果，该分子用于接受发热性中性粒细胞减少发生率很高的骨髓抑制化疗的非骨髓恶性肿瘤患者，以降低感染的发生率[187]。

巨噬细胞集落刺激因子

虽然巨噬细胞集落刺激因子（M-CSF）可影响多种器官系统，其主要的效果仍然是影响单核细胞/噬细胞的生长和功能的各个方面。

M-CSF 的生物学活性

M-CSF 刺激祖细胞的分化为成熟的单核细胞，并延长单核细胞的生存期。它增强了单核细胞和巨噬细胞的细胞毒、过氧化物生成、吞噬作用、趋化和二次细胞因子产生（G-CSF，IL-6，IL-8）的能力。除刺激造血此外，M-CSF 还促进破骨细胞祖细胞的分化和增殖，对脂质代谢具有深远的影响。

M-CSF 与恶性肿瘤

M-CSF 参与动脉粥样硬化错综复杂的发病机制，但有关它的作用仍然是有争议的。例如，应用 M-CSF 可降低胆固醇水平。自相矛盾的是，即使在高脂血症存在下，缺乏 M-CSF 对动脉粥样硬化的发生具有保护作用[188]。M-CSF 及在脑组织中表达。这种细胞因子诱导小神经胶质细胞的增殖、活化和生存。

在恶性肿瘤当中，据报道人类髓系恶性肿瘤（包括骨髓增生异常和 AML）约 10% 的病例有 Fms 基因（M-CSF 受体）密码子 969 的突变。

M-CSF 的临床应用

在一项大规模的研究中，已证实 AML 患者巩固化疗后应用 M-CSF 可缩短化疗后中性粒细胞减少和血小板减少的持续时间，并且可降低中性粒细胞减少性发热的发生率、缩短其持续时间[189]。据报道化疗或 BMT 后应用 M-CSF 可取得类似获益。M-CSF 可以提高儿童慢性中性粒细胞减少症患者的中性粒细胞计数。最后，非对照试验的初步结果表明，这种分子可以改善真菌感染后的结局[190]。

干细胞因子

干细胞因子（stem cell factor，SCF），也被称为 kit 配体，肥大细胞生长因子，或钢因子。它是一种造血细胞因子，通过与 c-kit（SCF 受体）结合触发其生物效应[191]。

SCF 的生物学活性

骨髓间质成分产生 SCF。现已明确 SCF 作用于造血干细胞，并作用于某些谱系的成熟细胞。

SCF 协同其他细胞因子（包括 EPO，IL-3，GM-CSF 和 G-CSF）在半固体培养基中直接促进 BFU-E、CFU-GM、CFU-粒/红/巨噬细胞/巨核细胞（GEMM）集落生长，并且目前的数据表明，SCF 可作用于能够生成直接克隆形成细胞的更原始的细胞（前 CFU-C）。SCF 还能促进祖细胞的存活，加速干细胞进入细胞周期，并可作为这些细胞的作为趋化和化学激动因子。当将 SCF 与 TPO 或 IL-3 联合应用时，还观察到对巨核细胞祖细胞的协同增殖作用[192]。SCF 也参与细胞黏附和运输的过程。SCF 诱导祖细胞黏附于纤维连接蛋白，在这个过程中，配体结合后 c-kit 受体激酶活化产生一个由内而外的信号，使整联蛋白亲和力发生了变化。或者，成纤维细胞 SCF 的跨膜部分直接与造血细胞表面的 c-kit 受体结合，这样有助于造血细胞在微环境中定殖[192]。

SCF 与 G-CSF 的联合应用时效果更加显著[193]。1 期临床研究显示，应用 SCF 可增加骨髓中多种类型细胞的祖细胞数量（包括 BFU-E、CFU-GM、CFU-Meg 和 CFU-GEMM）[194]。

恶性肿瘤中的 SCF 与 c-kit

正常人体血清中 SCF 的浓度平均为 3.3ng/ml。再生障碍性贫血，骨髓增生异常，慢性贫血，或清髓性治疗后血清 SCF 水平不升高[192]。与 EPO 水平不同，循环中 SCF 水平，不与血细胞比容成反比。

皮肤内 SCF 局部分布的改变与皮肤肥大细胞增多症的发病机制有关。c-kit 受体胞浆区的点突变已经在小鼠和人肥大细胞株以及肥大细胞疾病患者的造血干细胞中得以确定[192]。

kit 的活化突变是一种类型的平滑肌肉瘤—胃肠间质瘤的特点。

人类造血细胞肿瘤(AML,间变性大细胞淋巴瘤,霍奇金病)也表达 c-kit 受体。红白血病细胞株的受体密度最高,每个细胞可表达 50 000~100 000c-kit 的受体。实体瘤细胞系以及各种新鲜的人类肿瘤组织中也表达 c-kit 受体蛋白[192]。

SCF 的临床应用

已进行了许多项关于 SCF 的临床试验。SCF 似乎耐受性良好,主要的副作用是短暂的局限性红斑和注射部位的持久色素沉着。最令人担忧的不良反应是一种肥大细胞效应导致的过敏样反应,以荨麻疹为特征,伴或不伴呼吸道症状[192]。SCF 的副作用,包括过敏现象,似乎是剂量依赖性的。

特别有趣的是胃肠道间质瘤 SCF 受体(kit)的基因突变的作用。突变激活了 kit 激酶的活性。已发现靶向于 kit 的激酶抑制剂(STI571 或格列卫)是治疗这些众所周知的化疗抗拒肿瘤的显著有效的药物[195]。

血小板生成素

巨核细胞和血小板生成的体液基础一直比其他谱系的血细胞难以理解。目前认为至少在某些方面影响血小板发展的因素包括 IL-3、IL-6、IL-10、IL-11、G-CSF、GM-CSF、SCF、白血病抑制因子和 TPO。TPO 被认为对血小板生成发挥极为重要的生理调节作用。然而,不幸的是,与在中性粒细胞减少患者中粒细胞生成因子的显著效果相比,临床应用血小板生成分子的效果不太理想。

TPO 的生物学特征

有实验证实,消除 TPO 或其受体基因,导致可移植干细胞的数量减少 65%~95%。这一结果支持除了血小板生成 TPO 还在总体上参与造血过程。在循环中 TPO 的存活时间长于其他造血生长因子(半衰期=30 小时)。

TPO 与恶性肿瘤

已发现的常染色体显性遗传性血小板增多症患者血清 TPO 升高[196]。TPO 基因左拼接剪接突变,使 5′-非翻译区缩短,较其正常结构翻译效率更高,导致 TPO 过度产生[196]。由于血小板自身可调节循环 TPO 水平,所以在骨髓造血功能衰竭的患者也可发现高水平的 TPO。c-mpl(TPO 受体)纯合子缺失可导致先天性无巨核细胞性血小板减少症。

TPO 的临床应用

两种结构的 TPO 已进入临床试验阶段[197,198],分别为 TPO(全长多肽)和聚乙二醇(PEG)化的重组人巨核细胞生长和发育因子(PEG-conjugated recombinant human megakaryocyte growth and development factor,PEG-rHuMGDF)。因为 TPO 的生物学行为是长效的,所以肠胃外给药 TPO 连续 7~10 天,使 6~16 天后的血小板生成增加[199]。进行了一些临床试验评价 PEG-rHuMGDF 或重组人 TPO 治疗接受化疗的癌症患者的效果,虽然研究采用的方案仅导致中度血小板减少,但是研究结果显示血小板计数恢复至基线显著加快,血小板计数最低值也较高[200,201]。然而,清髓性治疗后应用这些分子加快血小板恢复的有效性尚不明确[202]。此外,在外周血造血干细胞移植或骨髓移植后血小板恢复延迟的患者,重组人 TPO 没有显著地提高大多数患者的血小板计数[203]。

对未来的展望

十年前对细胞因子早期的了解现在已转变为复杂的相互作用的刺激性和抑制性因子的相交织的景象。对这一过程有影响的许多分子已被克隆并已进入临床试验。现已明确,调节性细胞因子是多效性的,在同一时间,表现出显著的多功能性。

医学的历史充满了创新技术如何改善临床结果的例子。基因工程技术允许迅速克隆新确定细胞因子并将其转化为血液学和肿瘤学的临床治疗,是这种现象的一个令人振奋的例子[204]。但是,应该记住的是,不是全部,也是大多数,细胞因子及其各自的天然抑制剂被广泛表达,具有无数的生物学特性,影响几乎每一个器官系统(图 63-1)。已经很明显,这些分子可能在过敏性和炎症状态下也发挥作用。此外,对作用越来越清楚地认识以及对重组分子用于治疗的可获得性表明,这些药物的临床作用将继续扩大,并有可能最终影响医学的各个领域。

(张清媛 译)

参考文献

The complete reference list can be found on the Wiley Companion Digital Edition of this title (see inside front cover for login instructions).

1 Dinarello CA. Interleukin-1, interleukin-1 receptors and interleukin-1 receptor antagonist. *Int Rev Immunol*. 1998;**16**:457–499.

14 Grimm EA, Owen-Schaub LB, Loudon WG, et al. Lymphokine-activated killer cells. Induction and function. *Ann N Y Acad Sci*. 1988;**532**:380–386.

17 Rosenberg SA. IL-2: the first effective immunotherapy for human cancer. *J Immunol*. 2014;**192**:5451–5458.

21 Prieto PA, Yang JC, Sherry RM, et al. CTLA-4 blockade with ipilimumab: long-term follow-up of 177 patients with metastatic melanoma. *Clin Cancer Res*. 2012;**18**:2039–2047.

23 Saranga-Perry V, Ambe C, Zager JS, et al. Recent developments in the medical and surgical treatment of melanoma. *CA Cancer J Clin*. 2014;**64**:171–185.

27 Ribas A, Flaherty KT. BRAF targeted therapy changes the treatment paradigm in melanoma. *Nat Rev Clin Oncol*. 2011;**8**:426–433.

28 Frederick DT, Piris A, Cogdill AP, et al. BRAF inhibition is associated with enhanced melanoma antigen expression and a more favorable tumor microenvironment in patients with metastatic melanoma. *Clin Cancer Res*. 2013;**19**:1225–1231.

37 Kurzrock R, Talpaz M, Estrov Z, et al. Phase I study of recombinant human interleukin-3 in patients with bone marrow failure. *J Clin Oncol*. 1991;**9**:1241–1250.

56 Kurzrock R, Redman J, Cabanillas F, et al. Serum interleukin 6 levels are elevated in lymphoma patients and correlate with survival in advanced Hodgkin's disease and with B symptoms. *Cancer Res*. 1993;**53**:2118–2122.

62 Ebrahimi B, Tucker SL, Li D, et al. Cytokines in pancreatic carcinoma: correlation with phenotypic characteristics and prognosis. *Cancer*. 2004;**101**:2727–2736.

66 Blade J, de Larrea CF, Rosinol L. Incorporating monoclonal antibodies into the therapy of multiple myeloma. *J Clin Oncol*. 2012;**30**:1904–1906.

90 Akdis CA, Blaser K. Mechanisms of interleukin-10-mediated immune suppression. *Immunology*. 2001;**103**:131–136.

100 Trinchieri G. Interleukin-12: a cytokine at the interface of inflammation and immunity. *Adv Immunol*. 1998;**70**:83–243.

104 Ku CC, Murakami M, Sakamoto A, et al. Control of homeostasis of CD8+ memory T cells by opposing cytokines. *Science*. 2000;**288**:675–678.

116 Parrish-Novak J, Dillon SR, Nelson A, et al. Interleukin 21 and its receptor are involved in NK cell expansion and regulation of lymphocyte function. *Nature*. 2000;**408**:57–63.

119 Caudell EG, Mumm JB, Poindexter N, et al. The protein product of the tumor suppressor gene, melanoma differentiation-associated gene 7, exhibits immunostimulatory activity and is designated IL-24. *J Immunol*. 2002;**168**:6041–6046.

121 Ekmekcioglu S, Ellerhorst J, Mhashilkar AM, et al. Down-regulated melanoma differentiation associated gene (mda-7) expression in human melanomas. *Int J Cancer*. 2001;**94**:54–59.

128 Chen Q, Ghilardi N, Wang H, et al. Development of Th1-type immune responses requires the type I cytokine receptor TCCR. *Nature*. 2000;**407**:916–920.

130 Witte K, Witte E, Sabat R, et al. IL-28A, IL-28B, and IL-29: promising cytokines with type I interferon-like properties. *Cytokine Growth Factor Rev.* 2010;**21**:237–251.

133 Dinarello C, Arend W, Sims J, et al. IL-1 family nomenclature. *Nat Immunol.* 2010;**11**:973.

135 Nold MF, Nold-Petry CA, Zepp JA, et al. IL-37 is a fundamental inhibitor of innate immunity. *Nat Immunol.* 2010;**11**:1014–1022.

141 Talpaz M, O'Brien S, Rose E, et al. Phase 1 study of polyethylene glycol formulation of interferon alpha-2B (Schering 54031) in Philadelphia chromosome-positive chronic myelogenous leukemia. *Blood.* 2001;**98**:1708–1713.

146 Preudhomme C, Guilhot J, Nicolini FE, et al. Imatinib plus peginterferon alfa-2a in chronic myeloid leukemia. *N Engl J Med.* 2010;**363**:2511–2521.

148 Kurzrock R, Talpaz M, Kantarjian H, et al. Therapy of chronic myelogenous leukemia with recombinant interferon-gamma. *Blood.* 1987;**70**:943–947.

154 Ridolfi R, Chiarion-Sileni V, Guida M, et al. Cisplatin, dacarbazine with or without subcutaneous interleukin-2, and interferon alpha-2b in advanced melanoma outpatients: results from an Italian multicenter phase III randomized clinical trial. *J Clin Oncol.* 2002;**20**:1600–1607.

158 Kirkwood JM, Manola J, Ibrahim J, et al. A pooled analysis of eastern cooperative oncology group and intergroup trials of adjuvant high-dose interferon for melanoma. *Clin Cancer Res.* 2004;**10**:1670–1677.

169 Mickisch GH, Garin A, van Poppel H, et al. Radical nephrectomy plus interferon-alfa-based immunotherapy compared with interferon alfa alone in metastatic renal-cell carcinoma: a randomised trial. *Lancet.* 2001;**358**: 966–970.

170 Flanigan RC, Salmon SE, Blumenstein BA, et al. Nephrectomy followed by interferon alfa-2b compared with interferon alfa-2b alone for metastatic renal-cell cancer. *N Engl J Med.* 2001;**345**:1655–1659.

174 Hamming OG, Gad HH, Paludan S, Hartmann R. Lambda interferons: new cytokines with old functions. *Pharmaceuticals.* 2010;**3**:795–809.

175 Miller DM, Klucher KM, Freeman JA, et al. Interferon lambda as a potential new therapeutic for hepatitis C. *Ann N Y Acad Sci.* 2009;**1182**:80–87.

177 Adamson JW. Epoetin alfa: into the new millennium. *Semin Oncol.* 1998;**25**: 76–79.

182 Hubel K, Dale DC, Liles WC. Therapeutic use of cytokines to modulate phagocyte function for the treatment of infectious diseases: current status of granulocyte colony-stimulating factor, granulocyte-macrophage colony-stimulating factor, macrophage colony-stimulating factor, and interferon-gamma. *J Infect Dis.* 2002;**185**:1490–1501.

192 Broudy VC. Stem cell factor and hematopoiesis. *Blood.* 1997;**90**:1345–1364.

195 Demetri GD, von Mehren M, Blanke CD, et al. Efficacy and safety of imatinib mesylate in advanced gastrointestinal stromal tumors. *N Engl J Med.* 2002;**347**:472–480.

197 Kaushansky K, Drachman JG. The molecular and cellular biology of thrombopoietin: the primary regulator of platelet production. *Oncogene.* 2002;**21**: 3359–3367.

第 64 章　单克隆抗体血清治疗

Robert C. Bast Jr. , MD ■ Michael R. Zalutsky, PhD, MA ■ Arthur E. Frankel, MD

概述

单克隆抗体的出现深刻改变了癌症患者的治疗。美国食品药品管理局(Food and Drug Administration, FDA)已经批准了 22 种单克隆抗体、细胞毒偶联物、放射性核素偶联物及靶向毒素用于多种不同恶性肿瘤的治疗,虽然其中 3 种已经退出市场。有效的单克隆抗体大多数是针对肿瘤细胞表面的蛋白[利妥昔单抗(rituximab)针对 CD20,曲妥珠单抗(trastuzumab)针对 HER2]来抑制生长,诱导凋亡并增强化疗疗效。也有一些则针对细胞因子[司妥昔单抗(siltuximab)针对白介素 6]、生长因子[贝伐珠单抗(bevacizumab)针对血管内皮生长因子]以及生长因子受体[雷莫芦单抗(ramucirumab)针对 VEGFR2],从而影响肿瘤血管的内皮细胞。或者通过中和性的免疫检查点抑制剂[伊匹木单抗(ipilimumab)针对 CTLA4 及纳武利尤单抗(nivolumab)或帕博利珠单抗(pembrolizumab)针对 PD1]来改变免疫应答。以曲妥珠单抗及帕妥珠单抗为例,它们与 HER2 细胞表面受体的不同位点结合,可以较单药应用产生更强的抗肿瘤活性。通过抗体与细胞毒性药物[美坦辛(emtansine)与抗 HER2 曲妥珠单抗及 vendotin 与抗 CD30 本妥昔单抗]或放射性核素偶联(钇-90 与抗 CD20 替伊莫单抗)可以增强对肿瘤细胞的杀灭,为非偶联抗体治疗失败的患者带来了有效的治疗手段。单克隆抗体治疗发挥疗效仍然存在重重障碍,包括抗原特异性、抗原调变、抗原表达的异质性、有效输送抗体至肿瘤细胞、效应物机制的潜能及对外源性球蛋白的反应。其中最后一个问题可以通过嵌合结构、鼠抗体的人源化以及开发基因工程改造的老鼠使其具备产生完全的人源抗体的能力。随着我们关于肿瘤生物学及免疫学知识的增长,非偶联抗体的应用也在不断进步,发现新的靶点比如 OX-40 配体。应用更小的分子工程改造的结合物则可以进一步提高血清治疗的药代动力学及药效学。而由于抗原异质性的存在,抗体可能需要联合应用。抗体偶联物的研发也需要鉴别出能够针对肿瘤启动干细胞的单克隆试剂。预定位及 α 发射器的使用是改进抗体放射性核素偶联物的有效手段。靶向毒素的研发还需要更为深入的探索。

简介

自 Kohler 和 Milstein 初次报道之后[1],单克隆抗体技术就对实验室研究产生了迅速而重大的影响。在过去 40 年中,单克隆试剂的应用使得新型标记物的体外应用获得了发展,包括用于监测治疗反应、应用组织化学方法检测恶性细胞、区分预后良好和预后不良的患者亚群以及鉴别一些原发不明的肿瘤。虽然目前体内应用单克隆抗体治疗人类肿瘤的进展有所减缓,但单克隆抗体及其偶联物的血清治疗在众多血液系统肿瘤及实体瘤治疗中的地位已经确立[2-5]。截止到 2015 年,FDA 已批准 43 种非偶联单克隆抗体、偶联药物及放射性核素偶联物用于临床治疗,适应证包括移植排斥、冠状动脉血栓、呼吸道合胞病毒感染、类风湿关节炎、系统性红斑狼疮、阵发性睡眠性血红蛋白尿、黄斑变性、炎性肠病、牛皮癣、哮喘和肿瘤[6,7]。43 种中有 21 种被批准用于不同肿瘤的治疗,包括一种靶向毒素(表 64-1)。3 种之前被批准的抗癌单克隆抗体已经退市。而无修饰的单克隆抗体为急性及慢性淋巴细胞白血病、霍奇金淋巴瘤及非霍奇金淋巴瘤、Castleman 病、神经母细胞瘤、HER2 扩增的乳腺癌、非小细胞肺癌、头颈部肿瘤、结直肠癌及胃癌患者的治疗作出了贡献。这些药物的广泛应用显示出单克隆血清治疗已经在临床肿瘤学中建立了一定的地位。

为了在体内获得更强的抗肿瘤活性,单克隆抗体常常偶联上细胞毒性药物、放射性核素和免疫毒素。每一种免疫偶联物目前都已进行了大量的临床前研究和临床研究,其中几种已经获得 FDA 的批准用于多个瘤种的治疗[8]。本章将讨论单克隆制剂、放射性核素偶联物和靶向毒素目前的临床应用以及未来进一步发展的机遇与挑战。

表 64-1　美国批准的用于癌症治疗的单克隆抗体、放射性核素偶联物和靶向毒素

抗体	商品名	FDA 批准年份	类型	抗原靶位	适应证
利妥昔单抗	Rituxan	1997 年	嵌合	CD20	复发或难治性滤泡淋巴瘤和低度恶性非霍奇金淋巴瘤
曲妥珠单抗	Herceptin	1998 年	人源	HER-2	过表达 HER-2 的转移性乳腺癌
地尼白介素毒素连接物	Ontak	1999 年	人源	CD25	皮肤 T 细胞白血病

续表

抗体	商品名	FDA 批准年份	类型	抗原靶位	适应证
吉姆单抗	Mylotarg	2000 年[a]	人源 ADC	CD33	老年患者复发性急性髓系白血病
阿伦单抗	Campath	2001 年[a]	人源	CD52	B 细胞慢性淋巴细胞白血病
钇-90-替伊莫单抗	Zevalin	2002 年	小鼠 ARC	CD20	老年患者或利妥昔单抗耐药的复发或难治性滤泡淋巴瘤和低度恶性非霍奇金淋巴瘤
碘-131-托西莫单抗	Bexxar	2003 年[a]	小鼠 ARC	CD20	老年患者或利妥昔单抗耐药的复发或难治性滤泡淋巴瘤和低度恶性非霍奇金淋巴瘤
西妥昔单抗	Erbitux	2004 年 2006 年	嵌合	EGFR	与伊立替康联合治疗转移性结直肠癌 与放射治疗联合治疗头颈部肿瘤
贝伐珠单抗	Avastin	2004 年 2006 年 2008 年 2009 年 2009 年 2014 年	人源	VEGF	转移性结直肠癌 非小细胞肺癌 进展期乳腺癌[a] 肾细胞癌 胶质母细胞瘤 卵巢癌

[a] 从市场撤回。

无修饰的单克隆抗体淋巴瘤和白血病的血清治疗

除极少数例外，小鼠抗人肿瘤单克隆抗体可识别肿瘤相关抗原，这些抗原也在正常成人或胚胎组织中表达。不过，一些抗原仅仅在少数的正常细胞中表达，对患者的健康是无关紧要的。非偶联的单克隆抗体为淋巴瘤[3]及白血病[9,10]患者的治疗带来了显著的获益。

抗独特型抗体

在 20 世纪 80 年代早期，Levy 和他的同事制备了针对独特表位（unique idiotope）的肿瘤特异性小鼠单克隆抗体，这种独特表位与人 B 细胞淋巴瘤中表达的细胞表面膜免疫球蛋白相关，但至多只在很少量的正常 B 细胞亚群中表达[11,12]。18 例接受抗独特型抗体单独治疗的患者中，客观缓解率为 67%，几乎无毒性，一位患者完全缓解时间持续了 72 个月，生存时间超过 17 年[6]。在后续的试验中，抗独特型抗体与干扰素（IFN）-α、苯丁酸氮芥或 IL-2 联合。大多数在体内产生应答的抗体为小鼠免疫球蛋白 G1（IgG1）同种型（isotype），其结合补体或参与抗体依赖的细胞介导的细胞毒性反应（antibody-dependent cell-mediated cytotoxicity，ADCC）效果通常最弱。抗独特型抗体与 B 细胞受体复合物结合，似乎会通过发出死亡信号诱导凋亡（程序性细胞死亡）。在一小部分经抗独特型抗体治疗的患者中，淋巴瘤复发与肿瘤细胞丢失相关抗原有关。编码细胞表面膜免疫球蛋白的基因发生点突变，导致独特型决定簇丢失[13]。抗独特型抗体的使用已经为此理论提供了有力证据，但其广泛应用受制于为每一位患者提供个性化制剂的逻辑挑战。

抗 CD20 单抗

利妥昔单抗

不同患者的肿瘤细胞共享有一些相同的分化抗原（differentiation antigens），抗分化抗原的单克隆抗体也被用来治疗非霍奇金淋巴瘤（non Hodgkin lymphoma，NHL）以及急性和慢性白血病。CD20 就是经证实有用的靶位之一，它是一个分子量 35kDa 的钙通道磷蛋白，在所有正常 B 细胞和 80% NHL 细胞表面表达，但在其他正常组织中不表达。针对 CD20 不同抗原决定簇的特异性抗体可以分为 2 类，Ⅰ类将 CD20 易位至细胞膜内不溶于活性剂的脂筏中，从而促进补体依赖的细胞毒效应；Ⅱ类不诱导脂筏而是促进由 Fcγ 受体的自然杀伤（nature killer，NK）细胞及巨噬细胞介导的 ADCC 效应[3]。利妥昔单抗是一种属于Ⅰ类的嵌合性的小鼠/人抗 CD20 IgG1 抗体，每周重复给药一次治疗复发性低度恶性滤泡 NHL 的缓解率为 48%～50%，至中位进展时间为 10.2～13.2 个月[14,15]。在 37 例新诊断的患者中，使用利妥昔单抗治疗的总缓解率为 72%，其中完全缓解率 36%，中位至疾病进展时间 2.2 年[16]。所以，利妥昔单抗一开始被批准用于复发或难治的惰性滤泡性 NHL，并逐渐扩展至单药或与化疗联合治疗初诊的低级别非霍奇金淋巴瘤及其维持治疗[17]。利妥昔单抗也可用于弥漫大 B 细胞 NHL、慢性淋巴细胞白血病及自身免疫病的治疗。

滤泡性及惰性非霍奇金淋巴瘤

自从 1997 年被美国 FDA 批准用于治疗复发性或难治性滤

泡或惰性NHL,利妥昔单抗的使用已经从4周疗程扩展到8周,并可重复治疗之前对其有反应的患者[18]。60例复发患者再次采用相似疗程的利妥昔单抗治疗,总缓解率为38%,其中完全缓解率为10%,中位至进展时间延长至15个月[19]。40例低度恶性滤泡淋巴瘤,其中一些既往接受过化疗,采用利妥昔单抗联合环磷酰胺、阿霉素、长春新碱和泼尼松(cyclophosphamide,doxorubicin,vincristine,and prednisone,CHOP)治疗后,总缓解率达100%,其中完全缓解率58%,部分缓解率42%。中位至进展时间延长至40.5个月[20]。对包含1 943例滤泡淋巴瘤、其他惰性淋巴瘤和侵袭性更高的套细胞淋巴瘤的7项试验进行荟萃分析,化疗联合利妥昔单抗治疗后,总生存期延长,其中惰性淋巴瘤显著性好于套细胞组织类型[21]。环磷酰胺、长春新碱和泼尼松(cyclophosphamide,vincristine,and prednisone,CVP)方案联合利妥昔单抗治疗初治的滤泡性NHL可延长疾病进展时间,因而FDA在2006年批准了利妥昔单抗应用于一线治疗[22]。已经有4项随机试验证实利妥昔单抗维持治疗可延长无进展生存期(progression-free survival,PFS),但总生存期只在一些研究而不是全部研究中获得延长[23]。2011年,美国FDA批准了利妥昔单抗应用于维持治疗,主要基于一项随机对照研究,在1 018名既往接受利妥昔单抗治疗以及1/3接受了化疗获得完全或部分缓解的高瘤负荷的滤泡性NHL患者中,对比了利妥昔单抗维持治疗(最多12次8周方案)和不接受维持治疗。结果显示利妥昔单抗降低了46%的PFS事件风险($P<0.000\,1$)。在第3年,利妥昔单抗维持治疗组患者PFS率为74.9%,观察组仅为57.6%($P<0.000\,1$)[24]。

弥漫大B细胞NHL

侵袭性更高的弥漫大B细胞NHL对利妥昔单抗单药治疗反应较差。54例复发的患者使用利妥昔单抗治疗8周期,总缓解率为31%,其中完全缓解率9%。治疗缓解的患者中位至进展时间为8个月或更长时间[25]。成人淋巴瘤研究组开展了一项试验,399例老年患者,均罹患侵袭性较高的弥漫大B细胞NHL,随机接受CHOP联合利妥昔单抗治疗或CHOP单用。联合治疗组观察到的完全缓解率为76%,对比CHOP单用组为60%[26]。联合利妥昔单抗组无事件生存期($P<0.005$)和总生存期($P<0.01$)显著延长。在两项验证性试验中,年轻患者和老年患者均取得了相似结果[27,28],从而使FDA在2006年批准了CHOP联合利妥昔单抗方案应用于弥漫大B细胞淋巴瘤,也使弥漫大B细胞淋巴瘤的系统性治疗在过去20年中首次取得了进展。在近期一项包含1 470例复发或难治弥漫大B细胞淋巴瘤患者的7项试验的荟萃分析中,利妥昔单抗的维持治疗带来了无进展生存期及总生存期的延长,但未达到统计学差异。但在挽救治疗中引入利妥昔单抗,相较无利妥昔单抗的方案显著延长了总生存期($P=0.02$)及无进展生存期($P<0.05$)[29]。但感染相关的副作用在利妥昔单抗治疗组中也更高(RR=1.37,$P=0.000\,1$)。

慢性淋巴细胞白血病及华氏(Waldenstrom)巨球蛋白血症

利妥昔单抗单药及与氟达拉滨的联合方案,已经扩大到对慢性淋巴细胞白血病(chronic lymphoblastic leukemia,CLL)的治疗[30]。在早期研究中,使用标准低剂量的利妥昔单抗,只能观察到很低的缓解率(15%),这可能与CLL细胞表面CD20浓度较低(每个细胞8~15 000位点对比90 000位点)和可溶性CD20脱落产生"抗原沉降"有关[31,32]。不过,使用更高剂量的利妥昔单抗治疗或每周给药3次,在CLL中取得46%的总缓解率,在初治患者中缓解率甚至更高[31]。一项癌症和白血病研究组(Cancer and Leukemia Group B,CALGB)试验中,42例CLL患者接受氟达拉滨和利妥昔单抗治疗,缓解率达到100%,其中完全缓解率为48%[33]。在两项Ⅲ期随机对照试验中,利妥昔单抗与氟达拉滨及环磷酰胺联用延长了经治及初治的CLL患者的无进展生存期达10~19月[34,35]。基于此,美国FDA在2010年批准了利妥昔单抗与氟达拉滨及环磷酰胺的联合治疗。利妥昔单抗还与烷化物一起治疗华氏巨球蛋白血症。一项研究报告,利妥昔单抗联合地塞米松和环磷酰胺治疗,缓解率为74%,2年无进展生存率为67%[36]。

自身免疫病

B淋巴细胞的耗竭可被用于自身免疫病的诊治,利妥昔单抗已经被批准与地塞米松联用于抗肿瘤坏死因子(tumor necrosis factor,TNF)治疗失败的类风湿关节炎患者的诊治,也被批准与糖皮质激素联用治疗肉芽肿性多血管炎(韦格纳肉芽肿)及显微镜下多血管炎(microscopic polyangiitis,MPA)[37]。

毒副反应

利妥昔单抗治疗总的来说耐受良好。绝大多数的不良反应与输液相关,在治疗开始的前几个小时内发生。不良反应通常持续几分钟到几小时,包括畏寒、发热、恶心、呕吐、疲乏、头痛、瘙痒和喉部肿胀感[38]。尽管77%的患者会发生不良反应,但严重者仅占10%[39]。在首次用药后,正常B淋巴细胞计数即可降至零;在停药后第6个月时开始恢复,在第9~12个月时完全恢复。由于成熟浆细胞不表达CD20,因此免疫球蛋白水平保持不变。随访1年内,并发感染需要住院治疗的患者仅占2%。自1997年获得FDA批准之后至2002年,美国有超过125 000例患者接受了利妥昔单抗治疗。在这些患者中,只有8例死于与治疗相关的毒副反应,包括输液反应、副肿瘤性天疱疮、斯-约综合征(Stevens-Johnson syndrome)和中毒性表皮坏死松解症[40]。有超过120例间质性肺疾病被报道,通常出现在利妥昔单抗与化疗联用的情况下,但也有25%与单药治疗相关[41]。近年来,利妥昔单抗的治疗被发现与乙肝表面抗原阴性/核心抗体阳性患者的乙肝病毒(hepatitis B virus,HBV)再激活相关。一项包含578名患者15项研究的荟萃分析发现,再激活的风险大约为6.3%[42],提示之前有HBV感染证据的患者接受利妥昔单抗治疗前应当检测病毒并预防性抗病毒治疗。

作用机制及耐药性

利妥昔单抗杀死白血病和淋巴瘤细胞的机制尚不完全清楚,可能包括ADCC反应、补体介导的细胞毒作用和与CD20结合后的直接作用[43]。在肿瘤细胞中,偶联的CD20可诱导细胞周期停滞,抑制DNA合成,激活天冬氨酸特异性半胱氨酸蛋白酶,并诱导凋亡[33]。对化疗的敏感性可能与抑制了AKT的组成性激活、引起抗凋亡蛋白Bcl-XL下调有关[44]。NK细胞、巨噬细胞和多形核白细胞是ADCC的重要效应物[33],已经在一些研究中观察到利妥昔单抗的临床反应和介导ADCC所需的IgG的FcγRⅢa和FcγRⅢa受体的特异等位基因多态性之间存在相关性[45]。个体NK细胞可以"连环杀灭"各种淋巴瘤细胞,尤其在存在利妥昔单抗时,能在含有CD20、ICAM-1及微管组织中心的肿瘤细胞的一极形成"帽子",从而增强对NK细胞杀伤的敏感性[3,46]。C1q 遗传缺陷的小鼠具有完整的 ADCC，但缺少补体途径的第一成分，从而缺乏补体介导的细胞毒作用，因此对利妥昔单抗的反应减弱[47]。利妥昔单抗治疗的临床耐药与 CD20 表达缺失基本无关，但可能与补体耐受蛋白 CD55 和 CD59 的上调有关[48]。有趣的是，对治疗之前获取的淋巴瘤细胞分析发现，对利妥昔单抗有效者和无效者其基因表达模式不同[49]。对利妥昔单抗治疗无效的肿瘤细胞的基因表达类似于正常的淋巴组织，编码某些补体成分的基因和涉及细胞因子、T 细胞和 TNF 信号转导的基因都显现出过高表达。

奥法木单抗

奥法木单抗是一种Ⅰ型人抗 CD20 IgG1 抗体，其结合表位不同于利妥昔单抗所识别的位点，并且有更高的亲和力及更慢的解离速率，能促进 CDC 及 ADCC 效应。基于一项对比奥法木单抗联合苯丁酸氮芥与单药苯丁酸氮芥的多中心随机对照开放试验的结果，奥法木单抗在 2009 年被美国 FDA 批准用于治疗慢性淋巴细胞白血病[50]。这项研究纳入了 447 名被研究者认为含氟达拉滨方案不适用的患者，包括高龄（中位年龄 69 岁）或存在合并症（72%存在 2 个或更多的合并症）。接受奥法木单抗及苯丁酸氮芥联合治疗的患者中位无进展生存期为 22.4 个月，而接受单药苯丁酸氮芥治疗的患者为 13.1 个月（$P<0.001$）。

毒副反应

奥法木单抗与苯丁酸氮芥联合应用最常见的不良反应（>5%）包括输液反应、中性粒细胞减少、疲乏、头痛、白细胞减少、单纯疱疹、下呼吸道感染、关节痛及上腹痛。总体上，67%接受奥法木单抗治疗的患者会经历一次或多次的输液反应，10%的患者会出现 3 级及以上的输液反应。

阿托珠单抗

阿托珠单抗是一种Ⅱ型人源化的抗 CD20 IgG1 抗体，主要通过 ADCC 起效，并通过糖基化来增强与效应细胞 FcγR 的结合[3]。阿托珠单抗与 CD20 的结合能够启动胞内信号转导、肌动蛋白纤维重组、溶酶体膜通透性的增加以及导致非凋亡性细胞死亡[51]。阿托珠单抗在 2013 年被美国 FDA 批准用于治疗慢性淋巴细胞白血病，主要基于一项在 781 例初治的老年或有合并症的患者中开展的对比单药苯丁酸氮芥与苯丁酸氮芥联合阿托珠单抗治疗的开放多中心随机对照研究[52]。接受阿托珠单抗及苯丁酸氮芥联合治疗的患者平均无进展生存时间为 26.7 个月，较苯丁酸氮芥单药治疗的 11.1 个月有显著改善。

毒副反应

接受阿托珠单抗与苯丁酸氮芥联合治疗的患者最常见的不良反应包括输液反应、中性粒细胞减少、血小板减少、贫血、肌肉骨骼疼痛及发热。阿托珠单抗获批的同时也伴随一个黑框警告，包括在其他抗 CD20 抗体中观察到的 HBV 再激活以及在其他阿托珠单抗的试验中极少数受试者出现的进行性多灶性脑白质病。

苯丁酸氮芥与阿托珠单抗或奥法木单抗联用为可能无法耐受氟达拉滨方案治疗的老年有合并症的慢性淋巴细胞白血病患者提供了一个替代选择[10]。

抗其他淋巴细胞相关性细胞表面膜蛋白的抗体

在过去的 30 年中，在不同 B 细胞来源的肿瘤患者中开展了众多临床试验，以评估抗 CD22、CD23、CD40、CD74 和 CD80 的抗体作用[23]。在对 CD10 阳性急性淋巴细胞白血病（acute lymphocytic leukemia，ALL）的早期研究中发现，抗 CD10 抗体可诱导 ALL 共同抗原迅速调变，阻碍有效的治疗[53]。静脉输注抗 CD5 同样会产生抗原调变，仅在一部分 T 细胞白血病/淋巴瘤和 CLL 患者中产生一过性的部分缓解[54]。在最早的单克隆制剂血清治疗试验之一中就证实，有血清阻断因子阻止单克隆抗体同血液循环中的淋巴肿瘤细胞结合，这与肿瘤抗原壳的存在相一致[55]。

抗白介素 6 的抗体

Castleman 病是一种由白介素 6 或其他细胞因子释放所导致的淋巴组织增生性疾病，可以局限在一个单一的淋巴结，也可呈多中心型。感染人类疱疹病毒 8（HHV-8）可以刺激细胞因子的释放，但有一部分 Castleman 病为 HHV-8 阴性且没有确切的白介素 6 的来源。

司妥昔单抗

司妥昔单抗在 2014 年被美国 FDA 及欧盟批准用于治疗 HIV 阴性且 HHV-8 阴性的多中心型 Castleman 病，主要基于一项国际多中心Ⅱ期随机对照（2∶1）研究。其对比了 53 名静脉输注司妥昔单抗并接受最佳支持治疗的患者与 26 名接受安慰剂及最佳支持治疗的患者[56]。与安慰剂对照组相比，司妥昔单抗带来了更高比例的肿瘤及症状的持续缓解（18 周）（34% vs 0，$P=0.0012$），肿瘤退缩（38%∶4%，$P<0.05$），中位至进展时间的延长（>422 天 vs 134 天，$P<0.05$）及血红蛋白水平的升高（36% vs 0，$P<0.05$）。虽然在 Castleman 病的治疗中获得了成功，但司妥昔单抗在其他白介素 6 信号转导被认为起重要作用的恶性肿瘤中未能显示出临床获益，包括多发性骨髓瘤、肾细胞癌及前列腺癌[57]。

毒副反应

在司妥昔单抗治疗过程中常见的不良反应（与安慰剂相比>10%）包括皮肤瘙痒、体重增加、皮疹、高尿酸血症及上呼吸道感染。所以司妥昔单抗是一个针对驱动一种少见但耗竭性的淋巴组织增生性疾病的一个细胞因子进行靶向治疗的很好的范例。

无修饰的单克隆抗体实体瘤的血清治疗

跨膜酪氨酸激酶生长因子受体 HER 家族，为实体瘤的血清治疗提供了靶点。如第 107 章概述，肽类生长因子配体与 HER 家族受体相互作用，激活 Ras-丝裂原激活蛋白激酶（MAPK）途径和磷脂酰肌醇 3-激酶（PI3K）途径的信号转导，提高正常细胞和肿瘤细胞的细胞周期进程、增殖和存活。在 HER 家族的 4 种受体中，最受关注的为 HER-1（表皮生长因子受体或 EGFR）和 HER-2。

抗 EGFR 抗体

EGFR 分子量为 170kDa，它在许多肿瘤包括非小细胞肺癌、头颈部肿瘤、胰腺癌和结直肠癌中过度表达。目前针对 EGFR 的胞外区研发了几种单克隆抗体。

西妥昔单抗

西妥昔单抗是一种嵌合型 IgG1 单克隆抗体，可阻断 EGFR

配体结合位点，阻止受体激活，诱导内化并下调受体水平。在试验系统中，应用西妥昔单抗治疗人肿瘤细胞，可使细胞周期停滞在G0~G1期，诱导p21活化，引导Rb去磷酸化，抑制增殖和阻断血管生成因子的产生，如血管内皮生长因子（vascular endothelial growth factor，VEGF）[58]。另外，应用西妥昔单抗可增强阿霉素、紫杉醇、拓扑替康和伊立替康及放射治疗对裸鼠的人类肿瘤移植物的作用。对细胞毒化疗和放疗的增强可能与以下因素有关：通过诱导BAX引起MAP激酶和PI3激酶的抑制，激活caspase8，下调BCL-2和NFκB，赋予肿瘤细胞对凋亡刺激物更高的敏感性[59]。另外，在外周血单核细胞存在时西妥昔单抗可诱导ADCC。仅需极少量的EGFR表达即可介导肿瘤细胞死于ADCC[60]。如同利妥昔单抗一样，西妥昔单抗治疗的无进展生存期与FcγR多态性有关，这与ADCC作为一项杀灭肿瘤细胞的机制的重要性相一致[61]。

结直肠癌

57例化疗后复发的结直肠癌患者接受西妥昔单抗每周给药一次的治疗，获得了9%的部分缓解率[62]。两项更大规模的试验使用伊立替康和西妥昔单抗联合治疗450例结直肠癌患者。这些患者有经证实的转移灶，EGFR阳性，既往接受过伊立替康治疗[63]。西妥昔单抗和伊立替康联合治疗的部分缓解率为17%~23%，而使用伊立替康单药再治疗的部分缓解率仅为11%。在一项研究中，联合治疗使无进展生存期从1.1个月显著延长至4.1个月。在接下来的一项3期试验中，共有1 289例复发的EGFR表达的结直肠癌患者被随机分入西妥昔单抗加伊立替康组和伊立替康单药组。这些患者既往均接受过氟尿嘧啶和奥沙利铂一线方案治疗。西妥昔单抗明显延长了无进展生存期，但未能延长总生存期，这可能与47%的患者交叉到联合治疗组有关[64]。有趣的是，EGFR的表达水平与西妥昔单抗的治疗反应无关。16例经治的结直肠癌患者，其EGFR免疫组化阴性，接受西妥昔单抗和伊立替康联合治疗后有4例（25%）达到缓解，这与前面的观察结果相一致[60]。因此，不能根据EGFR的免疫组化结果将患者排除在治疗之外。在2004年，美国FDA加速批准了西妥昔单抗与伊立替康联合用于伊立替康耐药的结直肠癌患者的治疗。基于一项572例奥沙利铂和伊立替康方案治疗失败的晚期EGFR阳性结直肠癌患者对比接受最佳支持治疗与最佳支持治疗加西妥昔单抗直至疾病进展的试验，西妥昔单抗在2007年获得了常规批准，其使总生存期从4.6个月提高到6.1个月（P=0.004 8）[65]。西妥昔单抗也被批准用于单药治疗奥沙利铂和伊立替康方案治疗失败的结直肠癌患者。与其他与EGFR相作用的小分子抑制物或单克隆抗体类似，西妥昔单抗很少能在*KRAS*突变的患者中起效[66]。CRYSTAL研究其纳入了1 217例初治的转移性结直肠癌患者，不考虑KRAS突变状态，随机分为FOLFIRI及FOLFIRI联合西妥昔单抗组[67,68]。在回顾过程中，将*KRAS*突变的患者排除会显著的影响试验结果。联合西妥昔单抗将中位无进展生存期从8.1个月延长至8.9个月（P=0.036），但不影响总生存期。当肿瘤进行*KRAS*突变检测后，FOLFIRI联合西妥昔单抗延长了KRAS野生型肿瘤患者的总生存期（19.5至23.5个月）、无进展生存期（8.1至9.5个月）及客观缓解率（39%：57%）。在*KRAS*突变型的肿瘤患者中，在FOLFIRI基础上联合西妥昔单抗未带来总生存期、无进展生存期及客观缓解率的改善。另外两个随机试验的数据也支持只有KRAS野生型的肿瘤患者能受益[69,70]，使西妥昔单抗在2012年被批准与FOLFIRI联用于初治的结直肠癌患者。

头颈部肿瘤

西妥昔单抗还被批准用于头颈部鳞癌（squamous cell carcinoma of the head and neck，SCCHN）。在一项关键性的多中心Ⅲ期研究中，424例局部进展期头颈部肿瘤患者，被随机分为高剂量放疗组或放疗联合西妥昔单抗治疗组[71]。加用西妥昔单抗后，局部控制时间从15个月增加至24个月，总生存期从29个月增加至49个月。在3项前瞻性试验中观察到，头颈部鳞癌患者（n=103）在含铂方案治疗进展后给予西妥昔单抗可获得10%~13%的缓解率，疾病控制率为46%~56%[72]。中位至疾病进展时间介于2.2~2.8个月，中位总生存期介于5.2~6.1个月。西妥昔单抗也提高了含铂方案在头颈部鳞癌中的疗效，在2011年获美国FDA批准，主要基于一项多中心研究，共纳入442例局部复发或转移的头颈部肿瘤患者，随机分为接受顺铂（或卡铂）及氟尿嘧啶加或不加用西妥昔单抗的治疗[73]。在接受西妥昔单抗与化疗联用的患者中，总生存期（10.1个月 vs 7.4个月，P=0.34）、无进展生存期（5.5个月 vs 3.3个月，P<0.000 1）及客观缓解率（35.6% vs 19.5%，P<0.000 1）均有显著提高。

毒副反应

绝大多数患者的不良反应包括痤疮样皮疹，主要位于面部（图64-1）和躯干上部，以及由虚弱、乏力、不适或嗜睡组成的复合综合征。应用米诺环素治疗可减轻痤疮样皮疹的严重性[74]。荟萃分析皮疹的程度与总生存期、无进展生存期及客观缓解率相关[75]。低镁血症是由于西妥昔单抗对远端肾小管EGFR的直接作用引起镁的流失所致[76]。一小部分患者发生严重的过敏反应，通常发生在首次输注西妥昔单抗时，这可能是由于治疗前患者体内存在的一种IgE抗体有关，这种抗体针对的是西妥昔单抗重链Fab段上发现的半乳糖-α-1,3-半乳糖-低聚糖[77]。

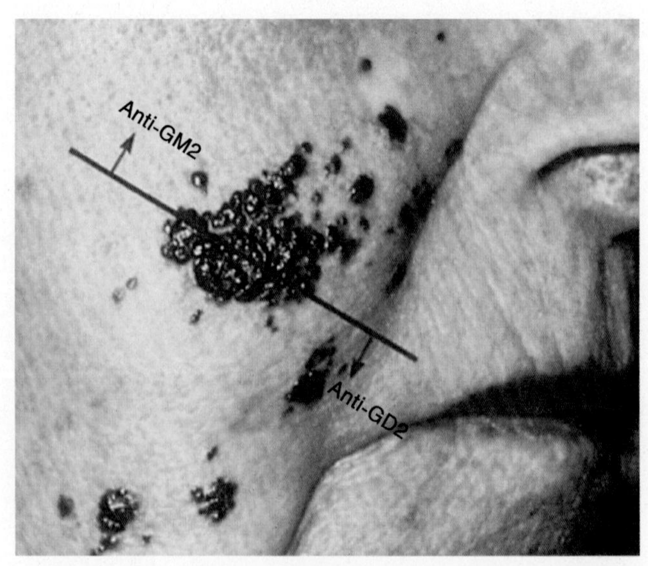

图64-1 复发黑色素瘤，之前放疗无效，在进行病灶内注射人抗GM2或GD2单克隆抗体的免疫治疗之前

帕尼单抗

帕尼单抗是一种完全人源化的抗 EGFR IgG2 型抗体。在一项试验中，463 例 EGFR 阳性、对标准治疗耐药的结直肠癌患者，被随机分入帕尼单抗单药治疗组或最佳支持治疗组。帕尼单抗治疗的客观缓解率为 10%，支持治疗对照组的客观缓解率为 0%，平均无进展生存期从 60 天延长至 96 天[78]。基于此项试验，美国 FDA 在 2006 年加速批准了帕尼单抗。与西妥昔单抗相同，缓解也仅限于 KRAS 野生型的患者[79]。有趣的是，近期的一项荟萃分析显示，在 HRAS 野生型但 BRAF 突变型的结直肠癌患者中，帕尼单抗与西妥昔单抗均不能带来总生存期、无进展生存期或客观缓解率的获益，提示 BRAF 测序也能识别出不能从抗 EGFR 治疗中获益的患者[80]。欧盟在 2007 年批准了帕尼单抗在结直肠癌患者中的使用。在初治的复发结直肠癌患者中曾尝试在贝伐珠单抗联合 FOLFOX-4 或 FOLFIRI 基础上加用帕尼单抗。对超过 1 000 例患者的中期分析显示，不含帕尼单抗的对照组具有显著的统计学优势，因此试验被终止[81]。

毒副反应

帕尼单抗观察到和西妥昔单抗相似的毒副反应谱。痤疮样皮疹和低镁血症最为显著[81]。到目前为止，帕尼单抗观察到的过敏反应较西妥昔单抗少。

抗 HER2 抗体

酪氨酸激酶生长因子受体 c-erbB2（HER-2）的分子量为 185kDa，在接近 20%～30% 的乳腺癌患者中存在过表达[82]。由于 HER-2 缺乏配体结合功能区，它成为其他 HER 家族成员理想的二聚体构成物，包括 EGFR、HER-3 和 HER-4[83]。乳腺癌细胞 HER-2 过表达与预后不良相关，尤其在淋巴结阳性的病例中，对紫杉醇、CMF 和他莫昔芬耐药，但对阿霉素的反应性提高[84,85]。对全身治疗的耐药、复发风险的增加以及生存期的缩短这些全部反映了 HER-2 过表达的生物学结果，包括增加增殖、增加细胞存活、增加侵袭和转移和增加血管生成。直接抗这些受体胞外区的单克隆抗体可抑制 HER-2 过表达肿瘤细胞的生长[86,87]。另外，应用抗 HER-2 抗体治疗可增加肿瘤细胞对铂类化合物、紫杉醇类、阿霉素和 4-氢过氧化环磷酰胺的敏感性[88,89]。有趣的是，抗 HER-2 抗体和 HER-2 受体胞内区[90]结合可激活酪氨酸激酶活性[87]，但是可能会阻止配体驱动的 HER-2 和 HER-3 的相互作用对 PI3 激酶通路的激活，降低磷酸-AKT 的抗凋亡活性[87,91,92]。与 HER-2 分子不同位点相结合的抗体已被研发。

曲妥珠单抗

曲妥珠单抗是一种人源化的小鼠 IgG1 抗体，能与 HER-2 胞外区的亚结构域 4 结合，阻止其他 HER-2 受体的同源二聚化并可下调 HER-2 受体的表达。在体内，对促血管生成因子的抑制和介导 ADCC 也可能发挥作用。曲妥珠单抗获 FDA 批准用于治疗转移性乳腺癌、早期乳腺癌、胃癌及胃食管连接处癌。

乳腺癌

在临床研究中，269 例既往接受过多程化疗的复发乳腺癌女性，应用曲妥珠单抗获得 12%～15% 的客观缓解率[93,94]。在之前的研究中，顺铂对乳腺癌显示出边缘性的作用，但顺铂联合曲妥珠单抗治疗 37 例患者获得了 24% 的客观临床缓解率，疗效中位持续时间为 8.4 个月[95]。一项关键性的国际多中心研究共入组了 469 例复发的乳腺癌女性患者[96]。既往未接受过阿霉素辅助化疗的患者随机接受阿霉素（或表柔比星）和环磷酰胺联合或不联合曲妥珠单抗的治疗。既往接受过阿霉素辅助化疗的患者则随机接受紫杉醇联合或不联合曲妥珠单抗的治疗。加用曲妥珠单抗的化疗组，至疾病进展时间更长（中位时间 7.4 个月 vs 4.6 个月；$P<0.001$），客观缓解率更高（50%～32%，$P<0.001$），缓解期更长（中位时间 9.1 个月 vs 6.1 个月；$P<0.001$），生存期更长（中位时间 25.1 个月 vs 20.3 个月；$P=0.01$）。此项研究使美国 FDA 及欧盟分别于 1998 年和 2000 年批准曲妥珠单抗用于治疗复发的 HER-2 过表达的乳腺癌。之后，又开展了 6 项大规模、多中心辅助化疗试验（见乳腺肿瘤章节），以评估联合曲妥珠单抗能否提高化疗预防原发 HER-2 阳性乳腺癌复发的作用。6 项试验中的 5 项中期分析显示出无病生存显著延长，因此终止临床研究，并推荐在此种情况下使用曲妥珠单抗[97-99]。在 5 项阳性结果的试验中，联合曲妥珠单抗使复发风险减低 46%～58%，第 3 年的复发率绝对值降低 8%～12%。相似地，死亡率降低 33%～59%，第 3 年的绝对值降低 2%～6%。

基于这些研究中的两项（NSABP B31 和 NCCTGN9831）纳入了 3 752 例女性患者的研究结果，FDA 在 2006 年批准在环磷酰胺、阿霉素及紫杉醇基础上联合曲妥珠单抗，用于 HER-2 过表达的女性乳腺癌患者的辅助治疗。

曲妥珠单抗可增加其他一些细胞毒性药物的缓解率，包括长春瑞滨、吉西他滨和铂类化合物[100-104]。一项随机试验中，81 例疾病复发后未接受过化疗的转移性 HER-2 阳性乳腺癌患者，长春瑞滨联合曲妥珠单抗治疗的缓解率为 51%，而紫杉醇联合曲妥珠单抗治疗的缓解率为 40%[105]。在大部分研究中，只有那些由于基因扩增驱动而高表达 HER-2 的乳腺癌才会对抗体单药或抗体与化疗的联合治疗发生反应。免疫组化可对 HER-2 的过表达进行初步筛查，但是 2+～3+的反应需经更可靠的原位荧光杂交技术证实[106]。乳腺癌进展时可出现获得性 HER-2 基因的扩增，因此有需要重复进行 HER-2 表达的检测[107]。由于仅有一小部分患者有效，因此 HER-2 过表达是确定对曲妥珠单抗发生反应的必要但非充分条件。对曲妥珠单抗缺乏反应与下列因素相关：缺乏 PTEN 磷酸酶的表达，此酶可从 PI3 上转移磷酸基团，阻断通过 AKT 的信号转导[108]。应用曲妥珠单抗治疗可增强 PTEN 在细胞膜上的定位，增强磷酸化酶的活性，后者通过抑制 Src 在 HER-2 受体上的锚定导致 PTEN 酪氨酸的磷酸化减低而实现。

胃癌及胃食管连接处癌

在 2010 年，FDA 批准了曲妥珠单抗与顺铂及一种氟尿嘧啶类药物（卡培他滨或 5-氟尿嘧啶）用于 HER-2 过表达的转移性胃或胃食管连接处癌初治患者的治疗。获批主要基于一项纳入了 594 例 Her2 过表达的局部晚期或转移性胃或胃食管连接处腺癌的国际多中心开放的随机对照临床试验 BO18255（ToGA 试验）[109]。患者随机分配至单纯化疗组或化疗加曲妥珠单抗组，当分析曲妥珠单抗的加入可以提高无进展生存期（13.5 个月 vs 11.0 个月，$P=0.0038$）时，试验在第二次中期分析后被终止了。更新的生存分析显示曲妥珠单抗能带来持续的优势（13.1 vs 11.7），最大获益出现在 HER-2 过表达的肿瘤中。

毒副反应

曲妥珠单抗治疗耐受良好,通常在首次给药时可观察到轻度的发热、畏寒和疲乏。在大部分研究中曲妥珠单抗每周给药,但曾经也采用过每 3 周给药方式,每次给予更高剂量的治疗,其毒性和谷浓度可以接受[110]。当曲妥珠单抗与阿霉素或紫杉醇联合使用时,观察到心脏毒性增加。在证实曲妥珠单抗对复发乳腺癌效果的关键性试验中,曲妥珠单抗联合蒽环类和环磷酰胺组中,Ⅲ级和Ⅳ级心功能不全(美国心脏协会分级)的发生率为 27%,而单纯给予蒽环类和环磷酰胺组的发生率为 8%[111]。相似程度的心功能不全在紫杉醇联合曲妥珠单抗组中发生率为 13%,单纯接受紫杉醇组发生率为 1%。218 例乳腺癌患者接受含曲妥珠单抗的方案长期治疗至少 1 年,Ⅲ级心功能不全的发生率为 11%[112]。在 6 项辅助化疗试验中,曲妥珠单抗联合紫杉醇或卡铂,没有阿霉素,序贯或同步给药,观察到Ⅲ/Ⅳ级心功能不全的发生率为 0.5%~4.1%[98,99]。心功能不全在曲妥珠单抗停药并予对症治疗后通常可以缓解。因此,心功能基线值正常的患者,应用曲妥珠单抗治疗疾病复发或作为辅助治疗的收益通常超过其风险。曲妥珠单抗导致心功能不全的机制仍不清楚。在心肌细胞上只发现低水平的 HER-2,但是曲妥珠单抗可定位于心肌,与 HER-2/HER-3 和 HER-2/HER-4 二聚体结合的配体,人表皮生长因子受体调节蛋白对胚胎发育和凋亡压力下心脏组织的生存具有关键作用[113]。选用心脏毒性较低的蒽环类药物与曲妥珠单抗联合使用可作为一种替代方法。一项新的辅助化疗试验报告,采用表柔比星、紫杉醇和曲妥珠单抗同步治疗较单纯化疗,获得显著更高的病理学完全缓解率(67% vs 25%),而且没有发生临床症状明显的充血性心力衰竭[114]。

帕妥珠单抗

帕妥珠单抗是在曲妥珠单抗的不同位点与 HER-2 二聚化结构域结合的一种 IgG1 人源化单克隆抗体,可阻断配体介导的 HER-2 与其他 HER 家族成员的二聚化[115,116]。帕妥珠单抗和曲妥珠单抗联合使用可协同抑制 HER-2 过表达的乳腺癌细胞系,这与增加凋亡、阻断通过 AKT 而非 MAP 激酶的信号转导有关[117]。基于一项临床研究 Cleopatra,美国 FDA 及欧盟分别在 2012 年及 2013 年批准帕妥珠单抗用于 HER-2 扩增的乳腺癌的治疗。研究纳入了 808 例 HER2 阳性的转移性乳腺癌患者,随机分为接受帕妥珠单抗、曲妥珠单抗和多西他赛治疗组和接受曲妥珠单抗、多西他赛和安慰剂治疗组[118]。接受帕妥珠单抗治疗的患者中位无进展生存期为 18.7 个月,而安慰剂组为 12.4 个月。在后续的随访中,在曲妥珠单抗及多西他赛基础上加入帕妥珠单抗使总生存期延长了 15.7 个月,从 40.8 个月延长至 56.5 个月($P<0.001$),并且使无进展生存期延长了 6.3 个月[119]。

在 2013 年,帕妥珠单抗成为了第一个 FDA 批准的用于复发和死亡风险高的 HER-2 阳性、局部晚期、炎性乳腺癌或早期乳腺癌(直径>2cm 或淋巴结阳性)患者新辅助治疗的药物。帕妥珠单抗被批准与曲妥珠单抗及其他化疗药在术前联合应用,术后的化疗方案可序贯术前使用的治疗方案。患者在术后需继续应用曲妥珠单抗至 1 年。帕妥珠单抗在新辅助治疗中加速获批是基于一项测定 pCR 率的研究,依照一项 FDA 的新建议,它可以作为替代终点指标。在 NeoSphere 研究中,417 例受试者随机接受 4 种方案之一的新辅助治疗:曲妥珠单抗联合多西他赛,帕妥珠单抗、曲妥珠单抗联合多西他赛,帕妥珠单抗联合曲妥珠单抗,或者帕妥珠单抗联合多西他赛[120]。接受帕妥珠单抗、曲妥珠单抗及多西他赛治疗的受试者中,39% 获得了 pCR,而接受曲妥珠单抗和多西他赛治疗的受试者 pCR 比例为 21%。这项加速审批的验证性试验正在接受过手术并具有高复发风险的 HER2 阳性乳腺癌患者中开展,共招募了超过 4 800 例受试者。试验会进一步提供有效性、安全性及长期结果的数据。结果预期 2016 年公布(译者注:2017 年已公布阳性结果,与曲妥珠单抗联合化疗相比,使用帕妥珠单抗联合曲妥珠单抗和化疗的术后辅助治疗方案能降低早期 HER2 阳性乳腺癌患者的乳腺癌复发或死亡风险)。

毒副反应

接受帕妥珠单抗、曲妥珠单抗和紫杉醇或多西他赛治疗的患者,最常见的不良反应包括脱发、腹泻、恶心及中性粒细胞减少。其他严重的不良反应包括心功能下降,输液相关反应及过敏。此外,针对心功能不全及胚胎受损有黑框警告。

抗神经节苷脂抗体

GD2 是在神经母细胞瘤、黑色素瘤以及正常神经元、黑素细胞和疼痛纤维上表达的一个双唾液酸神经节苷脂。在肿瘤细胞上的表达相对统一,并且在接受单克隆抗体治疗后 GD2 不会从细胞表面丢失[121]。

达妥昔单抗

达妥昔单抗是一种抗 GD2 的 IgG1 嵌合抗体,在 2015 年被美国 FDA 批准用于治疗对一线多药多学科综合治疗有效的高危神经母细胞瘤新发患儿。加用达妥昔单抗改善了接受粒细胞-巨噬细胞集落刺激因子、白介素 2 及顺式维 A 酸(retinoic acid,RA)维持治疗患者的疗效[122]。关键的 COG 研究将 226 例患者随机分为达妥昔单抗联合 RA 或 RA 单药治疗 6 周期。在随访及实验终止时,显示出无事件生存期(event-free survival,EFS)的改善(HR 0.57,$P=0.01$,log-rank 检验)。当时中位的无事件生存期还未达到[达妥昔单抗联合 RA 组 3.4 年,NR;RA 组 1.9 年(1.3,NR)]。3 年后针对总生存期的分析显示达妥昔单抗与 RA 联合治疗组较 RA 单药治疗组总生存期有所改善(HR 0.58),虽然两组的中位总生存期均未达到。

毒副反应

达妥昔单抗与 RA 联合治疗组最常见的不良反应包括疼痛、发热、血小板减少、输液反应、低血压、低钠血症、丙氨酸氨基转移酶升高、贫血、呕吐、腹泻、低钾血症、毛细血管渗漏综合征、中性粒细胞减少、荨麻疹、低蛋白血症、天冬氨酸氨基转移酶升高和低钙血症。达妥昔单抗与 RA 联合治疗组中最常见(>5%)的严重不良反应包括感染、输液反应、低钾血症、低血压、疼痛、发热及毛细血管渗漏综合征。

抗血管治疗

新生血管形成对正常胚胎发育和伤口愈合来说是非常关键的,肿瘤的生长和转移也同样需要血管生成[123]。正在针对肿瘤相关内皮上表达的抗原或由肿瘤细胞产生的促血管生成因子研发抑制血管生成的新方法。

贝伐珠单抗

贝伐珠单抗是一种人源化的 IgG1 抗体，可与促血管生成的 VEGF-A 结合。VEGF-A 也被认为是血管通透因子（vascular permeability factor, VPF）。阻断 VEGF/VPF 可以抑制异种移植物中肿瘤驱动的血管生成[124]。VEGF/VPF 的表达与小鼠卵巢癌异种移植模型中腹水的形成有关[125]。应用贝伐珠单抗治疗可完全抑制腹水的形成[126]。另外，肿瘤细胞本身也表达 VEGF 受体。VEGF 的自分泌刺激可增强肿瘤细胞的增殖和对化疗的耐药。贝伐珠单抗已通过 FDA 批准用于治疗结直肠癌（2004、2006 和 2013 年）、非小细胞肺癌（2006 年）、乳腺癌（2008 年；2011 年撤回）、肾癌（2009 年）、胶质母细胞瘤（2009 年）、宫颈癌（2014 年）及卵巢癌（2014 年），但是它在肿瘤治疗中的地位仍在完善中[127]。

结直肠癌

在初治的转移性结直肠癌患者中，在伊立替康、氟尿嘧啶和甲酰四氢叶酸基础上加用贝伐珠单抗，可增加总缓解率（34.8%~44.8%），显著延长中位无进展生存期（7.4~10.4 个月）和中位总生存期（15.6~20.3 个月）[128]。该研究使 FDA 最初在 2004 年批准了贝伐珠单抗与化疗联合用于结直肠癌的一线治疗。两项随机 2 期临床试验显示，在 5-FU 和甲酰四氢叶酸基础上加用贝伐珠单抗，可提高缓解率、无进展生存期和总生存期[129-131]。但一项 3 期临床试验结果表明，在更有效的一线方案如 FOLFOX4 和 XELOX 中加用贝伐珠单抗，缓解率、无进展生存期和总生存期没有显著提高[132,133]。在非劣效研究中，贝伐珠单抗和多种药物的组合也获得了类似的结果[134]。然而，在二线治疗中，FOLFOX-4 联合高剂量的贝伐珠单抗显著提高了缓解率（9%~23%）、无进展生存期（4.7~7.3 个月）和总生存期（10.8~12.9 个月），使贝伐珠单抗在 2006 年获批用于二线治疗[135]。在接受过含伊立替康或奥沙利铂方案的化疗与贝伐珠单抗联合治疗后进展的转移性结直肠癌患者中，继续应用贝伐珠单抗或与互补的化疗方案联用，可以提高总生存期（11.2 个月 vs 9.8 个月，$P=0.0062$）和无进展生存期（5.7 个月 vs 4.0 个月；$P<0.0001$），使贝伐珠单抗获批在二线治疗中可以继续应用[136]。

非小细胞肺癌

有三项 3 期试验研究了初治的转移性非小细胞肺癌采用贝伐珠单抗联合卡铂/紫杉醇[137,138]或吉西他滨/顺铂[139]的疗效。缓解率显著提高（14%~28.1%）无进展生存期（0.6~2.7 个月）及总生存期（0.5~2.0 个月）轻度改善[134]，但具有统计学意义。

乳腺癌

在复发转移性乳腺癌患者的一线治疗中，紫杉醇联合贝伐珠单抗可显著增加缓解率（21%~37%）和无进展生存期（5.9~11.8 个月）[140]。多西他赛联合贝伐珠单抗无进展生存期有轻度延长（8.0~8.9 个月），但具有统计学意义[141]。在二线治疗中，卡培他滨联合贝伐单抗显著提高了缓解率（9%~20%），但未增加无进展生存期（4.2~4.9 个月）或总生存期（14.5~15.1 个月）[142]。考虑到在验证性试验中贝伐珠单抗疗效有限，其乳腺癌适应证被撤回。

肾细胞癌

大部分散发性肾细胞癌都表现出 von Hippel Lindau（VHL）基因失活，继而导致 VEGF 过表达[143]。在一项 2 期随机试验中，针对既往治疗过的肾细胞癌患者，比较了两种不同剂量的贝伐珠单抗（3mg/kg 或 10mg/kg，每 2 周 1 次）和安慰剂的疗效，结果观察到高剂量贝伐珠单抗较安慰剂的无进展生存期显著延长（4.8 个月 vs 2.5 个月，$P<0.01$）[144]。α 干扰素（IFN-α）是肾细胞癌的标准初始治疗方案，在随机试验中显示出缓解率和生存期轻微获益。两项 3 期试验对比了初治的肾细胞癌患者中 IFN-α 联合贝伐珠单抗较 IFN-α 单药的疗效[145,146]。结果显示，无进展生存期从 5.2~5.4 个月显著增加至 8.5~10.2 个月。

多形性胶质母细胞瘤

在 2 项单臂试验，AVF3708g 和 NCI06-C-0064E 中，贝伐珠单抗显示出抗多形性胶质母细胞瘤（*glioblastoma multiforme*，GBM）的活性。在总共 141 例手术，放疗或替莫唑胺治疗后复发的患者中，单药贝伐珠单抗获得了 20%~25% 的缓解率及 3.9~4.2 个月的中位持续时间[147]。从而加速了 FDA 对这一适应证的批准。最近一项随机双盲试验评估了放疗和替莫唑胺基础上加用贝伐珠单抗是否能为 637 例初诊的 GBM 患者带来获益[148]。加用贝伐珠单抗时无进展生存期从 7.3 个月增加至 10.7 个月（$P=0.007$），但对总生存期没有影响。

卵巢癌

在既往接受过多程治疗的复发性卵巢癌患者中，给予贝伐珠单抗单药[149,150]或联合低剂量环磷酰胺每天口服，进行“节拍”疗法[151]，获得 16%~24% 的缓解率，无进展生存期为 4.4~7.2 个月。在约 40% 的卵巢癌患者中观察到 6 个月的疾病稳定期。4 项随机试验分别评估了标准化疗基础上加用贝伐珠单抗在一线治疗（GOG 218[152] 和 ICON7[153]）、铂类敏感（OCEANS[154]）及耐药（AURELIA[155]）的复发患者中的疗效[156]。在这些研究中，无进展生存分别提高了 3.8 个月（$P<0.001$），1.7 个月（$P=0.001$），3.3 个月（$P=0.001$）和 4.0 个月（$P<0.0001$），总生存期均没有改善。但在 COG 218 及 ICON7 中，预后不良的患者亚组似乎能有所获益。由于在总生存上缺乏获益，而且在一线和后线的患者中见到了类似的无进展生存期改善，因而产生了是否需要将贝伐珠单抗的治疗延后至疾病复发时的疑问[156]。基于 Aurelia 试验，贝伐珠单抗已获批与化疗联合用于复发性卵巢癌的治疗。

宫颈癌

在一项纳入 452 例复发、持续或转移性宫颈癌患者的随机试验中，卡铂联合紫杉醇或拓扑替康的基础上加用贝伐珠单抗可使总生存期增加 3.7 个月（从 13.3 个月至 17.0 个月，$P=0.004$），缓解率可从 36% 增加至 88%（$P=0.008$）[157]。

毒副反应

结直肠癌、非小细胞肺癌、乳腺癌、肾细胞癌、宫颈癌和卵巢癌患者使用贝伐珠单抗，绝大多数人耐受良好。大约 20% 的患者发生 3 度高血压。虽然大多数情况下血压控制良好，但恶性高血压及致命的出血性卒中也有发生，因而支持更为积极的血压监测及管理。<5% 的病例会出现明显的蛋白尿，还可观察到鼻出血。手术后 60 天内给予贝伐单抗可观察到伤口愈合延迟和出血风险增加[158]。在一项非小细胞肺癌患者的早期研究中，可观察到大咯血，这导致了 35 例患者中的 4 例死亡。威胁生命的咯血最常发生在组织类型为鳞状细胞癌、肿瘤坏死形成

空洞以及病变邻近大血管的老年患者中。许多临床研究已经将具有这些特征的患者排除在外。在卵巢癌患者的随机试验中,5%~7.4%的患者出现血栓事件[156]。在大规模3期研究中,2%的患者发生动脉血栓栓塞。在既往多程治疗过的卵巢癌患者中,5%~7%的病例发生肠穿孔,通常见于部分小肠梗阻和受侵肠壁病变经治疗缓解的情况下。在一线辅助试验的卵巢癌患者中,2.6%~3%的病例发生肠穿孔[156]。当贝伐珠单抗与FOLFOX联合给药,结直肠癌患者只有1%发生肠穿孔[135]。

雷莫芦单抗

雷莫芦单抗是一种人IgG1单克隆抗体,与人VEGFR2结合从而阻止其与VEGF配体的相互作用。雷莫芦单抗被美国FDA批准用于胃及胃食管连接处癌(2014年)、肺癌(2014年)及结肠癌(2015年)的治疗。

胃及胃食管连接处癌

雷莫芦单抗可以单药或与紫杉醇联合用于治疗氟尿嘧啶或铂类耐药的胃或胃食管连接处肿瘤。雷莫芦单抗作为单药的获批主要基于一项跨国的随机双盲试验,其纳入了655例经治的进展期或转移的肿瘤患者,随机(2∶1)分至雷莫芦单抗或安慰剂联合最佳支持治疗。在紫杉醇基础上加用雷莫芦单抗显著改善了总生存期(9.6个月 vs 7.4个月,$P=0.017$)和无进展生存期(4.4个月 vs 2.9个月,$P<0.001$)[159]。

肺癌

雷莫芦单抗与多西他赛联用被批准用于治疗含铂方案或抗EGFR或抗ALK靶向治疗进展后肺转移性非小细胞肺癌的治疗。雷莫芦单抗与多西他赛联用的获批是基于一项纳入了1 253例经治的转移性非小细胞肺癌患者的双盲安慰剂对照试验[160]。多西他赛基础上加用雷莫芦单抗显著延长了总生存期(10.5个月 vs 9.1个月,$P=0.024$)和无进展生存期($P<0.001$)。

结直肠癌

雷莫芦单抗可以与FOLFIRI联合治疗一线含贝伐珠单抗、奥沙利铂及氟尿嘧啶方案治疗进展后的转移性结直肠癌患者。其获批是基于一项跨国双盲随机试验,纳入了1 072例患者,随机分至接受FOLFIRI加安慰剂组或FOLFIRI加雷莫芦单抗组[161]。FOLFIRI基础上加用雷莫芦单抗提高了总生存期(13.3个月 vs 11.7个月,$P=0.023$)和无进展生存期(5.7个月 vs 4.5个月,$P<0.001$)。

毒副反应

雷莫芦单抗的治疗可能会导致疲劳、虚弱、高血压、低钠血症、腹泻及鼻出血。当与紫杉醇或多西他赛联用时,出现过中性粒细胞减少、发热性中性粒细胞减少和贫血。其他在产品标签上描述的少见但重要的风险包括出血、动脉血栓栓塞事件、输液相关反应、胃肠梗阻、胃肠穿孔、伤口愈合延迟、肝硬化患者临床恶化以及可逆性后部白质脑病。在结直肠癌的患者中也出现过甲状腺功能减退。

免疫检查点抑制剂

抗CTLA-4

抗CTLA-4单克隆抗体已被用于免疫调节干预。$CD4^+CD25^+$调节性T细胞(Treg)表达细胞毒性T淋巴细胞抗原4(CTLA-4)。肿瘤组织中存在Treg细胞与几种人类癌症的不良预后相关,在临床前期动物模型中发现消除Treg细胞可以增强抗肿瘤反应。此外,抗原呈递细胞上的CD80/86与T淋巴细胞上的CTLA-4相互作用可以阻断肿瘤免疫的有效激活,使用CTLA-4单克隆抗体抑制这种相互作用可以增强肿瘤特异性免疫[162]。

伊匹木单抗

伊匹木单抗(Ipilimumab)是一种与CTLA-4作用的全人源性IgG1单克隆抗体,2011年美国FDA和欧盟基于一项国际研究批准其应用,该研究纳入676名对FDA已批或常规治疗无效的黑色素瘤患者,这些患者被随机分为使用Ipilimumab、Ipilimumab+gp100疫苗或单独疫苗治疗3组。结果显示接受Ipilimumab+疫苗联合治疗或单独Ipilimumab治疗的患者平均存活时间约10个月,而那些只接受实验性疫苗治疗的患者平均存活6.5个月。在人类黑色素瘤和肾细胞癌患者中应用Ipilimumab单药治疗的ORR为7%~15%[163,164]。预期使用Ipilimumab联合特定抗肿瘤疫苗可有更好的疗效。2015年JCO杂志上发表一项使用Ipilimumab治疗的1 861例无法切除或晚期黑色素瘤的Ⅱ/Ⅲ期临床研究,结果显示中位OS为11.4个月,其中254例患者至少有3年的生存随访。生存曲线在3年左右开始趋于平稳。所有患者、未接受治疗的患者和以前接受治疗的患者的3年生存率分别为22%、26%和20%[165]。在一项辅助治疗的研究中,951例完全切除的Ⅲ期黑色素瘤患者随机分为Ipilimumab或安慰剂组。Ipilimumab延长了中位无复发生存期(26.1个月 vs 17.1个月,$P=0.001\ 3$)。在Ipilimumab治疗组中有5例(1%)患者死于药物相关不良事件[166]。CTLA-4单抗的疗效与肿瘤突变负荷、新抗原和细胞学标记分子的表达有关[167,168]。

毒副反应

与使用Ipilimumab相关的自身免疫反应可能导致的常见副作用包括疲劳、腹泻、皮疹、葡萄膜炎、垂体炎、内分泌不足、肠道炎症(结肠炎)和肝炎[164]。约12.9%使用Ipilimumab治疗的患者出现严重甚至致命的自身免疫反应。当出现严重副作用时,停用Ipilimumab并开始皮质类固醇治疗。但不是所有的患者都对这种治疗有反应,在某些情况下,确实有反应的患者可能在几周内未看到显著好转。

抗PD-1

抗PD-1抗体靶向T细胞相关的PD-1抗原,为T细胞免疫的第二调节因子,可阻断PD-1与癌细胞和巨噬细胞上的PD-L1和PD-L2配体的相互作用。阻断这种相互作用,可解除癌细胞对T细胞的免疫抑制[169]。

帕博利珠单抗

帕博利珠单抗(Pembrolizumab),是一种人源化IgG4单克隆抗体,靶向PD-1抗原,阻断PD-1与PD-L1和PD-L2配体的相互作用。2014年,基于一项多中心、开放随机、剂量比较队列的研究,Pembrolizumab被美国FDA批准用于经Ipilimumab治疗后进展但尚未使用BRAF抑制剂治疗的黑色素瘤。该研究纳入173例无法切除或转移的黑色素瘤患者,这些患者随机接受2mg/kg(n=89)或10mg/kg(n=84)的pembrolizumab治疗,每 3 周为 1 个周期,直到疾病进展或出现不可接受的毒性。2mg/kg 组的 ORR 为 24%,包括 1 例完全缓解(CR)和 20 例部分缓解。在 21 例有客观反应的患者中,3 例(14%)在最初反应后的第 2.8 个月、2.9 个月和 8.2 个月出现疾病进展,其余 18 例(86%)患者持续反应 1.4~8.5 个月,其中有 8 例患者持续反应在 6 个月或更长时间。在 10mg/kg 组也观察到类似的 ORR 结果。在一项扩展的随机Ⅱ期试验中,6 个月 PFS 在 2mg/kg 组为 34%,10mg/kg 组为 38%,研究者选择的接受化疗组为 16%[170]。一项入组 834 例患者的临床试验比较 Pembrolizumab 每 2 周或每 3 周一次和 Ipilimumab 的疗效。Pembrolizumab 每 2 周、Pembrolizumab 每 3 周和 Ipilimumab 的 6 个月 PFS 分别为 47.3%、46.4%和 26.5%(P<0.001)[171]。

毒副反应

使用 Pembrolizumab 2mg/kg 每 3 周为 1 个周期治疗的患者,最常见(>20%)的不良反应是疲劳、咳嗽、恶心、瘙痒、皮疹、食欲缺乏、便秘、关节痛和腹泻。最常见(≥2%)的严重不良反应是肾衰竭、呼吸困难、肺炎和蜂窝织炎。其他临床上显著的免疫介导的不良反应包括肺炎、结肠炎、垂体炎、甲状腺功能亢进、甲状腺功能减退、肾炎和肝炎。

纳武利尤单抗

纳武利尤单抗(Nivolumab)(Opdivo®)是一种人源性 IgG4 抗 PD-1 单克隆抗体,于 2014 年基于一项单臂试验获美国 FDA 批准用于经 Ipilimumab 和 BRAF 抑制剂治疗失败的无法切除或转移性黑色素瘤患者。该试验纳入 120 名患者,结果显示 ORR 为 32%,其中约三分之一的有效者在 6 个月或更长时间内仍处于缓解状态。一项研究比较 Nivolumab 和达卡巴嗪在 418 例 BRAF 野生型黑色素瘤患者的疗效,Nivolumab 对比达卡巴嗪结果为>1 年 OS 率(72.9% vs 42%,P<0.001),PFS(5.1 个月 vs 2.2 个月,P<0.001)和 ORR(40% vs 13.9%,P<0.001)[172]。另一项研究,在抗 CTLA-4 治疗进展的患者中,与研究者选择的化疗相比,Nivolumab 提高了 ORR(37.7% vs 10.6%)[173]。

非小细胞肺癌

2013 年,FDA 基于一项随机试验批准 Nivolumab 用于铂为基础治疗失败的 NSCLC 患者。该试验纳入含铂化疗方案期间或之后进展的转移性鳞状 NSCLC 患者,随机给予 Nivolumab(135)或多西紫杉醇(137)治疗[174]。结果显示 Nivolumab 较多西紫杉醇显著提高 OS(9.2 个月 vs 6 个月,P=0.000 25)。另一项在接受以铂为基础的治疗和至少一种二线及以上的化疗方案后进展的转移性鳞状 NSCLC 患者中进行的单臂、多国、多中心试验支持了该批准,结果显示接受 Nivolumab 治疗患者(n=117)的 ORR 为 15%。所有患者均为部分,但 17 例治疗有效的患者中有 10 例(59%)的缓解持续时间为 6 个月或更长。

毒副反应

在上述单臂试验中,接受 Nivolumab 的 117 名患者中最常见(>30%)的不良反应是疲劳、呼吸困难、肌肉骨骼疼痛、食欲下降和咳嗽。至少 5%的患者中观察到最常见的 3 级和 4 级药物不良反应为呼吸困难、疲劳和肌肉骨骼疼痛。临床上显著的免疫相关不良反应包括肺炎、结肠炎、肝炎、肾炎/肾功能障碍、甲状腺功能减退和甲状腺功能亢进。

Nivolumab 和 Ipilimumab 联合治疗

在 142 名先前未治疗的 BRAF 野生型黑色素瘤患者中,Nivolumab 和 Ipilimumab 联合治疗比 Ipilimumab 单药提高了客观缓解率(61%∶11%, P<0.001)。在联合治疗中观察到 22%的完全缓解,而 Ipilimumab 单药治疗的患者中观察到的完全缓解为 0%。此外,联合组具有更长的 PFS(P<0.001)。在有 BRAF 突变的黑色素瘤的患者中观察到类似的结果[175]。另一项随机的Ⅲ期研究将 Nivolumab 联合 Ipilimumab 与 Ipilimumab 或 Nivolumab 单药治疗之前未治疗的Ⅲ或Ⅳ期黑色素瘤患者进行了比较。PFS 分别为 11.5 个月、2.9 个月和 6.9 个月(联合组 P<0.001)。联合治疗组中 55%的患者发生 3~4 级治疗相关的不良事件,而 Ipilimumab 单药组的发生率为 27.3%[176]。

双特异性抗体

免疫球蛋白可以被设计成含有两个不同特异性的结合位点。也可在含有相关结合位点并且具有更好的组织穿透性的较小的单链可变区片段(ScFv)上做同样的设计。由可识别仅存在于 B 细胞决定簇的 scFv 片段和另一个可识别仅存在于 T 细胞的决定簇的 scFv 片段构建成的双特异性抗体,可以增强细胞毒性 T 细胞和恶性 B 细胞之间的接触,增强免疫杀伤肿瘤细胞的作用。

Blinatumomab

Blinatumomab(Blincyto)是一种含 ScFv 片段的双特异性抗体,可结合到急性淋巴细胞白血病(ALL)上的 CD3 T 细胞决定簇和 CD19 B 细胞决定簇。基于一项纳入 185 名费城染色体阴性的复发或难治性前体成人 B 细胞 ALL 的研究,Blinatumab 于 2014 年获得美国 FDA 批准用于治疗所有对常规治疗无效的 ALL。参与研究的患者至少接受 4 周的 Blinatumab 治疗,随访 6.7 个月,其 CR 率为 32%[177]。

毒性

Blinatumomab 具有一些黑框警告的风险,一些参与临床试验的患者在第一次治疗开始时发生了炎症因子释放综合征,并出现短暂的脑部病变。使用 Blinatumomab 治疗的患者中最常见的副作用是发热、头痛、外周水肿、发热性中性粒细胞减少、恶心、低血钾、疲劳、便秘、腹泻和震颤。

无修饰单克隆抗体治疗成功的障碍

抗原特异性

几乎没有或仅有很少的单克隆抗体只作用于肿瘤细胞,而不作用于正常组织。抗独特型抗体的显著效果和轻微毒性,至少部分反映出它们与绝大多数人 B 细胞的反应性是有限的。现在已经退市的 Campath-1 的毒性对正常淋巴细胞和单核细胞产生作用。治疗某些器官的肿瘤,如卵巢或甲状腺,由于相应的全部正常组织在治疗伊始即被切除,组织特异性抗体而非肿瘤特异性抗体可能就足够了。

抗原调变

抗原调变和抗原脱落至血液循环中,如 ALL 中的 CD10,通常被证实为血清治疗的不良靶位。此种情况普遍存在，唯一例外是曲妥珠单抗治疗 HER-2 过表达的乳腺癌。HER-2 的胞外区截断脱落到血液中，可作为受体过表达的标志物。

抗原表达的异质性

在不同患者的肿瘤内或肿瘤之间观察到抗原表达的异质性。缺乏抗原表达的细胞无法被有效地锁定。对于缺乏“旁观者”活性的非结合型抗体，可能需要联合数种制剂来靶定所有细胞。联合使用 5 种单克隆制剂可使>90%的乳腺癌患者中>90%的细胞成为靶点[178]。

有效输送抗体至肿瘤细胞

绝大部分有效的血清治疗都采用 IgG 抗体，分子量为 150kDa。相反，大部分传统的细胞毒性药物分子量<1kDa。因此，单克隆抗体较传统药物分布动力学更缓慢、组织穿透性更低[179]。例如，静脉注射抗 250kDa 黑色素相关硫酸软骨素蛋白聚糖核心蛋白小鼠单克隆抗体 IgG2a，结果抗体选择性地定位于恶性黑色素瘤的转移结节中[180]。对活检组织的免疫组织化学检查显示，给予抗体的剂量越大，则小鼠免疫球蛋白的累积越多。甚至在输入 500mg 抗体后，所有患者的抗原位点仍未达到完全饱和，这与抗体达到血管腔外肿瘤细胞非常有限是一致的。抗体成功定位到肿瘤取决于一些因素。单克隆抗体到达肿瘤细胞的能力受限于异常的血管、间质压力升高以及免疫球蛋白通过间质运输的距离相对过长[181,182]。肿瘤血管的异常允许白蛋白和其他血浆蛋白渗漏入肿瘤细胞周围的间质内。肿瘤细胞阻断淋巴外流，妨碍了间质蛋白的清除，增加了渗透压和液体积聚。间质压力升高妨碍了抗体的有效移位。生物分布研究显示距血管的距离是影响抗原识别和结合的重要因素。肿块的中心区不仅液体压力高，而且很难渗透，使抗体很难接近这些区域[183]。另外，大肿瘤团块可成为抗原沉积槽，减少药物输送至其他肿瘤部位[184]。Juweid 和他的同事通过模型研究提出了结合位点屏障假说，假设正是由于抗体分子与肿瘤周围抗原的成功结合，妨碍了其渗透到肿瘤中[185]。接下来的实验研究支持了这一假说。曾尝试使用腔内治疗促进抗体接近肿瘤细胞，但抗体通常只能穿透至浆膜下几毫米。

对外源免疫球蛋白的免疫应答

人们进行了大量努力使人免疫球蛋白具有更小的免疫原性，但是其滴度、特异性、独特型和亲和力仍然限制了这些制剂的临床使用[186-188]。由于临床使用的抗体很大一部分来自小鼠，它们可以诱导产生人抗小鼠抗体。人抗小鼠抗体的存在可以妨碍小鼠单克隆抗体有效运送至肿瘤细胞，尤其当必须给予成倍的剂量以获得最佳抗肿瘤活性时。对小鼠单克隆抗体进行基因修饰可以获得免疫原性更小的制剂。嵌合型抗体（60%人成分）和人源化抗体（95%人成分）通过基因工程保留小鼠抗原结合互补决定区，与人免疫球蛋白构架区连接[186]。尽管这样的抗体可大大降低免疫原性，限制 HAMA 反应，但是它们注射给药仍可激起抗独特型抗体反应。通过噬菌体展示技术，从组合文库中分离出的完全人源化的抗体，改革了治疗策略[188]。含有人免疫球蛋白基因的基因工程的转基因小鼠也被研发以产生完全的人抗体。不同于小鼠抗体，包含人类抗体 Fc 段的人或人源化抗体，可激发 ADCC 和补体依赖的细胞毒反应。一系列新型的亲和力成熟技术，如细菌细胞表面 scFv 展示和无细胞核糖体展示正在不断涌现，以分离稀有的高亲和力克隆[189]。基因工程还被用于生产单链抗原结合蛋白，较完整的免疫球蛋白或 Fab 段可能具有更佳的药代动力学属性[190]。

效应物机制的效能

无修饰单克隆抗体可抑制肿瘤生长的程度，与其抗肿瘤作用相关的一些重要机制包括直接抑制生长、诱导凋亡、抑制血管生成、补体依赖性溶解和 ADCC 反应，还可能干扰宿主特异性免疫调节网络。在体外，当缺乏补体成分或宿主效应细胞时，与 EGFR 或 HER-2 作用的抗体可抑制肿瘤细胞生长[87,191]。阻断 EGF 与 EGFR 结合的抗体如西妥昔单抗，较与受体其他位点结合的抗体，更易影响生长。抑制配体结合似乎对抑制锚定依赖性生长，而不是非锚定依赖性生长很重要。抗体可在淋巴细胞系、激活的 T 细胞和某些肿瘤细胞系中引发凋亡[192]。小鼠 IgM、IgG2a 和 IgG3 独特型抗体可固定人补体，但作用通常很弱。当人细胞带有适当抗原、人补体成分存在时，抗体可介导人细胞的溶解，但大鼠单克隆抗体 Campath-1G 是一个很重要的例外[193]。小鼠 IgG3、IgG2a 和 IgG2b 抗体可介导 ADCC 反应，当抗体与肿瘤细胞表面特异性抗原决定簇结合后，大颗粒淋巴细胞、单核细胞、巨噬细胞或多形核白细胞通过 Fc 受体与肿瘤细胞结合。IgG3 似乎对大颗粒淋巴细胞参与的 ADCC 反应特别重要，而 IgG2a 可能在与人单核细胞相互作用时更有效[194]。在某些情况下，在与肿瘤靶位相互作用前，用抗体武装单核白细胞已成为可能。在体内，肿瘤患者由于缺乏适当的效应细胞或由于存在循环免疫复合物占据或下调了 Fc 受体，ADCC 反应可能被削弱。与黑色素瘤细胞 GD3 反应的抗体还可与 T 细胞表面 GD3 结合，增强其细胞毒反应或增殖反应[195]。一个结合位点为 T 细胞相关抗原、一个结合位点为肿瘤相关抗原的复合抗体已经产生[196]。这样的复合抗体可能通过增强效应细胞与肿瘤靶位的接触而增强 IL-2 激活的 T 细胞对肿瘤细胞的杀灭[197]。

药物-单克隆抗体偶联物治疗

单克隆抗体已与多种传统细胞毒性药物结合，包括抗叶酸类、蒽环类、长春碱类和烷化剂类药物。一些药物如阿霉素在形成偶联物前预聚合可获得更高的药物抗体比。如果在抗原结合位点未找到最具活性的残基，药物可以与赖氨酸残基的氨基侧链结合。小鼠免疫球蛋白碳水化合物基团与药物的连接是一种位点特异性偶联，通常不妨碍抗体的结合[198,199]。

由于观察到许多细胞表面抗原数量不足每细胞 10^5 拷贝数，一些研究者担心在细胞表面释放（1~3）×10^6 个药物分子可能或不足以消除肿瘤。另一担心与大免疫球蛋白载体偶联物通过肿瘤毛细血管的转运能力有关。然而，临床前研究证实药物-单克隆抗体偶联物较游离单药更加有效。仅有部分偶联物的疗效更好，不过大部分毒性降低，使得治疗指数提高。当与单克隆制剂相连时，治疗优势可能与药物的摄取率或摄取模式改变有关。在某些情况下，新设计的连接方式使偶联物在低

pH 或只有在溶酶体蛋白酶存在时才释放出药物。

吉姆单抗奥佐米星

吉姆单抗奥佐米星(gemtuzumab ozogamicin,Mylotarg®)属于卡奇霉素类,可以与抗 CD33 偶联[200]。CD33 是一个分子量为 67kDa 糖蛋白,在 90%以上的 AMLs 和早期髓系祖细胞表面表达,但在正常多能干细胞上不表达。吉姆单抗奥佐米星,是人源化抗 CD33 抗体和细胞毒性卡奇霉素类抗生素的偶联物,可被成髓细胞迅速内化并诱导其凋亡[201]。3 项多中心试验对吉姆单抗奥佐米星在 142 例 $CD33^+$ AML 患者中进行了评估,在首次复发后于第 1 天和第 15 天分别以 $9mg/m^2$ 的浓度给药两次[202],30%的患者得到完全缓解。

毒副反应

由于造血前体细胞表达 CD33,在 101 位 60 岁及 60 岁以上患者中,99%的观察到 3 度或 4 度中性粒细胞减少症和血小板减少症。感染(27%)和黏膜炎(4%)较少见[203]。不过,在 119 例接受吉姆单抗奥佐米星的患者中,14 例(12%)发生静脉闭塞性疾病,包括 5 例之前未接受干细胞移植的患者[204]。尽管有这些毒性,吉姆单抗奥佐米星于 2000 年获得 FDA 的加速批准。但由于中期分析中因未取得生存获益而于 2004 年停止了试验,并于 2010 年自愿撤出市场。近期的荟萃分析结果显示尽管吉姆单抗奥佐米星改善了 PFS,但并未改善 OS[205]。

本妥昔单抗

本妥昔单抗(brentuximab vedotin,Adcetris®)是抗 CD30 嵌合 IgG1 抗体和一种有丝分裂的小分子抑制剂 3~5 单位瑞他汀(单甲基乙基澳瑞他汀 E)的结合物,在 2011 年和 2012 年分别获得了美国 FDA 和欧盟的加速批准上市,用于治疗复发性霍奇金淋巴瘤(Hodgkin lymphoma,HL)和间变性大细胞淋巴瘤(anaplastic large cell lymphoma,ALCL)。在一项涉及 102 例 HL 患者的临床试验中评估了本妥昔单抗的疗效,其中 73%的患者得到完全或部分缓解,其平均治疗时间是 6.7 个月。

本妥昔单抗在全身性 ALCL 患者中的疗效在一项单臂临床试验中进行了评估,58 例患者中 86%的患者得到完全或部分缓解,其平均治疗时间为 12.6 个月[206],获批试验是基于移植前因素的随机、双盲、安慰剂对照,在经过人类干细胞移植(human stem cell transplant,HSCT)的 329 名具有复发或较高进展风险的经典 HL 的患者中的Ⅲ期临床研究[85]。在进行自体 HSCT 后,患者被随机分配了本妥昔单抗或安慰剂组,每 3 周一次,最多进行 16 个周期。结果显示,本妥昔单抗组的中位 PFS 为 42.9 个月,而安慰剂组为 24.1 个月($P=0.001$)。

毒副反应

使用本妥昔单抗治疗的患者中最常见(>20%)的不良反应是中性粒细胞减少、周围感觉和运动神经异常、血小板减少、贫血、上呼吸道感染、疲劳、恶心和腹泻。有 25%的患者报告了严重的不良反应,包括肺炎、发热、呕吐、恶心、肝毒性和周围感觉神经异常。在注册试验中,32%的患者因严重不良反应导致中止治疗。

曲妥珠单抗-美坦新偶联物

曲妥珠单抗-美坦新偶联物(ado-trastuzumab-emtansine,TDM-1,Kadcyla®)是人源化抗 HER-2 IgG1 抗体曲妥珠单抗和结合微管蛋白的细胞毒性药物氨丹宁(DM1)的结合物。该药物于 2013 年获得美国 FDA 和欧盟的批准上市,用于治疗 HER-2 阳性复发性乳腺癌患者,基于一项纳入了 991 例紫杉类和曲妥珠单抗治疗失败患者的随机,多中心,开放性临床试验。患者被随机分配至接受静脉输注 TDM-1 组或口服拉帕替尼和卡培他滨组。与口服拉帕替尼和卡培他滨组相比,TDM-1 组患者具有更长的 PFS(9.4 个月 vs 6.4 个月,$P<0.0001$)和 OS(30.9 个月 vs 25.1 个月,$P=0.0006$)[207]。

毒副反应

在接受 TDM-1 治疗的患者中观察到的最常见的不良反应是疲劳、恶心、肌肉骨骼疼痛、血小板减少、头痛、转氨酶升高、贫血和便秘。最常见的 3~4 级毒副反应(>2%)是血小板减少、转氨酶升高、贫血、低钾血症、周围神经病和疲劳。导致药物停用最常见的不良事件是血小板减少症和转氨酶血症。TDM-1 的临床试验已经报道了严重的药物引起的肝胆疾病,包括至少两例药物性肝损伤和相关性肝性脑病的死亡病例。其他重大不良反应包括左心室功能不全,间质性肺疾病和输注相关反应。

肿瘤的放射免疫治疗

放射免疫治疗(radioimmunotherapy,RIT)是一种肿瘤治疗方法,将发射细胞毒性射线的放射性核素标记抗体或抗体片段选择性地输送至肿瘤细胞。虽然通过抗体使放射性核素定位于肿瘤细胞的概念长期以来都被接受,但这一方法直到单克隆制剂的出现才得以实现,单克隆制剂可进行特异性的定位并允许临床试验用偶联物大批量生产。外照射治疗时,躯体只有有限部位受到照射,设计的照射野与肿瘤的范围相匹配。尽管常规放射疗法可有效治疗局部疾病,但由于正常组织的毒性问题以及放疗野外的肿瘤可以逃逸射线的照射,因此通常难以对弥散性的肿瘤进行放射治疗。对于 RIT,如果靶向抗原或受体也存在于转移灶上,则原则上也可以对其进行治疗,即使在治疗时尚不清楚它们的存在。

接受 RIT 的最大障碍也许来源于医师和患者对放射性物质的恐惧,而如果接受更好的教育可以改善这一情况。另一方面,与本章中讨论的其他基于抗体的策略相比,RIT 具有一些重要的优势。首先,可以用小剂量的治疗性放射性核素或类似的放射性核素标记抗体,然后可以通过核医学成像确定 RIT 患者的 RIT 药代动力学。这些信息随后可用于选择最有可能从 RIT 中受益的患者,并确定个体特异的治疗肿瘤所需要的放射性剂量水平[208]。其次,与仅杀死靶细胞的 ADC(抗体药物结合物)和免疫毒素不同,综述[209]中总结的放射性核素的细胞毒性作用可以扩展到靶细胞之外,包括自照射、交叉辐射和旁观者的作用。交叉辐射源于大多数治疗性辐射的范围是多细胞的,而旁观者效应可以通过目前尚不了解的机制杀死未被辐射直接穿过的邻近细胞[210,211]。两者均可导致不摄取标记抗体的邻近细胞的破坏,有助于弥补抗体递送、靶分子表达的异质性,或两者皆有的异质性。

放射性核素的作用

RIT 的一个优势在于,在临床具体应用时,可使放射性核素的作用范围与正常组织的毒性限制与肿瘤剂量均匀分布最大化之间的平衡相匹配。在选择 RIT 放射性核素时必须考虑的其他因素包括:①物理半衰期与抗体药代动力学的兼容性;②存在相应的标记方法使标记抗体具有足够的稳定性;③适合临床使用的商业化供应。放射性核素的特性在 RIT 及其他靶向放疗中的应用进展已在综述中有了很广泛的探讨[212]。

绝大部分 RIT 研究采用衰变发射 β 粒子或 α 粒子的放射性核素,其组织穿透距离分别为 1~10mm 和 50~90μm。近期对发射亚细胞径程(<1keV)的俄歇电子的放射性核素进行了评估,最初被认为仅位于细胞核附近时才具有细胞毒性[213]。但是,至少有一项研究表明,俄歇电子发射体也可通过非内化抗体传送而发挥作用[214]。

β 放射源

绝大部分 RIT 试验和唯一获得 FDA 批准的两种 RIT 产品,均采用发射 β 粒子的放射性核素。辐射剂的细胞毒性作用在很大程度上取决于它们的线性能量传递(linear energy transfer,LET),这是它们在给定距离内沉积的能量。β 粒子的 LET 约为 0.2keV/μm,被认为是稀疏电离辐射,主要导致易于修复的单链 DNA 损伤[207]。考虑到它们的治疗路径长度,β 射线最适合治疗直径大于 0.5cm 的肿瘤,因为在此情况下,大部分的衰变能量被肿瘤而不是邻近的正常组织吸收。短距离 β 放射源如碘-131、镥-177 和铜-67 可用于治疗微转移灶,它们衰变能量中的大部分将沉积于小的肿瘤细胞簇中。相反,能量更大、距离更长的 β 放射源如钇-90 和铼-186 可破坏更大的肿瘤病灶,消灭因缺乏抗原表达或血管不良而逃过直接靶向治疗的肿瘤细胞。肿瘤中剂量沉积均匀性的程度高度依赖于抗体分子靶位的特点、肿瘤血流动力学和放射性核素的性质。

α 放射源

α 粒子通常较 β 粒子具有更高的能量,在组织内的治疗路径长度非常短(<100μm)。α 粒子的 LET 约为 100keV/μm,密集电离并产生 DNA 损伤簇,发生不易修复的双链 DNA 断裂[207]。此外,α 粒子的细胞毒性作用在很大程度上与剂量率和氧合作用无关,从而提供了治疗乏氧肿瘤区域的可能性。由于治疗距离短,α 放射源可能在 RIT 直接治疗血液循环中的肿瘤细胞、微转移灶和邻近腔室表面的肿瘤细胞如卵巢癌及脑膜肿瘤中最为有效。被广泛研究用于 RIT 的发射 α 粒子的放射性核素包括半衰期为 61 分钟的铋-212,半衰期为 46 分钟的铋-213,半衰期为 7.2 小时的砹-211,半衰期为 10 天的锕-225 和最近被研究的半衰期为 18.7 天的钍-227[215,216]。铋-212 和铋-213 的半衰期太短,在抗体标记方法和患者处理上产生逻辑问题。另外,半衰期过长的锕-225 和钍-227,虽然在逻辑上存在益处,但却对放射化学未来提出很大挑战,因为必须设计出策略以保持放射性核素和抗体之间的连接在多周疗程内保持稳定。更为复杂的是,需要将多种发射 α 射线、具有不同化学性质的子放射性核素局限在肿瘤内,以避免对正常组织的剂量限制性毒性。由于这些原因,应用最广泛的标记抗体 α 放射源为砹-211[217]。采用 α 放射源的临床试验已经开始,将在本章稍后部分中叙述。

淋巴瘤的放射免疫治疗

血液恶性肿瘤,尤其是淋巴瘤,由于其天然的放射敏感性以及在淋巴瘤细胞表面存在分化抗原可以作为靶点,是 RIT 极具吸引力的治疗靶位。目前唯一获得 FDA 批准的两种 RIT 药物,主要临床适应证为治疗复发性或难治性低级别 B 细胞 NHL(表 64-2)。它们是钇-90-伊替莫单抗和碘-131-托西莫单抗,分别于 2002 年和 2003 年获得批准。靶点均为细胞表面抗原 CD20,其不仅在约 95% 的 B 细胞淋巴瘤中表达,也见于正常 B 细胞。由于此原因,治疗方案的一个基本部分为,在给予放射性标记抗体前,先给予相对大剂量的冷抗体使正常 B 细胞结合位点饱和。RIT 试剂的标准的操作流程和其他使用实践方面的注意事项也被描述[218,219]。

表 64-2 获批准的非霍奇金淋巴瘤放射免疫治疗

性质	钇-90-伊替莫单抗	碘-131-托西莫单抗
产品名称	Zevalin	Bexxar
标记抗体	伊替莫单抗	托西莫单抗
类型	小鼠 IgG1	小鼠 IgG2a
用于阻断的抗体	嵌合利妥昔单抗	小鼠托西莫单抗
计量	$250mg/m^2$	450mg
治疗用放射性核素	钇-90(^{90}Y)	碘-131(^{131}I)
半衰期	2.7 天	8.1 天
最大 β 射线能量	2.28MeV	0.61MeV
最大组织距离	11.3mm	2.3mm
γ 射线发射	否	是
标记方法	双功能螯合剂(tiuxetan)	亲电子放射卤化
放射性核素显像	铟-111(^{111}In)	碘-131(^{131}I)
显像作用	显示可接收的生分布	确定全身清除动力学
患者特异性计量测量	否	是
给药活性	20~30mCi	50~200mCi
计量参数	mCi/kg	计算全身剂量
血小板>150 000/m^3 的基准点	0.4mCi/kg	75cGy
血小板在 100 000~149 000/m^3 之间的基准点	0.3mCi/kg	65cGy

钇-90-伊替莫单抗

钇-90-伊替莫单抗(^{90}Y-ibritumomab tiuxetan,Zevalin®)包含抗 CD20 小鼠单克隆抗体和发射纯 β 射线的放射性核素钇-90,两者通过 MX-DTPA(tiuxetan)螯合物共价连接。治疗方案为先采用另一种放射性金属铟-111 标记的伊替莫单抗对患者显像,在钇-90 治疗前明确可接收的抗体生物分布[220]。很多早期的研究表明,钇-90-伊替莫单抗与利妥昔单抗治疗相比,可以显著增加复发型滤泡性淋巴瘤的治疗效果。在 143 例复发淋巴瘤患者中进行的一项随机试验，比较钇-90-伊替莫单抗和利妥昔单抗的治疗效果，钇-90-伊替莫单抗的缓解率为 80%，利妥昔单抗为 56%（$P=0.002$）[221]。应用钇-90-伊替莫单抗治疗 54 例利妥昔单抗难治性滤泡淋巴瘤，总缓解率为 74%，其中完全缓解率为 15%[222]。对 211 例患者进行长期随访，37%的患者达到长期缓解且时间大于 12 个月，其长期应答组的中位进展时间为 29.3 个月[223]。更多的近期研究评估钇-90-伊替莫单抗联合大剂量化疗方案的治疗潜力[224]，在诱导治疗后巩固，包括其他形式的 B 细胞淋巴瘤[225-228]，以及作为一种滤泡性淋巴瘤患者的前线单药治疗[229,230]，在大多数研究中均观察到 PFS 和 OS 的明显改善。

碘-131-托西莫单抗

碘-131-托西莫单抗（^{131}I-tositumomab，Bexxar®）临床使用流程与钇-90-伊替莫单抗的操作流程相似，不同之处在于，为使放射性碘标记的抗体脱落后造成的甲状腺辐射剂量最小化，给予甲状腺保护剂量的碘化钾饱和溶液（或卢戈尔液）[231]。此外，由于碘-131-托西莫单抗清除动力学在个体患者中变化较大，治疗策略的一个基本部分就是确定药物的全身清除半衰期，在注射相当于 5mCi 剂量的碘-131-托西莫单抗后的 1 周内通过一系列三核药物扫描获取。然后根据血小板计数高于或低于 150 000/m^3，计算产生 65cGy 或 75cGy 全身剂量所需要的碘-131 活性。在对 250 例经过充分预处理的惰性淋巴瘤患者进行的长期分析中，报告了碘-131-托西莫单抗治疗后的客观缓解率为 47%～68%，其中完全缓解率为 20%～38%[232]。对于完全缓解者，中位缓解期在最近一次合格的化疗后是 6.1 个月，而 RIT 后的中位缓解期超过 47 个月。这些结果与^{131}I 标记的嵌合抗 CD20 抗体利妥昔单抗进行治疗获得的结果相似[233]。在长期随访中发现经碘-131-托西莫单抗治疗的 12 例惰性淋巴瘤患者中有 6 例发生复发，其中位 DFS 达到 9.8 年[234]。应用 RIT 在复发/难治的 NHL 患者中，使用清髓剂量的碘-131-托西莫单抗治疗后进行自体干细胞输注，结果显示的总缓解率为 87%，中位进展时间为 47.5 个月，OS 为 101.5 个月[235]。最后，两项近期的Ⅲ期研究单用碘-131-托西莫单抗和多剂量利妥昔单抗联合 BEAM 和 CHOP 方案化疗分别治疗复发性 DLBCL[236] 和先前未治疗的滤泡性 NHL[237] 时，显示出相似的令人鼓舞的结果。

尽管使用 Zevalin 和 Bexxar 获得了令人信服的反应数据，但两种 RIT 药物均未成为淋巴瘤患者的标准一线治疗药物。由于销售不佳，葛兰素史克（Glaxo-SmithKline）于 2014 年 2 月停止出售 Bexxar，有人猜测 Zevalin（Spectrum Pharmaceuticals）可能会遭受类似的命运，这种情况可能归因于许多因素。当前的法规要求放射性药物必须由核医学或放射肿瘤学人员管理，而不是由负责 NHL 患者治疗的肿瘤学家管理。肿瘤医师需要承担化疗和利妥昔单抗的费用管理，而不是 RIT 药物的费用，从而进行肿瘤医师的财务控制。此外，RIT 是在医院而不是在门诊设施中执行的，执行低辐射剂量成像研究来确定患者特定的剂量会使其他程序的安排变得复杂。最后，尽管在这些经过大量预处理的人群中，其他药物可能会导致这些不良反应，但使用这些 RIT 治疗后，存在继发性恶性肿瘤，白血病和骨髓增生异常的风险[238]。

实体瘤的放射免疫治疗

应用 RIT 对实体瘤进行治疗更加难以获得成功，这源于许多因素，其中最重要的是它们对放射线的敏感性较低。在外部射线照射下，低至 4Gy 的剂量可有效治疗淋巴瘤，而对于包括乳腺癌、肺癌、前列腺癌、结肠直肠癌和胰腺癌以及成胶质细胞瘤的实体瘤，临床反应通常需要 50～80Gy 的剂量[239]。在 NHL 中杀死细胞的主要机制是细胞凋亡，而在实体瘤中却是不同的，它们对放射线的反应有所不同[207]。RIT 治疗实体瘤的其他障碍包括肿瘤间质压力影响了完整抗体的可达到性和异质性血流，肿瘤缺氧。最近的两项综述[240,241]中概述了实体瘤患者的试验结果，观察到的肿瘤反应不一，并且不如血液系统恶性肿瘤令人印象深刻。最令人鼓舞的结果来源于对微小残留病灶的治疗，最大限度减小了因剂量分布不均带来的不利影响，而这些微小病灶用常规手段治疗存在困难。有前景的应用领域包括结直肠癌，前列腺癌和外科减瘤术后的脑瘤。

结直肠癌

实体瘤患者中最令人鼓舞的 RIT 试验之一也许是一项 2 期试验，结直肠癌患者肝转移灶姑息性切除后，应用放射性碘标记的抗癌胚抗原（anticarcinoembryonic antigen，CEA）人源化单克隆抗体拉贝珠单抗进行辅助治疗[242]。采用^{131}I 作为放射性标记是因为其 β 粒子的穿透距离相对较短，与微转移灶的大小正好匹配。23 例患者接受了 40～60mCi/m^2 ^{131}I 标记的拉贝珠单抗，对其中 19 例进行了疗效评估，并与未接受 RIT 的同期对照组进行比较。在 91 个月的中位随访中，接受 RIT 患者的中位生存期为 58 个月，对照组为 31 个月，其 5 年生存率为 42.1%。

前列腺癌

J591 是对前列腺特异性膜抗原（prostate-specific membrane antigen，PSMA）胞外域具有特异性的人源化单克隆抗体，已被^{90}Y[243]和^{177}Lu[244]标记，并在Ⅰ期研究中被评估为转移性去势抵抗性前列腺癌患者的靶向放射治疗药物。选择^{177}Lu 标记的 J591 进行Ⅱ期评估，是因为其较低的 β 粒子能量，从而降低了骨髓毒性，并释放出可以成像的 γ 射线[245]。共有 47 例患者接受了 65 或 70mCi/m2 的治疗^{177}Lu-J591；在较低的剂量下有 13.3%的患者 PSA 下降 30%，中位生存期为 11.9 个月，而在最大耐受剂量水平，有 46.9%的患者的 PSA 下降 30%，中位生存期为 21.8 个月。^{177}Lu 活性分布的伽马相机成像显示，在 93.6%的患者中药物靶向了转移部位。

脑肿瘤

由于成年人的脑肿瘤几乎不转移至颅外，因此可以使用 RIT 局部疗法，将标记抗体直接注射到肿瘤手术切除后形成的空腔内。到目前为止，已有超过 300 例脑肿瘤患者接受了与细胞黏合素-C 结合的放射性标记抗体治疗，细胞黏合素-C 为一种细胞外基质糖蛋白，在超过 90%的 GBM 中过表达，随肿瘤的发展其表达水平增加[246]。一系列Ⅰ、Ⅱ期临床试验报道了令人鼓舞的疗效，这些试验经 FDA 授权，在复发和新诊断患者中，给予固定放射活性的^{131}I 标记抗细胞黏合素 81C6 抗体。近期很多试验研究了^{131}I 标记的 81C6 的效果，注射的^{131}I 的剂量使手术切除形成的 2cm 空腔内平均放射剂量达到了 44Gy 的目标剂量[247]。44Gy 的目标剂量是根据之前固定活性水平方案的结果分析得出的，此剂量可提供最大的肿瘤控制而不伴放射性坏死。在新诊断的患者中（16 例 GBM，5 例间变型星形细胞瘤），所有患者及 GBM 患者的中位 OS 分别为 97 周和 91 周。

改进的放射免疫治疗策略

特别是对于实体瘤患者的治疗，要提高 RIT 的治疗效果，就需要在基于抗体的载体系统和放射性核素的特性方面开发更复杂的策略。已评估了各种酶和遗传衍生的大小不同的抗体片段[248,249]，目的是在更好的肿瘤渗透性和更快速的正常组织清除之间寻求最佳平衡，这可通过较小的构建体和更长的肿瘤停留时间来实现，而通常在保持完整 IgG 抗体的情况下会更好。肿瘤脉管系统起着重要的作用，因为它阻碍了均质抗体的传递，这可以通过使用血管破坏剂（例如康培他汀）来克服[250]。另一方面，肿瘤脉管系统为 RIT 提供了诱人的靶标，因为破坏肿瘤血管可以提高治疗的效率和均一性[251]。改善 RIT 的两种方法受到了特别关注，即预靶向和发射 α 粒子的放射性核素。

在预靶向中，首先使用抗体，并在一段延迟时间后实现对肿瘤的充分摄取和正常组织清除，然后注射放射性标记的低分子量化合物。通过将标记物从抗体转移到较小的分子，可以提高肿瘤与正常组织的比率和肿瘤放射剂量[252]。最初的方法是使用抗体-链霉亲和素偶联物，然后使用放射性标记的生物素，有或没有中间清除剂[253]。然而，免疫原性和内源性生物素的干扰是混杂因素。已进入临床研究阶段的第二种预靶向策略涉及使用与肿瘤相关分子靶标以及含有放射性金属螯合物的小分子或肽结合的双特异性抗体[254]。这种方法的可行性已经在复发性甲状腺髓样癌患者中进行了评估。患者首先接受了双特异性抗 CEA 抗体，然后在 4 天后用 ^{131}I 标记的肽携带了两个半抗原组。中位 OS 为 110 个月，显著长于未经治疗的患者（61 个月）。

发射 α 粒子的放射性核素对于 RIT 的最吸引人的特点是，与其他类型的辐射相比，它们的效力显著提高。细胞培养研究表明，只需少量的 α 粒子穿过，人类肿瘤细胞就可能被杀死[256]。此外，α 粒子的细胞毒性几乎与剂量率，氧气浓度和细胞周期无关[207]。α 粒子在 RIT 方面的概念优势已广为人知，对患者的实际研究需要放射性核素生产，蛋白质标记化学和辐射剂量学方面的发展。

第一项使用发射 α 粒子的放射性核素进行的 RIT 临床试验涉及 ^{213}Bi 标记的 HuM195，HuM195 是一种与 CD33 抗原反应的人源化抗体，在人白血病细胞中过表达[257]。Ⅰ期试验在 18 例复发性和难治性 AML 或慢性粒细胞性白血病进行。由于 ^{213}Bi 的半衰期为 46 分钟，因此为了获得治疗所需的活性水平（602~3 515MBq），应多次给药（3~7 次）。潜在的肿瘤部位（骨髓、肝脏和脾脏）与全身之间的吸收剂量比，比以前用该 β 发射体标记的抗体高出约 1 000 倍。很多患者的白血病肿瘤细胞负荷大幅减少，不过尚未观察到完全缓解。一项后续的Ⅰ/Ⅱ期临床试验评估了 ^{213}Bi 标记的 HuM195 用于阿糖胞苷部分减瘤性化疗后的疗效，该研究结果显示，25 例患者中有 6 例完全缓解和部分缓解。最近启动了半衰期为 10 天的 α 粒子发射器 ^{225}Ac 标记的 HuM195 的Ⅰ期试验[258]。

最近报道了一项Ⅰ期试验，将 ^{211}At 标记的嵌合型 81C6 抗细胞黏合素单克隆抗体输入复发胶质瘤患者手术切除后形成的胶质瘤空腔内，以确定其药代动力学和治疗疗效[259]。患者包括 14 例 GBM 患者，3 例间变性星形细胞瘤和 1 例间变性少突胶质细胞瘤。连续的伽马照相机成像和血液计数表明，^{211}At 标记的免疫偶联物在体内是稳定的，其中 96.7%±3.6% 的衰减发生在切除腔中。复发性 GBM 患者的中位生存期为 54 周，明显优于常规治疗（31 周）。其中两个复发性 GBM 患者中的生存时间达到了 150 周和 151 周，尤其令人鼓舞，已经计划在初诊断的 GBM 患者中使用 ^{211}At 标记的 81C6 抗体进行临床试验。

靶向毒素治疗

靶向毒素是包含细胞结合域和毒素域的杂合蛋白药物。细胞结合结构域将药物递送至细胞表面。在加工和/或内化后，毒素域触发细胞死亡。毒素可使细胞表面出现穿孔（蛋白水解作用）或催化失活胞质蛋白的合成（白喉毒素，假单胞菌外毒素或皂苷）。在某些情况下，通过将蛋白酶特异性切割序列添加至毒素来产生特异性。构建靶向毒素的最大挑战是鉴别出靶向受体或蛋白酶，以选择性杀灭肿瘤细胞。尽管一些正在研制中的复合物已经具备了独立的细胞结合肽段和效应物/毒素肽段，但大部分药物仍由单个多肽组成。设计靶向毒素是为了对标准的细胞毒性药物耐药的恶性肿瘤产生临床作用。由于任何一种靶向毒素都不具有绝对的肿瘤特异性，因此根据结合或活化的特异性以及特殊的毒素可观察到不同的毒副反应。尽管合成这种复杂蛋白质复合物具有挑战性，但一些药物在一些人肿瘤治疗中已显示出出色的临床获益，并仅伴有轻、中度的不良反应。我们将讨论已获批准或正在进行中后期临床试验的抗肿瘤药物。每一种药物我们都将单独描述其药代动力学、免疫反应、毒性和临床反应，尽管许多药物的药代动力学和毒理学性质相同。

用于白血病和淋巴瘤的靶向毒素

地尼白介素毒素连接物

白喉毒素是一个分子量 58kDa Mr 的蛋白质，包含 3 个结构域。N 末端区催化 ADP 核糖基化延长因子（EF-2），可使细胞蛋白质合成失活，导致细胞死亡。中间区为疏水区，协助催化区转移至细胞质。C 末端区为 β 折叠富集区，可与细胞结合。地尼白介素毒素连接物（denileukin diftitox）是用人 IL-2 代替了白喉毒素正常的细胞结合区。在关键性Ⅲ期试验中，IB 到 IVA 皮肤 T 细胞淋巴瘤（cutaneous T-cell lymphoma，CTCL）患者给予药物 9μg/（kg · d）或 18μg/（kg · d），静脉输注，连续 5 天，每 3 周一次，共 8 周期[260]。药物半衰期为 30 分钟，不良反应包括急性细胞因子反应（发热、畏寒、恶心、呕吐、肌痛和关节痛、胸痛、背痛）、一过性肝酶异常（高转氨酶血症）和血管渗漏综合征（低血压、低白蛋白血症、呼吸困难和水肿）。大部分患者发生了针对药物的免疫反应，但这与药物的毒性或临床反应无关。临床缓解率为 30%，其中部分缓解 20%，完全缓解 10%，中位缓解期 6 个月。基于这些结果，地尼白介素毒素偶联物被批准用于治疗难治性 CTCL。在随后的随访中，有许多患者在 2 年内仍然维持缓解状态[261]。地尼白介素毒素偶联物还可以应用于 T 细胞 NHL（48%应答）、CLL（27%）、B 细胞 NHL（25%）及全身性肥大细胞增多症，以及结外 NK/T 细胞淋巴瘤、外周

T-细胞淋巴瘤、皮下脂膜炎样 T 细胞淋巴瘤和成人 T 细胞白血病[262-269]。此外,甲状腺毒症和视力丧失的罕见毒性也得到了报道[270,271]。丹尼白二氟乙酸与其他药物如细胞毒性药物、利妥昔单抗、贝沙罗汀或电子束辐射联合应用可能会增强疗效[272,273]。目前,由于制造问题,无法使用地尼白介素毒素偶联物。

假单胞菌外毒素

假单胞菌外毒素(moxetumomab pasudotox)是一个分子量 68kDa Mr 的多肽,包含 N 末端细胞结合区,两亲性含螺旋转运区和 C 末端 ADP 核糖基化区。假单胞菌外毒素通过去除 1~252 号和 365~380 号氨基酸残基改造假单胞菌外毒素,阻断其与正常组织的结合,将二硫键稳定性抗 CD22 Fv 段与一个分子量 38kDa Mr 的修饰毒素(PE38)融合。然后使用热点诱变来增加分子的亲和力,苏氨酸-组氨酸-色氨酸在重链的抗原结合位点取代了丝氨酸-丝氨酸-酪氨酸。应用假单胞菌外毒素治疗 28 例毛细胞性白血病患者,以 5~30μg/kg 隔日一次的剂量给药,共 3 次,持续 1~16 个周期,未产生剂量限制性毒性[274]。毒副作用包括 2 级溶血性尿毒症综合征、低白蛋白血症、转氨酶异常、水肿、头痛、低血压、恶心和疲劳。在第 1 周期之后,只有 5%的患者出现中和抗体。总缓解率为 86%,完全缓解率为 46%。中位无病生存时间超过 2 年。所有接受假单胞菌外毒素的患者均得到了疾病缓解。

SL-401

白喉毒素的催化和易位结构域通过一个 Met-His 接头与人 IL-3 融合。45 例高危,复发或难治性的急性髓细胞性白血病或骨髓增生异常的患者接受 SL-401 不超过 6 次的治疗,每隔 15 分钟静脉输注一次[275]。半衰期为 30 分钟,且峰浓度呈剂量依赖性。在患者间进行剂量递增,剂量范围为 4~12.5μg/(kg·次)。没有观察到剂量限制性毒性,但副作用包括短暂的转氨酶血症、低白蛋白血症、发热、寒战、恶心和呕吐。大多数患者在第 15 天到 30 天之间出现抗融合蛋白抗体。疗效显示 1 例完全缓解,持续 8 个月,两例部分缓解,持续 3 个月和 4 个月。另外,使用 SL11 的 10 例浆样树突状细胞瘤患者,每天给予 SL401 12.5μg/kg,静脉输注 15 分钟,最多 5 次[276]。9 例可评估患者中有 7 例(78%)有效,包括 5 例完全缓解和 2 例部分缓解。中位缓解期为 5 个月,且 2 例患者缓解期超过 2 年。

DT2219

将白喉毒素的催化和易位域与靶向人 CD19 和人 CD22 的抗体的双特异性 scFv 融合,产生了 DT2219。该药在临床研究中,以 0.5~80μg/(kg·d)静脉输注 2-h 隔日一次共 4 次的方式给药,纳入 25 例表达 CD19 和/或 CD22 的成熟或前体 B 细胞淋巴恶性肿瘤患者[277]。药物半衰期为 1~2 小时。1 周后,有 30%的患者出现了中和抗体。剂量限制性毒性是血管渗漏综合征。其他副作用包括短暂的体重增加、水肿、低白蛋白血症、发热、疲劳和转氨酶血症。最大耐受剂量超过 80μg/kg。两例患者获得部分缓解,分别持续了 2 个多月和 8 个多月。

免疫再塑

白喉毒素的催化结构域和易位结构域与两个单链抗体片段融合,该片段与 CD3ε 细胞外结构域上的酸性环具有反应性。实验纳入 CD3 阳性淋巴瘤患者,剂量递增范围 2.5~11.25μg/kg,连续 15 分钟静脉输注,每天两次,最多 4 天,以进行免疫重塑[278]。剂量限制性毒性为 EBV 活化和血管渗漏综合征。最大耐受剂量为 7.5μg/kg。其他常见的不良事件是发热、寒战、低血磷和转氨酶血症。在 25 例 CTCL 患者中,有 9 例缓解,缓解率为 36%。中位完全缓解期超过 5 年。

针对实体恶性和良性肿瘤的靶向毒素

PRX302

以气单胞菌溶素原前体蛋白加工酶的切割位点修饰前列腺特异抗原(prostate-specific antigen, PSA)选择性切割位点形成 PRX302。气单胞菌溶素原是形成通道的细菌原毒素,可与多种细胞表面受体结合。24 例首次放疗失败后局部复发的前列腺癌患者及 92 例良性前列腺增生(benign prostate hyperplasia, BPH)患者,通过组织间隙给药,给予重组修饰的气单胞菌溶素 PRX302[279,280]。在每项研究中,该药物耐受性良好,仅轻度不良反应包括在开始的几天内出现短暂的局部不适和刺激性的泌尿症状。对于前列腺癌,剂量范围为 0.03~3μg/g 组织,对于 BPH,剂量范围为 0.6μg/g 组织。通过超声引导的经会阴前列腺内注射完成药物输入。63%的前列腺癌患者的 PSA 降低,而 BPH 患者的前列腺症状得到改善。BPH 患者的中位反应持续时间超过 1 年。

SS1P

将用于构建莫妥昔单抗假单抗的结合位点缺失的假单胞菌外毒素 PE38 片段与间皮素抗体二硫键稳定的 Fv 融合,以形成重组免疫毒素 SS1P。晚期间皮瘤、卵巢癌和胰腺癌患者接受 SS1P 治疗,18~45μg/(kg·次),静脉输注 30 分钟,隔日一次,共 3~6 次[281]。

剂量限制性毒性是荨麻疹,血管渗漏综合征和胸膜炎。3 次给药方案的最大耐受剂量为 45μg/kg。4/33 例轻微反应,19/33 例稳定疾病。在另一项研究中,24 例间皮瘤,卵巢癌或胰腺癌患者以 4~25μg/(kg·d)的剂量连续输注 10 天的 SS1P[282]。最大耐受剂量为 25μg/(kg·d),剂量限制性毒性为血管渗漏综合征。在 75 例患者中观察到了免疫原性。SS1P 血浆水平维持稳定时间达到 10 天,中位峰浓度为 153ng/ml。一例患者表现出部分缓解。与喷司他丁联合环磷酰胺或甲氨蝶呤联合顺铂联合使用时,SS1P 具有显著的抗间皮瘤活性[283,284]。在前者,3/10 例患者获得了重大反应。后者,12/20 例患者获得部分缓解。

IL13-PE

IL13-PE 是一种重组人细胞毒素,由人 IL-13 与截短形式的假单胞菌外毒素融合而成。8 例转移性肾上腺皮质癌的患者接受 1 或 2μg/kg 的 IL13-PE 静脉输注治疗[285]。平均血清峰浓度为 21ng/ml,半衰期为 30 分钟。8 例患者中 4 例在 14~28 天内产生中和抗体。毒性反应是血小板减少症和肾功能不全。1 例患者疾病稳定。

癌症相关疾病的靶向毒素

SP-SAP

神经肽 P 物质化学耦合到重组皂苷。SP-SAP 的给药方式是通过对癌症患者进行腰椎穿刺给予单一鞘内剂量完成[286]。目前,患者已经接受的剂量范围为 1~16μg,正在逐步增加剂量,但已经观察到了短暂的疼痛减轻和使阿片类药物的使用减少。

关于靶向毒素的结论

靶向毒素的毒性似乎可以预测。如正常组织中存在被目标毒素识别的受体/抗原，则预期可观察到与该正常组织受损有关的副作用。SS1P 结合正常的胸膜表面间皮素并产生胸膜炎。其他毒性与配体结合无关，由与肝细胞，血管内皮和巨噬细胞蛋白受体的结合而介导。这些正常组织对靶毒素的非特异性摄取会导致转氨酶升高（高转氨酶血症）、血管渗漏综合征和急性输注反应。预防性皮质类固醇可缓解其中一些毒性。

大多数靶向毒素的循环半衰期为 30~120 分钟，主要在肾脏和肝脏清除。这些药物由于体积大而无法渗透到血管外部，因此在药物更易进入的血液系统肿瘤中观察到更高的反应率。在某些研究中，靶向毒素的免疫原性影响了药代动力学和再治疗的反应率。

这些药物中某些药物的反应率极佳，尤其对细胞毒性药物耐药的疾病。毒素激发的灾难性死亡可激活免疫反应，是有的患者获得长期缓解的原因之一。靶向毒素联合具有非交叉耐药作用机制和毒性不重叠的其他手段，为患者提供了额外的获益希望[287,288]。因此，该领域在抗癌药强有力的武器库中保持着重要地位。

（瞿望　龚彩凤　钟巧凤 译，周爱萍 审校）

参考文献

The complete reference list can be found on the Wiley Companion Digital Edition of this title (see inside front cover for login instructions).

1 Kohler G, Milstein C. Continuous cultures of fused cells secreting antibody of predefined specificity. *Nature.* 1975;**256**:495–497.

3 Teo EC, Chew Y, Phipps C. A review of monoclonal antibody therapies in lymphoma. *Crit Rev Oncol Hematol.* 2016;**97**:72–84.

6 Levy R. Karnofsky lecture: immunotherapy of lymphoma. *J Clin Oncol.* 1999;**17**:7–12.

7 Reichart, JM. http://www.antibodysociety.org/news/approved_mabs.php (accessed 11 December 2015).

11 Miller RA, Maloney DG, Warnke R, Levy R. Treatment of B-cell lymphoma with monoclonal anti-idiotype antibody. *N Engl J Med.* 1982;**306**:517–522.

23 Cheson BD, Leonard JP. Monoclonal antibody therapy for B-cell non-Hodgkin's lymphoma. *N Engl J Med.* 2008;**359**:613–626.

26 Coiffier B, Lepage E, Briere' E, et al. CHOP chemotherapy plus rituximab compared with CHOP alone in elderly patients with diffuse large B-cell lymphoma. *N Engl J Med.* 2002;**346**:235–242.

35 Robak T, Dmoszynska A, Solal-Celigny A, et al. Rituximab plus fludarabine and cyclophosphamide prolongs progression-free survival compared with fludarabine and cyclophosphamide alone in previously treated chronic lymphocytic leukemia. *J Clin Oncol.* 2010;**28**:1756–1765.

36 Dimopoulos MA, Anagnostopoulos A, Kyrtsonis MC, et al. Primary treatment of Waldenstrom macroglobulinemia with dexamethasone, rituximab, and cyclophosphamide. *J Clin Oncol.* 2007;**25**:3344–3349.

42 Mozessohn L, Chan KKW, Feld JJ, Hicks LK. Hepatitis B reactivation in HBsAg-negative/HBcAb-positive patients receiving rituximab for lymphoma: a meta-analysis. *J Viral Hepat.* 2015;**22**:842–849.

50 Hillmen P, Robak T, Janssens A, et al. Ofatumumab + chlorambucil versus chlorambucil alone in patients with untreated chronic lymphocytic leukemia (CLL): results of the phase III study complement 1 (OMB110911). *Blood.* 2013;**122(21)**:528a.

52 Goede V, Fischer K, Busch R, et al. Obinutuzumab plus chlorambucil in patients with CLL and coexisting conditions. *N Engl J Med.* 2014;**370**:1101–1110.

56 Van Rhee F, Wong R, Nikhil M, et al. Siltuximab for multi-centric Castleman's disease: a randomised, double-blind, placebo-controlled trial. *Lancet Oncol.* 2014;**15**:966–974.

63 Cunningham D, Humblet Y, Siena S, et al. Cetuximab monoclonal and cetuximab plus irinotecan in irinotecan refractory metastatic colorectal cancer. *N Engl J Med.* 2004;**351**:337–345.

65 Jonker DJ, O'Callaghan CJ, Carpetis CS, et al. Cetuximab for treatment of colorectal cancer. *N Engl J Med.* 2007;**357**:2040–2048.

68 Van Cutsem E, Köhne CH, Láng I, et al. Cetuximab plus irinotecan, fluorouracil, and leucovorin as first-line treatment for metastatic colorectal cancer: updated analysis of overall survival according to tumor KRAS and BRAF mutation status. *J Clin Oncol.* 2011;**29**:2011–2019.

71 Bonner JA, Harari PM, Giralt J, et al. Radiotherapy plus cetuximab for squamous-cell carcinoma of the head and neck. *N Engl J Med.* 2006;**354**:567–578.

73 Vermorken JB, Mesia R, Rivera F. Platinum-based chemotherapy and cetuximab in head and neck cancer. *N Engl J Med.* 2008;**359**:1116–1127.

78 Giusti RM, Shastri K, Pilaro AM, et al. US food and drug administration approval: panitumumab for epidermal growth factor receptor-expressing metastatic colorectal carcinoma with progression following fluoropyrimidine, oxaliplatin, and irinotecan containing chemotherapy regimens. *Clin Cancer Res.* 2008;**14**:1296–1302.

82 Slamon DJ, Godolphin W, Jones LA, et al. Studies of the HER-2/neu protooncogene in human breast and ovarian cancer. *Science.* 1989;**244**:707–712.

85 http://investor.seattlegenetics.com/phoenix.zhtml?c=124860&p=irol-newsArticle&ID=2080061 (accessed 11 December 2015).

96 Slamon DJ, Leyland-Jones B, Shak S, et al. Use of chemotherapy plus a monoclonal antibody against HER2 for metastatic breast cancer that overexpresses HER2. *N Engl J Med.* 2001;**344**:783–792.

109 Bang YJ, Van Cutsem E, Feyereislova A. Trastuzumab in combination with chemotherapy versus chemotherapy alone for treatment of HER-2 positive advanced gastric or gastro-esophageal junction cancer (ToGA): a phase 3, open label, randomized controlled trial. *Lancet.* 2010;**376**:687–697.

119 Swain SM, Baselga J, Kim S-B, et al. Pertuzumab, trastuzumab and docetaxel in HER-2 positive metastatic breast cancer. *N Engl J Med.* 2015;**372**:724–734.

122 Yu AL, Gilman L, Oskaynak MF, et al. Anti-GD2 antibody with GM-CSF, interleukin-2, and isotretinoin for neuroblastoma. *N Engl J Med.* 2010;**363**:1324–1334.

128 Hurwitz H, Fehrenbacher L, Novotny W, et al. Bevacizumab plus irinotecan, fluorouracil, and leucovorin for metastatic colorectal cancer. *N Engl J Med.* 2004;**350**:2335–2342.

137 Sandler A, Gray R, Perry M, et al. Paclitaxel-carboplatin alone or with bevacizumab for non-small cell lung cancer. *N Engl J Med.* 2006;**355**:2542–2550.

144 Yang JC, Haworth L, Sherry RM, et al. A randomized trial of bevacizumab, an anti-vascular endothelial growth factor antibody, for metastatic renal cancer. *N Engl J Med.* 2003;**349**:427–434.

148 Gilbert MR, Dignam JJ, Armstrong TS, et al. A randomized trial of bevacizumab for newly diagnosed glioblastoma. *N Engl J Med.* 2014;**370**:699–708.

152 Burger RA, Brady MF, Bookman MA, et al. Gynecologic Oncology Group. Incorporation of bevacizumab in the primary treatment of ovarian cancer. *N Engl J Med.* 2011;**365**:2473–2483.

155 Pujade-Lauraine E, Hilpert F, Weber B, et al. Bevacizumab combined with chemotherapy for platinum-resistant recurrent ovarian cancer: the AURELIA open-label randomized phase III trial. *J Clin Oncol.* 2014;**32**:1302–1308.

156 Monk BJ, Pujade-Loraine E, Burger RA. Integrating bevacizumab into the management of epithelial ovarian cancer: the controversy of front-line versus recurrent disease. *Ann Oncol.* 2013;**24(supplement 10)**:53–58.

159 Wilke H, Muro K, Van Cutsem E, et al. Ramucirumab plus paclitaxel versus placebo plus paclitaxel in patients with previously treated advanced gastric or gastro-oesophageal junction adenocarcinoma (RAINBOW): a double-blind, randomised phase 3 trial. *Lancet Oncol.* 2014;**15**:1224–1235.

165 Schadendorf D, Hodi FS, Rovert C, et al. Pooled analysis of long-term survival data from phase II and phase III trials of ipilimumab in unresectable or metastatic melanoma. *J Clin Oncol.* 2015;**33**:1889–1894.

167 Snyder A, Makarov V, Merghoub T, et al. Genetic basis for clinical response to CTLA-4 blockade in melanoma. *N Engl J Med.* 2014;**4**:2189–2199.

172 Robert C, Long GV, Brady B, et al. Nivolumab in previously untreated melanoma without BRAF mutation. *N Engl J Med.* 2015;**372**:320–330.

175 Postow MA, Chesney J, Pavlick A, et al. Nivolumab and ipilimumab in untreated melanoma. *N Engl J Med.* 2015;**372**:2006–2017.

176 Larkin J, Chiarion-Sileni V, Gonzalez R, et al. Combined nivolumab and ipilimumab in untreated melanoma. *N Engl J Med.* 2015;**373**:23–34.

177 Przepiorka D, Ko CW, Deisseroth A, et al. FDA approval: Blinatumomab. *Clin Cancer Res.* 2015;**21**:403555–403559.

202 Sievers EL, Larson RA, Stadtmauer EA, et al. Efficacy and safety of gemtuzumab ozogamicin in patients with CD33-positive acute myeloid leukemia in first relapse. *J Clin Oncol.* 2001;**19**:3244–3254.

207 Amiri-Kordestani L, Blumenthal GM, Xu QC, et al. FDA approval: ado-trastuzumab emtansine for the treatment of patients with HER2-positive metastatic breast cancer. *Clin Cancer Res.* 2014;**20**:4436–4441.

208 Sgorous G, Hobbs RF. Dosimetry for radiopharmaceutical therapy. *Semin Nucl Med.* 2014;**44**:172–178.

209 Pouget JP, Navarro-Teulon I, Bardies M, et al. Clinical radioimmunotherapy—the

role of radiobiology. *Nat Rev Clin Oncol*. 2011;**8**:720–734.

211 Prise KM, O'Sullivan JM. Radiation-induced bystander signaling in cancer therapy. *Nat Rev Cancer*. 2009;**9**:351–360.

215 Huclier-Markai S, Alliot C, Varenot N, Cutler CS, Barbet J. Alpha-emitters for immuno-therapy: a review of recent developments from chemistry to clinics. *Curr Top Med Chem*. 2012;**12**:2642–2654.

218 Macklis RM, Pohlman B. Radioimmunotherapy for non-Hodgkin's lymphoma: a review for radiation oncologists. *Int J Radiat Oncol Biol Phys*. 2006;**66**:833–841.

233 Leahy MF, Turner JH. Radioimmunotherapy of relapsed indolent non-Hodgkin lymphoma with 131I-rituximab in routine clinical practice: 10-year single-institution experience of 142 consecutive patients. *Blood*. 2011;**117**:45–52.

248 Steiner M, Neri D. Antibody-radionuclide conjugates for cancer therapy: hisorical considerations and new trends. *Clin Cancer Res*. 2011;**17**:6406–6416.

259 Zalutsky MR, Reardon DA, Akabani G, et al. Clinical experience with alpha-particle emitting 211At: treatment of recurrent brain tumor patients with 211At-labeled chimeric antitenascin monoclonal antibody 81C6. *J Nucl Med*. 2008;**49**:30–38.

260 Olsen E, Duvic M, Frankel AE, et al. Pivotal phase III trial of two dose levels of denileukin diftitox for the treatment of cutaneous T-cell lymphoma. *J Clin Oncol*. 2001;**19**:376–388.

262 Dang NH, Hagemeister FB, Pro B, et al. Phase II study of denileukin diftitox for relapsed/refractory B-cell non-Hodgkin's lymphoma. *J Clin Oncol*. 2004;**22**:4095–4102.

274 Kreitman RJ, Tallman MS, Robak T, et al. Phase I trial of anti-CD22 recombinant immunotoxin moxetumomab pasudotox (CAT-8015 or HA22) in patients with hairy cell leukemia. *J Clin Oncol*. 2012;**30**:1822–1828.

276 Frankel AE, Woo JH, Ahn C, et al. Activity of SL-401, a targeted therapy directed to interleukin-3 receptor, in blastic plasmacytoid dendritic cell neoplasm patients. *Blood*. 2014;**124**:385–392.

281 Hassan R, Bullock S, Premkumar A, et al. Phase I study of SS1P, a recombinant anti-mesothelin immunotoxin given as a bolus IV infusion to patients with mesothelin-expressing mesothelioma, ovarian, and pancreatic cancers. *Clin Cancer Res*. 2007;**13**:5144–5149.

第 65 章　疫苗与免疫刺激剂

Jeffery Schlom, PhD ■ James L. Gulley, MD, PhD, FACP ■ James W. Hodge, PhD, MBA

概述

随着前列腺癌治疗疫苗 sipuleucel-T、检查点抑制剂抗 CTLA-4 和抗 PD-L1/PD-1 单克隆抗体经美国食品药品管理局(Food and Drug Administration, FDA)批准上市，以及近期涉及癌症疫苗和其他免疫疗法的临床研究结果的发表，"免疫疗法"逐渐成为多种癌症治疗的主流方案。本章回顾了目前正在进行临床评估的各种癌症疫苗平台，可作为疫苗靶标的潜在肿瘤相关抗原种类，以及癌症疫苗与所谓的"非免疫标准护理疗法"或其他免疫疗法结合使用的情况。本文还从临床层面对癌症疫苗和更传统的细胞毒性疗法进行了比较。

美国食品药品管理局近期批准上市了：①前列腺癌治疗疫苗 sipuleucel-T；②用于治疗转移性黑素瘤的抗 CTLA-4 单克隆抗体(monoclonal antibody, MAb) ipilimumab；③用于治疗转移性黑素瘤和肺癌的针对程序性死亡配体 1(PD-L1)/PD-1 免疫抑制轴的单克隆抗体。同时也随着免疫疗法的相关临床研究结果的发表，"免疫疗法"逐渐成为多种癌症治疗的主流方案。

本章综述了目前正在进行临床评估的各种癌症疫苗平台，可作为疫苗靶标的潜在肿瘤相关抗原(tumor-associated antigen, TAA)种类，以及癌症疫苗与所谓的"非免疫标准护理疗法"或其他免疫疗法结合使用的情况。本文还从临床层面对癌症疫苗和更传统的细胞毒性疗法进行了比较。

疫苗治疗的靶点

如今已经确定出了多种用于肿瘤免疫治疗的潜在 TAA 靶标。疫苗治疗的目标不一定是细胞表面蛋白。当一个分子作为疫苗治疗的靶点时，疫苗诱导的活化 T 细胞能够识别出细胞表面的肿瘤抗原肽和主要组织相容性复合物(major histocompatibility complex, MHC)分子的复合物。TAA 疫苗靶标可分为几个主要类别(表 65-1)。

表 65-1　当前和潜在治疗性癌症疫苗靶标谱

靶标类型	举例
肿瘤相关抗原	
癌胚抗原	CEA, MUC-1
干细胞/EMT	Brachyury, SOX-2, OCT-4, TERT, $CD44^{high}$/$CD24^{lo}$, CD133+
原癌基因	MUC-1 C terminus, p53, EGFR, HER2/neu, WT-1
癌症-睾丸	MAGE-A3, BAGE, SEREX-defined, NY-ESO, 生存素
组织谱系	PAP, PSA, gp100, 酪氨酸酶, 肿瘤抗原
糖肽类	STn-KLH
抗血管生成	VEGF-R
肿瘤特异性抗原	
原癌基因	点突变的：ras, B-raf, 帧移位突变, 未定义的独特肿瘤突变
病毒类	HPV, HCV
B 细胞淋巴瘤	抗独特型抗体

BAGE, B 黑素瘤抗原；CEA, 癌胚抗原；EMT, 上皮-间质转化；gp100, 糖蛋白 100；HCV, 丙型肝炎病毒；HPV, 人乳头瘤病毒；MAGE-A3, 黑素瘤相关抗原-A3；MUC-1, 黏蛋白 1；NY-ESO, 纽约食管癌抗原 1；OCT-4, 八聚体结合转录因子 4；PAP, 前列腺酸性磷酸酶；PSA, 前列腺特异抗原；SOX-2, (性别决定区域 Y)-BOX-2；STn-KLH, 唾液 Tn 抗原钥孔虫戚血蓝蛋白；TERT, 端粒酶逆转录酶；VEGF-R, 血管内皮生长因子受体；WT-1, 野生型 1。

肿瘤特异性抗原

肿瘤特异性抗原(tumor-specific antigen, TSA)包括在肿瘤中唯一表达的基因产物，例如点突变的 *ras* 致癌基因、*p53* 突变以及核糖核酸(RNA)剪接变体和基因易位的产物。密码子 12 的 3 个突变代表了绝大多数 *ras* 的突变，这些突变在大约 20%～30%的人类肿瘤中均有发现[1]。虽然在细胞表面没有发现 ras 蛋白，但人们设想出了直接针对细胞表面的肽-MHC 复合物的疫苗治疗。事实上，现如今已经有了针对 ras 的胰腺癌方面的临床试验[2-3]。B 细胞淋巴瘤在其细胞表面过度表达了单一免疫球蛋白(Ig)变异体；因此，每个 B 细胞淋巴瘤作为靶标都表现出了对免疫治疗的特异性[4-6]。RNA 剪接变体和脱氧核糖核酸(DNA)易位的基因产物也产生了独特的融合蛋白，可以作为免疫治疗的特定靶点，包括 c-erb-B2 RNA 剪接变体和慢性粒细胞白血病 DNA 易位的产物 bcr/abl。

有几种病毒与一些肿瘤的病因密切相关，其中人乳头瘤病毒(HPV)与宫颈癌的联系便是一个很好的例子。这也是 FDA 批准上市 HPV 疫苗以防控宫颈癌的原因所在[7]。

肿瘤相关抗原

TAAs 可分为三大类：癌胚抗原、致癌基因产物和组织谱系抗原(表 65-1)。癌胚抗原通常在胎儿发育过程中发现，但在出生后会显著下调。这类抗原包括前列腺特异性膜抗原(prostate-specific membrane antigen, PSMA)、癌胚抗原(carcinoembryonic antigen, CEA)、癌黏蛋白 MUC-1 等，与正常组织相比，常在肿瘤中过度表达。MUC-1 TAA 通常在大多数的人类肿瘤和一些血液恶性肿瘤中过度表达。作为疫苗靶点之一的 MUC-1 N 端的低糖基化数目可变串联重复序列(variable number of tandem repeats,VNTR)部位已引起了广泛关注。虽然以前的研究将 MUC-1 描述为一种肿瘤相关组织分化抗原,但现在的研究已经确定 MUC-1 的 C 端是一种癌蛋白,其表达在许多肿瘤类型中是预后不良的标志[8]。

癌基因和抑癌基因产物,如非突变的 HER2/neu 和 p53 类似于癌胚抗原,因为它们可以在肿瘤中过度表达,并且也可能在某些胎儿和正常组织中表达。同样地,端粒酶作为一种对细胞复制和染色体稳定性非常重要的酶,与大多数正常细胞相比,在恶性细胞中也存在着过度表达的现象。来自人类端粒酶的表位已经被报道,并推测可能被肿瘤细胞过度表达[9]。

组织系抗原如前列腺特异性抗原(prostate-specific antigen, PSA)和黑素细胞抗原 MART-1/Melana A、酪氨酸酶、gp100 和 TRP-1/gp75 通常在给定类型的肿瘤和其来源的正常组织中表达。如果它们表达所在的正常器官/组织不是必需的(如前列腺、乳房或黑素细胞),则组织系抗原将会是免疫治疗的潜在的有效靶点。

疫苗治疗最具挑衅性的潜在靶点是那些与癌症"干细胞"和/或上皮-间充质转化(epithelial-mesenchymal transition, EMT)过程相关的分子,两者都与耐药性有关。EMT 的驱动因素也与肿瘤细胞向转移部位外渗和内渗有关。近期的研究描述了所谓的癌症干细胞的可塑性,以及正在经历 EMT 的细胞与获得"干细胞特性"之间的相似性[10]。与 EMT 和癌症"干细胞特性"相关的基因产物有 SOX-2,OCT-4,以及那些表型为 $CD44^{high}/CD24^{lo}$ 和/或 $CD133^{+}$ 的肿瘤细胞[11-15]。目前正在通过对这些基因产物在体外诱导人类 T 细胞产生免疫应答的研究来评估它们的免疫原性,但其中一些基因产物在一些正常成人组织中也会有相对广泛的表达。最近发现 T-box 转录因子 brachyury 是 EMT 的主要驱动因子[16]。它已被证明在几种癌症类型的原发和转移癌肿组织中都有选择性表达。现如今开发出的疫苗能够诱导产生足以裂解一系列人类癌细胞的 T 细胞[17]。目前正在进行临床试验的疫苗,其靶点为与 EMT 和具有"干细胞特性"的癌细胞相关的基因产物[18-20]。

疫苗的种类

许多疫苗供应平台已经完成了在实验模型中的分析,其中许多现在正在进行临床评估(见表 65-2)。这些平台有各自的优缺点,其中一些模式有望被证明在组合或联用时是最有益的。

全肿瘤细胞疫苗

使用全肿瘤细胞疫苗最主要的优点是,肿瘤细胞突变的 TSA 和 TAA 可能存在于疫苗制剂中,它们中目前只有一小部分已被确定。目前正在进行临床测试的两种全肿瘤细胞疫苗平台分别是:①自体疫苗(即对患者的肿瘤进行处理制成针对该患者的疫苗);②同种异体疫苗,这种疫苗使用的是来自其他患者的肿瘤细胞,通常来自已建立的肿瘤细胞系。制作自体肿瘤细胞疫苗工程繁琐,因为首先要在手术中获得新鲜的肿瘤细胞,并以类似的方式为每个患者制备他们各自的疫苗。考虑到不同患者肿瘤细胞之间有着很大的差异性,以及定制疫苗的高昂成本,目前大多数全肿瘤细胞疫苗的制备方法都集中在使用同种异体细胞系和细胞库上[21-26]。此外,该制剂中使用的细胞株可以感染表达细胞因子(如粒细胞-巨噬细胞集落刺激因子(granulocyte-macrophage colony-stimulating factor, GM-CSF)[27]或其他免疫刺激因子转导基因[28])基因的载体,以增强肿瘤细胞的免疫原性。利用转染的肿瘤细胞株表达 GM-CSF 来治疗了胰脏癌和其他肿瘤的研究已经获得初步进展[24-27,29,30]。

表 65-2 Ⅱ/Ⅲ期临床研究中现有疫苗平台的范围(种类)

疫苗平台	举例	癌症种类
多肽/蛋白质		
多肽	gp100,MUC-1,HER2/neu	黑素瘤、肺癌
蛋白质	MAGE-A3,NY-ESO	黑素瘤
抗体	抗独特型	淋巴瘤
糖肽类	sTn-KLH	黑素瘤
重组载体		
腺病毒	Adeno-CEA,alpha-CEA	恶性上皮肿瘤
痘病毒	牛痘病毒,MUA,禽痘	前列腺癌
酿酒酵母	Yeast-CEA	胰腺癌
肿瘤细胞		
同种异体	GVAX(+GM-CSF)	胰腺癌
树突状细胞/自体肿瘤细胞融合		骨髓瘤
自体同源	Adeno-CD40L,colon(BCG)	慢性淋巴细胞白血病,结肠癌,黑素瘤
树突细胞/APCs		
树突细胞-多肽类	神经胶质瘤肽	神经胶质瘤,黑素瘤
树突细胞-病毒感染	rV,rF-CEA-MUC1-TRICOM(Panvac-DC)	结肠直肠癌
APC-蛋白	Sipuleucel-T(PAP-GM-CSF)	前列腺癌

APC,抗原呈递细胞;BCG,卡介苗佐剂;CD40L,CD40 配体;CEA,癌胚抗原;gp100,糖蛋白 100;GM-CSF,粒细胞巨噬细胞集落刺激因子;MAGE-A3,黑素瘤相关抗原 3;MUC-1,黏蛋白 1;NY-ESO,纽约食管癌抗原 1;PAP,前列腺酸性磷酸酶;PSA,前列腺特异抗原;rF,重组鸡痘;rV,重组痘苗;sTn-KLH,唾液 Tn 抗原钥孔虫戚血蓝蛋白。

直接向肿瘤中注射细胞因子基因或共刺激分子基因(原位自体肿瘤细胞疫苗)要有效激活T细胞需要两种信号。第一个信号通过抗原呈递细胞(APC)表面的肽-MHC复合物介导,它与T细胞表面的T细胞受体(TCR)结合,第二个信号涉及APC表面的T细胞共刺激分子与T细胞表面的配体的相互作用。迄今为止,研究最多的T细胞共刺激分子是B7-1,它与T细胞表面的两个配体相互作用:与CD28作用上调T细胞功能,与CTLA-4作用下调T细胞功能。大量的临床前期研究表明,将B7-1添加到弱免疫原性的肿瘤中会使其获得更强的免疫原性[28]。当其他共刺激分子,如细胞间黏附分子(ICAM)-1和淋巴细胞功能相关抗原(LFA)-3加入肿瘤中时,也会发生这种现象。因此,我们可以设想,将表达一个或多个共刺激分子的载体直接注射到肿瘤块中,从而诱导抗肿瘤免疫应答。这种直接注射方法的优点是"疫苗"是患者自己的肿瘤,它可能表达出该患者独特的突变TSA或TAAs。在临床研究中,表达B7-1共刺激分子的基于牛痘和禽痘的重组体已被直接注射到黑素瘤或癌症病灶中[31]。一项临床研究在把包含共刺激分子的三联体(B7-1,ICAM-1,和LFA-3)的重组载体直接注入黑素瘤或癌症病灶中时曾报道了有趣的发现[32,33]。细胞因子也可以借由载体被引入到肿瘤组织中,如表达GM-CSF的重组牛痘苗病毒直接注射到黑素瘤组织中[34]。

多肽类

大多数用于诱发免疫应答的多肽类通常来源于TSA和TAA,它们大多为8~11个氨基酸长度。这些多肽类可以与APC表面合适类别的MHC分子相结合。因此,只有当患者中存在适当的MHC等位基因时,这些MHC限制性反应才有效。在人类人群中研究最多的MHC限制元件是MHC Ⅰ类等位基因,人类白细胞抗原(human leukocyte antigen,HLA)-A2,它存在于大约50%的高加索人群中。

使用多肽作为免疫原有以下优点:①制备相对方便且经济;②因为免疫原非常明确,所以可以通过多种方法对免疫反应效果进行定量分析;③当多肽类被修饰成激动肽的形式时,会获得更强的免疫原性。特异性是多肽类疫苗的优点,但同时也是其劣势所在。例如,CTL(细胞毒性T细胞)表位肽可能诱导由于缺少辅助肽提供的帮助而短暂存在的CTL反应。另外,多肽类疫苗也只有在被治疗的患者拥有特定的等位基因时才能起效。目前投入研究的多肽类疫苗包括HPV[35]、ras[36,37]、HER-2/neu[38]、MAGE[39]、MART-1、酪氨酸酶[40]、gp100[41,42]、CEA[43]、MUC-1[44]和PSMA[45,46]等[47]。

激动肽

肽激动剂分为两大类。在第一类,与MHC结合的肽的氨基酸被修饰。越有活力的MHC结合位点(即对MHC分子有更高的亲和力)通常就会诱发越强的T细胞反应。这方面的例子是brachyury,gp100黑素瘤和MUC-1肽的改变[8,41,48]。第二类激动剂被称为TCR激动剂。

在这种情况下,与T细胞上的TCR相互作用的肽的氨基酸被修饰,这也可以诱导出更强烈的T细胞反应。这方面的一个例子是CEA的TCR激动剂的生成[49]。

抗独特型

独特型网络参与免疫调节的控制。B细胞淋巴瘤在细胞表面呈现独特的免疫球蛋白,为免疫治疗提供了精确的靶点。对于这种恶性肿瘤,抗独特型(Id)单克隆抗体疫苗在临床上已经相当成熟[4,5,50-55]。但这些疫苗策略中固有的特异性既是优势也是劣势;不同的B细胞淋巴瘤将在其细胞表面显示独特的Ids,这使得为每一位患者准备其特定的疫苗的工作量大大增加[56]。

载体

载体是更灵活的疫苗递送手段之一。目前几个主要的病毒载体和细菌载体平台现在已在临床上投入使用(表65-2)。每一种载体都有其自身的优缺点。目前已有综述这些载体各自潜在优点的文章发表[57-63]。总的来说,经载介导的疫苗有以下几点优点:①部分载体中可以插入多种基因(包括共刺激分子和细胞因子的基因);②与制备和纯化蛋白质或全肿瘤细胞疫苗相比,生产成本相对较低;③许多载体具有感染专职APC的能力,从而加工其表达的抗原;④病毒和细菌载体由原核蛋白组成,在刺激宿主免疫反应中起天然疫苗佐剂的作用。有一部分(非全部)载体的缺点是,载体疫苗由宿主诱导的对载体的自身免疫建立起来的,这一点限制了它的继续使用。

病毒载体

研究最多的疫苗载体群之一是痘病毒组,痘苗病毒源自良性痘病母牛,已被接种给10亿多人,并帮助在全世界范围内根除了天花[64]。因此,美国和大多数西方国家在大约40年前就停止了小痘疫苗接种,但大多数癌症患者年龄都超过了40岁,因此对痘苗病毒具有一定程度的预先存在的免疫力。因此,重组痘苗病毒不能在疫苗方案中多次接种。痘病毒家族中包括一种无复制能力的改良安卡拉痘苗病毒(MVA),痘苗病毒的一种衍生物[57]。MVA被认为是天花疫苗的更安全的替代品,因为它可以感染哺乳动物细胞,但不能复制[65]。痘病毒家族的其他复制缺陷成员是禽痘载体(禽痘和金丝雀痘/ALVAC)[58]。这些禽痘载体能够感染人类细胞,在细胞死亡前可表达其转基因2~3周;同时它们不能重新感染别的细胞。临床研究表明,以禽痘为基础的CEA载体可以多次注射给患者,从而增加CEA特异性T细胞应答[47,66]。临床前和临床研究[47,67-69]表明,最佳的重组疫苗或MVA使用方法可能是,激发免疫反应,然后用其他载体(如无复制能力的痘病毒,多肽类或DNA)进行增强接种。使用痘苗病毒或不具复制能力的MVA痘病毒的优点是:①可以将大量外源DNA插入载体中;②痘病毒中表达的蛋白质比天然蛋白具有更强的免疫原性,这很可能是针对高免疫原性痘病毒蛋白触发的炎症反应的结果。如今,几个包含TAAs(如CEA,MUC-1,PSA和HPV)的重组痘病毒的临床试验已经完成,其他研究还在进行中。

腺病毒也被提议作为重组疫苗设计的载体,因为它的病毒基因组可以通过改造而可以接受稳定整合的外源基因。在生产重组腺病毒载体过程中,通常要把内源性病毒DNA序列从复制能力区域中删除,从而使病毒减毒,提高其安全性。研究者命名了一种新的病毒载体基因传递平台,腺病毒血清型-5型(Ad5)[E1-,E2b-][70-79]。该平台由复制缺陷的Ad5组成,其中早期1(E1)、早期2(E2b)和早期3(E3)基因区域的部分已被删除;据报道删除这些基因会导致晚期基因表达显著减少,这会引起宿主炎症反应和抗Ad宿主反应显著减少。与其他腺载体平台相比,转染了这些腺病毒结构的人体细胞可以在体内更长时间地表达编码的转基因。在Ⅰ期和Ⅱ期的临床试验中,研究者对转移性结直肠癌(metastatic colorectal cancer,mCRC)患者队列接种了递增剂量的携带 CEA 基因的腺病毒平台的疫苗,这诱导了针对 CEA 的 T 细胞反应,同时也获得了患者有较高的生存概率的证据[80]。

酵母和细菌载体

重组酿酒酵母作为疫苗载体的一个优点是它没有毒性。除了其固有的非致病性外,这种特定种类的酵母可以在给药前被高温灭杀,已有几个临床试验证实了它对人体的安全性,这些试验均未达到其最大耐受剂量[63,81,82]。酿酒酵母很容易通过改造,大量表达一种或多种抗原,可以快速繁殖和纯化,并且非常稳定[83]。此外,重组酵母已被证明能诱导对非自身抗原的强烈的宿主免疫反应[19,63,83-86]。细菌载体,如沙门菌[87,88]和李斯特菌[62]具有对专职 APC(如巨噬细胞)的嗜性优势。虽然这些载体在人类中具有潜在的毒力,但已经开发了几种供人类使用的减毒菌株。从临床角度来看,基于重组沙门氏菌和重组李斯特菌细胞基因的载体都可以口服。

质粒 DNA

多核苷酸疫苗很容易制备,但这些载体诱导免疫反应的作用方式还不完全清楚,因为大多数研究都涉及肌肉接种,并且尚不清楚抗原如何到达专职 APCs。如今,许多使用感染性疾病制剂和癌症抗原的临床前和临床研究都已经用 DNA 载体进行介导了[89-92]。

树突状细胞疫苗

树突状细胞(dendritic cell,DC)被认为是最有效的 APC,因此是最受欢迎的免疫手段之一[93,94]。DCs 可以通过:①装载肽、蛋白质或抗-ID 抗体;②感染病毒载体;③装载来自肿瘤细胞的凋亡小体;④与肿瘤细胞融合[95-98]。这种方法的主要缺点是其高昂的制作成本。患者的外周血单个核细胞(peripheral blood mononuclear cell,PBMC)必须通过白细胞采集术获得。然后,PBMC 必须在有 GM-CSF、IL-4 和/或 TNF-α 等细胞因子存在的环境下培养几天,然后回输到患者体内。每个患者都需要经历此操作。目前已有一项成功策略获得 FDA 批准,它涉及用负载有重组融合蛋白的自体 DC 来免疫转移性前列腺癌患者,该融合蛋白由肿瘤抗原前列腺酸性磷酸酶(prostatic acid phosphatase,PAP)连接 GM-CSF 组成,如下所述。

疫苗组合

虽然所述的各种免疫方法各有优缺点,但最有效的免疫方案可能是用一种免疫原引发并用另一种免疫原增强。这种方法的潜在优点如下:①可以通过使用两种不同的免疫模式(即先是 $CD4^+$ 介导的免疫过程然后是 $CD8^+$ T 细胞介导的免疫过程)来增强免疫系统的两端;②一种免疫方法可能在刺激幼稚细胞的方面更有效,而另一种模式可能会更有效地增强记忆细胞功能;③一些最有效的免疫方法,如使用重组痘苗病毒或腺病毒,由于宿主的抗载体反应,可使用的次数有限。如果将这些载体用作引发剂,然后用其他试剂来助推,可能获得更好的效果。大量的临床前研究和临床研究证明了多样化的“引发-助推”方案的优势所在[47,66,67,99-103]。

非特异性免疫刺激剂

根据定义,TAA 和 TSA 是弱免疫原,因为肿瘤在完整的免疫系统存在的情况下仍能发展、持续和生长。诸如不完全弗氏佐剂(incomplete Freund's adjuvant,IFA)等传统佐剂将允许免疫原保持在注射部位(所谓的仓库效应),以便使浸润的 APCs 和效应细胞可以启动更强烈的免疫反应。免疫刺激剂也通过跨膜屏障发挥作用。在这种情况下,蛋白质必须被专业的 APC 吞噬,并在有 MHC 分子存在的环境中被呈递,以便有效地将抗原信息呈递给免疫系统。具有亲脂性成分和脂质体[104]的佐剂促进了这一过程。

某些佐剂(如 IFA)、卡介苗(bacillus Calmette-Guerin adjuvant,BCG),甚至病毒载体中存在的微生物产物也是 DC 的有效激活剂,部分原因是它们含有 Toll 样受体(Toll-like receptor,TLR)的激动剂。TLR 由 DC 和其他先天免疫细胞类型表达,包括大约 10~15 个受体[105,106]。通过其 TLR 激活 DC 增强了黏附、趋化因子和趋化因子受体分子的表达,这些分子反过来调节细胞向炎症和致病相遇部位的运输。因此,TLR 参与的生物学效应会导致炎症,其特征是募集关键的免疫和非免疫效应细胞来介导病原体的破坏。关于 TLR 激动剂,CpG 基序是这些序列中被研究的最多的[107-110]。

此外,已经证明某些细胞因子和趋化因子能够局部或系统地增强 APC 和/或效应细胞功能的水平。例如,据报道 GM-CSF 可以增强抗原特异性 T 细胞反应,延迟型超敏反应,和抗肿瘤细胞反应[111-120]。使用了 GM-CSF 和蛋白免疫原的临床研究显示,其抗原特异性免疫应答能力大大增强[50,121]。不管是动物模型还是临床试验都显示,注射 Flt-3L 能够系统性增加 DCs 的数量。最终结果显示,一些细胞因子和趋化因子再提高 T 细胞功能的方面起着重要的作用[124-128]。这方面研究得最多的是 IL-2[129,130]。当用作单一制剂时,IL-2 已被证明对黑素瘤和肾细胞癌(RCC)患者具有抗肿瘤作用[129,131],并且如最近报道的那样,可以增强基于黑素瘤的多肽疫苗的有效性[41]。其他细胞因子,如 IL-7、IL-12 和 IL-15,在实验模型中被证明可以增强 T 细胞反应和抗肿瘤活性,甚至可能比 IL-2 更具有潜在的临床应用价值[125,132-134]。

提高促炎细胞因子(如 IL-2 和 IL-12)安全性的一种策略是通过与导向肿瘤靶向抗体融合,将它们输送到肿瘤部位。这种抗体-细胞因子融合蛋白或“免疫细胞因子”以前已经在临床前模型中证实,能够增强抗肿瘤免疫的能力[135]。为了最大限度地提高免疫细胞素的耐受性,被选为载体的抗体必须特异性地与肿瘤中的抗原结合。通过将两个人 IL-12 异源二聚体基因融合到 NHS76 抗体重链的 C 末端,可构建出一种肿瘤靶向 IL-12 免疫细胞因子,称为 NHS-IL12。在 3 种小鼠肿瘤模型中,NHS-IL12 作为抗肿瘤药物评价优于重组 IL-12。在临床前研究中,将 NHS-IL12 治疗与癌症疫苗、放疗或化疗相结合,其抗肿瘤效果比单独使用任一种治疗都要大[136]。

疫苗临床试验

下面是对以往和正在进行的疫苗临床试验的代表性描述。

前列腺癌

PAP 在超过 95% 的前列腺癌细胞上表达，已被用作疫苗 sipuleucel-T 的靶标，也被称为 Provenge®（PAP-GM-CSF-pulsed APCs）。在 sipuleucel-T 疫苗的早期临床试验被证明是安全的后，在无症状或轻微症状的无转移去势抵抗性前列腺癌（MCRPC）中进行了更大规模的试验。

在Ⅲ期临床试验中[137]，以总生存期（overall survival，OS）作为终点，募集了 500 多名患者。研究显示，患者肿瘤的进展时间（time to progression，TTP）并没有发生变化，但疫苗组的 OS 却有所改善（疫苗组：25.8 个月，对照组：21.7 个月；$P=0.032$）。2010 年 4 月，FDA 批准 sipuleucel-T 用于治疗微小或无症状的 mCRPC。第二种前列腺癌疫苗也在同一前列腺癌人群中展开了评估。这个“现成”的平台（PROSTVAC）由重组牛痘初免疫苗和多种禽痘增强疫苗组成。每个载体包含 PSA 和 3 个共刺激分子（B7-1，ICAM-1 和 LFA-3，特指 TRICOM）的转基因[138,139]。随机安慰剂对照的 43 个中心的Ⅱ期试验招募了 125 名微小症状的 mCRPC 患者[140]。与 sipuleucel-T 相似，PROSTVAC 没有使 TTP 延长，但相对于安慰剂组相比改善了中位 OS（疫苗组：25.1 个月；对照组：16.6 个月）。接受 PROSTVAC 治疗的患者与对照组相比死亡率也降低了 44%（$P=0.0061$）[140]。第二次单臂Ⅱ期研究中的中位 OS[141] 为 26.6 个月，与更大的 PROSTVAC 随机试验相似。一项全球Ⅲ期安慰剂对照试验在 1 298 名微小症状的前列腺癌患者中进行，现在已经完成。该研究的观察终点为 OS。

最近的一篇综述[142]分析了前列腺癌患者使用 PROSTVAC（PSA-TRICOM）所引起的免疫影响。在 104 名接受 T 细胞反应测试的患者中，57% 的患者在疫苗接种后 4 周表现出 PSA 特异性 T 细胞的增加，68% 的患者对疫苗中不存在的 TAA（抗原扩散/抗原级联）产生了疫苗后免疫反应。对 PSA 的系统免疫反应的测量可能低估了真正的治疗性免疫反应（因为这并不包括已被转运到肿瘤组织的细胞），并且不包括抗原扩散/抗原级联（如下所述）。此外，虽然整个 PSA 基因都作为疫苗，但是只评估了针对一个 PSA 表位的 T 细胞应答。因为这种疫苗是针对产生细胞/Th1 免疫反应的，只有不到 0.6% 的接受测试的患者在接种疫苗后有 PSA 抗体诱导的证据。在诊断为“低风险”前列腺癌的男性中，积极的监测逐渐被越来越广泛地应用。目前也有一项随机、多中心、安慰剂对照的研究正在比较“前列腺癌预防接种”与“积极监测”这两种方法对新诊断为临床局限性前列腺癌的患者的效果。这项研究的终点将是 12 个月后活检与初始活检时免疫浸润和肿瘤范围的变化。

GVAX，一种 GM-CSF 分泌疫苗，是两种前列腺癌细胞系的混合物，这两个前列腺癌细胞系已经用复制缺陷反转录病毒转导了 GM-CSF 的表达。在两个单独的多中心阶段Ⅱ试验中，给予 GVAX 的无症状 CRPC 患者的中位生存期为 26.2～35.0 个月[24,143]。通过基于常用的诺模图估计预测的生存率，两个试验中的 144 名患者超过了预期生存期 6 个月以上[145]。

19 例 HLA-A2 阳性患者接受了含有 11 个 HLA-A ∗ 0201 限制性和两个来自前列腺癌肿瘤抗原皮下（subcutaneous，s. c.）的 HLA-Ⅱ类合成肽的疫苗。这些患者的特点是 PSA 升高但未检测到转移疾病或局部复发。给药时间持续 18 个月或一直到 PSA 进展。在接种期间，19 名患者中有 4 名（占比 21%）的 PSA 倍增时间从 4.9 个月增加到 25.8 个月[146]。对复发或激素难治性前列腺癌患者，进行了Ⅱ期腺病毒/PSA 疫苗试验。大多数患者表现出高于注射前水平的抗 PSAT 细胞反应。64% 的患者表现出 PSA 倍增时间的增加[147]。临床试验也使用负载了人 PSMA[148-150] 多肽的多肽脉冲树突细胞，以及与 PSA 肿瘤 RNA 转染的树突细胞[151]。在这些研究中，研究者观察到了抗原特异性免疫反应，血清 PSA 也有部分降低。

黑素瘤

绝大多数疫苗临床试验都是在黑素瘤患者身上进行的，因为：①干扰素（interferon，IFN）和 IL-2 在黑素瘤中都能表现出临床反应；②黑素瘤病变易获得，因此可以研究免疫浸润，来自黑素瘤病变的细胞可以在体外环境中培养中生长从而获得肿瘤细胞和肿瘤浸润性淋巴细胞（tumor-infiltrating lymphocyte，TIL）；③如今已经确定出多种与黑素瘤相关的抗原。

目前已经有许多使用来自黑素瘤的相关抗原制成的各种多肽进行的临床试验，包括酪氨酸酶，MART-1，gp100，Melan-A（修饰的 gp100 表位[152]），以及 MAGE 家族中的成员[152-157]。研究报道了疫苗诱导的免疫应答以及其临床益处。一种新的方法是将这些多肽与在 Montanide ISA-51[158] 中乳化的 GM-CSF 结合。另一种与多肽有关的方法是用自体肿瘤衍生的热休克蛋白/肽复合物进行疫苗接种[159]。使用黑素瘤多肽疫苗结合抗 CTLA-4[160]、黑素瘤多肽致敏的树突细胞[94,154]、肿瘤 RNA 转染的树突细胞[161]和瘤内注射自体树突细胞，均可观察到免疫应答和临床应答[162]。根据一项随机Ⅲ期试验显示，与使用达卡巴嗪进行一线治疗转移性黑素瘤的患者相比，使用自体多肽冲击的树突细胞疫苗对转移性黑素瘤患者没有任何益处[163]。

有 185 名Ⅳ期或局部晚期Ⅲ期皮肤黑素瘤患者参加了一项随机Ⅲ期试验，这些患者均有 HLA ∗ A0201 的表达，且适合大剂量 IL-2 治疗。患者被随机分配为两组，一组单独接受 IL-2 另一组先接受 gp100 加 IFA，然后接受 IL-2。与单用 IL-2 组相比，疫苗-IL-2 组在总体临床反应方面有显著改善（16% vs 6%，$P=0.03$）。疫苗-IL-2 组的中位 OS 也比单用 IL-2 组长（17.8 个月 vs 11.1 个月，$P=0.06$）[164]。在一项多中心随机试验中，175 名Ⅳ期黑素瘤患者被纳入四个治疗组。在 148 名可评估的患者中有 7 名患者（4.7%）临床反应良好但在两个研究间无显著差异。在另一项试验中，3 种 HLAI 类多肽以析因 2×2 设计给予：肽疫苗单独或联合 GM-CSF，或与干扰素-α2b 联合，或两者联合使用[165]。在另一项试验中，3 种 HLAI 类多肽以析因 2×2 设计给予：单独多肽疫苗注射，多肽疫苗联合 GM-CSF，多肽疫苗联合 IFN-CSFα2b，或与两者联合。在中位 25.4 个月的随访中，有疫苗免疫应答的患者的中位 OS 明显长于没有免疫应答的患者（前者 21.3 个月，后者 13.4 个月；$P=0.046$）[166]。

Vitespen 是一种自体的，肿瘤衍生的热休克蛋白 gp96 肽疫苗。322 名Ⅳ期黑素瘤患者按照 2∶1 的比例被随机分配到接受 Vitespen 或医生选择的治疗。Vitespen 组的 OS 值与医生选择治疗组的 OS 值无统计学差异[167]。随机试验证据表明与肿瘤细胞疫苗相比，DC 疫苗有更长的生存期，这一点也与既往研究中所证明的特异性免疫疗法的生存益处结果一致[168]。在一项对主要为 HLA-A24 基因型的转移性黑素瘤患者给予 DC 疫苗的Ⅱ期临床试验中,OS 分析显示接受 DC 疫苗的患者具有显著的生存延长效应[169]。还有研究检测了预测转移性黑素瘤患者对 MAGE-A3 疫苗反应的预处理基因表达特征。表达特征与患者的临床反应有关[170]。一项Ⅱ期试验研究了针对 survivin 的肽疫苗在治疗难治性Ⅳ期转移性黑素瘤患者中的应用(survivin 是肿瘤细胞存活的关键蛋白)。Survivin 特异性 T 细胞反应活性与肿瘤反应和患者生存密切相关[171]。

一些临床研究已经采用自体黑素瘤细胞作为疫苗。并观察了在使用环磷酰胺后再给予这些黑素瘤细胞疫苗的临床反应[172,173]。当用 GM-CSF 转导自体黑素瘤细胞并作为疫苗给予时也观察到了临床反应[174,175]。此外,据报道,在皮肤黑素瘤患者瘤内注射编码了 GM-CSF 的重组痘苗病毒可诱导抗肿瘤免疫反应[31,32,176]。一些随机Ⅱ期试验在已切除的黑素瘤患者中使用自体[177,178]或同种异体[179,180]黑素瘤疫苗。在这些试验中,有证据表明,与对照组或不治疗组相比,疫苗组的无病存活率(disease-free survival,DFS)有所提高。最近的研究表明,用肿瘤细胞和 APC 的混合免疫可以在各种啮齿动物模型中诱导保护性免疫和对已建立的肿瘤的排斥[95,181,182]。最近报道了新的临床试验策略包括基于 DC 的疫苗[183-185]。从 DC 和肿瘤细胞(树突瘤)融合而来的纯化杂交瘤已被证明是安全的,当与低剂量 IL-2 结合时,可以诱导免疫学和临床反应[184]。

T-VEC 是一种病变内溶瘤免疫疗法,包括通过改造 1 型 HSV 以制造 GM-CSF。在随机Ⅲ期试验中,436 名ⅢB～Ⅳ期黑素瘤患者被随机分成 2∶1 两组,分别接受病灶内 T-VEC 与 s. c. GM-CSF。与 s. c. GM-CSF 相比,T-VEC 组反应时间≥6 个月者比例显著增加(实验组 16%,对照组 2%),总有效率也有显著增加(实验组 26%,对照组 6%)。许多患者在经过中位数超过 18. 4 个月的随访后仍处于缓解状态[186,187]。

结肠癌

采用自体肿瘤细胞疫苗联合术后卡介苗灌注治疗Ⅱ期和Ⅲ期结肠癌,对 254 例患者进行前瞻性随机对照Ⅲ期临床试验。中位 5. 3 年的随访结果显示,对照组有 40 例复发,疫苗组有 25 例复发。该疫苗在手术切除的Ⅱ期结肠癌患者中显示出统计上显著的无复发生存(recurrence-free survival,RFS),但Ⅲ期结肠癌没有[188]。进一步的随访显示,与纯手术组相比,疫苗组仍具有显著的生存益处[189]。

已经使用基于 CEA 的疫苗进行了几项临床试验。对患者接种重组痘苗病毒疫苗[69]、重组禽痘病毒疫苗[66,190,191]或使用重组疫苗(rV)-CEA 进行初免并使用禽痘-CEA 多次增强的结果表明,晚期胃肠(GI)癌和其他表达 CEA 的癌症患者产生了 CEA 特异性免疫反应。一项使用含有 TRI-COM 的痘苗和禽痘-CEA 疫苗的试验表明,接受初免-加强免疫接种策略加 GM-CSF 的患者的存活率有所提高;40%的患者转入疾病稳定期(stable disease,SD)至少 4 个月[47,79,192,193]。在一项多中心Ⅱ期研究中,结直肠癌患者接受了肝和肺转移瘤切除术后的 PANVAC 疫苗(rV-,rF-CEA-MUC1-TRICOM)治疗[192]。接受了 PANVAC 或 PANVAC 感染的 DC 的两组患者,其临床结果没有统计学差异。接种疫苗的患者(n=74)与接受当下临床常用方案(接受转移性切除术及标准护理疗法)的"对照"(未随机)组(n=161)进行了比较。对照组和 PANVAC 疫苗组都有相似的预后特征,两组的 TTP 几乎相同,中位数 TTP 约为 24 个月[20,192]。然而,PANVAC 疫苗接种的患者 2 年时的 OS 为 95%,40 个月时为 90%,而对照组 2 年时 OS 为 75%,40 个月时为 47%。对照组的 OS 值与其他 5 个临床研究中该人群的 3～5 年生存数据相似[194-199]。这是迄今为止又一个 TTP 不增加而 OS 值增加的例子(同见于易普利姆玛,sipuleucel-T 和 PROSTVAC)。

CEA 多肽冲击的树突细胞也被应用于使用修饰的 CEA 激动剂肽的临床研究[200]。12 例晚期结直肠癌患者中有 2 例经历了肿瘤消退,1 例患者出现混合反应,2 例产生 SD。临床反应与 CEA 特异性 T 细胞的扩增相关。26 例接受了结直肠转移瘤切除术的患者接受了结内注射自体肿瘤裂解物脉冲调制的 DC 疫苗和对照蛋白脉冲调制的 DC 疫苗。患者被随机分配随机接受 CD40L 激活或未激活的 DC。所有患者都进行了至少 5. 5 年的随访。疫苗接种后 1 周有证据表明有肿瘤特异性 T 细胞增殖反应或干扰素-γ 反应的患者在 5 年时的 RFS 明显好于无反应者(实验组 63%,对照组 18%,$P=0.037$)[201]。

临床研究中也会使用针对抗 CEA 单克隆抗体的抗 Id 抗体。这些研究已经证明其可诱发免疫反应[202,203],延缓疾病进展,延长生存时间[204]。含有一种常见于多种肿瘤的癌胚抗原基因(5T4)的 MVA,已经被研究试用于多种癌肿(TroVax,牛津,英国)。在一项纳入了 22 名 mCRC 患者的试验中,免疫应答似乎与疾病控制相关,免疫应答患者的免疫应答时长长达 18 个月[205-207]。

胰腺癌

同种异体全肿瘤细胞毒素修饰的混合物 GM-CSF 也已用于胰腺癌患者。疫苗诱导的免疫应答的证据通过延迟型高敏感性测量被观察到[25,208]。一项在佐剂环境下设置的,对使用同一疫苗 60 名受试者的Ⅱ期试验显示,化疗后诱导的特异性 CD8 细胞与无进展生存率相关[209]。在同一机构的同一患者群中,中位 OS 大约为 26 个月,而单独化疗仅 21 个月[210]。GVAX 和 CRS-207 癌症疫苗在研究胰腺导管腺癌(pancreatic ductal adenocarcinoma,PDA)的过程中得到了评估。GVAX 由两种经辐射的 GM-CSF 分泌的同种异体 PDA 细胞系组成,在用低剂量的环磷酰胺(cyclophosphamide,Cy)处理 24 小时后,再施用,以抑制调节性 T 细胞。CRS-207 是重组活减毒、双缺失单核细胞增生李斯特菌,经过改造以表达间皮素。GVAX 针对广泛的 PDA 抗原诱导 T 细胞,并且已经显示出与存活率相关的肿瘤特异性 T 细胞应答。间皮素是大多数 PDA 中过度表达的 TAA。在既往的研究中,接受 Cy/GVAX 治疗的,并且先前已接受过 PDA 治疗的患者对间皮素特异性 $CD8^+$ T 细胞的诱导效果优于单独使用 GVAX 治疗的患者。中位存活期分别为 4. 3 个月和 2. 3 个月。将先前治疗过转移性胰腺癌的患者按照 2∶1的比例分别给予两剂的 Cy/GVAX,后跟四剂 CRS-207 或单独给予 Cy/GVAX。在接受至少三剂治疗(两剂 Cy/GVAX 加一剂 CRS-207 或三剂 Cy/GVAX)的患者的预先指定的方案分析中,前者 OS 为 9. 7 个月而后者为 4. 6 个月。无论是否为治疗组,增强的间皮素特异性 $CD8^+$ T 细胞反应都与较长的 OS 相关[211]。

乳腺癌

Sialy1-Tn(STn)是含有与癌相关的黏蛋白的糖肽。患者随机接受含有或不含有环磷酰胺的疫苗[STn与钥匙孔血蓝蛋白(keyhole limpet hemocyanin,KLH)]。据报告显示,接种含有环磷酰胺的疫苗的患者比接种不含有环磷酰胺的疫苗的患者的寿命要长得多[212]。此外,STn KLH疫苗已用于接受高剂量化疗后进行自体干细胞移植的乳腺癌和卵巢癌患者。接种疫苗的患者更容易存活并且不太可能复发,但要需要进一步研究进行证实[213]。在一项关于STn与KLH疫苗结合使用的多中心随机双盲Ⅲ期试验中,纳入了1 028名在一线化疗后患有非进展性疾病或没有疾病的证据的转移性乳腺癌的女性。和单独接受KLH的女性对照组相比,接受伴随性内分泌治疗和STn-KLH治疗的女性TTP和OS均较长。此外,在接受伴随性内分泌治疗的女性中,那些对STn-KLH疫苗具有中等或更高水平抗体反应的女性患者,她们中位OS显著高于那些具有低于中等水平的抗体反应的女性患者[214]。

目前已有几项临床试验将MUC-1作为靶标开展,包括使用MUC-1肽疫苗[215-217]、编码MUC-1和IL-2[218]重组痘病毒,表达人MUC-1的MVA[219]和甘露聚糖-MUC-1融合蛋白[220,221]。在使用或不使用GM-CSF的HER2/neu肽进行的研究中,患有乳腺癌的患者能够产生对HER2的特异性免疫应答[222-224]。一项Ⅰ/Ⅱ期临床试验使用了E75(一种HLA-A2/A3限制性HER2/neu肽疫苗)和GM-CSF分别接种乳腺癌患者。经过24个月的分析DFS在接种组中为94.3%,在对照组中为86.8%($P=0.08$)。在子集分析中,从疫苗接种中获益最多的患者表现有淋巴结阳性、HER2 IHC 1+至2+或1至2级肿瘤,并且这些患者接受的是最适剂量[225]。对转移性乳腺癌和肾癌患者的融合细胞(DCs和肿瘤细胞)疫苗接种显示其可同时诱导免疫和临床反应[226]。模拟人乳脂肪球抗原的抗Id抗体也被用作乳腺癌疫苗与自体干细胞移植(autologous stem cell transplantation,ASCT)结合使用。这项研究表明,3年OS占比48%,而无进展生存率为32%[227]。基于HER2肽的疫苗(nelipepimut-S)已经在195名患有局部乳腺癌并且具有高复发风险的患者中进行了Ⅱ期试验。HLA-A2-/A3阳性患者接受GM-CSF疫苗,而非HLA-A2或-A3阳性患者则接受对照治疗。接种疫苗组的患者的5年DFS为89.7%,未接种疫苗的患者为80.2%。在接受最佳剂量的患者中,5年DFS高达94.5%。如今已进入了Ⅲ期试验[228]。

肺癌

非小细胞肺癌(non-small cell lung cancer,NSCLC)患者的3项Ⅲ期研究未能达到其主要终点。基于MAGE-A3肽的疫苗在ⅠB、2和3A期肿瘤切除的NSCLC患者中进行了评估,这些患者的肿瘤表达MAGE-A3基因[229,230]。L-BLP25疫苗由MUC-1基因的串联重复区的肽组成。对无法切除其肿瘤的3期NSCLC患者进行放化疗后使用该疫苗的Ⅲ期试验未达到OS增加的主要终点[231]。Lucanix是一种由4种TGF-β2反义修饰的,经照射的同种异体NSCLC细胞系组成的疫苗。对于那些在ⅢA,ⅢB和Ⅳ期的Ⅲ期试验中和一线化疗后没有进展的NSCLC患者来说,在疫苗组中没有观察到OS的显著增加;然而,随机化和一线化疗的结束之间的时间差造成了生存率上的显著落差($P=0.002$)[232,233]。目前还在针对NSCLC患者评估其他疫苗。将编码了MUC-1和IL-2基因的修饰疫苗病毒(MVA)与一线化学疗法组合后,在患有晚期NSCLC的患者(n=74)中进行了评估。添加疫苗化疗组的6个月PFS为43.2%,而单独化疗组为31.5%[234]。在经过化学放射后NSCLC患者(n=23)中开展了对端粒酶肽疫苗的Ⅱ期临床试验[235]。免疫应答者的中位PFS为371天,而无免疫应答者为182天。

卵巢/宫颈癌

一些临床研究使用了一种由特异性针对肿瘤抗原CA125的Mab制成的疫苗对晚期卵巢患者进行治疗[236]。一项Ⅱ期研究测试了功能上模仿CA125抗原的抗独特型抗体疫苗,并报告了生存获益;疫苗组的中位OS为19.4个月,而对照组为4.9个月[237]。

另一项Ⅱ期单组临床试验的目的是评估低剂量环磷酰胺预处理是否能够改善复发性卵巢癌患者p53合成长肽疫苗的免疫原性。该研究在20.0%(2/10)的患者中观察到SD[238]。研究人员对组合免疫疗法进行了两项独立的连续性研究,包括基于DC的自体全肿瘤抗原疫苗接种与抗血管生成疗法的组合。其中,31名患者复发了进展Ⅲ期和Ⅳ期卵巢癌。在两项研究中,疫苗接种均具有良好的耐受性并引发了针对各种卵巢肿瘤抗原的肿瘤特异性T细胞应答,并且65%的临床益处是与部分正在延长的PFS免疫应答相关的[239]。一项Ⅱ期临床试验在22例有高度复发和进展可能性的上皮性卵巢癌(EOC)患者中进行,采用的是重组牛痘-NY-ESO-1(rV-NY-ESO-1)后加重组鸡痘-NY-ESO-1(rF-NY-ESO-1)进行强化。中位PFS为21个月,且中位OS为48个月。接种疫苗后患者产生的$CD8^+$T细胞,被发现可以溶解表达NY-ESO-1的肿瘤靶点。这些数据初步证明,基于重组痘苗病毒的多元化初免-加强免疫接种策略在卵巢癌中具有临床意义[240]。

进一步的研究确证了给予终末期宫颈癌患者的人乳头瘤病毒16(HPV16)E6和E7长肽疫苗的毒性,安全性和免疫原性。HPV16 E6和E7是基于长肽的、具有良好的耐受性的疫苗,能够诱导广泛的IFN-γ相关T细胞反应,哪怕是对晚期宫颈癌患者也有效[241]。外阴上皮内瘤变是由高危型HPV引起的慢性疾病,其中最常见的是HPV16型(HPV-16)。20例HPV-16阳性,3级外阴上皮内瘤变患者均接种了来自HPV-16病毒癌蛋白E6和E7的长肽混合物[242]。一组20名患有HPV16诱导的外阴上皮3级内瘤变的患者中,有一半在治疗性疫苗接种后,显示出完全消退的情况。这提示一组确定的疫苗引发的特异性免疫应答和治疗性疫苗接种的临床疗效之间存在很强的相关性[243]。

白血病/淋巴瘤

淋巴瘤上B细胞受体Igs的可变区是疫苗的优良靶标。这些Ids现已成功用于治疗B细胞淋巴瘤[50,244-247]。在化疗诱导的第二次完整临床症状消退后,对25名滤泡性淋巴瘤(follicular lymphoma,FL)患者使用了Id蛋白疫苗。接种疫苗后,25名患者中的20名出现了肿瘤特异性体液或细胞免疫应答[246]。

所有具有足够随访期的反应者第二个 CR 比第一个 CR 维持的时间更长,而没有产生免疫反应的 5 名患者则如预期的那样,第二次 CR 短于第一次 CR。用与 KLH 缀合并与 GM-CSF 一起施用的杂交瘤衍生的自体肿瘤 Ig Id 接种后可诱导 FL 特异性免疫应答。在对该疫苗的一项双盲多中心对照Ⅲ期试验中,入组的 234 名患者有 177 名(81%)在化疗后达到 CR/CRu 并呈现随机分布状态。对于这 177 名随机分布的患者,Id-疫苗和对照组之间的中位 DFS 分别为 23.0 个月和 20.6 个月(P=0.256)。对于接种了 Id 疫苗的患者,随机化后的中位 DFS 在 Id-疫苗组为 44.2 个月而对照组为 30.6 个月。在因化疗产生 CR/CRu 后的 FL 患者接种特异性杂交瘤的 Id 疫苗可延长患者的 DFS[248]。

现已开发出一种多发性骨髓瘤疫苗,这种疫苗源自患者的肿瘤细胞,这些肿瘤细胞与自体 DC 融合,产生了可以刺激产生广泛抗肿瘤反应的杂交瘤。在Ⅱ期试验中,患者在 ASCT 后接种疫苗以靶向治疗微小残留病。78%的患者达到 CR 或 PR 的最佳反应状态,47%达到 CR/近 CR(nCR)状态。值得注意的是,24%在移植后获得部分反应的患者在接种疫苗后和移植 3 个月以上后转为 CR/nCR,这与疫苗介导的对残留疾病的影响一致。多发性骨髓瘤患者的移植后期为细胞免疫治疗提供了独特的平台,其中接种 DC/骨髓瘤融合疫苗导致骨髓瘤特异性 T 细胞显著扩增,同时微小残留疾病的细胞减少[249]。在多发性骨髓瘤患者中使用 Id 疫苗也观察到临床反应[52,250]。

对于慢性粒细胞白血病患者,接种 bcr-abl 致癌基因断裂点融合肽能够产生特异性免疫反应[251]。一项研究调查了表达 WT1 的急性髓性白血病(AML)中 Wilms 肿瘤基因产物 1(WT1)-肽疫苗接种的免疫原性。接种的疫苗由 GM-CSF 和 WT1 肽和 KLH 组成。AML 患者(n=17)的接种中位数为 11 次。AML 患者的客观反应为:10 名进入疾病稳定期,其中 4 名进入稳定期的患者出现了 50%以上的骤降,两名有血液学改善。另外 4 名患者在初始进展后呈现出临床改善,其中一名完全缓解,3 名疾病稳定[252]。Ⅰ/Ⅱ期试验研究了 10 名 AML 患者自体 DC 疫苗接种的效果。化疗后病情得到部分缓解的两名患者在皮内施用完整 WT1 mRNA 电穿孔的 DC 后,病情得到彻底缓解。在这两名患者和其他三名完全缓解的患者中,AML 相关肿瘤标志物在 DC 疫苗接种后恢复正常,这与分子缓解的诱导相吻合。WT1 特异性 $CD8^+$T 细胞频率的临床反应与其疫苗相关的增加密切相关[253]。

其他肿瘤类型

膀胱内 BCG 已成功用于治疗膀胱癌,这其中涉及免疫机制问题[254]。野生型痘苗病毒的膀胱内给药现已被证明是安全的,4 例患者中有 3 例在 4 年的随访中没有发病[255]。肾癌对高剂量 IL-2 和 IFN-α 的反应也侧面表现了治疗反应中的免疫机制[256]。采用了经遗传修饰以表达 B7-1、从而共刺激反应性 T 细胞的自体 RCC 肿瘤细胞的疫苗[257]。在这项单组临床Ⅱ期试验中,66 名患者入组,39 名患者接受了至少一剂低剂量 IL-2 的疫苗。最佳反应为 CR(3%),PR(5%),SD(64%)和 PD(28%)。事后分析表明,通过活组织检查确定疫苗位点的淋巴细胞浸润与存活直接相关(28.4 个月,对照组 17.8 个月,P=0.045)。DC 疫苗的Ⅰ期试验评估了其在转移性 RCC 患者(n=21)中的可行性、安全性和有效性。用 HLA-A2 结合的 MUC1 肽脉冲自体成熟 DCs。在 6 名患者中,接种疫苗后检测到了转移部位的消退,其中 3 名患者实现客观反应(一个完全反应,两个部分反应,两个混合反应和一个 SD)。另外 4 名患者在长达 14 个月的治疗期间保持稳定状态[258]。

已经显示用肿瘤裂解物脉冲 DCs 对小儿实体瘤患者进行疫苗接种可以诱导特异性 T 细胞的扩增并介导一些肿瘤消退[259]。除了转移性乳腺癌和肾癌患者的 DC 融合疫苗接种之外,临床试验已经检查了用于 DC/神经胶质瘤融合的神经胶质瘤患者的疫苗接种[226,260]。早期临床试验显示 DC 疫苗、自体甲醛溶液修饰[262]或 TGF-β 修饰全肿瘤细胞疫苗[263]均可在原发性脑肿瘤患者体内诱导产生免疫反应和客观反应[261]。一项关于与神经胶质瘤相关的抗原(GAA)表位肽 s.c. 的接种疫苗的初步研究在患有新诊断的脑干神经胶质瘤(BSG)和高级别神经胶质瘤(HGG)的 HLA-A2 阳性儿童中进行。共纳入了 26 名儿童,其中 14 名新诊断的 BSG 用辐射治疗,12 名新诊断的 BSGs 或 HGGs 用辐射和同步化疗治疗。五名儿童出现假性症状进展,对地塞米松有反应,并与延长的生存期相关。在前两个疫苗疗程中,只有两名患者患有进行性疾病;19 例有 SD,2 例有部分反应,1 例有轻微反应,2 例手术后其无病状态期延长[264]。

疫苗临床试验结果分析的考虑因素

现在已经证明,适当的疫苗递送系统和配给策略可以引发一系列癌症患者机体对 TAA 的免疫应答,并且在一些情况下,可以介导其存活期的延长和无患病间隔时期的延长、血清中肿瘤标志物比例的下降和/或转移性疾病的消退。患有晚期癌症的有可能是证明癌症疫苗功效的最不合适的人群。因此,未来的临床试验应该在肿瘤负荷转移性疾病较少或所占比例较低或处于患病过程早期的患者中进行。疫苗的最佳使用时机应在即将进行辅助治疗之前,期间或之后立即进行。目前已有一系列相关的研究正在开展。其总体目标在于,通过将疫苗治疗与一线癌症治疗方法相结合,从而缩短了疾病诊断与开始注射疫苗之间的时间间隔;这将使癌症疫苗的使用更接近最初的意图——在患有微小疾病的群体中使用。

联合疗法

有许多方法可以将疫苗疗法与所谓的非免疫疗法(表 65-3)以及其他免疫疗法结合使用。癌症疫苗疗法的主要优点之一是它们的毒性比较低。目前正在被重新评估的医疗界传统观点之一是,癌症疫苗不能与化学疗法或放射疗法组合使用。人们不应该擅自忽略一些疫苗潜在的降低疗效的可能性,这部分降低的疗效可能会导致一些在联合疗法的化疗步骤之前经历过多次既往化疗并且失败了的患者再次接受不必要的联合疗法中的化疗步骤。临床前研究和现在的几项临床研究表明,当与某些细胞毒性药物、激素或肿瘤局部放疗联合使用时,患者可以对癌症疫苗产生增强的免疫应答。研究表明,当肿瘤细胞暴露于低于致死剂量的辐射或某些化学治疗剂中时,肿瘤细胞的表型实际上受到了调节从而使其更容易受到 T 细胞介导的杀伤(图 65-1)。事实上,治疗性癌症疫苗与其他免疫治疗药物以及所谓的非免疫性常规癌症治疗药物的结合使用仍处于早期发展阶段并且具备完整的临床潜力。

疫苗接种配合其他免疫疗法

最近，研究人员采用针对检查点抑制剂PD-L1/PD-1免疫抑制轴的MAb的临床研究已将癌症免疫疗法作为癌症治疗的主流策略考虑在内。检查点抑制剂在治疗大多数转移性黑素瘤和亚型肺癌的患者中有着令人振奋的结果[266-271]。PD-L1/PD-1检查点抑制剂使用在少数患有其他肿瘤类型(例如膀胱癌)的患者中时可显示出一些活性，而在其他癌症例如结肠直肠癌和前列腺癌中则显示出极低水平的活性。在几乎所有PD-L1/PD-1检查点抑制剂研究中，其临床反应的主要相关性都是肿瘤中存在T细胞。看来这些TIL在诱导肿瘤细胞上的PD-L1并使之重新发生作用，从而重现身体防御自身免疫的过程。施用抗PD-L1/PD-1剂将通过减少或消除这种免疫抑制现象从而“释放T细胞上的制动物”，导致TIL的活化和随后的肿瘤细胞破坏(图65-2)。一些肿瘤疫苗临床试验的结果缺乏成功的一个潜在原因可能是由于其在TILs存在的情况下反应时引起了肿瘤细胞上PD-L1含量的上升。因此，似乎在使用抗PD-L1/PD-1试剂之前或同时使用治疗性疫苗，会诱导肿瘤中T细胞的产生，随后通过抑制肿瘤中PD-L1的表达而活化，最终导致肿瘤细胞的裂解(见图65-2)。当然，我们需要进行更加严格控制的随机临床试验来验证这一假设。

表65-3 疫苗联合其他治疗方案

方法	提高疫苗效力的作用机制
放疗	肿瘤细胞表型的改变
化疗	“免疫”肿瘤细胞死亡 改变肿瘤细胞表型 富集效应物：调节细胞比例
激素疗法	胸腺再生和诱导幼稚T细胞改变肿瘤细胞表型
小分子靶向疗法	调节肿瘤细胞微环境 改变肿瘤细胞表型
单克隆抗体	增强抗体依赖细胞介导的细胞毒性 免疫调制检查
Imidsa*(母乳喂养)	刺激T细胞增殖

* Imidsa是一类新型的免疫调节剂。

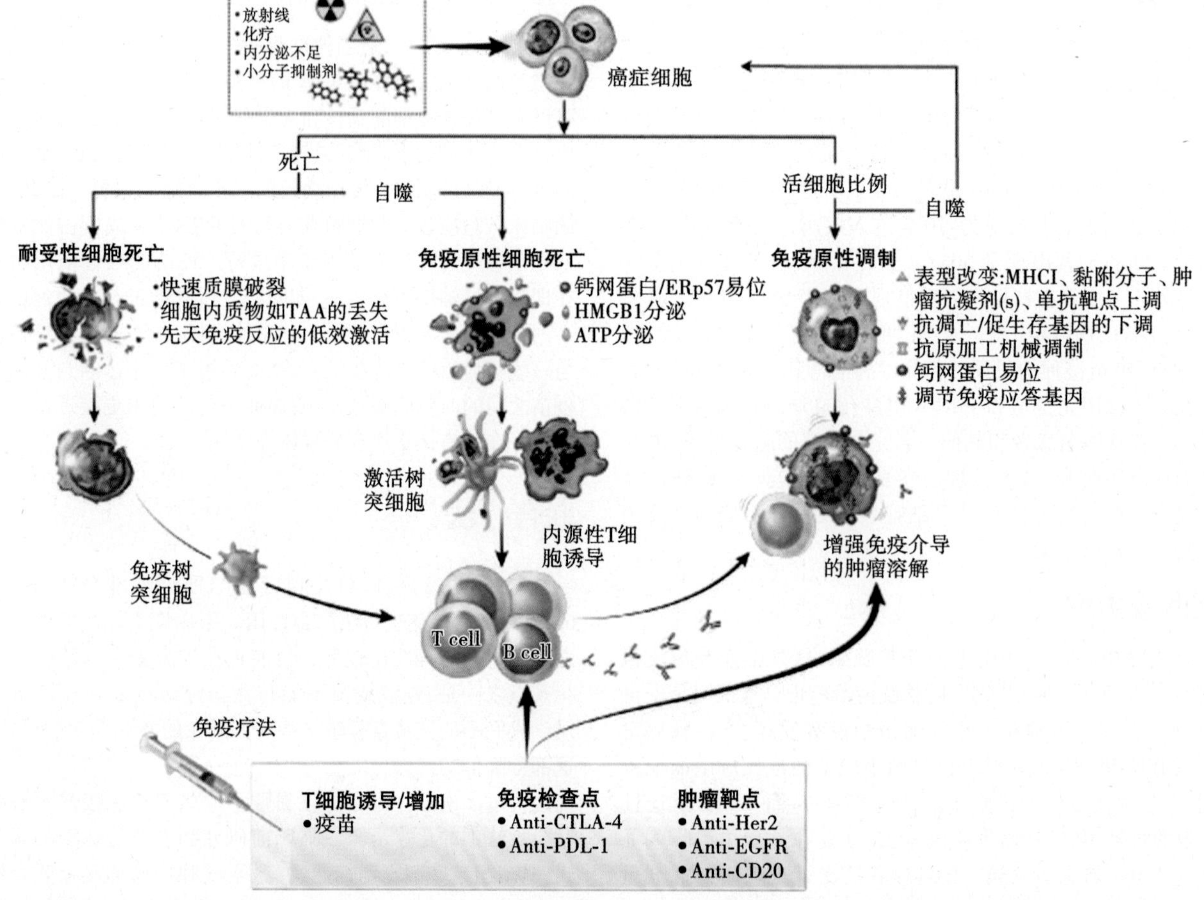

图65-1 放射治疗、化疗、内分泌剥夺或小分子抑制剂的多重免疫原性后果，可用于促进与免疫治疗方案的协同作用。抗癌治疗的这些免疫原性后果，从免疫原性细胞死亡到免疫原性调节，可以被利用来实现与肿瘤疫苗的最佳协同作用

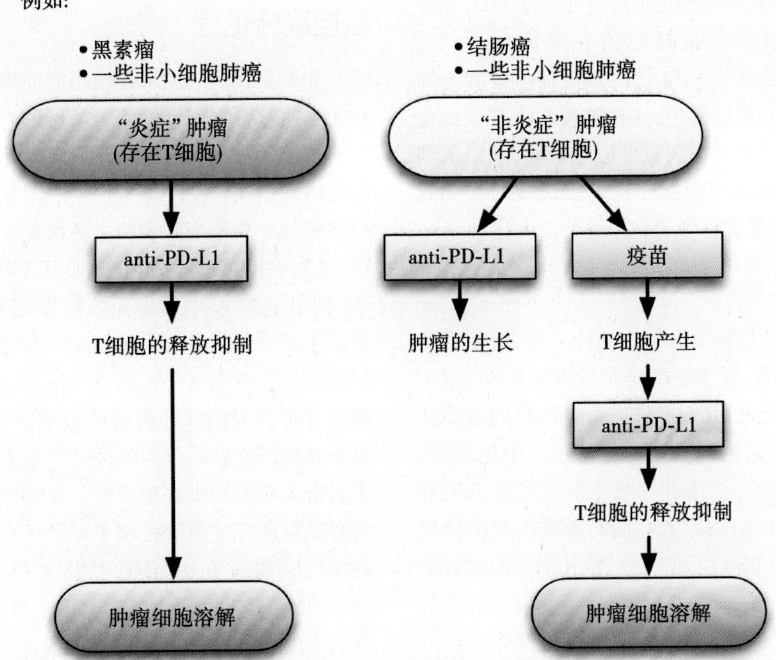

图 65-2　便于理解 T 细胞发炎与非发炎肿瘤微环境及其对疫苗治疗的影响的工作模型。一部分肿瘤即便在缺乏 T 细胞浸润的情况下仍缺乏自发免疫反应的潜在原因包括免疫激活的失败(A)通过 PD-L1/PD-1 相互作用的外源性抑制。这种局部抑制可以通过用抗 PD-L1/PD-1 检查点抑制剂单克隆抗体阻断来克服,产生临床收益。其他被称为"非炎性"的肿瘤类型,由于缺乏潜在的浸润反应性 T 细胞,通常对 PD-L1 抑制不起反应。这种模型表明,这些肿瘤可以通过疫苗方案转化为"炎症"的 T 细胞浸润表型(B)这些 T 细胞可能被 PD-L1/PD-1 阻断进一步激活

临床前研究表明,疫苗和检查点抑制可以起协同作用。抗-CTLA4 MAb 加入 CEA-TRICOM 疫苗可以增加 T 细胞反应的亲合力,进而提高疫苗的抗肿瘤活性[138,272]。当与 GVAX 疫苗联合使用时,PD-1 和 CTLA-4 的阻断将会导致 $CD8^+$ TIL 功能障碍的逆转和抗肿瘤活性的增强[273]。

在一个Ⅰ期临床试验中[274],30 名转移性前列腺癌患者接受了 PROSTVAC 疫苗与增加剂量的易普利姆马(抗-CTLA4)联合使用。其中,58%的患者 PSA 下降。虽然该试验未随机分组,但接受该组合疗法的患者的中位 OS 为 34.4 个月,而接受 PROSTVAC 的患者为 26.3 个月(Halabi 预测存活率[144]在两个试验进行到约 18 个月时相似)。在最近完成的使用易普利姆玛 plus 的 mCRPC 患者群体的辐射试验显示中值 OS 为 17.3 个月。此外,在疫苗加易普利姆玛治疗的患者中没有观察到比单独用易普利姆玛更多的额外毒性。在另一项研究中,DNA/肽疫苗诱导黑素瘤患者的 T 细胞反应,这些反应在 CTLA-4 阻断后被"加强"[275]。9 名先前已接受免疫的晚期癌症患者也被注射了 CTLA-4 MAb[276];研究者在一些黑素瘤和转移性卵巢癌患者中观察到了肿瘤免疫增加的证据。

疫苗和单克隆抗体可以通过多种方式组合使用。这些方法包括:①使用治疗性抗体如赫赛汀或利妥昔单抗与疫苗联合使用,但是两种成分会独立发挥作用。②使用抗肿瘤抗体细胞因子融合蛋白,如抗肿瘤抗体/IL-12 可增强肿瘤部位的 T 细胞活性[277-281]。③使用针对性调节 T 细胞的 MAb 或融合蛋白[282-284]。疫苗也可以与抗原特异性 T 细胞的过继转移组合使用。在临床前研究中,将点突变的 ras 特异性 T 细胞过继转移到免疫耗竭的宿主中。供体抗原特异性 T 细胞应答在接受肽促进剂(含有或不含有 IL-2 的受体)的受体小鼠中反应最为强烈。以上这些结果表明,T 细胞转移后的疫苗接种,比外源性 IL-2 更能具有强制性地维持过继转移的 T 细胞[285]。

免疫原性细胞死亡和免疫原性调节

某些癌症治疗方案具有诱导癌细胞死亡的能力,这引导了针对肿瘤的内源性免疫应答的刺激;这种刺激被称为"免疫原性细胞死亡"(见图 65-1)[286-293]。免疫原性细胞死亡的主要迹象是:①濒死细胞表面的钙网蛋白暴露;②高迁移率组 1 (HMGB1)的释放;③ATP 释放;④细胞死亡[289](最重要)。这些分子作用于 DC 以促进肿瘤表面抗原向免疫系统的递呈[287]。当被暴露在垂死细胞表面时,钙网蛋白是钙网蛋白伴侣和钙离子调节剂,会作为 DC 的吞噬信号[291,294]。当 HMGB1 (一种非组蛋白染色质结合蛋白)从濒死细胞中释放出来时,它会与 DC 上的 TLR-4 结合,导致 DC 成熟[289]。濒死细胞分泌的 ATP 与 DC 上的受体结合,进一步支持 T-细胞活化[288]。此外,治疗后存活的肿瘤细胞已被证明可以改变其生物学特性,使其对免疫介导的杀伤更敏感;这种现象被称为"免疫原性调节"

（见图 65-1）[295-302]。免疫原性调节包括癌细胞生物学特性中的一系列分子改变，其独立地或共同地使肿瘤更易于 CTL 介导的破坏。这些特性包括：①下调抗凋亡/存活基因[297,298,303]；②抗原加工装置元件的调制[299,302]；③钙网蛋白易位至肿瘤细胞表面（见图 65-1）[265,299]。可以设想，这种抗癌疗法产生的免疫原性效果从免疫原性细胞的死亡到免疫原性调制，可以被利用以达到治疗性癌症疫苗和其他免疫疗法方案最佳的协同效果，从而使接受联合疗法的患者得到的临床益处最大化。

疫苗联合放疗

放射治疗方法是多种恶性肿瘤的标准治疗方法，旨在直接杀伤并破坏肿瘤细胞。然而，对于一些全身性肿瘤疾病，鉴于肿瘤对于放射治疗的治疗抗性，我们或许需要将治疗剂量降低至略低于致死剂量，以使正常组织受到的毒作用最小化，这些全身性肿瘤细胞通常转化为存活的肿瘤细胞群或者是进展肿瘤细胞[304,305]。辐射可以在死亡和/或存活的肿瘤细胞中诱导连续的免疫原性改变（见图 65-1）。据报告，致死剂量的放射治疗可以诱导免疫原性细胞死亡[306]。虽然单独接受放射治疗的癌症患者的免疫反应通常很弱并且很少转化为保护性免疫，但是可以利用放射疗法的免疫原性效应来促进接受免疫疗法联合治疗患者的协同临床效益[304,305,307]。已经证明的是，使用相对低剂量的外部辐射治疗是不足以杀死肿瘤细胞，诱导免疫原性调节，改变这些肿瘤细胞以使它们更易受 T 细胞介导的裂解的。MHC Ⅰ类分子和钙网蛋白在肿瘤上的细胞表面的表达以辐射剂量依赖性的方式增加，它们的表达最终使肿瘤细胞对 T 细胞介导的杀伤更敏感[265,298,302]。在临床前研究中已经证明，与单独使用任何一种方式相比，放射治疗联合癌症疫苗可以引发更大的肿瘤抗原特异性 $CD8^+$T 细胞反应和/或减少肿瘤负担[298,308-310]。重要的是，在联合治疗（抗原级联）后，观察到对疫苗不编码的多种 TAA 特异性的 $CD8^+$T 细胞的诱导。这种多克隆 T 细胞反应功能性地介导了在皮下或肺部的 TAA 阴性转移灶[310]。

以上这些发现在临床试验中证实了癌症患者接受疫苗治疗联合放疗的可观收效[304,305,307,311,312]。Ⅰ期试验评估了 14 例晚期/转移性肝癌患者接受放疗联合注射自体 DC 疫苗的组合疗法[311]。患者首先接受单次放射治疗，随后连续两次向瘤内注射自体未成熟 DC。这种组合疗法在 7/10 名可评估的患者中产生了肿瘤特异性免疫应答，6 名患者具有客观的临床反应。在一项患者接受使用痘病毒疫苗的局部前列腺癌的随机Ⅱ期研究中，接受放射治疗联合痘病毒疫苗治疗的患者与单独接受放射治疗的患者相比，PSA 特异性 T 细胞反应显著增加[312]。在多中心Ⅱ期研究中，mCRPC 患者（n=44）被随机分配[153]单独接受 Sm-EDTMP（Quadramet®，FDA 批准靶向骨转移放射性药物）或与 PSA-TRICOM 疫苗联合使用。联合治疗组与单独使用 SM-EDTMP 组相比，TTP 显著改善（前者 3.7 个月，后者 1.7 个月，$P=0.03$）[313]。此外，一些正在进行的临床试验正在研究这种组合策略[314]，包括 sipuleucel-Tplusradiation 疗法的Ⅱ期研究[62]，sipuleucel-T 加立体定向消融体放疗的Ⅱ期研究[63]，和 sipuleucel-T 加高剂量单次分割放疗[64]治疗激素难治性前列腺癌的初步研究。

疫苗联合化疗

如果要在疾病的早期使用癌症疫苗，它们很可能需要与某些化学治疗方案联合使用。虽然这有些违背直觉，但最近已经证明疫苗疗法不仅可以与某些化学疗法相容，并且可能具有实际的协同作用（见图 65-1）[296,315]。现在已经显示，各种化学治疗剂通过上调癌细胞表面上各种免疫相关蛋白的含量（包括多种 TAA，钙网蛋白，黏附分子如 ICAM-1 和 MHC Ⅰ类蛋白），在不同来源的肿瘤中诱导免疫原性调节[295,298-300,303,316,317]。这在暴露于亚致死剂量的顺铂/5-FU[317]多烯紫杉醇[299]紫杉醇[299]和顺铂加长春瑞滨[317]后，这些表型变化转化为小鼠和/或人肿瘤对 CTL 介导的体外裂解的敏感性增加。这些临床前研究结果和其他研究已转化为各种可以提出假设的临床试验，现在有了振奋人心的初步实验数据。在随机Ⅱ期试验中，接受多烯紫杉醇联合治疗性癌症疫苗 PANVAC（基于痘病毒的疫苗，编码肿瘤抗原 CEA 和 MUC-1，以及 3 种 T 细胞共刺激分子；TRICOM）的转移性乳腺癌患者相比于单独使用多烯紫杉醇的患者有更好的 FPS（前者 6.6 个月，后者 3.8 个月）[318]。最近的一份报告[319]表明，对于大多数患有转移性前列腺癌或乳腺癌的患者以及采用顺铂加长春瑞滨治疗 NSCLC 的患者，多烯紫杉醇注射显著增加了效应 T 细胞和 Tregs 的比例，并降低了后者的免疫抑制活性。这些研究为在癌症患者中选择性使用主动免疫疗法联合特定的标准疗法，以获得最佳的临床结局提供了理论依据。考虑使用疫苗化疗的几个重要因素是：①在疾病过程早期联合使用疫苗和化疗的组合疗法，不应与晚期疾病时在接受多种不同化疗药物治疗后使用疫苗的疗法相混淆，因为免疫系统最有可能受损；②并非所有化学治疗药剂都与疫苗相容；③与化疗一起使用时，疫苗的剂量安排可能非常重要。显然，未来的研究将需要优化疫苗和化疗的联合使用方案。最近已经发表了一些有关抗肿瘤药物与肿瘤疫苗联合的综述[320]。

疫苗联合激素治疗

含有抗雄激素的疫苗疗法有望使得治疗前列腺癌成为可能。先前已经表明雄激素消融疗法能够诱导前列腺中的 T 细胞浸润。在治疗 1~3 周后，T 细胞浸润很明显[321]。雄激素剥夺的免疫原性调节潜力已经用第二代雄激素受体拮抗剂（androgen-receptor antagonist，ARA）——恩杂鲁胺——治疗前列腺癌的小鼠 TRAMP 模型进行了描述[322]。TRAMP-C2 前列腺肿瘤细胞体外暴露于恩杂鲁胺可显著增强细胞表面 Fas 和 MHC Ⅰ类的表达，从而提高其对免疫介导的裂解的敏感性。恩杂鲁胺的这些免疫调节性质被应用于在与针对与转移过程相关的转录因子的治疗性癌症疫苗组合中。与未接受治疗或单独使用恩杂鲁胺的小鼠中观察到的水平相比，联合治疗显著增加了抗原特异性 T 细胞的增殖和 OS。此外，恩杂鲁胺或阿比特龙（一种雄激素生物合成抑制剂）都能够使雄激素受体阳性 LNCaP 患者的前列腺肿瘤细胞对 T 细胞介导的裂解更敏感[316]。这些研究和其他研究的结果为 ADT 联合主动免疫治疗提供了理论依据。一项临床试验对已经接受过激素治疗的前列腺癌患者进行了研究,这些患者血清 PSA 增加,且并没有癌症转移的影像学证据。该试验随机进行二线激素治疗(尼鲁米特)与疫苗治疗,并在疾病进展期进行交叉互换,以便每组可以接受联合疫苗加激素治疗。在最初接种疫苗而后接种疫苗联合尼鲁米特的患者中,治疗方案宣告失败的时间和存活 4 年以上[323]的比例相较于对照组延长了。显然,需要进一步的研究来验证这些观察结果,这些进一步的研究正在进行中(NCT01867333,NCT01875250)。

疫苗联合小分子抑制剂

最近的一些研究表明,抗血管生成的酪氨酸激酶抑制剂(tyrosine kinase inhibitor,TKI)靶向抑制肿瘤生存必需的微环境的多种成分,是与癌症疫苗协同作用的理想药物[324]。众所周知,TKI 可调节肿瘤内皮细胞,致使血管正常化;然而,这些药物最近也被证明可以降低肿瘤紧密度和紧密连接的密度,从而改善肿瘤引发的压迫情况,改善塌陷血管的灌注能力,还能增加肿瘤氧合作用[325]。此外,选择 TKI 能够诱导免疫原性调节(见图 65-1)。当抗血管生成 TKI 与免疫疗法结合时,免疫情况会得到改善,这些对肿瘤细胞的直接修饰效果和改善的血管灌注能力致使抗肿瘤效力得到增强。这些数据支持多靶点抗血管生成 TKI 的临床组合,包括但不限于卡博替尼[326]、舒尼替尼[325,327-329]和索拉非尼[325],以及其他抗血管生成的疗法,如抗 VEGF 抗体贝伐单抗,以及用于改善实体瘤治疗的癌症疫苗。

用其他疗法配制的疫苗的剂量

可以说,癌症疫苗疗法最独有的特征是疫苗能够启动宿主免疫反应的动态过程,这种特性可以在后续疗法中加以利用(表 65-4)。在Ⅰ期研究中,晚期进展期癌症患者接种了针对细胞色素 P4501B1 的疫苗。他们中的大多数对疫苗产生免疫力,但需要进行其他补救治疗的患者对其下一次治疗方案有显著反应;这些反应大多数持续>1 年以上[331]。在对处于广泛期小细胞肺癌患者的研究中[332],疫苗治疗后立即进行化疗的客观临床反应率很高。这些临床反应也与诱导或增强对疫苗的免疫应答密切相关。

表 65-4　治疗性疫苗与传统疗法

	治疗性疫苗	传统疗法
靶点	免疫系统	肿瘤或其微环境
药效动力学	延迟作用(适应性强,随着时间的推移可能会变得更好)	通常立即起作用
是否有记忆效应	是	否
肿瘤进化/新的突变	新的免疫原性靶点	对治疗产生耐药性
缺点	需要足够的免疫系统功能(包括系统和肿瘤部位)	毒性

前列腺癌的 3 项随机临床试验提供了证明这种现象的进一步证据。在第一项试验中,患有转移性 CRPC 的患者被随机接种疫苗或在使用疫苗的同时联合应用每周一次的多烯紫杉醇[333]。单独接种疫苗的患者被允许在出现癌症进展时交叉治疗方案接受多烯紫杉醇。接种疫苗后,多烯紫杉醇的中位 PFS 为 6.1 个月,而同一机构的采用多烯紫杉醇的方案的患者 PFS 为 3.7 个月。使用 sipuleucel 疫苗也可以观察到类似的结果[334]。在一项随机多中心研究中,疫苗组和安慰剂组的患者在癌症进展时接受了多烯他赛。先前疫苗与安慰剂相比,使用多烯紫杉醇的 OS 的增加具有统计学意义($P=0.023$)。

在Ⅱ期试验中[335],患有非转移性 CRPC 和血清 PSA 升高的患者随机接受疫苗或尼鲁米特(一种 ARA)。6 个月后,PSA 升高的患者被允许联合使用两种疗法。宣告治疗失败的中位时间在疫苗组和 ARA 组相似。然而,对于首先接种疫苗然后接种疫苗加 ARA 的患者来说,宣告治疗失败的时间是从使用 ARA 开始的 13.9 个月。如果要从给与治疗手段开始计算,到宣告治疗失败的时间是 25.9 个月。在最初的随机人群中,对于首次接受单独使用尼鲁米特或先使用尼鲁米特再接种疫苗的患者,5 年 OS 为 38%,而首次接种疫苗或尼鲁胺加疫苗的患者的中位 OS 为 59%[336]。

对于传统的具有细胞毒性的药物,人们普遍认为改良后的 TTP 是改善 OS 的先决条件。最近的一项研究[337]评估了 4 项化疗试验和一项疫苗试验中 mCRPC 患者的肿瘤消退和增长率。细胞毒性剂仅在给药期间影响肿瘤;药物停药后不久,由于耐药性或毒性,抗肿瘤活性停止增加,肿瘤生长速度增加(图 65-3)。疫苗治疗的临床反应的作用机制和动力学似乎有

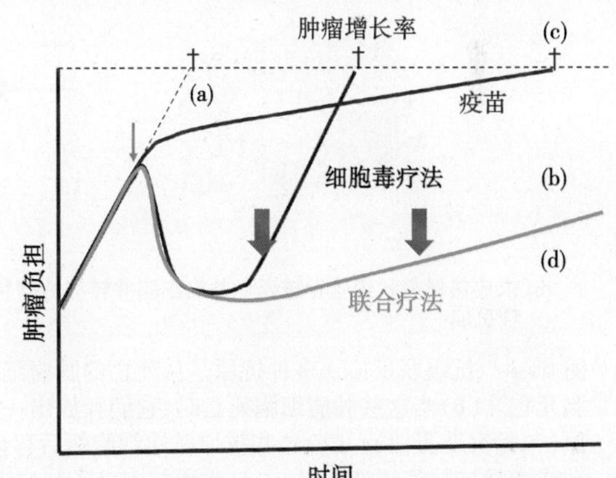

图 65-3　转移性前列腺癌患者的肿瘤增长率,来自 4 次化疗试验和 1 次 Prostvac(PSA-TRICOM)试验(改编自参考文献[337-339]中的数据)。无治疗的肿瘤生长率(a,虚线)。化疗诱导的初始肿瘤减少,但由于毒性或耐药而停止治疗时的肿瘤生长速率与治疗前的肿瘤生长速率相似(b,蓝线)。Prostvac 疫苗降低治疗后的肿瘤生长速率(c,红线)。因此,接受疫苗的患者几乎没有肿瘤消退(几乎没有进展时间的增加),但总体生存率有所增加。对同时接受疫苗和细胞毒疗法治疗的患者的总体生存率的提高的预测(d,绿线)。联合治疗,细胞毒治疗减少了肿瘤负担,免疫治疗降低了增长率,最终达到客观的临床反应和总存活率的提高。如果在低肿瘤负担患者的疾病处理中更早启动疫苗,这种现象可能会进一步加强。箭头表示治疗的开始;交叉表示癌症死亡的时间

很大不同(见表 65-4)[337]。治疗性疫苗不直接针对肿瘤发挥作用,而是针对免疫系统。免疫反应通常需要时间来发展,并且可以通过持续的加强免疫接种来增强这种反应;任何由此产生的肿瘤细胞裂解都可导致其他 TAA 的交叉发展,从而通过一种被称为抗原级联或表位扩散的现象扩大免疫库(图 65-4)。这种更广泛的,可能具有更高相关性的免疫反应也可能需要一些时间来发展。尽管疫苗可能不会引起肿瘤负荷的任何显著性的降低,但作为单独使用的疫苗,有可能通过长期影响抗肿瘤活性,致肿瘤生长速度较慢(见图 65-3)。这种增长速度的减缓可能持续数月或数年,更重要的是,会贯穿于后续的治疗中。该过程可以导致临床上 OS 的显著改善,通常在 TTP 中具有很小的差异或没有差异,抑或是低的或完全没有客观反应[340];因此,用疫苗治疗具有较低肿瘤负荷的患者可以产生更好的结果。据推测,联合使用疫苗和细胞毒性治疗可能导致肿瘤消退(通过细胞毒性治疗)和降低肿瘤生长速度(通过疫苗治疗)(见图 65-3)[337,338]。早期接种疫苗的临床试验可能已经在给予足够的疫苗增强剂之前,因观察到肿瘤进展而提前终止。这种现象实际上导致了现在设计疫苗临床试验的方式和免疫疗法的"新免疫应答标准"的改变[341]。

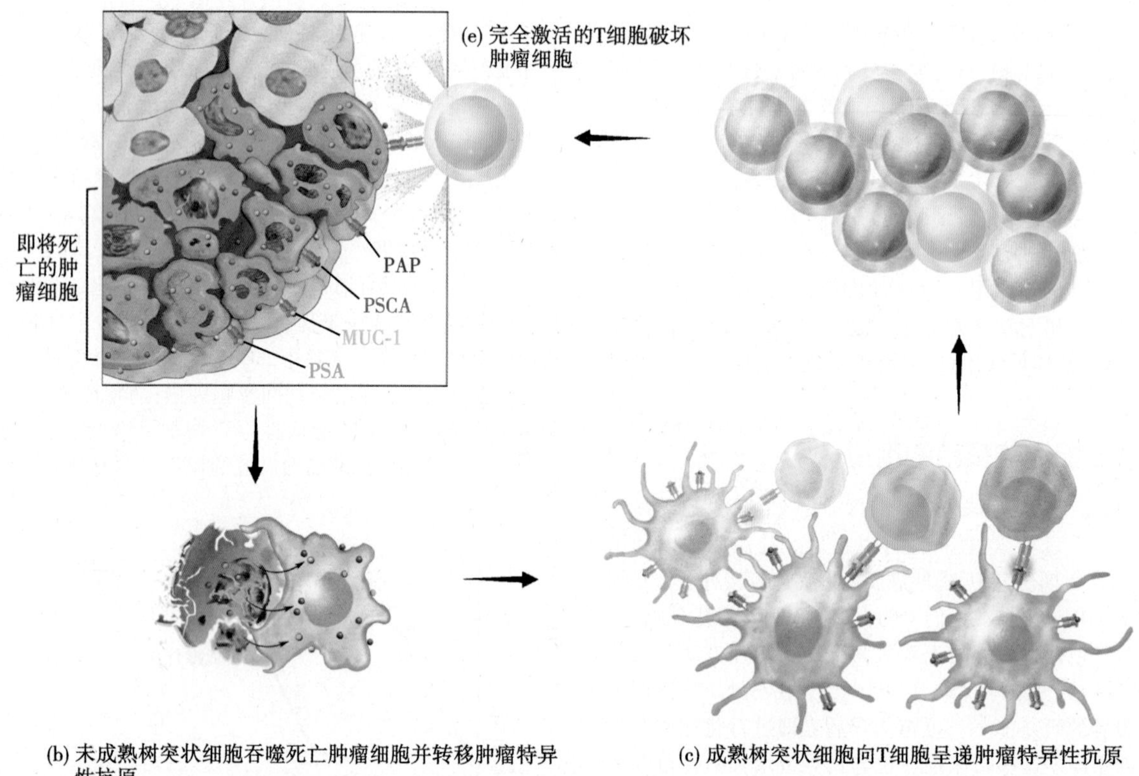

图 65-4 抗级联反应。多种抗原是从死亡的肿瘤细胞中释放出来的,可以激活免疫反应。(a)癌症治疗导致癌细胞死亡。(b)当这些肿瘤细胞死亡时,它们释放出一系列被称为由抗原呈递细胞的清道夫细胞吸收的肿瘤蛋白抗原(包括突变蛋白)。(c)这些抗原呈递细胞然后移动到区域淋巴结,在那里它们将这些多个抗原呈递给 T 细胞,启动或增强抗肿瘤免疫反应。(d)激活的多克隆肿瘤特异性 T 细胞然后可以运输到肿瘤区域,参与免疫介导的肿瘤杀伤,摧毁更多的癌细胞并进一步增强级联(e)

涉及疫苗活动的机制

最近的研究表明,一系列效应细胞可能参与了抗肿瘤作用。在大多数临床前研究中,$CD8^+$ CTL 参与抗肿瘤作用,$CD4^+$辅助 T 细胞对于通过细胞因子提供帮助以进一步激活 CTL 非常重要。其他效应细胞也可能参与其中,例如巨噬细胞和自然杀伤(NK)细胞。研究还表明,在某些情况下,抗肿瘤抗体的产生可通过抗体依赖性细胞介导的细胞毒作用,进一步介导抗肿瘤作用[342]。T 细胞活化已被证明是一种复杂现象,涉及 APC 上的肽-MHC 复合物与 T 细胞上的 TCR 的相互作用;对于弱抗原如 TAA 来说,必须有辅助分子才能有效活化 T 细胞。这些辅助分子被称为 T 细胞共刺激分子。到目前为止。已经鉴定了十几种这样的共刺激分子。刺激分子仅仅存在于专属的 APC 上,例如 DC,但在绝大多数实体瘤中未被发现。最近还有研究显示,这些共刺激分子的组合可以产生协同作用以进一步增强 T 细胞活化[139]。最近的研究还表明,生成的 T 细胞数量不一定是必需的,但它们的质量或亲和力[138,343,344]是必须得到保障的。这是通过不同隶属于种群的T细胞实际杀死其对应靶标的能力来衡量的。最近已经证明,使用具有T细胞共刺激和某些细胞因子的疫苗实际上可以增强T细胞活性[138]。

现在已经确定了几种不同类型的调节性T细胞[345-348]。它们存在的进化层面的原因最有可能减少自身免疫现象。由于TAA大部分是自身抗原,因此调节性T细胞似乎在减少对TAA的免疫应答中起主要作用。现已鉴定的几种类型的调节性T细胞是$CD4^+CD25^+$ $FoxP3^+$(Tregs),未成熟巨噬细胞和$CD4^+$,NKT^+细胞[347,348]。正在进行的研究使用了可能会减少这些调节性T细胞活性的试剂,包括融合蛋白Ontak[349]、环磷酰胺[212,221,350]和抗CD25 Abs[351,352]。这些细胞的抑制很可能是未来癌症疫苗治疗的一部分。

抗原级联反应

抗原级联现象(图65-4)现在正在发展成为癌症疫苗评估的重要指标。这首先使用了术语表位扩散定义,其中将给定的肽用作疫苗,疫苗接种后的宿主免疫应答不仅仅针对该表位,还针对同一肿瘤抗原的其他表位。这一现象现在已经使用抗原级联这一术语进行了扩展,其中给定的抗原被用作疫苗,接种后的宿主免疫反应不仅针对疫苗中的抗原,还针对肿瘤中的其他抗原[308,352,353]。对这些现象的解释是,由于疫苗诱导的一些肿瘤细胞被破坏,呈递给T细胞APC将吞噬肿瘤碎片,然后将这些肿瘤碎片交叉分布于细胞中,从而引发抗原级联现象。一些研究还表明,1/8接受放射治疗的前列腺癌患者产生了一系列TAA的抗体,而接受PROSTVAC加辐射的15/33患者产生了此类抗体[354,355]。现在已经在临床前模型中观察到抗原级联[356],并且一些试验已经显示抗原级联与抗肿瘤活性相关[142,357-361]。抗原级联的这种现象本身,同时也是宿主指导肿瘤中许多突变基因产物的免疫应答的机制。一些研究还表明,对于对疫苗中未发现的表位具有更广泛免疫应答的患者,临床结果将有所改善[359,362-364]。

免疫监测

人们总是要求在治疗性癌症疫苗的临床研究中获得患者临床益处的免疫相关性,详情见参考文献[365]的精选评论部分。人类免疫系统的极端复杂性、人口的遗传多样性以及癌症患者在疾病类型和阶段方面的多样性使这成为一项真正艰巨的任务。除了抗原特异性CD4和CD8免疫细胞亚群的分析之外,许多其他免疫亚群可能在患者反应中起重要和/或相互依赖的作用;调节性T细胞和髓源性抑制细胞是这些免疫亚群细胞的实例。现在已经鉴定了超过130种不同的人免疫细胞亚群。由肿瘤或肿瘤微环境产生的可溶性因子也可以影响免疫应答,这些因子包括TGF-β、IL-8、VEGF、IFN-γ、TNF、CD40L和sCD27。除了上述那些之外的混杂因素包括先前疗法的数量和类型,患者的年龄和性别,以及肿瘤病变的大小。外周免疫细胞与肿瘤内不同位置的差异是极其重要的。在黑素瘤患者中更容易获得这些类型的数据,但是在大多数实体瘤患者中,不容易获得转移性病变的活组织检查结果。

目前正在采用较新的技术来研究患者的免疫反应;这些新技术包括肿瘤和外周血样品的基因芯片RNA阵列,接种前和接种后TCR克隆的变化分析,以及通过多激光FACS分析的100多个免疫细胞亚群的变化。此外,在治疗前对患者的众多免疫细胞亚群的分析正在成为确定哪些患者更有可能从疫苗治疗中受益的有价值的工具[318,366]。

范式转变

在临床试验中对癌症疫苗的评估可能需要新的范式[20,315]。癌症疫苗和细胞毒性药物在作用动力学模式和局限性方面表现不同(见表65-4和图65-3)。细胞毒性药物可能能够但也可能不能杀死肿瘤细胞。疗效不佳的原因可能是由于肿瘤细胞的耐药性、向肿瘤输送的药物量不足和/或药物对宿主的毒性停用。因此,如果患者的疾病在细胞毒性药物的作用下进展,则该药物会被立即停用。癌症疫苗的使用涉及一个动态过程的启动,在这个过程中患者自身的免疫系统被激活。从几十年的临床前研究和现在的临床试验中可以清楚地看出,为了最大限度地提高宿主的免疫反应,不仅必须进行一次免疫接种,而且还必须在几周或几个月的时间内进行多次加强疫苗接种,以进一步提高免疫反应的水平。而由于肿瘤可能会释放出削弱免疫反应的因素,接种多类型的疫苗显得尤为重要。因此,在早期接种疫苗后看到疾病进展,多次接种后疾病稳定或肿瘤负担减少的情况并不少见。因此,随着癌症疫苗的使用,"肿瘤进展即停药"的范式需重新讨论。

使用新药的临床试验传统上是在那些先前细胞毒性治疗失败的晚期肿瘤(通常是负担较重的肿瘤)患者中进行评估的。客观的临床反应由RECIST标准评估,寻找目标病变最长直径总和的持续性大于30%的减少。根据RECIST标准,通过减少肿瘤负担,可以观察到细胞毒性药物或小分子靶向疗法的抗肿瘤活性,但在生存率方面未见统计学差异。不幸的是,仍然一些人坚持使用一种"范式麻痹",将对免疫治疗药物的评估作为评估疗效的唯一手段。

由于对疫苗的免疫应答的产生是一个动态的过程,在这个过程中T细胞可以在增强疫苗上持续产生,因此更合适的评估终点应该是TTP,更重要的,应该是存活。由于疫苗只能产生有限数量的T细胞,因此可能不适合通过显著降低肿瘤负担的能力来评估癌症疫苗;这在由于多次化疗而导致免疫系统受损的患者中尤其如此。更合适的方案应当是在疾病状态早期(例如,新辅助治疗或辅助治疗时)即评估癌症疫苗的效果,或在具有小肿瘤负担的转移性患者中进行评估。当在癌症疫苗的使用中出现的相对较低的毒性水平时应当特别考虑这一点。

小结

随着前列腺癌治疗疫苗 sipuleucel-T、检查点抑制剂抗 CTLA-4 和抗 PD-L1/PD-1 单克隆抗体经 PDA 批准上市，以及近期涉及癌症疫苗和其他免疫疗法的临床研究结果的发表，"免疫疗法"逐渐成为多种癌症治疗的主流方案。如今已经确定出了多种用于肿瘤免疫治疗的潜在 TAA 靶标和疫苗平台。在临床试验中对癌症疫苗的评估可能需要新的范式。癌症疫苗和细胞毒性药物在作用方式和动力学方面表现不同。细胞毒性药物要么杀死或不杀死肿瘤细胞；由于肿瘤细胞的耐药性，向肿瘤输送的药物不足，和/或在宿主中药物诱导的毒性使其疗效不佳。癌症疫苗的使用涉及一个动态过程的启动，在这个过程中患者自身的免疫系统被激活。因此，在早期接种疫苗后看到疾病进展，多次接种后疾病稳定或肿瘤负担减少的情况并不少见。因此，应该通过使用癌症疫苗来重新审视"早期进展时停药"的范式。临床前研究以及现在的几项临床研究表明，当患者与某些细胞毒性药物、激素或肿瘤的局部辐射联合使用时，患者可以对癌症疫苗产生免疫反应。研究表明，当肿瘤细胞暴露于亚致死剂量的辐射、某些化疗药物、激素操纵疗法或小分子靶向疗法时，肿瘤细胞的表型实际上受到调节，使它们更容易受到疫苗介导的 T 细胞介导的杀伤。在使用抗 PD-L1/PD-1 药物之前或同时使用治疗性疫苗似乎会诱导肿瘤中 T 细胞的产生，随后通过抑制 PD-L1 在肿瘤上的表达而激活 T 细胞，从而导致肿瘤细胞溶解。

致谢

作者谨在此感谢 Debra Weingarten 在本章节中的协助。

（由婷婷 译，赵方辉 审校）

参考文献

The complete reference list can be found on the Wiley Companion Digital Edition of this title (see inside front cover for login instructions).

7 The Future II Study Group. Quadrivalent vaccine against human papillomavirus to prevent high-grade cervical lesions. *N Eng J Med*. 2007;**356**:1915–1927.

10 Polyak K, Weinberg RA. Transitions between epithelial and mesenchymal states: acquisition of malignant and stem cell traits. *Nat Rev Cancer*. 2009;**9**:265–273.

17 Palena C, Polev DE, Tsang KY, et al. The human T-box mesodermal transcription factor Brachyury is a candidate target for T-cell-mediated cancer immunotherapy. *Clin Cancer Res*. 2007;**13**:2471–2478.

20 Schlom J. Therapeutic cancer vaccines: current status and moving forward. *J Natl Cancer Inst*. 2012;**104**:599–613.

25 Jaffee EM, Hruban RH, Biedrzycki B, et al. Novel allogeneic granulocyte-macrophage colony-stimulating factor-secreting tumor vaccine for pancreatic cancer: a phase I trial of safety and immune activation. *J Clin Oncol*. 2001;**19**:145–156.

38 Disis ML, Grabstein KH, Sleath PR, et al. Generation of immunity to the HER-2/neu oncogenic protein in patients with breast and ovarian cancer using a peptide-based vaccine. *Clin Cancer Res*. 1999;**5**:1289–1297.

50 Bendandi M, Gocke CD, Kobrin CB, et al. Complete molecular remissions induced by patient-specific vaccination plus granulocyte-monocyte colony-stimulating factor against lymphoma. *Nat Med*. 1999;**5**:1171–1177.

51 Kwak LW, Campbell MJ, Czerwinski DK, et al. Induction of immune responses in patients with B-cell lymphoma against the surface-immunoglobulin idiotype expressed by their tumors. *N Engl J Med*. 1992;**327**:1209–1215.

98 Kugler A, Stuhler G, Walden P, et al. Regression of human metastatic renal cell carcinoma after vaccination with tumor cell-dendritic cell hybrids. *Nat Med*. 2000;**6**:332–336.

115 Dranoff G. GM-CSF-based cancer vaccines. *Immunol Rev*. 2002;**188**:147–154.

132 Waldmann TA, Dubois S, Tagaya Y. Contrasting roles of IL-2 and IL-15 in the life and death of lymphocytes: implications for immunotherapy. *Immunity*. 2001;**14**:105–110.

136 Fallon J, Tighe R, Kradjian G, et al. The immunocytokine NHS-IL12 as a potential cancer therapeutic. *Oncotarget*. 2014;**5**:1869–1884.

137 Kantoff PW, Higano CS, Shore ND, et al. Sipuleucel-T immunotherapy for castration-resistant prostate cancer. *N Eng J Med*. 2010;**363**:411–422.

138 Hodge JW, Chakraborty M, Kudo-Saito C, et al. Multiple costimulatory modalities enhance CTL avidity. *J Immunol*. 2005;**174**:5994–6004.

140 Kantoff PW, Schuetz TJ, Blumenstein BA, et al. Overall survival analysis of a phase II randomized controlled trial of a Poxviral-based PSA-targeted immunotherapy in metastatic castration-resistant prostate cancer. *J Clin Oncol*. 2010;**28**:1099–1105.

142 Gulley JL, Madan RA, Tsang KY, et al. Immune impact induced by PROSTVAC (PSA-TRICOM), a therapeutic vaccine for prostate cancer. *Cancer Immunol Res*. 2014;**2**:133–141.

158 Markovic SN, Suman VJ, Ingle JN, et al. Peptide vaccination of patients with metastatic melanoma: improved clinical outcome in patients demonstrating effective immunization. *Am J Clin Oncol*. 2006;**29**:352–360.

166 Kirkwood JM, Lee S, Moschos SJ, et al. Immunogenicity and antitumor effects of vaccination with peptide vaccine+/-granulocyte-monocyte colony-stimulating factor and/or IFN-alpha2b in advanced metastatic melanoma: Eastern Cooperative Oncology Group Phase II Trial E1696. *Clin Cancer Res*. 2009;**15**:1443–1451.

167 Testori A. Phase III comparison of vitespen, an autologous tumor-derived heat shock protein gp96 peptide complex vaccine, with physician's choice of treatment for stage IV melanoma: the C-100-21 Study Group. *J Clin Oncol*. 2008;**26**:955–962.

170 Ulloa-Montoya F. Predictive gene signature in MAGE-A3 antigen-specific cancer immunotherapy. *J Clin Oncol*. 2013;**31**:2388–2395.

181 Rosenblatt J, Kufe D, Avigan D. Dendritic cell fusion vaccines for cancer immunotherapy. *Expert Opin Biol Ther*. 2005;**5**:703–715.

186 Andtbacka RHI, Kaufman HL, Collichio F, et al. Talimogene laherparepvec improves durable response rate in patients with advanced melanoma. *J Clin Oncol*. 2015;**33**:2780–2788.

192 Morse MA, Niedzwiecki D, Marshall JL, et al. A randomized phase II study of immunization with dendritic cells modified with poxvectors encoding CEA and MUC1 compared with the same poxvectors plus GM-CSF for resected metastatic colorectal cancer. *Ann Surg*. 2013;**258**:879–886.

211 Le DT, Wang-Gillam A, Picozzi V, et al. Safety and survival with GVAX pancreas prime and Listeria monocytogenes-expressing mesothelin (CRS-207) boost vaccines for metastatic pancreatic cancer. *J Clin Oncol*. 2015;**33**:1325–1333.

222 Disis ML, Gooley TA, Rinn K, et al. Generation of T-cell immunity to the HER-2/neu protein after active immunization with HER-2/neu peptide-based vaccines. *J Clin Oncol*. 2002;**20**:2624–2632.

225 Mittendorf EA. Clinical trial results of the HER-2/neu (E75) vaccine to prevent breast cancer recurrence in high-risk patients: from US Military Cancer Institute Clinical Trials Group Study I-01 and I-02. *Cancer*. 2012;**118**:2594–2602.

226 Avigan D, Vasir B, Gong J, et al. Fusion cell vaccination of patients with metastatic breast and renal cancer induces immunological and clinical responses. *Clin Cancer Res*. 2004;**10**:4699–4708.

248 Schuster SJ, Neelapu SS, Gause BL, et al. Vaccination with patient-specific tumor-derived antigen in first remission improves disease-free survival in follicular lymphoma. *J Clin Oncol*. 2011;**29**:2787–2794.

253 Van Tendeloo VF. Induction of complete and molecular remissions in acute myeloid leukemia by Wilms' tumor 1 antigen-targeted dendritic cell vaccination. *Proc Natl Acad Sci U S A*. 2010;**107**:13824–13829.

264 Pollack IF, Jakacki RI, Butterfield LH, et al. Antigen-specific immune responses and clinical outcome after vaccination with glioma-associated antigen peptides and polyinosinic-polycytidylic acid stabilized by lysine and carboxymethylcellulose in children with newly diagnosed malignant brainstem and nonbrainstem gliomas. *J Clin Oncol*. 2014;**32**:2050–2058.

269 Pardoll DM. The blockade of immune checkpoints in cancer immunotherapy. *Nat Rev Cancer*. 2012;**12**:252–264.

273 Duraiswamy J, Kaluza KM, Freeman GJ, et al. Dual blockade of PD-1 and CTLA-4 combined with tumor vaccine effectively restores T-cell rejection function in tumors. *Cancer Res*. 2013;**73**:3591–3603.

274 Madan RA, Mohebtash M, Arlen PM, et al. Ipilimumab and a poxviral vaccine targeting prostate-specific antigen in metastatic castration-resistant prostate cancer: a phase 1 dose-escalation trial. *Lancet Oncol*. 2012;**13**:501–508.

298 Hodge JW, Ardiani A, Farsaci B, et al. The tipping point for combination therapy: cancer vaccines with radiation, chemotherapy, or targeted small molecule

inhibitors. *Semin Oncol*. 2012;**39**:323–339.

305 Formenti SC, Demaria S. Combining radiotherapy and cancer immunotherapy: a paradigm shift. *J Natl Cancer Inst*. 2013;**105**:256–265.

306 Kroemer G, Galluzzi L, Kepp O, et al. Immunogenic cell death in cancer therapy. *Annu Rev Immunol*. 2013;**31**:51–72.

337 Stein WD, Gulley JL, Schlom J, et al. Tumor regression and growth rates determined in five intramural NCI prostate cancer trials: the growth rate constant as an indicator of therapeutic efficacy. *Clin Cancer Res*. 2011;**17**:907–917.

353 Ribas A, Timmerman JM, Butterfield LH, et al. Determinant spreading and tumor responses after peptide-based cancer immunotherapy. *Trends Immunol*. 2003;**24**:58–61.

365 Butterfield LH. Cancer vaccines. *BMJ*. 2015;**350**:h988.

第 66 章　肿瘤细胞免疫治疗

Krina K. Patel, MD ■ Judy S. Moyes, MA (Cantab), MB, BChir, FRCPC, FRCPCH ■
Laurence J. Cooper, MD, PhD

概述

近几十年来，科学家们开始应用细胞免疫疗法治疗肿瘤。供体或自体来源的多克隆 T 细胞的成功应用部分建立在对效应细胞成分的精确定义和肿瘤相关抗原的识别。靶向这类抗原有助于安全地获得抗肿瘤效应而不产生脱靶其他组织的毒性，如移植物抗宿主病(graft versus host disease, GvHD)。T 细胞的过继转移可以重建或增强宿主的免疫力，这与内源性免疫系统可能对免疫原无反应的疫苗策略的局限性形成对比。其他溶细胞的循环淋巴细胞群也可以用于输注。这些淋巴细胞包括可以介导抗肿瘤作用的同种异体自然杀伤(natural killer, NK)细胞，无需预先限定肿瘤相关抗原(tumor associated antigen, TAA)，可能不存在 GvHD 的风险。在某些情况下，一种 TAA 可以被淋巴细胞识别，例如 B 细胞 TAA CD19，但是宿主免疫耐受阻止有效的免疫反应发生。基因工程结合 T 细胞治疗，通过强制表达嵌合抗原受体(chimeric antigen receptor, CAR)在体外产生抗原特异性细胞。CD19 特异性 CAR-T 细胞治疗已在多个针对常规治疗无效的 B 细胞恶性肿瘤患者的临床试验中凸显疗效。在这里，我们将阐述肿瘤细胞免疫治疗的现状。

引言

异基因造血干细胞移植(hematopoietic stem-cell transplantation, HSCT)是血液系统恶性肿瘤细胞治疗的第一种有效形式。同种异体 HSCT 患者的成功治疗与供体免疫细胞介导的移植物抗肿瘤(graft versus tumor, GvT)效应直接相关。移植物的相关细胞免疫成分包括 T 细胞、NK 细胞和 B 细胞，它们是执行 GvT 效应的潜在效应细胞。移植的 T 细胞可以清除残留的肿瘤细胞，这一观察结果导致使用供体淋巴细胞输注(donor leukocyte infusions, DLI)治疗复发的白血病，这为 GvT 反应提供了直接证据[1]。虽然细胞毒性 T 细胞是 GvT 效应的主要效应细胞，但是因为恶性细胞和正常细胞之间共享主要和次要组织相容性抗原，因此，它们也与移植物抗宿主病(graft-versus-host-disease, GvHD)[2]的发生密切相关。实际上，GvHD 一定程度上抵消了 GvT 效应的获益，从而限制了 DLI 和异基因 HSCT 的应用。

近几十年来，科学家们应用细胞免疫疗法治疗肿瘤。供体或自体来源的多克隆 T 细胞的成功应用部分建立在对效应细胞成分的精确定义和肿瘤相关抗原的识别。靶向这类抗原有助于安全地获得抗肿瘤效应而不产生脱靶其他组织的毒性，如 GvHD。T 细胞的过继免疫可以增强患者的免疫功能，这与内源性免疫系统可能无法对免疫原作出反应的疫苗策略的局限性形成对比[3,4]。

其他淋巴细胞也可用于输注。如异体 NK 细胞可以介导抗肿瘤作用，无须识别 TAA，也无 GvHD 发生[5-7]。在某些情况下，CD19 等 TAA 可以被识别，但是免疫耐受会阻止有效免疫反应的发生。基因工程与 T 细胞治疗相结合，通过强制表达 CAR，在体外产生抗原特异性细胞。实际上，CD19 特异性 CAR-T 细胞治疗已在多个常规治疗无效的 B 细胞恶性肿瘤患者的临床试验中凸显疗效，如表 66-1 所示。在本章中，我们将介绍肿瘤细胞免疫治疗的现状。

表 66-1　CD19 CAR-T 细胞临床试验

嵌合抗原受体类型	共刺激结构域	肿瘤类型	疗效	总患者数	毒副反应	参考文献
慢病毒	4-1BB	ALL	27 CR	30	严重 CRS	Maude et al.[8]
γ 逆转录病毒	CD28	ALL, NHL	14 CR	19	严重 CRS	Lee et al.[9]
γ 逆转录病毒	CD28	ALL	14 CR	16	严重 CRS	Davila et al.[10]
γ 逆转录病毒	CD28	DLBCL, 惰性淋巴瘤, CLL	8 CR, 4 PR, 1 SD, 2 无法评估	15	神经毒性，谵妄	Kochenderfer et al.[11]
慢病毒	4-1BB	CLL	3 CR, 5 PR, 6 无治疗反应	14	发热	Porter et al.[12]

ALL，急性淋巴细胞白血病；NHL，非霍奇金淋巴瘤；DLBCL，弥漫大 B 细胞淋巴瘤；CLL，慢性淋巴细胞白血病；CR，完全缓解；PR，部分缓解；SD，稳定病变；CRS，细胞因子释放综合征。

细胞治疗产品的产生

T 细胞

肿瘤患者的免疫系统可以通过输注淋巴细胞和旨在增强内源性 T 细胞杀肿瘤的适应性免疫调节途径来调控。这两种方法都有抗肿瘤作用。输注特异性抗体阻断 CTLA4 和 PD-1/PDL-1 免疫检测点轴，从而激活内源性抗肿瘤免疫效应，相关临床试验提示患者取得了显著的长期反应[13-15]。活检标本分析显示，在转移性黑色素瘤患者治疗中，阻断 PD-1/PDL-1 轴的抗肿瘤作用与 T 细胞在肿瘤组织中的基线密度和位置有关[16,17]。对于某些肿瘤，肿瘤微环境中没有足够数量或具备功能的浸润性 T 细胞，因此可以输注外源的效应细胞使之在体内扩增，从而达到抗肿瘤效应。因此，过继性细胞治疗（adoptive cellular therapy，ACT）已经成为一种非常有效的治疗方法，使得某些血液系统恶性肿瘤和实体肿瘤患者获得了持续的临床反应，如表 66-2。

表 66-2　针对实体瘤的细胞疗法临床试验

肿瘤类型	过继性细胞转移类型	靶抗原	疗效	总患者数	毒副反应	参考文献
黑色素瘤	TCR	MART-1; gp-100	8PR；1CR	36	皮肤，眼部，耳部	Johnson et al. [18] and Morgan et al. [19]
黑色素瘤，滑膜肉瘤及食管癌	TCR	MAGE-A3	1 CR，4 PR，4 无治疗反应，2 死亡	9	检测到 MAGE-A12 在脑部表达并导致神经毒性：3 例患者出现精神状态改变，其中 2 例患者发生昏迷并随后死亡	Morgan et al. [20]
黑色素瘤，高危多发性骨髓瘤	TCR	MAGE-A3	2 名患者均出现发热，进展性低氧，低血压，并在输注 4~5 天后死亡	2	与心肌细胞中的肌联蛋白发生交叉反应导致心力衰竭并最终死亡	Linette et al. [21]
滑膜肉瘤；黑色素瘤	TCR	MY-ESO-1	2CR；7PR	17	无	Robbins et al. [22]
肾细胞癌	1 代 CAR	CAIX	无客观治疗反应	11	肝脏毒性	Lamers et al. [23,24]
结直肠癌	TCR	CEA	1PR	—	结肠炎	Ma et al. [25]
结直肠癌	3 代 CAR	ErbB2	1 死亡	1	正常肺部中检测到 ErbB2 表达，导致致命性肺毒性和器官衰竭	Morgan et al. [26]
卵巢癌	1 代 CAR	αFR	无客观治疗反应	14	IL-2 相关性毒性反应	Kershaw et al. [27]
神经母细胞瘤	1 代 CAR	GD2	3CR	19	疼痛	Pule et al. [28] and Louis et al. [29]

总的来说，有 5 种形式的 T 细胞被用于人类治疗。这些细胞是：①淋巴因子激活的杀伤（lymphokine activated killer，LAK）细胞；②细胞因子诱导的杀伤（cytokine-induced killer，CIK）细胞；③肿瘤浸润性淋巴细胞（tumor-infiltrating lymphocyte，TIL），来源于肿瘤活检组织中扩增的淋巴细胞；④抗原特异性 T 细胞；⑤基因工程 T 细胞，其表达一种 TAA 特异性 T 细胞受体（T cell receptor，TCR）或 CAR。

外周血与大剂量白细胞介素-2（interleukin-2，IL-2）共培养后产生的 LAK 细胞输注是 ACT 的首次应用之一[30]。但是，大剂量的 IL-2 可导致终末分化和效应器功能的循环障碍。此外，LAK 细胞早期临床试验的阳性反应可能是与 IL-2 共输注的结果[31]。然而，与 LAK 细胞相关的临床数据导致了 TIL 的发展。TIL 具有抗肿瘤活性，尤其是对黑色素瘤患者。CIK 细胞是体外扩增 T 淋巴细胞的异质性亚群，呈现混合 T/NK 表型，具有主要组织相容性复合物（major histocompatibility complex，MHC）非限制性抗肿瘤活性[32]；这类细胞表达 T 细胞（$CD3^+TCR\alpha^+\beta^+$）和自然杀伤 T 细胞（$CD3^+CD56^+$）的表面标记[33]。由 αβ 异二聚体组成的 TCR 的 T 细胞是外周血中最普遍的 T 细胞群，它们广泛用于 ACT 研究。效应 T 细胞（$CD8^+$）和辅助 T 细胞（$CD4^+$）都能应用于 ACT 治疗，如制备抗原特异性克隆或在基因修饰后表达 TAA 特异性受体。

肿瘤浸润淋巴细胞

动物实验表明 TIL 比 LAK 细胞具有更强的杀瘤效应[34]，这促使研究者发起临床试验输注体外扩增 TIL 治疗转移性黑色素瘤患者[35,36]。这些试验最初由 NIH 主导，目前在全世界范围内进行[37-39]。这些临床数据表明，输注的淋巴亚群能识别含有突变表位的 TAA，突变表位基于肿瘤标本全外显子测序分析所得[40,41]。

Rosenberg 和 National Cancer Institute(NCI)外科分院的同事们开创了 ACT TIL 扩增的标准方法[42]。首先，在扩增前阶段，将手术切除的肿瘤标本消化为单细胞悬液，培养在含有 IL-2 的培养基中，检测其生长和反应性，然后进一步进行扩增和表型鉴定。早期研究显示，TIL 治疗转移性黑色素瘤的客观缓解率约为 50%，具有良好的疗效[35]。但是，最初注册这些临床试验的患者只有一部分接受了 TIL 的输注[43]。诸多原因限制这种治疗策略的应用，比如缺乏可用于手术切除的肿瘤，难以从切除的肿瘤中分离 TIL，TIL 无法扩增或扩增的 TIL 缺乏特异的效应细胞功能。治疗相关毒性如低血压、心律失常和血管渗漏综合征是为维持 TIL 的持久作用而输注的大剂量重组 IL-2 所致。在后续的临床试验中，选择合适的患者及给予大剂量 IL-2 治疗均改善了临床试验结果。约有五分之一的患者获得了完全缓解(complete remission，CR)且无病生存时间达三年或以上[44]。进一步，其他临床试验似乎显示在 TIL 输注时不需要给予高剂量的 IL-2，这可能会扩大该疗法的应用范围[45,46]。

为了改善 TIL 的治疗效果，可在 TIL 输注前给予淋巴细胞清除方案[47-49]。淋巴细胞清除通过抑制细胞因子谱、髓源抑制细胞和调节 T 细胞，为 TIL 提供利于其增殖的环境、增强它在体内的持久性[50]，从而改善临床疗效。但是淋巴细胞清除方案导致免疫防御系统抑制，从而导致了机会性感染增加。

淋巴细胞清除的程度可影响抗肿瘤效应。环磷酰胺和氟达拉滨联合应用的非清髓性淋巴细胞清除方案有效率可达 51%[51,52]。当全身照射(total body irradiation，TBI)的剂量需要自体造血细胞移植来挽救造血时，总有效率可增加到 70%，CR 为 40%，但清淋治疗的强度增加导致了更严重的副作用，如发热性中性粒细胞减少、感染和血栓性微血管病[44,48]。

在等待 TIL 制备期间，由于疾病进展或身体状况下降而导致患者失去治疗机会是 TIL 治疗策略的一个限制。因此，研究者改进方法以减少从 TIL 收集到输注的培养时间[53]。在最近的一次临床试验中，缩短预扩增期使 TIL 制备在 28 天内完成，这导致注册率达到 74%。因为这些“年轻的 TIL”含有未经终末分化的 T 细胞，避免复制衰老，可能有更好的杀瘤效应[54]。使用活化和繁殖细胞作为饲养细胞来扩增 TIL 的方法正被采用[55]，这些饲养细胞使得肿瘤特异性 T 细胞不需要采集肿瘤标本而得以制备，可使更多患者从 TIL 治疗中获益。

随着免疫治疗知识的迅速增长，目前采用 TIL 治疗的临床试验数量也在增加。

这些临床试验包括比较淋巴细胞清除方案(NCT01807182；Fred Hutchinson Cancer Center)，CTLA-4 联合免疫治疗(NCT01701674；Moffitt Cancer Center)，PD-1/PDL-1 轴抑制剂或疫苗(NCT00338377；MD Anderson Cancer Center)，评估 TIL 在非黑色素瘤肿瘤中的疗效(NCT01174121；National Cancer Institute)。

外周血 T 细胞

利用含肽表位的 MHC 多聚体可以从外周血中收集 TAA 特异性 T 细胞。荧光标记循环 T 细胞后，目标自体效应细胞群可在体外进行分选、激活和扩增，然后输入患者体内以杀灭肿瘤细胞并提供长期免疫保护[45,56]。TAA 特异性效应 T 细胞在外周血中的比例很低，约为 0.2%；然而，几项黑色素瘤研究显示，针对 gp100、酪氨酸酶和 MART-1 等黑色素细胞抗原的特异性 T 细胞比例达到 2%[57]。这项体外研究还表明，尽管 TAA 特异性 T 细胞应答可在癌症患者中发生，但抗原特异性无反应解释了此类细胞无法控制肿瘤生长的原因。因此，需要共刺激分子激活 TCR，然后细胞因子诱导扩增，以富集 TAA 特异性效应 T 细胞[58]。TCR 识别抗原肽-MHC 复合物，该复合物将抗原呈递给 T 细胞。

T 细胞低频识别常见表达抗原，限制了这种方法的应用。为了克服该问题，Pollack 等[59]在体外运用 IL-21 刺激经四聚体引导分选的细胞来产生 TAA 特异性细胞毒性 T 淋巴细胞。用肿瘤相关抗原 NY-ESO-1 四聚体引导经单次临床级分选后，TAA 特异性 T 淋巴细胞比例即从 0.4%富集到大于 90%。所有纳入研究的患者均产生 NY-ESO-1 特异性 T 细胞，最终的寡克隆产物平均扩增 1 200 倍，含有 67%～97%的 $CD8^+$ 四聚体 $^+$T 细胞，并具有识别内源性 NY-ESO-1 的记忆表型。

外周血树突状细胞

自体树突状细胞(dendritic cells，DCs)是一类专职抗原呈递细胞(antigen-presenting cells，APCs)，通过体外共培养可以选择性增殖自体 T 细胞。为了获取树突状细胞，将外周血单核细胞在含 IL-4 和粒-巨噬细胞集落刺激因子(granulocyte macrophagecolony stimulating factor，GM-csf)的培养液中培养，去分化为未成熟树突状细胞。这些未成熟的树突状细胞可以负载肿瘤抗原或裂解物，在细胞因子中培养促使其成熟并介导 CD80 和 CD86 等共刺激配体上调。或者，利用肽刺激成熟树突状细胞产生高亲和力的 $CD8^+$ 和 $CD4^+$T 细胞，仅识别单一抗原表位。来源于人类红白血病细胞系 k562 的人工 APCs 也被开发为树突状细胞的替代品。这些细胞表达人类白细胞抗原(human leukocyte antigen，HLA)c 等位基因，不表达其他经典的 HLA Ⅰ类或Ⅱ类分子，可以通过基因修饰来表达 TAA、HLA 和共刺激分子，以优化抗原特异性 T 细胞的生成[55,60]。

TIL 和抗原特异性 T 细胞为恶性实体肿瘤患者的治疗提供了互补策略，在 ACT 作为治疗手段的发展中具有广阔的前景。它们不仅为患者提供了有效的治疗，而且为免疫生物学的发现提供了丰富的数据源。

基因工程 T 细胞

随着免疫学和基因工程的发展，可通过改变受体特异性和信号功能来增强 T 细胞功能[61]。对 T 细胞进行基因修饰的一个重要原因是，内源性 TAA 特异性 T 细胞由于免疫耐受介导，使之无法识别或有效地对恶性细胞作出应答。目前，已有两种类型的基因修饰 T 细胞通过强制表达特定的 TCR 或 CAR 来增强其靶向特异性，并用于肿瘤治疗临床试验中。

有效的 T 细胞基因修饰是制备 TCR 和 CAR 细胞制剂的必要条件。γ-反转录病毒和慢病毒转导技术基于这些病毒可与宿主基因组永久整合。GMP 级病毒载体生产是一项成本高、耗时长、专业化的技术。尽管早期人们已开始关注基因修饰过程中可能产生的插入突变，但几十年的原代 T 细胞转导经验中并没有发现这种并发症的例子[62]。非病毒的基因转移是另一种相对经济的方法。最常用的方法是转座子系统，如睡美人系统。该系统可使 CAR 在 T 细胞上持续表达，抗 CD19 转座子 CAR T 细胞尚处于早期临床试验阶段[63]。另一种新方法是 T 淋巴细胞体外电转 RNA[64]，这可以导致 CAR 高效但仅瞬时的表达。除 mRNA 电转技术外，T 细胞的基因转移通常是在体外培养和刺激的开始阶段进行的，这导致更有效的转导和大量的 T 细胞用于随后的过继转移。

T 细胞受体(TCR)

植入高亲和力 TCR 的根本原因是，内源性 TCR 靶向自身 TAA 时通常亲和力较低。因此，有学者提出假说，这种低亲和力 TCR 链不能控制恶性肿瘤，而增加亲和力将引发有效的抗肿瘤反应[65]。事实上，已有动物研究数据支持该假说[66]。提高 TCR 亲和力的方法一般有三种：①在硅化过程中改变抗原结合结构域，特别是 CDR3[67]；②使用组合平台，如 XPRESIDENT 技术，它使用质谱分析、基因表达谱分析、基于文献的功能评估、体外人 T 细胞试验和生物信息学筛选最合适的肿瘤相关肽[68]；③在限制 HLA 分子的背景下识别肽的 CAR[69,70]。TCR 由六条多肽链(α、β、γ、δ、ε 和 ζ)组成，它们作为免疫突触的一部分连接在细胞表面，启动 T 细胞激活信号。α 和 β 链组成一个异二聚体，形成 TCR 的主要结合域，该结合域识别由经典 HLA Ⅰ类和Ⅱ类分子呈现在靶细胞表面的细胞内处理肽。免疫突触的其他成分，如共刺激分子和黏附分子，增加了 TCR-HLA-肽结合的强度和质量，导致一系列 T 细胞激活事件，具体被定义为：①连续杀灭；②持续增殖；③Tc1 细胞因子产生；④对活化诱导细胞死亡的保护。经基因修饰后 TCR 表达增强的 T 细胞已经从实验室[71]应用到临床。最初的临床尝试是将基因修饰的特异性自体 T 细胞用于黑色素瘤治疗[19]。结果提示临床反应低于非基因修饰的 TIL。但是，这些数据证实了 T 细胞可以被设计为靶向 TAA，并为靶向黑色素瘤以外的肿瘤治疗提供了依据。但同时研究者也注意到，表达高亲和力 TCR 的 T 细胞还靶向识别内耳和视网膜中正常表达黑色素的细胞[18]。

人类广泛应用经基因修饰表达 TAA 特异性 TCR 的 T 细胞面临两大挑战。首先是引入的 αβTCR 与内源性 αβTCR 之间不必要的错配，这可能导致：①能够识别 HLA-肽的合适成对链的数目减少；②产生未经胸腺选择和耐受的 TCR 异二聚体，从而导致对正常结构的有害识别。这已经在小鼠动物试验[72,73]中得到证实，但在临床试验中并未观察到相应副作用。表 66-3 列出了消除引入 TCR 和内源性 TCR 之间错配的方法。第二个面临的问题与 TCR 亲和力有关。增加亲和力的方法不受胸腺选择和耐受机制的影响，当对其特异性不完全了解时，会使患者暴露于靶向抗原但缺乏组织选择性的副作用。目前大多数方法依赖于靶向非突变的自身抗原，其中最有希望的可能是癌-睾丸基因家族的基因产物[22]。在黑色素瘤和滑膜细胞肉瘤患者中尝试一种亲和力增强的 NY-ESO-1 特异性和 HLA-A2 限制性的 TCR，未发现严重毒性[22]。然而，输注表达亲和力增强的[21] HLA-A1 限制性 MAGE A3 特异性 TCR 的自体 T 细胞，导致了两名患者出现致死性心脏毒性，原因是对肌联蛋白的非靶向识别。在另一项临床试验中[20]，给黑色素瘤患者输注表达亲和力增强的 HLA-A2 限制性 MAGE A3 特异性 TCR 的自体 T 细胞，由于脑细胞表达 MAGE A12，输注后出现了脑细胞交叉反应而发生显著神经毒性；特别是 3 个患者出现精神状态改变，两人昏迷死亡。全身系统性应用糖皮质激素并没有逆转毒性。虽然这些事件说明基因改造自体 T 细胞可以显示抗肿瘤潜能，但同时提示迫切需要改进临床前系统，以便在开始临床试验之前发现脱靶不良事件。

表 66-3　用于消除被导入的和内源性的 α/β TCR 之间错配的典型方法

促进引入 TCR 配对的各种方法	参考文献
使用完全或部分的老鼠 TCR α 和 β	Cohen et al.,[74] Sommermeyer and Uckert,[75] and Cohen et al.[76]
在恒定区链接二硫键	Kuball et al.[77] and Cohen et al.[78]
使用柞白构型	Voss et al.[79]
在 TCRαβ 恒定区应用短发夹 RNA(shRNAs)以抑制内源性 TCRαβ 表达	Okamoto et al.[80,81]
引入锌指核酸酶(ZFNs)或其他人工核酸酶以完全破坏内源性 TCRαβ 在基因组水平的表达	Provasi et al.,[82] Poirot, et al.,[83] Torikai et al.[84]

尽管基于 TCR 的 ACT 策略具有很大的潜力，但它们确实存在固有的局限性。基因修饰 TCR 的 HLA 限制性将潜在的患者数量限制为表达 T 细胞识别的相关 HLA 等位基因的患者。此外，肿瘤常常下调 HLA 等位基因表达，蛋白酶体处理受阻，抗原逃逸均降低该治疗策略的完全缓解率。

嵌合抗原受体

典型的 CAR 将抗体的胞外单链可变片段(single chain variable fragment, scFv)与 T 细胞信号复合物分子的跨膜(TM)结构域和胞内信号结构域结合起来。一般临床上有吸引力的 CAR 将 CD3-ζ 链的信号基序和参与细胞激活或共刺激分子的信号域结合[85,86]。由于 scFv 结构域直接与靶细胞表面表位结合，CAR 可以绕过 MHC 限制性抗原呈递的需要，而不受 HLA 下调的肿瘤逃逸机制影响。同时，scFv 对 TAA 有很高的亲和力，CAR 可以克服与表位密度相关的 T 细胞激活限制。多代 CAR 已经被开发出来，它们将信号结构域与胞浆激活域相结合。这些 CAR 的设计使其在肿瘤微环境中能够发生完全的免疫应答反应。具有信号传导和磷酸化 CD3-ζ 中免疫受体酪氨酸激活基序的 CAR，可以提高其在体内的持久性[87]，从而提高抗肿瘤效应。两种第二代 CAR 在 $CD19^+$ 恶性肿瘤患者中产生了显著的抗肿瘤作用。具有嵌合 CD137 信号结构域(即 4-

1BB)的 CAR-T 细胞在急慢性 B 淋巴细胞白血病患者中产生了显著的抗瘤效应[88-90]。此外,具有嵌合 CD28 信号结构域的 CAR-T 细胞对 B 淋巴细胞白血病和 B 细胞淋巴瘤患者亦具有强效的抗瘤作用[9,10,91]。对常规治疗无效的 B 系急性淋巴细胞白血病患者对 CAR-T 治疗有非常高的应答率,90%以上达到 CR[8]。这两种 CAR 的持续抗肿瘤作用与以下因素可能有关:基因修饰 T 细胞的体内增殖,以及患者复发是否因为白血病细胞 CD19 表达缺失。

以 CD19 为靶点的急慢性白血病临床数据显示,自体 CAR-T 细胞清除这些恶性血液肿瘤的能力存在差异。与在慢性淋巴细胞白血病治疗中的疗效相比,通过 CD28 或 CD137 激活 CD19 特异性 CAR 的靶向急性淋巴细胞白血病的治疗获得了更高的缓解率。这些临床数据提示,需要了解基因修饰 T 细胞和非基因修饰 T 细胞参与一系列 T 细胞激活事件的微环境。

具有 CD28 信号域的靶向 CD19 的 CAR-T 细胞在急性淋巴细胞白血病患者中显示出明显的疗效[6];然而在慢性淋巴细胞白血病患者中疗效不显著[92]。与 4-1BB 信号域的 CAR 不同,这些 CD28 信号域的 CAR 不能在体内持久增殖。基于 CD28 信号域的第二代 CAR 与第一代 CD3ζ CAR-T 细胞相比,存活时间有所提高,但在 Memorial Sloan Kettering Cancer Center 接受治疗的急性淋巴细胞白血病患者的 CAR-T 细胞平均存活时间仅约 28 天[10]。NCI 的第一阶段试验也显示,在大多数患者中,具有 CD28 信号域 CD19 特异性 CAR 在 28 天后无法存活[9]。然而,这两项试验都显示在输注的前 14 天内 CAR-T 细胞发生急剧的扩增,同时具有治疗反应患者的外周血原始细胞消失。值得注意的是,大多数患者在第 28 天再次出现正常 B 细胞,与那些持续存在 CD19 特异性 CAR-T 细胞并且 B 细胞发育不良的试验患者相反。CAR-T 细胞在体内存活时间短,更利于其作为移植的桥接治疗。第三代 CAR,如 CD20 特异性的 CAR-T 细胞,具有 CD28 和 4-1BB 共刺激域,也显示初期潜力,但需要进一步评估[93]。最近 Long 等发现在持续刺激的 CAR-T 细胞中,CD28 信号可能增强 CAR-T 细胞耗竭,4-1BB 减少 CAR-T 细胞耗竭,提示 4-1BB 促进 CAR-T 细胞在患者体内持久存活。他们正在实施进一步研究,以阐明参与 CAR-T 细胞耗竭的潜在机制[94]。CAR-T 细胞是否会取代异基因 HSCT,或者它们是否会成为移植的桥接治疗,或者作为一种巩固治疗的手段仍需要长时间观察与研究。目前尚不清楚在缓解的患者体内是否所有肿瘤细胞都被清除,或者是否存在由持续存活的 CAR-T 细胞所控制的休眠肿瘤细胞。由于肿瘤细胞生物负荷程度的不同,可能需要针对性地设计不同的 CAR。

多个早期临床试验也强调了 CAR-T 细胞疗法的潜在毒性。非肿瘤的靶向毒性是由于正常组织不同程度地表达肿瘤相关抗原。重定向的 T 细胞对表达低水平肿瘤相关抗原的正常组织具有高度亲和力和毒性。位于 Rotterdam 的 Erasmus 大学在 2006 年便提出这可能极其有害[95]。在这项研究中,由于碳酸酐酶 9 在胆管上皮细胞上有生理表达,输注经此抗原特异性 CAR 修饰的 T 细胞后,患者发生明显的胆汁淤积。非肿瘤的靶向细胞毒性的严重程度取决于表达靶向抗原的组织是否对生存至关重要,以及这种损伤是否可由其他途径控制。例如,在 CD19 特异性 CAR-T 细胞的临床试验中,丙种球蛋白作为一种有效的替代手段成功地控制 CAR-T 细胞治疗后产生的重度 B 细胞再生不良[89]。相反,据 NCI 在 Bethesda 的报告,一个经淋巴细胞清除预处理后接受高剂量的第三代 ERBB2 特异性 CAR-T 细胞治疗的结肠癌患者,其肺上皮细胞 ERBB2 低水平表达可能导致了致命的肺毒性[26]。Baylor 医学院靶向 ERBB2 治疗多发性胶质母细胞瘤患者,目前为止,未经淋巴细胞清除预处理并用更低剂量的第二代 CAR-T 细胞治疗的患者中尚未观察到显著毒性。当设计 CAR/TCR 时,详细分析靶抗原在正常组织的表达和验证正常细胞被基因靶向的 T 细胞杀伤的易感性是至关重要的。体外实验并不总能准确地预测这些重要数据,因为有些靶抗原只在特定的分化阶段表达(如 CD123),或可被环境信号改变(如 CD44v6)。因此,应考虑在适当的临床前模型中进行体内实验。

目前在 CAR-T 细胞治疗的患者中观察到的最严重的毒性是细胞因子释放综合征(cytokine release syndrome,CRS),表现为一种快速、大量细胞因子释放的免疫反应,包括 γ 干扰素和 IL-6[96]。高水平的 γ 干扰素源于 CAR-T 细胞强有力的效应功能,而 IL-6 的增加可能是巨噬细胞活化综合征(macrophage activation syndrome,MAS)的结果。在不同的临床试验中,输注第二代 CD19 特异性 CAR-T 细胞的患者出现与 MAS 相似的临床表现(发热、低血压、噬血细胞综合征)。由于 IL-6 受体拮抗剂托珠单抗的应用可改善患者的临床症状[96],因此认为巨噬细胞异常活化可能是 CRS 背后的驱动力。为降低危及生命的 CRS 风险,一系列预防措施被提出来,包括将 CAR-T 细胞的初始剂量分 3 天给予,在输注后的前几个小时密切监测重要参数,早期发现提示 CRS 的临床和实验室标志,如 C 反应蛋白[97],以及给予适当的治疗干预,如高剂量糖皮质激素和托珠单抗。尽管这些措施取得了不同程度的效果,但 CRS 仍然是 CAR-T 细胞治疗的整体安全中需重点关注的问题。同时,CRS 也可以作为一种提示 CAR-T 细胞起作用的生物标志。有趣的是,并不是所有的临床试验报告了 CRS,输注时的疾病状况和输注的 CAR 类型可能是影响 CRS 风险的因素。

用于过继 T 细胞免疫治疗的 T 细胞亚群的类型与各种临床结果有关[56]。最初,效应 T 细胞(effector T cells,Teff)由于其高细胞毒性被认为是过继 T 细胞免疫治疗细胞制备的较好选择。然而,早期的临床试验证明,与异质性的肿瘤浸润淋巴细胞群相比,高度分化、肿瘤抗原特异性的 $CD8^+$ Teff 抗肿瘤效应较低,并且当输入患者体内后,与那些输入分化程度较低细胞的患者相比,临床疗效更差。动物研究已经揭示过继分化程度较低的 T 细胞群有更好的体内扩增性、持久性和抗肿瘤活性[98]。给灵长类动物过继来源于中央记忆 T 细胞(central memory T cells,Tcm)的 $CD8^+$ Teff,与过继效应记忆 T 细胞不同,该细胞在体内长期存活并重新获得记忆 T 细胞功能[87]。进一步证实,与 Tcm 来源的 Teff 相比,来自初始 T 细胞亚群的 Teff 显示出更强的抗肿瘤活性和更长的体内存活时间[99]。最近,一个干细胞记忆 T 细胞(stem cell memory T-cell,Tscm)亚群被发现,它被描述为具有自我更新和衍生为其他记忆 T 细胞亚群能力的长寿记忆 T 细胞[100]。体内实验证明 Tscm 的抗肿瘤效应优于其他所有记忆 T 细胞亚群[100],而最近的临床观察提示 CAR-T 细胞在患者体内的扩增仅与类似 Tscm 的细胞亚群的比例相关[51],推测 Tscm 是细胞工程的理想 T 细胞亚群。

基于利用低分化的 T 细胞亚群并保持它们的记忆特征，目前正在研究几种方法来生产最优质的用于过继免疫的 T 细胞。一个主要的方法是通过从 γ 链细胞因子受体家族选择细胞因子，形成不同的组合，来改变细胞培养条件。IL-7、IL-15 和 IL-21 已成为产生理想 Tcm 和 Tscm 亚群的关键因素[51,101-103]。深入研究信号转导通路的细节，越来越多的证据揭示了几个信号通路在决定基于刺激强度的 T 细胞分化上的重要性。PI3K/Akt/mTORC1 通路的活化以渐进的方式诱导 T 细胞分化，使用 AKT 和 mTOR 抑制剂能增强记忆 T 细胞的产生[104-107]，而激活 Wnt 信号通路可以促进包括 Tscm 亚群在内的 $CD8^+$ 记忆 T 细胞形成[108]。尽管这些通路与营养感知和信号整合密切相关，但最近出现了更多证据表明这些代谢通路影响 T 细胞记忆形成。例如，可以通过增强 T 细胞中的脂肪酸氧化或抑制糖酵解代谢来增强 CD8 T 细胞的记忆形成[107,109,110]。这种具有记忆特征的 T 细胞有重要的价值，因此应用于临床生产的培养方法在持续提高 T 细胞治疗潜力方面是至关重要的。

γδT 细胞

γδT 细胞（$CD3^+TCR\gamma^+\delta^+$）是一个独特的 T 细胞亚群，它们占外周血中 T 细胞比例为 1%～5%。这类特殊的 T 细胞以 MHC 非限制性方式广泛识别靶点，表现为溶解活性和促炎性细胞因子分泌。异基因骨髓移植后，较好的 γδT 细胞恢复，与白血病无病生存率增加有关，而未增加 GvHD 的风险[111]。氨基双膦酸盐，例如唑来膦酸，可导致 γδT 细胞在体内增殖。因此，氨基双膦酸盐已用于体外培养 γδT 细胞[112]；然而，只有 vγ9vδ2 T 细胞亚群能用这种方法扩增出来。利用固定化抗原、激动性单克隆抗体、肿瘤源性人工 APC 或激活性单克隆抗体与人工 APC 联合应用已成功地扩增表达寡克隆或多克隆 TCR 的 γδT 细胞[113,114]。这些细胞正在用于 ACT 试验[115,116]，在体外扩增[117]后作为未修饰细胞进行试验，或如前所述使用基因工程修饰 CAR 进行试验[118]。

NK 细胞

大约 10% 的外周血淋巴细胞为 NK 细胞（$CD56^+CD3^-$）[119]，是先天性免疫系统的主要细胞毒性成分。NK 细胞同时具有细胞毒性和调节活性，可识别表达危险信号（应激配体和抗体）和/或缺乏 MHC-Ⅰ分子[120]的病毒感染细胞或恶性肿瘤细胞，是抗体依赖性细胞毒性作用（antibody dependent cell cytotoxicity，ADCC）[121]的有效介质。NK 细胞被用于各种 ACT，最常见的是被采集和激活的供体来源的外周血 NK 细胞[122]。为增加过继性转移的 NK 细胞的数量和功能，已经开发出许多体外扩增方案[123-126]。除了作为 ACT 发挥抗肿瘤作用外[127-132]，NK 细胞在 HSCT 中可能具有调节感染和 GvHD 的潜力[133-137]。

NKT 细胞

NKT 细胞为更小的淋巴细胞亚群，表型介于典型 NK 细胞和 T 细胞之间，已用于 ACT 试验。NKT 细胞（$CD3^+CD56^+$）、恒定自然杀伤细胞（Invariant natural killer T cell，iNKT）（$CD3^+CD56^+$Va24-Ja18）和 CIK 细胞（$CD3^+CD56^+$）都是具有潜在优势的效应淋巴细胞亚群。NKT 细胞具有调节抗恶性肿瘤细胞的免疫应答并刺激效应细胞的功能。此外，NKT 细胞可在肿瘤细胞和肿瘤相关巨噬细胞（tumor associated macrophages，TAMs）产生的趋化因子作用下转移至实体瘤中[138,139]，与 TAMs 共区域化，能够以 CD1d 依赖的方式杀死或抑制这些肿瘤细胞[140,141]。Heczey 等[142]在小鼠模型中发现，GD2 特异性 CAR 使 NKT 细胞对神经母细胞瘤细胞有强效的抗肿瘤效应，而无 GvHD 发生。iNKT 细胞可识别 CD1d 提呈的特异性糖脂类分子 αGalCer，从而在体内和体外特异性扩增。其他的 NKT 细胞亚群已经被定义，但是还未用于 ACT。

调节 T 细胞

天然存在的调节 T 细胞（regulatory T cells，Treg）具有预防 GvHD 的潜能[143,144]。近年来发现了新的 Treg 扩增方式，可用于产生满足临床需求数量的细胞[145,146]。此外，在 GvHD 的异种模型中，预防性注射第三方脐带血来源并体外扩增的 Treg 可预防 GvHD，改善 GvHD 评分、降低循环炎症细胞因子并显著提高总体生存率[147]。通过输注调节 T 细胞预防和治疗 GvHD 的早期临床试验正在进行，例如旨在评估造血干细胞移植[148]后输注调节 T 细胞对 GvHD 的作用的临床试验。目前还有其他早期临床试验正在进行，如 Treg 的输注对 1 型糖尿病[149]的作用（NCT01210664）。

树突状细胞

Sipuleucel-T 是一种促进表达抗原前列腺酸性磷酸酶（prostatic acid phosphatase，PAP）的前列腺癌的免疫应答的自体细胞免疫疗法，FDA 批准用于治疗无症状或症状轻微的转移性激素不敏感的前列腺癌（hormone refractory prostate cancer，HRPC）患者。通过白细胞去除术收集患者的外周血，然后再分离出外周血单个核细胞（peripheral blood mononuclear cells，PMBCs）。APC 前体由 CD54 阳性细胞（包括树突状细胞）组成，从外周血单个核细胞中分离出。然后用重组人融合蛋白 PAP-GM-CSF 在体外活化 APCs，培养 40 小时。最终产物被重新回输患者体内，诱导 T 细胞对表达 PAP 的肿瘤细胞产生免疫反应。完整的治疗包括三次输注，每两次输注之间间隔两周。

在 D9901、D9902a[150]、IMPACT[151]三项双盲随机Ⅲ期临床试验中，Sipuleucel-T 疗法使患者获得了总体生存率的获益。IMPACT 试验是 FDA 批准 sipuleucel-T 的基础。该试验招募了 512 例无症状或症状轻微的转移性 HRPC 患者（随机比例为 2∶1）。接受 sipuleucel-T 的患者中位生存时间为 25.8 个月，接受安慰剂的患者中位生存时间为 21.7 个月（$P=0.032$）。

Sipuleucel-T 曾被预测会轰动一时。然而，发明这项创新疗法的 Dendreon 公司在 2014 年 11 月宣告破产。该药的销售受到了一系列因素的阻碍，包括一个疗程 93 000 美元的高昂花费，为每位患者定制治疗方案的复杂性，以及最近获得 FDA 批准的前列腺癌口服新药带来的竞争。

通用型疗法

为了消除 ACT 产品对患者特异性的需要，减少生产细胞所需要的时间，产生"通用型供者 T 细胞"成为了科学家研究的焦点。常用手段包括使用人工核酸酶清除内源性的 TCR 的表达，例如，锌指核酸酶（zinc finger nucleases，ZFNs）[84,152]或转录激活因子样效应物核酸酶(transcription activator-like effector nucleases,TALENS)[153]。此外,降低工程T细胞的同种异体识别能力,为开发通用型疗法提供可能,即通过从单个供者生产通用型同种异体TAA特异性T细胞以供给多个受者。

脐带血

脐带血(cord blood,CB)越来越多地用于缺乏合适的HLA相合供者的造血干细胞移植患者的造血重建。与骨髓或动员外周血相比,CB具有较低GvHD发生率的优点。CB移植受到细胞剂量低从而致中性粒细胞、血小板植入延迟的限制;然而,与未经处理的CB相比,移植前在体外扩增CB祖细胞可提供更快的造血和免疫重建,以及更低的植入失败率。输注扩增后的CB产品是安全的,并且发生严重反应的可能性低。近期的研究表明,CB在体外岩藻糖基化可增强其在小鼠模型中的植入,移植前对CB使用体外岩藻糖基转移酶处理正在进行临床试验[154-157]。

CB也为细胞治疗提供了一种细胞来源。病毒感染是干细胞移植后最常见的死亡原因之一,尤其是脐带血移植(cord blood transplantation,CBT)后,因为CB中不含有足量的可保护受者免受感染的T细胞。Hanley等开发了一种方法以产生特异性抗巨细胞病毒和腺病毒的自体CB T细胞。在这种方法的基础上,Bollard等发起一项临床试验评估靶向EBV、CMV和腺病毒的CB来源多病毒特异性T细胞在预防和治疗移植后病毒感染的作用[158]。

如前所述,NK细胞和Treg也都可从CB中扩增并用于细胞治疗。有学者报道静息的CB NK细胞相比外周血NK细胞具有明显降低的细胞毒性。然而,在细胞因子刺激后,CB NK细胞的细胞毒性可迅速提高到外周血NK细胞相当的水平。Brunstein等从第三方CB中获取Treg并扩增,然后输入到接受双倍剂量CBT的23名患者体内。没有观察到严重的Treg相关急性毒性反应,而且GvHD发生率有所下降[159]。进一步的研究表明,在Treg输注的前30天内,病毒感染的发生率更高;然而,并没有远期的不良反应[160]。

安全性

以防发生不良事件,需要一种安全机制确保ACT所需输注的细胞能够迅速被消除,尤其是那些经过基因修饰的细胞。其中一种机制是利用一种可诱导的安全开关,这种开关是将人caspase 9融合到人FK结合蛋白上形成的一种条件性的二聚体[161]。当暴露于合成的二聚药物时,可诱导的caspase 9被激活,导致表达该结构的细胞迅速死亡。在2014年美国血液学年会上,Bonini等[162]报告了一项评估表达HSV-TK自杀基因T细胞的Ⅲ期临床试验的初步数据。在该试验的Ⅱ期研究中,他们发现,这些细胞在T细胞清除性半相合移植时可安全地诱导早期免疫重建,并且在GvHD发生时可以使用一个剂量的更昔洛韦杀灭[163]。

结论

细胞治疗作为一种有效的抗癌治疗的潜力正在逐渐实现,因此,免疫疗法被誉为2013年度的科学突破[164]。基因工程T细胞通过使难治患者获得完全和深度的缓解,在临床研究中展现出令人印象深刻的疗效。而ACT主要的障碍包括对TAA的不完全了解及对更安全的TAA的需要。目前,每年有数百名患者在各个医学中心接受ACT治疗。随着ACT的商业化,在全世界范围内为成千上万的患者提供ACT医疗服务的基础设施仍然是必要的[165]。

(洪振亚 译,周剑峰 校)

参考文献

The complete reference list can be found on the Wiley Companion Digital Edition of this title (see inside front cover for login instructions).

2 Weiden PL et al. Antileukemic effect of graft-versus-host disease in human recipients of allogeneic-marrow grafts. *N Engl J Med*. 1979;**300(19)**:1068-1073.

3 Rapoport AP et al. Restoration of immunity in lymphopenic individuals with cancer by vaccination and adoptive T-cell transfer. *Nat Med*. 2005;**11(11)**:1230-1237.

4 Walter EA et al. Reconstitution of cellular immunity against cytomegalovirus in recipients of allogeneic bone marrow by transfer of T-cell clones from the donor. *N Engl J Med*. 1995;**333(16)**:1038-1044.

5 Ruggeri L et al. Effectiveness of donor natural killer cell alloreactivity in mismatched hematopoietic transplants. *Science*. 2002;**295(5562)**:2097-2100.

8 Maude SL et al. Chimeric antigen receptor T cells for sustained remissions in leukemia. *N Engl J Med*. 2014;**371(16)**:1507-1517.

9 Lee DW et al. T cells expressing CD19 chimeric antigen receptors for acute lymphoblastic leukaemia in children and young adults: a phase 1 dose-escalation trial. *Lancet*. 2014;**385**:517-528.

10 Davila ML et al. Efficacy and toxicity management of 19-28z CAR T cell therapy in B cell acute lymphoblastic leukemia. *Sci Transl Med*. 2014;**6(224)**:224ra25.

19 Morgan RA et al. Cancer regression in patients after transfer of genetically engineered lymphocytes. *Science*. 2006;**314(5796)**:126-129.

21 Linette GP et al. Cardiovascular toxicity and titin cross-reactivity of affinity-enhanced T cells in myeloma and melanoma. *Blood*. 2013;**122(6)**:863-871.

22 Robbins PF et al. Tumor regression in patients with metastatic synovial cell sarcoma and melanoma using genetically engineered lymphocytes reactive with NY-ESO-1. *J Clin Oncol*. 2011;**29(7)**:917-924.

30 Rosenberg SA et al. Observations on the systemic administration of autologous lymphokine-activated killer cells and recombinant interleukin-2 to patients with metastatic cancer. *N Engl J Med*. 1985;**313(23)**:1485-1492.

35 Rosenberg SA et al. Use of tumor-infiltrating lymphocytes and interleukin-2 in the immunotherapy of patients with metastatic melanoma. A preliminary report. *N Engl J Med*. 1988;**319(25)**:1676-1680.

36 Schwartzentruber DJ et al. In vitro predictors of therapeutic response in melanoma patients receiving tumor-infiltrating lymphocytes and interleukin-2. *J Clin Oncol*. 1994;12(7):1475-1483.

40 Robbins PF et al. Mining exomic sequencing data to identify mutated antigens recognized by adoptively transferred tumor-reactive T cells. *Nat Med*. 2013;**19(6)**:747-752.

41 Tran E et al. Cancer immunotherapy based on mutation-specific CD4+ T cells in a patient with epithelial cancer. *Science*. 2014;**344(6184)**:641-645.

45 Yee C et al. Adoptive T cell therapy using antigen-specific CD8+ T cell clones for the treatment of patients with metastatic melanoma: in vivo persistence, migration, and antitumor effect of transferred T cells. *Proc Natl Acad Sci U S A*. 2002;**99(25)**:16168-16173.

48 Dudley ME et al. Adoptive cell therapy for patients with metastatic melanoma: evaluation of intensive myeloablative chemoradiation preparative regimens. *J Clin Oncol*. 2008;**26(32)**:5233-5239.

49 Rosenberg SA, Spiess P, Lafreniere R. A new approach to the adoptive immunotherapy of cancer with tumor-infiltrating lymphocytes. *Science*. 1986;**233(4770)**:1318-1321.

56 Hunder NN et al. Treatment of metastatic melanoma with autologous CD4+ T cells against NY-ESO-1. *N Engl J Med*. 2008;**358(25)**:2698-2703.

57 Lee PP et al. Characterization of circulating T cells specific for tumor-associated antigens in melanoma patients. *Nat Med*. 1999;**5(6)**:677-685.

60 Huls MH et al. Clinical application of Sleeping Beauty and artificial antigen presenting cells to genetically modify T cells from peripheral and umbilical cord blood. *J Vis Exp*. 2013;**72**:e50070.

62 Scholler J et al. Decade-long safety and function of retroviral-modified chimeric antigen receptor T cells. *Sci Transl Med*. 2012;**4(132)**:132ra53.

70 Hwu P et al. In vivo antitumor activity of T cells redirected with chimeric antibody/T-cell receptor genes. *Cancer Res*. 1995;**55(15)**:3369-3373.

80 Okamoto S et al. Improved expression and reactivity of transduced tumor-specific

TCRs in human lymphocytes by specific silencing of endogenous TCR. *Cancer Res.* 2009;**69**(**23**):9003-9011.

82 Provasi E et al. Editing T cell specificity towards leukemia by zinc finger nucleases and lentiviral gene transfer. *Nat Med.* 2012;**18**(**5**):807-815.

84 Torikai H et al. A foundation for universal T-cell based immunotherapy: T cells engineered to express a CD19-specific chimeric-antigen-receptor and eliminate expression of endogenous TCR. *Blood.* 2012;**119**(**24**):5697-5705.

87 Xu Y et al. Closely related T-memory stem cells correlate with in vivo expansion of CAR.CD19-T cells and are preserved by IL-7 and IL-15. *Blood.* 2014;**123**(**24**):3750-3759.

89 Grupp SA et al. Chimeric antigen receptor-modified T cells for acute lymphoid leukemia. *N Engl J Med.* 2013;**368**(**16**):1509-1518.

90 Porter DL et al. Chimeric antigen receptor-modified T cells in chronic lymphoid leukemia. *N Engl J Med.* 2011;**365**(**8**):725-733.

94 Long AH et al. 4-1BB costimulation ameliorates T cell exhaustion induced by tonic signaling of chimeric antigen receptors. *Nat Med.* 2015;**21**(**6**):581-590.

96 Maude SL et al. Managing cytokine release syndrome associated with novel T cell-engaging therapies. *Cancer J.* 2014;**20**(**2**):119-122.

97 Lee DW et al. Current concepts in the diagnosis and management of cytokine release syndrome. *Blood.* 2014;**124**(**2**):188-195.

100 Gattinoni L et al. A human memory T cell subset with stem cell-like properties. *Nat Med.* 2011;**17**(**10**):1290-1297.

107 Gattinoni L, Klebanoff CA, Restifo NP. Pharmacologic induction of CD8+ T cell memory: better living through chemistry. *Sci Transl Med.* 2009;**1**(**11**):11ps12.

151 Kantoff PW et al. Sipuleucel-T immunotherapy for castration-resistant prostate cancer. *N Engl J Med.* 2010;**363**(**5**):411-422.

158 Hanley PJ et al. Functionally active virus-specific T cells that target CMV, adenovirus, and EBV can be expanded from naive T-cell populations in cord blood and will target a range of viral epitopes. *Blood.* 2009;**114**(**9**):1958-1967.

161 Straathof KC et al. An inducible caspase 9 safety switch for T-cell therapy. *Blood.* 2005;**105**(**11**):4247-4254.

163 Ciceri F et al. Infusion of suicide-gene-engineered donor lymphocytes after family haploidentical haemopoietic stem-cell transplantation for leukaemia (the TK007 trial): a non-randomised phase I-II study. *Lancet Oncol.* 2009;**10**(**5**):489-500.

164 Couzin-Frankel J. Breakthrough of the year 2013. Cancer immunotherapy. *Science.* 2013;**342**(**6165**):1432-1433.

165 Rosenberg SA, Restifo NP. Adoptive cell transfer as personalized immunotherapy for human cancer. *Science.* 2015;**348**(**6230**):62-68.

第 67 章　癌症免疫疗法

Padmanee Sharma, MD, PhD ■ Sumit K. Subudhi, MD, PhD ■ Karl Peggs, MD, MA, MRCP, FRCPath ■ Sangeeta Goswami, MD, PhD ■ Jianjun Gao, MD, PhD ■ Sergio Quezada, PhD ■ James P. Allison, PhD

概述

癌症免疫学的基本原理包括免疫监视、免疫编辑和免疫耐受。对于这些基本原理具体机制的认识快速进展,已经应用于临床上成功治疗癌症。本章我们将讨论基础和临床免疫治疗领域的基本原理和最新进展,这些理论、试验和案例已经证明了长久以来的理念:自身免疫系统可以用来治疗癌症。我们也将重点讨论不同类型免疫疗法与其他治疗方法的联合应用在癌症治疗中的作用。

免疫监视

免疫系统可以识别和抵御癌症的观点由来已久。以 Paul Ehrlich(1854—1915 年)为代表的早期学者便推测机体的免疫系统在抑制肿瘤生长过程中发挥重要作用,指出若免疫系统不能识别并清除新生肿瘤细胞,癌症的患病率将会明显增加。这一观点直到 50 年后被 F. Macfarlane Burnet 和 Lewis Thomas 重新重视时,才得以形成广为人知的免疫监视(immune surveillance)假说[1-3]。然而,要确切地证明这一观点依然很困难。虽然在小鼠模型中已证明化学致癌物诱导的肿瘤具有免疫原性(immunogenicity),然而,天然自发的肿瘤细胞表现迥异,且不被相似的实验系统排斥[4]。这些实验资料促成了一种共识:天然发生的肿瘤不具有免疫原性,而化学致癌物诱发的可被免疫系统识别的肿瘤抗原仅限于小鼠实验模型。另外,在化学致癌物诱导的条件下,无胸腺小鼠的肿瘤发生率并未提高[5]。尽管因接受器官移植而免疫抑制的患者表现出各种癌症发生率增高,但令人沮丧的是,一直到 20 世纪 80 年代早期,依然缺乏小鼠实验模型的确切证据来支持免疫监视假说[3]。此外,即使在免疫抑制个体中某些肿瘤的发生率提高了上百倍(例如某些皮肤癌、卡西波肉瘤、淋巴瘤等),非皮肤来源或非病毒诱发的癌症的发生率则并无升高,这提示免疫监视可能对致癌病毒相关的恶性肿瘤有潜在的独特作用[6,7]。就在此时,获得性免疫缺陷综合征(AIDS)得以确诊,AIDS 患者的恶性肿瘤发生率明显增高,这为免疫监视在人体内发挥作用这一假说提供了进一步的证据[8,9]。然而,免疫监视与病毒诱导癌症的显著相关性同样令人瞩目。

多种证据交织,人们重新燃起基于免疫的治疗策略的热情。Aline van Pel、Thierry Boon 和 Pierre van der Bruggen 的工作奠定了免疫治疗的重要基础。他们首次证明,给小鼠接种诱变处理的肿瘤细胞,可以诱导针对自发肿瘤的特异性免疫应答[10],并进一步鉴定出可为人类细胞毒 T 细胞所识别的肿瘤特异性抗原[11]。这些研究表明,自发性肿瘤并非缺失肿瘤抗原,而是肿瘤抗原不能激发机体免疫应答,但这一不能激发免疫应答的状态在小鼠模型中可以通过接种肿瘤抗原加以克服。肿瘤抗原的分子鉴定给肿瘤免疫研究领域带来了革命性的变化,适应性免疫系统如何辨别正常和新生肿瘤细胞的机制研究普遍开展。在人体中检测到的肿瘤特异性反应促使人们有了新的假设:这种特异性反应可以人为地诱导或放大,以彻底清除肿瘤[12]。与此同时,在肿瘤免疫研究中迅速拓展出一个专门寻找肿瘤相关抗原的新领域。自此,大量肿瘤抗原得以克隆,大体上可分为 5 类:①分化抗原:例如黑色素细胞分化抗原、酪氨酸酶、gp-100 以及 Melan-A/MART-1;②突变抗原:例如抑癌基因 P53 的异常表达形式;③过量表达的正常抗原:例如 HER-2/neu、galectin-9;④肿瘤—睾丸抗原(CTAs):例如 MAGE、LAGE 及 NY-ESO-1;⑤病毒抗原:例如 EBV、HERV[13,14]。

免疫编辑

自发性肿瘤的肿瘤特异性抗原可以被机体免疫系统识别,这一发现进一步增加了免疫监视理论的可信度,但依然缺乏确凿的证据。事实上,就免疫原性而言,抗原性仅仅是必要条件,而非充分条件。2001 年,Robert Schreiber 与 Lloyd Old 合作发表了一篇文章,他们发现,T 细胞和免疫刺激因子 IFN-γ 协同作用,共同阻止了在基因工程制造的免疫系统缺陷(RAG-2-/-)小鼠中自发性和致癌物诱导发生的肿瘤的进展[15]。某些逃避了免疫监视的肿瘤细胞最终导致癌症的发生。他们提出以下假设:在机体免疫系统的选择性压力下,肿瘤细胞群处于一种类似于达尔文理论的环境选择的变化过程之中,因此经历了“免疫编辑(immunoediting)”的过程,使其免疫原性相比开始时不断下降。也有实验结果表明,免疫缺陷小鼠中分离出的肿瘤细胞比免疫功能正常小鼠体内分离出的肿瘤细胞免疫原性更强。这些实验结果虽然支持免疫监视理论,然而在临床应用时却遇到障碍:当患者患有的癌症被查出时,也就意味着机体的免疫系统已经失去了清除这种肿瘤的能力。然而,从治疗的角度出发,他们证明可通过增加肿瘤抗原的表达来促进免疫系统对肿瘤细胞的识别。类似的发现见于 RAG-1$^{-/-}$ 小鼠的报道[16]。此外,αβT 细胞或 γδT 细胞特异性缺陷的小鼠实验证明,这两类细胞在免疫监视过程中发挥重要但却不同的作用[17-19]。NK 和 NKT 细胞也在免疫监视中起到免疫保护作用,实验中在化学致癌物刺激之前,必须通过抗 NK1. 1 单克隆抗体或抗去唾液酸基鞘糖脂 GM1,来预先清除 NK 或 NKT 细胞[16]。干扰素 δ 和穿孔素的研究结果进一步阐明了机体抵御化学致癌物诱导性肿瘤及自发性肿瘤的效应机制,这些关键免疫调节分子的缺失会增加肿瘤生长机会[15,20-26]。与最初提出免疫编辑概念相比,免疫编辑假说的实质内容已略有演变,可认为是由三个同时或序贯的阶段组成的过程[27-33]。第一,“清除”阶段。作为肿瘤的一种外在抑制因素,免疫系统体现其清除肿瘤的功能(等同于原始的免疫监视概念);第二,“平衡”阶段。在此阶段,肿瘤细胞虽然能够存活,但是一直处于免疫系统的控制之下;第三,“逃逸”阶段。肿瘤细胞通过降低免疫原性,或灭活、破坏免疫应答等方式,逃脱机体免疫系统的控制,最终演变为临床症状明显的癌症。支持平衡阶段的证据一直较罕见,大多为基于临床观察的推测。例如,观察到接受异体肾移植的两个受者发生了黑色素瘤,他们移植的肾脏来源于同一个供者,而此供者在 16 年前就患有黑色素瘤,且被治愈了[31]。较新的,Schreiber 研究小组发现,在化学致癌物诱导发生原发癌症的小鼠模型中的确存在一个平衡阶段,该阶段的状态明显有别于“清除”和“逃逸”状态[32]。在暴露于化学致癌物的小鼠中,大约 20%的小鼠长出了致命的肿瘤,但是一些小鼠却没有明显的肿瘤生长表现(显然肿瘤被清除了)。然而,对这些小鼠进行免疫抑制处理,则发现这些小鼠体内处于休眠状态的肿瘤重新生长起来,并发生扩散,最终导致小鼠死亡。这种效应主要见于 T 细胞缺失,或干扰素 γ 和白介素 12(IL-12)活性被中和的小鼠模型中,而非缺失 NK 细胞的小鼠模型,由此可见适应性免疫应答在维持平衡阶段所发挥的特殊作用。此外,进一步研究发现,稳定休眠的肿瘤细胞与处于进展期的肿瘤细胞相比,其形态无差异,但是增殖能力下降,凋亡现象增加。在肿瘤部位有 T 细胞浸润,提示宿主免疫系统与肿瘤存在持续的相互作用。将这些休眠的肿瘤细胞在体外进行短期培养后接种于免疫缺陷的小鼠体内,肿瘤细胞可以继续生长。相反,如果这些肿瘤细胞接种于免疫功能正常的小鼠,就不能生长。最后,在免疫功能正常的小鼠中,可偶见肿瘤细胞历经一段休眠期后再度生长,而且将这些肿瘤细胞接种于其他免疫功能正常的小鼠,也可观察到肿瘤生长的现象。这表明这些肿瘤细胞的免疫原性已被弱化。这些资料支持以下观点:在平衡阶段,肿瘤细胞并未被编辑,而一旦完成编辑过程便可以自发逃逸机体免疫系统的控制。

免疫耐受

2005 年,Gerald Willimsky 和 Thomas Blankenstein 提出,小鼠中偶发的肿瘤并非是免疫编辑假说推测的肿瘤细胞免疫原性的降低所造成的,而是通过诱导免疫耐受(immune tolerance)来逃逸机体免疫监视[33]。这种观点本身并非新颖,而且事实上已经成为原始免疫编辑理论中的一部分,其传递的信息也很简单,但是对以免疫为基础的治疗方法的成功实施却有重要的启示。肿瘤的生长也许并不是仅仅依赖于肿瘤细胞对机体的内在适应而逃逸机体的免疫监视,更重要的是通过影响机体的免疫系统,进而诱导机体免疫系统出现无功能的状态。这些机制并非相互排斥或者完全分离的,因为上调肿瘤细胞表面的免疫抑制配体可以像下调免疫刺激因素一样有效消除机体的免疫应答。他们的研究基于病毒肿瘤促进基因(SV40 大 T 基因)小鼠模型。虽然最初在该小鼠体内可测到对 SV40 大 T 蛋白的免疫应答,但是后来该小鼠对 SV40 大 T 蛋白产生免疫耐受。然而,如果把这种蛋白接种于同种品系且无肿瘤负荷的小鼠中,可以诱导出很强烈的免疫应答(没有明确证据显示与免疫编辑有关)。

这个实验与其他支持肿瘤内在编辑理论研究相矛盾,也许反映了肿瘤免疫原性本身的固有差异。从定义上说,有较强免疫原性的肿瘤可诱发出更加强烈的免疫应答,部分原因是因为树突状细胞(dendritic cell,DC)呈递肿瘤碎片的能力是基于免疫原性的,这也反映了二级危险信号导致的活化。在这种情况下,如前文所述的进化压力可能较高,而免疫编辑对肿瘤细胞可以进行免疫逃逸的重要性就凸显了。对于那些免疫原性较弱的肿瘤细胞,由于并未有效地活化细胞的抗原呈递机制,所诱导的免疫应答强度较弱,其逃逸变异株因此较少经过免疫编辑。在这些情况下,免疫耐受或者说免疫忽略(immune ignorance)就可能发挥它们的作用。也就是说,当肿瘤细胞本身免疫原性强,诱发强烈免疫反应并因此面临较大的进化压力时,免疫编辑发挥主要作用,帮助肿瘤细胞进行免疫逃逸;而当被研究的肿瘤细胞本身的免疫原性较弱,则不会诱发较强的免疫应答,因此免疫编辑发挥的作用小,此时免疫耐受机制是帮助肿瘤进行免疫逃逸的主体。这也就是为什么有的实验发现了肿瘤的免疫编辑,而有的实验则认为肿瘤依靠免疫耐受进行免疫逃逸。

早期的失败——汲取的经验

免疫监视假说被普遍认可,促使人们以极大的热情开发了基于免疫的众多抗肿瘤疗法。然而,与初始预期相比,人类肿瘤免疫治疗的尝试结果并不成功,从而导致了免疫治疗在肿瘤治疗主流领域内被边缘化。肿瘤患者自身抗肿瘤免疫效能低下,不足以清除肿瘤。肿瘤过度生长的一个原因可能是免疫忽略,然而这些患者中很多也可以检测出抗肿瘤应答。通过小鼠模型详细研究免疫编辑的实验已明确:即使免疫监视功能失效了,机体免疫系统和肿瘤的关系也并未结束。因此,免疫系统不能清除肿瘤有可能与肿瘤特异性 T 细胞的效应功能受限有关。若想使抗肿瘤应答效应最大化,携带 T 细胞受体(T cell receptor,TCR)的效应细胞应具有肿瘤靶向性、适度活化、可迁移至肿瘤部位,且在免疫抑制的肿瘤微环境中能够发挥免疫效应的特点。TCR 转基因小鼠表明,即使所有 T 细胞均可识别肿瘤抗原,肿瘤依然可以不受限制地生长。这说明即使有大量能识别肿瘤抗原的 T 细胞存在,仍然不足以抑制肿瘤生长[34]。主动免疫相关的临床研究表明,即使肿瘤细胞反应性 T 细胞扩增到占循环 $CD8^+$ T 细胞群的 40%,肿瘤的生长依然不受限制[35]。大量的实验证据表明,由于在肿瘤组织中缺乏 T 细胞的浸润[36],或肿瘤微环境的免疫抑制效应,全身性抗肿瘤功能并不能导致肿瘤的清除。尽管荷瘤小鼠肿瘤特异性免疫应答不能有效发挥,但这些小鼠中也并不存在普遍的免疫缺陷[37]。这提示肿瘤组织可以诱导特异地抑制抗肿瘤免疫效应。这一概念也许在伴随免疫中体现突出:当一只小鼠接种某种肿瘤之后,虽然初始接种部位的肿瘤不断生长,但是却可抑制接种的同种肿瘤在其他远处部位的生长[38-40]。然而有趣的是,众所周知,一开始产生的伴随免疫,最终将会被原发性肿瘤进展过程中建立的 $CD4^+$ T 细胞介导的免疫抑制所克服[41,42]。尽管有这些发现,肿瘤免疫治疗的方法依旧停留在基于防治传染性疾病的原理水平。早在20世纪80年代就已证明，抗原特异性$CD8^+$细胞毒T细胞（cytotoxic T cell，CTL）能够诱导抗流感病毒的保护性免疫，进而推动了有效疫苗的发展[43]。Ralph Steinman以及其他研究者关于DC介导免疫应答起到关键作用研究成果问世，随后获得普遍认同[44]。不断积累的证据表明，肿瘤细胞所表达的抗原可为专职的抗原呈递细胞（antigen-presenting cell，APC）所识别，并且可以诱导产生肿瘤特异性CTL。基于上述发现，肿瘤免疫学家希望能够复制研发传染性疾病疫苗的成功。相关策略包括接种抗原肽、DNA及负载抗原的树突状细胞等。此外，其他替代性的方法，如直接增加效应细胞数量或强化其功能也在探索之中，包括过继转移扩增的肿瘤浸润淋巴细胞（tumor-infiltrating lymphocyte，TIL）和体外细胞因子活化的T细胞，T细胞过继治疗与细胞因子联合应用，以及最近开展的过继表达识别肿瘤相关抗原特异T细胞受体的基因工程T细胞（TCR或嵌合型抗原受体）[45-49]。虽然这些方法已获得令人印象深刻的效果（见后叙述），但其效果均有限，原因与肿瘤局部的免疫抑制微环境有关。相关试验已证明，如果减少免疫细胞数量，或进行非髓系细胞调节，可以增强免疫应答。既然肿瘤可以借助免疫忽视、免疫无能、免疫抑制等方式避免机体的免疫应答，进而在免疫功能正常的宿主体内建立独立的免疫豁免区，那么，肿瘤发生就是类似于结核分枝杆菌、单核细胞增多性李斯特菌、利什曼原虫等建立慢性感染性疾病的过程。在这种背景下，要实施有效的疫苗接种或免疫治疗，就应更多地借鉴慢性传染性疾病的免疫治疗方法，而不是采用针对急性传染性疾病的预防免疫接种策略。深入阐明肿瘤期免疫编辑模型的机制，将会启迪我们采用相关策略来加强免疫治疗的效果。

免疫逃逸的介导者

如前所述，目前普遍认为在肿瘤免疫逃逸（immune escape）过程中有两个重要变化：肿瘤细胞本身内在改变和局部肿瘤微环境的变化，两者相互交叉重叠。前者的经典例证包括：肿瘤细胞可下调协同刺激分子（例如B7分子）表达，使肿瘤反应性T细胞失去协同刺激分子刺激的活化条件，导致其无能[50]；或者通过肿瘤抗原丢失、下调主要组织相容复合物（major histocompatibility complex，MHC）分子等方式，使免疫系统不能识别肿瘤细胞[51]。进一步的例证包括通过突变的方式增加对诱导凋亡及细胞介导细胞毒性的抵抗能力，例如过表达抗凋亡分子（如FLIP和BCL-XL）[52,53]，FAS突变，或TRAIL受体死亡受体5（DR5）突变[54-56]。程序性死亡配体1（PD-L1）、B7-H3、B7x、HLA-G以及HLA-E等T细胞抑制性分子在肿瘤细胞表面及周围组织（间质细胞或抗原呈递细胞）的表达增加可以直接抑制效应T细胞功能。在许多病例中发现，这些分子在肿瘤细胞及其微环境中的表达水平与肿瘤治疗效果呈负相关[57-65]。据推测，局部免疫抑制介导分子还包括一些肿瘤和间质细胞产生的可溶性抑制因子，如白细胞介素（IL）-10、转化生长因子（TGF）-β、VEGF或神经节苷脂类物质[66-72]。表达在肿瘤细胞及浆细胞样DC（plasmacytoid dendritic cell，pDC）等抗原呈递细胞表面的吲哚胺2,3二氧化酶（IDO），同样可诱导获得性免疫耐受，主要通过直接抑制T细胞的功能和增强局部调节性T细胞（Treg）的能力来介导免疫抑制效应[73,74]。IDO是色氨酸降解过程中的限速酶。局部色氨酸水平的下降（可能通过介导效应性T细胞的应激反应状态）与色氨酸代谢物免疫调节作用相协同，导致免疫耐受。此外，表达IDO的pDC主要定居在肿瘤引流淋巴结内。它们可以直接活化成熟的Treg，进而通过Treg来上调其他DC表面PD-1的表达，继而抑制效应T细胞的增殖[75]。这些调节网络很复杂，但也已经日趋明了[76]。肿瘤和引流淋巴结中存在着一系列可主动抑制免疫应答的细胞，例如$CD4^+CD25^+$ Treg，分泌IL-10的Treg，CD1d限制性（NKT）T细胞，未成熟树突状细胞（immature dendritic cell，iDC）和pDC，以及髓系来源抑制细胞（myeloid-derived suppressor cell，MDSC）（非细胞-自发性抑制），这些细胞对诱导和维持局部免疫豁免发挥十分重要的作用[74,77]。这些细胞也许是选择性地被募集到这些部位，进行数量扩增或诱导相关抑制活性。

非细胞的自发性抑制

若干具有调节或抑制功能的$CD4^+$T细胞亚群已经得到确认，主要分两类：一类起源于胸腺，表达CD4、CD25、GITR、OX40和细胞毒性T淋巴细胞相关抗原4（cytotoxic T-lymphocyte-associated-antigen 4，CTLA-4），同时在发育过程中非常依赖于X连锁的叉头翼状螺旋转录因子（Foxp3），此类调节性T细胞就是所谓天然发生的Treg[78-84]；另一类来源于外周初始$CD4^+$ T细胞，在环境中遭遇"耐受原"后，进而分化为Treg，称为"诱导性"或"适应性"调节性细胞，其中包括分泌IL-10而不分泌Foxp3的Tr1细胞[85-87]，分泌TGF-β的Th3细胞[88,89]，以及胸腺外产生的$CD4^+$ $CD25^+$ $Foxp3^+$ iT_{reg}细胞[90-95]。此外，$CD4^+$ $CD25^-Foxp3^+$ T细胞的调节性作用也已得到确认[96]。在某些情况下，传统的非调节性$CD4^+$ T细胞与抗原接触，可获得调节T细胞的表型和功能。这种方式被认为是维持T细胞自身稳定和控制炎症的一种主要途径。特别值得关注的是，相对于小鼠而言，人类的胸腺退化较早，人类Treg的端粒长度也相对较短。因此，与小鼠Treg相比，有可能外周来源的人类Treg在维持免疫耐受（也许还包括肿瘤导致的免疫损害）方面发挥更加重要的作用[97-99]。而且，如果抗原接触对调节性T细胞的产生是必备条件的话，既然一旦前体T细胞识别肿瘤抗原就会朝着抑制表型而非活化表型分化，那么很有可能调节性T细胞库的产生需要牺牲潜在效应T细胞为代价[96,100,101]。这种表型转化的条件还在研究之中，但是一些因素，例如用最适量的抗原刺激联合TGF-β似乎相当重要，而且两者可能与肿瘤微环境相关[93,102]。肿瘤细胞或间质组织（例如pDC）产生的IDO也有利于调节性T细胞的形成[75,103,104]，同时维A酸似乎也是建立肠道耐受的一个关键因素[105-108]。调节性T细胞只有经过TCR刺激之后才能够获得功能，至少部分肿瘤相关调节性T细胞可以特异识别肿瘤抗原[109]，但是一旦活化，这些细胞便以一种抗原非依赖的形式发挥抑制功能。适应性Tr1和Th3主要通过分泌可溶性因子（IL-10和/或TGF-β）发挥抑制作用，$Foxp3^+$ T_{reg}则通过一系列机制来发挥抑制功能，这些机制在所有特定环境下的相对重要性仍有待阐明。可能涉及的机制包括：CTLA-4、与膜结合的TGF-β以及细胞外周腺苷的产生[110-116]。这些因素可以抑制多种免疫效应细胞的功能，包括$CD4^+$和$CD8^+$ T细胞、B细胞和NK细胞[117]，使得它们成为在免疫抑制网络中用于干预治疗的潜在新靶点。具有抑制功能的 $CD8^+$ T 细胞的研究发现使这个网络更加复杂[118-121]。在恶性肿瘤小鼠模型中，调节性 T 细胞的主要抑制功能已获证实[122]。而且，最近其在人类癌变中的重要作用也有证明[123]。癌症患者体内调节性 T 细胞扩增并积累的机制尚未明了，但是很可能与预先存在的调节性 T 细胞的增殖以及初始 T 细胞向调节性 T 细胞的转化有关[101,124,125]。在小鼠模型中，依据调节性 T 细胞的相对丰度可预测到肿瘤生长的结果[126,127]，调节性 T 细胞丰度与某些上皮癌生长状态呈负相关，包括卵巢癌[123,128]、乳腺癌[129]以及肝细胞癌[130]。有意思的是，在血液肿瘤中，上述关系却完全颠倒了，高水平的调节性 T 细胞似乎更有利于预后（例如皮肤性 T 细胞淋巴瘤、滤泡状淋巴瘤以及霍奇金淋巴瘤[131-133]）。单独看肿瘤组织中浸润调节性 T 细胞的水平，似乎并不能成为判断预后的最好指标。霍奇金淋巴瘤中存在大量的调节性 T 细胞，主要包括分泌 IL-10 的 Tr1 以及 $CD4^+$ $CD25^+$ T_{reg}，这些细胞可以诱导彻底的免疫抑制微环境[134]。表达 Foxp3 细胞和表达 TIA-1（细胞毒性颗粒相关性 RNA 结合蛋白）细胞的联合评估提供了一个更好预测指标[133]，提示了评估多种浸润细胞的重要性。事实上，在现代临床医疗中，确定可以预测预后、指导治疗原则或监测疗效的特异性免疫指标（依靠流式细胞技术，PCR 或微点阵分析技术[135]）是十分重要的。例如，在肿瘤组织中，如果只有少量肿瘤浸润性 T 细胞，包括调节性 T 细胞，那么这种肿瘤就可能对以提高 CTL 数量、功能和迁移能力为目标的治疗有良好的反应性，而那些有大量调节性 T 细胞浸润的肿瘤则会从针对降低调节性 T 细胞数量或功能的治疗中获益。此外，调节性 T 细胞代表了另外一种免疫治疗干预的调节机制，可以通过加强调节性 T 细胞的作用来降低免疫治疗的效果。例如，IL-2 已经被用于包括黑色素瘤、肾细胞癌、横纹肌肉瘤、卵巢癌等在内的多种人类癌症的治疗。开始使用 IL-2，就是基于可以直接加强固有免疫和适应性免疫的效应功能的想法。然而，在体内环境中，IL-2 在维持 $CD4^+CD25^+$ 调节性 T 细胞稳态和功能方面发挥十分重要的作用[136-138]。给癌症患者使用 IL-2，发现可以导致外周调节性 T 细胞的增加，刺激 T_{reg} 表达 CXC-趋化因子受体 4（CXCR4）和 CCR4，进而促进这些细胞向表达 CXCL12 和 CCL2 的肿瘤微环境中迁移[139-141]。因为肿瘤免疫接种策略的靶标都是一些自身抗原，因此这种“治疗性”的癌症疫苗也可以诱导肿瘤特异性调节性 T 细胞的扩增[142,143]。所以，在免疫接种过程中，既然常规意义上的“成熟”树突状细胞也可以活化并扩增自身抗原特异性的调节性 T 细胞，那么树突状细胞的“免疫原性”或“耐受原性”就显得尤为重要[144,145]。具有多重抑制功能的抗原呈递细胞已有报道，而且这些 APC 在肿瘤局部免疫豁免的产生中可能扮演重要角色。处于生长状态的肿瘤细胞可能像对待抑制性 T 细胞那样选择地募集具有抑制性的 APC，或者将刺激性 APC 转化为抑制性 APC。树突状细胞和髓系来源细胞造成主动免疫抑制的分子机制尚未完全阐明，其中包括 IL-10 和 TGF-β 的分泌，FAS 配体 PD-L1 表达以及胞内 IDO 的加工[146-150]。如前所述，合成 IDO 的树突状细胞可以诱导活化性 T 细胞凋亡和 T 细胞无能以及将效应 T 细胞转化为调节性 T 细胞[75,103,151,152]。在这些部位，刺激性和抑制性 APC 的平衡可能在很大程度上决定了 T 细胞接触抗原后的最终结局。目前已经证实，树突状细胞与调节性 T 细胞的相互作用是一个双向过程[153-155]。MDSC 具有异质性，由巨噬细胞、粒细胞和树突状细胞的前体细胞以及分化早期的骨髓细胞组成。小鼠 MDSC 表达髓系分化抗原 Gr-1（Ly6G 和 Ly6C）和 CD11b，人类 MDSC 具有 CD14-$CD11b^+$ 细胞表型（表达 CD33 但是却缺少成熟髓系和淋巴系细胞的标志）[156-158]。MDSC 特异抑制表型标志尚未确定[159]。小鼠主要包括 $Ly6G^+Ly6C^{low}$ 粒细胞和 Ly6G-$Ly6C^{high}$ 单核细胞两个细胞亚群。在人类癌症中，MDSC 数目可能与预后相关[160]。多种来源于肿瘤的细胞因子参与 MDSC 的扩增，包括 VEGF、IL-1β 和 GM-CSF[161-163]。MDSC 介导的免疫抑制机制是复杂的，其中涉及 iNOS 或者精氨酸酶 1[147,164-167]。这两种物质可以通过诱导凋亡、抑制增殖或诱导调节表型等方式来抑制 T 细胞应答。尽管 TCR-CD8 复合物中酪氨酸的硝化反应具有对非特异刺激信号的应答能力，但是这一反应似乎可以导致 $CD8^+$ T 细胞不能与抗原肽-MHC 复合物的结合以及对特异抗原肽的应答[168]。在肿瘤组织中的 2 型巨噬细胞不仅参与了抑制肿瘤免疫，而且似乎拥有未成熟的髓系细胞某些功能特点[169,170]。

尽管在一些癌症的免疫治疗中已经成功地诱导出全身免疫反应，但转化为显著的临床治疗效果的例子依然很罕见。为了提升治疗效果，这其中的机制需要阐明。但我们依然不清楚，这一目标要达成多少，以及还有多少分散的靶标需要被发现、解决，才能产生对局部有疗效的免疫应答。

向临床有效的免疫疗法前进

免疫监视的基本概念已不再新颖，尝试利用免疫系统来治疗肿瘤同样有很长的历史。1891 年，纽约肿瘤医院（后来成为纪念 Sloan-Kettering 癌症中心的一部分）的骨外科医生 William Coley（1862—1936 年）从医院一份病历记录中发现，7 年前一个颈部长有不宜手术的恶性肿瘤的患者，在一次皮肤细菌感染后肿瘤消失了。这次感染是由化脓性链球菌引起的丹毒[171]。Coley 医生推断这次感染可能是奇迹般痊愈的主要原因。他还发现，在 1890 年前，就有超过 20 例将丹毒和抗肿瘤反应联系起来的报道。在这一背景下，加上当时无如今严格管理条文的束缚，Coley 医生开始用活菌进行临床试验，并在出现几例因感染而死亡的病例后，转而利用热灭活的细菌[172,173]。即使只有很少部分的患者被治愈，其结果仍然是令人瞩目的。他用感染丹毒法治疗的第一个肿瘤患者明显治愈了，10 年后死亡，原因不详。Coley 用混合毒素治疗的第一位患者，25 年后因为心脏病发作而死亡。这种抗肿瘤作用可能是通过细菌内毒素诱导产生的肿瘤坏死因子（TNF）介导的[174,175]。尽管 TNF 本身由于毒性过大不宜用于临床，但其他 TNF 超家族成员及其受体仍然是当前免疫疗法的重要靶点。接下来的章节中会讨论前面提及研究的各种策略，促进 DC 功能的方法，并主要讨论过继性细胞免疫治疗和免疫刺激性单克隆抗体。

过继细胞治疗和个体化免疫疗法的发展

荷瘤宿主通常确实可产生抗肿瘤反应，而且肿瘤特异性细胞可能集中于瘤体内（即使被局部的免疫因素抑制），对这一观点的认同逐渐增加，促进了过继细胞治疗（adoptive cell therapy，

ACT)的发展。而且主动免疫在临床上未见到显著疗效并不总是因为全身抗肿瘤免疫反应的缺失。虽然有人认为这种失败至少与低亲和力效应T细胞的刺激有部分相关性但更多的是反映了抗自身的T细胞库的缺失耐受。这些细胞尽管能被传统的免疫检测技术识别,但是基本不能抑制已经存在的肿瘤,特别是如何进入并在肿瘤微环境内起作用也是限制因素。过继免疫疗法可鉴定出少量但对肿瘤抗原有相对高亲和力的细胞,通过在体外选择、扩增,然后再回输患者体内。这些细胞可以在体外进行激活,然后直接施用,可避免受到肿瘤局部耐受因素影响。起初认为,大量扩增肿瘤反应性T细胞可以避开所有外周和局部的调节机制,达到冲击肿瘤并抑制肿瘤的效果。现在的治疗方法进一步关注对宿主进行调整的重要性,进而尽量提高治疗成功的可能性。随着对抗肿瘤免疫抑制因素有关研究认识的深化,现代治疗方法也得到了发展。在部分恶性肿瘤病例中,尤其是黑色素瘤,给淋巴细胞耗竭的宿主输注大量活化的高亲和力肿瘤特异T细胞,能克服抑制因素,出现有效的癌症治疗效果。到目前为止,获得T细胞的方法大多基于体外扩增肿瘤浸润性T细胞,小部分经由外周血和淋巴结活检获得。细胞过继治疗通常联合T细胞生长因子IL-2使用。如果与免疫刺激性抗体研究进展相结合,这种方法可能有望得到进一步发展(如下所述)。

早在20世纪50年代,Nicholas Mitchison便做了大量的开拓性工作[176,177],为后续经由ACT的被动抗癌免疫疗法奠定了基础。这些开创性的工作证明,宿主接受的辐射剂量越强,产生的能够引起免疫应答的抗原量越显著[178-180]。ACT的进一步发展主要归功于华盛顿大学的Alexander Fefer、Martin Cheever和Philip Greenberg团队,以及美国国家癌症研究所的Steven Rosenberg和Nicholas Restifo团队。在19世纪60年代晚期,Fefer发展了化学免疫疗法的概念,证明同基因淋巴瘤(FBL-3或者韦林德病毒诱导的淋巴瘤)可以通过联合使用大剂量烷化剂环磷酰胺及来源于同种肿瘤致敏的小鼠免疫细胞转输的方法达到根治[181]。进一步的研究阐明了一些关于这种抗肿瘤活动的机制,证实此类免疫应答主要由T细胞介导[184],可以直接作用于肿瘤或病毒抗原[182,183],并且相似活性的T细胞可以从非致敏的小鼠中分离出来,尽管其免疫活性很低[185]。这一点非常重要,因为提示未免疫的动物体内也有肿瘤反应性T细胞。进一步的工作证明,在体外接受辐射并增殖和再次致敏的细胞中,抗肿瘤活性增强了[186-192]。甚至那些仅仅在体外初步致敏的细胞中,抗肿瘤活性也增强了[189]。该项工作的一个重要进展是将IL-2引入体外扩增体系,这可以进一步扩增肿瘤反应性T细胞[189]。最后,研究显示肿瘤反应性T细胞可以在体外培养很长一段时间,并在过继输注后,能够继续增殖并特异地抑制肿瘤生长,而体内联合应用IL-2能明显增强这种反应效果[190-192]。这些研究首次强调了体内外应用IL-2在促进效应细胞增殖和增强肿瘤抑制方面的潜力。

同时,Rosenberg也证实了IL-2在肿瘤免疫治疗方面的作用。当时,关于利用"T细胞生长因子"(TCGF或IL-2)来克隆和扩增T细胞的研究成果纷纷发表[45,193,194],其中包括分离和扩增实体肿瘤的浸润性T细胞方面[195]。这些研究成果成为ACT的基础之一。重要的是,在TCGF存在的情况下生长的人类淋巴细胞,在体外能够杀死自体肿瘤细胞[196]。这个最初的观察带来了一系列研究成果的发表,包括IL-2在淋巴因子激活的杀伤细胞(lymphokine-activated killer,LAK)中的作用[197],以及这些细胞在体外杀伤新鲜肿瘤细胞的能力,和诱导在过继转移的动物模型中建立的弥散性抑制淋巴瘤细胞的能力[198]。这些研究并不只限于淋巴瘤,后续研究很快转向对黑色素瘤鼠类模型的研究[199]。Rosenberg的免疫治疗方法的一个显著特征就是能很快转化为临床试验。早在1984年,首次应用LAK细胞进行人体临床Ⅰ期试验的研究成果就已发表[200]。临床试验结果表明,从外周血中获得的淋巴细胞在体外可以扩增至非常大的数目;这些细胞可以安全地回输到癌症患者体内。该项研究也证实,这些细胞能够迁移到一些器官和组织中,包括肿瘤组织。另外两个关于IL-2在小鼠模型体内作用的实验研究促进了ACT在临床应用方面的进展[201,202]。通过Ⅰ期临床试验评估了IL-2在人类全身用药的安全性后[203],进行了更大规模的联合应用LAK和IL-2的研究[204,205],在研究中,超过100名患者使用了不同剂量的IL-2和大量的自体LAK细胞(高达18.4×10^{10}个细胞)。在21%的患者中可以看到完全或部分反应[205]。尽管这些早期临床试验得到了一些不错的结果,但小鼠模型得到的一些实验数据还是使研究方向从回输LAK细胞转向回输高度特异的肿瘤反应性T细胞。新方法以体外分离和应用IL-2扩增TIL为基础[195]。扩增的TIL杀伤不同类型的肿瘤细胞的能力比LAK细胞高了50~100倍,而且在联合环磷酰胺和IL-2进行体内回输时,它们的抗肿瘤能力也得到明显增强[45]。临床试验得到了类似动物实验的结果,在联合应用环磷酰胺、TIL和IL-2时,31%的已转移黑色素瘤患者出现完全或部分的治疗应答[206]。

这些早期研究促进了ACT作为个体化免疫疗法的发展[207-209]。当然,ACT在转化临床应用方面也不是没有困难。这些困难主要包括两方面:生产合适的过继产品的困难以及宿主或肿瘤对过继细胞的抵抗。

细胞治疗药物的生产

一个主要的限制因素是难以获得含有足够数量且可成功分离和扩增TIL的肿瘤样本。这一困难是60%~70%的病例的限制性步骤[210]。分离肿瘤反应性淋巴细胞(tumor-reactive lymphocyte,TRL)的替代策略将能促进细胞疗法得到更广泛的应用。这些方法包括利用来源于外周血或淋巴结活检组织的T细胞[211-214]。现在广泛应用的方法是联合CD3和T细胞表面的协同刺激受体CD28的抗体在间接体内(ex vivo)刺激并扩增出大量的TRL,而近来4-1BB(见下)在活化和选择方法的应用引起了更多关注[215-218]。通过肿瘤细胞过量表达或者较少表达的某些特异抗原分子(NY-ESO-1、MART-1、酪氨酸酶、gp-100、p53)来鉴定和克隆抗原特异性的T细胞大大地促进了TIL分离替代方案的发展。通过这些方法从外周血中获得的TRL(肿瘤反应性淋巴细胞,TIL的替代者)可以在体外富集,并通过前文叙述的方法扩增。我们已经了解很多回输细胞的理想特征,包括最长存活时间和最强抗肿瘤活性。已经证明,长期体外培养的T细胞是有害的,并且T细胞分化程度也是关键因素[219]。此外,因为Il-2也可扩增Treg以及具有明显毒性,因此,IL-2可能不是用来增强体内活性的最佳细胞因子。第一个替代方案是使用 IL-7、IL-15 和 IL-21。在这些因子单独或联合应用时，能更特异地扩增效应 T 细胞[220]，这可以较少产生耐受性 $CD8^+$ T 细胞[221]，而且能产生具有更强抗肿瘤活性的低分化免疫细胞[222-224]。过继回输 T 细胞的扩增和维持长时间存活似乎都需要 IL-2。近期更多的小鼠模型研究提示，联合回输 $CD4^+$ T 细胞能够提供 IL-2 并维持 TRL 长期存在，进而可以增强 ACT 的抗肿瘤效应[225-227]。大量研究证实，记忆性 $CD8^+$ T 细胞的产生和/或维持需要 $CD4^+$ T 细胞参与。除了提供细胞因子支持，它们也参与了 DC 细胞的功能塑化，同时还可以募集和活化具有介导抗瘤作用的巨噬细胞和嗜酸性粒细胞[224,228,229]。

近来大量的努力聚焦于 T 细胞基因修饰，以期增强其抗肿瘤效应。此类方法之一包括转入 CAR（chimeric antigen receptor，嵌合抗原受体），CAR 是具有基于抗体的外部受体结构和胞内区编码 TCR 信号转导的结构域[230]。这可以允许 T 细胞实现非 MHC 限制性的特异性重新定向，并传输等同于 TCR 配体触发的细胞内信号。此外，还可对胞内结构域进行改造，用模仿 CD28、4-1BB 或者 OX40 的配体，提供仿制性协同刺激信号，从而增强 CAR 的触发强度。尽管加入 CD28 组分可导致 IL-2 的释放，不利于增殖（增加对 T_{reg} 抑制作用的抵抗[231]），但为了活化 T 细胞还是要加；虽如此，T 细胞的活化仍然是不完全的，整合入 4-1BB 或 OX40 信号结构域能进一步增强其活化[232,233]。早期的一些试验表明，转基因细胞在回输体内后生存时间只能维持数天到数周[49,234-237]。这可能与 CAR 潜在的免疫原性有部分关系。从早期 ACT 研究中获得的经验依然是有用的，现在人们集中研究中央记忆型 T 细胞和疱疹病毒特异性 T 细胞，而非效应性记忆细胞[238,239]。因为疱疹病毒作为一个潜伏病毒储存池，会不断刺激相应初始 T 细胞的 TCR，进而使疱疹病毒特异性 T 细胞维持一个相对高的水平[49]。中央记忆型 T 细胞是幼稚 T 细胞经历抗原刺激后最大程度未分化的细胞，保留了幼稚 T 细胞发育选择，包括很强的克隆扩增能力。一种重塑 T 细胞特异性的替代性策略是转入来自肿瘤反应性 T 细胞克隆的 TCR 基因，但是这种方法有一定的 MHC 限制性[48,240-242]。在应用此方案的第一个临床试验中，将 MART-1 反应性的 TCR 转导入人类淋巴细胞中，这些转导后的淋巴细胞与 MART-1^+ 肿瘤细胞共孵育，可分泌效应性细胞因子，并表现出溶细胞活性。在去除患者体内淋巴细胞后，将这些转基因淋巴细胞输入到黑色素瘤患者体内，并注射 IL-2，结果显示在 17 名患者中，有 2 名患者输注 T 细胞后产生临床有效应答[48]。一些潜在的因素限制了这项实验的效应，包括基因修饰细胞存在的差异以及转导 TCR 的相对低水平表达。与后者相关的可能原因有：外源性 TCR 链和内源性 TCR 链在与 CD3 组分组装时存在竞争；内源性及外源性 TCR 链形成混合二聚体限制了亲和力[243]。事实上，只要通过基因优化使 TCR 的表达适度增加，就可以显著增强抗肿瘤活性[244]。另一种可能形成互补的替代方法是增强基因修饰细胞的存活，例如向细胞转导 GM-CSF-IL-2 受体（基于结合 GM-CSF 时可传递 IL-2 信号，形成一个自分泌环路的设计[245]）、CD28[246] 或端粒末端转移酶的催化亚基[247]。转导编码失活 TGF-β 的基因或抑制性 RNA，以阻止抑制性分子如 CTLA-4 和 PD-1 的表达，这些方法会使淋巴细胞更少被肿瘤微环境中的抑制因素所影响，可能会更进一步增强回输细胞的抗肿瘤活性[248]。另外，一些选择性协同刺激配体的过表达可以诱导自发协同刺激或转导协同刺激，以产生有效的抗肿瘤活性[249]。

淋巴清除的作用

向未处理的个体输注肿瘤特异的 T 淋巴细胞，常不能确定转导的细胞是否成功输入，或其存活时间的长短，或对庞大的肿瘤是否表现出抗肿瘤活性[250-252]。人们也许需要进一步关注内在和外在的抑制性因素，这对临床治疗方案的成功与否至关重要。宿主的淋巴清除（lymphodepletion）能极大地促进细胞过继疗法的有效性，其中可能与多种机制相关，包括消除细胞因子池（淋巴细胞与转导细胞竞争内环境中的细胞因子，如 IL-7 和 IL-15），消除 T_{reg} 和骨髓来源抑制性细胞，形成促进平稳增殖的内环境[225,238,253-255]。过继回输的细胞中的 T_{reg} 细胞含量可能也很重要[225]。除了作用于免疫细胞以外，对宿主进行放射治疗也能致敏肿瘤周围的间质细胞[256]，上调肿瘤血管系统黏附分子的表达[257,258]。最后，对宿主进行放射治疗也能使肠道共生微生物释放 LPS，从而促进 DC 成熟，活化肿瘤反应性 T 细胞[259]，而且伴随造血干细胞恢复，能进一步促进过继转移的 $CD8^+$T 细胞的扩增和功能[260]。

T 细胞过继回输的现状

尽管 ACT 所获经验令人鼓舞，但是，应认识到 TIL 也许更适用于自身免疫系统介导较强抗肿瘤能力的患者。许多人类恶性肿瘤研究显示，肿瘤的 TIL 浸润水平与肿瘤的预后相关，因此从 TIL 中获得治疗性细胞的能力可以作为预测肿瘤预后的一个生物标志物。从这个角度出发，CAR 或 TCR 转导的 ACT 治疗可以在不经严格选择的患者中获得更高的临床反应率，这将是此领域内的一大进步，但是目前结果显示其他单一药物的临床治疗效果却更好。由于未进行大量随机研究，因此不能确定淋巴消除、化疗放疗、IL-2 及 ACT 在整体结果中的相对贡献多少。在这个领域的随机研究还太少（在参考文献 212 中有所综述），且只有一例有阳性结果。有意思的是，这阳性结果发生在肝癌患者身上，而不是通常用 ACT 法治疗的黑色素瘤和肾癌。患者在外科切除原发肿瘤后辅以输注 CD3 抗体和 IL-2 体外扩增的外周血 T 细胞治疗（$n=150$）。接受 ACT 治疗的患者肿瘤复发率下降 41%，并具有更长无进展生存期（$P=0.01$）及总生存时间有延长的趋势（$P=0.09$）[261]。但是，最近一个在Ⅲ期黑色素瘤患者中进行的临床试验，患者随机接受 TIL 加 IL-2 或者单独 IL-2 治疗，并没有观察到如上的疗效[262,263]。ACT 应用的主要问题在于，作为一种高度个体化的治疗方法，不易成为现代肿瘤治疗的常规模式。获得合适的细胞制品需要密集的劳动及严格的实验室操作技术。而且，基本上需要为每个患者都生产新的制剂，这限制了简单商品化的可能性。这意味着 ACT 是服务导向性的，而不是产品（如大部分药品）。在此方面，人们意识到尽量减少 T 细胞的离体操作，可能有利于临床效果。上述实践与认识推动了当今临床疗法的改进。免疫疗法的最佳靶点是共用的还是特异性的问题逐渐成为争论的焦点。长久以来，我们主要关注肿瘤共同抗原或多种肿瘤共有抗原，如 MART-1 和 gp-100。结果发现，抗肿瘤效能不可避免地与组织特异性毒副作用相关联。然而,肿瘤专有抗原或者患者特异抗原的产生与恶性肿瘤表型演变以及固有遗传不稳定性相关[264,265],肿瘤特异性抗原因其优势更获关注[266]。随着对组织特异性毒副作用的认识产生了一个新概念,即"非必需组织"[267],如治疗黑色素瘤导致的白癜风,应用CD20抗体治疗后伴随的B淋巴细胞缺陷等,都是可接受的。但是,当治疗靶点同时也为一重要生命器官所共有时,就是一个难题了[235]。同时为增强免疫效果开发的"现成"试剂为提高ACT的效能提供了许多有趣的途径。最近报道的基因修饰T细胞疗法在临床上的成功[268],以及制药公司对制定策略以推进ACT最终可以被批准用于治疗患者的热情重燃,这些都让T细胞过继回输的未来有着乐观的前景。

促进树突状细胞的功能

本章节简要叙述促进抗原呈递以提高抗肿瘤免疫的一些观点,但不会深入详细讨论。DC可以独一无二地呈递加工过的抗原并刺激抗原特异性效应细胞产生应答。对DC产生促进免疫应答而不是免疫耐受相关因子的认识促进了临床治疗的进步,同时也认识到,即使是传统的成熟DC(高表达协同刺激分子)也能介导免疫抑制反应[142,269-271]。可增强DC免疫原性的细胞因子(如IFN、IL-15、TNF和IL-1)单独使用时一般不能有效地诱导强烈的主动免疫反应[272]。

相比之下,在临床研究中,尤其是联合其他临床治疗方案时,Toll样受体(Toll-like receptor,TLR)激动剂已经显示出某些潜力。非甲基化CpG-寡聚脱氧核苷酸(oligodeoxynucleotide,ODN)能结合pDC和B细胞上的TLR9,诱导产生Th1型免疫应答,在小鼠模型及Ⅰ、Ⅱ期临床试验均能抑制已经发生的肿瘤[273-280]。TLR9活化的APC,可活化NK细胞,提高多核淋巴细胞Fc受体的表达,并促进CTL的活化。然而,也要认识到某些TLR配体也可以诱导免疫抑制或免疫耐受应答[281,282]。TLR信号转导途径十分重要,有待于进一步研究,比如免疫系统如何区分病理性炎症和"有益性"炎症,并产生相应的免疫活化或者抑制反应。"有益性"炎症与共生性微生物或伤口愈合相伴随。Imid-azoquinolone化合物咪喹莫特能结合TLR7(以及较低程度的TLR8)。当使用时,能活化并募集pDC和骨髓来源的DC至肿瘤部位,参与抗肿瘤反应[283]。这可能直接诱导血管E-选择素的上调、抑制Treg功能(包括Treg和新γδ抑制亚群)[284-286],而且已证明有利于激发外阴上皮肿瘤的临床治疗反应[287,288]。在多个小鼠类模型中,CD1d反应性α-半乳糖酰基鞘氨醇及其类似物α-半乳糖酰基鞘氨醇能活化NKT细胞,通过另一种途径促进DC成熟,增强抗肿瘤反应[289-291]。CpG和咪喹莫特也都可以在接种过重组蛋白肿瘤抗原NY-ESO-1的黑色素瘤患者中诱导肿瘤抗原特异性T细胞水平升高[292,293]。

另一个促进APC功能的靶点是CD40。CD40属于TNF受体(tumor necrosis factor receptor,TNFR)超家族(见下文),其与配体结合对细胞免疫非常重要,至少体现在诱导DC分泌IL-12的过程中。CD40对体液免疫反应的亲和力成熟和重链类别转换也有重要影响[228,294]。CD40在B细胞和DC细胞上持续表达,在巨噬细胞、T细胞和非造血细胞如血管内皮细胞表面也有表达[295]。CD40的配体CD40L主要表达于活化的$CD4^+$ T辅助细胞,pDC、活化的NK细胞和血小板也有CD40L表达。DC上的CD40与配体结合后使之成为"条件性"DC(增强了活化和共刺激能力),为$CD4^+$ T辅助细胞诱导$CD8^+$ CTL的产生提供短暂的桥梁作用。这个功能可能依赖于CD27与CD70的相互作用,因为在一个小鼠淋巴瘤模型中,阻断CD70便可消除CD40抗体的保护作用[296]。刺激CD40能通过多种途径影响抗肿瘤反应[297,298]。首先,很多淋巴瘤和肿瘤细胞表面表达CD40,CD40抗体可以诱发补体或抗体依赖的细胞毒反应(CDC或ADCC)。其次,据报道,在一些肿瘤细胞,尤其是高等级的B细胞非霍奇金淋巴瘤(NHL)和上皮癌中CD40信号途径能直接诱导肿瘤凋亡反应[299-301]。最后,CD40结合配体后可以直接提高抗原呈递能力,尤其在B细胞淋巴瘤中;或间接促进对免疫系统呈递肿瘤抗原,至少能部分替代$CD4^+$T辅助细胞以产生有效持久的抗肿瘤CTL应答[302-304]。CD40与配体或刺激性单抗结合后,能在体外或在多种恶性肿瘤小鼠模型体内促进抗肿瘤疫苗的效能[297,305]。利用DC疫苗或者通过重组腺病毒载体使B细胞肿瘤如慢性淋巴细胞白血病,过表达CD40配体,可以增强T细胞的抗肿瘤应答,诱发一定水平的临床效应[306,307]。当然,这些反应可能短暂且不稳定,并可能快速触发机体免疫抑制环路(例如调节性T细胞),这提示联合多种方法可能会更有效[143]。联合应用CD40配体三聚体或CD40抗体的临床试验证明,靶向肿瘤细胞和/或APC上的CD40能在少数患者,尤其B细胞淋巴瘤或黑色素瘤患者体内诱发抗肿瘤反应,但同时也记录到包括全身炎症反应及静脉血栓形成在内的毒副作用[308-310]。一种新方法可利用电穿孔,将编码CD40配体、活化TLR4、CD70和多种黑色素瘤肿瘤抗原的mRNA导入自体DC(TriMix-DC)。17例接受干扰素-α-2b联合TriMix-DC治疗的患者中,有6例观察到肿瘤的消退[311]。另外,联合使用抗CD40抗体和化疗药吉西他滨,在小鼠模型和临床试验中都观察到了肿瘤的消退[312]。这些抗肿瘤效应是因为浸润肿瘤基质的巨噬细胞被激活了。上述试剂可作为将来联合治疗策略非常有价值的组成部分[313]。

直接促进T细胞功能

免疫活化主要受到T细胞表达的两个主要共受体家族的调节:免疫球蛋白(Ig)样超家族和TNFR超家族[314,315]。前者包括CD28和可诱导T细胞共刺激因子(ICOS),而OX40、CD27、4-1BB、CD30、GITR(glucocorticoid-induced TNFR family related gene,糖皮质激素诱导的TNFR家族相关基因)和HVEM(herpes-virus entry mediator,疱疹病毒侵入介质)属于后者。最广为人知、研究最充分的的免疫球蛋白"共刺激"家族的抑制因子包括CTLA-4和程序化细胞死亡因子1(programmed cell death 1,PD-1)。B和T淋巴细胞衰减因子(B-and T-lymphocyte attenuator,BTLA)是近期阐述最多的家族成员,同样表现出对T细胞活性的抑制作用[316]。B7配体家族新成员(B7-H3和B7x/B7-H4)的受体的特性尚不明了,但是这些受体同样可以介导重要的抑制活性。考虑到这些新确认的配体在组织内的分布,其受体的抑制活性在外周组织中或许更强。因为可提高T细胞数量和功能以及维持免疫记忆性的作用,刺激性或阻断性单克隆抗体(图67-1)得到了广泛的研究[317,318]。

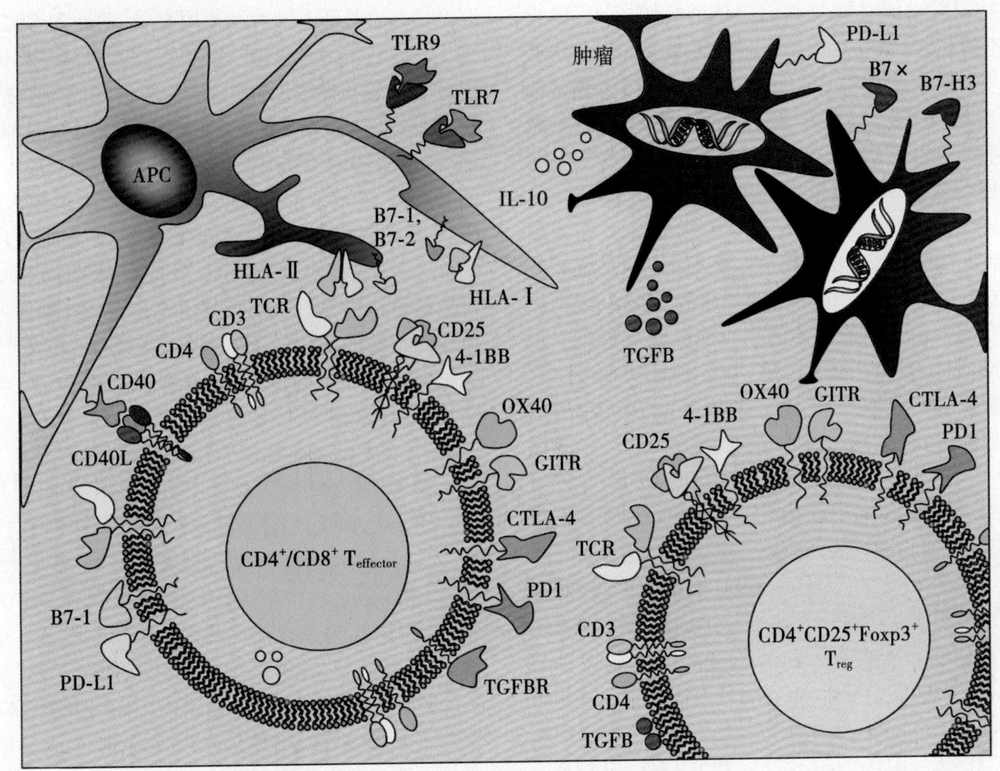

图 67-1 免疫刺激治疗的潜在靶点。大多数在激活效应细胞时被上调的 T 细胞共受体也由调节性 T 细胞群体表达，这两种细胞类型都可能是治疗干预的重要靶点

4-1BB(CD137)、OX40(CD134)和 GITR 的刺激性抗体—强化阳性作用?

TNFR 家族的许多成员都是靶向治疗极具吸引力的候选对象。迄今为止，尽管竞争性抗 CD27 抗体确实表现出可能成为提高抗肿瘤免疫性靶点的潜能，但其在小鼠肿瘤模型中的资料还不多见[296]。更多的关注集中在 4-1BB 和 OX40 上。4-1BB 表达在活化的 T 细胞(包括 Treg 和 NKT 细胞)、活化的 NK 和 DC 细胞、嗜酸性粒细胞、肥大细胞和一些转移性肿瘤的上皮细胞中[315,319-321]。4-1BB 的配体 4-1BBL 表达在活化的 DC、B 细胞和巨噬细胞表面。4-1BBL 与 T 细胞连接后导致抗凋亡基因的上调，保护细胞免于活化诱导的细胞死亡(activation-induced cell death，AICD)[322]，增加持久记忆性 CTL 的生成[323]。经过抗原刺激的 T 细胞中 4-1BB 的表达上调，提示抗 4-1BB 抗体可不同程度地靶向这些致敏的 T 细胞，优先影响那些带有高亲和力受体的 T 细胞，这部分解释了 4-1BB 在产生用于过继性治疗的抗原特异性细胞上优于 CD28 共刺激因子的原因[217]。anti-4-1BB 的作用除了最主要的 $CD8^+$ T 细胞的共刺激外，还有其他许多免疫调节作用。因此，从我们对免疫共刺激抗体功能的理解得出一个结论：抗体的功能具有多样性，这反映了受体在细胞分布上的不同。这些功能主要包括：①活化 APC[324]；②降低 Treg 的抑制能力[325]或者提高效应细胞的抗抑制能力[326]；③对 $CD4^+$ 和 $CD8^+$ T 细胞的共刺激。以上功能都有实验数据支持。而且，活化的 NK 细胞(可能相当于产生 IFN-γ 的杀伤性 DC)、IKDC[327-329]和 NKT 细胞或许可以成为抗肿瘤治疗的靶向细胞[320,321,330,331]。最近，在这些分子免疫调节功能研究中，另一个关注点是对表达 Ig 或 TNFR 超家族成员(见下述 GITR：GITRL、CTLA-4：B7 和 PD-1：PD-L1)配体的细胞信号进行逆转。就 4-1BBL 来说，这样可以提高炎症介质的产量，增强细胞的黏附能力，帮助效应细胞迁移到达炎症位点[332,333]。关于 4-1BB 连接到 T_{reg} 后，究竟是引起免疫抑制作用的增强还是减弱尚存在争议[325,334,335]，其抗肿瘤活性与其他可靶向 T_{reg} 数量/功能的方法协同作用可作为证据，证明 4-1BB 介导的 T_{reg} 的抑制作用相对来说是温和的[336-338]。4-1BBL 在小鼠肿瘤中的高表达在提高肿瘤免疫原性的同时降低了免疫活化受体的移植率，而在相对低免疫原性的肿瘤中，未转染细胞的生长只受到了轻微的影响[320]。竞争性抗 4-1BB 单克隆抗体(即人工制造的配体)提高了 CTL 的抗肿瘤反应，使其可以抑制同源肿瘤细胞系[339-341]。这种抗肿瘤活性严重依赖 $CD8^+$T 细胞(多数研究均证明这一点)和 NK 细胞，而 $CD4^+$T 细胞在不同的肿瘤模型中发挥不同的作用[320,340-343]。就像与其他免疫刺激抗体联合应用一样，与免疫疫苗联合应用可以使低免疫原性肿瘤模型中 CTL 的活性得以提高[344,345]。与转基因的肿瘤特异性 CTL 联合注射能够提高抗肿瘤活性，而且这种提高是通过降低 AICD 而不是通过提高增殖来实现的[346]。这些研究证实了即使在缺少正常调节机制的免疫缺陷宿主(RAG2-/-)体内，没有 $CD4^+$T 细胞的帮助，抗 4-1BB 抗体同样可以发挥作用。早期使用人源化的临床级别抗体(BMS-603513)靶向黑色素瘤和肾细胞癌的患者[347]，抗体产生了很好的耐受，并观察到一些抗肿瘤效应(在 6%的黑色素瘤患者中出现部分应答)，再次证明了评价组合方法效果(以及确定合适剂量的策略)的必要性[336,348,349]。

抗 4-1BB 单抗有两个有趣而且看似矛盾的特点：可以改善

小鼠的自身免疫[350-352],同时抑制它们的体液免疫[353]。尽管确切的机制仍不清楚,但是存在以下几种可能性:对 Treg 功能的作用,干扰 $CD4^+$ T 细胞活性(可能通过介导分泌 IFN-γ 的 $CD^{11c+}CD^{8+}$ T 细胞增殖[354]),或者 IFN-γ 依赖的 IDO 诱导[351,352]。这突出了免疫调节干预时间的重要性,因为如果与抗原相遇后立即与抗 4-1BB 抗体结合,引起的 AICD 可导致 CD4 的下调,同样的情形也会发生在 $CD8^+$T 细胞身上[355,356]。就减少抗体介导毒性来说,这种抑制活性具有一定的优点,但对抗肿瘤免疫的发展却是不利的。在小鼠模型中联合应用抗 CD137 抗体和直接靶向肿瘤的抗体的临床前试验观察到了很有前景的抗肿瘤活性。最近,抗 CD-137 抗体被证实在小鼠移植模型中可以增加西妥昔单抗(一种靶向 EGFR 的单抗)的效力[357],这使其成为了联合治疗的又一个合适的靶点。在 B 细胞淋巴瘤中联用 PF-05082566(辉瑞公司开发的 CD137 单抗)和利妥昔单抗,以及在实体瘤中联用 PF-05082566 和 MK-3475(一种 PD-1 抑制剂)的临床试验都在进行中。

OX40 瞬时表达在活化的 $CD4^+$ 和 $CD8^+$ T 细胞上,起到后期共刺激受体的作用[315,358]。NKT 细胞和 T_{reg} 上也可以表达 OX40,但在 NKT 细胞上的表达需要通过 a-Galcer 的适当活化来激发[359]。OX40 的配体 OX40L 的表达分布类似于 4-1BBL,主要在活化的 DC、B 细胞和巨噬细胞,以及活化 T 细胞和内皮细胞表面[315]。OX40 与配体的结合可以调节 $CD4^+$ 和 $CD8^+$T 细胞的存活和记忆产生,阻止 T 细胞耐受[360-363]。OX40 与配体相互作用也可以削弱 T_{reg} 抑制功能[364,365]。而且,激发 OX40 可拮抗抗原反应性幼稚 $CD4^+$ T 细胞中 Foxp3 的诱导,有效地抑制 iT_{reg}($CD4^+$ T 细胞在外周被诱导表达 FOXP3,进而获得免疫抑制功能,就成为 iT_{reg} 细胞)的产生[366,367],并阻止分泌 IL-10 的 Tr1 细胞的产生[368]。这些都说明 OX40 可以阻断多种不同的被诱导出的调节性 T 细胞。4-1BB 和 OX40 可以独立地辅助强化 $CD8^+$和 $CD4^+$细胞的记忆应答,它们的细胞内信号通路存在部分重叠[369]。然而,4-1BB 或者 GITR 都不能阻断 Th1 细胞的产生[368]。目前,尚无报道阐明它们是否可以影响 $Foxp3^+$ iTreg 的诱导和产生。与 4-1BBL 一样,在肿瘤细胞中强制表达 OX40L 可以增强其免疫原性,产生依赖于 $CD4^+$和 $CD8^+$ T 细胞的免疫排斥[370]。而且,在肿瘤内部注射高表达 OX40L 的 DC,可以在小鼠模型中产生依赖于 $CD8^+$CTL 应答的肿瘤排斥,它们本身依赖于 $CD4^+$ T 细胞和 NKT 细胞[359]。在一些移植肿瘤模型中,竞争性抗 OX40 抗体可提高抗肿瘤活性[371]。效应和调节部分的伴随作用也许是对肿瘤产生有效排斥的先决条件[81]。在临床前模型中,联合使用 OX40 可以提高其他几种免疫刺激方案的效果[372-376]。在一项 I 期临床试验中,使用鼠源单抗(mAb)对晚期癌症患者的 OX40 信号传导进行阻断,观察到用一个疗程的抗 OX40 mAb 治疗的患者,毒理学是可接受的,而且在 30 例患者中,有 12 个患者至少一个转移灶消退了[377]。

与 4-1BB 和 OX40 一样,GITR 瞬时表达在活化的 T 细胞上[378,379]。它也高表达在 T_{reg} 细胞上,活化后其表达量进一步提高[380,381]。它的配体 GITR-L 在 B 细胞、巨噬细胞和一些 DC 细胞上低水平表达,活化后瞬时表达增加。GITR 结合可以刺激 $CD4^+$和 $CD8^+$ T 细胞的增殖和功能[382],然而,它对 T_{reg} 的作用一直存在很大的争议[383,384]。在 $CD4^+$ $CD25^-$效应细胞和 $CD4^+$ $CD25^+$ T_{reg} 共培养中,抗 GITR 抗体可降低抑制作用,但这究竟是与降低 T_{reg} 的抑制作用有关,还是与增强了效应细胞抵抗 T_{reg} 抑制作用有关,或者是两者的结合作用,仍然没有阐明。$GITR^{+}/^{+}$效应细胞和 $GITR^{-}/^{-}$调节性细胞混合培养实验提示,GITR 与效应细胞而非调节细胞的结合对解除抑制是至关重要的[384]。这表明,对于体外分析而言,增强效应细胞对抑制作用的耐受是十分关键的。向 B16 黑色素瘤组织内注射表达重组 GITR-L 的腺病毒,可以提高 T 细胞的浸润能力,缩小肿瘤体积[385]。已经证实,在经 B16 黑色素瘤激发后,竞争性抗 GITR 抗体既可以增强对甲基胆蒽诱导产生的纤维肉瘤的作用,又可以提高系统的抗肿瘤反应和伴随免疫功能[386,387]。而且,同样的抗体也可以提高 DNA 疫苗所产生系统免疫功能的效果,提高小鼠对黑色素瘤接种的抵抗[388]。

通过阻断 CTLA-4(CD152)、PD-1(CD279)和 PD-L1(CD274)关键作用点的刺激——消除负性作用

与 TNFR 超家族相反的是,一直以来,人们认为共抑制受体的存在可以介导淋巴细胞活性和功能下调,是 Ig 超家族的一个特征。事实上,在 Ig 超家族中,共抑制受体—配体的数目要多于共刺激成员的数目。10 余年前,Jams Allison 由此提出了把调节或者阻断抑制性检查点(checkpoint)作为治疗性抗肿瘤的一个策略[389]。阻断抑制性免疫检查点为治疗效果带来了极大的希望,特别是当其与其他一些可以提高抗肿瘤免疫交叉致敏的方法联合应用时,可能获得额外或者协同作用。在小鼠模型和临床上的首要策略就是应用 CTLA-4 抗体带来肿瘤的消退[389,390]。

CTLA-4 表达在活化的 $CD4^+$和 $CD8^+$ T 细胞上,其表面表达受到严格调控,半衰期很短。尽管在静息 T 细胞上很难检测到 CTLA-4,但是它也会影响到 T 细胞活化的一些早期事件[391,392]。TCR 交联后,它被快速地从靠近微管组织中心的细胞内囊泡转移到免疫突触[393]。在非磷酸化状态下,一个细胞内定位元件介导它与 AP-2 迅速结合,内吞并靶向到溶酶体[394]。CTLA-4 表达在自然和诱导产生的 $Foxp3^+T_{reg}$ 上。即便是在活化后,CTLA-4 仍多数分布在细胞内。CTLA-4 同一个重要的共刺激分子 CD28 共同分享 B7-1(CD80)和 B7-2(CD86)两个配体。CD28 结合与 TCR 刺激配合,可以通过诱导产生 IL-2 和抗凋亡因子来增强 T 细胞增殖,降低某一既定生物反应所需交联 TCR 的数量[395]。CTLA-4 交联可以选择性地阻断 CD28 介导的共刺激所致基因调控的升高,但它不能阻断 TCR 诱导的基因调控[396]。CTLA-4 作为一个 CD28 依赖型 T 细胞应答的负向调控因子,其作用是通过 CTLA-4 敲除的小鼠证实的,这种小鼠在出生 3~4 周后就会由于 CD4 依赖的多克隆增殖而死亡[397,398]。CTLA-4 与 B7 配体的亲和力要远高于 CD28,它与 B7-1 的亲和力高于 B7-2,而 CD28 与 B7-2 的亲和力大于 B7-1[399]。最初的检测提示,CTLA-4 与 B7 结合的亲和力提高了 100~1 000 倍。近期通过表面等离子体共振实验显示,由于快速的分离速率,这两种分子结合的亲和力比最初的检测低 10 倍。CD28 和 CTLA-4 在突触中累积受到配体结合的影响。在没有 B7-1 和 B7-2 结合的情况下,CD28 可以被募集到突触,但没有很好的稳定性,会被 CTLA-4 破坏。CTLA-4 在突触的集中

则依赖于配体的结合[400]。因此,CTLA-4 会在与 CD28 的配体竞争中胜出,特别是当配体的浓度有限时。它可以通过与 B7-1 产生高亲和力的同型二聚体来将免疫突触中的 CD28 清除[401]。因此,CTLA-4 在时间和空间上的严格调控对于决定 CD28 所介导的信号是至关重要的。而且,CTLA-4 的结合会引起细胞因子(特别是 IL-2 及其受体)产生量的下降,导致细胞周期停止在 G_1 期,提示结合依赖和非结合依赖机制都会对它的负性调控起作用。最后,CTLA-4 还在 T_{reg} 介导的免疫抑制中扮演重要角色。最近的实验表明,在条件敲除(conditional knock-out,CKO)小鼠中,T_{reg} 特异性 CTLA-4 的缺乏与其免疫抑制能力的严重下降相关[112]。CKO 小鼠产生致命的自身免疫性淋巴细胞增生综合征的时间稍慢于 CTLA-4$^{-/-}$小鼠。CTLA-4 介导的与 T_{reg} 相关的效应机制尚不清楚,但它或许与表达 B7 的细胞中的信号逆向传导有关[110,111]。CTLA-4 与 DC 相关 B7 结合后,某些 DC 亚群可被诱导表达 IDO[110,402],可诱导的 cAMP 早期抑制因子和 cAMP 反应调控因子(ICER/CREM)的表达降低了 IL-2 在活化的 CD25$^+$Foxp3$^-$效应 T 细胞中的表达,机制与 B7 介导的信号通路相似[111]。而且,通过对体外抑制作用的分析发现,T_{reg} 介导的抑制作用与 APC 活性的降低有关(证据是 B7 分子在表面表达降低[112])。

用抗体阻断 CTLA-4 在提高二次免疫应答方面特别有效,尤其对于 CD4$^+$T 细胞。抗 CTLA-4 抗体在免疫源性较弱的肿瘤临床前模型中单独应用,其作用效果有限,通常与其他的一些抗肿瘤免疫疗法联合应用[314,318]。这些很有前景的临床试验结果促进了两款人源化 CTLA-4 单抗的开发:ipilimumab (IgG1)和 tremelimumab(IgG2)。Tremelimumab 在早期临床试验中表现出持久的应答[403-405];然而,在晚期黑色素瘤患者中进行的Ⅲ期随机临床试验中,与化疗(达卡巴嗪或替莫唑胺)相比,未能表现出总体生存优势(overall survival advantage)[406]。这一结果主要与临床试验设计有关,而不是 tremelimumab 本身缺乏生物活性。Ipilimumab 的临床进展就相当成熟了,在黑色素瘤、前列腺癌、卵巢癌、肾癌、结直肠癌和肺癌患者中都观察到了反应。在晚期黑色素瘤患者中进行的两项Ⅲ期随机对照临床试验中,ipilimumab 都提高了生存率[407,408]。更值得注意的是,约 20%的患者生存获益超过 4 年,部分患者生存获益超过 10 年[409]。这些临床试验的成功,促使 FDA 批准 ipilimumab 成为晚期黑色素瘤治疗的一线和二线用药。值得注意的是,在最近报道的用 ipilimumab 治疗化疗难治性晚期前列腺癌的Ⅲ期临床试验中,与安慰剂组相比,ipilimumab 改善了中位无进展生存期;然而它并未改善总生存期(P=0.053)[410]。第二项临床试验比较了 ipilimumab 和安慰剂在未接受化疗的转移性前列腺癌患者中的疗效。该Ⅲ期试验已完成,结果将很快报告。

目前已经发现了许多因子,可以作为 ipilimumab 治疗后产生应答的生物标志物。最近的研究表明,TIL 的增加与抗 CTLA-4 治疗的临床应答相关[411]。另外,CD4 T 细胞持续表达 ICOS 也与接受抗 CTLA-4 治疗的黑色素瘤患者的生存相关[412,413]。与此观察结果一致的是,ICOS$^+$ CD4T 细胞频率的增加,也可以作为抗 CTLA-4 治疗的药效学生物标志物[414]。如上所述,ICOS 是 T 细胞的共刺激受体之一。临床前研究表明,ICOS 途径的参与显著增强了抗 CTLA-4 治疗在癌症免疫治疗中的效力[415]。

PD-1 的表达比 CD28 或 CTLA-4 更广泛。在活化的 CD4$^+$、CD8$^+$ T 细胞、B 细胞和单核细胞中都能检测到其表达,在 NKT 细胞中也有低水平表达。它可以结合到两个具有独特表达谱的配体 PD-L1 和 PD-L2 上[150]。PD-L1 广泛表达,在静止和活化的 T 细胞(包括 CD4$^+$CD25$^+$Foxp3$^+$ T_{reg} 细胞)、B 细胞、巨噬细胞、DC 细胞和肥大细胞中均能检测到。此外,PD-L1 在非造血细胞(包括角膜、肺、胰岛、胎盘绒毛合体滋养细胞、角质细胞和血管内皮细胞)中的表达或许与其他受体-配体的功能有关。这种在非造血细胞中的广泛表达,提示 PD-L1/PD-1 的抑制作用或许并不仅仅局限在与 T 细胞和 APC 的相互作用上,也许它与外周组织免疫反应的效应期有关,直接在组织表面协助阻止免疫介导的组织损伤。相比之下,PD-L2 的表达谱十分有限,它在初始和活化的 T 细胞中均不表达,而仅限于活化的巨噬细胞、髓系 DC 和肥大细胞。这说明 PD-L2 扮演着与 PD-L1 完全不同的角色。PD-1$^{-/-}$表型的小鼠提供了这个受体抑制功能的最直接证据[416,417]。这种小鼠能够发展出一系列以高浓度自身抗体为特点的自身免疫疾病,这与它对 T 和/或 B 细胞的负向调节作用相一致。PD-L1 和 PD-L2 或许也能通过逆向信号来调节 T 细胞反应。PD-L2 的交联抗体可以直接诱导 DC 产生免疫调节因子,比如 IL-6 和 TNF-α[418,419],同时保护 DC 避免死亡[420]。另外,PD-1-Ig 可以不受任何 IDO 的影响来抑制 DC 活性,同时提高 IL-10 的产量[421]。

近期的研究证实,PD-L1 可以与 B7-1 结合,而且其亲和力介于 CTLA-4 和 CD28 之间[422]。这种结合比较特异,而且是双向的,可以通过 B7-1 或者 PD-L1 来抑制 T 细胞的增殖和因子产生。因此,通过 TCR 和 CD28 传递的 T 细胞活化信号便可以与通过 CTLA-4 和 PD-L1(通过 APC 上的 B7-1,也可能通过其他 T 细胞上的 B7-1 和 PD-1),PD-1 和 B7-1(通过 APC 上的 PD-L1,也可能通过其他 T 细胞上的 CTLA-4,PD-1 和 PD-L1)传递的共抑制信号。最后,通过 PD-1 和 B7-1(通过非造血组织上的 PD-L1)介导的抑制性信号转导可能影响外周接触抗原的最终结果。这将导致受各种受体和配体瞬时表达谱的影响,一个本来就令人困惑、复杂的细胞固有抑制信号变得更加错综复杂。其中各种元素相对重要性的等级仍不清楚,它们可能在不同 T 细胞亚群中有所区别。这个如此复杂和明显交叉的体系中有一些是备份重复。这些发现在生理学上的联系仍不确定,但 PD-1:PD-L1/PD-L2 确实已经成为提高肿瘤免疫尝试中一个有吸引力的治疗靶点。同时阻断 CTLA-4 和 PD-L1 或许可以通过 CTLA-4、B7-1、PD-L1 和 PD-1 来清除细胞固有的负向信号,而利于 CD28 的正向信号。最近的实验结果突出了这种途径与 T 细胞对病原体的慢性反应之间的联系[423-426]。在慢性 LCMV 感染中,抗原特异性的 CD8+T 细胞受到损伤。这些受损 T 细胞中的 PD-1 选择性上调,体内注射抗 PD-L1 抗体可以提高 T 细胞增殖和因子产生,恢复它们的活性,同时降低病毒负荷[423]。与上述类似,在人体中,HIV 特异性 CD8+T 细胞中 PD-1 的上调与 T 细胞损伤和疾病进展有关[424]。最后,近期的报道证实,处于疾病进展期的 HIV 患者,其病毒特异性 CD4$^+$ T 细胞中的 PD-1 和 CTLA-4 均上调,两者的表达与疾病进展及再次刺激无法产生 IL-2 直接相关[427]。所有这些资料提示,阻断 PD-1 和/或 PD-L1 能够恢复 T 细胞的功能。这种方法不仅可以应用于恢复 T 细胞对慢性感染的反应,还可以用于提高 T 细胞对其他慢性疾病比如肿瘤的活性。

PD-L1 在各种人类和小鼠肿瘤中都有表达，PD-1 同样可以在 TIL 中表达。这带来一种假说：PD-L1 分子或许在限制肿瘤内效应 T 细胞应答中起到重要作用。从人类卵巢癌患者的肿瘤或者淋巴结中分离得到的髓系 DC 中高表达 PD-L1。只有将 PD-L1 阻断后，这些 DC 才能提高 T 细胞的活性[428]。同样地，肿瘤引流淋巴结中的 pDC 产生的高水平的 IDO 可以活化 T_{reg}，上调 DC 中的 PD-L1，并负调控 T 细胞应答[75]。PD-L1 在多种人类肿瘤（乳腺癌、子宫颈癌、肺癌、卵巢癌、结肠癌、肾癌）以及黑色素瘤、恶性胶质瘤中和一些造血系统恶性肿瘤中都有表达[57,429-433]。它的表达与膀胱癌、乳腺癌、肾癌、胃癌、胰腺癌等预后较差直接相关[59,431,434]。在小鼠肿瘤细胞系中，强制表达 PD-L1 能够削弱 T 细胞在体外的活性和对肿瘤的杀伤能力，显著地促进肿瘤在体内的生长，抗 PD-L1 抗体能够阻断这种效果[435,436]。在 4T1 乳腺癌模型中，PD-L1 在体内的表达被肿瘤上调，使肿瘤难以被抗 4-1BB 抗体免疫治疗治愈。同时注射抗 PD-L1 抗体会引起显著的肿瘤抑制[437]。同样的，抗 PD-L1 抗体可以延缓表达 PD-L1 的小鼠骨髓瘤细胞在体内的生长。已证实，阻断 PD-L1 可以与 ACT 协同作用，抑制鳞状细胞癌的生长[436]。而且，过继性回输 $PD1^{-}/^{-}$肿瘤反应 $CD8^{+}$T 细胞可抑制 B16 黑色素瘤生长，而野生型和 CTLA-$4^{-}/^{-}$肿瘤反应性 CD8T 细胞均不能产生这种作用[429]。在上述研究中，在效应 T 细胞阶段而非致敏 T 细胞阶段封闭 PD-L1 能产生与 $PD1^{-}/^{-}$肿瘤反应性 $CD8^{+}$ T 细胞介导的类似的抗肿瘤效果。这说明 CTLA-4 在调控 $CD4^{+}$ T 细胞免疫反应中发挥了重要作用[438]，而 PD-1 对调节 $CD8^{+}$效应性 T 细胞对肿瘤细胞的攻击是至关重要的。

尽管阻断 PD-L1 已被证实能有效促进 T 细胞抗肿瘤反应，然而，关于阻断 PD-1 是否能直接促进体内 T 细胞抗肿瘤效应的研究尚不多见。研究发现，当把抗 PD-1 抗体注入脾脏（以及遗传学上去除）能延缓 B16 黑色素瘤向肝脏的转移。在相同的研究中，给予抗 PD-1 治疗显示能阻断静脉注入的 CT26 结肠肿瘤转移至肺脏[439]。新近一项研究发现，封闭 PD-1 以及 PD-L1 能小幅度延缓小鼠胰管肿瘤的生长速度，且这种下调具有统计学意义[440]。

这些临床前的成功已经转化为临床应用。一项在复发或难治性霍奇金淋巴瘤患者中进行的Ⅰ期临床试验，使用人 IgG4 抗 PD-1 单抗（nivolumab），20 名（87%）患者中观察到了临床应答，并在 17%的患者身上观察到了完全的应答[441]。单独使用 nivolumab 的Ⅰ期临床试验中，nivolumab 对晚期 NSCLC、RCC 和黑色素瘤患者的客观缓解率分别为 18%，27%和 28%[442]。一项随机对照Ⅲ期临床研究比较了 nivolumab 与化疗（达卡巴嗪）用于未经治疗的黑色素瘤患者（无 BRAF 突变型）的效果，nivolumab 组的整体反应率更好（40% vs 14%）[443]。在 ipilimumab 难治性晚期黑色素瘤患者中进行的另一项Ⅲ期临床试验比较了 nivolumab 与化疗（达卡巴嗪或卡铂加紫杉醇），总体反应率分别为 32%和 11%[444]；这些试验结果促使 FDA 加速批准 nivolumab 用于不可切除的或转移性黑色素瘤患者，这些患者用其他药物治疗都是无效的。

与这些研究结果一致，另一种靶向 PD-1 的药物 pembrolizumab（人源化 IgG4 单抗）在Ⅰ期临床试验中，治疗 ipilimumab 难治性晚期黑色素瘤患者的总体反应率为 26%，这一结果促使 FDA 加速批准了 pembrolizumab[445]。对于 brentuximab vedotin（FDA 2017 年批准的一种治疗霍奇金淋巴瘤的抗体药）治疗失败的霍奇金淋巴瘤患者，pembrolizumab 治疗的总体反应率为 53%[446]。这些研究表明，nivolumab 和 pembrolizumab 在多种恶性实体瘤患者中有显著的临床作用，且对相当比例的血液系统恶性肿瘤患者也有很好的疗效。

针对 PD-1 的配体 PD-L1 的药物也观察到很有希望的临床结果。用抗 PD-L1 的单抗（人 IgG4 单抗，BMS-936559）在晚期 NSCLC、黑色素瘤和 RCC 患者中进行的Ⅰ期临床试验的客观缓解率为 6% ~ 17%[447]。另一种靶向 PD-L1 的单抗（MPDL3280A，人 IgG1），在 Fc 段做了修饰，可以消除 ADCC。MPDL3280A 在包括 NSCLC、黑色素瘤、RCC、结直肠癌、胃癌和头颈部鳞状细胞癌在内的多种恶性实体瘤中的客观缓解率为 13%~26%[448]。值得注意的是，MPDL3280A 在膀胱癌中的客观缓解率为 26%，而膀胱癌是一种在过去 30 年中治疗方法都没有进展的恶性肿瘤[449]。目前正在评估其他靶向 PD-1 的药物如 pidilizumab（人源化 IgG1 单抗）和 MEDI0680（人源化 IgG4 单抗），以及靶向 PD-L1 的药物 MEDI4736（人源化 IgG1 单抗）和 MSB0010718C（人源化 IgG1 单抗）在多种恶性肿瘤中的作用。这些结果表明，靶向免疫检查点（CTLA-4，PD-1，PD-L1）的单一疗法，有望成为黑色素瘤和其他多种恶性肿瘤的标准治疗。

其他 Ig 超家族抑制性成员分子也可能成为协同免疫抑制的靶点，尽管目前这种抗肿瘤效应尚停留在假设阶段。迄今为止尚未鉴定出的 B7x（B7-H4）[450-452]配体的受体则可能为研究对象[453,454]。目前，对 B7-H3 及其抗肿瘤效应的解释仍存在一定的矛盾[314]。BTLA（B 和 T 细胞衰减因子，CD272）同样是一个潜在的靶标分子，由于 BTLA 是 Ig 超家族成员之一，其配体又是 TNFR 家族成员之一[455]，因此 BTLA 可能在两类重要的协同刺激分子家族间建立起一种关联[456]。

靶向 T_{reg} 的抑制功能

由于 T_{reg} 可以在肿瘤局部介导免疫豁免的重要性，因此下调 T_{reg} 的数量或削弱其抑制性功能的免疫治疗策略颇具吸引力。针对 T_{reg} 功能的小分子抑制剂可以成为我们目前治疗策略的有益补充。从以前的讨论可知，直接靶向 Ig 和 TNFR 超家族成员的治疗，对免疫调节功能和效应功能均有影响。这种双重功能可在增强正向免疫效应的同时下调抑制功能（和/或增强对抑制效应的抵抗），这对临床前和临床治疗应用来说十分重要。激发 TLR8 能逆转 T_{reg} 介导的抑制性功能，并对抑制性 γδT 细胞亚群产生抑制作用[284,285]。

另一类下调 T_{reg} 功能的替代方法是通过耗竭 T_{reg} 来实现的。破坏 T_{reg} 对建立并维持瘤内耐受具有重要作用，而这一认识部分是基于对 CD25 缺失时肿瘤的发生发展的研究得来的。抗 CD25 单抗（如 PC61）在一系列小鼠肿瘤模型中都具有抗肿瘤活性[122,457-460]。这种抗肿瘤活性只有在肿瘤接种前给予该单抗才有明显效果，当肿瘤一旦形成，上述活性就有限了。此外，目前认为，抗体在肿瘤生长部位缺乏有效的浸润及浓度积累，也是导致临床治疗失败的原因之一，这进一步验证了一个原理：全身性免疫应答的产生不足以发挥有效的抗肿瘤活性[36]。再者，T_{reg} 耗竭可能只是短期的，涉及 T_{reg} 天然状态下

的快速增殖及外周 $CD4^+Foxp3^-$ 前体细胞的转变[97,100]。而 T_{reg} 耗竭持续时间又与参与耗竭的因子发挥功能的半衰期相关。在人体的研究中，使用 IL-2 或抗 CD25 作为介导不同毒素的载体，地尼白介素-2（Ontak）作为融合蛋白，将白喉杆菌用来结合受体的结构域替换为 IL-2，从而介导白喉毒素杀伤过表达 IL-2 受体的细胞。体外实验证实，这种融合蛋白能与细胞表面高、中等亲和力 IL-2 受体相互作用并完成内吞过程。在后续的裂解过程中，将白喉毒素释放入胞质，抑制胞内蛋白的合成，导致细胞快速死亡。与单克隆抗体相比较，其特点是半衰期短（60 分钟左右）。对卵巢及肾癌进行的初步研究表明，给予白喉毒素治疗后可在早期引起循环系统中 T_{reg} 数量降低，维持 $CD4^+CD25^{int}$ 记忆性 T 细胞库[461]，而在长期反复给予白喉毒素时可耗竭 $CD25^+$ 效应性 T 细胞[462]。在使用肿瘤 RNA 转染 DC 疫苗前，给予地尼白介素-2 治疗，可增强肿瘤免疫，这一点在随后的体外 DC 疫苗特异性细胞因子分泌水平的检测中得到证实[461]。而关于体内的抗肿瘤效应目前仍处于临床前研究中。然而，在已建立的小鼠模型中，维持抗肿瘤活性与增强系统性免疫功能相比更为困难，而且耗竭 T_{reg} 的持久性似乎也很重要[463,464]。此外，通过其他一些方法也可实现上述耗竭 T_{reg} 的目的，如将抗 CD25 单抗与截短形式的假单胞菌外毒素 A[465] 或蓖麻毒素[466] 进行融合。这些改进方法都意在调控 T_{reg} 的功能而非其数量。如果这些方案能针对肿瘤微环境可发挥作用，那么由免疫治疗引发的一些危险如自身免疫损伤等将得到一定程度的控制。根据我们对 T_{reg} 的产生及增殖方面已具备的认知，目前可以考虑更多的免疫治疗手段，抑制 IDO 信号通路或 TGF-β，以下调外周 T_{reg} 转化的速率，同时影响肿瘤内免疫豁免的状态[125,467-470]。

细胞因子——免疫应答的细胞间介质

在过继细胞治疗部分中，已论述了细胞因子（cytokine）在免疫治疗中的应用。在体内免疫治疗中较少涉及关于细胞因子的抗肿瘤活性研究成果，部分原因在于多数细胞因子具有多效性，以及高剂量的细胞因子治疗时会出现副作用（如 IL-2 和 IFN-α）。IL-15 和 IL-21 两者均属于 γ-链家族的细胞因子，目前都备受关注。IL-15 在调节小鼠和人类 $CD4^+$ 记忆性 T 细胞稳定性中发挥着不同的作用，给予 IL-15 刺激时人类 $CD4^+$ 记忆性 T 细胞产生并发生增殖，而小鼠 T 细胞对 IL-15 却没有明显反应[471,472]。其他有关 IL-15 的生理性活性见于对单核细胞、巨噬细胞、树突状细胞及基质细胞的作用。IL-15 还有激活 NK 细胞，参与维持 $CD8^+$ 记忆性 T 细胞高水平应答，促进 DC 表达 MHC-Ⅰ类分子等作用[473,474]。给予外源性 IL-15 或通过接种肿瘤疫苗而分泌的内源性 IL-15 还可增强 $CD8^+$ T 细胞对疫苗接种的免疫应答效应，促进其抗肿瘤活性，因而 IL-15 在临床应用前景较乐观[220,223,475]。基于 IL-15 的超激动剂 ALT-803 促进了记忆性 $CD8^+$T 细胞从抗原非依赖型向着天生性效应细胞转变，后者在小鼠癌症模型中有抗肿瘤活性[476]。目前 ALT-803 正在血液和实体恶性肿瘤中做Ⅰ期临床试验。IL-21 主要由 NKT 细胞及 $CD4^+$T 细胞产生，IL-21 能促进 $CD8^+$T 细胞、NK 细胞和 NKT 细胞的增殖及功能活性，并影响 B 细胞的分化[477]。此外，IL-21 还能削弱 T_{reg} 的抑制功能[478]。在许多小鼠模型中，IL-21 无论是单独给予或联合其他细胞因子（IL-15、IL-2、凋亡诱导抗体、CD1d 反应性糖脂或协同刺激剂），均可促进免疫细胞的抗肿瘤活性[479-482]。在早期临床试验中，重组的人 IL-21 在患者体内的耐受性较好，尽管目前肯定 IL-21 的抗肿瘤效应尚为时过早，但 IL-21 确实能够激活 NK 细胞、$CD8^+$T 细胞的免疫活性[483,484]。

并非所有细胞因子都发挥免疫激活作用，如肿瘤细胞可分泌免疫抑制性细胞因子或通过调节基质细胞使其分泌这类抑制性细胞因子。IL-10 和 TGF-β 均为免疫治疗中涉及的抑制性细胞因子，靶向 TGF-β 的疗效在小鼠肿瘤模型中已被证实[67,69]，在多发性硬化症的临床治疗中 IL-10 也得到了相应的应用。

联合免疫治疗

临床前期模型及早期临床研究均显示，多种方法组合形成的联合治疗方案能有效清除低免疫源性的肿瘤。最近的文献证明了许多组合治疗可能产生协同或累加效应。虽然确定哪种组合治疗会达到最佳效果依然很具有挑战性，但从基本的治疗原则出发，有助于找出效果最佳的组合。我们可简化设计免疫治疗方案，如：①增强抗原呈递或增强其免疫原性（如疫苗、CpG）；②直接促进效应 T 细胞的功能、增加其数量和延长其活性维持时间（如竞争性抗 TNFR 抗体、细胞因子等）；③清除或关闭细胞内在及外在的免疫检查点（如阻断 CTLA-4 或 PD-1，T_{reg} 耗竭，以及使用竞争性抗 INPR 抗体）；④“重塑”免疫系统，利用淋巴细胞微环境促进其免疫细胞增殖（如 ACT）；⑤增强抗原特异性或促进 T 细胞受体与肿瘤抗原的亲和力（如 CAR 和 TCR 基因治疗）。一些免疫制剂可将不同治疗方案联系起来，增强免疫正向功能，同时减少免疫抑制效应，如单一药物可通过同时阻断 CTLA-4 和刺激 OX40，既然近期资料强调在调控性免疫检查点上施加影响，可直接限制免疫刺激治疗的效果，那么联合治疗策略中至少包含一种使免疫检查点抑制剂在理论上是具有吸引力的。如联合抗 CTLA-4 与疫苗[466,485,486]、T_{reg} 耗竭[487] 或抗-4-1BB[488] 治疗能显著地增强治疗活性。类似的联合应用还见于抗 4-1BB 抗体与其他方式的组合[330,348,372]。以下为联合三种免疫治疗方案的一个例证：在临床前研究的模型中，应用抗体直接针对死亡诱导 TNF 相关凋亡诱导配体受体（TRAIL-R）、CD40 及 4-1BB，可在 TRAIL 敏感的小鼠肿瘤模型中观察到抗肿瘤活性增强[313]。诱导肿瘤细胞凋亡、抗原释放，并通过抗 DR5 抗体（抗 TRAIL-R）募集固有免疫细胞到肿瘤位点，同时增强抗 CD40 诱导的 DC 功能，并通过抗 4-1BB 抗体加强肿瘤特异性 CTL 的诱导、活化和存活，这都是有利于增强抗肿瘤活性的重要方法[489,490]。此外，利用 CpG 替代抗 CD40，通过 NKT 细胞活化来放大 DC 的功能，亦可达到类似的效果[331]。利用多种策略协同治疗方案的另一个优势在于能减少单一药物高剂量使用所致的毒副作用（如免疫反应可限于针对肿瘤相关抗原而非广泛的自身抗原）。为不同的疗法安排合适的顺序和时机，是联合治疗中需考虑的一个重要方面。

临床前研究表明，同时靶向 CTLA-4 和 PD-1，与单一疗法相比可以显著提升治疗效果[491]。一项Ⅰ期临床试验评估了在晚期黑色素瘤患者中联用不同剂量的 ipilimumab(CTLA-4 抑制剂)和 novolumab(PD-1 抑制剂)的治疗效果(一共 4 个队列)。总体客观缓解率 40%,4 个队列中最大剂量且毒性可控的一组客观缓解率为 53%[492]。这一队列的一年期和两年期总生存率分别为 94%和 88%,这也是从未见过的好结果。

在患有转移性肾细胞癌的患者中,联用 ipilimumab 和 nivolumab 的最佳疗法可以在 6 个月治疗后达到 40%的缓解率[493]。同样在转移性肾细胞癌患者中,联用 PD-1 抑制剂(nivolumab)和靶向药酪氨酸激酶抑制剂 sunitinib/pazopanib,六个月治疗后,缓解率也能分别达到 52%、45%[494]。联用抗 CTLA-4 和抗 PD-1 的Ⅲ期临床试验正在进行中。

免疫治疗药物引发的不同毒性

与临床反应的情况一样,抗 CTLA-4 和抗 PD-1 疗法的不良事件与常规化疗不同,更多地表现为与免疫系统的全身激活和炎症样状态有关,例如结肠炎、葡萄膜炎、垂体炎和皮炎等[495-500]。这些不良事件有一个特定的名字,叫免疫相关不良事件(immune-related adverse events),或者简写为 irAEs。大多数 irAEs 都可以自发或在使用皮质类固醇的情况下实现可控或逆转。之前批准的细胞因子疗法,如高剂量 IL-2,由于可能发生严重的毛细血管渗漏综合征,需要与重症监护病房相当的医疗条件[501],而抗 CTLA-4 治疗不需要这么高的监护条件,在临床试验中可以在门诊完成每次的静脉输注。治疗后出现的大多数 irAEs 可以在门诊环境下管理。使用皮质类固醇治疗 irAEs 不会影响抗 CTLA-4 抗体的抗肿瘤作用[502]。

范式的转变——从免疫辅助治疗到免疫支持疗法?

近期对于免疫疗法的关注点集中于免疫疗法提高常规化疗或放疗效果的潜力[503],并致力于最大化肿瘤细胞死亡后的免疫原性提升。细胞毒性化疗似乎可以诱导一个适合呈递肿瘤抗原的环境[504]。更多的益处包括可能增加抗原交叉呈递[505],DC 的部分激活[506],以及细胞毒 T 细胞介导的肿瘤细胞溶解的部分致敏作用[507]。虽然目前的人体研究很少有证据表明上述因素对免疫治疗效果的重要性,但增强体内细胞死亡后免疫原性,以及诸如 CpG 等药物的一个共同作用就是,肿瘤可能转变为自身多价细胞疫苗,可以呈现某种肿瘤自己的抗原表位,并有利于肿瘤特异性免疫。这就解决了以往必须充分了解相关目的抗原再进行相应的抗体设计和生产的问题,因为目的抗原非常多,在用抗体治疗之前,也并不知道具体针对哪一种效果好,会造成人力物力的极大浪费后依然难以探索出有效的治疗方法。我们开始利用肿瘤细胞因其基因不稳定性带来的潜在的新免疫原性的优势[508,509],从传统的抗肿瘤治疗转变为免疫治疗,而不是将肿瘤免疫治疗仅仅视为一种辅助方法。

未来,我们将面临诸多艰巨的挑战。我们需要在小鼠模型中仔细研究相关机制,以确定最理想的联合免疫治疗方案;寻找治疗过程中可靠的预测分子,就像根据肿瘤的遗传轮廓和基质浸润情况制定化疗方案那样。最后,对患者的状态进行调整,以获得有利于治疗的免疫学状态,这一想法还需要在比较性研究中证明它对肿瘤免疫治疗的价值,和远超目前生物标志物的预后意义。

(岳圆 译,王孟昭 审校)

参考文献

The complete reference list can be found on the Wiley Companion Digital Edition of this title (see inside front cover for login instructions).

11 van der Bruggen P et al. A gene encoding an antigen recognized by cytolytic T lymphocytes on a human melanoma. *Science*. 1991;**254(5038)**:1643-1647.

13 Boon T, van der Bruggen P. Human tumor antigens recognized by T lymphocytes. *J Exp Med*. 1996;**183**:725-729.

15 Shankaran V et al. IFN-gamma and lymphocytes prevent primary tumor development and shape tumor immunogenicity. *Nature*. 2001;**410**:1107-1111.

25 Smyth MJ et al. Perforin-mediated cytotoxicity is critical for surveillance of spontaneous lymphoma. *J Exp Med*. 2000;**192(5)**:755-760.

27 Dunn GP et al. Cancer immunoediting: from immunosurveillance to tumor escape. *Nat Immunol*. 2002;**3(11)**:991-998.

34 Overwijk WW et al. Tumor regression and autoimmunity after reversal of a functionally tolerant state of self-reactive CD8+ T cells. *J Exp Med*. 2003;**198(4)**:569-580.

35 Rosenberg SA et al. Tumor progression can occur despite the induction of very high levels of self/tumor antigen-specific CD8+ T cells in patients with melanoma. *J Immunol*. 2005;**175(9)**:6169-6176.

45 Rosenberg SA, Spiess P, Lafreniere R. A new approach to the adoptive immunotherapy of cancer with tumor-infiltrating lymphocytes. *Science*. 1986;**233(4770)**:1318-1321.

48 Morgan RA et al. Cancer regression in patients after transfer of genetically engineered lymphocytes. *Science*. 2006;**314(5796)**:126-129.

57 Dong H et al. Tumor-associated B7-H1 promotes T-cell apoptosis: A potential mechanism of immune evasion. *Nat Med*. 2002;**8(8)**:793-800.

82 Fontenot JD, Gavin MA, Rudensky AY. Foxp3 programs the development and function of CD4+CD25+ regulatory T cells. *Nat Immunol*. 2003;**4(4)**:330-336.

83 Gavin MA et al. Foxp3-dependent programme of regulatory T-cell differentiation. *Nature*. 2007;**445(7129)**:771-775.

84 Zheng Y, Rudensky AY. Foxp3 in control of the regulatory T cell lineage. *Nat Immunol*. 2007;**8(5)**:457-462.

126 Quezada SA et al. CTLA4 blockade and GM-CSF combination immunotherapy alters the intratumor balance of effector and regulatory T cells. *J Clin Invest*. 2006;**116(7)**:1935-1945.

171 Hall SS. A commotion in the blood: Life, death and the immune system. New York: Henry Holt and Company; 1997.

172 Coley WB II. Contribution to the Knowledge of Sarcoma. *Ann Surg*. 1891;**14(3)**:199-220.

173 Coley WB. End results in Hodgkin's disease and lymphosarcoma treated by the mixed toxins of erysipelas and Bacillus prodigiosus, alone or combined with radiation. *Ann Surg*. 1928;**88(4)**:641-667.

174 Old LJ. Tumour necrosis factor. Another chapter in the long history of endotoxin. *Nature*. 1987;**330(6149)**:602-603.

217 Zhang H et al. 4-1BB is superior to CD28 costimulation for generating CD8+ cytotoxic lymphocytes for adoptive immunotherapy. *J Immunol*. 2007;**179(7)**:4910-4918.

265 Segal NH et al. Epitope landscape in breast and colorectal cancer. *Cancer Res*. 2008;**68(3)**:889-892.

268 Maude SL et al. Chimeric antigen receptor T cells for sustained remissions in leukemia. *N Engl J Med*. 2014;**371(16)**:1507-1517.

357 Kohrt HE et al. Targeting CD137 enhances the efficacy of cetuximab. *J Clin Invest*. 2014;**124(6)**:2668-2682.

371 Weinberg AD et al. Engagement of the OX-40 receptor in vivo enhances antitumor immunity. *J Immunol*. 2000;**164(4)**:2160-2169.

389 Leach DR, Krummel MF, Allison JP. Enhancement of antitumor immunity by CTLA-4 blockade. *Science*. 1996;**271(5256)**:1734-1736.

397 Waterhouse P et al. Lymphoproliferative disorders with early lethality in mice deficient in Ctla-4. *Science*. 1995;**270(5238)**:985-988.

407 Hodi FS et al. Improved survival with ipilimumab in patients with metastatic melanoma. *N Engl J Med*. 2010;**363(8)**:711-723.

409 Schadendorf D, et al. Pooled analysis of long-term survival data from phase II and phase III trials of ipilimumab in metastatic or locally advanced, unresectable melanoma. Presented at the 38th Congress of the European Society for Medical Oncology (ESMO), Amsterdam, Netherlands, September 27-October 1, 2013.

415 Fan X et al. Engagement of the ICOS pathway markedly enhances efficacy

of CTLA-4 blockade in cancer immunotherapy. *J Exp Med*. 2014;**211**(**4**): 715–725.

441 Ansell SM et al. PD-1 blockade with nivolumab in relapsed or refractory Hodgkin's lymphoma. *N Engl J Med*. 2015;**372**(**4**):311–319.

443 Robert C et al. Nivolumab in previously untreated melanoma without BRAF mutation. *N Engl J Med*. 2015;**372**(**4**):320–330.

492 Wolchok JD et al. Nivolumab plus ipilimumab in advanced melanoma. *N Engl J Med*. 2013;**369**(**2**):122–133.

508 Gubin MM et al. Checkpoint blockade cancer immunotherapy targets tumour-specific mutant antigens. *Nature*. 2014;**515**(**7528**):577–581.

509 Linnemann C et al. High-throughput epitope discovery reveals frequent recognition of neo-antigens by CD4+ T cells in human melanoma. *Nat Med*. 2015;**21**(**1**): 81–85.

第 68 章　肿瘤基因治疗

Haruko Tashiro, MD, PhD ■ Malcolm Brenner, MB, PhD

概述

肿瘤基因治疗显现出越来越多令人鼓舞的结果，即将进入主流的肿瘤治疗体系。基因转移能够修饰恶性肿瘤细胞或宿主免疫细胞的细胞表型和行为，从而调节肿瘤对治疗的反应。在这一章中，我们将分别讨论上述两种方法，并描述能够产生预期遗传修饰的载体系统。我们在叙述当前基因治疗的临床成功案例的同时，也指出了它尚未克服的挑战。每一种方法的成功都依赖于有效、安全的基因转移，基因转移的载体有的能够整合至人类基因组（如逆病毒、慢病毒、腺相关病毒或转座子），有的不能整合至人类基因组（如腺病毒、疱疹病毒或非病毒载体）。到目前为止，我们还无法实现逆转肿瘤中所有干细胞的表型，而且感染性溶瘤病毒治疗也尚未成功应用于临床。虽然可能多种方法的联合治疗最终会产生最佳的治疗结果，但通过强制表达抗原和细胞因子来提高肿瘤免疫活性，或通过采用特异性 T 细胞受体和嵌合抗原受体来修饰 T 淋巴细胞以提高获得性免疫治疗的疗效已经显示出了较好的短期疗效。

引言

最近，在手术、化疗和放疗这些传统的肿瘤治疗方法的基础上涌现出一系列的肿瘤靶向性和免疫调节性抗体。在本章中，我们将描述基因转移的方法，这是另一种已经被研发出的治疗方法，虽然这一方法目前仅用于少数疾病的治疗，但现在已经取得了显著的成效。基因转移的目的是对正常细胞或肿瘤细胞的细胞学表型或行为进行修饰，从而达到控制或清除肿瘤的目的。新的遗传物质可以通过细胞输入的方式在体外进行转移，也可以直接在体内转移至细胞内。这一修饰可以是永久的，也可以是暂时的。

将遗传物质递送至靶细胞

理想的基因递送系统（载体）要求安全、高效而且有比较广的应用范围，但这样的载体目前还不存在。相反，基因传递载体，无论是病毒来源还是非病毒来源的，都有它们各自的优势与局限（表 68-1），在特定的应用中应权衡它们的预期特性和局限性后再进行选择。

病毒载体

病毒通过高效地将其遗传信息插入靶细胞来实现它们的繁殖。研究者们利用这一特性对病毒进行了改造，使它们能够把治疗性遗传物质导入细胞，却不能在宿主体内致病。为此，已经有几种不同的病毒载体被应用到肿瘤基因治疗中。

表 68-1　肿瘤基因治疗载体的优缺点

	优点	缺点
载体序列整合到基因组		
逆病毒	基因组整合稳定	仅整合分裂期细胞
	基因长期表达	潜在插入突变
	低免疫原性	体内基因传递低效
	插入片段较大：7~8kb	
慢病毒	感染非分裂期细胞	潜在插入突变
	基因长期表达	体内基因传递低效
	低免疫原性	
腺相关病毒	基因长期表达	潜在插入突变
	感染非分裂期细胞	插入片段有限：4kb
载体序列不整合到基因组		
腺病毒	效价高	瞬时表达
	感染效率高	累积免疫相关毒性
	感染非分裂期细胞	插入片段有限：7~8kb（第一代）
	低免疫原性	
疱疹病毒	插入片段较大：30kb	细胞毒性
	神经嗜性	瞬时表达
非病毒 DNA 传送	插入片段较大	瞬时基因表达
	低免疫原性	体内传递低效
	可重复使用	

整合载体

逆病毒载体

逆病毒是有包膜的单链 RNA 病毒，有几种不同的逆病毒家族成员已经被改造成为载体，包括 γ-逆病毒［如鼠白血病病毒（murine leukemia virus）MLV，是最早改造成功并仍然广泛应用的逆病毒载体之一］[1] 和人免疫缺陷病毒（human immunodeficiency virus，HIV）（HIV-1，也在广泛应用中[2,3]）。其他一些逆病毒也已经被发展为潜在的载体，包括猴免疫缺陷病毒（simian immunodeficiency virus，SIV）、牛免疫缺陷病毒、猫免疫缺陷病毒、马传染性贫血病毒(equine infectious anemia virus, EIAV)、泡沫病毒、牛白血病病毒、Rous 肉瘤病毒(Rous sarcoma virus, RSV)、脾坏死病毒和鼠乳腺肿瘤病毒。这些载体能够整合入宿主 DNA,因此即使在分裂细胞中它们也能够稳定表达。

γ-逆病毒(如 MLV)

野生型 MLV 逆病毒包含 5′和 3′长末端重复序列(long-terminal repeats, LTRs),它们负责病毒整合并发挥启动子的功能。在 LTRs 之间是病毒复制和包装所必需的 3 段基因序列:*gag* 基因,编码 3 个病毒结构蛋白;*pol* 基因,编码病毒复制必需的逆转录酶、整合酶和核酶 H(RNaseH);*env* 基因,编码包膜糖蛋白。重组逆病毒载体通过从病毒核酸骨架上去除 *gag*、*pol* 和 *env* 基因序列,并代之以一段含有目标治疗性序列的核酸,这样就生成了复制缺陷型逆病毒。这些"无肠"载体是在工程细胞系中产生的,缺失的病毒基因以反式整合的方式产生非复制性的病毒颗粒,这些病毒具有传染性,并且含有足够多的逆转录酶,从而启动双链 DNA 分子的合成,将目标核酸序列整合到靶细胞中。

如前所述,逆病毒序列稳定整合到宿主细胞基因组中意味着逆病毒中的任何修饰都是稳定表达的[4],并会遗传给所有子代细胞。尽管对于快速分裂的细胞群,这种稳定性具有极大的优势,但 γ-逆病毒载体也存在其局限性。首先,稳定的感染和整合发生在细胞分裂的 S 期,且整合的前体复合物并不稳定,因此只有在分裂活跃的细胞中,γ-逆病毒才能有效地整合。其次,逆病毒载体的整合从定义上讲是一个突变事件,整合有利于活性基因的调控,插入突变可以实现——并且已经实现——导入的靶细胞的转化[5,6]。再次,插入序列的长度是有限的。由工程细胞系产生复制功能不全的 γ-逆病毒载体只含有逆病毒 LTR 和包装信号。因此,这些载体理论上可以容纳 7~8kb 的目标序列。然而,外源序列插入的包装限制大大降低了这一容量[7]。最后,逆病毒在灵长类靶体中是不稳定的,不适用于体内基因转移。由于这些局限性,通常来说,逆病毒在用于患者体内的基因转移之前会被用于特异性靶细胞的体外基因转移。

慢病毒载体

源于艾滋病毒的慢病毒载体是最早被开发出来的病毒载体,已广泛应用于实验室和临床。慢病毒载体的设计来自 HIV-1 基因组,该基因组包含 *gag-pro-pol* 基因、*env* 基因以及病毒复制所需的两个调节基因 *rev* 和 *tat*。HIV-1 基因组有编码关键的毒力因子的 4 个辅助基因,分别是 *vif*、*vrp*、*vpu* 和 *nef* 基因。这些基因两侧各有一个 LTRs,重组慢病毒载体通过去除大部分远离 LTRs 的 HIV 基因、包装信号和其他调控元件设计而成[8]。第一代包装质粒具有完整的 gag 和 pol 序列、病毒调控基因和辅助基因。在第二代慢病毒载体中,4 个辅助基因被去除。为了进一步降低基因修饰的感染性慢病毒的重组和生产的风险,第三代载体是分离载体组成的基因组包装系统,其中 *rev* 基因在一个单独的质粒中表达,而 5′LTRs 在转移骨架质粒中表达[9];而且,在最新一代载体中,*rev* 和 *tat* 基因由第四个质粒提供[10]。与用于包装 γ 逆病毒所使用的稳定细胞系不同,要想大规模生产由多质粒系统构建成的慢病毒包装载体或降低其生产成本来满足更多的临床实验需求,是十分困难的。科学家正不断努力以期建立一个稳定的安全生产线来生产高滴度载体。虽然很难大规模生产,但相对于 γ 逆病毒,慢病毒具有以下优势:尽管稳定的整合复合物前体只有在进入细胞周期后才能被高效的整合,但分裂期和非分裂期细胞均易被感染[11]。不同病毒包膜的替换改变并扩大了靶细胞的病毒亲和性[12]。最初的针对慢病毒载体的临床研究评估了抗 HIV 包膜反义基因在 HIV 患者中的安全性,但最近的研究集中于用慢病毒载体感染 T 细胞来表达肿瘤定向受体[13]。

腺相关病毒载体

腺相关病毒(adeno-associated viruses, AAV)是一种体积小、无包膜的单链 DNA 病毒,对人类及动物没有致病性[14],需要辅助病毒(腺病毒、单纯疱疹病毒或牛痘病毒)来复制产生新的病毒颗粒[15]。腺相关病毒基因组由 *rep*(用于病毒复制)和 *cap*(编码病毒衣壳)组成。AAV 至少有 11 个血清型,它们的区别主要在于衣壳蛋白的不同,这些不同的衣壳蛋白可结合不同的细胞受体,从而感染不同的靶细胞。重组 AAV 载体去除了 *rep* 和 *cap* 基因,但是保留了目标基因两侧的反向末端重复序列(inverted terminal repeats, ITRs)。虽然 rAAV 广泛并成功应用于单基因疾病的治疗,但其运载能力有限,且生产规模难以扩大,目前该病毒很少用于临床中的肿瘤基因治疗[16,17]。

非整合病毒载体

腺病毒载体

腺病毒是无衣壳的线性双链大分子 DNA 病毒。早期基因(*E1A*、*E1B*、*E2A*、*E2B*、*E3* 和 *E4*)编码调节蛋白,用于启动细胞增殖、DNA 复制和下调宿主免疫防御。晚期基因(L1~L5)编码结构蛋白。重要的是,腺病毒根据衣壳的组成分为不同的种属(A~F)和血清型,其旋钮/纤维附着在一个或多个细胞受体上;细胞受体的类型与物种和血清型相关[18]。这些分子相互作用,在受体介导下完成病毒内吞、内化及脱衣壳[19]。腺病毒可以感染多种正常和恶性细胞,无论细胞是处于分裂期还是非分裂期,但它们不整合在宿主细胞 DNA 中,因此遗传修饰在子代细胞中会逐渐丢失。

重组腺病毒载体是通过去除一个或多个早期基因(包括调节复制的 *E1* 基因和减少免疫识别的 *E3* 基因)设计而成的。缺失的 *E1* 基因由包装/辅助细胞系反式提供,产生可携带 7~8kb 新的遗传物质的复制能力不全的腺病毒[20]。已被开发出来的第二代腺病毒,里面的 *E2* 和 *E4* 连同 *E1* 和 *E3* 一起被去除,可提供高达 14kb 的插入域。然而,该重组腺病毒生产的腺病毒滴度较低[21]。由于腺病毒载体无法整合到宿主细胞基因组中,不会发生插入突变,在分裂的细胞中的基因表达是短暂的。腺病毒载体有较强的促炎作用,会增强针对被感染的细胞及其表达基因的免疫反应[22,23]。尽管这两种特性都使腺病毒载体不适合长期用于治疗单基因疾病,但它们在肿瘤治疗方面很有应用前景,比如对于肿瘤疫苗,具有免疫原性的转基因的短暂表达及高表达可能是非常必要的。

腺病毒载体的两个主要变种目前正在临床开发中[22,23]。去除包装和复制所需的基因之外的所有病毒基因就制成了辅助依赖性("无肠")腺病毒载体,这种载体具有较低的免疫原性和较大的运载能力。相反,对上述去除的那些基因进行限制或修饰就可以产生有一定复制能力的腺病毒载体(conditionally replication-competent adenoviral vectors, CRAD),这种 CRAD 腺病毒载体可以特异地在恶性肿瘤细胞中进行复制并将其杀死,但对正常细胞则没有杀伤作用。由于 CRAD 所需的转录调节因子在恶性肿瘤细胞中的表达水平远高于正常细胞，或由于研究者使用肿瘤特异性启动子替代关键的复制基因的病毒启动子，使得这些溶瘤病毒对肿瘤细胞具有选择性[24,25]。

其他非整合病毒载体

疱疹病毒(Herpes viruses，HSV)是具有衣壳包被的大分子(~186nm)线性双链DNA病毒。其基因组由独特的长编码区和短编码区组成，两侧都有末端重复序列[26]。虽然HSV可编码多达90个基因，但许多基因的缺失并不影响基因组复制或病毒包装。因此，在去除这些基因后，HSV载体能够携带很长的DNA序列(长达30kb)[27]。具有复制能力的HSV也已被研发出来，针对不同肿瘤类型的溶瘤病毒也正在研发中[28-30]。痘苗病毒是可以在细胞质中复制的大型DNA病毒。改良痘苗病毒Ankara(modified vaccinia virus Ankara，MVA)从亲本基因组中删除了31kb，包括调节先天免疫应答的*k1l*、*n1l*和*a52r*基因[31]，而MVA和哥本哈根衍生疫苗株目前正被用作治疗肿瘤的溶瘤病毒进行研究[32]。终止溶瘤反应的高免疫原性是临床应用要解决的问题之一[33]。

非病毒载体

虽然病毒载体传递基因的效率很高，但它们有几个缺点，包括成本高且生产复杂，以及一些制剂(如慢病毒和rAAV)生产的可扩展性受限。此外，抗体或细胞介导的免疫对病毒蛋白的识别可能会限制载体的全身性给药和/或重复给药，或限制转基因表达的持久性。病毒载体的其他局限性包括由一些病毒载体产生的插入突变和编码的转基因的长度限制。

因此，人们致力于提高质粒DNA的非病毒传递效率，从而有效地使DNA逃脱核酸酶介导的降解[34]。质粒传递可通过物理方法(例如电穿孔、超声波和流体动力注射)破坏细胞膜或通过化学物质(例如阳离子聚合物或脂质)诱导内吞作用来实现[35]。与传统的非病毒载体不同，将转座子/转座酶元件添加到目的基因的质粒中，可将其整合到宿主细胞DNA中，目前这个研究方法在体外用来在T淋巴细胞中产生稳定的基因转移和表达。非病毒基因递送方法通常具有较低的免疫原性和毒性，但在体内基因递送的效率不高，而且转基因的表达水平一般。迄今为止，这些方法还没有被广泛应用于肿瘤治疗。

基因治疗的靶点

由于癌症是一种获得性遗传疾病，理论上，基因疗法可以用来治疗这种疾病。例如，用一个活性基因替换一个无活性的基因或中和一个功能亢进的基因。尽管在一些报道中基因治疗已被证明对治疗*p53*缺陷的肿瘤是成功的[36]，但由于种种原因，直接针对癌细胞的工程基因疗法是十分困难的。与单基因遗传病不同，针对癌细胞的基因疗法需要修饰整个肿瘤细胞群，而这个细胞群通常是非常巨大的。如上所述，目前还没有高效的基因传递系统。即使基因传递系统可用，纠正单个基因异常可能并不足以修复转化的细胞表型。因此，针对正常宿主组织进行抗肿瘤治疗的替代策略也正在探索中。

直接攻击肿瘤的基因治疗策略

前体药物-代谢酶

编码前体药-代谢酶的基因的导入可在一定程度上克服基因转移效率低的问题，这些基因编码的酶将无毒的小分子前体药转化为致死的细胞毒素，然后释放到肿瘤的广泛区域。单纯疱疹病毒衍生的胸苷激酶(HSV-tk)基因已被广泛研究用于此目的。由导入的基因编码的HSV-tk可将无毒的前体药物，如阿昔洛韦、伐昔洛韦和更昔洛韦，磷酸化成抑制细胞DNA合成和复制的有毒代谢产物。由于代谢物可以通过缝隙连接等细胞间通讯从感染的细胞运输到邻近的非感染的细胞，因此除了对感染的癌细胞有直接的细胞毒性作用外，这种方法也具有间接的旁观者细胞毒性作用[37-39]。一项针对神经胶质瘤患者的HSV-tk基因治疗的随机3期临床试验采用了这一方法，即向瘤体周围注射腺病毒载体[40]。由于病灶周围注射并不总是可行的，肿瘤细胞也可以通过其他方法被靶向，例如使用只能感染分裂细胞的载体，使用仅在分裂细胞中具有药理活性的酶——前体药系统，或使用靶向肿瘤特异性分布的受体的载体[41]。

病毒治疗或病毒溶瘤

一些病例报告记录了病毒感染后自发的肿瘤消退的现象[42,43]。随着对病毒和癌症分子生物学更详细的了解，人们已经设计了仅能进入肿瘤细胞或只能在肿瘤细胞中复制的溶瘤病毒。这些溶瘤病毒中的一些是可以选择性感染和杀死癌细胞的天然病毒物种。例如，H1自主复制细小病毒、呼肠孤病毒、新城疫病毒、腮腺炎病毒和莫洛尼白血病病毒，这些都是肿瘤特异性的。其他病毒，如麻疹、腺病毒、水疱性口炎病毒、牛痘和单纯疱疹病毒，需要进行基因修饰才能成为肿瘤特异性病毒[44]。例如，腺病毒E1B区域通常与*p53*基因结合并使其失活以允许病毒复制，在ONYX-015中E1B区域是缺失的。因此，ONYX-015不能阻断*p53*的功能，这样它就只能在*p53*功能缺陷的恶性细胞中复制[45]。

溶瘤病毒不仅可以通过直接裂解(其细胞病变效应)杀死肿瘤细胞，还可以通过间接机制，比如破坏肿瘤血管或增强特定的抗肿瘤免疫应答，来杀死肿瘤细胞。因此，可进一步修饰溶瘤病毒以递送诱导T细胞趋化性(例如Rantes)或免疫调节的治疗基因[例如GM-CSF(粒细胞-巨噬细胞集落刺激因子)、IL-2、IL-12或IL-15][46-50]，或者递送一种前体药物转化酶，其在肿瘤中将惰性药物转化为细胞毒性药物并富集(参见标题为“前体药物-代谢酶”部分)[51]。

虽然几种溶瘤病毒临床试验证明了溶瘤病毒的安全性，但几乎无一例外[52]，溶瘤病毒的临床疗效却并没有达到临床前研究所设想的那样好的预期。有许多阻碍病毒扩散到靶细胞的障碍。当全身注射病毒时，它们可以通过中和抗体、补体或网状内皮系统，在到达肿瘤细胞之前就被从血液中清除[53-55]。此外，最初的肿瘤感染率可能不足以有效地进行后续的病毒复制。为了克服这些障碍，人们已经研究了几种应对方案，例如使用间充质干细胞传递溶瘤病毒以帮助它们逃避免疫应答[56]，以及预先使用免疫抑制药物[57]。

通过疫苗诱导宿主对肿瘤的免疫力

与针对传染性病原体的疫苗不同，肿瘤疫苗不用于预防疾病，而是用于治疗疾病，通过增强患者自身的免疫系统来识别和攻击癌细胞。虽然人类研究肿瘤疫苗已经研究了100多年，但并未发现有效的制剂，并且只有不到10%的肿瘤疫苗接种者从中获益[41]。尽管如此，仍有充分理由继续探索肿瘤疫苗。

许多癌细胞表达肿瘤相关抗原(tumor-associated antigen,TAA),但由于免疫逃逸,缺乏对 TAA 的有效免疫(图 68-1)。肿瘤逃逸机制包括共刺激分子的下调、免疫抑制受体/配体(如 PD-L1)的表达、多种可溶性免疫抑制因子[如转化生长因子 β(TGF-β)、IL-10]和免疫抑制配体(如 FasL、TRAIL)的分泌,以及诱导调节性 T 细胞(T_{reg})或髓源性抑制细胞(MDSC)[58]。接种疫苗旨在通过抗原与强效免疫刺激信号结合来诱发宿主对已耐受的 TAA 的免疫反应。靶抗原包括癌蛋白、癌胚抗原、分化相关蛋白和病毒蛋白,科学家也在努力识别每个患者机体针对独特的肿瘤相关新抗原(由每种肿瘤特异性突变产生的抗原)产生的免疫应答[59]。因此,可以通过以下方法引入 TAA:①伴随免疫佐剂注射肽或蛋白质[60];②重组病毒或其他重组微生物的成分,以利用由这些生物诱导的促炎性固有免疫应答和适应性免疫应答[61];③蛋白质、肽段激活的树突状细胞[62];④来自肿瘤细胞的 mRNA 或肿瘤细胞自身经修饰可表达免疫刺激基因,两者都旨在产生针对新抗原的免疫反应[63]。对于最后一个应用,研究人员经常将免疫调节基因(包括 IL-2[63]、GM-CSF[64]和 CD40L 等共刺激分子)组合来诱导更强的 T 细胞反应[63-65]。

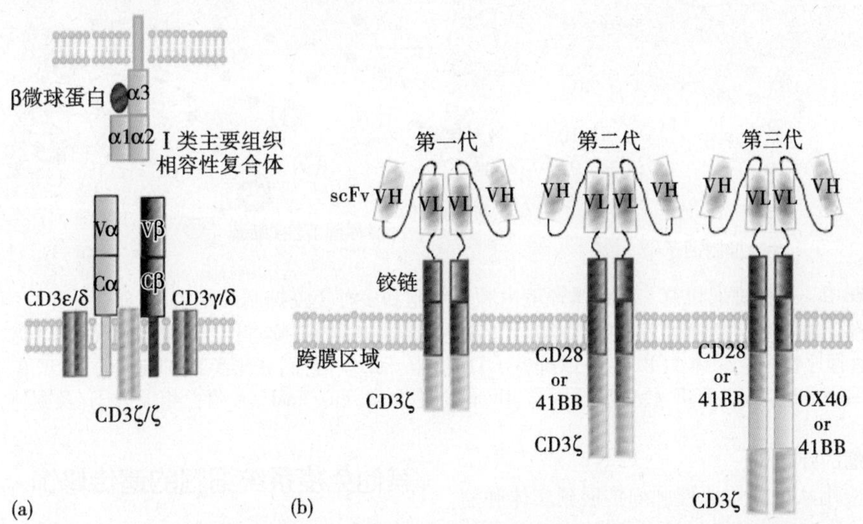

图 68-1 转基因 T 细胞受体。(a)需要 HLA 辅助识别靶抗原的转基因 α 和 βT 细胞受体;(b)嵌合抗原受体,识别抗原时不受 HLA 限制。对于内域,第一代 CAR 只有 CD3ζ,第二代和第三代 CAR 同时含有 CD3ζ 和共刺激分子。scFV,单链可变片段

尽管经过多年的努力,FDA 仍然只批准了一种癌症疫苗(Provenge)。这种疫苗表达前列腺酸性磷酸酶与 GM-CSF 的融合蛋白,用于治疗晚期前列腺癌。Provenge 是在患者的外周血中经自身抗原呈递细胞群体外转化后产生的。虽然单独的疫苗治疗很少足以引发治愈性免疫反应,但是疫苗和 T 细胞免疫检查点抗体(如 CTLA4mAb 或 PD-1mAb)的联合应用可能会增强疗效,取得令人满意的效果。

修饰宿主免疫效应细胞

癌症疫苗的一个局限是它们在体内诱导的免疫反应可能会被恶性细胞的免疫逃逸以及这些细胞产生的肿瘤微环境阻断或破坏(见图 68-1)。另一种方法是体外制备针对肿瘤的,尤其是针对肿瘤的免疫逃避机制的效应细胞。这些经过修饰的效应细胞可以被回输入患者体内。

产生肿瘤特异性

通过将编码标准化 TAA-特异性受体的序列转移到大量 T 细胞群中,T 细胞被工程化为肿瘤特异性 T 细胞。特异性受体包括两种类型:"天然"α 和 βT 细胞受体(T-cell receptor,TCR)或人工嵌合抗原受体(chimeric antigen receptor,CAR),之所以这么命名,是因为它们是肿瘤抗原结合域和 TCR 信号域的嵌合体。TCRα 和 β 链由 TRA 和 TRB 基因编码并已被用于克隆几种不同的 TAA 表位[66]。这些合成的 TCR 在修饰后具有较高的亲和力,一旦转移到 T 细胞即可提高 T 细胞的有效性[67],但有时会产生不必要的交叉反应[68-71]。已经开展了几项临床试验[68-70],其中一些已经显示出显著的功效,例如在黑色素瘤、结直肠癌和骨髓瘤中,但"脱靶"导致的毒性仍然是个问题。

TCR 基因治疗的主要局限性在于每个 TCR 只能识别整个肿瘤抗原的一小部分(表位)。肿瘤中不但可能存在这部分表位的丢失("编辑"),并且此表位的识别还受 MHC 多态性的限制,使 TCR 基因治疗只能在具有相同人类白细胞抗原(HLA)的个体之间产生效应。TCR 可识别 9~14 肽段,与之相比,CAR 转导的 T 细胞可识别的抗原肽段更大。CAR-T 细胞还可以克服 HLA 限制的局限性,识别碳水化合物和其他非蛋白抗原。CAR 由一个与靶抗原结合的细胞外结构域(外域)、一个跨膜结构域和一个或多个细胞内信号结构域组成(图 68-2)。通常情况下,细胞外结构域由靶向预期抗原的单克隆抗体的抗原结合部位构成,细胞内信号域(内域)则来自 TCR 的 CD3ζ 成分[41]。最初的 CAR-T 细胞效果并不明显,因为单独的 CAR 刺激不足以完全激活 CAR-T 细胞,在体内产生的扩增和持久性有限。第二代 CAR 增加了 T 细胞克服多个激活障碍物所需的一个或多个共刺激信号,例如来自 CD27、CD28、41BB、OX40 或 ICOS 的信号转导结构域。当这些二代 CAR 与 CD19(一种存在于大多数正常细胞和许多 B 细胞源性肿瘤细胞上的抗原)的外域结合时,CAR-T 细胞在 B 细胞恶性肿瘤治疗中产生了显著的疗效。例如,CD19 CAR-T 细胞治疗复发/耐药的 B 细胞型急性淋巴细胞白血病,完全缓解率可达 90%[13,72]。

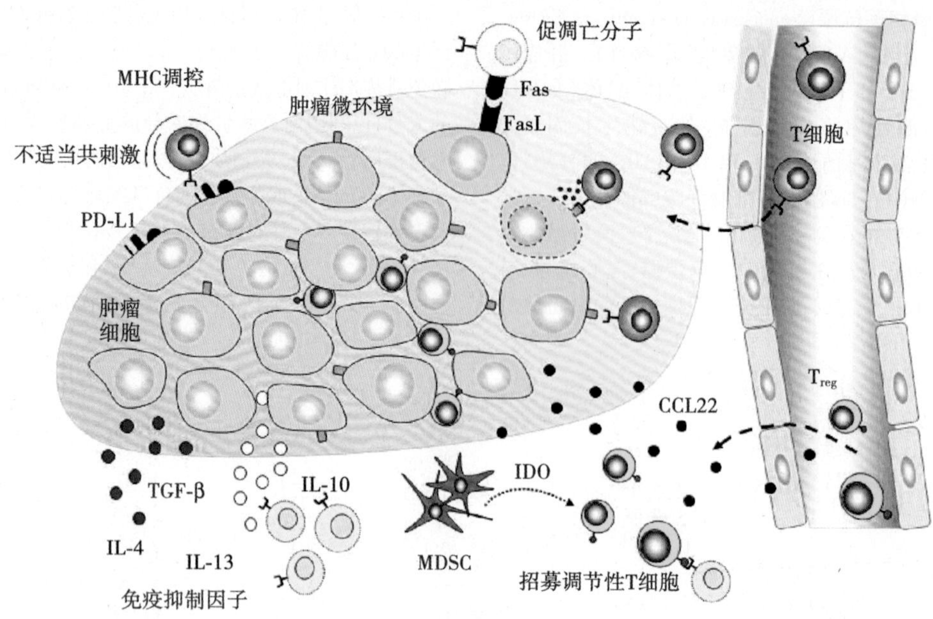

图 68-2 肿瘤逃逸机制。肿瘤微环境由肿瘤细胞和多种免疫抑制细胞组成,如 T_{reg} 和骨髓来源的抑制性细胞(MDSC)。肿瘤细胞自身表达 FasL 以诱导细胞毒性 T 淋巴细胞(CTL)凋亡,表达程序性死亡受体 1(PD-L1)以抑制 CTL 功能。此外,它们分泌免疫抑制分子 TGF-β、IL-10、IL-4 和 IL-13。TGF,转化生长因子;IL,白细胞介素;Fas/FasL,人凋亡相关因子/及配体

工程 T 细胞抗实体肿瘤的疗效

将 CAR-T 细胞的应用从 B 细胞恶性肿瘤扩展到实体肿瘤是具有挑战性的。CD19 CAR-T 细胞的不良作用之一是会破坏也表达 CD19 的正常 B 细胞,但这种副作用可以通过输注免疫球蛋白制剂来缓解。实体瘤与其他器官也存在共同抗原,与 B 细胞不同,实体器官中的正常细胞大多承担着不可或缺的功能。只有极少数的真正独特的 TAA 可以被抗体或其他适合包含在 CAR 中的抗原识别结构域所识别。此外,T 细胞在许多肿瘤部位的运动能力较差。T 细胞运动到肿瘤部位时,会进入一种免疫抑制性的肿瘤微环境(见图 68-1)[73]。这种肿瘤微环境是通过抑制性细胞(如髓样抑制细胞和调节性 T 细胞)的募集、抑制分子(例如,PD-L1 和 FasL)的表达和可溶性抑制分子/Th2-极化细胞因子(如腺苷、IDO、TGF-β、IL-6、IL-10 和 PGE-2)的产生而形成。因此,研究人员正在改造 T 细胞以提高过继输注的 T 细胞在肿瘤中的迁移能力、在体内的增殖和存活能力。例如,为了拮抗 TGF-β,可以在肿瘤靶向的 T 细胞中表达一类具有显性负活性的 TGF-β Ⅱ型受体。这种 TGF-β Ⅱ型受体的表达导致 T 细胞对肿瘤分泌的 TGF-β 不敏感,并显示出良好的临床获益[74,75]。目前,针对肿瘤免疫逃逸的其他对策正在研究中(表 68-2)。

表 68-2 肿瘤免疫逃逸的策略

靶基因	基因修饰	参考文献
TGF-β	显性负活性的 TGF-β 受体	74
FasL	下调 Fas	76
IDO,精氨酸酶	敲降 GCN2	77,78
IL-10	IL-10 受体 1/IgG1-FC 融合蛋白	79
IL-4	IL-4/IL-7 嵌合受体	80

其他免疫系统细胞的遗传修饰

自然杀伤(natural killer,NK)细胞和恒定链或自然杀伤 T(natural killer T,NKT)细胞都能在体外被激活和扩增。这些细胞是先天免疫和适应性免疫反应之间的桥梁,一旦重新定位到肿瘤中,可能具有显著的抗肿瘤活性。针对 T 细胞进行的所有研究也正在 NK 和 NKT 细胞群中进行;未来几年,它们的效力、安全性和抗肿瘤活性的持久性将得以揭示。

安全性

尽管用过继转移的 T 细胞进行免疫治疗的疗效已经取得了惊人的成果,但是跟其他任何有效的治疗一样,其风险还是要考虑的。据报道,除了与正常组织发生致命的交叉反应外,一些 T 细胞疗法,尤其是 CD19 CAR-T 细胞治疗有可能诱发细胞因子释放综合征(或全身炎症反应综合征)。由于这些不良反应可能是致命的,研究人员正在研发和尝试该疗法的安全系统或自杀系统,使这一治疗过程可以准确可控。这些系统包括细胞毒性抗体、前体药物-代谢酶和可诱导型凋亡基因[81-84]。

结论:肿瘤基因治疗如何进入临床实践?

现在,基因治疗在癌症治疗中的作用越来越明确,制药行业和医疗保健行业不得不开始评估开发、制造和提供这些个性化疗法的高成本。由于只有多种生物疗法(例如,工程 T 细胞、溶瘤病毒和检查点抗体)联合使用时才能获得最佳结果,健康保健服务专家们需要仔细地对药物经济学进行评估,提供能够广泛替代传统疗法的合理方案。尽管我们相信这种情况终将

实现，但在肿瘤基因治疗真正成为癌症一线治疗之前，这仍然是众多挑战中的一大挑战。

（王海娟　钱海利 译）

参考文献

The complete reference list can be found on the Wiley Companion Digital Edition of this title (see inside front cover for login instructions).

1 Miller AD. Retroviral vectors. *Curr Top Microbiol Immunol*. 1992;**158**:1-24.

2 Reiser J, Harmison G, Kluepfel-Stahl S, Brady RO, Karlsson S, Schubert M. Transduction of nondividing cells using pseudotyped defective high-titer HIV type 1 particles. *Proc Natl Acad Sci U S A*. 1996;**93**(**26**):15266-15271.

3 Goyvaerts C, Kurt de G, Van Lint S, et al. Immunogenicity of targeted lentivectors. *Oncotarget*. 2014;**5**(**3**):704-715.

7 Mann R, Mulligan RC, Baltimore D. Construction of a retrovirus packaging mutant and its use to produce helper-free defective retrovirus. *Cell*. 1983;**33**(**1**):153-159.

8 Liechtenstein T, Perez-Janices N, Bricogne C, et al. Immune modulation by genetic modification of dendritic cells with lentiviral vectors. *Virus Res*. 2013;**176**(**1-2**):1-15.

10 Escors D, Breckpot K. Lentiviral vectors in gene therapy: their current status and future potential. *Arch Immunol Ther Exp (Warsz)*. 2010;**58**(**2**):107-119.

11 Durand S, Cimarelli A. The inside out of lentiviral vectors. *Viruses*. 2011;**3**(**2**): 132-159.

12 Naldini L, Blomer U, Gallay P, et al. In vivo gene delivery and stable transduction of nondividing cells by a lentiviral vector. *Science*. 1996;**272**(**5259**):263-267.

13 Porter DL, Levine BL, Kalos M, Bagg A, June CH. Chimeric antigen receptor-modified T cells in chronic lymphoid leukemia. *N Engl J Med*. 2011;**365**(**8**): 725-733.

14 Basner-Tschakarjan E, Mingozzi F. Cell-mediated immunity to AAV vectors, evolving concepts and potential solutions. *Front Immunol*. 2014;**5**:350.

15 Flotte TR, Carter BJ. Adeno-associated virus vectors for gene therapy. *Gene Ther*. 1995;**2**(**6**):357-362.

16 Nathwani AC, Tuddenham EG, Rangarajan S, et al. Adenovirus-associated virus vector-mediated gene transfer in hemophilia B. *N Engl J Med*. 2011;**365**(**25**): 2357-2365.

20 Berns KI, Giraud C. Adenovirus and adeno-associated virus as vectors for gene therapy. *Ann N Y Acad Sci*. 1995;**772**:95-104.

26 Wadsworth S, Jacob RJ, Roizman B. Anatomy of herpes simplex virus DNA. II. Size, composition, and arrangement of inverted terminal repetitions. *J Virol*. 1975;**15**(**6**):1487-1497.

27 Lentz TB, Gray SJ, Samulski RJ. Viral vectors for gene delivery to the central nervous system. *Neurobiol Dis*. 2012;**48**(**2**):179-188.

32 Gomez CE, Najera JL, Krupa M, Esteban M. The poxvirus vectors MVA and NYVAC as gene delivery systems for vaccination against infectious diseases and cancer. *Curr Gene Ther*. 2008;**8**(**2**):97-120.

33 Whitman ED, Tsung K, Paxson J, Norton JA. In vitro and in vivo kinetics of recombinant vaccinia virus cancer-gene therapy. *Surgery*. 1994;**116**(**2**):183-188.

34 Al-Dosari MS, Gao X. Nonviral gene delivery: principle, limitations, and recent progress. *AAPS J*. 2009;**11**(**4**):671-681.

35 Niidome T, Huang L. Gene therapy progress and prospects: nonviral vectors. *Gene Ther*. 2002;**9**(**24**):1647-1652.

36 Atencio IA, Grace M, Bordens R, et al. Biological activities of a recombinant adenovirus p53 (SCH 58500) administered by hepatic arterial infusion in a Phase 1 colorectal cancer trial. *Cancer Gene Ther*. 2006;**13**(**2**):169-181.

37 Freeman SM, Abboud CN, Whartenby KA, et al. The "bystander effect": tumor regression when a fraction of the tumor mass is genetically modified. *Cancer Res*. 1993;**53**(**21**):5274-5283.

40 Westphal M, Yla-Herttuala S, Martin J, et al. Adenovirus-mediated gene therapy with sitimagene ceradenovec followed by intravenous ganciclovir for patients with operable high-grade glioma (ASPECT): a randomised, open-label, phase 3 trial. *Lancet Oncol*. 2013;**14**(**9**):823-833.

41 Brenner MK, Gottschalk S, Leen AM, Vera JF. Is cancer gene therapy an empty suit? *Lancet Oncol*. 2013;**14**(**11**):e447-e456.

43 Taqi AM, Abdurrahman MB, Yakubu AM, Fleming AF. Regression of Hodgkin's disease after measles. *Lancet*. 1981;**1**(**8229**):1112.

44 Russell SJ, Peng KW, Bell JC. Oncolytic virotherapy. *Nat Biotechnol*. 2012;**30**(**7**): 658-670.

45 Heise C, Sampson-Johannes A, Williams A, McCormick F, Von Hoff DD, Kirn DH. ONYX-015, an E1B gene-attenuated adenovirus, causes tumor-specific cytolysis and antitumoral efficacy that can be augmented by standard chemotherapeutic agents. *Nat Med*. 1997;**3**(**6**):639-645.

48 Senzer NN, Kaufman HL, Amatruda T, et al. Phase II clinical trial of a granulocyte-macrophage colony-stimulating factor-encoding, second-generation oncolytic herpesvirus in patients with unresectable metastatic melanoma. *J Clin Oncol*. 2009;**27**(**34**):5763-5771.

51 Agarwalla PK, Aghi MK. Oncolytic herpes simplex virus engineering and preparation. *Methods Mol Biol*. 2012;**797**:1-19.

54 Bessis N, GarciaCozar FJ, Boissier MC. Immune responses to gene therapy vectors: influence on vector function and effector mechanisms. *Gene Ther*. 2004;**11**(**Suppl 1**):S10-S17.

55 Muharemagic D, Zamay A, Ghobadloo SM, et al. Aptamer-facilitated protection of oncolytic virus from neutralizing antibodies. *Mol Ther Nucleic Acids*. 2014;**3**: e167.

58 Whiteside TL. Immune suppression in cancer: effects on immune cells, mechanisms and future therapeutic intervention. *Semin Cancer Biol*. 2006;**16**(**1**):3-15.

59 Schlom J. Therapeutic cancer vaccines: current status and moving forward. *J Natl Cancer Inst*. 2012;**104**(**8**):599-613.

61 Moss B. Genetically engineered poxviruses for recombinant gene expression, vaccination, and safety. *Proc Natl Acad Sci U S A*. 1996;**93**(**21**):11341-11348.

62 Kantoff PW, Higano CS, Shore ND, et al. Sipuleucel-T immunotherapy for castration-resistant prostate cancer. *N Engl J Med*. 2010;**363**(**5**):411-422.

65 Dessureault S, Noyes D, Lee D, et al. A phase-I trial using a universal GM-CSF-producing and CD40L-expressing bystander cell line (GM.CD40L) in the formulation of autologous tumor cell-based vaccines for cancer patients with stage IV disease. *Ann Surg Oncol*. 2007;**14**(**2**): 869-884.

67 Li LP, Lampert JC, Chen X, et al. Transgenic mice with a diverse human T cell antigen receptor repertoire. *Nat Med*. 2010;**16**(**9**):1029-1034.

72 Maude SL, Frey N, Shaw PA, et al. Chimeric antigen receptor T cells for sustained remissions in leukemia. *N Engl J Med*. 2014;**371**(**16**):1507-1517.

73 Han EQ, Li XL, Wang CR, Li TF, Han SY. Chimeric antigen receptor-engineered T cells for cancer immunotherapy: progress and challenges. *J Hematol Oncol*. 2013;**6**:47.

74 Bollard CM, Rossig C, Calonge MJ, et al. Adapting a transforming growth factor beta-related tumor protection strategy to enhance antitumor immunity. *Blood*. 2002;**99**(**9**):3179-3187.

81 Marin V, Cribioli E, Philip B, et al. Comparison of different suicide-gene strategies for the safety improvement of genetically manipulated T cells. *Hum Gene Ther Methods*. 2012;**23**(**6**):376-386.

第 69 章　癌症纳米技术

Yanlan Liu, PhD ■ Danny Liu ■ Jinjun Shi, PhD ■ Robert S. Langer, ScD

概述

抗癌药物药代动力学不佳、治疗效果有限、副作用大以及产生耐药性和肿瘤转移等因素，导致癌症死亡率和复发率高，先进纳米材料的发展为克服抗癌药的这些难题提供了振奋人心的机遇。在此，我们重点介绍临床阶段的纳米技术在传统癌症治疗中的应用以及新型抗癌疗法的开发。我们还讨论了该领域最新的前沿研究进展，这些进展可能发展为用于癌症治疗的更有效的纳米颗粒。

引言

尽管在癌症生物学、癌症诊断及治疗方面取得了令人欣喜的进展，但癌症作为全球最具破坏力的疾病之一，仍在以惊人的速度持续蔓延，已经成为全球人类共同的负担。根据《2014年世界癌症报告》预测，新增癌症病例将在未来 20 年内从 2012 年预估的每年 1 400 万增加到每年 2 200 万，同期癌症死亡人数从每年 820 万增加至每年 1 300 万[1]。由于常规癌症疗法有很大的局限性，如药代动力学不理想、副作用大以及产生耐药性等[2]，发展能改善治疗效果的癌症治疗新策略，对缓解日益增加的癌症负担至关重要。

自 FDA 批准第一个抗癌纳米颗粒脂质体多柔比星（Doxil）以来的 20 年间，纳米技术在提升癌症治疗效果方面已显示了巨大潜力[3-5]。例如，纳米颗粒能很好地调节药物分子的药代动力学和体内分布，达到改善治疗效果或减少副作用的目的[6]。有些纳米材料由于具有独特的物理化学特性，其本身就具备治疗作用，如用于肿瘤热疗的氧化铁纳米颗粒[7]。迄今为止，约有 10 种纳米抗癌药物已被批准用于临床，还有许多纳米抗癌药物处于临床试验阶段（表 69-1）[8]。本章概述了癌症治疗中临床阶段的纳米技术，并讨论了癌症纳米技术领域的最新前沿研究。

临床阶段的癌症纳米技术

纳米技术独特的药物递送特性使得它在癌症治疗中尤其重要。利用纳米技术，①可改善药物分子（例如，疏水性药物）的递送，并保护药物分子不会被过早地降解、清除或与生理环境相互作用[9,10]；②通过对纳米颗粒进行靶向配体修饰，可将药物选择性地递送至肿瘤细胞[11,12]；③将成像试剂与治疗药物同时装载，可对药物递送进行实时反馈和患者选择[13]；④可穿过致密的内皮和上皮屏障[14,15]；⑤可实现多种药物的共递送，通过协同效应提升治疗效果，克服药物耐药性[16,17]；⑥可实现药物缓释，降低给药频率；⑦能保护核酸免受酶催化降解，促进其细胞内吞及内涵体逃逸[18]；等等。此外，有些纳米颗粒能在局部环境刺激下被激活，具有热疗能力，能够克服肿瘤细胞对化疗药物的耐药性，并避免全身系统性副作用的出现。鉴于这些优点，纳米技术能克服传统癌症治疗中存在的障碍，发展新一类癌症治疗方法，具有极大的潜力。在此，我们将讨论用于不同癌症治疗法的临床阶段的纳米技术，如化学疗法（chemotherapy）、放射疗法（radiotherapy）、热疗法（hyperthermia therapy）、基因治疗（gene therapy）和主动免疫治疗（active immunotherapy）（表 69-1）。

表 69-1　癌症治疗中代表性的临床期纳米技术

类型		产品	描述	适应证	临床状态
化学疗法	被动靶向	Doxil 阿霉素脂质体	载阿霉素的 PEG 化脂质体	卵巢癌、卡波西肉瘤、多发性骨髓瘤	1995 年 FDA 批准
		DaunoXome 柔红霉素脂质体	载柔红霉素的脂质体	晚期 HIV 相关卡波西肉瘤	1996 年 FDA 批准
		Mepact 米伐木肽	胞壁酰三肽磷脂酰乙醇胺脂质体	肺转移性可切除骨肉瘤	欧洲批准，美国临床Ⅲ期
		Myocet 柔比星	载阿霉素的脂质体	转移性乳腺癌	欧洲及加拿大批准
		Abraxane 白蛋白结合紫杉醇	白蛋白颗粒结合紫杉醇	转移性胰腺癌、非小细胞肺癌、乳腺癌	2005 年 FDA 批准
		Genexol-PM 紫杉醇胶束	紫杉醇结合型聚合物胶束	乳腺癌	韩国批准，美国临床Ⅳ期

续表

类型		产品	描述	适应证	临床状态
	主动靶向	BIND-014	结合 PSMA 靶向性小分子配基的载多西他赛聚合物纳米颗粒	非小细胞肺癌、转移性去势抵抗性前列腺癌	临床Ⅱ期
		MM-302	肿瘤抗原靶向性抗体片段修饰的载阿霉素脂质体	HER2 阳性乳腺癌	临床Ⅲ期
		MBP-426	转铁蛋白受体靶向性转铁蛋白修饰的载奥沙利铂脂质体	胃癌、食管癌、胃食管腺癌	临床Ⅰb/Ⅱ期
	刺激响应性靶向	MTC-DOX	载多柔比星的活性炭-铁微球,其中多柔比星结合在活性炭上,铁微球作为磁靶向载体	成人原发性肝癌	临床Ⅲ期
		ThermoDox(脂质体)	包埋阿霉素的热敏脂质体	肝细胞癌	临床Ⅲ期
放射疗法		NBTXR3	氧化铪纳米颗粒	软组织肉瘤、局部晚期口腔或口咽鳞状细胞癌	临床Ⅰ期
高热疗法		NanoTherm	氨基硅烷包覆的氧化铁纳米颗粒	恶性胶质瘤	欧盟批准
		AuroLase	纳米金壳包覆的硅核	难治性头颈癌,原发性和/或转移性肺癌	临床Ⅰ期
基因治疗		CALAA-01	转铁蛋白修饰型环糊精聚合物纳米颗粒,包埋了抗核糖核酸还原酶 M2 亚基的 siRNA	实体瘤	临床Ⅰ期
		ALN-VP02	脂质纳米颗粒,包埋了抗纺锤体驱动蛋白和 VEGF 的 siRNA	实体瘤	临床Ⅰ期
		Atu027	脂质体,包埋了抗蛋白激酶 N3 修饰的 siRNA	晚期或转移性胰腺癌	临床Ⅰ/Ⅱ期
		SGT53-01	载 *p53* 基因脂质体,表面用靶向转铁蛋白的抗体片段修饰	实体瘤	临床Ⅰb 期
主动免疫治疗		Lipovaxin-MM	载黑色素瘤抗原的脂质体疫苗	黑色素瘤	临床Ⅰ期
		dHER2+AS15	HER2/neu 肽和免疫激动剂 AS15 组成的脂质体疫苗	转移性乳腺癌	临床Ⅰ/Ⅱ期
		DPX-0907	载多肿瘤相关抗原的脂质体	HLA-A2 阳性晚期卵巢癌、乳腺癌和前列腺癌	临床Ⅰ期
		Tecemotide	载 MUC1 抗原的脂质体	非小细胞肺癌	临床Ⅲ期

化学疗法

化学疗法的一个主要优点是在于其系统性攻击癌症的能力。然而,由于药代动力学缺陷,只有一小部分药物能够被递送至肿瘤部位。药物向健康细胞的非特异性递送会不可避免地产生严重的副作用。因此,纳米技术已成为将药物有效递送至肿瘤组织、同时降低副作用的最有前途的一种方式[19,20]。人们已经认识到,肿瘤周围密布着有漏洞的血管,再加上功能性淋巴引流的缺乏,纳米颗粒能够从血液循环中渗出并富集在肿瘤组织内(图 69-1a),这种现象被称为高渗透性与滞留效应(enhanced permeability and retention effect,EPR 效应)[21]。研究人员在 EPR 效应的基础上开发了多种纳米颗粒递送体系,其中大约有 10 种已进入市场，包括 Doxil、Abraxane 和 Genexol-PM[8]。

为进一步提高纳米颗粒递送的特异性，主动靶向的方式被提出并进入临床研究。这种主动靶向是通过在纳米颗粒表面修饰靶向基团，可选择性识别肿瘤细胞的特异性受体。靶向配体可以是抗体、适配体、肽、糖类、小分子或其他基团[22]。通过受体介导的内吞作用，靶向递送可提高纳米颗粒的滞留和细胞的摄取，从而显著提高治疗效果(图 69-1b)[23]。最近有一个代表性实例 BIND-014，这是一种用抗前列腺特异性膜抗原(prostate-specific membrane antigen，PSMA)小分子修饰的聚合物纳米颗粒，其中装载了多西紫杉醇，由 BIND Therapeutics 公司研发，目前处于实体瘤治疗的Ⅱ期临床试验。在用 BIND-014 治疗的移植瘤动物模型中，静脉注射 12 小时后，肿瘤中的多西紫杉醇浓度比常规多西紫杉醇(Taxotere)治疗的肿瘤中药物浓度高出了 7 倍。转移性胆管癌患者的临床数据显示，能使肿瘤缩小的 BIND-014 多西紫杉醇剂量仅为常规多西紫杉醇用药剂量的 20%[24]。

除了增加药物的靶向性外，避免药物在到达肿瘤之前的过早释放对于使治疗效果最大化和使副作用最小化，也是同样重要的。刺激响应的纳米颗粒在这方面显示出了巨大的潜力，因为它们只在肿瘤微环境(tumor microenvironment，TME)中被激活(图 69-1f)[25]。通常来说，这类纳米颗粒能够识别与肿瘤病理相关的微妙的环境改变(例如 pH、氧化还原、酶)，或者可被外加刺激(例如，热、光、磁场、超声)激活[26]。在某种程度上，外部刺激可通过控制释放时间、空间和剂量很好地控制所设计的药物释放曲线[27]。尤其是非侵入性磁场和超声响应的纳米颗粒递送系统，由于具有不受组织穿透的限制的优点，已获得了广泛关注[25,26]。目前，装载阿霉素的热响应脂质体已用于结直肠癌肝转移、骨转移和乳腺癌治疗的Ⅱ期试验，并进入肝癌治疗的Ⅲ期试验[26]。

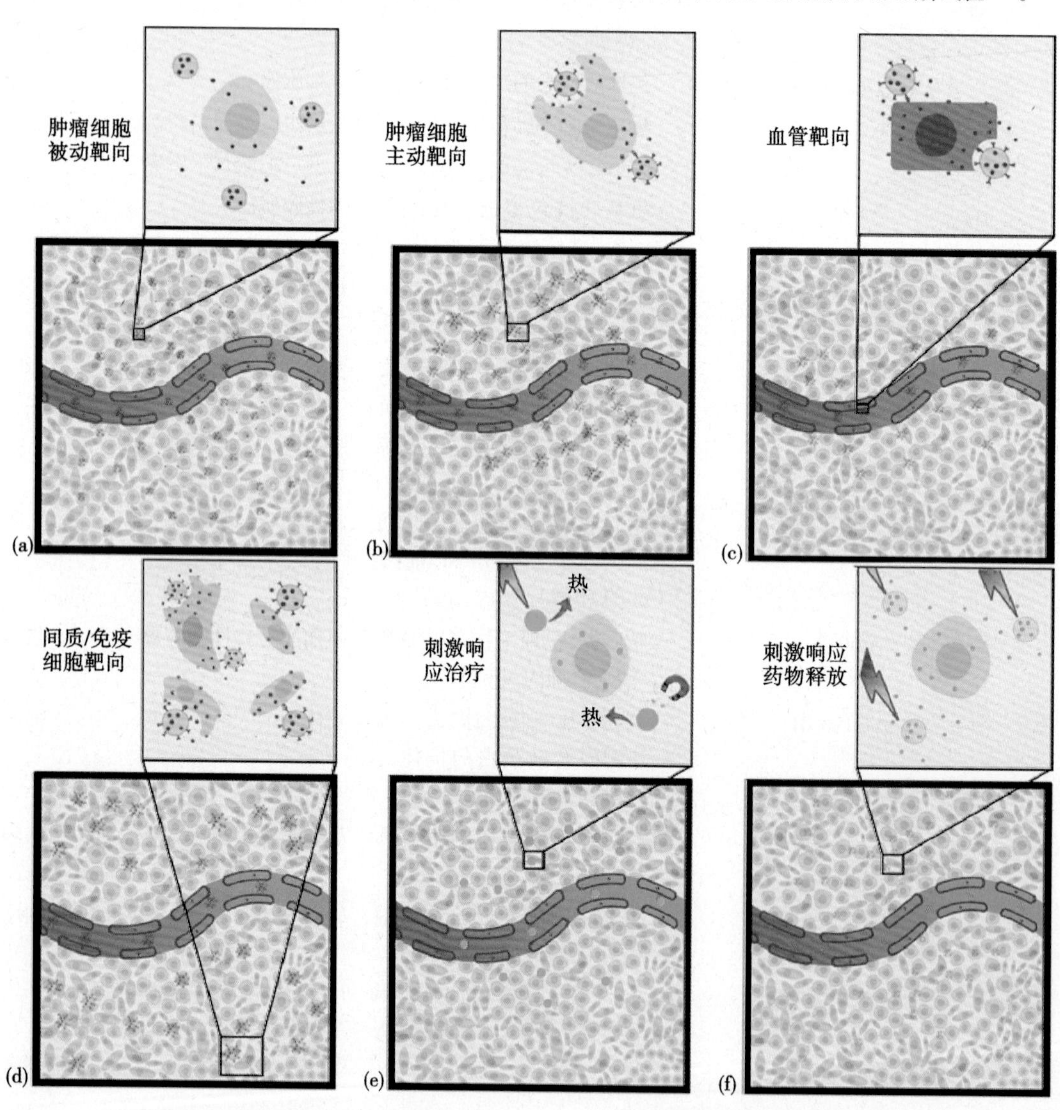

图 69-1 癌症治疗中不同纳米治疗策略的示意图。(a)非靶向纳米颗粒通过 EPR 效应从有漏洞的血管系统被动渗出，在肿瘤部位聚积。药物分子可以从纳米颗粒中释放并在整个组织中扩散以获得生物活性。(b)对肿瘤细胞的主动靶向，用靶向配体修饰纳米颗粒，可识别肿瘤细胞表面上的受体。受体介导的内吞作用能增强纳米颗粒的积累和细胞摄取。(c,d)通过导入与内皮细胞(c)或间质/免疫细胞(d)表面上的受体结合的配体，纳米颗粒可以主动靶向肿瘤微环境，利于癌症治疗。(e)一些纳米颗粒可以在交变磁场或激光照射下产热，利于癌症的热疗。(f)一些纳米颗粒通过在内源刺激(例如，pH、酶和氧化还原)或外源刺激(例如，光、热、磁场或超声)下释放药物而产生治疗活性

放射疗法

在常规的放射治疗中，通常使用高能电离辐射，如 γ 射线和 X 射线，使细胞内组分和/或水分发生电离，产生自由基，对肿瘤细胞的 DNA 造成损伤。然而，由于正常组织对电离辐射剂量的耐受性不佳、肿瘤细胞对辐射会产生抗性等原因，放疗的效果十分受限[28]。如今已发展出了几种解决的策略，将放射增敏纳米材料（如金、钆和氧化铁纳米粒）引入 X 射线路径中，被认为是在较低辐射剂量下根除肿瘤的有效方式[29]。这些材料的电子密度高于组织中的水，可以与 X 射线发生强烈的相互作用，会对肿瘤产生更多的局部性和加强性损伤。目前，基于氧化铪纳米颗粒的新型辐射剂 NanoXray（由 Nanobiotix 开发）正针对患有不同软组织肉瘤的患者进行临床测试。

增强放疗效果的另一种方法是保护周围的健康组织免受放射损伤或降低健康组织对辐射的敏感度。研究者对添加了具有辐射保护作用小分子（如，半胱氨酸、胞磷胆碱、氨磷汀）的纳米颗粒进行了研究。在哺乳动物细胞和大鼠实验中，添加或口服这些纳米颗粒药物后，辐射暴露期间都显示出了辐射保护作用[30-32]。此外，装载生物抗辐射药物（如存活蛋白和表皮生长因子受体）的纳米颗粒也显示出了克服肿瘤对放射治疗抗性的能力[33,34]。以上这些纳米颗粒的策略可以使临床的放疗效果得到进一步改善。

热疗法

光热疗法（photothermal therapy，PTT）和磁热疗法（magnetothermal therapy）等热疗法由于其低毒性、易控性和低抗性等优势，被用于癌症治疗，尤其是耐药性癌症的治疗。与传统的癌症治疗方法不同，PTT 依靠光敏剂吸收光能，并将其转化为热能来杀死周围的细胞[35]。和传统化疗相比，其关键优势在于光敏剂在未受光照时毒性极低，因此即使光敏剂在体内累积，对健康组织的损害也很小。与放疗不同的是，PTT 所使用的光是非电离的（通常为近红外光），因此对组织的损伤要小得多。考虑到大多数肿瘤为乏氧的，临床上用 PTT 治疗癌症比光动力治疗（photodynamic therapy，PDT）更有吸引力，这是因为 PTT 不需要氧气，而 PDT 则要在氧气存在的条件下利用紫外光或可见光激活光敏剂产生有毒的活性氧[36]。而且，PTT 使用的近红外光比 PDT 使用的紫外或可见光具有更深的组织穿透性[37]。但是，低分子量的 PTT 试剂也有很多局限，比如在水溶液中易聚集、会非特异性地结合蛋白、缺乏靶向性等。因此，大量纳米颗粒被研究用作 PTT 试剂，包括碳基纳米材料、半导体纳米晶体、金属纳米颗粒、稀土离子掺杂的纳米晶体和有机纳米颗粒等。体内临床前结果表明，这些 PTT 纳米颗粒制剂能够在对周围健康组织产生最小损伤的同时缩小肿瘤体积[38]。目前，AuroLase（由 Nanospectra 研发的一种金纳米壳二氧化硅纳米颗粒）正用于难治性头颈癌和原发性/转移性肺肿瘤的光热治疗 I 期临床试验。除了光热治疗，磁热治疗也显示出了巨大的潜力。一个成功的例子是 Nano Therm（氧化铁纳米颗粒），作为胶质母细胞瘤治疗的医疗设备，最近已获得欧盟监管机构的批准。有趣的是，这些纳米颗粒也可用于 X 射线 CT 或核磁成像，实现诊断、患者选择及/或响应示踪。

基因治疗

对肿瘤发展/转移至关重要的癌症遗传学以及肿瘤特异性信号通路的研究已取得了新进展，并已应用于癌症的基因治疗。与其他抗癌策略相比，基因治疗的优点在于原则上我们可以合理地对核酸进行设计（如 DNA、siRNA、反义 RNA 和 mRNA），从而特异性地调节任何目的基因的表达。可以特异性沉默靶基因表达的 RNA 干扰（RNA interference，RNAi）技术代表了基因治疗的一场革命，为癌症的研究和治疗带来了巨大的希望[39-41]。例如，许多癌症的基因变异被认为是“无成药性的”靶标和/或需要复杂、耗时的有效抑制剂的开发，而 RNA 干扰技术为研究人类癌症基因变异提供了一种快速的方法[42,43]。然而，RNAi 制剂递送的安全性和有效性（如 siRNA 向肿瘤的递送）阻碍了 RNAi 在癌症治疗中的普遍应用。由于 siRNA 分子易被内源酶降解，并且由于其聚阴离子和大分子特性而不易穿透细胞膜，研究者广泛探索了多种纳米颗粒载体来保护 siRNA 并促进其向肿瘤细胞质内递送[18,44]。迄今为止，有几种基于阳离子脂质体或聚合物的 siRNA 纳米颗粒，包括 CALAA-01、ALN-VSP02、Atu027 等已进入临床 I 期或 II 期试验，用以治疗不同类型的癌症[18]。RNAi 纳米技术也显示出了逆转耐药性的潜力。通过下调过表达的抗细胞凋亡调节剂（例如 Bcl-2）和转运蛋白（例如 P-糖蛋白），或通过抑制 DNA 修复通路，可以重新敏化耐药的肿瘤细胞[45-47]。

与 siRNA 或反义导致的基因沉默不同，DNA 介导的基因治疗旨在用功能性治疗基因取代肿瘤细胞中的突变基因。然而，与 siRNA 递送类似，限制基因治疗在体内应用的主要难题是将脆弱、分子量大、带负电的 DNA 分子递送到肿瘤细胞内的细胞核。在过去的几十年里，研究者们设计了大量带正电的材料，提高了 DNA 递送的安全性和有效性[48]。如今，一种装载 *p53* 基因、表面用转铁蛋白修饰的脂质体 SGT53-01 正在进行实体肿瘤治疗的 I 期临床试验[49]。除了 DNA 之外，mRNA 近年来也被作为有前途的治疗性核酸药物得到研究。mRNA 的治疗机制与 DNA 介导的基因治疗类似，但在某种程度上来说，mRNA 更有效，因为它不需要核定位/转录。此外，mRNA 几乎没有机会与宿主基因组相互作用，因此不会发生潜在的有害基因组整合[50]。未修饰的、以及用鱼精蛋白保护的 mRNA 目前正进行癌症治疗的临床试验[51,52]。虽然目前尚无临床试验，但大量研究表明，纳米颗粒制剂中的 mRNA 表现出了翻译增强的现象，并且由于增强了胞内摄取/内涵体逃逸，产生了更强的免疫应答[53]。

总之，用核酸作为药物进行癌症治疗的思路是直接有效的，但基因治疗的成功应用还面临着体内安全性和基因递送有效性的挑战。虽然机制尚不完全明确，但纳米颗粒递送载体具有血液循环时间长、肿瘤富集多、组织渗透均一、细胞摄取和内涵体逃逸高效等特点，给基因治疗领域带来了巨大机遇。

主动免疫治疗

与上述几种治疗法不同，主动免疫疗法（或称肿瘤疫苗）通过激发患者的免疫系统来攻击肿瘤细胞，为癌症治疗提供了一种独特的策略。由于免疫系统非常强大，具有记忆性，并有精准的特异性，因此主动免疫治疗可以实现完全、持久的癌症治疗，而且对健康组织细胞的损害最小[54]。然而，只有少数疫苗被证实具有足够的临床应用功效。肿瘤微环境、宿主衍生的免疫抑制作用导致的物理障碍、肿瘤免疫逃逸效应等原因限制了大多数癌症疫苗的临床效应[55]。纳米技术在该领域势头正旺，并且作为能有效递送疫苗抗原和佐剂的载体，越来越具有吸引力。首先，纳米颗粒经设计后可被免疫细胞快速内吞，并可以保护抗原(例如肽、蛋白质和核酸)免于过早地被酶解[56]。尤其是与游离抗原相比，纳米颗粒可使一些免疫细胞(如树突状细胞 DCs)更有效地摄取抗原[57]。靶向脂质体疫苗 lipovax-in-MM(目前处于Ⅰ期研究)是在脂质体表面修饰上能靶向 DCs 的特异性抗体片段，可利用配体-受体相互作用有效地将多种抗原递送至 DCs。其次，纳米颗粒可将装载的抗原和佐剂同时运送至靶点，这对获得理想的免疫疗效至关重要。例如，通过将肿瘤相关抗原 HER2/neu 及佐剂 AS15(具有潜在的免疫激活和抗肿瘤活性)装载到脂质体中制备成疫苗，可刺激宿主的免疫应答，产生细胞毒性 T 淋巴细胞应答，使肿瘤裂解，目前已处于转移性乳腺癌的Ⅱ期临床研究中。与脂质体相比，生物可降解聚合物纳米颗粒不仅能调节抗原/佐剂的药代动力学和体内分布，而且还表现出其他的独特性能，例如无需反复给药就可在靶点持续释放抗原/佐剂[58]。Selecta Biosciences 公司一项最近的研究进一步表明，携带佐剂的聚合物纳米颗粒可以增强对所装载抗原的免疫应答，并表现出强烈的局部免疫激活，同时并不会诱导系统性细胞因子的释放[59]。

癌症纳米技术最新进展

对于癌症纳米技术，尽管前面介绍了许多令人欣喜的成就，但其潜力远未实现。在下一节中，我们将简要讨论该领域内最新取得的一些令人兴奋的进展，在我们看来，这些进展将有助于开发更有效的癌症纳米治疗药物。

有效地将系统性药物递送至肿瘤组织的一个主要挑战是如何使纳米颗粒药物逃避肝脏和脾脏中单核吞噬细胞系统(mononuclear phagocyte system，MPS)的识别，从而实现血液长循环。这样，纳米颗粒才能有足够的时间通过渗漏的肿瘤血管系统向肿瘤组织外渗，实现药物在肿瘤部位的有效富集。研究证实，纳米颗粒的物理化学性质，如粒径、形状、表面电荷和表面修饰(如聚乙二醇修饰)，会影响纳米颗粒的循环和肿瘤富集[60-64]。最近，通过在纳米颗粒表面包覆细胞膜来有效规避 MPS 系统的新思路成为人们关注的焦点。用天然红细胞膜包覆的纳米颗粒在血液中的循环半衰期比 PEG 涂覆的纳米颗粒延长了 2.5 倍[65]。与此同时，细胞膜仍可以保持其固有功能，使纳米治疗药物能够向肿瘤主动递送。例如包覆白细胞膜的新一代纳米治疗药物已被证实可以避开调理素作用，延缓肝脏的清除，并活跃地识别和结合肿瘤内皮细胞[66]。另一个意义深远的抑制吞噬清除的策略是用“自身标记”配体，如 CD47 或其多肽变体来修饰纳米颗粒[67]。这类配体可以通过吞噬细胞受体 CD172a 的信号传导来阻止“自身”细胞或纳米颗粒的内吞，从而延迟巨噬细胞介导的纳米颗粒清除，促进血液长循环，从而更有效地将药物递送至肿瘤。

肿瘤微环境已逐渐被认为是导致肿瘤生长、发展和转移的关键因素，因此被视为能有效治疗癌症的潜在靶点[68]。血管内皮具有很多关键性的功能，例如将氧气和营养物质从血液运送到组织，控制血液流动和运输血细胞等。血管内皮的异常与肿瘤发展和转移的发病机制密切相关[69]。因此，用纳米颗粒携带能靶向功能障碍性肿瘤血管内皮的药物或 siRNA 进行癌症治疗，越来越受到关注(图 69-1c)[70]。最近，一种特定的聚合物纳米颗粒平台得到开发，它可以向肺内皮细胞选择性地递送 siRNA，使 5 种内皮基因(*Tie1*、*Tie2*、*VEcad*、*VEGFR-2* 和 *ICAM-2*)有效沉默，同时并不会显著降低肺部免疫细胞、肝细胞或腹膜免疫细胞的基因表达[71]。另一种策略是靶向肿瘤相关炎症，可以此来抑制肿瘤相关巨噬细胞等的浸润(图 69-1d)[72-73]。靶向癌细胞和肿瘤微环境之间的通讯也受到关注，一个最近的例子是使用生物可降解的 PLGA-PEG 聚合物主动靶向递送硼替佐米 Bortezomib，以此增强成骨分化和结合强度，从而显著抑制骨骼中肿瘤的生长，而骨是许多癌症中最常见的转移部位[74]。此外，一些高细胞毒性的化疗药物可制备成“前药”进行给药，通过肿瘤微环境(如 pH、酶和乏氧环境)活化后，成为细胞杀伤性药物[75]。

经口服、鼻腔或眼部途径进行非侵入性给药的纳米治疗药物的研究虽然还处于早期阶段，但其正在不断地发展，并显示出许多系统性注射给药所不具备的优点。经鼻给药的药物递送有利于肺癌的治疗，因为这种给药方式可以绕过肝富集且无需多次给药。最近，载阿霉素的可吸入纳米颗粒被用于肺癌治疗的体内研究，与静脉注射组相比，存活率得到显著改善[76]。另一方面，口服药由于给药方便，需要频繁给药的癌症患者能从中受益，但这种给药方式受到由肠黏膜屏障导致的药物肠吸收不足的限制。最近，有研究者将 IgG Fc 片段与聚合物纳米颗粒连接，可以有效靶向新生的 Fc(FcRn)受体，并在口服给药后通过肠上皮转运至全身循环，平均吸收率比非靶向纳米颗粒高 10 倍[15]。这些靶向纳米颗粒为癌症治疗中的口服递送纳米治疗药物的开发提供了新希望。

总结

癌症纳米药物的临床成功已成为开发新纳米颗粒技术的驱动力，这种纳米颗粒新技术可用于更安全、更有效及具有个性化的纳米治疗。同时，我们也认识到由于癌症的复杂性、异质性以及临床转化中的难题，癌症纳米技术领域仍具有很大的挑战。因此，纳米技术与肿瘤生物学和其他生物/生物医学科学的融合对于充分发挥癌症纳米技术的潜力至关重要。我们希望本章能够激励不同专业领域的医生、科学家、工程师和其他人一同参与到这一令人兴奋的领域中来，共同促进纳米技术在癌症治疗中的广泛应用。

(吕岩霖　马光辉　译)

参考文献

The complete reference list can be found on the Wiley Companion Digital Edition of this title (see inside front cover for login instructions).

1 Stewart BW, Wild CP. *World Cancer Report 2014*. IARC: Lyon; 2014.

4 Hubbell JA, Langer R. Translating materials design to the clinic. *Nat Mater*. 2013;**12**:963–966.

9 Farokhzad OC, Langer R. Impact of nanotechnology on drug delivery. *ACS Nano*. 2009;3:16–20.

11 Langer R. Drug delivery and targeting. *Nature*. 1998;**392**:5–10.

15 Pridgen EM, Alexis F, Kuo TT, et al. Transepithelial transport of Fc-targeted nanoparticles by the neonatal fc receptor for oral delivery. *Sci Transl Med*. 2013;5:213ra167.

18 Kanasty R, Dorkin JR, Vegas A, et al. Delivery materials for siRNA therapeutics. *Nat Mater*. 2013;**12**:967–977.

21 Matsumura Y, Maeda H. A new concept for macromolecular therapeutics in cancer chemotherapy: Mechanism of tumoritropic accumulation of proteins and the antitumor agent SMANCS. *Cancer Res*. 1986;**46**:6387–6392.

22 Peer D, Karp JM, Hong S, et al. Nanocarriers as an emerging platform for cancer therapy. *Nat Nanotech*. 2007;**2**:751–760.

24 Hrkach J, Hoff DV, Ali MM, et al. Preclinical development and clinical translation of a PSMA-targeted docetaxel nanoparticle with a differentiated pharmacological profile. *Sci Transl Med*. 2012;**4**:128ra39.

26 Mura S, Nicolas J, Couvreur P. Stimuli-responsive drug-delivery systems in clinical trials. *Nat Mater*. 2013;**12**:991–1003.

29 Kwatra D, Venugopal A, Anant S. Nanoparticles in radiation therapy: a summary of various approaches to enhance radiosensitization in cancer. *Transl Cancer Res*. 2013;**2**:330–342.

38 Jaque D, Maestro ML, Rosal B, et al. Nanoparticles for photothermal therapies. *Nanoscale*. 2014;**6**:9494–9530.

41 Whitehead KA, Langer R, Anderson DG. Knocking down barriers: advances in siRNA delivery. *Nat Rev Drug Discov*. 2009;**8**:129–138.

56 Smith DM, Simon JK, Baker JR Jr. Applications of nanotechnology for immunology. *Nat Rev Immunol*. 2013;**13**:592–605.

65 Hu CMJ, Aryal S, Cheung C, et al. Erythrocyte membrane-camouflaged polymeric nanoparticles as a biomimetic delivery platform. *Proc Natl Acad Sci U S A*. 2011;**108**:10980–10985.

67 Rodriguez PL, Harada T, Christian DA, et al. Minimal "self" peptides that inhibit phagocytic clearance and enhance delivery of nanoparticles. *Science*. 2013;**339**:971–975.

68 Albini A, Sporn MB. The tumour microenvironment as a target for chemoprevention. *Nat Rev Cancer*. 2007;**7**:139–145.

71 Dahlman JE, Barnes C, et al. In vivo endothelial siRNA delivery using polymeric nanoparticles with low molecular weight. *Nat Nanotechnol*. 2014;**9**:648–655.

第 70 章　造血干细胞移植

Roy Jones, MD, PhD ■ Elizabeth Shpall, MD ■ Richard Champlin, MD

概述

造血干细胞移植是多种血液系统肿瘤和某些实体肿瘤、免疫缺陷病以及遗传性疾病的有效治疗方法。随着移植技术的不断改进，高龄患者和接受人类白细胞抗原不匹配供体造血干细胞的患者也能从中获益。虽然移植治疗（包括药物）毒副作用明显，但具备治愈高危肿瘤的潜能；也就是说，异基因造血干细胞移植是目前治愈某些恶性肿瘤的最有效手段，甚至是唯一的方法。异基因造血干细胞移植的核心是异基因免疫排斥反应（移植物抗肿瘤效应），其治疗获益和风险为未来的肿瘤免疫治疗提供了宝贵经验。

造血干细胞移植（hematopoietic cell transplantation, HSCT）涉及干细胞的植入，这些干细胞可以从骨髓、外周血或者脐血中获取。异基因造血干细胞移植（allogeneic HSCT, allo-HSCT）所用的干细胞来自其他人，自体造血干细胞移植（autologous HSCT, AHSCT）所用的干细胞，通常是患者自身冻存的造血干细胞，同基因造血干细胞移植是同卵双生的双胞胎之间的移植。

造血干细胞移植是许多致命的血液病、免疫、代谢和肿瘤性疾病的有效治疗方法（表 70-1）[1,2]。AHSCT 的基本原理是用来源于患者的造血干细胞防止预处理所致的致死性骨髓抑制。为了探索产生增强免疫效应的方法，有些学者对自体造血干细胞进行了体外处理的研究。Allo-HSCT 的基本原理是供体来源的干细胞在受体中植入，重建造血和免疫功能，移植成功后受体成为含有来自供体造血细胞和免疫细胞的嵌合体。近年来，人们已经认识到造血干细胞能够有限的分化为非造血组织[4]，包括间充质细胞[5,6]、肝脏[7,8]、心血管组织[9]、还可能有神经组织[10]。造血干细胞移植对恢复受损或患病的器官和组织具有极大的益处[11,12]。

表 70-1　造血干细胞移植适应证

恶性病	非恶性病
急性髓系白血病	再生障碍性贫血及相关的骨髓衰竭状态
骨髓增生异常综合征	血红蛋白病：地中海贫血、镰状细胞性贫血
急性淋巴细胞白血病	先天性造血功能障碍
慢性粒细胞白血病和骨髓增殖性疾病	Fanconi 贫血及相关综合征
淋巴瘤和慢性淋巴细胞白血病	先天性免疫缺陷：重症联合免疫缺陷、Wiskott-Aldrich 综合征、慢性肉芽肿和相关综合征
多发性骨髓瘤和淀粉样变性	先天性代谢异常
实体瘤：乳腺癌、睾丸癌、卵巢癌和小细胞肺癌	自身免疫病
小儿实体瘤：神经母细胞瘤、尤文氏肉瘤、髓母细胞瘤、肾细胞癌、黑色素瘤	

移植方法

大多数情况下，移植的造血干细胞在强烈的化疗、放疗和其他治疗（如抗体）后输注。随着研究的不断进步，许多化疗药物用于移植预处理，尤其是烷化剂类药物，如环磷酰胺、白消安、美法仑、噻替哌和卡莫司汀。全身放疗（total body radiation, TBI）也被应用于移植。Allo-HSCT 中除使用这些药物外，还往往需要联合应用同时具有杀伤肿瘤细胞和免疫抑制作用的药物，如氟达拉滨[13]。

移植物抗肿瘤（graft-versus-malignancy, GVM）效应作为 allo-HSCT 治疗的重要组成部分已经获得公认[14]。这种介导移植物抗肿瘤的同种异基因免疫效应，通常与移植物对正常组织的毒性相关，称为移植物抗宿主病（graft-versus-host disease, GVHD）。Allo-HSCT 研究的一个主要焦点是探索在没有 GVHD 的情况下，可能产生 GVM 的特定细胞类型和技术[15]。移植后的供体淋巴细胞输注（donor lymphocyte infusions, DLI）可用于增强 GVM 效应[16]。

造血干细胞移植治疗恶性肿瘤

造血干细胞移植已经用于治疗多种血液系统恶性肿瘤[17]。许多化疗药物（主要是烷化剂[18]）和放疗有剂量依赖的抗肿瘤反应，同时具有剂量限制性毒性骨髓抑制，从而限制其加大剂量使用。预处理后移植自体或异体造血干细胞恢复造血,可以把化疗药物的剂量提高到最大耐受剂量的 3~5 倍(图 70-1)。

自体造血干细胞移植(AHSCT)

一般来说,AHSCT 对常规化疗敏感的恶性肿瘤患者疗效最好[19]。治疗失败的已知因素包括残留较大的肿瘤病灶[20,21]、量效关系不明确的肿瘤类型[22]、推荐治疗方案具有高毒性风险的患者。移植后免疫增强的策略正在被积极探索,以免移植后的免疫功能恢复时间过长,进而增加肿瘤复发风险[23]。另一个导致复发的可能因素是采集的造血干细胞中混有肿瘤细胞。尽管有个别研究使用基因标记的肿瘤细胞,证明冻存造血干细胞中的肿瘤细胞可以植入并导致复发,但其重要性在 AHSCT 的临床应用中尚未被明确证实[24]。AHSCT 可以治愈某些血液系统肿瘤,其中包括危险度分组中等的及某些特定病理类型的非霍奇金淋巴瘤[25]、霍奇金淋巴瘤[26]、急性淋巴细胞白血病(acute lymphoblastic leukemia,ALL)[27,28]、急性髓系白血病(acute myelogenous leukemia,AML)[29,30]。尽管未能证实 AHSCT 可以治愈多发性骨髓瘤(multiple myeloma,MM),但接受 AHSCT 的患者生存期明显延长,使得该技术被作为有适应证患者的标准治疗方法[31,32]。生殖细胞肿瘤[33]、淋巴瘤[34]和多种小儿实体瘤的患者也可从 AHSCT 中获益[35]。

异基因造血干细胞移植(allo-HSCT)

Allo-HSCT 是化疗与免疫介导的 GVM 效应的结合。供体来源的淋巴细胞可以攻击并清除在大剂量细胞毒性药物治疗后残存的肿瘤细胞[36,37]。急性或慢性 GVHD 可以降低患者复发风险,表明 GVM 效应与 GVHD 之间存在一定的关联[38,39]。GVM 效应最直接的证据是 DLI 可以使移植后复发的肿瘤患者再次达到临床缓解[40,41]。

恶性肿瘤对 GVM 效应的易感性存在显著差异。Allo-HSCT 后复发的肿瘤患者,通过减量或停用免疫抑制剂或 DLI 治疗后,患者病情持久缓解,证明了惰性髓系和惰性淋巴系统恶性肿瘤对 GVM 效应高度敏感,GVM 效应在 allo-HSCT 治疗的慢性髓系白血病(chronic myelogenous leukemia,CML)患者中得到了最好的证明。

接受 allo-HSCT 的其他血液系统恶性肿瘤患者,包括 AML、MM、霍奇金淋巴瘤和中危非霍奇金淋巴瘤,也存在 GVM 效应,但强度较弱。Allo-HSCT 治疗这些疾病比同基因造血干细胞移植或 AHSCT 能产生更高的持久缓解率,但它们对 DLI 的反应较小,并且通常是短暂的。ALL 和高危淋巴瘤对 GVM 效应相对不敏感[42],尽管某些研究中显示,allo-HSCT 后伴发 GVHD 的 ALL 和高危淋巴瘤患者肿瘤复发风险会有所降低[43]。

GVM 效应可以作用于许多潜在的靶抗原。探索分离 GVM 效应和 GVHD 的方法以及诱导抗原特异性抗肿瘤反应是当前研究的主要目标。例如,自然杀伤(natural killer,NK)细胞可以产生低风险 GVHD 的 GVM 效应[44],调节性 T 细胞(regulatory T cells,T_{reg})可以抑制 GVHD 而对 GVM 效应影响较小[45]。

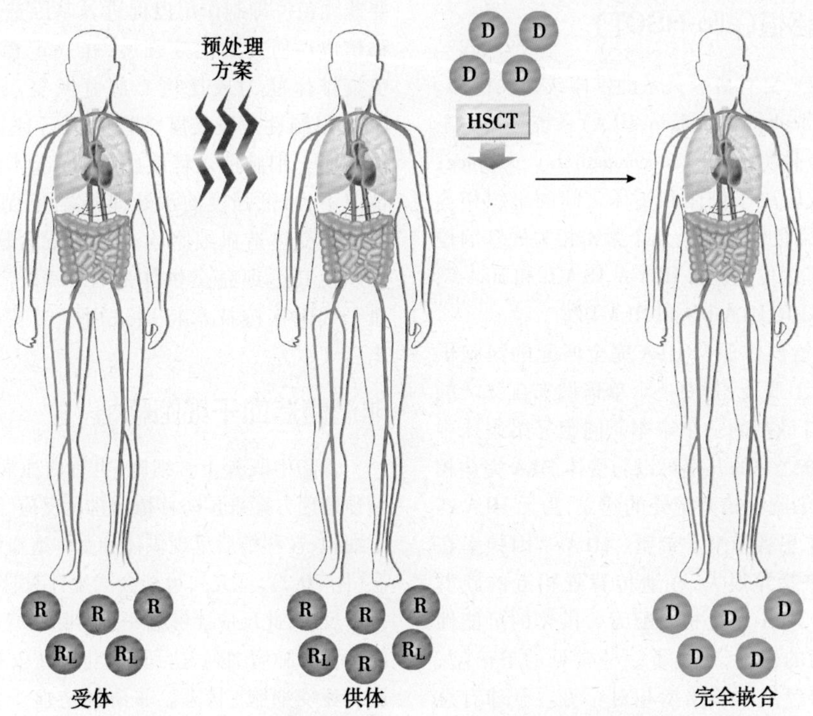

图 70-1　异基因造血干细胞移植流程。患者接受可同时清除体内肿瘤细胞和正常细胞的清髓预处理方案,然后输注供体造血干细胞,恢复造血。D,供体造血干细胞;HSCT,造血干细胞移植;R,受体正常骨髓细胞;RL,受体骨髓中的白血病细胞

供体选择

自体造血干细胞移植(AHSCT)

AHSCT患者的供体通常是患者自己,特殊情况下,遗传学完全相同的同卵双胞胎也可作为AHSCT患者的供体。AHSCT不需要考虑组织相容性匹配的问题,但由于患者既往接受的大剂量化疗造成骨髓造血干细胞的损伤,使得采集足够的干细胞比较困难。AHSCT所需的造血干细胞,既可从骨髓采集,也可用粒细胞集落刺激因子(granulocyte colony-stimulating factor,G-CSF)或化疗药物做造血动员后从外周血采集。为了达到满意的造血植入,需要采集的$CD34^+$细胞数按患者公斤体重计算至少为2×10^6/kg。若采集的造血干细胞中混有肿瘤细胞,称为肿瘤细胞污染干细胞。肿瘤细胞污染可能是AHSCT后疾病复发的一个来源。因此,那些骨髓有明显肿瘤细胞浸润的患者不是AHSCT治疗的理想选择[46,47]。为了减少或消除肿瘤细胞污染,多种体外"净化"技术正在研究中。

采集的患者骨髓或外周血干/祖细胞在存活状态下被冻存。患者接受清除恶性肿瘤的大剂量清髓性化疗后输注冻存的干/祖细胞以重建造血。自体造血干/祖细胞也可以作为潜在的基因治疗载体,用于纠正免疫功能缺陷。

异基因造血干细胞移植(allo-HSCT)

Allo-HSCT的干细胞来自有血缘关系的供体或无关供体。人类白细胞抗原(human leukocyte antigen,HLA)系统是人类主要的组织相容性复合体(major histocompatibility complex,MHC),allo-HSCT的疗效取决于供体和受体之间的组织相容性。HLA系统是由6号染色体短臂上几个紧密相关的基因位点编码组成[48,49],Ⅰ类基因位点包括HLA-A、HLA-B和HLA-C,Ⅱ类基因位点包括HLA-DR、HLA-DQ和HLA-DP。

Allo-HSCT初期,移植供体源自HLA完全匹配的同胞供体。HLA基因作为单倍型遗传,其中一个单倍型来自父亲的一个亲本,另一个则来自母亲的一个亲本。同胞兄弟姐妹中的任何一位,大约有四分之一的几率可以与受体HLA完全相匹配。无关供体造血干细胞移植登记处的建立,为无HLA匹配同胞供体的allo-HSCT患者带来了希望。HLA基因频率在不同种族和民族群体中差异很大,在遗传背景相近的族群中,allo-HSCT患者获得HLA完全相匹配无关供体的可能性最大。因为连锁不平衡的发生,产生了一些常见的单倍型,但也有接近半数的人群产生的单倍型相对罕见。全球有总计超过1 800万个无关供体造血干细胞移植志愿者登记,他们有可能作为无关供体造血干细胞的捐献者。因此,大约一半的allo-HSCT患者,可以有HLA-A、HLA-B、HLA-C、HLA-DR-和HLA-DQ相匹配的供体。目前,10个位点相匹配的无关供体造血干细胞移植与组织相容性的同胞供体造血干细胞移植相比,已经达到了相似的移植成功率和近/远期临床疗效[50,51]。

患者接受一个或多个HLA基因位点不匹配的移植会有更高的移植排斥、GVHD和其他移植相关并发症的风险。对大多数allo-HSCT的患者而言,单倍型相合的供体最容易找到。在单倍型相合造血干细胞移植的临床实践中,移植后应用大剂量环磷酰胺能够降低GVHD风险,使得单倍型相合造血干细胞移植的成功率和临床疗效也得到进一步提高[52]。除单倍型相合造血干细胞移植供体外,脐血也经常被用于allo-HSCT的干细胞来源[53,54]。脐血移植的HLA匹配限制远小于其他供体来源的造血干细胞移植,脐血移植时,HLA-A、HLA-B和HLA-DR的6个基因位点中2个不匹配是可以接受的[55]。由于儿童患者体重低,移植所需的造血干细胞数量相对较少,单份脐血移植在儿童患者中最为成功。当单份脐血的造血干细胞数量足够或使用多份脐血时,成人患者的脐血移植也可成功。免疫重建延迟和高发的机会性感染率仍然是单倍型造血干细胞移植和脐血移植的主要并发症。

与AHSCT一样,allo-HSCT通常在清髓性强化疗预处理后进行回输。移植预处理除了尽可能杀伤肿瘤细胞之外,还要兼顾免疫抑制作用以促进异基因造血干细胞的顺利植入。移植成功所需的化疗强度,在一定程度上与患者的移植物免疫排斥能力成比例。造血恢复后,通过PCR对供体的DNA限制性片段长度多态性进行评估,是最常用的判定供体造血干细胞植入程度(称为嵌合体)的检测方法。在某些情况下,减低强度的预处理方案用于降低治疗相关的毒性,建立供受体造血细胞均存在的混合嵌合状态。后续的DLI可以使其达到完全供体嵌合状态[56]。这种减低强度的造血干细胞移植技术特别适用于需要接受移植治疗的老年患者[57,58]。

非清髓造血干细胞移植

骨髓中既有正常细胞,也有白血病细胞的患者,接受非清髓预处理方案来预防移植物排斥反应,再接受来自供体的造血干细胞,在移植后呈现供体和受体造血细胞共存的混合嵌合状态(图70-2)。随后,可能会产生针对骨髓造血组织的移植物抗排斥反应,此反应能够进一步清除非清髓预处理后残留在受体的正常和肿瘤细胞,达到完全嵌合(仅存在供体衍生的造血细胞和免疫细胞)状态。非清髓造血干细胞移植后,也可通过DLI达到增强GVM效应的目的。

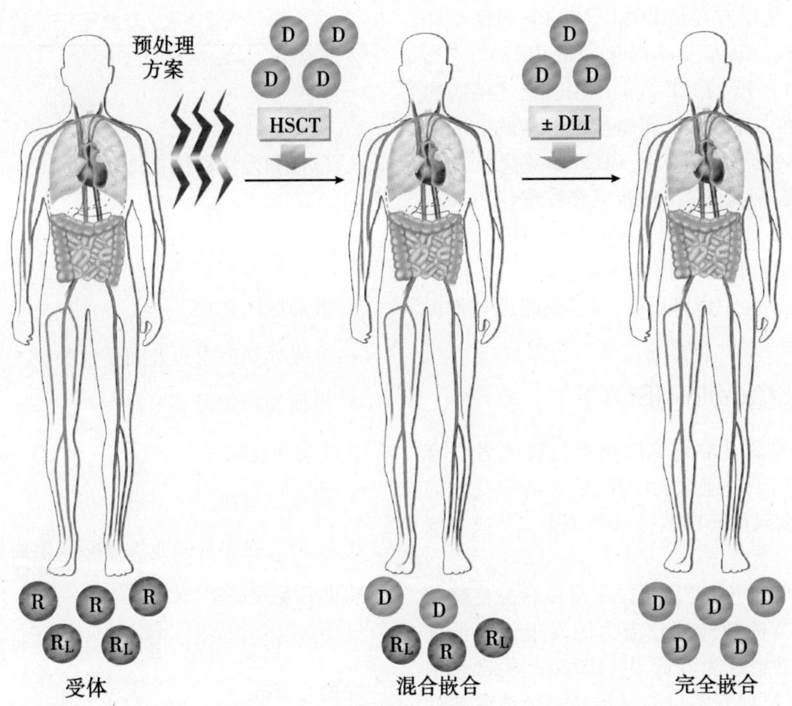

图 70-2 非清髓异基因造血干细胞移植流程。D,供体造血干细胞;HSCT,造血干细胞移植;DLI,供体淋巴细胞输注;R,受体正常骨髓细胞;RL,受体骨髓中的白血病细胞

自体造血干细胞移植(AHSCT)或异基因造血干细胞移植(allo-HSCT)的选择

患者选择 AHSCT 还是 allo-HSCT 治疗,取决于恶性肿瘤的类型、受体的年龄、可用的合适供体、能否采集无肿瘤污染的自体移植物、疾病的分期和状态(骨髓受累、疾病的严重程度、对常规化疗的敏感性)以及恶性肿瘤对 GVM 效应的易感性。

AHSCT 的实施相对简单,而且不需要 HLA 匹配的供体。AHSCT 发生危及生命并发症的风险较低,无 GVHD 风险,不需要用免疫抑制剂来防治 GVHD 和移植排斥。AHSCT 后的免疫重建比 allo-HSCT 更快,并且机会性感染的风险更低,移植失败很少发生。在大多数临床研究中,AHSCT 相关死亡率低于5%,老年患者可以相对较好地耐受治疗[59,60]。然而,AHSCT 也有一些缺点,克隆性肿瘤细胞侵犯血液或骨髓可导致复发。AHSCT 只能通过大剂量化疗达到根除肿瘤的目的,缺乏 allo-HSCT 后免疫介导的 GVM 效应。尽管 AHSCT 治疗多数血液系统恶性肿瘤的复发率高于 allo-HSCT,但其治疗相关死亡率较低,这是 AHSCT 被选择的重要原因。AHSCT 后,先前接受过大剂量化疗的患者发生骨髓异常增生和继发性急性白血病的风险较高[61,62]。

Allo-HSCT 具有移植物无肿瘤细胞污染的优点,以及供体衍生的免疫活性细胞可能产生的 GVM 效应。Allo-HSCT 可能发生许多潜在的致命并发症,如预处理相关的器官毒性,移植失败和 GVHD。Allo-HSCT 后免疫重建较慢,机会性感染更常见,治疗相关的死亡率明显高于用 AHSCT。

通常情况下,allo-HSCT 多用于治疗白血病和骨髓增生异常综合征(myelodysplastic syndrome,MDS)。AHSCT 则更多地用于实体瘤、淋巴瘤和骨髓瘤,然而,非清髓性 allo-HSCT 在这些疾病中作为诱导 GVM 效应的手段也正在被评估。

移植的临床疗效不仅与患者选择有关,也与移植时机有关。疾病早期,恶性肿瘤细胞对放、化疗反应敏感时,以及肿瘤负荷较低时,进行移植疗效最佳。相反,移植作为挽救治疗手段时,不仅肿瘤复发率高,治疗相关毒性的发生率也显著升高。对常规剂量化疗的治疗反应是造血干细胞移植疗效的主要预测因素。复发后化疗敏感的患者,或巩固治疗阶段的高危患者,特别是肿瘤负荷降到最低的时间点进行移植,疗效最为理想。诱导治疗不能达到缓解的急性白血病、霍奇金淋巴瘤或 MM 患者经大剂量强化治疗,部分患者能够克服原发耐药而降低肿瘤负荷。强化治疗后肿瘤负荷依然很大,或难治复发或多次复发的恶性肿瘤,移植的临床疗效尚不理想。

移植前治疗

自体造血干细胞移植(AHSCT)

早期 AHSCT 的预处理方案参照 allo-HSCT 的经验,并使用环磷酰胺加 TBI 或白消安。TBI 应同时做到精确剂量治疗和保护易损器官(例如肺和肾)这两点。然而,深部肿瘤细胞因缺氧而对放疗不敏感;相反,化疗药物如白消安可以渗透肿瘤血管并更有效地到达深部肿瘤,因此,TBI 对于体积较大的肿瘤是次选的。

烷化剂是造血干细胞移植预处理方案中最常用的药物,其剂量通常与清除的肿瘤细胞负荷成正比。最常用的烷化剂包括环磷酰胺、美法仑、白消安、卡莫司汀(BCNU)和噻替哌。铂类衍生物卡铂[63]和顺铂[64]也被使用。其他常用的非烷化剂有依托泊苷(VP-16)、阿糖胞苷和氟达拉滨。霍奇金淋巴瘤和非霍奇金淋巴瘤最常用的化疗方案是BCNU、VP-16、阿糖胞苷和美法仑(BCNU, etoposide, Ara-C, and melphalan, BEAM)[65]。含有异环磷酰胺、卡铂和VP-16的ICE方案也用于上述疾病的治疗。近年来,已经证明在白血病和非霍奇金淋巴瘤的标准治疗方案中联合单克隆抗体,疗效更佳。抗CD20单克隆抗体利妥昔单抗与含有环磷酰胺、阿霉素、长春新碱和泼尼松(cyclophosphamide, doxorubicin, vincristine, and prednisone, CHOP)的化疗方案联合化疗,可提高中危淋巴瘤患者的生存率。同样,单克隆抗体联合BEAM方案治疗中危淋巴瘤,似乎也能进一步提高疗效[66]。

异基因造血干细胞移植(allo-HSCT)

Allo-HSCT的预处理方案通常是单用化疗药物或者联合TBI。经典的"清髓"方案用于白血病的治疗,旨在清除受体的造血和免疫系统,通常是大剂量环磷酰胺联合TBI[67,68]或大剂量白消安[69,70]。

大剂量清髓方案的毒性,使其应用局限于身体状况良好的年轻患者。免疫介导的GVM效应治疗潜力的发现使得低剂量、减低强度的预处理新方案成为降低allo-HSCT相关毒性的一种手段。减低强度的预处理方案目的并不是完全清除恶性肿瘤细胞,而是提供足够的免疫抑制以实现造血干细胞植入并诱导GVM效应[71,72](图70-2)。老年或有合并症无法接受清髓方案的患者,可以耐受减低强度的预处理方案。大多数减低强度的预处理方案含有嘌呤类似物,例如氟达拉滨,它可以与烷化剂(环磷酰胺,美法仑或白消安)或与低剂量TBI联合使用。减低强度的预处理方案对恶性血液病是有效的,大多数患者可以实现造血干细胞植入。为了显著增强对受体的免疫抑制作用,通常可以联合使用抗胸腺细胞免疫球蛋白。

造血干细胞移植的并发症

高强度放化疗和造血干细胞移植可能发生表70-2中列出的一些严重并发症,这些包括免疫介导的病理损伤,如移植排斥和GVHD、预处理相关毒性、中性粒细胞减少引起的感染和移植后免疫缺陷等。

表70-2 造血干细胞移植后并发症

免疫相关并发症
• 移植排斥
• 急性和慢性移植物抗宿主病
预处理相关毒性
• 黏膜炎和肠胃炎
• 肝静脉闭塞病
• 弥漫性肺泡出血及间质性肺炎
• 出血性膀胱炎
血液学并发症
• 溶血性贫血
• 血栓性血小板减少性紫癜和溶血性疾病
感染和免疫缺陷
• EBV感染相关的淋巴组织增生性疾病
晚期并发症
• 生长障碍
• 甲状腺功能减退
• 不育及性腺功能减退
• 白内障
• 缺血性坏死
• 继发恶性肿瘤

移植排斥和移植失败

移植失败的定义为未能实现造血干细胞植入(原发移植失败)或造血干细胞植入后丧失(继发移植失败)。移植失败很少发生在AHSCT,通常与输注的有造血能力的干细胞数量不足有关。

Allo-HSCT后移植失败是由移植免疫排斥反应引起的[73,74]。根据目前的治疗方案,HLA匹配的同胞供体造血干细胞移植中,只有不到2%的患者发生移植排斥反应。HLA不匹配会增加患者发生移植排斥的风险[75,76]。供体$CD8^+$ T淋巴细胞具有促进造血干细胞植入效应,去除供体T淋巴细胞,会增加移植失败的风险[77,78]。因脐带血中$CD34^+$和$CD8^+$T细胞含量较少,更容易发生造血干细胞植入失败。

髓系抑制药物的使用、GVHD和移植后早期感染,可能引起继发性移植失败和移植物功能不良。更昔洛韦或甲氧苄啶-磺胺甲噁唑可能会引起全血细胞减少,但在停药后通常是可逆的。巨细胞病毒[79]、细小病毒[80]、人疱疹病毒[81,82]及分枝杆菌和真菌感染也可能损害移植物。植入不良也可能由患者的潜在疾病或既往治疗相关的微环境或骨髓基质功能障碍引起。

除移植排斥引起的移植失败外,其他原因导致的植入失败通常可以通过使用G-CSF或输注来自相同供体或者替代供体的二次造血干细胞来治疗。

移植物抗宿主病(GVHD)

GVHD是allo-HSCT治疗中可能危及生命的一个主要并发症。急性和慢性GVHD有不同的临床病理特征,但两者又相互关联。急性GVHD通常发生在移植后100天内,是移植物中存在的成熟供体T淋巴细胞对抗受体(宿主)主要或次要组织相容性抗原反应的结果[83]。急性GVHD的主要靶器官是皮肤、胃肠道和肝脏,也可以累及造血和免疫系统。皮肤急性GVHD通常首先出现斑丘疹,表现为典型的瘙痒和融合,严重时可能会出现全身性红皮病、大疱和脱屑。肝脏急性GVHD累及胆管上皮导致胆汁淤积性肝炎,可使胆红素和碱性磷酸酶明显升高。GVHD可以影响整个胃肠道上皮细胞。胃肠道GVHD特征性的表现为分泌性腹泻、腹痛以及罕见的肠梗阻。单纯上消化道GVHD而无下消化道和其他组织受累时会出现恶心、呕吐和厌食[84]。急性GVHD也可表现为结膜炎和其他眼部症状、贫血和血小板减少。

严重 GVHD 与预后不良相关，因为 GVHD 本身和治疗 GVHD 使用的免疫抑制药物都会导致组织损伤、受体体质衰弱和严重的免疫缺陷。

预测 GVHD 风险最重要的因素是供受体之间 HLA 匹配的差异[85-88]。通过应用目前的免疫抑制剂进行预防，HLA 匹配的同胞供体造血干细胞移植急性 GVHD 的发生率为 25%～50%，这可能与次要组织相容性抗原不合有关。据报道，HLA 不匹配的同胞供体和无关供体造血干细胞移植急性 GVHD 的发生率可高达 61%～90%。通过使用更精确的分子组织相容性配型来选择供体，可以改善无关供体造血干细胞移植的临床疗效。高龄与急性和慢性 GVHD 的高发生率密切相关。减低强度的非清髓预处理方案也可以减轻 GVHD 的严重程度，可能是由于组织损伤的减少，缩短了炎性反应的持续时间，进而限制了 GVHD 的发展。

移植后前 6 个月使用药物加强免疫抑制，可以降低 GVHD 的发生率和严重程度。目前 GVHD 的标准预防方案是环孢素或他克莫司联合短程甲氨蝶呤[89,90]。皮质类固醇是急性 GVHD 患者的一线治疗药物。大约一半的患者对皮质类固醇治疗有效[91]，并且皮质类固醇剂量可逐渐减少，皮质类固醇耐药的 GVHD 患者预后不良。局限于皮肤的 GVHD 预后最佳，累及肝脏或多个器官的急性 GVHD 预后不良。除了上述 GVHD 防治方案外，还有其他多种免疫抑制药物用于防治 GVHD。最近研究表明，针对不匹配移植物，移植后使用环磷酰胺可以降低 GVHD 的风险，并且可使有血缘关系的单倍型造血干细胞移植风险控制在可接受范围内[92]。

慢性 GVHD 是 allo-HSCT 后期合并的相关综合征，移植后存活超过 6 个月的患者中，有 25%～60% 的患者发生慢性 GVHD[93]。慢性 GVHD 最常发生于移植后的 80～200 天，但发病也可能延迟到移植后第二年。慢性 GVHD 通常在老年患者和既往有急性 GVHD 的患者中更为常见，但也有大约三分之一的慢性 GVHD 患者既往无急性 GVHD 病程[94]。与骨髓干细胞移植相比，外周血干细胞移植后慢性 GVHD 的发生更为多见[95]。

慢性 GVHD 有多种临床表现，与一些自身免疫性疾病相类似，如进行性系统性硬化症、干燥综合征和原发性胆汁性肝硬化。慢性 GVHD 伴有重度免疫抑制，是患者发生机会性感染的主要危险因素。慢性 GVHD 可以没有其他症状而仅表现为闭塞性细支气管炎，肠道受累时可能出现厌食、吞咽困难、吸收不良和消瘦。多发性肌炎、浆膜炎和自身免疫症状很少出现。慢性 GVHD 可能成为一种影响生活质量的慢性衰弱性疾病，并且仍然是影响晚期移植相关并发症的主要决定因素。全身性进行性慢性 GVHD 由急性 GVHD 发展而来，血小板减少是慢性 GVHD 预后不良的因素（表 70-3）[96]。

表 70-3 GVHD 的临床分期与分级

分期	急性 GVHD					
	皮肤[a]			肝脏[b]		胃肠道[b]
1	皮疹<25%			胆红素 2～3mg/dl		腹泻 500～1 000ml 或持续呕吐[c]
2	皮疹 25%～50%			胆红素 3～6mg/dl		腹泻 1 000～1 500ml
3	全身皮疹			胆红素 6～15mg/dl		腹泻>1 500ml
4	皮肤剥脱和水疱			胆红素>15mg/dl		严重腹痛或肠梗阻
总分级[d]	严重程度	皮肤		肝脏		胃肠道
0	无	0	和	0	和	0
Ⅰ	轻	1～2	和	0	和	0
Ⅱ	中	3	和/或	1	和/或	1
Ⅲ	重	0～3	和	2～3	和/或	2～3
Ⅳ[e]	危重	4	和/或	4	和/或	4
慢性 GVHD						
局部性	局部皮肤受累和/或肝功能障碍					
广泛性	1. 全身皮肤受累					
	2. 局部皮肤受累和/或肝功能障碍，加上以下列任何一项：					
	（a）肝脏组织学显示慢性进行性肝炎、桥接性坏死或肝硬化					
	（b）眼部受累（Schirmer 试验<5mm 润湿）					
	（c）累及黏膜腺或口腔黏膜					
	（d）累及任何其他靶器官					

注：[a] 范围按九分法或者烧伤面积图计算。[b] 有其他导致胆红素升高或腹泻的原因时降低一个分期。[c] 需要胃或十二指肠 GVHD 的组织学证据。[d] 确定分级所需的最小器官分期。[e] 单一器官受累但器官功能严重受损时也可确定为Ⅳ级。

资料来源：引自参考文献 117、118、137。

皮质类固醇是治疗慢性 GVHD 的一线药物[97]。慢性 GVHD 通常需要使用最小剂量的皮质类固醇维持治疗至少 6~9 个月才能控制。隔日用药可能对减少由长期应用皮质类固醇治疗引起的并发症更为有益。环孢素或他克莫司联合皮质类固醇可用于高危患者的治疗[98,99]。联合应用免疫抑制剂会更好控制慢性 GVHD 的临床症状,但会增加患者感染和死亡风险。体外光化疗对控制慢性 GVHD 有一定作用,可减少皮质类固醇的用量[100]。

预处理相关毒性

用于清除恶性肿瘤细胞的清髓性预处理方案的毒性接近以下几种组织的耐受极限。胃肠道、肾脏、肺和肝脏最容易发生毒性损伤,毒性严重时也可能累及心脏、膀胱、神经系统和其他组织,但实际的毒性风险因方案和相对剂量强度而异。具体的决定因素包括所使用的药物毒性特征及其相互作用,而药物之间的相互作用又与受累器官数量、疾病本身和既往治疗以及感染等因素密切相关。大多数毒性反应发生在移植后的前 30 天,但预处理相关的肝损伤[肝静脉闭塞性疾病(VOD)]、肺毒性和神经系统损伤可能会延迟几个月。

肝脏 VOD 通常发生在使用含有 TBI、白消安、BCNU、噻替派、卡铂和 VP-16 的治疗方案后[101],临床表现主要为肝肿大、腹水、全身性体液潴留、胆红素明显升高。目前,除了支持治疗之外,还没有发现对此有确切疗效的治疗方案,预测致命 VOD 的风险因素也有报道[102]。与药物损伤直接相关的肺毒性最常由 BCNU 引起,随着剂量的增加,发生率在 5%~60%不等[103]。实际上,用于移植的每种烷化剂都有肺毒性,但与 BCNU 相比,肺毒性发生率要小得多。这种损伤通常发生在移植后 3~12 周,临床表现为渐进性呼吸困难和咳嗽,胸片或 CT 表现为弥漫性肺间质异常。如果排除感染,皮质类固醇治疗后这种改变可以完全逆转[104]。预处理方案中的多种烷化剂引起的心脏毒性,通常表现为短暂性心肌损伤和心脏射血分数下降。心脏毒性通常无症状,且仅持续 1~3 个月,但在某些方案中,发生率达 20%~40%[105]。此外,不可逆性心力衰竭也可能发生,但不常见。

血液学并发症

供受体 ABO 血型不合可导致溶血反应[106],但 ABO 血型不合并不是 allo-HSCT 的禁忌证。为防止急性溶血反应的发生,对主要 ABO 血型不合者,应去除供体移植物中的红细胞,而次要 ABO 血型不合者,应去除移植物中的血浆。

造血干细胞移植后可能会发生非典型血栓性血小板减少性紫癜(thrombotic thrombocytopenic purpura,TTP)[107],TTP 的发生与化疗药物、放疗、他克莫司和环孢素、巨细胞病毒和真菌感染及细胞因子释放综合征引起的血管内皮损伤有关。

免疫缺陷和感染

接受造血干细胞移植的患者会有严重的 T 细胞及 B 细胞相关的免疫缺陷[108]。HLA 不匹配或无关供体和脐血移植会有更严重且较长时期的免疫缺陷和机会性感染的风险。自体或同基因造血干细胞移植也有免疫缺陷期,但恢复较快。造血干细胞移植患者更易并发少见病原菌的机会性感染和急性暴发性感染。制定一系列预防潜在感染的措施和快速识别并及时抗感染治疗是移植成功的关键[109]。对于免疫球蛋白缺乏的患者应给予免疫球蛋白替代治疗。疫苗再接种应该在患者机体免疫功能恢复后或移植后 6 个月进行。

移植后淋巴组织增生性疾病(posttransplant lymphoproliferative disease,PTLD)是 allo-HSCT 的一种危及生命的并发症[110],其在不匹配供体造血干细胞移植或脐血移植中更易发生,特别是接受高强度免疫抑制剂治疗(包括大剂量抗胸腺细胞免疫球蛋白)的患者。造血干细胞移植患者发生 PTLD,是由 EB 病毒(Epstein-Barr virus,EBV)感染引起的供体源性 B 淋巴细胞转化所致。PTLD 的治疗包括停用免疫抑制剂和使用利妥昔单抗。供体或 EBV 致敏淋巴细胞[111]输注疗法在控制 PTLD 方面疗效显著[112]。EBV-DNA 水平升高的患者发生 PTLD 的风险最高,可预防性使用利妥昔单抗。

晚期并发症

造血干细胞移植晚期并发症包括大剂量药物治疗后的延迟反应、隐性感染、输血相关并发症及慢性 GVHD。大剂量药物治疗后的晚期毒性可导致白内障、肺纤维化、牙齿异常、甲状腺功能减退、性腺功能减退、生长迟缓、骨质疏松和股骨或其他骨骼的缺血性坏死,大部分患者还会并发永久性不育。造血干细胞移植后患者并发实体瘤和血液系统继发肿瘤的风险也会增加。接受含 TBI 治疗方案的患者并发实体瘤(如头颈癌、鳞状细胞癌、黑色素瘤以及脑瘤、乳腺癌和甲状腺癌)更为常见,其 15 年累积发病率高达 7%~10%。骨髓增生异常和继发性白血病在 AHSCT 后患者更常见,移植后 2.5~8.5 年内发生率为 4%~18%[113,114]。

造血干细胞移植适应证

急性髓系白血病(AML)

造血干细胞移植用于 AML 患者的治疗已得到广泛认可[115,116],清髓性移植主要用于年轻 AML 患者。然而,AML 在老年人中更为常见,因此,以白消安/氟达拉滨为基础的减低强度的预处理移植方案,已经广泛应用于有移植适应证的 70 岁以下的老年 AML 患者。大多数患者在大剂量药物治疗和造血干细胞移植后可达到完全缓解。治疗失败的主要原因是 GVHD、预处理相关毒性、感染及白血病复发。为达到更好的抗白血病效应而增加 TBI 剂量或额外化疗药物的方案,除了增加额外的毒性并没有提高患者的总体存活率[117]。Allo-HSCT 后的临床疗效主要取决于疾病状态(缓解与复发)、白血病的细胞遗传学特征和异常突变、患者年龄以及供受体之间的组织相容性[118]。处于缓解期的患者移植后长期无病生存率可达 40%~65%[119,120]。越来越多的中危或高危患者,有完全匹配的供体时在第一次完全缓解后就进行造血干细胞移植。预后良好的患者[如有 t(8;21),t(15;17)及 inv 16 异常],通常在复发再诱导缓解后进行造血干细胞移植。

无 HLA 匹配供体的患者 allo-HSCT 风险会增加，有亲缘关系的不匹配供体或脐血移植，通常用于复发的年轻患者、高危细胞遗传学异常的患者或者由 MDS 等其他血液病转化而来的 AML 患者[121]。

骨髓增生异常综合征

MDS 是一组以外周血细胞减少和高风险转化 AML 为主要表现的克隆性血液疾病，国际预后评分（International Prognostic Score，IPS）根据骨髓原始细胞比例、血细胞减少程度和核型将其分为低危、中危和高危组[122]。IPS 评分低危患者中位生存期为 5.7 年，而高危患者中位生存期仅 0.4 年。

Allo-HSCT 是治愈 MDS 的潜在治疗手段[123,124]，但是移植时机尚存在争议。高危、原始细胞过多、严重的中性粒细胞减少、输血依赖及高风险细胞遗传学异常的 MDS 患者可实施 allo-HSCT。疾病稳定的低危患者，可以通过保守治疗延长生存期，通常在疾病进展前不进行移植。MDS 预处理方案与 AML 相似，移植后的长期缓解率等于或可能略优于 AML。

急性淋巴细胞白血病

强化化疗方案在儿童 ALL 患者中治愈率已达到 80%～90%，但成人 ALL 患者治愈率只有 30%～35%[125]。与 AML 相同，预后不良的成人 ALL 患者如有 t(9;22)ph 染色体和其他高危的遗传学标志，一般在首次缓解后移植，其他的成人 ALL 患者则在一次或多次复发后移植。成人 ALL 患者若出现化疗耐药，预后极差。

ALL 患者最常用的预处理方案是大剂量环磷酰胺和 TBI，可以联合或不联合其他化疗药物。含 TBI 的预处理方案无病生存率可能高于不含 TBI 的预处理方案[126]。单用化疗药物作为 ALL 预处理方案的临床疗效正在积极探索中。

慢性髓系白血病

在过去十年中，由于 BCR-ABL 酪氨酸激酶抑制剂（tyrosine kinase inhibitor，TKI），如伊马替尼在 CML 中的成功应用，接受 allo-HSCT 治疗的 CML 患者数量已明显减少。这些药物可使大多数患者获得长期缓解，新一代 TKI 还能够从分子生物学机制上克服常见的一代 TKI 耐药。因此，通常只有应用两种或两种以上 TKI 治疗无效、药物不耐受、加速期或急变期的 CML 患者才选择进行移植。

临床常用的 AML 移植方案也用于 CML 的移植治疗，并且 CML 移植疗效与 AML 相似或略优于 AML。早期移植失败的患者通常可以通过 DLI 达到完全缓解[127,128]，尽管该治疗有并发 GVHD 的风险，但 CML 对 DLI 治疗非常敏感。CML 或许是最早使用以 PCR 为基础的分子检测微小残留病变（在本例中为 BCR-ABL）的典范，这在当时提高了 DLI 免疫疗法的应用价值。

造血干细胞移植已被用于治疗其他骨髓增殖性疾病[129,130]，但合适的移植时机尚不明确。大多数研究者需要根据患者对输血的依赖性确定造血干细胞移植的受益与风险[131]。

慢性淋巴细胞白血病

慢性淋巴细胞白血病（chronic lymphocytic leukemia，CLL）是一种惰性的淋巴系统恶性肿瘤，其中位生存期在 10 年以上[132,133]。美国国立癌症研究院工作组建议将最初的 Rai 五期分期系统修改为“3 级危险分组”[134]，低危、中危和高危组的中位生存期分别为大于 14 年、8 年和 4 年。不良预后因素包括免疫球蛋白基因重排丢失、表达 CD38 和高水平的β2-微球蛋白[135]。

如果 CLL 患者出现相关症状或体能下降，通常建议进行化疗[136]。化疗用药包括氟达拉滨、利妥昔单抗、环磷酰胺和新药伊布替尼，其可显著改善临床症状和延长生存期，但使用上述的标准治疗方案 CLL 仍然不可治愈。目前 CLL 有关的 allo-HSCT 研究越来越多[137,138]，并且结果表明化疗敏感的 CLL 患者移植后有较好的疗效。国际骨髓移植登记处（International Bone Marrow Transplant Registry，IBMTR）资料分析显示，移植后 CLL 患者 3 年总生存率仅为 46%，而移植相关死亡风险却很高[139]。但令人欣喜的是，GVM 效应在 CLL 中也得到了证实[140]，这促使研究者们使用非清髓预处理方案来减少毒性，并将 allo-HSCT 应用到 75 岁以下的 CLL 患者。通过使用非清髓预处理方案，很多团队取得了令人鼓舞的初步结果。

CLL 患者 allo-HSCT 的最佳时机是有争议的。考虑到 allo-HSCT 的风险和初诊患者的疾病慢性进展过程，一般建议只有在初始治疗失败后才考虑移植，多次复发或化疗无效后才进行移植，预后相对较差。

非霍奇金淋巴瘤

非霍奇金淋巴瘤是一组高度异质性的血液系统肿瘤，常伴随着惰性至高度侵袭性的自然病程。非霍奇金淋巴瘤的治疗方案包括标准化疗和造血干细胞移植，具体选择取决于每个患者的组织亚型和预后因素。淋巴瘤可分为低危、中危、高危 3 个级别。低危淋巴瘤常与 t(14,18) 导致的 BCL2 基因重排有关，其中位生存期为 7～15 年[141]。影响预后的主要因素包括疾病分期、乳酸脱氢酶和β2-微球蛋白水平。

大剂量化疗联合 AHSCT 已广泛应用于淋巴瘤，完全缓解率可超过 80%。许多研究通过使用抗 B 细胞单克隆抗体清除骨髓或外周血移植物中的肿瘤细胞延长缓解期[142,143]。AHSCT 后，PCR 检测 BCL2 基因重排阴性，即分子学完全缓解的患者无病生存期更长。尽管 AHSCT 在治疗淋巴瘤中疗效尚好，然而，有关 AHSCT 在淋巴瘤中的应用还是有争议的。有研究认为淋巴瘤 AHSCT 和标准剂量化疗的保守治疗有着相似的远期生存疗效[144]。淋巴瘤 AHSCT 后有并发继发性骨髓增生异常和急性白血病的风险，尤其是治疗前病情严重的患者[145,146]。与此相反，最近也有研究显示，少数经过初始系统治疗失败后接受 AHSCT 的患者，获得了长期无复发生存，提示 AHSCT 疗效可能优于传统化疗。

异基因骨髓移植曾经在淋巴瘤治疗中进行了尝试。大剂量环磷酰胺和 TBI 或 BEAM 联合利妥昔单抗是最常用的预处理方案。很多研究报道，晚期淋巴瘤患者经 allo-HSCT 治疗后无病生存期有所延长。Allo-HSCT的复发率明显低于AHSCT，这很有可能与GVM效应相关[147,148]。最近应用的非清髓预处理方案也取得了令人振奋的结果，不仅降低了治疗相关死亡风险，并且大多数患者可获得长期完全缓解，使其越来越多地被用于初始治疗失败的年轻高危患者[149]。套细胞淋巴瘤预后不良，特别是套细胞淋巴瘤国际预后指标(MIPI)评估为中危或高危的患者[150]。化疗敏感的套细胞淋巴瘤患者，首次化疗缓解后接受AHSCT有较好的疗效。然而，复发的套细胞淋巴瘤患者大多需要使用减低强度的预处理方案进行allo-HSCT治疗。与CLL和其他淋巴瘤一样，GVM效应也有助于提高套细胞淋巴瘤allo-HSCT的疗效。

中高危淋巴瘤是侵袭性恶性肿瘤，若化疗治疗无效其自然病程短暂。若中高危淋巴瘤对联合化疗有反应，其中一小部分患者可获得持久缓解。标准化疗方案可治愈约40%~60%初诊的弥漫性大细胞淋巴瘤患者。

大剂量化疗和AHSCT能提高对挽救性化疗有反应的复发大细胞淋巴瘤患者的治愈率[151,152]。Parma等的研究将60岁以下复发的化疗敏感的大细胞淋巴瘤患者随机分为常规化疗组或AHSCT组，结果证实AHSCT疗效更好[153]。化疗耐药和多次复发的患者传统AHSCT效果不佳，但可以考虑采用改良预处理方案的AHSCT或清髓的allo-HSCT。

也有许多研究对中高危淋巴瘤患者采用大剂量化疗联合allo-HSCT治疗。有研究表明，与AHSCT相比，虽然allo-HSCT可以降低患者的复发率，但也同时增加了治疗相关的死亡率，并未显示出allo-HSCT的治疗优势[154]。化疗相对不敏感的患者或AHSCT不可行的患者，很多医师将allo-HSCT作为备选治疗方案。

霍奇金淋巴瘤

大约三分之一的患者，在初次化疗未能完全缓解时，可通过AHSCT进行挽救性治疗。复发的霍奇金淋巴瘤患者，尤其是获得再次缓解尽早移植的患者，大剂量化疗和AHSCT可使移植后3~5年的完全缓解率达到50%~80%，无病生存率达40%~60%[155,156]。BEAM、环磷酰胺、卡莫司汀及VP-16是最常用的预处理方案。许多Ⅱ期临床研究表明，与标准化疗相比，大剂量化疗可提高患者的无病生存率，并可能提高患者的总生存率。

非清髓allo-HSCT主要用于AHSCT后疾病进展的患者，或自体骨髓中造血干细胞数量缺乏的患者[157]。

多发性骨髓瘤

MM的标准化疗方案可以用于治疗不同分期的疾病，但即使是含有来那度胺和/或蛋白酶体抑制剂的新方案，也只有20%~30%的患者达到完全缓解。越来越多的随机性和回顾性对照临床试验研究均表明，标准化疗联合AHSCT可提高MM患者的无病生存率和总生存率。目前，大剂量化疗联合AHSCT被认为是中危或高危MM的标准治疗方案。大剂量化疗和AHSCT可以延缓疾病的复发但无法治愈，几乎所有的MM患者最终都会复发。

肿瘤的化疗敏感性是影响AHSCT疗效的主要因素。化疗敏感的患者，在一年内接受AHSCT有更好的疗效，约40%~50%的患者可达到完全缓解。原发难治性MM患者，如果在疾病早期进行移植也可获得显著的疗效[158,159]，但对于晚期耐药尤其是难治复发患者，AHSCT的治疗价值有限[160]。高β2-微球蛋白和几种细胞遗传学异常是最突出的不良预后因素[161,162]。MM的AHSCT预处理方案通常使用单药美法仑，即使在老年患者中也只有1%~2%的毒性死亡风险。连续双次(续贯)AHSCT也常常被应用，这可使MM患者获得更高的总生存率和无复发生存率[163]。大多数研究表明，MM患者缓解早期进行AHSCT疗效更好。一项法国的随机临床研究显示，MM患者早期和晚期移植的生存时间无差异，但早期接受移植的患者可有更长的时间不需要接受化疗[164]。

Allo-HSCT可以治愈30%~40%的MM患者，但预处理相关毒性和感染率也较高。减低强度的预处理及GVM效应可提高allo-HSCT的疗效，但其在AHSCT失败后的应用仍处于研究阶段。其他浆细胞肿瘤，通过应用大剂量美法仑和AHSCT也可得到有效治疗。正如近期的多项研究结果一样，AHSCT治疗淀粉样病变也可能有效，但治疗相关死亡率远高于MM，可高达8%~12%。

实体瘤

大剂量化疗联合AHSCT在乳腺癌和卵巢癌的治疗中也得到了研究，但结果是有争议的，目前这项技术还不是这些疾病常规治疗的一部分。

同样，大剂量化疗联合AHSCT也被用于治疗化疗敏感的其他成人实体瘤，包括睾丸或纵隔生殖细胞肿瘤，最近的研究数据显示，该治疗方法可提高复发和难治性疾病患者的无复发生存率[165]。

AHSCT在神经母细胞瘤和尤因肉瘤等一系列儿童实体瘤中也有研究，这些肿瘤对化疗和放疗高度敏感，但晚期肿瘤患者预后较差[166,167]。

再生障碍性贫血

重型再生障碍性贫血(aplastic anemia，AA)的诊断标准为：骨髓细胞增生程度小于正常的25%，中性粒细胞数小于$0.5\times10^9/L$，血小板数小于$20\times10^9/L$，或网织红细胞总数小于$40\times10^9/L$。如果不能得到有效治疗，50%以上的重型AA患者可能在诊断后6个月内死亡。AA有效的治疗方法包括免疫抑制疗法(如环孢素和抗胸腺细胞免疫球蛋白)[168]和allo-HSCT。

免疫抑制剂治疗无反应的患者，allo-HSCT是一种有效的治疗方法。多次输血可能使受体对供体致敏，增加移植排斥的风险。根据目前的治疗方案，早期移植、合理的输血策略及完善的护理，只有不到10%的人会发生移植排斥，更重要的是，接受HLA匹配的同胞供体骨髓移植的患者中，80%~90%的患者可获得长期生存。无关或不匹配供体的allo-HSCT正在积极研究中，但其发生并发症的风险较高。

先天性代谢和免疫紊乱

Allo-HSCT是一种潜在的治疗先天性造血和免疫系统疾病的有效方法。地中海贫血[169]和镰状细胞性贫血[170]是最常见的可通过移植治愈的非恶性血液病。Fanconi贫血的治疗与

AA 相似,但由于这些患者对放疗和烷化剂敏感性较高,因此,只需要很小剂量的药物预处理[171,172]。Allo-HSCT 已经用于重度联合免疫缺陷婴儿的治疗[173]。即使在没有预处理的情况下,很多患者也可以实现异基因造血干细胞的植入。Allo-HSCT 治疗还可以逆转骨硬化症[174]。Allo-HSCT 治疗脂质贮积病的效果不一[175],无匹配同胞供体的患者,无论是无关供体还是单倍体相合的亲缘 allo-HSCT 都有成功的报道[176]。对大多数疾病而言,早期接受 allo-HSCT 效果更好。未来,自体细胞的基因修饰可能是治愈这些疾病的一种可行方法[177]。

在过去的几年里,人们越来越关注去除或不去除移植物中的 T 细胞在 AHSCT 治疗自身免疫性疾病的不同影响[178],目的是清除体内异常免疫反应,恢复造血干/祖细胞的免疫功能。在少数类风湿性关节炎、系统性红斑狼疮、多发性硬化、重症肌无力和其他疾病患者中,AHSCT 也取得了很好的疗效。

展望

在过去十年中,造血干细胞移植在多种疾病中应用,治疗了数以万计的患者,已成为一种安全有效的治疗方法。造血干细胞移植的应用可能会随着肿瘤分子靶向治疗的发展而发展,并通过改进方法选择性地靶向治疗和免疫调控。靶向放射治疗,如单克隆抗体-放射性核素免疫偶联物和骨靶向同位素,其作为靶向放射治疗肿瘤的一种手段正在被深入研究,这种方法除了骨髓抑制外很少有全身毒性。未来可以通过使用克服耐药性机制的方法,如使用 DNA 修复抑制剂、谷胱甘肽结合剂或其他制剂进一步改善疗效。目前,AHSCT 技术的改进将着重纳入新疗法,特别是靶向药物和补充性的免疫增强技术。

与 allo-HSCT 相伴随的 GVM 效应,阐明了机体免疫系统清除肿瘤的独特能力。因此,增强 allo-HSCT 和 AHSCT 免疫抗肿瘤机制的方法正在被积极探索,主要目的是将有益的 GVM 效应与 GVHD 分离。通过体外基因转染肿瘤细胞产生的肿瘤疫苗(增加抗原的表达)、共刺激分子和多种细胞因子,都可以增强抗肿瘤免疫反应。在 Allo-HSCT 中通过调节某些淋巴细胞亚群[NK 细胞、调节性 T 细胞和嵌合抗原受体 T 细胞(CAR-T 细胞)]提高抗肿瘤免疫反应,同时降低 GVHD 风险的研究也在积极进行中。在 allo-HSCT 研究领域,正在努力扩大供体库并降低 allo-HSCT 的相关毒性。大多数需要 allo-HSCT 的患者没有 HLA 匹配的同胞供体,未来进一步扩充国际上骨髓、造血干细胞和脐血的无关供体登记,将会增加获得匹配良好供体的可能性,特别要注意登记中的少数民族。提高组织相容性匹配精确度的新分子方法,可降低移植排斥和 GVHD 的发生风险。Allo-HSCT 供体的另一个选择是使用有血缘关系的不完全匹配供体,即单倍体相合造血干细胞移植,这项技术加上大量储备可用的脐血有望使大部分需要 allo-HSCT 的患者获得合适的供体移植物。预防感染和移植相关并发症等支持治疗的进展,使得 allo-HSCT 更加安全。GVM 是 allo-HSCT 治疗潜力的主要原因,这一发现使得非清髓预处理方案得以应用,不仅可使供体细胞植入而且又能减少毒性。要证实 GVM 的主要治疗作用,还需要进一步做前瞻性的临床研究,以确定 GVM 的作用、适应证和受益患者。

(宋永平 张兵雷 译,周健 孙恺 审校)

参考文献

The complete reference list can be found on the Wiley Companion Digital Edition of this title (see inside front cover for login instructions).

1 Thomas ED, Storb R, Clift RA, et al. Bone-marrow transplantation (second of two parts). *N Engl J Med*. 1975;**292**:895–902.

2 Thomas ED, Buckner CD, Banaji M, et al. One hundred patients with acute leukemia treated by chemotherapy, total body irradiation, and allogeneic marrow transplantation. *Blood*. 1977;**49**:511–533.

4 Anderson DJ, Gage FH, Weissman IL, et al. Can stem cells cross lineage boundaries? *Nat Med*. 2001;7:393–395.

11 Korbling M, Katz RL, Khanna A, et al. Hepatocytes and epithelial cells of donor origin in recipients of peripheral blood stem cells. *N Engl J Med*. 2002;**346**:738–746.

13 de Lima M, Couriel D, Thall PF, et al. Once-daily intravenous busulfan and fludarabine: clinical and pharmacokinetic results of a myeloablative, reduced-toxicity conditioning regimen for allogeneic stem cell transplantation in AML and MDS. *Blood*. 2004;**104**:857–864.

17 Thomas ED. Karnofsky Memorial Lecture. Marrow transplantation for malignant diseases. *J Clin Oncol*. 1983;**1**:517–531.

18 Frei E 3rd, Holden SA, Gonin R, et al. Antitumor alkylating agents: in vitro cross-resistance and collateral sensitivity studies. *Cancer Chemother Pharmacol*. 1993;**33**:113–122.

24 Brenner MK, Rill DR, Moen RC, et al. Gene marking to trace origin of relapse after autologous bone marrow transplantation. *Lancet*. 1993:34185–34186.

25 Ferrara JL, Deeg HJ. Graft-versus-host disease. *N Engl J Med*. 1991;**324**:667–674.

31 Attal M, Harousseau J-L, Stoppa A-M, et al. A prospective, randomized trial of autologous bone marrow transplantation and chemotherapy in multiple myeloma. *N Engl J Med*. 1996;**335**:91–97.

37 Champlin R, Khouri I, Shimoni A, et al. Harnessing graft-versus-malignancy: non-myeloablative preparative regimens for allogeneic hematopoietic transplantation, an evolving strategy for adoptive immunotherapy. *Br J Hematol*. 2000;**111**:18–29.

39 Sullivan KM, Weiden PL, Storb R, et al. Influence of acute and chronic graft-versus-host disease on relapse and survival after bone marrow transplantation from HLA-identical siblings as treatment of acute and chronic leukemia. *Blood*. 1989;**73**:1720–1728.

41 Kolb HJ, Schattenberg A, Goldman JM, et al. Graft-versus leukemia effect of donor lymphocyte transfusions in marrow grafted patients. European Group for Blood and Marrow Transplantation Working Party Chronic Leukemia. *Blood*. 1995;**86**:2041–2050.

48 Hansen JA, Choo SY, Geraghty DE, et al. The HLA system in clinical marrow transplantation. *Hematol Oncol Clin N Am*. 1990;**4**:507–515.

49 Kernan NA, Bartsch G, Ash RC, et al. Analysis of 462 transplantations from unrelated donors facilitated by the National Marrow Donor Program. *N Engl J Med*. 1993;**328**:593–602.

52 Bayraktar UD, Champlin RE, Ciurea SO, et al. Progress in haploidentical stem cell transplantation. *Biol Blood Marrow Transplant*. 2012;**18**:372–380.

54 Rocha V, Labopin M, Sanz G, Arcese W, et al. Transplants of umbilical cord blood or bone marrow from unrelated donors in adults with acute leukemia. *N Engl J Med*. 2004;**35**:2276–2285.

62 Armitage JO. Myelodysplasia and acute leukemia after autologous bone marrow transplantation. *J Clin Oncol*. 2000;**18**:945–946.

64 Martelli M, Vignetti M, Zinzani PL, et al. High-dose chemotherapy followed by autologous bone marrow transplantation versus dexamethasone, cisplatin, and cytarabine in aggressive non-Hodgkin's lymphoma with partial response to front-line chemotherapy: a prospective randomized italian multicenter study. *J Clin Oncol*. 1996;**14**:534–542.

67 Clift RA, Buckner CD. Marrow transplantation for acute myeloid leukemia. *Cancer Invest*. 1998;**16**:53–61.

71 Giralt S, Estey E, Albitar M, et al. Engraftment of allogeneic hematopoietic progenitor cells with purine analog-containing chemotherapy: harnessing graft-versus-leukemia without myeloablative therapy. *Blood*. 1997;**89**:4531–4536.

83 Ferrara JL, Deeg HJ. Graft-versus-host disease. *N Engl J Med*. 1991;**324**:667–674.

90 Przepiorka D, Ippoliti C, Khouri I, et al. Tacrolimus and minidose methotrexate for prevention of acute graft-versus-host disease after matched unrelated donor marrow transplantation. *Blood*. 1996;**88**:4383–4389.

92 Bolaños-Meade J, Fuchs EJ, Luznik L, et al. HLA-haploidentical bone marrow transplantation with post-transplant cyclophosphamide expands the donor pool for patients with sickle cell disease. *Blood* 2012;**120**:4285–4291.

93 Sullivan KM, Agura E, Anasetti C, et al. Chronic graft-versus-host disease and other late complications of bone marrow transplantation. *Semin Hematol*. 1991;**28**:250–259.

101 Shulman HM, Hinterberger W. Hepatic veno-occlusive disease—liver toxicity syndrome after bone marrow transplantation. *Bone Marrow Transplant*. 1992;**10**:197–214.

105 Gottdiener JS, Appelbaum FR, Ferrans VJ, et al. Cardiotoxicity associated with high-dose cyclophosphamide therapy. *Arch Intern Med*. 1981;**141**:758–763.

112 Heslop HE, Slobod KS, Pule MA, et al. Long-term outcome of EBV-specific T-cell infusions to prevent or treat EBV-related lymphoproliferative disease in transplant recipients. *Blood*. 2010;**115**:925–935.

117 Appelbaum FR, Fisher LD, Thomas ED. Chemotherapy v marrow transplantation for adults with acute nonlymphocytic leukemia: a five-year follow-up. *Blood*. 1988;**72**:179–184.

129 Anderson JE, Sale G, Appelbaum FR, et al. Allogeneic marrow transplantation for primary myelofibrosis and myelofibrosis secondary to polycythaemia vera or essential thrombocytosis. *Br J Haematol*. 1997;**98**:1010–1016.

138 Khouri IF, Keating MJ, Vriesendorp HM, et al. Autologous and allogeneic bone marrow transplantation for chronic lymphocytic leukemia: preliminary results. *J Clin Oncol*. 1994;**12**:748–758.

154 Chopra R, Goldstone AH, Pearce R, et al. Autologous versus allogeneic bone marrow transplantation for non-Hodgkin's lymphoma: a case-controlled analysis of the European Bone Marrow Transplant Group Registry data. *J Clin Oncol* 1992;**10**: 1690–1695.

159 Alexanian R, Dimopoulos MA, Hester J, et al. Early myeloablative therapy for multiple myeloma. *Blood*. 1994;**84**:4278–4282.

163 Moreau P, Hullin C, Garban F, et al. Tandem autologous stem cell transplantation in high-risk de novo multiple myeloma: final results of the prospective and randomized IFM 99–04 protocol. *Blood*. 2006;**107**:397–403.

165 Nieto Y. Transplantation for refractory germ cell tumors: does it really make a difference? *Curr Oncol Rep*. 2013;**15**:232–238.

167 Fraser CJ, Weigel BJ, Perentesis JP, et al. Autologous stem cell transplantation for high-risk Ewing's sarcoma and other pediatric solid tumors. *Bone Marrow Transplant*. 2006;**37**:175–181.

168 Bacigalupo A, Bruno B, Saracco P, et al. Antilymphocyte globulin, cyclosporine, prednisolone, and granulocyte colony-stimulating factor for severe aplastic anemia: an update of the GITMO/EBMT study on 100 patients. European Group for Blood and Marrow Transplantation (EBMT) Working Party on Severe Aplastic Anemia and the Gruppo Italiano Trapianti di Midolio Osseo (GITMO). *Blood*. 2000;**95**:1931–1934.

170 Walters MC, Storb R, Patience M, et al. Impact of bone marrow transplantation for symptomatic sickle cell disease: an interim report. Multicenter investigation of bone marrow transplantation for sickle cell disease. *Blood*. 2000;**95**: 1918–1924.

176 Filipovich AH, Shapiro RS, Ramsay NK, et al. Unrelated donor bone marrow transplantation for correction of lethal congenital immunodeficiencies. *Blood* 1992;**80**: 270–276.

178 van Bekkum DW. Autologous stem cell therapy for treatment of severe inflammatory autoimmune diseases. *Neth J Med*. 1998;**53**:130–133.

第十篇

特 殊 人 群

第 71 章　儿童肿瘤的诊治原则

Teena Bhatla, MD ■ William L. Carroll, MD

概述

儿童恶性肿瘤的相对发病率、病理类型、临床表现和预后方面与成人恶性肿瘤均不同。20 世纪后期，儿科癌症研究领域取得了巨大成就，这些成就的取得离不开多个国家和国际团体精心设计并开展的临床试验，这些临床实验的结果一直在不断完善和提高。本章旨在概述儿童肿瘤学的发展和阐述儿童群体几种常见癌症类型。

流行病学

肿瘤是儿童期相对罕见的疾病，但仍是仅次于意外伤害，是导致儿童死亡的第二大原因。与成人相比，儿童肿瘤类型明显不同。成人肿瘤谱中上皮源性肿瘤（癌）占主导地位，但儿童肿瘤多来源于造血系统（如白血病和淋巴瘤）、间叶细胞（肉瘤）和神经外胚层（如神经母细胞瘤、神经胶质瘤和成神经管细胞瘤）。急性淋巴细胞白血病（Acute lymphoblastic leukemia，ALL）和脑肿瘤是最常见的儿童肿瘤，分别占 25% 和 20%。最常见的儿童肿瘤的发生率如图 71-1 和表 71-1 所示，但儿童肿瘤发病率因种族和地域的不同而不同。例如，Burkitt 淋巴瘤占非洲赤道地区所有儿童肿瘤的 50%。

有人认为儿童肿瘤的发病率有所上升，特别是其中的某些亚型，但其实是因为更详尽的病例报道和影像学诊断技术的提高所致[1]。大多数儿童肿瘤的病因仍然不确定。儿童肿瘤的发生很少会受到环境因素的影响，但辐射是目前较为确定的致癌危险因素。此外，二代测序技术的突破性进展也表明，与成人恶性肿瘤相比，儿童肿瘤的突变频率要低得多，这也证实环境因素在儿童肿瘤发生中并未发挥很重要的作用[2]。

随着二代测序不断揭示出肿瘤易感基因中的未知突变，遗传易感性占儿童所有致癌病因的 5%，这一数字随着技术的发展可能还会增加。大约三分之一的视网膜母细胞瘤（retinoblastoma，RB）是由生殖细胞 *RB1* 基因突变引起的，唐氏综合征（Down syndrome，DS）患儿发生白血病（淋系和髓系）的概率增加了 20 倍，其他遗传综合征如神经纤维瘤病 1（与脑肿瘤发病相关）、Beckwith-Wiedemann 综合征［与 Wilm 肿瘤、肝母细胞瘤（hepatoblastoma，HB）、横纹肌肉瘤（rhabdomyosarcoma，RMS）发病相关］、Li-Fraumeni 综合征（与某些肉瘤和癌发病相关）、Gorlin 综合征（与成神经管细胞瘤、皮肤癌发病相关）和共济失调性毛细血管扩张症（与白血病和淋巴瘤发病相关），虽仅占儿童疾病的一小部分，但却是重要的致癌因素。这些家族性遗传性综合征往往为某些散发型肿瘤性疾病重要致癌基因的发现提供了依据。

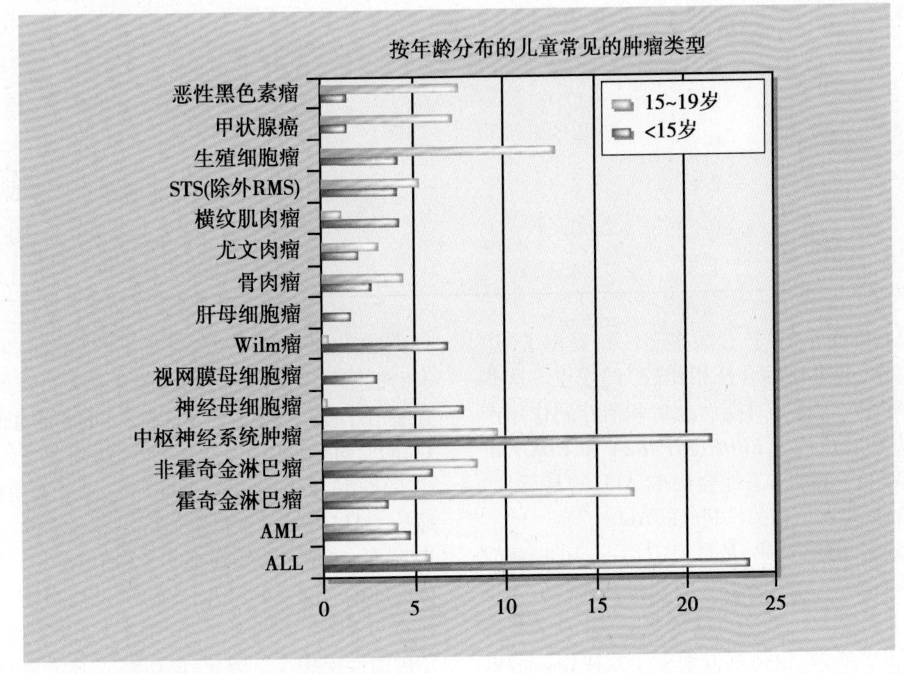

图 71-1　儿童肿瘤依年龄的分布情。ALL，急性淋巴细胞白血病；AML，急性髓性白血病；RMS，横纹肌肉瘤；STS，软组织肉瘤

表 71-1 2007—2011 年每百万儿童中特定年龄相关的癌症年发病率

肿瘤类型(ICCC 分组)	诊断时年龄/岁						
	0~14	0~19	<1	1~4	5~9	10~14	15~19
所有肿瘤(包括良性中枢神经系统肿瘤)	172.8	191.2	253.4	228.1	137.2	150.9	246.2
白血病	54.4	49.4	51.7	95.0	44.5	33.9	34.5
急性淋巴细胞白血病	41.9	35.9	20.3	79.7	37.1	22.1	18.2
急性髓细胞白血病	8.0	8.5	18.9	10.6	4.5	7.4	9.9
中枢神经系统肿瘤	44.3	45.1	48.8	49.4	43.1	40.6	47.8
室间隔膜瘤和脉络丛神经瘤	4.0	3.7	8.8	6.9	2.6	2.4	2.8
星状细胞瘤	16.7	15.6	15.5	18.7	17.1	15.2	12.2
胚胎肿瘤	7.6	6.4	12.5	11.3	7.4	4.1	2.7
霍奇金淋巴瘤	5.9	12.4	—	1.1	5.0	11.6	31.8
非霍奇金淋巴瘤(除外伯基特淋巴瘤)	6.8	8.6	—	4.5	6.9	9.5	14.1
伯基特淋巴瘤	2.6	2.6	—	1.7	3.4	3.0	2.4
神经母细胞瘤和节细胞神经母细胞瘤	10.6	8.1	51.0	20.9	4.3	1.2	0.9
视网膜母细胞瘤	4.2	3.1	27.7	8.7	—	—	—
Wilm 瘤和其他非上皮性肾肿瘤	8.4	6.8	15.3	19.8	5.8	1.1	1.9
肝母细胞瘤	2.9	2.5	10.1	6.4	0.8	0.9	1.5
骨肉瘤	4.2	5.1	—	—	3.3	8.5	7.7
尤文肉瘤	2.5	2.8	—	1.1	2.2	4.3	3.5
软组织肉瘤	11.2	12.4	19.6	11.0	8.8	12.2	15.6
横纹肌肉瘤和胚胎肉瘤	5.4	4.9	5.8	7.7	4.9	4.1	3.5
生殖细胞瘤	6.0	12.2	18.9	4.0	3.2	7.8	30.7
癌	6.8	17.6	—	1.8	4.0	14.3	49.7
肾上腺皮质癌	0.3	0.2	—	—	—	—	—
甲状腺癌	2.8	8.3	—	—	1.3	6.8	24.6
鼻咽癌	0.3	0.6	—	—	—	0.8	1.4
恶性黑色素瘤	1.8	4.3	—	0.9	1.3	3.1	11.7

此外,通过识别遗传变异(单核苷酸多态性),提出了"患病个体因素"遗传变异(与上述综合征相比较)的观点。这些变异可导致癌症发病风险增高并对疾病预后和治疗副作用产生影响。例如,*ARID5B*、*IKZF1*、*CEBPE*、*PIP4K2A* 和 *CDKN2A-CDKN2B* 基因的胚系单核苷酸多态性会影响 ALL 的易感性,*GATA3* 变异与 ALL 的特定亚型相关("Ph 样"ALL)[3]。

儿童癌症研究取得的显著成果,是自 1971 年以来"癌症战争"最伟大的事件之一。那时,20 岁以下的儿童自确诊后 5 年存活率只有约 60%,而今天这一数字超过 80%(见图 71-2 和表 71-2)。这些进步有很多原因,包括致力于多学科协作诊治以及由国家和全球性团体(如儿童肿瘤学协会 COG)开展的高质量的临床试验。有趣的是,许多几十年前研发的化疗药物至今仍在使用,但经过几十年发展,人们意识到随着支持治疗的改善,增加化疗强度可改善几乎所有肿瘤的生存结局。最终,专家们根据与疾病预后相关的临床和实验室研究,制定了危险度分层治疗方案,该方案允许部分可能受益的患者进行强化治疗,同时对于采用标准化疗即可达到理想治疗效果的患儿,减少了化疗的毒副作用。肿瘤研究的进展使得最常见的恶性肿瘤——ALL——的存活率显著提高(20 世纪 60 年代存活率为 10%,目前的生存率超过 90%),但对于某些脑肿瘤、转移性实体瘤和肿瘤复发的患儿,存活率仍然很低。此外,虽然患儿的死亡率下降了大约 50%,但在美国每年仍有近 2 000 名儿童死于肿瘤性疾病[4]。因此,迫切需要制定更有效的治疗方案,并且高昂的治疗费用、短期或长期的副作用也是需要解决的问题,因此更针对性、更强效且毒性更小的治疗方案仍是肿瘤治疗的首选。

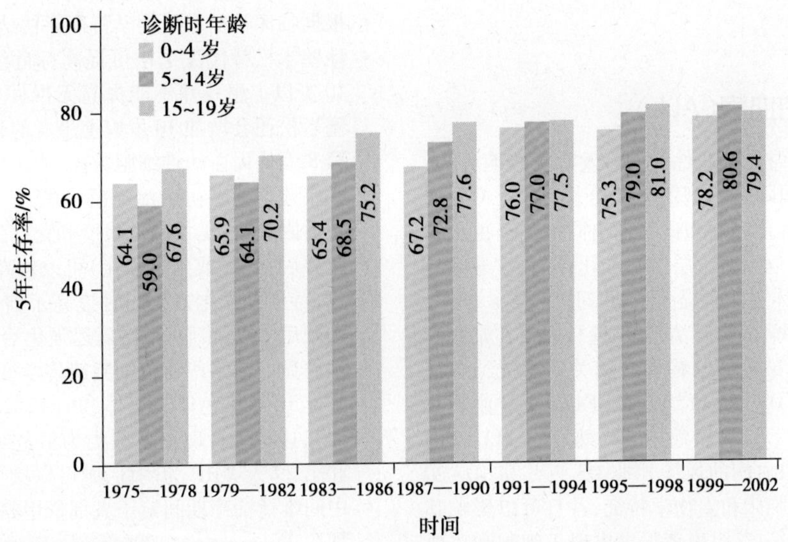

图 71-2　从 1975 年到 2002 年，不同年龄组和不同时期内的所有癌症的 5 年存活率。Source：Smith et al. 2010.[5] Reprinted with permission. © 2010 American Society of Clinical Oncology. All rights reserved.

表 71-2　儿童不同类型肿瘤的 5 年生存率（%）（SEER. cancer. gov/csr/1975_2011）

年龄按照 0~14 岁	1975—1977	1978—1980	1981—1983	1984—1986	1987—1989	1990—1992	1993—1995	1996—2002	2004—2010
所有儿童肿瘤总体生存率	58	62. 6	66. 7	68. 2	71. 4	75. 4	77. 0	79. 4	83. 1
骨和关节肿瘤	51. 3	48. 7	56. 8	59. 4	66. 8	66. 8	73. 9	71. 6	78. 9
脑和中枢神经系统肿瘤	56. 9	57. 7	56. 0	61. 8	63. 8	64. 0	70. 1	74. 1	74. 1
霍奇金淋巴瘤	80. 3	87. 7	87. 7	90. 8	87. 1	96. 7	94. 6	95. 3	97. 6
急性淋巴细胞白血病	57. 6	66. 4	71. 3	72. 5	77. 7	83. 0	83. 8	87. 0	91. 8
急性髓细胞白血病	18. 8	25. 8	26. 7	30. 0	36. 2	41. 0	41. 0	53. 1	66. 3
神经母细胞瘤	52. 4	56. 9	54. 5	52. 0	61. 9	76. 6	67. 2	68. 7	76. 6
非霍奇金淋巴瘤	42. 6	52. 7	66. 9	70. 3	70. 7	75. 9	80. 6	86. 0	85. 6
软组织肿瘤	61. 0	74. 3	69. 2	73. 4	65. 4	79. 2	76. 4	71. 7	81. 3
Wilm 瘤	73. 1	78. 6	86. 4	90. 7	92. 2	91. 9	91. 4	92. 1	91. 7
年龄按照 0~19 岁	**1975—1977**	**1978—1980**	**1981—1983**	**1984—1986**	**1987—1989**	**1990—1992**	**1993—1995**	**1996—2002**	**2004—2010**
所有儿童肿瘤总体生存率	61. 5	65. 2	68. 0	70. 6	73. 3	76. 0	77. 4	79. 5	83. 5
骨和关节肿瘤	51. 1	48. 4	51. 2	57. 2	63. 5	68. 2	68. 6	68. 0	75. 5
脑和中枢神经系统肿瘤	58. 7	58. 1	57. 6	64. 0	65. 9	66. 1	71. 0	75. 1	74. 0
霍奇金淋巴瘤	86. 0	88. 7	85. 4	90. 8	88. 9	94. 2	93. 9	95. 1	97. 3
急性淋巴细胞白血病	54. 1	62. 4	67. 1	70. 1	75. 0	79. 7	81. 3	83. 5	90. 0
急性髓细胞白血病	18. 7	26. 2	26. 4	31. 7	36. 9	41. 0	39. 4	48. 4	65. 1
神经母细胞瘤	52. 7	57. 0	53. 4	52. 0	60. 5	76. 3	67. 0	69. 0	76. 3
非霍奇金淋巴瘤	43. 4	53. 9	63. 5	68. 1	70. 3	72. 1	77. 8	81. 9	83. 9
软组织肿瘤	65. 2	68. 8	68. 2	72. 4	67. 2	68. 9	73. 8	70. 9	78. 1
Wilm 瘤	72. 6	78. 0	86. 5	91. 0	92. 2	91. 3	91. 5	92. 1	91. 5

血液系统肿瘤

儿童急性淋巴细胞白血病(ALL)

ALL是美国儿童中最常见的恶性肿瘤。发病高峰期为2~6岁,以男性为主。通过国际间大型团队的合作,儿童ALL的预后逐步改善,这与其他儿童肿瘤相比呈现出同等甚至更大幅度的提升。修订后的根据危险度分层治疗和化疗剂量/方案的增加,使得儿童ALL的总体存活率提高到90%以上[6]。

虽然儿童ALL的确切病因尚不清楚,但遗传因素在某些病例中起着重要作用。多种染色体结构异常相关的遗传综合征与儿童ALL发病相关,如DS、Bloom综合征、Fanconi贫血和共济失调性毛细血管扩张症。这些疾病中,DS继发的ALL特别值得关注。DS患儿发生白血病的风险比非DS患儿高10~20倍。此类患儿具有独特的临床和生物学特征,并且可以影响其治疗和预后。值得注意的是,这组患者很少出现T细胞和成熟B细胞免疫表型以及预后相对较好的变异如超二倍体和*ETV6-RUNX1*易位等。在大约20%的DS-ALL中发现了新的体细胞突变,例如*JAK2*激活突变,而50%的DS-ALL病例中出现*CRLF2*突变(*P2RY8-CRLF2*融合)[7,8]。DS-ALL儿童发生氨甲喋呤相关毒性反应,黏膜炎和感染性并发症也更常见。

一般而言,DS-ALL的预后比非DS-ALL更差,但是支持治疗水平的提高改善了患儿的生存结局。最近,全基因组关联研究(GWAS)已经确定*GATA3*位点的遗传变异与青少年和青年(AYAs)人群中的ALL相关[9]。

ALL患儿通常会出现骨髓浸润的体征和症状,表现为发热(60%),出血(50%)和骨痛(30%),可能会出现跛行或拒走。大约1/2到2/3的病例存在无症状的肝、脾、淋巴结肿大。极少数情况下,患者可能出现髓外受累症状,如中枢神经系统受累、睾丸增大和眼球改变。骨髓穿刺和/或骨髓活检可以诊断儿童ALL。此外,白血病细胞多种膜表面抗原标记物、细胞遗传学改变和较少用的组织化学染色异常可用于ALL分型和制定特异性治疗决策[10]。约85%的儿童ALL患者表达的膜标记物与前体B细胞一致,约15%表达前体T细胞的膜标记物。在ALL中,虽然发病年龄和初始白细胞计数是预测预后的重要因素,但其他因素如白血病细胞的免疫表型、细胞遗传学特点、中枢神经系统是否受累以及对化疗的早期反应等其他因素目前也被用于危险度分层中。在脑脊液(CSF)中找到白血病细胞是诊断白血病中枢神经系统受累所必需的。ALL标危人群定义为1~9岁且初始白细胞(WBC)计数小于50 000/mm^3;而年龄超过10岁且WBC计数大于50 000/mm^{3}则定义为高危人群。危险度评估还包括是否存在预后良好或预后不良的细胞遗传学变异[前者包括超二倍体(特别是4和10号染色体三倍体)或*EVT6/RUNX1*融合基因,后者包括亚二倍体或iAMP21]、初诊时是否有明确的中枢神经系统受累、睾丸受累、第8天和诱导化疗结束时微小残留(MRD)值。费城染色体阳性(Ph$^+$)的ALL或t(9:22)染色体易位发生在2%~3%的儿童ALL患者中,以往观点认为和疾病预后不良相关,现在认为化疗联合酪氨酸激酶抑制剂(TKI)治疗可以取得较好的疗效。

现在儿童ALL的治疗分为以下几个阶段,即诱导期治疗、症状前期或中枢神经系统预防性治疗、诱导后强化治疗和维持治疗。目前治疗方案可治愈80%~90%的ALL患者。儿童ALL治疗的其他最新进展包括:

- 根据临床特征和生物学特征评估结果制定一线治疗方案;
- 地塞米松替代泼尼松可提高标危组患者的生存率,而对于10岁以上患儿并不能提高无事件生存率(EFS)。此外,地塞米松还会增加10岁以上患者的骨坏死发生率[11]。
- 第8天外周血幼稚细胞数和/或诱导缓解后(第29天)骨髓微小残留值是初始治疗反应的评判指标,它不仅是重要的预后因素,也是目前危险度和化疗强度调整的重要参考[12]。
- 诱导后强化(或延迟强化)可改善高危组和标危组患儿的疗效,特别是强化方案同时提高了前体B-ALL和T-ALL患者的预后[13]。然而,二次延迟强化治疗并无更多益处。
- 预后良好与某些特定细胞遗传学变异有关,包括超二倍体、4号、10号染色体三倍体和t(12:21)(*ETV6-RUNX1*融合基因),这些患者现在被归类为低危组,如果这类患者第8天和第29天MRD为阴性,则可以接受较低强度化疗[14]。
- 中间维持治疗期间给予大剂量甲氨蝶呤可改善高危患者的预后[15]。
- 除了那些在诊断时即有明显CNS受累的患者外,目前全身性化疗可以使所有患者不用再接受头部放疗[16]。
- AYAs人群中使用儿童或成人ALL方案的患者,并对其预后进行回顾性分析,发现使用儿童ALL方案可以改善该类人群预后。然而,AYAs人群与年幼儿童相比,前者治疗相关死亡率在不良事件中所占的比例更高[17,18]。
- 儿童Ph$^+$ ALL可采用强化疗方案并联合靶向药酪氨酸激酶抑制剂(如伊马替尼或达沙替尼),可以显著提高EFS并且不需要进行造血干细胞移植[19]。
- 造血干细胞移植(HSCT)在新诊断的ALL治疗作用有限,但是难治性ALL、具有亚二倍体和持续高MRD的患者中可以进行HSCT。早期复发的ALL(初诊后36个月内或化疗中骨髓复发)通常需行HSCT,而晚期复发患者可选择化疗,或根据个体情况选择HSCT。

除了疾病和治疗相关的预后因素,最近研究发现患病个体因素在疾病控制方面的重要性。患病个体因素是患者在药物吸收、代谢、药物敏感性方面的差异。不同患病个体硫嘌呤和长春新碱的药理学作用具有显著遗传学差异[20,21]。此外,已经确定单核苷酸多态性与多种白血病化疗药物的不利药代动力学相关,这表明药物性质的不同也会影响疾病复发风险[22]。

随着基因组学和表观遗传学研究逐渐兴起,儿童ALL的异质性得以揭示。在编码B细胞发育调节因子的基因中可检测到DNA拷贝数异常,该类基因包括*CDKN2A/B*、*PAX5*、*IKZF1*和*EBF1*[23]。此外,*JAK2*体细胞突变、RAS通路基因突变(*NRAS*、*KRAS*、*PTPN11*、*NF1*)和*CRLF2*基因组变异在高危患者中的检出率增加[24,25]。*JAK1*和*JAK2*突变先前也已在DS-ALL和T细胞-ALL中被检测到。此外,基因表达谱分析发现了一组特殊ALL患者,他们与Ph$^+$ ALL患者具有相同的基因表达谱,但是却缺乏BCR-ABL1融合蛋白,这类患者被称为"Ph样"ALL[26]。"Ph样"ALL患者的预后更差。*IKZF1*的缺失或突变是Ph$^+$ ALL和"Ph样"ALL都有的典型特征[27]。该亚群含有除*BCR-ABL*以外的酪氨酸激酶基因融合,包括*ABL1*、*ABL2*、*CSF1R*和*PDGFR*融合,该类患儿可应用酪氨酸激酶抑制剂治疗[28],而携带JAK突变的患者是JAK抑制剂的适用人群[29]。COG目前正在开展高危ALL患者的靶向药物临床试验。

尽管在过去40年中新发ALL的预后已取得明显改善,但婴儿 ALL 和早期复发的 ALL 这两个亚组的预后仍然较差，对这类人群而言，仍迫切需要研制新型治疗方案。由于婴儿 ALL 中 *FLT3*（一种酪氨酸激酶）的表达增加，目前正在开展在白血病标准强度化疗方案基础上联用 *FLT3* 抑制剂来他替尼的研究。同样，鉴于婴儿 ALL 的独特生物学特征，大多数患者在 11q23 上存在 *MLL* 基因重排，蛋白质 DOT1L 被募集到 *MLL* 靶基因上，导致 *MLL* 基因的异常表达。DOT1L 抑制剂正在临床试验中。

对于复发性 ALL，出现了多种新型治疗策略，包括分子靶向药物和细胞疗法。最近，双特异性 T 细胞嵌合抗体获得了相当大的关注。这类抗体同时具有 T 细胞特异性和 B 细胞特异性，从而将患者自身的细胞毒性 T 细胞驱动到恶性肿瘤细胞周围。博纳吐单抗是一种 CD19/CD3 T 细胞双特异性抗体，在多次复发和难治性 B-ALL 儿童中，该药表现出单一用药活性和安全性，并且目前 COG 正开展应用此药治疗首次复发 B-ALL 患者的临床试验。细胞学治疗和免疫治疗的发展对复发和难治性 ALL 来说是一个重大飞跃。此外，嵌合抗原受体（CARs）修饰的 T 细胞经遗传学修饰后，可以表达针对肿瘤抗原（在 B-ALL 中是 CD19）和 T 细胞活化分子的抗体。CAR-T 细胞免疫疗法为 ALL 患者实现长期缓解带来了希望，并且可用于治疗部分预后极差的 ALL 患者[30]。

儿童急性髓性白血病（AML）

AML 占儿童白血病的 20%，慢性粒细胞白血病约占儿童白血病的 1%~2%。与 ALL 相似，AML 的发生也与多种遗传性和获得性肿瘤易感综合征有关，如 DS 和骨髓衰竭综合征［如范可尼贫血、先天性角化不良、重型先天性中性粒细胞减少症（Kostmann 综合征）、Diamond-Blackfa 贫血及获得性再生障碍性贫血］。接受化疗（特别是烷化剂和拓扑异构酶抑制剂）和放疗的患儿有发展为治疗相关性 AML（t-AML）的风险。AML 临床表现和 ALL 类似，少见的临床表现是皮肤或牙龈上出现紫红色凸起的斑块样病变，称为绿色瘤，这是 AML 的一种髓外表现。急性早幼粒细胞白血病（APL）是一种特殊的 AML 亚型，以 t(15;17) 或 *PML-RARA* 融合为特征，常伴有严重的凝血功能障碍和高白细胞血症。

与 ALL 相比，儿童 AML 对化疗反应较差。目前 AML 存活率有所改善，儿童 AML 的治愈率接近 60%~70%[31]，这得益于化疗剂量增强和支持性治疗的改进，也源于大量临床试验和对该病生物学和异质性的深入理解。与 ALL 不同，年龄和 WBC 计数并未被视为分层的独立预后因素。事实上，目前的危险度分层治疗方案综合考虑了细胞遗传学、分子特征及对诱导化疗的治疗反应[32,33]。而且，16 号染色体倒位、t(8;21) 和 t(15;17)、*CEBPA* 双等位突变和 *NPM1* 突变被认为是预后良好的遗传学特征，而 7 号染色体单倍体、5 号染色体单倍体或 del(5q) 和 *FLT3-ITD* 融合伴高比例等位基因被认为是预后不良因素。AML 疗法包括诱导缓解治疗、CNS 预防性治疗和缓解后治疗。由于化疗方案强度大，需要长时间住院和积极的支持治疗。在最初 1~2 个疗程诱导化疗并获得形态学缓解（骨髓中原始细胞小于 5%）后即开始缓解后治疗，包括巩固强化化疗或 HSCT，具体取决于细胞遗传学危险因素和对诱导化疗的反应强度（MRD 状态）。现已证实延长维持治疗疗程疗效较差，因此目前未被纳入除 APL 外的 AML 治疗方案中。治疗 APL 需尽快使用全反式维 A 酸（ATRA）（一种分化诱导剂），同时予以积极的对症支持治疗，之后进入 ATRA、6-巯基嘌呤、甲氨蝶呤联合用药的长期维持化疗阶段。该方案能在首次完全缓解且未行 HSCT 的情况下，使 EFS 达到 70%~80%[34]。此外，三氧化二砷也是一种治疗 APL 的有效药物，早期用药预后更好。

由于诱导化疗强度已达最大，因此急需新的有效药物和治疗策略。目前，COG 正在开展在标准化疗方案基础上加用新型治疗药物的随机临床试验，包括对 *FLT3-ITD* 阴性患者应用一种蛋白酶体抑制剂—硼替佐米并观察疗效，对等位基因 *FLT3-ITD* 高比例阳性的 AML 患者应用索拉非尼（一种针对 *FLT3*、*c-KIT*、*PDGF*、*VEGF* 和 *MEK/ERK* 的多靶点酪氨酸激酶抑制剂）并观察疗效。此外，目前还包括表观遗传修饰因子相关药物研究（如伏立诺他和 5-氮杂胞苷）、抗骨髓细胞表面抗原的单克隆抗体研究、各种移植预处理方案和移植物来源研究，都旨在提高儿童 AML 的远期预后。

儿童非霍奇金淋巴瘤（NHL）

淋巴瘤占美国儿童肿瘤的 15%。NHL 占儿童淋巴瘤的 60%，在 5 岁以下儿童所有恶性肿瘤中占 3%，在 5~19 岁儿童和青少年恶性肿瘤中占 8%~9%。成人中，大多数 NHL 是低度或中度恶性的，但几乎所有儿童 NHL 都是高度恶性的。儿童 NHL 有 3 种主要亚型：①成熟 B 细胞淋巴瘤为主的 Burkitt 淋巴瘤（典型和非典型）或弥漫性大 B 细胞淋巴瘤（DL-BCL）；②前 T 细胞淋巴瘤或淋巴母细胞淋巴瘤；③成熟 T 细胞或裸细胞淋巴瘤，间变性大细胞淋巴瘤（ALCL）。世界卫生组织（WHO）将 ALCL 归类为外周 T 细胞淋巴瘤。这些组织学亚型包括约 40% 的 Burkitt 淋巴瘤，30% 的淋巴母细胞淋巴瘤，20% 的弥漫大 B 细胞淋巴瘤和 10% 的 ALCL。Burkitt 淋巴瘤肿瘤细胞以 t(8;14) 为特征（*c-myc* 癌基因和免疫球蛋白基因位点调控元件发生异位），少见 t(8;22) 或 t(2;8)。类似地，超过 90% 的儿童 ALCL 可检测到 *ALK* 基因 t(2;5) 特征性染色体重排。

NHL 肿瘤体积较大，容易造成两种潜在的危及生命的情况。首先是肿瘤溶解综合征，主要表现为电解质紊乱，典型表现包括高尿酸血症、高钾血症和高磷血症。此时除其他支持治疗外，还需进行积极的水化治疗、使用别嘌醇或拉布立酶（尿酸氧化酶）进行治疗。其二是纵隔大肿块，尤其见于淋巴母细胞性淋巴瘤，此时会因上腔静脉综合征出现心脏或呼吸骤停的危险。

儿童 NHL 所有组织学类型和不同分期的主要治疗方式都是多药联合化疗。精准的化疗方案（含或不含鞘内注射）、化疗强度、治疗疗程通常取决于疾病的严重程度和组织学亚型。虽然 Burkitt 淋巴瘤、DL-BCL 及 ALCL 可采用短期加强化疗方案，但淋巴母细胞性淋巴瘤的治疗是基于 ALL 的长期维持化疗方案。手术组织病理活检在淋巴瘤诊断和分期过程中至关重要，但在儿童 NHL 的整体治疗中作用有限。在儿童 NHL 的整体治疗中，放疗的作用微乎其微，甚至没有作用。

在过去的 20 年中，早期和晚期儿童和青少年 NHL 预后有了显著改善。除罕见亚型外，早期和晚期 B-NHL 总体生存率和 5 年无病生存率分别为 95% 和 80%[35]。儿童和青少年晚期淋巴母细胞 NHL 的生存率已提高到 85% 以上[36]。然而，晚期儿童和青少年 ALCL 患者 7 年总体生存率仍低于 70%[37]。

目前，儿童 NHL 的治疗方案包括细胞表面、细胞内和分子靶向治疗，不仅可以提高晚期 NHL 的整体治愈率，而且最大限度地降低化疗药的副作用。利妥昔单抗（Rituximab）是一种针对 CD20 抗原的单克隆抗体，该抗原在儿童 Burkitt 淋巴瘤和 DLBCL 中表达。COG 已证实了利妥昔单抗加至儿童和青少年 NHL 标准化疗方案中，具有安全性及可耐受性，且结果证实可以使晚期成熟B细胞淋巴瘤（骨髓和中枢神经系统受累）患者的3年EFS达到90%[38]。同样地，在初诊复发ALCL患儿中将克唑替尼（*ALK*靶向抑制剂）[39]和本妥昔单抗（抗CD30单克隆抗体）[40]同时联合化疗可发挥有效作用，目前正进行2期随机临床试验。

霍奇金淋巴瘤（HD）

在发达国家，霍奇金淋巴瘤占儿童恶性肿瘤的5%左右。Reed-Strengberg（RS）多核巨细胞是HD的标志，它存在于由嗜酸性粒细胞、小淋巴细胞、浆细胞、中性粒细胞、组织细胞和成纤维细胞组成的炎症细胞背景中。RS细胞几乎全表达CD30，而只有大约70%的病例表达CD15。HD的两大病理类型是经典型霍奇金淋巴瘤和以结节性淋巴细胞为主型霍奇金淋巴瘤。经典型霍奇金淋巴瘤占儿童HD的大多数，而结节性淋巴细胞为主型霍奇金淋巴瘤仅占5%～10%。

儿童HD患者的治愈率超过90%。儿童HD的标准治疗包括联合化疗和低剂量局部放疗（RT）。儿童HD的临床研究旨在发现能治愈疾病的化疗药物最低剂量，并消除或减少晚期后遗症。

PET扫描已被证明可用于发现早期治疗反应相关的生物标志物，在基于治疗反应的治疗方案中，可用于检测哪些患者适于单纯化疗，哪些患者需要加强治疗。最近结束的COG HD临床试验表明局部放疗可使肿瘤缩减，但这并不包括某些中危HD患者，该类患者应用两个周期的ABVE-PC方案（阿霉素、博莱霉素、长春新碱、依托泊苷、强的松、环磷酰胺）后即很快出现疗效（PET-CT阴性患者），于4个周期后疾病可得到完全缓解[41]。对于复发/难治性HD的治疗仍然具有挑战性，目前大剂量化疗后自体HSCT被认为是大多数患者的标准治疗方法。最近，对于复发/难治性HD患者，正在研究本妥昔单抗（CD30定向抗体结合物）与化疗联合用药。RS细胞生物学特性相关研究可有助于探索新型靶向药物，因此此类研究也受到了较多关注。

肾肿瘤

肾母细胞瘤（WT）

肾母细胞瘤占儿童肾肿瘤的90%以上，占儿童肿瘤的6%。如今，肾母细胞瘤患者的生存率超过90%，即使是存在肿瘤转移的患者，其2年无事件生存率也可达80%[42]。该病典型的临床表现是外观正常的儿童偶发腹部肿块。超过90%的患者是单侧肿块。单侧肿瘤患者平均发病年龄是36.5个月（男性）和42.5个月（女性），而双侧肿瘤的WT患者平均发病年龄是33～35个月，且具有一定的遗传倾向[43]。

许多先天性综合征与WT有关，通过对这些临床综合征的基因分析，人们逐渐发现了一些遗传性以及与散发性WT发病相关的抑癌基因。WAGR综合征（WT、虹膜缺失、泌尿生殖系统畸形和精神发育迟滞）患儿患WT风险大大增加，并且这种综合征与11p13胚系原发性结构性缺失突变有关。*WT1*基因是WT的致病基因（*PAX5*是虹膜缺失相关基因），该基因位于基因缺失区域内。疾病的发病机制符合典型的“二次打击”模型即两个*WT1*等位基因均丢失。同样地，Denys-Drash综合征（假两性畸形、肾脏退行性病变）也与*WT1*原发性突变有关，肿瘤包含*WT1*的两个等位基因的突变。*WT1*的体细胞突变见于10%～20%散发WT病例[44]。

第二个抑癌基因*WT2*已被定位到11p15。这一区域的异常与Beckwith-Wiedemann综合征（巨舌、脐膨出、内脏肿大和单侧肢体肥大）相关。该区域包含大量的印记基因，包括胰岛素样生长因子2（*IGF2*）和*H19*，后者编码一种非编码RNA，并作为抑癌基因[45]。*WT2*的体细胞杂合性缺失是散发性WT最常见的突变类型，发生率高达80%。其他突变包括*WTX*（32%）、*CTNNB1*（15%，可编码β-连环蛋白）和*T53*（5%）。

WT典型表现为起源于肾脏的边界清楚、不均匀强化的肿块（图71-3a）。病理学上，WT通常由胚细胞、上皮细胞和基质细胞三种细胞类型组成，尽管在某些情况下，这些细胞类型中只有一种或两种可以被观察到。间变性WT的肿瘤细胞核明显增大、核具有多形性和多倍体有丝分裂特征，提示预后不良。间变性WT可以是局部病变，也可以表现为弥漫性病变，可见于5%的肿瘤[46]。除间变性WT之外，其余WTs被归为“预后良好的组织学类型”。肾源性残余是初期病变，提示持续存在未完全分化的肾母细胞组织[47]。肾源性残余患者（30%散发性和100%双侧WTs）有发展为WT的风险。根据起病位置的不同分为两种肾源性残余：小叶周围型和小叶内型。大多数肾源性残余会逐渐消退。

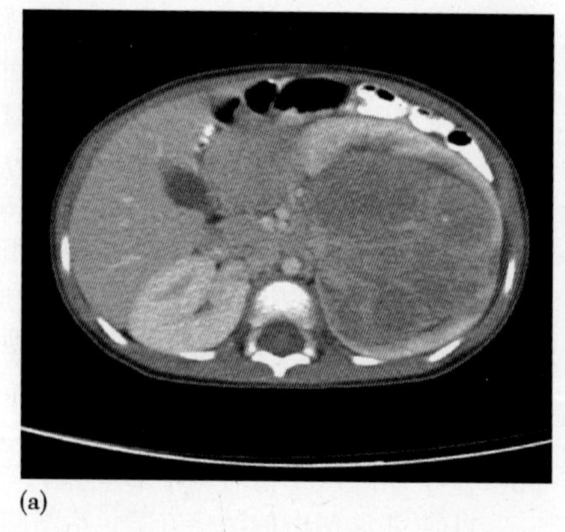
(a)

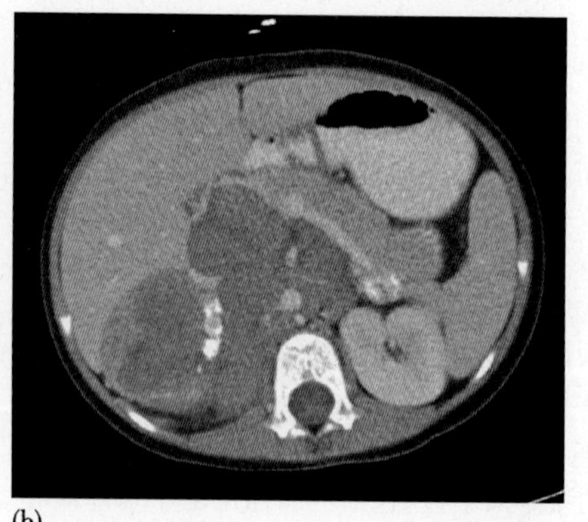
(b)

图71-3 常见儿童腹部肿瘤的计算机断层扫描（CT）成像特征。（a）Wilm瘤：腹部增强CT横断面图像显示，右肾出现较大肿块，肿块呈异质性，边界清楚，不跨中线。（b）神经母细胞瘤：腹部增强CT横断面图像显示右上象限出现一较大的分叶状、异质性肿块，跨中线，主动脉被肿块包裹，肠系膜静脉、脾静脉和胰腺出现位移。肿块中有致密的钙化点

WT 的治疗包括手术切除和化疗,放疗只用于晚期 WT 患者。在世界范围内,有两种预后相近的不同治疗方法。在北美(GOS 协会),大多数病例采用初始手术(肾切除术和淋巴结活检)之后进行化疗[42]。在欧洲(SIOP 协会),提倡新辅助化疗,并推迟手术治疗时间。北美方案的优点是,它可以对所有肿瘤组织进行完整、准确的评估并进行精准分期,而欧洲方案术前可使肿瘤体积缩小,从而更易切除瘤灶,减少肿瘤播散风险[48,49]。

经腹大切口根治性肾切除术是 WT 常用的术式,包括肾上腺的切除和局部淋巴结的切除活检。最新的术式是一种侧路式,但是是否需切除肾上腺仍存在争议[50]。考虑到 WTs 的复发风险,肾部分切除术或"保留肾单位"手术可用于双侧肿瘤患者,此外,预后良好组织学类型的单侧 WT 也可以采用这种术式,尤其是在新辅助化疗作用下,由于化疗效果显著可以保证切缘阴性。最后,一些外科医生正在探索腹腔镜/机器人辅助切除术。

WT 的治疗包括肾切除术和分期化疗,伴或不伴腹部和/或肺部放疗。COG 和 SIOP 的分期方法略有不同,但总体而言,肿瘤分期如下:Ⅰ期:肿瘤被完整切除并且包膜完整,未扩展至肾窦;Ⅱ期:肿瘤可被完全切除,但肿瘤扩散到包膜外或肾窦内;Ⅲ期:不能完全被切除、有淋巴结受累、肿瘤播散和/或手术切缘肿瘤残留;Ⅳ期:肿瘤血源性转移播散(通常为肺,但也包括肝、脑或骨)。术前评估包括腹部和骨盆的 CT 检查和多普勒超声检查,以确定是否存在下腔静脉癌栓。磁共振成像(MRI)有助于发现肾源性残留,并有助于针对双侧肿瘤患者制定手术计划。

肿瘤切除后及时做病理学检查,以明确疾病预后、检测是否存在间变性改变。此外,某些分子标记物可能提示预后不佳,如 1p 和 16q 体细胞杂合性缺失,最新的治疗方案对这些遗传学改变进行了统一的评述[42]。

小于 2 岁的Ⅰ期 WT 患者(肿瘤为预后良好组织学类型且重量小于 550g)的患者进行肾切除,如有小部分患儿复发,应进行补救性放化疗。Ⅰ期和Ⅱ期肿瘤患儿(无 1p 和 16q 体细胞杂合丢失)接受长春新碱和放线菌素 D(疗程 18 周),而Ⅲ期患者应接受长春新碱、放线菌素 D 和阿霉素化疗加腹腔放射治疗(疗程 24 周)。1p 和 16q 体细胞杂合丢失的患者需要追加化疗。对于预后良好组织学类型的Ⅳ期患者,多药物联合用药正在接受治疗评估,但上述三种化疗药联合用药同时辅以胸腹部放疗,似乎并没有提高患者生存率。那些在治疗过程中转移性病变较早恢复的患者不需要接受胸部 X 线放疗,而那些病变在早期未恢复的患者则需要胸部放疗,并可能受益于加强化疗。间变性肾母细胞瘤预后差,根据是弥漫性还是局灶性以及肿瘤分期调整治疗方案。且至今未有最佳治疗方案因此需根据是弥漫性还是局灶性以及肿瘤分期调整治疗方案,如Ⅱ~Ⅳ期弥漫性间变性肾母细胞瘤需采用包括长春新碱、阿霉素、环磷酰胺、卡铂、依托泊苷在内的联合化疗。

双侧肿瘤患者和单侧肿瘤患者以及易患肿瘤性疾病的某些先天性综合征患者面临着特殊的挑战,因为这些患者存在继发第二肿瘤的风险。这些患者可以在术前接受化疗[长春新碱、放线菌素 D(单侧肿瘤合并某些先天性综合征)±阿霉素(双侧肿瘤)],根据最佳反应在第 6 周或第 12 周进行保留肾单位手术。由于该病有典型的临床和影像学表现,这些患者病初通常不需要活检。切除后的治疗由肿瘤的分期和组织学特点来定。

所有良好分化的 WT 预后均较好,10 年无复发生存率分别为 91%(Ⅰ期)、85%(Ⅱ期)、84%(Ⅲ期)和 75%(Ⅳ期),而间变性肿瘤预后较差,10 年无复发生存率为 43%(Ⅰ~Ⅲ期),18%(Ⅳ期)。双侧肿瘤患者预后一般,10 年无复发生存率为 65%(总生存率 78%)[42]。

其他肾肿瘤

肾细胞癌、肾透明细胞肉瘤和恶性横纹肌样肿瘤分别占儿童所有肾肿瘤的 5.9%、3.5%和 1.6%。肾细胞癌患儿常出现腹痛、血尿和腹部肿块。许多疾病与肾细胞癌有关,包括 von Hippel-Lindau 病、家族性肾细胞癌以及之前接受过恶性肿瘤治疗。儿童肾癌与成人的不同之处在于儿童乳头状肾细胞癌占比高,而其他特殊型、透明细胞型、嫌色细胞型不太常见[51,52]。大多数儿童肿瘤中常见转录因子 E3 基因(*TFE3*)位点的易位,该基因位于 XP11.2,可有多种融合形式。与成人相比,儿童肾癌往往处于高危分期。根治性肾切除术同时行淋巴结清扫仍然是主要治疗方法。Ⅰ、Ⅱ和Ⅲ期肾癌患儿的 4 年的存活率分别是 92%、85%和 73%,而Ⅳ期生存率较差仅为 14%[42,53]。对于不可切除或转移性疾病患者的最佳治疗方案尚未确定,在易位突变阳性的肾细胞癌患儿中,可以尝试使用酪氨酸激酶抑制(舒尼替尼)[42]。

透明细胞肉瘤是一组特殊的肿瘤,其组织学表现为肿瘤细胞成巢分布,癌巢由细薄的网状纤维组织分割。该病发病机制不清楚,但是可在少数患者中检测到 t(10;17)(q22,p13)。除肺和肝外,透明细胞肉瘤还可以转移到骨和大脑,但大多数癌灶为局限性。既往认为该病预后不良,但经过 NWTS(美国肾母细胞瘤研究组)连续性临床试验,提高了患儿生存率。应用长春新碱、阿霉素、环磷酰胺、依托泊苷等多种化疗以及放疗,使得该病的 5 年的 EFS 可达 79%[42,54]。

恶性横纹肌样肿瘤与 WT 相比发病年龄较小,症状包括发热和严重血尿[55]。大多数患者进展为疾病晚期,高达 15%的患者有相关的中枢神经系统病变。组织学上,肿瘤细胞体积较大,核仁明显,可见嗜酸性胞质颗粒。这些肿瘤是由 *SMARCB1* 基因(又称为 *INI1*)的双等位基因突变和/或缺失引起的,该基因编码染色质重塑复合体中一个功能蛋白分子[56]。三分之一的患者可检测到 *SMARCB1* 胚系突变,这些患儿发病年龄较早(发病中位年龄为 5 个月)。大多数患者可通过手术、放疗和多药联合化疗进行治疗,但最佳化疗方案尚未确定。发病年龄小、肿瘤晚期和中枢神经系统受累是疾病预后不良的因素。疾病Ⅰ、Ⅱ、Ⅲ期和Ⅳ期的患儿 4 年疾病无复发生存率分别为 50%、33%、33%和 21%。

先天性中胚层肾瘤往往在婴儿期发病,表现为单侧腹部肿瘤。存在两种类型:经典型和细胞型。细胞型中胚层肾瘤以 *ETV6/NTRK* 基因融合[t(12;15)(p13,q25)]为特征,t(12;15)(p13,q25)也可见于婴儿纤维肉瘤[57]。这些肿瘤以完整的手术切除治疗为主,因为该肿瘤很少出现转移,故无需化疗。该病总存活率约为 95%[58]。

神经母细胞瘤(NB)

NB 是儿童最常见的颅外实体瘤,占所有儿童肿瘤的 8%~10%。它来源于前体神经嵴细胞,正常情况下,这些前体神经嵴细胞会分化为交感神经节和肾上腺髓质细胞。NB 是婴儿期最常见的肿瘤,平均发病年龄为 18 个月[59]。值得一提的是该病具有多种不同的临床和生物学特征,婴儿期尽管疾病累及范围广,但可以自愈;而较大儿童容易出现持续性、侵袭性疾病进展。约 2%的病例是家族性的,50%的患者携带有间变性淋巴瘤激酶基因(*ALK*)的胚系突变,而少部分家族性病例是由于 *Phox2b* 突变所致,*Phox2b* 突变与其他神经疾病相关如 Hirschsprung 病[60-62]。发展为肿瘤性疾病可能还需要另一条件,因为只有 50%携带 ALK 胚系突变的患者发展为 NB[63]。事实上,GWAS 已经确定了一些易感基因位点,但相对而言大多数散发病例却较少能检测到易感基因突变位点[64]。在散发 NB 患者中,*ALK* 基因突变占 8%~12%,*ALK* 基因扩增占 2%~3%,*Phox2b* 突变占 2%[65]。

NB 的临床表现取决于肿瘤的原发位置,但大多数患者因初诊时疾病累及范围广而出现全身症状如发热、体重减轻、易怒、骨痛和血细胞减少。三分之二病例与腹部原发病有关,绝大多数 NB 位于肾上腺(图 71-3b)。患儿可能出现腹痛、便秘和腹胀。体格检查时可发现腹部的较大肿块,可穿过体正中线。Horner 综合征可能与颈部和胸部肿瘤(后纵隔)有关。骶前和椎旁肿瘤可出现脊髓受压症状,如尿潴留、运动无力和阵挛。最后,NB 可能出现一种罕见的副肿瘤综合征,其特征是眼阵挛肌阵挛综合征(OMS),具体表现为眼球不自主运动和肌阵挛,伴或不伴有共济失调[66]。值得注意的是,OMS 通常提示肿瘤预后良好,但神经系统症状经治疗后仍可持续存在。

NB 的初步评估包括胸部、腹部和骨盆的 CT 或 MRI 横截面成像,以确定是局灶性、区域性(包括硬膜外区域)还是存在远处病变。碘苄胍(MIBG)是一种去甲肾上腺素类似物,可被交感神经组织选择性摄取,并用于评估 CT 或 MRI 未检出的受累部位。大多数肿瘤可以摄取 MIBG,但对于不摄取 MIBG 的肿瘤,FDG-PET 可协助发现肿瘤部位。该病的诊断依赖原发或远处转移部位组织活检,或骨髓中可见典型肿瘤细胞同时伴有尿香草基杏仁酸(VMA)和尿高香草酸(HVA)水平升高。

组织学上,肿瘤细胞可表现为多种细胞分化形式,从分化良好的神经节细胞瘤到节细胞神经成纤维细胞瘤,再到典型的神经母细胞瘤。典型的肿瘤细胞呈蓝色小圆形细胞,形似玫瑰。组织学上,肿瘤可以根据年龄、分化程度(高分化提示预后较好)、Schwannian 基质含量和核碎裂指数方面分成不同的亚类。核碎裂指数是指每 5 000 个细胞中有多少有丝分裂数和核碎裂数,指数小于 100 或 200 提示疾病预后良好(取决于细胞基质、年龄、分化程度)[67]。

国际神母细胞瘤分期系统(INSS)的制定是为了协助该病的治疗和疗效分析(表 71-3)[68]。值得注意的是,尽管疾病累及范围广泛,但 4S 期 NB 患儿仍有很大可能自愈。最近,这个分析系统被国际神母细胞瘤风险协作组(INRG)的分层系统取代,INRG 分层系统基于放射学特征,具体为:L1(局部单一体腔的局部肿瘤),L2(单一局部肿瘤,可累及肿瘤附近的结构),M(远处转移)和 MS(年龄在 18 个月以内,转移仅限于皮肤、肝脏和/或骨髓)[69]。

表 71-3 国际神母细胞瘤分期系统(INSS)

1 期	完全切除的局灶性肿瘤,同侧淋巴结阴性
2A 期	不完全切除的局限性肿瘤,非粘连同侧淋巴结阴性
2B 期	完全或不完全切除的局限性肿瘤,同侧淋巴结阳性,对侧淋巴结阴性
3 期	不完全切除的单侧肿瘤横穿中线,有双侧淋巴结转移
4 期	肿瘤转移至远处的淋巴结、皮肤、肝脏、骨、骨髓和其他器官
4S 期	病程属 1 期或 2 期局部性肿瘤,发生于 1 岁以下的婴儿,有皮肤、肝脏和/或累髓受累(肿瘤细胞数量<10%的有核细胞)

分层治疗是指基于一些临床和生物学因素,将疾病分为低、中、高危组。两个最重要的危险因素是年龄和疾病分期,18 个月以下儿童的预后明显优于较大年龄组儿童。INSS 1、2、3 和 4S 期儿童的总生存率为(91±1)%,而Ⅳ期儿童的总生存率为(42±1)%[70]。NB 是人类最早出现的肿瘤之一,且受遗传变异影响。20%的患者可见 *MYCN* 基因扩增,并预示为侵袭性疾病。染色体倍数也可作为生存结局预测指标,尤其是对于婴儿和局灶性病变患者,其中超二倍体提示疾病预后良好。COG 根据年龄、分期、组织学特点、*MYCN* 变异和染色体倍数将患者分为低危组、中危组和高危组,三组患儿占比分别为 40%、20%和 40%,三组的 EFS 分别为>95%、80%~95%和 40%~50%[65]。其他的遗传突变也影响疾病预后,包括 17q 等位基因扩增和 1p36 和 11q 的杂合性缺失。所有这些均提示疾病预后不良。除了用于 COG 风险分类外,11q 杂合性缺失也纳入 INRG 分类系统[70]。新版的分类方法还包括染色体片段的扩增或删失。虽然整个染色体的扩增提示疾病预后良好,但染色体片段的扩增或删失提示疾病预后不佳,特别是 1p、3p、4p、11q 染色体片段删失,或 1q、2p 或 17q 染色体片段的扩增。未来的研究将会把这些纳入低危组疾病的分类中[71]。

对于低危患者(INSS 1 期或生物学行为良性的 INSS 2A/2B 期),可只行手术切除,对那些有生命危险的或少数病情进展甚至复发的患者则需要进行化疗[71]。有一小部分年龄小于 6 个月、存在微小肾上腺原发病变的患者,其肿瘤可消退[72]。大多数 4S 期患者都会自发消退,但一些肝脏肿大导致呼吸窘迫的患儿,需要立即进行低剂量化疗和/或放疗。中危患者(例如:INSS 3 期和大多数年龄大于 18 个月的 4 期患者,年龄小于 18 个月的 INRG L2 期患者)则需接受手术和中度强化化疗,化疗药物通常包括卡铂/顺铂、依托泊苷、环磷酰胺和阿霉素,约 2~8 个疗程,疗程长短通常取决于初始治疗反应和其他预后相关标志物(如染色体结构异常)。在某些情况下,可以不需手术和化疗(如 18 个月内的 L2 期患儿)。

治疗高危组 NB 仍然是一个挑战,但通过清髓治疗方案、诱导分化治疗和免疫疗法,疾病的诊治逐步取得了改善[73,74]。初始治疗包括用环磷酰胺、拓扑替康、顺铂、依托泊苷、阿霉素和长春新碱或类似物进行 6 个周期的大剂量化疗。手术(巩固治疗前,同时行用清髓性化疗)和放疗(巩固治疗后)联合可以将肿瘤负荷降至最低,这是高危人群的常用治疗方法。多项研究表明,巩固治疗联合清髓性化疗后再输注自体外周血干细胞可改善预后[75]。研究表明,净化干细胞来源没有益处,干细胞通常是在两个化疗周期后采集的[76]。已有数据表明,使用 Busulfan-Melphalan 法清髓优于其他方案,并且大剂量化疗与干细胞移植的联合治疗在单疗程中是有益的[77]。对新确诊的 NB 患者,COG 正开展研究,旨在揭示巩固治疗之前使用^{131}I-MIBG 靶向治疗的疗效[71]。

生物学方法的使用也改善了高危组患者的预后。顺式维甲酸在研究中被认为可以分化肿瘤细胞,但早期用于治疗复发或难治性疾病的效果却不佳。然而,一项随机试验表明,对于高危患者(存在微小残留病)在接受细胞毒药物治疗后加用该药后,病情得到改善。目前正在评估该药在低危患者中的疗效[78]。此外,抗 GD2 单克隆抗体(mab)与粒细胞-单核细胞集落刺激因子和白细胞介素-2 联合用药,可以显著增加 NB 患儿的 2 年生存率(mab 组为 66%±5%,无 mab 组为 46%±5%)[74]。

对难治、复发 NB 患者的治疗仍无显著疗效。全基因组拷贝数分析和测序发现 12%的患者存在 *ALK* 基因突变,这些患者使用 *ALK* 抑制剂(如 crizotinib)可能有效,这也是目前早期研究的重点。但是,包括 *ATRX*、*ARID1A* 和 *PTPN11* 基因(调控 ras 通路的基因)在内的其他体细胞来源基因突变率要低很多,但到目前为止还没有针对这些基因的靶向治疗。高危 NB 肿瘤细胞膜表面可以表达神经促性腺激素受体 TrkB,这是可能的治疗靶点之一,尽管没有使用来妥替尼的早期经验[79]。与其他转录因子一样,核转录因子 MYCN 一直很难作为靶点进行靶向治疗,但针对调控染色质的溴域和额外终端域(BET)溴域蛋白的新方法可以有效治疗含 Myc 扩增的肿瘤,该药物的研究正处于早期阶段[80]。

儿童骨肿瘤

对于年轻和老年患者来说,恶性原发性骨肿瘤的发病机制、临床表现和治疗方面存在显著差异。虽然原发性骨肿瘤很少见,但它们是儿童第六常见的恶性肿瘤,也是青年中第三常见的肿瘤。在美国 20 岁以下的儿童和青少年中,每年恶性骨肿瘤的发病率约为 8.7/1 000 000。儿童骨肿瘤中只有一半是恶性的,其中骨肉瘤(OS)最为常见,约占所有原发性恶性骨肿瘤的 35%。尤文肉瘤(EWS)是第二常见的原发性恶性骨肿瘤,10 岁以下儿童中 EWS 比 OS 更常见。

骨肉瘤

骨肉瘤(OS)是最常见的原发性恶性骨肿瘤,由产生类骨质的梭形细胞组成。它是一种高度侵袭性肿瘤,在过去的几十年里,该病在治疗和预后方面取得了显著提高。虽然老年人也可患 OS,但该病主要发生在青壮年人群中。OS 的发病年龄呈双峰分布,第一个高峰出现在 10~20 岁,即青少年生长高峰期,第二个高峰出现在老年期。据估计,美国每年约有 400 名 20 岁以下的儿童和青少年被确诊为骨肉瘤。该病在 5 岁之前非常罕见。最常见的临床表现是骨受累部位的疼痛,伴或不伴有软组织包块。在年轻患者中,长骨干骺端是最常见的受累位置。大约有一半的 OS 以膝关节周围骨病变为首发表现。

该病发病高峰年龄与年轻人骨骼快速生长期相吻合,这提示骨骼快速生长与骨肉瘤的发生存在相关性。此外,有证据表明辐射暴露是该病的另一个病因。视神经母细胞瘤存活者中 OS 的发生率显著增加。而且,在遗传型 RB 患儿中常检测到 *RB* 基因突变。这可能是这类患儿继发第二肿瘤的几率增加的原因,因为单侧散发性视神经母细胞瘤存活者的 OS 发病率要低很多。*P53* 基因胚系突变可能会导致恶性肿瘤(包括 OS)发病率明显升高,Li-Fraumeni 综合征患儿中也可出现。大多数 OS 患者,包括儿童和青少年的 OS,都属于成骨细胞亚型。目前 WHO 根据肿瘤细胞的主要分化类型,将 OS 分为两种亚型:软骨母细胞型和成纤维细胞型。毛细血管扩张性 OS 是一种罕见的亚型,在骨骼平片上表现为单纯的溶骨性病变,因此可能与动脉瘤性骨囊肿或巨细胞瘤混淆。

在年轻患者中,骨肉瘤与其他肉瘤(通常为高级别肉瘤)类似,在其演变过程中很早就会转移。大约有 20%的患者通过影像学可发现转移,最常见转移部位是肺,而几乎所有新诊断的患者都至少有肺内转移性微小病灶,如果单靠手术切除治疗,2 年内 80%的患者会出现肺肿瘤复发[81]。死于肺转移的患者,几乎都是由于呼吸衰竭、肺出血、气胸或上腔静脉阻塞引起的。通常根据受累部位影像学表现疑诊 OS,可表现为溶解性、硬化性或溶解-硬化混合病变。OS 的确诊依赖于组织活检并进行病理诊断。骨肉瘤是一种由多形性梭形细胞构成的肿瘤,形成以类骨质为主的细胞外基质。免疫组织化学和细胞遗传学对骨肉瘤的诊断没有太大帮助。骨肉瘤患者应进行肿瘤分期,以确定疾病的严重程度,检查内容包括骨及其邻近关节的平片和核磁、胸部 CT、骨扫描和/或 PET-CT。

该病常规治疗方案包括全身多药联合化疗、局部和转移灶的手术切除[81]。对于未出现肿瘤转移的 OS 患者来说,尽管化疗方案有多种,但是其标准化疗方案一般包括顺铂和阿霉素,以及大剂量的甲氨蝶呤。外科技术的进步极大地改变了医学发展,也帮助患者实现了肢体功能性修复。Rosen 等人提出了在手术切除前进行化疗的理念[82]。尽管新辅助化疗与手术后辅助化疗在预后上没有差异。但新辅助化疗确实提供了一些潜在的优势,包括可使肿瘤体积缩减,更易切除,改进手术计划和内支架方案以及微转移疾病的治疗,最重要的是可以评估化疗反应。观察发现,骨坏死程度与治疗后的无病生存率具有很强的相关性[83],随后的多项临床试验也证实这一点。诱导化疗后骨坏死程度可以判断预后情况,建议对骨坏死较少的患者修订化疗方案。对于化疗效果不佳的患者,包括异环磷酰胺和依托泊苷在内的强化疗方案尽管早期有治疗有效的报道,但并没有改善其预后[84]。由于完整的手术切除对于骨肉瘤的治疗非常重要,能否手术切除是一个重要的预后影响因素,因此中轴骨肿瘤患者比四肢骨肿瘤患者的预后要差。

在诊断初期,无论是否有转移,总体治疗原则相同。OS 患者的预后取决于多个因素。最重要的预后影响因素是是否存在转移,肿瘤转移往往提示预后不良。对于初诊时出现转移的患者,肺结节的数目以及单侧或双侧肺受累对判断预后也有重要意义。在目前治疗方案下,大约 60%~70%的非转移性骨肉瘤患者可存活,并且不会出现复发。在大多数已报道的临床研究中,转移患者的存活率只有 10%~20%。OS 对放疗不敏感,因此标准治疗方案中不包括放疗，仅在姑息治疗中用于缓解疼痛。

近年来，骨肉瘤患者的存活率无显著提高。目前，正在进行早期临床试验的化疗药物已证实均不推荐用于骨肉瘤的一线治疗。但目前的研究倾向于疾病相关分子的靶向药物，其中抗 GD2 抗体和抗 RANKL 抗体尤为重要。

尤文肉瘤（EWS）

EWS 是儿童和青少年中第二常见的原发性恶性骨肿瘤。EWS 是外周原始神经外胚层肿瘤（PPNETs）的一部分。在 20 世纪 80 年代早期，发现 EWS 和 PPNET 在染色体 11 和 22 号之间含有相同的相互易位，t（11；22）（q24，q12）[86,87]。十年后，在这些肿瘤中发现了相同的癌基因表达模式（*c-myc*、*N-myc*、*c-myb* 和 *c-mil/raf1*）。相同的易位、细胞生理学和治疗反应，使这些肿瘤都被归为尤文肉瘤肿瘤家族（EWSFTs）。EWSFT 包括 EWS、PPNET、神经上皮瘤、非典型 EWS 和 Askin 肿瘤（胸壁 EWSFT）。

大多数病例都是散发的，但 EWSFT 患者的家庭成员患神经外胚层恶性肿瘤和胃恶性肿瘤的几率明显增加[88]。尽管确切的细胞来源尚未确定，但目前认为 EWSFT 起源于神经外胚层，可能是神经节后胆碱能神经元。EWSFT 的免疫组化特征为弥漫性 $CD99^+$（MIC2），90%以上的 EWSFT 中均有 $CD99^+$。除波形蛋白和 FLI1 外，未分化型肿瘤其他标志物均为阴性，而分化程度较高的肿瘤可表达其他标志物，如神经元特异性烯醇化酶、S-100、神经丝、CD57 和突触素。EWSFT 肿瘤细胞不含肌肉细胞和淋巴细胞标记物。95%以上的 EWSFT 中可见 t（11：22）（q24，q12）易位或其他相关易位。一些人认为这种易位是该病的发病原因，对于 EWSFT 的诊断是十分必要的。经典的 t（11；22）（q24，q12）易位将位于 22 号染色体上的 *EWS* 基因与位于 11 号染色体的 ets 家族基因上的 *FLI1* 基因连接起来。Ets 家族的其他成员包括 *ERG* t（21；22）、*ETV1* t（7；22）和 *E1AF* t（17；22）。标准细胞遗传学和荧光原位杂交（FISH）可以揭示这种异常的、额外的核型改变，包括 8 号、12 号染色体三体，以及 1 号、16 号染色体的异常。一些易位（如 t（21；22））通过标准的细胞遗传学技术仍然难以发现，需要反转录聚合酶链反应或 FISH 来检测。

EWSFT 的发病高峰在 10~20 岁，但不同人种发病率不同，白人的发病率至少是黑人的 9 倍。EWS 最常见于骨骼，但也可起源于骨外软组织。常见的原发部位包括骨盆（25%）、股骨（16%）、肋骨（12%）和脊柱（8%）。大约 25%的患者会出现转移，其中 37%的转移局限于肺或胸膜，其余患者会有骨和/或骨髓转移，伴或不伴有肺/胸膜转移。骨髓转移的患者很少有广泛浸润和全身症状。该病的诊断通常依赖肿瘤组织病理活检。肿瘤分期相关检查通常包括原发部位的 MRI/CT、胸部 CT 以评估肺转移情况、骨扫描以及骨髓穿刺和活检。近些年，FDG-PET/CT 逐渐取代骨扫描用于 EWS 转移灶的筛查。肿瘤转移是预后不良的重要因素，其他预后不良因素包括中轴骨肿瘤、发病年龄较大、原发肿瘤体积较大、诱导化疗后组织学反应差。

ESFT 患者需要局部和全身治疗，局部治疗采用手术和放疗，全身治疗采用化疗。与骨肉瘤不同，EWS 具有很强的放疗敏感性，明确指出放疗是局部治疗的标准方案，可作为截肢手术的替代治疗。烷基化剂（环磷酰胺、异环磷酰胺、马法兰和白消安）和多柔比星是 EWS 治疗最常用的化疗药物，而异环磷酰胺和依托泊苷的加入使得无病生存率和完全缓解率显著增加，尤其是对于非转移性患者而言[89]。最近，COG 研究表明，对于没有转移的患者，每 2 周一次的非格司亭及其他化疗药物的联合加强化疗比传统每 3 周一次的化疗具有更好的疗效[90]。总体而言，这些措施已将非转移性 EWS 的 5 年无事件生存率提高到 75%。

在诊断早期就存在转移的 EWS 患者预后较差，多处转移的患者存活率极低。局限于肺转移的患者，其预后比存在骨或骨髓转移的患者要好。尽管采用了包括异环磷酰胺和依托泊苷在内的标准化疗方案，并利用手术和放疗对原发和转移部位进行局部治疗，但转移性 EWS 的总治愈率仍为 20%。清髓化疗后自体干细胞移植并没有明显的改善整体生存情况[91]。

目前，COG 正在对局限性 EWS 患者进行 3 期随机临床试验，该实验旨在探究拓扑替康/环磷酰胺联合化疗的可行性。胰岛素样生长因子Ⅰ型受体（IGF-1R）对 ESFT 的转化和生长都至关重要[92]，目前对于治疗新诊断的转移性 EWS 患者，COG 正开展抗 IGF-1R 抗体联合巩固强化治疗的疗效研究。此外，研究还包括 mTOR 抑制剂对于复发和难治性 EWS 的疗效研究[85]。

软组织肉瘤

软组织肉瘤是一组广泛的异质性恶性肿瘤，在 19 岁以下儿童和青少年肿瘤中占 7.4%。美国每年约有 800~900 例新发病例[1]。最常见的软组织肉瘤是横纹肌肉瘤，大部分起源于横纹肌，其余的起源于纤维结缔组织（纤维肉瘤）、平滑肌（平滑肌肉瘤）和脂肪（脂肪肉瘤）。滑膜细胞肉瘤目前被认为起源于非滑膜细胞前体细胞。

横纹肌肉瘤

横纹肌肉瘤（RMS）占 14 岁以下儿童软组织肿瘤的 50%。尽管有报道发现，该病可能与 Costello 综合征、Beckwith-Wiedemann 综合征和 Li-Fraumeni 综合征相关，但到目前为止，大多数为散发病例。RMS 肿瘤细胞呈蓝色、小圆形，其组织学特征和免疫组化（肌 D 蛋白、肌原蛋白、肌特异性肌动蛋白、肌红蛋白和肌间线蛋白）均证实其由骨骼肌分化而来的。RMS 可以分为胚胎型 RMS 和腺泡 RMS 两种组织学亚型。胚胎型 RMS（ERMS，约占 60%~75%）以梭形细胞和黏液样结构为特征，而腺泡 RMS（ARMS）的典型特征是由卵圆形细胞形成的腺泡腔，周围可见纤维间隔[93]。大多数 ARMS 的特征是存在 *PAX3*（55% ARMS）、*PAX7*（20% ARMS）、*FOXO1* DNA 结合区域之间的易位。大约 15% ERMS 的融合基因是阴性的。ERMS 的预后要好于 ARMS，而融合基因阴性的 ARMS 预后优于融合基因阳性的 ARMS[94]。有趣的是，ERMS 与 RAS 通路基因的高频率、高丰度突变相关[95]。

RMS 的临床表现取决于发病部位。大约 40%的 RMS 发生在头部、颈部和眼眶。症状包括无痛性肿块（原发头颈部的浅表肿瘤）、眼球突出、眼球内斜视（眼眶肿瘤）、打鼾、反复单侧鼻出血、鼻窦炎和脑神经麻痹（鼻咽癌和副鼻咽癌）。泌尿生殖系统 RMS 占 20%，膀胱/前列腺病变可导致尿路梗阻。四肢

RMS 占 20%，通常表现为无痛性肿块。肢体肿瘤多为腺泡亚型，而头颈部和泌尿系部位的肿瘤多为 ERMS。ERMS 的葡萄状肉瘤出现在黏膜表面（如阴道、鼻咽部），可出现葡萄样突起。

RMS 的临床评估包括原发肿瘤的断层成像（CT 或 MRI）和可能的转移部位的影像学检查（胸部 CT、双侧骨髓穿刺和活检以及骨扫描）。大约 15%的患者在诊断时就有转移，最常见的是肺，其次是骨髓、淋巴结和骨骼。RMS 根据预后相关因素（年龄、原发肿瘤的位置、疾病的程度或分组情况、组织学亚型和分期）进行分类。分期评估内容包括原发部位（预后良好部位和预后不良部位）、肿瘤大小（局限于器官的 T_1 期和出现肿瘤扩散的 T_2 期；肿瘤≤5cm 或>5cm）、淋巴结情况（N_0 未受累、N_1 受累、N_X 未知）及有无转移（M_0 或 M_1）。预后良好部位包括眼眶、脑膜外、胆道和除膀胱/前列腺外的泌尿生殖部位。根据手术的可切除性可以将 RMS 分为四组：组 1 为完全切除，组 2 为大体切除但有局部扩散的依据，组 3 为残留病灶，组 4 为远处转移。原发部位位于四肢的 RMS 患者应进行区域淋巴结活检。值得注意的是，COG 研究表明初始化疗反应与预后无明显相关性。这些因素被用于 COG 临床试验的危险度分层中（表 71-4）[96]。

表 71-4　横纹肌肉瘤的 COG 危险度分层

危险等级分组	分期	分组	组织类型	占比	无事件生存率
低危，组 1	Ⅰ	Ⅰ-Ⅱ	胚胎型 RMS	27%	85%～95%
	Ⅰ	Ⅲ（眼眶）	胚胎型 RMS		
	Ⅱ	Ⅰ-Ⅱ	胚胎型 RMS		
低危，组 2	Ⅰ	Ⅲ（非眼眶）	胚胎型 RMS	5%	70%～85%
	Ⅲ	Ⅰ-Ⅱ	胚胎型 RMS		
中危	Ⅱ-Ⅲ	Ⅲ	胚胎型 RMS	27%	73%
	Ⅰ-Ⅲ	Ⅰ-Ⅲ	腺泡型 RMS	25%	65%
高危	Ⅳ	Ⅳ	胚胎型 RMS	8%	35%
	Ⅳ	Ⅳ	腺泡型 RMS	8%	15%

来源：引自 Hawkins et al. 2013[96]。

RMS 的治疗需要多学科综合治疗，最有效的化疗药物是长春新碱、放线菌素和环磷酰胺（VAC）。低危组（组 1）患者，VAC 短期治疗有效，其中环磷酰胺的推荐剂量应最小化，以避免影响生殖功能，而组 2 患者则需要更大剂量的药物[97]。同时组 2 和组 3 患者还需要接受放疗。许多研究人员想通过在 VAC 中加用其他药物如依托泊苷、卡铂、异环磷酰胺和托泊替康等，以改善中危患者的预后，但是收效甚微。COG 最近完成的一项研究着眼于在 VAC 中添加长春新碱/伊立替康（V/I），虽然患者无病生存率没有得到改善，但血液毒性更低，并且环磷酰胺的总剂量更低。因此，VAC/VI 可作为中危患者的标准化治疗方案[98]。高危患者的预后几乎没有改善，但间断使用异环磷酰胺/依托泊苷和长春新碱/阿霉素/环磷酰胺可以使高危患者受益。目前正在考虑或研究一些针对分子靶点的药物，如 IGF-1R（自分泌激活）、ALK（扩增）、C-Met（过表达）和 RAS（*ERMS* 突变）[96,99]。

非横纹肌肉瘤软组织肉瘤

非横纹肌肉瘤软组织肉瘤（NRSTS）是一类具有独特的遗传、病理和临床表现的肿瘤。它们好发于老年患者，大多数病变位于四肢。许多肿瘤都有不同的基因异常，且具有诊断意义，如滑膜肉瘤 t（X；18）（p11，q11）（*SYT-SS1* 和 *SYT-SSX2*）。手术切除是主要的治疗方法，放疗则用于高级别肿瘤和切缘阳性的患者。化疗的作用是不确定的，但新辅助化疗可以提高手术切除的机会。对于体积较大的肿瘤，放疗的同时是否使用辅助化疗仍存在争议，但在最近的 COG 方案中推荐使用辅助化疗[100]。表 71-5 总结了不同危险度分组及预后情况[101]。

表 71-5　非横纹肌肉瘤软组织肉瘤的预后分组

危险度分组	完全切除	分级	大小	远处转移	在 NRSTS 中的占比	5 年生存率
低危	是	低	不限	否	60%	90%
	是	高	<5cm	否		
中危	是	高	>5cm	否	30%	50%
	否	不限	不限	否		
高危	不限	不限	不限	是	10%	15%

来源：数据来自参考文献 96 和 100。

中枢神经系统肿瘤

婴幼儿中枢神经系统肿瘤与成人中枢神经系统肿瘤在流行病学、分子遗传学和生物学上有着显著差异。由于这些差异，使得儿童中枢神经系统肿瘤在临床表现、治疗和预后方面有着独特的表现。

恶性中枢神经系统肿瘤是儿童时期最常见的实体肿瘤，美国每年都有 2 200 例新发病例。在整个儿童期和青春期，儿童脑肿瘤的组织学、形态学和性别分布上有很大差异。在所有年龄组中，男孩比女孩更容易患病，但这种差别主要表现在髓母细胞瘤、PNET 和室管膜瘤上。儿童中枢神经系统肿瘤 90%以上为原发性脑肿瘤。其生存率已经由 1975—1984 年的 60%提高到 1985—1994 年的 65%，再到 1995—2011 年的 73.3%。存活率随着年龄的增加而增加，1 岁患儿生存率低于 45%，1～4 岁为 59%，5～9 岁为 64%，10～14 岁为 70%，15～19 岁为 77%。儿童中枢神经系统肿瘤组织学分型中最主要的是毛细胞星形细胞瘤（23.5%），其次是髓母细胞瘤（16.3%）、室管膜瘤（10.1%）、间变性星形细胞瘤和胶质母细胞瘤（各 7.2%）和颅咽管瘤（5.6%）[102]。成人脑部肿瘤的绝大多数为高级别胶质细胞瘤、间变性星形细胞瘤、胶质母细胞瘤，其次为脑膜瘤和其他间叶细胞瘤。

在美国，中枢神经系统肿瘤是儿童期肿瘤患者死亡最常见的原因，占肿瘤相关死亡的 24%。由于越来越有效的治疗，患者虽然存活下来，但是仍可出现认知、记忆和学习障碍、神经内分泌缺陷、听力缺陷、不孕不育和继发第二肿瘤等后遗症。

中枢神经系统肿瘤的病因尚不清楚。已知的危险因素包括：性别（男性）、头部放疗治疗剂量（如白血病或先前的脑肿瘤）和遗传综合征，如神经纤维瘤病、结节性硬化症、痣样基底细胞癌综合征(Gorlin 综合征)、Turcot 综合征和 Li-Fraumeni 综合征。

中枢神经系统胚胎性肿瘤是一组组织学相似、形态未分化的肿瘤,是儿童最常见的恶性脑肿瘤(约占 21%)。从婴儿时期到 3 岁,发病率呈逐步下降趋势。中枢神经系统胚胎性肿瘤包括原始神经外胚层肿瘤(PNETs)、室管膜细胞瘤和非典型畸胎样横纹肌样瘤(AT/RT)。PNETs 是一组高度恶性肿瘤,由神经外胚层来源的蓝色小圆形细胞组成。根据发病位置的不同可将 PNET 进一步细分为髓母细胞瘤(后颅窝)和幕上 PNET。幕上 PNET 和髓母细胞瘤的分类一直存在争议,但分子遗传学、生物学和临床表现证实了这一分类[103]。

髓母细胞瘤是儿童时期最常见的恶性脑肿瘤,发病年龄呈双峰分布,首先是 3~4 岁,其次是 8~10 岁。典型的影像学表现是后颅窝中线的实性肿块,起源于小脑,占据第四脑室(图 71-4a)。手术(首选肿瘤全切)和颅脑脊髓放疗是成功治疗髓母细胞瘤的关键。然而,为了减少晚期副作用,特别是对非常年幼的儿童,同时加用化疗可以减少放疗剂量。最近发现大剂量化疗联合造血干细胞移植可以取得更好的疗效,并且不影响高危髓母细胞瘤的存活率。

目前,通过转录图谱可以将髓母细胞瘤分为 4 类:WNT、Sonic Hedgehog(SHH)、C 组和 D 组[104]。WNT 通路激活的肿瘤占总数的 10%,而 *PTCH1* 或 *SMO* 基因突变导致 SHH 通路激活约占 30%,两者均预后良好。无论其是否存在转移,C 组预后都较差。目前有研究正在评估分层治疗疗效,和发掘更有效且毒副作用更小的新型靶向治疗。

AT/RT 是一种恶性侵袭性肿瘤,常发生在 2 岁以下儿童。由于这些肿瘤在组织学上与 PNET 相似,其中三分之二的肿瘤在形态学上与 PNET 表现相同,因此直到最近才被确认是与 PNET 不同的肿瘤。大约一半的 AT/RTs 发生在幕下,并有侵犯小脑-桥脑角的倾向。由于其与 22 号染色体的缺失和 *SMARCB1/INI1*(抑癌基因)的突变有关,在可疑髓母细胞瘤/PNET 的婴儿和儿童中,对这些标记物进行分析已成为一种分子生物学诊断工具。尽管经过积极的治疗,但这类疾病通常会导致死亡。

室管膜瘤约占儿童中枢神经系统肿瘤的 10%,大约三分之二发生在幕下。超过一半的肿瘤发生在 5 岁以下的儿童,该病在 2 岁时发病率达到高峰。尚未证实在手术和放疗的基础上加用化疗,会对儿童室管膜瘤总体生存率有影响,该方案目前还在进一步研究中。

神经胶质瘤的种类包括良性低级别胶质瘤和恶性高级别胶质瘤,前者可切除和/或长期随访,后者预后极差。低级别胶质瘤泛指包括毛细胞型星形细胞瘤(WHO 1 级)和弥漫性纤维型星形细胞瘤和绒毛膜样星形细胞瘤(WHO 2 级),而高级别胶质瘤包括间变性星形细胞瘤(WHO 3 级)和胶质母细胞瘤(WHO 4 级)。脑皮质星形细胞瘤的发病率随着年龄的增长而增加,两次发病高峰为 5 岁和 13 岁。在儿童中,脑干和小脑星形细胞瘤与脑皮质星形细胞瘤一样常见。小脑星形细胞瘤几乎只发生在儿童中,好发年龄在 4~9 岁之间。幼年毛细胞型星形细胞瘤(JPA)是最常见的亚型,占小脑星形细胞瘤的 85%(图 71-4b)。弥漫性星形细胞瘤是第二常见的,而恶性星形细胞瘤很少会出现在小脑。全手术切除的治愈率为 95%~100%。JPAs 可能长期稳定,甚至会自发消退。然而,患有Ⅰ型神经纤维瘤病(NF-1)的儿童,小脑星形细胞瘤可能更具有侵袭性。视觉通路、下丘脑和丘脑胶质瘤是儿童星形细胞瘤的一种相对常见的形式。视交叉和下丘脑的肿瘤通常是低级别的,而丘脑肿瘤有多种类型。大约 20% NF-1 患儿在儿童时期会发展成视路胶质瘤,主要是 JPA。这些肿瘤最常见于 5~10 岁儿童。最近的研究强调了 MAPK/ERK 通路在肿瘤发生中的作用。虽然 *IDH1* 突变是绝大多数成人低级别和继发性高级别胶质瘤的特征[105],但大多数儿童低级别胶质瘤都有 *BRAF* 基因突变,表现为重排、融合和/或点突变[106,107]。目前,有研究正在利用这些通路对儿童低级别胶质瘤进行分子靶向治疗。

脑干胶质瘤(BSG)占所有儿童中枢神经系统肿瘤的 10%~15%,在成人中比较罕见。发病高峰在 5~9 岁之间,但在儿童的各个时期都可以发病。BSGs 最常发生在脑桥(实质内弥漫病变),其位置与成人多形性胶质母细胞瘤(GBM)相似,预后都较差(图 71-4c)。相反,发生在中脑或髓质的病变很可能是低级别病变,进展更缓慢,预后更好。手术和术后放疗是治疗儿童高级别胶质瘤的主要方法。最近测序研究表明,在约 30%~40%的儿童胶质母细胞瘤中,组蛋白 H3F3A 和 IDH1 存在重复发生但互斥的基因突变[108],表明表观遗传调节机制被破坏,这可以进一步用于靶向治疗。

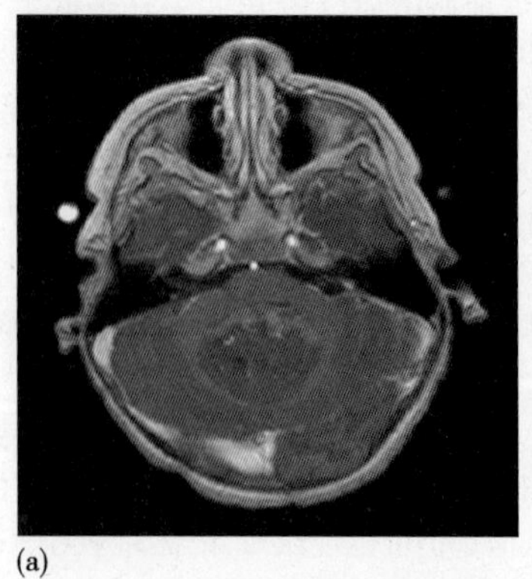
(a)

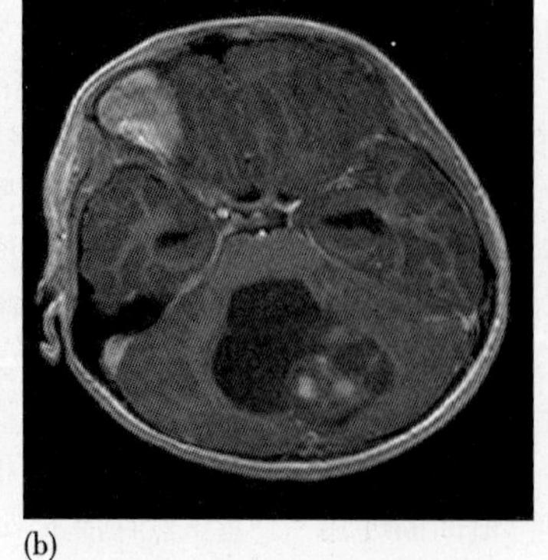
(b)

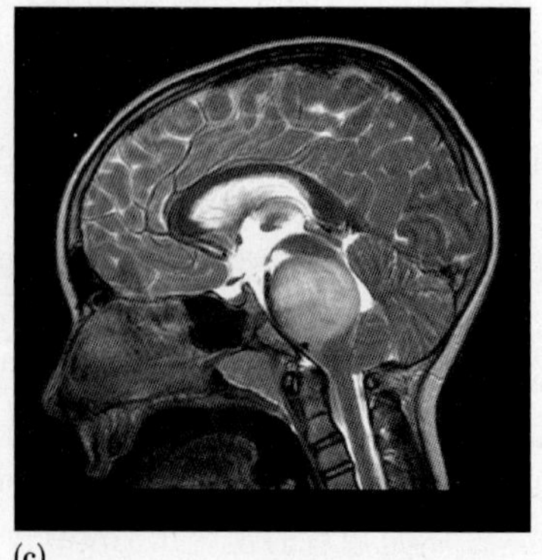
(c)

图 71-4 常见儿科脑肿瘤的 MRI 成像结果。(a)T1 像显示小脑中线肿瘤,病理确诊为成神经管细胞瘤。(b)T1 加权像显示一 5 岁儿童典型的小脑毛细胞星形细胞瘤,壁结节和肿瘤内囊肿异质性强,双侧扩张的颞角提示脑积水。(c)T2 加权像显示弥漫扩大的脑胶质瘤,使得患儿脑桥明显扩大

颅内生殖细胞肿瘤(IGCTs)在儿童中枢神经系统肿瘤中所占比例不到 5%,但主要见于儿童和青少年,其中 90% 发生在 20 岁以内,发病高峰在 10~12 岁,占儿童松果体肿瘤的 50%。生殖细胞瘤约占 IGCTs 的三分之二,其余三分之一为非恶性生殖细胞瘤(GCTs),包括卵黄囊瘤、绒毛膜癌、混合非恶性生殖细胞瘤、成熟和未成熟畸胎瘤。血清和脑脊液肿瘤标记物(如 AFP 和 β-HCG)及影像学检查可作为替代性诊断依据,但当肿瘤标记结果模棱两可的时候,需要行肿瘤活检以明确诊断。生殖细胞瘤对放疗高度敏感,放疗后 5 年的总生存率超过 90%。COG 目前正开展反应性放疗后加化疗的疗效研究,以最大限度地减少辐射剂量和长期副作用。

罕见肿瘤

从个体角度来讲,视网膜母细胞瘤(RB)、生殖细胞瘤(GCT)、肝脏肿瘤及癌在儿童中罕见,但是从整体来讲,上述肿瘤在儿童和青少年肿瘤中占 18%。此外,某些肿瘤(如生殖细胞恶性肿瘤和某些癌)在 15~19 岁的年长儿中发病率更高,但此类人群在全国前瞻性合作性临床试验中所占比例较少。

视网膜母细胞瘤

视网膜母细胞瘤是儿童期最常见的眼部肿瘤,占所有儿童肿瘤的 3%。据估计,每年有 200~300 名儿童新发视网膜母细胞瘤,多数患者(约 2/3)在 2 岁以内婴儿期发病,95%在 5 岁以内发病。肿瘤起源于视网膜,常生长至玻璃体腔内[109]。常见症状包括白瞳症和斜视。RB 有两种不同的临床表现形式:①遗传性双侧或多灶性病变(约占所有 RB 患者的 25%):特征是存在 *RB1* 基因胚系突变,该突变可遗传自某一发病亲本(约占 25%),也可为新的胚系突变(约占 75%);②单侧病变(约占所有 RB 的 75%):大约 90%的单侧病变患儿为非遗传性。双侧病变患儿发病年龄(<1 岁)早于单侧非遗传性病变患儿(2~3 岁)。

基于该病的临床表现形式,Knudsen 在 1971 年提出了经典的"二次打击"假说,在假说中,视网膜细胞存在两个突变事件并可进行转化[110]。进一步研究表明,这两次突变需要发生在同一个抑癌基因的双等位基因上。1986 年,位于染色体 13q14 的 *RB1* 基因被发现和克隆[111]。*RB1* 的编码产物(pRb)是一种 110kd 的细胞核磷酸化蛋白分子,该蛋白通过影响细胞周期中某些基因的转录来发挥作用。在整个细胞周期中,pRb 磷酸化的水平不断变化,失活时可消除 pRb 对细胞周期的限制作用,导致细胞增殖失调。

遗传性 RB 患者出生时即存在某一 *RB1* 胚系突变,另一 *RB1* 等位基因失活为体细胞突变,而单侧病变或非遗传性患者则为双等位基因体细胞失活性突变。

RB1 基因较大,为约 200kb,包括 27 个外显子,该基因的所有的外显子均可发生突变。无义突变和移码突变是最常见的胚系和体细胞突变(>80%),缺失突变也可见到(10%~20%)[112]。尽管 *RB1* 缺失是肿瘤发病机制中的关键步骤,但是其他突变事件也是肿瘤发展所需的。所有 RB 患者均需接受遗传咨询和基因检测。尽管目前没有突变热点基因,但是随着检测技术的提高,几乎所有致病倾向的胚系突变均可被检测出来。

疑诊 RB 的患者需由经验丰富的眼科医师接诊后,通过麻醉后扩瞳进行诊断,眼部 MRI、CT 和超声等影像学检查有助于将 RB 和其他引起白瞳症的疾病相鉴别(如:晶状体后纤维发育不良(晶状体后纤维组织增生)、Coats 病、弓蛔虫和弓形虫病),并且可用于评估眼外病变累及范围。由于遗传型 RB 患者可出现放疗相关性继发肿瘤,故应谨慎使用眼 CT。目前许多分期系统用于预测预后、指导治疗[113]。

治疗目标是根除肿瘤,保持视力,避免长期并发症(尤其是继发第二种肿瘤)。通常来讲,单侧肿瘤患者瘤体较大,很难保全视力。对于超过 90%的单侧病变患者,摘除术是有效的。同时需要由经验丰富的眼科病理学家对切除的标本进行仔细地病理学检查,以确定是否存在任何转移性特征:玻璃体播散、脉络膜大部受累、肿瘤超过筛板或侵及巩膜/巩膜外。这些特征提示需要开始化疗,通常为多种有效药物联合应用,包括长春新碱、多柔比星、环磷酰胺、卡铂和依托泊苷。对于瘤体较小的肿瘤,往往能保全视力,可以考虑化疗和激光凝固法、冷冻治疗、热疗等局部治疗方法[114]。直接通过眼动脉给药进行化疗的方法使用得越来越多[115]。RB 对放疗特别敏感,但是考虑到放疗会继发第二肿瘤,放疗常作为补救性治疗。双侧病变的患者进行化疗(全身±眼周或眼筋膜囊内给药)可减少肿瘤负荷,之后再辅以局部控制治疗[116,117]。这可使眼球保留下来的几率更高,减少并推迟放疗。

遗传型 RB 患者继发第二肿瘤的风险明显更高,放疗后这一风险会进一步增加[118]。骨肉瘤(OS)和软组织肉瘤、鼻腔肿瘤和黑色素瘤是最常见的继发性肿瘤。许多肿瘤起源于头颈区与辐射相关性,但是大多数发生在放疗(化疗)区域外的肿瘤,可能与生殖细胞突变相关。

生殖细胞瘤

生殖细胞瘤(GCTs)约占儿童和青少年肿瘤的 3.5%,60%起源于性腺外部位。这一分布与原始生殖细胞在发育过程中的异常迁移和持续定位于卵巢或睾丸外的其他部位有关。生殖细胞肿瘤临床表现多样,取决于原发部位及良恶性的病理特征。单个肿瘤可表现出多种组织类型以及良、恶性成分。其年龄分布符合双峰模型,即第一个高峰出现在 3 岁之前,第 2 个高峰出现在青春期后期。一般来讲,女性的总体发病率更高,但是男性发生恶性 GCTs 的风险更高。隐睾症是继发睾丸 GCT 的危险因素,但是需要注意的是,这种高风险往往出现在对侧已降至阴囊的睾丸[119]。手术或激素治疗可降低但不能消除这种风险。Klinefelter 综合征(47,XXY)也是发生 GCT 的高危因素,所有患有纵隔 GCT 的男性患者均需进行筛查[120]。46 XY 性腺发育不全的患者(Swyer 综合征)同样易患 GCTs。

GCTs 的病理分类可以部分预测他们的组织病理学起源(胚细胞瘤或非胚细胞瘤)以及是否为恶性肿(成熟畸胎瘤,不成熟畸胎瘤和恶性生殖细胞瘤)[121]。畸胎瘤含有来源于多个胚层的组织(内胚层、中胚层和外胚层),并且具有不同程度的分化。畸胎瘤可分为 3 类:良性畸胎瘤、未成熟畸胎瘤和恶性畸胎瘤。良性畸胎瘤包含有分化良好的组织,如软骨、鳞状上皮细胞、平滑肌以及某些复杂结构,如牙齿、唾液腺等。成熟畸胎瘤可见于骶尾区和卵巢。未成熟畸胎瘤含有未成熟组织,往往是神经上皮,也可为未成熟间质瘤或肾脏胚芽。未成熟畸胎瘤多见于卵巢,很少发生在卵巢以外部位。根据成熟度将未成熟畸胎瘤分为四级。0~2级通常具有良性生物学行为。另一种良性GCT是仅发生于性腺发育不良的性腺母细胞瘤。

恶性畸胎瘤包括表71-6中总结的一系列肿瘤。症状与肿瘤的原发部位有关。经细胞遗传学和分子学研究证实,儿童GCTs由异质性成分构成的实体肿瘤。成人GCT中常见的染色体畸变是12号染色体短臂异常,即i(12p)。然而在儿童中,i(12p)几乎只见于青春期男性的性腺和性腺外(通常是纵隔)肿瘤患者[122]。染色体1q、2号、3号、7号、8号、12号和14号获得性突变已有报道,多发生在青春期前期的女性患者中,而在青春期前期男性肿瘤患者中已发现1q、7号和21号染色体获得性突变和1p染色体缺失[122]。最后,1p36染色体缺失是卵黄囊肿瘤(YST)幼儿出现性腺外肿瘤和睾丸肿瘤的常见突变[123]。最近研究发现,BLIMP1的重要调节因子LIN28在GCTs中过表达[124],后者对胚胎生殖细胞的发育至关重要。骶尾骨是儿童GCTs最常见的发病部位[125],大多数发生在出生后两年。其中有三分之二是成熟或未成熟的畸胎瘤,症状包括肉眼可见的肿块、尿潴留、便秘以及由于压迫引起的下肢无力。卵巢是第二常见的发病部位,腹痛是最常见的症状。卵巢扭转可引起急性疼痛。几乎70%的卵巢GCTs是良性畸胎瘤。无性细胞瘤和混合组织形态的恶性瘤占卵巢恶性GCTs的80%,其余多数是卵黄囊肿瘤。大约10%GCTs发生在睾丸,此类患者肿瘤生长缓慢,其中三分之二是卵黄囊肿瘤。纵隔GCTs占全部GCTs的4%,患者表现为喘息,咳嗽和气促。多见于男性,大多数病例发生于10岁以上的儿童。约3%的GCTs发生在中枢神经系统中。

表71-6 恶性生殖细胞肿瘤

肿瘤类型	发生率	临床特征	组织学类型	好发部位	肿瘤特异性分子表达
单潜能性					
生殖细胞瘤	12%	年长患儿多见	大细胞性伴有清除过的胞浆	卵巢,前纵隔,大脑,睾丸(年龄较大患儿)	阴性(部分病例可见轻度升高)
精原细胞瘤(睾丸)					
无性细胞瘤(卵巢)					
性腺外的生殖细胞瘤					
多潜能性					
胚胎癌	8%		与卵黄囊肿瘤相似,但细胞较大,主要上皮生长模式	睾丸	阴性或轻度升高
卵黄囊(真皮内窦瘤)	55%		假乳头状(Schiller-Duval小体),网状,多囊性和均质状	卵巢,睾丸(近骶尾部)	AFP升高,HCG正常
绒毛膜癌	1%(非妊娠)	多见于转移癌	细胞滋养层和合体滋养层	卵巢,睾丸,性腺外部位	HCG升高
恶性生殖细胞瘤(多组织学类型)	24%		由不成熟或成熟畸胎瘤组成,包含一种或多种恶性GCT类型	卵巢,睾丸,性腺外部位	AFP和/或HCG升高

横断面成像和肿瘤标志物可协助GCTs诊断,前者用于评估原发病灶的严重程度及可能的肿瘤播散(淋巴结、腔内种植、肺、肝及中枢神经系统)。GCTs存在许多分期系统,目前正在努力制定儿童、成人和妇科肿瘤医师共用的分期共识[126]。目前大多数肿瘤分期主要依赖于年龄和疾病严重程度,后者包括是否可手术切除,是否有淋巴结受累以及是否出现转移[126]。该病的治疗基于个体肿瘤生物学亚型和分期[127]。成熟畸胎瘤和未成熟畸胎瘤以只通过手术切除治疗。对未能完全切除的未成熟畸胎瘤患者使用化疗是有争议的。对于Ⅰ期可完全切除的睾丸和卵巢(无性细胞瘤)肿瘤可仅采用手术治疗并观察(包括肿瘤标志物水平减低),因为大多数患者(>80%)可以治愈,并且化疗对少数复发患者的救治率很高。一般而言,睾丸GCT患儿不需进行腹膜后淋巴结清扫术。需注意的是,Ⅰ期卵巢非生殖细胞瘤也可以通过手术治疗,然后观察病情。其复发率明显高于卵巢无性细胞瘤,但救治率也很高[128]。对于Ⅱ~Ⅳ期卵巢和睾丸肿瘤,建议进行手术和化疗。标准化疗药物包括顺铂、依托泊苷和博来霉素(PEB),根据肿瘤分期和对化疗药物的反应(包括二次探查术后的评估),治疗可进行4~6个疗程。此类肿瘤的治愈率大于90%。同样的,所有性腺外的生殖细胞瘤患者也能从手术和化疗(Ⅰ~Ⅱ期2个疗程,Ⅲ~Ⅳ期6个疗程)中受益,完全存活率为90%。发生纵隔转移的Ⅰ~Ⅱ期及Ⅱ~Ⅳ期的生存率分别为80%和70%[129]。

肝脏肿瘤

肝脏恶性肿瘤占所有儿童肿瘤的1%,其中肝母细胞瘤(HB)占所有肝脏肿瘤的43%,其次是肝细胞癌(HCC)。HB多发生于年幼儿,4 岁以后很少发生。HB 的发病率上升可能与早产和低出生体重有关[130]。HB 与某些综合征有关,包括家族性腺瘤性息肉病和 Beckwith-Wiedemann 综合征等。父母或儿科医生常发现患儿出现无症状腹部肿块。HB 是一种胚系来源肿瘤,组织学上囊括了肝脏发育的不同阶段,有 4 种公认的亚型:上皮细胞来源(胚胎和胎儿型,67%)、间叶细胞来源(上皮和间质,21%)、单纯高分化胎儿型(7%)和小细胞未分化型(5%)[131]。胎儿组织型可能预后良好。HB 中最常见的体细胞突变是 *CTNNB1*(β-连环蛋白)的外显子 3 的缺失或突变,从而导致 Wnt 通路激活[132,133]。

由于手术技术的提高和以铂类为基础的化疗方案的引入,HB 患儿的预后有所改善。目前,5 年总体生存率约为 70%。疾病预处理程度(PRETEXT)目前已用于 HB 的分层治疗,因此必须对肝脏原发病变进行详细评估以确定是否可行手术切除[134]。由于 20%~30% 的患者可能出现肺转移,因此肺横断面影像学检查也是分期依据之一。甲胎蛋白是一种非常敏感的诊断性标记物,对评估疗效至关重要。PRETEXT 基于 4 个主要肝区的受累程度以及肝静脉、门静脉和肝外组织是否受累以及是否出现肿瘤转移。边缘清晰的手术切除是治疗的主要目标。虽然 PRETEXT Ⅰ和Ⅱ期的肿瘤适合前期切除,但许多中心倾向于对所有 PRETEXT 阶段的患者使用新辅助治疗。肿瘤通常对化疗敏感(通常为顺铂、5-氟尿嘧啶和长春新碱±多柔比星)。目前正在对高危患儿使用剂量密度疗法和包括对伊立替康和西罗莫司在内的新药联合用药进行评估[127]。PRETEXT Ⅳ期或静脉和/或门静脉受累的患者化疗后建议进行肝移植,但在进行器官移植之前,通过化疗和/或手术,所有转移病灶均需要完全缓解。

肝细胞癌(HCC)常见于年长儿和成人。虽然成人 HCC 与先存肝病(乙型肝炎和丙型肝炎、炎症性肝病、肝硬化(酪氨酸血症所致肝硬化、胆汁性肝硬化))有关,但在西方国家确诊患者中不到三分之一的患者有肝病史[135]。与 HB 患者相比,HCC 患者通常有一些综合征,如体重减轻,厌食和呕吐。在显微镜下,HCC 与 HB 的不同之处在于前者肿瘤细胞较大,具有明确的边界,核仁明显,并且肿瘤的血管侵袭度高。过渡型肝脏肿瘤同时存在 HB 和 HCC 的两种病理学和遗传特征。HCCs 的整体突变负荷较 HB 高,但 CTNNB1 突变少得多并且具有多拷贝数变异[136]。*TP53* 和表观遗传修饰因子突变频繁发生。HCC 的预后并不理想,在过去 20 年内其预后没有任何提高,这与其他儿童肿瘤的治疗进展形成了鲜明对比[137]。完整的手术切除是最重要的预后影响因素,但多数患者仍会进展至晚期。对于早期肿瘤,建议完全切除,然后进行辅助化疗,对于更晚期的患者,建议进行新辅助化疗(以期提高切除率)(例如 PRETEXT Ⅲ期)。出现肿瘤转移的患者预后不佳。

癌和黑色素瘤

癌和黑色素瘤占所有儿童肿瘤的 9%左右。在 SEER 数据库中,这些恶性肿瘤的比例如下:甲状腺癌 35%,黑色素瘤 31%,肾上腺皮质癌 1.3%,鼻咽癌 4.5%,其他皮肤癌 0.5%。大多数癌症(75%)发生在 15~19 岁。在 15~19 岁的患者中,甲状腺癌和黑色素瘤占该年龄组中恶性肿瘤的 14%以上。

约 90%的甲状腺癌为乳头状癌,成人中可见的 *BRAFV600E* 突变在儿童中很少见[138]。这些肿瘤通过手术切除和放射性碘消融治疗,10 年生存率超过 90%[139]。患者需要终身甲状腺激素替代治疗。甲状腺髓样癌通常是家族性(多发性内分泌肿瘤Ⅱ)并且具有侵袭性[140]。患者可以选用 RET 激酶抑制剂。大多数黑色素瘤患者(90%)在初始评估时有局部病变,最常见的部位是躯干,尽管 20 岁以下患者比成人更容易出现原发于头颈部的疾病[141]。与成人相似,大多数儿童黑色素瘤存在 $BRAF^{V600E}$ 突变。年龄小于 20 岁组与大于 20 岁的患者的生存率相近,且预后似乎与分期有关[142]。1973 年至 2006 年,在 15~19 岁年龄组中,皮肤黑色素瘤的发病率以每年 2%的速度增长,但最近的报告显示儿童发病率呈减少趋势[1]。

晚期后遗症和生存质量

通过多模式和基于风险的肿瘤治疗,美国每年 12 500 多名儿童和青少年(0~19 岁)肿瘤患者的 5 年总体生存率接近 80%(SEER)。生存率的提高导致 20 岁以下人群每 810 人中约有 1 人为肿瘤存活者,20~39 岁人群每 640 人中有 1 人为肿瘤存活者。

肿瘤治疗的后遗症可能导致慢性医学问题,涉及全身器官及系统。儿童期肿瘤存活者的总体死亡率为一般人群的 10 倍。儿童癌症幸存者研究(CCSS)在一项回顾性队列研究中评估了 20 227 名五年存活者的总体死亡率和特殊病因死亡率,并显示总死亡率超过 10.8 倍[143]。女性、在 5 岁前确诊肿瘤疾病、初步诊断为白血病或脑肿瘤的个体死亡风险在统计学上显著升高。高死亡率是由原发肿瘤、继发第二肿瘤、心脏毒性和非肿瘤性死亡所致,并且可持续至初诊后 25 年。

较为常见的第二原发肿瘤包括乳腺、骨和甲状腺肿瘤、治疗相关的骨髓增生异常和急性髓系白血病。胸部或斗篷式放疗儿童恶性肿瘤的女性存活者患乳腺癌的风险显著增加。

首次提出遗传易感性对遗传型 RB 患者继发肉瘤的风险有显著的影响。放疗可进一步增加这种风险,并且随着总辐射剂量的增加而增加。具有早发型肿瘤家族史的患者继发第二肿瘤的风险也增加。据报道,患有 Li-Fraumeni 综合征的家族成员继发多种肿瘤的风险增加,其中儿童期肿瘤存活者的发病风险最高[144]。此类人群已报道的肿瘤以 Li-Fraumeni 综合征为特征。因此,抑癌基因的胚系突变(如在 Li-Fraumeni 综合征中发生)可能与治疗相关暴露相互作用,导致继发第二肿瘤的风险增加。

已经检测了几种酶的遗传多态性,如 NADPH、醌氧化还原酶(NQO1)、谷胱甘肽 S-转移酶(GST)-M1 和-T1,以及 CYP3A4,这些酶能够代谢性激活或消除抗癌药物毒性,在与治疗相关的白血病或骨髓异常增生症的发展中发挥了作用。这些研究表明,NQO1 多态性与治疗相关的急性白血病和骨髓增生异常的遗传风险具有显著相关性。此外,具有 *CYP3A4-W* 基因型的个体出现治疗相关白血病的风险更高,可能与损害 DNA 的活性中间体产生增多有关[145,146]。

由于继发的恶性肿瘤仍然是儿童期肿瘤存活者健康的重大威胁,因此对高危人群进行有效筛查非常重要。继发急性髓系白血病的风险与拓扑异构酶Ⅱ抑制剂(即表鬼臼毒素和蒽环霉素)接触有关(长达 10 年)并且与烷化剂的接触(长达 15

年)有关。此外,对于接受放疗的霍奇金病存活者,患乳腺癌(女性)和其他实体瘤的风险显著增高。

儿童肿瘤治疗的神经认知后遗症是由于全脑放疗、高剂量甲氨蝶呤或阿糖胞苷全身化疗、或鞘内注射甲氨蝶呤和其他药物引起的。有脑肿瘤、ALL 或 NHL 病史的儿童最有可能受到影响。危险因素包括增加辐射剂量、发病年龄小、颅脑放疗和全身或鞘内化疗联合治疗及女性患者[147-149]。严重神经系统功能缺陷最常见于脑肿瘤放疗以及发病小于 5 岁的儿童。

慢性心脏毒性通常表现为心肌病、心包炎和充血性心力衰竭。与普通美国人群相比,接受胸部或脊髓放疗的 CCSS 儿童癌症存活者心脏疾病相关的死亡风险增加了两倍[150]。蒽环类药物、多柔比星和正定霉素是引发心肌病的常见病因[151,152]。心肌病的发病率呈剂量依赖性,蒽环类药物累积剂量超过 300mg/m^2 的患者发病率可能超过 30%。与低于 300mg/m^2 相比,蒽环类药物累积剂量大于 300mg/m^2 时临床出现心力衰竭的风险增加(相对危险度 11.8)。临床心力衰竭的预计风险随着时间的推移而增加,并在 15 年后接近 5%。这些研究和其他研究指出,心肌病可发生在治疗结束 15~20 年,并且发病可能是自发性的,也伴发劳累或妊娠。

肺纤维化和肺炎可由肺部放疗引起。因此,这些问题最常见于患有胸部恶性肿瘤的患者,特别是霍奇金病。除放疗外,越来越多的化疗药物也可导致长期存活者出现肺部疾病。博来霉素毒性是引起化疗相关肺损伤的经典药物。虽然间质性肺炎和肺纤维化在儿童中已有报道,但临床上典型的博来霉素相关肺病在老年患者中最常见。慢性肺毒性通常在治疗后 3 个月内持续存在或进展。烷基化剂也可引起慢性肺损伤。进行 HSCT 后,患者会出现包括闭塞性细支气管炎在内的限制性和阻塞性肺部疾病[153]。

肝脏的慢性纤维化与辐射有关。即使在没有放疗的情况下,化疗也可能是慢性肝病的原因之一。在 1992 年之前,病毒性肝炎最常见于血制品输注,现在认为病毒性肝炎是长期存活者发生慢性肝病的另一个原因[154]。

化疗引起的近端肾小管损伤可引起范可尼肾综合征(低钾血症、低磷血症、糖尿、蛋白尿、肾小管酸中毒和佝偻病)。高危因素包括接受一种以上肾毒性药物治疗、并发手术或放疗相关肾损伤[155]。与异环磷酰胺治疗相关的电解质消耗和与顺铂治疗相关的低镁血症似乎在某些儿童中持续存在。环磷酰胺和异环磷酰胺均可因代谢产物丙烯醛在膀胱内积聚而引起出血性膀胱炎。对骨盆或膀胱的放疗可导致膀胱纤维化,形成瘢痕,导致膀胱容量降低且易出现尿路感染。一些在儿童期肿瘤治疗期间接受膀胱毒性药物治疗的患者可发生膀胱癌。对这些患者,每年应进行尿液分析,评估是否存在镜下血尿。

身高增长减慢是癌症患儿治疗期间的常见问题。尽管可能发生追赶性生长并恢复至患病前生长状态,但在某些情况下,身材矮小是永久性的甚至是进展性的。严重的生长迟缓被定义为站立高度低于第五百分位,已发现多达 30%~35%的儿童脑肿瘤存活者[156]和 10%~15%的接受了某些抗白血病治疗的患者存在这一问题[157]。全脑放疗是身材矮小的主要危险因素,特别是在剂量超过 18Gy 时。

观察研究表明,在接受常规治疗或 BMT 治疗的 ALL 和脑肿瘤患儿会出现通过体重或体重指数(BMI)测定的肥胖症[158]。这一问题多在治疗期间或在停止治疗后的第一年内出现,可呈进行性进展也可维持在稳定状态。此外,甲状腺功能减退症是一种常见晚期后遗症,通常是由于非甲状腺恶性肿瘤接受颈部放疗所致,这也会导致肥胖。

所有治疗方式(放疗、手术或化疗)都会导致男性肿瘤存活者的生殖细胞耗竭以及性腺内分泌功能异常[159]。目前已知,睾丸放疗会导致生发组织功能丧失,睾丸体积和精子产生减少,卵泡刺激素水平(FSH)升高。该影响为剂量依赖性,通常发生在 0.1~6Gy 的分次暴露之后。尽管阴囊有铅屏蔽,但是所有使用倒 Y 辐射治疗 HD 的男性患者,接受 1.4~3.0Gy 累积剂量后会出现无精症,并且随访 2~40 个月后仍无法恢复。剂量 4~6Gy 时,无精症可持续至少 3~5 年,而剂量高于 6Gy 时,无精症似乎是不可逆转的。对于肿瘤长期存活者,烷化剂可减少的精子发生,其作用具有剂量依赖性。在 HSCT 中使用的氮芥累积剂量低于 7.5mg/m^2 或环磷酰胺累积剂量小于 200mg/kg,对 70%的患者来讲,其造成的性腺损伤在数年停药间隔后是可逆的。

性腺毒性是患者及其家庭密切关注的问题。这种担忧推广了治疗前精子建库的实行。与男性不同,生殖细胞衰竭和卵巢内分泌功能丧失在女性中常同时发生。在放疗中,表现为年龄依赖性和剂量依赖性。青春期前卵巢是相对抗放射性的,因为原始卵泡数量较多。卵巢衰竭也与化疗有关,如单一烷化剂(环磷酰胺、白消安和氮芥)或联合化疗。CCSS 报道了 1915 年 4 029 例女性儿童期肿瘤 5 年存活者妊娠时未发现化疗药物过量相关不良预后[160]。对 1 427 名男性存活者的 2 323 名伴侣妊娠相关研究报道,69%为活产婴儿,死产率 1%,自然流产率 13%,人工流产率 13%(5%的结果未计入)[161]。女性以活产婴儿结束妊娠的比率显著少于男性同胞伴侣对照组($RR=0.8$,$P=0.007$)。

在治疗结束后生育的患者可能需要在高危产科医院进行护理,特别是那些接受过腹部或盆腔放疗未储存精子的患者。由于儿童癌症存活者所生子女的问题仍然未知,因此应强调长期随访。

几种潜在的耳毒性药物通常用于治疗恶性肿瘤患儿,包括铂类化疗、氨基糖苷类抗生素、袢利尿剂和 RT。这些药物都能引起感觉神经性听力受损。在癌症治疗期间接受耳毒性药物治疗且言语尚未发育的幼儿应接受听力评估,确定是否需要干预。因肿瘤治疗而导致听力受损患儿的干预措施包括使用助听器和其他辅助设备,以及选择教室前面的优势座位。儿童期肿瘤后期的肌肉骨骼问题包括骨质异常,如脊柱侧凸、萎缩或发育不全、缺血性坏死(AVN)、骨质疏松症(骨密度低于平均值 2.5SD)/骨质缺乏(骨密度低于平均值 1~2.5SD),特别是在 ALL 治疗中使用激素。

为肿瘤存活者提供合适的医疗服务将成为医学上的主要挑战之一。儿童期肿瘤存活者是高危人群,需要寻求和接受多领域医疗专业人员的帮助,包括肿瘤学家、医学和儿科专家、外科医生、初级保健医生、妇科医生、护士、心理学家和社会工作者。这一挑战源于这一群体的异质性,他们在这个时代可以快速了解晚期后遗症,并以多种治疗方式进行治疗。COG 最近更新了基于风险的、暴露相关的指南,专门用于指导随访确诊儿童恶性肿瘤并接受治疗的患者。这些指南提出了一系列临床相关的全面筛查建议，可用于标准化治疗和监测，并且对于该组人群中有专业医疗护理需求的肿瘤存活者，可以指导后续护理。

（张利平 译，王天有 审校）

参考文献

The complete reference list can be found on the Wiley Companion Digital Edition of this title (see inside front cover for login instructions).

1 Siegel DA, King J, Tai E, Buchanan N, Ajani UA, Li J. Cancer incidence rates and trends among children and adolescents in the United States, 2001–2009. *Pediatrics*. 2014;**134(4)**:e945–e955.

2 Vogelstein B, Papadopoulos N, Velculescu VE, Zhou S, Diaz LA Jr, Kinzler KW. Cancer genome landscapes. *Science*. 2013;**339(6127)**:1546–1558.

4 Smith MA, Altekruse SF, Adamson PC, Reaman GH, Seibel NL. Declining childhood and adolescent cancer mortality. *Cancer*. 2014;**120(16)**:2497–2506.

6 Hunger SP, Lu X, Devidas M, et al. Improved survival for children and adolescents with acute lymphoblastic leukemia between 1990 and 2005: a report from the children's oncology group. *J Clin Oncol*. 2012;**30(14)**:1663–1669.

10 Schultz KR, Pullen DJ, Sather HN, et al. Risk- and response-based classification of childhood B-precursor acute lymphoblastic leukemia: a combined analysis of prognostic markers from the pediatric oncology group (POG) and children's cancer group (CCG). *Blood*. 2007;**109(3)**:926–935.

12 Borowitz MJ, Devidas M, Hunger SP, et al. Clinical significance of minimal residual disease in childhood acute lymphoblastic leukemia and its relationship to other prognostic factors: a children's oncology group study. *Blood*. 2008;**111(12)**:5477–5485.

16 Pui C-H, Campana D, Pei D, et al. Treating childhood acute lymphoblastic leukemia without cranial irradiation. *N Engl J Med*. 2009;**360(26)**:2730–2741.

19 Schultz KR, Carroll A, Heerema NA, et al. Long-term follow-up of imatinib in pediatric Philadelphia chromosome-positive acute lymphoblastic leukemia: children's oncology group study AALL0031. *Leukemia*. 2014;**28(7)**:1467–1471.

31 Gamis AS, Alonzo TA, Perentesis JP, Meshinchi S. Children's oncology group's 2013 blueprint for research: acute myeloid leukemia. *Pediatr Blood Cancer*. 2013;**60(6)**:964–971.

35 Cairo MS, Gerrard M, Sposto R, et al. Results of a randomized international study of high-risk central nervous system B non-Hodgkin lymphoma and B acute lymphoblastic leukemia in children and adolescents. *Blood*. 2007;**109(7)**:2736–2743.

38 Goldman S, Smith L, Galardy P, et al. Rituximab with chemotherapy in children and adolescents with central nervous system and/or bone marrow-positive Burkitt lymphoma/leukaemia: a children's oncology group Report. *Br J Haematol*. 2014;**167(3)**:394–401.

39 Mosse YP, Lim MS, Voss SD, et al. Safety and activity of crizotinib for paediatric patients with refractory solid tumours or anaplastic large-cell lymphoma: a children's oncology group phase 1 consortium study. *Lancet Oncol*. 2013;**14(6)**:472–480.

40 Gopal AK, Chen R, Smith SE, et al. Durable remissions in a pivotal phase 2 study of brentuximab vedotin in relapsed or refractory Hodgkin lymphoma. *Blood*. 2015;**125(8)**:1236–1243.

41 Friedman DL, Chen L, Wolden S, et al. Dose-intensive response-based chemotherapy and radiation therapy for children and adolescents with newly diagnosed intermediate-risk hodgkin lymphoma: a report from the Children's Oncology Group Study AHOD0031. *J Clin Oncol*. 2014;**32(32)**:3651–3658.

42 Dome JS, Fernandez CV, Mullen EA, et al. Children's oncology group's 2013 blueprint for research: renal tumors. *Pediatr Blood Cancer*. 2013;**60(6)**:994–1000.

49 Lemerle J, Voute PA, Tournade MF, et al. Effectiveness of preoperative chemotherapy in Wilms' tumor: results of an International Society of Paediatric Oncology (SIOP) clinical trial. *J Clin Oncol*. 1983;**1(10)**:604–609.

59 London WB, Castleberry RP, Matthay KK, et al. Evidence for an age cutoff greater than 365 days for neuroblastoma risk group stratification in the children's oncology group. *J Clin Oncol*. 2005;**23(27)**:6459–6465.

64 Maris JM. Recent advances in neuroblastoma. *N Engl J Med*. 2010;**362(23)**:2202–2211.

70 Cohn SL, Pearson AD, London WB, et al. The International Neuroblastoma Risk Group (INRG) classification system: an INRG Task Force report. *J Clin Oncol*. 2009;**27(2)**:289–297.

71 Park JR, Bagatell R, London WB, et al. Children's oncology group's 2013 blueprint for research: neuroblastoma. *Pediatr Blood Cancer*. 2013;**60(6)**:985–993.

74 Yu AL, Gilman AL, Ozkaynak MF, et al. Anti-GD2 antibody with GM-CSF, interleukin-2, and isotretinoin for neuroblastoma. *N Engl J Med*. 2010;**363(14)**:1324–1334.

81 Link MP, Goorin AM, Miser AW, et al. The effect of adjuvant chemotherapy on relapse-free survival in patients with osteosarcoma of the extremity. *N Engl J Med*. 1986;**314(25)**:1600–1606.

85 Gorlick R, Janeway K, Lessnick S, Randall RL, Marina N, on behalf of the COG-BTC. Children's oncology group's 2013 blueprint for research: bone tumors. *Pediatr Blood Cancer*. 2013;**60(6)**:1009–1015.

89 Grier HE, Krailo MD, Tarbell NJ, et al. Addition of ifosfamide and etoposide to standard chemotherapy for Ewing's sarcoma and primitive neuroectodermal tumor of bone. *N Engl J Med*. 2003;**348(8)**:694–701.

90 Womer RB, West DC, Krailo MD, et al. Randomized controlled trial of interval-compressed chemotherapy for the treatment of localized Ewing sarcoma: a report from the children's oncology group. *J Clin Oncol*. 2012;**30(33)**:4148–4154.

93 Pappo AS, Shapiro DN, Crist WM, Maurer HM. Biology and therapy of pediatric rhabdomyosarcoma. *J Clin Oncol*. 1995;**13(8)**:2123–2139.

96 Hawkins DS, Spunt SL, Skapek SX. Children's oncology group's 2013 blueprint for research: soft tissue sarcomas. *Pediatr Blood Cancer*. 2013;**60(6)**:1001–1008.

97 Walterhouse DO, Pappo AS, Meza JL, et al. Shorter-duration therapy using vincristine, dactinomycin, and lower-dose cyclophosphamide with or without radiotherapy for patients with newly diagnosed low-risk rhabdomyosarcoma: a report from the Soft Tissue Sarcoma Committee of the Children's Oncology Group. *J Clin Oncol*. 2014;**32(31)**:3547–3552.

98 Hawkins DSAJ, Mascarenhas L. Vincristine, dactinomycin, cyclophosphamide (VAC) versus VAC/V plus irinotecan (VI) for intermediate-risk rhabdomyosarcoma (IRRMS): a report from the Children's Oncology Group Soft Tissue Sarcoma Committee. American Soceity of Clinical Oncology ASCO annual meeting abstract. *J Clin Oncol*. 2014;**32**:5s(suppl; abstr 10004).

100 Spunt SLML, Anderson JR. Risk-based treatment for nonrhabdomyosarcoma soft tissue sarcomas (NRSTS) in patients under 30 years of age: children's oncology group study ARST0332. American Soceity of Clinical Oncology ASCO annual meeting abstract. *J Clin Oncol*. 2014;**32**:5s(suppl; abstr 10008).

102 Rickert C, Paulus W. Epidemiology of central nervous system tumors in childhood and adolescence based on the new WHO classification. *Childs Nerv Syst*. 2001;**17(9)**:503–511.

104 Northcott PA, Korshunov A, Witt H, et al. Medulloblastoma comprises four distinct molecular variants. *J Clin Oncol*. 2011;**29(11)**:1408–1414.

109 Rodriguez-Galindo C, Orbach DB, VanderVeen D. Retinoblastoma. *Pediatr Clin North Am*. 2015;**62(1)**:201–223.

126 Frazier AL, Hale JP, Rodriguez-Galindo C, et al. Revised risk classification for pediatric extracranial germ cell tumors based on 25 years of clinical trial data from the United kingdom and United States. *J Clin Oncol*. 2015;**33(2)**:195–201.

127 Rodriguez-Galindo C, Krailo M, Frazier L, et al. Children's Oncology Group's 2013 blueprint for research: rare tumors. *Pediatr Blood Cancer*. 2013;**60(6)**:1016–1021.

128 Billmire DF, Cullen JW, Rescorla FJ, et al. Surveillance after initial surgery for pediatric and adolescent girls with stage I ovarian germ cell tumors: report from the children's oncology group. *J Clin Oncol*. 2014;**32(5)**:465–470.

134 Brown J, Perilongo G, Shafford E, et al. Pretreatment prognostic factors for children with hepatoblastoma—results from the International Society of Paediatric Oncology (SIOP) study SIOPEL 1. *Eur J Cancer*. 2000;**36(11)**:1418–1425.

147 Mulhern RK, Merchant TE, Gajjar A, Reddick WE, Kun LE. Late neurocognitive sequelae in survivors of brain tumours in childhood. *Lancet Oncol*. 2004;**5(7)**:399–408.

149 Krull KR, Brinkman TM, Li C, et al. Neurocognitive outcomes decades after treatment for childhood acute lymphoblastic leukemia: a report from the St Jude lifetime cohort study. *J Clin Oncol*. 2013;**31(35)**:4407–4415.

152 van der Pal HJ, van Dalen EC, van Delden E, et al. High risk of symptomatic cardiac events in childhood cancer survivors. *J Clin Oncol*. 2012;**30(13)**:1429–1437.

第 72 章　癌症与妊娠

Jennifer K. Litton, MD

概述

妊娠期癌症的诊断对患者和照护者来说都是一个医学上和情感上的挑战。一个包括肿瘤内科医师、外科医师、放射肿瘤医师和产科医师在内的多学科团队对于协调母亲的治疗和胎儿的监测至关重要。本文回顾了有关妊娠期癌症治疗的现有数据，详细介绍分期、手术、放疗和全身化疗，以及患者和受化疗影响胎儿的生存结局等方面。

妊娠期癌症的诊断对患者、家属和医生是一个复杂的挑战。由于对疾病、诊断和治疗的担忧，以及希望避免对胎儿造成伤害，妊娠期患者的福利可能受到影响。许多人认为癌症治疗需要综合考虑对患者和胎儿的影响。然而在某些特殊情况下，癌症治疗可能不可避免地导致胎儿死亡。但是明智的决策往往不仅可以为孕妇提供适当的癌症治疗，而且还可以通过成功的助产来保护胎儿。

妊娠合并恶性肿瘤带来了很多问题（表 72-1）。目前关于特定肿瘤类型、诊断程序、治疗手段和长期预后等方面的数据主要来源于病例报告、小的病例系列报告和回顾性研究。这方面的对照研究很少，前瞻性研究数据更少。而关注完成妊娠的患者分娩结局，以及胎儿期暴露于癌症治疗的儿童长期生长和发育的数据仍然很少。在过去的十年中，妊娠期癌症的治疗已经有了长足的进展。基于已发表的队列研究和前瞻性病例系列研究，妊娠期多种癌症的治疗已经有章可循[1]。与此同时，虽然目前关于患者结局以及暴露于化疗的胎儿的结局的数据仍然很少，但关注这一方面的研究层出不穷。

表 72-1　与妊娠及癌症相关的问题

问题
癌症对妊娠的影响
妊娠对癌症的影响
癌症治疗导致妊娠终止或胎儿死亡
妊娠期癌症诊断手段及分期
癌症治疗对母亲的影响
癌症治疗对胎儿的影响
胎盘部位转移
跨胎盘转移
对儿童的长期影响
伦理、道德、法律问题
其他未知问题

妊娠期癌症的流行病学

妊娠期间诊断的癌症较为罕见，探究真正的发病率仍然很困难。目前包括妊娠相关乳腺癌在内的大部分数据表明，妊娠期癌症应定义为怀孕期间和分娩后 1 年内诊断的癌症。最新研究表明，肿瘤的生物学行为和患者的结局可能受到诊断时间的影响，因此评估妊娠期每一种癌症的发病率可能尤为重要。Smith 等人[2]使用加利福尼亚癌症登记系统中 4 846 505 名女性的数据，发现其中 4 539 人在妊娠期或分娩后 12 个月内确诊为恶性肿瘤。在这项分析中，从 1991 年到 1999 年，每 1 000 次分娩中就有 1 位女性诊断了妊娠相关性癌症。然而，64%的病例发生在分娩后的 12 个月内。每 1 000 例活胎中，妊娠期女性诊断的最常见的肿瘤类型为乳腺癌（0.19）、甲状腺癌（0.14）、宫颈癌（0.12）、黑色素瘤（0.09）、霍奇金淋巴瘤（0.05）、卵巢癌（0.05）和急性白血病（0.04）。此外，澳大利亚一项 1994 年和 2008 年之间的研究表明[3]，在 1 309 501 例分娩中发现了 1 798 例妊娠相关癌症。同样地，这些癌症的诊断时间包括分娩期间和分娩后 1 年内。其中 495 例癌症是在妊娠期间诊断的。在孕期，该队列中发现的最常见癌症为黑色素瘤（15.1/100 000）、乳腺癌（7.3/100 000）、甲状腺（3.2/100 000）和妇科肿瘤（3.9/100 000）。然而，几乎任何部位的癌症都可以在妊娠期发生。

有趣的是，无论是这项澳大利亚的研究还是其他国家的研究均表明与妊娠相关的乳腺癌发病率一直在上升。这可能继发于产妇年龄的增加以及其他流行病学危险因素。在澳大利亚队列中，从 1994 年到 2007 年，妊娠相关乳腺癌的发病率从 112.3/100 000 增加到 191.5/100 000。瑞典癌症登记系统的数据也表明，这一趋势可以部分归因于产妇年龄的增加。该队列的数据显示，从 1963 年到 2002 年，妊娠相关乳腺癌的发病率已从 16.0/100 000 增长至 37.4/100 000[4]。由于辅助生殖技术的发展，高龄孕妇比例不断升高，妊娠相关乳腺癌的发病率可能也随之升高。

诊断和分期

妊娠期间任何恶性肿瘤的诊断都需要活检，以进行细胞学和组织学评估。活检的类型取决于病变部位的可及性和诊断所需组织的体积。

如果需要手术取病理，术前应充分评估活检部位及胎儿的胎龄。既往的研究表明，手术活检可以安全进行[1,5,6]。获取足够体积的组织进行病理诊断是必要的，如乳腺癌的准确评估需要考虑激素受体及 HER-2/neu 的表达，淋巴瘤和白血病组织细胞的形态学检查和免疫组织化学染色对准确的评估与治疗尤为重要。

分期为讨论癌症的预后、推荐局部治疗或全身治疗、治疗的潜在风险及患者获益提供了指导。通常情况下，对未怀孕患者癌症的分期评估需要进行有电离辐射的检查，但在怀孕期间应尽可能避免电离辐射。电离辐射对胎儿的影响与胎龄有关。胚胎着床前和及胎儿器官形成期对电离辐射的负面影响最为敏感[7]。小于 5cGy 的暴露对胎儿来说是无害的[8]。而腹部 CT 的辐射可高达 30mSv。由于我们已知妊娠期间暴露于电离辐射会对胎儿造成巨大影响，因此在进行检查时应尽可能使用腹部防护或采用无电离辐射的检查[8]。超声对乳房、肝脏和其他腹部器官的成像不需要电离辐射。必要时，磁共振成像可用于评估骨骼和肝脏疾病，以及胎儿异常[9,10]。在妊娠期使用钆作为磁共振成像的造影剂仍有争议。虽然多个病例报告没有显示钆会对胎儿产生不良影响，但由于缺乏毒性信息，往往尽可能避免使用钆[11-13]。准确评估癌症分期对于癌症治疗至关重要，分期的结果也可能影响妇女对是否继续维持妊娠的决定。

PET/CT 的应用已成为淋巴瘤治疗和评估的标准程序，在转移性实体瘤评估中的应用也有所增加。关于 PET/CT 在妊娠期乳腺癌患者中的应用的数据非常有限。动物实验已经证实了 FDG 能通过胎盘并可在胎儿大脑、膀胱和心脏组织中沉积[14]。Zanotti-Fregonara 等[15]推测，早孕期行 PET/CT 检查胚胎组织摄取的 FDG 至少为 3.3×10^{-2}（文献中实际为 3×10^{-2}）mGy/MBq。此外还有少量病例报告。如 Hove 等人[16]报告了一位 18 岁的妊娠期霍奇金淋巴瘤患者，她接受了 PET/CT 检查。胎儿心肌有明显的摄取。患者出现 HELLP 综合征，胎儿在 31 周时经剖宫产娩出。因此，目前尚没有足够的安全数据支持在妊娠期间可使用 PET/CT 扫描，应该尽可能推迟到分娩后。

妊娠期癌症的治疗

妊娠期间癌症的最佳治疗决策的制定需要一个配合默契的多学科团队。在妊娠过程中，必须详细且多次咨询产科医生及母婴医学专家。在制定治疗计划之前，必须对胎儿的胎龄、成熟度和预产期进行准确的评估。妊娠患者的治疗选择与非妊娠癌症患者没有区别，但治疗手段的应用可能更复杂。Stensheim 等人[17]调查了瑞典健康登记中心的数据，发现妊娠期和哺乳期诊断的癌症总体死亡率大致相同。然而有趣的是，哺乳期诊断的乳腺癌和卵巢癌死亡率高于妊娠期。大的队列研究的结果表明，不同肿瘤类型、诊断时间、治疗手段都对患者的结局产生重要影响。

手术

手术仍然是治疗实体瘤的主要手段，妊娠并不是癌症手术的禁忌。Mazze 和 Kallen[6]报道了一项纳入 5 405 名进行了急诊手术的妊娠患者的研究。他们没有观察到胎儿先天畸形或死产的发生率的增加。但低出生体重儿和极低出生体重儿的数量有所增加。他们把这一现象归因于早产和胎儿宫内生长迟缓，并认为可能受到导致手术的潜在原因的影响。手术类型或麻醉方式与妊娠结局无关。在一项病例对照研究中，相比于妊娠期未接收手术的对照组患者，Duncan 等人[18]发现在 2 565 名在妊娠期间接受手术的孕妇中，胎儿先天性畸形的发生率并不增加。如果需要根据肿瘤类型和肿瘤分期进行手术，应与产科医生、麻醉师和新生儿医师充分协调。

放射治疗

妊娠是癌症放疗的绝对禁忌。妊娠期宫颈癌放疗常导致胎儿死亡和自然流产[19]。妊娠 2~8 周的胎儿暴露于辐射环境中最容易产生畸形，而妊娠 8~25 周的胎儿暴露于辐射环境中可能有较大的智力发育迟缓风险[7]。然而，也有成功的放疗治疗妊娠女性霍奇金淋巴瘤的报道[20]。如果确实有必要进行放疗，需进行适当的胎儿防护、严格的剂量计算并预估胎儿暴露剂量。但是，由于安全性非常有限，只能在特定的情况下才考虑放疗[21-25]。乳腺癌的术前放射治疗，不管接下来是进行乳房全切术或保乳手术，通常都可以推迟到产后，尤其是在已经进行了化疗的情况下。

全身化疗

已有多种不同的制剂被报道可用于妊娠期。表 72-2 列出了具有代表性的化疗药物、激素和生物制剂。

表 72-2　妊娠期间被报道过使用的药物

化疗方案	全身化疗药物	
MACOP-B	羟基脲	α-干扰素
MOPP-ABVD	全反式维 A 酸	利妥昔单抗
FAC	甲氨蝶呤	曲妥珠单抗
CMF	多柔比星/表柔比星	拉帕替尼
AC	环磷酰胺及氮芥	伊马替尼
VACOP-B	长春新碱及癌宁	泼尼松
CHOP	博来霉素	他莫西芬
BEP	顺铂	促红细胞生成素
	长春瑞滨、长春碱及长春新碱	非格司亭
	紫杉醇	达沙替尼
	多西他赛	
	依托泊苷	
	伊达比星及柔红霉素	
	胞嘧啶-阿糖胞苷	
	5-氟尿嘧啶	
	白消安	
	替尼泊苷	
	6-巯基嘌呤	
	达卡巴嗪	
	氨蝶呤	
	放线菌素 D	
	丙卡巴肼	
	安丫啶	
	门冬酰胺酶	

ABVD：多柔比星（阿霉素）、博来霉素、长春地辛、氮烯唑胺；AC：多柔比星（阿霉素）、环磷酰胺；CMF：环磷酰胺、甲氨蝶呤、5-氟尿嘧啶；FAC：5-氟尿嘧啶、多柔比星（阿霉素）、环磷酰胺；MACOP-B：甲氨蝶呤、多柔比星（阿霉素）、环磷酰胺、长春新碱、泼尼松、博来霉素；MOPP：氮芥、长春新碱、丙卡巴肼、泼尼松；VACOP-B：依托泊苷、多柔比星（阿霉素）、环磷酰胺、长春新碱、泼尼松、博来霉素

由于全身化疗可能对胎儿产生不良影响，需引起重视。妊娠相关的生理变化（如血容量增加、心输出量增加、肾小球滤过率增大、循环蛋白水平变化）使得我们很难准确预测药物的药代动力学[26]。此外，全身性药物大多有抑制细胞增殖的作用，在妊娠期使用它们会对发育中的胎儿造成较大的风险。潜在的风险包括死产、自然流产、胎儿畸形、器官特异性毒性、低出生体重、宫内生长迟缓和早产[27]。

除了细胞毒药物治疗，也有很多报道关注支持治疗。Scott等人[28]和其他研究人员均报告了妊娠期促红细胞生成素的使用。他们没有发现孕产妇毒性或胎儿毒性。FDA黑框警示提示促红细胞生成素在乳腺癌女性中的使用也适用于孕妇，即使目前对妊娠期女性的用药尚无具体的风险数据。Dale等人[29]发现，在妊娠期间是否使用非格斯亭不影响新生儿结局。目前有少量关于在妊娠期乳腺癌大剂量化疗后安全使用培非格司亭的案例报道[30]。地塞米松和劳拉西泮也被报道为无明显毒性的术前用药[9]。

受化疗影响胎儿的结局

在早孕期，化疗可能对胎儿产生更大的影响。Doll等人[27]回顾了抗肿瘤药物及胎儿畸形与不同孕期的关系。他们发现14%暴露于烷基化剂和19%暴露于抗代谢药物的胎儿有畸形风险。另一项研究得出相似的结论：在中孕期和晚孕期使用这些药物，仅有1.3%的胎儿畸形发生率。因此，他们认为单药或多药联合化疗在中晚孕期使用致畸风险低，但应避免在早孕期化疗。在另一项相似的研究中，Ebert等人[26]从1983年到1995年发表的多篇文献中选取了其中217个患者。他们根据不同的疾病来对药物使用进行分组，并分析了药物种类、剂量、使用时的孕周数等因素对妊娠结局的影响。这些患者中，有94例白血病患者，57例淋巴瘤患者，26例乳腺癌或卵巢癌患者，16例因风湿免疫病接受细胞毒性药物治疗的患者以及其他恶性肿瘤患者。18位患者分娩的新生儿有先天性发育畸形，其中的15人在早孕期使用细胞毒性药物。两个新生儿存在染色体异常，其母亲均在早孕期使用细胞毒药物[26]。在早孕期暴露于抗代谢药物的新生儿有50%的概率发生先天性畸形。回顾既往的案例，82.3%的妊娠相关白血病患者、75.4%的妊娠相关淋巴瘤患者、75%的妊娠相关乳腺癌或卵巢癌患者都能娩出正常发育的新生儿。Germann等人[31]收集了160例孕期接受蒽环类药物的患者的临床信息。他们发现，有5(3%)个胎儿存在先天异常，其中3个胎儿的母亲在早孕期接受了化疗。剩下的2个胎儿的母亲在中孕期接受化疗：其中一个胎儿患有与化疗无关的唐氏综合征，另一个胎儿存在无临床意义的先天性虹膜与角膜的粘连。多药联合化疗中的阿糖胞苷及环磷酰胺可能与胎儿畸形的发生有关。较多的案例提供了孕期蒽环类药物及紫杉醇在全身化疗中的安全性信息，少量研究关注中晚孕期使用铂类药物的安全性[32-34]。除特殊情况外（如急性白血病患者不及时治疗可能危及生命），全身化疗，尤其是在早孕期使用抗代谢药物化疗是不合适的。

Aviles和Neri[35]对孕期患有多种血液系统肿瘤并接受化疗的患者的后代进行了长期的随访。他们的研究纳入84个孩子，中位随访18.7年。38个孩子在早孕期暴露于化疗。他们的生育功能不受影响，有些后代已为人父母。这些母孕期暴露于化疗的孩子并无智力、神经、心理问题。Van Calsteren等人[36]报道了9名妊娠期患有不同癌症并接受化疗的患者的10个孩子的情况。其中早产（孕33周前出生）的孩子存在严重程度不一的发育异常，如语言发育迟缓、智力及运动系统发育迟滞等。心电图提示这些孩子往往心室壁较薄。Abdel-Hady等人[37]的研究发现，母孕期接受化疗的118个孩子的生存结局与对照组正常女性的后代没有明显差异。

目前大多数关于暴露于化疗的胎儿的数据都来源于在孕期诊断并治疗乳腺癌的患者。Murthy等人[38]汇报了暴露于化疗的胎儿的生存结局。新生儿并发症包括早产、中性粒细胞减少、新生儿呼吸过快、呼吸窘迫综合征。一个婴儿患有可治愈的自发性隐匿性颅内出血。三个婴儿患有先天性异常，分别为：唐氏综合征一例、先天性输尿管反流一例、内翻足一例[38]。Cardonick等人[39]总结了一项暴露于化疗的胎儿自愿登记的研究结果，他们发现有3.8%的胎儿出现先天性畸形，这一结果与全国平均值一致。

Loibl等人[40]进行了一项欧洲多国妊娠期乳腺癌患者的登记研究。在2003年到2011年间随访的447名患者中，有197人在妊娠期接受了化疗。22个胎儿出现合并症，并在37周前早产，其中4人有先天性畸形（18三体、直肠闭锁、多指、颅缝早闭）。9个37周后分娩的胎儿有如下三种先天畸形：头颅不对称、多趾、Moebius综合征。为了评估这些后代的长期结局，Amant等人[41]对70名儿童进行了随访，发现尽管存在早产，但其神经认知、心血管系统发育、整体健康水平与正常人无差。这些研究都强调需要尽可能避免医源性早产，治疗应尽可能在孕35周后进行以避免患者血细胞数下降，并尽可能维持至足月产。

特殊类型癌症

乳腺癌

妊娠相关乳腺癌的诊断往往较晚，可能是由于妊娠期乳房的解剖学变化和生理反应[42]。然而，各个期别的妊娠相关乳腺癌患者的生存率与未怀孕的乳腺癌患者相同[34,43,44]。目前已有大量关于妊娠期乳腺癌影像学、成功的局部治疗及系统治疗的报道。

对于乳腺可触及肿块或腺体增厚的女性进行乳房影像学检查是必要的，特别是它持续了2周或更长时间。乳腺钼靶和超声检查可以确认恶性肿块的存在。尽管Max和Klamer报告说，8名患有乳腺癌的女性中有6人的乳腺钼靶结果是正常的，但其他人的研究显示，大多数妊娠相关乳腺癌患者的钼靶检查呈现异常(18/23,5/8)[45-47]。关于超声的研究有限。Liberman的研究显示6例患者均呈超声阳性，而在Samuels的研究中，在4例患者中有2例为阳性[46,47]。Yang等人[48]的研究中，20名患者均能通过超声诊断乳腺癌，其中18例可以发现腋窝转移。超声也被证明可用来对化疗后乳腺癌进行再分期，来评估化疗反应[48]。超声可用于指导进行细针穿刺（FNA）或锥形活检来明确诊断[49-51]。胸片、肝脏超声和胸椎/腰椎MRI可用于评估其他器官转移[1,9]。

是否进行淋巴结的评估需根据临床表现综合考虑。如果在体格检查或影像学检查发现临床可疑的局部淋巴结，可在直视下或超声引导下进行细针穿刺来确定转移。经计算，患者接受前哨淋巴结活检，胎儿所吸收的理论辐射剂量小于 5cGy[52,53]。Khera 等[54]报道了他们在孕妇前哨淋巴结手术中的经验。他们进行了 10 例前哨淋巴结活检手术，6 例使用蓝色染料和^{99m}Tc，2 例单独使用^{99m}Tc，2 例单独使用蓝色染料。其中 9 例新生儿无不良后遗症。一位妇女进行了流产手术。Gropper 等人[55]发表了他们的一项纳入 25 例妊娠期接受前哨淋巴结活检手术妇女的研究，他们并没有发现术后并发症。Gentilini 等人也在 12 名患者身上进行了这项操作，其中有 1 名患者的孩子患有先天性室间隔缺损[10]。

保乳手术可配合产后乳房放疗。术前或术后化疗的选择标准与非妊娠患者相同。然而，只有在产后能及时给予放射治疗时，才应考虑保乳手术。通常，考虑到化疗的时机，常进行产后放疗。Dominici 等人[49]的单中心研究阐述了进行乳腺切除术、保乳手术或活检手术在伤口并发症、细针穿刺或锥形活检并发症方面并无差异。其他治疗乳腺癌的药物包括长春瑞滨、紫杉醇、多西他赛和顺铂[56,57]。有报道在中孕期和晚孕期使用紫杉类药物，如紫杉醇、多西紫杉醇，随访数据表明儿童健康不受影响[56,58-65]。长春瑞滨已被报道用于乳腺癌的辅助治疗和转移性乳腺癌的治疗，在 6~35 个月的随访中，6 名儿童中有 5 名健康状态良好。一名儿童的数据不详。新生儿并发症包括 1 例 4 级中性粒细胞减少和出生后第 6 天短暂性血细胞减少[63,66-68]。多项研究报道妊娠期间使用曲妥珠单抗。有些病例报道称使用曲妥珠单抗可能与羊水过少或无羊水有关[62,66,69-73]。有 1 例报道称母亲患有可逆性心力衰竭，但胎儿未发生羊水过少[71]。还有一例新生儿出现呼吸衰竭、毛细血管渗漏综合征、感染和坏死性小肠结肠炎，在分娩 21 周后死于多器官衰竭[73]。此外，Bader 等人[62]还描述了一例胎儿患有可逆性肾功能衰竭。还有一例妊娠期间使用拉帕替尼的患者。尽管服用了大约 11 周的药物，但没有生下了一个健康的婴儿[74]。妊娠期不推荐常规使用生物制剂，曲妥珠单抗现在已被 FDA 列为 D 类药物。

他莫西芬是绝经前激素受体阳性乳腺癌患者的标准治疗方案。虽然有些病例报告显示使用他莫西芬对新生儿没有影响。但也有其他报告显示使用他莫西芬会导致多种出生缺陷，包括 Goldenhar 综合征（小鼻畸形、耳前皮肤赘皮和半面短小）[75]、外生殖器发育异常等。此外，还有患者阴道出血和自然流产的报告[75-79]。Braems 等人[80]报道了 44 例活产和 3 例死产中有共 11 例有先天性畸形。芳香化酶抑制剂单药、或与卵巢功能抑制剂联用均不在妊娠期患者中使用。内分泌治疗应推迟到分娩后。

中孕期和晚孕期的乳腺癌患者如果接受合适的治疗，预后似乎与非妊娠期患者相似。一项由利顿等[81]完成的得克萨斯大学 MD 安德森癌症中心的单中心队列称，自 1989 年以来，所有中孕期及晚孕期诊断早期乳腺癌的患者均接受了 FAC 方案（5-氟尿嘧啶、多柔比星、环磷酰胺）的化疗。Rouzier 等人[82]回顾了 48 例妊娠相关乳腺癌患者的数据，他们得出的结论为在妊娠和非妊娠乳腺癌患者中，药物敏感性和治疗反应率相似。Amant 等人比较了 311 名妊娠期乳腺癌女性和 865 名非妊娠期乳腺癌患者，发现两组患者在总体生存期方面无统计学差异。

Azim 等人[33]的一项囊括了 30 项研究的荟萃分析并未发现妊娠相关乳腺癌高复发率和高死亡率。但这一研究并不是只纳入了妊娠期间诊断的乳腺癌，这可能进一步强调了区分妊娠期间和妊娠后诊断的重要性。该分析还包括多个较早的研究，这些研究要么治疗较晚，要么治疗不标准，这些都可能影响患者的生存结局。

甲状腺癌

在孕妇中，甲状腺癌最常表现为颈部的无症状结节。超声检查可以确定结节的大小和其他特征。在妊娠期间，细针穿刺活检是最可靠的诊断检测，并且是安全而准确的[83-85]。最常见的妊娠相关甲状腺癌是分化型甲状腺癌（DTC）。放射碘核素扫描和核素治疗不应在妊娠期间进行，这可以安全推迟到分娩后。对许多患者，尤其是晚孕期诊断的患者，甲状腺手术可以推迟到分娩后进行[86,87]。如有必要，可在局部麻醉下行甲状腺切除术[88]。Moosa 和 Mazzaferi[89]报道了一项包括 61 名患有甲状腺癌的孕妇和 528 名年龄匹配的对照组甲状腺癌患者的病例对照研究。他们回顾了两组患者的诊断、治疗和临床结局。74%的妊娠甲状腺癌患者通过常规体检发现了无症状的甲状腺结节。20%的孕妇在中孕期接受了甲状腺手术，而 77%的孕妇在分娩后接受了手术。30%的患者术后接受^{131}I 治疗。是否妊娠或手术时机并不影响肿瘤复发率、远处转移率及死亡率。基于这些发现，Moosa 和 Mazzaferi[89]得出结论，对大多数患者来说，妊娠期甲状腺癌的治疗可以推迟到分娩后。此外，Yasmeen 等人[90]回顾了加州癌症登记中心的 595 名在产前 9 个月至产后 12 个月内被诊断为甲状腺癌的妇女，并与相应的非妊娠妇女进行了比较，研究发现两组患者在总体生存率、母婴结局方面没有发现显著差异。Alves 等人[91]进行了一项纳入四项研究的系统回顾（包括前面提到的两项研究），他们发现妊娠和非妊娠分化型甲状腺癌患者的长期生存结果没有区别。

宫颈癌

评估宫颈癌需要结合体格检查和 MRI 结果。有报道称妊娠期宫颈癌患者可进行腹腔镜淋巴结清扫手术[92]。妊娠期宫颈癌的治疗方案因疾病分期、诊断时的孕周数和患者的意愿而异。对于Ⅰ期宫颈癌，Sorosky 等人的报道称，随访观察到妊娠晚期再进行治疗也能有比较好的结果。他们纳入了 8 例病灶小于 2.5cm 的Ⅰ期妇女，平均随访时间为 109 天。所有患者均行先剖宫产，再行全子宫切除术。2 名患者采用多次核磁共振检查来进行随访，没有发现疾病进展。治疗后，经过平均 37 个月的随访，所有患者均存活并无疾病复发。

在一项纳入了 22 例妊娠期或产后 12 月内诊断宫颈癌的患者的综述中，Allen 等人[94]发现其中 20 例患者产下活胎，只有一例患者出现疾病复发。11 名微小浸润性癌的患者中 9 例只接受了锥切手术。10 例ⅠB 或ⅡA 期的患者接受了子宫全切术，1 例ⅢB 期的患者接受了放化疗及单纯子宫切除术。Allen 建议所有妊娠期宫颈癌的妇女进行宫颈细胞学评估。在妊娠期锥切是安全的，对微小浸润性宫颈癌可能是足够有效的[94]。

对于妊娠期或产后 6 个月内诊断的宫颈癌来说，分娩方式对患者结局及复发风险的影响已得到充分的评估。Sood 等人[95]随访了 83 名宫颈癌孕妇，其中 56 例为妊娠期诊断，27 例为产后诊断。由于经阴道顺产的患者产后复发风险高，Sood 等人得出结论，妊娠期宫颈癌患者应采用剖宫产。然而，van der Vange 等人[96]在一项病例对照研究中报道分娩方式对患者生存没有影响。总的来说，他们注意到与未怀孕组相比，妊娠的宫颈癌患者的生存期没有差异。宫颈癌的全身化疗在妊娠期间也是有效的。目前报道的大多数治疗方案都是以铂为基础，联用长春新碱、博来霉素等其他药物[97]。此外，也有些采用新辅助化疗的报道，如紫杉醇联合卡铂或顺铂[97-99]。许多案例报道证实，使用以铂为基础的，联合紫杉醇或长春瑞滨的新辅助化疗方案能够很好地保护妊娠，产生良好的母婴结局[100-102]。

妊娠期宫颈癌患者的治疗需仔细评估癌症分期和胎龄。妊娠早期诊断的早期宫颈癌患者，终止妊娠后再进行治疗可能是合适的。另一种选择是，在密切随访的情况下，也可先完成妊娠再进行治疗[93]。放疗通常导致胎儿死亡及自然流产[19]。

由于有相当一部分患者在育龄期被诊断为宫颈癌，出于对保留生育功能的考虑，在部分Ⅰ期宫颈癌患者中，可采用根治子宫颈切除术联合盆腔淋巴结清扫，而不采取根治性子宫切除术。Burnett 等人[103]在 6 年的时间里对 21 名患者实施了这一手术，21 名患者中有 18 人接受了根治性子宫颈切除术以保留生育功能。在这一组中，一名患者在接受超排卵处理后，经过 24 周的妊娠，产下了健康的双胞胎。1 例患者行剖宫产后子宫切除术分娩 1 例单胎足月婴儿并且宫颈未见残余病变。另有一个患者可能在行根治性宫颈切除术前一周怀孕。她在孕 20 周时出现了自发破膜，紧急行全子宫切除术娩出胎儿，但随后新生儿死亡。许多其他研究也已经证实了这种保存生育能力的手术可以成功实施[104,105]。但目前关于在妊娠期间进行这种手术的病例报道很少，因此它的使用仍有争议[98,106]。

对于在妊娠期间诊断为宫颈癌患者的生存结局的研究仍然很少。Nguyen 等人[107]认为，妊娠对肿瘤的生物学行为和产妇生存结局没有不利影响，反之宫颈癌对妊娠也没有不利影响。van der Vange 在一项病例对照研究中也得出了类似的结论。他们纳入了 23 名在妊娠期间确诊宫颈癌的患者和 24 名在产后 6 个月内确诊的患者。其中 39 名患者疾病为早期。与对照组相比，病例组患者的生存率没有差异。他们指出，分娩方式对生存没有影响，进而得出结论：妊娠期和非妊娠期宫颈癌的预后相似[96,108]。

Zemlickis 等人[109]的一项关于妊娠期女性的长期随访的病例对照研究表明，妊娠期与非妊娠期患者生存率没有差别。和对照组相比，微小浸润宫颈癌患者更可能产下低出生体重儿。妊娠对宫颈癌的负面影响很小。

霍奇金淋巴瘤和非霍奇金淋巴瘤

临床表现上，妊娠期霍奇金淋巴瘤患者与非妊娠期患者无明显不同，通常表现为淋巴结肿大[110]。诊断需要进行淋巴结活检获取足够的组织标本来鉴别淋巴瘤的亚型[111]。病史、体格检查、进行腹部保护的胸片、腹部超声、核磁等检查有助于确定疾病分期，指导疾病的治疗。病变局限在膈以上时，进行子宫部位防护的放疗可以起到治疗效果，并且保护胎儿[20,22,111-113]。Woo 等人的一项研究报道了妊娠期ⅠA 及ⅡA 期霍奇金淋巴瘤患者中接受放疗的情况[20]。16 例患者接受了放疗，部位包括颈部（2 例）、颈部及纵隔（3 例）、斗篷野放疗（11 例）[114]。根据对 9 名患者的分析，估算的胎儿接受辐射的剂量范围是：1.4～5.5cGy（光子治疗）及 10～13.6cGy（钴治疗）。这些患者共娩出了 16 个正常足月儿，患者的 10 年生存率为 71%[20]。这一结果与 Jacobs 等人[113]的研究相似。Jacobs 的研究关注中孕期和晚孕期行颈部及纵隔放疗的患者。他们发现，膈上放疗能够在不影响胎儿的情况下起到治疗效果。霍奇金淋巴瘤对妊娠的影响以及妊娠对霍奇金淋巴瘤预后的影响尚不得而知。Anselmo 等人[115]的结论是霍奇金淋巴瘤的预后不受怀孕的影响。Tawil 等人[112]报告了他们对 12 例妊娠期霍奇金淋巴瘤患者治疗的经验，他们的结论是妊娠对肿瘤的病程没有显著影响，肿瘤也不影响妊娠结局。在回顾妊娠结局时，Zuazu 等人[116]发现在 56 例白血病或淋巴瘤患者中妊娠相关并发症的发病率没有增加。在接受全身化疗的患者中，胎儿畸形的发生率没有增加。在 Gelb 的研究中，患者接受多种方案的全身联合化疗，包括 MOPP（氮芥、长春新碱、丙卡巴肼、泼尼松），ABV（多柔比星、博莱霉素、长春碱），COP（环磷酰胺、多柔比星、泼尼松），CHOP（环磷酰胺、多柔比星、长春新碱、泼尼松）[110]。他的研究无胎儿畸形的报告。15 名患者活了下来，没有疾病复发或进展。Gelb 和他的同事得出结论，除特殊情况外，全身化疗不应该因为怀孕而推迟。

相比于霍奇金淋巴瘤，妊娠期非霍奇金淋巴瘤通常期别更高，生物学行为更恶劣[110,117,118]。孕期非霍奇金淋巴瘤患者的临床表现与非孕期相同。因为大多数患者的疾病都属于晚期，所以需要全身化疗。多药联合化疗方案可发挥疗效。使用的药物包括表柔比星、长春新碱、泼尼松、依托泊苷、环磷酰胺、多柔比星和博莱霉素（VACOP-B 方案和 MACOP-B 方案）[119-121]。也有许多孕期使用利妥昔单抗的报道。Herold 等人[122]使用联合利妥昔单抗、多柔比星、长春新碱和泼尼松龙的方案治疗一名巨块型ⅡA 期非霍奇金淋巴瘤女性患者。在开始治疗时，患者已经怀孕 21 周。她对治疗的反应良好，35 周时通过剖宫产生下了一个健康的婴儿。这个孩子的 B 细胞数量正常。Kimby 等人[123]治疗了一位ⅡB 期非霍奇金淋巴瘤患者，连续 4 个周期每周使用利妥昔单抗。患者在前两次注射利妥昔单抗之间发生怀孕。她在孕 40 周时产下了一个健康的女婴。婴儿出生时粒细胞计数较低，血象在 18 个月时恢复正常。从那时起，有多个关于使用 R-CHOP 方案（利妥昔单抗、环磷酰胺、多柔比星、长春新碱和泼尼松）在妊娠期间治疗弥漫性大 B 细胞淋巴瘤的报告，有的胎儿患有白细胞减少，妊娠期并发症只有早产[124,125]。

在最大的一项多中心回顾性研究中，Evens 等人[125]纳入了 90 例妊娠期诊断霍奇金淋巴瘤或非霍奇金淋巴瘤的患者。6 例患者选择终止妊娠。56 名患者接受了 R-CHOP 方案或其他包括依托泊苷、博莱霉素、达卡巴嗪、阿糖胞苷和顺铂的改良化疗方案。治疗前使用激素、生长因子诱导。一个患者产下小头畸形的宝宝。引产、剖宫产发生率、NICU 转运率均增高。患者的生存期和非孕期患者相似。Aviles 等人[126]介绍了 16 例孕期治疗非霍奇金淋巴瘤患者的结局。没有发现先天畸形，分娩都很顺利。所以他们得出结论，妊娠不是治疗非霍奇金淋巴瘤的禁忌，但远期复发也是有可能的。此外，间变性淋巴瘤、Burkitt 淋巴瘤及 T 细胞淋巴瘤均有妊娠期诊断的报道[127-131]。

卵巢癌

在对妊娠期间发现附件肿块患者的回顾中，125 例患者中有 1 例卵巢癌，40 例皮样囊肿，15 例子宫内膜样瘤，14 例单纯囊肿，13 例囊腺瘤，9 例输卵管囊肿，4 例肌瘤，恶性肿瘤发生率为 0.8%[132]。在一项回顾性研究中，Sayedur 等人[133]在 24 年中诊断了 9 例卵巢癌，发病率为 0.08/1 000 名孕妇。对于孕妇来说，附件包块发生率高，而且可能是良性的，因此对妊娠期附件肿物的诊断及治疗也变得越来越复杂。超声、经皮穿刺和手术治疗均可能发生。在 Platek 等人的一项研究中[134,135]，43 372 名孕妇中有 31 人在妊娠 16 周后发现>6cm 的附件肿块，但没有人被诊断为卵巢癌。当发现恶性肿瘤时，生殖细胞肿瘤和低度恶性的上皮性肿瘤是最常见的。Dgani 等回顾了妊娠期卵巢癌的病理结果[136]。他们记录了 24 年间 23 名患者的数据。交界性癌最为常见(35%)，其次是侵袭性上皮性肿瘤(30%)、无性细胞瘤(17%)和颗粒细胞瘤(13%)。早期疾病很常见：74% 的患者处于 Ⅰ 期。在 Sayedur 等人的系列研究中[133]，9 例患者中有 7 例 Ⅰ 期上皮性肿瘤。5 例行附件切除术，3 例行经腹全子宫切除双侧大网膜切除术。Ⅰ 期疾病患者生存率为 100%，5 年总体生存率为 78%。早期卵巢癌患者可行保留生育功能的手术。在 Dgani 的研究中，23 例患者中的 4 例可娩出活胎[136]。Dgani 总结道，妊娠期卵巢癌患者由于诊断时疾病多处于早期、肿瘤多为低度恶性的病理类型，因此预后比全人群普遍要好。

个案报道中，化疗可被用于治疗进展期卵巢癌的患者。顺铂、卡铂、多柔比星、博来霉素、环磷酰胺以及近年来常用的紫杉醇都被报道可用于治疗妊娠期卵巢癌[99,137-139]。

急慢性淋巴瘤

急性白血病

由于骨髓抑制及随之而来的血细胞减少，妊娠期白血病患者临床表现很有特色。髓系白血病比淋巴系白血病更常见。其症状和体征与非妊娠患者无明显差异。诊断采用骨髓穿刺，分型采用标准分型。在 Mayo 诊所的一项研究中，37 年中共有 17 名患者诊断有急性白血病。其中 15 人被诊断为急性髓系白血病。白血病大多诊断在早孕期或晚孕期。9 名患者妊娠期间接受了化疗，5 名实现了长期完全缓解。而在分娩后才开始治疗的 4 名患者中，有 3 名死于白血病。在妊娠期间接受化疗的患者中没有胎儿畸形的报道[140]。

Cardonick 和 Iacobucci[141]分析了包括 63 例淋巴系和 89 例髓系急性白血病的孕妇的临床特征及母婴结局。他们发现 6 名新生儿有先天性异常，12 名新生儿出现宫内生长迟缓。宫内胎儿死亡 11 例，新生儿死亡 2 例。上述异常病例均在早孕期以单药或联合用药的形式使用过阿糖胞苷或硫鸟嘌呤。然而，在妊娠的各个时期使用长春新碱、巯基嘌呤、多柔比星或柔霉素、环磷酰胺、泼尼松和甲氨蝶呤的联合用药似乎是合适的。

特别地，全反式维 A 酸是急性早幼粒白血病的标准治疗方案。维 A 酸有已知的致畸性[142]。然而，也有一些个案报道证实患有早幼粒白血病的患者使用全反式维 A 酸对母婴结局无明显影响[143,144]。

慢性白血病

妊娠期慢性淋巴细胞白血病患者极其罕见[145,146]。Welsh 等人[146]报告了一例病例，这位患者产后白细胞数目大幅下降。但他们注意到这种整体血象上的缓解并不伴随着白细胞的克隆缓解。Gurman 报道了一例诊断慢性淋巴细胞白血病后不久便怀孕的患者，她没有接受细胞毒性药物的治疗，在孕 39 周时产下一健康的婴儿[31]。她在妊娠晚期伴有妊娠期糖尿病和先兆子痫。尽管 Welsh 报道的病例绒毛间隙淋巴细胞的数目明显升高，本例患者的胎盘未见淋巴细胞浸润。Ali 等人[147]治疗了一例孕 17 周诊断为慢性淋巴细胞白血病的患者。患者在孕 25 周、30 周和 38 周接受了三次降白治疗，使得白细胞数可以降至 $100×10^9$/L 以下。她在孕 39 周时成功娩出一活婴。

妊娠期慢性髓系白血病可采用降白治疗联合 α-干扰素、羟基脲，或单纯采用降白治疗[148-151]。这些治疗方式对胎儿的生长发育无明显影响，也不增加产科合并症的发生率。

维持妊娠至分娩是可行的。有限的研究表明，妊娠对慢性髓系白血病的长期预后无影响，但这些研究没有一项是病例对照研究。虽然少量动物实验表明，伊马替尼有致畸毒性，但也有越来越多的妊娠期使用伊马替尼的报道。Yilmaz 等人[152]报道了三例服用伊马替尼的孕妇，都产下了健康的婴儿。Prabhash 等[153]报道了两例全孕期持续采用伊马替尼疗法的女性仍能产下正常胎儿。Ault 等人的研究中，19 例患者中的 18 例均在服用伊马替尼期间怀孕。所有患者都在发现妊娠时中断了伊马替尼的治疗。3 例患者出现自然流产，1 例选择人工流产。16 个婴儿中的 2 个有先天缺陷：一例患有尿道下裂，一例出现小肠扭转。考虑到中断伊马替尼的治疗可能对疗效产生负面影响，他们建议在服用伊马替尼期间严格避孕。另一项案例报道中，由于母亲使用伊马替尼，胎儿出现了脑脊膜膨出进而胎死宫内[154]。Yadav 等人[155]也报道了一位晚孕期接受羟基脲和伊马替尼治疗的女性，妊娠期间出现了胎儿宫内发育迟缓及羊水过少等并发症。然而该胎儿在分娩后发育良好。

Alizadeh 等人[156]报道 14 例孕妇(或其性伴侣)服用酪氨酸激酶治疗 CML，其 22 次孕产仅 1 例有房间隔缺损。因此，由于这些少量但互相矛盾的研究，妊娠期慢性白血病患者应在服用伊马替尼期间持续避孕。但是也有些患者在妊娠期并未中断伊马替尼的治疗。在充分告知风险的情况下，这也可能为少部分患者提供一种治疗选择。

黑色素瘤

手术是妊娠期诊断的黑色素瘤的主流治疗手段。已有不少妊娠期诊断的黑色素瘤的报道。Johansson 等人[157]总结了瑞典疾病登记中心 1 019 例妊娠相关黑色素瘤患者的特点。研究发现妊娠期黑色素瘤患者与非妊娠期诊断的黑色素瘤患者的疾病死亡率无明显差异。然而澳大利亚的研究者 Bannister-Tyrell 等人[158]的一项纳入 577 例妊娠相关黑色素瘤患者(包含 195 个妊娠期诊断的病例)的研究中,妊娠相关性黑色素瘤诊断时期别更高。

跨胎盘转移和胎盘部位转移

大量案例报道证实癌症可通过胎盘由母亲转移给胎儿[159-167]。Catlin 等人[159]报道了一项由于母亲自然杀伤细胞淋巴瘤转移给胎儿致胎儿死亡的案例。也有报道称可成功治愈母亲跨胎盘转移给胎儿的小细胞肺癌[166]。另有 Teksam 的案例中,母亲诊断肺癌后紧急引产一 33 周胎儿。由于存在胎盘部位转移,婴儿接受了脑 MRI、胸腹 CT 检查,无明显异常发现。不幸的是,后续检查还是发现存在婴儿存在脑部肿瘤,虽然对化疗敏感,但数月后疾病进展。活检证实这一肿瘤为肺癌转移灶,后续的随访中也发现了更多的位于额叶和颞叶的病灶[167]。

另一项研究中,在母亲患有急性淋巴细胞白血病的新生儿外周血中,可检测出白血病细胞,但尚不足以诊断白血病[164]。另一项研究表明,急性单核细胞白血病也能经母亲转移给胎儿[162]。

Alexander 等人[163]回顾了 87 例发生胎儿转移或胎盘转移的案例,他们发现恶性黑色素瘤占 31%,是发生胎儿胎盘转移的最常见的肿瘤类型。

Dildy 等人在 1989 年发表了一篇回顾了 52 例发生胎盘转移患者的文章。研究发现实体瘤和血液系统肿瘤都能发生胎盘转移(表 72-3)[129,168-176]。妊娠期女性分娩后往往未对胎盘进行系统的评估,然而新技术的使用正在使对胎盘的评估变得更加简便。

表 72-3 胎盘转移

肿瘤类型	大细胞肺癌[171]
小细胞肺癌[166]	B 细胞淋巴瘤[172]
黑色素瘤[166]	T 细胞淋巴瘤[173]
胰腺癌	非霍奇金淋巴瘤[174]
乳腺癌[169]	大细胞淋巴瘤[129]
成神经管细胞瘤[170]	

结论

妊娠期癌症的诊断及治疗需要多学科的肿瘤医师及产科团队密切配合。产科、外科、麻醉科医师通力合作能更好地收集患者的信息,指导诊断治疗。为了母亲和胎儿的健康,医师的首要职责是在患者做决定时为其提供足够的支持。母亲和胎儿都可能有很大获益。表 72-4 列出了多学科团队管理妊娠相关性癌症的流程纲要。

表 72-4 妊娠期癌症患者的多学科管理

诊断及治疗计划	考虑的因素
明确诊断	细胞学及组织病理学
评估疾病程度	分期、体格检查、器官功能、转移灶
妊娠以外的疾病诊断	
评估妊娠	合并症—年龄、糖尿病、心功能
	胎龄
	预产期
回顾治疗选择	对患者
	对患者的潜在好处
	"治愈"延长生命、改善症状、推迟疾病进展
	对胎儿
	可能的结果
	维持妊娠
	潜在风险
制定并实施治疗方案	
多次再评估患者和胎儿	
多学科治疗团队成员	患者
	产科医师
	肿瘤医师-外科、放疗科、内科
	护理团队
	伦理专家
	社会服务机构
	宗教治疗师

(邵禹铭 向阳 译)

参考文献

The complete reference list can be found on the Wiley Companion Digital Edition of this title (see inside front cover for login instructions).

1 Peccatori FA, Azim HA, Orecchia R, et al. Cancer, pregnancy and fertility: ESMO Clinical Practice Guidelines for diagnosis, treatment and follow-up. *Ann Oncol.* 2013;**24**:vi160–vi170.

5 Dominici LS, Kuerer HM, Babiera G, et al. Wound complications from surgery in pregnancy-associated breast cancer (PABC). *Breast Dis.* 2010;**31**:1–5.

6 Mazze R, Kallen B. Reproductive outcome after anesthesia and operation during pregnancy: a registry study of 5405 cases. *J Obstet Gynecol.* 1989;**161**:1178.

9 Hahn K, Johnson P, Gordon N, et al. Treatment of pregnant breast cancer patients and outcomes of children exposed to chemotherapy in utero. *Cancer.* 2006;**107**:1219–1226.

11 De Santis M, Straface G, Cavaliere AF, et al. Gadolinium periconceptional exposure: pregnancy and neonatal outcome. *Acta Obstet Gynecol Scand.* 2007;**86**:99–101.

17 Stensheim H, Moller B, van Dijk T, et al. Cause-specific survival for women diagnosed with cancer during pregnancy or lactation: a registry-based cohort study. *J Clin Oncol.* 2009;**27**:45–51.

20 Woo S, Fuller L, Cundiff J, et al. Radiotherapy during pregnancy for clinical stages IA-IIA Hodgkin's disease. *Int J Radiat Oncol Biol Phys*. 1992;**23**:407.

27 Doll D, Ringenberg Q, Yarbro J. Antineoplastic agents in pregnancy. *Semin Oncol*. 1989;**16**:337–346.

30 Cardonick E, Gilmandyar D, Somer RA. Maternal and neonatal outcomes of dose-dense chemotherapy for breast cancer in pregnancy. *Obstet Gynecol*. 2012;**120**:1267–1272.

31 Germann N, Goffinet F, Goldwasser F. Anthracyclines during pregnancy: embryo-fetal outcome in 160 patients. *Ann Oncol*. 2004;**15**:146–150.

32 Cardonick E, Bhat A, Gilmandyar D, et al. Maternal and fetal outcomes of taxane chemotherapy in breast and ovarian cancer during pregnancy: case series and review of the literature. *Ann Oncol*. 2012;**23**:3016–3023.

33 Azim HA Jr, Santoro L, Russell-Edu W, et al. Prognosis of pregnancy-associated breast cancer: a meta-analysis of 30 studies. *Cancer Treat Rev*. 2012;**38**:834–842.

34 Litton J, Warneke C, Hahn K, et al. Case control study of women treated with chemotherapy for breast cancer during pregnancy as compared with non-pregnant breast cancer patients. *Oncologist*. 2013;**18**(**4**):369–376.

35 Aviles A, Neri N. Hematologic malignancies and pregnancy: a final report of 84 children who received chemotherapy in utero. *Clin Lymphoma*. 2001;**2**:173–177.

36 Van Calsteren K, Berteloot P, Hanssens M, et al. In utero exposure to chemotherapy: effect on cardiac and neurologic outcome. *J Clin Oncol*. 2006;**24**:e16–e17.

37 Abdel-Hady el S, Hemida RA, Gamal A, et al. Cancer during pregnancy: perinatal outcome after in utero exposure to chemotherapy. *Arch Gynecol Obstet*. 2012;**286**:283–286.

38 Murthy R, Theriault R, Barnett C, et al. Outcomes of children exposed in utero to chemotherapy for breast cancer. *Breast Cancer Res*. 2014;**16**:3414.

39 Cardonick EMD, Dougherty RMD, Grana GMD, et al. Breast cancer during pregnancy: maternal and fetal outcomes. *Cancer J*. 2010;**16**(**1**):76–82.

40 Loibl S, Han SN, von Minckwitz G, et al. Treatment of breast cancer during pregnancy: an observational study. *Lancet Oncol*. 2012;**13**:887–896.

41 Amant F, Van Calsteren K, Halaska MJ, et al. Long-term cognitive and cardiac outcomes after prenatal exposure to chemotherapy in children aged 18 months or older: an observational study. *Lancet Oncol*. 2012;**13**:256–264.

48 Yang WT, Dryden MJ, Gwyn K, et al. Imaging of breast cancer diagnosed and treated with chemotherapy during pregnancy. *Radiology*. 2006;**239**:52–60.

54 Khera SY, Kiluk JV, Hasson DM, et al. Pregnancy-associated breast cancer patients can safely undergo lymphatic mapping. *Breast J*. 2008;**14**:250–254.

56 Mir O, Berveiller P, Ropert S, et al. Emerging therapeutic options for breast cancer chemotherapy during pregnancy. *Ann Oncol*. 2008;**19**:607–613.

58 Mir O, Berveiller P, Goffinet F, et al. Taxanes for breast cancer during pregnancy: a systematic review. *Ann Oncol*. 2009;**21**:425–433.

62 Bader AA, Schlembach D, Tamussino KF, et al. Anhydramnios associated with administration of trastuzumab and paclitaxel for metastatic breast cancer during pregnancy. *Lancet Oncol*. 2007;**8**:79–81.

70 Pant S, Landon MB, Blumenfeld M, et al. Treatment of breast cancer with trastuzumab during pregnancy. *J Clin Oncol*. 2008;**26**:1567–1569.

71 Shrim A, Garcia-Bournissen F, Maxwell C, et al. Favorable pregnancy outcome following Trastuzumab (Herceptin(R)) use during pregnancy – Case report and updated literature review. *Reprod Toxicol*. 2007;**23**:611–613.

72 Shrim A, Garcia-Bournissen F, Maxwell C, et al. Trastuzumab treatment for breast cancer during pregnancy. *Can Fam Physician*. 2008;**54**:31–32.

98 Amant F, Halaska MJ, Fumagalli M, et al. Gynecologic cancers in pregnancy: guidelines of a second international consensus meeting. *Int J Gynecol Cancer*. 2014;**24**:394–403. doi: 10.1097/IGC.0000000000000062.

126 Aviles A, Diaz-Maqueo JC, Torras V, et al. Non-Hodgkin's lymphomas and pregnancy: presentation of 16 cases. *Gynecol Oncol*. 1990;**37**:335–337.

171 Dildy GA 3rd, Moise KJ Jr, Carpenter RJ Jr, et al. Maternal malignancy metastatic to the products of conception: a review. *Obstet Gynecol Surv*. 1989;**44**:535–540.

第 73 章　癌症与老龄化

Arti Hurria, MD ■ Hyman B. Muss, MD ■ Harvey J. Cohen, MD

概述

癌症是一种与老龄化相关的疾病。大约 60%的癌症以及 70%的癌症相关死亡发生于 65 岁以上人群。随着美国人口的老龄化，罹患癌症的老年人人数逐渐增加。但是，老年人的健康状况存在很大异质性，这可能会影响癌症治疗的决策和疗效。本章节将回顾老年医学评估和衰弱的原理，癌症和老龄化的生物学，以及在治疗和生存期期间护理老年癌症患者的特有问题及需考虑的因素。

癌症是一种严重影响老年患者的疾病。几乎 60%的癌症发生在 65 岁及以上人群。与 65 岁以下人群相比，65 岁及以上人群的癌症发生率增加 9 倍，癌症相关死亡率增加 18 倍（表 73-1）[2]。随着人口老龄化，罹患癌症的老年人数也在逐渐增长。1900 年美国 65 岁以上老年人约有 310 万。在过去的一个世纪里，这一数字增长了约 10 倍，2000 年美国 65 岁以上老年人约有 3 500 万。预计该数字还会再翻一番，截至 2030 年，预计 65 岁以上的人口将达到 7 150 万人，占总人口的 20%（表 73-2）。

表 73-1　年龄≥65 岁人群相比于年龄<65 岁人群癌症发生率增加 9 倍，癌症相关死亡率增加 18 倍

年龄	发生率（每 100 000 人）	死亡率（每 100 000 人）
<65 岁	223.8	56.1
≥65 岁	2 095.8	1 008.4

来源：Data derived from SEER for 1975—2011 Incidence and 1975—2010 for Mortality.[1]

表 73-2　美国 65 岁及以上人群逐渐增多

年份	百万	人群比例/%
1900	3.1	4.1
2000	35.0	12.4
2030	71.5	19.7

在 65 岁以上的人群中，年龄会随着时间而发生改变，导致老年人口的增加。例如，20 世纪 90 年代 85 岁及以上老年人口增长 38%，75～84 岁人口增长 23%，65～74 岁人口增长不足 2%。截至 2030 年，85 岁及以上人口有望翻倍[3]。"百岁老人"，即 100 岁及以上老年人，是老年人口中增长最快的。基于这些数据，肿瘤科医生不可避免地需照看大量的老年患者。对于"老年"，目前尚无标准的"实足年龄"界限。一般定义为≥65 岁，理由如下：

1. 传统的退休年龄
2. 在美国有资格获得福利项目（社会保障，医疗保险）

随着人口年龄的增长，我们看到≥65 岁人群存在很大异质性，许多个体可以像年轻人一样继续生活。因此，本章侧重于以"功能年龄"，而非"实足年龄"来定义老年人的特征。本章还专门讨论护理老年癌症患者的独特问题和注意事项。

预期寿命和老龄化

在护理老年患者时，关于平均预期寿命的统计数据很有意义。出生时人的平均预期寿命是 76.5 岁。随着个体年龄的增长，平均预期寿命也会增加。例如，一个 65 岁的人的平均预期寿命是 19.1 岁，预期死亡年龄是 84.1 岁。活到 80 岁的人的平均预期寿命是 9.1 岁，预期死亡年龄是 89.1 岁。即使活到 100 岁的老人，平均预期寿命也有 2.3 岁，平均预期死亡年龄为 102.3 岁。有人可能认为这是"适者生存"现象，其中绝对预期寿命随着年龄的增长而增加（表 73-3）[5]。

表 73-3　平均预期寿命

目前年龄/岁	预期寿命/年	死亡年龄/岁
65	19.1	84.1
70	15.5	85.5
75	12.1	87.1
80	9.1	89.1
85	6.6	91.6
90	4.7	94.7
95	3.3	98.3
100	2.3	102.3

来源：Data derived from the National Vital Statistics Report 5.

癌症和老龄化的生物学

老龄化可被定义为"将健康成人转变为虚弱的人的过程，在大多数生理系统中，这些人的生理储备减少，对疾病和死亡的脆弱性呈指数增长"[6]。尽管这一定义具有普遍性，但老龄化显然是一个异质的过程。每个个体都以各自独特的步伐逐渐衰老，并表现出多样的虚弱表现。尽管已经取得了很大的进展，但对老龄化和肿瘤的机制尚不完全了解，因此关于这两个过程的理论关联仍是研究的热点[7,8]。有人认为，癌症和老龄化可以被认为同一枚硬币的两个面，这枚硬币是调控组织更新和修复的关键点，如过度增殖可导致肿瘤的形成，如细胞增殖

和功能下降可导致衰老[9,10]。P16[INK]表达可能在该分支点起关键作用,可能通过新陈代谢抗性途径和自噬途径进行废物管理控制[11,12]。

与老龄化和肿瘤相关的其他理论[13,14]包括:更长时间的氧化应激和致癌物的暴露(时间)和对其可能增加的敏感性;年龄引起的增加的 DNA 不稳定性,可导致更高的突变潜力,可能导致致癌基因活化或扩增,或抑癌基因缺陷;随着年龄的增长 DNA 修复能力下降,这可能会增加遗传缺陷的易感性;年龄相关的端粒缩短,可能增加上述的 DNA 不稳定性;免疫失调,可能会降低免疫监视,导致恶性克隆,但也可能会形成促炎环境,有利于恶性细胞的生长;最后是微环境的改变,包括可能分泌促炎因子和致癌因子的衰老细胞的出现[14-16]。这些理论不能解释为何人口老龄化人群的癌症发病率下降。在一项针对 507 名 75 岁以上患者的尸检研究中,尸检时癌症的患病率随着年龄的增长而降低(75~79 岁 35%,95~99 岁 20%,百年老人 16%)。一项详细的人口统计学研究已证实了这一点,并表明针对这一现象成因的研究可能对老龄化和癌症的总体关系具有启发性[17]。

老龄化引起的生理变化

每个器官系统都会随着年龄的增长而发生生理变化,而与疾病无关。大多数器官系统从 30 岁开始出现线性生理衰退。不同个体和器官间的生理衰退速度不同。正常活动期间这些变化的影响很小;但是,在应激状况下,储备量的减少就变得更加明显了[18]。

随着心血管系统老化,运动后心输出量下降,最大心率下降及恢复时间延长。在应激状况下,对儿茶酚胺的反应下降。随着肺部老龄化,对低氧血症或高碳酸血症的反应下降,肺组织弹性减低,通气-血流不匹配增加,用力呼气量减少。随着年龄的增长,内分泌也会发生变化,包括某些激素水平的下降和其他激素水平的升高。比如,胰岛素样生长因子、生长激素、肾素、醛固酮、脱氢表雄酮和性激素水平下降,胰岛素、去甲肾上腺素、甲状旁腺激素、血管升压素和心房利钠肽水平升高。随着年龄的增长,神经系统的变化包括神经元丢失、脑重量减轻、视力下降、高频和低频听力丧失以及味觉和嗅觉的改变。免疫系统的变化主要表现为胸腺实质减少,胸腺激素产生减少,幼稚淋巴细胞减少,以及抗体反应降低[18]。

随着年龄的增长,肝脏和肾脏的实质减少。尸检研究表明,随着年龄的增长,肝脏实质会减少约 25%~50%。此外,在肝脏实质减少的基础上,随着年龄的增长,肝血流量也随之约下降 10%~15%[19-21]。整个寿命期间肾脏实质减少 25%~30%,导致功能性肾单位数量减少。50 岁以后肾脏血流每年减少 1%,40 岁以后肾小球滤过率每年下降 1ml/(min·年)[19,21]。

老龄化相关的造血改变,包括骨髓量减少和骨髓脂肪增多。尽管如此,健康的老年患者的外周学细胞浓度与年轻的患者相似[22]。

体弱的老年患者

"体弱"一词用于描述由于功能储备严重降低而面临依赖,机构化,疾病,住院和死亡等风险的一类老年患者[23]。体弱被用于定义"由于体内平衡能力受损和机体承受压力的能力降低而导致相应的年龄相关的生理脆弱性状态。"因此,临床上体弱综合征被认为是能量平衡失调的动态结果。例如,起初为营养不良导致肌肉和骨骼含量下降,进一步导致活动水平和强度的进一步下降。结合储备水平下降,导致体弱患者脆弱性增加。最终导致发育停滞,即难以解释的体重下降,肌肉含量减少,代谢异常,包括白蛋白、肌酐、胆固醇及血红蛋白减低等综合征。免疫功能障碍和慢性炎症可能在体弱中发挥着作用。与老龄化和体弱相关的炎性标志物包括:白介素 6(IL-6)和急性期反应物,C 反应蛋白(CRP)[24-26]。此外,血浆 D 二聚体升高也可能与年龄相关。IL-6 和 D 二聚体均可预测死亡和功能减退[23,27,28]。

在针对 5 317 例≥65 岁的社区男性和女性的一项前瞻性观察性研究中,建立了一种体弱表型。"体弱的表型"被定义为存在以下 3 个或以上标准的临床综合征:①过去 1 年内体重意外下降≥10lbs;②自诉疲惫;③虚弱,即性别和体重指数调整的握力器强度在人群的最低的百分之二十;④步速慢,即步行 4.5m 的时间在人群的最低的百分之二十;⑤低体力活动,即每周的热量在人群的下五分之一。具有以上一项或两项标准的个体被归类为"中度和前期体弱表型"。与非体弱患者相比,体弱或前期体弱患者的 3 年和 7 年死亡率,住院率及事件发生率,日常生活活动能力下降率和行动能力下降率都增加。根据这些标准,有 7%的 65 岁及以上的社区个体为体弱,47%个体为前期体弱。体弱和前期体弱的患者中女性的发病率较男性高,并随着年龄的增长而增加[29]。体弱也与反复跌倒、髋部骨折及非脊柱骨折风险增加相关[30]。

Rockwood 及其同事建立了另一种衡量体弱的方法,即用缺陷累积来评价体弱[31]。体弱指数基于以下前提:个体缺陷可能不会对死亡率(或其他结局)产生明显的威胁,但这些个体的缺陷累积可能会导致老年患者预后更差。比如,在老年人群中,缺陷累积已被证明可预测住院、机构化和死亡[32,33]。与 Fried 和同事建立的表型模型相比,该模型需了解特定的参数,如能收集足够多的变量,缺陷累积方法几乎可用于捕获老年评估变量的任何数据集。目前仍需进一步研究来确定不同的体弱衡量方法在预测老年癌症患者预后中的效用。

体弱的老年癌症患者是一类独特的在治疗决策上很有挑战性的患者群。前述的老年体弱测量方法仍未在老年癌症患者中广泛应用,而这些人群当中可能有其他令人感兴趣的结果。比如,关于老年癌症患者的专家研究共识指出对于体弱的肿瘤学定义应该评估患者癌症治疗相关的毒性风险[34]。评估体弱患者首要一步就是明确癌症是否会缩短患者的预期寿命。Balducci 和 Stanta[35]提出的模型中指出如果癌症会影响患者的预期寿命或者引起生活质量下降,则应考虑针对癌症的治疗。治疗目标必须明确:延长生存和减轻痛苦。治疗决策包括权衡患者和护理人员的风险和获益。随着人口老龄化,年老体弱的癌症患者数目将逐渐增加。仍需要针对这类患者的治疗有效性和耐受性的临床研究[36]。

老年患者的评估:老年评估

1989 年在一次共识会议上,"老年评估"一词被定义为"多学科、跨学科、可识别患者问题的患者评估”[37]。该评估包括评估老年患者的功能状态（在家和社区中独立生活的能力）、合并症、认知、心理状况、社会功能和支持、药物审查及营养状况（表 73-4）。这项全面的评估可以确认薄弱环节，并制定针对这些领域的多学科计划。此外，老年评估还提供了有关老年患者发病和死亡预后因素的有价值信息[38]。下一节将回顾老年评估的各个领域。

表 73-4　全面的老年评估的关键因素

功能状态	社会功能与支持
并存的医学状况	社会经济学问题
认知	药物评价
心理状态	营养状态

功能状态

功能状态的评估包括对个体在家庭和社区中独立生活能力的评估。传统的评估方法是“日常生活活动”（activities of daily living，ADL）和“日常生活辅助活动”（instrumental activities of daily living，IADL）（表 73-5）。ADL 是基本的自理能力，如洗澡、穿衣、上厕所、转移、保持身体健康和自给自足的能力。这些活动对维持在家中的生活自理能力至关重要。ADL 的辅助需求已预示着认知障碍和更多的资源需求[39]，疗养院的安置[40]，住院时间的延长，以及在医院中功能恶化[41]。

表 73-5　功能状态评估

日常生活活动	日常生活辅助活动
洗澡	打电话
穿衣	旅行
如厕	购物
转移	做饭
大小便	做家务
吃饭	吃药
	理财

日常生活辅助活动包括哪些使其在社区中独立生活的自理技能。其中包括打电话，购物，旅行，做饭，做家务，吃药和理财的能力。在 *Reuben* 及其懂事对 282 例 64 岁及以上人群中进行的一项研究中，IADL（如家务、购物、开车，按照连续变量评分）的独立性是死亡率的独立预测因素（$P<0.0001$）[42]。对 IADL 的辅助需求可预测发生认知障碍的风险[43]。需要 IADL 辅助的个体通常需要帮助以维持社区的独立性。

老年患者中癌症与日常活动中辅助需求量增加相关。在一项针对老年患者的大型研究中，与非癌症患者相比，癌症患者在 ADL 和 IADL 中的局限性更大，且需要更多的医疗保健服务[44,45]。在老年癌症患者中，IADL 的辅助需求与更差的总生存期[46,47]和化疗毒性风险增加相关[48-50]。例如，老年肺癌患者的 IADL 辅助需求和较差的生活质量与较差的总生存期相关[47]。在一项关于老年卵巢癌的研究中，化疗毒性的预测因子包括不良的工作状态（ECOG 评分<2）和功能依赖性（定义为在家中生活需要协助或在专业机构中生活需要协助）[51]。

合并疾病

合并症定义为同时发生的与发病和死亡有关的医学问题。在 *Yancik* 及其同事的一项研究收集了 7 600 例≥55 岁患者的合并症汇总数据。最常见的合并症包括高血压（42.9%），心脏相关疾病（39.1%）和关节炎（34.9%）。合并症随着年龄的增长而增加。55~64 岁的患者平均患有 2.9 种合并症，65~74 岁的患者患有 3.6 种合并症，75 岁及以上的患者患有 4.2 种合并症（表 73-6）[3]。癌症患者合并症与生存的相关性与患者的功能状态无关[52]。因此，每个都是重要的评估领域。随着年龄的增长及预期寿命下降，新疾病致死亡率的潜在影响也随之降低[53]。比如，可以想象下 5 年内预期死亡率为 50% 的疾病对 65 岁以下人群或者 85 岁的人的影响。这种疾病会使 65 岁的人的平均寿命减少大约 10 年，而由于 85 岁的人的绝对预期寿命比 65 岁的人短，它仅会使 85 岁的人的平均预期寿命降低约 2 年[53]。*Piccirillo* 等[54]进行的一项研究对 27 000 多名患者进行了评估，结果表明，在癌症患者中，合并症的平均数量和严重程度随着年龄的增长而增加。

表 73-6　主要条件的等级顺序，大于研究样本量的 10%

条件	百分比
高血压	42.9
心脏相关条件	39.1
关节炎	34.9
胃肠道疾病	31.0
贫血	22.6
眼睛疾病	19.0
尿道	18.0
癌症史	15.4
膀胱疾病	14.9
慢性阻塞性肺疾病	14.5
糖尿病	12.8
骨折	10.8
腺疾病	10.6

来源：Yancik 1997.[3] Reproduced with permission from John Wiley & Sons.

合并症的水平已被证实会影响乳腺癌手术治疗后的功能恢复。在一项针对老年乳腺癌妇女的研究中，患有 2 种以上合并症的妇女在手术后独立完成 IADL 的可能性较小，并且在完成需要上身力量的任务时遇到困难的可能性更大[55]。

合并症也影响接受化疗的可能性和化疗耐受性。来自监测、流行病学和结果数据库（SEER 数据库）的数据表明，合并心力衰竭，糖尿病或慢性阻塞性肺病的老年结肠癌患者接受辅助化疗的可能性较小[56]。在老年患者的临床试验中，合并症多的成年肺癌患者更有可能中断化疗[57]。

营养

营养状况差是功能依赖性和生存的独立预测因子。在一项针对214位社区老年人的前瞻性队列研究中，低体重指数(定义为体重指数<22kg/m^2)与ADL依赖相关[比值比1.21；95%置信区间1.01~1.45]。调整可能的混杂因素(包括年龄，性别，心理状况，合并症和功能依赖性)后，体重指数<22kg/m^{2}与1年生存率降低相关[相对风险比(RR)0.85，95%CI 0.74~0.97][58]。但是，也有数据得出相悖的结果，住院的成年人中，BMI≥30与较好的4年全因死亡率相关，而BMI较低与死亡率升高无关[59]。

在一项针对4 714名65岁及以上社区老年人的研究中记录了其3年间的体重变化。体重变化(定义为3年内体重减少或增加5%或以上)可见于34.6%的女性和27.3%的男性。受试者中体重减轻的比例高于体重增加的比例。体重减轻与死亡风险增加相关(危险比=1.67，95%CI=1.29~2.15)[60]。

一项针对美国东部肿瘤协作组(Eastern Cooperative Oncology Group，ECOG)化疗试验的3 047名患者的研究评估了癌症患者无意的体重减轻的预后影响。化疗前6个月内体重减轻与生存期较差相关(在12种肿瘤的9种中具有统计学意义)。此外，体重减轻与化疗反应率低有关(仅在乳腺癌患者中显著)。在除胰腺癌和胃癌外的其他类型肿瘤中，体重减轻均与体力状况下降有关[61]。

认知

痴呆是生存的独立预后因素[62,63]。Wolfson和同事的一项研究中，对10 263名65岁以上老年人进行了痴呆筛查。其中，有821人被诊断出阿尔茨海默病，可能患有阿尔茨海默病或患有血管性痴呆。这些患者的中位生存期为3.3年(如果诊断为阿尔茨海默病，则为3.1年；如果为可疑的阿尔茨海默病，则为3.5年；如果为血管性痴呆，则为3.3年)[63]。

对老年癌症患者的认知基线评估很重要，原因有几个。首先，如果一个人的记忆力快速变化或出现新的认知缺陷，则应排除脑转移性疾病。其次，在制定治疗计划时需要考虑认知障碍的程度。例如，认知障碍患者应谨慎使用任何口服药物，尤其是化疗药物。口服化疗药物的正确剂量与静脉化疗一样重要，因此，如果患者服用剂量不正确，可能发生严重的副作用，甚至是致命的。患者家人或护理人员在维持患者安全方面发挥着至关重要的作用。认知障碍患者可能需要帮助来记住止吐药等支持性药物的说明。护理人员需意识到需要医疗关注的治疗的潜在副作用。认知障碍的存在与住院风险增加和化疗耐受性较弱相关[49,64]。

心理状态和社会支持

与年轻患者相比，老年癌症患者通常表现出更好的心理功能。在诊断乳腺癌后，与年轻女性相比，老年女性心理状态更健康、更幸福[65]。对于65岁以下女性，与最近的乳腺癌相比，近期诊断乳腺癌相比于诊断乳腺癌5年，可显著增加焦虑和抑郁，并打击自信心。相比之下，对于年龄≥65岁的女性，近期诊断乳腺癌，与诊断乳腺癌5年的女性相比，并没有影响其焦虑、抑郁或自信心[66,67]。

社会支持在老年患者的心理功能中起着重要作用。所有年龄段乳腺癌女性严重心理困扰的重要预测指标包括离婚或分居以及社会支持减少[68]。社会支持可以缓解压力性生活事件对心理的影响。

此外，社交孤立是死亡率的独立预测因子。Seeman及其同事进行的一项研究证明了这一观点，他们研究了4种社会支持措施的重要性：①婚姻状况；②与两个或更多亲密朋友/亲戚的亲密接触；③定期去教堂做礼拜；④参加其他类型的团体。社会关系的存在与生存有关，无关年龄。在3个社区的群体中，与参与4个社交关系相比，没有社交关系的男性和女性的五年死亡率的相对危险度增加1.97~3.06倍[68]。在另一项针对282名65岁及以上患者的研究中，独自生活是独立的死亡预测风险[42]。

药物审查：复方用药评估

审查患者的药品清单是老年医学评估的重要组成部分。此外，必须考虑新开的药物是否会引起不良反应或药物间相互作用。老年患者比年轻患者更容易发生药物不良事件[19]。老年患者中约有五分之一的入院是由于药物不良事件。部分原因是老年患者使用药物比年轻患者多。老年癌症患者使用药物的平均数目为5±4个[69]。

随着年龄增长而发生的药代动力学和药效学变化，增加了药物不良反应的风险。这些变化应考虑药物(包括化疗)的剂量。胃肠道会随着年龄变化，如胃酸分泌减少和黏膜绒毛减少。体积分布也发生显著变化，包括体内脂肪增加(导致脂溶性药物的代谢减慢)，体内总水分减少(导致水溶性药物的血浆水平升高)，干体重减少，血清白蛋白减少，血红蛋白减少。继发于肝脏容量减少和肝血流量减少，肝代谢随着年龄的增长而变化。Ⅰ期肝反应(氧化，脱氨基，羟基化)随老龄化而降低。这些包括通过细胞色素P-450介导的反应，在老年患者中减少约30%。随着年龄的增长，Ⅱ期肝反应(结合：乙酰化，葡萄糖醛酸化，硫酸化)没有显著变化[19-21]。肾质在整个寿命期内减少25%~30%，从而导致功能性肾单位数量减少。因此，随着年龄的增长，肾小球滤过、肾小管分泌和重吸收减少。因此，依赖肾脏清除的药物在老年患者中具有更长的半衰期，并且可能需要根据肌酐清除率调整药物剂量。

综合的老年医学评估

老年评估是对老年患者进行全方位评估的方法，针对上述领域评估：功能状态，合并症，认知，营养状态，心理状态和社会支持，以及药物审查。关于这项评估价值的研究一直存在争论。但是，Stuck及其同事对对照试验进行的荟萃分析表明，老年医学评估是有益处的。28项对照研究的荟萃分析包括4 959名受试者和4 912名对照者，随机分配到五个综合的老年病评估项目之一，证实老年医学评估和管理(老年医学评估和康复的住院单元)降低6个月内死亡率35%，家庭评估服务(在家中的老年医学评估)通过早期发现和治疗，降低36个月内死亡率14%[70]。最近发表的一项有关住院和门诊老年医学评估和管理多中心随机对照试验表明,老年医学评估和管理减少功能下降并改善心理健康,但对生存没有影响[71]。

在老年癌症患者护理领域,老年医学评估是研究的热点。老年癌症患者的老年医学评估相关的系统评价表明,在肿瘤实践中,老年医学评估是可行的,并且可以辨别有风险的老年患者的不良预后;然而,还需要对老年医学评估对肿瘤学决策和干预措施的影响进行进一步的研究以改善其结局[72,73]。Balducci[74]研究了老年癌症患者评估中的老年医学评估,发现该评估通过识别以下受损来辨别同龄老年癌症患者的特征:功能状态的依赖性(18% ADL,72% IADL),严重的合并症[Charlson量表为36%,累积疾病评定量表(老年病)为94%],记忆障碍(22%),营养不良(19%),多重用药(41%)。Garman[75]等对老年病学评估和管理住院部收治的老年癌症患者进行了回顾性图表综述,其中使用了全面的老年病学评估来确定治疗目标。这些目标在超过75%的病例中得以实现:73%的症状管理、79%的功能改善和100%的处理和护理支持。其他研究已经表明,老年评估领域可以预测癌症老年患者的生存和化疗毒性[47,51]。老年评估和干预可以改善癌症老年患者的疼痛控制、心理健康和情绪健康[76]。

从老年评估中获得的信息可能对肿瘤科医生有价值,有以下一些原因。首先,这将有助于临床医生了解患者的"功能年龄"。其次,它可以识别出功能衰退或治疗毒性高风险的患者,针对性的干预可能对其有益。最后,它将在临床试验中,提供有价值的老年患者信息,使我们能够标准化研究中的患者特征,并控制可能导致死亡的混杂因素。

传统的全面老年医学评估是一项多学科评估,可能需要2小时完成。由于费时,在繁忙的肿瘤学实践中通常是不可行的。因此,其他老年医学评估手段也正在研究中。B组癌症和白血病(Cancer and Leukemia Group B,CALGB)正在开发一种简短的老年医学评估工具。试点数据表明,这种简短而全面的,主要自我管理的老年医学评估问卷对于门诊肿瘤诊所[77]和合作组[78]是可行的。老年评估将在随后的临床试验中作为基线信息收集。其他作者报告了在就诊之前,邮寄问卷给患者进行老年评估的可行性[79,80]。目前有几种简单的老年评估筛查工具可供使用。但是,关于识别受益于更详细的老年医学评估的患者的最佳筛查工具尚无共识[34]。

在*Cohen*和DeMaria[81]开发的"综合老年医学模型"中一个拟议的框架描述了决策者对老年癌症患者需要考虑的因素。该模型总结了对老年患者护理至关重要的方面,包括可能影响患者、疾病和预后的社会、心理和生物学因素。在此模型中,实足年龄在随着老龄化而发生的功能储备下降中发挥着作用,但是随后的因素,包括个体患者特有的生物学、社会和心理因素,会被纳入决策制定。这是一个动态过程,其中一个域的改变随后会影响模型中的其他域。

有关老年癌症患者的知识:临床试验中代表性不足

尽管人口老龄化以及癌症与衰老的关系,有关治疗老年癌症患者的治疗获益和风险的数据仍然有限。这个源于参与临床试验的老年患者有限。西南肿瘤小组分析了从1993年到1996年的164项临床试验,包含了16 396例患者。他们发现临床试验中只有25%的患者年龄在65岁以上。这一代表性不足的结果,包含除淋巴瘤外的15种癌症。老年乳腺癌患者的情况最少,只有9%的患者年龄在65岁以上[82]。

在加拿大的试验中,也发现了有关老年患者代表性不足的类似数据。分析了从1993年到1996年按年龄划分的临床实验。58%的加拿大癌症患者,年龄≥65岁,而接受试验的患者中只有22%的年龄≥65岁[83]。

随着年龄的增长临床试验的代表性越差。美国国家癌症研究所分析了≥65岁的患者和≥75岁的患者的入组情况。分析了500项治疗试验中的23 000例患者数据。他们发现在临床试验中,65岁以上的患者代表性不足;但是对于≥75岁的患者,这一点更为明显。在临床试验中,只有11%的男性年龄在75岁以上,而只有5%的女性年龄在75岁以上。值得注意的是老年乳腺癌患者中,只有2.7%是年龄在75岁以上的。这项研究表明,随着年龄的增长,临床试验的代表性越差[84]。2001年至2011年的NCI成人合作组临床试验总结,结果显示老年人的代表性持续下降[36]。

了解临床试验入选的阻力

CALGB老年癌症委员会开展了一项研究,以了解老年患者参与癌症治疗试验的障碍。年龄小于65岁和≥65岁的乳腺癌女性患者通过医师和分期进行配对。该试验试图确定对每个组参与临床试验的频率以及在试验中接受治疗的可能性。结果表明,与年轻女性相比,老年女性被邀请参与临床试验的可能性较小(51%<65岁 vs 35%≥65岁;$P=0.06$),但是如果被邀请的话,老年女性患者接受的可能性与年龄较小的女性患者接受的可能性差不多(56%<65岁与50%≥65岁;$P=0.67$)。医师未邀请老年患者参与临床试验的原因:①医师担心老年患者治疗的毒性;②医师担心合并症的影响[85]。最常见医师建议的改善老年患者增加临床试验的方法包括:提供临床人员向老年患者及其家人解释试验;提供有关临床试验的教育材料给患者及其家人;以及提供交通工具使老年患者更易参加到临床试验中[86,87]。

老年人癌症筛查

国家组织发布了整个公众的筛选建议;但是很少有人提供老年人癌症筛查的指南。此外,干预筛查相关的随机试验很少包括有意义的老年人样本。美国老年医学会(American Geriatrics Society,AGS)建议癌症筛查应根据患者个性化,而不是严格按照年龄来指导,需考虑到患者的个性化,预期寿命以及筛查测试的风险和获益。在"明智选择"运动的近期意见中,他们建议不要对预期寿命少于10年的前列腺癌,结肠癌或乳腺癌患者进行例行的筛查[88]。帮助引导与患者讨论癌症的平均风险的指南在下节进行了概述。

乳腺癌

传统上,乳腺癌筛查包括乳房X线摄影,临床乳房检查以及乳房自我检查。美国癌症协会(American Cancer Society,

ACS)建议,只要女性身体健康并且是接受治疗的候选人,就应继续进行乳腺癌筛查[89]。AGS 建议不要对预期寿命少于 10 年的女性进行筛查。在最近对老年女性进行乳房 X 线筛查的综述中,建议停止对预期寿命少于 10 年的女性进行乳房 X 线筛查[90]。我们建议仅对估计生存期至少为 10 年的老年女性进行年度或每两年一次筛查。

宫颈癌

ACS 宫颈癌筛查指南建议,如果女性过去 10 年内(有最近 5 年的最新试验)有 3 次或 3 次以上有记录的连续的正常的巴氏涂片或两次或多次连续的巴氏涂片和 HPV 检测,则 65 岁及以上的女性可以停止巴氏涂片筛查[91]。美国预防服务工作队建议停止对经过足够筛查且结果正常的 65 岁及 65 岁以上女性进行细胞学筛查[89]。

前列腺癌

前列腺癌的筛查包括直肠指检和前列腺特异性抗原(prostate specific antigen,PSA)检测。ACS 建议对一般风险的预期寿命至少为 10 年的男性患者,从 50 岁开始进行前列腺癌年度筛查,同时进行直肠指检和 PSA 检测。应与患者讨论检测的益处和局限性,以便做出有关筛查的知情决定。美国预防服务工作在 2012 年更新的指南中建议不考虑年龄进行前列腺癌 PSA 筛查[92]。我们同意 AGS 的建议,建议仅在预期寿命超过 10 年的男性中讨论筛查的风险和益处[93]。

结肠癌

ACS 建议一般风险的成年人从 50 岁开始筛查大肠癌。结肠癌筛查有很多选择,包括每年的粪便潜血测试,每 5 年一次乙状结肠镜检查,每年的粪便潜血测试加每 5 年一次乙状结肠镜检查,每 10 年一次结肠镜检查或每 5 年一次结肠钡剂双对比造影[89]。美国预防服务工作队认为停止大肠癌筛查的合适年龄是不明的,因为筛查研究通常仅限于 80 岁以下的患者[94]。他们建议在年龄或合并症限制预期寿命的患者中停止筛查[95]。我们支持 AGS,不建议对预期寿命少于 10 年的患者进行筛查[93]。

肺癌

ACS 建议在 55~74 岁健康且有 30 年包的现吸烟者和前吸烟者进行肺癌筛查[91]。在这一人群中,应仔细说明筛查的风险和益处[96],应将戒烟作为重中之重。美国胸外科协会和 USPSTF 将筛查的年龄上限分别提高到 79 岁和 80 岁[97,98]。我们同意将年龄上限提高到 80 岁。

老年患者的治疗耐受性

手术

手术是大多数实体瘤的主要治疗方法。无论年龄大小,不能进行明确的手术治疗都会增加疾病死亡率。例如,在英国癌症研究乳腺癌试验小组进行的一项研究中,将 455 名年龄在 70 岁以上且患有可手术的乳腺癌的妇女,随机分配到单独接受他莫昔芬治疗与他莫昔芬联合手术治疗。在 12.7 年的随访中,未接受手术的女性乳腺癌死亡率增加(危险比 1.68;95% CI 1.15~2.47)[99]。因此,如果可能的话,老年妇女应进行乳腺癌的初级手术切除以降低其乳腺癌死亡的风险。

几项研究表明,高龄不应成为拒绝接受结直肠癌手术治疗的理由[100-103]。腹腔镜手术或在紧急情况下进行的手术会增加手术并发症发生率和死亡率的风险;但是,即使在这些高风险情况下,老年患者也可以从手术管理中获益。在一项紧急结直肠手术研究中,年龄较大和较年轻的患者具有相似的初级切除率(95%>70 岁,89%≤70 岁;$P=0.70$)和初级吻合率(84%>70 岁,78%≥70 岁;$P=0.64$)。老年患者术后心肺并发症的发生率较高,但死亡率无统计学差异(9%>70 岁,5%≥70 岁;$P=0.48$)[100]。PACE 工具利用老年评估项目来识别有手术并发症风险的癌症老年患者[104,105]。

放射治疗

放射治疗通常用于老年患者的可治愈的和姑息的治疗。研究表明,年轻和老年患者的治疗耐受性相似[106,107]。在对 1 208 例接受胸腔照射的患者的研究中,年龄对急性或迟发的放射毒性没有影响。患者被分为 6 个年龄段,范围从<50 到>70。在急性放射毒性影响下并无显著差异,如恶心、呼吸困难、食管炎或虚弱,各年龄组的生存也无显著差异($P=0.82$)。老年患者比起年轻患者更容易出现体重减轻($P=0.002$)[107]。因此,应密切注意接受放射治疗的老年患者的营养状况。

放射治疗的的耐受性和疗效在"最老的"患者中也被证实了。在对 191 名≥80 岁的患者进行的回顾性研究中,有 94%的患者能够完成治疗且没有并发症。77%接受可治愈性治疗的患者和 81%接受姑息治疗的患者对治疗均得到了缓解反应。6%的患者因腹泻、吞咽困难或疾病进展导致体重减轻而需要中断治疗。这种情况更常见于接受大范围治疗的患者。在接受消化道癌症治疗的患者中,20%的患者患有 3 级黏膜炎,2%的患者患有 4 级黏膜炎,这增加了对老年患者的营养状况和体重减轻的关注需求[108]。

其他研究试图确定是否有某一亚组低危老年患者可以免除放射治疗。CALGB 进行的一项研究将 636 名年龄在 70 岁及以上、临床Ⅰ期、雌激素受体阳性进行了肿块切除术的乳腺癌老年患者,对患处的乳腺进行了放射治疗和他莫昔芬治疗或单独使用他莫昔芬。仅接受他莫昔芬治疗的妇女在 5 年的随访中局部复发率更高:单独使用他莫昔芬组的患者复发率为 4%,而他莫昔芬和放疗组的患者复发率为 1%($P<0.001$);然而,乳腺癌特异性死亡率或 5 年总生存率没有差异[109]。

化学疗法

几项研究试图确定化学疗法是否对于老年患者毒性更大[110]。皮埃蒙特肿瘤学协会的一项研究是一项纳入转移性乳腺癌女性的病例对照研究。按年龄将女性分为 3 组:<50 岁,50~69 岁和>70 岁。研究表明,临床试验中接受治疗的老年妇女中毒性作用,给药剂量或延迟给药的发生率与年轻女性相比并无显著差异。此外,治疗反应、疾病进展时间或生存率也无差异。因此,在临床试验中接受治疗的老年妇女不仅可以耐受治疗,而且同样可以从治疗中获益[111]。伊利诺伊州癌症中心进行的Ⅱ期临床试验的分析也发现了相似的结果。老年患者和年轻患者的毒性反应无差异,无需降低剂量、中断治疗或延迟治疗[112]。此外,对治疗的反应没有差异。反之,3 项 CALGB 临床试验的分析表明,对于淋巴结阳性的乳腺癌患者进行辅助治疗的老年人更有可能出现 4 级血液学毒性,并且而更可能因毒性反应中止治疗。此外,老年人更有可能死于急性骨髓性白血病或骨髓增生异常综合征[113]。

这些研究结果解读的局限性在于未收集老年评估信息。因此,尚不清楚参加这些临床试验的老年患者是否代表日常接受护理的患者。由于很少有老年患者参加临床试验,因此参加临床试验的老年患者可能具有较年轻的“功能年龄”。因此,将老年医学评估纳入临床试验将是一种有价值的方法使拥有相同实足年龄这一混杂因素的患者标准化,有助于确定患者所代表的“功能年龄”。针对老年人的临床试验是必要的,以优化对该患者群体的护理。选择罹患某些疾病(乳腺癌、结肠癌、中级淋巴瘤等)的老年患者的建立登记表,并对其进行以治愈为目标的化学治疗,这将提供一个用于评估护理模式和疗效的数据库。

幸存者

随着越来越多的老年人罹患癌症以及治疗的改善,老年癌症幸存者的数量也在增加。据估计,到 2020 年,三分之二的癌症幸存者将超过 65 岁。老年癌症幸存者正面临其老年生理学,多种慢性病累积,老年综合征,癌症的同时和交互影响,癌症后遗症以及癌症治疗后遗症[114]。后者对多器官系统的影响可能在一定程度上模仿了老龄化的表型[114]。要应对这一棘手的情况,需要肿瘤学家和初级护理人员间进行有效的信息交换。以共享的、全面的老年医学评估为基础的面向老年医学生存护理计划可能是实现此目标的最有效方法[115,116]。患者也可以发挥作用,并以癌症生存状况作为指导,除了仔细随访之外,还可以通过针对生活方式的干预来改善预后[117]。

总结

癌症是一种严重影响老年患者的疾病。临床试验中的老年患者代表性不足,导致有关这类患者护理的数据有限。从发展的角度,应努力将老年患者纳入临床试验,以更加了解护理这类不断增多的人群的最理想方法。在老年患者的护理中引入老年医学评估将提供有关区分两个实足年龄相同患者预后的信息,从而帮助我们理解“功能年龄”和化疗副作用的风险。综合来说,已开发出针对老年肿瘤患者的全面的老年医学评估筛选工具。

(谷俊杰 译,白春梅 审校)

参考文献

The complete reference list can be found on the Wiley Companion Digital Edition of this title (see inside front cover for login instructions).

3 Yancik R. Cancer burden in the aged: an epidemiologic and demographic overview. *Cancer*. 1997;**80**:1273–1283.

11 Liu Y, Johnson SM, Fedoriw Y, et al. Expression of p16(INK4a) prevents cancer and promotes aging in lymphocytes. *Blood*. 2011;**117**:3257–3267.

12 Finkel T, Serrano M, Blasco MA. The common biology of cancer and ageing. *Nature*. 2007;**448**:767–774.

13 Irminger-Finger I. Science of cancer and aging. *J Clin Oncol*. 2007b;**25**:1844–1851.

16 Campisi J. Aging, cellular senescence, and cancer. *Annu Rev Physiol*. 2013;**75**: 685–705.

24 Leng SX, Xue QL, Tian J, Walston JD, Fried LP. Inflammation and frailty in older women. *J Am Geriatr Soc*. 2007;**55**:864–871.

25 Walston J, Mcburnie MA, Newman A, et al. Frailty and activation of the inflammation and coagulation systems with and without clinical comorbidities: results from the Cardiovascular Health Study. *Arch Intern Med*. 2002;**162**:2333–2341.

26 Cohen HJ, Pieper CF, Harris T, Rao KM, Currie MS. The association of plasma IL-6 levels with functional disability in community-dwelling elderly. *J Gerontol A Biol Sci Med Sci*. 1997;**52**:M201–M208.

27 Cohen HJ. In search of the underlying mechanisms of frailty. *J Gerontol A Biol Sci Med Sci*. 2000;**55**:706–708.

28 Cohen HJ, Harris T, Pieper CF. Coagulation and activation of inflammatory pathways in the development of functional decline and mortality in the elderly. *Am J Med*. 2003;**114**:180–187.

29 Fried LP, Tangen CM, Walston J, et al. Frailty in older adults: evidence for a phenotype. *J Gerontol A Biol Sci Med Sci*. 2001;**56**:M146–M156.

31 Rockwood K, Mitnitski A. Frailty in relation to the accumulation of deficits. *J Gerontol A Biol Sci Med Sci*. 2007;**62**:722–727.

33 Song X, Mitnitski A, Rockwood K. Prevalence and 10-year outcomes of frailty in older adults in relation to deficit accumulation. *J Am Geriatr Soc*. 2010;**58**:681–687.

34 Decoster L, Van Puyvelde K, Mohile S, et al. Screening tools for multidimensional health problems warranting a geriatric assessment in older cancer patients: an update on SIOG recommendationsdagger. *Ann Oncol*. 2014;**26**(**2**):288–300.

36 Hurria A, Dale W, Mooney M, et al. Designing therapeutic clinical trials for older and frail adults with cancer: U13 conference recommendations. *J Clin Oncol*. 2014;**32**(**24**):2587–2594.

38 Wildiers H, Heeren P, Puts M, et al. International Society of Geriatric Oncology Consensus on Geriatric Assessment in Older Patients With Cancer. *J Clin Oncol*. 2014;**32**:2595.

44 Mohile SG, Xian Y, Dale W, et al. Association of a cancer diagnosis with vulnerability and frailty in older Medicare beneficiaries. *J Natl Cancer Inst*. 2009;**101**:1206–1215.

47 Maione P, Perrone F, Gallo C, et al. Pretreatment quality of life and functional status assessment significantly predict survival of elderly patients with advanced non-small-cell lung cancer receiving chemotherapy: a prognostic analysis of the multicenter Italian lung cancer in the elderly study. *J Clin Oncol*. 2005;**23**:6865–6872.

48 Hurria A, Togawa K, Mohile SG, et al. Predicting chemotherapy toxicity in older adults with cancer: a prospective multicenter study. *J Clin Oncol*. 2011b;**29**:3457–3465.

50 Extermann M, Boler I, Reich RR, et al. Predicting the risk of chemotherapy toxicity in older patients: the Chemotherapy Risk Assessment Scale for High-Age Patients (CRASH) score. *Cancer*. 2012;**118**:3377–3386.

51 Freyer G, Geay JF, Touzet S, et al. Comprehensive geriatric assessment predicts tolerance to chemotherapy and survival in elderly patients with advanced ovarian carcinoma: a GINECO study. *Ann Oncol*. 2005;**16**:1795–1800.

53 Welch HG, Albertsen PC, Nease RF, Bubolz TA, Wasson JH. Estimating treatment benefits for the elderly: the effect of competing risks. *Ann Intern Med*. 1996;**124**:577–584.

56 Gross CP, Mcavay GJ, Guo Z, Tinetti ME. The impact of chronic illnesses on the use and effectiveness of adjuvant chemotherapy for colon cancer. *Cancer*. 2007;**109**:2410–2419.

57 Frasci G, Lorusso V, Panza N, et al. Gemcitabine plus vinorelbine versus vinorelbine alone in elderly patients with advanced non-small-cell lung cancer. *J Clin Oncol*. 2000;**18**:2529–2536.

67 Kornblith AB, Dowell JM, Herndon JE 2nd, et al. Telephone monitoring of distress in patients aged 65 years or older with advanced stage cancer: a cancer and leukemia group B study. *Cancer*. 2006;**107**:2706–2714.

70 Stuck AE, Siu AL, Wieland GD, Adams J, Rubenstein LZ. Comprehensive geriatric assessment: a meta-analysis of controlled trials. *Lancet*. 1993;**342**: 1032–1036.

71 Cohen HJ, Feussner JR, Weinberger M, et al. A controlled trial of inpatient and outpatient geriatric evaluation and management. *N Engl J Med*. 2002;**346**: 905–912.

73 Puts MT, Santos B, Hardt J, et al. An update on a systematic review of the use of geriatric assessment for older adults in oncology. *Ann Oncol*. 2014;**25**:307–315.

76 Rao AV, Hsieh F, Feussner JR, Cohen HJ. Geriatric evaluation and management units in the care of the frail elderly cancer patient. *J Gerontol A Biol Sci Med Sci*. 2005;**60**:798–803.

78 Hurria A, Cirrincione CT, Muss HB, et al. Implementing a geriatric assessment in cooperative group clinical cancer trials: CALGB 360401. *J Clin Oncol*. 2011a;**29**:1290–1296.

79 Ingram SS, Seo PH, Martell RE, et al. Comprehensive assessment of the elderly cancer patient: the feasibility of self-report methodology. *J Clin Oncol*. 2002;**20**:770–775.

82 Hutchins LF, Unger JM, Crowley JJ, Coltman CA Jr, Albain KS. Underrepresentation of patients 65 years of age or older in cancer- treatment trials. *N Engl J Med.* 1999;**341**:2061–2067.

85 Kemeny MM, Peterson BL, Kornblith AB, et al. Barriers to clinical trial participation by older women with breast cancer. *J Clin Oncol.* 2003;**21**:2268–2275.

86 Dale W, Mohile SG, Eldadah BA, et al. Biological, clinical, and psychosocial correlates at the interface of cancer and aging research. *J Natl Cancer Inst.* 2012;**104**:581–589.

87 Kornblith AB, Kemeny M, Peterson BL, et al. Survey of oncologists' perceptions of barriers to accrual of older patients with breast carcinoma to clinical trials. *Cancer.* 2002;**95**:989–996.

90 Walter LC, Schonberg MA. Screening mammography in older women: a review. *JAMA.* 2014;**311**:1336–1347.

95 U.S. Preventive Services Task Force. Screening for colorectal cancer: recommendation and rationale. *Ann Intern Med.* 2002;**137**:129–131.

104 Audisio RA, Participants P, Pope D, Ramesh HSJ, Gennari R, Van Leeuwen BL. Shall we operate? Preoperative assessment in elderly cancer patients (PACE) can help - A SIOG surgical task force prospective study. *Crit Rev Oncol Hematol.* 2008;**65**:156–163.

113 Muss HB, Berry DA, Cirrincione C, et al. Toxicity of older and younger patients treated with adjuvant chemotherapy for node-positive breast cancer: the Cancer and Leukemia Group B Experience. *J Clin Oncol.* 2007;**25**:3699–3704.

117 Demark-Wahnefried W, Morey MC, Sloane R, et al. Reach out to enhance wellness home-based diet-exercise intervention promotes reproducible and sustainable long-term improvements in health behaviors, body weight, and physical functioning in older, overweight/obese cancer survivors. *J Clin Oncol.* 2012;**30**: 2354–2361.

第 74 章　癌症的健康差异

Otis W. Brawley, MD, MACP

概述

在过去的 50 年里,临床治疗疗效的差异越来越明显,这种差异在癌症中尤为凸显。肿瘤学是一门发展天翻地覆的学科,但是由于社会经济的差异,部分人群可能并没有享受到该学科所取得的进步。健康差异已发展成为流行病学的一个分支,它包含依据种族、地理地区、社会经济地位等划分的各类人群间差异,主要着眼于癌症风险、死亡风险、生存率和生存经历的不同。

许多研究表明,无论是按种族、社会经济学或其他主要因素对人群进行分类,同等治疗在相同患者中都会产生一样的效果。如果对具有相同遗传标记的人进行比较,种族在一般情况下不能作为研究转归的分类因素。许多医疗模式的研究表明,美国依然存在种族不平等。目前,健康差异这一分支已取得进展,包括对能够减少差异的干预措施进行评估。

精准医学和个体疗法的发展,使利用基因和多态性进行分类的方法更为重要。大致的种族和族裔的分类,甚至社会经济地位只有在涉及获取医疗服务和平等待遇等社会问题上才会产生一定的影响。

克服差异和实现公平的社会干预措施包括:①提高卫生保健者文化水平以及他们对患者的了解;②增加获得护理的机会;③增强沟通且对需要服务的人进行培训。

引言

在过去的 50 年里,医学领域特别是癌症的预防和治疗取得了巨大的进展,这使得人们越来越重视不同人群之间的治疗结果差异。20 世纪 60 年代末进行的第一项研究讨论了某些人群死于某些癌症的比率较高这一事实,并于 70 年代初发表[1,2]。这些研究指出,美国黑种人的死亡率高于白种人。随着这一问题得到更广泛的理解和相关学科的逐渐成熟,健康差距和健康公平成为一个政治问题。事实上,这对医疗改革立法以及美国政府资助的临床试验的设计和招募立法产生了影响。

报告和了解人群的癌症发病率和预后的差异非常重要。癌症的原因既有遗传因素,也有环境因素。当真正了解人口间差异,才能对导致或预防癌症的因素提出合理假说。通过对特定人群的研究,人们还可以增加对预防和治疗等干预性措施进行更深入的认识。

学科起源

美国国家癌症研究中心在 20 世纪 70 年代早期建立了监测、流行病学和终点结果(Surveillance, Epidemiology, and End Results, SEER)计划,将其作为国家癌症法案实施的一部分。这个项目从美国各地的人口登记处收集癌症发病率和死亡率数据。在 SEER 之前,癌症发病率数据非常有限。即使在今天,SEER 也没有提供一个具有充分代表性的国家样本来计算发病率。SEER 每年按种族和性别发布癌症发病率和死亡率数据以及 5 年生存率。数据可在 www. cancer. gov/statistics 上公开获取。

通过 20 世纪 80 年代和 90 年代的"黑白研究",SEER 清楚地记录了黑种人和白种人在癌症发病率、死亡率和生存率方面的种族差异。SEER 研究还显示,黑种人和白种人在治疗模式上存在差异,黑种人接受不适当癌症治疗的比例较高。

随着癌症差异的研究,心血管疾病特别是高血压的差异正在消除。人们对镰状细胞贫血这种遗传性血液病的兴趣正在增加。

这一学科最初被称为"少数人群健康研究",后来又被称为"特殊人群的研究"。现在它已经演变成"健康差异"的领域,有些人甚至把它称为"健康公平"。随着该领域的成熟,问题变得更加明确,一些解决方案也得到了更好的阐述。如今,健康差异已经是基础科学、临床科学、流行病学和社会科学的交叉学科。

健康差异的定义

美国国家癌症研究所(National Cancer Institute, NCI)将美国特定人群中存在的癌症的发病率、癌症罹患率、死亡率、存活率以及癌症负担或相关健康状况的差异定义为健康差异。换言之,即有些人比其他人的情况更糟。

衡量指标

健康差异是不同人群之间的差异。许多结果可以用来衡量和比较,最常见的有:

发病率——通常表示为人口中每 10 万人在某一年内被诊断为该病的人数。发病率相当于人口患病的风险。发病率较高的群体中的个人患这种疾病的风险较高。

死亡率——通常表示为每 10 万人口中某一年因某一疾病死亡的人数。死亡率相当于人口死于这种疾病的风险。来自疾病死亡率较高的群体死于该疾病的风险较高。

发病率和死亡率根据标准人群进行"年龄校正",以消除两个人群因年龄分布不同而产生的影响。通过年龄校正也可以消除随着时间的推移人口老龄化的影响。年龄是许多癌症的一个危险因素。1990 年人群按年龄调整的发病率比 1960 年高，并不是因为 1990 的人群存在更多的老年人。

生存率——一个队列从诊断到死亡的中位时间或 5 年生存率。

患病率——存在疾病或疾病危险因素的人口比例。

同时也对治疗模式（筛查和治疗）的差异进行了衡量。它指的是两个或两个以上组得到标准治疗的比例。在更复杂的分析中，这可能指的是一个组与另一个组相比获得高质量治疗的比例。

比较不常用的并且不在 NCI 定义中的衡量指标还包括病死率、并发症和生活质量方面的差异。

人群分类

虽然研究是从黑种人和白人开始的，但已经发展到了“人口”可以由种族、民族和文化、地理起源地区、社会经济地位（socioeconomic status，SES）和其他因素来定义的程度。很明显，明确界定人口在开展健康差异研究方面极为重要。

350 年前首次提出种族的概念。最初的分类是白种人、黑种人、非洲人、蒙古人或亚洲人[3]。这些分类与肤色、面部特征和生源地有关，不存在明显的种族群体，纯粹基于可见的特征，种族群体是重叠的群体。人类学界从未接受种族作为生物学范畴的分类方法。

美国行政管理和预算局（Office of Management and Budget，OMB）定义了种族概念，以用于政府数据收集。在十年一次的人口普查中，最重要的是使用 OMB 对种族的定义，但根据立法，它也用于描述联邦资助的临床试验中登记的人群。

OMB 指令特别指出，其种族类别反映了美国所承认的一种社会对种族的定义，这种定义并不是试图从生物学、人类学或遗传学上对一个种族进行定义。OMB 的种族定义随着时间的推移而改变。一个来自亚洲印度次大陆的人在 1950 年人口普查前移民到美国，在过去 65 年里被认为是 3 个不同的种族。目前使用的定义于 1997 年公布（表 74-1）。

在收集种族数据时，OMB 有一个“种族”问题。OMB 将种族划分为简单的“西班牙裔”或“非西班牙裔”。

美国国家癌症研究所 SEER 计划和疾病控制与预防中心的国家健康统计中心使用 OMB 定义发布健康数据。它们通过美国人口普查数据来计算发病率和死亡率。NCI SEER 发布的根据 OMB 种族/民族标准的死亡率趋势如图 74-1 所示。该图使用了 1990 年人口普查中的定义。

如果将种族视为社会定义，种族认定为收集数据有用类别的话，有些人口确实承受着不平等的负担。社会中确实存在公民权利问题，例如歧视和获得护理机会的差异。

学术研究中使用的种族和文化是一个非常宽泛的术语，涵盖了人类身份。它不是静态的或互斥的。它是动态的，没有明确的界限。在社会研究中，族群的区别在于明确了人类变异的性质和来源（例如行为、生活方式习惯和其他环境影响）及其与健康的关系。如果使用得当，一个民族的人口可以具有许多种族。

表 74-1　美国政府对 2000 年人口普查中种族和民族的定义

白种人	起源于在欧洲、中东或北非的人。包括那些表明自己的种族为“白种人”或者报告以下条目的人，如爱尔兰人、德国人、意大利人、黎巴嫩人、阿拉伯人、摩洛哥人或高加索人
黑种人或非裔美国人	起源于非洲任何一个黑人种族的人。包括那些表明自己的种族为“黑种人或非洲人”或报告以下条目的人，如非洲裔美国人、肯尼亚人、尼日利亚人或海地人
美国印第安人和阿拉斯加原住民	起源于北美和南美（包括中美洲）原始民族并保持部落关系的人。包括那些表明自己的种族为“美国印第安人或阿拉斯加原住民”或报告以下条目的人，如纳瓦霍人、黑脚人、因纽特人、尤伊克人，中美印第安人或南美印第安人
亚洲人	起源于远东、东南亚或印度次大陆（包括柬埔寨、中国、印度、日本、韩国、马来西亚、巴基斯坦、菲律宾群岛、泰国和越南）的原始民族的人。包括那些表明自己的种族为“亚洲印度人”“中国人”“菲律宾人”“韩国人”“日本人”“越南人”和“其他亚洲人”或者提供其他详细属于亚洲人回答的人
夏威夷土著和其他太平洋岛民	起源于夏威夷、关岛、萨摩亚群岛或其他太平洋岛屿的原始民族的人。包括那些表明自己的种族为“夏威夷土著人”“关岛人或查莫罗人”“萨摩亚人”和“其他太平洋岛民”或提供其他详细属于太平洋岛民回答的人

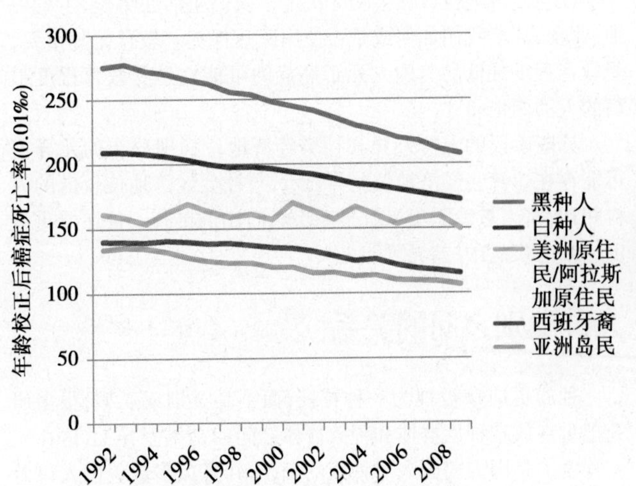

图 74-1　1990—2010 年经年龄调整的癌症死亡率（按 1990 年 OMB 种族/民族分类）。注：过去 20 年中，除美洲原住民/阿拉斯加原住民外，所有原住民的年龄调整死亡率均显著下降。美洲原住民/阿拉斯加原住民、西班牙裔和亚洲岛民的死亡率低于白种人，而白种人的死亡率低于黑种人。这个图表使用亚太岛民这一类别，这是 2000 年以前使用的类别。夏威夷土著人属于美洲土著/阿拉斯加土著

相较于种族，它是一种更科学的分类，因为它与环境因素有关，例如饮食可能增加或减少患病可能性的其他外部影响。种族和文化甚至也影响着诸如抽烟或从事性活动等习惯。

尽管种族和文化与导致癌症的因素有关，但种族和文化也影响着人们对疾病的接受程度以及人们寻求和接受治疗的方式。

按地理区域分类比种族更科学。许多人混淆了种族和地理起源区域这两个概念，这两者之间存在一些重叠。由于几个世纪以来人口的混合，许多人可能有几个地理起源地区。

许多遗传特征与地理起源区域相关。例如，镰状细胞病是地中海盆地和撒哈拉以南非洲地区人群的遗传病。来自西班牙、意大利、希腊、叙利亚、土耳其和黎巴嫩的人患有镰状细胞病。南部非洲人没有镰状细胞病。我们认为的白种人也可能会患此病，而黑种人也可能不会。

虽然某一遗传性状在某一特定地理区域的人群中可能具有较高的患病率，但更要认识到，一个地区较高的患病率并不意味着该地区人群会垄断该遗传性状。例如，囊性纤维化在北欧人群中更常见，但不限于北欧人群；酒精脱氢酶缺乏症也很常见，但不限于日本人群。

血统是另一种对人口进行分类的方法。血统当然与种族和地理起源有关。当人们跨越种族界限的时候，用种族分类可能会产生一些问题。在考虑血统的情况下，比较容易理解家庭和其他因素的作用。遗传的影响常常与血统同步。

在乳腺癌和前列腺癌中，黑种人和白种人的一些差异可能是基因上的差异，这种差异与血统或地理起源更相似，而不是种族。

社会经济地位由教育、收入和职业定义。虽然健康的社会是重要的决定因素，但对于如何利用社会经济地位来定义人类状态却争议很大。欧洲文学使用了一个叫做“剥夺”的概念。“剥夺指数”是在苏格兰十年一次的人口普查中计算出来的，它考虑了许多财富、教育和社会地位的指标[4]。

社会经济地位或社会剥夺决定了我们生活在哪里、生育习惯、饮食，甚至我们如何或是否使用医疗保健。教育尤其重要，受教育程度最低的美国人死于癌症的可能性是受教育程度最高的人的两倍多[5-7]。

诊断阶段的人群差异和社会经济地位病理分布的差异也可能存在。社会经济地位差异显示，与社会经济地位较低的人群相比，富人被诊断出患有早期疾病的比例更高。且在严重过度诊断的疾病中，差异可能更大。

人口类别之间的关系

种族更应该被视为一种特征，而不是类别或亚型；很多研究把重点放在种族群体和种族群体之间的结果差异上，这在一定程度上是因为美国人对种族的痴迷，并且大多数美国人口差异数据是基于美国政府对种族的定义来收集的。基于种族，SES或血统很难获得数据。尽管种族类别并非基于生物学，但它们确实有关，这是一种社会政治构造，可能与种族、地理区域和SES有关。

不幸的是，医学文献充斥着“种族医学化”。有许多论文表明遗传学定义了种族之间的差异，而这些差异是造成其他许多差异的原因[8]。但一些研究忽略了与种族相区别的血统，也忽略了种族和SES之间存在的明显关联。低SES可能是造成差异的原因，种族也可能与文化相关，从而影响行为习惯。而一些行为习惯会增加患病的风险。

尽管种族与癌症的发生之间可能存在相关性，但这种相关性不一定意味着因果关系。种族差异通常是由于社会问题，例如教育和医疗保健中的歧视。医学上的许多人错误地认为种族是一种生物学分类，认为种族是由基因定义的，镰状细胞病是遗传病。在美国，它曾经并且仍然被错误地视为“黑色疾病”。这有助于加强关于种族、遗传学和疾病风险的许多观点。在关于前列腺癌发病率和死亡率的讨论中，或者在黑人女性患三阴性乳腺癌的患病率高于白人的讨论中，我们经常听到种族是影响疾病的生物类别。

在描述上述类别时，由于缺乏明确的通用术语，从而难以收集有关不同/服务不足的人群的信息。SES通常包括教育和收入，甚至包括财富指标，但忽略了在社会等级中的地位。在欧洲社会科学概念中，贫困和贫困指数考虑了社会等级和社会经济地位。它是比SES更精确的衡量社会状况工具。

即使粗略的度量SES，种族和SES之间也存在明显的相关性。因此，SES对健康不良的结局的影响很容易被误认为是种族。事实上，研究人员经常在没有考虑潜在原因或贡献作用的情况下，将社会经济地位的测量结果放入模型中，或者在控制了一两个社会经济地位的测量结果后，得出种族/民族差异一定是遗传或文化的结论。

社会经济地位往往与某些癌症的高风险相关，因为穷人的患病风险与患病率较高。这些习惯往往是由于贫穷造成的。例如：

- 习惯性的高热量摄入、缺乏体育活动和肥胖与十几种癌症有关[9]。在美国，三分之一的癌症都是由这种三联症引起的，这在国际上是个日益严重的问题。在美国，社会经济地位低的人更容易肥胖[10]。受教育程度低和贫穷的人确实倾向于每天摄入更多的卡路里，因为加工过的高热量碳水化合物食物比低热量富含蛋白质的食物便宜[11]。
- 肺癌和一些与吸烟有关的癌症在穷人和中产阶级中更常见。与美国中产阶级的成年人相比，生活在贫困线以下的成年人更有可能吸烟（30%的美国人吸烟，有大学学位的美国人占6%）[12]。
- 穷人或社会经济地位较低的人不太可能获得医疗预防服务。调查显示，他们接受乳腺癌或结肠癌筛查的可能性较低[13]。社会经济地位、种族和文化可以共同增加风险，可以导致癌症像传染病一样在人群中流行。这可能导致该人群患癌症的风险增加。在人类乳头状瘤病毒导致的宫颈癌中，无法获得预防服务的女性已出现这种情况。东南亚人患肝癌的风险增加是另一个例子。肝癌与乙型肝炎有关，乙型肝炎的流行率很高[14]。也有研究表明，从亚洲低癌症风险地区迁移到美国的人群，在两代内增加了患癌症的风险[15]。

治疗模式的差异

许多早期健康差异研究的重点在于，在所接受的治疗质量方面存在显著差异。在最初的研究中，接受高质量治疗的白种人比例高于黑种人。研究表明，很多因素导致治疗的差异[16,17]。贫困、缺乏保险或社会剥夺公民权使患者面临接受质量低劣的医疗保健或得不到充分服务的风险[18]。

有些患者：

- 拒绝治疗，因为他们的文化拒绝接受或他们与医疗服务提供者存在文化差异。
- 由于文盲或缺乏医疗经验，难以坚持规范的治疗方案。
- 因为不方便获得护理而不能够坚持规范的治疗。
- 由于在不同人群中更常见的共病，不能接受首选的更积极的治疗。
- 由于种族主义或基于社会经济地位的歧视而得不到必要的照顾。

认识到这些问题是极其重要的，也是克服这些问题的最大障碍。对这些问题敏感的医疗保健提供者往往能够提供更好的服务[19]。有一种趋势是培训医生提供“满足文化背景”的护理[20]。美国临床肿瘤学协会和其他机构为来自不同背景的患者提供交流课程。

在乳腺癌研究中，研究发现一些群体更有可能接受质量较差的治疗。Lund 等[21]对亚特兰大大都市的治疗模式进行了研究。在两年（2000 年及 2001 年）中，通过评估被诊断为局限性乳腺癌的女性，他们发现 7%的黑种人和 2%的白种人在确诊后的第一年没有接受治疗。

其他研究表明，少数民族、缺乏教育、缺乏保险和较低的社会经济地位是变量，预示着患者更有可能不能够得到充分的护理[17,22]。当这些研究用逻辑回归评估时，无论种族，受教育较少的乳腺癌患者更有可能接受非标准的乳腺癌治疗方案，较少接受足够的化疗剂量[10,23]。肥胖乳腺癌患者接受足够剂量化疗的可能性也较低。

医疗质量的差异导致在预后和治疗上的差异

虽然种族似乎不是造成这些差异的直接原因，但确实黑种人或非裔美国妇女接受不规范癌症治疗的比例较高。这是因为与白种人相比，黑种人或非裔美国女性中接受高中教育程度以下的比例更高，肥胖比例也更高。大约 50%的黑种人女性肥胖，而白种人女性的肥胖比例为 34%。对受教育程度较低的人、穷人和肥胖者的不同对待，导致黑种人接受不到最佳医疗照顾的比例高于白种人。同样，相关性和因果关系之间的区别也很重要。

不同种族获得高质量医疗服务的机会不同，可能会导致结果的差异，而且这种差异不仅会引起结果差异，还会导致错误的假设。例如，美国的黑种人和白种人在癌症死亡率上存在差异。与白种人相比，黑种人在肿瘤每个阶段的死亡率都更高，5 年生存率更低。这使得一些人认为，结直肠癌在黑种人中更具有侵袭性。值得注意的是，黑种人和白种人结直肠死亡率在 20 世纪 70 年代非常相似，而自 1981 年以来，死亡率的差距逐年扩大。尽管两个种族的死亡率都在下降，但 2011 年的死亡率差距比以往任何时候都要大。

Patterns of care 研究表明，患有Ⅲ期癌症的黑种人接受辅助化疗的可能性更小，Ⅲ期疾病的部分差异可能是由于治疗的差异。但进一步看，有研究表明，黑种人往往在医院接受治疗，医院人满为患，资源有限[24]。他们在手术中切除的淋巴结更少，对这些淋巴结进行彻底的病理检查的可能性也更小。也就是说，如果黑种人患者接受了适当的手术和病理检查，那么他们中被诊断为Ⅰ期和Ⅱ期癌症的比例将会被诊断为Ⅲ期结肠直肠癌。通过纳入这些真正的Ⅲ期患者会提高黑种人Ⅲ期患者的生存率，通过排除他们也会提高黑种人Ⅰ期和Ⅱ期患者的生存率。

这是威尔・罗杰斯的一个经典现象[25]。由于治疗和分期的差异，每个分期的 25 名黑种人患者的 5 年生存率较低。在平等机会制度下评估时，结果的种族差异会显著减少[26]。

基因表达：种族、血统、种族和文化

结直肠癌仍处于良好治疗的阶段，但在结果上存在差异。黑人的存活率略低于白人。

在结直肠癌领域，即使治疗得当，预后仍存在差异。黑种人生存率略低于白种人生存率。EMAST 是微卫星不稳定性的标志，预后较差，在黑种人或非裔美国人中更为常见。EMAST 似乎是一种与炎症相关的后天缺陷[27]。饮食、微生物组和脂肪积累在研究黑种人-白种人结肠癌病患差异中起着重要作用。这是一个饮食的例子，一个种族和文化的元素，与种族或祖先平行并影响肿瘤的基因表达和生物行为。

一些与种族、民族、文化甚至社会经济学相关的外在因素会影响恶性肿瘤的基因表达，其中，美国白种人女性中产阶级和受过大学教育的比例更高，中产阶级、受过大学教育的女性常常为了事业而推迟生育。第一次怀孕在 30 岁以后对乳腺癌来说是危险因素，尤其是对雌激素受体阳性的乳腺癌。事实上，这可能就是美国白种人女性乳腺癌发病率高于黑种人女性的原因，此外也是白种人女性雌激素受体阳性疾病发病率较高的原因[28]。

对美国和苏格兰白种人乳腺癌患者的研究表明，童年时的中产阶级社会地位与成年后雌激素受体阳性乳腺癌的高风险相关。儿童时期的贫困与之后雌激素受体阴性疾病相关[29,30]。儿童期饮食和体重增加模式的差异被认为是原因。母乳喂养期间、儿童母乳喂养的数量和母乳喂养的时间长短都与基底样乳腺癌风险的降低有关，但与预后较好的 luminal A 乳腺癌风险的降低无关[31]。

在美国，超重和肥胖的黑种人和西班牙裔女性比例过高，这可能是由于种族和文化以及社会经济地位的不同。肥胖，或者更确切地说成年期体重增加，被认为是绝经后乳腺癌的一个危险因素[32]。美国黑种人和白种人妇女不同的病理趋势可能是由于这些影响[31]。

在比较的群体中，了解与社会经济地位、种族和文化相关的环境影响十分有用。了解与地理起源有关的遗传多态性和突变（标记）以及由于种族和文化而被保存下来的遗传标记也很有帮助。随着表观遗传学领域的发展，外部影响的作用将会得到越来越多的认同。

种群和遗传差异

虽然有证据表明，广泛且定义不明确的种群类别之间的差异被过分强调,但在定义明确的种群之间确实存在固有的遗传差异。种族不是定义这些群体的合适方式。内在遗传标记与祖先、地理起源地区,有时与种族和文化有更好的相关性。与种族相关或联系的遗传差异通常被认为是家族性的或祖传的。一个基因或一系列基因可以在家族中保存。即使这样,多态性或基因的患病率在特定人群中可能更高,但该人群不太可能独占该基因[33]。

一个封闭的社群会保留社群中的遗传特性。基于种族、民族和文化、地理起源地区或其他因素的不同可能导致在隔离的人群中保留特定的基因或一系列基因。这在一些遗传性疾病如 Tay Sachs 病、囊性纤维化和镰状细胞病中得到了证实[34]。这其中的每一种疾病在某一特定群体中发病率较高,但不限于该群体。

也许最好的例子就是 *BRCA* 突变。*BRCA-1* 和 *BRCA-2* 基因发生某些突变的女性患乳腺癌和卵巢癌的风险高于平均水平。在所有种族的女性身上都发现了 *BRCA-1* 和 *BRCA-2* 的突变,但是有 3 种特定的突变对于那些认为自己是德系犹太人后裔的人来说是常见的,但不是唯一的[33,35]。人口模型表明,这些特定的突变与生活在 1 000~1 200 年前的小部分个体有关。这些突变被认为是祖传的,而且由于家庭之间的种族隔离,在犹太家庭中很常见。

药物基因组学

由于药物代谢酶的不同,药物反应存在临床相关的变异性。这些差异可以根据种族、民族、祖先、地理起源地区甚至有时因社会经济地位的不同而有所不同。外源性因素如饮食和某些药物的使用可上调或下调肝酶的表达。同样的药物代谢途径也常常涉及环境毒素和致癌物的解毒,因此解毒酶的变化可能导致癌症风险的变化。

当然,医生感兴趣的是患者如何代谢处方药。有时可以使用"人口概况"的形式来评估一个人的某些常见药物治疗问题。例如,大约 10%来自亚洲某些地区的人在使用卡马西平时出现严重的皮肤不良反应,如斯蒂文斯-约翰逊综合征[36]。这可能是祖先的地理起源在马来西亚、新加坡、泰国或印度的人应避免使用卡马西平的合理理由。如果必须使用卡马西平,则应仔细监测或检测 HLA-B*1502 的某些等位基因频率。

他克莫司在肾移植患者中得到了很好的研究。该药物在结构上与几种抗癌药物相关,由 CYP3A 代谢。在临床应用中,一些黑种人或非洲裔美国肾移植患者需要更高的他克莫司剂量才能达到与白种人患者相似的最低浓度。这是由于 CYP3A 的多态性不同。即使在一个特定的群体中,药理学也会有很大的变化。在黑人中,他克莫司 12 小时后的浓度范围是 3~5 倍[37]。所有用这种药治疗的患者都需要特别注意药代动力学。

在癌症药物中,*UGT1A1* 基因多态性的人群差异影响伊立替康的剂量和疗效[38]。确实,有些人建议在使用这种药物之前进行基因检测。*ABCG2* 的差异影响拓扑替康、伊立替康、米托蒽醌、阿霉素和甲氨蝶呤的剂量和疗效[36]。

这并不是一个新概念,事实上在基因组时代,它是一个被重新应用的旧概念。几十年来,我们已经认识到葡萄糖-6-磷酸脱氢酶(G6PD)缺乏症在其祖先包括地中海或非洲血统的人中更为常见。事实上,这是人类最常见的酶缺陷。当服用磺胺类抗生素、抗疟药或某些其他药物时,缺乏维生素 D 的患者有溶血的风险。

美国政府对少数族裔参与临床试验的规定

美国政府的规定是担心"少数族裔和女性没有从联邦资助的研究中受益,因为他们没有参与其中"。

由美国国立卫生研究院(National Institute of Health, NIH)资助进行研究的临床试验人员必须每年报告涉及试验的患者的种族和性别。虽然美国国立卫生研究院在法律义务上只要求所有三期临床试验提供这些信息,但美国国立卫生研究院和其他政府机构在涉及人类受试者的所有试验中往往都要求提供这些信息。

1993 年美国国立卫生研究院的振兴法案(第 103-43 号公法)规定,临床研究必须纳入妇女和少数族裔。具体来看,这是说,"国立卫生研究院负责人应确保试验的设计和实施足以提供有效的分析,以确定在试验中研究的变量是否对妇女或少数群体产生影响,因为案例可能与试验中的其他受试者不同。"该法案的目的是获得用以增进所有美国人的健康和疾病治疗的重要信息,以及发现并解释存在的性别或种族和民族群体之间的显著差异,并确定可能需要在目标研究中进一步探索更细微的差异[39]。

振兴法案要求在联邦资助的试验,特别是三期试验中有不同的代表性。受资助的研究人员必须做出真诚的努力,使少数民族和妇女与美国人口成比例[39]。

这项立法存在争议,因为它在科学上存在缺陷。它要求用子集分析来评估种族和民族差异。它使用种族和民族来定义生物类别。另一个问题是立法要求进行子集分析。临床试验的一个基本原则是,子集分析常常是错误的,应该只用于建立一个假设,以便在更严格的研究中进行检验。子集分析是事后的、回顾的和功能不足的。权可以通过对少数民族的过度采样来增加,但这引发了伦理上的担忧,因为与占人口多数的白种人相比,更大比例的少数民族将承担到这项研究的风险。

有趣的是,这项法律是在一项研究的子集分析表明齐多夫定在黑种人或非洲人中效果较差后制定的。其结果是许多携带艾滋病病毒的黑人停止服用或拒绝开始抗病毒治疗[40,41]。后来的研究表明,同等的治疗在同等的患者中产生了同等的结果,但这并没有得到广泛的认可。在最初的研究中,更高比例的黑人参与者开始治疗更严重的艾滋病毒疾病,并且由于社会原因不太可能坚持规范的治疗方案[42]。与社会经济地位相关的因素再次导致了结果的差异,一些人认为这是由于固有的种族-生物差异造成的。

撰写振兴法案的议员们认为,由于用于治疗重大疾病的药物和疗法尚未在少数族裔和妇女中进行测试,因此存在着差异;有些人甚至认为,像癌症这样的疾病在不同的种族中是不同的;另一些人认为药物或疗法对黑种人和白种人有不同的影响[43]。一个被忽略的重要事实是,许多种族差异是由于少数民族和贫穷的患者没有得到已知的对他们有益的治疗,而且不给予治疗肯定不起作用。

如果要克服健康差异,实现公平,最好将与健康差异相关的研究问题纳入癌症治疗、预防、筛查和控制试验,这可以提供更强大的统计功效来解决重要的问题。

临床试验的多样化参与是重要的。在干预措施和结果的研究中,存在效能和有效性的概念。效能是指在理想的临床环境中,干预的效果如何。有效性是指干预在"现实世界"情况下的效果。来自所有社群的人员参与临床试验是必要的。在大多数人得到了癌症治疗的社群进行研究是为了使结果更广泛地相关。一段时间以来,对 NCI 资助的治疗研究的累积性研究显示,在临床试验参与率和拒绝率方面存在相对的种族/民族平衡[44,45]。事实上,将老年人、共病患者纳入临床试验,将会得到更真实的结果[46]。

总结

卫生差异或卫生公平研究和规划很重要。而且至关重要的是,我们要仔细确定我们对结果和正在比较的人群的衡量标准。无论如何定义,发病率和结果在人群中存在差异。

许多精心设计的研究和研究的荟萃分析表明,同等的治疗在同等的患者中产生同等的结果。如果对具有相同遗传标记的人进行比较,除非允许,否则种族不是影响结果的因素。很少讨论的事实是,许多模式的护理研究表明,没有平等的治疗;人们常常讨论的焦点是一种特定的乳腺癌药物对黑人和白人同样有效,但人们忘记了有相当比例的黑人没有得到足够的治疗,包括手术、化疗和放疗。

随着科学的进步,我们对癌症的了解也越来越多。现在我们更好地了解了它的病因、生物学行为和治疗方法。我们正迅速进入个性化医疗时代,在这个时代,遗传学和基因组学变得非常重要。精准医疗和定制治疗的出现,将使利用基因和遗传多态性进行分类变得更加重要。种族和民族甚至社会经济地位的粗略分类只在诸如获得保健和平等待遇等社会问题方面影响比较大。

旨在克服差异和实现公平的社会干预措施包括:

- 提高医护人员的文化能力和对患者的了解
- 增加获得治疗的机会
  - ■ 提供保险
  - ■ 配备社区卫生中心人员
  - ■ 关注患者的社会状况
- 改善沟通,培训并教育那些需要服务的人
  - ■ 目标信息
  - ■ 患者导航

(吴建中 译,冯继锋 审校)

参考文献

1 Fontaine SA, Henschke UK, Leffall LD Jr, et al. Comparison of the cancer deaths in the black and white U.S.A. population from 1949 to 1967. *Med Ann Dist Columbia*. 1972;**41**:293–298.

2 Burbank F, Fraumeni JF Jr. U.S. cancer mortality: nonwhite predominance. *J Natl Cancer Inst*. 1972;**49**:649–659.

3 Witzig R. The medicalization of race: scientific legitimization of a flawed social construct. *Ann Intern Med*. 1996;**125**:675–679.

4 Brewster DH, Black RJ. Breast, lung and colorectal cancer incidence and survival in South Thames Region, 1987-1992: the effect of social deprivation. *J Public Health Med*. 1998;**20**:236–238.

5 Siegel R, Ward E, Brawley O, Jemal A. Cancer statistics, 2011: the impact of eliminating socioeconomic and racial disparities on premature cancer deaths. *CA Cancer J Clin*. 2011;**61**:212–236.

6 Jemal A, Siegel R, Xu J, Ward E. Cancer statistics, 2010. *CA Cancer J Clin*. 2010;**60**:277–300.

7 Jemal A, Simard EP, Xu J, Ma J, Anderson RN. Selected cancers with increasing mortality rates by educational attainment in 26 states in the United States, 1993-2007. *Cancer Causes Control*. 2013;**24**:559–565.

8 Goldson A, Henschke U, Leffall LD, Schneider RL. Is there a genetic basis for the differences in cancer incidence between Afro-Americans and Euro-Americans? *J Natl Med Assoc*. 1981;**73**:701–706.

9 Calle EE, Rodriguez C, Walker-Thurmond K, Thun MJ. Overweight, obesity, and mortality from cancer in a prospectively studied cohort of U.S. adults. *N Engl J Med*. 2003;**348**:1625–1638.

10 Griggs JJ, Culakova E, Sorbero ME, et al. Effect of patient socioeconomic status and body mass index on the quality of breast cancer adjuvant chemotherapy. *J Clin Oncol*. 2007;**25**:277–284.

11 Harrington J, Fitzgerald AP, Layte R, Lutomski J, Molcho M, Perry IJ. Sociodemographic, health and lifestyle predictors of poor diets. *Public Health Nutr*. 2011;**14**:2166–2175.

12 Jamal A, Agaku IT, O'Connor E, King BA, Kenemer JB, Neff L. Current cigarette smoking among adults—United States, 2005-2013. *MMWR Morb Mortal Wkly Rep*. 2014;**63**:1108–1112.

13 Cancer screening—United States, 2010. *MMWR Morb Mortal Wkly Rep*. 2012;**61**:41–45.

14 Characteristics of persons with chronic hepatitis B—San Francisco, California, 2006. *MMWR Morb Mortal Wkly Rep*. 2007;**56**:446–448.

15 Shimizu H, Ross RK, Bernstein L, Yatani R, Henderson BE, Mack TM. Cancers of the prostate and breast among Japanese and white immigrants in Los Angeles County. *Br J Cancer*. 1991;**63**:963–966.

16 Simon MS, Lamerato L, Krajenta R, et al. Racial differences in the use of adjuvant chemotherapy for breast cancer in a large urban integrated health system. *Int J Breast Cancer*. 2012;**2012**:453985.

17 Wu XC, Lund MJ, Kimmick GG, et al. Influence of race, insurance, socioeconomic status, and hospital type on receipt of guideline-concordant adjuvant systemic therapy for locoregional breast cancers. *J Clin Oncol*. 2012;**30**:142–150.

18 Shavers VL, Brown ML. Racial and ethnic disparities in the receipt of cancer treatment. *J Natl Cancer Inst*. 2002;**94**:334–357.

19 Moy B, Polite BN, Halpern MT, et al. American Society of Clinical Oncology policy statement: opportunities in the patient protection and affordable care act to reduce cancer care disparities. *J Clin Oncol*. 2011;**29**:3816–3824. doi: 10.1200/JCO.2011.35.8903. Epub 2011 Aug 1.

20 Betancourt JR, Green AR, Carrillo JE, Park ER. Cultural competence and health care disparities: key perspectives and trends. *Health Aff*. 2005;**24**:499–505.

21 Lund MJ, Brawley OP, Ward KC, Young JL, Gabram SS, Eley JW. Parity and disparity in first course treatment of invasive breast cancer. *Breast Cancer Res Treat*. 2008;**109**:545–557.

22 Short LJ, Fisher MD, Wahl PM, et al. Disparities in medical care among commercially insured patients with newly diagnosed breast cancer: opportunities for intervention. *Cancer*. 2010;**116**:193–202.

23 Griggs JJ, Hawley ST, Graff JJ, et al. Factors associated with receipt of breast cancer adjuvant chemotherapy in a diverse population-based sample. *J Clin Oncol*. 2012;**30**:3058–3064.

24 Breslin TM, Morris AM, Gu N, et al. Hospital factors and racial disparities in mortality after surgery for breast and colon cancer. *J Clin Oncol*. 2009;**27**:3945–3950.

25 Feinstein AR, Sosin DM, Wells CK. The Will Rogers phenomenon. Stage migration and new diagnostic techniques as a source of misleading statistics for survival in cancer. *N Engl J Med*. 1985;**312**:1604–1608.

26 Bach PB, Schrag D, Brawley OW, Galaznik A, Yakren S, Begg CB. Survival of blacks and whites after a cancer diagnosis. *JAMA*. 2002;**287**:2106–2113.

27 Grady WM, Carethers JM. Genomic and epigenetic instability in colorectal cancer pathogenesis. *Gastroenterology*. 2008;**135**:1079–1099.

28 Chu KC, Anderson WF, Fritz A, Ries LA, Brawley OW. Frequency distributions of breast cancer characteristics classified by estrogen receptor and progesterone receptor status for eight racial/ethnic groups. *Cancer*. 2001;**92**:37–45.
29 Gordon NH. Association of education and income with estrogen receptor status in primary breast cancer. *Am J Epidemiol*. 1995;**142**:796–803.
30 Thomson CS, Hole DJ, Twelves CJ, Brewster DH, Black RJ. Prognostic factors in women with breast cancer: distribution by socioeconomic status and effect on differences in survival. *J Epidemiol Community Health*. 2001;**55**:308–315.
31 Millikan RC, Newman B, Tse CK, et al. Epidemiology of basal-like breast cancer. *Breast Cancer Res Treat*. 2008;**109**:123–139.
32 Brawley OW. Health disparities in breast cancer. *Obstet Gynecol Clin North Am*. 2013;**40**:513–523. doi: 10.1016/j.ogc.2013.06.001.
33 Berman DB, Wagner-Costalas J, Schultz DC, Lynch HT, Daly M, Godwin AK. Two distinct origins of a common BRCA1 mutation in breast-ovarian cancer families: a genetic study of 15 185delAG-mutation kindreds. *Am J Hum Genet*. 1996;**58**:1166–1176.
34 Liu E. The uncoupling of race and cancer genetics. *Cancer*. 1998;**83**:1765–1769.
35 Offit K, Gilewski T, McGuire P, et al. Germline BRCA1 185delAG mutations in Jewish women with breast cancer. *Lancet*. 1996;**347**:1643–1645.
36 Yasuda SU, Zhang L, Huang SM. The role of ethnicity in variability in response to drugs: focus on clinical pharmacology studies. *Clin Pharmacol Ther*. 2008;**84**:417–423.
37 Vadivel N, Garg A, Holt DW, Chang RW, MacPhee IA. Tacrolimus dose in black renal transplant recipients. *Transplantation*. 2007;**83**:997–999.
38 McLeod HL, Sargent DJ, Marsh S, et al. Pharmacogenetic predictors of adverse events and response to chemotherapy in metastatic colorectal cancer: results from North American Gastrointestinal Intergroup Trial N9741. *J Clin Oncol*. 2010;**28**:3227–3233.
39 Freedman LS, Simon R, Foulkes MA, et al. Inclusion of women and minorities in clinical trials and the NIH Revitalization Act of 1993—the perspective of NIH clinical trialists. *Control Clin Trials*. 1995;**16**:277–285; discussion 86–89, 93–309.
40 Hamilton JD, Hartigan PM, Simberkoff MS. The effect of zidovudine on patient subgroups. *JAMA*. 1992;**267**:2472–2473.
41 Rothenberg R, Woelfel M, Stoneburner R, Milberg J, Parker R, Truman B. Survival with the acquired immunodeficiency syndrome. Experience with 5833 cases in New York City. *N Engl J Med*. 1987;**317**:1297–1302.
42 Easterbrook PJ, Keruly JC, Creagh-Kirk T, Richman DD, Chaisson RE, Moore RD. Racial and ethnic differences in outcome in zidovudine-treated patients with advanced HIV disease. Zidovudine Epidemiology Study Group. *JAMA*. 1991;**266**:2713–2718.
43 Brawley O. Response to "inclusion of women and minorities in clinical trials and the NIH Revitalization Act of 1993—the perspective of NIH clinical trialists". *Control Clin Trials*. 1995;**16**:293–295.
44 Wendler D, Kington R, Madans J, et al. Are racial and ethnic minorities less willing to participate in health research? *PLoS Med*. 2006;**3**:e19.
45 Langford AT, Resnicow K, Dimond EP, et al. Racial/ethnic differences in clinical trial enrollment, refusal rates, ineligibility, and reasons for decline among patients at sites in the National Cancer Institute's Community Cancer Centers Program. *Cancer*. 2014;**120**:877–884.
46 Unger JM, Coltman CA Jr, Crowley JJ, et al. Impact of the year 2000 Medicare policy change on older patient enrollment to cancer clinical trials. *J Clin Oncol*. 2006;**24**:141–144.

第 75 章　获得性免疫缺陷综合征中的肿瘤

Jeremy S. Abramson, MD, MMSc ■ David T. Scadden, MD

概述

多种病因的免疫缺陷可增加恶性肿瘤,特别是淋巴瘤的风险,这种风险与免疫异常的严重程度和范围有关。继发于免疫缺陷病毒1型(HIV-1)感染的获得性免疫缺陷综合征(acquired immunodeficiency syndrome, AIDS)中,肿瘤的类型更广泛。肿瘤通常与致癌病毒有关,被认为可能是继发的机会性肿瘤。造成这种情况的因素包括对致癌病毒控制不佳、HIV 对免疫细胞的影响而改变细胞因子的调节以及来自其他获得性免疫缺陷综合征相关事件的组织刺激。免疫、感染和肿瘤发生的相互作用是获得性免疫缺陷综合征相关恶性肿瘤的核心。

免疫缺陷背景下的肿瘤类型谱超出淋巴瘤的范围,但相当有限。在一般人群和免疫缺陷人群中,上皮性恶性肿瘤的发病差别不大。相反,免疫缺陷肿瘤包含的肿瘤亚型相对较少见,其中一些在普通人群中发病率非常低。例如,原发中枢神经系统(primary central nervous system, PCNS)淋巴瘤和卡波西肉瘤(Kaposi sarcoma, KS)在整体人群中非常罕见,但在免疫缺陷人群中占很大比例。

此外,具体肿瘤类型的发病率因免疫缺陷状态而异。非霍奇金淋巴瘤(non-Hodgkin lymphoma, NHL)是所有免疫缺陷患者中一个共同的主题,但获得性免疫缺陷综合征与其他免疫缺陷状态相比,肿瘤的组织学亚型范围更广。在 HIV 相关和药物诱导的免疫缺陷患者中,KS 的发病率增加。皮肤肿瘤常见于多种免疫缺陷状态中,但皮肤鳞状细胞瘤在实体器官移植后的人群中比在获得性免疫缺陷综合征相关的免疫缺陷人群中要高。后者与乳头瘤病毒相关肛门-生殖器区域的鳞状细胞瘤为主(表 75-1)。

与免疫缺陷状态相关的肿瘤共有的是与传染性病原体关系密切。免疫缺陷相关淋巴瘤中存在 EB 病毒(Epstein-Barr virus, EBV)为大家熟知。很可能是病毒直接刺激 B 细胞增殖的结果。表达 EB 病毒潜伏期基因产物的细胞,可过度生长不受抑制,随后就会出现细胞转化。病毒直接诱导细胞增殖的模型可能也适用于乳头状瘤病毒(human papilloma virus, HPV)相关肿瘤。然而,这种模型不太适用于 KS 相关的疱疹病毒/人疱疹病毒-8(KSHV/HHV8)相关的肿瘤。更多的变化以及与病毒基因产物的病理生理关系不明,这将在更深入的章节中讨论。一般来说,肿瘤可在免疫缺陷时出现,而这种情况与次生病原体的出现也有关(表 75-2)。

免疫缺陷进一步导致先天宿主肿瘤监视的失败。本质上,免疫控制不足的概念提供了一个统一的机制。这些肿瘤可认为是机会性恶性肿瘤,如同特异性感染被认为是机会性感染的途径一样。确实,免疫不足患者的机会性恶性肿瘤,体现了感染和肿瘤的重叠,为免疫功能和肿瘤发展的交叉提供了独特的视角。

表 75-1　HIV 中发病率增加的肿瘤类型

卡波西肉瘤
非霍奇金淋巴瘤
弥漫大 B 细胞淋巴瘤
伯基特淋巴瘤
淋巴母细胞性淋巴瘤
原发性渗出性淋巴瘤
原发中枢神经系统淋巴瘤
鳞状细胞异常增生
霍奇金淋巴瘤
平滑肌肉瘤(儿童)
浆细胞瘤
精原细胞瘤
皮肤癌
肺癌
口咽癌
肝癌
前列腺癌

表 75-2　艾滋病相关恶性肿瘤的继发性病毒感染

病毒	肿瘤
EBV	NHL(PCNSL;DLBCL;PBL)
	HL
	平滑肌肉瘤(儿童)
KSHV/HHV8	KS
	NHL(PEL);多灶性 Castleman 病(恶性前期)
HPV	鳞状细胞异常增生

缩写:EBV,EB 病毒;HL,霍奇金淋巴瘤;HPV,人类乳头状瘤病毒;KS,卡波西肉瘤;KSHV,卡波西肉瘤疱疹病毒;NHL,非霍奇金淋巴瘤;PCNSL,原发中枢神经系统淋巴瘤;PBL,淋巴母细胞性淋巴瘤;PEL,原发渗出性淋巴瘤;DLBCL,弥漫大 B 细胞淋巴瘤。

流行病学

HIV-1 感染相关肿瘤谱与危险因素以及是否使用现代联合抗反转录病毒治疗(combination antiretroviral therapy, cART)相关。

cART 治疗前时代

直到 1996 年随着蛋白酶抑制剂类治疗获得性免疫缺陷综合征药物的出现，cART 才开始使用。在美国、西欧和澳大利亚，蛋白酶抑制剂的迅速广泛使用，改变了获得性免疫缺陷综合征的死亡率和并发症发生率。机会性疾病的谱系也随之改变[1,2]，对相关恶性肿瘤也有影响，这将在“cART 治疗后时代”部分进行探讨。在很多发展中国家，cART 的获得仍然缺乏，相当数量的患者无法接受 cART 治疗或者 cART 治疗失败。因此，cART 治疗前时代与获得性免疫缺陷综合征有关的恶性肿瘤仍然是相当重要的。

获得性免疫缺陷综合征流行的最初表现之一是在美国的沿海城市与男性发生性关系的男性中，发现了罕见恶性肿瘤的病例。这个肿瘤就是 KS，疾病预防控制中心(Centers for Disease Control and Prevention，CDC)首次尝试对免疫缺陷综合征进行分类时，将 KS 认定为一种定义获得性免疫缺陷综合征的疾病[3]。在获得性免疫缺陷综合征流行早期患者中 KS 大约占 20%，但在传播危险因素为男性与男性发生性关系患者中最高[4]，在通过血液制品或非肠道药物使用传播患者中比较低[5]。随后的行为研究表明性行为的具体类型，包括滥交、经口粪接触者中风险最高[6]，这提示 KS 可能是一种继发性的、可传播病原体的表现。事实上，强有力的流行病学数据显示，对识别病原体的激发导致了 KSHV 分子克隆，也称为 HHV8[7]。第二种最常见的恶性肿瘤是 NHL。1984 年发现与男性发生性关系的男性中 NHL 发病增加。这种疾病在 CDC 首次尝试对免疫缺陷综合征进行分类时，列入获得性免疫缺陷综合征并发症的名单。值得注意的是，这个人群中发生的淋巴瘤通常是高度恶性的，临床过程极具侵袭性。与 KS 不同，这种并发症在 HIV 感染的不同危险因素组都广泛存在。所有组都有较高的相对风险，估计约为一般人的 60 倍以上[6,8-10]。不同受感染个体的亚群风险不一，如其中至少有一项研究指出血友患者群的风险增加[6,10]。同样，人们也注意到了静脉注射吸毒者或来自加勒比盆地的人可能风险较低，但对于护理和监测混淆因素的担心使这种分析复杂化。然而，这些人群中仍然存在引起淋巴瘤生成的潜在重要因素。对这种可能性的关注可能会提供有关淋巴细胞转化过程的重要信息。

HIV 病中第三种最常见的恶性肿瘤是肛门-生殖器鳞状细胞瘤，这与 HPV 感染的致瘤血清型有关。然而，大多数是原位癌或高级别上皮内瘤变。同时，侵袭性癌发生率的增加仍然是有争议的[11,12]。HPV 相关的头颈部癌的患病率可能也在增加，与 HPV 高血清阳性率以及导致头颈部癌额外伴随风险因素包括免疫抑制、烟草和酒精的使用有关。

cART 治疗后时代

cART 的出现对获得性免疫缺陷综合征的病程产生了深远而巨大的影响。在蛋白酶抑制剂联合治疗的情况下，免疫功能的下降及其伴随的继发感染，以及肿瘤均出现停止，甚至逆转。晚期疾病患者病情的改善导致这些药物的广泛使用，包括在新近获得 HIV-1 感染的人群中，导致能获得药物的获得性免疫缺陷综合征患者中，死亡率急剧下降。虽然获得性免疫缺陷综合征引起的死亡和衰弱急剧下降，HIV 感染新患者数没有出现类似的下降。因此，西方 HIV 感染的总人数在增加，感染者的生存期更长；在全球范围内，获得性免疫缺陷综合征的流行势头有增无减。自 cART 出现以来，HIV 感染中恶性肿瘤的流行病学出现了明显的改变，较长时间中度的免疫功能障碍或者抗反转录病毒药物本身的影响直到现在才被了解。一项对晚期 HIV 患者临床护理的观察发现，在 cART 成功抑制获得性免疫缺陷综合征病毒之后，KS 发生率出现立即下降。对 KS 新病例的影响也很快被发现，而且流行病学数据证实了这些临床上明显的现象。来自美国、欧洲和澳大利亚的多项研究显示出 KS 的普遍下降，发病率下降估计高达 80 倍[13-16]。无论是 cART 治疗前时代还是 cART 治疗后时代，KS 发生风险都与 CD4 细胞计数抑制程度直接相关[17]。在 cART 治疗后时代，CD4 细胞计数增加的 KS 患者报道越来越多[18,19]，这些患者疾病可能更局限于下肢皮肤，较少内脏播散，较多见于地中海盆地非 HIV 感染者的地方性 KS 中。

与 KS 一样，原发性中枢神经系统淋巴瘤(primary central nervous system lymphoma，PCNSL)的发病率也出现了急剧下降。这种并发症在晚期 HIV 的发病率远低于 KS，因此，它的下降并没有被很好地记录下来。但对临床方面的影响同样是意义重大的。除了在那些接受抗反转录病毒治疗失败或从未接受过抗反转录病毒治疗的人中间，很少见到这种病例。这是严重免疫抑制的并发症，就像移植后的环境一样。几乎一致地与肿瘤组织中检测到的 EB 病毒有关。一般来说，这些肿瘤中表达的 EBV 潜伏基因是第Ⅲ类或淋巴增生性疾病相关(EBNA1-6，LMP1 和 LMP2)[20]。这些特征和其他特征可区分 PCNS 淋巴瘤和其他获得性免疫缺陷综合征相关淋巴瘤(AIDS-related lymphoma，ARL)。在 cART 时代，系统性获得性免疫缺陷综合征相关 NHL 的发生率也有所下降，淋巴瘤亚型的模式也在进化[21-24]。在 cART 时代的早期，cART 对淋巴瘤亚型的影响存在显著的变异性，PCNSL 以及免疫母细胞弥漫性大 B 细胞淋巴瘤(DLBCL)的风险降低最大，伯基特淋巴瘤(BL)和霍奇金淋巴瘤(HL)的发生率没有下降[22,25]。最近美国一项对 23 050 例 HIV 阳性个体进行的研究发现，476 例(2%)患者在 1996 年至 2010 年发生淋巴瘤，其中 83% 为 NHL，17% 为 HL[26]。cART 时代最常见的亚型为 DLBCL，占病例的 42%，这也是非 HIV 感染者中最常见的 NHL 类型。BL 占全部病例的 12%，明显高于普通人群。与 cART 前时代相比，PCNSL 的发病率有最显著的下降，这一人群只占 NHLs 的 11%。大多数 HIV 相关淋巴瘤发生的风险与 CD4 细胞计数下降直接相关，但与其他类型相比，BL 和 HL 关系不大[17]。中位 CD4 细胞计数在现代 DLBCL 和 BL 中分别为 68 个细胞/μl 和 118 个细胞/μl。在 cART 治疗前时代，感染获得性免疫缺陷综合征病毒的患者人群中，CD4 细胞计数中位数在 PCNSL 最低，中位 14 个细胞/μl。cART 在淋巴瘤亚型中的差异影响突出这些肿瘤类型之间的生物学差异和提示差异免疫参与肿瘤的发展。

卡波西肉瘤(KS)

1981 年，洛杉矶和纽约报道的 KS 爆发，首次把获得性免疫缺陷综合征的流行带到了公众视野[27]。1872 年，匈牙利皮肤科医生莫里茨卡波西首次把 KS 描述为一种惰性的肿瘤[28]，通常发生于老年地中海男性,或者器官移植免疫抑制药物的情况下。后者帮助人们把注意力集中在城市中心的各个小区之间的免疫变化传播上。KS 在与男性发生性关系的 HIV 阳性男性常见,但在具有其他 HIV 感染风险因素(如血液制品暴露)的群体中却并不常见[5,25],因此长期以来人们一直怀疑 KS 与第二个因素有关[29]。在鉴定出 KSHV/HHV8 之前,没有任何证据证明调查的若干可能因素是站得住脚的。这种病毒最初是通过对有 KS 和无 KS 个体的组织进行遗传学比较而被识别出来的。人们观察到其脱氧核糖核酸(DNA)片段与伽玛疱疹病毒家族的其他成员具有部分同源性。疱疹病毒的这一亚群包括几种具有致癌潜能的病毒,如与许多肿瘤有关的 EBV,与转化 T 细胞能力有关的疱疹病毒(herpesvirus saimiri,HVS)。由于 KS 病变中可检测到 KSHV/HHV8 及其特征性的 DNA 高频序列,该病毒迅速而合理地成为 KS 病理生理学基础研究的焦点。

病毒流行病学

KSHV/HHV8 是一种 165kb 双链 DNA 病毒,其特征强烈支持其在 KS 临床中的致病作用。有资料表明,KSHV/HHV8 感染先于肿瘤形成[29,30],具有 KSHV/HHV8 高血清价的人群也是 KSHV/HHV8 的高发生率人群[25],病毒可感染肿瘤内的细胞[29]。

KSHV/HHV8 暴露的定义取决于对该病毒特异性反应的抗体的记录。已有的一些检查结果各不相同。数据显示,在北美,血清阳性率估计为 3.5%,在地中海盆地的人民高达 25%,在撒哈拉以南非洲人民高达 89%[31-33]。

在旧金山进行的一项历时 10 年的男性纵向研究,令人信服地证明了性传播这一备受怀疑的角色。在纯异性恋男性中,未检测到 KSHV/HHV8 阳性;然而,在与男性发生性关系的男性中,血清转化的发生率与男性性交接触者的数量有关[34]。前两年有超过 250 个性伴侣的男性中血清阳性率为 65%。然而,性传播并不是病毒传播的唯一途径。KSHV/HHV8 可在唾液中发现,人们认为口腔传播很少发生[35]。在 KS 流行地区,KSHV/HHV8 在家庭成员中较高的发病率以及撒哈拉以南非洲儿童经常受到感染,表明确实发生了非性传播手段,但具体依据仍有待充分确定。

临床表现

KS 的特征性表现为黏膜表面色素沉着的斑丘疹性病变(图 75-1 和图 75-2)。典型为紫罗兰色或红斑,可能伴有瘀斑。通常,病变是多灶的,没有可预测的顺序或进展速度。病变可能表现为孤立的结节或斑块,但也可能集群出现或在多个位置同时出现。虽然典型的或地方性的 KS 通常发生于下肢,但在 HIV 感染的情况下,这种受累模式是很难预测的。几乎所有的黏膜和皮肤部位都可能受到影响。在面部,耳朵和鼻子经常受累,导致严重的毁容。除了 KS 的毁容作用外,病变有时会变厚,形成不舒服的斑块,并可能并发溃疡。然而,病变通常不具有破坏性。覆盖在病变上的表皮或黏膜通常是完整的,通常不会发生深部的肌肉或骨骼浸润。

KS 通常伴随病变局部或远处依赖部位的水肿(图 75-3)。水肿可表现为肢体活动严重受损,有时伴有眶周、耻骨周围或生殖器水肿。有两种机制被认为与水肿的发生有关。一种是

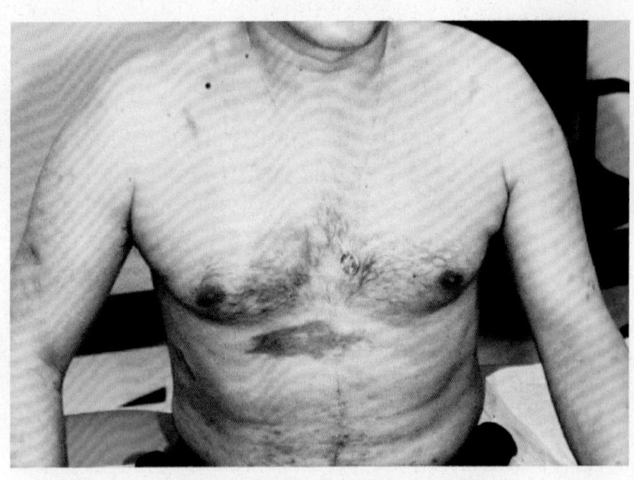

图 75-1　一例白人晚期获得性免疫缺陷综合征患者的皮肤卡波西肉瘤。胸部具有特征性的紫色斑块。这些病变在紫杉醇化疗和抗反转录病毒药物治疗后完全消失了

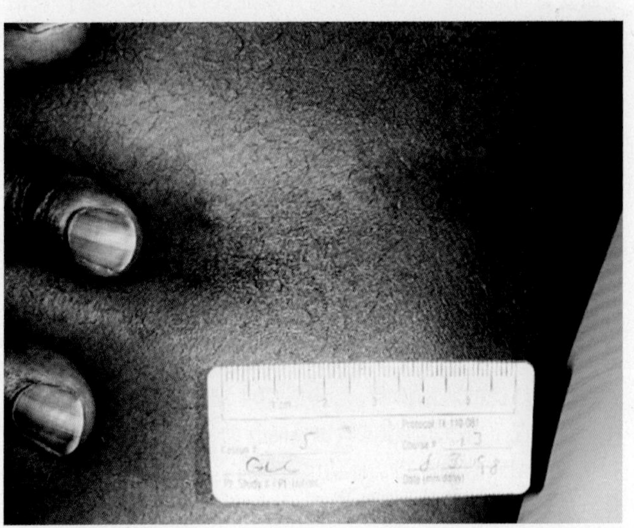

图 75-2　一名感染 HIV-1 的非裔美国男性卡波西肉瘤。肤色使病变不易与其他皮肤病变区分,并与浅肤色个体的外观截然不同

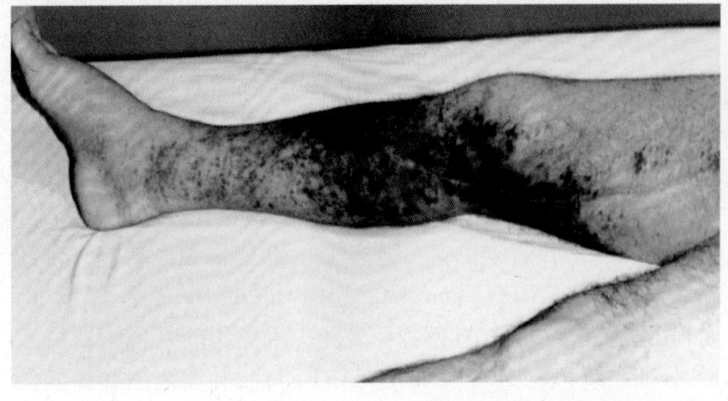

图 75-3　卡波西肉瘤累及下肢可导致明显水肿和活动受限。尽管该患者化疗后卡波西肉瘤有明显改善,但足部水肿无明显变化

KS 引起的淋巴管或淋巴结受累,从而对淋巴管流动造成机械阻塞。二是 KS 病变对渗透性因素的影响。构成 KS 病变的血

管本身是渗漏的，血浆蛋白和细胞外渗进入周围软组织。此外，KS 病变产生的血管内皮生长因子（vascular endothelial growth factor，VEGF）可以改变周围正常血管的完整性，增加血管的通透性，从而增加血管对间质液的渗出。淋巴引流需求的增加和淋巴出口的减少导致局部皮肤增厚和远处明显水肿。

淋巴结和皮肤以外的器官受累是经常发生的。最常见的部位是胃肠道，在内镜检查过程中常见以黏膜为基础的病变。然而，这些病变的生理学意义往往是最小的。大多数患者不知道胃肠道受累，偶然发现的黏膜 KS 病变不应进行积极治疗。然而，对有些人来说，胃肠道 KS 可能具有症状甚至危及生命的并发症。可出现大量出血和肠套叠。

肺受累有多种形式。胸膜表面的 KS 病变可导致胸腔积液，这种积液通常是血性的，但没有特征性的实验室检查或细胞学异常。支气管黏膜可能被累及，与胃肠道黏膜表面一样，在支气管镜检查中可能被偶然发现。病变一般不具破坏性；但根据不同的部位，它们可能引起支气管刺激、咳嗽和咯血。肺实质受累可以说是 KS 最严重的并发症，因为如果不能有效治疗它可引起危及生命的呼吸损害，死亡率高[36]。在放射学上，受累常表现为计算机断层扫描（CT）上的支气管周围病变。病理上，这种浸润可扩展至细小的间质组织，影响肺功能。这在 X 射线上导致斑片状或弥漫性网状结节外观。如果缺乏实质的胸腔镜检查或开放活检，通常很难确定肺部 KS 累及的诊断。

支气管镜检查有助于鉴别具有相同临床表现的其他感染性疾病，并可鉴别黏膜病变。然而，黏膜病变并不一定与实质浸润同时发生，经支气管活检往往不能显示。值得注意的是，支气管黏膜 KS 可能与肺实质的机会性感染共存，如卡氏肺孢菌、巨细胞病毒（CMV）等，因此临床医生必须对 HIV 患者的肺表现进行广泛的鉴别诊断，尤其是 CD4 细胞计数较低的患者。在某些情况下，使用治疗试验也可能有助于确立一个假定的诊断。如果彻底的微生物学评估没有异常，下文讨论的化疗药物具有良好的耐受性，且缓解率高，因此在选定的患者中使用这些药物可作为检测肺实质浸润化疗有效性的一种方法。这种策略通常用于下列患者：①已经从其他受累部位明确了 KS 的诊断；②没有感染的症状；③积极评估感染为阴性，没有其他细胞毒性化疗的禁忌证。

除了肺、消化道和淋巴结外，上气道的特殊部位也值得关注。口腔、鼻窦、咽部和喉部的黏膜受累可导致软组织的变形，从而导致气道损害或食物摄入的改变。这些病变通常对治疗反应迅速，不会侵入更深的结构。治疗方法将在“治疗”一节中讨论。

考虑到常见超出皮肤或口腔黏膜的累及，需考虑系统的分期评估。除了肿瘤体积确实影响预后，获得性免疫缺陷综合征临床试验组织（AIDS Clinical Trials Group，ACTG）基于 cART 前时代 KS 患者的数据，将患者免疫和一般健康的其他特征纳入 KS 分期系统（表 75-3）[38]。在 cART 时代，肿瘤范围和伴随的系统性疾病似乎是这个模型中最有力的预后预测因子。肿瘤侵犯有限，没有机会性感染的患者 3 年预测总生存约为 90%，而有广泛或内脏疾病或其他获得性免疫缺陷综合征相关并发症的患者，3 年预测总生存只有 50%[39]。基于 326 例获得性免疫缺陷综合征相关 KS 患者多变量分析提出的 cART 时代预后模型中，多因素分析确定了 4 个有利预后变量：①KS 为定义获得性免疫缺陷综合征的疾病；②CD4 细胞计数增加；③年龄<50 岁；④无其他获得性免疫缺陷综合征相关疾病[40]。这些变量预测的 5 年总体生存率风险评分，从最有利队列的 98% 到最低的 8% 不等。

表 75-3 艾滋病相关卡波西肉瘤的分期和分类

	好的因素[a]	差的因素(1)[b]
肿瘤(T)	肿瘤负荷小，1 个或以上部位局限受累	肿瘤负荷大
	淋巴结	口腔
	皮肤	胃肠道
	其他[c]	肺
		其他内脏侵犯，伴水肿或溃疡
免疫系统(I)	CD4⁺ 细胞计数大于 200 个/mm³	CD4⁺ 细胞计数小于 200 个/mm³
系统性疾病(S)	无机会性感染（包括鹅口疮），或 B 症状[d]	机会性感染史、鹅口疮、B 症状
		其他 HIV 相关疾病（如 NHL 或其他恶性肿瘤，神经系统疾病、消耗综合征）

[a] 所有列出参数。
[b] 任一所列参数。
[c] 局限于上颚并且无结节生成的口腔疾病。
[d] B 症状包括无法解释的发热，盗汗，体重减轻至少 10%，腹泻持续超过 2 周。
缩写：HIV，人类免疫缺陷病毒；NHL，非霍奇金淋巴瘤。
来源：Krown 1989.[3]

诊断时的分期通常基于临床表现，X 线检查仅限于胸部 X 线，除非另有症状。粪便潜血检测是一种合理的胃肠道受累筛查方法，但特异性较差。如果局部症状确实提示器官受累，那么更广泛的放射学检查和程序干预是适当的，但不能常规推荐。分期标准包括对潜在获得性免疫缺陷综合征病毒感染的评估，所有患者都应该有关于药物治疗、获得性免疫缺陷综合征病毒感染的其他并发症和血液中 CD4 细胞计数的详细记录。

确定 KS 的诊断通常依赖于皮肤的简单穿刺活检或黏膜表面的切取活检。CDC 对于定义获得性免疫缺陷综合征的 KS 诊断标准中提到，如果经由有经验的临床医师评估，不要求对 KS 进行组织学确认。然而还是强烈推荐活检，用于广泛鉴别类似 KS 的非白化性病变[38]，包括细菌性血管瘤病（通常由巴尔通体感染引起，在晚期 HIV 感染患者中发病率增加）、血肿、紫癜、肉质的斑块、扁平苔癣、化脓性肉芽肿、蕈样真菌病、二期梅毒、玫瑰糠疹、与药物有关的多形性红斑、结节性痒疹、痣、噬菌体病的血管病变、类上皮血管内皮瘤、血管肉瘤、黑色素瘤和基底细胞癌。

病理学和病理生理学

KS 的组织学表现掩盖了其与“肉瘤”一词的不明确联系。未见间充质来源细胞的单形排列。病变是由内膜细胞、外周血管壁细胞、梭形细胞、单核免疫细胞、外渗红细胞等组成。正是红细胞为 KS 病变提供了色素，它们的破坏导致了在活跃生长的病变中可见的瘀斑。局部沉积的含铁血黄素会产生色素沉着病变，即使有效治疗逆转了梭形细胞和内皮细胞成分的增殖，这种病变仍可能存在。皮肤病变一般在真皮内，一般不会侵犯深部的肌肉。

内皮细胞和梭形细胞成分的起源仍有争议。KS 病变的内皮细胞表达淋巴管内皮特征性的 VEGF-C 受体，检测不到通常存在于血管内皮的一氧化氮合酶[41,42]。梭形细胞表达甘氨酸结合受体和 CD68 表明其起源可能是巨噬细胞样细胞类型，可能起源于次级淋巴器官并在血液中循环，最后才在 KS 病变中发挥作用[43]。

界定细胞起源的困难源于其复杂的组织学结构和现有的体外或体内模型的局限性。已经建立了一些细胞类型的体外培养，并记录了细胞株的生长，尽管与原发疾病过程的关系尚不清楚。将 KS 组织移植到免疫缺陷小鼠体内可导致肿瘤，这些肿瘤为小鼠起源。细胞因子精细化驱动病变发展的潜能已被提出假说，研究已广泛描述了 KS 病变产生的细胞因子特点[44-46]。细胞因子，尤其是 VEGF 和碱性成纤维细胞生长因子（basic fibroblast growth factor, bFGF）可能在 KS 的旁分泌或自分泌中发挥作用。即使存在外源性生长因子如白介素（IL）6-IL-6R 复合物、IL-10、肿瘤坏死因子（TNF）-α 和制瘤素 M，bFGF 抗体可拮抗 KS 细胞增殖和阻止它们进入细胞周期 S 期[47]。但外源性生长因子并不能完全解释 KS 细胞的表型和增长潜能，不论细胞条件培养基中含有什么成分，它可过度表达抗凋亡的 Bcl-2 基因[48]。

无论是 HIV 相关、器官移植，还是地方性 KS，KSHV/HHV8 对于诱导 KS 似乎是必要的，并且可在 KS 病变中发现。然而，病毒参与致癌过程的具体机制尚不清楚，也不符合其他病毒相关肿瘤疾病所确立的模式。参与 EBV 诱导转化的潜伏基因与 KSHV/HHV8 不具有同源性。HVS 的基因是已知的转化细胞，只有在 KSHV/HHV8 基因 K1 的基因组中才有同源性，K1 能够转化细胞系使其永生[49]。然而，该基因在 KSHV/HHV8 生命周期的潜伏期没有表达。同样，趋化因子受体样的 KSHV/HHV8 基因产物可读框（ORF 74）具有结构性激活，当作为单个基因转导时能够转化细胞，但它也是一种溶相基因[50]。编码的病毒 G 蛋白偶联受体可激活多种信号通路，包括磷脂酰肌醇-3 激酶（phosphatidylinositol-3 kinase, PI3K）/AKT、丝裂原活化蛋白激酶（mitogen-activated protein kinase, MAPK）、Janus 激酶/信号转换器和转录激活因子（Janus kinase/signal transducer and activator of transcription, JAK/STAT）通路[51-53]。这些通路发挥多种抗凋亡和增殖作用，促进肿瘤的发生。另外两个基因产物，K9（干扰素调节因子家族的同源基因）和 K12（没有明确的基因家族同源性）在转导时能够转化细胞株，但在潜伏期不表达[54-57]。与潜伏期缺乏明确的关联，提示这些基因产物不是顺式转化，但是否可能是反式转化不能排除。已经提出了若干 KSHV/HHV8 可能的其他机制，包括可能在远处发挥作用的机制。这些包括与化学激酶相关的基因产物，vMIP-Ⅰ（K6）和 vMIP-Ⅱ（K4），或 IL-6 同源物 K2。每一种受体都能与靶细胞上的同源受体相互作用，要么作为激动剂（K2 和 K6），要么作为拮抗剂（K4）[58,59]。最后，KSHV/HHV8 基因产物还具有抗凋亡作用，可能增强致瘤性。

ORF 16 编码 bcl-2 相关基因产物[60]，ORF 71（K131）编码 FASO 相关死亡域样 IL-10 转化酶抑制蛋白（FLIP）家族抗凋亡基因的功能成员[61]。KSHV/HHV8 的 vFLIP 可保护细胞免受 FASO 介导的细胞死亡，并可促进体内移植细胞系的肿瘤进展。KSHV/HHV8 进一步诱导缺氧诱导因子 1（hypoxia-induced factor 1 alpha, HIF1α）和 HIF2α 的转录，导致促血管生成因子 VEGF 以及其他促血管生成和抗凋亡因子的上调[62,63]，VEGF 和 VEGF 受体在 KS 病变内表达丰富，在致病机制中似乎发挥重要作用[64,65]。KSHV/HHV8 被进一步证明可以编码一种下调血小板反应蛋白 1（血管生成和肿瘤抑制的负调节因子）的 microRNA[66]。因此，KSHV/HHV8 编码了一系列具有改变受感染细胞生长、死亡和免疫特性潜力的基因产物。目前尚不清楚这些机制中哪些在肿瘤发生中起主导作用，对这一过程的进一步研究必将对病毒引起的肿瘤产生新的认识，并为治疗开辟新的途径。

KS 在以下人群中流行：①获得性免疫缺陷综合征病毒感染；②接受实体器官移植；③老年人；④地中海来源，或生活在热带非洲的经济欠发达地区，这表明 KS 疾病表型的表达需要一定程度的免疫抑制。cART 用于获得性免疫缺陷综合征病毒感染治疗的出现为免疫抑制的中心作用提供了巨大的支持：在 cART 导致 CD4 细胞计数增加和 HIV 病毒载量下降的背景下，皮肤和肺的 KS 得到了完全缓解[67,68]。虽然 HIV 诱导的免疫缺陷只是一种可能易患 KS 的免疫异常类型，但是 HIV 和 KSHV/HHV8 共感染人群的相对风险非常高，提示这两种病毒在肿瘤发病机制中可能存在相互作用。HIV 基因产物 *tat* 可影响 KSHV/HHV8 自身复制[69]，改变靶细胞的细胞因子和细胞因子受体表达，导致促血管生成效应[70,71]。*tat* 的表达可能诱发 KSHV/HHV8 的裂解，导致病毒转录增加，白细胞介素 6 产生，以及 JAK/STAT 增殖通路的激活，在 HIV 病毒感染者与实体器官移植者和其他免疫抑制人群相比，它提供了一个 KS 更容易出现的基本病理生理背景[51]。对接受抗疱疹病毒药物治疗的 HIV 感染者中 KS 发生率的回顾性分析显示 KSHV/HHV8 的复制在病理过程中起直接作用。在几项研究中，使用更昔洛韦或膦甲酸治疗的患者中，KS 的发生率有所下降[72-75]。因此，抑制病毒复制似乎可以降低 KS 的风险。一项在 HHV8 血清阳性个体中使用缬更昔洛韦的随机对照临床试验也显示，该药物显著降低了 HHV8 的复制[76]，尽管尚未确定其对临床有意义终点的益处。虽然转化通常与疱疹病毒感染的潜伏期有关，但对裂解期（抗疱疹病毒药物已知的唯一活性时间）的控制可能会限制转化的潜力。

通过免疫手段控制病毒似乎也与发生 KS 的风险高度相关。长期以来，人们都知道，在多种类型的免疫缺陷的背景下，KS 的风险增加。由细胞毒性 T 淋巴细胞（cytotoxic T lymphocyte, CTL）识别病毒表位的定义将进一步确定这一重要观点，并可能因此产生针对性的疫苗。

治疗

KS 的治疗应以肿瘤对患者的影响为指导。治疗这种疾病的目的是减轻症状，减轻器官损害，减少水肿，提高患者的生活质量，并最终提高患者的总体生存期。HIV 感染的 KS 患者病程的变异性以及肿瘤控制与死亡率之间缺乏明确的联系,这表明积极治疗可能并不总是对KS的合理治疗。这在晚期获得性免疫缺陷综合征或未经治疗的获得性免疫缺陷综合征患者中尤其如此。在这种情况下,细胞毒性治疗的毒性可能是令人生畏的,而抗HIV药物的潜在治疗效果是相当可观的。抑制HIV病毒复制与CD4细胞计数的增加有关,并伴随免疫功能的改善,相关病理生理学的改变都应予以恢复。最终的结果是,cART治疗KS患者带来临床改善的可能性很高,有时甚至完全根除。因此,如果KS对患者的影响不是器官威胁或严重症状,单独抗反转录病毒治疗是适当的一线治疗(图75-4)。在撒哈拉以南非洲进行的Ⅲ期安慰剂对照试验验证了这种策略,该实验中59个受试者被随机分配到cART单独用药或cART联合化疗[77]。接受化疗的患者1年总有效率较高(66% vs 39%),但总体生存率无差异。两组的CD4细胞计数和生活质量均有改善,但无统计学显著性差异。

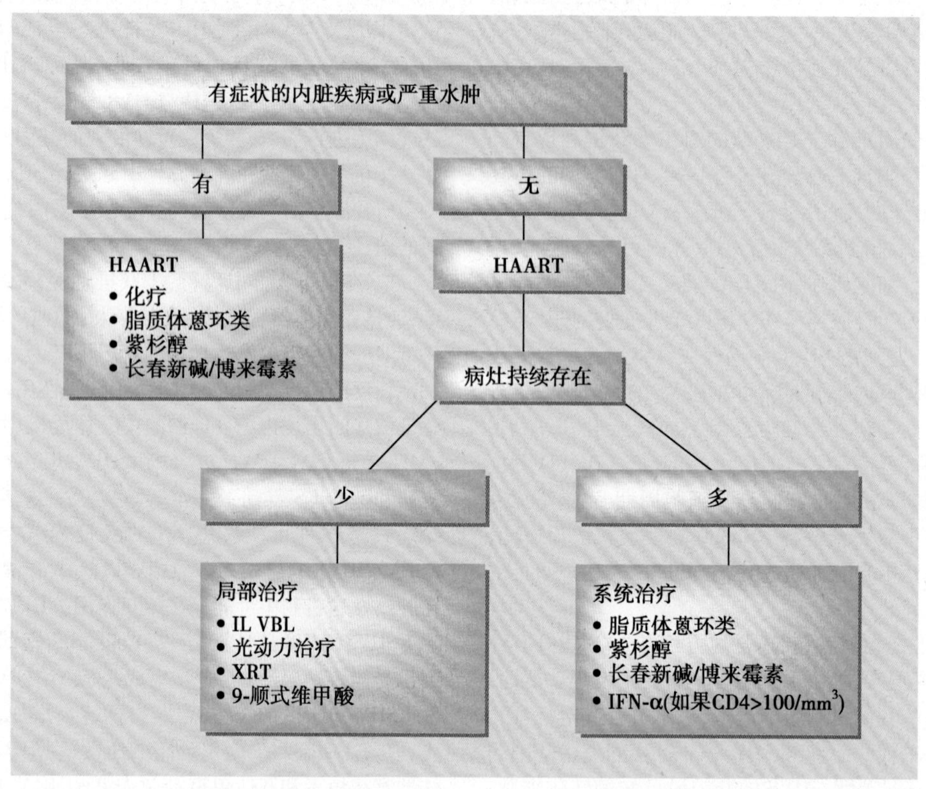

图75-4　卡波西肉瘤患者的治疗流程。缩写:HAART,高活性抗反转录病毒治疗;IFN-α,干扰素-α;,IL,白介素;VBL,长春碱;XRT,放射治疗

在有严重症状或器官威胁疾病的患者,一个更积极的方法与cART联合是必要的。虽然抗HIV治疗是治疗与HIV相关的KS的一个重要组成部分,但应该认识到,并不是所有患者都能通过抗反转录病毒治疗改善其KS,而且只有在4~8周的治疗后才能出现这种改善。如果患者在开始抗HIV治疗的12周内没有显示出KS的改善,他们的疾病将不太可能仅通过干预得到控制,然后必须考虑其他治疗方案。另一个重要的现象是,一些患者在开始使用cART后不久就会出现KS复燃,这可以从KS病变的大小和数量迅速增加得到证明。这种复燃可能是自限性的,继续cART治疗会出现肿瘤退缩;然而,这需要治疗医生的密切关注,如果复燃变得临床显著,需考虑额外的KS治疗。与针对HIV的抗反转录病毒药物相比,抗疱疹病毒药物在活动性KS方面似乎没有治疗作用,更昔洛韦和缬更昔洛韦还没有观察到有缓解的病例。因此,目前可用的抗疱疹病毒药物不能推荐作为抗KS治疗。

局部抗肿瘤化疗

针对KS肿瘤的治疗分为局部治疗和全身治疗。局部治疗的好处是,可以推迟全身化疗,后者可增加本已脆弱的患者群体免疫抑制的风险。局部治疗的选择可能受到某些因素的影响,如病变的范围和位置(如躯干或肢体上小的、单一的病变)和临床进程的快慢(如新病变在数月而不是数周内缓慢发展)。局部治疗方案包括病灶内注射长春碱、局部类维生素A、放疗和冷冻治疗等。

对于病灶数目少、抗HIV药物无效,或需要比抗HIV药物更快改善的患者,病灶内注射长春碱是一种合理的一线治疗方法。特别是腭或颊黏膜病变对病灶内长春碱反应迅速[78]。最常用的长春碱剂量为0.1~0.4mg/ml,在1cm^{2}病灶内注射约0.1~0.2ml。局部不适可能相当严重,因此长春碱可与利多卡因1:1混合以提高耐受性。局部反应一般是温和的,但皮肤也可能发生破损。不幸的是,这种肿瘤缓解通常是短暂的,大多数病变在几个月后就会进展。

基于139名患者的随机安慰剂对照试验,外用9-顺式维A酸(alitretinoin)凝胶也已被批准用于治疗皮肤KS。该试验表明,与安慰剂治疗组相比,维A酸治疗组的缓解率高6倍[79]。这种药物的困难之处在于,当应用于正常皮肤时,可能会引起刺激性的局部反应。因此，必须建议患者要非常小心地将这种化合物仅用于受影响的皮肤。即使这样的护理，一些患者也会产生局部反应，这可能会带来麻烦。肿瘤缓解不是立即的，而且可能在治疗后 1~2 个月内观察不到，所以需要耐心。值得注意的是，当系统性给药时，同样的化合物似乎具有活性。在两项开放标签多中心试验中，肿瘤的缓解率接近 40%[80]。明显的毒性为头痛、皮肤干燥、高脂血症和胰腺炎。

放疗

即使是相对低剂量，使用正压或电子束的放射治疗可以给 KS 带来高度有效的局部控制，绝大多数接受治疗的患者会出现肿瘤缓解，其中许多会完全缓解。法国一项针对 643 名与获得性免疫缺陷综合征相关的 KS 患者的研究发现，在 2 周内每周给予 20Gy 照射，之后 2 周每周给予 10Gy 照射，完全缓解率为 92%[81]。剂量计划的修改可能会降低患者的复杂性。一项 36 人参与的研究，在两周内以每周 3 次进行总量 21Gy 的治疗，总有效率为 91%，完全缓解率为 80%[82]。据报道，仅用 8Gy 的照射就能使大约四分之三的患者出现缓解[83,84]。治疗的耐受性较好，尽管可能发生急性和晚期毒性，包括水肿加重、溃疡和慢性皮肤损伤。当照射黏膜时必须谨慎，因为获得性免疫缺陷综合征患者对放射治疗引起黏膜炎的敏感性似乎提高了，并可能发生使人衰弱的并发症。

光动力疗法是一种利用光活化光敏药物引起局部肿瘤坏死的实验方法。对近 350 例 KS 病变光敏剂的研究显示，缓解率为 96%，其中三分之一是完全缓解[85]。

冷冻疗法

Ⅱ期临床试验已评估液氮冷冻治疗用于控制皮肤局部 KS[86]。有 2~4 个病灶的 20 例患者，每 3 周治疗一次，直到达到最大反应。80%的病例出现完全缓解，每个病变平均治疗 3 次（范围 1~8）。随后一项对 30 例患者的回顾性分析显示完全缓解率为 63%，大多数为持续缓解[87]。这种疗法常常会引起水泡发生，但出血、疼痛和感染并不常见。因此，液氮冷冻治疗可被认为是一种有效和耐受性良好的局部治疗，用于分散的、有症状的 KS 病变。然而，应该考虑对于可见部位病变的治疗对容貌的影响，因为水泡可能几天到几周都是难看的。

系统性抗肿瘤化疗

全身治疗适用于晚期有症状性疾病的 KS，特别是对于水肿、广泛黏膜皮肤病变和肺部或症状性胃肠道受累的患者。1 型干扰素由于其抗病毒、抗增殖、抗血管生成和促免疫活性而具有疗效，但由于起效缓慢且耐受性差，很少采用这种治疗方法[88]。单药和联合细胞毒化疗最为有效。通常用于有症状或器官威胁疾病的患者，这些患者不适合单独使用局部治疗或 cART。该疾病的有效药物包括阿霉素、博来霉素、依托泊苷、紫杉类、长春花生物碱和吉西他滨。博来霉素联合长春新碱（BV）或多柔比星（阿霉素）、博来霉素和长春新碱（ABV）的联合一线治疗肿瘤的缓解率为 57%~88%[89,90]。由于二维测量对皮肤、黏膜和内脏病变的局限性，KS 对化疗缓解的定义与大多数其他肿瘤相比更加模糊。KS 可以在组织学上出现可识别肿瘤的完全消退，但是色素沉着过度的区域大小可能不会改变。改变的是病变的结节性，颜色特征（从紫罗兰色或橙红色到灰褐色含铁血黄素染色），以及最初出现时相关的水肿。由于缺乏统一的缓解标准，早期文献中的缓解难以评估，而最近的研究受益于 ACTG 最初定义的、并通过获得性免疫缺陷综合征恶性肿瘤协会、国家癌症研究所和美国食品药品管理局（Food and Drug Administration，FDA）的共同努力改进的标准反应评价标准。

ABV 联合细胞毒治疗已成为与新治疗方案进行比较的标准治疗方案。虽然这种方案带来了相当大的缓解率，但副作用很常见，最突出的是恶心、脱发、疲劳、周围神经病变、肢端发绀、雷诺现象、血细胞减少和感染[91]。这些毒性可使许多患者非常虚弱。需要其他的药物治疗处理许多其他医疗问题。

因此，在 KS 中，对有效且更容易耐受的治疗方案的需要尤为急迫。脂质体包裹的蒽环类已经成为一种高效且可耐受的治疗选择。构成 KS 病变的渗漏脉管系统有利于药物沉积，并且已经显示药物在病灶的浓度比非病灶组织高几乎一个数量级[92]。此外，这些药物的副作用更小。两项Ⅲ期研究各入组大约 250 名 HIV 相关 KS 患者，均显示脂质体多柔比星单药优于 ABV 或 BV 的传统细胞毒性组合。脂质体多柔比星治疗的缓解率为 46%~58%，相比之下，传统的两药和三药组合的缓解率为 25%[93,94]。尽管存在生存差异，脂质体多柔比星治疗患者的至缓解时间、耐受性、与健康相关的生活质量均得到改善[95]。一项大型随机研究比较了传统的 ABV 与脂质体柔红霉素的组合，发现脂质体药物的毒性较小，但肿瘤缓解率相当，并没有之前发现的那么高[96]。

一项小型试验比较了阿霉素和柔红霉素的脂质体制剂，脂质体多柔比星看起来更好，但试验太小而无法得出明确的结论[97]。整体证据支持使用脂质体多柔比星作为晚期症状性 KS 的首选化疗，标准剂量为每 2~3 周 20mg/m^2，直至最大缓解或不可接受的毒性。

紫杉烷通过稳定微管作用于肿瘤细胞，已经成为治疗 KS 的高效且耐受良好的药物。在Ⅰ期试验中显示出令人鼓舞的疗效和安全性之后[98]，对先前接受过治疗的 KS 患者进行了Ⅱ期研究，结果显示缓解率为 56%~71%，中位缓解持续时间为 9~10 个月，这长于任何其他治疗[99]。在蒽环类药物治疗过的患者中，低剂量紫杉醇（100mg/m^2 每 2 周 1 次，）仍有疗效，耐受性好。鉴于紫杉醇具有优异的疗效和耐受性，在一项随机对照试验中将其与脂质体多柔比星作为初始治疗进行了比较[100]。入组了 73 名患者，其中四分之三的患者同时接受 cART 治疗。紫杉醇和脂质体多柔比星的总体缓解率分别为 56%和 46%，统计学无显著性差异。两组中大部分有疼痛或 KS 相关性水肿的患者接受各自的治疗后出现了临床改善。中位无进展生存期在紫杉醇组为 18 个月，脂质体多柔比星组为 12 个月（$P=0.66$）。两组的总体生存期相同，两种药物总体耐受性良好。根据汇总数据，脂质体多柔比星或紫杉醇均可被用于 KS 的一线全身治疗，如果复发进展后可使用另一种药物。在我们中心，如果没有使用蒽环类药物的禁忌证，我们通常使用脂质体多柔比星作为一线治疗，紫杉醇用于后线治疗。对于停止治疗后快速进展的患者，可以继续使用紫杉醇作为维持治疗；一些患者在我们中心接受治疗超过 2 年，并且肿瘤一直控制很好。较新的紫杉烷，多西他赛，也已证实在晚期 KS 中有效,包括先前接受过蒽环类药物甚至紫杉醇治疗的患者,但是中性粒细胞减少是一个问题[101,102]。我们目前不建议在临床试验之外使用多西紫杉醇。

新的治疗方法

KS病变的富血管性及其研究的可及性使其成为评估抗血管生成药物的候选疾病。涉及一系列不同药物的临床试验已经或正在进行中。贝伐单抗是一种针对VEGF-A的单克隆抗体,在Ⅱ期临床试验中对HIV相关的KS患者进行了评估,这些患者对cART单药没有反应[103]。这是一个总体高危人群,大多数患者以前接受过化疗(最常见的是脂质体阿霉素),中位距末次化疗时间为3个月。共17名受试者接受贝伐单抗的治疗,剂量为15mg/kg静脉注射,每21天为一周期。总有效率为31%,其中3例患者达到完全缓解。中位治疗周期数为10次(范围1~37),中位至疾病进展时间为8个月。考虑到研究人群都为高危且之前接受过治疗,这些结果表明贝伐单抗在HIV相关的KS中具有令人鼓舞的活性。贝伐单抗联合其他药物的研究正在进行中。沙利度胺具有多种特性,包括抑制血管生成,并已在KS患者的早期研究中得到评估。一项对20名患者进行的Ⅱ期研究显示,8名患者出现部分缓解,中位至疾病进展时间为7个月[104]。显著的毒性包括营养不良、抑郁、嗜睡和神经病变。病例报告显示第二代药物来那度胺具有疗效,来那度胺治疗KS的前瞻性试验正在进行中[105,106]。

膜金属蛋白酶(Membrane metalloproteinase,MMP)在KS细胞中过表达,可能促进肿瘤的侵袭和转移[107]。在75名患者的随机Ⅱ期临床试验中,MMP抑制剂COL-3显示了有效性和安全性[108]。总有效率在COL-3低剂量组为41%,高剂量组为29%,其缓解与血浆MMP水平下降有关。皮疹和光敏性是最常见的不良事件。

KSHV/HHV8诱导PI3K/AKT/mTOR通路,产生促增殖和抗凋亡作用,促进KS发病[53]。因此,靶向mTOR通路作为一种合理的治疗靶点引起了人们的关注。对这一策略的热情来自15例肾移植术后KS患者的报告,当免疫抑制药从环孢霉素改为西罗莫司时,这些患者的完全缓解率达到惊人的100%[109]。AIDS恶性疾病联盟对7名HIV相关KS患者进行了一项小型研究,发现3名患者出现肿瘤缓解,他们都接受了含有蛋白酶抑制剂的治疗,这导致了更高的西罗莫司暴露[110]。该药物耐受性良好,没有导致HIV病毒载量的显著变化或CD4细胞计数的显著下降。更多的数据有望进一步说明这一药物在获得性免疫缺陷综合征相关KS中的作用。

由于血小板衍生生长因子(PDGF)和c-KIT活化在KS生物学中的作用,酪氨酸激酶抑制剂作为一种可能的KS治疗策略引起了人们的关注[111,112]。AIDS恶性疾病联盟进行了一项30人参与的甲磺酸伊马替尼治疗HIV相关KS的Ⅱ期试验[113]。77%的患者之前接受过cART治疗,57%之前接受过针对KS的化疗。总体缓解率为33%,全部为部分缓解,中位至缓解时间为21周。在缓解者中,中位缓解持续时间为9个月。

KS的病毒过程及其与免疫功能的关系也表明,免疫学方法可能最终具有治疗价值。KSHV/HHV8可以改变巨噬细胞和CTL的功能。巨噬细胞抑制趋化因子由病毒编码,在KSHV/HHV8感染细胞中产生。这些细胞还产生一种被称为K-14的OX-2同源物。OX-2受体存在于单核/巨噬细胞上,抑制巨噬细胞被其他刺激激活的能力。K14能够减少活化的巨噬细胞产生炎症细胞因子,可能限制宿主对KSHV/HHV8的反应[114]。此外,KSHV/HHV8可编码具有改变受感染细胞被CTL靶向能力的基因。K3和K5病毒基因产物限制MHC Ⅰ类分子的CTL参与,K5还抑制与激活CTL所必需的共受体(B7)复合物的相互作用[115]。然而,一些报道已经定义了可被CTL识别的KSHV/HHV8基因产物中的表位[116,117]。对特定表位是否有反应的定义与预防疾病有关,以及免疫抑制通路是否可行疫苗或过继细胞治疗。

非霍奇金淋巴瘤(NHL)

淋巴细胞增殖发生在许多不同类型的免疫缺陷的背景下。它是先天性T细胞功能异常的个体、接受器官移植免疫抑制药物治疗的个体和感染获得性免疫缺陷综合征病毒个体的常见并发症。其中一个共同的主题是EBV在诱导B细胞增殖方面的作用不受抑制。然而,只有少数ARL与先天性或移植后环境下的淋巴增生性疾病相似。ARL包括一组具有挑战性临床过程的复杂肿瘤。它一直是,而且仍然是获得性免疫缺陷综合征病毒感染中最致命的并发症,需要新的方法和对其病理生理学基础的新理解。最常见的ARL为DLBCL,其次为BL、PCNSL、原发性渗出性淋巴瘤(primary effusion lymphoma,PEL)、浆细胞性淋巴瘤(plasmablastic lymphoma,PBL),还有很少见的外周T细胞淋巴瘤(peripheral T-cell lymphomas,PTCL)。基于HIV相关免疫抑制的深度,这些类型的发病率有显著的差异。

流行病学

NHL与HIV感染的关系在获得性免疫缺陷综合征流行的前5年就很明显了,当时在加州的癌症注册中,年轻男性中淋巴瘤的数量异常多。美国疾病控制与预防中心在1987年首次修订了对获得性免疫缺陷综合征的定义,将NHL包括在内,NHL仍然是获得性免疫缺陷综合征病毒感染的重要和破坏性表现。与KS不同的是,在KS中,HIV感染者的特定亚群具有独特的风险,而NHL在不同HIV危险因素组上的分布更为均匀,几乎没有差异。目前的差异可能部分归因于治疗。

获得性免疫缺陷综合征病毒感染者发生NHL的风险部分由免疫抑制水平决定,CD4细胞计数低的人患NHL的风险较高;然而,特定的淋巴瘤亚型与严重的免疫抑制有较强的相关性。PCNSL的发生仅限于那些免疫缺陷非常严重的患者,系统性ARLs的PEL和PBL亚群也是如此。自cART出现以来,这些严重的免疫功能障碍的发病率显著降低了。在其他的ARL中,DLBCL的发生率因cART而下降,但仍是最常见的ARL。与其他亚型的ARL不同,BL最常发生在免疫功能保留的时候,在HIV控制良好生存期长的患者中,随着时间的推移占ARLs的比例越来越高[26,118]。中位CD4细胞计数在大多数ARLs治疗报告都在50~100个细胞/mm^3的范围,BL组CD4细胞计数通常>200个细胞/mm^3。相反,PCNSL患者的报告显示CD4细胞计数严重下降[26,119]。因此,非霍奇金淋巴瘤可能发生在HIV疾病的不同过程中,包括那些几乎没有其他免疫抑制表现的情况,并且可能是HIV感染的首发表现。因此,任何有非霍奇金淋巴瘤组织学表现的人都应考虑可能发生的未被确认的HIV 感染。持续免疫抑制的持续时间和严重程度对确定发生ARL 的风险很重要,CD4 细胞计数每下降 50%,相对危险度约为 1.4。令人欣慰的是,随着 CD4 细胞计数对 cART 的反应,淋巴瘤的风险降低,但有大约 1 年的延迟时间,比其他机会性疾病的延迟时间稍长[21]。有趣的是,风险的降低似乎是随着cART 治疗时间的延长而同时进行的,这可能反映了长期 cART治疗带来免疫功能的逐渐修复。免疫功能与艾滋病毒核糖核酸酸(RNA)水平有关,后者为 ARL 风险的预测因子。EuroSIDA 研究表明,每一 log HIV RNA 的相对危险度为 1.51[21]。因此,控制 HIV 是 ARL 的关键因素,可能是因为其产生的免疫改变或其他病理生理机制。

病理和发病机制

HIV 感染相关淋巴瘤的进展实质上总是伴随着 B 细胞的转化,而 HIV 本身并不感染 B 细胞。因此 HIV 在 ARL 进展中并不起直接作用,只是为病毒转化或者 B 细胞功能不减弱的启动增殖提供了一个免疫抑制的环境。然而,PTCL 作为 T 细胞肿瘤的一个亚型,对此却是一个罕见的例外。

HIV 导致的外周 T 细胞淋巴瘤虽然少见,但是却包含一系列临床病理特征[24,120-122],一方面,HIV 的基因组在 T 细胞和肿瘤相关的巨噬细胞中都被发现,HIV 的基因融合位点清晰准确地定位于癌症驱动基因 C-fes 的上游,这个发现充分地说明了HIV 直接导致了 T 细胞肿瘤疾病的发生[123]。

虽然,HIV 仅仅在罕见的 PTCL 中存在,但是对于其他的淋巴瘤来说,仍然有其他的病毒存在且起到关键作用。例如,EB病毒是一个与免疫缺陷相关淋巴瘤高度相关的病毒,也是导致PCNSL 的必然因素。γ-疱疹病毒发挥的生物学作用通过分子分析正在被揭开,很可能是在 PCNS 淋巴瘤和移植后淋巴组织增生性疾病(post-transplantation lymphoproliferative diseases,PTLD)中发挥重要作用。在这种情况下,这些潜伏病毒表达的具体基因具有所谓的Ⅲ型模式的特征。这些基因包括 *LMP1*、*LMP2* 和 *EBNA1* 至 *EBNA6*。*LMP1* 基因已被广泛研究,作为一个 B 细胞增殖的介质,且已被证明参与到肿瘤坏死因子受体(tumor necrosis factor receptor,TNFR)的信号通路[124,125]。*LMP1* 基因在 PTLD 和 ARL 患者的原发肿瘤组织中都有表达,参与了NFκB 通路的激活,也在调控正常 B 细胞和恶性 B 细胞存活中发挥关键作用[126]。LMP1 是一个具有细胞质羧基的六层跨膜分子,羧基能够与 TNFR Ⅱ相关因子(TNFR Ⅱ-associated factor,TRAF)相互作用,进而介导下游转录因子激活[125,127,128]。LMP1 的细胞质结构域的聚集活化了 TNFR Ⅱ,激活途径类似于 TNFR 家族成员 CD30,CD30 是一个参与到 NFκB 和 cjun 通路的细胞因子[129,130]。这些调控因子的下游靶点是促增殖细胞的因子,如 IL-6 和 IL-10。

LMP1 的羧基末端内有许多突变已经被发现,并且有一些数据支持这些突变与 HIV 相关的 NHL 或 HIV 相关的 HL 相关[129,131-133]。然而,其他研究表明,淋巴增生性疾病患者中此类突变的发生频率并不高于未发生淋巴增生性疾病的患者[132]。EBV 及其诱导的分子改变促使 B 细胞感染并逐步恶变的假说目前广泛引人关注。

EBV 感染比例在不同类型肿瘤中比例不同。EBV 几乎存在于所有的 PCNSL 和 PBL 患者体内,在 HIV 相关 DLBCL 和BL 中分别是 30%和 80%[134-137]。目前研究没有发现与 ARL 发生发展密切相关的病毒;然而,其中一小部分研究提示可能与KSHV/HHV8 有一定相关性。PEL 是一种独特的 ARL 亚型,通常见于患有严重免疫抑制的患者,一般不形成明显肿块,主要表现为腔隙恶性积液,如:胸膜腔,腹膜或心包[138]。肿瘤细胞通常不表达大多数 B 细胞,T 细胞或甚至造血细胞表面标志物(CD45、CD3 和 CD19 阴性)。细胞的分子分析证明了这一点它们经历了与 B 细胞谱系起源一致的免疫球蛋白基因重排。迄今为止,这种肿瘤迄今为止包括 *KSHV/HHV8* 基因组,大多数都证实与 EBV 感染相关。值得注意的是,几乎所有的 PEL 病理都表达了 CD30 表面抗原。CD30 是本妥西单抗的靶点,CD30单克隆抗体共价结合 MMAE(microtubule toxin monomethyl auristatin E)。目前 FDA 已经批准本妥西单抗用于治疗复发的CD30 表达的淋巴瘤、HL 和间变性大细胞淋巴瘤。由于 PEL 中的 CD30 表达阳性,细胞研究中发现:CD30 抗体本妥西单抗可抑制 PEL 细胞增殖和促进其凋亡[139]。在小鼠 PEL 细胞异种移植瘤体实验中:本妥西单抗对肿瘤进展和延长生存期方面,发现本妥西单抗有良好的效果但是目前并不能满足临床的需求。

体外细胞试验已经发现 KSHV/HHV8 可以感染 B 细胞,但这种感染对细胞的影响在体外细胞水平比较难以观察。目前没有证据表明 B 细胞生长动力学与病毒感染有关,如 EBV 与KSHV/HHV8 之间的联系。然而,KSHV/HHV8 与 PEL 之间密切的临床和病理联系,为 KSHV/HHV8 与 B 细胞肿瘤发生提供了强有力的证据。PEL 细胞被 KSHV/HHV8 感染,导致潜伏的基因激活进一步促进肿瘤的发生发展。具体而言,LANA-1、LANA-2、v-cyclin、v-FLIP 和病毒 IL6 都是由同一个共同的启动子转录而来的,在 PEL 细胞中异常表达,进一步通过各种机制促进肿瘤细胞生长[140]。

病毒导致恶性肿瘤的发生主要是因为病毒改变了肿瘤细胞的免疫反应性。具体机制包括 EBV EBNA1 改变了抗原加工过程,从而掩盖了 EBV 感染的细胞,逃避细胞毒性 T 淋巴细胞的杀伤作用[141]。虽然该机制的具体细节仍有待阐明,但是KSHV/HHV8 在对感染细胞的转化中发挥类似的作用。此外,病毒基因产物可以被感染的细胞精心包装,并可能影响免疫效应细胞。例如,EBV 编码的病毒 IL-10 类似物(BRCF-1)具有生物活性,具有内源性 IL-10 的作用[142]。在 AIDS 患者和 ARL 肿瘤动物模型中发现了 IL-10 的存在[142-145],在辅助 T 细胞(TH1)的反应中发挥抑制作用。IL-10 通过抑制效应细胞 TH1的应答有效抑制了干扰素-α 和 IL-2 的产生,同时 IL-10 还是促细胞分裂剂。

其他的一些细胞因子也参与肿瘤细胞的发生。例如 IL-6,除了促进 B 细胞的增殖外,同时其可能会改变对肿瘤细胞的敏感性免疫杀伤。具体而言,在 HIV 感染个体中,IL-6 已经证明可以降低抗原特异性 CTL 细胞对 EBV 阳性细胞的裂解能力[146]。IL-6 水平在患有艾滋病的患者的血清中升高,并且可能与 NHL 发生发展有关[147]。CD40 和 CD40 配体(CD40L)相互作用也可能参与艾滋病相关淋巴瘤的发展。TNFR 家族通路参与细胞增殖、分化和 B 细胞的存活,激活 TNFR 家族通路激活是 B 细胞和 T 细胞介导的免疫机制之一。感染来自骨髓和

CNS 的微血管内皮细胞可改变 CD40 的表达，增加与 B 细胞的相互黏附作用，这一机制可能解释 HIV 感染者的结外淋巴瘤[148]。

趋化因子途径也可能有助于 HIV 感染患上淋巴瘤。具有 *SDF-1* 基因(stroma-derived growth factor-1)(CXC 趋化因子)突变患者更容易患 BL 亚型 ARL[149]。这个趋化因子是已知的促 B 细胞分裂剂，并通过促进化学动力学效应，可能促进携带 *SDF-1* 基因变异患者的增殖。*SDF-1* 基因突变增加患者淋巴瘤的风险，*SDF-1* 基因突变成为筛查淋巴瘤易感性因素之一。

研究已经发现某些特定的基因突变与特定亚型的淋巴瘤有关。DLBCL 患者肿瘤标本中，33%存在 *Bcl-6* 重排，40%存在 *c-myc* 重排。大约 25%存在 *TP53* 突变[150,151]。相比之下，在艾滋病相关 BLs 中发现 *c-myc* 重排，但没有发现 *Bcl-6* 重排，很少发现 *TP53* 突变[152-154]。EBV 分别与 BL 和 DLBCL 中的 *c-myc* 或 *Bcl-6* 重排相关。*c-myc* 基因与免疫球蛋白基因并列链开关区域重排表明：恶性转化发生在接近免疫球蛋白类转换的时间。这一 B 细胞发育中的晚期事件表明这个转化发生在相对成熟的生发中心 B 细胞阶段。

临床表现

ARL 通常是高度侵袭性淋巴瘤，ARL 患者的临床特征与高度侵袭性 NHL 类似，HIV 感染相关的 ARL 表现为更晚的分期及结外病灶。ARL 患者大多数出现结外累及[155]，且大约一半患者病灶局限在结外病灶。特定淋巴瘤亚型易出现特定部位累及，如：BL 患者，四分之一左右患者出现骨髓和软脑膜侵犯，而 DLBCL 容易出现胃肠道、肝脏、脑实质及软脑膜侵犯。

系统性“B”症状包括：明显减轻体重，发热及盗汗很常见。由于此类患者多伴随免疫抑制，因此需要进行微生物检测排除合并的细菌、分枝杆菌、病毒、真菌或寄生虫病等感染。KSHV/HHV8 相关的多中心 Castleman 病(multicentric castleman disease，MCD)患者也应该考虑病毒检测，详细情况见后面章节。

Primary Effusion Lymphoma(PEL)通常发生在艾滋病感染患者的终末期，通常发生 CD4 细胞计数<50 个细胞/mm^3 时，偶尔也会发生在器官移植相关的免疫抑制患者。这种淋巴瘤通常累及腹膜腔，胸膜腔和心包，部分进展期患者可以出现骨髓受累[156]，很少累及腔外，但可以出现其他结外累及[157-159]，对这一类型淋巴瘤的处理方法与其他亚型 ARL 相似，包括中枢神经系统评估。

在 HIV 感染患者中，浆细胞瘤发生率明显增加，并且相当异质。罕见的高度侵袭性的发生于下颌骨和口腔的 PBL 通常发生于严重免疫缺陷患者，通常 CD4 细胞计数低于此值 50 细胞/mm^3，但也可以发生在不太严重的免疫功能障碍患者[136]。这部分淋巴瘤细胞标记为浆细胞相关 MUM1，CD138 和 CD38 标记，而不表达典型的淋巴标记物如 CD45、LCA(白细胞共同抗原)和 CD20。部分也可以 EBV 感染阳性和频率更低的 KSHV/HHV8 感染。PBL 是一种高度侵袭性的淋巴瘤，Ki67 增殖分数通常>90%，大约一半的患者检测到 C-MYC 易位[160]。有报告发现：髓外浆细胞瘤和多发性骨髓瘤表达 HIV 抗原特异性的蛋白。针对此类浆细胞瘤和多发性骨髓瘤的治疗应该参照标准指南进行，同时应该考虑此类患者的艾滋病背景。目前仍没有针对 PBL 患者的最佳治疗方案，采用 DLBCL 患者常用的 CHOP 方案(环磷酰胺、多柔比星、长春新碱和泼尼松)，效果很差。由于高度增殖活性及存在且 MYC 易位，Burkitt 淋巴瘤(Burkitt lymphoma，BL)患者，若考虑采用这些治疗方案应充分考虑患者的耐受性。

PCNSL 占所有 HIV 相关淋巴瘤的 15%～20%，并且表现为严重的免疫抑制。通常 CD4 细胞计数<30 个细胞/mm^3，多数患者既往存在艾滋病相关的并发症，以及 EBV 相关基因可以在淋巴瘤细胞中检测到[161]。组织学上，此类型淋巴瘤临床表现与免疫母细胞使用大 B 细胞外观并表达一种类型 EBV 潜伏基因产物的Ⅲ型[162]。这些患者的临床方法将在后面的章节中详述。

MCD 或血管滤泡性淋巴结增生可能发生在晚期 HIV 疾病患者中，表现为 ARL 或传染病[163]。MCD 是一种多克隆疾病，进而在 HIV 感染患者中均与 KSHV/HHV8 相关，可表现为快速进展威胁生命。已报道 MCD 的透明血管和浆细胞亚型均存在 AIDS 感染，浆细胞亚型更为常见。KSHV/HHV8 被发现在相应淋巴结中，并且共同发生或随后的 KS 患病率很高[163]。几乎所有患者都存在发热，淋巴结肿大，肝脾肿大和贫血；IL-6 在 MCD 中大量产生并在疾病发生发展中发挥关键作用，通过激活 JAK/STAT 途径，促进血管生成和增殖[164-166]。抗 IL-6 的单克隆抗体已显示出临床疗效。治疗 HIV 阴性且 HHV8 阴性 MCD[167]，但与 HIV 相关的 MCD 的临床疗效尚未明确。MCD 患者可能同时出现 ARL 或随后发生 ARL；因此对于考虑复发或进展，临床症状发生任何变化的时候，有必要进行重复活检，明确是否类型发生转变。

临床方法

ARL 患者的评估遵循其他类型 NHL 的分期系统。但其中包括几个针对 HIV 感染患者的警告。第一，与 HIV 阴性患者相比，HIV 阳性患者 CNS 的累及概率更高，要求对 CNS 进行更彻底的评估，包括诊断时大多数患者的脑脊液(cerebrospinal fluid，CSF)取样，以及脑影像学检查，尤其是在有神经系统体征或症状时候。在没有神经系统症状和低风险特征的患者中可以不进行脑脊液取样，包括分期局限、无结外累及 LDH 正常患者。第二，在评估患有“B”症状或可疑影像学检查结果的患者时，必须牢记同时发生机会性感染的可能性。对于 CD4 细胞计数<200 个细胞/mm^3 的人群，微生物学评估尤其重要，机会性感染的风险增加，并且对于<50 个细胞/mm^3 的人群是必需的。根据临床情况，应特别关注活跃的卡氏肺孢子虫、CMV、弓形虫、鸟分枝杆菌复合体、结核分枝杆菌和隐球菌的可能存在。应该在所有患者中评估乙型肝炎和丙型肝炎血清学，因为可能发生共感染。第三，评估艾滋病的状况对于确定治疗方法至关重要。应测量 CD4 细胞以及血浆 HIV RNA，并应获得先前抗反转录病毒治疗和既往机会性感染的详细病史。

对于那些终末期表现的 NHL 患者，复发难治性 HIV 患者应考虑用于姑息治疗。然而，对于大多数患者，采用 cART 的病毒抑制为 HIV 感染提供了更好的预后，重点应该是治愈淋巴瘤。这个概念在 cART 治疗时代之前并未实际考虑，但具有重要意义。但自 1996 年 cART 治疗时代之后，选择适合患者的 cART 方案包括评估患者可能处于 HIV 疾病哪一期，以及考虑药物-药物相互作用，并应与传染病专家合作进行。

预后因素

ARL 患者的预后一般较差；但随着 cART 的出现，HIV-1 本身预后的改善，以及化疗耐受性的提高，ARL 患者的远期疗效已大大改善。在 cART 出现之前，HIV 相关 DLBCL 患者的中位生存期为 8 个月，而 cART 出现后患者中位生存期为可长达 43 个月[168]。引入 cART 前 ARL 预后不良因素包括：年龄 >35 岁，静脉注射药物和Ⅲ/Ⅳ期疾病，预测总生存期从最有利亚组的 46 周到最少的 18 周[169]。国际预后指数（International Prognostic Index，IPI）是最常用的风险分层工具，采用于评估非 HIV 相关侵袭性淋巴瘤的风险分型[170]，已在 ARL 中进行了评估。在 pre-cART 时代，所有 IPI 小组的结果都很差；而 cART 问世以来，IPI 将风险评分分别为 0~2、3 和 4~5 的 3 个风险组分开，预测的 3 年总体生存率分别为 64%、50% 和 13%[171]。当然这个早期研究的患者，虽然大部分 CD20 阳性，仅采用单纯化疗，并没有接受利妥昔单抗治疗。另一项基于利妥昔单抗联合化疗的前瞻性临床试验治疗的 487 例 ARL 患者分析发现：在 cART 和利妥昔单抗时代已经开发出新的预后评分[172]。大多数患者是 DLBCL（70%），大多数患者同时有 BL。中位 CD4 数为 174 个细胞/μl，40% 的患者先前诊断为 AIDS。最常见的化疗方案是 R-CHOP（49%），其次是 EPOCH-R（19%）、GMALL 方案（16%）和 CDE（环磷酰胺、多柔比星和依托泊苷，15%）。对于预后相关明显因素进行生存多因素分析，开发了一个新的预后模型，结合传统的年龄调整 IPI 风险因素（晚期、PS 评分差和 LDH 升高），再加上 CD4 细胞计数，HIV 病毒载量，艾滋病病史和结外累及的数量。这些预后因素产生了 3 个风险组，其中低、中、高风险组的 5 年总生存率分别为 78%、60% 和 50%，这似乎优于传统 IPI 评分的预测模型。这些数据证明了使用现代疗法联合 cART 治疗明显提高了 ARL 的治愈率。

其他的研究发现表达非生发中心标志物的患者（BCL-6 和 CD10 阴性，MUM1/IRF4 或 CD138 阳性）无病生存率更短，这个结果与 HIV 阴性 DLBCL 类似[173]。以往研究发现 BL 患者治疗上采用 CHOP 等传统 DLBCL 治疗方案大多治疗效果不佳，但新的研究结果表明，采用新的联合方案治疗后，HIV 相关 BL 患者的治疗效果与 HIV 阴性患者一样好[171,174-176]。在考虑 ARL 患者的预后时，必须整个过程都要考虑 HIV 疾病本身的状况，因为对于抗反转录病毒治疗失败的晚期艾滋病患者，治疗耐受性明显变差。

治疗

在艾滋病流行的早期，侵袭性高的淋巴瘤治疗上也多采用高强度的临床治疗方法，这样会导致严重的毒性和很高的治疗相关的死亡率。然而，随着造血生长因子的问世，对于机会性感染的预防性治疗得到了很大改善，提高了化疗的耐受性。低剂量强度化疗方案的出现也减少艾滋病患者的治疗相关毒性，但在前 cART 时代，低剂量强度化疗方案均疗效差。但 cART 时代后，由于 cART 和支持治疗，患有 HIV 相关的 ARL 的患者可以使用与 HIV 阴性对应物相同的标准剂量化疗方案进行治疗，与 cART 前时代相比，疗效大大改善。因此，目前在 ARL 治疗中很少用低剂量强度方案。

ARL 最常用的治疗方案是 CHOP 和 EPOCH 化疗方案，对于 CD20 阳性患者联合利妥昔单抗（见下文进一步讨论）（表 75-4）。

表 75-4　艾滋病相关淋巴瘤的常用治疗方案。

治疗方案	剂量和时间表
CHOP（基于 CD20 表达的+/-利妥昔单抗）[a]	
环磷酰胺	750mg/m²，IVPB，第 1 天
阿霉素	50mg/m²，IVPB 第 1 天
长春新碱	1.4mg/m²（不超过 2mg），IVPB，第 1 天
泼尼松（每个周期 q21~28d）	100mg，po，第 1~5 天
利妥昔单抗（如果包括在内）	375mg/m²，第 1 天
支持性护理包括并发 cART 和预防 P. jiroveci 和疱疹病毒	
EPOCH 方案（+/-基于 CD20 表达的利妥昔单抗）[a]	
依托泊苷	50/m²，CI，第 1~4 天
长春新碱	0.4mg/m²，CI，第 1~4 天
多柔比星泼尼松	10mg/m²，CI，第 1~4 天
	60mg/m²，po，第 1~5 天
环磷酰胺	375mg/m²，iv，第 5 天
利妥昔单抗（如果包括在内）	375mg/m²，iv，第 1 天（SC-EPOCH-RR 采用第 1 天和第 5 天用药）

支持性护理包括应用 cART 治疗和预防卡氏肺孢菌和疱疹病毒以及质子泵抑制剂。

缩写：G-CSF，粒细胞刺激因子；SC-EPOCH-RR，短程 EPOCH，每周期 2 剂利妥昔单抗。

[a]对于大多数患者，应包括鞘内注射甲氨蝶呤的 CNS 预防，但在选择的低风险患者中可能会遗漏，这些患者的分期早，LDH 正常，且无结外累及。

标准化疗药物加抗反转录病毒治疗

早期因为 cART 的相关药物较少，临床将抗病毒治疗和化疗的联合应用很受争议，因为两者联合很难在临床推广，其主要原因是药物和药物的相互作用及毒性反应叠加（如骨髓移植及外周神经毒性）。随着 cART 新的药物不断问世，药物毒性降低及药物-药物相互作用减少并且易于控制。同样明显的是，应用 cART 治疗后减少了 AIDS 的并发症，并且提高了全剂量化疗的耐受性。因此，在 ARL 治疗中，cART 联合化疗是标准治疗 ARL 方案。

这种方法在 CHOP 方案联合抗 HIV 药物英地那韦，d4T 和 3TC（艾滋病恶性联合会指导下）试验中得到验证，研究中一组患者接受低剂量，另一组接受全剂量 CHOP 加上相同的抗反转录病毒治疗方案的队列[177]。该研究表明该组合不会导致更严重的或更频繁的毒性。药理学分析测试了抗肿瘤药物对蛋白酶抑制剂水平的影响和代谢的抗病毒药物对化疗药物代谢的影响。没有观察到英地那韦或多柔比星水平的改变，但观察到环磷酰胺清除率降低约 50%。

美国国家癌症研究所测试了无伴随 cART 治疗的剂量调整 EPOCH 方案[178]。依托泊苷，长春新碱和多柔比星以 96 小时连续给药输注，然后在第 5 天推注环磷酰胺；环磷酰胺剂量基于前一周期中的基线 CD4 细胞计数和中性粒细胞减少症进行了修改。每个周期使用鞘内注射甲氨蝶呤用于预防 CNS 转移。持续抗病毒治疗导致癌症化疗期间 HIV RNA 升高，当化疗完成后恢复抗病毒药物时，恢复到入门水平。临床结果是迄今为止在 ARL 患者中报告最好的，74%的患者达到完全缓解，5 年无疾病和总体存活率分别为 92%和 60%。连续输注化疗方案联合抗病毒治疗也用于 ARL 的初始治疗。在 98 例患者采用 CDE 方案（环磷酰胺 800mg/m^2，多柔比星 50mg/m^2，依托泊苷 240mg/m^2，连续 96 小时输注）联合 cART 治疗（采用测试在前 43 名患者中使用地达诺新治疗），导致完全缓解率为 45%，2 年生存率 43%[179]。与达诺新对比，联合 cART 治疗的患者由于血液学毒性降低及治疗相关死亡率降低，总生存率提高。这些试验均显示：抗病毒药物联合抗肿瘤治疗是安全有效的。在免疫功能抑制低风险的患者中，进行短期的抗反转录病毒治疗似乎是可以接受的；但这应该谨慎进行，一旦可行就启动 cART。

以往研究，BL 患者被纳入其他 ARL 的临床研究中，其治疗效果并不像 HIV 相关 DLBCL 治疗效果那么差。尽管大多数临床试验是在 cART 时代之前进行的，这些研究结果治疗效果较差。近期的新的临床研究证据表明，艾滋病相关 BL 患者在接受强化多药联合化疗同样可以取得与非 HIV 感染患者一样令人鼓舞的效果[174,175]。

单克隆抗体治疗

人源化抗 CD20 抗体利妥昔单抗出现改善艾滋病相关的淋巴瘤患者的预后，利妥昔单抗在 HIV 阴性 DLBCL 中与 CHOP 化疗联合使用时显示出生存获益[180]。一项多中心随机Ⅲ期试验 CHOP 与 CHOP 联合利妥昔单抗（R-CHOP）相比，证明在艾滋病的情况下，加入利妥昔单抗后，患者的总体结果没有改善[181]。利妥昔单抗的反应有改善的趋势（58% vs 47%）没有达到统计学意义；然而，与感染相关的死亡率增加（14% vs 2%）。利妥昔单抗组的大多数死亡发生在 CD4 细胞计数<100 个细胞/mm^3 的患者中，60%的死亡发生在 CD4 细胞计数<50 个细胞/mm^3。该试验的进一步复杂分析是在最初的 R-CHOP 后 3 个月维持利妥昔单抗期，在此期间发生了 40%的感染相关死亡。然而，随后的Ⅱ期研究表明艾滋病相关的淋巴瘤治疗中标准化疗联合利妥昔单抗，可以提高临床治疗效果[175,182-185]，和 1 060 名艾滋病相关的淋巴瘤患者的荟萃分析，这些患者均接受利妥昔单抗联合化疗或单独化疗的前瞻性临床试验，发现利妥昔单抗治疗的患者中生存率提高[186]。因此，目前 ARR 患者治疗中纳入利妥昔单抗被认为是标准治疗，但 CD4 细胞计数低的患者应用利妥昔单抗，应密切警惕治疗相关并发症的风险，必要时给予最佳支持治疗，包括预防性抗生素和生长因子支持。

最佳的化学免疫治疗策略仍然是一个争论的主题。R-CHOP 和 EPOCH-R 均被认为是 HIV 相关 DLBCL 的标准方案。对艾滋病恶性肿瘤联盟研究中治疗的 150 例艾滋病相关 CD20$^+$NHL 患者的汇总分析发现，EPOCH-R 方案提高无事件生存率（HR 0.40；95%CI，0.23，0.69；P<0.001）和总体而言生存（HR，0.38；95%CI，0.21，0.69；P<0.01）[187]。对 EPOCH-R 的研究还表明，与序贯应用 EPOCH 及利妥昔单抗相比，在每个化疗周期的第 1 天用利妥昔单抗似乎改善疾病控制，并且如果利妥昔单抗是每个周期给药两次（短程 EPOCH-RR 方案），则可以用较少的化疗周期治疗艾滋病相关的淋巴瘤患者[184,185]。标准 EPOCH-R 和短程 EPOCH-RR 均可作为 CD20$^+$艾滋病相关的淋巴瘤患者的合适方案。虽然早期研究没有联合 cART 治疗，但 EPOCH-R 联合 cART 治疗可安全地作为标准治疗方法。EPOCH-R 的常规预防还包括常规白细胞生长因子支持，以及用质子泵抑制剂预防卡氏肺孢菌、疱疹病毒感染和胃溃疡。

HIV 相关的 BL 患者可以使用与非 HIV 感染的 BL 患者相同的强化化疗方案加利妥昔单抗治疗[174]。HIV 感染患者采用中高强度方案的安全性得益于有效的抗病毒治疗，使 HIV 感染有效控制和 CD4 细胞计数的普遍改善。最近，在 11 例 HIV 相关 BL 中评估了短程 EPOCH-RR 方案（利妥昔单抗每周期两次）的疗效，6 年总生存率为 90%[175]，这个令人鼓舞的数据需要在更大规模的 HIV 相关 BL 患者中验证。PBL 是一种高度侵袭性的淋巴瘤，通常还包括 MYC 易位，治疗上通常参考 BL 的治疗。浆母细胞淋巴瘤患者治疗上多采用 EPOCH 方案。利妥昔单抗通常没有作用，因为这些病例通常是 CD20 阴性，但是对于罕见的 CD20 阳性病例应该包括利妥昔单抗。多个病例报告已证实对蛋白酶体抑制剂硼替佐米的反应，因此硼替佐米可以作为 HIV 相关的 BL 患者复发后的治疗选择[188-192]。与其他艾滋病相关的淋巴瘤一样，建议所有患者同时联合 cART 治疗。

CNS 预防

CNS 预防的作用一直备受争议。虽然早期研究表明中枢神经系统受累的发生率非常高，常规 CNS 预防的有效性从未经过严格的研究证实。CNS 预防的方法目前没有统一共识，很多肿瘤中心对所有此类患者进行全身化疗联合鞘内化疗（最常采用甲氨蝶呤），有些肿瘤中心的做法是对于高危患者采用全身化疗联合鞘内化疗，其中包括：BL 或骨髓、睾丸或魏氏环受累或多发结外累及和 LDH 升高的患者。我们的做法是将鞘内注射甲氨蝶呤作为中枢神经系统预防用于大多数 DLBCL 患者的治疗方案，但在具有极低风险特征的患者中省略，包括有限期疾病，无结外受累和正常的 LDH。所有具有高度侵袭性 BL 和浆母细胞淋巴瘤组织学的患者都需要 CNS 预防。

治疗复发或难治性疾病

在非 HIV 感染者中治疗复发性侵袭性淋巴瘤包括使用大剂量化疗和自体干细胞移植（ASCT），这种方法已被证明比单独使用标准剂量化疗治愈率更高[193]。大剂量清髓化疗在艾滋病毒感染的情况下，发病率和死亡率的风险大大增加，尽管有证据表明它可以在 cART 时代有效地发挥作用。在一项包括 50 例复发性艾滋病相关的淋巴瘤患者的研究中，27 例进行了外周血干细胞移植，4 年无进展总生存率分别为 76%和 75%。所有 50 名患者的总生存率为 50%，反映了未行骨髓移植的患者的预后不良[194]。未行骨髓移植的原因主要是化疗耐药性（14 例），干细胞动员失败（6 例），早期毒性引起的死亡（2 例）。其他多个研究亦发现：自体干细胞移植在复发艾滋病相关的淋巴瘤患者中取得类似的令人鼓舞的治愈率[195,196]。值得注意的是，在 HIV 感染或非感染人群中，CXCR4 拮抗剂 plerixafor 都可促进干细胞动员，从而降低骨髓动员失败的风险[197]。因此，ASCT 应被视为复发的能够耐受高剂量化疗的艾滋病相关的淋巴瘤患者的治疗选择。对于这种独特的高风险患者群体，这种移植手术应该仅建议在具有丰富干细胞移植经验的中心。

已有研究发现：HIV 感染患者采用大剂量化疗完全清髓

后，进行同种异体干细胞移植（alloSCT），除了会出现移植物抗宿主病外，还会出现明显的感染相关毒性及淋巴瘤进展[198-200]。使用强度降低的非清髓性预处理方案的同种异体干细胞移植（alloSCT）适用于一小部分 HIV 感染和复发性血液系统恶性肿瘤患者，毒性降低，似乎是可行的[201,202]。采用同种异体干细胞移植在一例患者中治愈了 HIV。这个患者是 Timothy Ray Brown（也称为柏林患者）的特殊病例，他同时患有 HIV 及急性髓性白血病（AML）[203]。他被给予了 alloSCT，其供体干细胞在 *CCR5* 基因存在 32 碱基对缺失，通过阻止病毒进入而赋予对 HIV 感染的抵抗力。此患者到目前为止，在没有接受所有抗反转录病毒治疗下，在血液或组织中仍然没有发现 AML 及 HIV。使用 alloSCT 和同时 cART 治疗复发性血液系统恶性肿瘤的另外两例艾滋病患者，使用来自 CCR 野生型供体的干细胞，移植后刚开始没有发现持续存在 HIV 感染的证据，但随后在 12 周和 32 周时发现两名患者复发病毒[204]这些患者证明 alloSCT 和 cART 可能显著减少 HIV 储库，但在使用 CCR 野生型干细胞时不会根除它，可能是由于病毒在移植后的组织库中持续存在。通过这个柏林患者提示：在采用基因工程方法使供体干细胞中产生 CCR5 突变的可以防止 HIV 病毒进入移植患者，从而治愈 HIV，当然这一设想仍需要进一步实践证实。

支持性护理

所有患者应预防机会性感染的可能。在化疗期间大约一半患者会出现 CD4 细胞计数减少。并且即使 CD4 细胞计数超过 200 个细胞/mm^3 情况下，也推荐 *P. jiroveci*（原发卡氏肺孢子虫）预防。标准用于晚期 HIV 疾病的其他预防性治疗也适用于该人群。

鉴于 HIV 患者对骨髓抑制的敏感性增加，通常需要使用生长因子。CHOP 与 CHOP 加 GM-CSF 的单一随机试验发现，接受预防性生长因子的队列中发热和中性粒细胞减少的发生率和住院天数显著减少[205]。该试验设计较早，在蛋白酶抑制剂问世之前的临床试验，目前认为蛋白酶抑制剂通常可以改善患者对化疗的耐受性。鉴于 HIV 患者中性粒细胞减少和化疗感染的发生率增加，我们建议在接受艾滋病相关的淋巴瘤联合化疗方案的大多数患者中常规使用 G-CSF 支持。

与 HIV 并发的恶性肿瘤的治疗也值得注意，尤其要考虑药物-药物相互作用。许多蛋白酶抑制剂如地瑞那韦，茚地那韦，利托那韦和沙奎那韦抑制 CYP3A4 代谢活性，长春生物碱和紫杉烷类药物通过 CYP3A4 代谢。因此，同时使用这些抗反转录病毒药物的患者体内药物代谢受阻，是体内暴露于高浓度化疗药物，因此必须监测骨髓毒性和外周神经毒性，并且相应降低药物剂量。而非依赖核苷酸反转录酶抑制剂如依法韦仑和奈韦拉平将诱导 CYP3A4 活性，理论上导致化学药物代谢加快，降低化疗药物作用。然而，不推荐在这种情况下增加化疗药物剂量。一般情况下，由于骨髓毒性，应避免使用 cART 和齐多夫定，并且由于周围神经病变也应谨慎使用司他夫定和去羟肌苷。

原发性 CNS 淋巴瘤

在 HIV 感染的情况下，脑部肿块可能由许多感染和肿瘤过程引起，从而增加了诊断难度。最常见于艾滋病患者是弓形虫脓肿、PCNS 淋巴瘤、分枝杆菌或细菌性脓肿和进行性多灶性白质脑病（PML）。在没有活检病理的情况下，区分这些 CNS 性质仍然不完美，但对于有些患者活检是不可能的或被拒绝，某些参数可能会提高或降低淋巴瘤诊断的可能性，以及使用 CSF 中 EBV DNA 的 PCR 分析大大改善了没有组织学确认的诊断的可靠性。

一般来说，PCNSL、PML 和弓形虫病都是免疫抑制（CD4 细胞计数<50 个细胞/mm^3）的晚期并发症。该患者群体通常使用甲氧苄氨嘧啶磺胺甲噁唑预防卡氏肺孢菌，其可提供针对弓形虫的极好保护。对于弓形虫抗体滴度为阴性并且已进行此类预防的患者，中枢神经系统肿块诊断淋巴瘤的可能性为 74%[206]。PCR 分析中获得 CSF 样本中的 EBV 基因组，检测脑脊液中的 EBV 诊断淋巴瘤的特异性接近 100%[206,207]，敏感度为 80%。CSF 中 EBV+患者很少出现没有诊断出淋巴瘤的情况，但这个 PCR 检测 EBV 的方法非常适用于没有办法获取组织学活检患者。

提示淋巴瘤的影像学特征包括：中枢位置，非多灶性，大小>2cm[208]。此外，穿过中线的占位病灶很可能是恶性肿瘤性质病灶。单光子发射计算机断层扫描（SPECT）或正电子发射断层扫描（PET）也可以用来帮助区分脓肿和淋巴瘤。如果上述影像学检查其中之一发现典型占位，且 PCR 方法检测 CSF 样本 EBV 的阳性，都可以考虑开始治疗。如果影像学检查和 PCR 检查两者都是阴性，并且无法进行 CNS 病灶活检，可考虑经验性抗弓形虫治疗用作诊断和治疗工具。用乙胺嘧啶引发磺胺嘧啶或克林霉素，通常 5 天左右会使进展停止，14 天左右出现临床症状或影像学改善[209,210]。若治疗无效的话，则感染弓形虫病的可能性很低。

PCNSL 的治疗方法有限，且效果仍然很差。放疗联合或不联合化疗是主要的治疗方法，治疗客观缓解率从 60% 到 79% 不等，但持久缓解并不常见。在 cART 时代后，疗效似乎有所改善[161,211-213]。甲氨蝶呤为基础的大剂量化疗一直是非 HIV 感染患者 PCNSL 的主要治疗方法，其缓解率很高，并且会持续缓解。但在 cART 时代之前，因为高病毒复制和感染性并发症，这种大剂量化学应用受到限制，导致治疗效果很差[213]。然而，即使在 cART 时代，PCNSL 患者通常也有晚期 HIV 和 CD4 细胞计数非常低，因此也应该高度警惕感染风险。在与 CD4 细胞计数>100 细胞/mm^3 和健康状况良好的 HIV 相关的 PCNSL，可以考虑甲氨蝶呤为基础的大剂量化疗联合利妥昔单抗。目前已经发现化疗联合放疗，毒性很大，且疗效不佳。尽管 EBV 基因组与 PCNSL 相关，但它通常处于潜伏期，因此不太可能对溶解相特异性抗病毒剂敏感。尽管如此，使用更昔洛韦与齐多夫定联合使用的经验有限，IL-2 提示抗肿瘤活性[214]。这些药物或其他 EBV 指导的遗传或化学操作的最终用途有待于进一步临床试验证实。淋巴瘤与 HIV 引起的不良免疫功能之间存在明显关联，所以强调优化抗 HIV 疗法作为抗肿瘤疗法的重要组成部分。这些患者的总体治疗效果不佳，因此应鼓励积极参加新药临床试验。

由于类固醇激素可以引起免疫抑制，在该患者群体中使用类固醇激素需引起关注，目前缺乏关于这一方面的数据。类固醇激素用于减少水肿和肿块效应时仍可以考虑应用类固醇激素，但类固醇激素的减量应该尽可能快，并且要密切注意并发感染的可能。在 cART 之前的时代，死亡通常由肿瘤等继发性事件引起[215]。对于那些未接受 cART 的 PCNSL 患者，应首先考虑启动抗 HIV 病毒治疗，因为有研究发现 HIV 有效控制患者有可能长期生存[216,217]。

多中心 Castleman 病

MCD 是一种与 KSHV/HHV 相关的淋巴组织增生性疾病，通常见于晚期 HIV 感染。患者通常表现为发热，全身乏力，弥漫性淋巴结肿大，肝脾肿大，水肿，积液和贫血等全身综合征。虽然不是克隆过程，但部分 MCD 可以转化为 DLBCL，因此在初次诊断和随后的复发时应该注意 MCD 向高级 DLBCL 转化的可能。患者还可能出现其他伴随的 HHV8 相关恶性肿瘤，KS 或 PEL，或者在诊断时 CD4 细胞计数通常较低的机会性感染。所有患者均应接受 cART 治疗，但单独使用抗反转录病毒药物不太可能产生疾病缓解。虽然抗 HIV 的抗病毒治疗尚未显示成功治疗 MCD，但抗 HHV8 的抗病毒治疗可能是有效的，因为 HHV8 裂解复制在 MCL 中很常见，因此 HHV8 可能是 MCD 的治疗方向。14 例有症状的 HIV 和 HHV-8 相关性 MCD 患者接受高剂量齐多夫定加缬更昔洛韦的前瞻性研究发现，总体临床和完全缓解率分别为 86% 和 50%[218]。单独的传统化疗药物疗效有限，虽然有研究报道使用单药物烷化剂，长春碱类，口服依托泊苷，沙利度胺或脂质体多柔比星有一定疗效[163,219-223]。因 MCD 中存在 CD20⁺B 细胞，采用利妥昔单抗治疗也进行了探索。

一项关于利妥昔单抗单药治疗的前瞻性试验，入组了 24 例 HIV 相关 MCD 患者，1 年缓解率为 1%。还报道了既往接受过利妥昔单抗治疗的患者再次应用利妥昔单抗的效果[224,225]。值得注意的是，患有 MCD 和伴随 KS 的患者在使用利妥昔单抗可能会出现突发的 KS，这需要临床医生的注意。对于具有高度侵袭性疾病或利妥昔单抗单药治疗疾病的患者，利妥昔单抗联合依托泊苷或脂质体多柔比星具有很多的效果[226,227]。利妥昔单抗联合脂质体多柔比星对于合并 KS 的 MCD 患者具有更好的疗效。最近，基于一项随机试验，抗 IL-6R 单克隆抗体 siltuximab 已被 FDA 批准用于 HIV 阴性 HHV8 阴性 MCD，结果显示 34%的患者接受 siltuximab 治疗获得了持久的临床缓解和放射学反应，而安慰剂组未见到治疗缓解患者[167]。这个数据不容易外推至 HIV 相关的 MCD，这是因为病毒 IL-6 由 HHV8 产生，但其不能被 siltuximab 抗体靶向。目前靶向 IL-6 药物需要在临床试验的背景下对 HIV 患者进行尝试。

对于 MCD 的一线治疗，我们建议患者使用利妥昔单抗联合 cART 抗病毒。可以添加脂质体多柔比星或依托泊苷用于快速进展或耐药患者，其中更加强化的治疗方案，如 CHOP[228] 保留用于罕见的暴发性进展或伴随高级别转化的患者。也可考虑使用含有缬更昔洛韦的高剂量齐多夫定。

霍奇金淋巴瘤(HL)

虽然不是特定的艾滋病相关肿瘤，但在艾滋病病毒感染者 HL 发生率增高，同时在艾滋病背景下，具有一些独特的不同于非 HIV 的 HL 的特征。

流行病学

感染 HIV 的患者发生 HL 风险大约比未感染人群高 2.5~8.5 倍[9,229-231]。这种风险似乎在 HIV 感染的风险组中均匀增加，与年龄或性别无关[232]。尽管如此艾滋病病毒感染人群的相对患 HL 风险增加，但与 NHL 相比，这种相对风险仍较小。与大多数艾滋病相关的 NHL 不同，HIV 感染中 HL 的发病率在 cART 时代并没有减少，甚至可能增加[123,233,234]。这种惊人增加的原因推测可能是由于宿主体内发挥关键作用的 CD4⁺T 细胞信号传导在 HL 的微环境中起作用。实际上，与严重免疫缺陷患者相比，HL 更可能发生在中度降低的 CD4⁺细胞计数患者身上。

病理和发病机制

在 HIV 感染的背景下，HL 具有不同于血清 HIV 阴性群体的病理特征。HIV 感染的 HL 患者中，混合细胞亚型的比例很高，结节性硬化型患者的比例相应较低。混合细胞和淋巴细减少型的总比例占 HIV-1 阳性患者的 2/3，而未感染 HIV 患者仅为 29%[235]。此外，与 HIV 阴性人群相比，EBV 阳性感染在 HIV 感染的 HL 患者组织中显著增加，估计范围为 80%~100%[234,236]。值得注意的是，EBV LMP1 而非 EBNA2，潜伏基因的表达属于 2 型模式。因此，EBV 基因组在 HIV 感染的 HL 中被高频率鉴定，并且被认为可能与发病相关。

除 EBV 的存在外，还有 HIV 感染人群 HL 的特有的其他分子特征。在生发中心 B 细胞中表达的转录因子 Bcl-6 存在于来自 HIV-1 感染和未感染个体的 Reed-Sternberg 细胞上，而 syndecan-1 仅在 HIV-1 阳性人群中表达[237,238]。因此，末端后中心(postminminal-center)B 细胞可能是 HIV-1 相关 HL 的起源细胞；而不是生发中心细胞，被认为是在未 HIV 感染的人群中 Reed-Sternberg 细胞的起源细胞。

临床表现

HIV 患者的 HL 通常处于晚期并且与 B 症状相关[239,240]。诊断时大约 80%的 HIV 相关 HL 患者存在Ⅲ期或Ⅳ期疾病，而无 HIV 的 HL 患者中Ⅲ期或Ⅳ期患者比例不到一半。与艾滋病相关的淋巴瘤一样，HL 在 HIV-1 感染环境中的病灶部位通常是在结外，大于 50%的患者伴有骨髓侵犯，其他部位包括舌、直肠、皮肤、肺和结外等部可能是表现的部位。疾病分期与无 HIV-1 的 HL 患者相同，同时应该特别注意跟 B 症状可能相关的微生物学原因。

治疗

HIV 感染 HL 患者的临床治疗方法与其他非 HIV 感染的 HL 治疗方法相似，根据不同采用放射治疗，化疗或联合放化疗，具体参照相应通用指南。虽然 cART 抗病毒时代之前，HIV 相关 HL 的治疗效果非常差，中位生存期<2 年[241]，现在 cART 抗病毒时代，目前治疗效果已经明显改善，显示出较高的治愈率[240]。据报道晚期 HIV 感染的 HL 患者，采用标准的 ABVD 方案(多柔比星+博来霉素+长春碱+达卡巴嗪)联合 cART 抗病毒治疗，87%的病例获得完全缓解，5 年无事件率和总生存率分别为 71%和 76%[242]。cART 治疗联合 BEACOPP 或 Stanford V 同样取得好的效果[243,244]。

在开始这些疗法之前，必须考虑患者的潜在免疫抑制水平和整体一般状况，并且一般而言，无论 CD4 细胞计数如何，建议对所有患者预防卡氏肺孢菌。

通常在晚期艾滋病的患者中，骨髓抑制和机会性感染等并发症可能更严重；然而，HIV 感染的 HL 患者仍以治愈为目标。只有在已证明对标准剂量方案不耐受的晚期艾滋病患者中才应考虑减少抗肿瘤剂量。与 NHL 的治疗一样，临床医生必须警惕化疗和 cART 之间的药物-药物相互作用。

鳞状细胞瘤

与 HPV 相关的疾病日益受到关注有几个原因，包括：①感染 HIV 病毒的妇女比较逐渐增加；②世界上高宫颈癌易发且缺乏宫颈疾病筛查地区，近年来出现明显增高的新发 HIV 感染；③HIV 感染者的总体存活期延长。异常的肿瘤谱相当广泛，包括肛门生殖器、结膜、口咽和皮肤瘤形成。

流行病学

已经发现：HIV 感染者中鳞状细胞癌发生率增加，即使引入 cART 后，发生率也没有减少，可能较前增加[12,245,246]。HPV 相关肿瘤中单一的艾滋病定义疾病是浸润性宫颈癌。虽然关于宫颈癌在 HIV 感染环境中的发生频率增加，但仍存在争议。然而，非常明确的是子宫颈和肛门的上皮内瘤变发生率增加。感染 HIV 的男性患者因男男性关系鳞状细胞癌的发生率特别高，并且颅内上皮内瘤变和肛门癌的风险也显著增加，这是 cART 时代所有恶性肿瘤中发病率最快的肿瘤类型[12]。免疫抑制增加这种癌症风险的间接证据来自对艾滋病和癌症登记的分析。在一项针对超过 30 万名艾滋病患者的回顾性研究中，艾滋病定义疾病发病后 5 年内原位癌和侵袭性癌症的发病率明显高于其前 5 年[245]。女性主要是宫颈、外阴/阴道和肛门癌增加，而男性主要是肛门、阴茎、扁桃体和结膜癌增加。

病理和发病机制

HPV 某些亚型与表皮细胞转化相关已经得到认可。早已确立，据报道 HPV-16，HPV-18 和 HPV-19 感染率在 HIV 感染者中增加[247]。多种亚型 HPV 被发现在 HIV 感染人群中感染比例显著增加（HIV-1 感染男性中 73%感染，而未感染 HIV 男性为 23%感染）[247,248]。据估计，在 4 年间隔期间与男性发生性关系的 HIV-1 阳性男性中，肛门高级别上皮内瘤变的发生率高达 48%，这与多种 HPV 亚型的存在相关，持续性肛门感染和致癌 HPV 亚型的高水平感染有关[249]。在 HIV-1 感染的男男性接触者中筛查上皮内瘤变已表现出高度肛门上皮内瘤变或原位癌的患病率为 36%，而与 HIV-1 阴性男性发生性关系的为 7%[250]。肛门和子宫颈上的这些病变通常不是孤立的，而是代表不典型增生的多个区域之一，因此难以令人满意地治疗，特别是在肛门。具有高级别上皮内瘤的患者可能经常在切除，冷冻疗法或局部治疗的尝试后反复复发，这是因为 HPV 感染的普遍存在及病毒对局部组织的持续刺激。评估这一问题严重程度的一个关键问题是上皮内瘤变进展为高侵袭性癌症的风险。目前这个问题仍然不明确，备受争议。如果风险估计为≥1%，则成本效益分析表明目前进行的筛查是合理的[251]。HIV 感染患者中侵袭性肛门生殖器癌的发病率没有大幅增加，表明风险相对较小，但风险不是零，因此，在患者中警惕 HIV 是很有必要的。

在积极治疗 HIV 和抑制 HIV 复制的情况下，一些机会性肿瘤的风险明显减弱。关于改进的抗 HIV 治疗有效抑制 HIV 复制后，是否可以改善 HPV 相关肿瘤目前仍存在矛盾。一些报告表明，一些人可能会出现 HPV 相关瘤变的改善[252]；然而，大部分数据表明，抗反转录病毒治疗对不典型增生或侵袭性肛门癌的发病率几乎没有影响[253]。目前，完全抑制 HIV 不应被视为对抗 HPV 相关肿瘤发展的自动防御措施。

临床表现

HPV 疾病可能存在于从尖锐湿疣到侵袭性肛门癌的任何地方。患有肛门不典型增生的患者可能有或没有与之相关的症状。具有严重肛门不典型增生的患者一般需要进行内窥镜检查和必要的活检，即使病变部位位于肛门边缘，也可以考虑内窥镜检查发现可能的恶性肿瘤。一些中心对 HIV 感染者进行肛门巴氏染色法，已经证明这种方法可以有效识别癌前病变。一项针对 245 名男性的研究发现，96%的肛门子宫颈涂片检查发现其中 2/3 的男性筛查出细胞学检查异常[254]。高分辨率的肛门镜检查和活检显示：96%的细胞学筛查阳性可发现肛门不典型增生。尽管早期病变可能受益于局部治疗，但早期细胞学检测的临床相关性仍不清楚。鉴于 HIV 感染者中 HPV 相关肛门癌的发病率不断上升，可能会在高风险人群中考虑肛门子宫颈涂片检查，如男男性接触者。

对于感染 HIV 的妇女，应严格遵循宫颈筛查的标准做法，尤其需要高度警惕严重免疫抑制患者。对于 $CD4^+$ 细胞计数 <200 个/mm^3 的 HIV 感染女性，建议每半年进行一次子宫颈涂片检查。

HPV 疫苗接种是预防宫颈癌的重要工具，已经证明它可以降低与 HPV 相关的宫颈高级别上皮内瘤变的发生率[255]，现在被认为是年轻女孩的标准疫苗。男孩的 HPV 疫苗接种一直存在争议，尽管它可能降低 HPV 相关肿瘤的发生率以及防止 HPV 交叉传播给女性，从而有助于降低宫颈癌的发病率。在一项随机安慰剂对照试验中，对 4 065 名年龄在 16~26 岁的男性进行了四价 HPV 疫苗的检测，发现 HPV 感染率以及 HPV 相关外生殖器病变减少[256]。男男性行为人群的一项亚组研究也发现了该疫苗在这些人群中有效，可减少肛门高级上皮内瘤变的发生率。根据以上研究数据，目前建议所有 21 岁以下的男性及 26 以下的男男性行为人群都接种 HPV 疫苗。

治疗

子宫颈不典型增生和宫颈癌的治疗方法在相应指南中已经明确，但对于 HIV 患者同时应考虑艾滋病毒感染的情况。肛门疾病的治疗目前仍不太明确。

肛门边缘的癌前病变（高级别上皮内瘤变和原位癌）可以用局部咪喹莫特或 5-氟尿嘧啶治疗，而肛管中的病变可以用手术切除,冷冻疗法或激光消融治疗。鉴于癌前病变进展为浸润性癌的风险目前未知,并且肛门上皮内瘤变可能出现自发消退,这些病变也可以选择密切随访观察[257]。对于非 HIV 感染的肛门浸润性癌患者,治疗指南推荐联合放化疗,同样在 HIV 感染人群也可以很好地耐受联合放化疗[258,259]。HIV 感染患者对黏膜损伤非常敏感,因此需要肿瘤内科和放射科医生之间密切沟通。但对于非常晚期的 HIV 患者,需要根据实际情况,可能需要选择保守治疗恶性肿瘤的方法。

其他非艾滋病定义癌症

cART 时代艾滋病被有效控制,但许多其他非艾滋病定义的恶性肿瘤发生在 HIV 感染者的风险仍然较高,这些包括肺癌,口咽癌,肝癌,前列腺癌,睾丸癌和皮肤癌[231,260-263]。在皮肤癌中,黑色素瘤,基底细胞癌和鳞状细胞癌均具有较高发生率。

默克尔细胞癌(Merkel cell carcinoma,MCC)是一种非常罕见的神经嵴衍生的皮肤癌,在艾滋病以及实体器官移植受者中也被证明有所增加[264,265]。虽然 MCC 一般发生于老年患者,但免疫抑制患者的 MCC 患者倾向于发生在更年轻患者,并且多伴其他恶性肿瘤病史。这种罕见的皮肤癌与免疫抑制患者的相关性促使寻找潜在的感染性病原体,最近研究鉴定发现了一种以前未知的多瘤病毒,现在称为 Merkel 细胞多瘤病毒(Merkel cell polyomavirus,MCV)[266]。发现 MCV DNA 被整合在大多数 MCC 肿瘤细胞基因组中,但在对照组织中没有发现。提示这种整合模式先于肿瘤细胞的克隆扩增。这些数据表明这种新型多瘤病毒在 MCC 发病机制中的关键作用,尽管这一作用的确切机制尚未明确。

MCV 的成功发现及鉴定提示:其他未知病毒在其他免疫抑制相关恶性肿瘤中的潜在作用,仍需要进一步探索。

(刘欣 张晓伟 译,罗志国 审校)

参考文献

The complete reference list can be found on the Wiley Companion Digital Edition of this title (see inside front cover for login instructions).

1 Palella FJ Jr, Delaney KM, Moorman AC, et al. Declining morbidity and mortality among patients with advanced human immunodeficiency virus infection. HIV Outpatient study investigators. *N Engl J Med*. 1998;**338**:853–860.

7 Chang Y, Cesarman E, Pessin MS, et al. Identification of herpesvirus-like DNA sequences in AIDS-associated Kaposi's sarcoma. *Science*. 1994;**266**:1865–1869.

12 Simard EP, Pfeiffer RM, Engels EA. Spectrum of cancer risk late after AIDS onset in the United States. *Arch Intern Med*. 2010;**170**:1337–1345.

14 Buchbinder SP, Holmberg SD, Scheer S, et al. Combination antiretroviral therapy and incidence of AIDS-related malignancies. *J Acquir Immune Defic Syndr*. 1999;**21(Suppl 1)**:S23–S26.

17 Biggar RJ, Chaturvedi AK, Goedert JJ, Engels EA. AIDS-related cancer and severity of immunosuppression in persons with AIDS. *J Natl Cancer Inst*. 2007;**99**:962–972.

20 Young L, Alfieri C, Hennessy K, et al. Expression of Epstein-Barr virus transformation-associated genes in tissues of patients with EBV lymphoproliferative disease. *N Engl J Med*. 1989;**321**:1080–1085.

24 Gibson TM, Morton LM, Shiels MS, et al. Risk of non-Hodgkin lymphoma subtypes in HIV-infected people during the HAART era: a population-based study. *AIDS*. 2014;**28**:2313–2318.

25 Kedes DH, Operskalski E, Busch M, et al. The seroepidemiology of human herpesvirus 8 (Kaposi's sarcoma-associated herpesvirus): distribution of infection in KS risk groups and evidence for sexual transmission. *Nat Med*. 1996;**2**:918–924.

38 Krown SE, Testa MA, Huang J. AIDS-related Kaposi's sarcoma: prospective validation of the AIDS Clinical Trials Group staging classification. AIDS Clinical Trials Group Oncology Committee. *J Clin Oncol*. 1997;**15**:3085–3092.

40 Stebbing J, Sanitt A, Nelson M, et al. A prognostic index for AIDS-associated Kaposi's sarcoma in the era of highly active antiretroviral therapy. *Lancet*. 2006;**367**:1495–1502.

50 Bais C, Santomasso B, Coso O, et al. G-protein-coupled receptor of Kaposi's sarcoma-associated herpesvirus is a viral oncogene and angiogenesis activator. *Nature*. 1998;**391**:86–89.

69 Harrington W Jr, Sieczkowski L, Sosa C, et al. Activation of HHV-8 by HIV-1 tat. *Lancet*. 1997;**349**:774–775.

77 Mosam A, Shaik F, Uldrick TS, et al. A randomized controlled trial of highly active antiretroviral therapy versus highly active antiretroviral therapy and chemotherapy in therapy-naive patients with HIV-associated Kaposi sarcoma in South Africa. *J Acquir Immune Defic Syndr*. 2012;**60**:150–157.

93 Northfelt DW, Dezube BJ, Thommes JA, et al. Pegylated-liposomal doxorubicin versus doxorubicin, bleomycin, and vincristine in the treatment of AIDS-related Kaposi's sarcoma: results of a randomized phase III clinical trial. *J Clin Oncol*. 1998;**16**:2445–2451.

100 Cianfrocca M, Lee S, Von Roenn J, et al. Randomized trial of paclitaxel versus pegylated liposomal doxorubicin for advanced human immunodeficiency virus-associated Kaposi sarcoma: evidence of symptom palliation from chemotherapy. *Cancer*. 2010;**116**:3969–3977.

125 Mosialos G, Birkenbach M, Yalamanchili R, et al. The Epstein-Barr virus transforming protein LMP1 engages signaling proteins for the tumor necrosis factor receptor family. *Cell*. 1995;**80**:389–399.

126 Liebowitz D. Epstein-Barr virus and a cellular signaling pathway in lymphomas from immunosuppressed patients. *N Engl J Med*. 1998;**338**:1413–1421.

136 Delecluse HJ, Anagnostopoulos I, Dallenbach F, et al. Plasmablastic lymphomas of the oral cavity: a new entity associated with the human immunodeficiency virus infection. *Blood*. 1997;**89**:1413–1420.

156 Nador RG, Cesarman E, Chadburn A, et al. Primary effusion lymphoma: a distinct clinicopathologic entity associated with the Kaposi's sarcoma-associated herpes virus. *Blood*. 1996;**88**:645–656.

161 Uldrick TS, Pipkin S, Scheer S, Hessol NA. Factors associated with survival among patients with AIDS-related primary central nervous system lymphoma. *AIDS*. 2014;**28**:397–405.

163 Oksenhendler E, Duarte M, Soulier J, et al. Multicentric Castleman's disease in HIV infection: a clinical and pathological study of 20 patients. *AIDS*. 1996;**10**:61–67.

172 Barta SK, Xue X, Wang D, et al. A new prognostic score for AIDS-related lymphomas in the Rituximab-era. *Haematologica*. 2014;**99**:1731–1737.

174 Barnes JA, Lacasce AS, Feng Y, et al. Evaluation of the addition of rituximab to CODOX-M/IVAC for Burkitt's lymphoma: a retrospective analysis. *Ann Oncol*. 2011;**22**:1859–1864.

175 Dunleavy K, Pittaluga S, Shovlin M, et al. Low-intensity therapy in adults with Burkitt's lymphoma. *N Engl J Med*. 2013;**369**:1915–1925.

181 Kaplan LD, Lee JY, Ambinder RF, et al. Rituximab does not improve clinical outcome in a randomized phase 3 trial of CHOP with or without rituximab in patients with HIV-associated non-Hodgkin lymphoma: AIDS-malignancies consortium trial 010. *Blood*. 2005;**106**:1538–1543.

185 Dunleavy K, Little RF, Pittaluga S, et al. The role of tumor histogenesis, FDG-PET, and short-course EPOCH with dose-dense rituximab (SC-EPOCH-RR) in HIV-associated diffuse large B-cell lymphoma. *Blood*. 2010;**115**:3017–3024.

187 Barta SK, Lee JY, Kaplan LD, et al. Pooled analysis of AIDS malignancy consortium trials evaluating rituximab plus CHOP or infusional EPOCH chemotherapy in HIV-associated non-Hodgkin lymphoma. *Cancer*. 2012;**118**:3977–3983.

194 Re A, Michieli M, Casari S, et al. High-dose therapy and autologous peripheral blood stem cell transplantation as salvage treatment for AIDS-related lymphoma: long-term results of the Italian Cooperative Group on AIDS and Tumors (GICAT) study with analysis of prognostic factors. *Blood*. 2009;**114**:1306–1313.

203 Hutter G, Nowak D, Mossner M, et al. Long-term control of HIV by CCR5 Delta32/Delta32 stem-cell transplantation. *N Engl J Med*. 2009;**360**:692–698.

212 Hoffmann C, Tabrizian S, Wolf E, et al. Survival of AIDS patients with primary central nervous system lymphoma is dramatically improved by HAART-induced immune recovery. *AIDS*. 2001;**15**:2119–2127.

224 Gerard L, Berezne A, Galicier L, et al. Prospective study of rituximab in chemotherapy-dependent human immunodeficiency virus associated multicentric Castleman's disease: ANRS 117 CastlemaB Trial. *J Clin Oncol*. 2007;**25**:3350–3356.

227 Uldrick TS, Polizzotto MN, Aleman K, et al. Rituximab plus liposomal doxorubicin in HIV-infected patients with KSHV-associated multicentric Castleman disease. *Blood*. 2014;**124**:3544–3552.

234 Biggar RJ, Jaffe ES, Goedert JJ, et al. Hodgkin lymphoma and immunodeficiency in persons with HIV/AIDS. *Blood*. 2006;**108**:3786–3791.

242 Xicoy B, Ribera JM, Miralles P, et al. Results of treatment with doxorubicin, bleomycin, vinblastine and dacarbazine and highly active antiretroviral therapy

in advanced stage, human immunodeficiency virus-related Hodgkin's lymphoma. *Haematologica*. 2007;**92**:191–198.

245 Frisch M, Biggar RJ, Goedert JJ. Human papillomavirus-associated cancers in patients with human immunodeficiency virus infection and acquired immunodeficiency syndrome. *J Natl Cancer Inst*. 2000;**92**:1500–1510.

246 Palefsky JM, Holly EA, Efirdc JT, et al. Anal intraepithelial neoplasia in the highly active antiretroviral therapy era among HIV-positive men who have sex with men. *AIDS*. 2005;**19**:1407–1414.

255 The FUTURE II Study Group. Quadrivalent vaccine against human papillomavirus to prevent high-grade cervical lesions. *N Engl J Med*. 2007;**356**:1915–1927.

256 Giuliano AR, Palefsky JM, Goldstone S, et al. Efficacy of quadrivalent HPV vaccine against HPV Infection and disease in males. *N Engl J Med*. 2011;**364**:401–411.

257 Tong WW, Jin F, McHugh LC, et al. Progression to and spontaneous regression of high-grade anal squamous intraepithelial lesions in HIV-infected and uninfected men. *AIDS*. 2013;**27**:2233–2243.

261 Clifford GM, Polesel J, Rickenbach M, et al. Cancer risk in the Swiss HIV Cohort Study: associations with immunodeficiency, smoking, and highly active antiretroviral therapy. *J Natl Cancer Inst*. 2005;**97**:425–432.

第 76 章　癌症生存:癌症的新挑战

Julia H. Rowland, PhD

概述

随着癌症人群的持续增多,治疗后癌症患者的生存状况和长期康复受到越来越多的关注。一部分患者治疗后的副作用会慢慢消失而很好地适应生活,个别患者治疗后的副作用会持续存在导致恢复和适应困难。本章节我们列出几种常见的后遗症及处置方法,综述一下新的康复指南,讨论一下随访计划和模式,以及个别少见癌症的支持治疗方法,为未来的康复研究指明方向。

引言

纵览《癌症医学》(第 9 版)的全部内容,我们可以看到癌症治疗的技术和模式有了很大的进步,其中最重要的判断标准就是生存期的明显延长。在取得可观的治疗效果的同时,这些人群仅仅限于治愈癌症和延长生存期是不够的,我们必须关注他们的生活质量。在首次治疗后,如何使无瘤残存的患者完全康复是医务人员面临的重要挑战。

本章节我们列举出临床医生以及患者和家属共同面对的重要挑战。

由于儿童癌症治疗取得了巨大进步,儿童癌症患者的生存状况在美国受到广泛关注,这些患者的长期康复计划非常详细[1-8]。本章我们将重点关注成人肿瘤患者的康复与保健。

癌症生存:简史

20 世纪 70 年代以前,患者确诊癌症后非常恐惧和悲观,可选择的治疗手段非常有限,一些治疗方法的副作用非常难于控制[9,10]。这一时期治疗的重点就是患者最终死于癌症而不是与癌症共存。在这一时期癌症患者的角色只是一名痛苦的家庭成员而不是独立的自我。随着我们治疗和控制癌症的能力的增强,这种局面发生了巨大变化。

关于癌症生活质量问题的推动归因于两个重要事件。第一个是 1985 年《新英格兰杂志》发表了一位年轻医生菲茨休·穆兰(Fitzhugh Mullan)的文章《生存季》(*Seasons of Survival*)[11],在这篇文章中穆兰医生描述了作为一个癌症生存者的亲身经历,接下来几年,包括穆兰在内的 23 个人在新墨西哥的阿尔伯克基成立了国际癌症生存者联盟(National Coalition for Cancer Survivorship,NCCS),该组织提出了癌症生存的新概念,

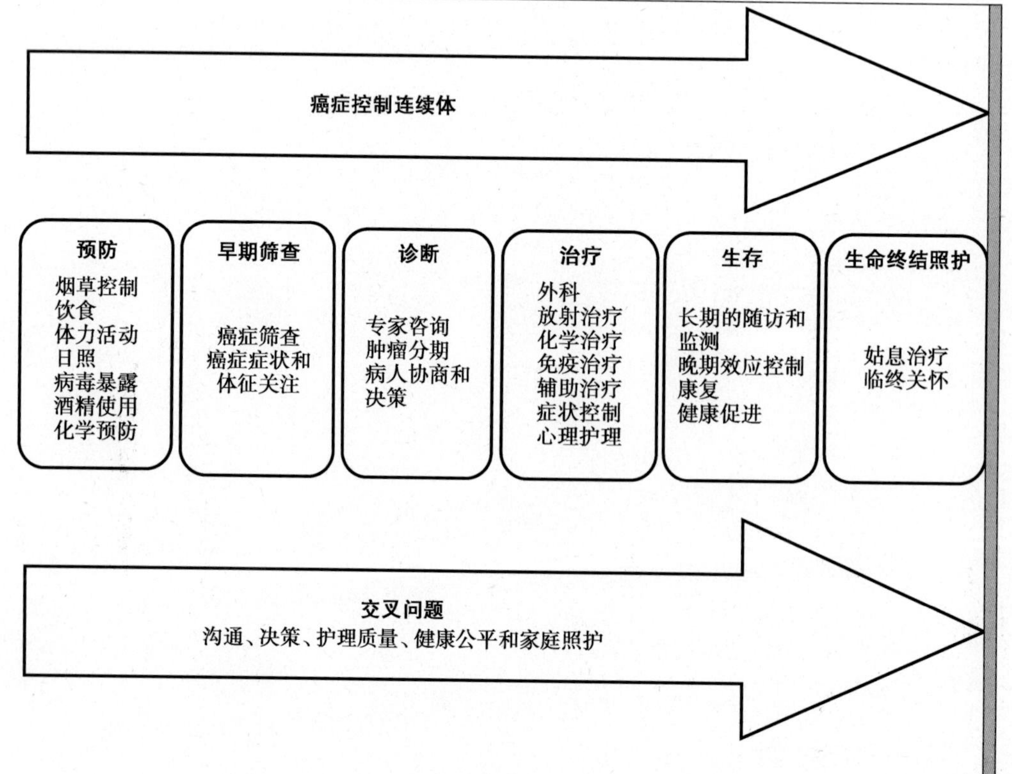

图 76-1　阐述了癌症控制连续体。资料来源:修改自 http://cancercontrol.gov/od/continuum.html

当时的癌症生存特指生存 5 年以上的患者,后来该组织讨论认为所有癌症患者从诊断癌症到后来的与癌症共存的整个过程为癌症生存。该组织的成立不在于个人的目的,而是为所有的癌症患者从诊断的那一刻起,提供了一个饱含希望的信息——诊断癌症不等于死亡,同时提出了患者之间以及患者与医生之间对话的重要话题,探讨不同治疗手段的选择对于患者今后身体状况和生理功能的影响,确立以患者为主导的选择。虽然部分患者身患癌症后不将自己视为癌症生存[12,13],但是这些概念从整体上推动了癌症生存运动。

从 1986 年开始,癌症生存成为一个独立的领域,过去的几十年间,政府部门开始关注癌症生存,主要体现在美国国家科学院(Institute of Medicine,IOM)两份关于癌症生存[1]和康复研究的报告[14],还有美国疾病预防控制中心及兰斯阿姆斯特朗基金一份关于儿童和成人癌症生存的报告[15],以及总统癌症计划的两份报告[16,17]。大多数癌症杂志或非癌症杂志设有癌症生存专栏[18-21],来汇总在癌症生存研究中的成果以及循证医学中的证据[22,23],这一领域得到蓬勃发展[24]。重要的是癌症生存与癌症控制成为一个连续的不可分割的整体,成为独特的关注点和新的挑战,其中这一领域发展的重要推动力是非常可观的癌症人群(图 76-1)。

重要问题

癌症流行病学

据统计截至 2014 年 1 月,仅美国就有 1 450 万癌症生存者[25],虽然部分国家仅统计 5 年内的癌症生存者,全球大约有 3 260 万癌症生存者[26]。图 76-2 反映了在过去的 45 年,癌症的生存者的数量呈稳步增长。在 1971 年,尼克松总统签署总统计划向癌症宣战时,美国大约有 300 万癌症生存者,到 2024 年这一数字将攀升至 1 900 万,这一数字增长归因于癌症早期诊断的进步和有效治疗手段以及支持治疗的进步。尽管出现了一些突破性的进展,但是最重要的因素是人口老龄化的问题[28]。

今天大约超过 60%诊断为癌症的患者年龄超过 65 岁。由于历史上“婴儿潮”的影响,从 2011 年起,每天大约有 11 000 人步入 65 岁以上老年人的行列。据估计到 2020 年将有 1 100 万癌症生存者为老年人,这一比例在 10 年内(2010—2020 年)增长了 42%[29]。

此外,现在癌症患者生存期延长也增加了癌症人群的数量。2014 年,41%的癌症生存者生存期超过 10 年,15%的癌症生存者生存期超过 20 年(见图 76-2)。至 2020 年癌症生存者的 5 年生存率目标要超过 72.8%[30],在儿童癌症患者(小于 15 岁)的 5 年生存率已经超过这一目标达到 77%,目前成人癌症生存者的 5 年生存率为 68%,这一目标确实是成人癌症生存的巨大挑战。此外,癌症生存者的身体状况和疾病状态是未知的,诊断癌症 1 年内的死亡率也不详。SEER(Surveillance Epidemiology and End Result)登记的关于健康状况的信息也有限,是我们基础认知的缺陷。健康 2020 也有一个目标就是提高癌症患者的精神和身体的生活质量(health of quality,HOQ)[30],但是尚没有具体的标准。

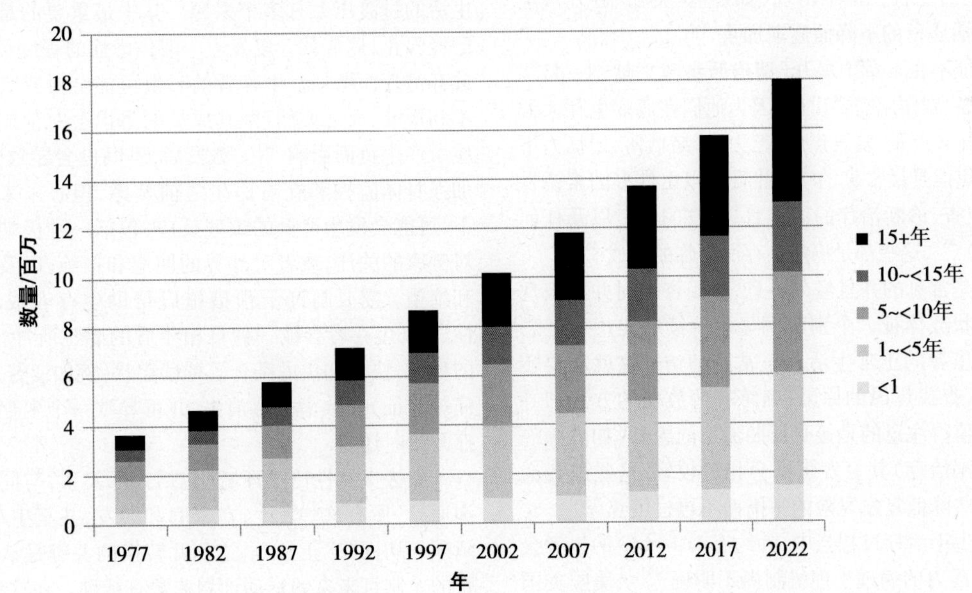

图 76-2　1997 年至 2022 年间美国癌症生存者的估计和预测数量(按照诊断年份)。资料来源:DeMoor 2013.[27]

癌症的长期和晚期副作用

随着癌症生存者的增多,有关癌症生存者的研究也增多,有证据表明告知癌症患者癌症去除并不等于从癌症中真正解放出来,有一名患者表述为“结束时并没有真正结束”。

癌症可以影响身体和生活的各个方面:生理、心理、社会、经济和人类生存(表 76-1)。有些副作用随着治疗结束而消失(如恶心、呕吐、脱发),另外一些成为慢性的持续存在(如乏力、性功能下降、记忆力减退,以及膀胱和直肠的问题),有一些症状可以通过一段时间的治疗而痊愈,有一些则永久存在(如

表 76-1　癌症及其治疗的潜在的长期和晚期影响

机体和疾病(例如:第二原发癌/复发、心功能不全、疼痛,疲劳,记忆问题,睡眠障碍,性功能障碍,不孕不育,肠道/膀胱功能失控)
心理(例如:害怕复发、抑郁、焦虑、自卑,以及身体形象改变)
社交(例如:人际关系变化、家庭状况改变、社会关系变化、工作/返学情况)
经济(例如:关于健康和人寿保险的准入/覆盖问题,医疗费用,失业造成的经济压力)
人文和精神问题(例如:精神幻灭、信仰丧失、意识变化,目的意义改变,生命欣赏,利益得失和痛定思痛)

不育症、残疾)。

另外随着癌症生存者生存期的延长,会受到后续治疗的副作用影响(如放疗和化疗的副作用)。第三类副作用为迟发反应,定义为 6 个月以上发生的副作用。此外,癌症复发和第二原发[31,32]以及其他慢性病的发生风险也会增加(如心血管疾病、糖尿病和骨质疏松)[33,34],随着癌症生存者年龄的增长,这些情况的关注度甚至超过癌症本身[35]。

总之,大部分癌症生存者随着治疗的结束而完全恢复,但是有相当多的一部分患者的紧张状态会持续 1 年甚至更长时间。大部分癌症生存者报告的精神健康状况不差于无癌症病史的人[36],但是身体的健康状况则大不相同,有癌症病史的人则会有身体功能障碍,能力丧失和失业[37-39]。更进一步的研究表明,慢性的持续的症状会集中出现(如疼痛、失眠、乏力),这些症状会随着生活质量的下降而逐渐加重[40]。

具体的综合征不在本章中展开(请参照参考文献 41~43)。然而,有 4 类常见的副作用需要讨论,因为他们在癌症生存人群中普遍存在而且比较严重:复发焦虑、乏力、情绪低落、记忆力下降。或许复发的焦虑是最常见的[44],并且可以由许多因素诱发加重(如常规的复查、诊断治疗的周年日、癌友的死亡以及任何无法解释的疼痛)[45],这些都是癌症生存所面临的挑战[46]。

复发焦虑症是常见的并且经久不息,接受咨询时并不表现为一个明确的症状或体征。个别案例显示持续的焦虑甚至恐惧严重地影响了患者的正常生活和正常的随访。这就需要转变为简短的咨询,查找焦虑的原因,训练一些放松的方法和寻求社会的支持。值得注意的是接受长期治疗的患者(如乳腺癌患者的辅助内分泌治疗)其复发焦虑会相对较轻,这些患者会因为主动采取一些降低复发风险的举措而不再过度焦虑。

乏力经常发生于治疗过程当中,大约有 1/4~1/3 的患者会出现乏力[47,48]。乏力的病理生理机制尚不明确[49]。美国美国临床肿瘤学会(American Society of Clinical Oncology,ASCO)指南在评估癌症治疗副作用时非常重视乏力[50]。时至今日,除了锻炼外并没有更好的缓解癌症乏力的方法,坚持锻炼的癌症患者在癌症治疗的过程中和治疗后乏力的程度会减轻[51]。排除几项病理性的乏力因素(如贫血、感染),会有助于乏力症状的逐渐改善。

抑郁在癌症人群中发生率明显高于普通人群,特别是在治疗后的 1~2 年内[52]。抑郁不仅仅是痛苦,而且与延迟工作和不接受治疗有关[53]。年轻患者、女性、有抑郁史的人均是癌症抑郁发生的危险因素,也有诊断癌症后首次发生抑郁的[54-56]。癌症生存者和临床医生均应意识到癌症治疗会诱发抑郁的发病,尤其是由于癌症的紧张状态一些副作用难于处理[55]。由于癌症抑郁与死亡相关,常规辨识抑郁的症状并予以处理很重要,许多癌症生存者单纯从心理治疗中获益很大[57,58]。

尽管临床上被忽略,但是人们越来越意识到记忆力减退和注意力下降这一副作用,出现精神系统异常(如记忆困难,细致思考能力下降,注意力不集中,被称作"化疗脑"或"精神迷雾")。这是癌症的一种真实而持久的影响,最近的研究表明,其可能影响 15%~25%的生存者。在神经细胞再进入早期,受影响比例高达 61%[59]。癌症相关认知障碍的病因是多因素的,可能涉及全身性促炎细胞因子穿过血脑屏障,以及化疗、激素及生物治疗和直接治疗毒性(如手术,对大脑的放射治疗)[60,61]。老年人和认知能力较低的人化疗后认知问题的风险增加,印证了癌症治疗加速衰老过程的假说发现[61]。采取一些有益的干预措施来帮助儿童癌症生存者解决由癌症引起的认知问题[62],最近,认知行为治疗干预在成年生存者中也进行探索[63]。

生存护理

过渡到康复

对于许多生存者来说,完成治疗的解脱感可能会减弱对未来的担忧。癌症后(而非癌症时)进入康复阶段,向康复和正常生活的过渡压力有多个来源。其中最重要的是担心既然治疗已经停止,癌症就会复发。一般焦虑症的程度可能会随着患者放弃治疗而增加。生存者的恐惧可能会对家庭生活质量产生不利影响;反之亦然,家庭成员的恐惧会对他们生存者的生活质量产生负面影响[64]。激发后,恐惧也会导致破坏性行为,如加强身体监控和在看医生之前焦虑,担心未来。在某些情况下,可能会发生严重的致残反应,包括一种极端的忧郁症般的对健康的关注,或者对外界的回避和拒绝,以及无法计划未来和绝望。需要制订干预措施以帮助生存者成功应对不确定性[65]。生存者会被一种自相矛盾的感觉所冲击,对结束治疗的反应,快乐和焦虑杂合。持续症状(例如疲劳、记忆困难和疼痛综合征)导致幸福感消失,并可导致一个生存者感觉她比治疗开始时还差。

失去支持性治疗环境(包括人际关系,与同事和其他病友沟通)。所有这些发生,在家庭和朋友,甚至生存者他们自己,亟须一切回归"正常"。达到此转换的关键是认同它可以是紧张的。制订未来的行动计划非常有帮助。在这种背景下,目前的发展需要制订一个生存护理计划(survivorship care plan,SCP),借此提供一个现成的解决方案,协助协调治疗后护理。

生存护理标准

癌症的总统计划的关键建议之一,就是实行来自癌症患者到癌症生存者的癌症生存者小组报告[16]和国际移民组织报告:在转变中迷失(其题目恰当地描述了当治疗结束时生存者的困境,临床医生应该为患者提供全面的治疗,总结并制订后续护理康复计划。这些文件还包括所谓的生还者护理计划或SCP。尽管关于 SCP 标准格式和内容尚未达成共识,但是建议使用几个常规内容。治疗总结应提供特定癌症内容(如诊断、分期、病理学和相关遗传标记),接受的治疗类型(如化疗,放射治疗剂量和靶区的,激素治疗,以及生物制剂的使用),发生的药物毒性、副作用和后期迟发反应的风险,以及经治医生的姓名和联系信息。这些信息用于生成独特的治疗后护理计划。IOM14 作为本文件的一部分,可以归纳出 11 个要素,4 大类:①复发监测或新发癌症,包括这些检查的性质和时间;②社区资源的评估、处理或转介帮助癌症的持续影响,包括心理以及生理上的后遗症,生存者的心理影响常常被忽视[66];③预防未来癌症或不良健康状况的建议,包括生活方式建议和基因检测的预测;④关于后续护理组成部分的规范,以及负责的临床医生的联系方式提供后续护理(表 76-2)。

表 76-2 生存护理的基本要素

监测复发或新癌症(例如,将要进行的检查及其周期性和需要监测的变化)
长期副作用的评估和治疗或转诊,包括医疗问题(如抑郁症、淋巴水肿、性功能障碍和功能性损伤)、症状(如疼痛和疲劳)和癌症生存者及其护理者的心理困扰;关注就业、保险和残疾相关问题;以及进行康复治疗
预防晚期效应(例如,第二癌症、心脏问题和骨质疏松症),伴随着基因检测的使用;包括注重健康促进(如饮食、体重、体力活动和防晒)和合并症的管理
护理协调(例如,包括随访频率、检查和执行者),在专家和一线护理者之间保持有效沟通,以确保所有生存者的健康需求都得到满足

资料来源:Adapted from Hewitt 2006. [14]

尽管在两份国家报告中强烈建议使用,但是对 SCP 的研究进展缓慢。Mayer 等[67]在他们的文献回顾中总结了关于 SCP的使用情况,得出了几个总体结论:SCP 得到了患者和护理者的广泛认可,但在实践中仍然没有得到充分利用,大量的临床医生调查显示报告未能提供患者也未接受这样的计划;而护理者和患者之间就 SCP 内容、交付时间和交付人也未能达成一致;最后,关于 SCP 影响的数据有限。其实施未能引起人们的关注,对于生存结果影响的资料也有限,SCP 实施使用的压力正在增加,面临诸多挑战。

制订治疗总结和护理计划是优质护理的一部分,ASCO 决定采取相关措施,作为肿瘤学实践活动质量(quality oncology practice initiative,QOPI)的一部分。2006 年向 ASCO 成员开放的自愿项目,QOPI 被创建以促进癌症治疗的飞跃。通过帮助肿瘤学家创造一种自我检查的文化改进。2008 年,ASCO 在其核心部分中增加了 3 项关于化疗治疗总结完成后,给患者提供了一份复印件,一份发送或传达给另一个医生,全部在 3 个月的化疗结束。乳腺癌、结直肠癌和前列腺癌的癌症监测模板设置为 AscoWeb 站点上的常规功能。最近,ASCO 发布了一个简短的 SCP 模板[68]。健康保险公司和倡导团体与肿瘤专家创建了一个用于构建 scp 的在线工具“继续前行”(http://journeyforward.org/)。一些重要的肿瘤学电子软件供应商已经开始为此目的开发软件工具,尽管存在平台间的屏障,妨碍了他们信息共享和护理协同的目的。SCP 使用的主要障碍是人员难以进行简单的 IT 集成,完成数据整合和共享,难于生成循证的护理指导意见[69]。由于时间和预算有限,临床医生很难使用这些软件并提供高质量的护理。同时 SCP 的时效有限,患者和护理者之间的内容和使用没有预期的对话,这些信息只是一张纸。

尽管对它们的使用有顾虑,美国外科学院癌症委员会于 2015 年对包括 SCP 的开发和交付标准进行认证[70]。理想情况下,这一行动将促进深入的研究,内容涉及谁应该创建和交付这些文档,在护理过程中应该启动什么样的程序,谁来支付这项活动的费用。了解 SCP 的使用是否提高了患者、护理者和系统功能将至关重要。

生存护理模式

虽然人们越来越认识到癌症生存者需要在治疗后的生活中护理康复和随访,关于应该如何做。肿瘤学提供者的预期短缺[71],再加上越来越大的新患者的压力,解决谁应该提供癌症相关的后续治疗是最重要的关注点。一些文献考虑施行共同照顾初级保健模式的初级保健医师(primary care physician,PCP)负责随访,并根据需要转诊回肿瘤科或其他专家[72-74]。在这个模式中,必须由肿瘤学家为 PCP 提供一个 SCP 来传递密钥访问关于生存者病史的信息,监视建议,以及需要监测的潜在晚期并发症。一项大型调查显示,许多美国 PCP 更喜欢共享医疗模型;很少有人喜欢肿瘤学家主导的模型、PCP 主导的模型,或者其他专业生存者诊所[75,76]。同一研究报告 PCP 对其生存护理知识的信心可能不足[77]。然而,国际研究表明发现在肿瘤随访的生存者的复发时间、生活质量和心理生理状况,以及实施指南内容上,初级保健与肿瘤专家有一定的差异(例如,一页后续说明)[78,79]。其他后续护理模式也已推出。其中最常见的是发展大范围的多学科的综合性癌症中心,设立专门的生存者诊所[80]。它们往往提供两种模式:①计划咨询,患者可以在治疗后的任何时候来复查,它们的病史、当前身体功能状态和未来问题的风险,以及当前问题的处理建议和与护理者拟议共享的未来护理大纲;②一个完整的服务项目,生存者可以在癌症后特定时间段(如 2~5 年)的定期就诊。第三种模式为护理导的,在护理团队和生存者之间架构的沟通渠道[81-83]。给定模式的演化通常反映诊所的硬件设施、所服务的患者群体等内容。一般来说,一个或多个关键领导的热情共同为团体争取资金支持。生存护理计划的可持续性是一个中心问题。目前还没有明确的制度来补偿这种工作。主要支持模式来自融资包括服务费、保险费、研究补助金、慈善事业和专项基金。一些较大的中心将生存诊所视为为他们的运营“增值”手段,耗资支持的目的在于希望他们能带来更多新患者(以及生存者)到他们机构中来。

因为癌症及其治疗的复杂性,患者的癌症经历千变万化(例如,关于既往病史、功能状况以及心理社会资源),很明显一个生存者的护理模式不能千篇一律。有关团体已呼吁制定风险分层治疗后护理方法。在这种方法中,临床医生的专业和访问频率取决于生存者的需要和复发风险晚期影响[84,85]。低风险生存者(如早期乳腺或结直肠只接受手术的癌症)可以在治疗结束后不久进行初级保健。高风险生存者(例如,接受干细胞移植或更多复杂的护理需求)将定期由肿瘤科专业人员按照PCP处理的常规护理[72,73]。一项风险分层模型目前正在英国进行护理测试(http://www.ncsi.org.uk/what-we-are-do/risk-layedized-pathways-of-care/风险分层/)。为了让这种护理模式变得更加普遍,生存者最需要基于证据的预测模型防止在癌症后出现后遗症。不管采用何种模式,生存的两个核心原则保持不变:生存者接受最佳的治疗后随访,以及生存者自己在他们的康复中扮演着重要的角色。目前美国的生存者护理涉及多个专业供应商[86],无专门的部门协调管理[87]。此外,护理者的主体责任,护理技术以及基本的护理要素尚未达成共识[77,88,89]。癌症生存者可能面临重复的、不适当的护理风险(例如,在没有证实用性的情况下进行过度检查或肿瘤标志物监测),或对降低癌症发生率无效。甚至一些肿瘤学家也对癌症治疗的晚期效应进行不实报告[90]。夸大生存护理的有效性。患者和护理者以及专家之间在癌症治疗的结束后的PCP必须职责明晰,沟通顺畅,如谁来提供什么样的服务,服务时间,什么情况下转诊。对于护理人员的培训工作需要加大力度,同时制定癌症最佳生存指南。为了实现后1个目标,美国国家综合癌症网络(National Comprehensive Cancer Network,NCCN)[91,92]、ASCO[68,93]和美国癌症协会(American Cancer Society,ACS)[94]已经在全球范围内推进生存者护理。类似的努力正发生[95]。

对于生存者来说,在治疗多年后他们持续看到他们的肿瘤学家依然在为他们提供服务[96]。除了临床医生应用外,SCP可以促进生存者对自己的角色教育。在管理治疗后,康复方面自我管理干预可以提高生存者的生活质量身体功能和健康行为。当积极参与治疗相关决策时,生存者得到与需求和目标一致的关怀也更多[97]。

康复与健康促进

癌症治疗的目标不仅仅是治愈或控制疾病以优化功能和生活质量,在癌症之后,另外两个方面的护理已经成为中心目标,分别时是:康复和健康促进。随着时间的推移,使用的美国与癌症相关的康复已经减少,部分反映了早期诊断(因此更激进的治疗手段应用减少)和更多的保留肢体和器官功能的手术方法得以广泛的应用。长时间的对于癌症和其治疗的关注,临床医生需要重新审视这些治疗手段。这些治疗手段仍然是美国以外许多国家的标准治疗[98,99]。生存者报告显示癌症后有多种康复需求[100],研究表明,无论是预防性的还是患病后[101],加强康复可以减少癌症相关的发病率和死亡率。为满足康复需要而设专项,已经有几个地方开始为癌症生存者进行康复治疗[102]。2013年,康复设施认证委员会(Commission on Accreditation of Rehabilitative Facilities,CARF)对于癌症的康复制定了认证标准[103]。一些大型癌症中心的康复诊所迅速出现。

过去十年受多种因素的驱动,包括生存者自身的需求,人们对癌症后康复治疗的兴趣增加了。大多数癌症生存者年龄较大,常伴有因癌症治疗或会增加合并症的健康问题(如心脏病的风险问题,肥胖,骨质疏松),同时在治疗期间养成不良的健康习惯(久坐和不良饮食),年龄增长,进行生活方式干预可能使生存者受益。重要的是,生存者经常问他们的护理团队他们能做什么,如何降低癌症复发的风险,恢复健康。由于这些因素,研究人员认为癌症生存者的康复过程是一种"可教的"时间"[104]。

在本卷其他部分,健康生活方式对于癌症预防具有重要意义。对癌症生存者的观察性研究表明:戒烟、增加体力活动、控制体重可能会减少癌症复发的风险、癌症相关死亡率及总死亡率[105-107]。尽管仍需要随机临床试验,验证关于行为改变影响癌症生存者的因果关系的论断。但是有足够的证据让临床医生推荐患者努力做到保持或加强在癌症期间和之后进行更多的体力活动。ACS就推荐并定期更新癌症生存者营养以及癌症后的体力活动指南[108]。有一些生存者自发的改变他们的行为[109],有相当一部分癌症生存者没有做到[110]。生存者护理为临床医生提供治疗癌症的重要机会,努力帮助生存者改变饮食行为、体力活动、戒烟和压力管理,降低复发和第二肿瘤风险,以及共同管理健康状况,这些方面既往被许多人忽略了[111,112]。更多研究亟须开展,藉以了解护理者如何有效地提供健康促进服务以及生存者如何成功实施和保持有益的变化。

家庭和非正式照料者

有关团体倡导认为非正式的护理人员与癌症生存者是共同生存者,不考虑家庭照顾者参与的生存护理的讨论是不完整的。现在大多数癌症护理在门诊提供,癌症作为一种慢性病,癌症后长期生活的个人越来越多,癌症家庭的负担也越来越重。研究表明家人常常对癌症生存者的需求感到力不从心。其一,很少或根本没有关于该做什么的指导,而且经常会因竞争的氛围而紧张,包括保住工作,管理孩子,关心他们自己的健康[113]。一项研究发现2/5的护理者有中度的心理问题,1/5的人渴望得到正式的支持[114]。护理者可能比生存者更担心复发。不切实际的渴望尽快恢复生活导致焦虑,持续的症状导致复发的担忧,导致家庭气氛紧张。

为癌症生存者及其护理人员提供治疗后前6个月的预期信息,对于减少双方的痛苦至关重要。并研究表明患者及其护理者的健康状况是相辅相成的[115-117]。因为家庭护理者,同他们的护理对象一样,往往是老年人,他们自身的健康状况(包括癌症)通过接受健康的生活方式教育有利于护理者自身的保健,尽管这种效果仍然有待验证。此外,家庭照顾者的参与是至关重要的。有助于生存者接受推荐的辅助疗法,随访检查,症状控制报告。因此,这个重要的支持系统运行良好,可以辅助医疗机构有效管理患者。许多癌症中心已经在努力为照顾者提供服务,并作为其综合护理的一部分[118]。

结论

越来越多的癌症生存者为我们提供了许多经验教训。第一,癌症生存期定义为从完成治疗到复发或死于癌症或其他事件,在癌症控制连续体中的一个独立阶段。它具有独特的一系列生存和康复的挑战和机遇。第二,大多数生存者初步诊断后会生活很长一段时间。儿童、青少年或年轻人诊断癌症后一生很长时间与癌症相伴。然而,我们目前的治疗方法很少是完全无副作用的;大多数有一定程度的相关毒性,会产生严重的身体和心理上的不良后遗症。第三,所有这些慢性和晚期的影响必须跟踪并积极解决。第四,一部分生存者在癌症治疗结束后仍在继续斗争,生存者的生活质量是提供优质服务的医疗机构和癌症生存者的共同目标，两者之间需要密切交流和合作。定义和提供高质量生存护理，尽管是一个高端问题，却构成了一个重大的癌症医学的挑战。我们努力的目标就是减少因癌症造成的过度痛苦和过早死亡。继续资助癌症生存研究。它还需要加强多学科协作，和一代一代癌症护理人的共同努力。在迅速发展中，如何实现这些崇高的目标，一些基于满足生存者的治疗后需要的循证研究项目正在开展，已经制订了一些初步计划，这些都足以开始传播产生影响[119]。尽管如此，仍需要更多关注老年癌症生存者的急速增长，为被忽视的老年癌症生存者量身定做护理计划[120]。在癌症生存领域，国内外科学家和实践者都在稳步发展[121,122]。越来越多的人意识到像癌症这样的慢性病的生存护理的重要性。倡导社区癌症的生存需求依然强烈。未来十年，我们共同推进和检验我们对生存者和他们的家人的健康所付出的努力。

总结

- 美国有癌症史的人数在接下来的 20 年里，将继续增长，主要是由于人口老龄化。到 2022 年，将有 1 800 万癌症生存者，其中约 2/3 将是 65 岁或以上的。
- 癌症生存期定义为从完成治疗时起，到癌症复发或死亡或非癌症死亡，代表了癌症控制的独特连续体，以及与之相伴的康复挑战。
- 癌症及其治疗可导致多种持久性疾病（例如，疼痛、疲劳、记忆困难和性功能障碍）迟发性疾病（如第二癌症、心脏病、糖尿病，骨质疏松和抑郁）不良后遗症。经常合并存在，这些效应会影响生存者的方方面面：生理的、心理的、社会的、经济的和生存的。
- 大多数癌症生存者在癌症后都表现出非凡的适应能力。然而，有相当一部分人在为他们疾病困扰。治疗结束时早期应用系统评估的手段，识别和推荐需要额外支持的人群很重要的。
- 使用 SCP 提高治疗后护理质量和沟通的需求正在增长。除了治疗总结，SCP 的基本要素包括：①监督计划复发或新发癌症；②持续性癌症的评估和治疗以及癌症的影响；③预防晚期效应，包括使用基因检测和健康促进手段；④护理协同。
- 对提供的后续护理最佳模式没有达成共识。目前，多个模型正在研究中。人们对发展模型，包括：①初级保健医生和肿瘤专家之间的共享护理；②以风险为基础的测算法（例如，有早期疾病和简单治疗的生存者会很快回归到他们的 PCP，而那些高复发风险与肿瘤治疗团队和中心保持密切联系）。
- 生存可能为临床医生提供一个"可教的时刻"来帮助癌症生存者追求健康的生活方式和行为。
- 在康复过程中，必须注意家庭护理者的心理和身体健康。非正式照料者，被视为"次要生存者"，在生存者康复中发挥着重要作用，与癌症生存者共同"获得新生"。

（林华 译）

参考文献

The complete reference list can be found on the Wiley Companion Digital Edition of this title (see inside front cover for login instructions).

1 Hewitt M, Weiner SL, Simone JV (eds.). *Childhood Cancer Survivorship: Improving Care and Quality of Life.* Washington, DC: The National Academies Press, 2003.

4 Phillips SM, Padgett L, Leisenring W, et al. Survivors of childhood cancer in the United States: prevalence and burden of morbidity. *Cancer Epidemiol Biomarkers Prev.* 2015;**24**:653–663.

7 Children's Oncology Group Guidelines (2015) *Long-Term Follow-up Guidelines,* http://www.childrensoncologygroup.org/index.php/survivorshipguidelines (accessed 12 January 2015).

11 Mullan F. Seasons of survival: reflections of a physician with cancer. *N Engl J Med.* 1985;**313**:270–273.

14 Hewitt M, Greenfield S, Stovall E (eds.). *From Cancer Patient to Cancer Survivor: Lost in Transition.* Institute of Medicine, National Academies Press: Washington, DC, 2006.

16 National Cancer Institute. *President's Cancer Panel, 2003–2004 Annual Report: Living Beyond Cancer: Finding a New Balance* (NIH publication No. P986). Washington, DC: National Institutes of Health; 2004.

25 *American Cancer Society.* Cancer Treatment & Survivorship. Facts & Figures *2014-2015.* Atlanta, GA: American Cancer Society, 2014.

29 Parry C, Kent EE, Mariotto AB, Alfano CM, Rowland JH. Cancer survivors: a booming population. *Cancer Epidemiol Biomarkers Prev.* 2011;**20**:1996–2005.

36 Reeve BB, Potosky AL, Smith AW, et al. Impact of cancer on health-related quality of life of older Americans. *J Natl Cancer Inst.* 2009;**101**:860–868.

37 Smith AW, Reeve BB, Bellizzi KM, et al. Cancer, comorbidities, and health-related quality of life of older adults. *Health Care Financ Rev.* 2008;**29**:41–56.

39 Farley Short P, Vasey JJ, Moran JR. Long-term effects of cancer survivorship on the employment of older workers. *Health Serv Res.* 2008;**43(1 Pt 1)**:193–210.

44 Koch L, Jansen L, Brenner H, Arndt V. Fear of recurrence and disease progression in long-term (≥5 years) cancer survivors – a systematic review of quantitative studies. *Psychooncology.* 2013;**22**:1–11.

47 Bower JE, Ganz PA, Desmond KA, et al. Fatigue in long-term breast carcinoma survivors: a longitudinal investigation. *Cancer* 2006 ;**106**:751-758.

53 Mitchell AJ, Ferguson DW, Gill J, et al. Depression and anxiety in long-term cancer survivors compared with spouses and healthy controls: a systematic review and meta-analysis. *Lancet Oncol.* 2013;**14**:721–732.

57 Andersen B, DeRubeis RJ, Berman BS, et al. Screening, assessment and care of anxiety and depressive symptoms in adults with cancer: an American Society of Clinical Oncology guideline adaptation. *J Clin Oncol.* 2014;**32**:1605–1619.

58 Faller H, Schuler M, Richard M, et al. Effects of psycho-oncologic interventions on emotional distress and quality of life in adult patients with cancer: systematic review and meta-analysis. *J Clin Oncol.* 2013;**31**:782–793.

59 Ahles TA, Root JC, Ryan EL. Cancer- and cancer treatment-associated cognitive change: an update on the state of the science. *J Clin Oncol.* 2012;**20**:2675–3686.

66 Adler NE, Page AEK (eds.). *Cancer Care for the Whole Patient: Meeting Psychosocial Health Needs.* Institute of Medicine, Committee on Psychosocial Services to Cancer Patients/Families in a Community Setting, Academies Press: Washington, DC, 2008.

67 Mayer DK, Birken SA, Check DK, Chen RC. Summing it up: an integrative review of studies of cancer survivorship care plans (2006-2013). *Cancer.* 2014;**121**:978–996 [Epub ahead of print].

68 Mayer DK, Nekhlyudov L, Snyder CF, et al. American Society of Clinical Oncology clinical expert statement on cancer survivorship care planning. *J Oncol Pract.* 2014;**10**:345–351.

72 Howell D, Hack TF, Oliver TK, et al. Models of care for post-treatment follow-up of adult cancer survivors: a systematic review and quality appraisal of the evidence. *J Cancer Surviv.* 2012;**6**:359–371.

73 Oeffinger KC, McCabe MS. Models for delivering survivorship care. *J Clin Oncol.* 2006;**24**:5117–5124.

75 Potosky AL, Han PKJ, Rowland J, et al. Differences between primary care physicians' and oncologists' knowledge, attitudes and practices regarding the care of cancer survivors. *J Gen Intern Med.* 2011;**26**:1403–1410.

78 Grunfeld E, Levine MN, Julian JA, et al. Randomized trial of long-term follow-up for early-stage breast cancer: a comparison of family physician versus specialist care. *J Clin Oncol.* 2006;**24**:848–855.

90 Nekhlyudov L, Aziz NM, Lerro C, Virgo KS. Oncologists' and primary care physicians' awareness of late and long-term effects of chemotherapy: implications for care of the growing population of survivors. *J Oncol Pract.* 2014;**10**:e29–e36.

91 Denlinger CS, Carlson RW, Are M, et al. Survivorship: introduction and definition. *J Natl Compr Canc Netw.* 2014;**12**:34–45.

92 Denlinger CS, Ligibel JA, Are M, et al. Survivorship: screening for cancer and treatment effects Version 2.2014. *J Natl Compr Canc Netw.* 2014;**12**:1526–1531.

93 McCabe MS, Bhatia S, Oeffinger KC, et al. American Society of Clinical Oncology statement: achieving high-quality cancer survivorship care. *J Clin Oncol.* 2013;**31**:631–640.
94 Skolarus TA, Wolf AM, Erb NL, et al. American Cancer Society prostate cancer survivorship care guidelines. *CA Cancer J Clin.* 2014;**64**:225–249.
95 Cancer Journey Survivorship Expert Panel, Howell D, Hack TF, Oliver TK, et al. Survivorship services for adult cancer populations: a pan-Canadian guideline. *Curr Oncol.* 2011;**18**:e265–e281.
98 Stubblefield MD, Hubbard G, Cheville A, et al. Current perspectives and emerging issues on cancer rehabilitation. *Cancer.* 2013;**119**:2170–2178.
99 Alfano CM, Ganz PA, Rowland JH, Hahn EE. Cancer survivorship and cancer rehabilitation: revitalizing the link. *J Clin Oncol.* 2012;**30**:904–906.
104 Demark-Wahnefried W, Aziz NM, Rowland JH, Pinto BM. Riding the crest of the teachable moment: promoting long-term health after the diagnosis of cancer. *J Clin Oncol.* 2005;**23**:5814–5830.
108 Rock CL, Doyle C, Demark-Wahnefried W, et al. Nutrition and physical activity guidelines for cancer survivors. *CA Cancer J Clin.* 2012;**62**:243–274.
110 Underwood JM, Townsend JS, Stewart SL, et al. Surveillance of demographic characteristics and health behaviors among adult cancer survivors—behavioral Risk Factor Surveillance System, United States, 2009. *MMWR Surveill Summ.* 2012;**61**:1–23.
113 Van Ryn M, Sanders S, Kahn K, et al. Objective burden, resources, and other stressors among informal cancer caregivers: a hidden quality issue? *Psychooncology.* 2011;**20**:44–52.
117 Waldron EA, Janke EA, Bechtel CE, et al. A systematic review of psychosocial interventions to improve cancer caregiver quality of life. *Psychooncology.* 2013;**22**:1200–1207.
118 Matson M, Song L, Mayer DK. Putting together the pieces of the puzzle: identifying existing evidence-based resources to support the cancer caregiver. *Clin J Oncol Nurs.* 2014;**18**:619–621.
119 Earle CC, Ganz PA. Cancer survivorship care: don't let the perfect be the enemy of the good. *J Clin Oncol.* 2012;**30**:3764–3768.
122 Stein K, Mattioli V. Dialogues on cancer survivorship: a new model of international cooperation. *Cancer.* 2013;**119(Suppl 11)**:2083–2085.

第十一篇

肿瘤部位

第 77 章　成人中枢神经系统原发性和转移性肿瘤

Lisa M. DeAngelis, MD, FAAN

概述

原发性脑肿瘤并不常见，即使组织学级别较低、仍然有侵袭性。继发性或转移性脑肿瘤是原发性脑肿瘤总和的 3 倍以上。借助磁共振成像（MRI），脑肿瘤很容易明确诊断；手术切除可以获得组织学确诊和颅内减压。对于低级别和多数轴外肿瘤（如脑膜瘤），单纯手术足以获得满意疗效；而对于原发性或转移性脑实质内肿瘤，通常需要联合放疗和化疗以改善神经功能和控制肿瘤发展，但往往难以治愈。

前言

中枢神经系统（CNS）肿瘤包括颅内和椎管内的各种良恶性肿瘤。颅内肿瘤分为两类：脑内肿瘤和颅内脑外肿瘤。同样的，椎管内肿瘤分为两类：髓内肿瘤和椎管内髓外肿瘤。以往 CNS 肿瘤对标准治疗（手术切除、放疗、化疗）的疗效欠佳。近几十年里，由于影像诊断、手术技术和肿瘤放疗学的进步，患者生存期和生活质量得到了改善。重要的是，随着对脑肿瘤恶性表型相关的分子事件更深入的理解，出现了几种治疗脑肿瘤的新化疗方法。

流行病学

原发颅内肿瘤不是常见病。在美国，脑肿瘤（包括良性和恶性肿瘤）总的年发病率约为 21.03/10 万，估计每年有 63 000 例新发病例［美国脑肿瘤登记中心统计报告（CBTRUS）2006—2010 年］[1]。其中，超过 26% 是胶质瘤，其中 3/4 是高级别肿瘤，而且胶质瘤的年发病率男性（7.76/10 万）高于女性（5.60/10 万）[1]。

颅内肿瘤的发病率和病理组织类型因种族、性别、年龄而不同[1]。脑肿瘤总发病率（尤其是胶质瘤）白人高于黑人。但是，脑膜瘤发病率黑人高于白人。垂体腺瘤也是黑人较白人多见。性别差异也很明显，男女比在少突胶质瘤为 1.7，星形细胞瘤为 1.38，恶性脑膜瘤为 0.77，良性脑膜瘤为 0.44。淋巴瘤和生殖细胞肿瘤在男性中更常见，男女比分别为 1.31 和 2.33。

CNS 肿瘤可发生于任何年龄，各年龄段肿瘤发病率和病理类型有差异。10 岁前发病率有一个小高峰，15 岁以后呈稳定上升趋势。原发脑肿瘤发病平均年龄是 54 岁，胶质母细胞瘤（GBM）和脑膜瘤为 62 岁，少突胶质瘤为 16 岁。CBTRUS 资料显示，75～84 岁年龄组脑肿瘤发病率最高，GBM 在年龄大于 65 岁患者中发病率最高。生存期与患者年龄和肿瘤组织类型直接相关。例如，毛细胞星形细胞瘤（一类常见的儿童肿瘤）的 5 年相对生存率为 94.4%，而 GBM 只有 4.7%。其他重要的预后因素包括肿瘤部位、大小和切除程度。

危险因素

有大量关于环境因素和脑肿瘤发病关系的研究，但只有 2 个明确的危险因素得的确认：电离辐射和免疫抑制（表 77-1）。低或高剂量治疗性电离辐射作为脑肿瘤发病的一个重要危险因素已在多项研究中得到证实。颅内肿瘤（如髓母细胞瘤、脑外头颈部癌）放疗，包括白血病预防性放疗，在生存期超过 3 年的患者中，使胶质瘤和肉瘤的发病率增加了 7 倍。脑部放疗患者继发性脑肿瘤的累积相对危险为 5.65～10.9；其中 2/3 为胶质瘤，1/3 为脑膜瘤[2]；脑部放疗后，高级别胶质瘤中位潜伏期为 9.1 年，脑膜瘤为 19 年。用于治疗头癣（一种头皮真菌感染）、儿童皮肤血管瘤的低剂量放疗增加了脑肿瘤发生风险；神经鞘瘤、恶性脑膜瘤和胶质瘤的相对风险分别为 18、10 和 3。

表 77-1　神经上皮、脑膜及淋巴细胞来源的原发性脑肿瘤的危险因素

明确的危险因素
电离辐射
遗传性综合征
脑肿瘤的家族史
免疫抑制

先天性或获得性免疫缺陷，如人类免疫缺陷病毒（HIV）感染，或器官移植后使用免疫抑制性药物，增加原发性中枢神经系淋巴瘤（PCNSL）的发病率[3]。HIV 感染可能也增加胶质瘤和颅内平滑肌肉瘤的发生率。免疫缺陷患者的 PCNSL 是由预先潜伏于 B 淋巴细胞的 EB 病毒（Epstein-Barr virus，EBV）感染引起的。当免疫缺陷患者发生淋巴瘤，脑内发生的概率几乎是身体其他部位的 2 倍。

其他环境危险因素的研究，缺乏电离辐射和免疫抑制研究结论的说服力；这包括饮食中含有 N-亚硝基脲化合物、杀虫剂和肥料的职业暴露、人工橡胶生产、氯乙烯合成以及石化工业等。其他研究评估了脑肿瘤与头部外伤、吸烟、癫痫病史、母亲酗酒、感染的关系，但没有得到明确的结论。

电磁场暴露（EMF），特别是手机使用，引起了极大的研究兴趣。大多数研究认为，手机使用与脑肿瘤发生无关，但可能存在剂量相关风险[4,5]。最近的研究数据提示，变态反应性或过敏性疾病史，可能会降低胶质瘤发生风险。此外，大基因组相关性研究发现，在 7 个基因中的 8 个 DNA 单核苷酸多态性与胶质瘤发生或特定胶质瘤的级别和分型有关，但是相关机制不明[6]。

分子遗传学

有证据表明体细胞突变通过不同的分子通路导致了相同的 GBM 发生。GBM 至少有四个不同的分子亚型：①经典型，以 EGFR 扩增/突变和 *P53* 突变为特点；②前神经元型，以 PDGFRA 改变和异构橼酸脱氢酶(IDH)突变为特点；③间质型，以 NF1 功能障碍为特点；④神经元型，以 EGFR 过度表达和神经元标志物表达为特点[7]。但是现在，这项分子分型方案还未能推进治疗选择和预后。具有星形细胞或少突胶质细胞特点的低级别胶质瘤以 IDH 突变为特点，IDHR132H 突变发生率达 70%[8]。这个突变引起肿瘤代谢产物 2-羟基戊二酸酯(2HG)形成，而 2HG 是磁共振波谱分析(MRS)诊断和新型 IDH1 抑制剂治疗的靶点。IDH1 突变在胶质瘤发生早期升高，但在原发 GBM(即高龄、新发 GBM)中明显缺乏。

除了致癌基因扩增和抑癌基因的失活，恶性肿瘤具有侵袭邻近神经结构和通过血管生成形成新血供的能力。胶质肿瘤是极具侵袭性的肿瘤，往往侵袭到肉眼所见或影像学边界之外。血管生成引起血管增生，是 GBM 的病理学特征。血管表皮生长因子(VEGF)是胶质瘤的血管生成中重要的刺激因子之一。VEGF 在正常脑血管内皮中不表达，但在胶质瘤中因局部低氧状态影响而表达增加。VEGF 也增加血管通透性，因而在恶性胶质瘤的瘤周水肿形成中发挥作用。

CNS 相关的家族性肿瘤综合征

家族性脑肿瘤综合征是一组不同种类的疾病，以脑肿瘤伴发皮肤疾病为主的全身性病变为特点(表 77-2)。

表 77-2 CNS 肿瘤综合征

疾病	CNS 肿瘤	其他器官或组织肿瘤	皮肤病变	基因	染色体
神经纤维瘤病 1 型	胶质瘤，神经纤维瘤	虹膜错构瘤，骨病变，嗜铬细胞瘤，白血病	咖啡牛奶斑，腋窝皮肤雀斑，神经纤维瘤	*NF1*	17q11.2
神经纤维瘤病 2 型	前庭神经鞘瘤，脑膜瘤	晶状体后浑浊，视网膜错构瘤	无	*NF2*	22q12.2
VHL 病	血管母细胞瘤	视网膜母细胞瘤，肾细胞癌，嗜铬细胞瘤，内脏囊肿，内淋巴囊肿瘤	无	*VHL*	3p25-p26
结节性硬化病	室管膜下巨细胞星形细胞瘤	心脏横纹肌肉瘤，十二指肠和小肠的腺瘤样息肉，肺和肾囊肿，淋巴管肌瘤病，肾血管肌脂瘤	皮肤血管纤维瘤(皮脂腺瘤)，鲨革样皮，甲周纤维瘤	*TSC1*，*TSC2*	9q34.14，16p13.3
Li-Fraumeni 综合征	胶质瘤(10%)	乳腺癌，骨和软组织肉瘤，肾上腺皮质、肺及胃肠道的癌，白血病	无	*P53*	17p13.1
考登病	小脑肿物(Lhermitte-Duclos 病)	眼、结肠、甲状腺的错构瘤性息肉病，乳腺癌，甲状腺癌	毛根鞘瘤，纤维瘤	*PTEN*	17q22.3
脑肿瘤-息肉病综合征 1 型	恶性胶质瘤	结直肠腺瘤，结肠癌，无息肉		*MLH1* *MSH2* *MSH6* *PMS2*	3p21.3 2p21~22 2p16 7p22.1
脑肿瘤-息肉病综合征 2 型	髓母细胞瘤	结肠癌，结肠息肉		*APC*	5q21
痣样基底细胞综合征(Gorlin 综合征)	髓母细胞瘤(间变性)	颌骨囊肿，卵巢纤维瘤，骨骼异常	多发基底细胞癌，掌和足底小坑	*PTCH*	9q22.3~31
视网膜母细胞瘤	松果体肿瘤	视网膜肿瘤，骨肉瘤及其他肿瘤	无	*RBI*	13q14
布卢姆综合征(Bloom syndrome)	髓母细胞瘤，脑膜瘤	特征性的脸和声音，性腺衰竭，糖尿病，免疫缺陷	阳光敏感性，色素沉着过多或不足斑	*BLM*	15q26.1
范科尼贫血(Fanconi anemia)	星形细胞瘤，髓母细胞瘤	贫血，骨骼畸形，脑室扩大，胃肠畸形，AML	咖啡牛奶斑，色素沉着和不足	*FANCA*	16q24.3

续表

疾病	CNS 肿瘤	其他器官或组织肿瘤	皮肤病变	基因	染色体
家族性黑色素瘤	星形细胞瘤	黑色素瘤,胰腺,乳腺	痣	*CDKN2A* *P16(INK4)*	9p21.3
横纹肌易感性综合征	PNET,脉络丛肉瘤	肾肿瘤,肾外恶性横纹肌样瘤	无	*HSNFA/INH1*	22q11
多发内分泌腺肿瘤(MEN-1carey 综合体)	垂体腺瘤	甲状旁腺功能亢进,胃泌素瘤,胰岛素瘤,甲状腺/支气管类癌	面部血管纤维瘤,脂肪瘤,胶原瘤	*MEN1*	11q13
共济失调毛细血管扩张症	星形细胞瘤,髓母细胞瘤,小脑性共济失调	淋巴瘤,性功能减退症,辐射敏感性,胰岛素抵抗性,过早老化,身材矮小	毛细血管扩张	*ATM*	11q22-q23

PNET:原始外胚层肿瘤;AML:急性粒细胞白血病。

神经纤维瘤病 1 型

神经纤维瘤病 1 型(NF-1),又称为 von Reckling-Hausen 病,是最常见的有伴发 CNS 恶性肿瘤发生倾向的遗传性疾病,发病率为 1/4 000,男女无差别。它是常染色体显性遗传病,外显率达 100%;但疾病表现度差异很大,同一家族的不同个体可能表现轻微或严重。NF-1 基因定位于染色体 17q11.2,其编码一个抑癌基因,产物为神经纤维瘤蛋白。

NF-1 最常见的 CNS 肿瘤是视觉通路和脑干的胶质瘤。视觉通路胶质瘤常见为毛细胞星形细胞瘤,脑干胶质瘤为星形细胞瘤。典型的外周神经肿瘤是丛状的神经纤维瘤,常发生于脊髓旁神经和脑神经。其他 NF-1 相关肿瘤包括恶性神经鞘瘤、横纹肌肉瘤和 GBM。

神经纤维瘤病 2 型

神经纤维瘤病 2 型(NF-2),又称中央型神经纤维瘤病,是常染色体显性遗传病,仅占神经纤维瘤病总数的 10%。NF-2 基因是抑癌基因,位于染色体 22q12.2,其编码肿瘤抑制蛋白 Merlin。NF-2 主要的 CNS 肿瘤是听神经瘤(常为双侧)和脑膜瘤。

结节性硬化症

结节性硬化症(TS)是常染色体显性遗传病。TS 定位于 2 个不同的基因位点:*TSC-1* 位于染色体 9q34.14,编码蛋白 hamartin;*TSC-2* 位于染色体 16p13.3,编码蛋白 tuberin。典型的临床三联征(智力发育迟缓、癫痫和面部血管纤维瘤)只发生于最严重的病例。皮肤损害见于 96% 的患者,包括血管纤维瘤、甲周纤维瘤、皮肤色素脱失斑又称"灰叶斑"及牙齿凹陷。其标志性的 CNS 肿瘤是室管膜下巨细胞型星形细胞瘤(SEGA),在病理学上属于良性肿瘤;SEGA 是帕雷霉素靶蛋白(mTOR)过度表达驱动的,最近的研究发现利用药物(如依维莫司)阻断 mTOR 通路能够使肿瘤消退并改善癫痫控制效果[9]。

Von Hippel-Lindau 病

Von Hippel-Lindau(VHL)病是一种肿瘤综合征,涉及多个器官系统的多种肿瘤,包括小脑、脊髓和视网膜的血管母细胞瘤,嗜铬细胞瘤和肾细胞癌。其他少见的病变包括胰腺和肾脏囊肿、内淋巴囊肿瘤。血管母细胞瘤与 VEGF 的过表达有关。VHL 病是一个常染色体显性遗传病,位于染色体 3p25-p26,其外显率高但表现多样。

Li-Fraumeni 综合征

Li-Fraumeni 综合征是一种少见的常染色体显性遗传病,见于儿童和青年人,可引起多种不同肿瘤。它是由于 *P53* 的种系突变引起的。然而,一些家族并没有 *P53* 突变,他们的基因缺陷不明。30 岁前总的基因外显率约 50%,60 岁前约 90%。常见肿瘤包括乳腺肿瘤、骨肉瘤和脑肿瘤(主要是高级别胶质瘤);还有髓母细胞瘤和幕上原始神经外胚层肿瘤(PNET)。其他少见肿瘤包括软组织肉瘤、白血病和肺、肾上腺、胃和结肠肿瘤。

脑肿瘤-息肉病/胃肠道(GI)癌综合征

这类遗传性综合征以伴发/或不伴发息肉病的结肠癌和恶性脑肿瘤为特点。这两型脑肿瘤-息肉病综合征不同之处在于与恶性脑肿瘤的关系:1 型与恶性胶质瘤有关,2 型与髓母细胞瘤有关。这类综合征包括常染色体显性和隐性。由于某一错配修复基因突变,1 型脑肿瘤-息肉病综合征可能没有息肉病,也称为 Turcot、Lynch、Muir-Torres 或 Gardner 综合征。2 型脑肿瘤-息肉病综合征是由于 APC 基因的胚系突变造成的,也称为 Turcot 综合征。

CNS 肿瘤组织学分类

WHO 肿瘤分类是以肿瘤起源细胞及分化模式来进行分类的。大多数原发性 CNS 肿瘤是神经上皮来源的,起源细胞是胶质细胞(通常为星形胶质细胞)(表 77-3)[10]。其他来源于脑膜、垂体、淋巴细胞或生殖细胞。神经元占脑细胞不到 10%,不是 CNS 肿瘤的常见来源。

总的来说,儿童最常见的是原始神经外胚层肿瘤(PNET)、低级别星形细胞瘤和室管膜瘤;其中 70%位于幕下和中线附近。与儿童相比,成人倾向于发生远离中线的幕上肿瘤和较高级别的星形胶质细胞肿瘤。GBM 是 WHO 4 级,细胞丰富伴核多形性、分裂象、内皮细胞增殖和坏死。胶质肉瘤有特征性的 GBM 病理学特点,同时伴有鲱鱼骨样密集排列的纺锤形细胞。胶质肉瘤的预后和治疗与 GBM 类似。间变星形细胞瘤(AA)是 WHO 3 级,有细胞成分增多、核不典型

表 77-3 部分常见神经上皮肿瘤的 WHO 分类列表

Ⅰ. 星形细胞肿瘤
1. 弥漫星形细胞瘤,WHO 2 级
2. 间变性星形细胞瘤,WHO 3 级
3. 胶质母细胞瘤(巨细胞型,胶质肉瘤型),WHO 4 级
4. 毛细胞星形细胞瘤,WHO 1 级
5. 多形性黄色星形细胞瘤,WHO 2 级
6. 室管膜下巨细胞型星形细胞瘤,WHO 1 级
Ⅱ. 少突胶质细胞肿瘤
1. 少突胶质细胞瘤,WHO 2 级
2. 间变性少突胶质细胞瘤,WHO 3 级
3. 少突星形细胞瘤,WHO 2 级
4. 间变性少突星形细胞瘤,WHO 3 级
Ⅲ. 室管膜肿瘤
1. 室管膜瘤,WHO 2 级
2. 间变性室管膜瘤,WHO 3 级
3. 黏液乳头型室管膜瘤,WHO 1 级
4. 室管膜下瘤,WHO 1 级
Ⅳ. 脉络丛肿瘤
1. 脉络丛乳头状瘤,WHO 1 级
2. 脉络丛癌,WHO 3 级
Ⅴ. 神经及混合神经-胶质肿瘤
1. 神经节细胞瘤,WHO 2 级
2. 神经节胶质瘤,WHO 2 级
3. 间变性神经节胶质瘤,WHO 3 级
4. 胚胎期发育不良性神经上皮肿瘤(DNET),WHO 1 级
5. 中枢神经细胞瘤,WHO 2 级
Ⅵ. 松果体肿瘤
1. 松果体细胞瘤,WHO 1 级
2. 中间分化状态的松果体实质肿瘤,WHO 2 级
3. 松果体母细胞瘤,WHO 3 级
Ⅶ. 胚胎性肿瘤
1. 髓母细胞瘤(促纤维增生型,大细胞型,黑色素细胞型,髓肌母细胞瘤型)
2. CNS 原始神经外胚层肿瘤(PNET)
a. 神经母细胞瘤
b. 神经节神经母细胞瘤
c. 室管膜母细胞瘤
d. 髓上皮瘤

性和分裂象,但无坏死和微血管增殖。WHO 2 级的星形细胞瘤,通常由纤维基质中相当一致的星形胶质细胞组成,其细胞多形性和有丝分裂少见无血管增生和坏死。伴有 IDH 突变的 2~3 级胶质瘤较无突变的同级别、同类型肿瘤预后更好。

胶质瘤可具有明显异质性,同一肿瘤可能有不同的病理级别,甚至在同一肿瘤中出现星形细胞瘤和少突胶质细胞瘤的组织学特征。这给诊断带来很大的挑战,同时也突出了获得足够病理标本进行检查的必要性。病灶中发现的最高病理级别肿瘤,决定了诊断和治疗。青少年型毛细胞星形细胞瘤(JPA)是 1 级肿瘤,几乎全部发生于儿童;组织学特征包括少细胞成分、Rosenthal 纤维、囊肿形成,不会广泛地侵犯周边组织。它们可能会有稀少的核分裂和浓染的核,但不是该肿瘤的恶性特征。在儿童,该肿瘤最常发生于小脑半球;手术全切后,有约 95%的 5 年无进展生存(PFS)率。其他低级别胶质肿瘤也倾向于良性和低浸润性,这些肿瘤包括多形性黄色星形细胞瘤(PXA)、神经节细胞胶质瘤、神经细胞瘤和胚胎发育不良性神经上皮肿瘤(DNET)。这些肿瘤的诊断通常需要经验丰富的神经病理医师来完成。

少突胶质细胞瘤的特征是伴有核周晕的小圆形细胞相对均匀一致地分布在呈铁丝网样的纤细毛细血管的背景中,通常描述为"荷包蛋样"特征。偶尔,少突胶质细胞瘤有间变、多形性和坏死,而被归类于 3 级间变性少突胶质细胞瘤(AO)。少突胶质细胞瘤比星形细胞肿瘤预后更好。有些少突胶质细胞瘤有染色体 1p 和 19q 碱基易位而导致的杂合性缺失。有 1p19q 联合缺失的肿瘤预后更好、治疗反应更好。有 IDH 突变和 1p19q 联合缺失的肿瘤预后最好。

PNET 是以未分化的小蓝细胞 Homer-Wright 菊形团样(细胞环形分布形成一真腔)排列为特征的一组肿瘤。PNET 通常生长迅速,倾向于沿脑脊液通路播散,儿童最为常见,常见于小脑(髓母细胞瘤)和松果体(松果体母细胞瘤)。虽然这类肿瘤在组织学上类似,但髓母细胞瘤相对更容易治疗、预后更好。

室管膜瘤起源于脑室与脊髓中央管的室管膜细胞。室管膜瘤可来源于任何部位的室管膜细胞,但好发于第四脑室。室管膜瘤是脊髓中最常见的神经上皮肿瘤,占儿童和成人脊髓胶质瘤的 50%以上。室管膜瘤组织学特征包括血管周围的假菊形团(肿瘤细胞围绕血管呈放射状排列)及 Homer-Wright 菊形团。室管膜瘤通常为低级别肿瘤,可具有侵袭性、沿脑脊液通路播散。

临床表现

脑肿瘤患者可表现为全身非局灶性的症状和体征,或表现为与肿瘤在脑内的特殊位置有关的局灶性症状[10]。临床症状体征的影响因素包括肿瘤位置、大小、生长速度。幕上肿瘤更易于出现癫痫,而幕下肿瘤以头痛、恶心呕吐更为常见。表浅的皮质肿瘤更易出现癫痫,而深部肿瘤更易于引起性格和认知的改变。约 20%的恶性脑肿瘤患者发病症状是癫痫,而大概 90%低级别肿瘤患者的首发症状是癫痫。脑功能区的肿瘤会导致局灶性症状,如失语、偏瘫或感觉障碍。脑干肿瘤典型的表现是脑神经损伤,如复视或面肌无力。小脑肿瘤可引起同侧共济失调、步态不稳和眼球震颤。

症状通常在几周内进展，有时可能因转移性或胶质肿瘤卒中出血或癫痫发作而急性发病。任何级别的 GBM 和少突胶质细胞瘤都有 5%～10%出血风险。任何颅内转移瘤都可能出血，特定类型的肿瘤如黑色素瘤、甲状腺癌、肾癌和脉络膜癌更易出血；但由于肺癌 CNS 转移高发，肺癌是最常见的出血性脑转移灶来源。有时，局灶性癫痫可能导致无法完全缓解的神经症状。

神经影像诊断

症状体征提示可能有颅内病变的患者应进行 MRI 检查。MRI 是 CNS 肿瘤检查的首选方式，只有无法进行 MRI 的患者才进行 CT 检查。

高级别肿瘤（如 GBM）的血脑屏障受损，增强后呈中央低信号、周边不规则高信号环绕的特征性表现（图 77-1）。几乎 95%的 GBM 注药后强化；间变胶质瘤并不明显强化，尤其是在年轻成年患者，容易与低级别胶质瘤混淆（图 77-2）。GBM 有明显的沿白质传导束浸润的倾向，尤其是通过胼胝体浸润至对侧大脑半球。相反，低级别肿瘤血脑屏障完整，通常无强化。但 JPA 例外，它虽然是 1 级肿瘤、但可以有明显强化区。液体衰减反转恢复（FLAIR）序列能快速鉴别正常脑组织、脑肿瘤或脑水肿，提供了勾画病灶影像学范围的最佳图像（图 77-3）。然而，在 FLAIR 图像中，无法区分侵袭性肿瘤和水肿。弥散加权成像（DWI）可评估水分子的运动，可以鉴别缺血和肿瘤。灌注成像可评估血容量和血管分布，与肿瘤级别和 FDG-PET 研究有关。

在 MRI 图像上，转移瘤通常呈球形，较原发肿瘤边界更规则。转移瘤通常位于脑分水岭区域的灰白质交界区。较小的转移瘤往往均匀强化，而较大的转移瘤常呈环状强化；瘤周水肿通常非常明显。非常小的转移灶可能表现为点状强化伴或不伴 FLAIR 像高信号，往往没有瘤周水肿。50%的患者是单发脑转移，20%有 2 个转移灶，13%有 3 个转移灶，其余患者有多于 3 个的脑转移灶。MRI 也有局限性，脑肿瘤需要与放射性坏死、缺血性梗死、感染、炎症和脱髓鞘进行鉴别。

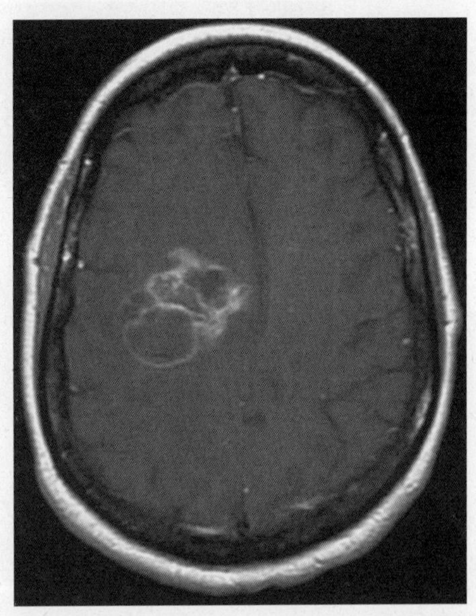

图 77-1　胶质母细胞瘤。增强 T1 像显示右侧额叶后部胶质母细胞瘤，病灶不规则增强伴局部坏死

其他影像技术

PET 在脑肿瘤诊断中有一些有用之处。PET 能区分肿瘤复发和放射性坏死，能区分低级别和高级别病灶，能分辨出 MRI 上明显呈低级别肿瘤特征的病灶中的高级别肿瘤部分、而指导引导立体定向活检（图 77-4）。PET 是通过注射用正电子发射放射性核素如 O15、C11、N13 和 F18 标记的物质如葡萄糖、氨基酸（如蛋氨酸）或核苷酸来进行的。FDG 是评价脑肿瘤最常用的放射性核素，能界定所检测区域的代谢率。高代谢状态（FDG 摄入增加）在高级别肿瘤中常见，低代谢状态（FDG 摄入低）在低级别肿瘤中常见。

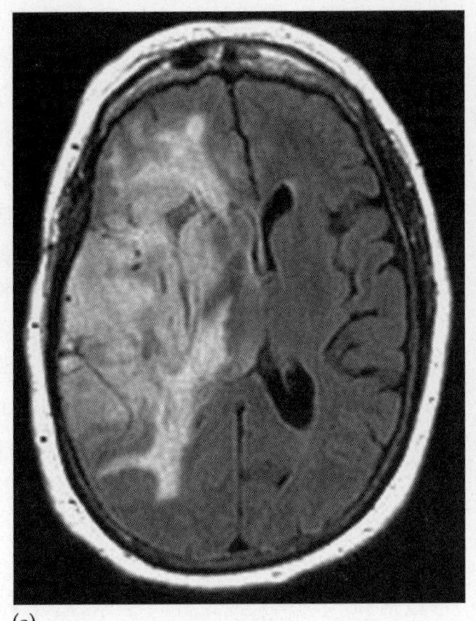

(a)

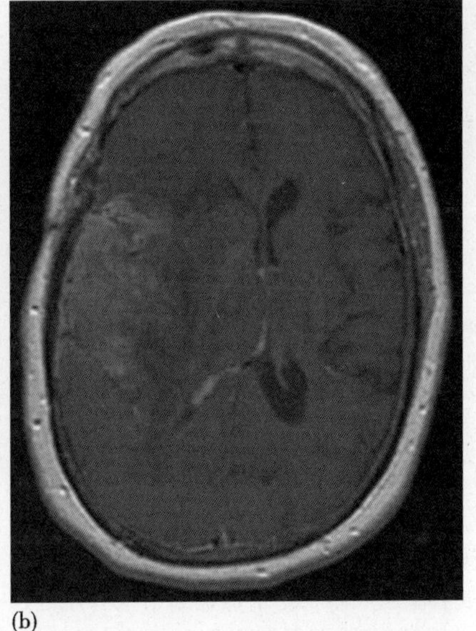

(b)

图 77-2　间变少突胶质细胞瘤。（a）FLAIR 像显示右侧半球广泛肿瘤浸润。（b）整个肿瘤呈斑片样强化

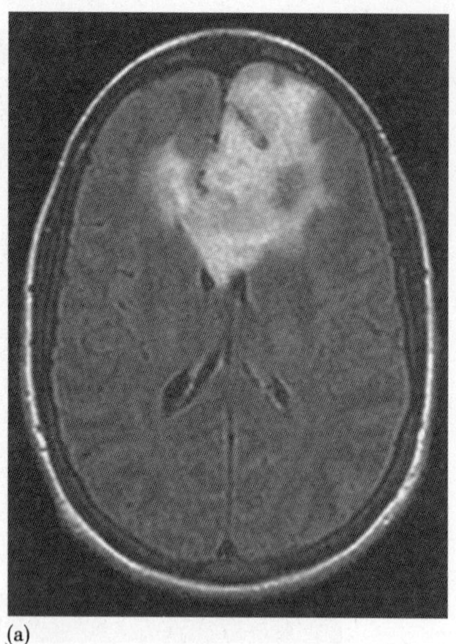
(a)

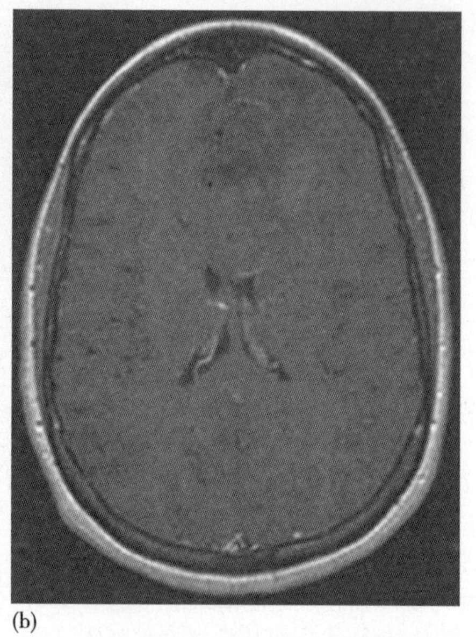
(b)

图 77-3 低级别胶质瘤。(a)FLAIR 像显示广泛的浸润性病变主要累及左侧额叶,经前胼胝体侵犯右侧额叶深部白质。(b)增强后未见病灶明显强化

FDG-PET 能区分放射性坏死和肿瘤复发。虽然在 MRI 成像上两者相似,典型的放射性坏死在 PET 上表现为低代谢状态,而复发的高级别肿瘤在 PET 上与正常脑组织相比呈等代谢状态或高代谢状态。

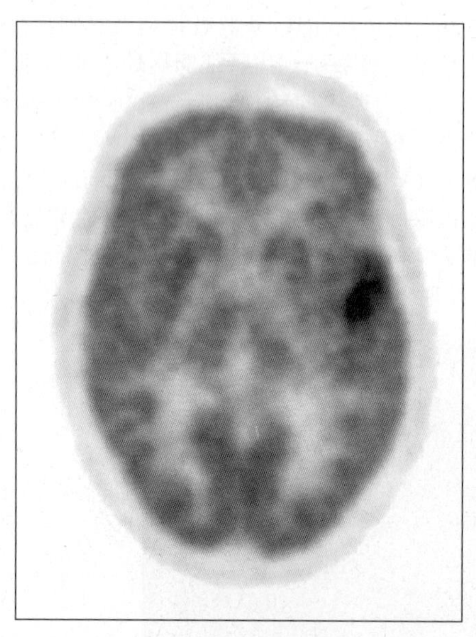

图 77-4 低级别胶质瘤。左侧颞叶低级别胶质瘤 FDG-PET 图像显示病变中呈局灶高代谢状态的间变性肿瘤病灶

功能 MRI(fMRI)用于定位脑功能结构,尤其是运动、感觉及语言皮质。fMRI 成像理论是神经元活动增加会引起脑血流量(CBF)增加,引起氧合血红蛋白与脱氧血红蛋白比率变化,从而在 MRI 成像中信号增加。fMRI 在术前计划中很有用处,它能让外科医生定位功能区皮质,规划切除病变的同时保护神经功能,有利于实现避免神经损伤前提下的最大限度病灶切除。

治疗原则

脑肿瘤的治疗包括针对性治疗和支持性治疗。针对性治疗包括手术、放疗和化疗。支持性治疗指对肿瘤症状的处理,如用皮质激素治疗局部或全身性症状,用抗癫痫药物控制癫痫,用抗凝剂治疗深静脉血栓(DVT)及必要时提供社会心理学支持。

支持性治疗

治疗的目标是延长患者生存期,除了手术、放疗和化疗,还需各种支持性治疗以缓解患者的神经症状、提高患者生活质量。

所有脑肿瘤导致的癫痫初始都是局灶性癫痫,甚至可能局部病灶临床上还没有被发现。脑肿瘤患者一旦发生癫痫,不管是属于发病症状还是治疗过程中发生,均需用抗癫痫药物(AED)治疗。最合适的抗癫痫药物不会影响肝脏微粒体系统、以致影响化疗药物代谢;常用的抗癫痫药物包括左乙拉西坦、妥泰、左尼沙胺。抗癫痫药物不能预防无癫痫病史的脑肿瘤患者发作癫痫,不建议预防性应用抗癫痫药物[10]。

皮质激素能显著缓解脑肿瘤引起的脑水肿相关症状,可降低颅内压。症状改善一般需要数小时,患者症状可在 24~48h 内得到缓解。皮质激素适用于所有症状的脑肿瘤患者;但可疑 PCNSL 的患者除外,因为皮质激素的溶淋巴细胞效应会导致肿瘤坏死,活检前使用激素会影响肿瘤的组织诊断。

皮质激素的最佳剂量并无定论。常用起始剂量是地塞米松 16mg/d,由于它是长效,每日剂量分两次给药。剂量应调整到可获得良好神经功能的最低剂量。患者使用皮质激素大于 6 周,应预防性治疗卡式肺囊虫感染。

深静脉血栓(DVT)是脑肿瘤的一种常见并发症。诱发因素包括:卧床不动、神经外科手术、脑中释放促凝血酶原激酶、与肿瘤和化疗相关的高凝状态。预防性和治疗性抗凝安全有效,不会增加瘤内出血的风险[11]。可选的抗凝药物包括低分子肝素和新的凝血酶或Xa 因子抑制剂。腔静脉滤器适合于有

绝对抗凝禁忌的患者。

手术

在脑肿瘤的治疗中，手术是最重要的治疗方式。手术目的具有多重性：明确病理诊断，减少肿瘤体积和占位效应，缓解症状，减少皮质激素剂量。手术的终极目标是全切除肿瘤。活检，尤其是立体定向穿刺活检，适用于以下情况：①不能手术切除的肿瘤，如脑干、基底核或丘脑的肿瘤；②多发肿瘤或大脑胶质瘤病；③患有其他疾病，手术/麻醉风险高的患者。穿刺活检有一些缺陷；由于组织标本有限，可能不能获得肿瘤类型和病理级别的准确诊断。良性或 1 级胶质瘤可能通过完全手术切除而治愈。对于不能治愈的肿瘤，如所有侵袭性胶质瘤，手术切除程度是一个重要的预后因素；仅行活检的患者比肿瘤更广泛切除者预后差。对 3 个前瞻性 RTOG 随机试验的 645 例 GBM 患者回顾性分析，发现全切除患者（中位生存期为 11.3 个月）比仅行活检的患者（中位生存期为 6.6 个月）的生存期有统计学意义的显著改善[12]；关于低级别胶质瘤（LGG）的结论相似。此外，切除肿瘤通常可以改善患者神经功能、而非使之恶化。在一项前瞻性多中心研究分析了新诊断恶性胶质瘤、进行开颅手术的 408 例患者，致残率为 24%，死亡率为 1.5%；53%的患者术后神经功能改善，近 8%神经功能恶化[13]。术前 fMRI（如前述）和术中唤醒皮质定位有利于避免神经损伤的前提下切除肿瘤。

放疗

放疗是恶性胶质瘤有效的辅助治疗方法。放疗可治愈某些肿瘤，如生殖细胞瘤。在前瞻性临床试验中，生殖细胞瘤患者行放疗比单纯手术或手术+化疗的生存期更长。在最早的 1978 年脑肿瘤研究组关于高级别胶质瘤的报道中，仅接受手术的患者中位生存期为 14 周，而接受术后 50~60Gy 剂量全脑放疗（WBRT）的患者为 36 周。不断进步的放疗技术使得肿瘤能够接受更高剂量照射而不损伤正常脑组织。局灶放疗照射野包括 MRI 中 Flair 序列异常信号区域及外侧边缘 2~3cm 范围，随后缩小至强化区域。标准的分割外照射治疗是将 60Gy 的最佳剂量在 6 周内每天分次进行，即 1.8~2.0Gy/d。现代放疗技术包括调强放疗（IMRT）能够使照射剂量与靶区体积形状相适应，从而保护临近重要结构。

立体定向放射外科（SRS）是用于治疗某些脑肿瘤（尤其是转移瘤）的另一种放疗技术。在典型的单次照射中，SRS 向明确定位的小靶区内发射高度聚焦的放射线。SRS 能通过 γ 刀（钴-60 来源）、直线加速器或射波刀实现等效的结果。为了保持陡峭的剂量梯度，靶直径要小于 4cm。放射外科主要用于治疗小的病灶，如转移性肿瘤、脑膜瘤、听神经瘤和垂体腺瘤。由于恶性胶质瘤不适用于聚焦放疗，放射外科很少用于治疗恶性胶质瘤。

质子、中子和带电重粒子也已用于治疗 CNS 肿瘤。质子束与原子的核相互作用，而不是与原子的电子相互作用，使大剂量射线累积于靶区而附近的组织不受损伤。带电重粒子射线速度能够陡然下降，从而使无法耐受治疗性照射的敏感组织免受损害。对颅底肿瘤（如脊索瘤、脑膜瘤、软骨肉瘤）和临近视神经、视交叉和脑干的病变的治疗来说是一种理想的方式。质子治疗也广泛用于儿童患者，以降低发育性器官的放射性暴露，但是与标准放疗相比，其优越性尚不明确[14]。

化疗

除了少数例外，包括 PCNSL、生殖细胞瘤和部分少突胶质细胞瘤，传统化疗药物治疗多数脑肿瘤并不太成功。在延长生存期方面，与单纯手术和放疗相比，化疗对星形细胞瘤的作用有限。没有合适的化疗药物可用于治疗听神经瘤、脑膜瘤。

脑肿瘤的化疗有几个特殊的问题，包括：血脑屏障的作用、脑内缺乏淋巴系统、胶质瘤的异质性、胶质瘤固有的耐药性和偏低的疗效/毒性比。由于完整血脑屏障的存在，许多化疗药物不能进入脑肿瘤。某些肿瘤，如转移瘤或高级别胶质瘤，存在血脑屏障的破坏，允许水溶性化疗药物不同程度的渗透进肿瘤。但是，某些肿瘤如低级别胶质瘤，血脑屏障完好，水溶性化疗药物不能到达病灶。在高级别胶质瘤的浸润边缘，血脑屏障是完好的，此区域的细胞最具活力。在治疗脑肿瘤过程中为开放血脑屏障，人们尝试了很多方法，例如用高渗药物（如动脉输注甘露醇）开放血脑屏障；其他方法包括动脉灌注、经导管瘤内注射、瘤腔内载药片植入、改造型药物。迄今，没有证据显示这些方法比常规途径更有效，而且某些方法毒副作用更大。

除了血脑屏障的阻碍外，多数脑肿瘤对化疗药物有固有的耐药性；因此，即使肿瘤组织中有足够的药物浓度，多数药物也是无效的。例外的是，全身性化疗治疗脑转移瘤的作用越来越重要。即使放疗或化疗能成功杀死肿瘤细胞，由于脑组织中缺乏淋巴系统，妨碍了治疗引起的细胞碎片清除。因此，坏死组织将成为脑水肿的发源地，加重神经功能损伤。特殊药物将按肿瘤类型讨论。

胶质母细胞瘤和间变性星形细胞瘤

GBM 多发于年长患者，中位发病年龄为 54 岁；而 AA 中位年龄为 45 岁。AA 中位生存时间为 3~5 年，而 GBM 大约为 18 个月。预后良好的因素包括：年龄较小，KPS 评分较高，病理为 AA 而非 GBM，手术切除而非仅行活检[10]。

对于新诊断的 GBM，术后标准治疗方案是每日口服替莫唑胺同步放疗（60Gy，分割剂量 1.8~2.0Gy），后至少进行 6 周期替莫唑胺辅助化疗。一项包括 573 例 70 岁以下新诊断 GBM 患者的前瞻性随机试验表明，放疗联合每日替莫唑胺［75mg/（m^2·d）］同步放化疗+6 周期替莫唑胺辅助化疗［150~200mg/（m^2·d），d1~5，28d/周期］方案的治疗患者中位生存期为 14.6 个月，而单纯放疗患者为 12.1 个月；更重要的是，2 年生存率为 26.5%和 10.4%[15]；而且放疗+化疗组治疗毒性很小。DNA 修复酶 MGMT 具有重要意义。Hegi 等分析了三期临床研究中近一半患者的 MGMT 启动子甲基化状态，发现启动子甲基化并失活的患者有明显的生存优势[16]。放疗联合替莫唑胺治疗的患者，有 MGMT 启动子甲基化患者的中位生存期为 21.7 个月，而无甲基化患者为 15.3 个月（$P=0.007$）。尽管肿瘤有 MGMT 启动子甲基化的患者服用替莫唑胺受益更大，但是无启动子甲基化的患者口服替莫唑胺也可受益。

手术联合 RT 的老年患者（>70 岁）生存期要长于单纯手术者，但预后仍然很差[17]。和延长的 RT 方案相比，减少 RT 的剂量和周期（45Gy/25 次）治疗效果相当。另外，单用替莫唑胺也能达到同样的治疗效果。目前，没有关于老年患者放化疗效果的明确结论。

即使进行标准治疗，几乎所有肿瘤仍会复发，复发通常发生在原部位。肿瘤复发时的治疗选择包括：再手术，少数情况下进行高聚焦放疗(如 SRS)联用/不联用贝伐珠单抗,全身性化疗方案调整。随机Ⅱ期临床试验结果表明:贝伐珠单抗单药治疗复发 GBM 的 6 个月无进展生存率为 30%、中位生存期 9 个月,效果与贝伐珠单抗联用伊立替康相当;因此,FDA 批准贝伐珠单抗可单药治疗复发 GBM[18]。基于上述初步结论,有两项大样本随机Ⅲ期临床试验主要研究标准放化疗联用或不联用贝伐珠单抗治疗新发 GBM[19,20]。两项研究均表明,联用贝伐珠单抗可以显著延长无进展生存期(PFS)(中位生存期由 6~7 个月延长至 10.7 个月),但对总生存期无影响(中位生存期 15~16 个月)。但是,两项研究关于生活质量的结论有所不同:一项研究认为联用贝伐珠单抗可以获得较好的生活质量,而另一项认为联用贝伐珠单抗加重了患者的症状、降低了其生活质量。基于上述结论,并不推荐贝伐珠单抗用于首次治疗的患者。此外,一项欧洲随机试验的初步结果显示:贝伐珠单抗联用洛莫司汀治疗复发 GBM 优于单用贝伐珠单抗,当肿瘤进展时单用贝伐珠单抗疗效不佳;但研究的最终结果尚不明确。恶性胶质瘤分子生物学研究主要集中在肿瘤生长的信号通路上。针对复发 GBM 正在进行的几项临床试验主要对 EGFR 抑制剂、mTOR 抑制剂、PKC 抑制剂和干扰 RAS 信号通路进行评估[21]。

鉴于在其他实体肿瘤治疗上的进展,免疫治疗成为一种新的胶质瘤治疗策略[22]。其包括了利用肿瘤抗原产生疫苗在内的一系列方式,而肿瘤抗原往往来自患者自身的肿瘤。利用树突状细胞或者多肽疫苗的免疫治疗可以产生抗肿瘤反应。关于 EGFRvⅢ疫苗的随机Ⅲ期临床试验的初步结果表明,初发患者在标准治疗基础上增加免疫治疗可获得生存受益;可惜的是,只有 20%的患者受益。树突状细胞疫苗接种可能增加肿瘤细胞对化疗的敏感性,从而改善生存期。其他免疫治疗方式,例如免疫检查点抑制剂,包括抗 CTLA4、抗 PD1、抗 PDL1 药物,均有相关研究在进行。

虽然肿瘤进展不可避免,GBM 中位生存期只有 18 个月,但有小部分患者从这些新的治疗方式中获益而生存达数年,并且能获得良好的功能状态。

间变性胶质瘤

Ⅲ级肿瘤 AA 较 GBM 少见,因此相关单独临床试验研究也较少。一项正在进行的关于放疗联合替莫唑胺的随机试验的结果值得期待,其研究终止标准基本参考了类似新发 GBM 患者的治疗方案。包括所有类型Ⅲ级胶质瘤的Ⅲ期临床试验结果表明,无论初始治疗是单放疗或单化疗,当肿瘤进展时增加其他治疗方式后,最终治疗结果并不受影响[23]。但是,多数患者在初始发病时就采用了放疗联合替莫唑胺方案。

低级别胶质瘤和少突胶质细胞瘤

低级别胶质瘤(LGG)包括星形细胞瘤、少突胶质细胞瘤和混合性少突星形细胞瘤[1]。LGG 的组织学多样性使得其治疗和预后很难一概而论。但是总体而言,LGG 生长缓慢,可能并不需要立刻进行治疗干预。然而,LGG 的主要的风险是有转变成高级别胶质瘤的倾向,而且一旦转变为高级别胶质瘤,预后就取决于新的病理类型。

LGG 约占原发性颅内肿瘤的 10%[1]。患者确诊中位年龄为 37 岁,低龄是重要的较好的预后因素。年轻成人的少突胶质细胞瘤常发生在额叶(40%)、顶叶(30%)和颞叶(20%)脑白质,约占成人 LGG 的 10%,占儿童 LGG 的 5%。

60%~80%的患者首发症状的为癫痫,大部分癫痫为局灶性发作。大部分患者就诊时神经功能良好,90%的患者在诊断时的 KPS 评分在 90~100 分。LGG 患者较其他恶性胶质瘤预后更好,但绝大多数都会死于该疾病。低级别少突胶质细胞瘤的中位生存期为 9.8 年,而低级别星形细胞瘤为 4.7 年。

目前,在诊治 LGG 中,唯一一致认可的干预措施是获得肿瘤组织进行组织学诊断。目前,越来越多的证据表明,在诊断时就彻底切除肿瘤是预后良好的影响因素。最近一项包括 216 例进行手术切除的 LGG 患者的回顾分析表明,在进行了年龄、KPS、肿瘤位置、组织类型因素的校正后,手术切除程度是影响总生存期和 PFS 的重要因素[24]。另外,切除程度和术后神经功能障碍无相关性。大多数研究报道,肿瘤全切除(术后即刻 MRI 证实)的患者的 5 年生存率达 80%以上。以上证据都强烈建议对 LGG 进行最大限度切除。

LGG 患者进行 RT 的时机也存在争议。欧洲癌症研究与治疗组织(EORTC)进行了一个关于成人幕上 LGG 的前瞻性Ⅲ期临床试验,随机把患者分成观察组和单纯 RT 组;RT 组的中位 PFS 为 5.3 年,而观察组只有 3.4 年($P<0.0001$);但是两组的总生存期相似(中位生存期 7.4 年和 7.2 年);2/3 的观察组患者最终接受了 RT[25]。因此,根据患者的临床状况,选择观察或延缓的 RT 都是合适,不会影响总生存期。但是,对于高风险患者,包括癫痫控制不佳、严重神经功能障碍、肿瘤残留大于 4~6cm 和高龄的患者,需要立即进行治疗。

两个前瞻性随机临床试验比较了低剂量(45~50Gy)和高剂量(59.4~64Gy)RT 疗效,PFS 和总生存期两组没有差别,但高剂量组的放射毒副作用增加;因此,低剂量 RT 成为治疗标准[26,27]。重要的是,最近辅助化疗的作用已经明确。一项大型前瞻性临床试验(RTOG9802)按照危险因素(年龄和切除程度)将患者分为低风险组和高风险组,低风险组随访观察(第 1 组),高风险组随机接受 RT±丙卡巴肼、CCNU、新长春碱(PCV 方案)(第 2、3 组);RT 增加 PVC 化疗显著延长了高风险患者的中位生存期(7.8 年增加至 13.3 年)[28]。

一些研究表明,对于放疗后进展的 LGG 患者,替莫唑胺治疗有效;47%~67%的肿瘤缩小(>25%),PFS 为 10~22 个月[29]。几项小的研究评估了首次术后即使用替莫唑胺治疗 LGG,有效率(包括轻微有效)为 31%~61%,肿瘤进展的中位时间为 31~36 个月[30]。基于上述结果,鉴于替莫唑胺的低毒性,有人建议:使用替莫唑胺替代 PCV 方案、联合 RT,作为 LGG 的初始治疗方案。

染色体 1p 和 19q 缺失的 LGG 对化疗敏感,染色体 IDH 突变、1p/19q 联合缺失的 LGG 化疗效果最好、患者生存期最长。越来越多的Ⅱ、Ⅲ级肿瘤的诊断分级是基于分子病理分析,而非易于混淆的组织学表现。1p/19q 联合缺失最早是在少突胶质细胞瘤中发现的,是间变性少突胶质细胞瘤(AO)的预后和疗效预测因素。无 1p/19q 缺失的 AO 患者的中位总生存期为 2~3 年,而有 1p19q 联合缺失者中位生存期为 6~7 年。有研究发现,PCV 方案化疗对 1p 缺失或 1p19q 联合缺失的 AO 患者

100%有效,而对染色体正常的患者有效率为 25%~31%[31]。有肿瘤 1p19q 缺失的患者 5 年生存率达到 95%,而肿瘤基因正常的患者仅有 25%。没有 PCV 方案和替莫唑胺的前瞻性对比研究报道,但有些回顾性数据提示 PCV 方案可能更好[32]。

有两项关于初次诊断 AO 患者的大型随机临床试验,都评估了 RT±PCV 方案的疗效:一项试验中,把 PCV 方案作为新辅助化疗(即 RT 前化疗);而另一项试验中,RT 后进行 PCV 化疗[33,34]。两项试验均提示化疗可以显著延长 PFS;而一项试验中,总生存期都得到延长;而两个试验均表明,RT 联合 PCV 化疗可以显著延长 1p19q 联合缺失组的中位总生存期(中位生存期 14.7 年:7.3 年)。因此建议 1p19q 联合缺失的 AO 患者的标准治疗方案是 RT 联合化疗。但是,鉴于替莫唑胺明确的疗效和低毒副反应,PCV 是否为必选方案尚不明确。

AO 的化疗敏感性使首选化疗更具有吸引力,以此推迟放疗、避免长期存活者的放疗副作用。目前,有些关于替莫唑胺治疗的小样本研究。一个首选替莫唑胺单药治疗的研究表明,没有 1p 缺失的患者无进展期为 8 个月,而有 1p 缺失的患者无进展期为 24 个月[35]。在一个包括 69 例新诊断 AO 患者的Ⅱ期临床试验中,治疗方案为强化 PCV、联合高剂量噻替哌(thiotepa)+自体干细胞移植,而未做 RT;其中 39 例接受自体干细胞移植患者的 PFS 为 78 个月,但总生存期并没有延长[36]。这些数据显示的关于 AO 患者最佳治疗方案的信息相互矛盾,但 RT+化疗的标准很明确。

室管膜瘤

室管膜瘤约占成人颅内肿瘤的 2%、儿童颅内肿瘤的 5%。室管膜瘤起源于室管膜细胞,一般生长在脑室表面,也可能发生在毗邻脑室的脑实质组织或在椎管的任何位置。超过 60%的室管膜瘤生长在后颅窝和第四脑室底部。典型幕上室管膜瘤发生在脑实质组织内而不在脑室中,以额叶和顶叶最多见。室管膜瘤能沿着蛛网膜下腔扩展,并沿脑脊液种植。

WHO 分类把室管膜肿瘤分为室管膜瘤(WHO Ⅱ级)、间变性室管膜瘤(WHO Ⅲ级)、室管膜下瘤(WHO Ⅰ级)和黏液乳头状室管膜瘤(WHO Ⅰ级)。尽管组织学相似,但室管膜瘤分子表现因位置而不同:幕上,后颅窝和脊髓。幕上室管膜瘤特点是致癌基因 RELA 与未知基因 *C11orf 95* 融合,其可自发驱动 NF-κB 通路[37]。颅内室管膜瘤预后良好的分子因素包括染色体 9、15q、18 增加和染色体 6 丢失;而染色体 1q 增加或 CDKN2A 纯合性缺失与 PFS 和总生存期缩短显著相关[38]。

临床症状取决于肿瘤所在的部位。幕下室管膜瘤最常见的症状是脑干受压或脑脊液梗阻引起的头痛、恶心和呕吐。幕上的肿瘤可能表现为癫痫发作或局灶神经功能缺损。在 MRI 上,肿瘤表现为 T1 像低或等信号、T2 像高信号,有或无增强。60%的幕下肿瘤有钙化,80%的肿瘤能有囊变和坏死。

室管膜瘤的初始治疗方式是手术切除。全切除肿瘤能延长生存期,但可能因肿瘤的部位而不一定总是能实现。Ⅱ级肿瘤全切除后无须辅助放疗;但是次全切除的Ⅱ级肿瘤和所有间变性室管膜瘤(Ⅲ级,无论切除彻底程度)都需进行局部 RT。RT 主要针对瘤床而非整个神经轴,除非术前脊髓 MRI 和脑脊液细胞学(为了分期需要,所有患者均应行这两项检查)证实肿瘤已通过脑脊液播散。室管膜瘤属于化疗耐药肿瘤,一般不进行常规辅助化疗。对于复发室管膜瘤,有报道认为铂类药物的有效率达 65%;有报道认为亚硝基脲、依托泊苷、甚至贝伐珠单抗都有效,但替莫唑胺无效[39]。

原发性中枢系统淋巴瘤(PCNSL)

PCNSL 是一类以弥漫大 B 细胞淋巴瘤为主的非霍奇金淋巴瘤,主要累及脑、脊髓、脑脊液或眼睛,约占 CNS 肿瘤的 2%[1]。在免疫抑制的人群中更常见,常与 EB 病毒有关。

PCNSL 的中位诊断年龄是 60 岁,免疫缺陷患者年龄更小。年龄越大、一般情况差的患者,生存期也越短。散发病例中有 30%~40%为多发病灶。PCNSL 生长迅速,因此从出现症状到诊断一般只有数周。最常见的症状是认知障碍或者性格改变,这与肿瘤常发生在额叶及肿瘤的多发倾向有关(图 77-5)。眼

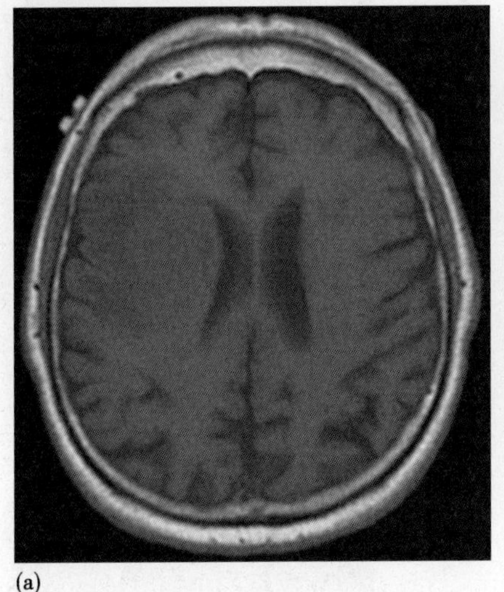

(a)

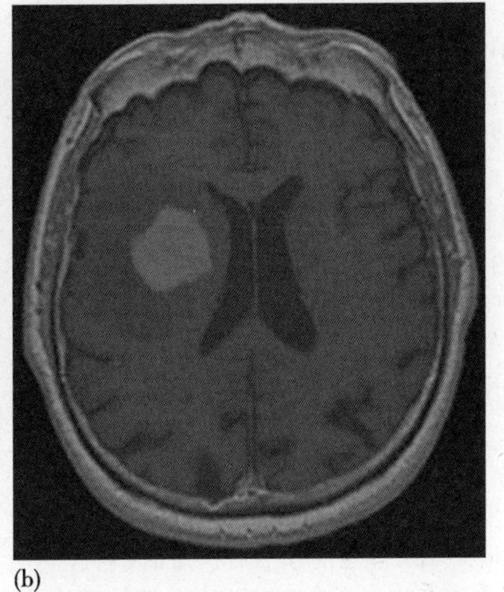

(b)

图 77-5　PCNSL。右侧额叶弥漫增强的 PCNSL 其增强前(a)和增强后(b)图像。注意增强肿瘤周边的水肿

部受累常见，可能是初发症状，也可能在肿瘤复发时发生。眼部淋巴瘤患者有50%~80%的可能发展为颅内淋巴瘤。孤立性眼部淋巴瘤的诊断十分困难，因为症状类似于良性炎症反应如葡萄膜炎。最常见的症状为飞蚊症和视物模糊。诊断依靠裂隙灯检查、眼部超声和玻璃体活检。所有PCNSL患者分级评估都应包括眼部检查、腰椎穿刺脑脊液细胞学检查和全身性检查。

PCNSL治疗预后良好。类似于全身性非霍奇金淋巴瘤，PCNSL对放化疗敏感。尽管对治疗敏感，但PCNSL有很高的复发率，5年生存率25%~50%。对于手术切除的治疗价值结论不一；由于手术切除往往不可行，因此多数患者是通过单纯活检确诊的。由于激素对恶性淋巴细胞有溶瘤作用，为了不干扰病理诊断，在手术活检前不应使用激素。

PCNSL的现代治疗策略是基于大剂量甲氨蝶呤的方案。全身性淋巴瘤的标准化疗方案，如CHOP（环磷酰胺、多柔比星、长春新碱、泼尼松），对PCNSL无效，应该避免使用。甲氨蝶呤是最有效、最常用的PCNSL治疗药物。大剂量的甲氨蝶呤（剂量3~8g/m^2）配合亚叶酸解救，无论是单一用药还是联合其他药物，有效率达60%~90%。文献报道，不同剂量范围的大剂量的甲氨蝶呤化疗方案能使患者的中位总生存期达30~60个月。其他配合甲氨蝶呤使用的药物包括阿糖胞苷、丙卡巴肼和替莫唑胺。以甲氨蝶呤为基础的治疗方案中，各种巩固性治疗包括：自体干细胞移植（特殊选择的患者）、低剂量全脑放疗（2 340cGy，理论上有潜在神经毒性）、依托泊苷和大剂量阿糖胞苷持续灌注化疗（严重的全身毒性）[40~42]。虽然美罗华穿过血脑屏障、进入CNS的能力很差，但是其有效性明确，被加入大多数治疗方案中。一项大型Ⅲ期临床试验表明，4 500cGy的最大剂量全脑放疗作为甲氨蝶呤方案的巩固性治疗并未使患者生存受益；由于长期生存患者（尤其是高龄患者）严重的神经毒性，这种方案被禁止使用[43]。

脑膜瘤

脑膜瘤约占颅内肿瘤25%，属于脑外肿瘤，起源于蛛网膜帽状细胞而非硬脑膜；女性比男性多见[1]。大约85%的脑膜瘤位于幕上，散发病例中约10%是多发脑膜瘤。电离辐射暴露是唯一明确的诱发因素；低剂量和高剂量的辐射都与脑膜瘤的发生有关，且非典型性或者恶性脑膜瘤更常见，而且常为多发。

最近的分子分析结果表明，肿瘤抑制基因NF2在半数患者中失活。大约25%的肿瘤有TRAF7突变合并转录因子KLF4的K409Q突变。大约20%有AKT1的E17K突变，常常伴随TRAF7突变。大约5%有SMO突变，与Hedgehog信号通路激活有关。后述几个突变都参与决定了肿瘤在颅底的解剖位置（通常是前颅底）；而NF2突变不同，其无遗传重叠，相关肿瘤主要位于后颅底[44,45]。这些有趣的生物学发现暂时还没有治疗性意义，但或许将来会有所不同。

脑膜瘤的预后主要取决于肿瘤组织学类型和肿瘤切除程度。确诊时年龄和肿瘤大小可能也对预后有一定的影响。年轻患者恢复情况要好于年老患者。典型脑膜瘤全切除后的5年复发率为20%，10年复发率为25%。未完全切除的脑膜瘤在没有接受RT的情况下，复发率为60%。Mc-Carthy等调查了在美国治疗的9 000多例脑膜瘤，包括美国癌症数据库的资料，得出结论：5年生存率超过60%，小于65岁的患者5年生存率为81%，大于65岁的患者5年生存率为56%；良性脑膜瘤的5年生存率为75%，恶性脑膜瘤为55%[46]。基于总人群的研究报道，脑膜瘤5年生存率接近90%。

典型的脑膜瘤压迫而非侵犯临近脑组织。但是，脑膜瘤可能会侵犯静脉系统，如上矢状窦。脑膜瘤的组织学表现各异，但只有横纹肌样或透明细胞特征的脑膜瘤有侵袭性、预后较差。非典型脑膜瘤具有较高的有丝分裂指数，同时瘤内可见细胞数增加、核/质比增高、核仁明显、坏死和无规律生长。恶性脑膜瘤必须具备的特征是：每10个高倍镜视野至少有20个有丝分裂或者组织学上有类似癌组织和肉瘤组织。仅1%的脑膜瘤会发生转移，但近50%的恶性脑膜瘤会发生转移，常见的转移部位有肝脏、骨骼和肺脏。

大多数脑膜瘤生长缓慢，且无症状；有些患者因其他原因检查而发现脑膜瘤。脑膜瘤产生临床症状或体征主要是由于压迫脑组织、引起水肿或脑积水。虽然大部分脑膜瘤不会引起明显的脑水肿，但分泌型脑膜瘤会引起水肿导致显著的神经功能障碍。凸面的脑膜瘤可能会引起癫痫。特定部位的脑膜瘤可能造成典型的临床综合征，如海绵窦脑膜瘤可引起复视、眼球突出和其他眼球运动障碍。

CT和MRI能诊断脑膜瘤。在CT上，脑膜瘤表现为高密度脑外肿块，其中25%可见钙化；增强后脑膜瘤表现为明显规则强化；非典型、恶性或者巨大脑膜瘤可引起周边脑组织水肿。在MRI的T1W和T2W成像上，大多数脑膜瘤的信号与周边灰质相似；在增强MRI上，肿瘤弥漫增强，可见到特征性的“脑膜尾”征（图77-6）。一些脑膜瘤可能有流空信号，提示肿瘤血供丰富。处理脑膜瘤患者，首先要决定的是肿瘤是否有治疗的必要。如果没有进展或未造成神经功能损害，许多脑膜瘤可以随

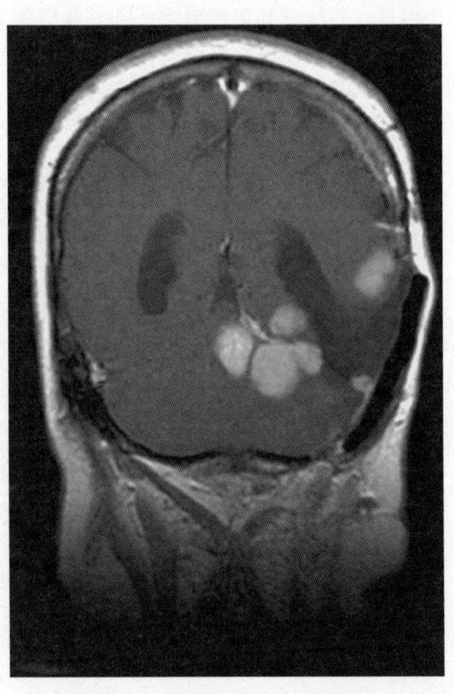

图77-6 脑膜瘤。冠状位强化MRI显示多结节样脑膜瘤累及幕上幕下，左侧颞枕叶皮质可见第二个病灶

访观察数年。如果癫痫是唯一症状而且药物控制良好，就没有必要进行手术切除。如果手术风险很高，许多脑膜瘤可不进行手术切除，主要是位于颅底和海绵窦的肿瘤；这些肿瘤可能包绕海绵窦段颈内动脉及多个脑神经。

手术切除是明确的治疗方式；如果能够完全切除肿瘤，患者能彻底治愈。最有可能手术全切除的脑膜瘤往往位于凸面。术前栓塞可能会使肿瘤体积缩小、血供减少，有利于手术切除。即使完全手术切除的患者，仍有 15%~20% 会复发，可能需要进一步手术或放疗。

放疗适用于某些部分切除术后复发而又无法切除的脑膜瘤和所有恶性脑膜瘤（无论切除彻底与否）[47]。在非典型性脑膜瘤中，放疗的作用仍不明确。最近的研究表明，放疗对非典型脑膜瘤有效，认为可以延长患者的 PFS；但实际只有少数患者 PFS 延长，对总生存期的影响还不明确。此外，新的 3D 放疗计划技术和立体定向引导共聚焦放疗有效减少了正常组织的辐射影响、降低了神经毒性。在一些脑膜瘤的治疗中，质子刀的运用能减少放疗毒副作用和延缓复发。

立体定向放疗是治疗非典型、恶性和复发脑膜瘤的一个重要手段。放射外科也已成为小于 3cm 的小典型脑膜瘤的治疗选择之一。对 198 例手术切除或者放射外科作为初始治疗手段的脑膜瘤患者进行的回顾性队列分析表明，这两种治疗方式的效果相似。在多数报道中，放射外科的肿瘤控制率高于 90%，并发症发生率低于 5%。

有一小部分患者，尽管进行了多次手术切除及放疗，但脑膜瘤仍然复发。这部分患者可以考虑进一步治疗，但通常无效[48]。孕激素受体拮抗剂米非司酮开始有一定效果，但其后没有得到进一步的证实。到目前为止，没有发现治疗脑膜瘤有效的化疗方案。有些应用多柔比星、顺铂和伊立替康等化疗药物的尝试，但没有成功。一些小型试验发现复发脑膜瘤对羟基脲治疗有效，但是大多数患者不能从中获益。有报道称，舒尼替尼对复发脑膜瘤有效[49]。帕瑞肽对肿瘤表达生长抑素受体的患者可能有效[50]。贝伐珠单抗可以减轻水肿或治疗潜在的脑放射性坏死，但不能使任何级别的肿瘤缩小。

脑转移瘤

转移瘤是最常见的脑肿瘤，每年因出现症状而诊断颅内转移的患者约 70 000 名。大多数脑转移发生在癌症广泛转移的后期，但少数情况下，脑转移可能是患者确诊癌症的最初证据；或者，被认为是局灶癌症的患者，可能有神经影像检查发现的无症状脑转移灶。随着全身性治疗效果越来越好，在其他部位癌症控制良好的患者中，脑转移瘤逐渐成为唯一的复发原因[51,52]。

脑转移瘤最常见来源包括肺癌、乳腺癌和黑色素瘤（表 77-4）。然而，任何恶性肿瘤都可以转移入脑，且来自传统意义上不常见部位的肿瘤转移至脑的病例也越来越多，比如卵巢和前列腺[51,52]。即使脑转移瘤的免疫组化分析可帮助判断肿瘤原发部位，但是仍有 10% 的脑转移瘤患者在最初筛查时无法找到原发病灶。在一些罕见情况下，甚至尸检也无法确定原发灶。

表 77-4　729 例脑转移瘤患者的原发部位[53]

原发肿瘤	总计	单发	多发
肺癌	288(39)	137	151
非小细胞	178	89	89
小细胞	110	48	62
乳腺癌	121(17)	59	62
黑色素瘤	80(11)	39	41
泌尿生殖器癌	81(11)	49	32
肾细胞癌	45	25	20
膀胱癌	14	9	5
前列腺癌	11	9	2
睾丸癌	11	6	5
妇科肿瘤	52(7)	28	24
子宫癌	38	20	18
卵巢癌	14	8	6
消化系统肿瘤	45(6)	30	15
未知来源肿瘤	33(5)	23	10
其他肿瘤	29(4)	19	10
总计	729	384	345

转移的病理生理过程

为进入脑内，全身性肿瘤需要形成自有的供血系统，侵入局部组织，通过侵犯小静脉或淋巴管（淋巴管最终汇入静脉循环）进入循环系统（图 77-7）[52,54]。由于进入静脉循环的肿瘤细胞最终回流入右心，因此肿瘤在肺部遇到首个毛细血管床。因此，大多数脑转移瘤患者在脑部病变出现症状时，有原发性肺肿瘤或肺转移癌。肿瘤进入动脉循环的途径：①在肺内生长并向肺静脉播散[14]；②经肺毛细血管床进入左心；③直接经未闭的卵圆孔到达左心。对未发生肺转移的患者，有人认为肿瘤是经脊椎静脉系统（Batson 静脉丛）转移入脑。

脑转移好发有两个原因：①在静息状态下，脑组织接受 15%~20% 的体循环血流，增加了循环肿瘤细胞进入脑内的可能性；②脑组织是某些肿瘤细胞（如小细胞肺癌）种植、生长的良好场所。一旦进入颅腔，肿瘤细胞会被毛细血管床捕获，然后穿过内膜和血管壁，在脑组织内生长并通过血管增生为自身供血，最后生长到足够大而导致临床症状。肿瘤细胞在转移过程中的每一步都可能失败，因此只有很小一部分进入循环系统的肿瘤细胞形成转移灶。

肿瘤可以转移至颅内的任何部位，但脑转移瘤的大体分布取决于部位大小和血管分布。因此，85% 以上脑转移瘤发生于大脑半球，10%~15% 发生于小脑，只有约 3% 发生于脑干，与这些部位的血流分布吻合。

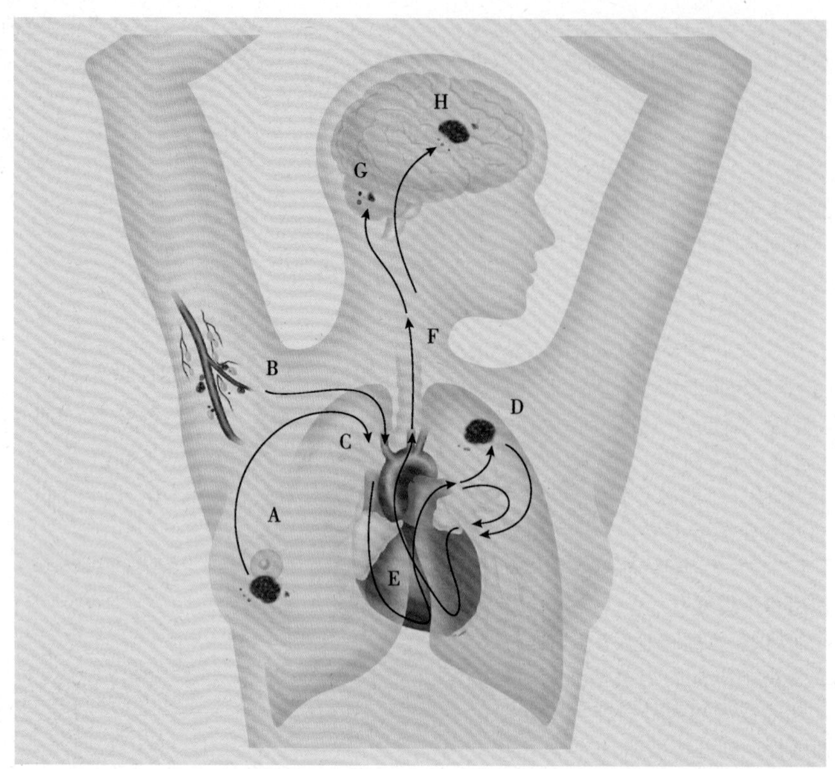

图 77-7 肿瘤转移的病理生理过程。转移是一个多步骤过程。如图所示：(A)恶性肿瘤在远离中枢神经系统的器官中形成，在其生长过程中、逐渐形成自有的供血系统。(B)具有转移潜能的恶性肿瘤细胞克隆侵入血管、淋巴管，最终进入静脉循环。(C)恶性肿瘤细胞经静脉循环进入右心，可经肺动脉进入肺(D)，或经未闭的卵圆孔(D)进入体循环。大多数进入肺部的肿瘤细胞，可被肺毛细血管床捕获，生长成为肺转移瘤，继而向肺静脉系统播散，或者两者交替进行。(E)经过肺血管床但未被捕获(E)，直接侵入肺静脉系统。肺静脉系统中的恶性肿瘤细胞克隆进入左心，与可能经未闭的卵圆孔进入左心的细胞一起(F)，进入体循环(F)。由于在静息状态下，心排血量的 15%~20% 供应中枢神经系统；因此，肿瘤细胞一旦进入体循环，进入脑循环系统的可能性就很大了。进入脑循环系统的肿瘤细胞必须被脑的毛细血管或小静脉捕获，穿过血管壁，然后在脑组织内生长(G、H)(图片来源：DeAngelis and Posner，2008[52]。经牛津大学出版社授权)

其他部位恶性肿瘤得到控制的患者，脑部往往是孤立的转移部位。血流和中枢神经系统(CNS)微环境都不能完全解释这一现象，但血脑屏障也许可以。无法穿透血脑屏障的水溶性药物能够有效控制乳腺癌、小细胞肺癌及其他癌症，不能控制脑转移瘤，CNS 是良好的“避难所”。当对化疗药物敏感的肿瘤在 CNS 复发时，并不意味着 CNS 的转移瘤对全身性肿瘤控制良好的化疗药物耐药，可能是血脑屏障使得药物无法达到控制肿瘤细胞的有效浓度，使得肿瘤细胞对药物的敏感性下降；或许可以通过改变药物剂量或用药方法来提高脑内药物浓度来证实这种理论。

治疗

治疗方案的制订应依据转移瘤的数量和部位、原发肿瘤的生物学特征以及全身性疾病的进展情况。

手术

两个对照临床试验明确指出，对于单发脑转移瘤，手术切除联合术后全脑放疗(WBRT)无论对预防复发还是改善生存质量都优于单纯 WBRT[55,56]。第三个临床试验并未提示两者的显著差异，但其中很多经随机分组单纯放疗的患者都因复发进行了手术切除[57]。全身性肿瘤无进展或控制良好的患者，经手术切除单发脑转移灶可显著提高生存率；2 年生存率为 15%~20%，因原发肿瘤而异；5 年生存率约 10%。回顾性分析结果支持对两个甚至三个脑转移瘤的切除，其结果与单发转移瘤手术治疗的结果类似。

一项随机对照临床试验显示，单发脑转移灶切除后接受 WBRT 的患者比仅手术的患者脑内复发率低，死于神经系统损害的可能性也减小[58]。然而，两组的总生存期大体相当，因为脑部肿瘤控制良好的患者往往死于全身性肿瘤的进展。以上结果表明，对适合手术切除的单发转移瘤患者，应手术切除转移瘤并进行术后 WBRT。鉴于 WBRT 的放射毒性，尤其是 60 岁以上人群，很多医生并不将其用于即刻的术后治疗，而是等到肿瘤复发时再进行，尽管 RT 对复发肿瘤的疗效可能不佳。

放疗

WBRT 是一种历史悠久的脑转移瘤治疗方法，通常 3 000cGy 的照射剂量分割为 10 次。对于有广泛的全身性肿瘤或多发脑转移患者，这一方案仍是最佳选择。大多数接受糖皮质激素治疗和 RT 的患者病情可以得到改善(图 77-8)，因神经系统病变而致死的可能性比未接受上述治疗的患者小。但由于多数患者死于控制不佳的全身性肿瘤，因此生存期仍较短，中位生存期为 4~6 个月。即使患者对 RT 有反应、脑转移瘤得到有效控制，仍有系统性肿瘤再次播散入脑的风险。个别患者，RT 确实能消灭脑转移瘤而未再复发。鉴于生存期大于 1

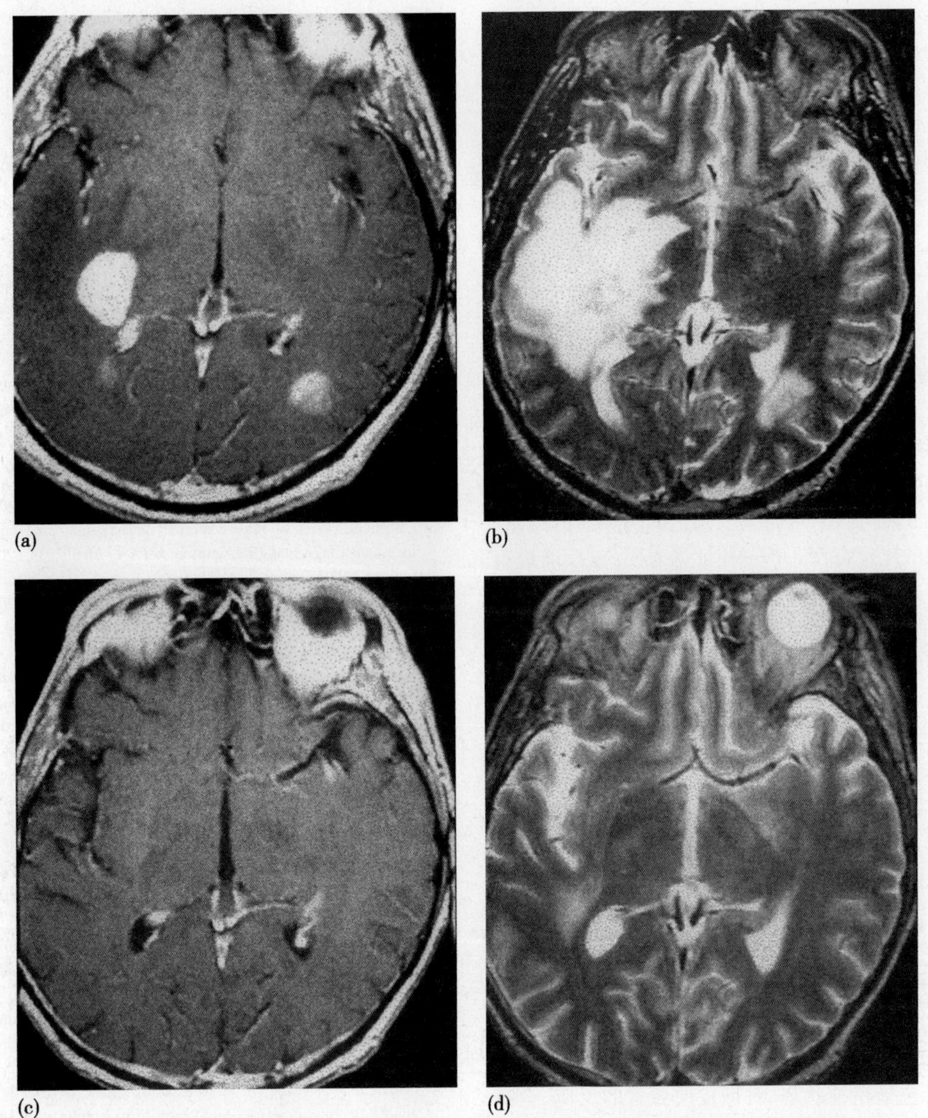

图 77-8　放疗前、后的肺小细胞癌脑转移瘤。(a)放疗前 T1 加权像显示了明显强化的多发转移瘤中的 2 个病灶；较大周边可见低信号脑水肿带。(b)放疗前 T2 加权像显示相对低信号的肿瘤周边的高信号水肿。(c、d)放疗后 MRI 显示放疗效果良好

年的患者的远期延迟放射毒性，我们推荐放疗剂量为 4 000～5 000cGy，分割剂量 180～200cGy。较小的分割剂量可以减少放射毒性的风险，但患者可能仍然会有认知功能障碍，特别高龄患者。RT 导致的认知功能障碍在 60 岁以上和接受大剂量化疗的人群中更为严重。但是，年轻人在接受 WBRT 后也常抱怨记忆力减退。

放射外科

放射外科(SRS)越来越多的用于替代手术治疗单发甚至多发的直径<3～4cm 的脑转移瘤[52,59～61]。SRS 可以通过伽玛刀、直线加速器或射波刀来完成，治疗效果类似；通常进行单次照射，也可以进行分割照射。这种方法对某些常规外照射 RT 抵抗的肿瘤特别有效，如黑色素瘤和肾细胞癌。多数报道认为约 80%的肿瘤可以得到控制，包括肿瘤消失、体积减小或经治疗的病变未进展。由于放射损伤或肿瘤坏死，放疗后 MRI 可能显示一过性的肿瘤体积增大，一般数月后可缓解。因此，SRS 后数周到数月内，肿瘤体积增大并不一定意味着肿瘤进展。60%的患者局部肿瘤控制可达 2 年，但随着生存期的延长，症状再发的可能性增加。SRS 较传统手术的优势在于相对无创、无须住院、可治疗手术无法达到的部位。SRS 的缺点是不适用于直径 3～4cm 以上的肿瘤，应避免用于广泛水肿控制不佳的肿瘤。

一项随机前瞻性临床试验对 331 名新诊断有 1～3 个脑转移瘤的患者进行 WBRT 和 WBRT+SRS，结果显示 WBRT 后增加 SRS 生存获益[62]。一项独立的随机对照临床试验对有 1～4 个脑转移瘤的患者进行 SRS 或 SRS＋WBRT 治疗；与术后 WBRT 的研究结果相似，WBRT 能有效地减少脑转移瘤复发，但对生存期无影响[63]。其次，研究者认为，采用 WBRT 来控制 CNS 肿瘤，患者的认知功能也因肿瘤控制而得到改善；而且他们确实观察到，WBRT 可改善一些长期生存患者的认知功能损害[64]。因此，术后或 SRS 后进行 WBRT 治疗需要根据个体情况决定。

目前还没有随机的前瞻性研究比较手术和 SRS 治疗孤立

性脑转移瘤。而一些回顾性研究的结果不一致，但多数认为两者可以达到相似的局部肿瘤控制效果。现在，对于手术可切除部位的>3~4cm、有严重的血管源性水肿或出血、原发肿瘤放疗不敏感或引起梗阻性脑积水的转移瘤，建议手术切除。对较小的或手术不可及部位的转移瘤，SRS 是最佳选择；对于有 3 处以上转移瘤的患者不建议进行 SRS，也不建议同时进行 WBRT。

化疗

化疗对药物敏感的全身性癌症来源的脑转移瘤的有效性越来越得到认可，其中包括生殖细胞肿瘤、乳腺癌、小细胞肺癌等[52,59,65,66]。化疗通常用于手术或 WBRT 后复发转移瘤患者的治疗；但对于经 MRI 发现的无症状脑转移瘤、计划接受全身性肿瘤化疗的患者，化疗也可考虑作为治疗选择。

RT 前进行化疗的原因包括：①有利于在放疗前判断肿瘤对化疗的反应。如果有效，可继续进行化疗。②放疗可减少肿瘤供血，但可能增加脑部血供，从而减少到达脑转移瘤的药量、而增加正常脑组织的化疗毒性。③一些证据表明，放疗前进行化疗比放疗后化疗减轻了药物的神经毒性；因为 RT 可以开放血脑屏障，使 RT 后给予的有潜在毒性的药物进入脑内。最好的证据就是甲氨蝶呤，但其他化疗药物也是如此。

除了标准的化疗药物，小分子抑制剂也能有效治疗脑转移瘤。例如，埃罗替尼对非小细胞肺癌、舒尼替尼对肾癌、舒尼替尼对黑色素瘤都有很好的疗效[67,68]。此外，将剂量方案更改为更利于药物进入 CNS 的每周大剂量方案，也能够提高 CNS 肿瘤的疗效。在一项Ⅱ期临床试验中，拉帕替尼治疗乳腺癌脑转移瘤的初步结果未能达到预期的治疗效果[69]。

预后

经 WBRT 治疗的患者中位生存期为 4~6 个月，经手术+WBRT 治疗的患者中位生存期约 9 个月。全身性肿瘤控制良好的转移瘤患者经手术和 RT 后，5 年生存率为 10%~15%。SRS 治疗后也可出现长期生存者[52]。

预后影响因素包括精神状态、对糖皮质激素的反应、全身肿瘤的情况和治疗方式。原发肿瘤的部位、年龄、脑转移瘤的数量也是预后影响因素，但影响程度较上述因素小。原发于肺癌患者，男性是预后不佳的重要因素。原发于乳腺癌的患者，原发肿瘤与脑转移瘤发生的间隔时间也有意义，间隔时间越长生存期越长。在 3 项放射治疗肿瘤协作组（RTOG）的临床试验中，采用递归分区分析了经 WBRT 治疗的 1 200 例脑转移瘤患者的预后因素[70]。将患者按照 KPS 评分、年龄和有无颅外转移分为三级：第一级患者 KPS≥70、年龄<65 岁、原发灶控制良好且没有颅外转移，中位生存期为 7.1 个月；第三级患者 KPS<70，中位生存期为 2.3 个月；第二级包括其余所有患者，中位生存期为 4.2 个月。这种分级方案可能同样适用于手术和 SRS 治疗的患者[71]。

（孟肖利 译 万经海 校）

参考文献

The complete reference list can be found on the Wiley Companion Digital Edition of this title (see inside front cover for login instructions).

1 Ostrom QT, Gittleman H, Farah P, et al. CBTRUS statistical report: primary brain and central nervous system tumors diagnosed in the United States 2006-2010. *Neuro Oncol*. 2013;**15**:ii1-ii56.

4 Coureau G, Bouvier G, Lebailly P, et al. Mobile phone use and brain tumours in the CERENAT case-control study. *Occup Environ Med*. 2014;**71**:514-522.

6 Ostrom QT, Bauchet L, Davis FG, et al. The epidemiology of glioma in adults: a "state of the science" review. *Neuro Oncol*. 2014;**16**:896-913.

7 Huse JT, Holland E, DeAngelis LM. Glioblastoma: molecular analysis and clinical implications. *Annu Rev Med*. 2013;**64**:59-70.

8 Cohen AL, Colman H. Glioma biology and molecular markers. *Cancer Treat Res*. 2015;**163**:15-30.

10 Omuro A, DeAngelis LM. Glioblastoma and other malignant gliomas: a clinical review. *JAMA*. 2013;**310**:1842-1850.

13 Chang SM, Parney IF, McDermott M, et al. Perioperative complications and neurological outcomes of first and second craniotomies among patients enrolled in the Glioma Outcome Project. *J Neurosurg*. 2003;**98**:1175-1181.

14 Merchant TE, Farr JB. Proton beam therapy: a fad or a new standard of care. *Curr Opin Pediatr*. 2014;**26**:3-8.

15 Stupp R, Hegi ME, Mason WP, et al. Effects of radiotherapy with concomitant and adjuvant temozolomide versus radiotherapy alone on survival in glioblastoma in a randomised phase III study: 5-year analysis of the EORTC-NCIC trial. *Lancet Oncol*. 2009;**10**:459-466.

18 Friedman HS, Prados MD, Wen PY, et al. Bevacizumab alone and in combination with irinotecan in recurrent glioblastoma. *J Clin Oncol*. 2009;**27**:4733-4740.

19 Chinot OL, Wick W, Mason W, et al. Bevacizumab plus radiotherapy-temozolomide for newly diagnosed glioblastoma. *N Engl J Med*. 2014;**370**:709-722.

20 Gilbert MR, Dignam JJ, Armstrong TS, et al. A randomized trial of bevacizumab for newly diagnosed glioblastoma. *N Engl J Med*. 2014;**370**:699-708.

21 Thomas AA, Brennan CW, DeAngelis LM, Omuro AM. Emerging therapies for glioblastoma. *JAMA Neurol*. 2014;**71**:1437-1444.

22 Reardon DA, Freeman G, Wu C, et al. Immunotherapy advances for glioblastoma. *Neuro Oncol*. 2014;**16**:1441-1458.

23 Wick W, Hartmann C, Engel C, et al. NOA-04 randomized phase III trial of sequential radiochemotherapy of anaplastic glioma with procarbazine, lomustine, and vincristine or temozolomide. *J Clin Oncol*. 2009;**27**:5874-5880.

25 van den Bent MJ, Afra D, de Witte O, et al. Long-term efficacy of early versus delayed radiotherapy for low-grade astrocytoma and oligodendroglioma in adults: the EORTC 22845 randomised trial. *Lancet*. 2005;**366**:985-990.

28 van den Bent MJ. Practice changing mature results of RTOG study 9802: another positive PCV trial makes adjuvant chemotherapy part of standard of care in low-grade glioma. *Neuro Oncol*. 2014;**16**:1570-1574.

31 Jenkins RB, Blair H, Ballman KV, et al. A t(1;19)(q10;p10) mediates the combined deletions of 1p and 19q and predicts a better prognosis of patients with oligodendroglioma. *Cancer Res*. 2006;**66**:9852-9861.

32 Lassman AB, Iwamoto FM, Cloughesy TF, et al. International retrospective study of over 1000 adults with anaplastic oligodendroglial tumors. *Neuro Oncol*. 2011;**13**:649-659.

33 Cairncross G, Wang M, Shaw E, et al. Phase III trial of chemoradiotherapy for anaplastic oligodendroglioma: long-term results of RTOG 9402. *J Clin Oncol*. 2013;**31**:337-343.

34 van den Bent MJ, Brandes AA, Taphoorn MJ, et al. Adjuvant procarbazine, lomustine, and vincristine chemotherapy in newly diagnosed anaplastic oligodendroglioma: long-term follow-up of EORTC brain tumor group study 26951. *J Clin Oncol*. 2013;**31**:344-350.

37 Parker M, Mohankumar KM, Punchihewa C, et al. C11orf95-RELA fusions drive oncogenic NF-κB signalling in ependymoma. *Nature*. 2014;**506**:451-455.

39 Green RM, Cloughesy TF, Stupp R, et al. Bevacizumab for recurrent ependymoma. *Neurology*. 2009;**73**:1677-1680.

40 Morris PG, Correa DD, Yahalom J, et al. Rituximab, methotrexate, procarbazine, and vincristine followed by consolidation reduced-dose whole-brain radiotherapy and cytarabine in newly diagnosed primary CNS lymphoma: final results and long-term outcome. *J Clin Oncol*. 2013;**31**:3971-3979.

41 Rubenstein JL, Hsi ED, Johnson JL, et al. Intensive chemotherapy and immunotherapy in patients with newly diagnosed primary CNS lymphoma: CALGB 50202 (Alliance 50202). *J Clin Oncol*. 2013;**31**:3061-3068.

42 Omuro A, Correa DD, DeAngelis LM, et al. R-MPV followed by high-dose chemotherapy with TBC and autologous stem-cell transplant for newly diagnosed primary CNS lymphoma. *Blood*. 2015;**125(9)**:1403-10.

43 Thiel E, Korfel A, Martus P, et al. High-dose methotrexate with or without whole brain radiotherapy for primary CNS lymphoma (G-PCNSL-SG-1): a phase 3, randomised, non-inferiority trial. *Lancet Oncol*. 2010;**11**:1036-1047.

44 Clark VE, Erson-Omay EZ, Serin A, et al. Genomic analysis of non-NF2 meningiomas reveals mutations in TRAF7, KLF4, AKT1, and SMO. *Science*. 2013;**339**:1077-1080.

48 Kaley T, Barani I, Chamberlain M, et al. Historical benchmarks for medical therapy trials in surgery- and radiation-refractory meningioma: a RANO review. *Neuro Oncol*. 2014;**16**:829-840.

51 Kastritis E, Efstathiou E, Gika D, et al. Brain metastases as isolated site of relapse

in patients with epithelial ovarian cancer previously treated with platinum and paclitaxel-based chemotherapy. *Int J Gynecol Cancer*. 2006;**16**:994–999.

52 DeAngelis LM, Posner JB. *Neurologic Complications of Cancer*, 2nd edition. New York: Oxford University Press; 2008.

53 Kleihues P, Cavenee WK (eds). *Pathology and genetics. Tumors of the nervous system. World Health Organization Classification of Tumors*. Lyon: International Agency for Research on Cancer (IARC) Press; 2000:6–7.

55 Patchell RA, Tibbs PA, Walsh JW, et al. A randomized trial of surgery in the treatment of single metastases to the brain. *N Engl J Med*. 1990;**322**:494–500.

56 Vecht CJ, Haaxma-Reiche H, Noordijk EM, et al. Treatment of single brain metastasis: radiotherapy alone or combined with neurosurgery? *Ann Neurol*. 1993;**33**:583–590.

58 Patchell RA, Tibbs PA, Regine WF, et al. Postoperative radiotherapy in the treatment of single metastases to the brain: a randomized trial. *JAMA*. 1998;**280**:1485–1489.

59 Bertolini F, Spallanzani A, Fontana A, Depenni R, Luppi G. Brain metastases: an overview. *CNS Oncol*. 2015;**4**:37–46.

62 Andrews DW, Scott CB, Sperduto PW, et al. Whole brain radiation therapy with or without stereotactic radiosurgery boost for patients with one to three brain metastases: phase III results of the RTOG 9508 randomised trial. *Lancet*. 2004;**363**:1665–1672.

63 Aoyama H, Shirato H, Tago M, et al. Stereotactic radiosurgery plus whole-brain radiation therapy vs stereotactic radiosurgery alone for treatment of brain metastases: a randomized controlled trial. *JAMA*. 2006;**295**:2483–2491.

65 Brastianos HC, Cahill DP, Brastianos PK. Systemic therapy of brain metastases. *Curr Neurol Neurosci Rep*. 2015;**15**:518.

68 Grommes C, Oxnard GR, Kris MG, et al. "Pulsatile" high-dose weekly erlotinib for CNS metastases from EGFR mutant non-small cell lung cancer. *Neuro Oncol*. 2011;**13**:1364–1369.

71 Regine WF, Rogozinska A, Kryscio RJ, et al. Recursive partitioning analysis classifications I and II: applicability evaluated in a randomized trial for resected single brain metastases. *Am J Clin Oncol*. 2004;**27**:505–509.

第 78 章　眼部肿瘤

Jasmine H. Francis, MD ■ Amy C. Schefler, MD, FACS ■ David H. Abramson, MD

概述

与肺癌、前列腺癌和乳腺癌相比，涉及眼睛的癌症较少见。然而因为它们可以影响患者的生活和视力，它们构成了一个特殊的挑战。眼科肿瘤学领域主要关注两个要素：一是提高治疗疾病和挽救生命的疗效，二是控制治疗的不良后果以维持视力。眼睛本身由各种不同的组织组成，并且眼科恶性肿瘤可以影响许多解剖区域。这使得眼部肿瘤的主题在起源、发病机制、预后和治疗方面是异质的。

前言

本章回顾了儿童及成人眼球、眼眶及眼睑的良恶性肿瘤，其中最常见的部分已在表 78-1 中列出。

表 78-1　最常见的良性和恶性眼部肿瘤

	良性	恶性	
		原发	继发
儿童			
眼内	—	视网膜母细胞瘤	白血病
眼眶	毛细血管瘤	横纹肌肉瘤	白血病
成人			
眼内	脉络膜痣	脉络膜黑色素瘤	转移癌（肺、乳腺）
眼眶	海绵状血管瘤	淋巴瘤	鼻窦恶性肿瘤
眼睑	睑板腺囊肿	基底细胞癌	淋巴瘤

儿童眼部肿瘤：眼内病变

良性疾病

儿童良性眼内疾病非常少见。在成人发病率超过 10% 的脉络膜痣，在青春期前极少发病，而在婴幼儿则几乎从不出现。结膜及虹膜痣在青春期前的儿童也异常罕见。儿童中发现的虹膜痣经常代表了 Lisch 结节，为 I 型神经纤维瘤病的主要表现。

良性视网膜肿瘤也很少见，发现的多为星形错构瘤或结节性硬化综合征的表现形式。在间接检眼镜下，星形错构瘤多有薄而透明的薄膜覆盖视网膜表面，以及典型的模糊不清的视网膜血管。随时间延长可伴有肿瘤增大及钙化，并可能与有髓神经纤维相混淆。后者为白色，随神经纤维层走行分布，且有模糊的视网膜血管。

RPE 层的错构瘤在儿童罕见，多靠近视盘，有色素分布，伴视网膜血管变形及轻度不透明的外观，不具有恶性倾向。

原发恶性肿瘤（视网膜母细胞瘤）

视网膜母细胞瘤简介

视网膜母细胞瘤为儿童最常见的原发眼内恶性肿瘤，起源于未分化的视网膜祖细胞[1]。尽管视网膜母细胞瘤相对罕见，然而因其研究较为详尽的遗传性及分子生物学特征，仍然成为关注的热点[2]。

世界范围内，视网膜母细胞瘤的年龄累计发病率为 1∶18 000～1∶30 000 活产婴儿[3]。流行病学调查显示了 20 世纪内其发病率相对稳定。在美国的发病率相对较低，15 岁以下儿童每百万人口有 3.58 例病例，且发病率随年龄增长而下降。在美国，视网膜母细胞瘤诊断的中位年龄为 18 个月，双眼视网膜母细胞瘤病例为 12 个月，而单眼视网膜母细胞瘤病例为 24 个月。在极少数情况下，视网膜母细胞瘤可在胎儿期经 B 超发现或在成年期发现。

在 20 世纪，发达国家的视网膜母细胞患儿生存率得到了极大提高。1897 年，报道经眼球摘除治疗的视网膜母细胞瘤患儿的死亡率为 83%，在 1916 年，这一数字在所有患儿中为 43%。相比之下，最近在欧洲及美国的癌症登记报告显示患儿的 5 年生存率分别为 90% 及 98%。肿瘤的早期发现及局部肿瘤控制手段的日益提高使得生存率得以显著提升。然而，相比较发达国家，发展中国家则报道了相当低的生存率，在这些国家中，患儿的典型表现为肿瘤的广泛转移。全世界大约 50% 的患者仍死于转移性视网膜母细胞瘤。

关于性别、种族及眼别的发病率并没有差别，有些数据显示了地区性聚集，但尚缺乏足够的证据支持，但全球范围内，视网膜母细胞瘤确实高发于贫困的患儿。

视网膜母细胞瘤的分子生物学

至今仍被普遍接受的传统视网膜母细胞瘤遗传学观点认为，该疾病以 2 种形式发生：生殖型和非生殖型。两种类型肿瘤的发生均由双等位视网膜母细胞瘤基因（*rb1*）的缺失或突变造成。在非生殖型病例中，*rb1* 双等位基因均在同一发育中的视网膜前体细胞中失活。而在生殖型病例中，第一次突变发生于生殖细胞中，仅第二次突变在体细胞中发生。非生殖型视网膜母细胞瘤多为单侧、单发病灶，尽管有时肿瘤可分散为数百个眼内子瘤。在过去的十年中，更多近期报道证明几乎所有视网膜母细胞瘤患者均显示了不同程度 *rb1* 基因突变的嵌合状态。而且近来的证据表示：基因不稳定性、微卫星不稳定性、DNA 错配修复系统缺陷及 DNA 甲基化、乙酰化、去乙酰化的改变可能均对 pRB 缺失后视网膜母细胞瘤的恶性转化起到了重要作用[4]。

经缺失及连锁分析研究推定，*rb1* 基因位于染色体 13q14。核磷酸蛋白（pRB）是细胞在 G1 期进入 S 期的细胞周期检查点的调节因子（图 78-1）。如同在肿瘤中发生的状况，失去正常 *rb1* 的功能，细胞将不受限的进入 S 期及更快地完成细胞分裂。最近，发现 *rb1* 野生型肿瘤可能在 MYCN 癌基因扩增的背景下发生[5]。

rb1 是首个被发现的抑癌基因，其肿瘤抑制作用通过在肿瘤组织标本中双等位基因缺失的相关研究得以证实。后续的研究显示生殖型 *rb1* 突变几乎在所有视网膜母细胞瘤家族中均有存在，遗传突变的 *rb1* 等位基因将具有疾病易感性[6]。该基因的肿瘤抑制作用在转染试验中得以进一步证实，该试验显示将野生型 pRB 的表达引入 pRB 表达缺失的细胞系，可以部分逆转其恶性表型。

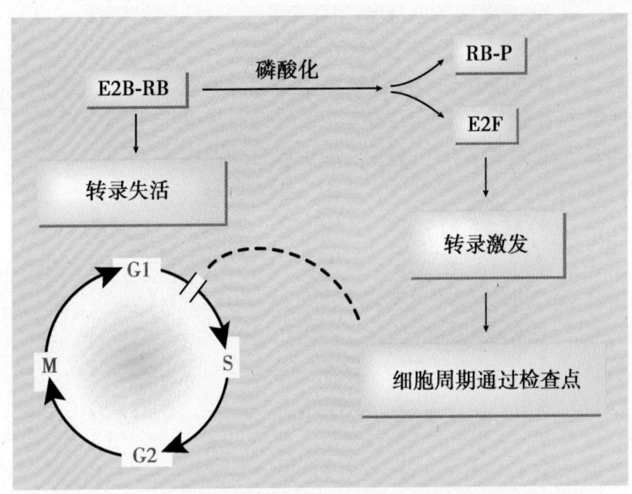

图 78-1　视网膜母细胞瘤基因功能的分子机制示意图

基因检测

家庭收集的人口数据及我们当前对于视网膜母细胞瘤遗传方式的分子机制的了解，使得我们能够预测家庭中新出生后代受影响并发展为视网膜母细胞瘤的可能性（表 78-2）。核型分析可以分析全部染色体的形态，但对于视网膜母细胞瘤的临床诊断一般没有作用。因其只能辨别超过 200 万～500 万碱基的缺失，而视网膜母细胞瘤患者中只有 3%～5% 携带如此大的缺失[7]。反之，更为复杂的直接或间接检测方法可检测更小的突变，正在得到应用。当前，因为突变的发生形式及位置多种多样，单独的基因检测无法检测所有视网膜母细胞瘤患者的生殖型 *rb1* 基因突变。但是，采用常规的临床试验规程，包括一系列基于观察到的大多数突变会导致蛋白大小改变及干扰口袋结构域的补充检测，可以快速发现大多数突变[8]。

表 78-2　视网膜母细胞瘤遗传咨询

如果父母是：	双侧患病				单侧患病				未患病			
后代患视网膜母细胞的概率	45% 患病			55% 未患病	7%~15% 患病			85%~93% 未患病	< 1% 患病			99% 未患病
单侧或双侧	85% 双侧	15% 单侧		0%	85% 双侧	15% 单侧		0%	33% 双侧	67% 单侧		0%
病灶数	100% 多病灶	96% 多病灶	4% 单病灶	0%	100% 多病灶	96% 多病灶	4% 单病灶	0%	100% 多病灶	15% 多病灶	85% 单病灶	0%
下一个兄弟姐妹患视网膜母细胞的概率	45%	45%	45%	45%	45%	45%	45%	7%~15%[a]	约6%[a]	约6%[a]	约6%[a]	< 1%

[a]如果父母是携带者，下一个兄弟姐妹患视神经母细胞瘤的概率是45%。

视网膜母细胞瘤的主要症状和体征

视网膜母细胞瘤最常见的症状和体征依据患儿所处的社会经济条件不同而各异。在发展中国家，儿童在诊断前常已出现眼外表现，多表现为眼球突出和眼眶肿物（图 78-2）。这些患儿的诊断年龄较美国患儿大（4～6 岁），并且只有少数存活。过去 25 年间的多项大型回顾性研究显示了在较大的发达国家视网膜母细胞瘤最常见的表现[8]。在美国，最常见的表现（60% 的病例）为白瞳症-白色瞳孔反光（图 78-3）。这种反射或由入射光在肿瘤表面形成或由视网膜下方的肿瘤造成的视网膜脱离导致。

在美国较为少见的表现包括斜视（眼位失调）、眼内炎症（伪装为眶内蜂窝织炎）、瞳孔不等（双侧瞳孔不等大）、虹膜异色症（双侧虹膜颜色不同）、前房积血（出血位于前房）、肿瘤发育不全（前房肿瘤）及眼球震颤。近来两个基于大量视网膜母细胞瘤患者的大型回顾性研究显示了视网膜母细胞瘤在美国的发现方式，绝大多数患儿的肿瘤由家庭成员（80%）而非儿科

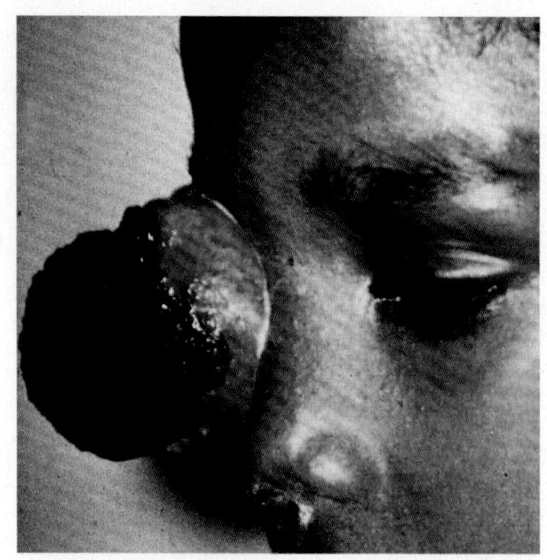

图 78-2 晚期视网膜母细胞瘤眼眶表现

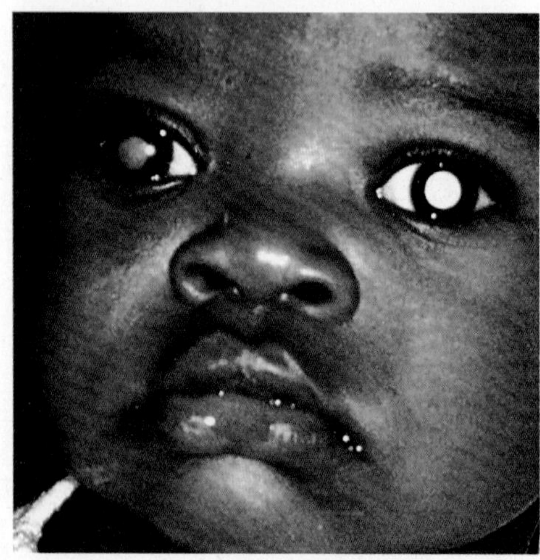

图 78-3 视网膜母细胞瘤导致的白瞳症(白色瞳孔反射)。玻璃体内可见肿瘤,虹膜前可见位于前房的子瘤

医师(8%)或眼科医师(10%)发现[8]。

诊断检查

视网膜母细胞瘤的鉴别诊断包括可模仿单个眼内肿瘤的肿物,包括星形错构瘤、弓形虫感染及能导致全视网膜脱离的疾病,如 Coat 病,早产儿视网膜病变及永存原始玻璃体增殖症(表 78-3)。疑似患有视网膜母细胞瘤的患儿应行间接检眼镜的检查、眼底照相及眼科 B 超检查。超声波检查可帮助显示具有高反射,可阻断声波导致典型肿瘤后声影的肿物。针刺活检在疑似视网膜母细胞瘤的患者中很少实施,眼内穿刺可导致肿瘤播散,眼眶转移,甚至导致因转移造成的死亡。

眼内视网膜母细胞瘤的分期

Reese-Ellsworth 分期方案是描述眼内肿瘤最常用的金标准(表 78-4a)[9],其并非一个真正的分期方案,因未治疗的患儿不会由组 I 进展到更高的分组,但其确实为比较不同的系列及治疗方案提供了一个出色的眼内依据。更高的分期提示肿瘤更为靠近前部,使用横向外放射线照射治疗肿瘤的成功率更低。近年来,这一分期系统的有用性遭到了许多眼科肿瘤学家的质疑,他们认为鉴于当今较少应用外放射治疗的趋势,该分期已不再适宜。近来,一个新的分期系统已经建立并且在数个合作研究中心得以临床应用(表 78-4b)[10]。经显示:该系统与当今最常用的眼内疾病治疗手段(化疗结合局部治疗)的疗效相一致。和 Reese-Ellsworth 分期系统一样,这一分期系统在将来随着治疗趋势不可避免的更改而逐渐变得过时。

表 78-3 与视网膜母细胞瘤相似的疾病

单个眼内肿瘤
星形错构瘤
弓形虫感染
全视网膜脱离
Coats 病
早产儿视网膜病变
永存原始玻璃体增殖症(PFV)

表 78-4 (a)眼内视网膜母细胞瘤的 Reese-Ellsworth 方案,(b)视网膜母细胞瘤新的国际分期

(a)	眼内视网膜母细胞瘤的 Reese-Ellsworth 方案
组 I	• 单个肿瘤,小于 4 个视盘直径,位于赤道部或赤道部后
	• 多个肿瘤,每个肿瘤大小均小于 4 个视盘直径,全部位于赤道部或赤道部后
组 II	• 单个肿瘤,4~10 个视盘直径大小,位于赤道部或赤道部后
	• 多个肿瘤,4~10 个视盘直径大小,位于赤道部后
组 III	• 任何肿瘤位于赤道部前
	• 单个肿瘤,大于 10 个视盘直径,位于赤道部后
组 IV	• 多个肿瘤,部分大于 10 个视盘直径
	• 任何肿瘤侵犯至齿状线前
组 V	• 大范围肿瘤累及一半以上视网膜
	• 玻璃体肿瘤
(b)	视网膜母细胞瘤新的国际分期
组 A	肿瘤基底径或厚度≤3mm
组 B	肿瘤>3mm 或有一项或多项以下表现:
	• 位于黄斑区(距离中心凹≤3mm)
	• 位于视盘旁(距离视神经≤1.5mm)
	• 视网膜下液(距离边缘≤3mm)
组 C	具有一项或多项以下表现的视网膜母细胞瘤:
	• 视网膜下种植≤3mm
	• 玻璃体种植≤3mm

续表

	• 视网膜下及玻璃体种植，均≤3mm
组 D	具有一项或多项以下表现的视网膜母细胞瘤：
	• 视网膜下种植≥3mm
	• 玻璃体种植≥3mm
	• 视网膜下及玻璃体种植，均≥3mm
组 E	广泛的视网膜母细胞瘤占据眼球的50%以上，或具有以下任何表现：
	• 新生血管性青光眼
	• 位于前房、玻璃体或视网膜下的来自玻璃体积血的不透明基质
	• 筛板后视神经、脉络膜（>2mm）、巩膜、眼眶或前房受累

眼内视网膜母细胞瘤的治疗

目前在发达国家，通过眼球摘除术、外放射治疗、敷贴治疗、经瞳孔温热治疗（TTT）、冷冻疗法和化学疗法（全身性，动脉内，眼周和玻璃体内）等综合治疗，患儿的生存率已超过95%。对于每个患儿治疗策略的选择取决于几个因素：双眼还是单眼患病，遗传性，年龄，肿瘤的体积和位置，疾病分期（包括Reese-Ellsworth 分期），是否伴眼球外病变[1]。

眼球摘除术

眼球摘除术是通过外科的手段摘除眼球，但不包括眼睑和眼外肌[1]。对于单眼或双眼进展期的视网膜母细胞瘤，丧失视力并伴有活肿瘤的患眼，青光眼伴疼痛。

外放射治疗

外放射治疗曾经被用于很多眼内视网膜母细胞瘤的治疗，但近些年由于它与生殖细胞突变的视网膜母细胞瘤发生眼外第二肿瘤有关而逐渐应用减少[1]。放射治疗通常被作为其他治疗失败后的最后补救治疗。

经瞳孔温热疗法（TTT）

TTT 是视网膜母细胞瘤的一种治疗方法，可通过对红外二极管激光器的硬件和软件进行改良来提供[1]。TTT 用于治疗选择性的小视网膜母细胞瘤，尤其是当肿瘤位于眼球后方。另一项研究是针对研究 TTT 作为单独的治疗方法治疗小的肿瘤，发现92%的基底≤1.5 视盘直径的小肿瘤由 TTT 单独成功治愈。

冷冻疗法

冷冻疗法是周边小肿瘤的主要治疗方法，或作为其他方式治疗后复发的肿瘤的次要治疗方法[1]。快速冷冻（-90℃）导致眼内冰晶形成，蛋白变性，pH 值改变，最终细胞膜破裂。所有的仅运用冷冻治疗的研究证实了对于直径小于 3mm，厚度小于 1mm 的肿瘤可以达到 90%~100%的治愈率，并发症很少。

敷贴治疗

巩膜外敷贴治疗于 1993 年由英国眼科医师 Henry Stallard 首先提出。在过去的几年中，为了避免外放射治疗，放射敷贴器被更多地作为主要治疗。放射敷贴器治疗的相对适应证包括：R-S5a 或更早，肿瘤大小在 4~10 个视盘直径内。敷贴治疗也可以作为其他治疗（包括动脉内化疗，外照射，光凝或冷冻疗法）失败后的补救措施。^{125}I 是目前视网膜母细胞瘤敷贴治疗中最常用的放射性核素，它的优势在于放射粒子可以放置于定做的适合病变大小的敷贴器中。

全身化疗

化疗被用于收缩这些肿瘤，然后局部治疗（敷贴治疗、经瞳孔温热治疗（TTT）、冷冻疗法等）可以继续控制[1]。自从 1996 年以来，大多数视网膜母细胞瘤化学减容治疗的研究运用长春新碱、卡铂、一种表鬼臼毒素（依托泊苷或替尼泊苷）。也有建议加入环孢素作为 P-糖蛋白抑制剂来降低肿瘤细胞对抗肿瘤药物的转运能力，对抗耐药[11]。药物的选择和治疗周期在不同的医疗机构不尽相同。

最新的研究表明对于 R-S 1~3 期的患眼化疗结合局部治疗是最有希望的。对于这些患者，有些作者已证实眼摘可100%成功避免。但 R-S 4~5 期患者的疗效就差得多。在一个荟萃分析中，化疗使得 37%的患眼避免了外放射治疗和眼球摘除。41%的患眼需要放疗但避免了眼球摘除，40%的患眼需要眼球摘除（先前用或未用放射治疗）[12]。由于担心短期和长期的毒性，许多中心已放弃全身化疗作为主要治疗手段治疗视网膜母细胞瘤，而更多地采用局部化疗技术。

经眼动脉化疗

日本医师最先提出另一种局部给药方法，经眼动脉注射化疗药，这种方法可以提高药物对于较小的眼内肿瘤的通透性，并降低全身副作用[13]。我们小组引入了一种技术，其中对眼动脉进行选择性插管，并在入口处注射多达三种药物（美法仑、托泊替康和卡铂）的组合[1]。其他进入眼动脉的技术还包括对脑膜中动脉进行导管插入术或使用球囊。治疗通常包括每月平均输注 3 次。该技术已被全球许多中心采用，它是我们治疗单侧和双侧视网膜母细胞瘤的主要方法。它可以用于治疗各种类型的肿瘤，无论是初治的还是先前治疗过的，双侧病例都可以在同一疗程中接受串联治疗。在 3 个月以下或 6kg 以下的儿童中，采用过桥疗法：给予单药卡铂，直到儿童达到适当年龄和体重以进行动脉化疗。两年的 Kaplan-Meier 估计，初治眼的无事件存活率分别为 82%和先前治疗的眼为 60%[14]，尽管最近采用玻璃体内化疗的情况下，这些数字可能更高（图 78-4）。

眼部副作用很小，可能包括眼周炎，前额内侧红斑和脉络膜视网膜改变[14]。视网膜电图对视网膜功能的监测表明卡铂和托泊替康对视网膜功能没有影响。尽管美法仑可能会产生影响，但这些变化微乎其微，可能与临床无关。大约 30%的儿童在治疗过程中（尤其当美法仑剂量超过 0.4mg/kg 时）至少发生 1 次 3 或 4 级血液毒性，因此建议监测血细胞计数。血管并发症是一种罕见的并发症，没有据报道该手术导致死亡。

眼周化疗

卡铂或托泊替康的眼周注射已被使用，特别是作为挽救或辅助治疗。但是，副作用，尤其是卡铂的副作用，包括瘢痕形成和视力丧失。此外，人们对这种方法的长期疗效存在质疑。

玻璃体内化疗

由于担心肿瘤通过针道眼外扩展，已经避免了通过眼壁进行玻璃体的注射。但是，采用安全性增强的技术以及计算得出的眼外扩散风险极低可以减轻了这些担忧。玻璃体内化学疗

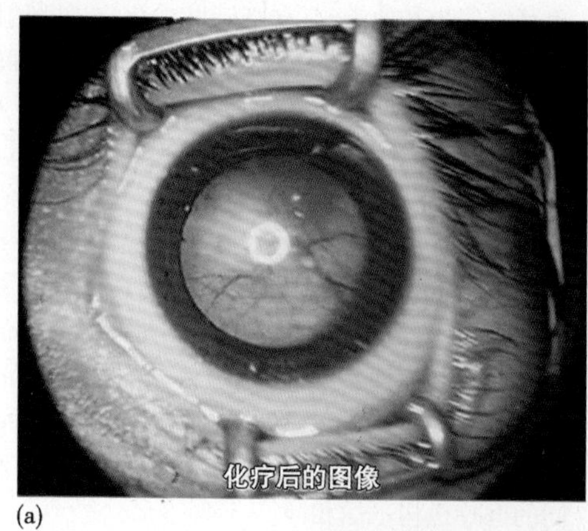

(a)

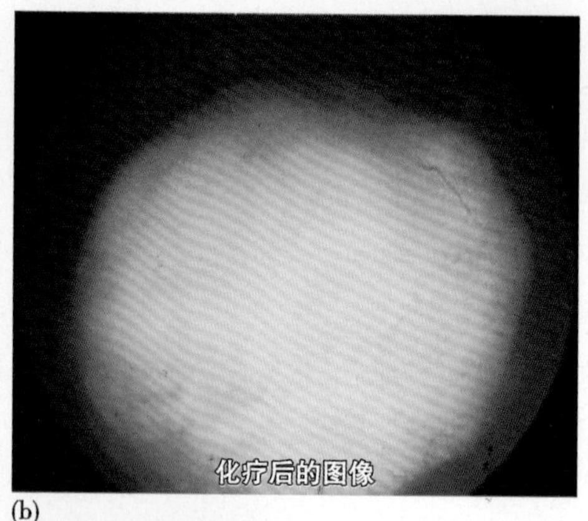

(b)

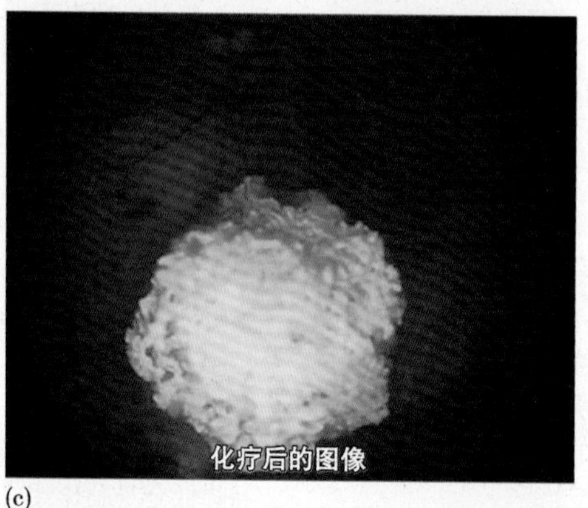

(c)

图 78-4 (a)典型病例进行经眼动脉化疗的例子。眼球布满了视网膜母细胞瘤,晶体后可以看到视网膜完全脱落;(b)经眼动脉化疗前的眼底图片。肿瘤使得视神经乳头模糊不清;(c)经眼动脉化疗后的眼底图片。肿瘤钙化,没有见到玻璃体种植。肿瘤上方可以清楚地看到视神经乳头,视网膜平坦

法注射主要是采用美法仑,但也包括卡铂和托泊替康,每周最多给药 8 次。这种方式正迅速成为治疗玻璃体内肿瘤的最佳方法,据报道其眼存活率高达 83%~100%。然而,视网膜电图记录显示,每注射 30μg 的美法仑,视网膜功能会下降 5%,将来的工作可能会减轻这种毒性,无论是使用其他药物还是改变给药方法[15]。

眼外视网膜母细胞瘤的治疗

在最发达的美国,眼外疾病仅在少数患者中发生。有关眼外视网膜母细胞瘤治疗的更完整信息,鼓励读者咨询更广泛的资源[16,17]。

第二肿瘤

1949 年,首次发现某些视网膜母细胞瘤的患者在成功治愈眼部肿瘤后多年发生了眼外第二肿瘤。自那之后就有研究广泛地回顾了 *rb1* 基因突变的视网膜母细胞瘤患者中眼外第二肿瘤的发生率[18]。已有研究显示在美国眼外第二恶性肿瘤是生殖细胞突变的视网膜母细胞瘤生存者的主要死因。关于生殖细胞突变的视网膜母细胞瘤生存者第二肿瘤的累积发生率的报道各家不尽相同,但多数长期随访的大型研究已报告发生率是每年 0.5%~1%[18,19]。

有一些临床危险因素和治疗相关的暴露与视网膜母细胞瘤生存者的眼外第二肿瘤发生有关(表 78-5)。外放射治疗以剂量依赖的方式增加第二肿瘤发生的风险。继发性急性粒细胞性白血病(AML)与依托泊苷(表鬼臼毒素)在视网膜母细胞瘤的全身化疗方案中的使用有关。

表 78-5 与视网膜母细胞瘤生存者的眼外第二肿瘤发生相关的危险因素

因素	与第二肿瘤发病率的相关度
rbl 基因存在生殖细胞突变	明确相关(必需的危险因子)
外放射治疗剂量	剂量相关(因果性)
不足 1 岁时接受外放射治疗	很可能相关
脂肪瘤	明确相关(非因果性)
吸烟	明确相关
化疗	可能相关
日晒	可能相关
生长激素	可能相关

按照常见度排序,在美国视网膜母细胞瘤生存者第二肿瘤包括:颅骨和长骨骨肉瘤、软组织肉瘤、成松果体细胞瘤、皮肤黑色素瘤、脑瘤、霍奇金病、肺癌、乳腺癌、涎腺癌和口腔癌。这

反映了一组曾接受大剂量外放射治疗的患儿。在英国，一项研究对于未接受外放射治疗的患者发生的恶性肿瘤提出了独特的观点[20]：研究中的患者在随访时年龄都已超过 25 岁，与在美国接受放射线治疗的患者相比，罹患上皮癌（尤其是肺癌，膀胱癌和乳腺癌）的风险要高于发展为肉瘤和其他早期癌症的风险。

继发性恶性病变（白血病）

儿童急性淋巴细胞白血病（ALL）是儿童眼部最常见的恶性肿瘤。白血病主要累及葡萄膜：虹膜、睫状体、脉络膜，也可以累及视网膜、视神经、眼眶。

白血病的虹膜浸润可以表现为虹膜表明漂浮的奶油样细胞团。当虹膜浸润出现时，它们可以表现为异色性、前房细胞、前房积血。前房积血可以伴随着青光眼和眼睛的疼痛与光敏感性。相对于虹膜受累，白血病的浸润很少发生于睫状体和脉络膜，因为 ALL 弥散地侵犯脉络膜血管。这种轻微的增厚一般通过 B 超能够发现[21]。白血病患者死后尸检可以发现 90% 的有脉络膜白血病浸润。视网膜浸润很罕见。

眼部白血病浸润可以发生在疾病的不同时期。通常，浸润出现在疾病的初始阶段。大多数 ALL 患者表现为 B 超发现眼内异常。当白血病被治愈时，脉络膜受侵通常很快消失。在诱导性治疗和中枢神经系统预防性放疗后，眼部白血病浸润也可以表现为复发的孤立病灶。在这些患儿中，CNS 通常接受了放射治疗，但眼睛则没有接受治疗因此充当肿瘤细胞的避难所。在这种情况下，单独治疗眼睛可能是合理的。最终，白血病浸润可以表现为 CNS 病变复发的信号，无论伴与不伴 CNS 肿物。这些患者经常在玻璃体后极部有白血病细胞。在这些病例中，肿瘤细胞通过视神经进入眼内，视神经内的肿瘤细胞是直接从 CNS 来的。在这些病例中，通常会考虑用化疗或外放疗治疗脑部病变。

儿童眼部肿瘤：眼眶病变

良性病变

毛细血管瘤

儿童眼眶良性肿瘤经常因双眼睑或者眼眶不对称行 CT 检查时被发现，大部分不需要治疗。毛细血管瘤是儿童时期最常见的眼眶良性肿瘤[22]。CT 表现与横纹肌肉瘤不同的是，毛细血管瘤经常伴有先天性眼眶扩张。

毛细血管瘤的治疗很困难，肿瘤对于低剂量的放射治疗有效，并且我们已经利用分次的剂量直至 800cGy 取得了治疗上的成功。同时还有报道利用重组干扰素进行治疗[23]。由于对视力要求以及极大地美容需求时，局部注射短效和长效的类固醇也是治疗选择之一。当皮肤出现毛细血管瘤时，也可以局部使用 β-受体阻滞剂。

皮样囊肿

皮样囊肿是良性的并且起源于先天性的外胚层发育不良。治疗方案是手术，但是需要引起特别注意的是，部分肿瘤可以分叶并往眼眶后部生长，甚至可以到达颅内。

淋巴管瘤

尽管眼内没有淋巴管，良性的淋巴管瘤依然存在[24]。通常认为这些肿瘤是先天性的，并且没有恶变倾向，与毛细血管瘤不同的是，肿瘤并不在出生时表现出来，它们通常在 6 岁的时候有所表现，同时伴有肿瘤出血至囊样组织（巧克力样囊肿）所导致的眼球突出。治疗起来很困难，类固醇类或者放射治疗无效，手术中激光电凝可作为治疗的选择。术后良好的美容效果很难达到。

恶性病变

横纹肌肉瘤

儿童眼眶最常见的恶性肿瘤是横纹肌肉瘤，平均诊断年龄为 6~10 岁，男女发病率相同，也无左右眼差别。尽管横纹肌肉瘤表现为病情发展迅速，进展快，无痛性眼球突出，患者也可以表现为不明显的病程，伴有进展缓慢的眼球突出，或者伴有上睑下垂、斜视或结膜下肉质肿物。在 20 岁之前如果有进展迅速的眼球突出，应该考虑横纹肌肉瘤的诊断。肿瘤在眼眶的常见位置是在鼻上。CT 及 MRI 扫描有助于确定肿瘤的范围。

及时对肿瘤组织进行活检是必需的，但要保证活检操作不要经由鼻窦及颅内组织，因为这样有可能在活检通路上造成肿瘤的播散转移。横纹肌肉瘤最常见组织学类型是胚胎型。当肿瘤生长于眼眶下方时，多为腺泡型。肿瘤并不是起源于眼外肌而是起源于眼眶软组织的未分化的多能造血干细胞间质。

外线束辐射最早运用于 20 世纪 60 年代中期，随后与化疗相结合，产生了极好的局部治疗效果，大于 90% 的长期生存率。20 世纪 80 年代多个组间的横纹肌肉瘤研究证明，针对局限位于眼眶的肿瘤最有效的联合治疗是长春新碱、放线菌素 D 以及放射治疗。放射线对于眼睛的作用并没有被隔离，长时间的随访证明平均 7 年之后，只有 14% 的眼球被摘除，但是其中 70% 的视力受到损害[25]。最近由四个国际合作组织完成的一次荟萃分析结果表明，单独运用化疗的患者与结合放射治疗的患者相比生存率没有显著差异[26]。

成人眼部肿瘤：眼内病变

良性病变

眼睑、结膜、虹膜以及脉络膜的良性肿瘤较常见，而视网膜及角膜的少见。晶状体及玻璃体不产生肿瘤。成人最常见的最重要的良性肿瘤是脉络膜痣。

脉络膜色素痣

脉络膜痣出生时无表现，常在青春期表现出来。在美国，10%~13% 的成人有脉络膜痣，具有种族相关性，在黑人中少见。

脉络膜痣表面扁平，是色素沉着性良性病变，边缘可以为羽毛状的和不规则的，或者圆形的（图 78-5），常为灰色或者浅巧克力色。数月或者数年后，运用检眼镜检查可见伴有的改变。其眼底表面被证实的改变包括玻璃疣，或者伴有视网膜下积液或者新生血管膜，这些易导致视野缺损。10% 的成人患者有脉络膜痣并且在美国每年仅有 1 500 例脉络膜黑色素瘤，由此可以推测由脉络膜痣发展到脉络膜黑色素瘤的概率小于 1/

6 000。如今很多的研究已经证实哪些色素痣较有可能转变为恶性，相关预测因素详见表 78-6。

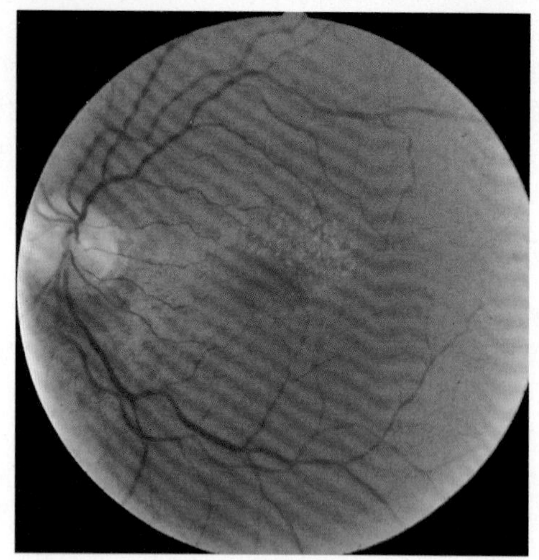

图 78-5 位于黄斑下面的脉络膜痣。黄色玻璃疣提示良性

表 78-6 色素痣转变为黑色素瘤的预测因素

• 体积：脉络膜痣越厚，发展成黑色素瘤的可能就越大。2. 5mm 厚的脉络膜痣，每个月约有 1%变为黑色素瘤
• 部位：眼后部的色素痣比前部的更容易变为黑色素瘤
• 橘色斑点：脉络膜痣表面出现橘色斑点，提示发展为黑色素瘤的概率大大增加
• 浆膜液：浆膜液叠加在视网膜但与其分离开，这种类型的色素痣更可能发展成黑色素瘤
• 玻璃疣缺失：玻璃疣是提示慢性和良性的有力指标，伴有玻璃疣的损害几乎不会转化
• 荧光血管造影出现热斑点
• 症状（视力下降，视野缺损）

虹膜痣及黑色素瘤

虹膜色素痣是虹膜良性病变，裂隙灯下表现是一扁平的色素沉着区域。虹膜色素痣很常见，多发，并且常见于蓝色眼睛的患者。与脉络膜痣相似，虹膜色素痣出生时无表现，常在青春期表现出来，其不表现为隆起型，并且不发展，不会出现其上的色素细胞脱落至前房，堵塞小梁网，导致严重的继发性青光眼，从而致盲。上述病变一般提示为虹膜黑色素瘤，但是广泛的转移几乎没有，即使有也不多见。许多临床医师提出虹膜黑色素瘤比脉络膜黑色素瘤侵袭力低的原因只是单纯因为其病变范围要小。但是，最近的研究表明，它们明显区分于脉络膜病变的一点在于 BRAF 基因的外显子 15 的活化变异具有显著差异，而这在皮肤黑色素瘤中很常见，但是在脉络膜病变中几乎看不到。虹膜色素瘤的治疗措施要根据青光眼是否存在，并且不应该以避免转移的需求为指导。起源于睫状体后来又发展至虹膜的色素瘤，被证明侵袭能力强并且容易转移。

恶性病变

脉络膜黑色素瘤介绍

脉络膜黑色素瘤是美国成人最常见（全球成人第二常见，仅次于视网膜母细胞瘤）的眼内恶性肿瘤，在美国每年有 1 500 个新发病例，平均诊断年龄在 55~65 岁，男女发病率相似，无眼别差别。在美国，99%的脉络膜黑色素瘤发生于高加索人。最常见发现肿瘤的方式为例行体检（41%）。男性更容易表现出症状，并且当有症状出现时，右眼常发现有肿瘤。最常见的症状是视力下降及随之而来的周边视野缺损。病变区无疼痛，不同于眼部转移性肿瘤，其疼痛并不罕见。

脉络膜黑色素瘤起源于脉络膜中的黑色素细胞，脉络膜位于巩膜和视网膜之间，富有高度流动性的血管小叶合体细胞，它们不仅能供给视网膜的光感受细胞（视锥和视杆细胞）血液，并且还可以作为一个散热装置来消散吸收可见光所释放的热量。

是否所有的脉络膜黑色素瘤都起源于脉络膜色素痣尚不清楚，但是患者有扁平，色素沉着并且未治疗的 20 年以上的色素痣可以经由之前处于静止状态的病灶发展成为黑色素瘤。脉络膜黑色素瘤起因不明，但是潜在的医学因素包括：眼球黑变病（Ota 痣），发育不良痣综合征。用药能致使肿瘤生长，包括雌激素替代治疗和左旋多巴。与职业相关包括农业畜牧工作和一些工业操作（如电焊）。GNAQ/GNA11 的相互排斥突变几乎发生在所有脉络膜色素痣和黑色素瘤中，额外的 BAP1 突变被认为是与这些病变的恶性转化相关的遗传事件[27]。

脉络膜黑色素瘤的诊断

脉络膜黑色素瘤的诊断可以直接由检眼镜检查得出，病变常表现为隆起、圆顶形、可突破 Bruch 膜（玻璃膜，图 78-6）。当 Bruch 膜被突破时，因为其特征性的形状，肿瘤被描述为蕈状生长。病变可以是多叶的，或者是扁平的和弥漫性的。不同患者及不同部位肿瘤病变部颜色不同。临床上高达 40%的肿瘤没有色素。当肿瘤含有色素时，其颜色常为暗灰色至炭色，偶尔也会表现为深褐色。

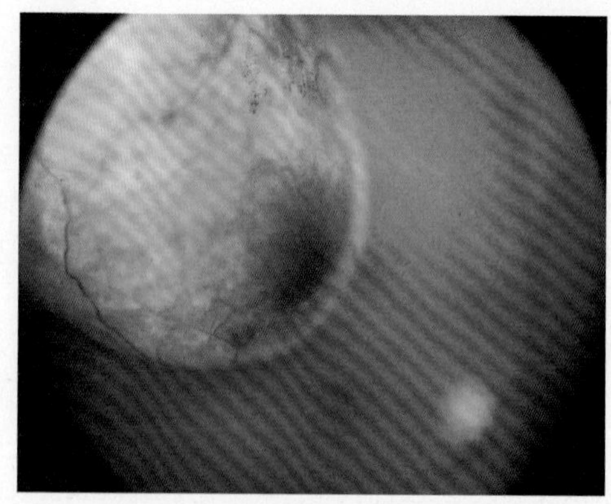

图 78-6 恶性脉络膜黑色素瘤

眼部超声检查以及荧光造影检查有助于诊断，所有的脉络膜黑色素瘤常伴有视网膜脱离，一些病例中用检眼镜观察很难察觉脱离，但是也有一些病例视网膜脱离范围广泛导致临床上检查不到黑色素瘤。典型的 B 超检查表现为隆起的实性肿瘤，

A 超检查表现为中至低的反射。多中心合作的眼科黑色素瘤研究(COMS)表明,采用严格而又标准的眼科以及系统检查,诊断精确率可以达到 99.7%[28],因此针吸活组织检查很少用于临床。

因为眼部及眼眶没有淋巴管组织,肿瘤通过血行扩散,大约 68%的单器官转移发生于肝脏,中位生存期为 6 个月~1 年[29]。

临床及病理风险因素

很多临床以及病理特征与患者预后密切相关[30]。第一,一些大的肿瘤更容易发生转移,采用高度和最大基底径来描述肿瘤大小;第二,肿瘤的位置影响预后,起源于虹膜的色素肿瘤预后最好,睫状体肿瘤是脉络膜肿瘤的死亡率的 3 倍。第三,60 岁以下的患者有较好的预后生存率。第四,发生眼外扩散患者死亡率要比没有发生扩散的死亡率高。第五,很多病理学特征(从一些摘除的眼球中得到)与预后相关,比较公认的是细胞类型,一些大的肿瘤常表现为上皮细胞型,并且预后不好。

COMS 团队包括了美国 44 家研究中心,进行了一系列随机的前瞻性的临床试验和其他研究,研究不同大小的肿瘤的预后和治疗。其分类标准详见表 78-7,研究结果详见表 78-8。

表 78-7　多中心协作脉络膜黑色素瘤研究(COMS)中脉络膜黑色素瘤的分类表

	小	中等大小	大
肿瘤高度	1~2.5mm	2.5~10mm 并且	>10mm 或者
最大的基底直径	5~16mm	<16mm	超过 16mm(当高度为 2mm 或更大)

表 78-8　多中心协作脉络膜黑色素瘤研究(COMS)的研究结果

	小	中等大小	大
文献	Arch Ophthalmol. December 1997;115(12):1537-1544	Arch Ophthalmol. July 2001;119(7):969-982	Am J Ophthalmol. June 1998;125(6):779-796
研究类型	非随机,前瞻性	前瞻性随机临床试验	前瞻性随机临床试验
患者样本量	204	1 317	1 003
研究中的黑色素瘤大小	高度:1~2.5mm 最大基底直径:5mm	高度:2.5~10.0mm 最大基底直径:5~16mm	高度:10mm 或更大 最大基底直径:16mm 或更大
研究目的	描述时间对肿瘤生长的影响以及小肿瘤生长特征的确定	比较 125I 近距离治疗与眼球摘除对中等大小肿瘤的治疗效果	比较眼摘前放射治疗与仅用眼摘对大的肿瘤的治疗效果
研究发现	21%在 2 年内增长 31%在 5 年内增长 与生长相关因素:肿瘤最初的厚度及直径,橘黄色色素的出现,玻璃膜疣的缺失,视网膜色素上皮质改变	12 年后两种治疗方案对于生存率在临床上及统计学意义上无明显差异	两种治疗方法在生存率上没有显著的差异 年龄和最大基底径是仅有的能影响预后的两个因素

基因分析

最近几年,有关分析脉络膜黑色素瘤的染色体变化以及基因表型的研究越来越多。在一些原发葡萄膜黑色素瘤中可见一些染色体异常,包括染色体 3/6/8 染色质缺失或者增加,并与肿瘤转移相关。统计学分析表明,染色单体 3 是肿瘤恶化以及生存重要的预测因素[31]。

采用基因芯片分析研究可以将患者分为两组:1 级(低级别肿瘤)和 2 级(高级别肿瘤)[32]。这个分类很好地预测了转移性死亡率,95%Kaplan-Meier 生存分析预测显示 95%的 1 级患者生存达 92 个月,而 2 级只有 31%。研究表明此分类优于其他的临床以及病理预测指标。已经证实特定的基因突变与生存相关。例如,体细胞 BAP1 突变被发现于 84%的高风险的 2 级肿瘤[32]。3%~5%的脉络膜痣或黑色素瘤患者可能发生生殖系细胞 BAP1 突变,并与遗传性癌症综合征相关,如间皮瘤和肾、胃癌。最近,两个其他突变(SF3B1 和 EIF1AX)据报道与更有利的预后相关,并且更常见于男性患者[33]。

最近几年,采用细针活检抽吸及眼摘样本进行核型分析、单核苷酸多态(SNP)分析、荧光原位杂交(FISH)分析、比较基因组分析研究的临床机构数量显著增加。一些组织也开始进行有关细针活检抽吸组织的 FISH 及微卫星矩阵分析研究。活检可以经由睫状体平坦部以及巩膜组织进行。因为对于转移性肿瘤目前尚无有效的治疗方法,还不清楚可以提供给活检组织发现有高转移风险的患者什么样的转移干预措施以及筛选程序。但是,随着针对转移性肿瘤的新的治疗措施(如塞来替尼[34])和预防性药物的发展以及临床试验的可行性增加,确定哪些患者可以进行相应的临床试验是很重要的。

小肿瘤的治疗与预后

COMS 对于小肿瘤定义为病变范围高度在 1~2.5mm,最大基底径为5~16mm。观察性研究发现,对于脉络膜黑色素瘤最初采用观察的方法治疗,21%的肿瘤在2年的时间里生长至中到大肿瘤,而31%在5年的时间里可以长至中到大肿瘤。但是,目前没有确定的治疗标准。此组可能还包括那些病变范围不再扩大并且没有高风险因素的患者。研究中统计学分析一些因素与肿瘤生长密切相关,包括最初肿瘤的厚度及最大基底径数值高、橘黄色色素的出现,玻璃膜疣的缺失,邻近肿瘤区域的视网膜色素上皮质改变(表78-6)。

黑色素细胞瘤是一种特殊类型的色素痣,常见于地中海起源的深色皮肤的高加索人。黑色素细胞瘤是一种常见起源于视盘的棕黑色损害,但是也可由脉络膜、睫状体或者虹膜发展而来。病变可能有几毫米高,生长缓慢,影响视野及视敏度。病理学上,病变是大细胞性的痣伴有黑色素。经过没有死亡的病例,但是仍有少量良性病变恶性转化。

脉络膜痣的鉴别诊断包括:先天性视网膜色素上皮增生(CHRPE),视网膜色素上皮的错构瘤和视网膜出血,尤其是视网膜色素上皮下出血(最常见伴有年龄相关性黄斑变性)。检眼镜所见,血管荧光造影结果以及超声检查可鉴别相关疾病。

因为有关COMS的近距离放射治疗试验已经公布,大部分的美国眼科医师继续基于COMS关于肿瘤大小的认定指南从而对肿瘤开展近距离放射治疗,但是一些研究者提出了一个问题,是否小肿瘤应该做放射敷贴治疗或者活检进行基因测序。尽管COMS研究表明对于这些患者,长期死亡率很低(8年全因死亡率为14.9%)[35],施行放射敷贴治疗的考虑还是具有足够的意义。只有一项研究调查了小原发肿瘤的转归,然后在其生长或者发现新的橘黄色素之后对其施行了标准化的近距离放射治疗方案。COMS对于小肿瘤的研究表明黑色素瘤相关的5年死亡率为1%[35],但是这个数值的计算包括一些疑似肿瘤,这些肿瘤不生长并且没有治疗过。未来的随机前瞻性试验研究,可以通过对比观察和及时治疗后的患者的视力以及存活率,有助于回答这个关键问题。

中等大小肿瘤的治疗与预后

COMS完成了一项前瞻性的随机的临床试验,纳入1 317名中等大小肿瘤的患者,这些患者被随机分为眼球摘除或者放射敷贴治疗(^{125}I,剂量为10 000cGy)[36]。研究表明,治疗后的12年,放射敷贴治疗死亡率(5年生存率为81%)与眼摘死亡率(5年生存率为82%)无明显变化。根据这些结果,具有中等大小肿瘤的患者均可以进行眼摘或者放射敷贴治疗。^{125}I放射治疗剂量在肿瘤最高点可以为7 500~10 000cGy。放疗剂量分割方案的变化对局部控制、转移和并发症没有明显影响。并发症包括放射性视网膜病变和视神经乳头病变,由于并发症,43%的患者只有20/200的视力或者随访3年视力变得更差。

大肿瘤的治疗和预后

在过去,大肿瘤的患者通常进行眼球摘除,伴有或者不伴术前放疗。COMS前瞻性随机临床试验研究发现单纯进行眼摘的患者与术前进行放射治疗的患者两组5年生存率无明显变化(57% vs 62%)[37]。眼摘前进行放疗的患者接受了5次分割200cGy外线束放射治疗并且于72h内进行眼球摘除手术。现在的大肿瘤患者一般只单独进行眼球摘除术。

眼球表面鳞状细胞肿瘤(OSSN)

眼球表面鳞状细胞肿瘤(OSSN)是指结膜/角膜的皮内新生物和鳞状细胞癌。这类疾病的发病率具有明显地域性,如部分病种在非洲发病率最高。紫外线辐射是一个重要的危险因素,但病毒,特别是人乳头瘤病毒,和遗传病因也被认为是致病因素之一。鳞状细胞癌在HIV患者中更具攻击性。

OSSN的表现各异,但通常表现为缓慢进行性的眼睛发红或眼睛刺激症状伴有黏膜白斑。病变可以是孤立的,但随着病变进展,它们可以侵入邻近的皮肤、眼眶、巩膜和眼睛内部。边界清楚的病灶可以通过切除活检进行治疗,同时切除足够的组织边缘,并辅助冷冻疗法和/或局部化疗。在更广泛和更晚期的病例中,放疗或者眼眶及其内容物摘除是有指征的。鳞状细胞癌发生转移的风险从小于1%到8%不等,但在黏液表皮/梭形细胞亚型、具有高线粒体指数的肿瘤或复发或侵入眼睑和眼眶的肿瘤中更为常见。转移通常首先在相邻的淋巴结中发现。

转移性病变

儿童及成人眼内及眼眶最常见的转移性肿瘤是脉络膜转移癌,在美国每年仅有350例视网膜母细胞瘤和1 500例脉络膜黑色素瘤,但据估计每年有30 000~100 000例患者发生眼部转移性肿瘤。

大部分的肿瘤转移至葡萄膜(虹膜、睫状体以及脉络膜),以脉络膜最常见。眼睑、结膜、视神经、眼眶、眼外肌和眶骨的转移性肿瘤也有报道,转移至视网膜的肿瘤几乎没有。脉络膜转移性肿瘤常为无色素的、多发,双眼发病、隆起度不高并且疼痛位于视神经周围或者侵犯巩膜时。相反,眼内黑色素瘤典型的具有色素、单发、单眼发病、显著隆起并且不伴疼痛。转移性肿瘤和眼内黑色素瘤相似,经常伴有严重的视网膜脱离,脱离的程度与转移的程度密切相关。转移性肿瘤在B超检查中有强回声。大部分的眼内肿瘤在例行的检查中被发现,然而眼部转移性肿瘤的表现很典型,因为由于严重的视网膜脱离,视野缺损以及视敏度下降的症状表现突出。

眼内转移性肿瘤成人多发生于55~65岁,与眼内黑色素瘤年龄分布相似。眼部转移性肿瘤原发第一位器官是肺癌,第二位是乳腺癌。34%的表现为脉络膜转移癌的患者没有原发肿瘤的病史[38]。其他转移性肿瘤转移至眼内包括胃肠道、前列腺(最常见转移至眶骨)、甲状腺、卵巢、皮肤黑色素瘤。事实上所有的恶性肿瘤都可以转移至眼内。

眼内转移性病变最显著的特点是同时伴随有中枢神经系统的转移,这两种病变的一致性尚不清楚,大约有75%的眼部转移性病变伴有CNS病变,尽管最初的影像学尚不能经常发现CNS疾病。因此推测部分眼部转移性病变并不是通过血液途径,CNS转移可能是经由蛛网膜下腔途径导致脉络膜的种植,如同儿童白血病一样。

当出现视力下降、疼痛、复视等症状时,要考虑进行治疗。治疗对于生存率几乎没有影响,除非是类癌的转移性病变,但是可以显著地改善患者的生存质量。与其他系统的转移瘤一样,化疗、靶向治疗及生物治疗对许多眼内转移性肿瘤有效。化疗和/或激素性疗法结合抗VEGF注射可致使肿瘤和视网膜下积液的退变。外线束放射治疗和光动力治疗也可用来减轻转移瘤的症状。除了类癌以及乳腺癌,脉络膜转移癌患者的平均生存率只有6个月。

肿瘤相关性视网膜病(CAR)

肿瘤相关性视网膜疾病(CAR)是一种副肿瘤性疾病,以癌症患者的视力丧失为特点。患者常有明视或者内视现象,以及光敏感性和夜盲。检查可以发现有视力下降、色彩感下降及暗点。CAR 抗体,一种血液中可检测的分子量为 23kDa 的蛋白,是一种特异性结合光感受器和双极细胞钙结合蛋白。潜在的肿瘤被认为表达视觉恢复蛋白并且激发抗体反应,循环抗体再与视网膜作用引发光感受器退化。尽管视觉恢复蛋白的抗体占大部分病例,另外一些分子量为 46kDa、45kDa、60kDa 和 65kDa 蛋白抗体也有报道。肺癌、子宫内膜肉瘤、淋巴瘤和前列腺癌都与症状相关。治疗起来很困难。一直在努力尝试甾体类药物、血浆、静脉注射免疫球蛋白(IVIG)等治疗潜在的肿瘤。尽管有报道个体治疗成功,但是大部分患者没有改善,而且到目前为止没有弄明白最佳的治疗方案[39]。

眼部淋巴肿瘤

非霍奇金淋巴瘤可以偶发浸润眼内组织,并且早于全身其他系统就可出现明显的临床表现。免疫受损的患者,特别是患有病毒性疾病(如 HIV/AIDS)的患者,该病的发病率升高。

眼部原发恶性淋巴瘤,之前被称为网状细胞肉瘤或者小神经胶质细胞瘤病,患者玻璃体中可见肿瘤细胞,常累及视网膜及视神经。玻璃体切除活检或者腰椎穿刺术可明确诊断。治疗方法有全身应用甾体类药物以、眼部 2 400cGy 外线束放射治疗和/或化疗。患者经常伴有 CNS 病变,但是很少有其他系统性疾病。现在仍然有争论的是当腰椎穿刺以及 MRI 影像学检查提示 CNS 没有疾病时,脑部是否需要治疗。该病的中位生存期为 3.5 年,通常脑部累及的程度决定了患者的预后。眼内病变的治疗似乎并不会影响后期眼外病灶的出现。

葡萄膜淋巴系统浸润不常见,以淋巴细胞局限性或者弥漫性浸润葡萄膜为特征。患者的典型表现为无痛性、进展性视力缺损。脉络膜结节性无色素性增厚或者渗出性视网膜脱离导致的继发性青光眼可以出现。活检部位要位于最易接近的组织。治疗上强调保留眼球,目的是保存视力,包括口服激素和/或外线束放射治疗。生存预后很好,并且与全身累及程度有关,较少累及 CNS。

成人眼部肿瘤:眼眶病变

眼眶肿瘤简介

幸运的是眼眶的恶性肿瘤并不常见,眼眶肿瘤大约占眼眶疾病的 20%~25%,常见的发病年龄是 60 岁或者 60 岁以上。眼眶恶性原发肿瘤通常需要活检,并且外科处理指征包括泪腺肿瘤和眼眶淋巴瘤。所有可疑眼眶肿瘤的患者都应行影像学检查,包括眼科超声、CT 平扫(增强)和/或 MRI 平扫(增强),以便更清楚地显示肿瘤的位置及特征。

良性和恶性病变

边界清楚的眼眶病变

成人眼眶最常见的良性肿瘤是海绵状血管瘤,患者常有缓慢的进展性无痛性眼球突出,伴有视网膜上出现条纹和影像学表现为扁平的眼球。治疗方法为手术治疗,全部摘除肿瘤是可行的。其他边界清楚的病变包括神经纤维瘤、神经鞘瘤、血管外皮细胞瘤、脑膜瘤以及神经胶质瘤。

黏液囊肿或者黏液鞘膜积脓是一种囊样,起源于鼻旁窦(常是额窦),有包膜的肿块,鼻窦炎常反复发作而导致眶蜂窝织炎。这是儿童时期眼球突出的最常见原因。影像学检查骨壁是不完整的。治疗方法可选择抗生素治疗。如果抗生素治疗不能解决积脓的问题或者视神经受到压迫,则需要进行外科引流。

弥漫性眼眶病变

弥漫性眼眶病变通常需要活检,包括眼眶淋巴瘤、眼眶蜂窝织炎、纤维组织细胞瘤(良性以及恶性的)、神经纤维瘤和肉瘤。淋巴细胞增生性肿瘤大约占所有眼眶肿瘤病变的 20%。非霍奇金淋巴瘤的发病率一直以来每年以 3%~4%的速度增长,而眶淋巴瘤的发病率更高,但具体的发病增长因素尚不明了。淋巴样瘤曾经被分为活跃的淋巴组织增生或者恶性淋巴瘤。近来,人们逐渐认识到淋巴组织增生病变是一个连续的过程,最终的肿瘤行为学很难预测。如今以分子基因学研究以及单克隆细胞表面标志物为依据,70%~90%眼部淋巴组织增生病变被定性为恶性淋巴瘤。

典型的淋巴组织增生性病变表现为逐渐发展的无痛性肿物,可以位于眼眶的前面或者结膜下。眼眶影像学检查能显示位于正常组织结构周围的特征性肿瘤组织,骨损害少见,但可见于病变严重区域。高达 50%的病变出现在泪腺窝,约 17%的患者为双眼发病。早期活检对于诊断有重要作用,并且可以根据 REAL 分类标准反映不同肿瘤的形态学、免疫学、细胞遗传学和分子学特性[40]。这个分类可以被用来预测临床上病变区损害的不同情况,它将淋巴瘤分成了 5 类:边缘区域的淋巴瘤(MALT)、淋巴质浆细胞淋巴瘤、滤泡中心淋巴瘤、弥漫性大 B 细胞淋巴瘤和其他少见淋巴瘤。

对于肿瘤科医师而言,眼附属器淋巴瘤的治疗涉及转移性病灶的处理。眼部疾病一般运用 2 000~3 000cGy 的外线束放射治疗,几乎在所有的病例中均可以局部控制并且可能避免全身性传播,但是,至少 50%的患者最终检测到全身系统性淋巴瘤,其治疗要根据肿瘤病变的病理分级及其侵袭程度。一些惰性淋巴瘤对化疗药物不敏感,长期生存率高,然而一些迅速进展的淋巴瘤则有可能被积极的化疗药物和/或放射治疗治愈。

一些研究发现双侧眼眶受累的患者预后不好,结膜病变进而导致全身系统性疾病的概率最小(20%),而眼睑部淋巴瘤的概率最高(67%),眼眶病变则介于两者之间(35%)。

泪腺肿瘤

泪腺肿瘤通过眼科超声很容易被诊断,但是对于明确的肿瘤定位,特别是骨质破坏,需要 CT 扫描确定。当影像学上显示泪腺肿瘤为双侧时,它们通常与肉瘤样病变、眼眶炎性假瘤或者淋巴瘤相类似。这些泪腺肿瘤不表现出相关感染症状,大多数表现为淋巴组织增殖性病变,50%的眶部淋巴瘤可发展至泪腺窝,只有少数泪腺窝区病变为原发泪腺上皮肿瘤。当有可疑病例需要做出病理诊断时,活检是必需的。

大约 50%的原发泪腺上皮肿瘤是良性多形性腺瘤(多形性

腺瘤)，还有50%的为恶性肿瘤。其中近一半的恶性肿瘤为腺样囊性癌(图78-7)，其余包括恶性多形性腺瘤、原发腺癌、黏液表皮样癌和鳞状细胞癌。对于原发恶性泪腺肿瘤的治疗主要为手术切除以及放射治疗。除了多形性腺瘤可以不需要初步活检而进行手术摘除(活检会引起肿瘤壁破损，从而增加复发风险)，这类肿瘤的临床病程多为多次疼痛复发，最终死于颅内转移或全身其他转移，经常发生于初诊的10年之后或者更长时间。

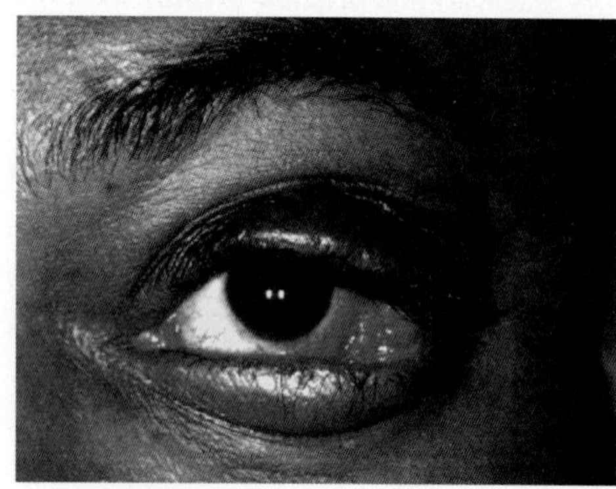

图78-7 泪腺腺样囊性癌，病变取了2次活检均无法明确诊断，随后肿瘤转移到腮腺，患者最终死亡

(王嘉炜 译　万经海 校)

参考文献

1 Abramson DH. Retinoblastoma: saving life with vision. *Annu Rev Med.* 2014;**65**:171–184.
2 Xu XL, Singh HP, Wang L, et al. Rb suppresses human cone-precursor-derived retinoblastoma tumours. *Nature.* 2014;**514**:385–388.
3 Albert DM. Historic review of retinoblastoma. *Ophthalmology.* 1987;**94**:654–662.
4 Dimaras H, Khetan V, Halliday W, et al. Loss of RB1 induces non-proliferative retinoma: increasing genomic instability correlates with progression to retinoblastoma. *Hum Mol Genet.* 2008;**17**:1363–1372.
5 Rushlow DE, Mol BM, Kennett JY, et al. Characterisation of retinoblastomas without RB1 mutations: genomic, gene expression, and clinical studies. *Lancet Oncol.* 2013;**14**:327–334.
6 Dunn JM, Phillips RA, Becker AJ, Gallie BL. Identification of germline and somatic mutations affecting the retinoblastoma gene. *Science.* 1988;**241**: 1797–1800.
7 Harbour JW. Overview of RB gene mutations in patients with retinoblastoma. Implications for clinical genetic screening. *Ophthalmology.* 1998;**105**:1442–1447.
8 Abramson DH, Beaverson K, Sangani P, et al. Screening for retinoblastoma: presenting signs as prognosticators of patient and ocular survival. *Pediatrics.* 2003;**112**:1248–1255.
9 Reese AB. *Tumors of the Eye*, 3rd ed. New York: Harper and Row; 1976.
10 Murphree AL. The case for a new evidence-based group classification of intraocular retinoblastoma: linking natural history with clinical outcomes. In: *International Conference of Ocular Oncology*, September 3, 2005; Whistler, Canada.
11 Chan HS, DeBoer G, Thiessen JJ, et al. Combining cyclosporin with chemotherapy controls intraocular retinoblastoma without requiring radiation. *Clin Cancer Res.* 1996;**2**:1499–1508.
12 Abramson DH, Schefler AC. Update on retinoblastoma. *Retina.* 2004;**24**:828–848.
13 Yamane T, Kaneko A, Mohri M. The technique of ophthalmic arterial infusion therapy for patients with intraocular retinoblastoma. *Int J Clin Oncol.* 2004;**9**:69–73.
14 Gobin YP, Dunkel IJ, Marr BP, Brodie SE, Abramson DH. Intra-arterial chemotherapy for the management of retinoblastoma: four-year experience. *Arch Ophthalmol.* 2011 Jun;**129(6)**:732–737.
15 Francis JH, Schaiquevich P, Buitrago E, et al. Local and systemic toxicity of intravitreal melphalan for vitreous seeding in retinoblastoma: a preclinical and clinical study. *Ophthalmology.* 2014;**121(9)**:1810–1817.
16 Chantada G, Fandino A, Davila MT, et al. Results of a prospective study for the treatment of retinoblastoma. *Cancer.* 2004;**100**:834–842.
17 Dunkel IJ, Aledo A, Kernan NA, et al. Successful treatment of metastatic retinoblastoma. *Cancer.* 2000;**89**:2117–2121.
18 Abramson DH. Second nonocular cancers in retinoblastoma: a unified hypothesis. *The Franceschetti Lecture Ophthalmic Genet.* 1999;**20**:193–204.
19 Moll AC, Imhof SM, Schouten-Van Meeteren AY, Kuik DJ, Hofman P, Boers M. Second primary tumors in hereditary retinoblastoma: a register-based study, 1945–1997: is there an age effect on radiation-related risk? *Ophthalmology.* 2001;**108**:1109–1114.
20 Fletcher O, Easton D, Anderson K, Gilham C, Jay M, Peto J. Lifetime risks of common cancers among retinoblastoma survivors. *J Natl Cancer Inst.* 2004;**96**:357–363.
21 Abramson DH, Jereb B, Wollner N, Murphy L, Ellsworth RM. Leukemic ophthalmopathy detected by ultrasound. *J Pediatr Ophthalmol Strabismus.* 1983;**20**:92–97.
22 Haik BG. Vascular tumors of the orbit. In: Hornblass A, ed. *Ophthalmic and Orbital Plastic Reconstructive Surgery.* Baltimore: Williams and Wilkins; 1989:509–517.
23 Teske S, Ohlrich SJ, Gole G, Spiro P, Miller M, Sullivan TJ. Treatment of orbital capillary haemangioma with interferon. *Aust N Z J Ophthalmol.* 1994;**22**:13–17.
24 Jones IS. Lymphangiomas of the ocular adnexae: an analysis of 62 cases. *Am J Ophthalmol.* 1961;**51**:481–509.
25 Raney RB, Anderson JR, Kollath J, et al. Late effects of therapy in 94 patients with localized rhabdomyosarcoma of the orbit: report from the Intergroup Rhabdomyosarcoma Study (IRS)-III, 1984–1991. *Med Pediatr Oncol.* 2000; **34**:413–420.
26 Oberlin O, Rey A, Anderson J, et al. Treatment of orbital rhabdomyosarcoma: survival and late effects of treatment–results of an international workshop. *J Clin Oncol.* 2001;**19**:197–204.
27 Harbour JW, Onken MD, Roberson EDO, et al. Frequent mutation of BAP1 in metastasizing uveal melanomas. *Science.* 2010;**330**:1410–1413.
28 Collaborative Ocular Melanoma Study Group. Accuracy of diagnosis of choroidal melanomas in the Collaborative Ocular Melanoma Study. COMS report no. 1. *Arch Ophthalmol.* 1990;**108**:1268–1273.
29 Collaborative Ocular Melanoma Study Group. Assessment of metastatic disease status at death in 435 patients with large choroidal melanoma in the Collaborative Ocular Melanoma Study (COMS): COMS report no. 15. *Arch Ophthalmol.* 2001;**119**:670–676.
30 Shields JA, Shields CL, Donoso LA. Management of posterior uveal melanoma. *Surv Ophthalmol.* 1991;**36**:161–195.
31 Prescher G, Bornfeld N, Hirche H, Horsthemke B, Jockel KH, Becher R. Prognostic implications of monosomy 3 in uveal melanoma. *Lancet.* 1996;**347**:1222–1225.
32 Onken MD, Worley LA, Ehlers JP, Harbour JW. Gene expression profiling in uveal melanoma reveals two molecular classes and predicts metastatic death. *Cancer Res.* 2004;**64**:7205–7209.
33 Martin M, Maßhöfer L, Temming P, et al. Exome sequencing identifies recurrent somatic mutations in EIF1AX and SF3B1 in uveal melanoma with disomy 3. *Nat Genet.* 2013;**45**:933–936.
34 Carvajal RD, Sosman JA, Quevedo JF, et al. Effect of selumetinib vs chemotherapy on progression-free survival in uveal melanoma: a randomized clinical trial. *JAMA.* 2014;**311**:2397–2405.
35 Collaborative Ocular Melanoma Study Group. Mortality in patients with small choroidal melanoma. COMS report no. 4. The Collaborative Ocular Melanoma Study Group. *Arch Ophthalmol.* 1997;**115**:886–893.
36 Diener-West M, Earle JD, Fine SL, et al. The COMS randomized trial of iodine 125 brachytherapy for choroidal melanoma, III: initial mortality findings. COMS Report No. 18. *Arch Ophthalmol.* 2001;**119**:969–982.
37 Collaborative Ocular Melanoma Study Group. The Collaborative Ocular Melanoma Study (COMS) randomized trial of pre-enucleation radiation of large choroidal melanoma II: initial mortality findings. COMS report no. 10. *Am J Ophthalmol.* 1998;**125**:779–796.
38 Shields CL, Shields JA, Gross NE, Schwartz GP, Lally SE. Survey of 520 eyes with uveal metastases. *Ophthalmology.* 1997;**104**:1265–1276.
39 Keltner JL, Thirkill CE, Tyler NK, Roth AM. Management and monitoring of cancer-associated retinopathy. *Arch Ophthalmol.* 1992;**110**:48–53.
40 Coupland SE, Krause L, Delecluse HJ, et al. Lymphoproliferative lesions of the ocular adnexa. Analysis of 112 cases. *Ophthalmology.* 1998;**105**:1430–1441.

第 79 章　内分泌腺肿瘤：垂体肿瘤

Chirag D. Gandhi, MD, FACS, FAANS ■ Margaret Pain, MD ■ Kalmon D. Post, MD, FACS, FAANS

概述

垂体肿瘤是涵盖了多种临床表现和病理分型的一类肿瘤。由于这类肿瘤的症状可能来自异常的激素分泌或对邻近神经结构产生的压迫，还有部分肿瘤是罕见的转移性肿瘤。根据不同的患者及肿瘤情况，其治疗和分类都有特异性。经蝶手术是一种常见的治疗方式，绝大多数垂体腺瘤都有良好的耐受性；然而，放射和化学疗法的进展增加了治疗的选择，提高了治疗效果和可行性。

垂体腺瘤为腺垂体来源的上皮性肿瘤。一方面因其占位效应可以导致患者出现神经系统症状，如头痛、视野障碍、颅内压逐渐增高、脑神经麻痹；还会因激素分泌异常导致各种临床症状。少数病例（小于 1%）会出现尿崩症。垂体腺瘤占颅内肿瘤的 10%~15%，而尸检的发病率高达 24%。常见发病年龄为 30~40 岁，总体好发性别方面无明显差异，但在某些亚型中有性别差异，例如库欣病常好发于女性，泌乳素腺瘤常好发于年轻女性，而无功能腺瘤、嗜酸细胞肿瘤及促性腺激素释放激素腺瘤则好发于男性。

随着病理学及生物化学的发展，以及对垂体腺的研究深入，对垂体肿瘤亚型的分类方法也在逐步改进。经典的分型是根据显微镜下肿瘤细胞的特征和占优势的胞质，分为嗜酸性肿瘤、嗜碱性肿瘤及嫌色细胞肿瘤。一般认为嗜酸性肿瘤会分泌过量生长激素（GH）从而导致肢端肥大症及巨人症。嗜碱性肿瘤会分泌促肾上腺皮质激素（ACTH），导致库欣病。嫌色细胞肿瘤通常无激素活性，多为无功能腺瘤。但该分型系统由于未充分说明激素分泌及细胞分化，因此应用价值有限。现在已有研究证明，嗜酸性肿瘤及嗜碱性肿瘤均可分泌其他的激素，而嫌色细胞肿瘤也可有激素活性，可以分泌激素，如生长激素（GH）、泌乳素（PRL）、ACTH、促甲状腺素（TSH）、卵泡刺激素（FSH）、促黄体素（LH）及 α 亚基[1]。

从临床角度出发，垂体腺瘤常根据肿瘤细胞分泌激素的不同来进行分类[2,3]。这种分型中，不管肿瘤细胞是否有分泌能力及分泌何种激素，仅根据临床是否有激素分泌过量及与激素过量相关的临床症状来进行分型。非分泌型腺瘤的细胞从细胞内结构上看可能具备分泌功能，但生化检查时激素分泌量不超过正常水平，也没有激素过多而导致的临床症状。该机制目前尚不完全清楚，但普遍认可的假说包括：过量增殖的肿瘤细胞分泌能力下降；或肿瘤分泌的激素不被常规的免疫抗体所识别，细胞基因逐步获得性缺失导致丧失分泌能力[4]。随着分子生物学及免疫组化的研究进展，垂体腺瘤功能分型的方法也在不断改进。

从解剖学及影像学的角度，垂体腺瘤可依据与海绵窦的位置关系及侵犯海绵窦的程度分型。专门针对垂体的磁共振（MRI）检查，是首选的影像诊断检查方法。垂体磁共振要包含垂体的冠状位及矢状位薄层扫描（图 79-1）。由于 T2 加权像对颅内病变显示的敏感性较高，如果存在视交叉移位或瘤内有囊变和出血，都可以在冠状 T2 加权像上清晰辨认。钆造影剂增强扫描对提高微腺瘤（<10mm）的诊断率至关重要，在界定大腺瘤的病变与正常组织边界方面也很有用（T1 加权像注射钆造影剂前后）[5]。一般情况下，垂体腺瘤在 T1 加权像上表现为低密度病变，而在 T1 强化序列像上其强化程度低于正常垂体组织。Jules Hardy 和 Engelbert Knosp 依据影像学表现将鞍旁侵袭性垂体瘤进一步分型（图 79-2），Knosp 分型已成为术前预测海绵窦侵犯的相关策略，简而言之，磁共振影像上肿瘤对海绵窦内侧壁以及对海绵窦内颈内动脉位置的影响，是用来评估肿瘤是否侵袭海绵窦的依据。海绵窦内侧壁肿瘤占位效应越多说明肿瘤侵袭性越大，与非侵袭性肿瘤相比，侵袭性肿瘤更易表现出侵犯行为[7]。

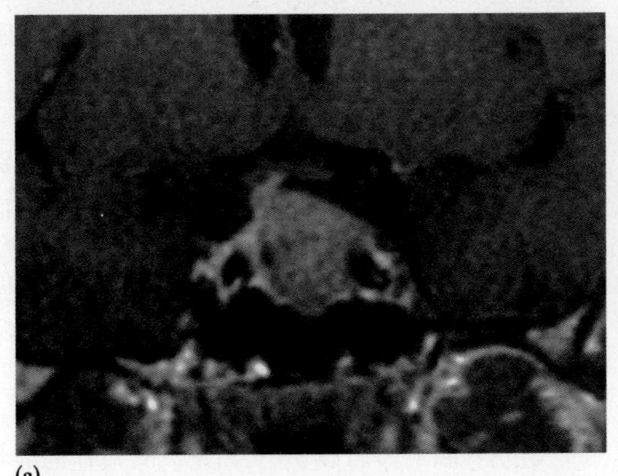

(a)

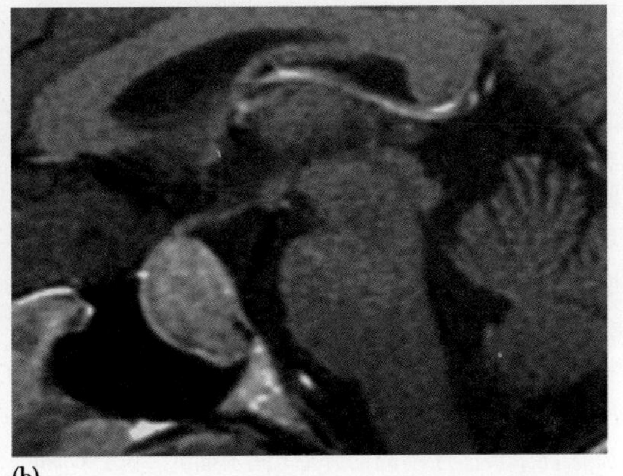

(b)

图 79-1　一位 38 岁女性，患有促肾上腺皮质激素腺瘤。（a）磁共振冠状位 T1 增强像显示鞍内的大腺瘤，延伸到左海绵窦并包裹颈动脉的一部分。（b）磁共振矢状位 T1 增强像显示鞍内有强化的大腺瘤

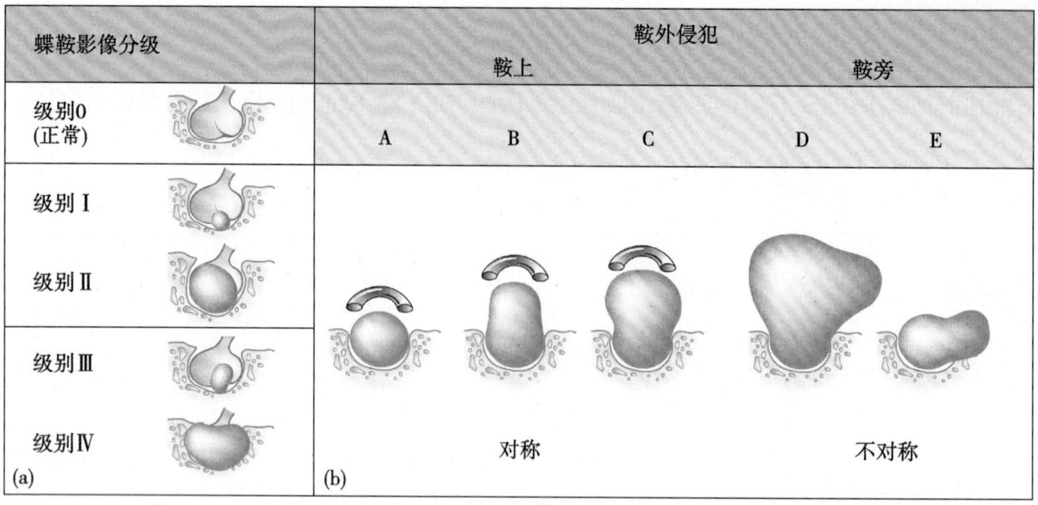

蝶鞍影像分级	鞍外侵犯				
	鞍上			鞍旁	
级别0（正常）	A	B	C	D	E
级别Ⅰ					
级别Ⅱ					
级别Ⅲ					
级别Ⅳ	对称			不对称	
(a)	(b)				

图 79-2 （a）Hardy 对垂体腺瘤的分级。一级和二级在鞍内。三级和四级具有侵袭性。鞍外分类 A、B 和 C 是直接向鞍上侵犯，但侵犯程度不同。D 是向上不对称生长，E 是向一侧海绵窦生长。改编自 Hardy J 和 Somma M[6]。（b）Knosp 海绵窦侵犯分类。摘自 Woodworth，GF et al. J. Neurosurgery 120：1086-1094，2014

垂体肿瘤发生的分子生物学研究表明腺瘤是单克隆增殖的结果[8~10]，肿瘤的进展与癌基因和机体肿瘤抑制功能障碍有关。虽然垂体肿瘤发生学研究牵涉到几个突变，但只有一个突变被证实会显著影响到患者的发病。10%~40%生长激素腺瘤中检测到 GTP 结合蛋白 α 链上出现点突变，从而激活环磷腺苷（cAMP）途径，据此推测是 cAMP 的升高导致了生长激素分泌增多和肿瘤生长[11]。虽然理论上认为，具有 *gsp* 癌基因突变的腺瘤较小且对药物治疗敏感，但最近的研究未能证实具有该突变的患者与未发生该突变的患者之间存在任何表型差异[12]。许多其他因素已被认定会影响肿瘤进展。其他与肿瘤生长相关的致癌基因包括环磷腺苷（cAMP）效应的核转录因子，*Gsα* 过度表达从而促进 CREB 的增加；在侵袭性泌乳素腺瘤中可检测到 *ras* 癌基因突变[13]；最新研究进展表明，垂体肿瘤转化基因（*PTTG*）可能是侵袭性分泌型腺瘤的标记物[14,15]。其他研究包括肿瘤抑制基因如 *Rb*、*menin*、*TP53*、*p27*、*p16*[16,17]，激素促进因子如下丘脑神经激素，以及局部产生的生长因子和细胞因子等与腺瘤生长的相关性[18]。有研究发现半乳凝素-3（Gal-3），作为一种靶向治疗的靶点在 PRL 及 ACTH 分泌型腺瘤中有表达，还有作为核受体的过氧化物酶增殖子活化受体-γ（PPAR-γ），也在多项垂体腺瘤的研究中被分离出来，这些发现让人们看到了开发治疗垂体瘤新型药物的前景[19~21]。

对可疑或确诊的垂体腺瘤患者进行评估，需要在初始治疗前进行完整的放射学和内分泌学以及潜在的遗传学评估[22]。内分泌评估应包括完整的激素代谢项目，包括妊娠试验、血清生长激素、胰岛素样生长因子（IGF-1）、TSH、游离 T4、T3、泌乳素、ACTH、皮质醇、LH、FSH 和睾酮。通过这些测试，才能决定进一步的药物或手术治疗方案。

手术是所有垂体腺瘤的首选和明确的治疗方法，除了泌乳素瘤以及无症状且激素活性不高的肿瘤（偶发瘤）。基于 Cushing、Guiot 和 Hardy 的革新工作，经蝶入路是大多数垂体腺瘤的首选手术方式，其并发症发生率低且康复快[23,24]。手术目的包括减少肿瘤对邻近结构的占位效应，中止内分泌亢进，保留或恢复正常垂体功能。然后，根据组织病理学和免疫化学结果、术后激素分泌状况和鞍外肿瘤扩展程度，可以展开辅助治疗。相对以上需手术治疗的肿瘤，泌乳素腺瘤通常对药物治疗反应良好，偶发瘤只需要临床观察，直到它们产生相关的症状。

最后，极少一部分垂体肿瘤会表现出侵袭性行为或发生癌变。有激素活性的肿瘤通常还需要针对激素的特异性治疗，但这可能不足以控制疾病。替莫唑胺作为一种口服烷基化剂，已成为这些患者的有效的辅助治疗手段[25]。其疗效可以通过在侵袭性垂体肿瘤中经常发现的 O^6-甲基鸟嘌呤-DNA 甲基转移酶（MGMT）的表达降低来解释[26]。

垂体泌乳素腺瘤

泌乳素腺瘤是最常见的垂体腺瘤，约占总例数的 30%[27]。虽然很少危及生命，但可表现临床症状，可出现与高泌乳素血症（生殖或性功能异常）相关的临床表现，或生长增大而对邻近结构造成占位影响。由于这型肿瘤对药物反应较好，药物治疗往往是这型肿瘤的一线治疗（图 79-3）。然而，外科手术也被证明同样有效，并可作为对某些特定病例的主要干预性治疗。

临床表现

虽然尸检研究表明，泌乳素腺瘤的发病率无性别差异，但女性患者出现症状的可能性是男性的四倍。在育龄妇女中，高泌乳素血症可引起月经减少、继发性闭经、溢乳和不育。其他少见症状包括性欲下降、雌激素缺乏引起的阴道黏膜干燥、体重增加及抑郁和焦虑等精神症状。约有 5%原发性闭经和 25%继发性闭经（不包括怀孕）的患者存在垂体泌乳素腺瘤[28]。当闭经同时伴有溢乳时，泌乳素腺瘤的发生率可增加到 70%~80%[29]。

在男性和绝经后妇女中，高泌乳素血症的症状要轻微得多，肿瘤可能会长得很大，只有当肿瘤开始产生占位效应时才会被发现。巨大腺瘤的占位效应可导致头痛、视觉障碍（典型的是视交叉受压迫导致的双眼颞侧偏盲）、垂体功能减退、眼肌

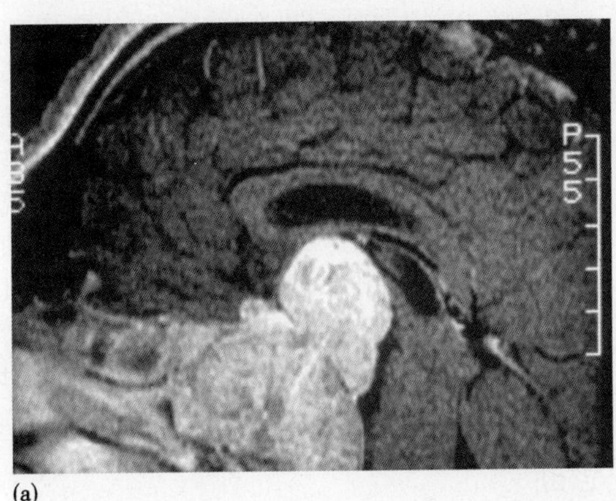

(a)

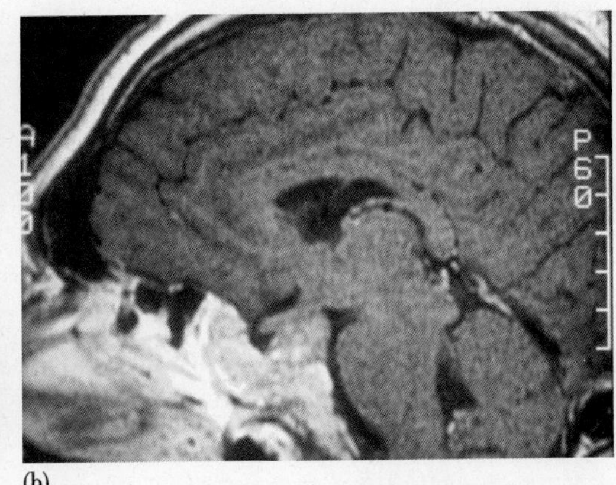

(b)

图 79-3　一位 52 岁男性，性欲减退，并伴有巨大泌乳素腺瘤。(a)磁共振矢状位 T1 增强像显示巨大的鞍内/鞍上腺瘤伴视交叉压迫。(b)矢状位 T1 增强像显示用溴隐亭治疗后肿瘤体积显著减少

麻痹，以及少见的因孟氏孔阻塞而导致的非交通性脑积水。男性也可能引起性欲减退、勃起功能障碍、男性乳房发育，以及由于雄激素分泌减少而导致的不育。高泌乳素血症引起性功能低下的机制仍有争议。一种可能性是，泌乳素通过抑制多巴胺影响下丘脑释放促性腺激素释放激素(GnRH)，进而导致黄体生成素(luteinizing hormone，LH)正常的脉冲性分泌中断[30]。虽然在月经正常的高催乳素血症妇女中，骨密度是正常的，但长时间的高泌乳素血症会由于性腺功能减退途径导致骨质脱钙[31]。

诊断

除泌乳素腺瘤外，高泌乳素血症还可能与多种原因有关，如妊娠、甲状腺功能减退、促泌乳素释放药物(如吩噻嗪、丁丙酚和甲氧氯普胺)和肾衰竭，这些都需要作为鉴别诊断。此外，由于心理和生理上的压力，如运动、手术和低血糖，也可以引发生理性的高泌乳素血症，但泌乳素水平很少超过 40ng/ml[32]。明确诊断泌乳素腺瘤较困难，通常除了泌乳素升高外，还需要影像学的证据。在男性中，基础泌乳素水平大于 100ng/ml 通常提示为泌乳素腺瘤。在女性中，泌乳素水平在 100~200ng/ml 时应可疑患有泌乳素腺瘤，而超过 200ng/ml 则高度提示为泌乳素腺瘤[33,34]。最难确定诊断的是泌乳素水平在 50~100ng/ml 之间的患者。在这个范围内，高泌乳素血症也可能与“垂体柄效应”有关，即肿瘤压迫影响来自下丘脑的泌乳素抑制因子(PRIF)的传递。虽然有多种内分泌刺激试验用来鉴别这两种可能性，但都还没有被证实是可靠的[35]。

血浆泌乳素水平是肿瘤分泌活性的一个指标，并且与肿瘤的大小相关(除囊性或坏死成分外)。泌乳素小于 200ng/ml 的肿瘤中有 80%是微腺瘤，而大于 200ng/ml 的肿瘤中只有 20%是微腺瘤。对于巨大肿瘤(>4cm)则不一定，虽然总泌乳素水平通常与大小有关，甚至可能大于 1 000ng/ml，但由于一种称为“Hook 效应”的现象，实验室检测值可能出现偏低结果(25~150ng/ml)，不能反映实际血清浓度[36,37]。简单地讲，Hook 效应是由于抗体结合位点在放射免疫分析过程中饱和，从而扭曲了结合曲线。这可以通过连续稀释来解决，对于所有巨大垂体腺瘤都患者都应考虑到这一点。

治疗

对泌乳素腺瘤患者的治疗选择包括观察、药物治疗、手术和放疗。决定治疗方案前应综合考虑肿瘤的大小、泌乳素水平、临床表现、药物治疗耐受性和生育要求。绝大多数的泌乳素微腺瘤(<10mm)不会增长[34]。尸检研究显示，人群中微腺瘤的发病率较高，而大多数未被临床发现。许多临床医生和患者在没有临床高泌乳素血症、垂体功能正常和没有怀孕意愿的情况下，选择观察而反对治疗微腺瘤。

由于下丘脑分泌的多巴胺是泌乳素的内源性抑制剂，多巴胺激动剂在抑制肿瘤生长和泌乳素分泌方面有高效的作用。溴隐亭是第一种用于治疗泌乳素腺瘤的多巴胺激动剂，其他新的药物如卡麦角林、奎那格列得、利尿苷和特古里特也得到了广泛的认可。在分子水平上，多巴胺激动剂选择性地激活 D2 型多巴胺受体，从而阻断了泌乳素基因的转录[38]。泌乳素细胞的收缩导致肿瘤淀粉样变和纤维化[39]。多巴胺激动剂有效率较高，高达 70%~80%的患者泌乳素水平可恢复正常，80%~90%的肿瘤可缩小，80%~90%的患者可恢复排卵[40]。基于以上结果，有些人认为除了 10%有明显副作用的患者外，所有的患者都应该接受药物治疗[41]。此外，有证据表明，有相当多的患者应用卡麦角林后泌乳素恢复正常，肿瘤缩小缓解，而在停药 2 年后仍能保持效果[42,43]。然而，即使对卡麦角林敏感有效(泌乳素恢复正常、肿瘤体积缩小、关键结构无侵犯且无视交叉压迫)的患者，大多数仍会复发，因此停药后的密切随访是至关重要的[43]。

多巴胺激动剂也有阻碍其应用的因素。首先对许多患者来说，药物疗效是可逆的，因此选择通过药物控制泌乳素腺瘤需要长期甚至终身服药。其次，药物有显著的副反应，如恶心、呕吐、直立性低血压、头痛、抑郁和焦虑。再有，在垂体卒中和肿瘤囊变的患者中，由于肿瘤的大小与肿瘤细胞的数量无关，多巴胺激动剂不能有效地使肿瘤缩小。还有更多的关于多巴胺激动剂副反应的报道，如大剂量的卡麦角林的使用会引起心脏毒性。虽然有报道用卡麦角林治疗泌乳素腺瘤可引起亚临床瓣膜纤维化和二尖瓣反流，但没有患者因此而出现临床上显著的心功能改变[44,45,136]。最后，多巴胺激动剂并非对所有泌乳素腺瘤都有效，溴隐亭效果不佳既可能与肿瘤耐药有关，也

可能提示肿瘤具有侵袭性[46]。

目前,手术治疗泌乳素腺瘤仍有争议。与长期服药和频繁随访相比,有些人认为手术才是一线治疗,只有在手术没有缓解的情况下才用药物作为辅助治疗[47]。术后的长期缓解率随术前泌乳素水平和肿瘤大小变化而差异显著。对于术前泌乳素水平低于 200ng/ml 的微腺瘤,缓解率最高,可达 50%~80%[40,47~49]。对于大腺瘤和泌乳素水平为 200~500ng/ml 的患者,缓解率显著下降。对于巨大腺瘤和泌乳素水平大于 500ng/ml 的肿瘤,由于完全切除几乎是不可能的,因此手术的效果不好,而对这些患者,多巴胺激动剂似乎是有效的,数据分析发现,有 3/4 的患者肿瘤体积显著缩小,60%~70%的患者泌乳素恢复正常水平[50]。有证据表明,当多巴胺激动剂被用作新辅助治疗时,手术效果更好[51]。此外,有研究表明,对多巴胺抵抗患者,行肿瘤部分切除术后能更好地控制激素水平,并且降低需要服药的剂量[52,53]。总的来说,泌乳素分泌水平与肿瘤缓解率呈负相关。

常规放射治疗通常不作为是主要的治疗方式[54]。立体定向放射外科作为一种主要[55]或辅助[56]治疗手段正变得越来越普遍。放射外科已被证实在降低泌乳素水平方面是有效的(在一项研究中,30%的患者获得了内分泌治愈)[57]。由于放射治疗很少单独使用,这些数据可能因混杂因素而出现偏差。

用多巴胺激动剂进行药物治疗仍是大多数泌乳素腺瘤的一线治疗方法[58]。对于所有患者,包括那些希望怀孕和有原发性闭经的患者,都应该考虑药物治疗。

对于大于 2cm 或泌乳素水平在 200~500ng/ml 之间的肿瘤,可以用多巴胺激动剂做新辅助治疗,使肿瘤体积缩小后再行手术,残留的肿瘤再用药物治疗。对于泌乳素水平超过 500ng/ml 的巨大或侵袭性肿瘤,应以药物治疗为主[50]。对于妊娠期泌乳素腺瘤的患者应特别注意,停药后肿瘤有迅速扩大的风险,发生率虽低但后果很严重,这种并发症大多发生在向鞍上扩展的大腺瘤,而微腺瘤的发生率更小[59]。一旦这些患者出现症状,可以使用多巴胺激动剂。溴隐亭和卡麦角林都是美国 FDA 批准的妊娠 B 类药物,这表明动物研究没有显示胎儿有风险,但对人类使用的风险评估尚缺乏随机对照试验的支持[60,61]。在怀孕期间,只有当肿瘤对药物治疗无效且有进行性神经系统症状时才行手术。为了降低妊娠相关并发症的风险,希望怀孕的大腺瘤患者应在怀孕前接受经蝶入路肿瘤切除手术,或在整个怀孕期间服用溴隐亭。

垂体生长激素腺瘤

生长激素的分泌受下丘脑生长抑素和促生长素释放素(GHRH)的调控。生长激素释放后,经肝脏代谢产生 IGF-1,从而促进骨骼和组织生长,并反馈性抑制 GH 和 GHRH 的分泌。肢端肥大症是生长激素腺瘤的临床表现,它是由于 GH 的自主分泌增加和负反馈抑制丧失而导致的。而且,研究发现生长激素腺瘤的临床表现与 IGF-1 水平的相关性比与 GH 水平的相关性更强。

临床表现

生长激素腺瘤约占所有分泌性垂体腺瘤的 30%,大多数患者在 30~50 岁发病,多为巨大腺瘤,通常有 4~10 年亚临床病史[62]。生长激素分泌过量典型地表现为肢端肥大症或巨人症,两者的特点都是具有前额隆起和颌骨前突、巨舌症和夸张的肢端肥大等粗糙的面容特征。患者也会合并有内脏器官肿大、高血压、心肌病、充血性心力衰竭、限制性肺病、睡眠呼吸暂停和关节病。此外,这些患者中有很高比例的出现糖耐量异常和糖尿病。常见症状还包括疲乏、头痛、关节痛、油性皮肤和多汗症。对于部分泌乳素也有异常分泌的患者,也可能同时出现闭经、溢乳和性欲丧失。由于发病隐匿,并发症的发病率很高,如未经干预有较高的可能性会早亡,有高达 50%的患者在 50 岁前死亡,是普通人群的 2~3 倍[63]。

诊断

肢端肥大症经常由于外观和亚临床病史的变化被发现。激素分泌异常可通过抽血化验来评估,常用的是晨起空腹血生长激素数值或血 IGF-1 数值,血 IGF-1 数值需根据年龄和性别调整为标准值。空腹生长激素数值高于 2.5ng/ml 提示肢端肥大症。然而,由于生长激素半衰期短且以脉冲方式分泌,用 IGF-1 的数值评估生长激素的异常分泌通常更准确[64]。动态测试通常用于监测治疗效果,如口服糖耐量试验(OGTT),口服葡萄糖(75~100g),抽血测量服糖前后生长激素的数值,正常患者在服糖后生长激素分泌发生抑制,水平降至 1ng/ml 以下,如果服糖后未发生生长激素分泌抑制,可以诊断为生长激素腺瘤。一项对 92 名肢端肥大症患者的研究表明,生长激素的最低值在年龄和性别上都没有显著差异[65]。

尽管罕见,异位促生长素释放素也有报道,约占肢端肥大症的 1%。胸部或腹部的肿瘤通常可分泌异位 GHRH,导致 GH 过量。为避免不必要的手术,在临床和生化诊断后需要做影像学检查来确诊垂体腺瘤。

治疗

自 20 世纪 60 年代引入生长激素测定以来,肢端肥大症的治愈标准已被多次修正。目前,治愈的生化指标是基础生长激素水平低于 2.5ng/ml,IGF-1 恢复正常,OGTT 试验生长激素最低水平低于 1ng/ml[66]。一个彻底痊愈的概念应该能恢复正常的垂体功能,并且在大多数情况下,可以缓慢地逆转美容和生理上的异常。

经蝶入路手术仍是生长激素腺瘤的一线治疗方法[63]。手术的优势包括迅速降低生长激素水平和得到组织病理诊断。在我们的研究中心,对 115 名患者进行的 14 年回顾显示,单纯手术可使 61%的患者达到生化指标缓解[67],其中微腺瘤为 88%,大腺瘤为 53%。手术预后与肿瘤大小及术前生长激素水平呈负相关,术后即刻生长激素水平与远期预后相关,在术后生长激素水平低于 3ng/ml 的病例中,有 89%的患者长期预后较好。术后放疗 32 例,缓解率 31%。另有三名患者通过联合手术、放疗和药物治疗获得缓解。总体并发症发生率为 6.9%,无脑脊液漏、脑膜炎、永久性尿崩症及新发垂体功能减退,复发率为 5.4%。其他发表的研究也反映了类似的结果[68,69]。

放射治疗和放射外科治疗也都被用来治疗肢端肥大症。在 50%~70%的病例中,使用传统的外照射可以将生长激素水平降低到 5ng/ml 以下,但这种疗效可能需要长达 10 年才能显现[70]。放射治疗 10 年后,50%的患者开始出现垂体功能减退,此后的发病率逐年上升[71]。放射外科在3~5年内能使生长激素水平恢复正常[72],发生垂体功能减退的可能性也是相似的。并且,放射线对邻近敏感结构(如视交叉)的损伤仍然是个问题,一般建议对所有垂体腺瘤保留4mm的安全边界进行放射治疗。通常在经蝶手术失败后,把放射外科作为一种辅助治疗[68,73,74]。但手术成败的结果有些难以界定,因为治愈标准并不一致[57]。一些小样本研究中报道内分泌治愈率在0~96%,改善率在0~67%。在回顾的20项研究中,有6项没有提到他们的治愈标准,另14项中有11项使用了不同的治愈标准。而且,在这些关于放射外科治疗的研究中,患者同时使用生长抑素类似物的情况也不一致,导致进一步混淆了研究结果。目前对放射外科疗效的研究也缺乏长期的随访。因此还需要更多的随机研究。最近的一项回顾性研究接受辅助放射外科的患者,通过OGTT试验结果正常来定义内分泌治愈,发现65%的患者在61.5个月时达到缓解,并且在之后的时间观察点出现缓解增加的趋势[75]。尽管口服糖耐量正常化,但放射治疗后仍有一部分患者出现持续性IGF-1升高,显示为持续性垂体轴功能障碍和轻微的肢端肥大症的临床症状[76]。

药物治疗作为肢端肥大症的主要或辅助治疗仍有争议。如果患者没有视力缺损的症状,一些内分泌学家提倡使用生长抑素类似物作为一线治疗[77]。但是,由于肢端肥大症患者可能会引起相应的长期并发症,大多数医生建议手术作为一线治疗,如果再需要的话辅助药物或放射治疗。治疗肢端肥大症的药物有三类:多巴胺激动剂、生长抑素类似物和生长激素受体阻滞剂。多巴胺激动剂如溴隐亭和卡麦角林已被证实能缓解某些肢端肥大症患者的症状[78]。尽管这些药物疗效有限,但由于其低成本和口服给药,仍然是治疗肢端肥大症的常用药物。相比之下,生长抑素类似物更有效,奥曲肽能使大约50%的患者IGF-1恢复正常,并将生长激素水平降低到小于5ng/ml[79]。长效类似物如兰利肽和奥曲肽缓释剂则更有效,可以使70%的患者生长激素降至2.5ng/ml以下,88%的患者IGF-1恢复正常[80~82]。另一类治疗肢端肥大症的药物是生长激素受体拮抗剂,目前,培维索孟(pegvisomant)是该类药物中唯一获得FDA批准的药物。这类药物的独特之处在于作用部位不是垂体,而是生长激素受体。通过阻止生长激素受体的二聚化,培维索孟类药物抑制了IGF-1的产生,而IGF-1是导致肢端肥大症的主要激素。由于它不影响肿瘤大小或生长激素的产生,这种药物通常被用来处理其他方法难以治愈的肢端肥大症。该药物有显著的副作用,包括转氨酶肝炎和罕见的肿瘤增长[83],因此,建议服用此类药物的患者要监测肝功能,并常规复查磁共振。

药物治疗在控制生长激素过量的临床症状方面显示出良好的效果,可以缓解头痛和多汗症的症状,改善关节病和心功能。如果药物治疗能够使OGTT试验中IGF-1和GH水平恢复正常,患者左室射血分数会显著改善。因为值得注意的是,肢端肥大症患者往往也伴有左室射血分数恶化[84,85]。与泌乳素腺瘤不同,药物不能治愈肢端肥大症。虽然目前的药物治疗具有良好的耐受性和良好的疗效,但为了避免复发,仍需要终身治疗。这给药物治疗带来了严重的负面影响,因为治疗成功的先决条件是昂贵的费用和长期的依从性。正因为如此,许多医生和患者把药物治疗作为手术或放疗的辅助手段。生长抑素类似物的新辅助治疗在统计学上没有显著的受益[86]。

少数(20%~30%)生长激素分泌腺瘤也分泌泌乳素,也可能会出现闭经、溢乳、阳痿或性欲丧失等症状。多巴胺激动剂在治疗这种生长激素和泌乳素混合腺瘤方面特别有效,但经蝶手术仍然是一线治疗方法[87]。

促肾上腺皮质激素腺瘤

库欣病或"库欣综合征",是皮质醇增多症在临床上最常见的表现。促肾上腺皮质激素腺瘤刺激肾上腺增生并最终导致皮质醇增多症。许多人认为库欣病在诊断和治疗方面都是最具挑战性的垂体内分泌疾病。肿瘤通常很小,无法被影像学检查发现。大腺瘤常具有侵袭性,复发率高。人口统计学发现库欣病在女性中的发病率是男性的9倍,发病高峰出现在30~40岁。

临床表现

只有10%~20%的促肾上腺皮质激素腺瘤大到足以产生占位效应,从而出现视野缺损、脑神经病变或垂体功能减退。绝大多数肿瘤小于5mm,但皮质醇增高,临床表现包括向心性肥胖、满月脸、水牛背、多毛症、腹部皮肤紫纹和痤疮。其他临床表现包括高血压、骨质疏松、近端肌肉肌病、糖尿病,以及较常见的精神类疾病。有这些临床症状的患者发病率极高,如不治疗5年死亡率为50%[88]。由于体内皮质醇的增涨,导致了分泌型库欣病患者特有的高发病率和死亡率。临床皮质醇增高的持续时间、术前促肾上腺皮质激素水平和抑郁症被证实是与库欣病患死亡率显著相关的风险因素[89]。

诊断

库欣病的明确诊断依赖于同时有高皮质醇血症的内分泌证据和垂体病变的病理定性。结合以上全面检查,诊断准确率接近100%[90];但单凭某一个检查都有10%~30%的误诊可能(表79-1)[91]。

24h尿游离皮质醇和17-羟基糖皮质激素检查可显示皮质醇升高,午夜唾液皮质醇的检测对高皮质醇血症的敏感性和特异性也很好[92]。高皮质醇血症的病因应首先用低剂量地塞米松抑制试验进行评估,这项试验能评估下丘脑-垂体-肾上腺皮质醇分泌负反馈回路的功能。库欣病患者在应用低剂量地塞米松后,仍会有皮质醇持续升高,而当使用大剂量地塞米松时,95%的库欣病患者的血浆皮质醇会下降50%。血浆促肾上腺皮质激素水平的评估,用以鉴别库欣病和肾上腺原因导致的高皮质醇血症[93]。如果能做促肾上腺皮质激素释放激素(CRH)刺激试验,可以进一步提高对库欣病诊断的敏感性[94]。最后,如果之前的检查结果仍不能确诊,可以进行岩下窦采样检验(IPSS)以提高诊断的特异性。对于直径大于3mm的肿瘤,磁共振是一项敏感的定位诊断检查,虽然有很高比例的肿瘤常规序列无法检测出[95],但通过优化后T1序列增强扫描或利用扰相梯度回波序列(SPGR),可以侦测到更多的肿瘤[95,96]。IPSS和海绵窦采样检查在这些情况下是有帮助的,因为它们可以确认垂体病理,但也有25%~30%偏移误差[97]。

表 79-1 库欣综合征的生化学评估

A. 库欣综合征的筛查
1. 在两个或三个样本中测量 24h UFC。如果在两或三个样本中皮质醇水平是正常值的四倍，那么可以明确是高皮质醇血症。如果结果不明确，继续进行低剂量的 DST。唾液皮质醇水平也具有高度的敏感性和特异性
2. 低剂量 DST。1mg 地塞米松在下午 11 点给药，第二天早上 8 点取血清皮质醇，试验通常需要 2 天
如果<5μg/dl：排除库欣综合征
如果 5~10μg/dl：不确定，需要重新测试
如果>10μg/dl：很可能是库欣综合征
B. 原发性库欣病与异位或肾上腺肿瘤的鉴别试验
1. 肾上腺肿瘤患者血清 ACTH 水平较低。血浆 ACTH（大于 10pg/ml 表示 ACTH 依赖性疾病；小于 5pg/ml 表示 ACTH 非依赖性疾病）
腹部 CT 可帮助鉴别 ACTH 依赖性的单侧肾上腺肿块或双侧肾上腺增大
2. 大剂量 DST。8mg 地塞米松在下午 11 点开始，第二天早上 8 点抽取血清皮质醇，试验通常也需要 2 天
95%的库欣病患者血浆皮质醇抑制率为 50%
异位或肾上腺来源的患者则未见抑制
3. CRH 刺激试验。可在高剂量 DST 不确定时使用
库欣病对 CRH 有反应，血浆皮质醇水平进一步升高
异位和肾上腺肿瘤对 CRH 无反应
4. IPSS 在反复检测仍不能确诊的患者，及之前没做过 IPSS 需再次手术的患者中应用
CRH 给药后，岩下窦/血浆 ACTH 梯度>3∶1提示库欣病以及提示病变侧别

DST，地塞米松抑制试验；UFC，尿游离皮质醇；CRH，促肾上腺皮质激素释放激素；IPSS，岩下窦采样检验。

治疗

经蝶入路手术是库欣病的一线治疗方法。术后总缓解率为 76%~91%[98]。微腺瘤预后稍好，缓解率在 84%~94%[98]，手术成功的主要决定因素是在磁共振上能否准确定位肿瘤[99]。而不同的是，大腺瘤的手术缓解率似乎主要取决于肿瘤侵袭的程度。回顾研究表明 64%的患者仅通过手术就能得到缓解，而结合辅助放疗或放射外科治疗，缓解率分别提高到 83%和 70%[98,100]。

虽然每个患者的术后过程有所不同，但成功切除肿瘤的患者，其血清皮质醇和 ACTH 水平能够快速下降，这可能会引发危及生命的低皮质醇症（艾迪森危象）。大多数患者需要长达 1 年的激素替代治疗，使他们的下丘脑-垂体-肾上腺轴从慢性 ACTH 过度刺激中恢复。术后缓解良好的预后因素包括血浆皮质醇和 ACTH 低于正常水平。但在血清皮质醇水平立即改善的患者中，仍有 15%~25%会复发[21,101]。根据我们的经验，即使皮质醇正常，地塞米松抑制试验反应正常，也不能保证长期缓解。因此，长期随访对这些患者至关重要。

在手术切除不完全时，放射治疗和放射外科治疗常作为辅助治疗。常规放射治疗的 5 年治愈率高达 90%[102]。然而，这些患者中的很大一部分在晚年开始出现垂体功能减退，5%发展为 Nelson 综合征[102]。传统的放射治疗并不是首要的治疗手段，主要是因为治疗的效果需要几年的时间才能显现出来，而且库欣病的症状和危险会持续存在。相对而言，放射外科治疗库欣病的效果要快得多。能有 35%~90%的患者达到缓解，而垂体功能减退的发生率较低[103,104]。但对这些数据的全面解释较为复杂，因为构成“治愈”的因素存在差异，而且缺乏长期随访。

虽然不推荐将药物治疗作为库欣病的主要治疗方法，但药物治疗可能适用于术后没有改善或不适合手术的患者。2012 年，美国食品药品管理局（FDA）批准了帕西罗肽作为药物治疗的适应证。帕西罗肽是一种生长抑素类似物，对生长抑素受体 5 具有高度特异性，已被证明在降低皮质醇水平方面具有临床疗效，应被视为治疗库欣病的首选药物[105]。此外，化疗可以在等待手术期暂缓皮质醇增多症的严重症状。在这方面酮康唑通常是首选药物，因为它可以阻断肾上腺类固醇的合成。高达 90%的患者服用酮康唑后血浆皮质醇和 ACTH 恢复正常。但这类药物在停药后药效会立即停止，并且服药期间必须密切监测它的肝毒性[106]。其他治疗库欣病的药物包括氨基谷氨酰胺、甲吡酮、米托坦和赛庚啶。多巴胺激动剂如卡麦角林在治疗促肾上腺皮质激素腺瘤方面也显示了一定的疗效。卡麦角林治疗 3 个月后，60%的患者出现皮质醇抑制，40%的患者皮质醇恢复正常。这一点可以解释之前大多数促肾上腺皮质激素腺瘤的多巴胺受体（D2）免疫染色阳性的发现[107]。

对上述治疗效果不佳的患者，可以选择更激进的手术方案。肾上腺全切除术可以完全控制皮质醇的分泌，但需要终身依赖外源性糖皮质激素和盐皮质激素替代。Nelson 综合征是一种由于皮质醇负反馈抑制丧失而导致垂体腺瘤迅速扩大的疾病，其发生率为 10%~30%[108]。Nelson 综合征典型表现为促肾上腺皮质激素升高刺激黑色素细胞引起的色素沉着。大多数 Nelson 综合征患者都发展为巨大的侵袭性垂体腺瘤。神经外科治疗 Nelson 综合征的有效性的研究表明，各组所报道的成功率的数据范围很大[109~111]。在行肾上腺切除术前，对垂体进行放射外科治疗预防 Nelson 综合征似乎有一定的价值[112]。

如果术后促肾上腺皮质激素和皮质醇水平仍然升高，对垂体的进一步探查通常是有效的[113]。为了增加第二次手术的成功率，术前应做 IPSS。如果先前治疗均不成功的患者，可以考虑进行完整的垂体腺体切除术，但真正提及的极少。

静止期垂体 ACTH 腺瘤

垂体腺瘤有一个亚型，免疫组化染色提示会产生 ACTH，但患者没有高皮质醇血症的临床证据。这种情况的准确发生率尚不清楚，但据报道在 6%~43%[114]。有证据表明，这些肿瘤比其他促肾上腺皮质激腺瘤更具侵袭性，复发率为 37%[115,116]。然而，与 ACTH 阴性的无功能垂体腺瘤相比，这些肿瘤的复发率相似[117]。此类肿瘤患者有部分也会在术后出现下丘脑-垂体-肾上腺轴功能障碍，需要术后类固醇替代[114]。

促性腺激素和无功能垂体腺瘤

大约 1/3 的垂体瘤是无功能腺瘤。发病率高峰出现在

40~50 岁，患者通常表现为垂体功能减退症状、视野缺损和视力问题。尽管它们的临床表现相似，但这些肿瘤的病理构成有异质性。超微结构检查经常显示有分泌颗粒，染色提示可能分泌 FH、LSH 和 α 亚基。更小的一组亚群中，肿瘤可能产生其他垂体前叶分泌的激素但无临床表现[118]。由于这组肿瘤的异质性，没有明确或一致的治疗或预后评估。

临床表现

由于肿瘤无激素的异常分泌，这些患者通常表现为肿块的占位效应症状。这可以从垂体功能减退到视力改变或头痛。大多数病例表现为大腺瘤。

治疗

手术仍是无功能腺瘤的主要治疗方法。手术目的是减轻占位效应，恢复垂体功能，并获得组织病理诊断。同其他垂体腺瘤一样，经蝶入路通常是首选，除非有明显的鞍外扩展。由于没有明确的治愈标准，相较其他类型肿瘤，手术疗效难以评估。很多患者表示术前的症状在术后有所改善，70%~80% 的患者视觉功能显著改善[119]，近 100% 的患者头痛症状能改善[120]，15%~57% 的患者垂体功能改善[119]。然而，这些改善主要是由于减瘤术后占位效应的缓解，并不能代表肿瘤被根治。由于术后早期的影像常常会因水肿或其他正常的术后改变所混淆，切除范围通常需术后 3~4 个月行磁共振检查来评估。66%~86% 的患者中会发现残余肿瘤，但各文献报道的复发率不同且差别较大[121,122]。

放射治疗或放射外科越来越多地用于无功能腺瘤的初治或辅助治疗。最近的一项多中心研究分析了放射外科治疗残存病灶的安全性和有效性，发现随访过程中肿瘤的总体控制率超过 90%，且副作用发生率较低[123]。同组后续研究将放射外科作为不适合手术的患者的主要治疗方式，他们发现患者的 10 年肿瘤控制率为 85%，24% 的患者出现新的或加重的垂体功能减退[124]。由于放射线对垂体的危害，许多临床医生主张只对术后随访的影像表现为持续增长的肿瘤进行放射治疗[125,126]。对这些肿瘤的病程研究表明，年轻患者和 61 岁或以上患者的肿瘤生长模式及增殖指数（MIB-1）存在差异[127]。对于老年患者，肿瘤的倍增时间明显更长，表明了对老年患者可能并不总是需要辅助治疗。

此外，药物治疗对这类肿瘤的疗效有限。在一项对 9 例无功能腺瘤患者应用卡麦角林治疗 1 年的研究中，67% 的肿瘤有多巴胺受体的表达，但只有 56% 的患者表现出对卡麦角林有反应[128]，这其中仅在两名患者的疗效具有临床意义。其他药物如溴隐亭、其他多巴胺激动剂、奥曲肽和 GnRH 激动剂或拮抗剂也已被使用，但结果不好。

垂体促甲状腺素腺瘤

促甲状腺素腺瘤是垂体瘤中最少见的一种，仅占 1%~2%[129]。

临床表现

患者表现出甲状腺功能亢进的症状和体征，如不耐热、腹泻、视力改变、体重减轻、震颤、疲劳和眼球突出。这常导致患者在早期诊断为格雷夫斯病（Graves disease）。因此，促甲状腺素腺瘤患者通常在发病后期，肿瘤较大且有局部侵袭性时才被诊断。所以，他们也可能有肿瘤占位效应的相关症状，如头痛、视力改变和垂体功能减退[130]。

诊断

不管 T3 和游离 T4 是否升高，大多数促甲状腺素腺瘤的 TSH 水平都会升高。随着 α 亚基/TSH 比值的增加，诊断的敏感性也增加。最后，超灵敏的 TSH 免疫测定可以区分原发性甲状腺功能亢进和中枢性甲状腺功能减退以及甲状腺素抵抗的患者。

治疗

甲状腺功能亢进由于对心率和心功能的影响使其具有很高的麻醉和手术风险。因此，术前控制甲状腺功能亢进的治疗是必不可少的。常用药物是贝塔受体阻断剂，如非急诊手术，也可以添加抗甲状腺药物（丙硫氧嘧啶或甲巯咪唑）。经蝶手术是这类肿瘤的主要治疗方法，但缓解率较低（35%~62%）。联合辅助药物治疗或放射治疗，缓解率增加到 55%~81%[131~134]。目前尚没有确立的缓解标准，通常以甲状腺功能亢进临床症状的缓解作为缓解指标。放射治疗虽然不能作为一线治疗，但对单独手术不能获得临床缓解的患者可以使用外照射。

奥曲肽在 92% 的病例中具有临床疗效，能使大多数患者的 TSH 恢复正常，并使肿瘤缩小[135]。尽管奥曲肽作为辅助药物有效，但其长期服药的巨大成本，以及对持续服药依从性的要求，使得奥曲肽很难被采纳为主要的治疗方式。最近的报道表明，一种长效的奥曲肽类似物兰诺肽，在避免奥曲肽的某些缺点的同时，可能也有类似的功效。

结论

垂体腺瘤是一组异质性肿瘤，需要针对其病理学分型进行治疗。经蝶手术仍然是最常见的治疗措施，而药物和放射治疗在长期控制疾病中发挥着重要作用。随着我们对分子生物学、药物开发和放射外科等领域的不断发展，毫无疑问，患者的临床预后和满意度将进一步提高。

总结

垂体肿瘤起源于腺垂体，可根据细胞类型和影像学表现进行分类。经蝶手术是除泌乳素腺瘤外所有腺瘤的首选治疗方法，泌乳素腺瘤的主要治疗方法是药物治疗。激素特异性药物治疗和放疗已被证明对许多肿瘤亚型有临床疗效。预后在很大程度上取决于激素的控制，因为激素分泌过量导致的全身效应往往比肿瘤的占位效应更严重。遗传学及其肿瘤生物学的研究进展，为未来垂体肿瘤的治疗带来了许多有希望的靶点。

（钱海鹏　译　万经海　校）

参考文献

The complete reference list can be found on the Wiley Companion Digital Edition of this title (see inside front cover for login instructions).

4 Kovacs K, Horvath E, Vidal S. Classification of pituitary adenomas. *J Neurooncol*. 2001;**54**:121.

7 Knosp E, Steiner E, Klaus K, Matula C. Pituitary adenomas with invasion of the cavernous sinus space: imaging classification compared with surgical findings. *Neurosurgery*. 1993;**33(4)**:610.

10 Yu R, Melmed S. Oncogene activation in pituitary tumors. *Brain Pathol*. 2001;**11**:328.

15 Mete O, Ezzat S, Asa SL. Biomarkers of aggressive pituitary adenomas. *J Mol Endocrinol*. 2012;**49**:R69.

18 Salehi F, Agur A, Scheithauer BW, Kovacs K, Lloyd RV, Cusimano M. Biomarkers of pituitary neoplasms: a review. *Neurosurgery*. 2010;**67**:1790.

22 Syro LV, Builes CE, Di Leva A, Sav A, Rotondo F, Kovacs K. Improving differential diagnosis of pituitary adenomas. *Expert Rev Endocrinol Metab*. 2014;**9(4)**:377.

25 Syro LV, Ortiz LD, Scheithauer BW, et al. Treatment of pituitary neoplasms with temozolomide: a review. *Cancer*. 2011;**117**:454.

26 McCormack A, Kaplan W, Gill AJ, et al. MGMT expression and pituitary tumors: relationship to tumor biology. *Pituitary*. 2013;**16**:208.

43 Kharlip J, Salvatori R, Yenokyan G, Wand GS. Recurrence of hyperprolactinemia after withdrawal of long-term cabergoline therapy. *J Clin Endocrinol Metab*. 2009;**94(7)**:2428.

44 Boquszewski CL, dos Santos CM, Sakamoto KS, Marini LC, de Souza AM, Azevedo M. A comparison of cabergoline and bromocriptine on the risk of valvular heart disease in patients with prolactinomas. *Pituitary*. 2012;**15**:44.

50 Maiter D, Delgrange E. The challenges in managing giant prolactinomas. *Eur J Endocrinol*. 2014;**170**:R213.

53 Vroonen L, Jaffrain-Rea ML, Petrossians P, et al. Prolactinomas resistant to standard doses of cabergoline: a multicenter study of 92 patients. *Eur J Endocrinol*. 2012;**167**:651.

58 Bloomgarden E, Molitch ME. Surgical treatment of prolactinomas: cons. *Endocrine*. 2014. PMID: 25112227.

59 Molitch ME. Pregnancy and the hyperprolactinemic woman. *N Engl J Med*. 1985;**312**:1364.

63 Melmed S, Casanueva FF, Cavagnini F, et al. Guidelines for acromegaly management. *J Clin Endocrinol Metab*. 2002;**87**:4054.

67 Freda PU, Wardlaw SL, Post KD. Long-term endocrinological follow-up evaluation in 115 patients who underwent transsphenoidal surgery for acromegaly. *J Neurosurg*. 1998;**89**:353.

76 Elias PCL, Lugao HB, Pereira MC, Machado HR, de Castro M, Moreira AC. Discordant nadir GH after oral glucose and IGF-1 levels on treated acromegaly: refining the biochemical markers of mild disease activity. *Horm Metab Res*. 2010; **42**:50.

82 Ayuk J, Stewart SE, Stewart PM, Sheppard MC. Long-term safety and efficacy of depot long-acting somatostatin analogs for the treatment of acromegaly. *J Clin Endocrinol Metab*. 2002;**87**:4142.

83 Van der Lely AJ, Hutson RK, Trainer PJ, et al. Long-term treatment of acromegaly with pegvisomant, a growth hormone receptor antagonist. *Lancet*. 2001;**358**:1754.

85 Colao A, Cuocolo A, Marzullo P, et al. Is the acromegalic cardiomyopathy reversible? Effect fo 5-year normalization of growth hormone and insulin-like growth factor I levels on cardiac performance. *J Clin Endocrinol Metab*. 2001;**86**:1551.

86 Fougner SL, Bollerslev J, Svartberg J, Oksnes M, Cooper J, Carlsen SM. Pre-operative octreotide treatment of acromegaly: long-term results of a randomized controlled trial. *Eur J Endocrinol*. 2014;**171**:229.

87 Freda PU, Reyes CM, Nuruzzaman AT, Sundeen RE, Khandji AG, Post KD. Cabergoline therapy of growth hormone & growth hormone/prolactin secreting tumors. *Pituitary*. 2004;7:21.

89 Lambert JK, Goldberg L, Fayngold S, Kostadinov J, Post KD, Geer EB. Predictors of mortality and long-term outcomes in treated Cushing's disease: a study of 346 patients. *J Clin Endocrinol Metab*. 2013;**98**:1022.

96 Chowdhury IF, Sinaii N, Oldfield EH, Patronas N, Nieman LK. A change in pituitary magnetic resonance imaging protocols detects ACTH-secreting tumours in patients with previously negative results. *Clin Endocrinol*. 2010;**72**:502.

100 Sheehan JP, Xu Z, Salvetti DJ, Schmitt PJ, Vance ML. Results of gamma knife surgery for Cushing's disease. *J Neurosurg*. 2013;**119**:1486.

101 Bochicchio D, Losa M, Buchfelder M. Factors influencing the immediate and late outcome of Cushi'g's disease treated by transsphenoidal surgery: a retrospective study by the European Cushing's Disease Survey Group. *J Clin Endocrinol Metab*. 1995;**80**:3114.

104 Sheehan JM, Vance ML, Sheehan JP, Ellegala DB, Laws ER Jr. Radiosurgery for Cushing's disease after failed transsphenoidal surgery. *J Neurosurg*. 2000;**93**:738.

105 Colao A, Petersenn S, Newell-Price J, et al. A 12-month phase 3 study of pasireotide in Cushing's disease. *N Eng J Med*. 2012;**366(10)**:914.

107 Pivonello R, Ferone D, de Herder WW, et al. Dopamine receptor expression and function in corticotroph pituitary tumors. *J Clin Endocrinol Metab*. 2004;**89**:2452.

112 Mehta GU, Sheehan JP, Vance ML. Effect of stereotactic radiosurgery before bilateral adrenalectomy for Cushing's disease on the incidence of Nelson's syndrome. *J Neurosurg*. 2013;**119**:1493.

117 Ioachimescu AG, Eiland L, Chhabra VS, et al. Silent corticotroph adenomas: Emory University cohort and comparison with ACTH-negative nonfunctioning pituitary adenomas. *Neurosurgery*. 2012;**71**:296.

118 Black PM, Hsu DW, Klibanski A, et al. Hormone production in clinically nonfunctioning pituitary adenomas. *J Neurosurg*. 1987;**66**:244.

122 Colao A, Cerbone G, Cappabianca P, et al. Effect of surgery and radiotherapy on visual and endocrine function in nonfunctioning pituitary adenomas. *J Endocrinol Invest*. 1998;**21**:284.

123 Sheehan JP, Starke RM, Mathieu D, et al. Gamma knife radiosurgery for the management of nonfunctioning pituitary adenomas: a multicenter study. *J Neurosurg*. 2013;**119**:446.

124 Lee C, Kano H, Yang H, et al. Initial gamma knife radiosurgery for nonfunctioning pituitary adenomas. *J Neurosurg*. 2014;**120**:647.

128 Pivonello R, Matrone C, Filippella M, et al. Dopamine receptor expression and function in clinically nonfunctioning pituitary tumors: comparison with the effectiveness of cabergoline treatment. *J Clin Endocrinol Metab*. 2004;**89**:1674.

134 Malchiodi E, Profka E, Ferrante E, et al. Thyrotropin-secreting pituitary adenomas: outcome of pituitary surgery and irradiation. *J Clin Endocrinol Metab*. 2014;**99**:2069.

136 Schade R, Andersohn F, Suizza S, Haverhamp W, Garbe E. Dopamine agonists and the risk of cardiac-valve regurgitation. *N Eng J Med*. 2007;**356**:29.

第 80 章　甲状腺肿瘤

Steven I. Sherman, MD ■ Maria E. Cabanillas, MD ■ Stephen Y. Lai, MD, PhD

概述

甲状腺肿瘤，通常为甲状腺乳头状癌，近年来的发病率逐年上升，但是死亡危险程度较低。确诊甲状腺肿物的最佳方法主要依靠超声性质和对具有可疑恶性风险的病灶进行针吸细胞学检查。鉴于缺乏前瞻性研究，分化型甲状腺癌的最佳初始治疗策略仍存在争议，包括甲状腺切除范围和颈部清扫范围以及是否行放射性碘同位素治疗。甲状腺髓样癌患者应该首先接受全甲状腺切除术、中央区淋巴结清扫，必要时行侧颈淋巴结清扫，并进行早期评估以区分散发性髓样癌和家族遗传性髓样癌。近年来靶向治疗的最新进展显示多种抗血管生成药物可用于治疗进展期转移性分化型甲状腺癌或甲状腺髓样癌，可显著延长无进展生存期，但改善总体生存率的证据不足。与此形成鲜明对比的是，甲状腺未分化癌仍然是最具侵袭性的恶性肿瘤之一，即使通过手术、放疗和化疗的多学科综合治疗模式，获得的治疗益处有限且通常是姑息性的。

历史回顾

历史上，甲状腺肿瘤并不是一个常见病，但是随着世界范围内发病率逐年上升，已经成为最常见的恶性肿瘤之一。尽管大多数患者仅需要局部治疗，但随着靶向治疗的出现，晚期甲状腺癌的治疗已经得到改善。即使是首次治疗的方案在逐渐变化，人们逐渐认识到相对保守的治疗方法可达到有效的治疗。

发病率和流行病学-美国和全球

2015 年，美国约有 62 450 人被诊断患有甲状腺癌，与疾病相关的死亡率接近 2 000 例[1]。在全球范围内，发病率增加了 6 倍，而疾病相关死亡率则增加了约 20 倍[2]。女性发病率大约是男性的两倍，在韩国甲状腺癌是女性的主要恶性肿瘤。新发的病例主要是局限于腺体内的微小癌，与甲状腺超声筛查的增多有关，且与社会经济地位提高和“过度诊断”有关[3]。

源自产生激素的滤泡上皮细胞的分化型甲状腺癌（DTC）占甲状腺癌的 96%，包括乳头状甲状腺癌（PTC），滤泡性甲状腺癌（FTC）和嗜酸性癌（分别占 88%、6%、2%）[4]。另外 2% 是来自神经内分泌“C”细胞的甲状腺髓样癌（MTC），其余 1% 是低分化甲状腺癌（PDTC）以及高度侵袭性、未分化型甲状腺癌。

危险因素-遗传，行为和环境

分化型甲状腺癌的病因尚不明确，已知最明确的危险因素是辐射暴露，特别是在儿童期和青春期。在 0.1～10Gy 的辐射暴露之间，相对风险为 7.7/Gy，20 岁后暴露时，每 10Gy 风险上升一个水平[5]。肥胖也与 DTC 的发病有相关性（相对风险约为 1.3）[6]。碘缺乏与甲状腺滤泡癌发病升高有关，并可能导致甲状腺未分化癌[7]。分化型甲状腺癌是某些遗传综合征的表现之一，包括家族性腺瘤性息肉病、Cowden 综合征和 Carney 综合征[8,9]。家族性非髓样癌表现为家族中至少两个一级亲属发病，据报道约占所有乳头状癌患者的 5%，目前基因位点和机制尚不清楚[10]。遗传性甲状腺髓样癌综合征，包括多发内分泌肿瘤（MEN）2A 型和 MEN2B 亚型，占所有甲状腺髓样癌病例的 25%。尚未发现环境因素会影响 MTC 的发生[11]。

预防

除了在核事故时使用碘化钾预防，或者在外辐射时屏蔽保护甲状腺，目前尚没有预防分化型甲状腺癌发生的方法[12]。对遗传性 MTC 高风险儿童进行前瞻性筛查后进行甲状腺切除术可预防髓样癌的发生[13]。

病理

经典的甲状腺乳头状癌的特征具有由肿瘤细胞包围的纤维血管核心的乳头状结构，细胞核大而呈椭圆形，通常重叠，其包含低密度粉末样染色质、细胞质假包含体和核沟（图 80-1）。滤泡亚型约占 PTC 的 10%，具有 PTC 的核型特征，但形态呈滤泡状而不是乳头状。相对罕见的高细胞亚型是一种更具侵袭性的甲状腺乳头状癌，其特征是肿瘤细胞呈嗜酸性特征，高度是宽度的两倍。原发性肿瘤较大，侵袭性更强且经常发生转移。

甲状腺滤泡癌与滤泡性腺瘤的区别是侵袭性，滤泡癌通常沿着包膜或者血管内皮质出现一个或多个的浸润灶。根据浸润程度将甲状腺滤泡癌分为微小侵袭和广泛侵袭两种，微小侵袭的滤泡状癌只有散在包膜浸润或血管侵袭灶。细胞学不能可靠地区分滤泡病变的良恶性。嗜酸性（或 Hürthle 细胞）肿瘤由含有大量线粒体的细胞组成，因此具有颗粒状、嗜酸性粒细胞质的特征[14]。大多数嗜酸性肿瘤具有滤泡结构，因具有侵袭性而被诊断为癌。

通常认为分化差的甲状腺癌是介于分化型甲状腺癌和未分化癌中间的类型，表现出部分去分化状态。细胞倾向于以实性岛状结构形成细胞巢，没有甲状腺乳头状癌的核特征。诊断标准还包括：①形态复杂的核；②肿瘤坏死；或③每高倍视野至少三个有丝分裂象[15]。甲状腺未分化癌通常表现为肉眼下向周围组织广泛浸润，显微镜下肿瘤表现为异质性，多型性核，呈梭

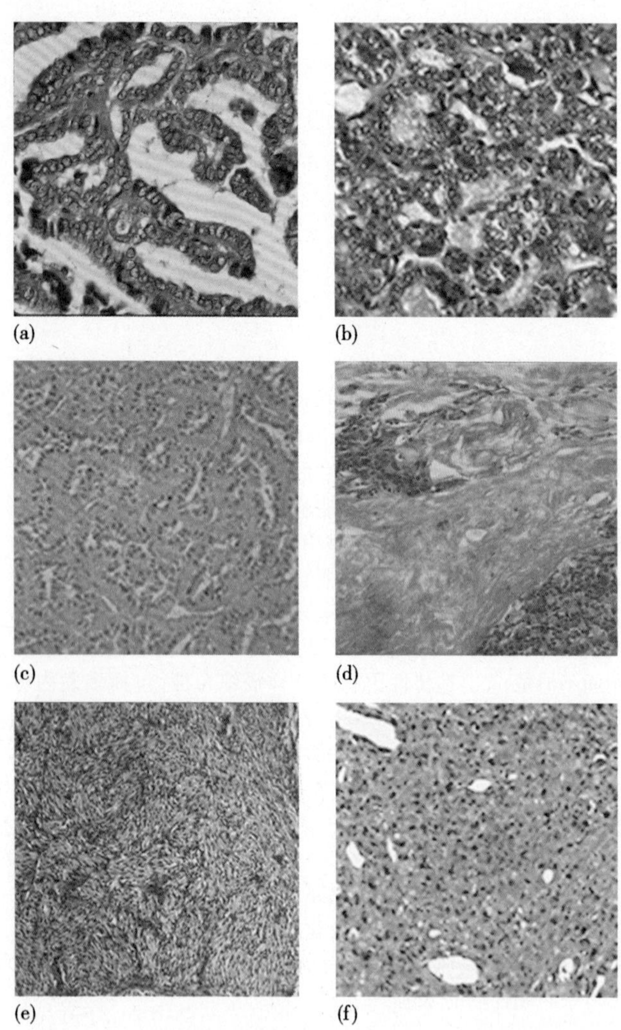

图 80-1　分化型甲状腺癌的病理特点。(a)乳头状癌：具有特征性的纤维血管乳头形成、拥挤的细胞核和核沟。(b)乳头状癌的滤泡亚型：形成的滤泡中有典型的乳头状癌细胞的核特征。(c)乳头状癌的高细胞亚型：细胞的高度是宽度的两倍，具有嗜酸性粒细胞质。(d)滤泡癌：显示肿瘤穿过厚包膜侵入邻近的甲状腺。(e)甲状腺髓样癌：呈现梭形细胞巢。这种巢通常以圆形卵圆形细胞簇而散布在。(f)未分化癌：大且分散的多形性肿瘤细胞。资料来源：Michelle D. Williams M. D. 提供

形片状，有上皮样细胞或巨细胞，大量坏死区域和广泛的炎性浸润。甲状腺乳头状癌，甲状腺滤泡癌甚至分化差的甲状腺癌通常呈现出甲状腺球蛋白(Tg)和其他滤泡细胞特异性抗原染色阳性，甲状腺未分化癌只有细胞角蛋白和 PAX8 染色阳性[16]。

MTC 通常由纤维血管基质包围的片状或巢状圆形或纺锤形神经内分泌细胞组成。细胞核表现有斑点染色质，细胞质通常呈颗粒状和嗜酸性。基质内的淀粉样蛋白沉积是其特异性的特征。甲状腺髓样癌通常可检测降钙素和神经内分泌免疫组化标记物。遗传性综合征中的甲状腺髓样癌起源于 C 细胞增生。

病理和自然病程

分子病理

与甲状腺乳头状癌相关的癌基因包括 *BRAF* 突变(62%)，*RAS*(13%)和 *RET/PTC* 染色体重排(7%)，均位于丝裂原活化蛋白(MAP)激酶的上游[17]。*BRAF* 突变是在经典型甲状腺乳头状癌和高细胞亚型中最常见的突变。在甲状腺乳头状癌滤泡亚型和甲状腺滤泡癌的滤泡变体中可见 *RAS* 突变。综合分析基因组、转录组、表观遗传组和小 RNA 的变化可以较明确地界定 *BRAF* 突变型和 *RAS* 突变型[17]。在甲状腺滤泡癌中，染色体重排导致甲状腺特异性转录因子与过氧化物酶体增殖物激活受体 γ-1 融合形成 *PAX8-PPARγ* 原癌基因[18]。在分化差的甲状腺癌和甲状腺未分化癌(可能来自预先存在的分化型甲状腺癌)中，共存突变更常见，包括 *RAS*、*BRAF*、*TP53*、*CTNNB1*、*PIK3CA* 和 *PTEN* 突变以及杂合性缺失。导致分化型甲状腺癌进展的其他因素包括细胞内激酶过表达、脱氧核糖核酸高甲基化和组蛋白脱乙酰化导致肿瘤抑制基因沉默，以及细胞周期失调[17,19]。

酪氨酸激酶受体 *RET* 的外显子 8，10，11 和 13~16 的突变几乎发生在所有遗传性甲状腺髓样癌的家族中。在 40%~50% 的散发性甲状腺髓样癌中也发现了体细胞突变，特别是与较差预后相关的高活化密码子 918 突变[20]。基因型和表型的强相关性允许以突变分层来预测疾病侵袭性[21]。在缺乏 *RET* 突变的散发性髓样癌中，有 20%~70%具有 *RAS* 突变。

筛查

遗传性 MTC 中的 *RET* 突变以常染色体显性遗传方式遗传，通常具有较高的外显率。约 6%散发性 MTC 的患者中携带胚系 *RET* 突变，从而被鉴定为新的遗传家族[22]。应对所有临床上表现为散发性甲状腺髓样癌的患者进行遗传咨询和 *RET* 原癌基因突变检测，包括对已知遗传家族的儿童和成人进行筛查[21,23]。在散发性 MTC 的患者中，*RET* 胚系突变的假阴性率小于 1%，如果家族史提示常染色体遗传性疾病，可以考虑 *RET* 基因测序，并且应该对该家族的成员进行临床和生物化学筛选以寻找潜在的髓样癌。对于家族性腺瘤性息肉病或 Cowden 综合征患者，乳头状癌的患病风险较高，建议进行年度检查和甲状腺超声检查[24]。

诊断

大约 5%的人有可触及的甲状腺结节，触诊无结节的患者通过超声检查约有一半可发现甲状腺结节，只有 5%的结节是恶性的[25,26]。大多数是无症状的，临床症状很少是恶性肿瘤的特征之一。超声判断恶性的标准包括微钙化、边缘不规则、纵横比大于 1[27]。有 1%~2%甲状腺结节可见于氟脱氧葡萄糖-正电子发射断层扫描(FDG-PET)检查时，其中是恶性肿瘤的比例为 40%[28]。细针穿刺活检(FNA)适用于单个直径大于 1cm 的结节。当有多个结节时，可对可疑恶性的结节(如果没有可疑的，选最大的结节)进行细针穿刺[29]。根据细胞学标准易于诊断乳头状癌，髓样癌和未分化癌[30]。细针穿刺的假阳性率和假阴性率均小于 5%。然而，由于滤泡癌(以及乳头状癌的滤泡亚型)具有不同于良性滤泡性肿瘤的突破包膜或侵入血管壁的特征，这些结节通常在细胞学报告上表现为不确定的滤泡病变或肿瘤，此类型细胞学报告的总体恶性率为 20%[30,31]。通过基因检测可以将这种细胞学中间类型的总恶变风险降低到 5%。尽管不常在细胞学不确定的结节检测 *BRAF* 突变，但 *BRAF* 突变具有较高的阳性预测价值[32~35]。随机血清降钙素水平>100pg/ml 对诊断髓样癌具有很高价值，但不推荐用于甲状腺结节的初始

评估。一旦怀疑有恶性肿瘤,建议在手术前对颈部的淋巴结进行超声检查;计算机断层扫描(CT)或磁共振成像(MRI)可对侵袭性或者巨大的甲状腺肿瘤手术计划制订提供一定帮助。

患有侵袭性甲状腺癌的患者,特别是分化差的甲状腺癌和甲状腺未分化癌,通常伴有广泛的局部侵袭和远处转移[36]。肺和胸膜是远处转移的最常见部位,可见于高达 90%的远处转移患者中,其次是骨骼、大脑、皮肤、肝脏和肾脏。颈部和纵隔的 CT 可以准确地确定甲状腺肿瘤的范围,并能识别肿瘤是否侵犯大血管和上呼吸消化道。有必要评估是否发生远处转移,但不应延误治疗[37]。

一半的 MTC 患者初诊时可见颈部淋巴结转移。在散发性髓样癌中有多达 15%的患者出现压迫或侵犯上呼吸消化道的症状。最常见的远处转移是肝脏转移。肿瘤过度分泌降钙素,偶尔也分泌其他肽类物质和生物胺如促肾上腺皮质激素或降钙素基因相关肽,可导致许多患者出现不明原因的腹泻或库欣综合征。

TNM 分级分期

推荐第 7 版美国癌症联合委员会(AJCC)/UICC(国际抗癌联盟)分期系统用于标准临床病理分期和甲状腺癌死亡风险评估(表 80-1)[21,37,38,40]。然而,有学者担心该分期系统可能会高估微小癌的风险并低估年轻分化型甲状腺患者的风险[41,42]。有重要预后价值的甲状腺癌组织学亚型也没有包括在其中。在完成初始治疗后,一些其他的评估方法可以更好地预测 DTC 复发的风险[40,43,44]。

表 80-1 TNM 分期:美国癌症联合委员会(AJCC)甲状腺癌分期(第 7 版)

T:肿瘤大小			
T0	无原发肿瘤		
T1a	肿瘤≤1cm,无腺体外侵犯		
T1b	肿瘤最大直径>1cm 但≤2cm,无腺体外侵犯		
T2	肿瘤最大直径>2cm 但≤4cm,无腺体外侵犯		
T3	肿瘤最大直径>4cm 且局限于腺体内或		
	任何大小有腺体外微小侵犯(如侵犯到带状肌或甲状腺旁软组织)		
T4a	任何大小,突破甲状腺被膜外并侵犯皮下软组织,喉,气管,食管或喉返神经		
T4b	任何大小,侵犯椎前筋膜或包绕颈总动脉或纵隔血管		
Tx	肿瘤状态未知		
N:区域淋巴结			
N0	无淋巴结转移		
N1a	转移到Ⅵ区淋巴结(气管前、气管旁、喉前/Delphian 淋巴结)		
N1b	转移到同侧、双侧或对侧侧颈部淋巴结(Ⅱ、Ⅲ、Ⅳ、Ⅴ区)或咽后或上纵隔(Ⅶ区)		
Nx	淋巴结状态未知		
M:远处转移			
M0	无远处转移		
M1	远处转移		
Mx	远处转移状态未知		
		<45 岁	≥45 岁
分期:分化型甲状腺癌			
Ⅰ期		任何 T,任何 N,M0	T1,N0,M0
Ⅱ期		任何 T,任何 N,M1	T2,N0,M0
Ⅲ期			T3,N0,M0
			T1~3,N1a,M0
Ⅳ期			A:T4a,任何 N,M0
			任何 T,N1b,M0
			B:T4b,任何 N,M0
			C:任何 T,任何 N,M1
分期:甲状腺髓样癌			
Ⅰ期		T1,N0,M0	
Ⅱ期		T2~3,N0,M0	
Ⅲ期		T1~3,N1a,M0	
ⅣA 期		T4a,N0,M0	
ⅣB 期		T4a,N1b,M0	
		任何 T,N1b,M0	
ⅣC 期		任何 T,任何 N,M1	
分期:甲状腺未分化癌			
所有分为Ⅳ期			

预后影响因素

在包含15 700名患者的美国SEER数据库中，经年龄和性别矫正后，甲状腺乳头状癌的总体10年生存率为98%，滤泡癌为92%，髓样癌为80%，未分化癌为13%[45]。较大的年龄和较重的病情（包括肿瘤体积较大，甲状腺外侵犯和远处转移）与较差的预后有关，在各种肿瘤类型中均如此。在甲状腺乳头状癌中，*BRAF*突变可能是局部复发以及死亡的预后影响因素。在MTC中，*RET* M918T突变与较差的预后相关[20,46~48]。

多学科诊疗

手术-标准术式，并发症，预后

大多数甲状腺乳头状癌患者首选甲状腺全切除术，因为：①PTC的病灶通常是双侧的[49,50]；②5%~10%接受单侧手术的患者会出现对侧复发；③全切除术后可使放射性碘治疗效果最大化。早期队列研究认为，对乳头状癌直径大于1cm的患者行单侧腺叶切除术后复发率比行甲状腺全切除要高2~3倍，在多因素分析中，全切除的总生存率也有所提高[51~53]。最近，更大规模的研究对这些结论提出质疑，甲状腺全切除术后的存活率没有改善[54,55]。对于某些局限于腺体内的微小癌患者，甚至主张进行积极监测，因为连续的超声观察提示肿瘤往往不进展[56]。在没有随机前瞻性研究的情况下，推荐对原发肿瘤>4cm，或术前临床证据表明有甲状腺外侵犯或淋巴结转移或远处转移的乳头状癌患者行甲状腺全切除术。甲状腺全切除术或同侧腺叶切除术适用于没有淋巴结转移或低侵袭性的原发性肿瘤，而腺叶切除术或者密切随访适用于小于1cm的微小癌。

尽管有高达80%的乳头状癌患者出现局部区域的微转移灶，但只有约35%的患者临床可见颈部或纵隔淋巴结转移，通常在侧颈部[57]。若临床上表现出侧颈部转移，则应该进行颈清扫术（Ⅱ~Ⅴ区）[58,59]。对临床上发现转移的患者行中央区淋巴结清扫（Ⅵ区和上纵隔淋巴结）可提高生存率，因此推荐对这部分患者行中央区淋巴结清扫。但对于预防性中央区淋巴结清扫，只有经验丰富的外科医生来操作才可能使得潜在益处超过潜在的外科手术并发症[60]。在肿瘤侵犯上呼吸消化道的情况下，完全手术切除和削除大体肿瘤仅残留微观病灶相比，患者的生存率类似[61]。然而，在气管软骨破坏或腔内受累的患者中，有一半患者在削除术后4年内死亡。因此，广泛侵袭性甲状腺癌患者的手术应该旨在切除所有肿瘤，同时最大限度地保护器官功能，除非肿瘤无法切除或患者拒绝建议的手术方式[62]。

对于新诊断的髓样癌，应监测血清钙和血浆游离肾上腺素，以排除共存的甲状旁腺功能亢进和嗜铬细胞瘤，此外需要通过胚系*RET*检测以排除MEN2。所有MTC患者均应该行甲状腺全切除术，因为散发性和家族性疾病髓样癌患者有较高的双侧腺叶发生率，全切除术与生存率提高有关[21,63]。即使没有临床可检测的淋巴结转移，也应在所有患者中行中央区淋巴结清扫。当原发肿瘤>1cm或存在中央区淋巴结转移时，强烈推荐行同侧侧颈部和/或纵隔淋巴结清扫。根治性颈部淋巴结清扫术式不会改善预后，因此不推荐使用。在侵袭性病变中，可考虑扩大切除受累及的颈部结构，但仍推荐尽量保留功能。

对于家族性*RET*突变的携带者，最早在6岁时就可确诊是否患有恶性肿瘤，因此建议在5岁时行预防性甲状腺切除术。鉴于有早期发生淋巴结转移的可能性，建议对MEN2B患儿应在1岁时进行手术。对50个*RET*突变携带者在接受预防性甲状腺切除术后5~10年进行评估，发现88%的患者中血浆降钙素水平正常[13]。含有*RET*基因中危险度最小的突变点（768、790、791、804和891密码子），并且其家族史提示肿瘤进展缓慢的儿童，可通过降钙素监测、甲状腺超声密切随访，从而延迟手术治疗[23]。

微创手术方法，包括从腋窝远端切口入路行甲状腺切除，可达到美容的目的，且可减少术后不适[64,65]。通过使用内镜器械可为外科医生清晰显示关键解剖结构。机器人技术为甲状腺提供了最新的手术方法，包括真正的三维可视化，高度清晰的内镜转动功能和运动缩放。正在开发经自然孔道手术技术，包括用于经口机器人辅助内镜甲状腺切除术[66,67]。实施这些新的手术方法时应该比较并记录相对于传统开放手术而获得的手术效果提高[68,69]。

除肿瘤小且完全局限于甲状腺内的患者外，完全切除肿瘤的甲状腺全切除术并不能延长甲状腺未分化癌患者的生存期[70,71]。由于肿瘤生长速度快，远处转移率高，因此不完全切除通常没有治疗作用。

放射性碘同位素治疗——标准流程，方式，并发症和预后

放射性碘同位素治疗

DTC初次手术后的辅助放射性碘治疗旨在消除甲状腺床或区域淋巴结中残留的微小病灶，并应通过消除残余甲状腺细胞以提高血清甲状腺球蛋白（Tg）对检测复发或转移性疾病的预测价值（即所谓"消融"）。多项关于放射性碘治疗疗效的回顾性研究报告了相互矛盾的数据[72]。在最近的多中心甲状腺癌登记研究中，在校正甲状腺切除术范围后，对Ⅱ~Ⅳ期患者行术后放射性碘治疗和改善生存率有关，其中在Ⅲ~Ⅳ期患者中还校正了促甲状腺素抑制治疗[52]。对残留疾病或远处转移的患者，建议进行放射性碘治疗。然而，对于较小的单灶肿瘤，如果没有甲状腺外侵犯或转移的证据，不应行放射性碘治疗。由于MTC和ATC缺乏浓聚碘的能力，放射性碘在其治疗中没有任何作用。

放射性碘的功效取决于患者的准备工作、肿瘤特异性特征、疾病部位和放射性碘活性。甲状腺组织对碘化物的吸收受促甲状腺素（TSH）的刺激，并受到内源性碘化物的抑制。可通过停用甲状腺素或使用外源性重组人TSH而充分升高TSH水平[73]。在消融或治疗前经常进行诊断性全身放射性碘扫描以定位摄取病灶，在给予2~5mCi的^{123}I或^{131}I后24~72h，大多数甲状腺切除术后的患者显示甲状腺床内放射性碘的显著摄取，可能来自正常的残留甲状腺[74,75]。然而，对于明显没有严重转移的患者，放射性碘治疗前并不是必须行碘扫描[40,76]。

如果甲状腺床摄取在诊断扫描中可见，则常规使用30~100mCi的^{131}I，如果没有进行治疗前扫描，则根据经验选择剂量。如果扫描显示局部或远处转移性病灶的摄取，则给予更高

的量，如 150~200mCi。^{131}I 治疗区域淋巴结转移在 80%的患者中有效，但对残留的大块肿瘤可能效果不理想[77]。5%的分化型甲状腺癌患者有可摄碘的肺转移灶，这些患者的 5 年生存率为 60%~80%，而不摄碘的患者生存率仅为 30%[78,79]。仅通过^{131}I 扫描确诊的小结节性肺转移患者的长期生存率最高[78]。使用 200mCi 的^{131}I 治疗骨转移可以在不到 10%的治疗患者中达到完全缓解（CR），部分缓解（PR）仅有 35%[80]。对颅内转移患者，手术切除转移灶后，也可以应用放射性碘治疗[81]。

放射性碘的短期并发症包括唾液腺炎、精量减少、白细胞减少症和卵巢功能衰竭[82,83]。继发性肿瘤与放射性碘的剂量呈现剂量依赖相关性，包括结肠直肠癌、唾液肿瘤和急性白血病（绝对风险：在 10 000 人·年的随访中每 GBq ^{131}I 有 14.4 例实体癌，0.8 例白血病）[84]。因弥漫性肺转移而反复接受放射性碘治疗的患者很少发生肺纤维化。

外照射放射治疗（EBRT）

对于侵袭性 PTC 的老年患者，EBRT（外照射放射治疗）用于预防局部复发可能有效[85,86]。对 282 例接受 EBRT 治疗的患者进行回顾性研究发现，155 例有显微镜下残留的 PTC 患者的 10 年局部控制率降低（93% vs 78%），疾病特异性生存率降低（100% vs 95%）[87]。辅助 EBRT 对年龄小于 45 岁的患者几乎没有益处，老年患者因食管和气管的治疗副作用而耐受性变差[88]。调强放疗（IMRT）可能与短期毒性降低有关。推荐对大体腺外侵犯切除后留有显微镜下残留及呼吸消化结构旁切除不净的患者，可使用 40~50Gy 的 EBRT 照射甲状腺床。

甲状腺髓样癌患者，因严重的腺外侵犯或广泛的大块淋巴结转移导致术后局部复发风险较高，对于这类患者，最大范围手术切除可考虑 EBRT。在一项研究中，辅助 EBRT 后 10 年局部无复发率为 86%，而在未接受此类治疗的患者中为 52%[89]。采用 60Gy 治疗 30 次的适形放疗或 IMRT，即使在有远处转移的情况下仍可获得比较好的局部控制率，且治疗毒性在可接受的范围内[90]。

甲状腺未分化癌的患者初始治疗选择常规剂量 ERBT，尽管最多 40% 的患者有初始治疗反应，并不能延长患者生存期[91,92]。超分割放疗联合放射增敏化疗，可将局部反应率提高至约 80%，中位生存期为 1 年，但患者最终死于远处转移。

甲状腺素替代治疗

DTC 患者需要终生服用甲状腺素来治疗术后甲状腺功能减退，并尽量减少 TSH 对肿瘤生长的刺激。使用 TSH 抑制性治疗，总生存期和无病生存期可提高 2~3 倍，尤其是Ⅲ期和Ⅳ期患者[52]。较低程度的抑制也可改善Ⅰ期和Ⅱ期患者的总体生存率[52,93]。但是，过度激进的甲状腺素治疗的潜在并发症包括骨质疏松症[94]、心房颤动[95]及可能发生的心脏肥大和心脏功能障碍以及生活质量下降[96]。在初始随访期间，对甲状腺癌复发和死亡风险较低的患者，TSH 水平维持在 0.1 和 0.5mU/L 之间，而高风险患者应将 TSH 水平抑制到<0.1mU/L[40]。无疾病复发已有 5~10 年的患者可通过降低甲状腺素剂量来降低 TSH 抑制程度。然而，在可耐受的范围内那些患有转移性疾病的患者 TSH 水平应保持在 0.1mU/L 以下[97]。在髓样癌手术后，也应进行甲状腺素替代治疗，但不适合 TSH 抑制，因为 C 细胞缺乏 TSH 受体。

复发监测

血清标志物监测

考虑到肿瘤大小和 Tg 水平之间的相关性，测量血清 Tg，即滤泡细胞的特征性产物，有助于检测残留、复发或转移性分化型甲状腺癌。在甲状腺切除术和残余灶行放射性碘消融治疗后，血清 Tg 浓度应该接近检测不到，但在初次治疗后可能需要几年时间才能降低到检测不到[98]。血清 TSH 的升高可刺激 Tg 的产生，从而提高了检测残留肿瘤的敏感性。TSH 刺激后 Tg 的敏感性为 85%~95%，但在 TSH 抑制期间或在去分化甲状腺癌中的 Tg 敏感性低至 50%[99]。功能敏感性低至 0.1ng/ml 的 Tg 检测可无需 TSH 刺激[100]。在 1 年内 Tg 水平翻倍升高的患者，复发率和死亡率均较高[101,102]。

血清降钙素和癌胚抗原（CEA）水平是髓样癌同样有价值的生物标志物。大多数术后可检测到血清降钙素的患者都有肿瘤残留。降钙素<150pg/ml 时可进行密切随访治疗，降钙素>150pg/ml 时应该重新评估是否有颈部残留的可切除病灶或存在远处转移灶。术后降钙素水平分别在>24 个月、6~24 个月和<6 个月内翻倍的患者其五年生存率分别为 100%、92%和 25%[103,104]。

影像诊断

大多数分化型甲状腺癌和髓样癌患者的随访都依赖于颈部超声，其可准确地识别局部区域转移和直径几毫米的复发灶。超声有助于对可疑病变进行细针细胞学穿刺，通过测量针头洗脱液中的 Tg 或降钙素可提高其敏感性[105~108]。应通增加其他影像学检查以识别可手术切除或可使用其他方式治疗的病灶。对于 DTC 患者，放射性碘扫描可以检测对进一步治疗有反应的残留或转移性疾病。在随访期间 Tg 水平升高时，颈部和胸部的增强 CT 是合适的影像学检查。在 Tg 水平>10ng/ml 且放射性碘扫描呈阴性或富含线粒体的嗜酸性肿瘤中，FDG-PET 成像可能很有帮助[109,110]。对于髓样癌，当降钙素水平超过 150pg/ml 时，应进行颈部、胸部和肝脏增强 CT（三相增强）和躯干骨的 MRI[21,111]。

复发或转移性疾病的治疗

手术

对于直径>1cm 的转移淋巴结的 DTC 患者，应进行全面的颈部清扫术（Ⅱ~Ⅴ区），但只有不到一半的患者术后甲状腺球蛋白水平检测不到[112,113]。即使因先前的手术导致手术区域纤维化，有更高并发症的风险，在疾病复发时也需要再次探查甲状腺术床以及中央和/或侧颈淋巴结[114]。呼吸消化道受侵犯时，彻底切除肿瘤可以提高生存率，但需要切除更广泛的组织，如气管切除吻合术或部分下咽切除术。气管支架、气管切开术和激光消融或部分切除有姑息治疗的价值。在脑转移患者中，行手术切除或外放射切除可以提高生存率[81,115]。在 MTC 中，再次手术切除淋巴结或可触及的病变很少能使血清降钙素水平正常化，因此只有颈部转移较严重的患者才考虑进行二次颈部手术。

放射性碘治疗

^{131}I 的重复治疗对于通过放射性碘成像明确的转移性 DTC 患者是有益的，但累积^{131}I 活性>600mCi 后很少有效[78]。放射

性碘难治性甲状腺癌的特征是可在 CT 上检测病变，该病变之前摄入了放射性碘，但是在目前的放射性碘成像中没有摄取，或者在影像学上存在进展。

电子线外照射治疗

颈部无法切除的侵袭性甲状腺癌患者可从 EBRT 中获益，5 年局部控制和疾病特异存活率约为 65%[87]。EBRT 还可以减轻骨转移引起的疼痛。对于单个病灶，可以给予 25 次、50Gy 的放射剂量，但是应该对脊椎病灶降低剂量。

化疗

多靶点激酶抑制剂可用于一个或多个器官有可测量病灶的进展期分化型癌和髓样癌患者。这些药物的靶点包括促血管生成受体，如血管内皮生长因子受体（VEGFR）和成纤维细胞生长因子受体（FGFR）[116]。除了促血管生成外，这些受体激酶也位于肿瘤细胞本身上，发挥促进肿瘤增殖的作用。BRAF 突变的 PTC 和 *RET* 突变的 MTC 中细胞信号转导通路过度激活，提示有更多选择性激酶抑制剂的靶标。

乐伐替尼（lenvatinib）和索拉非尼（sorafenib）均可延长进展性放射性碘难治性分化型甲状腺癌患者的无进展生存期（PFS）[117,118]。在乐伐替尼的 SELECT Ⅲ期试验中，与安慰剂相比，中位 PFS 从 3.6 个月显著延长到 18.3 个月（*HR* 0.21，99%*CI* 0.14~0.31，*P*<0.000 1）[117]。对乐伐替尼的反应率为 65%，其中 4 例患者完全缓解。常见的与乐伐替尼相关的不良事件包括高血压、腹泻、疲劳、食欲下降、恶心、呕吐、体重减轻和口腔炎。在索拉非尼的 DECISION Ⅲ期试验中，与安慰剂相比，中位 PFS 从 5.8 个月延长到了 10.8（*HR* 0.59，95% *CI* 0.45~0.76，*P*<0.000 1）[118]。索拉非尼的反应率为 12%，所有患者均为部分反应。常见的索拉非尼相关不良事件包括手-足综合征、腹泻、脱发、皮疹、疲劳、体重减轻和高血压。在晚期 DTC 中具有疗效证据的其他激酶抑制剂包括多靶点药物凡德他尼（vandetanib）[119]、培唑帕尼（pazopanib）[120]，BRAF 抑制剂维莫非尼（vemurafenib）[121]和达拉非尼（dabrafenib）[122]。

在进展期 MTC 患者中，卡博替尼（cabozantinib）和凡德他尼（vandetanib）均可延长 PFS[123,124]。在进展期 MTC 患者的卡博替尼 EXAM Ⅲ期临床试验中，与安慰剂相比，中位 PFS 从 4.0 个月延长至 11.2 个月（*HR* 0.28，95% *CI* 0.19~0.40，*P*<0.001），应答率为 28%，所有患者均为部分反应。在亚组分析中，肿瘤含有 *RET* 或 *RAS* 突变的患者更有可能获益，而缺乏这些突变的患者 PFS 没有改善[125]。常见的卡博替尼相关不良事件包括腹泻、手掌-足底红斑感觉减退、体重下降、恶心、疲倦。在 MTC 患者中使用凡德他尼的 ZETA Ⅲ期试验中，与安慰剂相比，中位 PFS 延长从 19.3 个月延长至 30.5 个月（*HR* 0.46，95%*CI* 0.31~0.69，*P*<0.001）。亚组分析表明，疾病处于进展期以及有 *RET M918T* 突变患者的 PFS 得到改善。常见的凡德他尼相关不良事件包括腹泻、皮疹、恶心、高血压和头痛；心脏 QT 间期延长，需要在治疗期间密切观察电解质和心电图（ECG）。

针对分化型癌和髓样癌的细胞毒性化疗价值有限[126]。在转移性分化型癌的随机试验中，联合多柔比星和顺铂与单用多柔比星进行了比较，联合治疗仅有 16% 的客观反应，包括两例患者有持久的完全反应（CR），而 31% 的患者对多柔比星单药治疗有部分反应[127]。在 MTC 中，达卡巴嗪联合其他药物包括长春新碱、氟尿嘧啶、环磷酰胺或多柔比星可达到高达 30% 的治疗反应率[128]。

在 ATC 中，紫杉醇可能在少数患者中产生短期稳定病情的益处或姑息性治疗益处[129]。虽然缺乏有效性的正式临床试验，但共识指南推荐包括紫杉醇、蒽环类和含铂化合物的联合方案[37]。一项随机Ⅲ期试验提示，福莫布菌素、紫杉醇和卡铂联合用药对比紫杉醇和卡铂联合用药，总生存率没有改善，但入组还没有完成[130]。尽管索拉非尼和培唑帕尼有临床试验前的疗效提示，但两者没有表现出单药治疗效果[131,132]。

（王健 朱一鸣 译 刘绍严 校）

参考文献

The complete reference list can be found on the Wiley Companion Digital Edition of this title (see inside front cover for login instructions).

3 Davies L, Welch HG. Current thyroid cancer trends in the United States. *JAMA Otolaryngol Head Neck Surg*. 2014;**140**:317–322.

11 Wells SA Jr, Pacini F, Robinson BG, et al. Multiple endocrine neoplasia type 2 and familial medullary thyroid carcinoma: an update. *J Clin Endocrinol Metab*. 2013;**98**:3149–3164.

13 Skinner MA, Moley JA, Dilley WG, et al. Prophylactic thyroidectomy in multiple endocrine neoplasia type 2A. *N Engl J Med*. 2005;**353**:1105–1113.

15 Volante M, Collini P, Nikiforov YE, et al. Poorly differentiated thyroid carcinoma: the Turin proposal for the use of uniform diagnostic criteria and an algorithmic diagnostic approach. *Am J Surg Pathol*. 2007;**31**:1256–1264.

17 Cancer Genome Atlas Research Network. Integrated genomic characterization of papillary thyroid carcinoma. *Cell*. 2014;**159**:676–690.

20 Elisei R, Cosci B, Romei C, et al. Prognostic significance of somatic RET oncogene mutations in sporadic medullary thyroid cancer: a 10-year follow-up study. *J Clin Endocrinol Metab*. 2008;**93**:682–687.

21 Wells SA Jr, Asa SL, Dralle H, et al. Revised American Thyroid Association guidelines for the management of medullary thyroid carcinoma. *Thyroid*. 2015;**25(6)**:567–610. Epub Mar 26 2015.

28 Cibas ES, Alexander EK, Benson CB, et al. Indications for thyroid FNA and pre-FNA requirements: a synopsis of the National Cancer Institute Thyroid Fine-Needle Aspiration State of the Science Conference. *Diagn Cytopathol*. 2008;**36**:390–399.

30 Baloch ZW, LiVolsi VA, Asa SL, et al. Diagnostic terminology and morphologic criteria for cytologic diagnosis of thyroid lesions: a synopsis of the National Cancer Institute Thyroid Fine-Needle Aspiration State of the Science Conference. *Diagn Cytopathol*. 2008;**36**:425–437.

32 Alexander EK, Kennedy GC, Baloch ZW, et al. Preoperative diagnosis of benign thyroid nodules with indeterminate cytology. *N Engl J Med*. 2012;**367**:705–715.

33 Nikiforova MN, Wald AI, Roy S, et al. Targeted next-generation sequencing panel (ThyroSeq) for detection of mutations in thyroid cancer. *J Clin Endocrinol Metab*. 2013;**98**:E1852–E1860.

34 Nikiforov YE, Carty SE, Chiosea SI, et al. Highly accurate diagnosis of cancer in thyroid nodules with follicular neoplasm/suspicious for a follicular neoplasm cytology by ThyroSeq v2 next-generation sequencing assay. *Cancer*. 2014;**120**:3627–3634.

37 Smallridge RC, Ain KB, Asa SL, et al. American Thyroid Association guidelines for management of patients with anaplastic thyroid cancer. *Thyroid*. 2012;**22**:1104–1139.

43 Tuttle RM, Tala H, Shah J, et al. Estimating risk of recurrence in differentiated thyroid cancer after total thyroidectomy and radioactive iodine remnant ablation: using response to therapy variables to modify the initial risk estimates predicted by the new American Thyroid Association staging system. *Thyroid*. 2010;**20**:1341–1349.

45 Gilliland FD, Hunt WC, Morris DM, et al. Prognostic factors for thyroid carcinoma: a population-based study of 15,698 cases from the Surveillance, Epidemiology and End Results (SEER) program 1973–1991. *Cancer*. 1997;**79**:564–573.

47 Xing M, Alzahrani AS, Carson KA, et al. Association between BRAF V600E mutation and mortality in patients with papillary thyroid cancer. *JAMA*. 2013;**309**:1493–1501.

52 Jonklaas J, Sarlis NJ, Litofsky D, et al. Outcomes of patients with differentiated thyroid carcinoma following initial therapy. *Thyroid*. 2006;**16**:1229–1242.

53 Bilimoria KY, Bentrem DJ, Ko CY, et al. Extent of surgery affects survival for papillary thyroid cancer. *Ann Surg*. 2007;**246**:375–381; discussion 381–374.

54 Adam MA, Pura J, Gu L, et al. Extent of surgery for papillary thyroid can-

cer is not associated with survival: an analysis of 61,775 patients. *Ann Surg*. 2014;**260**:601–605; discussion 605–607.

56 Ito Y, Miyauchi A, Inoue H, et al. An observational trial for papillary thyroid microcarcinoma in Japanese patients. *World J Surg*. 2010;**34**:28–35.

61 Gillenwater AM, Goepfert H. Surgical management of laryngotracheal and esophageal involvement by locally advanced thyroid cancer. *Semin Surg Oncol*. 1999;**16**:19–29.

71 Haigh PI, Ituarte PHG, Wu HS, et al. Completely resected anaplastic thyroid carcinoma combined with adjuvant chemotherapy and irradiation is associated with prolonged survival. *Cancer*. 2001;**91**:2335–2342.

73 Pacini F, Ladenson PW, Schlumberger M, et al. Radioiodine ablation of thyroid remnants after preparation with recombinant human thyrotropin in differentiated thyroid carcinoma: results of an international, randomized, controlled study. *J Clin Endocrinol Metab*. 2006;**91**:926–932.

76 Cailleux AF, Baudin E, Travagli JP, et al. Is diagnostic iodine-131 scanning useful after total thyroid ablation for differentiated thyroid cancer? *J Clin Endocrinol Metab*. 2000;**85**:175–178.

77 Maxon HR, Englaro EE, Thomas SR, et al. Radioiodine-131 therapy for well-differentiated thyroid cancer – a quantitative radiation dosimetric approach: outcome and validation in 85 patients. *J Nucl Med*. 1992;**33**:1132–1136.

78 Durante C, Haddy N, Baudin E, et al. Long-term outcome of 444 patients with distant metastases from papillary and follicular thyroid carcinoma: benefits and limits of radioiodine therapy. *J Clin Endocrinol Metab*. 2006;**91**:2892–2899.

84 Rubino C, de Vathaire F, Dottorini ME, et al. Second primary malignancies in thyroid cancer patients. *Br J Cancer*. 2003;**89**:1638–1644.

96 Biondi B, Cooper DS. Benefits of thyrotropin suppression versus the risks of adverse effects in differentiated thyroid cancer. *Thyroid*. 2010;**20**:135–146.

97 Carhill A, Litofsky D, Ain K, et al. Long-term moderate thyroid hormone suppression therapy is associated with improved outcomes in differentiated thyroid carcinoma: National Thyroid Cancer Treatment Cooperative Study Group Registry analysis 1987–2012. *Thyroid*. 2014;**24(S1)**:A6.

98 Pacini F, Agate L, Elisei R, et al. Outcome of differentiated thyroid cancer with detectable serum Tg and negative diagnostic 131I whole body scan: comparison of patients treated with high 131I activities versus untreated patients. *J Clin Endocrinol Metab*. 2001;**86**:4092–4097.

99 Haugen BR, Pacini F, Reiners C, et al. A comparison of recombinant human thyrotropin and thyroid hormone withdrawal for the detection of thyroid remnant or cancer. *J Clin Endocrinol Metab*. 1999;**84**:3877–3885.

100 Castagna MG, Tala Jury HP, Cipri C, et al. The use of ultrasensitive thyroglobulin assays reduces but does not abolish the need for TSH stimulation in patients with differentiated thyroid carcinoma. *J Endocrinol Invest*. 2011;**34**:e219–e223.

102 Pacini F, Sabra MM, Tuttle RM. Clinical relevance of thyroglobulin doubling time in the management of patients with differentiated thyroid cancer. *Thyroid*. 2011;**21**:691–692.

103 Giraudet AL, Al Ghulzan A, Auperin A, et al. Progression of medullary thyroid carcinoma: assessment with calcitonin and carcinoembryonic antigen doubling times. *Eur J Endocrinol*. 2008;**158**:239–246.

109 Leboulleux S, Schroeder PR, Schlumberger M, et al. The role of PET in follow-up of patients treated for differentiated epithelial thyroid cancers. *Nat Clin Pract Endocrinol Metab*. 2007;**3**:112–121.

117 Schlumberger M, Tahara M, Wirth LJ, et al. Lenvatinib versus placebo in radioiodine-refractory thyroid cancer. *N Engl J Med*. 2015;**372**:621–630.

118 Brose MS, Nutting CM, Jarzab B, et al. Sorafenib in radioactive iodine-refractory, locally advanced or metastatic differentiated thyroid cancer: a randomised, double-blind, phase 3 trial. *Lancet*. 2014;**384**:319–328.

123 Elisei R, Schlumberger MJ, Muller SP, et al. Cabozantinib in progressive medullary thyroid cancer. *J Clin Oncol*. 2013;**31**:3639–3646.

124 Wells SA Jr, Robinson BG, Gagel RF, et al. Vandetanib in patients with locally advanced or metastatic medullary thyroid cancer: a randomized, double-blind phase III trial. *J Clin Oncol*. 2012;**30**:134–141.

129 Ain KB, Egorin MJ, DeSimone PA. Treatment of anaplastic thyroid carcinoma with paclitaxel: phase 2 trial using ninety-six-hour infusion. *Thyroid*. 2000;**10**:587–594.

第 81 章　肾上腺皮质肿瘤

Tito Fojo, MD, PhD

概述

肾上腺皮质癌(ACC)是一种具有多种临床表现并且预后不良的罕见恶性肿瘤。影像学已成为核心诊断方法,在大多数情况下,诊断肾上腺皮质癌无需进行组织活检,并且也不建议为了确诊而进行穿刺活检。利用 Weiss 标准的病理检查对于区分小腺瘤和癌非常有价值。其治疗方法多种多样,主要包括手术切除、口服米托坦、化疗和姑息性放疗。手术仍然是唯一经过验证的治疗方法,应在症状出现或确诊复发时首先考虑,且应尽量避免使用腹腔镜。米托坦被批准用于治疗不能手术的功能性和非功能性肾上腺皮质癌,其治疗原理主要表现为一种抗激素药物。在肿瘤产生过量激素的患者中,米托坦的作用是不可替代的,但是,它应用于辅助治疗的效果是不确定的。类固醇替代治疗是必需的。系统性化疗,即米托坦与依托泊苷、多柔比星和顺铂(EDP-M)或链脲佐菌素(S-M)联合应为优先选择方案。不应该为了"新型的靶向治疗"而放弃这些传统的治疗方式,因为目前并没有任何证据显示新型靶向治疗的疗效。越来越多的证据显示姑息性放疗对转移性肿瘤患者有益。对于复发患者来说,射频消融(RFA)或冷冻消融术已经成为一种外科辅助或独立的治疗方式。和大多数罕见疾病一样,肾上腺皮质癌需要更多的临床试验研究。

简介

肾上腺皮质癌(ACC)是一种罕见的恶性肿瘤,发病率为 1.5/100 万~2/100 万人每年。患者可以毫无临床症状,某些较大、局部侵袭性的原发肿瘤可以表现为局部症状,某些高分泌型肿瘤可表现为全身症状。这种疾病的治疗仍面临很多挑战,因此多学科治疗显得尤为重要。

综述

患者五年生存率为 10%~25%,平均生存期约为 14.5 个月。约 50%的患者存在激素过度分泌,其中 10%~20%的患者表现为库欣综合征,其他症状包括女性多毛症和男性乳房发育。有些综述进行了更深入的总结[1~5]。

综合评估

初步评估应包括病史、体格检查、血液和尿液检测,以确定肿瘤是否有功能。计算机断层扫描(CT)和磁共振成像(MRI)都具有诊断意义,两者都可以帮助区分良性腺瘤与恶性病变[6~9]。MRI 在识别肝脏肿瘤转移及血管受侵程度(尤其是下腔静脉)方面具有更大优势。^{18}F-脱氧葡萄糖正电子发射断层扫描(FDG-PET)可以帮助评估疾病的范围,在手术前也许有一定价值,然而它无法监测疾病的进展,不应该作为主要的评估手段[10~13]。

活检

大多数具有肾上腺可疑恶性肿瘤的患者应该进行手术而不是诊断性活检,因为活检有播散肿瘤的风险,而且通过小体积活检,区分良性与恶性肿瘤比较困难[14~16]。以下两种情况,可以在没有活组织检查的情形下进行手术:①有激素过量分泌的证据,肾上腺皮质细胞癌诊断明确;②没有激素过量产生的证据,但是在评估或者偶然影像学扫描过程中发现了孤立的肾上腺占位。只有在肿瘤广泛转移使得手术切除获益较小,或者其他疾病提示肾上腺占位非原发肿瘤时,才应该进行组织活检。

病理

Weiss 标准,于 1984 年第一次被提出,用于区分没有局部扩散或远处转移的小肾上腺皮质癌与良性腺瘤[17~22]。Weiss 发现了九个最有用的标准以鉴别恶性肿瘤:①核Ⅲ/Ⅳ级;②核分裂率>5 个每 50 高倍视野;③非典型核分裂;④透明细胞≤25%的肿瘤;⑤结构弥散;⑥镜下坏死;⑦静脉侵犯;⑧窦状小管侵犯;⑨包膜侵犯。当出现≥3 个标准时,即诊断为恶性肿瘤。

Weiss 标准被用来区分小腺瘤与癌,但在预测较大肿瘤的预后上意义还不明确。在 42 例诊断为肾上腺皮质癌的患者中,仅核分裂率与预后有较强的统计学相关性[18]。肿瘤质量>250g、大小>10cm、非典型核分裂和包膜侵犯几项参数与较差生存率有临界统计学意义($P<0.06$)。与此同时,其他标准与生存无相关性。最近的一项研究同样证实了核分裂率的重要性[22]。

肾上腺皮质癌的治疗

主要包括外科切除或消融、口服米托坦、化疗和姑息性放疗。虽然缺少对照试验用于指导治疗方式的选择,但这并不意味选择毫无根据,也不意味某种治疗方式是固定的选择。

外科切除

手术仍然是唯一经过验证的治疗方法,在初发和复发时均可进行。初发患者应考虑选择完全性切除局部病灶,当不能完全切除时,患者生存期<1 年[2,23,24]。由经验丰富的肿瘤外科医生行开放手术是治疗初发患者的关键。虽然有些人认为腹腔镜手术可以在某些患者中使用,但是更易发生一种致命的手术并发症——肿瘤腹膜转移,因此不鼓励除开放式切除以外的其他手术方式。对于不会种植转移于腹腔的肾上腺偶发瘤来说,腹腔镜手术是合适的。但是,有文献报道,尽管是经验丰富的外科医生,术中肿瘤散落率同样可高达 50%[25,26]。一项纳入 152 名肾上腺皮质癌患者[27]的研究指出,对于直径≤10cm 的肾上腺皮质癌患者,腹腔镜并不比开放性肾上腺手术切除效果差。但是,经过广泛的预选后,仅 23%的患者接受腹腔镜手术,且其中 1/3 转为开放手术。对于一般社区来说,这些专业治疗中心的研究结果适用性有限。另外,腹腔镜切除术的切缘阳性率更高,且复发更快。一项针对腹腔镜手术的系统评价总结说,“没有前瞻性随机研究支持使用腹腔镜切除术治疗肾上腺皮质癌”[28]。

肿瘤复发时,积极的手术治疗可能是更好的选择,尤其适用于临床症状较轻或肿瘤生长速度较慢的患者[29,30]。我们应该认识到,采用这种途径进行治疗的研究有一个固有的选择性偏倚:接受手术的患者可能疾病更加局限性、有着更好的身体状态以及肿瘤可能具有更惰性的生物学特征。

米托坦

作为一种抗肾上腺素能药物,米托坦最初被批准用于治疗不能手术的功能性和非功能性肾上腺皮质癌。然而,它杀伤肿瘤的活性有限,其临床应用价值主要是作为一种抗激素药物。有数据表明米托坦能够改变类固醇的外周代谢。对于肿瘤产生过量激素的患者,米托坦是不可替代的,即使疾病进展,也必须尽早且持续使用。

米托坦在辅助治疗中的价值尚不明确。有几个小的和一个大的研究指出,辅助性持续应用米托坦能够延迟或预防疾病的复发,但这些研究都是回顾性研究,有一定的偏倚存在[31,32]。因为只有一小部分患者对米托坦的耐受性良好,所以识别那些能够受益的人群显得尤为重要。米托坦的治疗应该被视为一场马拉松而不是短跑冲刺,而且其用药方式也应该根据情况有所调整。初始计量应该从 1~2g/d 开始,之后逐步增加,直到 2~3 个月后达到最大剂量 4~6g/d,最后将用药剂量降低至 0.5~1g/d,可以根据血清米托坦水平调整用药剂量。类固醇替代药物可以与米托坦同步使用,或当临床或实验室数据提示早期肾上腺皮质功能不全时使用。给予氢化可的松和氟氢可的松时,应当指导患者佩戴标有肾上腺皮质功能不全的手环。停药后,米托坦可能需要数月才能从体内完全清除,激素补充治疗需要额外 6~12 个月。

系统性化疗

米托坦联合依托泊苷、多柔比星、顺铂(EDP-M)及米托坦联合链脲佐霉素(S-M),这两种治疗方案已成为治疗肾上腺皮质癌的首选化疗方案。目前,新型靶向治疗尚未被证明有效,因此传统的化疗不应该被丢弃。两种方案均在 FIRM-ACT[33]试验中进行了评估,发现同样作为一线用药,跟 S-M 相比,EDP-M 表现出了明显更好的反应率(23.2% vs 9.2%,$P<0.001$)和无进展生存期(PFS)(5.0 个月 vs 2.1 个月,HR 0.55,$P<0.001$),且两者的毒性事件发生率相似。总生存率没有显著差异,可能是由于交叉分组的原因。重要的是,虽然 185 名接受 EDP-M 二线治疗的患者具有相似的中位无进展生存期,但在招募进实验组的时候,存在一个窗口期。FIRM-ACT 试验也提示治疗方案不具备交叉耐药性,因而可以接连采用两种方案。

最后,≥50%的肾上腺皮质癌患者接受了肾切除术,促使卡铂代替了顺铂。然而,鉴于在其他癌症中,两者活性分布并不相同,因此建议仍应坚持使用顺铂。

放疗

越来越多的证据表明姑息性放射治疗对于转移性患者是有益的。除了缓和症状,已有的数据并不支持放疗的使用,术后放疗也同样不被支持。最开始的研究发现辅助性放疗并无获益,虽然后面一些使用更好的放疗技术的研究声称放疗有更低的毒性,但也不建议常规应用[34,35]。获益不确定,但副作用却是明确的,包括放疗的急性并发症,而且可能也会增加之后的手术难度。只有在患者经过高资历肿瘤外科医生手术切除之后仍存在切缘阳性的情况下,才应考虑术后放疗,或者当患者同时存在其他相关疾病,无法再次手术时,才应该使用放射治疗。

介入放射学作为一种治疗方式

鉴于外科处理方式在肾上腺皮质癌治疗中的价值,射频消融(RFA)或冷冻消融术已成为复发患者外科手术的辅助或者一种独立的治疗方式[36]。虽然侵入性较小,但消融治疗应被视为一种外科干预方式。虽然缺少随机对照试验的数据支持,但栓塞的价值在于能够减少肿瘤的体积,减少肿瘤相关血管的供应,使得后续的外科干预能够更加顺利进行。

治疗激素过分泌和缺乏

因为任何一个有功能的肿瘤均可抑制促肾上腺皮质激素的分泌,使得对侧肾上腺萎缩,因此在术前应该评估患者的激素水平,以确定术后类固醇替代治疗的剂量。

我们必须认识到不受控制的激素分泌所带来的严重后果,必须严密且持续监测[37]。不建议使用化疗去解决激素过量的问题。为了控制激素分泌,除了米托坦,单独或联合应用酮康唑、甲吡酮或依托咪酯也是重要的方法。激素的管理必须积极主动,具有前瞻性。

结论

手术仍然是治疗肾上腺皮质癌的关键,射频消融和冷冻治疗也有一定的价值。化疗在许多患者中也有一定作用,但是需要新的治疗方案以及开展更多的临床试验。放疗主要用于缓解症状。激素过度分泌能够严重影响患者的生存质量,因此必须多加注意。最后,疾病的治疗需要多学科的共同努力。

(刘飞 译　邢念增 校)

参考文献

1 Fassnacht M, Kroiss M, Allolio B. Update in adrenocortical carcinoma. *J Clin Endocrinol Metab*. 2013;**98**:4551 - 4564.

2 Ayala-Ramirez M, Jasim S, Feng L, et al. Adrenocortical carcinoma: clinical outcomes and prognosis of 330 patients at a tertiary care center. *Eur J Endocrinol*. 2013;**169**:891 - 899.

3 Else T, Kim AC, Sabolch A, et al. Adrenocortical carcinoma. *Endocr Rev*. 2014;**35**:282 - 326.

4 Terzolo M, Daffara F, Ardito A, et al. Management of adrenal cancer: a 2013 update. *J Endocrinol Invest*. 2014;**37**:207 - 217.

5 Ronchi CL, Kroiss M, Sbiera S, et al. EJE prize 2014: current and evolving treatment options in adrenocortical carcinoma: where do we stand and where do we want to go? *Eur J Endocrinol*. 2014;**171**:R1 - R11.

6 Korobkin M, Brodeur FJ, Yutzy GG, et al. Differentiation of adrenal adenomas from nonadenomas using CT attenuation values. *AJR Am J Roentgenol*. 1966;**166**:531 - 536.

7 Mitchell DG, Crovello M, Matteucci T, et al. Benign adrenocortical masses: diagnosis with chemical shift MR imaging. *Radiology*. 1992;**185**:345 - 351.

8 Outwater EK, Siegelman ES, Huang AB, et al. Adrenal masses: correlation between CT attenuation value and chemical shift ratio at MR imaging with in-phase and opposed-phase sequences. *Radiology*. 1996;**200**:749 - 752.

9 Goldfarb DA, Novick AC, Lorig R, et al. Magnetic resonance imaging for assessment of vena caval tumor thrombi: a comparative study with venacavography and computerized tomography scanning. *J Urol*. 1990;**144**:1100 - 1103.

10 Groussin L, Bonardel G, Silvéra S, et al. ^{18}F-fluorodeoxyglucose positron emission tomography for the diagnosis of adrenocortical tumors: a prospective study in 77 operated patients. *J Clin Endocrinol Metab*. 2009;**94**:1713 - 1722.

11 Nunes ML, Rault A, Teynie J, et al. ^{18}F-FDG-PET for the identification of adrenocortical carcinomas among indeterminate adrenal tumors at computed tomography scanning. *World J Surg*. 2010;**34**:1506 - 1510.

12 Ansquer C, Scigliano S, Mirallié E, et al. ^{18}F-FDG PET/CT in the characterization and surgical decision concerning adrenal masses: a prospective multicentre evaluation. *Eur J Nucl Med Mol Imaging*. 2010;**37**:1669 - 1678.

13 Takeuchi S, Balachandran A, Habra MA, et al. Impact of ^{18}F-FDG PET/CT on the management of adrenocortical carcinoma: analysis of 106 patients. *Eur J Nucl Med Mol Imaging*. 2014;**41**:2066 - 2073.

14 Mazzaglia PJ, Monchik JM. Limited value of adrenal biopsy in the evaluation of adrenal neoplasm: a decade of experience. *Arch Surg*. 2009;**144**:465 - 470.

15 Osman Y, El-Mekresh M, Gomha AM, et al. Percutaneous adrenal biopsy for indeterminate adrenal lesion: complications and diagnostic accuracy. *Urol Int*. 2010;**84**:315 - 318.

16 Williams AR, Hammer GD, Else T. Transcutaneous biopsy of adrenocortical carcinoma is rarely helpful in diagnosis, potentially harmful, but does not affect patient outcome. *Eur J Endocrinol*. 2014;**170**:829 - 835.

17 Weiss LM. Comparative histologic study of 43 metastasizing and nonmetastasizing adrenocortical tumors. *Am J Surg Pathol*. 1984;**8**:163 - 169.

18 Weiss LM, Medeiros LJ, Vickery AL Jr. Pathologic features of prognostic significance in adrenocortical carcinoma. *Am J Surg Pathol*. 1989;**13**:202 - 206.

19 Gicquel C, Bertagna X, Gaston V, et al. Molecular markers and long-term recurrences in a large cohort of patients with sporadic adrenocortical tumors. *Cancer Res*. 2001;**61**:6762 - 6767.

20 Lau SK, Weiss LM. The Weiss system for evaluating adrenocortical neoplasms: 25 years later. *Hum Pathol*. 2009;**40**:757 - 768.

21 Jain M, Kapoor S, Mishra A, et al. Weiss criteria in large adrenocortical tumors: a validation study. *Indian J Pathol Microbiol*. 2010;**53**:222 - 226.

22 Volante M, Bollito E, Sperone P, et al. Clinicopathological study of a series of 92 adrenocortical carcinomas: from a proposal of simplified diagnostic algorithm to prognostic stratification. *Histopathology*. 2009;**55**:535 - 543.

23 Henley DJ, van Heerden JA, Grant CS, et al. Adrenal cortical carcinoma—a continuing challenge. *Surgery*. 1983;**94**:926 - 931.

24 Pommier RF, Brennan MF. An eleven-year experience with adrenocortical carcinoma. *Surgery*. 1992;**112**:963 - 970.

25 Leboulleux S, Deandreis D, Al Ghuzlan A, et al. Adrenocortical carcinoma: is the surgical approach a risk factor of peritoneal carcinomatosis? *Eur J Endocrinol*. 2010;**162**:1147 - 1153.

26 Miller BS, Ammori JB, Gauger PG, et al. Laparoscopic resection is inappropriate in patients with known or suspected adrenocortical carcinoma. *World J Surg*. 2010;**34**:1380 - 1385.

27 Brix D, Allolio B, Fenske W, et al. Laparoscopic versus open adrenalectomy for adrenocortical carcinoma: surgical and oncologic outcome in 152 patients. *Eur Urol*. 2010;**58**:609 - 615.

28 Angst E, Hiatt JR, Gloor B, et al. Laparoscopic surgery for cancer: a systematic review and a way forward. *J Am Coll Surg*. 2010;**211**:412 - 423.

29 Wängberg B, Khorram-Manesh A, Jansson S, et al. The long-term survival in adrenocortical carcinoma with active surgical management and use of monitored mitotane. *Endocr Relat Cancer*. 2010;**17**:265 - 272.

30 Bellantone R, Ferrante A, Boscherini M, et al. Role of reoperation in recurrence of adrenal cortical carcinoma: results from 188 cases collected in the Italian National Registry for Adrenal Cortical Carcinoma. *Surgery*. 1997;**122**:1212 - 1218.

31 Terzolo M, Angeli A, Fassnacht M, et al. Adjuvant mitotane treatment for adrenocortical carcinoma. *N Engl J Med*. 2007;**356**:2372 - 2380.

32 Huang H, Fojo T. Adjuvant mitotane for adrenocortical cancer—a recurring controversy. *J Clin Endocrinol Metab*. 2008;**93**:3730 - 3732.

33 Fassnacht M, Terzolo M, Allolio B, et al. Combination chemotherapy in advanced adrenocortical carcinoma. FIRM-ACT Study Group. *N Engl J Med*. 2012;**366**:2189 - 2197.

34 Markoe AM, Serber W, Micaily B, et al. Radiation therapy for adjunctive treatment of adrenal cortical carcinoma. *Am J Clin Oncol*. 1991;**14**:170 - 174.

35 Fassnacht M, Hahner S, Polat B, et al. Efficacy of adjuvant radiotherapy of the tumor bed on local recurrence of adrenocortical carcinoma. *J Clin Endocrinol Metab*. 2006;**91**:4501 - 4504.

36 Wood BJ, Abraham J, Hvizda JL, et al. Radiofrequency ablation of adrenal tumors and adrenocortical carcinoma metastases. *Cancer*. 2003;**97**:554 - 560.

37 Veytsman I, Nieman L, Fojo T. Management of endocrine manifestations and the use of mitotane as a chemotherapeutic agent for adrenocortical carcinoma. *J Clin Oncol*. 2009;**27**:4619 - 4629.

第 82 章　弥漫性神经内分泌和胃肠胰系统肿瘤

Evan Vosburgh, MD

概述

弥漫性神经内分泌系统(DES)由一类散布在全身的数量不多的细胞组成。起源于这类细胞的肿瘤非常有趣,这些细胞产生的肿瘤呈现出广泛的流行病学、病理学、生物学特征。对遗传性多发性内分泌肿瘤(如 MEN-1、MEN-2)综合征以及由于特异性肽分泌引起的各种独特临床综合征(如胰岛素瘤、高血糖素瘤、VIP 瘤)的临床和科学研究具有挑战性。有的肿瘤很典型,但更多情况下临床表现无特异性,或肿瘤很小(小于 1.0cm)难以发现而无临床症状和体征,但却可以在尚不能界定其是否为肿瘤时而已经发生远处转移。癌症登记数据显示神经内分泌系统肿瘤的 5 年生存率在过去数十年中没有改善,仍保持在 30%~60%。相同的注册数据记录了这些肿瘤,特别是胃肠道胰腺系统的神经内分泌肿瘤(GEP-NET)的发病率上升和无法解释的发病率,当加上长期平均存活率,其发病率与睾丸、卵巢和多发骨髓瘤等癌症相似。最近在遗传学、生物学、临床特征和对治疗反应的理解方面的进展是神经内分泌肿瘤的更好的定义亚型,一旦聚集并研究为“类癌”。修订后的组织学分组和分期正在通知正在进行的临床试验,并为这些不同的肿瘤提供更明智的临床护理。最近对几种有无进展生存益处的靶向治疗的批准表明,DES 肿瘤的现状正在改变。

弥漫性神经内分泌系统(DES)由一类散布在全身的数量不多的细胞组成。起源于这类细胞的肿瘤非常有趣,原因是它们的流行病学、病理学、生物学和临床特征令人困惑不已。这类少见的肿瘤复杂多样,包括遗传性多发性内分泌腺瘤病(如 MEN1 或 MEN2),常伴继发于特殊肽类激素(如胰岛素瘤、高血糖素瘤、血管活性肠肽瘤等)的临床独特综合征,加之有的患者可以长期生存,这些为临床和科研研究工作带来了极大挑战。有的肿瘤很典型,但更多情况下临床表现无特异性,或肿瘤很小(小于 1.0cm)难以发现而无临床症状和体征,但却可以在尚不能界定其是否为肿瘤时而已经发生远处转移。以上特点在一定程度上解释了为什么在过去数十年的癌症数据库中,这类肿瘤的 5 年生存率始终为 30%~60%,没有取得进步,以致众多学者强烈质疑将神经内分泌肿瘤统称为良性肿瘤的合理性。相同的登记数据记录了这些肿瘤,特别是胃肠道胰腺系统的神经内分泌肿瘤(胃肠胰神经内分泌肿瘤)的发病率上升和无法解释的发病率,当加上长期平均存活率,其发病率与睾丸、卵巢,多发性脊髓瘤等相似。

最近在遗传学、生物学、临床特征和治疗反应方面的研究进展是神经内分泌肿瘤的更好的定义亚型,一旦聚集并研究为“类癌”。经修订的组织学分组和分期正在通知正在进行的临床试验,并正在提供对这些不同的肿瘤进行更有效的临床治疗。最近对几种有无进展生存益处的靶向治疗的批准表明,DES 肿瘤的现状正在改变。

这章所讨论的 DES 肿瘤重点包括胃肠胰腺神经内分泌肿瘤(GEP-NET),代表了所有 DES(弥漫性神经内分泌系统)肿瘤的绝大部分。包括以下特殊亚型:

- 类癌,属分化好的 GEP-NET,占所有 GEP-NET 的一半以上。
- 胰腺神经内分泌肿瘤(PENT),是发生率仅次于类癌的 GEP-NET,分为非分泌型肿瘤和分泌型肿瘤。分泌型肿瘤有独特的临床和免疫化学表现,分泌相关的特殊肽类激素(如胰岛素瘤)。
- 多发性内分泌腺瘤病(MEN)综合征 1、2a、2b 和家族性甲状腺髓样癌(FMTC),是特征明确的(家族性)癌综合征,往往累及有 DES 细胞分布的多种组织。
- 嗜铬细胞瘤和甲状旁腺肿瘤,散发性或伴随 MEN 综合征。

流行病学

过去一个世纪里,类癌和相关神经内分泌肿瘤的分类系统所面临的挑战之一是,组织学并不是特别具有信息性,而且对于良性和恶性的生物表型往往是相似的。随着时间的推移,胃肠道典型类癌肿瘤与胰岛细胞瘤或 PNET 的分离是一致的。

在对类癌肿瘤的全面流行病学回顾中,Modlin 等人[1]和 Yao 等人[2]报道了 SEER(监测、流行病学和最终结果)癌症登记数据,其发病率和患病率跨越了半个世纪。对 13 000 多例和 35 000 多例病例的十年分析表明,过去 30 年的总发病率有所增加。超过 65%的 NET 主要是两大类肿瘤,即类癌(重命名为 GI-NET)和胰岛细胞瘤(重命名为 PNET),统称为 GEP-NET(图 82-1)。在胃肠 NET 中,小肠仍是最常见的部位,随着时间的推移发病率保持稳定,而胃和直肠类癌在近几十年中有所增加。PNET 大致分为非功能 PNET 和功能 PNET。功能性 PNET 的发病率依次为胃泌素瘤、胰岛素瘤、VIP 瘤、高血糖素瘤,以及非常罕见的神经紧张素瘤、生长抑素瘤和其他异位症。PNET 大致分为非功能 PNET 和功能 PNET。功能性 PNET 的发病率依次为胃泌素瘤、胰岛素瘤、VIP 瘤、高血糖素瘤,以及非常罕见的神经紧张素瘤、生长抑素瘤和其他分泌异位激素的肿瘤[1]。胃和直肠发病率的变化被认为是随着上消化道和上消化道内镜的使用而增加的检出率。同一时期,阑尾类癌的发病率下降,可能反映了开放性腹部手术和旁观者阑尾切除术的减少。胃、直肠和阑尾 NET 常被偶然诊断为浅表性病变,本章不讨论其处理方法。

超过 50 年的数据表明,总体生存率、T 特定部位的生存率和不同疾病程度的生存率几乎没有变化,包括诊断时即为转移性疾病,相对恒定 10%~12%。值得注意的是,GEP-NET 肿瘤的低发病率具有欺骗性,正如 Yao 等[2]人所证明的,超过许多

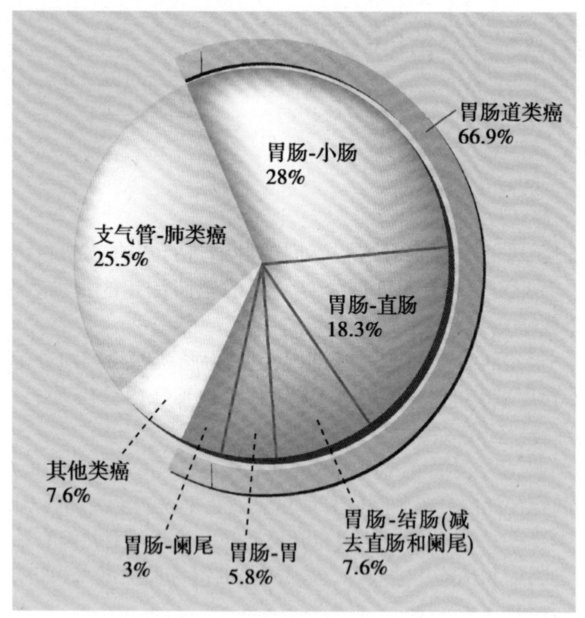

图 82-1 按解剖部位估计神经内分泌肿瘤(NET)的相对发病率。为说明目的从许多出版物中汇编,并通过结合随时间和来源而变化的分类系统进行估计

其他肿瘤类型的总生存率转化为 GEP-NET 的患病率超过了其他胃肠道肿瘤,包括食管、胃、胰腺和肝胆。

弥漫性神经内分泌系统

弥漫性神经内分泌系统(DES)在早期组织学和细胞生物学中有其描述性起源,定义了广泛分布于肠道(肠嗜铬细胞)和其他器官包括大脑、甲状旁腺、垂体、甲状腺、肺、肾上腺(嗜铬细胞或透明细胞)的一组正常的嗜铬上皮细胞[3]。在胃肠道中,从胃到直肠都能发现 DES 的细胞,并且不到周围细胞群的1%。消化道道 DES 细胞与神经细胞具有一样的表型和生化特征。这些 DES 细胞不仅包含内分泌细胞所具有的致密核心大囊泡(LCDV),也包含神经细胞突触区域特征性的突触样微小囊泡(SLMV)。Weidenmann 等详细讨论了 DES 细胞生化的复杂多样性以及 LCDV 和 SLMV 分泌的调控机制[4]。DES 的细胞可能共享或不共享一个胚胎起源。然而,众所周知,肠道内分泌细胞是由肠内胚层产生的[5],肠道的四种上皮细胞类型,包括神经内分泌细胞,是由在肠腔中发现的一种常见的多潜能干细胞衍生而来的[6],这种干细胞以富含亮氨酸的重复包含的G 蛋白偶联受体 5(IGR 5)为特征[7]。胰腺神经内分泌细胞来源于胰岛的多能干细胞,期起源细胞的遗传、表观遗传和生物学特性以及 NET 的众多表型的确定才仅仅是个开端。

神经内分泌的标志物

神经内分泌标志物被用于 NET 的组织学和免疫组化分类,并在一定程度上作为诊断和评估反应和复发的临床标志物。标记包括:

血清素和代谢物-NET 合成和分泌血清素的限速步骤是色氨酸转化为 5-羟色胺(5-HTP)。5-HTP 迅速转化为 5-羟色胺,该 5-羟色胺储存在神经分泌颗粒中,或可直接分泌到血管室,在那里转化为尿代谢物 5-羟基吲哚醋酸(5-HIAA)[8]。对于合成和分泌 5-羟色胺的 NET,24h 尿液中 5-羟色胺的定量分析是诊断和随访的最佳特征和最常用的临床分析[9]。

嗜铬粒蛋白 A(CgA)是糖蛋白类嗜铬粒蛋白家族的一员,与许多肽激素一起储存在内分泌和神经内分泌细胞的大而密的核心囊泡(LDCV)中[10]。因此,它可以作为组织染色的免疫组织化学标记物和血浆标记物。CgA 已被公认为是对于 GEP-NET 患者最有用的诊断标志物,敏感性高于 90%[11]。CgA 水平与转移性与非转移性疾病相关,可用于术后复发患者的随访[12]。

突触蛋白(P38)是一种主要的神经元蛋白,主要集中在神经细胞小突触囊泡膜上[13]。Weidenmann 等人[14]证实了突触蛋白在广泛的正常神经内分泌细胞和神经内分泌肿瘤中的存在。

Bishop 及其同事证实,神经元特异性烯醇化酶(NSE)存在于所有可识别的胃肠道和胰腺内分泌和神经细胞中[15]。NSE已经取代了早期的组织嗜银染色作为正常神经内分泌细胞和肿瘤的细胞溶质标志物。

生长抑素和生长抑素受体

生长抑素及其受体(SSTR)的生物学特点及它们在 GEP-NET 上的表达为这类肿瘤诊断和治疗带来了重要的信息。生长抑素类似物作为早期癌症靶向治疗的成功典范,极大地提高了内科和外科手术治疗的疗效,并且提高了患者的生活质量。与放射性物质耦连的生长抑素类似物为临床提供了很有价值的影像学信息,目前已将其发展为针对多肽受体的放射疗法(PRRT)。

生长抑素是一种多肽,可以抑制多种生理活动,治疗最相关的作用是抑制激素分泌。生长抑素存在于中枢神经系统、下丘脑-垂体系统、胃肠道、胰腺的外分泌和内分泌细胞以及免疫效应细胞中。生长抑素包括 28 肽和 14 肽两种形式[16]。

生长抑素及其类似物和分布于细胞质膜表面,与不同 G 蛋白耦联受体亚型 SSTR 1~5 的亲和力不同。从而导致细胞增殖减少和凋亡诱导[17,18]。

GEP-NET,尤其是小肠和胰岛的肿瘤,表达多种 SSTR 亚型,最常见和密度最高的是 SSTR2,在 80%以上的病例高表达,其次是 SSTR5[19-21]。SSTR2 表达生长抑素类似物为治疗、诊断和核医学成像随访以及新出现的 PRRT 的治疗的发展至关重要。

神经内分泌的组织学和分期

Modlin[22]详述了网络的丰富历史,可追溯到 Siegfried Oberndorfer 在 1907 年独立描述的一类表现一致的胃肠道肿瘤,命名为类癌或癌样肿瘤,以区别于侵袭性更强的腺癌。近 100 年来,类癌被广泛用于所有 DES 肿瘤,这类肿瘤有相似的组织学形态,直到今天仍被描述为一类单一的细胞核小且形态规则,以岛状小梁样、腺样、未分化和混合性方式生长的肿瘤[23]。随着对 DES 认识的深入,尤其是 GEP 细胞,正常细胞和相应肿瘤细胞具有共同之处,已经试图根据生物学特点对类癌进行分类和描述。

组织学和分期

认识到原发部位和分化程度的重要性，由 Solcia 等人于 2000 年发表的修订后的 WHO 分类采用了神经内分泌的术语以避免过去各种各样的关于类癌的定义[24]。在 2000 版的 WHO 分类中引入了 GEP-NET 的术语，并基于分化程度将之分成 3 类，将原发部位作为最主要描述特征以适应广泛的 NET 的亚型。UICC/AJCC/WHO[25]的最新改进和欧洲神经内分泌学会（ENES）[26]和北美神经内分泌肿瘤学会（NANETS）[27]的修改认识到组织分化的共性和重要性，并进一步强调由有丝分裂率和/或 Ki67 百分比决定的分级（表 82-1）。TMN 分期于 2010 年首次应用[28]，判断其预后的价值的前瞻性和回顾性验证正在进行中。

表 82-1　GEP-NET 的分类

WHO 2010 命名	AJCC/ENET 命名
神经内分泌肿瘤 1 级	神经内分泌瘤 1 级
神经内分泌肿瘤 2 级	神经内分泌瘤 2 级
神经内分泌癌 3 级	神经内分泌癌 3 级
小细胞癌	小细胞癌
大细胞神经内分泌癌	大细胞神经内分泌癌

DES 肿瘤的临床特点

一般来说，DES 在早期阶段很难识别。在取得病理结果之前，肺结节、胰腺肿块、肝脏转移、内镜下胃和直肠的病变往往被认为是普通的常见恶性肿瘤。早期症状通常是非特异性的（如腹痛和腹泻），即使出现了更多的激素分泌相关的症状，原发肿瘤往往仍然很小并且难以定位。患者通常有长期持续的症状，但往往在发展至局部晚期或远处转移引起相关症状时才被诊断。一旦考虑该诊断，非特异性（如 CgA）和特异性的（如 5-HIAA，促胃液素）肿瘤标志物检查以及联合影像学手段如放射性生长抑素类似物显影、B 超、CT、MRI 和 PET 扫描，都将提供有力的诊断依据以指导内科或外科治疗。受肿瘤位置的多变性、分泌状态及生物学行为的影响，对这类肿瘤开展临床研究十分困难。尽管缺乏比较性临床试验的结果，对 NET 的处理原则已有一致的认识[29]。

影像学

生长抑素受体闪烁显影法（SRS）在大多数 GEP-NET 诊断和定位中是中心地位。OctreoScan™（111In-DTPA 喷曲肽）数十年来一直是首选的扫描方法，最近在一些机构中被特异性和敏感性更高的 68Ga-PET/CT 的增强所取代[30]。神经内分泌肿瘤的低增殖活性使得 18FDG-PET 对类癌及相关肿瘤的敏感性很低[31]。CT 和 MRI 通常为 SRS 诊断的疾病提供进一步的解剖学信息，在肿瘤生长或反应中比 SRS 更有用[32]。大多数文献报道支持 SRS 作为首选的成像方式来定位确诊和怀疑 GEP-NET 患者的原发性和转移性病变（包括骨），胰岛素瘤患者除外[33,34]。一项欧洲的多中心临床试验共纳入 350 例经组织学或生物化学证实的胃肠胰腺伸进内分泌肿瘤患者。常规方法的肿瘤定位阳性率为 88%，SRS 的阳性率为 80%。大多数 GEPNET 中 SRS 阳性，高血糖素瘤阳性率为 100%，血管活性肠肽瘤阳性率为 88%，类癌阳性率为 87%，非功能性胰岛细胞瘤阳性率为 82%。胰岛素瘤的检出率较低（46%）与其低表达 SSTR2 相关。空腹胰岛素水平加上内镜超声（EUS）是胰岛素瘤术前定位最敏感的方法[35]。

胃肠神经内分泌肿瘤（GI-NET）

分化良好的小肠神经内分泌肿瘤（GI-NET）是最常见的神经内分泌肿瘤。一般来说肿瘤很少见于小肠，GI-NET 占所有小肠肿瘤的 13%～34%，占所有小肠恶性肿瘤的 17%～46%[36]。

GI-NET 已经报道近百年。Modlin 等人[1]报道在过去几十年里诊断平均年龄从 59.9 岁增加到 61.4 岁。除了少数未分化神经内分泌癌的患者外[37]，GI-NET 通常生长缓慢，通常延误诊断多年，有时仅通过与淋巴结、肝脏和不太常见骨相关的转移症状来诊断。

小肠 GI-NET 可出现小肠梗阻、腹痛、腹泻或胃肠道出血。在大多数病例中肿瘤定位于远端小肠呈较低的壁内生长方式（图 82-2），许多肿瘤超过 2cm 却仍然不能被诊断就不足为奇了。小肠肿瘤是否会引起明显的局部症状，与受累肠段的缺血、绞窄及纤维化反应相关。远处转移的发生和肿瘤大小相关。回肠肿瘤小于 1cm 时远处转移发生率小于 15%，但是当肿瘤增大到 2cm 时转移率升高到 95%。如果在外科手术或内镜检查中没有被顺带诊断出来，只有在对腹部主诉或缺铁性贫血进行长时间评估，或对类癌综合征进行敏锐识别后，才能确认

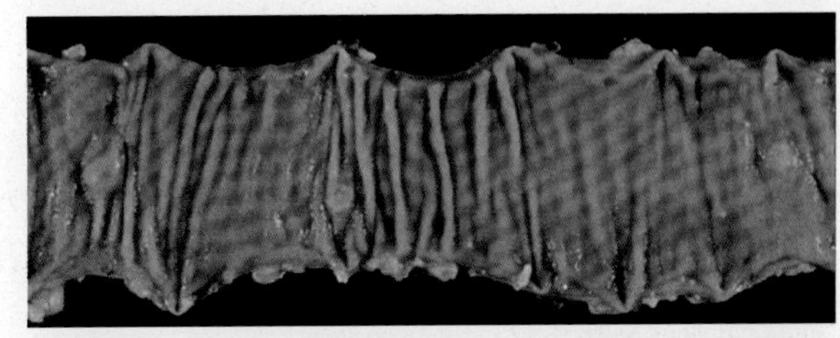

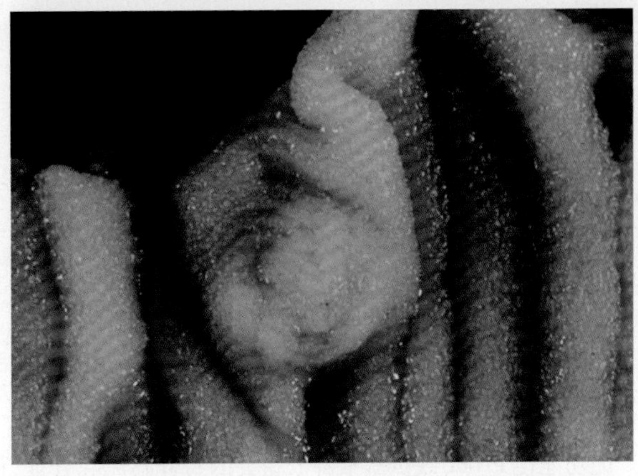

图 82-2　小肠多发类癌。一名年轻男性患者在结肠镜检查时发现 3 枚小于 1cm 小肠类癌（Courtesy of Ed Uthman，MD）

GI-NET。

类癌综合征

发生类癌综合征的小肠 GI-NET 患者不到 10%，但小肠 GI-NET 占类癌综合征患者的 90%以上[38]。90%以上的类癌综合征仅发生在转移扩散到肝脏后，主要特征为腹泻（83%），潮红（49%），喘息（6%），腹痛，很少见的还有糙皮病[37,39]。5-羟色胺及其代谢产物被认为是引起类癌综合征的主要原因，但是其他生物活性物质如前列腺素类 SP、胰腺血管舒缓素、多巴胺和神经肽 K 也参与其中[9]。没有一个单一的检测方法能检测到所有类癌综合征病例。虽然尿 5-HIAA 似乎是最好的筛查程序，但仅 84% NET 相关的类癌综合征患者检测到尿 5-HIAA[40]。摄入富含 5-羟色胺的食物可能会出现假阳性，如坚果、鳄梨、猕猴桃、菠萝和香蕉[41]。已发现 CgA 在 100%的类癌综合征患者中升高，但缺乏肿瘤定位的特异性，因为它在 PNET 和其他神经内分泌肿瘤中升高[42]。

类癌心脏病

1/2~2/3 的类癌综合征患者会发展成类癌心脏病[43,44]。大部分以右侧瓣膜损害为主，表现为肌成纤维细胞增生、致密的细胞外胶原以及黏液沉积[45]。心脏的瓣膜增厚挛缩引起反流导致结构性疾病（然后纤维化融合导致狭窄），最终可因右心充血性心力衰竭[46]。Moller 等[47]随访了超过 100 名患者的系列超声心动结果或者根据初始超声心动图进行手术治疗，并且发现类癌性心脏病患者的中位生存期为 1.6 年，而无类癌性疾病患者的中位生存期为 4.6 年。5-HIAA 的峰浓度及既往化疗是预示类癌性心脏病进展的独立预测因子。间接证据包括类癌心脏病患者的心脏出现了类似减肥药芬氟拉明-芬特明这类药物引起的心脏瓣膜组织学损伤[48]。已有的研究表明在发生类癌心脏病之后控制 5-HIAA 水平不能阻止瓣膜损伤的进展[47,49]。人们普遍接受但未证实，在诊断时尽早应用生长抑素类似物控制 5-羟色胺分泌能降低症状性类癌心脏病的发病率。

胰腺神经内分泌肿瘤（PNET）（胰岛细胞瘤）

第二种最常见的 GEP-NET 发生在胰腺。作为一个群体，他们具有与其他 GEP-NET 类似的组织学特征[50]。PNET 占所有 GEP-NET 的约 15%，但仅占所有胰腺肿瘤的 1%~2%。非功能性 PNET 和胃泌素瘤是最常见的 PNET，其次是胰岛素瘤和由其特定分泌产物相关的临床综合征定义的罕见的一些肿瘤（表 82-2）。

表 82-2 临床综合征

临床症状	肿瘤类型	部位	激素
潮红/腹泻/哮鸣音	类癌	中前肠 胰腺/前肠，肾上腺髓质	血清素，P 物质 NKA，TCT，PP，CGRP，VIP
溃疡疾病	胃泌素瘤	胰腺（85%）、十二指肠（15%）	促胃液素
低血糖症	胰岛细胞瘤肉瘤 肝细胞瘤	胰腺/子宫 腹膜后肝脏	胰岛素、TNF IGF、BP
皮炎/痴呆 糖尿病/DVT	高血糖素瘤	胰腺	高血糖素
糖尿病/脂肪泻	生长抑素瘤	胰腺	生长抑素
胆结石/神经纤维瘤病	生长抑素瘤	十二指肠	生长抑素
无症状/肝脏转移胰	多肽瘤	胰腺	PP
肢端肥大症	GEP	胰腺	GH（GHRH）
库欣综合征	GEP	胰腺	ACTH/CRF
高钙血症	血管活性肠肽瘤 GEP	胰腺 胰腺	VIP PTHrP
色素沉着	GEP	胰腺	MSH

ACTH，促肾上腺皮质激素；BP，结合蛋白；CGRP，降钙素基因相关肽；CRF，促肾上腺皮质激素释放因子；DVT，深部静脉血栓形成；GEP，胃肠胰的；GH，生长激素；GHRH，促生长素释放素；IGF，胰岛素样生长因子；MSH，促黑细胞激素；NKA，神经肽 A；PP，胰多肽；PTHrP，甲状旁腺激素相关肽；TCT，降钙素；TNF，肿瘤坏死因子；VIP，血管活性肠肽。

无功能性胰腺神经内分泌肿瘤

无功能性 PNET 缺少激素释放相关的特异临床综合征，但可以有一种或几种肽或胺染色阳性，甚至血清中可定量检测到相应的神经内分泌标志物。无功能性 PNET 共占 PNET 的 15%~30%。由于没有相应的激素分泌症状，患者大多由于在 40 岁或 50 岁以后被诊断，36%的患者主诉为腹痛，28%为黄疸，另有 16%为术中探查发现[51]。因此，60%~90%的患者在确诊时就已经发生局部或者远处转移。无功能性 PNET 近 100%均有血清 CgA 的升高[42]。CT 和 MRI 可以用来确定肿瘤分期和随访肿瘤的复发和远处转移。

手术是多数 GEP-NET 的治疗选择，也是唯一可以达到根治的治疗方法。但对于无功能性 PNET 患者来说，由于症状出现较晚，很大比例的患者在确诊时已经有了远处转移，因而无法手术。但手术可以减轻瘤负荷、解除胆道梗阻而达到姑息的目的。由于影像诊断使用的增加导致早期诊断影响尚未证实。

胃泌素瘤

胃泌素瘤综合征，也称佐林格-埃利森综合征，最早见于一份描述了两个严重消化道溃疡，同时伴有胰腺非 β 细胞来源肿瘤的患者的报告[52]，随后发现这种肿瘤还分泌促胃液素[53]。胃泌素瘤以严重的溃疡体质以及基础胃酸分泌持续升高为特征。高胃酸分泌可导致常见的症状腹泻。高达 20% 的患者腹泻是唯一症状[54]。胃泌素瘤占了各类 PNET 的大约 25%，好发部位为十二指肠（70%）、胰腺（25%），约 50% 为恶性[55,56]。大约 20% 的胃泌素瘤患者最终在 MEN-1 中发现了种系突变[54]，其表现和病程与散发病例不同（见 MEN-1 综合征）。

空腹血清促胃液素升高以及基础胃酸水平升高是诊断胃泌素瘤重要的两项指标。这两者升高也见于 Hp 感染、抗胃酸分泌治疗（如奥美拉唑）、慢性胃炎、恶性贫血、萎缩性胃炎和迷走神经切断术后状态[57]。敏感性和准确性最高的检测方法是肠促胰液素激发试验[58]。

用药物治疗（即奥美拉唑）治疗胃泌素瘤综合征的成功率约为 95%[59]，因此，生长缓慢的胃泌素瘤患者的长期生存率现在主要取决于肿瘤的最终恶性行为，而不是溃疡体质和腹泻[60]。手术已经从胃切除术发展到控制溃疡病，到使用术前和术中成像的复杂手术，以定位和切除通常较小的局部和区域转移性疾病。除去 MEN-1 的患者，胃泌素瘤患者的 5 年总生存率在 60%~80%，10 年总生存率在 45%~75%[56,61,62]。

胰岛素瘤

Whipple 在 1938 年报道了 30 名胰腺腺瘤伴有低血糖症的患者，从而最早描述了胰岛素瘤[63]。胰岛素瘤是第二常见的功能性 PNET，发病率大约为（0.8~0.9）/100 万。总体上看，胰岛素瘤转移的发生率为 5%~15%，低于其他的 PNET[64]。发现多发性胰岛素瘤应及时检测 MEN-1[65]。在胰岛素瘤患者的前瞻性数据库中，88% 的 MEN-1 患者有多灶性病变，而非 MEN-1 患者只有 4%[66]。

几乎所有的胰岛素瘤患者都表现出低血糖症，同时伴有低血糖相关的神经症状（视物不清、意识障碍、虚弱），这些表现比单纯的交感兴奋症状（出汗、颤抖）更加常见[64]。对于怀疑病例可通过严密监控下的禁食试验而得到确诊。超过 90% 的患者在禁食 48h 内血糖会降至 50mg/dl 以下，而相应的胰岛素在低血糖状态下则大于或等于 5μU/ml[67]。

经过手术，80%~90% 的患者能被治愈。超声内镜（EUS）据报道的敏感性可达到 80%，可以定位小于 1cm 的肿瘤[68]。当超声内镜无法定位，术中超声（IOUS）进行肿瘤定位可以避免盲目的胰腺切除。少食多餐的饮食联合直接阻断 β 细胞胰岛素释放的药物二氮嗪和奥曲肽可以控制多达 60% 的术前患者或不可切除的病变患者的症状[69]。

血管活性肠肽瘤

血管活性肠肽瘤（VIPomas）首先由 Verner 和 Morrison[70] 描述，并随后在一篇综述中回顾性分析了 55 名有 WDHA 综合征（水样腹泻、低钾血症、胃酸缺乏症）的患者的资料[71]。VIPomas 相当少见，约只占 PNET 的 5%，与其他 PNET 不同，VIPomas 有明确的成人和儿童亚组患者。在成人中，90% 的肿瘤在胰腺中发现，大多数是孤立性结节，60% 以上的病例出现或发展为转移性疾病。在儿童中，大多数儿童分泌血管活性肠肽的肿瘤发生于胰腺外且为神经起源，最常见的病理类型为节神经母细胞瘤和神经节瘤[72]。疾病的诊断依靠血液中 VIP 水平的升高和大量的分泌性腹泻症状[73]。

奥曲肽对临床症状的控制率超过 80%，同时可降低血浆 VIP 水平[69]。Long 等[72]报道了 52 例胰腺 VIPomas，平均直径为 9cm，凭借 CT 或超声就能够准确定位。有些 VIPomas 需要通过血管造影或不加选择性静脉取血标本检测 VIP 水平才能够准确定位[73]。手术完整切除可以使 30%~50% 的成年患者的症状得到长期缓解[74]。

高血糖素瘤

高血糖素瘤首先在 1966 年由 McGavran 等报道[75]。当时 McGavran 等呼吁关注一种伴获得性糖尿病合并高血糖素升高的综合征。这种罕见肿瘤占全部 GEP-NET 的 1%，并随后被发现伴有特征性皮疹和坏死松解性游走性红斑（necrolytic migratory erythema，NME）[76,77]。这种肿瘤几乎只发生在 40 岁以上的成年患者，并且少数病例中伴 MEN-1 综合征[78]。

最大的单中心报道来自 Mayo Clinic 在 1975—1991 年诊治的 21 例病变[79]。主要的临床表现包括：体重下降（71%）、特征性 NME 皮疹（67%）、轻度糖尿病（38%）、腹泻（29%）、疼痛性舌炎和口角炎（29%）。

几乎所有的肿瘤都表现为胰腺（胰尾多于胰体）处单发结节，平均直径 5~10cm。超过 60% 的患者在确诊时就发生了远处转移，肝转移最常见[80]。如果诊断时肿瘤仍然局限，手术切除可以治愈[81]。由于肿瘤生长缓慢和有可用的治疗方法，转移患者 10 年生存率为 51.6%，无转移患者为 64.3%[82]。在 50% 以上的患者中，NME 皮疹和腹泻（但一般不是葡萄糖不耐症/糖尿病）对奥曲肽有反应，大约 30% 的患者症状完全消失[69]。

生长抑素瘤

生长抑素瘤是非常罕见的 PNET，到目前仅有 50 多例病例报告。第一例由 Ganda[83] 及 Larsson 等[84] 在 1977 年报告。Krejs 等[85] 在 1979 年又报告了系列 8 个病例，Vinik 等[86] 在 1986 年发表了迄今为止最大的综述，包括 48 例患者。生长抑素瘤患者很少出现 MEN-1 综合征[78]。

尽管定义了糖尿病、腹泻、脂肪泻、胆囊疾病、低氯血症和体重减轻的临床综合征[87]，但大多数病例在剖腹手术或腹腔镜检查时被诊断，或在腹部不是或黄疸的影像学检查时被发现。血浆中生长抑素水平的显著升高被认为是导致大多数症状的原因。肿瘤通常表现为较大的实性肿块，释放高水平的生长抑素，并引起相关症状。确诊时，大约 85% 原发于胰腺和 50% 原发于小肠的肿瘤已经发生转移[88]，尽管相关数据不多，但由于其转移率高，生长抑素瘤的预后差。文献中，接近一半的患者在诊断后一年内死亡，而有的患者可以生存超过 5 年[87]。

GEP-NET 的治疗

总体来讲,GEP-NET 均生长缓慢,其临床症状多与分泌的激素类物质有关或者巨大肿物引起的疼痛。对于那些无法手术切除或已发生远处转移的患者,治疗重点在于控制症状。使用长效生长抑素类似物可以减少有血管活性作用的激素及其他激素的分泌,结合减轻瘤负荷的其他治疗手段(主要针对肝脏转移瘤),GEP-NET 患者在相当长的时间生活质量不会受到影响。最近的数据表明,对于选择的患者,生长抑素类似物、舒尼替尼和依维莫司可以延长转移性疾病患者的无进展生存期。

首选手术

在对 GEP-NET 患者进行所有手术之前使用生长抑素类似物预防性治疗以避免类癌综合征或其他分泌性危象的出现[89]。对发生于胃和十二指肠的小于 1cm 的经选择的 GEP-NET 可以经内镜下切除[90]。局限性的小肠 GEP-NET 可以连同淋巴结完整切除以及同时切除肠系膜[91]。小于 2cm 的阑尾 GI-NET 可以行阑尾切除,大于 2cm 的可以行根治性切除术[92]。

肝定向治疗

鉴于转移扩散到肝脏的频率很高,许多肝脏定向治疗已用于 GEP-NET 的治疗。超过 90%的患者由于肝转移灶过大、过多或广泛转移以至于无法切除。肝脏切除:Que 等[93]于近期发表了一篇荟萃分析关于 GEP-NET 行半肝切除、三段式切除、楔形切除。局部肝切除术后患者的死亡率为 2.3%。超过 80%的病例由激素分泌引起的症状得到了改善(如类癌综合征),缓解期为 4~120 个月。

射频消融术

对于这类患者,射频消融术可以用来减轻瘤负荷并控制相关症状。目前最大的关于射频消融术用于转移性神经内分泌瘤治疗的文献报道了单中心十年间的结果。文中围术期死亡率小于 5%,症状部分缓解率为 90%,完全缓解率为 72%,中位缓解期约为一年[94]。

肝动脉栓塞治疗

总体来说,肝血管栓塞治疗后的生化反应率可高达 50%,40%的患者肿瘤缩小,但持续时间较短[95]。肝动脉栓塞后序贯化疗的反应率可高达 80%,中位缓解期约 18 个月或更长[96~98]。

肝移植

最近的涉及欧洲 103 例神经内分泌肿瘤肝移植的综述显示,接受肝移植的患者 5 年生存率为 46%,5 年无病生存率为 24%[99]。但严格的移植适应证、较高的并发症及死亡率以及肝源的普遍缺乏,导致肝移植的开展受到限制。

生长抑素类似物

生长抑素类似物对于转移性神经内分泌肿瘤和类癌综合征引起的面色潮红、腹泻以及喘息等症状效果明显,可以控制各种 NET 引起的激素分泌相关症状。Yao 对 SEER 数据的分析显示,1998 年[2]奥曲肽在美国应用后,GEP-NET 的生存率有所提高,这可能反映了抗增殖作用和降低手术风险,使患者能够从更积极的转移性疾病治疗中获益。Janson[100]和 Kvols[101]等人发现 SRS 阳性预示在使用奥曲肽后症状均得到改善。奥曲肽是一种长效制剂(生长抑素 LAR)[102]和最近批准的兰诺肽,在美国可获得[103]。SOM 230 是一种能够与 1~5 型生长抑素受体广泛结合的药物,目前正在进行治疗 GEP-NET 的Ⅲ期临床试验,最近在美国被批准治疗库欣病[103]。

几十年来使用生长抑素类似物(短效和长效制剂)[104,105]与 70%~80%患者的生化反应、80%以上患者腹泻和潮红的症状控制以及 70%以上患者 5-HIAA 水平(如果在基线时升高)的降低有关[106,107]。最新研究生长抑素类似物在无症状具有明显肿瘤负荷的 GEP-NET 患者中的研究显示,其临床疗效超出症状控制。PROMID 试验是一项Ⅲ期、随机、安慰剂对照、双盲的研究,对微小或无症状转移性的小肠 GI-NET 患者进行了疾病的治疗,并将长效奥曲肽与安慰剂进行了比较。奥曲肽的中位进展时间为 14.3 个月,安慰剂为 6.0 个月,奥曲肽的 6 个月病情稳定率为 67%,安慰剂为 37%。由于交叉设计,中位总生存率没有评估[108]。CLARINET 试验是一项Ⅲ期、随机、安慰剂对照、双盲的研究,对无症状但进行性转移的高分化 GI-NET 和 PNET 患者进行研究。试验比较了长效 lanreotide 和安慰剂。与安慰剂组相比,lanreotide 组主要终点无进展生存期的(未达到)显著高于安慰剂组 18 个月,总体生存期无显著差异[109]。

生物制剂

Oberg 等人首先使用白细胞干扰素治疗 GEP-NET 类癌患者[110],并回顾了 2000 年的一些早期研究[112],结果显示生化指标缓解率可达到 63%~77%,超过 50%的患者肿瘤大小保持稳定,但很少出现完全或部分缓解。一项多中心随机对照研究对此进行了探索,但结果显示客观有效率方面联合用药组与单药组相比并没有提高[111]。尽管联合治疗组在症状及生化指标的缓解率方面更高,但这是以毒性增加为代价。

多肽受体介导的放射性核素治疗(PRRT)

生长抑素类似物可以靶向过度表达的 SSTR,从而使 PRRT 治疗 GEP-NET 有了发展前景。据此奥曲肽扫描定位的肿瘤表达 SSTR2、SSTR5,也是放射性药物作用的目标[112]。在Ⅰ、Ⅱ期临床试验中研究了几种不同的放射性核素生长抑素类似物组合,但尚未完成Ⅲ期试验。据报道有效率(CR+PR)在 10%~30%,40%~60%的患者病情稳定[113,114]。目前还没有 PRRT 批准用于治疗,它们只能通过临床试验或在欧洲选定的中心慈善性的使用。

GEP-NET 的细胞毒性化疗

一些作者回顾总结了过去单药或多药联合方案治疗类 GEP-NET 的历史[9,115]。在没有包含无治疗组的随机试验的情况下,没有可靠的证据表明单剂或联合化疗对转移性 NET 患者的疾病进展或生存率有任何显著影响。经批准的药物 DTIC 和链霉素具有显著的毒性和可疑的获益。最近关于替莫唑胺、沙利度胺联合用药[116]或卡培他滨回顾性研究[117]的结果令人鼓舞。化学药物通常只用来缓解激素过多分泌引起的以及肿瘤压迫相关的症状。

靶向治疗

一些新型靶向药物的早期临床试验已经完成。在酪氨酸激酶抑制剂伊马替尼[118]和吉非替尼[119]的Ⅱ期试验中，只观察到轻微疗效或完全无效。VEGF 拮抗剂贝伐单抗的Ⅱ期试验结果令人鼓舞[120]。一系列的临床试验使得 FDA 在 2011 年批准了依维莫司和舒尼替尼用于 PNET 的治疗。GI-NET 患者也被纳入试验并有反应，然而尚未达到能够批准的水平。

依维莫司是 M-TOR 的口服抑制剂，在随机、安慰剂对照的Ⅲ期临床研究 RADIANT-3 试验中，对晚期和进展性疾病的高分化 PNET 使用依维莫司的中位 PFS 为 11.0 个月，而安慰剂为 4.6 个月[121]。更早的随机、安慰剂对照的Ⅲ期临床研究 RADIANT-2 中，对晚期和进展期的高分化 GI-NET 或者类癌综合征患者，使用依维莫司的中位 PFS 为 16.4 个月，而安慰剂为 11.3 个月[122]。

舒尼替尼和口服多重酪氨酸激酶抑制剂在一项针对局部进展期或转移且近期进展的高分化 PNET 的Ⅲ期、随机、安慰剂对照研究中显示，其 PFS 为 11.4 个月，而安慰剂为 5.5 个月。尽管数据安全委员会的早期关闭和研究者对反应评估的可能偏倚使结果混杂，但 FDA 在独立的数据审查后批准了舒尼替尼用于该适应证[123]。

MEN 综合征

MEN-1 和 MEN-2 综合征起初被命名为维尔纳综合征，是因为该学者报道了一组常染色体显性遗传的多发腺瘤[124]。然而 MEN-1 综合征及 MEN-2 综合征在遗传学、临床表现和某些内分泌组织被累及的频率、预防性及治疗性手术及患者的随访以及家族成员方面均存在差异。MEN 综合征范畴内的神经内分泌肿瘤与其相对应的散发性肿瘤既有相似之处也存在差异。

MEN-1 综合征

由约 20 个不同组织学类型的神经内分泌肿瘤和非内分泌肿瘤组成了 MEN-1 综合征家族（表 82-3）。尽管所有的神经内分泌肿瘤的类型没有典型的组合，但来自多个家族的数据表明最常见的肿瘤为甲状旁腺来源的，其中增生占 90%，及胰腺来源（70%）和垂体前叶来源（25%）[126]。按目前的临床指南诊断 MEN-1 个体患者必须确认该患者患 3 种主要肿瘤中的 2 种，而要诊断 MEN-1 家族则需要至少有一个家族成员患有上述疾病，并至少有一个一级亲属患有至少一种主要相关肿瘤。

表 82-3 MEN-1 肿瘤类型分布及 40 岁前预计外显率（%）

内分泌肿瘤（常见）	内分泌肿瘤（不常见）	非内分泌
甲状旁腺腺瘤（90%）	胸腺类癌（2%）	胶原瘤（70%）
胃泌素瘤（40%）PP（无功能）瘤（20%）	支气管类癌（2%）PNET（VIP 瘤、高血糖素瘤等）（2%）	面部血管纤维瘤（85%）
催乳素瘤（20%）	ACTH，GH（2%）	脂肪瘤（30%）
胰岛素瘤（10%）	嗜铬细胞瘤（<1%）	
肠嗜铬细胞瘤（10%）	TSH（罕见）	

MEN-1 患者中非功能性肾上腺肿瘤的发生率可高达 25%。
来源：数据来源于 Giusti 等。

大约 80% 的家族性 MEN-1 和 50% 的散发性 MEN-1 患者有胚系 MEN-1 基因的杂合性突变[127,128]。目前已检测到的 1 336 种突变分布于 MEN-1 基因的编码区。MENIN 是 MEN-1 的产物，MEN-1 是一种抑癌基因，多数 MEN-1 基因的突变会导致其功能的丧失。尽管有多种基因型，但未发现基因型与可预测的临床表型之间有明确联系，故对具有特定基因突变的患病家族成员推荐预防性手术及进行特别筛查尚无充足的根据[129]。

MEN-1 综合征和甲状旁腺病变

多数患者以甲状旁腺功能亢进（HPT）、有症状的高钙血症起病，MEN-1 家族成员往往在接受筛查时发现生化异常或甲状旁腺肿瘤而诊断本病。平均发病年龄为 25~30 岁，到 50 岁时接近 100% 的 MEN-1 患者会出 HPT。与之相反，只有 2%~4% 的散发性甲状旁腺功能亢进患者有 MEN-1 基因的突变[130]，并且平均发病年龄为 55~60 岁。

MEN-1 综合征和胃泌素瘤

胃泌素瘤是 MEN-1 患者继 HPT 之后第二个最常见的“肿瘤”。

约 20% 的胃泌素瘤与 MEN-1 综合征有关[54]，起病较早、肿瘤多发、较小或初诊不易被发现、相对于散发胃泌素瘤较少恶性（7%~12%）。胃泌素瘤无远处转移及血生化检查表明肿瘤较局限时，摘除术（胰头）或切除术（胰体或胰尾）可能有较好的姑息治疗效果，但很少治愈[9]。一般建议避免手术，使用药物进行治疗并定期评估肿瘤的放射进展情况。

MEN-1 的内科和外科治疗

MEN-1 的临床表现完全取决于肿瘤的自然病程及内分泌功能的亢进情况。MEN-1 综合征的治疗依赖于患病个体的表型。多数需要手术干预的 MEN-1 胰腺疾病可表现出特定激素（如促胃液素、胰岛素、VIP 或高血糖素）分泌亢进引起的症状。总之，家族性 MEN-1 肿瘤患者的生存优于散发性胰腺内分泌肿瘤患者[9]。不论初始病变在何处，MEN-1 患者必须终身随访，对垂体腺体、甲状旁腺、胰腺或十二指肠、肾上腺及肺脏（支气管类癌）进行监测。家族成员如果 MEN-1 基因检测阳性的应接受类似的终身监测[131]。

MEN-2

MEN-2综合征代表几种不同的神经内分泌肿瘤群，其特异的RET原癌基因突变与表型有一种关联。MEN-2A综合征中甲状腺髓样癌占95%，嗜铬细胞瘤占50%，甲状旁腺增生/腺瘤占15%～30%[132]。MEN-2B患者100%发生甲状腺髓样癌，50%发生嗜铬细胞瘤，黏膜神经瘤及马方综合征样体型的发病率报道不一（表82-4）[133,134]。世界范围内已报道1 000个MEN-2家族，其中MEN-2B亚型约占80%[135]。已经鉴定出70多个不同的RET突变，并且随着大家族数据的增加，每个突变的基因型-表型关系变得不如最初报道的那样明显[136]。

表82-4 MEN-2综合征的分类

	MEN-2	MTC	Pheo	甲状旁腺增生/腺瘤
MEN-2A	60%～90%	95%	50%	20%～30%
MEN-2B	5%	100%	50%	不常见
FMTC	5%～35%	100%	0%	0%

FMTC，家族性甲状腺髓样癌；MTC，甲状腺髓样癌；Pheo，嗜铬细胞瘤。

来源：数据来源于Moline等。

甲状腺髓样癌

MTC占甲状腺癌新发病例的5%～10%，在美国每年有1 000例新发患者。其中，约75%无MTC家族史（即为散发型MTC），诊断时年龄多为50～60岁[137]。MEN-2A和2B患者均有患甲状腺髓样癌的高风险。MEN-2A患者常在患嗜铬细胞瘤或甲状旁腺疾病前就发现MTC。MEN-2A的家族成员常在5～25岁就出现早期MTC的生化证据[138]。同MEN-2A患者相比，MEN-2B患者起病年龄较早，甲状腺髓样癌的侵袭性更强、预后更差[139,140]。幸运的是，能够对马方综合征及黏膜神经瘤进行基因筛查或者能够临床识别，在发生MTC前就被识别诊断[141]。约30%的MTC患者不能被基因检测或者生化筛查中被诊断，最终可出现颈部肿块（有痛性）和/或高降钙素引起的腹泻。这些患者大多已经有局部或远处肿瘤播散[137]。

家族性甲状腺髓样癌

家族性甲状腺髓样癌（FMTC）不同于MEN-2A、MEN-2B及散发性MTC，指一个家族中有4个或4个以上成员患有MTC且没有嗜铬细胞瘤或甲状旁腺增生/腺瘤。FMTC中RET基因的突变约90%[142]。考虑到有些FMTC后来被诊断为MEN-2A或MEN-2B[143]，建议对所有FMTC患者行定期的嗜铬细胞瘤及甲状旁腺疾病筛查。FMTC的临床病程及预后较好，与MEN-2A、MEN-2B相关的MTC相似[142]。

甲状腺髓样癌的治疗

预防性甲状腺切除术（及甲状旁腺自体移植）适用于所有具有胚系RET基因突变的MEN-2患者。关于手术的时机仍存在争议，特定的RET密码子受累对治疗有一定的指导意义[126]。MTC的治疗包括甲状腺全切及淋巴结切除术，并给予终身甲状腺素替代治疗。患者术后复发率约50%[144]，推荐每年进行降钙素刺激试验检查。化疗和放疗的临床研究没有显示出任何持久的反应[145]。然而，对各种靶向多激酶抑制剂的临床研究已显示出有希望的结果，并导致最近FDA批准了两种新的MTC药物。凡德他尼是一种口服的VEGF2～3、RET、EGFR抑制剂，在一项Ⅲ期、随机、安慰剂对照的临床试验中，无进展生存率提高了30.5个月，而安慰剂组为19.3个月[146]。部分缓解率为45%，降钙素和CEA的生化缓解更高。到目前为止，还没有显示出总体生存效益。在2011年FDA批准时，显著的毒性包括QTc间期延长需要未知警告[147]。

卡波扎替尼是一种口服的VEGF2～3、RET、MET抑制剂，在一项对患者进行的Ⅲ期/随机、安慰剂对照试验（有近期进展的记录）中，达到了主要终点：无进展生存期增加11.2个月（与安慰剂的4.0个月相比）。部分缓解率为28%，未显示总体生存效益。除对QTc的影响外，毒性与万德他尼相似[148]。

万德他尼、卡博扎丁尼和其他几种多重激酶抑制剂单独或联合的临床试验正在进行中[149]。

嗜铬细胞瘤

嗜铬细胞瘤来源于肾上腺髓质的嗜铬细胞。副神经节瘤来源于交感神经及副交感神经系统。交感神经系统的副神经节瘤常被称为肾上腺外嗜铬细胞瘤，最常见于腹膜后。副交感神经系统的副神经节瘤最常见于主动脉弓、颈部及颅底（如颈动脉体副神经节瘤）[150]。梅奥诊所的数据估计美国每年有大约800例嗜铬细胞瘤[151]。0.1%～0.5%的高血压患者发现患有嗜铬细胞瘤[152]。

临床表现与诊断

嗜铬细胞瘤诊断和治疗应考虑“大体十定律”：10%发生于儿童，10%散发病例为双侧，10%发生于肾上腺外，10%为恶性。以前，该定律还包括约10%的嗜铬细胞瘤是家族性的，但最近更新的数据表明无个人史或相关内分泌肿瘤家族史嗜铬细胞瘤患者中40%以上的患者体细胞有以下易感基因之一的突变：*VHL*，*RET*，*NF-1*，*MEN-1*及琥珀酸脱氢酶亚单位D（*SDHD*）、B（*SDHB*）、C（*SDHC*），*SMAD4*，*ENG*，*ALK1*，*TMEM127*，*MAX*，*HIF2A*[153,154]。目前推荐所有嗜铬细胞瘤患者尤其是诊断年龄小于50岁伴有家族史或病灶呈多发（基因突变风险超过10%）的患者进行遗传咨询或遗传检测[155]。

嗜铬细胞瘤可表现为血压正常、无任何症状，也可出现严重的致死性高血压危象。嗜铬细胞瘤的诊断基础是临床表现高度怀疑，通过生化检测血浆中的儿茶酚胺或儿茶酚胺代谢产物测定甲氧基肾上腺素。也可采用更广为流行的检测24h尿液儿茶酚胺、甲氧基肾上腺素或3-甲氨基4-羟扁桃酸（VMA）含量的方法[156]。对生化检测提示嗜铬细胞瘤的患者如行CT或MRI检查，90%可发现肾上腺嗜铬细胞瘤[157]。

良性或复发可切除病变的手术治疗

几乎所有的良性嗜铬细胞瘤均可通过外科手术切除治愈。由于肿瘤虽生长缓慢但并发症状严重，对局部复发病灶及恶性嗜铬细胞瘤的局限性转移应尽可能完全切除。对不能完全切除的肿瘤行减瘤术的价值尚未完全确定，但是有报道称减瘤术有助于控制症状[158]。一项关于术前管理的国际共识总结了术前准备的关键点，控制血压、控制心率和心律、规范液体状态和预防侵入性手术和手术时"儿茶酚胺风暴"[159]。

复发或转移疾病的内科治疗

据估计只有 5%～25% 的嗜铬细胞瘤是恶性的[151]。对晚期儿童神经母细胞瘤有效的 CVD 方案（环磷酰胺、长春新碱及达卡巴嗪）被认为是症状性、播散性嗜铬细胞瘤的首选治疗方法[160]。

MEN-2 和嗜铬细胞瘤

MEN-2 相关嗜铬细胞瘤患者的诊断年龄多在 20～30 岁，早于散发性嗜铬细胞瘤的诊断年龄 35～45 岁[161]，部分原因是 MEN-2 患者筛查积极。大约 25% 的 MEN-2A 患者以嗜铬细胞瘤为首发肿瘤[162,163]。75% 的患者常同时伴有甲状腺髓样癌[161]。MEN-2 相关嗜铬细胞瘤患者可有双侧肿瘤，出现恶性转化的概率比散发性肿瘤低[164]。鉴于 MEN-2 患者的嗜铬细胞瘤恶性概率较低，可行单侧或双侧次全肾上腺切除术以保留肾上腺皮质功能，从而避免终身肾上腺功能替代治疗。MEN-2A 患者常常无症状，但在因甲状旁腺功能亢进或甲状腺髓样癌而进行的手术过程中，可出现高血压危象。因此，所有 MEN-2 患者在行任何手术或侵袭性检查前均应仔细检查有无嗜铬细胞瘤的存在。如有，可应用 α-肾上腺能受体阻断剂来控制血压[159]。

在 MEN-2 家族中，RET 基因的第 634 位密码子突变与嗜铬细胞瘤的发生有非常密切的联系，因此在这些患者的随访中应加以密切关注。总之，建议对所有 MEN-2 患者每年进行嗜铬细胞瘤的筛查[155]。

（马福海 译　田艳涛 校）

参考文献

The complete reference list can be found on the Wiley Companion Digital Edition of this title (see inside front cover for login instructions).

2 Yao JC, Hassan M, Phan A, et al. One hundred years after "carcinoid": epidemiology of and prognostic factors for neuroendocrine tumors in 35,825 cases in the United States. *J Clin Oncol*. 2008;**26**:3063–3072.

7 Clevers H. The intestinal crypt, a prototype stem cell compartment. *Cell*. 2013;**154**:274–284.

11 Oberg K. Biochemical diagnosis of neuroendocrine GEP tumor. *Yale J Biol Med*. 1997;**70**:501–508.

12 Nehar D, Lombard-Bohas C, Olivieri S, et al. Interest of Chromogranin A for the diagnosis and follow-up of endocrine tumors. *Clin Endocrinol* (Oxford). 2004;**60**:644–652.

16 Lamberts SW, van der Lely AJ, de Herder WW, et al. Octreotide. *N Engl J Med*. 1996;**334**:246–254.

22 For a definitive historical discussion on carcinoid tumors, the reader is encouraged to read:Modlin IM, Shapiro MD, Kidd M. Siegfried Oberndorfer: origins and perspectives of carcinoid tumors. *Hum Pathol*. 2004;**35**:1440–1451.

27 Klimstra DS, Modlin IR, Coppola D, et al. The pathologic classification of neuroendocrine tumors. A review of nomenclature, grading, and staging systems. *Pancreas*. 2010;**39**:707–712.

36 Moertel CG, Sauer WG, Docherty MB, Baggenstoss AH. Life history of the carcinoid tumor of the small intestine. *Cancer*. 1961;**14**:291–293.

37 Kulke MH, Mayer RJ. Carcinoid tumors. *N Engl J Med*. 1999;**340**:858–868.

45 Simula DV, Edwards WD, Tazelaar HD, et al. Surgical pathology of carcinoid heart disease: a study of 139 values from 75 patients spanning over 20 years. *Mayo Clin Proc*. 2002;**77**:139–147.

52 Zollinger RM, Ellison EH. Primary peptic ulceration of the jejunum associated with islet cell tumors of the pancreas. *Ann Surg*. 1955;**142**:709–723.

59 Metz DC, Strader DB, Orbuch M, et al. Use of omeprazole in Zollinger-Ellison: a prospective nine-year study of efficacy and safety. *Aliment Pharmacol Ther*. 1993;**7**:597–610.

60 Norton JA, Fraker DL, Alexander HR, et al. Surgery increases survival in patients with gastrinoma. *Ann Surg*. 2006;**244**:410–419.

65 Marx S, Spiegel AM, Skarulis MC, et al. Multiple endocrine neoplasia type 1: clinical and genetic topics. *Ann Intern Med*. 1998;**129**:484–494.

71 Verner JV, Morrison AB. Endocrine pancreatic disease with diarrhea: report of a case due to diffuse hyperplasia of non-beta islet tissue with a review of 54 additional cases. *Arch Intern Med*. 1974;**133**:492–499.

75 McGavran MH, Unger RH, Recant L, et al. A glucagon secreting alpha-cell carcinoma of the pancreas. *N Engl J Med*. 1966;**274**:1408–1413.

84 Larsson LI, Hirsch MA, Holst J, et al. Pancreatic somatostatinoma clinical features and physiologic implications. *Lancet*. 1977;**1**:666–668.

86 Vinik AI, Strodel WE, Eckhauser FE, et al. Somatostatinomas, PPomas, neurotensinomas. *Semin Oncol*. 1987;**14**:263–281.

93 Que FG, Nagnorney DM, Batts KP, et al. Hepatic resection for metastatic neuroendocrine carcinomas. *Am J Surg*. 1995;**169**:36–43.

94 Mazzaglai PJ, Berber E, Milas M, Siperstein AE. Laparoscopic radiofrequency ablation of neuroendocrine liver metastases: a 10-year experience evaluating predictors of survival. *Surgery*. 2007;**142**:10–19.

98 Del Prete M, Fiore F, Modica R, et al. Hepatic arterial embolization in patients with neuroendocrine tumors. *J Exp Clin Canc Res*. 2014;**33**:43–51.

101 Kvols LK, Reubi JC, Horisberger U, et al. The presence of somatostatin receptors in malignant neuroendocrine tumor tissue predicts responsiveness to octreotide. *Yale J Biol Med*. 1992;**65**:505–18.

111 Faiss S, Pape UF, Bohmig M, et al. Prospective, randomized, multicenter trial on the antiproliferative effect of lanreotide, interferon alfa, and their combination for therapy of metastatic neuroendocrine gastroenteropancreatic tumors—the International Lanreotide and Interferon Alfa Study Group. *J Clin Oncol*. 2003;**21**:2689–96.

114 Kwekkeboom DJ, Bakker WH, Kam BL, et al. Treatment with Lu-177 DOTA-Tyr3-octreotate in patients with neuroendocrine tumors: interim results. *Eur J Nucl Med Mol Imaging*. 2003;**30**:S231.

117 Strosberg JR, Fine RL, Choi J, et al. First-line chemotherapy with capecitabine and temozolomide in patients with metastatic pancreatic endocrine carcinomas. *Cancer*. 2011;**117**:268–275.

121 Yao JC, Shah MH, Ito T, et al. Everolimus for advanced pancreatic neuroendocrine tumors. *N Engl J Med*. 2011;**364**:514–523.

123 Raymond E, Dahan L, Raoul J-L, et al. Sunitinib maleate for the treatment of pancreatic neuroendocrine tumors. *N Engl J Med*. 2011;**364**:501–513.

126 Brandi ML, Gagel RF, Andeli A, et al. CONSENSUS: Guidelines for diagnosis and therapy of MEN type I and type 2. *J Clin Endo Metab*. 2001;**86**:5658–5671.

129 Lemos MC, Thakker RV. Multiple endocrine neoplasia type I (MEN1): analysis of 1336 mutations reported in the first decade following identification of the gene. *Hum Mutat*. 2008;**29**:22–32.

131 Thakur RV. Multiple Endocrine neoplasia, type I (MEN1). *Best Practice & Res Clin Endocrinol & Metab 2010*. 2013;**24**:355–370.

138 Lips CJ, Landsvater RM, Hoppener JW, et al. Clinical screening as compared with DNA analysis in families with multiple endocrine neoplasia type 2A. *N Engl J Med*. 1994;**331**:828–835.

146 Wells SA, Robinson BG, Gagel RF, et al. Vandetinib in patients with locally advanced or metastatic medually thyroid cancer: A randomized, double-blind phase III trial. *J Clin Oncol*. 2013;**30**:134–141.

148 Eisei R, Schulmberger MJ, Muller SP, et al. Cabozantinib in progressive medullary thyroid cancer. *J Clin Oncol*. 2013;**31**:3639–3646.

152 Pacak K, Linehan WM, Eisenhofer G, et al. Recent advances in genetics, diagnosis, localization, and treatment of pheochromocytoma. *Ann Intern Med*. 2001;**134**:315–329.

第83章　头颈部癌

Renata Ferrarotto, MD ■ Merrill S. Kies, MD ■ Adam S. Garden, MD ■ Michael E. Kupferman, MD

概述

头颈部癌包括影响上呼吸消化道的多种恶性肿瘤。最常见的肿瘤类型是鳞状细胞癌。虽然头颈部癌的主要危险因素仍然是烟草和酒精的滥用,但人类乳头状瘤病毒和EBV病毒等致癌病毒在口咽和鼻咽肿瘤中起着重要的致癌作用。不同部位和病理类型的头颈部恶性肿瘤治疗策略是不同的,需要多学科团队综合诊治。在本章中,我们回顾了头颈部癌的理论知识,以鳞癌和涎腺癌为重点,并讨论时下和未来在治疗和预后改善方面的热点研究。

引言

2016年美国新诊断的头颈部癌患者有大约62 000例,死于该病者超过13 000例。尽管头颈部癌仅占美国每年新发癌症总数的4%、癌症死亡总数的2%[1,2]。吸烟和饮酒是头颈部癌的首要的流行病学因素,因而通过控制烟酒进行预防是公共卫生领域的首要目标[3]。此外,越来越多的头颈部癌(特别是在口咽部位)的发生可能源于致癌性人乳头瘤状病毒(HPV)[4],广泛进行的人乳头瘤状病毒接种对该病发病率导致的影响尚待评估。头颈部癌对那些流行吸/嚼烟草致癌物的地区造成更为明显的影响,从而成为全球癌症死因的重要原因[1,5,6]。综合治疗的广泛采用可能提高了某些部位头颈部癌(鼻咽和口咽)[7]的生存率,但是对其他部位的头颈部癌而言长期生存率并无改善[8]。

尽管在重建手术和康复治疗、调强放疗和对某些癌症的保护性手段方面取得了很大的进展,头颈部鳞癌患者仍然存在明显的功能缺乏和生活质量的下降。这些问题使新辅助化疗、戒烟、化学预防以及语言/吞咽功能重建显得更为重要。化疗和放疗的联合治疗是目前针对不能手术的局部晚期头颈部癌的标准治疗方式,同时还能够保护器官功能。通过对头颈部癌的生物学行为的进一步了解,分子靶向治疗药物的研发进行得如火如荼,分子靶向化学预防的研究也正在进行中。这些新的治疗和预防手段对于提升我们对头颈部癌及其后遗症的控制能力极具前景。本章将主要就头颈部癌的流行病学、生物学、化学预防、诊断和治疗的现状以及未来的研究方向进行讨论。

描述流行病学

发病率

在美国,2015年新发的口腔癌和咽癌约为45 780例,喉癌13 560例,鼻咽癌3 200例,恶性涎腺肿瘤3 100例,鼻腔鼻旁窦肿瘤2 000例[2]。虽然美国已从20世纪60年代开始控烟并卓有成效,其大部分头颈部癌的发病率自20世纪80年代开始下降,但近来其口咽癌的发病率呈上升趋势[9]。大约1/2的口腔癌发生在女性,而在咽癌和喉癌中这一比例为1/4。1993—2017年间,白种人和黑种人的口腔癌及咽癌患者死亡率有效下降,其中黑种人的变化较大,这得益于长期的健康教育。而喉癌男性患者中,黑种人的死亡率是白种人的两倍,女性患者中黑种人的死亡率则比白种人高40%。西班牙裔口腔癌/下咽癌的发病率最低,而亚裔的喉癌发病率则是最低的[10]。头颈部鳞癌的中位诊断年龄大约为60岁,但是它在年轻成人(<45岁)中的发病率正在增长,这种增长可能与致癌性人乳头瘤病毒相关性口咽癌的增多有关[4]。致癌性人乳头瘤病毒相关性口咽癌在白种男人中更常见,据推测这与口交行为的流行有关[9]。

2011年全世界头颈肿瘤的发患者数约550 000例。美拉尼西亚人口腔癌的患病率最高(36∶100 000),中南亚、中欧和东欧地区紧随其后[10]。虽然在亚欧地区大多数国家,口腔癌的致死率得到了控制,但是在东欧国家患者尤其是女性中仍在持续升高,这与这些地区的烟草滥用有关。在中南亚地区80%的头颈部癌是口腔癌和咽癌(不包括鼻咽癌),但在其他地方,喉癌和鼻咽癌所占的比例更大。例如,喉癌在发达国家约占头颈部癌的1/3,这一数字在东欧和南欧达到约40%。在如马来西亚、印度尼西亚和新加坡等东南亚国家中鼻咽癌占所有头颈部癌的70%左右,在男性所有癌症发病率中排第六位[10]。

患病率

在2007年11个月,美国有大约350 000例曾患头颈部癌的患者仍存活(其中240 176例为口腔/咽部癌症患者,93 096例为喉癌患者)。这些患病人群的性别分布能够反映出患者群的特点。然而,非洲裔美国人仅占喉癌患者的11.5%,占口腔/咽部癌症患者的7.3%。如此低的比例可能反映了诊断为头颈部鳞癌的非洲裔美国人生存期更差。在过去的十年中,非洲裔美国人口腔/咽部癌症的生存率比白种人要低大约20%,在喉癌中则为15%[11]。

死亡率

2015年在美国有8 650例患者死于口腔癌和口咽癌,3 640例患者死于喉癌[2]。综合治疗的广泛应用和发展使鼻咽癌、口咽癌和下咽癌患者的生存率得到显著提高,生存率在口腔癌患者中也有升高的趋势,但是在喉癌患者中却在下降。死亡率不仅能体现疗效/生存情况的进展,还能反映出控烟所带来的发病率的下降[7,8]。正如其他部位的肿瘤一样,头颈部癌在发展中国家的死亡/发病比无论在男性还是女性都明显高于美国[1,10]。

危险因素

烟草

在 20 世纪 50 年代末期，一项里程碑式的病例对照研究由 Dr Ernst Wynder 完成，它阐述了吸烟和口腔癌之间的关系。其后一年的另一项队列研究分析了超过 180 000 名男性，发现在头颈部鳞癌男性患者中，吸卷烟比从不吸烟者的死亡风险更高[12]。在这些研究中同样发现吸雪茄和烟斗的头颈部鳞癌患者也具有更高的死亡风险。1964 年，美国普通外科顾问委员会发布的吸烟与健康的报告指出吸烟与癌症发病有关[13]。大量病例对照研究和队列研究完全一致地证明了吸烟与头颈部鳞癌发病的关系，其相对危险度或优势比在 5～25 倍之间[14,15]。这些研究还表明吸烟量与头颈部鳞癌的发病风险呈正相关，在戒烟后发病风险下降。头颈部的其他黏膜性恶性病变，例如鼻咽癌和鼻窦恶性肿瘤则与吸烟关系不太密切[16]。

虽然对于支气管来源的肿瘤而言，抽雪茄或烟斗者的危险性比吸卷烟者要低，但对于头颈部鳞癌来说，这几种吸烟方式均能导致其发病风险的增加[17]。在不同的烟草消费模式中，含有致癌物的唾液在重力的作用下分布部位不同，从而可能导致头颈部鳞癌发生于特定部位。事实上在美国，口底癌、喉癌和下咽癌几乎都发生于吸烟者[27]。无烟烟草及其相关产品的使用者和吸烟斗者常常有咀嚼烟草或用烟斗吸烟的习惯，而这些烟草产品同样与口腔癌有关[28]。中南亚正是常用这类产品的地区，龈颊区的头颈部鳞癌在这儿就最为常见[6,18]。

虽然在发达国家吸烟率正在下降，但在发展中国家这一数据却在上升。1965 年美国成人中有 42.4% 的烟民，而到了 2013 年已降至 17.8%[19]。虽然在最近 3 个 10 年中其男性吸烟者下降的幅度更大，但目前仍有 20.5% 的男性和 15.3% 的女性吸烟，而对于本土美国人来说，烟民比例达到 26.1%[20]。在全球范围，头颈部鳞癌的发生部位及发病率在不同地区、不同文化、不同人口学特征的人群中有着显著的差异，而这很大程度上取决于不同的烟草使用模式和某些药物滥用的情况[2,9,14,15]。例如，在中南亚地区，人们常咀嚼“pano”（槟榔，含有蒌叶、石灰、阿仙药和槟榔子），这是口腔癌独立于烟草以外的一个强危险因子，而口腔癌正是这一地区男性和女性的最常见癌症之一[10,21]。

酒精

酒精同样也在癌症发生过程中起着重要的促进作用，它对至少 30% 的头颈部鳞癌的发生有影响[10,22]。它对头颈部鳞癌的发病风险还具有独立于烟草以外的影响，但这种影响仅在最大量的酒精消费群体中才表现得显著[23]。那些试图寻求酒精饮料种类与特定肿瘤发生风险之间联系的研究并未得到一致的结论，但大多数研究者相信酒精本身就是发病的主要原因。然而，酒精最主要的临床意义在于它会加强烟草的致癌作用，吸烟和酒精的协同作用可以使头颈肿瘤的患病风险升高 30 倍[22,24]。

感染因素

虽然有很多感染因素可能在头颈部癌的发生过程中起作用，但基于现有的科学证据，只有 EB 病毒（Epstein-Barr virus，EBV）和 HPV 能够被看作头颈部癌癌变的致病因子。有人认为单纯疱疹病毒可能是口腔癌的危险因素之一[25]，而幽门螺旋杆菌可能是喉癌的危险因素[26]，但这些均未获证实。

人乳头状瘤病毒

与非口咽癌不同，口咽鳞状细胞癌的发病率在近几十年内逐渐升高，在年青群体中尤为明显[27~31]。这与 HPV 感染相关的口咽癌发病率上升密切相关[32,33]。在美国 HPV 与大约 70% 的口咽鳞癌相关[34]。HPV 与鼻腔鼻窦鳞状细胞癌的发病也可能有关[35]。

HPV 是对人上皮细胞具有独特亲和力的脱氧核糖核酸（DNA）病毒，HPV 相关的癌症起源于缺少上皮覆盖的扁桃体隐窝。HPV 已知为宫颈癌及肛管癌的致病因子[36]，在过去几十年的研究中一些研究者也表明 HPV 对于口咽癌也是重要的危险因素[37~44]。至今已有超过 120 种不同的 HPV 亚型被分离出来，其中低风险的类型（如 HPV6、11）可以诱导上皮的良性过度增殖，导致诸如乳头状瘤和疣等病变。而高风险类型（如 HPV16、18、31、33、35）则有致癌的作用[45]。典型的致癌类型 16 和 18 型占 HPV 相关口咽鳞癌的 90% 以上，并且能使生殖器或上呼吸道上皮细胞来源的原代人角质形成细胞发生恶变[46]。HPV-16 的主要癌蛋白由 E6 和 E7 基因编码。E6 蛋白能够使抑癌基因 *p53* 的蛋白泛素化并被降解。E7 癌蛋白与 pRb 的功能抑制有关[47,48]。这些病毒癌蛋白不仅是转化必需的，同时也诱导细胞增殖、延迟细胞分化、增加自发突变和诱导突变的频率、使转染细胞系的染色体不稳定性增加[49]。此外，为了维持恶性表型，具有转录活性的病毒基因组可能是必需的[50~53]。

HPV 相关口咽鳞癌的危险因素包括口交性行为及大麻的使用等，与 HPV 阴性肿瘤是不同的。此外，已经证实 HPV 阳性口咽鳞癌发生风险与口交性伴侣数量及联合使用大麻的时间存在剂量-反应关系[54]。虽然是在没有烟草暴露的口咽癌患者才常常伴有 HPV-16 型相关的肿瘤[37]，但烟草和酒精作为口咽癌传统的危险因素仍可能与 HPV-16 型存在协同作用[41]。用以预防宫颈癌的 HPV-16 型免疫接种治疗在预防口咽癌方面也很有潜力[4]。

EBV

EBV 与鼻咽癌之间的流行病学联系是十分紧密的[42,43]。有研究在鼻咽癌前病变中发现了 EBV DNA，进一步证实了两者的联系。EBV 除了在 WHO 分型为Ⅱ型和Ⅲ型的鼻咽癌表现为强阳性，与分化良好的鼻咽癌（WHO Ⅰ型）也有关系[46]。在鼻咽癌流行的地区，通过血清和黏膜刷检检测 EBV 病毒感染已用于筛查[42]。对于原发灶不明的颈部转移癌进行 EBV DNA 检测可用于鉴定是否原发于鼻咽。最近发现，在外周血（无论含细胞成分或不含细胞成分）中进行 EBV DNA 检测能够预测生存及远处转移情况，这一方法有可能成为鼻咽癌患者随访的标准生物标志物[51]。

遗传易感性

但是在吸烟者中也只有一部分人发生癌症，遗传易感性的差异在其发病过程中可能同样重要。大规模的家庭研究发现头颈部鳞癌患者的一级亲属患头颈部鳞癌的风险要提高 3～8 倍[53,55]。根据这个假设，致癌物代谢系统、DNA 修复系统和/或细胞周期控制/凋亡系统性能的遗传差异将影响烟草所诱发癌症的发病风险[56,57]。在普通人群中可以通过这些生物标记物检测发现发病的高危个体，这将对一级预防、早期检测和二级预防策略产生影响。近期在3篇关于全基因组关联研究的高影响因子的文献中都发现了肺癌在不同人群中的同一个的易感性部位[54,58,59]。在不远的将来全基因组头颈部鳞癌的关联研究将继续跟进，并有望将烟草相关癌症的个体化预防变为现实。

环境性吸烟

一项对象为173例头颈部鳞癌患者和176例健康对照的研究，发现环境性吸烟(二手烟)与超过2倍的头颈部鳞癌发病风险相关，而且还发现其中具有量效关系[60]。在另一项研究中，观察了44例非吸烟的头颈部鳞癌患者和132例非吸烟健康对照，研究发现环境性吸烟导致头颈部鳞癌发病风险的显著上升，这一点在女性和暴露于工作场所者尤为明显[61]。

咽喉反流

无对照的观察性研究早就发现胃食管反流可能与喉癌的发病有关[62,63]。而且大量的研究通过24h pH监测观察到在喉癌患者中很多伴有咽喉部位的消化道反流[64]。此外还有一项针对喉癌和咽癌的回顾性病例对照研究，分析了美国退伍军人事务部数据库中患病的共计10 140例住院病例和12 061例门诊病例，并以其他的40 561例住院病例和48 244例门诊病例作为对照[65]。该研究发现，患胃食管反流性疾病者喉癌(住院患者 $OR=2.4$，门诊患者 $OR=2.3$)和咽癌(住院患者 $OR=2.4$，门诊患者 $OR=1.9$)的发病风险显著升高。而这种风险的提高还受年龄、性别、人种、烟酒嗜好的影响。但是瑞典的一项大型队列研究通过对66 965例出院诊断为胃灼热、食管裂孔疝或食管炎患者随访共计376 622人年后认为，无证据表明胃食管反流与喉癌或咽癌存在因果关系[66]。

大麻

吸大麻比吸烟所带来的焦油负担高4倍，而苯并芘和芳香烃的浓度也要高出50%。非对照研究早就认为大麻可能是头颈部鳞癌的危险因素之一，但由于吸食大麻者大多嗜好烟酒，很少有关于大麻作为头颈部鳞癌病因的直接证据的报道[67,68]。近来有一项病例对照研究分析了240例头颈部鳞癌患者以及322例健康对照，发现吸食大麻者患HPV相关头颈部鳞癌的风险超过正常人5倍，而且也具有量效关系[69]。但另一项对64 855例保健组织(HMO)成员进行的大型的回顾性队列分析则未发现大麻与烟草相关癌症的关系[70]。由于统计漏报问题以及重度吸食者样本量有限，很难对吸食大麻与头颈部鳞癌发病风险得出结论[71]。

饮食

源于传统病例对照研究的流行病学证据表明高动物脂肪少蔬菜水果的饮食习惯可能是头颈部鳞癌的危险因素[72,73]。数个病例对照研究分析了腌鱼消费水平与鼻咽癌发病风险之间的联系，这种风险可能由于腌制食品中所含的亚硝胺类化合物所致[74,75]。有证据表明类胡萝卜素缺乏可能是头颈部鳞癌和肺癌的危险因素之一，而多吃蔬菜水果能起到的保护作用可能就源自其中的维生素A和β-胡萝卜素[76]。但是，类胡萝卜素有超过500种，我们并不知道哪一种具有保护作用，不知道会发生什么样的化学反应，我们也不知道在富含类胡萝卜素的食物中的其他微量元素是否会起到保护作用。有人就发现同时服用维生素C和E也有保护作用[73]。但对膳食进行评估及验证是很困难的，特别是很难准确地将每种食物都转换为营养成分来进行分析。以后的研究需要能更精确的鉴定出膳食和各种类胡萝卜素成分的血清水平之间的联系。我们从大量的化合物中寻找到最具保护作用的成分还是有可能的，但对其他饮食变量和混杂危险因子的控制在方法学上仍是个难题。

职业/空气污染

虽然职业暴露可能在头颈部鳞癌的总体发病中作用很小，但它却是鼻窦区域恶性肿瘤的主要危险因素[77~79]。最主要的职业暴露来自金属加工、炼油、木工、皮革/纺织工业[77,78]。室内空气污染在大部分使用生物质或矿物燃料作为烹饪和取暖的首选方法的发展中国家都是个显著的问题。虽然有些证据并不支持石棉作为头颈部鳞癌的危险因素，但美国科学院专家委员会认为已有充分证据表明石棉是喉癌的一个显著的独立危险因素[80]。

放射线

目前，还未发现电离辐射和头颈部鳞癌发生之间有明显的联系。但嘴唇的鳞癌，像皮肤癌一样，是与紫外线辐射有关的。此外，伽马射线的暴露与甲状腺癌、头颈部肉瘤、唾液腺恶性肿瘤以及鼻窦癌相关。头颈部恶性肿瘤的治疗性照射并不诱发呼吸消化道第二原发鳞癌，但却与头颈部肉瘤的发病风险升高有关[81]。对于接受治疗性照射的儿童更需特别关注。而且环境性辐射、医学诊断性辐射以及治疗性照射对头颈部的暴露均与唾液腺恶性肿瘤有显著的关系[82,83]。一些研究发现这种致病风险随辐射量的增加呈显著的量效关系，而黏液表皮样癌则是其中最常见的类型[82,83]。职业病研究发现室内氡气暴露和挥发性化学物质暴露均可导致头颈部鳞癌的发病风险增加[79]。

公共卫生体系应通过控制烟酒，针对HPV高危型进行预防性接种，发现和避免其他致病因素，鉴定遗传易感性等手段来更好的预防和早期发现这些恶性肿瘤。但遗憾的是由于患病人数和相关专家较少，头颈部鳞癌还没有有效的筛查手段[84]。但在有些头颈部鳞癌高发的地区，预防和筛查项目已被有效实施[6]。

病理评估和生物学

病理学家除了要说明某个特定的肿瘤是鳞癌之外，还常常需要提供肿瘤分级或分化程度等信息。肿瘤分化程度的级别并不能准确反映鳞癌的生物学侵袭性[85]。其预后情况除了肿瘤分级以外还受到很多因素的影响[86,87]。这些影响因素包括：肿瘤大小、形态、部位、表皮生长因子受体的表达情况、宿主免疫反应、年龄以及一般情况等。对于口咽鳞癌患者的生存率来说，P16的表达情况/HPV状态是最强的独立预后因素[88]。

反映侵袭性疾病的特征包括：淋巴管侵犯，神经周围浸润，淋巴结转移和肿瘤穿透受侵淋巴结被膜情况(结外侵犯)。本章将不在分子病理学方面进行深入的讨论，这个领域有大量的文献可供读者参考[89,90]。目前对细胞和基因改变的复杂的相互作用正在进行大量探索，这种作用是头颈部鳞癌发生发展和转移的原因。对p53、下调受体的酪氨酸激酶信号、抗凋亡、血管生成和化疗耐药的原理正在很多实验室进行研究。

解剖学

头颈部癌是由上呼吸消化道(UADT)的不同解剖部位发生

的各种不同病理类型的肿瘤的合称。本章主要讨论在其中占大约 90%的鳞癌。上呼吸消化道是一个食物和空气所通过的由黏膜覆盖的管道，它由嘴唇表面直到颈部食管。头颈部癌通常指的是唇、口腔、咽、喉和颈段食管起源的癌症，但也包括其他重要部位包括鼻窦和鼻旁窦、唾液腺、甲状腺和甲状旁腺以及皮肤(包括黑色素瘤和非黑色素瘤皮肤癌)来源的癌症。在这一区域还有些肿瘤并不归入头颈部癌的范畴，比如中枢神经系统肿瘤、眼部肿瘤以及淋巴系统原发的肿瘤。

由于发病部位和组织的多样性，肿瘤生长的生物学方式、转移的模式、肿瘤发展的自然边界以及疾病的症状体征都有着很大的不同。这个区域的解剖情况决定了该类疾病最佳的诊断治疗和评价需要由多学科的专家达成共识，需要有从事神经外科、耳鼻喉科、头颈外科、口腔及颌面外科、整形美容以及放射、病理、放疗和化疗的专家共同协作。该类疾病的临床表现多种多样，但都对头颈部区域的整体外形和功能产生很大的影响。声带癌很少发生转移且治愈率很高，而在解剖学距离声带只有几毫米的梨状窝，情况则恰恰相反，这里发生的癌症在相同疾病分期会很早出现远处播散，预后很差[91]。不同部位癌症的临床差别并不能单独用解剖性因素来解释，还要考虑到它们主要的生物学差异。可惜的是头颈部癌的患者总量较少，而进行各种临床研究需要大量的受试者。病情和治疗会不同程度的影响器官功能，尤其是语言、吞咽、嗅觉、呼吸和咀嚼功能，它们对于社交，生活质量和生存非常重要。

口腔

口腔的定义是从唇边开始向后延伸包括颊黏膜、舌前部、口底、硬腭和上、下牙龈的区域。舌在口腔中占了主要的部分并与口底相连。牙龈黏膜在上、下颌骨的牙槽嵴上，其下与骨膜相连。硬腭位于口腔顶部，由上牙槽嵴到与软腭交接处的上颌骨硬腭部分以及其上覆盖的黏膜组成，软腭则位于口咽部。虽然口腔和口咽的区分主要是人为的，但由于这些部位疾病不同的自然病程、治疗手段以及许多功能性问题，把它们分开是很有意义的。

咽部

咽部是起始于颅底至第 6 颈椎水平的一段肌膜性管道，它由重叠的括约肌(上、中、下组)和其他起自颅底和茎突的肌肉所支撑。这一段肌膜性管道向前与口咽相连，向上与鼻咽相连，向下与下咽和喉部相连。它分为四部分：扁桃体区，作为咽侧壁的主要部分并与舌底、软腭、磨牙后三角相连；舌底区；软腭区；咽后壁区。咽部的神经分布来自咽丛神经，含有舌咽神经(感觉)和迷走神经(感觉和运动)。

下咽分为三个区域：梨状窝、喉的后表面(环后区)以及下、后、侧咽壁。梨状窝是对称的黏膜窝位于喉的两侧，进食时呈漏斗状张开使食物进入食管。其上方与咽会厌襞相连，下方为环状软骨。它们在 C6 水平与颈段食管和食管入口汇合。

喉部

喉部是个黏膜覆盖的软骨结构(甲状软骨和环状软骨)，起自甲状舌骨膜下的舌骨，下方与气管相连。喉的入口与咽部气道相连。与咽部不同，喉黏膜主要由呼吸型柱状纤毛上皮组成。在会厌、杓状会厌襞和真声带部位还有复层鳞状上皮。值得注意的是淋巴组织存在于喉的上部，但在声门和声带处却十分稀少。

喉被分为三个解剖部位：声门上区、声门区和声门下区。声门上区包括会厌、杓状会厌襞、杓状软骨的喉面、假声带和喉室。声门区起源于支气管，由真声带和前后联合的黏膜构成。它从喉室最外侧端延伸至声带游离缘以下 1cm 处，且很少含有淋巴组织。声门下区是位于声门下方以环状软骨为下界的区域。该区域的淋巴引流于两侧广泛分布。声门下的淋巴引流是通过环甲膜到达颈部淋巴结，而在声门上的则是通过甲状舌骨膜。

鼻和鼻旁窦

鼻和鼻旁窦是指前至鼻前庭，后至后鼻孔的覆以鳞状上皮的区域。鼻旁窦恶性肿瘤的定义不包括鼻咽部位在内，直接侵犯的情况除外，它的范围包括上颌窦、筛窦、额窦、蝶窦这些鼻旁窦区域。虽然鼻和鼻旁窦区域恶性肿瘤最常见的病理类型就是鳞癌，但这个区域有一系列需要特殊对待的情况，将在后面专门的章节中进行说明。此外，此区域的非鳞状细胞癌也可能以特殊的肿瘤进展模式发生，需要进行有效的治疗。

颈部

头颈部癌的治疗需要对该部位的神经、血管，尤其是颈部淋巴结构有透彻的了解。解剖学研究已细致地了解了上呼吸消化道的淋巴引流情况。对于头颈部的特定部位以及这些部位原发的肿瘤，它们的淋巴引流情况是一致且可以预测的。头颈部主要有 12 组淋巴结(左右各 6 组)(图 83-1)[92]，但只有Ⅰ~Ⅴ组在头颈部鳞癌起到主要的作用。头颈部黏膜的每个主要区域的淋巴引流的第一站和第二站都已被确定。经验表明任何区域的动脉供应均可预示该区域的淋巴引流情况。嘴唇、颊部、牙龈前部的淋巴引流至颌下和颏下淋巴结。此外，颊部和上唇的淋巴还引流至腮腺下和面淋巴结，而牙龈后部和腭部的淋巴引流至颈内静脉链和咽后组的外侧。舌的淋巴引流至颈内静脉链、二腹肌下、肩胛舌骨、颌下和颏下组淋巴结。中线病变的淋巴大多引流到双侧。口腔来源的转移性淋巴结很少位于下颈部，但通常肿瘤生长部位在舌上越往前，就越有可能出现颈内静脉下组的淋巴结转移。口底的淋巴引流与舌是类似的。咽上部的淋巴沿着颈内静脉链引流至颈内静脉上组淋巴结。口咽和扁桃体的淋巴引流通过咽旁间隙至中颈内静脉区，常常到颈内静脉二腹肌淋巴结，也会引流至咽后、咽侧淋巴结。下咽和喉部区域的淋巴引流则主要沿着供血路线到达颈内静脉中组的颈深淋巴结(咽上部及喉)或颈内静脉下组及气管旁的淋巴结(咽下部、喉)。

为了治疗需要对颈部的各组淋巴结进行了分区。Ⅰ区淋巴结包括：颏下淋巴结(ⅠA 区)，位于二腹肌前腹与舌骨所形成的三角中；颌下淋巴结(ⅠB 区)，位于下颌骨和二腹肌前后腹之间。Ⅱ区淋巴结由颈内静脉上组淋巴结构成，它位于颈内静脉的上 1/3 处，上界为颅底，下界为颈动脉分叉水平，前界为胸骨舌骨肌侧缘，后界为胸骨锁乳突肌后缘。Ⅱ区淋巴结还根据与脊副神经的位置关系分为ⅡA 和ⅡB 区，ⅡA 位于脊副神经的前下方，ⅡB 位于其后上方。Ⅲ区为位于颈内静脉中 1/3

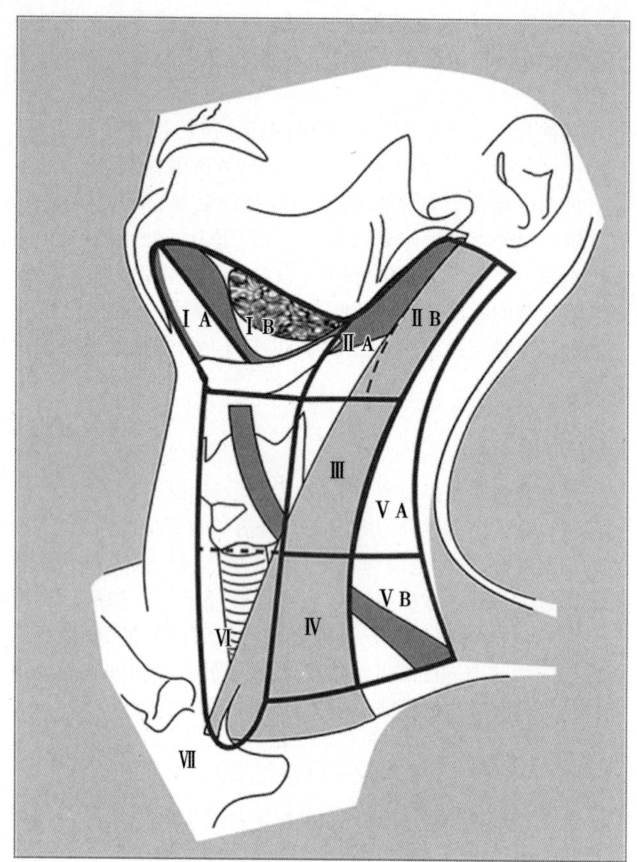

图 83-1 头颈部的淋巴结分区

处的淋巴结，上界为颈动脉分叉水平，下界为肩胛舌骨肌与颈内静脉交叉水平（环状软骨水平）。前后界与Ⅱ区相同。Ⅳ区淋巴结为颈内静脉淋巴结下组，上界为肩胛舌骨肌，下界为锁骨。Ⅴ区淋巴结在颈后三角内，这个区域内还有脊副神经和颈横动脉。前界为胸锁乳突肌后缘，后界为斜方肌前缘，下界为锁骨。Ⅴ区也被分为Ⅴa 和Ⅴb 区，Ⅴa 区淋巴结在环状软骨下缘水平以上，在脊副神经的上方，胸锁乳突肌后方。Ⅴb 区淋巴结则在环状软骨水平以下，在脊副神经下方，并包括了沿颈横动脉走行的淋巴结和锁骨上淋巴结。

诊断和分期

疾病在诊断时的分期是头颈部鳞癌治疗最重要的预后因素，因此对早期癌症进行早期诊断和治疗能获得很好的疗效。口腔黏膜的大多数不典型增生或原位癌可以很容易由视诊发现，它们常表现为红斑（增殖性红斑）或白斑（黏膜白斑病）。在难以直接看到的部位，比如喉和下咽，早期病变常伴有慢性声嘶、咽喉疼痛，并会逐渐发展至耳痛或吞咽困难。这些症状需要我们对喉和下咽进行可视性检查，电子纤维喉镜是目前的常用手段。

吞咽困难、吞咽疼痛、耳痛、声嘶、黏膜不规则和溃疡、口咽疼痛、体重下降以及颈部无法解释的肿物等症状是在侵袭性头颈部鳞癌中最常见的。发病部位不同，其主要症状也不同。出现慢性吞咽困难或疼痛需要进行口咽、下咽及食管的镜检；慢性声嘶则需行喉部镜检；成人的慢性单侧浆液性中耳炎有可能是由于鼻咽癌阻塞咽鼓管所致；单侧鼻息肉、鼻塞、鼻出血则是鼻腔或鼻旁窦恶性肿瘤的常见症状。颈部单侧的质硬包块也常常提示恶性病变，在 20 岁以上的患者中，这种症状有 80% 以上都由恶性肿瘤所致，而且其中 60% 是由于原发上呼吸消化道肿瘤转移所致。

对于存在颈部可疑肿物的患者，进行头颈部的全面检查常常能发现原发病灶（图 83-2），若未能明确原发部位，则还应对锁骨上下部位进行彻底的检查。光纤技术和软、硬式内镜技术的发展可以很好地为临床提供气道上部的可视化诊断以及进行常规活检[93]。内镜技术能对包括鼻咽、口咽、下咽、喉以及食管上段等部位进行诊断。内镜检查还需与胸片以及头颈部的轴向影像相配合。如果这些手段都未能找到原发病灶，则还应考虑进行食管镜检查，它对食管黏膜病变比计算机断层扫描技术（CT）的敏感性更高。大多数情况下，原发隐匿的颈部转移来源于鼻咽、舌底、扁桃体或下咽部位。如果不伴有可用于诊断的肿块，则可直接对上述部位进行内镜下活检，而对有肿块却无法确认原发灶的情况则还应进行双侧扁桃体切除术以寻找证据。孤立的左锁骨上淋巴结（魏尔啸淋巴结，Virchow 淋巴结）转移有时会来源于锁骨下的癌症，尤其是结肠癌。而孤立的锁骨上转移（Ⅳ期）还会来源于乳腺癌、肺癌或横膈下肿瘤。甲状腺恶性肿瘤也可能转移到这个部位。

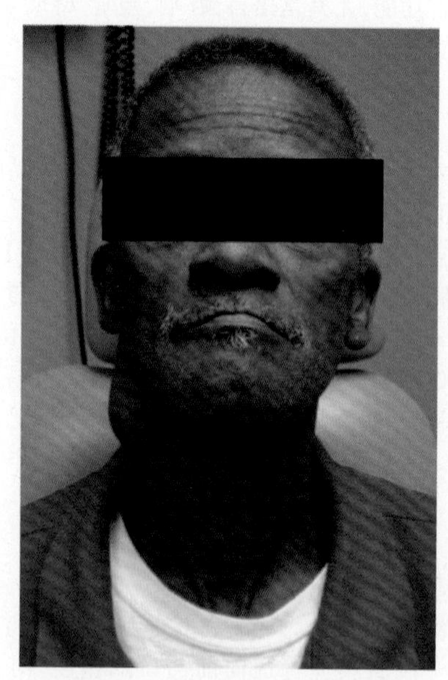

图 83-2 1 例头颈鳞癌患者的 N3 病变治疗前

计算机断层扫描（CT）和磁共振成像（MRI）技术经常用于对原发肿瘤和区域淋巴结进行临床评估和分期。超声成像与细针抽吸活检（fine-needle aspiration，FNA）相结合是对颈部、甲状腺和唾液腺进行分期的有效手段。开放性活检应仅在可疑结节经 FNA 后未明确的情况下进行。对于需要进行切除活检进行诊断的情况，若被高度怀疑为转移性鳞癌，则术者和患者应作好准备进行颈淋巴结清扫术。细针抽吸很明显可能存在假阴性的情况。而穿刺活检学诊断的准确性则取决于超声大夫和病理医生的技术和经验。

正电子发射成像（PET）技术在头颈部癌的应用取得了可喜的成果。原发病灶的氟脱氧葡萄糖标准摄取值（FDG SUV）

越高可能预示着肿瘤的侵袭性更高，预后更差[94~96]。FDG-PET 对于提前进行原发灶及颈部淋巴结分期的敏感性和特异性均能达到 90% 以上[97]，并能找到组织成像或体检不能发现的隐匿性的原发病灶[98,99]和远处转移灶[100]。FDG-PET/CT 技术则能进一步提高颈部淋巴结分期的准确性[101,102]。FDG-PET 相对于单独的 CT 或 MRI 在颈淋巴结分期上的优势经近期一项荟萃分析所确认。这项荟萃分析对多项回顾性及前瞻性研究的数据进行了分析，其中包括超过 1 200 个进行 FDG-PET 检查的病例，它们均经过颈部淋巴结清扫的病理结果进行证实[103]。根据对这些数据的分析，FDG-PET 对颈淋巴结分期的敏感性为 79%，特异性为 86%。近来对 T 分期为早中期的口腔癌和口咽癌患者的前瞻性研究发现，FDG-PET 结合 CT 和前哨淋巴结活检[104]或者 CT/MRI 检查[105]，可能更好的指导 N0 患者的治疗。

近来 FDG-PET 的研究热点集中在监测放疗和化疗的疗效方面。许多研究组织发现使用 FDG-PET 进行疗后分期有很强的阴性预测能力[106~108]，因此，对于放疗后没有 FDG 摄取升高的残存淋巴结已开始有不再进行全颈淋巴结清扫术的倾向[109]。但也有人认为，通过对疗程中一系列 CT 片的专业性临床判读也能达到类似的效果[61,110]。FDG-PET/CT 还可能对更好进行放疗计划的靶区勾画有意义[111]。但挑战仍有很多，尤其在如何通过设定阈值来精确区分癌组织和癌旁组织方面[112,113]。在 MD Anderson 癌症中心，FDG-PET/CT 已作为解剖影像和临床检查以外的补充，常规用于制订放疗计划，但若体检或常规诊断技术发现了化疗后的可疑病灶，其治疗计划不会因阴性的 FDG-PET 结果而推迟。

上呼吸消化道、鼻旁窦及唾液腺原发肿瘤的分期标准已由美国癌症联合委员会（AJCC）建立（表 83-1）。这个分期标准定期进行重新评估和修改。在本章节中提及是最新版本第 7 版[114]。头颈部癌的分期包括 T（原发肿瘤）、N（区域淋巴结）、M（远处转移）分期。由于不同原发部位的头颈部癌的生长方式、生物学行为和预后各不相同，它们的分期标准也不尽相同，不同的原发部位有各自的分期方法。但除了鼻咽和甲状腺原发的肿瘤以外，其他头颈部癌的 N 分期的标准都是一致的（表 83-2）。

表 83-1　AJCC 头颈部癌的临床肿瘤分期和分组[114]

0 期	Tis	N0	M0
Ⅰ期	T1	N0	M0
Ⅱ期	T2	N0	M0
Ⅲ期	T3	N0	M0
	T1	N1	M0
	T2	N1	M0
	T3	N1	M0
ⅣA 期	T4a	N0、N1 或 N2	M0
	任何 T	N2	M0
ⅣB 期	任何 T	N3	M0
	T4b	任何 N	M0
ⅣC 期	任何 T	任何 N	M1

来源：Edge 2010[114]，获得 Springer 授权。

表 83-2　AJCC 区域淋巴结和远处转移的临床肿瘤分期特征[114]

区域淋巴结	
Nx	区域淋巴结不可评价
N0	无区域淋巴结转移的证据
N1	同侧单个区域淋巴结转移，最大径<3cm
N2a	同侧单个区域淋巴结转移，最大径 3~6cm
N2b	同侧多个区域淋巴结转移，最大径均不大于 6cm
N2c	双侧或对侧区域性淋巴结转移，最大径均不大于 6cm
N3	区域淋巴结转移，最大径>6cm
远处转移	
Mx	远处转移的存在无法评价
M0	无远处转移的证据
M1	存在一个或更多部位的远处转移

来源：Edge 2010[114]，获得 Springer 授权。

记录精确的肿瘤范围和分期对于对比不同治疗方案的疗效是十分重要。要想对某种治疗方法或一项新治疗手段的有效性进行准确的评估，就需要在具有相同的肿瘤范围及行为的患者组之间进行比较。疗后再分期或复发肿瘤的分期应与未治疗时的首次分期区别对待。术后或病理分期对于头颈部癌的初始治疗十分重要，因为对于有局部侵袭性的肿瘤、周围软组织中有包膜外扩散或切缘阳性、有神经侵犯等情况时越来越多的需要进行术后放疗（PORT）和/或辅助化疗[154]。

值得注意的是，虽然 AJCC 分期系统已被广泛应用于头颈部癌的分期，但它仍不能很好体现深部浸润性肿瘤和表浅的外向性生长的肿瘤的差异。而经验告诉我们，这种差异会对生存情况产生很重要的影响。另外，由于 HPV 阳性的癌症患者代表了一类特殊的分组，较早的基线分期并不适用在这类患者中[115]。将来 AJCC 标准修订时会加以考虑，尤其是口咽部肿瘤。

基本治疗原则

在确定了肿瘤组织学类型和范围后，对于特定肿瘤选择合适的治疗取决于一系列因素，包括肿瘤部位和分期、HPV 感染状态、预后情况、不同治疗方法的相对死亡率、患者的一般状况和营养状态、伴随疾病、社会和心理因素、对潜在复发或第二原发癌的治疗方案以及患者的选择。这些因素还需要与已知不同治疗方案的预期疗效综合在一起进行考虑。

头颈部癌患者的总体治疗目标是获得最佳疗效的同时，尽可能减少对功能和外观的影响。要达到这个目标需要能早期发现和诊断、进行有效的康复治疗和选择恰当的姑息治疗方式；还需要多专业团队的紧密协作，要包括外科、放疗、肿瘤内科、化疗、口腔修复、牙科、语言病理、社会服务、营养学、物理和康复医学、病理学和护理方面的从业人员，还常常要有精神病学方面的专业人士。

有效的康复治疗是头颈部癌整体治疗的重要组成部分。手术重建、微血管游离组织转移和口腔修复学的新进展已大大改善了治疗后的器官功能情况[116]。康复治疗需要在最初制订治疗计划时与各种治疗形式很好地整合到一起。疗前的牙科评估以及语言和吞咽功能的评价是需要常规进行的。在放疗前要进行必要的牙科护理和/或拔牙以减少牙科相关黏膜炎和放射性骨坏死的发生率。肿瘤治疗和康复对患者的生活质量十分重要，它还可能需要由特殊的社会精神支持体系对患者及其家庭进行帮助。而且，营养支持也需要重视，在某些患者中需要早期行胃造口术以给予肠内营养支持治疗。目前的化放疗联合治疗手段就对患者的身体造成了长远的负担。正是对营养支持治疗的重视才使这种联合治疗方案的实施成为可能。而进展性疾病需要进行长期的治疗，有时长达数月，作出治疗决定需要考虑到患者、患者家庭和患者职业生涯等社会经济方面的影响因素。

若不能达到充分的局部控制，则只对原发肿瘤进行活检不需要进行全切除术。肿瘤外科的切除原则不包括那些计划不周的重建手术，或为了降低功能或外观性影响而缩减必要的切除范围。肿瘤残存或肿瘤切除后切缘阳性预示着高概率复发。恰当的治疗还应包括对经过选择的患者用现代技术进行精确的保守性手术切除（如喉部分切除术和功能性颈清扫术），这能达到与那些激进治疗手段相似的疗效。

口腔癌前病变

高度怀疑黏膜白斑病和黏膜红斑病的，尤其是在具有高危因素的个体中，需要合理的管理。尽管这两者同属癌前病变，但黏膜红斑病需要更多的医学关注，因为红斑病变中约有一半包含原位癌（CIS）或浸润癌的成分。黏膜红斑病可通过活检除外浸润癌。对黏膜红斑病和黏膜白斑病的处理要根据其位置、范围和组织学情况。而上皮癌癌变过程弥漫多灶性的特点提示有效预防的必要性。在不典型增生的口腔上皮内瘤变（IEN）中，多种分子标志物，如非整倍体、杂合性丢失（LOH）和平足蛋白的表达预示着将有高风险出现恶性转化[117~119]。白斑病变可能与黏膜炎、扁平苔藓、局部组织的机械、热、化学刺激所致的损伤、组织胞浆菌病、念珠菌病及其他感染性病变相混淆。

对于活检组织的诊断或对高危人群进行筛查时，通过甲苯胺蓝局部染色能够进行有效的鉴别。甲苯胺蓝染色可能与不典型增生、微小不典型增生或非不典型增生的口腔上皮内瘤中的杂合性丢失有关，这提示甲苯胺蓝可用于鉴别伴癌变高风险的口腔上皮内瘤变，可指导确定手术切缘的宽度[120,121]。无论是否存在局部刺激因素的持续病变，以及那些与溃疡有关的、垂直生长的、硬结性的、近期大小有变化的或是有疼痛的病变，都需要进行活检和/或切除。但即使进行了充分的局部治疗，比如对非整倍体的黏膜白斑进行完全切除（定义为切缘不存在不典型增生的情况）并不能预防口腔恶性肿瘤的发生[118]。针对该情况，一种靶向治疗预防方法目前已处于Ⅱ期试验。该研究在口腔癌前病变伴杂合性丢失的高危患者中比较了表皮生长因子抑制剂厄洛替尼和安慰剂的效果。尽管总体人群中为阴性结果，但在未罹患口腔癌症的患者中有提升无癌生存期的趋势[122]。未来这一领域的研究将着眼于评估外科切缘的最佳宽度，以及经分子检测确认的完全性切除在降低高危口腔上皮内瘤变的癌变风险方面的作用和地位。

不同部位病变自然史和治疗情况概述

口腔

不论肿瘤还是肿瘤的治疗都显著影响了语言和吞咽功能，尤其是在肿瘤侵犯到舌、口底或下颌骨时。尽管口腔部位很容易经过视诊和触诊进行检查，但超过50%的患者初诊时即为晚期。目前口腔原发肿瘤的T分期见表83-3。

表 83-3 口腔癌的原发肿瘤分期特征

Tx	原发肿瘤不能评价（如切除性活检后分期）
T0	无原发肿瘤的证据（如原发灶不明的肿瘤）
Tis	原位癌
T1	肿瘤最大径≤2cm
T2	肿瘤最大径介于2cm和4cm之间
T3	肿瘤最大径>4cm
T4	A：肿瘤侵犯邻近结构（穿过骨皮质、上颌窦、皮肤、舌肌、深部组织、神经）
	B：侵入咀嚼肌间隙、翼突板，颅底、颈动脉

唇

唇黏膜的鳞癌是口腔肿瘤中最常见的类型。唇黏膜鳞癌与唇周围皮肤的癌症的区分是十分重要的，而后者被认为是皮肤恶性肿瘤。超过90%的唇癌发生于下唇，常常位于外露的唇红部，并在中线和口角的中部。上唇肿瘤则大多为基底细胞癌[123]。分化好的癌以及疣状癌极少出现转移。而分化差的癌和梭形细胞癌则常常侵袭性生长并转移。主要神经的受侵则意味着病变具有侵袭性，需要积极的治疗，大多数情况下需要联合治疗。

唇癌的治疗需要考虑以下几个方面：①病变的控制；②具有功能的口腔括约肌；③可接受的外貌改变。在肿瘤小于2cm或非常表浅时，不论通过放疗还是手术都能很好地达到上述目标。但对于大病变而言，外科切除和重建是最佳选择，因为这样能够更准确的评估肿瘤的范围，包括神经和淋巴受侵的情况。肿瘤周围常常存在癌前病变，可以通过手术（予以处理以预防第二原发癌的出现[124,125]。对于大病变的首次重建治疗，使用局部皮瓣，游离组织皮瓣可以避免因放疗而组织缺失所致的缺陷，为未来的重建和治疗提供选择，并降低下颌骨的放射性骨坏死的风险。而对于广泛的浸润性病变，侵犯骨骼或出现淋巴转移等情况则需要进行包括术前放疗和手术的综合治疗。

治疗唇癌的放疗技术包括外照射、组织植入物和这两者的联合治疗。放疗的局部控制率超过80%[126,127]，5年存活率（包括外科补救）超过95%。原发手术切除报告的局部控制率和生存率与放疗类似[128]。局部转移使生存率降低到 55% 左右[129,130]。上唇癌患者的 5 年生存率要比类似的下唇癌患者低,在 40% ~ 60%[131]。上下唇及口角同时受累的情况很少。口角癌的预后没有其他唇部肿瘤的好。

舌

舌癌占口腔鳞癌超过 25%的比例,最常发生的部位在舌前 2/3 的外侧和腹侧。舌的肌层受累发生较早。T1 和 T2(<4cm)病变的生物学侵袭性是值得注意的,相较于其他类似分期的口腔病变,它们具有更高的隐匿局部转移的概率。隐匿的淋巴结转移发生在 30% ~ 40%的早期病变中[132]。舌尖或舌中线发生的肿瘤可能有双侧淋巴结受累。局部复发是 60% ~ 70%舌癌患者的肿瘤相关死亡的原因。远处转移所致的死亡占 15%,上呼吸消化道的第二原发癌则占 20% ~ 40%[132,133]。人们越来越认识到舌癌病变范围虽小却侵犯程度很深,还有着很高的隐匿性淋巴结转移概率,另外在软组织及骨的重建方面有很多进展,这都大大影响了舌癌的治疗模式。尽管单纯外科切除仍是治疗的主要方式,联合外科和术后针对原发部位和区域淋巴结的辅助放疗已常规用于治疗大多数晚期病变(Ⅲ、Ⅳ期),并越来越多地用于病理结果显示有淋巴结转移或神经侵犯的Ⅱ期病变的治疗(图 83-3)。术后的同步化放疗则建议用于有神经侵犯、淋巴结包膜外生长或者外科切缘过近等情况[134]。

对于Ⅰ期病变的治疗,手术切除是迅速有效的,且能够很好地保存器官功能。对于浸润性Ⅱ期病变,半舌切除术或部分舌切除术能够获得很好的肿瘤控制率,但必须联合对有转移风险的颈部淋巴结清扫术(肩胛舌骨肌上清扫术)以获得准确的分期信息,从而决定是否需要辅助治疗,特别是术后放疗。游离组织转移重建能够显著改善半舌切除术所致的功能障碍。

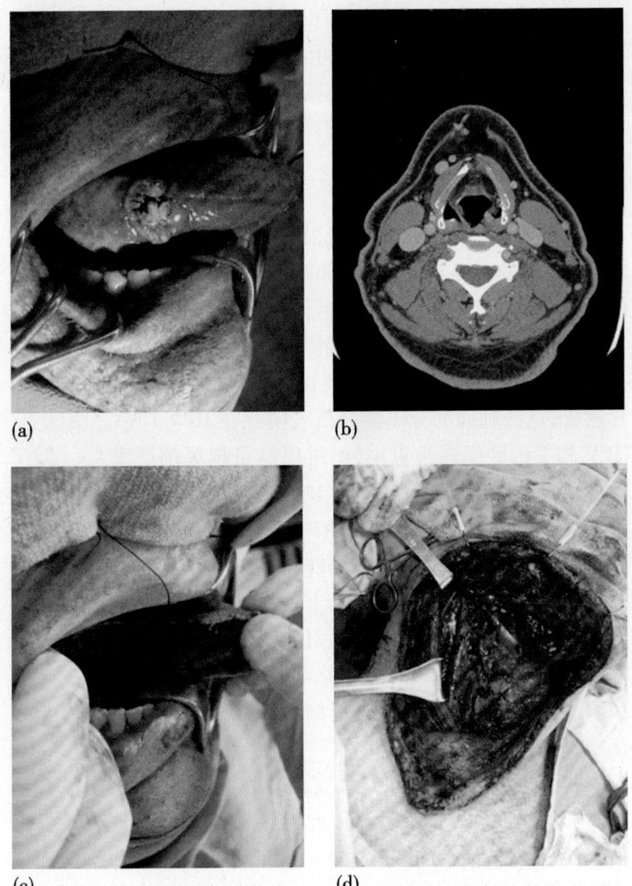

图 83-3　(a)口腔鳞癌 T1N0。(b)CT 扫描提示无淋巴转移。(c)半侧舌切除术。(d)肩胛舌骨上颈淋巴结清扫术

肿瘤侵及口底或下颌骨时可能需要行下颌骨切除术或部分下颌骨切除术。现代重建技术使用带吻合血管的合成骨和软组织游离皮瓣,钛金属假体和牙科植入物等已能大大改善下颌骨切除后对功能及外观的影响。对于浸润深度超过 4mm 的具有隐匿淋巴结病变风险者应行选择性颈清扫术治疗。

对于晚期原发病变(Ⅲ、Ⅳ期),手术加术后外照射已被普遍应用。目前尚无前瞻性的对照研究证实在没有淋巴结转移时联合治疗相对于单纯手术的优势,但有回顾性研究表明联合治疗能获得更好的局部控制率[135~138]。但远处转移和第二原发癌的发生率的增加部分抵消了联合治疗的这种优势。手术治疗主要包括部分舌切除术和颈部淋巴结清扫,下颌骨若未被直接侵及则可以保留。如果有局部骨膜受侵,可行皮质和其他部分下颌骨切除以保留下颌骨的主要功能和连续性。如果肿瘤侵犯到中线或舌根,则可能需要进行全舌切除术或次全切除术。重建技术的不断发展大大提高了这些手术所可能导致的功能问题。作好临时气管切开和长期肠内营养的准备是十分必要的。全舌切除术或不保留双侧舌下神经时常需要进行造瘘术以进行永久性肠内治疗。现有的经验表明,在高选择性患者中,全舌切除时可以不进行喉切除术,但可能需要进行长期甚至永久性的肠外营养治疗[139]。术后放疗应在术后 4 ~ 6 周内开始。对于高危外科切缘或包膜外侵犯可给予高剂量放疗或同步化放疗。晚期口腔癌放疗时,双侧颈部都需要进行照射,其剂量取决于病变范围。因为术后舌内肿瘤即使残余很少也难以被根除,手术切缘较近时需要进行高剂量放疗(66 ~ 70Gy)。即使进行联合治疗,晚期疾病的 2 年无病生存率(DFS)和总生存率大约只有 50%。Ⅰ期和Ⅱ期病变的 5 年生存率在 50% ~ 70%,而Ⅲ期和Ⅳ期病变则为 15% ~ 30%[140~144]。

口底(FOM)

口底癌的发生率与舌癌类似。它早期常播散至邻近区域(牙龈和下颌骨骨膜)。下颌骨骨膜对于肿瘤侵袭是一道自然屏障。舌固定就是肿瘤深度浸润的体征之一。口底癌可能蔓延到或穿透下颌舌骨肌,而后者正是对于舌骨下直接播散的一道自然屏障。大约 40%的患者表现出淋巴结转移性病变。隐匿性淋巴结转移率随着原发灶 T 分期的上升而升高:T2 病变为 40%,而 T3 病变则为 70%[145,146]。

口底癌淋巴引流的首站是颌下淋巴结和二腹肌淋巴结(Ⅰ区和Ⅱ区)。早期下颌骨受侵易于通过触诊发现。颏下淋巴结受侵相对少见。由于固定到下颌骨即意味着骨膜受侵,而且这类肿瘤中有 50% ~ 60%存在直接骨受侵的情况。另外也可通过 CT 的骨窗进行鉴别。

肿瘤较小时(T1、T2)经过广泛切除普遍能获得较好的效果。外侧口底癌常常能经口切除,手术缺损的修复依靠邻近黏膜的推进、皮肤移植或二期愈合来达到。对于表浅的病变,可对离断的下颌腺管行唾液管成形术。T1 病变伴有超过 4mm 浸润深度以及所有的 T2 ~ 4 的病变可进行选择性颈清扫术。口

底前部病变应进行双侧颈清扫，因为该区域的淋巴引流致使双颈部均有隐匿性转移的风险。若已出现淋巴结转移，则应进行治疗性颈淋巴结清扫术。对于早期口底癌，手术治疗仍是主要手段，并能够获得很好的疗效。

较晚期的口底癌（T3、T4）普遍使用联合治疗手段，与前文舌癌治疗中所述的治疗手段类似（图 83-4）。保留下颌骨连续性和功能的皮质切除术仍常常被用到。在这些病例中，我们发现筋膜皮瓣在口底和舌的重建中很有潜力。大的黏膜和软组织缺损常规以游离组织皮瓣来进行重建，而下颌骨缺损的重建如今是用腓骨或肩胛骨皮瓣来进行。

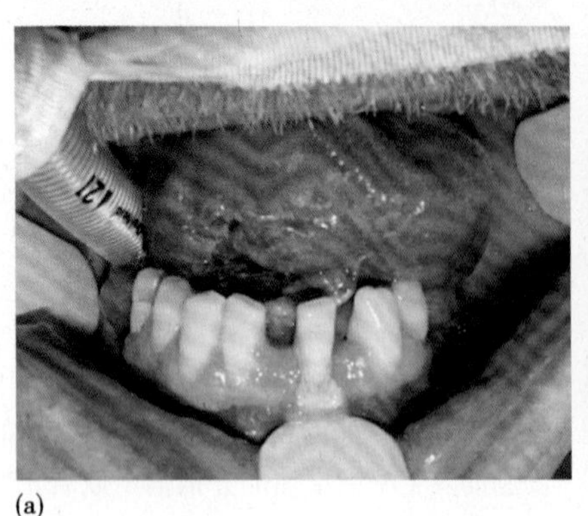

(a)

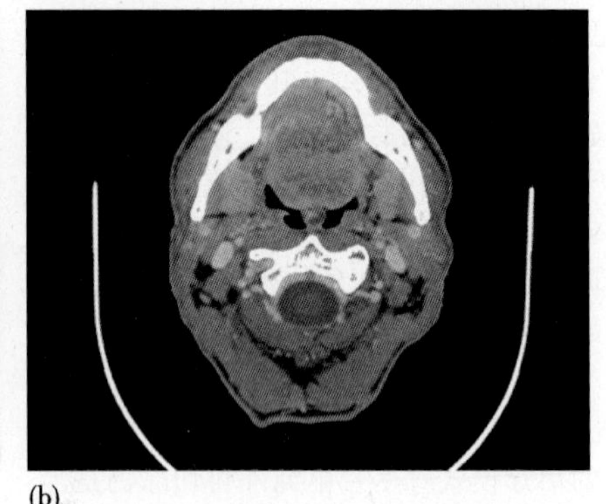

(b)

图 83-4 （a）T3N0 的口底鳞癌。（b）舌内肌深部浸润的轴状位显像

治疗效果受原发肿瘤大小、是否有淋巴结转移、下颌骨的受侵程度、切除是否充分等因素的影响。局限的Ⅰ期和Ⅱ期口底癌的 5 年生存率在 80%[146]。肿瘤跨中线、侵及舌或下颌骨时，5 年生存率为 50%～60%[147]。更晚期的病变（Ⅲ期和Ⅳ期）的 5 年生存率则不到 50%。联合治疗（手术和放疗）的主要优点在于对同侧及对侧颈部病变的更好控制。颈部临床检查阴性仅进行手术治疗后失败的患者中，颈部是最常见的复发部位[148]。对于有多发淋巴结转移的患者，其晚期远处转移风险高，诱导化疗（IC）正在研究中[149]。推荐持续监测头颈部、食管和肺部发生第二原发癌的可能[150,151]。

牙龈和颊黏膜

牙龈癌大多（80%）发生在下龈，位于前磨牙的后方。对牙龈癌和颊黏膜癌来说，牙关紧闭的症状都预示着肿瘤侵及了咬肌或翼外肌。据文献报道隐匿性淋巴结转移在颊黏膜癌中发生率高达 30%。除了最早期的癌症外，所有患者均应进行选择性颈清扫术[152]。外生性肿瘤的外观为乳头状或疣状，容易与良性的过度角化症相混淆。

小而表浅的牙龈癌经手术切除达到有效治疗，且可完好保留功能。即使较大病变需要进行局部上颌骨切除或牙槽骨切除时也能不经过外部切口完成手术。而对于更大的病变（T3 和 T4），需要进行部分下颌骨切除和/或上颌骨切除，而辅助放疗通常是被推荐的（图 83-5）。下颌牙龈的晚期病变易发生隐匿性转移，需要进行选择性颈清扫术。关于上颌脊和硬腭的癌症只有很少的资料，但它们能转移到侧颈淋巴结，进行颈清扫术或颈部放疗是很有必要的[153]。临床表现颈部淋巴结增大的患者则应在进行原发肿瘤切除的同时进行颈清扫术。

牙龈和颊黏膜癌的总生存率与肿瘤大小、骨受侵和淋巴结转移的情况有关。当有骨受累时，手术治疗效果明显优于放疗。

磨牙后三角

发生于磨牙后三角的肿瘤很少只局限于这里的牙龈黏膜，它常常侵及附近的颊黏膜、咽腭弓、口底和/或后牙龈。当侵及咽腭弓时其行为更倾向于口咽癌的表现。其发生临床阳性或隐匿的淋巴结转移的风险要比其他部位牙龈癌更高。由于常常出现骨膜受侵，即使针对小病变也应进行部分（边缘性）下颌骨切除术。对于表浅的覆盖面积较大和处于移动状态的病变，比如蔓延至软腭或颊黏膜时，可行初始放疗。中度进展或侵犯程度较深的病变的最佳治疗方案是进行手术（下颌骨切除和颈清扫），并推荐进行术后辅助治疗。

口咽

口咽癌的临床分期主要是根据肿瘤的大小，与口腔癌分期是类似的（表 83-3）。虽然口咽癌可以从口咽的任何部位发生，但最常见的位置是在舌腭弓，舌腭弓包括扁桃体窝和舌根。近期证明 HPV 作为口咽癌发生的主要病致病因素引导了对于一类特定疾病表现的认识。许多相对年轻的患者没有典型烟草暴露史，这些肿瘤的分子学分析表明存在 HPV DNA。临床上，HPV 相关的肿瘤通常更小，但淋巴结负担更加严重[37]。除了颈部出现原因不明的肿物外，口咽癌的症状最常见的就是慢性吞咽痛（常为单侧）和耳痛。而声音改变、吞咽困难和牙关紧闭则是后继的体征。区域淋巴结转移在口咽癌经常发生，它与肿瘤侵犯深度和肿瘤大小有关。上颈部淋巴结一般被最先累及，但也会出现跳跃式的转移而先出现下颈部淋巴结的受侵。口咽癌也会发生双侧淋巴结转移，特别是在肿瘤位于软腭、舌根和中线咽壁的时候。咽后淋巴结也常常出现转移，在制订治疗计划时需要对此进行评估。

鉴于该解剖部位在呼吸、言语和吞咽中的重要作用，口咽癌的管理非常具有挑战性。因此，治疗的目标不仅是实现肿瘤治疗，还要保持口咽的多重功能。口咽部的传统手术方法与显著的发病率相关，这促使在 20 世纪 90 年代转向非手术方式，特别是利用放疗或化放疗，是过去 15～20 年的主要治疗方法[155,156]。然而，最近的技术创新通过经口机器人方法（TORS），逐渐转向重新选择手术治疗，其允许基于疾病的病理学发现来修改辅助治

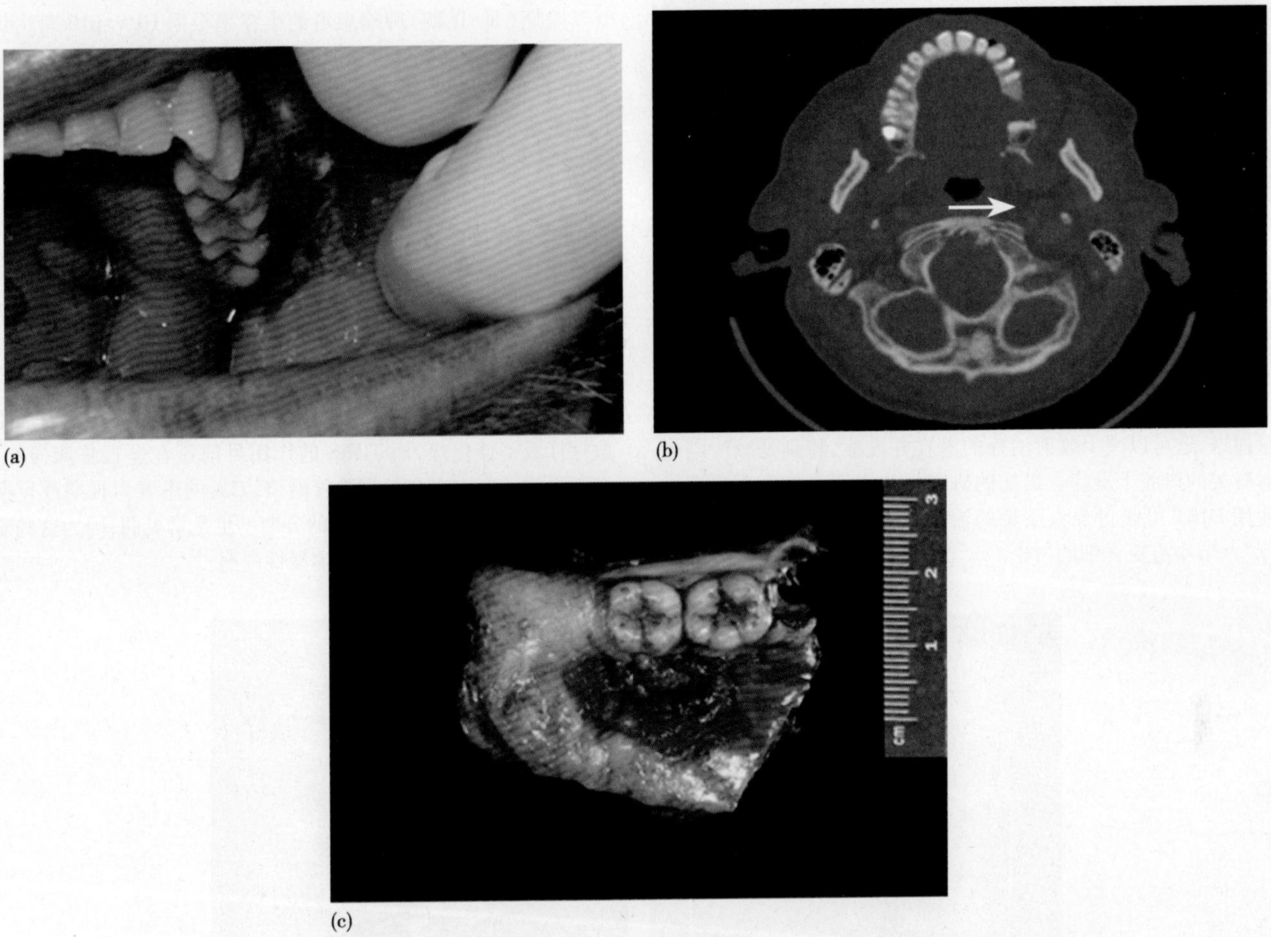

(a)　(b)

(c)

图 83-5　(a)口腔(颊黏膜)的 T4N0 鳞癌。(b)CT 扫描显示硬腭的骨破坏。(c)上颌窦切除术标本

疗。这种新颖的范例可以减少辐射剂量,并且理论上可以减少长期副作用。考虑到新出现的 HPV 相关癌症患者群体,这些优势势在必行。

TORS 的肿瘤相关禁忌证包括不可切除的颈部肿大淋巴结、下颌骨侵犯、咽壁或舌根受累,需要切除超过 50% 以上部位,颈动脉受累以及肿瘤固定于椎前筋膜。TORS 的另一个限制是入路,因此必须对患者和肿瘤特征进行彻底的术前评估。这应该包括牙列的评估,是否存在牙关紧闭或凸起、舌头大小、颈部伸展程度、先前治疗的后遗症和肿瘤范围。迄今为止,机器人手术的肿瘤学结果一直受到青睐,OS 和 DFS 分别为 82%~100% 和 86%~96%。虽然 TORS 的作用仍待确定,但几个病例对照研究显示早期肿瘤治疗效果与放疗或同步放化疗的结果相当[157]。

扁桃体

早期扁桃体肿瘤(Ⅰ期和Ⅱ期)的治疗常常以放疗作为单一治疗手段。针对表浅的小病变进行经口广泛的局部切除术能够获得较好的局部疗效,但却无法明确高发的隐匿性淋巴结转移的具体情况。对于小肿瘤的情况,尽管手术治疗和放疗的局部控制效果是相当的,HPV 阴性的肿瘤患者通常需要进行术后放疗[158]。对于早期 HPV 阳性的肿瘤患者,TORS

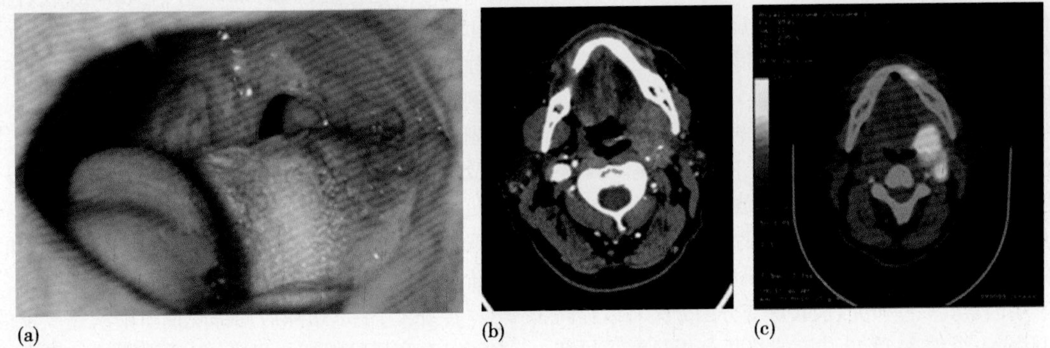

(a)　(b)　(c)

图 83-6　(a)口咽鳞状细胞癌 T2N2b,临床小病灶。(b)CT 扫描明确显示已深侵达咽旁间隙。(c)在 PET-CT 显像上,有明显的两个病灶,原发肿瘤和后方的淋巴结转移

加颈部淋巴结清扫术可有效实现局部控制，而无需辅助放疗[157]。晚期病变手术治疗常导致功能不全，所以需要联合放疗、化疗(图 83-6)。对于存在淋巴结转移(N1～2)的患者，TORS 联合术后放疗、无同步化疗可达到很好的肿瘤治疗效果和功能保全。不进行术后放疗的临床证据越来越多，特别是在 p16 阳性(HPV 相关)小肿瘤(T1、T2)和小体积颈部疾病(N1)患者中，这种治疗方案目前正在多个研究中进行评估(ECOG 3311)。

放射治疗早期扁桃体癌的优势在于能够同时对原发肿瘤周围的前哨淋巴结进行治疗。除非肿瘤侵及舌根或者软腭的中线部位，放疗只需要进行单侧照射[159]。照射范围可以不包括对侧的黏膜和唾液腺。现代治疗技术，如 IMRT，允许连续剂量递送，这可以减少放射治疗的潜在并发症，特别是减少与辐射有关的口腔干燥症。最初的研究报告表明在口咽癌患者中使用 IMRT 可获得令人鼓舞的治疗效果[160～164]；这在“放射治疗”一节中有更详细的讨论。

晚期(Ⅲ/Ⅳ期)肿瘤患者的生存率根据 HPV/p16 表达状态和吸烟史而不同。化疗和放疗联合治疗、HPV 阳性肿瘤和低于 10 包年吸烟史(低风险)的患者 3 年生存率为 93%，超过 10 包年的吸烟史和接受放化疗的 HPV/p16 阴性肿瘤的 3 年生存率为 46.2%[88]。一般来说，除非下颌骨严重受侵，否则很少推荐手术治疗晚期扁桃体肿瘤。计划手术时，应在适当选择的患者中采用术后同步放化疗。

舌根

舌根癌比扁桃体癌更难治疗，特别是对于 HPV 阴性的恶性肿瘤。大多数 HPV 阴性肿瘤患者由于这些肿瘤的隐匿性而导致原发灶病情很晚，局部转移多，导致更大的治疗致残率和较差的生存期。由于 HPV 阴性肿瘤具有侵袭性，大多数采用放疗伴或不伴化疗，而 TORS 的作用目前正在进行临床研究。由于舌根部存在丰富的淋巴管网络，75%的患者为Ⅲ期或Ⅳ期疾病(图 83-7)。原发性肿瘤的分期不足是常见的，因为这些癌症往往在其临床表现之外有弥漫性浸润[165]。

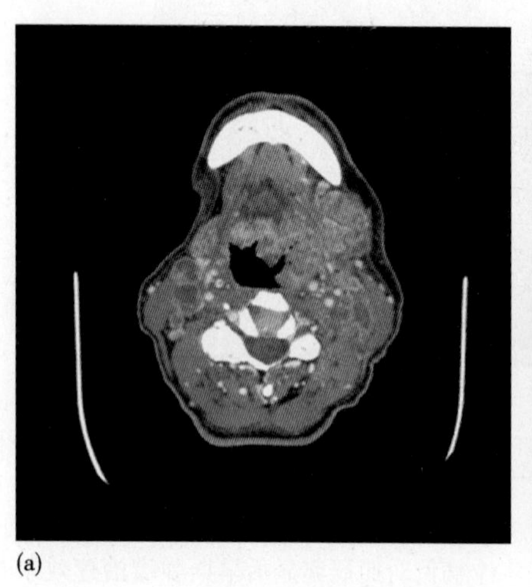

(a)

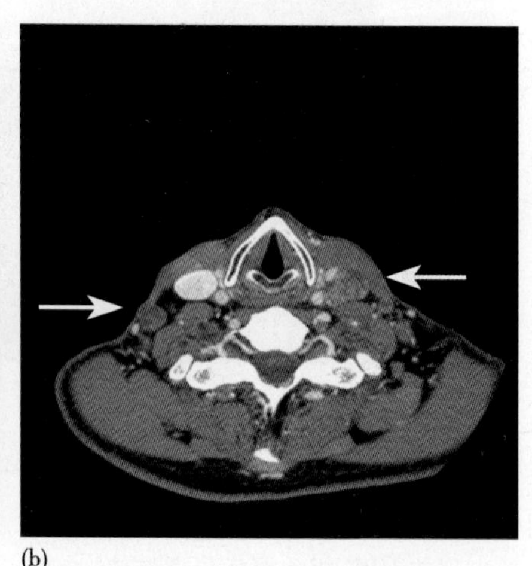

(b)

图 83-7　(a)口咽部巨大鳞癌 T4N2c(左舌底)。(b)存在多区淋巴结转移

单纯放疗作为小原发肿瘤(T1、T2)的确定性治疗对于外生性肿瘤比对于深部侵袭性肿瘤更好[166]。单纯放疗通常适用于没有临床淋巴结转移的患者，但对于具有临床阳性淋巴结的患者可在完成放疗的基础上联合颈部清扫术。

早期原发性舌根肿瘤(T1、T2)的手术治疗取得了与单独放疗相似的效果。机器人手术的进展使这项技术可应用于舌癌的治疗，现在已成为 HPV 阳性人群中一种成熟的治疗手段[167]。选择性颈部清扫术可作为淋巴结分期手术，从而为辅助放疗提供依据。迄今为止，还没有前瞻性随机试验比较单纯手术与手术联合术前或术后放疗的效果。

放射治疗是对口咽癌进行根治性治疗的标准方法，因为其结合了肿瘤治疗和器官保存的双重目标。目前的放疗方案来自几项大型随机临床试验，这些试验表明放疗可提高患者 OS 和 DFS[168]，虽然永久性吞咽困难和永久性胃造口率仍然很高[156]。总辐射剂量和总治疗时间被认为是肿瘤学反应和组织毒性的重要影响因素。一些研究表明，可变分割方案可以提高局部区域控制率，一个纳入 15 项试验的荟萃分析显示了可变分割方案具有生存优势[169]。由于口咽癌与几个关键结构相邻，理想的剂量分布将与目标区域紧密符合而周围组织不受影响，这导致 IMRT 作为头颈鳞癌的标准治疗[170]。

在口咽鳞癌中 RT 后复发的典型模式是局部复发，归因于治疗后持续存在的放疗耐受的肿瘤细胞。为了克服这种抗性，联合化疗以使肿瘤细胞对电离辐射的破坏作用敏感。对于患有局部晚期口咽癌的患者，法国 GORTEC 组进行的一项关键性随机Ⅲ期临床试验显示，接受联合治疗的患者(42%和 51%)患者的无进展生存期(PFS)和 5 年 OS 较单独放射治疗(22.4%和 15.8%)均有改善，化放疗组局部控制率(66%)与单独放射治疗(42%)相比有所改善。尽管有这些益处，但在两组中均观察到相似的远处转移率(11%)，并且在化疗组中观察到更显著的副作用，包括血液学毒性和 3 级和 4 级黏膜炎[171,172]。与单独放射治疗组相比，这些毒性导致联合组中临时胃造口术使用率更高。总之，这些结果表明，在放疗中加入同步化疗可以改善局部区域控制，这可以转化为这些患者的 PFS 和 OS 益处，但代价是更严重的毒性。

传统上，手术切除后局部晚期口咽鳞癌复发的风险很高。对于具有高风险特征的患者，包括周围神经浸润，多个淋巴结阳性和 T 分期晚期，PORT 已被证明可减少局部区域复发。此外也已经证明同步放化疗可以提高高风险患者的局部控制率，特别是当手术切缘阳性或 ECS 存在时[134,173]。因此,接受口咽鳞癌手术切除的患者当存在不良病理特征时,考虑用辅助放化疗。目前正在审查这种治疗模式是否对 HPV 阳性患者是必要的。

软腭和咽壁

原发于软腭和咽壁的癌症比其他的口咽部位肿瘤少见。许多软腭癌和后壁癌症位置比较表浅。晚期病变可浸润深达椎前筋膜、颞下窝以及颅底,并与伴临床跳跃区域的广泛黏膜下播散有关。

在大多数情况下,即使是原发病变达 T3 时,放疗为基础的手段是治疗的首选。软腭病变的手术治疗常常带来严重的功能残疾。隐匿性局部转移的发生率的高低很难评估,因为双侧淋巴结包括咽后部分均在初治时就进行了照射。临床发现有阳性淋巴结的患者大约占到 30%[174]。原发病灶小并且伴有阳性淋巴结时,原发灶及颈部的根治性放疗是有效的手段。如果颈部病变在经过外照射后 6~8 周仍然存在,应进行颈部淋巴结清扫术。咽壁癌或软腭癌范围很广侵及扁桃体并伴有晚期局部转移时,常常以同步化放疗进行治疗,但这在出现明显的下颌骨受侵时并不适用。软腭和腭弓癌的 5 年总生存率是 60%~70%,T1 和 T2 病变的 5 年生存率在 80%~90%,而在Ⅲ期和Ⅳ期病变则为 30%~60%[221]。局部复发是治疗失败的最常见原因[175]。

下咽

下咽癌是头颈部鳞癌中致死率最高的部位之一。在诊断时就有 70%~80%的患者伴有明显的淋巴结转移[176]。双侧和对侧淋巴结转移发生于 10%~20%的患者,这在肿瘤生长过中线时尤为明显。下咽癌具有在黏膜下层播散的倾向而影响到口咽和食管。深溃疡以及跳跃性的病变很常见,导致难以确定确切的肿瘤边界,而且导致了即使联合了辅助放疗,这个部位病变的局部控制情况也很糟糕。超过 75%的下咽癌源自梨状窝,而另外有大约 20%发生于咽后壁(图 83-8),发生于环状软骨后的很少(小于 5%)。由于下咽癌位置的特点及其生物学行为,其手术治疗通常需要进行全咽喉切除,若侵及食管则还需要进行颈段食管切除。

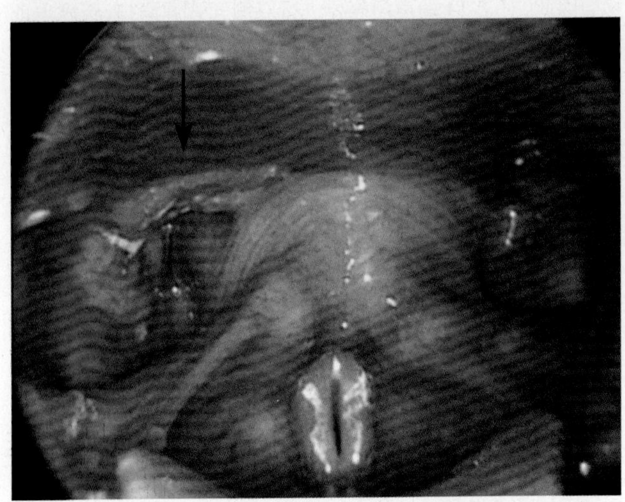

图 83-8　下咽鳞癌 T1,侵及咽后壁并蔓延至食管入口

下咽癌的分期基于其侵及的部位、肿瘤的大小、是否有声带固定以及淋巴结转移的范围[114]。确定分期对于指定治疗方案是十分关键的,进行内镜下评估是必需的[178]。

由于大多数下咽癌的手术治疗范围较大,需要进行喉切除,人们对 T1 及 T2 病变进行放疗,对 T3 病变进行化、放联合治疗进行了研究[179]。回顾性研究数据都反映出单纯放疗不论在生存率还是在局部控制率方面均劣于手术或手术加放疗[180,181]。

尽管如此,由于手术所致的功能性影响即使在最早期病变亦十分突出,放疗还是有它的一席之地。对于 T1 病变较小的下咽癌以及原发于咽后壁的表浅病变,单纯放疗效果不错,而手术可作为其补救措施[182]。放疗对于双侧隐匿性淋巴结转移的治疗是有优势的,其中也包括了常常出现于原发在咽后壁肿瘤的咽后淋巴结。但大多数患者(T3、T4)的局部晚期并伴有淋巴结转移,对于他们来说,单纯放疗的局部控制率只有 50%,而手术补救很少能成功。因此,手术治疗是最主要的手段。对于诊断时状态较差的患者也是如此。

发生于下咽下部或环状软骨后黏膜的肿瘤常常播散至食管。食管远端的黏膜下播散可能范围较广,需要进行部分或全部食管切除术。用胃、游离空肠或者管形游离皮瓣来重建食管功能是目前的主要选择[183~185]。随着咽喉全切除术的出现以及术后放疗的应用,肿瘤的局部控制改善,复发部位常常位于远处(如肺部)。手术联合术前或术后放疗显著提高了局部控制率,但生存率的数据较单纯手术却没有实质性的上升,这是由于远处转移的发生率升高了。目前术后放疗相对于术前放疗来说是首选,因为前者的局部复发更少、并发症发生更少,而且更易于精准地确定肿瘤边界[180,186]。淋巴结转移的发生、包膜外淋巴结受侵以及原发肿瘤直接侵及颈部软组织,这些都是预后不良的指标,同时也是进行术后化放疗的适应证[187,188]。

咽后壁癌总体的 5 年生存率在 10%~30%,而在梨状窝癌则在 20%~40%。远处转移的发生率在 20%~50%[123,127],它随着淋巴结病变范围的增大而升高[176,189~191]。

喉癌

由于喉这个部位在我们的沟通交流、吞咽、呼吸、对下呼吸道的保护等会影响生活质量的许多方面具有十分突出的意义,在喉癌治疗时,我们常常进退两难:治疗会导致明显的功能障碍而疾病则威胁着生命。对生活质量的考虑在头颈部癌治疗策略制订时十分重要,而在喉癌的治疗上最为明显。

喉癌分为声门上、声门、声门下三部分,它们有着不同的局部扩散情况、淋巴结转移风险以及疾病控制率。关于喉的血管淋巴引流进行的大量解剖学研究,发现了喉部肿瘤扩散天然解剖屏障。这使某些特定部位的肿瘤能够进行选择性的部分喉切除术[192,193]。

真声带是声门上区和声门下区不同淋巴引流的分界。这一解剖屏障在肿瘤侵及前后联合或垂直生长侵犯真假声带时(贯声门癌)作用就不明显了。甲状软骨内部的软骨膜通常也是肿瘤扩散的屏障之一。但肿瘤侵及前联合或范围贯声门时,出现甲状软骨侵犯的概率达 40%~60%[194]。

早期发现及诊断对于提高生存率和保存喉功能至关重要。声门癌大多能够早期发现,这是由于肿瘤生长所致的声带振动的微小改变就能体现出声音嘶哑或发音困难的症状。声门上癌发现时常常分期较晚,因为它并不引起类似的早期症状。事实上,声门上癌最早的体征表现为咽喉痛、吞咽困难、耳痛或者代表了局部转移的颈部包块的出现。而气道阻塞则可能是声门下癌的早期症状。

当代临床诊断技术包括纤维喉镜、直接喉镜、喉及颈部的CT和MRI以及喉镜分析(图83-9)。放射学手段在评估肿瘤对会厌前和声带旁间隙的侵犯以及针对软骨、软组织和颈部淋巴结进行评估时很有价值。但要精确评估肿瘤范围时仍需行麻醉下的直接喉镜,若肿瘤巨大有阻塞性改变则还需进行气管造口。在有些患者,直接喉镜时进行减瘤术可以避免进行气管造口,从而减少引起种植转移的风险。尽管进行了这样的精确评估,但仍有30%~40%的病例的结论并不准确,而且常常是被低估[195,196]。

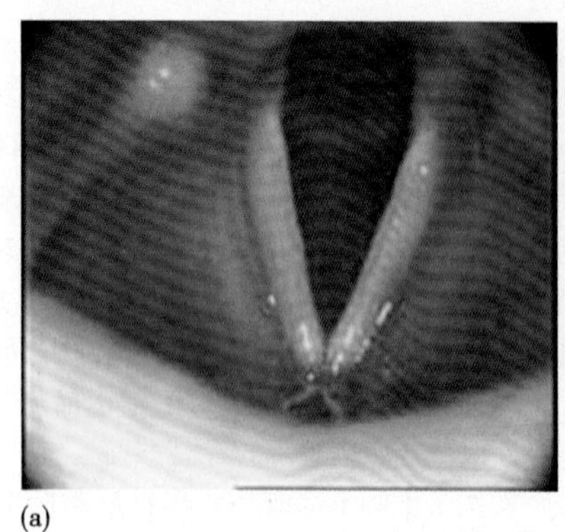
(a)

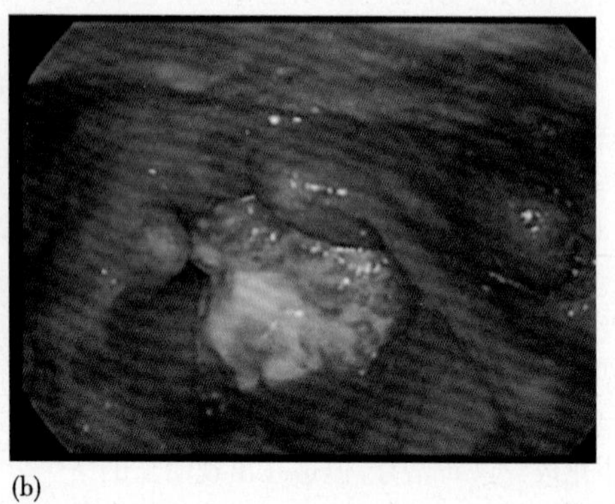
(b)

图83-9 (a)正常喉部。(b)T3期左声门区鳞癌,正常声带解剖结构闭塞,明确蔓延至声门上区和杓状软骨

声门上癌占喉癌总数的35%[8]。声门上癌的分期是基于受侵部位,包括假声带、杓状软骨、会厌的舌面和喉面以及杓会厌襞。会厌本身也被分为舌骨上和舌骨下两部分。除了肿瘤侵犯杓状会厌襞并侵及梨状窝时,会厌舌骨上的肿瘤预后都要好于舌骨下的。这是由于会厌的舌骨下部分具有更为丰富的淋巴网络。早期(T1和T2)病变可以包括上述的一个或多个部位,但声带活动是正常的。肿瘤导致杓状软骨固定或侵犯到环状软骨后区、梨状窝内侧壁以及会厌前间隙时分期为T3。肿瘤范围超出喉部或侵犯了甲状软骨时分期为T4。

声门型喉癌的分期也是由解剖和功能性特征来决定的。肿瘤局限于真声带时为T1,肿瘤侵犯到一个邻近结构或声带活动受损时分期为T2。杓状软骨固定和声带固定的分期为T3,有软骨受侵或肿瘤范围超出喉部分期为T4。

声门下癌中局限于声门下区者分期为T1,范围在声门下和真声带者分期为T2,均属于早期癌症。声带固定属于T3,而软骨受侵或范围达到喉外属于T4,这些意味着预后更差。喉癌的淋巴结分期与其他头颈部鳞癌是一致的。

尽管喉癌的最佳治疗手段还存在很大的争论,在得克萨斯大学MD Anderson癌症中心,根治性放疗已通常作为早期喉癌的治疗选择。对于中期病变,则需要在根治性放疗与根治性手术之间权衡,根治性放疗可以将补救手术作为备选治疗,而根治性手术在最近也开始联合化疗及放疗手段进行综合治疗。除了分期以外,在决定治疗策略时还有些因素应当考虑:年龄、并发症、喉的功能和它康复的潜力。晚期T4病变要进行手术和术后放射治疗。

早期声门癌的治疗手段主要为放疗,但在某些情况下,可以选择保喉的手术治疗,比如局限性病变内镜下激光切除或部分喉切除术。这两者都需要进行切缘的冷冻病理检查。另外,对于Ⅰ期和Ⅱ期病变外照射效果不佳时,补救性的保喉手术有效率在10%~20%。

更晚期喉癌(T3和T4)的治疗在历史上既有单纯手术也有手术联合放疗。前瞻性随机研究已有力地证明了化疗加放疗(包含外科补救治疗)对于T3喉癌患者的长期生存与手术联合或不联合放疗是等同的,这就使大约60%的患者的生活质量显著提高[197~199]。非手术组患者的语言交流情况有明显的优势,但并未对吞咽功能进行评估[200]。对于T4病变而言,局部控制情况很差。对它们是否以保喉治疗作为标准手段还有争议,有观点认为诊断时就功能很差的晚期患者保守治疗后喉功能仍会很差。对于出现明显误吸症状的患者,进行手术应该是很有意义的。此外,对于那些有着呼吸系统和心血管系统并发症的患者,由于化放疗的毒性,他们的治疗强度受限,手术加放疗可能是最佳的手段。

喉癌的许多外科手术方式都会建立一个气管造瘘,这个区域有时是肿瘤复发的高危部位,复发大多是气管旁淋巴结转移。因此,对于T4的声门癌要进行双侧气管旁清扫,若病理证实有阳性淋巴结,则术后还应进行放疗。一旦气管造瘘处复发,则无论作何补救治疗都很难影响预后。一项研究显示他们的5年生存率仅为17%[201]。因此,若存在气管造瘘复发的风险,在初始治疗过程中要加入该部位的放疗。

声门上型喉癌

影响声门上型喉癌选择治疗方案的主要因素有肿瘤位置、声带是否固定和会厌前间隙是否受累。肿瘤局限于会厌舌骨上区时应进行放疗,放疗野包括有转移风险的颈部淋巴结。另外,微创支持者们建议行内镜下的激光切除术,与颈部淋巴结的治疗分开。肿瘤侵犯到杓会厌皱襞、梨状窝或者会厌舌骨下区时,侵袭性更明显,浸润程度更深,而且常常侵及会厌前间隙。单纯放疗的疗效不如手术治疗,前者的局部复发机会更高,需要进行手术补救。同步进行系统性化疗能够改善预后。声门上区放疗后持续性的水肿是常见的,给诊断复发造成一些困难,而复发的发生率在40%~50%[202,203]。绝大多数患者复发后最终将接受全喉切除的挽救治疗。

对于任何进行部分喉切除的患者，术前需完成全喉切除的知情同意，因为术中可能因病变需要进行更广泛的切除。大约 20%的患者需要延长气管造口的时间，这常常是由于术后放疗继发的水肿所致。持续吞咽困难的发生率较低，而由于持续误吸所需进行的补充喉切除术仅发生于 0~5%的病例中[204,205]。

T2 及以上病变发生颈部淋巴结转移的概率至少有 20%。颈部淋巴结临床阴性时治疗可选手术或放疗[206]。放疗患者的治愈率大多报道为 73%~75%，若再行补充手术则治愈率上升至 80%~85%[207~209]，大多数复发位于颈部淋巴结，接受补充手术的患者中，65%~70%能保留正常发音功能[207]。

针对更晚期病变（T3、T4）的治疗还有着争议，其焦点之一在于是否保喉（图 83-10）。化放疗联合治疗有效率高，但毒副作用十分明显。因而，T4 病变患者进行喉切除术加放疗是最佳选择，因为软骨和骨的受侵单靠放疗很难控制。在一些有经验的医院，针对喉骨架的微小侵犯病例进行化放疗联合治疗取得了很好的疗效。另一个有争议的是针对 T3 大肿块且疗前一般情况较差患者的治疗。这些患者最终可能需要进行长期或永久的肠内营养，也会由于严重的误吸需要进行气管造口，还可能最终为了避免肺部并发症进行喉切除。一种新出现的方案建议行诱导化疗，以评估肿瘤和器官功能对药物的反应。一周期化疗后有明显功能改善者可能可以耐受同步化放疗，从而避免进行喉切除。而那些化疗无效或效果很不明显者则最好选择手术加术后放疗。

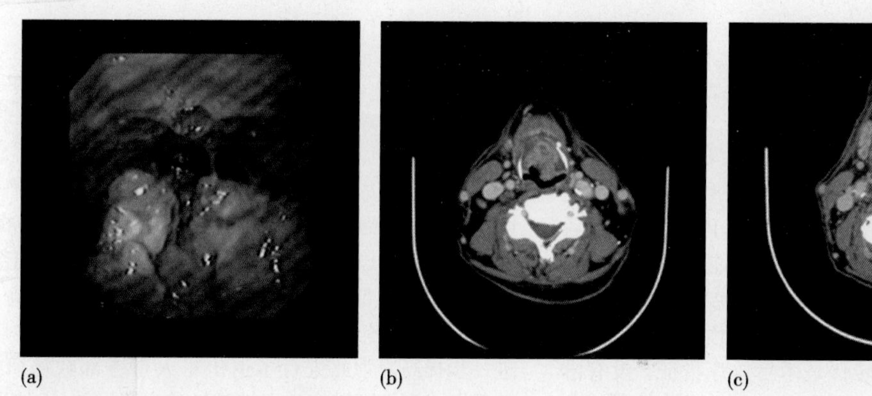

图 83-10　（a）声门上 T3N0 鳞癌。明显破坏会厌。（b）CT 扫描可见会厌前区侵犯，同步化放疗前。（c）治疗后显像，显示原发病灶完全缓解

虽然全喉切除术造成器官功能损失，但术后的功能康复治疗已能达到不错的效果。气管食管穿刺术（TEP）以及相应的康复练习显著改善了喉切除患者术后的功能。人工喉发音能在手术后两周内实现。对于挽救性手术而言，为了术后充分恢复，进行 TEP 置入要推迟至少 3 个月。置入过早会导致瘘管形成以及伤口愈合不佳。

N2 或 N3 病变，治疗的最后常常仍需要行颈淋巴结清扫术。对于临床评估阴性的颈部行预防性颈清扫，发现 15%~30%的患者有颈部淋巴结转移，因此双侧预防性放疗是必要的。颈部淋巴结转移的治疗失败是声门上型喉癌的主要死因之一。大多数报道中认为单纯放疗对存在 N2 或 N3 淋巴结的声门上喉癌的疗效明显劣于联合治疗。声门上型喉癌的 5 年总生存率为 40%~50%，局部复发约为 10%，区域淋巴结复发为 15%~20%，远处转移的概率为 11%~18%，Ⅳ期患者远处转移率接近 30%。第二原发癌是本病的主要死因之一，占 20%~25%，而并发疾病也导致了大约 20%的患者死亡[209~211]。

声门型喉癌和声门下型喉癌

声门癌的治疗很大程度上取决于是否要保留发音功能。对于病变较小（T1、T2）且声带可活动的患者，单纯放疗即可获得 80%~95%的良好局部控制效果，生存数据则与手术治疗相似[212,213]。虽然放疗也会影响发音质量，但比起手术来说要好得多[214]。根治性放疗后的局部复发常常能通过手术挽救。肿瘤侵犯至前联合或杓状软骨时，单纯放疗的局部复发率很高，这可能与临床分期不足有关。“放疗加随访观察”这样的治疗策略需要进行密切随访以早期发现复发，这样能够进行手术挽救。但相较于声门上型喉癌，声门癌放疗后复发的情况常常发现较晚，此时只能行全喉切除。激光部分喉切除术也可作为声门癌的初治或挽救治疗选择。

因肌肉受侵导致声带固定时属于 T3 病变，单纯放疗的预后较差[215~218]。贯声门癌和范围达声门下者区域性转移的机会很高，经常需要进行全喉切除术（图 83-11）。对部分这样的晚期患者，可选择扩大声门上部分喉切除术或环状软骨上部分喉切除术治疗，能避免永久性气管造口[219]。这些治疗会严重影响发音质量，也可能需要进行永久性气管造口。而且这类手术难度较大，需要有高水平的培训和大量的临床经验。

放疗计划针对患者情况不同因人而异，但也具有一些共性。早期（T1、T2，N0）声门病变治疗范围仅需覆盖喉部的常规区域；对于明确声门下扩散的 T2 肿瘤，治疗范围也包括上段气管。T1 期肿瘤治疗频率为每日一次，总剂量为 6 300~6 600cGy，而 T2 肿瘤治疗更为积极，采用每日两次或同步加量治疗[220]。T2 期肿瘤如有明显声门上扩散或向前侵犯可疑突破甲状软骨时，治疗失败的风险增加，可考虑同时进行放化疗。最近的热点是使用调强放疗来减少对邻近颈动脉血管的照射剂量，对于非常早期的病变，也有报道通过单侧声带照射[221]以进一步减少照射范围。T3 声门癌的治疗传统上主要有全喉切除或全喉切除加术后放疗。较早的研究发现单纯放射治疗非选择的 T3 和 T4 患者控制率（20%~35%）、生存率（10%~50%）均不理想。如今，针对 T3 患者，放疗联合含铂方案化疗

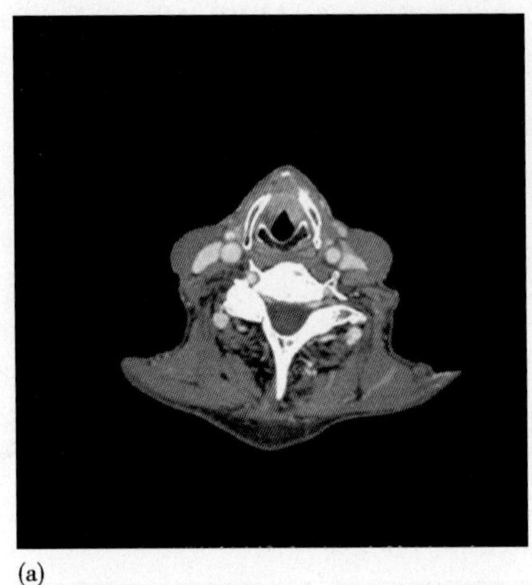
(a)

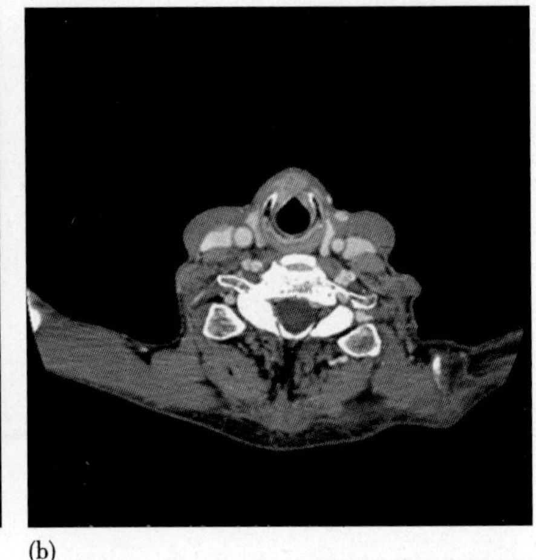
(b)

图 83-11 小体积喉鳞癌伴有声门(a)和声门下(b)累及。由于广泛的软骨侵犯,蔓延入颈部软组织,病灶分期为 T4

的控制率可达 70%~80%[222,223]。没有区域性转移的患者,其单纯手术的局部肿瘤控制就很高,再联合放疗并未发现能够显著提高局控率。但对于有区域性转移的患者,单纯手术的预后不佳,颈部复发是主要的问题,术后辅助放疗能够提高区域性肿瘤控制率[224]。隐匿性区域淋巴结转移在晚期声门癌(T3、T4)患者中接近 30%,在原发灶手术时应进行预防性颈清扫或择区清扫以明确分期。淋巴结转移是术后放疗指征。没有淋巴结转移的患者单纯手术的治愈率在 50%~80%[216,225~228],若存在转移则不到 40%[216,229,230]。

由于 T3 期和 T4 期肿瘤更容易出现淋巴结转移,所以放疗野应包括颈部Ⅱ~Ⅳ区。对术后患者而言,放射野包括肿瘤床和引流淋巴组织,包括上段气管旁淋巴结。气管造口应包括在放射野内,特别在侵犯声门下或淋巴结转移(尤其是包膜外侵犯)或在肿瘤治疗之前先做急诊气管切开的情况下。

同时累及声门及声门上区的喉癌(跨声门)是要特别对待的。这类肿瘤常常分期较晚并伴有较高的区域淋巴结转移率(30%~50%)[231,232]。单纯放疗很难解决这种情况,应该考虑联合化疗进行治疗。

声门上型喉癌发生远处转移的机会大约是声门癌的 4 倍[233]。随着联合治疗在声门癌中的应用,远处转移的发生率有所上升,有报道大约 20%的晚期患者可出现。远处转移发生率可能与淋巴结转移程度直接相关,有报道在 N2 或 N3 患者中远处转移率可高达 40%~50%[234]。

声门下型喉癌很罕见,但其气管旁转移、局部复发和致死率很高。除了早期表浅型病变都应首选手术治疗[235,236]。原发于声门下或侵犯到声门下的喉癌可扩散至上段气管旁淋巴结以及侧颈部淋巴结。因此,这种情况下放疗范围必须包括上纵隔[237]。

原位癌(CIS)

声带原位癌的治疗有一些特殊。通常是进行声带剥脱术,但如果进行充分的连续切片检查,还是能够发现浸润病变。声门的弥漫性原位癌建议进行放疗,因为其转化为恶性的风险很高且手术很难清除。局限于声带游离缘非常表浅的肿瘤或原位癌可用常规手术或激光有效的切除,对发音的影响很小[238]。范围更广的病变则需要进行声带切除术,垂直半喉切除术或环状软骨上喉切除术。

非手术治疗

各期喉癌的治疗中,化疗越来越受到重视。随机研究已证明局部晚期头颈部鳞癌患者进行同步化放疗能够提高局控率和生存期。早已发现诱导化疗方案有效率较高,局部晚期头颈鳞癌患者中部分缓解和完全缓解的比例高达 80%~90%[239~241]。有人假设初始化疗有效者,手术或放疗的效果将进一步提高。为此进行了退伍军人事务部喉癌研究[155],332 例Ⅲ期或Ⅳ期喉鳞癌患者被随机分为两组,一组接受顺铂加氟尿嘧啶诱导化疗后序贯以放疗,一组进行手术加术后放疗。化疗无效,局部肿瘤残留或复发者进行挽救性全喉切除术。两组的两年生存率均为 68%,试验组中 41%的患者两年时存活且具有喉功能。可见,化疗联合后续放疗(可加挽救性手术)的有效性与手术加放疗相似,以治愈为目标的非手术治疗有效且能够达到保存器官的目的。Lefebvre 等[179]后来报道了一项在欧洲进行的临床研究,其中入选了下咽癌患者,研究发现诱导化疗序贯以放疗可能是有效的。

在那些退伍军人事务部的研究,还观察了肿瘤复发的模式,在化疗组中 20%的患者出现局部复发,而手术组为 7%。远处转移的发生率则在手术组较高,为 17%,化放疗组为 11%。分析需要挽救手术的发生情况,发现声门癌比声门上型喉癌更多(43%:31%),声带固定的比声带活动的更多(41%:29%),侵犯甲状软骨者比未侵犯的更多(41%:35%)。挽救手术在 T4 病变患者发生率为 56%,而在其他较小原发病变患者为 29%($P=0.001$)。

退伍军人事务部的喉癌研究还对中间分期的喉癌的化疗和放疗进行了进一步的研究,这些临床研究证实,对于中间分期的喉鳞癌来说,综合治疗能达到根治肿瘤和保存喉功能的目的。同样我们要认识到,该项多中心研究并未纳入局部晚期的喉癌患者,这类患者的治疗应考虑全喉切除以控制原发肿瘤和保留吞咽功能。

鼻咽

简介和分期

在美国,鼻咽癌占所有头颈部鳞癌的 2%。其具有特殊的流行病学及自然病史特点,其中包括早期就出现区域性和远处播散的趋势。鼻咽癌对放疗和细胞毒药物化疗很敏感。

鼻咽部前界是鼻腔的后鼻孔,上界是斜坡,下界为软腭,其后壁是覆盖于咽上部括约肌和 C1、C2 椎体的黏膜,其外侧壁包含有咽鼓管开口。这个区域的淋巴引流丰富,引流至咽后和颈深淋巴结。

鼻咽的恶性肿瘤主要为上皮来源,角蛋白的表达意味着预后更差。其组织病理分类根据 WHO 标准分为三型:1 型,分化型鳞状细胞癌(有着不同分级);2 型,非角化癌;3 型,未分化淋巴上皮癌。混合型也比较常见。

大约 1/3 的患者仅表现为颈部肿物,70%~75%的患者发病时存在颈部淋巴结肿大。其他常见的症状有鼻出血、鼻塞、头痛、听力下降(多为单侧)。肿瘤会向外侧和上方侵犯而破坏颅底骨质。脑神经症状很常见,尤其是第 6 对脑神经最常受侵。与鼻咽癌相关的脑神经综合征主要有两种:①腮腺后综合征,受侵脑神经为Ⅸ、Ⅹ、Ⅺ、Ⅻ;②岩蝶交叉综合征,受侵脑神经为Ⅲ、Ⅳ、Ⅴ、Ⅵ(有时肿瘤经破裂孔侵犯中颅底时可累及脑神经Ⅱ)。鼻咽部病变的评估要进行内镜下直视观察,MRI 对于评价颅底受侵情况和发现隐匿性淋巴结转移十分重要。

最新修订的 AJCC/UICC 分期系统也指出了鼻咽癌在头颈部肿瘤中的特殊性。

治疗

早期和局部晚期的鼻咽癌标准治疗分别为放疗和同步放化疗。即使对于早期病变,手术治疗都十分困难,因为其解剖结构特殊,还常常伴有双侧颈部及咽后的淋巴结转移。手术的作用仅限于:获取组织以确诊,根治性放疗后残存淋巴结切除,罕见的非 WHO 组织病理类型病变的手术治疗,比如腺样囊性癌[242]。放疗前要进行牙科检查,因为放疗会照射双侧腮腺而导致口干症,这会诱发严重的口腔问题。

近年来,IMRT 技术被用于鼻咽癌放疗以期提高疗效。考虑到治疗位置附近有一些重要的血管、神经以及软组织,使用该技术的目的之一就是功能保护。

颈部淋巴结转移的程度与随后远处转移的发生有明确的相关性,双侧淋巴结转移者 5 年内有约 80%的可能发生远处转移。远处转移常常发生于肺、骨和肝脏。在部分患者中,原发灶治疗失败可由外照射联合腔内植入物来补救治疗[243,244]。残留病灶者的 5 年局部控制率(87.2%)比起首次复发者(62.7%)或二次复发者(23.4%,$P=0.0004$)都高,而 5 年生存率则分别为 79.1%、53.6%和 42.9%。

目前,系统性化疗的有效性和安全性评估的相关研究都是把鼻咽癌作为一个独立病种进行的,根据 WHO 分类分配患者队列。将鼻咽癌和其他头颈部鳞癌同时纳入临床研究会导致研究结论难以评判,一部分原因是鼻咽癌对化疗和放疗都很敏感,还因为鼻咽癌有其独特的人口学特征和肿瘤复发模式。

顺铂、卡铂、氟尿嘧啶、博来霉素、甲氨蝶呤、蒽环类抗生素、长春碱类和紫杉类药物的单药有效性已经有很多Ⅱ期临床研究数据[245,246]。有效率在 20%~60%。在最近的报道中,以顺铂为基础的联合方案有效率 50%~80%,完全缓解率为 20%~25%[247~250]。此外,Fandi 等[251]还报道了经多年随访的一组患者获得了长期病情缓解。Chan 等[252]最近报道既往有多程治疗史的鼻咽癌患者,使用西妥昔单抗(一种针对 EGFR 的单克隆抗体)联合卡铂有时也有效(总的疾病控制率为 60%)。

对于诊断时即为Ⅲ期和Ⅳ期的患者,同步放化疗是标准的治疗方式。在美国,一项合作研究(IG0099)以单纯放疗作为对照,试验组先进行放疗并在第 1、22、43 天同步进行顺铂化疗,放疗后再行 3 周期顺铂加氟尿嘧啶联合化疗[253]。研究入选Ⅲ期和Ⅳ期鼻咽癌患者,共 147 例患者可进行评价,其中约 1/3 为 WHO 1 型,这与太平洋周边地区大多报道的超过 95%为 WHO 2/3 型不同。在试验组,3 年无病生存率(69% vs 24%,$P=0.001$)和 3 年总生存率(76% vs 46%,$P=0.005$)均得到提高,远处转移发生率降低(13% vs 35%,$P=0.002$)。这项研究确立了美国鼻咽癌的标准治疗模式。这些数据也在另一项Ⅲ期随机研究中得到确认,这项针对局部晚期鼻咽癌(WHO 分期 N2 和 N3 病变,或淋巴结≥4cm 的 N1 病变)的研究纳入 350 例患者,比较了与顺铂同步(每周 40mg/m^2)的放疗和单纯放疗这两种方式[254]。该研究发现同步放化疗延长了无病生存。疗效与肿瘤分期存在明显的协变量相互作用,在亚组分析中发现,分期为 T3 的患者接受同步放化疗能显著获益($P=0.0075$),首次远处转移的发生时间也显著晚于单纯放疗组($P=0.016$)。其后续报道[255]结论是同步放化疗在 T3/T4 患者中的总生存获益比较明显($P=0.013$)。Lin 等进行了另一项前瞻性随机的Ⅲ期临床研究,单纯放疗为对照,放疗联合 2 周期顺铂加氟尿嘧啶(分别在第 1 周和第 5 周)为试验组,总生存仍然是在联合治疗组有优势(表 83-4)。

表 83-4　局部晚期鼻咽癌经选择的同步化放疗试验

研究	n	治疗组	结果
Al-Sarraf 等[253]	78 69	cddp 100mg/m^2,第 1、4、7 周-RT+辅助性 cddp/fu RT	CM 组 5 年 PFS 58%,OS 67% RT 组 29%和 37% ($P<0.001$)
Lin 等[256]	141 143	cddp 20mg/(m^2·d)+fu 400mg/(m^2·d)96h 输注,第 1、5 周-RT RT	CM 组 5 年 PFS 72%,OS 72% RT 组 53%和 54% ($P=0.001+0.002$)
Chan 等[254,255]	174 176	cddp 40mg/m^2,每周一次-RT RT	CM 组 5 年 PF S60%,OS 70% RT 组 52%和 59% ($P=0.06+0.05$)
Hui 等[257]	34 31	doc 75mg/m^2+cddp 75mg/m^2×2→CRT CRT	3 年 PFS 88%,OS 94% 对照组 60%($P=0.12$)和 68% ($P=0.01$)

cddp,顺铂;CM,联合治疗;doc,多西他赛;fu,氟尿嘧啶;OS,总生存;PFS,无进展生存;RT,放疗。

由于鼻咽癌全身播散的风险很高，先进行诱导化疗的治疗策略更有吸引力。然而这一方式是否真正具有生存优势还不明确。Chua 等[258]分析了两项大型Ⅲ期研究的数据来研究鼻咽癌中诱导化疗的作用。在这些研究中，总共 784 例患者随机分为接受 2～3 周期顺铂为基础的联合化疗之后再放疗或进行单纯放疗。5 年无复发生存率分别为 50.9%和 42.7%（$P=0.014$），疾病特异生存率分别为 63.5%和 58.1%（$P=0.029$）。而总生存则在两组间无显著性差异（$P=0.092$）。Hui 等[257]最近报道了一项Ⅱ期临床研究，选用多西他赛加顺铂作为诱导化疗方案进行化放疗，其无进展生存和总生存数据较理想。目前验证诱导化疗价值的Ⅲ期临床试验正在进行中。NRG-HN001 是一项正在进行的Ⅱ/Ⅲ期临床研究，旨在探索血浆 EBV DNA 作为同步放化疗疗效标志物的价值。该实验将检测不到 DNA 的患者随机分配到对照组或辅助化疗组，将放化疗后可检测到 DNA 的患者单独设组接受额外治疗，观察由紫杉醇和吉西他滨/顺铂和氟尿嘧啶组成的用药方案。

鼻窦和鼻旁窦

鼻和鼻旁窦有一系列独特的问题与其他部位的鳞癌不同。鼻旁窦肿瘤最常见的三种病理类型为鳞癌、腺癌和腺样囊性癌，另外还有不少病理类型也很普遍，如鼻窦未分化癌（SNUC）、神经内分泌癌和嗅神经母细胞瘤。

鼻窦和鼻旁窦癌相对少见，它们占比在 UADT 来源的肿瘤中只有大约 3%，最常发生于 50～60 岁[259]。鼻窦和鼻旁窦肿瘤没有明显症状而且常常同时存在于鼻腔和窦室中。较早出现的症状有鼻气道阻塞、鼻溢液、鼻窦炎、鼻出血，有时还有牙科症状如牙齿疼痛、麻木和松动。较晚出现的症状有脑神经症状、眼球突出、面部疼痛肿胀、溃疡穿透上腭和牙关紧闭症，这些都是不良的征象（图 83-12）。

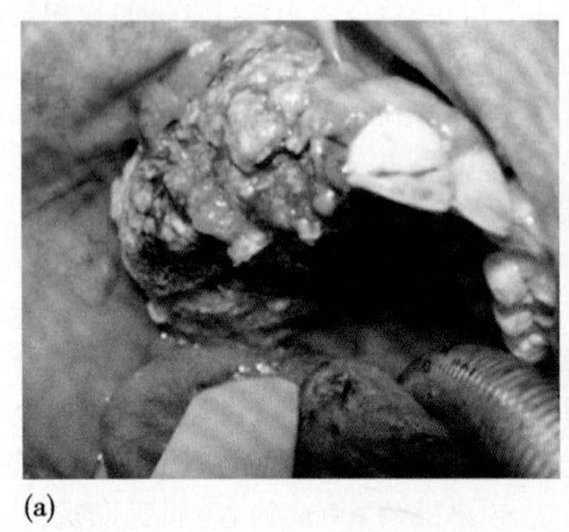
(a)

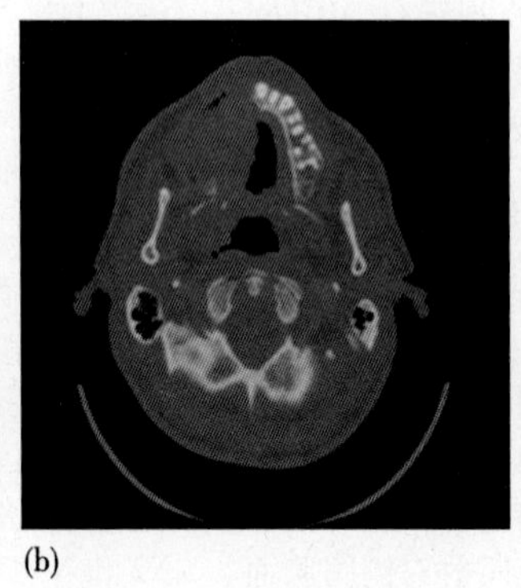
(b)

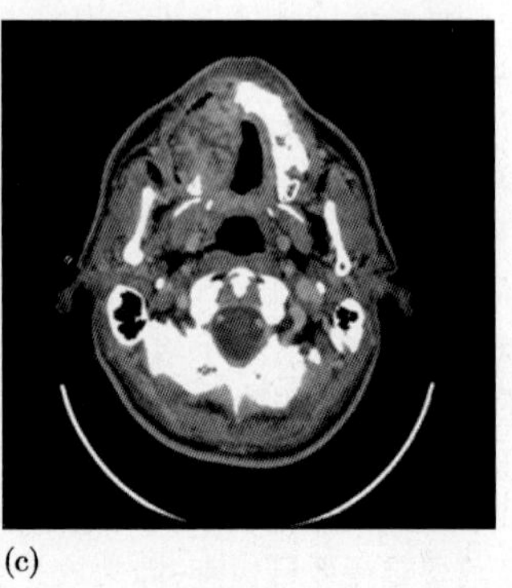
(c)

图 83-12 （a）上颌窦 T4 期鳞癌，蔓延入口腔。（b）CT 扫描骨窗发现上颌窦完全被肿瘤组织替代，翼状板破坏。（c）软组织窗发现肿瘤侵犯面中部的骨外组织

鼻气道阻塞和鼻腔肿物的患者要高度怀疑为鼻窦和鼻旁窦癌。确诊的关键是对整个鼻腔进行彻底的内镜或纤维鼻镜检查，以除外良性的鼻息肉或不复杂的急慢性鼻窦炎，当发现肿物时应进行活检。活检时要注意病变可能出血，尤其是神经内分泌癌和嗅母细胞瘤本身就容易导致鼻出血。如果在手术室给患者进行内镜检查和活检，必须进行冷冻切片检查。必须注意要尽量减少未受侵结构的暴露，活检操作时不能同时进行 Caldwell Luc 手术、鼻中隔成形术或进入到未受侵窦腔。影像学检查对于诊断、分期和制订手术计划都很重要。CT 和 MRI 能提供大量有价值的信息，这在病变侵及颅底时尤为重要。

因为这类恶性肿瘤很少为早期，所以常用的分期系统在临床实践中很少用到。Ohngren 线是值得关注的分期方式，它是从内眦至下颌角的连线，并穿过眶下孔。在该线“之下”或“之前”的肿瘤预后较好，Ohngren 线“之上”或“之后”的肿瘤，预后不佳。

治疗

鼻窦肿瘤的治疗方式多种多样，主要取决于组织学类型。手术切除加术后放疗通常被推荐用于许多此类肿瘤。对某些组织类型的不太大的肿瘤，传统治疗方式效果较好，但对于晚期肿瘤，特别是侵及了眼眶、颅底和面部软组织的肿瘤疗效较差。针对晚期患者进行诱导化疗的模式正在研究中，患者将根据诱导化疗的疗效分为同步化放疗组和手术加术后放疗组进行治疗。（临床试验注册号 NCT00707473）[260]。

鼻旁窦癌手术治疗的详细讨论不在本章的范围内，但我们可以谈谈关于手术最重点的是什么。在这里的手术术式包括：①揭面手术；②面中部掀翻入路/唇下入路；③内镜手术。手术切除方式包括：①内侧上颌骨切除术；②下部上颌骨切除术；③上颌骨全切除术伴或不伴眶内容物摘除；④颅颌面切除术。这些术式和切除方式的应用是个体化的，要根据肿瘤部位、范围、组织学类型、是否美观以及患者的偏好来决定。

内镜入路在鼻旁窦癌中的应用日益广泛。这一方法采用成角镜管时可提供很好的视野，采用高速钻头能够移除骨质，采用切吸器可以去除软组织，也可以使用术中手术导航作为补充。然而，这一方法对技术熟练程度、内镜技术的经验和必要时转做开放性手术的能力都提出了很高的要求。这一方法的部分局限性包括：不能修复大的缺损、不能达到眼眶，并且双手操作时需要有经验的外科助手。

放疗在鼻窦恶性疾病的处理中占主要地位。放疗在术前和术后都可使用，并且在经选择的病例中作为小的 T1 和 T2 病灶的根治性治疗，尤其是那些局限于鼻前庭和前鼻腔的病变[261]。在此情况下，应保证高局部控制率和好的美容效果。随着放疗越来越多地与手术联合使用，局部控制率已经取得了持续改善。手术联合术后放疗仍然是晚期鼻窦腔肿瘤的标准治疗。如上所述，同步化放疗能用于经选择的患者。对于不可

手术肿瘤的患者或被认为不适合手术的患者，采用单纯放疗进行局部控制或姑息治疗可能是最好的选择。

鼻旁窦和颅底放射治疗相关后遗症比较常见。急性并发症包括皮肤脱屑、鼻腔干燥、黏膜炎、干眼症和瘘管形成。慢性副作用包括鼻腔干燥、干眼症、视力损害、萎缩性鼻炎、放射性骨坏死和垂体功能异常。眼干程度不等，从轻微干燥，到角膜溃疡甚至失明。由于眼肌麻痹致人衰弱，甚至必须采取眼球摘除术。尽管视网膜像多数神经结构一样对放疗不敏感，但由于晶状体损伤和/或支持视网膜和视神经的微血管损伤，可能发生视力损害。额叶坏死是毁灭性的并发症，可能需要神经外科干预。

尽管化疗是同步化放疗的组成部分，这在一个单独的章节中将更详细涉及，化疗的一些方面应得到特别关注，并将在此简要提及。在保全眼眶方面，对部分眼部受累的患者使用诱导化疗有一定潜力[262]。Choi 和同事报告了同步化放疗的结果，Chicago 大学的研究者采用顺铂和输注氟尿嘧啶诱导化疗改善了局部控制并保全了眼球[262,263]。不同中心正进行研究以验证诱导化疗对晚期鼻窦恶性肿瘤的作用。一些研究者已使用动脉内化疗继以手术和/或放射治疗晚期鼻窦恶性肿瘤[264~266]。尽管这些研究已经显示出局部控制的益处，动脉内治疗的死亡率似乎不支持其合理性。对不可切除的颅底肿瘤患者，同步化放疗是合理的手段，局部控制率可高达 50%[262]。SNUC、神经内分泌癌和嗅神经母细胞瘤都由神经内分泌细胞分化而来，组织学上鉴别困难。准确诊断这些病变经常需要免疫组织化学，这些疾病也可能与鼻窦黑色素瘤、横纹肌肉瘤、PNET 或淋巴瘤混淆。在决定治疗计划前应请有经验的头颈病理学家会诊。

SNUC 是罕见但致死性的肿瘤，通常见于老年患者，表现为晚期肿瘤。传统治疗是手术继以术后放疗，但长期控制差。这些肿瘤可能对化疗敏感，诱导化疗有反应者可以采用同步化放疗作为根治性治疗[267~269]。挽救性手术普遍预后差，也考虑到传统手术加术后放疗的局部区域控制差，多数专家认为有理由进行同步化放疗的研究。

嗅神经母细胞瘤是鼻腔的罕见肿瘤，来源于筛状板的嗅神经丝。在病程中早期侵入前颅窝，最终累及脑实质(图 83-13)。患者经常表现为鼻塞和鼻出血。治疗围绕着手术切除和术后放疗进行，这些治疗手段能达到有效的局部区域控制和总生存[270]。化疗保留给广泛颅内或眶内病变并且若不化疗则需要广泛切除的患者使用。在诱导治疗时，化疗可以作为细胞减灭手段，使完全手术切除成为可能[271]。

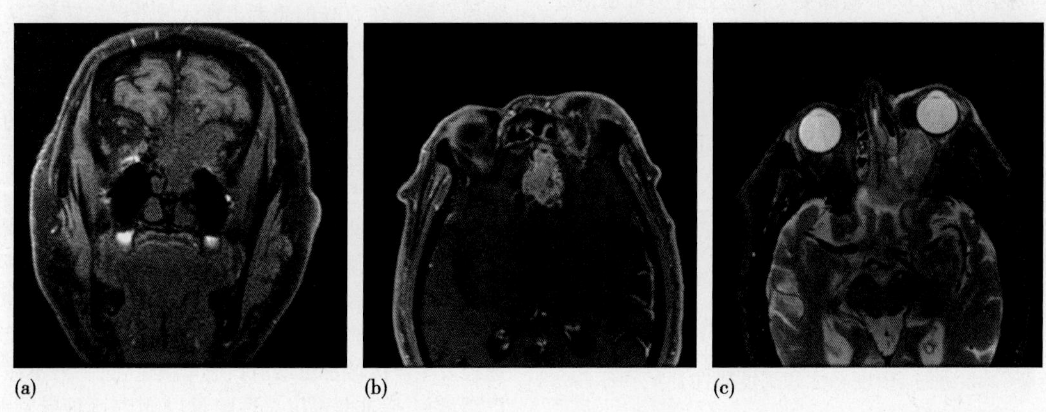

图 83-13　(a)嗅母细胞瘤累及颅底中部，伴颅内侵犯。(b)MRI 示左前叶受侵。(c)左眶尖侵犯

唾液腺

解剖学

唾液腺组织广泛分布于上消化道的黏膜下层各处，分为 3 组大唾液腺：腮腺、下颌下腺和舌下腺。最常发生小唾液腺癌的部位是腭部、舌底和颊黏膜[272]。

大多数唾液腺肿瘤发生于腮腺，尽管近 80%的腮腺肿瘤为良性，但大多数唾液腺恶性肿瘤来源于腮腺。下颌下腺、舌下腺或小唾液腺的肿瘤更可能是恶性的。

最大的唾液腺为腮腺，位于外耳道和耳郭前方的颊部。此腺体围绕下颌骨分布，当面神经穿过腮腺时，将其分为浅叶(或外侧叶)和深叶。约 80%的腺体位于面神经的外侧，而 20%位于此神经的深面，下颌骨的后面和内侧。颈内动脉、颈内静脉、颈交感神经链和第Ⅸ、Ⅹ和Ⅺ对脑神经紧邻腮腺的深叶。腮腺的淋巴引流为腮腺内淋巴结、颈外淋巴结和颈上淋巴结(第Ⅱ和第Ⅲ区)。其余的淋巴引流为邻近区，包括颈后三角或第Ⅴ区。腮腺中存在神经，尤其是面神经和三叉神经的耳颞支，可能被肿瘤侵及，尤其是腺样囊性癌和鳞癌。任何腮腺的肿瘤都必须进行评价，并且手术切除经常是唯一的解决方法，因为即使是良性肿瘤也会导致面部不对称，也可能影响面神经。而且，良性病灶可能随时间推移转化为高度恶性肿瘤，正如多形性腺瘤恶变。

第二大唾液腺是下颌下腺，位于二腹肌的两腹和下颌骨组成的三角区内。这一位置的恶性肿瘤可以扩散到Ⅱ、Ⅲ和Ⅳ区的淋巴结，也可沿神经生长，尤其是舌神经分支，偶尔有面神经的下颌支。

舌下腺在大唾液腺中是最小的，由口底黏膜下腺体集合而成，围绕下颌下腺的外分泌管(Warton 管)。

诊断

恶性唾液腺肿瘤的临床表现各有不同，取决于部位和组织学类型。面神经麻痹不常见，但常提示病灶为恶性。腮腺深叶的肿瘤可导致吞咽困难和软腭黏膜下畸形。当咽旁部位发生明显侵犯时，可出现第Ⅸ、Ⅹ、Ⅺ甚至是Ⅻ脑神经的受侵。颌下腺常见的表现为下颌下无痛性肿胀，这类肿瘤需要与更常见的颌下腺细菌性唾液腺炎相鉴别。

体格检查时，不伴皮肤或黏膜浅表溃疡的可触及肿物是最常见的表现。细针穿刺是重要的诊断方法，可通过细胞学明确是否为肿瘤。这一诊断方式，尤其对于腮腺和下颌下腺，接受度已经越来越高，而且只要获取的细胞学信息会对治疗或预后产生影响，就应该考虑穿刺检查。肿瘤的准确分型经常不那么重要，可以推迟至决定性的病理检查。该项检查应该审慎选择，尽管专家报告的准确率已经很高（即敏感性 94%，特异性 97%，准确性 95%）[273]。

组织学

良性病变是腮腺最常见的肿瘤。多年来，唾液腺恶性肿瘤的分类被多次审议并扩展到包括一些更少见的恶性肿瘤，最常援引的是现今的 WHO 分类（表 83-5）[274]。黏液表皮样癌是腮腺是常见的癌症，分为高度恶性、中度恶性和低度恶性肿瘤（图 83-14）[275,276]。分化良好，低度恶性黏液表皮样癌的特点是生长率慢，完全手术切除后复发率低（约 15%），罕见转移。高度恶性肿瘤侵袭性更强，单纯手术后局部复发率达 60%[277]。局部复发和远处转移可以在治疗后许多年发生。约 50% 的高度恶性黏液表皮样癌患者表现为区域性转移，30% 出现远处转移[275,278]。腺泡细胞癌通常分化良好，在腮腺癌中约占 13%。淋巴结转移的发生率为 15%。局部复发和远处转移可在治疗完成多年后发生[279]。腺样囊性癌占腮腺恶性肿瘤的约 10%，而占颌下腺或小唾液腺恶性肿瘤的 60%[272,280]。已确定了 3 种与生物学行为相关的亚型：筛状型、管样型和实质型（侵袭性最强）。这一肿瘤显著的特征是其侵袭主要神经和沿神经内膜和神经外膜蔓延的倾向。这对预后具有重要意义，会影响治疗方案的确定，特别是考虑是否需要术后放疗。尽管这些肿瘤发展倾向惰性，但多达 40% 的患者最终发展为区域或远处转移[280]。

表 83-5　唾液腺最常见的恶性肿瘤

唾液腺最常见的恶性肿瘤
黏液表皮样癌（低度恶性、中度恶性和高度恶性）
腺泡细胞癌
腺样囊性癌
腺癌
恶性多形性腺瘤（多形性腺瘤恶变）
鳞状细胞癌

腺癌在小唾液腺中更为常见，且大多数为高度恶性肿瘤。约 36% 的患者表现为或随后出现区域淋巴结转移；因此，在高度恶性腺癌的治疗策略中，应将区域淋巴结包括在内[281]。肺和骨是远处转移的常见部位。

多形性腺瘤恶变由良性多形性腺瘤发展而来。恶变的风险随时间和患者年龄而增高。持续时间小于 5 年的腺瘤中 1.6% 去分化，而出现 15 年以上的腺瘤中 9.4% 去分化[282]。真正的恶性混合肿瘤非常罕见，在所有恶性唾液腺肿瘤中仅占 2%～5%。这些是典型的侵袭性肿瘤。一种值得一提的组织学类型是唾液导管癌，在显微镜下类似乳腺癌。唾液腺的原发性鳞癌罕见，在腮腺肿瘤中不足 3%。这一病灶必须与由皮肤癌或其他部位肿瘤转移至腮腺淋巴结的转移性鳞癌相鉴别。腮

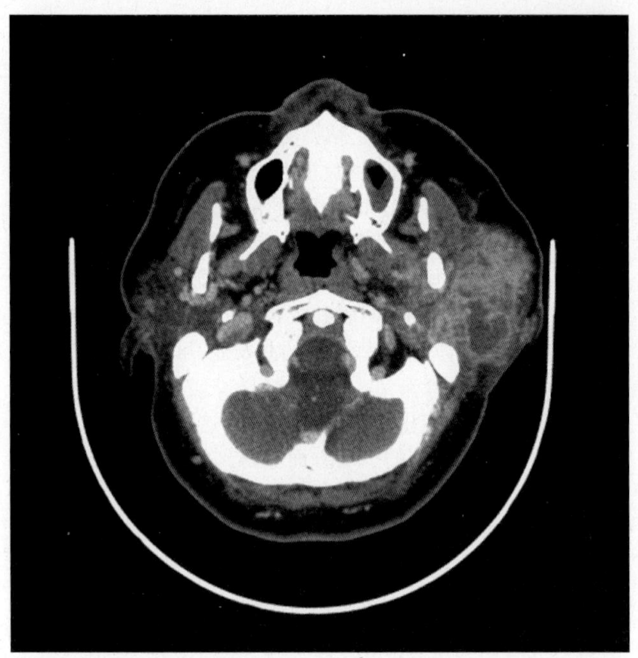

图 83-14　左侧腮腺的黏液表皮样癌

腺原发鳞癌在 50% 的患者出现区域淋巴结转移，这是患者接受手术和术后放疗时必须考虑的临床特征。

治疗

关于唾液腺肿瘤的分期系统，AJCC 和 UICC 的专著受到广泛认可[114]。良性和恶性唾液腺肿瘤的治疗都是手术。早期（T1 或 T2）尤其是低度恶性肿瘤应进行完整切除，并确保切缘阴性。腮腺的此类肿瘤通常使用保留面神经的腮腺切除术。任何组织学类型的早期高度恶性肿瘤都应手术切除原发部位，并努力实现切缘阴性。但这经常是不可能的，微扩散，尤其是腺样囊性癌的微扩散，可能沿组织平面、黏膜下区域和神经旁途径发生。区域淋巴结清扫应审慎进行；一般不做预防性颈淋巴结清扫，除非是高度恶性肿瘤，尤其是唾液导管癌、黏液表皮样癌和鳞癌[283]。唾液腺恶性肿瘤曾被认为对传统光子照射不敏感，但多年来的研究已证实术后照射对根除亚临床病灶是有效的[280,284,285]。

存在以下任一情况的大唾液腺或小唾液腺癌都需要术后放疗：①肿瘤为高度恶性或为转移性鳞癌，无论手术切缘如何；②手术切缘近或显微镜下阳性；③已经对复发性癌进行了切除，无论组织学类型或切缘状态如何；④肿瘤已侵犯至腺体包膜外，进入皮肤、骨、神经或腺组织；⑤区域淋巴结转移；⑥肿瘤有大体残留或未切除病灶。此外，计划性的术前放疗有利于晚期病例的手术切除，并有助于保留面神经功能[284,286]。如果面神经在就诊时已受侵，则倾向于手术加术后放疗。

对于 T3 和 T4 腮腺癌，除非面神经被肿瘤环绕包围或由于肿瘤明显增大，可以使用保全神经的手术，继以放疗。原发部位和受累结构的放疗剂量为 55～65Gy 不等。一般而言，对于低度恶性的黏液表皮样癌和腺泡细胞癌，颈部无临床转移时不需要治疗。对于所有其他高度恶性组织学类型，颈淋巴引流区通常用 50Gy 的剂量治疗。对于腺样囊性癌，放疗野应包括指定的神经干至颅底的解剖学范围[280]。面神经的处理是腮腺癌治疗中有争议和更为复杂的问题。切除此神经会导致严重的

面容改变和功能缺陷。即使切除一个分支，尤其是额支，也会导致明显的功能异常。因此，关于神经的术中处理，必须在术前与患者进行广泛的讨论。术前的功能受损预示功能转归差，即使是进行神经移植。当术中发现功能正常的面神经受到肿瘤侵犯并且不能保留时，应进行手术切除和一期神经移植。可以对移植神经进行术后放疗，尽管长期功能恢复仍不理想。

治疗的结果取决于组织学类型和肿瘤部位这两个方面。在得克萨斯州立大学 MD Anderson 癌症中心的一组研究序列中，腺泡细胞癌患者的 5 年生存率为 100%，腺样囊性癌者为 95%，低度恶性黏液表皮样癌者为 90%，高度恶性黏液表皮样癌者为 80%，腺癌者为 70%，恶性混合肿瘤者为 59%[281,284]。在 Princess Margaret 医院，单纯手术对原发腮腺疾病的控制率为 24%，手术和放疗的控制率为 74%[287]。

小唾液腺肿瘤，尤其是鼻旁窦肿瘤，经常表现为晚期疾病。在 MD Anderson 中心统计的患者中，单纯手术治疗的患者中 2 年局部控制率为 47%，手术和术后放疗的患者中为 76%[284,288,289]。

对于唾液腺肿瘤巨大不可切除或完全切除术后局部复发风险高的患者，快中子放疗是标准放疗外的另一选择。快中子具有不同于标准照射的放射生物学特性，Batterman 等[290]开展的体内研究是关于肺转移对分割放疗的反应，数据显示唾液腺肿瘤的相对生物效应（RBE）因子在 8.0 范围内，而大多数正常组织的后效应 RBE 在 3.0~3.5 范围内。基于这一结论，如果给予腮腺肿瘤 20 中子 Gy 的剂量，黏膜和颞颌关节的生物效应将等同于 60~70 光子 Gy，但对肿瘤的生物效应将等同于 160 光子 Gy——理论治疗增益因子为 2.3~2.6。

美国的放射治疗肿瘤学协作组（RTOG）和英国的医学研究理事会（MRC）进行了一项 3 期随机临床研究，比较快中子放疗和传统光子照射治疗不可手术的唾液腺肿瘤。快中子组的原发部位和区域淋巴结的肿瘤清除都得到显著改善。在 2 年终点指标上，中子组的局部/区域控制率为 67%，而光子组为 17%（$P<0.005$），中子组的生存率为 62%，而光子组为 25%（$P=0.1$）。由于快中子组的局部区域控制率显著更高，研究由于伦理学原因早期关闭。10 年的数据继续显示中子组的局部区域控制改善（56% vs 17%，$P=0.009$），但由于远处转移造成的死亡，总生存率无差异[291]。

由于中子疗法仅在极少数中心可用，并且中子治疗的结果仍有不确定性，而且疗效取决于疾病的部位，因此不具备手术条件的唾液腺癌的其他替代方案也多有研究，尽管目前的报告多为较小的回顾性研究。Samant 等人[292]报道了无法手术切除的腺样囊性癌患者接受同步化放疗后，取得了较好的疗效。麻省总医院[293]的一个研究小组描述了侵及颅底的腺样囊性癌患者，接受质子治疗后获得了令人鼓舞的结果。为了研究高能粒子的治疗作用，德国研究人员进行了一项结合 IMRT 和碳离子增强的小型Ⅱ期试验（COSMIC）。目前只获得了非常初步的结果，但在 16 例不可切除的恶性唾液腺肿瘤患者中缓解率为 69%[294]。

系统治疗

唾液腺癌的全身治疗仍旧是探索性的，并无普遍接受的标准方案。对局部晚期和不可手术切除病灶的患者可以联合使用化疗和放疗。对远处转移复发的患者而言，化疗是治疗选择之一。以往的研究已经显示以下单药的抗肿瘤活性：甲氨蝶呤、多柔比星、顺铂、氟尿嘧啶、长春碱类和最近的紫杉醇类。缓解率介于 15%~20%。联合化疗在一定程度上提高了缓解率，但并无明确的生存优势。在采用环磷酰胺、多柔比星和顺铂的方案（CAP）的患者中，缓解率为 40%~50%，缓解持续时间为 4~6 个月[295]。顺铂和长春瑞滨联用的方案缓解率为 44%~54%[296,297]。腺癌患者更有可能疾病缓解，腺样囊性癌患者则不易缓解。VEGF 抗体如舒尼替尼和阿西替尼在转移性腺样囊性癌中表现出最低的活性，最多只能稳定疾病[298,299]。

在作出进行全身治疗的决定时，需要关注肿瘤组织学类型，分期，首次治疗后至疾病进展的时间，患者状态评分和疾病进展的速度。分子标志物的研究也是当下努力的方向，有助于提高我们的个体化治疗能力。大多数头颈肿瘤学家倾向于在制订治疗策略时将腺样囊性癌患者与其他患者分开。由于转移性腺样囊性癌的进展通常为惰性的，一般需要一段短时间的观察。有时，在数年内都维持缓慢进展。然而，如果评价结果显示为更具侵袭性的肿瘤，则应该考虑进行临床试验或化疗[295,300~303]。在高度恶性黏液表皮样癌或唾液导管腺癌的患者中，传统的含顺铂联合化疗可能更有效。紫杉类作为单药是有效的，现正在联合化疗方案中接受检验[304]。

大约 70%的唾液腺恶性肿瘤会过表达 EGFR。我们研究组在进行吉非替尼（一个小分子 EGFR 酪氨酸激酶抑制剂）治疗晚期唾液腺癌的临床试验，但没有明显疗效[305]。目前已确定腺样囊性癌中 c-KIT 高水平表达，但甲磺酸伊马替尼（针对 KIT 的酪氨酸激酶抑制剂）的初步试验未显示临床获益[306]。多达 50%的唾液导管腺癌患者中有 HER2 过表达，约 20%会有 HER2 扩增[307]。雄激素受体过度表达可见于 80%的唾液导管腺癌中可见。已有关于曲妥珠单抗（一种针对 HER2 的单克隆抗体）和雄激素阻断剂的疗效报道[308~311]。一项研究激素调控在雄激素受体阳性唾液导管腺癌中的作用的临床试验正在规划中（临床试验编号 NCT01969578）。鉴于唾液腺癌在总体上相对罕见，正规的试验可能需要多个、大型中心的合作，或通过肿瘤协作研究组的机制来实现。

放射治疗

放疗在多数头颈部癌的治疗中起不可或缺的作用。在经选择的早期疾病中作为唯一的治疗模式，其治疗结果与手术切除相似，通常死亡率更低。放射治疗是早期鼻咽癌的治疗选择。它对于早期口咽癌也是一种非常有效的疗法，尽管经口微创手术的出现后，选择手术还是放疗出现了一些争议。放疗（结合外部放射和近距离放射治疗）也是口腔早期癌症的手术替代方案，特别是舌活动部癌，这种治疗选择虽然在美国不常用，但在一些国际中心较常见。起源于咽部的肿瘤，放疗与手术相比更被接受，因为可以保留功能和发声的质量。

对于体积较大的病变，放疗是联合治疗的组成部分。对于计划进行手术的患者，通常使用放疗作为辅助以改善局部区域控制。与手术相结合的放疗时机一直是一个争论的话题，因为术前和术后放疗都有各自的优点和缺点。RTOG 进行了一项比较术前和术后放疗的随机试验，结论是术后放疗可以改善局部区域的疾病控制，并显示生存率有所改善[312]。该研究的结果，加上常用的治疗顺序，使术后放疗成为较好的选择。首先进行手术的一个主要优点是可以评估病理。目前使用的是三分法风险评估系统，将患者分为“低”“中”和“高”风险类别。对于低风险患者，复发并不常见；因此，可能无法保证辅助治疗的益处。高风险患者通常是那些手术切缘不足或侵犯淋巴结被膜外的患者，复发率非常高，因此现阶段的研究重点是评估通过改变放射分次或进行化学增敏来增强辅助放射治疗疗效的方法[313]。

当作为辅助治疗时，重要的是外科医师和放射医师间应进行良好的沟通，以避免因为治疗不及时影响疗效。部分研究组强调应该尽可能压缩整体治疗时间，即从手术到术后放疗的时间，来最大化原位和局部控制效果[314,315]。

对于在某些部位出现的晚期肿瘤，例如咽和喉，可以考虑由联合放疗和化疗的非手术治疗。联合放化疗是晚期鼻咽癌和局部晚期口咽癌的首选治疗方法。值得注意的是，已经证明口咽的 HPV 相关癌症对化疗和放疗非常敏感，接受联合放化疗的患者存活率很高[88]。晚期喉癌和下咽癌的最佳治疗（见上文）仍然是一个争议话题。喉保留的观点仍然是引人关注的；然而，几十年的研究使研究人员更加谨慎，认识到喉保留可能伴随着吞咽困难和误吸风险的增加。此外，一些人质疑喉保留的趋势是否导致癌症的患者的存活率降低[8]。

电离辐射（高能量光子、电子、中子、质子、和其他带电粒子）与其他物质进行微观相互作用，不应被认为只是一种形式的烧灼[316]。肿瘤和正常组织修复电离辐射所致的细胞损伤的能力存在巨大差异。这令我们可以使用诸如化疗和热疗这样的治疗手段来降低肿瘤组织的修复能力，并设计方案来扩大肿瘤控制和正常组织损伤之间治疗窗。头颈鳞癌一般被描述为“中度放射敏感”，意味着必须给予很大量的照射才能达到高的肿瘤控制概率。幸运的是，需要的剂量在头颈部大多数组织的耐受范围内。

特定剂量照射的有效性取决于给予照射的方式[317]。过去的 30 年中，治疗头颈部癌的不同“标准”治疗方案已经发生了演变。在美国，传统的“治愈性”治疗方案包括给予 180~200cGy 每次，每日一次，每周 5 天，总剂量为 6 500~7 400cGy；在英国和加拿大，每日给予一次更高的剂量，为 220~250cGy，每周 5 天，总剂量为 5 000~5 500cGy。这两种方案是根据经验产生的，回顾文献似乎表明它们均实现了较好的肿瘤控制，主要的争议在于并发症的差异。临床研究中已经将各种改变剂量的方案和标准方案进行比较，其中一些看起来正演变为新的“标准”。

放射会破坏皮肤和黏膜基底层的干细胞，数周后，更表浅的保护层在正常生理过程中丢失而未被充分更新。这使表皮裸露进而导致黏膜反应，可能会明显抑制患者的吞咽功能。这个过程并不会立即发生，而是在放疗后数周出现进展。使用同步化疗和/或改变分割的治疗方案可使此反应发生更快，更为严重。应密切观察患者，以确保他们在治疗中的充分营养，这通常需要饲管。与停止治疗相比，使用饲管营养更值得推荐，因为前者可因肿瘤细胞再增殖而降低肿瘤控制能力[318~320]。在皮肤治疗野可发生类似的反应，导致严重的晒伤样反应。头颈区域的放射可导致唾液腺功能和味觉的严重改变[321~323]。辐射防护剂和唾液分泌刺激类药物已经被大量研究，但在减轻口干症方面取得的成功有限。在减轻口干症方面更为重要的进展是通过使用最新的保形技术来减少唾液腺接受的辐射[324]。这些变化的严重程度和持续时间取决于剂量。当使用 1 000~1 500cGy 剂量时，出现一过性唾液缺乏和味觉减退，但是低剂量的治疗量不会导致永久性的后果。而使用 7 000cGy 剂量时几乎总会导致永久性改变。Michigan 大学和 Utrecht 大学的研究[325]显示导致腺体损伤的辐射量并没有明显的阈值，但对腮腺而言，其 TD(50)，即有 50%的可能导致并发症的剂量为 40Gy。

无论是唾液量减少还是化学成分的变化都使口腔微生物的分布发生变化，继而显著增高龋齿的风险。对于有牙齿的患者，必须在开始放疗前进行积极的牙科预防，因为相对治疗后对严重照射过的组织进行处理，修复和/或拔牙在治疗前进行可以显著降低放射性骨坏死的发生率[326]。如果必须拔除，在拔牙和开始放疗间有 2~3 周的间期是必要的，以使组织充分愈合。如果在高剂量放疗后需要拔牙或进行其他有创性操作，高压氧治疗对降低放射性骨坏死是有用的，尤其是在下颌骨受累的情况下[327,328]。

技术进步

现代放疗中心使用精密复杂的直线加速器产生不同能量光子束和高压电子线，可以容易地治疗后颈淋巴结而不带来脊髓损伤的风险。计算机控制的多叶光栅有助于定制遮挡技术以保全未受侵的正常组织，使用 CT 和 MRI 来定位肿瘤，许多肿瘤放疗中心有模拟和制订治疗计划的专用复杂扫描机。结合 CT、MRI 和 PET 以提供临床医师对肿瘤播散风险的区域定位的更全面。

强度调整放疗（调强放疗，IMRT）

放射治疗（放疗）的主要目标是向癌症病灶区域提供适当的辐射剂量，同时避免对邻近正常组织的损伤。这个概念被称为适形治疗。IMRT 是在 20 世纪的最后发展起来的，目前是头颈部肿瘤适形治疗的公认标准。该方法使用许多个不同的处理区域，每个区域又被分成多个区段，并且每个区段接受的辐射量都可以预先设置[329]。该技术近期又有了进一步发展，可以将治疗加速器和计算机断层扫描单元相结合，或者结合电弧旋转技术（体积调制电弧治疗），实现动态治疗。

软件系统的创新带来了逆向治疗计划手段，使得 IMRT 系统得到进一步增强。这种计划方式可以实现给予治疗靶区充足的辐射剂量同时，限制正常组织接受的辐射剂量。在头颈部肿瘤中，肿瘤附近通常会有重要的解剖结构，在为靶区提供高剂量辐射的同时限制附近正常组织接受的辐射量可以带来显著的治疗收益。该技术的另一个好处是可以减少腮腺受辐射剂量而降低口干症的可能，这项优势已经被包括随机Ⅲ期 PARSPORT 试验在内的多项临床试验所证实[324]。除此之外，未来的 IMRT 剂量划分策略还会将喉和咽缩肌等对吞咽功能影响较大的解剖结构纳入在内，以改善治疗后的功能恢复[330]。

肿瘤显像改善的优势是显而易见的，“边缘遗漏”应该比以前少了。另一优势是这有助于安全地给予肿瘤更高的放射剂量。在其他条件相同的情况下，更高的放射剂量可能导致更好的肿瘤控制。对于头颈鳞癌，剂量-效应曲线通常有一个陡峭区域，此时较小的放射剂量提升可以显著改善结果[331~333]。以口咽癌为例，Sloan-Kettering 纪念癌症中心的 Setton 和同事报告 IMRT 治疗 442 例原发性口咽癌患者(73%为Ⅳ期)并经中位随访时间 37 个月的结果[334]。推算 3 年无局部进展率、无区域进展率、无远处转移和总生存率分别为 95%、94%、87%和 85%。2 度及以上口干程度的患者占 29%。Garden 和同事报告了我们 MD Anderson 癌症中心在 2000 年至 2007 年使用 IMRT 治疗的 776 例口咽癌患者的初步结果[163]。中位随访期为 54 个月。5 年局部区域控制率、无复发率和总生存率分别为 84%、90%和 82%。其他的研究也证实了上述口咽癌局部区域控制率[160,162,164]。鼻咽癌由于邻近重要神经结构而增加了治疗的复杂性，但该疗法也取得了较好的结果。RTOG 编号 0225 的Ⅱ期试验尝试了将使用 IMRT 治疗鼻咽癌转化为多中心试验的可行性，预期的 2 年无进展生存率大约为 93%[335]。最近一些大型临床试验也报道了类似的较好的疾病控制率，特别是来自中国的试验，在该国鼻咽癌属于地方病[336]。

由于 IMRT 治疗计划和实施的复杂性，严格的质量和技术支持，以及充分的临床经验对于 IMRT 的最终有效性是十分重要的[337]。

手术与放疗联合治疗

放疗常用于局部晚期肿瘤手术切除后的辅助治疗。多数头颈 T3 或 T4 原发肿瘤或颈淋巴结有转移时，给予辅助放疗可改善局部控制。

放疗可以在手术前或手术后进行。术前放疗的目的在于清除手术区域外的镜下病灶，以及缩小瘤体，利于手术切除。理论上，术前放疗也可以降低肿瘤细胞术中播散的风险。通常给予的剂量是 5 000cGy，治疗周期为 5 周至 5.5 周，此剂量不会导致显著的伤口愈合问题。目前术前放疗使用较少。

在术后，手术操作已经破坏了区域血液供应。传统观点认为这需要更高的放疗剂量，因为肿瘤细胞乏氧的可能性增大，这些细胞较氧供充分的肿瘤细胞对放疗抵抗性更强。通常，给予镜下残存病灶 5 500～6 000cGy 总剂量，分次剂量 180～200cGy。若手术切缘阳性或有肉眼残存病灶的风险，则使用更高的剂量。Peters 等[338]的研究已经显示若手术标本中发现淋巴结被膜外侵犯，至少应给予 6 300cGy 剂量。术后放疗的优势在于可以根据病理学结果，只治疗有显著局部区域复发风险的患者。它另外的一项优势是不延误手术，而手术是晚期可切除肿瘤患者的最重要的治疗方式。

尽管通常认为减瘤手术并无太大的作用，但有些情况下，减瘤手术继以高剂量放疗优于单纯放疗。头颈协作组的一项分析(IG0034)显示，被排除入组的手术切缘阳性的患者，与 RTOG 数据库中相匹配的接受单纯放疗患者相比，局部区域肿瘤控制得到改善[339]。随访第 4 年，两者局部区域控制率分别为 44%和 24%(P=0.007)。因为这并非随机研究，作者未主张改变传统的可切除标准，而是提出应在随机临床试验中检验这一概念。

手术后的局部区域复发在手术切缘阳性、淋巴结包膜外侵犯或多个淋巴结阳性的患者中尤为常见。基于回顾性研究[340,341]，辅助放疗可以降低相对约 50%的复发风险。然而，研究患者的局部区域复发率仍高达 35%～60%[342]。两项里程碑多中心Ⅲ期试验显示在术后高复发风险的患者中，使用同步放化疗可以改善预后。在第一项试验中[173]，EORTC 将 334 例受试者随机分配到 66Gy 放疗联合或不联合 3 周期顺铂 100mg/m^{2}化疗组。加入顺铂改善了估算的 3 年局部控制率(85% vs 70%)，无病生存率(60% vs 40%)和总生存率(65% vs 50%)。化疗加重了急性毒性，但远期副作用的严重程度基本相同。RTOG 进行了一项补充性研究[134]，将 459 例患者随机分入与 EORTC 试验几乎相同的两个治疗组：60～66Gy 放疗联合或不联合 3 周期顺铂 100mg/m^2 化疗。化疗改善了估算的 2 年局部控制率(82% vs 72%，P=0.01)和无病生存率(70% vs 60%，P=0.05)。与 EORTC 相同，这一改善的代价是 3 度和 3 度以上急性毒性的发生率更高。这两项研究具有不同的纳入标准、研究人群和随访间隔。然而，此两项研究的合并分析强烈提示对手术切缘阳性或淋巴结包膜外侵犯的患者，给予联合辅助治疗有显著临床获益[173]。

全身治疗

局部晚期疾病的化疗和放疗

诱导化疗

在手术或放疗前使用化疗-称为诱导化疗或新辅助化疗-具有潜在的优势。它具有可行性。此时药物活性可能是最佳的，因为正常血管分布未受到扰乱。在这种情况下，有效的全身治疗可能可以诱导肿瘤缓解，并降低远处复发风险[155,199,343,344]。诱导化疗对手术后放疗后局部疾病控制的潜力仍在研究中。早期的研究显示 PF 是高度有效的方案[345]；对化疗的有效反应预示着肿瘤对放疗敏感；并且似乎对手术和放疗副作用的发生率没有影响[344]。

前文已述，VA 喉癌研究组[155]的研究显示 PF 方案诱导化疗继以放射治疗喉部Ⅲ/Ⅳ期鳞状细胞癌的可行性。患者随机分为两组，一组接受标准治疗，即喉切除术加术后放疗，另一组接受 2～3 周期 PF 方案，继之以放疗。手术仍保留为病程持续或进展的患者的挽救治疗方案。3 年随访后，诱导治疗组中 66%的生存患者保留了有功能的喉。而且，在治疗组间没有总生存的差异。随后的一项研究由 EORTC 在下咽鳞癌患者中进行，比较 PF 方案诱导化疗缓解的继以放疗的患者和喉咽切除术联合放疗的患者[179]。两组之间未观察到生存的差异，而在化疗组中 28%的患者生存并且保留了喉部功能。3 年的喉保全率为 42%。这些研究显示序贯化疗和放疗具有成为有效治疗策略的潜力，并且对许多患者解剖器官保全是合理的治疗目标。

作为 VA 研究的后续[199]，头颈部协作组开展了一项前瞻性 3 组的研究，将序贯 PF 方案和放疗作为对照组，与同步使用顺铂和放疗，以及单纯放疗对比。对肿瘤持续存在或进展的患者施行挽救性手术。入组标准为患Ⅲ/Ⅵ期疾病的患者，但除外 T1 和晚期 T4 患者。结果显示同步治疗组显示出了更好的局部疾病控制率，10 年喉保全率为 82%，序贯化放疗的患者为 68%，单纯放疗的患者为 64%。然而，疾病控制的增加似乎已被同时出现的非癌症相关死亡人数增加所抵消；因此，在同步和顺序治疗组之间没有观察到显著的生存差异[346]。一系列研究集中于在 PF 方案基础上加入紫杉类，以增强抗肿瘤活性。EORTC 在一项前瞻性试验中对 358 例患者开展研究(TAX323)[347]，比较 PF 诱导方案和多西他赛、顺铂和氟尿嘧啶联合方案(TPF)。在 4 周期诱导化疗后，所有患者接受单纯放射治疗。中位随访 32 个月时，TPF 组产生了更佳的肿瘤缓解、PFS(HR=0.72)、生存率增加(HR=0.73)。在 TAX324 的Ⅲ期试验中[348],501 例患者随机接受以下任一诱导方案治疗:多西他赛($75mg/m^2$)、顺铂($100mg/m^2$)和氟尿嘧啶($1\ 000mg/(m^2 \cdot d)×4d$)或标准 PF 方案。3 个周期后,给予同步放化疗(含每周卡铂)。部分患者因淋巴结进展接受了手术。结果表明 DFS 和 OS 有显著差异,在 36 个月时接受 TPF 方案的有 62%的患者生存,对照组有 48%的患者生存。

为了建立更新的包含紫杉类的诱导化疗方案,GORTEC 进行了 TREMPLIN Ⅱ期随机试验,比较同步顺铂与同步西妥昔单抗对 TPF 诱导后部分反应的情况[349]。OS 在两组中未显示出差异,作者得出结论,他们无法确定与诱导化疗加单纯放疗作对照的最佳测试方案。

虽然多西他赛加入 PF 化疗方案改善了 TAX323 和 324 的结果,但三药诱导化疗方案是否优于同步化放疗仍未确定。至少有四项临床试验试图回答这个问题。PARADIGM 研究随机分配 145 例不能切除的Ⅲ期或Ⅳ期头颈鳞癌患者接受 TPF,然后同时给予卡铂(对诱导化疗有反应的患者)或多西他赛(对诱导化疗无反应),与顺铂同步放射治疗($100mg/m^2$,每 3 周×2 剂)。3 年 OS 在两组之间无统计学差异(诱导化疗组为 73%,同步化放疗组为 78%)。在诱导化疗组中观察到较高的血液学毒性和一例与治疗相关的死亡。由于入组缓慢,该研究未达到其目标入组患者数量,限制了其结果解读的权效[350]。DeCIDE 试验纳入了 285 名 N2 或 N3 淋巴结分级的患者(因此,远处转移的复发风险较高)。患者随机分组为接受两个疗程的 TPF,然后序贯 DFHX(多西他赛,氟尿嘧啶和羟基脲)同步化放疗,TPF 同步化放疗组。再次,由于入组缓慢,曾调整入组量,并且提前终止了研究。两组的 3 年 OS 率相似,诱导化疗组为 75%,同步化放疗组为 73%。接受诱导化疗治疗的患者远处转移率明显降低(10% vs 19%,$P=0.025$),接受诱导化疗治疗的 N2c 和 N3 患者存在生存获益的趋势($P=0.19$)[351]。PARADIGM 和 DeCIDE 的研究效力都不足。患者预后优于历史对照,很可能是因为大多数人群患原发性口咽癌,且可能是 HPV 相关。Hitt 等[352]在一项随机Ⅲ期诱导化疗试验中进行了评估,该试验使用 PF 或 TPF 进行诱导化疗,序贯使用高剂量顺铂进行同步化放疗,对比原方案同步化放疗。两组之间中位 PFS、治疗失败时间或 OS 无差异。在 2014 年 ASCO 会议上提交的Ⅱ/Ⅲ期欧洲试验的初步结果,在 415 名患者中评估了诱导 TPF 与无诱导化疗,序贯使用西妥昔单抗或 PF 进行化学放射治疗。诱导组的中位生存期为 53.7 个月,而前期化放疗组的中位生存期为 30.3 个月($HR=0.72$,$P=0.025$),接受诱导化疗的患者的远处转移风险降低。在该试验中观察到的结果与 DeCIDE 和 PARADIGM 的差异可能是由于不同的患者人群和纳入标准[353]。

根据这些试验的结果,结合 MACH-NC 荟萃分析[168],同步顺铂放化疗仍作为局部晚期头颈鳞癌的治疗标准。鉴于远处转移率的降低,基于 HPV 状态、吸烟史、N 分期和分子标记相关的风险分层人群中的进一步研究,可能确定从诱导化疗策略中获益最多的人群。在我们的机构中,诱导化疗用于保留喉及特定的口咽癌病例、N2c/N3 颈部大肿块的患者、下颈部转移且具有良好功能评分的患者。

同步化疗和放疗

一系列随机试验[171,199,354-361]和荟萃分析[362]显示在局部晚期鳞状细胞癌,尤其是口咽癌,同时给予化疗和放疗可以达到局部控制和 OS 的改善。然而,大多数研究包括各个部位的侵袭性鳞癌患者。建议仔细阅读原文进行鉴别,因为口腔、咽和喉部原发部位患者的百分比可能因不同中心而异,这会显著影响研究结果。应该强调的是,同步放化疗与明显的急性皮肤黏膜毒性有关,需要专业的对症治疗。语言和吞咽的康复治疗应常规进行。有很大一部分患者接受了胃造瘘术。骨坏死或口咽纤维化等长期并发症的风险尚在研究当中。

如果没有禁忌证,口腔原发性肿瘤大多数是通过外科手术治疗的。根据肿瘤组织学、大小、切缘病理和淋巴结转移程度,给予术后放疗。如前所述,具有阳性手术切缘或淋巴结包膜外侵的患者更有可能从辅助性同步化放疗中获益,而不是进行单纯放疗[134,173,313]。

关于毒性,通常在放化疗时会更快地出现皮肤黏膜反应,需要使用漱口液进行清洁、镇痛,并注意液体和卡路里摄入,同时需要语言和吞咽康复专家的参与。此外,人们担心同步化放疗比单纯放疗更容易在远期出现口干症、纤维化和相关的吞咽功能障碍。大多数患者的长期功能数据尚未报道。在 Intergroup 研究[199]和术后放化疗研究[134,173,313]中,与单纯放疗的对照组相比,同步治疗的慢性副作用似乎没有更高的风险。Setton 等[363]报道了近 1 500 例口咽癌患者接受了同步放化疗。2 年胃造瘘管的依赖率为 4.4%。在 MD Anderson 癌症中心进行的一项前瞻性研究评估了 47 名接受诱导化疗的患者的长期预后,序贯进行了风险调整的局部治疗,包括放射治疗,同步放化疗或口腔原发部位的手术,在 2 年的时候吞咽效率没有显著性的降低,相对于基线平均降低 13%($P=0.191$),慢性吞咽困难率为 7.1%,胃造瘘依赖性为 4.8%[364]。

在一项具有里程碑意义的研究中,Bonner 等[365]进行了一项前瞻性随机试验,其中先前未治疗的局部晚期鳞癌患者(包括口咽,下咽或喉部)接受了有或没有西妥昔单抗的放射治疗。西妥昔单抗是针对 EGFR 的嵌合人和鼠单克隆抗体。在该Ⅲ期试验中,纳入了 424 名患者,随访时间中位数为 38 个月。值得注意的是,严重级放疗相关的皮肤黏膜毒性没有增加。此外,中位生存期(28 个月对 54 个月)和 3 年生存率(44% vs 57%)提示联合治疗组在局部肿瘤控制方面具有显著优势。该研究促成西妥昔单抗被批准与放疗同步应用治疗局部晚期头颈鳞癌。

后续Ⅲ期研究 RTOG 0522 纳入 891 例Ⅲ期或Ⅳ期头颈鳞癌患者,评估西妥昔单抗加入标准顺铂同步放化疗的效果。患者在接受放疗和顺铂治疗的同时,随机分为使用或不使用西妥昔单抗。使用西妥昔单抗导致治疗中断显著增加,急性 3 级和 4 级毒性发生率增加,并且没有提高患者的预后[366]。Concert 1、2 试验进一步探讨了帕尼单抗的生物放射治疗(表 83-6)[367,368],结果显示在调整了新增或替换的抗体后,没有 OS 或局部疾病控制的优势。

表 83-6 基于 EGFR 的生物放射治疗与帕尼单抗(P)

	数量	2 年局部控制率/%
研究 1		
化疗-放疗	63	68
化疗-放疗+帕尼单抗	87	61
研究 2		
化疗-放疗	61	61
帕尼单抗-放疗	90	51

因此，目前对于不适合手术的Ⅲ期和Ⅳ期头颈鳞癌患者的治疗标准，将明确采用同步放化疗进行治疗。目前广泛使用的方案为：在第 1、4 和 7 周使用顺铂 100mg/m^2 同时每日一次放疗或每周 40mg/m^2 顺铂。使用西妥昔单抗同步放射治疗是不适合接受顺铂（如肾功能不全、听力丧失、高龄或一般情况较差）的患者的替代方案。

鉴于 HPV 相关口咽鳞癌患者的预后和治疗效果较好，因此降级治疗研究正广泛地在该患者人群中进行。正在进行的 RTOG 1 016 试验正在将患有 HPV 相关口咽鳞癌的患者随机分组，放射治疗同步使用顺铂或西妥昔单抗。目前已完成入组，正在等待结果。

复发和转移性疾病：细胞毒素

在Ⅱ期试验中已证实使用单一药物进行细胞毒性化疗的疗效，表 83-7 中列出了多种药物的预期应答率。更有可能获益的群体包括：ECOG 评分为 0 或 1；初始治疗后大于 6 个月后复发；受累部位之前未接受过放疗。

Ⅲ期研究直接比较了顺铂和甲氨蝶呤（随机，双臂设计）。这些研究之一，Hong 等[369]在每月的第 1 天和第 8 天给予顺铂 50mg/m^2，另一组每周给予甲氨蝶呤 40mg/m^2。应答率分别为 28.6%和 23.5%。紫杉烷类药物在头颈鳞癌中构成了一类独特的活性药物[370~372]。在之前未接受过姑息性化疗的患者中使用多西他赛的Ⅱ期研究中产生了 21%~42%的应答率[370,372]。

表 83-7　单药在头颈复发性肿瘤的活性

试剂	预期反应率/%
甲氨蝶呤	25
博来霉素	15
顺铂	25
卡铂	20
氟尿嘧啶	15
紫杉醇	30
多西他赛	30
异环磷酰胺	20
西妥昔单抗	13

联合化疗可能在 30%~40%的患者中产生应答，但与单药治疗相比没有显著的生存优势，生存期通常在 6~9 个月（表 83-8）。Gibson 等[378]进行了一项前瞻性Ⅲ期试验，比较了 218 例使用顺铂和静脉氟尿嘧啶与顺铂和紫杉醇的患者。他们的应答率（分别为 27%和 26%）或中位生存期（8.7 个月和 8.1 个月）没有差异，毒性相似。

表 83-8　选择在头颈部复发或转移性鳞状细胞癌化疗的随机Ⅲ期试验

试验	患者数量	方案	应答率/%	生存（P 值）
Jacobs 等[373]	79	顺铂/氟尿嘧啶	32	不显著
	83	顺铂	17	
	83	氟尿嘧啶	13	
Forastiere 等[374]	87	顺铂/氟尿嘧啶	32	不显著
	86	卡铂/氟尿嘧啶	21	
	88	甲氨蝶呤	10	
Clavel 等[375]	127	顺铂/甲氨蝶呤/博来霉素/长春新碱	34	不显著
	116	顺铂/氟尿嘧啶	31	
	122	顺铂	15	
Schrijvers 等[376]	122	顺铂/氟尿嘧啶/α2b-干扰素	47	不显著
	122	顺铂/氟尿嘧啶	38	
Forastiere 等[377]	101	顺铂/紫杉醇（高剂量）	35	不显著
	98	顺铂/紫杉醇（低剂量）	36	
Gibson 等[378]	104	顺铂/氟尿嘧啶	22	不显著
	100	顺铂/紫杉醇	28	
Vermorken 等[347]	215	铂类/氟尿嘧啶	20	中位生存期 7.4 个月
	219	铂类/氟尿嘧啶-西妥昔单抗	36	中位生存期 10.1 个月（P=0.04）

在一项随机Ⅲ期前瞻性试验中，Vermorken 等[379]评估了442 例复发或转移性头颈鳞癌患者中西妥昔单抗联合铂类-氟尿嘧啶治疗的效果。结果呈现出更好的应答率，中位生存期从7.4 个月增加到10.1 个月。该方案没有异常的毒性，且已成为适合患者标准治疗的一线方案。

复发或转移性头颈鳞癌患者的 OS 仍然很差，只有约 30%的患者存活 1 年，目前对新药开发和更有效全身治疗策略的需求仍十分迫切。

新疗法

随着多个基因组事件的积累，出现了侵袭性鳞癌。似乎存在具有生物学意义的必需分子改变，其赋予癌细胞生存优势并且构成癌发生过程[380]。随着我们更好地了解深层的癌症生物学，已经确定了潜在的治疗目标，并且正在制订创新的治疗策略。

表皮生长因子受体

EGFR 是一种跨膜糖蛋白，其激活引发的下游细胞内信号转导的级联事件，对于上皮细胞生长的调节很重要[381~385]。EGF 和转化生长因子-α（TGF-α）是受体的配体。大约在 90%的头颈鳞癌可以观察到 EGFR 或 TGF-α 的表达[384]。

吉非替尼和厄洛替尼是 EGFR 的小分子抑制剂。两种药物均已在复发或转移性头颈鳞癌中作为单一药物进行测试，显示出最低的临床活性[386,387]。阿法替尼和达克替尼，第二代 EGFR 抑制剂，正在铂类难治性转移性头颈鳞癌中进行研究。初步结果显示一些活性，应答率约为 10%[388]。

西妥昔单抗是针对 EGFR 细胞外部分的单克隆抗体。单克隆抗体与配体竞争性的结合阻止受体二聚化，进而阻碍多个下游信号。Vermorken 等[389]报道了用西妥昔单抗单药治疗铂类难治性患者的应答率为 13%。如前所述，Vermorken 等[379]在Ⅲ期试验中证明西妥昔单抗加入顺铂或卡铂和氟尿嘧啶方案中可提高肿瘤应答率，并使总体中位生存期提高 2.7 个月（从 7.4 个月到西妥昔单抗组的 10.1 个月）。如前所述，Bonner 等[365]还报道了放射治疗加西妥昔单抗联合治疗组较单纯放疗组可以达到更好的局部肿瘤控制和 OS。

已经反复观察到皮疹和肿瘤应答之间的关联[343,390]并且需要进一步探索，可能可以通过提高西妥昔单抗剂量直至出现皮疹或剂量限制性毒性。迄今为止，西妥昔单抗是唯一被美国食品药品管理局批准的用于治疗头颈鳞癌的靶向治疗。

血管生成

新血管形成是肿瘤生长的必要过程。血管内皮生长因子（VEGF）是一种多功能细胞因子，是内皮细胞生长的有效刺激物。包括头颈鳞癌在内，许多癌症中观察到 VEGF 蛋白表达的增加[391,392]。

贝伐单抗阻止 VEGF 与受体酪氨酸激酶（VEGFR1 和 VEGFR2）结合，从而抑制肿瘤细胞生长。Argiris 等[393]在单臂Ⅱ期试验中评估了西妥昔单抗和贝伐单抗治疗 46 例复发或转移性头颈鳞癌患者的活性，这些患者接受了一系列全身治疗。整体应答率为 16%，中位 PFS 和 OS 分别为 2.8 和 7.5 个月。目前针对患有复发性或转移性头颈鳞癌的患者，在使用铂和多西他赛或铂和氟尿嘧啶的基础上，使用或不使用贝伐单抗的大型Ⅲ期试验（E1305）正在进行且等待结果中（临床试验参考号 NCT00588770）。目前正在临床研究新一代小分子 VEGFR 抑制剂阿西替尼和培唑帕尼。索拉非尼和舒尼替尼是小分子泛受体酪氨酸激酶抑制剂，具有多种靶标，其中包括 VEGFR。他们已经在转移性头颈鳞癌中进行了测试，并表现出了一定的活性[394,395]。

磷脂酰肌醇-3 激酶（PI3K）

新一代测序的进展揭示了头颈鳞癌中反复发生的遗传改变。最常见的潜在靶向改变包括激活 PI3K（磷脂酰肌醇-3 激酶）途径，不论是 PIK3CA 突变或扩增（约 35%）或 PTEN 缺失（约 5%）[396,397]。PI3K/AKT/mTOR 通路在调节细胞周期中很重要，其失调与癌细胞增殖相关。在头颈鳞癌中正在使用 PI3K 抑制剂作为单一药剂或与其他靶向疗法（如 EGFR 抑制剂或 MEK 抑制剂）组合的各种临床试验正在进行中。

基因治疗

利用腺病毒介导的野生型 TP53 基因转导治疗在一部分肿瘤患者中产生了令人兴奋的结果[398]。Khuri 等[399]进行了一项多中心Ⅱ期试验，通过 ONYX-015，一种选择性复制腺病毒，联合顺铂和氟尿嘧啶治疗晚期头颈鳞癌患者。在 30 名可以完整评估的肿瘤患者中观察到 52%的应答率。在可向肿瘤注射和因不能达到肿瘤部位而不能进行瘤体注射的亚组分析中，观察到肿瘤缓解存在明显差异，给予化疗和 ONYX-015 后更常出现肿瘤缓解（$P=0.006$）。正在继续进行采用 TP53 替代策略治疗可瘤体注射头颈鳞癌或作为化疗预防的试验。

免疫治疗

最近，出现了一类增强抗肿瘤免疫力的新药，正在改变医学肿瘤学领域。最有希望的操作途径之一涉及程序性死亡配体 1（PD-L1）。PD-L1 可在实体瘤中过表达，并且在与表达 PD-1 的肿瘤浸润性 T 细胞结合后，抑制其活性并促进免疫耐受，保护肿瘤细胞免于凋亡。阻断 PD-1-PD-L1 相互作用、增强免疫功能显示了有临床意义的活性[400~402]。帕博利珠单抗（pembrolizumab）和纳武单抗（nivolumab），靶向 PD-1 的人源化单克隆抗体，已被批准用于治疗转移性难治性黑素瘤；并且最近，纳武单抗被批准作为肺鳞癌的二线治疗。这些抗体的活性似乎与肿瘤和/或基质细胞中的 PD-L1 表达相关。

KEYNOTE-012 Ⅰ期试验的头颈部队列的初步结果显示，104 例难治性转移性/复发性头颈鳞癌的患者中有 78%在肿瘤微环境中至少有 1%的细胞中表达 PD-L1。在可评估反应的 51 名患者中，51%的患者肿瘤负荷减轻，RECIST 评分总体应答率为 20%，与 HPV 状态无关[403]。8 名患者超过 6 个月疾病稳定，当提交研究的初步数据时有七人仍在接受治疗。整体治疗耐受性良好，主要副作用是乏力、瘙痒和皮疹。

鉴于这些令人鼓舞的早期结果，许多免疫疗法临床试验与检查点抑制剂、共刺激激动剂、疫苗和过继性 T 细胞转移正在头颈鳞癌进行，并在不久的将来有很大的希望（图 83-15）。

目前的方向

全身治疗是 HNC 治疗的一个组成部分。许多局部晚期疾

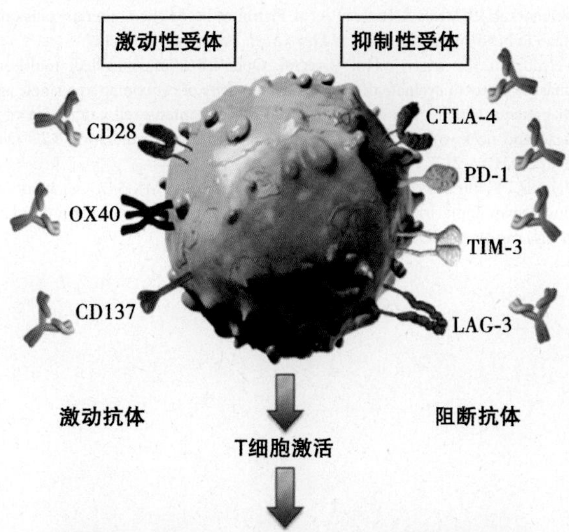

图 83-15　T 细胞的激动性与抑制性受体[404]

病的患者接受化疗和放疗治疗。HPV 作为病因,其有利预后因素的价值可望影响患者的治疗,目前降级治疗临床研究正在进行中。现在,治疗复发性疾病的方案包括再次放疗、细胞毒性化疗和分子靶向治疗。随着对 HNC 基因组学的深入了解,多项靶向治疗试验正在特定亚组中进行。检查点抑制剂在转移性头颈鳞癌中的初步结果具有前景,并可能在不久的将来加入到全身治疗当中。

(廖理达　王健　朱一鸣 译　刘绍严 校)

参考文献

The complete reference list can be found on the Wiley Companion Digital Edition of this title (see inside front cover for login instructions).

4 Sturgis EM, Cinciripini PM. Trends in head and neck cancer incidence in relation to smoking prevalence: an emerging epidemic of human papillomavirus-associated cancers? *Cancer*. 2007;**110**:1429–1435.

29 D'Souza G, Kreimer AR, Viscidi R, et al. Case-control study of human papillomavirus and oropharyngeal cancer. *N Engl J Med*. 2007;**356**:1944–1956.

42 Chien YC, Chen JY, Liu MY, et al. Serologic markers of Epstein-Barr virus infection and nasopharyngeal carcinoma in Taiwanese men. *N Engl J Med*. 2001;**345**:1877–1882.

88 Ang KK, Harris J, Wheeler R, et al. Human papillomavirus and survival of patients with oropharyngeal cancer. *N Engl J Med*. 2010;**363**:24–35.

94 Allal AS, Dulguerov P, Allaoua M, et al. Standardized uptake value of 2-[(18)F] fluoro-2-deoxy-D-glucose in predicting outcome in head and neck carcinomas treated by radiotherapy with or without chemotherapy. *J Clin Oncol*. 2002;**20**:1398–1404.

103 Kyzas PA, Evangelou E, Denaxa-Kyza D, Ioannidis JP. 18 F-fluorodeoxyglucose positron emission tomography to evaluate cervical node metastases in patients with head and neck squamous cell carcinoma: a meta-analysis. *J Natl Cancer Inst*. 2008;**100**:712–720.

119 Lippman SM, Hong WK. Molecular markers of the risk of oral cancer. *N Engl J Med*. 2001;**344**:1323–1326.

134 Cooper JS, Pajak TF, Forastiere AA, et al. Postoperative concurrent radiotherapy and chemotherapy for high-risk squamous-cell carcinoma of the head and neck. *N Engl J Med*. 2004;**350**:1937–1944.

144 Schiff BA, Roberts DB, El-Naggar A, Garden AS, Myers JN. Selective vs modified radical neck dissection and postoperative radiotherapy vs observation in the treatment of squamous cell carcinoma of the oral tongue. *Arch Otolaryngol Head Neck Surg*. 2005;**131**:874–878.

152 Diaz EM Jr, Holsinger FC, Zuniga ER, Roberts DB, Sorensen DM. Squamous cell carcinoma of the buccal mucosa: one institution's experience with 119 previously untreated patients. *Head Neck*. 2003;**25**:267–273.

155 Hong WK, Wolf GT, Fisher SG, et al. Induction chemotherapy plus radiation compared with surgery plus radiation in patients with advanced laryngeal cancer. The Department of Veterans Affairs Laryngeal Cancer Study Group. *N Engl J Med*. 1991;**324**:1685–1690.

156 Machtay M, Moughan J, Trotti A, et al. Factors associated with severe late toxicity after concurrent chemoradiation for locally advanced head and neck cancer: an RTOG analysis. *J Clin Oncol*. 2008;**26**:3582–3589.

157 Hinni ML, Nagel T, Howard B. Oropharyngeal cancer treatment: the role of transoral surgery. *Curr Opin Otolaryngol Head Neck Surg*. 2015;**23**:132–138.

166 Weber RS, Gidley P, Morrison WH, et al. Treatment selection for carcinoma of the base of the tongue. *Am J Surg*. 1990;**160**:415–419.

168 Pignon JP, le Maitre A, Maillard E, Bourhis J, Group M-NC. Meta-analysis of chemotherapy in head and neck cancer (MACH-NC): an update on 93 randomised trials and 17,346 patients. *Radiother Oncol*. 2009;**92**:4–14.

169 Bourhis J, Overgaard J, Audry H, et al. Hyperfractionated or accelerated radiotherapy in head and neck cancer: a meta-analysis. *Lancet*. 2006;**368**:843–854.

170 Marta GN, Silva V, de Andrade CH, et al. Intensity-modulated radiation therapy for head and neck cancer: systematic review and meta-analysis. *Radiother Oncol*. 2014;**110**:9–15.

171 Calais G, Alfonsi M, Bardet E, et al. Randomized trial of radiation therapy versus concomitant chemotherapy and radiation therapy for advanced-stage oropharynx carcinoma. *J Natl Cancer Inst*. 1999;**91**:2081–2086.

172 Denis F, Garaud P, Bardet E, et al. Final results of the 94-01 French Head and Neck Oncology and Radiotherapy Group randomized trial comparing radiotherapy alone with concomitant radiochemotherapy in advanced-stage oropharynx carcinoma. *J Clin Oncol*. 2004;**22**:69–76.

173 Bernier J, Domenge C, Ozsahin M, et al. Postoperative irradiation with or without concomitant chemotherapy for locally advanced head and neck cancer. *N Engl J Med*. 2004;**350**:1945–1952.

197 Hong WK, Lippman SM, Wolf GT. Recent advances in head and neck cancer—larynx preservation and cancer chemoprevention: the Seventeenth Annual Richard and Hinda Rosenthal Foundation Award Lecture. *Cancer Res*. 1993;**53**:5113–5120.

199 Forastiere AA, Goepfert H, Maor M, et al. Concurrent chemotherapy and radiotherapy for organ preservation in advanced laryngeal cancer. *N Engl J Med*. 2003;**349**:2091–2098.

251 Fandi A, Bachouchi M, Azli N, et al. Long-term disease-free survivors in metastatic undifferentiated carcinoma of nasopharyngeal type. *J Clin Oncol*. 2000;**18**:1324–1330.

253 Al-Sarraf M, LeBlanc M, Giri PG, et al. Chemoradiotherapy versus radiotherapy in patients with advanced nasopharyngeal cancer: phase III randomized Intergroup study 0099. *J Clin Oncol*. 1998;**16**:1310–1317.

255 Chan AT, Leung SF, Ngan RK, et al. Overall survival after concurrent cisplatin-radiotherapy compared with radiotherapy alone in locoregionally advanced nasopharyngeal carcinoma. *J Natl Cancer Inst*. 2005;**97**:536–539.

256 Lin JC, Jan JS, Hsu CY, Liang WM, Jiang RS, Wang WY. Phase III study of concurrent chemoradiotherapy versus radiotherapy alone for advanced nasopharyngeal carcinoma: positive effect on overall and progression-free survival. *J Clin Oncol*. 2003;**21**:631–637.

297 Airoldi M, Pedani F, Succo G, et al. Phase II randomized trial comparing vinorelbine versus vinorelbine plus cisplatin in patients with recurrent salivary gland malignancies. *Cancer*. 2001;**91**:541–547.

314 Ang KK, Trotti A, Brown BW, et al. Randomized trial addressing risk features and time factors of surgery plus radiotherapy in advanced head-and-neck cancer. *Int J Radiat Oncol Biol Phys*. 2001;**51**:571–578.

329 Leibel SA, Fuks Z, Zelefsky MJ, et al. Intensity-modulated radiotherapy. *Cancer J*. 2002;**8**:164–176.

346 Forastiere AA, Zhang Q, Weber RS, et al. Long-term results of RTOG 91-11: a comparison of three nonsurgical treatment strategies to preserve the larynx in patients with locally advanced larynx cancer. *J Clin Oncol*. 2013;**31**:845–852.

347 Vermorken JB, Remenar E, van Herpen C, et al. Cisplatin, fluorouracil, and docetaxel in unresectable head and neck cancer. *N Engl J Med*. 2007;**357**:1695–1704.

348 Posner MR, Hershock DM, Blajman CR, et al. Cisplatin and fluorouracil alone or with docetaxel in head and neck cancer. *N Engl J Med*. 2007;**357**:1705–1715.

350 Haddad R, O'Neill A, Rabinowits G, et al. Induction chemotherapy followed by concurrent chemoradiotherapy (sequential chemoradiotherapy) versus concurrent chemoradiotherapy alone in locally advanced head and neck cancer (PARADIGM): a randomised phase 3 trial. *Lancet Oncol*. 2013;**14**:257–264.

351 Cohen EE, Karrison TG, Kocherginsky M, et al. Phase III randomized trial of induction chemotherapy in patients with N2 or N3 locally advanced head and neck cancer. *J Clin Oncol*. 2014;**32**:2735–2743.

360 Staar S, Rudat V, Stuetzer H, et al. Intensified hyperfractionated accelerated radiotherapy limits the additional benefit of simultaneous chemotherapy—results of a multicentric randomized German trial in advanced head-and-neck cancer. *Int J Radiat Oncol Biol Phys*. 2001;**50**:1161–1171.

361 Wendt TG, Grabenbauer GG, Rodel CM, et al. Simultaneous radiochemotherapy versus radiotherapy alone in advanced head and neck cancer: a randomized mul-

ticenter study. *J Clin Oncol.* 1998;**16**:1318–1324.

362 Pignon JP, Bourhis J, Domenge C, Designe L. Chemotherapy added to locoregional treatment for head and neck squamous-cell carcinoma: three meta-analyses of updated individual data. MACH-NC Collaborative Group. Meta-Analysis of Chemotherapy on Head and Neck Cancer. *Lancet.* 2000;**355**: 949–955.

365 Bonner JA, Harari PM, Giralt J, et al. Radiotherapy plus cetuximab for squamous-cell carcinoma of the head and neck. *N Engl J Med.* 2006;**354**:567–578.

366 Ang KK, Zhang Q, Rosenthal DI, et al. Randomized phase III trial of concurrent accelerated radiation plus cisplatin with or without cetuximab for stage III to IV head and neck carcinoma: RTOG 0522. *J Clin Oncol.* 2014;**32**:2940–2950.

379 Vermorken JB, Mesia R, Rivera F, et al. Platinum-based chemotherapy plus cetuximab in head and neck cancer. *N Engl J Med.* 2008;**359**:1116–1127.

389 Vermorken JB, Trigo J, Hitt R, et al. Open-label, uncontrolled, multicenter phase II study to evaluate the efficacy and toxicity of cetuximab as a single agent in patients with recurrent and/or metastatic squamous cell carcinoma of the head and neck who failed to respond to platinum-based therapy. *J Clin Oncol.* 2007;**25**:2171–2177.

403 Seiwert TY, Burtness B, Weiss J, et al. A phase Ib study of MK-3475 in patients with human papillomavirus (HPV)-associated and non-HPV-associated head and neck (H/N) cancer. *ASCO Meeting Abstracts.* 2014;**32**:6011.

第 84 章　肺癌

Charles Lu, MD, SM ■ Daniel Morgensztern, MD ■ Anne Chiang, MD, PhD ■ Amir Onn, MD ■ Boris Sepesi, MD ■ Ara A. Vaporciyan, MD ■ Joe Y. Chang, MD, PhD ■ Ritsuko K. Komaki, MD ■ Ignacio I. Wistuba, MD ■ Roy S. Herbst, MD, PhD

概览

在世界范围内，肺癌在癌症相关死亡人数中位居首位，减少吸烟率是降低肺癌死亡率的最有效方法。标准治疗手段包括手术、放疗和/或化疗。由于肺癌是一种异质性疾病，因此希望蛋白质组学和基因组学的转化研究能够促进我们对驱动分子通路的理解，并开发更有效、毒性更小的靶向治疗。免疫疗法最近取得了令人鼓舞的进展，作为一种新的治疗策略，已经影响了当前的标准治疗方案。

病因学和流行病学

肺癌是最常见且致死性很强的恶性肿瘤。全世界每年新发生的 1 270 万例癌症病例中有 161 万例是肺癌，760 万例癌症死亡中有 138 万是肺癌[1]。近期发表的美国 2015 年癌症统计数据显示，美国男性和女性肺癌发病率均位于第二位，分别占男女性癌症新发病例总数的 14%和 13%。但肺癌死亡率在美国此前癌症统计中均居男女性首位：男性 86 380 人，占所有癌症相关死亡人数的 28%，女性 71 660 人，占所有癌症相关死亡人数的 26%。事实上，美国死于肺癌的人数多于紧随其后的三种癌症相关死亡之和，即前列腺癌，乳腺癌和结直肠癌[2]。1920 年报告的肺癌病例总数还不到 1 000 例，当时被认为是一种罕见的恶性疾病。但自 20 世纪 50 年代以来肺癌一直被公认为主要的公共卫生问题。首先是男性肺癌新发病例数攀升，在 20 世纪 80 年代中期达峰值之后稳定降低；女性肺癌的发病率则一直上升至 20 世纪 90 年代末，近期趋于平缓。上述变化与男女性吸烟的普遍程度相平行，男性肺癌发病率和死亡率的下降可以被吸烟率的降低解释[3]。

吸烟与肺癌

吸烟是世界上最有可能避免的致死原因。肺癌是烟草致死疾病中最常见的癌症：每吸 300 万支纸烟就有 1 人死于肺癌。正如 Proctor 所述[4]，烟草是最早发现的环境致癌物。在 18 世纪和 19 世纪，欧洲最早发表了吸烟与口腔癌和唇癌间有关联的报告。60 多年前，德国 Muller 首先确认吸烟与肺癌可能的正相关。随后大量的流行病学研究证实了这些观察，阐明吸烟致癌的分子机制，提供了充足的证据明确吸烟与呼吸消化道、膀胱、肾脏、子宫颈癌以及髓样白血病之间存在强烈的因果关系。一项对 50 多个非吸烟者研究的荟萃分析表明，接触环境烟草烟雾与肺癌发病风险显著相关[4]。

到目前为止，吸烟占男女两性肺癌死亡人数的 85%～90%，肺癌发生的频率与接触烟草的时间有强烈的关联。持续吸烟 45 年、30 年和 15 年的肺癌年发病率分别为 0.5%、0.1%和 0.01%，即吸烟时间延长 3 倍，肺癌的年发病率升高 50 倍。随着吸烟停止，此后每年的风险大致保持不变。例如，吸烟 30 年后，风险约为 0.1%，若此后不再吸烟，该风险将保持稳定，15 年后的年均风险仍然为 0.1%，而非继续吸烟的风险 0.5%。因此，通过戒烟可以避免大约 80%的风险[5]。

被动吸烟

不但吸烟者具有烟草接触风险，在环境中"被动吸烟"也可增加肺癌死亡风险。据环境保护署（EPA）报告，每年大约 3 000 名非吸烟成人因吸入他人吸烟产生的烟雾而死于肺癌。分析表明，从吸烟者排出的烟雾当中能够检测到吸烟者吸入的主流烟雾中已识别出的所有致癌化合物。

家族易感性

值得关注的是，包括重度吸烟在内的大多数吸烟者并不都发展成肺癌，这表明癌症的形成依赖于遗传的易感性或辅助因子，如其他致癌物质。对经组织学证实的肺癌病例与吸烟相关的其他癌症进行比较，发现肺癌的家族史不增加肺癌风险，但会增加某些部位癌症的风险[6]，提示个体对致癌物的反应具有遗传的差异。呼吸系统疾病也具有肺癌的易感性。研究家族的肺癌易感性表明，年轻个体（小于 50 岁）的肺癌发生与 Mendelian 共显性遗传或罕见常染色体基因相似[7]。

其他环境原因

除烟草外，接触职业性和环境性致癌物也与发生肺癌有关。国际癌症研究中心确定为致癌物 1 组的职业因素包括无机砷、石棉、二氯甲醚、铬（六价）、镍及镍的化合物、多环芳烃化合物、氡、氯乙烯。确定为可能致癌物 2A 组的有乙酰，铍、镉、甲醛、丙醛、合成纤维、硅、焊接烟雾。据估计，目前职业性暴露约占全世界肺癌病例的 5%～15%（表 84-1）。

表 84-1　建档在册的职业性致癌物

物质	职业性接触
砷	冶炼工，农药制造工
石棉	采矿工，碾磨工，绝缘体工，铁道工和造船工
氯甲醚	离子交换树脂制造工
铬	铬盐和染料制造工
烃类	煤气工，烟囱清洁工
芥子气	毒气制造工
镍	精炼工
辐射	铀矿和其他矿工

改编自 Roth 1989。

分子病理机制

近年来，随着分子生物学技术的迅速发展，使导致肺组织癌性病变的多基因鉴定成为可能。有趣的是，这些基因以可转变的形式正常存在于真核细胞中。受烟草和其他致癌物诱导产生的多种形式的基因变异和信号通路的激活决定了肺癌的异质性，这种作用与其他实体瘤相比十分显著。在这方面，必须明确某些特定肿瘤是以特殊的遗传变异为特征的，从正常上皮组织转变为侵袭性肿瘤是一个基因变异逐渐积累的结果。表 84-2 罗列了肺癌发生的相关基因。有关肿瘤生物学方面的综述将在本书的其他章节中详述。

表 84-2 与肺腺癌和肺鳞癌相关的主要遗传变异

基因	分子改变	肺腺癌	肺鳞癌
MYC	突变	10%~40%	极少
	扩增/CNG	15%	40%
	IHC 过表达	15%~39%	~58%
KRAS	突变	10%~30%	极少
BRAF	突变	2%	3%
EML4-ALK	易位	13%	极少
ROS1	易位	1%	极少
RET	易位	1%	极少
LKB1	突变	8%~30%	0%~5%
HER2	突变	2%~4%	极少
	扩增	8%	2%
	IHC 过表达	35%	1%
DDR2	突变	Very rare	4%
TP53	LOH 和突变	50%~70%	60%~70%
FGFR1	扩增	1%~3%	8%~22%
PIK3CA	扩增/CNG	2%~6%	33%~35%
	突变	2%	2%

CNG，拷贝数增加（copy number gain）；IHC，免疫组化（immunohistochemistry）；LOH，杂合性缺失（loss of heterozygosity）。

癌前病变的分子异常

上皮细胞结构和基因的改变是不断积累的过程，侵袭性的肿瘤从气道最初的损伤后（图 84-1），经过 5~20 年的时间逐渐形成。在肺癌和暴露于烟草等致癌物的支气管上皮中常可以检测到特殊染色体的单一等位基因的缺失［杂合性缺失（LOH）］。最早和发生频率最高的等位基因缺失的区域位于 3q21、3P22~24、3p25 和 9p21[9]。值得注意的是，在吸烟者的正常支气管上皮组织中可观察到以上基因的多种变异，而非吸烟者并未见到类似改变[10,11]。然而，随着癌前病变的进展，这些染色体缺失变异变得更加频繁和广泛。在某些情况下，这些分子改变是不断重复并独立出现的。肿瘤抑癌基因启动子的甲基化序列可以在肿瘤、吸烟损伤的正常肺（癌前改变）、痰和血液中检测到。这些改变可作为有效的生物标志物用于早期检测和监测化学预防、戒烟及对治疗的反应。随着 DNA 和 RNA 高通量二代测序技术的发展[12,13]，肺癌分子特征取得许多新的进展，许多参与浸润性肺鳞癌和肺腺癌发病机制的新的分子通路被报道，并被扩展应用于分析参与肺气道癌前病变的分子变化[14]。有研究表明，在携带表皮生长因子受体（EGFR）突变的肺腺癌中，可以在邻近肿瘤的支气管正常上皮中检测到这些突变[15]。在鳞状细胞癌中，在支气管发育不良合并侵袭性鳞状细胞肿瘤患者中能够检测到细胞谱系基因 SOX-2 的基因扩增和蛋白质过表达[16,17]。肺呼吸道的高通量芯片分析研究表明，正常上皮细胞基因表达的全局变化可以预测吸烟者的癌症发展[18]，识别信号通路的激活（如 PI3K）并作为靶向治疗的潜在化学预防策略[19]以及更好地定义和解释不同组织学肺癌发生发展的分子谱特征[14,20,21]。

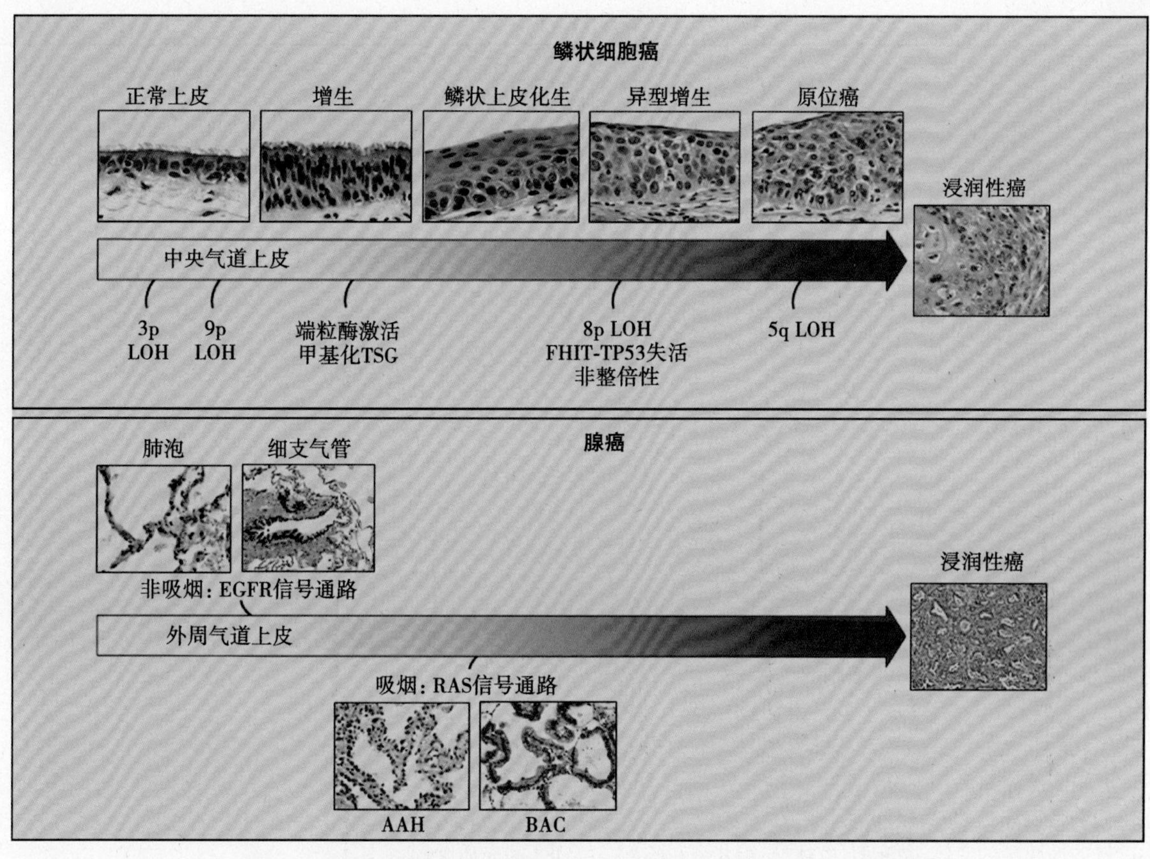

图 84-1　肺鳞状细胞癌和肺腺癌发病机制的组织病理学和分子变化总结

肺癌的病理学

从组织病理学和生物学角度来看，肺癌是一种复杂的肿瘤。2004 年世界卫生组织（WHO）肺癌组织学分类最近在国际肺癌研究协会（IASLC）病理学小组的支持下进行了修订[22]。新的分类基于使用标准组织学技术下的光学显微镜分析和代表分化标志物的蛋白免疫组化分析（表 84-3）[22,23]。肺癌组织学类型分为非小细胞肺癌（NSCLC）和小细胞肺癌（SCLC），其中最常见的是非小细胞肺癌，包括鳞状细胞癌（SCC）、腺癌（包括微浸润腺癌）和大细胞癌[24]。肺肿瘤一般按肿瘤的最佳分化区域分类，并由其分化程度最差的部分进行分级。

癌前病变

肺癌被认为是呼吸道黏膜发生一系列循序渐进的病理变化（癌前病变）后引起的。新的 WHO 组织学分类中，将肺的癌前病变列为三种主要的形态学形式：①鳞状上皮不典型增生和原位癌（CIS）；②不典型腺瘤样增生（AAH）；③弥漫性特发性肺神经内分泌细胞增生（DIPNECH），与肺类癌的发生有关[22,23]。然而已经确定的序列发生的癌前病变主要引起鳞状细胞癌，对于大细胞癌、腺癌和小细胞癌的癌前病变报道很少[25,26]。

浸润性肿瘤

微浸润腺癌（MIA）

该病变定义为小的（≤3cm）孤立性腺癌，以贴壁生长为主，浸润的最大直径≤5mm[22,27]。MIA 通常由非黏液细胞组成，但少数情况下也可为黏液性的。浸润区域的测量应该包括组织学亚型而不只是贴壁模式（即腺泡型、乳头型、微乳头型和/或实体型），或者鉴定明确恶性细胞浸润基质[22]。如果肿瘤侵入淋巴管、血管或胸膜或含有肿瘤坏死，则应将其诊断为侵袭性腺癌。

腺癌

这种肿瘤类型占所有肺癌的近 40%（图 84-2a、b）。大多数腺癌呈现组织学异质性，并且根据新的 WHO 分类，腺癌可以基于存在的主要组织学模式（即腺泡、乳头状、伴黏液产生的实体型、微乳头型及附壁型）进行细分[22]。当肿瘤细胞以纯粹的附壁方式生长而没有浸润证据时，被认为是 AIS[22]。实体型腺癌分化差，这些低分化肿瘤被证实有黏液产生，可通过黏液卡红或过碘酸雪夫染色显示。肺腺癌通常对甲状腺转录因子 1（TTF-1），Napsin A 和细胞角蛋白 7 进行免疫染色。腺癌肿瘤有四种变体，包括黏液型，胶体型，胎儿型（低级和高级）和肠型。虽然肺腺癌主要通过淋巴和血源性途径传播，但是在黏液性肿瘤中经常发生气道播散，这时播散的肿瘤细胞通过气道形成远离主体肿瘤的病变[28]。

鳞状细胞癌（SCC）

SCC 约占所有肺癌的 30%。细胞间桥、角化珠的形成和单个细胞的角化是这种肿瘤类型鳞状分化的特征（图 84-2c）。虽然这些特征在高分化鳞状细胞癌中非常明显，但在分化差的肿瘤中很难发现。WHO 新的鳞癌组织学亚型分为角化型、非角化型和基底细胞型[29]。对于具有角化特征的肿瘤，不需要进

表 84-3 WHO 肺癌分类

Ⅰ. 上皮性肿瘤	c. 基底细胞癌型
A. 良性	3. 腺鳞癌
1. 乳头状瘤	4. 肉瘤样癌
a. 鳞状细胞乳头状瘤	a. 多形性
b. 腺乳头状瘤	b. 纺锤细胞
c. 混合性鳞状细胞和腺体乳头状瘤	c. 巨细胞癌
2. 腺瘤	d. 癌肉瘤
a. 硬化性肺细胞瘤	e. 肺母细胞瘤
b. 肺泡腺瘤	5. 大细胞癌
c. 乳头状腺瘤	6. 神经内分泌肿瘤
d. 黏液性囊腺瘤	a. 典型的类癌
e. 肺细胞腺肌上皮瘤	b. 非典型类癌
f. 黏液腺瘤	c. 大细胞神经内分泌癌 LCNEC
B. 浸润前病变	d. 小细胞癌 SCLC
1. 非典型肺泡增生 AAH	7. 其他和非分类癌
2. 原位腺癌 AIS	a. 淋巴上皮瘤样癌
3. 鳞状上皮异常增生和原位癌	b. NUT 癌
4. 弥漫性特发性肺神经内分泌细胞增生	8. 唾液腺肿瘤
C. 恶性	• 黏液表皮样癌
1. 腺癌	• 腺样囊性癌
a. 微浸润腺癌 MIA	• 上皮-肌上皮癌
b. 侵袭性腺癌	• 多形性腺瘤
c. 侵袭性腺癌的变体:黏液型、胶体型、胎儿型和肠型	Ⅱ. 间充质肿瘤
2. 鳞状细胞癌	Ⅲ. 淋巴组织细胞肿瘤
a. 角化型	Ⅳ. 异位起源的肿瘤
b. 非角化型	Ⅴ. 转移性肿瘤

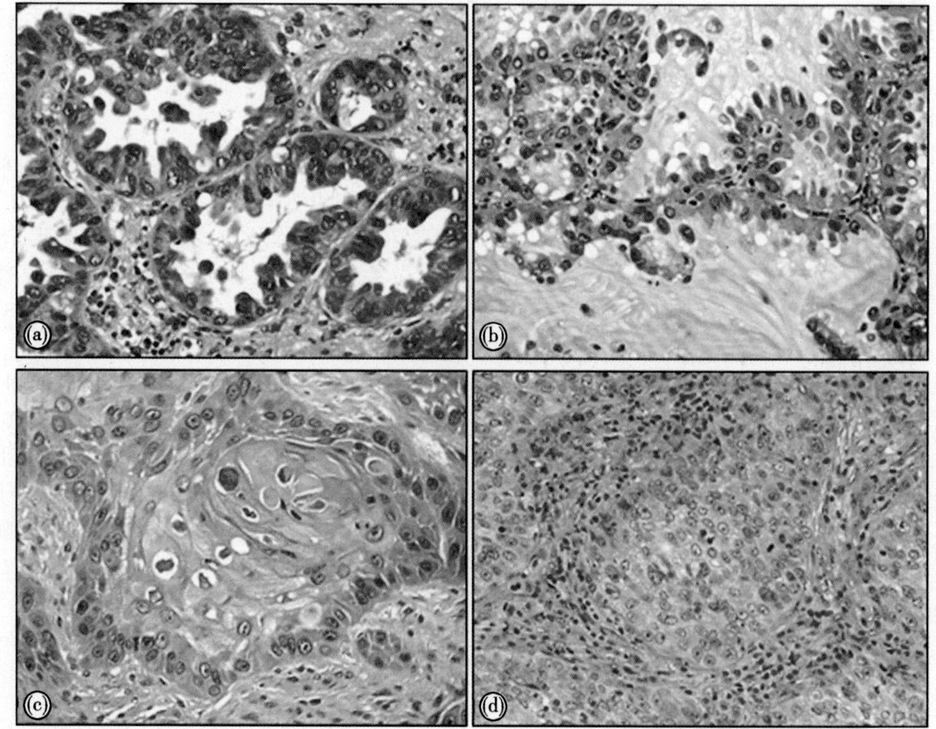

图 84-2 NSCLC 主要形式的组织病理学特征。(a)具有腺泡模式的浸润性腺癌。(b)附壁型(非浸润性)腺癌。(c)角化型鳞状细胞癌。(d)大细胞癌

行免疫组化分析。对于非角化型肿瘤需要进行免疫组化检查从而与手术切除标本无免疫表型的大细胞癌及其他类型的低分化 NSCLC 进行区分。对于此类肿瘤，可用 p40、p63 和/或 CK5 或 CK5/6 的弥漫性阳性染色证实它们的鳞状表型并分类为非角化 SCC。同时 TTF-1 和黏蛋白染色均应为阴性或仅为局部阳性(<10%的细胞具有微弱染色)。

大约 70%的肺鳞状细胞癌是中央型肺癌[30]。肿瘤体积可以很大，并且继发于坏死的中央空洞的形成常在大体检查中发现[31]。

腺鳞癌

肺腺鳞癌的特点是同时存在鳞状细胞癌和腺癌，且每种肿瘤成分至少占 10%[32]。它们占肺癌的 0.4%~4%，通常位于肺部周围，可以有中央瘢痕。扩散和转移的途径与其他非小细胞肺癌相似。

肉瘤样癌

肺部肉瘤样癌是一组分化差的 NSCLC，包含肉瘤或肉瘤样(梭形和/或巨细胞)分化成分。目前，已经鉴定出 5 种变型：多形性癌、梭形细胞癌、巨细胞癌、癌肉瘤和肺母细胞瘤[33,34]。肉瘤样癌是罕见的肿瘤(占肺肿瘤的 0.3%~1.3%)[33,35]。

大细胞癌

大细胞癌是一种缺乏鳞状细胞癌、腺癌或小细胞癌细胞学、结构和免疫组织化学特征的未分化癌(图 84-2d)。因此，大细胞肺癌的诊断是一种排除诊断。大细胞癌占所有肺癌的 10%左右，代表着一个形态学谱系，大多数大细胞癌由胞质丰富、细胞核大且核仁显著的大细胞组成(图 84-2d)[31]。2004 年 WHO 分类列出了大细胞癌的四种组织学变型：大细胞神经内分泌癌(LCNEC)、基底细胞癌、淋巴上皮瘤样癌、透明细胞癌和含有横纹肌样成分的大细胞癌。然而，在修订的 WHO 分类中，LCNEC 被重新划分为神经内分泌癌，并且基底细胞癌被归类为 SCC 的变体。具有透明细胞或含有横纹肌样成分的纯大细胞癌非常罕见。如果在大细胞癌中检测到这些成分，则应在描述中呈现。

神经内分泌癌

肺神经内分泌肿瘤约占所有肺癌的 15%。它们由神经内分泌分化的恶性细胞组成，代表广泛的肿瘤类型：包括低度恶性的典型类癌、中度恶性的不典型类癌以及高级别的 LCNEC 和 SCLC(图 84-3a~c)。

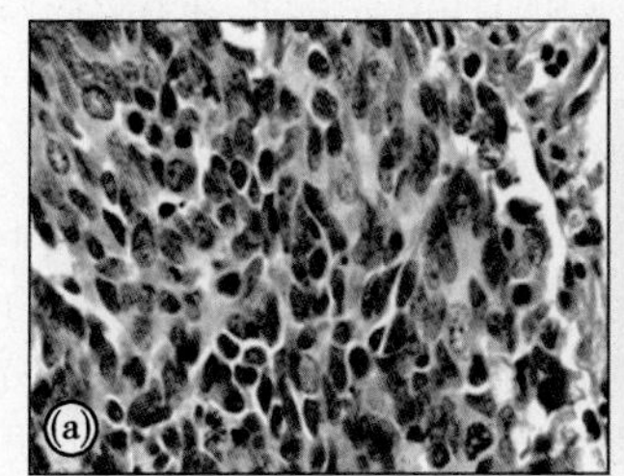

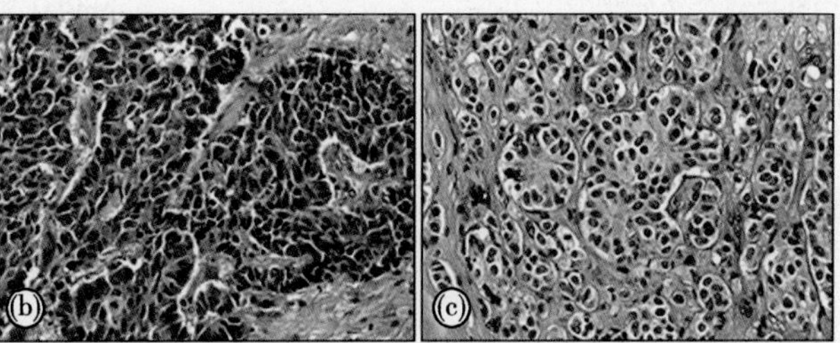

图 84-3　肺的神经内分泌肿瘤。(a)SCLC。(b)LNEC。(c)典型的类癌

类癌

类癌肿瘤的特征在于器官生长模式，均匀的细胞学特征和神经内分泌标记物的免疫组化阳性，例如嗜铬粒蛋白和突触素(图 84-3c)[36]。类癌根据其临床行为和病理特征分为典型和不典型两类，不典型类癌具有更多的恶性组织学和临床特征[37]。典型和不典型类癌也分别指低度和中度神经内分泌癌。组织学上，典型类癌显示每 $2mm^2$ 视野少于 2 个核分裂象，且缺乏坏死，而不典型类癌每 $2mm^2$ 视野显示 2~10 个核分裂象，和/或伴有坏死灶[36]。典型类癌均匀分布于整个肺，而不典型类癌更常见于周围肺。与典型类癌相比，不典型类癌体积更大，转移率更高，其生存期显著缩短[38]。就诊时，10%~15%的典型类癌和 40%~50%的不典型类癌已证实有区域性淋巴结转移[36]。

大细胞神经内分泌癌(LCNEC)

这种肿瘤类型是指存在大量含有明显核仁、神经内分泌生长模式、大量核分裂象的大的未分化细胞，并经免疫组化证实具有神经内分泌分化的肿瘤(图 84-3b)。它们通常是周围型的、伴有坏死的结节状肿块。LCNEC 被认为是一种预后与 SCLC 类似的侵袭性恶性肿瘤[39]。复合性 LCNEC 是指伴有其他分化较好的 NSCLC 成分，主要是腺癌的肿瘤。

小细胞肺癌(SCLC)

这种肿瘤类型占全部肺癌的大约 15%，其特征是由小的、具有细颗粒状染色质、核仁缺乏或不明显的上皮样肿瘤细胞组成(图 84-3a)。坏死频繁且广泛，且核分裂象多。没有一个确切的上限来定义多大的细胞为小细胞，但是有人认为细胞的直径大约应为 2 或 3 个小的成熟淋巴细胞大小[40]。光学显微镜下诊断的 SCLC，在电子显微镜下至少 2/3 的病例存在神经内分泌颗粒，并且在大多数(近 90%)病例中，神经内分泌标志物(嗜铬粒和突触素蛋白)免疫组化染色阳性[40,41]。不到 10%的 SCLC 被证实混有 NSCLC 组织学类型，通常是腺癌、鳞状细胞癌或大细胞癌，它们被称为复合性 SCLC。

NSCLC 小活检和细胞学标本的组织学分类

在这些肿瘤样本中，NSCLC 诊断已经集中在一起，而没有关注更具体的组织学分型。最近肺癌病理学的一个主要变化是在小组织学活检和细胞学检查中开发了肺癌病理诊断的标准化标准和术语。除了标准和术语之外，病理学家在肿瘤分类和标本管理方面也存在范式转变，指出需要进行免疫组织化学以进一步对原先被诊断为“非特异性的”(NOS)NSCLC 进行分类。目前，如果 NSCLC 在小组织学活检或细胞学标本中未显示清晰的腺体或鳞状形态，则将其归类为 NSCLC-NOS。对于这些标本推荐有目的的特殊免疫组化标记检查用于更精准的分类。建议使用单个腺癌标志物(即 TTF-1)，单个鳞状标记物(p40 或 p63)和/或黏蛋白染色[42]。对腺癌标志物或黏蛋白呈阳性的肿瘤被归类为 NSCLC，支持为腺癌。对 SCC 标志物阳性伴腺癌标志物阴性的肿瘤被归类为 NSCLC，支持为 SCC。细胞学也是一种强大的诊断工具，在大多数情况下可以准确地对

NSCLC进行分型,并且如果将细胞学样品制备成细胞块,则可以容易地获得免疫组化结果。

临床表现

临床症状

一些患者表现为胸部影像偶然发现的无症状病灶。然而,大多数肺癌被发现是由于出现新的症状或体征,或症状体征的恶化。尽管没有一组体征或症状是肺癌的特异性表现,但它们可以分为四类:局部肿瘤生长和胸内扩散导致的表现、远处转移导致的表现、非特异性全身症状和副肿瘤综合征。

局部肿瘤生长和胸内扩散的表现

原发肿瘤的体征和症状取决于肿瘤的部位和大小。中心型肿瘤引起咳嗽、局限性哮鸣音、咯血,以及气道阻塞和阻塞性肺疾的症状和体征,如呼吸困难、发热和排痰性咳嗽。偶尔,大的肿瘤团块,通常是鳞癌和大细胞癌,形成空洞,表现为恶性肺脓肿。外周型肿瘤当体积小且局限于肺内时,更易是无症状性的,偶尔有明显的咳嗽和胸膜炎性胸痛。

肺癌的胸内扩散,无论是通过直接蔓延或经淋巴道转移,均与各种体征和综合征相关。纵隔侵犯可能表现为模糊的、定位不明确的胸痛,合并神经卡压、血管阻塞和/或食管压迫或侵犯的其他表现。纵隔受累引起的最常见神经障碍之一是喉返神经卡压引起的声音嘶哑。左侧喉返神经由于胸内行程更长,较右侧喉返神经更易导致声嘶[43]。肿瘤所致的食管压迫也可造成吞咽困难。气管食管瘘或支气管食管瘘的发生率为0.16%,可以表现为剧烈咳嗽,尤其在吞咽时发生的剧烈咳嗽,和反复发作的吸入性肺炎[44]。膈神经受侵在早期与呃逆相关,更晚时产生偏侧膈肌的麻痹和上抬,以及由此所致的呼吸困难。

肺癌纵隔内蔓延所致的主要血管综合征是上腔静脉(superior vena cava,SVC)综合征,最常由于肿瘤对静脉的侵犯和外压引起,但腔内血栓形成也能导致[45]。肺癌在所有SVC综合征病例中占65%~90%,而在这些肺癌病例中,原发肿瘤85%位于右肺,主要是右上叶或右支气管主干。在开始治疗之前建立组织学诊断很重要,因为SVC综合征不再被认为是放射治疗的紧急情况。

存在肺尖肿瘤时,可以由于局部侵犯下臂丛(C8和T1神经根)、星状神经节和胸壁而逐渐出现明显的典型Pancoast综合征[下臂丛神经病变、霍纳综合征(Horner syndrome)和肩痛][46]。肿瘤可以因侵犯第一或第二肋、第一或第二椎体和其他神经根而引起症状。放射学征象是非对称性肺尖帽或肺尖肿物的表现。大多数肺上沟癌是鳞癌,尽管也可以是腺癌,甚至1%~2%的病例为SCLC,这强调了建立组织学诊断的重要性。

大约15%的肺癌患者在初次就诊时有胸膜受累,50%的播散性肺癌患者在患病期间发生胸腔积液。胸腔积液可能导致呼吸困难,咳嗽或胸痛[47]。已经提出了许多胸腔积液的发病机制,尽管已有证据显示肺癌肺切除术时胸腔冲洗液中存在恶性细胞对生存有不利影响,但细胞学标本中存在恶性细胞与否并不显著影响生存转归[48]。

心包受累起因于肿瘤的直接延伸或由纵隔和心外膜淋巴管逆行扩散。肺癌是心包转移最常见的一个来源[49]。临床发现包括心律失常、胸部X线片上心影增大和少见的心脏压塞(表84-4)。

表 84-4 局部肿瘤生长和胸内扩散导致的临床表现

临床表现	频率/%	
	SCLC	NSCLC
咳嗽	50~76	40
呼吸困难	34~40	30~40
胸痛	35~36	25~40
咯血	15~23	15~35
肺炎	21~25	13~24
SVC综合征	12	<10
胸腔积液	10~15	15
Pancoast综合征	罕见	3
心包积液	少见	罕见

NSCLC,非小细胞肺癌(non-small cell lung cancer);SCLC,小细胞肺癌(small cell lung cancer);SVC,上腔静脉(superior vena cava)。

远处转移的表现

约60%的SCLC患者和30%~40%的NSCLC患者表现为Ⅳ期转移性疾病。尽管肺癌可以转移至几乎所有器官部位,临床上明显的最常见血行播散部位是中枢神经系统(central nervous system,CNS)、骨、肝和肾上腺。许多此类患者没有可归因于特定远处转移部位的症状。

全身性、非特异性体征和症状

如表84-5所示,全身性、非特异性体征和症状在SCLC和NSCLC中均常见。纳差发生率为30%,很可能这一数字是被低估的,实际发生率更高。体重减轻通常但不总是伴随着纳差出现,发生于约半数的患者,1/3的患者全身乏力。发热和贫血更少发生,见于不足20%的患者。在肺癌患者中,发热通常不认为是副肿瘤综合征;如果出现发热,通常与经证实的感染(如阻塞性肺炎)或肝转移相关。

表 84-5 就诊时全身效应导致的临床表现

临床表现	频率/%	
	SCLC	NSCLC
纳差	30	30
体重减轻(≥10磅)	35~52	45~52
疲乏	23~42	35
发热	11~15	7~16
贫血	11~15	16~20

NSCLC,非小细胞肺癌;SCLC,小细胞肺癌。

副肿瘤综合征

表84-6列出了21种副肿瘤综合征,它们导致了原发肿瘤或其转移之外的体征和症状。副肿瘤综合征的主要类型包括:内分泌、神经、皮肤和骨骼肌肉,以及心血管和血液的表现[50]。

表 84-6 肺癌主要副肿瘤表现

综合征	临床频率/%	备注
内分泌综合征		
抗利尿激素异常	5~10	主要为 SCLC
心房利钠因子	?	—
异位 ACTH	3~7	最常见于 SCLC
恶性肿瘤高钙血症	10	最常见于鳞癌
男性乳房发育症	6	更常见于大细胞癌
其他激素	—	无显著临床表现
神经综合征		
Eaton-Lambert	6	主要为 SCLC
亚急性感觉神经病变	罕见	主要为 SCLC
亚急性小脑变性	罕见	主要为 SCLC
边缘性脑病	罕见	主要为 SCLC
视觉副肿瘤综合征	罕见	主要为 SCLC
亚急性坏死性脊髓病	罕见	主要为 SCLC
皮肤/肌肉骨骼综合征		
肥大性肺性骨关节病	<10	更常见于腺癌
黑棘皮症	罕见	—
胼胝症	罕见	—
皮肌炎	罕见	—
心血管/血液综合征		
非细菌性血栓性心内膜炎	少见	更常见于腺癌
游走性血栓静脉炎	少见	更常见于腺癌
高凝状态	10~15	肾
肾小球肾炎	罕见	—
肾病综合征	罕见	—

ACTH,促肾上腺皮质激素(adrenocorticotropic hormone);SCLC,小细胞肺癌(small cell lung cancer)。

内分泌综合征

抗利尿激素异常分泌综合征

精氨酸升压素过量分泌伴低钠血症是抗利尿激素异常分泌综合征(syndrome of inappropriate secretion of anti-diuretic hormone,SIADH)的特征性表现。主要的临床发现是低钠血症伴随着相应的血清和细胞外液低渗;肾脏持续外排钠;缺乏体液容量不足的临床证据;尿渗透压高于平时血浆渗透压对应的合适水平,即尿未被最大限度地稀释;并且肾脏、肾上腺和甲状腺的功能正常。SIADH 可以由各种恶性肿瘤导致,而 SCLC 是最常见的(可多达 15%,尽管其中仅有 1/3 有症状)。限水经常足以控制症状,直至全身抗肿瘤治疗开始,后者通常可以改善或消除低钠血症。少见情况下需要输注盐水、使用呋塞米或给予去甲金霉素。

异位促肾上腺皮质激素综合征

肾上腺皮质功能亢进伴异位促肾上腺皮质激素(adrenocorticotropic hormone,ACTH)产生(>200pg/ml)是肺癌中常见的激素综合征,尤其是在 SCLC 中。血清 ACTH 水平在 30%~72%的 SCLC 患者中升高,皮质醇分泌失调见于 51%的 SCLC 患者,但仅有 3%~7%的 SCLC 患者有相应症状。伴异位 ACTH 综合征的患者通常符合肺癌患者的人口学特征,罕有典型的类库欣症表征向心性肥胖或满月脸。异位促肾上腺皮质激素综合征与化疗并发症和 SCLC 患者的生存期缩短有关[51]。

其他激素产生

肺癌(尤其是 SCLC)时水平升高的其他激素包括降钙素、生长因素、催乳素、血清素(5-羟色胺)、胰岛素、促胃液素和促黑色素细胞因子。然而,在大部分病例中,这些激素异常只有很小的临床意义。

恶性肿瘤高钙血症

很久以来,我们已知道癌症患者即使无明确的骨转移,也可存在高钙血症。据报道高达 30%的癌症患者在其病程中会出现高钙血症。随着双膦酸盐类在多发性骨髓瘤或乳腺癌患者中的广泛使用,这一发生率可能正在下降,尽管尚缺乏相关数据。高钙血症产生进行性的精神损害(包括昏迷)和肾衰竭。这些并发症在癌症患者中是极其常见的终末事件。检测到癌症患者的高钙血症预示其预后极差;约 50%的此类患者在 30 天内死亡。甲状旁腺激素相关蛋白已被证明是大多数恶性高钙血症的原因。鳞癌是肺癌中最常出现高钙血症的类型,而 SCLC 罕有发生。当有效治疗基础肿瘤时,高钙血症是完全可逆的,同时双膦酸盐类可以作为特异性治疗手段使用[52]。denosumab,一种结合骨吸收介质 RANKL 的单克隆抗体,最近被批准用于治疗对双膦酸盐治疗无效的难治性恶性肿瘤高钙血症[53]。

神经综合征

肺癌相关神经综合征的发生可能是由于自身免疫机制,通常见于 SCLC 患者。其症状可能在诊断肿瘤数月前出现,或是肿瘤复发的首发征象。神经症状的严重程度与肿瘤大小无关,尽管有致残症状,但在死亡前仍可能未发现原发性恶性病变。大多数此种情况不是肿瘤特异性的。

Eaton-Lamber 综合征

这是一种重症肌无力样异常,最初认为其与 SCLC 相关,后来发现其他肿瘤亦可出现。此综合征以近端肢体肌无力和肌肉疲劳为特征,是由于形成了一种 IgG 抗体,此种抗体针对肿瘤和神经接头均存在的钙通道。已确定一种 1 型抗神经元核自身抗体(type 1 anti-neuronal nuclear auto anti-body,ANNA-1,亦称"抗-Hu")是神经自身免疫标志物,与 SCLC(97%)和其他副肿瘤神经异常高度相关[54]。

亚急性感觉神经病

这是 SCLC 最特征性的外周神经病变。临床症状的特征为各类感觉的进行性损害,首先是反射消失和显著的感觉性共济失调,继而在数周后稳定,可在诊断 SCLC 数月前出现。可伴有更广泛的副肿瘤脑炎证据,如小脑脑干功能障碍和痴呆。

皮肤和肌肉骨骼综合征

杵状指和肥大性肺性骨关节病(hypertrophic pulmonary osteoarthropathy,HPO)也是肺癌的主要副肿瘤综合征,最常见于

NSCLC。杵状指比 HPO 更常见,后者通常类似于类风湿关节炎,其特征在于对称性多关节炎(通常涉及脚踝、手腕和膝盖)、长骨的增生性骨膜炎和手和脚的神经血管变化。肺癌占成人 HPO 病例的 80%以上[55]。放射性核素骨扫描通常显示受累长骨的远端摄取增高,并且此结果可能被平片上新骨形成的证据所证实,而脊柱不受损害。HPO 的发病通常是急性的,可先于癌症的诊断。已提出了各种基础机制,包括巨核细胞或绕过肺毛细血管网的血小板凝块释放血小板衍生生长因子。当肿瘤在治疗后缓解时,此综合征可消退。尚未发现有效的治疗,包括阿司匹林或非甾体抗炎药均未被证明有效。

心血管和血液表现

动脉血栓形成和更常见的静脉血栓形成,是癌症频繁出现的并发症,有时也预示隐匿性肿瘤。并且,新的抗肿瘤治疗增高了血栓形成的风险。肺癌最值得关注的两个心血管表现是非细菌性血栓性心内膜炎(non-bacterial thrombotic endocarditis, NBTE)和静脉血栓栓塞(venous thromboembolism, VTE)。

诊断与分期技术

准确的临床分期包括无创和有创策略。无创性方法包括痰细胞学和影像学;最常用的是胸片,计算机断层扫描(computed tomography, CT)和正电子发射断层扫描(positron emission tomography, PET)。对于纵隔或脊柱病变,考虑磁共振成像(magnetic resonance imaging, MRI)。有创检查包括支气管镜检查、CT 或超声(ultrasound, US)引导的细针抽吸活检(fine-needle aspiration, FNA)或活检、淋巴结活检以及纵隔镜或胸腔镜检查。对于临床或影像学证据支持广泛疾病(extensive disease, ED)的患者,需要采用创伤最小的方式建立诊断和临床分期。通过 FNA 或活组织检查获得的细胞学或组织学证据通常足以证实对 N3 或 M1 疾病的怀疑。积液患者可采用胸腔穿刺或心包穿刺以评估恶性细胞学。对肿瘤的分子评估以更好的选择化疗方案可能需要组织标本。因此,在某些情况下需要重复活检。

无创检查

痰细胞学

痰、气管镜灌洗、气管镜刷片和细针抽吸活检标本的细胞学检查有很高的诊断率,但是各项检查的阳性预测值、阴性预测值和诊断的准确性与取材、样本的保存、制片质量及诊断者的经验密切相关。痰细胞学检查操作简便、特异性可高达 99%。但其敏感性在中心型肺癌仅 70%左右,在周围型肺癌低于 50%。要提高痰细胞学检查敏感性,通常需要收集三次痰标本。临床工作中,对大多数病例获得诊断要采取创伤较大的检查方法。

影像学检查

肺癌通常先进行胸片检查。CT 扫描、PET 扫描和偶尔施行的 MRI(脑 MRI 现已经成为肺癌术前分期的常规方法-译者注)用于对已知的或可疑的病变进行分期和治疗反应监测。

胸片

后前位和侧位胸片仍然是发现肺癌患者的最简便的方法,且普及、价格便宜、辐射剂量低,但是大多数病例发现时已经处于进展期。标准的胸片能够发现直径小至 3mm 的病变,但是,除非直径大于 5mm,否则未被怀疑的结节常常容易被漏诊。伴随的肺不张、阻塞性肺炎、肺脓肿、支气管肺炎、胸膜反应、肋骨受侵、胸腔积液或纵隔淋巴结显著肿大,胸片都可能检出,这些都能增加对原发肺部恶性肿瘤的怀疑程度。

胸片可以检出异常的肺结节。尚无根据影像学表现判断病变属于良性的绝对标准,但 2 年内体积无变化以及特定形式的钙化(多发灶状、中央密集巢状、爆米花状或层状"牛眼"征)提示良性病变。然而,一些肿瘤,例如细支气管肺泡癌和典型的类癌有时也可稳定 2 年或更长时间没有变化[56]。

CT 检查

作为一项更进一步的检查,CT 扫描仍然是评估可疑或已知肺癌、纵隔及其相关转移病变最有效的无创技术。但是,CT 扫描对于纵隔淋巴结转移的准确性变化较大,其敏感性介于 51%~95%。准确性变化如此之大的原因是淋巴结异常的诊断标准的不同,而这些标准则源于淋巴结的大小和形状,不同 CT 扫描机以及淋巴结密度不均。通常将短径≥1cm 作为异常淋巴结肿大的标准。8%~15%的患者,其 CT 扫描纵隔淋巴结未见肿大,淋巴结短径≤1cm,而手术证实纵隔淋巴结转移。纵隔淋巴结直径大于 2cm,90%以上病例存在转移。纵隔淋巴结直径 1.5~2cm,50%以上病例存在转移,纵隔淋巴结直径 1~1.5cm,15%~30%的病例存在转移。对于纵隔淋巴结转移,CT 扫描的阴性预测值为 85%~92%。由于这些原因,许多医学中心已经在使用 PET-CT 成像。

MRI

MRI 并不常规用于肺癌患者的评估,但其与 CT 扫描相比有着特殊的优势。由于其具有较好的显示神经和血管结构的能力,使用 MRI 评估邻近神经和血管结构的肿瘤可能比 CT 扫描更加准确。MRI 用于评估肺上沟瘤患者最有价值。

PET

在过去的数年中,使用 18F 脱氧葡萄糖(FDG)的 PET 扫描越来越广泛地被应用于肺癌的诊断、分期和治疗监测。这项检查能够检出糖代谢水平升高的区域,而糖代谢升高正是肺癌的特点。商业化的 PET 扫描机在其轴向视野的中央部分空间分辨率能够达到 4.5~6.0mm,因此基于 FDG 的摄取增加甚至可以检测直径≤1cm 的病变。尽管最初被认为是肺部肿瘤定性和分期的可靠的非侵入性手段,但是一些局限性已逐渐显现出来。许多炎症过程,例如脓肿和活动性肉芽肿疾病,以及诸如放疗后存在的低氧条件,可能引起高 FDG 摄取并导致假阳性结果。治疗引起的高代谢炎性改变也能对鉴别治疗反应与肿瘤残存造成困难。假阴性结果主要见于一些糖代谢水平较低的肿瘤(类癌和细支气管肺泡癌)和较小的肿瘤,后者是由于目前 PET 扫描机空间分辨率的限制[57]。

集成 PET-CT

PET 对具有准确的空间位置的局灶性病变提供了不精确的信息。因而,即便 PET 和 CT 扫描的结果在视觉上能够融合起来,病变的准确位置有时候还是很难确定。为了克服这个缺点,出现了融合的 PET-CT[58]。最近的研究发现,融合的 PET-CT 能够改善非小细胞肺癌诊断的准确性。与单独的 CT($P=0.001$)、单独的 PET($P=0.001$)或 PET 与 CT 的视觉融合($P=$

0.013）相比，PET-CT 对肿瘤分期的准确性显著提高；与单独的 PET（$P=0.013$）相比，PET-CT 对淋巴结分期的准确性也显著提高[58]。在可切除的 NSCLC 患者中，PET-CT 对纵隔分期仍然不够准确，纵隔淋巴结的病理评估仍然是金标准方法[59]。随机临床试验（RCT）表明 PET-CT 有助于术前评估远处转移，从而避免不必要的手术[60]。

有创性检查

获取组织标本可用于病理学诊断、分子检测和基因检测。在大多数情况下，细针抽吸活检标本并不能满足检测所需，建议进行核心活组织检查。支气管内和中央型肺癌通常采用支气管镜进行诊断，而外周病变则采用 CT 或超声引导的活检。在许多情况下，活组织检查的目标是明确疾病的诊断和分期。例如，当对侧淋巴结会影响 N 分期时应当考虑对侧淋巴结活检，肝脏病变的活检能够进一步证实原发肿瘤并有助于准确的 M 分期。另外，必须考虑原发性肿瘤与其转移灶之间基因表达的潜在差异，并避免骨转移病变的活组织检查，因为脱钙过程可能改变肿瘤的基因表达。

细针抽吸活检

经胸经皮穿刺活检（transthoracic percutaneous needle biopsy，TPNB）显著提高了胸内肿瘤的病理诊断能力。在 CT 或超声引导下，穿刺针可以达到肺内、纵隔、腹腔以及腹膜后某些其他技术难以触及的位置，从而获得病变组织标本。该手术在局部麻醉下使用小规格针进行抽吸或活组织检查。穿刺过程应用细径穿刺针可在局麻下完成，穿刺针吸到的组织及细胞最好能在细胞病理学者的协助下立即完成处理。在许多医学中心，该过程均有细胞病理学者在床旁协助处理标本，如果穿刺组织量或细胞量不足，可立即重复穿刺一次。已经证明 TPNB 在建立最终诊断方面有 90%以上的确诊率，假阳性率低于 1%，而假阴性率 23%～29%[61]。

纤维支气管镜检查

纤维支气管镜检查（fiberoptic bronchoscopy，FOB）是肺部肿瘤患者一项必需的标准检查，对于判定病变在支气管内浸润的范围起着至关重要的作用。FOB 可以观察声门上、声门、气管、支气管以及更亚段的支气管情况。通过观察病变与隆突的距离，病变在支气管树中的位置，以及发现未被检查出的隐性病灶提示多发肿瘤从而判定肿瘤 T 分期。90%支气管镜下能够观察到的病变最终可以获得准确的病理组织学诊断。对于中央型的病变，通过支气管镜下针吸、灌洗、刷检等细胞学检查以及结合病变部位活检病理检查确诊率可达 95%以上。而周围型肺癌支气管镜下无法直接观察到，但仍可通过刷检以及支气管肺泡灌洗（BAL）等细胞学检查方法，达到 50%～60%的确诊率。此外经支气管镜针吸细胞学技术（transbronchial fine-needle aspiration，TBNA），也极大地提高诊断效率。

经支气管细针针吸活检

经支气管细针针吸活检（TBNA）技术是由 Wang 与 Terry[62]最先在纤维支气管镜下应用。现在已广泛应用于支气管内以及肺周围病变的组织获取，同时与传统的诊断方法（灌洗、刷检及活检）联合使用极大地提升了肺部病变诊断的能力。在透视的条件下进行 TBNA 可以提高定位病变的准确度，有助于 TBNA 的更好完成。评价纵隔肿大淋巴结性质是 TBNA 最重要的一个临床应用，其灵敏度与特异度分别为 14%～50%与 96%～100%。因此 TBNA 为阴性的结果仍需要最终的手术来证实，但出现假阳性概率却极低[63]。

支气管镜检查的进展

线性超声内镜的出现为肺癌患者提供了一项新的诊断方法。经食管内镜超声引导下细针针吸活检（transoesophageal endoscopic ultrasoundguided FNA，EUS-FNA）以及经气管超声内镜引导下细针针吸活检（endobronchail ultrasound-guided transbronchail，needle aspiration，EBUS-TBNA）均具有微创的优点，可以对纵隔淋巴结以及中央型肺癌进行针吸组织操作。相关报道表明 EBUS-FNA 比 TBNA 具有更高的敏感性，EUS 与 EBUS 联合可以在微创的条件下对疑诊肺癌的患者进行几乎所有的纵隔淋巴结分期。这些新的诊断技术可作为疑似肺癌患者纵隔分期的替代方法[64]。电磁导航诊断支气管镜是结合了虚拟支气管镜、三维 CT 影像以及导向探头辅助用于肺部病变组织活检的一项新技术，但其诊断病变的效果以及安全性仍在进行多中心临床研究进行验证[65]。

纵隔镜检查

经颈部纵隔镜检查是侵入性中纵隔到气管周围和隆突下淋巴结活检的最好方法。纵隔镜检查的适应证是术前 CT 扫描发现纵隔内有大于 1cm 的肿大淋巴结的患者。在这些已被证实的肺癌患者中，淋巴结转移的可能性超过 7%。如果淋巴结增大到 1.5～2cm 甚至更大，那么淋巴结转移的风险将超过 30%。经颈部纵隔镜检查的准确性达 80%～90%，假阴性率为 10%～12%。在所有淋巴结中，最不容易取样的是隆突下淋巴结，并且它也很难定性，所以，在绝大多数患者中需要完全将其切除活检才能定性。标准纵隔镜是不能检查主动脉下和主肺动脉窗淋巴结的[66]。扩展的颈部纵隔镜检查（标准纵隔镜检查的一种改良方法）对左上叶病变的分期有一定的作用。目前已经开展的标准纵隔镜下切开可以在水平面上从前面一直切到无名动脉和主动脉，在横断面上可以切到主肺动脉窗水平。起初被 McNeil 和 Chamberlain 命名的“前纵隔镜检查”可以通过第二、第三或者第四前间隙（移除或者不移除一小部分邻近的软骨）直接观察前纵隔。对于右侧病变，这种方式可以检查到近侧的肺动脉和上腔静脉的区域。对于左侧病变，这种方式可以检查到主动脉下和主动脉侧面的区域。

胸腔镜检查

胸腔镜和电视辅助胸腔镜（thoracoscopy and video-assisted thoracoscopic surgery，VATS）检查有很广泛的应用范围，包括切除技术。VATS 技术用于许多胸部疾病，其在肺癌的评估和管理方面的作用不断发展。目前，它被广泛用于胸膜肿瘤和胸腔积液的评估和治疗中，以及一些不明确性质的肺结节的诊断中，并且在纵隔淋巴结分期方面起到对标准纵隔镜检查的互补作用。目前，VATS 已经被很多医院接受成为切除周围型早期肺癌的一种手术方式[67]。

手术分期

手术分期使我们有机会经组织学证实肿瘤在大体上和镜下的侵犯范围。外科医师负责实施完全淋巴结清扫或淋巴结取样，这是开胸手术的必需组成部分。手术清除淋巴结并按其在区域淋巴结图上的分区位置给予标志（图 84-4）。

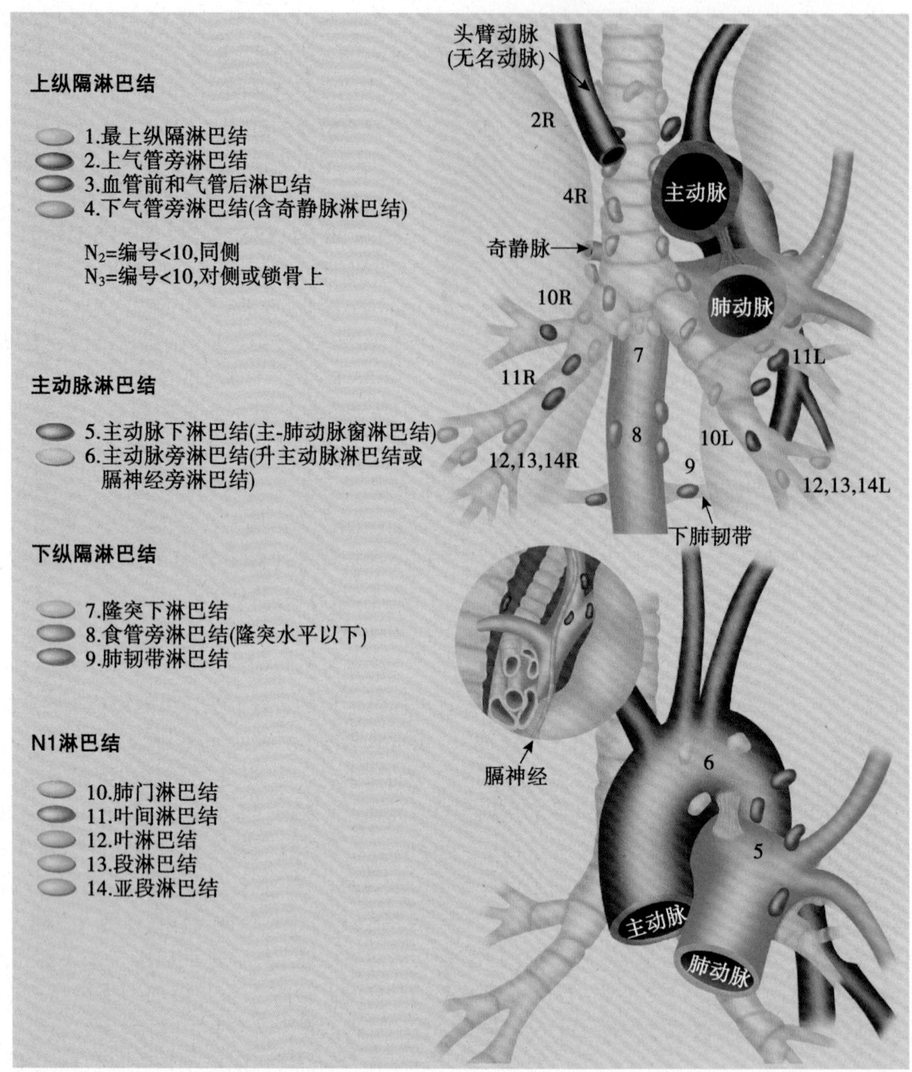

图 84-4 肺癌分期中的区域淋巴结分区。淋巴结的位置及其被分配的数字由外科医师在手术时决定。改编自参考文献 68

癌症的筛查和早期发现

由于早期的、局限性的病变的症状隐匿且不特异,它们常常被认为是吸烟引起的。当患者寻求医学处理的时候,疾病常常已经进展,因此只有不到 30% 的病例能够手术切除,并且总的 5 年生存率小于<17%。显然,理想的目标是在更易治疗的阶段对癌症进行筛查和早期发现。

20 世纪 70 年代,美国国立癌症研究院(NCI)资助了三项独立的随机临床试验来评估肺癌筛查在男性吸烟者中的效能(45 岁及以上,每天至少吸 1 包烟)[69]。到 1978 年,共有 31 360 名患者入组,这三项研究的最终结果均未能证明能够降低疾病特异性死亡率(disease-specific mortality)[70]。

低辐射剂量螺旋 CT(LDCT)的引入重新引起了医学界对高危人群早期肺癌筛查的兴趣[71]。NCI 随后资助了全国肺部筛查试验(NLST),该试验在 2002 年至 2004 年期间在 33 个医疗中心招募了 53 454 名肺癌高危人群。符合条件的参与者年龄在 55~74 岁之间,吸烟史至少为 30 包年,包括在随机分组前 15 年内戒烟的重度吸烟者。对入组人群随机分组进行每年一次的 LDCT 或者胸片筛查,连续三年。该临床试验发现 LDCT 筛查组的受试者肺癌特异性死亡率降低 20%(95% *CI*, 6.8~26.7; P=0.004)[72]。美国预防服务工作组(USPSTF)建议对年龄在 55~80 岁之间且至少有 30 包年吸烟史的无症状成人进行年度 LDCT 肺癌筛查[73]。

分期

分期是为了确定病变的范围,目的是将处于疾病同一阶段的患者进行分类,以便对其分析、治疗、判断预后。肺癌的分期也适用于由其他原发性肺恶性肿瘤引起的一系列疾病。准确的分期对判断手术的可能性、选择合适的治疗策略、预测生存以及提供具有可比性的结尾数据而言是至关重要的。

准确的分期依赖于获得的临床信息、手术前的评价和在后续疾病进程中的准确评价:临床诊断分期(c),手术评估分期(s),术后病理分期(p),治疗后再分期(r)和尸检分期(a)。

NSCLC 分期

目前第七版 AJCC 和 UICC 肺癌分期系统于 2009 年更新,基于 1990 年至 2000 年接受治疗的 67 725 例病例,来自 19 个国家的 46 个来源[74]。这一修订进一步改善了 TNM(肿瘤、淋巴结和远处转移)分期与预后和治疗的一致性(表 84-7~表 84-9)。

表 84-7 TNM 定义

原发肿瘤	
TX	原发肿瘤不能评价;或痰、支气管冲洗液找到癌细胞,但影像学或支气管镜无可视肿瘤
T0	无原发性肿瘤的证据
Tis	原位癌
T1	肿瘤最大径≤3cm,周围为肺或脏层胸膜包绕,气管镜检查肿瘤没有累及叶支气管[a] 近端以上位置(即没有累及主支气管)
	T1a 肿瘤最大径≤2cm[a]
	T1b 肿瘤最大径>2cm 且≤3cm
T2	肿瘤最大径>3cm 且≤7cm;或具有以下任何特征的肿瘤:
	• 累及隆突远端≥2cm 的主支气管
	• 累及脏层胸膜
	• 肿瘤扩展到肺门区伴肺不张或阻塞性肺炎,但不累及全肺
	T2a 肿瘤最大径>3cm 且≤5cm
	T2b 肿瘤最大径>5cm 且≤7cm
T3	肿瘤最大径>7cm 或直接侵犯下述部位之一者:胸壁(包括上沟瘤)、膈肌、纵隔胸膜、壁层心包;肿瘤位于距隆突 2cm 以内的支气管,但未侵及隆突;全肺的肺不张或阻塞性炎症
T4	任何大小的肿瘤直接侵犯了下述部位之一者:纵隔、心脏、大血管、气管、食管、椎体、隆突;原发肿瘤同侧不同肺叶出现卫星结节
区域淋巴结(N)	
NX	区域淋巴结不能评价
N0	没有区域淋巴结转移
N1	转移至同侧支气管淋巴结和/或同侧肺门淋巴结;肿瘤直接侵犯肺内淋巴结
N2	转移至同侧纵隔和/或隆突下淋巴结
N3	转移至对侧纵隔、肺门淋巴结,同侧或对侧斜角肌或锁骨上淋巴结转移
远处转移(M)	
MX	远处转移不能评价
M0	没有远处转移
M1	存在远处转移
	M1a 原发肿瘤对侧肺叶出现卫星结节及胸膜播散(恶性胸腔积液、胸膜结节或心包积液[b])
	M1b 有远处转移

[a] 对于罕见的浅表肿瘤,无论肿瘤大小,如果其累及范围局限于支气管壁,尽管延伸到主支气管附近,也被分类为 T1a。

[b] 大多数与肺癌相关的胸腔积液是由肿瘤引起的。然而,有少数患者对胸腔积液进行多次细胞病理学检查未显示肿瘤。这时积液一般为非血性的漏出液。当这些因素和临床判断表明积液与肿瘤无关时,应排除积液作为分期因素,患者的肿瘤分期应为 M0。

资料来源:参考文献 75,经 Springer 许可转载。

表 84-8 肺癌分期:TNM 亚组[a]

分期	TNM 亚组	分期	TNM 亚组
0	原位癌	ⅢA	T1a~T3N2M0
ⅠA	T1a~T1b N0M0		T3N1M0
ⅠB	T2a N0M0		T4N0~N1M0
ⅡA	T1a~T2a N1M0	ⅢB	T1a~T4N3M0
	T2b N0M0		T4N2M0
ⅡB	T2bN1M0	Ⅳ	任意 T,任意 N,M1a~M1b
	T3N0M0		

[a] 隐匿性肿瘤并未列入分期,定义为 TxN0M0。

资料来源:参考文献 75,经 Springer 许可转载。

表 84-9 淋巴结的定义

淋巴结分站	解剖标记
N2 淋巴结,均在纵隔胸膜内	
1. 最上端纵隔淋巴结	位于头臂静脉(左侧为无名静脉)上缘水平线以上的淋巴结,头臂静脉在此跨过气管中线升入左侧
2. 上段支气管旁淋巴结	位于主动脉弓上缘切线的水平线和第一组淋巴结下缘之间
3. 血管前和气管后淋巴结	也称 3A 和 3P 组,位于中线的淋巴结视为同侧淋巴结
4. 下段气管旁淋巴结	右侧的下段气管旁淋巴结位于气管中线的右侧,在主动脉弓上缘切线水平和右上叶支气管上缘与主支气管连线之间,纵隔胸膜内。左侧的下段气管旁淋巴结位于气管中线的左侧,在主动脉弓上缘切线水平和左上叶支气管上缘与主支气管连线之间,动脉韧带中间,纵隔胸膜内。为了研究的目的,研究者愿意把下段气管旁淋巴结分为上组(No. 4s)和下组(No. 4i)。上组定义为奇静脉头端的切线与气管连线水平以上,而下组为上组淋巴结界限以下的淋巴结
5. 主动脉下淋巴结(主肺动脉窗)	主动脉下淋巴结位于动脉韧带或主动脉或左肺动脉的侧面,靠近左肺动脉第一分支,位于纵隔胸膜内
6. 动脉旁淋巴结(升主动脉或膈神经)	位于主动脉弓上缘切线以下,升主动脉和主动脉弓或无名动脉的前方及侧面
7. 隆突下淋巴结	位于气管隆突角下方,但不包括肺内动脉或下叶支气管周围淋巴结
8. 食管旁淋巴结(低于隆突)	位于食管壁周围,中线左侧或右侧的淋巴结,但不包括隆突下淋巴结
9. 肺韧带淋巴结	肺韧带以内,包括下肺静脉后壁和低位的淋巴结
N1 淋巴结,均在纵隔胸膜反折远端,脏层胸膜内	
10. 肺门淋巴结	包括近端肺叶,纵隔胸膜返折远端,以及右侧中间端支气管周围的淋巴结。影像学上,肺门阴影可由增大的双侧肺门和叶间淋巴结构成
11. 叶间淋巴结	两叶之间的淋巴结
12. 叶淋巴结	叶支气管远端的淋巴结
13. 段淋巴结	段支气管周围的淋巴结
14. 亚段淋巴结	亚段支气管周围的淋巴结

SCLC 分期

TNM 分期系统最早于 20 世纪 60 年代用于 NSCLC,但却发现其用于 SCLC 时不能提示预后。最大的可能是由于 SCLC 中分期为Ⅰ期、Ⅱ期的太少,而且如果不进行化疗,所有 SCLC 患者的生存期都很短。在一个环磷酰胺和安慰剂对照的临床实验中,美国退伍军人肺癌治疗组(VALG)首次提出把 SCLC 分为两期:他们把患者分为两组,根据病变部位是否能被单个放射野包括在内定义为局限期和广泛期[76]。局限期包括恶性胸腔积液;有远处转移的则都归为广泛期。这种分期方法在临床实验中表现出预后价值,局限期的患者的中位生存时间是广泛期的 2 倍。过去的 20 年中,对局限期的定义限于找到适合做根治性放化疗的患者。

正如 NSCLC,SCLC 的分期也是决定治疗和预后的重要因素。完善分期的主要目的就是确定可以接受根治性放化疗的合适患者。临床上有明确转移的患者(广泛期)不要求对所有潜在转移灶进行完善分期。分期的主要目的是选择治疗方案,由于脑转移是脑部放疗的指证,因此所有的患者都应该做脑部扫描。

肺癌分期的总指南

患者出现了一个新的肺部病灶并且通过病史、体格检查,胸片都未找到转移的证据时,患者应该进行胸部 CT 检查,范围包括肝脏和肾上腺。当临床上怀疑恶性肿瘤为Ⅰ期而需要进行有创性检查以确诊时,可以直接切除肿物达到诊断和治疗的目的。但如果手术范围超过肺叶切除或者患者有手术高危因素,则最好在术前确诊。如果患者需要切除一侧肺,则术前必须确诊为癌症。

体格检查无异常且无症状的患者和那些临床分期Ⅰ期、Ⅱ期和ⅢA 期(N0 或 N1)的患者可进行手术治疗。胸部 CT 提示转移,尤其是 N2 或 N3 的患者,应行包括纵隔镜在内的有创检查。某些情况下也需要做细针抽吸活检。对有可能进行手术治疗的Ⅲ期患者,纵隔淋巴结是决定能否手术的最重要因素。如果影像学检查提示淋巴结增大(最大径>1cm),那么在行开胸术之前需做组织学或细胞学评估。

一旦确诊为 SCLC,应立即寻找转移灶,进而选用合适的治疗策略:化疗或者化放疗。仅有极少数(5%)的 SCLC 患者可采用手术干预,比如极早期的患者,即病变仅限于肺部,无淋巴结和远处转移。

如果病史和体格检查提示转移灶存在,必须对可疑转移区域进行其他无创检查。除胸部CT还包括PET-CT,脑CT或脑MRI,骨扫描,腹部CT(如果胸部CT没有包括肝脏和肾上腺)。

大约10%的肺癌患者在确诊时伴发中枢神经系统的转移,这在SCLC患者中尤其常见。隐匿的脑转移灶在NSCLC中占3%~6%。脑CT发现胸部病灶可切除的患者中约13%存在脑转移,他们当中有21%无明显的神经系统体征。由于隐匿性脑转移的低发生率,尤其是早期患者,不需要常规行脑MRI或CT扫描。脑MRI在诊断无症状脑转移方面敏感性较脑CT高[77,78]。

非小细胞肺癌的治疗

肿瘤分期是非小细胞肺癌最重要的预后因素[79]。手术是Ⅰ期和Ⅱ期肿瘤患者的标准治疗方式。部分选择的Ⅲ期患者也可手术切除,并需要联合术前新辅助化疗(或放化疗)或术后辅助化疗和放疗。局部晚期的Ⅲ期非小细胞肺癌患者联合治疗模式是临床研究的热点领域,将在本章后面进行讨论。Ⅳ期患者的治疗为化疗、姑息性放疗或单纯支持治疗。对于病理明确且不能切除或不可手术的非小细胞肺癌患者,首先要评估根治性同步放化疗方案的可行性。如果出现症状的压迫症状需要缓解,如呼吸道完全阻塞、咯血、上腔静脉压迫、承重骨的疼痛性转移或者出现有症状性的脑转移,主要的治疗应该采用放疗联合或者不联合化疗。如果有证据显示肿瘤已经播散,且不需要放疗缓解的压迫症状则应考虑给予全身化疗,或如果患者的一般状况不适合全身化疗可只进行支持治疗。肺癌的三大主要治疗方式:手术、放疗、化疗会在后面分别论述。小细胞肺癌与非小细胞肺癌虽然都是肺癌,但是两者的治疗模式截然不同,将其在其他章节论述。

手术治疗

术前评估

对于任何一个准备行肺切除术的患者均应接受胸外科医生的术前评估。在专业的胸外科医生的诊治下,肺癌疗效能够得到改善[80]。影响患者肺部切除术式的选择、手术入路和手术步骤的因素有很多。常见的可能增加围术期并发症发生率和死亡率的因素包括:高龄、长期吸烟、心脏疾病、肺功能障碍和全肺切除。另外,东部肿瘤协作组(Eastern Cooperative Oncology Group,ECOG)的PS评分是另一个常见的围术期预后和对积极治疗的耐受能力的评价指标[81]。

手术技术

麻醉的实施

肺部切除术需要在全身麻醉下进行选择性单肺通气。通常首先进行纤维支气管镜检查以确保气管导管的正确放置并检查气道中支气管腔内病变范围以及其他位置未预料到的病变。

切口

有多种外科技术和手术入路被用于肺部肿瘤切除术。关于手术入路和技术的抉择是基于肿瘤的大小、位置以及与其他胸腔内结构的关系;患者的并发症和外科医生的经验也被考虑在内。手术技术的选择包括传统的开胸手术、电视辅助胸腔手术(video-assisted thoracic surgery,VATS)或机器人辅助胸腔手术(robotic-assisted thoracic surgery,RATS)。

后外侧切口(有或无背阔肌切开)通常可获得最佳的胸膜腔暴露,并可以直接触诊半侧胸腔内的所有结构。当病变位于上叶或者两侧均有病变需要探查双侧胸腔时,可采用胸骨正中劈开切口或者"蚌壳样"切口。

VATS已经成为胸外科医生非常成熟的工具[82]。多名研究者已经证明可以在VATS下行解剖学肺叶切除术甚至全肺切除术。有足够的数据表明,与标准的牵开肋骨的开胸手术相比,大量数据表明VATS大大缩短了术后的恢复时间。其他优点包括减少术后漏气、肺炎、心房颤动、住院时间和死亡率。由于这些优势,一些研究者猜测,胸腔镜肺叶切除术后比传统的开胸术后能更好地耐受辅助化疗,从而提高总体存活率(OS)。这些观点尚未被随机临床研究所证实。

机器人技术RATS的出现进一步扩大了无胸廓切开和肋骨牵引的肺切除术适应证,并且RATS肺叶切除术的早期预后表现出很大的潜力[83]。目前,机器人手术的成本相对较高,这项技术是否比传统的电视胸腔镜手术有显著获益还有待观察。

标准手术步骤

全肺切除,即完全切除该侧肺,适用于中心型病变侵及主支气管或主肺动脉、同时位于上叶和下叶的肿瘤。手术多经后外侧切口开胸充分暴露术野。全肺切除术后围术期死亡率约为5%,在一些接受新辅助化放疗的局部晚期患者的研究中,围术期死亡率在2%~26%。右侧全肺切除术被认为是风险最高的肺部手术。心肺相关并发症(肺炎、急性呼吸窘迫综合征、肺不张、误吸、房颤和心肌梗死)是全肺切除术后最常见的并发症,出现于20%~30%的患者中[84~87]。

肺叶切除是肺癌手术最常用的术式。它被认为是肺癌切除的肿瘤学标准,因为这种解剖性切除既可以切除原发肿瘤、伴随的病变和引流区域的淋巴结,同时又保留大部分有功能的肺组织。对于不同分期的肺癌患者来说,根治性肺叶切除和全肺切除的肿瘤相关生存是相同的。肺叶切除需要分离、结扎、切断供给肺叶的动脉和静脉分支以及叶间裂。接近肺叶支气管起源的肿瘤需要采用袖状切除才能获得阴性切缘;这种术式可以在不影响手术效果的情况下尽可能保留功能性肺实质(图84-5)。在部分患者中,支气管袖状切除可以安全、有效地保留肺组织,而且肿瘤相关生存率与全肺切除术后相当[88]。

局部切除术包括段切除、楔形切除和肿物切除术。肺段是根据命名的动脉、静脉和支气管划分的不同解剖区域,尽管肺段的实质边界不明显。每个肺段贡献了5%~6%的肺功能,因此功能性肺实质的丢失远小于肺叶切除术。在分离支气管血管结构后,肺段的肺实质用吻合器分开。肺段切除适用于肺功能不能耐受肺叶切除或者肿瘤最大径小于2cm的患者。对于T1A患者肺段切除和肺叶切除的疗效是否相同尚不清楚,但已经有两个正在进行的随机对照试验尝试回答这个问题。

楔形切除是不需要识别支气管血管解剖标志的部分肺叶切除。这是一种简单快捷的外周病变手术方式。吻合装置被用于移除病变。目的是获得至少与肿瘤大小相当的正常组织边缘。通过激光或电烙术辅助进行的精确局部切除,可以消除

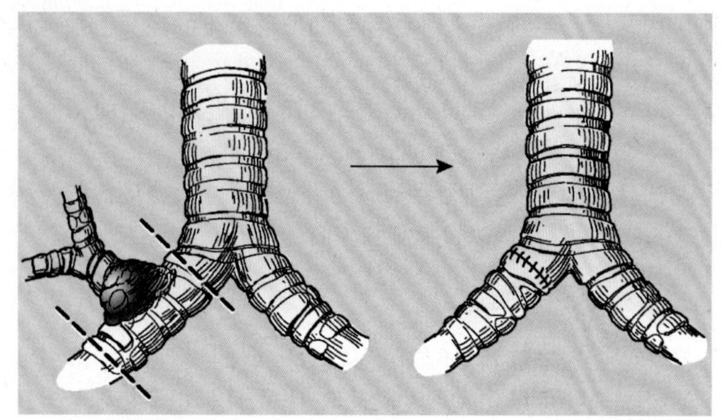

图 84-5 在图示的情况下，标准的右肺上叶切除术，不能完全切除肿瘤，支气管上还有肿瘤残余。此时，行袖状切除，与全肺切除相比，既可以保证切缘阴性，又能保留右肺中下叶

肺组织内更深的病变。直接切开肺组织并移除病变，同时保留周围的肺的手术方式更适用于肺良性病变，或选择切除肺转移灶而不是肺原发肿瘤。

切缘阳性（支气管和肺实质）

行肺切除术时，支气管切缘应当行冰冻病理检查以保证根治性切除。如果切缘有癌残留，则应当尽量采取适当的方式保证切缘干净。但也有部分研究认为，支气管切缘阳性也可以达到一定的生存率。当黏膜内有镜下病变残留或原位癌（CIS）时，5 年生存率可以达到 24%[89]。Shields 等也发现支气管黏膜有癌残留患者的生存率是可观的[90]。虽然如此，在这组病例中，当病变侵出支气管黏膜外或者累及支气管周围淋巴结时，预后较差，这与其他研究的结果相一致[89,91]。

放射治疗

在过去的十年中，肺癌的放射治疗发生了迅速的变化。随着四维（4D）CT 和 FDG-PET 扫描技术的进步，靶区定义的准确性和正常器官的保护都有了很大的提高。现在，我们可以个体化测量肺内肿瘤的活动度。治疗计划系统中算法的优化也实现了根据不同组织的放疗耐受度来给予剂量，同时优化了靶区的剂量分布。通过使用国际辐射单位和测量委员会（ICRU）对体积和剂量的定义，常规实现三维适形放射治疗（3D CRT）。调强适形放疗（IMRT），包括体积调强电弧疗法（VMAT）和立体定向消融放疗（SABR）已在临床上实施，质子疗法也已成为现实。我们还期待将新的生物疗法（包括生物标志物、信号通路靶向治疗和免疫治疗）合理地整合到标准治疗中。

高达 60%的肺癌病例在其治疗过程中需要行放射治疗，这其中 45%的病例使用放疗为初始治疗手段，而 17%的病例需要采用放疗进行姑息治疗[92]。这就意味着在美国，每年接受放疗的肺癌患者高达 10 万以上。我们需要经验丰富的放疗团队来实施放疗，尤其是在综合治疗模式中放疗经验尤为重要，观察结果也显示疗效与放疗医生的经验有着直接关系，当患者接受有经验的医生治疗时，结果明显更好[93,94]。

肺癌的放疗技术及靶区确定

ICRU 对于现代肺癌的放疗定义了一系列重要的靶区：大体肿瘤靶区（gross tumor volume，GTV），临床靶区（clinical target volume，CTV），计划靶区（planning target volume，PTV）和内靶区（internal target volume，ITV）。

大体肿瘤靶区（GTV）

在影像学中可视的病灶范围。FDG-PET 扫描在放疗计划的制订过程中起着非常重要的作用[95]。譬如，第一，它可以减少不同的勾画者之间勾画 GTV 的误差[96]，可以协助判断可疑的纵隔肿物的良恶性、最高标准摄取值（SUV）同时可以预测是否存在转移。第二，FDG-PET 可以分辨出肺不张和肿瘤区域，从而减少正常肺的照射。第三，由于 FDG-PET 可以诊断出远处转移（转移率约为 30%，尤其是在一些病期偏晚的病例），所以有助于选择最佳的治疗模式[97]。

临床靶区（CTV）

CTV 包括可见肿瘤区及微小病灶区。为了将肿瘤包括在 CTV 中并保证准确性达到 95%以上。GTV 到 CTV，在鳞癌外扩 6mm，腺癌外扩 8mm[98]。其他病理类型的肿瘤外扩多少目前尚无定论，目前较为保守的倾向是外扩 8mm。纵隔淋巴结区域的 GTV 到 CTV 的外扩程度尚无一个严格的界定。我们经验性的在受侵淋巴结（转移淋巴结或者 FDG-PET 上阳性的淋巴结）外扩 8mm。临床对 CTV 边缘的调整需要考虑解剖学边界和复发模式。

计划靶区（PTV）

PTV 为 CTV 加摆位误差及靶区活动度。PTV 的定义中涉及了摆位的不确定性和肿瘤的活动。应用不同的技术，或是在不同的治疗单位实施治疗，摆位误差各不相同，所以应该根据不同的治疗技术和治疗单位来进行个体化测量误差。

为了解决由呼吸导致的肿瘤位移这一艰巨的任务，人们探讨出了一系列的方法。显而易见的是二维（2D）测量（如荧光透视）肿瘤的活动是不够的。肿瘤的运动不仅是不可预知的，还会随着肿瘤的大小、位置、PFT 结果的变化而变化[99]。应根据每位患者的疾病状态、呼吸模式和其他临床情况个体化测量肿瘤运动。最近四维 CT 显示在呼吸过程中，大约 40%的肺癌活动度超过 5mm，10%的肺癌运动超过 10mm。对于活动度小于 5mm 的肿瘤，单独在轴位外扩 PTV 是足够的。但是，对于肿瘤运动幅度在 5mm 以上的肿瘤，尤其是活动度超过 10mm 的肿瘤，可以在治疗设施上配套呼吸门控装置，或是利用一个呼吸屏气协助设施，或者在计划制订中附加一个内靶区（ITV）来解决呼吸活动度大的问题。

内靶区

根据 ICRU62，ITV 事实上是 CTV+肿瘤活动度。目前，可以采用新的治疗技术，如多层探测器及快速成像重建技术，可以在患者治疗过程中，在 4 维 CT 上实时显影器官随呼吸的运动[100]。为了在 4 维 CT 上确定 ITV 的界限。除了在呼气相勾画之外，还需要在 4 维 CT 的每个时相都将肿瘤出现的区域勾画出来，以创建包围目标所有可能位置的区域。同样的，这一规则也应用于呼气和吸气相屏住呼吸时所采集到的图像。此外，需要密切注意治疗过程中的非正常呼吸，呼吸变异，以及上述情况所引起的 ITV 界限的变化。即便是使用了 4 维 CT 之后，自由呼吸时，我们获得的 ITV 也仅仅是在患者进行 4 维 CT 扫描时随机扫取到的一个单独的呼吸时相的图像抓取。因此，真实的 ITV 界限应该在此基础上进一步扩大，也就是在此基础上，将患者在治疗过程中的呼吸动度的不确定在考虑在内。

调强放疗（IMRT）

IMRT，包括 VMAT，可以改善剂量的可适性并保证剂量波动和剂量覆盖在 PTV 内。总的来说,这导致向肿瘤的高风险区域(如肿瘤、缺氧区域或 PET-CT 上显示高 SUV 的区域)发射更高的辐射剂量,而不增加治疗总辐射剂量,同时最大限度减少正常组织暴露[101,102]。然而,IMRT 在肺癌中的应用一再被推迟,因为 IMRT 的多野照射增加了正常肺组织受照的低剂量区域。此外,肿瘤随着呼吸运动的活动也会增加 IMRT 的剂量分布和技术实施的复杂性。

尽管调强放疗也许对于降低正常组织毒性和提高肿瘤的适形度,高剂量覆盖度是有益有效的,但因为其剂量跌落快,适形度好,在剂量实施和肿瘤位置确定方面的要求也更加精确。同时,我们也必须意识到在实施调强放疗时,肿瘤活动度所带来的复杂性。与三维适形放疗不同的是,调强放疗在特定的时间只实施特定方向,特定的区域的照射。人们经常关注,能否让准直器随着靶区的活动而相应的移动,从而使得计划中的剂量分布与实际实施过程中之间的误差达到最小化。为了使调强放疗在治疗非小细胞肺癌更为合理和有效,应该开发一些可以减少呼吸活动的方法,例如呼吸屏气装置,肿瘤追踪装置等。我们初步的临床数据表明:调强放疗在特定的病例中,可以减少正常组织的受量,这样我们才有可能在后期增加肿瘤区域的处方剂量[103]。如果使用得当,IMRT 是肺癌剂量递增放疗的首选放射治疗方式[104]。

立体定向消融放疗(SABR)

SABR,也称为立体定向放射治疗(stereotactic body radiation therapy,SBRT),实现精确放疗的同时将高剂量放疗疗程缩短至 2 周以内。肺癌的立体定向放疗采用三维适形放疗系统,并常常与其他可以控制肿瘤活动度、减少摆位的不确定性的技术联合应用。这一系列装置可以实现大分割放疗,提高每日剂量(>10Gy),显著缩短了治疗时间。应用多野照射,可以使得剂量跌落快,获得较陡的剂量线,高精确度的定位。在颅外的组织进行每次大剂量照射,称为立体定向放疗。单次剂量的增加使得靶区的生物有效剂量(biological effective dose,BED)增加,同时正常组织毒性最小化。这些将转化为局部控制率和生存率的提高。

来自日本的 Onishi 和他的同事们多中心回顾性报道入组Ⅰ期的非小细胞肺癌 245 例,所有病例的中位年龄 76 岁。155 例分期为 T1N0M0,90 例分期为 T2N0M0,在 13 个中心接受了大分割治疗[68]。立体定向的三维适形放疗采用非共面动态弧或者多静态接口,给予总量 18~75Gy,分 1~22 次。中位等效生物剂量为 108Gy,(57~180Gy),中位随访 24 个月(7~78 个月)。根据美国癌症中心急性不良事件评估标准,6 例出现了 2 度以上的肺炎,占据 2.4%。33 例(14.5%)出现了局部进展。BED=100Gy 和<100Gy 者局部复发率分别为 8.1%和 26.4%($P<0.05$)。在原本可以手术切除的病例,BED=100Gy 和<100Gy 者 3 年生存率分别为 88.4%和 69.4%($P<0.05$)。以上数据表明对于Ⅰ期非小细胞肺癌,根治性立体定向放疗中 BED>150Gy 比较适宜。对于所有的治疗模式来讲,BED=100Gy 者和 BED<100Gy 者,局部控制率和生存率都是前者更好。在部分病例,如原本可以切除但因为其他原因不能手术的病例,行立体定向放疗 BED=100Gy 之后,生存率非常好,几乎可以获得和手术同等的效果。

一项纳入超过 2 000 例患者行图像引导下 SABR(4 维 CT 模拟定位,每日行 CT,确定肿瘤位置和摆位准确性)的研究显示:当给予总剂量为 50Gy,分 4 次(每日一次)或 70Gy 分 10 次时,与原发部位的局部控制率高于 95%相关,且毒性最小,即使对于中心位置的病灶限制正常组织照射剂量结果也一样[105]。

质子治疗

质子是一种带电粒子,与光子相比,它拥有确定的剂量射程,这一特点由射线的能量和它穿梭的组织密度共同决定。质子射线进入体内后发生减速,并于临近射程末端释放出巨大的能量,这一现象称为布拉格峰。通过将布拉格峰调整至肿瘤靶区,质子射线可以形成一个完整的局限于特定的局部的剂量区域,使得周围正常组织不受照射。当器官保护至关重要时(如肺癌),这种疗法是非常理想的。采用梯度加速的质子治疗对于ⅠA 期的非小细胞肺癌可以取得和手术类似的效果[106,107]。需要再次强调的是,无论是光子治疗还是质子治疗,精确地靶区勾画和肿瘤活动度都是至关重要的。解剖结构的位移,位置的不确定性和组织异质性对质子治疗的影响更大[108]。

Ⅰ~Ⅱ期 NSCLC 的根治性放疗

手术可切除的 NSCLC 但在医学上无法手术或拒绝手术的患者应考虑进行根治性放疗。早期 NSCLC 的根治性放疗被认为是标准治疗,并且一些研究报道表明剂量递增可带来早期 NSCLC 患者生存和局部控制获益[109~112]。由于早期 NSCLC 在诊断时本身并不是一种全身性疾病,并且由于常规放疗后局部控制并不乐观,所以如果要提高生存率,必须密切注意放疗后的局部控制情况。

需要注意的是,行放疗的肺癌患者的分期往往是临床分期,而手术患者得到的往往是病理分期,放疗疗效与术后疗效往往难以作分期对应性的比较。部分研究显示临床分期Ⅰ~Ⅱ期者,手术后 24%~37%的病例病理分期都要高于临床分期[113],这在一定程度上解释了为什么临床早期的病例行放疗后结果并不是特别理想。随着对早期 NSCLC 的更好的筛查工具的开发,可以检测出的小病灶但不宜手术切除的病例数目将有所提升[71]。

术后放疗

根据术后放疗(postoperative radiotherapy,PORT)荟萃分析的结果,目前术后放疗不常规应用于Ⅰ期完全切除的非小细胞肺癌[114]。Ⅱ期以上的非小细胞肺癌在完全切除术后是否行立体定向放疗暂无特殊的推荐或不推荐(因为 *HR* 为 1.0),尽管术后放疗显著改善了区域控制率。

术后放疗最早应用于Ⅱ~Ⅲ期的非小细胞肺癌首先由 LCSG 报道,入组了 210 例患者,随机分为观察组和放疗组,放疗组给予 50Gy,25 次[115]。两组对比,术后放疗显著降低了局部复发率(3% vs 41%),但两组的总生存和无病生存无差别,因为两组的远处转移率都很高。然而,最近的一项Ⅲ期临床研究(ANITA),这一研究目的是为了检测根治术后化疗的作用,它的亚组分析显示术后放疗在 N2 的病例可以提高生存率。

对于可切除或者边缘可切除的 N2 非小细胞肺,5 年生存率为 14%~30%。许多临床 N0 或者纵隔镜检查确定为 N0 的病例,最后发现有隐匿性的纵隔淋巴结转移。将近 15%的 T1 病例 N 分期为 N2,40%~45%的 T2~3 病例 N 分期为 N2。未全切的病例,包括切缘阳性者,多为淋巴结转移者、包膜外侵者和

N2病例,局部控制率一般较差,推荐术后放疗。

术前化疗及术前同步放化疗

对于确诊为N2且病灶体积较大的病例,能否行根治性手术尚不能确定,可以考虑术前化疗联合手术治疗。根据Rosell等人的研究显示,越来越多的Ⅲ期疾病患者接受术前诱导化疗[116]。美国西南肿瘤协作组(SWOG)开展了一项Ⅱ期临床试验,入组了74例经活检证实为ⅢA(N2)期的非小细胞肺癌,给予术前同步放化疗,化疗采用顺铂+依托泊苷方案;这一研究结果提示术前同步放化疗可以进一步延长患者的生存,并且毒副作用在可以接受的范围内[117]。随后NCI开展了一项Ⅲ期多中心临床研究,入组了有病理证实的且有手术机会的N2病例。

未经活检证实的N2疾病和可切除的NSCLC(NCI Protocol INT 139)的患者启动了Ⅲ期多中心临床试验。根据PS评分和T分期对患者进行分层,随机分为2组,第1组接受术前同步放化疗+手术,第2组接受术前同步放化疗+根治性放疗。结果显示,手术治疗组OS无差异,但无进展生存期(progression-free survival,PFS)更好。亚组分析提示了三点:第一,肺叶切除术者生存最优($P=0.002$);第二,对于接受了术前放化疗的病例,不推荐行手术风险大且死亡率较高的全肺切除;第三,术中N0往往预示着更好的生存率。作者指出:同步放化疗后的病例若可行肺叶切除术,提示可以考虑手术[119]。

Ⅲ期不可切除的非小细胞肺癌的放疗

不可切除的非小细胞肺癌病例,单独放疗后的中位生存期为10个月,5年生存率为5%。研究者考虑用放化疗相结合的手段来提高疗效。可以采用的方式有序贯放化疗和同步放化疗。最著名的研究是CALGB报道的结果。对比了放疗与序贯放化疗的疗效。放疗总量均为60Gy,化疗采用长春瑞滨+顺铂方案。放化疗组的中位生存期和5年生存率较之单独放疗组有明显提高(13.8个月vs 9.7个月,19% vs 7%)[120]。

鉴于以上结果,RTOG开展了RTOG8808研究,将病例随机分为3组,第1组行常规分割放疗,第2组行序贯放化疗(具体方案参照CALGB研究),第3组行69.6Gy的大分割治疗。结果显示,序贯放化疗组的效果优于两个单独放疗组[121]。

Schaake-Koning等[122]对比了单独放疗及放疗联合顺铂治疗的结果。两组的远处转移率无明显差异,但是放疗联合顺铂组的1年、2年、3年生存率均优于单独放疗组(54% vs 46%,26% vs 13%,16% vs 2%,$P=0.009$)。因此,该研究提示局部控制率的提高在一定程度上可以转化为生存的获益。

Furuse等人对比了同步放化疗和序贯放化疗的效果。化疗采用丝裂霉素、长春碱和顺铂,28天1个周期,放疗常规分割56Gy。同步放化疗组的5年生存率明显高于序贯放化疗组[123]。

RTOG进行了一项三臂RCT(RTOG9410),分析以顺铂为基础的同步放化疗与序贯放化疗相比能否改善Ⅱ~Ⅲ期不可切除的非小细胞肺癌患者的生存情况。第1组行化疗后放疗(化疗采用顺铂+长春新碱,放疗剂量60Gy),第2组行相同方案的同步放化疗。第3组行超分割同步放化疗,化疗方案为顺铂50mg/m^2+口服依托泊苷50mg,放疗方案每次1.2Gy,2次/日,总量69.6Gy。该研究提示采用同步放化疗较序贯放化疗能延长生存期[124]。

第3项对比同步放化疗和序贯放化疗的研究发表于2001年,在2005年进行了数据更新,这项研究同时还讨论了巩固化疗的作用[125]。这项来自法国的三期临床研究入组了205例,放疗剂量66Gy,化疗采用长春瑞滨联合顺铂,对比序贯放化疗和同步放化疗的疗效。序贯放化疗组在化疗2周期后行放疗,放疗后行同方案巩固化疗2周期;同步放化疗组在同步放化疗后行巩固化疗2周期。同步放化疗组的局部控制率更高(40% vs 24%),中位生存期和4年生存率也高于序贯放化疗组(16.3个月vs 14.5个月,21% vs 14%),但未达统计学差异。同时,同步放化疗组的3度以上食管炎的发生比率(32% vs 3%)和毒副作用相关死亡率也更高(9.5% vs 5.6%)。

以上三项Ⅲ期随机对照研究均提示同步放化疗较序贯放化疗可以提高生存,且其中两项研究显示有统计学差异。基于上述结果,自2001年起,同步放化疗被定位局部晚期不可切除非小细胞肺癌的标准治疗方案。值得注意的是,行同步放化疗所带来的毒副作用也随之增加。

RTOG9410中,同步放化疗后,局部复发率仍在34%和43%之间。为了进一步提高局部控制,RTOG,NCCTG及北卡大学分别进行了针对不可切除的非小细胞的放疗剂量爬坡试验。三项结果提示最高的放疗安全剂量为74Gy。北卡大学的Ⅰ/Ⅱ期临床研究显示行诱导化疗+同步放化疗,若放疗采用三维适形放疗,最高剂量可以达到60~74Gy[126]。全组3年生存率约36%,局部复发率约13%,完成全程放疗者的3年生存率约45%。

由于74Gy三维适形放疗在保证局部控制率,生存率的同时,毒副作用在可以耐受的范围之内,RTOG开展了另外一项Ⅲ期临床实验,对比了传统的放疗剂量60Gy与爬坡实验所得到的74Gy的结果。所有病例均采用同步放化疗,化疗采用紫杉醇+卡铂,有或没有西妥昔单抗(一种EGFR靶向药),用于ⅢA或ⅢB期NSCLC患者。令人惊讶的是,早期结果分析显示,接受较高辐射剂量患者的总生存并没有改善[127]。事实上,高剂量组的存活率更低,毒性更大。这可能是因为基于光子的辐射技术照射时74Gy的辐射剂量毒性太大。此外,西妥昔单抗的加入也没有改善生存。

随机临床试验未能确定同步化疗的最佳方案。几种常用的选择包括铂类(顺铂或卡铂)联合依托泊苷、紫杉醇或培美曲塞使用[128~130]。

无法根治的晚期NSCLC的全身治疗

对于Ⅳ期或不适合根治性手术或放疗的复发性NSCLC患者,全身治疗的目标是减轻症状并延长生存期。在一项荟萃分析中,2 714例患者纳入16项随机对照试验,将化疗与最佳支持治疗(best supportive care,BSC)进行比较,结果提示化疗患者能够显著获益,中位OS从4.5个月增加到6个月,1年总生存率从20%增加到29%($HR=0.77$;95%CI 0.71~0.83,$P<0.0001$)[131]。大多数试验包含以铂类为基础的两药联合化疗,这是唯一与OS显著改善相关的化疗方案。

一线化疗

三项大型随机对照试验将以铂类为基础的两药联合化疗与单药非铂化疗进行比较。瑞典肺癌研究组(Swedish Lung Cancer Study Group)纳入334名晚期NSCLC患者随机分入吉西他滨+顺铂组或单药化疗组[132]。与单药化疗组相比,铂二联化疗能够显著提高患者总体缓解率(30% vs 11%)、中位生存时间(10 个月 vs 8.6 个月)和 1 年总生存率(40% vs 32%)。Georgoulias 等[133]展开的一项纳入 324 例患者的临床试验发现,尽管与多西他赛和顺铂单药化疗相比联合用药能够改善患者的缓解率(36% vs 22%),但中位生存时间(10.5 个月 vs 8 个月)和 1 年总生存率(44% vs 43%)均无显著差异。同样,在纳入 565 名患者的 CALGB9730 研究中观察到类似的结果,其中卡铂+紫杉醇联合化疗组能够显著增加缓解率(30% vs 17%),但中位生存时间(8.8 个月 vs 6.7 个月)和 1 年总生存率(37% vs 32%)均没有达到统计学意义[134]。相比之下,两项大型临床研究显示,与单用顺铂相比,使用吉西他滨或长春瑞滨联合顺铂的联合化疗总体缓解率、中位生存时间和 1 年总生存率都有显著改善[135,136]。三项大型荟萃分析比较以铂为基础的两药联合化疗与单药化疗,结果显示联合化疗组缓解率和总生存都显著增加[137~139]。在铂类为基础的治疗方案中加入第三种药物能够提高缓解率,但患者生存并不能获益。根据这些数据,2009 年美国临床肿瘤学会指南推荐使用铂类为基础的二联化疗作为 PS 评分为 0/1 的晚期 NSCLC 患者的一线化疗方案[140]。

多项研究显示,对于特定的联合化疗方案,没有显著差异或只有很小的改善[141~143]。在一项大型随机对照试验中,将 1 725 名未接受过治疗的晚期 NSCLC 患者随机分为顺铂联合吉西他滨或培美曲塞[144]。与之前大多数比较铂类为基础的二联化疗的研究相似,中位 PFS 和中位 OS 均无显著差异。然而,这是第一项在组织学类型亚组中分析化疗结果差异的研究,顺铂+培美曲塞方案能够增加非鳞状细胞癌的中位生存时间(11.8 个月 vs 10.4 个月,*HR*=0.84,*P*=0.005),但在鳞状细胞癌中没有统计学差异(9.4 个月 vs 10.8 个月,*HR*=1.23,*P*=0.05)。在一项纳入 1 052 例患者比较卡铂+紫杉醇或纳米颗粒白蛋白结合型(nab)紫杉醇的Ⅲ期临床试验中,也对不同组织学亚组进行分析[145]。该研究显示缓解率增加(33% vs 25%,*P*=0.05),但中位 PFS 和 OS 相似。仅在鳞癌患者中观察到缓解率的改善(41% vs 24%,*P*<0.001),在腺癌中几乎相同(26% vs 27%)。

由于卡铂与顺铂具有相似的作用机制,因此两项荟萃分析分析了它们是否在 NSCLC 中具有相同的疗效。一项荟萃分析纳入了来自 8 项随机对照试验的 2 948 名患者,另一项纳入了来自 9 项随机对照试验的 2 968 名患者。尽管使用基于顺铂的二联化疗显示 OS 延长,但未达到统计学意义[146,147]。在亚组分析中,基于顺铂的二联化疗与ⅢB 期非鳞状细胞癌和使用第三代化疗药(包括紫杉醇、多西他赛和吉西他滨)治疗的患者的 OS 改善相关。卡铂与血小板减少症的发生率增加有关,而顺铂与恶心、呕吐和肾毒性的风险增加有关。与卡铂相比,基于顺铂的二联化疗在微小改善 OS 的同时带来毒性的也增加,这使得在接受姑息治疗的无法根治的患者群体中接受两种铂类药物。

单克隆抗体

贝伐单抗

贝伐单抗(bevacizumab)是抗循环血管内皮生长因子(VEGF)的重组人源化抗体。一项Ⅱ期临床研究,在晚期 NSCLC 患者中比较一线卡铂+紫杉醇与卡铂+紫杉醇+贝伐单抗的疗效,结果显示贝伐单抗能够改善缓解率和中位生存时间[148]。其中 6 名患者出现了危及生命的咯血,4 人因此死亡。所有 6 名患者均为中央型肺癌,5 名患者在治疗前或贝伐单抗治疗后肿瘤中出现空洞,4 名患者为鳞癌。ECOG 4599 试验纳入 878 例复发或晚期 NSCLC 患者,其患者主要为非鳞癌,单次咯血少于半勺且无脑转移。患者随机分配接受卡铂+紫杉醇±贝伐单抗联合治疗[149]。贝伐单抗组能够改善患者缓解率(35% vs 15%,*P*<0.001)、PFS(6.2 个月 vs 4.5 个月,*HR*=0.66,*P*<0.001)和中为生存时间(12.3 个月 vs 10.3 个月,*HR*=0.79),*P*=0.003)。贝伐单抗的加入增加了中性粒细胞减少症、血小板减少症、高血压、蛋白尿和出血的发生率。AVAiL(avastin in lung cancer)临床试验将 1 043 例患者随机分为顺铂+吉西他滨组、顺铂+吉西他滨+低剂量(7.5mg/kg)贝伐单抗组和顺铂+吉西他滨+高剂量(15mg/kg)贝伐单抗组[150]。低剂量和高剂量贝伐单抗组的缓解率增加(34.1% vs 30.4% vs 20.1%,*P*=0.003),但中位生存时间无显著差异[151]。

ramucirumab

ramucirumab 是一种针对 VEGF 受体 2 的人单克隆抗体。在一项随机试验中,对 130 例未接受治疗的晚期 NSCLC 患者进行了铂类+培美曲塞联合或不联合 ramucirumab 的比较,两组缓解率(49.3% vs 38%,*P*=0.18)和中位无进展生存期(7.2 个月 vs 5.6 个月,*HR*=0.75,*P*=0.13)均无统计学差异[152]。

西妥昔单抗

西妥昔单抗(cetuximab)是针对 EGFR 的嵌合单克隆抗体。在两项大型随机对照试验中评估了西妥昔单抗在化疗中的应用。在 BMS099 研究中,676 名未接受过治疗的晚期 NSCLC 患者被随机分配到化疗组(铂联合紫杉醇或多西他赛)或西妥昔单抗组(化疗+西妥昔单抗)[153]。虽然西妥昔单抗组的缓解率增加(25.7% vs 17.2%,*P*=0.007),但 PFS 和 OS 没有显著改善。在 FLEX 研究中,1 125 名患者被随机分为单独顺铂+长春瑞滨或与西妥昔单抗联合使用[154]。结果显示西妥昔单抗组的缓解率有所提高(36% vs 19%,*P*=0.01)但对中位 PFS 没有影响(两组均为 4.8 个月)。然而,接受西妥昔单抗治疗的患者中位 OS 显著增加(11.3 个月 vs 10.1 个月,*HR*=0.87,95% *CI*:0.76~0.99,*P*=0.04)。对 FLEX 研究的进一步分析显示,加入西妥昔单抗的获益仅见于免疫组化 H 评分(计算为每周 EGFR 表达为弱阳性的细胞百分比×1+中等阳性细胞的百分比×2+强阳性细胞的百分比×3,分布 0~300 之间)大于 200 的患者,其中位生存时间为 12.2 个月,而单独化疗的患者为 9.6 个月[155]。

化疗周期

对于能够达到临床获益(定义为无进展性疾病(PD)且能够耐受化疗无严重的毒性反应)的晚期 NSCLC 患者,应接受不超过 4~6 个周期的以铂类为基础的化疗。临床试验将三到四个化疗周期与六个周期的持续治疗直到肿瘤进展进行比较,结果显示更长周期的治疗并不能使患者获益[156~158]。

维持治疗

对于无肿瘤进展的患者,在接受 4~6 个周期以铂类为基础的化疗之后的持续治疗被称为维持治疗。维持治疗的主要类型包括:同药维持治疗,单克隆抗体维持治疗,以及换药维持治疗。许多研究评估了维持治疗在接受 4~6 个周期化疗后无肿瘤进展的患者中的作用(表 84-10)[164~168]。这些研究都是针对非鳞癌患者,维持期使用的主要两种化疗药为培美曲塞和贝伐单抗,前者表现出更好的有效性,后者安全性更高。培美曲塞维持治疗能够改善患者中位生存期,但单用贝伐单抗维持或者与培美曲塞联合维持的效果仍然不明确。

表 84-10　维持化疗

临床试验	诱导	维持	PFS/月	OS/月
JMEN[159]	铂两药化疗	培美曲塞 vs 观察	4 vs 2($P<0.001$)	13.4 vs 10.6($P=0.01$)
PARAMOUNT[160]	顺铂+培美曲塞	培美曲塞 vs 观察	4.4 vs 2.8($P<0.01$)	16.9 vs 14($P=0.01$)
AVAPERL[161]	顺铂+培美曲塞+贝伐单抗	培美曲塞+贝伐单抗 vs 贝伐单抗	7.4 vs 3.7($P<0.001$)	17.1 vs 13.1($P=0.29$)
PRONOUNCE[162]	卡铂+培美曲塞 卡铂+紫杉醇+贝伐单抗	培美曲塞 贝伐单抗	4.4 vs 5.5($P=0.6$)	10.5 vs 11.7($P=0.06$)
PointBreak[163]	卡铂+培美曲塞+贝伐单抗 卡铂+紫杉醇+贝伐单抗	培美曲塞+贝伐单抗 贝伐单抗	6 vs 5.6($P=0.01$)	12.6 vs 13.4($P=0.9$)
ECOG 5508	卡铂+培美曲塞+贝伐单抗	培美曲塞+贝伐单抗 培美曲塞 贝伐单抗	进行中	进行中

二线化疗

两项多西他赛的随机临床研究表明二线化疗能够带来获益。在 TAX320 研究中，373 名接受过治疗的患者被随机分配到多西他赛组或对照组（异环磷酰胺或长春瑞滨）[169]。多西他赛每 3 周以 100mg/m^2（D100）或 75mg/m^2（D75）给药。D100 组、D75 组和对照组的缓解率分别为 10.8%、6.7% 和 0.8%。与对照治疗相比，D75 组 1 年 OS 显著升高（32% vs 19%，$P=0.025$），而 D100 组 OS 没有改善。紫杉醇的预先使用对缓解率或生存均没有影响。第二项临床研究采用了类似的设计，纳入曾接受过治疗且无紫杉醇暴露的晚期 NSCLC 患者，随机将患者纳入多西他赛组（D75 或 D100）或最佳支持治疗（best supportive care，BSC）组[170]。与 TAX320 研究相似，与 D100 和 BSC 相比，D75 能够改善患者的 1 年 OS（37% vs 19% vs 19%），且较 D100 相比毒性更小。第二种批准用于二线化疗的药物是培美曲塞。一项大型 RCT 将多西他赛（75mg/m^2）与培美曲塞（500mg/m^2）进行比较，均每 3 周一次。缓解率和中位 PFS 相似，中位 OS（培美曲塞为 8.3 个月，多西他赛为 7.9 个月）和 1 年 OS 也没有显著差异[171]。与培美曲塞相比，接受多西他赛治疗的患者更容易发生 3 级或 4 级中性粒细胞减少、发热性中性粒细胞减少和脱发。在 REVEL 研究中，共纳入 1 825 名接受一线铂类为基础化疗的晚期 NSCLC 患者，随机分为多西他赛组或多西他赛与 ramucirumab 联合用药组[172]。结果显示加入 ramucirumab 能够增加 PFS 和中位 OS（10.5 个月 vs 9.1 个月，$HR=0.86$，95% CI：0.75～0.98，$P=002$）。在接受过治疗的 NSCLC 患者中，将两种 EGFR 酪氨酸激酶抑制剂（tyrosine kinase inhibitors，TKI）与 BSC 进行比较。在 ISEL（Iressa survival evaluation in lung cancer）研究中共纳入 1 692 名患者，并随机分配到吉非替尼（易瑞沙）组或安慰剂组[173]。吉非替尼组中位 OS 无明显改善（5.6 个月 vs 5.1 个月，$HR=0.89$，95% CI：0.77～1.02，$P=0.08$）。相比之下，将 731 例患者随机分配至厄洛替尼组或安慰剂组的 NCIC-BR21 研究显示，厄洛替尼组患者中位 OS 显著改善（6.7 个月 vs 4.7 个月，$HR=0.70$，95% CI 0.58～0.85，$P<0.0001$）[174]。目前批准的能够用于二线治疗晚期 NSCLC 的化疗方案包括多西他赛、培美曲塞、厄洛替尼以及多西他赛与 ramucirumab 联合用药。

老年患者的化疗

约 1/3 的非小细胞肺癌患者≥70 岁，虽然老年患者的并发症增多、器官功能下降，但是大多数研究显示年龄本身不应该成为单纯决定患者是否接受化疗的因素。对晚期非小细胞肺癌患者的治疗进行回顾性分析显示，≥65 岁患者与<65 患者之间并无显著区别[175]。以年龄作为危险因素分析化疗的研究显示，老年患者与非老年患者对化疗的疗效、毒性反应和生存率均相似[176]。国际专家小组发布了针对老年 NSCLC 患者推荐意见，建议进行老年综合性评估，以便更好地明确预后和预测治疗的耐受性。该小组认为对于非选择的老年晚期非小细胞肺癌患者应该推荐第三代化疗药物的单药方案（长春瑞滨，吉西他滨，紫杉烷类），一般状况好、器官功能好的老年患者可以选择含铂联合化疗方案[177]。

靶向治疗

表皮生长因子受体（EGFR）

吉非替尼是第一个被纳入进展期非小细胞肺癌（NSCLC）患者临床试验的表皮生长因子酪氨酸激酶抑制剂（TKI）。在 IDEAL 临床研究中，纳入吉非替尼单药治疗化疗失败后的晚期 NSCLC 患者，并随机分为吉非替尼低剂量组（250mg）和高剂量（500mg）[178,179]。该研究显示吉非替尼的总体缓解率为 10%～18%，两组间无显著差异，500mg 组的皮疹发生率增加。与药物缓解率较好相关的临床指标主要包括 PS 评分、腺癌、女性患者和日本族。EGFR 突变，主要是第 19 号外显子缺失突变和精氨酸取代第 858 位亮氨酸的错义突变（L858R），为 EGFR TKI 的药物有效率预测指标提供了生物学解释[180,181]。在其中一项研究中，在对吉非替尼应答的 9 位患者中，有 8 位患者存在 EGFR 突变，并且 EGFR 突变在从不吸烟的肺腺癌患者中更加常见[180]。在一项纳入 2 105 例非鳞癌 NSCLC 患者的西班牙研究中，350 例患者（16.6%）有 EGFR 突变，并且这些突变在从不吸烟的患者中最常见（37.7%）[182]。纪念斯隆-凯瑟琳癌症中心数据显示，EGFR 突变率在从不吸烟、既往吸烟和正在吸烟的肺腺癌患者中分别为 52%、15%和 6%，并且 EGFR 突变率与吸烟负担呈负相关[183]。

在一项 EGFR TKI 治疗结果的汇总分析中，EGFR 突变的患者能够达到 78%的缓解率，而在野生型 EGFR 患者中缓解率只有 10%[184]。为了在大型随机对照临床试验(RCT)中比较靶向治疗和传统化疗,开展了 IPASS(Iressa Pan Asia Study)研究,旨在比较吉非替尼与卡铂联合紫杉醇在未接受化疗的进展期 NSCLC 患者中的疗效[185]。结果显示,EGFR 野生型与吉非替尼的缓解率(23.5% vs 1.1%)和中位无进展生存期(HR=2.85,95%CI:2.05~3.98,P<0.001)的降低显著相关。相反,EGFR 突变患者在接受吉非替尼治疗后有更高的缓解率(71.2% vs 47.3%)和更长的中位无进展生存期(HR=0.48,95%CI 0.36~0.64,P<0.001)。另外还有几项类似的仅纳入了 EGFR 突变肿瘤患者的临床试验,在接受吉非替尼[186,187]或厄洛替尼[188,189]治疗的患者中得到类似的结果[188,189]。

最近更多的研究旨在比较第二代 EGFR TKI 阿法替尼与化疗的疗效。二代 EGFR TKI 能不可逆的与包括 HER-2 和 HER-4 在内的 HER 家族蛋白结合。Lux-Lung 3 和 Lux-Lung 6 研究表明,在未接受过治疗的进展期肺腺癌患者中,与传统的顺铂+培美曲塞/吉西他滨相比,阿法替尼治疗可使患者获得更长的疾病无进展生存期[190,191]。尽管这两个临床试验的联合分析表明,阿法替尼与化疗比较,患者总生存时间并无差异,但是亚组分析显示,存在 EGFR 第 19 号外显子缺失突变的患者接受阿法替尼治疗可获得更长的中位生存时间,而 L858R 突变患者 OS 并未从阿法替尼获益[192]。

尽管相比于标准的化疗,EGFR 突变的患者对 EGFR-TKI 治疗表现出较高的起始应答率并能够延长中位 PFS,但是几乎所有患者最终都会发生获得性耐药[193]。最常见的 EGFR TKI 耐药缘于第 20 号外显子 T790M 突变的发生[194]。其他潜在的原因有 Met 扩增、PIK3CA 突变、HER-2 扩增、BRAF 突变以及向小细胞肺癌转化[195,196]。第三代 EGFR TKI 是 T790M 突变的潜在抑制剂。有两种药物目前正处于研发阶段。CO-1618 的临床试验早期结果表明,T790M 突变患者的缓解率为 58%,中位 PFS 超过 12 个月[197]。类似的,T790M 突变患者对 AZD-9291 的缓解率为 64%,总体疾病控制率为 94%[198]。另外一项针对 EGFR TKI 获得性耐药患者的治疗措施是联合阿法替尼和西妥昔单抗。在一项ⅠB 期临床研究中[199],这项两药联用的治疗措施在 126 位对厄洛替尼或阿法替尼耐药的患者中试验,结果发现总体缓解为 29%,在 T790M 突变和野生型的患者中并无显著差异(分别为 32%和 25%,P=0.34)。

间变性淋巴瘤激酶(ALK)

间变性淋巴瘤激酶(anaplastic lymphoma kinase,ALK)与 EML4、KIF5B、TFG、KLC1 或其他基因融合会导致 ALK 及其下游通路的持续激活[200]。克唑替尼是一类口服的 ATP 竞争性的 AKL、MET 和 ROS1 酪氨酸激酶抑制剂。在一项纳入 82 例具有 ALK 融合突变患者的一期临床试验中,缓解率为 57%,并且另外有 33%的患者获得了疾病稳定(stable disease,SD)[201]。在观察截止时间,虽然中位 PFS 尚未达到,但预估可达到 6 个月 PFS 的患者可达 72%。在有 ALK 融合突变的患者中,与铂类联合培美曲塞相比,一线克唑替尼治疗可延长患者中位 PFS(10.7 个月 vs 7 个月;HR=0.45,95% CI:0.35~0.60,P<0.001),但是在中位 OS 上并无显著差异[202]。此外,与多西他赛或培美曲塞相比,二线克唑替尼治疗也可延长患者中位 PFS,但对中位 OS 并无显著影响[203]。对于克唑替尼获得性耐药的患者,二代 ALK 抑制剂可作为候选治疗方案。在第 1 阶段研究的剂量递增部分,色瑞替尼能够达到 58%的缓解率和 7 个月的中位 PFS,PFS 从之前接受过克唑替尼治疗患者的 6.9 个月到未接受过 ALK 靶向治疗患者的 10.4 个月不等[204]。

其他靶向治疗

有几个潜在的可作为治疗靶点的基因变异已在 NSCLC 中被发现,目前正处于临床试验阶段[205]。最近研究表明 ROS1 融合突变的患者可从克唑替尼治疗中获益[206]。在另外一项纳入 50 例 ROS1 融合突变患者的二期临床试验中,缓解率可达到 72%,中位 PFS 为 19.2 个月[207]。尽管目前没有直接针对 KRAS 突变的抑制剂,利用 MEK 抑制剂阻断下游通路可能在这类患者的治疗中具有重要作用。一项二期临床试验将之前接受过治疗的 KRAS 突变的晚期 NSCLC 患者随机分组,分别接受多西他赛单药治疗,或多西他赛和司美替尼联合治疗,结果发现,联合治疗可延长患者中位 PFS(5.3 个月 vs 2.1 个月,P=0.01)和中位 OS(9.4 个月 vs 5.2 个月,P=0.21)[208]。

免疫治疗

免疫检查点通路在调节 T 细胞免疫应答过程中起关键作用。程序性细胞死亡受体 1(PD1)是一种 T 细胞受体抑制剂,在肿瘤中能够与其配体 PD-L1 结合。临床前研究表明抑制 PD-1/PD-L1 相互作用可以促进 T 细胞应答并诱导抗肿瘤作用。设计用于阻断该通路的几种药物正在开发中,包括抗 PD1 抗体 BMS-936558[纳武单抗(nivolumab)]和 MK-3475[帕博利珠单抗(pembrolizumab)]以及抗 PDL1 抗体 MPDL-3280A 和 MEDI-4736[209]。在一项评估纳武单抗在 NSCLC、肾细胞癌和黑色素瘤患者中作用的一项 1 期临床试验中显示:122 例 NSCLC 患者中有 14 例缓解[210]。所有缓解均发生在接受 3 或 10mg/kg 治疗的患者中,包括 6 例鳞癌患者(共 13 例)和 7 例非鳞癌患者(共 44 例)。在一项评估 MPDL-3280A 在多种恶性肿瘤患者中疗效的研究中,53 例 NSCLC 患者的缓解率为 34%,其中 17%患者的 SD 持续 24 周或更长时间[211]。在两项研究中,PD-1/PD-L1 检查点抑制剂的治疗耐受性良好,肿瘤中 PD-L1 的表达与缓解率相关。

可根治 NSCLC 患者的全身治疗

辅助化疗

可根治的 NSCLC 手术切除后进行化疗以改善 OS 被称为辅助化疗。尽管接受手术切除,大多数肺癌患者仍然出现复发和/或转移性疾病,这些复发和转移中有 2/3 发生在全身。因此,化疗补充手术是一种合理的治疗策略[212]。1995 年的一项荟萃分析比较了单纯手术和术后行基于顺铂的化疗。该研究包括 8 项试验共纳入了 1 394 名患者,结果显示术后辅助化疗死亡风险降低 13%,表明辅助化疗在 5 年绝对生存获益 5%(P=0.08)[213]。随后的几项随机临床试验均表明辅助化疗可带来一定获益[214~217]。对 1995 年荟萃分析后进行的五项最大随机临床试验进行汇总分析,共纳入了 4 584 名患者。结果显示辅助化疗能够改善Ⅱ期和Ⅲ期患者的生存[218]。近期的 ASCO 临床指引推荐ⅡA、ⅡB 和ⅢA 期非小细胞肺癌患者常规行含铂方案辅助化疗,并且可选择性用于大于 65 岁的老年患者。尽管多个关于术后辅助化疗的随机研究均证实辅助化疗可改善患者总生存,但这些研究的亚组分析显示ⅠB 期不能从辅助化疗中获益,因此不推荐该期患者术后常规行辅助化疗。到目前为止,仅少数ⅠA期患者被纳入辅助化疗的研究中,该期患者亦不推荐行术后辅助化疗[219]。

新辅助化疗

在手术切除之前进行的化疗称为新辅助化疗或诱导化疗。与辅助化疗相比,新辅助化疗的潜在优势包括改善化疗依从性、降低肺切除率以及评估肿瘤对化疗的药物反应。尽管辅助化疗仍然是可切除的 NSCLC 的当前标准治疗,但临床试验数据表明新辅助化疗可以达到相当水平的获益[220~223]。一个纳入 13 项随机临床研究共 3 224 名患者的荟萃分析显示,新辅助化疗可提高患者生存率($HR=0.84$,$P=0.000\ 1$)[224]。虽然这些数据表明新辅助化疗是可切除的 NSCLC 患者的合理方法,但很少有研究对如何选择患者进行辅助治疗和新辅助治疗提供指导。

SCLC 的治疗

SCLC 与 NSCLC 的不同之处在于其快速生长速度、早期系统性扩散倾向以及较短的自然病程。随着 SCLC 作为一种系统性疾病的普遍接受和对多模式综合治疗优于单独局部治疗的优越性的认识,化疗成为 SCLC 治疗的基础[225]。

手术治疗

尽管手术切除通常不会在 SCLC 的治疗中发挥作用,但是在一些具体临床情况下手术可能具有潜在的获益,例如外周型 SCLC。尽管 2/3 的患者就诊时即为广泛病变,但有不到 5%的一小部分小细胞肺癌患者的病变仍局限于肺内,伴或不伴 N1 组淋巴结转移。这些患者常常是在偶然胸部影像检查时发现的孤立性肺结节。对于这些患者接受外科治疗后再加用辅助化疗,Ⅰ期患者的总体 5 年生存率在 28%~60%,T1N1 期患者为 20%~35%[226]。最近的一项回顾性研究显示,所有接受手术的 SCLC 患者的 5 年 OS 为 52.6%,T1N1 患者可达到 45%~51%[227]。个别报道中描述,病期非常局限的患者,五年生存率可高达 70%~80%。这些外周型小细胞癌患者与常见的中央型小细胞肺癌患者生存率之间巨大的差异导致了很多推论。一些研究者认为,这些肿瘤可能是伴有生物学改变的小细胞肺癌另外群体;然而另一些人认为,这些肿瘤的诊断上不确切,事实上它们可能是良性或者是中分化神经内分泌癌(典型或不典型类癌)[228]。

大多周围型小细胞肺癌患者是在开胸后获得诊断,只有很少一部分是通过术前细针抽吸活检而获得诊断。能明确诊断的周围型小细胞肺癌较少见,而且事实上非小细胞肺癌和类癌在针吸活检时可能被误诊为小细胞肺癌,促使临床医生继续考虑是否应该对患者实施手术治疗,而不是立即转向化疗。基于术前明确小细胞癌的诊断,分期时应该比常规分期更加详尽,因小细胞肺癌伴有高发的纵隔和全身性淋巴结隐匿性转移。在考虑手术治疗之前,除应该进行详尽的影像学分期外,也应包括纵隔镜检查。如已经出现纵隔淋巴结受累的情况,则不应行外科治疗,但是,影像学分期中已经出现肺门淋巴结肿大并不是外科手术的绝对禁忌证。如果为了明确肿瘤是否伴有肺门淋巴结转移,这些患者仍然可以考虑开胸探查。对于那些合适的患者,如果病变可以完全切除,对其行肺切除术也是可以的。无论术前、术中或术后有无确诊,所有接受手术治疗的小细胞肺癌患者均应接受术后化疗。美国退伍军人外科辅助治疗的研究报告指出:接受术后化疗组的预后要好于无化疗组。当对化疗时机进行研究时发现,似乎术前化疗并没有优势[225]。

放射治疗

局部手术仅仅适用于非常小的一部分的小细胞肺癌。除了全身治疗,小细胞肺癌患者需要另外一种局部治疗手段作为综合治疗的一部分,而放射治疗恰恰就是这样的一种治疗手段。两项采用不同研究方法的荟萃分析肯定了胸部放疗的价值,提示胸部放疗可以降低局部复发率,延长生存期。第一项荟萃分析纳入了 11 个研究结果,显示胸部放疗使 2 年总生存率增加 5.4%[229]。第二项荟萃分析选取了 13 项随机研究,共纳入了 2 140 例病例,对比了单独化疗和放化疗的结果,显示 3 年生存率提高了 5.4%,即从 15%提高到 20.4%[230]。值得一提的是,这些研究都不是最近的研究,都没有采用目前的标准化疗方案——EP 方案。此外,这些研究既包括了序贯放化疗也包括了同步放化疗。

胸部放疗的时间相对于化疗

虽然放疗目前对于局限期小细胞肺癌的应用还在继续发展,现今的随机对照研究结果,包括最近的荟萃分析结果显示同步放化疗或者尽早放疗(即化疗周期 1~3 期间)的结果最佳[231~237]。

同步放化疗中放疗的分割模式

由于小细胞肺癌是一种放疗敏感的肿瘤,在肿瘤的剂量效应曲线中有一个肩区,肿瘤倍增时间短,从这个理论上讲,降低剂量,提高每日治疗次数的超分割治疗能够提高疗效。这一特点同时有利于保护正常组织,尤其是对于剂量线上有一个肩区的组织,可以减少晚期毒副作用[238]。与常规分割的历史对照组相比,局限期 SCLC 患者的超分割和加速化放疗的几项Ⅱ期临床试验获得了令人鼓舞的 2 年生存结果[239,240]。INT-0096 研究对比了常规分割治疗(1.8Gy/次,25 次,5 周)和加速超分割治疗(1.5Gy/次,2 次/天,30 次,3 周),入组了 417 例局限期小细胞肺癌[241]。同步放化疗的化疗方案采用顺铂 60mg/m^2,d1,依托泊苷 120mg/m^2,d1~3,共 4 个周期。与每天一次的常规分割放疗相比,加速超分割放疗组的中位生存期更长(23 个月 vs 19 个月),5 年生存率更高(26% vs 16%,$P=0.04$)两组的毒性反应对比中,仅 3 度以上的食管炎在超分割组有着增加(27% vs 11%,$P<0.001$),其余无差异[242]。

最大耐受剂量

胸部放疗剂量是另外一个有争议的领域[243]。加拿大国家癌症研究所(NCIC)开展了一项研究来探讨胸部肿瘤的剂量效应。结果显示诱导化疗后,在 3 周内分 15 次给予 37.5Gy 放疗,对比在 2 周内分为 10 次给予 25Gy 放疗,无进展生存期显著延长[244]。Arriagada 等发表的一项 173 例局限期小细胞肺癌的多中心研究,在三个中心开展,总剂量为 45~65Gy 采用放化疗交替治疗放疗剂量并没有明显影响局部控制率和生存率[245]。提示同步放化疗可以提高局部控制率,同时食管毒性的增加在可以接受的范围内。可以考虑通过增加每日单次剂量来增大总剂量。鉴于加速超分割的结果,延长放疗疗程也许是有一定弊端的。

与常规的每日分割相比,同步补量的加速超分割治疗可以提高头颈部肿瘤的局部控制率[246]。这一方法先采用每天一次放疗,4~5周后每天两次放疗2周,前者为大野治疗,后者的补量为局部小野治疗。因此,这称为同步补量。由于该模式在头颈部肿瘤中取得了有效的结果,RTOG开展了Ⅰ期和Ⅱ期临床研究(分别为RTOG9712和RTOG0239)评估SCLC同步补量放疗联合EP方案化疗的疗效。结果显示,严重急性食管炎的发生率为18%(低于之前在INT 0096中指出的27%),2年生存率为36.6%(低于INT 0096中的47%)[247,248]。

理论上而言,超分割治疗的45Gy的实际剂量应该高于常规分割的45Gy剂量,所以CALGB对比了局限期小细胞肺癌常规分割放疗和超分割放疗的最大耐受剂量[249]。放疗在化疗前4个周期开始,推荐给Ⅱ期临床研究的常规分割剂量为70Gy。意料之中的是,超分割组的毒性限制性剂量为45Gy。随后的Ⅱ期临床研究CALGB39808显示在紫杉醇和托泊替康的诱导化疗之后,行70Gy放疗同步EP方案化疗是合理的[250]。中位生存期22.4个月,也就是说,常规分割的结果是非常好的。3~4度放射性食管炎发生率为21%,而在RTOG0239中,食管炎为17%,在样本量更大的INT0096中为32%。对3个CALGB临床试验(39808、30002、30206)患者进行的汇总分析采用高剂量(70Gy)每日分割放疗和两个诱导化疗周期后的同步化疗,显示中位生存期为19.9个月,2年和5年OS率分别为37%(95% *CI*:31%~44%)和21%(95%*CI*:16%~27%)[251]。

CALGB39808和RTOG0239报道中食管炎发生率更低,且效果较好。故而另一项Ⅲ期临床研究正在进行,将对比这两种放疗模式,其中对照组给予45Gy的超分割放疗,2次/天,同步EP方案化疗,放疗于化疗第一周期开始。

SCLC预防性颅内照射

大约10%的SCLC患者在初次就诊时检测到脑转移症状,另外10%的患者在MRI或CT成像中表现为隐匿性转移,随着生存期的延长,新生颅脑转移的可能性也会增加[252]。在没有针对中枢神经系统的特异性治疗的情况下,随访28个月时颅脑转移的累积概率达到80%,包括了尸检发现的中枢神经系统转移病例,而在24个月的随访中只发现了58%的临床脑转移。在尸检时,颅脑转移的发病率高得多,达到65%。由于寄希望于中枢神经系统是残留疾病的唯一部位,在20世纪70年代早期将预防性颅内照射(prophylactic cranial irradiation,PCI)作为SCLC治疗的初始部分[225]。一项荟萃分析得出结论,对于完全缓解的SCLC患者,PCI可延长OS和DFS[253]。在PCI前后评估局限期SCLC患者时,83%(25/30)的患者在PCI前发现有轻微的认知功能障碍,但在治疗前和治疗后神经心理学结果的比较中未发现显著差异[254]。一项RCT比较了720名患者接受照射剂量为25Gy或35Gy的PCI时神经认知功能和生活质量,发现两组之间没有显著差异[255]。这些数据表明,对PCI相关神经毒性的担忧不应阻止患者接受PCI。

PCI可以改善治疗后缓解的进展期SCLC患者的预后。最近一项在对化疗达到完全缓解的进展期小细胞肺癌患者中进行的随机对照研究显示,预防性头颅照射(PCI)能减少头部转移症状的发生,延长无病生存期及总生存期。相较于对照组,预防性头颅照射(PCI)将中位生存期从5.4个月提高到6.7个月($P=0.003$),1年生存率从13.3%提高到27.1%($P=0.003$),这些生存率上的差异部分是由于实验组患者额外的中枢神经系统治疗增加(68% vs 45%)以及对照组脑转移头部放射率低所致(59%)。收集PCI对健康相关生活质量的影响,3个月的短期结果显示PCI具有负面影响,尤其是脱发和疲劳,但认知和情绪功能无显著影响。长期生活质量的影响尚无法评估[256]。

化疗

小细胞肺癌最初发现时对于多种细胞毒性药物都很敏感,包括以下几类:烷基化物、蒽环类抗生素、喜树碱衍生物、表鬼臼毒素类、铂酸盐制剂、长春碱类和紫杉烷类。虽然氮芥衍生物、甲氨蝶呤、长春瑞滨、吉西他滨确实有效,但是其效果不及其他药物,也不常应用。药物的单剂反应率超过30%即被认为有效。

依托泊苷和顺铂联用(EP方案)起初是在20世纪80年代作为补救方案来研究,在过去25年中已成为局限期(LD)及进展期(ED)患者初次治疗的标准治疗。随机对照研究已经证实EP方案与其他毒性更强的药物对于进展期患者同样有效,因此成为基于较高疗效指数的标准治疗方案[257]。在局限期患者中采用EP方案联合同步胸部放疗,与使用环磷酰胺、表柔比星、长春新碱相比生存率受影响[258],部分原因可能由于EP方案可以全剂量发挥效应而没有蒽环类抗生素-烷基化物中出现的剂量限制及肺实质和骨髓毒性。

联合化疗

北美初始治疗的标准方案是EP的组合。东南癌症研究组(Southeastern Cancer Study Group)一项Ⅲ期临床试验中,将患者随机分为4个疗程的EP方案组和6个疗程环磷酰胺+多柔比星+长春新碱组(CAV)以及EP和CAV交替应用组,根据该研究结果建议SCLC患者至少接受4个疗程的EP方案化疗[257]。

日本临床肿瘤学组(JCOG)9511试验将ED患者随机分为EP组或伊立替康+顺铂(IP组)[259]。与依托泊苷相比,IP组患者的中位生存期和长期生存率均有所提高(中位生存期:12.8个月 vs 9.4个月,$P=0.002$,2年生存率:20% vs 5%)。其中实验组(IP组),给药4个周期,在第1天应用顺铂60mg/m²,在第1、8、15天应用伊立替康60mg/m²。北美将这一方案稍微改动后进行了一项实验,然而这项实验主要在高加索人群中进行,在IP组中没有发现获益,而且药物毒性也有差异,更多地表现为伊立替康所致的腹泻及EP组的骨髓抑制。从JCOG 9511复制IP剂量和时间表的SWOG 0124研究结果也未能证实进展期患者的IP方案优于EP方案[261]。有趣的是,随后对JCOG 9511和SWOG 0124患者的汇总分析显示,试验中IP组的反应率和存活率存在显著差异,但EP组没有。这些数据表明参与伊立替康代谢的基因多态性可以解释日本和美国患者之间毒性和功效的差异[262]。

已经在多项RCT和荟萃分析中研究了卡铂替代顺铂与依托泊苷联合的化疗方案[263]。最新的荟萃分析纳入了4项RCT,共纳入了663名局限期和进展期SCLC患者,并显示顺铂和卡铂在OS、PFS和缓解率方面均无差异[264]。顺铂和卡铂的中位OS分别为9.6和9.4个月(*HR*=1.08,$P=0.37$)。此外,卡铂在呕吐、肾毒性和神经毒性方面的毒性较低,而血液学毒性较高。目前的实践标准认为卡铂与依托泊苷联合是进展期患者的合理治疗方案,并且基于其有利的毒性特征,在 PS 评分和/或有显著并发症的患者中优先考虑。

卡铂联合伊立替康是进展期 SCLC 患者另一个一线化疗方案。一项随机Ⅱ期临床试验发现,卡铂+伊立替康与卡铂+依托泊苷相比,PFS 有所改善[265]。随后的一项Ⅲ期临床试验将卡铂+口服依托泊苷与卡铂+伊立替康进行比较,结果显示,OS 从 7.1 个月延长到 8.5 个月有所改善($P=0.04$)[266]。已发现包括卡铂与培美曲塞在内的其他方案疗效均不如卡铂联合依托泊苷[267]。

老年患者的治疗

目前的数据显示 1/3 以上 SCLC 患者为老年患者(年龄>70 岁),随着人群老龄化,老年患者的比例还将继续升高。尽管该组人群存在异质性,但是由于并发症发生率高、功能状况差、器官储备减低(尤其是骨髓),通常认为这一人群治疗相关并发症和死亡发生率高。尽管在该人群中进行的随机临床试验十分有限,但是结果均显示通过单药或减量来降低治疗强度可导致缓解率降低和生存期缩短,因此并不推荐这些治疗措施[268,269]。许多依托泊苷联合卡铂治疗老年 SCLC 患者的Ⅱ期临床试验显示,该方案耐受良好,缓解率较高[270,271]。在近期的一项随机临床试验中,老年患者在 G-CSF 支持下安全地接受了全剂量 EP 方案治疗,疗效与年轻患者相似[272]。

关于局限期老年患者的治疗,Yuen 等人报道了 INT-0096 研究中对 70 岁以上老年患者的分析结果。随机后 6 个月内,老年患者的死亡率逐渐升高,治疗相关死亡率达 10%,而 70 岁以下患者为 1%[273]。接受 4 周期 EP 方案化疗的老年患者的严重骨髓抑制发生率高于年轻患者,分别为 78%和 90%。两组的其他毒性发生率相似。老年患者的中位生存期更短(21.6 个月 vs 14.4 个月),5 年生存率更低(22% vs 16%),这一定程度说明在治疗阶段及随访早期,老年患者的死亡率升高。这些数据表明行为状况评分良好的局限期老年患者可从标准放化疗中获益。但是,需要根据行为状况仔细选择这类患者,并给予更强的支持治疗。

特殊临床情况——脑转移

既往的观点认为全身化疗对于脑转移患者的治疗作用十分有限,因为化疗药物很难到达脑组织。在 20 世纪 80 年代,一些研究组在前瞻性临床试验中观察到单纯采用全身化疗,不联合脑放疗,脑转移灶也可出现客观缓解。这些结果提示一旦 MRI 或 CT 上出现造影剂强化的转移病灶,表明血脑屏障已遭到破坏,脑内和 CNS 之外的病灶对化疗的反应率可达到一致[274,275]。脑转移患者一线治疗并非必须采用全脑放疗,尽管这一观点尚未获得临床试验的证实。但是,基于放疗可增加完全缓解率,建议最终应联合全脑放疗。一项纳入 3 个研究 192 名患者的荟萃分析显示:全脑放疗(WBRT)+托泊替康与单独 WBRT 相比,替尼泊苷+WBRT 与单独替尼泊苷相比,化疗方案为替尼泊苷+顺铂的续贯化放疗与同步化放疗相比,OS 均没有显著差异[276]。对于颅内复发患者,现有的数据表明二线化疗的有效率远远低于一线化疗患者,因此全脑放疗是标准治疗。相反,全脑放疗后复发的患者应试用全身化疗。目前正在进行探讨前期和复发环境中进行伽玛刀放射外科手术的小型研究。

SCLC 二线化疗

复发后接受二线治疗的 SCLC 患者预后不佳,中位生存期通常为 4~6 个月。治疗反应以及复发后生存期与一线治疗的疗效及无进展生存期相关。Giaccone 等人[277]在替尼泊苷的临床试验中首次观察到该现象,并在 1988 年报道。该研究中,7 例对一线治疗无反应的患者均对替尼泊苷无反应。16 例无进展生存期≤2.6 个月的患者中,仅 2 例(12%)替尼泊苷治疗有效。而一线治疗有效患者,二线治疗有效率达 42%(10/24);无进展生存期大于 2.6 个月者,二线治疗有效率达 53%(9/17)。尽管每个亚组的患者人数很少,但是 1990 年之后的许多临床试验证实了这一现象。一线治疗后 2~3 个月内复发的患者通常称为难治性患者,这些患者的缓解率低于 2~3 个月后复发者,后者称为敏感性患者。

尽管复发转移后无标准治疗方案,但托泊替康是研究最为广泛的药物,是 FDA 批准用于敏感性复发转移 SCLC 患者的唯一药物。该批准来源于一项临床试验,该试验比较了对一线化疗有效并且在化疗结束后≥60 天复发的患者中托泊替康与 CAV 的疗效[161]。托泊替康组 107 例患者,CAV 组 104 例患者,两组的缓解率分别为 24.3%和 18.3%($P=0.285$)。两组之间的中位进展时间或中位生存期均没有差异。评估的 8 个症状中,托泊替康组 4 个症状的改善情况优于 CAV 组,分别为呼吸困难、食欲缺乏、声音嘶哑和疲乏,托泊替康组对日常生活影响的改善程度也更佳($P=0.043$)。托泊替康组和 CAV 组 4 度中性粒细胞减少的发生率分别为 38%和 51%(0.001)。托泊替康组 4 度血小板减少和 3、4 度贫血的发生率均更高,托泊替康组分别为 10%和 18%,CAV 组分别为 1%和 7%(p 值均为 0.001)。随后的Ⅱ期和Ⅲ期随机临床试验对托泊替康口服和静脉用药剂型进行了比较,结果显示两者的有效率相当,口服剂型使用更为方便。托泊替康口服剂型的毒性有所不同,中性粒细胞减少的发生率更低,但是腹泻的发生率更高[159,160,162]。托泊替康每周给药尚有争议的,目前仍在研究中。

近期的一项临床试验对口服托泊替康和最佳支持治疗作为 SCLC 二线治疗进行了比较。不适合标准静脉化疗的难治性和敏感性复发患者随机分为接受最佳支持治疗或口服托泊替康($n=141$)。尽管托泊替康组缓解率仅 7%,但是 44%接受治疗的患者达到稳定,改善了症状和生活质量。托泊替康对难治或敏感性患者疾病进展和生存情况的影响相似。托泊替康和对照组中位生存期分别为 26 周和 14 周($P=0.0104$)。治疗组的 6 个月生存期优于对照组,分别为 49%和 26%。化疗对该患者人群作用的证据是极具有说服力的,将在临床研究范围内外影响化疗在该患者人群中的应用。

其他复发 SCLC 患者的治疗选择包括使用最初的诱导化疗方案,特别是诱导化疗后无进展生存期延长者,尤为无进展生存期≥6 个月者。尽管未能像托泊替康一样在复发患者中开展大规模的临床研究,伊立替康的疗效似乎与托泊替康相当[278,279]。紫杉类和蒽环类药物单独使用或与其他药物联合的临床研究较少,结果显示治疗复发患者疗效较差[280]。蒽环类药物氨柔比星(amrubicin)在二线化疗中显示出活性潜力,但是将氨柔比星与托泊替康相比较的Ⅲ期 RCT 的初步结果尚未达到其 OS 或 PFS 的主要终点,尽管缓解率得到改善

(31% vs 17%, $P=0.002$)[281~284]。胸、脑和骨的姑息性放疗同样有效,经常用于耐药的复发 SCLC 患者。

靶向治疗

采用了多种方法和努力对 SCLC 的基因组特征进行分析,包括对人和小鼠的肿瘤组织及循环肿瘤细胞(CTC)的全外显子测序、转录组分析、拷贝数及基因重排分析等[285~288]。SCLC 具有非常高的突变频率,尽管其中许多是“乘客”突变,而不是驱动突变。最常见的突变包括肿瘤抑癌基因 TP53 和 RB-1 的失活突变,其他值得注意的变异包括 PTEN 丢失、MYC 扩增以及参与 PI3K/AKT 和干细胞信号转导的基因的改变。尽管进行了相关的研究,但 SCLC 患者尚未从与其发生和进展相关的异常生物学机制中获益。

结论和未来前景

戒绝烟草消费无疑是降低肺癌发病率的最有效手段。然而,由于持续的社会和经济压力,这一目标依然遥不可及。此外,肺癌也发生于从不吸烟者。在 21 世纪的很长一段时间,肺癌将继续成为沉重的公共卫生负担。因此,需要研究早期诊断和新的治疗选择,以改善肺癌患者令人沮丧的生存率。最近的证据表明,低剂量螺旋 CT 扫描可以改善高危人群的肺癌死亡率,这是令人鼓舞的。在过去的 15 年中,在定义涉及肺癌致癌作用和治疗抗性的分子事件方面的进展很快,并且这种进展对患者的潜在益处可能是巨大的。

癌症治疗的中坚力量仍然是手术、放疗和化疗,而近年来联合使用这些手段并加以优化,已经改善了患者的转归(图 84-6)。通过增加生物疗法,致力于进一步改善肺癌的转归。这种方法利用构建的重组基因改变癌基因表达以实现逆转转化表型。此外,目前正在探索大量干扰肺癌发生发展过程中的信号转导事件的生物活性剂。这些治疗不是直接针对实际的遗传错误,而是纠正或干扰这些遗传变化引起的下游信号通路改变。例如,可以通过阻断受体本身或通过干扰其下游信号转导通路来靶向导致生长因子受体的表达或活性增加的基因突变。第一个被获批用于肺癌治疗的这类药物是 EGFR TKI。同时,VEGF 的单克隆抗体与常规化疗联合以改善肺癌、结直肠癌、乳腺癌和肾细胞癌等患者的生存。免疫疗法最近已成为一种非常有潜力的治疗策略,例如纳武单抗被批准作为治疗肺鳞癌的标准治疗方案,并且随着许多临床试验研究新的组合方案,其应用前景越发光明。

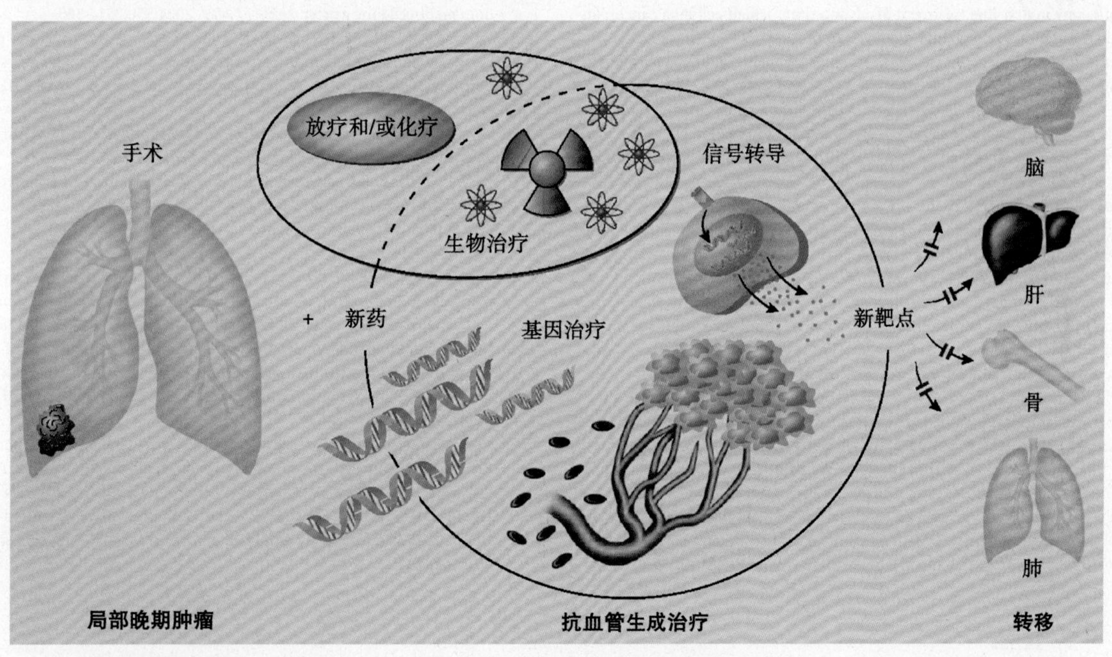

图 84-6 大部分非小细胞肺癌患者死于转移。局部晚期患者的治疗很可能需要化疗或放疗联合生物治疗,以提高其疗效并预防肿瘤转移播散

总之,近年来肺癌治疗领域的努力集中于癌症预防、早期发现和多学科治疗。全身治疗(化疗、分子靶向治疗和免疫治疗)的进展必将对所有期别的肺癌产生影响。由于肺癌是一种异质性疾病,因此鉴定和更好地理解特定的分子靶点并根据其肿瘤的生物学特征选择合适的患者进行治疗也是至关重要的。希望蛋白质组学和基因组学转化性研究的进展能成为鉴定可靠的、经验证的预测性生物标志物的关键。这些领域的进展有望产生成果,更好地控制疾病,并尽可能地减小治疗相关副反应。

(李嘉根 张帆 译 高树庚 校)

参考文献

The complete reference list can be found on the Wiley Companion Digital Edition of this title (see inside front cover for login instructions).

10 Mao L, Lee JS, Kurie JM, et al. Clonal genetic alterations in the lungs of current and former smokers. *J Natl Cancer Inst*. 1997;**89**:857-862.

11 Wistuba II, Lam S, Behrens C, et al. Molecular damage in the bronchial epithelium of current and former smokers. *J Natl Cancer Inst*. 1997;**89**:1366-1373.

13 Hammerman PS, Hayes DN, Wilkerson MD, et al. Comprehensive genomic characterization of squamous cell lung cancers. *Nature*. 2012;**489**:519-525.

14 Kadara H, Fujimoto J, Yoo SY, et al. Transcriptomic architecture of the adjacent airway field cancerization in non-small cell lung cancer. *J Natl Cancer Inst*. 2014;**106**:dju004.

46 Rusch VW. Management of Pancoast tumours. *Lancet Oncol*. 2006;**7**:997–1005.

64 Wallace MB, Pascual JMS, Raimondo M, et al. Minimally invasive endoscopic staging of suspected lung cancer. *JAMA*. 2008;**299**:540–546.

72 National Lung Screening Trial Research Team, Aberle DR, Adams AM, et al. Reduced lung-cancer mortality with low-dose computed tomographic screening. *N Engl J Med*. 2011;**365**:395–409.

73 Moyer VA. Screening for lung cancer: U.S. preventive services task force recommendation statement. *Ann Intern Med*. 2014;**160**:330–338.

74 Goldstraw P, Crowley J, Chansky K, et al. The IASLC lung cancer staging project: proposals for the revision of the TNM stage groupings in the forthcoming (seventh) edition of the TNM classification of malignant tumours. *J Thorac Oncol*. 2007;**2**:706–714.

104 Chang JY. Intensity-modulated radiotherapy, not 3 dimensional conformal, is the preferred technique for treating locally advanced lung cancer. *Semin Radiat Oncol*. 2015;**25**:110–116.

105 Chang JY, Li QQ, Xu QY, et al. Stereotactic ablative radiation therapy for centrally located early stage or isolated parenchymal recurrences of non-small cell lung cancer: how to fly in a "no fly zone". *Int J Radiat Oncol Biol Phys*. 2014;**88**:1120–1128.

119 Albain KS, Swann RS, Rusch VW, et al. Radiotherapy plus chemotherapy with or without surgical resection for stage III non-small-cell lung cancer: a phase III randomised controlled trial. *Lancet*. 2009;**374**:379–386.

124 Curran WJ, Paulus R, Langer CJ, et al. Sequential vs concurrent chemoradiation for stage III non-small cell lung cancer: randomized phase III trial RTOG 9410. *J Natl Cancer Inst*. 2011;**103**:1452–1460.

144 Scagliotti GV, Parikh P, von Pawel J, et al. Phase III study comparing cisplatin plus gemcitabine with cisplatin plus pemetrexed in chemotherapy-naive patients with advanced-stage non-small-cell lung cancer. *J Clin Oncol*. 2008;**26**:3543–3551.

147 Ardizzoni A, Boni L, Tiseo M, et al. Cisplatin- versus carboplatin-based chemotherapy in first-line treatment of advanced non-small-cell lung cancer: an individual patient data meta-analysis. *J Natl Cancer Inst*. 2007;**99**:847–857.

149 Sandler A, Gray R, Perry MC, et al. Paclitaxel-carboplatin alone or with bevacizumab for non-small-cell lung cancer. *N Engl J Med*. 2006;**355**:2542–2550.

155 Pirker R, Pereira JR, von Pawel J, et al. EGFR expression as a predictor of survival for first-line chemotherapy plus cetuximab in patients with advanced non-small-cell lung cancer: analysis of data from the phase 3 FLEX study. *Lancet Oncol*. 2012;**13**:33–42.

165 Ciuleanu T, Brodowicz T, Zielinski C, et al. Maintenance pemetrexed plus best supportive care versus placebo plus best supportive care for non-small-cell lung cancer: a randomised, double-blind, phase 3 study. *Lancet*. 2009;**374**:1432–1440.

166 Paz-Ares L, de Marinis F, Dediu M, et al. Maintenance therapy with pemetrexed plus best supportive care versus placebo plus best supportive care after induction therapy with pemetrexed plus cisplatin for advanced non-squamous non-small-cell lung cancer (PARAMOUNT): a double-blind, phase 3, randomised controlled trial. *Lancet Oncol*. 2012;**13**:247–255.

168 Patel JD, Socinski MA, Garon EB, et al. PointBreak: a randomized phase iii study of pemetrexed plus carboplatin and bevacizumab followed by maintenance pemetrexed and bevacizumab versus paclitaxel plus carboplatin and bevacizumab followed by maintenance bevacizumab in patients with stage IIIB or IV nonsquamous non-small-cell lung cancer. *J Clin Oncol*. 2013;**31**:4349–4357.

172 Garon EB, Ciuleanu TE, Arrieta O, et al. Ramucirumab plus docetaxel versus placebo plus docetaxel for second-line treatment of stage IV non-small-cell lung cancer after disease progression on platinum-based therapy (REVEL): a multicentre, double-blind, randomised phase 3 trial. *Lancet*. 2014;**384**:665–673.

180 Lynch TJ, Bell DW, Sordella R, et al. Activating mutations in the epidermal growth factor receptor underlying responsiveness of non-small-cell lung cancer to gefitinib. *N Engl J Med*. 2004;**350**:2129–2139.

186 Maemondo M, Inoue A, Kobayashi K, et al. Gefitinib or chemotherapy for non-small-cell lung cancer with mutated EGFR. *N Engl J Med*. 2010;**362**:2380–2388.

188 Rosell R, Carcereny E, Gervais R, et al. Erlotinib versus standard chemotherapy as first-line treatment for European patients with advanced EGFR mutation-positive non-small-cell lung cancer (EURTAC): a multicentre, open-label, randomised phase 3 trial. *Lancet Oncol*. 2012;**13**:239–246.

190 Sequist LV, Yang JC, Yamamoto N, et al. Phase III study of afatinib or cisplatin plus pemetrexed in patients with metastatic lung adenocarcinoma with EGFR mutations. *J Clin Oncol*. 2013;**31**:3327–3334.

196 Camidge DR, Pao W, Sequist LV. Acquired resistance to TKIs in solid tumours: learning from lung cancer. *Nat Rev Clin Oncol*. 2014;**11**:473–481.

202 Solomon BJ, Mok T, Kim DW, et al. First-line crizotinib versus chemotherapy in ALK-positive lung cancer. *N Engl J Med*. 2014;**371**:2167–2177.

204 Shaw AT, Engelman JA. Ceritinib in ALK-rearranged non-small-cell lung cancer. *N Engl J Med*. 2014;**370**:2537–2539.

207 Shaw AT, Ou SH, Bang YJ, et al. Crizotinib in ROS1-rearranged non-small-cell lung cancer. *N Engl J Med*. 2014;**371**:1963–1971.

208 Janne PA, Shaw AT, Pereira JR, et al. Selumetinib plus docetaxel for KRAS-mutant advanced non-small-cell lung cancer: a randomised, multicentre, placebo-controlled, phase 2 study. *Lancet Oncol*. 2013;**14**:38–47.

210 Topalian SL, Hodi FS, Brahmer JR, et al. Safety, activity, and immune correlates of anti-PD-1 antibody in cancer. *N Engl J Med*. 2012;**366**:2443–2454.

211 Herbst RS, Soria JC, Kowanetz M, et al. Predictive correlates of response to the anti-PD-L1 antibody MPDL3280A in cancer patients. *Nature*. 2014;**515**:563–567.

214 Arriagada R, Bergman B, Dunant A, Le Chevalier T, Pignon JP, Vansteenkiste J. Cisplatin-based adjuvant chemotherapy in patients with completely resected non-small-cell lung cancer. *N Engl J Med*. 2004;**350**:351–360.

222 Pisters KM, Vallieres E, Crowley JJ, et al. Surgery with or without preoperative paclitaxel and carboplatin in early-stage non-small-cell lung cancer: Southwest Oncology Group Trial S9900, an intergroup, randomized, phase III trial. *J Clin Oncol*. 2010;**28**:1843–1849.

256 Slotman B, Faivre-Finn C, Kramer G, et al. Prophylactic cranial irradiation in extensive small-cell lung cancer. *N Engl J Med*. 2007;**357**:664–672.

261 Lara PN Jr, Natale R, Crowley J, et al. Phase III trial of irinotecan/cisplatin compared with etoposide/cisplatin in extensive-stage small-cell lung cancer: clinical and pharmacogenomic results from SWOG S0124. *J Clin Oncol*. 2009;**27**:2530–2535.

267 Socinski MA, Smit EF, Lorigan P, et al. Phase III study of pemetrexed plus carboplatin compared with etoposide plus carboplatin in chemotherapy-naive patients with extensive-stage small-cell lung cancer. *J Clin Oncol*. 2009;**27**:4787–4792.

283 Jotte R, Conkling P, Reynolds C, et al. Randomized phase II trial of single-agent amrubicin or topotecan as second-line treatment in patients with small-cell lung cancer sensitive to first-line platinum-based chemotherapy. *J Clin Oncol*. 2011;**29**:287–293.

285 Peifer M, Fernandez-Cuesta L, Sos ML, et al. Integrative genome analyses identify key somatic driver mutations of small-cell lung cancer. *Nat Genet*. 2012;**44**:1104–1110.

286 Rudin CM, Durinck S, Stawiski EW, et al. Comprehensive genomic analysis identifies SOX2 as a frequently amplified gene in small-cell lung cancer. *Nat Genet*. 2012;**44**:1111–1116.

第 85 章　恶性胸膜间皮瘤

Daniel R. Gomez, MD ■ Anne S. Tsao, MD Anne S. Tsao, MD ■
Haining Yang, PhD Haining Yang, PhD ■ Harvey I. Pass, MD Harvey I. Pass, MD

概述

恶性胸膜间皮瘤是一种侵袭性恶性肿瘤，在未来的5~10年，其发病率在世界范围内可能达到顶峰。虽然大多数患者最终会死于这种疾病，但在过去十年该疾病的治疗和诊断均有了实质性提高，包括全世界对定义该疾病的早期检测生物标志物的兴趣逐渐增加，关于最佳手术方法的争论（胸膜外全肺切除术与肺保留方法，如胸膜切除术/剥脱术），进一步完善允许适形治疗领域的放射技术和辐射的传递与所涉及的肺完好无损，出现了针对性的全身治疗，并允许增加个体化治疗，这可能会改善患者的长期预后。实际上，评估新治疗方法的安全性和有效性的前瞻性临床试验对于建立标准化治疗至关重要，希望这些努力的成果会帮助寻找到最佳方法。早期患者将受益于多种方式协同控制，同时限制毒性，使得接下来十年或二十年的长期幸存者数量增加。

发病率和流行病学

人类统计数据库中低估了间皮瘤的发病率[1]。目前，全球每年有15 000~20 000人死于胸膜间皮瘤，主要集中在美国和其他工业化国家，如英格兰等国的石棉产品工厂和造船设施领域[2,3]，在美国每年大约诊断出3 000例病例，根据20~40年的潜伏期和石棉暴露率，预计发病率将在2010—2015年达到峰值[4]，与其他国家（如英国，澳大利亚、荷兰）的预测结果相似[5,6]。男性与女性之间的比例约为4∶1，80%来自胸膜[7]。在尸检中发现，恶性间皮瘤的发生率从0.02%到0.7%不等。在大多数医院中，胸膜多于腹膜，右侧多于左侧（60∶40），然而在一些流行病学监测研究发现石棉工人腹膜形式比胸膜更常见[8]。患者的平均年龄约为60岁，但该疾病可发生在任何年龄，包括儿童期[9,10]。

病因

众所周知，间皮瘤的主要发病原因之一是石棉暴露。据估计，从暴露发生后15年开始，6%~10%的35岁以上的石棉工人将死于中耳炎[11]。此外，从1940年到1979年，约有2 750万工人被职业暴露于美国的石棉，年度死亡率从1980年的大约2 000增加到20世纪90年代后期的3 000[12]。绝缘材料，建筑，造船业和汽车制动器是职业暴露的众多来源之一，虽然石棉暴露和吸烟的协同作用会产生肺癌，但实际上吸烟并不是间皮瘤的既定风险因素，尽管假设使用“微米级”过滤嘴的卷烟之间存在关联。妇女和儿童的家庭污染通常也会发生，通常是通过石棉工人的工作服[13]。其他不太常见的致病因子如：患肾母细胞瘤（WT）或纵隔淋巴瘤转移的年轻患者所接受的放射治疗（RT）。胸膜斑块的作用及其与神经胶质瘤的关系已争论数年，最近法国的一项研究通过针对曾接触过石棉的患者进行筛查初步解决了这个问题，该团队通过CT（计算机断层扫描）扫描对5 287名男性进行了7年随访，并评估了间皮瘤的发生率和随后的存活率[14]。结果发现，17例患者被诊断为恶性胸膜间皮瘤（MPM），胸膜斑块之间存在显著相关性，危险比为8.9。作者得出结论，胸膜斑块的存在可能是“间皮瘤的独立危险因素”[15,16]。

间皮瘤的分子机制

多种细胞遗传学和分子异常可导致MPM的发病。通常认为，吸入石棉使纤维沉积在肺实质中，最终迁移并在胸膜内层植入纤维，反复发作的炎症、愈合，炎症细胞产生的氧自由基、石棉中的铁以及纤维对DNA的直接损伤是石棉暴露的致病特征[17]。运用核型和比较基因组杂交（CGH）技术分析原发性MPM肿瘤和细胞系发现频繁的缺失，重复和易位，基因组损失比增益更常见[18]。染色体1p、3p、4p、4q、6q、9p、13q、14q和22q的缺失是常见的。值得注意的是肿瘤抑制基因*p16/CDKN2A*，*p53*和*NF2*的丢失位于这些位点内[19]。

HMGB1、肿瘤坏死因子α（TNF-α）和NF-κ信号在间皮细胞遗传受损后存活中起重要作用[20]。HMGB1是一种典型的DAMP（损伤相关分子模式）[21,22]，是炎症的关键介质，也是引发石棉介导TNF-α的释放和随后的NF-κB信号转导的关键调节因子[23]。炎症部位的巨噬细胞吞噬内化石棉并释放诱变与石棉相关致癌基因有关活性氧和多种细胞因子[24]，包括TNF-α和白介素-1（IL）-1，暴露于石棉时活性巨噬细胞释放大量HMGB1，其他炎症细胞和人间皮细胞（HMC）释放也可释放该因子[20,25]。在程序性坏死过程中，HMGB1结合几种促炎分子并引发炎症，从而将这种类型的细胞死亡与凋亡症区分开来，它刺激邻近炎症细胞如巨噬细胞上的RAGE，TLR2和TLR4（三种主要的HMGB1受体），并诱导TNF-α和IL-1β的释放。然后石棉介导的TNF-α信号转导诱导NF-κB依赖机制的激活，促进石棉暴露后HMCs的存活，因此可使石棉诱导遗传损伤的HMC存活、分裂、繁殖和遗传，最终导致恶性克隆的癌前细胞的畸变[26]。此外，HMGB1增强NF-κB的活性，促进肿瘤形成，进展和转移。已发现HMGB1在接触石棉的个体和MM（多发性骨髓瘤）患者的血清中升高，并且正在确认该分子是石棉暴露的生物标志物（图85-1）。

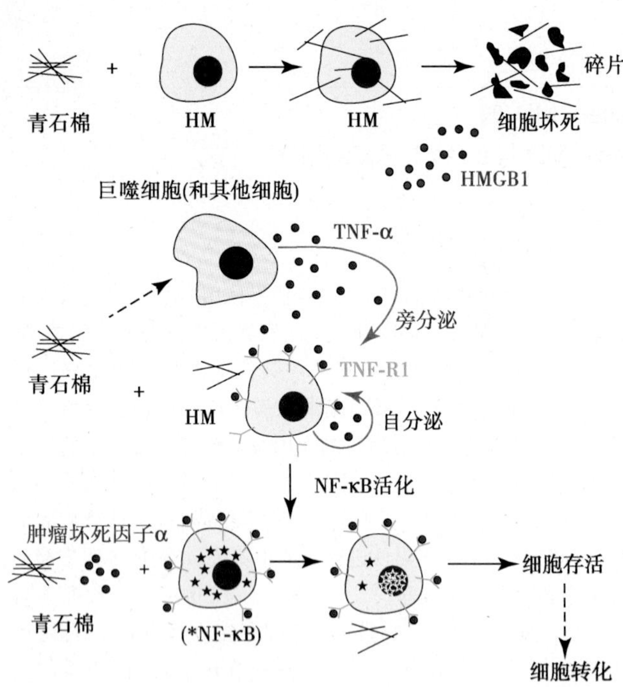

图 85-1 矿物纤维致癌作用(矿物纤维致癌。石棉和离子石导致 HM 细胞坏死死亡,导致 HMGB1 释放到细胞外空间,HMGB1 释放导致噬菌体堆积、炎症反应和 TNF-α 分泌,TNF-α 激活 NF-κB 通路,使 HM 在石棉/离子接触后存活率增加。如果基因变异累积,最终发展成 MM)

间皮瘤的遗传易感性:BAP1 家族的作用

最近一项美国研究,BAP1 家族似乎对石棉致癌作用具有特殊易感性,并且这些家族在其种系中具有 BAP1 突变基因[27],与其家族易感性相关,同时也存在于葡萄膜黑色素瘤和其他罕见的恶性肿瘤中。BAP1(BRCA 相关蛋白 1)已被鉴定为新型 MPM 肿瘤抑制基因,其位于 3p21,这是一个经常在 MM 中缺失的区域,并编码已知靶向组蛋白和其他蛋白质的去泛素化酶。Bott 等[28]人最初发现 23%的间皮瘤样本中体细胞突变与 BAP1 关联,在更大的一系列患者中,同一组确认体细胞 BAP1 突变发生在约 20%的胸膜 MM 中,并报道,有和没有 BAP1 突变的患者中唯一的临床变量显著不同是吸烟(前或当前),BAP1 突变在吸烟者中更为普遍(75%对 42%)[29]。最新研究报道,MM 中 61%具有 BAP1 基因改变(缺失或序列水平突变)[30],Arzt 等[31]人在 sep 52 例胸膜 MM 的 arate 队列报告中发现 60%的胸膜 MM 缺乏 BAP1IHC 染色,证实了以前的结果。在该研究中,BAP1 表达与石棉暴露之间没有相关性,且 BAP1 在肿瘤样本中的表达与存活率呈负相关。BAP1 似乎主要以不依赖 BRCA 的方式通过细胞表观基因组,调节组蛋白 H2A 泛素化和染色质可及性发挥其抗肿瘤活性[32]。然而,BAP1 与正常细胞和癌细胞生物学的相关性仍然很大程度上无法解释[33]。事实上,在癌细胞中操纵 BAP1 经常产生意想不到的甚至相互矛盾的结果。例如,MM 和葡萄膜黑色素瘤细胞系中 BAP1 的沉默导致细胞生长减少。Testa 等人最先报道 Germline BAP1 突变,发现于具有高频率 MPM 的两个国家家庭中[34]。在同一项研究中,22%的散发性 MM 肿瘤具有体细胞 BAP1 突变。这些发现促使人们推测 BAP1 种系突变可导致一种新的癌症综合征,其特征是胸膜和周围性 MM,葡萄膜和皮肤黑色素瘤以及可能的其他肿瘤均显著过量表达。

疑似间皮瘤患者的诊断和分期

症状与体征

间皮瘤的发病与胸痛、呼吸困难或咳嗽有关(图 85-2)。胸壁的逐渐侵入常导致难以承受的疼痛。胸腔积液最初存在于多达 95%的病例中,由于透明质酸含量高,液体通常是黏性的。随后,肿瘤生长通常导致胸膜腔完全闭塞和包裹肺部。晚期症状主要为纵隔浸润伴吞咽困难、膈神经麻痹、心包积液和上腔静脉综合征[35]。间皮瘤腹膜受累的特征是腹水和肠道功能紊乱导致的恶病质。

实验室诊断

多种实验室检测指标异常与神经胶质瘤相关,其中以血小板计数>400 000/μl 的血小板增多症最为常见,其他包括高人免疫球蛋白血症、嗜酸粒细胞增多症、慢性贫血、同型半胱氨酸水平升高、叶酸缺乏、维生素 B_{12} 和 B_6 缺乏[35]。

组织学亚型

间皮瘤有三种主要类型:上皮型,纤维形态型(也称为肉瘤样)以及双相混合型。大多数间皮瘤(50%~70%)属于上皮型,10%为肉瘤样,其余为混合型。区分转移性癌和间皮瘤必须采用免疫组织化学(IHC)标记,常见的标记物包括阳性角蛋白、角蛋白 5/6、钙结合蛋白和 WT-1,阴性标记物包括 CEA、CD15、Ber-EP4、Moc-31、TTF-1 和 B72.3[36]。这些标记物很重要,因为间皮瘤可能很难与其他恶性肿瘤区别开来,即来自癌肉瘤的双相间皮瘤或来自转移性胸膜肉瘤的纤维性间皮瘤。

一些研究已经验证了组织学亚型对预后的影响。事实表明,上皮型比双相或肉瘤样亚型具有更好的预后[37]。除了这些组织学外,还存在其他几种较低等级的间皮瘤,如乳头间皮瘤常发生于腹腔,多囊性间皮瘤常呈"簇"聚集并也可存在于腹膜中的腺瘤样间皮瘤中,其是泌尿生殖系统中的良性间皮损伤。这些亚型通常比上皮型、双相或肉瘤样组织更为无痛性的,但临床过程可能有所不同[38]。

肿瘤标志物

研究最为火热的两种间皮瘤肿瘤标志物是骨桥蛋白(osteo-pontin,OPN)和间皮素(mesothelin,SMRP)。OPN 是一种糖蛋白生物标志物,多种癌症可表达,包括肺癌、乳腺癌、结肠直肠癌、胃癌、卵巢癌和黑色素瘤。OPN 还参与石棉诱导的与癌症发生相关的细胞信号转导途径。最新一项研究对比了间皮瘤患者与非恶性石棉相关疾病患者的 OPN 水平,研究显示,OPN 可用于鉴别石棉暴露的间皮瘤患者与非恶性肿瘤的石棉暴露患者[39]。最近的一项荟萃分析研究了 7 项研究中骨质疏

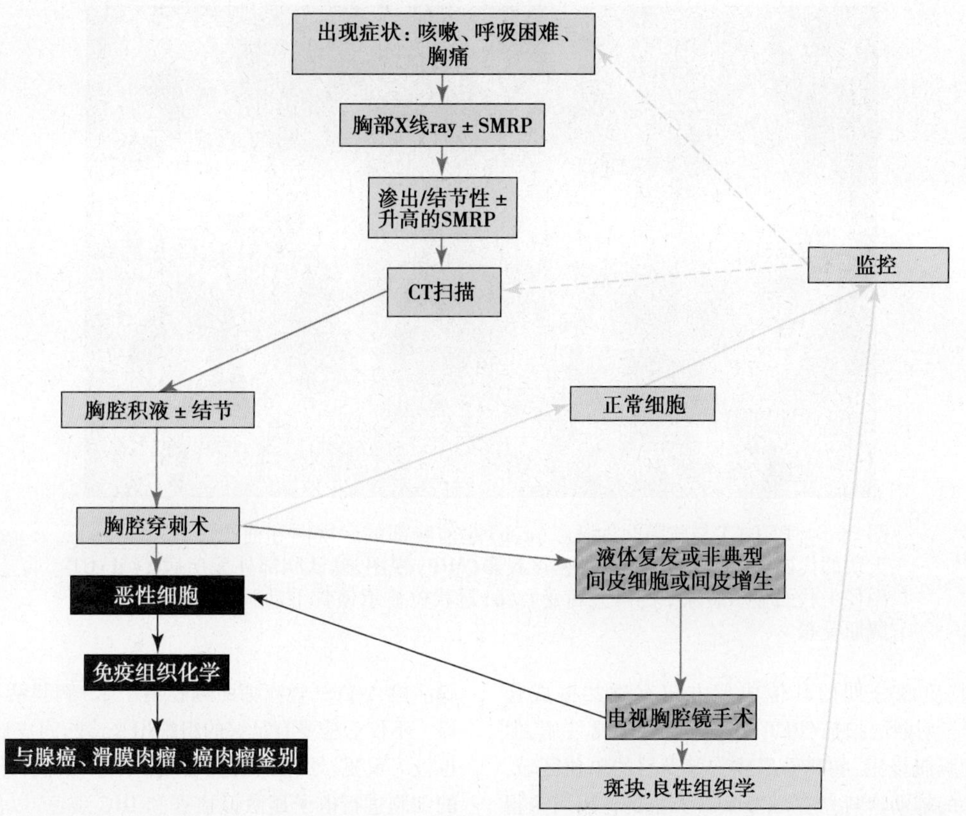

图 85-2　暴露在石棉中的个体出现新症状时的工作算法(新石棉暴露个体的治疗方法及新的胸膜穿刺术及免疫组化分析。如果发现非典型间皮细胞,应进行胸腔镜检查,以确定恶性肿瘤或炎症性疾病)

松症在间皮瘤诊断中的作用,发现其总敏感性为 0.57(95%*CI* 0.52~0.61),特异性为 0.81(95%*CI* 0.79~0.84),阳性似然比(*PLR*)为 3.78(95%*CI* 2.23~6.41),阴性似然比(*NLR*)为 0.51(0.38~0.67)。这些结果证明 OPN 与间皮瘤具有上述相关性。但 OPN 缺乏特异性,并且其性能在血浆中优于血清[40]。

最初由 Pastan 描述的 SMRP[41,42],也是一种糖蛋白,存在于间皮瘤、卵巢癌和胰腺癌中。Robinson 等[43]在 48 例患者中证实 SMRP 是一种血清生物标志物,敏感性为 83%,特异性为 95%,表明其有希望成为是血液和胸膜液中 MPM 的标志物[44]。MPM 患者血清 SMRP 水平高于肺癌患者,与良性胸膜液或其他非 MPM 胸腔积液相比,胸水中的 SMRP 水平也是如此。事实上,先前研究表明,胸水中的检测准确性优于血清,但是血清分析是衡量这一因素的一种更便捷的方法[45]。某研究试图寻找血清标志物组合作为间皮瘤的诊断工具,并确定其他标志物是否可提高单独使用 SMRP 的诊断率,该研究发现,结合 SMRP 和癌胚抗原(carcinoembryonic antigen,CEA)可提高间皮瘤和肺癌的鉴别率,以及间皮瘤和非患病石棉暴露患者之间的差异[46]。荟萃分析证实了该研究:SMRP 的敏感性和特异性在许多研究中是相似的[47]。除了用作诊断工具外,还有一些研究关注这些标志物来追踪疾病的进程。一项前瞻性研究向 41 名患者收集了 165 份样本,并使用实体瘤反应评估标准(response evaluation criteria in solid tumors,RECIST)对疾病状态进行了临时评估,研究发现,虽然 SMRP 与 RECIST 标准或改良 RECIST 标准测评的反应性显著相关,如绝对变化,但 OPN 没有发现这种相关性[46]。另一项 97 例患者的前瞻性研究发现可溶性 SMRP 的变化与放射反应、代谢活跃的肿瘤体积和中位生存期相关[48]。SMRP 作为预后标志物和检测肿瘤反应的方法正在进一步研究。

已经探索了几种其他潜在的肿瘤标志物在这种临床病例中具有实用性。最近广受关注的肿瘤标志物 fibulin-3,是一种位于脉管系统基底膜的细胞外蛋白。在评估血浆 fibulin-3 水平时,研究人员发现,该标记物可以区分 200 名患者队列中接触石棉的健康患者与恶性肿瘤患者,并且通过盲法研究证实了这一点[49]。此外,将血浆与胸膜积液中的 fbulin-3 检测结果进行对比分析,发现该标记物可有效地鉴别良性以及其他类型的恶性胸腔积液。fibulin-3 的诊断价值已在其他研究中得到证实[50]。在一项研究中,将可溶性 SMRP 和 fibulin-3 作为肿瘤标志物进行比较,研究人员发现虽然 SMRP 在诊断方面具有优势,但 fibulin-3 在评估预后方面更为出色。因此,这意味着两种标志物都能在实际中发挥作用[51]。

扫描方式

CT 扫描对诊断和评估疾病非常有用(图 85-3)[52]。CT 扫描结果包括胸腔积液、胸膜结节和向心性胸膜增厚。最近牛津大学的研究人员评估了大约 400 名患者在胸腔镜检查前进行 CT 扫描的阳性和阴性预测结果,发现 CT 扫描显示“恶性”的阳性预测值为 80%,而阴性预测值为 65%。因此,单独 CT 扫描似乎不足以确定哪些患者应进行侵入性胸膜活组织检查[53]。

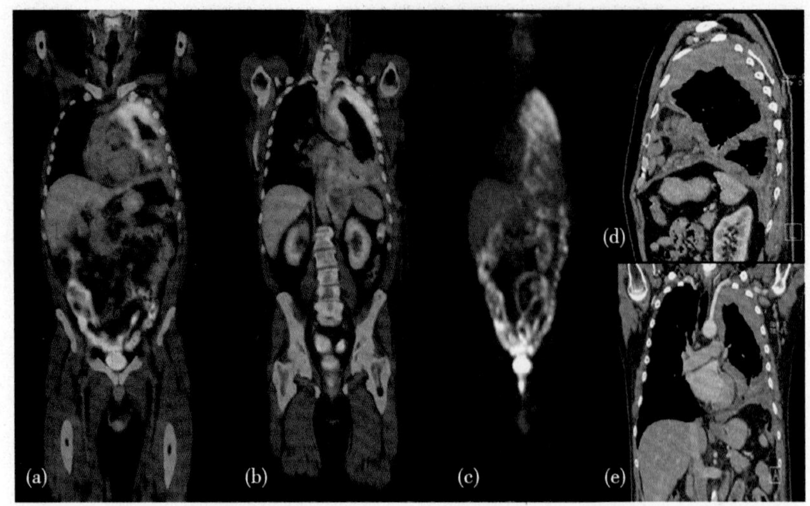

图 85-3 PET-CT 与胸膜间皮瘤。(a、b)左前胸部的后视图和前视图显示了一个大块的代谢过度的肿瘤(c)最大密度投影(MIP)视图,确认胸部外无疾病。(d)CT 图像矢状面显示裂隙中的巨大病变。(e)冠状位显示锁骨下动脉的桥接和可能的膈肌受累

可行神经胶质瘤分期的其他成像方式有磁共振成像(MRI)和正电子发射断层扫描(PET)扫描。MRI 不常使用,但可能有助于检测膈肌侵犯、胸膜受累或胸壁受累的单独区域,可能是手术切除的辅助诊断方法。PET/CT 扫描的作用尚未得到证实,2014 年美国综合癌症网络指南不建议 PET 成像用于诊断或分期。然而,许多先前的和正在进行的研究正在评估该技术,因为其可用于其他胸部恶性肿瘤,例如肺癌。在一项研究中发现 PET 在检测转移性淋巴结病中的敏感性仅为 11%[54]。然而,同一项研究发现,切除时的高标准摄取值(SUV)与 N2 疾病相关。最近,来自同一机构的研究表明,与 SUV 水平低于 10 相比,SUV 水平高于 10 的存活期更短以及死亡风险增高 3.3 倍[55],这表明 PET 可根据肿瘤新陈代谢活动结果对患者进行分类。CT-PET 联合比单独的 PET 更能提供有用的信息。在一项针对 29 名 MPM 患者的研究中,CT-PET 联合准确地对 72%的病例进行了整体分期,显示了其对 T4 疾病的敏感性,单独使用 PET 的患者敏感性为 19%,CT-PET 联合的敏感性为 67%,通过放射学诊断出 7 例常规漏诊的胸外疾病患者,并根据常规研究确定 12 名患者不用手术切除治疗[56]。此外,来自 Memorial Sloan-Kettering 癌症中心的研究人员验证 PET 扫描检测组织学亚型的准确性,在 100 例接受术前 PET 扫描的 MPM 患者中,发现相对于非畸形亚型患者,上皮样间皮瘤的混合亚型具有更高的 SUV,因此支持了更高的 SUV 与侵袭性疾病相关的结论[57]。另一项研究探索 50 例 MPM 可切除患者新辅助化疗后 PET 扫描对预后的意义,所有患者均接受 EPP(胸膜外全肺切除术)和术后胸腔放疗,结果显示新辅助化疗后的代谢反应与总生存率显著相关,作者得出结论,对治疗的反应有助于确定新辅助化疗后是否行手术切除[58]。

间皮瘤外科诊断和分期

可用于间皮瘤诊断目的的干预措施包括胸腔穿刺闭合胸膜活检、VATS(视频辅助胸腔镜手术)胸膜活检和开胸胸膜活检。不仅活检要有足够的组织用来诊断间皮瘤,间皮瘤的亚型也极为重要。虽然细胞学诊断可能很困难,但可以对胸膜液的细胞进行电子显微镜检查和 IHC 染色,以便将诊断率在疑似病例中提高 84%。直接活检的视频辅助胸腔镜检查和肺及胸膜受累的评估仍然是诊断的金标准。多项研究证实这项技术在接受间皮瘤手术的患者中实用性,但也指出该技术难以获得正确的组织学诊断[59]。开胸胸膜活检可能获得关于壁层、内脏和隔膜胸膜受损的信息,这可能对预后具有预测价值[60]。虽然其很少进行,但在没有自由胸膜空间时仍可能需要。

分期和预后指标

美国癌症联合委员会(AJCC)的间皮瘤分期系统已经在许多外科手术试验中得到验证[61],并且自 20 世纪 90 年代以来一直在使用。为了改进目前的分期系统,国际肺癌研究协会分析了国际数据库 2 000 多名 MPM 患者的分期,并且预测生存的协变量-最佳分期信息:年龄、性别、组织学(是否为上皮样)或外科手术的类型(姑息性与 EPP 或胸膜切除术剥离)[62]。为补充预后指标添加了血小板计数、白细胞计数和辅助治疗[63]。Gill[64]研究了 88 例 EPP 治疗对上皮 MPM 肿瘤体积的影响,这是 MPM 阶段独立的死亡风险模型,具有神经细胞减少的患者,如 Pass 等人最初描述的那样[65],Gill 的研究显示,肿瘤体积、血红蛋白浓度、血小板计数、病理性 TNM(肿瘤,淋巴结和转移)类别以及辅助化疗或 RT 的给药均与生存相关[64]。Richards 使用 Brigham 和 Women Hospital 系列中的与 Gill 相同的 MPM 队列,描述了使用血红蛋白、CT 体积、裂隙厚度和组织学亚型的细胞减少来验证 MPM 存活和复发时间的模型(表 85-1)[66]。

表 85-1　国际间皮瘤研究小组(IMIG)胸膜间皮瘤分期系统[61]

T1	
T1a	肿瘤局限于同侧壁层胸膜±纵隔±膈肌胸膜,不累及脏层胸膜
T1b	肿瘤局限于同侧壁层胸膜±纵隔±膈肌胸膜,累及脏层胸膜
T2	肿瘤累及同侧胸膜表面(壁层胸膜、纵隔胸膜、横膈胸膜、脏层胸膜),至少具有下列特征之一:
	• 侵犯膈肌
	• 通过脏胸膜侵及肺实质
T3	局部晚期但潜在可切除的肿瘤,肿瘤侵及单侧胸膜各表面(壁层胸膜、纵隔胸膜、横膈胸膜、脏胸膜),且至少侵及以下任一结构:
	• 胸腔内筋膜
	• 纵隔脂肪
	• 单个、完全可切除的肿瘤病灶侵及胸壁软组织
	• 非穿壁性心包膜受侵
T4	局部晚期技术上不可切除的肿瘤,肿瘤侵及单侧胸膜各表面(壁层胸膜、纵隔胸膜、横膈胸膜、脏胸膜),且至少具有以下一种情况:
	• 肿瘤弥漫性侵及胸膜或胸壁多发肿块,不论有无肋骨破坏
	• 肿瘤通过横膈直接侵及腹膜
	• 肿瘤直接侵及对侧胸膜
	• 肿瘤直接侵及纵隔器官
	• 肿瘤直接侵及脊柱
	• 肿瘤侵及心包膜内面,不论有无心包膜渗出或心肌受侵
N 分期	
NX	区域淋巴结不能确定
N0	无区域淋巴结转移
N1	同侧支气管周围和/或同侧肺门淋巴结转移
N2	同侧纵隔和/或气管隆突下淋巴结转移
N3	对侧纵隔、对侧肺门、同侧或对侧斜角肌或锁骨上淋巴结转移
M 分期	
MX	不能确定远处转移的存在
M0	无远处转移
M1	远处转移
Ⅰ期	
Ⅰa	T1a N0 M0
Ⅰb	T1b N0 M0
Ⅱ期	T2 N0 M0
Ⅲ期	任何 T3 M0
	任何 N1 M0
	任何 N2 M0
Ⅳ期	任何 T4
	任何 N3
	任何 M1

T,原发肿瘤;T1,仅限于同侧胸膜(壁层胸膜、脏层胸膜);T2,局部浸润(膈肌、胸内筋膜、同侧肺、肺间裂);T3,深局部浸润(胸内筋膜以上的胸壁);T4,广泛的直接侵袭(对侧胸膜、腹膜、腹膜后);N,淋巴结;N0,无淋巴结受累;N1,同侧肺门淋巴结转移;N2,同侧纵隔淋巴结转移;N3,对侧肺门淋巴结转移;M,远处转移;M0,无远处转移;M1,远处转移;血行传播或淋巴系统传播。

治疗

间皮瘤的治疗选择取决于几个参数，包括表现状态、临床并发症、肺功能、发病阶段、患者的年龄以及其他因素。只要可以在不留下严重疾病的情况下排除大部分疾病，就可考虑手术方案。如果无法实现，则可使用支持性缓解治疗（表 85-2）。

表 85-2 胸膜间皮瘤的治疗选择

支持治疗	
积液控制	滑石粉胸膜固定术
	VATS 辅助
	糊剂（slurry）
	置胸管（pleurex catheter）
	反复胸腔穿刺
控制疼痛	麻醉类药物
	永久硬膜外置管
	局部放疗
手术	胸膜剥脱术
	胸膜外全肺切除术
化疗[a]	培美曲塞（力比泰）和顺铂[a]
	吉西他滨和顺铂[a]
	长春瑞宾（诺维本）
	处于Ⅰ/Ⅱ期试验中的靶向药物
综合治疗	综合应用化疗、手术和术后放疗[b]
	手术和术后放疗
	手术和术后化疗
	手术和新的细胞毒/靶向药物[b]
新胸腔注射疗法	热灌注化疗[b]
	光动力疗法[b]
	基因疗法[b]
部分中心采用的新放射技术	调强放疗

[a] 目前常在Ⅱ/Ⅲ期试验中使用。
[b] 还在评估中。

支持性护理

选择支持治疗的 MPM 患者中位生存期仅为 4[67]～13 个月[68]，且受多种因素影响，包括肿瘤的生物学以及从症状发作时或从明确诊断时间开始记录的存活时间。控制胸腔积液有多种途径，包括反复胸腔穿刺术、滑石粉胸膜固定术或放置 Pleur X（Denver Biomedical，Denver，CO）导管[69]。这些技术的失败通常与肿瘤限制的肺有关，实体肿瘤体积较大、长期积液、年龄超过 70 岁等导致多个胸腔穿刺定位或表现不佳。在这种情况下，带有单向瓣膜的 PleurX 导管可以在局部麻醉下植入胸腔积液，患者可以使用现有的一次性引流装置在家中自行排液[70]。最近，一项随机试验验证了胸膜液体缓解对间皮瘤的影响。MesoVats 试验是随机选择在 2003 年至 2012 年未考虑最大细胞减灭术的 87 例 VAT 增殖性胸膜切除术或 88 例滑石粉胸膜固定术的患者，两者没有生存差异，但胸膜切除术患者胸腔积液得到了更好的控制，有利于提高生活质量[71]。

患有间皮瘤胸壁疼痛的患者应在专门的疼痛管理小组协商下进行，以考虑麻醉控制以及包括门诊硬膜外导管在内的新型疼痛控制技术。姑息性放疗与中位生存期相关，为 4～5 个月[72,73]。

胸膜间皮瘤的手术治疗

最全面的细胞减压术

MPM 细胞减压术的目标是切除所有可见或可触及的肿瘤（R0 或 R1）或“宏观完全切除术”（macroscopic complete resection，MCR），无论是否涉及 EPP 或肺保留手术。国际肺癌研究协会的间皮瘤领域已确定了胸膜间皮瘤切除术的统一命名法[74]，包括 EPP、扩大胸膜切除术和剥脱术（ePD）（切除膈肌和/或心包）以及胸膜切除术剥脱作为潜在的 MCR。怀疑和文献记载的半胸以外的疾病排除使用 MCR。ECOG 表现状态为 2 级或更高，或者具有不可逆心肌缺血或心室功能受损（射血分数<50%）的心脏储备受限患者通常不适合进行细胞减压术。此外，肺功能检查受损不应视为肺切除术适应证，必须仔细评估延长的 P/D，因为细胞减少不损害现有的肺功能，但可能会修复受损的肺，并可能改善呼吸困难。

胸膜外全肺切除术（EPP）

正如最近对 EPP 用于 MPM 的系统评价中所描述的那样[75]，中位总生存期从 9.4 个月到 27.5 个月不等，1 年、2 年和 5 年生存率分别从 36% 到 83%，5% 到 59% 和 0% 到 24% 不等（图 85-4）。总围术期死亡率从 0% 到 11.8%，并且通过改进术前分期、麻醉、切除、重建和手术相关并发症的围术期处理，常规手术中心的死亡率接近 3%[76]。围术期主要并发症为心房颤动、心肌梗死和肺部并发症[77]。单独使用 EPP 似乎不能延长生存期。在大多数 EPP 系列中，中位生存期<2 年，但 10%～20% 的患者是 5 年生存者。肉瘤样组织学和/或淋巴结受累的患者预后较差，不应被视为 EPP 的适应证[78]。

trimodality 疗法和向肺保留转变的技术

trimodality 疗法包括诱导化疗、EPP 治疗、作为半胸切除术到肺切除术腔或作为强度调节的 RT[79]。总体而言，MPM 三联疗法的研究证明 EPP 的疗效为 3.1%，完成所有项目中 60% 的患者中位生存期为 27.7 个月。Mesothe lioma 和 Radical Surgery（MARS）试图验证 EPP 为根治性治疗方案的一部分。最初设计 MARS 为随机试验，需比较 670 名进行诱导化疗、EPP 和术后 RT 与诱导治疗但没有 EPP 的患者[80]。当招募患者出现困难时，仅对 50 名接受 EPP 或未接受 EPP 治疗的患者进行初步可行性研究。该研究显示，手术组与非手术组的 6、12、18 个月和中位生存率无显著差异，中位生存期分别为 14.4 个月和 19.5 个月。MARS 中 EPP 的手术死亡率为 18%，其他Ⅱ期三联试验的手术死亡率为 3.1%。此外，研究缺乏效力、术前化疗

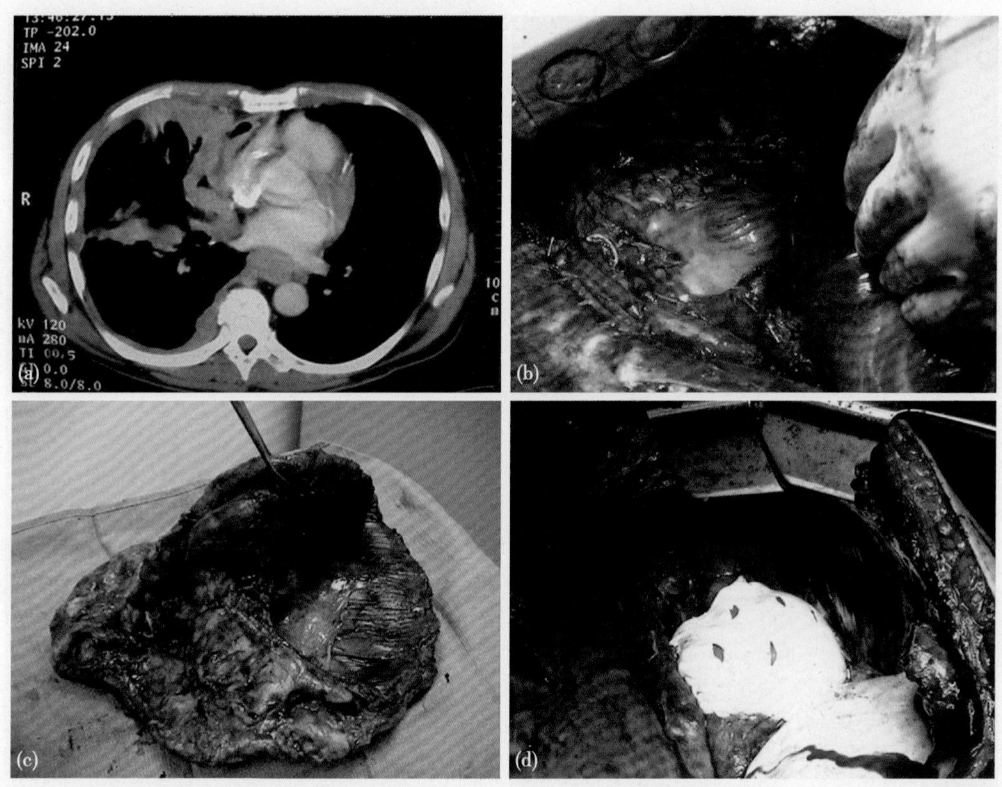

图 85-4　胸膜外肺切除术治疗间皮瘤：(a)计算机断层扫描显示胸膜增厚、心包增厚、裂隙中有疾病。(b)手放在肝上切除术后的术中观察。可见支气管残端、右心房及心包切开范围。(c)手术标本显示右侧膈肌切除和包裹肺的增厚胸膜。(d)用 gore-tex 补片重建膈肌和心包

的非标准化及只有 1/3 的人获得完全三联治疗，限制了 MARS 的影响[81]。

然而，MPM 的唯一手术 MCR 是 EPP 的这一观点正被逐渐淡化(图 85-5)。一项对 663 名连续患者(538 名男性和 125 名 MPM 女性在三个国家间皮瘤中心接受 EPP 或 P/D)的回顾性研究中，EPP(n=27/385)的手术死亡率为 7%，P 为 4%/D(n=13/278)[82]。多变量分析显示，EPP(P<0.001)控制分期、组织学、性别和多模式治疗的死亡概率增加 1.4 倍。这项研究是第一个假设接受 P/D 治疗的患者与接受 EPP 治疗的患者有相当的生存率。但是，这种结论的原因是多因素的并且受到选择偏差的影响。

其他研究显示，如果进行 P/D 以强制性方式排除所有肉眼可见的疾病，则总体存活率会翻倍[83~90]。在同一外科医生进行 EPP 和 P/D 直接比较的研究中，P/D 具有较低的死亡率、较低的发病率和与 EPP 相当的总体存活率。这些发现对于早期间皮瘤尤为突出。由于 ePD 是一种不太广泛应用的手术，其术后发病率和死亡率低于 EPP，因此新设计的 MARS-2 试验将试图证明这种手术是否能对 MPM 患者生存和/或生活质量有益[91]。在 MARS-2 注册的 MPM 患者将接受两个周期的铂-培美曲塞化疗，未进行 CT 扫描的患者将被随机分配至多达 4 个铂-培美曲塞化疗或 ePD 周期，随后进行多达 4 个周期的术后培美曲塞联合铂类化疗。EORTC(欧洲癌症研究和治疗组织)试验将研究与 ePD 联合化疗的时间[92]。MPM 患者将被随机分配到 ePD 之前或之后标准剂量顺铂或培美曲塞的 4 个周期。希望这项随机试验能够结合标准(新)辅助化疗解决手术的可行性，并为随后的Ⅲ期试验设置实验部门，探讨手术在 MPM 中的作用，或者可以成为未来 MPM 手术试验的标准方法。

新型手术策略

Cho 等[93]人已经研究了一种创新的Ⅰ/Ⅱ期方法(放射治疗后的间皮瘤手术，SMART)，使用短期加速的高剂量半胸强度调制放射治疗(IMRT)，随后进行 EPP。在完成新辅助 IMRT 的 1 周内，对于整个同侧半胸，在 1 周内每天五次 25Gy，5Gy 加速至风险区域，接着是 EPP。在 25 名患者中，IMRT 耐受性良好，没有 3 级以上的毒性，并且在完成 IMRT 后 6±2 天进行 EPP，没有任何围术期死亡率。中位随访 23 个月后，上皮亚型的累积 3 年生存率达到 84%，而双相亚型则为 13%(P=0.000 2)。计划采用多中心方法验证这些结果。

在宾夕法尼亚大学，计划进行 MCR 伴光动力治疗(PDT)对照 MCR 不伴 PDT 的Ⅲ期试验。随着 MCR 转换为肺保留技术(如标准或 ePD)，PDT 的结果与存活时间增加有关[94,95]。胸腔内热灌注现在更受欢迎，尤其是在欧洲，但与美国的研究不同，因为它们在灌注期间没有使用顺铂/吉西他滨，而是选择研究温暖的聚维酮碘，此外，灌注主要在接受胸膜切除术的患者中进行[96]。

间皮瘤的放射治疗

间皮瘤 RT 的放射治疗通常在 MPM 的辅助治疗中进行，RT 方法和风险主要决定所涉及的手术切除类型，可分为两类：EPP 后的 RT 和 P/D 后的 RT 或无手术。

胸膜外全肺切除术后的辅助放射治疗

由于间皮瘤是一种涉及胸膜的恶性肿瘤，人们普遍认为即

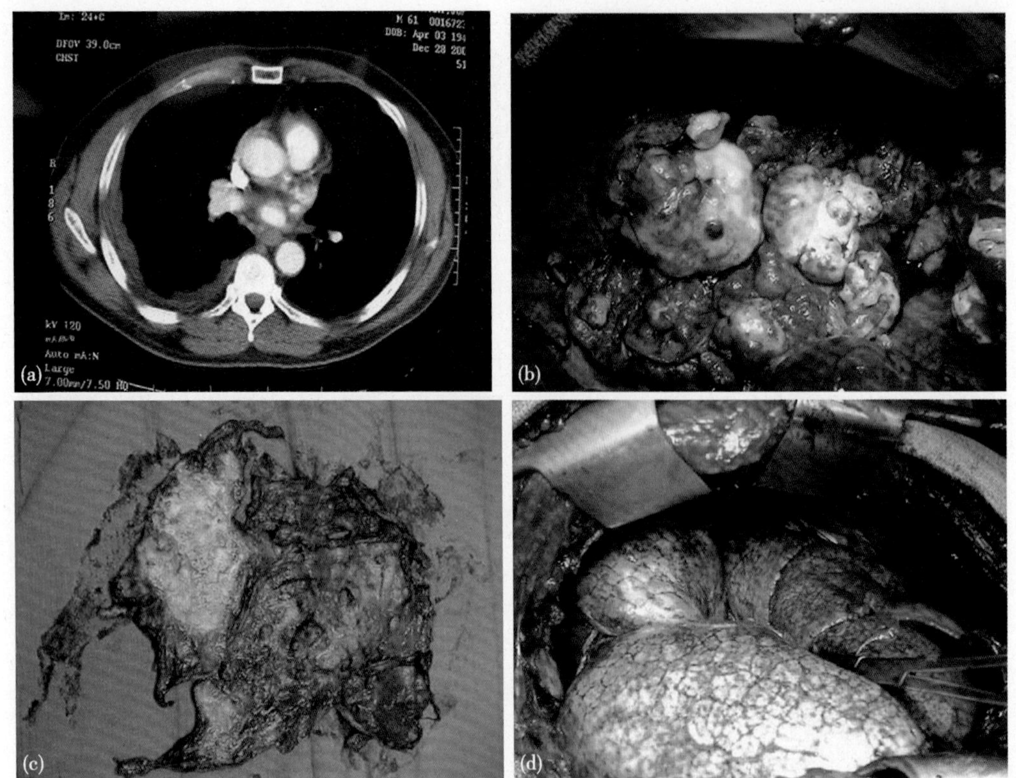

图 85-5　胸膜间皮瘤切除术：(a)典型的计算机断层扫描显示胸膜增厚。(b)手术视图显示疾病主要在顶胸膜上。(c)手术标本。(d)完成令人满意的细胞减少，同时保留肺和去肺皮

使发现特定区域与恶性肿瘤有关，整个胸膜腔也有患病的风险。因此，用 RT 控制微观疾病的尝试通常包括治疗整个半胸，特别是整个胸膜±同侧肺和心外膜。历史上，已经使用二维或"常规"技术给出了胸腔放射。这些方法使用有限数量的字段和非保形方法。因此，通常会发生大量的剂量异质性，例如靶区不足，且周围正常组织，例如食管，肺，心脏和脊髓，接受了增加的剂量或"热点"。Rusch 等进行了一项前瞻性Ⅱ期手术切除试验，随后采用常规方法进行了半球形放射治疗。从 1995 年到 1998 年，MSKCC(Memorial Sloan Kettering 癌症中心)大约 90 名患者接受了手术切除术(70%用 EPP)，然后 57 名患者接受了半胸外科手术，剂量为 41.4～54Gy，中位生存期为 17 个月，其中约 20%的患者在放射治疗边缘复发，大多数复发的患者远处转移[97,98]。

在过去十年中，IMRT 的适形技术已经发展并应用于临床，这种方法增加了保形性(图 85-6)。一些机构用以下方法报告了他们的结果：在安德森癌症中心的一项早期 MD 研究中，28 名患者在 EPP 后接受了胸腔 IMRT 治疗，剂量为 45～50Gy，一年的 OS 和 DFS 分别为 65%和 88%，65%的患者存在 2 级或 3 级恶心/呕吐副作用[99]，这些结果在 2007 年和 2013 已经更新两次[100,101,102]。最近的研究在选定的一组患者中，OS1 年时显示 90%，2 年时显示 71%。3 级毒性通常<20%，3 级皮炎和胃肠道副作用的发生率为 15%～20%。应该强调的是，遵守剂量限制对于最大限度地降低高级别和潜在致命毒性的风险至关重要。Dana-Farber 癌症研究所的研究人员早期报告显示，13 例 EPP 治疗后接受 IMRT 治疗的患者中有 6 例出现致命的放射性肺炎。虽然这些患者中有 11 例也接受了术中顺铂的加热，但剩

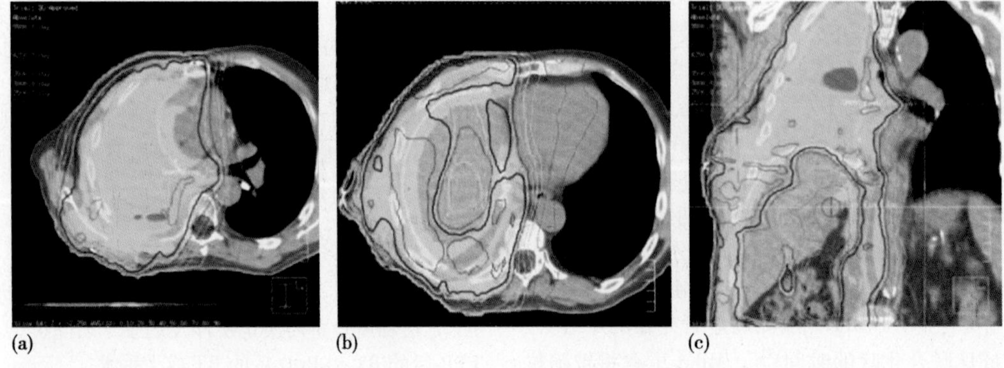

图 85-6　胸膜外肺切除术后 IMRT 的两个横向/水平切片和冠状视图。IMRT 可改善目标体积和关键正常结构的保形性，并提高剂量均一性

余肺部的低剂量区域(特别是接受 20Gy 或 V20 的肺部的百分比)高于我们目前可接受的水平[103]。因此,与 IMRT 的共形性伴随着"低剂量辐射浴"与剩余肺的权衡,需要在进行 RT 计划时密切监测。

胸膜切除术/剥脱术(P/D)或不可切除的疾病后的放射治疗

P/D 之后 RT 的作用尚未确定。实际上,当患者不接受 EPP 时,胸腔放射更具挑战性的原因有以下几点。首先,功能性肺部残留使患者暴露于双侧高度急性肺毒性的风险。其次,同侧肺对全肺功能有贡献,因为大部分肺将接受放射剂量,患者在放疗后肺功能显著降低的风险较高(与术后即刻相比)。最后,通过治疗大部分同侧肺并因此认为它不起作用,可以产生"分流"效应,从而在同侧肺中继续灌注,但发生很少的空气交换。因此,研究这种方法的初步研究表明结果不理想。在 Memorial Sloan Kettering 的一项分析中,123 例患者接受了保肺手术,并使用传统技术进行了胸腔放射治疗,中位总剂量为 42.5Gy,约半数患者也接受了近距离放射治疗。局部控制率约为 40%,38 例患者发生 3 级毒副作用,7 例患者发生 4~5 级毒副作用。因此,该技术与低水平的局部控制和相对高的毒性相关联[104]。

最近的研究已将现代技术纳入这一范畴。图 85-7 显示了已接受该治疗的患者,通过在治疗区产生"外皮"来保留同侧肺。Memorial Sloan Kettering 的一项研究报告了 67 名接受肺保留手术或单独活检患者的结果,发现 1 年和 2 年的精算失败率分别为 56% 和 74%。局部复发是主要的失败模式,接受 P/D 的患者延长了局部复发的时间(仅对活组织检查)[105]。MD Anderson 癌症中心最近也分析了 24 例在 P/D 后接受 IMRT 治疗患者的数据,并发现 1 年 OS 和 PFS 率分别为 76% 和 67%,2 年则分别为 56% 和 34%。术后观察肺功能的可测量变化[21% 用力肺活量(FVC),第 1 秒用力呼气容积 16%(FEV_1)],胸外后 IMRT 再次在观察为(31%FVC 和 25%FEV_1)。将这组患者与 EPP 和辅助 IMRT 治疗的历史对照组进行比较时,高级别毒性和中位 OS(28.4 个月 vs 14.2 个月,$P=0.04$)和 PFS(16.4 个月 vs 8.2 个月)均无差异[106]。总体而言,需要进行前瞻性试验来评估 P/D 后或在无法切除的疾病中加入 RT 这两种治疗方法,目前 Memorial Sloan Ket tering 和 MD 安德森癌症中心正在进行一项Ⅱ期试验。此外,诸如质子束治疗的辐射技术的进一步发展可改善肺功能的保留程度。

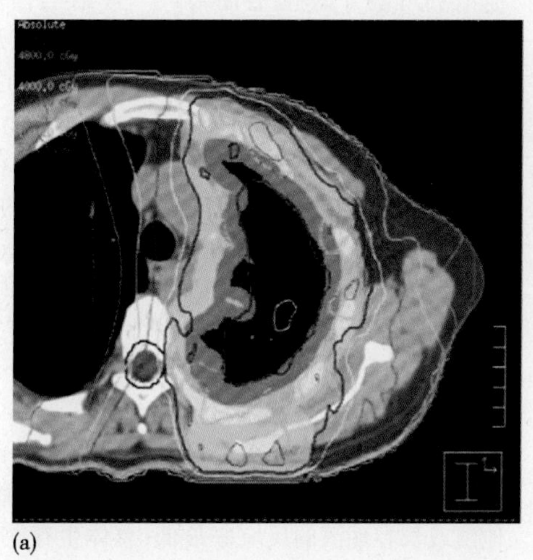
(a)

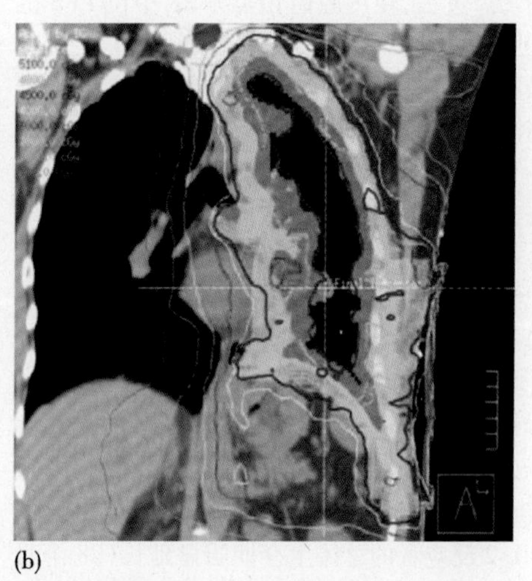
(b)

图 85-7　进行胸膜切除/剥脱术后接受 IMRT 治疗的患者的轴向和冠状视图。创建"外皮"以尝试保留肺的内部,尽管完全保留同侧肺通常是不可行的

间皮瘤的全身化疗

美国用于治疗可切除 MPM 的标准方案为:包含四个周期的新辅助或辅助顺铂-培美曲塞化疗的三联疗法。然而,关于三联疗法的最佳顺序和系统方案选择的若干问题尚不清楚。

新辅助或辅助全身治疗选择

关于新辅助或辅助全身治疗适应证的研究是在多学科环境中进行的。在切除前新辅助化疗有可能延迟手术切除而诱发并发症,此外,顺铂-培美曲塞对肿瘤缩小的显著反应率介于 29% 和 44% 之间[107,108]。据临床试验统计,在 42%~84% 时可完成新辅助化疗后 EPP。辅助化疗不会影响手术切除,但由于患者的性能状况下降,确实存在手术和放射后无法给药的风险[107~113]。迄今为止,没有比较新辅助治疗或辅助治疗的随机试验,这两种方法都是可接受的标准实践。一些前瞻性新辅助回顾性临床试验显示中位总生存范围为 16.6~25.5 个月[29~35],一项辅助试验($n=20$)报告,使用铂金-吉西他滨或铂-培美曲塞后 EPP 的中位总生存期为 17 个月[36,114]。美国的标准疗法是顺铂-培美曲塞,但是,其他国家更喜欢替代疗法。

对于可切除的 MPM 来说,最理想的全身性铂类双药治疗是未知的。顺铂-培美曲塞是美国普遍接受的护理标准;但是,其他国家更喜欢替代疗法。De Perrot 等[115]对其中心使用新辅助化疗进行了回顾性分析($n=60$),并报告生存结果无显著差异。评估的新辅助治疗方案包括顺铂-长春瑞滨,铂-培美曲塞,顺铂-雷替曲塞和顺铂-吉西他滨。考虑到风险,新辅助化疗具有为手术切除提供预后信息的能力。在迄今为止完成的最大的新辅助 EPP 试验($n=75$)中,Krug 等[107]人报告了响应患者(定义为完全或部分反应)与没有反应的患者相比,新辅助化疗的中位总生存期有所改善(29.1 个月比 13.9 个月,$P=0.076$)[107]。在本试验中,对于治疗人群的意图,中位数进展时间为 13.1 个月,总生存期为 16.6 个月。总之,新辅助铂-双联系统治疗试验表明,需要更好的全身性药物,具有更高的反应率,低毒性和作为维持治疗的能力。

得克萨斯大学安德森癌症中心探索新辅助达沙替尼的治疗窗口。本研究发现 MPM 细胞系和肿瘤细胞过度表达激活的 Src 激酶是达沙替尼的抗肿瘤机制,且证明生物标志物 Src kinaseTyr419 是一种药效学标志物,较高的基线水平可预测 PETCT 对新辅助达沙替尼治疗的代谢反应。此外,免疫组织化学中 PDGFRα 和 β 不同表达模式可预测肿瘤对达沙替尼治疗的敏感性或抗性。此外,西南肿瘤学组(SWOG)正在进行一项可切除 MPM 应用抗 PDL1 抑制剂的新辅助免疫治疗研究[116],并于三联治疗完成后将免疫治疗剂作为维持治疗。纪念斯隆凯特林研究中心一项由国防部赞助的临床试验率先使用佐剂 WT-1(Wilm Tumor-1)疫苗[117]。该疫苗激活宿主 T 细胞并消除 WT-1 阳性细胞,因此入组患者的间皮瘤肿瘤细胞上必须表达 WT-1。在正常细胞中,WT-1 是存在于幼儿中的转录因子,但是一旦到达成年期则消失。

胸膜内和免疫治疗策略

关于 MPM 的胸腔内给药化疗已有诸多重要研究,然而,它并不是标准治疗,建议仅在精心设计的临床试验中进行胸腔内治疗。使用胸膜内治疗的前提是使药剂与肿瘤细胞直接接触并输送高浓度的药物。过去,使用腔内铂类方案,中位 PFS 范围为 7.5~13.6 个月,中位 OS 为 11.5~18.3 个月[118~123]。这些研究中发现的最严重不良事件是全身吸收顺铂引起的肾衰竭。P/D 后给予高温胸腔内治疗,中位总生存期在 9~13 个月之间[122,124~126]。

使用含有疱疹病毒胸苷激酶(Ad-HSVtk)自杀基因[127~129]的腺病毒载体和含有免疫刺激剂,干扰素-β 的腺病毒载体进行胸膜内基因治疗(Ad. hu. IFN-β)[130]也已被探索,其中一些研究已取得初步阳性结果,可成功将基因转移到患者肿瘤细胞中。然而,这种方法似乎也只能使肿瘤体积较小的患者受益。在一些小型研究中也报道了胸膜内细胞因子给药具有潜在的抗肿瘤作用[131~134],γ-干扰素和重组人白介素-2(IL-2)是的最常见药物,主要的毒性作用包括发热,流感样症状和导管感染。Astoul 等[132]发现 IL-2 反应者的总体生存期明显延长(28 个月 vs 8 个月,$P=0.01$)。Lucchi 等[131]研究发现新辅助胸腔内 IL-2,P/D,辅助放射,全身 IL-2 和顺铂-吉西他滨化疗,然后维持皮下 IL-2 的试验,中位总生存期为 26 个月。尽管大多数患者出现局部复发,但在可切除的 MPM 中使用免疫调节剂有望成为一种有价值的治疗方法。

免疫疗法在可切除的间皮瘤中的作用也正在逐步探索中,间皮瘤被认为是一种免疫原性疾病,据推测,在新辅助治疗中加入顺铂-培美曲塞的抗 PDL1 抑制剂在临床上是可获益的。在手术切除和辅助放射治疗后,维持免疫疗法以增强针对微观疾病的 t 细胞活化将潜在地增加总体存活结果。在 ESMO 2014 上,Mansfield 等[135]小鼠单克隆抗人 B7-H1(克隆 5H1-A3)中发现,40%的 PD-L1IHC 表达在胸膜间皮瘤($n=224$)中。IHC 表达<5%为被认为是消极,PD-L1IHC 表达常意味着疾病负担更重,且患者从手术中获益更少,此外,PD-L1IHC 表达与存活率呈相关(6 个月 VS 14 个月,$P<0.0001$)[135]。因此,SWOG 开始在可切除的 MPM 患者中进行新辅助试验,分为顺铂-培美曲塞后使用和不使用 MPDL3280A(PD-L1 抑制剂)两组。

不可切除间皮瘤的全身治疗

在前线转移性环境中,顺铂-培美曲塞是美国食品药物管理局(FDA)批准的治疗方案[136]。Vogelzang 等对 456 名患者进行随机研究,将患者随机分为顺铂(每 3 周静脉注射 75mg/m²)单药治疗或顺铂(75mg/m²)和培美曲塞(500mg/m²),每 3 周静脉注射一次,最多 6 个疗程。顺铂-培美曲塞方案改善了反应率(41.3%对比 16.7%,$P<0.001$),进展时间(5.7 个月对 3.9 个月,$P<0.001$)和中位总生存期(12.1 个月对 9.3 个月,$P=0.02$))。在组合方案中超过 10%的患者主要 3/4 级副作用是中性粒细胞减少、恶心/呕吐和疲劳。培美曲塞的使用必须有维生素 B_{12} 和叶酸补充剂,此外,在培美曲塞给药期间使用糖皮质激素是必要的。虽然没有关于维持治疗的随机临床试验数据,但患者可接受铂-培美曲塞治疗 4~6 周治疗,然后接受培美曲塞维持治疗。在非鳞状非小细胞肺癌的治疗中,持续维持治疗是一种标准做法[137],对于无法切除的间皮瘤也表现良好。正在进行一项随机试验以评估间皮瘤中的这一问题,但由于经常使用培美曲塞维持治疗,现实中实施是有问题的。对于不能耐受铂的患者,常给予单药培美曲塞[138]。

在无法切除的情况下,卡铂是顺铂的一种非常合理的替代方法,并且已经证明具有相同的存活率[139,140]。既往已研究其他铂-抗叶酸方案(雷替曲塞)[141]或铂-吉西他滨[142,143]如果患者无法治疗,接受培美曲塞将是合理的替代方案。在环境中目前没有 FDA 批准任何药剂可用于间皮瘤的抢救,但鼓励患者参加新药和免疫疗法的临床试验。脱离药物指南,最常用的药剂包括吉西他滨、长春瑞滨,或吉西他滨-长春瑞滨的组合。据报道,在化疗初期,吉西他滨(在 28 天周期的第 1、8 和 15 天静脉注射 1250mg/m²)的反应率为 7%,中位 OS 为 8 个月[144]。据报道吉西他滨-长春瑞滨(1 000mg/m² 吉西他滨和 25mg/m² 长春瑞滨在第 1 天和第 8 天每 3 周一次,最多 6 个疗程)疗效较差,反应率为 7.4%,中位进展时间为 2.8 个月[145]。单剂长春瑞滨($n=63$)的Ⅱ期试验报告的反应率为 16%,总生存期为 9.6 个月[146]。回顾性分析在 Memorial Sloan Kettering 进行第二和第三线治疗的 60 例挽救性间皮瘤患者中的病例报告[147],吉西他滨或长春瑞滨的反应率最低,总体生存获益没有显著增加,但疾病显著稳定。吉西他滨($n=27$)中位 PFS 为 1.6 个月,中位 OS 为 4.9 个月,而长春瑞滨($n=45$)的中位 PFS 为 1.7 个月,中位 OS 为 5.4 个月。

生物和新型靶向药物

新型生物疗法的使用一直是 MPM 研究较为活跃的一个领域。最早的生物单药治疗研究基于临床前数据,发现表皮生长因子受体(EGFR)和血小板衍生生长因子受体(PDGFR)在 MPM 肿瘤细胞上的过度表达,并未显示 EGFR 酪氨酸激酶抑制剂(吉非替尼或埃罗替尼[69,70,148,149])或甲磺酸伊马替尼(一种 PDGFR 抑制剂)的显著反应率。在甲磺酸伊马替尼单药治疗试验中疾病稳定[150]。该领域已经扩大了几个新的目标和生物制剂。

靶向血管生成的药剂

间皮瘤肿瘤细胞通常分泌大量血管内皮生长因子(VEGF),并且患者血清的高 VEGF 水平与不良结局相关[151]。Bevacizumab 是 VEGF 配体的单克隆抗体,是间皮瘤迄今为止研究最多的。随机前线Ⅱ期临床试验比较 115 例使用顺铂-吉西他滨治疗和不使用贝伐单抗患者,结果显示贝伐单抗的生存期较短且反应率较低[152]。然而,对低于中位 VEGF 水平且接受贝伐单抗治疗的患者进行亚组分析,发现无进展($P=0.043$)和总生存($P=0.028$)均得到改善。另外两项Ⅱ期试验采用铂-培美曲塞联合贝伐单抗,然后贝伐单抗维持,但尚未在未选择的人群中证实可显著获益,也未提供对生物标志物信息[153,154]。Dowell 等人对用可治疗 53 例顺铂-培美曲塞-贝伐单抗的间皮瘤患者并且显示出 34%的反应率,6 个月中位无进展生存期为 6.9 个月,中位总生存期为 14.8 个月。Ceresoli 等[153]对 76 名接受卡铂-培美曲塞-贝伐单抗治疗的意大利患者发现,其反应率为 34%,中位无进展生存期为 6.9 个月,中位总生存期为 15.3 个月。两项试验都有 3~4 级小肠穿孔事件(Dowell 等人试验中有 1 例,Ceresoli 等人中有 3 例)。法国正在进行顺铂-培美曲塞治疗的Ⅲ期临床试验(IFCT-GFPC-0701MAPS)[155],结果表明抗血管生成治疗可能对某些 MPM 患者有益,并且靶向作用于 VEGF 配体并不是最佳疗法,还有更多抗血管治疗。

SWOG 正在对尚未接受化疗的 MPM 患者(SWOG 0905)进行顺铂-培美曲塞联合Ⅰ/Ⅱ期试验,分为接受和不接受西地尼嗪治疗两组。cediranib 是 VEGFR 和 PDGFR 酪氨酸激酶抑制剂。Ⅰ期试验的部分结果在 ASCO 2013 上公布,中位 PFS 为 13~14 个月,中位 OS 为 14~16 个月[156]。非维持治疗的顺铂-培美曲塞-甲磺酸伊马替尼的小Ⅰ期试验($n=17$)结果显示中位 PFS 为 7.9 个月,中位 OS 为 8.8 个月[157]。然而,在完成六个三联疗法周期的 6 名患者中,中位 PFS 为 9.6 个月,中位 OS 为 22.4 个月,在 p-PDGFRα 高表达的患者其存活率也较高。

包括 VEGF/VEGFR 抑制途径在内的多激酶抑制剂口服已得到广泛研究。迄今为止,大多数试验都是在经过大量预处理的患者中进行的,并且已将这些新药用作单一疗法药物。据推测,抗血管生成剂可能需要与其他疗法(新药或化学疗法)同时使用才能获得最大的益处。例如,作为单一药物的沙利度胺可以达到疾病的稳定性[158],但是当国际试验中 MPM 患者接受四个铂-培美曲塞循环,接着行沙利度胺或最佳支持治疗时,该试验结果为阴性[159]。

在其他挽救性试验中,单药 vatalanib 治疗(VEGFR-1,-2 和-3;PDGFR;和 c-Kit)的反应率为 11%,稳定疾病发生率为 66%,中位无进展生存期为 4.1 个月,中位总生存期为 10 个月[160]。CALGB 30307 给予 MPM 索拉非尼(VEGFR-2,PDGFR 和 Raf)400mg,每日两次,化疗或提前培美曲塞治疗,报告的疾病稳定反应率为 4.4%和 38.8%,中位无失败生存期为 4.1 个月,中位总生存期为 10.4 个月[161~163]。有趣的是,化疗患者的生存率低于先前培美曲塞治疗的患者。SWOG 0509 中的 54 例提前 ceritinib 单药治疗的 MPM 患者的Ⅱ期临床试验结果显示,其反应率为 9%,疾病稳定率为 34%[164]。中位无进展生存期为 2.6 个月,总生存期为 9.5 个月。

舒尼替尼(VEGFR-2,PDGFR-β,c-Kit 和 Flt-3)前线和补救治疗环境(加拿大国家癌症研究所,NCIC)中的活性有限[165]。北中央癌症治疗组正在对培唑帕尼(VEGFR-1,-2 和-3,以及 PDGFR)进行评估[166]。

核糖核酸酶抑制剂

ranpirnase(Onconase,Alfacell Corporation)对肿瘤细胞 tRNA 具有靶特异性并抑制蛋白质合成,这使得细胞周期停滞在 G1 期。评估 ranpirnase 的Ⅱ期 MPM 试验得出 5%的反应率,43% 的疾病稳定率,中位总生存期为 6 个月[167]。Ⅲ期试验($n=105$)将 ranpirnase(每周 480μg/m^2)与 doxoru bicin(每 3 周 60mg/m^2)进行比较,结果显示意向治疗分析的总生存率无差异。然而,患有 CALGB 预后组 1~4 和 EORTC 风险标准的患者在用多柔比星治疗时用多柔比星治疗时具有 2 个月的生存获益[168]。一项大型国际Ⅲ期试验(P30~302)对比多柔比星与多柔比星和 ranpirnase 的组合,结果未显示 ranpirnase 可使患者生存获益。

组蛋白去乙酰化酶抑制剂

组蛋白去乙酰化酶抑制剂(HDACI)是防止脱乙酰化并恢复对细胞周期控制的药剂。虽然临床前研究表明 HDACI 抑制细胞周期进程和/或诱导肿瘤细胞凋亡,但确切的抗肿瘤机制尚不清楚[169]。早期Ⅰ期试验对 13 例间皮瘤患者(12 例先前接受过治疗)进行了 Suberoylanilide hydroxamic acid(SAHA)或 vorinostat(一种口服 HDACI)并证实有两种临床部分反应[170]。国际随机安慰剂对照Ⅲ期试验(VANTAGE 14)累计治疗 660 名先前治疗的 MPM 患者,并将伏立诺他与安慰剂进行比较。遗憾的是,该试验结果表明任何总体生存获益均为阴性,并且该药物不会在间皮瘤治疗中进一步发展(未发表的数据)。

蛋白酶体抑制剂

蛋白酶体复合物处理无处不在的蛋白质并调节蛋白质降解,阻断蛋白酶体活性会 YIZHI NF-κB 并使肿瘤细胞凋亡,蛋白酶体抑制剂在细胞系和小鼠异种移植模型中均显示出抗肿瘤活性[171~173]。欧洲两项实验在评价硼替佐米疗效:单药硼替佐米(ICORG/GIME)和顺铂与硼替佐米(EORTC)联合治疗。

抗癌药物

SMRP 是在间皮瘤肿瘤细胞上表达的细胞表面糖蛋白,抗 SMRP 药物已被标记为有毒分子,并已显示出对 MPM 具有抗肿瘤活性[174,175]。SS1P(重组抗 SMRP 免疫毒素)在 1 期试验中与环磷酰胺和喷司他丁联合进行了评估,并报道了 10 例患者中有 3 例具有明显的抗肿瘤反应[176]。除 SS1P 外,还有其他抗 SMRP 疗法如 Morab009 和抗 SMRP 疫苗[177,177,178]。此外,CRS-207(一种单核细胞增生李斯特菌-SMRP 疫苗)正在Ⅰ期试验中进行评估[179]。

结论

间皮瘤仍然是一种难以治疗的整体生存率低的恶性肿瘤。更好分期方法可以帮助选择更适合手术治疗的患者,多模式治疗似乎是目前最可接受的治疗方法,几种新药和免疫疗法可能会改变这种疾病的病程,但已然需要医务工作者不断探索发现。

(陈先凯 译　高禹舜 校)

参考文献

The complete reference list can be found on the Wiley Companion Digital Edition of this title (see inside front cover for login instructions).

8 Hillerdal G. Malignant mesothelioma 1982: review of 4710 published cases. *Br J Dis Chest*. 1983;77(4):321-343.

17 Carbone M, Yang H. Molecular pathways: targeting mechanisms of asbestos and erionite carcinogenesis in mesothelioma. *Clin Cancer Res*. 2012;**18(3)**: 598-604.

20 Yang H, Bocchetta M, Kroczynska B, et al. TNF-alpha inhibits asbestos-induced cytotoxicity via a NF-kappaB-dependent pathway, a possible mechanism

for asbestos-induced oncogenesis. *Proc Natl Acad Sci U S A*. 2006;**103(27)**: 10397–10402.

24 Yang H, Rivera Z, Jube S, et al. Programmed necrosis induced by asbestos in human mesothelial cells causes high-mobility group box 1 protein release and resultant inflammation. *Proc Natl Acad Sci U S A*. 2010;**107(28)**:12611–12616.

27 Carbone M, Ferris LK, Baumann F, et al. BAP1 cancer syndrome: malignant mesothelioma, uveal and cutaneous melanoma, and MBAITs. *J Transl Med*. 2012;**10**:179.

28 Bott M, Brevet M, Taylor BS, et al. The nuclear deubiquitinase BAP1 is commonly inactivated by somatic mutations and 3p21.1 losses in malignant pleural mesothelioma. *Nat Genet*. 2011;**43(7)**:668–672.

34 Testa JR, Cheung M, Pei J, et al. Germline BAP1 mutations predispose to malignant mesothelioma. *Nat Genet*. 2011;**43(10)**:1022–1025.

39 Pass HI, Lott D, Lonardo F, et al. Asbestos exposure, pleural mesothelioma, and serum osteopontin levels. *N Engl J Med*. 2005;**353(15)**:1564–1573.

43 Robinson BW, Creaney J, Lake R, et al. Mesothelin-family proteins and diagnosis of mesothelioma. *Lancet*. 2003;**362(9396)**:1612–1616.

49 Pass HI, Levin SM, Harbut MR, et al. Fibulin-3 as a blood and effusion biomarker for pleural mesothelioma. *N Engl J Med*. 2012;**367(15)**:1417–1427.

54 Flores RM, Akhurst T, Gonen M, Larson SM, Rusch VW. Positron emission tomography defines metastatic disease but not locoregional disease in patients with malignant pleural mesothelioma. *J Thorac Cardiovasc Surg*. 2003;**126(1)**:11–16.

61 Rusch VW. A proposed new international TNM staging system for malignant pleural mesothelioma from the International Mesothelioma Interest Group. *Lung Cancer*. 1996;**14(1)**:1–12.

62 Rusch VW, Giroux D, Kennedy C, et al. Initial analysis of the international association for the study of lung cancer mesothelioma database. *J Thorac Oncol*. 2012;**7(11)**:1631–1639.

63 Pass HI, Giroux D, Kennedy C, et al. Supplementary prognostic variables for pleural mesothelioma: a report from the IASLC staging committee. *J Thorac Oncol*. 2014;**9(6)**:856–864.

64 Gill RR, Richards WG, Yeap BY, et al. Epithelial malignant pleural mesothelioma after extrapleural pneumonectomy: stratification of survival with CT-derived tumor volume. *AJR Am J Roentgenol*. 2012;**198(2)**:359–363.

65 Pass HI, Temeck BK, Kranda K, Steinberg SM, Feuerstein IR. Preoperative tumor volume is associated with outcome in malignant pleural mesothelioma. *J Thorac Cardiovasc Surg*. 1998;**115(2)**:310–317.

71 Rintoul RC, Ritchie AJ, Edwards JG, et al. Efficacy and cost of video-assisted thoracoscopic partial pleurectomy versus talc pleurodesis in patients with malignant pleural mesothelioma (MesoVATS): an open-label, randomised, controlled trial.. *Lancet*. 2014;**84(9948)**:1118–1127. doi: 10.1016/S0140-6736(14)60418-9. Epub 16 Jun 2014.

74 Rice D, Rusch V, Pass H, et al. Recommendations for uniform definitions of surgical techniques for malignant pleural mesothelioma: a consensus report of the international association for the study of lung cancer international staging committee and the international mesothelioma interest group. *J Thorac Oncol*. 2011;**6(8)**:1304–1312.

75 Cao CQ, Yan TD, Bannon PG, McCaughan BC. A systematic review of extrapleural pneumonectomy for malignant pleural mesothelioma. *J Thorac Oncol*. 2010;**5(10)**:1692–1703.

80 Treasure T, Lang-Lazdunski L, Waller D, et al. Extra-pleural pneumonectomy versus no extra-pleural pneumonectomy for patients with malignant pleural mesothelioma: clinical outcomes of the Mesothelioma and Radical Surgery (MARS) randomised feasibility study. *Lancet Oncol*. 2011;**12(8)**:763–772.

81 Weder W, Stahel RA, Baas P, et al. The MARS feasibility trial: conclusions not supported by data. *Lancet Oncol*. 2011;**12(12)**:1093–1094.

82 Flores RM, Pass HI, Seshan VE, et al. Extrapleural pneumonectomy versus pleurectomy/decortication in the surgical management of malignant pleural mesothelioma: results in 663 patients. *J Thorac Cardiovasc Surg*. 2008;**135(3)**: 620–626.

83 Cao C, Tian DH, Pataky KA, Yan TD. Systematic review of pleurectomy in the treatment of malignant pleural mesothelioma. *Lung Cancer*. 2013;**81(3)**:319–327.

97 Rusch VW, Rosenzweig K, Venkatraman E, et al. A phase II trial of surgical resection and adjuvant high-dose hemithoracic radiation for malignant pleural mesothelioma. *J Thorac Cardiovasc Surg*. 2001;**122(4)**:788–795.

98 Yajnik S, Rosenzweig KE, Mychalczak B, et al. Hemithoracic radiation after extrapleural pneumonectomy for malignant pleural mesothelioma. *Int J Radiat Oncol Biol Phys*. 2003;**56(5)**:1319–1326.

99 Ahamad A, Stevens CW, Smythe WR, et al. Promising early local control of malignant pleural mesothelioma following postoperative intensity modulated radiotherapy (IMRT) to the chest. *Cancer J*. 2003;**9(6)**:476–484.

105 Rimner A, Spratt DE, Zauderer MG, et al. Failure patterns after hemithoracic pleural intensity modulated radiation therapy for malignant pleural mesothelioma. *Int J Radiat Oncol Biol Phys*. 2014;**90(2)**:394–401.

107 Krug LM, Pass HI, Rusch VW, et al. Multicenter phase II trial of neoadjuvant pemetrexed plus cisplatin followed by extrapleural pneumonectomy and radiation for malignant pleural mesothelioma. *J Clin Oncol*. 2009;**27(18)**:3007–3013.

108 Van Schil PE, Baas P, Gaafar R, et al. Trimodality therapy for malignant pleural mesothelioma: results from an EORTC phase II multicentre trial. *Eur Respir J*. 2010;**36(6)**:1362–1369.

110 Weder W, Stahel RA, Bernhard J, et al. Multicenter trial of neo-adjuvant chemotherapy followed by extrapleural pneumonectomy in malignant pleural mesothelioma. *Ann Oncol*. 2007;**18(7)**:1196–1202.

117 Krug LM, Dao T, Brown AB, et al. WT1 peptide vaccinations induce CD4 and CD8 T cell immune responses in patients with mesothelioma and non-small cell lung cancer. *Cancer Immunol Immunother*. 2010;**59(10)**:1467–1479.

119 Rusch VW, Figlin R, Godwin D, Piantadosi S. Intrapleural cisplatin and cytarabine in the management of malignant pleural effusions: a Lung Cancer Study Group trial. *J Clin Oncol*. 1991;**9(2)**:313–319.

128 Sterman DH, Recio A, Vachani A, et al. Long-term follow-up of patients with malignant pleural mesothelioma receiving high-dose adenovirus herpes simplex thymidine kinase/ganciclovir suicide gene therapy. *Clin Cancer Res*. 2005;**11(20)**:7444–7453.

132 Astoul P, Picat-Joossen D, Viallat JR, Boutin C. Intrapleural administration of interleukin-2 for the treatment of patients with malignant pleural mesothelioma: a Phase II study. *Cancer*. 1998;**83(10)**:2099–2104.

136 Vogelzang NJ, Rusthoven JJ, Symanowski J, et al. Phase III study of pemetrexed in combination with cisplatin versus cisplatin alone in patients with malignant pleural mesothelioma. *J Clin Oncol*. 2003;**21(14)**:2636–2644.

140 Castagneto B, Botta M, Aitini E, et al. Phase II study of pemetrexed in combination with carboplatin in patients with malignant pleural mesothelioma (MPM). *Ann Oncol*. 2008;**19(2)**:370–373.

141 Van Meerbeeck JP, Gaafar R, Manegold C, et al. Randomized phase III study of cisplatin with or without raltitrexed in patients with malignant pleural mesothelioma: an intergroup study of the European Organisation for Research and Treatment of Cancer Lung Cancer Group and the National Cancer Institute of Canada. *J Clin Oncol*. 2005;**23(28)**:6881–6889.

143 Nowak AK, Byrne MJ, Williamson R, et al. A multicentre phase II study of cisplatin and gemcitabine for malignant mesothelioma. *Br J Cancer*. 2002;**87(5)**:491–496.

152 Kindler HL, Karrison TG, Gandara DR, et al. Multicenter, double-blind, placebo-controlled, randomized phase II trial of gemcitabine/cisplatin plus bevacizumab or placebo in patients with malignant mesothelioma. *J Clin Oncol*. 2012;**30(20)**:2509–2515.

156 Tsao A, Moon J, Wistuba I, et al. A phase I study of cediranib (NSC #732208) in combination with cisplatinum and pemetrexed in chemonaive patients with malignant pleural mesothelioma (SWOG S0905). *J Clin Oncol*. 2013. Ref Type: Abstract;**31**.

157 Tsao AS, Harun N, Lee JJ, et al. Phase I trial of cisplatin, pemetrexed, and imatinib mesylate in chemonaive patients with unresectable malignant pleural mesothelioma. *Clin Lung Cancer*. 2014;**15(3)**:197–201.

158 Baas P, Boogerd W, Dalesio O, Haringhuizen A, Custers F, van Zandwijk N. Thalidomide in patients with malignant pleural mesothelioma. *Lung Cancer*. 2005;**48(2)**:291–296.

170 Krug LM, Curley T, Schwartz L, et al. Potential role of histone deacetylase inhibitors in mesothelioma: clinical experience with suberoylanilide hydroxamic acid. *Clin Lung Cancer*. 2006;**7(4)**:257–261.

173 Fennell DA, McDowell C, Busacca S, et al. Phase II clinical trial of first or second-line treatment with bortezomib in patients with malignant pleural mesothelioma. *J Thorac Oncol*. 2012;**7(9)**:1466–1470.

176 Hassan R, Miller AC, Sharon E, et al. Major cancer regressions in mesothelioma after treatment with an anti-mesothelin immunotoxin and immune suppression. *Sci Transl Med*. 2013;**5(208)**:208ra147.

第 86 章 胸腺瘤和胸腺肿瘤

Ronan J. Kelly, MD ■ Alberto M. Marchevsky, MD

概述

胸腺瘤、胸腺癌和其他胸腺肿瘤是罕见的实体瘤，占比不到 1.5%。目前根据世界卫生组织（World Health Organization，WHO）最近更新的（2015）组织学分类标准进行分类。本章回顾了胸腺瘤和胸腺癌的组织学特征和分类标准，重点是各种诊断问题。胸腺瘤根据 Masaoka-Koga 系统进行分期，美国癌症联合委员会（American Joint Commission on Cancer，AJCC）目前正在制订分期指南。关于如何分期胸腺癌，目前存在一些不确定性。Ⅰ期和Ⅱ期胸腺瘤患者接受根治性胸腺切除术，而放疗和化疗则用于晚期患者。本章详细讨论了治疗胸腺瘤和其他胸腺肿瘤的现有技术。在没有大量随机临床试验的情况下，各种治疗选择的效果很难明确评估。事实上，对于患有罕见肿瘤，具有长的自然病史且需要随访多年的患者而言，Ⅰ级和Ⅱ级证据难以收集。国际胸腺肿瘤协作组织（International Thymic Malignancies Interest Group，ITMIG）为胸腺肿瘤的诊断，分期和治疗制订循证指南的努力在本文中进行了描述。

介绍

胸腺肿瘤很少见，在美国仅占所有实体肿瘤的 0.2%～1.5%，发病率为 0.13/（10 万人・年）[1]。因此，传统的临床研究在这类肿瘤中一直存在挑战。在过去几十年中，许多障碍也阻碍了我们进步，其中最主要的是缺乏适当国际公认的组织病理学和分期标准。已经有至少 15 种不同的分期分类系统被提出并使用[2]。这无疑导致了研究者之间的混淆，并且难以将一项临床试验与另一项临床试验进行比较。迄今为止，最广泛使用的分期分类系统是 Masaoka 和随后 Koga 修改的系统[3,4]。这些系统的模糊措辞和理解困难阻碍了临床研究，并使其难以在国际层面进行合作。国际胸腺肿瘤协作组织（ITMIG）和国际肺癌研究协会（International Association for the Study of Lung Cancer，IASLC）正在持续努力提出一种基于肿瘤，淋巴结，转移（TNM）的胸腺恶性肿瘤分期系统，作为官方的分期分类系统，正如由美国癌症联合委员会（AJCC）和国际癌症控制联盟（Union for International Cancer Control，UICC）提出的分期分类系统一样。

基于上皮肿瘤细胞的形态（A 型胸腺瘤到胸腺癌其异型程度增加）、淋巴细胞受累的比例和与正常胸腺组织的相似性，世界卫生组织（WHO）将胸腺瘤（A 型，AB 型，B1 型，B2 型和 B3 型）与胸腺癌（以前由 WHO 指定为 C 型）从组织学分类上区分开来。近年来，由于比较基因组杂交（CGH），表达阵列分析和下一代测序等先进技术的应用，我们对胸腺瘤和胸腺癌的分子生物学理解有了逐步的改进。越来越明显的是，A 型、AB 型、B1 型、B2 型、B3 型胸腺瘤和胸腺癌的亚类分类具有不同分子特征，这些可能在临床上相关。基因组分析能将 B3 型胸腺瘤和胸腺癌明显区分出来，就如同 A 型和 B2 型胸腺瘤的差别一样。此外，B2 型胸腺瘤可以与其他亚组分开，因为它具有更明显的淋巴细胞成分，而其他组上皮细胞更占优势[5]。最近的下一代 RNA 测序研究发现，在 A 型和 AB 型胸腺瘤患者的染色体 19q13.42 区域有一个大的 microRNA 簇，而 B 型胸腺瘤和胸腺癌患者中则不存在。该簇已被证明可导致 PI3K/AKT 通路的激活，这表明 PI3K 抑制剂可能在这些亚型中起作用[6]。部分胸腺癌患者也被发现存在 *KIT* 基因突变，尽管相对罕见，但它们可能会是成功的靶点。

手术切除仍然是早期疾病治疗的基石，而在晚期或复发性疾病中推荐采用多学科综合治疗的方法，包括手术，放疗和化疗。此外，人们现在非常关注的领域是最激动人心的肿瘤免疫系统靶向治疗。胸腺瘤与多种自身免疫疾病如重症肌无力（myasthenia gravis，MG）有关，其与 T 细胞介导的自身免疫有关。自身免疫疾病的理论中，已经提出诸如 T 淋巴细胞的阳性和阴性选择失败以及自身免疫调节基因（AIRE）缺陷的过程，但还需要进一步的研究。计划在不久的将来进行使用检查点抑制剂（如 PD-1 抑制剂）的研究，并且免疫治疗策略可能对那些化疗耐药的患者带来希望。

本章讨论了正在开发的新的组织学和分期系统，并重点介绍了一些促进我们对这些罕见肿瘤的理解的分子生物学突破。此外，我们还讨论了胸腺恶性肿瘤的治疗方法，重点是手术，放疗（RT）和全身治疗。强调了涉及化疗和靶向治疗最近的临床试验，并探讨未来的靶点等。

发病率和流行病学

虽然胸腺恶性肿瘤相对罕见，但它们是最常见的纵隔原发肿瘤，前纵隔肿块高达 50% 证明是胸腺退化[7]。男性患胸腺瘤的风险略高于女性，风险随之增加年龄，70 岁时达到顶峰，这与胸腺随年龄的逐渐退化成反比[8]。美国国立癌症研究所“监测、流行病学和结果数据库”（SEER）数据中，关于西班牙裔和亚洲太平洋岛民的数据是分别仅从 1992 年和 1998 年开始提供。美国的胸腺瘤发病率在非洲裔美国人尤其是亚洲/太平洋岛民中高于白人或西班牙裔。此外，胸腺瘤发病的年龄，非裔美国人比白人年轻（诊断时的中位年龄，48 岁与 58 岁；SEER 数据）。同样，MG 在非裔美国人中可能比在白人中更常见[9]。与其他相比，胸腺瘤患者在其生命中的某个时间点更容易患有自身免疫性疾病（32.7% 对 2.4%；$P<0.001$），MG 患者中最常见（24.5%），如系统性红斑狼疮（2.4%）或红细胞再生障碍（1.2%）[10]。发病率较高和诊断年龄较小的种族差异表明遗

传因素的作用。6 号染色体 *HLA* 基因座上的等位基因分布在不同种族群体中显著不同[8]。Ⅰ类和Ⅱ类 HLA 蛋白均在胸腺上皮细胞中高表达[11]。需要进一步研究以了解是否特定的遗传变异(在 HLA 或其他位点)更易患胸腺瘤。没有已知的胸腺恶性肿瘤病因,尽管少数病例是在对胸部进行放射治疗后发生的。爱泼斯坦-巴尔病毒(EBV)与胸腺淋巴上皮瘤有关,胸腺淋巴瘤是一种罕见的胸腺癌,通常在年轻患者中更常见[12]。少数患有多发性内分泌肿瘤Ⅰ型综合征(MEN Ⅰ)的患者与胸腺瘤或胸腺来源的神经内分泌癌相关。

解剖发病机制

胚胎学和解剖学

胸腺组织主要起源于第三咽囊的内胚层上皮(较低的一对甲状旁腺也发源于此),部分偶尔也可源于第四咽囊[13,14]。在胚胎发育中,左右胸腺原基向下移动至前上纵隔,合二为一但并不完全融合,形成双叶状的胸腺[1]。虽然胸腺主要位于前上纵隔,但下移过程中每一部位都可能遗留组织成分,所以在上至舌骨,下至膈肌的任何部位,都可能在大体或显微镜下发现胸腺组织。因此,在单纯胸腺瘤患者,以及合并或不合并胸腺瘤的重症肌无力患者的外科手术中,一旦需要清除全部胸腺组织,那么充分暴露纵隔和颈部是非常必要的。胸腺的净重在青春发育期达到峰值[10~15 岁时平均(34±15)g],以后正常情况下,一生中重量随着年龄增长逐渐减少,永不终结[1]。组织学上,正常胸腺由许多特异小叶组成,小叶外周部为富含淋巴细胞的皮质,深部为富含上皮细胞及特征性 Hassall 小体(胸腺小体)的髓质,两者间有明显分界。胸腺小体由成熟的上皮细胞向心排列而成。在骨髓来源淋巴细胞(B 细胞)成熟为 T 细胞的过程中,以及细胞介导的免疫中,胸腺起着决定性作用。胸腺血供丰富,没有输入的淋巴管,但导出的淋巴管明显起于血管周围间隙,流入纵隔和下颈部淋巴结。

表 86-1 原发性胸腺肿瘤

胸腺上皮肿瘤
胸腺瘤
胸腺癌
生殖细胞肿瘤
精原细胞瘤
胚胎癌
卵黄囊瘤
绒毛膜癌
畸胎瘤
混合生殖细胞肿瘤
生殖细胞肿瘤具有体细胞型恶性肿瘤
生殖细胞肿瘤伴有相关的血液系统恶性肿瘤
纵隔淋巴瘤
原发性纵隔 B 细胞淋巴瘤
黏膜相关淋巴组织(MALT)的胸腺额外边缘区 B 细胞淋巴瘤
T 细胞淋巴瘤
霍奇金淋巴瘤
其他
组织细胞和树突状细胞肿瘤
髓系肉瘤
间充质肿瘤
胸腺脂肪瘤
孤立性纤维瘤
肉瘤
其他

胸腺肿瘤

胸腺可以形成表 86-1 中列出的各种上皮细胞、生殖细胞、淋巴细胞、间充质细胞和其他肿瘤[13]。

胸腺上皮肿瘤的病理学

胸腺上皮肿瘤包括低度恶性病变,称为胸腺瘤和中度至高度恶性潜能的恶性病变,归类为胸腺癌[13,15,16]。

胸腺瘤的病理学

胸腺瘤大体形态呈现单个或多个有包膜的肿瘤,小者显微镜下可见,大者占据整个前纵隔,并挤压相邻的胸腔内结构[13,17~21]。肉眼上大多数胸腺瘤包膜完整(图 86-1),但是有些胸腺瘤可局部侵犯纵隔软组织、上腔静脉和其他血管、淋巴结、胸膜、心包、气管和/或其他胸腔内与胸腺毗邻的结构(图

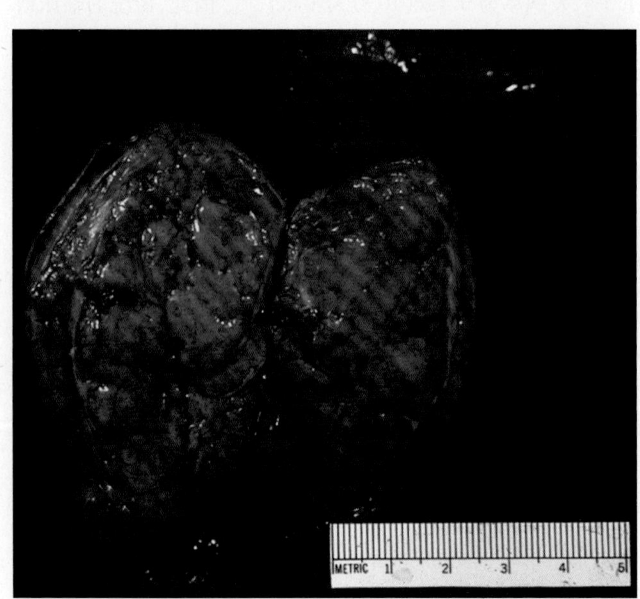

图 86-1 胸腺瘤的大体照片,显示一个被覆包膜、具有特征性纤维分隔的灰色、柔软的肿瘤

86-2)。显微切片上,胸腺瘤显示明显的纤维包膜以及由多条纤维分隔分割的特征性的小叶状外观(图 86-3)。它们通常是实体瘤,但可以进行囊性变性。囊性胸腺瘤由于局灶的实性区域存在,能显著区别于良性的胸腺囊肿。

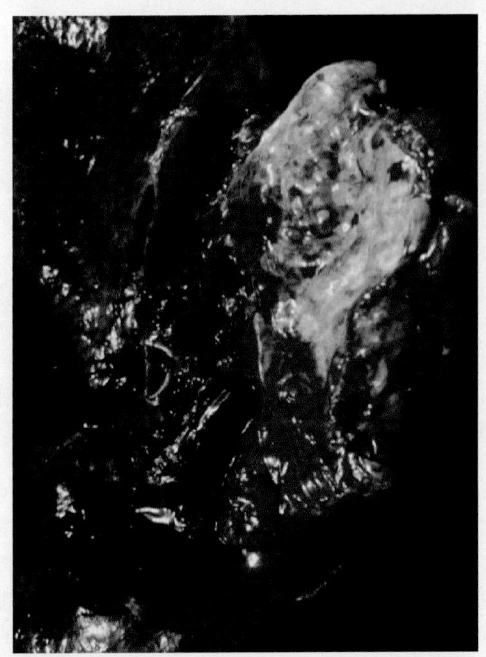

图 86-2 侵袭性胸腺瘤的大体照片,显示纵隔软组织和支气管壁被侵犯

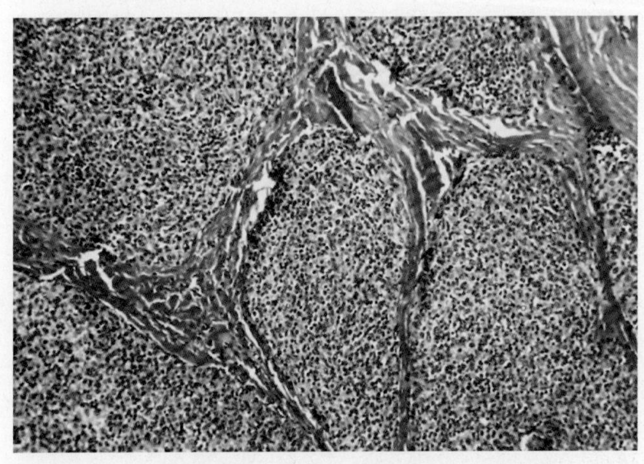

图 86-3 胸腺瘤显微照片显示了特征性的小叶状病变。上皮和淋巴细胞被薄的纤维分隔分割(HE,×40)

显微镜下,胸腺瘤由梭形、椭圆形或多角形细胞核的上皮细胞与多少不等的成熟淋巴细胞组成。胸腺瘤的上皮细胞和淋巴样细胞成实心片状结构排列,通常由纤维状隔膜分开,在大多数胸腺瘤中可以在低倍显微镜观察到呈略微分叶状(图 86-3)。

胸腺瘤的其他组织学特征包括血管周围间隙(图 86-4)、髓质区域、假玫瑰花团排列、腺体样结构、Hassall 氏小体、囊性变性区域,以及较少见的出血和/或钙化区域。胸腺瘤通常被附包膜,但可以侵及包膜并侵入相邻组织(图 86-5)。细胞有丝分裂,细胞异型性和坏死在胸腺瘤中是常见,如果出现应该怀疑是否是胸腺癌。

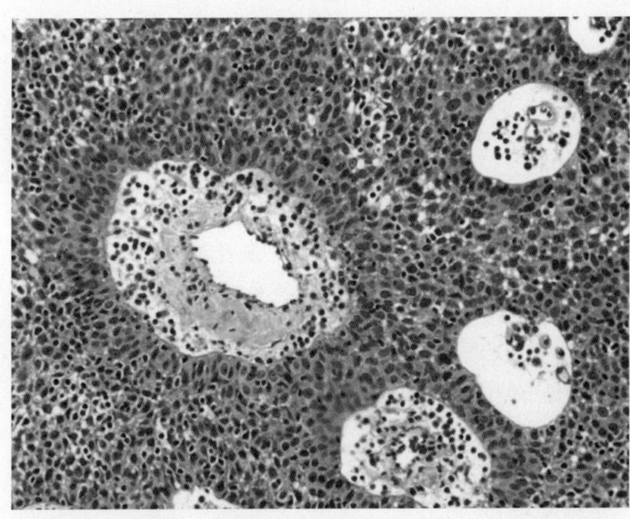

图 86-4 胸腺瘤高倍镜显微照片显示特征性的血管周生长方式,肿瘤细胞围绕血管排列。肿瘤细胞呈多角形,有轻度异型性,与小的成熟淋巴细胞混合(HE,×100)

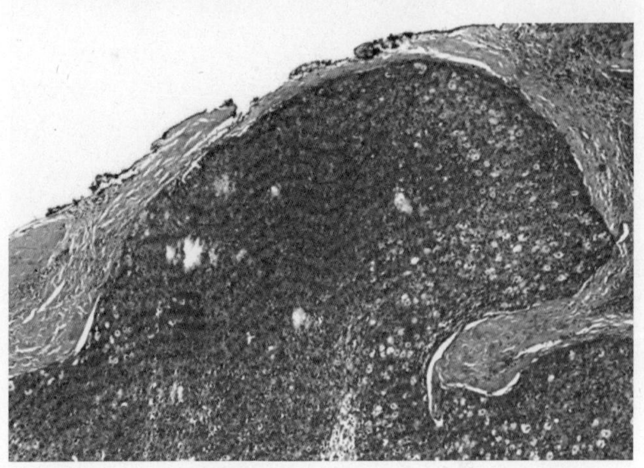

图 86-5 胸腺瘤显微照片显示包膜侵犯(HE,×40)

世界卫生组织对胸腺瘤的分类

已经提出了不同的分类方案用于胸腺上皮肿瘤的分类,但是使用最广泛的分类方案是由 WHO 在 1999 年提出并且在 2004 年和 2015 年进行了修改的方案(表 86-2)。

A 型胸腺瘤主要由梭形上皮细胞组成,淋巴细胞数量最少(图 86-6 和图 86-7)[19,20,22,23]。A 型胸腺瘤患者的 MG 发病率低于其他胸腺瘤组织学类型,但是再生障碍性贫血发生率更高。由多角形上皮细胞构成的胸腺瘤被命名为 B 型胸腺瘤,B1-B3 型胸腺瘤由 B 型胸腺瘤并进一步细分为 B1,B2 和 B3 型。B1 型胸腺瘤由不明显的多边形上皮细胞与大量成熟淋巴细胞混合组成。以前这种病变被命名为淋巴细胞为主型胸腺瘤,就是因为在苏木素和伊红染色的(HE)组织学切片上,只能找到稀少的上皮细胞,这些病变特征性地具有分散的圆形,低染色区域,称为髓质区域。B2 型胸腺瘤由比在 B1 型胸腺瘤中看到的更显著的多形性上皮细胞组成,这些细胞常常表现出轻微的核变化,局部可见突出的核仁(图 86-8)。B3 型胸腺瘤,在其他方案中被命名为"非典型胸腺瘤",是由在细胞大小和形状上中度改变(类似红细胞大小不等症),并出现局部核深染和细

表 86-2　世界卫生组织对胸腺瘤的分类和选择的肿瘤形态特征

A 型(梭形细胞)
非典型 A 型(具有局灶性异型的梭形细胞)
AB 型(混合纺锤和多角形上皮细胞)
B1 型(淋巴细胞丰富,散在的多角形上皮细胞)
B2 型(淋巴细胞丰富,多角形上皮细胞密度较高,局灶性,最轻异型)
B3 型(淋巴细胞贫乏,多角形上皮细胞伴轻度异型)
罕见的胸腺瘤
• 微结节型胸腺瘤
• 间变型胸腺瘤
• 显微镜下胸腺瘤
• 硬化型胸腺瘤
• 脂肪纤维瘤

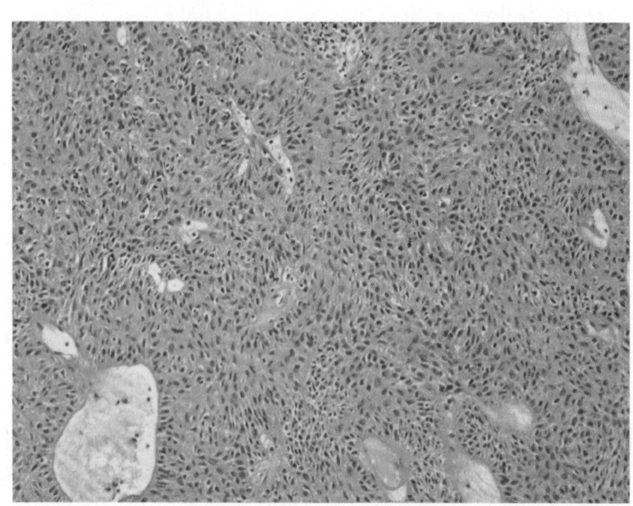

图 86-6　梭形细胞胸腺瘤(A 型胸腺瘤)的显微照片。肿瘤细胞具有细长的细胞核。注意其中成熟淋巴细胞的缺乏(HE,×100)

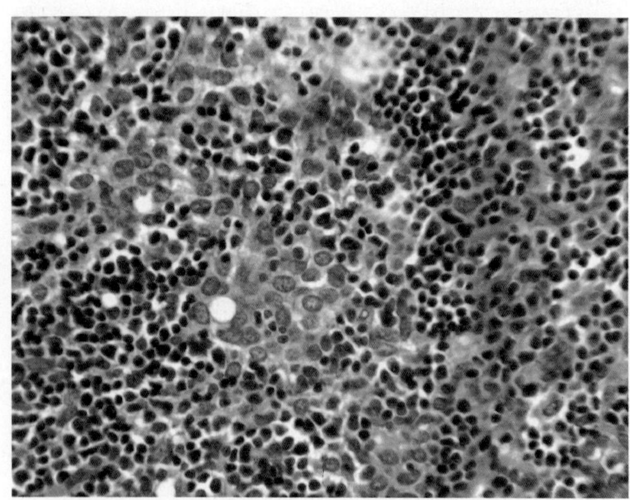

图 86-7　A 型胸腺瘤的显微照片显示小得多角形上皮细胞具有圆形细胞核,缺乏可见的核仁和缺乏细胞质,与大量淋巴细胞混合(HE,×200)

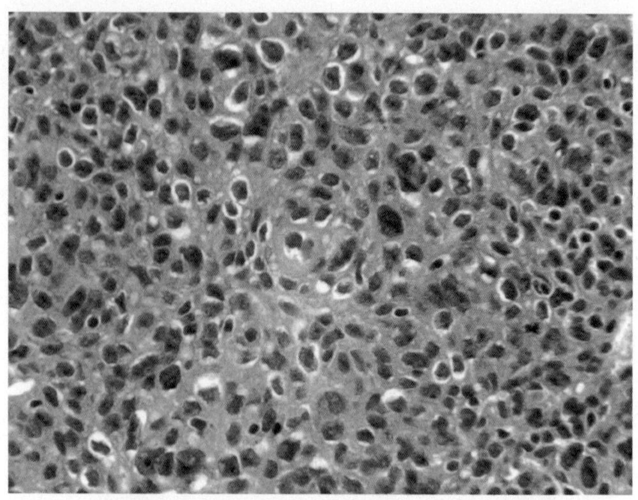

图 86-8　B3 型胸腺瘤显微照片(所谓不典型性胸腺瘤)。肿瘤细胞的大小及形状变化较大,核深染,核膜不规则。背景中淋巴细胞相对稀少(HE,×200)

胞异型的多角形或梭形上皮细胞组成。B3 型胸腺瘤中淋巴细胞的数量,比 B1 和 B2 型中的更少,使其和低级别的胸腺癌难以区分。AB 型胸腺瘤的淋巴细胞比例大于 5%,并且同时由纺锤体上皮细胞和多角形细胞组成。胸腺瘤通常是异质性肿瘤,并且可以在从同一病灶取得的不同切片上表现出不同的 WHO “类型”[24]。

免疫组织化学和其他辅助技术

胸腺瘤上皮细胞角蛋白 AE1/AE3 免疫反应胞质着色,这一特征通常对于确定穿刺活检标本和其他病理材料胸腺瘤的诊断是十分有用的(图 86-9)。许多其他的抗原表位也出现在胸腺瘤不同的 WHO 组织学类型中,诸如 CD5,层粘连蛋白,Ⅳ型胶原蛋白,金属硫蛋白,PE-53,细胞角蛋白(如 CAM5.2,

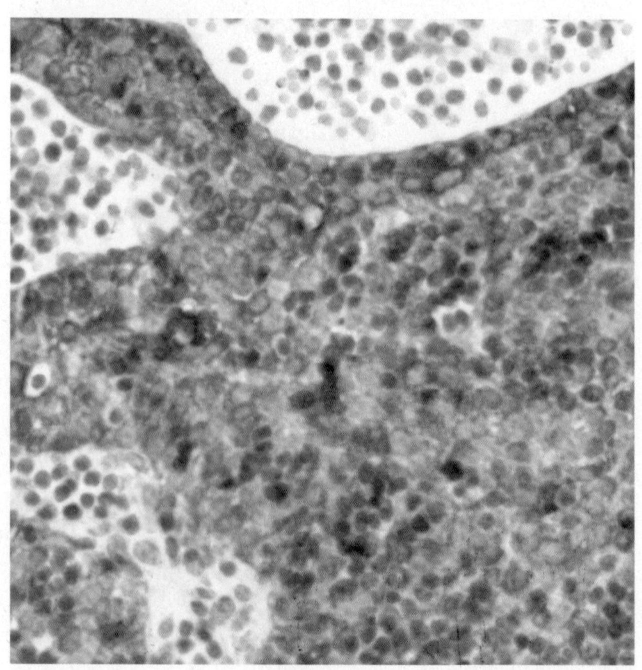

图 86-9　胸腺瘤的上皮细胞角蛋白 AE1/AE2 染色时,显示的细胞质免疫反应(免疫染色,×200)

CK7,CK14 和 CK18,CD57 等)。但是,它们的诊断价值有限,也不能帮助胸腺瘤的 WHO 分型和预后估计。CD5 是一种除了 C 型胸腺瘤外,通常在其他类型胸腺瘤阴性的免疫组化标志物。抗体 Foxn1,CD205 和桥粒芯糖蛋白 3 是新的胸腺上皮细胞标志物,可能对鉴别胸腺瘤和胸腺癌有帮助。

电子显微镜很少用于胸腺瘤的常规诊断[13]。肿瘤细胞的超微结构特征显示其具有上皮细胞的分化特性,如桥粒、张力微丝、伸长的细胞突起以及缺乏致密核心颗粒。恶性上皮细胞形成具有复杂交通空间和渠道的不规则的筛网结构,这种筛网中包含着成熟淋巴细胞,类似于胸腺的正常超微结构和微环境。

胸腺瘤的组织学预后特征

所有胸腺瘤均为低度恶性肿瘤[24~27]。A 型胸腺瘤(梭形细胞胸腺瘤)过去被认为是良性病变,但这些病变可在少数患者中复发或转移。A 型、AB 型与 B1 型胸腺瘤患者的预后似乎最好,而 B3 型胸腺瘤患者的复发和转移率更高,生存期更短。

胸腺瘤的分期系统

由于胸腺瘤是良性还是恶性一直存在争议,目前 AJCC 没有关于胸腺瘤的癌症 TNM 分期系统。用于其最广泛使用的分期系统是表 86-3 中给出的 Masaoka-Koga 分期系统[28~32]。

表 86-3 胸腺瘤的 Masaoka-Koga 分期

分期	疾病程度
Ⅰ	完全局限在包膜内
Ⅱ	侵入周围脂肪或纵隔胸膜显微镜下(Ⅱa)或肉眼可见(Ⅱb)
Ⅲ	侵入周围器官(心包,肺和大血管)
Ⅳ	(A)胸膜或心包植入
	(B)栓塞转移

胸腺癌

胸腺癌是上皮性肿瘤,约占胸腺肿瘤的 0.06%,由具有恶性细胞学特征的上皮细胞组成,如较多的核多形性、核浓染、核异型、核分裂象增多和/或坏死[22,28,31,31~38]。表 86-4 中描述了各种组织学类型。鳞状细胞癌可能是这些肿瘤中最常见的类型。胸腺淋巴上皮瘤是一种特别有趣的胸腺癌类型,常与 EBV 表达有关,并且与头颈部区域的此类肿瘤具有相似的组织病理学特征[16]。在影响儿童和年轻人的一种侵袭性胸腺癌类型中,最近描述其具有 *NUT* 基因的 t(15;19)易位[34]。

胸腺类癌和神经内分泌肿瘤

表 86-5 中的类癌和其他神经内分泌肿瘤可能出现在胸腺中[23,39~43]。胸腺中的此类肿瘤比肺部和其他器官中出现的更具侵袭性,在诊断时有 30%~40%的病例已经发生转移。当伴有异位促肾上腺皮质激素所致的库欣综合征患者同时有胸腺肿块时要考虑到胸腺类癌的可能性,因为 30%的胸腺类癌患者可伴有库欣综合征,而胸腺瘤的患者不会,胸腺类癌患者还可表现其他的伴癌综合征,如骨关节肥大,兰伯特-伊顿综合征(Lambert-Eaton syndrome),多发内分泌肿瘤(Ⅰ型和Ⅱ型)[[39,43]]。类癌综合征尚未见报道。所有的神经内分泌癌在低倍显微镜下均具有神经内分泌分化的组织病理学特征,包括细胞呈巢状、条索状和假玫瑰花团排列[13]。肿瘤细胞根据细胞不同类型而不同。类癌细胞的细胞核呈圆形或长条形,核染色质呈盐胡椒样,不同程度的深染和小量多形性。典型类癌通常缺乏核分裂和坏死,而不典型类癌具有低核分裂和灶状坏死。胸腺大细胞神经内分泌癌的细胞核呈大的、多形性的、深染的,由灶状多核的细胞组成,可以表现出局部突出的核仁。胸腺小细胞癌由染色质深的小细胞组成,细胞核折叠,核仁小。高级别的胸腺神经内分泌癌的各类亚型均表现高核分裂象,通常高于 10 个核分裂象/10 个高倍视野和广泛的坏死,胸腺神经内分泌癌的所有亚型的肿瘤细胞的细胞质与嗜铬粒蛋白和突触素呈免疫反应,电镜下有核心致密的神经内分泌颗粒。Ki-67 可用于评估病变的增殖比率。

表 86-4 世界卫生组织对胸腺癌的分类

鳞状细胞癌
基底细胞癌
黏液表皮样癌
淋巴上皮瘤样癌
透明细胞癌
肉瘤样癌
腺癌
NUT 癌
未分化癌
其他罕见的胸腺癌

表 86-5 胸腺神经内分泌肿瘤

典型的类癌
非典型类癌
大细胞神经内分泌癌
小细胞癌

胸腺淋巴瘤

淋巴瘤和胸腺瘤中最常见的胸腺肿瘤[13,33,44~46]。虽然胸腺是 T 细胞器官,但成人患者胸腺最常见的淋巴瘤是霍奇金淋巴瘤和 B 细胞淋巴瘤(表 86-3)。胸腺的原发性霍奇金淋巴瘤往往局限于腺体,并且通常是结节性硬化型,通常与相邻胸腺组织的囊性变化有关。纵隔的 B 细胞淋巴瘤经常累及胸腺和淋巴结,并且经常表现出其他位置的 B 细胞淋巴瘤不同的组织学特征,如硬化带对肿瘤细胞的分隔现象,透明样细胞,形成和上皮来源恶性肿瘤相似的细胞巢。临床行为通常呈侵袭性。儿童起源于胸腺和纵隔淋巴结的淋巴瘤包括 Burkitt 淋巴瘤,T 淋巴母细胞淋巴瘤。鉴别淋巴瘤和胸腺瘤非常重要,因为两者的治疗截然不同。对一些疑难病例,特殊染色和电镜可能会对诊断有帮助。

胸腺的生殖细胞肿瘤

胸腺是原发于性腺外的生殖细胞肿瘤的经典部位(表 86-1)。常见的胸腺生殖细胞肿瘤为精原细胞瘤(有时与胸腺瘤鉴别困难)和畸胎瘤(成熟或不成熟)。其他胚胎癌,卵黄囊肿瘤,畸胎癌和绒毛膜癌等也有报道。

其他胸腺肿瘤

其他胸腺肿瘤包括胸腺脂肪瘤,体积通常很大,胸腺囊肿,胸腺转移瘤和表 86-1 中列出的其他肿瘤。

TNM 分期-ITMIG/IASLC

如前所述,在过去的 40 年中,提出了至少有 15 种不同分期分类系统用于胸腺恶性肿瘤[47]。Masaoka 分期系统最初是在 1981 年提出的,主要关注胸腺包膜的完整性,是否存在微观或宏观周围结构的浸润,以及转移扩散。常使用的 1994 年的更新版本是 Masaoka-Koga 分期系统[4]。但是,长期以来人们认识到,对于胸腺肿瘤,非常需要美国癌症联合委员会/国际癌症控制联盟(AJCC/UICC)验证过的分期系统。从而会有一致的通用命名法促进多国协作临床研究。ITMIG 和 IASLC 的正在进行共同努力,全球已有超过 10 000 个回顾性和前瞻性病例组成的数据库[47]。这个分期系统的要求是它必须包含描述疾病解剖范围的命名法。仅适用于所有类型的胸腺肿瘤,并且符合 TNM(肿瘤,淋巴结,转移瘤)结构。拟议阶段分类的 T 部分根据受累结构的程度分为四期。如果侵及该分期中的一种或多种结构,则肿瘤被分类在该分期中,而不管是否侵及更低分期的其他结构。回顾性数据库所示,因为这对结果没有临床上显著的影响,T 分期中不涉及肿瘤的包膜。T1a 指包膜覆盖与否,不论是否侵及纵隔脂肪。病理证实的心包受累被指定为 T2 期,而 T3 期中侵及如下几种不同的结构,包括肺、头臂静脉、上腔静脉、胸壁、膈神经、肺门和肺血管。T4 期表明更广泛的局部受累,侵及如下结构,例如主动脉,肺动脉,心肌,气管和食管等。淋巴结状态“N”根据它们与胸腺的临近度分为两组,其中 N1 表示胸腺前(perithymic)受累,N2 疾病表示颈深部或胸部淋巴结受累。最后,转移性疾病将被分类为 M1a,表示单独的胸膜或心包结节,M1b 表示肺实质内结节或远处器官转移[48]。这一提出的分类系统将适用于胸腺瘤和胸腺癌,希望它能成为国际上统一的分期分类系统。

胸腺瘤和胸腺癌之间的分子差异

直到最近,我们对胸腺上皮肿瘤中发生的基因组变化的信息有限。一个重要的挑战是 AB,B1 和 B2 型含有大量的非肿瘤性胸腺细胞,其数量超过恶性上皮细胞,使得 CGH 和荧光原位杂交(FISH)分析具有挑战性。由于新技术如下一代测序和表达阵列分析,近年来我们对胸腺瘤和胸腺癌之间不同表型的肿瘤生物学知识有所改善。这些研究表明,按 2004 年 WHO 系统分类的胸腺肿瘤确实具有不同的分子特征。基因组分析将 B3 型和胸腺癌与 A 型和 B2 型胸腺瘤区分开来。此外,B3 型倾向于具有更明显的淋巴细胞成分,胸腺癌是 C-Kit 阳性。

最常见的遗传改变发生在染色体 6p21. 3(*MHC* 基因座)和 6q25. 2~25[35,49,50]。细胞遗传学研究已经证实所有组织学亚型中的染色体异常,包括 t(15;19)(q13:p13. 1)产生可在胸腺癌中发生的 *BRD4-NUT* 融合基因的易位[51]。分子相似性确实发生在胸腺癌和 B3 型胸腺瘤之间,其中 2q 的增加和 6 号染色体的丢失。这可能对未来几年的临床试验设计与 B3 型和胸腺癌一起治疗。来自胸腺癌的 CGH 分析的其他数据显示,17q 和 18 的拷贝数频繁增加,3p,16q 和 17p 的丢失 . 5,52 已有描述的进一步的畸变包括遗传物质的多次丢失和微卫星不稳定性(MSI)在不同的染色体【3p22~24. 3,3p14. 2(*FHIT* 基因座),5q21(*APC* 基因),6p21,6p21~22. 1,7p21~22,8q11. 21~23,13q14(*RB* 基因)和 17p13. 1(*p53* 基因)】[52,53]。除了 6 号染色体长臂的丢失外,5 号染色体(5q21)(*APC* 基因)杂合性缺失(LOH)可能是最重要的。已经证明染色体的改变根据 WHO 亚型(A 型 10%,AB 型 12%,B 型 20%~26%,胸腺癌 35%)和临床诊断阶段(Ⅰ期 7%,Ⅱ期 27%,阶段)而异(Ⅲ期 21%,Ⅳ期 24%)[50]。最常见的 LOH(48. 6%)发生在 6q25. 2 区域。另一个热点显示 LOH 在 32. 4%的肿瘤中是发生于 6q25. 2~25. 3。显示 LOH 的第三个热点(30%)出现在包括 *MHC* 基因座的区域 6p21. 31 中,并且在 6q14. 1~14. 3 上检测到第四个热点(26. 3%)。10%的胸腺瘤,特别是 B 型胸腺瘤中在 6 号染色体上发现了 MSI。这么多变化的生物学意义虽然尚未确定,但正意识到增量效益。6p23 区域包含 *FOXC1* 肿瘤抑制基因,并且染色体丢失与较低的蛋白质表达相关。FOXC1 阴性肿瘤患者肿瘤进展时间较短,患者相关生存期较短[54]。下一代 RNA 测序显示,A 型和 AB 型胸腺瘤与其他亚组明显不同。染色体 19q13. 42 上的大型 microRNA 簇已显示在这些组中显著过表达,而在 B 型胸腺瘤和胸腺癌中不存在[6]。该簇已显示通过下调 PTEN 激活 PI3K/AKT 途径,这表明 PI3K 抑制剂可能在这些亚型中发挥作用。

利用基因特征来判断胸腺肿瘤的预后

胸腺恶性肿瘤的主要预后指标是肿瘤分期,组织学亚型和手术切除范围。由于我们对基础分子生物学的理解定义的基因特征,被视为帮助肿瘤学家在临床和形态学特征的基础上,更好地确定下一步的预后,治疗积极性和监测复发程度。在一项优秀的研究中,作者将他们进行了全基因组表达的发现与 34 名胸腺瘤患者的结果相关联起来[55]。基因表达数据的无监督聚类分出了四组胸腺肿瘤,与组织学分类显著相关($P=0.002$)。此外,作者还发现了许多与胸腺肿瘤临床表现包括分期,复发和转移相关的基因,有一些基因使用 qRT-PCR 证实过。在所选择的最高基因中,Aldo-keto 还原酶家族 1B10(AKR1B10)和 junctophilin-1(JPH1)在Ⅲ期和Ⅳ期疾病中均被上调。刺猬靶(hedgehog target)基因 COL11A1 在晚期疾病中被下调。与非转移性疾病相比,AKR1B10 和 JPH1 在转移阳性肿瘤中显示出 5. 96 倍($P=0.05$)和 3. 01 倍($P=0.18$)的增加,并且在Ⅳ期肿瘤中 COL11A1 下调 12. 5 倍($P=0.11$)。这些基因的差异表达水平,通过 qRT-PCR 验证,证实了不同表型中的差异表达。作者提出了 *9* 基因特征,可用于鉴定胸腺瘤转移的高风险或低风险患者。还将进行更多的验证研究,以及临床试验环境中的前瞻性评估。为了区分胸腺癌和胸腺瘤,同一组已经提出一种 *12* 基因标记,可以帮助病理学家处理疑难病例。虽然目前临床上没有使用基因标记,但是经过验证的标记对胸腺瘤患者具有巨大的益处。这些标记在肿瘤可能有很大差异,许多被认为是惰性的肿瘤需要的临床监测可能比较具侵袭性的B3 型胸腺瘤要少。在罕见肿瘤中,随机研究的范围有限的,对不良预后指标的更好理解将在临床上产生巨大的益处。

胸腺瘤的临床特征

大多数肿瘤相关症状没有特异性(咳嗽、呼吸困难、胸痛)或继发于肿瘤局部和区域纵隔播散(胸腔积液、上腔静脉压迫综合征或心包积液),因此,通常显示肿瘤具有侵袭性。偶尔,胸腺瘤表现为弥漫的胸膜肿瘤,类似于恶性间皮瘤。半数左右的胸腺瘤患者没有任何症状,在做胸片检查时被偶然发现,胸片显示胸骨后肿物突出于心脏大血管的轮廓外,侧位片和斜位片上更为清晰。CT 在检测小的胸腺瘤方面没有价值,但是可以评价胸腺肿物是否侵及周围结构,例如纵隔、胸膜和心包。20%的胸腺瘤可见肿瘤中或外周钙化[57],但钙化与侵袭性无关。肿瘤的周围存在完整的脂肪层是肿瘤无局部侵袭的征象,相反,与周围组织存在纤维粘连显示可能受侵[58]。胸腺瘤在MRI 上表现为 T1 和 T2 加权像上高信号,但是 MRI 在检测是否存在包膜和血管侵犯方面,与 CT 相比是否具有优势仍需进一步研究[58]。PET 用于区分良性和恶性纵隔肿瘤的价值仍在研究[59]。胸腺癌和侵袭性胸腺瘤显示高摄取。但仍需要强调的是,手术探查和病理仍是评价胸腺瘤的侵袭性的最可靠方式。

相关的副肿瘤综合征

胸腺瘤可以伴发多种副肿瘤综合征。大多数与自身免疫机制相关,最常见 3 种特征性病症(表 86-3)。

重症肌无力

有 33%~50%的胸腺瘤患者会出现重症肌无力,约 10%的重症肌无力患者有胸腺瘤[60]。重症肌无力患者无论是否伴有胸腺瘤临床表现都是一致的,但伴有胸腺瘤的患者的年龄通常大于不伴有胸腺瘤的患者。组织学上的差别也很小,主要是伴有重症肌无力的胸腺瘤纺锤细胞型非常少见,50%的病例在周围的胸腺组织中存在具有生发中心的淋巴滤泡(而在不伴有重症肌无力的胸腺瘤患者中只占 5%~8%)[61]。重症肌无力是自身免疫性疾病,特征是血清中存在抗神经肌肉连接的烟碱乙酰胆碱受体抗体,约有 90%的重症肌无力患者的血清中含有这样的抗体。其发病机制仍不明确。正常胸腺中的肌样细胞可能引起原位致敏[62]。80%的合并胸腺瘤和重症肌无力患者和25%不合并重症肌无力的胸腺瘤患者的血清中可以检出针对肌小节成分的条纹状抗体,如肌动蛋白[58]。重症肌无力患者无论是否合并胸腺瘤均应行全胸腺切除术,而不是胸腺切除术(参见“手术”节)。

红细胞增生不全

也称为纯红细胞再生障碍(pure red cell aplasia,PRCA),红细胞增生不全是自身免疫性疾病,特征是网织红细胞显著减少和骨髓中成红血细胞缺乏造成的获得性贫血,常伴有白细胞和/或血小板计数的改变(增加或减少)[61,63]。约有 5%的胸腺瘤患者患有 PRCA,但有 50%的 PRCA 患者有胸腺瘤,2/3 的患者为纺锤细胞型胸腺瘤[61]。PRCA 通常发生在 40 岁以上的胸腺瘤患者,局部侵犯率与其他胸腺瘤没有差异,骨髓中通常细胞丰富,促红细胞生成素水平显著特征性增高[63]。一些患者的血清中发现了呈红血细胞生长的免疫球蛋白 IgG 型抑制剂[63]。胸腺切除可使约 30%的患者的贫血缓解[63]。糖皮质激素和免疫抑制剂也有效。近来有报道 1 例患者接受奥曲肽联合泼尼松治疗后出现长时间的完全缓解(伴有肿瘤减小)[64]。

低人免疫球蛋白血症

低人免疫球蛋白血症 1954 年由 Good 首次报道[65],这种获得性综合征导致患者非常容易反复出现严重感染。有 5%~10%的胸腺瘤患者会出现低人免疫球蛋白血症,约有 10%的低人免疫球蛋白血症患者有胸腺瘤[57,61]。低人免疫球蛋白血症患者的血中所有重要的免疫球蛋白均下降,特别是 IgG 和 IgA,骨髓中嗜酸性粒细胞下降,也可联合细胞介导的免疫缺陷。接近 1/3 的患者伴有 PRCA,和伴有 PRCA 的胸腺瘤患者相似,伴有低人免疫球蛋白血症的胸腺瘤患者多大于 40 岁,75%的患者为纺锤细胞型胸腺瘤[61]。低人免疫球蛋白血症的病理发生机制仍不清楚。骨髓中缺乏前 B 细胞、B 细胞,导致外周 B 细胞减少[66]。胸腺切除对症状没有改善,可以行补充免疫球蛋白的姑息性治疗[66]。

诊断前纵隔肿物

临床怀疑前纵隔肿物是致病因素时需要对前纵隔肿物的性质做出明确诊断。结构化的以临床导向的方法提高了效率并减少不必要的调查。年龄和性别是从一开始就考虑的两个最重要的特征,因为特定病变往往在某些人群中更常见。实验室检查包括 α-胎蛋白,β-人绒促性素和乳酸脱氢酶。前纵隔肿物由多种不同的疾病组成,其中最常见的包括:胸腺恶性肿瘤约 35%,淋巴瘤约 25%(霍奇金淋巴瘤 13%和非霍奇金 12%),甲状腺和其他内分泌肿瘤约 15%,良性畸胎瘤约占 10%,恶性生殖细胞肿瘤占约 10%(精原细胞瘤 4%,非精原细胞瘤 6%),良性胸腺病变约占 5%。对于胸腺瘤进行侵袭性切开活检,包括纵隔镜或纵隔切开术,均有可能破坏肿瘤包膜导致肿瘤细胞种植的风险[67]。而经皮细针穿刺、荧光镜或 CT 引导下粗针活检通常被认为安全有效。必要时联合特殊染色和电镜,诊断的敏感性可达 80%,特异性为 90%[57]。建立明确的病理诊断至关重要,因为许多其他类型的肿瘤需要特定的治疗。以下各节将讨论胸腺恶性肿瘤的治疗方法。

治疗

手术

由于胸腺瘤的恶性特征,组织学上缺乏公认的相应判定标准,胸腺瘤被认为具有潜在恶性。因此,即使是包膜完整的 I 期肿瘤,也应选择全胸腺切除术,而不是单纯的胸腺瘤切除术[57]。全胸腺切除术也适用于合并或不合并胸腺瘤的重症肌无力患者。通常切口采用胸骨正中劈开,有时或许要增加胸部或颈部切口。一些术者主张探查所有可能发现异位胸腺组织的区域,行最大胸腺切除术[68]。局部浸润作为最可信的恶性指征和最重要的预后因素,术中必须仔细探查纵隔以收集证据。为了寻找包膜浸润证据,以及鉴别浸润与单纯粘连,不应破损肿瘤包膜,并进行必要的系统性显微镜检查。完全胸腺切除后,包膜完整的Ⅰ期胸腺瘤的复发率一般较低(约2%)[61]。最近,一组49例包膜较完整的小胸腺瘤胸腔镜手术已完成,但长期结果还不得而知[67]。

重症肌无力(MG)合并胸腺瘤患者,胸腺切除术后肌无力的缓解率接近10%~30%,缓解时间可能延续到两年或更长。而不合并胸腺瘤的MG患者,术后缓解率为40%~80%[57,61,68,69]。另有一部分患者仅表现为MG症状好转。在MG出现后1年内早期手术患者中,所合并的胸腺瘤,非浸润性者所占比例较高[70]。在全胸腺切除术后,临床上所观察到的初发或再发的MG,实际上可能提示肿瘤的再生长或异位胸腺的持续存在[57]。过去,MG是胸腺瘤患者预后较差的信号。然而,从最近外科报道看,由于较好的手术和麻醉技术,较大程度地防止了术后MG导致的死亡,合并与不合并MG的胸腺瘤患者预后并无显著不同[3,71,72]。

术中发现胸腺瘤的局部浸润,占30%~40%[3,71,72]。但肿瘤较缓慢发展和较少远处转移的特性,使根治手术的努力更为可行。为了能够将严重局部浸润的肿瘤完全切除,需行扩大切除术。术中膈神经、喉返神经和迷走神经的识别非常重要[68]。必要时切除一侧肺、膈神经或心包,甚至切除和修补大血管,如无名静脉和上腔静脉。放射治疗适用于浸润性胸腺瘤患者,运用术前和术后现代放疗技术,外科治疗死亡率较低(0~5%),甚至在合并MG的患者中也同样如此[3,68,72]。

在总共744例的4个大研究组中,包膜完好的非浸润性胸腺瘤患者,5年和10年生存率分别为75%~85%和63%~80%[3,71,72]。浸润性胸腺瘤患者5年和10年生存率分别为50%~67%和30%~53%。因此,浸润性是胸腺瘤患者预后的一个主要因素。同时大多数研究还报告梭形细胞为主型胸腺瘤预后较好。淋巴细胞相对于上皮细胞比例越高,预后越好[3,71,72]。手术切除局部复发和/或转移(常在胸内)病灶,也可能适合手术切除。

放射治疗

胸腺瘤对放疗极为敏感,诸多报道中证实了其有效性。报道显示在活检术或局部切除术后的病例,放疗的生存期可以达到10年甚至10年以上[73]。大多数作者认为,不仅仅是淋巴细胞样胸腺瘤对放疗敏感,上皮样胸腺瘤同样对放疗非常敏感[73]。放疗在不同期别的胸腺瘤中的作用各不相同。Ⅰ期病例根治术后复发率极低,因此术后放疗不作为常规推荐。Ⅱ期及Ⅲ期病例即便是行根治术后,仍然建议行术后放疗[3,57,71,74]。Curran等的文献综述显示,单独手术胸腔内复发率分别为28%,而手术联合术后放疗则为5%[75]。然而,这一结果并没有得到一致的结论,其他研究认为完全切除术后,行术后放疗与否并不影响局部控制[76]。近年来,部分研究开始质疑术后放疗的价值,尤其是术后放疗对于Ⅱ期胸腺瘤是否获益。然而,这些研究均为小样本回顾性研究,暂缺随机对照研究的结果,所以至今尚不能得出确切结论。放疗范围包括纵隔及邻近纵隔的比较容易复发的区域,如锁骨上区等[73]。放疗总剂量在45Gy左右,部分研究的总剂量达到50Gy甚至以上,但总体上脊髓受量都在可以耐受的范围内[73,75]。可能的毒副作用包括放射性肺炎、纵隔炎、心包炎、冠脉纤维化、甲状腺功能减退等。

放疗亦可应用于手术后残留的病例,如仅行活检术后或者不完全切除的Ⅲ期病例。Curran等入组了20例这样的患者,4例出现纵隔复发,5例出现纵隔外复发,Ⅱ~Ⅲ期病例行根治术后,无局部区域复发[75]。对于Ⅲ~Ⅳ期病例,放疗前行局部减瘤术并无获益[77],5年生存率为45%,Ⅲ期和Ⅳ期病例分别为61%和23%。放疗计划制订至关重要,需要放疗医师和外科医师一起合作,勾画出肿瘤的侵犯范围。

化疗

化学疗法在可手术切除和已发生转移的情况下都具有作用(表86-6)。基于顺铂的化疗仍然是进展期疾病的标准治疗方法。联合化疗方案显示出比单药化疗更高的反应率。多柔比星,顺铂,长春新碱和环磷酰胺(ADOC)的四种药物联合治疗方案被认为是多年的治疗标准,报告的总体反应率为92%,中位生存期为15个月[79]。然而,一项组间试验证明了3种药物组合,顺铂、多柔比星和环磷酰胺(PAC),总体反应率为50%,中位生存期为38个月[78]。各种方案包括糖皮质激素,已被证明可减少所有组织学亚型的肿瘤体积。实际发生的作用可能在于肿瘤淋巴细胞成分中的类固醇诱导的反应,而不是对恶性上皮细胞的任何抗肿瘤作用。常用的第二种三药联合方案包括顺铂,多柔比星和甲泼尼龙(CAMP)。该方案在新辅助治疗中给药,并且在由17名患者组成的小型Ⅱ期试验中的结果总体反应率为93%,5年总体生存率为81%[84]。EORTC研究了16名患者的顺铂和依托泊苷双药联合方案并证实反应率为56%,中位生存期为4.3年[80]。在该双药联合方案(VIP)中加入异环磷酰胺,部分缓解率为32%,OS为32个月,但毒性较高[81]。最近发表的第二期临床试验显示,每3周检测一次卡铂AUC5和紫杉醇225mg/m^{2}的剂量,最多使用6个周期,在34名初治患者中,胸腺瘤的总体缓解率为33%,胸腺瘤的无进展生存期(PFS)为19.8个月,胸腺癌的无进展生存期为6.2个月,且耐受性非常好[82]。第二项多中心临床研究了在40名日本新诊断的胸腺癌患者中,卡铂/紫杉醇的疗效。总体RR为36%(95% *CI*:21%~53%;$P=0.031$),中位PFS为8.1个月,1年和2年生存率分别为85%和71%。卡铂/紫杉醇的组合是一种有效的治疗方案,如果不能使用蒽环类药物,那么这种双药联合方案在胸腺癌的一线治疗中是一个很好的选择[85]。

表86-6 用于胸腺恶性肿瘤的化疗方案的部分研究

方案	分期	完全缓解+部分缓解/%
PAC[78]	Ⅳ	50
ADOC[79]	Ⅲ/Ⅳ	90
PE[80]	Ⅳ	56
VIP[81]	Ⅲ/Ⅳ	32
Carbo-Px[82]	Ⅳ	35
Pemetrexed[83]	Ⅳ	17

PAC,顺铂,多柔比星,环磷酰胺;ADOC,多柔比星,顺铂,长春新碱,环磷酰胺;PE,顺铂,依托泊苷;VIP,依托泊苷,异环磷酰胺,顺铂;Carbo-Px,卡铂,紫杉醇。

二线化疗确实在胸腺恶性肿瘤中有作用。一项Ⅱ期研究评估了 27 例先前治疗过的不可切除的ⅣA 期($n=16$)或ⅣB 期($n=11$)复发性胸腺恶性肿瘤患者,每 3 周以 500mg/m[2] 剂量服用培美曲塞单剂[83]。中位数给药周期为 5(范围 1~6)。在 23 名完全可评估的患者中,有两个完全缓解和两个部分缓解(RECIST)。所有 4 名患者均为ⅣA 期胸腺瘤[83]。口服依托泊苷同样可能在治疗过的患者中有一定的作用,报告的反应率为 15%[86]。治疗过的患者中使用氨柔比星,剂量为 35mg/m^2,每三周的第 1~3 天使用,其疗效目前正在评估中[87]。

近年来,一些小型研究和病例报告评估了一线治疗进展后胸腺恶性肿瘤的靶向治疗。遗憾的是,结果有点令人失望。但考虑到这些肿瘤的罕见性以及选取特定的分子表型患者,这一极具挑战性事实,这种结果可能并非出乎意料。希望未来的分子分型分析的"篮子研究"能够选择具有特定的致癌驱动基因突变的肿瘤类型,以选取对靶向治疗具有显著敏感性的胸腺恶性肿瘤患者。

靶向治疗-KIT,EGFR/HER2,VEGF

尽管在胸腺恶性肿瘤中无法进行大规模的Ⅲ期随机临床试验,但许多小型Ⅱ期临床研究和病例报告(表 86-7)都显示了一部分患者确实能通过个性化医疗而获益。KIT 常常在胸腺癌中过表达,高达 73%~86%的肿瘤中 IHC 阳性,但在胸腺瘤患者中过表达有限,只有 2%证实为阳性[95,96]。遗憾的是,尽管胸腺癌中 KIT 过表达频率很高,*KIT* 突变率仍低至<10%。有病例报告显示特定的 *KIT* 突变类型决定了其对酪氨酸激酶抑制剂的敏感性。已经描述了许多突变,例如,11 号外显子中发现的 *V560* 缺失突变[97]和 *L576P* 替换突变[98],17 号外显子中的 *D820E* 突变[99],和 14 号外显子中的 *H697Y* 突变[52]。*V560* 突变的患者对舒尼替尼和伊马替尼都有较高的敏感度,*L576P* 突变的患者对舒尼替尼中度敏感和对伊马替尼的低度敏感,而 *D820E* 突变的患者对这两种 TKI 均有抗性。这说明在胸腺肿瘤中进行突变检测时"一种尺寸并不适合所有人"。由于突变的罕见性和敏感性,在一项小型Ⅱ期临床试验中,评估的 B3 胸腺瘤和胸腺癌患者令人失望地对伊马替尼均无反应[100]。

表 86-7 胸腺恶性肿瘤的靶向治疗

药物	患者数量	胸腺瘤	胸腺癌	反应率(RR/%)
吉非替尼[88]	26	19	7	4
厄洛替尼+贝伐单抗[89]	18	11	7	0
伊马替尼[90]	15	12	3	0
贝利司他[91]	40	24	16	5
西妥木单抗[92]	49	37	12	10
依维莫司[93]	35	23	12	11
舒尼替尼[94]	39	16	23	18

表皮生长因子受体(EGFR)在胸腺恶性肿瘤中同样过表达(70%的胸腺瘤和 50%的胸腺癌)[96,101],但遗憾的是,激活 EGFR 的体细胞突变极为罕见[98,102]。EGFR 表达和组织学类型之间没有相关性。FISH 检测到的 *EGFR* 基因扩增发生在大约 20%的胸腺恶性肿瘤中,最明显的是 B3 型胸腺瘤和胸腺癌,并且与分期较晚和包膜受侵相关[103]。不出意外的是,在一项治疗进展性恶性胸腺肿瘤的患者评估疗效的研究中,吉非替尼 250mg 或厄洛替尼和贝伐单抗联合,均没有治疗活性[88,89]。同样,尽管相关研究正在进行中,EGFR 单克隆抗体西妥昔单抗的疗效有限[90,104]。目前,文献中的证据表明不推荐 EGFR 酪氨酸激酶抑制剂和单克隆抗体治疗胸腺恶性肿瘤患者。类似地,目前没有通过 FISH 检测到 *HER2* 基因扩增的病例[105],所以在该疾病中没有数据推荐使用 HER2 的靶向治疗。

血管生成是被认为在胸腺发育中起重要作用,靶向血管生成可能是一种更成功的策略。血管内皮生长因子(VEGF)-A 和 VEGFR-1 和 VEGFR-2 在胸腺瘤和胸腺癌中均过表达[106,107]。虽然贝伐单抗的反应率较低,但有病例报告显示索拉非尼和舒尼替尼的这些多激酶抑制剂,在胸腺癌中作用突出。有报道说,在接受索拉非尼治疗有效的患者存在 *c-KIT* 基因的第 17 号外显子中具有错义突变(D820E)[99],并且第二位延长了疾病稳定期(>9 个月)的患者尽管没有突变,但是存在 KIT,*p53* 和 *VEGF* 基因的高 IHC 表达[108]。已经有包含 23 名胸腺癌患者的Ⅱ期临床试验,用于评估多激酶抑制剂舒尼替尼疗效。结果显示有效率相比于历史数据令人印象深刻的 26%,疾病控制率达到 91%[109]。

其他已经评估过的靶点包括胰岛素样生长因子-1(IGF-1)/IGF-1 受体(IGF-1R),它们已被确定为胸腺恶性肿瘤的不良预后指标[94,110]。IGF-1R 的不同表达量,胸腺瘤(4%)和胸腺癌(37%),表明其肿瘤生物学可能存在不同作用,进而可能作为靶点[94]。一项关于一种 IGF-1R 单克隆抗体西妥木单抗(cixutumumab)的Ⅱ期研究显示,49 例治疗过的晚期患者中,在胸腺瘤患者中表现出 14%反应率,但在胸腺癌中没有作用[92]。同样,组蛋白去乙酰化酶(HDAC)抑制剂也已经在胸腺肿瘤患者中进行了评估,特别是泛 HDAC 抑制剂贝利司他(belinostat),表现出适度的抗肿瘤活性。在贝利司他的Ⅰ期临床研究中,1 位胸腺瘤患者的治疗中取得了微并持续达 17 个月[111];因此,对 41 例(25 例胸腺瘤和 16 例胸腺癌)已经治疗过的胸腺恶性肿瘤患者,正在进行相关的Ⅱ期临床试验[91]。胸腺瘤患者中有两例部分有效(有效率为 8%),胸腺癌患者中无反应。目前正在进行针对 mTOR 信号通路的抑制剂研究[93]。已有计划针对 PD-1/PD-L1 轴的未来策略。在胸腺恶性肿瘤患者中,PD-L1 的表达范围从 60%到 90%,表明使用检查点抑制剂可能比针对单个基因突变更成功,但在 B3 型/胸腺癌中的自身免疫恶化现象的应首先进行关注并研究。

结论

随着分期分类系统的改进,以及对分子生物学理解的不断提升,希望通过提供国际分期的一致性,为更大的协作努力提供统一的命名和途径。正在开发和提出的 TNM 分期分类系统将为 2016 年发布的第 8 版 AJCC/UICC 分期分类提供基础。手术切除仍然是早期疾病治疗的基石,而对于晚期或复发性疾病,建议采用包括手术、放疗和化疗的多学科方法。基因表达谱和基因组聚类数据表明亚类的 A、AB、B1、B2、B3 和胸腺癌具有不同的分子特征,并可以选择特定的治疗方式。与 A 型和

B2 型胸腺瘤相比，胸腺癌和 B3 型胸腺瘤表现出现明显差异。未来对于临床医生来说，通过分子分类有希望可能比当前的分类系统更有用。使用预后和预测生物标志物或基因特征的未来策略，可以允许我们预先选择患者以进行最合适的治疗。此外，在这些最有趣的肿瘤中，人们现在非常关注对于免疫系统的靶向治疗。胸腺肿瘤与继发于 T 细胞介导的自身免疫的各种疾病有关，并且与高 PD-L1 表达相关，这表明检查点抑制剂如 PD-1 抑制剂可能给化疗耐药的患者带来希望。

（赵自然 译　薛奇 校）

参考文献

The complete reference list can be found on the Wiley Companion Digital Edition of this title (see inside front cover for login instructions).

1 Engels EA. Epidemiology of thymoma and associated malignancies. *J Thorac Oncol*. 2010;**5**:S260–S265.

3 Masaoka A, Monden Y, Nakahara K, et al. Follow-up study of thymomas with special reference to their clinical stages. *Cancer*. 1981;**48**:2485–2492.

4 Koga K, Matsuno Y, Noguchi M, et al. A review of 79 thymomas: modification of staging system and reappraisal of conventional division into invasive and non-invasive thymoma. *Pathol Int*. 1994;**44**:359–367.

13 Marchevsky AM, Wick MR. *Pathology of the Mediastinum*. Cambridge, UK: Cambridge Press; 2014.

15 Travis WD, Brambilla E, Muller-Hermelink HK. *Pathology and Genetics of Tumours of the Lung, Pleura, Thymus and Heart (IARC WHO Classifications of Tumours*. Lyon, France: IARC Press; 2004.

16 Marx A, Strobel P, Badve SS, et al. ITMIG consensus statement on the use of the WHO histological classification of thymoma and thymic carcinoma: refined definitions, histological criteria, and reporting. *J Thorac Oncol*. 2014;**9**:596–611.

17 Suster S, Moran CA. Histologic classification of thymoma: the World Health Organization and beyond. *Hematol Oncol Clin North Am*. 2008;**22**:381–392.

22 Moser B, Scharitzer M, Hacker S, et al. Thymomas and thymic carcinomas: prognostic factors and multimodal management. *Thorac Cardiovasc Surg*. 2014;**62**:153–160.

24 Marchevsky AM, McKenna RJ Jr, Gupta R. Thymic epithelial neoplasms: a review of current concepts using an evidence-based pathology approach. *Hematol Oncol Clin North Am*. 2008;**22**:543–562.

25 Gupta R, Marchevsky AM, McKenna RJ, et al. Evidence-based pathology and the pathologic evaluation of thymomas: transcapsular invasion is not a significant prognostic feature. *Arch Pathol Lab Med*. 2008;**132**:926–930.

26 Marchevsky AM, Gupta R, Casadio C, et al. World Health Organization classification of thymomas provides significant prognostic information for selected stage III patients: evidence from an international thymoma study group. *Hum Pathol*. 2010;**41**:1413–1421.

27 Marchevsky AM, Gupta R, McKenna RJ, et al. Evidence-based pathology and the pathologic evaluation of thymomas: the World Health Organization classification can be simplified into only 3 categories other than thymic carcinoma. *Cancer*. 2008;**112**:2780–2788.

30 Detterbeck FC, Nicholson AG, Kondo K, et al. The Masaoka-Koga stage classification for thymic malignancies: clarification and definition of terms. *J Thorac Oncol*. 2011;**6**:S1710–S1716.

31 Ruffini E, Detterbeck F, Van Raemdonck D, et al. Tumours of the thymus: a cohort study of prognostic factors from the European Society of thoracic surgeons database. *Eur J Cardiothorac Surg*. 2014;**46**:361–368.

32 Detterbeck FC. Clinical value of the WHO classification system of thymoma. *Ann Thorac Surg*. 2006;**81**:2328–2334.

34 Gokmen-Polar Y, Cano OD, Kesler KA, et al. *NUT midline carcinomas in the thymic region*. Vol. **27**. Mod Pathol: ; 2014:1649–1656.

36 Kelly RJ. Thymoma versus thymic carcinoma: differences in biology impacting treatment. *J Natl Compr Canc Netw*. 2013;**11**:577–583.

37 Okuma Y, Hosomi Y, Watanabe K, et al. Clinicopathological analysis of thymic malignancies with a consistent retrospective database in a single institution: from Tokyo Metropolitan Cancer Center. *BMC Cancer*. 2014;**14**:349.

38 Ruffini E, Detterbeck F, Van Raemdonck D, et al. Thymic carcinoma: a cohort study of patients from the European society of thoracic surgeons database. *J Thorac Oncol*. 2014;**9**:541–548.

42 Moran CA, Suster S. Thymic neuroendocrine carcinomas with combined features ranging from well-differentiated (carcinoid) to small cell carcinoma. A clinicopathologic and immunohistochemical study of 11 cases. *Am J Clin Pathol*. 2000;**113**:345–350.

53 Kelly RJ, Petrini I, Rajan A, et al. Thymic malignancies: from clinical management to targeted therapies. *J Clin Oncol*. 2011;**29**:4820–4827.

81 Loehrer PJ Sr, Jiroutek M, Aisner S, et al. Combined etoposide, ifosfamide, and cisplatin in the treatment of patients with advanced thymoma and thymic carcinoma: an intergroup trial. *Cancer*. 2001;**91**:2010–2015.

82 Lemma GL, Lee JW, Aisner SC, et al. Phase II study of carboplatin and paclitaxel in advanced thymoma and thymic carcinoma. *J Clin Oncol*. 2011;**29**:2060–2065.

83 Loehrer PJ Sr, Yiannoutsos CT, Dropcho S, et al. A phase II trial of pemetrexed in patients with recurrent thymoma or thymic carcinoma. *J Clin Oncol* (Meeting Abstracts). 2006;**24**:7079.

85 Yoshihito Kogure FH, Yamanaka T. A multicenter prospective study of carboplatin and paclitaxel for advanced thymic carcinoma: West Japan Oncology Group 4207L. O3.1. *J Thorac Oncol*. 2013;**8(Supplement 1)**.

86 Celine Boutros FF, Besse B. P2.03: oral etoposide in pretreated advanced thymoma and thymic carcinoma: a French experience. *J Thorac Oncol*. 2013;**8(Supplement 1)**.

87 Heather Wakelee JR, Pedro-Salcedo MS. Stage 1 results of a 2-stage phase II trial of single agent Amrubicin in patients with previously treated thymic malignancies. O3.2. *J Thorac Oncol*. 2013;**8(Supplement 1)**.

91 Giaccone G, Rajan A, Berman A, et al. Phase II study of belinostat in patients with recurrent or refractory advanced thymic epithelial tumors. *J Clin Oncol*. 2011;**29**:2052–2059.

92 Rajan A, Carter CA, Berman A, et al. Cixutumumab for patients with recurrent or refractory advanced thymic epithelial tumours: a multicentre, open-label, phase 2 trial. *Lancet Oncol*. 2014;**15**:191–200.

93 Wheler J, Hong D, Swisher SG, et al. Thymoma patients treated in a phase I clinic at MD Anderson Cancer Center: responses to mTOR inhibitors and molecular analyses. *Oncotarget*. 2013;**4**:890–898.

95 Pan CC, Chen PC, Chiang H. KIT (CD117) is frequently overexpressed in thymic carcinomas but is absent in thymomas. *J Pathol*. 2004;**202**:375–381.

96 Henley JD, Cummings OW, Loehrer PJ Sr. Tyrosine kinase receptor expression in thymomas. *J Cancer Res Clin Oncol*. 2004;**130**:222–224.

97 Strobel P, Hartmann M, Jakob A, et al. Thymic carcinoma with overexpression of mutated KIT and the response to imatinib. *N Engl J Med*. 2004;**350**:2625–2626.

98 Yoh K, Nishiwaki Y, Ishii G, et al. Mutational status of EGFR and KIT in thymoma and thymic carcinoma. *Lung Cancer*. 2008;**62**:316–320.

99 Bisagni G, Rossi G, Cavazza A, et al. Long lasting response to the multikinase inhibitor bay 43-9006 (Sorafenib) in a heavily pretreated metastatic thymic carcinoma. *J Thorac Oncol*. 2009;**4**:773–775.

100 Giaccone G, Rajan A, Ruijter R, et al. Imatinib mesylate in patients with WHO B3 thymomas and thymic carcinomas. *J Thorac Oncol*. 2009;**4**:1270–1273.

111 Steele NL, Plumb JA, Vidal L, et al. A phase 1 pharmacokinetic and pharmacodynamic study of the histone deacetylase inhibitor belinostat in patients with advanced solid tumors. *Clin Cancer Res*. 2008;**14**:804–810.

第 87 章　心脏和大血管肿瘤

Anthony F. Yu, MD ■ Sai-Ching Jim Yeung, MD, PhD, FACP ■ Carmen P. Escalante, MD ■ Sarina van der Zee, MD ■ A. P. Chahinian, MD ■ Valentin Fuster, MD, PhD

概述

心脏和大血管的原发性肿瘤很少见，而继发性肿瘤明显更常见。心脏肿瘤的临床表现取决于肿块的位置和大小，而不取决于肿瘤的组织病理学。目前有几种无创的成像方式，包括超声心动图，心脏 MRI，心脏 CT 和 PET，可提供有关心脏肿瘤的位置、范围和组织特征的信息。根据不同的肿瘤类型，临床症状和总体预后，心脏肿瘤患者的临床治疗而不同。

介绍

心脏原发性肿瘤很少见，尸检报告的发生率<0.1%～0.3%[1~4]，超过 75%心脏原发性肿瘤为良性（表 87-1）[5,6]。大多数原发性心脏恶性肿瘤是肉瘤和淋巴瘤，即使治疗预后也很差[7,8]。成人心脏转移瘤比原发性心脏肿瘤更常见[2,9~11]。大多数原发肿瘤来自心内膜，其次是心肌，心外膜最少见[2]，而后者是转移瘤最常见的发生部位[12]。

表 87-1　来自军队病理研究机构的两项研究中心脏和心包原发性肿瘤的种类和发病率

类型	1976—1993 年的研究		1977 年前的研究	
	例数	百分比	例数	百分比
良性肿瘤				
黏液瘤	114	27.9	130	29.3
乳头状纤维弹性组织瘤	31	7.6	42	9.5
横纹肌瘤	20	4.9	36	8.1
脂肪瘤	2	0.5	45	10.1
纤维瘤	20	4.9	17	3.8
血管瘤	17	4.2	15	3.4
房室结瘤	10	2.4	12	2.7
畸胎瘤	4	1.0	14	3.2
房间隔脂肪瘤肥厚	12	2.9	0	0.0
颗粒细胞瘤	4	1.0	3	0.7
淋巴管瘤	2	0.5	2	0.5
良性纤维瘤	3	0.7	0	0.0
神经纤维瘤	0	0.0	3	0.7
Histiocytoid 心肌病	2	0.5	0	0.0
炎性假性肿瘤	2	0.5	0	0.0
肌细胞错构瘤	2	0.5	0	0.0
副神经节瘤	2	0.5	0	0.0
上皮样血管内皮瘤	1	0.2	0	0.0
共计	248	60.6	319	71.8
恶性肿瘤				
血管肉瘤	37	9.0	39	88

续表

类型	1976—1993 年的研究		1977 年前的研究	
	例数	百分比	例数	百分比
未分类的肉瘤	35	8.6	0	0.0
横纹肌肉瘤	6	1.5	26	5.9
间皮瘤	8	2.0	19	4.3
纤维肉瘤	9	2.2	14	3.2
骨肉瘤	13	3.2	5	1.1
恶性纤维组织细胞瘤	16	3.9	0	0.0
淋巴瘤	7	1.7	7	1.6
平滑肌肉瘤	12	2.9	1	0.2
黏液肉瘤	8	2.0	0	0.0
关节肉瘤	5	1.2	1	0.2
恶性畸胎瘤	0	0.0	4	0.9
神经元肉瘤	0	0.0	4	0.9
胸腺瘤*	0	0.0	4	0.9
脂肪肉瘤	2	0.5	1	0.2
恶性神经鞘瘤	2	0.5	0	0.0
卵黄囊瘤	1	0.2	0	0.0
共计	161	39.4	125	28.2
肿瘤合计	409	444	0	0.0

*来自心包腔胸腺壁。

摘自 Refs. 4and 5. Cysts are excluded。

临床特征

心脏肿瘤的临床特点常常反映心脏结构受累和肿瘤的脱落，而不是肿瘤的组织学情况[12]。导致临床症状的潜在机制多种多样，可能包括栓塞、心内或瓣膜阻塞、心肌或邻近器官直接受侵等。心脏常见肿瘤的主要发生部位如图 87-1 所示。

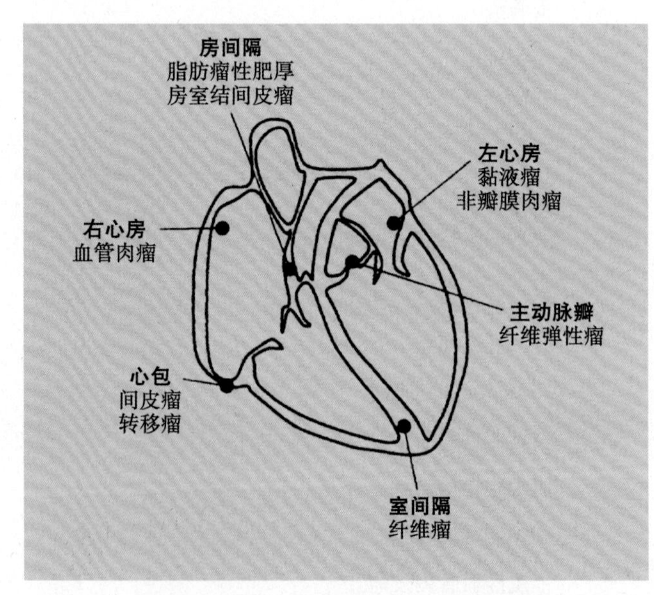

图 87-1　常见心脏肿瘤的主要发病部位

心内膜表面的肿瘤表现为瓣膜功能障碍或腔内阻塞。右房肿瘤可导致三尖瓣梗阻和右心衰竭的症状（即疲劳、外周性水肿、腹水、肝大、颈静脉扩张等）。左房肿瘤倾向于通过阻塞血流引起症状并且通常伴有左心衰竭症状（即呼吸困难、端坐呼吸、肺水肿或咯血等）。心肌受侵可能表现为心律失常、传导异常、收缩或舒张功能障碍。完全的空腔阻塞很少见，但可能导致猝死。心包受累可表现为胸膜炎性胸痛或心脏压塞。易脱落的肿瘤如一些黏液瘤和乳头状纤维弹性组织瘤会有脑动脉、肺动脉、颈动脉和外周动脉栓塞的表现。全身表现常见于黏液瘤和恶性心脏肿瘤，包括发热、体重下降、肌痛、关节痛、疲劳和虚弱。

心脏肿瘤的患者可以出现上面描述的症状，也可能没有症状而偶然在影像学检查时发现肿瘤，尤其是当肿瘤很小时。体格检查提示收缩期或舒张期杂音，如果肿瘤为活动性，杂音会随体位的改变而变化。活动性肿瘤如黏液瘤可以在舒张期第二心音后出现典型的肿瘤扑落音，其原因与黏液瘤在舒张期随血液进入左室、瘤蒂突然紧张产生振动或肿瘤碰撞房室壁和瓣膜有关[10]。肿瘤扑落音可能被误以为第三心音或二尖瓣开瓣音。心电图表现为非特异性 ST-T 改变、房性或室性心律失常、束支传导阻滞或出现心包积液时的 QRS 波群低电压。胸部 X 线表现包括心脏肥大和肿瘤钙化影。实验室异常包括贫血(可能是溶血性)或红细胞增多症、白细胞增多、血小板减少、血清免疫球蛋白水平升高以及急性期反应物如红细胞沉降率和 C 反应蛋白水平升高[10]。

诊断评估

有几种心脏成像技术可用于评估怀疑心脏肿瘤的患者。二维经胸超声心动图(TTE)提供了良好的心脏肿瘤的空间和时间分辨率,并且通常是首选的成像模式[13]。然而,TTE 可能受到声学窗口不良和缺乏组织特征的限制。经食管超声心动图(TEE)允许更好的肿瘤定位和特征以及心内和心外受侵程度的评估。使用造影剂增强的超声心动图可能有助于提高超声心动图的分辨率,并提供有关肿瘤血管的信息[14]。实时三维超声心动图可以提供二维超声心动图的增量值,通过准确评估肿物的大小和形状,更好的肿瘤附着点的定位[15]。

心脏计算机断层扫描(CT)和磁共振成像(MRI)提供具有时间和空间高分辨率的心脏的横截面图像。两种方式都能够描绘心内和心外肿物,以及心肌或心包受累的程度,而不受身体习性或声学窗口不良的限制。心脏 CT 提供有关组织学特征的信息有限,其缺点包括辐射暴露和造影剂的潜在肾毒性[16]。心脏 MRI 提供任何成像模式的高纬度的软组织对比,并同时有杰出的肿瘤定位、相邻结构的可视化、心肌运动和灌注评估的优点(图 87-2)[17~19]。此外,定制的成像序列允许对特定肿瘤进行更具体的特征描绘[18]。心脏肿块的组织特征可以使用 T1 和 T2 加权图像进行评估[20],虽然增强 CT 的空间分辨率大于 MRI,但 CT 的软组织特征描绘不如 MRI,因此,CT 可被认为是适合某些患者的中间模式[16]。正电子发射断层扫描(PET)也可以帮助确定恶性肿瘤患者的心脏受累情况[21]。心脏病血管造影一度是心脏肿瘤诊断的主要方式,但由于手术过程中存在栓塞风险,因此已停止使用。

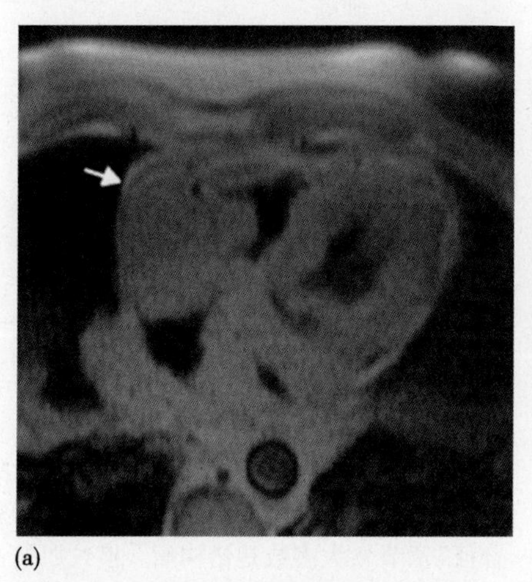

(a)

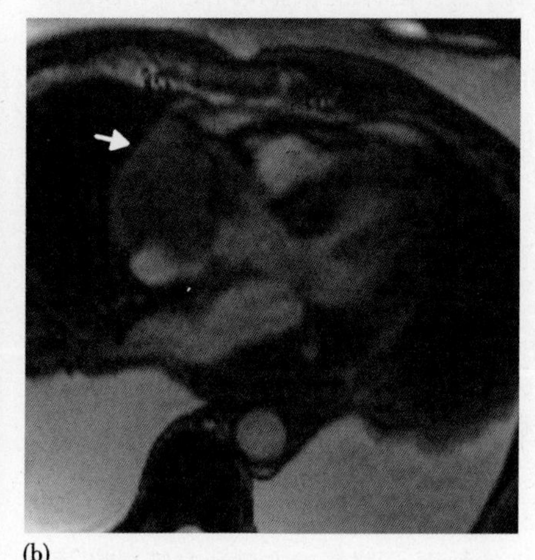

(b)

图 87-2　一例 69 岁男性淋巴瘤患者的心脏 MRI 影像,箭头所示处可见一大块均质肿块影,占据大部分右房并延伸至右室和后纵隔。(a)T2WI HASTE 序列所见的四腔心血液高信号。(b)稳态进动成像获得的四腔心血液低信号,注意大面积双侧胸膜渗出

当在成像研究中发现心脏肿物时,需要与包括血栓和赘生物相鉴别,以及需要鉴别是原发性还是继发性肿瘤[22,23]。血栓通常见于有血栓形成倾向的患者,包括心律失常(如心房颤动或心房扑动),心肌病或心肌梗死等。正常的解剖变异,如明显的欧氏瓣或希阿里网可以表现为心脏肿物[24]。

心脏肿瘤

心脏原发性良性肿瘤

黏液瘤

在成人群体中,黏液瘤最常见的原发性心脏肿瘤。目前认为这些柔软的凝胶状肿瘤的组织学来源是心内膜下间质,含有多角至星形黏液细胞(“胚层细胞”),常在嗜伊红基质中围绕血管,伴有不同面积的出血[5]。这些细胞Ⅷ因子阳性,也能表达神经元特异性烯醇化酶和 S-100 蛋白[25]。大多数源于左房的黏液瘤常附着在卵圆窝,对共计 1 029 例患者的 32 项报告进行的荟萃分析中,83%的黏液瘤出现在左房[26]。其余部分位于右心房,或者位于不常见的右心室或左心室。黏液瘤多表现为活动性肿物,由瘤蒂附着在心内膜表面[27]。出现症状的平均年龄是 50 岁,女性患者多于男性[26]。典型的临床表现包括全身基础情况、瓣膜阻塞和血栓栓塞三联征[12]。栓塞可见于 30%~40%的患者,当肿瘤表面不规则(息肉状或黏液样)而且不光滑时更容易出现。因为有栓塞的风险,所以一旦确诊应尽快手术治疗,对肿瘤和与正常组织交界处及卵圆窝进行全部切除。黏液瘤复发少见,但仍有必要进行长期随访[28~30]。

尽管大多数黏液瘤为散发,但也有家族性病例的报告。Carney 综合征是一种多发性内分泌肿瘤综合征,除了皮肤和黏膜色素沉着,还包括心脏、内分泌、神经和皮肤的肿瘤[31~33]。位于染色体 17q22~24、编码 cAMP 依赖蛋白激酶 A 调节亚单位的 *PRKAR1A* 基因突变与大约一半患者有关[34~37]。一类伴有远端关节弯曲的黏液瘤被发现与位于染色体 17p12-p13.1 的

肌球蛋白重链基因上的错义突变有关[38]。家族性黏液瘤多在年轻时发病，同散发病例相比，多发和手术切除后复发更常见[39]。对一级亲属的识别有助于发现有栓塞风险的黏液瘤。

乳头状纤维弹性组织瘤

乳头状纤维弹性组织瘤是心脏瓣膜中最常见的原发性肿瘤，由与正常腱索相似的乳头状叶组成。它们通常来自心内瓣膜，最常见的是主动脉瓣，并且发生在很多年龄段[40,41]。纤维弹性组织瘤可能无症状(约30%的患者)或可能出现短暂性脑缺血发作、卒中、心力衰竭、心绞痛、心肌梗死或猝死。对于发生过栓塞事件的及具有高栓塞风险的或者直径叫大(1cm)或活动肿块的患者，建议进行手术切除[40,42,43]。

其他良性肿瘤

横纹肌瘤几乎都见于儿童，将在随后进行介绍。脂肪瘤间隔肥厚是房间隔内正常脂肪的过度堆积[44]。出现腔静脉阻塞、房性心律失常和充血性心力衰竭时建议手术[45,46]。脂肪瘤和血管瘤可以发生在心脏的任何位置，纤维瘤常出现在室间隔，更常见于左心室[47]。心包囊肿最常见于右肋膈角，支气管源囊肿可以出现在心肌中[5]。副神经节瘤和间皮瘤可以是良性也可以是恶性。间皮瘤可以是原发或心包的转移瘤，或者发生在房室结，表现为房室传导阻滞、心律失常或猝死[48]。

心脏原发性恶性肿瘤

肉瘤

软组织肉瘤是最常见的心脏原发性恶性肿瘤[49]。尽管其他房室腔也可以累及，但血管肉瘤常发生在右房房室沟附近，伴有出血、心包受累和渗出[50]。血管肉瘤的高发年龄在20~50岁，男性发病率是女性的2~3倍[5]。临床表现包括心悸、呼吸困难和胸痛(胸膜或心包受累所致)或与心力衰竭或血栓栓塞相关的症状和体征。心脏血管肉瘤与累及心脏的卡波西肉瘤(Kaposi sarcoma，KS)的关系仍需深入研究[51,52]。横纹肌肉瘤是第二常见的心脏恶性肿瘤，同样影响右侧和左侧心腔[53]。从心内膜生长的肉瘤常伴有平滑肌或肌纤维细胞分化，常位于左房并含有多种亚型，包括未分化的多形性肉瘤、骨肉瘤、平滑肌肉瘤、纤维肉瘤和黏液纤维肉瘤。

心脏肉瘤的总体预后很差，并且局部侵袭性生长和转移性扩散很常见。中位生存期为6~12个月[54,55]。完全手术切除的心脏肉瘤是首选治疗方法，尽管许多患者会出现复发。在一些小型系列和病例报告中，已经有了原位心脏移植，有时联合双侧肺移植的报道。在大多数情况下，心脏移植之后采取化疗并不会影响长期预后[56]；但是，选择化疗的特定患者可能会有良好的移植效果[57,58]。

淋巴瘤

原发性心脏淋巴瘤很少见，应与全身性淋巴瘤继发心脏受累的相鉴别[8]。典型的发病部位是心房，心房壁浸润常见，心包也可以受累。心脏淋巴瘤可见于免疫缺陷患者或获得性免疫缺陷综合征以及器官移植相关的免疫抑制的患者。同其他心脏肿瘤不同，淋巴瘤的主要治疗是化疗，单独应用或联合放疗，偶尔也采用自体干细胞移植[59,60]。

心脏转移性肿瘤

心脏继发性肿瘤明显多于原发性心脏肿瘤[61]。转移机制包括直接侵袭，血源性扩散，淋巴扩散和心房或肺静脉扩散。心包是心脏转移最常见的部位，其次是心外膜和心肌。表87-2显示了可能转移至心脏的恶性肿瘤[27]。在最近对7 289例恶性肿瘤病例进行的尸检中，心脏转移的发生率为9.1%[11]。心脏转移的发生率按降序排列为间皮瘤(48.4%)、黑色素瘤(27.8%)、肺腺癌(21%)，低分化肺癌(19.5%)、鳞状细胞肺癌(18.2%)和乳腺癌(15.5%)。然而，几乎任何癌症都可以转移到心脏。恶性胸膜间皮瘤患者可见高频率的心脏转移和/或侵犯[62]。19例尸检中，14例(74%)发现心脏浸润，超过一半转移到心包，超过1/4转移到心肌[63]。治疗通常是姑息性治疗。

表87-2 可能转移至心脏的肿瘤

肿瘤
黑色素瘤
恶性生殖细胞肿瘤
白血病和淋巴瘤
乳腺癌
肺癌
肝细胞癌
肾细胞癌
肉瘤
食管癌和胃癌
间皮瘤(可以是心包原发或转移瘤)

小儿心脏肿瘤

和成人不同，小儿心脏转移瘤少见。发生在儿童的许多心脏肿物多是家族遗传性综合征的一个表现(见前文“Carney综合征”章节)，大多数是错构瘤。横纹肌瘤占儿童心脏肿瘤的大部分64，伴有结节性硬化症，该疾病是以心脏、肾脏、脑、肺和皮肤的良性肿物为特征的常染色体显性疾病[65]。横纹肌瘤大多数发生在心室，是家族遗传性综合征的表现之一，可自行好转，只有在出现流出道梗阻时才需要手术切除[66~68]。心脏纤维瘤主要存在于室间隔，并且可以长得很大，通常有中央钙化区域。纤维瘤发生在少数Gorlin综合征的患者，该疾病也是一种常染色体显性遗传疾病，表现为多发的肿瘤，包括基底细胞癌和髓母细胞瘤以及牙源性角化囊肿和骨骼异常[69,70]。Von Recklinghausen疾病的患者有神经纤维瘤的报道[27]。

大血管的肿瘤

累及主动脉、肺动脉和腔静脉的原发性肿瘤很少见，文献中报告的主要是病例报告或小样本的回顾性病例研究[71~73]。发生大血管肿瘤的危险因素尚不清楚。推测既往射线接触史可能是原因之一[74]。动物研究发现塑料聚合物如Dacron与主动脉肿瘤有关，但临床患者主动脉肿瘤发生在Dacron移植物附近，虽有报道但很少见[75]。大血管肿瘤的典型表现是血栓栓塞事件或阻塞综合征[71]。TEE和MRI有助于鉴别大血管肿瘤和腔内血栓、纵隔淋巴结病或邻近的肺部肿瘤。

主动脉良性肿瘤包括发生在主动脉窦的内皮乳头状纤维弹性组织瘤，表现为肿瘤间断脱出至主动脉或者心脏或脑的血栓形成[76]。主动脉内的黏液瘤也有报告，表现为反复动脉栓塞[72]。

主动脉和肺动脉的恶性肿瘤常常是侵袭性的低分化肉瘤，起源于内膜细胞，表现为肌成纤维细胞分化型（"内膜型"）。少数情况下，大血管肿瘤表现为血管肉瘤、平滑肌肉瘤、血管内皮瘤、神经鞘瘤和纤维组织细胞瘤[71,77~79]。下腔静脉肉瘤趋向于分化较好的平滑肌肉瘤[80]。但主动脉肉瘤平均发病年龄为 62 岁，肺动脉肉瘤平均发病年龄为 41 岁。对 60 例患者的汇总分析发现，平均发病年龄为 52 岁，男女患者的比例为 1∶2，平均症状持续时间为 10 个月[81]。临床表现提示肺栓塞，包括呼吸困难（70%）、胸痛（48%）、咳嗽（34%）、咯血（30%）和晕厥（25%）。肺转移（67%）和淋巴结转移（20%）常见。

患者表现为进展性疾病且预后不良，极少数患者能进行手术和化疗[82]。大血管肿瘤的核心治疗是彻底手术切除[83]。术中可以使用各种移植物[84]，同时术后放疗和化疗，化疗以蒽环类药为基础[71,77]。大血管肿瘤患者的平均生存时间只有 10 个月，肺动脉肉瘤的预后好于主动脉肉瘤（分别为 23 个月和 5 个月）[71,84,85]。长期存活率虽然极为罕见，但已有报道[86]。对于无法切除的患者，血管内支架置入可提高生活质量[87]。

（赵自然 译 高禹舜 校）

参考文献

The complete reference list can be found on the Wiley Companion Digital Edition of this title (see inside front cover for login instructions).

1 Bruce CJ. Cardiac tumours: diagnosis and management. *Heart*. 2011;**97**:151–160.

2 Lam KY, Dickens P, Chan AC. Tumors of the heart. A 20-year experience with a review of 12,485 consecutive autopsies. *Arch Pathol Lab Med*. 1993;**117**:1027–1031.

5 McAllister HA, Fenoglio JJ. *Tumors of the Cardiovascular System*. Washington: Armed Forces Institute of Pathology; 1978.

7 Shanmugam G Primary cardiac sarcoma. *Eur J Cardiothorac Surg*. 2006;**29**:925–932.

8 Simpson L, Kumar SK, Okuno SH, et al. Malignant primary cardiac tumors: review of a single institution experience.. *Cancer*. 2008;**112(11)**:2440.

11 Bussani R, De-Giorgio F, Abbate A, et al. Cardiac metastases. *J Clin Pathol*. 2007;**60**:27–34.

12 Burke A, Jeudy J Jr, Virmani R. Cardiac tumours: an update: Cardiac tumours. *Heart*. 2008;**94**:117–123.

13 Auger D, Pressacco J, Marcotte F, et al. Cardiac masses: an integrative approach using echocardiography and other imaging modalities. *Heart*. 2011;**97**:1101–1109.

14 Mulvagh SL, Rakowski H, Vannan MA, et al. American society of echocardiography consensus statement on the clinical applications of ultrasonic contrast agents in echocardiography. *J Am Soc Echocardiogr*. 2008;**21**:1179–1201; quiz 1281.

15 Zaragoza-Macias E, Chen MA, Gill EA. Real time three-dimensional echocardiography evaluation of intracardiac masses. *Echocardiography*. 2012;**29**:207–219.

16 Kassop D, Donovan MS, Cheezum MK, et al. Cardiac masses on cardiac CT: A review. *Curr Cardiovasc Imaging Rep*. 2014;7:9281.

19 Fussen S, De Boeck BW, Zellweger MJ, et al. Cardiovascular magnetic resonance imaging for diagnosis and clinical management of suspected cardiac masses and tumours. *Eur Heart J*. 2011;**32**:1551–1560.

20 Hoey ET, Mankad K, Puppala S, et al. MRI and CT appearances of cardiac tumours in adults. *Clin Radiol*. 2009;**64**:1214–1230.

21 Rahbar K, Seifarth H, Schafers M, et al. Differentiation of malignant and benign cardiac tumors using 18 F-FDG PET/CT. *J Nucl Med*. 2012;**53**:856–863.

24 Kim MJ, Jung HO. Anatomic variants mimicking pathology on echocardiography: differential diagnosis. *J Cardiovasc Ultrasound*. 2013;**21**:103–112.

27 Burke A, Virmani R. *Tumors of the Heart and Great Vessels, Atlas of Tumor Pathology*. Washington, DC: Armed Forces Institute of Pathology; 1996.

30 D'Alfonso A, Catania S, Pierri MD, et al. Atrial myxoma: a 25-year single-institutional follow-up study. *J Cardiovasc Med (Hagerstown)*. 2008;**9**:178–181.

31 Carney JA, Gordon H, Carpenter PC, et al. The complex of myxomas, spotty pigmentation, and endocrine overactivity. *Medicine (Baltimore)*. 1985;**64**:270–283.

33 Stratakis CA, Kirschner LS, Carney JA. Clinical and molecular features of the Carney complex: diagnostic criteria and recommendations for patient evaluation. *J Clin Endocrinol Metab*. 2001;**86**:4041–4046.

37 Carney JA. The complex of myxomas, spotty pigmentation, and endocrine overactivity. *Arch Intern Med*. 1987;**147**:418–419.

39 Carney JA. Differences between nonfamilial and familial cardiac myxoma. *Am J Surg Pathol*. 1985;**9**:53–55.

40 Sun JP, Asher CR, Yang XS, et al. Clinical and echocardiographic characteristics of papillary fibroelastomas: a retrospective and prospective study in 162 patients. *Circulation*. 2001;**103**:2687–2693.

41 Gowda RM, Khan IA, Nair CK, et al. Cardiac papillary fibroelastoma: a comprehensive analysis of 725 cases. *Am Heart J*. 2003;**146**:404–410.

46 Cale R, Andrade MJ, Canada M, et al. Lipomatous hypertrophy of the interatrial septum: report of two cases where histological examination and surgical intervention were unavoidable. *Eur J Echocardiogr*. 2009;**10**:876–879.

49 Yusuf SW, Bathina JD, Qureshi S, et al. Cardiac tumors in a tertiary care cancer hospital: clinical features, echocardiographic findings, treatment and outcomes. *Heart Int*. 2012;**7**:e4.

53 Castorino F, Masiello P, Quattrocchi E, et al. Primary cardiac rhabdomyosarcoma of the left atrium: an unusual presentation. *Tex Heart Inst J*. 2000;**27**:206–208.

54 Truong PT, Jones SO, Martens B, et al. Treatment and outcomes in adult patients with primary cardiac sarcoma: the British Columbia Cancer Agency experience. *Ann Surg Oncol*. 2009;**16**:3358–3365.

55 Hudzik B, Miszalski-Jamka K, Glowacki J, et al. Malignant tumors of the heart. *Cancer Epidemiology*. 2015;**39**:665–672.

57 Grandmougin D, Fayad G, Decoene C, et al. Total orthotopic heart transplantation for primary cardiac rhabdomyosarcoma: factors influencing long-term survival. *Ann Thorac Surg*. 2001;**71**:1438–1441.

61 Goldberg AD, Blankstein R, Padera RF. Tumors metastatic to the heart. *Circulation*. 2013;**128**:1790–1794.

64 Careddu L, Oppido G, Petridis FD, et al. Primary cardiac tumours in the paediatric population. *Multimed Man Cardiothorac Surg*. 2013;**2013**:mmt013.

65 Hinton RB, Prakash A, Romp RL, et al. Cardiovascular manifestations of tuberous sclerosis complex and summary of the revised diagnostic criteria and surveillance and management recommendations from the international tuberous sclerosis consensus group. *J Am Heart Assoc*. 2014;**3**.

66 Tao TY, Yahyavi-Firouz-Abadi N, Singh GK, and Bhalla S. Pediatric cardiac tumors: clinical and imaging features. *Radiographics*. 2014;**34**:1031–1046.

67 Sciacca P, Giacchi M, Mattia C, et al. Rhabdomyomas and tuberous sclerosis complex: our experience in 33 cases. *BMC Cardiovasc Disord*. 2014;**14**:66.

77 Blackmon SH, Rice DC, Correa AM, et al. Management of primary pulmonary artery sarcomas. *Ann Thorac Surg*. 2009;**87**:977–984.

80 Hollenbeck ST, Grobmyer SR, Kent KC, and Brenan MF. Surgical treatment and outcomes of patients with primary inferior vena cava leiomyosarcoma. *J Am Coll Surg*. 2003;**197**:575–579.

82 Mayer F, Aebert H, Rudert M, et al. Primary malignant sarcomas of the heart and great vessels in adult patients—a single-center experience. *Oncologist*. 2007;**12**:1134–1142.

83 Park BJ, Bacchetta M, Bains MS, et al. Surgical management of thoracic malignancies invading the heart or great vessels. *Ann Thorac Surg*. 2004;**78**:1024–1030.

86 Mattoo A, Fedullo PF, Kapelanski D, et al. Pulmonary artery sarcoma: a case report of surgical cure and 5-year follow-up. *Chest*. 2002;**122**:745–747.

87 Totaro M, Miraldi F, Ghiribelli C, et al. Cardiac angiosarcoma arising from pulmonary artery: endovascular treatment. *Ann Thorac Surg*. 2004;**78**:1468–1470.

第 88 章 原发纵隔生殖细胞肿瘤

John D. Hainsworth, MD ■ F. Anthony Greco, MD

概述

胸部原发性生殖细胞瘤(primary germ cell tumors, GCT)通常在年轻人群中发病,其中良性畸胎瘤占 60%~70%,其患病率虽低但绝大多数可以通过手术切除治愈。恶性纵隔 GCT 的高发人群为年轻男性,组织学上可将其分为精原细胞瘤(约 52%的病例)和各种非精原细胞瘤。精原细胞瘤对化疗高度敏感,其中睾丸癌中经博来霉素、依托泊苷和顺铂(bleomycin, etoposide and cisplatin, BEP)三周期化疗治愈率可达 80%以上,原位小精原细胞瘤(<6cm)经单独放射治疗即可达到较高的治愈率。非精囊纵隔 GCT 与克氏综合征(占 5%~10%)和各种急性白血病具有相关性。目前非精囊纵隔 GCT 最佳治疗方案为 BEP 四周期化疗(或等效方案)联合手术治疗,其预后相对较差,治愈率仅 45%。

纵隔生殖细胞瘤虽很罕见,但其影响年轻男性且多数可治愈,因此引起了广泛关注。

纵隔良性畸胎瘤

纵隔良性畸胎瘤(成熟的囊性畸胎瘤或皮肤样瘤)仅占所有纵隔肿瘤的 3%~12%,但占纵隔 GCT 的 60%~70%[1,2],7 月龄婴儿以及 65 岁老年人均可发病,但以年轻人为主,男女发病率大致相等[2,3]。

纵隔良性畸胎瘤的组织学改变与良性畸胎瘤相同,均起源于卵巢,来自外胚层、中胚层和内胚层生殖细胞层的成熟组织是其典型病理表现,肿瘤组织中可出现任何成熟组织,但以表皮成分(即皮肤、皮脂组织、神经组织)为主[3]。

大约 95%的良性畸胎瘤位于前纵隔,其余的发生在后纵隔[2,3]。良性畸胎瘤生长缓慢,50%~60%无症状的患者是行常规胸部 X 线检查发现的[3]。早期呼吸困难和胸骨后胸痛最为常见,晚期时畸胎瘤自发破裂进入肺,气管支气管树,胸膜或心包膜可导致急性发作,由于气管支气管树破裂导致咳出头发或皮脂等组织是纵隔畸胎瘤的特异性表现,但发生率较低。上腔静脉综合征也很罕见,且主要为晚期表现。良性畸胎瘤患者的血清人类绒毛膜促性腺激素(HCG)和甲胎蛋白水平始终正常。

纵隔良性畸胎瘤可经手术切除,但瘤体较大或侵犯邻近组织时手术切除比较困难,10%~15%的患者需要进行其他手术(如肺叶切除术,心包切除术)才能将肿瘤完全切除。良性畸胎瘤对放疗和细胞毒性药物有抵抗力,疗效较差。

肿瘤完整切除后复发率较低[2~4],肿瘤侵犯到重要纵隔结构无法完整切除的患者,行肿瘤次全切除也能够延长患者的生存期。

恶性生殖细胞肿瘤

病因学

最初认为纵隔 GCT 是一个隐匿性性腺原发部位的孤立转移灶,如今,已有充足的临床证据证实该肿瘤并非起源于生殖腺[1,5]。

流行病学

纵隔恶性生殖细胞肿瘤发病率较低,占纵隔肿瘤 3%~10%,在全部恶性生殖细胞肿瘤中仅占 1%~5%[6]。以 20~35 岁男性为主,女性很少发病,其肿瘤组织学和生物学特征与男性患者一致。

生殖腺外非精原性生殖细胞肿瘤患者患睾丸癌风险的增高(10 年患病率约为 10%),表明该肿瘤可能是生殖细胞肿瘤的癌前病变[7]。

组织病理学

纵隔生殖细胞肿瘤与来源于睾丸的生殖细胞肿瘤组织学形态相似,并包含相同组织学亚型,但是在纵隔生殖细胞肿瘤中,卵黄囊瘤和畸胎癌较常见,而胚胎性癌较少见。分析陆军病理研究所 1960 年到 1994 年间 229 例纵隔恶性生殖细胞肿瘤发现,单纯的精原细胞瘤是最常见的组织学类型,大约占到 52%[8],其他非精原细胞瘤包括畸胎瘤(20%)、卵黄囊瘤(17%)、绒毛膜癌(3.4%)、胚胎性癌(2.6%)和混合性非精原细胞瘤性肿瘤(5.2%)。

临床表现

恶性纵隔生殖细胞肿瘤与良性纵隔生殖细胞肿瘤不同,在诊断时通常已有临床症状。绝大多数恶性纵隔生殖细胞肿瘤体积大,通过压迫或侵犯邻近组织器官(如肺、胸膜、心包以及胸壁)造成一定的临床表现。与含有非精原细胞成分的纵隔生殖细胞肿瘤相比,单纯的精原细胞瘤生长相对慢,早期转移的可能性较低。尽管单纯精原细胞瘤和含有非精原细胞成分的生殖细胞肿瘤在临床特征方面存在较多的重叠,以下也分别对这两种类型的肿瘤临床特征进行阐述。

精原细胞瘤

精原细胞瘤生长相对慢,其直径为 20~30mm 时仅出现轻微的临床症状,20%~30%的精原细胞瘤是在无临床症状时通过常规胸片检查发现的[9]。最常见的早期临床表现是胸部压迫感或胸骨后钝痛,还可出现劳力性呼吸困难、咳嗽、吞咽困难、声音嘶哑,约 10%患者出现上腔静脉综合征,转移后所致的全身症状较为罕见。

纵隔生殖细胞肿瘤可分为两类,一类是没有其他组织学成分的精原细胞瘤（或女性生殖细胞瘤），一类是精原细胞瘤及非精原细胞瘤组织的非精原细胞性生殖细胞肿瘤。确诊精原细胞瘤时仅有 30%～40%患者病变局限，大部分为一处或多处远处转移[10]。区域淋巴结（颈部、上腹部）是最常见的转移部位；肺、骨是最常见的内脏转移部位[11]。

约 40%纵隔精原细胞瘤患者的血清 HCG 水平升高[11]，但仅为轻度升（2～10ng/ml）；血清 HCG 超过 100ng/ml 通常提示有非精原细胞瘤成分的存在。单纯精原细胞瘤患者的血清 AFP 通常在正常范围，任何水平的 AFP 升高均表明有非精原细胞瘤成分的存在。

非精原细胞瘤

纵隔非精原细胞瘤生长迅速，85%～95%的患者在诊断时即至少存在一处转移，临床症状常见为肿瘤压迫或侵犯纵隔结构所引起的症状，与精原细胞瘤相同[12～14]。纵隔非精原细胞瘤常见转移部位包括肺、胸膜、淋巴结（尤其是锁骨上淋巴结和腹膜后淋巴结）和肝脏。HCG 水平升高患者常出现男性乳房发育，体重下降、虚弱和发热症状较精原细胞瘤患者中更常见。

纵隔非精原细胞瘤患者血清肿瘤标志物 HCG 和 AFP 表达异常，74%～90%患者 AFP 升高，30%～38%患者 HCG 升高[15～17]。

5%～10%纵隔非精原细胞瘤患者合并克氏综合征[18～20]，两者的关联具有特殊性，但潜在的机制尚未研究明了，推测生殖细胞缺陷可能与 XXY 染色体异常有关[21]。在性腺的生殖细胞肿瘤中未发现与克氏综合征有相关性[18,19]。

纵隔非精原细胞瘤也常合并有多种血液系统肿瘤，包括急性髓细胞性白血病、急性非淋巴细胞白血病、急性淋巴细胞白血病、红白血病、急性巨核细胞白血病、骨髓增生异常综合征和恶性组织细胞增生症[22～28]。这些血液系统肿瘤并非放化疗引起，而是恶性淋巴母细胞、成髓细胞或含有生殖细胞肿瘤的体细胞的异常增殖所致[25～27]。

治疗前评估与分期

年轻男性发现纵隔肿块均需考虑纵隔生殖细胞肿瘤，行体格检查、常规实验室检查外、胸腹 CT 以及血清 HCG 和 AFP，有提示远处转移症状者还需行相应影像学检查。疑似纵隔生殖细胞瘤者必须给予组织病理学检查，某些肿瘤组织分化差，细针穿刺活检获得的标本通常不能满足确诊的要求，则行正中胸骨切开术或开胸术进行手术活检。由于纵隔生殖细胞瘤对放化疗反应良好，因此不需要完全手术切除纵隔肿瘤。

精原细胞瘤的治疗

精原细胞瘤对放疗和联合化疗高度敏感，即使诊断时已发生转移，大部分纵隔精原细胞瘤均可治愈。其治疗方案主要取决于疾病分期、纵隔肿瘤体积以及治疗过程中的毒副反应。

化疗

纵隔精原细胞瘤患者可选择治疗晚期睾丸癌的顺铂联合化疗方案。国际 GCCC[29]表示未出现肺外转移的生殖细胞肿瘤风险较小，可采用三期联合化疗，其中博来霉素、依托泊苷和顺铂（BEP）联合化疗应用最为广泛[30]。有肺部疾病的或曾接受过放射治疗的患者，应该避免使用博来霉素，采用四期依托泊苷/顺铂化疗。出现肺外转移的患者需选用四疗程顺铂治疗（BEP），如有博来霉素毒性风险，则选用四期ⅥP 治疗（依托泊苷、异环磷酰胺、顺铂）[31]。所有系列报道中均显示，用现代顺铂方案治疗的患者的治愈率固化率均高于 80%[10～12,14,30,32～36]，在最大的回顾性分析中，51 个中有 47 个患者完全康复，之后的复发率只有 14%[11]。

放疗

放疗也对纵隔精原细胞瘤有效[4,10,37,38]。局部肿瘤直径<6cm 的患者，放、化疗治愈率均较高，因此需个体化治疗，对于没有禁忌证的年轻患者，应当给予有效的化疗，避免纵隔放疗的远期危害（如冠脉疾病、瓣膜病、限制性心包炎、第二原发癌）[39,40]。不适合化疗的患者给予纵隔放疗（30～50Gy）。放疗后复发患者，经化疗后仍可获得较高的缓解率[12,30]，但应当避免使用含博来霉素方案，以降低肺损伤风险。

残余病灶

体积较大的精原细胞瘤化疗后，CT 扫描可见残余异常影。多数情况下，残余病灶直径<3cm 则仅包含纤维化和坏死性肿瘤，如果残余病灶直径>3cm，则残留组织活检显示为癌组织的可能性高达 30%[41,42]。因此，建议残余病灶<3cm 的患者进一步观察，暂无须手术治疗，病灶较大但 PET 扫描显示阴性的患者也可进一步观察[43,44]，即第一年每三个月做一次 CT 检查，第二年每六个月做一次检查直到完全恢复，只有明显增大的肿瘤需要干预治疗。当残余病灶>3cm 时建议行手术切除，同时行挽救性化疗，必要时行纵隔放射治疗。

非精原细胞瘤的治疗

目前，大多数纵隔非精原细胞性生殖细胞瘤患者可选用联合化疗后外科手术等多种治疗方案。

化疗

在以顺铂为基础的化疗方案出现之前，纵隔生殖细胞非精原细胞瘤并没有有效的治疗手段，由于远处转移的发生率高且肿瘤对放疗不敏感，局部治疗效果也不明显。以顺铂为基础的强化化疗稍微改善了晚期睾丸非精原细胞瘤患者的生存状态，但总生存率仍低于睾丸癌[12～17,32,33,36,45～48]。

据报道，晚期睾丸生殖细胞肿瘤患者接受以顺铂为基础的化疗方案治疗后，其长期生存率为 40%～50%[29]，纵隔和睾丸 GCT 之间固有的生物学差异决定了其相对治愈率较低。

纵隔非精原细胞性生殖细胞瘤患者具有较高的恶性肿瘤患病风险，因此，一线治疗应包括四期 BEP 或等效治疗方案[50]。完成治疗后，患者需定期行血清肿瘤标志物检查及胸腹部 CT 检查以重新分期。

残余病灶

后续治疗方案由初始化疗的疗效决定（图 88-1）。CT 结果及肿瘤标志物正常的患者无须进一步治疗，此类患者中近 20%的人会出现复发，几乎所有的复发均出现于化疗结束的前 2 年之内。标准的随访检查为：第一年每月进行体格检查、胸部 X 线片、血清肿瘤标志物，第 2 年则每 2 个月进行一次上述检查。大多数患者化疗后影像学上可见纵隔残余病灶[16]。对这些患者，如果技术上可行，应切除残余肿物。此种情况下血清肿瘤标志物的持续增高并不是手术禁忌证，因为对残存肿瘤的补救化疗通常无效[51,52]。不同研究报道中病理结果差异较大，可能是由于患者选择的标准不同。多数患者术后可见残余病灶（25%～66%）[53～56]，一小部分术后患者残余多种类型的非精原细胞瘤（如肉瘤、腺癌、神经内分泌癌）[55]，其余为良性畸胎瘤、坏死和纤维化，而没有活跃的癌细胞。

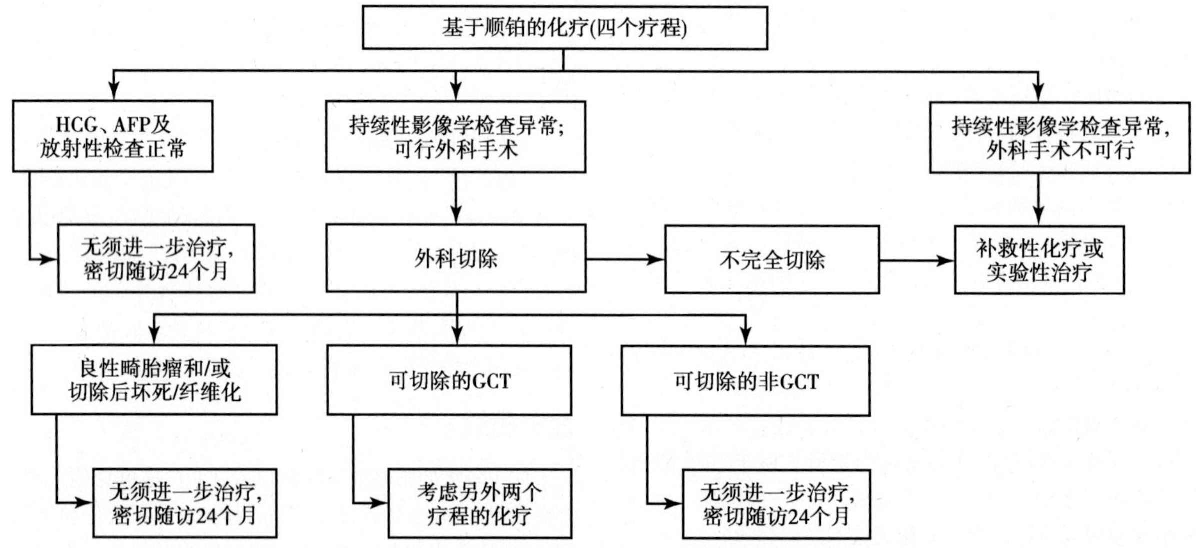

图 88-1 一线化疗完成后非精原性纵隔生殖细胞肿瘤的处理

多数残余病灶患者可经手术切除得到缓解。良性肿瘤患者（如坏死、纤维化和/或单纯良性畸胎瘤）与化疗后达到完全缓解患者的复发率均比较低（大约 20%）[53,55]。切除良性畸胎瘤可使患者获益，如不切除，这些肿瘤会缓慢生长或发生恶变。有术后生殖细胞癌残存的患者将来复发的风险高，其中有 20%～30%的患者需行两次手术切除[54,55]，对这部分患者，2 周期额外的术后化疗可能减少其复发率。对于大多数非生殖细胞残留的患者而言，即使把残存肿瘤完全切除疗效仍不理想，尽管偶有长期生存的个例报道[55]，对这部分患者术后进行进一步全身治疗是无效的。

复发/进展性疾病

无法肿瘤全切的患者预后很差，术后复发率较高。复发性睾丸癌患者可采用标准二线治疗即以顺铂为基础的高剂量化疗，有效率为 20%～50%，而在转移性非精原细胞瘤患者中有效率仅为 11%[51,52,57]。

预后

一项大型多中心研究对接受多种治疗方案的 287 名患者进行了回顾性研究[17]。化疗完全缓解率为 19%；另外 45%患者肿瘤标志物正常但伴有纵隔肿块，143 例（50%）患者仍需手术切除残留的纵隔肿块。5 年无进一步恶化的概率和总生存期率分别为 44%和 45%。

（陈先凯 译 王大力 校）

参考文献

The complete reference list can be found on the Wiley Companion Digital Edition of this title (see inside front cover for login instructions).

3 Lewis BD, Hurt RD, Payne WS, Farrow GM, Knapp RH, Muhm JR. Benign teratomas of the mediastinum. *J Thorac Cardiovasc Surg*. 1983;**86(5)**:727–731.

4 Dulmet EM, Macchiarini P, Suc B, Verley JM. Germ cell tumors of the mediastinum. A 30-year experience. *Cancer*. 1993;**72(6)**:1894–1901.

8 Moran CA, Suster S. Primary germ cell tumors of the mediastinum: I. Analysis of 322 cases with special emphasis on teratomatous lesions and a proposal for histopathologic classification and clinical staging. *Cancer*. 1997;**80(4)**:681–690.

9 Polansky S, Barwick K, Ravin C. Primary mediastinal seminoma. *AJR Am J Roentgenol*. 1979;**132**:17–21.

10 Jain KK, Bosl GJ, Bains MS, Whitmore WF, Golbey RB. The treatment of extragonadal seminoma. *J Clin Oncol*. 1984;**2(7)**:820–827.

11 Bokemeyer C, Droz JP, Horwich A, et al. Extragonadal seminoma: an international multicenter analysis of prognostic factors and long term treatment outcome. *Cancer*. 2001;**91(7)**:1394–1401.

13 Israel A, Bosl GJ, Golbey RB, Whitmore W Jr, Martini N. The results of chemotherapy for extragonadal germ-cell tumors in the cisplatin era: the Memorial Sloan-Kettering Cancer Center experience (1975 to 1982). *J Clin Oncol*. 1985;**3(8)**:1073–1078.

15 Nichols CR, Saxman S, Williams SD, et al. Primary mediastinal nonseminomatous germ cell tumors. A modern single institution experience. *Cancer*. 1990;**65(7)**:1641–1646.

16 Ganjoo KN, Rieger KM, Kesler KA, Sharma M, Heilman DK, Einhorn LH. Results of modern therapy for patients with mediastinal nonseminomatous germ cell tumors. *Cancer*. 2000;**88(5)**:1051–1056.

17 Bokemeyer C, Nichols CR, Droz JP, et al. Extragonadal germ cell tumors of the mediastinum and retroperitoneum: results from an international analysis. *J Clin Oncol*. 2002;**20(7)**:1864–1873.

20 Nichols CR, Heerema NA, Palmer C, Loehrer PJ Sr, Williams SD, Einhorn LH. Klinefelter's syndrome associated with mediastinal germ cell neoplasms. *J Clin*

Oncol. 1987;**5**(**8**):1290–1294.

21 Carroll PR, Whitmore WF Jr, Richardson M, et al. Testicular failure in patients with extragonadal germ cell tumors. *Cancer*. 1987;**60**(**1**):108–113.

22 Nichols CR, Hoffman R, Einhorn LH, Williams SD, Wheeler LA, Garnick MB. Hematologic malignancies associated with primary mediastinal germ-cell tumors. *Ann Intern Med*. 1985;**102**(**5**):603–609.

23 Nichols CR, Roth BJ, Heerema N, Griep J, Tricot G. Hematologic neoplasia associated with primary mediastinal germ-cell tumors. *N Engl J Med*. 1990;**322**(**20**):1425–1429.

25 Orazi A, Neiman RS, Ulbright TM, Heerema NA, John K, Nichols CR. Hematopoietic precursor cells within the yolk sac tumor component are the source of secondary hematopoietic malignancies in patients with mediastinal germ cell tumors. *Cancer*. 1993;**71**(**12**):3873–3881.

27 Ladanyi M, Samaniego F, Reuter VE, et al. Cytogenetic and immunohistochemical evidence for the germ cell origin of a subset of acute leukemias associated with mediastinal germ cell tumors. *J Natl Cancer Inst*. 1990;**82**(**3**):221–227.

28 Hartmann JT, Nichols CR, Droz JP, et al. Hematologic disorders associated with primary mediastinal nonseminomatous germ cell tumors. *J Natl Cancer Inst*. 2000;**92**(**1**):54–61.

29 International Germ Cell Cancer Collaborative Group. International germ Cell Consensus Classification: a prognostic factor-based staging system for metastatic germ cell cancers. *J Clin Oncol*. 1997;**15**(**2**):594–603.

30 Loehrer PJ Sr, Birch R, Williams SD, Greco FA, Einhorn LH. Chemotherapy of metastatic seminoma: the Southeastern Cancer Study Group experience. *J Clin Oncol*. 1987;**5**(**8**):1212–1220.

31 Nichols CR, Catalano PJ, Crawford ED, Vogelzang NJ, Einhorn LH, Loehrer PJ. Randomized comparison of cisplatin and etoposide and either bleomycin or ifosfamide in treatment of advanced disseminated germ cell tumors: an Eastern Cooperative Oncology Group, Southwest Oncology Group, and Cancer and Leukemia Group B Study. *J Clin Oncol*. 1998;**16**(**4**):1287–1293.

35 Mencel PJ, Motzer RJ, Mazumdar M, Vlamis V, Bajorin DF, Bosl GJ. Advanced seminoma: treatment results, survival, and prognostic factors in 142 patients. *J Clin Oncol*. 1994;**12**(**1**):120–126.

36 Gerl A, Clemm C, Lamerz R, Wilmanns W. Cisplatin-based chemotherapy of primary extragonadal germ cell tumors. A single institution experience. *Cancer*. 1996;77(3):526–532.

38 Bush SE, Martinez A, Bagshaw MA. Primary mediastinal seminoma. *Cancer*. 1981;**48**(**8**):1877–1882.

39 Majewski W, Majewski S, Maciejewski A, Kolosza Z, Tarnawski R. Adverse effects after radiotherapy for early stage (I,IIa,IIb) seminoma. *Radiother Oncol*. 2005;**76**(**3**):257–263.

40 van den Belt-Dusebout AW, Nuver J, de Wit R, et al. Long-term risk of cardiovascular disease in 5-year survivors of testicular cancer. *J Clin Oncol*. 2006;**24**(**3**):467–475.

41 Schultz SM, Einhorn LH, Conces DJ Jr, Williams SD, Loehrer PJ. Management of postchemotherapy residual mass in patients with advanced seminoma: Indiana University experience. *J Clin Oncol*. 1989;**7**(**10**):1497–1503.

42 Puc HS, Heelan R, Mazumdar M, et al. Management of residual mass in advanced seminoma: results and recommendations from the Memorial Sloan-Kettering Cancer Center. *J Clin Oncol*. 1996;**14**(**2**):454–460.

43 De Santis M, Bokemeyer C, Becherer A, et al. Predictive impact of 2-18fluoro-2-deoxy-D-glucose positron emission tomography for residual postchemotherapy masses in patients with bulky seminoma. *J Clin Oncol*. 2001;**19**(**17**):3740–3744.

44 Hinz S, Schrader M, Kempkensteffen C, et al. The role of positron emission tomorgraphy in the evaluation of residual masses after chemotherapy for advanced stage seminoma. *J Urol*. 2008;**179**(**936**).

47 Hidalgo M, Paz-Ares L, Rivera F, et al. Mediastinal non-seminomatous germ cell tumours (MNSGCT) treated with cisplatin-based combination chemotherapy. *Ann Oncol*. 1997;**8**(**6**):555–559.

48 Fizazi K, Culine S, Droz JP, et al. Primary mediastinal nonseminomatous germ cell tumors: results of modern therapy including cisplatin-based chemotherapy. *J Clin Oncol*. 1998;**16**(**2**):725–732.

49 Toner GC, Geller NL, Lin SY, Bosl GJ. Extragonadal and poor risk nonseminomatous germ cell tumors. Survival and prognostic features. *Cancer*. 1991;**67**(**8**):2049–2057.

50 Williams SD, Birch R, Einhorn LH, Irwin L, Greco FA, Loehrer PJ. Treatment of disseminated germ-cell tumors with cisplatin, bleomycin, and either vinblastine or etoposide. *N Engl J Med*. 1987;**316**(**23**):1435–1440.

51 Saxman SB, Nichols CR, Einhorn LH. Salvage chemotherapy in patients with extragonadal nonseminomatous germ cell tumors: the Indiana University experience. *J Clin Oncol*. 1994;**12**(**7**):1390–1393.

52 Hartmann JT, Einhorn L, Nichols CR, et al. Second-line chemotherapy in patients with relapsed extragonadal nonseminomatous germ cell tumors: results of an international multicenter analysis. *J Clin Oncol*. 2001;**19**(**6**):1641–1648.

53 Kesler KA, Rieger KM, Ganjoo KN, et al. Primary mediastinal nonseminomatous germ cell tumors: the influence of postchemotherapy pathology on long-term survival after surgery. *J Thorac Cardiovasc Surg*. 1999;**118**(**4**):692–700.

54 Vuky J, Bains M, Bacik J, et al. Role of postchemotherapy adjunctive surgery in the management of patients with nonseminoma arising from the mediastinum. *J Clin Oncol*. 2001;**19**(**3**):682–688.

55 Schneider BP, Kesler KA, Brooks JA, Yiannoutsos C, Einhorn LH. Outcome of patients with residual germ cell or non-germ cell malignancy after resection of primary mediastinal nonseminomatous germ cell cancer. *J Clin Oncol*. 2004;**22**(**7**):1195–1200.

56 Radaideh SM, Cook VC, Kesler KA, Einhorn LH. Outcome following resection for patients with primary mediastinal nonseminomatous germ-cell tumors and rising serum tumor markers post-chemotherapy. *Ann Oncol*. 2010;**21**(**4**): 804–807.

57 Broun ER, Nichols CR, Einhorn LH, Tricot GJ. Salvage therapy with high-dose chemotherapy and autologous bone marrow support in the treatment of primary nonseminomatous mediastinal germ cell tumors. *Cancer*. 1991;**68**(**7**): 1513–1515.

第 89 章 食管肿瘤

Max W. Sung, MD ■ Virginia R. Litle, MD ■ Steven J. Chmura, MD, PhD ■
Stephen G. Swisher, MD, FACS ■ David C. Rice, MB, BCh, BAO, FRCSI ■
Jaffer A. Ajani, MD ■ Ritsuko K. Komaki, MD ■ Mark K. Ferguson, MD

概述

食管癌是世界上重要的癌症死亡原因之一，占男性癌症死亡原因第六位，女性第九位。过去的约 1/4 世纪里，在北美和欧洲，食管癌主要病理类型已经从鳞癌转为腺癌。发病率逐渐增高的食管胃结合部腺癌也被列入 AJCC TNM 食管癌分期系统，治疗上出现了早期食管癌的内镜下黏膜切除和中期食管癌术前新辅助放化疗，外科已经实现微创胸腹腔镜技术，化疗联合激素治疗和靶向治疗食管腺癌已经屡见报道。对确诊为晚期的患者，预测和治疗技术在分子层面的研究也不断取得进步。

历史回顾

人们早在 12 世纪就对食管癌有了认识，16 和 17 世纪对其病理学进行了描述[1]。最初的外科治疗手段出现在 1877 年一例颈段食管癌的手术切除和 1913 年一例经胸的食管癌切除[2,3]。自 20 世纪 40 年代起，外科手术切除成为治疗食管癌的主要手段。放射治疗始于 20 世纪 20 年代，但是直到 50 年代高能量级的射线技术出现才开始经常使用。有效化疗成分在 20 世纪 60 年代才被筛选出来，在晚期肿瘤的应用越来越广。

解剖和组织学

食管是一个从环咽肌到胃食管接合部（EGJ）的肌性器官。根据解剖学和发生肿瘤的倾向不同，食管可分为不同的区域（图 89-1）。颈段食管从环咽肌到胸廓入口（距门齿 15～18cm），胸上段食管自胸廓入口到气管分叉水平，即在主动脉弓下方水平（距门齿 18～24cm）。胸中段食管自气管分叉至隆突和胃食管结合部的中点（距门齿 24～32cm），胸下段食管从上述的中点到胃食管结合部（32～40cm），食管胃结合部以及胃贲门部肿瘤和食管远端腺癌在病理生理学上相似，因此常放在食管癌中一起讨论[4]。胃食管结合部肿瘤根据肿块中心位置的不同分为不同类型（即 Ⅰ 型，EGJ 上方 >1cm；Ⅱ 型，EGJ 上方 1cm 到下方 2cm；Ⅲ 型，EGJ 下方 2～5cm）[5]。

食管肌肉组织呈外纵内环排布。食管的上 1/3～1/2 固有肌层来自支气管弓肌层，主要是骨骼肌，具有发生横纹肌肉瘤的可能（表 89-1），其余的食管肌层和上消化道一样由平滑肌组成，平滑肌瘤或平滑肌肉瘤都可能发生在这些部位。食管壁散布的脂肪、纤维结缔组织也可能恶变为肉瘤。

大部分的食管内壁被覆鳞状上皮，所以发生在食管的肿瘤中最常见的是鳞状细胞癌，在世界多数国家鳞癌也是食管癌最常见的肿瘤类型。这些肿瘤最常发生于颈段及胸中上段食管，而鳞癌的亚型——癌肉瘤和梭形细胞癌在这些部位比较罕见。食管远端 2～3cm 处和贲门披覆柱状上皮细胞，这些部位容易发生腺癌[5]。食管肠化生，即 Barrett 食管，是由于胃食管反流及其他因素，在个别情况也可以导致胸中上段食管腺癌。其他在黏膜层、黏膜下层和固有肌层的细胞成分也可能发生少见的肿瘤如小细胞癌、恶性黑色素瘤、颗粒细胞肿瘤、黏膜表皮样癌和腺样囊性癌[6,7]。食管良、恶性肿瘤类型见表 89-1。

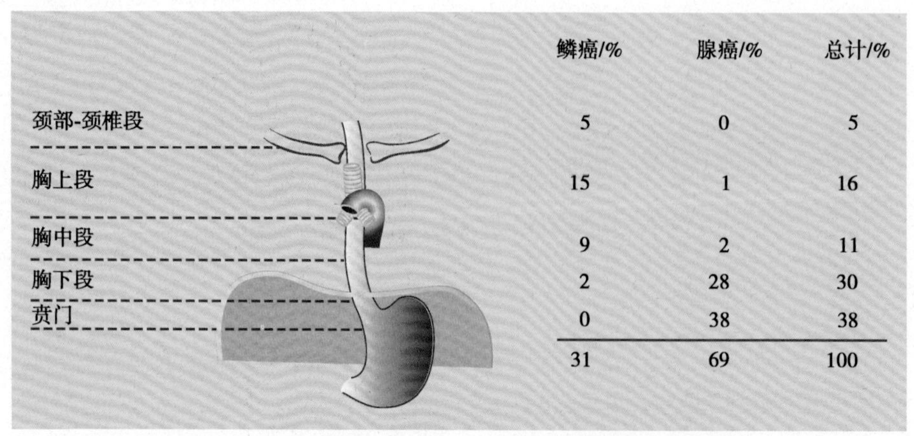

	鳞癌/%	腺癌/%	总计/%
颈部-颈椎段	5	0	5
胸上段	15	1	16
胸中段	9	2	11
胸下段	2	28	30
贲门	0	38	38
	31	69	100

图 89-1 根据肿瘤类型和发生部位划分的食管恶性肿瘤分布

表 89-1　食管肿瘤

上皮性
• 鳞状细胞癌
• 梭形细胞癌
• 癌肉瘤
• 腺癌
• 腺鳞癌
• 黏膜表皮样癌
• 腺样囊性癌
• 小细胞癌
非上皮性
• 平滑肌瘤
• 平滑肌肉瘤
• 恶性黑色素瘤
• 横纹肌瘤
• 横纹肌肉瘤
• 颗粒细胞瘤
• 恶性淋巴瘤

病因学

多数国家认为饮食和营养是食管癌最常见的病因,尤其是和鳞癌有关。最常见的致癌因素是亚硝胺,在中国北方某些地区的食物中含量较高[8]。食物中的真菌污染抑制硝酸盐向亚硝酸盐转化,使这种情况更恶化。其他致癌因素包括饮用烫食、食用含二氧化硅的食物或者对食管有刺激的粗糙谷物等[8,9]。缺乏叶酸、维生素 A、维生素 C、维生素 B_2、微量元素如钼、硒等也是食管肿瘤发生的因素[10~12a]。荟萃分析表明多摄入水果蔬菜会降低食管鳞癌风险[12]。

在西方国家,社会因素在食管癌的发生发展中起到重要作用。酗酒增加了 15~20 倍的致癌风险,依饮料中酒精度数,致癌倍数有所变化[13]。吸烟与鳞癌和腺癌的发生均有关[14]。同时暴露于低水平烟酒环境中,食管癌发生风险增加 10~20 倍,而同时暴露于高水平烟酒环境中可增加 100 倍[15]。由胃食管反流所致的慢性食管损伤也是腺癌发生的一个危险因素,有长期严重反流症状的致癌风险增加 40 倍[16]。慢性胃食管反流在病因学上与 Barrett 食管有关,后者多发于男性白人,可使食管腺癌发生风险增加 40 倍[17]。人们已经认识到食用高亚油酸食物的人群胃食管反流与食管鳞癌发生有关[18]。贲门失弛缓症患者一生有 5%~10%的发生食管鳞癌风险,发生风险为 15 倍,可能由于残留食物对食管的慢性刺激导致[19~21]。

在西方国家,不同种族和性别的食管癌发生率不同。男性较女性易发生,黑人较白人易发生食管鳞癌,而白人男性较女性或其他种族更易发生腺癌[22]。然而,发生率增高与遗传因素的关系还没有更多资料,更多的解释是之前描述的不同的社会经济状态和对应的社会习惯。唯一证实的基因异常是胼胝症 A 患者一生有 25%的食管鳞癌风险,这种患者以迟发的、以手掌和足底过度角化为特点[23]。许多基因突变与食管肿瘤形成有关,包括染色体 3p、5q、9p、9q、13q、17p、17q 和 18q 上等位基因缺失。TP53、Rb、cyclinD1 和 c-myc 的异常也与食管癌发生有关[24]。

传染性因素包括人乳头瘤病毒(HPV),已证实与食管肿瘤发生有关。来自高危 HPV 亚型 16、18 的转换蛋白导致肿瘤抑制基因 TP53 及 Rb 功能丧失,会导致异常增殖状态[25]。HPV 已被证实在将近 50%的食管癌患者中存在,在食管癌高发区似乎更普遍[26]。然而这些发现还未被完全证实[27a]。一项包含了 66 项病例对照研究回顾性荟萃分析证明 HPV 与食管鳞癌有关[27b]。但是各项研究结果差异较大,缺乏一致性,国际癌症研究中心(IARC)也指出这些结论还缺乏足够的流行病学资料[27c]。

流行病学

世界范围内最常见的食管恶性肿瘤是鳞癌(占 90%);而在美国和欧洲,腺癌发生率已经超过鳞癌(图 89-2)。食管癌的发生率比其他癌症地域差异都要大。在美国,食管癌的发生率大约是 7/100 000,而在高发区如中国、伊朗和俄罗斯,它可以高达 100/100 000[27d]。在中国林县,食管癌是主要的死亡原因[29,30a]。这些地域差异提示局部环境致癌物在食管癌发生中扮演着重要角色。食管癌的远期生存率低于 10%,很大程度上在于这些肿瘤在被发现时已处于晚期。2012 年,世界范围内食管癌新发生和死亡例数分别是 455 800 和 400 200[30b]。美国 2015 年食管癌新发和死亡例数分为预计为 16 890 和 15 590(贲门癌不计算在内)[31]。美国食管癌年龄调整的死亡率从 1975 到 2012 年上升了 11%[32]。

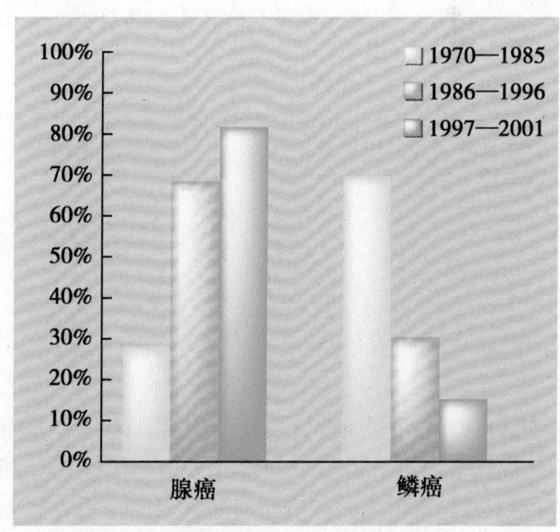

图 89-2　随时间推移腺癌和远端食管癌病例已经增加。摘自 Hofsetter 2002[28a]。Reproduced with permission of Wolters Kluwer

除了地域差异,在西方国家还有一些其他重要的差异。食管癌发病率男性高于女性(不区分组织学类型);相比白人而言,黑人更多是食管鳞癌。另外,虽然鳞癌发生率保持稳定,欧美国家腺癌的发生率却明显上升[33]。自 20 世纪 70 年代中期,食管远端及贲门部腺癌在白人男性中发生率增加了 350%,比其他任何实体瘤的增长速度都快(图 89-2)[22,34~38]。西方国家这些显著变化的具体原因并不清楚,但可能与增加的 Barrett 食管、胃食管反流、肥胖、药物过度使用及烟酒习惯有关[16]。在世界的其他地方(除欧洲及北美)食管鳞癌占主要地位,而腺癌发病率并未增加。

患者常表现为吞咽困难,这是由于肿瘤侵犯整个食管全周或肿瘤本身较大堵塞管腔所致。吞咽困难首先表现为吞咽硬质食物困难,随着病情进展可出现吞咽软质食物甚至液体困难。伴随呕吐和反流症状很常见。胃灼热症状与胃食管反流(40%)在食管腺癌更易发生[39]。除了吞咽困难最常见的症状是疼痛(25%患者)[39]。疼痛可能是吞咽疼或者肿瘤侵犯邻近组织如椎体、胸膜或纵隔引起。在某些情况则是由于全身播散引起的骨转移。由于吞咽困难和疾病的全身表现,超过 70%的患者表现为消瘦[39]。在许多研究中,出现体重下降的患者预后显著不良[40,41]。

肿瘤组织学类型很大程度上取决于发生部位。腺癌主要位于食管下段,而鳞癌主要位于颈段、上中段食管(图 89-1 和图 89-2)。遗憾的是,由于食管可扩张的特性,直到肿瘤长到很大或者侵透食管才出现临床症状。

相对于出现吞咽困难而被确诊的患者,在欧美一些早期食管腺癌患者在内镜监测胃食管反流症或 Barrett 食管时被诊断出来。这些患者多是早期的肿瘤,更易于治疗。另外,在中国鳞癌高发区,常规细胞学筛查提示可疑癌症或者细胞学直接能确诊,则进一步行内镜诊断。这些大规模的筛查活动带来的早期诊断,使中国食管癌 5 年生存率超过 90%[30a]。然而在世界大部分低发区,这种大规模的筛查并不现实,从公共健康的角度来看性价比较低。

治疗概述

疑似食管癌的患者,不管是因为出现症状还是肿瘤筛查结果提示,首先需要病理学确诊(见“诊断”部分)。一旦病理学诊断确立,患者需做肿瘤临床分期评估(见“分级评估”)和生理状态评估(见“治疗前评估”)。有了这些信息,才能优化出疾病的治疗方案,并尽可能降低治疗相关死亡率(见“治疗”)(图 89-3)。

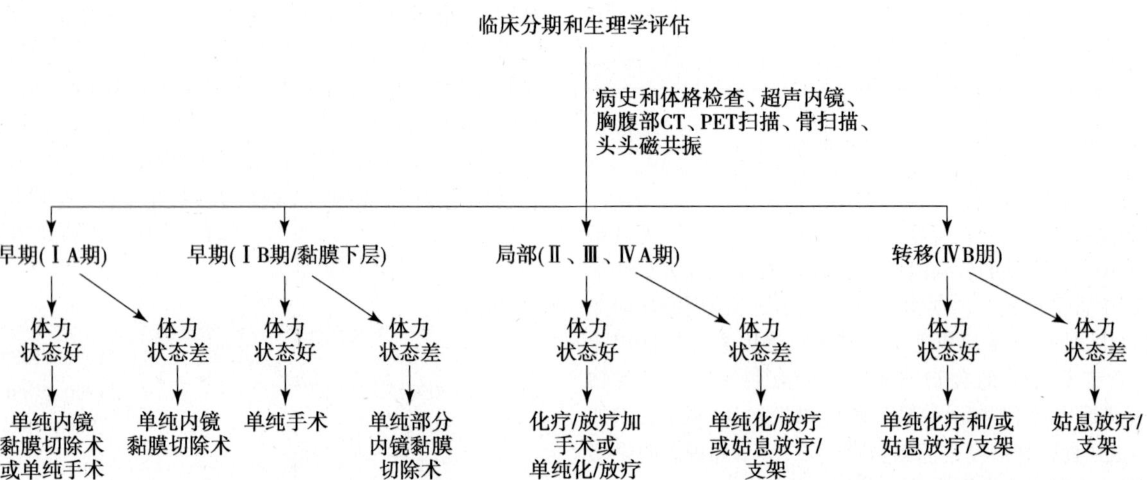

图 89-3 目前基于体力状态和临床分期的食管癌治疗策略建议

诊断

有症状或筛查时发现食管肿块的患者需要进一步行组织学或刷片细胞学检查。内镜取活检对食管癌的病理诊断总体的精确性约 80%[42,43]。内镜引导的细胞学刷片检查诊断精确性超过 90%。联合检测手段则可达到 98%[42]。如果软质内镜不能确诊,可考虑施行硬质内镜取活检,诊断精确性接近 100%[43]。对于筛选出来的有症状或体格检查提示有远处转移的患者,对可疑转移部位取活检不仅能提供组织学诊断,还能明确临床分期。

治疗前评估

除了详尽的病史询问和体格检查,对食管癌患者要注重评估。与治疗并发症及死亡率的相关因素包括患者年龄、近期烟酒滥用史、近期体重改变、营养状态、体力状态、肝功能和肾功能情况。还需要一些检查项目,评估食管癌术前的一些特别的危险因素如:肺部并发症预测指标包括年龄、术前动脉氧分压、胸部 X 线、第一秒用力呼气量(FEV1)[44];术中死亡率预测指标包括年龄、中臂围、吸烟史、诱发性肺计量、体力状态和医疗机构手术量[44,45]。心脏的评估可用心电图、超声心动图、压力试验和冠状动脉造影来完成。有严重冠状动脉疾病的患者,其并发症的发生及死亡风险明显增加,在食管癌手术前应该做心脏介入手术。这些生理学评估将患者风险状态分组,以便量身制订治疗方案。

分期评估

分期评估让医师可以精确讨论每个患者的病情,对治疗有充分的了解，也让患者及家属获知必要的预后信息。通常对大部分患者的分期评估检查包括上消化道内镜、食管造影、胸腹部 CT、超声内镜(EUS)和正电子发射断层显像(PET)。其他一些检查则基于不同患者特殊的症状，如神经系统症状(头颅磁共振)、肌肉骨骼症状(骨扫描)或锁骨上淋巴结肿大(颈部超声检查和活检)。分期评估可使患者精确地分到不同的治疗组，得到最好的治疗。

检查

食管造影

食管造影常是吞咽困难患者的首要检查。它可以表现黏膜紊乱，并且可以指导随后的内镜检查。在内镜使用受限情况下可以用来做食管或胃狭窄远端的评估。

内镜

上消化道内镜可以在大部分患者行病理学诊断。肿瘤的大体表现可分为进展型和表浅型，肿瘤范围可精确测定。另外，如果临床症状典型，内镜检查可以发现有将近 20%为鳞癌。内镜还能评估肿瘤的活动度，看它是否固定在纵隔。

超声内镜

超声内镜(EUS)提高了原发肿瘤和局部和非局部转移的淋巴结的准确分期。它已经成为帮助鉴别是否需要综合治疗的早期食管癌患者的必需手段(图 89-3)。EUS 将正常食管显示为 5 个不同的高低回声层，分别代表黏膜、黏膜固有层、黏膜肌层、黏膜下层、固有肌层和外膜。肿瘤侵犯的深度取决于瘤体延伸的层次。EUS 也可用于评估肿瘤是否侵犯主动脉，但由于气道内空气的干扰，不能精确评估是否侵犯气道。EUS 对原发灶的分期精确性与肿瘤病理学分期有关，进展越快的精确性越高，总体精确性约 80%[46~48]。放、化疗后 EUS 分期精确性下降，不能鉴别治疗所致纤维化和残余肿瘤，这种情况下总体精确度约 45%[49a,b]。

评估淋巴结时应用三个标准：大小、边界特征和内部结构。淋巴结增大、边界较清、回声均匀内部低回声常常提示恶性。运用这种标准，EUS 评估淋巴结状态总的准确度大约 75%[47,50]。放、化疗后 EUS 对淋巴结的分级准确性降低，略超过 50%[49a]。细针穿刺技术可用于局部或远处肿大淋巴结得到病理学确诊[48~51]。

胸腹部 CT

CT 由于可以更好地鉴别肿瘤转移(M1b)和局部侵犯(T4)，自 20 世纪 70 年代晚期开始应用于食管癌分期，很快变成食管癌分期的标准手段。CT 确定肿瘤原发灶(T)侵犯深度并不精确，但有助于明确邻近器官(如主动脉或大气道)侵犯，如有侵犯就不考虑外科手术[46]。当超过 25%的主动脉周被食管癌所占据则要考虑主动脉侵犯。

由于纵隔和腹部正常淋巴结在大小上常有变化，且单一淋巴结大小标准不易建立，CT 不能精确地确定淋巴结状态。另外，转移淋巴结常常并不增大[52~55]。所以 CT 检测受累淋巴结灵敏度很低(30% ~ 60%)，检测淋巴结总体准确度低于 60%[56~58]。

CT 对于检查远处转移性病灶很有用。除了局部淋巴结转移，最常见的转移部位(以递减顺序排)有肝脏、肺脏、腹膜、肾上腺、骨和肾脏。胸腹 CT 几乎都涵盖了这些器官，检测肝脏转移准确率超过 90%[52,57,59,60]。

气管镜

拟手术的患者或者肿瘤靠近气管或主支气管的患者都应该行气管镜检查，尤其是中段食管鳞癌，气管镜可以直接评估肿瘤是否侵犯气管腔或黏膜下。

磁共振

磁共振(MRI)由于价格昂贵且操作繁琐，与 CT 相比并无优势，作为食管肿瘤的分期应用较少。在评估肿瘤直接侵犯主动脉和大气道的灵敏度、特异度和可切除性的总体精确度方面 MRI 和 CT 两种检测手段相似[53,54,57]。两种手段对于局部或转移性淋巴结都不能提供更有用的信息。在评估肝转移方面，MRI 评估能力与 CT 相比并无优势，所以还未发现 MRI 技术在评估分期方面有何优势。

正电子发射断层技术(PET)

自 20 世纪 90 年代中期 PET 扫描通过^{18}氟脱氧葡萄糖代谢增加来评估转移淋巴结和转移灶被引进临床。PET 对于确定原发灶不明的转移性疾病最有意义。鉴于炎症假阳性的可能，对于 PET 阳性患者仍需活检来明确转移性病灶。PET 常用于引导可疑转移性部位进行活检。PET 的另一个潜在角色可能在于评估放化疗的效果，当然放化疗诱发炎症所致的假阳性仍然是个问题[61~63]。PET 通过检测高代谢部位还能鉴别食管癌是否复发[64]。

骨扫描

骨扫描在食管癌分期中已使用了数十年，但其意义尚未被证实。PET-CT 基本可以代替骨扫描，在没有骨痛或其他转移证据的患者，检出骨转移的概率低于 5%[65]。

颈部超声检查

高达 30%的胸段食管癌患者有颈部和锁骨上淋巴结转移，而大部分在体格检查时不能发现。在查体未触及淋巴结肿大的患者行常规颈部超声检查，仍可发现淋巴结转移率超过 10%[66]。用超声行颈部及锁骨上淋巴结评估总精确性超过 90%[67,68a]。超声引导的细针穿刺活检学检查是一项有价值的技术[68a]。然而现在穿刺并不常用，仅仅在淋巴结确诊是否转移时才使用。

微创手术分期

腹腔镜在 20 世纪 80 年代早期，胸腔镜在 90 年代早期都已被用于食管癌分期评估。1995 年一项 CALGB 研究表明电视胸腔镜外科(VATS)分期技术可行并且准确率达到 88%[68b,c]。目前由于 PET-CT 和 EUS 联合应用，外科分期技术已经不再常用。有时候在患者放化疗前用腹腔镜置放空肠造口管可以同时做分期的手术。

生物学分级

一些生物标志物已在评估食管肿瘤预后方面被证实有效，包括：生长因子(表皮生长因子 EGF、转化生长因子 TGF-β、血小板源性生长因子 PDGF)，癌基因(*c-myc*、*int-2*、*hst-1*、*cyclinD*、*EGFR*、*HER-2/neu*、*h-ras*)，抑癌基因(*Rb*、*TP53*、*p73*、*APC*、*MCC*、*p27*)，细胞黏附分子 E-钙黏素，肿瘤标志物 CEA，DNA 含量和整倍性[69~71]。但是到目前为止，这些评估技术还没有得到普及。

TNM(肿瘤、淋巴结、转移)分期系统

通过临床TNM(cTNM)分期系统对患者进行分期,帮助患者得到最佳治疗(图89-3)。目前食管癌分期系统包括颈段、胸段、腹内段和食管胃结合部癌(表89-2)[72a,b]。根据临床非侵入性和侵入性病理结果进行分期。通过活检和手术明确转移淋巴结具体位置非常重要,对区域淋巴结和非区域淋巴结的区分可以明确食管癌的分期(图89-4)。食管癌患者的预后由以下因素决定:原发肿瘤浸润深度(透壁性和非透壁性),是否有淋巴结转移,转移淋巴结相对数目,是否有远处转移[28,72,74~81,82~87]。分期中加入了非解剖性分级,如组织学类型(腺癌、鳞癌),组织学分级(G1~4),肿瘤的位置。食管癌患者的长期生存与病理学分级密切相关(图89-5)[74,80]。随着内镜超声、胸腹部CT、PET应用,临床分期越来越接近病理分期[28a]。

表89-2 食管肿瘤TNM分期

肿瘤原发灶(T)	
Tx	原发肿瘤无法评估
T0	无原发肿瘤证据
Tis	原位癌
T1	肿瘤侵犯黏膜固有层、黏膜、肌层或黏膜下层
T2	肿瘤侵犯固有肌层
T3	肿瘤侵犯外膜
T4a	可切除的肿瘤侵犯邻近的结构,如胸膜、心包和隔膜
T4b	不可切除的肿瘤侵犯邻近的组织,如主动脉、椎体和气管
区域淋巴结(N)	
从颈部到腹腔的所有食管周围淋巴结	
Nx	区域淋巴结无法评估
N0	无区域淋巴结转移
N1	1~2阳性区域淋巴结
N2	3~6阳性区域淋巴结
N3	≥7阳性区域淋巴结
远处转移(M)	
Mx	远处转移无法评估
M0	无远处转移
M1	有远处转移
增加非解剖性癌特征、组织病理细胞类型、腺癌、鳞状细胞癌组织学分级	
G1	高分化
G2	中分化
G3	低分化
G4	未分化
肿瘤位置	
胸上段	距门齿20~25cm
胸中段	距门齿25~30cm
胸下段	距门齿30~40cm
食管胃结合部	包括肿瘤中心在远端食管、食管胃结合部,或在胃近端5cm(贲门)扩展到食管胃结合部或远端食管胸(Siewert Ⅲ)

续表

腺癌分期				
0	Tis	N0	M0	G1
ⅠA	T1	N0	M0	G1~2
ⅠB	T1	N0	M0	G3
ⅡA	T2	N0	M0	G1~2
	T2	N0	M0	G3
ⅡB	T3	N0	M0	任何 G
	T1~2	N1	M0	任何 G
ⅢA	T1~2	N2	M0	任何 G
	T3	N1	M0	任何 G
	T4a	N0	M0	任何 G
ⅢB	T3	N2	M0	任何 G
ⅢC	T4a	N1~2	M0	任何 G
	T4b	任何 N	M0	任何 G
	任何 T	N3	M0	任何 G
Ⅳ	任何 T	任何 N	M1	任何 G

鳞状细胞癌分期					
分期	T	N	M	G	位置
0	Tis	N0	M0	G1	任何
ⅠA	T1	N0	M0	G1	任何
ⅠB	T1	N0	M0	G2~3	任何
ⅡA	T2~3	N0	M0	G1	下段
	T2~3	N0	M0	G1	中上段
ⅡB	T2~3	N0	M0	G2~3	下段
	T2~3	N0	M0	G2~3	中上段
	T1~2	N1	M0	任何 G	任何
ⅢA	T1~2	N2	M0	任何 G	任何
	T3	N1	M0	任何 G	任何
	T4a	N0	M0	任何 G	任何
ⅢB	T3	N2	M0	任何 G	任何
ⅢC	T4a	N1~2	M0	任何 G	任何
	T4b	任何 N	M0	任何 G	任何
	任何 T	N3	M0	任何 G	任何
Ⅳ	任何 T	任何 N	M1	任何 G	任何

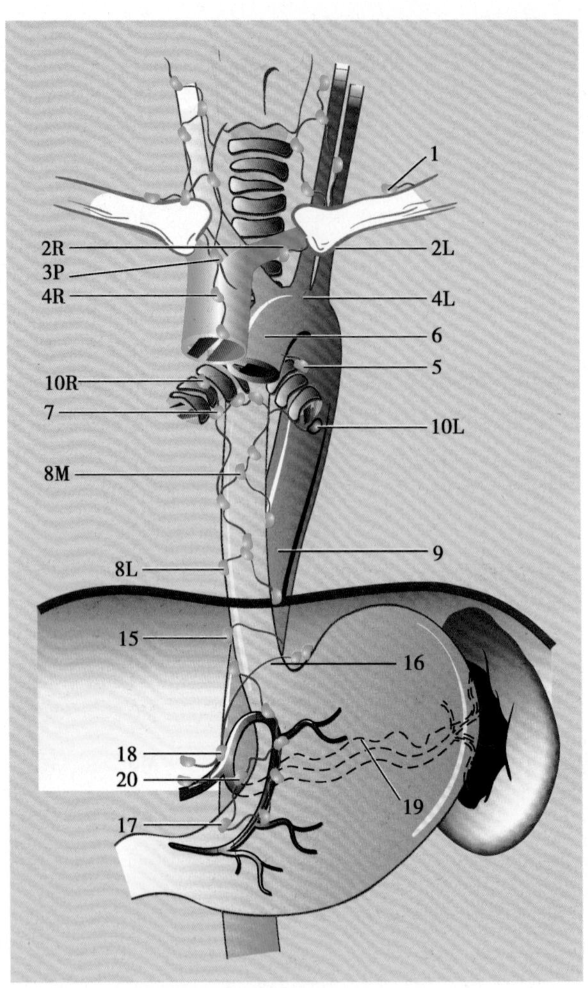

图 89-4　食管肿瘤的淋巴结分级图。摘自 Ferguson 2010[73]. Reproduced with permission of Elsevier

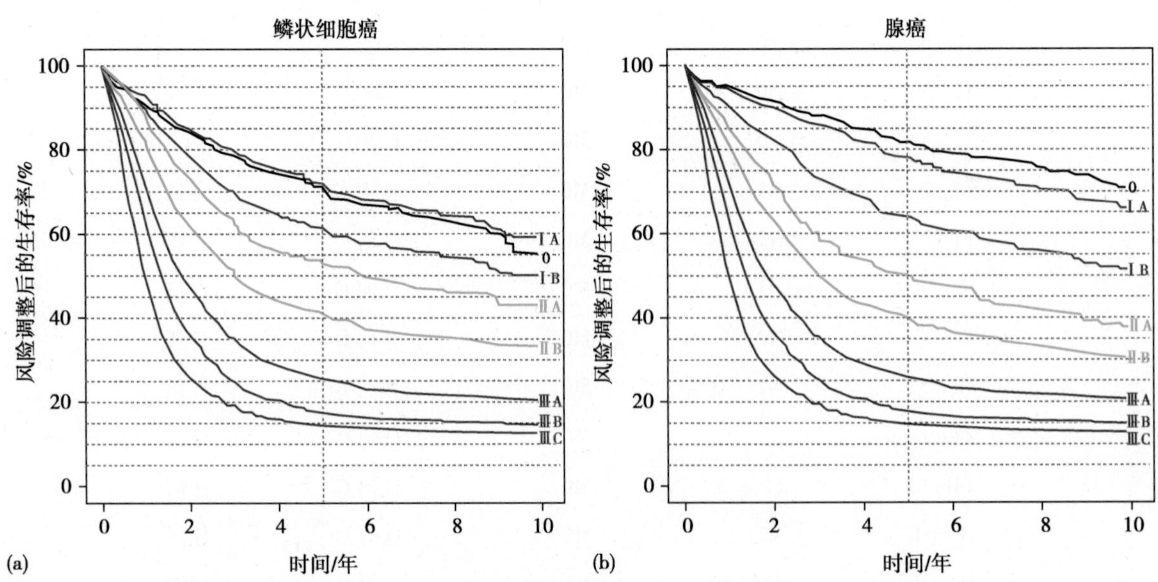

图 89-5　(a)根据第 7 版 ANCC 癌症分期手册,鳞状细胞癌的风险调整生存期。摘自 Rice 2010[72a]. Reproduced with permission of Springer。(b)根据第 7 版 ANCC 癌症分期手册,腺癌的风险调整生存期。摘自 Rice 2010[72b]. Reproduced with permission of Springer

治疗

食管癌的标准治疗包括手术切除、放疗、化疗或联合其中两种或三种治疗手段。由于这些疗法的前瞻性随机对照试验很少，到底哪一种治疗方法更优还无定论。另外，临床研究常常病例数不充分，历时较长，在研究时期内治疗手段可发生明显的变化(如放疗设备、剂量和照射野的变化，手术技术的改变和化疗药物的进展)。临床分期标准的也会随着时间推移出现分期转变，与病理学分期并不一致，尤其是在 CT 扫描、超声内镜、PET 检查出现前的研究[28a]。这些问题导致不同试验或治疗措施难以对比优劣。各地依区域性经验又有不同的治疗策略。为了指导现有治疗策略，我们采用一种基于患者生理状态和临床分期的综合治疗策略的食管癌治疗算法(图 89-3)。这种算法综合不同观点，期望在食管癌治疗领域给出一些指导或建议。

在食管癌的治疗策略方面，首要的治疗目标是控制局部病变和治愈疾病。这是由于食管肿物进行性生长和管腔阻塞所致的吞咽困难会带来机体的消耗虚弱。早期食管癌(0 期，Ⅰ期)患者首选手术治疗，不能耐受手术的患者则给予放疗和/或放疗增敏(化疗)。最新的微创手段包括内镜黏膜切除术和消融疗法。然而大部分患者由于长期无症状肿瘤增长表现为局部进展性食管癌。这些Ⅱ、Ⅲ和ⅣA 期的患者应用单一治疗手段如手术或放疗常由于远处转移或局部复发的出现而预后不佳，因此治疗常常集中于联合局部治疗(手术或放疗)手段和全身系统性治疗(化疗)的综合治疗手段。北美的肿瘤专家建议对这些患者进行单纯放化疗或术前新辅助放化疗联合手术进行治疗，但是这个观点也存在争议，就像结果相互冲突的众多随机临床研究结果一样，这种治疗策略也没有明确数据支持(表 89-3)，一些治疗中心认为更积极的肿物整块切除和三野淋巴结清扫更重要。身体状况评分较差的局部进展期患者由于治疗相关死亡率较高而常常不采用手术或化疗。在这些患者可采用辅助支架置入和/或放疗进行局部姑息治疗。对于初诊即为进展期(转移性)患者，化疗和/或姑息性放疗是治疗的主要手段。食管支架的发展提供了局灶姑息手段，并且减少了外科姑息性手术干预，甚至对于食管气管瘘也有很好的疗效(图 89-3)。

表 89-3　局部进展期食管癌联合放化疗的随机临床试验结果

作者	年份	治疗	技术	组织学	病例	中位生存期/月	P
放化疗 vs 单纯放疗							
Roussel 等[88]	1989	甲氨蝶呤+56Gy	C-RT	鳞癌	77	9	NS
		56Gy			73	8	
Araujo 等[89]	1991	5-FU，博来霉素，丝裂霉素+50Gy	C/RT	鳞癌	28	18	NS
		50Gy			31	16	
Hatlevoll 等[90]	1992	顺铂，博来霉素+53Gy	C-RT	鳞癌	46	6	NS
		53Gy			51	6	
Slabber 等[91]	1998	顺铂，5-FU+40Gy	C/RT	鳞癌	34	6	NS
		40Gy			36	5	
Smith 等[92]	1998	丝裂霉素，5-FU+40Gy	C/RT	鳞癌>腺癌	60	15	0.04
		40Gy			59	9	
Cooper 等[93]	1999	顺铂，5-FU+50Gy	C/RT	鳞癌>腺癌	61	13	0.01
		64Gy			62	9	
化疗/放疗(高剂量)vs 化疗/放疗(低剂量)							
Minsky 等[94]	2002	顺铂，5-FU+50Gy	C/RT	鳞癌>腺癌	10	18	NS
		顺铂，5-FU+50Gy	C/RT		9	13	
Stahl 等[95]	2005	顺铂，5-FU，依托泊苷+40Gy-手术	C-C/RT-S	鳞癌	86	16.4	NS
		顺铂，5-FU，依托泊苷-顺铂，依托泊苷+65Gy	C-C/RT		86	14.9	
Bedenne 等[96]	2007	顺铂，5-FU+46Gy-手术	C/RT-S	鳞癌>腺癌	129	17.7	NS
		顺铂，5-FU，66Gy	CRT		130	19.3	
化疗/放疗(5-FU 增敏)vs 化疗/放疗(无 5-FU 增敏)							
Ajani 等[97]	2008	顺铂，5-FU，紫杉醇-5-FU，+50.4Gy	C-RT	鳞癌>腺癌	41	28.2	NS
		顺铂+紫杉醇-顺铂+紫杉醇+50.4Gy	C-RT		43	14.9	

C，化疗；5-FU，氟尿嘧啶；RT，放疗；S，手术。

手术

食管癌切除术是局部进展期食管癌的主要治疗手段。过去 10~15 年里最重要的一个改变是对临床早期表浅食管癌(cT1aN0)进行内镜下 EMR 手术。早期食管癌手术死亡率也高达 7%,所以 20 年以前人们就开始对高级别上皮瘤变和早期食管癌尝试用更微创的方法治疗[28b]。在一项大型早期的研究中,Christian Ell 和同事发表了一组 61 例早期食管癌 EMR 手术患者,平均随访 12 个月,86%患者仍无病生存[28c]。此后,多项研究证实 EMR 和消融对 Barrett 食管癌前病灶和早期癌根治性治疗 5 年生存期可以达到 80%~90%[28d,e]。

外科手术切除在局部进展期食管癌综合治疗中仍占据必不可少的地位,经历了新辅助治疗后的食管癌患者仍有 75%的比例局部残留。但也有一些专家认为,只有局部复发患者适合手术干预。这种挽救性手术针对根治性放化疗后复发的患者,但是比较新辅助治疗后手术有更高的瘘发生、手术失败、住院时间长、手术死亡率高,所以挽救性手术的观点正在逐渐转变为非手术治疗[28f]。

切除方法

外科手术切除的方法包括经胸手术切除,经食管裂孔切除,胸腔镜/腹腔镜切除术(表 89-4,图 89-6)。

表 89-4 食管癌手术切除的方式

经胸廓手术
• Ivor-Lewis(腹部切开术、右胸切开手术、胸腔内高位吻合术)
• McKeown 改良 Ivor-Lewis 手术(颈部吻合术)
• 左胸开胸行胸廓内吻合术
• 左胸开胸行颈部吻合术
• 胸腹切开术
经食管裂孔手术
微创手术
• 胸腔镜下手术
• 腹腔镜下手术
• 胸腔镜下/腹腔镜下手术

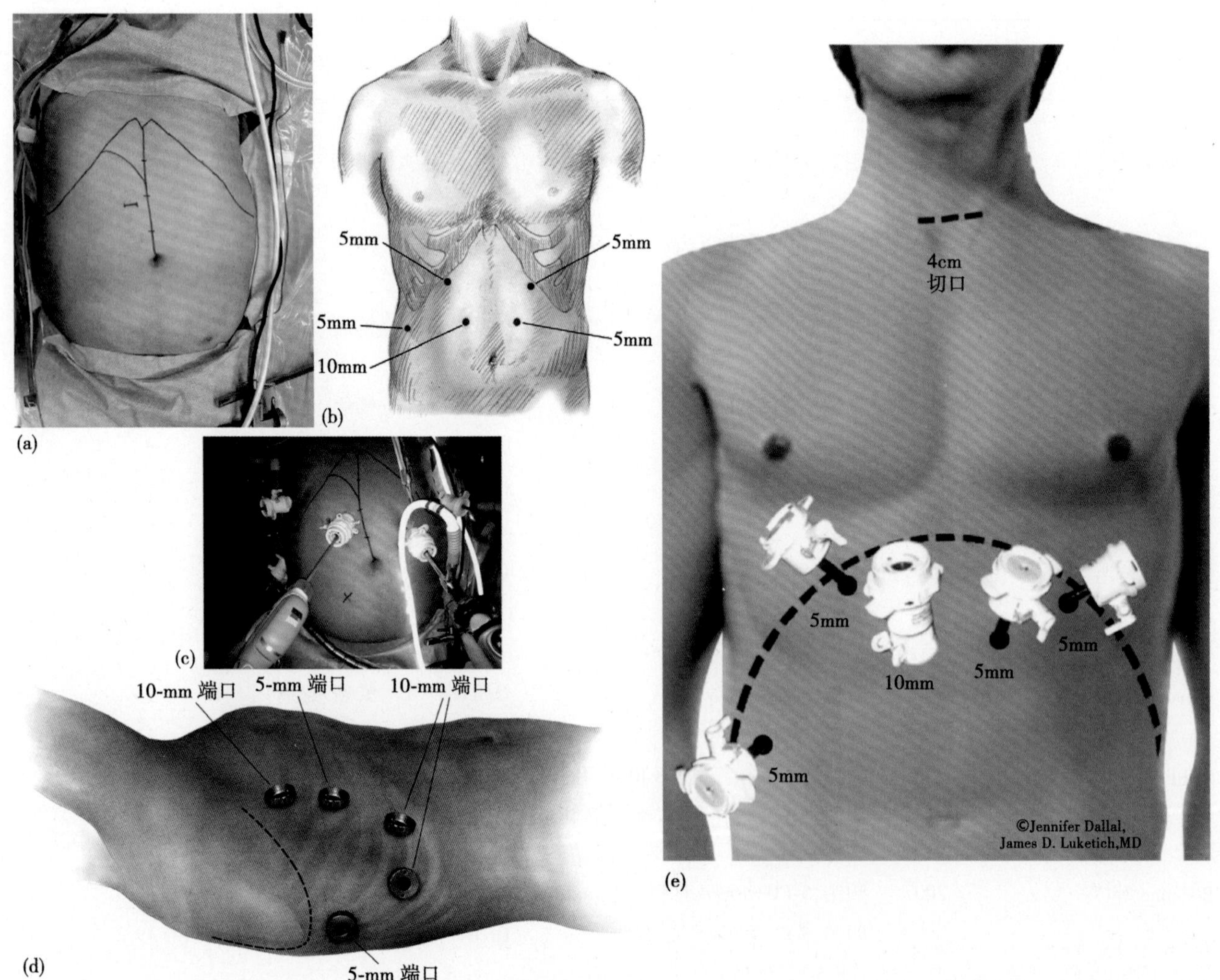

图 89-6 食管癌手术切除方式。(a)右侧开胸开腹联合胸内(Ivor Lewis 手术)或颈部吻合(McKeown 改良 Ivor Lewis 食管切除术)。(b)左侧开胸,通过横膈膜周围切口进入腹部,行胸内或颈部吻合。(c)经纵隔食管癌切除颈部吻合术。(d)胸腔镜食管癌切除术:戳卡放置(MIE Ivor Lewis)。(e)腹腔镜食管癌切除术:戳卡放置

与经食管裂孔的手术切除方法相比，开胸的手术可以更大程度地切除原发肿瘤和淋巴结。但经裂孔手术可以使创伤更小，手术也更快，肺部并发症更少。20 世纪 90 年代中期腹腔镜技术应用于良性疾病治疗，也被引进到肿瘤的微创治疗领域。90 年代末，9 例经腹腔镜膈裂孔手术被报道[28g]。随后完全胸腹腔镜治疗证明能缩短住院时间，死亡率低于 2%[28h]。另外的研究也证实肺部并发症从开式手术的 60% 降低到腔镜的 44%[28i]。微创食管癌切除（MIE）已经从三切口（McKeown）进展到 Ivor-Lewis 手术，优点是能减少喉返神经损伤和颈部吻合口瘘。

MIE 手术优越性已经被长期随访所证实。并且微创手术清扫淋巴结平均个数不少于 AJCC 规定的 20 枚淋巴结，用于明确肿瘤分期[28i,j]。一项研究包含了 95 例患者，证实 MIE 三年生存率达 60%，局部复发率低于 7%[28k]。

手术方法选择依赖于肿瘤的位置和外科医生偏好。鳞癌常位于食管中上段，常选择开式或者微创的经胸手术颈部吻合。腺癌多位于食管远端或贲门，经胸和经纵隔手术都适合。鳞癌几乎在 20% 的患者中是多原发的，建议全食管切除减少复发风险[81]。这就要求必须颈部吻合。而腺癌多原发不常见，但常侵及黏膜下层。理论上，术中冰冻证实上下切缘阴性，则表明切除范围已够。

从 44 例公开报道的经胸或食管裂孔食管癌切除术的结果表明，后者食管吻合口瘘并发症的发生率较高。但除此之外，在手术并发症发生率、死亡率和 5 年生存率方面，两者没有显著差异[83~87,98a]。目前，选择食管微创还是开式切除术很大程度上取决于培训、经验和外科医师的个人喜好。一些报道机器人食管癌切除术（TATE），比起其他外科方法，在住院时间、并发症和淋巴结个数方面各有差异[98b,c]。这个手术方法可能在未来仅保留在少数专业中心。

术前治疗的效果

术前治疗可能增加围术期发病率和死亡率。一项随机临床研究报道术前化疗与单纯手术的患者相比，其感染并发症、呼吸并发症和手术死亡率均较高[99]。但是一些研究表明，新辅助化疗和放化疗在术后并发症和手术死亡率方面没有显著差异[40,100~104]。食管手术的复杂性要求手术在高水平的中心进行，以降低手术并发症和死亡率[45]。医疗保险资料显示，高水平治疗中心手术切除术死亡率为 3%，而相对经验较少的中心死亡率为 19%[45]。如果加上术前治疗，食管癌手术并发症和死亡率会更高。在经验少的治疗中心，治疗中的并发症和死亡率可能远远大于患者受益，尤其是局部进展期的患者本来治愈可能性就很小。

颈段食管癌的手术治疗

颈段食管癌的手术治比较特殊。对侵犯至环咽肌或邻近气管的肿瘤，如果想切缘阴性，就有必要切除喉部。这就增加了并发症，并且这种手术方式也常常是姑息的手术。因此，相对于其他部位的食管癌，颈部食管癌的患者大部分采用非手术治疗。切除术可以缓解吞咽困难，但是对于长期生存并没有大的影响，而且切除术会导致大量并发症，所以更多的人选择放化疗治疗[105~108]。

食管切除术后重建

食管癌手术以合适的方式行消化道重建，使得食物顺利进入消化道消化吸收，这是食管癌外科治疗的一项重要内容。食管重建可以选择胃部作为替代或者在食管和邻近的胃部（当胃全切除术后选择十二指肠）之间接上空肠或者结肠。迄今为止，最常用的技术是利用胃进行术后重建，因为胃部有充足的血液供应，而其他的任何替代品不具备这个特点，同时跟插入肠段造成的三个部位吻合相比，胃部一个部位的吻合已经足够。有些外科医师喜欢食管颈部吻合术，因为它降低了术后胃酸反流入食管，同时一旦发生吻合口瘘更易做引流处理。但是它的缺点是喉返神经损伤和吻合口瘘的发生率比较高。颈部吻合术近端切除范围更多，是不是具有更高的生存率还没有得到证实[109]。后纵隔切除行重建术（食管床）利于重建器官的排空，但是如果切除不完全，可能会造成肿瘤的浸润[110]。

放射治疗

放射治疗应用于食管肿瘤的治疗已经有几十年，像手术一样更针对肿瘤的局部治疗，而并非全身治疗。放疗和手术一样，最初被认为是局部病变的治愈手段或者是晚期患者的姑息治疗。但是结果令人失望，因为肿瘤对射线并不是完全反应并且放疗导致的食管狭窄也会减弱放疗的姑息治疗作用。最近，放疗用于新辅助综合治疗能进一步提高局部病变的控制率。

放疗计划要同时照射肿瘤本身和周围可疑的微病灶，并且要最大限度减少对周围器官的损伤，如肺、心脏、脊髓。区域淋巴结要包括在照射野内，颈段食管癌要包括颈部淋巴结和锁骨上淋巴结；胸上段食管癌要包括锁骨上淋巴结和隆突下淋巴结；下段和贲门部分的肿瘤要包括腹部淋巴结。最初的治疗是对立的，前面-后面、后面-前面的照射野均需要高的能量（6~24MV）。对于高剂量可以治愈的患者来说，最后的治疗照射野应该有一个倾斜度以降低脊髓的受量。之前采取的方案是总量为 60~70Gy，每次用量为 1.8~2Gy，但是最近的试验表明降低总量至 50.4Gy，不仅有同样的疗效，而且毒性反应减少[94]。姑息治疗用量更低，进一步减少了并发症（30~40Gy）。

单纯放射治疗模式

单纯放疗用于当患者不能耐受手术或者根治性同步放化疗以及患者拒绝手术。单独放疗的无远处转移患者 5 年生存率为 0%~20%，绝大多数都低于 10%。但是生存率低可能是由于患者选择治疗方式偏差造成的，因为 PS 评分较好的患者通常选择手术，相反 PS 评分较差的患者就会选择放疗保守治疗。局部无法切除的肿瘤采取放射治疗，与可手术切除患者的 5 年生存率相似，也是低于 10%[88~93,111,112]。一项小型随机试验已经表明，单独手术比单纯放疗比，能够提高生存率[113]。

辅助放疗模式

为了提高食管癌的局部控制率，我们在术前或术后采用辅助放疗（表 89-5）[114~116,118,122]。手术与放疗间隔通常为 3~5 周（放疗剂量 10Gy/周），这是为了减少围术期并发症，例如出血、放射性纤维化等。在大的医学中心，程序得当，术前放疗并不会增加手术并发症和死亡率[45]。但多数随机对照临床研究并没有证明比单纯手术有更好的生存优势，虽然可能由于放疗硬件的陈旧[114~116,118,122]。将所有随机试验数据进行荟萃分析，也没有表示术前放疗有生存获益[123]。

表 89-5 局部进展期食管癌患者术前术后放疗的随机试验结果

作者	年份	治疗	组织类型	患者/例	5 年生存率	*P*
术前放疗	VS	单纯手术				
Launois 等[114]	1981	单纯手术	鳞癌	57	11.5%	NS
		手术+40Gy		67	7.5%	
Gignoux 等[115]	1988	单纯手术	鳞癌	106	10%	NS
		手术+33Gy		102	9%	
Wang 等[116]	1989	单纯手术	鳞癌	102	30%	
		手术+40Gy		104	35%	
Arnott 等[117]	1992	单纯手术	鳞癌	86	17%	NS
		手术+20Gy		90	9%	
Nygaard 等[118]	1992	单纯手术	鳞癌	41	4%	0.08
		手术+35Gy		48	18%	
术后放疗	VS	单纯手术				
FUASR 等[119]	1991	单纯手术	鳞癌	119	18%	NS
		手术+45~55Gy		102	20%	
Fok 等[120]	1993	单纯手术	鳞癌	65	11%(4 年)	NS
		手术+49~52.5Gy		65	11%(4 年)	
Ziernan 等[121]	1995	单纯手术	鳞癌	35	20%(4 年)	NS
		手术+56Gy		33	23%(4 年)	

术后患者可以采用高剂量放疗,比术前放疗相比更易做到,但是会带来吻合口狭窄,延迟患者术后康复,影响生活质量[117,120,121]。有研究指出,比起单纯手术来说,术后追加放疗中位生存期更短,这是由于早期发生远处转移或者放疗相关性死亡,所以在选择上可能有偏差[120]。术后放疗看似降低了局部复发率,但是对长期生存没有明显改善。腔内近距离照射配合外部照射在一些中心开展,用于改善局部控制率。外部照射完成之后,再加一个近距离 10~20Gy 的 ^{192}Ir 照射。对于潜在治愈可能的病灶采用近距离照射提高了局部控制率,但是有更高的食管狭窄发生率[119,124,125]。减少近距离放射剂量有可能减少局部并发症发生率[126]。对于局部不可切除或者复发的患者应用近距离照射还在研究当中,但是可能会取得比其他治疗手段更好的缓解效果,比如胃分流手术、化疗、激光治疗和支架植入[127~129]。

全身治疗

讨论化疗就不得不提起过去 50 年食管癌流行病学的变化。20 世纪 70 年代,化疗药物开始在临床试验应用,食管癌主要是鳞癌,多位于食管上 2/3 部位,化疗药物对头颈部鳞癌都证实有效,所以毫无悬念地,对食管鳞癌也取得了好的疗效。

过去 20 年里,美国和其他西方国家发生变化,多数食管癌是腺癌,位于食管远端 1/3 部位或者食管胃结合部癌延伸的胃和贲门。对胃癌治疗有效的药物对食管腺癌治疗也有效,并且出现了靶向药物治疗,如 Her-2 受体拮抗剂(曲妥珠单抗)、血管内皮生长因子受体拮抗剂(贝伐单抗和雷莫芦单抗)。食管鳞癌在非西方国家仍占据主要地位,如在中东、非洲和南亚。

单药化疗

之前Ⅱ期临床研究证实了许多单药成分治疗食管癌有 15%~30%的有效率。这些药物包括:顺铂、丝裂霉素、氟尿嘧啶、紫杉醇、长春新碱[130a]。这些药物的效应是对短暂的,对于延长生存期来说是没有意义的。

多药综合化疗

多药联合相对于单药来说,有更高的有效率,最高达 50%(图 89-3)。博来霉素联合长春新碱和顺铂有效率达 53%并且取得平均 7 个月的有效反应期。

更常用的和更易耐受的方案如氟尿嘧啶加顺铂,Ⅱ期随机临床研究证实比起顺铂单药有更高的有效率(35%对 19%),但是中位生存期没有区别(33 周对 28 周)。上述两药方案再加上紫杉醇,在Ⅱ期临床研究中有 48%的有效率和 5.7 个月的中位反应期以及 10.8 个月的中位生存期,在鳞癌和腺癌中的有效率分别为 50%和 46%[130b]。

单纯紫杉醇和顺铂的两药方案在Ⅱ期临床研究中对鳞癌和腺癌都有效,有效率达 40%临床获益率 70%(吞咽困难减轻、体重恢复)[130c]。紫杉醇联合卡铂在Ⅱ期临床研究中有效率 43%,中位反应期 2.8 个月,中位生存期 9 个月,1 年生存率 43%。联合用药方案耐受性好,没有相关死亡事件[130d]。

表柔比星、顺铂及氟尿嘧啶(ECF)以前被认为对胃腺癌有效。在Ⅲ期临床研究中,这个方案和丝裂霉素、顺铂及氟尿嘧啶方案对比对食管鳞癌/腺癌效果类似(44.1%对 42.4%;中位生存期 9.4 个月对 8.7 个月)[130e]。用奥沙利铂和口服卡培他滨替代顺铂和氟尿嘧啶(EOX)方案在Ⅲ期临床研究中(REAL-2)964 例可评估患者参与其中,证实 EOX 方案可以提高生存率,但是无疾病进展期和反应率 EOX 和 ECF 相似[130f]。

伊立替康联合顺铂的周化疗方案在Ⅱ期临床研究中对食管癌有效率达 57%,中位反应期 4.2 个月,中位生存期 14.6 个月,并且对腺癌(52%)和鳞癌(66%)都有效[130g]。

靶向治疗

曲妥珠单抗,是一个单克隆抗 Her-2 受体抗体,已经进行了Ⅲ期临床研究(ToGA),方案为氟尿嘧啶/卡培他滨和顺铂加或者不加曲妥珠单抗[130h]。胃和食管腺癌的患者经 IHC(1~3+)或者 FISH 检测 Her-2 阳性的患者入组,曲妥珠单抗组反应率较高(47%;35%),中位生存期 13.8 个月和 11.1 个月。进一步研究发现对于 IHC3+患者最有效。

雷莫芦单抗是一个单克隆抗体,通过抑制 VEGF-2 受体发挥作用,已经进行Ⅲ期临床研究(REGARD),对照组选择经治后的胃和食管腺癌,给予安慰剂对照[130i]。结论为中位无进展生存期为 2.1 对 1.3 个月;总生存期为 5.2 对 3.8 个月;反应率为 8%对 3%,疾病控制率(疾病反应加稳定率)为 49%对 23%。在另外一项Ⅲ期临床研究(RAINBOW)中,雷莫芦单抗加紫杉醇和安慰剂加紫杉醇治疗转移的胃癌和食管胃交界部癌取得了更好的生存[130j],中位生存期(9.6 对 7.4 个月),无疾病进展期(4.4 对 2.9 个月),反应率(28%对 16%)都取得了很好的效果。

贝伐单抗是一个单克隆抗体,直接抑制 VEGF。已经进行Ⅲ期临床研究(AVAGAST),联合卡培他滨加顺铂和安慰剂联合卡培他滨加顺铂治疗首治的胃和食管胃结合部腺癌,反应率和中位无进展生存期分别为 46%对 37%和 6.7 对 5.3 个月,但是并没有生存上的差别(12.1 对 10.1 个月)[130k]。

同样,Ⅲ期临床研究没有证据表明化疗加上抗 EGFR 成分能在胃癌和食管胃结合部癌患者中取得生存获益。Ⅲ期临床研究(EXPAND)卡培他滨加或者不加西妥昔单抗中位无疾病进展期为 4.4 个月对 5.6 个月(对照组)[130l]。Ⅲ期临床研究 REAL3 中,食管胃结合部癌随机分到表柔比星-奥沙利铂-卡培他滨加或不加帕尼单抗两组中[130m],中位生存期 8.8 对 11.3 个月,对照组更获益,研究被终止。

多模式治疗

对于局部进展期食管癌患者,我们正在研究化疗与放疗以及手术联合治疗,以降低单独放疗或者手术造成的较高的全身复发率。手术联合化疗包括术前和术后化疗,通常是以铂类化疗药物为基础的多药联合。这些随机试验通常采用术前化疗 2 个或者 3 个周期后再手术。有些研究也在手术后追加化疗。化疗在疗效上与组织学类型关系并不大。当在经验丰富的中心术前化疗并没有增加围术期的并发症。如表 89-6 所示,最近的随机试验已经显示术前化疗可以使患者生存获益,研究样本越大,研究结果越明显[41,101,104,105,123,131~133,135]。大多数试验失败可能是因为研究的患者样本量较小。荟萃分析已经显示,大样本量分析显示明显的获益,尤其在食管腺癌的术前化疗组[136]。

表 89-6　局部进展食管癌术前和术后化疗随机化研究的对比结果

作者	年份	治疗方法	组织类型	患者	手术切除率	手术死亡率	中位生存期/月	*P*
手术前化疗								
Roth 等[41]	1988	顺铂+博来霉素+长春地辛+手术	鳞癌>腺癌	19	—	10	9	NS
		单纯手术		20	—	0	9	
Nygaard 等[118]	1992	顺铂+博来霉素+手术/单纯手术	鳞癌	50	58%	10	NS	
		单纯手术		41	69%	13	7	
Schlag 等[100]	1992	顺铂+5-FU+手术	鳞癌	21	69%	—	6	NS
		单纯手术		24	79%	—	8	
Malpang 等[131]	1994	顺铂+博来霉素+长春地辛+手术	鳞癌	24	—	—	17	NS
		单纯手术		22	—	—	17	
Ancona 等[132]	1995	顺铂+5-FU+手术	鳞癌	35	78%	7	—	NS
		单纯手术		43	86%	5	—	
Law 等[103]	1997	顺铂+5-FU+手术	鳞癌	73	95%	9	13	NS
		单纯手术		74	89%	8	17	
Kelsen 等[104]	1998	顺铂+5-FU+手术	鳞癌>腺癌	213	76%	7	15	NS
		单纯手术		227	89%	6	16	

续表

作者	年份	治疗方法	组织类型	患者	手术切除率	手术死亡率	中位生存期/月	*P*
Clarke 等[133]	2002	顺铂+5-FU+手术	鳞癌>腺癌	400	78%	10	17	<0.05
		单纯手术		402	70%	10	13	
Cunningham 等[134]	2006	表柔比星+顺铂+5-FU+手术	腺癌	250	69%	6	23	<0.01
		单纯手术		253	66%	6	20	
术后化疗								
Ando 等[123]	1997	顺铂+长春地辛+手术	鳞癌	105	—	—	58	NS
		单纯手术		100	—	—	47	

NS,无意义;5-FU,氟尿嘧啶。

术后应用顺铂和氟尿嘧啶化疗没有证实患者生存获益,比单纯手术并无差异,可能是由于化疗增加了患者并发症(表89-7)[137]。在荟萃分析中也没有证据表明术后化疗使患者获益[143]。

表 89-7 局部进展期食管癌患者术前放化疗的随机试验结果

作者	年份	治疗方法	组织类型	患者/例	技术	手术死亡率	中位生存期/月	*P*
LePrise 等[137]	1994	顺铂+5-FU+20Gy+手术	鳞癌	41	序贯	9%	10	NS
				45		7%	10	
Walsh 等[138]	1996	顺铂+5-FU+40Gy+手术	腺癌	58	同时	12%	17	0.01
				55		3%	12	
Bosset 等[139]	1997	顺铂+37Gy+手术	鳞癌	143	同时	12%	19	NS
				139		4%	19	
Walsh 等[138]	2001	顺铂+5-FU+45Gy+手术	腺癌	50	同时	4%	18	0.15
				50		2%	17	
Burmeister 等[141]	2005	顺铂+5-FU+35Gy+手术	腺癌,鳞癌	128	同时	5%	22	NS
				128		5%	19	
Tepper 等[142]	2008	顺铂+5-FU+50.4Gy+手术	腺癌>鳞癌	30	同时	0%	54	0.002
				26		4%	22	
Van Hagen 等[96c]	2012	紫杉醇+卡铂+41.4Gy+手术	腺癌,鳞癌	178	同时	4%	49	0.003
				188		4%	24	
Mariette 等[96d]	2014	顺铂+5-FU+45Gy+手术	腺癌,鳞癌	98	同时	11%	32	0.99
				97		3%	41	

NS,无意义;5-FU,氟尿嘧啶。

根治性放化疗和选择性手术期望能够提高局部进展期食管癌的预后。这些研究多是序贯治疗或者同步治疗。同步放化疗理论上是有前景的,因为除了化疗全身作用外,药物也会成为放疗的增敏剂。随机同步研究证实比单纯放疗更有效(表89-4)[88,90~92,111~113]。放化疗联合手术治疗鳞状细胞癌的有效率高于腺癌,腺癌的生存期相对较短[105]。欧洲已经对鳞状细胞癌进行了两项随机试验,包括根治性放化疗或者术前放化疗[95,96a]。这些研究表明,两组之间的生存率无明显差别,说明根治性化放疗对于中上段食管癌来说也是个好的选择。目前根治性放化疗方案中放疗的剂量是 50.4Gy,一项随机试验表明增加放疗的剂量会增加放疗相关的死亡率,但并无生存获益[94]。有意思的是,高剂量放疗对局部放疗失败没有任何影响,临床研究表明在 24 个月的随访后,发现高剂量也同样有 50%的局部放疗失败率。

术前放化疗意在控制局部进展期食管癌的局部复发和全身复发比率,尤其是对比单纯手术和术前新辅助化疗的患者。理论上来讲,与术后放化疗相比,术前放化疗具有以下优势:①术前更易控制亚临床全身转移,因为手术会引起免疫抑制;

②减小肿瘤大小，降低肿瘤分期，增加手术根治的机会；③可以给予足量的放、化疗剂量，术后往往由于围术期患者体质虚弱，不能给予足够的剂量。正如表 89-7 所示，结果并不是一致的，序贯放化疗并没有显示出优势[95,137~141]。有些试验的结果表明，术前同步放化疗对于局部进展期食管癌患者，尤其是腺癌患者更有较，但是并没有统计学差异。荟萃分析表示尽管受临床前分期技术差异和肿瘤患者异质性的限制，术前放化疗和术前化疗是比较好的治疗策略（图 89-7）[136]。多数研究证实，手术标本病理完全缓解的患者，术前经历了放化疗，获得明显生存改善。因为单纯手术或者单纯放疗预后较差，很多肿瘤学家建议对于无远处转移局部进展的患者，根治性放化疗或者术前新辅助放化疗联合手术治疗（图 89-3）。欧洲两项随机临床试验，对比食管鳞癌根治性放化疗与术前放化疗联合手术进行了对比，初步结论手术组提高了局部病变控制率，但是远期生存没有差异[95,96a]。手术组死亡率比预期要高，在一些死亡率比较高的机构根治性放化疗对于食管中上段鳞癌是一个更好的选择[95,96a]。临床研究中新辅助放化疗后病理完全缓解的患者，生存率是否获益并没有定论。多数临床研究会被认为设计上有缺陷或者对生存率没有分析。最新的荟萃分析对 12 项新辅助放化疗联合手术的研究进行总结，包含 1 854 例患者，死亡风险比已经得到改善（0.78，95%CI = 0.70～0.88；P<0.000 1）；鳞癌和腺癌都有获益（0.80，CI = 0.68～0.93；P = 0.004 和 0.75，CI = 0.59～0.95；P = 0.02）。但是术后并发症和死亡率仍比较高，生存率还是没有定论。

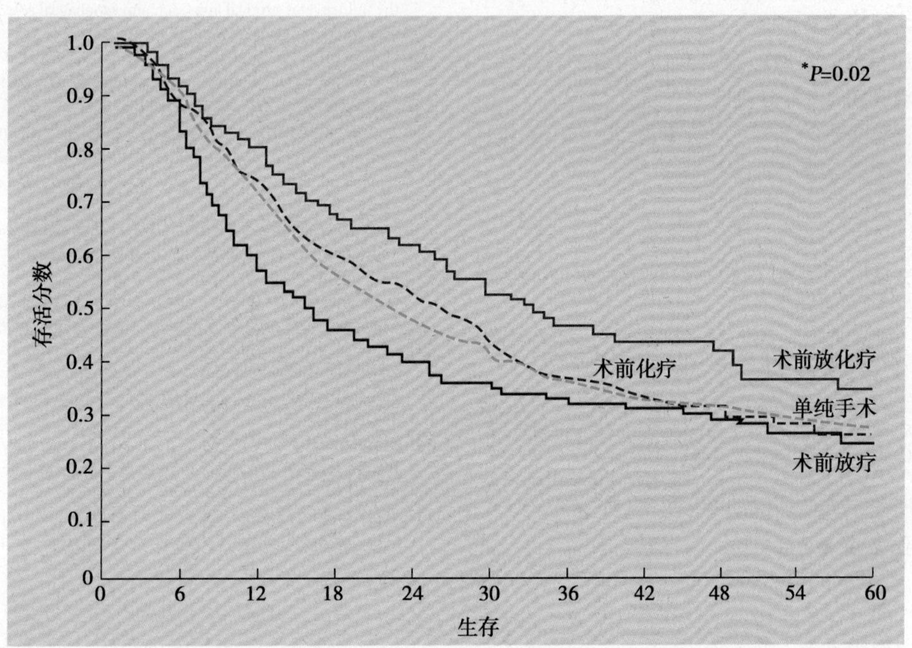

图 89-7 术前放化疗患者的长期生存率相比单纯手术患者得到改善（得克萨斯大学 Anderson 癌症中心的研究数据）。摘自 Hofsetter 2002[28a]. Reproduced with permission of Wolters Kluwer

一项Ⅱ期临床研究，旨在降低手术死亡率和提高手术切除率，用紫杉醇和卡铂联合放疗证实有较低的并发症和 100% 的完全切除率[96b]。Ⅲ期临床研究结论在临床分期 T1N1M0 或者 T2～3N0～1M0 不推荐单纯手术[96c]。一项包含 366 例患者的研究发现新辅助放化疗组 92% 例腺癌患者得到 R0 的切除，而单纯手术组 R0 切除率 69%（P<0.001），术后并发症两组没有区别。放化疗组生存率明显优于外科组，中位随访 45 个月，放化疗组中位生存期 49.4 个月，外科组 24 个月（P = 0.003），五年生存率 47% 对 34%，这个生存优势在鳞癌腺癌中都有获益。

基于这些临床研究和资料，NCCN 指南 3.2015 版建议合适的食管癌患者进行术前放化疗。

来自欧洲的一项研究比较早期食管癌（临床分期Ⅰ或者Ⅱ期）新辅助放化疗（4500cGY 加氟尿嘧啶顺铂方案）和单纯手术组，结果发现 3 年生存率没有区别（47.5% 对比 53%，HR = 0.99）；R0 切除相同，93.8% 对 92.1%（P = 0.749），但术后死亡率新辅助化疗组死亡率较高，11.1% 比 3.4%（P = 0.049）[96d]。

治疗选择

治疗策略如图 89-3。如果病变局部早期，PS 评分好的患者建议内镜下切除或者食管癌切除手术；PS 评分差的患者或者拒绝手术者建议根治性放化疗或者单纯放疗。而局部晚期患者，如果 PS 评分好，单纯的手术或者放疗很难取得好的治疗效果，建议根治性放化疗或者新辅助放化疗后手术。PS 评分差的局部晚期患者，给予放化疗或者姑息放疗加/不加支架置放。发生转移的食管癌患者，PS 评分好的可以给予单纯化疗加姑息性放疗加/不加支架术来控制局部进展。PS 评分差的患者不给予化疗，应专注姑息治疗。

食管梗阻的姑息治疗

进展期患者如果不能耐受根治性治疗手段，那么主要的治疗就是减轻吞咽困难的症状[144]。姑息性手术切除有较高的并发症和死亡率，并且延长了患者康复时间，所以必须评估其临床意义，目前多数肿瘤学家不建议姑息手术。外放疗，可以单独或者联合化疗进行，是无创的治疗，但是需要较长治疗周期，并且狭窄率高达30%。腔内近距离放射治疗也是一个治疗选择[145,146]。光凝激光治疗也是一个选择，通常选铷雅克激光，初始治疗有效率约85%，但是中位缓解时间低于1个月；光动力治疗有相似的有效率但是缓解时间更长，但是皮肤光过敏是一个副作用[147]。

食管支架是另一个姑息治疗的不错选择。对于晚期局部有梗阻患者，支架植入可以迅速持久改善吞咽困难症状。自膨性金属网状支架的使用，使支架植入更容易简单，相比塑料支架，减少了并发症[148,149]。这些姑息治疗手段侵袭性不强，可以较好改善患者症状，已经逐渐取代外科姑息治疗手段。

食管癌患者有时候发生恶性食管气管瘘，以前要依赖手术改流，但是并发症多，预期寿命短[150]。覆膜网状支架是一个更好的治疗选择，可以封堵瘘口，减轻梗阻，而不需要外科干预，通常这些患者也比较衰弱，PS评分较低[151,152]。

（李勇 译 李印 校）

参考文献

The complete reference list can be found on the Wiley Companion Digital Edition of this title (see inside front cover for login instructions).

4 Dolan K, Sutton R, Walker SJ, et al. New classification of oesophageal and gastric carcinomas derived from changing patterns in epidemiology. *Br J Cancer*. 1999;**80**:834–842.

13 Kjaerheim K, Gaard M, Andersen A. The role of alcohol, tobacco, and dietary factors in upper aerodigestive tract cancers: a prospective study of 10,900 Norwegian men. *Cancer Causes Control*. 1998;**9**:99–108.

24 Montesano R, Hollstein M, Hainaut P. Genetic alterations in esophageal cancer and their relevance to etiology and pathogenesis: a review. *Int J Cancer*. 1996;**69**:225–235.

31 Siegel RL, Miller KD, Jemal A. Cancer Statistics, 2015. *CA Cancer J Clin*. 2015;**65**:5–29.

35 Hesketh PJ, Clapp RW, Doos WG, et al. The increasing frequency of adenocarcinoma of the esophagus. *Cancer*. 1989;**64**:526–530.

39 Swisher SG, Hunt KK, Holmes EC, et al. Changes in the surgical management of esophageal cancer from 1970–1993. *Am J Surg*. 1995;**169**:609–614.

45 Swisher SG, DeFord L, Merriman KW, et al. Effect of operative volume on morbidity, mortality and hospital use after esophagectomy for cancer. *J Thorac Cardiovasc Surg*. 2000;**119**:1126–1134.

46 Tio TL, Coene PPLO, Luiken GJHM, et al. Endosonography in the clinical staging of esophageal carcinoma [abstract]. *Gastrointest Endosc*. 1990;**36**:S2–S10.

64 Flamen P, Lerut A, Van Cutsem E, et al. The utility of positron emission tomography for the diagnosis and staging of recurrent esophageal cancer. *J Thorac Cardiovasc Surg*. 2000;**120**:1085–1092.

70 Shimada Y, Imamura M, Shibagaki I, et al. Genetic alterations in patients with esophageal cancer with short-and long-term survival rates after curative esophagectomy. *Ann Surg*. 1997;**226**:162–168.

79 Tabira Y, Okuma T, Kondo K, et al. Indications for three-field dissection followed by esophagectomy for advanced carcinoma of the thoracic esophagus. *J Thorac Cardiovasc Surg*. 1999;**117**:239–245.

82 Jacobi CA, Zieren HU, Muller JM, et al. Surgical therapy of esophageal carcinoma: the influence of surgical approach and esophageal resection on cardiopulmonary function. *Eur J Cardio-Thorac Surg*. 1997;**11**:32–37.

83 Hulscher JBF, van Sandik JW, De Boer AGEM, et al. Extended transthoracic resection compared with limited transhiatal resection for adenocarcinoma of the esophagus. *New Engl J Med*. 2002;**347**:1662–1669.

94 Minsky BD, Pajak TF, Ginsberg RJ, et al. INT 0123 (Radiation Therapy Oncology Group 94–05) phase III trial of combined-modality therapy for esophageal cancer: high-dose versus standard-dose radiation therapy. *J Clin Oncol*. 2002;**20**:1167–1174.

101 Walsh TN, Noonan N, Hollywood D, et al. A comparison of multimodal therapy and surgery for esophageal adenocarcinoma. *N Engl J Med*. 1996;**335**:462–467.

117 Arnott SJ, Duncan W, Gignoux M, et al. Preoperative radiotherapy in esophageal carcinoma: a meta-analysis using individual patients data (Oesophageal Cancer Collaborative Group). *Int J Radiat Oncol Biol Phys*. 1998;**41**:579–583.

123 Ando N, Iizuka T, Kakegawa T, et al. A randomized trial of surgery with and without chemotherapy for localized squamous carcinoma of the thoracic esophagus: the Japan Clinical Oncology Group study. *J Thorac Cardiovasc Surg*. 1997;**114**:205–209.

141 Burmeister BH, Smithers BM, Fitzgerald L, et al. Surgery alone versus chemoradiotherapy followed by surgery for resectable cancer of the esophagus: a randomized controlled phase III trial. *Lancet Oncol*. 2005;**6**:659–668.

142 Tepper J, Krasna MJ, Niedzwiecki D, et al. Phase III trial of trimodality therapy with cisplatin fluorouracil, radiotherapy, and surgery compared with surgery alone for esophageal cancer; CALGB 9781. *J Clin Oncol*. 2008;**26**:1086–1092.

第 90 章 胃癌

Carl Schmidt, MD ■ Mariela Blum Murphy, MD ■ James C. Yao, MD ■ Christopher H. Crane, MD

概述

胃癌是全球癌症相关死亡的第二大常见原因，其风险因素包括自身免疫性胃炎，慢性幽门螺杆菌感染，肥胖和其他原因。虽然一些发病率较高的国家已经建立了筛查计划，但方法和资质仍然存在争议。尽管我们已经了解了胃癌的风险因素并筛查了高危人群，但识别早期潜在可治愈的胃癌仍然存在挑战。

多种基因突变参与胃癌的发病机制，细胞黏附蛋白 CDH1 的突变导致家族性弥漫性胃癌。胃癌转移的某些模式与特定的分子改变有关。我们对胃癌相关的分子途径的认知不断加深，使得在进展期胃癌中可以有效地使用靶向生物疗法联合细胞毒性化疗，例如在 HER2/neu 过度表达的胃癌患者中使用曲妥珠单抗。

手术切除是对未发生转移的患者的主要治疗方法。手术切除方式和淋巴结清扫范围并不统一，需要最佳实践标准。化疗和放疗在辅助治疗中起重要作用，因此，决定采取何种治疗及何时治疗需要通过内镜检查，横断面成像以及在某些情况下需要内镜超声或正电子发射断层扫描的全面评估来准确判断分期。

姑息性干预和治疗对于出现转移或复发后症状的患者往往很重要，因为胃癌的转移和复发都无法治愈。最近的临床试验结果令人鼓舞，在过去 10 年中进行了多项有关胃癌的辅助治疗及转移的有意义的Ⅲ期临床试验。尽管如此，大多数被诊断患有胃癌的人最终会死于胃癌，因此我们需要进行更多的研究。

发病率和流行病学

尽管胃癌发病率在世界范围内下降，但胃癌仍然是癌症相关死亡的第二大常见原因。胃癌在中国（占全球病例的 42%），南美，东欧，日本和韩国尤为常见，在韩国是最常见的恶性肿瘤[1]。过去的 30 年里，美国胃癌年龄标准化死亡率持续下降，2005 年的数据为每 100 000 人中有 3.8 人[2]，而胃癌发病率下降是这一现象发生的主要的原因。确诊胃癌的患者生存率仍然很低，多年来改善不大。根据调查、流行病学研究和终末登记（surveillance, epidemiology, and end results, SEER）的数据，胃癌患者五年的存活率仅从 1975 年到 1979 年的 16.3%提高到 2000 年的 23%[2]。需要说明的是这些数据发表早于有阳性结果的、被广泛认可的多学科综合治疗研究结果的发布。

风险因素

环境因素造成的胃黏膜损害可能最终导致萎缩性胃炎引起化生，是胃癌的癌前病变[3]。与胃癌风险增加相关的其他因素包括血清铁蛋白水平低，恶性贫血，消化性溃疡远端胃切除史，以及顽固性幽门螺杆菌感染[4~6]。虽然有些证据具有启发性，但根除幽门螺旋杆菌感染是否可以降低胃癌的发病率尚不明确[7]。长期以来人们一直认为与胃癌相关的行为包括饮食中接触硝酸盐、亚硝酸盐和食物中细菌或真菌污染，考虑到随着冷藏的出现其发生率逐渐降低[8]。研究还表明，近端胃癌的发病率增加与肥胖有关，并且体育锻炼对胃癌总体发病率有保护作用[9,10]。多项观察性研究发现，红肉消费与胃癌风险增加有关[11,12]。一些研究表明，红肉消费量和患癌风险之间存在剂量-反应关系，从而进一步支持了这种可能性。相反，食用水果可以降低患胃癌的风险[13]。

研究者已经注意到在约 1%的胃癌病例中发生家族聚集。种系突变仅占这些病例的一小部分。遗传性弥漫性胃癌（hereditary diffuse gastric cancer, HDGC）综合征由 *CDH1* 基因的种系突变引起；然而，*CDH1* 突变仅占具有弥漫性胃癌病史的家族的一小部分。*CDH1* 基因参与细胞黏附，该基因缺陷也与小叶性乳腺癌有关[14]。受影响的胃癌个体遗传了一份有缺陷的 *CDH1* 基因，而体细胞突变，缺失或启动子甲基化使另一份拷贝失活。胃癌遵循具有高外显率的常染色体显性遗传模式。

预防性胃切除术是受 HDGC 综合征影响的家庭成员的考虑选项。当进行预防性胃切除术时，在切除的标本中几乎总能找到多灶性的早期胃癌[15]。考虑家族中已知胃癌病例的外显率和发病年龄，以及缺乏预防性胃切除术的长期预后数据，建议在疑似病例中进行遗传咨询。Worster 等人[16]研究了预防性全胃切除术对健康相关生活质量（health-related quality of life, HRQOL）的影响。32 名接受全胃切除术的患者的 HRQOL 与 28 名未接受全胃切除术的 HDGC 风险患者进行了比较。虽然手术后 12 个月身体功能和精神状态恢复到基线水平，但仍存在一些症状，特别是稀便（70%），疲劳（63%），进食不适（81%），反流（63%），饮食受限（45%）和身体形象（44%）。

在患有结直肠家族性腺瘤性息肉病（familial adenomatous polyposis, FAP）的个体中，27%~70%出现胃息肉[17,18]。虽然胃底息肉通常被认为是错构瘤，但会经常发现凹陷性异常增生和侵袭性腺癌。遗传性非息肉病性结直肠癌（hereditary nonpolyposis colorectal cancer, HNPCC）是一种遗传性疾病，其特征在于一组错配修复基因中的种系突变，包括 *hMSH2*、*hMLH1*、*hMSH6*、*hPMS1* 和 *hPMS2*。这些基因的缺陷导致以微卫星不稳定性（microsatellite instability, MSI）为特征的基因组不稳定性。虽然结直肠癌和子宫内膜癌是 HNPCC 最常见的表现，但是胃癌也是其中的一种表现。对韩国遗传性肿瘤登记处的分析显示，

携带 *HNPCC* 突变基因的家族胃癌相对风险增加了 3.2 倍[19]。然而,其中错配修复基因的种系突变仅占 MSI 胃癌的一小部分。

- 胃癌是全球癌症相关死亡的第二大原因
- 风险因素包括自身免疫性胃炎,幽门螺杆菌感染和肥胖
- *CDH1* 基因中的种系突变与遗传性胃癌有关

病理学

腺癌是胃癌的主要组织学类型。Lauren 和 WHO 分类是主要使用的两个系统。Lauren 分型法将癌症分类为肠型、弥漫型或混合型[20]。因为简便,所以该分型法被广泛采用。肠型胃癌又称流行性胃癌。它的特点是保留了腺体结构和细胞极性。大体标本表现为肿瘤边缘清晰。肠型胃癌起源于胃黏膜,与慢性胃炎、胃黏膜萎缩以及肠上皮化生相关。弥漫性胃癌特点是侵袭性生长方式。大小一致的癌细胞形成的细胞簇星罗棋布,常侵袭到黏膜下层,很少形成腺体样结构,而癌细胞多表达黏蛋白(图 90-1)。

对无临床疾病的胃切除标本的研究发现,外表正常的上皮组织下出现了早期弥漫型胃癌[15]。这一类型的胃癌似乎起源于黏膜固有层的浅层。弥漫型胃癌的浸润式生长方式往往表现为没有肿块。使用内镜检查可能难以识别癌症,但胃褶皱增厚和胃扩张受限是弥漫性胃癌的标志。恶性细胞可以明显浸润到肿瘤边缘以外。在晚期病例中最终会导致皮革胃,其特征是整个胃受累,进展迅速,对治疗产生抵抗力,并且预后不良。

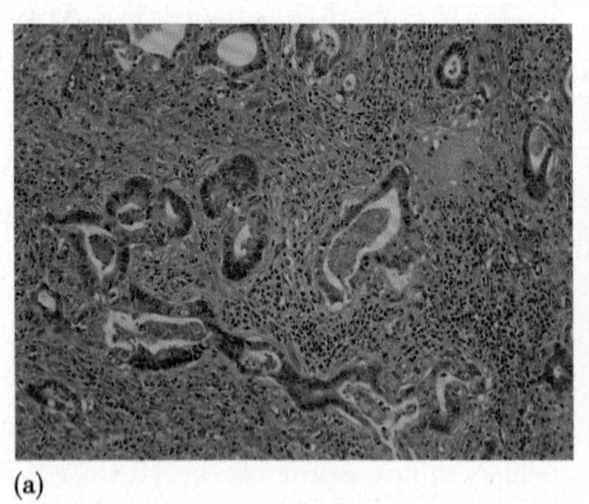
(a)

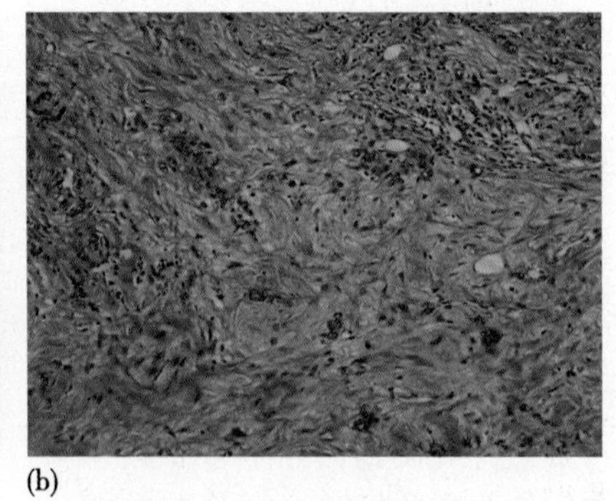
(b)

图 90-1 来自肠型(a)和弥漫型(b)胃癌的组织切片照片

发病机制与自然史

分子变化

多种分子改变在胃癌的发病机制中起重要作用(表 90-1)。表观遗传现象包括 *CDH1*、*hMLH1* 和 *p16* 在内的许多基因的启动子区域的高甲基化,这些基因可能参与早期癌变[21~27]。此外,据报道 DNA 修复基因突变引起的 MSI 高达 39%[28]。肿瘤抑制基因如 *p53*、*APC*、*MCC* 和 *DCC* 在胃癌中也发生突变,其发生率通常随组织学和分期而变化[29~31]。

细胞间黏附性缺失是人体恶性肿瘤形成过程中的重要特征,并且在胃癌的遗传改变中普遍存在。弥漫型胃癌的重要特征是细胞黏附性失调,成簇或者单个的肿瘤细胞浸润性生长。细胞表面的钙黏蛋白复合体在细胞黏附和极性中起关键作用,高达 90%的胃癌病例至少有其中一种复合体异常,包括 CDH1 和 α-、γ-连环蛋白[32,33]。CD44 跨膜糖蛋白在 31%~72%的胃癌中表达,其可能参与调节胃癌的侵袭和转移[34]。

表 90-1 与临床、病理相关的分子标志

分子标志	所占比例	主要组织学类型	临床相关性
表观遗传学改变			
超甲基化	普遍存在	肠型和弥漫型	
MSI	31%~39%	肠型	与生存率的关系不一致,有利或无显著差别
肿瘤抑制因子			
p53	47%~74%	两者都有:肠型(早期事件)、弥漫型(晚期事件)	与弥漫型胃癌的临床分期相关
APC	8%~34%	肠型	—
MCC	24%~33%	弥漫型	—
DCC	12%~49%	肠型	—

续表

分子标志	所占比例	主要组织学类型	临床相关性
FHIT	49%~67%	—	与临床分期和生存率相关
肿瘤黏附			
E-cadherin	54%~83%	弥漫型	—
α-catenin	83%~92%	弥漫型	—
γ-catenin	91%~100%	弥漫型	—
β-catenin	—	肠型(GSK3β 的区域)	生存率较低
CD44	31%~72%	CD44v6-与肠型	表达 CD44v6 的肠型胃癌病例生存率较低
酪氨酸激酶			
EGFR	35%~81%	肠型和弥漫型	与临床分期有关;和生存的关系不确定
HER2/neu	10%~38%	肠型	生存率较低
PDGF α	42%~45%	肠型和弥漫型	与临床分期和生存率较低相关
c-Met	34%~71%	弥漫型胃癌	与临床分期和腹膜高转移相关
血管生成			
VEGF	—	肠型胃癌	与胃癌肝转移相关
bFGF	—	肠型胃癌	增加肿瘤复发风险

与其他腺癌相似,胃癌中发生了细胞信号转导途径的改变,并为生物疗法提供潜在的靶点。*HER2/neu* 是膜受体酪氨酸激酶 erbB 家族中的一种致癌基因,在 10%~38%的胃癌病例中过度表达,与肠型远端胃癌和较差预后有关[30,35]。其他细胞受体在胃癌中的表达与致癌行为相关,例如跨膜受体表皮生长因子受体(epidermal growth factor receptor,EGFR)与侵袭有关,c-Met 与腹膜转移有关[36]。血管生成对胃癌和其他实体瘤的生长至关重要,而胃癌标本中血管生成的增加预示着不良的预后[37]。血管内皮生长因子(vascular endothelial growth factor,VEGF)和碱性成纤维细胞生长因子(basic fibroblast growth factor,bFGF)是血管生成的主要调节因子,具有预后评估价值,并且是胃癌患者抗血管生成治疗的潜在靶点[38,39]。胃癌细胞表达多种转录因子,如 Sp1 和 mTOR,可促进异常细胞生长、存活以及血管生成[40,41]。

胃癌转移过程与模式

胃癌可以通过多种方式转移。可通过直接侵犯而累及邻近的肝脏、横膈、胰腺、脾脏以及结肠(或肠系膜)等器官。胃癌很有可能通过淋巴系统扩散到区域和远端淋巴结。血源性转移常见于肝脏。腹膜转移在胃癌转移中也很常见,可能导致腹痛,肠梗阻,恶病质或三者都有。日本研究者提出,胃癌的组织学类型和患者年龄可能影响胃癌的扩散方式。通过对 173 例的尸检研究发现,弥漫型胃癌倾向于发生腹膜转移,而肠型胃癌则倾向于发生肝转移[42]。他们还发现腹膜转移在年轻患者中更为常见。在另一项研究中,分析了 216 例同时发生腹膜转移或肝转移的胃癌患者,发现组织学分化较差的病例倾向于发生腹膜转移,而组织学中-高分化的病例易于发生肝转移[43]。

分子水平的研究发现,VEGF 及其受体 KDR 的表达水平与胃癌肝转移相关[37,44]。VEGF-C 的表达可引起淋巴管的新生,与淋巴结转移有关[45,46]。细胞黏附失调可能是腹膜转移发展的核心。在动物模型中,CD44H 和促进胃癌细胞与间皮细胞黏附以及促进腹膜转移有关[47]。C-met 扩增也与腹膜转移有关[36,48]。进一步的分子生物学转化研究可能帮助我们发现不足之处,制订更合理的治疗策略。

- 胃癌的发病机制涉及许多基因和细胞通路的分子改变,包括启动子甲基化,MSI,细胞黏附,生长因子和血管生成的修饰
- 区域淋巴结转移受累非常常见
- 腹膜表面和肝脏是常见的转移部位

胃癌筛查

在一些胃癌发病率较高的国家,包括日本、韩国、委内瑞拉和智利,已经建立了大规模的筛查计划。可用的筛查试验包括上消化道内镜检查和使用口服造影剂,如钡餐造影。哪种筛查方法最有效仍然存在争议,在推荐年龄、时间间隔或筛查类型方面没有统一标准。目前比较缺乏比较不同筛查方法的大型对照试验。在胃癌风险较低的国家,如美国,对无症状人群进行筛查既不可行,也不具成本效益。

重要的是，胃癌的症状通常是非特异性的，导致到了进展期才诊断胃癌。这在很大程度上是由于胃和腹腔容积都很大且伸缩性好。在没有癌症的患者中，一些早期症状，例如不明部位的不适，发作性恶心、呕吐或厌食症是常见的。因此，医生可能很长时间不会将这些症状归因于胃癌。事实上，在诊断为胃癌之前，患者可能会接受几个月的经验性消化性溃疡治疗。因此，即使在胃癌发病率较低的国家，也需要开展更多研究以开发更好的早期筛查方法。

诊断

诊断胃癌时常见症状包括腹痛和体重减轻。虽然贫血也是常见发现，但明显的上消化道出血并不常见。吞咽困难可能主要发生在近端胃癌的患者中，而恶心和呕吐在非近端胃癌患者中更常见。早饱感在患有皮革胃的患者中尤其突出。异常的体格检查结果通常表明胃癌进入进展期，例如可触及的上腹部肿块，可能提示局部较大晚期肿瘤。黄疸通常提示有肝转移或门静脉区淋巴结转移。

胃癌的临床分期有几个方面，应逐步进行。潜在有益的实验室检查包括全血细胞计数、电解质、血尿素氮、肌酐、碱性磷酸酶、转氨酶和胆红素。可以考虑评估肿瘤标志物 CEA、CA19-9 和 CA125。在转诊给外科医生或肿瘤科医生时，通常进行上消化道内镜检查并进行诊断。内镜检查的结果应由初诊外科医生审查，复核肿瘤大小和位置，尤其是食管胃结合部肿瘤(gastroesophageal junction，GEJ)，因为其中一些种类可能更适合按照远端食管癌来治疗。对胸部，腹部和骨盆进行计算机断层扫描，以提供有关原发肿瘤的进一步信息，并检测恶性淋巴结或癌症转移的证据。甚至少量腹水的发现可能表明腹膜转移。

内镜超声(endoscopic ultrasound，EUS)可以准确评估 T 分期，并且能够对胃周可疑淋巴结甚至肝左叶肿物进行针刺活检。当 CT 扫描结果提示进展期胃癌时，可能并不需要做 EUS。对于进入新辅助治疗试验的患者和评估为可接受内镜黏膜切除术(endoscopic mucosal resection，EMR)的小肿物或考虑手术而不进行新辅助治疗的早期胃癌，应考虑使用 EUS。正电子发射断层扫描(positron emission tomography，PET)在胃癌诊断中的作用正在发展；有一些证据表明 PET 可用于评估胃癌患者对治疗的反应[49]。腹腔镜检查是有争议的，但被许多人认为是胃癌准确分期的必要检查。腹腔镜检查导致 1/5~1/4 的患者分期升级，通常是因为发现了 CT 扫描未见的腹膜转移[50~52]。

胃癌的 TNM 分期

表 90-2 显示了美国癌症联合委员会分期手册第 7 版(Springer，New York 2010)中当前胃癌分期系统的一部分。此表适用于未发生转移，即 M0 的患者。在目前的分期系统中，Ⅰ至Ⅲ期由 T(肿瘤)和 N(淋巴结)的各种组合来确定，且没有发生转移。过去的分期系统将一些广泛淋巴结转移的患者分为Ⅳ期。在当前系统中，只有存在远处转移时才能分为Ⅳ期。

表 90-2 AJCC 胃癌分期标准

T 分期	淋巴结分期			
	N0	N1	N2	N3
Tis	0			
T1a/b	ⅠA	ⅠB	ⅡA	ⅡB
T2	ⅠB	ⅡA	ⅡB	ⅢA
T3	ⅡA	ⅡB	ⅢA	ⅢB
T4a	ⅡB	ⅢA	ⅢB	ⅢC
T4b	ⅢB	ⅢB	ⅢC	ⅢC

以下定义用于对 T 和 N 进行分类：

- Tis：上皮内肿瘤，未侵及固有层
- T1a：肿瘤侵犯固有层或黏膜肌层
- T1b：肿瘤侵犯黏膜下层
- T2：肿瘤侵犯固有肌层
- T3：肿瘤穿透浆膜下结缔组织，无浆膜浸润
- T4a：肿瘤侵犯浆膜
- T4b：肿瘤侵入邻近的器官或结构
- N1：1~2 个区域淋巴结有转移
- N2：3~6 个区域淋巴结有转移
- N3a：7~15 个区域淋巴结有转移
- N3b：16 个或 16 个以上区域淋巴结有转移

- 在具有筛查计划的国家中，通过筛查可以发现早期胃癌
- 胃癌的可能症状包括腹痛、出血、吞咽困难、恶心、纳差、体重减轻和早饱感
- 临床分期基于内镜检查和胸部，腹部和骨盆的横断面成像(通常为 CT 扫描)
- 其他可能对分期有帮助的检查包括腹腔镜检查、EUS 和 PET

胃癌的多学科治疗

对于肿瘤体积较小和低组织学分级的患者，EMR 正逐渐被接受为局部治疗的主要方法。这种治疗的前提是这类肿瘤的淋巴结阳性率非常低[53]。T1 肿瘤的淋巴结阳性率约为 10%，而具备其他特征的原发肿瘤患者其风险甚至更低。局限于黏膜的肿瘤的淋巴结阳性率为 1%~3%，而侵犯黏膜下的肿瘤的阳性率高达 15%[54]。增加淋巴结阳性率的其他因素包括分化差，印戒细胞癌，淋巴管侵犯，肿瘤大小>2cm[55]。因此，对于肿瘤较小，局限于黏膜且分化良好的 T1 期患者，考虑行 EMR 是合理的。然而，一些大型临床中心的专家已经提出了使用内镜黏膜下剥离这一新技术的扩展标准[56]。更大的甚至溃疡肿块的切除已被实现。我们认为，这种更激进的方式需要术后标本必须经过仔细的病理检查，以确定病灶属于 T1 期(仅限于黏膜)。

手术治疗

胃癌手术的选择取决于肿瘤的位置，组织学类型和疾病分期。胃切除术是侵袭性胃癌最广泛的手术方式，最常见的术式有全胃切除术，远端胃大部切除术和近端胃大部切除术。节段性切除较少用于侵袭性胃癌，但对于其他胃恶性肿瘤，例如胃肠道间质瘤则非常常见且适用。前瞻性和随机研究显示，当所有病变都以足够的切缘移除时，对于远端胃癌，全胃切除术与远端胃大部切除术相比没有生存优势。这两种技术具备相似的死亡率(1%~3%)，并发症和 5 年生存率(约 60%)[57,58]。在大多数病例中，胃大部切除术后的生活质量优于全胃切除术后[59,60]。

近端胃癌和 GEJ 肿瘤通常需要考虑更复杂的切除和重建方式。Siewert 的分类法非常有用，通常用于描述 GEJ 肿瘤[61,62]。

- Ⅰ型：远端食管腺癌，通常发生于 Barrett 食管，从上方浸润食管胃交界处
- Ⅱ型：贲门癌，位于食管胃交界处上 1cm 到下 2cm
- Ⅲ型：贲门下癌，从下方浸润食管胃交界处

在涉及 GEJ 肿瘤的进展期肿瘤患者中，肿瘤起源部位(食管或胃)可能不清楚。Ⅰ型肿瘤的患者通常以远端食管癌进行治疗，考虑术前放化疗治疗更晚期的肿瘤，以及在颈部或胸部使用管状胃进行吻合的手术切除。在某些情况下，空肠或结肠被用来代替胃而重建消化道。根据肿瘤的范围，通常是经腹部采用全胃切除或近端胃大部切除来切除Ⅱ型和Ⅲ型肿瘤[63,64]。在美国全胃切除术通常比近端胃切除更受欢迎，因为在 Roux-en-Y 食管空肠吻合重建后，反流性食管炎很少发生，而大约 1/3 的患者在近端胃大部切除术后会出现明显的反流[59,65,66]。此外，近端胃大部切除术可能无法从胃小弯处移除足够的淋巴结组织，而胃小弯又是常见的淋巴结转移部位。然而，一些外科医生仍提倡近端胃大部切除术[64]。

淋巴结清扫的范围是胃癌治疗中最具争议的外科手术主题之一。根治性淋巴结清扫术涉及清扫超出常规胃切除术范围的淋巴结。日本胃癌协会使用字母“D”来定义淋巴结清扫的范围[67]。一般来说，D1 清扫包括胃周淋巴结。D2 清扫扩大了淋巴结清扫范围，包括沿肝动脉、胃左动脉、腹腔动脉和脾动脉的淋巴结(图 90-2)。D3 清扫包括沿肝门的淋巴结，以及位于胰腺后和主动脉周围区域的淋巴结。

检验扩大淋巴结清扫术潜在益处的最大前瞻性研究是荷兰 D1D2 淋巴结清扫试验，该试验将 1 000 多名患者(其中 711 例进行的是 R0 切除)随机分为 D1 或 D2 淋巴结清扫胃切除术，手术质量得到严格控制[68,69]。接受 D2 清扫术的患者术后并发症率和死亡率远高于 D1 清扫术(D2 术后并发症率和死亡率分别为 43%和 10%，D1 术后并发症率和死亡率分别为 25%和 4%；$P<0.01$)。然而，死亡率的增高大多发生在 D2 清扫的男性患者上，或为了完全清扫淋巴结而接受脾切除和胰尾切除的患者上。保留脾和胰尾的 D2 清扫术的患者的死亡率与保留脾和胰尾的 D1 清扫术的患者相近。中位随访 15.2 年后，D2 淋巴结清扫组与 D1 组相比具有更高的疾病特异性生存率(disease-specific survival，DSS)，以及更低的局部复发率(D2：12%，D1：22%，$P=0.02$)和区域复发率(D1：13%，D2：19%，$P=0.02$)[70]。

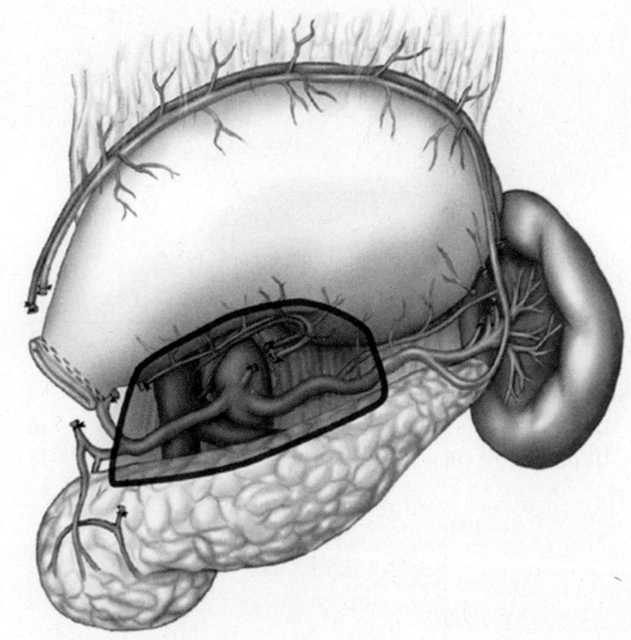

图 90-2　严格改良的 D2 淋巴结清扫区域，包括腹腔动脉，肝动脉，胃左动脉和脾动脉淋巴结(阴影区域)

意大利胃癌研究小组最近的一项试验评估了改良保留器官的 D2 淋巴结清扫术的作用[71]。可能被治愈的胃癌患者术中被随机分配为 D1 清扫或 D2 清扫。仅在怀疑发生局部侵袭时才进行部分胰腺切除术或脾切除术。共有 267 名患者被随机分组，D1 组的发病率和死亡率分别为 12%和 3%，D2 组为 18%和 2%。D1 和 D2 组的五年 DSS 分别为 71%和 73%；亚组分析显示，在淋巴结转移患者中，D2 组的 5 年 DSS 为 61%，而 D1 组为 46%。此外，在 T2-T4 期和淋巴结阳性的患者中，D2 组的 5 年 DSS 为 59%，而 D1 组为 38%(图 90-3)。美国综合癌症网络(NCCN)的胃癌专家组建议如果是大型临床中心经验丰富的外科医生的话，考虑在胃癌切除中行改良的 D2 淋巴结清扫术，并保留远端胰腺和脾脏[72]。

皮革胃是一种非常恶性的胃癌形式，许多临床医生认为其无法治愈。有些人认为患有皮革胃的患者不应该接受胃切除术，因为患者的 5 年生存率不超过 10%[73]。治疗皮革胃患者的一种方法是先进行腹腔镜分期评估，在没有发生转移的情况下，首先进行新辅助治疗，以期对未发生转移的患者行胃切除术。如果患皮革胃患者的术后切缘阳性，则应谨慎判断这是否值得考虑或采取具体的治疗措施，因为与发生广泛转移的风险相比，孤立的局部复发并不常见且很少影响生存。来自美国胃癌合作组织的最新证据表明，传统教学认为切缘应距肿瘤 5cm 以上，而这可能是不必要的[74]。在他们的回顾性队列研究中，结合了七个学术医疗中心的数据，发现切缘距离不是与总生存期(overall survival，OS)相关的独立因素。相反，T 和 N 分期是主要的相关因素，大多数患者保留 3cm 的切缘就已足够。

虽然前面提到的研究表明，在淋巴结清扫时不应常规进行多脏器切除，但有时候因原发肿瘤或严重受累的淋巴结而需要

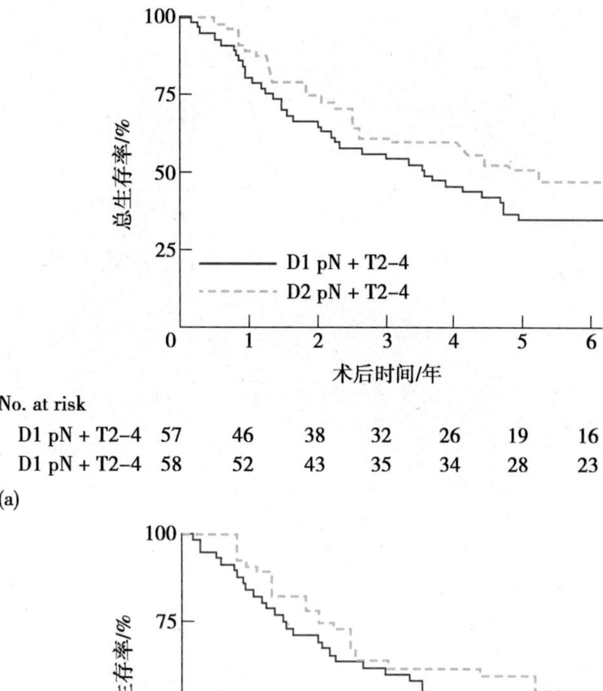

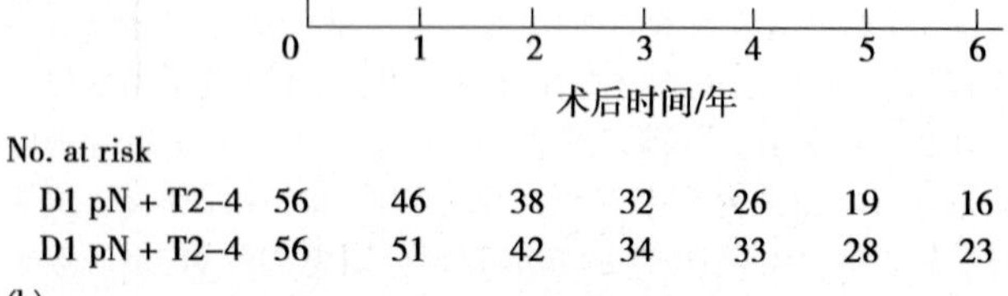

图 90-3　意大利胃癌研究组 D1D2 淋巴结清扫术试验中病理分期 T2-T4 和淋巴结转移的患者的总生存率(a)和疾病特异性生存率(b)的生存曲线

切除其他器官。来自纪念斯隆-凯特琳癌症中心研究人员发现,在 15 年内接受 R0 手术的 800 多例患者中,约 1/3 的患者接受了伴有其他器官切除的胃癌切除手术[75,76]。术后的总死亡率为 4%,与荷兰局限性切除术试验的术后死亡率接近,显著低于伴有邻近器官切除的 D2 清扫术的患者。有趣的是,最终的病理学检查发现邻近脏器浸润的可能性很低(约为 14%),这些患者术后 5 年生存率为 32%,低于接受不伴有联合脏器切除的 R0 清扫术的患者的术后 50%的生存率。这些数据表明,在手术死亡率低的医学中心实施 R0 切除术时,应合理利用伴有多器官切除的胃癌切除术。

近几年来,使用腹腔镜、计算机辅助(机器人)手术或混合手术进行胃大部或全胃切除的微创手术有所增加。这些技术与开放手术的前瞻性高质量比较尚未完成。有多项回顾性研究进行了比较,研究提示患者的短期和长期预后得到了改善或者并没有受到微创技术的不利影响[77,78]。虽然这些技术可能会增加手术时间和成本,特别是在外科医生的学习曲线早期,但是可能会被其他节省的成本所抵消,比如患者的住院时间更短,整体恢复更快。然而,迄今为止所有的没有实现随机化的研究都受到患者选择偏倚的影响,因此我们需要谨慎解释任何可能的益处。

- 肿瘤较小、没有不良的病理特征的 T1a 胃癌可以考虑行 EMR
- 手术切除方式通常是部分或全胃切除术,伴 D1 或改良 D2 淋巴结清扫
- 当有局部侵犯时,联合其他脏器切除是合适的
- 腹腔镜和机器人技术的使用值得进一步研究

胃癌的放射治疗

组间试验(INT 0116)的结果支持术后放化疗用于胃癌[79]。胃癌患者接受完整的切除手术后随机进入术后放化疗(45Gy 的氟尿嘧啶)组或观察组。556 例可评估的患者中,大多数(85%)已发生了淋巴结转移,68%的患者有 T3/T4 肿瘤病变。3 年后,辅助放化疗组患者的生存率为 50%,而对照组为 41%($P<0.01$)。但治疗组 33%的患者有严重的胃肠道反应(3/4 级),54%的患者有严重的血液系统症状(3/4 级)。该试验确立了术后辅助放化疗作为美国胃癌切除术后的标准治疗方案。虽然在胃癌切除中清扫哪些淋巴结目前尚无一致意见,但治疗剂量应根据每个个体的肿瘤位置进行调整。有关淋巴结清扫术后淋巴结转移风险的详细数据可以指导内科医生治疗[80]。根据原发肿瘤在胃中的位置,胃周、胃网膜、腹腔、肝门、幽门下、胃十二指肠、脾脏-胰腺后及胰腺十二指肠处淋巴结可能存在转移扩散的风险。所有残胃、胃周淋巴结及腹腔干旁淋巴结转移的患者均应进行治疗。

胃癌的新辅助治疗

术前化疗

近期发布的医学研究委员会辅助胃癌灌注化疗(MAGIC)的一项试验改变了局部晚期胃癌患者治疗选择的前景[81]。该项随机 3 期试验对比了单纯手术和进行了 3 个疗程术前和术后的表柔比星、顺铂和氟尿嘧啶(ECF)化疗的两组患者的疗效。总共 503 位患者参与了该试验,氟尿嘧啶的化疗毒性是可控制的,单纯手术治疗组和 ECF 组的术后并发症率和死亡率相似。与 ECF 组患者相比,单纯接受手术治疗组患者切除的肿瘤较小(3cm vs 5cm),而且肿瘤的 T 和 N 分期较早。在中位随访时间为 4 年的术后随访中,ECF 组患者较单纯手术组患者 5 年总体生存率(36% vs 23%,$P=0.009$)和无病生存率(DFS)明显改善。该试验明确地建立了围术期患者选择 ECF 治疗方案的可行性。但必须注意只有 42%的患者完成了该治疗方案。

法国消化肿瘤学临床行动坐标(ACCORD-07)研究证实术前化疗对 GEJ 肿瘤患者有益,尽管该研究因入组率低而提前结束[82]。总共 224 例食管下段腺癌,GEJ 肿瘤或胃癌(25%)患者进行随机分配,化疗组接受 2~3 个周期的氟尿嘧啶/顺铂的术前化疗,术后再进行 3~4 个周期的相同化疗,与单纯手术组进

行比较。中位随访时间为 5.7 年。只有 50%的患者接受了术后化疗。化疗/手术组的五年生存率为 38%，而单纯手术组为 24%。相比之下，欧洲癌症研究和治疗组织（EORTC）的一项研究将患有局部晚期胃腺癌或 GEJ 肿瘤的患者随机分配到单纯手术组和化疗/手术组，术前化疗方案为顺铂、甲酰四氢叶酸和氟尿嘧啶。该试验没有发现这两种治疗方案之间存在生存差异，但由于入组率差，可能结果不佳[83]。

术后辅助化疗

过去许多有关胃癌患者系统性辅助化疗试验已被实施。早期的许多试验有些缺点，如对照组设置不合理或化疗药物选择不当。这些缺点和不同的纳入标准使得所产生的结果不具有可重复性[84]。因此，很难通过荟萃分析对这些研究结果进行总结整理而找到理想的治疗方式。而两项大型的研究却得到了相反结论[85,86]。每项研究结果都推荐了针对亚组的治疗方案，如淋巴结转移患者和亚洲患者。Win 等人汇总了几项前瞻性研究的数据，以比较胃癌 R0 切除后的化学放疗与辅助化疗效果[87]。基本发现是放化疗与较好的无病生存率相关，而总生存期没有差异。

已有研究报道了大多数的化疗药物对晚期胃癌有效，但在应用单一化疗药物进行治疗时，单药的反应率只有 15%~20%，这使得使用单一药物辅助治疗的可能性存疑。尽管如此，一些研究人员对长期持续口服氟尿嘧啶前药（S-1）充满兴趣，并取得了一些有希望的结果。研究人员在一项研究中将 1059 例Ⅱ或Ⅲ期胃癌患者，在 R0 切除及 D2 或更大范围的淋巴结清扫术后，随机分为了单纯手术组和术后应用 S-1 化疗组[88]。在 S-1 化疗组中患者的无病生存率和总生存期得到改善。S-1 治疗组的 3 年总生存率为 80.1%，单纯手术组为 70.1%（$P<0.01$）。5 年后更新分析显示，S-1 治疗组的 5 年生存率为 71.7%，单独手术组为 61.1%。

需要注意的是，S-1 的安全性在西方和亚洲患者之间不同，并且 S-1 目前在美国不可用。在一项韩国的卡培他滨和奥沙利铂在胃癌中的辅助治疗研究（CLASSIC）中，胃切除术及 D2 淋巴结清扫术后使用卡培他滨和奥沙利铂辅助化疗 6 个月与单纯手术组进行了比较[89]。该研究证明术后辅助化疗对无病生存率和总生存期有益，尤其是治疗组的 3 年 OS 为 83%，而观察组为 78%。在亚组分析中发现 N0 期患者缺乏生存获益。一项对 17 个胃癌辅助化疗随机对照试验的荟萃分析显示，与单纯手术相比，使用氟尿嘧啶辅助化疗的患者在 OS 和 DFS 上有统计学意义的显著益处[90]。

多模式治疗整合

手术是原发性胃癌治愈性治疗的基石，但怎么强调辅助治疗的重要性都不过分。除了最早期的胃癌（T1N0M0）之外，单纯手术的长期存活率仍然不是很理想。如前所述，多中心随机研究表明，与仅手术相比，两种辅助治疗具有显著的生存获益（表 90-3）。无论患者人群，肿瘤位置或淋巴结清扫程度如何，单独手术对于适合辅助治疗的早期胃癌患者而言都不再适用。由于研究设计，患者人群，淋巴结转移患者比例和淋巴结清扫程度的差异，不建议直接比较不同研究。比较有趣的是，许多辅助治疗和扩展淋巴结清扫通常与 10%左右的生存获益相关。

表 90-3 备选化疗方案

术后化疗和化放疗（INT0116 研究）
化疗（28 日，一个周期）
氟尿嘧啶 425mg/(m²·d) IV，第 1~5 日
亚叶酸 20mg/(m²·d) IV，第 1~5 日
放化疗（5 周）
氟尿嘧啶 400mg/(m²·d) IV，第 1~4 日和放疗的最后 3 日
亚叶酸 20mg/(m²·d) IV，第 1~4 日和放疗的最后 3 日
外放射治疗 总照射剂量 45Gy，每次 1.8Gy/d，5 次/周
休息恢复 1 个月
化疗（28 日，两个周期）
氟尿嘧啶 425mg/(m²·d) IV，第 1~5 日
亚叶酸 20mg/(m²·d) IV，第 1~5 日
围术期化疗（MAGIC 研究）
ECF 化疗方案（21 日/周期，3 个周期）
表柔比星 50mg/(m²·d) IV，第 1 日
顺铂 60mg/(m²·d) IV，第 1 日
氟尿嘧啶 200mg/(m²·d) CIV 1~21 日
手术前休息恢复 3~6 周的时间
手术（胃切除术/淋巴结清扫）
术后休息恢复 6~12 周的时间
ECF 化疗（21 日/周期，3 个周期）
表柔比星 50mg/(m²·d) IV，第 1 日
顺铂 60mg/(m²·d) IV，第 1 日
氟尿嘧啶 200mg/(m²·d) CIV 1~21 日

IV，静脉注射；CIV，持续静脉滴注。

我们建议考虑采用以下方法行辅助治疗。具有明显早期胃癌（IA 期）的患者或急需行手术切除（急性出血或梗阻）的患者应首先进行胃切除术，包括改良的 D2 淋巴结清扫术。在此之后，如 INT0116 研究中那样，最终病理诊断为 IB 至ⅢC 期的患者应行术后放化疗。如 MAGIC 研究中所述，进展期胃癌的患者应考虑进行围术期化疗。在任一组中，在选择初始治疗之前，应考虑使用细胞学冲洗的诊断性腹腔镜检查。对于该检查不常规的机构，如果有任何其他检查表明患者可能发生转移，则应考虑腹腔镜检查或 PET。对于亚洲患者，如果可行且时机允许应考虑使用 S-1 进行术后化疗。我们应鼓励任何符合临床试验资格的患者参加试验，包括非治疗性肿瘤标记物及其他研究。

- 事实证明，大多数行辅助治疗的胃癌患者与单独手术切除的患者相比治愈率更高
- 随机Ⅲ期试验支持行围术期化疗或术后辅助化疗联合放化疗

复发监测

NCCN 胃癌专家组推荐对所有进行治愈性治疗后的胃癌患者进行监测[91]。推荐的检查项目仅包括定期门诊随访及体格检查,实验室检查,内镜和影像学检查仅限于对特定症状或问题的评估。这种方法可能受到复发或转移情况下任何治疗的相对有限益处的影响。在复发监测中重要的是评估胃切除术后患者的营养缺乏情况,特别是维生素 B_{12}、铁和钙的水平。

转移性胃癌的治疗

晚期病例的系统治疗

对于晚期,复发或转移性胃癌患者,治疗方式主要是姑息治疗。尽管进行了大量随机试验,但这些患者的生存率仍然很低。较差的临床分期或多病灶的转移通常与很差的预后相关。对于 SEER 登记处的分析显示,在过去 30 年中,胃癌转移患者的 OS 仅有轻微改善[92]。2004 年的一项研究显示,诊断时有转移的胃癌患者平均生存期不到 5 个月[93]。临床试验报道上述患者中位生存期为 7~10 个月。考虑到这种令人沮丧的预后,一些学者观察了全身化疗对胃癌晚期患者的疗效。

4 项随机分组试验评估了姑息化疗对患者生存期和生存质量的影响[94~97]。这四项试验的结果都显示,与单纯接受最佳支持疗法(best supportive care,BSC)的患者相比较,接受姑息性治疗的患者有显著的生存优势。BSC 治疗组患者的中位生存期为 3~5 个月,而姑息性化疗组患者的平均生存期为 8~12 个月。姑息性化疗组患者的症状和生存质量也有明显改善。这些研究结果与胃癌是化疗药物敏感性疾病是一致的。化疗的副作用必须与耐药肿瘤生长产生的症状相鉴别,需平衡利弊。对于一般情况好且有营养支持的患者,应考虑姑息性化疗。

对于无症状(如那些有少量腹腔转移的患者)且肿瘤难以评估的患者,其治疗比较困难,而且有争议。虽然一些学者主张立即实施化疗,但也有人建议只做观察。只做观察的原因在于仅有 30%~40%的患者对特定的化疗方案敏感。延期治疗直至患者出现早期症状或可评估的情况,可以使患者免受不必要的毒性作用并保持生存质量。这些患者需要密切观察病史,体检,必要的时候还需 CT 检查。一旦患者的病情被评估或症状出现,就可开始治疗。但是如果出现梗阻症状(由腹膜疾病引起),则全身性治疗可能是不可行的。

基于已知治疗胃癌的单一药物活性,很多联合化疗方案逐渐发展起来。其中一项关键性试验将 ECF 与 FAMTX(氟尿嘧啶、多柔比星和甲氨蝶呤)进行了比较[98]。在该Ⅲ期试验中,274 名患者接受了治疗。ECF 组的反应率为 46%,而 FAMTX 组的反应率为 21%。此外,ECF 组的中位生存期更长(9 个月 vs 6 个月;$P<0.01$)[99]。在先前未经治疗的 GEJ 肿瘤的患者中,ECF 还和丝裂霉素,顺铂和长期静脉输注氟尿嘧啶的方案(MCF)进行了比较[100]。在该试验中,580 名患者接受了 ECF 或 MCF。ECF 的总反应率为 42%,MCF 的总反应率为 44%($P=0.69$)。只有两人因化疗毒性死亡。ECF 的中位生存期为 9.4 个月,MCF 为 8.7 个月($P=0.32$)。该研究证实了 ECF 的反应率和生存益处。

在 ECF 方案取得成功的基础上,一项Ⅲ期临床试验 REAL-2 用 2×2 的设计方法分析了卡培他滨和奥沙利铂联合治疗胃食管癌的疗效[101]。1 002 例胃癌患者随机接受了或 ECF 治疗方案,或表柔比星、顺铂、卡培他滨(ECX)治疗方案,或表柔比星、奥沙利铂、氟尿嘧啶(EOF)治疗方案或表柔比星、奥沙利铂、卡培他滨(EOX)治疗方案。约 65%的患者为胃癌或是 GEJ 肿瘤,88%为腺癌。患者对这四种治疗方案反应率和总体中位生存时间分别如下:ECF 方案,41%和 9.9 个月;ECX 方案,46%和 9.9 个月;EOF 方案,42% 和 9.3 个月;ECX 方案,48% 和 11.2 个月。研究者推断,与氟尿嘧啶对比,卡培他滨有非劣势性;与顺铂相比,奥沙利铂有非劣势性。两项临床Ⅲ期试验证实了卡培他滨和奥沙利铂在治疗胃癌方面的作用。其中的一项研究中,220 例患者随机分组接受了氟尿嘧啶、亚叶酸钙、顺铂(FLP)或氟尿嘧啶、亚叶酸钙、奥沙利铂(FLO)方案的治疗[102]。虽然 FLO 治疗组患者的反应率高于 FLP 治疗组(34% vs 25%;$P<0.01$),但两种方案的疗效随着时间的进展没有显著差别。同期进行的另外一项Ⅲ期临床研究对比卡培他滨、顺铂(XP)方案与氟尿嘧啶、顺铂(FP)方案的疗效[103]。316 例患者随机分组后接受了 XP 方案或 FP 方案的治疗。XP 组的反应率较高(41% vs 29%;$P=0.03$)。然而,无进展生存期(progression-free survival,PFS)及 OS 无显著差异。

基于多西他赛的化疗方案也已在胃癌患者中进行了广泛研究。一项随机分组的Ⅲ期临床研究对比了多西他赛、顺铂联合氟尿嘧啶(DCF)方案与氟尿嘧啶联合顺铂治疗方案的疗效差异,该研究纳入了 445 例胃癌患者[104]。DCF 治疗组患者的反应率较高(37% vs 25%;$P=0.01$),PFS 较长(中位数 5.6 个月 vs 3.4 个月;$P<0.01$),OS 也较长(9.2 个月 vs 8.6 个月;$P=0.02$)。但是,DCF 化疗方案产生了大量的治疗相关的毒性作用。确切地讲,82%的患者有 3 级或 4 级的中性粒细胞减少,69%的患者至少有一种 3 级或 4 级治疗相关的不良事件。

S-1 已经在使用不同化疗方案的若干试验中测试了其在晚期胃癌中的作用。日本学者在一项Ⅲ期临床研究(SPIRITS)中测试了 S-1 和顺铂联合治疗的疗效[105]。在该项研究中,305 例患者随机分组后接受了 S-1 联合顺铂治疗或单纯的 S-1 治疗。患者对这两种治疗方案的反应率分别为 54%和 31%,中位 PFS 分别为 6 个月和 4 个月($P<0.01$),中位 OS 分别为 13 个月和 11 个月($P=0.04$),总体上,S-1+顺铂疗效优于单用 S-1。同样,S-1 的药物代谢差异,S-1 的化疗毒性在欧洲和亚洲患者中有区别。一项全球性的Ⅲ期临床试验通过对超过 1 000 例患者的研究对比了 S-1 和氟尿嘧啶的疗效,该项目使用了 S-1 联合顺铂或氟尿嘧啶联合顺铂的化疗方案,S-1 的剂量更低,而且给药的时间也不同。遗憾的是,该研究未能良好达到总生存期的主要终点[106]。

一项研究比较了伊立替康联合氟尿嘧啶(IF)与顺铂联合氟尿嘧啶(CF)这两种化疗方案在未经化疗的胃腺癌或 GEJ 肿瘤患者中的疗效[107]。与 CF 方案相比,IF 方案并没有延长 OS,并且 IF 的非劣效性结果是临界的。在一项日本的研究中,与单用 S-1 相比,伊立替康联合 S1 仍未能延长 OS[108]。然而,最近一项对 416 名病例的Ⅲ期临床研究显示,FOLFIRI 方案的治疗失败中位时间显著长于 ECX 方案(5.1 个月 vs 4.2 个月;$P<0.01$)[109]。而在 PFS、中位 OS(9.5 个月 vs 9.7 个月)或反应率方面没有差异。总之,伊立替康联合氟尿嘧啶方案是可接受的一线治疗方案。

在二线方案中,已经证明三种药物可以提高最佳支持疗法的生存率。德国肿瘤内科工作组(AIO)研究中将伊立替康联合最佳支持疗法与单独应用最佳支持疗法在晚期胃癌或 GEJ 腺癌患者中进行了比较[110],伊立替康能延长 OS。在 COUGAR-02 研究中,186 名患者被随机分为多西他赛联合 BSC 和单独使用 BSC 两组,化疗组的中位 OS 为 5.2 个月,而 BSC 组为 3.6 个月($P=0.01$)[111]。

分子靶向药物

尽管有新的化疗药物问世并应用于胃癌治疗,但由于化疗药的毒副作用,患者的中位生存时间很难超过 1 年。靶向药物的使用使患者的 OS,PFS 及反应率得到适度的改善。靶向治疗药物也在二线治疗方案中进行了探索。EGFR 家族是研究最广泛的受体之一。一些研究已经研究了在细胞毒性化学疗法中加入 EGFR 抑制剂。初步的Ⅱ期试验产生了有希望的结果。然而,Ⅲ期试验结果令人失望,将西妥昔单抗(针对 EGFR 的嵌合单克隆抗体(mAb))添加到卡培他滨和顺铂(XP)的化疗方案中,与单独应用 XP 相比并没有提供额外的益处[112]。此外,与表柔比星、奥沙利铂和卡培他滨(EOC)相比,帕尼单抗(一种完全人源化的抗 EGFR 单克隆抗体)加入 EOC 方案后导致 OS 较差(8.8 个月 vs 11.3 个月)[113]。故不建议在胃癌治疗中使用这两种药物。

一些研究已经报道了其他分子靶向药物更有希望的结果。HER2/neu(也是 EGFR 家族的成员)在 20%的胃癌和 30%的 GEJ 肿瘤中过表达。该受体已被证明是治疗这些肿瘤的关键靶点。曲妥珠单抗(人源化单克隆抗体)已被证明可以延长生存期,当加入化疗时可使 OS 从 11.1 个月增加至 13.8 个月($P<0.01$)[114]。与其他实体瘤一样,血管生成已被证明是胃癌进展的重要组成部分。血管内皮生长因子抑制剂贝伐单抗在Ⅲ期临床试验中进行了研究[115]。共有 774 名患有晚期胃癌或 GEJ 肿瘤的患者被随机分配接受贝伐单抗或安慰剂加顺铂联合卡培他滨的化疗方案[115]。三联疗法组的中位 OS 为 12.1 个月,而安慰剂组为 10.1 个月($P<0.01$)。贝伐单抗组的 PFS(6.7 个月 vs 5.3 个月)和反应率(46%对 37%)也有所改善。然而,该研究未达到其主要终点。进一步的亚组分析显示,北美和拉丁美洲患者似乎在添加贝伐单抗后具有生存获益(中位数为 11.5 个月,而安慰剂组为 6.8 个月),而在亚洲注册的患者(90%来自日本和韩国)似乎没有效益。欧洲的患者的疗效处于中间水平。

REGARD 试验是一项随机Ⅲ期临床试验,比较了雷莫芦单抗与安慰剂在未经治疗的进展期胃癌患者中的疗效,最近这项试验的结果已发表[116]。雷莫芦单抗是一种结合 VEGF-R2 并阻止其活化的单克隆抗体,与安慰组相比其改善了 OS(5.2 个月 vs 3.8 个月,$P=0.05$)。在随后的 RAINBOW 试验中,紫杉醇联合雷莫芦单抗与单独应用紫杉醇相比,显示了雷莫芦单抗在进展期胃癌患者中的生存优势[117]。665 名患者被分配接受紫杉醇加安慰剂或紫杉醇加雷莫芦单抗。雷莫芦单抗加紫杉醇组的中位 OS 明显延长(9.6 个月 vs 7.4 个月,$P=0.02$)。这种组合已被提议作为进展期胃癌患者二线治疗的新标准。

在未经治疗的转移性胃癌患者中,有关靶向药物疗效的研究结果令人失望。GRANITE-1 研究将 656 名患者随机分配到依维莫司联合最佳支持疗法组和安慰剂联合最佳支持疗法组[118]。依维莫司没有改善 OS(依维莫司中位数为 5.4 个月,安慰剂组为 4.3 个月)。同样,在 420 例 HER2/neu 阳性胃癌患者中,拉帕替尼联合紫杉醇与单独使用紫杉醇进行了比较[119]。拉帕替尼联合紫杉醇组中位 OS 为 11.0 个月,而单独使用紫杉醇组为 8.9 个月($P=0.21$)。尽管采用不同的治疗策略并将新靶向药物纳入标准化疗,但晚期胃癌患者的预后仍然很差。当然我们也需要进一步的研究。

支持治疗

胃癌患者可能出现的症状包括出血、梗阻、疼痛、早饱和体重下降。在考虑胃癌手术切除的适应证时必须仔细考虑手术意图,是为了治愈还是缓解症状或者解决其他与癌症相关的问题。没有发生转移但出现严重症状的患者应考虑先进行胃切除术,然后进行辅助治疗。对于在纽约纪念医院斯隆-凯特琳癌症研究中心接受非根治性切除的 307 例胃癌患者,大约有一半的患者进行了姑息性切除,最常见的原因是出血(20%)、梗阻(43%)或疼痛(29%)[120]。在发生转移的患者中,姑息性切除与术后高死亡率(14%)和并发症(27%)有关[121]。在最近的系列研究中,死亡率降至<5%,但实施手术时应非常谨慎。短路手术在姑息性治疗中也与高死亡率相关,并且经常不能达到预期的效果[122,123]。

在考虑姑息性切除时,外科医生应确定患者症状的程度。例如,虽然完全阻塞的患者可能仅受益于手术切除,短路手术或内镜下支架置入等干预,但在化疗患者中,高达 80%的患者可能会出现不完全阻塞的症状[124]。因此,梗阻可能是手术的相对指征,而不是绝对的。疼痛可能由于癌细胞在腹腔神经丛浸润生长,肠道梗阻或癌细胞的骨转移而引起。消化道梗阻使疼痛的治疗更加复杂。在没有梗阻的情况下,可以早期口服长效麻醉镇痛药。然而,一旦患者有梗阻症状,必须利用其他的方法来缓解疼痛。

大量的危及生命的出血需要动脉栓塞或内镜来处理,但在一些情况下也要考虑手术切除以控制出血。胃癌大量出血的患者应考虑切除,但在缺乏完整的分期评估时,必须作好在术中发现转移而改变手术意图的心理准备。在发生转移时,医生必须确定大量出血的患者是否考虑手术,如果不考虑手术,则专注于最佳支持治疗。偶尔,内镜和栓塞操作可以争取必要的时间来进行这些复杂情况的讨论。对于慢性渗血,每 1~2 周需要一次输血的患者,可以进行内镜治疗。一系列的研究表明,50%~75%患者的出血、胃出口梗阻和疼痛可以得到改善[125,126]。

梗阻的治疗方法包括激光再通、支架置放、放射疗法、短路手术、放置胃管或手术切除。在过去的二十年里,可扩张支架技术已有了很大的发展。Dormann 回顾分析了 136 例对内扩展支架的报道,其中 32 位患者是胃十二指肠恶性肿瘤,超过 90%的患者成功地接受了支架置入治疗,并且没有发生手术操作相关的死亡，并发症也相对较少[127]。但缓解症状可能是暂时的，在18%的病例中，由于瘤体的增长再次发生了梗阻。一般来说，由于无法切除的原发性肿瘤或发生转移而导致严重胃出口梗阻的患者存活率较低（中位数约为2个月），但内镜支架或手术短路等干预措施与提高术后生活质量有关[128]。对于具有状态良好和较长预期寿命的患者，应考虑采用短路手术。阻塞位于幽门或上端十二指肠，阻塞长度短且为单个阻塞部位是内镜支架术的最佳适应证。身体状态不好的患者，快速进展的癌症，癌病，恶性腹水，多个梗阻部位以及非常短的预期寿命可能最好采用经皮胃造瘘术或不进行干预。

胃癌治疗的不足与展望

临床医生和研究人员有很多机会为胃癌患者的治疗做出改进。近年来发表了许多令人兴奋的研究来探索改善胃癌治疗的新方法，例如静脉注射利多卡因以更好地控制术后疼痛[129]，前哨淋巴结定位[130,131]，术后早期肠内免疫营养[132]，以及通过使用外科体外解剖以改进病理分期[133]。胃癌治疗的进一步发展必须继续建立在我们对胃癌的分子发病机制的理解，强大的高质量的临床结果，以及疗效比较研究的基础上。

在预防和筛查领域，仍存在几个问题。我们是否应该促进根除幽门螺杆菌的努力？是否应该为西方高风险患者开发上消化道内镜筛查项目？就胃癌的正确分期而言，我们尚未确定哪些患者从治疗前的EUS或PET中受益最大。随着包括EMR和微创手术在内的许多方法可用于胃癌的手术切除，制订被广泛接受的手术实施标准、大规模临床研究以及关于术前质量和长期随访的公开研究势在必行。虽然姑息性胃切除术等一些决定总是需要考虑患者的个体差异，但其他考虑因素如淋巴结清扫范围可能最好通过证据和最佳实践来定义，而不是个别外科医生的偏见。

哪些患者应选择术前化疗或术后放化疗这两种基本辅助治疗，目前尚无定论。此外，对于术前化疗后无反应或出现进展的患者，术后应采取何种治疗，是替代化疗方案还是放化疗？关于胃癌最佳治疗的这些问题只是这个难题的一部分。对于新的研究来说，处理具有挑战性的术后症状，如胃排空延迟或胃功能低下，这方面的研究已经非常成熟。胃癌治疗有许多尚未解决的问题，但幸运的是，正在进行的一些研究对此很有兴趣。

结论

幸运的是，全世界胃癌的发病率正在下降。然而，许多人的治疗结果仍然很差，整体治愈率很低。虽然在胃癌治疗（包括手术，化疗和放疗）方面取得了令人鼓舞的进展，但是许多胃癌患者仍然会出现症状，健康相关生活质量降低，并且尽管有最好的治疗，但最终还是会死于胃癌。在未来，我们希望早期确定胃癌高危人群的能力将有助于制订具有成本效益的筛查方案和预防措施。随着我们进入分子靶向治疗和个性化医疗的时代，我们对分子生物学和胃癌的分子分型的认识不断提高，可能导致新的治疗策略的发展。我们希望，在我们的一生中，胃癌治疗的面貌发生变化，使得大多数胃癌患者在治疗后获得痊愈。

（胡海涛 徐泉 译 田艳涛 校）

参考文献

The complete reference list can be found on the Wiley Companion Digital Edition of this title (see inside front cover for login instructions).

7 Ford AC, Forman D, Hunt RH, Yuan Y, Moayyedi P. *Helicobacter pylori* eradication therapy to prevent gastric cancer in healthy asymptomatic infected individuals: systematic review and meta-analysis of randomised controlled trials. *BMJ* (Clinical research ed.). 2014;**348**:g3174.

14 Caldas C, Carneiro F, Lynch HT, et al. Familial gastric cancer: overview and guidelines for management. *J Med Genet*. 1999;**36**(**12**):873–880.

15 Huntsman DG, Carneiro F, Lewis FR, et al. Early gastric cancer in young, asymptomatic carriers of germ-line E-cadherin mutation. *N Engl J Med*. 2001;**344**(**25**):1904–1909.

20 Lauren P. The two histological main types of gastric carcinoma: diffuse and so-called intestinal-type carcinoma. An attempt at a histoclinical classification. *Acta Pathol Microbiol Scand*. 1965;**64**:31–49.

35 Lee EY, Cibull ML, Strodel WE, Haley JV. Expression of HER-2/neu oncoprotein and epidermal growth factor receptor and prognosis in gastric carcinoma. *Arch Pathol Lab Med*. 1994;**118**(**3**):235–239.

45 Yonemura Y, Endo Y, Fujita H, et al. Role of vascular endothelial growth factor C expression in the development of lymph node metastasis in gastric cancer. *Clin Cancer Res*. 1999;**5**(**7**):1823–1829.

49 Lordick F, Ott K, Krause BJ, et al. PET to assess early metabolic response and to guide treatment of adenocarcinoma of the oesophagogastric junction: the MUNICON phase II trial. *Lancet Oncology*. 2007;**8**(**9**):797–805.

52 Burke EC, Karpeh MS, Conlon KC, Brennan MF. Laparoscopy in the management of gastric adenocarcinoma. *Ann Surg*. 1997;**225**:262–267.

56 Gotoda T. Endoscopic resection of early gastric cancer. *Gastric Cancer*. 2007;**10**(**1**):1–11.

57 Bozzetti F, Marubini E, Bonfanti G, Miceli R, Piano C, Gennari L. Subtotal versus total gastrectomy for gastric cancer. Five year survival rates in a multicenter randomized Italian trial. *Ann Surg*. 1999;**230**:170–178.

62 Siewert J, Bottcher K, Stein H, Roder J, Busch R. Problem of proximal third gastric carcinoma. *World J Surg*. 1995;**19**:523–531.

66 Spector NM, Hicks FD, Pickleman J. Quality of life and symptoms after surgery for gastroesophageal cancer: a pilot study. *Gastroenterol Nurs*. 2002;**25**(**3**):120–125.

68 Bonenkamp JJ, Hermans J, Sasako M, van de Velde CJ. Extended lymph-node dissection for gastric cancer. Dutch Gastric Cancer Group. *N Engl J Med*. 1999;**340**(**12**):908–914.

69 Hartgrink HH, van de Velde CJ, Putter H, et al. Extended lymph node dissection for gastric cancer: who may benefit? Final results of the randomized Dutch gastric cancer group trial. *J Clin Oncol*. 2004;**22**(**11**):2069–2077.

70 Songun I, Putter H, Kranenbarg EM, Sasako M, van de Velde CJ. Surgical treatment of gastric cancer: 15-year follow-up results of the randomised nationwide Dutch D1D2 trial. *Lancet Oncol*. 2010;**11**(**5**):439–449.

74 Squires MH 3rd, Kooby DA, Pawlik TM, et al. Utility of the proximal margin frozen section for resection of gastric adenocarcinoma: a 7-Institution Study of the US Gastric Cancer Collaborative. *Ann Surg Oncol*. 2014;**21**(**13**):4202–4210.

78 Lee JH, Lee CM, Son SY, Ahn SH, Park do J, Kim HH. Laparoscopic versus open gastrectomy for gastric cancer: long-term oncologic results. *Surgery*. 2014;**155**(**1**):154–164.

79 Macdonald JS, Smalley SR, Benedetti J, et al. Chemoradiotherapy after surgery compared with surgery alone for adenocarcinoma of the stomach or gastroesophageal junction. *N Engl J Med*. 2001;**345**(**10**):725–730.

81 Cunningham D, Allum WH, Stenning SP, et al. Perioperative chemotherapy versus surgery alone for resectable gastroesophageal cancer. *N Engl J Med*. 2006;**355**(**1**):11–20.

82 Ychou M, Boige V, Pignon JP, et al. Perioperative chemotherapy compared with surgery alone for resectable gastroesophageal adenocarcinoma: an FNCLCC and FFCD multicenter phase III trial. *J Clin Oncol*. 2011;**29**(**13**):1715–1721.

83 Schuhmacher C, Gretschel S, Lordick F, et al. Neoadjuvant chemotherapy compared with surgery alone for locally advanced cancer of the stomach and cardia: European Organisation for Research and Treatment of Cancer randomized trial 40954. *J Clin Oncol*. 2010;**28**(**35**):5210–5218.

87 Min C, Bangalore S, Jhawar S, et al. Chemoradiation therapy versus chemotherapy alone for gastric cancer after R0 surgical resection: a meta-analysis of randomized trials. *Oncology*. 2014;**86**(**2**):79–85.

88 Sakuramoto S, Sasako M, Yamaguchi T, et al. Adjuvant chemotherapy for gastric cancer with S-1, an oral fluoropyrimidine. *N Engl J Med*. 2007;**357**(**18**):1810–1820.

89 Bang YJ, Kim YW, Yang HK, et al. Adjuvant capecitabine and oxaliplatin for gastric cancer after D2 gastrectomy (CLASSIC): a phase 3 open-label, randomised controlled trial. *Lancet*. 2012;**379(9813)**:315–321.

94 Glimelius B, Ekstrom K, Hoffman K, et al. Randomized comparison between chemotherapy plus best supportive care with best supportive care in advanced gastric cancer. *Ann Oncol*. 1997;**8(2)**:163–168.

98 Waters JS, Norman A, Cunningham D, et al. Long-term survival after epirubicin, cisplatin and fluorouracil for gastric cancer: results of a randomized trial. *Br J Cancer*. 1999;**80(1–2)**:269–272.

101 Cunningham D, Starling N, Rao S, et al. Capecitabine and oxaliplatin for advanced esophagogastric cancer. *N Engl J Med*. 2008;**358(1)**:36–46.

104 Van Cutsem E, Moiseyenko VM, Tjulandin S, et al. Phase III study of docetaxel and cisplatin plus fluorouracil compared with cisplatin and fluorouracil as first-line therapy for advanced gastric cancer: a report of the V325 Study Group. *J Clin Oncol*. 2006;**24(31)**:4991–4997.

105 Koizumi W, Narahara H, Hara T, et al. S-1 plus cisplatin versus S-1 alone for first-line treatment of advanced gastric cancer (SPIRITS trial): a phase III trial. *Lancet Oncol*. 2008;**9(3)**:215–221.

110 Thuss-Patience PC, Kretzschmar A, Bichev D, et al. Survival advantage for irinotecan versus best supportive care as second-line chemotherapy in gastric cancer – a randomised phase III study of the Arbeitsgemeinschaft Internistische Onkologie (AIO). *Eur J Cancer* (Oxford, England : 1990). 2011;**47(15)**:2306–2314.

111 Ford HE, Marshall A, Bridgewater JA, et al. Docetaxel versus active symptom control for refractory oesophagogastric adenocarcinoma (COUGAR-02): an open-label, phase 3 randomised controlled trial. *Lancet Oncol*. 2014;**15(1)**:78–86.

112 Lordick F, Kang YK, Chung HC, et al. Capecitabine and cisplatin with or without cetuximab for patients with previously untreated advanced gastric cancer (EXPAND): a randomised, open-label phase 3 trial. *Lancet Oncol*. 2013;**14(6)**:490–499.

113 Waddell T, Chau I, Cunningham D, et al. Epirubicin, oxaliplatin, and capecitabine with or without panitumumab for patients with previously untreated advanced oesophagogastric cancer (REAL3): a randomised, open-label phase 3 trial. *Lancet Oncol*. 2013;**14(6)**:481–489.

114 Bang YJ, Van Cutsem E, Feyereislova A, et al. Trastuzumab in combination with chemotherapy versus chemotherapy alone for treatment of HER2-positive advanced gastric or gastro-oesophageal junction cancer (ToGA): a phase 3, open-label, randomised controlled trial. *Lancet*. 2010;**376(9742)**:687–697.

117 Wilke H, Muro K, Van Cutsem E, et al. Ramucirumab plus paclitaxel versus placebo plus paclitaxel in patients with previously treated advanced gastric or gastro-oesophageal junction adenocarcinoma (RAINBOW): a double-blind, randomised phase 3 trial. *Lancet Oncol*. 2014;**15(11)**:1224–1235.

118 Ohtsu A, Ajani JA, Bai YX, et al. Everolimus for previously treated advanced gastric cancer: results of the randomized, double-blind, phase III GRANITE-1 study. *J Clin Oncol*. 2013;**31(31)**:3935–3943.

119 Satoh T, Xu RH, Chung HC, et al. Lapatinib plus paclitaxel versus paclitaxel alone in the second-line treatment of HER2-amplified advanced gastric cancer in Asian populations: TyTAN – a randomized, phase III study. *J Clin Oncol*. 2014;**32(19)**:2039–2049.

120 Miner TJ, Jaques DP, Karpeh MS, Brennan MF. Defining palliative surgery in patients receiving noncurative resections for gastric cancer. *J Am Coll Surg*. 2004;**198(6)**:1013–1021.

121 Lasithiotakis K, Antoniou SA, Antoniou GA, Kaklamanos I, Zoras O. Gastrectomy for stage IV gastric cancer. a systematic review and meta-analysis. *Anticancer Res*. 2014;**34(5)**:2079–2085.

127 Dormann A, Meisner S, Verin N, Wenk LA. Self-expanding metal stents for gastroduodenal malignancies: systematic review of their clinical effectiveness. *Endoscopy*. 2004;**36(6)**:543–550.

第 91 章　原发肝脏肿瘤

Junichi Shindoh, MD, PhD ■ Kristoffer W. Brudvik, MD, PhD ■ Jean-Nicolas Vauthey, MD

概述

原发性肝癌是导致男性癌症死亡的第二大原因，也是导致女性癌症死亡的第六大原因。肝细胞癌(HCC)占原发性肝肿瘤的 70%~85%，其次是肝内胆管癌(ICC)(10%~15%)和其他较少见的肝恶性肿瘤(5%)，如肝血管肉瘤、上皮样血管内皮瘤以及肝淋巴瘤。原发性肝恶性肿瘤通常预后较差，目前系统性治疗的循证医学证据有限，预防、监测、早期诊断和多学科治疗能最大限度提高治疗效果。此外，大多数原发性肝肿瘤与慢性肝病或肝硬化有关，肝功能储备的减少往往影响对肿瘤的积极治疗。因此，在选择治疗方案时，应充分考虑可治愈性和安全性这两个内在矛盾因素。目前，在制订 HCC 的治疗方案时，有几种临床分期系统和治疗流程可供选择。治疗方案的制订要根据患者的肿瘤负荷、潜在肝病的严重程度、患者的自身状态治疗副作用以及并发症的发生率与可接受的结局的平衡进行个体化选择。治疗方案应结合当前的专业知识，由多学科联合制订。在没有禁忌证的情况下，包括手术切除、射频消融术和原位肝移植(OLT)在内的最具疗效的治疗方案应是首选。对于其他肝脏恶性肿瘤，目前临床证据有限，手术切除或 OLT 被认为是一线治疗。

肝脏是所有内脏静脉血在回流到心脏之前经过的一个特殊脏器。因此，肝脏是胃肠道恶性肿瘤转移的最常见部位，这种肿瘤被称为继发性肝肿瘤。然而，肿瘤也可能由肝内的细胞产生，被称为原发性肝肿瘤。原发性肝肿瘤中，肝细胞癌(HCC)是最常见的恶性肿瘤，占原发性肝癌的 70%~85%，其次是肝内胆管癌(ICC)(10%~15%)和其他不太常见的肝脏恶性肿瘤(5%)，如肝血管肉瘤，上皮样血管内皮瘤(EHE)，血管外皮细胞瘤，或肝淋巴瘤。由于原发性肝恶性肿瘤通常预后较差，而且目前已有的系统性治疗证据十分有限，因此早期诊断和多学科综合治疗对于改善患者长期预后十分重要。本章将回顾和讨论 HCC、ICC 和其他不太常见的原发性肝癌的临床特征和目前的治疗方法。

肝细胞癌

发病率和流行病学

原发性肝癌在男性常见癌症中发病率位居第五，女性常见癌症中发病率位居第六，是男性癌症死亡的第二大原因，女性癌症死亡的第六大原因，全球每年约有 69.55 万人死于原发性肝癌[1]。近 85%的病例发生在发展中国家，特别是撒哈拉以南非洲和东亚以及东南亚，其典型发病率高于 20/100 000。发达国家的发病率普遍较低，但日本除外，在日本丙型肝炎病毒(HCV)感染是 HCC 最常见的病因。

在全球范围内，一些既往发病率较低的地区，肝癌的发病率在正在增加，包括大洋洲、中欧和北美的部分地区[2,3]。2009 年的一项研究表明，1975—2005 年，美国 HCC 年龄标准化发病率增加了两倍，从每 10 万人 1.6 例增至每 10 万人 4.9 例[2]。相比之下，在中国和新加坡等既往高发地区，肝癌的发病率正在下降，这很可能是由于公共卫生的改善减少了乙肝病毒(HBV)感染。

在不同的地理区域，男性的 HCC 发病率是女性的两倍多[4]。HCC 的发病率随年龄增长而增加，但由于 HCC 的主要病因不同，各国的年龄阈值有所不同。当主要危险因素是 HBV 母婴垂直传播时(如东南亚和非洲)，HCC 的年龄阈值通常较低，而当成年期获得性 HCV 感染是 HCC 最常见的原因(如日本和美国)，HCC 的年龄阈值更大。

危险因素

肝硬化是主要的危险因素，在 80%的 HCC 患者中存在。据推测，多种原因引起的慢性肝细胞损伤和炎症可导致肝硬化和 HCC，这是肝细胞再生和增生导致基因突变和恶性转化的结果。

病毒性肝炎(HBV 和 HCV)

据估计，75%~80%的 HCC 与 HBV(50%~55%)或 HCV(25%~30%)的慢性感染有关[5]。HBV 的传播主要发生在分娩(垂直传播)、输血、性交或经静脉注射毒品期间。丙型肝炎病毒也可通过肠外途径传播，主要传播途径是输血和经静脉注射毒品。

HBV 是一种双链 DNA 病毒，慢性 HBV 感染是 HCC 最常见的病因，尤其是在中国和韩国。乙型肝炎表面抗原(HBsAg)阳性患者患肝硬化和 HCC 的风险很高。然而据报道，即使 HBsAg 在血清学上呈阴性，抗乙肝核心抗体(HBcAb)阳性的患者也有较高的 HCC 风险[6]。与 HCV 相关的 HCC(通常发生在伴有严重纤维化或肝硬化的肝脏中)相比，约 20%的 HBV 相关 HCC 发生在没有肝硬化改变的情况下。HBV 具有直接致突变作用，可导致癌变。HBV DNA 与细胞癌基因相邻的宿主基因组整合或 HBx 蛋白对细胞基因表达的反活化作用可能是未发生肝硬化的 HCC 发生的原因[7~9]。事实上，HBsAg 阳性患者在肿瘤发生前肝细胞中就已经检测到 HBV-DNA 的整合，这可能会增强染色体的不稳定性，促进 HCC 的发生[10,11]。

丙型肝炎病毒是一种小型单链 RNA 病毒。丙型肝炎病毒感染的流行因地理区域的不同而有很大差异。一项对 21 例病例对照研究的荟萃分析显示，HCV 阳性个体患 HCC 的风险是 HCV 阴性个体的 17 倍[12]。氧化应激是 HCV 感染患者炎症相关肿瘤发生的机制之一[13]。在病毒抗原的作用下，活化的巨噬细胞和其他募集的白细胞释放活性氧，导致局部坏死和代偿性细胞分裂[14]。当这些氧化剂超过邻近细胞的抗氧化防御能力时，对生物分子的破坏，特别是对致癌基因或抑癌基因的破坏，可能会增加肝脏的致癌风险。HCV 表现出高度的遗传变异。根据核苷酸序列同源性，将全序列丙型肝炎病毒分离株分为 1a、1b、2a 和 2b 四种基因型。这些基因型有不同的地理分布特点，1a、1b 和 2a 型在西方国家和东亚占主导地位，而 2b 型在中东占主导地位[15]。据报道，丙型肝炎病毒 1b 基因型更具侵袭性，与肝硬化和 HCC 等晚期慢性肝病关系更密切。这些观察结果部分解释了病原体对抗病毒治疗的耐受，最近的研究表明，无论 HCV 的基因型如何，HCV 病毒载量的降低与肝癌手术切除后生存率的提高有关[16,17]。

酒精

酗酒是慢性肝病和 HCC 的主要危险因素，可导致从单纯脂肪堆积到肝硬化的不同程度的肝损害。多项研究表明，过量饮酒是 HCC 发生的重要危险因素。美国的一项病例对照研究显示，每天饮酒超过 60ml 的重度饮酒者 HCC 风险增加了约三倍[18]。HCC 在没有肝硬化的情况下很少发生；然而假如伴随 HBV 或 HCV 感染，这种风险会增加[19,20]。一篇纳入 1995—2004 年间发表的 20 项回顾性研究，涉及 15 000 名慢性丙型肝炎患者的荟萃分析表明，与不饮酒或少量饮酒相比，过量饮酒导致肝硬化的相对风险为 2. 33[19]。因此，病毒性肝炎患者应避免饮酒。

黄曲霉毒素

黄曲霉毒素（AF）是一种由黄曲霉和寄生曲霉产生的强效肝脏致癌物，在温暖、潮湿的环境下，黄曲霉很容易在玉米和花生等食物上生长。AF 有 B_1、B_2、G_1、G_2 四种化合物，其中最常见、毒性最大的 AF 化合物为 AFB_1。当摄入 AFB_1 时，它会代谢成一种高度活跃的 8,9-环氧化合物代谢物，这种代谢物可以与 DNA 结合并破坏 DNA。在肿瘤抑制基因 *p53* 的 249 密码子中发现了一个一致的基因突变，并且与 AF 的暴露呈正相关[21,22]。虽然 AFB_1 增加肝癌发生的风险，但其在 HCC 发病中的作用主要是通过其与慢性乙型肝炎的协同作用介导的，因为存在 AFB_1 暴露的环境问题的地区也有很高的慢性 HBV 感染率。一项来自中国的前瞻性研究表明，尿液排泄 AF 代谢物使 HCC 发生风险增加高达 4 倍，而 HBV 感染作为一个独立因素增加了 7 倍的风险。然而，尿液中排泄出 AFB_1 代谢物并同时感染 HBV 的患者发生 HCC 的风险增加了 60 倍[23]。这些结果表明，预防 HBV 相关 HCC 可降低 AF 对 HCC 发生风险的影响。

肥胖

肥胖与许多肝胆疾病（包括脂肪肝、肝脂肪变性、脂肪性肝炎和不明原因的肝硬化）密切相关[24,25]。在美国的一项大型前瞻性队列研究中，90 多万人进行了为期 16 年的跟踪调查，基线体重指数最高的男性（范围 35 ~ 40）的肝癌死亡率是正常体重指数男性的 5 倍，而女性患肝癌的风险没有那么高，相对风险为 1. 68[26]。来自北欧的另外两项以普通人群为基础的研究也表明，肥胖与 HCC 风险增加有关[27,28]。

糖尿病

近年来，糖尿病被认为是慢性肝病和 HCC 的危险因素。虽然在横断面和病例对照研究中调整潜在的偏差是困难的，但有几项研究明确表明糖尿病和 HCC 之间呈正相关[29~33]。2 型糖尿病引起肝细胞损伤的机制包括胰岛素抵抗和高胰岛素血症两种假说[34,35]。据报道，高胰岛素血症降低了肝脏合成和血液中胰岛素样生长因子结合蛋白-1（IGFBP-1）的水平，从而增加了：①胰岛素样生长因子-1（IGF-1）的生物利用度；②促进细胞增殖；③抑制细胞凋亡[36]。过量的胰岛素与胰岛素受体结合，激活其固有的酪氨酸激酶，导致胰岛素受体底物-1（IRS-1）磷酸化[37]，高胰岛素血症也与活性氧的产生有关，而活性氧的产生可能会对 DNA 造成损伤。过度的 IRS-1 与细胞凋亡的减少有关，这一过程通过转化生长因子 β 介导[38]。在基础研究和病理检查中均有证据表明，HCC 肿瘤细胞过度表达 IGF-1 和 IRS-1[39]，糖尿病可能是肝细胞损伤和 HCC 发生发展的原因之一。

血红蛋白沉着症

血红蛋白沉着症是一种与铁代谢相关的常染色体隐性遗传疾病，在高加索人群中患病率为 2. 5‰。在这种遗传性疾病中，6 号染色体上的 *HFE* 基因（Cys282Tyr［C282Y］和 His63Asp［H63D］）、1 号染色体上的 *HFR-2* 基因和 7 号染色体上的 *HFE-3* 基因均发生了突变。*C282Y* 突变是最常见的检测突变，*C282Y* 纯合子或 *C282Y/H63D* 复合杂合子[40~42]与膳食中铁的吸收增加和皮肤、心脏、肝脏等组织铁元素的积累有关，可导致心力衰竭或肝硬化。越来越多的证据表明，即使是微量的铁积累也对肝脏有害，尤其是当存在慢性病毒性肝炎或大量饮酒等其他肝毒性因素时。铁元素的累积增强了微生物的致病性，对巨噬细胞和淋巴细胞的功能产生不利影响，促进了组织纤维化[43]。丙型肝炎病毒感染与肝组织中铁元素超负荷之间存在协同关系[44]，而铁元素的缺乏已被报道可改善慢性丙型肝炎患者的肝功能[45]。虽然血红蛋白沉着症的诊断相对困难，但在肝硬化发病前采用治疗性放血或铁螯合疗法，对预防肝硬化和 HCC 的发生可能是有效的。

α_1-抗胰蛋白酶缺乏

α_1-抗胰蛋白酶缺乏（AATD）是一种常染色体显性遗传疾病，由丝氨酸蛋白酶抑制剂（Pi）基因突变引起。超过 75 个不同的 Pi 等位基因已经被鉴定，其中大多数与疾病无关[46]，然而 Pi 表型与血清中 α_1-抗胰蛋白酶浓度有关。AATD 患者的典型临床表现包括肺气肿、肝坏死性炎症、肝硬化和 HCC。由于没有有效的药物治疗，肝移植被应用于失代偿期肝硬化患者以纠正潜在的代谢紊乱。

其他潜在风险因素

男性肝癌的发生率高于女性，提示激素因素对肝癌发生的影响。长期口服避孕药被认为是肝癌的潜在危险因素；然而，对 12 项病例对照研究的回顾显示，总体调整优势比为 1. 6（95%*CI*：0. 9 ~ 2. 5）[47]，口服避孕药与 HCC 风险之间的相关性仍不确定。

甲状腺功能减退也被报道为 HCC 的潜在危险因素，尤其是在女性中[48,49]。甲状腺功能减退患者可能会出现体重增加[50]和胰岛素抵抗[51,52]，两者都是非酒精性脂肪性肝炎的重要因素。虽然其作用机制尚不清楚，临床证据也很有限，但这些激素因子可能在一定程度上影响慢性肝病和肝癌的发生发展。

预防

肝癌的预防主要取决于避免危险因素、对潜在的慢性肝病给予足够的治疗和早期诊断癌前病变。由于 HCC 最常见的病因是与病毒性肝炎相关的肝硬化，因此预防 HBV/HCV 感染和抗病毒治疗慢性肝炎是预防肝癌最重要的措施。对于乙型肝炎，在发展中国家，肠外接触是最常见的传播原因，改善卫生条件和公共教育对避免病毒传播至关重要。此外，乙肝病毒的疫苗接种和有效的抗病毒治疗目前是可行的预防手段。乙肝疫苗接种开始后，在中国台湾等高风险地区，HCC 的发病率有显著下降[53]。HBV 感染被确诊后，目前已有多种有效的抗病毒药物可使用，据报道，病毒载量的减少与慢性乙型肝炎患者 HCC 风险的降低和生存结局的改善有关[54~56]。

对于丙型肝炎，以干扰素（IFN）为基础的联合治疗已成为标准的疗法，并且可以降低 HCC 的发病风险，特别是在实现了持续病毒应答（SVR）的患者中[57~60]。然而，HCV 的遗传变异严重影响抗病毒治疗的有效性。虽然目前仅有少量的临床证据，但最近研发的新型直接作用抗病毒药物（DAA）已经显著提高了病毒学应答率，在不久的将来可能有助于预防慢性丙型肝炎患者中的 HCC[61~63]。

病理学

肝细胞向 HCC 的恶性转化被认为是一个多步骤的过程，与基因突变、等位基因丢失、表观遗传学改变和分子细胞通路的扰动有关。然而，肝癌在分子水平癌变过程尚不清楚。这些潜在的多步骤改变的性状表现为前体病变，其大小、颜色、质地和切面隆起程度可与周围肝硬化再生结节相鉴别。肿瘤血供的变化对应于从前驱病变到典型 HCC 的多步骤过程的每一步，有助于 CT 或 MRI 动态研究的鉴别诊断。（图 91-1）

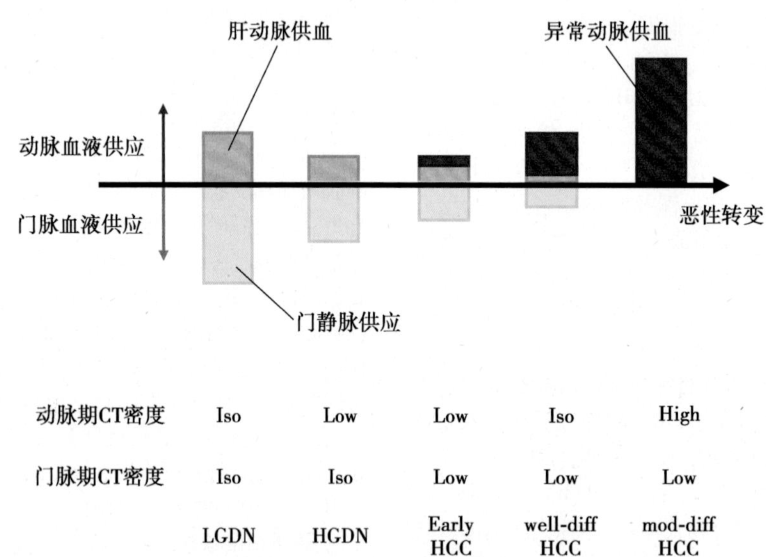

动脉期CT密度	Iso	Low	Low	Iso	High
门脉期CT密度	Iso	Iso	Low	Low	Low
	LGDN	HGDN	Early HCC	well-diff HCC	mod-diff HCC

图 91-1 一个血液供应从前体病变到典型肝细胞癌的动态变化模型。动脉和门静脉供应的动态变化和异常动脉供应的指数增长与动态 CT 或 MRI 的典型增强模式相关。LGDN，低级别发育不良结节；HGDN，高度发育不良结节；HCC，肝细胞癌；well-diff 分化良好；mod-diff，中度分化

增生结节

一般认为，肝硬化结节到 HCC 有一个逐步发展的过程。世界胃肠病学大会国际工作组最近对这类肝结节的统一命名法进行了审查[64]。发育不良结节（DN）是一种直径为>5mm 的明显结节性病变，分为低级别发育不良结节（LGDN）和高级别发育不良结节（HGDN）。LGDN 仅表现为轻度发育不良，无结构上的异型性，而 HGDN 以结构和/或细胞学异型性为特征，但不足以诊断 HCC。HGDN 常表现为细胞密度增加，小梁形态不规则。小细胞改变（小细胞发育不良）是 HGDN 中最常见的细胞异型性。

早期肝癌

早期肝细胞癌呈模糊的结节状，直径约为 2cm，主要表现为以下几种主要组织学特征的不同组合。

1. 细胞密度增加超过周围组织的两倍，核/细胞质比例增加，呈不规则的薄小梁状。
2. 结节内不同数量的门静脉分支（瘤内门静脉分支）。
3. 假腺管型模式。
4. 分散脂肪变化。
5. 不同数量的未配对动脉。

区分早期肝细胞癌和 HGDN 是一个尚未解决的挑战。间质浸润，定义为肿瘤细胞侵入门静脉或纤维间隔，被认为是鉴别早期 HCC 与 HGDN 最主要的特征。然而，这种特征可能很难识别，尤其是在活检标本上。在此背景下，一个由三个恶性转化的免疫组织化学标志物组成的组合，包括热休克蛋白 70，谷氨酰胺合成酶和 glypican 3，已经被用来区分 HCC 和 HGDN，以及用于早期 HCC 间质浸润识别的 CK 7 免疫染色[65,66]。

HCC 的宏观表现

肝细胞癌是肉眼外观不均匀的软组织肿块，有多种颜色的出血或坏死病灶（图 91-2）。1901 年 Eggel 所描述的三种主要生长模式目前仍然被广泛使用[67]。结节型由边界清楚的肿瘤结节组成。巨大的肝细胞癌呈局限性生长，巨大的肿瘤块占据了大部分或全部的肝叶。这种类型在没有肝硬化的患者中很

常见。弥漫型十分罕见，以无数模糊的小结节点缀整个肝脏为特征。不同的生长模式与肝内和肝外的各种传播风险有关[68]。日本肝癌研究组（LCSGJ）提出了一种改良分型，将结节型分为单结节型、瘤周生长的单结节型、融合多结节型三种亚型[69]。

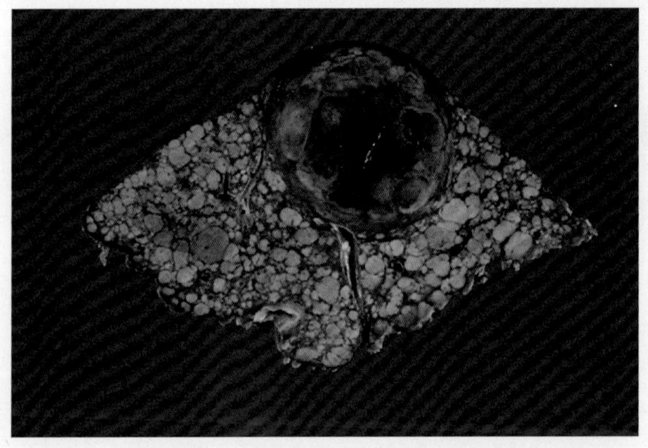

图 91-2　肝细胞癌的大体表现

从肝硬化肝脏切除的肝细胞癌中，有 16.74%的肿瘤具有多中心性[68~72]。虽然有时很难从多中心的新生癌变区别肝内转移瘤和肝细胞癌，但当出现以下情况时考虑肝转移瘤：①表现为门静脉肿瘤血栓或与血栓相邻生长；②围绕较大肿瘤的多个小卫星结节；或③单个病灶与肿瘤相邻，但大小明显变小，组织学相同[73]。

在低分化的 HCC 或巨大肿瘤中，血管侵犯和血栓形成是常见的。门静脉是最常见的血管侵犯部位，其次是肝静脉、胆道和胆动脉。肿瘤通过血管结构的延伸程度与预后密切相关。当门静脉肿瘤血栓向上延伸至门静脉左右蒂（Vp3）或门静脉主干（Vp4）时，大多数患者 2 年内复发死亡[74]。

HCC 的镜下表现

HCC 的分级多年来一直依赖于 Edmondson 和 Steiner 分级，根据组织学分化将 HCC 分为Ⅰ~Ⅳ级[75]。分化良好的肝癌细胞排列在薄小梁内的肿瘤符合Ⅰ级。在Ⅱ级，较大且不典型的肿瘤细胞有时呈腺泡状排列。结构上和细胞层面的发育不良在Ⅲ级表现突出，但这些肿瘤细胞在起源上很容易被识别为肝细胞。当明显的间变性肿瘤细胞不容易被识别为肝细胞来源时，该肿瘤被划分为Ⅳ级。

HCC 的组织学变异

纤维板层样肝癌

纤维板层状变是一种罕见的实体，占所有原发性肝癌病例的不到 1%，常见于无慢性肝病的年轻人群。纤维板层状癌是一种坚固的、界限清楚的肿瘤，通常为单个肿瘤，大小从 5cm 到 20cm 以上。组织学上，它的特征是存在核仁突出的大型多角形嗜酸性肿瘤细胞巢周围的层状基质带。即使纤维板层样肝癌患者出现肝外复发，扩大根治性手术可提供长期生存的机会[76]。

肝细胞癌合并胆管癌

肝癌合并胆管癌（HCC-CC）包含 HCC 和 ICC 的明确成分。这些肿瘤表现出 HCC 的特征（如胆汁生成、细胞间胆管或小梁生长）和 ICC 的特征（如腺结构、细胞内黏液素生成或 MUC-1、CK7 和 CK19 的免疫反应活性）的随机组合[77~79]。虽然合并 HCC-CC 的手术结果仍不确定，但有几项研究报道了 HCC 和 ICC 术后中期长期生存率[80,81]。

发病机制及自然史

肝硬化型 HCC 的发病机制是一个多步骤的去分化过程，从再生结节到发育不良边缘结节再到症状明显的 HCC。DNs 和早期 HCC 通常无症状，通常是影像学检查的偶然发现或筛查的结果。早期 HCC 通常是一种生长缓慢的病变，在表现出典型 HCC 的肿瘤特征之前无明显的侵袭性。小肝癌随着血管生成、肿瘤体积增大、侵入血管结构并在肝内转移，逐步获得侵袭能力。这些微小的肿瘤扩散过程可以演变为肉眼可见的血管肿瘤血栓形成或多种其他肿瘤表现。肝细胞癌的特点是早期发生肝内转移，而远处的器官通常在晚期发生。在肝脏包膜被拉伸、胆管结构受压或肿瘤随着体积增大而破裂之前，HCC 通常无明显症状。然而，在某些病例中，尽管没有证据显示存在胆道梗阻或骨转移等副肿瘤综合征，仍然出现高胆红素血症或高钙血症。

肝外转移发生在肿瘤晚期，主要通过血液向肺部、骨骼和大脑扩散。肝外转移患者的预后较差，根据肿瘤累及程度和其他预后因素，总生存期约 1 年。

筛查和诊断

HCC 筛查和监测的首要目标应该是在可接受的成本效益范围内尽可能降低实际发展为肝癌患者的死亡率。一般人群不建议进行监测，因为没有危险因素的个体中 HCC 的发病率较低。因此，HCC 筛查的第一步应该是识别有 HCC 发展风险的患者。传统上，肝癌高危患者的监测采用两种方法：肿瘤标志物测定、血清甲胎蛋白（AFP）浓度测定和诊断影像学检查。美国肝病研究协会（AASLD）根据现有的最佳证据，制订了关于使用这些筛选技术的指南[82]。目前，AASLDD 推荐在高危人群（如任何肝硬化患者）中每 6~12 个月进行一次肝脏超声和血清 AFP 测定。同样，日本肝病学会也推荐对非常高危人群（HBV 相关肝硬化或 HCV 相关肝硬化）每 3~4 个月检查一次肝脏超声和血清 AFP/血浆 des-γ 羧原凝血酶（DCP），每 6~12 个月进行一次动态 CT 或 MRI 检查，每 6 个月对高危人群（HBV 相关慢性肝炎、HCV 相关慢性肝炎或其他病因肝硬化）进行一次肝超声和肿瘤标志物检查，并酌情每 6 个 12 个月进行一次动态 CT 或 MRI 检查[83]。中国的一项随机对照试验报告，肝脏超声和血清 AFP 检测的应用可以早期发现 HCC，并将乙肝患者的 HCC 相关死亡率降低 37%[84]。多项非随机研究也证实，通过定期监测 HCC 高风险患者，可改善预后[85~87]。在筛查间隔方面，最近的荟萃分析显示，在 HCC 的早期发现方面，每 6 个月的监测效果明显好于每 12 个月的筛查。

Sant 等[88]报道，对于每 6 个月或更短间隔筛查的患者，70%的新诊断 HCC 符合米兰标准（孤立的肿瘤≤5cm 或 3 个以内肿瘤与每个肿瘤≤3cm）[89]，而每 6~12 个月进行一次筛查的患者，符合米兰标准的 HCC 比例为 57%，并且总生存率较低。当在常规筛查中发现可疑结节时，需要进一步检查动态增强 CT 或 MRI。由于 HCC 主要由动脉供血，早期增强和扫描延迟期的对比度降低是典型的 HCC 表现（图 91-3）。这些增强特征使扫描的特异性提高到>95%[90]。

最近发表了 AASLD 对 HCC 诊断的最新建议（图 91-4）[91]。

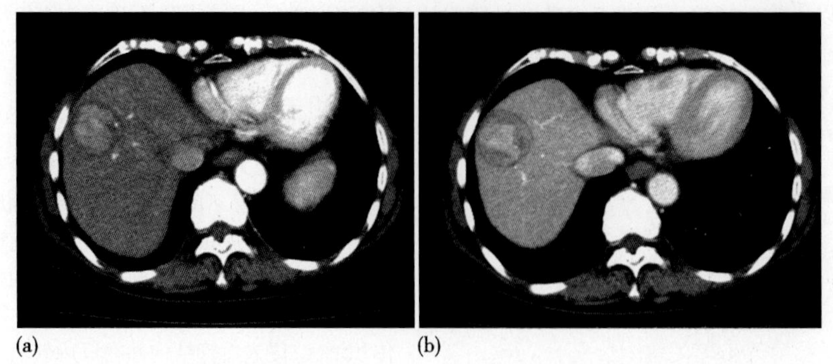

图 91-3 动态 CT 扫描肝细胞癌典型增强模式。在中分化肝癌中，动脉期早期增强(a)和晚期冲洗(b)是典型的表现

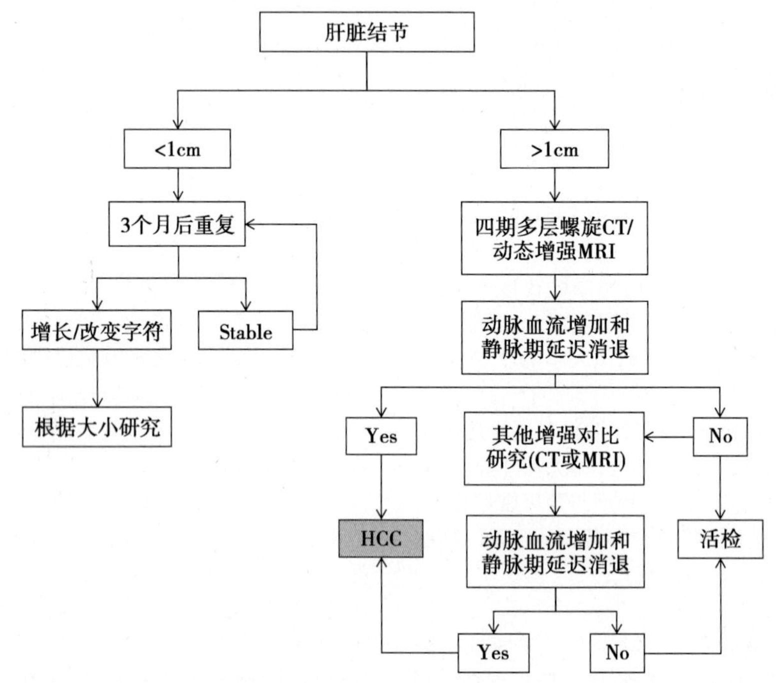

图 91-4 美国肝病研究协会(AASLD)对可疑 HCC 的诊断算法。摘自 Bruix 2005.82，经 Wiley 允许转载

这些指导方针建议，对于肝硬化患者，只要肝脏病变在 CT 扫描或 MRI 动态成像检查中表现出典型的血管增强模式(直径 >1cm)，影像学检查中发现的肝脏肿块不需要活检证实即可诊断为 HCC。直径小于 1cm 的病灶应每 3 个月超声检查一次。如有肿瘤生长或性质改变，建议根据肿瘤大小作进一步检查。

分期

由于 HCC 与潜在的慢性肝病密切相关，因此 HCC 患者的预后既取决于恶性程度，也取决于慢性肝病的严重程度。因此，目前可用的 HCC 分期系统大致分为临床分期系统和病理分期系统。临床分期系统在指导治疗选择方面非常有用，包括 Okuda 分期系统[92]，意大利肝癌项目(CLIP)评分[93]，巴塞罗那临床肝癌(BCLC)分期系统[94]。病理分期系统是建立在手术结果的基础上的，包括 LCSGJ 分期系统[95]，日本综合分期(JIS)评分[96]，中国大学预后指数(CUPI)[97]，以及美国癌症联合委员会/国际抗癌联盟(AJCC/UICC)分期系统[97]。每个分期系统都有优缺点，然而，将癌症分期与治疗原则相结合通常是困难的，导致在某些情况下对一种治疗过于保守，而在另一些情况下对其他治疗过于激进。因此，应将肝功能储备与肿瘤的肿瘤状态分开进行分类。根据 Child-Turcotte-Pugh(CTP)评分对肝功能储备和治疗风险的总体状况进行分层，CTP 评分由脑病的存在、腹水的存在、血清胆红素浓度、血清白蛋白浓度和凝血酶原时间计算(表 91-1)。CTP 评分目前已被纳入多种肝脏肿瘤的治疗原则中[82,98,99]，肝切除通常适用于 CTP A 类患者或高选择性 CTP B 类患者。CTP C 类患者围术期死亡率高，不应行手术切除已成为共识[98]。

AJCC/UICC 第 7 版 TNM 分期系统(表 91-2)是第 6 版 TNM 分期系统的修订版，该系统基于国际肝癌合作研究小组

(International Cooperative study Group on Hepatocellular Carcinoma)的一项研究,包括来自美国、日本和法国的数据,这些患者均接受了手术切除[100]。AJCC/UICC 分期系统的一个主要优势是使用了统一的病理检查标准。虽然 AJCC/UICC 分期系统是使用以丙肝相关 HCC 为主的人群制订的,但它也在乙肝患病率较高的中国人群中得到了独立验证[101]。最近,一项新的国际多中心研究报道,微血管侵犯或肿瘤分化并不影响 2cm 以下小肝癌的手术结果,这类特殊的患者可被归入预后良好的新分组[102]。

表 91-1　Child-Turcotte-Pugh(CTP)分级

	分级		
	1	2	3
白蛋白/(g/dl)	>3.5	2.8~3.5	<2.8
胆红素/(mg/dl)	<2.0	2.0~3.0	>3.0
凝血酶原时间	—	—	—
秒	<4	4~6	>6
国际标准化比率(INR)	<1.7	1.7~2.3	>2.3
腹水	无	轻度	重度
脑病	无	Ⅰ-Ⅱ级	Ⅲ-Ⅳ级
CTP A 级	5~6		
CTP B 级	7~9		
CTP C 级	10~15		

表 91-2　AJCC/UICC 第 7 版肝癌分期系统

T 分期	
T1	单发,无血管侵犯
T2	单发,有血管侵犯或多灶性≤5cm
T3a	多发性肿瘤>5cm
T3b	单个或多个肿瘤,大小不限,累及门静脉或肝静脉的主干
T4	邻近器官的侵犯或内脏腹膜穿孔
分期	
Ⅰ期	T1N0M0
Ⅱ期	T2N0M0
ⅢA 期	T3aN0M0
ⅢB 期	T3bN0M0
ⅢC 期	T4N0M0
ⅣA 期	任意 T N1M0
ⅣB 期	任意 T 任意 N M1

治疗

HCC 治疗方案的选择取决于肿瘤的负荷、潜在肝病的严重程度、患者的体力状态、治疗副作用或并发症的总体发生率与可接受的结果之间的平衡。BCLC 分期系统[94]被广泛用于对患者进行充分的分层以进行特定治疗(图 91-5)。然而,BCLC 分期系统的局限性在于,它在手术治疗的应用上比较保守(图 91-5,红色)。尽管本组患者的手术切除经验不断增加,并且预

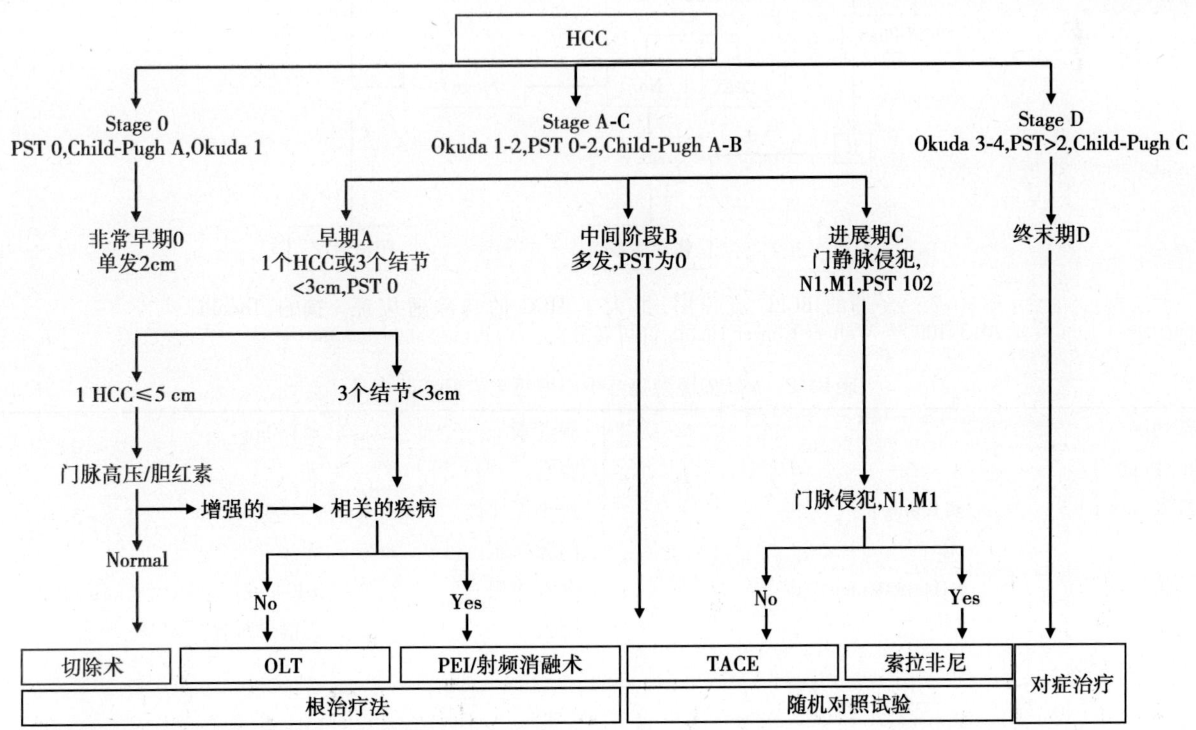

图 91-5　BCLC 流程图用于 hcc 患者的治疗选择。根据 BCLC 流程图,红色表示患者可能需要切除。来源:Llovet(2003)。经 Elsevier 许可复制

后可接受(图 91-6),但较大的孤立性肿瘤患者不被认为适合手术治疗[102~104]。研究人员已经认识到 BCLC 分期系统限制了切除标准,并提出了一种改进的 BCLC 分期系统,以扩大 HCC 切除的适应证(图 91-7)[105]。MD 安德森癌症中心目前使用的切除指南见表 91-3。在日本肝病学会提出的肝癌治疗指南中[99],对于 HCC≤3 个结节的 CTP A 类或 B 类患者,不论肿瘤大小,均建议手术切除,而肝移植仅限于符合米兰标准的 CTP C 类患者。治疗方案的选择应考虑到当地的专业知识,采用多学科方法确定。然而只要条件允许,手术切除、射频消融术(RFA)和原位肝移植(OLT)等最有效的治疗方法就应该首先考虑。

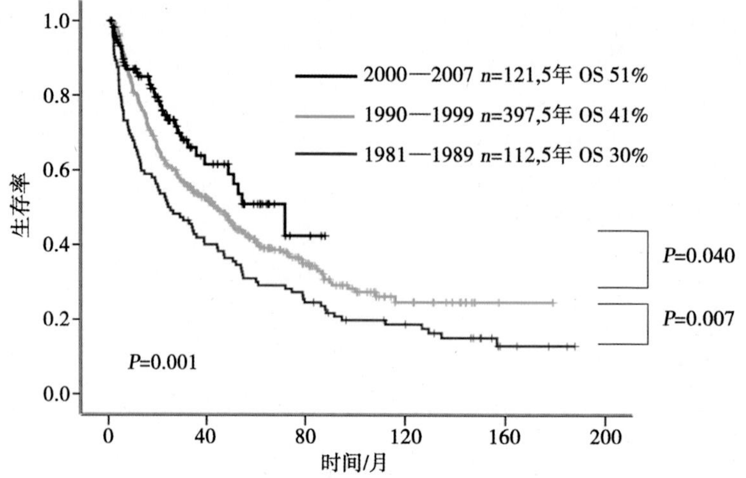

图 91-6 Kaplan Meier 绘制的 HCC 患者 4 节段切除后的生存曲线($n=630$),按 3 个不同时间段分层。摘自 Andreou,2013,经 Springer 许可转载

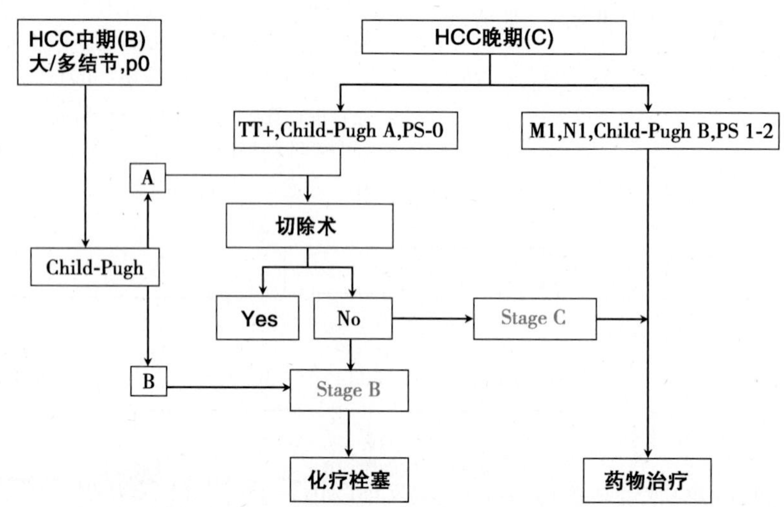

图 91-7 改进的 BCLC 流程图,扩大了 HCC 的切除适应证。摘自 Torzilli 2013. 109,经 Wolters Kluwer Health 许可转载

表 91-3 MD 安德森癌症中心肝癌患者肝切除标准

局部切除		胆红素	≤1.0mg
Child Pugh 分级	A	腹水	无
胆红素	≤1.0mg	血小板计数	>100 000/mm
腹水	无	门脉高压	无
血小板计数	>100 000/mm	余肝体积	>40%或门静脉栓塞的适应证
扩大切除		肥大	门静脉栓塞后>5%
Child Pugh 分级	A		

手术切除

对于肝切除,由于肝细胞癌通常发生在损伤的肝脏中,因此需要严格评估 HCC 患者肝功能储备,谨慎估计最大切除范围。为了更好评估慢性肝病严重程度,提出了一些肝功能研究方法。测定 15min 时吲哚菁绿滞留率(ICG-R15)是最常用的方法。对于梗阻性黄疸或先天性吲哚菁绿耐受不良的患者,^{99m}Tc-半乳糖

基人血清白蛋白(GSA)闪烁成像可敏感地估计肝功能储备。肝切除仅适用于腹水可控、血清总胆红素水平<2.0mg/dl 的 CTP A 类或 B 类患者,通过 ICG-R15 测定可确定最大切除范围[106]。

在东京大学,对于 ICG-R15<10%的患者,最大切除范围设定为 60%(右肝切除或肝三叶切除),对于 ICG-R15<20%的患者,最大切除范围为 50%(左肝切除或肝部分切除),ICG-R15<30%的患者行节段切除,ICG-R15>30%的患者仅限于局部切除。严格按照这一计算方法,1 056 例患者中没有因肝功能不全而死亡的报道[107]。在 MD 安德森癌症中心,门静脉栓塞(PVE)已被用于提高 HCC 患者接受肝大部切除术的可能性,并改善术后患者的预后和安全性[108]。该手术已被证明是安全的,并且具有良好的耐受性同时增加患者的生存率[109]。事实上,PVE 在 HCC 中还有另一个重要的好处。大多数 HCC 患者都有潜在的肝硬化,评估肝功能并做出有效的治疗决定在临床上是具有挑战性的,尤其是在需要进行大范围肝脏切除的情况下。PVE 后细胞的肥大程度与肝脏的再生潜能呈负相关。随后,细胞肥大程度提供了潜在漏诊肝损伤的有价值信息:PVE 术后小于 5%的肥大与肝切除后死亡率增加有关[110]。

原位肝移植(OLT)

肝移植是另一种理论上有较高机会消除肿瘤负担的手术方法,尤其是对严重肝功能障碍患者。既往肝癌肝移植治疗的临床效果较差。然而,在 Mazzaferro[89]等人进行了里程碑式的研究后,人们普遍认为,在有限规模和数量的肝癌患者中,可以预期较好的生存结果(米兰标准)。Mazzaferro 等[89]人使用的移植选择标准是单发 HCC 患者肿瘤直径为 5cm 或更小,如果患者有 2 或 3 个病灶,则肿瘤直径为 3cm 或更小。目前,在一些大规模移植中心,不论有无肿瘤标志物或活检结果,这一标准都得到了推广[111~122]。

局部区域消融治疗

对于早期 HCC 患者,在排除手术治疗的情况下,影像学检查引导下消融被认为是最佳治疗选择。近 20 年来,一些局部肿瘤破坏的方法得到了发展和临床应用。在随机对照试验的荟萃分析中,与传统的经皮酒精注射技术相比,RFA 具有更好的消融效果和更大的生存获益[123~127],目前已被确立为标准的消融模式。目前,包括微波烧蚀和不可逆电穿孔在内的热烧蚀或非热烧蚀方法正在研究作为 RFA 的潜在替代品。

肝动脉化疗栓塞术(TACE)

正常肝脏接受来自肝动脉(25%)和门静脉(75%)的双重血液供应。HCC 在发展过程中表现出强烈的新生血管活性,主要依赖于肝动脉供血。这为肝细胞癌的治疗提供了一种伴或不伴局部化疗的动脉阻塞治疗方案。经动脉治疗通常被认为是姑息性的,应该提供给没有肝外转移和足够的肝功能储备的中期疾病患者。经动脉化疗栓塞(TACE)最常用的药物是多柔比星和顺铂,其次是表柔比星,在随机对照研究中没有发现药物之间的显著差异[128,129]。在栓塞材料方面,明胶海绵(gelfoam)的使用较为常见。然而,它只能提供 2 周以内的短期动脉阻塞。目前,聚乙烯醇(PVA)颗粒被广泛应用于许多中心,它不仅具有永久性的动脉闭塞作用,而且由于其颗粒尺寸小,远端栓塞效果更好[130]。药物涂层珠是近年来发展起来的一种结合局部缺血和细胞毒性作用的治疗手段。尽管其相对于传统 TACE 的优越性仍存在争议,但已有多项研究表明其疗效和安全性至少与传统 TACE 相当[131,132]。

系统治疗

全身化疗通常是晚期和/或弥漫性 HCC 患者的唯一选择。几十年来,各种系统疗法都被探索用于治疗晚期肝癌。但迄今为止,细胞毒性的化疗仍未取得令人满意的结果。索拉非尼是一种多价分子,已在 HCC 细胞系中被证明可抑制丝氨酸苏氨酸激酶 raf1 和多种受体酪氨酸激酶,如血管内皮生长因子受体(VEGFR2)、血小板衍生生长因子受体(PDGFR)、FLT3、Ret 和 c-Kit。两项三期研究:SHARP 试验[133]和 Asia-Pacific 试验[134],分别证明索拉非尼在 HCC 患者中具有生存优势,这是目前唯一被批准用于 HCC 全身治疗的生物制剂。但总体有效率仅为 3%,目前尚未建立有足够的肿瘤反应率的治疗方法。最近,我们团队的研究已经表明,对于无肝炎或肝硬化患者,顺铂/α_{2b}-干扰素/多柔比星/5-氟尿嘧啶(PIAF)联合治疗可改善最初不可切除 HCC 患者的反应性、可切除性和患者生存率[135]。因此,这种传统的化疗方案可能为进展为不可切除 HCC 的非肝硬化患者提供一种选择(图 91-8 和图 91-9)。

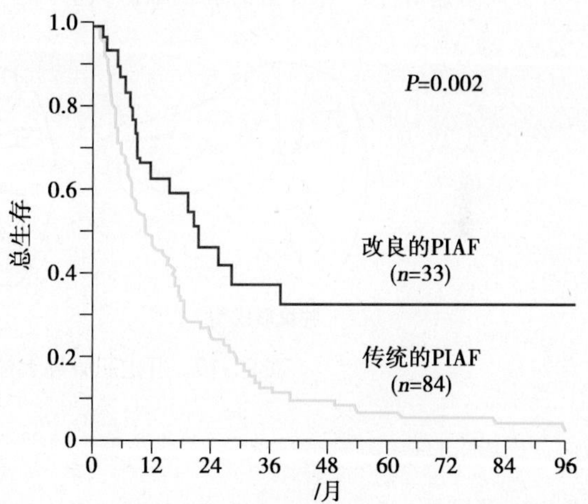

图 91-8　Kaplan-Meier 曲线与最初的生存不可切除的肝细胞癌($n=117$)分层治疗 PIAF(顺铂/α_{2b}-干扰素/多柔比星/5-氟尿嘧啶方案)。摘自 Kaseb 2013.135,经 wiley 许可转载

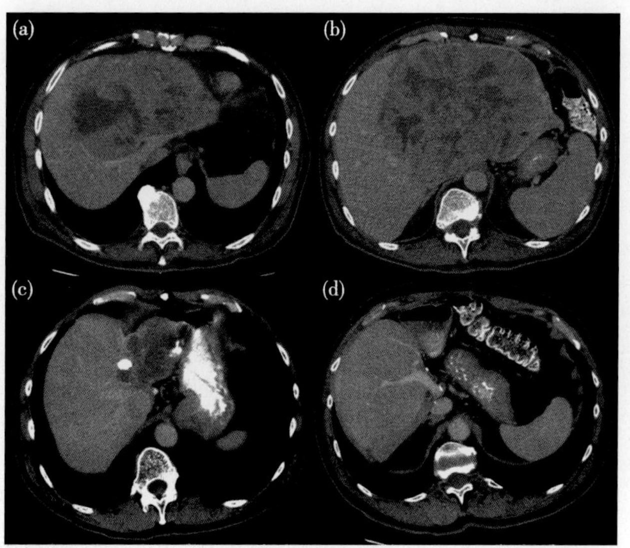

图 91-9　一位 60 岁男性巨大肝癌的计算机断层扫描。(a、b)直径 15cm 的 HCC,累及左肝叶、右肝前区,毗邻右肝静脉。(c)铂干扰素、多柔比星、氟尿嘧啶治疗后,经动脉化疗栓塞。(d)延长的左肝切除术后,包括尾状叶和下腔静脉切除。患者在手术后 8 年仍然活着,没有任何复发的迹象

肝内胆管细胞癌

发病率和流行病学

ICC 是仅次于 HCC 的第二大原发性肝脏肿瘤。ICC 的发病率存在较大的地理差异，东亚地区发病率较高[136]。在美国，经年龄调整的 ICC 发病率从 1975 年的 0.32/10 万人上升到 2000 年的 0.85/10 万人，并且仍有上升趋势[137]。不可切除肿瘤的总体生存率较低，5 年生存率为 5%～10%。由于对 ICC 的系统治疗尚未建立，手术切除是唯一的治愈机会。然而，治疗性手术后的总体生存率令人失望，5 年生存率为 20%～35%[138]。

危险因素

ICC 被认为起源于一种常见的肝祖细胞，也可能导致 HCC[139]，有时可观察到具有肝细胞癌和肝内胆管细胞癌组织病理学特征的联合肝细胞癌。虽然慢性肝病和肝硬化与 ICC 相关，但目前还没有确定 ICC 的危险因素。诱发条件包括影响胆道的感染，如病毒性肝炎、后肝吸虫病或华支睾吸虫病，以及硬化性胆管炎、胆总管囊肿、肝结石或肝硬化[140]。由于缺乏常见的诱发条件和肿瘤的稀缺性，很难确定常规监测的目标人群，便于早期诊断。

病理学

ICC 有三种形态亚型，可通过切面表现来鉴别：肿块形成、导管周浸润和导管内生长（图 91-10）。肿块形成型是 ICC 最常见的亚型。与 HCC 不同，ICC 在没有肿瘤包膜的情况下显示浸润性肿瘤生长。因此，当肿瘤附着在主要的血管结构上时，应警惕肿瘤对血管壁的显微侵犯，手术时通常需要整体切除。

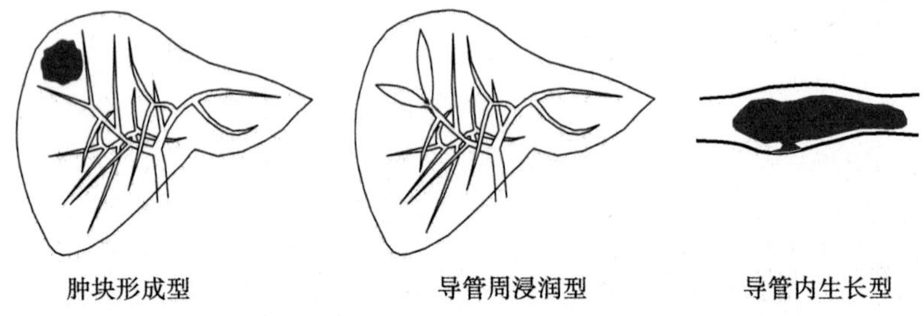

图 91-10　肝内胆管癌大体分级。改编自 2008 年日本肝癌研究组

诊断

在动态成像研究中，ICC 由于其乏血管性而没有得到增强。然而，病变周围可见不同程度的环形增强，反映了肿瘤周围常见的纤维结缔组织（图 91-11）。在实验室检测中，原发性实性肝损害中 CEA 或 CA19-9 升高提示 ICC。

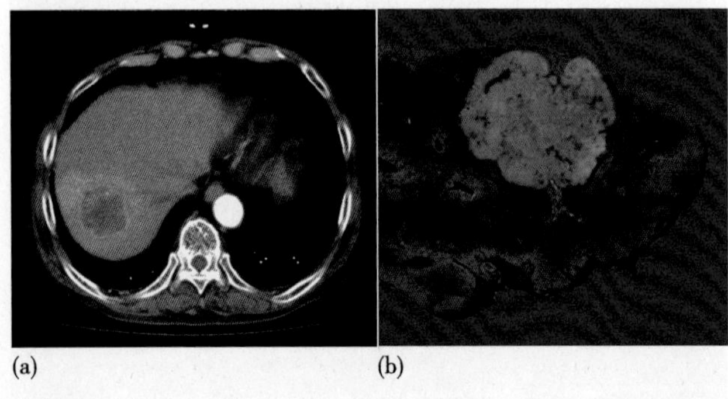

图 91-11　(a)增强 CT 扫描典型环形强化。(b)肝内胆管癌大体外观

分期

在第 6 版之前，ICC 的 AJCC 分类系统与 HCC 的分类系统是相同的。然而，在第 7 版中，基于 SEER 数据库中 598 例肝切除 ICC 患者的生存结果，采用了原始分期系统（表 91-4）[141]。法国外科协会（AFC）-IHCC 2009 研究小组已对外独立验证了这一修订的分期系统[142]。

表 91-4　AJCC/UICC 第 7 版肝内胆管癌分期系统

T 分期	
Tis	原位癌
T1	无血管浸润的孤立性肿瘤
T2a	孤立性血管侵犯
T2b	多发肿瘤，有或没有血管侵犯
T3	肿瘤直接侵及内脏腹膜或累及局部肝外结构
T4	肿瘤伴导管周围浸润
分期	
0 期	TisN0M0
Ⅰ期	T1N0M0
Ⅱ期	T2N0M0
Ⅲ期	T3N0M0
ⅣA 期	T4N0M0 或任何 TN1M0
ⅣB 期	任何 T 任何 NM1

治疗

对于 ICC 来说，只有手术切除才有治愈的机会，因为还没有确定的其他治疗方案。ICC 的手术治疗包括肝切除、肝外胆管切除以及根据肿瘤的程度进行系统性淋巴结清扫。系统淋巴结清扫的意义仍有争议。然而，淋巴结受累是影响 ICC 预后的重要因素[141]，据报道，多达 30% 的患者会有淋巴结转移[143]。OLT 治疗 ICC 的 5 年生存率为 23%，平均复发时间为 9 个月[144]，与肝细胞癌相比，这两项结果都明显较差且不足。然而，有报道称 OLT 联合新辅助放化疗的 1 年、3 年、5 年生存率分别为 92%、82%、82%，而单独手术的生存率分别为 82%、48%、21%[145]，OLT 可能对部分患者有优势。

对于晚期 ICC 患者，在过去的十年中，全身化疗取得了一定的进展。单剂氟尿嘧啶或吉西他滨全身治疗的有效率仅为 10%~30%[146,147]。ABC-02 三期随机对照试验研究了 510 例局部晚期或转移性胆道癌患者，结果显示，吉西他滨联合顺铂治疗的无进展生存率和总生存率（11.7 个月 vs 8.1 个月）均优于单纯吉西他滨治疗[148]，现在，吉西他滨和顺铂的双重治疗被认为是治疗晚期胆管癌和胆囊癌的第一线标准治疗。近年来，基于对胆道肿瘤分子致癌机制的现有认识，人们对检测新型靶向抗癌药物的兴趣日益浓厚[140]。

肝血管肉瘤

肝血管肉瘤是一种罕见的由肝内皮细胞恶性转化而来的肿瘤，已报道的研究显示与环境致癌物如二氧化钍（20 世纪 40 年代和 50 年代使用的造影剂）、氯乙烯、砷化合物和雄激素合成代谢类固醇密切相关。由于没有明确的病因或与慢性肝病的关系，肝血管肉瘤通常一经诊断已是晚期。虽然完整的手术切除或 OLT 可能提供延长生存的机会，但预后一般较差，即使接受了肝移植[149]。对于这种肿瘤，化疗的疗效还没有很好的报道。

上皮样血管内皮瘤

EHE 是一种非常罕见的低级别内皮源性恶性肿瘤，报道发病率<0.1/10 万人[150]。EHE 表现为异质性的临床特征、非特异性的放射学特征和多变的自然史[151]。EHE 的治疗方案包括肝切除、OLT、化疗和放疗。然而，由于这种疾病的罕见性，很难比较这些治疗方案的临床结果。肝切除术后 EHE 的预后良好，1 年和 5 年生存率分别为 100% 和 75%[152]。但由于该病常呈弥漫性表现，多数病例不宜行肝切除。OLT 的结果也令人鼓舞，1 年和 5 年生存率分别为 96% 和 54.5%。最近的一项研究也显示，OLT 术后长期效果良好，5 年和 10 年生存率分别为 83%和 74%，无论有无淋巴结累及或肝外疾病[153]。由于该疾病缺乏侵袭性，最近的一项研究得出结论，对仍有手术适应证的患者进行手术切除或 OLT 后的初步观察，可能有助于对治疗方案进行分层[154]。然而，由于该病的罕见性，很难建立强有力的基于临床证据的治疗指南，大型多中心前瞻性试验可能对提高对 EHE 的认识是必要的。

（康文哲 译　田艳涛 校）

参考文献

The complete reference list can be found on the Wiley Companion Digital Edition of this title (see inside front cover for login instructions).

1 American Cancer Society. *Global Cancer Facts & Figures*. Atlanta, GA: American Cancer Society; 2007.

8 Moroy T, Marchio A, Etiemble J, et al. Rearrangement and enhanced expression of c-myc in hepatocellular carcinoma of hepatitis virus infected woodchucks. *Nature*. 1986;**324**:276–279.

9 Wang J, Chenivesse X, Henglein B, Brechot C. Hepatitis B virus integration in a cyclin A gene in a hepatocellular carcinoma. *Nature*. 1990;**343**:555–557.

10 Brechot C. Hepatitis B virus (HBV) and hepatocellular carcinoma. HBV DNA status and its implications. *J Hepatol*. 1987;**4**:269–279.

11 Brechot C, Pourcel C, Louise A, et al. Presence of integrated hepatitis B virus DNA sequences in cellular DNA of human hepatocellular carcinoma. *Nature*. 1980;**286**:533–535.

12 Donato F, Boffetta P, Puoti M. A meta-analysis of epidemiological studies on the combined effect of hepatitis B and C virus infections in causing hepatocellular carcinoma. *Int J Cancer*. 1998;**75**:347–354.

15 Dusheiko G, Schmilovitz-Weiss H, Brown D, et al. Hepatitis C virus genotypes: an investigation of type-specific differences in geographic origin and disease. *Hepatology*. 1994;**19**:13–18.

16 Shindoh J, Hasegawa K, Matsuyama Y, et al. Low hepatitis C viral load predicts better long-term outcomes in patients undergoing resection of hepatocellular carcinoma irrespective of serologic eradication of hepatitis C virus. *J Clin Oncol*. 2013;**31**:766–773.

18 Hassan MM, Spitz MR, Thomas MB, et al. Effect of different types of smoking and synergism with hepatitis C virus on risk of hepatocellular carcinoma in American men and women: case–control study. *Int J Cancer*. 2008;**123**:1883–1891.

19 Hutchinson SJ, Bird SM, Goldberg DJ. Influence of alcohol on the progression of hepatitis C virus infection: a meta-analysis. *Clin Gastroenterol Hepatol*. 2005;**3**:1150–1159.

20 Ikeda K, Saitoh S, Suzuki Y, et al. Disease progression and hepatocellular carcinogenesis in patients with chronic viral hepatitis: a prospective observation of 2215 patients. *J Hepatol*. 1998;**28**:930–938.

25 Tolman KG, Fonseca V, Tan MH, Dalpiaz A. Narrative review: hepatobiliary disease in type 2 diabetes mellitus. *Ann Intern Med*. 2004;**141**:946–956.

26 Calle EE, Rodriguez C, Walker-Thurmond K, Thun MJ. Overweight, obesity, and mortality from cancer in a prospectively studied cohort of U.S. adults. *N Engl J Med*. 2003;**348**:1625–1638.

30 El-Serag HB, Tran T, Everhart JE. Diabetes increases the risk of chronic liver disease and hepatocellular carcinoma. *Gastroenterology*. 2004;**126**:460–468.

40 Edwards CQ, Griffen LM, Goldgar D, et al. Prevalence of hemochromatosis among 11,065 presumably healthy blood donors. *N Engl J Med*. 1988;**318**:1355–1362.

61 Kumada H, Suzuki Y, Ikeda K, et al. Daclatasvir plus asunaprevir for chronic HCV genotype 1b infection. *Hepatology*. 2014;**59**:2083–2091.

62 Lawitz E, Poordad FF, Pang PS, et al. Sofosbuvir and ledipasvir fixed-dose combination with and without ribavirin in treatment-naive and previously treated patients with genotype 1 hepatitis C virus infection (LONESTAR): an open-label, randomised, phase 2 trial. *Lancet*. 2014;**383**:515–523.

63 Lawitz E, Sulkowski MS, Ghalib R, et al. Simeprevir plus sofosbuvir, with or without ribavirin, to treat chronic infection with hepatitis C virus genotype 1 in non-responders to pegylated interferon and ribavirin and treatment-naive patients: the COSMOS randomised study. *Lancet*. 2014;**384(9956)**:1756–1765.

64 International Consensus Group for Hepatocellular Neoplasia. The International Consensus Group for Hepatocellular N Pathologic diagnosis of early hepatocellular carcinoma: a report of the international consensus group for hepatocellular neoplasia. *Hepatology*. 2009;**49**:658–664.

69 Liver Cancer Study Group of Japan. *The General Rules for the Clinical and Pathological Study of Primary Liver Cancer*, 5th ed. Tokyo: Kanehara; 2008.

75 Edmondson HA, Steiner PE. Primary carcinoma of the liver: a study of 100 cases among 48,900 necropsies. *Cancer*. 1954;**7**:462–503.

82 Bruix J, Sherman M. Practice Guidelines Committee AAftSoLD Management of hepatocellular carcinoma. *Hepatology*. 2005;**42**:1208–1236.

83 Kudo M, Izumi N, Kokudo N, et al. Management of hepatocellular carcinoma in Japan: Consensus-Based Clinical Practice Guidelines proposed by the Japan Society of Hepatology (JSH) 2010 updated version. *Dig Dis*. 2011;**29**:339–364.

91 Bruix J, Sherman M. American Association for the Study of Liver D Management of hepatocellular carcinoma: an update. *Hepatology*. 2011;**53**:1020–1022.

93 The Cancer of the Liver Italian Program (CLIP) Investigators. A new prognostic system for hepatocellular carcinoma: a retrospective study of 435 patients: the Cancer of the Liver Italian Program (CLIP) investigators. *Hepatology*. 1998;**28**:751–755.

94 Llovet JM, Bru C, Bruix J. Prognosis of hepatocellular carcinoma: the BCLC staging classification. *Semin Liver Dis*. 1999;**19**:329–338.

95 Makuuchi M, Belghiti J, Belli G, et al. IHPBA concordant classification of primary liver cancer: working group report. *J Hepatobiliary Pancreat Surg*. 2003;**10**:26–30.

97 Edge S, Byrd D, Compton C, et al. *AJCC Cancer Staging Manual*, 7th ed. New York: Springer; 2010.

100 Vauthey JN, Lauwers GY, Esnaola NF, et al. Simplified staging for hepatocellular

carcinoma. *J Clin Oncol*. 2002;**20**:1527–1536.

102 Shindoh J, Andreou A, Aloia TA, et al. Microvascular invasion does not predict long-term survival in hepatocellular carcinoma up to 2 cm: reappraisal of the staging system for solitary tumors. *Ann Surg Oncol*. 2013;**20**:1223–1229.

121 Yao FY, Ferrell L, Bass NM, et al. Liver transplantation for hepatocellular carcinoma: expansion of the tumor size limits does not adversely impact survival. *Hepatology*. 2001;**33**:1394–1403.

124 Lencioni RA, Allgaier HP, Cioni D, et al. Small hepatocellular carcinoma in cirrhosis: randomized comparison of radio-frequency thermal ablation versus percutaneous ethanol injection. *Radiology*. 2003;**228**:235–240.

133 Llovet JM, Ricci S, Mazzaferro V, et al. Sorafenib in advanced hepatocellular carcinoma. *N Engl J Med*. 2008;**359**:378–390.

134 Cheng AL, Kang YK, Chen Z, et al. Efficacy and safety of sorafenib in patients in the Asia-Pacific region with advanced hepatocellular carcinoma: a phase III randomised, double-blind, placebo-controlled trial. *Lancet Oncol*. 2009;**10**:25–34.

138 Mavros MN, Economopoulos KP, Alexiou VG, Pawlik TM. Treatment and prognosis for patients with intrahepatic cholangiocarcinoma: systematic review and meta-analysis. *JAMA Surg*. 2014;**149(6)**:565–574.

141 Nathan H, Aloia TA, Vauthey JN, et al. A proposed staging system for intrahepatic cholangiocarcinoma. *Ann Surg Oncol*. 2009;**16**:14–22.

151 Makhlouf HR, Ishak KG, Goodman ZD. Epithelioid hemangioendothelioma of the liver: a clinicopathologic study of 137 cases. *Cancer*. 1999;**85**:562–582.

第 92 章　胆囊癌和胆管癌

Ahmed O. Kaseb, MD ■ Marc Uemura, MD ■ Melanie B. Thomas, MD, MS ■ Steven A. Curley, MD, FACS

概述

原发性胆囊癌和胆管癌是相对罕见的胃肠道肿瘤。原发性胆囊癌和胆管癌的主要病理类型是腺癌，由胆囊和胆管黏膜内层异常增生所致。胆管癌根据其位置是在肝内或肝外，可进一步分为两类。两种类型肿瘤具有不同的病理生理学特征和肿瘤发生机制。例如，胆囊癌与胆囊结石、慢性胆囊炎和瓷化胆囊有关。它们常常在胆囊切除术标本中被偶然发现。另外，胆管癌常常与寄生虫感染和引起胆管慢性炎症的其他疾病（原发性硬化性胆管炎）有关。对可切除的胆囊癌和胆管癌，手术是可以治愈的，但是不可切除或进展期肿瘤的预后较差，通常需要辅助全身化疗。

胆囊癌

在美国，胆囊腺癌在常见的消化系统恶性肿瘤中排第 6 位。然而，在美国等西方国家，肝细胞癌（HCC）的发生率较低，胆囊癌的发生率相对较高。美国癌症协会估计，2016 年美国大约 10 910 例新发病患者被诊断为胆囊癌和胆管癌（不包括肝内胆管）。2015 年，美国约有 3 700 例患者死于胆囊癌或胆管癌。在这些新发病例和死亡病例中，约有一半的患者死于胆囊癌[1]。1980—1995 年，美国、加拿大、澳大利亚和英国的胆囊癌患者的死亡率呈明显下降，而日本、意大利和智利等国家胆囊癌患者的死亡率逐渐升高。与肝细胞癌和胆管癌不同，胆囊癌的女性发病率明显高于男性[2]，尤其是年龄小于 40 岁的女性更易发病，女性和男性发病率之比可高达 20 : 1[3]。

美国西南部土著居民的胆囊癌发病率相对于美国其他人群明显增高。美国不同人群中胆囊癌的年发病率（每 10 万人例数）分别为：美国男性白人 0.4、美国男性黑人 0.6、新墨西哥洲土著居民男性 3.8，而相应的女性人群发病率分别为：1.0、0.8 和 10.3[2]。在美国西南部土著居民胆囊癌患者中，有 6% 的患者曾经接受过胆道外科手术[4]。在美国西南部土著居民中，胆囊癌是第 2 常见的消化道恶性肿瘤，曾报道过的最年轻的胆囊癌患者是一名叫 Navajo 的 11 岁女孩[5]。

在其他人群中，胆囊癌的发病率呈逐渐上升趋势。在智利，胆囊癌的发病率逐渐上升，并且成为智利女性癌症患者中死亡的首位病因[6]。胆囊癌在不同地理和人群中的发病率差异表明环境因素是胆囊癌发病的危险因素，包括致癌物质、感染微生物（如伤寒沙门菌、幽门螺杆菌）、不良饮食习惯等环境因素在胆囊癌的发生、发展过程中发挥重要的作用。

致病因素

胆囊癌和乙型或丙型肝炎病毒感染、肝硬化或者真菌毒素感染之间没有明确的关系。同样，肝癌的化学性致癌因子亦没有被证明在增加胆囊癌发病风险方面发挥作用。然而，有研究表明长期暴露于致癌物质（如甲基胆蒽和亚硝胺）的工作人员，与对照人群相比，不仅胆囊癌的发病率高，而且发病的年龄更早[7]。研究证实胆囊结石和胆囊癌之间有明确的关系，74%～92%胆囊癌患者患有胆囊结石[8,9]。胆囊癌发生的风险与胆囊结石的大小呈正相关[10]，胆囊结石直径为 2.0～2.9cm 的患者发生胆囊癌的风险升高 2.4 倍，结石直径超过 3.0cm 的患者发生胆囊癌的风险升高 10.1 倍。长期慢性胆囊炎患者的胆囊壁可发生钙化，也称为瓷性胆囊。有研究显示，胆囊壁钙化的患者中有 22%患者患有胆囊癌，这也表明胆囊的慢性炎症或感染可以增加发生胆囊癌的风险[11]。此外，胆囊癌患者的胆囊培养出致病细菌的概率显著高于单纯胆囊胆石患者的胆囊[12]。胆石症和胆囊炎在女性中更常见，这也正是女性胆囊癌发病率高的原因所在[13]。

胆囊癌前病变的患者亦会发展为侵袭性胆囊癌。在因胆石症或胆囊炎接受胆囊切除的患者中，胆囊黏膜上皮发育不良、上皮不典型增生和原位癌的检出率分别为 83%、13.5%和 3.5%[14]。在侵袭性胆囊癌患者中，超过 90%的患者可以观察到黏膜异型增生[15]。亦有证据表明，胆囊黏膜的腺瘤样息肉也属于癌前病变。一篇关于胆囊切除术的综述报道发现，在 1 605 例胆囊切除标本中有 11 例良性腺瘤、7 例腺瘤发生了癌变和 79 例侵袭性胆囊癌[16]。从慢性胆囊炎、胆囊上皮异型增生，直到发展成为侵袭性胆囊癌的过程中，表皮因子和原癌基因，如 *ras* 基因的表达水平明显增加[17]。胆胰汇合异常的患者发展为胆囊癌的风险也增高，同时慢性炎症也可导致胆囊上皮的异型增生[18]。在一部分胆囊上皮高级别不典型增生中，发现了 *K-ras* 基因突变，而这一现象表明该原癌基因的突变是胆囊黏膜增生的早期事件，并最终导致癌症发生。针对侵袭性胆囊癌患者的研究发现，大部分患者确实存在异常的或突变的肿瘤抑制基因（*p53* 和 *P16*），以及细胞周期调节基因（*cyclin E*）和细胞凋亡基因（*Bcl-2*），同时细胞内血管内皮生长因子（VEGF）的表达水平亦明显增加[19,20]。最近，全基因组图谱显示，侵袭性胆囊癌患者中细胞周期调节所需的其他蛋白质（CDKN2B），染色质重组（ARID1A）和重要的生长途径，特别是表皮生长因子受体家族（ERBB2）和 PKI3CA/MTOR 都存在突变[21]。

病理

根据胆囊癌的分期和浸润程度不同，胆囊癌的大体病理表现呈多样化。胆囊癌早期，因肿瘤没有浸润胆囊壁的全层，此时病理表现很难和慢性胆囊炎区别。少数情况下，单发无蒂或带蒂的肿瘤也提示为胆囊癌[22]。进展期胆囊癌大体病理表现多为肿瘤细胞已经浸润肝脏或周围毗邻的器官，如十二指肠或胃等[23]。

90%以上的胆囊癌镜下病理诊断为腺癌，其余为腺鳞癌、鳞癌和未分化癌，少数为类癌或胚胎横纹肌肉瘤[8,22]。原位癌属于早期肿瘤，此时癌细胞仅侵袭胆囊壁的黏膜层。胆囊腺癌通常会出现乳头状或管腔样的细胞排列结构[22]。乳头状腺癌的特征是延伸的间质覆盖有柱状的细胞。管状腺癌的管腔通常是由高柱状细胞或立方上皮排列而成。胆囊腺癌常可以发现黏蛋白生成和印戒细胞[22]。分化程度较差的癌多表现为肿瘤质地较硬，呈片状或巢状结构，体积较小的癌细胞浸润细胞间质，破坏了正常的胆囊壁组织结构。另外，胆囊癌常常导致邻近血管、淋巴和周围神经的受累。

当诊断胆囊癌时，疾病通常已发展为局部进展期。仅有10%的胆囊癌患者，病变局限于胆囊壁[8]。69%～83%的胆囊癌患者，癌组织已经直接侵犯胆囊床邻近的肝脏组织[23-25]。患者一旦出现肝脏受累，通常提示其他部位亦可能存在转移病灶，因为仅有不到12%的肝脏受累患者没有合并身体其他部位的转移。57%病例合并肝外胆道受累；40%病例合并十二指肠、胃或横结肠受累；23%病例合并胰腺受累；15%病例出现肝动脉或门静脉被肿瘤包裹。另外，42%～70%病例存在胆囊、胆总管或胰十二指肠淋巴回流区域淋巴结的转移[23]，大约25%的病例存在腹主动脉旁或下腔静脉旁淋巴结等远处转移。值得注意的是，胆囊癌可以在没有肝脏或者其他邻近器官转移的情况下，直接出现远处淋巴结转移。

通过对胆囊淋巴回流的解剖学研究，可以预测胆囊癌淋巴结转移方式。胆囊周围的淋巴回流主要有三种途径（图92-1）[26]，其中主要的途径是胆囊-胰腺后方途径，即胆囊前后表面的淋巴管汇集后流入门静脉后方的大淋巴结，同时与胆总管和胰十二指肠淋巴结相互交通。胆囊-腹腔干途径主要是由胆囊前、后表面淋巴液向左流至门静脉的前方，与胰十二指肠淋巴结或与左肾静脉附近的主动脉腔静脉淋巴结相交通。胆囊癌的最终扩散方式与血管受侵犯相关。在胆囊癌患者中，发现非邻近的肝脏、肺和骨转移的比例分别为：66%、24%和12%[23]。

胆囊癌分期系统是基于肿瘤局部侵犯和淋巴结转移的病理学特征。在美国癌症联合委员会（AJCC）制订胆囊癌的肿瘤-淋巴结转移（TNM）分期方法之前，Nevin分期系统应用广泛[27]。而日本对胆囊癌的研究多采用日本胆道外科协会的分期系统[28]。但是，目前世界范围内的大多数临床研究都是根据TNM分期标准对患者进行临床分期的。AJCC分期系统中原位癌对应为T1aN0M0。胆囊癌三种不同的分期系统所对应关系如表92-1所示。

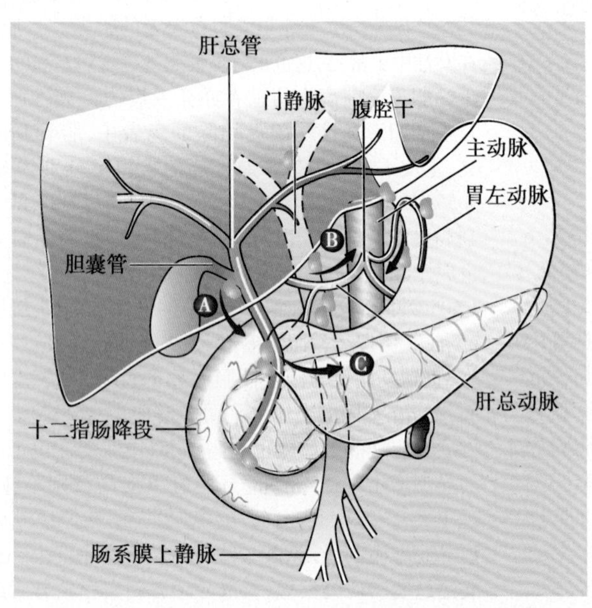

图92-1 胆囊淋巴回流途径。（A）淋巴回流的主要途径，同时也是胆囊癌主要的淋巴结转移途径。该途径从胆囊经胆囊管、胆总管之后汇入十二指肠和胰腺头部后方淋巴结。（B）胆囊-腹腔干途径，起自胆囊，经肝胃韧带，到达腹腔干淋巴结。（C）第三条淋巴回流途径：即胆囊-肠系膜途径，经胆囊、胰腺后方到达主动脉腔静脉淋巴结

表92-1 胆囊癌最常用的三种分期系统比较

分期	Nevin 分期	日本胆道外科协会分期	美国癌症联合委员会-TNM 分期
Ⅰ	肿瘤局限在黏膜层	肿瘤局限于浆膜下层	T1aN0M0，T1bN0M0
Ⅱ	肿瘤侵犯黏膜层和肌层	直接侵犯肝脏和/或胆道，肝门淋巴结出现转移	T2N0M0
Ⅲ	肿瘤侵犯浆膜层	肿瘤直接侵犯更远处的肝脏组织，更远处区域淋巴结出现转移（肝胃、胰腺后淋巴结）	T1N1M0，T2N1M0，T3 任何 NM0
Ⅳ	肿瘤突破胆囊壁全层，伴有胆囊淋巴结转移	肝脏、腹膜、和/或远处肝脏转移	T4 任何 NM0，任何 T 任何 NM1
Ⅴ	肿瘤直接侵犯肝脏和/或任何远处器官出现转移	无	无

T，原发肿瘤；Tx，原发肿物无法评估；T1，肿瘤浸润黏膜层或肌层；T1a，肿瘤侵犯黏膜层；T1b，肿瘤侵犯肌层；T2，肿瘤浸润肌层周围结缔组织，但没有突破浆膜层或侵犯肝脏；T3 肿瘤突破浆膜层，或侵犯一个邻近的器官，或包含以上两者情况（浸润肿瘤周围2cm范围以内的肝脏组织）；T4，肿瘤浸润超过肿瘤周围2cm范围的肝脏组织，和/或侵犯2个或2个以上的邻近器官（胃、十二指肠、结肠、胰腺、网膜、肝外胆道）；N，区域淋巴结；Nx 区域淋巴结无法评估 N0，区域淋巴结没有转移；N1，区域淋巴结转移；N1a，胆囊管，胆总管周围，和/或肝胃淋巴结转移；N1b，胰腺周围、十二指肠周围、肝门周围、腹腔干和/或肠系膜上动脉淋巴结转移；M，远处转移；Mx 远处转移无法评估；M0，没有远处转移；M1，出现远处转移。

临床表现

胆囊癌患者最常见的症状和体征不具有特异性，75%～97%的患者主诉右上腹部疼痛，但是进食脂肪是否会加重疼痛尚不确定[2,8,29]。少数患者会出现右上腹部压痛。这些症状和体征通常缘于胆石症或胆囊炎。另外，40%～64%的患者出现恶心、呕吐和纳差，45%患者存在不同程度的黄疸，37%～77%的患者体重减轻超过 10%。

尽管只有 45%的胆囊癌患者合并明显的黄疸，但是 70%的患者血清胆红素水平要比正常值升高至少 2 倍[29]。2/3 的胆囊癌患者血清碱性磷酸酶水平升高，1/3 患者伴随着肿瘤进展侵犯肝脏和出现肝转移，血清中的谷丙转氨酶和谷草转氨酶水平亦升高。超过 80%的 TNM 分期为Ⅲ或Ⅳ期的胆囊癌患者，血清中的 CEA 水平明显升高[29]，但是该病早期血清 CEA 升高的比例目前尚不清楚。

诊断方法

在超声和 CT 广泛应用之前，胆囊癌术前诊断率仅为 8.6%～16.3%[2]。目前，对于有临床症状的患者，当考虑为胆石症或胆总管结石时，超声检查为首要的影像学检查方法。高分辨率超声能够检测出早期和局部进展期的胆囊癌[30]。大小 5mm 的早期胆囊癌可表现为向胆囊腔内突出的息肉样肿块或胆囊壁的局部增厚[31]。对于局部进展期胆囊癌患者，超声检查可表现为肝外和肝内的胆管梗阻、肝门部淋巴结肿大以及肝脏肿瘤浸润和肝脏的转移病灶。术前超声诊断胆囊癌的确诊率为 75%[31,32]。然而，超声检查不能精确检测腹腔的或主动脉旁淋巴结病变以及腹膜种植的肿瘤[33]。彩色多普勒超声对胆囊癌的诊断有一定意义，90%的胆囊癌可发现高流速动脉血流，而良性肿瘤表现为较低流速[34]。近年来，随着内镜超声不断发展，尤其是对比-增强剂的应用，大大提高了胆囊癌 T 分级评估的诊断准确性[35]。

当临床考虑为良性胆道疾病时，则很少有患者会接受 CT 检查，然而当怀疑为胆囊癌时，88%～95%患者可以通过 CT 检查得到明确诊断[36,37]。胆囊癌的 CT 表现包括：95%的患者胆囊壁弥漫或局限性增厚超过 0.5cm，95%的患者胆囊壁出现对比强化表现，90%的患者表现为腔内肿块，85%的患者发现肿瘤已经直接侵犯了邻近肝脏组织（图 92-2），65%的患者合并区域淋巴结的病变，52%的患者同时存在胆石症，50%的患者肝内或肝外胆道扩张，12%的患者出现非邻近肝脏组织的转移，8%的患者胆囊毗邻的胃肠道器官受到侵犯已经 4%的患者发现了胆囊腔内有气体存在[36]。CT 也能显示钙化的胆囊壁（图 92-3）。

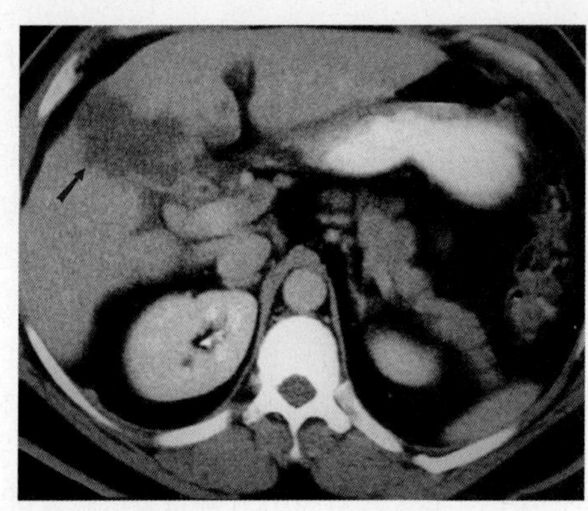

图 92-2 一例胆囊癌患者的高分辨率、螺旋 CT 扫描。明显地看到肿瘤直接侵犯肝脏实质

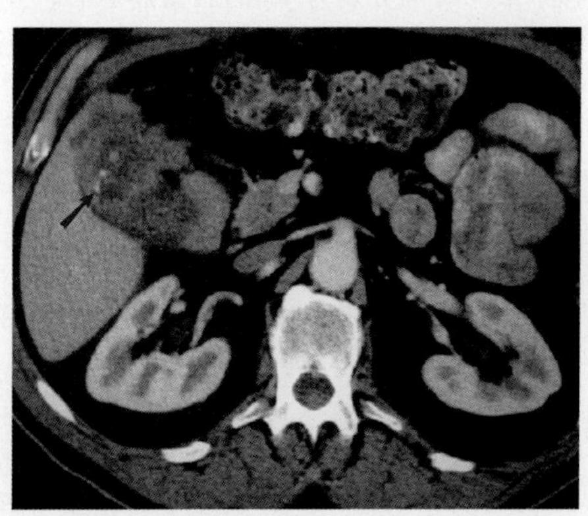

图 92-3 一例胆囊癌患者的高分辨率、螺旋 CT 扫描。局部浸润的肿瘤表现为增厚的胆囊壁出现钙化区域（箭头）

治疗

手术切除

胆囊癌根治性切除率为 10%～30%[38]。多数胆囊癌患者因为肿瘤局部浸润、非邻近肝脏组织的转移，和/或其他脏器远处转移，而无法行根治性切除手术。尽管可切除的胆囊癌患者可获得长期生存，但扩大性切除仍存在争议。

对于病灶局限于黏膜层的胆囊癌患者（T1aN0M0），单纯行胆囊切除已经足够，术后 5 年生存率为 57%～100%[39,40]。而对于这种肿瘤分期为 T1aN0M0 的胆囊癌患者行单纯胆囊切除术是否是唯一的治疗手段，目前尚未达成一致。一些学者推荐对于非常早期胆囊癌患者施行扩大的胆囊切除术，切除范围除了胆囊外，还包括距胆囊窝边缘 3～5cm 范围的肝脏实质，以及胆囊、胆总管周围、肝胃、胰十二指肠和主动脉旁淋巴结清扫[41,42]。

另外，这些学者也建议，对所有切除的胆囊标本都应该剖开，对任何可疑黏膜区域行冰冻切片检查。如果冰冻切片检查诊断为胆囊癌，或最终病理诊断为 T1aN0M0 分期的胆囊癌，均建议行扩大胆囊切除术。这种激进的外科治疗观点是基于少数胆囊癌患者在接受单纯胆囊切除术后出现区域淋巴结复发。但是，目前仍没有合理证据支持行肝脏切除，因为接受单纯胆囊切除术后复发的患者，通常发生转移的部位是胆总管及胆囊周围的淋巴结，并不是肝脏的复发和转移。再者，对于分期为 T1aN0M0 患者，术后出现淋巴结转移也只是在病例数为 32 和 36 的小样本量的研究中出现，且发生比率均小于 10%[41,42]。一项对 201 例病变仅局限于黏膜的胆囊癌患者施行胆囊及区域淋巴结切除的研究表明，淋巴结转移的比例仅为 2.5%[39]。另外，接受扩大切除手术的胆囊癌患者死亡率为 2%～5%，相关的手术并发症发生率为 13%～40%[39,40,43]。因此，对于病例不到 5%的 T1aN0M0 的早期胆囊癌患者，扩大胆囊切除术直接导致的死亡率和并发症发生率，确实需要和潜在的生存获益进行认真评估。

对于分期为 T1b，或 AJCC-TNM 分期Ⅱ期和Ⅲ期的胆囊癌患者，已有证据支持可行扩大胆囊切除术（图 92-4）。在 165 例分期为 T1b 的胆囊癌患者中，15.6%的患者发生了区域淋巴结转移[39]。867 例分期为 T2 的胆囊癌患者，56.1%发生了区域淋巴结转移[39]。453 例分期为 T3 的胆囊癌患者，74.4%发生了区域淋巴结转移。AJCC 分期为Ⅱ期和Ⅲ期的胆囊癌患者接受扩大胆囊切除术后，5 年生存率为 7.5%～71%[39,40,43,44]。区域淋巴结转移和/或肿瘤直接侵犯肝脏实质均提示患者预后较差，且与术后 5 年生存率显著降低密切相关[45,46]。另外，镜下肝脏切缘阳性提示患者预后较差，其平均生存期为 8.9 个月，与此相比，切缘阴性患者的平均生存期可达 67.2 个月[45]。术前螺旋 CT 扫描和术中超声检查有助于评估肝脏实质的受累范围，帮助决策为达到根治性切除而需要行切除部分肝脏的范围。研究表明，对于胆囊癌患者行右肝叶切除、扩大右半肝切除、右三叶切除和中肝切除可获得相似的术后长期生存时间，这一结果表明，如果术中能够保证肿瘤切缘阴性，进一步的扩大肝脏切除并不能延长生存时间[39,40,47~49]。目前，AJCC 系统将 T1b 期胆囊癌患者归为Ⅰ期尚有争议，因为该类患者中，有 15.6%的患者存在着区域淋巴结转移，而且，其中不少患者是可以从扩大胆囊切除术中获益的，术后可以长期生存（图 92-4）。

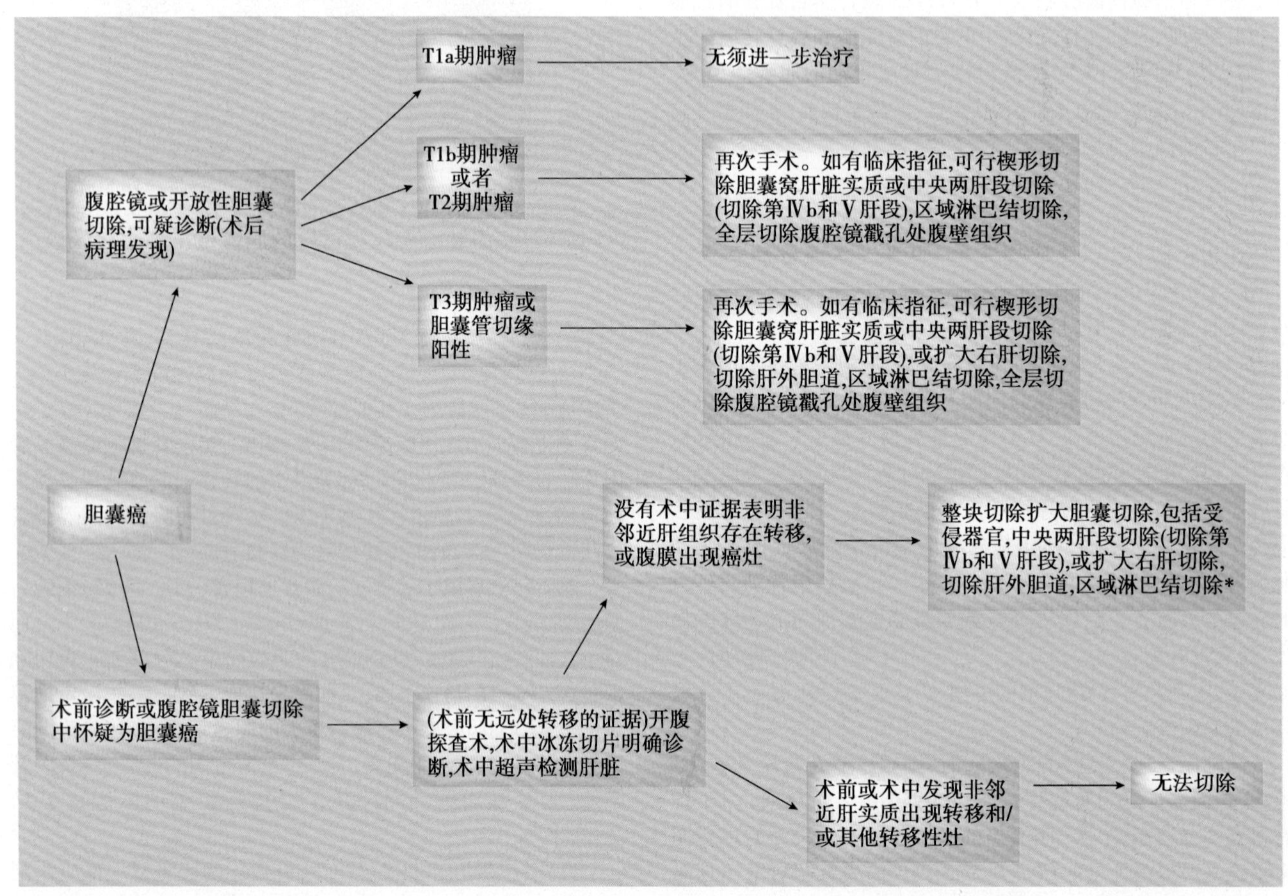

图 92-4　胆囊癌患者外科治疗选择的决策图。* 区域淋巴结切除包括完整移除胆囊、胆总管周围、胰十二指肠、肝胃韧带和主动脉旁淋巴结

所有的学者都不会把肝外胆管整体切除作为扩大胆囊切除手术的一部分，这是因为 57%的胆囊癌患者合并了肝外胆管受累，且大多数为期为 T3 或 T4 期，而对于这部分已经浸透了黏膜层的侵袭性胆囊癌的扩大切除应该包括适当的肝胆管、胆总管整块切除，以及肝胆管空肠的 Roux-en-Y 吻合术。另外，对于临床表现不考虑胆囊癌仅接受了单纯胆囊切除术，而术后病理诊断为胆囊癌，而且胆囊管切缘为阳性的患者也应该考虑行扩大切除术。胆囊癌通常累及胆囊管和胆囊颈部，并沿肝总管和右肝管浸润生长，此时有必要行右半肝或扩大右半肝切除，同时切除受累的肝外胆道，从而达到根治性切除[50]。

目前已有学者提出对分期为 T3N1M0 或 T4N01M0 的胆囊癌患者，应施行扩大根治性手术，手术方法包括肝胰十二指肠切除，以及针对局部进展期的胆囊癌患者行腹部器官移植[39,51,52]，但是，报道也显示这些扩大根治性手术最低死亡率为 15%，而手术重大并发症发生率高达 90%。为完全切除所有肉眼可见的肿瘤，通常需要行门静脉和/或肝动脉的切除和血管重建。因胆囊癌而行肝胰十二指肠切除术的大宗病例报道是来自日本的 150 例，其报道称该手术的术后 5 年生存率为 14%[39]，即使幸免于术中、术后并发症的患者，最终也不能免于肿瘤本身的复发和/或转移。

据统计，美国每年大约有 80 000 例腹腔镜胆囊切除手术。术前考虑为良性胆道疾病而接受胆囊切除的患者中，平均有 2%的患者最终被确诊为胆囊癌。因此，每年大约 1 600 名因接受腹腔镜胆囊切除的患者无意中发生了胆囊癌的扩散[53~56]。实际上,腹腔镜确实有播散肿瘤细胞的潜在可能,但是并没有显著影响大多数胆囊癌患者的自然病程。得克萨斯大学安德森癌症医疗中心对胃肠道恶性疾病诊断和腹腔镜治疗的经验回顾研究提示,胆囊癌很少存在孤立的复发部位,95%的胆囊癌患者肝门部复发是肿瘤广泛转移的前期征兆[57]。此外,美国癌症数据库 1989—1995 年报道,在此期间腹腔镜胆囊切除手术极大程度的取代了开放性胆囊切除手术,作为胆囊良性疾病的主要选择术式[58],而胆囊癌的发病率和生存率并没有明显变化。然而,鉴于目前绝大多数胆囊切除术是在腹腔镜下完成的,尽管腹腔镜导致肿瘤细胞播散的可能性很小,但对于以下几种情况:①术前临床或影像学诊断标准怀疑为胆囊癌的患者,无论采用腹腔镜、开腹探查或经皮活检等,外科医师应有施行扩大胆囊切除术的能力;②拟行腹腔镜胆囊切除,但手术探查怀疑为胆囊癌,应转为开放胆囊癌根治性手术,或者果断终止探查,无须活检,直接转而为更加恰当的外科治疗[53]。对于接受了腹腔镜胆囊切除的患者,术后病理诊断为胆囊癌,应为患者进一步提供积极的再次外科手术,因为这其中一部分患者因再次扩大切除后可长期无瘤生存[59]。

姑息治疗/化疗

大部分的胆囊癌患者在明确诊断时,已经处于肿瘤的进展期,而无法行手术切除。对于合并肝门部胆管癌的患者,应首先考虑缓解黄疸症状。无法手术切除的胆囊癌患者,通常情况肝外胆道广泛受累,肝门部淋巴结病变严重,使得内镜下放置内支架亦非常困难。如果在腹腔镜探查时,发现胆囊癌无法手术切除,应积极考虑行外科的胆道旁路手术,例如肝内胆管与肠道吻合,可以缓解 90%以上的患者临床症状[60]。当影像学检查以及经皮穿刺活检诊断胆囊癌无法切除时,可考虑经皮经肝放置胆道支架,以减轻黄疸。

与肝门部胆管癌相比,胆囊癌患者出现胃十二指肠梗阻症状相对较少,研究表明,30%~50%的进展期胆囊癌可出现胃十二指肠梗阻的临床症状[61]。当初出现胃十二指肠梗阻时,可以通过外科旁路,如胃空肠吻合术、内镜放置金属膨胀支架或放置胃肠减压管及空肠营养管来缓解梗阻症状。对于预期生存时间很短的进展期胆囊癌患者,可直接选择经皮内镜下胃造瘘。

化疗治疗研究发现,少数无法切除,包括肝门部胆管癌,或已经发生远处转移的进展期胆囊癌患者通过化学药物治疗可以延长生存时间。进展期胆囊的主要化疗方案包括基于氟尿嘧啶和吉西他滨的化疗方案。一项针对 53 名接受系统化疗的进展期胆囊癌患者的临床研究表明,接受氟尿嘧啶(5-FU)或氟尿嘧啶联合其他药物化疗,抗肿瘤反应率不超过 12%[62],而接受氟尿嘧啶类药物联合多柔比星类系统治疗的抗肿瘤反应率可达 30%~40%[63,64]。对三项随机实验研究作荟萃分析显示,对于进展期胆囊癌和胆管癌接受双重化疗,患者的中位总生存期为 3.8 个月($P<0.001$),中位无进展期生存期为 3.3 个月($P<0.001$),这三项随机研究主要比较吉西他滨单独化疗与吉西他滨联合铂类化疗治疗患者的中位总生存期和中位无进展生存期[65]。极少数患者能够获得完全缓解,大多数接受研究的患者中位生存期为 11 个月或者更短。然而,关于某种药物的治疗效果的相关文献存在着自身的局限性,因为多数研究报道的病例数仍较少,而且诸多研究还混杂了胆管癌、胆囊癌、胰腺癌或者肝细胞癌等。与之相关的近期临床实验研究的结果将在胆管癌章节中详述。

放射治疗

对胆囊癌切除术后失败的病例进行分析研究,结果发现导致超过一半以上病例治疗失败的原因就是局部复发[66]。总剂量为 45Gy 的体外放射治疗可使 20%~70%的肿瘤出现影像学证据上的缩小,并可暂时缓解 80%患者的黄疸症状[67~69]。总体来说,体外放射治疗应属于姑息治疗。接受放射治疗的局部进展期胆囊癌患者的平均生存时间约为 10 个月[66~69]。偶尔有报道,通过更高剂量的放疗或在体外放射治疗的同时,注入放疗增敏化疗药物,如氟尿嘧啶等可使患者获得长期生存[66]。虽然,通过更高剂量的体外放射治疗,患者获得更长的生存时间,但有些患者治疗后出现了不同程度的肝外胆管狭窄[70]。

多学科综合治疗

大多数接受扩大胆囊切除,或 AJCC 分期为Ⅱ,Ⅲ或Ⅳ期而接受更大范围根治性手术的胆囊癌患者,最终还是出现了肿瘤复发,并直接导致患者死亡。非随机对照研究和个案报道,对于分期为Ⅱ、Ⅲ或Ⅳ期的胆囊癌患者,术后接受辅助放疗和/或化疗可以显著地延长患者总体生存时间[71-73]。遗憾的是,临床治疗中只有少数患者术后接受了辅助治疗,而且辅助治疗的方法又是五花八门。在一项非随机对照研究中,9 例Ⅳ期的胆囊癌患者仅接受了完整的外科手术切除,另外 17 例患者除了接受完整的外科手术切除外,还辅以 20~30Gy 的术中放射治疗[74]。另外,17 例患者还有 10 例患者接受了 36.4Gy 的术后体外放射治疗。这两组患者均接受了完整外科手术治疗,即扩大胆囊切除以及范围更广的肝胰十二指肠切除的根治手术。这项研究结果表明,仅接受外科切除治疗的 9 例患者均未获得 3 年生存期,但是那 17 例既接受外科切除又接受放疗的患者中,10.1%的患者获得了 3 年生存期。此外,一项单中心研究报道 18 例胆囊癌患者行外科切除之前接受放、化疗(共计 4 500cGy,每次 180cGy,每周 5 天,氟尿嘧啶 350mg/m^2/1~5d,氟尿嘧啶 350mg/m^2/21~25d)[75]。18 例患者中的 13 例接受了手术治疗,1 例患者拒绝手术治疗,1 例患者未完成术前放化疗,1 例患者放化疗后,疾病进展恶化,2 例患者开腹探查后发现肿瘤无法切除。其中施行手术切除的 13 例胆囊癌患者实际 5 年生存率为 57%。

虽然,胆囊癌切除术后辅助治疗的文献报道主要来自单中心的回顾性研究,但近期一项非随机 2 期临床实验报道了辅助化疗和同步放化疗在 79 例胆囊癌术后患者辅助治疗中的作用,研究对象主要是行根治性手术后病理诊断为肝外胆管癌或胆囊癌(非壶腹癌)的 T2~4 期、N1 或者切缘阳性患者[76]。该项研究中,每 21 天每个患者接受 4 个周期的吉西他滨(第 1 天和第 8 天各 1 000mg/(m^2·d))和卡培他滨(1 500mg/(m^2·d),第 1~14 天),然后同时接受卡培他滨(1 330mg/(m^2·d))和放射治疗(局部淋巴结的照射剂量 45Gy,肿瘤床的照射剂量 54~59.4Gy)。研究结果显示,所有患者的 2 年生存率为 65%,R0

和 R1 患者的 2 年生存率分别为 67%和 60%；中位总生存时间为 45 个月（R0，34 个月；R1，35 个月）。

此外，一项包括 6 712 例胆囊癌或胆管癌患者的 20 项研究荟萃分析显示，接受辅助化疗或放化疗的患，特别是淋巴结阳性的患者没有明显的生存获益[71]。然而，由于临床数据不足，胆囊癌切除术后患者的最佳辅助治疗方案仍需进一步研究。

胆管癌

胆管癌是起源于肝内或肝外胆管上皮的恶性肿瘤。在美国，每年约有 3 000 名患者被诊断为肝内或肝外胆管系统的胆管癌[77]。胆管癌男性发病率稍高于女性。胆管癌可起源于肝内或肝外胆管系统的任何部位，但主要是来源于肝门部位，可占胆管癌总病例数的 2/3（图 92-5）[78]。

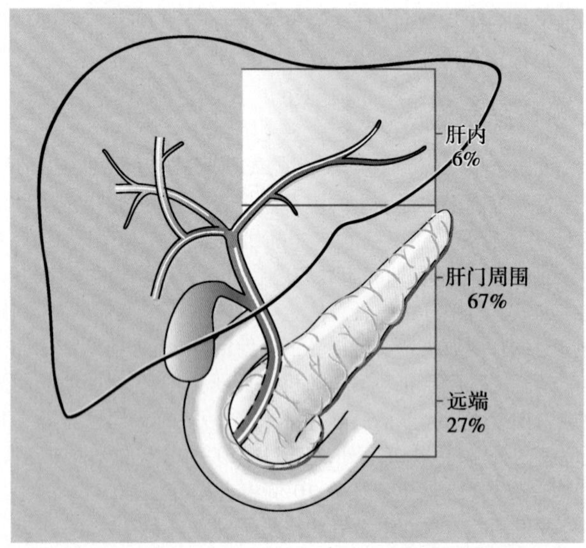

图 92-5 根据位置分布不同，294 例胆管癌可分为肝内、肝门周围和远端三个亚组。摘自 Aretxabala 1999[75].
Reproduced with permission of Elsevier

致病因素

胆管癌与肝癌的致病因素显著不同（表 92-2）。胆管癌中仅有 10%～20%的胆管癌患者合并存在肝硬化，然而，在肝癌中有高达 70%～90%的患者合并肝硬化[77,79,80]。丹麦的一项关于 11 605 例肝硬化患者的队列研究发现，肝硬化患者发生 HCC 的风险增加了 60 倍，发生胆管癌的风险增加了 10 倍[80]。一般来说，肝硬化是由于恶性肿瘤阻塞胆管引起长时间的胆管梗阻、胆管破坏而引起的，因此，与其说肝硬化是胆管癌的病因，不如说是胆管癌导致了肝硬化的发生。

东南亚国家胆管癌的发病率显著高于世界其他地区，而导致其高发的原因主要与肝吸虫华支睾吸虫（*Opisthorchis sinensis*）和麝猫后睾吸虫（*Opisthorchis viverrini*）的感染有关[81,82]。肝吸虫感染后可以引起胆管上皮细胞增生、组织纤维化和胆管上皮腺瘤样变，同时与肝内胆管结石的形成密切相关。目前，肝吸虫感染被认为是胆管癌发生的直接致病因素，但两者之间的确切关系尚不明确。

表 92-2 胆管细胞癌与肝细胞癌发病危险因素对比

胆管细胞癌	肝细胞癌
肝吸虫病感染	肝硬化
华支睾吸虫	慢性乙肝病毒感染
麝猫后睾吸虫	慢性丙肝病毒感染
先天性/慢性胆管扩张	黄曲霉素 B1
胆总管囊肿	慢性酒精肝
先天性肝内胆管扩张症	原发性胆汁性肝硬化
肝内胆管结石	血红蛋白沉着病
原发性硬化性胆管炎	α1 抗胰蛋白酶缺乏症
溃疡性结肠炎	糖原储积症
二氧化钍接触史	高血钙症
胆石症	血卟啉症
石棉接触史	遗传性酪氨酸血症
二噁英接触史	Wilson 综合征
多氯联苯接触史	肝毒素暴露史
亚硝胺接触史	二氧化钍
异烟肼接触史	聚氯乙烯
甲基多巴接触史	四氯化碳

其他可以引起胆道系统慢性炎症的疾病与胆管癌的发生关系亦非常密切，如多发性肝囊肿、胆总管囊肿、先天性肝内胆管扩张（Caroli 症）、原发性硬化性胆管炎（通常与炎症性肠病有关）、肝内胆管结石和胆总管结石等[83～88]。胆囊癌患者合并肝内胆管结石比较少见，仅有 5%～7%的肝内胆管结石患者最终发展成了胆管癌[87,88]。研究报告表明，在胆总管囊肿和 Caroli 症等先天性胆管扩张性疾病高发的地区，胆管癌的发病率为 3%～30%[89,90]。原发性硬化性胆管炎是导致胆管癌的另一个危险因素，9%～40%的硬化性胆管炎患者可发展成胆管癌[91,92]。溃疡性结肠炎也可以引起原发性硬化性胆管炎，但仅有 0.4%～1.4%的溃疡性结肠炎患者发生胆管癌[91]。在原发性硬化性胆管炎患者中，无论是否伴有溃疡性结肠炎，硬化性胆管炎和胆管癌影像学检查的鉴别诊断意义并不是很大。一项研究结果显示，血清肿瘤标志物 CA19-9 在原发性硬化性胆管炎合并胆管癌的诊断中敏感性和特异性分别为 89%和 86%[93]。联合应用 CA19-9 与 CEA 可能进一步提高硬化性胆管炎合并胆管癌诊断的正确率[94]。

患者接受过静脉注射造影剂 thorotrast（二氧化钍），原发性肝细胞癌、恶性血管内皮细胞瘤及胆管癌的发病率显著升高[95]。在由造影剂 thorotrast 引起的肝脏恶性肿瘤中，胆管癌是最常见的。服用或接触一些药物或致癌物质同样可以增加患胆管癌的风险（表 92-2）。由于胆管癌是一种相对少见的恶性肿瘤，因此我们还不能确切地了解每种致病因素导致胆管癌的致癌机制，但是可以肯定的是，任何可以引起胆道系统慢性炎症性疾病均可以增加患胆管癌的风险。

胆道系统的慢性炎症或胆汁中有毒成分浓度过高均可以引起胆管上皮细胞 DNA 的损伤,从而导致胆管癌的发生。胆管癌患者往往存在抑癌基因 *p53* 或 *K-ras* 的突变[96,97]。虽然 *p53* 或 *K-ras* 的突变率可能因地理或种族的不同而存在差异,但在绝大部分胆管癌患者中均存在着上述两种基因的突变(表 92-2)。*c-erbB-2* 是一种原癌基因,它编码一种跨膜蛋白,与表皮生长因子受体(EGFR)具有高度的同源性。胆管癌细胞和一些良性疾病增生的胆管上皮中,如肝内胆管结石、原发性硬化性胆管炎、肝吸虫病均发现 *c-erbB-2* 基因高表达[98]。突变的 *c-erbB-2* 可能在胆管慢性炎症疾病的早期就出现高表达,从而引起胆管上皮细胞的增殖并向胆管癌转变。胆道的慢性炎症还可以引起原癌基因 *Bcl-2* 的高表达,它可以通过抑制正常细胞凋亡从而导致胆管癌的发生[99]。

最后,最近的全基因组图谱还显示,肝内外胆管癌在细胞周期调节(CKDN2B)和染色质重塑方面有着许多相同的基因突变(*ARID1A*)[21]。肝内胆管癌还可表现为 *FGFR* 基因融合、IDH1/2(异枸橼酸脱氢酶)替换、*BRAF* 基因替换和 *MET* 基因扩增,而肝外胆管细胞癌可出现 PIK3CA/MTOR 通路频繁改变。

临床表现

胆管癌的临床表现缺乏特异性,但与肿瘤发生的部位关系密切。肝门部胆管癌常见的临床表现为无痛性黄疸,有些患者还可同时伴有疲劳、皮肤瘙痒、发热、不明原因的腹痛、纳差等症状。90%以上的肝门部胆管癌患者肝功能检查会出现碱性磷酸酶及总胆红素异常升高等梗阻性黄疸的表现[77]。肝内胆管癌往往在瘤体较大时才会出现临床症状。这些患者常表现为肝大、上腹部包块、腹部或背部疼痛及体重减轻等症状[77]。黄疸或腹水往往是肝内胆管癌晚期的临床表现。巨大肝内胆管癌出现的黄疸通常是肿瘤组织压迫左右肝管或两者汇合部引起的。

90%以上的肝内胆管癌患者可出现血清碱性磷酸酶水平升高[78]。大多数患者还同时伴有血清胆红素水平升高,特别是肿瘤组织发生于肝脏中心部位、肝外胆管或肝门部胆管部位的患者[100]。与原发性肝细胞癌不同的是,仅有不到5%的患者出现甲胎蛋白的升高[78]。40%~60%的患者伴有血清癌胚抗原的异常[78,101]。80%以上的患者可出现 CA19-9 的异常[101]。

病理

肝内胆管癌往往是孤立的实质性肿块,偶尔会出现微卫星灶结节[102]。肿瘤组织侵犯粗大的门静脉或肝静脉的概率远远低于原发性肝癌。肝内胆管癌体积大小和周围出现微转移灶对患者预后有重要的提示作用,因为肿瘤细胞的导管旁浸润往往提示淋巴结及肝内转移的概率增加[103]。胆管癌发生区域淋巴结、肺及腹腔转移较原发性肝细胞癌更常见。肿瘤压迫导致长期的胆道梗阻时可引起继发性胆汁性肝硬化。

显微镜下胆管癌细胞呈矮立方体状,与正常胆管上皮细胞相似。在同一肿瘤组织中可以看到肿瘤细胞不同程度的异型性、不典型性、核分裂象、细胞核深染以及核仁突出等异常表现。胆管癌细胞偶尔呈透明细胞状,此时应与肾脏透明细胞癌肝转移相鉴别[104]。胆管腺癌细胞可以分泌黏液,在肿瘤细胞内及胆管腔内常常可发现黏液素的存在,黏液素可作为胆管癌与原发性肝细胞癌的鉴别要点。另外,胆管癌细胞不能分泌胆汁,这一特征同样可以用于上述两种肿瘤组织的鉴别。通过免疫组化染色,如果上皮细胞膜抗原和组织多肽抗原阳性亦可支持胆管癌的诊断[105,106]。细胞角蛋白亚型免疫组化染色可帮助胆管癌与结肠癌肝转移相鉴别[107]。胆管癌以局部浸润为主,肿瘤细胞沿着神经纤维束和黏膜下层生长、浸润。

诊断

肝内胆管癌常常很难从病理学和影像学上与肝内转移性腺癌相鉴别。尽管腹部超声检查可以发现直径大于 2cm 的肝内恶性肿瘤,但很难区分究竟是肝内胆管癌、肝外腺癌肝内转移还是多发性肝细胞癌[108]。胆管癌的 CT 主要表现为不规则或分叶状低密度肿块(图 92-6),肿瘤周围可能出现微卫星灶,特别是在增强 CT 的动脉期会更为明显。约 25%的肿瘤组织可出现钙化现象,30%的肿块中心部会出现瘢痕组织[109]。胆管癌的 MRI 表现为边界不规则的非包裹性肿块,通常在 T1 加权像表现为低信号,在 T2 加权像表现为高信号。一般肿瘤组织在增强 MRI 往往表现为边缘强化肿块。相比 T1 加权像而言,肿瘤内瘢痕组织在 T2 加权像中更为明显,但肝内胆管癌在 CT 或 MRI 的表现同样也可以出现在其他肝脏肿瘤中[109]。

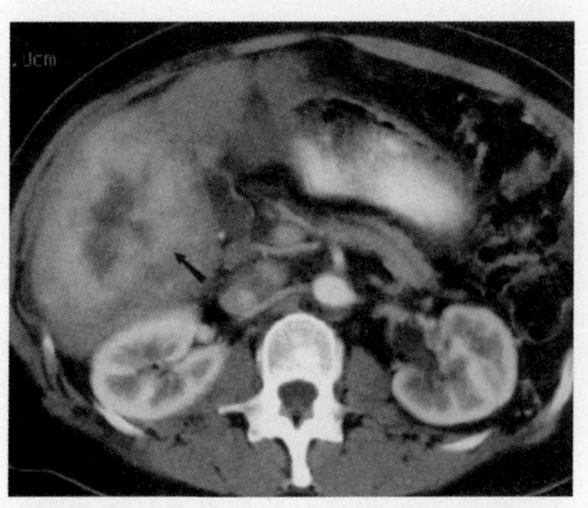

图 92-6 肝内胆管癌螺旋 CT 动脉期表现。肝内胆管癌(如箭头所示)边界不清并且在动脉期强化,在肿瘤的中心部位可见密度较低的瘢痕组织及肿瘤坏死组织

当患者表现为无痛性黄疸,且 CT 检查提示肝内胆管扩张而肝外胆管及胆囊大小正常时应考虑肝门部胆管癌。高分辨率螺旋 CT 可以明确胆道梗阻的部位及肿瘤侵犯肝脏及肝门部的范围(图 92-7)。多排螺旋 CT 可以准确地显示 63%~90%的肝门胆管癌患者胆道梗阻的部位[110,111]。术前螺旋 CT 检查还可发现由于胆道梗阻、门静脉栓塞而造成的肝叶或肝段萎缩(图 92-8)[111]。然而,术前 CT 并不能准确地判断肝门胆管癌是否可切除,因为 CT 对于评估肿瘤组织的胆管内浸润及门静脉、肝动脉的受累情况的准确性还有限[110,111]。

与 CT 扫描一样,肝门部胆管癌在超声下同样表现为肝内胆管扩张而胆囊及胆总管正常。随着超声影像技术的不断进步,65%~90%的肝门部胆管癌患者在 B 超检查下就可以发现病灶[112]。肝内胆管癌的 CT 或超声检查可发现肿瘤的局部浸润、远处转移以及门静脉周围转移的淋巴结[113]。术中超声检查也很难明确肝门部胆管癌沿胆管腔内的浸润程度,仅有 18%的患者可以明确肝门部胆管癌的局部浸润范围[114]。术中超声

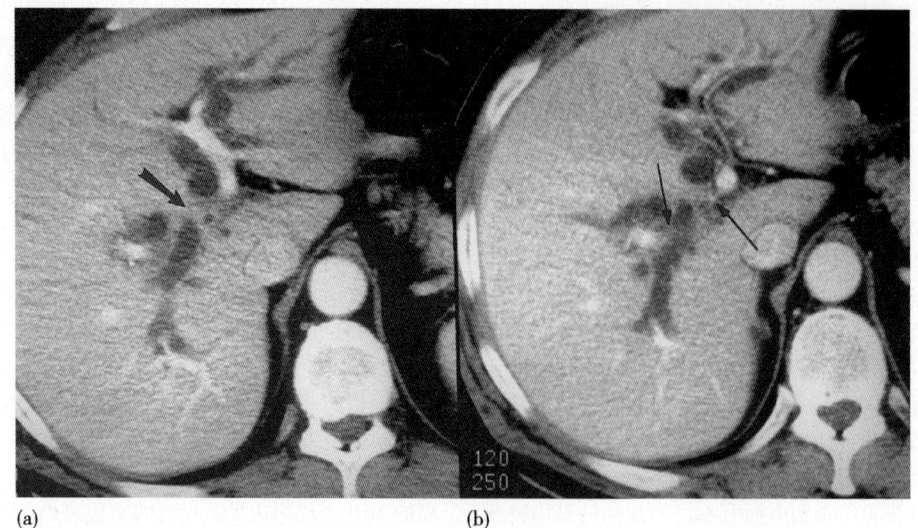

(a)　(b)

图 92-7　梗阻性黄疸患者高分辨率螺旋 CT 表现。图(a)显示肿瘤组织(粗箭头所指)导致肝内胆管显著扩张。图(b)显示(细箭头所指)肿瘤组织侵及门静脉,而且影像学检查结果在手术时得到了证实

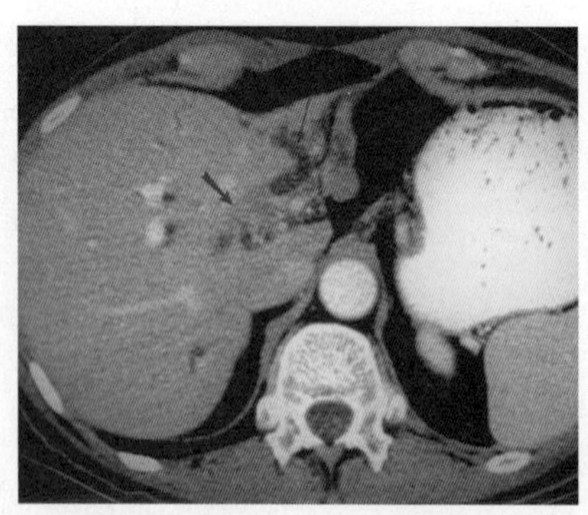

图 92-8　黄疸伴皮肤瘙痒数月患者的螺旋 CT 扫描。肿瘤呈低密度灶(大箭头)、肝内胆管扩张、肝左叶萎缩(小箭头),仅存少部分肝实质

可以用于发现肿瘤在肝内的微转移灶,并且可以准确判断肿瘤对门静脉及肝动脉的浸润情况,其准确率分别为 83.3%和 60%[114]。

与其他肝脏肿瘤类似,肝门部胆管癌在 T1 加权像表现为低信号和 T2 加权像上表现为高信号。肝门部胆管癌造成的梗阻时,可出现肝内胆管扩张的表现,若伴有门静脉栓塞时,还可出现肝叶的萎缩的表现。冠状位 MR 增强扫描可以显示胆管癌的浸润深度,同时还能很好地将血管及胆管组织区分开[115]。磁共振胰胆管成像(MRCP)及磁共振内镜技术可显示肿瘤组织阻塞肝门胆管而造成的肝内胆管扩张程度[115,116]。相比之下,MRCP 优于胆管造影的地方就是在于它是一种非侵入性的检查方式,并可以清晰地显示出孤立的胆管。

胆管造影能明确显示肝门部胆管癌引起的左右肝管梗阻(图 92-9),经皮肝穿刺胆道造影(PTC)及逆行性胰胆管造影(ERCP)对明确肝外胆道梗阻很有帮助。一项前瞻性的随机对照研究发现,上述两种技术在诊断梗阻性黄疸的准确率上基本一致[117]。PTC 在诊断左右肝管汇合部梗阻时的准确率为100%,而 ERCP 的准确率为 92%,不过 ERCP 的优点在于它在明确胆管是否存在梗阻的同时还可以使胰管显影,从而可以排除因微小的胰头部肿瘤而造成的胆道梗阻。另外,在行 PTC 或 ERCP 过程中还可以获得患者的细胞学标本,约 50%的患者在胆汁或胆管脱落细胞中可以发现肿瘤细胞[112,117~119]。

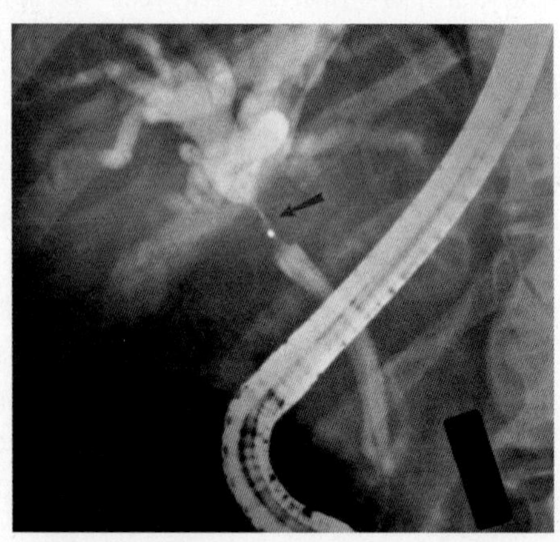

图 92-9　逆行性胰胆管造影显示肝外胆管局限性狭窄(箭头所示)及肝内胆管扩张,此例肝门部胆管癌行肿瘤切除,胆管空肠 Roux-en-Y 吻合来重建胆道

通过 PTC 置管引流可以部分或全部缓解由于胆道梗阻而引起的梗阻性黄疸等症状。随着引流技术的不断进步,引流管亦可以绕过肿瘤梗阻的部位进入十二指肠从而达到内引流的目的[120]。值得注意的是,临床工作中不能单纯为了缓解患者梗阻性黄疸的症状而一味地行胆道减压引流术。一项前瞻的随机对照研究结果显示,术前对梗阻性黄疸行胆汁引流并不能降低患者的死亡率[121],但术中置管造影不仅可以帮助辨别和解剖左右肝管汇合部位,还可以帮助肿瘤切除后的胆管重建[122,123]。

目前,正电子发射计算机断层显像(PET)已经被广泛地用于多种恶性肿瘤的临床诊断。PET 利用正电子发射放射性核素来标志一些生理需要的化合物如氟化脱氧葡萄糖(^{18}F-FDG),它

是一种葡萄糖的类似物，由于恶性肿瘤组织糖代谢非常快，因此造成该物质在肿瘤细胞内的堆积，从而可以被检测出来。PET 检查不能提供肝门胆管癌或肝内胆管癌的解剖结构来判断肿瘤的可切除性，但 PET 检查可以发现肿瘤组织远处转移灶，从而避免不必要的根治性手术。PET-CT 检查可以发现原发性硬化性胆管炎患者肝门或肝内胆管内微小的肿瘤病灶，从而为其治疗或器官移植提供决策依据[124]。目前，PET-CT 检查还为胆管癌的诊断与临床分期提供依据[125]。在 26 例行 PET-CT 检查的胆管癌患者中，有 24 例出现异常表现（敏感性为 92.3%），而 8 例胆管良性疾病的患者中（胆管腺瘤、硬化性胆管炎、先天性肝内胆管扩张）PET-CT 检查也提示为恶性病变。10 例经病理学证实存在远处转移的胆管癌患者中有 7 例 PET-CT 检查发现异常，而在 15 例伴区域淋巴结转移的患者中仅 2 例出现异常（13.3%）。

腹腔镜检查已经成为肝门部胆管癌诊断和临床分期的方法之一，我院正在对其应用价值作进一步评估。很多认为肿瘤可完整切除术的患者，通过腹腔镜检查时往往发现腹腔转移，从而避免了开腹探查更大的创伤。此外，具有腹腔种植风险的患者常在腹腔镜腹腔冲洗时发现肿瘤细胞。腹腔镜超声检查还可以发现肿瘤肝内转移灶以及肝门部胆管癌组织向肝内的浸润程度[126]。

肝内胆管癌的治疗

手术切除

30%～45%的肝内胆管癌患者可以在发生远处转移或出现梗阻性黄疸前得到明确诊断[127,128]，而对于这部分患者，手术切除当然是最佳的治疗方法，因为相关的研究结果显示，部分肝内胆管癌患者行部分肝切除术后可以长期存活[79,124,128,129]。另外一项对 19 例接受手术切除的肝内胆管癌患者的临床研究结果显示，不伴有肝门淋巴结转移的肝内胆管癌 3 年生存率为 64%，而伴有肝门淋巴结转移的患者 3 年生存率为 0[124]。一项对 32 例行肝切除术的肝内胆管癌患者的研究结果显示，区域淋巴结转移及肿瘤直径大于 5cm 是直接影响患者预后的危险因素[129]。切缘阴性的肝内胆管癌患者 5 年总体生存率为 20%～48%，伴有区域淋巴结转移、肝内微转移灶或门静脉浸润的患者往往预后较差[124,128,129]。肿瘤直径过大也提示患者预后较差，因为随着肿瘤的增长，肿瘤侵犯周围血管、淋巴管及胆管的概率也会增加[130]。

多学科综合治疗

与胆囊癌类似，由于缺乏临床试验数据，肝内胆管癌术后合理的辅助治疗方案尚未确定。尽管缺乏循证依据，但临床上术后是可以考虑行辅助放疗或化疗，尤其是对于淋巴结阳性或切缘阳性患者[71]。一些小样本量的回顾性研究均证实，对于不切除的肝门部胆管癌，实施射频消融（RAF）、经动脉化疗栓塞（TACE）、药物洗脱珠 TACE、EBRT、经动脉放射性栓塞（TARE）等局部治疗是安全有效的[131]。最近，MD 安德森癌症中心开展了一项研究，对 79 例不可切除的肝内胆管癌患者进行大剂量放射治疗 3～30 次，放射剂量为 35～100Gy（中位剂量 58.05Gy），其中中位生物当量剂量（BED）为 80.5Gy（43.75～180Gy）[132]。研究结果显示，中位总生存期为 30 个月。放射剂量是最重要的预后因素，且较高剂量的照射可见改善局部病灶控制率和提高总生存率，如当患者接受 BED>80.5Gy 时，3 年总生存率为 73%，而接受低剂量患者为 38%（$P<0.017$）；EBD>80.5Gy 时，3 年的局部控制率为 78% 显著高于低剂量患者（45%，$P=0.04$）[132]。

此外，对于不可切除和转移的肝门部胆管癌患者，传统的治疗是采用氟尿嘧啶或基于吉西他滨的方案进行全身化疗。关于肝门部胆管癌的化疗将在肝门部胆管癌治疗部分详细叙述。

肝门胆管癌

Fardel 于 1890 年首次提出了肝外胆管癌。1957 年一篇报道描述了 3 例起源于左右肝管汇合部的小腺癌[133]，这种起源于左右肝管汇合部的肝外胆管癌通常被称为 Klatskin 瘤。随后，该作者于 1965 年又报道了一组病例数更多的肝门部胆管癌[134]。

影响预后的因素

肝门部胆管癌患者预后的最重要因素是肿瘤的可切除性，但相关文献报道，肝门部胆管癌术后生存时间长短不一。文献报道，行肿瘤根治性切除的患者（肿瘤切缘阴性）3 年生存率为 40%～87%，5 年生存率为 10%～73%[60,135]。患者生存时间差别之大，究其原因可能是掺杂了其他因素影响患者预后。通常情况下，肝门部胆管癌根治性切除术后提示患者具有较好预后的因素包括：肿瘤组织高分化、不伴有淋巴结转移及肝内浸润、肿瘤细胞呈乳头状（而非结节型或硬化型）、血清胆红素水平<9mg/dl 以及患者一般情况正常或接近正常等。肿瘤的姑息性切除、外科胆管切除重建以及各种插管引流等保守治疗术后 3 年生存率仅为 0～4%[135]。肝门部胆管癌较中段或下段胆管癌的预后差，其直接原因在于肝门部胆管癌发现时往往已处于进展期，肿瘤组织浸入肝实质内，从而导致手术切除率明显下降[136]。与肝门部胆管癌相似，伴有淋巴结转移的中段或下段胆管癌术后较无淋巴结转移的患者，5 年生存率由 65%下降至 21%。

胆管癌术后的病理特征患者预后的重要因素。如果肿瘤浸润至浆膜或直接侵犯至肝实质时往往提示肿瘤已侵及血管或伴有淋巴结转移，通常提示预后不良。肿瘤的组织类型及分化程度同样是影响患者预后的重要因素。胆管乳头状癌虽然十分少见但预后最好，其 3 年生存率可达 75%[135,137]。与乳头状癌相比，胆管更多见的为结节型及硬化型，但 3 年生存率不到 30%。病理学通过研究各种组织类型胆管癌的扩散转移方式来解释其生存时间长短的差异。乳头状和表浅的结节型胆管癌主要局限在黏膜层，很少浸润到胆管壁的深层或淋巴管，但结节型胆管癌可以通过侵入淋巴管或直接在黏膜下浸润的方式向周围扩散[138]。肿瘤细胞从原发灶浸润至黏膜层或黏膜下层，最深多可达 30mm，但术中如可获得 5mm 阴性切缘便不会出现局部或吻合口的复发。胆管高分化或中分化腺癌 3 年生存率可达 51%，但低分化腺癌患者生存时间一般不超过 2 年[139]。

肝门部胆管癌治疗

手术切除

肝门部胆管癌手术切除是使患者获得长时间生存的首选的治疗方案。文献报道，肝门部胆管癌手术切除后 5 年生存率最高可达 40%，最低仅为 10%或更低。中段或下段胆管癌（往往需要行胰十二指肠切除术）患者生存率一般高于肝门部胆管癌[78]，这主要是由于中段或下段胆管癌术后较为容易获得阴性切缘且不容易发生肝内浸润有关。

肝门部胆管癌肝外胆管切除术后失败可表现成不同的形式(表 92-3)[139]，相当一部分肝门部胆管癌患者会出现肿瘤的局部复发，其中肝脏内肿瘤复发占 62%，肿瘤原位复发占 42%，区域淋巴结肿瘤复发占 20%。肝尾状叶是肝内复发的最常见部位。区域淋巴结复发包括肝门淋巴结、十二指肠后淋巴结及肝胃韧带内的胃周淋巴结群。大多数局部复发的患者往往伴有肿瘤的远处转移，但是有 24%的患者可直接发生远处转移。

表 92-3 肝门部胆管癌手术切除术后肿瘤复发部位

复发部位	频率(%)
肝脏	62
瘤床	42
区域淋巴结	20
腹膜	16
肺	71
骨骼	31
皮肤	7

对解剖学进行详细的研究，可以帮助我们了解肝门部胆管癌术后发生肝内及局部复发率高的原因。在 25 例行手术治疗的肝门部胆管癌患者中，有 12 例(46.2%)存在肿瘤肝内浸润，11 例(42.3%)肿瘤已同时侵入引流肝尾状叶的胆管中或直接侵入尾状叶肝实质内[140]。一项对 106 名成人的尸检结果显示，有 97.2%人存在引流尾状叶的胆管，该胆管可直接汇入左肝管、右肝管或同时汇入左右肝管。这些引流尾状叶的小胆管常直接汇入左右肝管汇合部 1cm 范围内，因此，发生于左右肝管汇合部附近的胆管癌很容易就浸润引流尾状叶的胆管。

通常认为胆管癌细胞沿着胆管壁呈浸润生长，而尾状叶和邻近的肝脏组织又常常是胆管癌切除术后肿瘤复发最为常见的部位，因此一些学者倾向于更为积极的手术方式，扩大切除的范围即包括尾状叶和肝门部肝脏实质[141~145]。肝门胆管癌的 Bismuth-Corlette 分型在临床中广泛应用，了解 Bismuth-Corlette 分型可以帮助确定肝切除的位置和范围(图 92-10)[146]。胆管癌扩大根治术后的中位生存时间为 10~37 个月，5 年生存率为 20%~44%，10 年生存率可达 14%[141~145]。虽然切除范围包括部分肝的肝门胆管癌扩大根治术可以给患者带来更长期生存的机会，但该术式风险很大，手术死亡率为 5%~12%，最常见的死亡原因是肝切除的体积过大而造成的术后肝衰竭[141~145]。据报道，手术后幸存的患者中，25%~45%的患者出现术后并发症，常见的是术后感染，而术前胆管支架置入引起的胆道感染更增加了患者术后发生感染的风险[147]。

我们近期回顾性分析了 1983—1996 年在得克萨斯大学安德森癌症医疗中心接受治疗的 91 例肝外胆管癌患者的资料[148]，其中 51 例(56%)患者已经失去手术机会，其余 40 例(44%)接受了手术治疗。手术患者术后中位生存时间为 22.2 个月，而非手术患者为 10.7 个月(P<0.001)。9 例(5 例肝门胆管癌和 4 例远端胆管癌)术前接受了放化疗(持续静脉滴注氟尿嘧啶 300mg/(m^2·d)联合体外放疗)，其中 3 例患者对放化疗反应良好，达到病理学完全缓解，剩余 6 例也出现了不同程度的缓解。9 例接受术前放化疗的患者术后病理学检查切缘均为阴性，而未接受术前放化疗的患者中仅有 54%的患者手术切缘阴性(P<0.01)。此外，术前接受放化疗的患者均未出现术中或术后并发症。因此，新辅助放化疗对于肝外胆管癌是安全的，可以达到抗肿瘤的作用，此外还有利于获得手术阴性切缘。

肝移植

肝门部胆管癌患者接受全肝切除后行原位肝移植(orthotopic liver transplantation，OLT)的病例已有报道[149~154]，这些患者在移植后 90 天内死于出血、脓毒血症及移植排斥反应的比例为 23.1%。1992 年的一项报道显示，对于原位肝移植后生存时间大于 3 个月的患者，其中位生存时间为 11 个月，而最近的一项调查显示其中位生存时间延长至 23 个月。研究系显示，对老年胆管癌患者行肝移植术后 5 年生存率为 5.0%，在移植术后三个月内死亡的患者中，85.4%的患者死于肿瘤复发。最近的研究显示，肝外胆管癌行 OLT 术后的 5 年生存率为 25%，对于一些处于Ⅰ、Ⅱ期的早期患者，其 5 年生存率可达 73%。大多数研究报告显示肝门胆管癌术后接受 OLT 效果不理想，因此大多数移植中心不再为肝门胆管癌患者行 OLT。肝移植治疗肝门胆管可作为一种评估多学科综合治疗的前瞻性治疗手段之一。

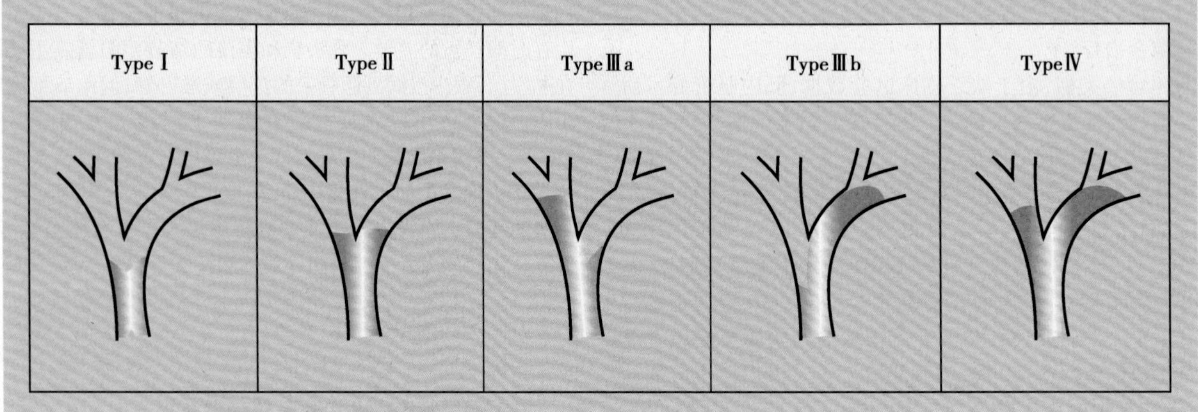

图 92-10 肝门胆管癌的 Bismuth-Corlette 分型。Bismuth Ⅰ型和Ⅱ型肝门胆管癌可行肝外胆管癌切除术(可酌情将肝门部肝实质和尾状叶一并切除)。Bismuth Ⅲa 和Ⅲb 型应分别将肝左叶或肝右叶一并切除。Bismuth Ⅳ型肝门胆管癌应放弃手术治疗

姑息治疗

一般而言，临床上只有不到30%的肝门胆管癌患者可以行手术切除[60,135,136]。对于那些已经失去手术机会的患者，可以通过经皮或经内镜胆道引流从而避免不必要的开腹手术[155,156]。传统的10-或12-聚乙烯支架容易出现支架闭塞和引起胆管炎[156]。然而，一种新型的扩张型金属支架可以达到长期通畅引流的目的，此外它还可以起到放疗定位作用[157,158]。当肝门胆管癌开腹探查发现已经失去手术机会时，此时必须决定是行转流手术还是行外科置管引流术。对于70%～100%的患者来说，无论是行转流术、外科置管还是经皮胆汁引流，均可使梗阻性黄疸得到部分或完全缓解[60]。与经皮胆汁引流相比，外科转流术的唯一好处在于患者不必携带外置的引流管，而体内没有内、外引流管是评价化疗后生活质量的重要指标。另外，对不可切除的肝门部胆管癌患者，全身化疗也无特殊的疗效。

放疗

目前，放疗对胆管癌的疗效尚不确定。不同放射性粒子、放疗剂量及照射路径在可切除和不可切除术的胆管癌患者治疗中均有少量报道。应用^{169}Ir射线内照射或粒子植入可以使梗阻性黄疸得以缓解，但由此引起的胆管炎发作次数或频率并没有得到改善，因此其放疗的总体价值尚不明确[159]。胆管癌体内放疗可以使患者的生存时间平均延长16个月，尤其是对于有些失去手术机会的患者通过体内放疗可以使生存时间延长至5年以上[160～162]。虽然单纯应用体外放疗治疗肝门胆管癌并没有显著改善患者的总体生存率，但仍有长期存活的个案报道[163]。目前，有研究对术中体内放疗治疗肝门胆管癌的疗效进行了评估[164,165]，它可以使失去手术机会的患者生存时间得到略微的延长，但目前人们对术中放疗最为感兴趣的就是直接对术后肿瘤最容易复发的部位进行放射治疗。

化疗

大多数肝门部胆管癌和肝内胆管癌患者就诊时就已经失去手术机会，因此目前有很多放、化疗方案可用于缓解患者症状、延长患者生存时间。前期研究结果显示，化疗效果明显优于单纯的营养支持治疗。这项研究对随机抽取的90例进展期胰腺癌或胆管癌患者(n=37)应用氟尿嘧啶为主的化学药物进行化疗，而对照组仅进行对症营养支持治疗。结果显示，化疗组患者中位生存时间为6个月，而对症支持治疗组中位生存时间为2.5个月[166]。随后，一项对23例局部进展期或远处转移的胆管癌患应用吉西他滨单药化疗治疗的研究结果显示[167]，中位随访13.4个月后，23例患者的肿瘤中位进展时间为8.1个月，总生存时间为13.1个月。这项实验研究表明，进展期胆管癌可以从吉西他滨的治疗中获益。目前，胆管癌常见的化疗药物包括氟尿嘧啶、吉西他滨、卡培他滨、顺铂和奥沙利铂[168]。

联合化疗方案正在应用于胆管癌，以期提供单药的疗效。对35例胆管癌患者应用氟尿嘧啶联合干扰素-2b进行化疗的研究结果显示，部分缓解率为34%(32例患者有11例缓解)，肿瘤中位进展时间为9.5个月，中位生存时间为12个月[169]。一项对75例患者(45例胆管癌，3例壶腹癌，27例胆囊癌)采取吉西他滨联合卡培他滨治疗研究结果显示，所有患者耐受性良好，有效率为29%，中位无进展生存期为6.2个月，总生存时间为12.7个月[170]。另一项对一般状态良好、胆红素小于正常值得2倍和自愿接受吉西他滨联合奥沙利铂作为一线化疗的患者予以吉西他滨联合奥沙利铂联合化疗(GEMOX)研究结果显示，有效率为33%，中位无进展生存期5.7个月，中位生存期为15.4个月[171]。

一项包括104项临床试验的荟萃分析显示，对2 810例进展期胆管癌联合吉西他滨和顺铂方案化疗较单药化疗的有效率最高，肿瘤控制更加稳定[172]。但这一结果并不意味着在肿瘤的任何时期行上述两种药的联合化疗方案均可控制肿瘤进展时间和延长总体生存率。一项包括410例不可切除或转移的胆管癌、胆囊癌或壶腹癌的ABC-02研究显示吉西他滨联合顺铂方案化疗较吉西他滨单药化疗疗效好[173]，总生存时间(11.7个月 vs 8.1个月；HR=0.64；95%CI：0.52～0.80；P<0.001)和无进展生存期延长(8.0个月 vs 5.0个月；HR=0.63；95%CI：0.51～0.77；P<0.001)。患者不仅对联合化疗的耐受性良好，而且临床获益显著。此后，另一项包括84例进展期胆管癌也显示类似的结果[174]。因此，吉西他滨联合顺铂仍然是不可切除的转移性胆囊癌或胆管癌的一线化疗方案，二线化疗方案包括联合氟尿嘧啶或联合吉西他滨的化疗方案。这些二线化疗方案得到了大量的Ⅱ期临床试验支持[175～179]。

近期，胆管癌中已经几种靶向药物治疗的研究报道。一项包含42例患者的临床研究结果显示，患者口服酪氨酸激酶抑制剂埃罗替尼拮抗表皮生长因子受体可以获得良好的疗效[180]，其中3例患者得到部分缓解，7例患者获得6个月的无进展生存。最新的靶向药物治疗试验报道了150例使用GEMOX方案化疗联合或不联合西妥昔单抗治疗进展晚期胆道癌[181]。研究结果显示，试验组总的生存率和无进展生存期无差异。其他靶向药物(包括索拉非尼和帕尼单抗)联合化疗药物治疗胆管癌研究结果显示，与单独化疗药物治疗相比没有显著改善结果[182～186]。

介入放疗及体内放疗

由于单纯体外放疗不能有效延长患者生存时间和改善治疗效果，体外放疗联合辅助腔内放疗成为一种人们广泛关注的治疗方案。最佳的治疗顺序是首先行体外放疗，使癌组织萎缩，然后进行辅助腔内放疗进一步杀伤存留的癌组织。目前已有对于无法行手术切除的肝门部胆管癌患者单独应用[170]Ir进行腔内放射治疗的报道[187]。腔内放疗联合体外放疗(45～50Gy)时的剂量应为15～35Gy，若单独应用时剂量可上调为60Gy，体内放疗的剂量参考点的范围是中央导管周围的0.5～1cm。体外放疗联合体内放疗的总剂量应控制在60～70Gy，尽管这一剂量已经超过了肝和小肠的最大耐受能力，但辐射剂量主要集中在一小块组织范围内。接受体内放疗的胆囊癌患者，其中包括是否或联合应用体外放疗的，其总体的中位生存时间为15～18个月，个别患者存活时间超过4年，但大多数患者最终还是发生了肿瘤的局部复发。

(李维坤 钟宇新 译 田艳涛 校)

参考文献

The complete reference list can be found on the Wiley Companion Digital Edition of this title (see inside front cover for login instructions).

9 Khan ZR, Neugut AI, Ahsan H, Chabot JA. Risk factors for biliary tract cancers. *Am J Gastroenterol*. 1999;**94**:149–152.

12 Csendes A, Becerra M, Burdiles P, et al. Bacteriological studies of bile from the gallbladder in patients with carcinoma of the gallbladder, cholelithiasis, common bile duct stones and no gallstones disease. *Eur J Surg*. 1994;**160**:363–367.

14 Albores-Saavedra J, Alcantra-Vazquez A, Cruz-Ortiz H, Herrera-Goepfert R. The precursor lesions of invasive gallbladder carcinoma. Hyperplasia, atypical hyperplasia and carcinoma in situ. *Cancer*. 1980;**45**:919–927.

20 Quan ZW, Wu K, Wang J, et al. Association of p53, p16, and vascular endothelial growth factor protein expressions with the prognosis and metastasis of gallbladder cancer. *J Am Coll Surg*. 2001;**193**:380–383.

23 Fahim RB, McDonald JR, Richards JC, Ferris DO. Carcinoma of the gallbladder. A study of its modes of spread. *Ann Surg*. 1962;**156**:114–122.

26 Ito M, Mishima Y, Sato T. An anatomical study of the lymphatic drainage of the gallbladder. *Surg Radiol Anat*. 1991;**13**:89–104.

44 Groot Koerkamp B, Fong Y. Outcomes in biliary malignancy. *J Surg Oncol*. 2014;**110**:585–591.

53 Fong Y, Brennan MF, Turnbull A, et al. Gallbladder cancer discovered during laparoscopic surgery. Potential for iatrogenic tumor dissemination. *Arch Surg*. 1993;**128**:1054–1056.

62 Falkson G, MacIntyre JM, Moertel CG. Eastern Cooperative Oncology Group experience with chemotherapy for inoperable gallbladder and bile duct cancer. *Cancer*. 1984;**54**:965–969.

65 Yang R, Wang B, Chen YJ, et al. Efficacy of gemcitabine plus platinum agents for biliary tract cancers: a meta-analysis. *Anticancer Drugs*. 2013;**24**:871–877.

69 Kopelson G, Harisiadis L, Tretter P, Chang CH. The role of radiation therapy in cancer of the extra-hepatic biliary system. An analysis of thirteen patients and a review of the literature of the effectiveness of surgery, chemotherapy and radiotherapy. *Int J Radiat Oncol Biol Phys*. 1977;**2**:883–894.

71 Horgan AM, Amir E, Walter T, Knox JJ. Adjuvant therapy of biliary tract cancer: a systemic review and meta-analysis. *J Clin Oncol*. 2012;**30**:1934–1940.

76 Ben-Josef E, Guthrie KA, El-Khoueiry AB, et al. SWOG S0809: a phase II intergroup trial of adjuvant capecitabine and gemcitabine followed by radiotherapy and concurrent capecitabine in extrahepatic cholangiocarcinoma and gallbladder carcinoma. *J Clin Oncol*. 2015;**33(24)**:2617–2622.

82 Kurathong S, Lerdverasirikul P, Wongpaitoon V, et al. *Opisthorchis viverrini* infection and cholangiocarcinoma. A prospective, case-controlled study. *Gastroenterology*. 1985;**89**:151–156.

84 Voyles CR, Smadja C, Shands WC, Blumgart LH. Carcinoma in choledochal cysts. Age-related incidence. *Arch Surg*. 1983;**118**:986–988.

86 Wee A, Ludwig J, Coffey RJ Jr, et al. Hepatobiliary carcinoma associated with primary sclerosing cholangitis and chronic ulcerative colitis. *Hum Pathol*. 1985;**16**:719–726.

95 Ito Y, Kojiro M, Nakashima T, Mori T. Pathomorphologic characteristics of 102 cases of thorotrast-related hepatocellular carcinoma, cholangiocarcinoma, and hepatic angiosarcoma. *Cancer*. 1988;**62**:1153–1162.

98 Terada T, Ashida K, Endo K, et al. c-erbB-2 protein is expressed in hepatolithiasis and cholangiocarcinoma. *Histopathology*. 1998;**33**:325–331.

101 Jalanko H, Kuusela P, Roberts P, et al. Comparison of a new tumour marker, CA 19–9, with alpha-fetoprotein and carcinoembryonic antigen in patients with upper gastrointestinal diseases. *J Clin Pathol*. 1984;**37**:218–222.

104 Yamamoto M, Takasaki K, Yoshikawa T, et al. Does gross appearance indicate prognosis in intrahepatic cholangiocarcinoma? *J Surg Oncol Suppl*. 1998;**69**:162–167.

108 Colli A, Cocciolo M, Mumoli N, et al. Peripheral intrahepatic cholangiocarcinoma. Ultrasound findings and differential diagnosis from hepatocellular carcinoma. *Eur J Ultrasound*. 1998;**7**:93–99.

111 Han JK, Choi BI, Kim TK, et al. Hilar cholangiocarcinoma. Thin-section spiral CT findings with cholangiographic correlation. *Radiographics*. 1997;**17**:1475–1485.

114 Kusano T, Shimabukuro M, Tamai O, et al. The use of intra-operative ultrasonography for detecting tumor extension in bile duct carcinoma. *Int Surg*. 1997;**82**:44–48.

119 Tanaka M, Ogawa Y, Matsumoto S, Nakayama F. The role of endoscopic retrograde cholangiopancreatography in preoperative assessment of bile duct cancer. *World J Surg*. 1988;**12**:27–32.

122 Cameron JL, Broe P, Zuidema GD. Proximal bile duct tumors. Surgical management with silastic transhepatic biliary stents. *Ann Surg*. 1982;**196**:412–419.

125 Kluge R, Schmidt F, Caca K, et al. Positron emission tomography with [(18)F]fluoro-2-deoxy-D-glucose for diagnosis and staging of bile duct cancer. *Hepatology*. 2001;**33**:1029–1035.

128 Lieser MJ, Barry MK, Rowland C, et al. Surgical management of intrahepatic cholangiocarcinoma. A 31-year experience. *J Hepatobiliary Pancreat Surg*. 1998;**5**:41–47.

129 Pichlmayr R, Lamesch P, Weimann A, et al. Surgical treatment of cholangiocellular carcinoma. *World J Surg*. 1995;**19**:83–88.

132 Tao R, Krishnan S, Bhosale PR, et al. Ablative radiotherapy doses lead to a substantial prolongation of survival in patients with inoperable intrahepatic cholangiocarcinoma: a retrospective dose response analysis. *J Clin Oncol*. 2015. pii: JCO.2015.61.3778.

134 Klatskin G. Adenocarcinoma of the hepatic duct at its bifurcation within the porta hepatis. *Am J Med*. 1965;**38**:241–248.

136 Burke EC, Jarnagin WR, Hochwald SN, et al. Hilar cholangiocarcinoma. Patterns of spread, the importance of hepatic resection for curative operation, and a presurgical clinical staging system. *Ann Surg*. 1998;**228**:385–394.

138 Ouchi K, Suzuki M, Hashimoto L, Sato T. Histologic findings and prognostic factors in carcinoma of the upper bile duct. *Am J Surg*. 1989;**157**:552–556.

142 Bengmark S, Ekberg H, Evander A, et al. Major liver resection for hilar cholangiocarcinoma. *Ann Surg*. 1988;**207**:120–125.

145 Baer HU, Stain SC, Dennison AR, et al. Improvements in survival by aggressive resections of hilar cholangiocarcinoma. *Ann Surg*. 1993;**217**:20–27.

149 Ringe B, Wittekind C, Bechstein WO, et al. The role of liver transplantation in hepatobiliary malignancy. A retrospective analysis of 95 patients with particular regard to tumor stage and recurrence. *Ann Surg*. 1989;**209**:88–98.

150 Yokoyama I, Sheahan DG, Carr B, et al. Clinicopathologic factors affecting patient survival and tumor recurrence after orthotopic liver transplantation for hepatocellular carcinoma. *Transplant Proc*. 1991;**23**:2194–2196.

159 Meyers WC, Jones RS. Internal radiation for bile duct cancer. *World J Surg*. 1988;**12**:99–104.

166 Glimelius B, Hoffman K, Sjoden PO, et al. Chemotherapy improves survival and quality of life in advanced pancreatic and biliary cancer. *Ann Oncol*. 1996;**7(6)**:593–600.

172 Eckel F, Schmid RM. Chemotherapy in advanced biliary tract carcinoma: a pooled analysis of clinical trials. *Br J Cancer*. 2007;**96(6)**:896–902. Epub 2007 Feb 27.

173 Valle J, Wasan H, Palmer DH, et al. Cisplatin plus gemcitabine versus gemcitabine for biliary tract cancer. *N Engl J Med*. 2010;**362(14)**:1273–1281.

第 93 章　胰腺外分泌肿瘤

Robert A. Wolff, MD ■ Christopher H. Crane, MD ■ Donghui Li, PhD ■ Douglas B. Evans, MD ■ Anirban Maitra, MD ■ Susan Tsai, MD

概述

胰腺腺癌是致死性最高的恶性肿瘤之一。在全球范围内,每年约有 33 万人死于胰腺癌。吸烟和肥胖是胰腺癌的危险因素,目前认为大约一半的病例是可以预防的。胰腺癌的遗传易感性包括 *BRCA1* 或 *BRCA2* 种系突变引发的综合征、波伊茨-耶格综合征(Peutz-Jeghers syndrome)以及遗传性非息肉病性结肠癌等。*KRAS*、*CDKN2A/INK4A*、*TP53* 和 *SMAD4/DPC4* 是常见的体细胞突变。胰腺癌经常在确诊时原发性肿瘤已不能手术或存在远处转移而失去根治性治疗的机会。目前,临床分期将胰腺恶性肿瘤分为可切除(潜在可治愈的),交界可切除、局部进展或转移性胰腺癌。对于可切除或交界可切除胰腺癌,手术具有治愈的可能性。对于局部进展期或转移性胰腺癌,化疗作为一种辅助治疗手段,已被证明可以延长生存期,但是放射治疗的作用还没有得到很好的定义,也没有被普遍接受。迄今为止,分子靶向治疗尚未显示出临床获益。辅助或新辅助治疗用于可切除和交界可切除的胰腺癌。胰腺癌的分子生物学研究越来越多的关注肿瘤微环境在侵袭、转移潜能和耐药性中的作用。关注基质修饰和免疫调控的新治疗策略成为临床和转化研究的前沿。

简介

通常所说的胰腺癌指胰腺导管腺癌。胰腺癌是恶性程度最高的实体肿瘤之一,极易出现局部侵袭,早期局部淋巴结转移,或血行远处播散。治愈只有在局部可切除胰腺癌的情况下才有可能而且约 80%的患者术后发生复发。在美国,胰腺癌是目前癌症相关的第四大死因[1]。在 2015 年,胰腺癌导致约 40 500 人死亡[1]。在全世界范围内,每年约 33 万人死于胰腺癌,预计到 2020 年,胰腺癌将成为癌症相关的第二大死因[3]。

在本章中,我们综述了现有的关于胰腺癌流行病学、病理学、分子细胞生物学,以及诊断和治疗方面的文献,进一步讨论了疾病预防、早期诊断、临床管理和涉及基因组学、表观遗传学、肿瘤代谢及肿瘤微环境的转化研究的未来发展方向。

流行病学

在世界范围内,胰腺癌发病率在常见恶性肿瘤中位列第十三,癌症相关死亡中位列第八[2]。胰腺癌的发病率在工业化发达地区和西方国家最高[4]。根据年龄调整后的发病率,在北欧,中欧和东欧部分地区每 10 万人中有 10~15 人,而非洲和亚洲地区发病率低于十万分之一[5]。基于 SEER(流行病学监测和最终结果)2001—2005 年数据,在美国,所有种族按年龄调整后的每年发病率(每 10 万人)分别为:男性 13.0,女性 10.3。根据年龄调整后年死亡率(每 10 万人)分别为:黑人男性 15.4,黑人女性 12.4,白人男性 12.1,白人女性 9.0。相对于非洲本土人群,非裔美国人的胰腺癌发病率明显增高,这就意味着胰腺癌的发病率可能与环境影响有关进而造成黑种人群和白种人群之间的差异。

大多数患者确诊时年龄在 60~80 岁之间[4,6]。以前胰腺癌发病率的男女比例为 1.2∶1,现在男女发病率大致相同。

病因学

和大多数其他类型的人类癌症一样,胰腺癌的病因学涉及遗传和非遗传因素(图 93-1)。

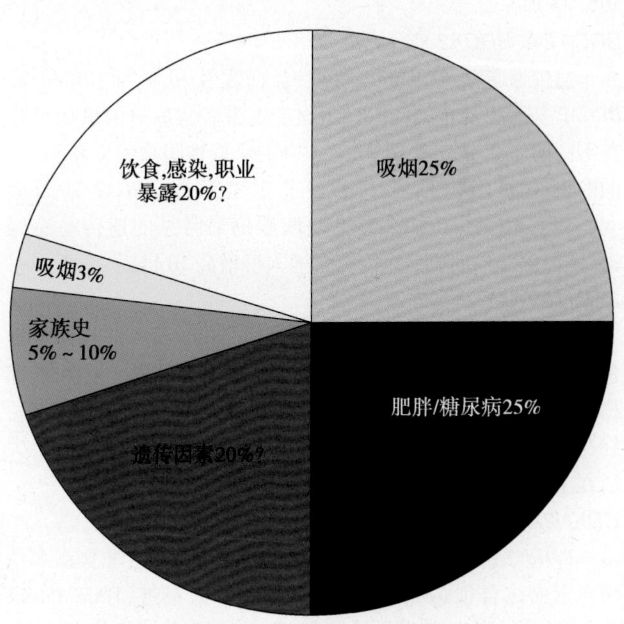

图 93-1　胰腺癌已知和可疑危险因素的示意图

遗传风险因素

遗传性或家族性胰腺癌大约占所有胰腺癌的 5%~10%[7]。家族性胰腺癌的高危人群为至少有两个直系亲属患胰腺癌[8]。虽然基因突变导致胰腺癌的大部分家族内遗传聚集类型尚未确定,少数几个与已知的癌症综合征或慢性炎性疾病有关的胰腺癌基因已被确定(表 93-1)[7]。

表 93-1 胰腺癌易感基因

基因	综合征	染色体位置	功能
PRSS1	遗传性胰腺炎	7q35	胰蛋白酶原、丝氨酸蛋白酶
SPINK1		5q32	丝氨酸肽(胰蛋白酶)抑制剂
CFTR	囊性纤维化	7q31.2	ABC 氯离子转通道
BRCA1	遗传性乳腺卵巢癌	17q21	DNA 损伤修复
BRCA2		13q12.3	
CDKN2A/P16	家族性非典型多痣黑素瘤	9p21	细胞周期蛋白依赖性激酶抑制剂
STK11/LKB1	黑斑息肉综合征	19p13.3	丝氨酸/苏氨酸激酶
MSH2,*MLH1*	遗传性非息肉性结直肠癌	2p21	错配修复
PMS1/2,*MGH6*		3p21.3	
APC	家族性腺瘤性息肉病	5q21	β-catenin 负性调节因子
PALB2	乳腺和胰腺癌	16p12.2	BRCA2 的定位协作基因
ATM	毛细血管扩张性失调	11q22-q23	DNA 损伤反应

PRSS1 和 *SPINK1*

PRSS1 和 *SPINK1* 基因的种系突变与遗传性胰腺炎相关。*PRSS1* 基因编码阳离子胰蛋白酶原蛋白,胰蛋白酶原蛋白过早激活导致急性胰腺炎。*SPINK1* 基因编码抑肽酶,该基因突变与慢性胰腺炎相关。研究表明遗传性胰腺炎患者胰腺癌的患病风险增加了 53 倍,胰腺癌的终身发病风险(70 岁)为 30%~40%[7]。

BRCA1 和 *BRCA2*

遗传性乳腺癌和卵巢癌综合征发生机制与 *BRCA1* 或 *BRCA2* 基因突变有关。*BRCA1* 突变携带者胰腺癌的患病风险在不同的研究中结果不同[7]。10%的家族性胰腺癌患者和 7%的散发性胰腺癌患者中出现了生殖系的 *BRCA2* 基因突变[9~11]。生殖系 *BRCA2* 突变是胰腺癌最常见的遗传易感因素,使得胰腺癌的患病风险比普通人群增高 10 倍[12]。

LKB1/STK11

波伊茨-耶格综合征(Peutz-Jeghers syndrome)是一种常染色体显性遗传,由 *LKB1/STK11* 抑癌基因突变导致。波伊茨-耶格综合征患者胰腺癌的患病风险比普通人群增高 96~132 倍,终身患病风险为 5%~36%[13,14]。双等位基因 *LKB1/STK11* 失活在手术切除的散发胰腺癌中占 4%[15]。

CDKN2A(p16)

CDKN2A(*p16*)抑癌基因的种系突变与家族性非典型多痣黑色素瘤综合征(FAMMM)高度相关。据报道,FAMMM 家族人群的胰腺癌患病风险增加了 13~22 倍[16],携带 *p16/CDKN2A* 突变的个体与普通人群相比,患病风险增加了 38 倍[17]。*CDKN2A* 基因失活在散发性胰腺癌中也经常发生。

HNPCC 和 *FAP*

遗传性非息肉病性结肠癌(HNPCC,也称为 Lynch 综合征),是由几种错配修复基因突变导致的种系突变引起的[18]。Lynch 综合征家族胰腺癌的患病风险增加了 8.6 倍[19]。也有研究表明:由于 *APC* 抑癌基因遗传缺陷导致的家族性腺瘤性息肉病家族,胰腺癌的患病风险升高[20]。

PALB2 和 *ATM*

PALB2 和 *ATM* 基因的突变已经在家族性胰腺癌患者中发现[21~23]。PALB2 蛋白与 BRCA2 蛋白结合后稳定存在于细胞核中,作用于双链 DNA 修复。ATM 是一个重要的细胞对 DNA 损伤的反应调节器。据估计,*PALB2* 突变可能占家族聚集胰腺癌的 1%~3%[21,22]。

最近在 727 个不相关的家族性胰腺癌先证者中进行的一项研究表明胰腺癌致癌突变占比分别为:*BRCA1*,1.2%;*BRCA2*,3.7%;*PALB2*,0.6%;*CDKN2A*,2.5%。大多数家族性胰腺癌具有 *BRCA2* 和 *CDKN2A* 基因突变[24]。

易感性变异

三项全基因组相关研究(GWAS)在美国开展,其中大多数研究人群具有欧洲血统[25-27]。*ABO*、*NR5A2*、*LINC-PINC*、*PDX1*、*BCAR1/CTRB1/CTRB2*、*ZNRF3* 和 *TERT* 基因多态性和非基因染色体区域 13q22.1 变异被确定为胰腺癌的易感因素且具有基因组显著性差异($P<5\times10^{-8}$)。另外两个 GWAS 研究在中国[28]和日本人群中进行[29]。GWAS 之后的分析表明参与胰腺发生途径的基因可能改变胰腺癌的发病风险[30~32]。对于基因和已知病因(如吸烟[33]、肥胖和糖尿病[34,35])的相互作用的进行初步分析为解释遗传因素导致的胰腺癌易感性提供有趣的线索。致病等位基因和功能特征的基因或变异研究可能涉及多种对表型影响微弱的基因[36,37]。

吸烟和饮酒

吸烟是胰腺癌最密切相关的危险因素。据估计,大约 25%的胰腺癌与吸烟相关,吸烟使患病风险增加 1.5~2.0 倍[38~41],且风险随着吸烟数量和持续时间而增加。长期戒烟(>10 年)比持续吸烟者的发病风险降低了大约 30%[38,42]。对于无烟烟草产品是否会增加胰腺癌患病风险仍有争议[43,44]。

吸烟诱发胰腺癌的机制包括烟草致癌物引起的脱氧核糖核酸损伤和胰腺组织伤害[45]。烟草致癌物可以被代谢激活引起脱氧核糖核酸损伤和基因突变[46,47]。烟碱在肿瘤发生、发展中通过乙酰胆碱烟碱型受体和肾上腺素受体介导的信号转导途径在导致胰腺损伤的多因素事件中发挥重要作用[45,46,48]。

酒精摄入和胰腺癌之间的联系也已被研究。一般来说，重度饮酒摄入（30~40g 酒精或≥3 杯/天），而不是轻度或中度酒精摄入，与胰腺癌风险增加有关[49~52]。饮酒引发的胰腺癌可能占所有胰腺癌的 2%~5%。

肥胖

与烟草相似，据估计在美国人群中，肥胖导致的胰腺癌占 25%[53]。几项大样本前瞻性研究和荟萃分析表明肥胖与胰腺癌发病率呈正相关[54~62]。除了体重指数之外，腹部脂肪（通过腰臀比例来测量），已被证明可以增加患胰腺癌的风险，并且在女性中更为明显[60,61]。年轻肥胖人群比年长者的胰腺癌患病风险更高。此外，肥胖与发病年龄越小和总体存活率降低有关[63]。肥胖与胰腺癌相关的生物学机制为胰岛素抵抗和炎症[64]。使用预测诊断的血样分析研究显示胰腺癌患病风险与高血糖和胰岛素抵抗标志物呈正相关[65~68]。胰岛素和胰岛素样生长因子是细胞内代谢和生长的关键调节剂，其信号转导的网络在肿瘤发生、发展中起着重要作用[69~71]。胰腺癌的发生机制可能与其他癌症相关炎症发生有相似之处。脂肪浸润可能导致脂肪性胰腺炎，这提示肥胖、非酒精性脂肪性胰腺疾病、非酒精性脂肪性胰腺炎和胰腺癌之间可能存在潜在联系[72,73]。

糖尿病和糖尿病治疗药物

糖尿病被认为是胰腺癌的早期表现和诱发因素[74]。三个大样本荟萃分析[75~77]和三个合并的数据（每个包括 1 500 以上胰腺癌患者）分析一致表明：长期糖尿病增加胰腺癌发病风险[68,78,79]。值得注意的是，胰腺癌可诱发外周胰岛素抵抗[80]和 3c 型（胰源性）糖尿病[81]。高糖血症可能在临床确诊胰腺癌两年前就已经发生，每 125 个新发糖尿病患者中有一人会在 3 年内患胰腺癌[82,83]。目前正在开发有助鉴别 2 型糖尿病和 3c 型糖尿病的生物标志物[84,85]。

自从发现最常用的糖尿病治疗药物双胍，在实验动物中[86]具有抑制胰腺肿瘤发生的作用后，糖尿病治疗药物降低胰腺癌发病风险的作用被深入研究。其他实验性证据亦支持二甲双胍的抗肿瘤作用[87,88]。二甲双胍具有多种调节作用，其主要分子靶点为肝激酶 B1（LKB1）-腺苷酸-活化蛋白激酶（AMPK）和西罗莫司激酶（mTOR）信号通路，其在细胞内能量稳态、细胞分裂和细胞增殖的调节中处于核心地位[89]。二甲双胍还抑制细胞转化相关的炎反应和选择性靶向作用于肿瘤干细胞[91-92]。在人群中，八项队列研究[92~98]和三项病例对照研究[99~101]报道了二甲双胍的使用对胰腺癌发病的影响。这些研究的荟萃分析估计相对危险度为 0.63[102]。另外两项研究显示二甲双胍用于胰腺癌并发糖尿病的患者可以延长生存期，降低死亡风险[103,104]。

胰腺炎

慢性胰腺炎是胰腺癌的一个危险因素，胰腺炎发作可能是隐匿性胰腺癌的征兆[105]。10 个病例对照研究汇总数据对肥胖和饮酒进行调整后，表明对于胰腺炎和胰腺癌诊断时间间隔超过 2 年的患者，胰腺癌的发病风险增加 3 倍[106]。

感染性疾病

幽门螺杆菌可能导致亚临床胰腺炎或增加患者体内促胃液素分泌水平，进一步影响胰腺的营养供给。多个研究报道了幽门螺杆菌和胰腺之间的联系；大样本的荟萃分析显示既往幽门螺杆菌感染与胰腺癌的发病关联比较微弱，但差异有统计学意义[107]。有假设认为 *ABO* 基因型/表型状态影响幽门螺杆菌的行为，进而影响胃和胰腺分泌功能。这些最终会影响饮食和吸烟相关的 N-亚硝胺暴露而对胰腺产生致癌性，从而导致胰腺癌患病风险[108]。

乙肝病毒同样也是胰腺癌的危险因素[109]。后续研究主要集中在亚洲进行，包括九项此类研究的荟萃分析报告慢性 HBV（乙型肝炎病毒）携带者总相对风险率为 1.39（95%*CI*：1.22~1.59），过去乙肝接触史的总相对风险率 1.41（95%*CI*：0.06~1.87）[110]。乙肝表面抗原在胰液和胆汁中均被检测到[111]，有证据表明 HBV 病毒在胰腺细胞中复制。乙型肝炎病毒通过炎症反应导致胰腺外分泌和内分泌上皮细胞的损伤[112,113]。

饮食因素

各种饮食因素在胰腺癌的发生、发展中有一定作用。一般来说，脂肪和肉类的大量摄入增加了胰腺癌的发病风险；而水果和蔬菜的大量摄入会降低胰腺癌发病风险[5]。哪种脂肪酸致癌作用最强还未能确定[114]。几项研究表明肉类的加工方法（油炸、烤或烧烤）及其产生的致癌物的摄入量可能与胰腺癌的发生有一定关联作用[115~117]。膳食碳水化合物、精制糖、血糖指数或胰腺癌负荷与胰腺癌相关性的研究已经进行了很多，但其研究结果并不一致。最近的一项包含八项前瞻性队列研究数据的荟萃分析表明，高糖饮食导致的高血糖指数、高血糖负荷及总碳水化合物或蔗糖与胰腺癌发病风险没有相关性[118]。

胰腺癌发病率与蔬菜、柑橘类水果、纤维和维生素 C[5]的高摄入量呈负相关。维生素 D 是否对胰腺癌发病有保护作用仍不确定[114]。

职业暴露

导致胰腺癌发病的职业或工业因素已经被广泛研究。那些暴露于特定化学物质（如有机氯、氯化烃和甲醛）或从事特殊职业（如石矿、水泥、园艺和纺织）的人群胰腺癌发病率明显升高[4,88]。迄今为止，氯代烃和多环芳烃碳氢化合物是公认的导致胰腺癌最强的职业风险因素[88]。

总体来说，吸烟和肥胖各与 25% 的胰腺癌患者发病相关，提示半数的胰腺癌病例是可以预防的[119,120]。相反，与已知肿瘤综合征相关的胰腺癌所占比例很小。发现高风险胰腺癌个体需要重点筛查[121~123]。迄今为止，筛查的益处仍然未能确定，除非是在高选择性的人群如高危家族性胰腺癌家族中。目前，对于那些确定具有结构性的[124]或血液异常[125]，提示癌前或早期阶段的肿瘤人群的处理仍然极具争议。目前的可选择方案从密切观察到积极外科手术都在演变中[126~128]。

胰腺癌的预防

前面描述的胰腺癌的流行病学为胰腺癌的预防提供了强有力的证据，可能导致全球胰腺癌死亡率大幅下降。一级预防包括生活方式和饮食习惯的改变，有望大幅降低胰腺癌发病风险。此外,许多非处方药物和常用处方药物有可能有助于降低胰腺癌的发病风险(表 93-2)[129~132]。

表 93-2 可能降低胰腺癌风险的干预措施

生活方式和营养因素
戒烟或者减少吸烟量
控制体重,减轻体重至体重指数<25mg/m²
健康饮食,高水果和蔬菜
潜在的化学预防制剂
二甲双胍
阿司匹林
姜黄素
塞来昔布
阿托伐他汀
HMG 辅酶还原酶抑制剂
β-胡萝卜素
维生素 C、D、E

病理学

胰腺外分泌肿瘤的组织病理学

胰腺导管腺癌约占胰腺来源肿瘤的 95%[133]。在手术切除肿瘤的组织学检查中,常常发现肿瘤细胞浸润到胰腺床之外的淋巴结构或神经末梢,这正是引起胰腺癌相关疼痛的原因。胰腺导管腺癌的另一个确定的组织学特征是肿瘤内丰富的宿主基质反应(结缔组织增生),其中表达平滑肌肌动蛋白的肌成纤维细胞产生丰富的细胞外胶原包绕在浸润性肿瘤腺体周围(图 93-2)[134]。其他促进宿主纤维增生的成分包括分泌的糖胺聚糖(如透明质酸),其可使间质压力升高并阻止从循环到肿瘤周围环境中化疗药物的被动流出[135]。

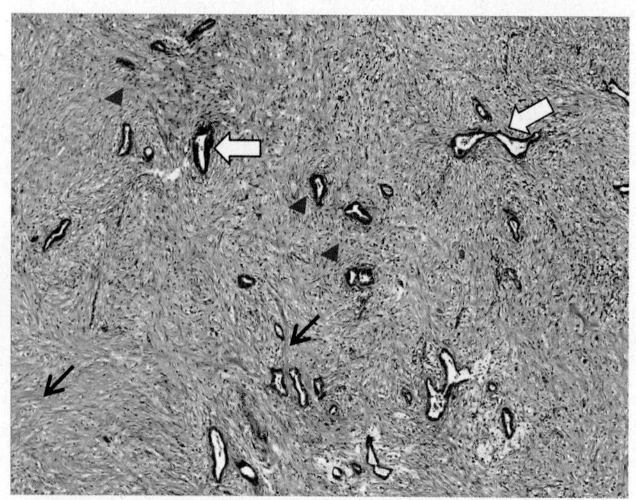

图 93-2 胰腺导管腺癌的间质结缔组织增生。浸润性肿瘤腺体(白色箭头)周围有明显的宿主反应,包括梭形肿瘤相关成纤维细胞和肌成纤维细胞(红色箭头)和细胞外基质,包括胶原蛋白 1(黑色箭头)

胰腺导管腺癌通过公认的癌前病变逐步发展而来。最常见的癌前病变是很微小病变,被称为胰腺上皮内瘤变,几乎总是存在于浸润性胰腺癌周围的胰腺实质。上皮内瘤变从低级别到高级别恶性风险逐步升高,其中高级别上皮内瘤变(以前称为原位癌),其中组成细胞在形态上类似胰腺导管腺癌,除了它们被限制在基底膜以内。高级别上皮内瘤变与浸润性癌有许多共同的遗传突变。值得注意的是,虽然低级和中级上皮内瘤变可能会偶然发生(尸检报告显示约 50%的老年人胰腺中存在低级和中级上皮内瘤变)[136],高级上皮内瘤变没有胰腺癌的情况下基本上从未被发现[137]。因此,高级别上皮内瘤变很可能提示胰腺导管腺癌在多步发展过程中。根据定义,与胰腺导管腺癌的囊性癌前病变不同(见下文),孤立的上皮内瘤变不能在腹部影像学检查中发现,尽管种系突变或家族性遗传倾向导致的胰腺结构性改变可能在超声内镜检查中发现(EUS)[128]。

胰腺导管腺癌囊性癌前病变包括两种不同的肿瘤-导管内乳头状黏液性肿瘤(IPMN)和黏液性囊性肿瘤(MCN)[138]。导管内乳头状黏液性肿瘤发生在主胰管或分支胰管,以宽的"手指状"乳头和丰富的细胞外黏液为特点。黏液性囊性肿瘤不太常见,而且女性发病率明显高于男性的(比例 9:1)。与导管内乳头状黏液性肿瘤不同,黏液性肿瘤与胰腺导管系统没有连通。类似于上皮内瘤变,囊性癌变病变的上皮内细胞也显示出组织学进展,从低度(腺瘤)到高度(原位癌)到侵袭性癌症。25%~33%的手术切除的囊性病变与侵袭性腺癌相关,并且侵袭的出现与显著降低的中位生存期有关[139,140]。虽然目前还不知道非侵袭性囊肿发展成侵袭性癌的时间跨度,但是囊性病变的中位发病年龄比胰腺导管腺癌的发病年龄小约 10 岁,这可能大概反映出囊肿癌变所需的时间。值得注意的是,因为非胰腺症状而进行的腹部影像检查的,使得囊性病变检出率增高,"人为"增加胰腺囊性病变发病率。鉴于大多数无症状囊肿不太可能发展成侵袭性肿瘤,已经提出了有助于区分"高风险"和"惰性"囊肿的影像学标准[141,142]。大量研究正在试图从囊液或血液中鉴定分子标记物从而进一步细化这种区别,并有助于预防不必要的手术和频繁的复查[123]。

其他不常见的外分泌肿瘤包括:①腺泡细胞癌,其在形态学上与胰腺腺泡相似,其中肿瘤细胞表达腺泡酶,如胰蛋白酶和糜蛋白酶[143];②实性假乳头状肿瘤,发生机制不明,好发于年轻人胰腺尾部,通常预后良好[122];③浆液性囊性肿瘤,一种以浆液性(水样)分泌物为特征的囊性肿瘤,与导管内乳头状黏液性肿瘤及黏液性囊腺瘤的黏液成分不同,很少发展成导管腺癌[144];④胰腺母细胞瘤,最常见的儿童胰腺肿瘤[145]。

大约 2%的原发性胰腺肿瘤来自内分泌细胞(朗格汉斯细胞团中的胰岛细胞),被称为胰腺神经内分泌肿瘤(PanNET)或胰岛细胞肿瘤[146]。约 1/4 的 PanNET 无分泌功能,而具有分泌功能的 PanNET 可以表达多种胰岛细胞激素如胰岛素或高血糖素,导致全身激素分泌量过多而引发全身性的症状。PanNET 不形成腺体结构,通常与旺盛的宿主纤维化增生反应无关。PanNET 可以通过鉴定组织切片中神经内分泌标记物,如色粒蛋白或突触素的表达来识别。

胰腺外分泌肿瘤的分子病理学

近 5 年来，由于肿瘤二代基因测序技术的出现，使得胰腺癌的基因组图谱[147]以及其他外分泌和内分泌肿瘤方面的研究取得很大进展[148,149]。国际癌症基因组联合会(ICGC)已经测序了数百个胰腺导管腺癌，且测序数据公开发表[150]。

到目前为止，在胰腺导管腺癌多步骤发病机制中最常见的遗传变异是癌基因 *KRAS* 的突变，其位于染色体 12p 上，编码 Ras，一种膜结合 GTP 酶[151]。*KRAS* 体细胞突变在 90%以上的胰腺癌细胞系和 75%~90%患者来源的异种移植瘤中被检出。大多数 *KRAS* 突变集中在 12 号密码子，13 号和 61 号密码子偶有突变。体细胞 *KRAS* 突变导致其编码的 Ras 蛋白，一种 GTP 酶活性的持续激活，进而激活多个下游效应途径[152]。体细胞 *KRAS* 突变即使在低级别上皮内瘤变中也存在，被认为是正常导管上皮发生转化的早期事件[153]。在基因工程小鼠模型中，*KRAS* 突变表达后，小鼠胰腺中出现了和人体胰腺上皮内瘤变高度类似的病变，甚至少数动物最终发展成侵袭性癌症[154]。其他的遗传事件，例如 *p53* 基因突变，或者 *Ink4a/Arf* 等位基因的表达缺失，显著加速了 Ras 诱导的胰腺瘤变的自然病程[155,156]。相反，在具有诱导型 *KRAS* 等位基因突变的 GEMM 中，在已建立的胰腺癌模型中，关闭 Ras，可逆转瘤变过程[157,158]。研究人员在胰腺癌及其他 *KRAS* 突变导致的肿瘤中探索了许多途径用于药理学抑制 Ras 活性[159~161]，但是总体临床结果令人失望。尽管如此，Ras 仍然是一个有吸引力的研究靶点，由联邦政府资助的大型“RAS 研究项目”目前正在美国癌症研究所进行以确定在胰腺癌及其他肿瘤中阻断 Ras 的治疗策略(http://www. cancer. gov/research and funding/priorities/ras)。

编码细胞周期调节剂 p16 的 *CDKN2A/INK4A* 基因的体细胞失活是胰腺癌多步发展病变的另一种早期遗传事件。p16 蛋白抑制细胞周期蛋白 D1/Cdk-4 复合物，该复合物通进而抑制视网膜母细胞瘤(Rb)蛋白磷酸化[162]。在大约 95%的胰腺癌中，*CDKN2A/INK4A* 基因是被几种机制之一灭活，包括纯合子缺失、等位基因及其他内部基因缺失以及启动子的甲基化导致表观遗传失活。一个潜在的治疗靶点即使用 Cdk4 功能的小分子抑制剂作用于 p16 的失活与 Cdk4 活性的依赖性有关的增殖失控[163]。

在胰腺癌的多步发展模型中，抑癌基因 *TP53*、*SMAD4/DPC4* 和 *BRCA2* 的失活被认为是病变的晚期事件[164]。*TP53* 的体细胞突变发现于大约 75%的人胰腺导管腺癌中，且免疫组织化学发现 p53 蛋白的细胞核内聚集发生在大多数高级别上皮内瘤变中，提示 *TP53* 基因的突变[165]。位于染色体 18q21 位置上的 *SMAD4/DPC4* 抑癌基因编码生长因子 β 信号通路的细胞内传感器，在生理条件下抑制细胞生长。*SMAD4/DPC4* 基因通过纯合子缺失或等位基因及其他内部基因缺失[166]。上皮 Dpc4 表达几乎总是存在低级别上皮内瘤变和非侵袭性胰腺癌的囊性癌前病变，表明 *SMAD4/DPC4* 异常通常伴随着病变进展到侵袭性癌症[167,168]。总体而言，*KRAS*、*CDKN2A/INK4A*、*TP53*、和 *SMAD4/DPC4* 是胰腺癌基因组谱中四个主要突变基因，每种突变发生于 50%以上的病例。同时具有 4 种突变基因的患者预后比具有 1 或 2 个突变基因的预后差的多，体现出这些突变基因在预后中的作用[169]。

BRCA2 基因突变(在上文对胰腺癌的家族遗传倾向部分提及)发生于大约 5%的胰腺癌患者。BRCA2 蛋白在同源重组介导的修复中的作用(HRR)起着至关重要的作用。具有 BRCA2 或其他 HRR 通路相关基因缺陷的肿瘤细胞对顺铂或丝裂霉素等药物诱导双链断裂非常敏感[170]。PARP(聚腺苷二磷酸核糖聚合酶)抑制剂是另一种新型的用于具有 *BRCA2* 突变的部分肿瘤的药物，其抑制了在 HRR 中受损细胞的 DNA 修复。PARP 抑制剂联合应用于 *BRCA2* 突变的胰腺癌中抑制 DNA 修复，有望产生一种“协同致死”作用，而具有一定治疗优势[171]。

尽管罗列一份全面的胰腺癌基因异常列表显然超出了本书的范围，但是许多细胞成分中都显示出显著的分子变异，包括 DNA 甲基化、组蛋白标记、编码和非编码 RNA(后者包括长非编码 RNA 和 microRNA)和蛋白质。这些异常如 *DNA* 突变、异常 DNA 甲基化或 microRNA 失调，常常存在于生物样本如血液或胰液中，故可作为诊断胰腺癌的生物标志物[172~175]。现在用 PCR 技术检测[178] cfDNA 及外泌体中的 DNA 等以发现新的肿瘤标志物用于胰腺癌的早期诊断和监测切除术后复发是近年来新兴的研究领域[176,177]。

胰腺外分泌肿瘤的分子生物学：转化应用

精选以下几个代表最新进展的例子，以了解胰腺癌的肿瘤生物学在癌症转化医学领域的应用。

胰腺癌进展的基因时间表：绝大多数胰腺癌患者表现为晚期疾病，因此早期诊断有助于提总高生存期。一份关于胰腺癌尸检案例报告比较了原发灶和同时性转移灶中基因变异类型，研究人员计算出从原发灶的突变克隆到晚期转移性疾病的过程可能需要 20 年的时间[179]。在有症状的患者中这种变化需要的时间不超过 2 年，提示开发应用于临床的胰腺癌发病前生物标志物的重要性。

胰腺癌间质：有利还是有害？传统上认为，胰腺癌中大量增生的结缔组织间质中的癌症相关肌成纤维细胞有助于肿瘤的侵袭性行为[180,181]。肿瘤和间质相互作用的途径之一是通过 Hedgehog 信号通路[182]，胰腺癌 GEMM 模型中，使用 Hedgehog 抑制剂造成胰腺癌间质中肌成纤维细胞的缺失后，增强了化疗药物的输送效果[183]。受此启示开展了一项 Hedgehog 信号抑制剂与吉西他滨联合应用的随机临床试验，结果却出乎意料，这种抑制反而促进了疾病进展。(www. businesswire. com/news/home/20120127005146/en/infinityreports-update-phase-2-study-saridegib)。最近的系列研究使用基因或药物消融胰腺癌 GEMM 模型的肌成纤维细胞，对阐释间质抑制肿瘤的作用具有指导意义[184~186]。具体而言，间质缺失导致肿瘤去分化并增加转移性，使得小鼠中位存活率降低，与临床发现类似。这些研究结酚酞致对间质在胰腺癌中作用的重新评估。一种新的研究方法不同于间质的消融缺失，而是在临床前模型中应用药理学策略使基质“重编程”，即肌成纤维细胞保留在原位但处于基本静止的状态[187]。

克服胰腺癌的免疫耐受：在过去的 5 年里，免疫检查点抑制剂药物的使用导致黑色素瘤患者存活率显著提高，肿瘤免疫治疗成为最有前景的治疗手段之一[188]。迄今为止，这些成功还没有转化到胰腺癌[189,190]。部分失败归因于胰腺癌特殊的

肿瘤微环境。与某些"免疫原性"肿瘤,如黑色素瘤不同,胰腺癌微环境中渗透的免疫性效应器T细胞很少,而具有大量免疫抑制性细胞,包括调节性T细胞、巨噬细胞和髓源抑制细胞[191~193]。这种免疫抑制微环境有助于免疫耐受并促进肿瘤进展。随着胰腺癌免疫治疗研究进展,联合用药方案的重要性逐渐被认知,例如诱导抗原特异性T细胞反应的疫苗联合免疫检查点抑制剂应用[194],或采用抗原特异性工程化T细胞的过继疗法联合免疫检查点抑制剂[195]。

胰腺癌的代谢紊乱:近一个世纪以前,由Otto Warburg[196]提出癌细胞大多依赖外源性葡萄糖的有氧糖酵解以满足其能量需求。除葡萄糖外,外源性谷氨酰胺是胰腺癌存活和增殖的关键物质[197]。摄取后,谷氨酰胺由谷氨酰胺酶转化为谷氨酸。*Ras*突变体是一个细胞内重编程的关键协调者。突变体*Ras*重新代谢谷氨酸通过与正常细胞不同的非经典氧化途径,不增加细胞内有害作用的活性氧水平[198]。在临床前模型中,这种独特的谷氨酰胺利用机制对癌细胞存活至关重要,因此激发了研究胰腺癌中谷氨酰胺酶或其代谢途径中其他酶的热情。第二,突变体Ras已被证明可促进对自噬的依赖,这种营养物质循环机制中溶酶体降解受损的蛋白质,大分子和细胞器,产生能量代谢的中间体[199]。自噬可以用氯喹等药物来阻断并且在临床前研究取得了很好的效果[200]。最后,突变体*Ras*显著增加了巨胞饮,一种原始的营养摄取机制,通过所谓的来源于细胞膜的巨噬细胞囊泡实现细胞外液和营养物质的内吞[201]。胰腺癌细胞中的巨胞饮可增加白蛋白和其他细胞外蛋白质的摄取,进而分解代谢成必需氨基酸再引入到各种合成代谢途径。因此,抑制巨胞饮作用可作为胰腺癌治疗的潜在靶点。或者,利用胰腺癌细胞摄取细胞外白蛋白的倾向,将治疗剂与白蛋白结合用作治疗。事实上,有一些证据表明,*KRAS*突变肿瘤细胞中,纳米白蛋白结合的紫杉醇疗效增强可能至少部分是由于巨胞饮诱导的药物摄取增多导致。

总之,这些结果有助于更好的理解胰腺癌复杂的潜在生物学机制包括长期的基因组进化,动态的微环境及正常和肿瘤细胞之间明显的代谢差异。这些观点提出了调节肿瘤细胞内和细胞外防御机制的策略。最近的一些基于实验室发现到临床转化的具体例子将在本章结尾的"未来方向"部分进行讨论。

诊断评估

患者在得到最终明确的胰腺癌诊断之前所接受的相关辅助性检查比较零散,而且效率较低。从分析腹痛原因到疑诊胰腺癌,再到组织活检证实为恶性肿瘤(已行或未行完整的分期评估)的整个诊断过程中,外科医师或亚专业的肿瘤科医师在任何时间点都要对患者进行病情评估。尤其是注意一些对治疗有直接提示作用的重要临床信息,是可以通过细致的问诊和查体而获得的,而且有些信息是无法从影像学检查中得到的,比如全身体力状态评估、心肺功能情况、有无锁骨上或脐周淋巴结肿大、静脉血栓等。

临床分期

临床分期使用标准化、客观的影像学标准至关重要。现代成像技术改变了胰腺癌的临床分期。精确和客观解剖影像学标准用于确定肿瘤-血管侵及的程度使临床分期更准确。胰腺癌的临床分期可以大致分为不能手术的病变(转移性或局部进展期)和局部病变(临界可切除或可切除);有关具体的影像学标准,请参见表93-3。大多数患者表现为转移性疾病,如腹水/腹膜种植,肝脏或肺转移。经皮活检或者超声内镜引导的细针穿刺活检可以确诊转移灶。在没有远处转移的情况下,临床分期由原发肿瘤与邻近的脉管系统侵及关系确定。影像学表现为可切除的胰腺癌(AJCC Ⅰ期或Ⅱ期):①无动脉侵犯或包绕②肠系膜上静脉(SMV)/门静脉(PV)受累<50%(图93-3)。一般而言,若肿瘤侵犯(肿瘤血管界面≤180°)或包绕(>180°)腹腔干、肝总动脉或肠系膜上动脉(SMA),被认为是立即手术的禁忌证。局部进展期,无法切除胰腺癌(AJCCⅢ期)定义为:①肿瘤包绕SMA或腹腔干>180°(图93-4),或②肠系膜上静脉-门静脉(SMPV)汇合处阻塞,没有静脉重建的可能性。交界可切除定义为:仅有局限血管侵犯而无SMA或腹腔干动脉包绕或肝总动脉部分包绕。此外,肿瘤导致SMV/PV>50%变窄或部分闭塞,具有切除重建可能的也被认为

表93-3 胰腺癌临床分期的影像学标准

可切除胰腺癌	
肿瘤-动脉关系	无影像学证据表明动脉受累(腹腔干、肠系膜上动脉或者肝动脉)
肿瘤静-脉关系	肿瘤引起的肠系膜上静脉、门静脉或肠系膜上静脉-门静脉狭窄≤50%
交界可切除	
动脉	肿瘤累及肠系膜上动脉或腹腔干≤180°。肿瘤侵犯或包绕(>180°)小段肝动脉
静脉	肿瘤引起的肠系膜上静脉、门静脉或肠系膜上静脉-门静脉汇合处狭窄>50%,或者以上静脉短段闭塞并且可以进行安全的血管重建
胰腺外疾病	影像学可疑,但不能确诊的,转移性疾病(如太小而不具有典型特征的肝脏小病灶)
局部进展	
动脉	肿瘤包绕(>180°)肠系膜上动脉或腹腔干
静脉	肠系膜上静脉、门静脉或肠系膜上静脉-门静脉汇合处闭塞,导致肿瘤上方和下方静脉切除后不能重建(近端或远端血管重建的长度不够)
胰腺外疾病	没有证据表明腹膜,肝脏和腹腔外转移
转移性	
腹膜或者远处转移的证据	

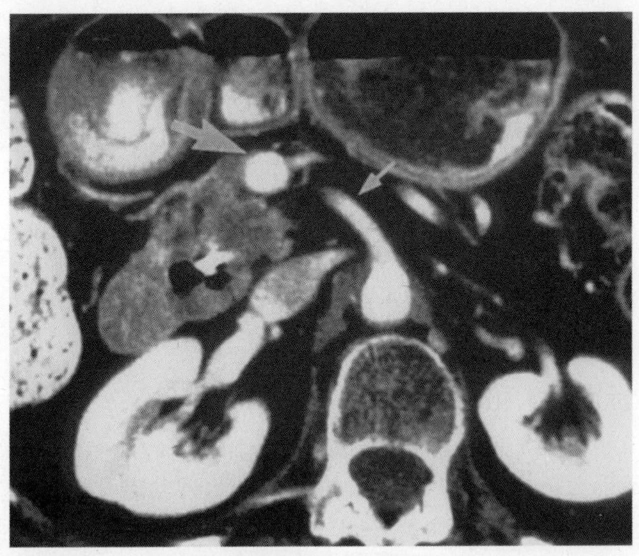

图 93-3 对比增强 CT 扫描显示胰头部一可切除的腺癌。胰头部低密度肿瘤可见。注意肿块并没有侵及肠系膜上动脉(小箭头);在肿块和肠系膜上动脉之间可见正常的脂肪平面。但是,肿块(低密度区)侵及了大箭头下方的肠系膜上静脉。这位患者可能需要在胰十二指肠切除术时进行静脉切除和重建。这种细微的发现在低质量的 CT 扫描中可能不明显。胆总管胰腺内段可见支架,是内镜下放置用于胆汁引流的

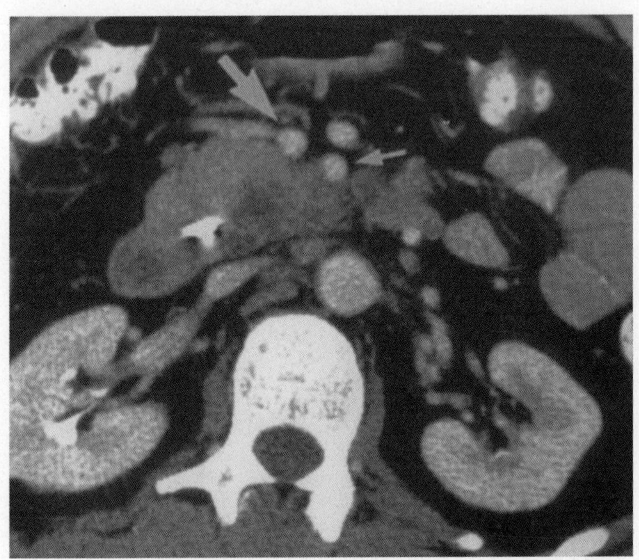

图 93-4 对比增强 CT 扫描显示为不可切除的胰头和钩突部的腺癌。该低密度肿瘤与肠系膜上动脉(小箭头)后壁不可分离。在手术中对于肿瘤在腹膜后与肠系膜上动脉毗邻关系的准确判断几乎是不可能的,除非是手术先将胃和胰腺横断,因此术前肿瘤-血管重要关系的准确成像是至关重要的。大箭头指示为肠系膜上静脉

是交界可切除。越来越多的共识,认为许多肿瘤静脉侵犯时为交界性可切除(特别是随着新辅助治疗越来越被广泛接受)。

影像学

准确表征肿瘤血管间的关系对于临床分期至关重要。EUS 和 ERCP(内镜逆行胰胆管造影,可以诱发胰腺炎并干扰疾病程度准确的评估)等干预措施应该暂时推迟到高质量的无创影像学检查之后。高分辨 CT 是胰腺癌的检查和分期的最重要的影像学检查[202,203]。目前的增强 CT 检测器使用双相技术。静脉快速注射造影剂后胰腺和肠系膜血管可以出现最大限度的增强[204]。第一期(动脉期)用于显示和评估原发肿瘤和肿瘤动脉的关系。第二期(静脉期)该期用来确定肿瘤和周围静脉血管(肠系膜上静脉、门静脉、脾静脉等)的相邻关系,以及局部区域淋巴结和远处器官(特别是肝脏)的转移情况。

如果在 CT 上未见低密度肿块,考虑胆道或胰管梗阻与恶性肿瘤有关时可以使用磁共振成像(MRI)检查。研究表明与 CT 相比,当胰腺病灶小于 2cm 时,MRI 检查可能更有优势[205,206]。在 CT 检查中,胰腺癌的乏血供特征可能在动脉期早期更容易发现[204]。如果怀疑胰腺癌仍没有发现病灶时可以行 EUS 检查。此外,与 FNA 结合的 EUS 可以提供恶性肿瘤的组织学证据。很少有患者在行 CT,MRI 或 EUS 后仍未发现病灶。如果患者出现黄疸,ERCP 检查可见典型的双管征或慢性胰腺炎时可见较长、光滑、逐渐变细的胆管狭窄征象(图 93-5)。这种情况下,胆道刷检可用于细胞学诊断。当没有反复发作胰腺炎或酒精滥用史的患者出现胆总管胰腺段恶性狭窄表现或没有胰腺占位出现胰管扩张时,仍然应该首先考虑胰腺癌的诊断。如果 CA19-9 水平升高,应考虑复查 EUS,如果细胞学诊断不能确诊,患者身体条件允许且没有腹部手术禁忌证时可考虑直接行手术治疗。

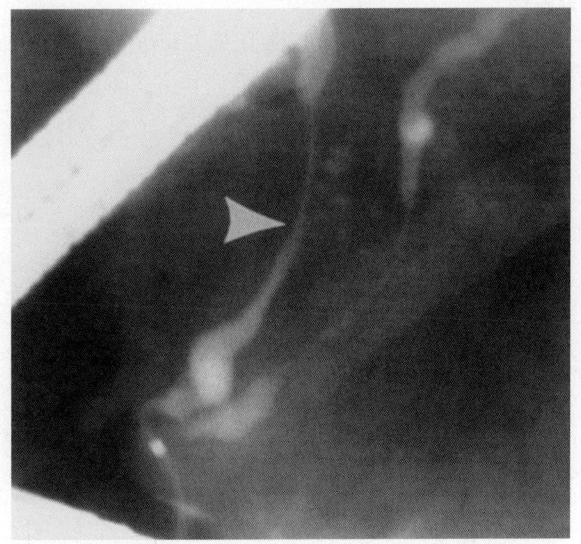

图 93-5 ERCP(内镜逆行胆胰管造影)显示光滑的逐渐变细的胆总管狭窄(箭头),见于慢性胰腺炎所致的继发性胆道梗阻

组织获取

在进行系统化疗或放疗前,所有局部进展或转移性疾病的患者都应取组织活检明确恶性病变。对于有影像学证据明确转移性病灶的患者,可以在超声或 CT 引导下经皮穿刺活检。对于局限期疾病的患者,可能行手术治疗时,我们更倾向于在 EUS 引导下进行活检,以降低肿瘤种植的风险。此外,当肿瘤较小或难以获得时,EUS 引导下组织活检优于 CT 引导下的经皮穿刺活检[207]。EUS 引导下组织活检阴性结果并不能完全除外恶性肿瘤的可能,再次穿刺活检可以提高诊断的准确性[208]。另外,只有影像学明确肿块部位后才考虑行细针穿刺活检,不宜在没有明确肿块部位时盲目的进行穿刺活检。

腹腔镜分期

过去,腹腔镜检查主要用于影像学资料表明为局限型的胰腺癌患者[209]。然而,随着高分辨率增强 CT 的出现,在分离麻醉诱导下的腹腔镜检查在分期中的应用越来越少。对于血浆 CA19-9 水平高的患者,腹腔镜检查分期可能会提高准确性,因此建议完善术前血浆 CA19-9 水平检测[210,211]。如果高度怀疑胰腺外侵犯,或者交界可切除患者容易出现并发症时,腹腔镜检查作为一种独立的检查操作可能比较合适。

胆汁引流

对于局限期胰腺癌患者,术前经内镜下放置胆道支架可缓解胆道梗阻症状,改善肝功能。肝功能的改善对将要接受新辅助治疗的患者尤其重要,因为高胆红素血症会影响系统治疗的安全性。对于计划行新辅助治疗的患者,在细胞学确诊为恶性肿瘤后可以置入短金属支架以最大限度地降低胆道并发症,包括支架阻塞和胆管炎[212]。对于局部进展期或者转移性胰腺癌患者,使用胆管内自膨胀的金属支架比塑料支架具有更好的长期通畅性[213,214]。

对于有临床症状的远端胆道梗阻患者,不应该直接置入金属支架。尽管覆膜金属支架也可以在内镜下移除[215],在没有明确组织病理学诊断情况下,不建议行覆膜支架置入术。

局限性、潜在可切除病灶的治疗

外科考虑

如果原发性肿瘤不能完全切除(肉眼下完全切除),胰腺癌手术(胰十二指肠切除术)就没有生存获益。接受不完全切除手术的患者,预期中位生存期小于 1 年[216]。即使镜下手术切缘阳性也对患者的总体生存期具有不利影响,因此切缘阴性对提高长期生存的具有重要意义[217]。

标准手术和辅助治疗

目前,早期可切除病灶的标准治疗是手术联合术后辅助治疗。近年来,随着手术技术、麻醉及重症监护医学的发展进步,经有经验的外科医师做胰十二指肠切除术,患者住院 30 天内死亡率可低至 2%以下[218~220]。研究数据表明手术量大的医院行胰腺手术,手术相关的死亡率更低[221]。标准的手术联合辅助治疗具有潜在治愈可能性。然而,这种治疗的中位生存期为 22~24 个月,在过去的 30 年里,基本没有改变[222,223]。

胰十二指肠切除术

胰头及壶腹部肿瘤标准的手术切除方式是胰十二指肠切除术。现行的胰十二指肠切除术的由 Whipple 及其同事最早在 1935 年提出的术式发展而来[224]。该术式包含了传统 Whipple 手术的部分步骤,更加强调去除 SMA 右侧所有软组织的重要性。手术切除分为 6 个明确的步骤(图 93-6):最重要和最困难的部分是第 6 步,此步骤需游离胰腺,并将标本自 SMPV 汇合处和 SMA 右侧缘分离[225]。

标准胰十二指肠切除术后局部复发率高,因此需要特别注意肠系膜上动脉切缘。肠系膜上动脉切缘(即腹膜后切缘或肠系膜切缘)是近端肠系膜上动脉右后侧的软组织切缘(图 93-7)[226]。病理医师对肠系膜上动脉切缘的鉴定及组织学评估至关重要。没有对腹膜后切缘进行组织学评估就不能确定残留胰腺的状态("R"因素)[220,227]。

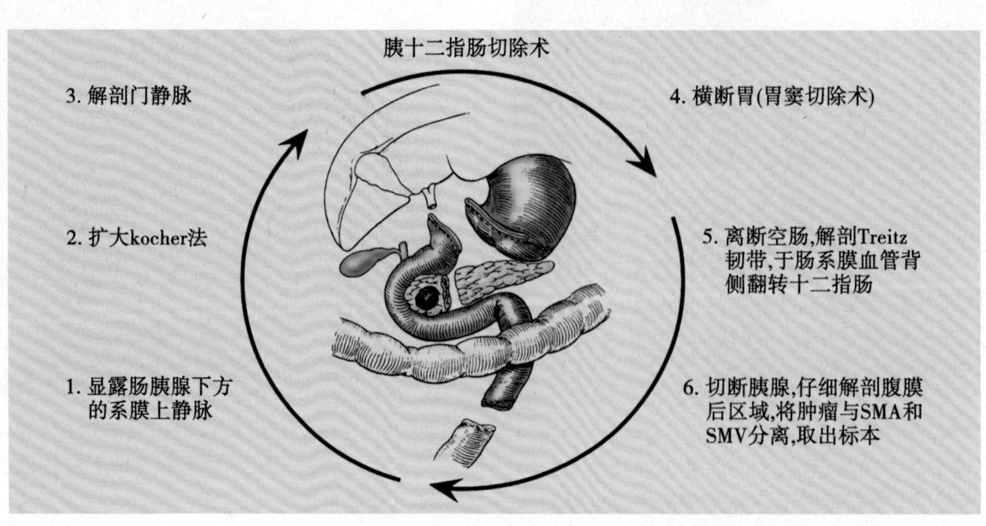

图 93-6 胰十二指肠切除术的六个手术步骤

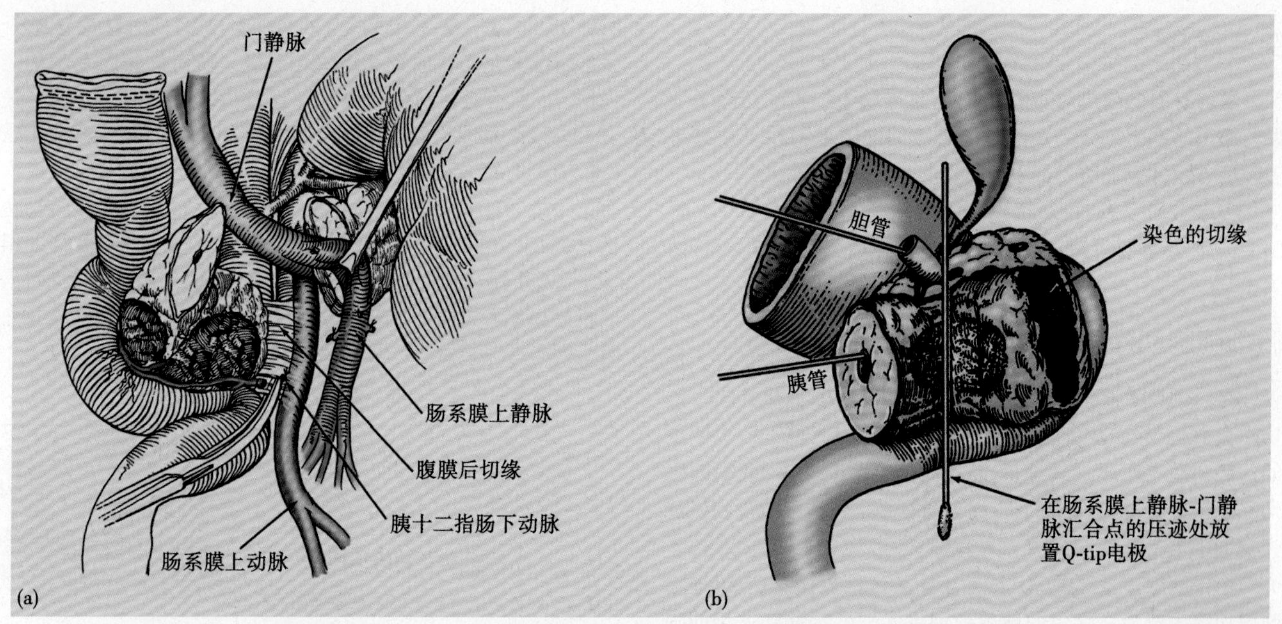

图 93-7　肿瘤切除时腹膜后切缘示意图(a)向内侧牵拉肠系膜上静脉(SMV)及肠系膜上静脉-门静脉汇合处,有利于解剖邻近肠系膜上动脉(SMA)近端外侧壁的软组织;这一区域即是腹膜后切缘。在对胰十二肠切除术的手术标本进行永久切片分析之前,需要与病理医师一起对腹膜后切缘进行定位和确认,确保能够准确评估腹膜后切缘及其他病理因素。(b)不能对腹膜后切缘进行回顾性评估。如图示,分别在胰管和胆管中插入探针,在肠系膜上静脉-门静脉汇合点的压迹处放置 Q-tip 电极。对邻近肠系膜上动脉(SMA)近端外侧壁的软组织进行标志(用于最终的病理评估);这一区域即代表腹膜后(肠系膜)切缘

血管切除

血管切除的目标是获得 R0 切除,需要从 SMV/PV 中完全分离切除肿瘤,并且暴露 SMA 以使肿瘤从动脉上锐性分离。对于侵犯 SMV 或 SMPV 汇合处(图 93-8)或者肿瘤未包绕 SMA 或腹腔干仅出现 SMV/PV 的短段闭塞的情况下应进行静脉切除和重建[202,225]。

对于部分患有局部进展期疾病(如目前所定义)的患者出现下列情况时可考虑在新辅助治疗后进行手术治疗:①使用 Appleby 手术(扩大的远端胰腺联合腹腔干切除术)可以完整切除包绕腹腔干或肝总动脉的肿瘤,②术前治疗出现影像学、生物化学(CA19-9)、生理(改善 PS)的反应。对这些患者,推荐行新辅助放化疗,并且在完成治疗后重新评估外科手术适应证。最常用的术式是远端胰腺切除术+脾切除术+整块腹腔干切除术(Appleby 手术)。在小部分患者中行联合动脉切除和重建的切除术,其结果令人鼓舞[228,229]。

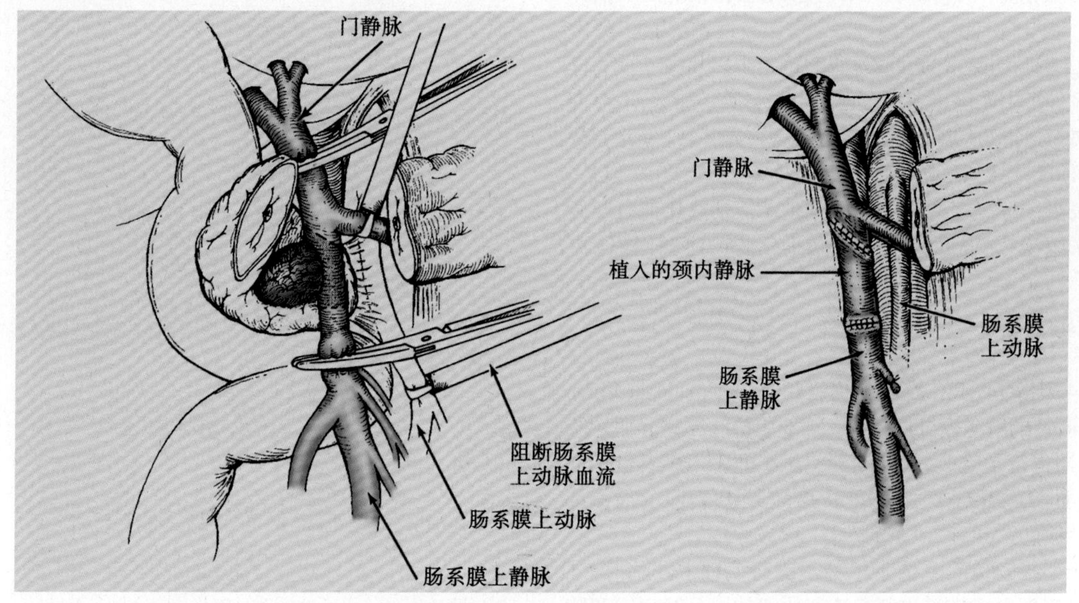

图 93-8　保留脾静脉而切除肠系膜上静脉(SMV)的手术示意图。由于脾静脉牵拉门静脉(PV),导致多数病例难以吻合。我们首选的 SMV 重建方法是植入颈内静脉。脾静脉牵拉造成暴露不足,而难以将肿瘤标本与 SMA 近端外侧壁分开。因此,可以在移出标本之前植入血管移植物,从而向内牵拉重建的 SMPV 汇合处;或者将肿瘤与肠系膜上动脉分离后再植入血管移植物。保留脾静脉的 SMV 节段性切除术的复杂程度大大增加

保留幽门

目前有限的随机对照研究表明，标准胰十二指肠切除术和保留幽门的胰十二指肠切除术两者之间的围术期并发症和患者预后方面并无显著差异[230~232]。

大多数研究表明，对于侵及十二指肠上部和降部较大的胰头或十二指肠肿瘤，不推荐采用保留幽门的胰十二肠切除术。

微创胰腺切除术

将微创技术应用于胰腺癌切除的兴趣来源于开放式手术切除会引起严重的生理应激和增加并发症的假说。尽管微创的优势和适应证还颇具争议，从 1998 年到 2009 年，微创胰腺切除术从 2.4%提高到 7.3%[233]。微创手术包括腹腔镜和机器人辅助手术。

由于胰腺体尾部肿瘤切除后不需要解剖重建，腹腔镜远端胰腺切除术成为最常用的胰腺微创手术。虽然没有进行前瞻性试验比较开腹与腹腔镜远端胰腺切除术，多项回顾性研究表明腹腔镜手术具有良好的围术期结果，减少失血，降低并发症，缩短住院时间[234,235]。比较开放性手术和腹腔镜手术在肿瘤学方面是否有差异的报道较少。只有三项腹腔镜下远端胰腺切除的研究描述了患者的肿瘤学结果[236~238]。最大的一项多中心，回顾性匹配的队列分析指出 R0 切除状态(74%比 66%)、淋巴结检出数目(14 比 12)或中位 OS(16 个月比 16 个月)在开腹和腹腔镜远端胰腺切除术之间无显著差异。

与腹腔镜远端胰腺切除术在许多大的肿瘤中心开展不同，胰十二指肠切除术尚未获得广泛认可。很少有中心报道超过 30 例手术的经验[239,240]。在这些研究中，中转开放手术的发生率为 6%~10%。

机器人辅助胰十二指肠切除术也是如此，据报道围术期并发症的发生率与腹腔镜手术接近[241~243]。与远端胰腺切除术相似，胰十二指肠切除术的肿瘤学研究也很少。其中一个大样本的研究报告了 108 例患者行微创胰十二指肠切除术，生存期与行开放胰十二指肠切除术的患者无显著差异[108]。研究者认为微创手术可以使更多的患者术后更及时地辅助治疗。但是，最近研究表明：患者是否接受所有预期的术后治疗比何时开始接受辅助系统治疗(从手术到开始辅助治疗的时间间隔)更重要[244]。

病理(手术)分期

表 93-4 列举了 AJCC 及国际抗癌联盟(International Union Against Cancer)的胰腺癌分期系统。第 6 版的胰腺癌分期系统对 TNM 分期进行了修改，使分期即使对于非手术患者也是准确的。T4(Ⅲ期)是指未发生远处转移、但无法切除的局部进展期原发肿瘤。

对胰十二指肠切除术的手术标本进行病理学评估时，外科医师和病理医师应该首先行冷冻切片评估胆总管切缘和胰腺切缘。然后通过标记肠系膜上动脉切缘，并垂直切缘制作永久切片以评估 SMA 切缘(即紧邻 SMA 近端 3~4cm 的软组织区域-图 93-7b)[220]。SMA 切缘未进行组织学评估就不能明确“R”状态。最重要的是，外科医师和病理医师应该结合手术情况和组织学对此切缘进行分级。所有的胰腺手术均应根据“R”状态进行分级：R0，无肉眼或镜下残余病灶；R1，镜下可见残余病灶(镜下可见阳性切缘但无肉眼可见病灶)；R2，肉眼可见残余病灶。“R”状态应该出现在手术记录或病历记录上，并与病理报告一致。永久切片的最终病理结论包括：肿瘤组织学和分化程度的描述、肉眼和镜下评估肿瘤的组织来源(胰腺、胆管、Vater 壶腹或十二指肠)、肿瘤最大横径、受侵淋巴结及总淋巴结检查、是否存在周围神经、淋巴管及血管受侵。

表 93-4 TNM 分期系统

指标			
原发肿瘤(T)			
Tx	原发肿瘤无法评估		
T0	无原发肿瘤的证据		
Tis	原位癌		
T1	肿瘤局限于胰腺，最大径≤2cm		
T2	肿瘤局限于胰腺，最大径>2cm		
T3	肿瘤扩展至胰腺外，但未累及腹腔动脉和肠系膜上动脉		
T4	肿瘤侵犯腹腔动脉和肠系膜上动脉(不能切除的原发肿瘤)		
区域淋巴结(N)	区域淋巴结无法评估		
Nx	无区域淋巴结转移		
N0	区域淋巴结转移		
N1			
远处转移(M)	远处转移无法评估		
Mx	无远处转移		
M0	远处转移		
区域淋巴结(N)	区域淋巴结无法评估		
Nx	无区域淋巴结转移		
N0	区域淋巴结转移		
分期			
0 期	Tis	N0	M0
1A 期	T1	N0	M0
1B 期	T2	N0	M0
2A 期	T3	N0	M0
2B 期	T1~3	N1	M0
3 期	T4	N0/1	M0
4 期	T1~4	N0/1	M1

预后因素

研究人员已经对胰腺癌标本的病理特征进行了研究，试图建立可靠的与患者不良预后相关的预后指标[218,245]，局部淋巴结转移、组织学低分化、原发肿瘤体积较大均与预后不良相关。然而，患者预后方面还存在很大差异。例如，一个研究报道45例切缘阴性、无局部淋巴结转移行根治性切除的胰腺导管腺癌患者，中位生存时间为32个月，5年生存率为40%[246]。然而另一项研究报道12例生存时间超过5年的患者（完整切除后）中，4例为组织学低分化，5例有局部淋巴结转移，9例出现胰腺外软组织侵犯，10例出现神经侵犯[247]。同样的，另一个研究指出生存时间达到5年的患者中有36%的患者淋巴结阳性，淋巴结阳性患者中有20%患者生存时间达到5年；最后一项研究中的患者在手术前接受了术前治疗[248]。

辅助（术后）治疗

1985年胃肠肿瘤研究小组（Gastrointestinal Tumor Study Group，GITSG）第一次报道了辅助治疗能使胰腺癌术后患者受益[249]。自此以后，开展了几项前瞻性随机试验并且研究结果已发表（表93-5）[250~254]。

表 93-5　可切除胰腺癌辅助治疗的随机试验的总结

研究（年份）	入组例数	R1 切除的患者	治疗 中位生存期/月	治疗 中位生存期/月	P	局部治疗失败率
GITSG[249]（1985）	49	0	氟尿嘧啶放化疗 21.0	观察 10.9	0.035	NR
EORTC[250]（1999）	114	19	氟尿嘧啶放化疗 17.1	观察 12.6	0.09	34
ESPAC-1[251]（2004）	289	18	氟尿嘧啶化疗 20.1	未化疗 15.5	0.09	60
			氟尿嘧啶放化疗 15.9	未放化疗 17.9	0.009	
RTOG 9704[252]（2011）	388（胰头病变）	≥35	先吉西他滨，再氟尿嘧啶放化疗，再吉西他滨 20.5	先氟尿嘧啶，再氟尿嘧啶放化疗，再氟尿嘧啶 16.9	0.09	26
CONKO 001[253]（2007）	368	19	吉西他滨 22.8	观察 20.2	0.005	>35%
ESPAC-3[254]	1 088	38	吉西他滨 23.6	氟尿嘧啶/叶酸 23.0	0.42	NR

NR，未报道

这些试验引发了很多疑问：术后放化疗是否优于单纯观察，包含放化疗的方案是否优于单纯化疗或者单纯观察，吉西他滨是否优于氟尿嘧啶（不论是单独系统治疗还是联合氟尿嘧啶为基础的放化疗）。

两项研究值得特别注意。CONKO-001，一个欧洲的大样本、多国家随机试验比较了术后应用吉西他滨化疗和单纯观察，结果表明随机接受吉西他滨治疗的患者具有明显的生存优势[253]。在该试验中，患者行根治性手术后被随机分组接受6个周期的术后吉西他滨化疗或单纯观察。虽然中位生存期非常接近（22.8个月 vs 20.2个月，$P=0.005$），但是3年和5年生存期（分别为26% vs 18%和20% vs 9%）显示出用吉西他滨治疗明显优于单纯观察。这个试验为术后单纯化疗可以改善无病生存期和总生存期提供了最佳的证据。ESPAC-3试验是有史以来最大样本辅助治疗试验，提供了许多有价值的信息[244]。本研究纳入了来自欧洲，澳大利亚，日本和加拿大的159个胰腺中心的1 088名患者。患者随机接受氟尿嘧啶425mg/m^{2}和亚叶酸（甲酰四氢叶酸）20mg/m^{2}静脉注射，连续5天，每28天一个周期，或吉西他滨1 000mg/m^2，输注时间超过30min，每周一次，连续3周，每28天一个周期。随机接受吉西他滨和接受氟尿嘧啶/亚叶酸两组之间中位生存期没有显著差异（分别为23.6个月 vs 23.0个月，$P=0.42$）。但是，基于氟尿嘧啶的化疗方案引发的毒性不良事件比吉西他滨更严重（14% vs 7.5%）。

总之，CONKO-01和ESPAC-3试验支持单独使用全身治疗作为胰腺癌的辅助治疗。ESPAC-3试验进一步比较了吉西他滨对比氟尿嘧啶/亚叶酸在药物毒性引发不良事件方面的差异。因此，目前，胰腺癌的标准辅助治疗方案是根治性手术后行6个周期的吉西他滨化疗，每周1次，连续3周静脉输注，每28天1个周期。

放射治疗在胰腺癌辅助治疗中的意义：没有作用?

尽管经过了多年的研究，放射治疗作为胰腺癌辅助治疗的意义仍然颇具争议。支持者认为作为辅助治疗的一个组成部分，术后放化疗的中位生存期无论是在GITSG的初步结果还是单中心SEER研究的数据中都与ESPEC-3结果基本一致[255]。

为了明确回答放射治疗在辅助治疗中的作用问题，放射治疗肿瘤学小组（RTOG）正在进行一项大样本随机试验（RTOG 0848），所有的入组患者均给予吉西他滨（有或无厄洛替尼）治疗，然后每隔一段时间根据有无转移重新分期[252]。对于没有转移的患者再次随机分组，一组接受两周期以上的吉西他滨单药治疗，另一组接受至少一个周期吉西他滨化疗以后行氟尿嘧啶为基础的放化疗(对术区行总剂量 50.5Gy 的放疗)。

其他辅助治疗方法

尽管放疗作为辅助治疗产生了阴性结果,基于氟尿嘧啶的放化疗仍然是已经完成的 2 期临床试验中辅助治疗的重要基石。一项强化放化疗的研究中生存期的结果令人鼓舞。试验包括外照射放疗(EBRT),剂量为 45~50Gy 和三药联合化疗:持续静脉泵入氟尿嘧啶,每周一次顺铂冲击以及皮下注射干扰素 α[256]。中位随访 31 个月,但可惜的是本试验未能达到中位生存期。随后一项更大样本的研究结果并不理想,研究中患者中位生存期为 24.7 个月,并且出现了显著治疗相关的毒性[257]。

另一种以免疫疗法为重点的新辅助治疗方法在约翰·霍普金斯医院(JHH)开展[258]。研究人员对 60 名胰腺癌术后的患者接种同种属的能够表达粒-巨噬细胞集落刺激因子(GM-CSF)胰腺癌细胞疫苗。首次接种时间为术后 8~10 周,之后患者接受基于氟尿嘧啶的放化疗。对完成放化疗后仍然没有复发的患者,再次行疫苗接种。最后的中位生存时间为 24.8 个月。虽然这些结果令人鼓舞,但仍需要更大样本的Ⅱ、Ⅲ期随机试验来验证,以期能够将免疫治疗包含在标准的胰腺癌综合辅助治疗方案中。

可切除胰腺癌的辅助治疗:正确的选择吗?

近 30 年来胰腺癌的辅助治疗逐渐细化,但是基本没有太大的进展。从辅助治疗定义的角度,辅助治疗效果的改善很大程度依赖于手术操作。然而,对可切除胰腺癌的标准手术存在许多问题。首先,即使原发肿瘤技术上可切除,手术切缘阳性也很常见。大量文献包括 ESPAC-3 研究也表明手术切缘阳性与不良预后相关[222,254,259~262]。第二,胰腺癌是一种系统性疾病,手术后超过 80%的患者最终会出现转移。一些研究表明大约 15%接受术前治疗的可切除胰腺癌患者在开始辅助治疗后的 6~12 周内出现影像学上明显可见的转移灶[263~269]。因此,据估计行手术治疗后的患者,可能至少有 20%患者在术后的影像学检查发现转移性疾病。最后,胰腺癌手术容易出现术后并发症,尤其在手术量小的中心,更易出现死亡。目前,胰腺癌手术后,约有一半的患者接受辅助治疗[270~272]。

鉴于胰腺癌容易局部侵袭和远处转移的特性,患者的长期生存需要手术联合多种治疗手段。然而,如果第一步手术后发现切缘阳性,许多其他治疗手段治疗效果就会明显降低。因此,对于局限性疾病行术前治疗即新辅助治疗可能比先手术,后行术后辅助治疗更具有优势。

术前(新辅助)治疗

局部进展期胰腺癌患者行新辅助治疗有许多实际的和理论上的优势。最重要的是所有确诊的胰腺癌患者都可以立即行系统性治疗。许多研究表明术前新辅助放化疗能增加术中切缘阴性的比例[273]。另一个重要的优势是新辅助治疗可以增加手术切除率。新辅助治疗完成后(拟行手术前)的重新分期评估会发现肿瘤快速进展或已经属于全身性疾病的患者。

1988 年以来,作者所在单位已经完成了 5 项新辅助治疗的前瞻性研究[263,264,267~269]。这些研究都根据 CT 扫描判断为可切除性病变(如前所述)作为入选标准,采用同样的胰十二指肠切除外科操作规范以及标准的手术标本和切缘的病理评价系统。我们两个最近的试验使用了基于吉西他滨的术前疗法。第一项试验使用快速分割联合连续 7 周吉西他滨静脉滴注。共有 86 名患者入组[268]。74%的患者接受了成功的胰十二指肠切除术。总体而言,86 名患者的中位生存期为 23 个月,实际 5 年生存率为 27%。64 例完成了包括胰十二指肠切除术在内全部治疗患者的中位生存时间为 34 个月,而另外 22 例由于疾病进展或并发症加重等原因未能行胰腺切除患者的中位生存时间为 7 个月。前者与后者的 5 年生存率分别为:36%和 0。我们接下来的新辅助治疗试验中在放化疗和手术前增加了系统性治疗。术前给予吉西他滨和顺铂每 2 周一次,连续 4 个周期,紧接着给予放化疗:持续静脉滴注吉西他滨每周一次连续 4 周,同时给予放射治疗(30Gy/10 次/2 周)[269]。

这项研究入组了 90 例患者,其中 79 例(88%)完成了"吉西他滨-顺铂-新辅助"治疗。79 例患者中有 62 例(78%)行手术,其中 52 例(66%)行胰十二指肠切除术。完成"吉西他滨-顺铂-新辅助"治疗的 79 例患者的中位生存时间为 19 个月,52 例进行手术切除患者的中位生存时间为 31 个月,而另外 27 例患者由于疾病进展未能切除原发肿瘤,其中位生存时间为 10.5 个月($P<0.001$)。这些结果基本上等同于术前仅应用吉西他滨化疗放疗但是没有应用诱导化疗。然而,这两个术前基于吉西他滨的放化疗试验足以有力的证明有必要对局限性Ⅰ/Ⅱ期胰腺癌的新辅助治疗进行更广泛的研究。

反对者担心新辅助治疗可能导致部分局限性肿瘤进展而失去了根治性手术的机会。在我们的研究中,术前新辅助治疗时出现了局部肿瘤进展的情况,但是很少同时伴随远处转移。单纯的局部肿瘤进展在所有入组患者中所占比例<4%。

如前所述,可切除胰腺癌的标准治疗是手术优先。这种方法的结果是导致 R1 切除比例高,约有 20%的患者很快出现远处转移,这其中几乎一半的患者无法行术后辅助治疗。因此,虽然可切除胰腺癌的新辅助治疗正在研究中,但更多的研究新辅助疗的试验是完全必要的。

交界可切除胰腺癌的新辅助治疗

随着多排螺旋 CT 的应用,以及对外科手术中阳性手术切缘更好的理解,越来越多的胰腺癌不能明确的被区分为是可切除性的还是不可切除的,而这类肿瘤现在被描述为交界可切除性肿瘤。相关的定义不尽相同,通常情况交界可切除性肿瘤被定义为肿瘤紧邻但非包绕主要动脉,如肠系膜上动脉、肝动脉、腹腔干,或者肿瘤不同程度的包绕肠系膜上静脉、门静脉和肠系膜上-门静脉的汇合处[274,275]。交界可切除性肿瘤患者直接行手术治疗发生切缘阳性切除(R1 或 R2)的风险较高,而阳性切缘被认为是影响预后的独立危险因素[218,259~262]。从可切除性患者结果方面考虑,先行新辅助治疗再手术的与直接手术的相比,R1 切除率明显降低[267~269],R1 切除术的风险降低[273]。

我们的研究结果为术前放化疗提供了进一步的支持证据,可能切除的胰腺癌患者接受新辅助治疗后约 40%最终进行了手术切除,这部分患者的中位生存时间约为 40 个月,且 R0 切除率高达 96%[276]。

鉴于上述研究结果,由于术后时常出现肿瘤切缘阳性,交界可切除胰腺癌患者不应直接手术切除。新辅助治疗可以使肿瘤消退,特别是肿瘤周围的癌细胞灭活使得肿瘤更有可能获得最终的根治性切除(如切缘阴性)。

目前的临床实践指南推荐对交界可切除胰腺癌患者应该

考虑术前行多手段的综合治疗(新辅助治疗)[277~279]。

关于可切除胰腺癌新辅助治疗的前瞻性试验正在开展。三个基本治疗方案正在研究中:系统治疗后手术,放化疗后手术,以及诱导化疗,随后放化疗,最后手术[280~282]。

放疗在交界可切除胰腺癌中的作用

与术后辅助治疗相比,术前放射治疗作为新辅助治疗的组成部分,对于交界可切除胰腺癌更具有意义。术前放射治疗在可切除及交界可切除胰腺癌治疗在之前已经讨论过,放疗在可切除胰腺癌中的作用逐渐彰显出来。

胰腺体尾部肿瘤

由于胰体尾腺癌不堵塞胆总管的胰内段,因此早期诊断较困难,大部分患者确诊时已经局部进展或发生远处转移。大多数情况下腹腔干或者肠系膜上动脉被肿瘤包绕。此外,腹膜转移容易发生,建议剖腹手术前进行腹腔镜检查[283,284]。

局部进展期胰腺癌

在 20 世纪 80 年代早期的研究表明:联合放化疗较单纯放疗能更好地延长局部进展期患者的生存期[285]。此后的 20 年来,对局部进展期患者,普遍推荐优先考虑放化疗。然而,在 1997 年批准吉西他滨用于胰腺癌后,对比单独使用吉西他滨和联合放化疗的试验显示不同的结果(表 93-6)。在一项法国研究中,局部进展期患者被随机分组,一组患者仅给予吉西他滨化疗;另一组患者吉西他滨化疗后给予放疗(总剂量为 60Gy)同步联合氟尿嘧啶和顺铂[286]。单药吉西他滨组与放化疗组中位生存期为:13.0 个月 vs 8.6 个月($P=0.03$)。值得注意的是,由于不良依从性及放化疗的毒性,这项试验过早地停止了。

表 93-6　局部进展期胰腺癌化疗,放疗及放化疗的部分临床试验

研究(年份)	例数	对照组中位生存期/月	实验组中位生存期/月	P
GITSG[285](1981)	194	XRT 40Gy(仅) 5.5	氟尿嘧啶+XRT 40~60Gy 10	<0.01
FFCD/SFRO[286](2008)	119	吉西他滨单药 13.0	先氟尿嘧啶/顺铂+XRT 60Gy,再吉西他滨 8.6	0.03
ECOG 4021[287](2011)	74	吉西他滨单药 9.2	吉西他滨+XRT 50.4Gy,再吉西他滨 11.1	0.017
LAP07[291](2013)	442(269 例 R2)	吉西他滨±厄洛替尼(R1)诱导治疗 4 个月,如果无进展继续吉西他滨治疗 2 个月 16.5	吉西他滨±厄洛替尼(R1)诱导治疗 4 个月,如果无进展继续卡陪他滨+XRT 54Gy 治疗 15.3	0.83

Gem,吉西他滨;XRT,放疗;R1,第一次随机化;R2,第二次随机化

相反,ECOG4201 显示基于吉西他滨的放化疗优于吉西他滨单药化疗。该试验将首先基于吉西他滨的放化疗,之后每周给予吉西他滨与标准的吉西他滨单药治疗方案进行比较。该研究原计划入组 316 例患者,虽然在入组 74 例之后就过早地结束了,但是放化疗组有明显的生存获益,放化疗组的中位生存时间明显长于单纯化疗组(11.0 个月 vs 9.2 个月,$P=0.034$)。这一生存获益的代价是胃肠毒副作用发生率升高(3 级及以上胃肠毒性作用发生率为:38% vs 14%,$P=0.03$;疲劳的发生率为:32% vs 6%[287]。因此,在标准的化疗之上联合放疗适度延长了中位生存时间,但同时也增加了可控的毒副作用。

与此同时,局部进展期胰腺癌的治疗方案开始转变。在 UTMDACC 进行的一项回顾性试验结果表明,先行化疗随后再行放化疗的患者与起初就给予联合放化疗的患者相比,中位生存期有明显提高(11.9 个月 vs 8.5 个月,$P<0.001$)[288]。研究者认为系统治疗作为一种选择手段有助于区分那些迅速出现疾病进展的患者。此后的两个前瞻性试验也支持上述观点,研究表明诱导化疗后行放化疗的中位生存期为 15~17 个月[289,290]。值得注意的是,在这两项试验中,大约 30%的患者全身诱导化疗 3~6 个月后出现疾病进展,这些患者没有继续接受后续的放化疗。

最近,对临床实践影响最大的 LAP07 试验是一个欧洲多个国家参与的试验。LAP07 试验的初步数据显示常规吉西他滨单药化疗之后进行附加的放化疗转化治疗没有明显的临床获益[291]。采用 2×2 随机设计,患者接受初始吉西他滨治疗(无论有无埃罗替尼)4 个月。对于那些没有出现转移的患者,第二次随机分组,继续接受 2 个月吉西他滨或卡培他滨为基础的放化疗(仅对肿瘤总量为 54Gy)。中位随访 36 个月后,化疗组和放化疗组之间中位生存期无明显差异(15 个月 vs 14 个月,$P=0.083$)。上述试验的更多细节在当本书出版时还未公布。

单独化疗还是化疗后再联合放化疗:如何选择患者?

类似于手术前的术前治疗,诱导化疗的一段时间间隔有助于发现肿瘤具有不良的生物学行为而很快出现转移的患者。就像可切除患者在术前治疗过程中出现转移,就不会从手术中受益一样,局部进展期胰腺癌患者具有能迅速远处播散的侵袭性疾病时,不能从局部的放化疗中获益。尽管 LAP07 通过 4 个月的系统性吉西他滨治疗,确实提供了一种识别具有高侵袭性肿瘤生物学行为的方法,却不能识别可能从强化放化疗中获益的患者。

将来,SMAD4 可能有助于选择接受系统治疗、标准剂量或剂量强化放射疗法的患者。目前,这是美国唯一正在进行的相关临床试验,用来评估吉西他滨和纳米白蛋白紫杉醇诱导化疗后行放射治疗的意义(RTOG1201)。*SMAD4* 表达状态是一个分层变量,患者随机接受六个周期的标准化疗,或者 4 个化疗周期后行 28 个分割总剂量 50.4Gy 的放疗,或者采用 4 个化疗周期后行 28 个分割总剂量 63Gy 的调强放射治疗(IMRT)。放疗的同时给予卡培他滨治疗。本试验将评估 SMAD4 作为放化疗预测标记物的价值,并进一步评估联合放化疗在更加有效的化疗中的意义。

基于吉西他滨与基于氟嘧啶的放化疗对比

吉西他滨的问世使得胰腺癌的治疗取得了很大进步。作为重要的胰腺癌系统化疗药物,吉西他滨能增强放疗的敏感性[292],使得人们开始对局限性胰腺癌患者进行吉西他滨与 EBRT(外照射放疗)联合应用的研究[293~297]。这些研究中的大部分结果表明胃肠道毒性是剂量限制性因素,另外也观察到血液系统毒性反应。目前关于吉西他滨和放射治疗联合应用尚无标准方案,但是一些变量可能对预测最大耐受剂量(maximum tolerated dose,MTD)具有重要意义,这些变量包括放射范围的大小,放射总剂量,每部分可能放射的剂量以及静脉给予吉西他滨的次数(一周一次还是两次)[298]。

比较局部进展期胰腺癌同步放化疗的最佳数据来自 SCALOP 研究,这项 2 期随机试验入组 114 名局部进展期胰腺癌,吉西他滨和卡培他滨治疗 12 周后,再行联合放化疗采用吉西他滨(每周 300mg/m^2)或卡培他滨(每天两次,每次 830mg/m^2 放射当天)的方案。与吉西他滨相比,使用卡培他滨治疗的中位生存期更长(15.2 个月 vs 13.4 个月,$P=0.012$),毒性更低[299]。

局部进展期胰腺癌的放射治疗

由于对区域淋巴结的放射治疗并不能使局部进展期胰腺癌患者获益,因此放射治疗的区域应局限于大体肿瘤部位。这种放疗方案可以减小放化疗的胃肠毒性。因此,正确的鉴定胰腺肿瘤位置非常重要,对比增强的 CT 片子应由有经验的放射科医师阅读,胰腺肿瘤与周围的胰腺组织对比呈现典型的低密度区,确定原发肿瘤的精确部位后,在仿真模拟检查的同时给予口服造影剂,能清楚地显示十二指肠的“C 环”结构。另外,胆道内的胆管支架亦可从 CT 片上显示,从而有利于胆总管位置的辨认。

胰腺和十二指肠位置随呼吸运动偏移幅度约为 1cm[300],如果对整个肿瘤进行放射,则必须控制呼吸运动或者调整放射治疗技术。这种技术调整通常通过在预定放射区域的头侧和足侧增加适当的附加边缘而实现。但是由于轴位的肿瘤运动可忽略,因此轴位的附加边缘可省略。由于呼吸周期调节放射治疗(呼吸门控)[301]是放射剂量渐增研究的必要组成部分,该研究的目的是寻求原发肿瘤给予大于 60Gy 的放射剂量而不引起十二指肠损伤的合理方案。因此,为不引起十二指肠损伤而将放射区域严格限定于原发肿瘤区域而不考虑对器官运动的校正会引起肿瘤靶点接受到的放射剂量低于预定的剂量或称作“边缘缺失”。推荐四区法即按等比例附加前、后及对边区域。放射位附 2cm 边缘,头侧和足侧分别附加 3cm。

放化疗新方案

分子药物作为放射增敏剂

正如分子药物与细胞毒性药物联合应用于化疗一样,分子靶向药物在实体瘤中用作放疗增敏剂正被广泛研究[302]。在局部进展期胰腺癌中,目前已有的抑制剂(吉非替尼、厄洛替尼或者西妥昔单抗)与放射治疗联合应用治疗胰腺癌的有效性尚无多中心试验报道。然而,小样本的试验应用分子放疗增敏剂,尤其是 EGFR 抑制剂的效果喜人[303~305]。遗憾的是,EGFR 抑制剂联合化疗未能明显延长局部进展期胰腺癌患者的生存期[306,307],因此研究 EGFR 抑制剂作为放疗增敏剂的试验随即停止了。

胰腺癌的三维定向体放射治疗(SBRT)

三维定向体放射治疗(stereotactic radiotherapy,SBRT)能精确地将高剂量的射线靶向体积较小的肿瘤。SBRT 用于局部进展期胰腺癌治疗的可行性已经在Ⅰ期和Ⅱ期试验中使用单分割方法研究[308,309]。鉴于效果不佳,毒性显著,研究方案调整为五次分割的方案。一项多中心的试验评估了五分割 SBRT 的效果(1 周内,5 次分割放射总剂量 33Gy)[310],结果表明耐受性良好,且中位生存期与标准分割的放化疗基本相当。因此,与标准放化疗方案相比,五分割的 SBRT 方案可能耐受性更好,更方便,并且具有相似的疗效。只有更好的控制局部肿瘤才能达到长期生存的目标。

不可逆电穿孔在局部进展期胰腺癌的应用

虽然不是放射治疗干预手段,但不可逆电穿孔(IRE)作为一种局部消融技术在肿瘤学领域受到越来越多的关注[311]。IRE 方法是在实体肿瘤中放置输送高压能量脉冲的电极。这些脉冲导致磷脂细胞膜中孔的形成,改变细胞渗透性进而导致细胞凋亡。相对于其他消融技术,电穿孔术的优势在于没有对周围组织,特别是血管和导管结构的热损伤[312]。在 27 例局部进展期胰腺癌应 IRE 的早期经验已有报道[313]。在 8 例患者中,IRE 联合手术切除(四个胰头病灶和四个体尾病灶)以保证切缘阴性。在其余的 19 例中,肿瘤原位进行了 IRE。所有 27 例患者出现淀粉酶和脂肪酶升高,48h 达到峰值,72h 后恢复正常。其他中心也开始报道他们的 IRE 操作经验包括经皮,影像引导的电极定位穿刺[314]。

根据目前的文献,研究人员对这种技术的兴趣不断增长,特别是应用于交界可切除和局部进展期疾病[315]。然而,需要更广泛的多中心经验来确定详细的标准以供患者选择及明确这种技术与其他治疗方法结合的先后顺序。如前面所强调的,鉴于胰腺癌是一种系统性疾病,强调系统性治疗应先于任何局部治疗包括(IRE、手术或放疗)。

局部进展期胰腺癌的治疗方法

无论何时,应尽可能地对功能状况良好的局部进展期胰腺癌患者进行临床试验治疗。预定的治疗程序包括先给予化疗,随后给予放化疗或给予替代方案为靶向药物联合放化疗，后续再进一步进行其他系统治疗。

临床试验之外，系统治疗的目的应该能改善疼痛及整体功能状况[316]，并且能避免放化疗相关的胃肠毒性。

胰腺癌系统性治疗的作用

虽然手术和放射治疗在胰腺癌的治疗中具有重要作用，但是这些方法在局限期疾病的中的应用受到一定限制。此外，本章前面章节已经讨论过，放射治疗可能对部分局部晚期胰腺癌患者有效。相比之下，系统治疗作为晚期胰腺癌的主要治疗手段[317]，已被证明在潜在治愈性手术[253]的患者中是有益的[291]。直到现在，吉西他滨仍然是局部进展期胰腺癌系统性辅助治疗的主要标准治疗药物。然而，随着 FOLFIRINOX 和吉西他滨联合白蛋白-紫杉醇方案的出现（在转移性疾病中两者都优于吉西他滨单药）[318,319]，需要进一步研究两种方案在疾病的较早阶段的应用，以便于：①提高行根治性切除患者治愈率和存活率；②增加交界性可切病患者行根治性手术的比例；③延长不能行手术治疗的交界性可切除患者的生存期；④改善局部进展期患者的总生存期。

系统治疗的发展

详细的介绍胰腺癌系统治疗的发展历史超出了本章的范围，在许多发表的综述中有很好的相关总结。

根据早期和近期的关于系统性细胞毒性药物的试验，可以得出如下的结论。首先，追加氟尿嘧啶在晚期胰腺癌中没有效果[316,320]。然而，输注氟尿嘧啶或口服卡培他滨单药在 7%～8%胰腺癌中有微弱的获益[321,322]。第二，吉西他滨单药治疗的客观反应率大约 10%，这一结果在不同时间及试验中基本一致。第三，吉西他滨双药联合与吉西他滨单药相比能提高客观缓解了。然而，这种效果只在吉西他滨联合纳米白蛋白紫杉醇中比较明显，将吉西他滨与奥沙利铂、顺铂、氟尿嘧啶或卡培他滨联合应用，生存期没有统计学上的显著提高（表 93-7）[319,323~331]。更重要的是，体能状况在各期胰腺癌中仍然是总生存期的重要预测指标。早在 1985 年，体能状况就被观察到可以影响各期胰腺癌的生存期[332]。现代的 CALGB 80803[333] 研究，比较吉西他滨与吉西他滨联合纳米白蛋白紫杉醇的随机试验，也印证了这一点[334]。

表 93-7　进展期胰腺癌患者单药对比吉西他滨双药联合的已完成随机临床试验总结

主要研究者	例数	转移性患者	对照组 中位生存期/月	实验组 中位生存期/月	*P*
Berlin[323]（2002）	322	90	Gem 5.4	Gem+氟尿嘧啶 6.7	0.09
Colucci[324]（2002）	107	58	Gem 4.7	Gem+顺铂 7.0	0.43
Rocha Lima[325]（2004）	342	80	Gem 6.5	Gem+伊利替康 6.3	0.79
Louvet[326]（2005）	313	70	Gem 6.0	Gem+奥沙利铂 9.0	0.15
Heinemann[327]（2006）	195	80	Gem 6.0	Gem+顺铂 7.5	0.15
Herrmann[328]（2007）	319	79	Gem 7.2	Gem+卡培他滨 8.4	0.14
Abou Alfa[329]（2007）	349	78	Gem 6.2	Gem+依沙替康 6.7	0.52
Cunningham[330]（2009）	553	71	Gem 6.2	Gem+卡培他滨 7.1	0.08
Colucci[331]（2010）	400	84	Gem 8.3	Gem+顺铂 7.2	0.38
Von Hoff[319]（2013）	861	100	Gem 6.7	Gem+纳米白蛋白紫杉醇 8.5	<0.001

Gem，吉西他滨

转移性疾病新治疗方案：FOLFIRINOX 和吉西他滨/纳米白蛋白紫杉醇

自本书最后一版以来，两种新的联合治疗方案已被提出。在转移性疾病中，这两种方案与吉西他滨单药相比，可以获得更长的生存期（表 93-8）。FOLFIRINOX 首次在一项 2 期临床试验中显示，47 名患者的客观 RR 为 26%，中位生存期为 10.2 个月[335]。随后在一项大型 3 期随机试验中比较了 FOLFIRINOX 和吉西他滨单药[318]。FOLFIRINOX 在 RR（32% vs 9%）、无进展生存期(PFS)(6.4 个月 vs 3.3 个月)和 OS(11.1 个月 vs 6.8 个月)方面均优于吉西他滨。两者死亡的危险比 0.57,P<0.001。值得注意的是,该试验入组患者仅限于首次接受化疗的晚期患者且 ECOG 体能评分为 0 或者 1 分。

表 93-8　进展期或者晚期胰腺癌患者细胞毒性药物或联合应用的随机试验总结

治疗	Burris 1996316		Conroy 2011[318](ACCORD)		Von Hoff 2013[319](MPACT)	
	氟尿嘧啶	Gem	Gem	FOLFIRINOX	Gem	Gem/nab-p
PS	Karnovsky PS≥50%		ECOG PS 0 或者 1		Karnovsky PS≥70%	
远处转移患者/%	70		100		100	
RR/%	0	10	9	32	7	23
MS/月	4.5	5.7	6.8	11.1	6.7	8.5
1 年生存期/%	2	18	21	48	22	35
中性粒细胞减少/%	5	25	21	46	27	38
乏力(3~4 级)	NS	NS	18	24	1	17
腹泻(3~4 级)	6	2	2	13	1	6
神经病变	NS	NS	0	9	7	17

PS,体能状况;Gem,吉西他滨;nab-p,纳米白蛋白结合紫杉醇;MS,中位生存期;NS,未说明;RR,反应率

随后,研究了纳米白蛋白结合型(NAB)紫杉醇在胰腺癌中的作用。在纳米白蛋白紫杉醇($125mg/m^2$)联合吉西他滨($1\,000mg/m^2$)的最大耐受剂量下,每周一次,连续 3 周,停药 1 周,每 4 周为 1 个周期,客观缓解率为 48%,中位生存期为 12.2 个月[336]。这一显著结果,促使更大样本的 3 期临床试验比较吉西他滨联合纳米白蛋白紫杉醇和吉西他滨单药[319]。该试验的入组标准为首次接受化疗的晚期患者且 KPS≥70%(大致相当于 ECOG PS 0~2),试验入组 861 例患者,证实了吉西他滨/纳米白蛋白紫杉醇在 RR(23% vs 7%),PFS(5.5 个月 vs 3.7 个月)和生存期方面优于吉西他滨单药。两药联合对比吉西他滨单药的中位生存期为 8.5 个月比 6.7 个月(死亡 HR 为 0.72;P<0.001)。不足为奇,与先前的临床试验结果一致,随后的分析显示,与那些 KPS 为 90%~100%的患者相比,KPS 为 70%~80%的患者生存率较低[334]。

根据这些良好设计的大型临床试验结果,两种方案 FOLFIRINOX 和吉西他滨/纳米白蛋白紫杉醇代表转移性胰腺癌系统性治疗的显著进步。并且,虽然两种方案都能引起粒细胞减少,但具体毒性反应谱有差异。因此临床肿瘤医师可以更灵活选择一线治疗方案[337]。

分子制剂抑制胰腺癌:没有明显效果

应用现代的分子治疗技术改善胰腺癌治疗方法的尝试令人失望,尽管分子制剂已经很大程度上改变了肝细胞癌[338]、进展期结直肠癌[339]、胃癌[340]等胃肠道肿瘤的治疗模式。多项随机临床试验对吉西他滨与吉西他滨联合其他靶向制剂的治疗疗效进行了比较[306,307,333,341~345]。只有吉西他滨和厄洛替尼的联合应用较吉西他滨单药显示出微弱的具有统计学差异的生存优势[306]。在加拿大国家癌症研究所进行的一项大型安慰剂对照、双盲、三期临床试验中,569 名患者随机接受吉西他滨联合厄洛替尼或吉西他滨联合安慰剂治疗。随机接受吉西他滨/厄洛替尼治疗的患者中位生存期为 6.24 个月,而接受吉西他滨/安慰剂治疗的患者中位生存期为 5.91 个月(死亡 HR=0.82,P=0.038)。

最近,激发性临床前实验表明,Hedgehog 通路抑制可调节胰腺癌肿瘤微环境,并增强细胞毒性药物向肿瘤递送[183]。这导致了一项安慰剂对照、双盲、随机 2 期试验的进行,该试验在 122 例初治转移性胰腺癌患者中比较吉西他滨联合 saridegib(一种 Hedgehog 抑制剂)和吉西他滨联合安慰剂治疗。根据一项中期分析显示,随机接受吉西他滨/saridegib 治疗的患者与接受吉西他滨/安慰剂治疗的患者相比生存期较低(www.businesswire.com/news/home/20120127005146/en/infinityreports-update-phase-2),因此该试验提前终止。未来成功的治疗胰腺癌的分子疗法临床试验除了多学科临床试验设计外,还需要严格和令人信服的临床前数据的支持。这将被更详细地在本章"未来发展方向"部分讨论。

系统治疗 *BRCA* 突变胰腺癌

临床医师已经认识到,胰腺癌患者具有异质性,部分患者生存期明显超过文献报道的各期胰腺癌的中位存活时间。此外,部分患者对化疗的客观反应有时也相当惊人。这些患者可能有潜在的生殖系或体细胞突变,使其对化疗药物,尤其是诱导 DNA 损伤药物(奥沙利铂、顺铂和丝裂霉素 C)及拓扑异构酶抑制剂等细胞毒性作用更加敏感。BRAC1、2 和 PALB2 生殖系基因突变的基因检测常为阴性,不能解释患者对药物高敏感性的原因。另外,散发性癌的亚群似乎定义不清,可能部分患者存在 DNA 修复途径存在缺陷的特征,对某些特异性细胞毒性药物治疗更为敏感。一些研究者将这些散发的胰腺癌描述为具有"BRCAness"表型,可能由调控 DNA 修复的基因突变、扩增或甲基化导致[346]。临床上有一些提示支持这一观点。对来自 JHH 患者的回顾性分析表明:与没有肿瘤家族史的患者相比,有胰腺、乳腺、口腔癌家族史的患者可从含铂方案中获益更多。重要的是,目前在胰腺癌中[347]发现了 *BRCA2* 基因的体细胞病变,这些肿瘤也可能对导致 DNA 损伤的化疗药物非常敏感。

将来,更好地研究 BRCAness 的特征可能会识别出更多可

能受益于铂类、丝裂霉素 C 和拓扑异构酶抑制剂治疗的患者。另外,PARP 抑制剂在胰腺癌中已经进入临床试验,可能特别适用于 BRCA 生殖系突变患者和/或具有 BRACness 的散发性胰腺癌患者。

转移性胰腺癌的治疗策略

系统性治疗的选择

基于先前提供的关于细胞毒性治疗在转移性胰腺癌中的作用的数据,对患者的 PS 进行准确评估对临床决策和推荐治疗方案至关重要。对于 PS 较差(ECOG>2,KPS<70%)或有明显转移性肿瘤负荷的转移性患者,应该避免进行系统治疗。如果可能的话,体能状态良好的患者应该鼓励参加临床试。当无法或不需要参加临床试验时,对于 ECOG PS 0~1 患者,使用 FOLFIRINOX 或吉西他滨/纳米白蛋白紫杉醇治疗是合适的一线选择。对于 ECOG PS 2 或 KPS 70%的患者,吉西他滨/纳米白蛋白紫杉醇是一个有效的选择,但应谨慎使用,密切随访并且将剂量/时间表调整到较低的阈值。对于不能准确判定是否适合系统性治疗的患者,可考虑使用吉西他滨单药治疗。在这种情况下添加厄洛替尼也是合理的。这种药物的预期益处不应被夸大,其作为系统治疗的一个组成部分在未来的应用可能会降低[306]。

目前,二线治疗仅限于体能状况良好的疾病进展期患者,并且明显依赖于先前的一线治疗方案。支持性治疗是一种可以持续进行的抗肿瘤治疗方案,后面章节有详细的讨论。

支持性和姑息性治疗

转移性胰腺癌患者表现为纳差、恶病质和疼痛,黄疸通常由原发肿瘤或肝内转移引起。局部的肿瘤浸润可以导致剧烈的疼痛、胃输出道梗阻和胃轻瘫。腹膜转移患者表现为难治性腹水、肠道蠕动障碍或机械性肠梗阻,便秘也很常见。患者通常也易发生静脉血栓,但发病风险是否较其他胃肠道肿瘤高目前仍不清楚[348]。姑息治疗通常是治疗的首选,而且需要多学科共同合作完成。在开始系统性治疗之前需要减轻胆道梗阻和疼痛症状。对于多数患者,不需过度使用镇静药物而仅通过长期或短期使用麻醉性止痛药物即可以控制疼痛[349]。但是通过口服和经皮使用麻醉药物效果不好,或患者无法耐受,则需考虑消融腹腔神经丛或内脏神经丛以控制顽固性疼痛。超声内镜引导下进行神经阻滞是否优于透视或 CT 引导下神经阻滞目前仍不清楚,但对于慢性胰腺炎患者,超声内镜引导下神经阻滞效果要好于 CT 引导下的神经阻滞[350]。

考虑到转移性胰腺癌患者预后较差,通常尽可能地通过非手术的方法缓解胆道梗阻。目前对于机械性胃输出道梗阻和预后不佳的患者使用十二指肠支架治疗已得到广泛认可[351]。对于有症状的难治性腹水进行腹腔穿刺抽液仍是最有效的办法[352],但这并非长久之计。腹腔置管引流适用于需要反复引流的患者,且总体感染风险较低[353]。

低分子肝素预防性治疗可降低接受化疗的晚期患者发生静脉血栓风险[354]。然而,这种干预对总生存期的是否有影响还不清楚。

未来发展方向

结合本章其他部分的论述,胰腺癌的治疗进展非常缓慢。随着对胰腺癌肿瘤生物学行为和微环境更深入的了解,加上更多种类肿瘤细胞杀伤药物,调节肿瘤微环境或增强宿主免疫反应的药物的应用,期待胰腺癌得到更好的治疗。目前,正在进行的工作可以分为三类:①直接提高对肿瘤细胞的非免疫杀伤;②调节肿瘤微环境促进细胞死亡;③增强对胰腺癌的免疫破坏。

肿瘤细胞的非免疫杀伤

细胞毒性药物联合

从使用 FOLFIRINOX 的早期经验中得到的最重要的教训之一可能是,联合使用细胞毒疗法可能比单一疗法或双药联合疗法更有效[355]。因此,目前正在对其他三种药物联合进行研究,包括吉西他滨、顺铂和纳米白蛋白紫杉醇(GAC)以及氟尿嘧啶、亚叶酸钙、奥沙利铂和纳米白蛋白紫杉醇(FOLFOX-A)的联合研究(www. clinicaltrials. gov)。

新型细胞毒性药物:重组伊立替康

MM398 是伊立替康(nal-IRI)的纳米脂质体包封物,与母体化合物相比具有更好的药代动力学和肿瘤生物分布。该药已作为单药在 40 例吉西他滨难治性胰腺癌患者中进行研究,其 RR 为 7.5%,中位 OS 为 5.2 个月[356]。随后,Napoli-1,一项三臂随机研究,比较了 nal-IRI 单独应用或 nal-IRI 与氟尿嘧啶/亚叶酸钙联合或氟尿嘧啶/亚叶酸钙单独应用,得出了一些初步结果。在吉西他滨难治性晚期胰腺癌患者中 Nal-IRI 加氟尿嘧啶/亚叶酸钙优于单独使用氟尿嘧啶/亚叶酸钙,中位生存期 6.1 个月 vs 4.2 个月,$P=0.012$[357]。期待最终的试验结果。

ruxolitinib

Janus 激酶/信号受体和转录激活剂(JAK/Stat)-3 通路被报道在胰腺癌中被持续性激活,体外试验应用该通路抑制剂可消除肿瘤细胞的生长[358]。ruxolitinib 是一种 JAK2 抑制剂,最近被批准用于治疗骨髓纤维化和其他骨髓增生性疾病[359]。在一组吉西他滨难治性胰腺癌患者的安慰剂对照试验中,研究了这种药物。患者随机分组接受 ruxolitinib/卡培他滨或者安慰剂/卡培他滨[360]。在这项预先设定研究对象为 C 反应蛋白(CRP)水平为>13 的患者试验中,与安慰剂/卡培他滨相比,ruxolitinib/卡培他滨延长了 PFS 和 OS。目前正在进行一项更大样本的三期临床试验,即用卡培他滨或安慰剂与 ruxolitinib 联合,且入组患者 CRP 水平>10(www. clinicaltrials. gov)。

PARP 抑制剂

如前所述,小部分胰腺癌患者具有 *BRCA1*、*BRCA2* 或者 *PALB2* 基因的生殖系突变。更大部分胰腺癌患者的肿瘤细胞可能存在 *BRCA1* 或 *BRCA2* 的体细胞突变[347]。理论上,这些突变的胰腺肿瘤更容易受到 PARP 抑制的影响,从而导致合成致死[361]。目前正在胰腺癌中对几种 PARP 抑制剂进行研究,包括 olaparib、veliparib、rucaparib 和 BMN-673[362]。

调节肿瘤微环境的药物

玻璃酸酶

透明质酸是胰腺癌赖以生长的细胞外基质的重要成分[363]。CD44 是一种表达于肿瘤细胞表面的跨膜糖蛋白,能够与透明质酸结合，导致细胞增殖和侵袭。在最近的研究基础上，人们对降解透明质酸作为调节肿瘤基质和增强细胞毒性化疗药物递送的手段重新产生了兴趣[135,364,365]。聚乙二醇化重组人玻璃酸酶PEGPH20的早期临床研究表明，与单药吉西他滨联合应用前景广阔[366]。因此，一项多中心研究正在研究在常规细胞毒治疗中添加玻璃酸酶，以提高化疗的细胞毒效果。这项试验目前正在招募以前未经治疗的转移性疾病患者，预期1~2年会得出试验结果(www.clinicaltrials.gov)。

调节胰腺癌微环境细胞成分的药物

除了试图操控胰腺癌的细胞外基质外，现在有一些药物可以调节胰腺癌微环境的细胞内成分。这些药物包括CD40激动剂，基于小鼠模型和临床研究，CD40激动剂具有释放原发性胰腺腺癌骨髓源性成分的能力[367]。其中一种单克隆抗体CP-870,893正在进入临床研究，这种药物与化疗联合使用似乎是安全的[368]。然而，目前还没有明确的疗效信息表明其可增强化疗或放疗的细胞毒性作用。

另一个有趣的化合物是PF-04136309，一种趋化因子受体2型(CCR2)拮抗剂。CCR2的激活可动员骨髓中的单核细胞和巨噬细胞浸润恶性肿瘤。这些炎症单核细胞可能具有促进肿瘤生长的特性。临床前模型显示，PF-04136309的递送降低了小鼠的循环单核细胞，减少了生长于小鼠的胰腺腺癌的单核细胞浸润[369]。此外，抑制CCR2可增强抗肿瘤免疫，抑制肿瘤生长，减少转移。已经有一些早期的临床研究该化合物与FOLFIRINOX联合应用。这种联合使用似乎是安全的，早期结果表明联合应用具有更好的抗癌效果[370]。

Salk研究所的研究人员提出了另一种调节胰腺癌间质的方法。他们发现维生素D受体(VDR)在恶性胰腺间质中表达，并与炎症和纤维化的标志物有关。应用VDR配体治疗导致转录改变、基质重构、炎症和纤维化标志物减少。当骨化三醇(一种维生素D的类似物)与吉西他滨联合使用时，研究人员在小鼠胰腺癌模型中发现肿瘤内吉西他滨的含量升高，进而延长了生存期[187]。一项新辅助化疗药物中添加帕利骨化醇(一种商业化的VDR激动剂)(www.ctrc.net/documents/pdf/vonhoff_2015.pdf)的临床试验正在开展。

扩大胰腺癌的免疫反应

整个免疫治疗学科正在迅速改变。这项工作包括开发更复杂和更具体的疫苗接种策略，递送检查点抑制剂，从患者身上分离和扩增T细胞亚群再回输，以及通过对T细胞进行分子调控来增强对肿瘤细胞免疫识别和免疫破坏。这些尝试的详细介绍可以在教科书的相关章节找到。本书的仅对一些新的免疫学方法的具体例子在以下章节中进行介绍。

疫苗治疗

利用疫苗策略提高胰腺癌免疫应答的研究已经进行了多年。来自JHH的研究人员一直致力于探索注射分泌GM-CSF的同种异体胰腺肿瘤细胞(现在叫GVAX)对胰腺癌患者的益处[371]。给胰腺癌患者注射GVAX的早期试验显示，患者出现了特异性免疫反应，提示具有临床相关的活性[372]。最近的一项2期临床研究[373]，为了提高GVAX的疗效，将低剂量环磷酰胺(用于抑制调节性T细胞)与GVAX和CRS 207(表达间皮素的减毒李斯特菌)的组合与低剂量环磷酰胺(Cy)和GVAX的治疗以2∶1随机分组进行比较。试验纳入了90例转移性胰腺癌患者(97%以前接受过治疗)。与只接受Cy和GVAX的患者相比，接受Cy、GVAX和CRS207的患者PFS和OS更长。Cy/GVAX/CRS 207组的OS为6.1个月，Cy/GVAX组为3.9个月($HR=0.59$；$P=0.02$)。此外，在对接受至少三剂(两剂Cy/GVAX加上一剂CRS 207或三剂Cy/GVAX)药物的患者进行的预先指定的每个方案分析中，两组的OS为9.7个月比4.6个月，表明应用CRS 207具有临床获益。这些结果令人沉思，并且为晚期胰腺癌的免疫治疗的临床获益提供了第一个强有力的证据。

检查点抑制剂

随着检查点抑制剂的发展，包括伊匹木单抗(ipilimumab)和纳武单抗(nivolumab)[188]，人们对免疫治疗可以显著增加目前用于胰腺癌的全身药物的作用的潜力产生了极大的兴趣。遗憾的是，伊匹木单抗作为晚期胰腺癌单一药物的早期试验令人失望[189]。其他检查点抑制剂目前正在研究中，包括纳武单抗和MEDI-4736，一种抗PD1单克隆抗体[374]。这些制剂不太可能作为单一制剂具有足够的活性来改变大多数胰腺癌患者的病程，因此期待它们在胰腺癌的未来研究中参与疫苗、细胞毒性药物、放射治疗、其他分子制剂或调节T细胞的递送[375]。

胰腺癌的另一个重要的潜在靶点是CD47，这是一种癌细胞表达的细胞表面蛋白。CD47向巨噬细胞和细胞毒性T细胞发出"不要吃我"的信号指令。研究人员合成了能抑制CD7的单克隆抗体，可以体内外试验中促进吞噬细胞功能，启动T细胞识别和杀死肿瘤细胞[376]。

针对胰腺癌的T细胞

许多研究小组正致力于降低调节性T细胞的抑制信号或者增强肿瘤浸润淋巴细胞(TIL)的细胞毒性作用。在胰腺癌的基础生物学和免疫学方面还有许多工作要做。但临床前和临床研究表明，这些方法具有调节肿瘤微环境的应用前景，进而成为我们治疗胰腺癌的武器。

准则，准则，准则

自从开展治疗胰腺癌的临床试验约50年以来，人们已经吸取了一些惨痛的教训，即需要在临床试验设计和胰腺癌患者的临床实践方面加强准则。

首先，从胰腺癌的前期试验中可以看出，试验登记的标准应该包括一个完整的评估指标，限制条件为KPS至少为70%或ECOG PS>2。其次，我们必须使用更严格的标准来区分胰腺癌不同临床阶段的患者：可切除的、交界可切除的、局部晚期和转移性疾病。如果不能做到这一点，就会阻碍对任何特定疾病阶段的快速学习和认识。

第三，我们需要更严格地评估临床前模型的价值，来预测任何单一用药或联合用药治疗的临床益处。最后，利用创新的成像技术、血液或组织分析技术进行的转化研究，应该被纳入几乎每一项早期临床试验中，以证明肿瘤细胞的杀伤、基质修饰或其他与临床获益相关的生物学变化。如果我们能够把对肿瘤生物学的基本认识跟以一定的准则相结合起来，进行临床前和临床试验检测新的药物或方法，我们就一定能够在不久的将来对胰腺患者治疗取得重大进展。

(金鹏 钟宇新 译 田艳涛 校)

参考文献

The complete reference list can be found on the Wiley Companion Digital Edition of this title (see inside front cover for login instructions).

1 Siegel R, Ma J, Zou Z, Jemal A. Cancer statistics, 2014. *CA Cancer J Clin.* 2014;**64**:9–29.

7 Klein AP. Genetic susceptibility to pancreatic cancer. *Mol Carcinog.* 2012;**51**: 14–24.

12 Klein AP, Hruban RH, Brune KA, Petersen GM, Goggins M. Familial pancreatic cancer. *Cancer J.* 2001;**7**:266–273.

31 Li D, Duell EJ, Yu K, et al. Pathway analysis of genome-wide association study data highlights pancreatic development genes as susceptibility factors for pancreatic cancer. *Carcinogenesis.* 2012;**33**:1384–1390.

41 Bosetti C, Lucenteforte E, Silverman DT, et al. Cigarette smoking and pancreatic cancer: an analysis from the International Pancreatic Cancer Case–control Consortium (Panc4). *Ann Oncol.* 2012;**23**:1880–1888.

68 Elena JW, Steplowski E, Yu K, et al. Diabetes and risk of pancreatic cancer: a pooled analysis from the pancreatic cancer cohort consortium. *Cancer Causes Control.* 2013;**24**:13–25.

89 Li D. Metformin as an antitumor agent in cancer prevention and treatment. *J Diabetes.* 2011;**3**:320–327.

126 Brand RE, Lerch MM, Rubinstein WS, et al. Advances in counselling and surveillance of patients at risk for pancreatic cancer. *Gut.* 2007;**56**:1460–1469.

134 Feig C, Gopinathan A, Neesse A, Chan DS, Cook N, Tuveson DA. The pancreas cancer microenvironment. *Clin Cancer Res.* 2012;**18**:4266–4276.

147 Jones S, Zhang X, Parsons DW, et al. Core signaling pathways in human pancreatic cancers revealed by global genomic analyses. *Science.* 2008;**321**:1801–1806.

159 Collisson EA, Trejo CL, Silva JM, et al. A central role for RAF— > MEK— > ERK signaling in the genesis of pancreatic ductal adenocarcinoma. *Cancer Discov.* 2012;**2**:685–693.

164 Maitra A, Hruban RH. Pancreatic cancer. *Annu Rev Pathol.* 2008;**3**:157–188.

176 Bettegowda C, Sausen M, Leary RJ, et al. Detection of circulating tumor DNA in early- and late-stage human malignancies. *Sci Transl Med.* 2014;**6**:224ra224.

183 Olive KP, Jacobetz MA, Davidson CJ, et al. Inhibition of Hedgehog signaling enhances delivery of chemotherapy in a mouse model of pancreatic cancer. *Science.* 2009;**324**:1457–1461.

184 Ozdemir BC, Pentcheva-Hoang T, Carstens JL, et al. Depletion of carcinoma-associated fibroblasts and fibrosis induces immunosuppression and accelerates pancreas cancer with reduced survival. *Cancer Cell.* 2014;**25**:719–734.

191 Vonderheide RH, Bayne LJ. Inflammatory networks and immune surveillance of pancreatic carcinoma. *Curr Opin Immunol.* 2013;**25**:200–205.

195 Beatty GL. Engineered chimeric antigen receptor-expressing T cells for the treatment of pancreatic ductal adenocarcinoma. *Oncoimmunology.* 2014;**3**:e28327.

197 Le A, Rajeshkumar NV, Maitra A, Dang CV. Conceptual framework for cutting the pancreatic cancer fuel supply. *Clin Cancer Res.* 2012;**18**:4285–4290.

202 Tamm EP, Balachandran A, Bhosale P, Szklaruk J. Update on 3D and multiplanar MDCT in the assessment of biliary and pancreatic pathology. *Abdom Imaging.* 2009;**34**:64–74.

217 Howard TJ, Krug JE, Yu J, et al. A margin-negative R0 resection accomplished with minimal postoperative complications is the surgeon's contribution to long-term survival in pancreatic cancer. *J Gastrointest Surg.* 2006;**10**:1338–1345.

225 Evans DB, Lee JE, Tamm EP, Pisters PWT. Pancreaticoduodenectomy (Whipple Operation) and total pancreatectomy for cancer. In: Fisher JF, ed. *Mastery of Surgery*, 5th ed. Philadelphia: Lippincott, Williams and Williams; 2007: 1299–1317.

227 Verbeke CS. Resection margins and R1 rates in pancreatic cancer – are we there yet? *Histopathology.* 2008;**52**:787–796.

228 Christians KK, Pilgrim CH, Tsai S, et al. Arterial resection at the time of pancreatectomy for cancer. *Surgery.* 2014;**155**:919–926.

233 Tran Cao HS, Lopez N, Chang DC, et al. Improved perioperative outcomes with minimally invasive distal pancreatectomy: results from a population-based analysis. *JAMA Surg.* 2014;**149**:237–243.

244 Valle JW, Palmer D, Jackson R, et al. Optimal duration and timing of adjuvant chemotherapy after definitive surgery for ductal adenocarcinoma of the pancreas: ongoing lessons from the ESPAC-3 study. *J Clin Oncol.* 2014;**32**:504–512.

248 Katz MH, Wang H, Fleming JB, et al. Long-term survival after multidisciplinary management of resected pancreatic adenocarcinoma. *Ann Surg Oncol.* 2009;**16**:836–847.

253 Oettle H, Post S, Neuhaus P, et al. Adjuvant chemotherapy with gemcitabine vs observation in patients undergoing curative-intent resection of pancreatic cancer: a randomized controlled trial. *JAMA.* 2007;**297**:267–277.

254 Neoptolemos JP, Stocken DD, Bassi C, et al. Adjuvant chemotherapy with fluorouracil plus folinic acid vs gemcitabine following pancreatic cancer resection: a randomized controlled trial. *JAMA.* 2010;**304**:1073–1081.

268 Evans DB, Varadhachary GR, Crane CH, et al. Preoperative gemcitabine-based chemoradiation for patients with resectable adenocarcinoma of the pancreatic head. *J Clin Oncol.* 2008;**26**:3496–3502.

274 Varadhachary GR, Tamm EP, Abbruzzese JL, et al. Borderline resectable pancreatic cancer: definitions, management, and role of preoperative therapy. *Ann Surg Oncol.* 2006;**13**:1035–1046.

277 Katz MH, Pisters PW, Evans DB, et al. Borderline resectable pancreatic cancer: the importance of this emerging stage of disease. *J Am Coll Surg.* 2008;**206**: 833–846.

291 Hammel P, Huguet F, van Laethem JL, et al. Comparison of chemoradiotherapy and chemotherapy in patients with a locally advanced pancreatic cancer controlled after 4 months of gemcitabine with or without erlotinib: final results of the international phase III LAP 07 study. *J Clin Oncol.* 2013;**31** (suppl):Late Breaking Abstract 4003.

309 Koong AC, Christofferson E, Le QT, et al. Phase II study to assess the efficacy of conventionally fractionated radiotherapy followed by a stereotactic radiosurgery boost in patients with locally advanced pancreatic cancer. *Int J Radiat Oncol Biol Phys.* 2005;**63**:320–323.

313 Martin RC 2nd, McFarland K, Ellis S, Velanovich V. Irreversible electroporation therapy in the management of locally advanced pancreatic adenocarcinoma. *J Am Coll Surg.* 2012;**215**:361–369.

318 Conroy T, Desseigne F, Ychou M, et al. FOLFIRINOX versus gemcitabine for metastatic pancreatic cancer. *N Engl J Med.* 2011;**364**:1817–1825.

319 Von Hoff DD, Ervin T, Arena FP, et al. Increased survival in pancreatic cancer with nab-paclitaxel plus gemcitabine. *N Engl J Med.* 2013;**369**:1691–1703.

334 Tabernero J, Chiorean EG, Infante JR, et al. Prognostic factors of survival in a randomized phase III trial (MPACT) of weekly nab-paclitaxel plus gemcitabine versus gemcitabine alone in patients with metastatic pancreatic cancer. *Oncologist.* 2015;**20**:143–150.

361 Ashworth A. A synthetic lethal therapeutic approach: poly(ADP) ribose polymerase inhibitors for the treatment of cancers deficient in DNA double-strand break repair. *J Clin Oncol.* 2008;**26**:3785–3790.

364 Jacobetz MA, Chan DS, Neesse A, et al. Hyaluronan impairs vascular function and drug delivery in a mouse model of pancreatic cancer. *Gut.* 2013;**62**: 112–120.

373 Le DT, Wang-Gillam A, Picozzi V, et al. Safety and survival with GVAX pancreas prime and Listeria Monocytogenes-expressing mesothelin (CRS-207) boost vaccines for metastatic pancreatic cancer. *J Clin Oncol.* 2015;**33(12)**:1325–1333.

第 94 章　小肠肿瘤、阑尾肿瘤、腹膜肿瘤和结直肠癌

Georgia M. Beasley, MD ■ Zhifei Sun, MD ■ Daniel P. Nussbaum, MD ■ Douglas S. Tyler, MD

概述

小肠、大肠和阑尾的肿瘤存在许多不同的病理类型和临床表现。小肠肿瘤并不常见，占消化道肿瘤比例不足 3%，占恶性肿瘤的 0.4%。结肠癌是全球第 3 大常见恶性肿瘤和第 4 大癌症死亡原因。腺癌是常见的病理类型，对其已有一定认识。目前我们在类癌、胃肠间质瘤的诊断和治疗方面也取得了很大程度进展，对其遗传学，新成像模式和微创手术的理解也较以前更为深入。本章将全面回顾小肠癌，大肠癌和阑尾癌的管理和治疗方法。

小肠肿瘤

2014 年美国新发小肠恶性肿瘤大概有 9 160 例。小肠占胃肠道（GI）总长度的 75%，占其黏膜表面积的 90%，但该区域很少进展为恶性肿瘤[1]。最近的数据显示，小肠肿瘤在所有的消化道肿瘤中占比不足 3%，在所有恶性肿瘤中约 0.4%[2]。

已有几种假说来解释小肠肿瘤低发病率的机制。其中最重要的是通过小肠快速转运内容物，使其黏膜较短地暴露于致癌物质。小肠内增加的淋巴组织，免疫球蛋白 A（IgA）的较高表达以及小肠中较低的细菌负荷，导致厌氧微生物将胆汁酸转化为潜在致癌物的能力下降[3,4]。此外，相比大肠中更多的固体内容物，小肠的液体含量可能导致较少的黏膜刺激。在小肠中还存在黏膜解毒酶，如苯并芘羟化酶[5]。

小肠恶性肿瘤中腺癌占 30%～50%，其次是类癌（25%～30%）、淋巴瘤（15%～20%），肉瘤较为少见。平滑肌瘤占所有良性肿瘤的 25%，其他良性肿瘤包括腺瘤、脂肪瘤等，纤维瘤、纤维瘤、神经纤维瘤、神经节细胞瘤、血管瘤和淋巴管瘤等较为少见[6]。

临床表现

由于小肠在常规内镜检查中相对难以达到，因此小肠肿瘤通常在症状出现后数月才得以诊断。许多小肠肿瘤直到病程晚期才出现症状，因为它们的生长相对缓慢，小肠的液体内容物通过容易，即使合并部分占位性病变，也可能不出现肠梗阻症状[6]。症状通常是由于发生部分阻塞而产生的，例如病变在近端时出现恶心、呕吐以及腹部疼痛，也可有体重减轻等非特异性表现。肿瘤侵及黏膜下层时常有出血，但以隐匿性居多，可表现为小细胞性贫血，愈创木脂粪检中可呈阳性。小肠肿瘤有一些特异性症状，如黄疸（壶腹癌），发热、腹泻和体重减轻（淋巴瘤）。肠道内分泌肿瘤（最常见的是类癌）可能出现一系列典型症状，如潮红、腹泻、发绀和间歇性呼吸窘迫。但仅少数类癌患者表现出这些症状，绝大多数患者无症状或出现肿瘤压迫症状。

最终，恶性肿瘤引起足够的症状从而被诊断。然而，在首发症状至确诊之前往往需要一段时间。一项研究显示，几乎 1/3 的患者在确诊前有 5 年或 5 年以上的症状[7]。另一项研究显示在诊断前有平均有 7 个月的持续症状[8]。许多最终诊断为小肠肿瘤的患者可能出现肠梗阻或穿孔等急症。

影像诊断

影像学通常有助于诊断这类病变，特别是在疾病晚期。然而，在许多情况下影像学检查难以早期发现可治疗的恶性肿瘤。针对小肠的影像学检查技术在过去的 20 年中有了巨大的发展。尽管腹部平片、小肠气钡双重造影在某些情况下有辅助诊断价值，但目前很大程度上已被可用来研究腔外异常和腔内变化的横断面成像技术，如计算机断层扫描（CT）和磁共振成像（MRI）所取代。在一些病例中，使用口服造影剂后进行 CT 检查可使小肠肿瘤的识别率接近 100%，但在鉴别肿瘤类型上仍有局限性[9]。这种方式在术前分期和转移评估相对常用[10]，一项研究结果标明，CT 检查对 T 分期的敏感性为 57%，对结肠癌和胃癌分别为 61% 和 42%[11,12]。MRI 技术能清楚呈现肠管腔内、体腔壁和肠腔外的细节，并可提供血管和功能信息，从而增强在小肠疾病中的诊断能力。MRI 提供详细的形态学信息和小肠疾病的功能数据，也能准确识别正常结构，从而有助于疾病的早期诊断或发现细微的结构异常，并指导患者护理中的治疗和决策。MRI 具有许多特性，使其成为小肠成像的理想选择：能够实现实时成像、功能成像，缺乏电离辐射，以及通过使用不同脉冲序列来改善的组织对比[13~15]。磁共振（MR）小肠造影在小肠肿瘤检测中的准确率为 96.6%[16,17]。除 CT 和 MR 外，血管造影和核素扫描在鉴别出血性肿瘤或血管瘤时有辅助诊断意义。内镜超声检查（EUS）用于检测小肠肿瘤及评价肿瘤分期，并可以进行实时的介入诊断（主要是在壶腹周围区域）。EUS 在预测血管侵犯和壶腹部肿瘤 T 分期的整体评估方面已被证明优于 CT 和 MRI[18,19]。在过去的 10 年中，小肠内镜作为诊断工具使用越来越广泛。小型内镜检查有三种主要类型：推进式小肠镜，术中或腹腔镜辅助小肠镜，以及最近出现的双气囊小肠镜。推进式小肠镜需要 220～250cm 的肠内插管，通常采用荧光镜辅助，可用于检查超过 Treitz 韧带以远平均 120cm 内的空肠[20]。在应用术中内镜检查时，外科医生手动操作使用推进式小肠镜（顺行）或结肠镜（逆行）通过小肠。外科医生通常可以通过缝合来标记可疑病变，并在肠镜检查完成时切除。这些技术特别适用于小肠大息肉（>15mm）的预防性息肉切除术，是用于 PJ 综合征患者的保守治疗方法[21]。新近出现的腹腔镜辅助肠镜检查侵入创伤小，不属于术中肠镜但仍需要全身麻醉，检查需外科医生和内镜医师共同操作[22]。双气囊小肠镜备有一个内镜和柔软灵活的球囊管外

套,每个外套管都有一个连接在其远端的可充气气囊。利用气囊的交替膨胀使两个管重复地相互推进以保持位置,允许深入推进到小肠中。整个小肠可以使用这种方法进行检查,与推进式小肠镜相比其不适程度要小[23]。在 2001 年获得食品药品监督管理局(FDA)的批准后,Swain 及其同事推出了一个小型可吞服的成像胶囊。通过肠道蠕动并将数据传输到捕获视频图像的接收器[24]。然而,使用胶囊内镜评估小肠肿瘤有一定的局限性,特别是对于黏膜下肿瘤[25,26]。此外,胶囊内镜检查在诊断占位性病变时有约 18.9%的漏诊率[27],有 10%~25%的患者检查时出现胶囊滞留。

治疗

小肠肿瘤的治疗通常是手术治疗,对良性病变进行局部切除,对恶性病变采取根治性的切除方式。总体而言,基于人群登记的 328 例患者统计,腺癌、类癌、淋巴瘤和肉瘤的生存率优于除乳腺、结肠、前列腺和子宫以外的所有其他器官的恶性肿瘤[29]。在极少数情况下,手术之前需进行新辅助放化疗。如果十二指肠肿瘤诊断为恶性,则可能需要进行胰十二指肠切除术,而回肠末端的肿瘤可能需要右半结肠切除术以确保完整切除和足够的边缘。

小肠恶性肿瘤

腺癌

腺癌是小肠恶性肿瘤中最常见的病理类型,约占所有恶性小肠肿瘤的 30%~50%[30,31],好发于 70~80 岁,男性多于女性[32]。队列研究表明,增加体重指数和饮酒可能会增加小肠癌的风险[33]。肿瘤常原发于十二指肠(48%~52%)和空肠(23%~25%),而较少见于回肠(13%~16%),这种分布的原因尚不明确[34,35]。有假说认为回肠中 IgA 分泌细胞的丰富程度可以通过中和腔内致癌物而使其相对免于腺癌[4],另有研究者认为丰富的酶苯并芘羟化酶可能通过解毒潜在的致癌物质起到保护作用[36]。小肠腺癌根据美国癌症联合委员会(AJCC)TNM 系统进行分期,仅有局部侵袭,无淋巴结转移并且分化良好时预后最好。然而,在小肠腺癌的治疗方面进展甚微。在诊断方式有所改进,对其分子机制的理解有所加深,但该病预后仍普遍较差。

小肠腺癌的组织发生很可能遵循最初描述的大肠癌的腺瘤-腺癌途径[37]。因此,小肠腺癌的最重要的单一危险因素是先前存在的腺瘤,无论是单个还是多个,并且与多发性息肉综合征相关[38]。小肠腺癌也与酒精(但与吸烟无关)、非热带炎性腹泻、局部肠炎、乳糜泻和尿路转流术(如回肠代膀胱术)有关[39~43]。

家族性腺瘤性息肉病(FAP)是腺癌已知的一种高危因素,其最容易发展为结肠癌,其次为小肠癌[44]。这些患者发生小肠癌的相对危险度(RR)超过 100[45]。其他与小肠肿瘤相关的遗传性综合征包括波伊茨-耶格综合征(空肠和回肠中的恶性息肉发病率增加),Gardner 综合征(腺瘤和腺癌)和 von Recklinghausen 病(副神经节瘤)。小肠炎性疾病与恶性肿瘤增加有关,特别是克罗恩病[46]。克罗恩病是小肠腺癌潜在的危险因素,在 2006 年的荟萃分析中报告了 $RR = 33$(95% CI: 15.9~60.9)[47]。与溃疡性结肠炎(UC)和结肠肿瘤一样,克罗恩病的诊断一般比小肠肿瘤的出现早大约 10 年。已发现克罗恩病患者发生小肠腺癌的几个危险因素:克罗恩病的持续时间、男性、瘘管形成、肠腔狭窄的存在以及外科旷置小肠手术[48,49]。其他与恶性肿瘤的风险增加的相关疾病为乳糜泻(淋巴瘤和腺癌)和免疫增生性疾病(弥漫性肠淋巴瘤和免疫增生性小肠疾病)[5]。

乳糜泻诱发小肠淋巴瘤的同时,也与小肠腺癌相关[40]。尽管相关文献报道中引用的病例数偏少,但在非典型部位的乳糜泻对谷蛋白介导的空肠回肠炎导致小肠腺瘤的发生有协同作用,谷蛋白介导的空肠回肠炎也是小肠腺癌和淋巴瘤发展的独立危险因素。小肠腺癌通常是侵袭性的,能够遗传下一代,通常与 PJ 错构瘤的退化有关[38]。

涉及小肠肿瘤作用的遗传机制仍然尚不明确,这主要是由于病例数量较少。来自德国的 Blaker 及其同事表明,尽管小肠癌显示出复杂的遗传变化,但大多小肠肿瘤表现出染色体核型不稳定和染色体 18q21-q22 的缺失。18q 缺失通常靶向 *SMAD4* 基因并通过 TGFβ 信号转导破坏肿瘤抑制[50]。Svrcek 及其同事使用组织微阵列分析确定 SMAD4/*DPC4* 基因的失活参与小肠腺癌的发生,TP53 过表达和 β-连环蛋白异常表达是小肠腺癌中的两种常见事件[51]。其他途径包括 Notch3 通路介导的 MUC5AC 表达等[52]。最近研究表明 DNA 错配修复基因也参与了小肠肿瘤发生过程,他们发现 dMMR 表型频率(5% 到 35%)是不同的[53]。

小肠腺癌的症状包括阻塞性症状(如十二指肠肿瘤患者的呕吐和黄疸)、腹部隐痛、体重减轻和远端病变时发生的贫血。体重减轻常见,超过 50%的患者发生。40%~70%的患者在以梗阻为首发症状。在收集的 Mayo 系列中,71%的患者有明显或隐形的失血证据[54]。腺癌,特别是十二指肠肿瘤,通常比其他小肠肿瘤更早出现症状,可以早期诊断和干预。尽管如此,30%~35%的小肠腺癌在诊断时已转移[34,35]。

全美外科医师联盟最近进行的一项 5 000 例研究中,小肠腺癌总体 5 年无病生存率(DFS)为 30.5%[55],中位生存期为 19.7 个月。腺癌的主要治疗方法是根治性手术切除,包括清扫淋巴结和血管根部结扎。切缘距肿瘤边距应为 5cm。但最近的报道表明,这种治疗方法未提高淋巴结转移的患者的生存率。在最近一项对 217 例小肠腺癌患者进行的研究中,患者均在 MD Anderson 癌症中心进行了 10 年的治疗,Ⅳ期患者 5 年总生存率(OS)差于Ⅰ~Ⅲ期疾病患者(5% vs 36%)[35]。阳性淋巴结比率(阳性淋巴结数/总淋巴结数)>75%与<75%(12% vs 51%)相比,前者 5 年生存率明显更差。

对于小肠肿瘤患者,应尽可能切除原发病灶以防止黏膜出血。对于在开腹手术时发现无法切除的患者,一些学者主张使用术中放射治疗[56~58]。由于缺乏相应的临床试验,这种治疗难以在专科医院以外的中心进行推广。关于辅助化疗作用的数据较少,无明确证据表明辅助化疗可使小肠腺癌患者存活有明显改善。2007 年的 Cochrane 综述没有发现任何可进行相应荟萃分析的研究[59]。尽管如此,因为辅助治疗对结肠癌有效,小肠癌还是会使用辅助化疗(类似于结直肠癌),因该病往往会复发。2009 年一项回顾性多中心研究表明,与其他方案治疗的患者相比,佐剂亚叶酸、氟尿嘧啶(氟尿嘧啶)和奥沙利铂(FOLFOX)方案使 OS 延长约 5 个月,但这项小型研究的结果无统计学意义[53]。对于晚期无法切除的疾病,近期一项Ⅱ期研究将改良 FOLFOX 作为晚期小肠腺癌的一线化疗方案,客观有效率为 48.5%[95% *CI*:31%~67%],其中晚期小肠腺癌患者的疗效评价为 CR(完全缓解)[60]。

类癌肿瘤

类癌约占小肠恶性肿瘤的 25%~30%[58~61]。1907 年,Obendorfer 使用了"karzinoide"一词,但是直到 1928 年 Masson 将肿瘤的起源描述为 chromaffin 细胞,肿瘤的确切性质才被发现[62,63]。在 CT 和内镜出现之前,约 85%的类癌患者直到尸检才被诊断。美国的数据显示,在过去的 30 年里,胃肠道类癌的发病率以每年 3%~10%的速度增长[64,65]。类癌最常见的部位是胃肠道(54.5%)和支气管肺系统(30.1%)。在胃肠道内,大多数发生在小肠(44.7%)、其次为直肠(19.6%)和阑尾(16.7%)。与腺癌相比,类癌往往发生在远端小肠,而不是在较近的部位。在 Moertel 报道的类癌病例(均经手术证实)中,3%在双肠,5%在空肠,32%在近端回肠,60%在远端回肠[66]。发现时的平均年龄为 60.9 岁,女性占 54.2%[67]。胃肠道类癌患者的总体 5 年生存率约为 58%,在过去 30 年几乎没有变化[64]。然而,在远处扩散的高分化类癌亚组中,5 年生存率从 15%提高到了 52%[64]。

组织切片中最有效的神经内分泌细胞标记物是嗜铬粒蛋白 A(CgA),它是一种储存在神经内分泌细胞分泌颗粒中的糖蛋白。血浆 CgA 水平与肿瘤负荷相关,可用于监测治疗[68]。尿中 5-羟基吲哚-3-醋酸(5-HIAA)(5-HT 的降解产物)的 24h 测定也有助于诊断。5-HIAA 作为类癌的标志物的特异性为 88%,但富含色氨酸/5-羟色胺的食物(香蕉、鳄梨、李子、茄子、番茄、大蕉、菠萝和核桃)也可以升高 5-HIAA 水平,一些药物可以导致 5-HIAA 水平的升高或降低[69]。尿液中 5-HIAA 浓度越高,预后越差,而持续低浓度的 5-HIAA 则预示着弥漫性疾病的预后较好。核分裂象增多和 Ki-67 指数(一种细胞增殖的标志物)也和预后相关[68]。

类癌的一个特征是它们能够产生多种蛋白质和肽产物,其中最常见的为 5-HT。系统性的 5-HT 被认为是引起类癌综合征的特殊物质,包括腹泻、面红、哮喘和右侧心脏病。类癌综合征见于 5%~7%的类癌患者,这些患者常肿瘤负荷较重和伴有肿瘤远处转移[54]。多数学者认为,转移灶对于确保类癌分泌的能引起类癌综合征的化合物进入全身循环十分重要,转移灶能提供大量肽类活性物质。

类癌往往症状不明确甚至无任何症状,往往术后才能明确的诊断。小肠类癌患者常在晚期才出现症状,一旦肿瘤侵及肠外,预后较差。在 145 例胃肠道类癌患者中,只有 12 例术前得到了正确的诊断,且这 12 例患者均有明确的类癌综合征症状[54,70]。大多数情况下,手术指征是患者出现肠梗阻征象,肠梗阻不是由肿瘤本身引起,而是由于纤维化和肠扭曲导致肠系膜萎缩的增生反应[71]。用放射性核素标记的奥曲肽进行显像成功地用于定位原发和转移灶[72],两项大型欧洲研究显示使用该诊断工具检测类癌病变,敏感性为 89%[73]。

类癌肿瘤的转移潜能与其大小密切相关。在 Moertel 进行的相关研究中,直径<0.5cm 的肿瘤中未见远处转移,直径 0.5~0.9cm 的肿瘤中 15%发现远处转移,直径 1.0~1.9cm 的肿瘤中 72%发现转移,>2cm 的肿瘤中 95%发现远处转移[66]。但是,当直径<1cm 时,小肠类癌仍有转移的可能。最近基于 5-HIAA 水平的证据表明,大多数原发灶不明确的转移性类癌的病例可能来自直径小的回肠肿瘤[74,75]。类癌病变的范围主要包括淋巴结局部扩散或肝脏转移,这是小肠腺癌明确的预后因素。在 Maggard 对 11 427 例类癌的分析中,小肠局限患者、区域扩散患者和远处转移患者的 5 年生存率分别为 70.4%、64.1%和 32.4%[65]。

手术切除原发肿瘤及区域淋巴结清扫是唯一可能治愈胃肠道神经内分泌肿瘤(GI NET)的方法,约 20%的患者通过该治疗方法可获得根治。手术仍然是唯一能够进行明确组织病理学分期、切除潜在转移淋巴结以及预防由于增生反应引起的局部并发症的方法[76]。手术治疗的进行不应受原发肿瘤无法定位的影响。肠道中部肿瘤难以通过影像学检查定位,但有研究发现,无论术前是否能够定位,大多数转移性 NET 患者术中可以确定原发肿瘤[77]。术中必须进行仔细探查,因为大多数文献报道 30%的该类肿瘤是多发的[66]。在美国,虽然他们认识到应更广泛使用上消化道内镜检查的重要性,但原发性十二指肠类癌仅占类癌的 2.6%[78]。由于这种疾病的罕见性,十二指肠类癌的管理建议只能从肠道中段和肠道下段类癌的经验中推断出来。最近,Mullen 及其同事进行的一项研究表明,6 名肿瘤<1.5cm 的患者成功进行了内镜治疗,切缘阴性[78]。有趣的是,这项研究发现 54%的十二指肠类癌患者存在淋巴结转移,其中 2 例肿瘤小于 1cm 且仅限于黏膜下层。然而,十二指肠类癌中淋巴结转移的影响因素尚不确定,因为在该研究中没有患者发生远处转移或类癌综合征。对于晚期患者,减瘤手术可能会使患者获益,目前仍存争议,因为肿瘤的大小与症状的程度不完全平行[54,79,80]。一些学者甚至建议对广泛转移性疾病患者进行积极的治疗,包括切除所有腹腔内肿瘤转移灶,必要时切除肝段,以及进行肝动脉栓塞,甚至还进行了胆囊切除术以防止肝栓塞期间的胆囊坏死。尽管尚未证实这种激进的外科手术方法是否能提高生存率,但已在高达 25%的患者中实现了生化缓解,长期随访发现肝转移灶消失[69,81]。在 MD Anderson 癌症中心,81 名接受肝动脉栓塞或化疗栓塞的类癌肝转移患者,67%获得部分缓解,平均反应时间为 17 个月。总体而言,63%的患者肿瘤相关症状减轻,OS 为 31 个月[82]。此外值得注意的是,许多被诊断患有类癌的患者常伴有其他恶性肿瘤。利用癌症监测、流行病学和结果(SEER)数据库随访终点结果确定 1973-2007 年间被诊断患有小肠类癌的患者,几乎 1/3 的小肠类癌患者合并相关的异时原发性肿瘤。最常见的部位是前列腺(26.2%),乳腺癌(14.3%),结肠癌(9.1%),肺/支气管(6.3%)和膀胱(5.3%)[83]。

生长抑素类似物或衍生物可有效缓解类癌综合征的症状,但证实肿瘤消退很少见。奥曲肽含 8 个氨基,是一种长效生长抑素类似物,结合 2、3、5 型亚型受体,已被广泛用于类癌的检测和治疗[84]。目前可用的 SSAs-Sandostatin LAR(奥曲肽;诺华)和 Somatuline Autogel(兰瑞肽;益普生)对受体亚型 2 和 5 显示高亲和力,对亚型 1 和 4 显示低亲和力,对亚型 3 显示中等亲和力。SOM230(帕瑞肽;诺华)是一种最近研发的生长抑素类似物,目前处于Ⅲ期试验阶段,可能具有更广泛的针对生长抑素受体活性的治疗优势,特别是在耐药性疾病中[85]。在一项研究中,奥曲肽以每天三次 150μg 的剂量皮下注射,88%

的患者症状得到改善,72%的患者尿液 5-HIAA 减少[86]。随着对肿瘤进展机制理解的深入,已经确定了几个潜在的治疗靶点(包括血管内皮生长因子(VEGF)和西罗莫司(mTOR)信号通路)。在一项随机Ⅲ期临床试验中,依维莫司加长效奥曲肽相比安慰剂加长效奥曲肽,改善了晚期神经内分泌肿瘤患者的无进展生存期。然而,依维莫司延长效奥曲肽组的无进展生存期仍为 16.4 个月(95% *CI*:13.7~21.2 个月),安慰剂加奥曲肽 LAR 组为 11.3 个月(95% *CI*:8.4~14.6 个月)[87]。其他几种正在研究的药物,包括使用新型生长抑素类似物,VEGF 和 mTOR 抑制剂,以及干扰胰岛素样生长因子 1(insulin-like growth factor 1,IGF-1)受体和 AKT 信号转导的药剂。另一种治疗方式是肽受体放射性核素治疗。该方法高度选择性地向类癌细胞施用杀肿瘤剂量的辐射,几乎没有副作用(恶心和偶发的骨髓抑制和肾毒性)。通过将放射性核素(^{111}铟、^{90}钇或^{177}镥)与生长抑素类似物相连接,类癌细胞(通常具有高密度的生长抑素受体)可能为其靶向目标。一些研究报道,肿瘤消退率高达 50%,无病生存接近 3 年[88]。

类癌患者的预后受多种因素影响。原发肿瘤的大小是转移和存活的重要预测因素。直径>2cm 的类癌肿瘤比<2cm 的预后更差[89]。在最近的一项 603 名患者的研究中,淋巴结转移对预后的影响符合预计[90]。在 Maggard 相关研究中,肿瘤大小与淋巴结转移可能性呈正相关[67]。杜克大学的类癌研究,发现原发肿瘤的大小与表现的疾病程度之间直接相关[91]。此外,相同分期患者根据原发肿瘤部位预测各组患者预后,发现为远处转移的患者肠道中段肿瘤患者的预后明显好于肠道上段或下段的患者。除传统的病理决定因素外,小肠类癌中可卡因和苯丙胺调节的转录物(CART)的表达与较差的存活率相关[92]。

复合肿瘤,可表现出类癌和腺癌的特征,在阑尾中较多,小肠中少见。这类肿瘤相对罕见,迄今为止的大多数报告仅包括 1 个或 2 个病例。复合肿瘤属于侵袭性肿瘤,具有与腺癌相似的转移潜能,应当作为腺癌进行治疗。淋巴结转移在组织学上由 2 例类似于腺癌,1 例类似于类癌。因此,这些肿瘤可能来自具有多种分化潜能的细胞[93]。

胃肠道间质瘤

胃肠道间质瘤(GIST)是目前对源自胚胎中胚层的多种胃肠道良性或恶性肿瘤的命名。GIST 有三种组织学亚型。梭形细胞样肿瘤最为常见(70%),由均匀的交叉束与嗜酸性粒细胞质组成。上皮样(20%)和稀有混合型(10%)由更多核异型的圆形细胞组成[94]。恶性 GIST 占小肠恶性肿瘤的 15%~20%[95]。据报道,美国每年发病约为 5 000 例,由于医疗意识和组织病理学诊断水平的提高,这一数字似乎还在上升[96,97]。GIST 在男、女性中发病率基本相同[98]。大多数被诊断患有 GIST 的患者年龄在 40~80 岁之间(中位数为 60.99 岁),大多为散发形式。家族性 GIST 发生由 KIT 或血小板衍生的生长因子受体 α(PDGFRα)原癌基因中的种系突变引起[100,101]。GIST 的细胞起源被认为是 Cajal 间质细胞,Cajal 是一种小肠起搏细胞[95]。GIST 的特点是原癌基因 *C-kit* 突变导致其糖蛋白产物 KIT 的组成性激活,之后又引起酪氨酸激酶活性的改变[102]。酪氨酸激酶抑制剂伊马替尼已经彻底改变了 GIST 的治疗方法。超过 95%的 GIST 表达 KIT,KIT 的生化证据可以在几乎所有的 GIST 中找到[103]。*KIT* 突变的最常见位点包括外显子 11(70%)和外显子 9(10%)[104,105]。其他常见表达的标志物包括 CD34(70%),平滑肌动蛋白(30%)和结蛋白(<5%)[106]。因为其他恶性肿瘤(包括转移性黑色素瘤,血管肉瘤和尤因肉瘤)也可以表现出 KIT 阳性,仅进行免疫组化诊断是不充分的[94],需同时基于形态学和免疫组化检查。GIST 也可发生在神经纤维瘤病 1 型(NF1)和部分年轻女性患者(包括副神经节瘤,肺软骨瘤和胃 GIST)中[107,108]。

GIST 可以发生在从食管到直肠的消化道的任何地方。胃是最常见的部位(60%),其次是小肠(30%)、直肠(约 5%)和食管(约 5%)[99]。高达 50%的患者在诊断时已发生远处转移。肝脏和腹膜是两个最常见的部位[109]。大多数 GIST 以腹部肿块的形式出现,引起肠梗阻,表现为恶心、呕吐和腹痛,或胃肠道出血。GIST 通常快速生长,常见直径 5cm 或更大的肿块[110]。这种快速的增长速度解释了胃肠道失血的倾向,因为这些肿瘤的增长速度可能超过他们的血液供应,因此可能出现坏死、溃疡。失血通常是慢性的,实验室检查可表现为小细胞性贫血[110]。瘘管和脓肿也可由肿瘤坏死引起。诊断和评估疾病程度的主要方式是通过腹盆腔的增强 CT 检查。其在 CT 上的特征性表现为与胃壁或肠壁紧密相关的增生性外生肿块。像其他肉瘤一样,GIST 倾向于外生而不是侵入邻近的结构。虽然正电子发射断层扫描(PET)不用于诊断 GIST,但它可用于评估对酪氨酸激酶药物治疗的反应。GIST 在内镜检查中表现为黏膜下肿块。对于计划新辅助治疗或怀疑有转移的病例,建议采用内镜或经皮穿刺活检[111]。

GIST 的主要治疗方法是根治性手术切除。然而,目前关于肿瘤<2cm 的 GIST 处理存在争议。目前的美国综合癌症网络(NCCN)对于胃 GIST<2cm、超声内镜检查无高危因素的处理为建议每 6~12 个月内镜检查[112]。对于>2cm 的肿瘤,提倡手术完整切除瘤体,如累及其他器官也要进行相应瘤体的完整切除。由于淋巴结受累并不常见,因此广泛的淋巴结切除术并不改善生存期。腹腔镜技术在 GIST 中的应用继续拓宽。在斯隆-凯特琳癌症中心行腹腔镜切除 GIST(最大直径为 8cm)的患者,其围术期和肿瘤预后与开放手术切除的病例对照组相当[113]。该研究的中位随访时间为 34 个月,两组肿瘤预后相似,镜下边缘均为阴性,各组各有 1 例复发。Bischof 等也报道,基于他们对近 400 名接受 GIST 手术切除患者的回顾,胃 GIST 的微创方法与低复发率和高 R0 切除率相关[114]。壶腹周围 GIST 的外科治疗更具挑战性。荟萃分析表明,只要技术上可行,局部切除应该是十二指肠 GIST 的首选治疗方法,因为与胰十二指肠切除术(PD)相比,该方法有良好的肿瘤学预后和更低的复发率。在十二指肠 GIST 患者中使用伊马替尼可能会使一部分需要 PD 的患者接受局部切除术[115]。

即使手术切除后,肿瘤也可能复发。一项对 16 年内 200 例 GIST 进行分析的研究发现,在接受完全切除的原发病患者中,5 年保险统计生存率为 54%[99]。即使做到整块切除,大多数肿瘤仍会复发,复发部位通常为肝脏和腹膜。在最大的 GIST 复发研究中,来自斯隆-凯特琳癌症中心的学者回顾性分析了 69 例此类患者[99]。76%的患者出现局部复发,其中一半合并同期肝转移。1/3 的复发性疾病患者完成了手术切除,中位生存期为 15 个月。酪氨酸激酶抑制剂的出现彻底改变了 GIST

的治疗方法。尽管认为肿瘤反应的机制主要是抑制 KIT 驱动的细胞,但最近的数据表明免疫系统对抗肿瘤作用有很大贡献。通过降低免疫抑制酶吲哚胺 2,3-双加氧酶的肿瘤细胞表达,伊马替尼治疗显示在肿瘤内诱导调节性 T 细胞凋亡[116]。该数据对于设计可能涉及免疫调节剂以增加反应的未来治疗策略至关重要。

由于该病的高复发率,多项临床试验对伊马替尼进行了研究。美国外科医师学会肿瘤学组(ACOSOG)进行了两项试验,研究了中危或高危复发风险患者手术切除后,甲磺酸伊马替尼辅助治疗的作用。ACOSOGZ9000 是第一个Ⅱ期试验,研究完全切除 GIST 后复发风险高的伊马替尼辅助治疗的疗效[117]。表达 KIT 的原发性 GIST 完全切除肿瘤后,如肿瘤大小>10cm,肿瘤破裂,或伴有腹膜转移灶被定义为高复发风险。切除后患者口服伊马替尼 400mg/d,持续 1 年。中位随访时间为 4 年,结果 1 年、2 年和 3 年 OS 分别为 99%、97%和 97%。1 年、2 年和 3 年无复发生存率分别为 94%、73%和 61%。这些结果优于历史对照的 RFS 和 OS。ACOSOG Z79001 是一项随访Ⅲ期试验,患者在接受手术后随机接受 1 年口服伊马替尼或安慰剂治疗[118]。手术后每天服用 1 次伊马替尼治疗局部原发性 GIST(≥3cm)与 713 例患者的安慰剂比较。与对照组(83%)相比,伊马替尼组 PFS(98%)显著更高,而 OS 无差异。随后的研究发现,相比于应用 1 年的伊马替尼,应用 3 年的患者生存时间更长[119]。然而,在安慰剂组中只有小部分的低风险患者出现复发,超过 70%的患者似乎仅通过手术治愈。因此,应仔细考虑切除的原发性 GIST 3cm 患者应用伊马替尼佐剂的价值。风险分层系统可用于识别没有指示辅助治疗的低复发可能性的患者;风险分层也可以确定应该接受治疗的患者[120]。例如,KIT 外显子 11 缺失的患者应用 1 年伊马替尼治疗后具有更长的无复发生存时间[121]。此外,已发现特定突变对伊马替尼具有耐药性;患有 PDGFRA *D842V* 突变的患者对伊马替尼无反应。另一项风险分层评分显示,具有核分裂象增多的非胃肠 GIST 患者复发风险很高[121]。

关于使用伊马替尼未来的研究重点是应该对哪些患者进行治疗以及治疗的最佳持续时间[122]。PERSIST5 试验是一项正在进行的Ⅱ期临床试验,研究中危至高危风险患者经 5 年伊马替尼辅助治疗后的复发风险(NCT00867113)。专家建议目前应进行肿瘤突变检测,以排除存在 *PDGFRAD842V* 突变或肿瘤为野生型的患者。对于其余患者,应该就辅助治疗的目标和并就当前已有的研究成果进行讨论[123]。

已经研究了新辅助伊马替尼在局部晚期疾病中的作用。新辅助甲磺酸伊马替尼具有很广阔的应用前景,因为它可以使肿瘤体积显著缩小,这可以在初始治疗后 2~4 周内通过 PET 扫描来预测。术前应用伊马替尼减瘤效应可使外科医师缩小切除范围,并获得 R0 切除。伊马替尼的新辅助治疗特别适用于食管胃连接部、壶腹部和直肠附近的病变。由放射治疗肿瘤学组(RTOG)领导的Ⅱ期试验的最新结果显示,伊马替尼在新辅助治疗中具有良好的耐受性[124]。该研究分成 A 组(局部进展且瘤体>5cm)和 B 组(复发/转移性且瘤体>2cm)。伊马替尼术前每天服用 600mg,连续 8 周然后进行手术,术后再进行 2 年的伊马替尼治疗。术前伊马替尼 8 周后的缓解率在 A 组和 B 组之间相似(4%~7%部分缓解,83%~90%疾病稳定,4%~5%疾病进展)[124]。另一项来自 MD Anderson 癌症中心的Ⅱ期临床试验中心对 19 名患者进行伊马替尼新辅助治疗,时间为 3 或 7 天[125]。这种方案耐受性良好,FDG-PET 检查发现缓解率为 69%。新辅助治疗持续时间和患者适应证选择仍有待进一步确定。目前的 NCCN 指南建议,对于新辅助伊马替尼患者,如连续两次 CT 扫描未显示影像学变化,应考虑手术切除。

在转移性 GIST 中,有强有力的证据表明甲磺酸伊马替尼的有效性。高达 80%的转移性 GIST 患者对伊马替尼有部分甚至完全缓解[118]。最近一项荟萃分析对两项大型随机研究进行回顾[126,127],比较了每天服用 1 次(400mg)或 2 次伊马替尼的疗效,结果显示,较高剂量组可使外显子 9 突变患者获得更长的无进展生存期[128]。伊马替尼耐药患者的二线药物是舒尼替尼[129]。舒尼替尼靶点为 KIT、PDGFRα 以及血管内皮细胞生因子受体(VEGFR)。在晚期伊马替尼耐药患者中,舒尼替尼是一种安全有效的二线药物[130]。分子研究表明,伊马替尼对外显子 11C-kit 酪氨酸激酶突变最有效,而舒尼替尼对外显子 9 突变可能更有效[128]。最近完成的其他研究还研发出了三线药物[131]。对于进行标准治疗后仍进展的转移性 GIST 患者,应用瑞格非尼组较安慰剂组延长了无进展生存期[131]。虽然 GIST 临床上相对少见,但其治疗方法仍不断发展并表现出积极的势头。

淋巴瘤

淋巴瘤占所有小肠恶性肿瘤的 15%~20%[132]。胃肠道淋巴瘤最常见的部位是胃(>60%),其次是大肠和小肠,两者占比相似[133]。男性发病率稍高,男女发病约为 1.5∶1,中位年龄低于其他小肠肿瘤患者(一个大型研究报道为 49 岁)[134,135]。淋巴瘤是移植受者中最常见的恶性肿瘤,在应用环孢素平均 20 个月后出现本病[135]。这样的患者有约 2/3 经手术切除、放疗、应用阿昔洛韦和减弱免疫抑制后,其预后要好于其他类型的小肠淋巴瘤[136,137]。小肠淋巴瘤也继发于艾滋病患者中,这类人群的所有病变均为 B 淋巴细胞来源,预后很差,但患者生存期主要取决于 HIV 相关疾病的轻重,这些患者的预期寿命并不显著低于没有淋巴瘤的单纯 HIV 阳性患者[136]。

胃肠道淋巴瘤的临床表现包括腹痛、恶心、呕吐、疲劳、体重减轻和胃肠道出血,可能隐匿性起病。CT 扫描显示较多肿大淋巴结时高度提示腹腔淋巴瘤可能[138]。已提出多种用于胃肠道淋巴瘤的分期系统,包括 Ann Arbor、Musshoff 和欧-美分期系统。每个分期系统都能将小肠淋巴瘤分为 4 个主要分期:Ⅰ期为局部病变,Ⅱ期伴有区域侵犯,Ⅲ期和Ⅳ期为伴有转移的晚期病变。2011 年第 11 届国际恶性淋巴瘤会议(ICML)之后,影像学检查也被纳入某些分期系统[139]。

切除小肠淋巴瘤对局部控制很重要,但极少能达到根治。疾病通常分期较晚,因此不到 30%的患者能够得到根治性切除[140]。辅助治疗是小肠淋巴瘤治疗的重要组成部分。应尝试对局部疾病进行手术切除,应尽力切除原发病灶,保证足够的切缘,切除受侵犯的肠管和受侵犯的肠系膜淋巴结。由于淋巴瘤可能在黏膜下层沿肠管长轴蔓延,因此需要保证切缘阴性。推荐对可能根治切除的患者术后进行辅助化疗[141]。对于无法切除的淋巴瘤患者,建议进行放射治疗和化疗[142]。此外,针对蛋白 CD20 的嵌合单克隆抗体利妥昔单抗在 B 细胞淋巴瘤治疗中也有一定的前景[143]。

据报道,40 年前一种平素罕见的免疫增殖性小肠病在中东地区尤为常见,特别是在伊朗南部。这种地中海淋巴瘤存在于儿童和年轻人中,并且预后较差[144]。患者倾向于来自社会经济较低的群体,营养背景不良。小肠淋巴瘤原始细胞一般认为是滤泡期的 B 细胞,这种细胞能够产生 IgA。小肠淋巴瘤过度表达 α 重链,α 重链可在血清中检测到[145]。然而,最近伊朗南部的流行病学报告表明,胃肠道非霍奇金淋巴瘤的分布与西方国家类似[146]。

转移性肿瘤

小肠的转移性肿瘤较小肠原发肿瘤更常见。结肠、卵巢、子宫和胃的原发性肿瘤均可侵犯小肠,最常见的方式是直接侵犯和腹膜种植。来自乳腺、肺和黑素瘤的癌细胞通常通过血行转移到小肠。斯隆-凯特琳癌症中心尸检回顾发现转移性黑色素瘤的胃肠道转移的发生率为 58%[147]。在胃肠道内,小肠是最常见的黑色素瘤转移部位,可能与其血供丰富相关。一项来自部队病理所的研究表明,他们对 103 例恶性黑色素瘤进行的回顾性分析,即使未发现明确的原发灶,小肠黑色素瘤通常也是转移性的[148]。如果可能的话,应该对小肠转移性肿瘤患者进行根治性手术。Ollila 等人对 John Wayne 癌症研究所 1971—1994 年 6 509 例胃肠道转移的黑色素瘤患者中的 124 例进行了回顾性研究[149]。在这 124 名患者中,69 名(56%)接受了腹部的探查术,其中 46 名(67%)行根治性切除,23 例(33%)进行了姑息性切除。69 例手术患者中几乎所有(97%)患者术后均出现症状缓解。接受根治性切除术的患者的中位生存期为 48.9 个月,而接受姑息治疗的患者仅为 5.4 个月,接受非手术干预的患者为 5.7 个月。小肠的转移性病变可以在选定病例和/或肿瘤特异性全身治疗时进行手术治疗。

阑尾肿瘤

急性阑尾炎患者进行阑尾切除术后,有 5%的患者被病理证实为阑尾肿瘤[150]。这些病变大部分是良性的,包括黏膜增生或化生、平滑肌瘤、脂肪瘤、神经瘤和血管瘤。阑尾恶性肿瘤较为罕见,在所有肠道肿瘤占比不到 0.5%[151]。Collins 在 40 年间的 71 000 例阑尾切除标本中发现了 958 例恶性肿瘤,占总体的 1.35%[150]。

一般来说,阑尾恶性肿瘤可分为神经内分泌来源(类癌)或上皮起源。上皮来源的恶性肿瘤包括黏液囊肿,腹腔假黏液腺瘤(PMP),杯状细胞癌和原发性腺癌。在 1973—2007 年期间从美国癌症研究所 SEER 数据库记录的 5 655 例阑尾肿瘤中,恶性类癌占标本的 11%,但 5 年疾病特异性生存率最高,为 93%[152]。

阑尾肿瘤常为阑尾炎的临床表现,可在阑尾切除术后有病理证实。然而,在穿孔性阑尾炎合并蜂窝织炎或脓肿的情况下,此种情况下一般采取二期阑尾切除术,此时先行非手术治疗。这一点十分重要,因为 2%的患者在进行非手术治疗时,可发现潜在癌症或克罗恩病,尤其对于 40 岁以上的患者[153]。

类癌

类癌是最常见的阑尾肿瘤,占所有阑尾肿瘤的 32%~85%,分为良性和恶性[154,155]。来自 SEER 研究,恶性类癌中有 11%的阑尾恶性肿瘤。一项基于 SEER 数据库的研究指出阑尾类癌不同性别间的发病率,女性占总病例数的 68%。这也可能由于女性盆腔手术数量较男性更多,从而导致更多的阑尾类癌的偶然发现。多发于 30~40 岁间,文献报道平均为 32~42 岁[156,157]。

大多数类癌发生在阑尾的远端 1/3 处,此处极少引起阻塞[158]。肿瘤较大且发生局部淋巴结以外转移时更容易表现出明显的临床症状。大约 10%的阑尾类癌位于阑尾底部,此时可造成管腔梗阻,引起阑尾炎[155]。与其他肠道类癌相似,阑尾类癌可产生血管活性物质,也可以导致类癌综合征。类癌综合征症状很少见,如有则提示可能存在远处转移,肝脏为其常见的转移部位[159]。

一般来说,直径<2cm 的阑尾类癌的转移并不常见。Moertel 及其同事在对 51 年间收录的 150 例阑尾类癌患者进行回顾后,发现 4.7%的病例合并转移,但<2cm 的肿瘤均未见转移灶[160]。阑尾系膜受累及与淋巴结转移存在相关性,肿瘤大小、核分裂象增多和 Ki67 阳性与肿瘤侵袭性相关[161,162]。

阑尾尖端小的类癌(<2cm)可以通过单纯的阑尾切除术治疗[163]。在开腹手术中,这些肿瘤表现为小的黄色结节,通常位于阑尾的远端 1/3 处。在组织学上,细胞小而均一,核分裂象少。几乎所有的类癌都显示出阑尾壁肌层受累,普遍存在肿瘤附近的淋巴管受累[163]。尽管有这种微观发现,但很少有患者会出现区域性侵犯。大的类癌(>2cm)和阑尾基底的类癌需要进行右半结肠切除术,这样可以切除引流淋巴结以及阑尾底部或阑尾系膜中的残留。

基于 2010 年和 2012 年来自北美神经内分泌肿瘤学会(NANETS)和欧洲神经内分泌肿瘤学会(ENETS)的共识指南,全结肠切除术在以下情况推荐:侵犯阑尾系膜 1~2cm 的肿瘤、切缘阳性或可疑阳性、高增殖率、血管侵犯、混合有杯状细胞类癌或腺癌的组织学类型[164,165]。

2010 年,AJCC 首次对阑尾癌进行了 TNM 分期,该分期与其他肠道和肺部来源的类癌 TNM 分期系统不同。早期阑尾类癌的总体结果是乐观的。根据对 SEER 数据库观察到的 900 例阑尾类癌的分析,如果肿瘤大小<3cm 而没有区域淋巴结或远处转移,则阑尾类癌的 5 年疾病特异性生存率为 100%,如果肿瘤大小在 2~3cm 伴有区域淋巴结转移、肿瘤大小>3cm 伴或不伴淋巴结或远处转移时 5 年疾病特异性生存率为 78%,如果有远处转移,则为 32%[166]。

黏液囊肿

阑尾黏液囊肿以阑尾腔扩张、黏膜走行改变,黏液分泌过多为常见表现,偶尔累及阑尾外层[167]。病理上可表现为增生性息肉、良性肿瘤例如囊腺瘤或恶性肿瘤如囊腺癌。多数学者支持使用基于组织学的分类系统,黏液囊肿带来损害的分类系统使用较少。在这个系统中,阑尾的黏液囊肿可分为单纯(梗阻性)黏液囊肿和伴有增殖上皮改变的黏液囊肿。良性肿瘤的增生性改变可表现为局限,如结肠腺瘤,也可表现为弥漫性,如黏液腺瘤或黏液囊腺瘤。恶性增殖组可分为结肠腺癌、黏液性囊腺癌和混合癌[168]。具有癌变潜能的增生上皮和腺瘤样增生的癌前病变特征为:增生性、腺瘤性上皮细胞和癌性上皮细胞在同一病变中可见共存[168]。阑尾黏液囊肿(囊腺瘤和囊腺癌)的一个转归结局是腹腔假性黏液瘤(PMP)。该病变以腹膜腔内大量黏液样物质为特征,被认为是黏液性囊腺癌在腹膜腔内的播散(见 PMP 部分)[169]。

阑尾黏液囊肿通常是开腹手术时偶然发现,但黏液性囊腺瘤和囊腺癌是少数几种可在术前诊断的阑尾肿瘤[163]。如果 CT 检查发现肿块位于右下腹,密度接近水,提示黏液性肿瘤可能。由于黏液和较多的无回声液体的结合,超声上显示为无回声暗区。尽管这两种影像学技术对诊断黏液囊肿都有帮助,但腹膜腔的其他囊性病变,如卵巢囊肿、附件囊肿、肠系膜和网膜囊肿或脓肿仍需再诊断过程中予以鉴别[170]。

即使对考虑为良性可能的阑尾黏液囊肿,也应进行手术切除,因为在影像学检查中看似良性的病变可能存在囊腺癌。切除方式取决于组织学病理检查结果。如为增生性息肉或囊腺瘤,单纯阑尾切除术即可达到根治目的。在 Higa 及其同事报道的研究中,46 例黏液性囊腺瘤患者中有 36 例行单纯阑尾切除术,术后随访未见复发[167]。多数黏液性囊腺癌患者有广泛的腹部转移或 PMP。原发性病变的治疗包括标准的右半结肠切除术,同时清扫引流区域淋巴结[171]。Stephenson 和 Brief 回顾了 53 例阑尾黏液性囊腺癌病例,这些患者均接受单纯阑尾切除术或右半结肠切除术。在术后第 10 年随访时,接受右半结肠切除术的患者生存率为 65%,而行单纯阑尾切除术的患者生存率为 37%[172]。除合适的切除范围外,也应对转移性沉积物和黏液进行清除。

腹腔假性黏液瘤

腹腔假黏液腺瘤(PMP)临床特征是弥漫的黏液类分泌物,可以位于腹部、盆腔,也可以表现为腹膜表面黏液样种植结节。PMP 与阑尾囊腺瘤扩散至腹腔内基本相似,随着肿瘤的生长和堵塞管腔,大量黏液聚集最后导致阑尾破裂,然后产生黏液的细胞在腹腔广泛种植,这些细胞继续增殖,并且产生黏液[173]。腹膜内黏液的聚集最终导致肠梗阻,出现恶心、呕吐和饥饿状态,甚至最终导致死亡。临床医生不仅使用术语 PMP 来表示良性囊腺瘤破裂后引起的腹膜内黏液性播散,也使用 PMP 来描述产生黏液的阑尾、大肠和小肠,甚至肺、乳腺、胰腺、胃、胆管、胆囊、输卵管/卵巢来源的囊腺癌在腹腔内的播散[174,175]。

PMP 多见于女性患者,在 10 000 例开腹手术中可偶然发现约 2 个 PMP[174]。该病最常见的症状是腹部增大;男性中第二常见的症状是腹股沟疝,而女性在常规骨盆检查时常可触及卵巢肿块[173]。CT 扫描中黏液物质密度与脂肪相似,密度不均匀。可见肝脏、脾脏和系膜移位,钙化也较常见。横膈下表面可有因囊腺性肿瘤堆积而成的较厚的团块。一个非常典型的特征是腹腔和盆腔内脏器(如小肠和系膜)的偏心性移位[173]。

PMP 的标准治疗是重复多次的减瘤手术[174]。这种治疗方式是姑息性的,旨在限制黏液的积聚,降低腹腔内压力。疾病复发需要再次手术时,往往会由于粘连和纤维化使手术更加困难。该病的 5 年生存率为 50%[176]。减瘤术和腹腔内化疗是相对积极的治疗方法,通过手术尽可能切除所有腹盆腔内的病灶,之后辅以腹腔内热化疗。通过加热含有化疗的灌注液来增强药物渗透能力,这种方法称为腹腔热灌注化疗(IPHC)[177~180]。这种方法最适合减瘤术后病灶微残留(残留物<2mm)的患者。然而,即使是加热的含有化疗的灌注液,也难于穿透较大体积的肿瘤。

Sugarbaker 等撰写了有关腹膜表面恶性肿瘤减瘤手术和 IPHC 的专著[179]。他的研究组使用四项临床评估来选择最有可能从联合治疗中获益的患者。第一,组织病理学评估哪些病例为非侵袭性恶性肿瘤。如真性 PMP 或囊性间皮瘤,一方面这类病灶可通过腹膜切除术获得根治,另一方面,这类病灶极少侵及其他组,转移到区域淋巴结、肝脏或其他全身部位的可能性较小。第二,术前进行胸部、腹部和盆腔的增强 CT 检查。该检查不仅可以确定有无肝脏或其他部位的全身转移,还可以确定是否存在小肠梗阻或直径大于 5cm 的肿瘤结节(这些指标提示预后不良)。另外两个临床指标,腹膜癌指数(PCI,腹膜表面结节大小和分布的预后定量指标)和肿瘤细胞减灭程度(经最大限度减瘤后肿瘤结节的大小)。Sugarbaker 及其同事 2001 年的报道了 10 年间(1983—1993)108 例 PMP 患者,这些患者均接受减瘤术+术中丝裂霉素腹腔热灌注化疗,术后第 1~6 天行氟尿嘧啶腹腔化疗,随后进行 3 周琦辅助化疗,方案为丝裂霉素静脉滴注+氟尿嘧啶腹腔化疗[181]。65 例真性 PMP 患者的 5 年生存率为 75%,10 年生存率为 68%。恶性肿瘤患者的预后较差,5 年和 10 年生存率分别为 26%和 9%。联合应用减瘤术和 IPEC,复发率较高(37.75%)[182]。然而,研究表明,这一比率在患者的成本-效益比方面是可接受的[176]。

腺癌

阑尾原发性腺癌是一种罕见的肿瘤,占原发性阑尾肿瘤的 4%~6%,通常起源于先前存在的腺瘤[183]。平均起病年龄为 50 岁,男性多见,依据文献不同,男女患者为 4∶1~2.8∶1[184~186]。根据文献报道,大多数患者的临床表现为急性阑尾炎或腹部肿块,术前很少能够确诊。高达 40%的病例发生穿孔,穿孔后临床表现更为复杂,单纯穿孔对 OS 影响较小[187]。

在组织学上,原发性腺癌区别于腺瘤在于肿瘤组织对肠壁的侵犯。约 25%的患者会发生淋巴结转移[188]。阑尾腺癌转移能力介于在阑尾类癌和结肠腺癌之间,20%的患者发生远处转移,最常见转移靶器官为卵巢[183]。远处转移的发生于组织学分级相关;高分化肿瘤患者有约 30%伴有远处转移,近 70%的低分化肿瘤患者在开腹手术时发现远处转移[184,185]。5 年总生存率为 55%,Dukes 分期亚组 5 年生存率分别为:A,100%;B,67%;C,50%;D,6%[189]。

文献表明,腺癌的外科治疗不应只包括阑尾切除术。Hesketh 报道阑尾腺癌患者行单纯阑尾切除术后 5 年生存率为 20%,而行右半结肠切除术的患者则为 63%[186]。Hopkins 等报告行单纯阑尾切除术后 5 年生存率为 20%,行右半结肠切除术的患者为 45%[190]。

结直肠癌

流行病学

结直肠癌(CRC)仍然是一个重要的全球健康问题。它是全球第三大常见恶性肿瘤和癌症死亡的第四位原因[191]。CRC在发达国家最为常见,仅在美国,2014 年估计有 130 000 人被诊断患有结直肠癌,大约有 50 000 人死于该疾病[192]。一般认为饮食、生活方式、遗传因素共同导致在发达国家中发病率增加。研究表明,人们从 CRC 发病低的地区迁移到高发地区,将沿袭东道国结直肠癌的发病风险[193]。

在不同性别、人种、族裔群体间,CRC 发病率和死亡率存在差异。虽然 CRC 是美国男性和女性中第三大常见恶性肿瘤,并且结肠癌的发病率在性别之间相似,但直肠癌在男性中更为常见。与男性远端肿瘤相比,右半结肠/近端结肠癌在女性中更为常见[191]。此外,男性的死亡率约高出女性 1/3[194]。与白人、亚裔美国人、美洲印第安人和西班牙裔人群相比,非裔美国人的发病率和死亡率最高[195]。导致差异的原因尚不完全清楚。然而据推测,获得高质量的定期筛查及时诊断和治疗、饮食和生活方式因素以及社会经济地位方面的差异是可能的原因[195,196]。

尽管美国 CRC 患病率很高,但几十年来 CRC 的发病率和总体死亡率都一直在下降,近些年来下降速度更快。无论男性或女性,发病率在 2008—2010 年间以约 4%的速度下降,同期死亡率下降约 3%[197]。研究表明,普及筛查和检查可以使结直肠癌的进展和死亡减少 10%~75%[198]。从解剖分布来看,筛查普及后 CRC 从直肠癌和左半结肠癌多见转变为右半结肠癌多见。来自 1988 年和 1993 年的美国国家癌症数据库的资料表明,CRC 中近端结肠到结肠脾曲的发病比例从 51%增加到 55%[199]。多项研究证实在美国和全球,近端结肠癌发病率高于远端结肠癌和直肠癌发病率[199~202]。

危险因素

年龄和种族背景

年龄是 CRC 的已知危险因素。绝大多数 CRC 病例发生在 50 岁以上的人群中,随后发病率继续增加[198]。事实上,不到 10%的新 CRC 诊断和死亡发生在年龄小于 50 岁的患者中[192]。如前所述,非洲裔美国人与其他种族和民族人群相比,CRC 的发病率和死亡率更高[195,198,199]。

个人史和家族史

有腺瘤性息肉或 CRC 癌前病变者其结肠癌的发病风险高。息肉的大小、数量和组织类型是重要的预后因素,其中息肉大小>1cm,绒毛状或管状腺瘤、多发息肉者 CRC 发病风险更高[203]。息肉单发、直径<1cm 的管状腺瘤患者不增加 CRC 的发病风险[203]。CRC 癌前病变者异时性 CRC 的发生率为 6%,异时性腺瘤的发生率为 25%[204]。

一级亲属中患 CRC 的家族史将 CRC 的发病风险增加 2~3 倍,而二级亲属有结肠癌家族史的人群发病风险增加 25%~50%[205,206]。此外,如果有 1 个以上的一级亲属患有结肠癌,或者如果他们在确诊时年龄小于 55 岁,那么他们罹患结直肠癌的风险还会更高[207]。结肠腺瘤的家族史也会增加 CRC 的风险,特别是腺瘤发生于年龄较小时。

炎症性肠病

溃疡性结肠炎(UC)和克罗恩病(CD)是众所周知的结肠癌的危险因素。对于 UC,疾病的程度和持续时间是影响预后的主要因素。患有全结肠炎的患者患结肠癌的风险增加 5~15 倍,而局限于左半结肠的结肠炎的癌变风险增加 3 倍[208]。风险也随着疾病持续时间延长而增加[209]。克罗恩病对结肠癌发病风险的影响与 UC 类似[210~212]。

饮食和生活方式

西方饮食习惯(包括红肉和脂肪的摄入增加,水果和蔬菜摄入减少)与 CRC 有相关性。水果和蔬菜对人群的保护作用有尚存争议,但普遍的共识是增加水果和蔬菜的摄入不会提高对人体的保护作用,但极低量的摄入确实会增加患 CRC 的风险[213~215]。混合性脂类和饱和脂肪的高脂饮食已被证明可以促进结肠癌的发生[216,217],高摄入量的家禽和鱼类有保护作用[218]。

肥胖增加男性和女性患 CRC 的风险,BMI≥30kg/m^2 的人群患 CRC 的风险增加了近 20%[219,220]。体力活动和锻炼能降低 CRC 发病风险[221]。

糖尿病和高胰岛素血症

越来越多的证据表明,糖尿病和胰岛素抵抗是 CRC 的危险因素。一项对 15 项研究的荟萃分析发现,糖尿病患者患 CRC 的风险比非糖尿病患者高 30%[222,223]。可能的解释是,与糖尿病相关的高胰岛素血症甚至糖尿病的长期胰岛素治疗导致结肠黏膜细胞通过胰岛素样生长因子 1 获得生长信号[223,224]。

酒精和烟草

大量饮酒轻度增加 CRC 的发病风险。这种相关是剂量依赖性的,而与是直接饮酒或是饮用酒精饮料无关[225,226]。吸烟与结直肠癌之间的关系较为复杂,吸烟对机体的影响依特定的体细胞多态性而不同[227]。

遗传学

结肠直肠肿瘤发生有独特的遗传学模式,在这个过程中基因突变不断累积,比祖细胞增殖能力更强的细胞克隆不断增加。在 CRC 的发展中涉及三大类基因,即癌基因如 *K-ras*,抑癌基因如 *APC* 基因(APC),结直肠癌缺失基因(*DCC*)、*p53*、*MCC*,和错配修复基因 *hMSH2*、*hMLH1*、*hPMS* 和 *hPMS2*。

CRC 的发展来自多步骤序贯性基因突变,称为杂合现象缺失(LOH)。这一现象在家族性和散发性 CRC 中均可观察到。Fearon 和 Vogelstein 在 1990 年第一次提出相关假说,他们认为如腺瘤发展为癌,至少需要有 5 个基因发生突变[228]。进一步的研究表明,在癌症发生之前至少有 7 个基因发生突变。LOH 模型中的重要基因包括 *APC*、*K-ras*、*DCC* 和 *p53*。另一种截然不同的癌症发展途径是由错配修复基因缺陷引发的。在这种情况下,错误复制(RER)增加导致微卫星不稳定和基因功能丧失,这种由于 RER 而导致肿瘤发生在结直肠肿瘤中占 20%[229]。

APC 基因

APC 基因位于 5 号染色体的长臂(5q)上。这种突变常见于在家族性腺瘤性息肉病(FAP)和 Gardner 综合征以及大多数

Turcot 综合征病例中。在 63% 的腺瘤和癌中能检测到突变的 *APC* 基因,但在癌旁组织中未检测到,表明这是体细胞突变。由于 APC 是一种抑癌基因,仅在第二等位基因的失活后,细胞才失去 APC 蛋白的肿瘤抑制活性。有大量证据表明 *APC* 突变发生在早期,可能是散发性结直肠癌的首发事件。

DCC 基因

DCC 基因位于 18 号染色体的长臂(18q)上。该基因产物参与细胞-细胞黏附作用和细胞-基质相互作用,这对于预防肿瘤生长、侵袭和转移可能是重要的。在散发性 CRC 中,DCC 似乎在决定肿瘤转移的能力中起关键作用。

p53 基因

p53 位于 17 号染色体的短臂(17p)上。*p53* 可能是结直肠肿瘤发生过程中最重要的恶性程度决定因素。作为四聚体,*p53* 结合其他基因的启动子区域中的 DNA 序列以增强其转录[230]。被 *p53* 激活的大多数基因被认为参与抑制生长。*p53* 的突变可以在超过一半的人类癌症中发现[231]。

K-ras 原癌基因

K-ras 是一种癌基因,通过经典途径发挥作用,位于 12 号染色体短臂(12p)上。K-ras 蛋白与特定的效应分子相互作用、传递生长信号。信号转导过程受到突变 K-ras 蛋白的干扰,导致肿瘤形成。在散发性结肠肿瘤中,大约 50% 的癌和大腺瘤中发现了 *K-ras* 突变[232]。

错配修复基因

细胞修复 DNA RER、自身发生的碱基修复缺失需要错配修复基因。在人类中发现的四种 DNA 错配修复基因是 *hMSH2*(染色体 2p),*hMSH6*(染色体 2p),*hMLH1*(染色体 3p),*hPMS1*(染色体 2q)和 *hPMS2*(染色体 7p)。这些错配修复基因共同导致了遗传性非息肉病综合征[233]。

遗传综合

尽管绝大多数 CRC 病例是散发性而非家族性,但遗传易感性导致 CRC 发生风险显著增加。遗传综合征通常为常染色体显性遗传,并且 CRC 的高发病风险相关。

FAP 是一种常染色体显性遗传病,其特征为儿童期出现的多发结肠腺瘤。该综合征接近 100% 显性表达,症状和诊断一般在 15 岁左右[234]。如果不及时治疗,FAP 将最终转归为 CRC,转归后平均 CRC 诊断年龄和死亡年龄分别为 39 岁和 42 岁[235]。轻表型家族性腺瘤性息肉病(AAPC)是 FAP 的轻度变异性表型,具有类似 FAP 发展为 CRC 的风险。AAPC 的特征是较少的腺瘤性息肉和较高的平均诊断年龄(通常在刚过 50 岁的时候)。这两种遗传综合征都是由同一 *APC* 基因中的不同种系突变引起的,该基因位于 5 号染色体上[236]。

遗传性非息肉性结直肠癌(HNPCC)是另一种常染色体显性遗传综合征,占所有结直肠癌的 1%~5%。也称为 Lynch 综合征,这种疾病的特征是早期发病(一些患者可以出现在 20 多岁,而平均诊断年龄是 48 岁),右侧多见,多发同时或异时结肠肿瘤,可伴发肠外肿瘤。结肠外肿瘤可包括子宫内膜癌、肾盂和输尿管癌、膀胱癌、小肠癌和皮肤病变[237]。HNPCC 也是由一种错配修复基因的突变引起的[238]。

与其他家族性息肉综合征相比,MYH 相关息肉病(MAP)是近期发现的常染色体隐性遗传性息肉病综合征,相比于其他家族性息肉病综合征,MAP 一定程度与弱显性表达相关[239]。*MYH* 突变,是一种缺失修复基因,与多发性腺瘤或多发性息肉病的发生风险相关。在没有发现 *APC* 基因突变的患者中,尤其是那些患有 10~15 或更多腺瘤的患者,需要进行 *MYH* 基因突变的检查以协助诊断[240,241]。此外,这些患者同样有胃肠道恶性肿瘤的高发病风险。

PJ 综合征是一种遗传性的错构瘤性息肉病综合征,具有向 CRC 转归的倾向。PJ 的两个主要临床表现是色素性黏膜皮肤病变和多发性结肠息肉,具有向恶性转化的能力。PJ 综合征与胃肠道和非胃肠道恶性肿瘤的发病风险增加相关,包括卵巢癌、乳腺癌、胰腺癌、子宫癌、睾丸支持细胞瘤和宫颈肿瘤[242~244]。幼年性息肉病(JP)是另一种遗传性错构瘤性息肉病综合征,可以恶变为 CRC。患有 JP 的人群患胃癌、十二指肠癌和胰腺癌的风险也增加[245,246]。

基因多态性

已发现许多基因多态性(正常的基因变异)与 CRC 的发生有关。致癌物代谢基因、甲基化基因和抑癌基因等变化可导致癌症风险的升高或降低。细胞色素 *P450* 基因、谷胱甘肽-S 转移酶基因、N-乙酰转移酶基因和抑癌基因都与 CRC 有关。细胞色素 P450A1(CYP1A1)是在烟草中发现的与致癌物相互作用的Ⅰ相酶[247]。Ile462Val 的 A 向 G 突变、*CYP1A1* 基因的外显子 7 出现等多态性使患者发生 CRC 的风险增加[248]。特别是吸烟患者如有上述基因的多态性,其 CRC 发病风险增高。

谷胱甘肽-S-转移酶是负责诱变亲电子物质(如多环芳烃等)解毒过程的Ⅱ相酶[247]。谷胱甘肽-S-转移酶 Mu(GSTM1)和 Theta(GSTT1)与 CRC 的关系都有过研究。此外,N-乙酰转移酶是参与解毒芳胺的Ⅱ相酶,这些酶在熟肉中被发现[247]。GSTT1 和 NAT2 快速乙酰化表型均被证实可增加 CRC 的发病风险[249]。

与 CRC 相关的最常见的肿瘤抑制基因是 *APC* 基因。主要在德系犹太人群中发现的 I1307K 多态性使 CRC 风险增加了两倍[250]。*APC* 基因的另一个多态性 I1317Q 也增加了 CRC 的风险[251]。

一些基因多态性也被证实有助于降低 CRC 的患病风险。那些吃低脂饮食的患者和 *APC* 基因密码子 *1822* 突变的患者,相对于野生型和高脂饮食患者,可以降低结直肠癌发病风险[252]。此外,亚甲基四氢叶酸还原酶(MTHFR)的甲基化基因突变被证实与 CRC 发病风险相关。患者带有 *MTHFR677TT* 基因型可以降低结直肠癌发生风险[253]。

临床表现、筛查和监测

症状和体征

大肠恶性肿瘤的表现通常分为三类:起病隐匿的慢性症状、急性肠梗阻、急性穿孔。最常见的临床表现是起病隐匿的慢性症状(77%~92%),其次是梗阻(6%~16%)和穿孔(2%~7%)[254~256]。

出血是结直肠恶性肿瘤最常见的症状。然而,患者和医生都经常认为出血是良性疾病引起的。出血可能是隐匿性的,也可能出现黑便,栗色或鲜红色的粪便,这取决于恶性肿瘤的位置。

排便习惯改变第二常见的主诉,患者可能出现腹泻或便秘等[257,258]。便秘通常见于左侧结肠病变,因为左侧结肠直径较右侧小,粪便在左侧大多已成形成。患者可能会主诉排便逐渐变细,如果肠腔进一步狭窄足以引起梗阻也可能会出现腹泻。右半结肠癌通常不伴有排便习惯的变化,但肿瘤产生的大量黏液可能引起腹泻,大的右半结肠病变或累及回盲瓣的病变可能引起阻塞。

腹部疼痛与排便习惯的改变同样常见[259]。左侧梗阻性病变可出现绞痛,可伴有恶心和呕吐,并随肠蠕动缓解。右侧恶性肿瘤可能出现隐痛,疼痛常难以定位。直肠病变可能伴有里急后重,肿瘤进展期如累及骶神经或坐骨神经,可出现盆腔疼痛。其他症状可有体重减轻、全身乏力、发热、腹部肿块和泌尿系症状等。链球菌引起的菌血症高度提示结直肠恶性肿瘤[260,261]。

体格检查通常难以发现阳性体征。一方面是由于腹部膨隆,另一方面无论原发性或转移性的肿物都是不易触及的。叩诊鼓音、腹水或腹部膨隆可能是腹部检查中的所见。直肠指检很少会发现肿瘤梗阻。表现为大肠梗阻的患者,均应考虑到结肠直肠恶性肿瘤的可能。可通过对比灌肠、内镜检查或腹盆腔CT 检查来确认诊断。

穿孔可能导致局限性或弥漫性腹膜炎,也可以形成肠梗阻或引起邻近器官出现瘘,比如膀胱。12%~19%的患者由于CRC 导致梗阻而发生穿孔[262,263]。当穿孔发生在阻塞性病变近端时,患者会出现弥漫性腹膜炎和败血症,应在充分的液体复苏后进行急诊手。然而,肿瘤穿孔(可能继发于肿瘤坏死)可能倾向于相对保守的方式,因其可能与其他诊断如阑尾炎、憩室炎或克罗恩病相混淆。

筛查和监测

CRC 癌症筛查适用于无明显症状的人群进行检测,以确定发生 CRC 的风险。监测是指持续监测具有高疾病发生风险的人群。对于 CRC,监测适用于炎症性肠病、家族性肿瘤相关综合征、有 CRC 或结肠直肠腺瘤病史的患者。多种筛查和监测方式可用于检测 CRC 和腺瘤性息肉。目前的筛查和监测建议如下(表 94-1)。

粪便筛查

大便潜血试验的优点包括可行性、便利性和低成本。局限性包括灵敏度差、特异性低、依从性低、无法鉴别腺瘤。敏感性受切片保存、维生素 C、测试时未出血以及结肠细菌对血红蛋白降解的影响。特异性受红肉和未煮熟的蔬菜中外源性过氧化物酶、药物(如阿司匹林和其他非甾体抗炎药等能引起非结肠部位的出血的药物)等影响。在一项纳入超过 300 000 名患者的五项大型病例对照研究中,正确使用粪便筛查证实可增加早期 CRC 的检出率[264,265],也显著降低了死亡率[264-268]。基于粪便的筛查技术包括高灵敏度愈创木脂检测、免疫化学检测以及新近出现的粪便 DNA 检测。DNA 检测可发现在 CRC 发生过程中已知类型的基因突变,文献报道中最高的灵敏度高达95%[269]。目前,DNA 测试尚未获得 FDA 批准,因此它不作为一线筛选方案。截至 2014 年,高灵敏度基于愈创木脂和免疫化学的粪便检测作为独立筛查方法被广泛认可,这项检查应每年进行一次的人,检查前要遵循规定的饮食。只要检查结果提示异常,则应进行后续有创筛查。最近研究表明,与愈创木脂测试相比,免疫化学已被证明具有更高的灵敏度[270]。粪便筛查为那些拒绝各类有创检查的人来说提供了一个很好的选择[271]。

表 94-1 美国国立综合癌症网络筛查建议

危险因素分类	推荐的检查项目
一般危险因素:	
无症状、≥50 岁,同时无以下病史:腺瘤、无蒂锯齿状息肉、结直肠癌	自 50 岁起,每 10 年行结肠镜检查,或每 5 年行可屈性乙状结肠镜检查并在其中的第 3 年行粪便检查,或每年行粪便检查(愈创木脂法或免疫化学法)
个人史外的危险因素:	
一级亲属≥60 岁时有结直肠癌或腺瘤样息肉,或 2 个二级亲属有结直肠癌,或 1 个二级亲属在<50 岁时有结直肠癌	从 50 岁开始或是比家族中患者诊断结直肠癌最早年龄早 10 岁开始,每 5 年行结肠镜检查
一级亲属<60 岁有结直肠癌或腺瘤样息肉,或 2 个及以上一级亲属有结直肠癌	从 40 岁开始或是比家族中患者诊断的最早年龄早 10 岁开始,每 3~5 年行结肠镜检查
基因携带者或有 FAP 风险	从 10~15 岁开始每年行可屈性乙状结肠镜检查
基因携带者或 HNPCC 风险	从 25~30 岁或比家族中最早诊断年龄提前 2~5 年开始每 1~2 年行结肠镜检查

可屈性乙状结肠镜检查

硬式和软质乙状结肠镜检查费用均较低。该检查无须麻醉,即可对息肉和癌组织进行直接观察和活组织检查[272]。可屈性乙状结肠镜相对于硬式乙状结肠镜的优点是它可以到达降结肠甚至结肠脾曲。乙状结肠镜检查的缺点是无法探查整个结肠,可能遗漏近端结肠病变。目前的美国综合癌症网络(NCCN)和美国癌症协会(ACS)指南建议乙状结肠镜检查每 5 年进行一次,粪便筛查可选做,如果发现腺瘤性疾病则应进行全结肠镜检查[273]。

钡剂灌肠

钡剂灌肠联合乙状结肠镜检查可以评估整个结肠和直肠。单一对比钡剂灌肠检查的敏感性和特异性明显低于气钡双重对比灌肠检查(DCBE),单一对比钡剂灌肠检查不宜用作 CRC 筛查。对于息肉<1cm,DCBE 的灵敏度为 50%~80%,息肉>1cm时为 70%~90%,Ⅰ期和Ⅱ期 CRC 分别为 55%~85%[274-276]。当与乙状结肠镜检查相结合时,对 CRC 敏感性达到 98%,对腺瘤敏感性达到 99%[277]。文献报道,因 DCBE 而导致穿孔的概率为 1/25 000[278]。目前的 ACS 筛查建议是每 5 年进行一次钡剂灌肠检查,如果检测结果为阳性,则进行结肠镜检查。NCCN不将钡灌肠剂作为筛查项目[273]。

结肠镜检查

通过结肠镜对整个结肠进行检查是筛查的金标准。由经过培训的内镜医师进行结肠镜检查是一种安全的方法,穿孔发生率为0.1%,出血发生率为0.3%,死亡率为0.01%~0.03%。98.6%的患者可探查到盲肠,如未能达到盲肠时,可辅以DCBE检查[279~284]。研究表明,结肠镜检查和切除息肉可降低结直肠恶性肿瘤的发生率,检测早期病变可降低与疾病相关的死亡率,结肠镜检查和息肉切除术患者的癌症发生率较低[285,286]。当病灶大小<1cm时结肠镜检查优于DCBE[276]。此外,在初诊时结肠镜即可进行组织诊断或治疗干预。结肠镜检查优于乙状结肠镜检查,因为前者可直接观察到整个结肠。一项研究报道,226人在乙状结肠镜检查1年内再接受结肠镜检查,有24%的人群检出新发腺瘤,有6%的人群发现了降结肠近端的进展期病变[287]。目前的ACS筛查建议每10年进行一次结肠镜检查。

CT结肠成像

CT结肠成像(虚拟结肠镜检查)是一项新兴技术,它利用CT对扩张的结肠的进行三维重建。在美国国家海军医疗中心,1 223名无明显危险因素的成人接受CT结肠成像检查,然后进行常规结肠镜检查,虚拟结肠镜检查在检测相关病变方面效果近似,在一些病灶检测方面甚至优于结肠镜检查[288]。然而,在监测人群中可能准确性较差,随后多次机构研究未能复现前述结果。该检查的主要局限性包括准确性差、检查前需要进行全肠道准备,以及如影像学发现异常,还需后续进行结肠镜检查以进行组织学诊断。CT结肠成像如作为筛选的主要方法也会导致对患者的重复射线暴露。因为从放射科医生的角度来看,虚拟结肠镜检查需要相当大的时间和工作量,所以正在积极研究自动化评估的方法。目前的ACS筛查建议是每5年进行一次虚拟结肠镜检查,如果发现病变,随后进行结肠镜检查。NCCN未将CT结肠成像认定为筛选方式。

术前评估和分期

常规体格检查仍然是评估患者术前局部侵犯程度、远处转移和手术风险的重要手段。应特别关注有无体重减轻、贫血貌,以及有无门静脉高压征象。此外,完整的检查应包括常规实验室检查、结肠镜检查、胸部X线检查,腹骨腔CT,直肠癌患者还应进行经直肠超声检查(TRUS)。

常规实验室化验

全血细胞计数(CBC)有助于贫血的诊断。如合并肝转移,肝功能检查(LFT)可能会提示异常。癌胚抗原(CEA)水平在治疗前监测可作为基线,治疗后可与之比较。发生肝转移性时CEA水平升至较高水平,治疗后复查如CEA超过10~20ng/ml,提示治疗可能失败[289]。

结肠镜

结肠镜检查仍然是结肠疾病评估中最重要的一项。它可以评估肿瘤大小、进行定位,但不能评估侵袭深度。结肠镜检查可对肿瘤组织进行活检,以行后续组织学病理检查,有助于发现同时性双原发或多原发肿瘤,如发现息肉可行同期切除。同时性双原发或多原发肿瘤发生率为2%~7%,结肠肿瘤伴发结肠息肉发生率约29.7%[290]。术前结肠镜检查改变了30%患者的手术方式[291]。

影像学评估

胸部X线检查可查见肺部占位,并可对心肺状态做粗略评估。结肠癌患者术前行腹盆腔CT检查尚存争议。进行CT检查以明确邻近器官有无累及,有无主动脉旁淋巴结转移和有无肝脏累及。只有15%的肝转移患者有异常LFT结果,然而无肝转移的时肝功能检查指标也可升高40%[292]。因此,LFT不能决定是否需加做CT检查。腹部超声有助于发现部分患者的肝转移、腹水和淋巴结转移。

PET和现在的PET-CT已经成为CRC的潜在重要的检查方式。使用氟代脱氧葡萄糖,代谢活性高的组织可被查见。标准摄取值对于区分良恶性疾病可提供一个半定量的参考,虽然这类检查对检查恶性肿瘤的复发有潜在的应用价值,但由于假阳性率高和费用昂贵,一般不用于结肠癌患者的初次评估。

TRUS已成为直肠癌患者术前评估的重要组成部分。TRUS可以辨认直肠壁的层次并确定侵犯深度。在不同的文献报道中,其敏感性为55%~100%,特异性为24%~100%。淋巴结的状态也可通过TRUS进行检查,发现率为73%~85%[293]。如果考虑局部切除,侵犯深度和淋巴结状态尤为重要。

近些年来MRI已被用于直肠癌的评估,特别是术前分期的评估。与TRUS相比,MRI在确定直肠层内侵袭深度方面具有类似的敏感性;然而,超声检查在检测周围组织和邻近器官累及方面具有优势[294]。MRI和TRUS在检测直肠周围淋巴结转移方面具有高度类似的敏感性,这两种方法都优于CT检查[294]。MRI的另一优势是可用于评估髂动脉、肠系膜和腹膜后淋巴结的情况。

此外,MRI在术前可以判断环周切缘(CRM)的情况,从而对预后风险进行分层,这是目前MRI在术前评估中新的应用。MERCURY研究术前利用MRI判断原发性直肠肿瘤与直肠系膜筋膜的关系,定义瘤体和系膜距离<1mm,则认为CRM可能受累[295]。研究结果表明CRM可能受累的患者,其5年总生存率、无病生存期缩短,这些患者术后局部复发可能性大。与AJCC的TNM分期方法相比,MRI的CRM术前评估对预后具有更高的预测价值。因此,MRI可能会继续在直肠癌患者的术前评估中发挥越来越大的作用。在未来它也可能成为新辅助治疗策略中不可或缺的部分,作为评估术前化疗或放化疗的反应的一种方法[296]。

分期

肿瘤分期对判断预后、为患者选择不同的治疗方案以及比较不同治疗方案的疗效非常重要。如果肿瘤要被认为具有侵袭性,一定要有浸透了黏膜肌层的证据。恶性细胞仅局限于黏膜上皮质时称为原位癌。1932年,Dukes提出了一种基于直接侵犯深度联合有/无区域淋巴结转移的直肠癌分期方法。由美国肿瘤外科医师协会结合开腹手术的情况提出的癌症TNM分期系统,目前很大程度上已经取代了Dukes在临床中的应用(表94-2)。

表 94-2　AJCC 第 7 版结直肠癌 TNM 分期

T-原发肿瘤分期			
TX	原发肿瘤不能评估		
T0	无原发肿瘤证据		
Tis	原位癌：局限于上皮内或黏膜固有层		
T1	肿瘤侵犯黏膜下层		
T2	肿瘤侵犯固有肌层		
T3	肿瘤穿透固有肌层进入结肠旁组织		
T4a	肿瘤穿透脏腹膜表面		
T4b	肿瘤直接侵犯周围脏器		
N-区域淋巴结分期			
NX	区域淋巴结不能评价		
N0	无区域淋巴结转移		
N1	1~3 个区域淋巴结转移		
N1a	1 个区域淋巴结转移		
N1b	2~3 个区域淋巴结转移		
N1c	无区域淋巴结转移，但在浆膜下、肠系膜或无腹膜覆盖的结直肠周围组织存在孤立性癌结节		
N2	≥4 个区域淋巴结转移		
N2a	4~6 个区域淋巴结转移		
N2b	≥7 个区域淋巴结转移		
M-远处转移			
M0	无远处转移		
M1	有远处转移		
M1a	单个器官或部位发生转移		
M1b	多个脏器发生远处转移		
分期	T	N	M
0	Tis	N0	M0
Ⅰ	T1，T2	N0	M0
ⅡA	T3	N0	M0
ⅡB	T4	N0	M0
ⅡC	T4b	N0	M0
ⅢA	T1~T2	N1/N1c	M0
ⅢB	T1	N2a	M0
	T3~T4a	N1/N1c	M0
	T2~T3	N2a	M0
	T1~T2	N2b	M0
ⅢC	T4a	N2a	M0
	T3~T4a	N2b	M0
	T4b	N1~N2	M0
ⅣA	任何 T	任何 N	M1a
ⅣB	任何 T	任何 N	M1b

改编自 Edge 2010[297]。已获 Springer 出版社授权。

AJCC 已经规定了两个分化程度，低危级（高分化和中分化）和高危级（低分化和未分化）。DNA 倍性分析是对细胞中 DNA 数目进行测量。二倍体与良好预后相关，而非整倍体与不良预后相关。肠穿孔和术前 CEA 升高与不良预后相关。

最近，随着对结肠癌的遗传决定因素理解的更加深入，人们对基因水平上描述疾病和判断预后更有兴趣。最初研究者评估了一些特定基因突变（主要是 *p53* 表达和 *K-ras* 突变状态）产生的结果，这些结论间存在着相互矛盾的地方。因此 *p53* 和 *K-ras* 无法作为标志物被列入常规的分期系统[296]。最近，利用阵列同时分析多个基因的方法成为热点。比如，Oncotype DX® 是一种多基因检阵列谱检测方法，它利用 PCR 定量测定来自单个肿瘤中 12 个基因的表达情况，目的是预测疾病术后是否复发[298]。这些基因的选择是基于 1 800 个结肠癌（Ⅱ期和Ⅲ期）患者的分析，这项研究是美国乳腺与肠道外科辅助治疗研究组项目的一部分[299]。随后，两项前瞻性研究验证了该方法预测Ⅱ期和Ⅲ期结肠癌患者复发风险的预后能力；然而他们没有证实其是否能预测化疗反应[300,301]。随着这些检测方法的改进，基因谱分析将会在不久的将来成为癌症分期的重要组成部分。虽然多基因检测的作用尚未确定，但在 2014 年，一项多中心前瞻性研究评估了提供 OncotypeDX® 复发评分对医生决策行为的影响（决定在Ⅱa 期结肠癌患者中使用辅助化疗），表明该评分已改变超过 40% 患者的治疗计划[302]。虽然这些结果并未证实 Oncotype DX 在做出治疗决策方面有临床获益，但他们有信心，肿瘤学治疗过程中，多基因分析可以提供有用的客观信息，最终可能有助于指导某些患者的治疗。

结肠癌的外科治疗

恶性息肉的处理

结肠癌可能为息肉部分恶变或有腺瘤性息肉（“恶性息肉”）产生的，这些恶性息肉局限在黏膜下层。它们的淋巴结转移倾向与较多组织病理学特征有关，包括分级、神经/血管是否累及、大体形态（如无柄与带蒂）。

Haggitt 分级系统用于确定恶性息肉的侵犯深度（表 94-3）。Haggitt 分级 1 级、2 级和 3 级病灶淋巴结转移的风险<1%，这些病变通常可以印度墨水标记后在内镜下完整[303]。这种情况下，建议对息肉切除部位进行仔细的结肠镜检查。脉管受累、地分化差或恶变部位距息肉切除边缘<2mm 时，应行结肠切除术，因为这种情况下淋巴结转移的风险较高。Haggit 4 级病灶的淋巴结转移发生率高（12%~25%），应行结肠切除术[303]。一般而言，有癌细胞的结肠无蒂息肉应行结肠切除术，这类病变属于 Haggit 4 级。

表 94-3　恶性息肉 Haggitt 分级

Haggitt 分级	癌变特征
0	原位癌
1	癌变侵及黏膜下层但局限于息肉头部
2	癌变侵及息肉颈部水平
3	癌变侵及息肉基底部
4	癌变侵及基底部以下黏膜层（但位于肌层以上）

结肠的大多数息肉可以在结肠镜下通过套圈结扎的方法切除。通过结肠镜观察息肉，并将圈套线环绕息肉并在施加电流时轻轻收紧。无论何时息肉都回收进行组织学检查。由经过培训的内镜医师进行内镜下息肉切除术是安全的，穿孔发生率为0.3%～1%，出血发生率为0.7%～2.5%[304]。

标准切除范围和技术

肠道准备

尽管最近的证据质疑肠道准备是否获益，但是肠道准备现在仍然是结直肠手术的常规的术前准备步骤。肠道准备一般使用强力的泻药和多次灌肠来完成，直至肠道清洁。最近，一种聚乙二醇高渗电解质口服肠道清洁药物（如GoLYTELY）被广泛使用。口服磷酸钠肠道清洁剂的使用也越来越多，上述肠道准备药物的应用可能导致水电解质紊乱。

抗生素使用

围术期抗生素可以采用口服和静脉注入的方式，前者通常与肠道准备制剂联用。静脉抗生素使用可以预防手术部位感染，在结直肠手术中尤为常见。虽然确切的抗生素使用方法仍有争议，但所用抗生素的抗菌谱应涵盖有氧和厌氧菌。快速康复（ERAS）倡导在手术前1h内应用1次抗生素，有1级证据支持该观点[305]。与多剂量方案相比，初始单剂用药有相同的预防效果，但手术时间延长的患者就需要追加使用抗生素[305]。口服抗生素的通常有两个作用，一是在机械性肠道准备时充当泻药，二是根除潜在的肠腔内致病菌。2014年Cochrane综述中指出，联合口服和静脉两种方式应用抗生素优于单独使用静脉注射抗生素（*HR*＝0.56）或单独使用口服抗生素（*HR*＝0.56）。如果在手术前已经结肠为空虚状态（肠道准备完毕），是否有必要进行口服抗生素预防尚不确定[306]。

右半结肠癌

右半结肠癌占原发性结肠癌的30%[307]。盲肠或升结肠的腺癌患者，如果没有HNPCC或其他同期病变，应行右半结肠切除术治疗（图94-1a）。结肠中血管的右侧分支，回结肠血管和右结肠血管应在其根部结扎，以确保能充分清扫淋巴结。与右半结肠延续的远端小肠应切除5～10cm，以确保在小肠的吻合口边缘有足够的血液供应。

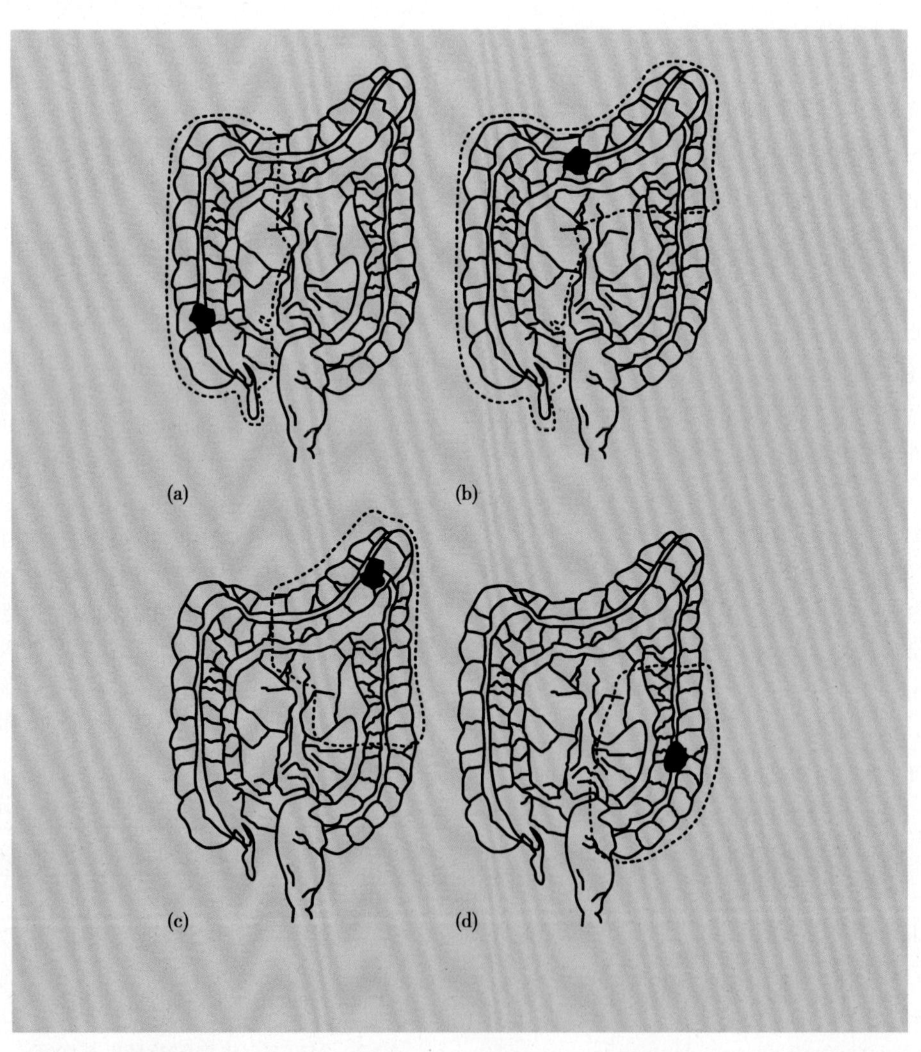

图94-1 结肠癌切除范围。（a）盲肠和升结肠癌。（b）横结肠癌。（c）结肠脾曲癌。（d）乙状结肠癌

横结肠癌

横结肠癌相对少见，仅占原发结直肠癌的 10%[307]。近端和中段的横结肠病变通常行扩大的右半结肠切除术，包括结扎回结肠血管、右结肠血管和结肠中血管（图 94-1b）。升结肠、结肠肝曲、横结肠和结肠脾曲被切除后，将回肠与降结肠吻合。因为考虑到吻合口血供和张力，应避免结肠肝曲和脾曲的吻合。

左半结肠癌

结肠脾曲和降结肠的病变也不常见，占原发性结直肠癌的 15%[307]。结肠脾曲的肿瘤处理方式可以是扩大的右半结肠切除术或者左半结肠切除术（图 94-1c）。降结肠癌可以通过左半结肠切除术进行治疗，左半结肠切除术包括分离左结肠动脉、保留结肠中动脉的左侧分支、远端横结肠和远端乙状结肠做吻合。另一种左半结肠切除术的方法是，结扎肠系膜下血管后并在横结肠和直肠上端进行吻合。

乙状结肠癌

乙状结肠癌占原发性结直肠癌的 25%。这些肿瘤通常行乙状结肠切除术，分离在左结肠动脉发出前或发出后结扎肠系膜下动脉，同时结扎直肠上动脉，行降结肠-直肠上段吻合（图 94-1d）。巨大的乙状结肠癌位于腹膜反折上方，但位于盆腔入口处，肿瘤会邻近输尿管、下腹下神经和髂血管，完善的术前准备方案是必需的，包括影像学检查和输尿管支架放置准备。

次全结肠切除术

该术式切除范围是全结肠切除，并进行回肠直肠吻合术（IRA）。该手术适用于同时性多原发结肠癌并且分布在结肠不同区域，特别是 FAP 但是直肠较少受累的患者（下文讨论）或部分 HNPCC 患者和部分结肠癌患者。

全直肠结肠切除术

FAP 的手术治疗取决于患者的年龄和直肠中的息肉密度。手术选择包括直肠结肠切除术加 Brooke 回肠造口术，全结肠切除术与回肠直肠吻合术（IRA），或直肠结肠切除术加回肠储袋肛管吻合术（IPAA）。目前，直肠结肠切除术加可控性回肠造口术已很少使用。全结肠切除术加 IRA 并发症发生率低，术后功能恢复良好，对于直肠中少于 20 个腺瘤的患者是一种可行的治疗方案。这些患者必须接受 6 个月的肠镜检查，以根治息肉并随访是否有新发癌变。如果直肠息肉太多，如条件允许则应行直肠切除术。克利夫兰诊所最近评估了已登记接受 IRA 或 IPAA 治疗的 FAP 患者。在对直肠息肉负荷较高的患者采取 IPAA 治疗之前，保留直肠的癌变风险为 12.9%，中位随访时间超过 17 年[308]。对于接受 IPAA 治疗或选择使用 IRA 治疗的患者（对于那些直肠息肉负荷较小的患者），在中位随访 5 年时，没有患者发生直肠癌。使用 IPAA 治疗的直肠结肠切除重建术的优点包括具有在保留肛门排便功能的同时，切除几乎所有肿瘤发生风险的大肠黏膜。在大型医学中心进行手术时并发症发生率较低，但并发症包括尿失禁、腹泻、阳痿、逆行射精、性交困难和储袋炎等。大约 7%的患者由于手术并发症必须转行永久性回肠造口术[308]。

直肠癌

直肠肿瘤的手术方法取决于侵犯深度和距肛门边缘的距离。这四种手术入路包括经肛切除，经骶前切除，低位直肠前切除（LAR）加全直肠系膜切除术（TME）和经腹会阴联合直肠切除术（APR）。

局部切除

局部切除的早期研究显示，适当选择的个体行该术式后局部控制率达 97%，DFS 达 80%[309]。局部治疗最适用于肛门边缘 10cm 内的 T1 期直肠癌，同时肿瘤直径<3cm、直肠壁累计不超过周长的 1/4、高活动度外生性肿瘤和组织学分化良好的肿瘤。决定单独使用局部切除或在局部切除后采用辅助治疗应基于原发性癌症的病理特征和引流淋巴结中微转移的可能性。T1 期病变在高达 18%的病例中存在淋巴结转移，而 T2 期和 T3 期病变的比率分别高达 38%和 70%。T2 肿瘤仅行局部切除其复发率可达 15%～44%[309]。因此，预后不良的 T1 病灶和对所有 T2 肿瘤均应行根治性手术。

局部切除远端直肠癌可通过经肛切除、后入路切除（Kraske 术）或经肛门内镜显微手术完成。经肛切除是最简单易行的方法，切除深度应达到肠周脂肪，并要求肿瘤距环周切缘至少 1cm。Kraske 术可用于直肠中部和直肠上部的肿瘤，与经肛切除相比，该方法更适合于较大的直肠病变。在该手术中，在肛门上方进行会阴切口，移除尾骨，分离筋膜，并进行直肠切除术。该方法的缺点是瘘管形成和切口肿瘤种植的可能性。经肛门内镜显微外科手术适用于直肠中段和上段肿瘤的治疗，如无法切除，则需要进行开腹手术或经骶前切除。这种方法可用于距离肛门边缘 15cm 的病变。该手术技术要求很高，需要特殊设备，该类设备价格昂贵，因此限制了它在美国的广泛引用。

低位直肠前切除术

由于直肠癌的外科治疗在过去的 20 年中得到了改进，有证据显示在保证肿瘤学安全的前提下保留括约肌是可行的。该手术要求切除乙状结肠和累及的直肠，肠系膜下动脉于根部进行结扎离断。常规游离结肠脾曲，行降结肠-直肠吻合进行重建。吻合不建议使用乙状结肠，因乙状结肠的肠壁较厚，肌肉顺应性差。随着圆形吻合器、牵开器的出现以及认识到距远端切缘 2cm 离断是足够的，LAR 的技术可行性得到了提高。然而，直肠系膜边缘应该在肿瘤下方远端至少 5cm 处或切到盆底的直肠系膜末端。TME 要求直视下锐性分离和切除直肠系膜，切除包括引流区域淋巴结和肠周脂肪组织和血管。在合适的患者中进行新辅助治疗，可有效地将潜在行 APR 的患者转化为可行保留括约肌的手术的情况[310]。

腹会阴联合直肠切除术

对于癌症累及括约肌（或与其重叠），或与括约肌邻接，或术前已有大便失禁的患者，应行腹会阴联合直肠切除术做完整切除。直肠切除后将会阴缝合并行永久性结肠造口术。

同时性和异时性病变

同时性结肠癌的发病率为 2%～11%，同时性腺瘤性息肉的发病率可能超过 30%[307]。对于弥漫性病变患者来说，只要满足肿瘤充分切除，通过多次吻合保证结肠长度是可取的。多次吻合的替代方案是次全结肠切除术并行回肠-直肠吻合或回肠-乙状结肠吻合。异时性结肠癌，定义为手术后 6 个月以上检测到的新发结肠肿瘤，由病变的位置所决定行部分或次全结肠切除术。

淋巴结清扫术

标准的淋巴结清扫应包括原发肿瘤引流区域的所有淋巴

结清扫。切除位于两个主要血管附近的淋巴结应该包括完整切除两根血管以及相关的淋巴结。肠系膜根部淋巴结应行常规清扫,并送病理科行病理检查。应切除区域外的可疑阳性淋巴结[311,312]。虽然并非总是可行,但病理科医生应该努力检查至少12个淋巴结。这可以使分期更为准确,为患者选择合适的辅助治疗提供依据[313]。此外,获检淋巴结的绝对数量本身与生存也有相关行[313]。尽管一些研究表明结肠癌患者的前哨淋巴结定位和活检是可行的,但其在结肠癌患者的真正临床应用尚需进一步研究[314]。

腹腔镜结肠切除术

腹腔镜结肠切除首次出现在1990年[315]。与传统开腹手术相比,腹腔镜结肠切除术的优势包括更短的恢复时间和更少的麻醉剂使用。腹腔镜辅助结肠切除技术包括腹腔探查和游离相关区域结肠。然后通过小切口将切除的结肠标本取出,肠管通过该切口进行体外切除和吻合。在腹腔镜结肠癌根治术刚开始应用时,大部分学者质疑腹腔镜辅助结肠癌切除术能否达到充足的切除范围和能否保证不增加结肠癌的复发风险[316]。但是,几项大型研究的结果为腹腔镜结肠切除术提供了可靠的证据。腹腔镜结肠切除术肿瘤学安全,围术期并发症发生率低于开放结肠切除术[317~326]。

五项前瞻性随机试验,即Barcelona试验,Australasian试验,COST试验,CLASICC试验,COLOR试验,已报告长期随访关于结肠癌患者腹腔镜结肠切除术与开放结肠切除术等效性的研究数据[317~322,324,325]。来自Barcelona试验研究的第一份长期随访数据显示,腹腔镜辅助组的癌症相关生存率明显高于开放手术组[317]。这研究发现Ⅲ期结肠癌患者行腹腔镜结肠癌根治术后生存率明显长于开放手术,而在Ⅰ期或Ⅱ期患者中两者没有显著差异。COST和CLASICC试验认为两组之间没有显著差异[318,319]。在最近的COST试验后续报告中,5年OS、5年DFS、复发率和首次复发的部位两组之间均相似[324]。同样,在近期CLASICC试验(也包括接受腹腔镜辅助切除直肠癌的患者)的随访报告中,腹腔镜辅助手术组在3年OS、DFS或局部复发无显著差异。COLOR试验显示手术切缘阳性率和检获区域淋巴结数量相似,3年DFS和OS两组无明显差异。腹腔镜检查的短期术后获益包括早期肠功能恢复、较少的镇痛药使用,以及缩短住院时间[322]。Australasian试验表明,5年OS和RFS两组无明显差异。在所有5项研究中,均报道住院时间缩短,而腹腔镜辅助结肠切除术的手术时间更长。在CLASICC和COST试验中,腹腔镜结肠切除术的回肠切除长度明显减少,而COST试验也观察到腹腔镜结肠切除术使用口服镇痛药的时间明显减少[318,119]。虽然观察到这些患者的近期获益,尚不清两组患者的远期预后。在CLASICC试验中,两组之间在3年内生活质量(QOL)量表评分上无显著差异。一项纳入超过1 500名患者的四项试验的荟萃分析表明,腹腔镜辅助或开放式切除后的3年DFS和OS相似,Ⅰ、Ⅱ和Ⅲ期的DFS和OS无明显差异。经验丰富的外科医生进行腹腔镜辅助结肠切除术,已被证明是一种和开放结肠切除术等效的肿瘤手术[327]。

腹腔镜结肠切除术技术更深入的研究需要更成熟更可靠的长期研究资料、合适的病例选择,以及对腹腔镜技术的成本效益分析。COLOR、COST和CLASICC试验的中转开腹比例分别为17%、21%和29%[318~320]。经过转化治疗的CLASICC试验患者的并发症发生率较高,合适的病例选择显得重要[319]。更长的手术时间和更高的外科技术要求,导致腹腔镜手术的成本效益比仍需更加深入的评估。

腹腔镜直肠癌切除术的调查结果不如腹腔镜结肠切除术的完整。手术切除是直肠癌的一种极其重要的治疗方式。如Heald[328]所描述,中位和低位直肠癌的标准手术是精准的TME。TME和充分的切除边缘与低复发风险和更长生存期相关[332]。腹腔镜直肠癌切除术必须能够达到相同的肿瘤学结果。腹腔镜直肠癌手术技术包括在体内离断远端肠管和分离直肠系膜,并在体外完成剩余的肠系膜和近端肠管的游离。通过将吻合器的砧座放置在降结肠中并将圆形吻合器插入直肠来进行体内端端吻合术[330,331]。对于需要腹腔镜辅助腹会阴联合直肠癌根治术(APR)的低位直肠癌,游离直肠和直肠系膜,并通过会阴切口切除剩余直肠和直肠系膜,并缝合会阴切口。目前腹腔镜辅助直肠癌根治术的肿瘤学效果尚未完全证实与开腹手术等同,但现有资料强烈支持腹腔镜辅助直肠癌根治术。

几个单中心腹腔镜辅助切除直肠癌报告了其安全性和可行性[331~334]。有几项前瞻性随机试验比较腹腔镜和开放手术切除直肠和直肠乙状结肠癌的应用,其中包括CLASICC试验中一个亚分组[319,325,330,335]。在CLASICC试验的初始观察数据中发现腹腔镜辅助经腹直肠癌根治术与经腹直肠癌根治术、经腹会阴直肠癌根治术的环周切缘(CRM)阳性率没有显著差异。但是,一份随访资料报道更高的CRM阳性率并不导致局部复发风险的增高[325]。这个结论可能是由于患者数量太少而且需要更长时间的随访。以上在腹腔镜结肠切除术讨论了部分该试验的其他结果。2004年对直肠乙状结肠癌患者进行的试验将患者随机分为腹腔镜辅助或开放性LAR(未包括APR)[330]。结果显示5年生存率,5年DFS或肿瘤复发中无显著差异[330]。腹腔镜组术后恢复明显更好,但手术时间明显更长,花费更高[330]。最近,腹腔镜手术对比直肠癌开放手术的(COLOR Ⅱ)试验是一项多中心随机、治疗的试验,比较腹腔镜和开腹切除术的近期围术期和肿瘤学结果[335]。该试验包括1100多名患者,并证实手术失血,肠功能恢复和住院时间有所改善。此外,两组有相似的根治切除率和CRM阳性情况。该研究尚未提供长期生存,但短期研究结果表明,与传统开放式手术相比,腹腔镜直肠癌切除术,在经过适当选择的患者和经验丰富的外科医生中,具有相同的肿瘤学结果。两项荟萃分析也对上述结论进行了验证[336,337]。学者Aziz等人共分析了2000多名患者,发现腹腔镜直肠癌手术、开腹直肠癌手术、腹腔镜APR术和开腹APR术的阳性切缘率和淋巴结清扫数目没有显著差别[336]。同时,造瘘口功能恢复时间、一次大肠蠕动和术后住院周期显著缩短,在腹腔镜辅助APR手术组术后伤口感染率也大大降低[366]。在另一项荟萃分析中,发现腹腔镜手术能够显著的降低并发症率但是需要更长的手术时间[337]。另外,在伤口愈合、吻合口瘘发生率或阳性切缘率方面,腹腔镜手术组和开腹手术组没有显著差异[337]。因此,越来越多的证据支持腹腔镜辅助切除直肠癌与传统开放手术疗效相同。

为了确定腹腔镜辅助切除癌症和开放性切除相等,需要更多有关癌症复发和生存的长期数据。而且,由于两个大型随机试验报道中转开腹率分别为23%和34%,选择合适的患者进行腹腔镜手术是必要的。腹腔镜手术还需要更长的手术时间和更先进的技术技能[325,326]。为了进一步研究腹腔镜辅助切除直肠癌的利弊，美国外科肿瘤学会开展了一项前瞻性随机Ⅲ期试验，验证腹腔镜直肠癌切除术时候在技术上和肿瘤根治上是否具有安全性(ACSOG-Z6051)[338]。该试验最近已经完成，预计很快就会有短期结果。随着该试验的长期数据的出现，将会对腹腔镜直肠癌切除术提供更多更深入的技术评估和腹腔镜在直肠癌根治术中的作用进行评价。

机器人结肠切除术

与腹腔镜或传统开放手术相比，关于机器人结肠直肠手术的数据有限。唯一的随机数据来自一项比较机器人右半结肠切除术与标准腹腔镜右结肠切除术的小型研究[339]，结果显示具有相同的淋巴结清扫数，切缘阳性率以及中转开腹率。大部分数据来自小型单中心研究。关于评估机器人与开放式结肠切除术的有效性的回顾性研究显示机器人手术(腹腔镜辅助手术)改善了围术期并发症和短期结果(如肠功能恢复，伤口并发症和住院时间)[340,343]。然而，在几乎所有研究中，机器人结肠切除术伴随更长的手术时间以及护理成本增加[340]。随着各中心在机器人手术系统积累更多经验，后两个缺点可能会有所改善。与腹腔镜结肠切除术相比，机器人手术具有类似的淋巴结清扫量，标本长度以及中转开腹率[344]。即使与腹腔镜设备相比，研究表明机器人结肠切除术增加了手术时间和手术室成本[344,345]。手术时间的延长可能与机器人结肠切除术中更多的体内吻合，以及腹腔镜系统的建立相关[345]。虽然缺乏随机研究数据，但迄今为止的研究表明，腹腔镜或开腹手术之间机器人结肠切除术的短期肿瘤学结果没有差异。

与传统的开放式和腹腔镜手术相比，机器人直肠手术具有几个理论上的优势。与开放手术相比，改善了并发症以及短期质量指标，例如住院时间和再入院率。与腹腔镜直肠切除术相比，机器人技术具有较低的中转开腹率。虽然迄今尚无随机研究，但一些单中心的评估表明，在经过选择的合适患者和经验丰富的外科医生的前提下，在机器人直肠癌手术是安全的[342,343,346]。最大的回顾性比较效果研究中，与腹腔镜 LAR 相比，机器人 LAR 具有更低的中转开腹率和严重的并发症发生率[342]。根治性 TME 手术也得到了改进。然而，鉴于该研究的回顾性，这些改善可能是患者选择偏倚的结果。目前，机器人与腹腔镜直肠癌切除术(ROLARR)试验正在进行中，这将为围术期并发症，短期死亡率，3 年 DFS 和 OS 以及性功能评估提供 1 级证据[347]。预计 2016 年会得出研究结果。在此期间，机器人直肠切除术应仅被视为一项正在研究的技术，最好交给具有先进微创手术经验的中心和外科医生处理。

结肠癌穿孔

结肠癌穿孔的患者常出现腹膜炎。在这种情况下，外科手术的目的只是为了切除病变的结肠肠管和阻止腹膜污染的进一步发展，并接着切除原发瘤并冲洗腹腔，后续处理方案可以有近端肠管造瘘/Hartmann 囊或者肠管一期吻合同时行回肠造瘘术。结肠癌伴肠穿孔与更高的局部复发率和更低的总生存期相关[348]。

梗阻性结肠癌

肿瘤是导致大肠梗阻的最常见原因[349]。右半结肠和横结肠梗阻需要行右半结肠切除术和一期吻合。左半结肠癌可以行单独的手术切除或者二期吻合[349]。一期手术的选择包括部分肠管切除或次全结肠切除术同期回直肠吻合。次全结肠切除术比较受人重视，因为这种术式切除了潜在可能坏死的肠管，但是这种手术方式创伤更大，并且术后每天大便次数可以达到 5~6 次。已经将术中灌洗用于梗阻性部分肠管切除术，但术后并发症率仍然是一个问题。分期手术包括首先切除原发肿瘤和近端结肠，然后行造瘘或 Hartmann 囊。二期手术在术后一段时间内完成，涉及结肠吻合。对于左半结肠梗阻的患者有一种可选择的方案，先行原发肿瘤切除术，再行回肠造口术[349]。

最近结肠支架植入术作为结肠癌梗阻患者的一种选择[350,351]。虽然它不是长期解决方案，但是支架对于那些远处转移或并发症较多的预后差的患者非常有益。支架一直用于短期内缓解梗阻症状和在准备手术切除前有或者无近端肠管结肠镜检查的术前准备[350,351]。

同期远处转移

肝脏是结肠癌转移的最常见部位，约 17%的患者会出现同期肝转移[307]。经过慎重选择的患者结肠病变和肝脏转移病变同期切除时安全的，肝脏转移性病灶切除也可以延期切除。全身化疗是结肠癌肝转移患者的必要治疗措施。

手术切除后的复查

结肠腺癌切除术后复查的目的是发现无症状复发病灶或新的原发灶，这将指导随后的早期治疗并延长患者的生存期。由美国临床肿瘤学会(ASCO)组建的专家小组分析总结了结直肠癌(CRC)术后各种扫描检查的途径(表 94-4)[352]。有趣的是，CBC、LFT、FOBT 和 CT 不被认为是必要的复查的组成部分。考虑到这些指导原则，复查应根据特定病例特有的因素进行个体化，包括患者本身其他疾病和患者心理状态。

表 94-4　ASCO 结直肠癌术后复查指南

检查项目	推荐
病史和体检	术后 5 年内每 3~6 个月 1 次，5 年后每年 1 次
血清 CEA	术后 5 年内每 3~6 个月 1 次
结肠镜	术后 1 年起复查，如第一次检查未见明显异常，每 5 年检查 1 次。直肠癌术后患者如未行放疗，直乙结肠镜检查应在术后 2~5 年内每 6 个月检查 1 次
CT	高危人群在术后 3 年内每 6~12 个月检查 1 次(直肠癌患者扫描范围必须包括盆腔)

局部复发

结肠腺癌术后局部复发在进展期肿瘤中最高可以达 4%[353]。尽管这些复发的患者预后差，但是外科切除复发病灶后仍然可以使 15%的患者得到长期生存[353]。在复发灶为单一的且肿瘤小于 5cm 的患者，如果能够保证切缘阴性，这些患者可以达到最佳的预后。

结直肠癌的新辅助化疗

基于氟尿嘧啶的方案

自 20 世纪 60 年代以来，叶酸拮抗剂氟尿嘧啶一直是 CRC

化疗的基本药物。氟尿嘧啶体内代谢物氟尿嘧啶脱氧核苷-磷酸盐（FdUMP）抑制胸苷酸合酶（TS）和干扰 DNA 的合成[354]。氟尿嘧啶也干扰 RNA 合成，进而破坏蛋白质合成[354]。然而，研究没有显示出单一使用佐剂氟尿嘧啶的生存优势。亚叶酸、左旋咪唑和甲氨蝶呤均作为氟尿嘧啶的调节剂[355-359]。LV 已被接受作为标准生物调节剂，并通过稳定 FdUMP/TS 复合物和增加氟尿嘧啶的细胞毒性，同时也能增加细胞内叶酸的量。

多项前瞻性试验显示术后氟尿嘧啶联合 LV 或左旋咪唑的临床益处[355,356,358,359]。全美外科乳腺癌和大肠癌辅助治疗 C-03 试验证实了输注氟尿嘧啶 6 个月加每周一次 LV 500mg/m² 滴注，持续 6~8 周（RoswellPark 方案）疗效优于氟尿嘧啶联合长春新碱+CCNU 方案[302]，无病生存期从 64%增加至 73%，总生存期从 77%增加至 84%，此报道与其他关于氟尿嘧啶+LV 的前瞻性随机试验结果一致。

有大量关于氟尿嘧啶剂量的规定。在辅助治疗方面，这些规定包括每四周连续 5 天快速静脉推注，这就是所谓的 Mayo Clinic 法；每 8 周连续静脉推注 6 天，或者 Roswell Park 法；静脉灌注法。与转移性癌治疗不同，连续静脉灌注氟尿嘧啶与辅助治疗中静脉推注方法相比较并没有显示出优越性。各种剂量使用方法没有证据显示出 DFS 或 OS 的差异，但是这些方法在毒性反应方面却有所不同[360,361]。

口服治疗的便利性和避免长期静脉通路并发症（如血栓形成和感染）的前景推动了口服氟哌利多的发展。卡培他滨是一种氟嘧啶氨基甲酸酯，其在三步酶促级联反应中转化为氟尿嘧啶。临床前研究表明，卡培他滨对肿瘤细胞具有选择性，因为最终的酶转化涉及胸苷磷酸化酶，与正常组织相比，优先在肿瘤中表达[362,363]。每日两次口服给药类似连续输注氟尿嘧啶泵，而费用和使用不便远次于静脉泵入。

X-ACT 试验表明，在辅助治疗方面卡培他滨疗效至少等同于静脉推注氟尿嘧啶[362]。这一项非劣效试验随机分配 1 987 名Ⅲ期结肠癌术后患者行卡培他滨 1 250mg/m² 每日两次，每三周连续两周停一周，持续 6 个月，或者每天静脉推注氟尿嘧啶 425mg/m²+LV 20mg/m²，28 天为一周期，每一周期第 1~5 天（Mayo 方案），卡培他滨组 3 年无病生存率为 64.2%，而静脉推注氟尿嘧啶组为 60.6%，$HR=0.87$，$P<0.001$。副作用特征略有不同，卡培他滨的手足综合征风险增加，但中性粒细胞减少和口腔炎的减少明显改善。

基于奥沙利铂的方案

奥沙利铂是第三代铂化合物，可交联 DNA 并诱导细胞凋亡。奥沙利铂具有与其他铂类化合物（如顺铂和卡铂）不同的特性。临床前试验模型表明奥沙利铂在顺铂抵抗的结直肠癌细胞和联合氟尿嘧啶方面具有独特的活性[360]。奥沙利铂几乎不引起肾毒性，耳毒性和脱发，但是骨髓抑制和其引起的神经毒性是可逆的、具有剂量累积效应，并且在患者受凉时加重[364~367]。

初步研究显示其在转移性分组中的功效后，奥沙利铂迅速转移至辅助治疗。MOSAIC 试验随机分配 2 246 例Ⅱ期（淋巴结阴性）和Ⅲ期患者接受奥沙利铂，亚叶酸和氟尿嘧啶（FOLFOX-4）联合或输注氟尿嘧啶/LV[364,366,367]。静脉灌注氟尿嘧啶以 28 天为一周期，每 2 周一次，滴注 LV 200mg/m² 超过 2h，静脉推注氟尿嘧啶 400mg/m²，然后在第 1、2 天静脉灌注氟尿嘧啶 600mg/m²。FOLFOX-4 包括相同的氟尿嘧啶/LV 方案，在 28 天周期内每 2 周加入奥沙利铂 85mg/m²，一次超过 2h[344]。FOLFOX-4 方案和氟尿嘧啶/LV 方案无病生存率分别为 78.2% 和 72.9%。亚组分析显示Ⅲ期患者通过两组方案在 DFS 获益方面（FOLFOX-4 方案和氟尿嘧啶/LV 方案 DFS 分别为 72%、65%）优于Ⅱ期患者（FOLFOX-4 方案和氟尿嘧啶/LV 方案 DFS 分别为 87%、84%，$P=ns$）。奥沙利铂方案使用仍然因其神经剂量毒性作用而受到限制，在试验期间 12%患者在试验期间出现严重神经毒性，但是 18 个月后严重神经毒性患者降至 0.5%[364,366]。2009 年，来自 MOSAIC 试验的长期结果，显示 5 年 DFS 的统计学显著改善（73.3% vs 67.4%）[368]。在Ⅲ期患者中，6 年 OS 有相应的改善（72.9% vs 68.7%）；然而，对于Ⅱ期患者，OS 没有统计学上的显著差异。此外，对 MOSAIC 试验的亚组分析表明，Ⅱ期和Ⅲ期的老年患者（70~75 岁）没有从奥沙利铂联合氟尿嘧啶/LV 中获益（OS 的风险比为 1.1）[369]。奥沙利铂的益处似乎不依赖于氟尿嘧啶/LV 的使用方法。NSABP C-07 试验将 2 407 名Ⅱ/Ⅲ期结肠癌患者随机分为每周注射氟尿嘧啶/LV（Roswell Park 方案）或 FLOX（双周奥沙利铂联合相同的氟尿嘧啶/LV 方案）[365]。在 *HR* 和 DFS 方面的提高两种方案与 MOSAIC 试验相似。奥沙利铂组 3 年总生存率和无病生存率的比例分别为 76.5%和 71.6%[365]。尽管 FLOX 的疗效与 MOSAIC 试验中使用的输注氟尿嘧啶相似，但是 FLOX 方案轻微的增加了毒性反应，且增加了腹泻和脱水的风险。

基于伊立替康的化疗方案

伊立替康是一种喜树碱衍生物，通过加速 DNA 裂解和提高 DNA 转录和复制时解螺旋化[370]。两个随机对照试验表明伊立替康联合氟尿嘧啶/LV 作为一线治疗方案治疗转移性结直肠癌疗效优于单独使用氟尿嘧啶/LV[371,372]。尽管在晚期结直肠癌治疗方面使患者获益得到改善，但三项大型试验的初步结果不支持在辅助治疗中使用伊立替康。CALGB C89803 比较推注伊立替康联合氟尿嘧啶/LV（IFL）和单独使用氟尿嘧啶/LV，发现Ⅲ~Ⅳ级毒性增加（中性粒细胞减少，中性粒细胞减少性发热和治疗期间死亡）而 DFS 没有改善[373]。PETACC-3 和 Accord02/FFCD9802 试验比较了 IFL 方案也发现Ⅲ结肠癌患者在实验组增加了毒性反应而没有提高 DFS[374]。在这些试验的基础上，基于伊立替康的方案不值得在辅助化疗中推荐[373,374]。

伊立替康在肝脏中被水解为其活性代谢物 SN-38，而后者又被尿苷二磷酸葡糖醛酸转移酶同种型 1A1（UGT1A1）葡萄糖醛酸化为无活性形式[370]。与伊立替康相关的不良事件，包括腹泻、骨髓抑制和恶心或呕吐，已在回顾性研究中显示与 UGT1A1 的多态性相关[370]。

FDA 已经批准了一个诊断试验，同时若干基于药物代谢酶类的基因药物组学的伊立替康剂量调整的试验也进行了相关研究，证实了上述机制的存在[370]。

生物制剂

最近 FDA 批准的治疗转移性结肠癌的两种药物是靶向生物制剂，而不是标准的细胞毒性药物。这两种药物都是单克隆抗体。贝伐单抗针对 VEGF 通路，西妥昔单抗针对表皮生长因子受体（EGFR）通路。

贝伐单抗是一种针对 VEGF 的人源化重组单克隆抗体。

贝伐单抗通过结合配体和阻止 VEGF 受体的信号传递，干扰肿瘤供血血管生长。两项Ⅲ期临床试验显示，在转移环境中，贝伐单抗与氟尿嘧啶联合奥沙利铂或伊立替康的方案，DFS 和 OS 均有改善[375,376]。这些临床试验发现贝伐单抗的副作用包括可逆性高血压和蛋白尿，罕见重度反应，但这两种副作用并不明显，其主要副作用包括胃肠道穿孔、伤口开裂、出血和凝血[375,376]。AVANT 试验比较了 FOLFOX4、FOLFOX4 联合贝伐单抗、XELOX 联合贝伐单抗对Ⅲ期或高危Ⅱ期结肠癌患者的疗效[377]。本试验发现，将贝伐单抗添加到以奥沙利铂为基础的辅助化疗药物中并没有改善 DFS，并提示可能导致 OS 降低。NSABP C-08 试验比较了在Ⅱ期和Ⅲ期结肠癌切除患者中，改良的 FOLFOX6 方案联合贝伐单抗与单独使用改良的 FOLFOX6 相比，发现加贝伐单抗不会增加 3 年 DFS[378]。

西妥昔单抗是一种作用于 EGFR 的单克隆抗体，参与多种生长信号通路。西妥昔单抗在 2004 年获得 FDA 批准用于治疗伊立替康抵抗的转移性疾病。在伊立替康抵抗性疾病中，使用西妥昔单抗/伊立替康治疗的患者的缓解率为 22%，而在随机Ⅱ期试验中，使用西妥昔单抗治疗的患者缓解率为 11%[379]。西妥昔单抗的副作用相对较轻，大多数患者在面部、胸部和背部出现痤疮样皮疹[379]。过敏反应也较常见，但不像贝伐单抗引发的过敏反应，西妥昔单抗过敏反应并不是全身的[379]。美国 N0147 试验比较有无西妥昔单抗的 FOLFOX-4 方案，发现无论患者是野生型或突变 KRAS，在切除的Ⅲ期结肠癌患者中未发现 3 年 DFS 存在差异[380]。此外，西妥昔单抗治疗的患者中三级不良事件和未能完成 12 个周期的治疗明显更多。

总结建议

辅助化疗获益大小总是与基于术后病理分期的复发和转移风险相关[381,382]。对于Ⅲ期（淋巴结阳性）患者，证据支持术后追加 6 个月辅助化疗。FOLFOX-4 具有最令人信服的疗效数据，但与氟尿嘧啶/LV 单药相比，其毒性增加。卡培他滨是静脉注射氟尿嘧啶/LV 的合理替代品。基于伊立替康的治疗方案在结肠癌辅助化疗方案的选择上并不值得推荐，但是贝伐单抗和西妥昔单抗用于结肠癌辅助治疗的效果有待于长期随访数据的证实。对于Ⅱ期（淋巴结阴性）患者，患者获益已被证实但获益并不多，目前的临床试验在Ⅱ期患者进行辅助化疗使患者获益方面的数据还不具有足够的说服力，因此Ⅱ期患者是否行辅助化疗有待进一步研究。根据 NCCN 实践指南，如果术后病理结果提示伴有高危因素例如分化程度低、淋巴管或血管见脉管瘤栓、术前伴有肠梗阻、淋巴结清扫数目少于 12 枚、肠穿孔或直接侵犯周围其他器官，推荐使用 FOLFOX-4 或氟尿嘧啶进行术后化疗[382]。对于没有高危特征的Ⅱ期患者，建议进行观察或参与临床试验[382]。

辅助化疗在老年患者中的作用仍然存在争议，特别是在基于氟尿嘧啶联合奥沙利铂的方案。虽然 MOSAIC 试验未能证实氟尿嘧啶/LV 联合奥沙利铂的益处[369]，三项随机临床试验荟萃分析提示基于氟尿嘧啶的辅助治疗的效果在老年患者（≥70 岁）仍然较好，毒性作用也与年轻患者相似，除了在一项研究中提示老年患者行辅助治疗中性粒细胞减少症发生率升高[383,384]。

直肠癌的新辅助和辅助治疗

对于结肠癌，外科手术切除仍然是治愈的根本治疗措施。然而，与结肠癌不同的是，在根治性手术切除术后，直肠癌局部复发导致治疗失败的比例更高，通过对外科手术标准的改进例如完整的 TME 切除术显著降低但并没有完全消除局部复发的风险。补救性外科手术难度非常大，常常失败并且伴有一定的手术死亡风险，因此，直肠癌辅助治疗规范与结肠癌显著不同的是通过放射治疗来降低局部复发的风险。

辅助化疗及放射治疗

二十世纪八九十年代的研究巩固了术后放化疗相对于单纯手术和术后放疗的优越性。放化疗能够降低局部复发的风险和远处转移的风险，并且能够降低死亡风险[385~387]。在这些研究中，放化疗主要使用司莫司汀+氟尿嘧啶，司莫司汀的副作用包括有较少的患者出现急性髓细胞性白血病，因而不在用于直肠癌辅助化疗[388]。北美组间试验证实，单用氟尿嘧啶而不联合司莫司汀患者获益不会有所提高，因此建议放疗的同时静脉持续灌注氟尿嘧啶[389]。对比持续静脉灌注氟尿嘧啶（每天 225mg/m^2，连续 5 周）和静脉推注氟尿嘧啶（500mg/m^2，第 1～3 天和第 36～39 天），4 年复发率由 63%降至 53%，生存率也由 60%提高至 70%。与结肠癌不同，用 LV 或左旋咪唑进行生物调节并没有提高氟尿嘧啶在直肠癌中的疗效。联合研究 0144 比较了持续全身治疗与放疗时灌注氟尿嘧啶、放疗前后 4 周、放疗时联合应用氟尿嘧啶和持续灌注氟尿嘧啶的疗效。研究发现，三组患者的无复发生存率和 OS 无差异[390]。2012 试验比较基于卡培他滨的放化疗（2 500mg/m^2，第 1～14 天，第 22 天重复一次，50.4Gy+卡培他滨 1 650mg/m^2，第 1～38 天，随后三周期卡培他滨）与基于氟尿嘧啶的放疗方案（2 周期氟尿嘧啶 500mg/m^2，第 1～5 天、第 29 天给药，放化疗 50.4Gy 联合滴注氟尿嘧啶，再给 2 周期氟尿嘧啶），发现卡培他滨在Ⅱ～Ⅲ期直肠癌患者中的 5 年 OS、3 年 DFS 和局部复发方面均不劣于氟尿嘧啶[391]。远处转移在卡培他滨组较少见。两组之间的不良反应有所不同，接受氟尿嘧啶的患者中白细胞减少症更常见，卡培他滨组中的手足皮肤反应，疲劳和直肠炎更常见。因此，在辅助放化疗方案中，氟尿嘧啶是一个合理的替代方案。一般来说，对于 T3 及更高或淋巴结阳性的肿瘤，推荐辅助治疗。放射治疗应针对肿瘤床，包括 2～5cm 的边缘以及骶前淋巴结和髂内淋巴结。如果进行 APR 手术，会阴伤口应包括在放射野中[392]。

新辅助化疗和放疗

新辅助治疗在直肠癌治疗中有重大作用，因为新辅助治疗可以使部分患者降期从而增加手术切除概率、增加保留肛门括约肌的概率、通过减少术后恢复时间而增加患者顺应度。瑞典的直肠癌试验首次表明，与单纯手术相比，短期高剂量术前放疗方案降低了局部复发率，提高了生存率[393]。德国Ⅲ期 EORTC 22921 研究是第一个比较新辅助氟尿嘧啶/放疗与术后辅助氟尿嘧啶/放疗疗效的研究[394]。肿瘤浸润深度达到或超过 T3 或者伴有淋巴结阳性（N1）的患者被随机分配到术前或术后辅助放化疗组。在第 1 周和第 5 周，用氟尿嘧啶（1 000mg/m^2/120h 以上）同时照射两组（5 040Gy/28F）。所有患者均接受 4 个月的额外全身氟尿嘧啶治疗。该研究没有发现 OS 的改善，但是术前治疗能够降低局部复发风险（术后 5 年复发率分别为 6%、13%），术前放疗联合氟尿嘧啶化疗能够减少急性和慢性毒性反应、增加血管顺应性、增加低位直肠癌保留肛门括约肌率。有趣的是,术后病理结果发现肿瘤退变显著或淋巴结阴性患者预后较好[394]。2012 年,德国试验的长期结果公布。在 10 年的研究中,术前放化疗与辅助放化疗相比,局部控制得到改善。然而,OS 并没有差异[395]。新辅助化疗有几个理论上的好处。首先,最终实施保留括约肌切除术的可能性增加。虽然有两项研究显示括约肌保存率较高[394,396],但其他大型荟萃分析对这些发现提出了质疑。在切除过程中,粘连可导致肠固定在骨盆内。术前和术后进行放疗相比,可以避免每天对同一段固定肠段进行放疗。第三个好处是切除前存在完整的血管系统,这可能导致更好的组织氧合和对放疗具有更好的反应。

短程放射治疗

短程放射治疗(如瑞典或欧洲方案)指的是 5 天的 25Gy 放射治疗并不匹配化疗方案。最初,试验显示,与单纯手术相比,短期术前放疗可提高局部复发率和 OS。然而,对该研究人群的一项后期分析表明,接受短程放射治疗的患者手术后胃肠道并发症的发生率更高,最明显的是肠阻塞[399]。在一项针对 1 300 多名患者的大型随机试验中,将没有任何辅助治疗的短期术前放疗与切缘阳性患者的术后放化疗进行比较[400]。短程放射治疗改善了局部复发率和 DFS,但 OS 无明显差异。最近,TME 试验比较了短期放疗患者和仅进行 TME 患者的局部复发改进情况(5% vs 11%),没有增加相应的 OS[401]。虽然用短期 RT 治疗的Ⅲ期周围边缘阴性、淋巴结阴性患者的 OS 明显改善,但患者中 CRC 特异性死亡率的改善可以通过其他死亡原因的增加来抵消。只有一项随机试验直接将短程高剂量放疗与常规术前放化疗进行比较,结果显示局部复发,RFS 或 OS 没有改善[402]。短疗程放疗与传统长疗程放化疗的局部控制率相同;然而,总生存率的改善尚未得到重视,对围术期毒性增加的担忧仍然存在。

总结建议

新辅助放化疗已被证明使近一半的患者肿瘤分期降低,病理完全反应高达 20%[403]。因此,尽管术前放化疗对比术后放化疗并没有延长患者生存期,但是相关研究结论提示术前放化疗仍然是局部进展期结直肠癌患者可选的治疗方案,术前放化疗能够提高肿瘤患者顺应率、改善局部控制率、减少毒副反应、改善相关术后脏器功能和增加低位直肠癌患者保肛概率。尽管没有相关试验证明行术前新辅助放化疗,手术后行基于氟尿嘧啶的化疗方案能够改善患者预后,NCCN 指南仍然推荐新辅助放化疗达到完全病理缓解(PCR)的患者术后有必要行含有氟尿嘧啶的方案进行化疗。

肝转移化疗

转化治疗

经慎重选择的肝转移患者初始不能进行手术切除的肝转移病灶,如果对化疗反应好,这些患者可能获得手术切除肝转移灶的机会。这种方法被称为“转化疗法”,以区别于“新辅助治疗”,后者适用于术前可切除化疗,给那些出现明显可切除疾病的患者。在这种情况下,选择特定方案的关键数不是生存率或改善的生活质量,而是缓解率。NCCN 目前推荐任何在转移情况下有效的化疗方案,因为转化疗法的目标不是治疗隐匿性疾病,而是获得将不可切除转移转化为可切除状态所需的肿瘤消退[404]。研究方案包括 FOLFIRI[405],FOLFOX[406],FOLFOXIRI[407,408]。12%~40%的初始不可切除的结直肠癌单发肝转移患者在进行转化治疗后肿瘤成功降期,能够完整切除肿瘤[404~408]。经转变治疗后手术切除肝转移灶患者 5 年生存率为 30%~35%,这一结果好于行单纯化疗的患者。在一项大型研究中,1 104 例最初无法切除的 CRC 肝转移患者中,138 例(12.5%)能够在化疗后进行切除,化疗主要包括氟尿嘧啶/LV 联合奥沙利铂(705)、伊立替康(7%)或两者联合(4%)[409]。5 年和 10 年生存率分别为 33%和 23%。靶向药物和生物制剂已在转化环境中与已建立的化疗方案联合进行测试。添加西妥昔单抗(EGFR 抑制剂)可显著提高野生型 KRAS 患者的可切除性;然而,对 OS 的影响仍然存在争议[410~412]。最近,贝伐单抗已与现有的化疗联合尝试应用于不可切除疾病[413~415]。虽然贝伐单抗联合伊立替康治疗方案在转化率上可能有一定的改善[413,414],但以奥沙利铂为基础的治疗方案没有观察到同样的效果[415]。综上所述,在这种情况下,单靠化疗是无法治愈的,因为大多数影像学上完全反应的病灶都含有活的肿瘤。因此,即使患者获得影像学完全临床反应,手术切除仍然是必要的措施。

肝转移的新辅助治疗

有证据表明,围术期化疗可改善初期可切除肝转移患者的无进展生存期和 DFS;然而,它对 OS 的影响还有待证实。患者从术前或术后的治疗中获益更多还不清楚[416]。新辅助化疗对可切除肝转移患者的理论获益包括保证这些患者将接受系统治疗(与无法耐受术后治疗的患者相比),以及与接受辅助化疗的患者相比更早开始系统治疗。EORTC 试验随机分配了 364 名患者,其中有多达 4 个转移瘤患者之前没有接触过奥沙利铂,他们接受了肝切除手术,同时接受了或没有接受 FOLFOX-4 围术期化疗[417]。术前化疗 6 个周期,术后化疗 6 个周期。182 名接受化疗的患者中有 67 人出现化疗客观反应,11 人疾病进展,其中 8 人认为是不可切除。总体而言,83%的患者成功手术切除,与单纯手术组成功切除的人数 84%相似。然而,化疗组术后并发症发生率明显高于对照组(25% vs 16%)。接受围术期化疗的患者肝功能衰竭、胆道瘘和腹腔内感染的发生率较高。两组术后死亡率相似。有越来越多的证据表明,对于可切除的肝转移患者,术前化疗,尤其是伊立替康或奥沙利铂方案与肝脏脂肪变性,血管损伤,结节状增生有关[409,418,419]。此外,有证据表明,在对新辅助治疗有完全放疗反应的患者,大多数转移部位都有活的癌细胞[420]。这对新辅助治疗后的手术计划提出了重大挑战。

肝切除后的辅助治疗

大多数学者认为结直肠癌肝转移瘤切除术后仍然需要行辅助治疗,虽然目前缺乏相应数据来支持这一观点。在这一方面仍有许多未知因素,包括切除的时间、最佳药物组合、治疗计划和疗程。由于结直肠癌一旦出现肝转移,则认为属于Ⅳ期,化疗方案多为期 4~6 个月的 FOLFOX-4 或者 FOLFIRI 化疗[421]。虽然目前缺乏相应数据支持,但是仍然推荐Ⅱ/Ⅲ患者化疗方案应加入靶向生物制剂。出于对伤口并发症和其他组织损伤的考虑,推荐在外科手术术前或术后进行非连续 8 周的贝伐单抗治疗[422]。

总结建议

关于哪些结直肠癌肝转移患者应该立刻行外科手术治疗、

合适进行新辅助治疗的问题，目前还没有一个统一的认识。但是，由于越来越多研究的发现新辅助化疗后肝损伤，促使越来越多的外科医师选择初始直接手术治疗，以降低手术风险，对于潜在可切除转移灶的患者，先进行手术治疗，然后进行辅助化疗[423]。另一方面，新辅助化疗适用于风险较高或有交界可切除或不可切除肝转移的患者。然而，化疗结束到手术治疗的间隔应该严格控制，应经常进行影像学检查评估治疗反应，一旦转移灶变得可以明确切除，就应立即进行手术。

转移性结肠癌

在过去二十年中，转移性结肠癌的治疗取得了前所未有的进展，但作为治疗其他实体肿瘤模型的进展并不十分迅速。在氟尿嘧啶为唯一治疗结直肠癌药物的时期，OS 为 11~12 个月，而现在，平均中位生存期已经延长至 2 年。这一巨大进步主要归功于新的治疗药物的问世。现在拥有了三种不同类型的具有显著抗肿瘤活性的一线化学疗法（氟嘧啶、伊立替康和奥沙利铂），以及多种靶向和生物疗法，在转移性结肠癌治疗中有新的作用（如西妥昔单抗、贝伐单抗、帕尼单抗和瑞格非尼）。对于大多数患者而言，治疗的目标将是姑息性治疗而不是治愈，治疗目标是延长 OS 并尽可能长时间地维持患者生活质量（QOL）。对于多数不可治愈性转移性 CRC 患者，合理设计的二联用药，如 FOLFOX 方案或 FOLFIRI 方案，应被视为一线姑息治疗的标准化疗方案。这些方案具有良好活性和可耐受的毒性反应。其他合适的方案包括 XELOX、氟尿嘧啶/LV、卡培他滨和 FOLFOXIRI。

FOLFOX 方案

第一个大规模随机Ⅲ期临床试验招纳了 420 患者，比较了氟尿嘧啶/LV 和 FOLFOX-4 疗效的差异[367]。患者接受静脉输注 LV 200mg/m^2 2h 后紧接静脉推注氟尿嘧啶 400mg/m^2，然后连续 22h 持续静脉输注氟尿嘧啶 600mg/m^2，上述药物每 2 周连续使用 2 天。一半的患者在第一天进行连续 2h 静脉输注奥沙利铂 85mg/m^2[367]。与对照组相比，接受 FOLFOX-4 的患者具有显著更长的 PFS（中位数 9.0m vs 6.2m；P=0.000 3）和更好的治疗缓解率（50.7% vs 22.3%；P=0.000 1）。然而，虽然可以看到有增长趋势，但 OS 的改善并没有达到统计学意义（中位数，16.2m vs 14.7m，P=0.12）[367]。由于这项欧洲试验中缺乏生存获益而推迟了 FOLFOX 在美国的批准。不久之后，NCCTG 和全美合作协会主导了 N9741 试验项目，该试验项目是一个Ⅲ期临床试验，将受试者分为三组[424]。奥沙利铂 85mg/m^2 联合伊立替康 200mg/m^2 即 IROX 化疗方案，或者奥沙利铂 85mg/m^2 联合氟尿嘧啶/LV 即 FOLFOX-4 化疗方案[424]。最终结果显示，接受 FOLFOX-4 治疗的患者的平均中位进展时间为 8.7 个月，应答率为 45%，中位生存时间为 19.5 个月。这些结果显著优于 IFL（分别为 6.9m、31% 和 15.0m）或 IROX（分别为 6.5m、35% 和 1.4m）[424]。FOLFOX-4 通常具有良好的耐受性，但它与如上所述的显著更高的感觉神经病变率相关。近期改良的 FOLFOX6 已经成为 FOLFOX 方案的首选给药方案[425]。

卡培他滨/XELOX 方案

卡培他滨是一种口服活性氟嘧啶，患者可以口服，免除了患者中央静脉置管和卧床静脉输注的痛苦。至少有 5 项随机Ⅲ期临床试验直接比较了 XELOX（卡培他滨、奥沙利铂）与 FOLFOX 对转移性 CRC 一线或二线化疗的影响[426,427]。没有证据显示 XELOX 方案在肿瘤缓解率、PFS 或者 OS 方面的效果次于 FOLFOX-4 方案。但是在几乎所有情况下，XELOX 的 PFS 和 OS 曲线均次于 FOLFOX。但是没有一项试验结果显示两种化疗方案肿瘤反应率、PFS 和 OS 有显著差异。因此，这些可靠的试验数据均支持 XELOX 作为 FOLFOX 非劣效替代方案。

FOLFIRI 方案

伊立替康的疗效最初在一项随机前瞻性临床试验联合或者不联合标准静脉推注氟尿嘧啶/LV 得到了证实[372]。联合方案被称为 IFL 方案，包括氟尿嘧啶 500mg/m^2，LV 20mg/m^2 和伊立替康 125mg/m^2，每 6 周一次，连续给药 4 周。伊立替康每周 125mg/m^2，每 6 周一次，连续 4 周，并且使用如上所述的标准 Mayo 方案给予氟尿嘧啶/LV[372]。三种药物方案优于氟尿嘧啶/LV 或单独使用伊立替康，后者产生与氟尿嘧啶/LV 方案相似的结果。在 IFL 和 Mayo 方案的比较中，中位 PFS 从 4.3 个月提高到 7.0 个月，并且中位 OS 从 12.6 个月提高到 14.8 个月[372]。FOLFIRI 方案是 IFL 方案的一个改进方案，FOLFIRI 方案同时也有大量改良类型，但是其中使用最多的方案为伊立替康 180mg/m^2 每周一给药，每周 LV 400mg/m^2 静脉推注后进行氟尿嘧啶 400mg/m^2 静脉推注，然后持续 46h 静脉灌注氟尿嘧啶 2 400mg/m^2，每 14 天作为一疗程。一项欧洲试验对比了 FOLFIRI 和 FOLFOX 方案作为转移性结直肠癌一线化疗方案。尽管多数学者认为该实验规模较小，但是该实验的结论仍然具有较高可信度，该实验结果认为这两种方案的肿瘤缓解率和平均生存期相似。这些数据得到了 Gruppo Oncologico Dell'Italia Meridionale 在 2005 年多中心试验的进一步支持，其中 360 名患者被随机分配到 FOLFIRI 而不是 FOLFOX4。缓解率，进展时间，缓解持续时间在两组之间没有差异。

在 XELOX 被广泛认为是 FOLFOX 方案的替代方案的同时，XELIRI 方案（联合卡培他滨和伊立替康）作为 FOLFIRI 方案替代方案的情况却有所不同。卡培他滨和伊立替康具有部分重叠的毒副反应，特别是在腹泻方面。伊立替康联合卡培他滨潜在的更重的毒副反是两者联合使用的不利条件，也使得在两者联合用药时剂量和使用时序方面困难重重。

FOLFOXIRI

最近有两项试验比较转移性 CRC 患者的 FOLFOXIRI 与 FOLFIRI。GONO 试验随机分配了 244 例未接受治疗的转移性、不可切除的 CRC 患者接受 FOLFOXIRI 或 FOLFIRI。每两周给予 FOLFOXIRI，在第 1 天给予伊立替康（165mg/m^2），奥沙利铂（85mg/m^2）和 LV（200mg/m^2），并且在第 1 天开始以 48h 连续输注给予氟尿嘧啶。FOLFIRI 组的部分缓解率较高（44% vs 66%），但是完全缓解率没有差异。FOLFOXIRI 组患者更有机会完全切除肝转移灶（12% vs 36%）。最重要的是，PFS 和 OS 在 FOLFOXIRI 组中均有显著改善（分别为 7m vs 10m 和 17m vs 23m）。HORG 试验还将 FOLFOXIRI 与 FOLFIRI 进行了比较，FOLFOXIRI 给药方案略有不同。在该试验中，各组之间的 OS，疾病进展时间或缓解率无差异。此外，FOLFOXIRI 与较高的毒副作用相关，包括脱发、腹泻和神经毒性。

贝伐单抗

在随机临床试验上，结直肠癌是第一个被发现抗 VEGF 有疗效的恶性肿瘤。在一项关键的早期试验中，静脉推注 IFL 方案联合贝伐单抗显著的提高肿瘤治疗反应率,由 35%上升至 45%;PFS 从 7.1 个月延长到 10.4 个月,更重要的是,总生存期从 15.6 个月提高到 20.3 个月。该试验中的不良事件在治疗中相似,但有一些明显的例外。接受贝伐单抗治疗的患者中有 11%出现 3 度高血压,1.5%患者出现肠梗阻。IFL 组中没有患者出现此类问题。ECOG 3200 试验比较了 FOLFOX 与贝伐单抗/FOLFOX 联合治疗的效果。联合治疗组的中位生存期为 12.5 个月,而 FOLFOX 组为 10.7 个月。这证实了贝伐单抗确实显著增加了基于奥沙利铂的方案的效力。从 2004 年开始,贝伐单抗成为大多数转移性结直肠癌患者一线化疗方案的标准用药,不管其化疗方案是 FOLFOX、XELOX 还是 FOLFOX。关于贝伐单抗在晚期中加入已建立的治疗方案,与未接受过预先辅助治疗的患者相比,FOLFOXIRI/贝伐单抗似乎与 FOLFIRI/贝伐单抗相比具有更高的无进展生存率和缓解率。FOLFOXIRI/贝伐单抗也被发现在肝转移患者的转化治疗中优于 FOLFOX/贝伐单抗(R0 切除率 49% vs 23%)。

抗 EGFR 单克隆抗体

CRYSTAL 试验和 CALGB 80203 试验均证实了西妥昔单抗联合含伊立替康的一线或二线治疗方案的疗效。在 CRYSTAL 试验中,1 198 名未经治疗的患者被随机分配到有或没有西妥昔单抗的 FOLFIRI 组。尽管西妥昔单抗的加入显著改善了 PFS,但增加仅为 0.9 个月。西妥昔单抗的加入也提高了缓解率,但仅提高了 8%。第二阶段 CALGB 80203 试验的早期结果,随机分配 283 名患者使用或不使用西妥昔单抗作为一线治疗的 FOLFOX 或 FOLFIRI,提供了支持 CRYSTAL 试验结果的确证数据。在一份初步报告中,有明确证明西妥昔单抗联合 FOLFOX 和 FOLFIRI 的缓解率增加,而对 PFS 的影响尚无定论。此外,回顾性分析 CRYSTAL 试验调查 *KRAS* 突变状态对 PFS 和缓解率的作用,结果显示,在 KRAS 野生型人群中,接受西妥昔单抗和 FOLFIRI 治疗的患者 1 年 PFS 率为 43%,而仅接受 FOLFIRI 的患者为 25%,联合治疗组的进展风险降低了 32%。然而,在 *KRAS* 突变体群体中,两组之间的 PFS 没有差异。该研究的长期结果应该很快就会公布。最近,对 14 项试验进行了荟萃分析,比较了使用或不使用抗 EGFR 单克隆抗体的效果,结果发现野生型 KRAS 患者的无进展生存期增加。在该分析中,具有 *KRAS* 突变的患者证明抗 EGFR 疗法没有临床获益。现在推荐所有转移性 CRC 患者进行 *KRAS* 基因分型。评估西妥昔单抗和帕尼单抗的其他试验已证实野生型 KRAS 患者的抗 EGFR 治疗有明显获益。建议不要在 *KRAS* 突变患者中使用抗 EGFR 治疗。最后,一些随机试验比较了贝伐珠单抗与抗 EGFR 治疗相比,在转移性野生型 KRAS CRC 患者的效果。这些数据对于两种组合的优越性益处仍然是不确定的。目前,对于患有野生型 KRAS 的转移性 CRC 患者,抗 EGFR 治疗或贝伐单抗作为一线方案的补充是可接受的治疗选择。

总结建议

对于不能手术的转移性结直肠癌患者,优先考虑综合治疗,对于姑息性治疗的患者,治疗策略应该是使患者尽可能多地接受所有的活性药物。实现上述目标的最佳策略是二联用药(如 FOLFOX、XELOX 或 FOLFIRI)作为基本化疗方案,这些方案只需增加另外一步即可作为二线治疗方案(如 FOLFOX 方案后再行 FOLFIRI 方案,或者 FOLFIRI 方案后再行 FOLFOX 方案)。无论选择何种方案,贝伐单抗都应被视为一线治疗的组成部分。野生型 KRAS 患者的西妥昔单抗治疗是贝伐单抗与化疗方案相结合的合理替代方案。

(马帅 李洋 译 田艳涛 校)

参考文献

The complete reference list can be found on the Wiley Companion Digital Edition of this title (see inside front cover for login instructions).

17 Van Weyenberg S, Meijerink MR, Jacobs MA, et al. *MR enteroclysis in the diagnosis of small-bowel neoplasms. Radiology.* 2010;**254(3)**:765–773.

21 Torroni F, Romeo E, Rea F, et al. *Conservative approach in Peutz-Jeghers syndrome: single-balloon enteroscopy and small bowel polypectomy. World J Gastrointest Endosc.* 2014;**16(6)**:318–323.

33 Boffetta P, Hazelton WD, Chen Y, et al. *Body mass, tobacco smoking, alcohol drinking and risk of cancer of the small intestine—a pooled analysis of over 500,000 subjects in the Asia Cohort Consortium. Ann Oncol.* 2012;**23(7)**:1894–1898.

52 Eom D, Hong SM, Kim J, et al. *Notch3 signaling is associated with MUC5AC expression and favorable prognosis in patients with small intestinal adenocarcinomas. Pathol Res Pract.* 2014;**210**:501–507.

53 Zaanan A, Meunier K, Sangar F, et al. *Microsatellite instability in colorectal cancer: from molecular oncogenic mechanisms to clinical implications. Cellular Oncology.* 2011;**34**:155–176.

60 Xiang X, Liu YW, Zhang L, et al. *A phase II study of modified FOLFOX as first-line chemotherapy in advanced small bowel adenocarcinoma. Anticancer Drugs.* 2012;**23(5)**:561–566.

77 Bartlett E, Roses RE, Gupta M, et al. *Surgery for metastatic neuroendocrine tumors with occult primaries. J Surg Res.* 2013;**184(1)**:221–227.

83 Amin S, Warner RR, Itzkowitz SH, Kim MK. *The risk of metachronous cancers in patients with small-intestinal carcinoid tumors: a US population-based study. Endocr Relat Cancer.* 2012;**19(3)**:381–387.

87 Pavel M, Hainsworth JD, Baudin E, et al. *Everolimus plus octreotide long-acting repeatable for the treatment of advanced neuroendocrine tumours associated with carcinoid syndrome (RADIANT-2): a randomised, placebo-controlled, phase 3 study. Lancet.* 2011;**378(9808)**:2005–2012.

96 Demetri GD, Antonia S, Benjamin RS, et al. *Soft tissue sarcoma. J Natl Compr Canc Netw.* 2007;**5(4)**:364–399.

113 Karakousis G, Singer S, Zheng J, et al. *Laparoscopic versus open gastric resections for primary gastrointestinal stromal tumors (GISTs): a size-matched comparison. Ann Surg Oncol.* 2011;**18(6)**:1599–1605.

114 Bischof D, Kim Y, Dodson R, Carolina Jimenez M, et al. *Open versus minimally invasive resection of gastric GIST: a multi-institutional analysis of short- and long-term outcomes. Ann Surg Oncol.* 2014;**9**:2941–2948.

115 Chok A, Koh YX, Ow MY, et al. *A systematic review and meta-analysis comparing pancreaticoduodenectomy versus limited resection for duodenal gastrointestinal stromal tumors. Ann Surg Oncol.* 2014;**11**:3429–3438.

116 Balachandran V, Cavna MJ, Zeng S, et al. *Imatinib potentiates antitumor T cell responses in gastrointestinal stromal tumor through the inhibition of Ido. Nat Med.* 2011;**17(9)**:1094–1100.

119 Joensuu H. *Twelve versus 36 months of adjuvant imatinib (IM) as treatment of operable GIST with a high risk of recurrence: final results of a randomized trial. J Clin Oncol.* 2011;**29(suppl; abstract LBA1)**.

122 Corless C, Ballman KV, Antonescu CR, et al. *Pathologic and molecular features correlate with long-term outcome after adjuvant therapy of resected primary GI stromal tumor: the ACOSOG Z9001 trial. J Clin Oncol.* 2014;**32(15)**:1563–1570.

139 Barrington S, Mikhaeel NG, Kostakoglu L, et al. *Role of imaging in the staging and response assessment of lymphoma: consensus of the International conference on malignant lymphomas imaging working group. J Clin Oncol.* 2014;**53**:5229.

146 Geramizadeh B, Keshtkar Jahromi M. *Primary extranodal gastrointestinal lymphoma: a single center experience from southern iran—report of changing epidemiology. Arch Iran Med.* 2014;**17(9)**:638–639.

165 Pape UF et al. *ENETS consensus guidelines for the management of patients with neuroendocrine neoplasms from the jejuno-ileum and the appendix including goblet cell carcinomas. Neuroendocrinology.* 2012;**95(2)**:135–156.

176 Andreasson H et al. *Outcome differences between debulking surgery and cytoreductive surgery in patients with Pseudomyxoma peritonei. Eur J Surg Oncol.* 2012;**38(10)**:962–968.

273 National Comprehensive Cancer Network (2014) *NCCN Clinical Practice Guidelines in Oncology (NCCN Guidelines®): Colorectal Cancer Screening. Version 1.2014.* May 19, http://www.nccn.org/professionals/physician_gls/pdf/colorectal_screening.pdf (accessed 24 March 2016).

295 Taylor FG, Quirke P, Heald RJ, et al. Magnetic resonance imaging in rectal can-

cer European equivalence study group. Preoperative magnetic resonance imaging assessment of circumferential resection margin predicts disease-free survival and local recurrence: 5-year follow-up results of the MERCURY study. *J Clin Oncol*. 2014;**32(1)**:34-43.

299 O'Connell MJ, Lavery I, Yothers G, et al. Relationship between tumor gene expression and recurrence in four independent studies of patients with stage II/III colon cancer treated with surgery alone or surgery plus adjuvant fluorouracil plus leucovorin. *J Clin Oncol*. 2010;**28(25)**:3937-3944.

300 Gray RG, Quirke P, Handley K, et al. Validation study of a quantitative multigene reverse transcriptase-polymerase chain reaction assay for assessment of recurrence risk in patients with stage II colon cancer. *J Clin Oncol*. 2011;**29(35)**:4611-4619.

301 Yothers G, O'Connell MJ, Lee M, et al. Validation of the 12-gene colon cancer recurrence score in NSABP C-07 as a predictor of recurrence in patients with stage II and III colon cancer treated with fluorouracil and leucovorin (FU/LV) and FU/LV plus oxaliplatin. *J Clin Oncol*. 2013;**31(36)**:4512-4519.

302 Srivastava G, Renfro LA, Behrens RJ, et al. Prospective multicenter study of the impact of oncotype DX colon cancer assay results on treatment recommendations in stage II colon cancer patients. *Oncologist*. 2014;**19(5)**:492-497.

335 van der Pas MH, Haglind E, Cuesta MA, et al. Laparoscopic versus open surgery for rectal cancer (COLOR II): short-term outcomes of a randomised, phase 3 trial. *The Lancet Oncology*. 2013;**14(3)**:210-218.

336 Aziz O, Constantinides V, Tekkis P, et al. Laparoscopic versus open surgery for rectal cancer: a meta-analysis. *Ann Surg Oncol*. 2006;**13**:413-424.

337 Gao F, Cao Y, Chen L. Meta-analysis of short-term outcomes after laparoscopic resection for rectal cancer. *Int J Colorectal Dis*. 2006;**21**:652-656.

339 Park JS, Choi GS, Park SY, Kim HJ, Ryuk JP. Randomized clinical trial of robot-assisted versus standard laparoscopic right colectomy. *Br J Surg*. 2012;**99(9)**:1219-1226.

340 Luca F, Ghezzi TL, Valvo M, et al. Surgical and pathological outcomes after right hemicolectomy: case-matched study comparing robotic and open surgery. *Int J Med Robot*. 2011;**7**:298-303.

342 Baik SH, Kwon HY, Kim JS, et al. Robotic versus laparoscopic low anterior resection of rectal cancer: short-term outcome of a prospective comparative study. *Ann Surg Oncol*. 2009;**16(6)**:1480-1487. doi:10.1245/s10434-009-0435-3.

343 Kim CW, Kim CH, Baik SH. Outcomes of robotic-assisted colorectal surgery compared with laparoscopic and open surgery: a systematic review. *J Gastrointest Surg*. 2014;**18**:816-830.

369 Tournigand C, André T, Bonnetain F, et al. Adjuvant therapy with fluorouracil and oxaliplatin in stage II and elderly patients (between ages 70 and 75 years) with colon cancer: subgroup analyses of the Multicenter International Study of Oxaliplatin, Fluorouracil, and Leucovorin in the Adjuvant Treatment of Colon Cancer trial. *J Clin Oncol*. 2012;**30(27)**:3353-3360.

371 Douillard J, Cunningham D, Roth A, et al. Irinotecan combined with fluorouracil compared with fluorouracil alone as first-line treatment for metastatic colorectal cancer: a multicentre randomized trial. *Lancet*. 2000;**255**: 1041-1048.

392 National Comprehensive Cancer Network (2014) *NCCN Clinical Practice Guidelines in Oncology (NCCN Guidelines®): Rectal Cancer. Version 1.2015*, http://www.nccn.org/professionals/physician_gls/pdf/rectal.pdf (accessed 24 March 2016).

394 Sauer R, Becker H, Hohenberer W, et al. German rectal cancer study group: preoperative versus postoperative chemoradiotherapy for rectal cancer. *N Engl J Med*. 2004;**351**:1731-1740.

400 Sebag-Montefiore D, Stephens RJ, Steele R, et al. Preoperative radiotherapy versus selective postoperative chemoradiotherapy in patients with rectal cancer (MRC CR07 and NCIC-CTG C016): a multicentre, randomised trial. *Lancet*. 2009;**373(9666)**:811-820.

401 van Gijn W, Marijnen CA, Nagtegaal ID, et al. van de Velde CJ; Dutch Colorectal Cancer Group. Preoperative radiotherapy combined with total mesorectal excision for resectable rectal cancer: 12-year follow-up of the multicentre, randomized controlled TME trial. *Lancet Oncol*. 2011;**12(6)**:575-582.

402 Ngan SY, Burmeister B, Fisher RJ, et al. Randomized trial of short-course radiotherapy versus long-course chemoradiation comparing rates of local recurrence in patients with T3 rectal cancer: trans-Tasman radiation oncology group trial 01.04. *J Clin Oncol*. 2012;**30(31)**:3827-3833.

403 Das P, Skibber JM, Rodriguez-Bigas MA, et al. Predictors of tumor response and downstaging in patients who receive preoperative chemoradiation for rectal cancer. *Cancer*. 2007;**109(9)**:1750-1755.

404 National Comprehensive Cancer Network (2014) *NCCN Clinical Practice Guidelines in Oncology (NCCN Guidelines®): Colon Cancer. Version 2.2015*, http://www.nccn.org/professionals/physician_gls/pdf/colon.pdf (accessed 24 March 2016).

第 95 章　肛周肿瘤

Bruce D. Minsky, MD ■ Jose G. Guillem, MD

概述

肛门癌是一种罕见的肿瘤，但是在过去的几十年里，肛门癌的发病率不断增加。这可能与人类乳头状瘤病毒以及人类免疫缺陷病毒的性传播相关。包括盆腔放疗和同时化疗（氟尿嘧啶联合丝裂霉素-C 或顺铂）在内的同步放化疗在保持大多数患者肛门括约肌功能的同时，也使患者的 5 年生存率达到了 80%左右。手术治疗适用于可予切除并可保留部分或全部的括约肌功能的 T1M0 患者，或同步放化疗之后可行腹会阴切除术（APR）的患者。

系统解剖学

肛门癌可发生于肛周皮肤或肛缘，肛管和直肠下部。肛管长 3~4cm，从肛缘延伸至盆底[1]。发生于肛管和肛缘的肿瘤有着不同的组织学起源。目前文献中对于“肛管”和“肛缘”的定义仍不一致。例如，有学者将肛管的末端界限定义为齿状线，所有发生在齿状线以下的肿瘤均定义为肛缘癌[2,3]，另有学者认为肛管的末端即为肛缘[4,5]，此外，另有学者将肛缘肿瘤定义为发生在距肛门边缘 5cm 以内的肿瘤[6]。

因此，解剖学分界不同，肛缘癌和肛管癌的发病率也不同。如果把肛管末端边缘定义为肛门外缘，则有 15%的肿瘤发生于肛缘部位，如果将齿状线作为肛管末端界限，则肛缘癌发病率会增长至 30%。为解决这一问题，美国癌症联合委员会（AJCC）和国际抗癌联盟（UICC）达成共识：肛管是从肛门直肠环（齿状线）延伸至肛门外缘[7,8]。这两个组织一致认为，肛缘癌的表现与皮肤癌相似，因此将其归类于皮肤肿瘤并予以治疗。

肛门周围有着广泛交通的淋巴系统。三个主要的途径包括：①主要沿直肠上血管至肠系膜下淋巴结；②从肛管上部到齿状线，沿直肠中血管和直肠下血管至下腹部淋巴结；③少数从肛缘和肛管至腹股沟浅淋巴结。

流行病学

在美国，肛门区域的癌症占全部大肠癌的 1%~2%，占肛门直肠癌的 4%。自 1997 年以来，肛门原位癌（CIS）和鳞状细胞癌（SCC）的发病率显著上升。然而，更多的男性则更有可能被诊断为 CIS[9]。2014 年，美国估计共有 7 210 例肛门区癌症病例，其中男性 2 660 例，女性 4 550 例[10]。这些患者中，预计将有 950 人死亡。

病因学

HPV 感染

肛门鳞状细胞癌与 HPV（人乳头瘤病毒）密切相关，其中最常见的类型为 HPV16 和 HPV18。来自斯堪的纳维亚的一项基于人群的病例对照研究中，共调查了 417 名肛门癌患者的一系列行为因素，包括：性活动、性病感染、烟草消费和肛门炎症病变[11]。通过单因素和多因素分析发现，性伴侣的数量与肛门癌的风险呈正相关。同时还提到了不论男女，性病感染与肛门癌也存在相关性。

肛门上皮内瘤变（AIN）在异性恋男性群体中少见，而在与 HIV（人类免疫缺陷病毒）阴性的男性同性恋群体中发生率为 5%~30%。而这种情况在 HIV 阴性的女性群体中少见。AIN 与 HPV 感染有关，在男性同性恋和免疫抑制的人群，特别是 HIV 阳性的患者中常见[12,13]。在 Surawicz 等[14]人的一份报道中，90 名肛管检查发现异常的男同性恋中，89%出现 HPV 相关的病变。最近的一项荟萃分析纳入了 53 项探讨 HPV 感染与男同性恋群体关系的试验，结果显示，肛门 HPV 与肛门 SCC 前体非常相似[15]。HPV-16 在艾滋病毒阳性患者中的总患病率为 35%，而在艾滋病毒阴性患者中的总患病率为 13%。然而，进展到癌症的比率远远低于宫颈癌前病变所报道的比率。

HIV（人体免疫缺陷病毒）

HIV 感染和肛门癌的发生有明确的相关性。将美国 AIDS 数据库同癌症数据库进行交叉比对发现，与普通人群中男性相比，同时或随后确诊为 AIDS 的男同性恋中肛管癌发生的相对危险度为 84.1[16]。在确诊为 AIDS 之前 5 年，肛门癌发生的相对危险度为 13.9。

肛管癌和 AIN 与湿疣相关[13]。HPV-16 感染与高级别 AIN 和肛门生殖区恶性肿瘤有很强相关性。然而，很多 HPV 细胞学检测阳性的患者没有发展为 AIN 或肛门癌，因此单纯 HPV 感染可能不足以导致恶变[17]。

分子因素

接受 CMT 的患者中 p53 蛋白的过度表达现象已经被研究。一项对包含参与肿瘤放射治疗组（RTOG）87~04 协议中近 20%的患者的分析发现，*p53* 过度表达的患者有预后较差的趋势（局部控制率和生存率下降）[18]。在一项包含 55 名患者的研究中，使用 MIB-1 小鼠单克隆抗体检测 KI-67 未能成功预测接受放疗±化学治疗患者的预后[19]。Patel 等人提出，可能通过

PI3K-AKT 通路激活的 AKT 是 SCCS 发生的一个组成部分[20]。一项包含 142 名接受 CMT 治疗的丹麦肛管 SCC 患者的队列研究中，p16 阳性率是影响疾病特异性和总体生存率的独立预后因素[21]。在 Williams 等人的报道中，174 例肛缘和肛管 SCC 患者血清 SCC 抗原的升高与获得临床完全缓解（cCR）、局部控制或更长生存期的机会降低有关[22]。Fraunholz 报道，EGFR 表达与预后相关[23]。一篇对 21 项已发表试验中 29 种生物学标志的系统综述认为，*p53* 和 p21 是在多个试验中发现的唯一可预测预后的标志物[24]。

其他因素

肛门癌和肛瘘之间的关系尚存在争议。在一项研究中，41%的肛管癌至少在 5 年前曾是良性肛门直肠疾病[25]。然而有两项研究表明这只是暂时的关联，但并没有因果关系的证据[26,27]。在另外一项研究中，曾有过肛裂或肛瘘的男同性恋者，患肛门生殖区鳞状细胞癌的危险性升高（相对危险度 9.1）[28]。但克罗恩病患者肛门癌的发生率低[29]。相比普通人群，肾移植免疫抑制的患者患肛门生殖区肿瘤的概率增加 100 倍[30]。在接受实体器官移植的 3 595 名患者中，肛门癌的发生率为 0.11%[31]。

病理学

肛门区域可发生多种组织类型的肿瘤[32]。其中主要为鳞状细胞癌（75%～80%）[33] 和腺癌（15%）。常见的肿瘤类型见表 95-1，此外，该区域还可出现其他罕见类型的肿瘤，如小细胞癌[35] 和淋巴瘤。黑色素瘤占所有肛门癌的 1%～2%[36]。

表 95-1　肛门癌的组织学分型

组织学分型	%
鳞状细胞癌	63
变异性（一穴肛原癌）	23
腺癌	7
基底细胞癌	2
黑色素瘤	2
佩吉特病（Paget disease）	2

摘自 Peters 1983[34]，经 MacMillan 出版社许可。

鳞状细胞癌可发生于肛管全程和肛缘。基底细胞癌是鳞状细胞癌的一种变异形式，通常称为一穴肛原癌。腺癌起源于齿状线处的腺体。小细胞癌是神经内分泌源性肿瘤，非常罕见。

肛缘癌包括鳞状细胞癌、基底细胞癌、鲍文氏病（鳞状 CIS）、佩吉特病（Paget disease）（原位腺癌）、疣状癌和卡波西肉瘤。恶性黑色素瘤可发生于任何部位，但发生在齿状线以下的黑色素瘤最常见。

鳞状细胞癌分为角化及非角化两种类型[37]，非角化肿瘤进一步细分为基底鳞癌，基底细胞癌，和一穴肛原癌。大多数临床医生认为，除黑色素瘤和肉瘤外，肿瘤分期对预后的影响比组织学类型更重要，并且，对于不同组织学类型的肿瘤，治疗原则一致[38,39]。相反，安德森癌症中心的 Das 医生和他的同事通过多变量分析发现，基底样组织类型的恶性肿瘤患者远处转移率更高[40]。

然而，流式细胞学分析的研究结果则相互矛盾，接近二倍体峰值的高增殖指数[41] 及非整倍体峰[42] 均被报道过。Shepard 等人通过多变量分析发现，渗透深度、腹股沟淋巴结受累情况和 DNA 倍体具有独立的预后意义[43]。

自然史

肛门癌最常见的转移途径是局部侵犯邻近的盆腔脏器。血行转移通常发生于齿状线及以上的肿瘤[44]。血行转移时，肿瘤细胞进入门脉系统，可导致 5%～8%的患者发生肝转移和肺转移[44]，2%的患者发生骨转移[45]。远处转移的发生率与肿瘤的组织学类型无关。肛缘肿瘤极少发生远处转移。

淋巴转移常见于腹股沟、盆腔和肠系膜淋巴结。有 15%～63%的患者可出现腹股沟淋巴结转移[46,47]。15%的患者在确诊的同时发现腹股沟淋巴结转移[44,48]。在一项包含 96 例患者的研究中，25%的患者发生异时性腹股沟淋巴结转移，发生转移的中位时间为 12 个月。盆腔淋巴结则较少受累，近端肿瘤的肠系膜淋巴结转移发生率（50%）比远端肿瘤肠系膜淋巴结转移（14%）更常见[49]。肛缘癌极少发生肠系膜淋巴结转移。

既往外科报道，同步阳性淋巴结清扫术后患者生存率为 0%～20%[50,51]。目前，同步放化疗（CMT）已经极大地改善这一局面。异时性淋巴结转移的患者行淋巴结清扫术后生存率可高达 83%[50,52]。其中大部分复发发生于 2 年之后，但也可能迟至 8 年出现复发[49]。

诊断

肛周肿瘤最早并且最常见的临床症状是出血，可发生在超过 50%的患者。其他常见的症状包括疼痛、里急后重、瘙痒、排便习惯改变、大便性状异常，少部分患者可出现异常的腹股沟淋巴结肿大[49,53,54]。这些症状大多与肛裂、肛瘘、痔疮、肛门瘙痒、肛门湿疣等肛门的良性疾病相关。60%的肛缘肿瘤和 6%的肛管肿瘤可能同时存在良性肛周病变[55]。

体格检查常可发现肛内肿物，易被误诊为痔疮[45,46]。内镜下，肿瘤表现为平坦或轻度隆起性病变，或边缘固定的隆起性病变，或息肉样病变（图 95-1）。必要时可进行经直肠超声检查，可明确肿瘤浸润深度及相邻器官的受累程度[56]。

为明确诊断，建议进行切取活检。切除活检应限于较小且表浅型的病变。临床可触及的腹股沟肿大淋巴结应进行针吸细胞学检查。由于淋巴结清扫后可能引起相关并发症、清扫术后对预后无改善作用，以及 CMT 治疗后对疾病有较好的控制率等原因，因此不推荐进行淋巴结清扫术。Garcia 及其同事的一项包含 46 名 HIV 阳性患者的研究显

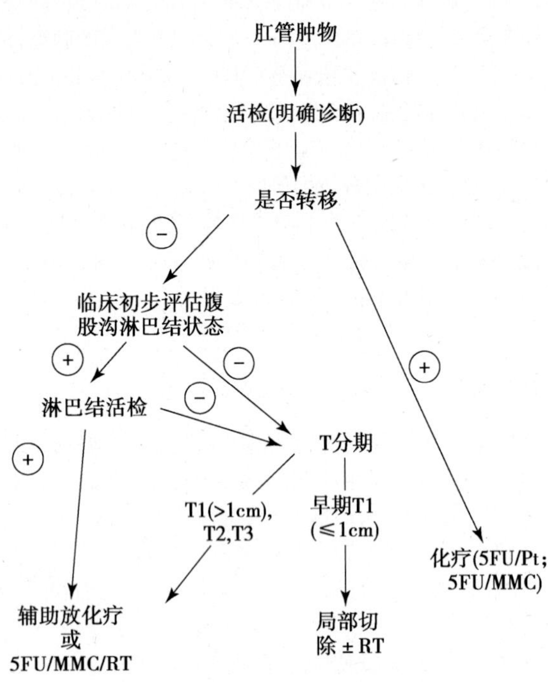

图 95-1　肛管鳞状细胞癌的治疗策略

示，相比较于内部病变，肛刷细胞学检查对外部病变的敏感性及特异性更高[57]。对于 HIV 阳性[58]和阴性[59]的患者，高分辨率的肛门镜检查有助于发现高级别上皮内瘤变和侵袭性病变。

即使相关针对远处转移的检查结果常为阴性，但是仍十分必要，腹部和盆腔电子计算机 X 线断层扫描技术(CT)可用来评估原发肿瘤并除外肝脏转移。胸部 X 线检查或胸部 CT 检查也是必要的。

大多数研究均显示了正电子发射断层成像(PET)对于肿瘤分期的优势[60~63]。在一项包含 41 例患者的研究中，^{18}F-脱氧尿苷葡萄糖正电子发射断层扫描(18FDG-PET)检查发现 91%的患者其原发病灶不可切除，而 CT 检查仅能发现 59%[64]。此外，17%的腹股沟淋巴结 CT 及体格检查为阴性，PET 检查则为阳性。Sveistrup 等[62]对 28 例 SCC 患者进行回顾性研究发现，与经直肠超声相比，经 PET/CT 检查后，14%的患者改变了肿瘤分期，17%的患者更改了治疗计划。Bannas 等[65]报道，与单独应用 PET 或 CT 检查相比，PET-CT 联合检查的患者中，有 23%的患者放射场设计发生了变化。

腹股沟前哨淋巴结活检虽然可行，但其优势尚不确定，在本疾病中的作用尚存在争议[66~68]。

分期

AJCC 和 UICC 于 1997 年提出一个通用的分期标准指南。这一分期标准也很好地解释了肛管癌的治疗首选 CMT，和治疗失败后行腹会阴联合切除术(APR)补救治疗的事实。临床工作中常用 TNM 分期。根据肿瘤大小、是否侵犯周围器官(如阴道、子宫、膀胱)对原发肿瘤进行评估。第 7 版 AJCC 分期指南见表 95-2[69]。

表 95-2　AJCC 肛管癌 TNM 分期(第 7 版)

原发肿瘤(T)			
Tx	原发肿瘤无法评估		
T0	无原发肿瘤证据		
Tis	原位癌		
T1	肿瘤最大直径≤2cm		
T2	肿瘤最大直径>2cm，但≤5cm		
T3	肿瘤最大直径>5cm		
T4	不论肿瘤大小，侵犯周围器官或组织(仅侵犯括约肌不属于 T4)		
区域淋巴结(N)			
Nx	区域淋巴结无法评估		
N0	无区域淋巴结转移		
N1	直肠周围淋巴结转移		
N2	单侧髂内及/或腹股沟淋巴结转移		
N3	直肠周围淋巴结和腹股沟淋巴结及/或双侧髂内及/或腹股沟淋巴结转移		
远处转移(M)			
Mx	远处转移无法评估		
M0	无远处转移		
M1	有远处转移		
分期组别			
0	Tis	N0	M0
Ⅰ	T1	N0	M0
Ⅱ	T2~3	N0	M0
ⅢA	T4	N0	M0
	T1~3	N1	M0
ⅢB	T4	N1	M0
	T1~4	N2~3	M0
Ⅳ	T1~4	N0~3	M1

注：肛缘癌归属于皮肤癌。

注：补充描述：补充的前缀表明需对肿瘤情况进行进一步分析，但不影响分期组别。

词缀	含义
m	同一部位存在多个原发肿瘤，记录在括号内：pT(m)NM
y	用于接受放疗或化疗期间或之后肿瘤的分期，并基于检查时肿瘤的数量，而不是治疗前对肿瘤的评估：ycTNM 或 ypTNM
r	用于复发性肿瘤：rTNM
a	用于尸检时：aTNM
淋巴管浸润(L)	
Lx	无法评估
L0	无淋巴管浸润
L1	有淋巴管浸润
脉管浸润(V)	
Vx	无法评估
V0	无脉管浸润
V1	镜下可见脉管浸润
V2	肉眼可见脉管浸润

摘自 Edge 2010[69]。经 Springer 许可转载。

预后因素

肛门癌最重要的预后因素是 T 分期和 N 分期，这与大多数的胃肠道肿瘤一致。在接受放疗或不接受化疗的患者中，T1～2（≤5cm）的原发肿瘤与 T3～4（>5cm）的原发肿瘤预后对比差异显著。原发肿瘤为 T3～4 的患者在 CMT 后，局部复发率近 50%，若治疗后肿瘤完全缓解，则局部复发率为 25%。

Peiffert 等[70]报道，随着肿瘤 T 分期的增高，局部复发率也会升高（T1：11%，T2：24%，T3：45%，T4：43%），5 年生存率则会相应下降（T1：94%，T2：79%，T3：53%，T4：9%）。Gerard 等[71]报道，对比 T1～2 的肿瘤与 T3～4 的肿瘤，5 年无造口生存率也有相似的下降（T1：83%，T2：89% vs T3：50%，T4：54%）。

与 T 分期相比，阳性淋巴结对预后的影响尚不明确。与直肠癌不同，肛门癌腹股沟淋巴结阳性是属于淋巴结转移（N），而不是远处转移（M），应用某种治疗方式，此时患者是可被治疗的。Cumming 等报道，接受 CMT 后淋巴结阴性的患者 5 年特异性生存率高于淋巴结阳性的患者（81% vs 57%）[72]。

RTOG 87～04 试验（表 95-3）报道，淋巴结 N1 的患者结肠造口率（局部复发的间接标志）比 N0 的患者更高（28% vs 13%）[73]。在淋巴结阴性和可疑淋巴结阳性的患者中，辅以丝裂霉素 C 治疗可降低结肠造口率。EORTC 随机试验（表 95-3）同样报道，对于接受 45Gy±氟尿嘧啶/丝裂霉素-C 治疗的患者，相较于淋巴结阴性者，淋巴结阳性患者的局部复发率更高（$P=0.035$），生存率则更低（$P=0.038$）[76]。

Allal 等报道，通过多变量分析，唯一可能对预后产生影响的变量是总体治疗时间（$P=0.09$）[80]。在 EORTC 随机试验中，多变量分析发现：阳性淋巴结、皮肤溃疡和男性性别是局部控制率和生存率的独立不利预后因素[76]。Goldman 等[81]研究也发现，相较于男性患者，女性患者预后更佳。Das 等一项关于 167 名患者的多变量分析发现，更高的 T 分期和 N 分期与更高的局部复发率相关[40]。N 分期和基底细胞样的组织学类型与远期复发转移相关，N 分期和 HIV 阳性则与较低的生存率相关。其他学者报道，T 分期、放射剂量和血红蛋白的百分比同样有意义。组间 RTOG 98～11 试验（表 95-3）多变量分析发现，男性（$P=0.04$），临床 N 分期阳性（$P<0.0001$）和肿瘤直径>5cm（$P=0.005$）是无病生存的独立预后因素[77]。

目前还未发现肛门鳞癌这种组织学类型（鳞状细胞癌与一穴肛原癌）对预后有重要影响。在一些研究认为一穴肛原癌的预后较好[38,82]。然而，一项入组 243 名可切除肛管癌患者的研究报道显示，与角化性病变相比，非角化性和基底细胞癌的预后较差[83]。肛门的小细胞癌罕见，同其他肺外小细胞癌一样，预后较差，远处转移率高[35,84]。原发肿瘤的位置对预后有一定的影响，如肛缘癌的预后优于肛门癌。

有三项研究对 DNA 含量（二倍体与非二倍体）进行了实验。其中 2 项研究未发现该因素对预后有影响[42,43]，另外一项研究对 184 名患者进行多变量分析[84]，发现 DNA 的倍性是患者生存的独立预后因素。另一项研究[42]显示，肿瘤分级是重要的预后因素，低级别肿瘤的 5 年生存率为 75%，而高级别肿瘤仅为 24%。Princess Margaret Hospital 的数据显示，在 CMT 失败的患者中，DT-硫辛酰胺脱氢酶突变不是影响治疗结果的一个强有力的决定因素[85]。

Tanum 和 Holm[86]报道，34% 的肛门癌患者 *p53* 过表达。采用免疫组化方法，对 RTOG 87～04 组间随机试验 CMT 组的 80 例患者进行预处理活检，检测 p53 表达[87]。所有实验组中，47% 的肿瘤中 p53 蛋白过度表达。通过多变量分析发现，这些肿瘤 p53 蛋白过表达的患者，4 年局部无病生存率显著下降（64% vs 88%，$P=0.027$）。然而，总无病生存期和总生存期并无显著差异。

Princess Margaret Hospital 的回顾性分析中，采用免疫组织化学方法对 49 例接受 CMT 治疗的患者进行了 *p53* 的检测[88]。p53 表达率为 82%。单因素分析显示，p53 表达≥5% 相较于 p53 表达<5%，是影响患者 5 年生存率的不利预后因素（78% vs 90%）。同时，也是影响无病生存期的独立不良预后因素（$P=0.01$）。

表 95-3 肛门癌综合治疗的随机试验

试验	患者数量	初始治疗	残余病变的评估/治疗		治疗组别	CR/%	结肠造口/%	局部控制率/%	精准控制率	%CFS	总生存期
Intergroup[73]	291	45Gy	残余	加量	RT/氟尿嘧啶	85	22	—	—	59	70(4 年)
RTOG87-04		氟尿嘧啶	阳性[a]	9Gy+氟尿嘧啶			*			*	
ECOG1289				CDDP	RT/氟尿嘧啶	92	9	—	—	71	75(4 年)
			阴性	观察	MMC						
		-vs-									
		45Gy									
		氟尿嘧啶/MMC									
ACT Ⅰ[74,75]	585	45Gy	≥50%CR[a]	15~20Gy EBRT	RT	—	—	41	34(5 年)	20	33(5 年)
				或近距离放射治疗				*	*		
					RT/氟尿嘧啶	—	—	64	59(5 年)	30	28(5 年)
		-vs-	<50%CR	解救手术	MMC						
		45Gy									
		氟尿嘧啶/MMC									
EORTC[78]	110	45Gy	PR/CR[a]	15~20Gy EBRT	RT	54	—	55	50(5 年)	40(5 年)	52(5 年)
				或近距离放射治疗				*	*	*	
		-vs-			RT/氟尿嘧啶	80	—	73	68(5 年)	72(5 年)	57(5 年)
			<PR	解救手术	MMC						
		45Gy									
		氟尿嘧啶/MMC									
Intergroup[77,78]	598	45Gy	阳性[b]	10~14Gy	氟尿嘧啶/CDDP		20	26	20	65(5 年)	71(5 年)

续表

试验	患者数量	初始治疗	残余病变的评估/治疗	治疗组别	CR/%	结肠造口/%	局部控制率/%	精准控制率	%CFS	总生存期
RTOG 98~11		氟尿嘧啶/CDDP	氟尿嘧啶/CDDP						*	
ECOG 1289			或 MMC	氟尿嘧啶/MMC	—	10	33	26	74(5 年)	78(5 年)
			阴性　观察	MMC						
		-vs-								
		45Gy								
		氟尿嘧啶/MMC								
ACT Ⅱ[79]	940	50. 4Gy	—	氟尿嘧啶/CDDP 90						72PFS(3 年)
		氟尿嘧啶/CDDP								
		±维持氟尿嘧啶/MMC		氟尿嘧啶/MMC 91						73PFS(3 年)
		-vs-								
		50. 4Gy	—							
		氟尿嘧啶/MMC								
		±维持氟尿嘧啶/MMC								

CFS,结肠造口无病生存期;*,差异有统计学意义($P\leqslant0.05$);MMC,丝裂霉素-C;CDDP,顺铂;CR,完全缓解;PFS,无进展生存期;EBRT,体外放射治疗。ACT Ⅰ试验包括 23%的肛缘癌。

[a]6 周时活检。

[b]8 周时活检。

原发肿瘤的治疗

一般原则

局部切除

局部切除适用于肿瘤直径小于2cm,分化较好,或肿瘤偶然发现于痔疮切除术时。于梅奥诊所治疗的188例肛管癌患者中,有19例患者行局部切除治疗[35]。12例患者肿瘤局限于上皮质和上皮下层组织,11例患者肿瘤<2cm,1例患者发现两处病灶。生存率为100%。12例患者中有1人复发,该患者行APR补救手术后,5年内无复发。肿瘤侵袭肌层且患者拒绝行结肠造口的患者复发率较高,这些患者可行补救的APR或CMT治疗。

综上所述,单纯局部切除适用于痔疮切除术中偶然发现的T1肿瘤,可于切除的同时保留括约肌功能。但这些患者需密切跟踪随访,局部复发后可予CMT治疗。

近距离放射治疗

与北美患者CMT治疗方案不同,在欧洲一些中心接受治疗的患者(最常见的是法国),仅行外照射治疗±近距离放射治疗。非随机数据表明,单独放疗的治疗效果与CMT相当;然而,放射相关毒性则更高[89]。近距离放射治疗通常利用^{192}Ir后负荷。常用的治疗方案是先行45Gy的外照射,然后补充15~20Gy的盆腔加量或近距离放射治疗。

Ortholan及其同事对66名肿瘤为T1/Tis的患者使用近距离放射治疗±小放射野外照射[90]。平均随访50个月,仅6例患者局部复发,其中4例复发发生在照射野范围之外。

经腹会阴联合切除术

APR是放射治疗失败或术前盆腔放疗患者的补救措施。治疗效果将在后面内容讨论。

同步放化疗

20世纪七十年代末以前,肛门癌的常规治疗是经腹会阴联合切除术。Nigro等人打破了这一“标准”。在他的早期报道中提到,3名鳞状细胞肛门癌的患者在术前接受了30Gy放射治疗同时予以氟尿嘧啶和丝裂霉素C化疗,手术时达到肿瘤病理完全缓解[91]。

从那时起,许多单组Ⅱ期实验表明,治疗初始行同时放化疗,加以APR作为补救治疗措施,可以获得80%~90%的完全缓解率。对于原发肿瘤较大(≥5cm)者,即使完全缓解率较低(50%~70%),大部分患者还是可以不行结肠造口术,而获较好的总生存率。

化疗

来自欧洲的两项前瞻性随机试验(表95-3)对比同步放化疗与单纯放射治疗(EORTC70和UKCCCR ACT174),结果支持应用同步放化疗。UKCCCR ACT1试验对患者进行了13年的随访,接受同步放化疗的患者与仅进行单纯放疗的患者相比,有更好的局部控制率(59% vs 34%)和无造口生存率(30% vs 20%)。然而,总生存率的提高(33% vs 28%)未能达到统计学差异74。在EORTC试验中,同步放化疗显示出更高的完全缓解率(80% vs 54%)和显著更高的精准局部控制率(68% vs 50%)与无造口生存率(72% vs 40%),但总生存期无显著差异(57% vs 52%)[76]。尽管两项试验在总生存期方面未能表现出优势,但提高了局部控制率和无造口生存率,帮助同步放化疗成为标准治疗方法。

结果与讨论

在北美,综合治疗已经得到普遍认可,许多随机试验关注于制订理想的治疗方案。组内试验RTOG 87~04证实了丝裂霉素C是综合治疗的一个必要组成部分[73]。患者被随机分为45Gy放射治疗加氟尿嘧啶持续灌注±无丝裂霉素C。在完成治疗后6周,未达到完全缓解的患者再给予包括原发肿瘤9Gy照射增量,同时加氟尿嘧啶或顺铂的补救方案。如果补救方案完成后6周仍未达到完全缓解将行APR。接受丝裂霉素C的患者有着更高的完全缓解率(92% vs 85%)和显著降低的结肠造口率(9% vs 22%),与相应增高的无造口生存率(71% vs 59%)(表95-3)。4年总生存率无明显差异(75% vs 70%)。丝分裂霉素C组早期4级以上毒性显著增加(23% vs 7%)。尽管总生存率无显著提高,但就其在无造口生存率方面的优势,丝裂霉素C被认为是综合治疗的必需组成部分。

丝裂霉素C与顺铂

接受以丝裂霉素C为基础的治疗方案的患者,完全缓解率为84%(81%~87%),局部控制率73%(64%~86%),五年生存率77%(66%~92%)。T1~2期患者完全缓解率大于90%,加之行补救性手术最终的局部控制率可达到80%~90%。对于T3~4期患者,近50%患者需接受补救性APR。如果接受完整综合治疗后达到完全缓解,仅25%的患者会再行补救性APR。

尽管氟尿嘧啶、丝裂霉素C同时联合45Gy放射治疗已经有令人满意的结果,但仍有提高的空间,特别是对于T3~4期的患者。很多的治疗方法已经证实。其中包括使用氟尿嘧啶与顺铂(作为初始治疗和/或联合放疗)和超过45Gy的增强剂量的外粒子束或近距离放射治疗。氟尿嘧啶联合顺铂是一种引人注目的治疗方案:①氟尿嘧啶/丝裂霉素C失败的患者仍然对氟尿嘧啶/顺铂有反应;②顺铂是一种放疗增敏剂。

RTOG98-11组内随机试验比较了传统的CMT联合氟尿嘧啶/丝裂霉素C方案和初始使用氟尿嘧啶/顺铂化疗,然后再使用联合氟尿嘧啶/顺铂的CMT方案(表95-3)[78]。试验将发生于肛管部位的包括T2~4期鳞状细胞癌(86%)、基底细胞癌和一穴肛原癌共682名患者随机分组,并根据性别、淋巴结状态和肿瘤大小进行分层,主要终点为无病生存期。最终,27%的肿瘤大于5cm,35%为T3~4期,26%淋巴结临床阳性。

具体分组情况治疗如下:传统综合治疗组:5FU(1 000mg/m^2,第1~4天和第29~32天)加丝裂霉素(10mg/m^2,第1~29天)和放射治疗(45~59Gy)。初始组:氟尿嘧啶(1 000mg/m^2,第1~4天、第29~32天、第57~60天和第85~88天)加顺铂(75mg/m^2,第1、29、57、85天)联合放疗(第57天起45~59Gy)。

放疗剂量和方法在两组中完全相同。全盆腔接受30.6Gy(1.8Gy/fx)继之以14.4Gy圆锥状照射真骨盆。对于N0患者,放疗36Gy后腹股沟区淋巴结排除在外。而对于T3~4期和/或N+的患者,或T2期病变行45Gy放疗后仍残有病变者,将针对原发肿瘤和淋巴结行二期10~14Gy圆锥形照射。

可触及的肿大淋巴结宜在治疗前行活检,若在综合治疗完成后8周仍有可触及的腹股沟肿大淋巴结,可选择切除活检。

局部复发是指综合治疗 8 周跟踪随访期间于放射野处出现肿瘤。

经过长期随访，接受丝裂霉素 C 治疗的患者 5 年无病生存率(68% vs 58%，$P=0.006$)、5 年无结肠造口生存率(72% vs 65%，$P=0.05$)和总生存率(78% vs 71%，$P=0.026$)均有显著改善。虽然局部-区域失败率较低(20% vs 26%)，但无统计学差异。3 级以上长期毒性无显著性差异(13% vs 11%)。与其他报道一致，另一项分析显示，较高的 T 和 N 分期对包括局部区域复发、远处转移、无结肠造口生存、无疾病生存和总体生存在内的预后有显著的负面影响[92]。

UKCCR ACTⅡ试验报道了相似的结果。这项 4 组对照试验对比顺铂和丝裂霉素 C 为基础的 CMT 方案(50.4Gy)，然后二次随机分为氟尿嘧啶/顺铂和观察组[79]。共 940 例患者(81%肛管，15%肛缘，43%T3~4，62%N+)被随机分组。与丝裂霉素 C 为基础的 CMT 相比，以顺铂为基础的 CMT 患者的 6 个月 CR 率(90% vs 91%)，3 级以上毒性(72% vs 71%)，接受维持化疗(72% vs 73%)或不接受维持化疗(74% vs 73%)的 3 年无进展生存期没有显著差异。

综上所述，基于丝裂霉素 C 的常规 CMT 仍是治疗的标准。尽管有这些结果，基于单中心的系列研究，一些研究人员仍然提倡基于顺铂的 CMT[93]。包括使用如卡培他滨、奥沙利铂和西妥昔单抗等细胞毒性药物的新的 CMT 方法已经被研究[94,95]。迄今为止，与氟尿嘧啶/丝裂霉素 C 为基础的 CMT 相比，这些方法以及 3 种药物方案[96]，还没有显示出获益。

剂量增强

传统外粒子束照射

为提高局部控制率及生存率，有人曾进行过两项放射剂量增强的平行试验。在两项试验中，患者接收 36Gy 盆腔照射(30.6Gy 全盆腔照射加 5.4Gy 真骨盆照射)然后休息两周，再对原发瘤及其边缘 2~3cm 范围内 23.4Gy 放射治疗，总剂量为 59.4Gy。两组试验主要区别在于化疗方案的不同。RTOG 9208 试验[97]使用氟尿嘧啶和丝裂霉素 C，而 ECOG4292 试验(2297)使用氟尿嘧啶和顺铂。

RTOG9208 试验显示了同 RTOG87-04 试验中使用的 45Gy 放疗联合氟尿嘧啶/丝裂霉素的标准方案相似的结果，但 2 年造口率有所增高(30% vs 7%)。同样，同传统治疗方法相比，ECOG4292 试验并未表现出更好的获益[98]。ECOG 4292 试验的长期随访显示，5 年 PFS 为 55%，5 年总生存率为 69%，这与其他以顺铂为基础的试验一致[99]。一项回顾性研究显示，大于 60Gy 的剂量改善了局部控制率和生存率[100]。RTOG98-11 试验增加 10~14Gy 的放疗剂量，然而却未表现出剂量反应关系[77]。

四臂 UNICANCER ACCORD 03 随机试验检测了诱导化疗和剂量递增的作用。307 例患者接受 5-Fu/顺铂 CMT+45Gy 放疗联合或不联合 5-Fu/顺铂诱导化疗。随后进行近距离治疗或外照射增强衰减 15 或 20Gy[101]。无论是诱导化疗(77% vs 75%)还是增强(78% vs 74%)对 5 年无结肠造口生存率都没有显著改善。

近距离放射治疗

近距离放射治疗是实现适形放疗同时不影响周围正常结构的理想手段。在大多数系列试验中，患者接受 30~55Gy 盆腔照射±化疗，继之以 10~25Gy 的 ^{192}Ir 后装导管作增强。大多数情况下使用低剂量率，但有些研究人员提倡高剂量率[102~104]。

综合各类实验，平均结果为完全缓解率 83%(73%~91%)，局部控制率 81%(73%~89%)，5 年生存率 70%(60%~84%)。主要存在的问题是肛门坏死，报道发生率从最低 2%到最高达 76%[103]，平均 5%~15%。尽管 Hannoun-Levi 等人[105]的回顾性分析显示，和外离子束增强相比，近距离放射疗法改善了局部控制率，同时另一项来自法国的研究认为，和没有增强相比，毒性从近距离放射增强中获益[106]，但前面讨论的 UNICANCER ACCORD 03 试验没有证实局部控制率的获益[101]。

调强放疗

IMRT 一种有较低的急性和较低长期毒副作用的盆腔放疗方法。通过识别原发肿瘤和盆腔淋巴结周围有剂量限制的组织并使用多放射野的方法来避开这些组织，IMRT 可以再增加剂量的同时有更少的毒副作用。Salama 和其同事使用 IMRT 为基础的 CMT 治疗了 53 名患者[107]。患者接受 45Gy 全盆腔照射随后补充增强，平均达到 51.5Gy。急性 3 级毒性主要是 15%发生血糖升高，28%出现皮肤反应。急性 4 级毒性包括 30%的白细胞减少和 34%中性粒细胞减少。平均中位随访时间 15 个月，局部无复发率：84%；无远处转移 93%，无造口生存率：84%；总生存率：93%。其他研究人员也报告了类似的急性毒性降低的结果[108~110]。

RTOG 0529 Ⅱ期临床试验在合作小组背景下检验了 IMRT[111]。采用氟尿嘧啶/丝裂霉素 C 联合以分期为基础的 IMRT(T2N0：50.4Gy 原发灶 PTV 和 42Gy 淋巴结 PTV，T3~4N0~3：54Gy 原发灶 PTV 和 45Gy 淋巴结 PTV))治疗了 63 例患者。与 RTOG 98~11 相比，接受 IMRT 治疗患者的治疗中断率低(49% vs 62%)，急性毒性低(2 级+血红素降低[73 vs 85，$P=0.032$]，3 级+GI[21% vs 36%，$P=0.0082$]，3 级+皮肤毒性低[23% vs 49%，$P<0.0001$])。另一项发现是 IMRT 计划的学习曲线陡峭。虽然医疗机构需要 IMRT 认证，81%的计划需要初始修改，46%需要再次修改。轮廓线向导现在是可行的[112]。在单医疗机构和 RTOG 数据的基础上，IMRT 已成为 CMT 治疗肛门癌的标准方法。

单纯放射治疗

单纯放射治疗加外粒子束或联合短程放疗可获得同 CMT 相当的局部控制率和生存率。然而，由于该方法即使由经验丰富者实施也会增加肛门坏死率，所以使用时应谨慎。

是否有必要 6 周后活检

对于在初始治疗结束后 6 周后行第一次活检的必要性尚有争议。来自玛格丽特公主医院的资料的显示，鳞状细胞癌衰退缓慢，CMT 结束后 3~12 周内肿瘤尺寸继续缩小[72]。ACT Ⅱ试验报告 CMT 治疗后 11 周的临床 CR 率为 66%，26 周时增加到 84%。

基于以上资料，越来越多的研究者提倡保守的治疗方法，不建议治疗后活检。RTOG87-04 试验中，对接受了 45Gy 和氟尿嘧啶/丝裂霉素 C 后再次进行 9Gy 加氟尿嘧啶/顺铂补救治疗的患者行剩余肿瘤的活检检查，6 周后(初始 45Gy 结束后的 12 周)55%获得了病理学完全缓解[73]。至于完全缓解是补救治疗的结果还是初始治疗后 6 周内肿瘤继续衰退的结果，尚无定论。

在许多研究机构,如果治疗后6周评估肿瘤仍有剩余,患者通常不接受1周的补救治疗。此后患者每6周定期复查,如果肿瘤继续缩小,则无须行补救治疗。然而,如果肿瘤进展或初始治疗后6周内肿瘤无反应,则需要行APR。除严格的体格检查外,肛门超声可以帮助观察肿瘤。在RTOG98-11肛门癌Ⅲ期组内试验中,初始45Gy放射治疗结束后6周内的活检是选择性进行的。

HIV阳性患者的治疗

通常来说,考虑到标准治疗方案可能无法耐受,HIV阳性患者需接受低剂量的放射治疗和化学治疗[16]。在更好地理解HIV阳性患者表现出的免疫缺陷的基础上,近期的许多研究报道建议,治疗的选择应根据临床和免疫学指标,如之前机会性感染的病史和CD4计数[113~115]。接受有效剂量抗病毒治疗的CD4计数>200μl的患者和没有HIV感染的患者结果相似,应当积极治疗[116]。CMT可导致CD4细胞计数长期下降,一个系列报告了晚期死人数的增加[117],而在另一个系列报告中,在CMT后6年内HIV相关发病率没有增加[118]。对于CD4计数<200μl或者有其他HIV相关疾病症状或体征的患者,推荐减量的放疗和/或化疗。

治疗相关的毒性反应

同其他肿瘤治疗中见到的一样,盆腔放疗与急性和长期毒副作用相关。急性毒性的反应是由于化疗和放疗联合导致的。这些反应包括白细胞减少、血小板减少、直肠炎、腹泻、膀胱炎和会阴皮肤红疹。长期毒性主要是排便急迫感的增加和大便失禁[119,120]。这是由于放疗对括约肌的影响,以及当肿瘤发生反应时,取而代之的是纤维化组织,而不是新的括约肌。与传统的三维放疗相比,IMRT的急性毒性较低[107~111,121]。然而,目前还没有长期毒性数据。

在关于肛门癌的文献中,关于功能性预后的报道有限。一项系列研究报道93%的患者全部功能得到保留[122],而另外一项系列研究使用直肠测压的方法报道括约功能完全者占56%[123]。另外还有报道称93%的患者至少一年内括约功能依然良好[124]。

肛缘癌的治疗

肛缘癌被认为是皮肤癌的一种。简单来说,一种合理的治疗方法是建议较小的肿瘤(≤4cm)并且不接触肛门外缘者可行局部切除。如果由于解剖限制需行APR,或局部切除会损伤括约肌功能,或肿瘤>4cm和/或淋巴结阳性,则适宜选择非手术治疗。根据来自UKCCCR的随机试验(包括23%的肛缘癌患者)推荐CMT。一项来自埃朗根的报道,肛缘癌行CMT,5年无造口率为69%,总生存率54%,均低于肛管癌。然而,这可能与T分期较高有关[125]。

治疗后随访

肛门癌治疗后的患者需密切随访,局部复发还可通过APR进行补救并能获得长期生存。患者需每6个月进行一次查体和肛门镜检查直到完全缓解,然后每3个月一次复查,共2年时间。接下来的三年,每6个月一次检查。5年后每年检查一次。综合治疗复发的患者,95%发生于治疗后3年内[126]。

腹盆腔CT和FDG-PET的使用在随访中尚不明确。Christensen和同事报道3D超声结合查体发现复发的敏感性为1.0,仅行3D超声为0.86,2D超声的敏感性只有0.57[127]。Goh等人对35例CMT后6~8周的患者进行了MRI检查,发现其对预测临床预后没有帮助[128]。由于大部分复发均在原发瘤的部位,因此查体是必须要做的项目。

腹股沟淋巴结的管理

在检查阳性淋巴结对局部控制和生存的影响时,重要的是确定淋巴结转移的位置,并区分同时性和异时性转移。遗憾的是,大多数系列研究未能区分N1、N2还是N3。但对同时性和异时性转移却有所研究。

关于同时性淋巴结转移患者接受CMT对预后的影响的报道不一。Allal等报道,同淋巴结阴性患者相比,淋巴结阳性局部复发率较高(N1~3:36%,N0:19%)[129],RTOG87-04组内试验报道造口率较高(N1:28%,N013%)[70]。尽管Cumming和他的同伴报道淋巴结阳性患者的局部复发率只有13%,但五年生存率却较低(N1~3:57%,N0:81%)[72]。EORTC随机试验通过多变量分析认为,淋巴结阳性是局部复发和远期生存一个负面独立预后因素[76]。

与此相反,Gerard等人进行的CMT加短程治疗方案中N1和N0患者的5年肿瘤特异生存期和总生存期相似[71]。同样,原发肿瘤的完全缓解率不受淋巴结状态的影响。Doci和同事报道患者接受以顺铂为基础的治疗方案,完全缓解率相似(N1~3:92 vs N0:100%)[130]。而另一项系列实验患者接受以丝裂霉素C为基础的方案,全部8名N1~3患者均获得完全缓解[131]。总的来说,单纯外粒子束照射[1,132~134]可以控制65%淋巴结阳性患者,而CMT[1,73,75,76]可以达到90%。

T2N0的患者应接受预防性放射治疗。在一项对T1N0期和T2N0期患者的回顾性研究中,腹股沟区淋巴结被排除在放射视野之外,其腹股沟区失败率分别为2%和13%[135]。当前对可以淋巴结转移患者建议细针吸取细胞学检查或活检病理检查。确认有肿瘤后,可以对受累侧腹股沟作增强45~50.4Gy的CMT。尽管淋巴结切除不作为首选治疗,但由于转移后的病死率具有显著性,因而对于谨慎选择的孤立淋巴结复发患者可以考虑切除。

单侧异时性淋巴结转移的进展同极差的预后不相关。梅奥诊所[6]的两项系列研究中,在治疗性腹股沟淋巴结切除后,5年和7年的生存率均超过50%[48],但却没有长期存活者。对于综合治疗后异时性孤立淋巴结转移患者,当前的治疗方法是完整切除后化疗。放疗与否取决于之前CMT中使用的剂量及放射野。

残余或复发肿瘤

1. 肛缘:局部复发的肛缘癌局部切除后的有效控制情况

较肛管癌好[136,137]。在一项 48 例复发后行局部切除的患者中，16 例出现复发，复发形式包括局部复发[11]，腹股沟淋巴结复发[4]，两处均复发[138]。无内脏器官复发。平均复发时间 26 个月。10 例接受再次切除，只有 1 例接受 APR。9 名患者生存期超过 5 年。全部 4 例腹股沟淋巴结转移患者接受腹股沟淋巴结切除术，其中 2 人获得长期存活。尽管关于局部复发行局部切除后接受放疗或 CMT 的报道资料较少，但对于除此之外将选择 APR 的患者来说是一个合理的选择，这取决于前次放疗剂量（如果有的话）。

2. 肛管：标准治疗方案是 APR。

转移后的治疗

由于肛管癌的发生率较低、综合治疗有效性高等原因，很少发展为转移者。许多研究者曾有过使用多柔比星单药和顺铂单药达到有限缓解的报道[139,140]。顺铂和氟尿嘧啶的联合化疗通过全身或局部（如肝动脉）途径，可使缓解率接近 50%[141-143]。再次治疗可选择氟尿嘧啶/丝裂霉素 C。伊立替康和西妥昔单抗等新药的临床应用经验有限[144]。

一项小的系列研究包含了 6 名局限于腹主动脉旁淋巴结转移患者，他们推荐包含淋巴结在内的扩大放射野的 CMT[145]。

其他类型肿瘤

黑色素瘤

肛门直肠部位的黑色素瘤相对罕见，不足全部肛管癌的 1%。肿瘤的分期取决于侵犯深度和淋巴结情况的，是决定生存期的主要的影响因素。远处转移常见[146~151]。

尽管 APR 可使患者获得较好的局部控制率，但同局部切除相比，大部分患者未表现出生存期方面的优势[146,147,152~154]。

Podnos 等人[155]报道了一项来自 SEER 数据库的回顾性分析，调查了从 1973 年至 2001 年的 126 名接受多种治疗方法的患者，在不同的疾病状态的 5 年生存率分别为：局部复发 32%，局部或区域复发 17%，远处转移 0%。

由于病例数的限制、选择偏倚和缺少随机研究治疗的限制，目前尚不能区分 APR 和扩大的局部切除术在生存期方面的优劣。辅助性的免疫治疗、化疗和放疗，其相关优势相互掩盖，很难区分。局部切除时应注意是否有至少 3mm 的镜下切缘。APR 具有潜在较高的局部控制率，是一种合理的选择[147~150,156,157]。

腺癌

原发于肛门腺体的肛门腺癌罕见。大部分肛门部位的腺癌来自直肠癌的局部侵犯。通常同直肠腺癌的治疗方法相同。如果肿瘤为 T3 期或淋巴结阳性，则应术前行 CMT，术后行 4 个月辅助治疗。放射野应包括腹股沟区淋巴结。Beal 和同事的一项 13 例患者的系列研究建议 CMT 和 APR 联合，其 2 年精确生存期可达 62%[158]。肛门腺鳞癌也很罕见，预后差[159]。由于鳞癌成分的存在，可选择氟尿嘧啶/丝裂霉素 C 同时放疗，并行 APR 作为补救措施。

肉瘤

目前仅有少数关于肛门平滑肌瘤肉的报道。对于此类疾病尚无合理治疗方案。标准的手术方法为 APR。借鉴肢体部位平滑肌肉瘤的治疗技术，可行局部切除+^{192}Ir 近距离放疗以保留括约肌功能[160~162]。这种方法可能在一些特定的患者中替代 APR。

其他

Bowen 病、Paget 病和卡波基肉瘤通常选用手术治疗，并保留肛门括约肌功能，很少有使用 CMT 的报道。

（邵欣欣　王杰 译　田艳涛 校）

参考文献

The complete reference list can be found on the Wiley Companion Digital Edition of this title (see inside front cover for login instructions).

10 Siegel R, Ma J, Zou Z, et al. Cancer Statistics, 2014. *CA Cancer J Clin*. 2014;**64**:9–29.

15 Machalek DA, Poynten M, Fairley CK, et al. Anal human papillomavirus infection and associated neoplastic lesions in men who have sex with men: a systematic review and meta-analysis. *Lancet Oncol*. 2012;**13**:487–500.

16 Melbye M, Cote T, Kessler L, et al. AIDS/Cancer Working Group. High incidence of anal cancer among AIDS patients. *Lancet*. 1994;**343**:636–639.

21 Serup-Hansen E, Linnemann D, Skovrider-Ruminski W, et al. Human papillomavirus genotyping and p16 expression as prognostic factors for patients with American Joint Committee on Cancer stages I to III carcinoma of the anal canal. *J Clin Oncol*. 2014;**17**:1812–1817.

24 Lampejo T, Kavanagh D, Clark J, et al. Prognostic biomarkers in squamous cell carcinoma of the anus: a systematic review. *Br J Cancer*. 2010;**103**:1858–1869.

58 Nahas CS, Lin O, Weiser MR, et al. Prevalence of perianal intraepithelial neoplasia in HIV-infected patients referred for high-resolution anoscopy. *Dis Colon Rectum*. 2006;**49**:1581–1586.

61 Bhuva NJ, Glynne-Jones R, Sonoda WL, et al. To PET or not to PET? That is the question. Staging in anal cancer. *Ann Oncol*. 2012;**23**:2078–2082.

62 Sveistrup J, Loft A, Berthelsen AK, et al. Positron emission tomography/computed tomography in the staging and treatment of anal cancer. *Int J Radiat Oncol Biol Phys*. 2012;**83**:134–141.

68 De Nardi P, Carvello M, Canevari C, et al. Sentinel node biopsy in squamous-cell carcinoma of the anal canal. *Ann Surg Oncol*. 2011;**18**:365–370.

72 Cummings BJ, Keane TJ, O'Sullivan B, et al. Epidermoid anal cancer: treatment by radiation alone or by radiation and 5-fluorouracil with and without mitomycin-C. *Int J Radiat Oncol Biol Phys*. 1991;**21**:1115–1125.

73 Flam M, John M, Pajak T, et al. Role of mitomycin in combination with fluorouracil and radiotherapy, and salvage chemoradiation in the definitive nonsurgical treatment of epidermoid carcinoma of the anal canal: results of a phase III randomized intergroup study. *J Clin Oncol*. 1996;**14**:2537–2539.

74 Northover J, Glynne-Jones R, Sebag-Montefiore D, et al. Chemoradiation for the treatment of epidermoid anal cancer: 13-year follow-up of the first randomised UKCCCR Anal Cancer Trial (ACT I). *Br J Cancer*. 2010;**102**:1123–1128.

75 UKCCCR Anal Cancer Trial Working Party. Epidermoid anal cancer: results from the UKCCCR randomised trial of radiotherapy alone versus radiotherapy, 5-fluorouracil, and mitomycin. *Lancet*. 1997;**348**:1049–1054.

76 Bartelink H, Roelofsen F, Eschwege F, et al. Concomitant radiotherapy and chemotherapy is superior to radiotherapy alone in the treatment of locally advanced anal cancer: results of a phase III randomized trial of the European Organization for Research and Treatment of Cancer radiotherapy and gastrointestinal cooperative groups. *J Clin Oncol*. 1997;**15**:2040–2049.

78 Gunderson LL, Winter KA, Ajani JA, et al. Long-term update of U.S. Intergroup RTOG 98–11 phase III trial for anal canal carcinoma: survival, relapse, colostomy failure with concurrent chemoradiation involving fluorouracil/mitomycin versus fluorouracil/cisplatin. *J Clin Oncol*. 2012;**35**:4344–4351.

79 James RD, Glynne-Jones R, Meadows HM, et al. Mitomycin or cisplatin chemoradiation with or without maintenance chemotherapy for treatment of squamous-cell carcinoma of the anus (ACT II): a randomized, phase 3, open-label, 2x2 factorial trial. *Lancet Oncol*. 2013;**14**:516–524.

91 Nigro ND, Vaitkevicius VK, Considine B. Combined therapy for cancer of the anal canal: a preliminary report. *Dis Colon Rectum*. 1974;**17**:354–358.

92 Gunderson LL, Moughan J, Ajani JA, et al. Anal carcinoma: impact of TN category of disease on survival, disease relapse, and colostomy failure in US gastrointestinal intergroup RTOG 98-11 phase III trial. *Int J Radiat Oncol Biol Phys.* 2013;**87**:638-645.

98 Martenson JA, Lipsitz SR, Wagner H, et al. Initial results of a phase II trial of high dose radiation therapy, 5-fluorouracil, and cisplatin for patients with anal cancer (E4292): an Eastern Cooperative Oncology Group study. *Int J Radiat Oncol Biol Phys.* 1996;**35**:745-749.

99 Chakravarthy AB, Catlano PJ, Martenson JA, et al. Long-term follow-up of a phase II trial of high-dose radiation with concurrent 5-fluorouracil and cisplatin in patients with anal cancer (ECOG E4292). *Int J Radiat Oncol Biol Phys.* 2014;**81**:e607-e613.

101 Peiffert D, Tournier-Rangeard L, Gerard JP, et al. Induction chemotherapy and dose intensification of the radiation boost in locally advanced anal canal carcinoma: final analysis of the randomized UNICANCER ACCORD 03 trial. *J Clin Oncol.* 2012;**30**:1941-1948.

102 Gerard JP, Mauro F, Thomas L, et al. Treatment of squamous cell anal canal carcinoma with pulsed dose rate brachytherapy. Feasibility study of a French cooperative group. *Radiother Oncol.* 1999;**51**:129-131.

105 Hannoun-Levi JM, Ortholan C, Resbeut M, et al. High-dose split-course radiation therapy for anal cancer: outcome analysis regarding the boost strategy (CORS-03 study). *Int J Radiat Oncol Biol Phys.* 2011;**80**:712-720.

107 Salama JK, Mell LK, Schomas DA, et al. Concurrent chemotherapy and Intensity-modulated radiation therapy for anal cancer patients: a multicenter experience. *J Clin Oncol.* 2007;**25**:4581-4586.

110 Kacknic LA, Tsai HK, Coen JJ, et al. Dose-painted intensity-modulated radiation therapy for anal cancer: a multi-institutional report of acute toxicity and response to therapy. *Int J Radiat Oncol Biol Phys.* 2012;**82**:153-158.

112 Ng M, Leong T, Chander S, et al. Australasian gastrointestinal trials group (AGITG) contouring atlas and planning guidelines for intensity-modulated radiotherapy in anal cancer. *Int J Radiat Oncol Biol Phys.* 2012;**83**:1455-1462.

118 Fraunholz I, Haberl A, Klauke S, et al. Long term effects of chemoradiotherapy for anal cancer in patients with HIV infection: oncological outcomes, immunological status, and the clinical course of the HIV disease. *Dis Colon Rectum.* 2014;**57**:423-431.

121 Das P, Cantor SB, Parker CL, et al. Long-term quality of life after radiotherapy foe the treatment of anal cancer. *Cancer.* 2010;**116**:822-829.

135 Tomaszewski JM, Link E, Leong T, et al. Twenty-five-year experience with radical chemoradiation for anal cancer. *Int J Radiat Oncol Biol Phys.* 2012;**83**:552-558.

158 Beal KP, Wong D, Guillem JG, et al. Primary adenocarcinoma of the anus treated with combined modality therapy. *Dis Colon Rectum.* 2003;**46**:1320-1324.

162 Grann A, Paty PB, Guillem JG, et al. Sphincter preservation of leiomyosarcoma of the rectum and anus with local excision and brachytherapy. *Dis Colon Rectum.* 1999;**42**:1296-1299.

第 96 章 肾细胞癌

Earle F. Burgess, MD ■ Stephen B. Riggs, MD ■ Brian I. Rini, MD, FACP ■
Derek Raghavan, MD, PhD, FACP, FRACP, FASCO

概述

在美国，每年有 64 000 名新发肾细胞癌患者，导致大约 14 000 人死亡。对于局限性疾病，可以通过肾切除来达到治愈目的，而精确的手术分期至关重要。随着成像技术的改进，主动监测已成为小的无症状肾肿瘤的一种选择。手术技术的改良，包括腹腔镜和机器人手术，有助于降低并发症发生率。在更晚期的疾病中，随着局部或远处转移扩散，免疫反应是患者结局与生存状况的调节者，而通过重组人白介素-2 或 PDL-1 抑制的免疫调节会导致持续的反应。细胞毒性化疗的活性可以忽略不计，但诸如酪氨酸激酶抑制剂和西罗莫司哺乳动物靶点抑制剂的靶向治疗往往会导致严重的退行性病变。罕见的肾癌约占突发病例的 10%，本章回顾了对其处理的一般方法。

简介

肾细胞癌（RCC）的发病率估计在美国每年约 64 000 例，其中 14 000 人死亡[1]。报道的 RCC 发病率随着时间的推移而增加，主要但不完全是因为其他指征而行腹部影像学检查偶然检测到的无症状肿瘤的数量增加所致[2,3]。

近年来在 RCC 方面取得了许多进展。已经开发了治疗局限性肾肿块的新方法，强调较少侵入性和保留肾单位的方法。此外，RCC 的生物学基础已经被阐明，并且针对相关生物通路的药物已经在转移性病例中显示出强大的临床效果。本章详细介绍了这些进展，并总结了 RCC 的流行病学、病理学、分期和治疗。

流行病学

RCC 通常在 60 岁到 70 岁发病，男性的发病率是女性的两倍。吸烟是 RCC 的确定危险因素，其相对风险为 2~3 倍[4]。肥胖也是一个危险因素，尽管具体的饮食关系没有很好的定义[5]。高血压，而非降压药物，与 RCC 的发生有关[6]。获得性多囊疾病也易发生 RCC[7]。一小部分患者（2%~3%）具有常染色体显性遗传综合征，这使得患者倾向所对应的各种 RCC 组织亚型，随后将会详细描述。一项澳大利亚的研究表明，止痛药的滥用与 RCC 有关，尽管更常见的是发现其与肾盂癌相关。

临床表现

在现今的患者中，超过 50% 的 RCC 患者都是由于无关原因行腹部 CT 扫描或超声检查发现而就诊，而并未表现出初始症状[8~11]。证据表明在 20 世纪 70 年代，只有 10% 的 RCC 是偶然发现，而在 1998 年，这一比例达到了 60%[3,12]，这表明了 RCC 的诊断在这些年所发生的变化。

RCC 最常见的局部症状包括血尿、侧腹疼痛和可触及的肿块，尽管这种典型的三联症目前并不常见。其他局部表现包括左侧阴囊精索静脉曲张，可能在高达 11% 的男性中观察到，这是因为左肾静脉中的肿瘤阻塞了直接汇入左肾静脉的生殖静脉。静脉受累也可导致下肢水肿、腹水、肝功能障碍和肺栓塞。特定器官的疼痛或功能障碍可能是转移性疾病患者的表现特征。

副肿瘤综合征的全身症状也可能是 RCC 的初始表现。高钙血症是 RCC 中最常见的副肿瘤综合征，在 13%~20% 的患者中表现出来。这是由肿瘤产生的甲状旁腺激素（PTH）或 PTH 相关肽介导的。红细胞增多症在 1%~8% 的病例中发生，并被认为是由高水平的促红细胞生成素介导的；贫血更常见，而且可能相当严重。铁含量的研究可以提示慢性贫血。Stauffer 综合征是无肝转移的 RCC 背景下的肝功能障碍。糖皮质激素不敏感的多肌痛风湿病偶尔会发生，并且通常在肾切除后得到解决。内分泌异常，包括 HCG 和 ACTH 升高也有报道。其他全身表现，包括体质症状如发烧、体重减轻和疲劳是常见的。

病理

世界卫生组织在 2004 年发表的肾肿瘤分类将恶性实质肾细胞肿瘤分为三种主要亚型和其他几种罕见亚型[13]。最常见的 RCC 组织学为传统透明细胞亚型，占所有 RCC 的 75%~80%。其余亚型包括乳头状癌（10%~15%），嫌色细胞癌（5%~10%），髓样癌（<1%）和集合管癌（CDC）（<1%）。最近，除了超出本综述范围的不太常见的变异体外，一些新的实体，包括与 Xp11.2/TFE3 易位和黏液性小管细胞癌和梭形细胞癌相关的 RCC 也被描述。传统肾透明细胞癌（ccRCC）起源于近曲小管，常规光镜下可见清晰的细胞质。ccRCC 中最常见的遗传改变是一种高度特异性的异常，涉及染色体 3p［*von Hippel Lindau*（*VHL*）基因］的沉默，35%~50% 的散发性病例中会发生这种异常[13]。非遗传性 ccRCC 倾向于出现较大的单侧肿瘤。遗传性 VHL 综合征（新生儿出现率为 1/36 000）是一种高度致病的常染色体显性遗传性疾病，患者在染色体 3p25 上遗传 VHL 基因缺陷，进而导致出现 ccRCC 和/或中枢神经系统、腹部内脏器官

的多发性囊肿和肿瘤[14]。中枢神经系统病变包括视网膜血管母细胞瘤，内淋巴囊肿瘤和颅脊髓血管母细胞瘤。这些患者的内脏病变包括 ccRCC、嗜铬细胞瘤、胰腺神经内分泌肿瘤、附睾囊腺瘤和阔韧带囊腺瘤。除了 *VHL* 的遗传畸变外，癌症基因组图谱研究网络对 400 多份 ccRCC 样本进行的综合基因组分析显示，除了染色质重塑基因外，*PI3K/Akt* 途径成分的突变是常见的，这与 ccRCC 肿瘤发生过程中的表观遗传失调有关[15]。已经明确定义的瘤内异质性[16,17]表明其分子学特征可能还需要多方面的努力，特别是这种特征是为临床服务为目的时。

乳头状 RCC 起源于远曲小管，由含铁血黄素沉积的管状毛细血管结构和纤维血管核心内的泡沫组织细胞组成。根据乳头状结构内衬肿瘤细胞的形态，将其细分为 1 型和 2 型乳头状 RCC[13]。乳头状癌没有 VHL 基因失活，但 7 号染色体、17 号染色体三体和 Y 染色体缺失是最常见的遗传改变。乳头状瘤倾向于具有多灶性，可能存在双侧肾脏受累。遗传性乳头状肾癌（HRPC）的特征是 c-Met 原癌基因激活（染色体 7q31～34）和 1 型乳头状肾癌的发生。遗传性平滑肌瘤病肾细胞癌（HLRCC）涉及富马酸水合酶基因（染色体 1q42～43）异常和 2 型乳头状肾癌、皮肤平滑肌瘤、子宫肌瘤和平滑肌肉瘤的发生[18]。

嫌色 RCC 起源于肾脏的插层细胞，其特征是细胞呈大片，胞质苍白或嗜酸性，细胞膜厚而清晰，细胞核多形，核膜不规则，核周清澈[13]。最常见的遗传改变是 1，2，6，10，13，17，21 染色体杂合性丢失和亚二倍体的出现。肾嫌色细胞癌的患者倾向于出现早期疾病，有不到 5%的患者表现为转移[19,20]。Birt-Hogg-Dube 综合征患者的 RCC 比例很高，组织学以嫌色为主。他们具有 17p 染色体上的 BHD 基因的功能突变缺失，有突出的皮肤表现（纤维滤泡瘤），并且易发生肺囊肿破裂引起的气胸[21]。最近，全面的全基因组分析发现，*TERT* 基因（端粒酶的催化亚基）的启动子区域内普遍存在基因组重排，导致 *TERT* 表达增加[22]。因此，通过结构启动子重排增强的端粒酶表达可能是嫌色性 RCC 发展过程中的早期致病事件。

预后特征

核分级

在局限性 RCC 患者中，核 Fuhrman 分级和 TNM 分期始终是最重要的预后因素[23]。Fuhrman 分级系统根据核和核仁大小、形状和含量对 RCC 的核等级进行 1（侵袭性最小）到 4（侵袭性最强）的评分[24]。较高的核级别与较差的 5 年总生存率相关。局限性肿瘤肾切除后 G1、G2 和 G3/4 肿瘤的 5 年肿瘤特异性生存率分别为 89%、65%和 46%[23]。Fuhrman 分级对嫌色 RCC 没有帮助[24]。

分期

在疑似 RCC 的患者中，需要进行分期检查以确定疾病的范围，包括胸部、腹部和盆腔的 CT。最常见的转移部位包括肺、腹部和纵隔淋巴结、肝脏和骨骼。除非患者有提示骨或脑转移的症状，最初的骨扫描和脑成像往往意义不大。

2010 年美国癌症联合委员会（AJCC）和 TNM 分期系统在之前已经进行了详细的报道[25]，它反映了肿瘤的范围（T）、淋巴结受累情况（N）及有无转移（M）。

局限性 RCC 的治疗

对于小的（<4cm）肾肿瘤，存在多种治疗选择。这些包括手术切除、射频消融（RFA）或冷冻疗法（统称为热消融），或在严格挑选的人群中进行主动监测和延迟干预。外科手术切除仍然是治疗局限性Ⅰ和Ⅱ期 RCC 的基本方法，通常不需要肾活检。只要可行，肾部分切除术是首选的，特别是对于肾功能受限的患者、双侧肿瘤和/或孤立肾的患者。尽管保留肾单位手术是治疗小肾癌的推荐方法，但与根治性肾切除（在选择性设置中）相比，其绝对益处受到质疑[26]。腹腔镜肾部分切除术侵袭性较小，而且看起来与开放手术的结果相似。通常腹腔镜手术是在机器人辅助下进行的，有助于克服一些固有的技术难点[27]。

对于较大的肿瘤（>7cm）和局部晚期肿瘤的首选治疗是根治性肾切除术，无论是行腹腔镜手术还是开放手术。这包括结扎肾血管系统、切除肾脏和 Gerota 筋膜。如果在术前影像学上发现肿瘤累及同侧肾上腺，肾上腺需一并切除。腹腔镜根治性肾切除术目前广泛使用，它减少了术后疼痛，缩短了住院时间和使患者更快的恢复。诸如冷冻消融和 RFA 等热消融治疗是一部分患者的额外选择，通常以经皮方式进行。最近对超过 1 400 名患者的队列进行有限的随访的回顾性数据表明，与肾部分切除术相比，经皮穿刺消融疗法的使用有着相似的局部无复发生存率[28]。遗憾的是，尚没有将这些无创方法与传统外科治疗进行比较的随机对照试验，而且与对照组相比，肾部分切除术具有获得完全病理评估和减少随访的优势。一般来说，希望选择手术以外治疗的小肿瘤（<4cm）患者或不适合进行侵入性手术的患者更倾向于经皮穿刺消融。主动监测是一种新兴的治疗小肾癌的方法，据了解，根据大小和分级，50%～60%的肿瘤将处于惰性状态。这部分肿瘤的平均生长速度约为 0. 3cm/年，转移率为 1%～3%[29~32]。然而，应该强调的是，发表的系列数据在随访方面是有限的，因此缺乏确定的结论[33]。重要的是，经皮肾活检的应用正在发展的过程中。历史上充满了不确定的研究结果，而更多现代的研究表明非诊断性活检发生的概率不到 10%[34]。遗憾的是，评级准确率仍然处于中等水平（50%～70%）[34~37]。

Ⅲ期肾癌涉及肾周组织、淋巴结和/或侵犯肾静脉或下腔静脉。对于这些人来说，选择的术式是为了治愈目的而进行的开放性根治性肾切除术。对淋巴结肿大的患者应进行淋巴结清扫。对没有可疑淋巴结转移的患者，常规行扩大淋巴结清扫术是有争议的[38]。虽然术前行靶向分子治疗可能是安全的[39]，但这些药物在非转移肾癌患者中的作用尚未确定。回顾性病例系列研究表明，在肾切除前使用目前可用的靶向药物并不会导致原发性肿瘤的频繁缩小[40~41]，同时使患者面临进展的风险[42]和随后手术难度的增加。在下腔静脉癌栓患者中，新辅助靶向治疗对瘤栓负荷也未显示出明显的细胞减少效应，不应常规应用而影响手术决策[43,44]。

局部和/或寡转移复发的治疗干预可改善患者预后，这强调了早期发现复发的重要性。在明确处理原发性肾肿瘤后，理想的监测策略应该平衡复发的风险和避免不必要的诊断检查的愿望。基于风险的个人监测准则已经提出[45,46]，但最佳的监测策略仍有待确定。

转移性疾病

预后因素

转移性肾细胞癌（mRCC）最广泛使用的预后因素是在 mRCC 患者主要接受免疫治疗的时代发展起来的。美国的 Memorial Sloan Kettering 癌症中心（MSKCC）标准是通过对接受 mRCC 治疗的患者进行多变量分析而制订的[47]。它开发了一种临床评分系统，并根据存在的不良风险特征的数量将患者分为良好、中等和不良预后类别。来自原始队列的患者存在显著的治疗异质性被用于建立这些标准，因此对另外接受干扰素（IFN）治疗的患者的最新分析仅将每个预后类别的中位总生存期分别定义为 30、14 和 5 个月（表 96-1）[48]。

表 96-1 转移性 RCC 的预后标准

MSKCC 标准[48]
预后不良因素
• Karnofsky 体能状态<80%
• 诊断治疗间隔<1 年
• 血红蛋白水平<正常值下限
• 血清校正钙水平>10g/dl
• LDH>1.5 倍正常值上限
危险度分级与临床结果
• 0 个预后因素（良好风险）：PFS 8.3 个月，OS 30 个月
• 1~2 个预后因素（中等风险）：PFS 5.1 个月，OS 14 个月
• 3~5 个预后因素（不良风险）：PFS 2.5 个月，OS 5 个月
IMDC 标准[49]
预后不良因素
• Karnofsky 体能状态<80%
• 诊断治疗间隔<1 年
• 血红蛋白水平<正常值下限
• 血清校正钙水平>正常值上限
• 中性粒细胞计数>正常值上限
• 血小板计数>正常值上限
危险度分级与临床结果
• 0 个预后因素（良好风险）：OS 43 个月
• 1~2 个预后因素（中等风险）：OS 23 个月
• 3~5 个预后因素（不良风险）：OS 8 个月

IMDC，国际转移性肾细胞癌数据库联盟；MSKCC，Memorial Sloan Kettering 癌症中心；OS，总生存期；PFS，无进展生存期。

当代患者在进行如下所述的分子靶向治疗后，新的预后因素又出现了。对使用舒尼替尼、索拉非尼或贝伐单抗治疗的 645 例 mRCC 患者进行多中心回顾性分析，建立了由三个风险组构成的修订预后模型（表 96-1）[50]。由国际 mRCC 数据库联盟（IMDC）进行的外部验证支持该预后模型与当前标准治疗的常规使用，并说明了由于治疗模式的演变而导致的生存改善，因为观察到的良好、中等和不良风险组患者的中位总生存期分别为 43、23 和 8 个月[49]。IMDC 风险分层在转移性非 ccRCC 患者中也有预后价值[51]，并可能有助于下一节讨论的减瘤性肾切除术的决策制订[52]。

转移癌患者的手术治疗

根治性肾切除术也适用于许多 mRCC 患者。来自两个Ⅲ期研究的结果表明，在使用 IFN 之前进行减瘤性肾切除术可提高总体生存率。在这些试验的联合分析中，单用干扰素 α 治疗的患者的中位生存期为 7.8 个月，而最初接受减瘤性肾切除术的患者为 13.6 个月[53~55]。体能状况较好的患者有更大的生存优势。尽管支持数据主要是经验数据，而且还没有与新的靶向药物相结合，但减瘤手术仍然占主导地位。尽管 1 658 名患者队列中 IMDC 预后标准的回顾性分析表明减瘤性肾切除术可能有益于预期寿命至少 12 个月且 IMDC 危险因素少于 4 个的患者，一项评估透明细胞 mRCC 患者在舒尼替尼使用之前行肾切除术是否有益的Ⅲ期临床试验正在进行中[52]。减瘤性肾切除术在非透明细胞 mRCC 患者中的作用尚未得到证实[56]。

虽然减瘤性肾切除术似乎对许多透明细胞 mRCC 患者有益，但它并不是治愈性的，不应该不加选择地进行。最有可能从减瘤手术中受益的患者包括：①受累肾脏的大量肿瘤负荷（如>75%）；②良好的体能状态和③无中枢神经系统或肝转移（极少特例除外）[57]。其他考虑因素与手术的可切除性有关，特别是如果靠近重要解剖结构、肾门包裹或其他复杂因素，则可能发生并发症。

伴有单发转移的 mRCC 患者可以考虑进行转移灶切除，尽管它们只占病例的 2%~3%。有利的预后因素包括从最初诊断到发生转移的长时间间隔、孤立的转移部位和具备完全切除已知转移灶的能力[58]。具有良好预后因素的患者可以预期转移灶切除术后高达 40%的 5 年生存率，因此在高度选择的 RCC 患者中应考虑手术切除转移性肿瘤。

转移性肾癌的系统性治疗

免疫治疗

由于早期试验表明化疗并不能产生明显的益处[59,60]，免疫治疗长期以来一直是 mRCC 治疗的标准治疗方法，试图利用 RCC 肿瘤的天然免疫反应，偶尔自发地消退转移病灶[61]。IFN 和高剂量重组人白介素-2（IL-2）产生的应答率为 10%~20%，使患者的总体生存期略有延长[62,63]。值得注意的是，这种治疗有明显的副作用，包括毛细血管渗漏综合征，这需要紧密的监测和偶尔的升压支持。大剂量 IL-2 的Ⅲ期临床试验未能证明其与替代低剂量细胞因子方案相比有显著的益处[64,65]。由于一小部分患者可以通过完全应答而显著受益，因此基于细胞因子的免疫治疗在 mRCC 中仍然是有意义的，尽管还未能预测哪些患者能够产生应答。

在一个小的Ⅱ期临床试验中，相对于具有不良风险因素的历史对照组患者，自体肿瘤细胞疫苗AGS-003与舒尼替尼的结合可以延长生存时间[66]，这也作为正在进行的ADAPTⅢ期随机临床试验的基础。通过调节抑制的PD-1/PD-L1轴激活细胞毒性T细胞也显示出显著的抗肿瘤活性[67~69]。这些新的免疫调节剂正在进行Ⅲ期临床试验，其结果令人期待。

靶向治疗

由于对RCC的生物学和遗传学有了更好的理解，新的治疗方法已经产生。如前所述，大多数ccRCC表现出VHL基因的异常(图96-1)。当失活时，VHL基因产物不能调节转录因子缺氧诱导因子(HIF)α的降解，从而导致许多缺氧调节基因的转录，包括血管内皮生长因子(VEGF)和血小板衍生生长因子(PDGF)。这些生长因子通过与各自的受体酪氨酸激酶(RTK)结合促进血管生成和肿瘤生长[14]。RTK的激活可通过*PI3K/Akt*通路诱导信号转导，并进一步激活哺乳动物西罗莫司靶点(*mTOR*)通路下游，通过调节mRNA翻译促进细胞增殖和存活。这些错综复杂的通路已被确定为治疗mRCC的关键治疗靶点(表96-2)。

***VEGF*配体导向治疗**

贝伐单抗是一种重组单克隆抗体，可结合并中和血液循环中的*VEGF*。该药物在晚期RCC一线治疗中的活性已通过两个随机的Ⅲ期临床试验确定。AVOREN研究将未经治疗的透明细胞mRCC患者和既往肾切除术患者随机接受IFN(每周3次，剂量为9MIU，长达1年)加用贝伐单抗(每2周1次，10mg/kg，静脉输注)治疗或安慰剂治疗，直至疾病进展[81]。IFN加用贝伐单抗显著增加了PFS(10.2个月vs 5.4个月)(HR=0.63；P=0.000 1)和客观肿瘤反应率(31% vs 13%；P=0.0001)。添加贝伐单抗治疗后可以看到OS改善的趋势[79]。一项类似设计的CALGB Ⅲ期试验证实了IFN加用贝伐单抗可以带来PFS的获益(8.5个月vs 5.2个月P<0.000 1)和客观反应率(ORR)的提高(25% vs 13%，P<0.000 1)[82]。尽管在两个试验中二线治疗的高比率混淆了生存分析，OS的改善仍然倾向于贝伐单抗治疗臂[80]。常见的毒性反应包括高血压和蛋白尿，少见但严重的毒性反应包括肠穿孔、动脉缺血事件和出血。由于在Ⅲ期试验中没有贝伐单抗单药治疗臂，目前尚不清楚贝伐单抗是否必须与干扰素联合使用。与mTOR抑制剂联合使用并不能提高疗效[83]，而与另外的VEGF靶向药物同时使用则与血栓性微血管病变的不可接受风险相关[84]。在使用其他靶向药物治疗后的患者中的使用这种药物仍未得到证实。

VEGF受体酪氨酸激酶抑制剂

RTK在*VEGF*和*PDGF*的信号传递级联中起到重要作用[85]。RTK有一个与它们各自配体结合的胞外区，它通过由细胞质激酶结构域调节的蛋白磷酸化事件来激活致癌的细胞内信号转导级联。小分子抑制剂靶向RTK已被证明是mRCC的一种有效的治疗策略，并已导致监管部门批准了这一类别的多种药物，详见下文。

舒尼替尼是一种口服多激酶抑制剂，可阻断*VEGFR-1*、*VEGFR-2*和*VEGFR-3*、*PDGFR-B*及相关RTK[86]。一项针对未经治疗的mRCC患者的关键Ⅲ期随机试验比较了一线舒尼替尼(50mg/d，6周中的4周)与干扰素的治疗效果，并证明其在客观缓解率(ORR)(47%对12%；P<0.001)、PFS(11个月vs 5个月，HR=0.54；P<0.001)和OS(26.4个月vs 21.8个月，HR=0.82；P=0.051)方面具有显著优势[71]。值得注意的是，大多数入选患者(94%)具有良好或中等风险的MSKCC预后标准。常见的毒性反应包括疲劳、手足综合征、腹泻、黏膜炎和高血压。基于这些结果，该制剂已成为mRCC一线标准治疗。通过改变剂量和给药时间表来改善毒性反应还未获得成功，或仍处于研究阶段[87,88]。

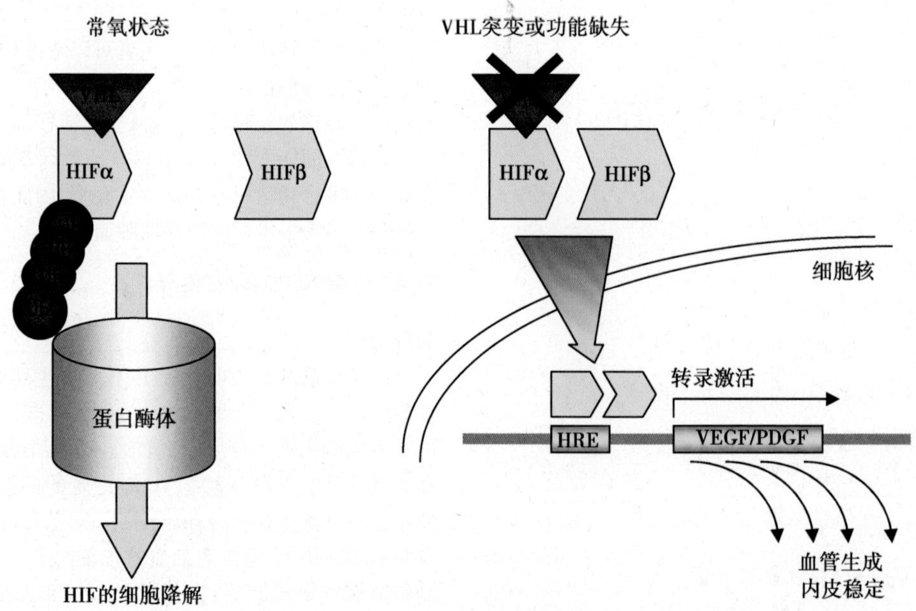

图96-1 常氧状态下*VHL*的正常功能与*VHL*异常状态或缺氧状态下功能的比较。在正常情况下，*VHL*与*HIFα*结合，并对其进行多泛素化反应，以标记其在细胞蛋白酶体中的破坏。在缺氧或VHL功能缺失时，*HIFα*与*HIFβ*结合，然后移位到细胞核内激活HIF反应元件(HRE)。这导致在血管生成和内皮稳定中重要的基因如*VEGF*和*PDGF*的转录激活

表 96-2 部分关于转移性肾细胞癌靶向药物的临床试验

药物	机制	效果			
		人群与试验臂	RR	PFS/月	OS/月
舒尼替尼[70,71]	VEGF 及其相关受体的酪氨酸激酶抑制剂	一线舒尼替尼 vs IFN	47%	11	26.4
			12%	5	21.8
			$P<0.001$	$P<0.001$	$P=0.051$
培唑帕尼[72,73]	VEGF 及其相关受体的酪氨酸激酶抑制剂	一线培唑帕尼 vs 舒尼替尼	31%	8.4	28.3
			25%	9.5	29.1
			$P=0.03$		NS
索拉非尼[74,75]	VEGF 及其相关受体的酪氨酸激酶抑制剂	难治性治疗,二线索拉非尼 vs 安慰剂	10%	5.5	17.8
			2%	2.8	15.2
			$P<0.001$	$P<0.01$	$P=0.146$
阿西替尼[76]	VEGF 及其相关受体的酪氨酸激酶抑制剂	难治性治疗,二线阿西替尼 vs 索拉非尼	19%	8.3	20.1
			11%	5.7	19.2
			$P=0.0007$	$P<0.0001$	NS
替西罗莫司[77]	mTOR 抑制剂	高危,一线替西罗莫司 vs IFN	8.6%	N/A	10.9
			4.8%	N/A	7.3
			NS		$P<0.008$
依维莫司[78]	mTOR 抑制剂	难治性治疗,二线依维莫司 vs 安慰剂	1.8%	4.9	14.8
			0%	1.9	14.4
				$P<0.001$	NS
贝伐单抗[79,80]a	VEGF 配体结合抗体	一线贝伐单抗+IFN vs 安慰剂+IFN	31%,25%	10.2,8.5	23.3,18.3
			13%,13%	5.4,5.2	21.3,17.4
			$P<0.0001$	$P<0.0001$	NS

IFN,干扰素;N/A,数据未能获得或数据还不成熟;NS,无统计学意义;PFS 的 P 值基于危险比。

[a]显示了两个Ⅲ期贝伐单抗试验的结果。

培唑帕尼是一种第二代口服多激酶抑制剂,可抑制 *VEGFR-1*、*VEGFR-2* 和 *VEGFR-3*、*PDGFR-A* 和 *PDGFR-B* 以及 *c-kit*[89]。对于未经治疗或细胞因子治疗失败的 mRCC 患者,一项比较培唑帕尼与安慰剂治疗的随机Ⅲ期试验表明培唑帕尼改善了 PFS(9.2 个月 vs 4.2 个月,$HR=0.46$;$P<0.0001$)和 ORR(30% vs 3%,$P<0.001$)[90]。常见的毒性反应包括高血压、腹泻、恶心、纳差和脱发。这种药物比同类药物更容易观察到肝毒性,并可能与 *UGT1A1* 基因多态性有关[91]。一项大型、非劣效性的随机Ⅲ期试验比较了先前未经治疗的具有透明细胞成分的 mRCC 患者培唑帕尼和舒尼替尼的治疗效果和耐受性,发现培唑帕尼可以导致相似的 PFS(8.4 个月 vs 9.5 个月,$HR=1.05$;95%*CI* 0.90~1.22),更高的 ORR(31% vs 25%,$P=0.03$)和类似的 OS(28.3 个月 vs 29.1 个月,$P=0.24$)[72,73]。尽管接受培唑帕尼治疗的患者的生活质量评分较好,包括疲劳和手足综合征这些毒性反应较少,但它有着和其他药物类似的停药率。在一项 PISCES 试验中,患者被随机分在一个双盲组接受一种药物治疗 10 周,然后再进行交叉治疗,它同样显示培唑帕尼的耐受性与舒尼替尼相比得到了改善[92]。

索拉非尼抑制包括 *BRAF*、*CRAF*、*VEGFR-2*、*-3*、*PDGFB*、*Flt-3*、*p38* 和 *c-kit* 在内的多种激酶[93]。在未经治疗的情况下,索拉非尼没有表现出比 IFN 更高的抗肿瘤活性,因此在这种情况下没有被证实的作用[94]。然而,在以前治疗过的患者中,索拉非尼优于安慰剂。肾癌全球评估试验(TARGET)中的治疗方法招募了 903 名以前治疗过的转移性 ccRCC 患者,并随机将患者分为服用索拉非尼(400mg,每天两次)和服用安慰剂[74,75]。所有入选的患者都有良好或中等风险的 MSKCC 预后标准,80%以上的患者以前接受过细胞因子治疗。和安慰剂组相比,索拉非尼组的 PFS 延长(5.5 个月 vs 2.8 个月,$P<0.01$),ORR 很小(有 10%的调查者评估),OS 相似(17.8 个月 vs 15.2 个月,$P=0.146$),尽管 OS 的获益可能被安慰剂组患者允许交叉治疗并在进展时接受索拉非尼所掩盖。

随后开发的阿西替尼是 *VEGFR-1*、*VEGFR-2* 和 *VEGFR-3* 的第二代抑制剂,其效力比以前的制剂更大[95],导致这种较新的制剂在很大程度上取代索拉非尼作为标准的二线选择。在AXIS试验中,以前接受过一系列系统性治疗[细胞因子(35%)、舒尼替尼(54%)、贝伐单抗(8%)或替西罗莫司(3%)]的700多名透明细胞mRCC患者随机接受阿西替尼(5mg,每日两次)或索拉非尼(400mg,每日两次)的治疗[96]。值得注意的是,1/3的登记患者具有MSKCC不良风险标准。虽然OS(20.1个月 vs 19.2个月,$P=0.3744$)和患者报告的结果在两组之间相似,但阿西替尼组的中位PFS明显更优(8.3个月 vs 5.7个月,$P<0.0001$)[76]。基于这些结果,许多人认为在先前治疗失败的患者中,阿西替尼比索拉非尼更可取。阿西替尼尚未被证明在一线治疗中优于索拉非尼[97]。一线剂量递增研究的结果表明阿西替尼剂量滴定可能发挥作用,尤其是在正常血压患者中,尽管最佳方法仍处于研究阶段[98]。

***mTOR* 抑制剂**

"*mTOR*"激酶由 *VEGFR* 下游的 *Akt* 和 *PI3K*,并通过调节mRNA翻译促进肿瘤生长和增殖。替西罗莫司是FDA批准的 *mTOR* 抑制剂,它与 *FKBP-12* 结合形成一种复合物,直接抑制 *mTOR*。一项Ⅲ期试验包含626名不良预后标准的先前未经治疗的患者,并将他们随机分为三组:第一组接受替西罗莫司,25mg静脉注射,每周1次;第二组接受干扰素α 18MU,每周注射3次;第三组接受替西罗莫司15mg静脉注射每周1次+IFN 6MU注射每周3次[77]。患者需要具有以下三种或三种以上的不良风险特征:Karnofsky表现状态<80%,乳酸脱氢酶>1.5倍实验室正常上限,血红蛋白<实验室正常下限,校正白蛋白的血钙>10mg/dl,从首次诊断RCC到开始治疗<1年的时间以及三个或更多转移部位。值得注意的是,有19%的入选患者是非透明细胞组织类型。与干扰素α相比,替西罗莫司单药治疗显示了总生存期的优势(10.9个月 vs 7.3个月,$P=0.008$)。基于这些结果,替西罗莫司已成为不良风险mRCC患者的一线治疗。在使用舒尼替尼进行治疗后的二线治疗中,一项INTORSECT的Ⅲ期研究结果显示,尽管其OS相对较低(12.3个月 vs 16.6个月,$P=0.01$),替西罗莫司与索拉非尼具有相似的PFS,因此替西罗莫司不应用于符合VEGF酪氨酸激酶抑制剂使用条件的患者[99]。

依维莫司是一种经美国FDA批准的口服mTOR抑制剂,基于将依维莫司与安慰剂进行比较的RECORD-1随机Ⅲ期试验的结果,依维莫司可用于舒尼替尼或索拉非尼治疗失败后的mRCC患者[78,100]。尽管没有OS的获益,依维莫司组显示出更好的PFS(4.9个月 vs 1.9个月,$P<0.001$),部分原因是安慰剂组患者的交叉治疗率较高。上述INTORSECT试验的结果是否适用于依维莫司的使用尚不清楚,因为在二线治疗中将依维莫司与VEGFR酪氨酸激酶抑制剂进行比较的研究尚未报道,并且鉴于阿西替尼和索拉非尼在二线治疗中的疗效,在RECORD-1试验中使用安慰剂对照不再被认为是适当的对照臂。RECORD-3试验研究了依维莫司与 *VEGFR* 酪氨酸激酶抑制剂序贯治疗的最佳顺序[101]。在这项随机Ⅱ期非劣效性试验中,未经治疗的患者要么先接受依维莫司治疗随后在疾病进展时接受舒尼替尼治疗,或者选择相反顺序进行治疗。一线治疗中使用依维莫司在中位PFS和OS上都劣于一线治疗中使用舒尼替尼,进一步证明在使用 *VEGFR* 酪氨酸激酶抑制剂之前不应使用依维莫司。

肾脏少见肿瘤

根据编辑要求,肾脏少见肿瘤的生物学行为和治疗方法并不在本章详细阐述之列,但在别处已有详述[102,103]。尽管如此,我们将介绍一种最近报道频率较高的肾脏少见肿瘤类型,因为其系统性治疗方法出现了较大的变化。

集合管癌

尽管在过去几年中病例报告越来越多,集合管癌在肾癌中所占比例不到1%[103~105]。它最初被认为起源于远端肾小管上皮细胞,但最近发现它出现在集合管中[102,104]。集合管癌通常见于肾髓质,大小不一,最大可超过10cm,通常边缘不规则并伴有局部浸润的证据。集合管常被结缔组织增生间质包绕,具有可变的管状-乳头状生长模式,具有高级别的细胞核和高的有丝分裂活性,可见黏蛋白和肉瘤样变,没有典型的免疫组织化学表现。

集合管癌是一种侵袭性肿瘤,经常发现时就已经在晚期[102,104,105]。常见的特征包括血尿、腰痛或腹痛,并且在第一次出现时经常有转移,包括肺、肝、骨、肾上腺或淋巴结。有2:1的男性比例优势,年龄范围较广。CT扫描的表现不是特异性的,主要由中心出现的浸润性病变组成,没有太多的对比强化。

集合管癌的诊断通常是在手术时作出,而且这也是局限性疾病的确定治疗方法。然而,这是一种侵袭性肾癌,因此通常伴有早期转移。几乎没有证据表明免疫治疗对集合管癌有任何显著的效用,因此大多数治疗转移性疾病的报道都涉及全身化疗的使用,大多是基于含顺铂的方案[106,107]。遗憾的是,这种治疗的缓解率相对较低,持续时间较短。有人认为顺铂和吉西他滨的联合使用具有持续疗效[106]。最近,来自法国的一个小样本研究报道了贝伐单抗、吉西他滨和顺铂联合治疗能对疾病持续和长期缓解[107],尽管值得注意的是贝伐单抗的额外影响尚未得到证实。这项工作表明,在这种疾病中,化疗和靶向治疗的结合可能会产生相加效应,并且需要确切证据才能将其视为标准。

结论

RCC发病率在全球范围内呈上升趋势。外科手术仍然是治疗局限性肿瘤的主要手段,也是转移性肾癌综合治疗的一部分。对RCC生物学基础的深入了解导致了许多靶向治疗方法的临床研发,这些治疗方法已经大大改变了治疗前景。未来的研究工作包括进一步完善小肾癌的治疗方法,更好地了解对靶向治疗反应与抵抗的生物学基础,mRCC靶向治疗的组合与序列的临床试验,以及新的免疫治疗方法的开发。

(范阳 译 张旭 校)

关键参考文献

The complete reference list can be found on the Wiley Companion Digital Edition of this title (see inside front cover for login instructions).

1 Siegel R, Ma J, Zou Z, Jemal A. Cancer statistics, 2014. *CA Cancer J Clin.* 2014;**64**(**1**):9–29.

3 Pantuck AJ, Zisman A, Belldegrun AS. The changing natural history of renal cell carcinoma. *J Urol.* 2001;**166**(**5**):1611–1623.

8 Lee CT, Katz J, Fearn PA, Russo P. Mode of presentation of renal cell carcinoma provides prognostic information. *Urol Oncol.* 2002;**7**(**4**):135–140.

9 Luciani LG, Cestari R, Tallarigo C. Incidental renal cell carcinoma-age and stage characterization and clinical implications: study of 1092 patients (1982–1997). *Urology.* 2000;**56**(**1**):58–62.

12 Nguyen MM, Gill IS, Ellison LM. The evolving presentation of renal carcinoma in the United States: trends from the Surveillance, Epidemiology, and End Results program. *J Urol.* 2006;**176**(**6**Pt 1):2397–2400; discussion 2400.

14 Cohen HT, McGovern FJ. Renal-cell carcinoma. *N Engl J Med.* 2005;**353**(**23**):2477–2490.

15 Cancer Genome Atlas Research Network. Comprehensive molecular characterization of clear cell renal cell carcinoma. *Nature.* 2013;**499**(**7456**):43–49.

19 Cheville JC, Lohse CM, Zincke H, Weaver AL, Blute ML. Comparisons of outcome and prognostic features among histologic subtypes of renal cell carcinoma. *Am J Surg Pathol.* 2003;**27**(**5**):612–624.

23 Tsui KH, Shvarts O, Smith RB, Figlin RA, deKernion JB, Belldegrun A. Prognostic indicators for renal cell carcinoma: a multivariate analysis of 643 patients using the revised 1997 TNM staging criteria. *J Urol.* 2000;**163**(**4**):1090–1095; quiz 1295.

24 Fuhrman SA, Lasky LC, Limas C. Prognostic significance of morphologic parameters in renal cell carcinoma. *Am J Surg Pathol.* 1982;**6**(**7**):655–663.

26 Van Poppel H, Da Pozzo L, Albrecht W, et al. A prospective, randomised EORTC intergroup phase 3 study comparing the oncologic outcome of elective nephron-sparing surgery and radical nephrectomy for low-stage renal cell carcinoma. *Eur Urol.* 2011;**59**(**4**):543–552.

30 Crispen PL, Wong YN, Greenberg RE, Chen DY, Uzzo RG. Predicting growth of solid renal masses under active surveillance. *Urologic Oncol.* 2008;**26**(**5**):555–559.

32 Rosales JC, Haramis G, Moreno J, et al. Active surveillance for renal cortical neoplasms. *J Urol.* 2010;**183**(**5**):1698–1702.

33 Chawla SN, Crispen PL, Hanlon AL, Greenberg RE, Chen DY, Uzzo RG. The natural history of observed enhancing renal masses: meta-analysis and review of the world literature. *J Urol.* 2006;**175**(**2**):425–431.

38 Blom JH, van Poppel H, Marechal JM, et al. Radical nephrectomy with and without lymph-node dissection: final results of European Organization for Research and Treatment of Cancer (EORTC) randomized phase 3 trial 30881. *Eur Urol.* 2009;**55**(**1**):28–34.

39 Chapin BF, Delacroix SE Jr, Culp SH, et al. Safety of presurgical targeted therapy in the setting of metastatic renal cell carcinoma. *Eur Urol.* 2011;**60**(**5**):964–971.

40 Abel EJ, Culp SH, Tannir NM, et al. Primary tumor response to targeted agents in patients with metastatic renal cell carcinoma. *Eur Urol.* 2011;**59**(**1**):10–15.

44 Cost NG, Delacroix SE Jr, Sleeper JP, et al. The impact of targeted molecular therapies on the level of renal cell carcinoma vena caval tumor thrombus. *Eur Urol.* 2011;**59**(**6**):912–918.

45 Donat SM, Diaz M, Bishoff JT, et al. Follow-up for clinically localized renal neoplasms: AUA guideline. *J Urol.* 2013;**190**(**2**):407–416.

47 Motzer RJ, Mazumdar M, Bacik J, Berg W, Amsterdam A, Ferrara J. Survival and prognostic stratification of 670 patients with advanced renal cell carcinoma. *J Clin Oncol.* 1999;**17**(**8**):2530–2540.

49 Heng DY, Xie W, Regan MM, et al. External validation and comparison with other models of the International Metastatic Renal-Cell Carcinoma Database Consortium prognostic model: a population-based study. *Lancet Oncol.* 2013;**14**(**2**):141–148.

54 Flanigan RC, Salmon SE, Blumenstein BA, et al. Nephrectomy followed by interferon alfa-2b compared with interferon alfa-2b alone for metastatic renal-cell cancer. *N Engl J Med.* 2001;**345**(**23**):1655–1659.

55 Mickisch GH, Garin A, van Poppel H, et al. Radical nephrectomy plus interferon-alfa-based immunotherapy compared with interferon alfa alone in metastatic renal-cell carcinoma: a randomised trial. *Lancet.* 2001;**358**(**9286**):966–970.

57 Rini BI, Campbell SC. The evolving role of surgery for advanced renal cell carcinoma in the era of molecular targeted therapy. *J Urol.* 2007;**177**(**6**):1978–1984.

62 Coppin C, Porzsolt F, Awa A, Kumpf J, Coldman A, Wilt T. Immunotherapy for advanced renal cell cancer. *Cochrane Database Syst Rev.* 2005;**1**:CD001425.

67 Brahmer JR, Tykodi SS, Chow LQ, et al. Safety and activity of anti-PD-L1 antibody in patients with advanced cancer. *N Engl J Med.* 2012;**366**(**26**):2455–2465.

71 Motzer RJ, Hutson TE, Tomczak P, et al. Overall survival and updated results for sunitinib compared with interferon alfa in patients with metastatic renal cell carcinoma. *J Clin Oncol.* 2009;**27**(**22**):3584–3590.

73 Motzer RJ, Hutson TE, McCann L, Deen K, Choueiri TK. Overall survival in renal-cell carcinoma with pazopanib versus sunitinib. *N Engl J Med.* 2014;**370**(**18**):1769–1770.

78 Motzer RJ, Escudier B, Oudard S, et al. Phase 3 trial of everolimus for metastatic renal cell carcinoma : final results and analysis of prognostic factors. *Cancer.* 2010;**116**(**18**):4256–4265.

79 Escudier B, Bellmunt J, Negrier S, et al. Phase III trial of bevacizumab plus interferon alfa-2a in patients with metastatic renal cell carcinoma (AVOREN): final analysis of overall survival. *J Clin Oncol.* 2010;**28**(**13**):2144–2150.

80 Rini BI, Halabi S, Rosenberg JE, et al. Phase III trial of bevacizumab plus interferon alfa versus interferon alfa monotherapy in patients with metastatic renal cell carcinoma: final results of CALGB 90206. *J Clin Oncol.* 2010;**28**(**13**):2137–2143.

82 Rini BI, Halabi S, Rosenberg JE, et al. Bevacizumab plus interferon alfa compared with interferon alfa monotherapy in patients with metastatic renal cell carcinoma: CALGB 90206. *J Clin Oncol.* 2008;**26**(**33**):5422–5428.

90 Sternberg CN, Davis ID, Mardiak J, et al. Pazopanib in locally advanced or metastatic renal cell carcinoma: results of a randomized phase III trial. *J Clin Oncol.* 2010;**28**(**6**):1061–1068.

96 Rini BI, Escudier B, Tomczak P, et al. Comparative effectiveness of axitinib versus sorafenib in advanced renal cell carcinoma (AXIS): a randomised phase 3 trial. *Lancet.* 2011;**378**(**9807**):1931–1939.

101 Motzer RJ, Barrios CH, Kim TM, et al. Phase II randomized trial comparing sequential first-line everolimus and second-line sunitinib versus first-line sunitinib and second-line everolimus in patients with metastatic renal cell carcinoma. *J Clin Oncol.* 2014;**32**(**25**):2765–2772.

103 Raghavan D. A structured approach to uncommon cancers: what should a clinician do? *Ann Oncol.* 2013;**24**(**12**):2932–2934.

106 Dason S, Allard C, Sheridan-Jonah A, et al. Management of renal collecting duct carcinoma: a systematic review and the McMaster experience. *Curr Oncol.* 2013;**20**(**3**):e223–232.

107 Pecuchet N, Bigot F, Gachet J, et al. Triple combination of bevacizumab, gemcitabine and platinum salt in metastatic collecting duct carcinoma. *Ann Oncol.* 2013;**24**(**12**):2963–2967.

第 97 章　尿路上皮癌

Derek Raghavan, MD, PhD, FACP, FRACP, FASCO ■ Richard Cote, MD, FRCPath, FCAP ■
Earle F. Burgess, MD ■ Stephen B. Riggs, MD ■ Michael Haake, MD

概述

尿路上皮恶性肿瘤是西方社会最常见的癌症之一，包括膀胱、尿道、输尿管及肾盂、肾盏肿瘤。尿路上皮恶性肿瘤的发生主要与吸烟、工业染料、血吸虫病、辐射暴露和患者所在地理区域有关。随着分子预后标志物的明确以及分期技术的进步，患者的预后得到了改善。对于非肌层浸润性尿路上皮癌，最好的治疗方法是手术切除，通常结合膀胱内免疫治疗或化疗。肌层浸润性尿路上皮癌最好采用以顺铂为基础的新辅助化疗，然后行根治性膀胱切除术；身体较弱的患者可适当采取顺铂为基础的化疗结合放疗。转移性尿路上皮癌对于 MVAC（甲氨蝶呤、长春碱、多柔比星和顺铂）或者 GC（吉西他滨、顺铂）化疗方案的反应率高达 70%，但却难以达到治愈效果。全身疾病治疗的新方法是以近期数据为基础的，反映了免疫功能检查点的重要性，并且与 PD-L1（程序性死亡配体 1）的表达相关。

简介及流行病学

膀胱癌是西方社会最常见的恶性肿瘤之一，年发病率男性为 16/100 000，女性为 5/100 000[1]。在美国，每年有 75 000 例新发病例，并约有 16 000 例患者死于该病[2]。另外每年还有约 3 000 例新发上尿路恶性肿瘤，及少量其他尿路上皮区域的肿瘤。在过去 50 年间，尽管由于吸烟人数减少，男性膀胱癌发病率已经趋于稳定，但是膀胱癌的总体发病率和死亡率都没有太大的变化。膀胱癌主要发生于老年男性，平均发病年龄为 60~65 岁。膀胱癌的发病率具有地区差异性，发病率升高的区域包括美国五大湖地区、中东沿海区域以及血吸虫病发病率升高的区域（多为鳞状细胞癌）。在巴尔干地区，地方性家族性间质性肾病可以将上尿路肿瘤的发病率升高 100~200 倍。在美国，白种人的尿路上皮癌发病率高于亚裔或非裔人群[2]。

膀胱癌的病因比较明确，最常见的相关病因是吸烟，其他因素包括接触染料和工业试剂、汽车尾气、水摄入减少（有争议）以及镇痛剂（对乙酰氨基酚）滥用[1]，此外还包括环磷酰胺及其他磷杂环己烷细胞毒性药物治疗史、高脂肪饮食、慢性泌尿系感染、截瘫以及盆腔放疗史。家族史也很重要，尤其对于有 Lynch 综合征及上尿路肿瘤病史的患者。

病理学及分子决定簇

膀胱癌主要为尿路上皮癌（urothelial carcinoma, UC），即过去所说的移行细胞癌[1,3]。尿路上皮癌可以发生于有尿路上皮生长的所有部位，并且可以多灶性起源，不同病灶具有相同的肿瘤组织学特点。膀胱癌中 90% 为尿路上皮癌，5%~10% 为鳞状细胞癌，4%~5% 为腺癌，此外还有一些少见癌，如未分化小细胞癌、肉瘤、黑色素瘤或淋巴瘤。偶尔可见其他肿瘤转移到膀胱。

越来越多的证据表明膀胱癌起源于肿瘤干细胞[4]，肿瘤干细胞具有通过不同通路分化的能力。因此，发现膀胱癌呈现多种类型细胞混杂的组织学生长方式就不足为奇了，但是尿路上皮癌仍然是其中最主要的组织类型。同样道理，转移灶有时也会表现出与原发病灶不同的组织学类型。这些肿瘤合并有区域性尿路黏膜缺陷，这可能与之前的致癌物刺激有关，因此肿瘤可同时或异时在多个位点发生。

尿路上皮癌可以表现为非浸润性或浸润性。在非浸润性肿瘤中，目前所知有 2 种不同的组织学亚型：乳头状癌与扁平的原位癌（carcinoma in situ, CIS）。非浸润性乳头状癌是膀胱癌最常见的病理类型，占膀胱癌发病率的 60% 以上。非浸润性乳头状癌被分为数级，从良性肿瘤（乳头状瘤）到具有浸润风险的高分级肿瘤（Ⅲ级和Ⅳ级）。分级系统通常仅限于非浸润性乳头状肿瘤的分级，而 CIS 属于高级别肿瘤，所有的浸润性肿瘤也属于高级别肿瘤[3]。

Ⅰ级（高分化）乳头状肿瘤的组织结构较为有序，类似于正常尿路上皮，其尿路上皮细胞具有极性且存在伞状细胞层，此外通常可见纤维血管蒂。而Ⅱ级肿瘤的核质比更高，并且核仁明显，伴有尿路上皮定位丢失和至少部分伞状细胞层丢失。Ⅲ级肿瘤表现为分化差或未分化，组织结构无序，并且有丝分裂指数高，伞状细胞层完全丢失。最新的 WHO 分级系统将肿瘤的分化程度整合后分为低级别和高级别两种，主要是因为这种分级方法比Ⅰ~Ⅲ分级方法能更准确地反应肿瘤的生物学特性[3,5]。尽管膀胱被厚实的脂肪及肌肉组织所包裹，但是上尿路的情况有所不同，因此，转移的阻碍和转移方式与膀胱癌不尽相同。

由于已经发现不同形态学亚型的膀胱癌（尤其是乳头状非浸润性肿瘤与扁平 CIS）之间在生物学行为上具有巨大的差异，这些亚型已经成为分子生物学研究的焦点[5]。最早的膀胱癌细胞发生学研究证实，第 9、11 和 17 号染色体发生了变异，这提示抑癌基因可能就存在于这些位置[5,6]。基于膀胱肿瘤中一贯和频繁的基因缺陷，膀胱癌的发生和发展已明确至少有两种不同的分子途径(图 97-1)。乳头状肿瘤常见 9 号染色体的变异,尤其是 INK4a/p16 位点。并且此类肿瘤常常表现出受体酪氨酸激酶-Ras 通路的组成性激活,表现出 HRAS 和成纤维细胞生长因子受体 3(fibroblast growth factor receptor 3,FGFR3)基因的激活突变。与之不同,扁平 CIS 和浸润性肿瘤常常表现出 *p53* 基因和蛋白(TP53)以及视网膜母细胞瘤(retinoblastoma,RB)基因的变异。在上尿路肿瘤中也发现了相似的基因变异,此外已发现的还有染色体 5q、1p、14q 和 8p 的变异。

RAS-MAPK 信号转导通路在非浸润性乳头状肿瘤中具有重要作用。绝大多数非浸润性乳头状 UC 都表现出这一通路的激活,其通常是通过激活 FGFR3 发生的,这也为新的治疗提供了潜在靶点。但是,其他受体酪氨酸激酶也参与了这一过程,如表皮生长因子受体(epithelial growth factor receptor,EGFR)和 Her2-neu[5]。

细胞周期调节是扁平 CIS 和浸润性 UC 的重要通路。这一通路的重要分子是 *p53* 这一肿瘤抑制蛋白,由 *p53* 基因编码。在三个决定簇(*p53*、*p21*、RB)中出现 2~3 个变异的膀胱癌患者的预后明显差于没有或单个决定性基因变异的患者(图 97-1)。

肿瘤血管生成和表观遗传变异也是 UC 的发生控制的重要因素。全面的全基因组测序已证实了染色质重塑基因突变的普遍性,并且强调了表观遗传失调在 UC 癌变中的重要性。目前所知的在 UC 中受甲基化影响的基因包括:RASSF1A、DAPK 和 INK4A[5]。

多元基因组表达分析在 UC 和其他肿瘤的研究中的重要性日益增加,该方法可以获得更加详尽的分子谱,具有组织发生、预后、治疗靶点和预测意义(图 97-2)[5,6]。

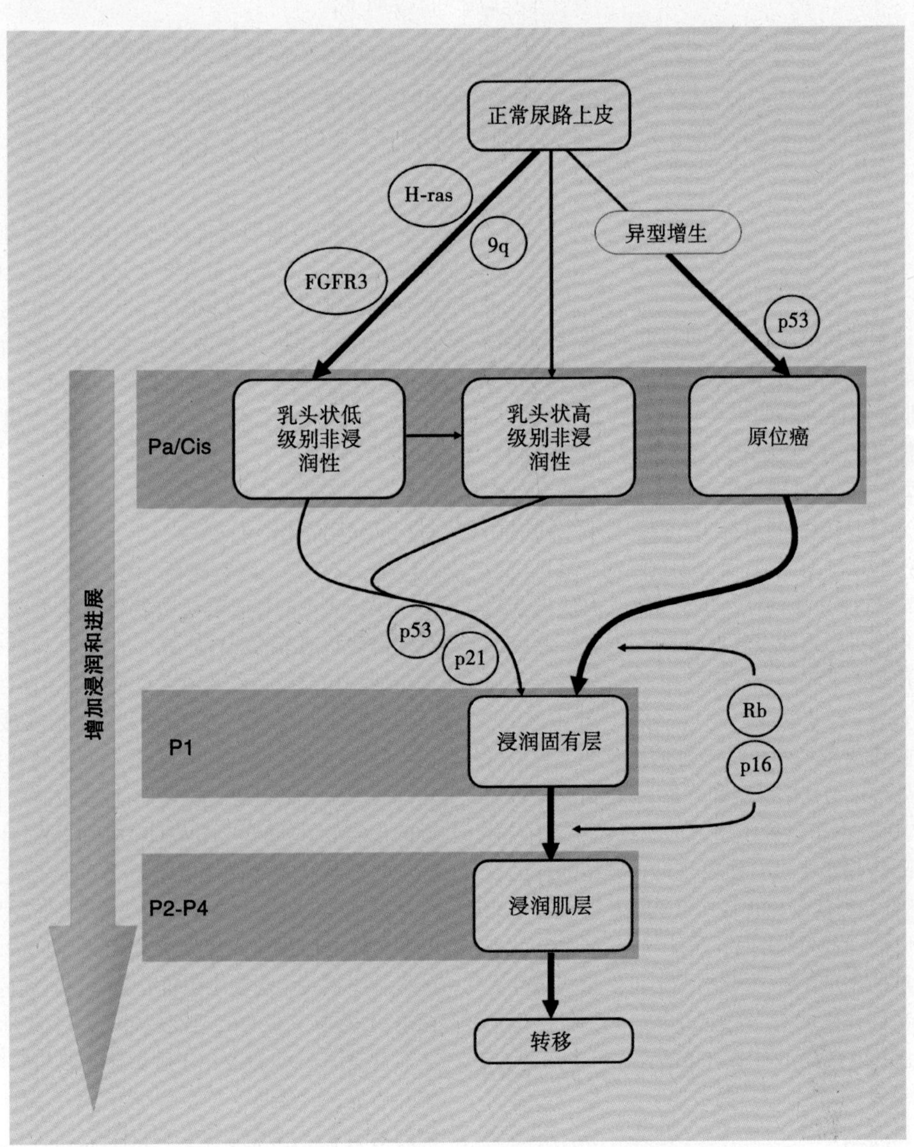

图 97-1　尿路上皮肿瘤发生发展模型。表浅性和侵袭性肿瘤具有特定的分子谱并来源于不同的通路。图中的分子:标识代表促进肿瘤进展为特定表型的风险事件。罕见的浸润性乳头状癌更有可能在关键位点发生基因突变。箭头的粗细表示发生的相对概率。来源:Mitra 2006

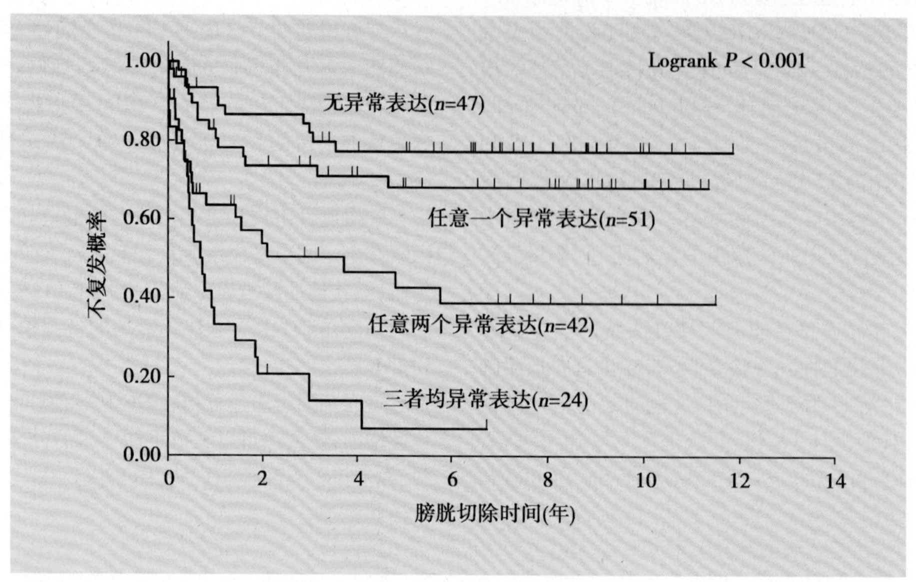

图 97-2 基于 *p53*、*p21* 和/或 *RB* 表达变化，得出 164 例接受根治性膀胱切除术的膀胱癌患者的无复发生存率。联合分析显示，随着异常表达数量的增加，复发风险增加（logrank $P<0.001$）来源：Chatterjee 2004

临床表现

膀胱癌的表现通常能反映疾病的严重程度，非肌层浸润性肿瘤、浸润性肿瘤、转移性和非转移性肿瘤的临床表现模式存在一些差异[1,8]。非浸润性肿瘤的患者可表现为无症状血尿（通过尿液常规检查诊断）、肉眼血尿以及刺激性症状如尿频、排尿困难、烧灼感或夜尿。有非肌层浸润性膀胱癌病史和经尿道电切病史的患者，膀胱刺激症状更突出。浸润性肿瘤患者的临床表现一般与非浸润性肿瘤类似，而分期更晚的肿瘤可以合并盆腔疼痛、尿流缓慢、性交痛，并且偶有气尿或大便失禁症状。肿瘤若侵犯三角区可导致输尿管梗阻，伴随腰痛。腰痛或更广泛的腹痛可能预示着上尿路肿瘤的存在，然而这些特性通常与局部晚期肿瘤有关。

转移性肿瘤的临床表现通常可反映肿瘤累及的部位。常见累及部位包括远处淋巴结、肺、肝脏和骨骼，少数情况下可累及脑、皮肤和其他内脏。由于影像学检查的积极应用，许多转移病灶是在常规的随访检查中被首次发现的。典型的肺部转移症状为咳嗽和呼吸困难，偶尔伴有咯血或胸痛。肝转移可表现为右上腹疼痛或肩痛，有时可出现肝功能损害，最常见的表现是黄疸。骨转移常常合并骨痛，少数情况下可发生病理性骨折，常见受累部位包括脊柱、肋骨、骨盆和颅骨。头痛、意识模糊或其他运动系统症状常常提示有脑转移的存在。头颅的 CT 或 MRI 检查通常能够发现问题，但是偶尔在影像学检查正常时需要行椎管穿刺抽液来诊断癌性脑膜炎（尤其对于有可疑症状，之前因转移性疾病接受过全身化疗的患者）。皮肤转移少见，通常表现为浸润性病变或孤立的皮肤或皮下结节。

肿瘤的非转移性表现主要是血清学的改变，但偶有患者会表现出常见于胃肠道腺癌的血栓栓塞综合征。膀胱癌偶尔会产生粒细胞-巨噬细胞集落刺激因子或其他细胞因子，表现为血液中白细胞计数的显著增加，与感染造成的白细胞增高有明显区别。鳞状分化的肿瘤有时可合并高钙血症，这与过量产生的免疫反应性甲状旁腺激素（PTH）类似物有关。总而言之，这些血清学改变要根据具体情况来处理，通常不需要特别治疗，除非导致了临床症状，如严重的高钙血症、明显的血栓栓塞等。

检查和分期

临床表现的特异性将决定检查的方式。表现为血尿或其他尿路症状通常需要行尿液常规检查，以除外感染或尿路结石的可能。如果排除了上述疾病或存在无菌性脓尿，通常需要进行尿细胞学和/或膀胱镜检查。在临床实践中，为了提高尿细胞学检查的敏感性，减少非肌层浸润性膀胱癌患者术后随访中定期膀胱镜检的需要，基于可溶性膀胱肿瘤抗原或以细胞为基础的标志物（NMP22、BTA-TRAK、BLCA-4、ImmunoCyt）的新型标志物检测试剂盒已经被研发[9]。分子学分析（urovysion）可探测染色体的非整倍性，以了解 3、7 和 17 号染色体的变化，这些染色体的变化与高级别肿瘤相关，而 *9p21* 位点的缺失与低分级肿瘤相关。病例对照研究和队列研究的结果提示，在上述标志物中，有一些的敏感性超过了尿细胞学，并且其中一些已经通过美国 FDA 批准用于肿瘤筛查或与膀胱镜联合应用于膀胱肿瘤复发的诊断[9]。在膀胱炎、尿石症、肠代膀胱或存在异物的情况下会出现假阳性。尿细胞学的特异性据称超过 95%，因此阳性结果提示需要进一步检查，但阴性结果的意义不大。近期出现了一种新的检查方式，是使用微过滤设备捕获和检查尿液中的膀胱癌细胞，该方法仍有待进一步验证[10]。近年来，随着更精密内镜摄像设备的应用，内镜检查技术得到了极大的改进，其包括：高分辨率影像、荧光膀胱镜及窄带成像膀胱镜检查，使检查的特异性和敏感性得到了提高[11,12]。这也促进了对于上尿路的检查设备的应用。

目前膀胱癌还没有特定的血清学检查方法。通过常规的血液学和生化检查可能发现由于肿瘤缓慢进展或失血、肾衰竭（继发于梗阻或导致肿瘤的潜在疾病）所导致的慢性贫血，偶尔也会发现转移的迹象，如碱性磷酸酶升高或肝功能检测。尚未发现膀胱癌特异性的血清学肿瘤标志物，虽然偶然会发现膀胱癌患者的癌胚抗原、HCG、CA19-9 或 CA125 升高，后者主要在有腺癌成分的情况下会出现。

泌尿系统的影像学检查可以在膀胱镜检查之前或之后进行。相对标准的方法是通过排泄性尿路造影来显示出泌尿道的解剖情况，包括膀胱和上尿路的肿瘤或肾积水[8]。CT 检查是现在最常应用的检查方法，因为它可以同时评价尿路上皮和肾实质的情况，并且检查过程比排泄性尿路造影更迅速。MRI 检查也有助于确定局部的解剖情况和浸润性肿瘤的侵犯范围，同时能提供淋巴结及远处转移等肿瘤分期信息。但需要强调一点，非肌层浸润性膀胱肿瘤的盆腔影像学检查的敏感性和特异性有限。另外很重要的一点，在膀胱肿瘤经尿道电切术（transurethral resection of bladder tumor，TURBT）后近期内进行 CT 和 MRI 检查，经常会由于电切后炎症性浸润导致影像学结果出现肿瘤侵犯深度增加的假象。正电子发射计算机断层扫描（positron emission tomography，PET）的作用尚不确定，但我们偶尔也会使用这一方法来辅助发现潜在的转移部位，如果其结果为阳性，则需要进一步检查，阴性结果意义不大。

确诊需要通过经尿道电切手术，其通常的目的是完整切除肿瘤和明确分期。经尿道电切（TUR）时行双合诊检查可以评价肿瘤的分期和膀胱外肿瘤侵犯情况。对于高分级肿瘤，明确是否存在逼尿肌受侵的情况是非常重要的。如果不准备进一步行膀胱全切术，在术后 4～6 周行二次 TUR 可发现 30%初始电切发现肌层受侵的患者和 60%初始电切未见肌层受侵的患者的病理分期增加。

预后

膀胱癌的预后与上文所讨论过的一些因素有关，包括肿瘤的分期和分级、多灶性、淋巴血管侵犯、合并 CIS、肿瘤形态、基因突变形式、贫血或肾积水。相似因素也决定着上尿路肿瘤的预后，其包括：分级、分期、血管淋巴受累、异倍体、EGFR 表达、肿瘤位置（输尿管肿瘤比肾盂预后更差）及术后肿瘤残余[1]。

AJCC 分期[13]与预后的相关性较好。膀胱由大量脂肪和肌肉包裹，然而上尿路的情况有所不同，因此两者的扩散障碍和转移模式有所不同。

此外，Bajorin 等人[14]研究的数学模型可评估晚期肿瘤患者的风险和预后，其主要关注内脏转移、体力状态及贫血；这些内容近期已被更新并提高了预后准确性[15]。还有一些修改建议也被提出，包括二线治疗和挽救性化疗的预后标准，但并没有改善生存数据。尽管他们可能有助于避免无作用的化疗（表 97-1）。

表 97-1　转移性膀胱癌的危险因子

变量	统计学显著性（*P*）	相对危险度
3 个变量		
内脏转移（是/否）	0.000 1	1.99
Karnofsky 体能状态评分（<80%或≥80%）	0.000 1	2.05
血红蛋白（正常/异常）	0.010 3	1.41
2 个变量		
内脏转移（是/否）	0.000 1	2.10
Karnofsky 体能状态评分（<80%或≥80%）	0.000 1	2.2

摘自 Adapted from Bajorin 1999。

非肌层浸润性膀胱肿瘤的治疗

非肌层浸润性膀胱肿瘤有效治疗的关键是膀胱镜检查和切除可见的膀胱肿瘤[16,17]，有时需要在术后进行膀胱内灌注治疗（免疫制剂或细胞毒性制剂）以减少复发的风险[8,16,17]。由于膀胱癌合并有黏膜区域性缺陷，对于尿细胞学阳性或高分级肿瘤且准备保留膀胱的患者，应该对外观正常的膀胱黏膜进行随机活检以除外 CIS 的存在。对于高分级和/或 T1 的肿瘤患者，通常在 4 周内进行重复电切，因为有超过 50%的患者在第二次活检时发现膀胱肿瘤侵犯肌层。

肿瘤的分级和分期决定了下一步的治疗。非肌层浸润、低分级乳头状膀胱癌进展为浸润性膀胱癌的风险较低，尽管其复发的风险高达 60%～80%。复发的风险取决于肿瘤大小、多灶性或是否曾有复发病史，有复发高风险的患者通常在电切后给予膀胱内治疗（通常每周灌注 1 次，持续 6～8 周），最常用的药物是卡介苗（bacillus calmette guerin，BCG），它可以使复发的风险减少约 40%[14]。BCG 的作用机制是局部免疫刺激，也可能与改变抑制性/辅助性 T 淋巴细胞的比值有关。这一治疗可使膀胱有效地"排斥"膀胱癌的种植和复发。这可能同时也是 PD-1 对于侵袭性和转移性肿瘤靶向效用的作用机制，因其释放了对 T 细胞功能的束缚。

随机试验结果提示，BCG 在预防肿瘤进展方面优于其他膀胱灌注药物，对于低分级肿瘤，包括 BCG 灌注的保留膀胱治疗远期效果与早期切除膀胱相似[17]。与单纯 6 周 BCG 诱导用药相比，BCG 维持治疗可减少肿瘤复发及膀胱全切的风险。BCG 的最佳灌注方案尚未确定，并且最佳的商品化 BCG 灌注制剂以及最理想的灌注周期也存在争议。

常用的膀胱内灌注药物的副作用包括刺激性症状和血尿。BCG 可导致流感样症状，并且由于 BCG 是减毒分枝杆菌，它可造成局灶性、区域性和系统性结核样感染。肉芽肿性感染可发生于膀胱外的部位，包括前列腺、附睾、睾丸、肾脏、肝脏和肺。BCG 脓毒症是最严重的并发症，有可能危及生命，通常需要接受三联抗结核治疗。

一些医学中心倾向于使用细胞毒药物膀胱内化疗,如丝裂霉素 C 或吉西他滨[18],因为据称可减少毒性反应,虽然这一观点尚未得到证实。对于肿瘤复发并且不愿接受膀胱全切术的非肌层浸润性膀胱癌患者,有多种免疫性或细胞毒性膀胱灌注药物可供选择,并且可以延迟肿瘤复发和进展。

治疗结束后,应对患者进行严格的监测,每 3~6 个月检查膀胱镜、选择性尿细胞学和/或肿瘤标志物评估,以及早发现肿瘤复发。高危非肌层浸润性肿瘤的患者(高分级 Ta、T1 或 CIS)发生浸润性膀胱癌的风险超过 50%,死于膀胱癌的风险达 35%。并且,如果患者在 1~2 个疗程的膀胱灌注治疗后持续或反复出现高分级肿瘤,约有 80%会发生肌层侵犯和肿瘤进展。因此我们建议对于复发的高分级肿瘤应及时行膀胱全切及尿流改道手术,尤其是当患者预期寿命较长时[19,20]。及时膀胱全切可使肿瘤治愈率达到 90%,如果延迟膀胱全切的时间,将会出现肌层侵犯,并且患者生存时间将缩短[19]。

肌层浸润性膀胱癌的治疗

根治性手术

在过去的 20 年间,根治性膀胱全切+双侧盆腔淋巴结清扫术逐渐成为局部浸润性膀胱癌的标准治疗方法[1,8,20,21]。这一术式要求将前盆腔脏器整块切除,包括男性患者的膀胱、前列腺和精囊,女性患者的膀胱、尿道、子宫、卵巢以及阴道穹窿加阴道前壁[20]。尿流改道则通过将输尿管与去管化肠管储尿囊连接来实现。可控性贮尿囊,如印第安纳膀胱和原位新膀胱,现在已经成为标准术式,因为控尿效果好,不需要外接尿液收集袋。原位新膀胱创造性地将贮尿囊与尿道相接,使患者可以像正常人一样排尿,不需要自我导尿。

根治性膀胱切除术如果不加辅助性治疗,根据分期和其他预后因素的不同,可治愈 60%的浸润性膀胱癌[20,21]。大宗病例研究中 T2~T3 期患者的五年总体生存率为 40%~65%。肿瘤复发风险与分期、分级、淋巴血管侵犯以及预后分子标志物表达情况相关。对于有盆腔区域淋巴结转移的患者,仅做根治性膀胱切除的治愈率仅为 20%~40%,治疗结果受肿瘤分期、受累淋巴结的数量以及结外侵犯情况影响[1,8,20,21]。扩大的淋巴结清扫可能提高治愈率[20,21]。但是,这一结论可能与病例选择偏倚、手术技巧或支持治疗及挽救性治疗的技术水平有关。

器械的进步

一些有腹腔镜手术经验的医学中心报道了腹腔镜伴/不伴机器人辅助的根治性膀胱切除术技术[22,23]。膀胱切除和淋巴结清扫通常在腹腔镜下完成,尿流改道通过在下腹正中做一较小切口在体外完成,这一小切口较传统手术明显减小。其可能的优势包括出血少、术后疼痛轻,恢复快。尽管现有的数据都是来自非随机研究,并且都是由腹腔镜经验丰富的外科医师操作,病例选择非常严格,随访时间也较短。最近,Bochner 等[24]报道了一项随机试验的初步结果,其表明腹腔镜根治性膀胱切除创伤相当,但花费更高。因为这是一个早期报告主要关注早期并发症,长期结果还有待报道。

另一技术的创新是保留前列腺的膀胱根治性切除术,其目的是为了减少损伤及其晚期并发症,但是其效果尚未得到随机研究的证实。这种技术对于侵犯前列腺的肿瘤或合并前列腺偶发腺癌的患者并不适用。

放疗的作用

对于浸润性、无临床转移的膀胱癌患者,如果由于患者的意愿、技术因素或其他并发疾病的影响而不适于手术治疗,可以选择进行放射治疗[25~27]。到目前为止,还没有设计非常好的随机研究对放疗和手术治疗膀胱癌的效果进行对比。适形放射治疗或调强放射治疗(IMRT)的最佳放射剂量仍存在争议[25]。适合放疗的预后因素包括:体积小、局限性、T2、无肾积水、经尿道最大限度切除肿瘤、肾功能正常以及无贫血表现[1,26,27]。

相对标准的放疗方法是:以大于 65~70Gy 的剂量治疗 6~7 周,通过诊断性扫描定位,将 40Gy 投射到膀胱区域,最高剂量能量主要聚焦于肿瘤及其周围。在行 TURBT 手术时,通过患者在俯卧位 CT 模拟成像进行放疗定位[26,27]。基于 RTOG 研究及加拿大国立肿瘤研究所[28]随机试验的结果,现在很少对患者进行单纯放射治疗,更常见的是放疗联合全身化疗。这些研究结果均显示放化疗可改善肿瘤的局部控制,但是生存获益的改善并不明显。在英国,一项临床随机试验表明放疗联合氟尿嘧啶和丝裂霉素 C 较单纯放疗能获得更好的局部控制和生存获益[29]。

放射治疗的毒性包括:皮肤炎症、偶伴出血和梗阻性直肠炎、膀胱炎或膀胱纤维化、勃起功能障碍、尿失禁以及放射区域周围继发恶性肿瘤。重要的是,如果放疗失败,由于放疗区域纤维化形成,将使挽救性手术变得非常复杂。

近年来提出了一些放疗计划和治疗方面的革新,包括可以追踪肿瘤随呼吸等生理性活动的位移并调整放射的仪器,和粒子治疗,如质子束,聚焦程度更高,对正常组织的毒性更小。这些新技术在膀胱癌治疗中的应用情况仍没有 1 级证据支持,尚有待进一步研究。

联合治疗策略

新辅助治疗

早在 30 年前,基于化疗可能减少局部肿瘤进展、控制隐匿的转移灶这一理论,笔者就发表了全身化疗联合局部治疗的研究结果[30]。我们前期试验证明:新辅助或预先全身化疗可以使膀胱原发肿瘤的体积缩小,导致肿瘤降期,有时可达到完全的临床和病理缓解[30]。虽然在早期的随机研究中单纯应用某一种化疗药物对于膀胱癌的生存并没有太大的影响。但是一些随机临床研究和荟萃分析的结果显示,将用于转移性膀胱癌的 MVAC 化疗方案(甲氨蝶呤、长春碱、阿柔比星和顺铂)和 CMV 化疗方案(顺铂、甲氨蝶呤和长春碱)用于新辅助治疗可以使患者生存获益(表 97-2)[31~33]。

因此,目前的一致观点是:MVAC 方案的新辅助化疗联合根治性膀胱切除术可使患者的绝对生存获益增加 7%~8%,中位生存时间可延长至 3 年。而初始治疗为放疗的生存获益并没有显著提高。最近美国国内的临床实践调查显示,只有极少的泌尿外科医师按照上述方法对患者进行治疗,临床治疗方法的改变非常缓慢[34,35]。

表97-2 侵袭性膀胱癌(分期:T1-T4)新辅助化疗临床随机试验结果

系列	新辅助化疗方案	根治性治疗	中位生存期/月 有/无新辅助化疗	长期生存率 有/无新辅助化疗
新辅助				
MRC-EORTC	CMV	放射治疗/膀胱全切	44/37.5	35%/30%10年
Intergroup	MVDC	膀胱全切	72/46	42%/35%10年
Nordic 1 trial	DC	膀胱全切	未达到/72	59%/51%5年
辅助				
EORTC	MVDC	膀胱全切	81/55	44%/39%5年
Stanford	CMV	膀胱全切	63/36	42%/38%5年
USC	CDCy	膀胱全切	52/30	44%/39%5年
Cognetti	GC	膀胱全切	38/58	44%/44%6.5年

C,顺铂;D,多柔比星;M,甲氨蝶呤;Cy,环磷酰胺;V,长春碱;G,吉西他滨;MRC-EORTC,药物研究委员会/欧洲癌症研究与治疗组织。

目前尚未发现其他多药新辅助化疗优于或等效于MVAC或CMV方案的新辅助化疗。但是,一些新的较温和的化疗方案如吉西他滨-顺铂或吉西他滨-卡铂在新辅助化疗中的应用日渐增多。这对于年老体弱的患者可能是一个合理的选择,但对于身体强壮没有其他并发疾病的患者可能会增加因肿瘤导致死亡的风险。希望能有更好的临床随机试验来验证这一问题。正如最初被EORTC开发测试时一样,剂量密度MVAC治疗转移性肿瘤的重要性仍然不明确且存在争议。尽管这种方法已被NCCN指南认可,可以降低治疗副作用,但是否能有相似的长期效果尚不明确。

辅助性化疗

对于T3~T4的肿瘤和/或淋巴结受累的患者,在根治性膀胱切除术后加用化疗可以提高无疾病进展的生存时间[36-41]。但是目前有关这一方面的研究都存在实验设计不合理和样本量小的缺陷,在总体生存上的统计学差异并不明显[42]。一个意大利团队进行了一项GC辅助方案化疗的试验,在化疗组中生存率并没有明显劣势[41]。有一项欧洲癌症治疗研究组织EORTC的随机试验考虑到了这些缺陷,并已经进行了数年,但由于病例累积速度较慢而被提前关闭。这项研究证实了对于没有淋巴结转移的患者,根治性膀胱切除术后辅助化疗提高了无病生存期,但没有总生存期获益[43]。这可能暗示辅助化疗对于没有完全的切除肿瘤能够达到补充治疗的效果。

虽然荟萃分析有时能有助于解决小规模试验无法解决的问题,但Cochrane组织发表的荟萃分析结果同样存在严重的缺陷[44]。这一分析集合了许多小规模的研究,这些研究存在实验设计不合理、操作不当或未对辅助化疗与复发后化疗进行对比等多种问题,因此分析结果并未提供有价值的信息,实际上只会使情况更混乱。通过对这些存在历史对照和操作不当等局限性随机试验的了解,笔者认为辅助性化疗可能使生存获益,不太可能使生存受损,因此最好将其选择性应用于高风险疾病的膀胱全切术后患者,或者是身体健康的患者。一个设计合理的随机试验也不太可能永远能回答这个问题。

转移性膀胱癌

化疗是转移性膀胱癌患者的一线治疗方法。自20世纪60年代至80年代早期,氟尿嘧啶、甲氨蝶呤、长春碱、多柔比星及顺铂的药物活性逐渐得到论证[45]。使用甲氨蝶呤、长春碱、顺铂联合[46]或不联合[47]多柔比星案可使患者的客观反应率超过60%,中位生存时间为1年。在一项由美国、加拿大及澳大利亚共同进行的国际多中心随机研究中发现,MVAC方案优于顺铂单药治疗,并且在平均随访6年后这一优势仍然存在[48]。MVAC方案的主要局限性是其比较严重的毒性反应,包括三到四级的胃肠道反应、口腔炎和骨髓抑制,偶尔也可见肾衰竭和心脏毒性[46,48]。有人尝试改进这一化疗方案,Sternberg等人通过随机研究发现,调整剂量的MVAC方案比原方案的反应率更高,毒性反应更低[49],但中位生存时间并没有显著的增加。但是5年患者生存人数高于标准剂量MVAC组,只是没有达到显著性统计学差异。

紫杉醇、吉西他滨、多烯紫杉醇、异环磷酰胺及培美曲塞单药治疗的反应率为20%~30%。这些药物与标准方案或其他研究药物联合使用的反应率可达50%~80%,有一些的毒性反应低于MVAC方案,但中位生存期仍然保持在12~20个月,并且对伴有其他内脏器官转移的患者的治愈率不超过10%~15%[45]。最初的一些研究发现吉西他滨+顺铂的联合治疗与MVAC相比具有相似的反应率和较低的毒性反应[50],而后一项随机试验对吉西他滨+顺铂联合治疗与MVAC方案进行了比较,再一次肯定了上述的发现,并且发现患者的生存率近似[51]。因此,在一个随机试验中,一个国际联合组织使用吉西他滨+顺铂+紫杉醇方案治疗未经治疗的转移性UC,试图改善治愈率,但结果显示对生存无明显影响[52]。一些Ⅰ~Ⅱ期试验比较了其他两联和三联治疗,但尚未发现更具优势的治疗方案。

在解释当今临床研究数据时需要特别注意的一点是,当今接受治疗的进展性膀胱肿瘤的分期已经出现了迁移,这是因为在术后使用CT、MRI及PET等更积极的影像学检查方法的比例增加了,并且对体积较小的、无症状的转移病灶进行全身化疗的比例也增加了。因此,对新的联合化疗方案进行评价时应考虑到,例如ITP方案(异环磷酰胺、紫杉醇和顺铂),其中位生存期是18个月,与现在使用的MVAC方案结果相似。在新的化疗方案被临床所接受和常规应用之前,需要通过随机试验将其与现在的标准治疗方案进行对比,以确定其安全性和有效性。尽管过去二十年有了一定进展,转移性膀胱癌的患者中仍然有大多数死于肿瘤进展。更重要的是,在一个成本意识和价值主张日益增强的时代,需要更加详尽地明确化疗的目的。不太可能延长生命或改善生活质量的患者或者被转到临终关怀中心,或者如果仍然足够健康可进入新治疗方法的临床试验。有症状的局部或转移性肿瘤的局部放射治疗也能给予这些患者缓解症状的益处。

由于细胞毒化疗并没有显著提高转移性膀胱癌的治愈率,已经开展其他治疗方法的研究。在过去的10年中,以控制细胞生长、分化和凋亡的基因和蛋白为目标的新药研究受到更多的关注。已经对具有调节EGFR功能的药物和其他酪氨酸激酶抑制剂进行了研究。这些新药被单独应用或与化疗联合使用。可以对HER-2/neu致癌基因、EGFR及其他可预测治疗效果的分子标志物进行检测,并据此调整个体的治疗方案。Hussain等人评价了赫赛汀(herceptin)联合化疗方案治疗表达HER-2/neu膀胱癌的效果,反应率达70%;但是14个月的中位生存期并不说明有显著的改善[53]。在这个研究中,表达EGFR的肿瘤可以获得更好的反应率。

酪氨酸激酶抑制剂,舒尼替尼(sunitinib)可使大部分经过治疗的膀胱癌获得部分缓解,但肿瘤的缓解仅能持续较短时间[54]。尽管这暗示抗血管生成途径的药物在膀胱癌中的应用价值,但其他研究发现这一类药物对膀胱癌没有明显作用。这种方法并没有获得足够的吸引力。

然而,两种新的方法似乎更有希望。最近的研究数据表明MET基因在尿路上皮癌和前列腺癌中高表达。早期的试验表明,它对前列腺癌有显著的治疗作用,而最近的一项研究表明对晚期尿路上皮癌有相似的抗肿瘤作用[55]。

初步研究表明,程序性死亡配体1(PD-L1)在尿路上皮恶性肿瘤中高表达。一期临床试验表明,PD-L1抑制剂(如MPDL3280A)有着较大的抗肿瘤作用[56]。二期临床试验正在进行中。尽管前期结果较理想,由于这些药物的长期作用仍不确定并且成本高昂,在进入临床常规使用前,这些药物应当严格依照既定的标准试验验证。

另一个被重新开始研究的治疗方法是,在化疗使肿瘤获得缓解后通过手术来巩固治疗成果[57]。膀胱癌这一治疗方法的研究始于20年前,先驱者是Alan Yagoda。其理论依据是,对化疗有反应性的肿瘤出现复发的比例很高,在对化疗有完全反应性并被切除的膀胱癌标本中发现活性强的肿瘤的概率高达33%。患者在接受基于顺铂化疗后完整切除转移灶,其5年生存率高达30%~40%,但是需要注意的是,这一方法对患者的选择非常严格,仅局限于单个转移灶的患者。

少见的组织学类型肿瘤

对膀胱腺癌、鳞癌、小细胞癌及肉瘤的详细论述不在本章的范围之内,详情可参考其他文献[58,59]。但是对于这些少见类型肿瘤的治疗原则是可以了解到的[60]。所有少见类型的肿瘤对化疗的抵抗性都强于单纯的尿路上皮癌,因此其治疗重心应该放在手术切除或根治性放疗上。如果诊断为少见组织学类型的肿瘤,应经肿瘤病理专家确诊,并除外在该部位存在第二原发肿瘤。一般情况下,我们建议患者转诊到级别更高的医学中心以确诊和征求多方面治疗意见[60]。

非移行细胞的转移性膀胱癌预后取决于肿瘤累及的部位、生长特点及肿瘤负荷。由于这些肿瘤的化疗效果不及UC[48,58,59],在计划对其进行化疗时应综合考虑患者的具体情况(年龄、预期寿命、并发疾病、转移部位)[60]。

通常认为鳞癌对包括铂类化合物、紫杉醇和吉西他滨的联合治疗比较敏感,偶尔也有联合使用甲氨蝶呤、博来霉素和异环磷酰胺获得反应的报道。我们前面提到MVAC方案对膀胱鳞癌并没有特别的效果[48]。目前临床治疗的模式多种多样,包括吉西他滨、异环磷酰胺、顺铂的联合治疗方案或紫杉醇、吉西他滨和顺铂的联合治疗方案,并且这些方案有时对于转移性肿瘤也能取得长期生存的效果。腺癌对应用于胃肠道肿瘤的化疗方案有短期反应,如联合使用奥沙利铂、伊立替康和氟嘧啶类药物(如氟尿嘧啶或卡培他滨),但是目前缺乏设计良好的Ⅱ期或Ⅲ期临床试验数据的支持。

MD安德森癌症中心报道了在治疗膀胱转移性未分化小细胞癌方面的大量经验,结果显示抗癌治疗对其有效,但很少能被治愈[59]。所用的药物与治疗肺小细胞癌类似,通常采用铂类化合物、依托泊苷、一种紫杉烷和一种烷化剂(oxazophorine)联合治疗。但是,与支气管来源的小细胞癌相比,膀胱来源的未分化小细胞癌对化疗的抵抗性更强,因此应更加重视对原发肿瘤的外科切除治疗。如果发生转移,相关性就很小。此外,有较好的2类证据证明化疗可增加手术切除临床非转移性疾病对生存的影响。

上尿路肿瘤

上尿路上皮癌的治疗方式与膀胱癌非常相似。需要提醒的是,上尿路周围的脂肪及肌肉支持组织较少,所以对于肿瘤转移的限制能力较差。此外那种“脱落转移”的现象可能会发生,即随着来源上尿路肿瘤的积聚,可能会种植到膀胱的尿路上皮。这是否是尿路上皮癌在时间和空间上多中心性的唯一机制仍不明确。关于病因学、流行病学、临床表现和体格检查的细节已经在相关章节讨论[61~63]。

手术治疗

上尿路肿瘤的手术入路与膀胱肿瘤有所不同[64~67]。局限性上尿路上皮癌的标准治疗方式是根治性肾输尿管切除术,完整地切除肾脏、周围脂肪及肾周筋膜,去除受累输尿管,以及膀胱袖状切除。笔者认为为了达到预测预后的目的,应行同侧淋巴结清扫或广泛取样,尽管没有一级证据支持这一操作的治疗效果。

腹腔镜肾输尿管根治性切除术正日益兴起,相比于开放手术腹腔镜手术被认为也是一个可行的选择,虽然长期结果的还有待证实。非随机系列试验已显示其结果与开放手术具有可比性,包括对于肿瘤控制,可能减少手术并发症[65,66]。

在某些情况下，应当考虑保留肾单位手术，例如，双侧肾脏疾病、孤立肾、肾功能受损或严重的并发疾病情况。这些技术包括肾部分切除术、输尿管部分切除术、肾盂部分切除术和经皮肾盂肿瘤切除术。这些治疗方法的选择实际是获益和风险的权衡，必须要考虑到肿瘤治疗效果和并发症以及对身体状况的影响。低级别肿瘤患者可选择内镜方法得到安全的、有效的治疗[67]。患者的选择是至关重要的，手术经验、使用的技术，仪器和预后决定因素决定了肿瘤术后复发率。

放疗和化疗

除了对无法手术的肿瘤患者姑息放疗，对于上尿路肿瘤的放疗仅仅有少量的1~2级证据支持。放疗剂量受正常组织对放疗敏感性的限制。此外，对于预后较差的肿瘤，在对局部肿瘤进行放疗的同时，实际上有很高概率存在同时或异时性淋巴结受累或远处转移，从而影响对放射治疗的作用。在结构化的临床试验中，辅助放疗并没有显示出对上尿路肿瘤患者的生存有较大影响[68,69]。

膀胱内治疗尿路上皮肿瘤的有效性使研究者将这些药物用于上尿路肿瘤的治疗。最常用的方法为双侧输尿管内置入支架管，然后像膀胱癌那样通过尿管灌注细胞毒性药物（通常为BCG）。然而如何保证药物能很好地向上传送到相应的部位，仍有很大不确定性。已有报道经皮插入可弯性导管至输尿管，然后灌入化疗药物。无对照研究数据表明，化学制剂和免疫制剂与肿瘤表面接触后可发生肿瘤消退。

内镜治疗后使用卡介苗（BCG）、多柔比星、丝裂霉素C作为辅助治疗均曾被报道。有证据表明对上尿路肿瘤有抗癌作用[70]。除膀胱内应用外，药物也通过经皮治疗后的肾盂引流管给药。包括长期随访的数据质量不尽相同，但目前一致认可的是这种治疗可以降低复发和进展。大约30%的上尿路上皮癌患者经治疗后会在膀胱内复发，因此需要对患者进行长期的膀胱镜随访[71]。

对上尿路上皮癌的全身化疗实际上与应用于膀胱的尿路上皮癌是相似的[45~52]。但在过去，上尿路肿瘤能对化学治疗反应比膀胱癌更差。然而，并没有多少证据支持这一观点。在多中心对顺铂相比于MVAC方案治疗转移性UC的研究中，发现上尿路和下尿路肿瘤患者的反应率和生存率是相近的[48]。因此，全身化疗的内容已在膀胱癌化疗的相关章节已做详细介绍。

总结

在过去的30年间，膀胱癌的治疗取得了非常显著的进步，包括对膀胱癌生物学行为的理解、基因表达及干细胞功能的相关性、分子学预测、手术方法的改进、手术并发症的减少及进展性肿瘤化疗的合理化。此外还有通过放化疗保留膀胱的治疗方法。尽管取得了很多进步，但仍有很多患者死于膀胱癌的转移，这促使我们研究新的全身治疗方法，包括新型的细胞毒性药物和靶向治疗，目前针对MET基因和PD-L1的药物最具前景。新药物在进入常规临床实践之前，应与目前标准方案在严格设计的随机对照研究中心进行比较。

（杨飞亚 译　邢念增 校）

关键参考文献

The complete reference list can be found on the Wiley Companion Digital Edition of this title (see inside front cover for login instructions).

1 Raghavan D, Shipley WU, Garnick MB, Richie JP, Russell PJ. Biology and management of bladder cancer. *N Engl J Med.* 1990;**322**:1129–1138.

2 Fleshner N, Kondylis F. Demographics and epidemiology of urothelial cancer of the urinary bladder. In: Droller M, ed. *American Cancer Society Atlas of Clinical Oncology: Urothelial Tumors.* London, Hamilton: BC Decker; 2004:1–16.

3 Cote RJ, Mitra AP, Amin MB: Bladder and urethra. In: Weidner N, Cote RJ, Suster S, Weiss LM eds. *Modern Surgical Pathology*, 2nd ed. Philadelphia, PA; Saunders; 2009, pp. 1079ff, Chapter 31.

4 Brown JL, Russell PJ, Philips J, Wotherspoon J, Raghavan D. Clonal analysis of a bladder cancer cell line: an experimental model of tumor heterogeneity. *Br J Cancer.* 1990;**61**:369–376.

5 Mitra AP, Cote RJ. Molecular screening for bladder cancer: progress and potential. *Nat Rev Urol.* 2010;7:11–20.

6 Chatterjee SJ, Datar R, Youssefzadeh D, et al. Combined effects of P53, P21, and PRb expression in the progression of bladder transitional cell carcinoma. *J Clin Oncol.* 2004;**22**:1007–1013.

7 Mitra AP, Datar RH, Cote RJ. Molecular pathways in invasive bladder cancer: new insights into mechanisms, progression, and target identification. *J Clin Oncol.* 2006;**24**:5552–5564.

8 Raghavan D, Huben R. Management of bladder cancer. *Curr Probl Cancer.* 1995;**19**:1–64.

11 Grossman HB, Gomella L, Fradet Y, et al. A phase III multicenter comparison of hexaminolevulinate fluorescence cystoscopy and white light cystoscopy for the detection of superficial papillary lesions in patients with bladder cancer. *J Urol.* 2007;**178**:62–67.

13 American Joint Committee on Cancer. Bladder cancer. In: Edge SB, Byrd DR, Compton CC, Fritz AG, Greene FL, Trotti A, eds. *AJCC Cancer Staging Handbook*, 7th ed. New York: Springer; 2010:569–577.

14 Bajorin DF, Dodd PM, Mazumdar M, et al. Long-term survival in metastatic transitional-cell carcinoma prognostic factors predicting outcome of therapy. *J Clin Oncol.* 1999;**17**:3173–3181.

15 Apolo AB, Ostrovnaya I, Halabi S, et al. Prognostic model for predicting survival of patients with metastatic urothelial cancer treated with cisplatin-based chemotherapy. *J Natl Cancer Inst.* 2013;**105**:499–503.

16 Cookson MS, Herr HW, Zhang ZF, et al. The treated natural history of high risk superficial bladder cancer: 15-year outcome. *J Urol.* 1997;**158**:62–67.

19 Herr HW, Sogani PC. Does early cystectomy improve the survival of patients with high risk superficial bladder tumors? *J Urol.* 2001;**166**:1296–1299.

20 Stein JP, Lieskovsky G, Cote R, et al. Radical cystectomy in the treatment of invasive bladder cancer: long-term results in 1054 patients. *J Clin Oncol.* 2001;**19**:666–675.

23 Kader AK, Richards KA, Krane LS, Pettus JA, Smith JJ, Hemal AK. Robot-assisted laparoscopic vs open radical cystectomy: comparison of complications and perioperative oncological outcomes in 200 patients. *BJU Int.* 2013;**112**:E290–E294.

24 Bochner BH, Sjoberg DD, Laudone VP, et al. A randomized trial of robot-assisted laparoscopic radical cystectomy. *N Engl J Med.* 2014;**371**:389–390.

25 Sondergaard J, Holmberg M, Jakobsen AR, Agerbaek M, Muren LP, Hoyer M. A comparison of morbidity following conformal versus intensity-modulated radiotherapy for urinary bladder cancer. *Acta Oncol.* 2014;**53**:1321–1328.

28 Coppin C, Gospodarowicz M, James K, et al. Improved local control of invasive bladder cancer by concurrent cisplatin and preoperative or definitive radiation. The National Cancer Institute of Canada Clinical Trials Group. *J Clin Oncol.* 1996;**14**:2901–2907.

29 James ND, Hussain SA, Hall E, et al. Radiotherapy with or without chemotherapy in muscle-invasive bladder cancer. *N Engl J Med.* 2012;**366**:1477–1480.

30 Raghavan D, Pearson B, Duval P, et al. Initial intravenous cis-platinum therapy: improved management for invasive high-risk bladder cancer? *J Urol.* 1985;**133**:399–402.

31 Grossman HB, Natale RB, Tangen CM, et al. Neoadjuvant chemotherapy plus cystectomy compared with cystectomy alone for locally advanced bladder cancer. *N Engl J Med.* 2003;**349**:859.

33 Griffiths G, Hall R, Sylvester R, Raghavan D. International phase III trial assessing neoadjuvant cisplatin, methotrexate, and vinblastine chemotherapy for muscle-invasive bladder cancer: long-term results of the BA06 30894 trial. *J Clin Oncol.* 2011;**29**:2171–2177.

35 Raj GV, Karavadia S, Schlomer B, et al. Contemporary use of perioperative cisplatin-based chemotherapy in patients with muscle-invasive bladder cancer. *Cancer.* 2011;**117**:276–282.

36 Skinner DG, Daniels JR, Russell CA, et al. The role of adjuvant chemotherapy following cystectomy for invasive bladder cancer: a prospective comparative trial. *J*

Urol. 1991;**145**:459–467.
37 Freiha F, Reese J, Torti FM. A randomized trial of radical cystectomy plus cisplatin, vinblastine and methotrexate chemotherapy for muscle invasive bladder cancer. *J Urol*. 1996;**155**:495–500.
39 Stockle M, Wellek S, Meyenburg W, et al. Radical cystectomy with or without adjuvant polychemotherapy for non-organ-confined transitional cell carcinoma of the urinary bladder: prognostic impact of lymph node involvement. *Urology*. 1996;**48**:868–875.
41 Cognetti F, Ruggeri EM, Felici A, et al. Adjuvant chemotherapy with cisplatin and gemcitabine versus chemotherapy at relapse in patients with muscle-invasive bladder cancer submitted to radical cystectomy: an Italian, multicenter, randomized phase III trial. *Ann Oncol*. 2011;**23**:695–700.
42 Raghavan D, Bawtinhimer A, Mahoney J, Eckrich S, Riggs S. Adjuvant chemotherapy for bladder cancer – why does level 1 evidence not support it? *Ann Oncol*. 2014;**10**:1930–1934.
43 Sternberg CN, Skoneczna I, Kerst JM, et al. Immediate versus deferred chemotherapy after radical cystectomy in patients with pT3–pT4 or N+M0 urothelial carcinoma of the bladder (EORTC 30994): an intergroup, open-label, randomised phase 3 trial. *Lancet Oncol*. 2015;**16**:76–86.
48 Saxman SB, Propert K, Einhorn LH, et al. Long-term follow up of phase III intergroup study of cisplatin alone or in combination with methotrexate, vinblastine, and doxorubicin in patients with metastatic urothelial carcinoma: a cooperative group study. *J Clin Oncol*. 1997;**15**:2564–2569.
51 von der Maase H, Sengelov L, Roberts JT, et al. Long-term survival results of a randomized trial comparing gemcitabine plus cisplatin, with methotrexate, vinblastine, doxorubicin, plus cisplatin in patients with bladder cancer. *J Clin Oncol*. 2005;**23**:4602–4608.
52 Bellmunt J, von der Maase H, Mead GM, et al. Randomized phase III study comparing paclitaxel/cisplatin/gemcitabine and gemcitabine/cisplatin in patients with locally advanced or metastatic urothelial cancer without prior systemic therapy: EORTC Intergroup Study 30987. *J Clin Oncol*. 2012;**30**:1107–1113.
53 Hussain MA, MacVicar GR, Petrylak DP, et al. Trastuzumab, paclitaxel, carboplatin, and gemcitabine in advanced human epidermal growth factor receptor-2/neu-positive urothelial carcinoma: results of a multicenter phase II National Cancer Institute trial. *J Clin Oncol*. 2007;**25**:2218–2224.
56 Powles T, Eder JP, Fine GD, et al. MPDL3280A (anti-PD-L1) treatment leads to clinical activity in metastatic bladder cancer. *Nature*. 2014;**515**: 558–562.
57 Lehmann J, Suttmann H, Albers P, et al. Surgery for metastatic urothelial carcinoma with curative intent: the German experience (AUO AB 30/05). *Eur Urol*. 2009;**55**:1293–1299.
58 Sternberg CN, Swanson DA. Non-transitional cell bladder cancer. In: Raghavan D, Scher HI, Leibel SA, Lange PH, eds. *Principles and Practice of Genitourinary Oncology*. Philadelphia: Lippincott-Raven; 1997:315–330.
59 Siefker-Radtke AO, Czerniak BA, Dinney CP, Millikan RE. Uncommon cancers of the bladder. In: Raghavan D, Blanke CD, Johnson DH, et al., eds. *Textbook of Uncommon Cancer*, 4th ed. Wiley-Blackwell: Hoboken; 2012:23–33.
60 Raghavan D. A structured approach to uncommon cancers: what should a clinician do? *Ann Oncol*. 2013;**24**:2932–2934.
63 Munoz JJ, Ellison LM. Upper tract urothelial neoplasms: incidence and survival during the last 2 decades. *J Urol*. 2000;**164**:1523–1525.

第 98 章　前列腺癌

Christopher J. Logothetis, MD ■ Jeri Kim, MD ■ John W. Davis, MD, FACS ■ Brian F. Chapin, MD ■ Deborah Kuban, MD, FACR, FASTRO ■ Eleni Efstathiou, MD, PhD ■ Ana Aparicio, MD

概述

在美国男性中，前列腺癌是皮肤肿瘤之外最常见的恶性肿瘤，也是癌症相关死亡的第二大原因。在筛查、诊断和治疗方面，特别是在晚期前列腺癌治疗方面，已经取得了相当大的进展，但在前列腺癌的诊断和治疗方面仍存在争议，特别是在筛查和治疗选择领域。晚期前列腺癌的争论已从预后判断转向疗效预测，目前的治疗焦点集中在优化现有治疗手段的续贯方案或联合方案，并需要判定局部治疗和骨保护剂的作用。预计通过对这些问题的研究和解决，将有助于制订出更加全面及有效的治疗策略。通过开发具有独特作用机制的新药以及将新药合理地整合到综合治疗中，可以实现治疗的进一步改善。

随着对前列腺癌认识的深入，临床活检方法的改进和影像学的发展，以及前列腺特异抗原（prostate specific antigen，PSA）的广泛应用，增加了前列腺癌的检出。在 2009 年首次公布了欧洲前列腺癌筛查随机研究（ERSPC）和美国的前列腺，肺，结直肠，和卵巢（PLCO）癌症筛查两项研究的结果[1]之前，没有相关研究证实应用血清 PSA 及其随时间的变化可以增加前列腺癌的检出。尽管这两项研究之间的许多差异可以通过试验设计和患者交叉污染来解释，但两项研究均提出了前列腺癌过度诊断和过度治疗的风险，迫切需要提高诊断有临床意义的前列腺癌的准确性。基于对前列腺癌生物学的进一步认识，希望用前列腺癌分子分类替代当前的形态学和解剖学分类，从而更加贴近对这种复杂疾病的个性化治疗。

前列腺癌区别于其他恶性肿瘤及相关疾病的主要特点有：发病率与年龄显著相关，其发病率随着年龄的增长而不断增加；病理形态相近的肿瘤死亡率却存在较大差异；雄激素信号转导的核心作用；其致死性进展中多见成骨性转移。在不远的将来，上述任一领域的重要进展都将改变目前预防、预测和治疗前列腺癌的方法。

前列腺癌生物学

前列腺的正常解剖学和组织学特征

前列腺位于盆腔内，被后方的直肠和上方的膀胱所包围，并固定于盆腔底部；尿道连同于膀胱和前列腺并通向阴茎（图 98-1）。前列腺由基质、导管和腺上皮细胞组成，每个腺体由沿腺导管分支分布排列的分泌上皮细胞和基底细胞组成[2]。分泌上皮细胞是腺体中的主要细胞类型。这些受雄激素调控的细胞产生 PSA 和前列腺酸性磷酸酶（prostatic acid phosphatase，PAP）。雄激素信号转导在前列腺癌生物学中的核心地位可能解释了临床上应用 PSA 和 PAP 确定疾病状态的作用。绝大多数前列腺癌具有与分泌上皮细胞相同特性的细胞。与上皮细胞不同，基底细胞不受雄激素信号转导的直接控制。有研究者认为基底细胞群含有前列腺干细胞，上皮细胞从中分化发展。如果这一观点是正确的（如果能证实这一观点），将对各期前列腺癌的防治产生重要的影响。

与其他人体组织相似，前列腺中也存在神经内分泌细胞。含有分泌颗粒的神经内分泌细胞呈树突样在相邻的上皮细胞之间延伸，或朝向腺泡或尿道腔凸入[3,4]。在分泌颗粒内可以发现多种分泌产物，包括血清素，降钙素，促胃液素释放肽和生长抑素。在分泌颗粒内可以发现多种分泌产物，包括血清素、降钙素、促胃液素释放肽和生长抑素[3,4]。神经内分泌细胞通常通过细胞质中存在如嗜铬粒蛋白 A 或突触素等标记物可进行免疫组织化学鉴定。神经内分泌细胞是终末分化的细胞，被认为可以调节前列腺细胞的生长、分化和功能，但它们的确切作用仍需要进一步证实。

前列腺具有分叶（腺叶）结构的观点已受到了挑战。McNeal 等人[5]对前列腺的正常和病理解剖学进行了详细的研究，并引入了解剖带替换腺叶的概念来描述前列腺腺体。正常前列腺中有四个主要区域：外周带、中央带、移行带（各占腺体组织的 70%、20%和 5%）和前纤维肌基质（图 98-2）。外周带自前列腺尖部延伸至底部，在后外侧围绕着腺体，是前列腺癌的最常发生的部位。中央带围绕着射精管结构并组成了前列腺底部的大部分。移行带由邻接尿道前列腺部的两个小叶组成，并且是良性前列腺增生（benign prostatic hypertrophy，BPH）的主要发生区域。有人认为起源于移行带的癌恶性潜能较低，但另外一些研究结果表明，对相同分级和分期的肿瘤，起源于移行带的肿瘤与起源于外周带的肿瘤相比，预后无显著差异。

腺体周围由间质包绕，含有成纤维细胞、平滑肌、神经及淋巴组织。间质-上皮细胞相互作用在前列腺生理及肿瘤发展中的作用正被逐渐阐明。最近的研究表明这些细胞组织成分之间相互作用在前列腺的正常功能中至关重要，越来越多的证据提示它们在前列腺癌变的过程中也发挥了重要作用。间质-上皮细胞相互作用可能同时发挥促进肿瘤生长和抑制癌变发生及进展两种作用。而且，在前列腺癌进展过程中参与肿瘤微环境发展的间质-上皮相互作用信号通路，可能在前列腺及骨骼的正常发育和功能中也发挥作用[8]。

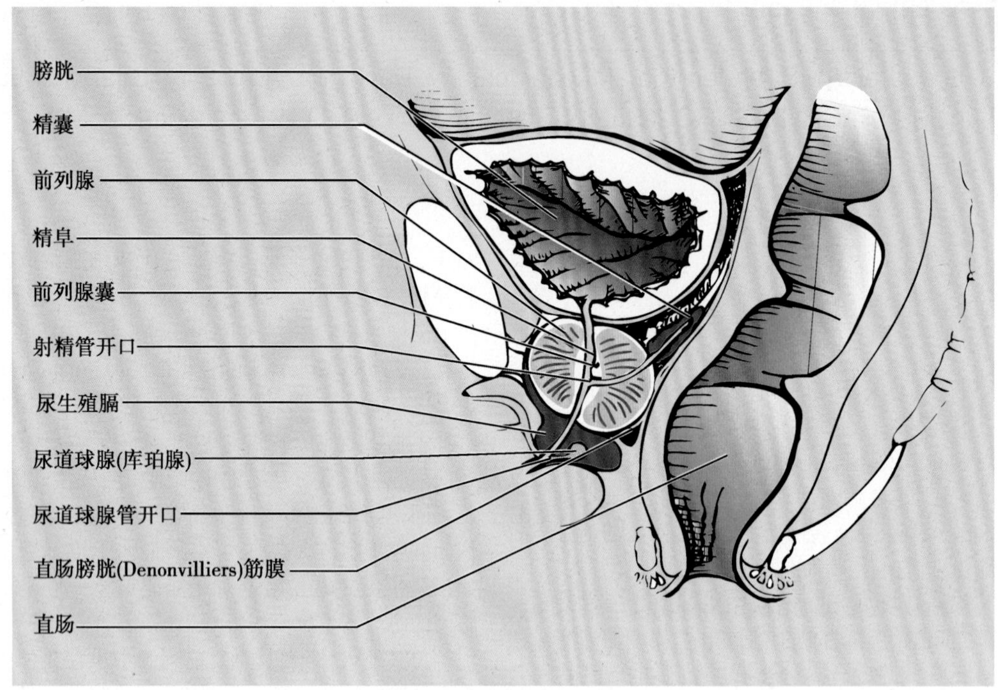

图 98-1 正常前列腺解剖

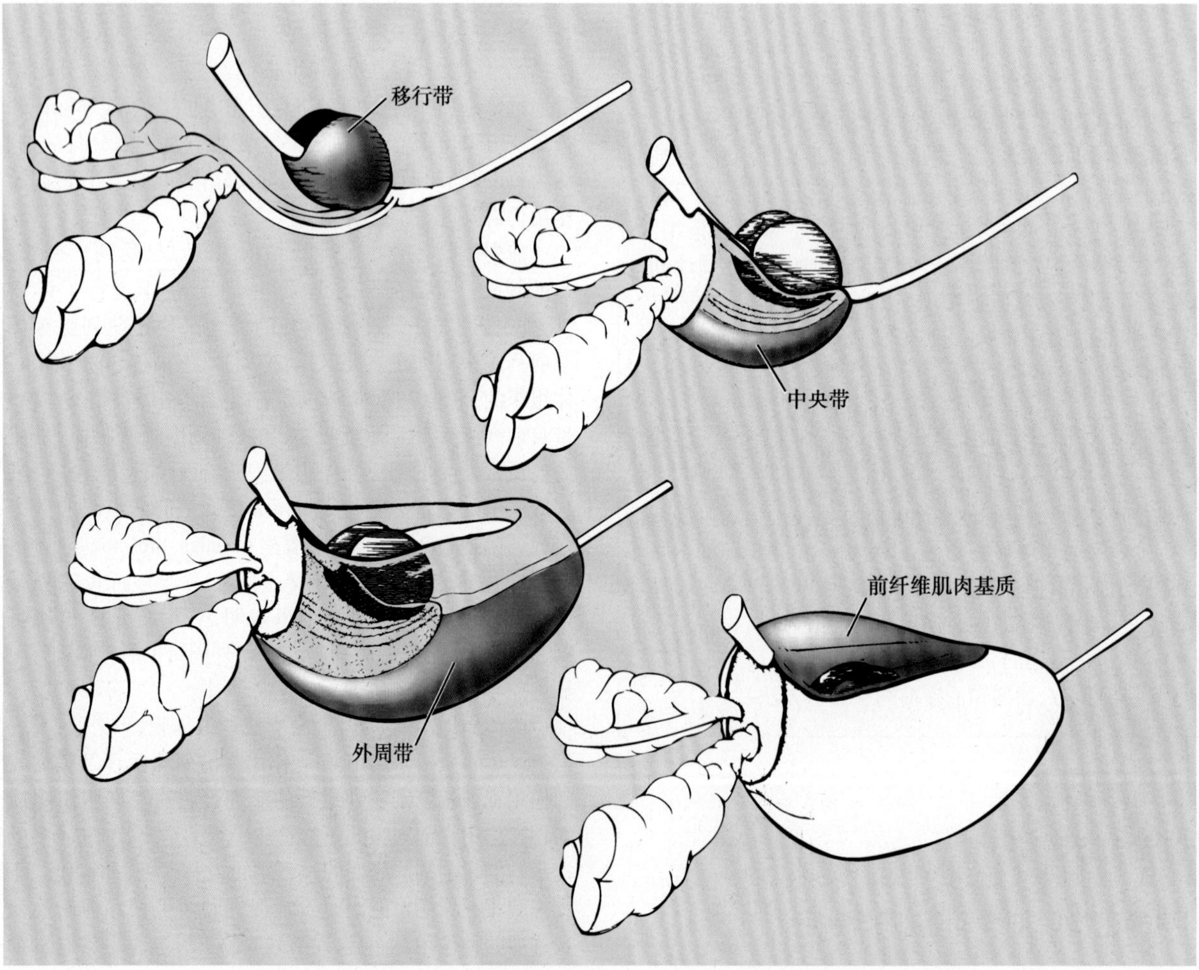

移行带
中央带
外周带
前纤维肌肉基质

图 98-2 前列腺的分区解剖:前列腺的三个腺性区带和前纤维肌肉基质

前列腺周围存在不同的解剖屏障。前列腺间质的平滑肌逐渐延伸到纤维组织中，然后终止于疏松结缔组织和脂肪组织中。特别具有意义的是，腺体的尖部和前方没有被覆包膜。这种对解剖细节的认识使床医师更有信心通过准确地界定手术切缘来确定前列腺手术的充分性。同时也可以将手术标本描述为“器官局限”或“标本局限”性肿瘤。器官局限性肿瘤是指肿瘤没有侵犯超出前列腺的范围，标本局限则是指手术切除充分并且没有肿瘤浸润超出切缘。这两个术语的区别在临床上有重要意义，因为它们被用于确定手术的充分性和在特定患者中术后放射治疗的应用。

有关前列腺解剖学的最后一条注解是 Walsh 和 Donker[9] 描述了紧邻前列腺两侧外后方通过的两条神经血管束。神经血管束穿行于前列腺筋膜后外侧，对于正常的勃起功能至关重要，Walsh 依据此解剖认识开展了一种“保留神经”的经耻骨后根治性前列腺切除术，从而改善了对性功能的保护[10]。

前列腺的癌前病变

用于解释其他实体肿瘤进展的理论可能不完全适于前列腺癌[11]。最近，人们取得了关于前列腺癌进展过程相关的遗传学和表观遗传学的大量信息，但尚未进入到真正的临床应用中。许多临床医师相信在癌症发生数年之前的前列腺组织中就可能存在癌前病变。但由于缺少对癌前病变发展的性质或速度的了解，在活检标本中对癌前病变形态学上的识别只能为密切监测患者提供依据。

形态学上多种不同的病变均被纳入到一个概念中：前列腺上皮内瘤（prostatic intraepithelial neoplasia，PIN）（图 98-3）[12]。PIN 被定义为在结构上呈良性表现的腺体和腺泡中存在细胞异型性或不典型增生的上皮细胞。它们被描述为三个不同的级别：1（轻度）、2（中度）、3（重度）。2 级和 3 级的 PIN 经常被合称为“高级别”。PIN 被推定为癌前病变，因为它通常出现于前列腺腺癌临近区域[13]。PIN 的发现提示在活检未取到的位置存在着癌或者在之后某时点发展出形态学上的癌的风险增加。如上所述，尚未确定或量化风险的程度和进展的时间。

现有的前瞻性研究虽然规模小，但是加强了这一假设：PIN 是前列腺癌的癌前病变的形态表现。研究表明高级别 PIN 的存在预示着其后癌症的发展，这或许是经过一种多步骤的癌变过程。然而，在仅诊断出高级 PIN 后，密切的临床随访仍然是标准治疗。

另一种可能的癌前病变是非典型性腺瘤样增生（atypical adenomatous hyperplasia，AAH），但是现有的关于该病变的研究比 PIN 的更为缺乏。AAH 的特征性表现是其符合恶性肿瘤的结构标准，主要为移行带基底细胞层被破坏，但是不具备诊断为癌的细胞学改变[14]。有些作者认为，慢性炎症相关的上皮萎缩［称为增生性炎症萎缩（proliferative inflammatory atrophy，PIA）］局部病灶所构成的前列腺病变，是 PIN 乃至最终的前列腺癌的先兆[15]。支持这一假设的证据包括：人们观察到 PIA 经常出现于 PIN 及前列腺癌的邻近区域[16]，并且见于 PIA 的遗传异常经常与前列腺癌中所见相似[17]。具有特别意义的是，PIA 与前列腺癌发展过程中的炎症反应相关。如果这一假设得到证实而且其在前列腺癌发展过程中的因果关联更加确定，那么这一发现可能将带来更有效的预防策略。

前列腺癌的组织学特征

起源于上皮的癌症占前列腺癌的 95% 以上（图 98-4）[19]。

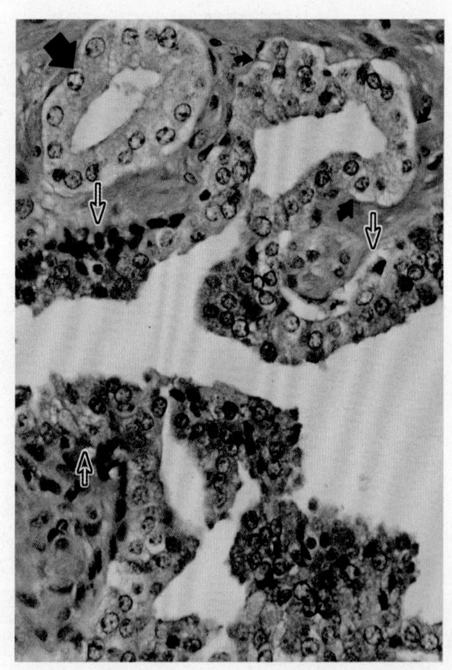

图 98-3　显微镜下高级别前列腺上皮内瘤（PIN）及基底细胞层（空心箭头所示）以及缺少基底细胞的芽生中的微腺泡（弯实心箭头所示）。在邻近的基质中可见浸润性 Gleason 3 分的前列腺腺癌的微腺泡（直实心箭头所示）。苏木精和伊红染色，160 倍镜下。资料来源：Thomas M. Wheeler 博士

其他病理类型肿瘤的发生率较低，这可能很大程度是由于仅检查前列腺原发肿瘤的病理标本，而其中主要为最常见的前列腺癌病理类型。其他少见病理类型，包括黏液或印戒细胞癌、腺样囊性癌、类癌、前列腺大导管癌（包括子宫内膜样癌）、腺癌和小细胞未分化癌。这些少见的肿瘤类型报道的发生率低，经常出现于临床进展性肿瘤，所以此类肿瘤接受手术治疗的可能性与最常见的前列腺癌相比是较低的。此外，此类肿瘤有时只是在疾病进展过程中出现在转移灶，而在原发部位不常被取到标本。因此，我们可能由于它们的表现形式而低估了它们的发生率。当人们试图估计前列腺小细胞癌的真实发生率时，上述事实可能尤其重要，有报道称其发生率正在增加[20]。然而，认识这些少见类型的前列腺癌是重要的，因为标准内分泌治疗可能对它们不太有效，但它们可能比常见的前列腺癌对化疗反应更敏感[17,21]。

具有神经内分泌表现的肿瘤（如类癌和小细胞未分化型），可能起源于 Kulchitsky 细胞，这种细胞位于前列腺上皮的基底区域[22]。前列腺小细胞癌与其他肺外小细胞癌具有相同的组织学和临床特点。这些肿瘤被描述为组织学上的连续体，可能在某些情况下反映了腺泡腺癌的进展[23]。因此，前列腺的这些“神经内分泌”肿瘤可能是发病机制和临床表现上的特殊形式。重要的是它们预示了一种肿瘤转移的特殊模式：伴有溶骨性转移的内脏器官转移，并且其对化疗可能具有一定的反应性。这些被认为是前列腺癌中一类独特的和具有侵袭性的病理类型，占晚期前列腺癌的很大一部分。累及前列腺的移行细胞癌也可能被误认为前列腺腺癌。起源于远端前列腺导管移行上皮的移行上皮癌和起源于膀胱上皮并浸润进入邻近前列腺导管的肿瘤，两者可能是难以区分的。

研究证实了前列腺腺癌的组织分化程度对其预后具有重

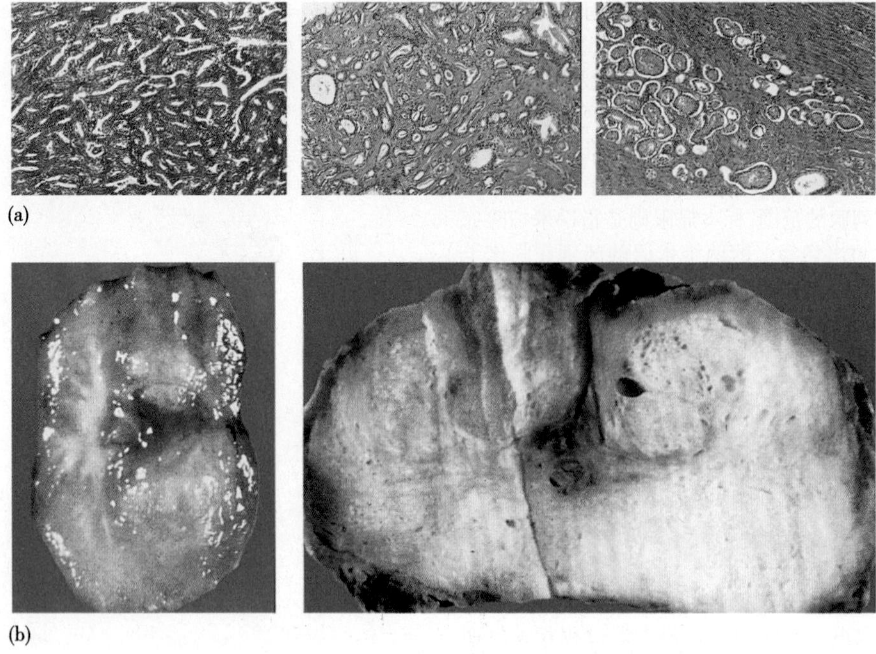

图 98-4 (a)前列腺腺癌的镜下表现。(b)前列腺腺癌的大体表现

要意义。这种分化程度通常是由腺体的组织学特点和细胞学特点决定的,其中后者居次要地位。最广为接受的前列腺腺癌分级方案是由 Gleason 制订的(图 98-5)[25]。这种前列腺癌分级体系以体现前列腺腺癌异质性的两级评分为基础。依据肿瘤的主要形态特征及其与正常表现的差异,对于主要分化类型进行评级(Gleason 1~5 级),次要类型也进行评级。两个数字相加组成最终的 Gleason 评分,例如:3+4=7。有人批评 Gleason 评分体系未能充分体现次主要形式在肿瘤中的构成比例,也未能充分区分 Gleason 5~7 分肿瘤患者(占大多数)的预后好坏。然而,Gleason 评分在不同病理学家之间一直表现出良好的可重复性和可靠性。Gleason 的原始研究证明高评分和高死亡率之间存在明确的相关性,此后其他人的研究也证实了这一点[26]。人们探索了前列腺癌临床行为的许多其他预测因子,但 Gleason 评分仍然是应用最广泛和最具预后价值的组织学分级体系。

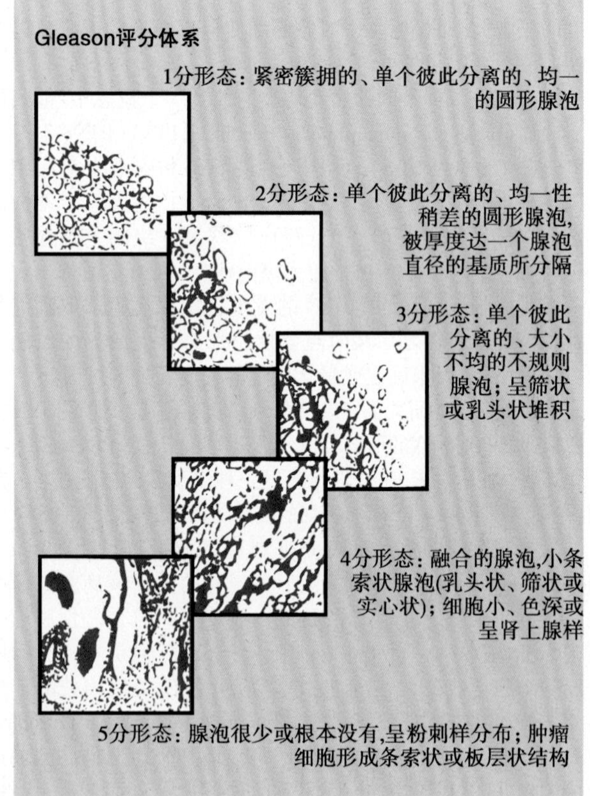

图 98-5 前列腺腺癌的组织学分级方案。摘自 Kattan 2007[24]。Reproduced with permission of Nature Publishing Group

分子发病机制

临床上乳腺癌的相关亚群已可根据其分子表达情况做出识别,与之不同的是,前列腺癌的形态学特征仍是其分类标准[27]。前列腺癌细胞携带了大量的体细胞突变,并且在进展的疾病中会增加其他的变异。影响前列腺癌发生和进展的改变包括激素和生长因子环境、激素和生长因子受体、细胞内信号通路以及细胞周期调节和凋亡。最近人们认定染色体 8q24 是一个易感基因,这支持了相当比例的前列腺癌具有遗传起源的假设[28]。

基因组测序的技术进步使得识别与前列腺癌风险增加有关的胚系突变成为可能。*HOXB13G84E* 变异体是首个被证实的前列腺癌易感基因。在一项对 94 名无相关性患者的研究中,*HOXB13G84E* 变异与显著增加的早发性遗传性前列腺癌的风险相关[29]。此外,*BRCA1* 和 *BRCA2* 胚系突变使前列腺癌具有更高的高风险和更具侵袭性的预后[30]。然而,这些胚系突变尚未转化为相关的治疗。

前列腺所处的激素和生长因子环境一直与其发病机制相关。在以大量人群为基础的研究中,发现两种激素与之相关:睾酮和胰岛素样生长因子Ⅰ(insulin-like growth factor Ⅰ,IGF-Ⅰ)。睾酮与前列腺癌进展的关系已众所周知。一些研究也表明 IGF-Ⅰ

可能在前列腺癌生长中有重要意义。首先,一些前列腺癌细胞系和前列腺癌异种移植模型均表达 *IGF-Ⅰ* 和 *Ⅱ* 及其受体[31,32]。其次,Chan 等人[33]报道了血浆 IGF-Ⅰ浓度与前列腺癌的相关性,其研究显示血浆 IGF-Ⅰ浓度最高四分位组的男性与最低四分位组相比,相对危险性为4.3。此外,有人注意到在诊断癌症5年之前取得的血浆标本中 IGF-Ⅰ浓度相对较高的患者其前列腺癌的发生率也较高[34],这支持了 IGF-Ⅰ可能在前列腺癌发生早期具有重要作用的观点。尽管这一观察尚未得到证实,但它确实提示 IGF-Ⅰ信号转导与前列腺癌进展相关。生长因子和其他基质-上皮相互作用通路可能在前列腺癌发展中协同作用。因此,针对单一信号通路的简单模型不可能完全解释人类对前列腺癌的发展情况。包括表皮生长因子、血管内皮生长因子(VEGF),血小板衍生生长因子(PDGF)和转化生长因子β(TGF-β)等在内的其他生长因子可能也在前列腺癌的发展过程中参与作用(表98-1)[35]。

表98-1 与前列腺癌有关的生长因子

转化生长因子β
成纤维细胞生长因子
表皮生长因子
胰岛素样生长因子
血小板衍生生长因子
血管内皮生长因子
神经降压素
内皮素
集落刺激因子

以内分泌方式出现的雄激素信号转导的核心作用在人们对前列腺癌信号通路的认识中占主导地位。人们清楚地认识到,雄激素是前列腺癌进展的重要介质,尽管它们在前列腺癌易感性中的作用尚很少被人所认识。事实上,在前列腺癌细胞中一些激素受体发生了改变。或许最好的例子就是雄激素受体(androgen receptor,AR)的改变。在早期癌中,AR 突变相对少见[36],但有证据表明 *AR* 基因的生殖细胞系变异(CAG 重复)是癌症侵袭性的预测因子[37],并且在非洲裔美国人前列腺癌的高发病率和侵袭性较高中可能发挥一定作用[38]。有趣的是,*AR* 突变更常见于雄激素非依赖性(去势抵抗性)前列腺癌[36~39],说明即使在对配体(雄激素)的需求减弱之后,*AR* 基因仍然在前列腺癌的生长和生存中发挥核心作用。一些解释雄激素非依赖性发展过程的理论框架已经被提出,其中大部分仍然假定癌细胞依赖于有功能的 *AR*,但它是扩增的、高敏感性的、紊乱的、被上调的共刺激因子或下调的共抑制因子所激活的 *AR*[40]。例如,LNCaP 前列腺癌细胞的一种 *AR* 突变,T877A,即877位点苏氨酸被丙氨酸替代,导致这种 AR 可被其他类固醇激素和雄激素拮抗剂氟他胺所激活[41]。这一 *AR* 突变可以帮助解释"抗雄激素撤退综合征"。然而,*AR* 突变发生频率太低以至于不能用来解释大多数转移性前列腺癌最终均演变到去势抵抗状态。

在前列腺癌中已经发现了 *AR* 剪接变异体。最初从单个患者的前列腺癌细胞系中分离出来的缺乏配体结合域(*ARV*)的 AR 剪接变异体,在正常和恶性的人类前列腺组织中可以检测到,并且在晚期去势抵抗性前列腺癌(CRPC)中观察到。目前已确定了大约20个 *AR* 剪接变异体,它们并非仅在前列腺组织中被发现。第一个 AR 剪接变异体是在胎盘中被发现的。"研究最多的变异体(称为 *AR-V7* 或 *AR3*)在没有配体的情况下激活 *AR* 报告基因,因此,可能在去势抵抗中起作用。"相关研究表明,*ARV7* 存在于前列腺癌浸润的骨髓活检和转移性 CRPC 患者的循环肿瘤细胞中,这些患者主要抵抗新型雄激素信号抑制剂醋酸阿比特龙(CYP17 抑制剂)和恩扎鲁胺(第二代抗雄激素药物)。

最近的观察支持了这样一种观点:通过自分泌和旁分泌两种方式进行"内在分泌"产生雄激素与前列腺癌的进展有关。一些证据表明 CYP17 裂解酶参与前列腺癌肿瘤微环境的重构:雄激素在微环境中的浓度高于其血浆浓度,CYP17 表达与肿瘤进展密切相关,临床上抑制 CYP17 后,去势抵抗性癌中会出现肿瘤缩小现象。这些数据支持了雄激素信号转导可以视为一种基质-上皮相互作用途径的假设。测量局部微环境中的雄激素浓度仍很困难,这使得上述观点虽吸引人,却仍未被证实。

真正的雄激素非依赖性可能来源于改变基质-上皮相互作用或其他信号通路。有人注意到一些骨和前列腺的发育通路参与了前列腺癌的进展并与较高分级肿瘤相关[44]。这一吸引人的假设可以解释了前列腺癌的骨归巢和骨形成表型及其以器官特异性方式表现出的对治疗的抵抗性。

改变细胞内信号通路的分子也可能在前列腺癌发病机制及进展到去势抵抗状态的过程中具有重要意义。迄今最明确的例证是肿瘤抑制因子基因 *PTEN*。该基因编码的磷酸酶对激活的生长因子受体所产生的信号具有重要调节作用。在前列腺癌细胞中,*PTEN* 的体细胞突变率很高,表明它是经常失活的靶点。一项研究记录到 *PTEN*60%的突变率,这些突变多数被发现于转移性疾病的细胞系中,尽管在原发肿瘤中也可发现突变[45]。事实上,另一团队证明了在晚期和高级别肿瘤中 *PTEN* 丢失或突变的概率较高[46]。在前列腺癌中另一可能被异常激活的通路是 hedgehog 通路。正常的 hedgehog 通路在前列腺上皮的早期发育和结构形成过程中非常重要。最近 Karhadkar 等人[47]的研究证明,hedgehog 通路的激活是前列腺癌区别于正常前列腺细胞之处,而且是转移性前列腺癌区别于局灶性癌之处。此外,他们还证明了抑制 hedgehog 通路会导致 PC3 种植形成的肿瘤体积的缩小。因此 PTEN 和 hedgehog 通路都是药物研发的热门靶点。

通常在 CRPC 进展过程中出现的小细胞前列腺癌,作为一种对 AR 定向治疗的原发性和可能继发性抵抗的模型,近来受到了广泛关注。大多数小细胞前列腺癌缺乏前列腺管腔分化的标志物,如 AR、PSA、PSAP、PSMA 和 p501s[48~56]。与之相反,它们通常表达神经祖细胞特征性的标记物,如 ASCL1、POU4F2 和 MYCN[50,57~59]。Re-1 沉默转录因子(REST)是一种神经细胞分化的主抑制因子,其表达的降低被认为是参与这种转分化的一种机制[60,61]。此外,小细胞前列腺癌具有高 Ki67 染色和参与细胞周期和有丝分裂的基因高表达水平的特征,包括 *AURKA*、*AURKB*、*PLK1* 和 *UBE2C*[58,60,62]。值得注意的是,在大约40%的小细胞前列腺癌[58]中发现了的 *AURKA* 和 *MYCN* 一致扩增,REST 导致前列腺癌模型中细胞周期基因[61]的释放,支持异常神经发育和有丝分裂程序之间的联系。最后,小细胞前列腺癌也被证明具有频繁的 *TP53* 突变[49~51,63~65],以及 *RB1* 和 *PTEN* 丢失和高拷贝数变化率[50,58,62,63,65,66]。

最后,调节细胞周期和凋亡的分子改变为进一步研究带来了希望。人们研究了 *TP53*、*p27*、*p21* 和 *Rb*,这些结果提供了不同等级的证据证明它们参与了前列腺癌的发病机制[67]。特别有价值的是,每一个这类分子都被某些研究者报道其可作为预后因子。应用这些分子作为独立预后因子或特征标志的一部分,尚未得到前瞻性研究证实。在临床上尚未找到可预测疾病术后复发情况的特征因子[68]。

前列腺癌的早期发现

在前列腺癌仍局限于前列腺内时,对其早期发现使得患者和医师面临这个富有争议的问题:局限性前列腺癌如何处理才会是最好的?换言之,患者如何能避免过度治疗而保留良好的生活质量同时免于威胁生命的疾病。

前列腺癌筛查和早期发现是存在争议的,因为每检出18个病例,只有3个将会死亡。根治性前列腺切除术,在没有转移的情况下去除了疾病的威胁,但可能使患者付出阳痿和尿失禁等严重影响生活质量的代价[69]。为了判定对前列腺癌和其他三种癌症的筛查是否降低了死亡率,1993年,美国国家癌症研究所癌症预防部在10个中心开展了随机、对照的PLCO筛查试验。前列腺筛查组发表了评论[1,70]。参加者进行了为期6年的每年一度PSA筛查检测和为期13年的随访[71,72]。

在样本量为76 685人,分配给干预组(38 340人)或对照组(38 345人),延长随访时间诊断了干预组的4 250例癌症和对照组的3 815例患者。这些事件相当于干预组158人死亡,对照组145人死亡。关键结论是PSA筛查提高了检出率,但不影响死亡率。Smith[70]对这项研究的一个常见评论是,干预组的不依从性筛查和对照组的机会性筛查都会对结果造成严重影响。

20世纪90年代也推出了ERSPC,它也在测试筛查是否能挽救生命。2009年,它与PLCO试验一起发布。更新后的结果在11年和13年时被截断[71,73]。在这项试验中,明显减少了污染。ERSPC结果显示,调整不符合项后,前列腺癌死亡率相对降低了21%和29%[74]。为了防止一人死亡,需要筛查的人数是1 055人,检测的人数是37人。额外的随访时间改善了预期的筛查指标。作者警告说,随着PSA的筛查,全因死亡率没有受到影响,而过度检测/过度治疗仍然是一个问题[75]。试验在设计上经常被批评为不是一个统一的多中心研究,而是几个筛选研究的合并,在方法和结果上存在差异。因此,美国预防服务特别工作组(USPSTF)发布了一个"D"级的PSA筛选评级(不鼓励使用该服务),但这仍然是存在高度争议的[76,77]。

应用PSA和PSAV识别早期前列腺癌

对诊断为局限性前列腺癌的处理策略包括主动监测、根治性前列腺切除术和放射治疗,并且早期干预将导致更好的无复发结果。早期发现前列腺癌的争论集中在应用绝对PSA截止值与PSA速率(PSAV)或PSA异构体。PSAV,一种用于监测局限性疾病患者的指标,现在已经应用于前列腺癌的诊断和预后预测。PSAV是利用2年内间隔不少于6个月至少三次PSA值的对数斜率来计算的[78]。PSAV可以在术前和术后用来评估前列腺癌进展的情况。研究者们有时依赖于测定时间彼此靠近的测量,考虑少于三次的测量并将纵向时期减低至少于2年。

前列腺癌筛查可能被过度简化为如下流程:PSA达到一定阈值(如2.5ng/ml或4.0ng/ml)或直肠指诊有异常发现的所有患者都提交到泌尿外科医师进行评估和可能的穿刺活检。然而,如果对患者进行更全面的评估,考虑到他们是否因为种族而增加患前列腺癌的风险(如非裔美国人的患病风险更高),年龄和/或家族史,以及由于他们的年龄更小,共存疾病较少的情况作出的前列腺癌的诊断是否可能影响他们的总体生存率,那么患者会得到更好的整体获益。一个完整的PSA病史可能有助于计算PSAV而复合PSA(cPSA)检验可能作为一线筛查工具发挥作用,因为它在诊断总PSA 2.5~4.0ng/ml范围内的前列腺癌特异性略优于总PSA检查结果[79]。

PSA血液检测是一项被称为"既不能排除良性疾病也不能完全预测有意义的恶性病变"的检测[78]。前列腺癌预防试验(prostate cancer prevention trial, PCPT)的首席研究员Ian Thompson和他的同事们研究了安慰剂组中的8 575名男性来估计PSA的受试者操作特性(receiver operating characteristic, ROC)曲线来预测无前列腺癌风险,结果他们没有发现一个截断值同时具有较高的敏感性和特异性。相反,他们认为应该综合考虑所有的PSA值视为连续性风险值[80]。

研究证实患者确诊前的血液PSA检查结果与前列腺癌发病风险水平在统计上有关,并因PSA检查简便性和有效性以及可对患者进行分层筛查的能力而受到极大关注,但PSA检查可靠性有待进一步验证[81,82]。这些研究结果是基于瑞典1974—1986年21 277名男性的血液样本和瑞典癌症登记处的数据得到。在这些样本中,一共诊断发现462例前列腺癌组织和血液样本,并与对照组进行匹配。在低风险组,PSA中位值约为0.6ng/ml。研究人员工作基础是依据人群40岁之前的单次PSA结果来预测癌症风险[82]。尽管根据"平价医疗法案"(Affordable Care Act),2012年USPSTF不建议对于50岁以上男性进行常规性PSA检查,但这项研究还是每12个月进行一次PSA检查。

PSAV是一种计算PSA水平上升速率的方法,最早于20世纪90年代初用来预测前列腺癌进展,它既能减少不必要前列腺癌活检,也能提高PSA检查结果特异性。然而,目前PSAV检查缩短了计算的最小检查周期并不断降低阈值水平[目前对于PSA<4ng/ml的男性患者PSAV阈值为3.5ng/(ml·a)],这实际上增加了前列腺活检的风险[83~86]。谨慎的研究者们认为,要用PSAV监测PSA<4ng/ml的男性,有必要有证据证明:这种测量能够保证有足够多的病例将被发现于"可治愈窗"之中,以使这些测定值得去做,并且过度诊断所带来的经济和情感成本不会削弱其他益处。他们还指出关于PSAV的认识尚非常缺乏,在未诊断病例中依赖它们将非常不同于依赖治疗后的PSAV发现并用于检查设置。他们和其他研究者们认为还需要进行前瞻性研究[85,87]。

关于PSAV的一项早期研究是对参加一个老年医学试验的男性患者进行的。Carter等[83]发现在PSA值<4ng/ml的人群中,PSAV<0.75μg/(ml·a)可以预测不存在前列腺癌,PSAV≥0.75μg/(ml·a)则表示预测有前列腺癌的发生可能。在此15年后发表的一篇研究中,Krejcarek等人[88]发现在PSAV<1.0ng/(ml·a)的人群中,只有6%的年龄小于70岁的cT1c患者中人患有高级别肿瘤;然而,他们发现中位PSAV值2.71ng/(ml·a)、年龄和临床T分期与肿瘤高危险度显著相关(Gleason评分4+3)。由于这些受试者接受过放射治疗,因此这些研究结果不适用于其他治疗方式的患者。Krejcarek等对这358名男性患者进行了回顾性研究来确定高风险人群,结果发现通过在放疗基础上增加雄激素剥夺治疗和改进放疗适用范围选择的方法来改善其结果。

2008年英国皇家马斯登医院(Royal Marsden Hospital)对初始中位值PSA为6.5ng/ml和中位值PSAV为0.44ng/(ml·a)

的 237 名患者进行了一项前瞻性主动监测试验[89]。研究人员发现在未治疗患者中 PSA 密度是一个独立于 PSAV 的具有统计学意义因素：PS 密度测量>0.185ng/ml 的患者 PSAV 中位值为 0.92ng/(ml·a)，而 PSA 密度测量<0.185ng/ml 的患者 PSAV 中位值为 0.35ng/(ml·a)。由于 PSA 密度在诊断之初即可检测，且不需要通过时间累及多次收集数据，因此如果其他研究也能证实这一观点，PSA 密度是比 PSAV 更高效的标志。

正如 Vickers 等[90]发表的一篇评论中指出，PSAV 在目前列腺癌早期检测和临床局限性前列腺癌管理中的应用价值受到质疑。目前反对 PSAV 检查的主要理由是缺乏临床实用性，它既没有增加前列腺癌预测准确性和方法灵活性，而且也不能较好的预测保守治疗和前列腺切除术后死亡率。

前列腺癌的分期

癌症的分期是决定后续治疗的重要参考依据，包括基于患者检查结果的初步临床分期和基于手术、病理结果的病理分期。临床分期主要依靠前列腺指诊结果，影像学检查结果（往往会遗漏低危和中危患者）和前列腺穿刺活检结果，因此不像病理分期那样准确。医生把临床分期与另外两个重要的预后因素（Gleason 评分和术前 PSA 值）结合起来，根据 D'Amico 分级系统可将前列腺癌分为临床低危、中危和高危型前列腺癌[91]。该系统最早在 1998 年发表的一想回顾性研究中提出，在该研究中 D'Amico 等人评估了 1 872 名前列腺癌患者，这些患者接受过根治性前列腺切除术、外放疗或放射性粒子治疗，并接受或不接受新辅助雄激素剥夺疗法。在该研究中，临床分期基于直肠指诊的结果（美国癌症肿瘤分期联合委员会[92]）。研究人员发现，在这个系统中，被划分为低风险或中等风险的男性，其结果在统计上与其他同龄人没有显著差异。大部分的可靠性可能是由于格里森评分和 PSA 水平。

医生主要依据肿瘤情况、淋巴结情况和远处转移情况即 TNM 系统进行前列腺癌的分期（表 98-2）。此 TNM 系统包括肿瘤（T）的范围，在区域淋巴结（N）是否有转移，和转移（M）的范围。根据 Gleason 评分结果与 TNM 分级结果相结合进行前列腺癌分级，包括Ⅰ、Ⅱ、Ⅲ或Ⅳ期，恶性程度随着分级增加而增加（表 98-3）。

表 98-2 前列腺癌的 TNM 临床及病理分期

临床分期	病理分期
原发肿瘤（T）	
Tx 原发肿瘤不能评价	
T0 无原发肿瘤证据	
T1 不能被扪及和影像学难以发现的临床隐匿肿瘤	
T1a 偶发肿瘤，体积<所切除组织体积的 5%	
T1b 偶发肿瘤，体积>所切除组织体积的 5%	
T1c 穿刺活检发现的肿瘤（如由于 PSA 升高）	
T2 局限于前列腺内的肿瘤[a]	pT2[b] 局限于前列腺
T2a 肿瘤限于单叶的 1/2（≤1/2）	pT2a 肿瘤限于单叶的 1/2
T2b 肿瘤超过单叶的 1/2 但限于该单叶	pT2b 肿瘤超过单叶的 1/2 但限于该单叶
T2c 肿瘤侵犯两叶	pT2c 肿瘤侵犯两叶 T1b 偶发肿瘤，体积>所切除组织体积的 5%
T3 肿瘤突破前列腺包膜[c]	pT3 突破前列腺
T3a 肿瘤侵犯包膜外（单侧或双侧）	pT3a 突破前列腺[d]
T3b 肿瘤侵犯精囊	pT3b 侵犯精囊
T4 肿瘤固定或侵犯除精囊外的其他临近组织结构，如膀胱颈、尿道外括约肌、直肠、肛提肌和/或盆壁	pT4 侵犯膀胱和直肠
区城淋巴结（N）	
临床	病理
Nx 区域淋巴结不能评价	Nx 区域淋巴结不能评价
N0 无区域淋巴结转移	pN0 无区域淋巴结转移
N1 区域淋巴结转移	pN1 区域淋巴结转移
远处转移[e]（M）	
Mx 远处转移无法评估	
M0 无远处转移	
M1	
M1a 有区城淋巴结以外的淋巴结转移	
M1b 骨转移	
M1c 其他器官组织转移	

[a] 穿刺活检发现的单叶或两叶肿瘤、但临床无法扪及或影像学不能发现的定为 Tlc。
[b] 没有病理 T1 分型。
[c] 侵入前列腺顶部或侵入（但不超过）前列腺包膜不是 T3 而是 T2。
[d] 阳性的手术切缘应用 R1 描述符（显微镜下残留的疾病）表示。
[e] 当存在多个转移位点时，使用最先进的分类（pM1c）。
摘自 Edge 2010[33]。Reproduced with permision of Springer。

表 98-3 前列腺癌分期

分期	TNM 分级和 Gleason 评分
Ⅰ	T1a、N0、M0,Gleason 评分 1
Ⅱ	T1a、N0、M0,Gleason 评分 2、3~4
	T1、T1b-T2、N0、M0,任何 Gleason 评分
Ⅲ	T3、N0、M0,任何 Gleason 评分
Ⅳ	T4、N0、M0,任何 Gleason 评分
	任何 T、N1、M0,任何 Gleason 评分
	任何 T 分级,任何 N 分级,M1,任何 Gleason 评分

摘自 Edge 2010[93]。Reproduced with permission of Springer。

前列腺癌是除了皮肤癌和原位癌以外美国男性最常见的癌症[94]。大约有 3/4 的男性患者至少接受过一次检查,早期前列腺癌因为没有明显症状,通常在门诊进行诊断。如何区分高危和低危的局限性前列腺癌,如何最大限度地控制疾病和提高生存,如何避免过度治疗特别是对可能死于手术并发症的男性,是医生每天都要面对的挑战[95]。

美国泌尿外科协会将局限性前列腺癌分为三类[96](表 98-4)。低危前列腺癌一般为 PSA 值≤10ng/ml,Gleason 评分≤6,无症状,无淋巴结和远处转移(如临床分期 T1c 或 T2a)。直肠指诊无法触及肿瘤,但是可以通过因前列腺增生行的经尿道前列腺电切术(TURP)或高 PSA 水平提示的穿刺活检而检测到肿瘤。PSA 值为>10ng/ml 且≤20ng/ml 和/或 Gleason 评分为 7(3+4 或 4+3)为中危前列腺癌。PSA 值为>20ng/ml 和/或 Gleason 评分为 8~10 表示为高危前列腺癌。

表 98-4 局限性前列腺癌的风险分层

危险分层	PSA 水平/(ng/ml)	Gleason 评分			临床分期
低危	≤10	和	≤6	和	T1c 或 T2a
中危	>10~20	或	7	或	T2b,但不符合高风险
高危	>20	或	8~10	或	T2c

摘自 Thompson 2007[96]。Reproduced with permission of Elsevier。

研究者采用多参数(mp)的直肠内螺旋磁共振成像(MRI)对前列腺癌进行分期[97]研究。有研究表明,MRI 上提示可疑的病变是根治性前列腺切除术后不良病理的独立危险因素[98]。mpMRI 提示病变正常或者恶性可能性较小,对于临床无意义前列腺癌具有很高的阴性预测价值[99]。但是 MRI 或任何其他影像学检查特点都未纳入局限性疾病的临床风险评估,也不作为原发肿瘤的分期手段。

有学者已经制订并验证了包含 PSA、Gleason 评分和临床分期的治疗前量表,以对病理分期做出预测,这对医生制订治疗计划是很有价值的[100~103]。在 2007 年对 Partin 量表的更新中,Markarov 等人[103]分析了在 2000—2005 年间于约翰霍普金斯医院接受过根治性前列腺切除术的 5 730 例患者,证实了此前这些研究者们曾揭示过的结论:临床分期和 PSA 水平及 Gleason 评分一样,具有重要的预测作用;它们组合的预测价值比任何单一因素更好。所有患者的临床分期均不高于 T2c,而术后有接近 75%的病变都局限于前列腺内。164 例临床 Gleason 评分≥8 的患者中有 123 例接受了相关检查,均未发现存在转移病灶。在他们的患者系列中,与其他研究一致,局限性前列腺癌的比例正在上升:1993 年为 54%[100],1997 年为 48%[101],2001 年为 64%[102],2007 年为 73%(年份为发表时间)[103]。这一患者系列的新颖之处是没有 Gleason 评分 2~4 分的病例,反映出病理学家认为这种评分代表了取样失误[104]。作者指出,2007 年的报道与 2001 年的相比,较高临床分期患者中存在着分期更为准确的趋势,而这或许意味着在这些具有较高临床分期和 Gleason 评分的患者中,手术治疗的需求进一步加大。2013 年更新的量表显示了相似的病理分期,更新的 Gleason 评分,以及更能反应目前状况的预后[67,68]。

通过对既往治疗后患者的随访,提高识别小体积、低级别肿瘤患者准确性的能力[105,106],得克萨斯大学安德森癌症医学中心的研究者优化了识别低肿瘤负荷、低级别肿瘤患者的量表,用于鉴别需要主动监测的患者[107]。该量表包括年龄、PSA 密度和活检组织中的肿瘤长度。量表引人注意之处在于其因子数量少,简便,因为确定它们的数值只需要实验室检查及穿刺活检,而且它们的非主观属性与曲线下面积(area under the curve,AUC)测量相结合意味着良好的鉴别效力(0.727)。研究者承认他们无法解释为什么他们的分析表明:较大年龄的患者低肿瘤负荷和低级别癌的可能性会降低,而一些较年轻患者预测数值较低,适合主动监测。不论如何,他们的工作提供了一种新型而实用的识别低危患者的工具。

将分子标志物作为一种预测因子纳入量表,是研究者尝试改善量表准确性的另一种方式。PCA3,一种前列腺特异性非编码 mRNA,当前列腺癌存在时则易于在尿液中检出,因为在 90%的情况下它会过度表达 60~100 倍[108]。Deras 等人[108]进行了一项多中心的前瞻性研究,对 570 名男性在行前列腺活检前即刻进行检测,发现对 PSA 值<4ng/ml 和>10ng/ml 的患者,对不同前列腺体积和不同穿刺活检次数的患者,PCA 均具有可靠的敏感性和特异性。总体来说,PCA3 的敏感性为 54%(95% *CI*:0.49~0.59),特异性为 74%(95%*CI*:0.71~0.77)。

分期是为了改善肿瘤终点风险预测,可以通过活检标本商业化的基因组预测生物标志物检测进一步完善。Cuzick 等人[109]报道了一组乳腺癌研究中已知的细胞周期进展(cell cycle progression,*CCP*)基因,这些基因在一组保守治疗的患者中进行了验证。CCP 评分是 CCP 基因平均表达水平与管家基因表达相比较的数值表征。与临床特征相比,CCP 评分在预测 10 年死亡率方面具有统计学优势。Klein 等人[110]验证了另一组基因,在一个小样本前列腺活检标本中混合了几种信号通路(基质反应、雄激素信号、增殖和组织)和相关元素,与前列腺切除术长期预后的关系。开发和验证工作构建了一个基因组评分,从活检结果良好的患者(Gleason 3+3~3+4)中,预估前列腺癌根治术后不良病理(Gleason≥4+3 和/或 pT3 分期)的情况。这两种生物标志物都有较强的统计学证据,但还需要临床应用方面的进一步研究,比如在主动监测和即刻治疗方面提供转变的建议,以及依据其建议所获得的最终肿瘤学以及生活质量方面的最终结果。从基因组学层面预测疾病预后,可以延续到根治性前列腺切除术后,CCP 评分和临床特征相结合将用于预测生化复发率,另一个基因组检测方法(商业名为 Decipher, GenomeDx 公司,圣地亚哥,加利福尼亚)可以预测病理高危患者的早期转移的风险。表 98-5 比较了临床关键终点、临床应用以及成本等问题。

表 98-5　三种商业化前列腺癌基因组检测方案要点比较[111]

	Decipher	Oncotype DX	Prolaris
检测组织	根治性前列腺切除 pT3,切缘阳性,PSA 升高	活检——NCCN 极低危至中危	活检或根治性前列腺切除
临床终点	早期局部淋巴结转移或骨转移	高危病理——pT3 和/或 Gleason 评分≥4+3	活检——保守治疗 10 年死亡率 根治性前列腺切除——生化复发风险
临床应用	辅助/挽救疗法	主动监测或立即治疗	活检-主动监测或立即治疗 根治性前列腺切除——辅助/挽救疗法
费用/美元	4 250	3 825	3 400

前列腺癌的影像学检查

骨扫描和 CT 扫描是诊断前列腺癌转移的标准影像学检查,但是,MRI 的 T2 加权检查可以在一定程度上帮助发现前列腺癌和明确分期。近期新的成像序列,如弥散加权成像和动态增强成像,联合 T2 加权成像,可以形成一个"多参数"(mp)序列。这也使得研究者对 MRI 再次产生了兴趣,MRI 对进一步筛查(如患者的 PSA 升高,但活检为阴性)或进一步分期(如评估低负荷/低级别病变患者能否存在未诊断的高级别/高负荷病变)可能有帮助[112]。

进行前列腺活检的医生可以利用商业化的新型软件包/硬件包,将 MRI 的可疑病灶与超声看似正常的图像"融合"[113]。这些额外的"有针对性的"活检增加了前列腺癌检测的方法,如提高了肿瘤的分期和/或增加穿刺标本中肿瘤组织的含量。然而,MRI/融合活检似乎不够敏感,目前尚无法替代标准的扩大核心活检(按区域随机选取穿刺点:右尖部和左尖部、中部、基底部和侧角至少 10~12 个穿刺点)。对于 MRI 难以发现的病变,进行这种系统穿刺活检似乎是有必要的,但是,有针对性的靶向穿刺更可能检测到高级别肿瘤,而舍弃低级别肿瘤。最近,一项纳入 1 003 名患者接受 MR/融合活检和标准(六点穿刺)活检的前瞻性队列研究中,靶向活检可以提高高危前列腺癌(Gleason 评分≥4+3)的检出率 30%,而降低低危前列腺癌检出率 17%[114]。

尽管这些结论令人兴奋,但是这一技术以及图像的标准化在该方法成为金标准之前还有相当一段路要走。正如 Emberton[115]所言,欧洲每年实施活检的例数超过一百万,如果每次都是需要 MRI 引导,那么就需要大量的后勤工作,包括购置合适的设备以及技术培训。此外,报告标准化也是新近提出的,并且临床正在实施中[116,117]。目前采用的方案是对主动监测或既往活检阴性/PSA 升高的患者进行 MRI/融合穿刺活检,泌尿放疗科医生和泌尿科医生联手推进这一令人兴奋的新领域。其意义在于,可以减少活检假阴性的患者,以及减少不该采用主动监测的发生。此外,还需要进一步的前瞻性研究来评估该技术对临床结果的预测价值(如主动监测患者疾病的重新分类、前列腺癌特异性死亡率)。

治疗方案选择与应用

主动监测

在前 PSA 时代,"等待观察"意指对积极治疗的一种替代,用来描述对患者进行监测但在疾病进展和/或症状出现之前不进行治疗的一段时间。随着 PSA 检测的出现,诊疗规范发生了变动,我们现在诊断出相当可观的更多的早期前列腺癌,包括那些一直在临床上无意义前列腺癌。人们需要新的策略来管理特定的低危前列腺癌,而不是立刻实施治疗。这种方法被冠以不同的术语,包括"带有选择性延迟干预的等待观察"[118]和"主动监测"[119]。这一新策略是对低危前列腺癌患者放弃即刻治疗而进行密切随访,在疾病仍可治愈时早期发现肿瘤进展并适时地开展确切的治疗。对于实现该策略的预期,两种临床工具是不可或缺的:一是在治疗前识别低分级、惰性肿瘤患者的方法,二是在疾病仍可治愈时能可靠地检出肿瘤进展的监测策略。从大样本研究和荟萃分析中收集到的数据支持对临床局限性前列腺癌病例进行保守处理[120-122]。在这些前 PSA 时代的研究中,高龄患者和有肿瘤临床表现的患者具有数量上的优势;因此,它们的结果不能被直接外推至接受了 PSA 筛查的人群。其他问题包括:诊断患者的方法——很多人没有进行对转移灶的全面检查,而且很多人的诊断是基于细针穿刺活检结果得出的[121]——而事实上研究者们并未集中进行病理学审查[120]。尽管它们存在这些局限,但这些观察性研究表明:患有低分级前列腺癌的患者疾病进展缓慢,即使经过 20 年的随访,其肿瘤特异性死亡的风险仍非常小[123]。

与之相反,Gleason 评分为 7~10 分的患者死于疾病进展的风险较高。瑞典研究者进行了一项重要的前瞻性研究比较等待观察和根治性前列腺切除术,在其初始报告 3 年之后进行了更深入的分析,并预估了 15 年的结果[81,124,125]。他们研究了 T1a、T1b、T1c 或 T2 期 695 例前列腺癌患者,将其随机地分配给行根治性前列腺切除术组($n=347$)或等待观察组($n=348$)。

2/3 的患者有可触及的肿瘤，但每组中有症状的患者均不足一半-行根治性前列腺切除术组为 43.8%，而等待观察组为 39.7%。在最近报道的延长随访(23.2 年)分析中[82]，研究者发现，在 18 年的随访中，前列腺切除组的患者和等待观察组后来接受去势治疗的患者之间统计学上存在显著差异[42.5%和 67.4%，*RR*=0.49(95%*CI*:0.39~0.60;*P*<0.001)]，发生远处转移[26%对 38.3%，*RR*=0.57(95%*CI*:0.44~0.75;*P*<0.001)]和疾病特异性死亡率[17.7%对 28.7%，*RR*=0.56(95%*CI*:0.41~0.77;*P*=0.001)]。仅 65 岁以下的患者可以从根治性前列腺切除术中获益。此外，值得注意的是，等待观察组中的大部分患者不需要任何姑息治疗。这些研究结论在美国的研究人群中是否可被重复是未知的，因为前列腺癌在美国通常比在瑞典诊断得更早[126]。

美国的前列腺癌干预与观察试验(Prostate Cancer Intervention versus Observation Trial，PIVOT)[127]在 731 例局限性前列腺癌患者中比较了前列腺切除术与观察等待的效果，他们的预期寿命不少于 10 年。中位随访时间 10 年，两组的全因死亡率和前列腺癌特异性死亡率没有显著性统计学差异。手术组中 PSA>10ng/ml 和高危亚组患者的前列腺癌特异性死亡率有降低的趋势。事实上，对于低危前列腺癌患者，手术后肿瘤特异性死亡率增加了 15%，虽然没有统计学意义。还有两项持续时间很久的前瞻性队列研究检验了主动监测或期待疗法的可行性。此外，其他大样本前瞻性队列研究正在进行中[128]。Carter 等人[129]对 81 名诊断为 T1c 期小体积前列腺癌的患者进行了中位随访时间为 23 个月(范围为 12~58 个月)的观察研究。他们的中位年龄是 65 岁(范围为 52~73 岁)。在基线水平上，所有患者的 PSA 密度≤0.15ng/ml，并且 Gleason 评分<7，这些患者游离 PSA 比例的中位值为 17%(范围为 4.3%~37%)。受试者每 6 个月进行一次(游离和总体)PSA 测定和直肠指诊。每 12 个月进行一次经直肠超声引导下穿刺活检，包含至少 12 针的取样评估。在研究 1 年后的时间里，患者中有 56 人(69%)未出现进展并仍在监测中。其余 25 名患者(31%)达到了疾病进展的标准，即在前列腺穿刺活检中发现不良病理结果，包括 Gleason 评分≥7，存在 Gleason 4 分或 5 分的组织形态，两针以上穿刺有癌组织浸润，或在任何一针中癌组织浸润超过 50%。他们的疾病进展中位时间为 14 个月(范围为 12~52 个月)。研究者发现，按照他们所定义的疾病进展的患者，与未经历进展的患者相比，前者的 PSA 密度统计学上显著高于后者，而前者游离 PSA 比值显著低于后者。

在一个更大规模的Ⅱ期临床研究中，Klotz 报道了[130]其对 299 例患者的研究发现，患者基线水平为分期 T2b 或以下的前列腺癌，PSA<15ng/ml，Gleason 评分≤7。所有受试者年龄均大于 70 岁。监测方法包括 PSA 测定、全身骨扫描、经直肠超声(最初 2 年每 6 个月一次，之后每年一次)以及进入试验后 1.5 或 2 年内进行的穿刺活检。疾病进展的标准是患者表现出 PSA、临床或组织学疾病进展。PSA 进展被定义为 PSA 倍增时间<2 年(在至少 6 个月的时间内测量至少 3 次)，末次 PSA>8ng/ml，并且 ln(PSA)对时间的回归分析 *P*<0.05。临床进展被定义为出现下述情况之一：原发病灶的最大垂直径乘积增大了两倍(以数字化方法测量)；因局部进展而需要 TURP；尿道梗阻；远处转移的临床或影像学证据。组织学进展被定义为在后续的穿刺活检中 Gleason 评分≥8。在 55 个月时，60%的患者仍在监测中；在 96 个月时，疾病特异性生存率为 99%，总生存率为 85%。35%的患者 PSA 倍增时间>10 年(中位倍增时间为 7.0 年)。放弃监测的原因包括患者的想法(16%)、快速的生化进展(12%)、临床进展(8%)和组织学进展(4%)。在最近公布的更新研究中，从第一次活检开始算起的中位随访时间为 6.4 年(范围为 0.2~19.8 年)，Klotz 等人[131]报告的主动监测患者中前列腺癌特异性死亡率为 1.5%。其他原因死亡风险是前列腺癌死亡风险的 9.2 倍。随着主动监测的方法转向影像学新技术和生物标志物的整合，研究者面临的挑战包括更多的早期前列腺癌患者，最大限度地降低癌症进展的风险，最大限度地提高生活质量。

前列腺癌的检查和治疗(ProtecT)研究是比较主动监测和积极治疗的优劣[132]。ProtecT 的研究者们自 2001 年开始该试验，预期在英国招收 1 500 名以上患者并将其随机分组分别接受适形放射治疗、前列腺切除术或主动监测。试验的结果预计将于 2016 年得出。这些试验将提供给研究者们关于经 PSA 筛查发现的局限性前列腺癌的更多信息，从而帮助医师和患者更好地理解各种策略的风险与获益，并在决策制订中更好地达成一致。

治愈性治疗-关于疾病控制和副作用最小化的解剖学讨论

患有早期疾病的患者可以在多种根治性治疗方案中选择进行一种，而每种方案都在技术上有其自身的多样变化。从根本上讲，可选方案包括根治性前列腺切除术和剂量升级的放射治疗。这两大类治疗方法的目标都是治疗整个腺体，只是分别通过手术切除或者以放射方法消灭肿瘤。其他科选择的治疗方法也已出现，例如冷冻治疗和高强度聚焦超声，这些方法针对腺体的全部或部分。所有这些针对前列腺癌的治疗，都会伴有一定的复发风险和不同程度的生活质量上的不良反应，包括：勃起功能障碍、尿失禁、尿路刺激症状和/或梗阻症状和肠功能紊乱。减少不良反应和治疗后复发的愿望，使本领域内出现了大量的技术更新、全新技术以及大量的对比研究。对每一个涉及疗效和不良反应的问题，患者和医师都希望知道平均的预期治疗效果，以及帮助预测患者个体可能出现有利或不利治疗结局的任何有用的特征。另外，研究也揭示了特定方法在不同治疗中心的可重复性如何[133~135]。现今被诊断的大部分患者都非常清楚潜在的治疗后不良反应，以及医师的经验可能会影响治疗效果。

针对患者的治疗选择通常取决于对前列腺癌缓慢的自然病程，老年人的预期寿命以及患者的个人意愿等方面的考虑。最广为接受的建议是如果患者有 10 年或更长的预期寿命，则他可能从治疗中获益。然而，这一估测可能存在一定的变化，因为随着对心脏疾病更好的治疗，该类疾病所致的死亡正在减少。患者不应该仅出于年龄的原因而放弃治疗[136]，Albertsen 等人[121]的研究表明当疾病诊断于 70 岁或更高年龄时，前列腺癌相特异性死亡率显著降低，尤其是对 Gleason 评分<7 的患者。在 Bill-Axelson 一项有关根治性前列腺切除术和观察等待的随机研究中的最新结果表明，随机选择根治性前列腺切除术和观察等待的患者在治疗决策的选择中明显获益[82]。根治性

前列腺切除术的患者队列研究显示,在根治性切除手术组大多数有生存获益的患者均小于 65 岁;然而,65~75 岁的患者在激素治疗、姑息治疗和转移进展方面有次要获益。

根治性前列腺切除术-早期前列腺癌治疗困境的范例

治疗早期前列腺癌的挑战可以通过根治性前列腺切除术的解剖学手术步骤来展示,而通过这些手术步骤也能重点显示出外科医生和放疗医生在控制肿瘤和最小不良反应两方面所考虑的问题。图 98-6 显示了前列腺周围非常复杂的解剖结构。

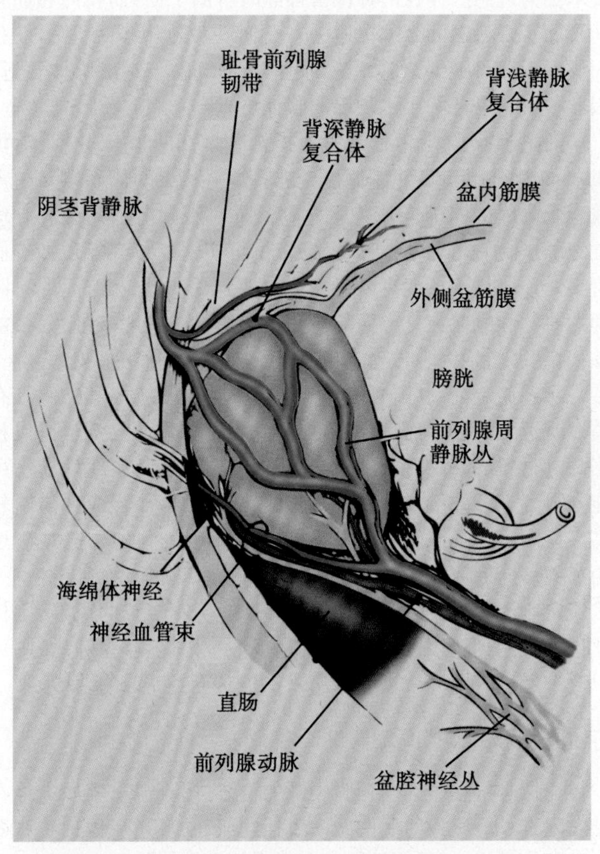

图 98-6 前列腺的外科解剖:与背深静脉复合体,神经血管束以及周围相关结构的关系(外侧观)

根治性前列腺切除术包括完整去除前列腺、精囊和远端输精管。从概念上讲,前列腺可以认为是一个两端开放(膀胱颈和尿道)的圆锥状结构。圆锥体的周围有一层包膜样结构(尽管不是真正的组织学包膜),并被两侧的盆内筋膜和后方的 Denonvilliers 筋膜所包围。在其尖部,前列腺被横纹括约肌和背静脉复合体所包绕,后者在尿道上方细窄,然后分散进入一个围裙样的结构以通过前列腺中部、底部并越过膀胱。不管采取何种路径和技术,切除前列腺都需要对将要遇到的复杂的解剖结构有深刻的理解,并且熟悉一系列明确的手术操作方法。

前列腺的入路

前列腺是手术较难达到的器官之一。它在前方覆有耻骨弓,远端有背静脉复合体和横纹括约肌,下方有直肠,侧下方覆有神经束,上方有膀胱。自耻骨至脐的下腹正中切口可以显露前列腺,该显露途径经过腹膜外间隙。其他可选的入路包括小切口手术、经下腹 5 或 6 穿刺孔的腹腔镜手术(经腹膜外或经腹)和经会阴入路。小切口手术的切口通常为 8~10cm,而标准开腹手术则需要 15~20cm 长的切口。在两种开腹入路中,对前列腺的显露相似,但在小切口手术中,外科医师将更依赖于器械解剖而非手工解剖。随着机器人手术系统投入使用,通过器械增加了腹腔镜术者操作的灵巧性,包括七维度动作和 3D 立体视觉,腔镜手术方式正变得越来越受欢迎。

手术方式的选择取决于术者的训练以及患者的特点。经耻骨后手术入路包含在全世界绝大多数住院医培训计划中,它提供了到达前列腺及淋巴结的入路,需要熟悉经腹的定位。经会阴入路可能所伴随的疼痛较轻,而且瘢痕更不明显。在病态肥胖的情况下该术式可能有其优势。然而,该术式不能显露淋巴结,且切除较大前列腺时(如>60g)可能存在困难。腹腔镜手术需要 100 例以上陡峭的学习曲线,而机器人辅助的腹腔镜手术所需例数较少[137~139]。在经耻骨后开放手术和腹腔镜手术之间并未确切地观察到术后疼痛和出院时间方面的差异[140~141],但经会阴入路手术的上述指标可能有所降低[142]。经会阴以及腹腔镜手术出血量均较少,但对熟练的外科医生来说,各术式的输血率可能并无显著差异[143]。非随机对照试验的结果显示,如果经耻骨后前列腺切除术的输血率超过 10%~15%。则该术式的输血率高于其他术式[144]。

继续围绕这个问题讨论,我们将只讨论经耻骨后开放手术和腹腔镜手术(包括和机器人辅助两种类型)。然而值得注意的是,尽管关于经会阴手术的历史讨论表明其结果可能增加切缘阳性率、降低性功能保留率并导致原发性排便失禁[145],但一些大样本量中心发表过截然相反结果[142,146],而且其相对于使用机器人的手术是否会节约成本尚有待商榷[147,148]。

其他可选择的治疗方法也必须考虑在其应用中进入前列腺的方法。近距离放疗是全腺体放射治疗的一种方式,在该疗法中放射性粒子在经直肠超声引导下,经会阴入路植入前列腺中。在 BPH 患者中,前列腺的前部可能延伸绕过耻骨弓,对穿刺针造成了干扰。因此,在应用近距离治疗和冷冻治疗(另一种经会阴入路的消融疗法)时,前列腺必须符合一定尺寸(一般来说为<60g)和形状以使其可以到达。与之相反,现代外照射放疗可处理的前列腺尺寸和形状的范围更加宽泛。例如,调强放射治疗(intensity-modulated radiation therapy,IMRT)技术使用来自不同角度的多个放射源以提高对前列腺的照射剂量同时限制前列腺外的照射剂量。最近流行的质子放射治疗,是可以限制正常组织照射剂量的另一种方法。

尖部的显露和分离

前列腺的前方和两侧表面覆有盆内筋膜。这层筋膜可以被锐性切开或电刀切开,需注意避开或结扎沿前列腺走行并经常于 11 和 1 点钟方向穿过尖部的变异繁多的静脉网络。多数外科医师会切开耻骨前列腺韧带以便于在远端结扎背静脉复合体。在这一区域的失误在开放手术中会导致严重的出血,而在腹腔镜和/或机器人手术中由于 CO_2 气腹的正压作用这样的出血会较少。

横纹括约肌在远端环绕于尿道周围,而前列腺的尖部没有包膜样结构。因此,在这一区域存在巨大的失误风险,而这也可能是手术中随着术者经验增加而改善最大的一步。从根本上讲,术者必须控制背静脉复合体的近端和远端结构,然后尽可能靠近尖部做横向切割以免损伤横纹括约肌复合体同时避免造成尖部阳性切缘。在这一方面有很多种不同的技术方法,在此无法完全列举,但是这一步对肿瘤控制(即手术切缘阴性)和尿控的手术目标影响巨大。

除手术外的其他可选择的治疗方法也必须充分覆盖尖部区域,同时避免不良反应。剂量递增的外照射和近距离放疗会不可避免地同时到达尖部和周围的横纹括约肌。然而,由于这些结构并没有被专门地破坏,因此其压力性尿失禁的发生率显著少于手术。冷冻治疗技术应包含在括约肌里的温度监测器,以避免对前列腺尖部以外括约肌结构的冷冻。

膀胱颈的显露和分离

在开放手术中,对膀胱颈的分离相对而言比对尖部的处理要简单得多。Foley 导尿管可以用作引导,而且电刀可以安全地使用。必须加以注意的是要保留好膀胱颈的后壁并将其与输尿管口分离开。保留膀胱颈的技术曾被报道称可能有利于避免尿失禁,但也可能与增加切缘阳性的发生率有关[149]。未保留膀胱颈的膀胱开口,可以通过缝合重建来使吻合口与尿道的尺寸相匹配。

对手术的替代性疗法必须充分治疗前列腺的基底部同时避免损伤膀胱。在对盆腔的传统剂量放疗中,对膀胱和直肠周边照射剂量通常是整个治疗的剂量限制因素。然而,剂量递增技术,不论是 IMRT、质子治疗还是近距离治疗,都有效地增加了对前列腺的照射剂量,同时把对膀胱的照射剂量控制在低水平上。然而,一部分照射剂量确实影响到膀胱,在不同程度上导致了排尿方面的不良反应,包括尿路刺激症状、尿频和血尿等。

精囊的显露和分离

精囊具有其自身的手术挑战。这些结构的位置紧邻膀胱后方,其尖部于侧方走行。精囊被数根小动脉分支所包绕,后者必须以夹闭或缝扎的方式进行控制。如未被控制,这些分支可能会引起严重的术后出血,甚至可能需要二次手术。然而,如果可能的话一定要避免电灼,因为精囊的尖部紧邻于血管神经束的内侧。一些研究者报道了保留精囊尖部完整以避免神经损伤的理念[150]。腹腔镜手术医师可以经 Douglas 陷凹于膀胱后方解剖精囊以应对这一挑战。对放疗医生而言,精囊无法通过粒子植入疗法得到充分的治疗,但可以通过外照射技术对其治疗。带有直肠内线圈的 MRI 可以用来评价精囊方面的分期以决定是否将其纳入治疗计划之中-治疗的代价是会增加膀胱毒性。

神经血管束的分离

神经血管束的分离方法在开放手术中通常是逆向进行(自尖部到底部),而在腹腔镜手术中通常是顺向进行(自底部到尖部)。在逆向进行方式中,在背静脉复合体和尿道的离断之后,用手指钝性分离出 Denonvilliers 筋膜后面的层面,然后即可触及两侧的神经血管束。直视下,神经血管束经过数层侧筋膜充分融合于前列腺的两侧。这里有一个筋膜三角,以前列腺筋膜为内侧界,盆内筋膜为外侧界,Denonvilliers 筋膜为后界。不论采用何种技法,在以下两个连接处必须松解神经束:前列腺筋膜和肛提肌筋膜的前外侧连接,以及前列腺筋膜和 Denonvilliers 筋膜的内后侧连接。

在分离神经血管束的过程中,必须避免使用电刀,否则热传导作用可能产生不可修复的神经损伤。神经血管束自中部至尖部的部分大多为平行走行的血管,有少部分穿支静脉,可以用夹子控制或仅直接切断而让其自行凝血。相反,神经血管束靠近底部的部分发出通往前列腺的穿支动脉,这些血管必须用夹子控制以避免出血。有报道指出其他替代性的止血装置产生的热量较少,但神经束对热损伤非常敏感,因而非热产生技术更为理想。存在两种保留神经时解剖平面:筋膜内和筋膜间平面。外科医师必须在这一方面加以斟酌,因为尽管自筋膜内层面入路可能会改善术后的性功能,但由于它离腺体更近,因此也就是染色的手术切缘离腺体更近[151]。

通过治疗前检测到的各项指标(如 PSA、临床分期、活检 Gleason 评分、穿刺活检阳性针数、活检中肿瘤的体积以及超声或直肠内线圈 MRI 等影像学检查),外科医师对前列腺外肿瘤侵犯的风险做出评估,并以此为依据可能选择放弃保留神经血管束。评分量表可能有助于完成这一评估[103,152,153],但外科医师的直觉和经验在这方面的作用很难衡量。一般来说,只要能够控制肿瘤,绝大多数患者更愿意选择保留神经的手术。

神经束和前列腺包膜的毗邻关系也与放疗方案的制订有关。就近距离治疗而言,在前列腺外周带内投放的剂量可以相当高,但在腺体外会陡然下降。其结果是,中危和高危疾病可能未得到充分的治疗,因为其前列腺外存在微小浸润的风险较高。许多中心会推荐剂量方案可以达到包膜外的放疗,或者近距离放疗与外放疗的联合方案。冷冻治疗医师也可以在这一区域定制治疗方案:如果存在前列腺包膜外侵犯的风险,则使冰球的范围到达该区域;而如果在某一侧别不存在肿瘤,则可以对神经血管束区域进行保温以保护其不受冰球的破坏。

尿道的分离

尿道必须在紧邻前列腺尖部的位置进行分离,实质上恰在精阜附近。应该保留周围的横纹括约肌,并且避免尿道扩张器和导管造成过度的创伤。

吻合

连续缝合和间断缝合方法均有人做过研究,后者在腹腔镜手术中更为普遍和可行。吻合的目标是使膀胱连接于尿道上,使吻合口不透水并使黏膜表面相互接触。应该尽量避免尿道缝合过多,从而可能导致尿道的有效功能长度缩短。吻合口瘘或者分离可能导致吻合口瘢痕形成和挛缩[154]。

高危肿瘤的技术改良

目前在手术患者中,已经观察到高危患者比例增加的趋势[155],这就需要额外的手术技巧保证切缘阴性的同时,在最大限度可行范围内保留神经束,通过盆腔扩大淋巴结清扫进一步获得分期的信息。正如 Yuh 等学者回顾分析[156],对高危前列腺癌者实施保留神经手术的比例存在很大变化,大约有 1/3 的患者中存在淋巴结转移。

早期疾病的治疗结果

肿瘤控制

现今的多数研究使用无 PSA 复发生存作为终点事件，因为可以在 5~10 年的时间框架内收集数据，而不是像肿瘤特异生存率和总生存率等较长期终点事件所需的 15~20 年的时间框架。然而，正如 AUA 指南所强调的，人们对 PSA 复发的定义并不一致，而且它与较长的生存并不直接相关。对手术患者 PSA 治疗失败最常用的定义是 PSA 水平>0.2ng/ml，而对放疗患者，美国放射治疗及肿瘤学会（American Society for Therapeutic Radiology and Oncology，ASTRO）更新的建议为 PSA 从低点增加 2ng/ml[157]。在不同研究中对风险分层的定义也不相同。AUA 指南推荐 D'Amico 标准及对各分层的选项：

- 低危组：PSA ≤ 10ng/ml，Gleason 评分 ≤ 6，且临床分期为 cT1c~cT2a
- 中危组：PSA>10~20ng/ml 或 Gleason 评分 ≤7 或临床分期为 T2b
- 高危组：PSA>20ng/ml 或 Gleason 评分 ≤ 8~10 或临床分期为 T2c

依据这些风险分组，图 98-7 显示了近距离治疗、外照射放疗和根治性前列腺切除术等治疗方法的 PSA 无复发生存率[96]。对各种治疗方式而言，5 年 PSA 无复发生存率：低危组 75%~95%；中位组 70%~90%；高危组 30%~80%。10 年 SA 无复发生存率：低危组 60%~90%；中危组 40%~80%；高危组 20%~60%。鉴于缺乏标准化的报告、对治疗失败的不同定义以及缺乏均衡随机对照试验所造成的局限，AUA 专家组认为目前没有充足的数据来得出一种治疗优于另一种的结论。对于选择放疗的患者，专家组援引了两个随机对照临床试验，表明较高剂量照射可能会降低 PSA 复发的风险[158,159]。

AUA 专家组还讨论了新辅助和/或辅助雄激素剥夺治疗的问题。关于新辅助雄激素剥夺治疗加根治性前列腺切除术的随机临床试验显示，无 PSA 复发生存并没有改善[160,161]。然而，对接受放射治疗的中危组患者，有研究显示为期 6 个月的新辅助和同期雄激素剥夺治疗可能延长放疗后的生存期[162]。对接受放射治疗的高危组患者，研究表明 2~3 年较长时间的辅助雄激素剥夺治疗具有生存获益。然而，值得注意的是，在这些试验中所使用的放疗为传统技术而非剂量递增放疗技术。

总而言之，AUA 指南列出了主动监测、近距离放疗、外放疗和根治性前列腺切除术作为低、中、高危前列腺癌患者可选治疗方案。就放射治疗而言，指南援引了关于放射剂量和雄激素剥夺治疗应用的随机对照试验。就高危患者而言，应注意其复发率很高，患者应该考虑“以改善疗效为目标，包括联合治疗在内的新形式的临床试验”。同样值得注意的是，AUA 专家组总结认为：一线内分泌治疗“在局限性前列腺癌患者中很少有应用指征”。

欧洲泌尿外科学会也发布了有关前列腺癌的指南，其中援

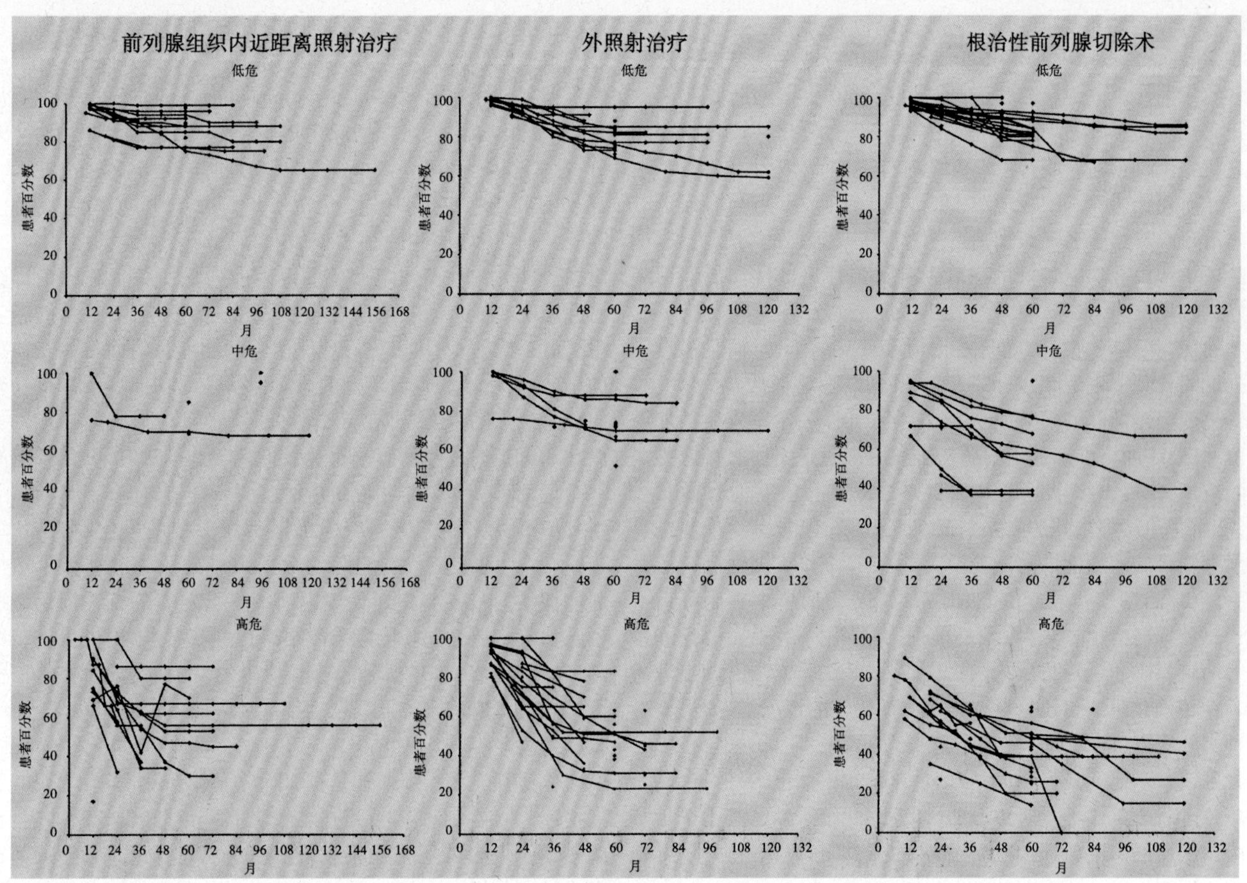

图 98-7 应用近距离放疗、外放疗和根治性前列腺切除的低危、中危或高危患者 PSA 无复发生存情况

引了关于等待观察、手术治疗和放射治疗的许多相同的随机临床试验[165]。指南中还引述了基于较低等级证据的补充建议。下面列出了一些有关早期肿瘤的相关建议:

- 近距离治疗"可以应用在 cT1~T2a,Gleason 评分<7 分(或为 3+4 分),PSA ≤ 10ng/ml,前列腺体积 ≤ 50ml,之前没有 TURP 手术史并且国际前列腺症状评分(International Prostate Symptom Score,IPSS)良好的患者(证据等级:2b)。"
- 对于不适合手术或者预期寿命<10 年的前列腺癌患者,冷冻治疗"已经由一种试验性治疗方式发展为一种可行的可选择的治疗方式(推荐等级 C 级)。"
- "所有其他的微创的治疗方案,如高强度聚焦超声(high-intensity focused ultrasound,HIFU)、间质肿瘤射频消融术(radiofrequency interstitial tumor ablation,RITA)、微波治疗和电外科手术,均仍处于试验性或研究性阶段。对所有这些方法而言,必须进行较长时间的随访,用以评估其在前列腺癌治疗中的真正作用(推荐等级 C 级)。"

另一项总结研究现状的大规模工作是为美国保健研究和质量机构(Agency for Healthcare Research and Quality)进行的,发表于《内科学年鉴》(*Annals of Internal Medicine*)[166]。研究者们再一次遇到了这些困难,由于在报告和定义中存在差异,而且只有三个随机对照试验比较了不同初始治疗的治疗效果(并非针对"由 PSA 检测最初发现"的患者),所以从本质上讲,无法得出任何结论。

治疗的并发症

概论

一般而言,根治性前列腺切除术会比放疗或主动监测导致更多的尿失禁。近距离放疗和外放疗会伴有更多的膀胱刺激症状和/或血尿等不良反应,但尿失禁较少。放疗导致直肠刺激症状的风险较高。所有治疗方式都有性功能障碍的副作用:根治性前列腺切除术的表现形式是早期丧失而逐渐改善,而近距离治疗或放疗的表现形式则是较为渐进和延迟的功能丧失。年龄较小和原有功能较好的患者则各种治疗后的性功能保留较好。

然而,在比较中存在着许多偏倚和变异的来源,而且没有证据证明任何一种治疗"并发症累积总风险显著较高"[164]。尽管患者们经常会询问某一个统计数字,如尿失禁率或性功能保留率,公认的更准确的生活质量研究应来源于下述工具或方法的应用:①提出多个问题并提供一系列潜在答案的有效量表;②由主治医师之外的人员管理的量表;③包含有治疗前基线水平测量的前瞻性纵向试验设计;④在整个研究期间保持应答率>70%的量表。最近由 Ferrer 等[167]进行的多中心研究评价了三种标准治疗方式(根治性前列腺切除术、近距离治疗和放射治疗),除了治疗方式未随机化而外,其试验方法已相当理想。在随机对照试验缺乏对副作用进行比较的情况下,如下不同种类的研究可以帮助我们认识治疗的不良反应:①来自多中心社区或学术研究系列(即对社区情况的自愿性报告)的结果;②单一术者的大样本量研究系列(即理想化结果);③基于医疗保险或索赔的研究(即非自愿性结果报告)。

多中心研究

Penson 等人[168]报道了前列腺癌治疗结果研究(prostate cancer outcomes study)的一些数据,该研究是在 6 个中心开展的基于社区的队列研究,患者们在 1994 年和 1995 年于这些中心进行了根治性前列腺切除术。在这一研究中,唯一相关的预测性信息是在社区中这些患者进行了根治性前列腺切除术,即没有给出任何技术描述或对术者和/或手术的质量分析。在所研究的 1 288 例患者中,频繁的漏尿在术前基线水平上见于 3% 的患者,在术后 6 个月时为 19%,在术后 1 年时为 13%,在术后 2 年时为 9%,在术后 5 年时为 11%。在术后 5 年时,对尿控水平的描述为:完全控制者 35%,偶尔漏尿者 51%,频繁漏尿者 11%,完全无控制者 3%。

此外还有人展示了有关尿垫使用、尿路刺激性症状和困扰等其他数据。在试验开始的基线水平上,87%的患者没有排尿困扰问题;在 5 年时,45%的患者报告称没有问题,42%的患者称有轻度问题,13%的患者称有中重度问题。报告称 81%的患者术前基线水平可以有足够的勃起完成正常性生活,在术后 6 个月时这一比例为 9%,在 1 年时为 17%,在 2 年时为 22%,在 5 年时为 28%。尽管在术后 2~5 年排尿功能和困扰评分有所改善,但无性活动的患者比例在基线上为 15%,在 1 年时为 44%,在 5 年时为 46%。保留双侧神经预示着在 5 年时勃起功能恢复较好:保留双侧神经者恢复率为 40%,而保留单侧神经者为 23%,未保留神经者为 23%。年龄也是一个预测因子:39~54 岁的患者,是功能保留最好的患者群,该组中有 61%报告称可以勃起。

Sanda 等人[169]报道了一个来自 9 个大学附属中心的多机构研究队列,患者接受了开放、腹腔镜或机器人辅助腹腔镜手术。在理论上,这一手术医师群体的手术量很大,但该研究也没有报道他们所采用的特定的手术技术。使用百分制前列腺癌扩展综合指数(expanded prostate index composite,EPIC)量表,接受根治性前列腺切除术的患者,尿控基线评分仅为 90 分,在 2 个月时下降至 50 分,在 6 个月时恢复至 70 分,在 12~24 个月间则稳定于 80 分。

然而,正如前述两个大型研究结果所表明的,文献中包含对尿失禁的各种不同定义。根治性前列腺切除术和放疗都会对性功能造成负面影响。在接受根治性前列腺切除术的患者中,保留神经技术可以更好地保留勃起功能。然而在接受放疗的患者中,用单一疗法治疗的患者保留勃起功能好于接受联合内分泌治疗的患者(即使 6 个月的短期治疗)。肠道功能受外放疗和近距离放疗的影响最为明显,即使经过 1 年之后,仍有 9%的患者有肠道功能相关的困扰。

AUA 指南专家组的综述报道称尿失禁的发生率在 3%~74%[96,164],并表明没有充足的数据来对排尿功能结果给出全面的评估。AUA 指南还大规模回顾了已发表的有关根治性前列腺切除术后勃起功能障碍的结果,这项综述未提供手术技术和经验的细节。1 年后勃起功能障碍的发生率高达 90%,而保留神经技术有利于降低其发生率。

专家系列

保留神经的手术最初是在 20 世纪 80 年代早期由 Walsh 等人描述[169],在引进 PSA 筛查之后该术式变得愈加普遍并且在肿瘤学上足够安全。我们可以想象,患者对 Walsh 服务的需求越来越高,对其他全身心致力于该术式的医师的服务需要越来越高。Walsh 等人发表了一项经过验证的生活质量调查研究,该研究表明在 1 年时 93%的患者恢复了尿控,在 18 个月时 86%的患者性功能正常[170]。一个大样本量的机器人辅助前列腺切除术系列也显示出极好的结果:在 1 年时 1 110 名患者中有 1 032 人(93%)每天只用一块尿垫或者不用,而且 79.2%的患者报告称性功能正常[171]。尽管其他一些研究密切关注于影响尿控或性功能保留率的因素,最近的趋势则是估测达到人们所希望的“三连胜”结果的概率:癌症控制、排尿控制和性功能。来自 Sloan-Kettering 癌症纪念中心的团队发布了一种用于这种估测的量表[172]。

专家比较研究已扩展到不同技术选择之间的比较。Touijer 等人[173]进行的一项单中心研究涉及两位手术量较多的外科医师,其中一位进行腹腔镜手术而另一位进行开放手术。人们超出预料地发现开放手术组的尿控恢复(定义为患者报告没有漏尿或不需要尿垫)更好:在 12 个月时,两组的尿控恢复率为 75%比 48%。文中引用了对手术技术的描述,但两者的真正差别并未详细描述。作者们怀疑这一结果可能是由腹腔镜手术方式中对尖部的解剖所导致的,他们表示还需要进一步的前瞻性研究。

因此,在早期疾病治疗效果的研究中一个明确的需要,就是要在技术和效果之间建立更好的联系。在 Masterson 等人[174]的研究中可以看到一个范例,该研究表明研究者可以描述在保留神经方面一个特定的技术改进并可以测定相应的结果。在标准手术技术中,尖部的分离起自背深静脉复合体,切断尿道,然后钝性游离后侧,最后松解后外侧的神经血管束。在改良的手术技术中,解剖顺序是先自尖部向精囊将整个神经血管束从前列腺的外侧面分离下来,再切断尿道并进行后方的解剖。这样避免了对神经血管束的过度牵拉。6 个月时的勃起功能恢复率由标准技术下的 40%提高到改良技术下的 67%。类似这样的比较还可见于有关近距离治疗的文献,在该研究中对植入粒子质量的 D90 分析是长期生化无疾病进展的重要预测因子[175]。

结果的变异与医疗保险数据库

在多中心研究和专家研究系列中,研究者们自愿地提交他们自己的结果,因此有能力决定是否参加研究。在其他研究中,往往使用了一些可获取的数据而无须每一个医师来决定是否参加研究。即使在熟练的外科医师之间,并发症的情况也存在差异[135]。医疗保险数据库和流行病学和最终结果(surveillance epidemiology and end results,SEER)的记录是这些研究的常用数据来源。这些研究的优势在于其患者数量大,并且提供了真实世界中一般社区患者人群的数据。它们的局限包括:仅选取年龄超过 65 岁的患者作为样本,其数据的观察终点更大程度上是为结算目的而非研究目的而设计的,因而其对结果的评估可能是不全面的。

这类数据库中的生活质量数据与专家系列中的数据看起来相当不同。Benoit 等人[176]发现尿道狭窄见于 19.5%的患者,尿失禁见于 21.7%的患者,而勃起功能障碍见于 21.5%的患者。Begg 等人[177]在 SEER-医疗保险联合数据库中检索了根治性前列腺切除术后的并发症情况,结果发现外科医师的手术量和并发症之间以及医院手术量和并发症之间有显著的相关趋势。最近,Hu 等人[178]分析了一个医疗保险数据库的患者样本,比较接受微创根治性前列腺切除术和开放手术的患者差异。数据趋势表明接受微创根治性前列腺切除术的患者围术期并发症较少并且住院时间较短,但是他们接受挽救治疗和发生吻合口狭窄的概率较高。然而,微创根治性前列腺切除术方法的术后不利并发症会随着术者手术量的增加而显著地减少。

PSAV 作为诊断后的预测因子

研究者们也依靠 PSAV 来预测疾病的进展、复发和治疗效果。在一项对接受了根治性前列腺切除术的 102 例患者的回顾性研究中,研究者们发现诊断前一年的 PSAV 值是否超过 2ng/(ml · a)与肿瘤体积之间在统计学上显著相关,发生生化复发者的肿瘤体积为 2.55cm^3,而术后 5 年无复发者的肿瘤体积为 0.94cm^3[3]($P<0.05$)。经历了复发的患者的中位 PSAV 值几乎是未经历复发者的两倍[1.98ng/(ml · a)和 1.05ng/(ml · a)]。尽管这些结果有助于识别高危患者,它们可能也会帮助医生识别那些更有可能根治的肿瘤患者。

发表于 2005 年的两项研究结果揭示了 PSAV 和治疗结果之间的关系。D'Amico 等人[180]在 1 095 例局限性前列腺癌患者中研究了诊断前一年的 PSAV,用以识别那些可能死于前列腺癌风险最高的患者。他们测定 PSAV>2.0ng/(ml · a)与较短时间死于前列腺癌($P<0.001$)显著相关,同时死于前列腺癌与死于其他任何原因相比($P=0.01$),统计学上也有显著意义。这些结果也受到 PSA 水平、肿瘤分期和诊断时 Gleason 评分的影响。预测死于前列腺癌时间的因素包括临床肿瘤分期达到 T2,Gleason 评分为 8、9 或 10,以及诊断时 PSA 水平处于上升中。

在一项随访超过 7 年的更大型的研究中,Sengupta 及其同事们[181]也发现死于前列腺癌的风险升高与术前 PSAV 和 PSA 倍增时间均显著相关。在进行了根治性前列腺切除术的 2 290 名患者中,460 名 PSAV>3.4ng/(ml · a)的患者与具有较低 PSAV 值的患者相比,前列腺癌死亡风险增加了 6 倍以上[危险比(HR)6.54;95%CI:3.51~12.91]。此外,506 名 PSA 倍增时间<18 个月的患者与 PSA 倍增时间较长的患者相比,也有类似的风险增加(HR 6.22;95%CI:3.33~11.61)。研究者认为,作为对生化进展的预测因子,PSAV 优于 PSA 倍增时间;而作为对临床进展和死亡的预测因子,PSA 倍增时间优于 PSAV。这一发现与前列腺癌的生长遵循指数模式而非线性模式的理念相符。

在 379 例根治性前列腺切除术后发生生化复发的患者中进行的一项研究,Freedland 及其同事们[182]发现 PSA 倍增时间以及病理 Gleason 评分和手术到复发的时间都是前列腺癌特异性死亡的统计学显著危险因子;在对 PSA 倍增时间<15 个月的人群的一项单独研究中,这些研究者们发现 90%的死亡可以归因于前列腺癌[183]。在对 PSAV 和 PSA 倍增时间的研究中,同样这些研究者们发现上述变量与病理学上的不良发现或根治性前列腺切除术后的生化复发之间没有关系[184]。

此外,尽管非洲裔美国男性比其他种族男性患前列腺癌的风险更高,但是研究者们发现 PSAV 或 PSA 倍增时间和白人、黑人、西班牙裔和亚裔等不同种族没有关系。正如人们所预料的那样,研究发现 PSAV 与前列腺体积也没有关系[179]。

前列腺癌化学预防:大规模试验

前列腺癌预防试验(prostate cancer prevention trial,PCPT)

入组 18 882 名男性，随机分成非那雄胺（5α 还原酶抑制剂）治疗组和安慰剂对照组[185]。因为数据安全和监察委员会认为试验已经达到了主要目的，所以 PCPT 比原计划提前了 1 年多结束。经历 7 年的观察，试验组比安慰剂组前列腺癌患病率降低了 24.8%（95%*CI*：18.6～30.6；*P*<0.001）。这个结果是令人鼓舞的，但治疗组高分级前列腺癌（Gleason 评分 7～10 分）的发生率却是安慰剂组的 1.67 倍（37.0% vs 22.2%，*P*<0.001）。

关于 PCPT 数据的最新研究结果提示，非那雄胺对于预防前列腺癌具有临床意义，也解释了非那雄胺组高级别前列腺癌较多的原因，并支持了它的应用。这些研究结果减轻了临床医师对非那雄胺导致侵袭性癌症的担忧，并鼓励将非那雄胺应用于更多的患者[186]。

对 PCPT 数据的重新分析表明，即使 PSA 小于 4.0ng/ml，前列腺癌的患病风险也开始增加[187]；对 PCPT 病理标本（非那雄胺 519 例，安慰剂组 716 例）重新分析以明确了肿瘤是否具有临床意义[188]。结果证明随着 PSA 值的增加，具有临床意义的肿瘤出现比例上升，无临床意义的肿瘤出现比例下降（表 98-6）。尽管如此，Gleason 评分小于 6 分的前列腺癌有 62%具有临床意义，相当于全部前列腺癌的 75%[188]。

表 98-6 有临床意义和无临床意义肿瘤的 PSA 和确诊

	PSA 值/（ng/ml）			
有危险的肿瘤类型	0～1.0	1.1～2.5	2.6～4.0	4.1～10.0
有临床意义肿瘤	15.6%	37.9%	49.1%	52.4%
无临床意义肿瘤	51.7%	33.7%	17.8%	11.7%

另一个 PCPT 数据的重新分析中，Pinsky 等[190]采用统计学模型来解决各组中病理学的误分类率以及如何识别高级别疾病中“真正”的相对风险。他们确定了一种函数，来判断从活检标本到根治性前列腺切除后的标本中，真正的低至高级别疾病的比率和误分类率。虽然与安慰剂组相比实验结果并没有统计学意义，高级别肿瘤的真实比率在非那雄胺组较低（*RR*=0.84；95%*CI*：0.68～1.05）；同样，低级别肿瘤的真实比率在非那雄胺组也较低且有统计学意义（*RR*=0.61；95% *CI*：0.51～0.71）。作者解释了这一矛盾，即尽管非那雄胺组降低了真正的低级别与高级别疾病的比率，使得误分类率降低，但两组中病变升期的比例类似。

PCPT 初步分析之后[187,189]，为了了解造成分析偏倚原因的影响，Redman 和她的同事[191]进行了重新分析，包括最终分析时被忽略的患者，应用最高标准（根治性前列腺切除术）估计了不同级别肿瘤的真正患病率和活检对前列腺癌诊断的敏感性。重新分析中一项是针对选择偏倚，其他则包括了 500 个癌症患者根治性前列腺术后病理分级的信息。与最初的分析相比，重新分析结果中前列腺癌的风险降低，且非那雄胺并没有增加癌高级别肿瘤的风险。在第一个重新分析研究中，风险降低了 30%（*RR*=0.70；95%*CI*：0.64～0.76；*P*<0.001），前列腺癌比率在安慰剂组中占 21%（4.2% 高级别），在非那雄胺组占 14.7%（4.8%高级别），高级别增加了 14%，但无统计学意义（*RR*=1.14；95%*CI*：0.96～1.35；*P*=0.12）。在 Redman 的第二个重新分析研究中，风险降低了 27%（*RR*=0.73；95%*CI*：0.56～0.96；*P*=0.02），高级别肿瘤在非那雄胺组更低（安慰剂组 8.2%；非那雄胺组 6.0%）。第三个重新分析研究中，病理敏感性可以影响风险比率的估计。作者认为使用非那雄胺治疗时不必担心高级别肿瘤的风险增高[191]。

更早的 PCPT 数据重新分析解释了非那雄胺引起的检出偏倚如何增加 PSA 对前列腺癌和高级别肿瘤（Gleason 评分 7～10 分）诊断的敏感性及直肠指诊的敏感性（非那雄胺组 21.3%；安慰剂组 16.7%，*P*=0.015）[187,189]。直肠指诊所探查到的高级别肿瘤比 PSA 更敏感，但结果并没有统计学意义[189]。

在这些新的分析公布之前，PCPT 主要的研究者 Ian Thompson 和他的同事已经部分回答了将非那雄胺增加 PSA 对前列腺癌和高级别肿瘤诊断敏感性的能力引入了结点时所遇到的问题[187]。PSA 升高或直肠指诊异常可提高高级别肿瘤的检出率，但非那雄胺组的活检的结果却并没有增加高级别肿瘤的检出率，研究者认为非那雄胺并没有引起相应组织学改变。Thompson 等[187]通过 AUC 研究证明非那雄胺组的总体肿瘤和高级别肿瘤的检出率显著高于安慰剂组，无论 Gleason 评分≥7 或≥8。此外，对 PCPT 研究的 18 年长期随访证实，非那雄胺对前列腺癌诊断后的总生存或生存没有显著影响[192]。

Thompson 和同事[187]对 PCPT 数据中的 PSA 进行了另一项研究，评估了 PSA 的 ROC 曲线，没有找到健康男性前列腺癌监测中，PSA 同时具有高敏感性和高特异性的切割点。在各个 PSA 水平都有患前列腺癌的风险。ROC 曲线对监测高级别肿瘤风险比总体风险好。但后续研究显示即使 PSA<4ng/ml，仍有检测到前列腺癌和高级别肿瘤的风险，既往认为 PSA<4ng/ml 属正常范围。虽然 PSA<4ng/ml 时也有患前列腺癌的风险，但如何应用于临床仍不清楚。这些资料阐明了：①需要更好的生物标志来判断前列腺癌风险和预后；②活检证实的阴性对照对前列腺癌风险、生物学行为以及预防的价值。

另一项重要的美国国家癌症研究所（National Cancer Institute，NCI）支持的化学预防、随机，安慰剂对照研究被称为硒和维生素 E 癌症预防试验（selenium and vitamin cancer prevention trail，SELECT）。该项研究评价单独或联合使用硒和维生素 E 对于预防前列腺癌的作用[193]。矛盾的是，研究人员在他们的第一份报告中报告了维生素 E 组前列腺癌风险在统计学上没有显著的增加，但随着随访时间的延长，这一风险变得显著，更多的前列腺癌事件出现[194,195]。SELECT 试验所有参与者中收集到的一系列生物样本将有助于构建风险模型，以帮助确定哪些男性最有可能患上前列腺癌，以及那些人可能会从硒和维生素 E 的补充中获益。

从 NCI 取得的其他样本最近刚刚公布，不论 NCI 是否同意，它们都向研究者开放[196]。

除非那雄胺外，其他可能的化学预防药物，包括已经研究的和正在开发的，有塞来昔布、舒林酸、托瑞米芬、大豆异黄酮、番茄红素和度骨化醇等。此外，正在探索新的预防策略，如免疫疗法和基于代谢的药物组合[197]。目前正在进行饮食和前列腺癌风险的分子流行病学研究，以及对杂环胺等特定饮食衍生化合物致癌性的基础研究。此外，他汀类药物也引起了人们的兴趣。2003 年 NCI 的癌症预防部门用 4 200 万美元资助 6 个研究，这些研究是由来自 6 个主要中心的肿瘤预防领域经验丰富的专家负责。这些研究的成员在预防研究和药物研究等方面有望成为美国的领先者，除感兴趣的药物外，他们研究的药物还包括以上曾经提到过的其他药物。

治疗流程：未来的方向

如果未来研究能够解决目前的综述中所提到的研究局限性，会对治疗策略产生极大的影响。这些研究必须：①设计采用随机的方法，包含一个无治疗的对照组；②应用癌症控制和生活质量结果的标准定义；③将特定技术与结果相联系；④证明特定技术可以被不同的操作者重复并得到类似的结论，就像处方一种药物一样，在不同的环境下在不同的患者群体之间产生类似的效果。科学标准达到后，研究设计需要有具体的措施以得到可能的进展，解决各种问题，如其他工作带来的问题以及潜在的可能使结论受到质疑的问题。

根据目前的知识，研究人员可以将局限性疾病患者的治疗流程概括如下：制订治疗方案，依据循证指南或者让患者加入临床试验，应用分子标志物以解决肿瘤异质性。第一，患者和他们的医师共同决定是否需要治疗，正如之前所说，期待治疗又被称为观察等待或者主动监测，使局限性疾病患者终止治疗，一些国家组织包括美国综合癌症网络（National Comprehensive Cancer Network，NCCN）已经制订了治疗方案[138]。但在一些主动监测研究中 75%选择观察等待的患者在 5 年内有选择了其他治疗，大部分是因为 PSA 升高[198]。通过预后因子如分子标志的组合对低危患者进行很好的识别以及密切的监测，可能会改变这一趋势。

为了使局限性前列腺癌患者免于不必要治疗的副反应，未来努力的关键方向是发展可以有效鉴别侵袭性和惰性肿瘤的工具。这样的工具，有一些还在发展中，例如之前所描述的图表形式、一种或多种分子标志与 PSA 结合、基因变异、辨别分子标签等[199~201]。通过这些组合我们找到的不是一个特定的指标，而是一组指标，不仅可以在手术前获取，还可以在活检前获得。通过这些信息我们可以预测治疗反应和疾病的自然进展[200]。

局部进展性肿瘤

临床表现

局部进展性前列腺癌以肿瘤突破前列腺包膜（T3a）或侵犯精囊（T3b）为标志。肿瘤可以两侧向盆壁生长、中央向尿道生长、上方向膀胱颈和三角区生长、下方向阴茎基底部生长或者后方向直肠生长。患者初诊时大部分没有任何症状，症状多与肿瘤生长的方向相关。

症状通常与 BPH 和尿道外口梗阻相似，如尿急、尿频、尿延迟、夜尿、排尿困难和尿线中断等。侵犯膀胱和尿道可能会产生血尿，尿道一旦梗阻还会引起肾功能损害。血精有时也会出现。虽然 Denvilliers 筋膜是防止肿瘤外侵的屏障，但直肠侵犯后会产生血便、便秘、梗阻、大便变细和盆腔不适等原发直肠癌的症状。肿瘤侵犯尿生殖膈或阴茎可能导致会阴部疼痛、阴茎持续勃起或勃起障碍等。

除了直肠指诊，盆腔 CT 或 MRI、经直肠超声、膀胱颈、直肠乙状结肠镜等检查手段也可以帮助确定肿瘤的范围以及邻近器官的情况。这些患者的 PSA 水平可能很高，但有些高分级的肿瘤、退行性肿瘤和导管变异等情况，PSA 水平并不高，或与疾病本身不平行。在 PSA 升高的肿瘤中，PSAV 是一项重要的指标，因为它衡量了肿瘤生长的速度和侵犯性。治疗（前列腺切除或放疗）前 PSAV 大于 2ng/（ml·y）与肿瘤造成的死亡密切相关[202]。PSA 倍增时间较短也是转移性肿瘤的标志。实验室检查可能会发现由于慢性出血所导致的红细胞下降以及由于尿道梗阻或肾功能障碍所导致的尿素氮、肌酐上升。

为了评估盆腔外的情况，同样推荐腹部 CT 或 MRI、骨扫描和胸片等检查。

治疗的选择和应用

根据 1990 年由美国外科医师学会完成的患者治疗的评估结果，局部进展性肿瘤最常用的治疗方法是放疗和内分泌治疗。12%的患者使用了联合治疗[203]。放疗和雄激素剥夺治疗[163,204~206]的疗效仍欠佳，因而在这些患者中采用了多模式的治疗方法。虽然外科手术可以有选择地用于局部晚期疾病，但术后通常会联合辅助放疗、化学内分泌治疗或者使用仍处于临床试验阶段的分子靶向治疗方法。

放疗和内分泌治疗

局部进展性肿瘤单独使用放疗很难完全去除肿瘤（概率<50%），而且不能降低转移的风险，因此放疗联合内分泌治疗成为标准的治疗方法。4 项随机临床试验——RTOG85-31、EORTC 22863、RTOG86-10 和 RTOG92-02 经过 10 年的随访，提供了令人信服的联合治疗的支持证据[207]。放射治疗肿瘤组（radiation therapy oncology group，RTOG）的患者主要是局部进展性肿瘤，欧洲癌症治疗研究组织（European Organization for Research on the Treatment of Cancer，EORTC）中的患者为 T3、T4 期肿瘤或高级别肿瘤。依据现在的标准，所有试验的放疗剂量都是较低的，为 65~70Gy。而采用的药物主要是促黄体素释放激素类似物（LHRH）。

RTOG85-31 试验放疗后进行内分泌治疗，内分泌治疗无明确时限。EORTC 试验放疗和内分泌治疗同时进行，内分泌治疗共持续 3 年。两个试验的结果显示，与单纯应用放疗相比，生化和临床终点（局部复发、远处转移、无疾病生存）、肿瘤相关死亡率和总生存率等指标都有显著改善。在对 RTOG85-31 试验的分层分析中，对于 Gleason 评分≥7 分的患者的优势善更为明显[204]。

RTOG86-10 试验将放疗前 2 个月开始 4 个月疗程的内分泌治疗与单纯放疗进行比较，研究的终点是生化复发、远处转移、无病和特异性生存。患者从联合治疗中获益较大[205,208]。最新的报道显示，仅 4 个月的辅助雄激素治疗对于肿瘤特异性生存率有着深远的影响。单纯放疗的患者中 1/3 在 9 年内死于前列腺癌[208]，而同样数量的患者在激素治疗 9 年后死于该疾病。但两组的总生存率仍没有显著差异。

RTOG92-02 试验将放疗联合 4 个月内分泌治疗（与 RTOG86-10 试验类似）和放疗联合 28 个月内分泌治疗（激素治

疗在放疗前 2 个月、放疗时 2 个月及之后的 24 个月）进行了比较。和其他研究的结果类似，除了总体存活率外，两组间都有差异。只有 Gleason 评分在 8～10 分的患者从长期内分泌治疗中获益[206,209]。

这些研究结果提示长时间的内分泌治疗联合放疗对局限性肿瘤和远处播散的患者都有意义，特别是 Gleason 评分较高的患者。

由 D'Amico 等做的一项研究[210]包括了中、高危前列腺癌患者（T1b～T2b 或直肠内线圈 MRI 证实的低危 T3，PSA10～40ng/ml 或 Gleason 评分 7～10 分），患者被随机分为两组，一组单独对前列腺和精囊进行 70Gy 的放疗，另一组再放疗前 2 个月开始共进行 6 个月的雄激素阻断治疗。结果也显示联合治疗对前列腺癌特异性死亡率有较大的改善：治疗后 8 年为 2% vs 8%。另外，总体存活率 74% vs 61%，提示联合治疗有更大的优势[163]。不伴或伴有轻微并发症的患者获益更高（90% vs 64%），但伴有中重度并发症的患者获益较少，虽然结果仍然比单独应用放疗好，但不具有统计学意义。D'Amico 和同事提出在该研究中内分泌治疗增加了心肌梗死的危险性[211]。

在另一项由 Trans-Tasman Radiation Oncology Group（96.01）开展的针对局部进展性肿瘤（T2b～T4）的随机试验中，66Gy 放疗前 5 个月进行共 6 个月的内分泌治疗显著改善了生化复发、局部复发、远处转移和前列腺癌特异性生存率[212]。增加激素治疗对高 PSA 值和高 Gleason 评分的患者中影响更大。因为内分泌治疗与心血管疾病、代谢综合征、骨密度降低等相关，目前仍趋于减少内分泌治疗的使用或者减少内分泌治疗的时间[211,213]，但激素治疗的理想持续时间还有待于评估最大治疗获益与损害比率的基础上确定[213]。

EORTC 的一项试验（22 961）旨在证明，对于局部进展前列腺癌患者（T2C-T4）和 T1c-T2b N1～2 期患者，放疗联合 6 个月的激素治疗不劣于放疗联合 3 年激素治疗。然而，这项试验在招募 990 名患者后提前结束，因为临时的分析显示该假设无法得到验证。接受激素治疗 6 个月的患者，5 年 PSA 和临床无进展生存率以及总体生存率均较低：78% vs 59%，82% vs 69%，85 vs 81%[214]。最新报道的试验（PCS Ⅳ）比较了 18 个月到 36 个月的雄激素剥夺联合中剂量放疗。随访时间中位数为 6.5 年，总生存和疾病特异性生存都无显著统计学差异[215]。此外，值得注意的是，目前标准的放疗比之前的剂量都要高，已经证明这既降低了局部复发、也降低了远处转移的风险[216,217]。因此，我们必须继续测试以确定最有益的雄激素剥夺治疗和放射治疗组合。

放疗与化疗

内分泌治疗联合放疗仍然有足够的改进空间，联合化疗也在进行临床试验。RTOG99-02 试验中，高危患者被随机分配到两组，一组放疗联合 2 年的内分泌激素治疗，另一组相同的治疗但放疗 8 周后，再联合四个周期的紫杉醇、雌莫司汀和依托泊苷化疗[218]。虽然因为过度的血栓毒性使该试验提前结束，但一项后续研究 RTOG05-21，已经获批，设计与 RTOG99-02 相同，化疗药物为多烯他赛和泼尼松，共化疗 6 个周期。未来的分析将提示这些药物与放疗联合的有效性。此外，类似于转移性前列腺癌的试验，人们也将注意力转向了新的靶向药物与放疗的联合。

根治性前列腺切除术

虽然根治性前列腺切除术可以用于局部进展性肿瘤，但报道的病例与放疗试验相比，通常是侵犯范围较小且能够切除的低级别肿瘤。前列腺切除术后 5～10 年 50%～60%的患者 PSA 无明显增长，60%～80%的患者需要接受辅助性放疗或补救性放疗或内分泌治疗[219～222]。和联合放疗不同，术前短期使用内分泌治疗的新辅助治疗并不能降低 PSA 进展的风险[161,223]。

到目前为止，手术并没有展现出比放疗联合内分泌治疗更大的优势。一项比较 T2b～T3 期患者使用已烯雌酚联合放疗或联合前列腺切除术的随机试验在生化复发、临床进展以及肿瘤特异性生存率等方面显示了类似的结果[224]。其使用的放射剂量仅在 60～70Gy 范围内，治疗相关并发症也是特异性的，如事先预期的一致。

虽然几个Ⅱ期研究均显示不同的化疗药物和内分泌治疗可联合作为手术的新辅助治疗，并且毒性在可接受的范围，但是否能减缓肿瘤进展仍有待观察[225～227]。最近开展的 CALGB（cancer and leukemia group B）90203 试验将患者随机分为两组，一组患者接受 6 个周期紫杉醇、泼尼松和内分泌治疗后进行根治性前列腺切除术，另一组只进行根治性前列腺切除术。

在 M.D 安德森癌症中心开展的一系列研究将手术用于局部肿瘤的概念扩展至进展性肿瘤综合治疗的一部分。虽然患者并没有达到前列腺切除的标准，但这些患者都具有盆腔和尿道梗阻症状的风险。在大型研究中仍没有关于该治疗方法有效性的评估。这种方法的好处是可以提供提出或验证假说的前列腺癌病理。术前平台增加了 sonic hedgehog 信号作为治疗靶点的证据，可以在体内进行调整[228]。这些发现可以进一步推动对抑制 sonic hedgehog 信号途径药物的研究。另外，我们认为，与前列腺癌进展有关的上皮-间质相互作用通路也是其在骨转移中进展的核心途径。手术治疗局部进展性前列腺癌的指征已经拓展至激素敏感性肿瘤，主要为寡转移灶的患者[229]。综合来看，这些临床观察提供了可行性的证据。

几项基于人群的研究分析了转移性肿瘤行局部治疗的效果，并表明接受原发灶放疗或手术治疗的患者生存率有所提高[230,231]。这种影响可能与减少肿瘤进展的局部症状及随后的局部并发症直接相关，但让人更感兴趣的是，局部治疗可能会破坏肿瘤的转移进程，从而改变肿瘤的生物学行为。一项研究证实了转移性肿瘤行前列腺癌根治术是可行的，并表明手术并发症的概率是可以接受的[232]。同时，两个临床试验正在评估局部治疗对去势敏感的 M1 期患者的作用。在欧洲进行的 STAMPEDE 试验评估 M1 期患者原发肿瘤放疗的价值[233]。同时，安德森癌症中心的一项试验正在评估去势敏感性疾病最佳系统治疗与局部治疗（手术或放射治疗）的结合（NCT10751438）。虽然转移性疾病的局部治疗的概念是耐人寻味的，但是直到我们有更明确的证据前，还不应该广泛采用这种方法。这些试验将有助于确定，在转移性肿瘤的综合治疗策略中，那些患者可能受益于将局部治疗。

前列腺切除术后放疗

三项随机试验的结果显示，前列腺切除术后的辅助放疗对突破包膜、侵犯精囊、切缘阳性具有相似的优势，其中切缘阳性是放疗最好的预测指标[234～236]。所有这三项研究现在都表明，在 10 年的随访中,PSA 无进展生存期至少有 20% 的获益。EORTC 和 SWOG 试验报告的局部复发率和临床进展也有下降[237]。在最新的更新中,中位随访期为 11.5 年,SWOG 试验证明两组间无转移生存率有统计学意义,这是主要的研究终点[235]。治疗 15 年后,54%辅助治疗组的患者发生了转移或死亡,而单纯手术组患者占 62%。辅助治疗组转移或死亡的危险性降低了 25%,总生存率也有了显著的改善[235]。

随着放疗剂量的提高、定位的改进,对手术的患者术前应用新的影像技术排除转移,辅助治疗的好处会越来越多。

去势抵抗局部进展性前列腺癌

位于前列腺内的巨大肿瘤在去势抗药性疾病患者中尤其成问题。通过对男性进展为去势抵抗性疾病的评估发现,未经治疗的原发性肿瘤患者出现随后局部症状的风险显著增加(根治术后 20%,外照射后 46.7%,前列腺完整 54.3%[238])。通常情况下保留原发灶的患者中,激素治疗并不能使肿瘤缩小达到预期的放疗效果。此外,最近的数据表明雄激素去除可与 DNA 修复酶结合,如果早期激素治疗不敏感可能也对放射治疗不敏感[239]。在转移性疾病患者中,仅仅放疗就可以达到姑息、缓解症状的目的,如血尿或复发性尿路梗阻。对于预期寿命较长的患者,化疗可在放疗前或联合放疗使用。但化疗应答的持续时间和程度没有得到充分的证实。另外,前列腺切除术可能是可行的,并将为这些患者中的许多人提供症状缓解[240]。

最近,前列腺癌的"间变性特征"被确认为临床特征,预示着预后不良,但对化疗反应增强。在这 7 个临床特征中,作者发现,体积巨大的原发性肿瘤是预后较差的重要预测因素,而神经内分泌特征并不预示生存或对全身化疗的反应[241]。虽然在后期对于原发灶行姑息性局部治疗是可能的,但通常意味着要采取更高侵袭性的手术(全膀胱前列腺切除或全盆腔脏器切除)[242]。这在为许多患者提供缓解的同时,这些手术往往伴随大量的并发症和必要的再手术的巨大风险,这使得这些推迟的干预措施不那么有吸引力。在 M. D. Anderson 癌症中心进行的临床试验中(NCT10751438),对于最初采取系统性雄激素去除治疗后早期出现进展者进行了进一步评估,以试图在局部治疗有可能对疾病进展造成潜在影响时,及时识别"间变性癌"。

治疗流程:未来的方向

为了应用最合适的治疗方法,临床医师应该最大限度地应用影像学、病理学、PSA 动力学和其他肿瘤标志评估肿瘤并采取个体化的治疗方案。需要强调的是,这种联合治疗将来不仅可以消除局部肿瘤,也能够预防和治疗远处的微小转移。应用分子靶向药物如酪氨酸激酶抑制剂及抗血管生成药物等与放疗或手术联合的临床试验仍在进行。必须探索这些药物的毒性和剂量以及它们对组织的分子效应。未来,分子标志可以预测肿瘤的生长和播散的形式(如局部区域转移和远处转移),使治疗更加个体化,达到最大疗效。新的分子靶向药物和它们对组织的影响(包括肿瘤和间质)必须具体明确,使治疗的方法与分子特点相适应。个体化、多学科的治疗方法为局限性或转移性肿瘤的治疗提供了更好的治疗策略。

转移性前列腺癌

在全世界癌症相关性死亡中,以成骨转移为特征的前列腺癌占据了相当大的一部分。尽管发病率和死亡率与骨转移灶的大小相关,但其中仍有 10%的变异,包括区域淋巴结的转移,以内脏为主(如肝和肺)的转移和一些并非骨转移的局部症状。神经内分泌肿瘤和小细胞肿瘤通常在长时间的内分泌治疗后出现,个别在治疗初期即为该性质的肿瘤。

在常规筛查的人群中,初诊为前列腺癌时 10%~15%的患者有明确影像学证据证明已有转移,而在未常规筛查的人群中,这一比例大于 70%。在对局限性前列腺癌治疗后,微转移的早期表现往往是血清 PSA 水平升高。而接近 1/3 的患者针对局限性前列腺癌的治疗会失败,据此可以估计每年大约有 70 000 人依据 PSA 水平升高诊断转移,而所有的出现转移的患者在美国可高达 100 万[243]。

前列腺癌生化复发的定义在不同的治疗后不同,手术后是 PSA≥0.2ng/ml[244],放射治疗后是比最低值增加 2ng/ml[245]。不同的定义可以帮助解释和评估不同治疗之后的效果。同时也应该意识到 PSA 升高并不是恶性肿瘤进展或需要治疗的绝对指征,也不能完全预测疾病的进展和疾病特异性死亡率。其原因为:①前列腺没有彻底切除和放射治疗之后一些良性的情况也可以引起 PSA 的升高;②前列腺癌本身进展缓慢;③早期的治疗在改善患者生存率和生活质量方面并没有明确的优势;④前列腺癌的患者通常为高龄老年,常合并其他疾病(诊断 PSA 上升的中位年龄为 70 岁),在 PSA 升高的较低风险患者中,其他死亡原因逐渐占优势。

局限性前列腺癌施行根治性前列腺切除术后转移的中位时间为 8 年,中位生存时间为 13 年[246]。一项随机研究选取了 695 例前列腺癌患者,一部分施行根治性前列腺切除术,另一部分等待观察,12 年后前者的累积转移率为 19%,后者为 26%[247]。

已经播散了但处于明显休眠状态的肿瘤细胞在合适的微环境比如骨髓中会持续存在,这些克隆被认为是处于非增殖期或者是增殖-凋亡平衡期而不易被检测到,直到从休眠状态激活表现为临床可检测的转移[248]。

PSA 倍增时间和 Gleason 评分可以用来评估转移及预后。比如 Gleason 评分高(8~10 分)的患者和 PSA 倍增时间小于两年的患者在 5 年内转移的可能性达 70%[246]。而倍增时间小于 3 个月的患者 5 年内因为前列腺癌死亡的可能性为 50%[182]。与之相比,PSA 倍增时间长(≥15 个月)的患者 10 年内因为前列腺癌死亡的可能性则不到 10%[182]。在那些年轻的预期寿命大于 15 年的患者中,这种 PSA 动力学的预测价值并不确定,持续的监测仍有必要。PSA 倍增时间是一个有用的工具,用于评估有意义的进展和以所谓"风险可接受方式"安排治疗和设计临床试验。

PSA 升高男性患者诊断时的中位年龄和伴随症情况影响治疗干预的时机。需要制订标准化的方法,将预后指标与年龄和医学上的伴随症结合起来,以指导今后的治疗[249,250]。未来需要能够将转移性疾病的异质性表型与特定治疗策略联系起来的生物标志物。

诊断

转移性前列腺癌可以根据症状、体征以及快速或明显升高的 PSA 浓度来考虑诊断。

转移的症状与体征

骨痛是转移性前列腺癌最常见的症状，对于疼痛原因恰当的判断是至关重要的，比如原先已有的"关节炎"的疼痛。如果疼痛性质、部位、严重程度的变化应该引起重视。恶性骨痛通常不间断并逐渐加重。颅底综合征可表现为枕部疼痛或脑神经麻痹；第六和第十二对脑神经经常受侵。神经系统症状可表现为下颌的麻木，这是由单侧或双侧下牙槽神经的侵犯和压迫造成的。如果侵及胸骨骨髓，则会有类似急性白血病的胸骨压痛。神经根侵犯造成的牵涉性痛可以类似一些良性疾病的症状；比如第二腰椎的疼痛可被误认为是腰椎的退行性疾病，下段胸神经的侵犯则有可能类似急腹症。莱尔米特征（Lhermitte sign）可能提示脊髓的侵犯。后背痛可以由腹膜后的病变导致而不一定是有脊髓的转移。在骨扫描中，像骨质疏松、严重的退行性变或者佩吉特病导致的椎骨压缩性骨折也可以出现类似恶性病变的浓聚灶。

咳嗽、气短或者胸部 X 线所示的间质水肿可能提示淋巴结的转移；卡氏肺孢子虫感染在前列腺癌的患者，甚至那些长期使用激素的患者中也不常见。肺转移较为罕见；肺部结节和胸水可能是由其他肺部疾病所致。高瘤负荷的肺转移虽然不常见，但若出现则提示可能已有脑部的转移。高瘤负荷肝转移、溶骨性的转移和脑转移可能提示神经内分泌或小细胞癌。

癌肿的局部进展症状可能是进展期前列腺癌比较明显的表现，而直肠指诊常常被忽略。晚期的刺激性或梗阻性尿路症状、里急后重、大便性状的改变或者会阴区的疼痛提示局部控制的失败以及周围组织的侵及。淋巴管的堵塞可以导致淋巴水肿，膀胱底部的受侵可以导致膀胱出口或输尿管梗阻、血尿、反复的泌尿系感染。阴茎和阴囊转移比较少见。

影像学诊断

影像学诊断对于转移性前列腺癌的分期有重要意义，包括骨扫描、腹部和盆腔 CT。胸片可以帮助鉴别一些不常见的肺部的临床表现，胸部 CT 有时则对肺部小结节性质的判断起到一定作用，除外一些淋巴结的病变。诊断有时会用到 CT 引导下的穿刺活检判断结节的性质；但取样错误和假阴性仍然存在，在这种情况下，随访是一种相对合适的解决办法。MRI 对于明确骨转移病灶的性质很有用处，同时可对脊髓压迫及脑部转移灶进行扫描，亦可评价骨盆转移灶的进展。PET-CT 在敏感性及特异性方面还有待提高，目前尚不能在临床中常规推荐应用。

病理研究

确诊转移病灶的病理诊断应该包括免疫组化检测 PSA 和 PAP 的表达，因为在雄激素去除治疗中 PSA 的表达有可能丢失。在未来，融合基因的分子诊断将有可能进一步明确诊断目前尚不能确定的情况。而那些 PSA 显著升高（如>100ng/ml）和有典型转移症状的患者几乎不需要活检就可以确诊。

目前的治疗手段

内分泌治疗

自从发现前列腺癌与激素的关系[251]，内分泌治疗在进展期前列腺癌的治疗中起重要作用。目前的内分泌治疗主要有手术或药物去势直接降低循环中雄激素的浓度，通过药物阻断雄激素与其受体结合[252]（图 98-8）。手术或药物去势联合雄激素受体阻断剂，被称为联合雄激素阻断。与单纯去势相比，某些分层患者是否可以通过联合雄激素阻断取得额外获益仍然需要确认[253]。联合雄激素阻断加 5α 还原酶抑制剂，以抑制睾酮转化为双氢睾酮，被称为三联雄激素阻断，支持这样应用的数据同样有限。更加高效和高选择性的雄激素受体拮抗剂（如 MDV3100）或雄激素合成抑制剂（如醋酸阿比特龙），是目前在Ⅰ～Ⅲ期临床试验中研究的新型激素疗法。

在 PSA 升高的人群中，没有证据表明在转移出现之前早期应用内分泌治疗可以改善患者的生存率和生活质量。对高危局限病灶的患者联合内分泌治疗和放疗生存率的改善可能与入组患者良好的局部控制有关[163,254]，而并非减少了微转移[255]。相反，在另外一个有关根治性前列腺切除术后淋巴结活检阳性的患者中即刻应用内分泌治疗的小型研究中，延迟内分泌治疗所得到的疗效比预期的要差[256]。正如既往医学研究会的一项比较转移性疾病即刻与延迟激素治疗试验的结果，均支持延迟激素治疗会导致不良预后[257]。目前严重缺乏高质量的研究，来评测激素治疗在高危患者术后辅助治疗中的原则或 PSA 升高状态对总生存率及生活质量终点的影响。

内分泌治疗的并发症包括潮热、体重增加、性欲减低、体力下降、失眠、情绪与智力障碍、骨质疏松、肌肉萎缩、代谢性疾病和心血管疾病进展[258]。这些并发症一部分归因于内分泌治疗，比如神经认知症状，但同时又跟年龄和疾病本身的进展有关[259]。对于低危疾病，单用非甾体类抗雄激素药物（如高剂量比卡鲁胺）可能与药物去势治疗有相同的生存结局[260]，但对骨量、肌肉力量和性欲的影响较小[261]。促黄体素释放激素间歇性去势治疗降低了费用和并发症，但对疾病本身的利弊尚不清楚，需要成熟的Ⅲ期临床试验来验证[262]。

PSA 升高或者出现转移的患者经去势治疗后，PSA 下降的最低值可以用来预测预后[263,264]。转移患者经过内分泌治疗 7 个月后如 PSA 最低值>4ng/ml，他们的中位生存时间为 13 个月，而 PSA 最低值<0.2ng/ml 的患者则为 75 个月[264]。这些数据表明，以这种方式可以识别致死表型，以便制订早期干预策略。

到目前为止，对新诊断的转移性疾病患者。随机研究还没有确定早期化疗联合内分泌治疗比延迟化疗联合内分泌治疗有生存或生活质量上的优势[265]。因此在这种情况下行内分泌联合化疗还只是试验性的。

非内分泌治疗

没有令人信服的证据支持化疗在治疗激素依赖性前列腺癌的价值。一些非内分泌治疗的药物，包括疫苗、免疫调节剂、血管生成因子、信号转导抑制剂以及其他种种不同的因子都在研究之中，以期应用于 PSA 升高和无症状的转移患者。这些研究在试验设计上面临特殊挑战，包括缺乏经过验证的可以较早用于替代生存的研究终点。目前尚没有证据证明非内分泌治疗对于疾病的转归有大的影响。

去势抵抗型疾病

前列腺癌激素控制的时间从无转移灶的 6 年[265]至有转移

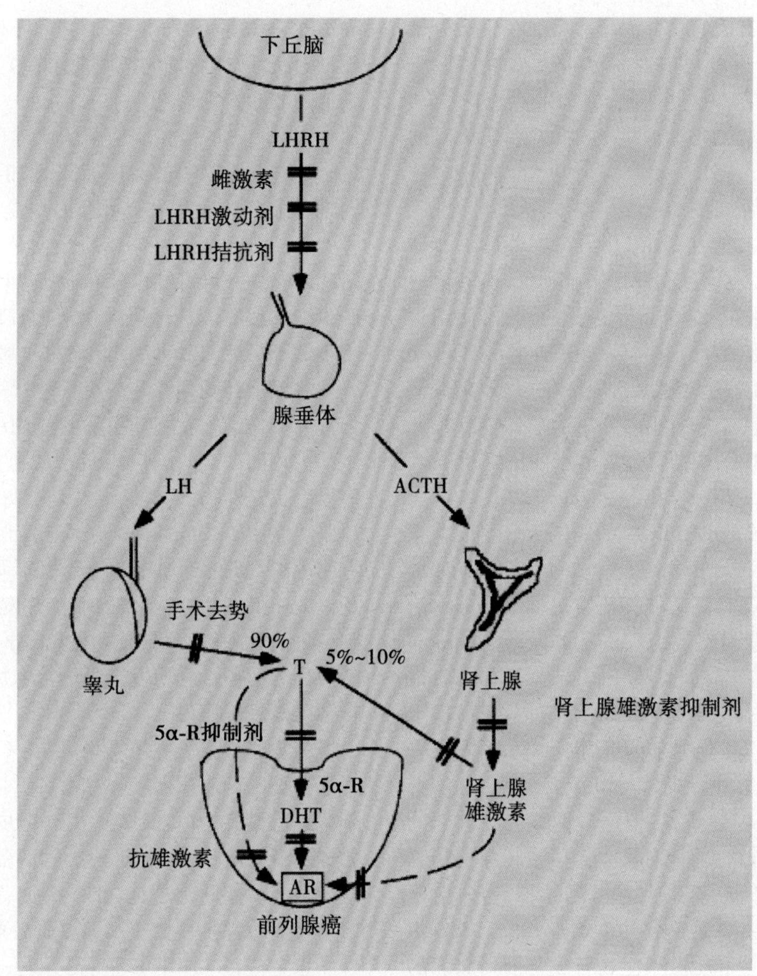

图 98-8　前列腺癌相关的激素轴和治疗靶点。LHRH,促黄体素释放激素;LH,促黄体素;ACTH,促肾上腺皮质激素;AR,雄激素受体;DHT,双氢睾酮;5α-R,5α-还原酶

灶的 18 个月不等[266]。当肿瘤在低睾酮水平下(<50ng/dl)[267]依然进展,我们可以将这种"激素难治型"或"雄激素非依赖型"前列腺癌称为"去势抵抗型前列腺癌"(CRPC)[268]。这些肿瘤可能对更换激素治疗药物有反应,因此它们并不是严格意义上的激素难治。即使去势后低水平的血清睾酮,也可以对"超敏感"的雄激素受体产生持续的信号,所以它们也并非真正意义上的雄激素非依赖。

预后

几乎没有研究报道单纯 PSA 水平升高的 CRPC 的预后,在对一个随机安慰剂对照的试验中,试验对象为 201 名睾酮为去势水平、PSA 升高、没有明确骨转移证据的患者,结果证明了骨转移需要经过很长时间才会逐渐出现,尤其是低 PSA 水平和倍增时间长的患者[269]。总的来说,这组患者 2 年内发生骨转移的可能性为 33%,骨转移中位时间 30 个月。而 PSA 倍增时间<6 个月的患者中,超过 50%在 18 个月内出现骨转移,而倍增时间>18 个月的患者中,只有 40%在 3 年内出现骨转移。

尽管无症状的非转移性 CRPC 中位生存时间为 4 年,但转移性 CRPC 的男性患者的预后是不同的,有症状[270,271]和无症状[272]的患者,中位生存时间则分别为 9~23 个月。一些预测模型根据容易确定的临床和生化参数预测 12~24 个月的生存率[273~275]。一种结合 PSA 倍增时间、去势治疗后 PSA 进展时间和转化为 CRPC 是否存在转移灶的模型确定了三种临床进展或无事件生存时间(EFS)[275]:低危组 PSA 倍增时间>10 个月(中位无事件生存时间 96 个月);中危组 PSA 倍增时间<10 个月,PSA 进展时间>13 个月(中位无事件生存时间 33 个月);高危组 PSA 倍增时间≤10 个月,在雄激素依赖性前列腺癌转化为 CRPC 后出现转移症状,PSA 进展时间≤13 个月(中位无事件生存时间 6 个月)。

鉴于 CRPC 自然病程上的这些明显变异,显然需要可靠的预后模型,用于常规临床实践以及试验研究中准确的分层与报告。临床试验中对生存结果差异的分析必须考虑到这些变异的潜在影响,这可能不完全能够通过随机化和预后分层策略来解释。

CRPC 的管理

CRPC 管理的一个关键原则是平衡治疗效益的局限性和疾病危害性的差异。目前的治疗可以通过改善症状、降低特定并发症发病率和改善生活质量以及总存活时间来控制疾病。雄激素剥夺治疗后患者的负担(雄激素剥夺综合征),以及患者的并发症,会影响治疗的选择。目前通行的治疗方法是基于对患者预后和耐受性的预测,顺序应用治疗方法。

未来的发展方向将是利用生物学的进步,应用预测标志物，选择不同的患者采取更有效的联合治疗。目前在分子分型方面已经取得了进展，用于区分可能对雄激素敏感的[42,43,276]或具有较高侵袭性的患者[241]。这些研究，是 CRPC 治疗[277]从目前普遍应用的预测模型转向基于生物学的预测模型的基础[278]。

二线治疗

二线内分泌治疗的反应，是由 CRPC 中雄激素受体的过表达或雄激素受体的旁路途径驱动肿瘤进展来解释的，但其内分泌机制未完全明确。总的来说，对于未经选择的人群，使用第一代抗雄药物行二线内分泌治疗，其中位无进展生存时间<6个月[279,280]。初次内分泌治疗有效期短、非最佳的 PSA 最低值和快速的 PSA 倍增时间的患者对二线内分泌治疗不会有很好的反应。在临床实践中，CRPC 二线内分泌治疗的选择受初次内分泌治疗、并发症和药物的相互作用等影响。

在抗雄激素治疗后进展的 CRPC 患者中有很小但很有意义的一部分，通过单独停用抗雄药物，PSA 水平可降低 50%伴疾病客观缓解；这个现象在泛甾体与非甾体类抗雄激素药物治疗中都被描述过。抗雄激素撤退反应（anti-antrogen withdrawal reaction，AAWR）的频率和持续时间不尽相同，但一项单中心最大规模的非甾体类抗雄药物（比卡鲁胺、氟他胺或尼鲁胺）撤退反应的前瞻性研究（n=132）表明，11%的患者 PSA 水平降低一半，2%有客观反应，中位 PSA 进展时间为 6 个月[281]。总体上讲，这些患者可取得中等程度的获益，但这一优势已经被新的证据所取代，包括更有效的改良的针对雄激素信号转导的药物（恩扎鲁胺）或雄激素生物合成抑制剂（醋酸阿比特龙）。对于 AAWR 仍然有兴趣的原因主要在于它的生物学意义。AAWR 现象表明，在雄激素受体改变和雄激素生物合成与前列腺癌的临床进展相关性之间新的机制[282]。在骨转移的患者中，有10%可以发现雄激素受体的突变，但他们与 AAWR 的出现并不相关[283]。在包括黄体酮和糖皮质激素在内的甾体类抗雄激素药物使用中亦存在撤退反应。这些数据说明 AAWR 尚未被完全了解，它的机制可能比最初预想的要复杂。最近，雄激素受体剪接变异体的出现，特别是 ARV 7 的出现，被认为与新的雄激素抑制剂，包括被称为不可逆性雄激素合成抑制剂的醋酸阿比特龙和第二代抗雄激素药物恩扎鲁胺的原发耐药密切相关。然而，目前尚不清楚剪接变异体的存在与去势抵抗间是否存在有机联系[42,43,284]。

新型雄激素抑制剂在 mCRPC 中的应用

阿比特龙是一种类固醇合成酶 CYP17 的抑制剂，通过选择性地抑制 17-α 羟化酶和 C17，20 裂解酶[285]，有效抑制肾上腺雄激素的合成。在两项化疗后和未经化疗的转移性 CRPC 的Ⅲ期临床试验中取得阳性结果后，醋酸阿比特龙目前被推荐用于转移性 CRPC 的治疗[286,287]。17a 羟化酶的抑制，可造成上游激素黄体酮和促肾上腺皮质激素的蓄积，引起高血压和低钾症，这一效应可以通过补充糖皮质激素泼尼松来抑制。

恩扎鲁胺是第二代抗雄激素药物，其与雄激素受体的结合亲和力约为抗雄药物比卡鲁胺的五倍。恩扎鲁胺可阻止雄激素受体向细胞核移位，此外，还可以阻止 AR 与 DNA 的结合，以及 AR 与共激活蛋白的结合。目前，基于在化疗后和未经化疗的转移性前列腺癌的两项Ⅲ期临床试验中取得阳性结果，恩扎鲁胺被推荐使用。疲乏是最常见的不良反应。在未经化疗的 mCRPC 的试验（PREVAIL）中[288]，高血压的发病率增加。此外，恩扎鲁胺与罕见的癫痫发作有关。

其他的雄激素抑制剂

大剂量的唑类抗真菌药酮康唑（400mg，每天三次）可以通过影响肾上腺来源的雄激素来增加去势的作用。肾上腺来源的雄激素自身是 AR 的弱配体，也是睾酮的来源。酮康唑所致肾上腺功能不全需要糖皮质激素替代。不良反应和并发症包括疲乏、恶心、肝毒性以及和通过 P450 酶系统代谢的其他药物产生交叉反应。这种药物在很大程度上已经被更有效和毒性更小的不可逆 CYP 17 抑制剂醋酸阿比特龙所取代。

雌激素在前列腺癌的治疗中有一定价值，部分由于其在去势方面的作用。在晚期疾病的控制中，雌激素显示了与 LHRH 激动剂相同的功效。但雌激素的血栓形成风险及心血管并发症风险也是广为人知的，尤其是当每日剂量大于 3mg 时。每日口服雌激素 1~3mg 对 mCRPC 的疗效曾经被报道[289,290]，但没有明确的剂量-效应关系的证据。雌激素的机制并不完全清楚。即使低剂量，雌激素的血栓并发症仍然存在。同时使用小剂量华法林和肠溶阿司匹林或低分子肝素可起预防作用。雌激素相关的男性乳房发育是非常麻烦的，建议在开始治疗前进行预防性乳腺照射。

糖皮质激素作为单一药物在 CRPC 的治疗中效能适中。不同种类的糖皮质激素间并没有直接比较，但小剂量地塞米松据报道有最高的单药活性[291]。糖皮质激素的作用机制很多，如抑制下丘脑-垂体轴，通过类固醇受体直接作用，或调节肿瘤的微环境。库欣综合征、体重增加、高血糖、骨质疏松、失眠和情绪障碍等都是长期应用糖皮质激素面临的问题。

患者应用 LHRH-α 进行持续去势治疗的原理尚未完全研究清楚。尽管回顾性数据表明持续性的去势治疗对患者的生存有潜在性益处，但没有随机的前瞻性的研究证明这一结论。基于此，PSAWG 这一机构规定去势治疗睾酮的水平应维持在小于 50ng/dl。在接受 LHRH-α 治疗的进展性去势抵抗性前列腺癌患者中关于进一步抑制睾酮水平的作用目前不再有任何异议。

在接受 LHRH-α 最佳治疗剂量或者在睾丸切除术后患者的血清睾酮水平大于 50ng/dl，常常与低水平的血清自由睾酮有关。然而，很少有 LHRH-α 抵抗的病例被报道，似乎与其免疫机制有关；这些病例都突出了规律监控血清睾酮浓度的重要性。近期一些研究已经呈现出把睾酮浓度降至更低的方法，并且建立了雄激素浓度与“细胞旁分泌/细胞内分泌”的相关性（睾酮水平小于 50ng/dl）。

尽管在前列腺癌患者中 PSA 降低和睾酮治疗的客观反应经常被提及，更深层次了解关于前列腺癌激素调节的生物学机制是很有必要的。

非激素治疗

对于没有接受过激素治疗的转移性病例，不同的非激素治疗都在临床试验中评估，以期应用于无症状或低危的 CRPC 中来代替二次激素治疗或化疗。在低危病例中，相比标准化疗所带来的明显有限的益处，应用试验性的治疗药物还是合理的。

化疗

尽管长期以来关于化疗在 CRPC 患者中的作用存在疑问，但最近几年几个随机对照临床试验的结果已经证明，化疗可以改善转移性 CRPC 患者的总生存和/或生活质量。

米托蒽醌，12mg/m²，每三周给药一次，联合泼尼松 5mg/d，两次，该治疗（MP）已经被美国 FDA 批准使用，因其对于有症状的 CRPC 患者的疼痛缓解要优于泼尼松单药治疗；然而在这项 160 例患者的随机试验中，并没有发现 MP 治疗可以改善患者生存。在另外一项 770 例患者的研究中，SWOG 对患者每 21 天给予 60mg/m² 的多西他赛，加连续五天每天三次 280mg 的雌氮芥，将之与 MP 治疗对比；结果证明多西他赛联合雌氮芥使无进展生存期增加了 3～6 个月，中位生存时间增加了 2 个月。然而，雌氮芥的临床毒性反应很明显，患者的生活质量并没有提高。

在一项跨国的 1 006 例患者的 TAX327 试验中，每天 10mg 泼尼松加上 6 周中每周 30mg/m² 的多西他赛持续 5 周，或者每天 10mg 泼尼松加上每三周 75mg/m² 的多西他赛，这两种给药方式与每天 10mg 泼尼松加上每三周 12mg 的米托蒽醌相比较。以上两种多西他赛组与 MP 组相比在 PSA 降低率、疼痛反应、整体生活质量方面均有类似的改善（图 98-9）；相反，客观反应在三组间无统计学差异。试验并未描述疾病无进展生存的结果。

研究结果促使美国 FDA 批准每天 10mg 泼尼松加上每三周 75mg/m² 的多西他赛作为 CRPC 的治疗方法。

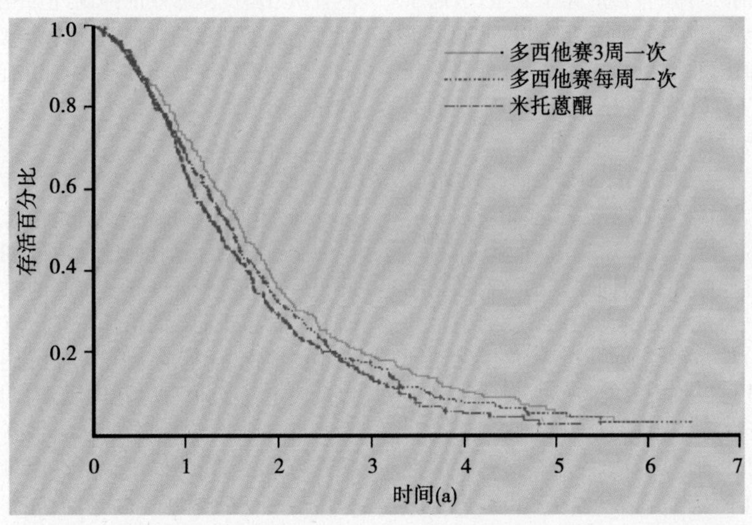

图 98-9 TAX327 试验结果更新。多西他赛化疗对于生存获益略有改善：中位生存时间仍在 2 年以下，哪种生物亚群的获益更大仍需进一步研究。经世界卫生组织许可复制

最近，卡巴他赛，一种新型的微管蛋白结合紫杉醇，对于紫杉醇和多西他赛耐药的临床潜伏期的病例仍具有活性。与 MP 治疗相比，对于含多西他赛治疗的进行中或者治疗后的转移性 CRPC 患者，卡巴他赛仍可以有效。在这项 775 例患者的随机试验中，每三周静脉注射一次 25mg/m² 的卡巴他赛，与 MP 治疗相比，使中位生存时间提高了 2.4 个月。两组间疼痛缓解相似。这些发现为系统性的化学治疗以期影响 CRPC 患者的总生存时间和生活质量提供了必要的动力。

CRPC 患者采取化疗的时机如何选择？最佳的初始化疗时间仍未明确。因为服用简单，费用相对较低，二线内分泌治疗对于无症状或者轻微症状或者低瘤负荷的转移性患者是一个合理的选择。等待观察对于 PSA 动力学惰性的和/或没有转移证据的患者也是合理的。在有症状的 CRPC 患者中，虽然多西他赛或者卡巴他赛化疗在患者生存和生活质量获益方面优于二线内分泌治疗，然而当单一的比较危险的区域发现转移灶时，由于重要且容易出现症状，比如脊柱和承重骨，可以先进行局部放疗来确保这个区域的安全，为接下来的化疗作好准备。而无症状的广泛转移的患者也应该进行基于多西他赛的化疗。

CRPC 最佳的治疗持续时间尚未确定。在观察到疗效最佳之后继续两个周期的治疗是合理和通常进行的，因为基于多西他赛的治疗有累积的效应。还有一种观点认为了保证患者的生活质量，可以给予间歇式的化疗，但是可能会出现停药期越来越短直到出现耐药。此外，维持化疗期间检测患者反应的指标仍待确定，必须做到平衡以对抗严重的毒性反应。

迄今为止包括多西他赛、卡巴他赛以及其他所有化疗药的获益都是有限的。化疗可以改善生存，但与乳腺癌化疗相比改善仍有限。另外的局限是，化疗高昂的花费和较大的毒性，CRPC 依然是不可治愈的，5 年生存率亦不是很高。

三线化疗方案通常在卡巴他赛失败后使用，但仍没有统一的标准。对于这部分患者，应强烈考虑参加临床试验。对于紫杉醇耐药的患者在选择治疗时，应考虑尚未使用过的其他内分泌治疗。

连续的数据都支持把微管作为 CRPC 的重要靶点，单药紫杉醇每周一次的给药被证明很有意义，在包含雌氮芥的联合治疗中同样如此。在多西他赛治疗失败后，MP 治疗通常优先于卡巴他赛，然而观察到的结果令人沮丧，只有大概 20% 的患者出现 50% 的 PSA 下降。关于卡巴他赛后续 MP 治疗作用的结果尚未发表。口服环磷酰胺在一些慢性 CRPC 患者中也可以有效，这种基于烷基化的机制与紫杉醇和蒽环类药物不同。

为了增加多西他赛使用的经验和更好了解疾病的生物学机制，过去十年中有很多随机三期临床试验在进行，以测试各种药物（包括内皮素受体拮抗剂阿曲生坦、多靶点抗血管生成受体酪氨酸激酶抑制剂舒尼替尼、Src 激酶抑制剂达沙替尼、

VEGF 抑制剂贝伐单抗和阿夫洛塞普、内分泌 A 受体拮抗剂齐博坦以及高剂量骨化三醇)。尽管多种上述组合相比单药多西他赛延长了疾病无进展生存,但并没有证据可以改善总生存。

近期一些Ⅱ期临床研究也评估了卡波铂在 CRPC 治疗组合中的作用,用于重点治疗侵袭性变异型的疾病,这些病例临床及表型特点以小细胞神经内分泌为主,基于这样一种假设:以铂类为主的化疗,同样的临床特征应该提示同样的敏感性。有人认为铂类敏感性可能是 CRPC 患者区分不同生物亚群的一个显著性特征,更多前瞻性研究仍需进行以证实这一假设。

骨的靶向治疗

上皮-间质相互作用是前列腺癌转移的典型表型,引起了广泛的兴趣。骨转移途径包括上皮-间质相互作用,可能会提供可以改变自然病程的治疗途径(图 98-10)。因为骨转移有较高的发病率和死亡率,器官特异性的治疗方法引起广泛的兴趣。骨肿瘤进展的病理标志特征是癌症细胞对增生结缔组织的浸润,包括成骨细胞的增生、大量编织骨和分散的破骨细胞。有许多研究模型是针对疾病进展早期的创立的,包括骨骼中转移微环境的成分和主要的生理特点。

骨骼高代谢部位选择性吸收并长时间保留的放射性药物指导了进展期前列腺癌骨转移灶早期的靶向治疗。放射性核素氯化锶-89(半衰期 50 天)作为钙类似物对骨骼的天然亲和力以及磷酸酯耦合的钐-153 可以将中等能量的 β 射线带到肿瘤和骨的交界处。这些药物可作为姑息治疗的选择方案,CRPC 患者在化疗联合放射性核素巩固治疗后存活率有所上升,进一步引发了对器官靶向治疗的研究热情。CRPC 患者中骨转移后骨质吸收增加证明了抑制破骨细胞二磷酸盐研究的合理性。大量Ⅲ期随机试验对 CRPC 患者联合化疗和唑来膦酸治疗的效果,证明了这种重要的二磷酸盐对减少骨疼痛和骨相关事件具有重要的意义。Denosumab 是核因子 κB 受体激动剂(receptor activator of nuclear factor κB,RANK)配体的抗体,应用于唑来膦酸治疗后仍有进展的患者中,能够有效降低骨质吸收。在 CRPC 患者中比较唑来膦酸和 denosumab 效果的Ⅲ期随机试验还在进行中。

血小板来源性生长因子受体(platelet-derivedgrowth factor receptor,PDGFR)与前列腺癌骨转移的进展有一定关系。应用 PDGFR 拮抗剂甲磺酸伊马替尼联合紫杉醇化疗的临床前期研究显示,以破骨为主的前列腺癌骨转移模型中有较好的效果。但在另一项多西他赛联合或不联合伊马替尼的随机研究中,虽然骨质溶解受到有效的抑制,但并没有获得明显的临床效益。准确描述前列腺癌成骨性骨转移模对其他器官分子靶向药物的前期临床研究是非常必要的,并促使临床观察向实验室研究转化。

未来的方向

在 CRPC 中细胞毒药物和骨靶向治疗药物具有较大的局限性。新的组合、剂量或计划不太可能显著改善前列腺癌患者的预后。对疾病进展分子机制的深入了解促使我们重新评估研究前景和开发新的治疗策略。新的方法需要探究恶性上皮细胞的独特生物学特性-包括血管生成、炎症、免疫微环境等,以及决定存活和疾病进展的无机基质的生理化学成分。

目前针对上皮细胞的研究主要以雄激素受体依赖或非依赖性为中心。组织内雄激素存在和雄激素受体信号通路在去势后依然存在提供了在去势抵抗患者中继续应用雄激素靶向治疗的依据。通过抑制或减少配体合成、阻断配体受体反应、增加雄激素受体分解、抑制雄激素受体核转移或干扰雄激素受体与反应元件之间的反应等方式使雄激素受体失活,可能会使

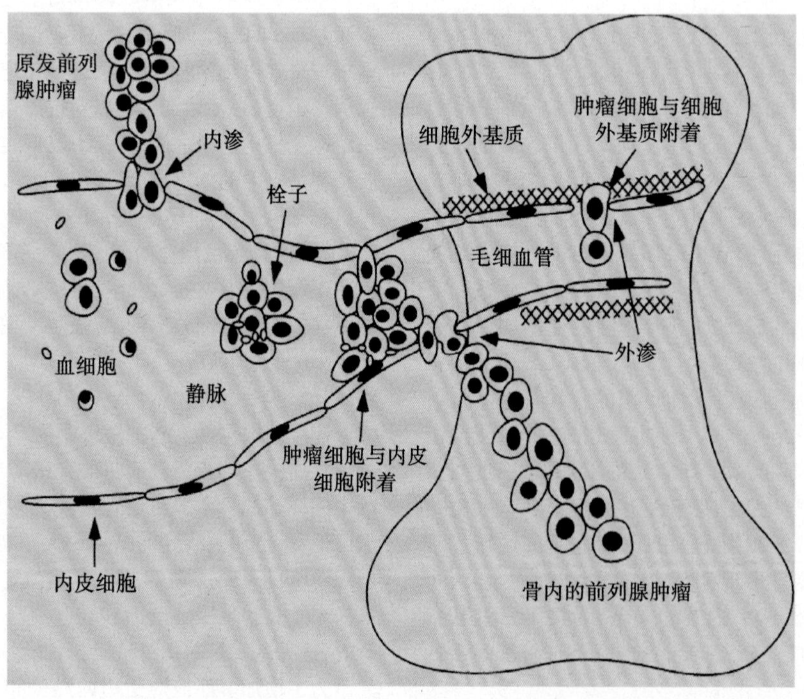

图 98-10　转移的多阶段过程:转移级联早期事件的病理生理学表现、未探测到的静止的微转移疾病、骨微环境的增生性疾病,很可能是由特别的事件所调节的,并伴有不同的治疗并发症

AR 阴性的干细胞避免死亡，这是肿瘤无法根治的原因之一。免疫组化方法对尸体解剖标本进行分析显示，虽然转移位点 AR 的表达仅占 10%以下，但 40%的转移位点表现出了 AR 表达的异质性。高级别肿瘤中抑癌基因 *PTEN* 的频繁失活和 PI3 激酶/Akt 信号通路激活及下游细胞存活增殖途径是定义致死分子表型框架的主题。针对 AR 和 PI3 激酶/Akt 信号通路的靶向治疗药物已经进入试验阶段[265]。2005 年报道了在原发前列腺癌标本中高频率的新基因融合。在目前研究的大部分标本中发现 TMPRSS2 基因 5′端的非翻译区和 ETS-1 家族成员 3′端融合。只在恶性上皮细胞中发现了这些新的融合基因，包括了任何 Gleason 评分的恶性上皮细胞。这些融合并不是随机的，而是该类肿瘤所独有的。TMPRSS25′端区域包含一个雄激素敏感性的启动子元件，这也提示该基因融合可能是肿瘤进展的中心环节。即使这一点得到证明，下游不依赖于融合基因的基因组仍可能导致晚期肿瘤，并且这些融合基因的转录因子难以确定，在治疗中的研究可能存在非常大的阻力。

对肿瘤血管共有和独特生物学性质的了解引发了 CRPC 中针对血管靶向治疗的研究。在 CRPC 治疗中联合应用血管内皮生长因子(vascular endothelialgrowth factor，VEGF)抗体贝伐单抗和多烯紫杉醇已进入Ⅲ期临床试验。对骨骼特异肿瘤血管内皮 PDGFR 激活的前期临床观察引起了在 CRPC 骨转移患者中应用 PDGFR 抑制剂联合化疗的研究。沙利度胺有抗肿瘤的活性，多烯紫杉醇联合沙利度胺的Ⅱ期随机试验可以改善治疗反应性和患者存活率。虽然到目前为止 VEGF、PDGF 和上皮生长因子等独立受体信号通路还没有表现出显著的抗肿瘤活性，但利用 VEGF 和 PDGF 受体的共同抑制剂舒尼替尼则表现了一定的抗肿瘤活性。据估计目前仅发现不到 10%的肿瘤血管生成决定因素。新的探索平台，如以噬菌体为载体和组织特异性内皮血管位点结合的肽链序列的体内注射、复原和鉴定等，可能会促使新的抗血管治疗药物的出现。

CRPC 免疫治疗的策略非常广泛，包括先天性和获得性免疫，可以使用疫苗和免疫辅助等手段。

通过药物阻断那些对生理免疫反应起负向调节和促进肿瘤血管生成的成分可能会改变患者对其他治疗的反应性。虽然Ⅱ期临床试验并没有观察到疫苗有任何抗肿瘤的活性，Ⅲ期临床试验的结果仍然备受期待。目前对于肿瘤间质的特殊作用了解仍较少。实验证据显示作用于破骨细胞的二磷酸盐如唑来膦酸或 PDGFR 抑制剂并没有改变进展性肿瘤的自然进程，但针对高危局限性肿瘤的大型随机辅助治疗试验仍在进行中，试验结果可能会改变既往的观点。使 RANK 配体失活的 denosumab 或使 Src 失活的达沙替尼可进一步增强针对破骨细胞的靶向性。因为破骨细胞在骨骼肿瘤进展的过程中起到重要作用，成纤维细胞生长因子抑制在以成骨细胞为主的骨转移模型中有明显的效果，相关临床试验已经在计划中。

无机基质的作用和肿瘤-基质相互作用决定恶性肿瘤细胞存活和肿瘤进展可能通过整合素、选择素、钙黏素等起作用，具体机制仍不完全清楚。这些作为治疗靶点也处于研究当中。

观点总结

我们对 CRPC 的生物学特性和转移行为了解较少，相关领域的进一步研究有赖于基础知识的深入研究和临床前期模型的进展。对于药物作用的研究和新药物的进展需要患者参与到临床试验中治疗目标的异质性导致不同组间获益和风险的差异，仍是实验设计时最大的挑战。获得有效的生物标志非常困难，不同的疾病可以有同样的表现。循环肿瘤细胞与转移灶肿瘤细胞的表型可能会有很大不同，消灭或控制微转移肿瘤的方法可能与控制临床转移的方法有所不同。

姑息治疗

CRPC 试验中对症状控制并没有太多关注。选择性的应用外放射治疗骨骼疼痛、脊髓压迫、骨折的预防在 CRPC 试验的治疗中非常重要，在早期，外放射或放射性核素应减少应用，因为骨髓抑制可能使系统的支持治疗前功尽弃。对脊柱和长骨的姑息手术治疗并不像乳腺癌和骨髓瘤那样重要，对于局部进展性的肿瘤进行手术治疗可以减少盆壁的侵犯。姑息治疗在疼痛和其他症状如食欲减退、恶心、便秘、抑郁、体重减轻和失眠、精神错乱等的治疗中有重要意义。美沙酮是一种有效且廉价的阿片类制剂，安全性可靠，在姑息性治疗中有重要意义，通常应用于需要硬膜外泵维持止痛的患者。在适当的时间临终讨论和转入收容机构对患者和家庭都是有好处的。

组织变异型

标志

WHO 前列腺肿瘤组织分型[270]列举了除腺泡腺癌外的超过 30 种的组织类型，这部分只讨论三种最常见的类型(表 98-7)。

管状腺癌

上皮肿瘤中管状腺癌最常见，最初由 Melicow 和 Pachter 描述为前列腺小囊内膜癌。曾经认为是来源于精阜(中肾旁管的残余部分)，但已有充分的证据证明其来源于前列腺，目前主要的争论集中在它们是否是前列腺腺癌中具有独特生物学特点的一个类别，而不仅仅是形态学的变异。前列腺管状腺癌占前列腺癌的 0.13%~6.3%。由单层或假复层高柱状上皮细胞组成的管状结构，这些细胞具有嗜酸性和双嗜性的细胞质，排列成乳头状、筛状、实性或腺状结构。超过 20%的肿瘤结构为单纯管状腺癌，大部分还混有腺泡腺癌的结构。管状腺癌不表达任何特异性的标志，因此很难和腺泡腺癌鉴别。管状腺癌 PSA 和 PAP 强阳性，通常会表达 α-甲基酰基辅酶 A 消旋酶(alpha-methylacyl coenzyme Aracemase，AMACR)，有时也表达癌胚抗原(carcinoembronic antigen，CEA)。大约 30%的管状腺癌有残存的基底细胞，免疫组化证明高分子量细胞角蛋白(high molecularweightcytokeratin，HM-WCK 或者 34βE12)和 p63 染色阳性。

肉瘤样癌

具有梭状细胞的前列腺癌，也被称为癌肉瘤或肉瘤样癌，非常罕见(只有大约 100 例病例报道)，以恶性高级别上皮和间质成分为主。上皮成分包括腺泡腺癌、管状腺癌、小细胞或鳞癌的成分。2/3 的病例间质成分为不典型的恶性梭状细胞增殖，另外 1/3 病例具有典型的间质成分，如骨肉瘤、软骨肉瘤或横纹肌肉瘤等。腺瘤成分角蛋白阳性，肉瘤成分波状蛋白阳性。75%病例的腺瘤成分 PSA 阳性。

表 98-7 WHO 对前列腺肿瘤的组织分型

肿瘤种类	肿瘤类型	肿瘤亚型
上皮	腺体肿瘤	腺癌(腺泡)
		萎缩
		假性增生
		泡沫状
		胶质
		疟原虫环状体
		嗜酸瘤细胞
		淋巴上皮瘤样
		癌伴梭状细胞分化(癌肉瘤)
		前列腺上皮内瘤(PIN)
		前列腺上皮内瘤,Ⅲ级(PINⅢ)
		导管腺癌
		筛状
		乳头状
		实体瘤
	泌尿道上皮肿瘤	泌尿道上皮癌
	鳞状上皮肿瘤	腺鳞状上皮癌
		鳞状上皮癌
	基底细胞肿瘤	基底细胞腺瘤
		基底细胞癌
神经内分泌肿瘤		腺癌内内分泌分化类癌瘤
		小细胞癌
		副神经节瘤
		神经母细胞瘤
前列腺间质肿瘤		不确定恶性潜力的间质肿瘤
		间质肉瘤
间叶肿瘤		平滑肌肉瘤
		横纹肌肉瘤
		软骨肉瘤
		恶性纤维组织细胞瘤
		恶性外周神经鞘肿瘤
		血管瘤
		软骨瘤
		平滑肌瘤
		颗粒细胞瘤
		血管外皮细胞瘤
		单个纤维瘤

神经内分泌肿瘤

前列腺癌的非上皮类型中,神经内分泌肿瘤最常见。WHO 分型中包括灶状神经内分泌良性肿瘤和小细胞神经内分泌癌。灶状神经内分泌良性肿瘤在免疫组化染色时神经分泌物如嗜铬蛋白 A、血清素或突触素在大部分腺泡腺癌中是阳性的,在雄激素去势治疗过程中会有所增加。

小细胞癌

只有 0.5%~2%的临床前列腺癌具有小细胞癌的成分,但 12%~20%的尸检病例中在腺泡腺癌的背景下会有小细胞癌的成分。42%~75%的病例首诊为腺泡腺癌,33%~74%的病例中会混有高等级腺泡腺癌的成分。

前列腺小细胞癌以小圆形的梭形恶性细胞为主,该类细胞胞质较少,细胞核脓染,染色质(黑白相间)较粗,核成型,核仁不明显。这些细胞成薄片状分布,通常坏死相和核分裂象较多见。大部分小细胞癌的组化染色细胞角蛋白 AE1/AE3 和 CAM5.2(点状细胞质)和一些神经内分泌标志如突触素、嗜铬蛋白 A 和 CD56 呈阳性。TTF-1 和 P504S 也经常阳性,CEA 有时阳性,PSA、PAP 或者 AR 很少阳性。

临床表现

管状腺癌

管状腺癌通常以血尿和尿路梗阻为主要表现,膀胱镜检查通常会发现前列腺尿道浸润或在精阜发现绒毛状的突起朝向尿道。诊断时已经体积较大和局部进展,55%~93%突破前列腺包膜,前列腺切除术后 20%~47%的病例切缘阳性。在进展性肿瘤的患者中,PSA 水平往往较高,但也有一些 PSA 的水平与肿瘤负荷不平行:在一个 23 名转移性前列腺癌的研究中,3 名患者(13%)PSA 小于 4ng/ml。部分前列腺管状腺癌向骨和淋巴结转移,和腺泡腺癌类似,也有不典型部位转移,如阴茎、睾丸和一些内脏器官。

肉瘤样癌

前列腺肉瘤样癌以向周围侵犯的局部大包块为主要特点,造成盆腔或会阴区的疼痛、下腹部包块和低 PSA 水平的下尿道梗阻症状。超过一半的病例曾被诊断为腺泡腺癌并经过去雄或放射治疗,两者的诊断间隔在 2 个月到 16 年不等。癌性成分和肉瘤成分都可以转移,通常在诊断时就已经有转移,最常见的非淋巴转移包括肺转移、骨转移和脑转移。

小细胞癌

大部分原发性小细胞癌在首次就诊时已经到了进展期,包块较大造成下尿路症状、膀胱出口梗阻、盆腔疼痛、输尿管梗阻和/或血尿。就诊时 75%的小细胞癌患者已经出现转移。之前可能被误诊为腺泡腺癌,诊断为腺泡腺癌和小细胞癌的时间间隔通常为 1.5 个月到 10 年不等。转移最常出现在淋巴结、肝脏、肺脏和骨骼,骨转移多为成骨反应,与腺泡腺癌骨转移的典型表现类似。转移到附睾、皮下组织、心包或网膜也有报道。在疾病进展过程中,20%以上的患者出现脑转移,因此头部的 MRI 和增强 CT 通常被用于临床分期。血清 PSA 和 PAP 水平通常在正常范围内,但血清 CEA 和乳酸脱氢酶分别在 53%~

65%和 39%~76%的患者中超过正常范围。循环中铃蟾肽、降钙素、肾上腺皮质激素和生长抑素的水平可上升。和肺小细胞癌类似,许多类癌综合征可能与前列腺小细胞癌相伴,包括高钙血症、肾上腺皮质激素升高、抗利尿激素不适当分泌综合征、肌无力综合征和高升糖素血症。

治疗方法和应用

管状腺癌

管状腺癌的自然进程仍存在很大争议,有些认为病程进展缓慢、生存期较长,有些则认为其具有侵袭性、5 年生存率较低。一些作者认为纯管状腺癌成惰性,而混合管状腺癌的预后通常受腺泡腺癌成分的影响,常为高级别。和腺泡腺癌类似,大部分管状腺癌对放疗和激素剥夺疗法敏感,除了腺泡腺癌的标准治疗方案外,还缺乏化疗的相关研究。

肉瘤样癌

不论肉瘤成分是哪种组织类型,前列腺肉瘤样癌的预后较差,对 21 名患者中位随访期 10 个月(1~107 个月)的研究显示,18 名患者在随访期内死于肿瘤,在最近的另一项 32 名患者的研究中,在第一年死亡率约 20%。去雄治疗通常用于针对恶性上皮成分,用于治疗肉瘤的化疗药物包括多烯紫杉醇、雌莫司汀、卡铂或顺铂,在 Hansel 等的研究中,9 名患者使用了化疗药物,包括多烯紫杉醇、雌莫司汀、卡铂或顺铂,3 名患者在诊断后的 1 年内死亡,5 名患者对化疗不敏感。因为该肿瘤局部侵犯所造成的死亡率较高,姑息手术(往往涉及尿流改道)联合或不联合辅助性放疗都是必要的。值得注意的是,Dundore 等报道的唯一长期存活者接受了全盆腔脏器取出术和肺转移灶的切除术。在他们的研究中,另外 2 名患者分别存活了 89 个月和 107 个月,在死亡前都接受了肿瘤内放射性碘 125 的治疗。

小细胞癌

虽然化疗药物对前列腺小细胞癌有一定的作用,但预后仍然较差,报道的中位生存时间从 5 个月到 17.5 个月不等。最近一个针对 83 名患者的回顾性分析显示,无转移的患者在初诊时表现较好(疾病相关存活期 17.1 个月 vs 12.5 个月),只有 20%的患者接受了除系统治疗外的局部治疗。该类肿瘤对放疗敏感,部分患者可以行根治性手术切除,此类患者的局部治疗仍然值得研究。Amato 等对 21 名患者进行的一项研究显示,8 名患者中有 4 名对长春新碱、阿柔比星和环磷酰胺的联合化疗有反应。在使用阿柔比星、依托泊苷和顺铂的Ⅱ期临床试验中,38 名已经通过病理检查证明为前列腺小细胞癌患者(单纯或混合有腺癌)接受了治疗,有效率为 61%,84%具有症状的患者疼痛减轻,但没有完全缓解,疾病进展和总生存中位时间很短,分别为 5.8 个月和 10.5 个月。多西他赛和标准剂量的依托泊苷-顺铂联合并没有提高疗效,反而增加了化疗的毒性作用。同样值得注意的是,13 名行激素治疗的患者对抗雄激素撤退治疗均无反应。虽然小细胞癌对去雄治疗反应较差,但大部分患者病理还表现有腺泡腺癌,因此仍然推荐使用内分泌治疗联合化疗。

治疗流程:未来的方向

最主要的问题是不同的组织类型是否具有真正的不同生物学特性并对腺泡腺癌的标准治疗方案反应不一,从而需要采用不同的治疗策略。小细胞癌看起来具有不同的生物学特性,问题在于:是什么原因导致的,又是什么因素推动疾病的进展?回答这些问题有助于发展特异的治疗策略。

局部治疗方法对三种组织类型的前列腺肿瘤的作用仍有待于研究。对小细胞癌而言,是否需要对系统性疾病已经得到控制的患者进行预防性的脑放射治疗仍然需要进一步证实。

(王栋 关有彦 韩苏军 陈羲 译 邢念增 校)

参考文献

The complete reference list can be found on the Wiley Companion Digital Edition of this title (see inside front cover for login instructions).

2 McNeal JE. Normal histology of the prostate. *Am J Surg Pathol*. 1988;**12**:619–633.

8 Logothetis CJ, Navone NM, Lin SH. Understanding the biology of bone metastases: key to the effective treatment of prostate cancer. *Clin Cancer Res*. 2008;**14(6)**:1599–1602.

10 Walsh PC. Anatomic radical prostatectomy: evolution of the surgical technique. *J Urol*. 1998;**160(6 pt 2)**:2418–2424.

15 De Marzo AM, Marchi VL, Epstein JI, Nelson WG. Proliferative inflammatory atrophy of the prostate: implications for prostatic carcinogenesis. *Am J Pathol*. 1999;**155**:1985–1992.

19 Bostwick DG. The pathology of early prostate cancer. *CA Cancer J Clin*. 1989;**39**:376–393.

20 Papandreou CN, Daliani DD, Thall PF, et al. Results of a phase II study with doxorubicin, etoposide, and cisplatin in patients with fully characterized small-cell carcinoma of the prostate. *J Clin Oncol*. 2002;**20(14)**:3072–3080.

25 Gleason DF. Classification of prostatic carcinomas. *Cancer Chemother Rep*. 1966;**50**:125–128.

33 Chan JM, Stampfer MJ, Giovannucci E, et al. Plasma insulin-like growth factor-I and prostate cancer risk: a prospective study. *Science*. 1998;**279**:563–566.

35 Ware JL. Growth factors and their receptors as determinants in the proliferation and metastasis of human prostate cancer. *Cancer Metastasis Rev*. 1993;**12(3–4)**:287–301.

39 Taplin ME, Bubley GJ, Shuster TD, et al. Mutation of the androgen-receptor gene in metastatic androgen-independent prostate cancer. *N Engl J Med*. 1995;**332**:1393–1398.

72 Lilja H, Cronin AM, Scardino PT, Dahlin A, Bajartel A, Berglund G. A single PSA predicts prostate cancer up to 30 years subsequently, even in men below age 40. *J Urol*. 2008;**179**(**206**:abstract 589. Presented 18 May 2008 at the American Urological Association's Annual Meeting in Orlando, Florida).

74 Schroder FH, Denis LJ, Roobol M, et al. The story of the European Randomized Study of Screening for Prostate Cancer. *BJU Int*. 2003;**92(Suppl 2)**:1–13.

75 Thompson I, Tangen C, Paradelo J, et al. Adjuvant radiotherapy for pathologically advanced prostate cancer: a randomized clinical trial. *JAMA*. 2006;**296(19)**:2329–2335.

80 Thompson IM, Ankerst DP, Chi C, et al. Operating characteristics of prostate-specific antigen in men with an initial PSA level of 3.0 ng/ml or lower. *JAMA*. 2005;**294(1)**:66–70.

85 Etzioni RD, Ankerst DP, Weiss NS, Inoue LY, Thompson IM. Is prostate-specific antigen velocity useful in early detection of prostate cancer? A critical appraisal of the evidence. *J Natl Cancer Inst*. 2007;**99(20)**:1510–1515.

91 D'Amico AV, Whittington R, Malkowicz SB, et al. Biochemical outcome after radical prostatectomy, external beam radiation therapy, or interstitial radiation therapy for clinically localized prostate cancer. *JAMA*. 1998;**280(11)**:969–974.

96 American Urological Association. *Guideline for the Management of Clinically Localized Prostate Cancer: 2007 Update*. Linthicum, MD: American Urological Association Education and Research, Inc.; 2007.

101 Partin AW, Kattan MW, Subong EN, et al. Combination of prostate-specific antigen, clinical stage, and Gleason score to predict pathological stage of localized prostate cancer. A multi-institutional update. *JAMA*. 1997;**277(18)**:1445–1451.

104 Epstein JI. Gleason score 2–4 adenocarcinoma of the prostate on needle biopsy: a diagnosis that should not be made. *Am J Surg Pathol*. 2000;**24(4)**:477–478.

105 Ochiai A, Troncoso P, Chen ME, Lloreta J, Babaian RJ. The relationship between tumor volume and the number of positive cores in men undergoing multisite extended biopsy: implication for expectant management. *J Urol*. 2005;**174(6)**:2164–2168.

119 Parker C. Active surveillance: an individualized approach to early prostate cancer. *BJU Int*. 2003;**92**:2–3.

120 Johansson JE, Holmberg L, Johansson S, Bergstrom R, Adami HO. Fifteen-year

survival in prostate cancer: a prospective, population-based study in Sweden. *JAMA*. 1997;**277**:467–471.

121 Albertsen PC, Hanley JA, Gleason DF, Barry MJ. Competing risk analysis of men aged 55 to 74 years at diagnosis managed conservatively for clinically localized prostate cancer. *JAMA*. 1998;**280**:975–980.

130 Klotz L. Active surveillance with selective delayed intervention: using natural history to guide treatment in good risk prostate cancer. *J Urol*. 2004;**172**:S48–S51.

140 Wood DP, Schulte R, Dunn RL, et al. Short-term health outcome differences between robotic and conventional radical prostatectomy. *Urology*. 2007;**70(5)**:945–949.

149 Marcovich R, Wojno KJ, Wei JT, Rubin MA, Montie JE, Sanda MG. Bladder neck-sparing modification of radical prostatectomy adversely affects surgical margins in pathologic T3a prostate cancer. *Urology*. 2000;**55(6)**:904–908.

157 Roach M III, Hanks G, Thames H Jr, et al. Defining biochemical failure following radiotherapy with or without hormonal therapy in men with clinically localized prostate cancer: recommendations of the RTOG-ASTRO Phoenix Consensus Conference. *Int J Radiat Oncol Biol Phys*. 2006;**65**:965–974.

158 Pollack A, Zagars GK, Starkschall G, et al. Prostate cancer radiation dose response: results of the M. D. Anderson phase III randomized trial. *Int J Radiat Oncol Biol Phys*. 2002;**53**:1097.

161 Gleave ME, Goldenberg SL, Chin JL, et al. Randomized comparative study of 3-versus 8-month neoadjuvant hormonal therapy before radical prostatectomy: biochemical and pathological effects. *J Urol*. 2001;**166**:500–506.

163 Bolla M, Collette L, Blank L, et al. Longterm results with immediate androgen suppression and external irradiation in patients with locally advanced prostate cancer (an EORTC study): a phase III randomised trial. *Lancet*. 2002;**360**:103–108.

164 Thompson I, Thrasher JB, Aus G, et al. Guidelines for the management of clinically localized prostate cancer: 2007 update. *J Urol*. 2007;**177(6)**:2106–2131.

180 D'Amico AV, Chen MH, Roehl KA, Catalona WJ. Preoperative PSA velocity and the risk of death from prostate cancer after radical prostatectomy. *N Engl J Med*. 2004;**351(2)**:125–135.

187 Thompson IM, Chi C, Ankerst DP, et al. Effect of finasteride on the sensitivity of PSA for detecting prostate cancer. *J Natl Cancer Inst*. 2006;**98(16)**:1128–1133.

188 Lucia MS, Darke A, Goodman PJ, et al. Pathologic characteristics of cancers detected in the Prostate Cancer Prevention Trial: implications for prostate cancer detection and chemoprevention. *Cancer Prev Res*. 2008;**1(3)**:167–173.

201 U.S. National Institutes of Health. *Finasteride in Treating Patients Undergoing Surgery for Stage II Prostate Cancer*. J Kim, principal investigator. Bethesda, MD: U.S. National Institutes of Health; 2008, http://clinicaltrials.gov/ct2/show/NCT00438464.

208 Roach M III, Bae K, Speight J, et al. Short-term neoadjuvant androgen deprivation therapy and external-beam radiotherapy for locally advanced prostate cancer: long-term results of RTOG 8610. *J Clin Oncol*. 2008;**26**:585–591.

216 Kuban D, Tucker S, Dong L, et al. Long-term results of the M. D. Anderson randomized dose-escalation trial for prostate cancer. *Int J Radiat Oncol Biol Phys*. 2008;**70**:67–74.

223 Aus G, Abrahamson P, Ahlgren G, et al. Three-month neoadjuvant hormonal therapy before radical prostatectomy: a 7-year follow-up of a randomized controlled trial. *BJU Int*. 2002;**90**:561–566.

225 Pettaway C, Pisters L, Troncoso P, et al. Neoadjuvant chemotherapy and hormonal therapy followed by radical prostatectomy: feasibility and preliminary results. *J Clin Oncol*. 2000;**18**:1050–1057.

246 Pound CR, Partin AW, Eisenberger MA, et al. Natural history of progression after PSA elevation following radical prostatectomy. *JAMA*. 1999;**281**:1591–1597.

254 Pilepich MV, Winter K, Lawton CA, et al. Androgen suppression adjuvant to definitive radiotherapy in prostate carcinoma—long-term results of Phase III RTOG 85-31. *Int J Radiat Oncol Biol Phys*. 2005;**61**:1285–1290.

257 The Medical Research Council Prostate Cancer Working Party Investigators Group. Immediate versus deferred treatment for advanced prostatic cancer—initial results of the Medical Council Research Trial. *Br J Urol*. 1997;**79**:235–246.

265 Millikan RE, Wen S, Pagliaro LC, et al. Phase III trial of androgen ablation with or without 3 cycles of systemic chemotherapy for advanced prostate cancer. *J Clin Oncol*. 2008;**26(36)**:5936–5942.

271 Tannock IF, Osoba D, Stockler MR, et al. Chemotherapy with mitoxantrone plus prednisone or prednisone alone for symptomatic hormone-resistant prostate cancer: a Canadian randomized trial with palliative endpoints. *J Clin Oncol*. 1996;**14(6)**:1756–1764.

274 Halabi S, Small EJ, Kantoff PW, et al. Prognostic model for predicting survival in men with hormone-refractory metastatic prostate cancer. *J Clin Oncol*. 2003;**21**:1232–1237.

第 99 章　阴茎和尿道肿瘤

James F. Holland, MD, ScD(hc) ■ Raymond S. Lance, MD ■ Donald F. Lynch, Jr., MD

概述

阴茎癌大多数为鳞癌，部分发病与人类乳头瘤病毒有关。阴茎癌在发达国家的经包皮环切后的男性中发生率很低，但在世界其他地区却十分常见。通过手术可以治疗阴茎癌，此外目前没有其他有效的治疗手段。从预防措施来说，目前认为通过免费向成年男性提供包皮环切术，可以降低感染人类免疫性病毒的可能性。尿道癌一般是移行上皮细胞癌，尽管发病相当罕见，但经常因诊断较晚而无法治愈。

阴茎鳞状细胞癌是一种基本上可以预防的疾病，取决于幼年时是否进行包皮环切、个人卫生状况、医疗水平和人类乳头瘤病毒(HPV)的预防。由于该病在发达国家并不常见，可见发达国家对 HPV 的预防十分有效。阴茎癌的早期发现和诊断，与更早的分期、更大的保留器官的可能性以及更低的死亡率相关。

在美国和欧洲，阴茎癌不太常见，其中美国每年的发病低于 2 000 人。但对于南美洲、非洲和亚洲的部分地区却并非如此。大约有 95%的原发性阴茎癌是鳞状细胞癌(squamous cell carcinoma, SCC)(图 99-1)。其他阴茎肿瘤主要包括阴茎疣状癌，表现为巨大湿疣或 Buschke-Lowenstein 瘤，是鳞癌的变异，不发生转移，但是局部浸润严重并破坏周围组织[1](图 99-2)。此外还有和艾滋病相关的传染性卡波西肉瘤，但现在较为少见(图 99-3)，阴茎黑色素瘤和基底细胞癌则更为罕见。上皮内的鳞状细胞原位癌侵犯阴茎和阴囊的基底时称为鲍恩病(Bowen disease)，临床表现为清晰的红色斑块。当其侵犯阴茎或包皮的腺体时称为红斑增生病，会显示出发亮的天鹅绒样红斑(图 99-4)。20%的原位癌有发展成浸润性鳞癌的可能，需要活检

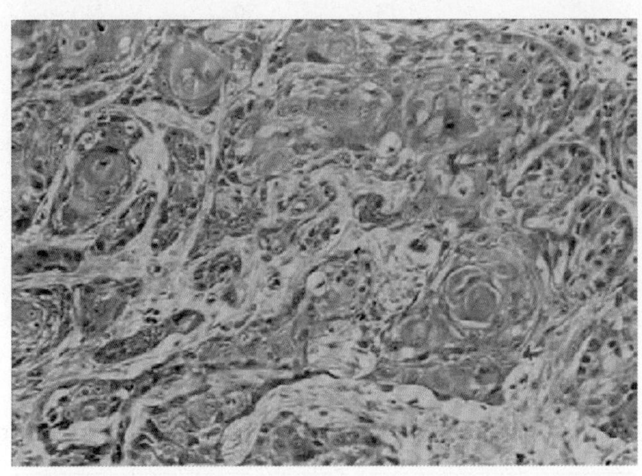

图 99-1　光镜：鳞状细胞癌，中等分化，具有特征性的角化珠形成

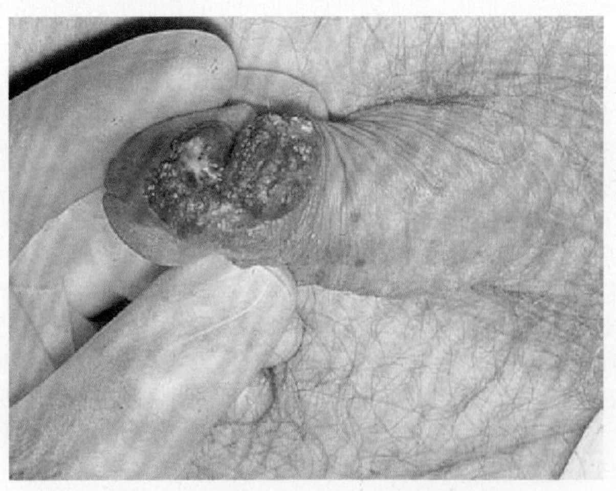

图 99-2　疣状癌(Buschke-Lowenstein 瘤)

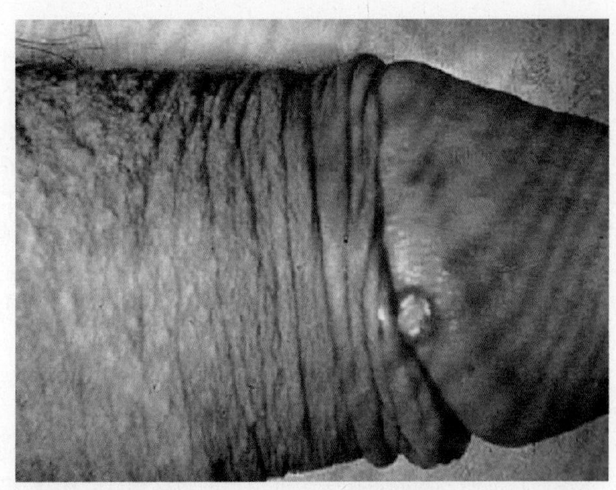

图 99-3　传染性卡波西肉瘤病变(AIDS 相关)累及阴茎头

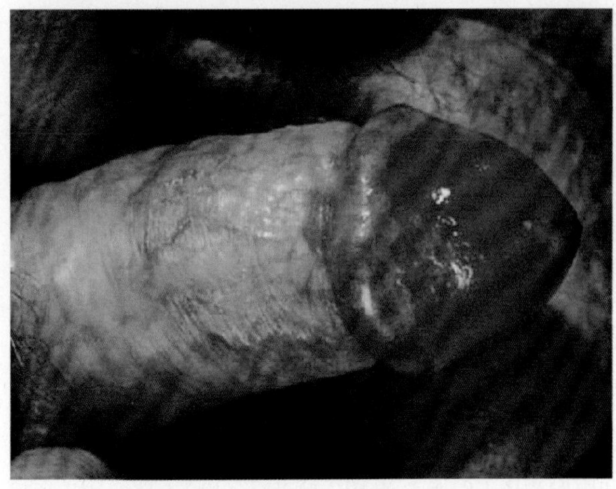

图 99-4　阴茎头部大面积病变，典型表现

确诊。此外,白血病和淋巴瘤会出现阴茎的异常勃起,需要进行系统性的诊断和治疗。

流行病学和病因学

在婴儿包皮环切盛行的国家,例如以色列和美国,阴茎鳞癌的发病率很低。婴儿期以后再做包皮环切似乎不能预防阴茎鳞癌,可能因为是在包茎和龟头已经产生炎症后才进行的包皮环切[2]。若没有进行包皮环切,包皮过长、腺体和包皮组织的长期慢性炎症刺激会使包皮的清洁变得困难。为了预防艾滋病感染,近期在非洲推行了廉价的成人包皮环切,可能会使之前的结论发生改变。

研究发现,一些宫颈癌的妇女其配偶患有阴茎癌,阴茎和宫颈鳞癌也与人类乳头状病毒(HPV[16、18、31])有关[3]。未行包皮环切的青春期男孩中,9%包皮中含有 HPV,这证实该病毒是普遍存在的[4]。未行包皮环切的男性感染 HPV 的风险是环切过的男性的 3 倍,而配偶未进行过包皮环切的女性更易患宫颈癌[5,6]。感染 HPV 的男性可能会罹患尖锐湿疣,或者为完全无症状的携带者,或者尿道内有病变,排出病毒并感染性伙伴。吸烟也与 HPV 感染、阴茎癌、宫颈癌的发生率升高相关。

诊断

早期浸润性肿瘤较小、不易察觉,有时表现为阴茎皮肤小的磨损和茧样增厚。阴茎鳞癌最早会发生在阴茎头和包皮上。它变化多端,从小的、光滑的、红色突起的斑丘疹到溃疡、角化过度的区域或外生生长的乳头状瘤。活检可以确诊,但需包括邻近的正常皮肤作为对照[1]。疾病进一步进展会外生性生长或出现溃疡,肿瘤发展到极致会完全毁损阴茎。疾病晚期肿瘤转移到腹股沟淋巴结会造成腹股沟的巨大溃疡。分化较好的肿瘤不易转移,分化差的肿瘤早期转移的机会很高。数项研究证实了肿瘤级别越高,腹股沟淋巴结转移的可能性越大[7]。

转移

浸润性的阴茎鳞癌遵循一个可预测的转移模式。阴茎头、冠状沟、包皮和阴茎远端的病变向深部的腹股沟淋巴结转移,而阴茎近端和基底部的病变则向更侧方、更浅表的腹股沟淋巴结转移。随后转移至髂内、髂外、闭孔淋巴结[8]。远处转移很罕见,一般都发生在疾病的晚期。如果放任阴茎癌进展而不治疗的话,大多数人将在 3 年内死亡。

原发性的腹股沟淋巴结病变可能是由于感染或慢性炎症引起的,继发性的炎性反应也经常出现,这些都很难与转移性的疾病进行鉴别。因此,在运用广谱抗生素治疗 4~6 周之后,应再次对腹股沟淋巴结进行仔细的检查,有利于鉴别炎症和癌症。

肿瘤的分期

一旦确诊了鳞癌,就需要进行完整的分期。要仔细触诊腹股沟淋巴结。其他用于分期的检查还应该包括胸部 X 线片,盆腔和腹股沟区 CT,或者是 MRI 检查[9]。PET-CT 和 MRI 在检出可疑结节性增大的病变方面,优于触诊。而淋巴造影技术已不再作为分期工具。MRI 不仅能良好地分辨阴茎结构,还可以确定阴茎海绵体或尿道海绵体是否受侵犯。

美国癌症联合会(AJCC)的第 7 版 TNM 系统,目前已被广泛接受为阴茎癌的分期系统(表 99-1)。

表 99-1 AJCC(2010)阴茎癌分期

原发肿瘤(T)			
Tx	原发肿瘤不能评估		
T0	未发现原发肿瘤		
Tis	原位癌		
Ta	非浸润性疣状癌[a]		
T1a	肿瘤侵犯皮下结缔组织,无淋巴血管侵犯,非低分化(即 3~4 级)		
T1b	肿瘤侵犯皮下结缔组织,有淋巴血管侵犯或低分化		
T2	肿瘤侵犯海绵体		
T3	肿瘤侵犯尿道		
T4	肿瘤侵犯相邻组织		
区域淋巴结(N)			
临床阶段定义[a]			
cNx	区域淋巴结无法评估		
cN0	未触及或未观察到腹股沟淋巴结肿大		
cN1	可触及单侧活动的腹股沟淋巴结		
cN2	可触及多个或双侧活动的腹股沟淋巴结		
cN3	可触及不活动的腹股沟淋巴结肿块,或单侧或双侧盆腔淋巴结转移		
解剖阶段/预后组			
0 期	Tis	N0	M0
	Ta	N0	M0
Ⅰ期	T1a	N0	M0
Ⅱ期	T1b	N0	M0
	T2	N0	M0
	T3	N0	M0
Ⅲa 期	T1~3	N1	M0
Ⅲb 期	T1~3	N2	M0
Ⅳ期	T4	任何 N	M0
	任何 T	N3	M0
	任何 T	任何 N	M1
ICD-O-3 形态学编码			
C60. 0	包皮		
C60. 1	阴茎头		
C60. 2	阴茎体		
C60. 8	阴茎多重病变		
C60. 9	阴茎,未特指		

[a] 临床阶段的定义基于触诊和影像。

摘自 Egde et al[10]。Reproduced with permission of Springer。

外科治疗

阴茎癌的治疗要基于对病变的活检病理来明确肿瘤进展的程度及分级。在活检前要开始抗生素治疗直至术后4~6周，还需评估淋巴结转移的情况。通过组织学确诊，一些小的浅表性肿瘤能通过局部手术切除、局部化疗、激光手术[11]、Mohs显微外科治疗[12]或者浅表性放疗治愈。

更大的侵袭性肿瘤有时能通过保留器官手术或放疗得到控制，但对于浸润较深，特别是已经造成阴茎头畸形或侵及阴茎体的肿瘤，不适合运用保守的手术治疗方式。对于侵及阴茎体远端或阴茎头的病变，通常是采用阴茎部分切除术，距肿瘤边缘2cm就能达到目的，这样给患者留下足够长度的阴茎，使其既能站立排尿，又保留了性功能[13,14]。对于已经进展至阴茎根部的病变或肿瘤，阴茎全切、会阴尿道造口术是最佳的治疗方法[14]。对于更广泛的或是侵及阴茎根部和尿道球部的病变，可能需要行膀胱前列腺切除术，甚至有时要行前盆腔或全盆腔脏器切除，这些都要同时行尿流改道。

在阴茎鳞癌的患者中，腹股沟或盆腔淋巴结是否有转移一直是最重要的预后因素之一。阴茎体和阴茎根部的淋巴回流至腹股沟浅表淋巴结。阴茎头、包皮和阴茎体远端的淋巴回流至腹股沟深部淋巴结。这些淋巴转移途径在阴茎根部存在交叉，因此，一侧的阴茎病变可能转移至对侧的腹股沟淋巴结。腹股沟深部淋巴结再引流至髂外和闭孔淋巴结，随后引流至主动脉、下腔静脉周围的髂总淋巴结和腹膜后淋巴结[15]。

数项临床研究表明，40%~60%的腹股沟淋巴结转移患者能从彻底的淋巴结清扫术中获益。然而，传统的淋巴结清扫术会导致一系列发生率很高的并发症，如皮瓣坏死、伤口感染、慢性淋巴管炎、淋巴囊肿和慢性下肢水肿。绝大多数外科医师已经采用经过改良、范围略有缩小的淋巴结清扫术，这能减少上述并发症的发生[16]。即便如此，也不应随意进行腹股沟淋巴结清扫术，必须进行临床和影像学的评估。50%~82%的患者在初诊时能触及腹股沟淋巴结。这些患者中仅有半数能通过淋巴结清扫发现癌细胞[17]。抗生素治疗4~6周后仍能触及腹股沟淋巴结为淋巴结清扫术的指征。此时应行PET-CT和MRI检查，前哨淋巴结活检也有一定作用。但是，大约有25%未触及淋巴结的患者已经存在转移，需要接受淋巴结清扫[18]。对于未触及淋巴结且影像上未观察到的患者，触诊和影像学的持续密切随诊非常重要。已经有腹股沟淋巴结转移的患者，若不进行适当的淋巴结清扫，会在3年内因阴茎癌而死亡。

肿瘤分级

肿瘤分级在评估淋巴结转移风险方面具有与分期同等的重要性。肿瘤局限于阴茎皮肤和浅表组织的G1患者，不大可能出现腹股沟淋巴结转移。而肿瘤分级为G2或G3的患者，无论肿瘤浸润阴茎的程度如何，出现腹股沟淋巴结转移的风险都会明显增加[19,20]。最近的研究建议对高级别和活检证实超出浅表浸润的肿瘤患者进行早期手术治疗。

盆腔淋巴结清扫术

已经发现有腹股沟淋巴结转移的患者需要接受患侧的盆腔淋巴结清扫术[21]。手术能通过经正中切口、改良的Gibson或腹股沟切口在腹膜外实施。在我们中心，盆腔淋巴结清扫与腹股沟淋巴结清扫同时进行，而在另一些中心，前者往往在后者的几周之后再次进行盆腔淋巴结清扫手术。盆腔淋巴结转移小于3个，并且都在髂内和髂外血管分叉以下的患者，预后会比较好。而出现血管分叉以上转移几乎都是致命的。

放疗

阴茎癌的放疗在欧洲比美国运用的更为广泛，适用于小的浅表性病变，或以保留器官为目标的患者，以及部分大体积肿瘤或拒绝手术治疗的患者[22]。但是对更具侵袭性的肿瘤，不宜进行保留器官的治疗。同时进行化疗可能会增强放疗的疗效。放疗可以选择应用补偿膜或蜡块补偿辅助下的常规外照射放疗，也可以在模板辅助定位下应用铱-192金属线进行近距离放射。对瘤体较大或过度角化的肿瘤，需要增大铱-192或铯-137的照射剂量。常规治疗剂量为30~50Gy持续3~5周。如果临床上有指征，可以通过各种近距离放疗技术将放射剂量增加至65~70Gy。放疗常常被用于治疗传染性(AIDS相关的)卡波西肉瘤所致的症状性肿瘤。对于局限性阴茎癌患者，放疗也可以作为主要的治疗方法[23]。适合放疗的此类患者很少，包括：年纪轻，肿瘤较小且局限于阴茎远端的表浅性非侵袭性阴茎癌患者；拒绝首先行手术治疗的患者。此外，放疗还用于无法手术治疗的患者。

外放疗和近距离放疗常见的急性放疗反应包括水肿和组织炎症反应，常伴有皮肤刺激、触痛和排尿困难。这些症状往往在治疗完成后很快消失。放疗带来的远期影响包括毛细血管扩张、色素沉着、感觉减退、瘢痕形成以及照射区组织萎缩等。放疗前已有明显组织破坏的大面积肿瘤病变还可能会发生纤维化改变或者形成窦道。虽然经过了明确可靠的放疗，照射部位仍有可能在10年后出现晚期复发，证实了密切随访的必要性。

由于阴茎癌少见，目前还没有随机对照研究来比较放疗和手术治疗的差异。在一项针对临床诊断为局限性阴茎癌患者的研究中，接受手术的患者中有13%出现局部复发，而只接受放疗的患者中有56%出现局部复发。在放疗失败的患者中，73%接受了挽救性手术治疗[24]。

腹股沟区术后进行辅助放疗存在争议。虽然有一些研究提示患者能从这些治疗中获益，但另有一些研究并未发现其疗效优于单独接受手术治疗的患者。对于手术无法切除的大体积转移性淋巴结，除非作为全身性化疗的联合方案，否则姑息性的放疗很难起效。

化疗

化疗在阴茎癌治疗中，通常是作为外科手术或放疗的辅助，或是放疗的增敏剂。由于阴茎癌相对少见，各种治疗方案的经验都比较有限。研究发现采用长春新碱、博来霉素和甲氨蝶呤(VBM)方案进行联合化疗，成功地为已经发生固定性淋巴结转移的患者争取到了手术切除的机会[25]。顺铂或卡铂与氟尿嘧啶、紫杉醇或多西他赛的联合化疗方案在治疗其他部位的鳞癌中显示出了有效性，如食管、头颈部、肛门。这些癌症大多也与HPV有关。目前认为鳞癌的分子特性比起源器官的相关性更大，因此阴茎鳞癌也可使用这些药剂。通过直接观察发现，新辅助化疗能够降低肿瘤负荷[26]。然而术后辅助化疗仍需要进行随机试验来证实其有效性。目前术后和放疗同步进行辅助化疗，是基于这种方式在其他位置的有效性而推定的。很多数据证实阳性结节被切除后，辅助化疗手段是有效的。但对于阴茎全切的鳞癌患者，如果活检甚至临床和影像学都显示腹股沟没有转移，采取辅助化疗仍然充满争议。

预后

毫无疑问，阴茎鳞癌患者若不接受治疗，其后果将是致命的，绝大多数患者将在3年内死亡。预后与诊断时疾病的发展程度以及是否有腹股沟淋巴结转移直接相关。局限性肿瘤的相对生存率为80%，存在区域淋巴结转移的5年生存率为50%，存在盆腔转移的5年生存率为10%。在一项对盆腔淋巴结阳性患者的回访性研究中，采用辅助化疗的患者生存时间中位数为22个月，而未使用的只有10个月[27]。而在另一项预期性研究中，对N2或N3M0的患者使用顺铂、氟尿嘧啶和一种紫杉类药物后，2年内的无病生存率仅为37%[26]。

尿道癌

男性尿道癌

男性的尿道平均长约18cm，被分为尿道阴茎部、尿道膜部和尿道前列腺部。自远端起，尿道阴茎部由尿道和舟状窝构成，覆盖复层鳞状上皮。尿道自舟状窝近端开始下垂，直至阴茎悬韧带，在韧带与尿生殖膈之间是尿道球部。膜部尿道为复层或假复层柱状上皮，是一段很短（1.5cm）的膜性尿道，由横纹肌组成的尿道外括约肌包含在内。尿道前列腺部穿过前列腺，为移行细胞上皮。

50%~75%的男性尿道癌发生于尿道球部（图99-5）。余下的主要发生于舟状窝。大约90%的肿瘤证实为鳞癌[28]。鳞癌经常合并有尿道狭窄。移行细胞癌或未分化肿瘤大多发生于膀胱颈部或尿道前列腺部。低分化的移行细胞癌可能会表现出鳞癌的特性。罕见的腺癌可能发生于Littre腺或前列腺囊。远处肿瘤转移至阴茎的很少见。

近端病变通常表现为排尿梗阻症状，而远端病变通常表现为尿道出血和可触及的尿道肿物。一般而言，肿瘤越靠近近端，发展就越晚，诊断时分期就越高。

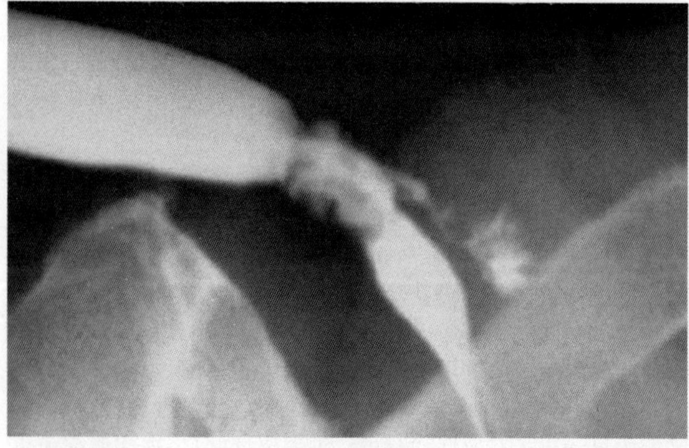

图99-5　逆行尿道造影显示起自尿道球部的鳞癌合并尿道狭窄

膀胱癌进行膀胱切除术后若保留尿道，后续复发的尿道肿瘤一般为移行细胞癌。若在膀胱切除术同时行尿道切除术，包括舟状窝在内的整个尿道都必须一并切除[29]。

男性远端尿道的淋巴回流类似于阴茎癌。舟状窝和尿道悬垂部的淋巴回流至腹股沟浅表淋巴结，而尿道球部、膜部、前列腺部的淋巴回流至髂血管、闭孔和骶前淋巴结。在耻骨前淋巴丛可能存在左右交叉。

分期

AJCC针对尿道癌的分期系统见表99-2。在老版的术语中，曾使用悬韧带的远端和近端肿瘤这样的名称。

表99-2　AJCC（2010）尿道癌分期

原发肿瘤（T）（男性和女性）			
Tx	原发肿瘤不能评估		
T0	未发现原发肿瘤		
Ta	非浸润性的乳头状、息肉状或者疣状癌		
Tis	原位癌		
T1	肿瘤侵犯皮下结缔组织		
T2	肿瘤侵犯尿道海绵体、前列腺和尿道周围肌肉组织		
T3	肿瘤侵犯尿道海绵体、前列腺包膜外、阴道前壁、膀胱颈		
T4	肿瘤侵犯相邻组织		
区域淋巴结（N）			
Nx	区域淋巴结无法评估		
N0	无区域淋巴结转移		
N1	转移至单个淋巴结，最大径不超过2cm		
N2	转移至单个淋巴结，最大径超过2cm，或者侵犯多个淋巴结		
解剖阶段/预后组			
0a期	Ta	N0	M0
0is期	Tis	N0	M0
	Tis pu	N0	M0
	Tis pd	N0	M0
Ⅰ期	T1	N0	M0
Ⅱ期	T2	N0	M0
Ⅲ期	T1	N1	M0
	T2	N1	M0
	T3	N0	M0
	T3	N1	M0
Ⅳ期	T4	N0	M0
	T4	N1	M0
	任何T	N2	M0
	任何T	任何N	M1

摘自Egde et al[10]。Reproduced with permission of Springer。

外科处理

低分级、分期的尿道肿瘤可以行经尿道切除或激光电灼术，但是这样的病变很少见。切除取活检是可行的，在激光电灼术前取活检明确肿瘤组织病理学和浸润深度非常重要。远端尿道病变可以行阴茎部分切除术，但这些病变不能侵及尿道海绵体或阴茎海绵体，并且切除必须距肿瘤边缘 2cm 以上[30]。进展期或更近端的病变需行阴茎全切、会阴尿道造口术。尿道膜部或前列腺肿瘤可能需行前盆腔脏器切除术和放疗。

腹股沟浅表或深部淋巴结转移经常会导致盆腔和全身性转移[31]。在尿道癌的随诊中，密切的进行临床和影像学评估十分重要。基于 MRI、PET/CT 或临床上怀疑淋巴结转移时，应该行淋巴结清扫。盆腔存在阳性淋巴结时也可行盆腔淋巴结清扫术，尽管这种手术在提高生存率方面还没有明确效果。

辅助治疗

由于大多术尿道癌仅行手术治疗的预后较差，所以只要不是浅表性和局限性肿瘤，化疗对尿道癌都是合适的辅助治疗手段，放疗也有使用。尽管未报道过任何对照组下的前瞻性研究，这些辅助治疗手段临床上已经取得了一些效果。对 T3 期或者有临床阳性腹股沟淋巴结转移的患者来说，开展新辅助化疗或同步放化疗后的手术结果比那些没有进行辅助治疗的要好[32]。

女性尿道癌

女性尿道大部分行走于阴道前壁内。成年女性尿道长 2~4cm。尿道远端表面是复层鳞状上皮，而近端表面是复层或假复层柱状上皮。膀胱颈部的黏膜为移行细胞上皮。发生于尿道憩室的尿道癌，往往位于尿道的远端，可能起源于沃尔夫管的遗迹，或来源于异位的泄殖腔上皮。

女性尿道癌的组织病理学取决于组织的起源。鳞癌是最常见的，大约占所有肿瘤的 50%。移行细胞癌和腺癌发生率居其次，两者发生率大致都是 25%。与男性尿道癌不同的是，女性尿道肿瘤的分级似乎对转移或预后没有太大影响。混合性肿瘤、未分化癌、黑素瘤、泄殖腔原癌（cloacogenic carcinoma）和透明细胞腺癌虽然少见，但偶有发生。

尿道癌的进展首先是局部扩散，然后是淋巴转移，最后是血道转移。远端尿道和阴唇的淋巴回流至腹股沟浅表淋巴结和深部淋巴结。近端尿道的淋巴回流至髂血管、闭孔、骶前、主动脉旁淋巴结链。目前，近半数的患者可触及异常肿大的淋巴结，绝大多数情况下，这意味着转移[33]。腺癌远处转移的部位主要有肝脏、肺、脑和骨骼。

分期

AJCC 提出的尿道癌 TNM 分期系统见于表 99-2。肿瘤一般会侵及女性尿道的全长。

外科处理

在女性患者中，绝大多数肿瘤临床表现为出血或尿道远端肿物。远端尿道即前尿道的病变通常出现得较早，在早期能得到诊断。这些肿瘤能通过局部切除、尿道部分切除、放疗、激光电灼得到满意的处理。对于少数高分期的局部肿瘤可能需要全尿道切除，保留膀胱后再进行管状的输出道手术，或采用 Mitrofanoff 法。多数近端病变表现得较晚，比远端病变分期更高。进行性的梗阻症状是近端即“后”尿道病变的典型表现。进展性或广泛性病变以及侵犯膀胱或阴道的病变需行膀胱切除或前盆腔脏器切除，然后进行尿流改道。这些高分期的肿瘤容易局部复发。若通过临床或者影像学发现阳性淋巴结，并确认肿瘤累及近端尿道，则需行盆腔淋巴结清扫术。

（李亚健　译　邢念增　校）

参考文献

1 Barnholtz-Sloan JS, Maldonado JL, Powsang J, Guiliano AR. Incidence trends in primary malignant penile cancer. *Urol Oncol*. 2007;**25**:31-367.

2 Albero G, Castellsagué X, Lin HY, et al. Male circumcision and the incidence and clearance of genital human papillomavirus (HPV) infection in men: the HPV Infection in men (HIM) cohort study. *BMC Infect Dis*. 2014;**14**:75.

3 Martinez I. Relationship of squamous cell carcinoma of the cervix uteri to squamous cell carcinoma of the penis among Puerto Rican women married to men with penile cancer. *Cancer*. 1969;**24**:777.

4 Balci M, Tuncel A, Baran I, et al. High-risk oncogenic human papilloma virus infection of the foreskin and microbiology of smegma in prepubertal boys. *Urology*. 2015;**86**(**2**):368-372.

5 Daling JR, Madeleine MM, Johnson LG, et al. Penile cancer: importance of circumcision, human papillomavirus and smoking in *in situ* and invasive disease. *Int J Cancer*. 2005;**116**:606-615.

6 Castellsague X, Bosch FX, Munoz N, et al. Male circumcision, penile human papillomavirus infection, and cervical cancer in female partners. *N Engl J Med*. 2002;**346**:1105-1112.

7 Ornellas AA, Correia AL, Marota A, Seixas ALC. Surgical treatment of invasive squamous cell carcinoma of the penis: retrospective analysis of 350 cases. *J Urol*. 1994;**151**:1244-1247.

8 Srinivas V, Morse MJ, Herr HW, Sogani PC, Whitmore WF Jr. Penile cancer: relation of extent of nodal metastasis to survival. *J Urol*. 1987;**137**:880.

9 Scardino E, Villa G, Bonoma G, et al. Magnetic resonance imaging combined with artificial erection for local staging of penile caner. *Urology*. 2004;**63**:1158-1162.

10 Edge, S., Byrd, D.R., Compton, C.C., Fritz, A.G., Greene, F.L., Trotti, A. (Eds.). *AJCC Cancer Staging Manual*. Springer New York, 2010.

11 Blastein LM, Finkelstein LH. Laser surgery for treatment of squamous cell carcinoma of the penis. *J Am Osteopath Assoc*. 1990;**90**:338.

12 Mohs FE, Snow SN, Messing EM, Kuglitsch MG. Microscopically controlled surgery in the treatment of carcinoma of the penis. *J Urol*. 1985;**133**:961-966.

13 Bevan-Thomas R, Slayton JW, Petaway CA. Contemporary morbidity from lymphadenectomy for penile squamous cell carcinoma: the MD Anderson experience. *J Urol*. 2002;**167**:1638-1642.

14 Culkin DJ, Beer TM. Advanced penile carcinoma. *J Urol*. 2003;**170**:359-365.

15 Ravi R. Correlation between the extent of nodal involvement and survival following groin dissection for carcinoma of the penis. *Br J Urol*. 1993;**72**:817-819.

16 Ravi R. Morbidity following groin dissection for penile carcinoma. *Br J Urol*. 1993;**72**:941-945.

17 Fraley EE, Zhang G, Manivel C, Niehans GA. The role of ilioinguinal lymphadenectomy and significance of histological differentiation in treatment of carcinoma of the penis. *J Urol*. 1989;**142**:1478.

18 Theodorescu D, Russo P, Zhang ZF. Outcomes of initial surveillance of invasive squamous cell carcinoma of the penis and negative nodes. *J Urol*. 1996;**155**:1626-1631.

19 Horenblas S, Van Tinteren H. Squamous cell carcinoma of the penis IV: prognostic factors of survival, analysis of tumor, odes, and metastasis classification system. *J Urol*. 1994;**147**:153-158.

20 D'Ancona CA, de Lucena RG, Querne FA, et al. Long-term followup of penile carcinoma treated with penectomy and bilateral modified inguinal lymphadenectomy. *J Urol*. 2004;**174**:498-501.

21 Lynch DF. Commentary on: Svinivas SV. Relation of extent of nodal metastasis to survival. *Semin Urol Oncol*. 1997;**15**:136-139.

22 Gerbaulet A, Lambin P. Radiation therapy of cancer of the penis. *Urol Clin North Am*. 1992;**19**:325-332.

23 Jakosbsen JK. A urologist's contemporary guide to penile cancer. *Scand J Urol*. 2015;**14**:1-6.

24 Ozsahin M, Jichlinski P, Weber DC, et al. Treatment of penile carcinoma: to cut or not to cut? *Int J Radiat Oncol Biol Phys*. 2006;**66**:674-679.

25 Tana S. Up-to-date management of carcinoma of the penis. *Eur Urol*.

1997;**32**:5–15.

26 Nicolai N, Sangalli LM, Necchi A, et al. A combination of cisplatin and 5-fluorouracil with a taxane in patients who underwent lymph node dissection for nodal metastases from squamous cell carcinoma of the penis: treatment outcome and survival analyses in neoadjuvant and adjuvant settings. *Clin Genitourin Cancer*. DOI: 10.1016/i, eigc, 2015.07.009, PMID 26341040 [ePub ahead of Print].

27 Sharma P, Djajadiningrat R, Zargar-Shoshtari K, et al. Adjuvant chemotherapy is associated with improved overall survival in pelvic node-positive penile cancer with lymph node dissection: a multi-institutional study. *Urol Oncol*. 2015;**33**:e17–e23.

28 Ray B, Canto AR, Whitmore WF Jr. Experience with primary carcinoma of the male urethra. *J Urol*. 1977;**117**:591–594.

29 Varol C, Thalmann GN, Burkhard FC, Studer UE. Treatment of urethral recurrence following radical cystectomy and ileal bladder substitution. *J Urol*. 2004;**172**:937–942.

30 Zeidman EJ, Desmond P, Thompson IM. Surgical treatment of carcinoma of the male urethra. *Urol Clin North Am*. 1992;**19**:359–372.

31 Gakis G, Morgan TM, Efstathiou JA, et al. Prognostic factors and outcomes in primary urethral cancer: results from the international collaboration on primary urethral carcinoma. *World J Urol*. 2015;**34(1)** 97–103. PMID: 25981402, [Epub ahead of print].

32 Gakis G, Morgan TM, Daneshmand S, et al. Impact of perioperative chemotherapy on survival in patients with advanced primary urethral cancer: results of the international collaboration on primary urethral carcinoma. *Ann Oncol*. 2015;**8**:1754–1759.

33 Dimarco DS, Dimarco CS, Zincke H, Webb MJ, Slezak JM. Surgical treatment for local control of female urethral carcinoma. *Urol Oncol*. 2004;**22**:404–409.

第 100 章　睾丸癌

Christian Kollmannsberger, MD, FRCPC ■ Craig R. Nichols, MD ■ Siamak Daneshmand, MD ■ Eric K. Hansen, MD ■ Christopher L. Corless, MD, PhD ■ Bruce J. Roth, MD ■ Lawrence Einhorn, MD

概述

睾丸癌是一种相对罕见的疾病，约占男性所有癌症的 1%。它是一种高度可治愈的肿瘤，主要发病人群为处于生育高峰的年轻男性。弥漫性非精原性生殖细胞肿瘤的治疗常结合手术和化疗。需要指出，初始治疗的目的绝不是减轻或延长生存期，而是治愈。

流行病学

发病率

睾丸癌的年龄相关发病曲线呈双峰分布[1]。主要发病高峰集中在 15~35 岁，该年龄段发病者主要为生殖细胞来源肿瘤，约占全部睾丸癌的 95%。35 岁以前，主要组织病理学诊断是胚胎癌，之后精原细胞瘤更为常见。2001—2005 年，睾丸癌诊断的中位年龄是 34 岁[2]。

睾丸癌发病率因地各异。北欧和北美地区发病率最高，而在亚洲和非洲地区最低。种族因素同样对睾丸癌发病率有显著影响，黑人和拉美裔的发病率远低于相应年龄段的白种人[3,4]。在美国，白人与黑人的发病率比例约为 4∶1~5∶1。在斯堪的纳维亚地区、英国及美国的年轻白人男性，其睾丸癌的发病率逐年升高[5]。尽管标准化发病率每年升高 2%~5%，但精原细胞瘤与非精原细胞瘤无显著差异。在美国，从 1989 年至 2005 年睾丸癌发病率每年增长约 0.8%。据估计，美国在 2008 年间约有 8 090 例患者被确诊为睾丸癌，约 380 人最终因癌病去世[6]。

危险因素

现已知与睾丸癌发生密切相关的最主要危险因素是隐睾。病例对照研究结果表明，其风险比(risk ratio)为 2.5~14[7]。未降睾丸的位置对睾丸癌发生也是一个重要的协同影响因子，因为隐睾位于腹腔者的睾丸癌发病率为隐睾位于腹股沟管者的四倍。然而，睾丸未降本身似乎并未导致了生殖细胞肿瘤的发生与发展：只有 10% 的睾丸癌与隐睾相关，而 10%~20% 的肿瘤癌患者其睾丸癌在对侧、正常下降的睾丸；即使在青春期前行睾丸固定术，也不能降低未降睾丸的睾丸癌发生风险；而且睾丸癌患者的一级男性亲属表现出隐睾、鞘膜积液和腹股沟疝以及睾丸癌的发病风险增加[8,9]。这些数据表明，某些遗传易感性和/或妊娠期内子宫内环境改变可能导致一系列泌尿生殖系统发育异常，包括睾丸未降和生殖细胞肿瘤。值得注意的是，似乎随着隐睾发生率的增加，并且睾丸癌的发生在时间和数量也相应增加，两者在一定程度上呈平行关系。睾丸生殖细胞肿瘤(testicular germ cell tumors，TGCT)的患者，其兄弟罹患睾丸生殖细胞肿瘤的风险要增高 8~10 倍，而其父亲和及儿子患病的相对风险约为 4 倍。这一家族性相对风险比大多数其他类型的癌症要高得多。一个全基因组连锁研究发现，睾丸癌易感基因位于染色体 Xq27 上，该基因也可能与睾丸下降不全有关[10]。

睾丸生殖细胞肿瘤在人类免疫缺陷病毒(human immunodeficiency virus，HIV)的男性中的发病率增加。在一项多中心研究中报道了此类特点。该研究共包含 35 例 HIV 相关的生殖细胞肿瘤患者。诊断年龄中位数为 34 岁(年龄范围 27~64 岁)。诊断时 CD4 细胞计数中位值为 315/mm^3(范围：90~960/mm^3)。有 26 例患者(74%)为精原细胞瘤，9 例患者(26%)为非精原细胞性生殖细胞瘤(nonseminomatous germ cell tumor，NSGCT)。21 例患者(60%)为Ⅰ期肿瘤，其余 14 例患者为转移性肿瘤。总体而言，6 例患者复发，3 例死于生殖细胞肿瘤，7 例死于艾滋病，2 年总生存率为 81%。精原细胞瘤的 HIV 感染患者，相对于年龄、性别匹配的非 HIV 感染人群，发病率增加，相对危险度为 5.4(95%*CI*：3.35~8.10)；然而，非精原细胞瘤的发病率并不高，并且在给予高剂量抗反转录病毒治疗后，生殖细胞肿瘤的发生率没有显著变化。最终得出结论，研究认为睾丸精原细胞瘤在 HIV 阳性的男性患者中发病率显著高于对照组人群。罹患 HIV 相关的生殖细胞肿瘤患者，其治疗原则与 HIV 阴性人群治疗相似。大多数死亡与 HIV 感染有关[11]。

另一类易患人群是纵隔非精原细胞瘤合并克兰费尔特综合征(Klinefelter syndrome)的患者。在患有纵隔非精原细胞瘤的患者中，约 10%合并克兰费尔特综合征，而原发肿瘤位于睾丸和后腹膜的生殖细胞肿瘤，则不存在这种相关性[12]。

相关研究报道，睾丸癌与痣发育不良综合征(dysplastic nevus syndrome)有关。罹患睾丸癌患者发生多发性非典型痣(mulitple atypical nevi)的风险增高 2 倍，同时黑色素瘤发生风险也有所增加[13]。

一侧患睾丸癌患者其对侧睾丸发生肿瘤风险增高。在一项包含 2 338 例睾丸癌患者的大样本研究中，有 2.7%患者在随访期间对侧睾丸发生肿瘤[14~16]。Royal Marsden 医院的一项研究指出，与前一研究结论相似，对 760 名睾丸癌患者进行了长达 15 年随访，其对侧睾丸肿瘤发生率为 2.75%[17]。

1950—2001 年，共有 3 984 例睾丸生殖细胞肿瘤患者在 Memorial Sloan Kettering 接受治疗，其中共确定 58 例为双侧睾丸生殖细胞肿瘤患者。中位随访时间为 60 个月。在这 58 例中 10 例(17%)为双侧同时发生肿瘤，而另 48 例(83%)双侧先后发生。总之,无论发生先后,精原细胞瘤是同双侧睾丸肿瘤中最常见的组织学类型。并且在同时性和异时性组肿瘤组中,大多数患者表现为低分期。在 58 例患者中,52 例(89%)没有疾病复发证据,6 例(11%)最终因该病死亡。在 16.7%的患者中,继发性肿瘤的治疗似乎受初次肿瘤治疗的影响[18]。

一些临床医生建议对诊断为单侧睾丸癌的患者进行对侧睾丸的常规活检。Fossa 等人在一项大量人群为基础(population-based)的队列研究当中,对 55 岁之前诊断为睾丸癌的男性患者其对侧睾丸发生癌变的风险进行评估和生存分析,该数据来自 SEER 数据库(Surveillance,Epidemiology and End Results)。该项目隶属于美国国家癌症研究所(National Cancer Institute,NCI)。自 1973 年至 2001 年,共有 29 515 例睾丸癌病例进入美国国家癌症研究所的 SEER 项目,该研究包括如下问题:双侧同时发生睾丸癌的流行病学结果,观察数与预期数比率(observed-to-expected ratio,O/E),对侧睾丸发生肿瘤的 15 年累积风险,以及双侧睾丸癌患者的 10 年总生存率。共有 175 例患者双侧同时诊断睾丸癌;287 例患者双侧先后发生睾丸癌(O/E = 12.4,95% *CI*:11.0%~13.9%);15 年累积风险 = 1.9%,95% *CI*:1.7%~2.1%)。在多变量分析中发现,初发肿瘤为非精原细胞瘤的患者,其对侧发生睾丸癌的风险降低,且有统计学意义(危害比(hazard ratio,HR) = 0.60;95% *CI*:0.46%~0.79%;P <0.001)。另外,睾丸癌初发年龄越大,其对侧发生非精原细胞瘤的风险越低(比值比(odds ratio) = 0.90;95% *CI*:0.86%~0.94%)。双侧先后发生睾丸癌的患者,其 10 年总生存率为 93%(95% *CI*:88%~96%),而双侧同时发生睾丸癌的患者为 85%(95% *CI*:78%~90%)。之所以前者的累积风险很低,且总生存率较好,可能与美国目前不推荐常规行对侧睾丸活检有关。

这些观察结果强调,对睾丸生殖细胞肿瘤患者进行持续长期随访,其意义十分重要。

病理

起源与分子遗传学

睾丸生殖细胞肿瘤分为若干大类。如表 100-1 所示。睾丸生殖细胞肿瘤的组织学分类一直以基于形态学特点,但根据最新的分子生物学研究结果,以不同细胞起源为依据,可将其分为五种不同的亚型[19]。相应地,发生于新生儿和幼儿的畸胎瘤(teratomas)和卵黄囊瘤(yolk sac tumors)起源于原始的生殖细胞或主要沿性腺嵴或睾丸/卵巢分布的早期生殖细胞。这些肿瘤保留了来自亲代基因组的大部分基因组印记。畸胎瘤仍保持二倍体,而卵黄囊瘤可表现为染色体 1q、12p13~14 和 20q 增益,1p、4 和 6q 减少[19]。

表 100-1 睾丸原发肿瘤

类型	相对频率	基因型/备注
生殖细胞肿瘤		
婴儿和幼儿	所有睾丸肿瘤约 1%	
卵黄囊肿瘤	青春期前 65%~80%	非整倍体
畸胎瘤	青春期前 20%~35%	两倍体;成熟成分;良性
青少年和成人	所有睾丸肿瘤约 95%	
未分类的导管内生殖细胞癌变(ITGCNU)	青春期后>90%	非整倍体(接近三倍体)
精原细胞瘤	青春期后约 45%	非整倍体(接近三倍体);iso12p
非精原细胞瘤(NSGCT)	青春期后约 55%	非整倍体(接近三倍体)iso12p
胚胎癌	NSGCT 中约 75%	
卵黄囊肿瘤	NSGCT 中约 50%	
畸胎瘤	NSGCT 中约 50%	恶性(即使有成熟成分)
绒毛膜癌	NSGCT 中约 10%	
成年人(年龄多>50 岁)		
精母细胞精原细胞瘤	青春期后<1%	染色体倍数不确定;9 号染色体获得
精母细胞精原细胞瘤伴肉瘤样变	非常罕见	
性索间质肿瘤		
Leydig 细胞瘤	所有睾丸肿瘤约 3%	7%~10%转移(青春期后)
Sertoli 细胞瘤	所有睾丸肿瘤<1%	

续表

类型	相对频率	基因型/备注
颗粒细胞瘤		
成人型	非常罕见	
幼年型	不常见	小于 6 个月的婴儿
混合型/不确定型	罕见	
混合性生殖细胞/性索间质肿瘤		
性腺母细胞瘤	非常罕见	

精母细胞精原细胞瘤是生殖细胞肿瘤的第二个独特亚型，起源于青春期后的精原细胞/精母细胞。因此，这些肿瘤有一个父方的基因组印记特征且染色体倍数不同，有时可伴有染色体的增益[10]。

在五个生殖细胞肿瘤的亚类中，有两类不会在睾丸中发生。卵巢皮样囊肿，被认为起源于卵原细胞/卵母细胞，可能是双倍体或四倍体，并且表现母方基因组印记。葡萄胎（妊娠滋养细胞疾病）是起源于胎盘的肿瘤，其染色体完全来自父方。

第五类生殖细胞肿瘤包括精原细胞瘤（seminoma）和非精原细胞瘤型生殖细胞肿瘤（nonseminomatous germ cell tumor，NSGCT），两者共同占原发性睾丸肿瘤的 95%。这类肿瘤的变异类型也可发生在卵巢（无性细胞瘤）、前纵隔和中线（生殖细胞瘤）。有学者认为，精原细胞瘤和非精原细胞瘤型生殖细胞肿瘤都起源于生殖细胞，这些生殖细胞在其发育过程中部分基因组的表达丧失，导致了婴儿畸胎瘤和卵黄囊瘤的发生。这些生殖母细胞呈多倍体（三倍体或四倍体），很可能是由于可能与减数分裂捕获（meiotic arrest）有关。由于这一事件在胚胎发育期确切时间不同，受影响的细胞可能分布单侧或双侧睾丸，这可以解释为什么有 2%～3% 的患者双侧同时罹患生殖细胞肿瘤。

精原细胞瘤和非精原细胞瘤型生殖细胞肿瘤有一个共同的癌前病变，称为未分类的导管内生殖细胞瘤（intratubular germ cell neoplasia，unclassified，ITGCNU）。在生精小管内原位生长的 ITGCNU 细胞表达与胚胎干细胞相同的分子标记，包括转录因子 *Oct3/4* 和 *NANOG*[20,21]。这些因子对于小鼠胚胎干细胞的发育必不可少，但在小鼠或人类的正常精原细胞中不表达。他们在 ITGCNU 的存在支持了一种理论，即多能性腺细胞是精原细胞瘤和 NSGCT 的起源细胞。此外，*Oct3/4* 在诊断 TGCT 外（表 100-2）中作为一种高度特异的免疫组织化学标志物[20,22]（表 100-2）。

表 100-2　睾丸生殖细胞肿瘤的标志物

形态学分类亚型	血清	免疫组化	FISH
未分类的导管内生殖细胞瘤变		PLAP，KIT，OCT3/4	
精原细胞瘤	HCG（低）	PLAP，KIT，OCT3/4	excess 12p
胚胎癌	HCG（低）	CD30，OCT3/4，PLAP	excess 12p
卵黄囊肿瘤	AFP	AFP，PLAP	excess 12p
绒毛膜癌	HCG（高）	HCG	excess 12p
畸胎癌			excess 12p

从 ITGCNU 进展为浸润性生殖细胞肿瘤，其过程可能涉及数个共同事件[23]。其中之一是从 12 号染色体的短臂上获取过量的遗传物质。在 80% 的病例中，存在 12q 的缺失和 12p 的复制（12p 等臂染色体），而在剩余的 20% 当中，额外的 12p 序列则附加在其他染色体上。有趣的是，胚胎干细胞基因 NANOG 位于 12p 上。在石蜡切片上进行 12p 荧光原位免疫杂交技术（FISH）已经进入临床应用，作为所有类型的生殖细胞肿瘤或非生殖细胞肿瘤的诊断标志物。

与 ITGCNU 恶性进展相关的其他事件包括同源框基因 *NKX3.1* 的表达缺失[24]，肿瘤抑制因子 *PTEN* 表达缺失[25]和细胞周期调节因子 *p21* 表达下调[26]。TP53 的突变罕见，但这一重要抑癌基因的作用可能是通过 *MDM2* 的过度表达的影响而削弱[26]或受到微小 RNA miR-372 和 miR-373 下调 *LATS2*。基因筛查表明 miRNA-372 和 miRNA-373 可能是睾丸生殖细胞肿瘤的原癌基因[27]。

虽然精原细胞瘤和非精原细胞瘤有共同的起源，但两者在临床病理上截然不同，但对此差异目前所知甚少。有趣的事，在 25% 的精原细胞瘤中发现 *KIT*（一种受体酪氨酸激酶）致癌突变，并且在非精原细胞瘤中基本上没有。这些突变可能在精原细胞瘤发生的早期就已经发生了，因为在 ITGCNU 中同样可以见到[28]，在卵巢、纵隔、大脑的无性细胞瘤/生殖细胞瘤也可以观察到这一现象。基于对小鼠的研究，*KIT* 基因的功能对于原始生殖细胞的发育和正常的精子发生是必不可少的；因此，这种激酶的结构性激活可能有参与精原细胞瘤发生。遗憾的是，KIT 激酶抑制剂，伊马替尼，对携带 *KIT* 突变肿瘤的精原细胞瘤患者并无获益，因为目前已知的突变大多存在耐药性。

精原细胞瘤

所有青春期后发生的睾丸生殖细胞肿瘤中约 45%为纯精原细胞瘤（“经典型”精原细胞瘤）。隐睾患者的该病的发病率增加到 60%。从大体标本上看，这些肿瘤通常质地均一，界限分明。可见明显分叶，瘤结节被致密的纤维条索隔开。偶可见坏死和出血的区。镜下，可见圆形细胞均匀分布，核仁大且位于细胞中样。细胞质呈透明状或颗粒状的，糖原、脂质和/或胎盘/生殖细胞碱性磷酸酶（PLAP）染色阳性。间质成分可见大量 T 淋巴细胞浸润，偶尔含有肉芽肿（图 100-1）。这些特征与肉芽肿性睾丸炎类似。

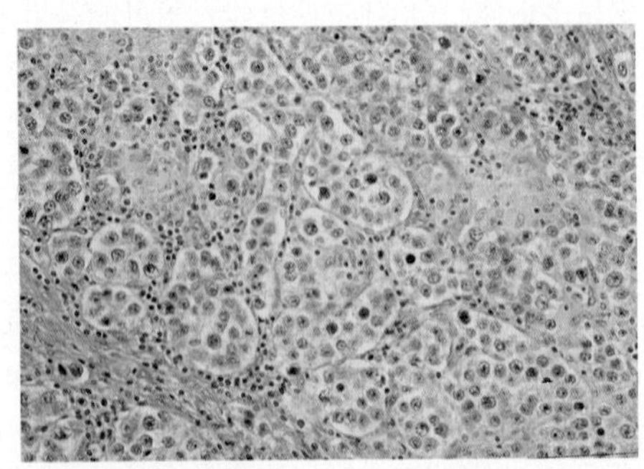

图 100-1　淋巴细胞浸润和肉芽肿性反应将精原细胞瘤细胞分隔成小的癌巢

精原细胞瘤最常见于 40～50 岁，常表现为睾丸无痛性肿大。约 70%的患者为临床Ⅰ期，20%的患者为了临床Ⅱ期，膈肌以上受累患者少见。淋巴转移途径是首先到腹主动脉旁（para-aortic，PA）淋巴结，然后转移到纵隔或锁骨上淋巴结。晚期可血行转移首先到肺、肝、骨或肾上腺。精原细胞瘤含有合体滋养层巨细胞，该细胞人类绒促性素（HCG）染色阳性。5%～10%的纯精原细胞瘤患者可见 HCG 轻度增高，可能反映肿瘤内存在的合体滋养细胞成分（表 100-2）。精原细胞瘤不分泌甲胎蛋白（α-fetoprotein）。

非精原细胞生殖细胞肿瘤

青春期后发生的睾丸生殖细胞肿瘤往往是由一种或多种成分混合组成，统称为“非精原细胞瘤”（non-seminomatous）。在这类肿瘤中，根据形态学可以大体分为四类，详见下文。在绝大多数情况下，这些成分以不同比例混合，并且逐渐地从一种成分过渡到另一种。肿瘤中也可能包含有精原细胞瘤成分（一些作者称为“混合性生殖细胞肿瘤”），但预后的好坏取决于其他成分的存在，而且总体来说，其预后要比纯精原细胞瘤差。

胚胎癌

胚胎癌在睾丸非精原细胞瘤中所占比例高达 90%。大体标本常表现为柔软肉样（fleshy）的不均匀肿块，可见坏死和出血的区域。易侵犯精索，附睾和白膜。镜下表现差异较大，可能包含乳头状，实性，管状和腺样结构，常见灶状坏死区域（图 100-2）。肿瘤细胞以较大的多角形细胞为主，胞质边界模糊（不同于精原细胞瘤），胞质呈灰色颗粒，核大，可见一个或多个位于中心的核仁。核分裂象和多核细胞多见。临床上，胚胎癌侵袭性强，2/3 的患者发生淋巴结转移。

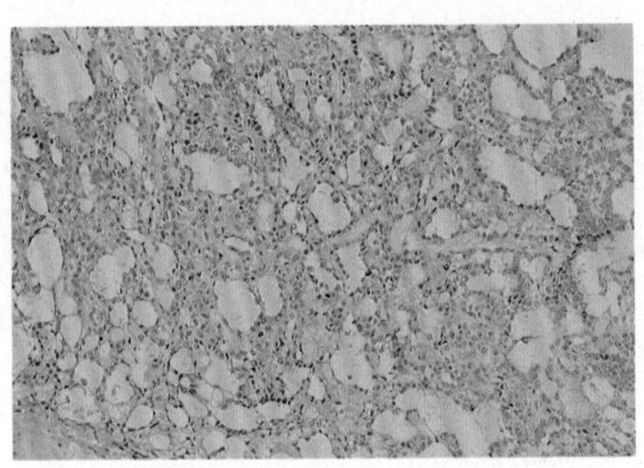

图 100-2　卵黄囊瘤。卵黄囊瘤最典型的病理学表现，伴有大量小囊形成

卵黄囊肿瘤

卵黄囊肿瘤，过去称内胚窦瘤，约半数非精原生殖细胞肿瘤中可见到该成分，但青春期后的患者，纯卵黄囊瘤罕见[29]。其典型特征是，肿瘤细胞呈簇状分布于中心小血管周围，该结构称为席勒-杜瓦尔体（Schiller-Duval body）（图 100-3）。该肿瘤形态学表现多种多样，包括微囊（蕾丝样），微乳头，实性以及肝细胞样形态。肿瘤细胞的细胞核略小于胚胎癌。胞质小球较常见，并且甲胎蛋白染色阳性，这解释了为什么此类肿瘤患者中血清甲胎蛋白升高（表 100-2）。

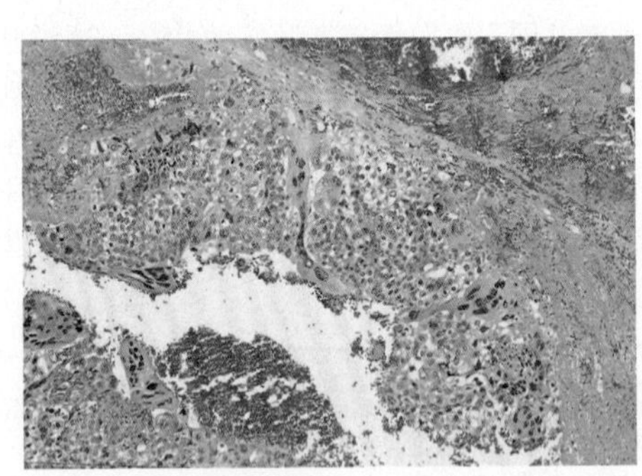

图 100-3　合体滋养细胞呈“帽”样覆盖数个岛状排列的单个细胞核的细胞滋养细胞，注意出血背景

应当指出，纯卵黄囊肿瘤是婴儿和幼儿睾丸肿瘤最常见的病理类型（表 100-1）。尽管在青春期后发生非精原生殖细胞肿瘤的患者也可发生形态相似的病理亚型，但小儿肿瘤从肿瘤学上来讲是一个截然不同的病理类型，而且预后较好。

绒毛膜癌

绒毛膜癌是非精原细胞生殖细胞肿瘤中是一种少见的成分（15%），纯绒毛膜癌罕见。肉眼观，绒毛膜癌特征为瘤内出血。显微镜下，需要同时看到细胞滋养层细胞和合体滋养层细胞才能诊断（图 100-4）。间质稀疏，但倾向于高度血管化。睾丸绒毛膜癌是非精原细胞生殖细胞肿瘤中最具侵袭性的亚型，常伴有多发内脏转移和/或脑转移。血清 HCG 水平的显著升高为其特征。

畸胎瘤

畸胎瘤包含所有三个胚层成分（内胚层，中胚层和外胚层），分化程度差异较大。约半数非精原生殖细胞肿瘤含有畸胎瘤成分，纯畸胎瘤少见。肉眼观，畸胎瘤多体积较大，呈多房囊性改变，囊内由血清等浆液成分以及软骨等实性成分组成。镜下，各种组织成分可能可见，包括鳞状上皮，呼吸道或肠上

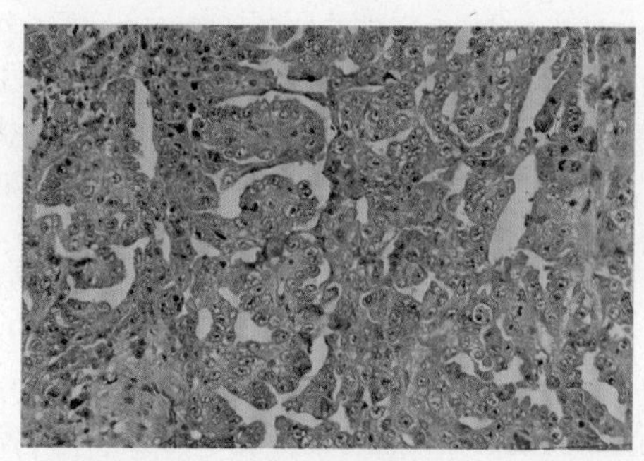

图 100-4　胚胎癌。由多形细胞形成不规则状腺体和乳头，胞核拥挤，呈小囊样，胞质染色欠佳

皮，成熟的软骨，肌肉和成纤维细胞间质（图 100-5）。而分化较差（“不成熟畸胎瘤”）的区域往往混合存在（图 100-6）。应当指出，无论分化程度如何，在青春期后发生的畸胎瘤都视为恶性。在化疗后的病理标本中（通常来自后腹膜淋巴结清扫标本），畸胎瘤是最常见的残余成分。当肿瘤中出现非畸胎瘤成分，提示患者可能需要其他治疗。

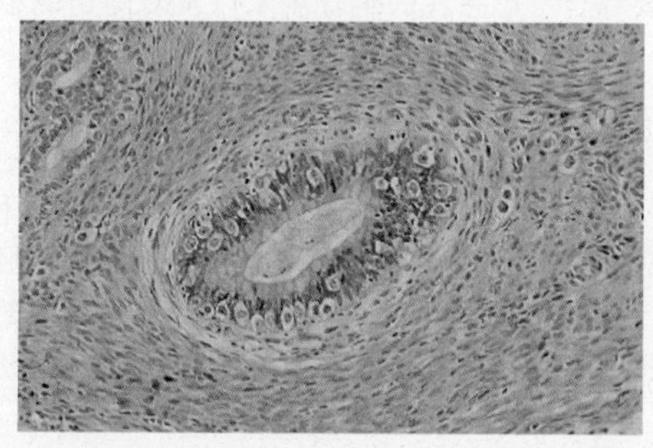

图 100-5　成熟畸胎瘤。有成熟形态的微小腺体，有一个皮脂腺单位，还有成束的平滑肌纤维

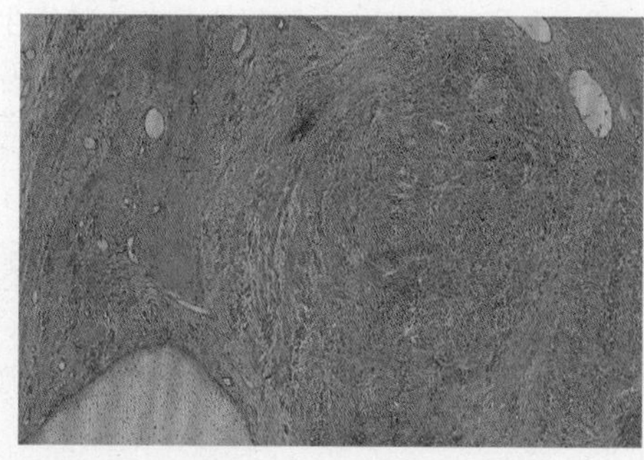

图 100-6　不成熟畸胎瘤。不成熟的神经上皮样组织呈岛状排列在透明软骨结节旁边

在四岁前的幼儿患者中，纯成熟畸胎瘤较为常见。虽然畸胎瘤与非精原生殖细胞肿瘤中成熟畸胎瘤成分形态相似，但两者起病途径不同，并且畸胎瘤本质上是良性的[30]（表 100-1）。少数情况下，肿瘤可能会含有非畸胎瘤成分，并可发生转移。

生殖细胞衍生的非生殖细胞癌

精原细胞和非精原生殖细胞肿瘤都被认为起源于生殖母细胞，鉴于生殖母细胞的多能性潜能，在青春期后的进展期睾丸癌病理中可能出现非生殖细胞成分，并且有可能成为其主要成分。这些肿瘤形态学上可能类似于胚胎性横纹肌肉瘤，腺鳞癌，平滑肌肉瘤，肾母细胞瘤，胶质母细胞瘤，原始神经外胚层肿瘤（primitive neuroectodermal tumor，PNET），所有这些可能都与化疗耐药有关[31]。非精原生殖细胞肿瘤也可能演变成骨髓增生异常与白血病[32]。

精母细胞精原细胞瘤

精母细胞精原细胞瘤只占睾丸生殖细胞肿瘤的 1%～2%。肉眼观，肿瘤呈浅灰色，质地与典型精原细胞瘤相比柔软。镜下，该类肿瘤由高度、大小不一的圆形瘤细胞构成，大小与正常精细胞相似，瘤细胞趋向于形成管簇状结构（图 100-7）。与典型精原细胞瘤相比，精母细胞精原细胞瘤少见间质淋巴细胞浸润。此肿瘤患者年龄大多在 50 岁以上，中位年龄 65 岁。术后预后良好，关于转移的报道极少。

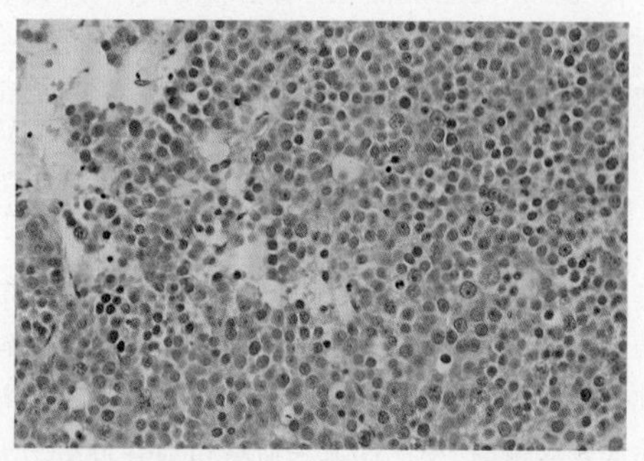

图 100-7　精母细胞精原细胞瘤。瘤细胞大小不一，呈薄片状弥散排列

性索-间质肿瘤

来自间质组织的肿瘤仅占所有成人睾丸肿瘤的 4%，但约占儿童睾丸肿瘤的 20%。这些肿瘤被认为起源于原始性腺间充质细胞，分为睾丸间质细胞瘤（Leydig 细胞瘤）、支持细胞瘤（Sertoli 细胞瘤）、性腺母细胞瘤、颗粒细胞瘤和混合/不确定型（表 100-1）。

睾丸间质细胞瘤

睾丸间质细胞瘤约占所有睾丸肿瘤的 3%，儿童也可发病，但中位发病年龄为 60 岁。组织学上，其典型特征是细胞质丰富具有嗜酸性圆形，核圆而规则。临床症状通常与肿瘤细胞产生雄激素和雌激素有关，导致儿童性早熟和成年女性乳房发育。大约 10% 的患者发生转移，仅见于成年患者。转移患者放化疗不敏感。腹膜后淋巴结清扫术（retroperitoneal lymph node dissection，RPLND）对该肿瘤分期有重要意义。对腹膜后转移淋巴结体积较小者，施行腹膜后淋巴结清扫术治疗作用尚不清楚，但转移灶较大者行后腹膜淋巴结清扫治疗效果较差。因此，临床Ⅰ期肿瘤患者应考虑预防性腹膜后淋巴结清扫术。

支持细胞瘤

支持细胞瘤的发病无年龄倾向性，症状上表现为睾丸肿块，可伴有继发于雌激素过量分泌导致的男性乳腺发育或阳痿。镜下可见该肿瘤由圆形细胞组成，细胞边界清晰，在纤维背景下呈条索状或薄层状生长。如同其他间质性肿瘤，治疗主要是切除原发病灶，为进行临床分期还需行腹部 CT 扫描和胸片。目前针对临床Ⅰ期病变是否应行腹膜后淋巴结清扫术目前仍存在争议。对于原发肿瘤较大,有丝分裂旺盛或有坏死区域的情况,可能提示需要进行腹膜后淋巴结清扫。与睾丸间质细胞瘤不同,睾丸支持细胞瘤能够对以铂类为基础的联合化疗产生反应。

临床表现

大多数患者因为睾丸肿胀而就诊。伴随症状包括在睾丸坠胀感或受累性腺疼痛。剧烈疼痛罕见,除非有相关的附睾炎或肿瘤出血。由于睾丸癌通常导致精子数量降低,部分患者可能会以不育症就诊。

约 25%患者由于肿瘤转移引起症状而就诊[33]。转移至腹膜后引起的严重背痛是最常见的,也可见于原发性腹膜后生殖细胞肿瘤患者。肺部症状如呼吸短促,胸痛和咯血通常是晚期肺转移的表现。原发性纵隔生殖细胞瘤是例外,因为此类肿瘤(如为恶性)会产生纵隔压迫症状如疼痛,吞咽困难,呼吸急促和上腔静脉综合征。纵隔畸胎瘤产生的症状很少,通常在常规胸片上发现,表现轻微的胸部症状。

诊断

如果要正确理解睾丸生殖细胞肿瘤的诊断和分期,首先要从解剖学上了解睾丸的血管和淋巴回流以及该疾病转移扩散的可能部位,睾丸的血供和淋巴回流位于精索内。在精索血管跨越至输尿管腹侧时,淋巴回流和血液供应在此处分开。右侧睾丸淋巴回流区域包括肾血管下方的血管间沟淋巴结(interaortocaval nodes)以及沿腹主动脉同侧分布的淋巴结,尤其是腔静脉周围(paracaval)淋巴结和腹主动脉前方(preaortic)淋巴结。而左侧睾丸的淋巴回流区域为同侧肾血管下方的腹主动脉旁(PA)淋巴结以及腹主动脉前方淋巴结。除非病灶体积较大,否则同侧髂总淋巴结很少受累。

对于既往有盆腔手术史的患者,如疝修补术,腹腔睾丸固定术,或阴囊受侵者,情况可能有些特殊[34]。需要强调的是,对于这类患者,经腹股沟睾丸根治性切除是最恰当也是唯一的诊断手段。经阴囊手术可能会使淋巴转移变得更为复杂且难以预测,一般不予推荐。

应从详细的病史采集和体格检查开始对睾丸肿瘤进行评估。睾丸检查的标准方法是将睾丸置于拇指与示指、中指之间,仔细触诊睾丸、附睾以及精索。睾丸肿瘤可呈多发结节样改变或呈弥漫浸润型(特别是精原细胞瘤和淋巴瘤)。对侧正常睾丸可以作为一个很好的参照物。如果怀疑睾丸肿物,应常规行经阴囊超声检查。如存在低回声占位,提示可能为睾丸肿瘤,经腹股沟睾丸根治性切除术后经病理学检查时确诊的手段,同时也实现了对原发肿瘤的局部控制。

值得注意的是,原发于腹膜后或纵隔的生殖细胞肿瘤(性腺外生殖细胞肿瘤,extragonadal germ cell tumors,EGT),需要特殊处理。对于这类患者,结合前纵隔和后腹膜肿物以及显著升高的肿瘤标志物水平,一般不难诊断。如果肿瘤标志物并不升高,则需行组织学活检确诊。诊断纵隔生殖细胞肿瘤,推荐采用经前方胸骨正中切开术。由于化疗是首选治疗,对于纵隔生殖细胞肿瘤的初始治疗不推荐行肿物完整切除或减瘤手术。对于后腹膜原发生殖细胞肿瘤,可能同时存在隐匿的睾丸原发病灶。对于这类患者,应该行系统的性腺检查,包括睾丸超声检查。如果能够发现睾丸肿瘤,行睾丸切除可作为诊断手段。否则,需要对腹腔肿物行针吸活检或行开腹探查术来获取组织学诊断。此外,有一例未分化癌患者通过发现 i(12p)染色体异常而诊断为生殖细胞肿瘤。

应绝对禁止经阴囊活检,因为这会导致瘤细胞阴囊内种植,并破坏区域淋巴回流,从而导致腹股沟淋巴结转移。对于有阴囊侵犯的患者,其处理原则取决于已经采取的治疗措施和下一步的治疗计划。如果在行经阴囊睾丸切除术时发现睾丸肿瘤,并且已将睾丸完整切除,那么唯一需要采取的措施就是继续切除腹股沟段的精索。可以在行腹膜后淋巴结清扫时进行,或者另行腹股沟切口切除。如果已经行睾丸活检,对于该侧阴囊的处理取决于原发肿瘤的治疗。如果选择化疗作为初始治疗,那么不需要行半阴囊切除。对于腹股沟区域可触及肿大淋巴结者需行腹股沟淋巴结清扫。对于早期的精原细胞瘤患者,如有阴囊受侵,有 5%~10%的患者会局部治疗失败。对于扩大局部治疗范围至腹股沟以及阴囊可减少局部治疗失败的风险,但会增加不育的风险。对于这类患者的治疗因人而异,需要综合考虑患者的生育需求以及对随访的依从性来决定。

肿瘤标志物

血清 HCG 和甲胎蛋白对 GCTS 患者的诊断、预后和治疗有重要价值。甲胎蛋白来源于卵黄囊或生殖细胞癌的胚胎癌细胞成分。正常成人未见甲胎蛋白升高。其在血清中的半衰期约为 5 天。在生殖细胞癌中,在生殖细胞癌中,合体滋养细胞成分产生 HCG。该蛋白包含一个 α 亚单位和一个 β 亚单位,每个亚单位都具有不同的抗原性。整个蛋白在血液中的半衰期是 18~30h。

在转移性非精原生殖细胞肿瘤患者中,约有 85%的患者血清 HCG 和/或甲胎蛋白升高。在转移性睾丸非精原生殖细胞癌的患者中,单纯甲胎蛋白升高者占 40%,而单纯 HCG 升高者占 50%~60%。乳酸脱氢酶(LDH)是一种特异性稍差的肿瘤标志物,其主要与肿瘤大小相关。

纯精原细胞瘤患者绝大多数甲胎蛋白和 HCG 正常,但约 10%的所有病例可以轻度增高,而晚期疾病患者可高达 30%(通常该数值<100mIU/ml)[35]。所以精原细胞瘤患者,一旦甲胎蛋白升高都必须被视为含有非精原细胞瘤成分,并应进行相应的处理。

睾丸切除术前后都应测定甲胎蛋白和 HCG,无论标志物水平升高与否,均应如此。但是,尽管标志物的持续升高意味着残留病灶,切除术后血清标志物的正常化并不能确保所有的病灶都被去除。肿瘤标志物的下降速率对于判断该病对化疗的反应性是非常有用的。在这方面 HCG 是最有参考价值的。例如,HCG 水平在三周时间内下降 10 倍,则高度提示该患者有可能通过化疗治愈。而如果 HCG 下降速度较慢的话,则提示肿瘤耐药性的发生。当肿瘤复发时,肿瘤标志物升高常先于影像学异常。

肿瘤标记物的存在虽然对诊断和治疗有着重要意义,但也可能导致误导临床治疗。首先,HCG 非特异性较高,并且在与促黄体素的放射免疫分析中存在一些交叉反应。此外,使用大麻的患者的 HCG 可能会呈假阳性。因此，出现如此情况，应重测定 HCG，以确保标高不是实验室错误。如果 HCG 水平仍然很高，应该询问患者的药物使用情况。睾酮应肌内注射 300mg，以确保睾丸切除术后性腺功能减退所致的促黄体素水平升高不会影响 HCG 测定。如果水平仍然增加，那么，需要对可能存在问题的区域（如脑和对侧睾丸）进行评估和再分期。印第安纳大学 Zon 等人进行了一项回顾性研究，对 HCG 显著升高患者的治疗问题进行了评估[36]。共有 41 例 HCG 水平大于 50 000mIU/ml 的患者被纳入。所有患者都接受了以顺铂为基础的化疗。在这 41 例患者中，有 2 例在行第四周期化疗时 HCG 水平降至正常，另有 8 例患者在完成 4 个周期化疗后一个月内 HCG 水平达到正常。在这 10 例患者中，有 7 例患者目前仍处于无瘤生存状态，有 3 例患者在接受挽救性治疗后达到无瘤生存。另外 31 例患者在 4 个周期化疗后 1 个月，血 HCG 仍然无法降至正常。其中 15 例尽管并没有采取进一步治疗措施，但目前仍然处于无瘤生存状态。该研究的亮点在于，对于 HCG 水平显著升高但治疗后下降并不十分满意的患者，如果仅仅考虑治疗后 HCG 水平下降情况来决定下一步治疗方案的话，可能会导致过度治疗或者不恰当的挽救性治疗。而我们采取的措施是，等到 HCG 再次升高后才开始实施挽救性治疗。

甲胎蛋白假性升高极其罕见。如果出现，应考虑系实验室检测误差，或者其他肿瘤（如肝细胞癌），或者肝硬化以及肝炎等引起的肝脏炎症。有一部分患者甲胎蛋白基线水平就高于正常（AFP 通常小于 100ng/ml），对于这类患者该数值保持稳定并不提示存在活动性病变。值得注意的是，部分患者血清 AFP 受到家族遗传性影响，血清 AFP 水平可能轻度升高，在 15~30ng/ml 范围内。对于临床Ⅰ期的患者，如影像学表现正常，对侧睾丸正常，AFP 水平轻度升高（<25ng/ml）的患者，仅当 AFP 明显增加和/或发展为转移时才进行治疗[37]。

分期

生殖细胞肿瘤大体分为Ⅰ期，肿瘤局限在睾丸内Ⅱ期，肿瘤转移至主动脉周围或腔静脉周围淋巴结，而没有肺或其他内脏器官转移。Ⅲ期，存在膈上或其他脏器转移。美国癌症联合委员会（American Joint Committee on Cancer，AJCC）对于该分期系统进行了改良，主要是将肿瘤标志物这一重要内容加入到了分期系统当中。这一新的 TNM 分期系统包括了一些重要的局部预后指标，诸如血管受侵，更多的区域淋巴结情况，包括淋巴结转移灶大小；以及内脏转移与否，还有肿瘤标志物升高情况。这一 AJCC 分类标准与世界卫生组织（WHO）分类法已经成为目前的国际标准（表 100-3）[39]。

确定临床阶段的标准程序包括体格检查、腹部和胸部 CT 扫描以及血清甲胎蛋白、βHCG 和 LDH 水平。只有在有临床症状和/或低风险疾病时，才应进行脑成像和骨扫描。正电子发射断层扫描（PET）在患者的初始分期中的作用仍处在研究阶段，尚不可用于分期。PET 扫描并非畸胎瘤或镜下病变的可靠检查手段。PET 扫描曾被用于精原细胞瘤患者化疗后残余病灶的评估，如果 PET 结果持续阳性，与复发风险存在相关性[40]。

表 100-3 AJCC 分期标准

TMN 临床分期系统	
T	原发肿瘤：原发肿瘤的侵犯范围在行睾丸根治性切除之后进行分期（见 pT）。如果未行睾丸根治性切除，则列为 Tx
N	区域淋巴结
Nx	区域淋巴结无法评价
N0	没有区域淋巴结转移
N1	区域淋巴结单个转移，最大径≤2cm，或多发淋巴结转移，且均不超过 2cm
N2	区域淋巴结单个转移，最大径>2cm，但≤5cm，或多发淋巴结转移，其中任一个大于 2cm，但均不超过 5cm
N3	转移淋巴结最大径>5cm
M	远处转移
Mx	远处转移无法评价
M0	无远处转移
M1	远处转移
M1a	区域淋巴结转移或肺转移
M1b	其他部位转移
pTNM 病理分期系统	
pT	原发肿瘤
pTx	原发肿瘤无法评价（未行睾丸切除则用 Tx）
pT0	无原发肿瘤的证据（如睾丸瘢痕）
pTis	生精小管内生殖细胞肿瘤（原位癌）
pT1	肿瘤局限于睾丸和附睾，不伴有血管/淋巴管浸润，可以浸润睾丸白膜但是无鞘膜侵犯
pT2	肿瘤局限于睾丸和附睾，伴有血管/淋巴管浸润，或者肿瘤通过睾丸白膜侵犯鞘膜
pT3	肿瘤侵犯精索，有或没有血管/淋巴管浸润
pT4	肿瘤侵犯阴囊，有或没有血管/淋巴管浸润
pN	区域淋巴结
pNx	区域淋巴结转移情况无法评价
pN0	没有区域淋巴结转移
pN1	转移淋巴结数≤5 个，且最大径≤2cm
pN2	单个转移淋巴结，最大径线>2cm，但≤5cm；或者 5 个以上≤5cm 的阳性淋巴结；或者存在扩散到淋巴结外的证据
pN3	转移淋巴结>5cm
pM	远处转移
	pM 与 M 相同
S	血清肿瘤标志物
Sx	无法评价标志物
S0	标志物水平不高
S1	AFP<1 000ng/ml，且 HCG<5 000IU/L，且 LDH<正常值上限的 1.5 倍
S2	AFP 1 000~10 000ng/ml，或 HCG 5 000~50 000IU/L，或 LDH 正常值上限的 1.5~10 倍
S3	AFP>10 000ng/ml，或 HCG>50 000IU/L，或 LDH>正常值上限的 10 倍

N，乳酸脱氢酶测定正常值上限。

摘自 Edge 2010[38]。经 Springer 许可复制。

治疗

原位癌

原位癌(CIS)或小管上皮内瘤变(TIN)是真正的癌前病变,未经治疗的患者中有50%可能进展为精原细胞瘤或非精原细胞瘤(图100-8和图100-9)[41]。对于这类病变的治疗,目前存在争议。对于诊断TIN的患者,密切观察可能是保留生育能力的最佳选择,这需要患者具有较高的依从性,同时存在疾病进展以及需要采取进一步治疗措施的风险。低剂量放疗(总剂量18~20Gy,每次照射量1.5~2.0Gy)有可能根除TIN,但导致生育能力降低甚至完全消失的风险很高。但如果Leydig细胞的功能能够得以保存的话,这一照射水平大多不会影响生育潜能[41,42]。对于受累睾丸行全睾丸切除显然能够根除TIN病变,但同时也损失了该侧全部的生殖细胞和Leydig细胞。对于一侧TIN病变而对侧睾丸正常的患者,行睾丸切除可能是较好的选择。不推荐行睾丸部分切除,因为TIN在受累睾丸中往往弥漫分布。不推荐对TIN行化疗[43]。

非精原细胞瘤:早期

对于早期非精原细胞瘤治疗方案的选择,关键是要正确理解睾丸原发病变的自然病程以及其淋巴回流途径。睾丸的淋巴系统在胚胎起源上非常靠近胚胎期睾丸,位于腰部较高位置的生殖脊(genital ridge)。尽管输入淋巴管与睾丸伴行下降至阴囊,但主要的引流淋巴结仍然位于后腹膜腔,包括一级腰淋巴结以及二级髂淋巴结链。

1910年,Jamieson和Dobson证明两侧睾丸肿瘤的淋巴回流方式不同,右侧病变引流到腔静脉周围淋巴结、血管间沟淋巴结和腹主动脉前淋巴结,左侧病变引流到腹主动脉周围淋巴结以及腹主动脉前淋巴结[44]。

Ⅰ期非精原细胞瘤

Ⅰ期非精原细胞瘤患者的治愈率接近100%。现有三种治疗选择包括腹膜后淋巴结清扫(RPLND)、辅助化疗和积极监测。无论哪种方案,预后都非常理想。因此,当前关注热点在如何减少毒副作用方面。治疗方案的选择基于对临床Ⅰ期肿瘤的准确诊断之上。在腹股沟睾丸切除术和确诊非精原细胞瘤之后,血清β-HCG和甲胎蛋白水平必须恢复正常(如果在切除术前升高的话),并且腹部CT、胸部X线摄影和/或胸部CT必须全部阴性才能将患者标记为临床Ⅰ期肿瘤。在这种情况下,如果不进行其他治疗,大约30%的患者将面临复发,尤其是腹膜后,仍是最高风险区域。8%~10%的患者会发生腹膜后以外其他区域转移,主最常见是在肺部[45]。

Freedman等基于睾丸癌四个预后危险因素的基础上开发了一个数学模型,根据此模型能够识别在2年时复发率为58%的患者[46]。而这四个因素包括睾丸静脉侵犯、睾丸淋巴管侵犯、病理不含卵黄囊成分以及肿瘤中存在未分化成分。其余影响因素如病理T分期高于Ⅰ,胚胎癌成分的存在,畸胎瘤占原发肿瘤的百分比等[46~48]。血管侵犯作为最主要的独立危险因素,其重要性被反复强调。临床上,如果原发肿瘤存在血管侵犯,则患者被归入"高危"组,其复发风险接近50%。与之相比,没有血管淋巴侵犯的"低危"组患者复发风险仅为15%~20%。

对于临床Ⅰ期非精原细胞瘤患者的最佳治疗方式,目前仍存在争议。三种治疗选择:腹膜后淋巴结清扫,辅助化疗和积极监测将在下文中予以讨论。

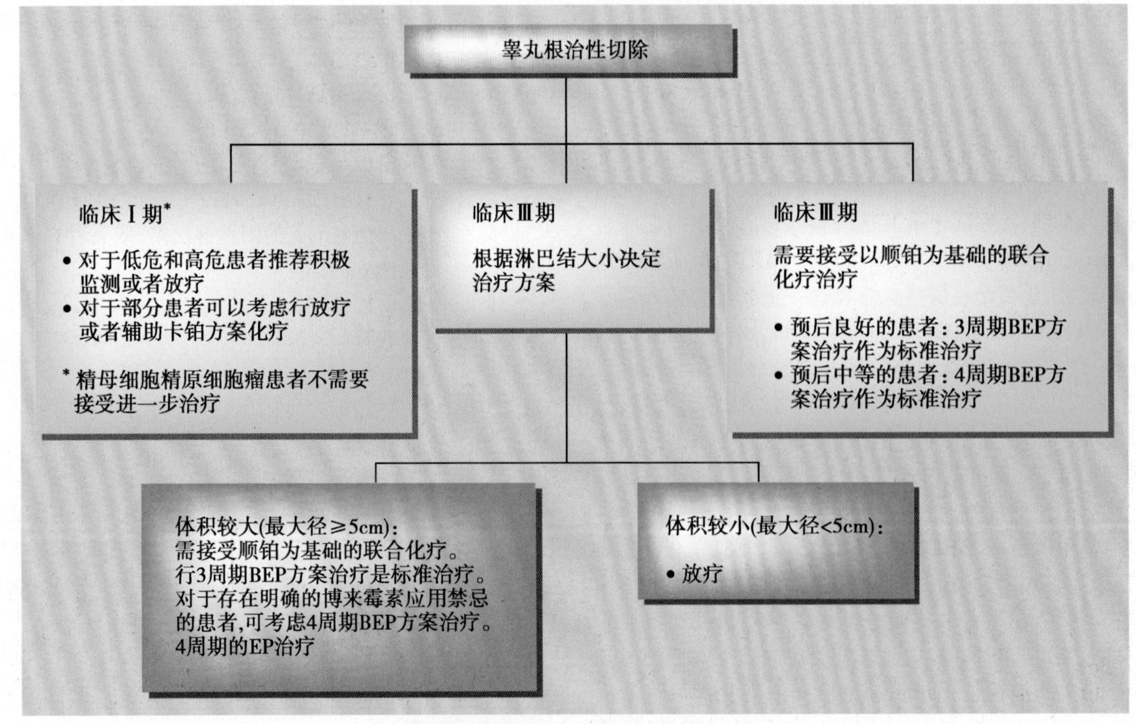

图100-8　精原细胞瘤治疗流程图

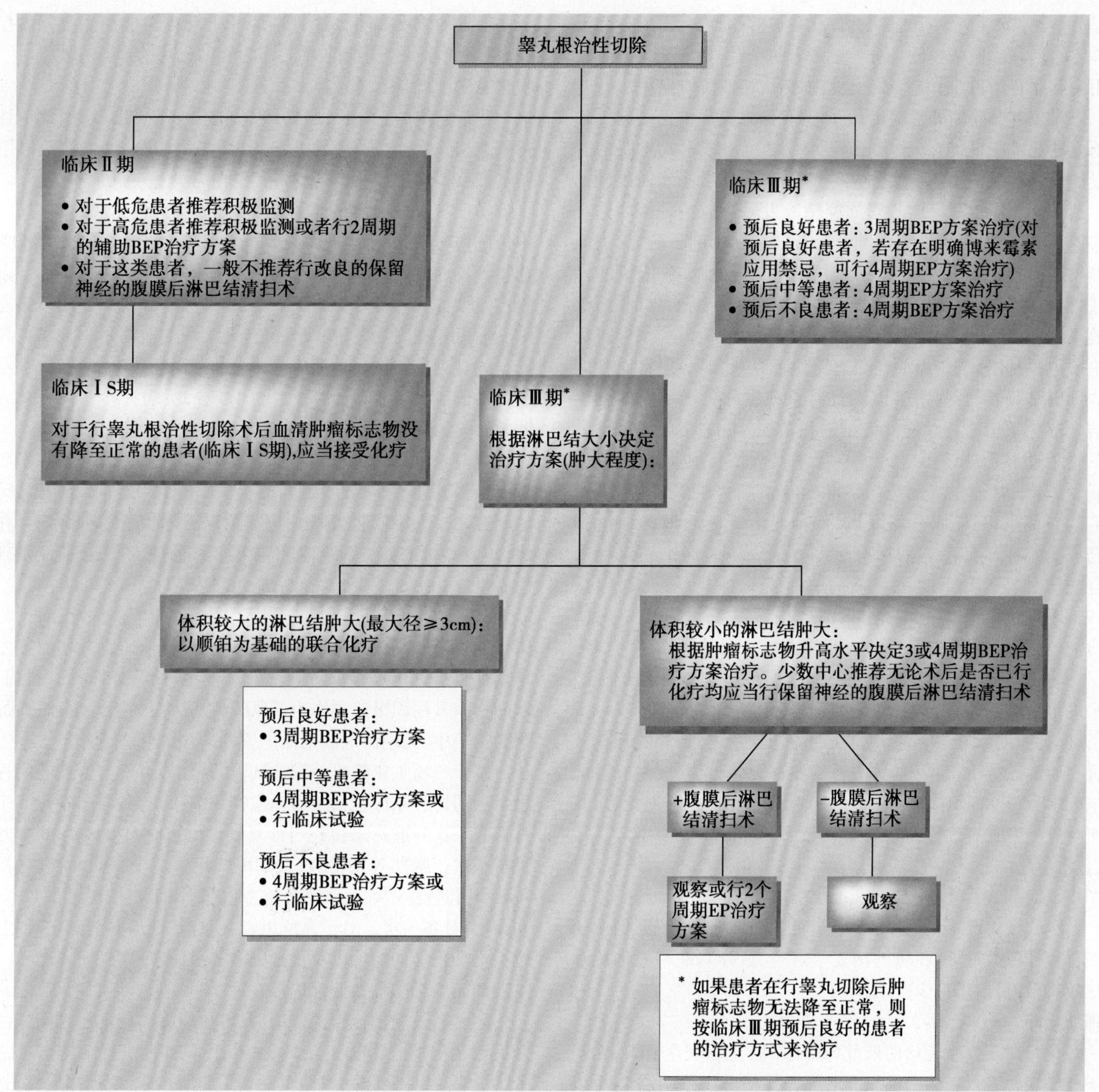

图 100-9 非精原细胞瘤治疗流程图

腹膜后淋巴结清扫

根据睾丸肿瘤的淋巴扩散途径，早在 1907 年间就已经有学者将腹膜后淋巴结清扫术用于睾丸癌的治疗[49~51]。在美国，腹膜后淋巴结清扫是临床Ⅰ期非精原细胞瘤患者的常规治疗方法。在欧洲和加拿大，共识指南目前并不提倡对早期病变行腹膜后淋巴结清扫[52,53]。然而，对于睾丸肿瘤而言，在初始转移部位中，超 90%位于腹膜后淋巴结，而行腹膜后淋巴结清扫是判断是否存在腹膜后淋巴结转移最为准确的方法。对于临床Ⅰ期但术后提示存在腹膜后淋巴结局限性病变的患者(pN1)，单纯行腹膜后淋巴结清扫可以治愈 50%~80%的患者。对于存在 5 个以上的转移淋巴结，淋巴结直径超过 2cm 以上，以及任何结外侵犯(pN2-pN3)的患者，需经过两个周期的辅助化疗，方可全部治愈[54]。另一个优势是能够去除腹膜后可能的畸胎瘤成分(畸胎瘤大多数对化疗耐药)，从而使后期畸胎瘤复发的风险降低[55]。然而，即使在纯畸胎瘤中，只有 20%的患者在诊断时会出现隐匿性腹膜后淋巴结转移[56]。对经验丰富的外科医生而言，腹膜后淋巴结清扫术后腹膜后复发者非常罕见。对于这类患者，如果术前病灶局限于睾丸，那么总体复发率约为 10%，且绝大多数复发发生在肺部。

早在 1950 年，就有学者报道采取经胸腹(腹膜外)入路行根治性淋巴结切除术于[57]，并由 Skinner 在 20 世纪 80 年代将这一技术推广[58]。20 世纪 70 年代最主流的术式是单纯经腹腔入路腹膜后淋巴结清扫(前入路)[59,60]。无论哪种入路方式，都有其自身的优点。胸腹联合入路的优点是尽管小肠梗阻的发生率较低，但同时也具有疼痛和胸部并发症等明显增多的缺点[58]。为了降低发病率，Donohue 等取前正中切口行经腹腔腹膜后淋巴结清扫术，采取该手术方式只能够行肾门下方的腹膜后淋巴结清扫[61]，但是对于临床Ⅰ期患者而言，发生肾门上淋巴结转移的概率极低。对于临床Ⅰ期患者，目前已经很少使用胸腹联合切口，基本上都已经被前正中切口所取代。

对于有经验的外科医生，经典的双侧腹膜后淋巴结清扫术围术期死亡率很低，甚至无围术期死亡[62]。该术式主要的并发症是顺行射精功能丧失，从而导致90%以上的患者需要辅助生殖技术才能生育。随着对支配精液发射和射精神经通路理解深入，以及对右侧和左侧肿瘤分布的精细解剖学研究，进而提出了改良的腹膜后淋巴结清扫术[63,64]。相对于传统的术式，保留神经的改良术式主要目的在于：在不影响分期/治疗效果的前提下，最大限度上减少对射精功能的影响[65~67]。无论采取哪种术式，均需要严格遵循如下原则，即必须将血管间沟淋巴结，同侧肾门水平以下至髂总动脉分叉区域内的淋巴结全部完整切除。对侧淋巴结清扫范围尽可能小，尤其是肠系膜下动脉（IMA）下方区域。为了最大限度地减少腹膜后复发，有学者主张双侧肾门下淋巴结清扫，仅保留对侧IMA下的对侧淋巴结[68]。如今，保留神经的腹膜后淋巴结清扫已成为临床Ⅰ期患者的标准治疗方式。如果能小心保存来自交感神经链和下腹神经丛的节后交感神经纤维，在保持99%以上治愈率的同时，绝大多数情况下都可以保持射精功能（96%~100%）[59,66,69]。

为了进一步降低手术的发病率，当前多已经使用腹腔镜技术进行腹膜后淋巴结清扫术[70]。虽然手术时间较开放手术长，但通过对550多名患者的长期随访显示，与传统的开放式腹膜后淋巴结清扫术相比，两者复发率无统计学差异。然而，绝大多数（>90%）淋巴结阳性的患者已经接受了辅助化疗，从而对这一术式有效性判断产生干扰。

放疗

尽管过去曾主张采用放疗治疗Ⅰ期非精原细胞瘤，但由于联合化疗疗效显著、积极监测安全可行，放疗对非精原细胞瘤疗效有限，目前已很少应用。

辅助化疗

化疗对于发生转移的低危（good risk）患者安全有效，而对于已经完整手术切除的临床Ⅱ期患者，两个周期的化疗也可以获得几乎完美的疗效。因此，对于存在血管侵犯的高危患者，研究人员正在考虑将化疗作为基础治疗来进行处理。

Ⅱ期临床试验的数据表明，两个周期的博来霉素、依托泊苷和顺铂（BEP）方案作为辅助治疗已足够，医学研究委员会（MRC）设计了一项前瞻性研究，向高危临床Ⅰ期NSGCTT[71]患者提供两个周期的BEP，以评估辅助化疗的疗效和长期毒性[71]。该项目共对114例患者进行了治疗和随访，中位随访时间为4年。2年无复发生存率为98%。实际复发率5%。在两个复发的患者中，一个被证实是睾丸腺癌而不是生殖细胞肿瘤。虽然中位随访时间只有4年，对于长期毒性而言并不足以得到结论性论断，但是在4年中确实没有发现显著临床差异。在不同的研究中，两个周期的BEP辅助化疗对临床Ⅰ期患者所取得疗效结论几乎一致，复发率从0%到2%不等，近乎治愈。

欧洲共识指南随后采用了两个周期的辅助BEP作为治疗血管侵犯患者的标准方法，而低风险疾病的患者采用积极监测作为治疗方案[52]。

最近的数据表明，1个周期的BEP化疗可能产生类似的疗效，目前推荐1个周期的BEP作为辅助化疗的推荐方案[72,73]。

积极监测

积极监测的主要理由是因为系统化疗非常有效，因此单纯行睾丸切除术治愈的患者，通过积极监测可以避免腹膜后淋巴结清扫或辅助化疗所带来的各种副作用。

早期曾有一项大型前瞻性随访研究，共包括373名患者，中位随访时间为5年[74]。复发率为27%，其中复发患者80%在第一年内复发。整个队列患者的总体治愈率超过98%。血管侵犯被证实为最重要的预后因素。包括1 139名Ⅰ期非精原细胞瘤患者在内的大量数据最近证实，积极监测是一种出色和安全的管理方式。在长期随访中，复发率为19%（淋巴血管侵袭阳性患者为44%，阴性患者为14%），疾病特异性存活率为99.7%，这一系列的监测强调了该方法的有效[75]。

目前全世界有超过3 000名临床Ⅰ期疾病患者在切除术后没有接受其他治疗，试验之间的复发率和存活率非常相似，无论研究规模大小或起源美国[76]。根据国际生殖细胞肿瘤合作组（IGCCCG）的分类系统，对于预后较好的患者，积极监测发现患者复发几乎都发生于确诊后2年之内[74,77]。

只有2%~3%的患者在2年后发生复发[75]。因此，对于临床Ⅰ期非精原细胞瘤患者的患者，采取严密的监测并在有复发早期征象给予化疗，可能是此类患者有效的治疗措施。目前，欧洲指南采用积极监测作为低风险疾病患者的治疗手段，而加拿大指南中，无论高危或是低危患者，均推荐积极监测[52]。

基于一项临床随机前瞻性试验的结果，对于血管侵袭阴性患者的随访计划应包括肿瘤标志物和临床检查：前2年每2个月检查一次肿瘤标志物并门诊复查，之后3~5年每4~6个月进行一次。胸部X线检查，最初前2年每4个月做一次，之后每6个月进行一次，直到第5年为止[78]。CT扫描在第3、12、24和56个月各一次。对于高危患者，还有其他不同的随访计划，包括更加密切的随诊以及更加频繁的影像学检查。

Ⅰ期非精原细胞瘤的治疗选择

随着有效辅助化疗的应用，保留神经腹膜后淋巴结清扫的开展以及积极监测的实施，现在对于Ⅰ期非精原细胞瘤的患者，尤其是那些高复发风险的患者，拥有了对后续治疗进行选择的机会。各种治疗措施如果选择得当的话，都会获得良好的生存预期，但是它们却存在着不同的缺点。

生存预期，但是它们却存在着不同的缺点。对于是否应行腹膜后淋巴清扫，目前仍然存在争议。主要在于，在美国或其他地区一些病例数很大的中心，手术治疗的效果非常好，不育以及其他并发症的发生概率非常低，而且这从根本上祛除了腹膜后这一区域发生复发的可能，使术后患者在随访时可以免于腹部影像学检查。然而，在接受手术治疗的患者中，70%最终病理结果为阴性，手术治疗可能并不能使这部分患者获益，即使是在最好的中心，术前评估也无法对此进行判断。此外，有25%~35%的患者由于广泛的腹膜后病变，术后还需要额外的两个周期的BEP化疗。最重要的是，尽管腹膜后淋巴结清扫可以将腹膜后复发率降至1%~2%，但其并不能够降低腹膜后区域以外复发的风险（8%~10%）。对于Ⅰ期非精原细胞瘤，在社区医院行腹膜后淋巴结清扫术患者，相比辅助化疗，复发率显著升高。而且不仅如此，术后阴囊复发以及腹腔复发患者的数量均有所升高,这说明,如果手术是由没有经验的医师实施,则无法实现对肿瘤的良好控制[72]。

辅助化疗,特别是针对高危患者的辅助化疗,是许多国家的标准治疗手段。虽然化疗可以讲复发率降低到 2%~4%,但至少 50%的患者存在过度化疗问题[76]。所有这些患者都会经历脱发;工作、学习和生活受到严重影响;严重的中性粒细胞减少症,罕见的致命并发症;其他并发症还包括血管并发症;急性化疗反应;至少对生育的暂时影响;以及所有接受化疗的患者所面临的焦虑和恐惧。潜在的长期并发症目前尚不清楚,复发仍有可能发生。因此,接受辅助化疗的患者仍然无法完全避免复发的可能,而且仍然需要进行烦琐的影像学检查。专家目前建议对高危Ⅰ期非精原细胞瘤进行一个周期的 BEP 治疗[73,79]。

对于积极监测,最为人诟病的地方在于患者往往缺乏依从性,尤其是对于高危的 CSI 非精原细胞瘤患者。目前尚没有关于依从性对于 CSI 非精原细胞瘤患者预后结局影响的相关研究[76]。目前没有证据表明不同区域依从性对存活率有实质性影响[76,80,81]。即使在依从性较差的研究当中,生存率也大都能够达到接近 100%。教育患者是至关重要的,强调病情发现较晚很可能会导致更复杂和烦琐的治疗,这是完全有必要的。未手术的腹膜后区域是否可能会在晚期发展成耐药的肿瘤病变或者出现畸胎瘤的晚期复发,这一问题在本文及其他研究中均未提及[76,80,82,83]。

在监测过程中,仅复发的患者才采取治疗措施。对这些患者的治疗,可能比单纯 2 周期 BEP 辅助化疗略长 BEP(分别是 6 周比 9 周)[84]。在我们看来,两个疗程和三个疗程的化疗的毒副作用差别甚微。然而,不化疗和 2 周期疗程之间有还是有着显著的差别,积极监测可以使 70%~75%的患者免于各种治疗负担,从而降低了各种治疗可能带来的副反应。

临床Ⅱ期病变

肿瘤标志物阳性和/或腹腔病灶较大(腹部 CT 提示病灶超过 2cm,ⅡB 期)的患者,应采用化疗。国际生殖细胞肿瘤合作组(IGCCCG)对于预后良好的患者的推荐意见是,标准治疗是方案为三个周期的 BEP[84]。只有在对博来霉素有明显禁忌证的情况下,才可以考虑使用四个周期的依托泊苷和顺铂(EP)[85]。基本上绝大多数ⅡA/B 期患者在化疗后将获得临床完全缓解,所有专一的淋巴结均消退,肿瘤标志物水平降至正常(缓解率:ⅡA 期的患者 80%~90%,ⅡB 期 65%~85%)[84,85]。只有在化疗后 CT 提示上有腹膜后残留病灶持续存在的患者才应接受腹膜后淋巴结清扫。采用这种策略,ⅡA 期复发率为 4%~9%,ⅡB 期为 11%~15%[86~88]。对于肿瘤标志物阴性ⅡA 期患者(淋巴结≤2cm),情况比较特殊。因为部分患者的肿大淋巴结可能为良性增生;而另一些会是畸胎瘤、纯胚胎癌或混合性肿瘤。目前还没有可靠的诊断工具来确定这些肿块的性质。这类患者治疗方案的选择,包括Ⅰ期腹膜后淋巴结清扫或积极监测,但监测期间应每 6~8 周就需要行影像学检查。如果病变缩小,则不需要进一步的治疗;对于稳定或生长的病变,大多数中心推荐化疗,少数选择的中心会考虑腹膜后淋巴结清扫。

精原细胞瘤,早期

20 世纪的大部分时间里,睾丸切除术后辅以放疗是早期精原细胞瘤的标准治疗[89~91]。采用腹股沟入路的根治性切除术是控制原发肿瘤部位疾病的高效疗法。由于精原细胞瘤对放疗敏感性极高,因此无论是隐匿或者是显著的腹主动脉旁淋巴结转移,在低剂量分割治疗(20~25Gy)后,达到根治效果的可能性非常之高。最近,一些临床试验的随访数据显示:绝大多数Ⅰ期精原细胞瘤患者的无病生存期显著延长,但如果以远期生活质量作为研究终点,可能会对治疗方案的选择产生显著的影响。

Ⅰ期精原细胞瘤:初始治疗及辅助治疗

精原细胞瘤患者最初诊断时,85%为临床Ⅰ期病变[92]。研究结果表明,睾丸切除术可以使 80%~85%的患者达到治愈。化疗和/或放射可以作为挽救治疗或预防的手段。但无论选择的何种治疗方法,5 年的疾病特异性存活率超过 99%[93~96]。对于未经辅助治疗复发的病变(treatment-naïve disease),治疗效果与原发病治疗一样有效。

共有四项临床研究证实,积极监测是一个可行的治疗措施[93~95,97~100]。综合四项研究的结论,可以更好地确定哪类患者适合积极治疗或密切观察[94]。4 项研究共 638 名患者,其中 6 例(0.9%)死于疾病或治疗复发相关的并发症。总的 5 年和 10 年无复发率分别为 82.3%和 78.7%。绝大部分(68.6%)复发发生在 2 年内,但仍有 7%的复发发生在 6 年后。两个最重要的预后因素是肿瘤大小和睾丸网侵犯。肿瘤直径超过 4cm 的患者复发的可能性是小肿瘤患者的两倍。睾丸网是一个横穿睾丸纵隔(mediastinum,或 hilum),使双侧生精管道能够互相沟通的网络结构。在所报道的病例中,睾丸网侵犯占 37%,一旦发现,则直接视为肿瘤侵犯睾丸纵隔,而并非一定侵犯小管管腔。对于同时具备两项危险因素的患者,其复发风险高达 33%。而对于不存在这些危险因素的患者,复发率约 13%。尽管肿瘤大小作为线性变量与风险相关,但在近发表的两组分析中,这一结论无法通过使用独立的数据集进行验证[101,102]。

对于随访监测需要进行的检查项目,一直在不停变化,但从总体趋势上来看,之前繁多的检查项目在逐渐减少[75]。许多中心将复查重点集中到风险最高的时期,并在随访时逐渐减少 CT 扫描。许多精原细胞瘤的随诊方案推荐 3-2-1 模式,即第一年有 3 个腹部/盆腔 CT,第二年有 2 次,之后不再行 CT 检查。因此,尽管密切观察是一个非常有吸引力的选择,但对于任何患者,各项影像学以及其他检测的频次都不能减少。因此,选择密切观察随访的患者需要良好的依从性顺并且可以信赖。

Ⅰ期精原细胞瘤患者,睾丸根治性切除和辅助放疗被证实成功有效,该策略已经沿用了 60 多年,目前的总体存活率超过 99%。辅助性腹主动脉旁放疗的复发率 3%~4%,其中绝大多数可以通过挽救性放疗和/或化疗来补救。近年来有许多学者提倡不进行积极治疗,仅采取密切随访观察,与此类似,许多研究者也提出减少放疗剂量和范围来降低辅助治疗的毒副作用。

放疗总剂量如今已逐渐减少到 20~25.5Gy(1.5~2Gy)。医学研究委员会 TE18(MRCTE18)/欧洲癌症研究与治疗组织

(EORTC)30 942 研究提出了这样一个问题:是否可以安全地将辐射剂量从 30Gy 降至 20Gy[103]。该研究中,绝大多数患者仅接受对腹主动脉旁淋巴结的放疗,他们被随机分为 2 组,一组放疗 15 次,剂量 30Gy;另一组次数和剂量分别是 10 次 20Gy。两组之间复发率为 0.7%,无统计学上差异。而低剂量组在 1 个月时发生嗜睡(Lethargy)和无法进行正常工作更少。

与此类似的是,放疗的范围也在缩小[104]。仅行腹主动脉旁淋巴结放疗的患者,3 年无复发生存率为 96%,而同时行同侧盆腔淋巴结照射者,结果并没有显著改善。然而,在仅行腹主动脉旁淋巴结放疗的患者中,有 9 名患者复发,其中 4 名患者复发部位包括盆腔淋巴结。因此,仅行腹主动脉旁淋巴结放疗的患者,在随访过程中,仍然需要常规行盆腔 CT 检查。目前的治疗方法是,对于腹主动脉旁淋巴结放疗,范围上至 T11 或 T12 水平,下至 L5 水平。既往有盆腔或腹股沟手术史的患者,其正常淋巴回流可能受到影响,所以仍然推荐行同侧盆腔淋巴结放疗。然而,对于睾丸淋巴回流未受影响的患者,单纯腹主动脉旁淋巴结放疗已经足够,而且生活质量更高,并发症更少。

睾丸切除后化疗

欧洲癌症研究与治疗组织/医学研究委员会主导展开了一项大型的随机试验,选取临床分期良好的Ⅰ期精原细胞瘤患者,随机分为两组,一组给予标准的预防性放疗(腹主动脉旁淋巴结放疗,剂量 20~30Gy),另一组给予单疗程、单剂卡铂(AUC7)治疗[105,106]。如果两年复发率绝对值增加超过 3%,则予以排除。根据 1∶2的随机方案中,共有 560 名患者被分配到单剂卡铂治疗,885 名患者被分配到标准放射治疗。中位随访时间为 4 年,3 年无复发生存率为 95.9%,而卡铂为 94.8%(P=0.31),卡铂治疗组患者复发绝大部分发生在腹部,几乎所有放疗治疗的复发都发生在放射野之外。与放疗组(10 例)相比,卡铂治疗(2 例),发生第二原发睾丸生殖细胞肿瘤的情况。作者的结论是,卡铂单药化疗是针对临床Ⅰ期精原细胞瘤安全有效的辅助治疗,但需要对患者长期随访(超过 4 年)。对这项研究的批评意见是,接受卡铂治疗的患者,复发主要部位在腹部,必须频繁进行腹部影像学检查,而如果随访时间过短的话,有可能会使真实的复发率被低估。2008 年这项试验进行了更新[106],中位随访时间为 6.5 年,5 年无复发生存率分别为卡铂(95%)和放疗(96%),两者没有显著差异。卡铂(2 例)与放疗(15 例)相比,第二睾丸原发生殖细胞肿瘤的发生率卡铂组(2 例)仍然低于放疗组(15 例)。

欧洲和加拿大编写的临床指南综合了有经验的放射肿瘤医师、肿瘤内科医生和泌尿科医生的经验及工作。欧洲的指南推荐对于所有的患者军采取随访观察治疗,与是否存在复发有危险因素无关。进行独立于个体复发风险的监测。只有在监测不适用的情况下,同样有效的替代方案要么是辅助性放射,要么是辅助性卡铂。关于如何根据个体风险来制订辅助治疗策略,即根据不同患者的危险因素调整治疗策略,目前仍然在研究当中,而且还停留在试验阶段[107]。

Ⅱ期精原细胞瘤

几种不同的分期系统,分别诠释了如何定义Ⅱ期精原细胞瘤,其主要区别在于淋巴结大小。然而无论采用哪种分期系统,膈上受累的可能性随着膈下病变的体积大小而增加。在绝大多数中心,全身系统化疗的界值为 5cm,淋巴结小于 5cm 的患者单纯放疗即可。与Ⅰ期病变不同,Ⅱ期患者并不推荐观察监测治疗。对于仅接受单独放射治疗的患者,预期 5 年无复发生存率下降至 89%~95%[108~110]。由于各种挽救疗法的高度有效,总体生存率仍然保持在 97%~99%左右。对于Ⅱ期精原细胞瘤患者,因为存在淋巴液逆流的可能,标准的放疗照射野包括腹主动脉旁淋巴结以及同侧盆腔淋巴结。Ⅱ期精原细胞瘤的放射治疗也在发展。以前,对于Ⅱ期精原细胞瘤的患者,放疗照射区域包括腹主动脉旁淋巴结,盆腔淋巴结,并且需要行预防性纵隔照射。采取这种治疗策略,尽管能够有效控制膈上病变,但却存在晚期心脏事件的风险。目前,对于膈上转移高风险的患者,推荐化疗。

对于体积较小或体积中等的Ⅱ期精原细胞瘤患者,以化疗作为一期治疗的相关经验也越来越多[111]。一项来自西班牙的多中心合作研究报道显示,共有 26 个中心参与,纳入 72 名患者。其中ⅡA 期患者 18 例,ⅡB 期 54 例。83%的患者到达完全缓解(CR),17%的患者获得部分缓解(PR),即存在残余病灶。中位随访时间为 71.5 个月,有 6 名ⅡB 期患者复发,其中 1 人死于精原细胞瘤。还有 3 名患者死亡,但与非精原细胞瘤无关。对于ⅡA 或ⅡB 期患者,预计 5 年无进展生存率分别为 100%和 87%(95%CI:77.5%~97%)。而总的 5 年无进展生存率和总生存率分别为 90%(95%CI:82%~98%)和 95%(95%CI:89%~100%);血液系统外最常见副反应包括,轻至中度呕吐,口腔炎和腹泻。这些经验表明,初级化疗可能是一种替代腹部放疗的有效方法。

转移性病变的治疗

化疗:前顺铂时代

1952—1972 年,人们曾尝试使用各种化疗药物来治疗转移性生殖细胞肿瘤。在 20 世纪 60 年代早期,长春碱(Vinblastine)也曾被用来治疗转移性生殖细胞肿瘤。在 30 名接受长春碱治疗的患者中,有 4 例诱导完全缓解[109]。尽管完全缓解状态持续时间很短,但它们为后续联合化疗方案提供了一个可供选择的合理构成成分。

还有一些其他抗生素类化疗药物被证实存在单药抗肿瘤作用,包括放线菌素 D(actinomycin D)。1970 年,博来霉素(Bleomycin)被证实存在显著抗肿瘤作用,甚至可诱导完全缓解[112,113]。

最早的联合化疗方案由 Li 等人在 1960 年描报道,包括甲氨蝶呤(methotrexate)、放线菌素 D 和苯丁酸氮芥(chlorambucil),这一方案一直沿用近十年[114]。根据 Li 的报告,该方案反应率能到达 52%,超过一半可以完全缓解。更为重要的是,他们第一次报道了治疗后持续缓解,有 5 名患者在治疗后存活了 9~39 个月(至报道时)。

更进一步的发展发是长春碱和博来霉素联合使用[115],使用该方案进行化疗的患者中,有 65%获得完全缓解,甚至可以达到持续缓解。

在转移性疾病的治疗的发展中,具有里程碑意义的事件为:1965 年 Rosenberg 等人报道铂类化合物具有抗菌作用[116]。在这些化合物中,顺二胺二氯铂(Ⅱ)(顺铂)也被发现具有显著的抗肿瘤活性。动物实验显示,顺铂可以使犬睾丸萎缩,当时认为是一种是副作用,但其促使一些研究人员意识到,这种化合物可以在临床上用于治疗睾丸恶性肿瘤。很快就有关于顺铂治疗睾丸肿瘤的报道,作为单药化疗药物,顺铂在治疗睾丸生殖细胞肿瘤上最为有效,有效率为 70%,完全缓解率为 50%[114]。三十年后,它仍然是治疗睾丸生殖细胞肿瘤上最为有效的药物。

印第安纳大学的研究

1974 年,印第安纳大学的研究人员开始研究长春碱(PVB)在治疗转移性睾丸癌中的作用。时至今日,该研究在现代肿瘤学中,仍具有里程碑意义[117]。这项研究主要研究联合化疗用药方案,同时也包括化疗后残留病灶手术治疗。诱导化疗时间短(3~4 个疗程),诱导治疗后维持化疗 2 年。在 47 例患者中,有 33 例(70%)通过化疗获得完全缓解。在剩下的 14 名患者中,有 5 名患者在切除残留病灶后获得了完全缓解。6 名获得缓解的患者复发。

最初的研究证明 PVB 是非常有效,但其毒副作用无法避免。因此,后续研究中,降低了长春碱的剂量(0.3mg/kg 与 0.4mg/kg),并与初期实验进行对比[118]。共 78 名患者进入这项研究,其中 70%的患者接受新治疗方案后持续无病,结果显示不同剂量的长春新碱具有相同的结果。然而,正如预期的那样,长春碱剂量的减少,相应脓毒症和粒细胞减少等情况也相应减少。因此,较低剂量的长春碱,连同顺铂和博来霉素,一起构成了 PVB 的标准方案。

另一项来自印第安纳大学的临床试验对上述试验结果进一步进行了证实,该试验名为 EORTC 试验[119]。该试验对比了高剂量长春碱(0.4mg/kg)与小剂量长春碱(0.3mg/kg)的治疗效果,并对长春碱维持治疗的价值进行评估。这项对 214 名患者进行的试验,高剂量长春碱并未显现出治疗优势,同样,长春碱维持化疗的患者也没有体现明显的治疗优势。

第三代研究始于 1978 年,由在印第安纳大学与东南癌症研究组(Southeastern Cancer Study Group,SECSG)联合进行[120]。在以前的研究中,在诱导治疗完成后的两年内,每月使用长春碱维持治疗。这项试验测试了维持化疗的有效性。本研究中,睾丸转移性肿瘤患者接受四个疗程的 PVB 诱导化疗。选取化疗后获得完全缓解的患者,或手术切除畸胎瘤后患者,随机分为两组,一组接受长春碱维持治疗,另一组不给予进一步治疗。这项研究结果显示,接受维持化疗的患者在结局上并无优势。

接下来的研究中,印第安纳大学与东南癌症研究小组一起,设计了一项随机试验,比对比顺铂+博来霉素与依托泊苷(BEP)联合化疗方案(PEB)与传统 PVB 化疗方案优劣[121]。共 261 例转移性生殖细胞癌患者入选,最早 244 例参与最终疗效评价。其中,123 人被随机分配至 BEP,83%达到无病生存状态。121 名患者被分配至 PVB,74%的患者达到无病状态。根据印第安纳大学的分类系统,在轻度或中度疾病患者的组合亚组中,90%的患者达到了无病生存状态,两个治疗组之间没有显著差异。然而,PVB 组患者,发生感觉异常,肌肉疼痛和腹部痉挛情况显著高于 PEB 组。由于 BEP 的神经肌肉毒性明显较小,具有同等或更好的治疗效果,顺铂、依托泊苷和博来霉素的组合仍然是标准联合化疗方案。

预后分级

一项国际协作研究收集了接受以铂类药物治疗的转移性睾丸肿瘤患者的资料,以建立一种新的关于转移性生殖细胞肿瘤患者的疾病预后模型[122]。该研究共收集非精原细胞瘤病例 5 202 例,和 660 例精原细胞瘤患者。通过单因素分析发现,能够预测最终结局的独立影响因子包括:纵隔原发非精原细胞瘤,甲胎蛋白、HCG 及 LDH 升高水平,和肺外脏器转移。根据这些独立影响因子,可以按照预后不同对患者进行分类。非精原细胞瘤低危(good-risk)患者包括:原发病灶位于睾丸或腹膜后,肿瘤标志不高或轻度增高,并且没有肺外脏器转移(预期无进展生存率 90%)。而高危患者(poor prognosis)包括:纵隔原发非精原细胞肿瘤,肺外脏器转移,或肿瘤标志物显著升高(预期无进展生存率 40%)。中危患者预期无进展生存率为 75%。而对于精原细胞瘤,仅列出了低危和中危组,而划分低危抑或中危主要取决于是否存在肺外脏器转移(表 100-4)。这一分类方法,应当作为标准的分类系统,用于比较不同中心的临床研究结果。

表 100-4　国际生殖细胞癌协作组预后因素分期系统

分组	非精原细胞瘤	精原细胞瘤
预后良好	睾丸或腹膜后原发	任何部位原发
	且无肺外器官转移	且无肺外器官转移
	且 AFP<1 000ng/ml,HCG<5 000IU/L,LDH<正常值上限的 1.5 倍	且 AFP 正常
		HCG 和 LDH 可以为任意值
预后中等	睾丸或腹膜后原发	任何部位原发
	且无肺外器官转移	且肺外器官转移
	且有下列之一者:AFP1 000~10 000ng/ml,或 HCG 5 000~50 000IU/L,或 LDH	且 AFP 正常
	高于正常值上限的 1.5~10 倍	HCG 和 LDH 可以为任意值
预后不良	纵隔原发	无
	或肺外器官转移	
	或 AFP>10 000ng/ml	
	或 HCG>50 000IU/L	
	或 LDH>正常值上限的 10 倍	

AFP,甲胎蛋白;HCG,绒促性素。

预后良好的转移性生殖细胞肿瘤患者的治疗

所有转移性生殖细胞肿瘤患者中，预后良好(good-risk)的患者约占56%。国际生殖细胞肿瘤预后分级系统(international germ cell consensus classification, IGCCC)对于低危患者的观点是，在该组患者当中，超过90%可以达到长期无病生存。

由于几乎所有这些患者都可以通过标准化疗达到完全缓解，所以这些试验目的在于减少化疗药物用量，进而减少急、慢性毒性反应，而同时仍然保持理想的治愈率。这些试验的结果有一些已经用于实际治疗，包括减少治疗持续时间，尽量使用单药毒性小的药物，以及减少化疗药物的用药种类。

东南癌症研究组(SECSG)开展了一项试验，将低危患者随机分为两组，分别接受3个周期和4个周期的BEP方案化疗[123]。两组患者获得了相同的完全缓解率，两组间没有差异，两组的无病生存率为92%，中位随访时间19个月。根据该研究结果，在印第安纳大学，采用3个疗程BEP方案化疗已经成为低危患者的标准治疗(顺铂20mg/m^2，依托泊苷100mg/m^2，静脉给药，第1天至第5天给药，每3周重复，博来霉素30单位每周静脉给药一次)。

东部肿瘤联合会(Eastern Cooperative Oncology Group, ECOG)完成了一项试验，将轻度或中度病变的患者随分为两组，分别给予3周期BEP方案，和EP方案进行化疗，以避免应用博来霉素带来的不良反应(也有可能是肺毒性)[124]。然而，接受博来霉素的患者有更高的存活率。欧洲癌症研究与治疗组织进行了一项试验，对于预后良好的非精原细胞瘤患者进行4个周期化疗，一组给予EP方案，另一组给予BEP方案[125]。在完全缓解率上，应用博来霉素组优于另一组(分别为95%和89%)，但两组复发率近似。在Memorial Sloan-Kettering癌症中心开展的一项随机试验中，预后良好的患者接受4个周期以VP-16(依托泊苷)为基础的联合化疗，一组为VP-16与顺铂联合(标准治疗组)，另一组为VP-16与卡铂联合[126]。需要补充的是，对于预后良好的患者，MRC/EORTC还对依托泊苷、博来霉素分别与顺铂和卡铂两种药物联合的治疗效果进行了对比[127,128]。在该研究中，卡铂的优势在于其较弱的肾脏毒性和神经毒性，而且该药可以用于门诊化疗，因为该药不需要水化预处理。试验结果显示，卡铂化疗组的生存率要低于顺铂组。Toner等人报道，与接受4个周期减量BEP化疗方案的患者相比，接受3周期标准剂量BEP化疗方案的患者生存率要明显占优[129]。总而言之，所有这些试图通过去除博来霉素或使用卡铂代替顺铂来达到进一步减少化疗毒性的临床试验，均得出一个同样的结论，即标准治疗方案的效果最好。

从预后良好患者的化疗方案中去除博来霉素的最后一次尝试来自法国的一项合作研究(French collabo-rative study)[130]。该试验招募了257名患者，他们被随机分配到三个周期的BEP或四个周期的EP(两种方案都使用5天的方案，每个周期500mg/m^{2}的依托泊苷)。该试验将257例患者随机分为两组，一组接受3周期BEP方案化疗，另一组接受4周期EP方案化疗(两种药物用法均为第一天至第五天给药，依托泊苷每个周期剂量为500mg/m^2)。在试验开始的时候，采用的是一项较旧的预后分级系统，导致该试验在生存分析方面略显不足，但是如果根据IGCCCC系统对患者重新进行分类的话，那4周期EP方案组患者发生不良结局的数量更多，死亡例数也更多。一个权威的临床试验，首先需要非常大的样本量，这样才能使两种方案之间的比较存在意义。实际上，在去除BEP组皮肤、神经毒性及EP组粒细胞减少和血小板减少的副反应之后，两组在化疗毒性方面并没有显著区别。在两组内均没有治疗相关死亡的发生，而且肺部毒性发生率也不存在显著差异。最终作者得出结论，对于预后良好的转移性生殖细胞肿瘤患者，采用标准"美国"剂量进行3个周期的BEP方案化疗(顺铂20mg/m^2，第1~5天；依托泊苷100mg/m^2，第1~5天；博来霉素30单位，第1、8、15天)，是目前最佳的治疗方案，而且完全没有必要进行更进一步的试验，单纯EP方案4周期化疗，在治疗效果上可能永远无法超过BEP方案。这一结论同样也体现在欧洲和加拿大的指南中，这些指南中，预后良好(IGCCC标准)的转移瘤患者的标准治疗是3周期BEP方案化疗。而且据我们所知，截至目前，对于预后良好的患者，已经没有其他大型的仍然进行中的临床研究继续对这一问题进行探讨。

即使更进一步减少药物剂量，也不太可能显著降低毒性，但却有可能降低治愈率。有学者曾尝试对BEP化疗方案给药时间做出调整。De Wit等人报道了一项来自欧洲癌症国际生殖细胞肿瘤预后分级系统研究与治疗组织和医学研究委员会的研究结果，患者分为两组，均接受3周期BEP方案化疗，一组依托泊苷用量为100mg/m^2，第1~5天；顺铂20mg/m^2，第1~5天。另一组依托泊苷用量165mg/m^2，第1~3天；顺铂用量50mg/m^2，第1~2天。两组的博来霉素均为每周给药。采用3日化疗方案的患者，耳毒性和胃肠道副反应轻度增高，长期生活质量评分和长期毒性作用无法评估。两种不同BEP给药方案的两年总生存率无显著差异，在HCG<1 000的患者当中，治愈率达到98%[131]。

预后中等的转移性病变治疗

1995年国际生殖细胞肿瘤预后分级系统Ⅰ对预后中等转移性病变进行了定义，但是当时可获得的研究很少。欧洲癌症研究与治疗组织(EORTC)开展了一项研究，比较了针对中等预后患者，使用EP加博来霉素(BEP)与使用异环酰胺(VIP)的疗效，发现二组的应答率和长期存活率相似，分别为83%和85%[132]。但是VIP方案容易导致导致急性血液毒性。通过与预后不良组对比分析，研究者发现相对BEP治疗方案，使用VIP方案治疗患者获益程度无显著差异，因而该研究中止于此[133]。在随后的研究中，研究者将紫杉醇加BEP(T-BEP)的组合与单独应用BEP方案进行了比较[134]，但遗憾的是该研究由于起效缓慢，未能显示出总体的生存益处，因而早早搁置了。总而言之，目前针对预后中等的转移性病变患者，由于没有开展其他大型研究，4个周期的BEP或4个周期的VIP仍然是治疗的标准。

"预后不良"的转移性肿瘤的治疗

对于预后不良的转移性睾丸癌患者，其治疗仍然是一个挑战对于此类患者究竟如何治疗，进行了各种各样的探索，其中一种方法是加大化疗剂量。

前临床前模型研究中发现，随顺铂剂量逐渐增加，患者的治疗反应也出现非常显著的变化。根据这一结果，设计了一系列临床试验，试图对于这类预后不良的转移性生殖细胞癌患者采用加大顺铂用量的方法来进行治疗。Ozols 等开展了项随机试验，对预后不良的睾丸癌患者采用高剂量顺铂方案化疗，并以标准 PVB 方案治疗组进行对照[135]。该研究中，共纳入 52 名预后不良患者，均进行了 2∶1的随机分配，具体方案为顺铂 40mg/m^2(标准剂量的 2 倍)，第 1~5 天，联合长春碱，博来霉素和依托泊苷，均采用标准剂量，对照组则采取经典 PVB 方案，顺铂剂量 20mg/m^2，第 1~5 天。在接受大剂量顺铂的治疗组，88%的患者达到完全缓解，而接受传统 PVB 方案治疗组患者，完全缓解率为 67%。而且，PVB 治疗组复发率较高，41%的患者病变复发，而在大剂量顺铂化疗组(联合博来霉素和 VP-16，PVeBV)复发率为 17%。最终，大剂量化疗组的患者有 68%能够维持无病生存状态，而标准治疗组仅 33%。遗憾的是，尽管治疗效果得到显著改善，但毒性作用发生率也显著增加。接受大剂量化疗的患者中，发生骨髓抑制和听力损害的患者显著增加，尽管治疗效果优于传统治疗，但究竟这一结局是由于增加了顺铂的治疗剂量，还是因为该治疗方案包含了依托泊苷，抑或其他原因，从该试验设计中无法得出结论。

对于采用高剂量顺铂治疗进展期转移性生殖细胞癌，有一项入选标准更为严格的试验，该试验由东南癌症研究会和西南肿瘤组(Southwest Oncology Group，SWOG)联合完成[136]。这项试验仅根据印第安纳分级系统对患者分级，并招募进展期患者。患者随机分为两组，所有患者都接受标准剂量依托泊苷和博来霉素治疗，但一组接受标准剂量顺铂(每天 20mg/m^2，连续 5 天)或大剂量顺铂(每天 40mg/m^2，连续 5 天)。共纳入 159 例晚期转移性生殖细胞癌患者，其中 153 个最终参与毒性反应评估。在接受大剂量化疗的 76 例患者中，52 例(68%)达到无病生存状态(仅单纯行化疗治疗，或者进行了后续手术治疗)。接受标准剂量治疗的患者 77 例，56 例(73%)达到无病生存(单纯化疗治疗或者通过手术切除残余病灶)。总而言之，接受大剂量顺铂治疗组的患者有 74%仍然存活，63%达到持续无病生存状态，相比之下，在标准治疗组，74%的患者存活，61%达到持续无病生存。需要指出的是，大剂量顺铂治疗组的患者，耳毒性、神经毒性、胃肠道毒性以及骨髓抑制发生率均显著增加。与 NCI 的研究结果正好相反，该试验的结果表明，与标准治疗方案相比，顺铂剂量的增加并不能带来治疗效果的获益。

在东南癌症研究会上述试验之后，东部肿瘤联合会(ECOG)又开展了另一项试验，试图用异环磷酰胺取代博来霉素[136]。共有 304 例进展期转移性睾丸肿瘤的患者进入该试验(均采用印第安纳分级系统)，患者随机分为二组，一组接受标准的四周期 BEP 方案化疗，另一组接受 4 周期 VIP 方案化疗，即依托泊苷(75mg/m^2，第 1~5 天)，异环磷酰胺(1.2g/m^2，第 1~5 天)，以及顺铂(20mg/m^2，第 1~5 天)。共有 290 例患者进行了毒性评估，286 例患者进行了治疗反应评估。完全缓解率 VIP 组 37%，BEP 组 31%反应较好(favorable response) VIP 组 63%，BEP 组 60%；2 年无复发率 VIP 组 64%，BEP 组 60%；2 年生存率(VIP 组 74%，BEP 组 71%)，两组之间无统计学差异。但 VIP 治疗组发生 3 级或更严重毒性作用的比例要显著高于 BEP 组，副反应主要集中于血液系统方面(P<0.000 1)。每组均有 5 例治疗相关性死亡发生。这一研究证实，对于高危生殖细胞肿瘤，VIP 方案的治疗效果并不优于标准的 BEP 治疗方案。

欧洲癌症研究与治疗组织(EORTC)和医学研究委员会(MRC)还有一项与此类似的试验，来评价异环磷酰胺在治疗高危生殖细胞肿瘤上的作用[137]。在这项试验当中，患者被随机分至 BEP/EP 组，或强化治疗组：即博来霉素，长春碱以及顺铂方案之后，再继续应用 VIP-B 方案。在疾病进展时间和总体生存率上两组之间并不存在差异。而在博来霉素，长春新碱和泼尼松(BOP)/VIP-B 组，发生 3 或 4 级骨髓抑制以及体重丢失的情况要更多一些。作者最终得出结论，强化 BOP/VIP-B 治疗方案毒性作用更大，但其治疗效果并无优越性。

还有一项高剂量强化治疗的方案的研究，包括顺铂、环磷酰胺、多柔比星、长春碱和博来霉素(CISCA-VB)，该研究将高危患者与包括中低风险患者进行随机试验，比较 CISCA-VB 与 BEP 方案。在高剂量的 ARM 中患者改善较少，但相反毒副作用较大[138]。

最近，GETUC 小组开展了一项随机试验，测试了在 BEP 化疗的第一个周期内的肿瘤标记物的下降。标记物下降慢于预期的患者被随机分为两组，一组接受标准 BEP 方案，另一组接受高剂量强化方案，包括博来霉素、紫杉醇、奥沙利铂、顺铂、异环磷酰胺和依托泊苷[139]。

结果提示高剂量组三年无进展生存率提高(59% vs 48%；P=0.05)。

对预后不良的患者采用高剂量化疗作为初始治疗

德国汉诺威和其他一些结构的研究人员，尝试对高危睾丸癌患者采用大剂量、重复性化疗，并联合应用生长因子(growth factors)及外周血始祖细(peripheral blood progenitor cell)支持治疗。

对于预后不良的转移性睾丸癌患者，给予顺铂 25~30mg/m^2，第 1~5 天；依托泊苷 100~250mg/m^2，第 1~5 天；异环磷酰胺 2g/m^2，第 1~5 天；每 22 天一个周期，共治疗 4 个周期[140]。在最大剂量水平时，需要同时给予生长因子和外周血祖细胞。在采取这些辅助治疗措施之后，大剂量化疗方案可以为患者耐受，同时避免出现导致减量的骨髓抑制、黏膜炎、肾毒性或神经毒性。然而，在最大剂量组的 32 名患者中，有 3 名患者为治疗相关性死亡。在 23 例可评价疗效的患者中，20 例(87%)达到无病状态，3 例复发。

在 Gustave Roussey 研究所开展的一项 115 例患者的随机试验中，对这些预后不良的睾丸癌患者进行随机分组，一组接受传统治疗，即顺铂、长春碱、依托泊苷以及伯莱霉素，而另一组也采取类似的治疗，但在上述方案结束之后，再给予一个周期的大剂量顺铂、依托泊苷和环磷酰胺疗程[141]。但最终结果显示，大剂量化疗组的治疗效果并不优于传统治疗组。

另有一项针对预后不良患者的大型临床试验，试验组患者接受 2 周期的标准 BEP 方案治疗后，再接受两个周期的极高剂量化疗，药物为卡铂、依托泊苷和环磷酰胺，对照组行 4 周期标准 BEP 方案治疗[142]。共 219 例患者参与该试验，其中标准 4

周期 BEP 治疗组患者 108 例,治疗中有 10 例死亡(大剂量组 6 例,标准 BEP 组 4 例)。大剂量组毒性较重。1 年持续完全缓解率大剂量组为 52%,标准 BEP 组为 48%($P=0.53$),两组间无显著性差异。

关于高危生殖细胞肿瘤,在欧洲有一项对比大剂量 VIP 方案与标准治疗的临床研究。该试验以 Schmoll 等人报道的 1/2 期临床试验结果作为基础[143]。共有 221 名患者纳入研究,其中以印第纳州"进展期肿瘤"为标准者 39 例,IGCCCG"不良预后"为标准 182 例。高剂量 VIP 组患者在接受 1 个周期的 VIP 方案化疗之后,继续给予 3~4 个周期的 6 梯度序贯高剂量 VIP 方案化疗,并每 3 周给予一次干细胞支持治疗。中位随访时间 4 年,对于"预后不良"组,2 年无进展生存率和疾病特异性生存率分别是 69%和 79%,5 年时为 68%和 73%,原发病变位于性腺/后腹膜者 76%,原发部位位于纵隔者 67%。严重的毒性作用包括,治疗相关死亡(4%),急性髓细胞性白血病(1%),长期肾功能损伤(3%),慢性肾功能不全(1%)。

化疗后手术治疗

介绍

转移性睾丸癌在化疗后通过手术切除残余病灶,是睾丸癌多学科联合治疗的重要组成部分。根据诊断时的分期结果,有 20%~50%接受化疗的转移性睾丸癌患者,存在明显的后腹膜残余病变,需要行手术治疗才能够达到完全治愈。这些较大的残余病变包绕在腹腔重要结构周围,而且由于化疗后严重纤维瘢痕的形成,使化疗后手术变得无比困难且充满挑战。所以这些手术应当在较大的中心由经验丰富的医师完成。

化疗后腹膜后淋巴结清扫(PC-RPLND)的适应证

只有当血清肿瘤标记物降至正常或持续稳定时,才应考虑化疗后手术。一般情况下,影像学证据提示化疗后尚有参与病灶是行 PC-RPLND 的典型适应证。尽管在适应证上精原细胞瘤与非精原细胞瘤尚有一些不同。一般而言,肿瘤标记物已降至正常,且腹膜后病完全缓解的患者被认为复发的风险较低,一般不需要手术[144]。但是一些学者也提倡,对所有非精原细胞瘤患者,都应行 PC-RPLND,因为即使肿瘤标志物正常,影像学提示完全缓解的患者,仍然有残存畸胎瘤和生殖细胞肿瘤的可能[145]。PC-RPLND 应该在最后一个化疗周期结束后 4~6 周进行,以使患者各项化验恢复正常。影像学检查需要包括胸部、腹部和骨盆的 CT 扫描,并尽量接近手术,以进一步确认腹膜后残留病的持续存在。

非精原细胞瘤

针对非精原细胞瘤,尽管虽绝大多数学者推荐化疗后切除"残余"病灶,但对于淋巴结大小标准尚无共识。化疗后判断残余淋巴组织确切大小往往非常困难,因为淋巴结往往已经与后腹膜融为一体。对于化疗后 C 扫描的结果,究竟什么样才算是"正常"仍无定论[146]。有研究报道,化疗后存留的微小病灶中(直径≤2cm),有高达 1/3 可能含有残存的畸胎瘤或者生殖细胞肿瘤成分[147]。目前尚缺乏可靠的影像学检查手段或预测模型,可以准确识别化疗后残余畸胎瘤或生殖细胞肿瘤成分残留[148]。氟-18 脱氧葡萄糖(^{18}F-FDG)正电子发射断层扫描(FDG-PET)在非精原生殖细胞肿瘤化疗后残余病灶的判断中作用有限,因为该检查不能区分纤维化和畸胎瘤。尽管 PET 扫描阳性高度提示肿瘤残留的,但据报道假阴性率高达 40%[149]。所以,一线化疗后如果影像学检查能够发现明确的病灶,目前绝大多数专家仍然同意行 PC-RPLND。对于睾丸根治性切除标本内发现畸胎瘤成分的患者,畸胎瘤残留的概率增加;针对这类患者,化疗后一旦发现残存病灶,均应考虑行 PC-RPLND[147]。针对血清 AFP 升高,原发肿瘤中的畸胎瘤含有畸胎瘤成分的患者,如果化疗后发现腹膜后囊性肿块,也应当行 PC-RPLND,而不是挽救性化疗。Beck 等证实,囊性畸胎瘤会导致不同程度的 HCG 和 AFP 水平升高,并这些标志物可能渗入血液,这解释了为什么此类患者肿瘤标志物会升高[150]。由于畸胎瘤很少会侵犯腔静脉并伴有肿瘤血栓,这不应被误认为是深静脉血栓[151]。

精原细胞瘤

精原细胞瘤患者在接受以顺铂为基础的化疗之后,再发现确切残余病灶的概率并不高。化疗后行 CT 扫描常显示包绕下腔静脉和/或腹主动脉周围的薄片样组织,并需要很长时间才能消退[152]。在残余病灶体积大于 3cm 的患者中,20%可能会含有不同成分的肿瘤残余,而在残余病变小于 3cm 的患者中,基本上无肿瘤残余[153]。由于在纯精原细胞瘤中不存在残留畸胎瘤成分,如果针对此类患者化疗后的残留疾病常规行 PC-RPLND,将导致约 80%的患者过度治疗。对泌尿科医生而言,在这种情况下,PC-RPLND 将极具挑战,并且导致术中联合脏器切除和并发症的发生率更高[154]。为了尽可能降低手术的并发症,许多学者致力于研究 FDG-PET 在判断 FDG-PET 的作用。在一项多中心研究("SEMPET"试验)中,对 51 例患者的 56 次 PET 扫描结果进行了分析,所有患者在化疗后都通过 CT 检查证实存在腹部残余病变,病灶大小在 1~11cm 之间。病变大于 3cm 的患者共 19 例,PET 检查全部判断正确,≤3cm 者 37 例,其中 35 例 PET 检查判断正确。PET 检查在残余病变判断中的敏感性、特异性以及阳性预测价值分别是 80%,100% 和 100%[155]。然而并非所有研究都证实了 PET 的可靠性,目前有一些关于 PET 假阳性的报告[156,157]。然而,要想探明化疗后参与组织中究竟有无肿瘤参与,PET 检查可能是目前最好的无创性检查手段。精原细胞瘤化疗后残留肿块是否切除仍有争议,应注定个体化治疗方案。对于 PET 扫描阳性患者,进一步处置方案包括积极监测、活检、手术切除或放疗。

手术范围

PC-RPLND 是一项对手术技巧要求很高的手术。目前手术切除的界限仍然存在争议。尽管对于分期较早的肿瘤,可能保留神经的改良术式更适用,但一些学者发现,在进展期病变患者中,有一些患者肿瘤已经超过该术式的切除范围。在一项包含 113 例患有巨大的腹膜后肿瘤患者的研究中,研究者发现如果仅行改良术式切除残余病变的话,9 例患者(8%)发生了腹膜后肿瘤残余。一项研究对比了 62 例患者的改良性和完全性双侧 PC-RPLND 的结果,该研究基于切除肿块的冷冻病理检查,冰冻切片提示坏死的患者(37 例中),行改良术式;对于那些有畸胎瘤或残余肿瘤成分的患者,行双侧完全性淋巴结清扫。中位随访 6 年,在行局限性切除的患者中,有一例发生腹膜后畸胎瘤复发。术中冷冻与最终病理结果的吻合率为 89%[158]。在一项纳入 50 个 PC-RPLND 标本的研究中,研究者发现发病变位于左侧且体积较小者,其回流途径仍遵循常规途径,按照左侧肿瘤切除范围行改良术式切除结果较为满意;而原发肿瘤位于右侧者,则有 20% 的概率转移至对侧。重要的是,在平均随访了 53 个月之后,并没有发现术区内复发[159]。Carver 等回顾了 532 例转移性非精原生殖细胞肿瘤而行 PC-RPLND 治疗的病例之后,发现 7%~32%的患者行改良术式后,发生手术区域外病变。有趣的是,残留肿块小于 1cm 的患者中有 2 例发生(8%)手术区域外转移[160]。因此,似乎最为稳妥的选择是在化疗后进行双侧完全淋巴结清扫,进而改良术式仅在原发病变位于左侧且体积较小时可以考虑。

手术入路应根据肿块的大小和位置来确定。对于大多数肿块,采用正中切口即可;而对于较大的病变以及需要清扫至肾门水平以上的病变,最好的入路可能是胸腹联合切口或将正中切口沿至肋软骨交界处。胸腹联合切口还可以同时切除同侧的肺部病灶。需要注意的是,PC-RPLND 的患者有 20%可能会需要联合脏器切除。最为常见的情况是术中同时切除左肾,偶尔也可能需要切除下腔静脉或腹主动脉并以人工移植物替代[161]。尽管行胸腹联合切口可以同时处理胸部病变和进行 PC-RPLND,但对于较为复杂的纵隔病变,推荐二期手术,以减少并发症。在腹膜后清扫标本中发现纤维化并不能排除胸部病变,因为高达 20% 的患者可能存在胸部畸胎瘤或者残余肿瘤[162]。

在手术量较多的中心,PC-RPLND 并发症发生率高于一般的腹膜后淋巴结清扫(7%~30%),死亡率约为 1%[163,164]。化疗后患者所发生的并发症最多见的还是与博来霉素相关的肺毒性。逆向射精仍然是个常见的并发症,尽管对于病变较小的患者可以行保留神经的手术(该术式能够使 80%的患者保留射精功能)[165,166]。

病理

通过对化疗后手术切除的标本进行组织病理学分析,决定了是否需要采取进一步治疗和今后的监测方案的。研究发现,标本内残余肿瘤的概率较之前有所降低,可能的原因包括:化疗方案的优化和对手术患者更为合理地选择。通过对进展期非精原生殖细胞肿瘤的患者行诱导化疗后手术切除的标本进行病理检查发现:坏死占 40%~50%,畸胎瘤为 35%~40%,癌细胞残余为 10%~15%[167]。行挽救化疗后的手术标本显示,癌细胞残存的概率增加至 50%[168]。对于术后在残余病灶内发现癌细胞的患者,推荐接受两个周期的术后化疗,2/3 的患者仍然能达到长期无病生存[136]。然而,对于手术无法切除的患者、部分切除或肿瘤标志物升高的患者应考虑进行全剂量挽救性化疗。

"绝望的"腹膜后淋巴结清扫

对于诱导化疗后肿瘤标志物升高的患者,在行挽救性化疗后仍进展但其腹膜后病变具备可手术条件时,有可能行所谓的"绝望 PC-RPLND"。这些患者通常对化疗耐药,因此手术切除可能是唯一获得治愈的办法。对于此类患者行 PC-RPLND,往往极具挑战性,常常需要切除邻近的器官,甚至腹部大血管,并且往往生存率很低。尽管肿瘤标记物升高,但高达 50%的患者的手术标本中出现成熟畸胎瘤成分或坏死/纤维化[169]。在切除标本中发现生殖细胞恶性肿瘤残余的患者,1/3 的患者可以长期无病生存[170]。但是,切除不完全的患者往往预后较差,所以行此类手术,对患者选择应慎重。

精原细胞瘤的化疗

当前的化疗研究表明,对于Ⅱ期或Ⅲ期转移性精原细胞瘤患者,化疗治愈率超过 90%[62]。与早期相关放疗研究相比,放疗的治愈率从 20%到 60%,因此基于顺铂的化疗是首选的治疗方法,标准的初始治疗仍然是顺铂组合。

累及肺外脏器的转移性精原细胞瘤治疗效果欠佳,属于中危组[126]。预后良好的患者一般需要接受 3 周期 BEP 方案化疗,而预后中等的患者需要接受 4 个周期的 BEP 方案化疗。

此外,当完成基于顺铂的联合化疗后,如影像学检查发现对有残余病灶,该如何处理这一问题,目前仍存在争议。Motzer 等报道,在 41 例占位型Ⅱ期、Ⅲ期或Ⅳ期病变的患者中,给予基于顺铂的联合化疗治疗后[171],有 23 例患者复查影像学,提示有明显的残余病灶,其中 14 例病灶≥3cm。在这 23 例患者中,有 19 例接受了手术探查,除了 5 例纤维化以外,还发现了 4 例精原细胞瘤和 1 例畸胎瘤。学者推荐,精原细胞瘤化疗后,如影像学提示病灶残余≥3cm,应穿刺活检。

印第安纳大学以及其他一些中心,选择不同的治疗策略。在这种情况下行手术治疗是极其困难的,因为一般情况下,术中都会遇到严重的瘢痕粘连。再者,这类患者往往年龄较大,有些时候除了化疗也可能接受过腹部放疗,在一些研究的结果中提到,这类患者手术死亡率更高[171]。一份印第安纳州的开展的关于精原细胞瘤回顾性研究报道,如果化疗后影像学提示残留病灶>3cm,此种情况患者仅有 10%的复发率[172]。但该研究指出,并没有证据表明复发风险与残余肿块的直径有关。印第安纳大学针对此种情况,给出的建议是密切观察。

对于使用 PET 扫描预测纯精原细胞瘤>3cm 患者化疗后残留的肿瘤仍存在争议[173]。目前广泛认可,相对保守的策略是,根据病变大小和活检结果进行评估并制订后续治疗方案。对于接受全身化疗后残余病灶<3cm 的患者,一般采取密切观察。而对于残余病变大于或等于 3cm 的患者,则需接受 PET 扫描。如果 PET 检查结果阴性,那么则选择密切观察,并不做过多的介入。而如果 PET 检查发现较大的阳性病变,则需要行活检或手术切除,之后根据病理结果来决定下一步治疗。

以往对于化疗后残留病灶,常考虑进行放射;然而,这些肿块中很少残留精原细胞瘤成分。此外,如果化疗尚且不能治愈患者的话,放疗的效果也需思虑再三。需要补充的是,当同时采用化疗和放疗时,包括白血病在内的长期并发症的风险也会增加。因此,不推荐对残余肿块进行放疗[40]。

挽救性化疗

对于转移性生殖细胞肿瘤,尽管化疗疗效显著,但仍有 20%~30%的患者无法通过一线治疗达到持续完全缓解[174]。这类患者,与那些达到完全缓解后再次复发的患者一样,适合接受挽救性化疗。由于二线化疗药物的效果降低，而毒性作用增加，因此对于这类患者，采用挽救性化疗是一项非常重要的决定；因为对这类患者的病情评估以及各种治疗选择错综复杂，所以对医师的治疗经验要求较高。

患者选择

有几种临床情况可能与持续，进展或复发性疾病相混淆。一种情况是，在化疗结束时或完成后不久，胸片或者胸部 CT 发现结节病变[1]。这些结节可能是由于博来霉素所导致的肺损伤，其特征是结节位于胸膜下区域。所以患者接受治疗后，血清学或影像学对治疗有反应，而在肺部却发现除原有病变外的新发病变，这时就要考虑到这种可能性。

另一种经常被误诊为肿瘤进展的情况是畸胎瘤增长综合征(syndrome of growing teratoma)[175]。在化疗过程中如果影像学检查发现持续增大的转移病灶，同时伴有正常或逐渐降至正常的血清肿瘤标志物，往往提示畸胎瘤。对此类患者，恰当的治疗手段是通过是手术切除影像学提示的残留病灶，而不是挽救化疗。

总之，在肿瘤标志物出现明确的持续升高之前，对于挽救性化疗应当持保守态度。肿瘤标志物轻度升高可能会有其他原因，有可能导致错误解读。因此，务必注意不要因为患者肿瘤标志物的假阳性升高而给予强烈的挽救性化疗。

在全身持续缓解但血清肿瘤标志物仍然升高的情况下，应考虑中枢神经系统(central nerve system, CNS)隐匿性转移病变的可能。在这种情况下，应进行 CT 扫描或 MRI 检查，同时评估睾丸侵犯情况。如果进展性疾病的唯一证据是上升的标记物，即使没有临床体征或症状，也应进行 CNS 评估。

对于生殖细胞肿瘤，睾丸本身也是化疗的一个重要的避难所。在绝大多数情况下，睾丸中的原发病变在诊断过程中已被手术根治性切除。然而，在一些进展期病变的患者中，有时在并没有取得病理学诊断的情况下就已经开始化疗了。在这种情况下，在化疗结束时应当切除睾丸，即便可能已经没有原发肿瘤存在的证据。同时，需要考虑到对侧睾丸发生肿瘤的可能性。

挽救性治疗的预后因素

二线治疗患者临床预后因素的重要性，在最近几年逐步为人们所认知[176,177]。迄今为止，由于各研究所选研究对象之间存在异质性，所以报道的常规剂量化疗和大剂量化疗最终结局差异很大。对于原发肿瘤位于性腺的患者，如果对顺铂化疗敏感，一线化疗后能够达到完全缓解而后再次复发，其在接受常规剂量的挽救性治疗后往往更有可能获得一个比较理想的治疗结果，反之，对于顺铂化疗耐药，或对一线化疗反应不完全，以及原发肿瘤位于纵隔者，其治疗结局要差些[178]。Einhorn 等最近报道了耐药性病变，原发肿瘤分期较晚，以及大剂量化疗(第三次或更晚)的时间，是不利的预后因素[179]。根据这些危险因素将患者分为低危、中位和高危预后组，其长期存活率分别约 80%、60% 和 40%。国际预后因素研究小组针对肿瘤复发患者，效仿针对尚未接受治疗的患者的 IGCCCG 分类系统，制订了相似的预后分类，其中包括从世界各地的高手术量中心收集的近 2 000 名复发患者的临床数据[180]。基于多变量分析中的七个重要因素：包括组织学(精原细胞瘤与非精原细胞瘤)，原发肿瘤部位(纵隔与腹膜后与性腺)，对一线化疗的反应(CR 与 PR 与其他)，一线化疗后的无进展时间，诊断复发时的 AFP 和 HCG 水平，以及是否存在非肺脏器转移，该模型能够很好地区分由非常低到非常高五个不同的风险组。由于该模型样本量大，囊括国际几大中心患者数据，因而该模型可以广泛运用，目前被认为是评估复发患者预后的新标准模型。

标准挽救性治疗

以顺铂为基础的一线化疗后复发的患者，相较于初发患者，治疗效果要更差一些，最主要的原因是：对于顺铂耐药的病变能起到治疗作用的药物很少。在引入顺铂治疗的最初 30 年里，仅少数药物可能对顺铂耐药患者有效，包括依托泊苷(VP-16)、异环磷酰胺(ifosfamide)、紫杉醇(paclitaxel)、吉西他滨(gemcitabine)以及奥沙利铂(oxaliplatin)。患者对传统挽救性治疗的反应率约为 50%，要明显低于一线治疗。仅 20%~30% 的患者能得到长期缓解。

挽救性化疗最初的治疗方案由印第安纳大学提出，即长春碱，异环磷酰胺和顺铂(VeIP 方案)[181]。共 13 例在以顺铂为基础的化疗期间无进展的患者接受了 VeIP 方案作为最初的挽救性化疗。在这些接受过化疗的患者中，再次化疗的毒性作用非常显著，有 71% 的患者发生了粒细胞减少相关发热。需要输注血小板(27%)和红细胞(49%)的情况很常见。有 7% 的患者发现肾功能不全(血清肌酐>4mg%)。有三名患者因治疗相关原因死亡。尽管毒性作用令人望而生畏，但治疗结果却相对满意。56 例患者(45%)达到无病生存状态，其中 34 例仅单纯行化疗治疗(25%)，15 例患者行残余畸胎瘤手术切除(12%)，7 例患者行残余癌灶切除(6%)。在这些患者中有 32 例(24%)达到持续无病生存状态，42 例(32%)目前仍为无病生存(最短随访时间为 5 年)。对于原发病变位于性腺以外的 31 例患者，仅 6 例达到无病生存状态，而且仅有 1 例为持续无病生存。这些结果已经被其他研究证实[182]。

Memorial Sloan-Kettering 癌症中心的研究人员对二线药物治疗进行了探索，选取预后良好的复发性睾丸肿瘤患者，进行紫杉醇联合异环磷酰胺及顺铂(TIP)方案化疗[183]。在该研究中，共 30 例患者，其中 23 例(77%)对单纯化疗完全反应(complete response)，有一例患者获得了持续部分缓解，且肿瘤标志物水平正常。仅有 2 例患者复发，而且绝大多数患者都能够耐受治疗。这项研究强调，对于标准挽救性治疗如果希望获得较理想的效果，患者的选择至关重要。接下来的研究进一步证实了这一结果，TIP 方案也逐渐成为一项广泛应用的标准挽救性治疗方案[184,185]。

其他研究结果表示，复发性精原细胞瘤可能对挽救化疗特别敏感。Miller 等报告在第一次行顺铂/依托泊苷化疗后复发的精原细胞瘤患者，给予 VeIP 方案化疗[186]，在 23 例患者中，19 例(83%)达到无病生存状态，13 例(56%)为持续无病生存。

高剂量化疗作为初始挽救性治疗

曾经有学者采取大剂量化疗作为挽救性化疗的初始治疗方案，此类研究最早见于英国哥伦比亚癌症中心(British Columbia Cancer Agency)Barnett 等人的报道。18 例接受以顺铂为基础化疗后生殖细胞肿瘤复发，或者未完全缓解的患者，首先给予每周常规化疗，包括顺铂、依托泊苷、长春新碱以及博来霉素，或者给予长春碱、异环磷酰胺以及顺铂方案治疗[187]。在常规挽救性化疗结束后，再给予大剂量化疗巩固疗效，同时给予自体造血干细胞移植治疗进行支(autologous bone marrow support)。大剂量治疗方案选择卡铂、依托泊苷、环磷酰胺或者异环磷酰胺。有 2 例患者因毒性作用死亡，还有 2 例患者因时间太短无法进行评估，在 14 例生殖细胞癌的患者中有 8 例仍然无病情进展。

Siegert 等报告了对患者使用大剂量卡铂、依托泊苷和异环磷酰胺的治疗情况[188]。患者在接受强化治疗之前，先接受两个周期常规剂量顺铂、依托泊苷和异环磷酰胺诱导治疗。74 例患者接受常规治疗，给予之后卡铂 1 500~2 000mg/m^2，依托泊苷 1 200~2 400mg/m^2，异环磷酰胺 0~10g/m^2。2 例(3%)因治疗相关原因死亡。在单纯化疗或化疗辅以手术治疗后，21 例患者(28%)完全缓解，14 例患者(19%)部分缓解但肿瘤标志物阴性。在这些患者中，有 25 例(34%)对治疗持续反应，维持时间 31~261 个月。

过去有一项关于常规诱导化疗后给予单周期高剂量化疗的随机试验。纳入患者为预后良好，其中绝大多数患者原发部位位于性腺或腹膜后，病理类型为生殖细胞肿瘤，并且所有患者之前都通过铂类联合化疗获得了完全或部分缓解。患者被随机分为 2 组，一组接受四个周期的 VIP 化疗或 VeIP 治疗，另一组首先接受三个周期的 VIP 治疗，然后给予一个周期的大剂量治疗，包括卡铂，依托泊苷和环磷酰胺。1 年无事件生存率和 3 年生存率(分别为 35%和 42%，结果更倾向于高剂量化疗组)，两组治疗结果均不令人满意，尤其是大剂量组[189]。

随着外周干细胞移植技术的发展，现在 2 或 3 个周期的大剂量化疗变得可行。Motzer[190]等人报道，在 37 例对顺铂耐药和预后不良的患者中，在接受两个周期的常规 TIP 化疗方案后，再给予三个周期的大剂量卡铂和依托泊苷治疗，长期无病生存率为 41%。

另有一项关于高剂量化疗的研究方案为，试验组在一个周期的 VIP 方案化疗后再给予 3 周期连续高剂量卡铂和依托泊苷治疗，对照组在 3 周期 VIP 方案化疗后给予单周期高剂量卡铂、依托泊苷和环磷酰胺治疗[191]。研究将患者随机分配至两个治疗组(不同预后因素的患者在两组间平衡分布)。生存率在两组之间并没有显著差别。对于这两种高剂量化疗方案能否适用于任何特殊人群，该试验无法给出答案。然而，与 3 种药物单周期治疗方案相比，2 种药物治疗方案的并发症发生率和死亡率均较低，而且有 10%对顺铂耐药的患者达到了长期生存。

在印第安纳大学，自 1989 年以来，共有 184 名患者接受了挽救性大剂量化疗。170 例患者接受了两个连续周期的高剂量卡铂和依托泊苷治疗，有 110 例患者在接受高剂量化疗之前接受了 1~2 周期的常规减瘤化疗，包括长春碱、顺铂和异环磷酰胺。只要技术上可行，所有患者化疗后残余病变均可以手术切除。总体上，长期无病生存率 63%。在 40 例进展期转移性病变且对铂类耐药的患者中，有 18 例仍然能够达到无病生存，中位随访时间 49 个月，更加进一步证实了对于相当一部分患者，高剂量化疗能够克服顺铂耐药这一问题。

国际预后因素小组开展了第二个大型的回顾性分析，共纳入 1 594 名接受 SCD-CT 或 SHD-CT 治疗的患者。在所有亚组的分析结果，都支持 SHD-CT 疗效[192]。

总而言之，高剂量化疗对复发的生殖细胞癌患者疗效很好，并且在年轻和健康的患者中，而且对于合适的患者，其并发症发生率尚能接受，且死亡率较低。虽然最佳的治疗药物仍然有待商榷，但进行 1~2 个周期的常规化疗之后序贯 2~3 周期卡铂/依托泊苷高剂量化疗，却是个很好的选择。高剂量化疗对于预后较差的患者是一项有效的治疗，但对于预后良好的患者，其治疗作用仍然存在争议。然而，考虑到并发症及死亡率均较低，而治疗效果显著，相对于传统挽救性治疗，高剂量化疗对于这类患者也是一个不错的选择。由于该疾病的复杂性以及治疗的特殊性，而且需要多学科紧密合作，包括内科肿瘤医师，泌尿外科医师以及放疗肿瘤医师，所有的患者都应当到专门的中心进行诊治。

多处复发生殖细胞肿瘤的治疗

生殖细胞肿瘤多处复发的高剂量化学治疗

对大剂量卡铂(CBCDA)和依托泊苷(VP-16)联合自体骨造血干细胞移植治疗的研究，最早于 1986 年开始。最初的研究对象，是那些已经经历过各种治疗，并且没有其他治疗选择的患者。

最初的 1/2 期高剂量治疗研究，探索了两个周期高剂量 CBDCA 和 VP-16 治疗在顺铂耐药的生殖细胞肿瘤患者(在最后一次顺铂治疗 4 周后或 4 周以内，发现疾病进展)或顺铂治疗后及异环磷酰胺-顺铂挽救性治疗后再次复发的患者中的应用[193]。共有 33 例患者，总体上，7 例患者(21%)因治疗原因死亡。死亡原因主要是感染，有 1 例患者死于肝脏静脉阻塞性疾病。需要指出的是，这类患者在之前都已经接受过各种治疗，有超过半数的患者在之前都已经接受过 3~4 种化疗药物治疗，而且有 67%的患者对顺铂耐药。结果显示，8 例患者获得了完全缓解，6 例患者部分缓解，对治疗的总反应率为 44%(95%*CI*:27%~63%)。在获得完全缓解的 8 例患者中，3 例达到长期无病生存，第 4 例患者在第 22 个月时死亡，但去世时并没有生殖细胞肿瘤复发的证据，而是死于治疗相关性急性髓细胞性白血病[194]。印第安纳大学一项总结研究发现，对 49 例肿瘤多发性复发并产生耐药的生殖细胞肿瘤患者，采取双重自体移植(double autologous transplantation)，结果长期无病生存率为 45%，中位随访时间 46 个月。

其他研究

关于睾丸癌多发行复发后使用高剂量化疗的其他研究结果，也得出了与此近似的几个结论。第一点，针对顺铂耐药或生殖细胞癌复发的患者，大剂量的化疗可以使治愈率达到 15%~20%。在经历了≥2 常规药物治疗方案失败后，大剂量的化疗可作为首选治疗。第二点，对于这类先前经过大量药物治疗的患者，目前死亡率<5%。第三点，对于高剂量挽救性治疗药物，目前没有统一标准。第四点，在所有这些研究中，纵隔原发非精原细胞瘤的患者预后极差，而且这类患者无法从高剂量化疗中获益。

挽救性(“绝望”)手术

对于一些患者而言,挽救性手术治疗可能比挽救性化疗更加有意义,尤其是对于那些晚期复发或者复发部位局限在某一个区域的患者。印第安纳大学曾经做过一项回顾性研究,研究对象为化疗耐药并且之后接受手术以期达到治愈性切除的患者[195]。所有的患者都有血清学或者其他肿瘤进展的证据。共48例患者,其中绝大部分只接受了腹膜后淋巴结切除(33例)。在这些患者中,38例(79%)通过手术去除了肉眼可见病变,29例(60%)达到血清学缓解。10例(21%)达到持续无病生存状态,随访时间31~89个月。只有那些病变局限在某一区域,而且在手术时能够达到完全切除的患者,通过这种治疗方法能够获益。对于有多发转移的患者,尽管可以通过手术切除,但无法达到治愈。Albers等人也曾经报道过,对于肿瘤标志物持续升高的患者,行挽救性手术治疗可以达到很高的长期无病生存率[196]。挽救性手术治疗可以达到一个非常不错的长期无病生存。这种治疗决策只能由对生殖细胞肿瘤富有经验的中心做出。总体来讲,挽救性手术患者的选择应当包含以下几点,在最初对治疗达到完全反应后(无论是一线治疗抑或是二线治疗)肿瘤标志物缓慢升高;影像学检查发现1~2处残余病变;试过所有化疗方案均无效,而且标志物持续升高、病变可以切除的患者[197]。

新药

新药的研发可能真正改变对复发或耐药性生殖细胞肿瘤患者的治疗预期,甚至包括预后不良的患者。已经有一些药物显示出了单药治疗作用,包括奥沙利铂[198],紫杉醇和吉西他滨。东部肿瘤联合会(ECOG)的一项Ⅱ期试验中,对30例耐药性生殖细胞肿瘤的患者,采取紫杉醇联合吉西他滨方案治疗[199]。治疗的总反应率为21.4%,有3例患者完全缓解,有2例患者达到持续无病生存,时间分别为15个月和25个月。关于奥沙利铂联合吉西他滨的方案目前共有3项研究,治疗的反应率分别为16%、32%和46%[200~202]。所有这些研究都有长期存活的病例,尤其是同时通过手术切除残余病变的患者。目前靶向药物治疗尚处于临床研究阶段。

特殊情况

晚期复发

经治疗后完全缓解的转移性睾丸癌患者,其复发大多数发生在治疗后的第一年,绝大多数发生在2年内。而关于晚期复发目前比较公认的标准是:治疗后无病生存期超过24个月,在此之后发生的复发。在完全缓解后,发生晚期复发的概率为2%~3%,目前已知在达到完全缓解后,晚期复发最迟者可长达32年。

总体来讲,复发为孤立成熟畸胎瘤者,手术治疗大多效果满意;而肿瘤标志物升高者、转移患者和/或肿瘤病理类型转变者,往往预后较差。至于从未接受过化疗的患者,无论是积极监测后的复发或事腹膜后淋巴结清扫后的复发,给予以顺铂为基础的化疗治疗都能获得较好的效果,即使复发超过3年[75]。

在印第安纳大学,对81名在无病生存达到2年或更长时间后复发的生殖细胞肿瘤患者进行了回顾性分析[203]。有60%的患者在5年以后复发(最大为32年)。可以发现血清肿瘤标志物升高,其中56%的患者AFP升高,27%的患者HCG升高。另外,15例(19%)畸胎瘤复发,8例持续无病生存,4例患者在接受进一步手术之后目前为无病生存状态(271~1 021个月)。7名患者复发为肉瘤样成分(伴或不伴畸胎瘤);4名患者为无病生存。59例患者复发为生殖细胞癌。在这些患者中仅10例(17%)为持续无病生存(101~781个月)。另有9例患者目前为无病生存。所有这些患者几乎都需要手术治疗。总体上,有65例患者接受了以顺铂为基础的化疗,17例(26%)达到无病生存状态(单纯化疗,或者化疗辅以手术治疗),17例中有12例发生复发。仅有2例单纯化疗的患者达到持续无病生存状态(这2例患者之前都没有接受过化疗)。在印第安纳大学还有另一项77例患者的研究,结果与此近似[204]。

Sharp等回顾了75例发生晚期复发生殖细胞肿瘤的患者。在此研究中,晚期复发的中位时间为6.9年(范围2.1~37.7年)。总的来说,56名患者(75%)复发部位在腹膜后。5年癌症特异性生存率为60%(95%*CI*:46%~71%)。在晚期复发时行完全手术切除的患者($n=45$)的,5年癌症特异性生存率为79%,而未完全切除的患者为36%($n=30$;$P<0.000\ 1$)。对于之前未行化疗的患者,5年肿瘤特异性生存率要显著优于曾接受化疗的患者(5年肿瘤特异性生存率分别为93%和49%)。该研究所选取的患者均为晚期复发患者,但该研究的结果究竟能不能代表所有晚期复发患者,目前并不清楚。尽管如此,这些和其他数据表明,这些患者在晚期复发后可以获得长期生存或达到治愈。在之前没有经历过化疗的患者,通过标准顺铂方案化疗并辅以化疗后手术治疗大多能够达到无病生存状态。这些研究的共同观点是,对于复发病灶含有非典型卵黄囊成分的晚期复发患者,如果AFP升高并且以前曾接受过化疗的话,且病变局限在某一区域,最佳治疗方法是手术治疗。

尽管晚期复发相对罕见(2年以上者1%~3%),但这些数据提示,目前对于睾丸癌患者仍然推荐终身随访。

化疗的长期毒性

自20世纪70年代中期以来,大多数转移性睾丸癌患者已经通过联合化疗达到治愈,无论是否接受辅助手术治疗或放疗。治愈型治疗的晚期并发症也常见于其他恶性肿瘤,最显著的是霍奇金病(如不孕症,与治疗相关的继发性恶性肿瘤)。关于顺铂治疗的晚期并发症的关注也在逐渐增加,而且,现在随着随访时间的延长,已经有大批随访超过10年的患者可供分析。

肾毒性

顺铂对肾小球和肾小管功能的急性毒性作用已广泛报道,该药物可造成肾小球滤过率(GfR)和有效肾血浆流量(ERPF)降低,同时伴有镁流失。当发现β2-微球蛋白水平升高时,提示近端小管功能障碍。大多数研究人员报道,GFR和ERPF的急性下降在化疗完成后的几个月到几年内不会进一步恶化;然而,长期亚临床损害经常出现[205~207]。

血管毒性

雷诺现象是睾丸癌化疗后最常见的血管毒性反应。自开始应用博来霉素单药治疗后，此现象就多有报道，但更常见于联合治疗。Vogelzang 等人发现，在长春碱联合博来霉素治疗的患者中，该现象发生率为 21%，在这两种药物基础上再加上顺铂，发生率为达到 41%[208]。研究发现，即使在无症状的患者当中，在冷刺激下，也可以激发血管收缩反应[208]。症状持续时间不一定，据一项研究的报道，49% 的患者化疗结束后症状持续存在一段时间后消退，中位时间 8.5 年。总体来讲，血管痉挛对治疗反应不佳，尽管曾有应用钙离子拮抗剂硝苯地平（nifedipine）治疗成功的报道[209]。将长春碱换为 VP-16，再与顺铂和博来霉素联合治疗，并没有降低雷诺现象的发生率[210]。

以顺铂为基础的化疗与大血管缺血事件的相关性，目前尚不清楚。曾经有长春碱单药治疗或联合博来霉素治疗后，发生心肌缺血和梗死以及脑血管事件的报道。还有一些年轻睾丸癌患者在接受化疗后发生重大心血管事件的报道，这提示化疗与这些事件之间可能存在相关性[122,211,212]。Weijl 等报道，肝脏转移及接受高剂量皮质醇治疗的患者，属于发生血栓栓塞并发症的高危人群[213]。在睾丸癌组间研究（testicular cancer intergroup study）中，为了评估患者在接受以顺铂为基础的化疗之后急性血管事件的风险，对该中心所有参与研究的患者分发了调查问卷，并从中收集化疗相关的毒性信息[213]。对于Ⅰ期的睾丸癌患者，在行腹膜后淋巴结清扫后，采取密切观察。而对病理Ⅱ期的患者进行随机分组，一组给予两个周期的术后辅助化疗（以顺铂为基础），而另一组选择观察。对于任何患者一旦出现复发迹象，则给予 4 个周期的辅助顺铂联合方案化疗。

对毒性作用进行回顾分析发现，接受辅助化疗（$n=97$）或因为复发接受化疗（$n=83$）的患者，没有急性心血管毒性事件发生。在中位随访时间 5.1 年之后，共寄出了 459 份问卷，收回了 270 份。对问卷做出回复的患者，在各个治疗组（观察组，辅助化疗组以及复发组）的分布比较平均（分别为 59%，54% 以及 64%）。在接受过化疗的两组患者中，发生肢端麻木的现象显著增多。在观察组有 2 例患者发生了致命性的心肌梗死，在辅助化疗组有一例心肌梗死报道，但属于非致命性的。在所有组里都没有患者发生脑卒中的报道。观察组 3 名患者，复发组 1 名患者，发生血栓栓塞事件。

其他以人群为基础的研究确实发现此类患者心血管疾病的发生风险增加，尤其顺铂累积剂量较高的患者。Fossa 等人对生存时间 1 年以上的 38 907 例睾丸癌患者进行了总结，该研究包括从 1943 年开始，北美和欧洲共 14 项以人群为基础的癌症研究[214]。他们利用这些研究的数据来计算非癌症死亡的标准化死亡比（standardized mortality ratios，SMR），并对病理结果、年龄、诊断时间及初始治疗与非癌症死亡的相关性进行评估。在中位随访时间 10 年之后，共有 2 942 例患者因各种原因导致非癌症死亡，超过了 6% 的总人群非癌症死亡率预期值（SMR＝1.06，95%*CI*：1.0～1.10）；无论患者诊断睾丸癌的时间在 1975 年之前还是之后，非癌症标准化死亡比并没有显著区别（1975 年之后以顺铂为基础的化疗方案才开始广为应用）。与总人群相比，睾丸癌患者非癌症相关死亡率更高，原因包括感染（SMR＝1.28，95%，*CI*：1.12～1.47）以及消化系统疾病（SMR＝1.44，95%*CI*：1.26～1.64）。在 35 岁之前诊断睾丸癌的患者，死于循环系统疾病的情况显著增加（1.23，95%*CI*：1.09～1.39）。但在年龄较大的男性患者中，却没有发现这一现象（SMR＝0.94；95%*CI*：0.89～1.00）。在 1975 年及 1975 年之后，接受化疗的男性（无论是否接受过放疗），死于癌症以外原因的比例增加（SMR＝1.34，95%*CI*：1.15～1.55），包括循环系统疾病（SMR＝1.58，95%*CI*：1.25～2.01），感染（SMR＝2.48，95%*CI*：1.70～3.50），以及呼吸系统疾病（SMR＝2.53，95%*CI*：1.26～4.53）。在 1975 年及之后，与总人群相比，年龄小于 35 岁并接受过放疗的睾丸癌患者死于循环系统疾病的概率增加（SMR＝1.70，95%*CI*：1.21～2.31）。

在对这些患者进行更长时间的随访后发现，高血压、糖耐量异常、血脂异常以及血管事件的发生都有所增加[215]。代谢综合征的发病与睾丸癌及接受顺铂联合方案化疗存在相关性[216]。

Haugnes 等在一项来自北欧国家的随访研究中，再次探索了这一问题（1998—2002）。该试验排除了所有大于 60 岁的患者，剩下 1 135 名患者符合条件。患者被分为 4 个治疗组：手术组（$n=225$）；放疗组（$n=446$）以及两个化疗组：顺铂累积剂量 850mg 组（$n=376$）和顺铂累积剂量大于 850mg 组（$n=88$）。并将来自 Tromsø 人群研究的 1 150 名男性作为对照组。根据改良的国际胆固醇教育计划（National Cholesterol Education Program）的定义来确定代谢综合征的诊断标准。与手术组相比，两个化疗组发生代谢综合征的概率均有所增加，顺铂剂量＞850mg 组发生率最高（OR 2.8，95%*CI*：1.6～4.7）。同样，顺铂＞850mg 组与对照组相比，发生代谢综合征的概率也有所增高（OR 2.1，95%*CI*：1.3～3.4）。在调整了睾酮、吸烟、体力活动、教育和家庭情况等影响因素后，代谢综合征和顺铂＞850mg 组间的相关性得到进一步加强。

睾丸癌患者需要进行终身随访。这类患者需要受到良好的医疗处置，包括体重控制，戒烟，监测血脂，以将血压控制在恰当范围内。患者和医师都需要认识到同一个问题，那就是在长期存活的睾丸癌患者中，心血管疾病的发生风险是持续存在的，不容乐观[217,218]。

神经毒性

睾丸癌患者的外周神经病变及耳毒性主要由顺铂副作用引起。在一些早期研究中发现长春碱可能也与神经毒性存在一定关系。外周神经病变在临床上表现为远端感觉性神经病变，包括麻痹和感觉异常，以及位置觉和振动觉失调，还有运动单位相对不足[219]。患者主观感觉这些症状可以长期存在。在一项研究中提到，有 43% 的患者在化疗结束后，仍感觉上述症状持续存在，时间为 6～12 年不等[220]。一项客观研究证实了这些神经病变是不可逆的，并且发现，背根神经节可能是顺铂导致损害的主要部位。

应用顺铂后导致的听力损害主要表现是高频听例丧失，并且主要与顺铂的累积剂量相关[221,222]。其他影响耳毒性的因素还包括，血清肌酐水平（高于 1.5mg/dl），年龄增加，以及既往存在基础听力损害等。

继发恶性肿瘤

继发性恶性睾丸肿瘤是目前排在首位的致死因素[223]。

Travis 等人总结了 14 项在欧洲和北美的存活时间超过 1 年以人群为基础的肿瘤学研究(1943—2001),共 40 576 例患者,在此生存期间,对新发的实体肿瘤均予以记录。在该研究中,共报道了 2 285 例继发性实体肿瘤。相对危险度以及年发病风险随着诊断睾丸癌的年龄增加而降低($P<0.001$);随着年龄增长,年发病风险逐渐增加($P<0.001$),但相对危险度逐渐降低。在 35 岁诊断睾丸癌并且存活超过 10 年的患者当中,发生继发实体肿瘤的风险增加($RR=1.9$,95%CI:1.8~2.1)。而且从统计学上看,这种发病风险增加可以持续 35 年($RR=1.7$,95%CI:1.5~2.0;$P<0.001$)。肺癌($RR=1.5$,95%CI:1.2~1.7),结肠癌($RR=2.0$,95%CI:1.7~2.5),膀胱癌($RR=2.7$,95%CI:=2.2~3.1),胰腺癌($RR=3.6$,95%CI:2.8~4.6),以及胃癌($RR=4.0$,95%CI:3.2~4.8)几乎占所有继发肿瘤的 60%。从总体上看,精原细胞瘤和非精原细胞瘤的发病情况近似,但在 1975 年之后诊治的非精原细胞瘤患者中,继发肿瘤的发病风险要稍微低些。从统计学上看,发生继发实体肿瘤的患者,可见于单纯行放疗者($RR=2.0$,95%CI:1.9~2.2),单纯行化疗者($RR=1.8$,95%CI:1.3~2.5),或曾经接受过两种治疗的患者($RR=2.9$,95%CI:1.9~4.2)。对于在 35 岁时诊断精原细胞瘤或非精原细胞瘤的患者,其 40 年后(如 75 岁时)罹患第二实体肿瘤的累积风险分别是 36%和 31%,而在总体人群中,这一数字是 23%。

从病例回顾中可以发现,对于采取高剂量依托泊苷治疗的患者,有可能会发生一种特殊类型的继发性白血病。

Nichols 等对印第安纳大学使用依托泊苷治疗的睾丸生殖细胞肿瘤患者进行了总结[194]。在 1982—1991 年间,共总结了 538 例患者,依托泊苷剂量 1 500~2 000mg/m^2,联合顺铂,再加上异环磷酰胺或者博来霉素。在这些患者中,有 348 例患者接受依托泊苷联合化疗作为初始化疗,另有 190 例患者依托泊苷是作为挽救性治疗的一部分。全算起来,共有 315 例患者存活,并且有 337 例患者随访时间超过 2 年。对于仍然存活的患者,中位随访时间是 4.9 年。有 2 名患者(0.37%)发现患有白血病。一例患者罹患急性未分化型白血病,伴有细胞遗传学异常 t(4;11)(q21;q23),该患者发生在依托泊苷治疗开始后 2.3 年;另有一例患者罹患的是急性髓单核细胞白血病,染色体分析正常,该病例发生在化疗开始后 2 年。在这段期间,有许多患者离开了临床试验,在这些患者中,我们注意到其中一些也发生了血液系统异常,包括有一例患者确诊为急性单核细胞白血病,t(11;19)(q13;p13)异常。对于化疗后继发白血病,即使采取常规剂量的依托泊苷,也有可能发生。然而,发生继发性白血病的概率很低,相较依托泊苷方案化疗对生殖细胞肿瘤的治疗作用而言,其风险-获益比是不受影响的。

生育能力

有睾丸癌病史的患者出现性功能障碍问题很常见,即使是行单侧睾丸切除术。过去有学者针对睾丸癌长期存活者进行横断面研究,评估了睾丸癌对生育和性功能的影响。1982—1992 年间,680 名接受治疗的患者完成了 EORTC Qly-C-30(qc30)问卷,该问卷是针对睾丸癌患者特别设计的关于一般健康问题和不育问题的问卷。根据患者接受治疗的不同进行分组:单纯睾丸切除组(观察组 S,$n=169$),术后辅助化疗组(C,$n=272$),术后辅助放疗组(R,$n=158$),或者术后既接受过化疗又接受过放疗组(C/RT $n=81$)。在观察组中,6%的患者 LH 水平升高,41%FSH 水平升高,11%睾酮水平降低(<10nmol/L)。随着附加治疗的实施,激素功能进一步恶化,但从总体上看,影响并不太大。在 C/RT 组中发生睾酮降低的情况更为常见(37%,$P=0.006$),而 FSH 异常则更多见于化疗后组(C 组 49%,C/RT 组 71%,$P<0.005$),LH 异常可见于放疗后组(11%,$P<0.01$)和化疗后组(10%,$P<0.001$)。有 367 例患者进行了性激素基线水平测定。在治疗之后,与基线水平相比,发现化疗组的患者 FSH 水平显著升高(平均升高 6IU/L(IQR 3~9.25),而观察组仅为 3IU/L(IQR 1~5);$P<0.001$),而且睾酮水平降低(分别为-2[IQR-8.0-1.5]和 1.0[IQR-4.0-4.0]$P<0.001$)。睾酮降低的患者(不伴 FSH 升高),在睾丸癌特异性量表上的生活质量评分更低,主要与性功能有关,而在 EORTC Qly C-30(qc 30)问卷当中,则主要表现为体力、社交以及社会角色的衰退与降低。睾酮降低的患者,同时会出现体重指数增加以及血压增高现象。治疗主要针对性活动减少,而接受化疗的患者更多的是关注生育的问题。据报道共有 207 例患者(30%)尝试生儿育女,其中 159 例(77%)获得成功,另有 10 例患者在接受辅助生殖措施后获得成功,总成功率 82%。在接受过化疗的患者中总成功率要低一些(化疗组 71%;化疗+放疗组 67%,而观察组为 85%,$P=0.028$)。FSH 升高与不育存在相关性(FSH 正常者 91%,升高者 68%,$P<0.001$)。

在考虑到各种治疗对生育的影响时,必须认识到,在任何治疗开始之前,高达 80%的睾丸癌患者在诊断时,就已经存在精子减少的症状了[224]。目前对少精子症的病因尚未完全了解,但有学者已经提出了几种机制,包括自身免疫过程或原发性内分泌功能障碍导致精子发生受损[225,226]。

化疗可能会对睾丸癌患者的生精细胞和 Leydig 细胞的功能产生急性损伤;绝大多数患者在治疗后的 12 个月内,持续出现精子缺乏并伴有血清促性腺激素水平升高。多于多数患者这一改变是可逆的,约 50%的患者在治疗结束后的第二年可以见到生精细胞和 Leydig 细胞的功能有所恢复[227,228]。影响生精功能恢复的可能因素包括:年龄大于 30 岁,治疗时间超过 6 个月,及之前接受过腹部放[229,230]。根据印第安纳大学的研究,至少有 1/3 单纯化疗的患者能够成功生育,而且无新生儿先天性异常,这进一步证实了先前的结果。Bohlen 等人报道,对于高危的 I 期生殖细胞肿瘤患者,行两个周期的以顺铂为基础的化疗,对生育功能以及性功能并不会产生影响[231]。Lampe 等人在一项对 170 例患者的分析中发现,在行睾丸切除并进行以顺铂为基础的化疗之后,2 年内恢复生精功能的概率为 48%,5 年内可增至 80%[232]。

肺毒性

博来霉素是各种针对睾丸癌患者化疗药物中唯一可能造成肺毒性的药物。接受博来霉素治疗的患者中,大约 5%的人可能发生肺纤维化,并且可能是致命[233]。这一毒性作用与累积剂量有关,超过 450 个单位以上,毒性显著增加。来霉素相关肺部损害在查体上最早的表现为吸气相延迟,一旦出现这种情况,应当立即停药。在此之后可能出现的症状与体征包括,双肺底湿啰音,干咳,以及呼气性呼吸困难。实验室检查异常包括，DLCO 下降，晚期改变包括低氧血症和高碳酸血症。影像学异常包括胸膜下基底部结节，可以通过胸片或者胸部 CT 发现。

超过 70 岁的患者，博来霉素相关肺病的发生风险随年龄而增加，而且还与下列危险因素相关，包括：胸部放疗史，或化疗同时行胸部放疗[113,234]，肾功能下降[235]和高浓度吸入氧，发生症状性博来霉素所致肺部疾病的风险增加。由于这类疾病的死亡率很高（约 50%），而且各种治疗手段，如应用皮质激素，效果往往不理想，所以对于无症状患者的早期诊断以及时停药就显得尤为重要。但是，如果仅行 3 个周期的 BEP 方案的话，博来霉素的临床毒副作用基本可以忽略不计。

放疗的长期毒性

放疗的毒性作用

急性

放疗的急性毒性作用，主要取决于哪些器官被照射到，放的剂量和范围。医学研究委员会（MRC）TE10 研究将患者随机分为单纯腹主动脉旁（PA）照射组以及腹主动脉旁联合同侧淋巴结照射组（dogleg[DL]）[104]。放疗的急性毒性反应包括：恶心/呕吐，二组发生率相似，但在 DL 组内稍高。诚如预期所示，因为 DL 照射野与 PA 区域相比，区域内所照射到小肠更多（$P=0.08$）。然而，在两组患者中，因恶心而需要药物治疗的比例均为 25%～30%。因为接受 DL 照射组的治疗野内，包含了更多的骨髓成分，因此该组内会发生更多白细胞减少症，与 PA 治疗组相比，发生白细胞减少症的患者几乎高出 1 倍。PA 治疗组发生白细胞减少症者为 19%，而同侧盆腔照射组的患者为 42%（$P<0.0001$）。需要补充的是，在 PA 治疗组仅有 7% 的患者发生腹泻，但在同侧盆腔照射的患者中有 14% 发生这一情况（$P=0.013$）。

在医学研究委员会的 TE18 研究中，将治疗剂量为分别为 30Gy 与 20Gy 的患者进行了对比。在该试验中，患者除每日由医师记录下他们的症状之外，还需要每天完成症状日记[103]。与接受较高剂量的患者相比，接受 20Gy 的患者，发生恶心的情况要少些（$P=0.06$），相应发生白细胞减少也较少（$P=0.02$）。比较重要的一点是，在接受 30Gy 治疗的患者中，更多的患者主诉中至重度的疲劳现象（20%，另一组仅 5%），以至于无法继续他们的正常工作（46%，另一组 28%）。但是在 12 周之后，两组间则比较接近。在该研究中，低剂量及较小治疗野的放疗发生急性毒性作用减少，同时并没有降低治疗效果，而且有可能会降低慢性及远期放疗后遗症的发生。

一项研究表明，约半数的精原细胞瘤患者存在不同程度的精子生成功能障碍，并且生育率降低[235]。因此，对于需接受辅助放疗而又有生育需求的患者而言，放疗前需要进行咨询并评价其基线生育能力，以及精液冷冻保存。

睾丸切除后剩余的对侧睾丸可能会受到 PA 及同侧盆腔淋巴结辅助放疗时内照射散射的影响，而影响将来的生育功能。对于生育功能的影响程度与剂量相关，有的数据表明，即便剂量水平仅仅为 40～50cGy（0.4～0.5Gy）时，也有可能发生一过性精子减少[236,237]。在剂量达到 2～3.5Gy 时，则有可能发生永久性不育症。对于仍然有生育需求的患者，很容易就可以将放疗剂量降低至不会产生永久性精子生成障碍的剂量水平。睾丸剂量的差异取决于治疗区域，在医学研究委员会 TE10 研究中通过对 DL+PA 照射野和单独 PA 照射野进行对比，发现睾丸受到照射的剂量与照射野不同有关。对于行 PA 放疗的患者，治疗后精子数量恢复正常的中位时间是 13 个月，而对于 DL 治疗的患者，则为 20 个月，尽管 63% 接受 DL 治疗的患者在治疗时对阴囊进行了防护，相比之下，行 PA 治疗的患者中仅有 3%[104]。对睾丸进行贝壳形遮挡防护可以使睾丸的照射剂量有效降低 3～10 倍。对于接受睾丸保护的患者，睾丸的累积放疗剂量约占全部处方剂量的 0.5%～2%，绝大多数患者都能够恢复到他们的基线精子水平[104,236,238]。研究发现，在更高的照射量下才可能影响激素水平，但睾酮水平基本不会受其影响，然而可能会导致 Leydig 细胞功能轻度受损，表现为血清 FSH 和 LH 浓度改变，这也取决于治疗剂量和照射野大小。还有可能出现一过性 FSH 和 LH 轻度升高（可能在正常范围之内变化），在 PA+DL 治疗组，这一异常有望在 3 年之内恢复正常，而单纯行 PA 放疗的患者，可能仅发生 FSH 轻度升高而 LH 不受影响[239]。

慢性

为尽量避免放疗所产生的慢性毒性和持久的远期毒性反应，许多年轻精原细胞瘤患者的首选积极监测作为治疗方案。在过去，由于精原细胞瘤的放射治包含纵隔区，因此许多患者出现了心脏毒性反应。Zagars 对 M. D. Anderson 内共 477 例Ⅰ期或Ⅱ期睾丸精原细胞瘤患者进行了总结，时间从 1951 年至 1999 年[240]。其中位随访时间 13.3 年，心脏特异性标准化死亡比为 1.61，而癌症特异性标准化死亡比为 1.91。这两种毒性反应都在随访 15 年之后才表现出来。15 年可能代表慢性毒性发展的潜伏期，但它也可能表明在 1990 年之前，放疗无论在剂量还是在照射野上，比现代做法所带来的毒性反应更强。

在一项基于人群的大型国际癌症注册研究中，对在顺铂治疗诞生前后，采取传统方法治疗发生继发恶性肿瘤的风险进行了定量分析[221]。在 1943—2001 年间，检索出共计超过 40 000 例睾丸癌患者。存活时间达到 10 年的患者，发生继发实体肿瘤的风险相较正常人群高出 2 倍，相对危险度（RR）为 1.9。精原细胞瘤和非精原细胞瘤的患病模式相似，在 1975 年之后治疗的非精原细胞瘤患者，其风险要低一些。在下述患者当中，发生继发恶性实体肿瘤的风险显著增加，包括：单纯放疗的患者（$RR=2.0$，95%CI：1.9～2.2），单纯化疗的患者（$RR=1.8$，95%CI：1.3～2.5），以及同时接受两种治疗的患者（$RR=2.9$，95%CI：1.9～4.2）。对于进行放疗的患者，在随访时间为 1～4 年，5～9 年以及超过 10 年的患者中，发病风险分别为 1.1，1.5 和 2.0。接受标准的单纯膈下放疗的患者，发生继发肿瘤的相对风险最高，包括：胃部（$RR=4.1$）、胰腺（$RR=3.8$）、肾脏（$RR=2.8$）、膀胱（$RR=2.7$）、结肠（$RR=1.9$）以及直肠（$RR=1.8$）。然而，在膈上器官发生继发恶性肿瘤的风险也是增加的，可能与过去经常进行膈上区域放疗有关。对于 35 岁诊断睾丸癌的患者，在 75 岁时发生实体肿瘤的累积风险，精原细胞瘤为 36%，非精原细胞瘤为 31%，而正常人群仅为 23%。尽管这些数据很有启示意义，但可能并不符合如今的情况，因为我们今天已经开始应用更低的放疗剂量以及更小的照射野。

肿瘤“庇护所”和中枢神经转移

睾丸癌患者发生中枢神经系统转移是相当少见的[52,53]，因而对晚期生殖细胞肿瘤患者并不推荐行中枢神经系统预防性治疗。然而，对于晚期血行转移或体积较大的绒毛膜癌的患者，临床应警惕中枢神经系统转移的发生，即使有轻微的中枢神经系统症状，也需要仔细检查。

对于存在中枢神经系统转移的患者，无论是首发症状还是复发性病变，都应尽可能采取治愈性治疗。所有患者均需接受全身治疗。表浅孤立性转移灶应考虑手术切除。多发性脑转移癌患者或晚期肿瘤伴随其他器官转移的患者应接受全脑放射治疗（30~50Gy 每 3~6 周，每次剂量<2Gy），并给予辅助全身化疗[52,53,241,242]。对无其他部位受累的孤立性中枢神经转移复发的患者，可以行手术接受切除，然后进行中枢神经放疗，并在术后进行两个疗程的以顺铂为主的“辅助”化疗。

就生殖细胞肿瘤的化疗而言，睾丸本身是一个重要避难所。在大多数情况下，患者一经诊断为睾丸癌，就会行睾丸根治性切除术。但是，某些晚期疾病的患者在开始实施化疗时并没有组织学诊断结果。在这种情况下，即使没有原发肿瘤存在的证据，在化疗结束后也必须切除睾丸。因为如果原发灶没有切除，当发现肿瘤标志物水平在化疗期间和化疗后出现升高时，会给我们带来困惑，且难以解释。如果原发灶没有切除，那么在治疗期间及治疗后，如果肿瘤标志物水平持续或进行性升高，一定要考虑到可能是原发灶的问题。

有时，必须考虑到对侧睾丸今后发生原发肿瘤的可能性。对于全身性疾病在治疗后已经达到血清学和影像学完全缓解的患者，如果再次出现肿瘤标志物水平升高，应当仔细检查对侧残余睾丸，并应行睾丸超声检查，以排除剩余睾丸中存在隐匿病灶的可能。目前，对于双侧睾丸先后发生癌变的病例，为了保留生育能力，可选择行保留器官的手术治疗（organ-sparing surgery）[243]。

性腺外生殖细胞瘤（EGCT）

虽然生殖细胞瘤多发于睾丸内，但原发于性腺外的生殖细胞瘤也是其重要类型之一。总体而言，5%~10%的生殖细胞癌发生于性腺外，特别是纵隔和腹膜后。除了这些部位，性腺外生殖细胞瘤（EGCT）也可发生于松果体，骶尾部，更少见区域有前列腺，阴道，眼眶，肝脏及胃肠道。

EGCT 曾经被认为是原发性肿瘤发生隐匿性转移。一项针对 20 例性腺外纵隔 GCTS 患者的尸检结果发现，仅有 1 例为睾丸原发肿瘤，另外一例为例睾丸瘢痕[244]。这两例均与临床隐匿性下腹膜后受累有关。这些病例都存在隐匿性的腹膜后侵犯。对于腹膜后原发生殖细胞肿瘤而言，可能更有可能发现隐匿性的睾丸原发病灶，特别是当肿瘤不是发生于中线时。

现在普遍认为，EGCT 是分布于上述区域的原始生殖细胞成分发生恶性转化所致，而这些成分本来应该集中分布于睾丸。

成年人中，纵隔是性腺外生殖细胞瘤最常见的发病部位[245,246]。常见症状包括，呼吸困难（25%），胸痛（23%），咳嗽（17%），其次为发热（13%），体重减轻（11%），腔静脉阻塞综合征和疲劳/虚弱（6%）[247]，纵隔部位最常见是成熟畸胎瘤[248]。提示存在大的外界性前纵隔肿块，血清 HCG 和 AFP 正常。成熟畸胎瘤需外科手术治疗，对化疗或放疗不敏感。虽然这些肿瘤在组织学上是良性的，但手术切除过程通常比较困难的。肿瘤与邻近结构发生一定程度粘连，如心包、肺和大血管。尽管如此，在当前的胸外科时代，卓越的疗效胜于一切[249]。在梅奥诊所治疗的一系列病例中，69 名患者中，有 64 名长期存活，其余患者中有 4 人死于手术并发症。

性腺外非精原生殖细胞肿瘤的治疗原则与睾丸生殖细胞癌的处理原则相同对于年轻患者，如果在中线结构上发现分化较差的肿瘤，应当考虑这一诊断。应对血清肿瘤标志物水平进行测定，如果临床情况允许的话，应当进行活检。在大多数情况下，手术切除不作为治疗的第一选择。与睾丸生殖细胞癌一样，应以顺铂为基础的化疗作为主要的治疗手段。但是，原发于纵隔的非精原生殖细胞肿瘤，其治愈率明显低于原发性睾丸癌。一项 635 例 EGCT 患者的国际性研究结果表明，不论原发灶位于何处，纯精原细胞瘤的治愈率几乎达 90%，但纵隔非精原生殖细胞肿瘤患者的 5 年生存率只有 45%[247]。除临床试验外，不推荐对这类患者采取大剂量化疗联合自体造血干细胞移植。

对于非精原 EGCT 患者，在化疗后影像学检查发现异常者，应当手术切除残余病灶，即使肿瘤标志物已经恢复正常，也应考虑手术治疗。Vuky 等报道了 32 例在化疗后辅以手术治疗的纵隔非精原生殖细胞肿瘤患者[250]，其中有 66% 发现残余肿瘤，其中 22% 为畸胎瘤。

纵隔非精原生殖细胞肿瘤与多种疾病存在相关性，其中克兰费尔特综合征的高发（高达 20%）[12,251]。

约 10% 的纵隔非精原生殖细胞肿瘤患者易发生血液系统恶性疾病。1976—1989 年间，在印第安纳大学的 40 例纵隔非精原生殖细胞肿瘤患者中，6 例生血液系统恶性肿瘤[32]。此外，还有 11 名患者被转到印第安纳大学，或仅仅提供了相关病例资料，以对这种关联性进行评价。在这组患者中，6 人发展为急性巨核细胞白血病，5 人患有急性非淋巴细胞白血病（非 M7），2 人发展为强性骨髓增生异常综合征，2 人被发现有髓外巨核细胞骨髓增多症，另 2 例患者表现为血小板计数显著升高及细胞遗传学异常，或骨髓过度增生。发现血液系统疾病的中位时间为 6 个月，有 5 名患者同时患有两种疾病。33 名类似的患者已被报道。本文中两个诊断的中位间隔时间为 5 个月，其中有 13 例同时发病。一项包含 287 例纵隔非精原生殖细胞瘤患者的回顾性研究显示，17 名血液病患者的中位发病时间为诊断为生殖细胞肿瘤后的 6 个月，且中位生存时间为诊断血液病后 5 个月[252]。

对这些病例进行仔细的临床和细胞遗传学分析，结果表明：这些肿瘤并不是由于对生殖细胞肿瘤进行治疗而导致的，但却呈现了这些疾病之间独特的重要的生物学相关性。在那些接受相同化疗的睾丸或腹膜后生殖细胞癌患者中，没有发现类似的病例。然而，最引人注目的是在一位患者的在纵隔生殖细胞瘤和其白血病母细胞中发现了等臂染色体 12p[31]。这意味着纵隔 GCT 和血液学恶性肿瘤来自一个共同的祖细胞。

患有 EGCT 的患者，尤其是病变位于腹膜后或病理类型为非精原细胞瘤者，以及原发性纵隔病变者，对侧睾丸发生癌变的风险增加[253]。腹膜后或非精原细胞瘤的 EGCT 患者诊断为 EGCT 后,其对侧睾丸今后发生癌变的十年累积风险约为 14%。纵隔非精原生殖细胞瘤与其他非血液系统疾病以及非生殖细胞肿瘤之间的相关性尚未得到证实。Ulbright 等回顾了美国印第安纳大学在 1974—1982 年间的生殖细胞肿瘤标本,结果表明,269 例畸胎瘤病例当中,有 209 例原发部位位于睾丸,28 例位于腹膜后,32 例位于纵隔[254]。在这组患者中,11 个例为恶性非生殖细胞成分,包括胚胎性横纹肌肉瘤、腺巨细胞癌、平滑肌肉瘤、肾母细胞瘤(Wilms tumor)和多形性胶质母细胞瘤。在 11 例患者中,有 10 例在开始治疗前即诊断。当能够获得患者多个病理标本时,往往可以发现组织学进展,从非典型病变逐渐过渡为明显的非生殖细胞特征。作者认为,这些恶性非生殖细胞成分可能是由肿瘤内畸胎瘤成分分化而成。尤其有趣的是,11 例患者中,有 3 例原发部位位于纵隔(27%),而在所有病例当中,纵隔原发肿瘤仅占病例总数的 12%。与此相反,在迄今为止规模最大的 EGCT 研究中,并未发现非血液病、非生殖细胞瘤与 EGCT 的发病率之间存在相关性[255]。

无法识别的生殖细胞肿瘤综合征

有时,患者的临床表现类似性腺外生殖细胞瘤(EGCT),但缺少能够证实生殖细胞瘤的血清学或组织病理学证据。Greco 等建议,对此类患者,应进行全面的组织病理学评估,有些患者还应当接受经验性顺铂化疗[168]。"未被识别的生殖细胞瘤综合征"的临床特征包括:患者年龄小于 50 岁;肿瘤主要累及中线(纵隔或腹膜后)、肺(以多个肺结节的形式)或淋巴结;或者是肿瘤生长迅速。在一项前瞻性研究中,根据上述标准,共挑选出 71 名符合条件的患者,这些患者主要为低分化癌或低分化腺癌,这些患者至少满足上述条件中的一条。血清学检查结果显示 51 例患者 AFP 和 HCG 正常,13 例患者有一项标志物升高,5 例患者两项标志物都升高。显微镜下观察结果显示:低分化癌有 48 例(68%),低分化腺癌有 18 例(25%),低分化大细胞癌有 5 例(7%)。根据电镜结果,在接受此手术的 33 例低分化癌患者中,有 17 例(52%)的诊断结果有所改变,其中多数被重新诊断为神经内分泌肿瘤。68 名患者接受了治疗,其中 62 名患者接受了以顺铂为基础的化疗。其中 15 例(23%)达到完全缓解,18 例(29%)部分缓解。对治疗有反应的普遍为青年患者,而且病灶多位于腹膜后中线附近、纵隔或颈部淋巴结。所有 15 例患者均诊断为低分化癌。Memorial Sloan-Kettering 癌症中心的 Motzer 等对 41 名原发灶不明的低分化癌患者进行了评价[107],发现 30%的肿瘤含有 i(12p),或 12p 拷贝增加,或 12 号染色体长臂缺失。对于明确存在染色体结构异常的患者中,有 75%对以顺铂为基础的化疗存在反应,而诊断不明的患者,缓解率仅 18%。

这些结果表明,原发灶不明的低分化癌对化疗药物反应良好,甚至可以治愈。其中部分患者可能表现出非典型生殖细胞癌的组织学和血清学表现。转移性低分化癌患者应进行调查,以确定其原发部位,同时测定血清 HCG 和 AFP。对于肺或纵隔存在明确肿物的患者应行纤维支气管镜检查。在行彻底的显微镜检后,应行免疫组化染色、细胞遗传学检查以进一步明确肿瘤特征。患者应接受以顺铂和依托泊苷为基础的化疗。

(范阳 宣云东 译 张旭 校)

参考文献

The complete reference list can be found on the Wiley Companion Digital Edition of this title (see inside front cover for login instructions).

6 Jemal A, Thomas A, Murray T, Thun M. Cancer statistics, 2002. *CA Cancer J Clin.* 2002;**52**:23–47.

13 Raghavan D, Zalcberg JR, Grygiel JJ, et al. Multiple atypical nevi: a cutaneous marker of germ cell tumors. *J Clin Oncol.* 1994;**12**:2284–2287.

17 Sokal M, Peckham MJ, Hendry WF. Bilateral germ cell tumours of the testis. *Br J Urol.* 1980;**52**:158–162.

20 Jones TD, Ulbright TM, Eble JN, et al. OCT4 Staining in testicular tumors: a sensitive and specific marker for seminoma and embryonal carcinoma. *Am J Surg Path.* 2004;**28**:935–940.

22 Cheng L. Establishing a germ cell origin for metastatic tumors using OCT4 immunohistochemistry. *Cancer.* 2004;**101**:2006–2010.

30 Brosman S. Testicular tumors in prepubertal children. *Urology.* 1979;**13**:581–588.

36 Zon RT, Nichols C, Einhorn LH. Management strategies and outcomes of germ cell tumor patients with very high human chorionic gonadotropin levels. *J Clin Oncol.* 1998;**16**:1294–1297.

41 Dieckmann KP, Skakkebaek NE. Carcinoma in situ of the testis: review of biological and clinical features. *Int J Cancer.* 1999;**83**:815–822.

47 Hoskin P, Dilly S, Easton D, Horwich A, Hendry W, Peckham MJ. Prognostic factors in stage I nonseminomatous germ-cell testicular tumors managed by orchiectomy and surveillance: implications for adjuvant chemotherapy. *J Clin Oncol.* 1986;**4**:1031–1036.

53 Krege S, Beyer J, Souchon R, et al. European consensus conference on diagnosis and treatment of germ cell cancer: a report of the second meeting of the European Germ Cell Cancer Consensus Group (EGCCCG): part II. *Eur Urol.* 2008;**53**:497–513.

59 Donohue JP. Retroperitoneal lymphadenectomy: the anterior approach including bilateral suprarenal-hilar dissection. *Urol Clin North Am.* 1977;**4**:509–521.

67 Richie JP. Clinical stage 1 testicular cancer: the role of modified retroperitoneal lymphadenectomy. *J Urol.* 1990;**144**:1160–1163.

76 Groll RJ, Warde P, Jewett MA. A comprehensive systematic review of testicular germ cell tumor surveillance. *Crit Rev Oncol Hematol.* 2007;**64**:182–197.

80 Colls BM, Harvey VJ, Skelton L, et al. Late results of surveillance of clinical stage I nonseminoma germ cell testicular tumours: 17 years' experience in a national study in New Zealand. *BJU Int.* 1999;**83**:76–82.

84 Mead G. for the IGCCCG. International germ cell consensus classification: a prognostic factor-based staging system for metastatic germ cell cancers. International Germ Cell Cancer Collaborative Group. *J Clin Oncol.* 1997;**15**:594–603.

89 Boden G, Gibb R. Radiotherapy and testicular neoplasms. *Lancet.* 1951;**2**: 1195–1196.

95 Schmoll H-J, Souchon G, Bokemeyer C. European consensus on diagnosis and treatment of germ cell cancer: a report of the European Germ Cell Cancer Consensus Group (EGCCCG). *Ann Oncol.* 2004;**15**:1377–1399.

99 von der Maase H, Specht L, Jackobsen GK, et al. Surveillance following orchidectomy for stage I seminoma of the testis [comment]. *Eur J Cancer.* 1993;**29A**:1923–1924.

106 Oliver RT, Mead GM, Fogarty PJ, Stenning SP, MRC TE19 and EORTC 30982 trial collaborators. Radiotherapy versus carboplatin for stage I seminoma: updated analysis of the MRC/EORTC randomized trial (ISRTN27163214). *J Clin Oncol.* 2008;**26**:May 20 suppl:abstr 1.

112 Warwick OH, Alison RE, Darte JM. Clinical experience with vinblastine sulfate. *Can Med Assoc J.* 1961;**85**:579–583.

118 Einhorn L, Donahue J. Cis-diamminedichloroplatinum, vinblastine, and bleomycin combination chemotherapy in disseminated testicular cancer. *Ann Intern Med.* 1977;**87**:293–298.

121 Einhorn L, Williams SD, Troner M, Birch R, Greco FA. The role of maintenance therapy in disseminated testicular cancer. *N Engl J Med.* 1981;**305**:727–731.

124 Einhorn LH, Williams SD, Loehrer PJ, et al. Evaluation of optimal duration of chemotherapy in favorable-prognosis disseminated germ cell tumors: a Southeastern Cancer Study Group protocol. *J Clin Oncol.* 1989;**7**:387–391.

128 Horwich A, Sleijfer DT, Fossa SD, et al. Randomized trial of bleomycin, etoposide, and cisplatin compared with bleomycin, etoposide, and carboplatin in good-prognosis metastatic nonseminomatous germ cell cancer: a Multi-institutional Medical Research Council/European Organization for Research and Treatment of Cancer Trial. *J Clin Oncol.* 1997;**15**:1844–1852.

135 Ozols RF, Ihde DC, Linehan WM, et al. A randomized trial of standard chemotherapy v a high-dose chemotherapy regimen in the treatment of poor prognosis nonseminomatous germ-cell tumors. *J Clin Oncol.* 1988;**6**:1031–1040.

140 Kaye SB, Mead GM, Fossa S, et al. Intensive induction-sequential chemotherapy with BOP/VIP-B compared with treatment with BEP/EP for poor-prognosis

metastatic nonseminomatous germ cell tumor: a Randomized Medical Research Council/European Organization for Research and Treatment of Cancer study. *J Clin Oncol*. 1998;**16**:692 - 701.

145 Sheinfeld J. Risks of the uncontrolled retroperitoneum. *Ann Surg Oncol*. 2003;**10**:100 - 101.

148 Vergouwe Y, Steyerberg EW, Foster RS, et al. Validation of a prediction model and its predictors for the histology of residual masses in nonseminomatous testicular cancer. *J Urol*. 2001;**165**:84 - 88; discussion 88.

151 Moore CJ, Daneshmand S, Kondagunta GV, et al. Management of difficult germ-cell tumors. *Oncology (Williston Park)*. 2006;**20**:1565 - 1570, 1575; discussion 1575 - 1576.

156 Ganjoo KN, Chan RJ, Sharma M, et al. Positron emission tomography scans in the evaluation of postchemotherapy residual masses in patients with seminoma. *J Clin Oncol*. 1999;**17**:3457 - 3460.

160 Carver BS, Shayegan B, Eggener S, et al. Incidence of metastatic nonseminomatous germ cell tumor outside the boundaries of a modified postchemotherapy retroperitoneal lymph node dissection. *J Clin Oncol*. 2007;**25**:4365 - 4369.

164 Baniel J, Sella A. Complications of retroperitoneal lymph node dissection in testicular cancer: primary and post-chemotherapy. *Semin Surg Oncol*. 1999;**17**:263 - 267.

169 Beck SD, Foster RS, Bihrle R, et al. Post chemotherapy RPLND in patients with elevated markers: current concepts and clinical outcome. *Urol Clin North Am*. 2007;**34**:219 - 225; abstract ix - x.

172 Friedman EL, Garnick MB, Stomper PC, et al. Therapeutic guidelines and results in advanced seminoma. *J Clin Oncol*. 1985;**3**:1325 - 1332.

177 Nichols CR. Treatment of recurrent germ cell tumors. *Semin Surg Oncol*. 1999;**17**:268 - 274.

184 Kondagunta GV, Bacik J, Bajorin D, et al. Etoposide and cisplatin chemotherapy for metastatic good-risk germ cell tumors. *J Clin Oncol*. 2005;**23**(**36**):9290 - 9294.

191 Lorch A, Kollmannsberger C, Hartmann JT, et al. Single versus sequential high-dose chemotherapy in patients with relapsed or refractory germ cell tumors: a prospective randomized multicenter trial of the German Testicular Cancer Study Group. *J Clin Oncol*. 2007;**12**(**19**):2778 - 2784.

198 Kollmannsberger C, Beyer J, Liersch R, et al. Combination chemotherapy with gemcitabine plus oxaliplatin in patients with intensively pretreated or refractory germ cell cancer: a study of the German Testicular Cancer Study Group. *J Clin Oncol*. 2004;**22**(**1**):108 - 114.

204 Meijer S, Mulder NH, Sleijfer DT, et al. Influence of combination chemotherapy with cis-diamminedichloroplatinum on renal function: long-term effects. *Oncology*. 1983;**40**:170 - 173.

209 Cantwell BMJ, Mannix KA, Roberts JT, et al. Thromboembolic events during combination chemotherapy for germ cell malignancy. *Lancet*. 1988;**2**:1086 - 1087.

214 Haugnes HS, Aass N, Fossa SD, et al. Components of the metabolic syndrome in long-term survivors of testicular cancer. *Ann Oncol*. 2007;**18**(**2**):241 - 248.

220 Reddel RR, Kefford RF, Grant JM, et al. Ototoxicity in patients receiving cisplatin: importance of dose and method of drug administration. *Cancer Treat Rep*. 1982;**66**:19 - 23.

224 Morrish DW, Venner PM, Siy O, et al. Mechanisms of endocrine dysfunction in patients with testicular cancer. *J Natl Cancer Inst*. 1990;**82**:412 - 418.

229 Bohlen D, Burkhard FC, Mills R, et al. Fertility and sexual function after orchiectomy and two cycles of chemotherapy for stage I high-risk nonseminomatous germ cell cancer. *J Urol*. 2001;**165**:141 - 144.

第 101 章　外阴、阴道癌

Summer B. Dewdney, MD ■ Jacob Rotmensch, MD

概述

外阴和阴道癌罕见，主要发生在绝经后女性，19%的外阴癌发生在 50 岁以上的女性。外阴癌的发病危险因素包括人乳头瘤病毒感染和慢性炎症。外阴上皮内病变的治疗以局部扩大切除术为主，以及其他多种治疗手段。大多数外阴癌是鳞状细胞癌，以局部扩大切除及放疗治疗为主。前哨淋巴结活检术降低区域淋巴结切除术后的并发症。对于多数晚期病变，采用放疗联合顺铂、5-Fu 和 MMC 的化疗。其他外阴恶性肿瘤包括巴氏腺癌、基底细胞癌、疣状癌和黑色素瘤等。阴道癌最常见是鳞癌，透明细胞癌见于年轻女性。在过去有认为，透明细胞癌与胎儿期的已烯雌酚暴露有关。阴道还可能发生黑色素瘤内胚窦肿瘤、横纹肌肉瘤、纤维上皮样阴道息肉等肿瘤。

外阴癌

流行病学

外阴癌占女性生殖道恶性肿瘤的 4%，占女性所有恶性肿瘤的 0.6%。它是第四常见的妇科恶性肿瘤[1]。美国癌症协会估计，2014 年预计有 4 850 例外阴癌新诊断病例，大约有 1 030 名女性将死于外阴癌[2]。

危险因素包括吸烟、人乳头瘤病毒（human papillomavirus, HPV）感染、外阴或宫颈上皮内病变、慢性免疫抑制性疾病、慢性外阴炎症（如硬化性苔藓或扁平苔藓）和南部欧裔人种[3]。大多数外阴癌发生于老年女性，大约有 50%的患者年龄在 60~70 岁之间。Kumar 等发现浸润性外阴癌在年轻女性中的发病率正在逐渐升高，尽管 SEER 数据库报道 19.3%的外阴癌诊断时患者年龄小于 50 岁，外阴鳞状细胞中，年轻患者和年老者的生存差异非常大（图 101-1）[4]。

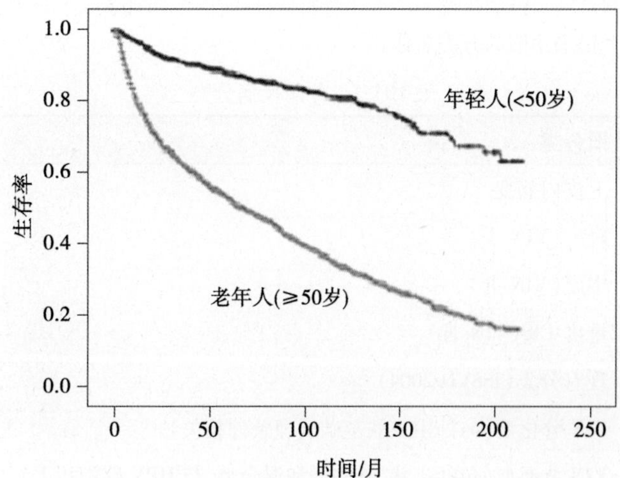

图 101-1　外阴鳞状细胞癌，1988—2005 年，比较年轻（<50 岁，蓝线）与老年人（≥50 岁，绿线）的生存率。Log-rank $P = 0.001$。摘自 Kumar 2009[4]，获 Elsevier 授权

在年轻女性中发病率升高的原因可能是由于在这一人群中 HPV 感染的增加，特别是某些亚型 HPV 相关的外阴上皮内病变可能进一步进展为癌。

外阴癌被发现有两种，第一种与 HPV 感染相关，第二种与慢性炎症进展有关[5]。几项流行病学研究结果显示性传播病毒是外阴癌的根本病因。在许多外阴癌前病变或者外阴恶性病变患者中均能发现与 HPV 相关的尖锐湿疣。据估计，在美国每年有超过 100 万的女性发生会阴湿疣，有 10%的女性发生 HPV 感染[6]。目前，HPV 6 型和 11 型是在良性湿疣中最常见的亚型；HPV16 型、18 型、31 型、33 型和 45 型更常见于上皮内瘤样病变或者浸润癌中[6~8]。在大约 50%的外阴癌患者中能发现 HPV 感染，这些病变通常为多灶，多与外阴间变性病变相关。HPV 阴性肿瘤通常见于患有外阴营养不良疾病的老年女性[9,10]。

虽然流行病学证据强烈显示病毒为发病病因，但是同时也提示了其他一些相关因素，例如外阴肉芽肿病变、糖尿病、高血压以及肥胖等也和外阴癌相关，但也许是因为这些因素也常见于高龄患者。Mabuchi 及其同事进行的一项病例对照研究发现在家仆、洗衣店工人或者清洁车间工人中的外阴癌发病率较高，这说明发病因素中有环境因素[11]。

外阴原位癌（carcinoma in situ, CIS）与外阴浸润癌之间的关系显示了从癌前病变到浸润癌的连续变化谱。Jone 等[12]报道了 405 例外阴上皮内病变（vulvar intraepithelial neoplasia, VIN）2~3 级中，经治疗后大约 3.8%的患者进展到浸润癌。而 10 名没有经过治疗的患者进展成癌的时间 3.9 年（平均）。然而在年轻患者和老年患者中的进展比例可能不同。一些作者提出在 30 多岁或者 40 多岁的妇女中的多灶外阴原位癌可能不会像老年妇女中的多灶外阴原位癌一样进展为浸润癌[13~15]。

外阴不典型增生

2004 年，国际外阴疾病研究协会颁布了现有的 VIN 疾病的分类系统（表 101-1）。过去是根据异常病变的程度分为 VIN1、2 和 3。现在，只有高度病变被定义为 VIN，还沿用此名词。VIN1 不再是癌前病变，因此不再描述位 VIN。在 2004 年，他们颁布了 VIN 的两个分类：普通型 VIN（包括以前的疣状或基底样和混合型的 VIN2 和 3）和分化型 VIN（与硬化性苔藓相关）[16]。除此之外，美国病理学家协会（College of American Pathologists）和 ASCCP 确定了采用下段肛门生殖器鳞状上皮学术用语（lower anogenital squamous terminology，LAST）最新系统的两分类系统方案[17]。VIN 病例在过去的 30 年中有大幅增加，美国妇产科大学和美国阴道镜和宫颈病理学会（ASCCP）组建了学会专门针对 VIN 疾病的治疗，并与国际外阴病变研究协会（ISVDD）就 VIN 分为普通型和分化型的分类达成共识，并讨论制订其治疗的建议。值得注意的是，目前许多病理学家和研究者仍采用旧的分类名称。

表 101-1 外阴疾病分类

旧分类：
上皮内病变
轻度（VIN Ⅰ）
中度（VIN Ⅱ）
重度-CIS（VIN Ⅲ）
现有分类（ISSVD 2004）
VIN 分化型（与外阴皮肤基础病理条件相关）
VIN 普通型（包括疣状、基底样和混合型，与 HPV 感染相关）

VIN，外阴上皮内病变；HPV，人类乳头瘤样病毒。

VIN 可以表现出多种症状。最常见的是刺激症状或者瘙痒；然而 20%的患者没有任何症状[18]。大体上病变可以为扁平的、外突的（斑丘疹样）或者疣状的。颜色上病变可以为褐色（过度色素沉着）、红色（增殖性红斑）、白色或者无色的。

白色病变可以表现为发白的增厚的角质层（黏膜白斑）或者弥漫的、白色易碎的纸样外观（硬化萎缩性苔藓）（图 101-2）。鳞状上皮增生区域（增生性营养不良）和间变性病变也可以表现为白色外观。然而与硬化性苔藓不同的是，组织通常为增厚的，病变倾向为局灶或者多灶而不是弥散边界不清的[15]。

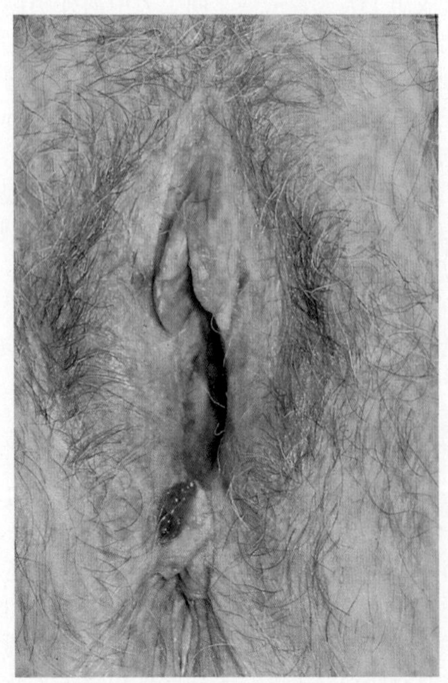

图 101-2 外阴白色易碎的纸样外观或外阴硬化苔藓

活检对于硬化性萎缩性苔藓很重要，因为可能存在潜在的外阴癌[19,20]。

在显微镜下外阴上皮不典型增生改变与癌前病变一致，通常表现为成熟鳞状上皮的缺失。有丝分裂像增加以及核浆比增加。

有学者认为外阴不典型增生和外阴癌有两类截然不同的病因。第一类与 HPV 感染和吸烟相关，见于年轻患者。这类病变表现为“疣状”增生。更常见的一类见于老年患者，与 HPV 或吸烟均不相关。这组患者多与邻近肿瘤的硬化性苔藓相关。据报道大约有 20%的外阴癌合并有外阴的间变性病变。

建立诊断的最好方法是高度警惕可疑的临床表现和早期活检。其他一些方法也能帮助评价这些病变，如细胞学、阴道镜和甲苯胺蓝 O 可以在活检前谨慎的使用。然而一般来说外阴细胞学检查不能作为一种筛查手段，因为外阴皮肤较厚，而且角质化。外阴的阴道镜检查比较困难，因为其病变不像宫颈病变那样容易分辨。因此阴道镜检查并不作为常规的外阴检查手段，而主要用于外阴不典型增生或上皮内癌患者的评价或随诊。甲苯胺蓝 O 试验是非特异性的，它能够将上皮的表层部分的核染色。在应用 1%甲苯胺蓝 O 水溶液染色 1min 后，用 1%醋酸脱色，随后进行阴道镜检查，对仍被染色的区域进行活检。然而阳性试验结果并不能总是说明存在癌前病变，因为 20%的外阴良性区域也可能出现染色阳性[19]。

为了取得皮肤全层以获得肯定的诊断，外阴活检通常使用凯氏皮肤钳（Keyes dermal punch）。有时候需要较大块的活检，就需要用利多卡因局部麻醉，然后用手术刀或者宫颈活检钳来取样[21]。

一旦通过活检确立了正确诊断，就可以进行合适的治疗。对于硬化性苔藓，一些局部方法例如穿棉质内衣，避免强力肥皂和洗涤剂常备用来减轻皮肤刺激症状。局部应用氟化皮质激素，每天 2 次，持续 1～2 周，可以帮助缓解瘙痒。但是长期应用这些激素制剂能够导致外阴萎缩或挛缩。如果需要长期治疗，可以使用非氟化制剂，如 1%的氢化可的松。一些硬化萎缩性苔藓患者在阴唇系带后部存在严重的挛缩，对于这类病变的治疗建议采用阴唇系带成型修复手术[22,23]。

VIN 能够通过多种方法治疗，多位作者报道通过局部扩大切除成功治疗了该病变[10,22]。局部扩大手术一定要达到充分的安全边界，然而由于这类病变的多灶性使得常常难以达到这一要求。Wallbillich 等[24]发现阳性切缘使复发率增加 11%～32%，复发还与吸烟和局部病灶大有关。

对于 VIN，还有一些其他治疗方法。二氧化碳激光气化和光动力治疗外阴[25]，可以达到 3mm 深度。现有证据显示激光治疗对于控制这类病变的效果与手术一样有效。然而在激光治疗之前，必须通过组织学检查除外浸润性病变。Leuchter 等治疗了 142 名外阴原位癌患者[26]，在那些接受激光治疗的患者中，17%出现复发，与通过病灶局部扩大切除治疗的患者接近。

咪喹莫特也一直被用于药物的保守治疗。一项系统回顾两项随机对照研究发现完全缓解率达 51%[27]。氟尿嘧啶（氟尿嘧啶）软膏也能够有效治疗外阴原位癌，据报道该方法的有效率能达到 75%。然而持续使用会导致水肿和疼痛。近来，一项多中心、随机 2 期研究比较西多福韦和咪喹莫特治疗 VIN3，显示两组患者大约 46%的反应率[28]。

佩吉特病

佩吉特病(Paget disease)是一种罕见的外阴皮肤上皮内病变,主要见于绝经后女性[29~31]。不像外阴上皮内病变的病变细胞是鳞状细胞,其病变细胞是上皮内的腺细胞。病变主要见于白人女性,平均发病年龄为 65 岁。大体上,病变表现为淡红色湿疹样病变。显微镜下,这类病变的特征性改变是灰白色大细胞,呈巢状浸润上皮组织。一旦作出诊断,需要注意除外潜在的浸润癌。浸润性外阴佩吉特病可见于大约 10% 的佩吉特病患者[20]。如果肛周区域受累,需要考虑合并肛门癌。Lee 等回顾性报道了 75 例外阴佩吉特病:16 例患者(22%)合并有附属器官的浸润癌,7 例患者(9%)合并有附属器官的原位癌[30]。

外阴佩吉特病通常以一种隐匿性的方式转移,其边界往往超过病变的外观边界[31]。如果没有证据证实存在潜在的浸润癌,通常采用局部扩大切除或外阴单纯切除术[32]。如果采用局部扩大切除术,切除深度需要略深一点达到皮下脂肪以确保切除表皮,从而确保切除皮肤的附属器官结构。由于该病变在皮下延伸,在术中冰冻病理检查可能有助于确保完全切除。

Bergen 及其同事评价了 14 例外阴佩吉特病患者,她们接受了外阴切除术、外阴皮肤切除及植皮手术或者单侧外阴切除术[32]。中位随访时间为 50 个月,所有患者均无瘤生存,然而其中有三例患者曾经出现局部复发。其他一些方法(如氟尿嘧啶软膏、激光等)并未用于治疗这类病变,这是因为存在局部和远处复发的风险,需要密切的随诊。

浸润性外阴癌

国际妇产科联盟(International Federation of Gynecology and Obsterics,FIGO)在 2009 年颁布了外阴癌的新的分期系统(表 101-2)。此手术分期系统自 1989 年形成,后在 1995 年曾经修订过一次。最近的分期系统指出之前的分期中对于病变尺寸、转移淋巴结的数目和大小的描述缺少预测预后的价值[32]。特别是 FIGO 根据基质浸润是否超过 1mm 将Ⅰ期细分为ⅠA 期和ⅠB 期。临床评价腹股沟淋巴结新的分期系统中,在Ⅲ期中还有三个病理分组(A、B 和 C):分别强调了阳性淋巴结的数目、大小和包膜外侵犯。另外,很多中心在使用关于肿瘤、淋巴结和转移的 TNM 分期系统。

表 101-2 外阴癌 TNM 分类及分期

TNM 分类	
T	**原发肿瘤**
Tis	原位癌(CIS)
T1	肿瘤局限于外阴和/或会阴,最大直径≤2cm
T2	肿瘤局限于外阴和/或会阴,最大直径>2cm
T3	肿瘤累及下列任何器官:尿道下段、阴道或者肛门
T4	肿瘤累及下列任何器官:膀胱黏膜、直肠黏膜、尿道上段或固定于肛门
N	**区域淋巴结**
N0	无淋巴结转移
N1	单侧区域淋巴结转移
N2	双侧区域淋巴结转移
M	**远处转移**
M0	无远处转移
M1	远处转移(包括盆腔淋巴结转移)

FIGO 分期(2019)		
ⅠA	T1AN0M0	肿瘤局限于外阴和/或会阴:最大直径≤2cm,间质侵犯≤1mm,无淋巴结转移
ⅠB	T1N0M0	肿瘤局限于外阴和/或会阴:最大直径≤2cm,间质侵犯>1mm,无淋巴结转移
Ⅱ	T2	肿瘤任何大小累及临近会阴结构(下 1/3 尿道和/或下 1/3 阴道和/或肛门),无淋巴结转移
ⅢA	T1 或 2,N1a 或 N1b,M0	肿瘤任何大小或累及临近会阴结构(下 1/3 尿道和/或下 1/3 阴道和/或肛门),合并单侧腹股沟区淋巴结转移:①1~2 个淋巴结转移(<5mm)或②1 个淋巴结转移(>5mm)
ⅢB	T1 或 2,N2a 或 N2b,M0	肿瘤任何大小或累及临近会阴结构(下 1/3 尿道和/或下 1/3 阴道和/或肛门),合并单侧腹股沟区淋巴结转移:①3 个及以上淋巴结转移(<5mm)或②2 个及以上淋巴结转移(>5mm)
ⅢC	T1 或 T2,N2c,M0	阳性淋巴结伴胞膜外扩散
ⅣA		肿瘤累及下列任何部分:尿道上段、膀胱黏膜、直肠黏膜、骨盆和/或双侧区域淋巴结转移
ⅣB		任何远处转移包括盆腔淋巴结转移

FIGO,国际妇产科联盟;TNM,原发肿瘤,区域淋巴结,远处转移。
摘自 Barakat 2013。

外阴癌能够通过直接浸润、淋巴及血道转移。曾有报道转移到股淋巴结而无腹股沟淋巴结受侵,但是这种现象很少见。有学者描述了从阴蒂通过淋巴途径直接转移到盆腔淋巴结,但是没有太多的临床意义。总的淋巴结转移率大约为30%。盆腔淋巴结转移不常见,总的发生率为9%。有腹股沟淋巴结转移的患者中大约有20%合并有盆腔淋巴结转移[33,34]。

鳞状细胞癌

鳞状细胞癌占原发外阴恶性肿瘤的90%。这类肿瘤大体上通常为外阴溃疡状或者多形性结节。活检能够揭示其特征性组织学表现:肿瘤表现为鳞状细胞呈巢状和索状浸润间质,通常合并有角蛋白岛。体格检查通常能发现溃疡样病变或者疣状病变。近年来,疣状癌的发病率有所增加,达到所有病例的20%。

对于这类病变既往报道了多种不同的临床预后。浸润深度小于5mm的肿瘤转移到区域淋巴结的比例从0%到10%[35~40]。例如Hoffman等报道了43例肿瘤浸润深度小于2mm的患者均没有淋巴结转移[38]。具有融合状舌结构浸润到基质内的肿瘤与仅有单个舌结构的肿瘤相比,转移到腹股沟淋巴结的风险更高。间质浸润深度≤1mm淋巴结转移风险<1%,因此肿瘤间质浸润深度<1mm者无须行腹股沟区淋巴结切除。肿瘤浸润深度1.1~3.0mm的淋巴结转移风险为6%~12%,浸润深度3.1~5mm的淋巴结风险则增加到15%~20%[41]。

如果病变同时合并有原位癌可能会降低淋巴结受累的风险。Rowley及其同事报道35例邻近有原位癌的病例中仅1例合并有淋巴结转移[39]。然而,27例浸润深度为2.1~5mm之间,邻近未见原位癌的Ⅰ期病变,有5例合并有淋巴结转移。

前哨淋巴结

前哨淋巴结活检(SLNB)正在用于外阴癌。临床检查未发现腹股沟淋巴结异常,SLNB可作为腹股沟淋巴结切除术的唯一选择。SLNB即可以检测淋巴结有无转移又可以减少手术后并发症。一项妇科肿瘤工作组研究(GOG173)比较了在452例肿瘤深度<1mm、肿瘤直径在2~6cm之间外阴鳞状细胞癌患者中行腹股沟淋巴结切除术和SLNB的结果[42]。本研究中SLNB的敏感度为92%、阴性预测值为96%。另一项多中心观察性的关于外阴癌前哨淋巴结GROnigen International研究(GROnigen INternational Study on Sentinel nodes in Vulvar cancer,GROINSS-V)分析了403例患者的623个腹股沟淋巴结,进一步确定了SLNB降低手术相关的近期和远期并发症。

与腹股沟淋巴结切除术相比,接受SLNB的患者较少反应治疗相关的并发症,而且整体生活质量没有受影响[43]。观察性研究GROINSS-Ⅶ中,SLNB发现阳性淋巴结患者继而行腹股沟淋巴结切除术、SLNB阴性者则观察,这项研究目前仍在进行中。

上述提到的研究均由丰富经验的外科医生进行SLNBS。目前仍建议如果SLNB经验缺乏,则直接经进行腹股沟淋巴结切除术,毕竟后者是外阴癌这种罕见肿瘤的常规治疗。

治疗

临床ⅠA期

肿瘤浸润深度小于1mm的患者发生淋巴结转移的风险很小。对于这些病例可以不行腹股沟淋巴结清扫术。经常采用广泛根治切除术治疗。这些患者的治愈率高,但是也需要定期随访监测以排除复发。

临床Ⅰ/Ⅱ期浸润癌

对于临床Ⅰ期或Ⅱ期外阴癌推荐广泛根治切除和单侧或双侧SLNB或腹股沟淋巴结切除术(淋巴结处理取决于肿瘤大小、位置和局部情况),既为了分期也为了治疗。切缘需要至少包括2cm的正常组织,切缘深度达会阴深筋膜层。病变的位置决定是否需要一侧还是双侧腹股沟淋巴结切除术(或SLNB)。一项GOG173的研究显示如果肿瘤大小于2cm位于中线位置,则双侧腹股沟淋巴结切除术。对于Ⅰ期和Ⅱ期,手术切除通常都会有很好的长期生存和局部控制效果。

部分肿瘤会通过外阴错综复杂的淋巴回流系统发生转移(图101-3)。肿瘤如果位于一侧阴唇,首先回流到同侧腹股沟淋巴结,而位于中线会阴区域的肿瘤能够回流到两侧淋巴结。Iversen和Aas将锝-99胶体这一放射示踪剂注射到外阴的一侧后,发现98%的示踪剂位于同侧淋巴结,不到2%位于对侧淋巴结[34]。位于阴蒂或尿道区域的肿瘤可以回流到两侧腹股沟区域。从腹股沟-股淋巴结链,淋巴会继续回流到深部盆腔髂血管和闭孔淋巴结。虽然以前曾注意到位于阴蒂和尿道区域的肿瘤能够直接转移到深部盆腔淋巴结,目前的证据表明这种情况非常罕见。

Ⅰ、Ⅱ和Ⅲ期浸润癌

外阴癌患者的预后与疾病分期(图101-4)相关[50]。区域淋巴结转移与原发病变的大小、厚度、肿瘤分化程度以及肿瘤是否侵犯血管相关(表101-3),以上结论最早来自Sedlis等的经典研究结果[44]。妇科肿瘤学组(Gynecologic Oncology Group,GOG)报道了272例患者有浸润性外阴癌的女性中,Ⅰ期患者区域淋巴结转移率为8.9%,Ⅱ期为25.3%,而Ⅲ期为31.1%[45,46]。对于厚度大于等于4mm的较大病变,淋巴结转移率为31%。Hacker等[47]报道对于淋巴结阴性的患者,5年实际生存率为96%。如果有一枚淋巴结转移,生存率降到94%。如果有两枚,生存率降到80%。而如果有大于等于3个淋巴结转移,则生存率为12%。

不仅淋巴结转移数目重要,转移灶的大小也很重要。Hoffman等[48]报道了15例合并有腹股沟淋巴结转移的外阴癌患者,转移灶大小均小于36mm,这15例患者中有14例无瘤生存达到5年。与之相对的是29例转移灶超过100mm的患者中,仅有12例无瘤生存达到5年。如果仅有1枚腹股沟淋巴结镜下转移,则不建议行辅助治疗,虽然关于这点仍有争议。Ⅰ期患者没有淋巴结转移。而Ⅳ期患者则有47.7%的患者有淋巴结转移。血管床受累也是一个预后影响因素,因为血管床受累的患者中72%会合并有区域淋巴结受累,而没有血管床受累的患者,仅有34%合并有区域淋巴结受累。淋巴结受累还和原发病变的位置相关[49]。病变位于阴唇的患者淋巴结转移率为7.4%;而阴蒂病变具有较高的淋巴结转移率,达到27.4%[50]。Boyce等[51]报道6例肿瘤直径在1cm以下的患者均无区域淋巴结转移,而29例肿瘤大小超过4cm的患者,淋巴结转移率升高到55%。

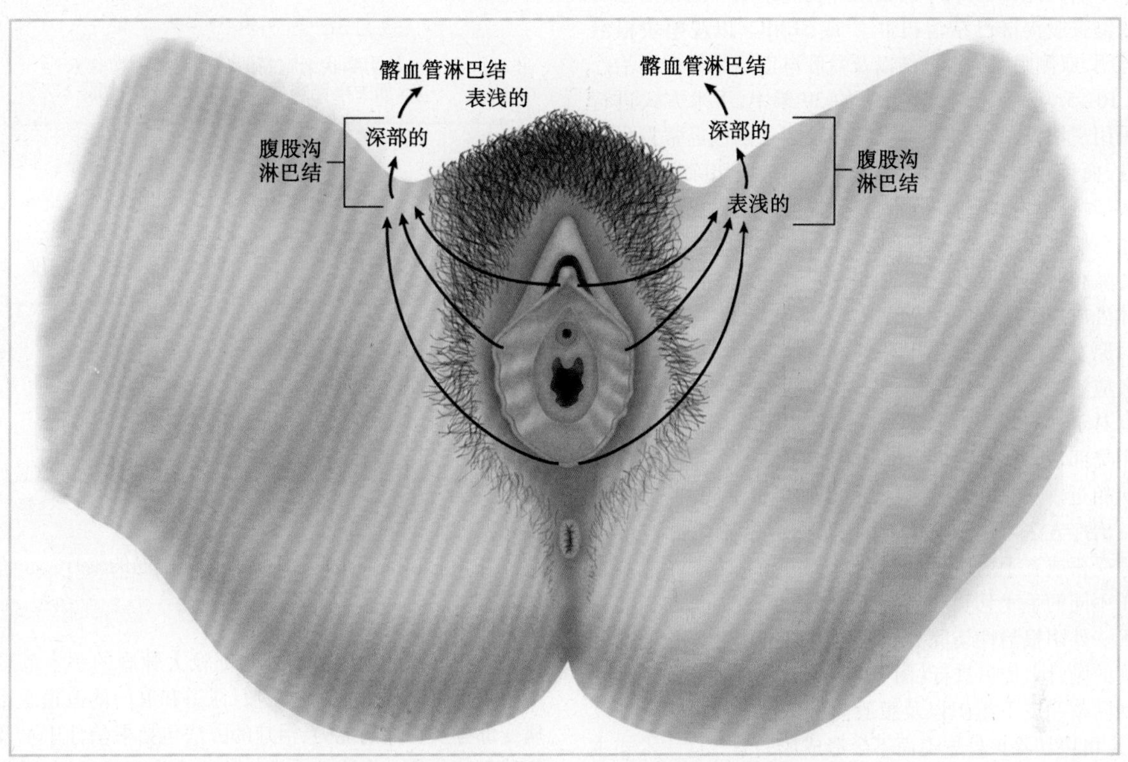

图101-3 外阴的淋巴引流

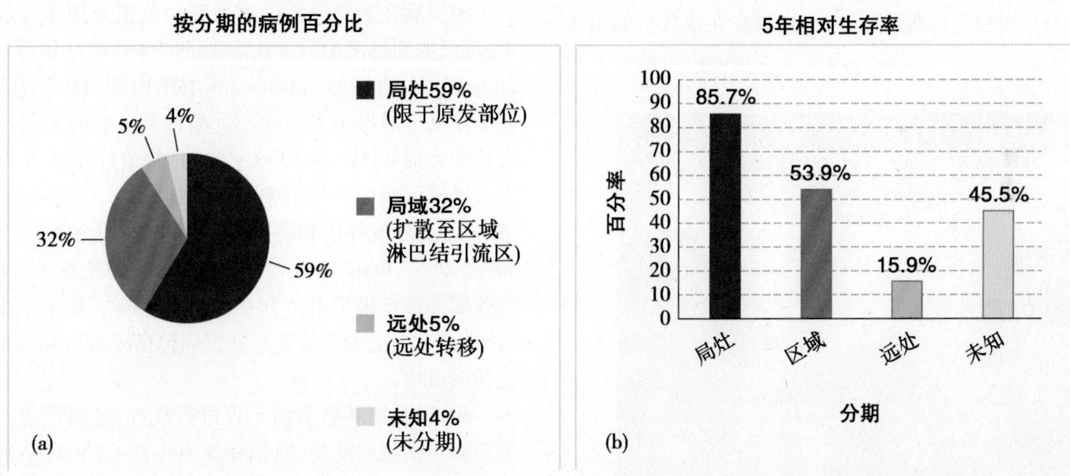

图101-4 (a)按分期的病例百分比。(b)外阴癌按照诊断时不同分期的5年相对生存率。摘自 National Cancer Institute, Surveillance, Epidemiology, and End Results Program(SEER) 2011. Stat Fact Sheets: Vulvar Cancer (reproduced from http://seer.cancer.gov/statfacts/html/vulva.html, accessed 12Feb 2015)

表101-3 分期、分级以及肿瘤厚度等预后因素与区域淋巴结转移的关系

分期	转移淋巴结/%	分级	转移淋巴结/%	肿瘤厚度/mm	转移淋巴结/%
Ⅰ	8.9	1	0	<1	3.1
Ⅱ	25.3	2	8.0	2	8.9
Ⅲ	31.1	3	24.6	3	18.6
Ⅳ	62.5	4	47.7	>4	31.0

摘自 Sedlis 1987[44]。Reproduced with permission of AJOG。

对于Ⅰ期、Ⅱ期以及较早的Ⅲ期外阴癌采用外阴根治性切除术加双侧腹股沟淋巴结清扫术[52]或SLNB。以往整块根治性切除外阴、双侧腹股沟淋巴结以及盆腔淋巴结是标准的治疗方法(图101-5为手术标本)。过去的30年中,手术方式进行了改良采用三切口,减少手术并发症。由于外阴癌经常发生于年轻女性,而且肿瘤直径较小,同时考虑到整块切除术的并发症发生率,对这一术式进行了改良。除非腹股沟淋巴结受累的情况下才会切除深部盆腔淋巴结。目前大多数肿瘤学家手术中仅仅切除腹股沟和股淋巴结,如果术后证实表浅淋巴结有受累则用体外放疗来治疗盆腔淋巴结。

针对原发肿瘤学者提出了许多种治疗选择。对于病变较小的患者应该采取个体化治疗。自从19世纪80年代早期,就有人建议对于肿瘤较小的患者采取局部根治性切除术。文献报道采用局部切除和其他更广泛根治性的术式,局部浸润性复发的比例相近。局部根治性切除术最适合于单侧、孤立的病灶。这一治疗方法可用于有危险因素的患者,如肿瘤大、淋巴脉管间隙受累或者手术切缘小于8mm。

对于不同的手术切口也进行了评价。经典的是进行的整块切除术。外阴根治性切除和腹股沟淋巴结均通过一个双侧髂嵴之间的耻骨上切口进行(图101-5)。这一手术切除了整个外阴包括阴蒂和皮下组织以及腹股沟淋巴结。如果病变累及尿道下段,可以切除该处尿道而不会造成尿失禁。这一术式主要的并发症就是伤口裂开和感染(发生率为50%)。最近,对该术式进行了改良从而减少了伤口裂开。这一改良包括通过独立的腹股沟切口行腹股沟淋巴结清扫术,然后再进行外阴根治性切除。当采用独立的腹股沟切口后,很少在皮肤桥处出现肿瘤复发[46,53]。

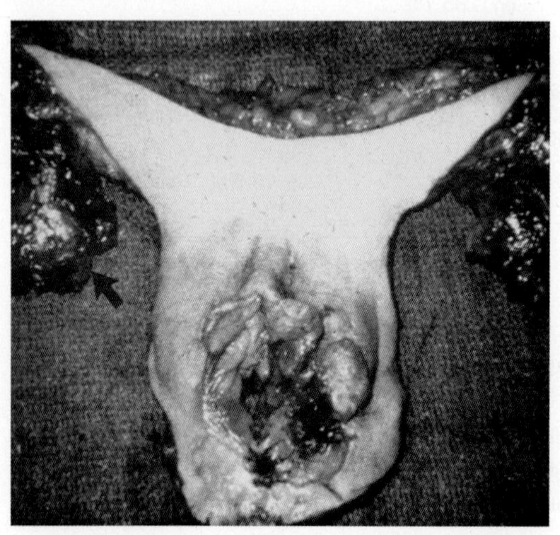

图101-5　大体外阴切除标本,外阴癌

还有报道针对Ⅰ期患者采用比标准的外阴根治切除术破坏性更小还同样有效的手术。对于Ⅰ期和Ⅱ期外阴癌患者,如果没有淋巴结转移,术后不需要辅助治疗。如果有淋巴结转移(特别是股淋巴结)则需要辅助盆腔体外放射治疗。一项随机分组研究中,Homesley等[45]报道在118名有淋巴结转移的患者中,接受4 500~5 000cGy放射治疗能够提高生存率(图101-6)。

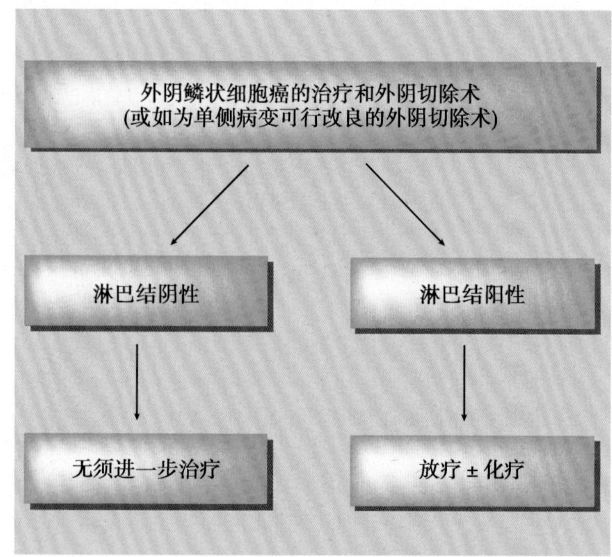

图101-6　外阴鳞状细胞癌的治疗

晚期外阴肿瘤

侵犯肛周区和尿道的外阴部较大肿瘤的手术范围要比外阴根治术更广泛,通常需要进行尿道和肛门的改道手术。根据病变部分及切除的能力,治疗的方法包括根治性手术及数钱的新辅助放化疗。根治性手术往往造成大面积组织缺损,需要皮瓣移植,如骨薄肌的肌肉皮瓣。据报道,如果淋巴结阴性,5年生存率为50%[49,54]。

根据病变的部位及手术切除的范围采用术前放疗联合手术,现已成为标准治疗方法。先进的体外放疗如适形调强放疗(intensity modulated radiotherapy,IMRT)常用在外阴癌根治术伴或不伴局部淋巴结术前缩小肿瘤体积。盆腔和腹股沟淋巴结区接受大约4 000~4 500cGy的照射,放疗结束5周后进行手术。这样可减少尿道和肛门的改道手术。Boronow等[55,56]报道了26名原发外阴和阴道癌患者进行如上治疗,5年生存率为80%。近来,Rotmensch等[57]报道了16例晚期外阴癌患者术前行外阴部放疗再手术,5年生存率为45%。如果手术切缘距肿瘤<1cm有可能发生复发。并发症包括尿道口和尿道狭窄以及直肠阴道瘘。

最近,晚期肿瘤术前不仅进行放疗,还可以进行化疗。常用药物包括氟尿嘧啶、顺铂和丝裂霉素-C(MMC),放化疗使可使肿瘤最多缩小46%;之前的研究发现最常见的毒性是急性皮肤反应和伤口损伤[58]。GOG一项Ⅱ期临床GOG101研究入组了局部晚期T3或T4不能通过根治性外阴切除术切除的患者,他们先接受化疗和每周一次的顺铂化疗,之后再接受手术切除残存肿瘤。研究发现放化疗的完全反应率为64%[59]。因外阴皮肤易发生放射性皮肤炎、纤维化和溃疡,放疗不作为唯一的治疗。但是,如患者因为内科并发症不能手术,放疗可作为外阴癌的主要治疗手段[60]。

复发性外阴癌

复发可发生在局部,也可远处转移。超过80%的复发发生在治疗后最初的2年内。分期越晚复发风险越高。一项包括502例外阴癌的研究中,作者报道了主要的复发发生在局部;53.4%的复发再会阴[61]。其他的复发部位包括腹股沟19%,

盆腔及盆腔外复发分别为 6% 和 8%。

局部复发可采用不同的治疗模式。放疗和手术均能有效控制病变，局部复发患者的 5 年生存率大约为 50%[61]。复发如果发生再腹股沟区域，生存率则锐减，5 年生存率仅为 27%。放化疗联合用于治疗复发外阴癌和某些病变较大的原发外阴癌。转移的病变需要化疗，但遗憾的是，没有化疗方案能完全有效。目前没有相关的前瞻性研究，更多的数据借鉴转移性宫颈癌的研究。因此，大多复发采用铂类为基础的联合方案，在宫颈癌研究中发现，较紫杉醇联合顺铂有更好的耐受性的是卡铂联合紫杉醇。对于不能耐受化疗者建议给予姑息治疗。复发患者总体预后差（图 101-7）。

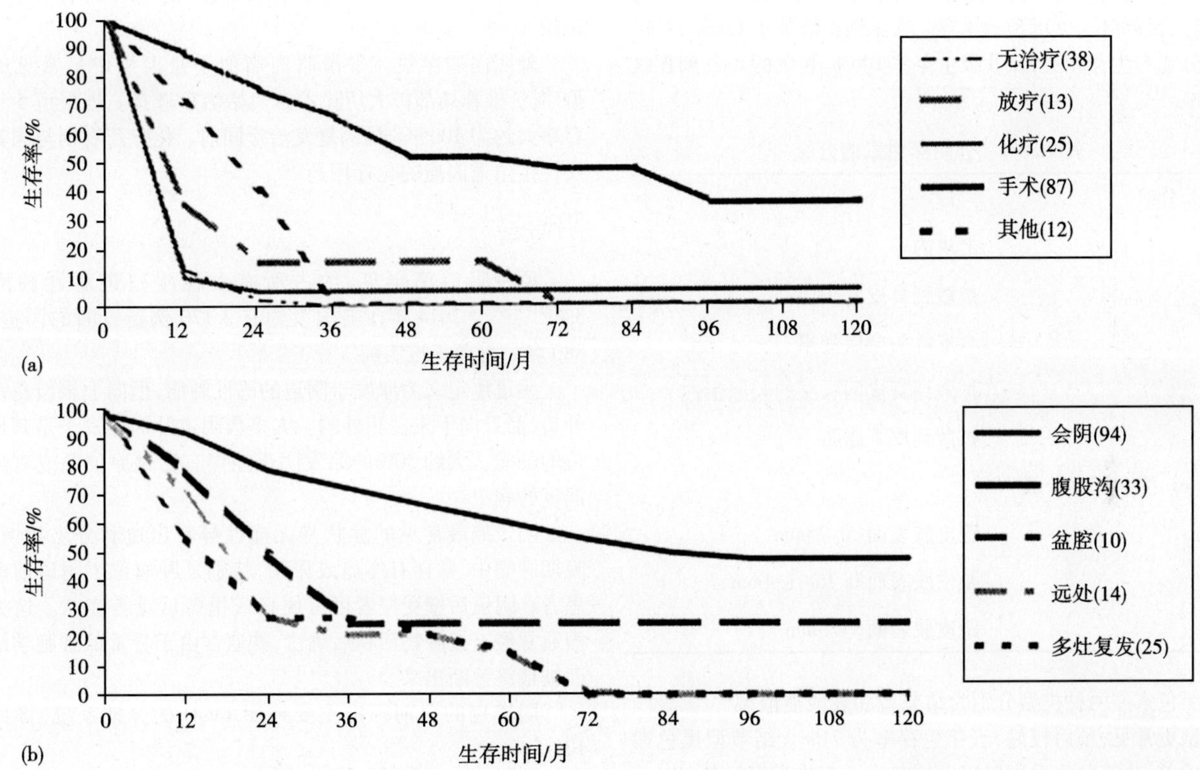

图 101-7　（a）复发外阴癌不同方式治疗的生存率。方框中显示了不同治疗方式患者的数目。手术和其他方式治疗有显著性差异（$P=0.000\,001$）。（b）不同复发部位的外阴癌的生存率（方框中显示了不同复发部位患者的数目）。摘自 Maggino 2000[61]。Reproduced by permission of John Wiley and Sons

巴氏腺癌

原发巴氏腺癌（Bartholin gland carcinoma）占全部原发外阴癌的 5%，已报道的有 200 余例[62]，其中大约有 50% 实际上为非表皮样肿瘤。巴氏腺癌如发生于腺管口附近为鳞癌，如发生于腺管转化上皮为乳头样癌，发生于腺体本身则为腺癌。绝经后巴氏腺体增大应警惕恶性可能。这种肿瘤的治疗与外阴原发鳞癌相似，需行根治性外阴切除和双侧腹股沟淋巴结切除术。5 年生存率大约为 70%，低于所有外阴癌，可能与其诊断常被延误有关。巴氏腺癌如果位于正确的解剖位置即大阴唇深部，下方皮肤完好，尚有正常腺体存在，则可以做出诊断。

巴氏腺的腺样囊腺癌病变局限、很少发生转移，发展缓慢，但易局部复发，侵犯周围组织。治疗上只需要扩大局部切除。Rosenberg 等报道了 5 例巴氏腺的腺样囊腺癌，其中 4 例治疗后无瘤存活 28~57 个月[63]。

基底细胞癌

基底细胞癌在女性生殖道罕见。肿瘤常侵犯局部，很少远处转移，多发生于大阴唇。局部淋巴结转移不常见。治疗为扩大的局部切除术。如果手术切缘净，病变则可治愈。

疣状癌

外阴的疣状癌是表皮样癌的一种。在临床上，外观类似较大的湿疣样病变。常局部侵犯，不转移，外观为真菌样肿瘤，逐渐长大，推挤而不是侵犯其下的结构组织。组织学上，由成熟的广泛角化的鳞状细胞组成。为明确诊断，充分的活组织检查很重要，大的疣状癌如不充分活检常常误诊为尖锐湿疣。

肿瘤缓慢生长、局部侵犯，很少扩散到局部的淋巴结。Japaze 等对 24 例疣状癌的报道中未发现淋巴结转移[64]。根据肿瘤的大小和部位进行治疗，局部扩大切除或单纯外阴切除术是有效的方法。根治性外阴切除联合腹股沟淋巴结切除术或放疗不适用于此病。放疗无效，甚至会导致肿瘤内恶变而恶化预后。Japaze 等报道的病例中有 17 例接受手术治疗的患者 5 年生存率达到 94%。此病可以局部复发，所以有必要进行密切的长期随访，特别当原肿瘤较大时。如果疣状癌内同时还有鳞状细胞癌，治疗上仅做局部切除则不够[65]。

黑色素瘤

是外阴的非鳞状细胞恶性肿瘤中最多见的一类，占外阴原发恶性肿瘤的 5%。目前已报道的外阴黑色素瘤有大约 400

例,无论治疗方式如何,5 年生存率大约为 33%。外阴恶性黑色素瘤患者的年龄分布广泛,从 10~96 岁,平均年龄 60 岁。此病多发于小阴唇和阴蒂[66]。

外阴黑色素瘤常使用 FIGO 分期。但是这种分期系统不能提示肿瘤深度,故不能提示预后。表 101-4 是外阴黑色素瘤的分级系统,类似于皮肤黑色素瘤的 Clark 系统。新的预后因素包括肿瘤厚度、溃疡、转移淋巴结的数目、前哨淋巴结微转移以及远处转移部位,可以预示生存。从Ⅰ到Ⅳ级基于 Clark 系统,浸润分级与生存相关,从Ⅱ级生存率 100%、Ⅳ级的 83%到Ⅳ级的 28%[67]。

表 101-4 外阴黑色素瘤分级

Clark 分级	
Ⅰ	上皮内
Ⅱ	扩散到真皮乳头层
Ⅲ	真皮乳头全层受累
Ⅳ	扩散到真皮网状层的胶原蛋白
Ⅴ	扩散到皮下脂肪
Breslow 浸润深度分级	
Ⅰ	距皮肤表面<0.75mm
Ⅱ	距皮肤表面 0.76~1.4mm
Ⅲ	距皮肤表面>1.5mm

黑色素瘤两种类型分别为结节型和表浅播散型[68]。表浅播散型更常见,预后较好,五年生存率为 71%。结节型黑色素瘤预后差,与其肿瘤垂直侵犯生长有关,5 年生存率仅有 38%。

肿瘤厚度有助于评价病变。Breslow 报道了从皮肤表面到肿瘤浸润深度的分级系统[69]。在这个分级系统中,Breslow 报道了深度小于 0.76mm(从皮肤表面到穿刺最深点)的黑色素瘤很少出现淋巴结受侵,总体预后较好。

Clark Ⅰ级和Ⅱ级病变如淋巴结未扪及肿大,推荐采用局部扩大切除术[70]。一项关于 36 例黑色素瘤报道中,Rose 等提到扩大切除术与外阴根治切除术一样有效[71]。年轻患者预后较好,可能是大多数为表浅播散型的原因。

如肿瘤厚度小于 2mm 则切除肿瘤保持 2cm 切缘,无须切除淋巴结。但是,亦有建议进行根治性局部切除术(距病变边缘 1~2cm)同时行同侧腹股沟淋巴结切除。后者建立于中等厚度皮肤黑色素瘤的选择性淋巴结切除与观察相比较的多中心非随机研究基础上。这项研究显示对于 1~4mm 的黑色素瘤,行选择性淋巴结切除的患者 5 年生存率比仅观察者高。

晚期黑色素瘤可以进行局部切除联合腹股沟淋巴结切除术,切缘为 2~3cm。对于病变为 Clark Ⅲ、Ⅳ和Ⅴ级的患者可选择进行外阴根治切除联合腹股沟、盆腔淋巴结切除术[72]。

有报道外阴的黑色素瘤通过腹股沟淋巴结可以转移到盆腔淋巴结,现有证据发现没有腹股沟淋巴结受累时盆腔淋巴结也不会发生转移。治疗时还要考虑到盆腔淋巴结转移的黑色素瘤患者一般不能治愈。

大宗黑色素瘤病例长期的生存结果尚无报道。大多数报道的总生存率大约在 50%[73]。相当于 Clark Ⅰ或Ⅱ级(病变厚度 0.76mm)的肿瘤接受局部扩大切除术,5 年生存率接近 100%。如病变厚度大于 3mm,预后则很差。如果局部淋巴结阴性,生存率接近 60%,如果淋巴结转移,生存率仅为 30%。

化疗的作用对于远处转移的病变还不明确。已有研究报道采用不同的多药联合方案的化疗和/或免疫治疗后,肿瘤可以缩小,但不是治愈。应尽可能鼓励这些患者参加临床研究。

肉瘤

外阴肉瘤罕见。平滑肌肉瘤似乎是肉瘤中最常见的类型[74]。推荐局部扩大切除术为初始治疗选择。据报道 5 年生存率大约为 100%。局部复发治疗同前。化疗药物则与同其他女性生殖道肉瘤的化疗用药[75]。

阴道癌

原发阴道癌罕见,约占所有女性生殖道恶性肿瘤的 3%[2,76~78]。2014 年在美国大约有 3 170 例新诊断的阴道癌,880 名妇女死于该疾病。

阴道癌定义为原发于阴道的恶性肿瘤,但向上未侵犯宫颈外口,而且向下未侵犯外阴。大多数阴道肿瘤继发于是其他部位的肿瘤。大约 30%的原发阴道癌伴有宫颈原位癌或宫颈浸润癌的病史。

阴道癌最常见的症状是无痛性异常出血和分泌物增多。晚期肿瘤中,常伴有疼痛或尿频,特别是肿瘤位于阴道前壁的患者。阴道后壁受侵者可有便秘或里急后重等症状。这类肿瘤通常经直接肿物活检后确诊,并通常由于异常的细胞学结果而被最终诊断出来。

阴道癌的分期标准主要按照 FIGO 的分期系统,详见表 101-5。

表 101-5 阴道癌的 FIGO 分期系统

分期	
0	原位癌
Ⅰ	肿瘤局限于阴道壁
Ⅱ	肿瘤累及阴道旁组织但未达盆壁
Ⅲ	肿瘤累及阴道旁组织达盆壁
Ⅳ	肿瘤超出真骨盆或侵犯膀胱或直肠黏膜
ⅣA	侵犯邻近器官和/或直接浸润范围超出真骨盆
ⅣB	侵犯远处器官

阴道癌前病变

阴道癌前病变一般都是通过阴道细胞学筛查发现。一旦发现细胞学异常,需要通过阴道镜下活检来确认病变的程度。因为阴道上皮内病变经常为多灶,仔细检查全段阴道壁很有必要[79]。

大多数病变发生于阴道穹窿。Audet-Laointe 等报道 66 例阴道上皮内瘤变中有 61 例发生在阴道上 1/3[80]。这些病变通常可进行局部切除。但由于病灶的多灶性特点,常需要切除较大区域,并需要联合皮瓣移植,所以也可以考虑其他治疗方式[81]。

该类病变的非手术治疗包括对于多灶病变进行激光消融或 5-Fu 软膏外敷。使用较多的是二氧化碳激光，如果作用深度控制在 2~4mm，可使病变组织汽化。Petrilli 等报道的采用此方法治疗的初步结果显示治疗成功率大约为 90%[82]。由于病变邻近膀胱和直肠，又有其他治疗方法可以选择，故现不推荐放疗治疗非浸润性病变。

另一种治疗阴道上皮内瘤变的方法是局部敷用 5% 5-Fu 软膏外敷，连用 7 天，如病变持续存在则每 3~4 周重复使用。角化病变似乎对该治疗不敏感，是因病变较厚而且角化不全。Kerbs 报道使用 5% 5-Fu 共 10 天，发现 20 例阴道湿疣患者中有 17 例治疗有效[83]。Petrilli 和 Ballon 等报道多周期用药治疗阴道上皮内瘤变的成功率达 80%~90%[82,84]。还有一种治疗药物是咪喹莫特，具体治疗方法和外阴病变的治疗方法相同（参见"外阴癌"）。

浸润性阴道癌

阴道的鳞状细胞癌可以表现为溃疡状或者息肉样肿瘤，并有可能外突脱出阴道口。该类病变是最常见的阴道恶性肿瘤，约占阴道原发癌的 90%。病变多发生于 50 岁以上的患者。大多数鳞癌发生于阴道上 1/3。检查患者时仔细检查整个阴道壁非常重要，因阴道后壁病变可能被窥器所遮挡[85]。这类肿瘤在镜下有典型鳞状细胞癌的表现，为多形性鳞癌细胞，有些具有角化珠。

肿瘤部位决定了淋巴引流区域（图 101-8）[86]。阴道中段和上段的淋巴引流向上与宫颈淋巴引流交汇并引流入盆腔的闭孔、髂内及髂外淋巴结。阴道下 1/3 淋巴引流到腹股沟和盆腔淋巴结，与外阴癌的淋巴引流相似。阴道后壁淋巴引流至直肠淋巴结系统。31.6% 的阴道下段肿瘤的患者发生腹股沟淋巴结转移。阴道癌的治疗应个体化。

根据病变位置，高剂量率近距离放疗和手术均是有效的治疗手段（表 101-6）。治疗方案通常根据肿瘤的大小、分期和位置来选择个体化的治疗[84,87]。如果肿瘤厚度<2cm，一些学者建议可以仅使用局部放疗[88,89]。如果肿瘤厚度<0.5cm，采用圆柱体容器进行阴道腔内放疗，黏膜表面给予 8 000cGy，可以使肿瘤控制率达到 90% 以上[90]。Spirtos 等研究了 23 例Ⅰ期患者，发现只有 2 例发生了局部复发，而这两例的放疗剂量均小于 7 500cGy[91]。对于较大的肿瘤，还需采用体外放疗，阴道局部近距离放疗剂量应该相应减少[92]。插植技术通常不用于肿瘤体积较大的Ⅲ期或Ⅳ期患者。对于这类者，仅采用体外全盆放疗 5 000cGy，然后进行中部加量[93]。

表 101-6　阴道癌的治疗方案

分期	体外放疗/cGy	组织间插植/cGy
Ⅰ		
Σ，小肿瘤（<2cm）	—	6 000~7 000
Σ，所有其他	全盆腔（4 000）	3 000~4 000
Ⅱ	全盆腔（4 000~5 000）	3 000~4 000
Ⅲ	全盆腔（5 000）	2 000
Ⅳ	全盆腔（5 000；如果不能进行插植，缩野后加量 1 000~2 000）	2 000（如果可能）

摘自 Nori et al[90]。经 Elsevier 公司授权复制。

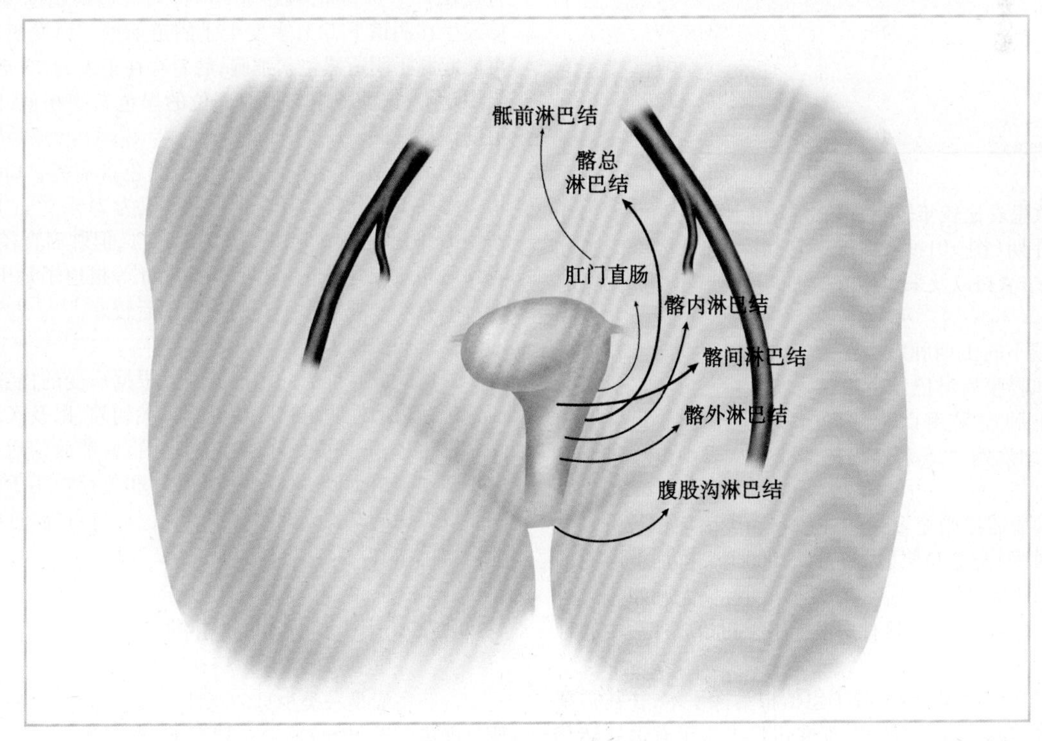

图 101-8　阴道的淋巴引流图

位于阴道上 1/3 较小的肿瘤通常可以行手术切除[94,95]。广泛子宫切除、部分阴道切除、盆腔淋巴结切除术对这类患者通常是有效的。年轻患者更倾向于选择手术。如果已发生远处转移，顺铂为基础的化疗对于复发的阴道鳞癌是否有效尚不清楚[96]。对于鳞状细胞癌，目前多采用与宫颈鳞癌类似的联合化疗方案。原发阴道癌总生存率与分期相关。

阴道透明细胞腺癌

阴道透明细胞癌与宫内已烯雌酚暴露有关，所以自从 1970 年之后年轻女性中发病率逐渐升高[97,98]。透明细胞癌有三种主要组织学类型，分别为囊管型、团块型及乳头状型[99,100]。大多数阴道透明细胞癌大体表现为红色息肉样或结节样。

透明细胞癌可局部扩散，或者经血液和淋巴管途径远处转移。大约 1/6 的Ⅰ期患者发生区域淋巴结转移。区域淋巴结转移在晚期患者中更多见。阴道透明细胞癌与其他类型的阴道癌一样，采用 FIGO 分期系统。80%的患者诊断时为Ⅰ期或Ⅱ期。

目前已确定了几个预后的相关因素。年龄较大的患者（如年龄超过 19 岁）比年龄小的患者预后好[101]。这种预后差异可能与年龄较大的患者的组织类型以囊管型为主有关。除此之外，肿瘤直径小、浸润表浅的肿瘤预后较好。预后还与肿瘤分期有关。在一项 547 例阴道透明细胞癌的研究中，Ⅰ、Ⅱ、Ⅲ及Ⅳ期的 5 年生存率分别为 93%、83%、37%和 0%（表 101-7）[101]。

表 101-7 547 例阴道和宫颈透明细胞癌患者的 5 年和 10 生存率

分期	生存率/%	
	5 年	10 年
Ⅰ	93	87
ⅡA	80	66
ⅡB	58	49
Ⅱ（阴道）	83	67
Ⅲ	37	12
Ⅳ	0	0

由于多数患者比较年轻，手术通常是主要治疗方式。对Ⅰ期和相早的Ⅱ期（图 101-9），广泛子宫切除、部分或全阴道切除、盆腔淋巴结清扫以及采用移植皮肤进行阴道再造是最常采用的术式[102]。

在肿瘤较小的Ⅰ期肿瘤中，已有学者尝试保留生育功能。在切除肿瘤和腹膜后淋巴结后进行局部放疗。Senekjian 等报道+了阴道小肿瘤采用以上治疗比传统治疗的生存率更好[102]。在这组病例中，5 名经局部治疗的患者中发生了 8 次妊娠。

较大的肿瘤需接受全盆腔体外放疗和腔内插植放疗。对于大于 2cm 肿瘤，全盆腔照射 4 000～5 000cGy，再加上腔内插植放疗 3 000～4 000cGy[103]。在有些情况下，较大肿瘤患者也可接受盆腔脏器切除术；但这种手术常用于初始放疗后中心性复发的治疗[104]。

肿瘤一旦出现复发，治疗方案包括根治性手术，往往需要盆腔脏器切除术或盆腔放疗。系统性化疗可用于有远处转移的患者。目前推荐方案是顺铂（75～100mg/m^2）联合 5-Fu

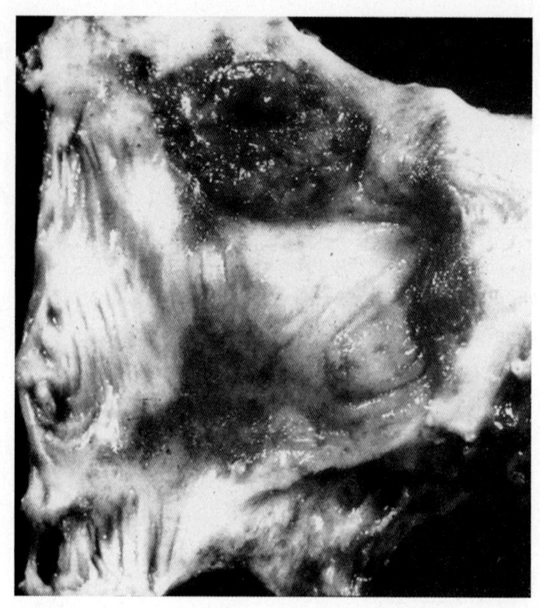

图 101-9 阴道前壁的透明细胞癌，后壁病变边缘伴有阴道腺病

（1g/m^2，第 3～5 天，每 4 周一次）持续静脉滴注方案。但是，没有发现任何单药或联合化疗非常有效[105]。长期随访很有必要，因为曾有报道在初始治疗后 19 年发生复发，特别是肺部和锁骨上区域的复发。

阴道黑色素瘤

阴道的恶性黑色素瘤罕见，占女性全部黑色素瘤的不到 1%。患者年龄从 26～98 岁不等[53]，中位年龄为 70 岁。大多数患者为绝经后，表现为阴道出血或排液，或阴道肿物。肿瘤直径在 0.5～7.5cm，大约有 30%患者肿瘤不超过 2cm。多数肿瘤发生在阴道下 1/3，多发生于阴道前壁。原发阴道黑色素瘤可能起源于阴道黑色素细胞，后者存在于大约 3%健康女性中。组织学上，这种肿瘤与其他部位的黑色素瘤相似，倾向于向阴道壁深部浸润。

阴道黑色素瘤的预后比外阴黑色素瘤差。Chung 等报道了一组共 19 例病例，其 5 年生存率仅为 21%[106]。Reid 等报道一组 15 例患者的 5 年生存率为 17.4%，但肿瘤直径不超过 3cm 者预后相对较好[107]。最近，Borazjani 等报道了每 10 个高倍镜视野下有丝分裂数小于 6 的病变预后较好[108]。与预后最相关的因素是病变的大小。

目前尚没有理想的治疗方案。根据病变的位置不同，治疗通常包括根治性阴道切除或局部扩大切除，以及区域淋巴结切除。近年来，一种更保守的方法是在行盆腔放疗后进行局部扩大切除术。由于该疾病预后差，放疗和化疗常用于治疗局部复发。该类疾病发生远处转移很普遍。如果可能，这些患者应参加临床试验。

年轻女性的少见阴道肿瘤

内胚窦瘤是一类少见的恶性生殖细胞肿瘤，最常发生的部位是卵巢[109]。肿瘤分泌 α 甲胎蛋白，可作为一种有效的肿瘤标志物来监测患者病情。常发生于年龄不超过 3 岁的婴儿和儿童[110,111]。患者常以阴道出血或血性分泌物就诊。查体可发现红色质脆或为粉白色息肉样肿物。肿瘤进展快,多数患者已死亡。治疗包括手术、放疗和化疗。Young 和 Scully 报道了6例患者在接受手术、放疗或手术联合放疗的局部治疗后接受 VAC(长春新碱联合放射菌素 D 和环磷酰胺)方案全身化疗,无瘤存活2~9年[112]。Copeland 等报道了联合化疗及手术取得相似结果[113]。Collins 等近来发现单纯化疗后肿瘤会消失[114,115]。这项报道中,一名5个月大的婴儿在使用 VAC 化疗后肿瘤消失。

另一种少见的发生于年轻女性的阴道肿瘤为葡萄状肉瘤或胚胎型横纹肌肉瘤[116]。这类肿瘤常发生于小于8岁的女童。和阴道内胚窦瘤一样,其最常见的症状是阴道出血。Hilgers 回顾了58例病例,症状出现时的平均年龄为38.3个月[50]。肿瘤外形似葡萄簇或多发息肉样物,起源于阴道表皮下层并很快膨胀性生长并充满阴道。组织学上,通过发现具有横纹的横纹肌母细胞可确诊为此类肿瘤。因为肿瘤为阴道表皮下浸润,常有一个明显的表皮下区带,称为形成层。过去经常采用脏器切除的治疗方法,5年生存率为10%~35%[117]。Hilgers 回顾了21例进行盆腔脏器切除术的胚胎横纹肌肉瘤病例,发现这种治疗方式并不能有效地治愈这些患者[118]。采用多药联合方案,如 VAC 方案化疗相对保守的手术或放疗的综合治疗方式能够有效地控制肿瘤。

Hayes 等最近报道了21例接受化疗的阴道横纹肌肉瘤病例[119]。其中7例出现复发,7例中有5例患者在手术时仅切除部分肿瘤而有肿瘤残存。21例中17例患者在术前接受新辅助化疗,然后进行手术切除。目前尚无大宗病例的长期生存数据,但联合多种治疗的综合治疗中虽然手术范围不那么广泛,但更有效。

一类少见的良性的纤维上皮性阴道息肉与阴道葡萄状肉瘤相似,可发生于婴儿或妊娠妇女的阴道[68,120,121]。尽管镜下存在大的非典型细胞,但缺乏上皮浸润、形成层和 strap 细胞。大体上,这些息肉并不会像葡萄状肉瘤那样聚集呈葡萄状。此种激素刺激的增生性病变称为葡萄状假性肉瘤,局部切除有效。

(安菊生 袁光文 译)

参考文献

The complete reference list can be found on the Wiley Companion Digital Edition of this title (see inside front cover for login instructions).

1 Whitcomb BP. Gynecologic malignancies. *Surg Clin North Am*. 2008;**88**:301–317.

10 Stroup AM. Demographic, clinical, and treatment trends among women diagnosed with vulvar cancer in the United States. *Gynecol Oncol*. 2008;**108**:577–583.

11 Mabuchi K, Bross DS, Kessler II. Epidemiology of cancer of the vulva: a case control study. *Cancer*. 1985;**55**:1843–1848.

13 Chafe W, Richards A, Morgan L, Wilkinson E. Unrecognized invasive carcinoma in vulvar epithelial neoplasia (VIN). *Gynecol Oncol*. 1988;**31**:154.

19 Raspollini MR, Asirelli G, Taddei GL. Analysis of lymphocytic infiltrate does not help in prediction of vulvar squamous cell carcinoma arising in a background of lichen sclerosus. *Int J Gynaecol Obstet*. 2008;**100**:190–191.

20 Armes JE, Lourie R, Bowlay G, Tabrizi S. Pagetoid squamous cell carcinoma in situ of the vulva: comparison with extramammary paget disease and nonpagetoid squamous cell neoplasia. *Int J Gynecol Pathol*. 2008;**27**:118–124.

21 Mulvany NJ, Allen DG. Differentiated intraepithelial neoplasia of the vulva. *Int J Gynecol Pathol*. 2008;**27**:125–135.

25 Campbell SM, Curnow A. Extensive vulval intraepithelial neoplasia treated with a new regime of systemic photodynamic therapy using meta-tetrahydroxychlorin (Foscan). *J Eur Acad Dermatol Venereol*. 2008;**22**:502–503.

29 Helwig EP, Graham JH. Anogenital (extramammary) Paget's disease. *Cancer*. 1963;**16**:387.

30 Lee SC, Roth LM, Ehrlich C, Hall JA. Extramammary Paget's disease of the vulva—a clinicopathologic study of 13 cases. *Cancer*. 1977;**39**:2540.

34 Iversen T, Aas M. Lymph drainage from the vulva. *Gynecol Oncol*. 1983;**16**:179.

37 Hacker NF, Nieburg RK, Berek JS, et al. Superficially invasive vulvar cancer with nodal metastases. *Gynecol Oncol*. 1983;**15**:65.

39 Rowley KC, Gallion HH, Donalson ES, et al. Prognostic factors in early vulvar cancer. *Gynecol Oncol*. 1988;**31**:43.

40 Berman ML, Soper JT, Creasman WT, et al. Conservative surgical management in superficially invasive stage I vulvar carcinoma. *Gynecol Oncol*. 1989;**35**:352.

46 Landrum LM, Lanneau GS, Skaggs VJ, et al. Gynecologic Oncolgy Group risk groups for vulvar carcinoma: improvement in survival in the modern era. *Gynecol Oncol*. 2007;**106**:521–525.

51 Boyce J, Fruchter RG, Kasambilides E, et al. Prognostic factors in carcinoma of the vulva. *Gynecol Oncol*. 1985;**20**:364.

52 Le T, Elsugi R, Hopkins L, Faught W, Fung-Kee-Fung M. The definition of optimal inguinal femoral nodal dissection in the management of vulva squamous cell carcinoma. *Ann Surg Oncol*. 2007;**14**:2128–2132.

53 Christopherson W, Buchsbaum HJ, Voet R, Lifschitz S. Radical vulvectomy and bilateral groin lymphadenectomy utilizing separate groin incisions: report of a case with recurrence in the intervening skin bridge. *Gynecol Oncol*. 1985;**21**:247.

54 Blotti F, Zullo MA, Angioli R. Incontinence after radical vulvectomy treated with Macroplastique implantation. *J Minim Invasive Gynecol*. 2008;**15**:113–115.

55 Boronow RC. Combined therapy as an alternative to exenteration of locally advanced vulvar vaginal cancer. *Cancer*. 1982;**49**:1085.

56 Boronow RC, Hickman BT, Reagan MT, et al. Combined therapy as an alternative to exenteration for locally advanced vulvovaginal cancer. *Am J Clin Oncol*. 1987;**10**:1711.

57 Rotmensch J, Rubin SJ, Sutton HG, et al. Preoperative radiotherapy followed by radical vulvectomy with inguinal lymphadenectomy for advanced vulvar cancer. *Gynecol Oncol*. 1990;**36**:181.

58 Moore DH, Thomas GM, Montana GS, et al. Preoperative chemoradiation for advanced vulvar cancer: a phase II study of the Gynecologic Oncology Group. *Int J Radiat Oncol Biol Phys*. 1998;**42**:1317–1323.

63 Rosenberg P, Simonsen E, Risberg B. Adenoid cystic carcinoma of Bartholin's gland: a report of 5 new cases treated with surgery and radiotherapy. *Gynecol Oncol*. 1989;**34**:145.

67 Phillips GL, Twiggs LB, Okagaki T. Vulvar melanoma: a microstaging study. *Gynecol Oncol*. 1982;**14**:80.

69 Breslow A. Thickness, cross-sectional areas, and depth of invasion in the prognosis of cutaneous melanoma. *Ann Surg*. 1970;**172**:908.

73 Podratz KC, Gaffey TA, Symmonds RE, et al. Melanoma of the vulva: an update. *Gynecol Oncol*. 1983;**16**:153.

75 Lieb SM, Gallousis S, Greedman H. Granular cell myoblastoma of the vulva. *Gynecol Oncol*. 1979;**8**:12.

80 Audet-Lapointe P, Body G, Vauclair R, et al. Vaginal intraepithelial neoplasia. *Gynecol Oncol*. 1990;**36**:232.

85 Gupta N, Mittal S, Dalmia S, Misra R. A rare case of primary invasive carcinoma of vagina associated with irreducible third degree uterovaginal prolapse. *Arch Gynecol Obstet*. 2007;**276**:563–564.

87 Beriwal S, Heron DE, Mogus R, Edwards RP, Kelley JL, Sukumvanich P. High dose rate brachytherapy (HDRB) for primary or recurrent cancer in the vagina. *Radiat Oncol*. 2008;**3**:7.

88 Andersen ES. Primary carcinoma of the vagina: a study of 29 cases. *Gynecol Oncol*. 1989;**33**:317.

89 Otton GR, Nicklin JL, Dickie GJ, et al. Early-stage vaginal carcinoma—an analysis of 70 patients. *Int J Gynecol Cancer*. 2004;**14**:304–310.

91 Spirtos NM, Doshi BP, Kapp DS, Teng N. Radiation therapy for primary squamous cell carcinoma of the vagina: Stanford University experience. *Gynecol Oncol*. 1989;**35**:20.

93 Prempree T, Viravathana T, Slawson RG, et al. Radiation management of primary carcinoma of the vagina. *Cancer*. 1977;**40**:109.

95 Basaran A, Ayhan A. Cancer of the vagina treated with wide local excision and modified Martius (labial) flap interposition. *Gynecol Oncol*. 2008;**108**:455–456.

96 Samant R, Lau B, Choan E, Le T, Tam T. Primary vaginal cancer treated with concurrent chemoradiation using Cis-platinum. *Int J Radiat Oncol Biol Phys*. 2007;**69**:746–750.

97 Herbst AL, Scully RE. Adenocarcinoma of the vagina in adolescence. *Cancer*. 1970;**25**:745.

102 Senekjian EK, Frey KW, Anderson D, Herbst AL. Local therapy in stage I clear cell adenocarcinoma of the vagina. *Cancer*. 1987;**60**:1319.

103 Senekjian EK, Frey KW, Herbst AL. Pelvic exenteration in clear cell adenocarcinoma of the vagina and cervix. *Gynecol Oncol*. 1989;**34**:413.

第 102 章　宫颈病变

Anuja Jhingran, MD ■ Ana M. Rodriguez, MD, MPH, FACOG

概述

宫颈癌是全球女性第三大常见恶性肿瘤及第四大恶性肿瘤死因，2008 年全球新发病例约 529 800 例，死亡 275 100 例。2015 年美国有 12 900 例新患者，发病率呈下降趋势，死亡 4 100 人。鳞状细胞癌是最常见的病理类型。人乳头瘤病毒（human papillomavirus，HPV）是最主要的病因。宫颈癌可以通过宫颈涂片和 HPV DNA 检查进行筛查，并有望以 HPV 疫苗进行预防。早期宫颈癌可手术治疗，包括保留生育的手术，治愈率较高。局部晚期宫颈癌通过放疗联合化疗可获得较高生存率，而晚期宫颈癌患者的生存率还有待治疗手段的进步得到提高。全身化疗可用于治疗复发和转移性疾病，应关注化疗毒副反应。发展中国家晚期宫颈癌最常见，治疗宫颈癌成功的关键仍然是提高发展中国家晚期宫颈癌的生存率。

流行病学

发病率和死亡率

宫颈癌是全球女性第三大常见恶性肿瘤及第四大恶性肿瘤死因，2008 年新发病例约 529 800 例，死亡 275 100 例[1]。发展中国家宫颈癌的发病率是发达国家的 2 倍，其中以非洲和中南亚地区发病率最高（每年 29/100 000），大洋洲和北美地区最低（每年 7.5/100 000）[2]。在发达国家，宫颈癌新发病例数占所有恶性肿瘤的 3.6%[2]。预计 2015 年美国的新发病例将达 12 900 人，死亡 4 100 人[3]。西班牙种族发病率较高（占 10.5%），其次为美国黑人（占 10.2%）、美国印第安人（占 9.5%）、白人（占 7.1%）和太平洋岛/亚洲地区居民（占 6.4%）[3]。

过去 40 年中，巴氏涂片筛查技术的应用使大多数发达国家宫颈癌的发病率和死亡率均明显降低[4]，其中美国降低了 70%。浸润性宫颈癌的发病率由 1998 年的每 100 000 名妇女 10.2 例降为 2002 年的 8.5 例[5]。但是，在发展中国家，由于筛查体系不完善以及癌前病变治疗不及时，宫颈癌一直严重威胁着妇女的健康。

宫颈癌前病变的患病率及发病率尚无确切数据。据美国国家癌症研究所估计，宫颈癌前病变的检出率为每年 300 000 例，而美国癌症联合委员会报道，2001 年宫颈原位癌患者约为 65 000 例。SEER 资料显示，1991—1995 年宫颈原位鳞癌的发病率为每年 41.4/100 000[6]。

宫颈病变的发病危险因素

人乳头瘤病毒和其他性传播病原体感染

流行病学资料早已提示，宫颈病变是由性传播病原体感染所致。多种性行为与宫颈病变的高发现象具有恒定的关系（如多个性伴侣，初次性生活过早和男性伴侣不良性习惯）证实了这个假说[7]。20 世纪 70 年代中期，首次提出了人乳头瘤病毒（human papillomavirus，HPV）与宫颈病变发病因果关系的假说[8]。此后，大量的实验室、临床和流行病学研究结果均证实某些 HPV 亚型在宫颈病变发生中具有重要的作用[9]。

在已经发现的 78 种 HPV 亚型中，35 种以上与肛门生殖道疾病相关，有 30 多种与恶性肿瘤相关[10]。宫颈癌前病变（cervical intraepithelial Neoplasia，CIN）中的 PCR 方法检测 HPV DNA 阳性率为 94%，细胞学正常者的阳性率为 46%[9,11]。

宫颈鳞状上皮内高度病变（high-grade squamous intraepithelial lesion，HSIL）（CIN Ⅱ 和 Ⅲ）标本中危型和高危型 HPV 的阳性率为 77%，浸润癌为 84%[12]。Bosch 等研究显示，HPV 16、18、31 和 45 型的阳性率为 80%[13]。HPV16 型是宫颈病变中阳性率最高的亚型，在高度病变和浸润癌中达 50%，也是细胞学正常者最常见的感染亚型[12,14,15]。

宫颈病变与 HPV 感染之间的相关性与研究人群、研究设计和 HPV 检测方法均无关[13]。发病的高危因素包括：某些 HPV 亚型感染（16、18、31、33、35 和 45 型）、病毒负荷高以及混合型感染[16,17]。HPV 高危型感染者发生高度 CIN 的风险上升 16~122 倍[17]。CIN 患者中 HPV 阳性率为 60%~92%[11]。此外，HPV 感染状态也反映了宫颈病变与性伴侣数和其他性行为之间的关系[11,16,17]。

尽管已经明确 HPV 感染与宫颈病变之间具有高度且恒定的相关性，但 HPV 感染率与宫颈病变发病率并不一致，提示宫颈病变的发生发展还有其他协同因素的参与。大量研究已表明 HIV 感染与宫颈癌相关[7]。1993 年，美国疾病控制和预防中心（Centers for Disease Control and Prevention，CDC）将浸润性宫颈癌列入 AIDS 相关疾病中[15]。有报道发现，HIV 病毒阳性妇女的宫颈病变发病率、病变范围广度和高度病变发生率以及复发率均高于 HIV 阴性者。此外，HIV 阳性妇女的 HPV 阳性率以及持续感染率显著升高。Mandelblatt 等的荟萃分析显示，HIV 是 HPV 导致宫颈病变的协同因素，这种协同作用与免疫功能水平有关[18]。

其他分子生物学指标

其他遗传学因素也可能在宫颈癌的发生发展中具有重要作用，但迄今认为这些因素的作用低于 HPV。宫颈癌中 *c-myc* 基因扩增是主要的激活途径，多数研究报道该基因激活率为 32%~34%[19,20]。基因激活与肿瘤大小、淋巴结转移以及复发风险具有相关性[21]。*ras* 基因家族也是恶性肿瘤中经常发生突变的基因。宫颈癌 K-ras 和 *H-ras* 基因突变率仅 10%~15%[22]。一项报道发现 *ras p21* 表达升高与淋巴结转移相关[23]。

表皮生长因子受体（epithelial growth factor receptor，EGFR）不仅在大多数宫颈癌组织中过度表达，在正常组织和癌前病变中也有同样改变。尽管有 2 项研究发现 EGFR 的表达水平与宫颈癌患者的总生存率及疾病特异性生存率具有相关性，EG-

FR 过度表达与宫颈癌预后的相关性目前尚有争议[24,25]。

凋亡抑制因子 Bcl2 阻止凋亡。有 2 项研究表明，61%～63%的宫颈癌细胞中有 Bcl2 的过度表达，与总生存率降低相关[26,27]，但其他研究没有发现这种相关性[28]。

血管生成是多数肿瘤进展的关键。最近发现血管内皮生长因子（vascular endothelial growth factor，VEGF）与宫颈癌相关[29,30]，但其在宫颈癌发生发展中的作用尚需进一步研究。

性行为

尽管曾有报道认为宫颈病变的发生与患者及其性伴侣的性行为有关，但最近有关 HPV 的研究结果认为此相关性并不强[16,31]。多数关于癌前病变的研究认为，校正了 HPV 感染因素后，性伴侣数目与病变发生间的相关性下降。但宫颈浸润癌的研究结果显示，性伴侣数目与宫颈癌有显著相关性。有趣的是，性伴侣数目与宫颈病变的相关性在 HPV 阴性的妇女中十分显著，而在 HPV 阳性者中则不存在此相关性。

初次性交的年龄与宫颈癌发生的风险没有太大相关性，控制了 HPV 感染和其他风险因素后，在一些研究中，初次性交的年龄与宫颈病变有一定相关，但是在其他研究中，结果相反[16,17,32]。初次性交的年龄与宫颈癌发生的风险相关提示在某一阶段，宫颈组织较高的易感性，暴露的可能性更高或暴露于致癌因素的时间更长。然而，不容易确定初次性交年龄作为独立高危因素是因为宫颈癌风险也与性伴侣数量相关。

宫颈癌发生的风险也与男性性伴侣相关[33]，男性 HPV 的感染率与性伴侣的数量及与妓女的性行为相关[34]，此外，宫颈癌发病率更高的地区男性 HPV 感染率高于宫颈癌发病率低的地区，这点支持了女性宫颈癌发生与其伴侣相关[34]。男性包皮环切术降低了男性 HPV 感染率，特别是对于有多个伴侣的男性，也降低了其现伴侣宫颈癌发生的风险[35]。

产次

宫颈病变与患者月经或生育特点，包括月经初潮或绝经的年龄、胎次、流产次数包括自然流产及人工流产、初次妊娠年龄、初次分娩年龄、末次分娩年龄，以及阴道分娩和剖宫产次数等因素无一致的相关性，同时，多次妊娠，初产年龄，多次分娩以及阴道分娩次数等因素与宫颈病变发生率相关[16,17,35,36]。尽管没有明确的生物学机制支持这种相关性，但分娩时宫颈的重复创伤被视为致病因素之一。

吸烟

一些流行病学研究为吸烟和宫颈病变之间的相关性提供了支持证据。大多数研究显示，吸烟者患病风险增加两倍，并且存在与吸烟年限和数量相关的剂量-反应关系[37,38]。而大部分校正了 HPV 因素的研究结果则结论不一。有些结果支持吸烟的独立效应，而另一些不支持[16,17,39]。尽管有人提出 HPV 和吸烟之间可能存在关联作用，检验这一联合效应的研究却甚少[21]。这些研究结果也不一致[39,50,51]。除了流行病学的研究，还有一些研究为这一相关性提供了生物学证据。在主动和被动吸烟者的宫颈黏膜中检测到高浓度的尼古丁、可替宁和烟草特异性 N-亚硝胺。在女性吸烟者的宫颈组织和脱落细胞已发现有 DNA 损伤。吸烟者的局部细胞免疫反应减弱。此外，在参加戒烟干预治疗的妇女中发现宫颈病灶的体积减小[40]。总之，尽管吸烟诱导宫颈组织肿瘤形成的机制尚不完全清楚，目前的生物学、流行病学和临床研究提示：吸烟可能是宫颈病变的一项危险因素。

宫颈腺癌的危险因素

宫颈腺癌占所有宫颈癌的 20%以上。但在大多数发展中国家，其发病率正在增加，尤其是在年轻妇女中。从 20 世纪 70 年代早期至 80 年代中期，腺癌在 35 岁以下妇女中的发病率增加了一倍以上[41]。腺癌与 HPV16，HPV18 感染具有更高的相关性，阴性率达 80%以上。宫颈腺癌患者中 HPV18 阳性率约为 50%，而鳞癌仅 15%[42]。与子宫内膜癌发生相关的危险因素也与宫颈腺癌具有相关性，如肥胖[43]和未产妇[6]。

总结

宫颈病变仍然是一个全球性的主要健康问题。发展中国家的发病率和死亡率较高。在较发达的国家，过去 50 年的发病率和死亡率明显下降，主要归功于筛查项目的引入。目前的流行病学数据支持 HPV 感染在宫颈病变致病中的重要作用。这一相关性满足流行病学研究的所有因果关系标准：相关性的强度、一致性和特异性，剂量-反应和时间关系以及生物学合理性[11]。HPV 感染似乎可以解释宫颈病变很多已确定的危险因素，包括性行为和吸烟。然而，HPV 感染在年轻健康妇女中的发生率高，而宫颈病变的发病率和未经治疗的宫颈上皮内瘤变（CIN）的病变进展速率均较低，这一事实支持在宫颈癌形成过程中其他辅助因素的存在[44]。未来流行病学研究需要进一步评估这些辅助因素的作用以及它们与 HPV 的相互关系。此外，需进一步评估 HPV 持续性感染和 HPV 变异株等病毒因素在宫颈病变进展中的作用，以及 HPV 持续感染的决定因素[45]。吸烟、外源性激素和饮食等环境因素近期得到重视，其影响也值得进一步的关注[7]。

上皮性肿瘤的组织学分类

宫颈上皮性肿瘤的 WHO 组织学分类包括三大类：鳞状细胞癌、腺癌和其他上皮性肿瘤（表 102-1）[46,47]。

表 102-1　宫颈上皮性肿瘤 WHO 组织学分类的修订版

鳞状细胞癌
微小浸润性鳞状细胞癌
浸润性鳞状细胞癌
疣状癌
湿疣状癌
乳头状鳞状细胞（移行细胞）癌
淋巴上皮瘤样癌
腺癌
黏液腺癌
宫颈型
肠型
印戒细胞型
子宫内膜样腺癌
子宫内膜样腺癌伴鳞状上皮化生

续表

透明细胞腺癌
微偏腺癌
宫颈管型(恶性腺瘤)
子宫内膜型
浆液性腺癌
中肾癌
分化良好的绒毛管状腺癌
其他上皮性肿瘤
腺鳞癌
毛玻璃样细胞癌
黏液表皮样癌
腺样囊性癌
腺样基底癌
类癌样肿瘤
小细胞癌
未分化癌

摘自 Blaustein pathology of the female genital tract, 4th ed。

鳞状细胞癌

大部分宫颈癌为鳞状细胞癌,可分为大细胞角化型和大细胞非角化型。大细胞非角化型鳞状细胞癌的特点是鳞状细胞的细胞核显示一定程度的浓染,并且在被间质分隔的癌巢中具有适量细胞质(图 102-1)。在某些癌巢的中心部位,鳞状细胞出现分化和退化现象。大细胞角化型鳞状细胞癌的特点是细胞核高度浓染且在不规则浸润癌巢中出现浓密的嗜酸性粒细胞胞质。这些癌巢中许多具有中心型"癌珠",其中含有大量角蛋白。鳞状细胞癌患者的平均年龄为 51.4 岁。我们将在以下章节中对鳞状细胞癌的一些变异型进行描述。

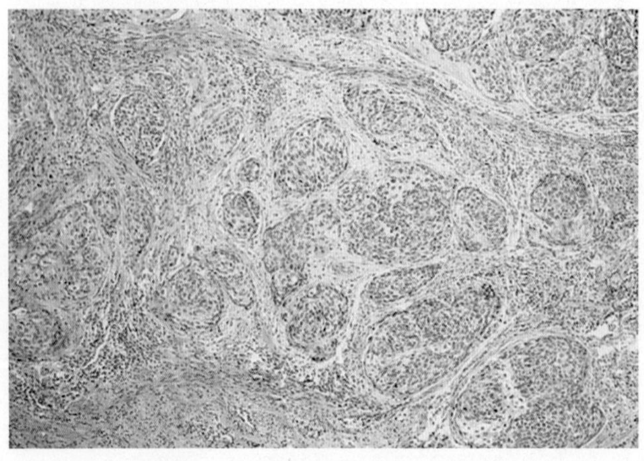

图 102-1 鳞状细胞癌,非角化型

疣状癌

疣状癌呈外生性生长,具有叶状乳头,外观像尖锐湿疣。虽很少转移,但局部可广泛浸润。患者多死于输尿管梗阻、感染或出血。组织学上,上皮缺乏细胞学异型性和有丝分裂活性,上皮乳头缺乏中心性纤维结缔组织核心。在肿瘤基底部细胞中可见明显的有丝分裂活动,可见浸润性生长的上皮细胞巢,也可见边界清楚的细胞巢,具有清晰可见或轮廓分明的肿瘤间质界面。上皮间质连接处的炎症反应明显。

这类肿瘤很少发生淋巴结转移,因此,对于早期的病变,治疗选择为Ⅱ型改良根治性子宫切除术,无须行淋巴结清扫术。

乳头状鳞状细胞癌

具有移行性或鳞状分化的宫颈乳头状鳞状细胞癌通常形似泌尿道的移行细胞癌(图 102-2)。具有移行细胞分化的肿瘤在女性生殖道各处均有描述。免疫化学检测细胞角蛋白多肽的细胞角蛋白 7 和细胞角蛋白 20 有助于区分原发性生殖道移行细胞癌与泌尿道移行细胞癌[48]。泌尿道移行细胞癌具有细胞角蛋白 20 强阳性的细胞角蛋白谱,而原发性生殖道移行细胞癌则细胞角蛋白 7 染色阳性。宫颈浸润性乳头状移行细胞癌潜在恶性程度高。将这些癌与良性鳞状乳头状瘤和尖锐湿疣正确鉴别非常重要[49]。活检标本必须包括上皮基底层之下的组织,以确定是否有间质浸润。

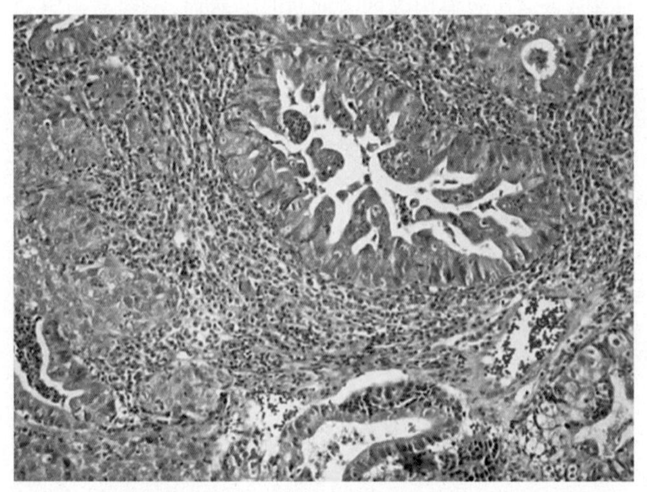

图 102-2 乳头状鳞状细胞(移行性)癌

淋巴上皮瘤样癌

淋巴上皮瘤样癌在组织学上与起源于鼻咽部和唾液腺的淋巴上皮瘤相似(图 102-3)。这些癌通常边界清楚,由未分化细胞构成。这些细胞被炎性细胞浸润包围,包括淋巴细胞、浆细胞和嗜酸性粒细胞[50]。Hasumi 等报道了东京癌症研究所医院的 39 例病例。这些患者中,72%年龄在 50 岁以下,他们接受了根治性子宫切除术和盆腔淋巴结清扫术。2 位患者淋巴结阳性。39 位患者中 38 位存活。1 例于手术后 5 个月死于血清性肝炎。

腺癌

腺癌目前占宫颈癌的 20%~25%,而在 1950—1960 年它们仅占 5%[51]。这种改变是一个全球性的现象[52]。浸润性腺癌患者确诊时的平均年龄为 47~53 岁。腺癌的亚型如下述。

黏液腺癌是最常见的宫颈腺癌类型[53]。在 WHO 的分类中,黏液腺癌的第一种类型由类似宫颈内黏膜正常柱状细胞的

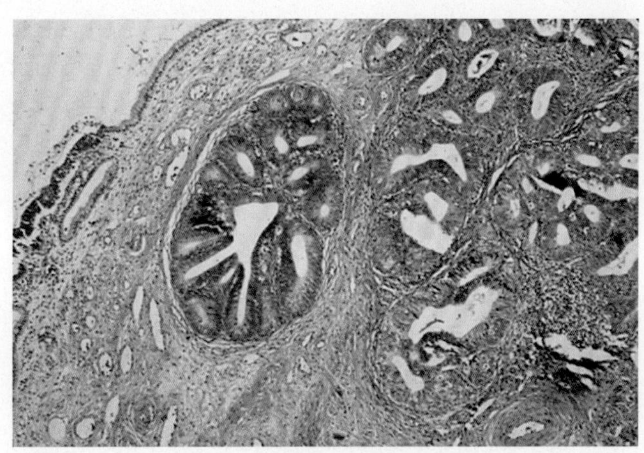

图 102-3　淋巴上皮瘤样癌

细胞构成，称为宫颈管型（图 102-4）。第二种类型称为肠型，因为它的组成细胞类似大肠腺癌中的细胞。第三种类型由印戒细胞构成，称为印戒细胞型。通常，黏液腺癌为这些类型的混合体。

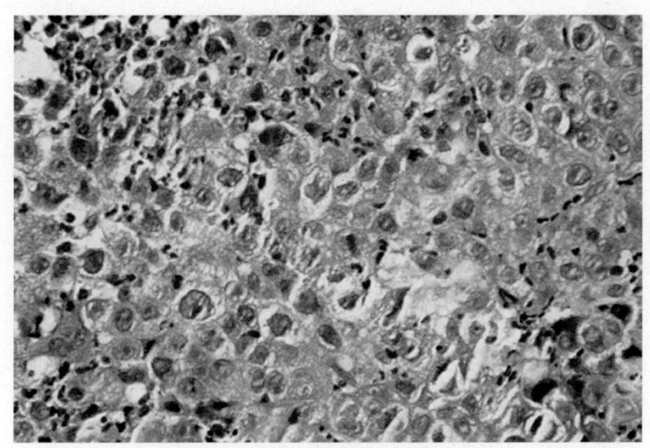

图 102-4　黏液腺癌，宫颈管型

子宫内膜样腺癌是宫颈管原发肿瘤的第二常见类型，占所有原发性宫颈管肿瘤的 30%。子宫内膜样腺癌类似来自宫腔内膜的典型子宫内膜腺癌（图 102-5）。原发部位的鉴别（如原发肿瘤是位于宫颈内还是子宫内膜）可能比较困难，但是正确的鉴别非常重要，因为病变部位或起源对治疗影响重大。

在细胞学上恶性腺瘤很难与正常宫颈内腺体进行区分（图 102-6）。因此，恶性腺瘤也称为微偏腺癌。恶性腺瘤的一个显著特点为奇异且不规则的腺体分支方式。这些不规则的腺体侵入深部间质，诊断需要大块组织的标本（如锥切活检标本），通常在子宫切除标本的基础上做出诊断。恶性腺瘤是一种极罕见的癌症，有时伴有 Peutz-Jegher 综合征[54]。如因其高分化的组织学形式导致治疗不充分，则生存率很低。

其他上皮性肿瘤

腺鳞癌是由恶性鳞状细胞和腺细胞构成的混合性肿瘤[55]。腺鳞癌占宫颈恶性肿瘤的 5%～25%[56,57]。其临床表现、流行病学及扩散方式与鳞状细胞癌和腺癌相似。鳞腺癌的低分化形式被称为毛玻璃细胞癌。这些癌由大而均匀的多角形细胞构成，细胞含有毛玻璃型细颗粒胞质，因此称为“毛玻璃细胞”（图 102-7）。与其他未分化肿瘤相似，毛玻璃细胞癌早期扩散且侵袭性高[57]。黏液表皮样癌也列于此类，包含大细胞非角化型或灶性角化型鳞状细胞癌，黏蛋白染色阳性，但是缺乏可识别的腺体。黏液组分包括杯状或印戒细胞，分布于鳞状细胞巢内。这类癌在有黏液性成分的癌中占 20%。

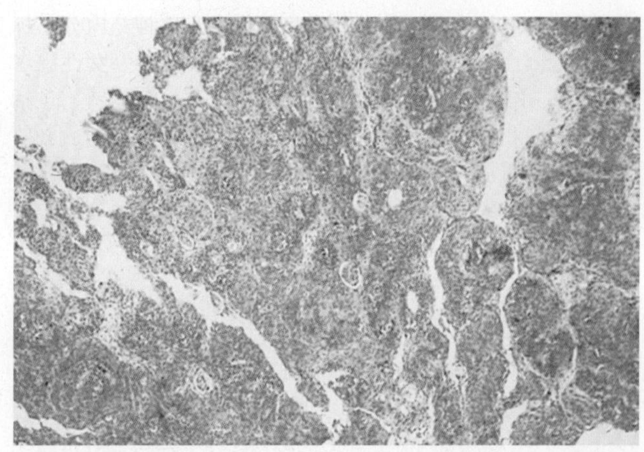

图 102-5　子宫内膜样腺癌

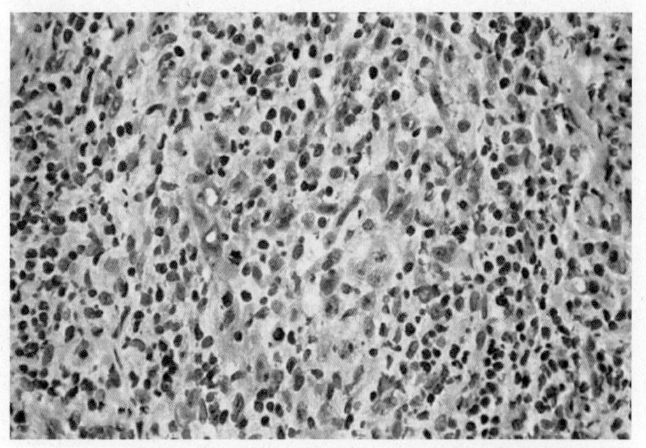

图 102-6　黏液腺癌，宫颈管型（恶性腺瘤）

小细胞癌在 WHO 宫颈肿瘤分类中的描述较明确，为胞质含量少的未分化的小细胞（图 102-8）。这些高度恶性的癌弥漫

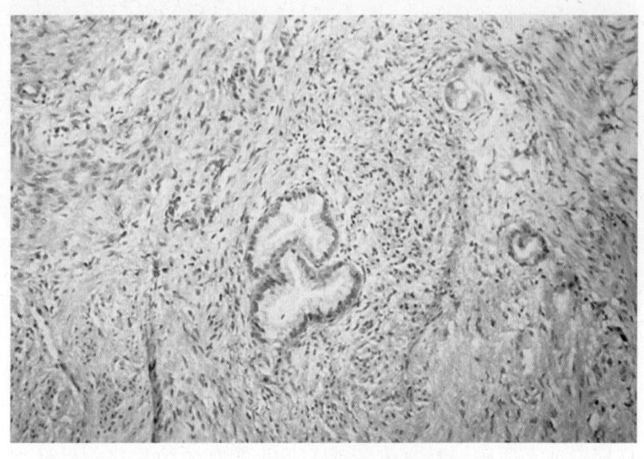

图 102-7　毛玻璃细胞癌

性浸润至宫颈基质[58]。在大部分病例中显示出神经内分泌标志物染色阳性。小细胞癌女性患者的年龄可比鳞癌女性患者小10岁。小细胞癌往往侵袭性强,常有广泛的多处转移,包括骨、肝、皮肤和脑。这一类肿瘤不应与小细胞鳞癌混淆,后者的预后更好。通常,在小细胞非角化性鳞癌中有些区域表现出鳞状上皮或腺体分化。用肺小细胞癌的经典方法治疗这类患者效果不一。

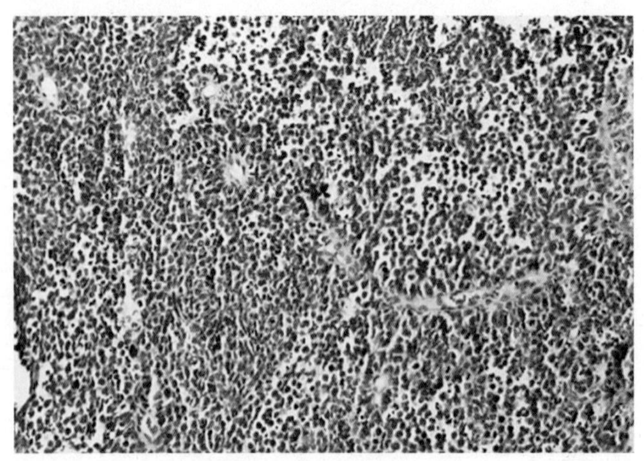

图 102-8 小细胞癌

非小细胞神经内分泌癌

已有宫颈非小细胞神经内分泌癌的报道,但是它们没被列入目前的WHO宫颈肿瘤分类中[59]。肿瘤包含中等至大的细胞,较多的核分裂象以及见于神经内分泌细胞中的嗜酸性胞质颗粒。通常呈小梁状,伴或不伴腺体分化(图102-9)。肿瘤通常对于嗜铬粒蛋白具有免疫反应性,其生存率与小细胞癌相似。

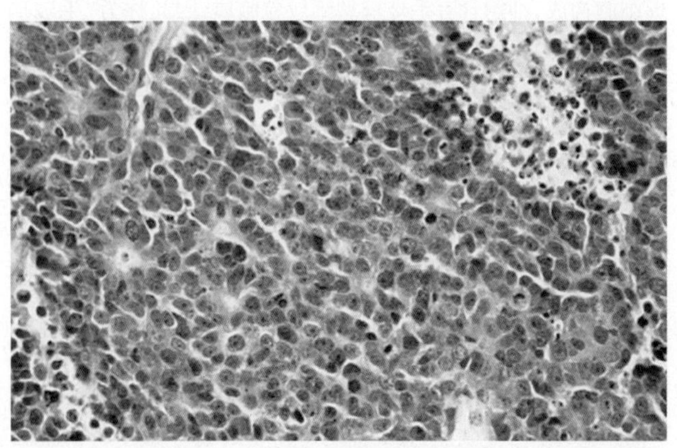

图 102-9 非小细胞神经内分泌癌

癌前病变的诊断和治疗

最新的宫颈癌筛查指南见图102-10[60]。CIN在性活跃的年轻妇女中是一个越来越普遍的疾病。自从Bethesda系统的引入以来,报告中轻度细胞学异常、意义不明的非典型鳞状细胞(atypia squamous cells of undermined significance,ASCUS)这样轻微或不明确细胞学改变或LGSIL的宫颈涂片比例已经增加[44]。美国每年约有5 000万次宫颈涂片检查,其中5%~10%报告为轻度细胞学异常。尽管关于宫颈涂片发现的HGSIL和癌的确诊和治疗已有基本共识,但对ASCUS和低度异常的治疗仍有争议[61]。争议包括疾病进展的风险、对患者造成的焦虑、对轻微病变患者过度治疗的风险,最新的问题包括立即治疗带来的经济负担[62]。

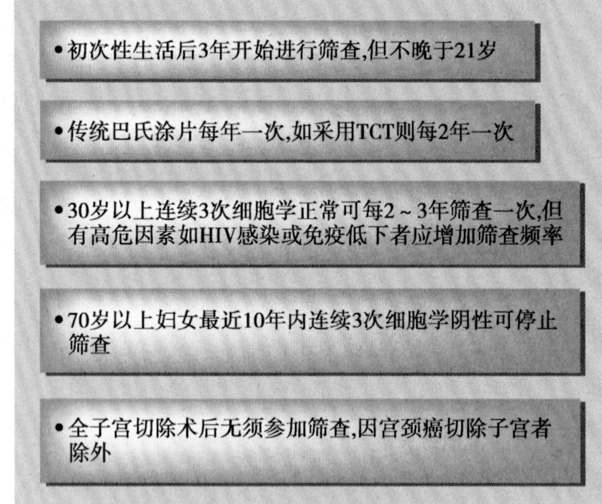

图 102-10 宫颈病变早期筛查指南

大量研究表明,5%~20%的轻度细胞学异常的患者有发生HGSIL以及更严重病变的风险[63]。此外,至少有1/3经常规筛查发现的HGSIL患者既往有细胞学为ASCUS的历史[64]。因此有些临床医生建议对细胞学ASCUS者行阴道镜检查更加安全且高效[65]。但是,由于轻度细胞学异常者大多没有明显宫颈病变,同时考虑到阴道镜带来的经济及精神负担,一些学者认为这些患者应重复细胞学检查而无需阴道镜检查。美国妇产科学会和NCI共识小组同意对于一次轻度不典型细胞学结果的妇女选择重复细胞学检查是可行的处理措施[61,66]。

治疗ASCUS和低度细胞学异常的主要目的是辨别那些具有发生HGSIL风险的妇女,主要是25岁以上、无随访条件、疑有或者已发现细胞学异常或有宫颈肿瘤治疗史的妇女[67]。目前推荐二种处理方法:①重复宫颈涂片,或直接进行阴道镜检查;②对ASCUS或低度病变但临床检查无异常以及无高危因素的妇女,可重复宫颈涂片,但不行阴道镜检查(图102-11)[61,67]。美国阴道镜及宫颈病理学会(ASCCP)还强调对细胞学提示ASCUS或LSIL者进行HPV检测。

低度细胞学异常的处理

大多数临床医师先用抗生素治疗潜在的外阴阴道感染,几个月之后重复细胞学检查。如果涂片结果恢复正常,则每年体检。宫颈细胞学仍然异常者行阴道镜检查,此后两年内每4~6个月检查一次宫颈细胞学。连续三次阴性者,可回归常规人群筛查[68,69]。在两年随访期内,临床怀疑癌的患者或宫颈涂片持续异常者,建议行阴道镜检查。ASCCP对于不同年龄段的ASCUS或LGSIL患者的处理方式有差异。21~24岁的ASCUS或LGSIL,建议12个月后重复细胞学检查,大于24岁的LGSIL且HPV阳性或无HPV检测,推荐直接行阴道镜检查(图102-12)[67]。

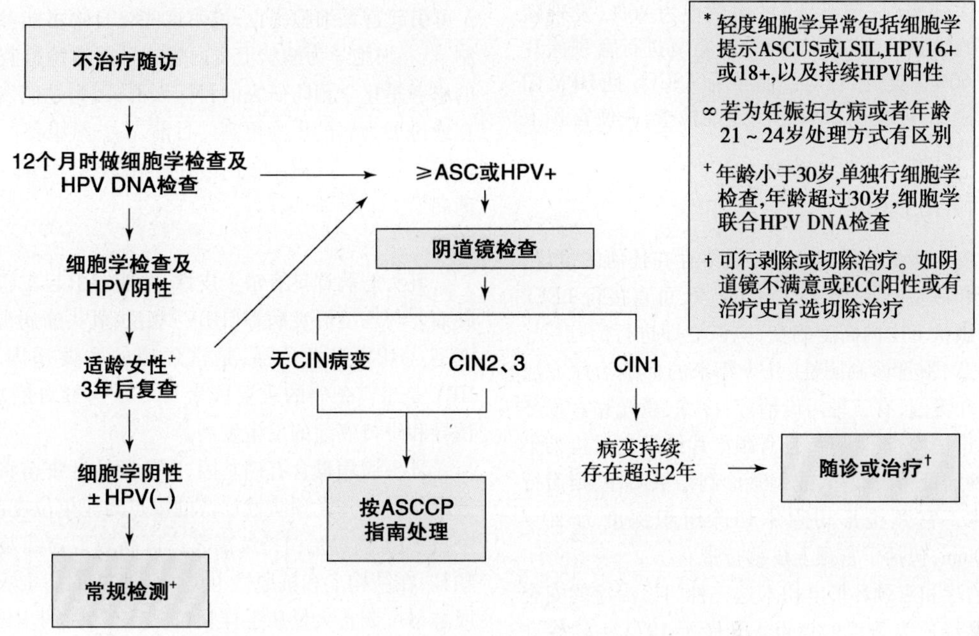

图 102-11　阴道镜活检病理诊断为 CIN Ⅰ患者的处理流程

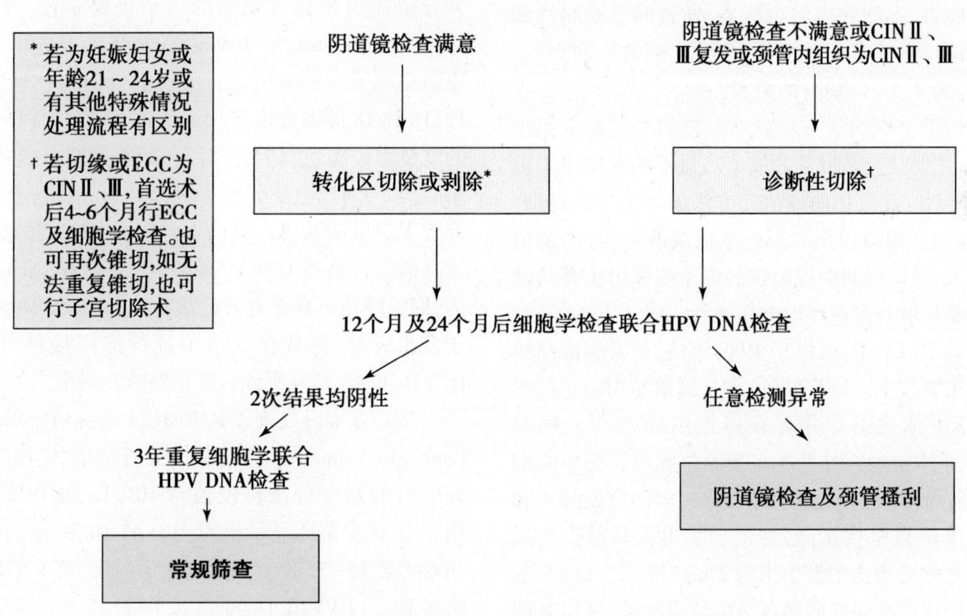

图 102-12　阴道镜活检病理诊断为 CIN Ⅱ和 CIN Ⅲ患者的处理流程

考虑行阴道镜检查及宫颈活检对患者造成的经济负担及情绪负担,学者们更倾向于寻找一种成本更低的检查方式用于诊断低度细胞学异常的患者。许多研究对 HPV DNA 检测的价值做出了评价,它可作为轻度细胞学异常者的替代检查和宫颈细胞学筛查的联合检测[70~73]。第二代 HPV DNA 检测方法,包括聚合酶链反应和杂交捕获,相较于早期 HPV DNA 检测都具有较高的敏感性,也能检测出更多型别的高危型 HPV,更支持其作为低度细胞学异常者的替代检查和宫颈细胞学筛查的联合检测[70~73]。

FDA 公布的 2014 年 ATHENA 临床研究结果表明单独 HPV 检测是优异的宫颈癌筛查手段[74],而还有更多正在进行中的临床研究结果将更有利于美国癌症联合委员会对单独宫颈癌检测在宫颈癌筛查中的作用进行评估。

医师和患者的选择和治疗成本应根据宫颈上皮内瘤变的治疗方法而决定,低度鳞状上皮内病变的正确处理仍然有较大争论。尽管治疗指南对于有随诊条件的低度鳞状上皮内病变者提出可以暂不治疗,但出于对病情进展所负法律责任的顾虑还是出台了密切随访方案，这一情况在美国尤为严重[75]。最近公开发布的指南可能对随访有帮助。Cox 等报道，HPV 检测对发现宫颈上皮内瘤变（任何级别）的敏感性为 86%，发现鳞状上皮高度病变的敏感性为 93%。而单独重复进行宫颈涂片检查的敏感性仅 60%。此外，仅对细胞学为 ASCUS 且 HPV 阳性者进行阴道镜检查，可减少 58% 的阴道镜检查，并使宫颈上皮内瘤变的检查费降低 38%。

高度细胞学异常的处理

高度鳞状上皮内病变的最佳处理方式不存在任何的争议，需行阴道镜检查和活检，或者年龄大于 24 岁，可直接行 LEEP 术。一旦诊断为鳞状上皮内高度病变，应该立即进行治疗[76]。如阴道镜检查满意、颈管诊刮阴性，几十年来的标准治疗方法为切除移行带。在美国，有三种门诊治疗：冷冻、激光和宫颈环形电切术。如阴道镜检查不满意，且宫颈涂片结果比活检结果更重，临床可见肿瘤疑为浸润癌，或颈管诊刮结果阳性，则需行宫颈锥形切除术。宫颈锥形切除术切除组织深度为 20～30mm，直径达 30mm，包括子宫颈上皮移行带。

冷冻、激光治疗和宫颈环形电切术这三种门诊治疗的安全性、疗效和费用已经成为争议的焦点。开展于 1972 年的冷冻治疗是宫颈上皮内瘤变的第一种门诊治疗手段，具有可靠性高、并发症发生率低、易操作和价廉的特点[77]。冷冻疗法的优势是可破坏细胞内残留的大量 HPV 病毒，从而提高宫颈上皮内细胞对病原体的免疫性。但主要缺点为缺乏对病变大小进行个体化治疗的能力、不能获得组织标本，导致漏诊浸润性病变的可能。冷冻治疗指征是阴道镜检查满意、颈管诊刮阴性，病变范围小（直径为 2.5～3.0cm）的患者。

激光治疗开始于 1997 年。它的优点是能够根据病变大小进行个体化治疗，主要缺点是设备的成本高且不能获得组织标本[77]。此外，激光治疗比其他两种治疗方法需要更多的培训，并有严重的安全隐患（眼睛损伤和因疏忽造成的烧伤）。适应证包括病变范围大，可疑浸润癌或原位腺癌希望保留生育功能的患者以及不接受局麻行宫颈环形电切术者。

宫颈环状电切术（LEEP）引进于 1989 年，它是目前治疗鳞状上皮内病变的主要技术。LEEP 既可靠又简单易用。它可根据病变大小进行个体化治疗并可获得组织标本[77]。同时 2%～4% 的 LEEP 手术标本意外发现宫颈原位腺癌及微小浸润宫颈鳞癌[67,77]，但 LEEP 也会无意识地切除过多的宫颈间质和正常组织。另一个缺点是费用高，并增加了出血和感染的风险。据报道，LEEP 术后出血的发生率为 2%～7%[77]。LEEP 的过度治疗往往与治疗前小病变的多点活检结果相关。LEEP 即诊即治方案已经表明，正确选择适应证可提高患者依从性。它在依从性欠佳的患者中的适用有巨大潜力[67]。

冷冻和激光治疗的成功率（基于复发率和病变持续存在）没有明显差异，但是在不同研究中这两项治疗的成功率有差异[77,78]。

预防

化学预防

宫颈上皮内瘤变治疗的最激动人心的研究领域之一是利用化学预防剂来进行治疗。化学预防剂的摄入可改变癌前病变的转归，并把组织恢复到正常状态。实验数据表明类维生素 A 可引起宫颈细胞凋亡，说明这些化合物可能参与细胞周期控制[79]。细胞学为鳞状上皮内病变且阴道镜检查看到明显异常的患者是化学预防研究的目标人群，因为她们发生病变持续存在或进展为癌的风险更高。目前，α-二氟甲基鸟氨酸和维 A 酸（维生素 A 的衍生物）是两种比较受美国和中国关注的药品[80,81]。

疫苗

乳头瘤病毒具有嗜上皮性，并能够引起皮肤和黏膜的良性肿瘤。与乙型肝炎病毒（HBV）相反，乳头瘤病毒有超过 100 种亚型。HPV 为性传播，是宫颈癌的主要病因。感染高危型 HPV 是患宫颈癌的重要因素[82,83]。病毒对癌基因进行编码，诱导和维持癌症的发生发展。

乳头瘤病毒含有癌基因，因此预防性疫苗将直接用于年轻健康妇女。开发预防性疫苗的重点为亚单位疫苗，类似于 HBV 疫苗。L1 病毒蛋白持续高表达可高效地自我装配成为病毒样颗粒，在结构上和抗原性上类似于真实的病毒衣壳。昆虫细胞或酵母可制备大量病毒样颗粒。具有免疫学阳性的构象表位，并可提高中和抗体的滴度。

目前有两种疫苗：一种是 Gardasil，为四价疫苗，包括 HPV 6、11、16 和 18[84]，另一种是 Cervarix，它是二价疫苗，包括 HPV 16 和 18[85]。这些疫苗已经在世界上超过 55 个国家批准使用，并有望成为预防宫颈癌的一个重要手段。FUTURE（Female United to Unilaterally Reduce Endo/Ectocervical Disease）Ⅱ研究小组完成了一项随机双盲的安慰剂对照实验，以评价 HPV6、11、16 和 18 的四价疫苗（Gardasil）预防 HPV16 和 18 感染导致的高度宫颈病变发生的作用。所有随机分组的妇女首剂接种后随访 3 年，以主要研究终点为评价指标分析显示，疫苗对研究方案定义的易感人群的保护率为 98%，对意向治疗人群（无论之前是否感染 HPV）的保护率为 44%。此项研究的结论认为，四价疫苗可非常有效地预防 HPV16 和 18 感染引起的高危子宫颈病变，将其在女孩中进行推广接种可能将显著降低 HPV16 和 18 感染所致的宫颈癌的发病率[84]。

2007 年 6 月发表了 PATRICIA 研究（Papilloma Trial against Cancer in Young Adult）的中期分析结果，这项随机双盲对照研究的目的是评价二价疫苗对 HPV16 和 18 型感染的预防作用[85]。该疫苗还显示出对 HPV45 和 31 型的交叉保护作用。18 644 名 15～25 岁女性分别在第一天、第 1 个月和第 6 个月随机接种了 HPV16/18 疫苗或甲肝疫苗。主要研究终点是 HPV16 或 18 型阳性的 CINⅡ及以上病变，并对基线期与疫苗相对应型别的 HPV 血清学和 DAN 检测均为阴性的妇女进行评估。当检出 23 例 HPV16 或 18 型阳性的 CINⅡ及以上病变患者时进行中期分析。中期分析时平均随访时间为 14.8 个月，疫苗组检出 2 例 HPV16 或 18 型 DNA 阳性的 CINⅡ及以上病变患者，对照组为 21 例。因此疫苗的保护率为 90.4%，且二组的安全性没有显著差异[85]。

HPV 疫苗推荐接种范围为 11～12 岁女孩。尽管可以在 9 岁开始接种，但对 13～26 岁尚无性生活史的女性也应接种。美国最近的数据表明，接种疫苗并从 24 岁开始每两年接受一次宫颈癌筛查，将使巴氏涂片的检查数量减少 43%，从而将大大降低性病诊所的工作量[86]。将 HPV 疫苗接种纳入英国宫颈筛查项目的模式将使宫颈癌死亡率降低 76%，高度病变的发病率降低 66%[86]。然而，在世界范围内推广疫苗的使用尚有很多问题，如疫苗价格较高、一些国家免疫机构缺乏无法进行接种以及保守派反对少女接种疫苗来预防所谓的性传播疾病[87]。

浸润性宫颈癌的诊断和治疗

在从原位癌到浸润性癌的转变过程中，肿瘤细胞穿透上皮基底层，浸润间质。一旦发生间质浸润，肿瘤细胞便易于进入淋巴管和血管，并可能扩散至宫旁组织。

宫颈、阴道和宫体的淋巴管合并形成主要的回流通路。主要淋巴干包括子宫卵巢（骨盆漏斗韧带）、宫旁和骶前淋巴道，它们回流入宫颈旁淋巴结、闭孔淋巴结、髂内动脉淋巴结、髂外动脉淋巴结、髂总动脉淋巴结、臀下动脉淋巴结、骶前淋巴结和腹主动脉淋巴结。208 例ⅠB-ⅡB 期宫颈癌患者行广泛性子宫切除及盆腔淋巴结切除术后发现腹膜后淋巴转移的发生率为 25%（53 例）[88]。转移率最高者为闭孔淋巴结 19%（39/208），作者认为闭孔淋巴结为宫颈癌的前哨淋巴结。闭孔淋巴结阴性提示可缩小盆腔淋巴结切除术的范围。

淋巴结转移、原发肿瘤大小和病变范围是宫颈癌最重要的预后因素。3 个以上淋巴结转移的早期患者 5 年生存率为 60%，而腹主动脉旁淋巴结转移者仅 25%～30%。原发肿瘤大小相同者的淋巴结转移率可不同，这取决肿瘤固有的侵袭性和组织学类型。宫颈癌可直接蔓延，随着肿瘤的生长可累及盆壁、膀胱、直肠或者侵及阴道。

目前已明确不同期别宫颈癌术后淋巴结转移的发病率[89~91]。Ⅰ期盆腔淋巴结转移率为 10%～25%，Ⅱ期为 25%～30%，Ⅲ～Ⅳ期为 30%～45%。肿瘤直径大于 3cm 的Ⅰ期患者淋巴结转移率上升[92,93]。由于巨块型宫颈腺癌患者多采用了放射治疗，故对其淋巴结转移率的了解不像鳞癌那样充分。低分化鳞癌和腺癌的淋巴结转移率均高于分化较好者。

宫颈癌的扩散具有顺序性。宫颈旁淋巴结首先受侵，跳跃性转移罕见。腹主动脉旁淋巴结阳性者通常均为盆腔淋巴结阳性。978 例ⅠB 期和ⅡA 期患者在进行广泛性子宫切除术前先进行了腹主动脉旁淋巴结取样，结果显示阳性率分别为 4.7%和 8.4%。肿瘤直径、分化程度、病变范围和分期均相同的腺癌与鳞癌患者的淋巴结阳性率可能相似。许多大样本研究报道腺癌患者生存率低于鳞癌患者，尤其是巨块型肿瘤[94,95]。小细胞癌和一些分类为其他上皮细胞癌的侵袭性非常高，这些宫颈癌可能含有高度恶性的细胞克隆，无论组织学分化程度和原发肿瘤大小如何，其病情进展不可预测，并发生广泛转移。

临床症状

宫颈癌的临床症状表现为阴道出血、排液和疼痛。临床症状与肿瘤的生长方式密切相关。性活跃患者中外生型肿瘤（因为性接触）比内生型更早出现阴道流血。向宫颈管内扩散形成的桶状肿瘤早期可不引起宫颈外口的鳞状上皮发生任何异常改变，直至肿瘤生长达直径 5～6cm。因此，这种方式生长的肿瘤症状隐蔽，在患者发生出血之前肿瘤已慢慢增大。如果进行宫颈细胞学取材时使用的不是颈管内毛刷采集器，将造成细胞学假阴性结果。溃疡型病变的宫颈外口组织较早发生损伤出血，因肿瘤生长过快而血供不足造成的组织坏死和感染导致阴道分泌物异味。

妇科检查时盆腔压痛提示可能伴有输卵管炎。放疗前应治疗输卵管炎，合并附件肿物者应先行手术切除肿物。

肿瘤向宫颈旁扩散直至其固定于盆壁之前可能患者无明显症状。盆壁受侵固定无论是否发生淋巴结转移均有可能造成输尿管梗阻。输尿管压迫梗阻的临床过程一般较为隐匿。患者可能出现双侧输尿管梗阻伴进行性肾衰竭而无肾脏疾病史可循。肿瘤直接压迫坐骨神经根可引起背痛，当盆壁静脉和淋巴管受压迫时则出现下肢水肿。背痛、下肢水肿和肾脏无功能三联征是晚期肿瘤侵达骨盆壁的表现。

膀胱毗邻子宫颈，宫颈肿瘤易于直接扩散至膀胱。尿频和尿急系早期临床表现，晚期患者可能出现血尿或尿失禁，提示肿瘤已直接侵入膀胱。此时应行膀胱镜检及活检以明确血尿或尿失禁的原因。

相反，肿瘤向后方侵向直肠甚至侵及直肠黏膜者较为少见。直肠子宫陷凹是直肠与宫颈的解剖学分隔。如就诊时已发生直肠黏膜受侵，阴道后壁大多已经广泛受侵而直接浸润至直肠。膀胱镜检查和乙状结肠镜检查对正确分期及制订治疗计划是十分必要的。

腹主动脉旁淋巴结转移性可穿透淋巴结包膜直接累及脊椎和临近的神经根。腰椎和腰大肌受侵引起的背痛提示淋巴结已经发生明显肿大。但也可能为血道转移至腰椎而不伴有明显淋巴结转移。

诊断

宫颈癌的诊断依据组织病理学检查。从肿瘤周边获取的活检标本往往更易于观察到完整的具有代表性的肿瘤细胞形态。在肿瘤中心进行活检标本可能多为肿瘤快速生长而血供不足产生的坏死性组织碎片，难以做出准确诊断。

临床检查肿瘤不明显或宫颈增粗、结节状或质地坚硬者，应行宫颈管内膜诊刮。老年腺癌患者还需行内膜活检，原发于宫颈管内的宫颈腺癌与子宫内膜癌侵及宫颈在临床上往往难以鉴别。

宫颈涂片异常但无肉眼可见病变的患者应行阴道镜检查及活检。组织标本可以是阴道镜指引的活检、宫颈管内膜诊刮或宫颈锥切标本。

FIGO 目前推荐ⅠA 期为镜下诊断的浸润癌。所有肉眼可见的肿瘤，哪怕为浅表生长，也列入ⅠB 期。淋巴脉管间隙受侵不改变分期。很多临床医师更喜欢用微小浸润这一名词，采用妇科肿瘤协会推荐的分期概念。微小浸润指从鳞状上皮或腺上皮的基底部开始测量浸润深度小于 3mm 的病变，不涉及淋巴脉管间隙受侵与否。钳取活检标本不足以诊断微小浸润，在包括全部病变组织的宫颈锥切标本上进行该诊断十分必要。锥切切缘阳性者还需再次切除，因为邻近阳性切缘处可能有隐匿的浸润癌病灶。

检查和分期

制订成功的治疗计划前需对患者的一般状况、肿瘤大小和扩散范围进行详细的评估。开始治疗之前，必须控制内科并发症并治疗贫血。对贫血患者的研究较为广泛，其局部复发率高于血红蛋白正常的患者（表 102-2）[96,97]。重视患者的既往手术史，从手术记录可看到对腹部器官的描述以及具体手术方式。对消化道溃疡性疾病、憩室炎和盆腔炎的诊断对制订治疗计划有重要意义。上述炎性疾病可导致肠管之间、肠管与邻近器官之间及与腹膜之间形成粘连，肠袢环形固定。

表 102-2　ⅡB 和Ⅲ期宫颈癌患者的复发率

血红蛋白/(g/dl)	患者人数	复发率/%		
		局部	远处	总计
<10	29	46	18	49
10~11.9	319	29	24	47
12~13.9	578	20	16	33
>14	129	20	18	33

ⅡB 期或Ⅲ期宫颈癌复发率与放疗期间平均血红蛋白水平相关。P=0.002（局部），P=0.1（远处），P=0.0007（总体）。

摘自 Bush 1986[96]。引用经编辑同意。

Ⅰ期患者治疗前需行胸部 X 线片、静脉肾盂造影、血常规、尿常规和血液生化检查。晚期患者还需行膀胱镜检查和直肠镜检查。采用 FIGO 分期十分重要（表 102-3）[98]，其分期系统中明确指出必要时可进行下列检查以便确定分期，包括：膀胱镜检查、阴道镜检查、宫颈管搔刮术（endocervical curettage，ECC）、宫腔镜检查、静脉肾盂造影、胸片和放射性骨显影[99]。尽管淋巴管造影术、剖腹手术、腹腔镜手术、电子计算机 X 线断层成像（CT）、磁共振成像（MRI）及其他未被 FIGO 列入的检查能够为制订治疗计划提供有价值的信息，但其检查结果不应改变临床分期。TNM 分期方法也被 FIGO 所接受[100]。FIGO 分期系统中未提及宫颈癌淋巴结情况，有三种放射成像技术可以评估淋巴结状态，即 CT、MRI 和正电子发射断层显像（FDG-PET）。

目前尚无检查淋巴结转移的最佳放射成像技术。CT 和 MRI 擅长识别肿大淋巴结，但无法发现较小的转移淋巴结，且许多肿大淋巴结是晚期肿瘤伴发的炎症所致，并无肿瘤转移，所以 CT 和 MRI 判断淋巴结转移的准确性不足。MRI 诊断淋巴结转移的准确率（72%~93%）与 CT 相近，但与术中所见相比较时，MRI 对肿瘤位置、肿瘤大小、宫颈间质浸润、阴道和宫旁受侵的判断比 CT、临床检查和超声检查更具有优势[101~104]。此外，研究表明，MRI 评估宫颈癌病变的成本-效益比更优[104]。图 102-13 为宫颈癌患者的 MRI 图像。

表 102-3　修订的 FIGO 分期[98]

分期	描述
Ⅰ期	肿瘤严格局限于子宫颈（子宫体受侵不予考虑）
ⅠA 期	浸润癌仅能在显微镜下确认。所有肉眼所见病灶，即使是表浅浸润，亦列入ⅠB 期。ⅠA 期仅限于间质浸润经测量的深度不超过 5.0mm，宽度不超过 7.0mm*
ⅠA1 期	测量的间质浸润深度不超过 3.0mm，宽度不超过 7.0mm
ⅠA2 期	测量的间质浸润深度大于 3.0mm，但不超过 5.0mm，宽度不超过 7.0mm
ⅠB 期	临床病灶局限于宫颈或临床前期病灶大于ⅠA 期
ⅠB1 期	临床病灶不超过 4.0cm.
ⅠB2 期	临床病灶大于 4.0cm
Ⅱ期	癌浸润阴道但未达下 1/3，浸润宫旁组织但未达盆壁
ⅡA 期	癌浸润阴道上 2/3，但无宫旁浸润
ⅡA1 期	临床病灶不超过 4.0cm.
ⅡA2 期	临床病灶大于 4.0cm
ⅡB 期	有宫旁浸润
Ⅲ期	肿瘤累及阴道下 1/3 或浸润达盆壁。凡有肾盂积水或肾无功能者，除非已知其因其他原因所致，均列入Ⅲ期
ⅢA 期	肿瘤累及阴道下 1/3，但宫旁浸润未达盆壁
ⅢB 期	癌浸润达盆壁，或肾盂积水，或肾无功能
Ⅳ期	癌扩散超出真骨盆或临床上累及膀胱或直肠黏膜
ⅣA 期	扩散至邻近器官
ⅣB 期	远处转移

FIGO，国际妇产科联合会。

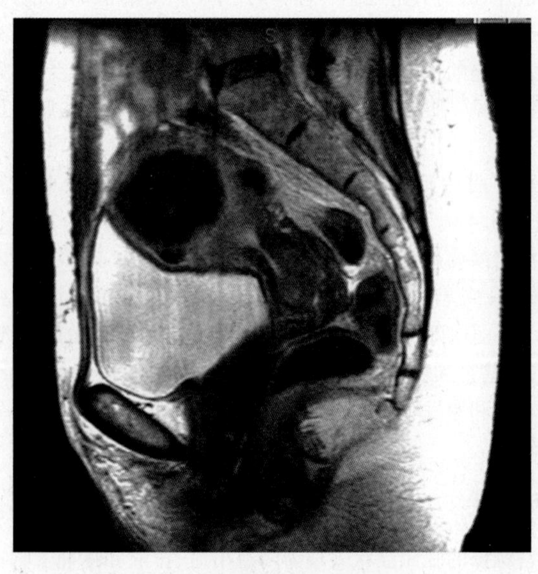

图 102-13　宫颈癌患者的 MRI 图像

PET 或 PET/CT 是肿瘤影像学的一个新兴技术，发展迅速(图 102-14)。在对 101 个宫颈癌患者的研究中，Grigsby 等分析了 101 例宫颈癌患者资料，CT 诊断盆腔和腹主动脉旁淋巴结肿大发生率分别为 20%和 7%，而 PET 显示 67%的盆腔淋巴结有异常增高的葡萄糖摄取，腹主动脉旁淋巴结为 21%，锁骨上淋巴结为 8%[105]。以腹主动脉旁淋巴结的状态为指标，CT 和 PET 检查均阴性者的 2 年无进展生存率为 64%，CT 正常而 PET 异常者生存率为 18%，CT 和 PET 均异常者为 14%。作者认为 PET 检查结果比 CT 更能准确判断预后。还需进一步研究来确证这些结果，并且需要进一步研究 PET 检查是否优于手术分期，尤其是对于可疑存在腹主动脉旁淋巴结转移的患者。

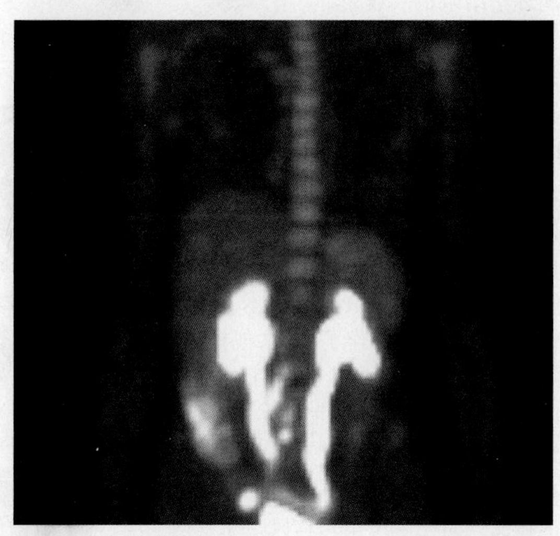

图 102-14　正电子发射断层扫描显示宫颈癌患者淋巴结肿大

有些患者可考虑手术探查淋巴结。已批准进行淋巴结外科检查。盆腔淋巴结显著肿大者的腹主动脉旁淋巴结隐匿性转移风险最高。这类患者也最适合行手术探查，切除单纯放疗无法控制的肿大淋巴结可获得生存获益[106]。腹膜外淋巴结切除术是目前首选术式[107]，其原因在于经腹手术后实施放疗可能导致较高的并发症发生率[108]。也可行腹腔镜淋巴结切除术，术后恢复快，日后放疗并发症少[109]。

预后因素

宫颈癌患者的生存率和局部控制率与 FIGO 分期密切相关，但预后也受其他因素影响，如未包括在 FIGO 分期中的患者和肿瘤的其他特征。

肿瘤大小和局部扩散

肿瘤大小是手术或放疗后局部复发率和死亡率最重要的预后因素(图 102-15)。FIGO 根据肿瘤直径对Ⅰ期进行了修订(≤4cm 为ⅠB1 期；>4cm 为ⅠB2 期)[98]。相关的预后因素有ⅡB 期宫旁受侵达中段还是外侧，ⅢB 期患者盆壁受侵为单侧还是双侧[111,112]。

对于已行广泛性子宫切除术的患者，宫颈旁受侵(≥10mm)和深部间质浸润(深度>70%)类同宫旁扩散，具有较高的淋巴结转移率、局部复发率和死亡率[91,113~115]。对于手术或放疗患者，子宫体受侵与远处转移率增加密切相关[116]。

淋巴结转移

淋巴结转移是另外一个重要预后因素，但不列入 FIGO 分期中。根治性子宫切除术后，盆腔淋巴结病理阳性者比阴性者的 5 年生存率低 35%~40%[89,91]。但最近研究表明，术后化疗可使之得到改善[117]。有些作者报道转移淋巴结的最大直径以及数目与生存率之间有显著相关性。相同期别患者中，腹主动脉旁淋巴结阳性患者的生存率仅为阴者的 1/2[89,91,114,118,119]。腹主动脉旁淋巴结转移的早期患者接受延伸野放疗后的治愈率为 40%~50%。

宫颈癌淋巴结转移与病理诊断淋巴脉管间隙受侵之间具有显著相关性。但淋巴脉管间隙受侵可能是独立预后因素，大量根治性子宫切除术治疗的临床资料已证实这一点[113,114,120,121]。Roman 等报道有淋巴脉管间隙受侵的病理切

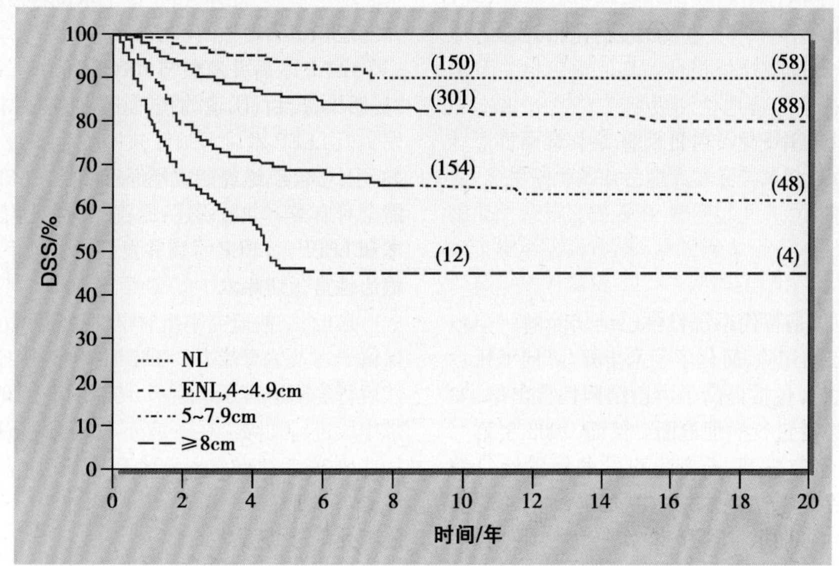

图 102-15　不同宫颈大小(NL，正常大小；ENL，直径 4~4.9cm)患者的疾病特异性生存率

片所占比例与淋巴结转移率之间具有相关性[122]。宫颈腺癌患者淋巴脉管间隙受侵是显著预后不良的因素[123,124]。

组织学类型

宫颈腺癌与鳞癌的预后是否相似一直有较大争议。一些回顾性研究发现宫颈腺癌患者与鳞癌患者放射治疗的预后相同[125,126]。但其他作者的结论相反，手术治疗的腺癌患者与鳞癌患者相比，前者的复发率异常地高于后者。在手术或放疗的患者中，腺癌患者的生存率低于鳞癌[110,127,128]。Eifel 等对 1 767 例放疗的ⅠB 期患者进行分析发现，腺癌患者复发和死亡风险显著高于鳞癌患者[127]，与患者年龄、肿瘤大小及肿瘤形态无关。巨块型腺癌（≥4cm）与鳞癌的盆腔复发率无明显差异，而前者的远处转移率几乎为鳞癌者的 2 倍。尽管鳞癌组织学分级对预后的影响一直存在争议，但腺癌的分化程度与临床行为之间有明显的相关性[123,124,129]。

其他肿瘤因素

治疗前血清鳞状细胞癌抗原（serum squamous cell antigen，SCCAg）水平与肿瘤分期具有较强相关性：30%~40%的Ⅰ期患者、60%~70%的Ⅱ期患者和 80%~90%的Ⅲ~Ⅳ期患者均出现 SCCAg 异常[130~132]。然而，治疗前 SCCAg 水平最重要的特性是能够预测临床结局。一些研究报道，治疗前 SCCAg 明显升高者的生存率显著低于 SCCAg 正常的患者，与分期无关[132~135]。应用 SCCAg 判断疗效尚需进一步研究，特别是 SCCAg 检测的频次和判断值、哪些患者可以此受益以及成本-效益比[136]。

一些研究报告了 HPV 亚型与预后之间的相关性[137~139]。有两项研究报告，组织学阴性的淋巴结，如果 PCR 检测淋巴结中 HPV DNA 强阳性，则复发率较高[140,141]。

其他与预后相关的分子标志物有 EGFR 和 COX-2[142]。但研究中样本量太小故而很难应用。为研究 EGFR 和环氧化酶-2 对预后判断的价值，研究人员对两者的其他特性进行了分析研究（包括宫颈间质炎症反应、腹腔细胞学、肿瘤血管以及 DNA 倍体或 S 期细胞比率），结论不甚一致[143,144]。

患者因素

一些研究已经报道了治疗前后及治疗过程中低血红蛋白水平与不良预后具有相关性[111,145]。据推测，贫血患者预后不良的部分原因是乏氧诱导的放疗抗拒性。其他预后相关因素有：年龄、血小板计数、社会经济地位和吸烟[93,146~150]。Kucera 等报道，吸烟患者 5 年生存率较低，在Ⅲ期患者中差异非常显著（20.3% vs 33.9%，$P<0.01$）[149]。

手术治疗

前哨淋巴结

前哨淋巴结检测最初是替代系统性淋巴结切除的一个步骤，仅行 1 个或几个淋巴结切除，简化了手术步骤，降低了死亡率，然而，它还有其他优势，包括提高了淋巴结阳性检出率，发现微转移，以及术中对患者进行病理诊断。然而，2008 年第一个大的、多中心的临床研究发现，前哨淋巴结的敏感性只有 77%，这对于此项操作在宫颈癌手术中的开展是一个大的挫折[151]。但是此项研究也存在很多问题，包括肿瘤大小，外科医生手术水平不一，以及病理超分期。随后的研究结果显示在肿瘤较小的宫颈癌行荧光淋巴显像后前哨淋巴结有非常高的敏感性，包括最近的法国 SENTICOL 临床研究报告显示前哨淋巴结的敏感性达到 92%，阴性预测值为 98%[152]。目前，前哨淋巴结假阴性率低，对于肿瘤体积较小的宫颈癌有很好的术中诊断作用。

宫颈锥切术和宫颈环形电切术（LEEP）

宫颈锥切术切除移行带，同时具有诊断和治疗的双重目的。顾名思义，宫颈锥切术的标本为圆锥体，其大小依病变范围的不同而不同。病变在宫颈表面时，锥形切除较表浅；当病变累及宫颈管，则切除较深。有下述情况之一者应行宫颈锥切术：阴道镜检查阴性但细胞学异常或宫颈管搔刮术（ECC）阳性；鳞柱交界或病变范围不能完全看到；宫颈活检病理为微小浸润癌；活检或 ECC 病理为原位腺癌；细胞学、阴道镜检查和组织病理学结果不一致。

锥切术是彻底切除鳞柱交界以及宫颈管下段组织。标本应包括整个病变，应测量病变的浸润深度和宽度。

另一种锥切技术是宫颈环形电切术。LEEP 刀（高频电波刀）中有一根细线回路电极，可切除鳞状上皮内高度病变患者的病变区域。LEEP 是门诊手术。虽然破坏性治疗（如激光烧灼和冷冻）可以有效治疗可疑病变；但最好选择可提供组织学标本的治疗方法，如宫颈冷刀锥切（cervical cold knife conization，CKC）、LEEP，或者激光锥切术。最近，Linares 等对 CKC、激光锥切术以及 LEEP 作了比较，他们发现 LEEP 与其他两种方法相比，其并发症较少且手术时间较短。LEEP 唯一的缺点是切除深度略浅，复发风险稍高[153]。

患者选择

单纯采用宫颈锥切术作为早期宫颈癌的治疗是一个相对较新的概念。对于淋巴结转移风险非常低，并且强烈希望保留生育功能的患者，宫颈锥切术可能是一个理想的选择[154,155]。得克萨斯大学安德森癌症医学中心建议，宫颈锥切术仅适用于宫颈鳞状上皮病变患者，且浸润深度小于 3mm，没有淋巴脉管间隙浸润，无切缘受累[156]。对于非鳞癌患者行宫颈锥切术治疗，目前资料较少，故不予推荐[157]。

CKC 的并发症包括出血、盆腔蜂窝组炎、宫颈管狭窄、宫颈机能不全[158]。此外，由于此手术过程需要全身麻醉，会有麻醉并发症和费用增加的可能。

LEEP 术后并发症与 CKC 相似，但又不完全相同，并发症有：感染，出血，阴道灼伤，宫颈管狭窄，宫颈功能不全，病变复发。但 LEEP 术后宫颈管狭窄发生率极低（1%），多见于未产妇、围绝经期、绝经期或绝经后妇女。LEEP 的另一个优点是不需全身麻醉。如前所述，比较三种宫颈锥切术（CKC、激光锥切术和 LEEP），LEEP 术后并发症较少且手术时间较短[153]。

根治性宫颈切除术

最近，一些研究小组对早期患者采用根治性宫颈切除术来保留子宫及生育能力。手术时先行腹腔镜下盆腔淋巴清扫术，然后行经阴道宫颈切除术，切除阴道长度 1~2cm，并于主、骶韧带中段进行切除。在子宫下段横断宫颈后行预防性环扎术。一些研究者建议，该手术仅限于肿瘤直径不超过 2cm 的患者[159,160]。

筋膜外子宫切除术

筋膜外子宫切除术切除完整的子宫底和子宫颈，而保留宫旁软组织和一部分阴道上部。可以经阴道或经腹或腹腔镜联合经阴道手术。

简单的筋膜外子宫切除术是ⅠA1 期子宫颈癌的标准治疗方法,有时对巨块型颈管型宫颈癌放疗后施行该手术。其是否适用于ⅠA2 期患者尚存争议。与ⅠA1 期相比,ⅠA2 期的淋巴结转移率为 3%~5%,复发率较高。因此,尽管一些数据表明,筋膜外子宫切除术可以有效治疗ⅠA2 期患者,但是许多国家妇科肿瘤学家还是将此手术仅限于ⅠA1 期患者[161,162]。目前一致认为,宫颈锥切术不应该是ⅠA2 期患者单一的治疗方法。

根治性子宫切除术

根治性子宫切除术包括整块切除宫体、宫颈、宫旁组织及阴道上部。在 20 世纪早期,维也纳的 Wertheim 对宫颈癌根治性术进行了描述。20 世纪 40 年代,美国的 Meigs 倡导此手术过程应该增加盆腔淋巴结清扫术。现在,包括盆腔淋巴结清扫术的根治性子宫切除术是ⅠA2~ⅡA 期患者的标准术式。

Ⅱ型子宫切除术(改良根治术)的切除范围较Ⅲ型(根治性)手术略小。Ⅱ型子宫切除术的主要适应证是早期浸润性癌,肿瘤直径小于 2cm。Ⅱ型手术应切除宽 2~3cm 的宫颈旁组织及部分阴道。手术标本包括宫旁组织的内 1/2 以及阴道上 1/3。该手术需解剖输尿管,切除主韧带以及宫骶韧带内 1/2,而不切除盆壁和盆底的韧带。Ⅱ型子宫切除术的膀胱和输尿管并发症的发生率低于Ⅲ型手术。Ⅱ型子宫切除术可以与改良的或完全的盆腔淋巴结切除术同时进行。

Ⅲ型(根治性)子宫切除术是经典的 Wertheim-Meigs 根治性子宫切除术。适用于ⅠB 期和阴道受侵长度不超过 1cm 的ⅡA 期患者。于盆壁处切除宫旁、主韧带和宫骶韧带,并切除阴道的 1/2。在髂内血管的起始处切断子宫血管。解剖输尿管隧道、分离远端输尿管破坏了来自子宫动脉和膀胱上动脉的血供。将输尿管推向外侧以便沿盆壁钳夹宫旁组织。从起始处切除主韧带和宫骶韧带破坏了远端输尿管血液供应将增加输尿管瘘的发生风险。恰当掌握手术适应证可获得较高的治愈率。年轻患者可保留卵巢。

根治性子宫切除术的术中和术后并发症包括:失血(平均 0.8L),输尿管阴道瘘(发生率为 1%~2%),膀胱阴道瘘(<1%),肺栓塞(1%~2%),小肠梗阻(1%~2%),术后发热,深静脉血栓形成,肺部感染,盆腔蜂窝织炎,尿路感染,或伤口感染(25%~50%)[163]。淋巴结切除的程度与亚急性并发症(包括淋巴囊肿的形成和下肢水肿)的发生有关。淋巴囊肿可能会压迫输尿管,随着淋巴囊肿引流量增多,肾积水多会改善[164]。术前或术后放疗者发生并发症的风险上升。

大多数患者在根治性子宫切除术后会出现短暂的膀胱神经功能下降,但只要给予适当的治疗,严重的长期膀胱并发症很少出现。尽管术后给予充分的膀胱引流,仍有 3%~5%的患者会出现慢性膀胱张力减退或收缩乏力[165]。膀胱麻痹可能是由于膀胱神经被破坏所致,可能与宫旁和阴道旁切除范围有关[166]。根治性子宫切除可能会引起压力性尿失禁,其发生率有很大差别,并可能受到术后放射治疗的影响[167]。根治性子宫切除术后的患者也可能会出现便秘,少数出现慢性便秘。

判断患者是否适合行根治性子宫切除术,应考虑患者是否可耐受大型手术以及肿瘤特点,如肿瘤体积和淋巴受累情况。对于早期患者选择手术或放疗时,患者因素十分重要。对于年轻女性来说,保留卵巢功能以及阴道是很重要的。同样,有严重健康问题的女性,如肥胖,放疗可能是更好的选择。

早期(ⅠA~ⅠB1)患者应根据肿瘤特点选择治疗方案。有复发高危因素者宜辅助放疗或加用同步化疗。多项研究发现,接受根治性手术和放疗二种治疗的患者并发症发生率较高[168]。高危因素包括肿瘤体积大,这与淋巴结转移相关,增加复发率,降低生存率。Eifel 等发现,肿瘤直径大于 5cm 的ⅠB 期患者的疾病特异性生存率显著降低(88% vs 69%,$P<0.0001$)[164]。其他高危因素包括淋巴结转移,宫旁受累和切缘阳性。

手术治疗疗效

有报道显示,ⅠB 期患者根治性手术治疗后 5 年生存率为 80%~90%(表 102-4)[89~91,168~176,208]。切缘阳性或淋巴结阳性者复发和预后不良的风险最高。Delgado 进行的大样本前瞻性研究显示,淋巴结阴性者的 3 年疾病特异性生存率为 85.6%,而淋巴结阳性患者仅 50%~74%[91]。在淋巴结阳性组中,受累淋巴结数目和髂总淋巴结转移均与生存率下降相关。最近的一项随机研究表明,术后放化疗可以提高淋巴结阳性,切缘阳性和宫旁受累患者的生存率[117]。

表 102-4　ⅠB~ⅡA 期宫颈癌患者行根治性子宫切除术和双侧盆腔淋巴结切除术的 5 年生存率

作者(参考文献)	分期	年份	例数	生存率/%
Sall[169]	ⅠB~ⅡA	1979	219	90.0
Kenter[170]	ⅠB~ⅡA	1989	213	87.3
Lee[171]	ⅠB~ⅡA	1989	343	87.2
Ayhan[90]	ⅠB~ⅡA	1991	270	80.7
Hopkins[129]	ⅠB	1991	213	92.5
Alvarez[172]	ⅠB	1991	401	85
Averette[89]	ⅡB~ⅡA	1993	726	90.1
Landoni[163]	ⅡB~ⅡA	1997	172	83

放射治疗

浸润性宫颈癌的初始放疗包括体外放疗(external beam radiation therapy,EBRT)和低剂量率(low-dose rate,LDR)或高剂量率(high-dose rate,HDR)的腔内放疗。治疗目标是获得最佳局部控制率和最低并发症发生率的平衡。所需的剂量根据宫颈肿瘤大小、宫旁参考点和局部淋巴结受累情况不同而不同。影响放疗耐受剂量的因素包括阴道和子宫的解剖学位置、受侵组织的破坏及感染程度以及患者特点(如体型、并发症、吸烟等)。

EBRT(体外放疗)

EBRT 通常作为肿瘤体积较大的患者的初始治疗。通常给予全盆腔剂量 40~45Gy。使中央部位的肿瘤和局部淋巴结受到均匀照射,以缩小原发肿瘤及区域淋巴结的微小病变,并破坏肿瘤邻近的淋巴脉管间隙,使原发肿瘤缩小以便达到更好的腔内照射剂量分布。

全盆外照射首选高能光子(15~18MV),可最大限度地保护正常的浅表组织。X 线平片、CT、MRI、PET 扫描、淋巴造影均有助于放射医师确定照射范围。典型的放疗区域如图 102-16 所示。标准治疗方法为全盆 EBRT 剂量 40~45Gy。淋巴结转移较大者还需进行缩野加量照射(图 102-16 和图 102-17),剂量增加 8~10Gy,肿大淋巴结及其 1~2cm 外放边界的总剂量为 60~66Gy,其中包括 2 次腔内近距离放疗的剂量贡献。对肿瘤体积有严格限定时,调强放射治疗(intensity modulated radiation therapy,IMRT)可以对限定的区域进行加量,提高肿大淋巴结的受照剂量(最高可达约 66Gy)。

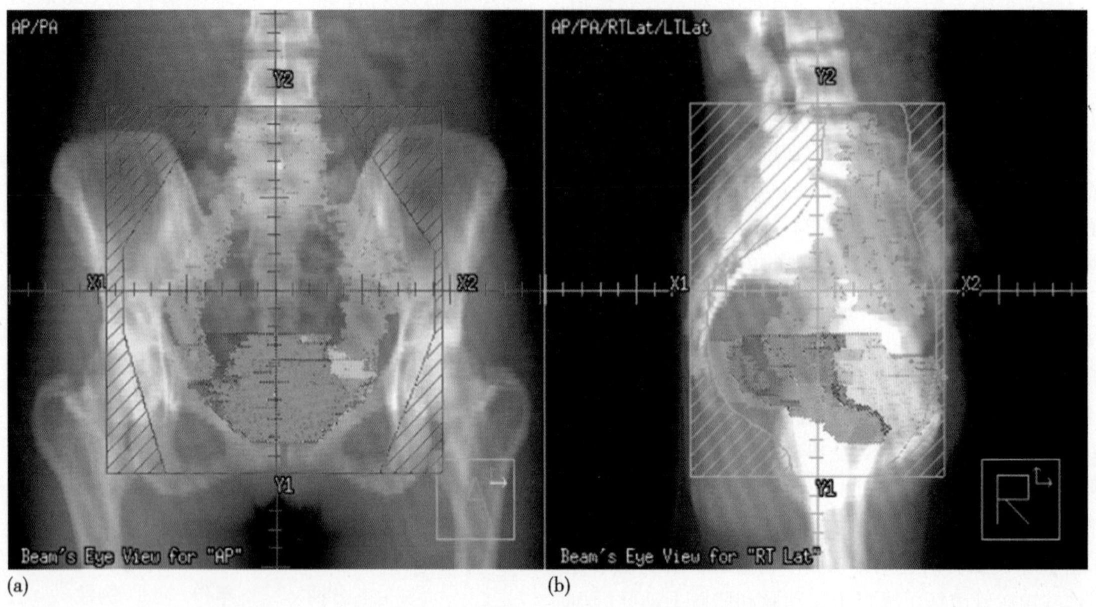

(a) (b)

图 102-16 宫颈癌的典型照射范围。(a)冠状位图。(b)矢状位图

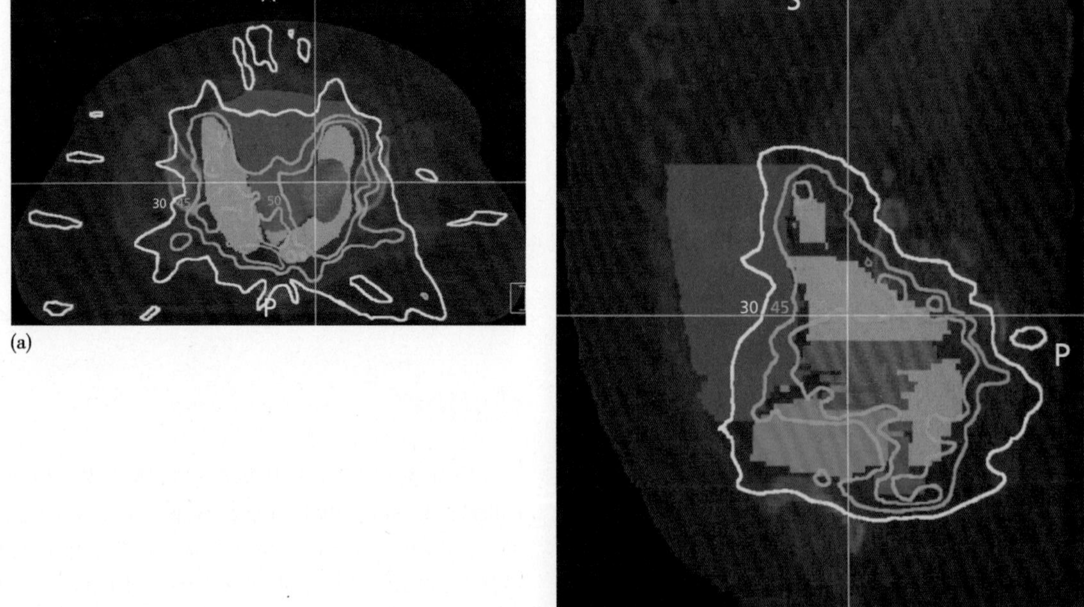

(a) (b)

图 102-17 经典的腔内放疗剂量分布,注意剂量迅速下降。(a)冠状位图。(b)矢状位图

最近调强放射治疗用于治疗宫颈癌。与传统治疗不同的是，调强放射治疗可使放射剂量集中于治疗区域，即对肿瘤给予更高的剂量，而周围正常组织受量较低，特别是小肠（图 102-17）。Mundt 等人报道[177]，对于子宫内膜癌或宫颈癌患者，术后调强放疗的急性和慢性[178]消化道不良反应发生率低于传统放疗。然而，调强放疗的高度适形性剂量分布也增加了误差空间，特别是内脏运动（特别是膀胱和直肠）以及肿瘤消退带来的误差，因此，调强放疗目前仍需进一步研究，特别是对初治根治性放疗的患者。许多关于评价宫颈癌调强放疗的多中心研究正在进行中。

腔内放疗

不可低估腔内放疗（intracavitary radiation therapy，ICRT）对子宫颈癌的重要性，虽然外照射至关重要：可以消灭盆壁肿瘤并改善肿瘤外形，但过度依赖外照射会降低局部控制率，并增加并发症的风险。

近距离放疗将施源器放入宫腔及阴道内。宫腔与阴道的放射源串联的最优驻留位置可使剂量分布呈梨形，使宫颈和宫颈旁组织得到较高剂量，并减少直肠和膀胱的受量。全球有多种系统用于确定宫颈癌的照射剂量和剂量率。在美国，中线旁剂量用 A 点表示（见上文定义）。A 点与肿瘤或靶体积无关，位于输尿管和子宫动脉的交叉点。其他系统的剂量体系包括国际原子能机构和测量委员会（ICRU）的 38 号报告（1985 年）以及 MG-H 系统的一些参考点。无论使用何种系统的剂量体系，关键在于优化施源器与宫颈肿瘤及其他盆腔组织之间的位置关系。放射源、强度和位置都应慎重选择，以提供最佳的剂量覆盖（图 102-18）。

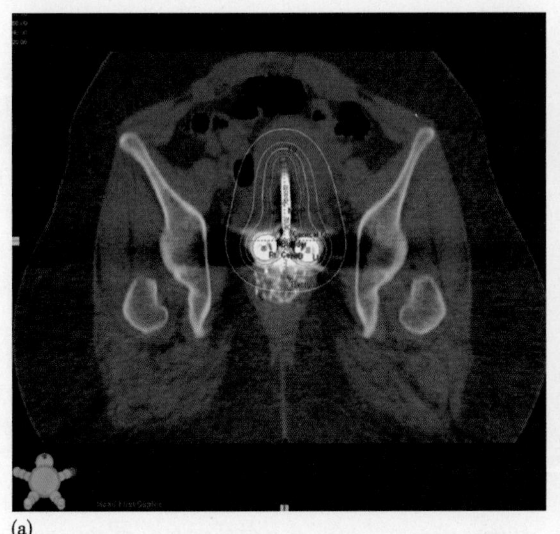
(a)

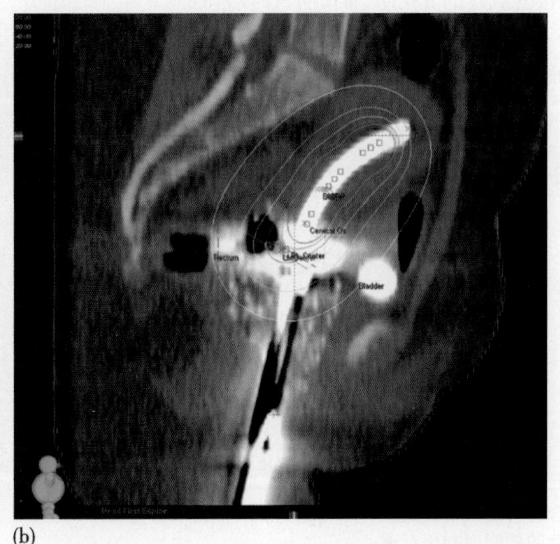

(b)

图 102-18 宫颈癌患者行全子宫切除术后接受放疗。需覆盖区域为淋巴结和阴道。调强放疗覆盖除小肠外的治疗区域。小肠剂量多低于 30Gy

过去，临床医师认为 LDR 腔内治疗的放射生物学优势（通常给予 A 点 40~60cGy/h 的剂量）是宫颈癌治疗取得成功的一大要素。低剂量率可使亚致死损伤修复，从而保护正常组织，提高治疗比。在过去的二十年里，计算机技术的发展使我们能够使用高活性钴-60 或铱-192 源并遥控施源器进行高剂量率治疗（<100cGy/min）。HDR 正在慢慢取代传统的 LDR 治疗，主要因为其辐射安全性较高。临床医师认为 HDR 不错，患者不用住院，对患者和医师来说都更方便。多项随机和非随机研究表明，高剂量率放疗的生存率和并发症发生率与传统的低剂量率治疗相似[179]。HDR 近距离放疗正在获得越来越多的认可，被认为是宫颈癌患者的标准治疗方法。2012 年，美国近距离放射治疗学会对 HDR 近距离放疗发布了指南[180]。该组织根据以往 LDR 成功治疗的经验提出，应优化施源器位置，权衡外照射与近距离放疗的比重，控制总治疗时间，对肿瘤给予足量照射，同时要考虑正常组织的最大耐受剂量。

图像引导的近距离放疗的应用越来越普遍，在欧洲尤其如此。多为 MRI 为基础的治疗计划系统确定肿瘤的照射剂量，同时避免破坏如膀胱和直肠等器官的结构，但在这类治疗手段成为标准治疗方法前，还需进行大量前瞻性研究。

组织间放射治疗

一些治疗团队建议在解剖结构变异或者宫旁受侵或者盆壁受侵的宫颈癌患者中可以使用会阴模板引导下的近距离插植放疗，插植针内多装载铱-192 源，通常经会阴以 Lucite 模板为引导，平行穿插于宫颈和宫旁间隙，倡导者认为这种方式能够在放置窥器困难的宫颈癌患者更容易放置施源器，同时施源器直接插植到宫旁，剂量相对均匀。近期的临床结果显示ⅡB 期和ⅢB 期宫颈癌生存率低，治疗相关副作用发生率高[181,182]。目前除了临床研究外，组织间放射治疗还仅适用于腔内放疗困难的宫颈癌患者以及远端阴道放射剂量需要加强的宫颈癌患者。

患者选择

ⅠB1 期患者治疗方法的选择主要取决于患者的意愿、麻醉和手术风险、医师的意愿以及对放疗和手术并发症的认识。年轻患者多选择手术治疗，因为手术治疗可保留卵巢功能并减少阴道缩短。而年长的绝经后患者则建议其选择放疗，以避免较大手术带来的并发症发生率。ⅠB2 期患者可手术后放疗或选择根治性放疗。患者异质性之大以至于 GOG 无法完成ⅠB2

期患者二种治疗方法的随机研究。大多数ⅡB~ⅣA期患者首选放疗。

结果

ⅠB~ⅡA期宫颈癌

ⅠB~ⅡA期患者采用放疗的生存率和盆腔控制率较高。Efiel等报道,宫颈肿瘤直径小于4cm、4~4.9cm和大于5cm的ⅠB期患者5年疾病特异性生存率分别为90%、86%和67%[164]。ⅡA期患者的5年生存率为70%~85%,与ⅠB期患者相似,ⅡA期的生存率也与肿瘤大小密切相关[112,183,184]。近来研究表明,巨块型肿瘤行同步化疗能进一步提高生存率[185,186]。

ⅡB~ⅣA期宫颈癌

单独接受放疗的ⅡB期、ⅢB期、Ⅳ期宫颈癌5年生存率分别为65%~75%、35%~50%、15%~20%(表102-5)[111,112,184,187]。联合顺铂的治疗有利于局部肿瘤的控制及生存率[186,188,189]。

表102-5 盆腔控制率与生存率

FIGO分期	例数	控制率/%	生存率/%
Ⅰ	229	93	89
ⅡA	315	88	85
ⅡB	314	80	62
ⅢA	266	63	62
ⅢB	216	57	50
Ⅳ	43	18	20

法国合作研究项目:根据Fletcher指南,1 383例根治性放疗的宫颈癌患者的盆腔控制率和生存率。

FIGO:国际妇产科联盟。

摘自Barillot et al. 1997[112]。

并发症

急性不良反应

盆腔放疗的急性不良反应包括肠道、膀胱和阴道的相关症状。多数患者出现轻度疲劳、轻中度腹泻,腹泻通常可服用止泻药和饮食调理得以控制。也可出现膀胱或尿路刺激征。进行尿液检验和尿液培养排除尿路感染后,可服用马洛芬或抗痉挛药物。延伸野放疗可引起恶心呕吐、胃激惹及外周血细胞计数降低。同时化疗会加重急性症状。所有绝经前患者接受盆腔放疗后都会发生卵巢功能衰竭,除非进行了卵巢移位。

腔内放疗鲜有致命并发症。腔内放疗较轻的并发症有血栓栓塞、子宫穿孔、发热、阴道撕裂及麻醉风险[190]。

远期不良反应

宫颈癌放疗后总的并发症发生率为5%~15%[191,192]。治疗后3年内远期并发症风险最高;然而,主要并发症可发生于治疗后30年甚至更晚。常见放疗并发症有直肠炎、膀胱炎和小肠炎。放射性直肠炎在放疗后3年内最为常见,患者出现便血、直肠狭窄、溃疡、瘘管形成。泌尿系统并发症平均发病时间略晚于肠道并发症,需要输血的血尿的5年发生率为2.6%[191]。消化道或泌尿系瘘的5年发生率为1.7%,而放疗后行辅助性子宫切除术或放疗前行经腹的腹膜后淋巴结切除术者发生并发症的风险更高。小肠阻梗的风险与患者的一些特性及治疗因素密切相关。消瘦、吸烟或有盆腔炎病史的患者患小肠阻梗的风险较高[150,191,192]。

宫颈癌放疗后阴道上1/3会出现不同程度的萎缩、毛细血管扩张或瘢痕化。也可能发生更为严重的阴道缩短。肿瘤范围大、高龄、性生活少或雌激素水平低下的患者阴道缩短幅度会更大[192,193]。规律的性生活和阴道扩张器的使用能防止阴道缩短。

不同分期宫颈癌的治疗方式

CIS和ⅠA1期宫颈癌

宫颈高度鳞状上皮内病变的治疗方法发展迅速。LEEP是一种有效方法。另外,冷冻和激光也是有效治疗方法。阴道镜满意且ECC阴性均可应用。ECC阳性则行冷刀锥切。上皮内病变所有切缘必须阴性。

ⅠA1期宫颈癌(微小浸润癌)间质浸润深度小于3mm且无淋巴脉管间隙浸润,肉眼观察不到,细胞学检查异常。需根据锥切标本作出诊断。对于有生育要求,鳞癌浸润深度小于3mm且无淋巴脉管间隙浸润的患者,锥切亦是一种潜在低风险治疗方法。锥切标本切缘必须为阴性。若切缘阳性,应再次锥切,因为浸润癌可能在阳性切缘附近。应当告知患者保守治疗也有风险。目前鲜有建议非鳞癌患者行锥切治疗的资料[155]。选择锥切治疗的患者须自愿接受密切随访,以便观察宫颈肿瘤残余或复发。

Ⅰ型全子宫切除(经腹筋膜外)是治疗ⅠA1期宫颈癌最传统的方法。年轻患者保留卵巢。患者也可选择单纯放疗,通常为腔内放疗。单纯放疗的10年疾病控制率为95%~100%[194]。

ⅠA2期宫颈癌

病变浸润深度3~5mm患者的淋巴结转移风险平均为5%。标准治疗方法为Ⅱ型子宫切除术和盆腔淋巴结切除术(改良根治术)。

近来一些研究显示,对于年轻患者欲保留生育能力,手术方式可考虑选择单纯全子宫切除术、单纯子宫颈切除术和宫颈锥切术,同时行或不行前哨淋巴结活检及盆腔淋巴清扫术。这些选择可以用于一些低风险早期宫颈癌患者,包括病理非神经内分泌肿瘤、肿瘤小于2cm、间质浸润小于10mm以及无脉管内癌栓。目前全球性有3项研究观察早期患者不同治疗方式的疗效。

若有手术禁忌证,可单纯放疗,通常为盆腔放疗加近距离放射治疗。然而,也有个别患者仅近距离放疗就能很好地控制病情。

ⅠB1期和ⅡA期肿瘤较小的宫颈癌

ⅠB期宫颈癌的治疗取决于肿瘤大小或淋巴结转移与否(图102-5)。

小于4cm的ⅠB1期肿瘤属于较小肿瘤,但其宫旁浸润或淋巴结转移的风险较高。美国 GOG 的前瞻性研究报告称,接受根治性子宫切除术者中,肿瘤直径小于 3cm 者的淋巴结转移率 16%(42/261)[195]。Landoni 发现,行根治性子宫切除术且肿瘤直径≤4cm 的ⅠB~ⅡA 期患者有 25%(28/114)为淋巴结阳性[163]。因此,ⅠB1 期或ⅡA 期小肿瘤(直径<4cm)患者可行Ⅲ型根治性子宫切除术及双侧盆腔淋巴结切除术或根治性放疗。这些治疗方案的目的均为消除宫颈恶性肿瘤细胞、宫颈旁组织和局部淋巴结转移。

接受手术或放疗的ⅠB1 期和ⅡA 期小肿瘤患者的总体生存率为 80%~90%,说明两种治疗方案疗效相同。然而,目前只有一项随机临床试验直接将两种治疗方案进行了比较[163]。接受两种不同治疗方案的患者复发率和生存率相似,但接受子宫切除术患者的Ⅱ、Ⅲ级并发症发生率较高。ⅠB1 期治疗方法的选择主要取决于患者意愿、麻醉和手术风险、医师的建议以及对放疗和子宫切除手术并发症本质和发生率的理解。根治性子宫切除术后放疗的价值仍不明确。GOG 临床试验中随机对根治性子宫切除术后有中危因素的ⅠB 期患者行盆腔放疗或不予进一步治疗[196]。满足以下任意两项条件的患者则符合入组条件:宫颈间质浸润>1/3、淋巴脉管间隙浸润、肿瘤直径≥4cm。结果显示,术后放疗患者的复发率可降低 47%(15% vs 28%,P=0.008)。该研究于 2006 年发表。最新研究结果表明,放疗能减少复发、病情恶化及死亡的风险,然而,尚无数据表明两组间总体生存率有何差异。本文作者得出结论,根治性手术后行盆腔放疗能大大减少ⅠB 期宫颈癌患者,尤其是宫颈恶性腺瘤或腺鳞癌患者的复发风险,并延长其无进展生存期[197]。美国西南肿瘤协作组报告了一项随机临床试验,比较根治性子宫切除术后放疗患者和顺铂同步放化疗患者疗效。入组条件为盆腔淋巴结转移、宫旁浸润或手术切缘阳性者。作者发现,相比仅接受放疗患者,接受放疗加化疗患者存活率较高[117]。

ⅠB2 期宫颈癌

肿瘤直径大于 4cm 且腹主动脉旁淋巴结阴性者行盆腔外照射加近距离放疗后存活率很高。但对临床判断肿瘤可切除者,其理想的处理方法仍有争议。由于不同癌症中心采用的治疗方案差异很大,且缺少手术联合放化疗与单纯放化疗两种治疗方案的比较研究,GOG 提前关闭了一项临床试验。

放疗对许多ⅠB2 期患者来说是有效的,但宫颈肿瘤大的患者复发率达 8%~10%以上[167,183,184]。文献中关于宫颈肿瘤大的患者放化疗后再辅助子宫切除术的报道较多。1991 年,Mendenhall 报道了佛罗里达州医院宫颈管肿瘤大(>6cm)患者的治疗结果[245],两种治疗方案的盆腔控制率和生存率差异不大,但接受子宫切除术患者的并发症发生率较高(18% vs 6%,P=0.027)。1999 年,GOG 报道对于ⅠB2 期患者筋膜外子宫切除术不能增加局部病灶的控制率或生存率,反而因联合放化疗而增加了毒性反应[185]。

有的学者推荐直接手术治疗,术后根据病理结果决定放疗或放化疗。Landoni 报道的随机临床试验将ⅠB2 期患者随机分为直接手术组和根治性放疗组[163]。虽然两组生存率相似,但 84%手术患者需要术后放疗,导致该组并发症发生率较高。

近来,许多临床试验开始研究新辅助化疗对肿瘤体积较大者的积极作用,新辅助化疗为其接受根治性子宫切除术提供了可能性[198,199]。一项荟萃分析[200]收集了 21 项局部晚期宫颈癌新辅助化疗临床试验。该项分析包括新辅助化疗后根治性放疗和单行根治性放疗疗效对比数据(2 074 例)及新辅助化疗后手术(±放疗)和单纯根治性放疗的比较(872 例患者)。由于临床试验的异质性,第一种对比无法正常进行,只能根据化疗周期长度和剂量强度进行分组,但得到相互矛盾的结果。然而,本文作者通过化疗周期长度和顺铂剂量强度分组的判断分析,对异质性作出了一定解释。本文作者发现,化疗周期长于 14 天者的相对死亡风险增加了 25%,相比周期较短化疗,其 5 年生存率减少了 8%,而周期较短化疗相对死亡风险减少了 17%,5 年生存率增加了 7%。他们还发现,每周顺铂剂量小于 25mg/m^2 的试验组死亡风险增加了 35%,5 年生存率降低了 11%,而高剂量组结果尚不明确,但可提高生存率。作者认为,辅助化疗不会影响单纯放疗的总生存率和疾病特异生存率。第二种比较说明,新辅助化疗患者死亡风险明显降低 35%(P=0.000 4),意味着 5 年总生存率提高 14%[201]。然而,该荟萃分析仅包括 1999 年之前的临床试验,当时的标准疗法是单纯放疗。此外,该分析包括两项临床试验,其中所有患者均接受了术后放疗,至少 30%的患者接受了放疗,50%的患者来自一项意大利临床试验,放疗技术差,治疗时间长。故而仍需将其与放化疗进行比较,从而最终找出最有效、毒性最小的治疗方法。为解决这一问题,欧洲癌症治疗研究组织目前正开展一项临床试验。ⅠB2 期宫颈癌患者随机接受新辅助化疗后放疗或同步放化疗。

2 项前瞻性研究显示,巨块型中心性宫颈癌患者可从顺铂增敏的同步放化疗中获益[185,186]。另一项研究也发现,手术病理有淋巴结转移或切缘阳性等复发高危因素者也可从同步放化疗中获益[117],具体内容详见本章“同步放化疗”一节。

ⅡB~ⅣA 期宫颈癌

放疗是绝大部分晚期患者(ⅢB~ⅣA 期)的初治手段。治疗成功与否取决于体外和腔内放疗合理结合使肿瘤和正常组织均达到最优照射剂量以及放疗的总天数。法国协作组根据 Fletcher 指南对 1 875 例患者进行了治疗,Barillot 等报道ⅡB、ⅢB 和ⅣA 期的 5 年生存率分别为 70%、45%和 10%[112]。

局部和远处复发一直是局部晚期宫颈癌患者面临的难题。新辅助化疗的疗效很好,但是随机临床研究结果显示生存率并未提高。事实上,有 2 项研究发现新辅助化疗后放疗使生存率下降。其他的方法,如中子治疗、高压氧治疗以及乏氧细胞增敏剂等,均以失败告终。

同步放化疗

1999 年,5 项大规模前瞻性随机研究结果明确显示[117,185,186,188,189],在放疗同时进行顺铂增敏的化疗可使复发率降低 50%,改善盆腔控制率和生存率(表 102-6)。

表 102-6 前瞻性随机对照临床试验：放疗同步联合顺铂化疗的疗效

作者(文献)	分期	例数	研究组	对照组	相对复发风险(90%*CI*)	*P*
Rose[188]	FIGO ⅡB~ⅣA	526	每周顺铂 40mg/(m²·w)(最多6周期)	HU 3g/m²×2/周	0.57(0.42~0.78)	<0.001
			顺铂 50mg/m²; 5-Fu4g/(m²·96h)×2/周(2周期)	HU 3g/m²×2/周	0.55(0.40~0.75)	<0.001
Morris[186]	FIGO ⅠB~ⅡA(≥5cm)ⅡB~ⅣA 或盆腔淋巴结转移	403	顺铂 75mg/m²; 5-Fu4g/(m²·96h)(3周期)	无[a]	0.48(0.35~0.66)	0.001
Keys[185]	FIGO ⅠB(≥4cm)	369	每周顺铂 40mg/(m²/w)(最多6周期)	无[b]	0.51(0.34~0.75)	0.001
Whitney[189]	FIGO ⅡB~ⅣA	368	顺铂 50mg/m²; 5-Fu4g/(m²·96h)(2周期)	HU 3g/m²×2/周	0.79(0.62~0.99)	0.03
Peters[117]	FIGO Ⅰ~ⅡA 根治性子宫切除术后淋巴结、宫旁或切缘阳性	268	顺铂 50mg/m²; 5-Fu4g/(m²·96h)(2周期)	无	0.50(0.29~0.84)	0.01
Pearcey[202]	FIGO ⅠB~ⅡA(≥5cm)ⅡB~ⅣA 或盆腔淋巴结转移	259	每周顺铂 40mg/(m²·w)(最多6周期)	无	00.91(0.62~1.35)[c]	0.43
Wong[203]	FIGO ⅠB~ⅡA(>4cm),ⅡB~Ⅲ	220	表柔比星 60mg/m²,然后 90mg/m²,每4周1次,≥5周期[d]	无	~0.65	0.02
Lorvidhaya[204]	FIGO ⅠB~ⅣA	926	丝裂霉素 C 10mg/m²d1,29 口服 5-Fu 300mg/d,d1~14 和 d29~42	无	0.001	

放疗同步联合顺铂化疗对局部晚期宫颈癌患者疗效的前瞻性随机临床试验结果。

[a]对照组患者接受了腹主动脉及预防性放疗。

[b]所有患者放疗后行筋膜外子宫切除术。

[c]生存率。

[d]第一天开始化疗,放疗期间及放疗结束后每四周化疗一次。

[e]该临床试验共分4组:1组,常规放疗;2组,常规放疗后辅助化疗,每天口服氟尿嘧啶(5-Fu)200mg,4周3个疗程,每6周休息2周;3组,常规放疗加同步化疗;4组,常规放疗加同步化疗及放疗结束后辅助化疗。辅助化疗不影响复发,但常规放疗组与常规放疗加同步化疗组之间复发率有显著差异。

CI,置信区间;FU,随访;HU,羟基脲。

GOG 的两项研究将接受体外放疗的ⅡB期~Ⅳ期宫颈癌患者根据其同步化疗方案随机分为两组:羟基脲组和顺铂组[188,189]。研究发现顺铂组(含3个以顺铂为主的方案)局部控制率和生存率较羟基脲组高。GOG 的另一项研究[185]将局部肿瘤≥4cm 的ⅠB期宫颈癌患者随机分为两组:一组在接受放射治疗后行筋膜外子宫切除术,一组在接受顺铂周疗的同步放化疗后行筋膜外子宫切除术。研究发现顺铂为主的同步放化疗组更易达到组织学上的完全缓解,在初步分析时其肿瘤消退率较高。GOG 和 SWOG 的一项研究将广泛子宫切除术后存在盆腔淋巴结转移、切缘阳性或宫旁受侵高危因素的宫颈癌患者随机分为两组:一组术后接受盆腔放疗,一组术后接受以顺铂+氟尿嘧啶为基础的同步放化疗[117]。初步分析结果表明接受同步放化疗的患者无瘤生存率更高。目前这项研究的最新数据表明同步放化疗组的5年生存率高于放疗组,然而,单因素分析发现肿瘤直经<2cm 或仅一枚淋巴结转移的患者增加同步化疗并没有获益[205]。增加同步化疗后,肿瘤直径≤2cm 患者的5年生存率仅提高了5%(77% vs 82%),而肿瘤直径>2cm 患者的5年生存率提高了19%(58% vs 77%)。同样,增加同步化疗后,仅1枚淋巴结转移患者5年生存率(79% vs 83%)的改善程度也明显小于至少2枚以上淋巴结转移的患者(55% vs 75%)[205]。

同时,放射治疗肿瘤协会(RTOG)的一项试验对盆腔放疗组和以顺铂+氟尿嘧啶为基础的同步放化疗组(包括预防性腹主动脉旁照射)进行了比较[186]。研究发现Ⅲ期或Ⅳ期以及

ⅠB2 期或Ⅱ期的宫颈癌患者行同步放化疗其结局有明显改善。两组患者治疗相关的晚期并发症的发生率无显著差异[194]。这项研究目前对生存患者的中位随访时间为 6.6 年，最新数据表明同步放化疗组的总体生存率较放疗组增高（67% vs 41%，8 年，$P<0.0001$），研究认为同步放化疗可改善局部晚期宫颈癌患者的生存，而不增加治疗晚期并发症的发生[206]。目前仅有一项大型随机试验未发现宫颈癌患者从同步放化疗中获益。这项试验于 2002 年由 Pearcey 等发表，作者认为其研究结果不同于上述 5 项试验可能归因于治疗技术的差异，尽管该试验对照组生存率的改善空间亦小于上述试验[202]。这项试验是 6 项试验中规模最小的。

综上所述，这些随机试验表明，盆腔放疗时同步加以顺铂为主的化疗可以使局部晚期宫颈癌患者获益。氟尿嘧啶是否起着重要作用尚不得而知。RTOG90-01、GOG85、GOG120 和 SWOG8797 这 4 个试验对顺铂和 FU 结合的方案作了比较。GOG120 试验表明顺铂/氟尿嘧啶和羟基脲联合组 3～4 度白细胞减少的发生率显著高于顺铂单药组和羟基脲单药组，但疗效相近。因此，尽管没有直接对这两种方案的比较，但单药顺铂与顺铂联合氟尿嘧啶相比，似乎疗效相近而毒性较小。

一项对 18 项同步放化疗研究（共 4 580 例患者）的荟萃分析发现，同步放化疗可以提高部分宫颈癌患者的总生存率和无进展生存期，并降低局部和远处复发率[207]。同步放化疗可使生存率提高 12%，这种作用在铂类为基础的化疗中较非铂类为基础的化疗中更为显著[207]。新近一项基于个体病例数据的系统性综述兼荟萃分析提示，同步放化疗可使 5 年生存率提高 7%，这种作用在铂类为基础的化疗和非铂类为基础的化疗中作用相似[208]。这项研究还提示化疗获益大小与肿瘤分期相关，但与患者的其他特征无关，表明早期患者与Ⅲ期和Ⅳ期患者相比，获益更大[208]。

2012 年，Duenas Gonzales 发表了一项大型的Ⅲ期临床研究结果，将局部晚期宫颈癌患者随机分为顺铂加放疗组和顺铂联合吉西他滨加放疗组[209]。患者在同步放化疗结束后继续接受系统性化疗，中位随访 3 年，接受顺铂加吉西他滨治疗的患者肿瘤消退率达到 32%，同时 3 年无瘤生存率高于单独接受顺铂的患者（74% vs 65%）。另外，顺铂联合吉西他滨能提高 32% 的生存率。然而，这项研究后续随访存在问题，之后发表的结果显示，各个亚组中两种方式的结果没有明显差异[210]。也有报道显示顺铂联合吉西他滨加放疗造成严重的毒副作用，目前在美国这种治疗方式比较少见[211]。

这些研究提出的一些有趣问题无疑将成为未来研究的主体。尽管北美的一些研究均强调以顺铂为基础的化疗，但东南亚的学者们发现放疗同时辅以表柔比星或丝裂霉素和氟尿嘧啶对患者结局有所改善[203,204]。其他一些在晚期宫颈癌中作为放疗增敏研究的药物包括紫杉醇、卡铂、奈达铂、拓泊替康和多种生物反应调节剂[212~215]。RTOG 刚刚发布了一项临床Ⅱ期研究结果，共纳入了 49 例患者，结果显示顺铂联合贝伐单抗加放疗者的 3 年 OS、DFS 以及 LRF 分别为 81.3%、68.7% 及 23.3%[216]。另一个治疗方案是抑制核糖核苷酸还原酶（RNR），RNR 水平升高降低了放化疗后肿瘤的反应率，同时增加了肿瘤复发的风险[217]。因此放疗联合 RNR 抑制剂靶向治疗或许能改善宫颈癌治疗效果。此外，也有将 3-氨基吡啶-2-羧醛硫半脲作为治疗靶点，一项Ⅱ期临床研究报道，中位随访 20 个月，25 例患者有 24 例达到临床缓解，24 例中有 23 例在 3 个月内接受 PET/CT 评估达到缓解[218]。今后期待更大的，多机构的临床Ⅱ期甚至临床Ⅲ期研究的结果。另外一些正在进行的靶向治疗的随机试验主要针对 EGFR 的表达和应用 PARP（腺苷二磷酸核糖）抑制剂。

腹主动脉旁淋巴结转移

腹主动脉旁淋巴结转移可以通过细针穿刺抽吸、腹腔镜或腹膜外途径开腹手术切除证实。腹腔镜和腹膜外途径开腹手术可以切除阳性淋巴结并对其他腹主动脉旁淋巴结进行取样，从而提高了放疗的控制率并有助于治疗靶区的勾画。

延伸野 EBRT 的上界应该位于阳性淋巴结顶端上 3cm，上界最高可达 T12。最近，盆腔淋巴结或髂总淋巴结阳性患者其放射野可延伸至 L1～L2 之间。

延伸野放射治疗对腹主动脉旁淋巴结阳性患者疗效显著，5 年生存率介于 25%～50%[219,220]。两项随机试验对预防性延伸野放疗的疗效进行了评估，但两组患者的无病生存率无差异[221,222]。

几项Ⅱ期研究对延伸野放疗+同步化疗的作用进行了评价[223]。尽管扩大放射野后副作用增加，但如果对化疗方案、照射体积和其他可能导致严重毒性的因素进行调整，患者仍可耐受联合治疗。总之，由盆腔放化疗的结果推测延伸野放化疗可达到较好疗效，但应该告知患者延伸野放疗+同步化疗的成本-效益比还未正式验证，但 IMRT 可能减轻急性毒性反应。

单纯子宫切除术后意外发现的浸润性宫颈癌

有些因为盆腔良性疾病行单纯子宫切除的患者在术后病理检查时可能会意外发现浸润性宫颈癌。许多因素可以导致这种意外的发生[224]。

单纯子宫切除后意外发现的浸润性宫颈癌患者根据疾病范围和表现可以分为 5 组：①微小浸润宫颈癌；②局限于宫颈、切缘阴性宫颈癌；③切缘阳性但无肉眼残存肿瘤；④病理证实的肉眼残存肿瘤；⑤单纯子宫切除术后 6 个月以后就诊的患者（往往因为疾病复发）[225]。治疗方案取决于残存肿瘤的大小。微小浸润或无残存肿瘤的患者只需对阴道残端进行腔内放疗；有切缘肉眼残存肿瘤的患者需要进行全方面的治疗。仅有微量残存肿瘤或无肉眼残存肿瘤的患者（组 1～3）其 5 年生存率可达 59%～79%，而有肉眼残存肿瘤的患者（组 4、组 5）5 年生存率较低（约 41%）[226]。

复发性宫颈癌

预后因素

许多临床病理因素与宫颈癌盆腔复发性相关。然而，在大部分研究中，由于患者数目少、临床治疗参数多样性，研究无法进行详细的统计学分析。复发部位（中心性 vs 盆壁复发）和盆腔复发肿瘤大小这两项临床因素与补救治疗是否成功有关[227]。转移淋巴结与盆腔复发 RC 融合者预后较差，其他临床不良因素包括：非鳞状细胞癌病理类型（尤其是腺癌）和原发肿瘤的高 FIGO 分期[228]。有争议的因素包括：初始治疗距复发的间隔时间和盆腔复发是否有症状[172,228,229]。

广泛子宫切除术

少数情况下，初始行放射治疗或广泛子宫切除术的复发患者补救治疗时经严格选择后行盆腔廓清术不失为一个较好的治疗措施。Coleman 等报道了 50 名放疗后肿瘤持续存在或复发行广泛子宫切除的患者[230]，5 年和 10 年生存率分别为 72%和 60%。64%的患者发生了严重并发症，42%的患者并发症持续存在。作者认为中心性复发灶较小的宫颈癌患者可以行广泛子宫切除术代替盆腔廓清术，但必须经过严格选择[230]。

盆腔廓清术

对于放射治疗后盆腔中心性复发或放射野内新发肿瘤的宫颈癌患者行盆腔廓清术是一种有潜在治愈可能的手段[231~233]。外科技术、麻醉和术后护理的发展减少了术中和术后并发症，从而大大降低了手术死亡率[224,232,233]。造瘘装置和护理的发展使患者术后可以接近正常生活、满足个人需求、履行个人职责。廓清术的种类取决于癌症的复发部位。(图 102-19)

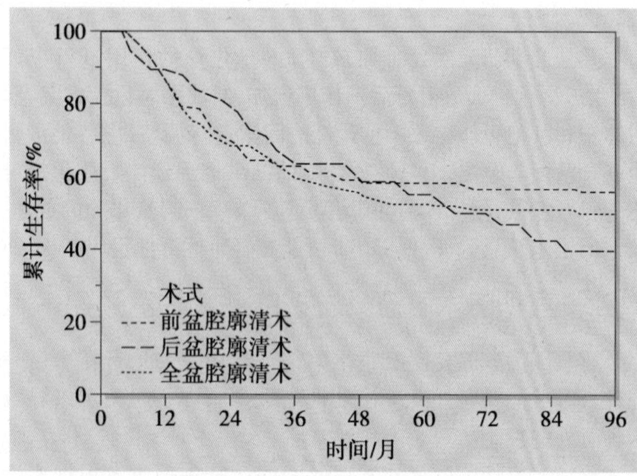

图 102-19 得克萨斯大学安德森癌症医学中心 1955—1984 年行盆腔廓清术患者三种术式的生存曲线。虽然 3 条曲线相似，但应注意，后盆腔廓清术多用于外阴和肛门直肠转移的患者，术后局部复发率更高

前盆腔廓清术

前盆腔廓清术包括子宫、附件、膀胱、尿道和阴道的切除。行这种术式的患者其肿瘤位于盆腔前部，未累及直肠、阴道顶端和阴道壁。根据情况行阴道重建。

后盆腔廓清术

后盆腔廓清术需要切除子宫、附件、肛门、直肠乙状结肠、肛提肌和阴道。许多妇科肿瘤医师会保留部分阴道前壁以支持尿道，从而减少术后尿失禁的发生。这种术式适用于肿瘤局限于阴道后壁和直肠阴道隔的患者。

全盆腔廓清术

全盆腔廓清术需要切除子宫、附件、膀胱、尿道、阴道、直肠乙状结肠、肛提肌和肛门。行该术式的患者其肿瘤位于中心或累及阴道上 1/2。膀胱底部和直肠阴道隔连续性肿瘤累及的患者无法选择较小范围的廓清术。阴道重建术能使患者术后恢复性功能并有助于盆底的重建。可通过网膜带蒂移植进行盆底重建，这种术式可以提供新的血供，从而减少了术后并发症[234]。在前盆腔和全盆腔廓清术中，均需要构建可控性尿路。

全盆腔廓清术目前被广泛应用，其 5 年生存率为 40%~50%。得克萨斯大学安德森癌症医学中心的 Rutledge 报道，1955~1984 年共进行了 448 例盆腔廓清术[231]。5 年生存率如图 102-19 所示。

放射治疗

初始行广泛子宫切除的宫颈癌患者如出现盆腔孤立性肿瘤复发可以行根治性放射治疗。Lanciano 的一项文献综述报道局部复发行放射治疗的无病生存率介于 20%~50%。复发肿瘤小和盆腔中心复发的患者其预后更好[227]。大部分患者可行体外放疗加或不加腔内放疗。无盆壁固定或局部转移的孤立性中心性复发宫颈癌患者的治愈率为 60%~70%[229]。如果盆壁受累，则预后更差(放射治疗后的 5 年生存率为 10%~20%)。

Ⅳ期或复发患者的治疗

化疗

单药化疗

化疗对于转移或复发宫颈癌相对无效。中位生存期位于 4~8 个月。顺铂被认为是宫颈癌最有效的化疗药，剂量为 50~100mg/m^2，反应率为 17%~21%[235,236]。Bonomi 等比较了不同顺铂剂量的疗效，发现高剂量与较高的部分缓解率(31% vs 21%)和轻度增高的完全缓解率(13% vs 10%)相关，但并不提高肿瘤缓解持续时间、PFS 和生存指数[236]。对 175 名患者采用卡铂化疗，340~400mg/m^2，28 天/周期，10 名患者肿瘤完全消退(5.7%)[237]。对一系列关于卡铂的研究总结发现其完全缓解率为 19%。

紫杉醇的化疗疗效较好，即使用于既往已行铂类化疗的患者(包括非鳞状细胞癌病理类型)，反应率也可达 17%~31%，中位生存时间 7 个月。其他 3 种药物，拓泊替康、长春瑞滨和异环磷酰胺[238~240]均可获得较好的肿瘤消退率，在一些Ⅱ期和Ⅲ期临床试验中用于联合化疗。

联合化疗

表 102-7 显示的 19 个单药化疗方案对宫颈癌有一定疗效，缓解率 15%以上定义为有效。然而顺铂化疗同时增加其他药物并未提高生存率。大量研究表明联合化疗可以提高缓解率，同时增加了毒性。异环磷酰胺得到了最多的关注。一些小型Ⅱ期研究对既往未行放射治疗的患者联合异环磷酰胺和顺铂或卡铂化疗进行了评估，缓解率为 50%~62%[241~244]。

顺铂联合氟尿嘧啶持续输注，顺铂联合紫杉醇，顺铂联合长春瑞滨和顺铂联合吉西他滨化疗在既往未治疗患者中均显示出较好的缓解率[245~252]。卡铂和脂质体多柔比星联合化疗的疗效中等[253]。同样，如果患者既往有盆腔放疗史则肿瘤缓解率明显下降[246,252]。

GOG 一项Ⅲ期随机临床试验显示，托泊替康与顺铂联合化疗的 *RR* 优于顺铂单药[254]。顺铂组的 *RR* 为 13%，联合化疗组的 *RR* 为 27%。中位生存期提高了 3 个月，且宫颈癌治疗功能评估(FACT-CX)量表表明生活质量也略有改善。他们发现既往的放射增敏化疗和从诊断至开始治疗的间隔时间可影响疗效。在放疗野外的部位反应率更高(70% vs 23%)。这促使

表 102-7　宫颈癌的单药化疗[235~240]

化疗药物	有效率/%
烷化剂	
环磷酰胺	38/251(15)
苯丁酸氮芥	11/44(25)
美法仑	4/20(20)
异环磷酰胺	35/157(22)
二溴卫矛醇	16/55(29)
重金属复合物	
顺铂	190/815(23)
卡铂	27/175(15)
抗肿瘤抗生素	
多柔比星	45/266(17)
博来霉素	19/176(11)
丝裂霉素	5/23(22)
抗代谢物	
氟尿嘧啶	29/142(20)
甲氨蝶呤	17/96(18)
羟基脲	0/14(0)
植物碱	
长春新碱	10/55(18)
长春花碱	2/20(10)
依托泊苷	0/31(0)
其他	
六甲密胺	12/64(19)
伊立替康(CPT-11)	36/192(19)
紫杉醇	14/74(19)
多西他赛	1/13(8)
拓泊替康	8/43(19)
六甲密胺	12/64(19)
丙二胺亚胺	5/28(18)

GOG 进一步开展针对原发性ⅣB 期或复发/持续宫颈癌的前瞻性临床试验。在该试验中，患者被随机分为四个组：第 1 组，紫杉醇和顺铂(PC)；第 2 组，长春瑞滨和顺铂(VC)；第 3 组，吉西他滨和顺铂(GC)；第 4 组，托泊替康和顺铂(TC)。这项研究由于结果差异明显而提前终止。但是，在 513 位患者中，就 OS 而言，VC，GC 或 TC 并不优于 PC，但 *RR*，PFS 和 OS 的趋势偏向于 PC[255]。在另一份报道，除 PC 具有较高的神经毒性发生率外，四组患者生活质量无显著差异，其最终结论是 PC 应该成为复发或转移性宫颈癌的治疗标准[256]。

最近 GOG 240 研究的结果使复发或转移性宫颈癌患者的治疗迈出了重要的一步，GOG 240 研究将患者随机分为 2 种化疗方案(顺铂加紫杉醇 vs 紫杉醇加托泊替康)，联合贝伐单抗或无贝伐单抗，不同化疗方案之间的结果没有差异[257]。与单纯化疗相比，联合贝伐单抗可显著改善 OS(17 个月 vs 13.3 个月)，PFS(8.2 个月 vs 5.9 个月)和 *RR*(48% vs 36%)，生活质量没有明显下降[258]。主要并发症包括瘘(3%)，血栓栓塞(8%)和易于控制的高血压(25%)[258]。自本文发表以来，顺铂-紫杉醇-贝伐单抗三联治疗已被美国国家综合癌症网络(NCCN)宫颈癌临床实践指南列为 2A 类[259]。

目前复发或转移性宫颈癌患者的预后仍然不理想，这也是世界范围内迫切需要解决的问题。因此，需要探索更好的治疗方法，包括确定预后因素，试用可能改善化疗疗效的新型药物以及各种免疫治疗方法。Moore 对 3 项 GOG 试验的 428 名患者进行了评估并确定了 5 个预后因素，包括种族，运动状态，骨盆疾病，既往放射增敏剂以及从诊断到首次复发的时间间隔(<1 年)，这些因素可能在临床上用于筛选出对顺铂的标准治疗方案没有反应但可能从研究试验中受益的女性[260]。

宫颈癌免疫治疗的基本原理是基于 HPV 感染在疾病中的致病作用。HPV 感染会引起细胞免疫反应，而调节性 T 细胞似乎在与 HPV 相关的肿瘤中的局部免疫抑制中发挥作用。能够中断涉及癌症免疫逃逸机制的新药也展示了不错的结果。Basu 在 2014 年美国临床肿瘤学会年会上发表了一项Ⅱ期随机试验结果，110 名印度复发/难治性宫颈癌患者随机接受了联合或不联合顺铂的减毒单核细胞增生李斯特菌活疫苗治疗，12 个月的 OS 为 36%，18 个月 OS 为 28%，总 *RR* 为 11%[261]，其中 6 例完全缓解，6 例部分缓解。联合顺铂并未改善 OS 或 *RR*[261]，这些有希望的结果报道后在美国进行了一项由 NRG 主持的相同减毒活疫苗的试验(GOG 265/NCT01266460)。

其他治疗方法包括限制机体对癌症的免疫反应调节，包括细胞毒性 T 淋巴细胞相关分子 4(CTLA-4)和 PD-1 的上调，均得到越来越多的研究。肿瘤浸润淋巴细胞的输入免疫疗法是晚期或转移性肿瘤患者的另一种潜在有用的方法。在这项技术中，选择肿瘤累及的淋巴细胞，进行选择性扩增，并回输患者体内。根据在恶性黑色素瘤等肿瘤中的治疗结果，NCI 正在进行一项用于复发性或转移性宫颈癌患者的研究(NCT01266460)。

作用于 HPV 影响的信号通路的新型靶向药物也可能发挥疗效。基因组数据记录了 *KRAS* 和 *P13KCA* 突变，目前有待于证明这些通路已激活且为宫颈癌发生过程中的必需机制。其他可能有效的新药包括西妥昔单抗、吉非替尼、厄洛替尼和丝美替尼。辐射是 DNA 损伤的主要原因，因此，PARP 的抑制为宫颈癌的治疗提供了另一个潜在的靶标，目前 NRG 有 2 项宫颈癌的临床研究(GOG 127W/NCT0101266447 和 GOG76HH/NCT01282852)。

总结

对于复发性宫颈癌患者首先应确定是否可行手术治疗或放射治疗，两种治疗的 5 年生存率均可达 20%~50%。系统性化疗可用于复发性和转移性宫颈癌患者，但需权衡受益与毒性。尚需进一步的研究以明确化疗对生活质量的影响、既往行同步化疗的患者对化疗的敏感性以及生物制剂的作用。

(李楠　吴忧 译　吴令英 校)

参考文献

The complete reference list can be found on the Wiley Companion Digital Edition of this title (see inside front cover for login instructions).

4 Coleman MP, Esteve J, Damiecki P, et al. Trends in cancer incidence and mortality. *IARC Sci Publ*. 1993;**121**:1–86.

7 Brinton LA. Epidemiology of cervical cancer—overview. In: Munoz FB, Bosch FX, Shah KV, Meheus A, eds. *The Epidemiology of Human Papillomavirus and Cervical Cancer*. Oxford (UK): Oxford University Press; 1992:3–23.

11 Munoz N, Bosch FX. Cervical cancer and papillomavirus: epidemiological evidence and perspective for prevention. *Salud Publica Mex*. 1997;**39**:274–282.

13 Bosch FX, Manos MM, Munoz N, et al. Prevalence of human papillomavirus in cervical cancer: a worldwide perspective. International biological study on cervical cancer (IBSCC) study group [comments]. *J Natl Cancer Inst*. 1995;**87**:796–802.

70 Cox JT, Lorincz AT, Schiffman MH, et al. Human papillomavirus testing by hybrid capture appears to be useful in triaging women with a cytologic diagnosis of atypical squamous cells of undetermined significance. *Am J Obstet Gynecol*. 1995;**172**:946–954.

74 US Food and Drug Administration. *Cobas HPV Test-P10020/S008. Parsippany*. NJ: US Food and Drug Administration; 2014. Accessdata.fda.gov/scripts/cdrh/cfdocs/cfTopic/pma/pma.cfm?num=P1000203008 (accessed 1 October 2014).

75 Cullen AP, Reid R, Campion M, et al. Analysis of the physical state of different human papillomavirus DNA's in intraepithelial and invasive cervical neoplasm. *J Virol*. 1999;**65**:606–612.

77 Mitchell MF, Tortolero-Luna G, Cook E, et al. A randomized clinical trial of cryotherapy, laser vaporization, and loop electrosurgical excision for treatment of squamous intraepithelial lesions of the cervix. *Obstet Gynecol*. 1998;**92**:737–744.

85 The HPV PATRICIA Study Group. Efficacy of a prophylactic adjuvanted bivalent L1 virus-like-particle vaccine against infection with human papillomavirus types 16 and 18 in young women: an interim analysis of a phase III double-blind, randomized controlled trial. *Lancet*. 2007;**369**:2161–2170.

87 Rogers LJ, Eva LJ, Luesley DM. Vaccines against cervical cancer. *Curr Opin Oncol*. 2008;**20**:570–574.

92 Piver MS, Chung WS. Prognostic significance of cervical lesion size and pelvic node metastases in cervical carcinoma. *Obstet Gynecol*. 1975;**46**:507–510.

93 Mitchell PA, Waggoner S, Rotmensch J, et al. Cervical cancer in the elderly treated with radiation therapy. *Gynecol Oncol*. 1998;**71**:291–298.

105 Grigsby PW, Siegel BA, Dehdashti F. Lymph node staging by positron emission tomography in patients with carcinoma of the cervix. *J Clin Oncol*. 2001;**19**:3745–3749.

117 Peters WAI, Liu PY, Barrett R, et al. Cisplatin, 5-fluorouracil plus radiation therapy are superior to radiation therapy as adjunctive therapy in high-risk, early-stage carcinoma of the cervix after radical hysterectomy and pelvic lymphadenectomy. Report of a phase III intergroup study. *Gynecol Oncol*. 1999;**72**:443.

152 Lecuru F, Mathevet P, Querleu D, et al. Bilateral negative sentinel nodes accurately predict absence of lymph node metastasis in early cervical cancer: results of the SENTICOL study. *J Clin Oncol*. 2011;**29**:1686–1691.

161 Lohe KJ, Burghardt E, Hillemanns HG, et al. Early squamous cell carcinoma of the uterine cervix. II. Clinical results of a cooperative study in the management of 419 patients with early stromal invasion and microcarcinoma. *Gynecol Oncol*. 1978;**6**:31–50.

185 Keys HM, Bundy BN, Stehman FB, et al. Cisplatin, radiation, and adjuvant hysterectomy for bulky stage IB cervical carcinoma. *N Engl J Med*. 1999;**340**:1154–1161.

186 Morris M, Eifel PJ, Lu J, et al. Pelvic radiation with concurrent chemotherapy compared with pelvic and paraaortic radiation for high-risk cervical cancer. *N Engl J Med*. 1999;**340**:1137–1143.

188 Rose PG, Bundy BN, Watkins J, et al. Concurrent cisplatin based chemotherapy and radiotherapy for locally advanced cervical cancer. *N Engl J Med*. 1999;**340**:1144–1153.

189 Whitney CW, Sause W, Bundy BN, et al. A randomized comparison of fluorouracil plus cisplatin versus hydroxyurea as an adjunct to radiation therapy in stages IIB–IVA carcinoma of the cervix with negative para-aortic lymph nodes: a Gynecologic Oncology Group and Southwest Oncology Group study. *J Clin Oncol*. 1999;**17**:1339–1348.

195 Delgado G, Bundy BN, Fowler WC, et al. A prospective surgical pathological study of stage I squamous carcinoma of the cervix: a Gynecologic Oncology Group study. *Gynecol Oncol*. 1989;**36**:314–320.

196 Sedlis A, Bundy BN, Rotman MZ, et al. A randomized trial of pelvic radiation therapy versus No further therapy in selected patients with stage IB carcinoma of the cervix after radical hysterectomy and pelvic lymphadenectomy: a Gynecologic Oncology Group study. *Gynecol Oncol*. 1999;**73**:177–183.

197 Rotman M, Sedlis A, Piedmonte MR, et al. A Phase III randomized trial of postoperative pelvic irradiation in stage IB cervical carcinoma with poor prognostic features: follow-up of a Gynecologic Oncology Group Study. *Int J Radiat Oncol Biol Phys*. 2006;**65**:169–176.

198 Sardi JE, Giaroli A, Sananes C, et al. Long-term follow-up of the first randomized trial using neoadjuvant chemotherapy in stage Ib squamous carcinoma of the cervix: the final results. *Gynecol Oncol*. 1997;**67**:61–69.

199 Eddy G, Bundy B, Creasman W, et al. Treatment of "bulky" stage IB cervical cancer with or without neoadjuvant vincristine and cisplatin prior to radical hysterectomy and pelvic/para-aortic lymphadenectomy: a phase III trial of the gynecologic oncology group. *Gynecol Oncol*. 2007;**106**:362–369.

200 Neoadjuvant Chemotherapy for Cervical Cancer Meta-Analysis Collaboration. Neoadjuvant chemotherapy locally advanced cervical cancer: a systematic review and meta-analysis of individual patient data from 21 randomised trials. *Eur J Cancer*. 2003;**39**:2470–2486.

201 Tierney JF, Vale C, Symonds P. Concomitant and neoadjuvant chemotherapy for cervical cancer. *Clin Oncol*. 2008;**20**:401–416.

202 Pearcey R, Brundage M, Drouin P, et al. Phase III trial comparing radical radiotherapy with and without cisplatin chemotherapy in patients with advanced squamous cell cancer of the cervix. *J Clin Oncol*. 2002;**20**:966–972.

204 Lorvidhaya V, Chitapanarux I, Sangruchi S, et al. Concurrent mitomycin C, 5-fluorouracil, and radiotherapy in the treatment of locally advanced carcinoma of the cervix: a randomized trial. *Int J Radiat Oncol Biol Phys*. 2003;**55**:1226–1232.

205 Monk BJ, Wang J, Im S, et al. Rethinking the use of radiation and chemotherapy after radical hysterectomy: a clinical-pathologic analysis of a Gynecologic Oncology Group/Southwest Oncology Group/Radiation Therapy Oncology Group Trial. *Gynecol Oncol*. 2005;**96**:721–728.

206 Eifel PJ, Winter K, Morris M, et al. Pelvic irradiation with concurrent chemotherapy versus pelvic and para-aortic irradiation for high-risk cervical cancer: an update of radiation therapy oncology group trial (RTOG) 90-01. *J Clin Oncol*. 2004;**22**:872–880.

207 Green JA, Kirwan JM, Tierney JF, et al. Survival and recurrence after concomitant chemotherapy and radiotherapy for cancer of the uterine cervix: a systematic review and meta-analysis. *Lancet*. 2001;**358**:781–786.

209 Duenas-Gonzalez A, ZarbaJJ PF, et al. Phase III, open label, randomized study comparing concurrent gemcitabine plus cisplatin and radiation followed by adjuvant gemcitabine and cisplatin versus concurrent cisplatin and radiation in patients with stage IIB to IVA carcinoma of the cervix. *J Clin Oncol*. 2011;**29**:1678–1685.

223 Varia MA, Bundy BN, Deppe G, et al. Cervical carcinoma metastatic to para-aortic nodes: extended field radiation therapy with concomitant 5-fluorouracil and cisplatin chemotherapy: a Gynecologic Oncology Group study. *Int J Radiat Oncol Biol Phys*. 1998;**42**:1015–1023.

227 Lanciano R. Radiotherapy for the treatment of locally recurrent cervical cancer. *J Natl Cancer Inst Monogr*. 1996;**21**:113–115.

231 Rutledge FN. Pelvic exenteration: an update of the U. T. M. D. Anderson Hospital experience and review of the literature. In: Rutledge FN, Freedman RS, Gershenson DM, eds. *Gynecologic Cancer: Diagnosis and Treatment Strategies*. Austin (TX): University of Texas Press; 1987:7.

254 Long HJ 3rd, Bundy BN, Grendys EC Jr, et al. Randomized phase III trial of cisplatin (P) vs cisplatin plus topotecan (T) vs MVAC in stage IVB, recurrent or persistent carcinoma of the uterine cervix: a Gynecologic Oncology Group study [abstract 9]. *Gynecol Oncol*. 2004;**92**:397.315.

255 Monk BJ, Sill MW, McMeekin DS, et al. Phase III trial of four cisplatin-containing doublet combinations in stage IVB, recurrent or persistent cervical carcinoma: a Gynecology Oncology Group study. *J Clin Oncol*. 2009;**27**:4649–4655.

256 Cella D, Huang HQ, Monk BJ, et al. Health-related quality of life outcomes associated with four cisplatin-based doublet chemotherapy regimens for stage IVB recurrent or persistent cervical cancer: a Gynecology Oncology Group study. *Gynecol Oncol*. 2010;**119**:531–537.

257 Tewari KS, Sill MW, Long HJ, et al. Improved survival with bevacizumab in advanced cervical cancer. *N Engl J Med*. 2014;**370**:734–743.

258 Penson RT, Huang HQ, Wenzel LB, et al. Bevacizumab for advanced cervical cancer: patient-reported outcomes of a randomized, phase 3 trial (NRG Oncology-Gynecologic Oncology Group protocol 240). *Lancet Oncol*. 2015:S1470–S2045.

259 NCCN (2014) Clinical Practice Guidelines in Oncology (NCCN guidelines). Cervical Cancer Version 1. NCCN.org.

260 Moore DH, Tian C, Monk BJ, et al. Prognostic factors for response to cisplatin-based chemotherapy in advanced cervical carcinoma: a Gynecologic Oncology Group study. *Gynecol Oncol*. 2010;**116**:44–49.

261 Basu P, Mehta AO, Jain MM, et al. ADXS11-001 immunotherapy targeting HPV-E7: final results from a phase 2 study in Indian women with recurrent cervical cancer. *J Clin Oncol*. 2014;**325s(suppl;abstr5610)**.

第 103 章　子宫内膜癌

Jamal Rahaman, MD ■ Karen Lu, MD ■ Carmel J. Cohen, MD

概述

子宫内膜癌是美国最常见的妇科肿瘤，每年诊断出新病例超过 50 000 例。超过 80%为Ⅰ型子宫内膜癌，具有典型的雌激素依赖性子宫内膜样组织学特征和良好的预后。Ⅱ型子宫内膜癌具有不同分子特征和更高的恶性度并且存活率降低，包括子宫浆液性乳头状癌(UPSC)和透明细胞癌。癌症基因组阿特拉斯计划(TCGA)近期基于体细胞突变，拷贝数改变和微卫星不稳定状态定义了四种子宫内膜癌分子亚型。超过 75%的患者出现不规则或绝经后出血。手术分期包括全子宫切除术，双侧输卵管卵巢切除术，盆腔和腹主动脉旁淋巴结取样，可通过剖腹手术，腹腔镜手术或机器人手术进行。在可能的情况下，手术是大多数子宫内膜癌患者的最主要治疗方法。放射治疗和激素治疗是不能手术患者的替代方案。Ⅰ期疾病的辅助治疗由年龄，肌层浸润深度，淋巴脉管间隙侵袭和肿瘤分级情况决定。晚期和复发患者则使用放射疗法，化学疗法和激素疗法。紫杉醇(T)、卡铂(C)、顺铂(P)和多柔比星(A)是最有效的单一药物，TC 和 TAP 是最有效的联合化疗方案。激素疗法包括孕激素、含黄体酮的宫内节育器、他莫昔芬，促性腺激素释放激素类似物和芳香酶抑制剂。具有活性的新兴生物制剂包括贝伐单抗和 mTOR 抑制剂。肿瘤分子谱分析、微创手术、前哨淋巴结评估以及新型生物疗法的整合将在未来发挥更大的作用。

流行病学

2015 年美国子宫体癌新诊断病例大约 54 870 例，10 170 名女性将死于这种癌症[1]。自 1991 年以来，美国子宫内膜癌的死亡率已超过宫颈癌，虽然宫颈癌是欠发达国家中最普遍的妇科癌症，也是全世界死亡率最高的妇科癌症[1,2]。子宫内膜癌的发病率从 1988 年开始每年增加约 0.6%，直到 20 世纪 90 年代末。挪威、捷克斯洛伐克和其他北欧国家也报告了子宫内膜癌发病率的显著增加。尽管发病率有所增加，但早期疾病预后良好[2]。FIGO 结果显示，85%～91%的Ⅰ期患者在 5 年内均存活，SEER 数据库中患有局部疾病的患者有 96%的 5 年生存率[2,3]。

黑人女性的子宫内膜发病率低于白人女性，但死亡率更高[1,4]。Hicks 和同事们观察到，黑人女性被诊断时出现组织学较差，疾病期别更晚，分化程度较差的肿瘤比白人女性更多[4]。黑人女性手术治疗率较低，经过手术治疗的晚期患者接受辅助放疗(RT)较少，但接受化疗比白人患者更常见。黑人女性的五年生存率较差，即使对于接受过外科手术治疗的Ⅰ期患者也是如此[1,4]。

风险因素

风险因素包括体型较大、肥胖、糖尿病、未生育、结肠和/或乳腺癌病史、排卵障碍、内源性雌激素暴露增加和外源性口服雌激素暴露。体内脂肪中雌激素前体的外周芳香化导致更高水平的循环雌激素，部分地解释了肥胖的风险。与包括 5 次以上的多产相比，53 岁以后绝经和超重 50 磅以上，这些都是重要的风险因素，能够增加女性罹患子宫内膜癌的概率 5～10 倍。

导致子宫内膜癌增加的风险因素的病理情况通常包括内源性雌激素水平升高或外源性雌激素补充剂的需求[5]。Gusberg 和 Kardon 回顾了 115 例卵巢颗粒细胞卵巢肿瘤患者的子宫内膜组织学，发现 21%的患者出现子宫内膜癌癌症，43%的患者有癌前期内膜增生。其他报道没有相当的内膜癌发病率，但发现子宫内膜非典型增生的发病率很高[6,7]。多囊卵巢综合征患者通常不排卵，因此暴露于无对抗的内源性雌激素的产生。当年龄小于 45 岁的女性发生子宫内膜癌时，通常患有多囊卵巢综合征[8,9]，并且病变组织周围最常见是非典型增生。卵巢发育不良的患者通过卵巢切除术和雌激素替代治疗后，可能在始基子宫内发生子宫内膜癌[10]。这种内源性雌激素或持续无对抗外源性口服雌激素的暴露和子宫内膜癌的关联已被广泛报道[11～19]。

美国疾病预防和控制中心[Centers for Disease Control and Prevention，CDC]报告说，与从未使用口服避孕药的妇女相比，使用口服避孕药至少 12 个月可使子宫内膜癌的风险降低 50%。未生育的女性似乎受益最多，并且在停止使用口服避孕药后，这种保护可持续十年[20]。Brinton 和 Hoove 的研究发现，之前使用口服避孕药并不能防止妇女在绝经后服用雌激素时患子宫内膜癌的相对风险增加，这提示了孕激素在联合口服避孕药中的作用对于预防子宫内膜癌至关重要[12]。

20 多年来，他莫昔芬被用于治疗乳腺癌，观察发现它能使转移性肿瘤消退，减少对侧乳腺癌的发病率，延迟复发时间，并提高患者亚组的存活率[21]。临床上，他莫昔芬降低血清胆固醇，增加性激素结合球蛋白[22]，保持腰椎骨密度[23]，可使部分患者的阴道上皮增厚[23,24]，可导致子宫肌瘤增大，子宫内膜息肉的生长，以及产生子宫内膜瘤变。这些都是类雌激素功能。矛盾的是，同一种药物与阴道萎缩的产生，血管舒缩症状的出现和临床性交困难的发展有关。这些是雌激素不足的特点。

他莫昔芬的作用可能是器官特异性的，正如它与实验动物肝肿瘤的联系是种特异性的。当把传代乳腺癌和子宫内膜癌细胞株植入无胸腺小鼠体内，两种癌症在同一动物中生长良好。当给予他莫昔芬治疗时，乳腺癌受到抑制，子宫内膜癌继续生长[25]。一些研究者描述了用他莫昔芬治疗的乳腺癌患者中子宫内膜癌发病率增加[26～31]。Killackey 和同事们是第一个报道了在接受抗雌激素治疗的三名乳腺癌患者发生子宫内膜癌的病例[28]。Fornander 和他的同事在瑞典癌症登记处对 1 846 名患有早期乳腺癌的绝经后妇女的新原发癌的发生频率进行了审查,并报告了表明他莫昔芬在子宫内膜癌的后续发展中起作用的最有力的初步数据。与对照组相比,931 名使用他莫昔芬治疗(40mg/d)患者的子宫内膜癌相对风险增加了 6.4 倍[26]。美国外科辅助乳腺和肠道项目(NSABP)描述了对 3 863 名患者的前瞻性研究的观察结果[27]。在 B-14 方案中,2 843 名淋巴结阴性,ER 阳性乳腺癌患者接受他莫昔芬(20mg/d)或安慰剂。另有 1 020 名服用他莫昔芬的患者在该项目中注册。与安慰剂组相比,他莫昔芬治疗组计算出的相对风险为 7.5,安慰剂组的年危险率为 0.2/1 000,随机的他莫昔芬治疗组为 1.6/1 000。最近,在 NSABP 的乳腺癌预防试验(P-1)中,13 388 名女性被随机分配接受安慰剂(6 707)或 20mg/d 的他莫昔芬(6 681)5 年[32]。他莫昔芬组的子宫内膜癌发病率增加(*RR*=2.53);这种增加主要发生在 50 岁或以上的女性身上。他莫昔芬组中的所有子宫内膜癌均为Ⅰ期,且未发生子宫内膜癌死亡。

加拿大的一项针对 304 名接受他莫昔芬治疗的乳腺癌患者的前瞻性纵向研究发现,对无症状患者进行子宫内膜常规超声检查无效[33]。在另一项研究中,Barakat 及其同事通过连续的子宫内膜活检评估了 159 例他莫昔芬治疗的患者。活检时间分别是他莫昔芬治疗的开始,和每 6 个月 1 次,为期 2 年,随后又进行了每年 1 次,为期 3 年[34]。尽管可行手术治疗,但仅在 3 名患者中观察到明显的病理需要进行子宫切除术,作者得出结论是,常规子宫内膜活检用于筛选他莫昔芬治疗的妇女作用是有限的。这些研究都没有为超声或子宫内膜活检的筛查提供强有力的支持[35]。要求及时评估任何阴道出血。然而对于有多种风险因素的患者,临床医生不应该不进行子宫内膜活检或阴道超声检查。

1980 年,Bokhman 首次提出Ⅱ型子宫内膜癌的概念,与经典的Ⅰ型雌激素依赖性子宫内膜样子宫内膜癌不同(表 103-1)。这些患者具有独特的表型,现在认为具有更高的恶性度和疾病相关的不同分子特征并且存活率降低[36,37]。Ⅰ型子宫内膜癌更多地与他莫昔芬治疗和无拮抗的雌激素使用相关。

表 103-1 子宫内膜癌的临床和分子特征

特征	Ⅰ型	Ⅱ型
临床[37]		
危险因素	非拮抗雌激素	年龄
种族	白人>黑人	白人=黑人
分化程度	分化好	分化差
组织学类型	子宫内膜样腺癌	非子宫内膜样
分期	Ⅰ/Ⅱ	Ⅲ/Ⅳ
预后	较好	较差
分子特征		
K-ras 过度表达	是	是
HER2/neu 过度表达	否	是
TP53 过表达	否	是
PTEN 突变	是	否
微卫星不稳定性	是	否

病理

子宫内膜增生

Gusberg 及其同事应用"腺瘤性增生"的专用术语,来描述与子宫内膜腺癌发展有关,且通常在子宫内膜腺癌发生之前,包括所有前体组织学的变异。这些排列范围从具有嗜酸性粒细胞的密集拥挤的腺体的温和排列,到更多无序排列,其特征是管腔内簇状和有丝分裂,假胞质化和奇异核的增加[38]。同样,Hertig 和 Sommers 研究了子宫内膜的浸润前变化。并描述了三种不同程度的异常情况,分别称为"腺瘤性增生""非典型增生"和"原位癌"[39]。Kurman 及其同事对 170 例子宫内膜增生患者进行了至少 1 年的随访;平均随访时间为 13.4 年[40]。他们建立了基于结构异常和细胞学异常来区分病变的标准。只有 1.6%没有细胞异型性的患者发展为癌症,相比之下,非典型细胞学检查的患者为 23%。结构异常对预后并不重要。表 103-2 列出了 Kurman 及其同事的分类和观察的详细信息。他们对简单或复杂的增生(有或没有异型性)的分类现在被用于描述这些病变。

表 103-2 170 例简单和复杂增生,单纯性和复杂性非典型增生患者的随访比较

	患者总数	逆转 n/%	病变持续 n/%	进展为癌症 n/%
单纯性增生	93	74[41]	18[19]	1[1]
复杂性增生	29	23[41]	5[17]	1[3]
单纯非典型增生	13	94[42]	3[23]	1[8]
复杂非典型增生	35	20[43]	5[14]	10[29]

改编自 Kurman et al,1985,40。经 John Wiley and Sons 许可转载。

子宫内膜样腺癌

子宫内膜样腺癌是最常见的子宫内膜癌组织学类型。它的特征是异常腺体之间的基质消失,其内衬的内层变成管腔,核染色质分布紊乱,核增大,以及不同程度的有丝分裂,坏死和出血。这种经典类型占腺癌的 80%~95%。

腺鳞癌

腺鳞癌既有鳞状成分,又有腺瘤成分。它通常占子宫内膜腺癌的 7%或更少。提示腺鳞癌表现与同分期、同分级的子宫内膜样腺癌无明显差异。

子宫乳头状浆液性癌

在 1982 年 Hendrickson 及其同事描述,子宫乳头状浆液性癌(UPSC)占Ⅰ期子宫内膜癌的 5%~10%,其特征是为乳头状结构扩张,伴纤维血管基质、明显的细胞异型性、怪异的细胞核和广泛的核多形性(图 103-1)[44,45]。这些特征可提示卵巢的乳头状浆液性囊腺癌。病变是高度致命的,通常在诊断时发现深肌层浸润,在临床早期患者中通常出现子宫外疾病,当疾病扩散到子宫外时几乎无法治愈[45~48]。

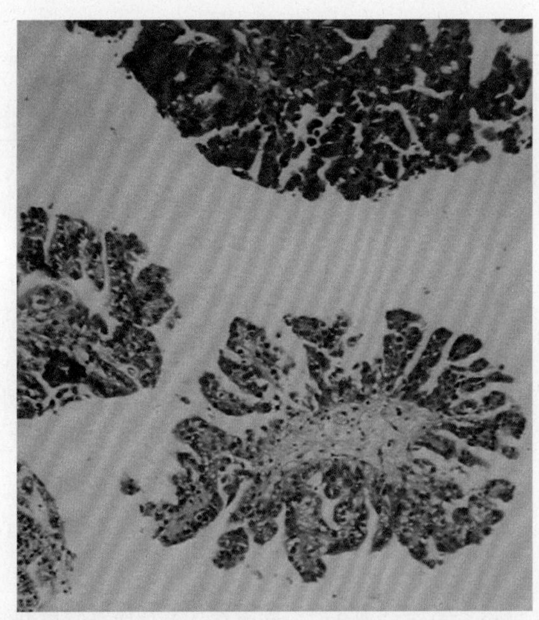

图 103-1　子宫乳头状浆液性癌。宽的茎支持乳头状叶，看起来像乳头状卵巢癌。由西奈山医学院医学博士 Diane Deligdisch 提供。CD-ROM 上提供了该图的四色版本。国际妇产科联合会（FIGO），Unio Internationale Contre Cancrum（UICC）和美国癌症联合委员会（AJCC）命名

子宫内膜乳头状腺癌

子宫内膜乳头状腺癌由于其不同的表现，必须与 UPSC 区分开来。组织学上，它们通常是分化良好的子宫内膜样腺癌，由非常细长的乳突，有序的肿瘤上皮细胞，少量有丝分裂和比 UPSC 更少的细胞病变组成。Chen 和同事详细描述了这两组之间的区别[49]。具有乳头状特征的子宫内膜癌与子宫内膜样腺癌的行为相同。

透明细胞癌

Kurman 和 Scully 详细描述了透明细胞癌[50]。在组织学上，虽然有多种模式，但是细胞质清晰的多边形或扁平细胞的呈现占细胞的一半以上。该类型约占子宫内膜癌的 6%，在老年女性中更常发生。5 年总生存率约为 40%[51]，但这可能是患者年龄偏大以及透明细胞癌通常在癌症期别较晚的患者中发现的结果。当肿瘤根据普遍的细胞类型划分到不同的类别时，透明细胞通常出现在组织学混合物中，并且它们的存在通常会使预后较差[52]。

基因组改变

癌症基因组阿特拉斯计划（TCGA）最近提供了子宫内膜样和子宫内膜癌中 DNA，RNA 和蛋白质改变的综合图谱[53]。在 TCGA 几十年的研究中，子宫内膜癌的发病机制涉及单个基因和蛋白质。子宫内膜癌。基于这些分子改变和临床特征，子宫内膜癌可分为Ⅰ型和Ⅱ型（表 103-1）。Ⅰ型肿瘤包括低至中等级的子宫内膜样肿瘤，表现出高雌激素和孕激素受体（PR）阳性和 PTEN 突变。Ⅱ型肿瘤包括高级别子宫内膜样和浆液性组织，其特征是 *TP53* 的高突变率。这种双重分类虽然过于简化，但仍具有一定的临床用途。

PI3K 通路是子宫内膜癌中最常见的失调通路，在多个关键成员中可见突变。PTEN（10 号染色体上缺失的磷酸盐和张力蛋白同源物）的丢失存在于子宫内膜样癌[54] 75%～85% 的肿瘤中，并导致 PI3K 途径的无对抗激活。突变是 PTEN 缺失的主要原因，可能发生在子宫内膜癌变的早期。然而，包括基因甲基化和蛋白质去稳定化的其他机制也可能导致 PTEN 丧失。在 PI3K 途径的其他成分也有突变，包括 PIK3CA、PIK3R1 和 AKT[55]。mTOR 是 PI3K 通路的关键下游效应器，它刺激蛋白质合成并进入细胞周期的 G1 期。针对 mTOR、AKT 和 PIK3CA 的疗法目前正在晚期和复发性子宫内膜癌患者中进行测试。

Ras/Raf/MEK/ERK 通路在子宫内膜癌中也经常发生失调。*K-ras* 基因突变在 18%～20%的子宫内膜样癌中发生。FGFR2 受体酪氨酸激酶的突变发生在大约 12%的子宫内膜样癌中，与 *K-ras* 突变的肿瘤不同时发生。在早期子宫内膜样癌患者中，*K-ras* 突变与预后更佳相关，FGFR2 突变与预后更差相关[56]。针对 FGFR2 的治疗效果有限[57]。针对 Ras/Raf/MEK/ERK 通路的治疗目前正在与 PI3K 通路抑制剂联合研究。ARID1A 已被证明在大约 25%的低级别和 44%的高级别子宫内膜样癌中发生突变[58]。WNT 通路是子宫内膜样癌中另一种重要的失调通路，其中 *β-catenin* 或 *CTNNB1* 突变发生在 10%～28% 的病例[59]。

微卫星不稳定性发生约占 35% 的子宫内膜样癌中[56]。MSI 表型主要来自 MLH1 通过启动子甲基化的体细胞沉默。在少数病例中，MSI 由 Lynch 综合征基因中的种系突变引起，包括 *MLH1*、*MSH2*、*MSH6* 或 *PMS2*。尚未发现 MSI 状态在子宫内膜子宫内膜癌患者中具有预后意义[43,60～63]。

TP53 突变发生在大多数浆液性癌症中。除突变外，蛋白质的稳定也可导致 *p53* 过表达。与高级别浆液性卵巢癌相似，*TP53* 突变发生在子宫浆液性癌症的发病机制的较早发生。子宫浆液性癌症中报道的其他改变包括 *PPP2R1A* 的突变，*ERBB2* 或 *Her2/neu* 的扩增和过表达，*FBXW7* 的突变和细胞周期蛋白的过度表达。TCGA 不是通过单基因方法，而是对子宫内膜样和浆液性子宫内膜癌进行了大规模的整合基因组分析[53]。基于体细胞突变，拷贝数改变和微卫星不稳定性，定义了四种子宫内膜癌分子亚型状态。这四组是：①POLE 超突变；②超突变/微卫星不稳定；③拷贝数低/微卫星稳定；④拷贝数高（浆液样）。第一组称为 POLE“超突变”肿瘤，包括具有子宫内膜样组织学的临床上最好的肿瘤。POLE 是指 DNA 聚合酶 epsilon，其涉及 DNA 复制并且在该类别的肿瘤中具有许多热点突变。POLE 亚型肿瘤中的拷贝数异常很少，但突变数量很多。*PTEN*、*PIK3R1*、*PIK3CA* 和 *KRAS* 的突变很常见。第二组称为 MSI“高突变”肿瘤，包括子宫内膜样肿瘤，由于 MLH1 启动子甲基化导致微卫星不稳定，几乎没有拷贝数异常，突变率低于“超突变”POLE 组但高于拷贝数低/MSS 组。KRAS 和 PTEN 的突变很常见。第三组是具有 PTEN 和 PIK3CA 突变的拷贝数低/MSS 组，但其特征在于频繁的 β 连环蛋白突变。第四组是拷贝数高（浆液样）肿瘤，具有广泛的拷贝数异常。除大多数浆液性肿瘤外，大约 1/4 的 3 级分化的子宫内膜样癌属于此类。需要验证这四种亚型，并确定其临床效用。另一种基于 TCGA

基因表达数据的子宫内膜样癌分类也被提出。在这种分类中，低级别子宫内膜样肿瘤中β连环蛋白突变的存在与预后不良有关[64]。我们的最终目标是将已知的临床和病理特征与分子数据相结合，以开发有用的分类以便更好地指导患者治疗。

诊断

子宫内膜腺癌患者的中位年龄为61岁，60～70岁中患病率最高。只有5%的人在40岁之前发展为腺癌，这些通常是先前讨论过的具有异常综合征的女性。80%的患者是绝经后的女性。至少75%的患者出现不规则或绝经后出血的症状，并且在诊断时，75%的患者疾病局限于子宫。因此，显而易见的是，不规则出血显然是一个关键的症状，通过组织学检查可证实，通过相对简单的治疗使其多数可治愈。

传统的诊断技术是子宫的分段诊刮，需要仔细取样子宫内膜腔和子宫颈管。这曾经是医院手术室的程序，现在作为门诊程序进行，准确率超过95%[65,66]。患者在医院通常需要全身麻醉，这是由于疼痛阈值非常低，宫颈管狭窄或并发其他并发疾病。

通过直接观察或视频摄像机放大，宫腔镜检查可以直接评估子宫内膜腔的形貌，可以进行更具选择性的取样，并确保不会遗漏任何隐匿性病变。许多人保留这种手术作为正式扩张和麻醉下刮除的辅助手段。但是，应该谨慎行事，因为在文献中已经描述了宫腔镜传播恶性细胞的报道[67,68]。

影像

无创射线照相成像技术，如磁共振成像[69]和超声检查[70]，对于筛查而言并不具有成本效益。对于诊断和记录复发，这些技术以及CT扫描和PET扫描可以达到80%以上的准确率[42,71~76]。

分期

从历史上看，子宫内膜癌分期是一种临床分期，基于体格检查，无创射线照相检查和子宫腔深度的测量。1988年，国际妇产科联合会(FIGO)介绍了GOG 33研究后对子宫内膜癌患者进行手术分期的要求，该研究表明，临床Ⅰ期的843名患者中有9.6%在综合手术分期中有淋巴结转移[77~80]。

2009年，FIGO更新了子宫内膜癌的手术分期分类，如表103-2所示[41]。此外，2009年子宫癌肉瘤将继续使用2009FIGO子宫内膜癌分期，并对平滑肌肉瘤、子宫内膜间质肉瘤和子宫腺肉瘤开发了新的特异性分期分类(表103-3)。

手术分期包括全子宫切除术，双侧输卵管卵巢切除术和盆腔冲洗液的细胞学检查。盆腔和腹主动脉旁淋巴结取样。对于那些非高分化，且浸润深于浅肌层的患者是首选方式。传统的手术方式是开腹手术(通常通过垂直中线切口)，微创技术越来越多地融入前沿，或是机器人辅助腹腔镜技术相结合[82]。已经有研究评估了前哨淋巴结识别的作用，通过比色和荧光成像识别前哨淋巴结，从而将广泛淋巴结清扫术的影响降到最低[83,84]。

最初，子宫内膜癌手术分期系统的采用引起了争议，包括如何构成合适的分期过程，哪些患者应该进行手术分期，广泛的手术分期或淋巴结切除术是否有治疗价值。

表103-3 子宫内膜癌分期

TNM分类	FIGO[a]分期	定义
原发肿瘤(T)		
Tx		原发肿瘤无法评估
T0		没有原发肿瘤证据
Tis[b]		原位癌(浸润前癌)
T1	Ⅰ	肿瘤局限于子宫体
T1a	ⅠA	肿瘤局限于子宫内膜或浸润深度<1/2肌层
T1b	ⅠB	肿瘤浸润深度≥1/2肌层
T2	Ⅱ	肿瘤侵犯宫颈间质，但无宫体外蔓延[c]
T3a	ⅢA	肿瘤累及子宫体浆膜层和/或附件(直接侵犯或转移)[d]
T3b	ⅢB	阴道受累(直接侵犯或转移)和/或宫旁受累[d]
	ⅢC	肿瘤转移至盆腔和/或腹主动脉旁淋巴结[d]
T4	ⅣA	肿瘤侵及膀胱和/或直肠黏膜(泡状水肿不能诊断为T4)
区域淋巴结(N)		
Nx		区域淋巴结无法评估
N0		没有区域淋巴结转移
N1	ⅢC1	肿瘤转移至盆腔淋巴结(盆腔淋巴结阳性)
N2	ⅢC2	肿瘤转移至腹主动脉旁淋巴结，有/无盆腔淋巴结转移
远处转移(M)		
M0		没有远处转移
M1	ⅣB	远处转移(包括腹股沟淋巴转移，腹腔内转移，或肺、肝、骨转移；不包括腹主动脉旁淋巴结转移、阴道转移、盆腔浆膜面或附件转移)

[a] 包括G1，G2，或G3。
[b] FIGO不再包括0期(Tis)。
[c] 宫颈腺体受累应视为Ⅰ期，而非Ⅱ期。
[d] 细胞学阳性需单独报告，但不影响分期。
摘自 Data from Pecorelli 2009[41] and Edge 2010[81]。

预后因素

在GOG组[77,78]进行的大型前瞻性手术病理分期研究中，最初诊断子宫外肿瘤播散和最终身存方面已经确定了几个因素。手术分期和年龄是非常重要的预后特征，在各种分析报告中都保持其重要性。

组织学类型

80%～95%的子宫内膜癌为典型的子宫内膜样腺癌，其余为一系列预后较差的组织学类型。包括浆液性乳头状腺癌、透明细胞癌、未分化癌和鳞癌。这些细胞类型与其他已知的预后因素无关，本身预后不良（表 103-1）[85]。

肿瘤分级

在经典的子宫内膜样腺癌中，肿瘤分级是一个非常重要的独立的预后因素（表 103-4）。此外，大量研究表明，总体来说分化程度较差的肿瘤更有可能与其他不良预后因素相关，包括深肌层浸润、血管侵犯和肿瘤分期的增加[80,86,87]。Salvesen 和他的同事表明，核形态的分级比主观的组织学分级更能预测预后[88]。

表 103-4　组织病理学：分化程度

G1	非鳞状或实体生长方式≤5%
G2	非鳞状或实体生长方式 6%～50%
G3	非鳞状或实体生长方式≥50%

肌层浸润

肌层浸润深度是Ⅰ期子宫内膜癌预后的一个非常重要的独立预后因素。肌层浸润深度越深，肿瘤复发和死亡的可能性越大[80,86,89]。虽然肿瘤浸润肌层深度的增加与肿瘤分级的增加相关，但肌层浸润深度是一个更重要的预后因素，可以预测在手术分期过程中发现的子宫外肿瘤的存在[77]。然而，无论肿瘤分级如何，局限于子宫内膜的患者仅有 1%出现子宫外肿瘤侵犯。而对于深肌层浸润者，盆腔淋巴结转移的发生率上升到 25%，腹主动脉旁淋巴结转移的发生率上升到 17%[77]。DiSaia 及其同事发现，仅子宫内膜受累的患者复发率为 8%，而浅表或中层肌层受侵的患复发率为 12%，而外 1/3 肌层受侵的患者复发率为 46%[89]。

毛细淋巴管间隙侵犯

血管间隙浸润是复发的重要危险因素，但其重要程度不如组织学分级和肌层浸润深度重要。大约 15%的子宫内膜腺癌具有毛细血管间隙侵犯，并且提高 5 倍的淋巴结转移概率，与盆腔淋巴结阳性（27%）和腹主动脉旁淋巴结受累（19%）相关[77,90]。

腹腔细胞学阳性

在 2009 年 FIGO 分期修订中，腹水细胞学阳性已不作为影响分期的因素[41]。但腹腔冲洗液细胞学阳性与复发风险增加有关[80]。约有 15%的患者腹水细胞学检查呈阳性[80]，这通常与其他不良预后因素有关，如高级别或深肌层穿浸润。因此，腹水细胞学阳性也与盆腔淋巴结转移（25%）和腹主动脉旁淋巴结转移（19%）的风险增加相关。在阐述腹水细胞学的独立预后因素意义方面，文献中的观点和数据存在冲突。大约 5%的腹水细胞学检查阳性的患者没有子宫外肿瘤的证据[77]，但约 1/3 的子宫外肿瘤患者的细胞学检查阳性。在一篇综述中，Wethington 根据低风险的子宫肿瘤特征（1～2 级，<50%浸润深度，无淋巴血管间隙浸润）与腹水细胞学阳性将患者分组。本组中，11%的病例细胞学检查呈阳性，复发率为 4%。高风险特征加上细胞学检查阳性的患者有 32%的复发风险[91]。

种族

刘及同事回顾了 1990—1993 年间 219 例子宫内膜癌患者的治疗模式、危险因素和生存率[92]。在本研究中，黑人女性与白人女性相比，组织学分级不良（38% vs 12%）、晚期疾病（51% vs 19%）、分化差（49% vs 18%）和存活率差的发生率更高。

激素受体状态

细胞质 ER-和 PR-结合蛋白（雌激素受体结合蛋白与孕激素受体结合蛋白）的存在与数量与更好的组织学分化[93]、好的组织学亚型和治疗反应相关[94~96]。与 ER 和 PR 结合的配体在高分化的病变中水平较高，相反在 G3 病变和非子宫内膜样癌中明显较低[96]。受体表达的改变、受体的组装和激活、反应要素的识别和/或受体的降解都是激素结合丧失的可能原因。此外，最近的证据表明，启动子位点高甲基化可能是 ER 丢失的部分原因[97]。同样，也有关于 PR-alpha（PRA）和 PR-beta（PRB）差异表达的报道[98]。PRA 似乎下调了 ER 的作用，而 PRB 是黄体酮反应基因的主要激活因子，两者中的任何一个缺失都会在理论上导致雌激素效应无对抗。在临床上，子宫内膜癌样本中配体与 ER、PR 或两者相互作用水平的降低与疾病的复发和死亡显著相关（$P<0.01$）[95,96]。

原发疾病的治疗

手术

初始的手术分期过程也是标准的治疗程序，参见图 103-2。当子宫外和腹膜后淋巴结有病变时，尽管缺乏临床试验验证其疗效，但我们有理由认为，积极的肿瘤细胞减灭术可能有助于减轻肿瘤负担。

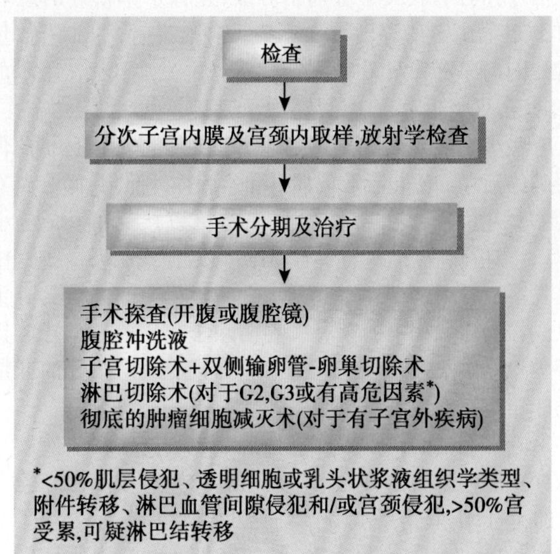

图 103-2　子宫内膜癌的手术治疗

有些情况下，在开腹分期手术中，发现宫颈或宫旁侵犯，并进行根治性(Wertheim)子宫切除术，伴盆腔和主动脉淋巴结清扫术，以便清除所有疾病。然而，术后增加体外放疗RT在很大程度上取消了此类手术的常规进行[99]。复发性疾病的手术治疗通常局限于那些有肠道或尿路梗阻症状或为局部孤立性复发或孤立的肺转移患者，这些患者对细胞毒性治疗或激素治疗没有反应。对于这类患者，手术可能有助于纠正功能缺陷或切除孤立复发病灶或耐药的转移性病灶。

经过几年的辩论和讨论，微创技术已被纳入子宫内膜癌的一个标准治疗方式[100]。用于子宫内膜癌早期治疗的技术包括腹腔镜辅助阴式子宫切除术(LAVH)[101~105]，全腹腔镜子宫切除术(TLH)[106~108]，和机器人子宫切除术[82]，伴盆腔和腹主动脉旁淋巴结清扫术。微创分期技术包括对淋巴结的经腹膜和腹膜外评估，可在子宫切除术时或在术后对分期不完全的患者进行重新手术分期。机器人手术可能代表着微创手术的下一步骤。自2005年FDA批准用于子宫切除和子宫肌瘤切除手术以来，机器人手术在妇科肿瘤领域的应用越来越多[82,109~113]。

前哨淋巴结(SLN)显像在子宫内膜癌分期中的作用目前正在评估中，但是还没有随机试验报告。根据目前NCCN的指导方针，当影像学检查未发现转移灶，且探查未发现明显疾病时，可考虑在手术分期时使用SLN(第3类)。外科医生的专业知识和对技术细节的关注是至关重要的[83,84,114]。

放射治疗(RT)

虽然手术是大多数子宫内膜癌患者的主要治疗方法，但很明显，放射治疗是治疗子宫内膜癌的第二最有效方法。

对无法手术患者进行精确放疗

现代外科技术和改进的术后护理减少了无法进行手术的患者的数量。然而，子宫内膜癌是一种常见的老年人疾病(65岁以上)，他们经常是肥胖的，有时患糖尿病或伴随其他疾病，手术并不总是可行的。一些相对较大的研究表明，无法手术时，盆腔放疗是子宫内膜癌的有效治疗方法[115~119]。

治疗存活率取决于肿瘤的分级，正像手术治疗的患者一样，1级肿瘤患者的存活率高于3级肿瘤患者[115]。当数量的患者死因与原发肿瘤无关[119]。未死于并发症且无法手术的患者，治疗后5年生存率中位数接近可手术的患者[119]。

有些小子宫的患者可能只需要腔内照射就可以治愈，但通常明确的治疗方法包括腔内照射和盆腔体外照射，因为具有更有利的辐射剂量。并发症发生率是可以接受的(通常小于10%)。在精确放疗后，与手术相比，失败模式主要由子宫中央型复发。这一观察结果对Ⅱ期患者治疗策略的制订具有重要意义。在治疗过程中的某一时刻摘除子宫比单独放疗能提供更好的总体中央控制。三组文献显示接受放射治疗的Ⅱ期患者的5年生存率约为50%[99,115,120,121]。

Kucera和他的同事报告了他们在228例患者中使用高剂量铱-192腔内近距离放射治疗而没有外照射放疗的经验[122]。5年的总生存率为59.7%。临床IA期患者5年生存率为88.6%，10年生存率为82.7%，与IB期患者5年的总生存率80.2%、10年生存率63.4%相比有显著性差异。其他也报道了高剂量率的近距离放射治疗，无论是否有外照射放疗[123,124]，美国近距离放射治疗协会(American brachytherapy Society)也发表了对此的指南和建议[124,125]。

Ⅰ期子宫内膜癌的辅助治疗

目前建议，Ⅰ期患者给予术后放疗取决于子宫内膜内原发肿瘤的组织学特征因素所定义的预后。大量的分期研究已经确定，上述几个因素预测了临床隐匿性子宫外疾病的存在[80]。

尽管具有高危复发因素的患者(如2~3级肿瘤，>50%的子宫肌层的浸润，通常术后需要辅助放疗，但目前仅有一个随机试验说明辅助放疗对于术后患者的好处(GOG-99)[126]。有三个随机临床试验说明患者在不完全手术分期后辅助放疗的好处。(Aalders[86]、Portec-1[127]和Portec-2[128])

GOG-99研究分层风险并验证了盆腔放疗(RT)可改善中高危险(HIR)组的无复发生存期。根据GOG 33，将HIR亚型患者(5年复发率增加25%)定义为[1]：中低分化肿瘤、淋巴血管浸润、外1/3肌层受侵[2]，年龄50岁或以上，并有上述任两项危险因素；或年龄不少于70岁[3]，并有任意上述风险因素的患者。治疗差异在HIR亚组中尤为明显(2年累计的复发率NAT和RT的分别为26%和6%；RH=0.42)。总的来说，放疗对盆腔和阴道复发有实质性影响(NAT有18例，RT有3例)[126]，但总生存率没有显著差异。

穹窿放疗

从理论上讲，如果患者接受了彻底手术分期，最好是进行双侧盆腔和低位腹主动脉旁淋巴结切除术，在没有淋巴结转移的情况下，盆腔侧壁复发的风险较低。其他未在手术中发现的隐匿性盆腔侧壁疾病，如宫旁或宫旁淋巴结的淋巴管，很少发生也不太可能成为复发来源。对于这些患者来说，盆腔内可能复发的主要部位是阴道穹窿，它可以通过近距离放射治疗减少发生率[129,130]。有几项回顾性研究表明，在高危患者(IB期、3级和IC期)已行盆腔淋巴结切除术后，在没有淋巴结转移的情况下，不做放疗[131,132]或仅行阴道穹窿的近距离放射治疗，盆腔复发率均很低[130,133~137]。此外PORTEC-2研究中有潜在的数据支持这一假设，在未分期且为HIR亚型的患者中，单独行阴道近距离放射治疗盆腔复发率较低，PORTEC研究中HIR特征定义(中度危险因素为外二分之一肌层受侵，3级肿瘤，或大于60岁；但除外深肌层受侵的3级肿瘤，而HIR患者被认为具有三种因素的两种)。中位随访45个月，5年阴道复发率仅做近距离放疗者为1.8%，体外放疗组为1.6%。淋巴结复发率有显著性差异，单纯近距离放疗组为3.8%，体外放疗组为0.5%。两组的远处转移、无病生存和总生存相似[128]。

Ⅲ期

2009年FIGO的子宫内膜癌的手术分期包括转移到盆腔和/或腹主动脉旁淋巴结的患者为ⅢC期。目前分期的分类涵盖了广泛范围的预后组，这些预后组在标准手术后接受或不接受辅助盆腔放疗出现了极不相同的预后。遗憾的是，许多发表文献没有区分包括镜下转移至附件的患者(ⅢA期)、腹水阳性患者(ⅢA期)，和盆腔侧壁肿瘤患者(ⅢA期或ⅢC期)的差别，导致生存数据差异很大。

Ⅲ期患者的治疗建议必须根据个人情况而定。对于那些已经完成明确手术分期但没有卵巢以外疾病证据的患者，应考虑在术后辅助盆腔体外放疗，尽管对于没有其他危险因素的患者，附件的镜下浸润的重要性尚不清楚。对于那些手术分期明确，有盆腔淋巴结转移，但未累及腹主动脉旁淋巴结的患者，术后应给予局限于盆腔的辅助体外放疗。接受了 45～50Gy 腹主动脉旁淋巴结外照射放疗的患者的无病生存率在 35%到 60%之间，通常伴有盆腔体外放疗。肉眼可见的腹主动脉旁淋巴结转移，若不先行完全的肿瘤细胞减灭术，几乎是无法治愈的[65,70,80,138～148]。来自约翰·霍普金斯医院的回顾性数据表明，在ⅢC 期子宫内膜癌患者中，除了定向放射治疗外，完整切除肉眼可见的转移淋巴结并给予辅助化疗均与提高生存率相关（图 103-3）[149]。部分Ⅲ期子宫内膜癌患者可能需要行细胞毒性化疗，无论是否行放疗，目前有两项Ⅲ期临床试验正在评估这一概念（GOG 258 和 Portec 3）。

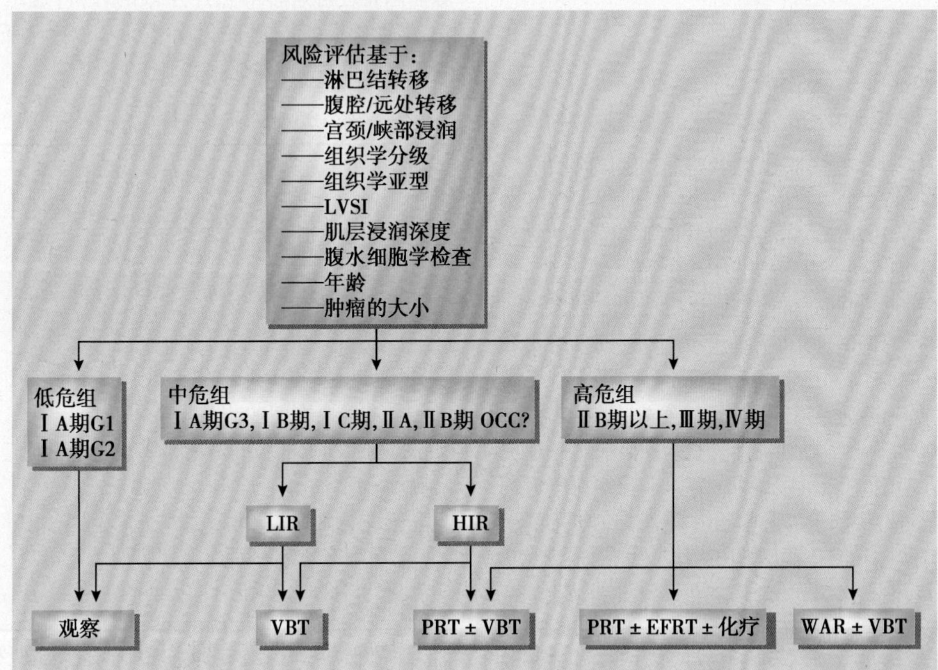

图 103-3　子宫内膜癌术后处理。EFRT，延伸野放射治疗；PRT，盆腔放疗；VBT，阴道近距离放射治疗；WAR，全腹放疗；LIR，中低危风险；HIR，中高危风险。根据 GOG99 定义：年龄<50、50～70、>70；LVSI，脉管间隙侵犯，外 1/3 肌层受侵，2～3 级肿瘤

早期高危疾病的辅助化疗

Stringer 等[150]研究了 31 例高危Ⅰ期子宫内膜癌患者和 2 例隐匿Ⅱ期子宫内膜癌患者。术后每 4 周分别给予顺铂 $50mg/m^2$，多柔比星 $50mg/m^2$，环磷酰胺 $500mg/m^2$（CAP）治疗，共 6 个周期。2 年无进展间隔率为 79%，2 年生存率为 83%。45 个月随访时患者的中位生存时间没有达到。这些结果被认为优于来自同一机构的历史对照。

GOG 将临床高危的Ⅰ期和Ⅱ期内膜癌术后患者随机分为两组，均行全盆腔照射，分别给予或不给予多柔比星，PFI 和 OS 无差异[151]。

日本的 GOG 设计试验旨在解决在 IC 至Ⅲ期 CAP 化疗相对于 WPRT 的相对疗效。尽管在整个队列中 PFS 和 OS 没有差异，但对 120 例 HIR 患者的亚组分析显示 PFR 和 OS 均有改善[152]。

GOG249 是一项Ⅲ期试验，针对高危但局限于子宫的内膜癌患者进行阴道断端近距离化疗，然后进行三个周期的紫杉醇/卡铂（TC）化疗对比体外放疗的研究。SGO 2014 的初步结果显示，两组患者的生存结果没有显著差异。

Kelly 等在一项对 74 例Ⅰ期子宫内膜浆液性乳头状腺癌（UPSC）患者的研究中发现，所有有残留病变（包括局限于子宫内膜的病变）的患者在辅助铂类化疗后，PRI 和 OS 均有所改善。接受阴道近距离放射治疗的患者无阴道复发[45,153]。由于透明细胞癌的表现与 UPSC 相似，尽管缺乏相关数据，但仍应采用类似的方式进行 TC 化疗和阴道近距离放疗[45,52]。

复发疾病的治疗

放疗

既往没有接受过放疗而出现局部阴道复发的患者，其放疗治愈率可达 80%。如果出现盆腔外复发的患者，则需要进行系统治疗。术后已行辅助盆腔放疗的患者中，除了存在孤立的盆腔中央型病灶，复发时可能应用间质治疗的作用。其他患者系统治疗可能是适用的。对于有其他部位疾病或骨、脑或淋巴结转移的患者，短期的姑息性放射治疗可能有助于缓解疾病症状。同样，对于罕见的Ⅳ期疾病患者（约占发病时的 3%），可以采用姑息性放射治疗[154]。

手术

与卵巢癌不同的是,关于复发性子宫内膜癌中行再次肿瘤细胞减灭术的作用知之甚少[155]。在一份来自意大利的文献中,20名复发的子宫内膜腺癌患者接受了最大限度的肿瘤细胞减灭术[156]。65%的患者肿瘤完全切除。无肿瘤残留与有肿瘤残留的妇女相比,无进展生存和总生存期明显增加;但是在这组患者中有10%的围术期死亡率。在一项对31例患者的四所机构的回顾性分析中研究了盆腔廓清术的作用[157]。20例患者均曾接受盆腔照射,均有手术治疗目的。5年无病生存率为45%。

细胞毒性化疗

1980年以前很少对子宫内膜癌患者进行细胞毒性化疗。Donovan在他1974年的文献中报告了126名患者接受了16种不同药物的治疗[158]。1977年,Muggia及其同事对11例复发性子宫内膜癌患者进行治疗,应用多柔比星(多柔比星,37.5mg/m^2)与环磷酰胺(500mg/m^2)静脉注射(IV),每21天1次,5个患者有效[159]。GOG研究了单药多柔比星,剂量率为每3周60mg/m^{2}静脉注射,43例患者的反应率为37%[160]。虽然最常见的不良反应是在造血系统,心脏毒性发生率12%,并有一个接受了超过500mg/m^{2}因心脏毒性死亡的患者。这项研究很重要,因为它明确地确立了多柔比星作为单一药物在子宫内膜癌化疗中的价值。GOG和东部肿瘤合作小组(ECOG)的研究表明,添加环磷酰胺并没有获益(表103-5)[175,176]。

表 103-5 子宫内膜癌联合化疗方案的随机试验

作者	年份	药物	可评估人数	RR/%	中位PFS/月	中位OS/月
Thigpen[176]	1994	A	132	22	3.2	6.7
		AC	144	30	3.9	7.3
Thigpen[176]	2004	A	150	25	3.8	9.2
		AP	131	42*	5.7*	9.0
Aapro[167]	2003	A	87	17	7.0	7.0
		AP	90	43*	8.0	9.0*
Gallion[179]	2003	AP标准	169	46	6.5	11.2
		AP昼夜	173	49	5.9	13.2
Fleming[180]	2004	AP	157	40	7.2	12.6
		AT	160	43	6.0	13.6
Fleming[181]	2004	AP	129	34	5.3	12.3
		TAP	134	57*	8.3*	15.3*

PFS,无进展生存;RR,反应率,完全缓解(CR)+部分缓解(PR);C,环磷酰胺;A,多柔比星(多柔比星);P,顺铂;F,五氟尿嘧啶;T,紫杉醇。

*有显著性差异。

GOG发现对严重患者先行单独使用顺铂并无疗效[177];但Trope观察到对11例化疗初治患者给予顺铂50mg/m^{2}化疗,4例有效(36%)[178]。顺铂联合多柔比星治疗晚期或复发性子宫内膜癌的有效率为33%~80%,这取决于之前接受化疗或放疗的患者比例[146,147]。

如果只选择参与的研究中能达到20%反应率的药物,且研究入组至少20名患者,则该名单很小(表103-6)。紫杉醇是治疗晚期或复发性子宫内膜腺癌的有效药物。GOG进行了紫杉醇应用于晚期或复发性子宫内膜腺癌患者的研究[144]。在28例可评估的患者中,观察到4例完全缓解和6例部分缓解,总体反应率为35.7%。Lissoni和他的同事对19例晚期子宫内膜腺癌患者进行紫杉醇化疗疗效的评价,这组患者之前应用顺铂、多柔比星、环磷酰胺化疗[145]。2例完全缓解和5例部分缓解,总体反应率为37%。

表 103-6 子宫内膜癌的单药细胞毒性化疗

药物	文献	人数	之前治疗	CR+PR数量	/%
紫杉醇	144	28	无	4+6	36
紫杉醇	145	19	是	2+5	37
顺铂	161,162	75	无	3+38	28
卡铂	163~165	76	无	5+18	28
多柔比星	160,166,167	280	无	31+49	29
表柔比星	168	27	无	2+5	26
氟尿嘧啶	169	34	NS	7	21
六甲蜜胺	170	30	无	10	33
多西他赛	171	35	无	3+4	21
托泊替康	172,173	42	无	3+5	20

注:报告的系列至少有20名患者,反应率至少为20%。

HMM=六甲蜜胺。

CR=完全缓解,PR=部分缓解,NS=未提及。

数据来源Muss[174],Thigpen[166]。

关于联合化疗的最佳信息来自表103-5所列的随机Ⅲ期试验。包括激素治疗的随机试验列于表103-7。

表 103-7 子宫内膜癌联合化疗+激素治疗的随机试验

作者	年份	药物	可评估人数	RR/%
Horton[182]	1982	CA+MA	55	27
		CAF+MA	56	16
Cohen[183]	1984	F-Mel+MA	126	38
		CAF+MA	131	36
Ayoub[184]	1998	CAF	20	15
		CAF+MPA/TAM	23	43*
Cornelison[185]	1995	APE+MA	50	54
		F-Mel+MPA	50	48

RR,反应率,完全缓解(CR)+部分缓解(PR);C,环磷酰胺;A,多柔比星(多柔比星);P,顺铂;F,五氟尿嘧啶;Mel,美法仑;MA,醋酸甲地黄体酮;MPA,醋酸甲羟黄体酮;TAM,他莫昔芬。

*有显著性差异。

表 103-5 列出了比较单一药物与一种或两种不同组合药物的随机试验。Van Wijk 和他的同事在欧洲癌症研究和治疗组织（EORTC）的研究中发现，多柔比星和顺铂联合化疗的生存率显著提高为 43%，而单药多柔比星的有效率为 17%（$P<0.001$）[148]。GOGw 则发现当多柔比星和顺铂按昼夜节律给药时，与标准给药方式相比，并无差异[179]。

GOG 还进行了一项Ⅲ期研究，对比多柔比星联合顺铂与多柔比星联合 24h 紫杉醇治疗原发Ⅲ期、Ⅳ期或复发性子宫内膜癌的疗效。本研究发现反应率、无进展生存期和总生存期两者并无差异[180]。另一组 GOG 的Ⅲ期前瞻性随机研究（GOG177）比较了标准多柔比星（$60mg/m^2$）联合顺铂（$50mg/m^2$），即 AP 方案与 TAP 方案（紫杉醇 $160mg/m^2$，每 3h 一次）、多柔比星（$45mg/m^2$）和顺铂（$50mg/m^2$）的疗效差异[181]。266 名患者被随机分组，结果显示 TAP 的反应率有显著提高（57% vs 34%；$P<0.01$），无进展生存期（中位生存期 8.3 个月 vs 5.3 个月；$P<0.01$）总生存期（中位 15.3 个月 vs 12.3 个月；$P=0.037$）。但接受 TAP 化疗的患者神经毒性更严重，有 12% 的 3 级和 27% 的 2 级周围神经病变。

GOG 随访了 GOG 209 方案，该方案将晚期（ⅣB 期）或复发性疾病患者随机分配应用 TAP 或 TC（紫杉醇和卡铂）方案化疗。2012 年的试验数据显示了类似的抗肿瘤疗效，但毒性和耐受性方面，TC 方案优于 TAP 方案[186]。

在Ⅲ期至ⅣA 期已行肿瘤细胞减灭术（残存肿瘤<2cm）的患者中，一项随机的Ⅲ期试验，GOG 122 方案表明与全腹放疗组比较，使用多柔比星（$60mg/m^2$）联合顺铂（$50mg/m^2$）化疗有较好的无进展生存期（0.71；95% CI：0.55～0.91；$P<0.01$），总生存率（0.68；95%CI：=0.52～0.89；$P<0.01$）[187]。

激素治疗

Kelly 和 Baker 在 1961 年描述了应用激素治疗 21 名患者中有 6 个客观缓解，持续时间从 9 个月到 4.5 年[188]。从那时起，许多报道描述了各种孕激素治疗：最常见的 17-羟黄体酮己酸酯，甲羟黄体酮醋酸酯（MPA），和黄体酮醋酸酯（MA）。Reifenstein 应用 113 名临床研究人员，对 992 例应用羟黄体酮己酸酯治疗的患者进行了分析[189]。他详细研究了 314 名患者的记录，发现在 7 周治疗前几乎没有反应，最长缓解出现时间则是至少 12 周的初始治疗之后实现的，对肿瘤分化进行校正后发现，临床反应情况与患者年龄无相关性。Kauppila 回顾了 17 个不同试验中使用 MPA（Provera）、MA 或羟黄体酮己酸酯治疗的 1 068 例患者，发现总有效率为 34%[190]。反应持续时间约 20 个月，平均生存时间约 25 个月。

孕激素治疗的最佳剂量尚未确定，最近 GOG 研究中使用的剂量是基于 Kohorn 和 Thigpen 寻求剂量的研究制订的[191,192]。

没有证据表明低剂量孕激素不同样有效，肠道外用药途径也无优势。因此，为了避免并发症，在特殊情况下选择较低剂量是允许的。Ramirez 和他的同事在回顾文献时发现[193]，大多数高分化子宫内膜腺癌患者，在使用孕激素保守治疗原发性内膜肿瘤（代替子宫切除）时，对孕激素治疗有效（62/81=76%）。当最初疗效没有出现或在有疗效后疾病出现复发（15/62=24%），子宫以外的肿瘤是罕见的。此外，Montz 和他的同事[194]还描述了使用含有黄体酮的宫内节育器来治疗围术期有高风险并发症的 FIGO 期 IA，1 级子宫内膜样癌患者的可行性。

综上所述，孕激素治疗可归纳如下[1]：晚期或复发性子宫内膜癌患者的反应率为 10%～30%，可能与肿瘤受体水平相关[2]；高分化肿瘤反应最好[3]；随着肿瘤级别的增加，PR 水平急剧下降[4]；在 7～12 周的治疗以前都可能不会发生临床疗效[5]；2/3 的患者没有疗效[6]；没有公开的证据表明在辅助模式中使用孕激素有任何获益[7]；根据 GOG 研究，适当的口服剂量为：孕烯醇 160mg/d 或 MPA 200mg/d；然而，低剂量治疗可以个体化；口服黄体酮和含黄体酮的宫内节育器是治疗可选择的早期低级别子宫内膜癌患者的首选方法。

他莫昔芬

除孕激素外，激素治疗已被许多研究人员研究。从乳腺癌的经验推断，研究人员使用他莫昔芬 20～40mg/d 剂量，用于晚期或复发性子宫内膜癌患者。对八项已发表的研究进行回顾中，摩尔和他的同事[195]描述了应用他莫昔芬总体反应率为 22%。正如人们预测的那样，报道的反应率范围很广，从 0 到 53% 不等[196]。Edmonson 和他的同事的报告可以解释这种大范围变化[197]，他们发现对既往无激素治疗的患者他莫昔芬有 21% 的反应率，而对黄体酮治疗失败的患者没有反应。与黄体酮的经验相似，他莫昔芬似乎对低级别肿瘤、受体阳性、没有激素治疗或以前对黄体酮治疗有反应的患者可能有效。

由于孕激素最终下调孕激素受体，而他莫昔芬在靶组织中诱导这些受体，因此这些激素的联合应用的概念已被 GOG 用两种不同的策略加以验证。在 Whitney 及其同事的报告中，58 例复发且或有可测量病灶的晚期子宫内膜癌患者中，枸橼酸他莫昔芬 40mg/d 联合 MPA 200mg/d 的每周交替周期治疗，应答率为 33%（10.3%的完全应答和 23.4%的部分应答），中位无进展间隔 3 个月，中位总生存期 13 个月[198]。在 Fiorica 研究中，56 例复发或有可测量病灶的晚期子宫内膜癌患者交替使用 MA（160mg/d）和枸橼酸他莫昔芬（40mg/d）3 周交替周期，产生 27%的应答率（21.4%的完全应答和 5.4%的部分应答），中位无进展期 2.7 个月，中位总生存期 14.0 个月[199]。

他莫昔芬、黄体酮和化疗的组合也已经过测试。Ayoub 和他的同事研究了 46 例转移性子宫内膜癌患者，随机分配他们接受环磷酰胺、多柔比星（多柔比星）、氟尿嘧啶（CAF）或 CAF+MPA 每日 200mg，持续 3 周之后与他莫昔芬循环使用，他莫昔芬用量 20mg/d，持续 3 周循环[184]。CAF 和 CAF 加激素治疗的客观反应率分别为 15%和 43%（$P=0.05$）。因为在之前引用的研究中孕激素并没有改善化疗的疗效[200]，将这种疗效差异归因于他莫昔芬的加入是合理的。Pinelli 和同事评估了序贯循环激素治疗（MA 和他莫昔芬枸橼酸盐）加单药卡铂的疗效[201]。在 13 例可评估的患者中，4 例完全缓解，6 例部分缓解，总体反应率为 77%。完全应答者的中位无进展间隔时间为 14 个月。所有患者的中位生存期为 11 个月，完全应答者为 33 个月。

其他激素治疗

促性腺激素释放激素类似物已在复发性子宫内膜癌患者的中进行了小规模的Ⅱ期试验测试，反应率从 0% 到 35% 不等[202~204]。芳香化酶抑制剂已经在有限试验中进行了测试。

在 GOG 的一项Ⅱ期试验中，阿那曲唑的反应率为 9%（2 例部分缓解/23 人）[205~207]，而加拿大美国癌症研究所报告中显示来曲唑的有效率为 9.4%（2 例部分缓解/28 例）[208]。

生物疗法

新的分子和生物疗法治疗复发或转移子宫内膜癌有正在评估的临床试验。在一项对 52 名可评估患者进行的Ⅱ期试验中（既往至多两种化疗方案治疗），贝伐珠单抗的反应率为 13.5%，总生存期为 10.5 个月[209]。一项Ⅱ期试验的初步结果显示 mTOR 抑制剂西罗莫司应用于 29 例可评价的化疗无效的复发或转移性子宫内膜癌患者中，5 例出现部分缓解（27%）[210]。一项Ⅱ期试验显示了 mTOR 抑制剂依维莫司联合芳香化酶抑制剂来曲唑治疗复发性子宫内膜癌患者，有 32% 的应答率（$n=35$；9 例完全缓解，2 例部分缓解）[211]。

未来

必须继续努力扩大分子特征的信息，以便更好地确定患者的更有效治疗的可能性。从外科的角度来看，腹腔镜和机器人手术目前被认为是标准技术，但是前哨淋巴结评估的作用还没有完全确定。对于早期疾病和预后差的患者，需要进一步的随机研究来比较放疗与系统治疗的必要。对于晚期或复发患者，必须确定包括生物制剂在内的更好的系统治疗方法。目前美国的治愈率约为 80%，有不良预后特征或复发或转移性疾病的患者必须进入合作试验，以便最大限度地提高生存机会。

（孙阳春 雷呈志 译 孙阳春 校）

参考文献

The complete reference list can be found on the Wiley Companion Digital Edition of this title (see inside front cover for login instructions).

18 Gusberg SB. Precursors of corpus carcinoma, estrogen and adenomatous hyperplasia. *Am J Obstet Gynecol*. 1947;**54**:905–27.

30 Cohen CJ, Rahaman J. Endometrial cancer. Management of high risk and recurrence including the tamoxifen controversy. *Cancer*. 1995;**76**(**10 Suppl**):2044–52.

32 Fisher B, Costantino JP, Wickerham DL, et al. Tamoxifen for prevention of breast cancer: report of the National Surgical Adjuvant Breast and Bowel Project P-1 Study. *J Natl Cancer Inst*. 1998;**90**(**18**):1371–88.

36 Bokhman JV. Two pathogenetic types of endometrial carcinoma. *Gynecol Oncol*. 1983;**15**(**1**):10–7.

40 Kurman RJ, Kaminski PF, Norris HJ. The behavior of endometrial hyperplasia. A long-term study of "untreated" hyperplasia in 170 patients. *Cancer*. 1985;**56**(**2**):403–12.

41 Pecorelli S. Revised FIGO staging for carcinoma of the vulva, cervix, and endometrium. *Int J Gynaecol Obstet*. 2009;**105**(**2**):103–4. Epub 2009/04/16.

43 Tashiro H, Isacson C, Levine R, Kurman RJ, Cho KR, Hedrick L. p53 gene mutations are common in uterine serous carcinoma and occur early in their pathogenesis. *Am J Pathol*. 1997;**150**(**1**):177–85.

44 Hendrickson M, Ross J, Eifel P, Martinez A, Kempson R. Uterine papillary serous carcinoma: a highly malignant form of endometrial adenocarcinoma. *Am J Surg Pathol*. 1982;**6**(**2**):93–108.

45 Boruta DM 2nd, Gehrig PA, Fader AN, Olawaiye AB. Management of women with uterine papillary serous cancer: a Society of Gynecologic Oncology (SGO) review. *Gynecol Oncol*. 2009;**115**(**1**):142–53. Epub 2009/07/14.

50 Kurman RJ, Scully RE. Clear cell carcinoma of the endometrium: an analysis of 21 cases. *Cancer*. 1976;**37**(**2**):872–82.

51 Christopherson WM, Alberhasky RC, Connelly PJ. Glassy cell carcinoma of the endometrium. *Hum Pathol*. 1982;**13**(**5**):418–21.

52 Olawaiye AB, Boruta DM 2nd. Management of women with clear cell endometrial cancer: a Society of Gynecologic Oncology (SGO) review. *Gynecol Oncol*. 2009;**113**(**2**):277–83. Epub 2009/03/03.

53 Cancer Genome Atlas Research N, Kandoth C, Schultz N, et al. Integrated genomic characterization of endometrial carcinoma. *Nature*. 2013;**497**(**7447**):67–73.

54 Djordjevic B, Hennessy BT, Li J, et al. Clinical assessment of PTEN loss in endometrial carcinoma: immunohistochemistry outperforms gene sequencing. *Mod Pathol : an official journal of the United States and Canadian Academy of Pathology, Inc*. 2012;**25**(**5**):699–708.

58 Mao TL, Ardighieri L, Ayhan A, et al. Loss of ARID1A expression correlates with stages of tumor progression in uterine endometrioid carcinoma. *Am J Surg Pathol*. 2013;**37**(**9**):1342–8.

65 Cohen CJ, Gusberg SB, Koffler D. Histologic screening for endometrial cancer. *Gynecol Oncol*. 1974;**2**(**2–3**):279–86.

77 Creasman WT, Morrow CP, Bundy BN, Homesley HD, Graham JE, Heller PB. Surgical pathologic spread patterns of endometrial cancer A Gynecologic Oncology Group Study. *Cancer*. 1987;**60**(**8 Suppl**):2035–41.

80 Morrow CP, Bundy BN, Kurman RJ, et al. Relationship between surgical-pathological risk factors and outcome in clinical stage I and II carcinoma of the endometrium: a Gynecologic Oncology Group study. *Gynecol Oncol*. 1991;**40**(**1**):55–65.

82 Boggess JF, Gehrig PA, Cantrell L, et al. A comparative study of 3 surgical methods for hysterectomy with staging for endometrial cancer: robotic assistance, laparoscopy, laparotomy. *Am J Obstet Gynecol*. 2008;**199**(**4**:360):e1–e9. Epub 2008/10/22.

83 Abu-Rustum NR. Sentinel lymph node mapping for endometrial cancer: a modern approach to surgical staging. *J Natl Compr Canc Netw*. 2014;**12**(**2**):288–97. Epub 2014/03/04.

86 Aalders J, Abeler V, Kolstad P, Onsrud M. Postoperative external irradiation and prognostic parameters in stage I endometrial carcinoma: clinical and histopathologic study of 540 patients. *Obstet Gynecol*. 1980;**56**(**4**):419–27.

91 Wethington SL, Barrena Medel NI, Wright JD, Herzog TJ. Prognostic significance and treatment implications of positive peritoneal cytology in endometrial adenocarcinoma: Unraveling a mystery. *Gynecol Oncol*. 2009;**115**(**1**):18–25. Epub 2009/07/28.

96 Mariani A, Sebo TJ, Webb MJ, et al. Molecular and histopathologic predictors of distant failure in endometrial cancer. *Cancer Detect Prev*. 2003;**27**(**6**):434–41. Epub 2003/12/04.

100 Walker JL, Piedmonte MR, Spirtos NM, et al. Recurrence and survival after random assignment to laparoscopy versus laparotomy for comprehensive surgical staging of uterine cancer: Gynecologic Oncology Group LAP2 Study. *J Clin Oncol*. 2012;**30**(**7**):695–700. Epub 2012/02/01.

106 Obermair A, Manolitsas TP, Leung Y, Hammond IG, McCartney AJ. Total laparoscopic hysterectomy for endometrial cancer: patterns of recurrence and survival. *Gynecol Oncol*. 2004;**92**(**3**):789–93. Epub 2004/02/27.

107 Nezhat F, Yadav J, Rahaman J, Gretz H, Cohen C. Analysis of survival after laparoscopic management of endometrial cancer. *J Minim Invasive Gynecol*. 2008;**15**(**2**):181–7. Epub 2008/03/04.

116 Grigsby PW, Kuske RR, Perez CA, et al. Medically inoperable stage I adenocarcinoma of the endometrium treated with radiotherapy alone. *Int J Radiat Oncol Biol Phys*. 1987;**13**(**4**):483–8.

125 Nag S, Erickson B, Parikh S, Gupta N, Varia M, Glasgow G. The American Brachytherapy Society recommendations for high-dose-rate brachytherapy for carcinoma of the endometrium. *Int J Radiat Oncol Biol Phys*. 2000;**48**(**3**):779–90. Epub 2000/10/06.

126 Keys HM, Roberts JA, Brunetto VL, et al. A phase III trial of surgery with or without adjunctive external pelvic radiation therapy in intermediate risk endometrial adenocarcinoma: a Gynecologic Oncology Group study. *Gynecol Oncol*. 2004;**92**(**3**):744–51.

127 Creutzberg CL, van Putten WL, Koper PC, et al. Surgery and postoperative radiotherapy versus surgery alone for patients with stage-1 endometrial carcinoma: multicentre randomised trial. PORTEC Study Group Post Operative Radiation Therapy in Endometrial Carcinoma. *Lancet*. 2000;**355**(**9213**):1404–11. Epub 2000/05/03.

128 Nout RA, Smit VT, Putter H, et al. Vaginal brachytherapy versus pelvic external beam radiotherapy for patients with endometrial cancer of high-intermediate risk (PORTEC-2): an open-label, non-inferiority, randomised trial. *Lancet*. 2010;**375**(**9717**):816–23. Epub 2010/03/09.

152 Susumu N, Sagae S, Udagawa Y, et al. Randomized phase III trial of pelvic radiotherapy versus cisplatin-based combined chemotherapy in patients with intermediate- and high-risk endometrial cancer: a Japanese Gynecologic Oncology Group study. *Gynecol Oncol*. 2008;**108**(**1**):226–33. Epub 2007/11/13.

153 Kelly MG, O'Malley DM, Hui P, et al. Improved survival in surgical stage I patients with uterine papillary serous carcinoma (UPSC) treated with adjuvant platinum-based chemotherapy. *Gynecol Oncol*. 2005;**98**(**3**):353–9. Epub 2005/07/12.

154 Huh WK, Straughn JM Jr, Mariani A, et al. Salvage of isolated vaginal recurrences in women with surgical stage I endometrial cancer: a multiinstitutional experience.

Int J Gynecol Cancer. 2007;**17**(**4**):886–9. Epub 2007/02/21.

166 Thigpen JT, Brady MF, Homesley HD, et al. Phase III trial of doxorubicin with or without cisplatin in advanced endometrial carcinoma: a gynecologic oncology group study. *J Clin Oncol*. 2004;**22**(**19**):3902–8.

167 Aapro MS, van Wijk FH, Bolis G, et al. Doxorubicin versus doxorubicin and cisplatin in endometrial carcinoma: definitive results of a randomised study (55872) by the EORTC Gynaecological Cancer Group. *Ann Oncol*. 2003;**14**(**3**):441–8.

181 Fleming GF, Brunetto VL, Cella D, et al. Phase III trial of doxorubicin plus cisplatin with or without paclitaxel plus filgrastim in advanced endometrial carcinoma: a Gynecologic Oncology Group Study. *J Clin Oncol*. 2004;**22**(**11**): 2159–66.

186 Miller DFV, Fleming G, et al. Randomized phase III noninferiority trial of first line chemotherapy for metastatic or recurrent endometrial carcinoma: A Gynecologic Oncology Group Study. SGO. *Gynecol Oncol*. 2012;**125**:771.

187 Randall ME, Filiaci VL, Muss H, et al. Randomized phase III trial of whole-abdominal irradiation versus doxorubicin and cisplatin chemotherapy in advanced endometrial carcinoma: a Gynecologic Oncology Group Study. *J Clin Oncol*. 2006;**24**(**1**):36–44. Epub 2005/12/07.

193 Ramirez PT, Frumovitz M, Bodurka DC, Sun CC, Levenback C. Hormonal therapy for the management of grade 1 endometrial adenocarcinoma: a literature review. *Gynecol Oncol*. 2004;**95**(**1**):133–8. Epub 2004/09/24.

198 Whitney CW, Brunetto VL, Zaino RJ, et al. Phase II study of medroxyprogesterone acetate plus tamoxifen in advanced endometrial carcinoma: a Gynecologic Oncology Group study. *Gynecol Oncol*. 2004;**92**(**1**):4–9. Epub 2004/01/31.

199 Fiorica JV, Brunetto VL, Hanjani P, Lentz SS, Mannel R, Andersen W. Phase II trial of alternating courses of megestrol acetate and tamoxifen in advanced endometrial carcinoma: a Gynecologic Oncology Group study. *Gynecol Oncol*. 2004;**92**(**1**):10–4. Epub 2004/01/31.

第 104 章 上皮癌、输卵管癌和腹膜癌

Jonathan S. Berek, MD, MMS, FASCO ■ Michael L. Friedlander, MD, MBChB, PhD ■ Robert C. Bast Jr., MD

概况

大多数卵巢癌对手术和辅助化疗的近期反应良好，因此卵巢癌是可以治疗的实体瘤之一。但是 70%的卵巢癌患者会复发，是死亡/发病比最高的妇科恶性肿瘤[1,2]。卵巢癌并非常见病，但也并不罕见。美国女性的卵巢癌终生患病风险为 1/70，绝经后女性的患病率为 1/2 500，这影响着卵巢癌早期诊断和预防的策略。*BRCA1* 和 *BRCA2* 胚系突变与 10%～15%的卵巢癌相关，显著增加卵巢癌发病风险。引起持续性排卵的因素明显增加散发性卵巢癌的发病风险，而口服避孕药可降低绝经后的发病风险。虽然卵巢上皮癌曾被认为是起源于卵巢表面上皮或卵巢表面下方的包涵囊肿，但目前认为高级别浆液性"卵巢癌"以及腹膜癌起源于输卵管伞，而非卵巢或腹膜[3-10]。卵巢上皮癌组织学类型有浆液性癌、子宫内膜样癌、黏液癌以及透明细胞癌。低级别的Ⅰ型卵巢癌生长缓慢，可起源于低度恶性潜能肿瘤，大部分存在 *Ras* 基因突变，*TP53* 呈野生型表达，常可在早期（Ⅰ～Ⅱ期）发现，并且对铂类联合紫杉类化疗药物不敏感。高级别的Ⅱ型卵巢癌生长迅速，起源于伴有 *TP53* 突变的前驱病变，发病由 DNA 拷贝数变异驱动，诊断时多为晚期（Ⅲ～Ⅳ期），常对联合化疗敏感。由于缺乏特异性症状以及有效的筛查手段，超过 70%的卵巢癌患者诊断时已是晚期（Ⅲ～Ⅳ期）。卵巢上皮癌的主要治疗手段包括肿瘤细胞减灭术和 6～8 周期卡铂联合紫杉醇化疗。对于残存肿瘤体积较小的患者，腹腔灌注化疗可以改善生存。复发性卵巢癌无法通过现有药物治愈，但是可以通过包括卡铂联合紫杉醇等细胞毒性药物的再次化疗延长生存。姑息治疗药物包括多柔比星脂质体、吉西他滨、托泊替康、贝伐珠单抗、培美曲塞、依托泊苷。低级别卵巢癌的试验药物包括 MEK 抑制剂，高级别浆液性卵巢癌的试验药物包括 PI3K 通路抑制剂和 PARP 抑制剂。有待开展靶向药物联合治疗的临床试验。

发病率、病因学、流行病学

发病率

卵巢癌、输卵管癌和腹膜癌主要发生于绝经后女性，只有 10%～15%发生于绝经前女性[1-3]，中位诊断年龄为 60～65 岁。不足 1%的卵巢上皮癌发生于 30 岁以前的女性，大多数年轻的患者为生殖细胞肿瘤（参见第 105 章）[2]。在美国，绝经后女性卵巢癌的患病率为 1/2 500，终生发病风险为 1/70（1.4%），是乳腺癌终生发病风险的 1/9～1/8。总人群的患病率对卵巢癌的预防和早期诊断策略有着实质性的影响。由于缺乏有效的风险评估标志物，卵巢癌的预防手段需没有严重的不良反应，而筛查方式需要有较高的特异性。卵巢癌的发生和遗传因素明确相关，*BRCA1* 和 *BRCA2* 胚系突变最常见，至少占 10%，错配修复基因（*MMR*）或 *P53* 突变少见。

在美国，2015 年预计卵巢癌新发病例 22 000 例，死亡 14 000 例[1]。卵巢癌患者的生存有改善的趋势[1,2]。基于美国监测、流行病学和最终结果（Surveillance, Epidemiology, and End Results, SEER）数据库，所有期别卵巢癌患者的整体 5 年生存率从 1975 年的 33.6%升至 2003—2011 年的 45.9%[2]。通过统计模型分析，卵巢癌在过去的 10 年发病率每年下降 1%，死亡率每年下降 1.6%。卵巢癌死亡率从 1976 年的 10/100 000 降至 2010 年的 7.8/100 000，总计降低了 22%[2]。卵巢癌的发病率在 55～64 岁（中位年龄 63 岁）的女性中最高，死亡率在 75～84 岁（中位年龄 71 岁）女性中最高[2]。

卵巢癌发病率在不同地区存在差别。包括美国和英国在内的西方国家卵巢癌的发病率是日本的 3～7 倍[10,11]。在亚洲卵巢生殖细胞肿瘤的发病率高于西方国家。但是，美国的日裔移民卵巢上皮癌发病率明显升高，接近美国白人女性。美国白人女性的卵巢上皮性肿瘤的发病率比黑人女性高 1.5 倍。

病因学和流行病学

既往认为大多数卵巢上皮癌起源于卵巢表面的单层上皮细胞或者紧邻卵巢表面下方排列的包涵囊肿。在过去 10 年间逐渐修正了这种观点。近 10%～15%的卵巢上皮癌患者存在 *BRCA1* 和 *BRCA2* 基因胚系突变，突变患者中大多数为高级别浆液性肿瘤。高达 80%合并 *BRCA1/2* 突变的高级别浆液性卵巢癌起源于输卵管伞端，至少占总体卵巢癌患者的 10%。约 20%的高级别浆液性癌累及卵巢表面，而非起源于卵巢，这些被定义为原发腹膜癌。大部分高级别浆液性原发腹膜癌很可能起源于输卵管伞端，而另一些可能起源于残存的 Müllerian 系统[12]。原发腹膜癌解释了仅接受卵巢切除而保留输卵管的患者多年后仍可能出现"卵巢癌"的原因[13-15]。1/3 甚至更多的高级别浆液性癌起源于输卵管伞，其余的起源于卵巢。卵巢、输卵管和腹膜高级别浆液性癌应当被认定为一种疾病，并且按照同样规范进行治疗。因此，国际妇产科联合会（International Federation of Gynecology and Obstetrics, FIGO）将输卵管癌纳入卵巢癌分期系统当中[4]。

卵巢癌的病因尚不明确[16,17]。吸烟和卵巢黏液癌相关，但和常见的浆液性癌没有相关性[17]。病例对照研究表明白种人、高脂饮食和食用半乳糖导致卵巢癌发病风险增加[16,18]。生育史、排卵周期和卵巢癌的发生有关，分娩次数少、不孕、初潮年龄早、绝经年龄晚可增加患病风险[16,19,20]。促排卵药物，如柠檬酸克罗米芬和促性腺激素诱导排卵被认为可能增加卵巢癌的风险，但是相关数据并不一致，也未能区分不孕本身和使用促排卵

药物对卵巢癌发生的影响[21~24]。包含 8 项病例对照研究、总计纳入了 5 207 例患者和 7 705 例对照人群的荟萃分析发现，促排卵药物和浆液性交界性肿瘤相关，但是和卵巢癌没有相关性[24]。许多病例对照研究和队列研究未能发现激素替代治疗增加卵巢上皮癌的发病风险[25]。一项大型队列研究再次引起了有关激素替代治疗是否和卵巢癌相关的争议[26]。在乳腺癌检测示范项目（Breast Cancer Detection Demonstration Project）中 44 241 例绝经后妇女，有 329 例发生了卵巢癌。仅接受雌激素替代而无孕激素治疗超过 10 年的女性卵巢癌的发病风险增加。雌激素单一替代治疗达 20 年时，这一风险增加 3.2 倍。最近的一项荟萃分析也支持这个结论。该研究纳入了超过 12 000 名绝经后女性，55%使用过激素治疗的女性发生了卵巢癌。对于末次随访时仍在接受激素替代的女性，即使治疗时间小于 5 年，发病风险（*RR*）仍然增加［*RR* 10.43，95%可信区间（CI）10.31～10.56，$P<0.0001$］。正在和近期接受激素治疗患者的发病风险为 10.37（95%CI 10.29～10.46，$P<0.0001$）；这和欧洲及美国的前瞻性研究结果类似，单用雌激素治疗和雌孕激素联合治疗的发病风险相当，但不同组织学类型发病风险有差异。激素替代治疗明确增加卵巢浆液性癌（*RR* 10.53，95%CI 10.40～10.66，$P<0.0001$）和子宫内膜样癌（10.42，10.20～10.67，$P<0.0001$）两种常见类型的发病风险。作者发现激素替代治疗和卵巢癌发病风险升高可能是有因果关系的，每 1 000 例在 50 岁左右开始使用激素治疗 5 年的女性中可多 1 例卵巢癌患者[27]。

预防

生育和卵巢癌呈负相关，生育一次可以至少降低发病相对危险 30%～40%，口服避孕药超过 5 年可以降低 50% 的风险[21]。生育两次并且使用口服避孕药超过 5 年的女性可降低 70%的发病风险。目前，口服避孕药是预防卵巢癌的唯一有效的药物，可以推荐给卵巢癌的高危个体。应向咨询避孕方式的女性强调口服避孕药降低卵巢癌风险（ROC）的作用。这对于存在卵巢癌家族史，但没有 *BRCA1* 或 *BRCA2* 突变的女性也十分重要[28]。预防性手术也很重要，但是应该严格把握适应证，仅对患病风险明确增加的女性实施预防性双卵巢输卵管切除术或全子宫双附件切除术。

遗传易感性

遗传性卵巢癌

有乳腺癌或卵巢癌家族史以及 Lynch 综合征家族史的女性罹患卵巢癌的风险显著高于普通人群[29~45]。尽管大多数卵巢癌为散发性，仍有至少 10%～13%的卵巢上皮癌患者存在 *BRCA1* 或 *BRCA2* 胚系突变[42]。

BRCA1 和 *BRCA2*

大多数遗传性卵巢癌是由位于 17 号染色体的 *BRCA1* 基因突变导致，另有部分是由位于 13 号染色体的 *BRCA2* 基因突变导致。这两个基因都参与 DNA 损伤修复，*BRCA1* 突变相关卵巢癌患者的发病年龄比无突变的患者要早大约 10 年[36,42]。卵巢上皮癌的中位发病年龄为 62～63 岁。如果一位女性的一级或二级亲属罹患卵巢癌且发病年龄较早，那么她携带 *BRCA1* 或 *BRCA2* 突变基因的概率较高。然而 44%存在基因突变的女性并没有明确的家族史。鉴于此，目前的指南推荐对所有 70 岁以下卵巢高级别浆液性癌患者，无论其有无家族史，均进行基因突变检测[44]。

德系犹太裔、冰岛女性和某些人种携带 *BRCA1* 和 *BRCA2* 突变基因的频率较高[35,36]。德系犹太人有 3 个先证者突变（founder mutation）：*BRCA1* 中的 *185delAG* 和 *5382insC*，*BRCA2* 中的 6174*delT*。德系犹太人后裔患者携带至少 1 种上述突变的频率为 1/40（2.5%），明显高于一般白人女性。先证者效应（founder effect）是德系犹太裔突变频率增高的原因。先证者效应是指在历史上某个族群的一个或多个祖先携带某个突变基因，由于地理或文化原因该族群和其他族群产生隔离，最终这个突变基因较多地传递给族群中的个体。

22 项不考虑家族史的研究结果汇总分析表明，携带 *BRCA1* 或 *BRCA2* 突变女性的卵巢癌终生患病风险分别为 39%（18%～54%）和 11%（2.4%～19%）[45]。携带 *BRCA1* 或 *BRCA2* 突变的女性发生乳腺癌的风险分别高达 65%和 45%，并且突变携带者乳腺癌发病年龄更早，可能为双侧发病。携带 *BRCA1* 突变的女性发生三阴性乳腺癌（*ER*-，*PR*-，*HER2*-）的风险更高。一项大型研究发现在 4q32.2 和 17q21.31 位点存在遗传风险调节因子，这些调节因子可显著增加 *BRCA1* 携带女性罹患卵巢癌的风险。这可能是 *BRCA* 突变患者发病风险报道不一的原因[46]。

Lynch 综合征

还有其他一些较少见的引起卵巢癌的遗传原因。Lynch 综合征，也被称为遗传性非息肉性结直肠癌综合征（HNPCC），是由错配修复基因（*MMR*）胚系突变导致，该综合征患者罹患结直肠癌及其他一些恶性肿瘤（如子宫内膜癌、卵巢癌和胃癌）的风险增加[39]。和 Lynch 综合征相关的基因有 *MSH2*、*MSH6*、*MLH1*、*PMS1* 及 *PMS2*。Lynch 综合征的女性患子宫内膜癌的风险与患结直肠癌风险相当甚至更高。Lynch 综合征人群中，罹患妇科恶性肿瘤者超过 50%，因此也将妇科恶性肿瘤称为 Lynch 综合征的“前哨癌”。Lynch 综合征的女性卵巢癌的终生发病风险为 6%～12%，诊断时平均年龄为 42.7～49.5 岁，其中子宫内膜样癌和透明细胞癌的发病风险较高，且多为Ⅰ～Ⅱ期疾病。

卵巢癌高风险女性的管理

对于有强烈卵巢上皮癌家族史的女性，需要根据年龄、生育计划和风险评估进行个体化管理。完整的家系分析十分重要。遗传学家应当评估至少三代以内的家系。对家系彻底分析之后再制定管理方案，并尽可能确定家系中卵巢癌患者的组织学类型、发病年龄和家系其他成员的肿瘤病史。尽管美国国立卫生研究院卵巢癌共识会议（National Institute of Health Consensus Conference on Ovarian Cancer，NIHCCOC）推荐经阴道超声联合 CA125 对高危女性进行卵巢癌筛查，但其价值并不肯定[47]。两项前瞻性研究表明，每年一次经阴道超声联合 CA125 筛查的获益十分有限，且可能仅体现在高危女性[48,49]。

一项由多个基因筛查中心协作的数据分析表明，口服避孕药可以降低 *BRCA1* 或 *BRCA2* 突变女性的卵巢癌发病风险[50]，但并未得到证实[51]。输卵管结扎似乎可以降低 *BRCA1* 突变女性卵巢癌发病风险，但不能降低 *BRCA*2 突变女性的风险，而且其预防效果比预防性双卵巢输卵管切除术（BSO）差[52]。

预防性 BSO 可使高危人群获益[53-58]。很多研究报道了预防性 BSO 后隐匿性卵巢/输卵管癌的发生率为 2.3%~23%。预防性双卵巢输卵管切除术可降低 96% *BRCA* 相关的妇科恶性肿瘤发生[56]。但也存在少部分患者 BSO 后发生腹膜癌的风险。在两个队列研究中,BSO 术后腹膜癌的发生率分别为 0.8%和 1%[54,55]。之前讨论过,一些所谓的卵巢癌实则起源于输卵管,因此预防性切除术必须同时切除双侧卵巢和输卵管,并且病理医生需要仔细寻找潜在的微小癌灶或癌前病变,尤其是输卵管伞端[6]。预防性双卵巢输卵管切除术可使绝经前女性患乳腺癌的风险降低 50%~80%[54,55]。Grann 等人报道了在一个虚拟的 30 岁携带 *BRCA1* 或 *BRCA2* 突变的女性队列中应用 Markov 模型进行质量调整生存预测分析的结果[59]。该模型预测在 30 岁女性队列中,相对于定期随诊,使用他莫昔芬可延长生存 1.8 年,预防性双卵巢输卵管切除术可延长生存 2.6 年,预防性双卵巢输卵管切除术联合他莫昔芬可延长生存 4.6 年,预防性乳房切除术可延长生存 3.5 年,预防性双卵巢输卵管切除术+预防性乳房切除术可延长生存 4.9 年。他莫昔芬可延长质量调整预期寿命 2.8 年,预防性双卵巢输卵管切除术可延长 4.4 年,预防性双卵巢输卵管切除术联合他莫昔芬可延长 6.3 年,预防性乳房切除术可延长 2.6 年,预防性双卵巢输卵管切除术+预防性乳房切除术可延长 2.6 年。另一项研究也支持上述结论,预防性乳房切除术可降低 *BRCA1* 和 *BRCA2* 突变的女性乳腺癌的发病风险,预防性双卵巢输卵管切除术可降低卵巢癌的发病风险,并且可降低全因素死亡率、乳腺癌相关的死亡率和卵巢癌相关死亡率[60]。

BRCA1 或 *BRCA2* 突变卵巢癌患者的生存期比无突变的患者长。一项研究报道,携带突变患者中位生存期为 53.4 个月,散发患者为 37.8 个月[61]。最近,以色列的 Chetrit 等人的一项基于人群的研究也证实了上述结果[62]。他们发现德系犹太女性卵巢癌人群中,携带 *BRCA1* 或 *BRCA2* 突变患者的远期生存率较高(5 年生存率 38% vs 24%)。肿瘤本身的生长特性或对化疗更敏感可能是突变携带者生存期较长的原因。

建议

推荐所有 70 岁以下非黏液性卵巢上皮癌、输卵管癌或腹膜癌的女性进行 *BRCA1* 或 *BRCA2* 基因检测[63]。卵巢癌高风险女性的管理建议总结如下[40,41,47,51~59,64]:

1. 卵巢癌和/或乳腺癌高风险女性应当进行遗传咨询:如果 *BRCA* 基因突变的概率大于 10%,推荐进行 *BRCA1* 和 *BRCA2* 检测。

2. 希望保留生育或推迟预防性切除手术的女性,推荐每 6 个月接受一次经阴道超声和 CA125 联合筛查,尽管现有证据并未证实该方法可降低死亡率。

3. 对于年轻的卵巢癌高风险女性推荐口服避孕药。

4. 推荐无保留生育功能愿望或已完成生育的女性接受预防性双卵巢输卵管切除术。对于有强烈卵巢癌或乳腺癌家族史的女性,推荐自 30 岁起每年接受乳腺钼靶和乳腺核磁筛查;如果家族中有早发乳腺癌的患者,筛查应当提前到 30 岁以前。

5. 由于患 Lynch 综合征女性存在子宫内膜癌和卵巢癌的风险,应当在完成生育后咨询是否接受预防性全子宫双附件切除术。尽管没有研究明确支持筛查,可考虑从 30~35 岁开始接受子宫内膜活检和经阴道彩超检查。推荐从 20~25 岁开始每 1~2 年接受一次结肠镜检查,或在家族中最年轻患者确诊年龄提前 10 年开始筛查[39,65,66]。

分子、细胞和临床生物学

和大多数上皮癌类似,超过 90%的卵巢上皮癌起源于单个细胞,这意味着卵巢癌是一种克隆性疾病[67]。尽管是单细胞起源,卵巢癌在分子水平、细胞水平和临床表现上存在显著异质性。卵巢癌存在基因激活或失活等异常事件(表 104-1)[68]。删除突变、杂合性缺失、失活突变(*BRCA1*、*BRCA2* 和 *TP53*)、启动子甲基化(ARHI)、组蛋白修饰或 miRNA 缺失等原因可造成抑癌基因功能丧失(表 104-2)。伴有 *Dicer* 和 *Drosha* 表达降低的 miRNA 加工异常见于 60%和 51%的卵巢癌患者,并且和预后较差有关[69]。癌基因可以扩增、转录过表达和/或因突变被激活(表 104-3)[68]。在细胞水平,增殖细胞的占比变异极大,自 1%至 90%[70]。卵巢癌分为浆液性癌、子宫内膜样癌、黏液癌和透明细胞癌,其中一部分和 *HOX* 基因异常表达有关,而 *HOX* 基因和女性生殖系统正常发育相关[71]。

表 104-1 卵巢上皮癌中基因型和表型异常

激活	
CGH 检测到的基因扩增	1q22(*RAB25*),3q26(*PKCiota*、*EVI1*、*PIK3CA*),5q31(*FGF-1*),8q24(*MYC*),19q(*PI3Kp85*、*AKT2*),20p,20q13.2(*BTAK*)
突变[a]	*K-Ras*,*BRAF*,*CTNNB1*,*CDKN2A*,*PIK3CA*,*KIT*,*MADH*
低甲基化	*BORIS*,*CLDN-4*,*IGF2*,*MCI*,*SAT2*,*SNCG*
组蛋白修饰 miRNA	cyclin B1,GATA4,GATA6,p21/WAF1,BAP1,DLK1,MSX2,PTEN,SIP1,VEGFA,ZEB1/2
抑制	
CGH 检测到的基因缺失	4q,5q,16q,17p,17q;Xp,Xq
杂合性缺失(LOH)	(>50%):17p13,17q21(>30%):1p,3p,5q,6q,7q,8q,9p,10q,11p,13q,18q,19p,20;Xp
突变	*ARID1A*,*TP53*,*Rb1a*,*APC*,*BRCA1*,*BRCA2*,*CDK12*,*NF1*,*PTEN*,*PP2R1A*
启动子甲基化	APC,ARHI,ANGPTL,ARLTS1,*BRCA1*,DAPK,FBX032,H-CADHERIN,hMLH1,HOXA10,HOXA11,Hsulf-1,ICAM-1,LOT-1,MCJ,MUC2,MYO188,OPCML,PACE-4,PALP-B,PAR-4,PEG3,p16,p21,RASSF1,SOCS1,SOCS2,SPARC,TMS/ASC,TUBB3,14-3-3σ
组蛋白修饰 miRNA	Adam 19,GATA4,GATA6,RASSF1
染色体异位导致的生长抑制	BCL2,FGF2,MMP13,PAR8,c-SRK,VEGFA 2、3、7、22

[a] www.Sanger.ac.uk。

表 104-2　卵巢上皮癌中可能的抑癌基因

基因	染色体	下调或失活	下调机制	功能
ARHI(*DIRAS3*)	1p31	60%的所有组织学类型	印记;杂合性缺失;启动子甲基化;通过 E2F1 和 E2F4 下调转录	26kDa 的 GTP 酶,抑制细胞增殖和活动,诱导自噬和休眠,下调 p21,抑制细胞周期蛋白 D1、PI3K、Ras-MAP、Stat3
ARID1A	1p35.5	49%的透明细胞癌,30%子宫内膜样癌	突变	染色质重塑
RASSF1A	3p21	—	超甲基化	在许多肿瘤中抑制增殖和降低致肿瘤性。和 *Ras* 基因相互作用抑制下调细胞周期蛋白 D,通过 JNK 信号通路、稳定微管、调节纺锤丝结合点和 fas 及肿瘤坏死因子介导凋亡
DLEC1	3p22.3	73%	启动子超甲基化和组蛋白低乙酰化	166kDa 的胞质蛋白抑制贴壁依赖性生长
SPARC	5q31	70%~90%表达下调;9%缺失	转录;超甲基化	32kDa 的钙离子结合蛋白,防止黏附
DAB-2(*DOC2*)	5q13	58%~85%缺失	转录	105kDa 的蛋白,与 GRB2 结合阻止 Ras/MAP 激活,阻止 c-fos 诱导和降低 ILK 活性,导致失巢凋亡并抑制增殖、贴壁依赖性生长,降低致肿瘤性
LOT-1(*ZAC1*)	6q25	39%	基因印记;超甲基化杂合性缺失;EGF, TPA 导致的转录下调	55kDa 的细胞核锌指蛋白降低增殖和致肿瘤性
RPS6KA2	6q27	64%	卵巢中单一等位基因表达;杂合性缺失	90-kDa 的核糖体 S6 丝氨酸-苏氨酸激酶抑制细胞生长,诱导凋亡,减少 pERK 和细胞周期蛋白 D1,抑制 p21 和 p27
PTEN(*MMAC-1*)	10q23	3%~8%突变;27%表达,尤其是子宫内膜样癌和透明细胞癌	启动子甲基化;杂合性缺失;突变	P13 磷酸酶;降低细胞增殖,移行和存活;降低细胞周期蛋白 D 和增加 p27 蛋白
OPCML	11q25	56%~83%	启动子甲基化;杂合性缺失;突变	GPI 锚定蛋白 IgLON 家族;诱导聚集;抑制增殖和降低致肿瘤性
BRCA2	13q12~13	3%~6%	突变;杂性缺失	结合 RAD51 进行 DNA 双链断裂修复
ARLTS1	13q14	62%	启动子甲基化	ADP 核糖基化因子介导凋亡
WWOX	16q23	30%~49%,特别是黏液癌和透明细胞癌	杂合性缺失;突变	降低贴壁依赖性生长和致肿瘤性;小鼠细胞凋亡所需
TP53	17p13.1	整体的 50%~70%;96%的高级别浆液性癌	突变	53kDa 的核蛋白诱导 p21 蛋白和暂停细胞周期,促进 DNA 稳定;诱导凋亡

续表

基因	染色体	下调或失活	下调机制	功能
OVCA1	17p13.3	37%	杂合性缺失	50kDa 蛋白;降低增殖和克隆性;减少细胞周期蛋白 D1
BRCA1	17q21	6%~8%	基因突变;杂合性缺失;启动子甲基化	Myc E3 泛素连接酶,通过同源重组直接参与 DNA 双链损伤修复;调节 c-Ab1;诱导 *TP53*,雄激素受体,雌激素受体和 c-Myc
PEG3	19q13	75%	基因印记;杂合性缺失;启动子甲基化;转录	介导 *TP53* 依赖的凋亡
PPP2R1A	19q13.44	7%的透明细胞癌	突变	蛋白磷酸酶 2 调节亚基抑制增殖

文献中报道过的潜在抑癌基因包括 *APC*、*BRMS1*、*CTGF*、*EPB41L3*、*MAP2K4*、*MKK4*、*RNF43*、*RP36RA7*、*PINX1*、*SFRP4*、*SLIT2*、*SOX11*、*TUSC3*、*53BP1*。

表 104-3 卵巢上皮癌相关的癌基因

癌基因	染色体	扩增/%	过表达/%	突变/%	功能
Rab25	1q22	54	80~90	—	胞质 GTP 酶/顶部血管运输
Evi-1	3q26	—	—	—	转录因子
eIF-5A2	3q26	—	—	—	延长因子
PKCi	3q26	44	78	—	胞质丝氨酸-苏氨酸激酶
PIK3CA(*PI3K p110α*)	3q26	9~80	32	8~12	胞质脂类激酶
FGF-1	5q31	—	51	—	肿瘤生长因子和血管形成
Myc	8q24	20	41~66	—	转录因子
EGFR	7p12	11~20	9~28	<1	酪氨酸激酶生长因子受体
Notch-3	9p13	20~21	62	—	细胞表面生长因子受体
K-Ras	12p11~12	5~53	30~52	2~24	胞质 GTP 酶
Her-2	17q12~21	6~11	4~12	—	酪氨酸激酶生长因子受体
P85PI3K	19q	—	—	—	胞质脂类激酶
Cyclin E	19q12	12~53	42~63	—	细胞周期蛋白
AKT2	19q13.2	12~27	12		胞质丝氨酸/苏氨酸激酶
BTAK/Aurora A	20q13+K11:L22	10~15	48	—	核丝氨酸-苏氨酸激酶/激活端粒酶

其他可在高级别浆液性卵巢癌中检测到的拷贝数>20%的基因:*AKT1*,*AKT3*,*CDK2*,*IL8RB*,*EPCAM*,*ERBB3*,*FGFR2*,*HDAC4*,*HSP90AB1*,*HSP90B1*,*IGF1*,*IGFR1*,*LPAR3*,*MAP3K6*,*MAPK15*,*MAPKAPK2*,*MAPKAPK5*,*MECOM*,*MSTN*,*MTOR*,*NCAM1*,*NOS1*,*NOS3*,*PIK3CD*,*POLB*,*POLE*,*RHEB*,*RICTOR*,*PPS6KC1*,*RAPTOR*,*SKI1*,*STAT1*,*STAT4*,*TERT*,*TGFB1*,*TGFB2*,*TGFBR3*,*TNFRSF9*,*VEGFA*。

低级别(Ⅰ型)和高级别(Ⅱ型)卵巢上皮癌在生物学和临床上存在较大差别[72]。低级别浆液性癌(占卵巢上皮癌<10%)来源于交界性肿瘤,多为早期(Ⅰ~Ⅱ期),其发生依赖 *Ras*(>50%)、*PIK3CA*(30%)和 *PTEN*(10%)基因突变以及胰岛素样生长因子受体(IGFR)的表达。IGFR 可以和肿瘤基质产生的 IGF 相互作用。高级别浆液性癌(占卵巢上皮癌的 60%)源于正常的卵巢和输卵管上皮,发现时多为晚期(Ⅲ~Ⅳ期),其发生依赖多种野生型癌基因的扩增和抑癌基因的功能缺失。*TP53* 基因突变极少见于低级别(Ⅰ型)卵巢癌,但几乎见于所有卵巢高级别浆液性癌(Ⅱ型)。*BRCA1/2* 胚系突变和体细胞突变和卵巢上皮癌相关,通常为高级别癌。DNA 同源重组修复缺陷(BRCAness)见于半数以上的卵巢高级别癌,但极少见于卵巢低级别癌,这可能是高级别癌对以铂类为基础化疗更敏感的原因。目前不论是否合并 *BRCA1/2* 突变,DNA 同源重组修复缺陷的患者可接受 PARP 抑制剂治疗。*PI3* 激酶通路的激活见于至少半数卵巢高级别癌,既是Ⅰ型也是Ⅱ型卵巢癌潜在的靶点[73]。

癌症和肿瘤基因组图谱计划(TCGA)对超过 300 例卵巢高级别浆液性癌标本进行了测序,*TP53* 和 *BRCA1/2* 突变频率分别为 98%和 15%~20%,除此之外有极少数基因突变频率超过 1%(*NF1*、*RB1*、*CSMD3* 和 *CDK12*)[74]。可见基因突变是卵巢低级别癌驱动因素,而 DNA 拷贝数异常是卵巢高级别癌的驱动因素。

透明细胞癌存在染色质处理酶 *ARID1A* 突变(49%)[75]和磷酸酶 *PP2R1A* 突变(6%)。卵巢子宫内膜样癌也存在 *ARID1A* 突变(30%)。在非上皮性卵巢癌中,97%的卵巢颗粒细胞瘤存在特征性 *FOXL2* 基因 *402C→G*(*C134W*)突变,*FOXL2* 编码颗粒细胞发育过程中重要的转录因子[76]。

卵巢癌组织产生的血管内皮生长因子/血管通透因子(VEGF/VPF)使毛细血管渗出蛋白液增多,以及肿瘤转移使膈肌淋巴管回流受阻共同导致腹水形成[77]。腹腔免疫生物学研究表明腹膜可能是一个免疫豁免区域,存在抑制分子和生长因子水平上调。卵巢癌组织中的血管形成依赖于多种因素,包括 VEGF 和 IL-8。多种血管源性因子的存在可以在一定程度上解释贝伐珠单抗耐药的原因。*ARHI*(*DIRAS3*)是抑癌基因,可以调节自噬和肿瘤休眠,其下调见于 60%的卵巢低级别和高级别癌[78,79]。在初始减瘤和化疗后二次探查手术的阳性病灶中发现休眠、耐药肿瘤细胞中 *ARHI* 上调和高度自噬现象,表明自噬可能是卵巢癌治疗的靶点[80]。

细胞外黏蛋白的上调和异常糖基化为肿瘤监测提供了标志物。黏蛋白 MUC-1 在超过 80%的卵巢癌中表达[81]。在转化细胞中,异常糖基化使肽决定因子被鼠单克隆抗体识别,用于血清治疗。CA125 也是一种黏蛋白(MUC16),和胚胎发育过程中被覆体腔上皮的细胞有关。80%的卵巢上皮癌细胞可产生 CA125[82,83],并且可通过鼠单克隆抗体 OC125 检测。

CA125 水平的降低或升高和肿瘤消退或进展具有良好的相关性。糖蛋白的准确功能尚不明确[84~86],敲除 *MUC16* 基因不影响小鼠的发育和生育功能[87]。在癌细胞中,CA125 的表达在转录水平上调,80%的 CA125 蛋白被降解。CA125 和间皮素在腹膜表面相互作用,这可能是卵巢癌腹腔种植转移最早接触的位置。

分类和病理

原发性卵巢癌根据它们所来源的卵巢结构进行分类[88]。上文提到,绝大部分来自覆盖卵巢表面的上皮细胞及包涵囊肿一层,但这种观点最近受到挑战,正如之前讨论的内容,多数高级别浆液性癌起源于输卵管伞。这些细胞最初来自中胚层起源的体腔上皮,和间皮层共享相同的细胞标志物。生殖细胞恶性肿瘤构成第二大类常见的卵巢恶性肿瘤,更少见的类型是起源自卵巢间质细胞的肿瘤(参见第 105 章)。颗粒-卵泡膜肿瘤是最少见的类型,起源于卵巢特殊的结缔组织(参见第 105 章)。

上皮性恶性肿瘤构成 85%~90%的卵巢癌。大部分上皮性癌见于 40 岁或以上的患者。40 岁以下的人群发生上皮性卵巢癌的情况少见,30 岁以下的女性最常见的恶性肿瘤是生殖细胞来源肿瘤。上皮性肿瘤的组织学类型列于表 104-4。大部分病变(约 75%)是浆液性癌,其次是黏液性癌、子宫内膜样癌、透明细胞癌、混合性癌、勃勒纳瘤及未分化的组织学类型[11]。

表 104-4 卵巢上皮性肿瘤

组织学类型	细胞类型
1. 浆液性	输卵管内皮样
(a)良性	
(b)交界性	
(c)恶性	
2. 黏液性	宫颈管内样
(a)良性	
(b)交界性	
(c)恶性	
3. 子宫内膜样	子宫内膜样
(a)良性	
(b)交界性	
(c)恶性	
4. 透明细胞“中肾管样”	中肾旁管样
(a)良性	
(b)交界性	
(c)恶性	
5. Brenner	移行细胞样
(a)良性	
(b)交界性(增殖的)	
(c)恶性	
6. 混合性上皮	混合性
(a)良性	
(b)交界性	
(c)恶性	
7. 未分化	
退行性	
8. 未分类	
(a)中肾管瘤	
(b)其他	

侵袭性癌的组织学类型

浆液性癌可能有复杂的囊性和伴大量乳头形成的实性区域，或可能由主要包含坏死和出血的实性成分组成（图 104-1）。分化差的肿瘤可能有乳头样的成分，但其他部分可能很难和下述其他组织学类型进行区分（图 104-2）。Ⅰ期或Ⅱ期的病变绝大部分是单侧的，大约 10%～20%累及双侧。相反，50%～70%的Ⅲ期浆液性癌是双侧的[11]。

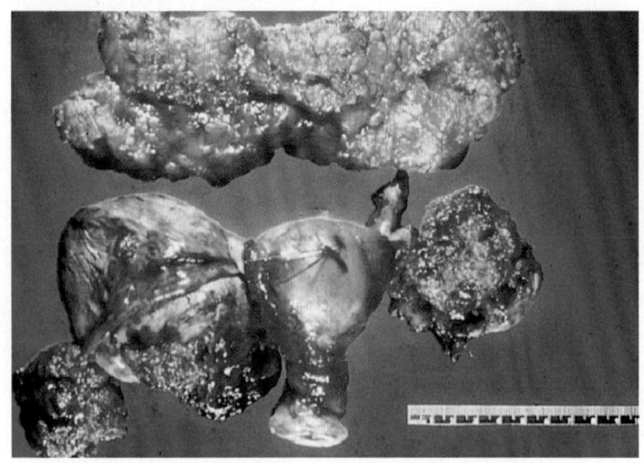

图 104-1　浆液性囊腺癌的肿瘤和大网膜

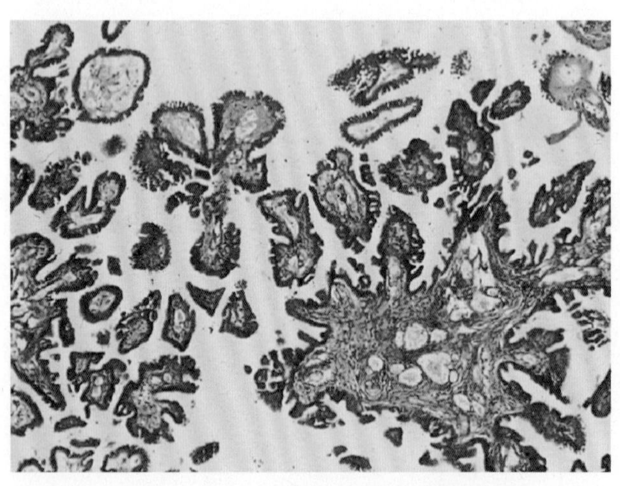

图 104-2　分化差的卵巢浆液性癌

黏液性肿瘤通常较大，很多直径可以超过 20cm（图 104-3）。组织学所见类似子宫颈管内腺体。病变部位通常包含坏死、出血和含量不等的黏液成分。约 10%～20%的病例肿瘤是双侧的。有时，黏液分泌进入腹腔，产生假性黏液瘤或腹膜黏液瘤。有时也可观察到伴发阑尾的黏液囊肿。

卵巢子宫内膜样癌与典型的子宫内膜癌相似。这些肿瘤也可能与子宫内膜癌同时存在，当二者同时出现时，可能都处于早期。卵巢子宫内膜样癌偶尔可能与盆腔子宫内膜异位症并存，可见良性病变向恶性病变的转化（图 104-4）[11]。与前文中子宫内膜癌相似，卵巢子宫内膜样癌与 *PTEN* 基因的失活突变进而激活 PI3K 信号通路相关。Ⅰ～Ⅱ期中约 10%～15%为双侧，Ⅲ期中约 30%为双侧。

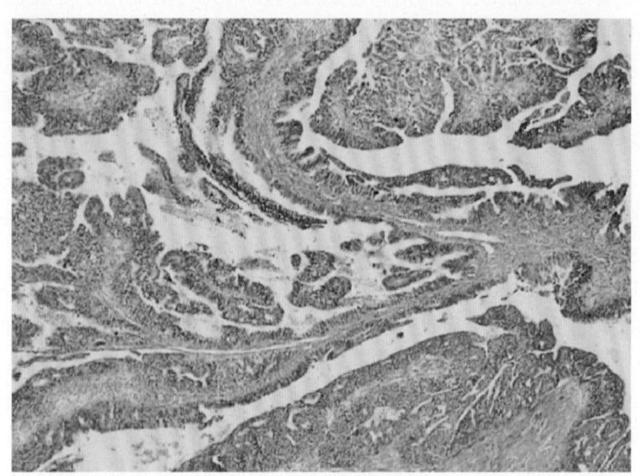

图 104-3　黏液性囊腺癌

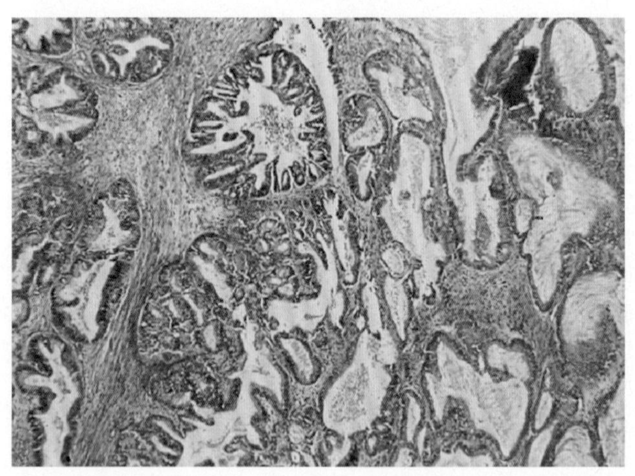

图 104-4　子宫内膜样癌

卵巢透明细胞癌的细胞中含有大量细胞内糖原并且在组织学处理过程中被洗脱。大约四分之一的透明细胞癌与子宫内膜异位症相关。双侧的透明细胞癌很少见[11]。

Brenner 瘤罕见，在上皮性肿瘤中约占不到 1%。混合性上皮性肿瘤可能含有一小部分 Brenner 瘤的组织学成分，其组织学所见与移行细胞癌类似。恶性 Brenner 瘤是单侧的[11]。

交界性肿瘤

交界性肿瘤或称低度恶性潜能肿瘤，需要和那些明确的侵袭性肿瘤进行鉴别，这一点很重要。交界性肿瘤的治疗和预后与侵袭性恶性肿瘤明显不同。交界性肿瘤在诊断时多局限于一侧卵巢，多见于更年轻的、绝经前女性（图 104-5）。它们容易和分化较好的侵袭性卵巢癌混淆，而二者的治疗可能不同。因此，如果在年轻女性中发现病变仅限于卵巢，怀疑是上皮性卵巢囊腺癌，一定要先排除交界性肿瘤的可能，因为对于交界性肿瘤切除双侧卵巢、子宫并进行化疗可能是不必要的。非良性卵巢肿瘤在小于 40 岁的女性中，60%～70%是交界性的，而在 40 岁以上的女性中，则仅有 10%是交界性的[11,89]。交界性肿瘤的组织学标准包括：①出现上皮细胞增殖并伴有细胞“堆积”的表现，即所谓的假性复层；②细胞异型性，但核分裂象罕见；

③没有间质浸润的证据。交界性肿瘤一般局限于卵巢,也可能合并腹膜病变,这代表了疾病播散或疾病的多灶性进展。在罕见的腹膜受累情况中,患者可能由于逐渐进展的肠梗阻而死亡。

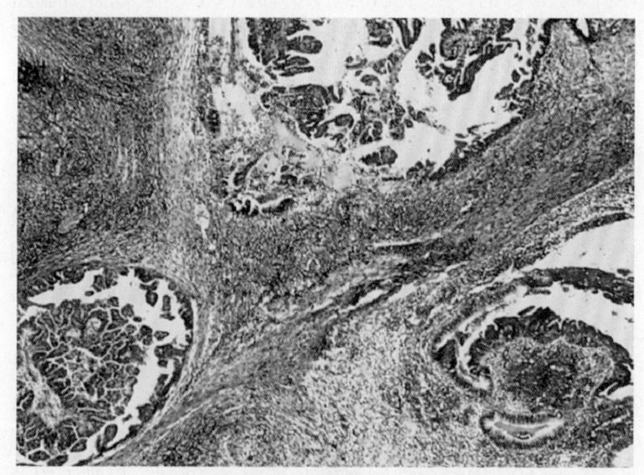

图 104-5 交界性浆液性肿瘤

腹膜癌

覆盖于卵巢表面和腹膜的恶性上皮肿瘤被称为腹膜癌[14]。这些癌和非常罕见的腹膜间皮瘤完全不同,间皮瘤有不同的疾病演化史和对化疗的反应[90]。尽管浆液性癌最为多见而其他类型的癌少见,但是腹膜细胞可模仿发展为卵巢癌中任何一种组织学类型。许多高级别浆液性原发腹膜癌可能来源于输卵管伞,但也有一些来源于次级 Müllerian 管系统的发育退化残留。

腹膜癌的发现可以解释双侧卵巢切除后发生的卵巢癌[91]。此外,腹膜癌可以累及卵巢表面,而卵巢体积并不增大。因此,在腹膜腔起源的癌变中卵巢可能是无辜的旁观者。从治疗角度看,腹膜恶性肿瘤应该和卵巢上皮癌接受相同的治疗。

播散模式

上皮性卵巢癌主要通过细胞在腹膜腔内的直接脱落和种植进行播散,也可通过淋巴和血行途径转移。GCT(参见第 105 章)更倾向于通过腹膜后淋巴途径转移,因此对这些似乎局限于卵巢的肿瘤进行分期时,应仔细评估[11,92]。

脱落的卵巢癌细胞直接播散到盆腔和腹腔的腹膜表面,可能随着腹腔积液的循环途径从右侧结肠旁沟向头侧到右半横膈膜。在初次手术时,脏层和壁层腹膜可能种植了数十至数百个转移性病灶。肠系膜也通过腹膜转移而受累。尽管小肠肠腔的直接受累十分罕见,小肠袢之间的粘连可导致机械性肠梗阻。肠功能的失调也可能是由于肿瘤侵犯肠肌层神经丛(肠系膜中发现的自主神经)导致的。这种情况被称作"癌性肠梗阻"。大的盆腔包块压迫直肠也可以导致肠梗阻。

上皮性卵巢癌常通过淋巴系统转移。据报道大部分情况下Ⅰ期和Ⅱ期的肿瘤腹膜后淋巴结转移率为 5%~10%,而在经过仔细检查的Ⅲ期患者中肿瘤淋巴转移高达 42%~78%[93]。这些淋巴结大部分并不增大,只是显微镜下可发现肿瘤细胞。通过腹膜后淋巴管系统和横膈淋巴管系统可分别导致左侧和右侧锁骨上淋巴结的转移。卵巢癌血行传播在诊断时并不多见,而多是疾病晚期的表现。确诊时发现血行传播到肝实质和肺的仅见于很少一部分患者。在晚期复发患者的脏器实质转移中,肺甚至脑转移常见。

临床表现

局限于卵巢的卵巢癌患者可能是无症状的,而且大部分患者的症状没有特异性,不一定能提示肿瘤来源于卵巢。一项针对 1 725 例卵巢癌患者的调查中,95% 的患者回忆起在诊断前出现症状,包括 89% 的Ⅰ~Ⅱ期患者和 97% 的Ⅲ~Ⅳ期患者[94]。70%的患者有腹部或消化系统症状,58% 出现疼痛,34% 出现泌尿系症状,26% 出现盆腔不适。有些症状至少能够体现盆腔脏器受增大卵巢的压迫。Goff 等建立了卵巢癌症状指数,并认为卵巢癌相关症状包括盆腔或腹腔疼痛、尿频或尿急、腹围增大或腹胀和进食困难或饱胀感,这些症状在一年内发生,并且每个月超过 12 天。这个指数对于早期卵巢癌的敏感性是 56.7%,对于晚期疾病是 79.5%[95]。有趣的是,一项来自澳大利亚以人群为基础的研究并没有发现早期和晚期卵巢癌患者在症状性质和持续时间上的不同[96,97]。

卵巢癌转移后极少没有症状。除了早期病变中可能出现的胃肠道和泌尿系症状外,腹水形成可以导致腹围增加。胸水形成可能引起呼吸困难并成为首发主诉。急性症状,包括附件肿瘤破裂或扭转,并不多见。阴道流血在绝经后卵巢癌女性中不多见,尽管绝经前女性可能有不规则出血或经量过多。盆腔检查发现附件包块有助于卵巢癌的早期诊断。由于恶性肿瘤发病较罕见且大部分可察觉的附件包块是良性的,盆腔检查发现的增大的卵巢一般不是恶性病变。在绝经前女性,卵巢癌罕见,在所有附件包块中占不到 7%[11]。即便在绝经后女性中,70%~80% 的附件肿瘤也是良性的。但是,在以腹部症状为主的患者中,盆腔检查通常被忽略而漏诊肿瘤。晚期病变的表现包括腹胀和与移动性浊音。这些症状并不特异,与腹腔内很多疾病有关,特别是其他部位原发的恶性病变,或者胃肠道和乳腺的转移性肿瘤。

诊断

卵巢癌通常经过开腹手术得以确诊,有时也可采用腹腔镜。如果出现可疑的盆腔包块,且很可能是卵巢癌,手术不应有不必要的延期。但是,在绝经前女性中,单纯卵巢囊性病变可监测 1~2 个月。病变活动性良好、单侧发生,且外形光滑者为恶性肿瘤的可能性小。绝经前患者的囊性病变如不到 8cm,可尝试口服避孕药治疗。对于绝经后的女性,如果囊肿超过 5cm,除非有慢性病史,都应切除。对于持续缩小的肿块可连续随访,而持续存在或增大的包块应该手术评估。相反,那些不规则、实性成分为主、活动度不同程度受限的包块,应进行开腹探查。

术前评估可以借助血液中的生物标志物。有三种算法可对良恶性盆腔肿块进行区分。联合超声检查、CA125 和绝经状态可计算恶性风险指数(risk of malignancy index,RMI),该指数预测盆腔肿物为卵巢癌的灵敏性为 71%～88%，特异性为 74%～97%[98]。OVA1 评价系统包含 CA125、载脂蛋白 A1、甲状腺素转运蛋白、转铁蛋白、B2 微球蛋白联合影像学及绝经状态，在绝经后女性中灵敏性可达 92%，特异性为 42%，在绝经前女性中灵敏性为 85%，特异性为 45%[99]。对于评价为低风险的女性阴性预测值为 94%～96%。不依靠影像，仅结合绝经状态，采用 CA125 和 HE4 数值计算出的恶性指数（罗马指数）可获得相似的灵敏性和更好的特异性。在转诊到研究中心的患者中进行的初步研究表明，预测恶性盆腔肿物的灵敏性为 93%，特异性为 75%，阴性预测值为 94%。在后续以社区人群为研究对象的试验中，灵敏性为 94%，特异性为 75%，阴性预测值为 99%[101]。罗马指数优于 RMI。OVA1 和罗马指数均获得 FDA 批准。使用这些评价方案可确保卵巢癌患者接受恰当的手术治疗。目前，在美国不足一半的卵巢癌女性接受的初始手术是经过培训的妇科肿瘤医师完成的满意肿瘤细胞减灭术。

超声提示恶性的指标包括盆腔附件区成分混杂的包块，如边界不规则；肿块内多种回声信号；致密的不规则分隔。尽管肿块的个体化特征更有意义，但是双侧的肿块更倾向于恶性。对于附件区的肿物，经阴道超声较经腹超声可以有更好的分辨率。多普勒彩色血流成像这种新技术可增强超声检查在诊断恶性病变方面的特异性。

影像技术，包括腹部平片、计算机成像（CT）扫描、PET-CT（正电子放射断层造影术）、磁共振成像（MRI），无法在手术前明确诊断为卵巢癌。有腹水但没有盆腔包块的患者可以用 CT 或 MRI 评估发现其他可能的腹水来源。不推荐穿刺，因为其增加种植转移和针刺道种植的风险。不必行头颅和骨扫描，除非有特别的症状提示转移到这些部位。

在绝经前女性，并不需要进行肠道的放射性检查，除非发现便潜血，或有症状提示上段或下段消化道梗阻。在绝经后女性中进行钡餐检查或内镜检查是合适的。乳腺钼靶可用于排除原发性乳腺癌，因为它可以和卵巢癌同时发生或转移到卵巢上。应行宫颈细胞学检查，尽管卵巢癌细胞很少经过子宫脱落到宫颈上。对于不规则阴道流血或月经过多的女性，应该行子宫内膜活检以排除原发的内膜病变。

附件包块的鉴别诊断包括多种卵巢功能改变、生殖道良性肿瘤及这些器官的炎性病变。输卵管积水、子宫内膜异位症、带蒂的子宫平滑肌瘤可类似卵巢肿瘤。非妇科疾病，如结肠和直肠的炎性病变，也应予排除。

筛查

目前没有良好的卵巢癌早期筛查策略。通过常规体格检查发现盆腔包块而手术则有助于在恶性病变转移前得到处理，但是传统的诊断技术仅发现不到 20%的处于Ⅰ期的病人。鉴于卵巢癌多发于绝经后人群，任何筛查策略必须是对早期病变高度特异（>99.6%）和高度敏感的（>75%），以达到 10%的 PPV（即 10 次开腹探查能够发现 1 例卵巢癌）。有研究正在评价超声和血清检查（如 CA125）用于卵巢癌早期诊断的意义。

超声

已经证实经阴道超声（TVS）对于盆腔包块的检测优于经腹超声（TAU）。在三项大规模研究中，66 620 例女性接受了 TVS 检查，565 例手术发现了 45 例卵巢癌，34 例是侵袭性的[102-104]。总体上发现早期病变的敏感性是 78%，但是特异性不足，因为每 12 例手术才能发现一例卵巢癌，而非预期的 10%的 PPV。最好的一项研究得到 9.9%的 PPV[103]。以多普勒超声进行确认检查的研究没有得到一致的结果。但是 3-D 超声的研究正在进行中，希望能改善从良性卵巢病变中鉴别恶性病变的特异性。

CA125

CA125 升高见于 50%～60%的Ⅰ期患者以及 90%的Ⅱ期患者[105]。CA125 能够在诊断前 10～60 个月开始升高，所有期别的肿瘤中平均在确诊前 1.9 年发生升高[106]。在前列腺、肺、结直肠和卵巢癌（PLCO）筛查研究中，37 500 位绝经后女性每年一次 CA125 和 TVS 检查，持续三年[107]。如果有任何一项异常，就被转诊给妇科肿瘤医师。单独 CA125 的 PPV 是 3.7%，单独 TVS 的 PPV 是 1%。如果两项均不正常，PPV 增加到 23.5%，但 60%的侵袭性卵巢癌会被漏诊。因此，单独 CA125 或 TVS 的特异性均不足以用于一般风险人群的筛查，但是在 CA125 升高的女性人群中序贯使用超声，这种两阶段的筛查方案可以提高特异性。根据 CA125 检测结果确定超声检查的策略已在瑞典和英国的研究中进行评价[108,109]。后者将 22 000 为女性随机分为传统监测组或实验组即每年监测 CA125，如果 CA125 升高则进行 TAU。如果 TAU 异常，则行手术。在 10 985 例筛查的女性中，29 例接受手术，发现 6 例卵巢癌，PPV 达 21%。在此后 7 年的随访中，实验筛查组又发现了 10 例卵巢癌，对照组诊断了 21 例。筛查组的中位生存期（72.9 个月）明显长于对照组（41.8 个月）（$P=0.0112$）。

卵巢癌风险评价

CA125 升高提示卵巢癌更具特异性。通过分析斯德哥尔摩和英国筛查研究中保存的 CA125 升高的血浆标本发现，持续随访个体数值随时间的变化可以提高 CA125 作为筛查方法的特异性[110,111]。未患卵巢癌的女性中升高的 CA125 水平保持不变，或逐渐降低，但是卵巢恶性病变的患者则倾向于持续上升。这一发现整合入应用年龄、CA125 变化速度和 CA125 绝对值的算法来计算个体的“卵巢癌风险”（risk of ovarian cancer algorithm，ROCA）。危险足够大的患者接受 TVS。在过去的 15 年间，MD Anderson SPORE 筹划了一项在卵巢癌患者中应用 ROCA 的研究。18 名患者基于上述评价方案接受手术治疗，6 名为良性病变，2 名为交界性病变（Ⅰ期），10 名为侵袭性卵巢癌，其中 7 名为早期（Ⅰ～Ⅱ）和 3 名为Ⅲ期。仅需要 3 例手术便可发现一例卵巢癌[112]。目前，一项已经完成的英国大型临床研究包含了 200 000 名绝经后女性，她们被随机分入三组：对照组（约 100 000 名）接受传统的盆腔检查；第二组（约 50 000 名）接受每年 TVS；第三组（约 50 000 名）接受至少每年一次 CA125 检查，基于 ROCA 的标准，第三组患者中部分接受 TVS 和/或手术。患者接受了三年的筛查并随访 7 年。在最初 3 年的“普查期”结果显示采用 ROCA 可更高比例的筛查出早期疾病（48%）并且仅需要进行 3～4 次手术便可发现一例病例[113]。研究的结果在 2015 年晚些时候公布，但是很显然与单纯采用

CA125 阈值的检测相比，使用 ROCA 可以使得筛查检测出的卵巢癌数量翻倍。随访第一年的结果显示 ROCA 联合 TVS 与单纯每年 TVS 相比特异性显著提高而不降低灵敏性。但是筛查是否改善患者的预后仍需要后续随访数据的支持。

无论目前英国的研究结果如何，基于单独 CA125 的诊断策略的灵敏性不太可能会超过 80%，因为 CA125 在 20% 的卵巢上皮癌中不表达。通过多种血清标志物的联合检测，在保证特异性不降低的情况下，可能实现更高的敏感性。其他两种生物标志物：HE4 和 CA72.4 可以发现一部分被 CA125 漏掉的病人。检测 *TP53* 的自身抗体可以发现 18% 被 CA125 漏诊的患者，并可提前 13~33 个月检出。

目前对一般风险女性的推荐

目前对整个女性人群进行除盆腔检查之外的卵巢癌筛查技术没有得到批准。单独使用 CA125 或超声的灵敏性和特异性不足。采用每年 CA125 检测联合 TVS 检测的方案似乎更有前景，但是在研究之外采用这种筛查方案仍需要 UKCTOCS 试验结果的支持。如果观察到生存时间和死亡率的显著改善，MD Anderson 的试验已经证明这个方案在美国可行。

目前对高危女性的推荐

尽管推荐采用超声和 CA125 对遗传 ROC 风险高的女性进行筛查，但是这种筛查对早期发现肿瘤和降低死亡率的效果未被验证。PBSO（预防性双侧输卵管卵巢切除）手术发现了许多隐匿于输卵管伞端的癌症，这个一致的发现提示对于遗传风险高的女性，卵巢超声可能无法早期发现癌症。由于这些高风险的人群主要包括绝经前女性，其 CA125 升高的假阳性率和 B 超异常的可能性更高，因而筛查方法可能出现问题。在这些高风险人群中，采用单纯 B 超或联合彩色血流多普勒进行初筛的假阳性率很高（2.5%~4.9%）。目前支持筛查的意见趋向于每 6~12 个月行一次超声检查，并且 3~6 个月行一次 CA125 检查。

目前有 5 项在高危人群中进行联合筛查的前瞻性研究[33,115~118]。在纳入 1 228 例有卵巢癌家族史的女性的三项筛查研究中，没有发现侵袭性卵巢癌，假阳性率为 0.4%~3.9%[33,48,49,115~119]。在余下的两项研究中，一项研究在接受筛查的 137 例高危女性中发现 1 例卵巢癌，假阳性率 0.7%；另一项研究筛查了 180 例女性，发现 9 例卵巢癌，假阳性率 3.9%[117,118]。两项针对荷兰 888 例 *BRCA1* 及 *BRCA2* 突变携带者及英国 279 例突变携带者采用每年经阴道超声和 CA125 筛查的前瞻性研究，结果并不乐观，提示在这些高危女性中筛查的获益很有限[48,49]。因此，通过每年筛查而降低 *BRCA1/2* 突变携带者死亡率的可能性很低。对要求进行筛查的高风险女性人群应充分知情，告知目前缺乏 CA125 或超声筛查的有效性证据及相关的假阳性率。尽管现有的策略存在这些风险和缺陷，许多人仍选择进行筛查。

分期

卵巢、输卵管和原发腹膜恶性肿瘤采用的手术病理分期依据 2014 版的新 FIGO 分期（表 104-5）。术前评估应除外腹腔外转移。疾病分期决定后续治疗，因此术中充分探查至关重要。对于剖腹探查术中经视诊和触诊整个腹腔未发现肉眼可见病灶的患者，应仔细探查寻找并活检，以发现镜下转移灶。在以往一组未接受标准手术分期的患者中，临床Ⅰ期卵巢上皮癌患者 5 年生存率仅约为 60%[4]。有报道经标准分期术后ⅠA 或ⅠB 期患者的生存率可达 90%~100%[4]。

表 104-5　卵巢癌、输卵管癌、腹膜癌 FIGO 分期（2014）

Ⅰ期	**肿瘤局限在卵巢或输卵管**
ⅠA	肿瘤局限在一侧卵巢（包膜完整）或输卵管；卵巢或输卵管表面无肿瘤；腹水细胞学或腹腔冲洗液无肿瘤细胞
ⅠB	肿瘤局限在双侧卵巢（包膜完整）或输卵管；卵巢或输卵管表面无肿瘤；腹水细胞学或腹腔冲洗液无肿瘤细胞
ⅠC	肿瘤局限在一侧或双侧卵巢或输卵管，同时合并以下任何一点 ⅠC1：肿瘤术中破裂 ⅠC2：肿瘤自发破裂或卵巢或输卵管表面有肿瘤 ⅠC3：腹水或冲洗液中有肿瘤细胞
Ⅱ期	**肿瘤累及一侧或双侧卵巢或输卵管同时合并盆腔扩散（真骨盆内）或原发腹膜癌**
ⅡA	侵犯和/或种植于子宫和/或输卵管和/或卵巢
ⅡB	侵犯其他盆腔腹膜内组织
Ⅲ期	**肿瘤累及一侧或双侧卵巢或输卵管或原发腹膜癌，合并细胞学或组织学证实的盆腔外腹腔种植和/或转移至腹膜后淋巴结**
ⅢA1	仅腹膜后淋巴结阳性（细胞学或组织学证实） ⅢA1（i）：转移淋巴结长径≤10mm ⅢA1（ii）：转移淋巴结长径>10mm
ⅢA2	盆腔外腹腔（真骨盆外）转移合并/不合并腹膜后淋巴结转移
ⅢB	临床可见盆腔外腹腔转移病灶最大径≤2cm，合并/不合并腹膜后淋巴结转移
ⅢC	临床可见盆腔外腹腔转移病灶最大径>2cm，合并/不合并腹膜后淋巴结转移（包括不侵犯脏器实质的肝、脾被膜转移）
Ⅳ期	**远处转移**
ⅣA	胸膜腔积液细胞学阳性
ⅣB	脏器实质转移和腹腔外器官转移（包括腹股沟淋巴结和腹腔外淋巴结转移）

FIGO，国际妇产科联合会（International Federation of Gynecology and Obstetrics）。

临床分期为Ⅰ~Ⅱ期的卵巢上皮癌患者发生转移并不少见。30%的肿瘤局限于盆腔的患者存在上腹部或腹膜后淋巴结的隐匿性转移[120]。组织学分级可预测隐匿性转移，组织分级为 G1、G2 和 G3 的患者中分期上升的比例分别为 16%、34%和 46%。

尽管文献强调彻底手术探查对于肿瘤局限于卵巢患者的重要性，但是如何理解肿瘤"侵犯"盆腔(如Ⅱ期)或腹腔器官(如Ⅲ期)仍有困难。如果存在独立于原发病灶的种植病灶或实性肿瘤侵犯邻近器官，对于手术医生不难确定分期。然而，肿瘤和邻近器官之间存在貌似良性的粘连，且无转移病灶或无明显侵犯邻近器官的情况更为常见。大量证据表明当卵巢肿瘤的良性粘连非常致密时，复发风险和Ⅱ期相当，这些患者更应被归为Ⅱ期而非Ⅰ期[120]。需要锐性解剖分离的粘连、分离粘连后存在粗糙区域、分离粘连时囊肿破裂，上述情况被认为是致密粘连。北美大多数中心临床实践中均将致密粘连的肿瘤分期升级为Ⅱ期，最近一项关于Ⅰ～Ⅱ期卵巢癌的多中心研究中也是这么做的[120]。

经全面分期术后为Ⅰ期或Ⅱ期的患者不足 25%。尽管Ⅰ期患者仅占 15%～20%，获得治愈的患者中将近 1/3～1/2 为Ⅰ期。由于Ⅰ期患者数量较少且远期预后较好(5 年无复发生存率超过 80%)，深入理解Ⅰ期患者的治疗存在困难。相应的，病例数量少和复发死亡率低都给开展Ⅲ期随机研究造成了困难。

预后

卵巢上皮癌的预后和诸多临床、病理因素相关。肿瘤期别、组织学分级、残存肿瘤大小均和预后密切相关[121,122]。如下文所述，分期较早的患者肿瘤组织学分级和预后相关(Ⅰ期患者中，与低级别患者相比，高级别患者的复发风险更高、生存更短)[122]。在晚期患者中残存肿瘤大小和预后明确相关[123]。完全切净肿瘤患者的预后最好。肿瘤复发距离末次化疗的时间同样和预后相关。大量研究表明 CA125 下降至一半的时间越短预后越好[124]。第 3 周期化疗后 CA125 降至正常患者的预后较好。恶性腹水提示预后不佳。

早期上皮癌的治疗

早期卵巢上皮癌和输卵管癌的治疗需要个体化。每个早期癌患者都应接受彻底的手术探查和准确分期。高复发风险的患者需接受辅助化疗。

手术

手术是Ⅰ期卵巢上皮癌的初始治疗，手术范围包括：经腹子宫切除、双附件切除和分期手术。某些情况也可行单侧附件切除，见后章节。

辅助化疗

GOG 报道了一项在早期卵巢癌患者中将卡铂联合紫杉醇 3 周期化疗对比 6 周期化疗的随机研究结果[125]。该研究中有大量患者(126，29%)手术分期结果记录不完整。6 周期化疗患者复发率较 3 周期化疗患者复发率降低了 24%，但无统计学差异(HR=0.76，95%CI 0.5～1.13 P=0.18)。6 周期化疗组和 3 周期化疗组 5 年复发率分别为 20.1%和 25.4%。该研究认为对于高复发风险的早期卵巢癌，特别是非浆液性癌患者，3 周期卡铂联合紫杉醇化疗是可选方案，而多数肿瘤学家仍推荐早期高级别浆液性癌患者接受 6 周期化疗。ICON1 和 ACTION 研究是两项关于早期卵巢癌的随机Ⅲ期研究[126,127]。将两项研究的数据合并分析，有 465 例患者随机至含铂方案辅助化疗组，460 例随机至观察组。在超过 4 年的中位随访期内，化疗组和观察组的总生存分别为 82%和 74%(HR=0.67，P=0.001)。化疗组和观察组无复发生存分别为 76%和 65%(HR=0.64，P=0.001)。鉴于大多数患者未接受彻底的分期手术，对于上述结果的解读仍需谨慎，但是对于未满意分期的患者应行含铂方案化疗。

浸润性早期低危肿瘤的处理(ⅠA 和ⅠB 期低级别肿瘤)

对于接受彻底手术探查没有卵巢外播散的患者，可选择行经腹子宫切除和双附件切除术。有生育需求的ⅠA 期二倍体病变(diploid lesions)患者，可保留子宫和对侧卵巢，但应通过规律的盆腔检查和 CA125 检测密切随访。通常在患者完成生育后应行子宫和对侧卵巢切除。最近 Guthrie 等报告了一项纳入 656 例早期卵巢上皮癌患者的研究结果，经标准分期为Ⅰ期、G1 的患者无一死于卵巢癌[129]。在标准分期的前提下，该组患者可获得 100%的生存。因此早期低危卵巢癌患者无须接受辅助化疗。

浸润性早期高危肿瘤的处理(ⅠA 和ⅠB 期高级别、ⅠC 和Ⅱ期肿瘤)

高危Ⅰ期是指ⅠA 或ⅠB 期 G3 的肿瘤、ⅠC 期肿瘤或透明细胞癌。对于组织学分化差或者腹水/腹腔冲洗液有肿瘤细胞的患者应接受辅助化疗。G2 和 G3、肿瘤致密粘连、大量腹水、腹水细胞学阳性的患者复发风险为 20%～45%，应接受术后辅助治疗。遗憾的是即使经过包括腹膜多点活检和腹膜后淋巴结取样这样的标准手术分期证实没有卵巢外病变，具有上述危险因素的患者仍有可能复发。早期高危卵巢上皮癌患者可接受卡铂单药或卡铂+紫杉类药物联合化疗。鉴于复发和死亡的风险超过 20%，推荐早期高危患者接受 6 周期卡铂[卡尔弗特公式的曲线下面积(AUC)5～6]联合紫杉醇化疗。

早期交界性肿瘤的处理

手术切除是卵巢交界瘤的主要治疗手段。术后化疗或放疗并不提高生存。冰冻病理诊断为交界性肿瘤，渴望保留卵巢功能的绝经前患者可行保守手术，如单侧附件切除，这可保留卵巢功能和生育功能。对于仅接受囊肿剔除术后病理明确为交界性肿瘤的患者无须补充手术。

关于局限性卵巢交界性肿瘤的治疗仍有争议。一定程度上是因为卵巢交界性肿瘤的诊断缺乏一致的标准。相对各期卵巢癌，交界性肿瘤的自然病程更缓慢。Ⅰ期和Ⅱ期交界性肿瘤患者接受辅助化疗并无获益。一项 GOG 大型研究中，有 51 例患者经病理复核诊断为交界性肿瘤，这组经标准分期后的患者无一死于交界性肿瘤。在这些研究中尽管大量患者的确接受了辅助化疗，但没有证据显示患者可获益。若间隔 1cm 连续切片排除了间质浸润，局限的交界性肿瘤患者不应接受辅助化疗。

晚期卵巢上皮癌的治疗

晚期卵巢上皮癌患者的治疗流程见图 104-6。具体治疗见后续章节。

肿瘤细胞减灭术

剖腹探查明确为晚期卵巢上皮癌的患者应接受肿瘤细胞减灭术，术中应尽可能切除原发肿瘤及转移病灶以提高后续治疗的效果。手术范围包括经腹全子宫双附件切除、网膜切除、腹膜表面及肠管等转移灶切除。盆腔肿瘤可能直接侵犯直肠、乙状结肠、末段回肠和盲肠。肿瘤局限于盆腔器官和网膜的患者，可切除这些器官达到无肉眼残存肿瘤，有机会获得完全缓解。

肿瘤细胞减灭术的基本原理是基于以下三点理论：①切除肿瘤可有潜在的生理获益；②改善肿瘤血液灌注、提高生长分数，增加对化疗或放疗的敏感性；③提高患者免疫力[131,132]。

肿瘤细胞减灭术的首要目的是切除全部原发肿瘤，如有可能也切除全部转移病灶。如果切除全部转移病灶难以实现，则应切除每个转移病灶至满意状态以减轻肿瘤负荷。“满意”的定义最早由 Griffiths 提出，他发现残存转移病灶最大径不超过

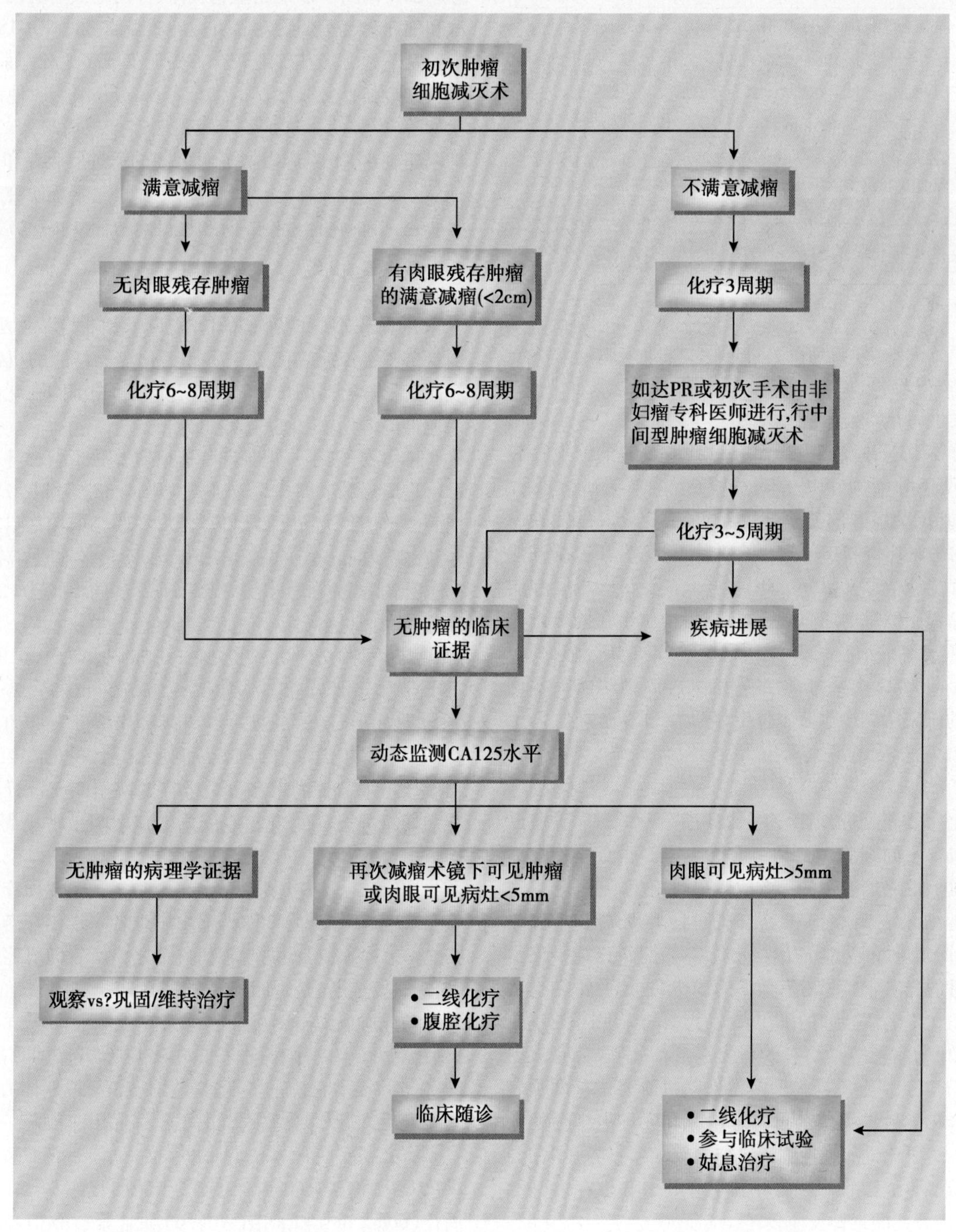

图 104-6　晚期卵巢上皮癌患者的治疗流程。在治疗以结果为基础的研究环境中进行。摘自 Berek 2015. Reproduced with permission of Wolters Kluwer Health

1.5cm 的患者生存显著优于残存病灶大于 1.5cm 的患者[133]。满意减瘤患者对化疗的有效率更高，无进展生存期更长(PFI)。后来 Hacker 等证实残存肿瘤最大径小于 5mm[定义为微小残存肿瘤(MRD)]患者的生存优于残存肿瘤最大径超过 5mm 的患者[134]。残存肿瘤<5mm 患者的中位生存期为 40 个月，而残存肿瘤>1.5cm 患者的中位生存期仅 18 个月(图 104-6)。转移灶的大小、腹膜转移瘤的范围、转移瘤的位置决定其是否可切除[135]。无肉眼残存肿瘤者的生存获益最大(表 104-6)。

表 104-6　卵巢癌残存肿瘤命名规则

残留病灶		状态
无	仅镜下可见	完全切除
镜下病灶		镜下残留
大体病灶	<5mm	微小残留
大体病灶	<1~2cm	满意减瘤
大体病灶	>1~2cm	不满意残留
大体病灶	>2~3cm	大块残留

根据化疗前残存病灶大小确定患者残存肿瘤状态的命名规则。

回顾既往数据表明妇科肿瘤医师施行肿瘤细胞减灭术的可行性为 70%~90%[131,134-143]。但仅 30%患者可达完全切除，主要并发症发生率在 5%左右，手术死亡率为 1%[136]。小肠切除并不增加总体手术并发症发生率。患者术后的中位生存和无铂间期与残存肿瘤大小相关。一项纳入 81 项研究共计 6 885 例Ⅲ期或Ⅳ期患者的荟萃分析提示，接受最大程度肿瘤细胞减灭术的患者比例和中位生存的对数正相关，在控制其他变量后依然有统计学意义($P<0.001$)[143]。接受最大程度肿瘤细胞减灭术患者比例每增加 10%，总体患者中位生存期可延长 5.5%。最大程度肿瘤细胞减灭术比例小于 25%的研究队列中患者中位生存期为 22.7 个月，而最程度大肿瘤细胞减灭术比例大于 75%的研究队列中患者中位生存期为 33.9 个月。

铂类联合紫杉类药物辅助化疗

系统性化疗是晚期卵巢上皮癌的标准治疗[144~169]。业已研究过多种包含不同细胞毒药物组合的方案。联合化疗在大多数晚期卵巢上皮癌患者中的疗效优于单药化疗。

荟萃分析结果表明顺铂和卡铂在卵巢上皮癌中疗效相当[164]。紫杉醇对卵巢癌十分有效[144,145]。Ⅱ期研究结果显示在既往化疗过的患者中紫杉醇有效率为 36%，这比顺铂初次治疗有效率高。在未满意减瘤的既往未化疗过的患者中，顺铂单药有效率为 70%，紫杉醇单药有效率为 42%，二者联合有效率为 70%(GOG132)[148]。三项大型前瞻性随机研究中有两项表明紫杉醇联合铂类较铂类单药可有总生存和无进展生存的获益[146,147,160]。两项随机前瞻性临床研究比较了紫杉醇+卡铂与紫杉醇+顺铂两种方案[157,158]，两种方案有效率和生存时间相似，但是含卡铂方案的毒性反应较轻。

多西他赛对比紫杉醇

多西他赛单药在铂耐药复发卵巢癌患者中有效率为 23%~28%。Ⅱ期研究中多西他赛联合顺铂或卡铂的有效率可达 66%~81%[168]。SCOTROC 研究将多西他赛(75mg/m^2 输注 1h)联合卡铂(AUC 5)和紫杉醇(175mg/m^2)联合卡铂(AUC 5)进行了比较[169]。两种方案疗效相当，但是多西他赛联合卡铂组神经毒性明显减少。因此，可考虑给因糖尿病等合并症而伴有明显神经病变的患者选用卡铂联合多西他赛。

其他双药和三药方案

铂类联合紫杉类药物可改善中位无进展生存期和总生存期，但是晚期卵巢癌患者的预后依然令人失望。最终绝大多数患者都将耐药。多柔比星脂质体、吉西他滨、拓扑替康、长春瑞滨和依托泊苷等药物对复发性卵巢癌有效。GOG182 研究探索卡铂及紫杉醇的基础上联合吉西他滨或多柔比星脂质体，以及卡铂联合拓扑替康序贯卡铂紫杉醇或卡铂吉西他滨序贯卡铂紫杉醇方案[170]。这是关于卵巢癌迄今规模最大的研究，共计纳入超过 4 000 例患者。各组之间的无进展生存和总生存无统计学差异，但各组间副反应存在差异。基于该研究以及其他一些研究，卡铂联合紫杉醇依然是目前的标准化疗方案。

剂量密集化疗

有临床前研究及临床研究表明卡铂联合紫杉醇剂量密集、剂量分割化疗疗效优于 3 周方案化疗。可能的机制包括每周规律紫杉醇给药的抗血管效应、降低肿瘤细胞在化疗间隔内的加速再群体化、减少获得性耐药[171,172]。

JGOG 开展了一项Ⅲ期临床研究比较了紫杉醇联合卡铂剂量密集周疗和 3 周疗。该研究共纳入 637 例 FIGO 分期Ⅱ~Ⅳ期的卵巢癌患者，患者随机至紫杉醇联合卡铂剂量密集周疗组(紫杉醇 80mg/m^2、卡铂 AUC 6)或紫杉醇联合卡铂 3 周疗组(紫杉醇 180mg/m^2、卡铂 AUC 6)[173]。中位随访 29 个月后，3 周疗组和剂量密集周疗组患者中位无进展生存分别为 17.2 个月和 28 个月(HR=0.71,95%CI 0.58~0.88,P=0.001 5)，三年总生存率分别为 65.1%和 72.1%(HR=0.75,95%CI 0.57~0.98,P=0.03)(图 11-19)。残存病灶超过 1cm 的患者中位生存期剂量密集周疗组为 17.6 个月，3 周疗组为 12.1 个月。残存病灶小于 1cm 的患者中位生存期两组间无统计学差异。残存病灶超过 1cm 的患者中位总生存期剂量密集周疗组优于 3 周疗组(51.2 个月 vs 33.5 个月)。

该研究认为相比常规化疗，接受剂量密集周疗患者可获得生存获益，可作为晚期卵巢上皮癌患者一线化疗潜在的标准方案之一。PFS 和 OS 的改善超过了之前所有卵巢癌Ⅲ期研究的结果。这些获益是否因日本人群在药物基因组学或药效动力学的差异所致尚不明确。一些研究提示亚洲人群卵巢癌患者预后显著好于白种人群[174]。一项 GOG 开展的Ⅲ期研究(Protocol 218)提示在校正了年龄、期别、残存肿瘤、体力状态和组织学类型后，亚洲卵巢癌人群的总生存优于白种人[175]。

有必要在白种人中验证 JGOG 研究。一项意大利的研究(MITO-7;NCT00660842)比较了卡铂周疗(AUC 2)联合紫杉醇周疗(60mg/m^2)和卡铂(AUC 6)联合紫杉醇(175mg/m^2)3 周方案。周疗方案并不显著改善 PFS(18.8 个月 vs 16.5 个月)，但患者生活质量更高、不良反应率更低[176]。GOG262 研究设计和 JGOG3016 类似[177]，主要区别在于两组患者可接受贝伐珠单抗治疗(15mg/kg,每 3 周重复)。经治医生和患者共同决定是否使用贝伐珠单抗。大部分患者(84%)接受了贝伐珠单抗治疗直至疾病进展。大部分入组患者存在肉眼残存病灶(63%),13%的患者接受过新辅助化疗。仅 24%的患者有镜下残存病灶。两组中位无进展生存期均为 14 个月。有 112 例患者没有接受贝伐珠单抗,两组间人数相当。剂量密集周疗组未接受贝伐珠单抗患者中位无进展生存期 14.2 个月,3 周疗组未接受贝伐珠单抗患者中位无进展生存期 10.3 个月。但这仅是亚组分析,无法得出确定的结论。

腹腔化疗

鉴于肿瘤组织在腹膜表面播散并经常在这些位置复发,研究者们探索了腹腔内给药以获得更高的局部药物浓度。SWOG 和妇科肿瘤学组 GOG 开展了一项随机前瞻研究,在残存肿瘤小于 2cm 的患者中比较顺铂($100mg/m^2$)腹腔给药和静脉给药,同时联合环磷酰胺($600mg/m^2$)的效果[178]。腹腔给药组患者较静脉给药组总生存有显著延长(49 个月 vs 41 个月,$P=0.03$)。在残存肿瘤小于 0.5cm 的患者中,两组的中位生存期无显著差异(51 个月 vs 46 个月,$P=0.08$)。

上述研究结论公布时正值紫杉醇开始用于临床实践。GOG 开展的后续研究中比较了顺铂($75mg/m^2$)联合紫杉醇($135mg/m^2$ 24h 持续输注)静脉给药和剂量强度方案。剂量强度方案具体为卡铂(AUC 9)诱导化疗 2 周期,随后予以顺铂 $100mg/m^2$ 联合紫杉醇($135mg/m^2$ 24h 持续输注)[179]。患者中位无进展生存期在剂量强度组和对照组分别为 27.7 个月 vs 22.5 个月($P=0.02$),但是两组患者总生存期无统计学差异(52.9 个月 vs 47.6 个月,$P=0.059$)。

2006 年 GOG 公布了一项重要标志性研究的结果,该研究对比了顺铂紫杉醇腹腔静脉联合化疗与顺铂紫杉醇静脉化疗的结果[180]。429 例患者参加随机,最终 415 例患者可进行分析。中位无进展生存在腹腔化疗组和静脉化疗组分别为 23.8 个月和 18.3 个月($P=0.05$)。中位总生存在腹腔化疗组和静脉化疗组分别为 65.6 个月和 49.7 个月($P=0.03$)。静脉化疗组 90%的患者完成了既定 6 周期化疗,而腹腔化疗组仅有 42%的患者完成了既定 6 周期化疗,其余患者均转换至静脉化疗组。导管相关并发症是腹腔化疗组中断治疗的主要原因。但腹腔化疗组其他不良事件的发生率更高,大多数患者出现严重乏力、腹痛、血液学毒性、恶心呕吐和代谢及神经毒性。通过经验积累、合适的剂量调整和更好的止吐药物有可能减轻不良反应。连同之前的研究结果,NCI 临床公告推荐经满意减瘤的Ⅲ期卵巢癌患者可考虑腹腔化疗,这在美国已广泛开展。

Cochrane 综述及另外一篇荟萃分析提示,腹腔化疗较静脉化疗可获得更好的效果[181,182]。这篇荟萃分析纳入了 6 项随机临床试验共计 1 716 例卵巢癌患者,结果提示顺铂腹腔化疗组较静脉化疗组患者复发风险降低 20.8%($HR=0.792$,95%CI 0.688~0.912,$P=0.001$),死亡风险降低 20.1%($HR=0.799$,95%CI 0.702~0.910,$P=0.0007$)。作者认为这些证据强烈支持满意减瘤的Ⅲ期卵巢癌患者在一线化疗中采用顺铂腹腔化疗可以改善生存。Cochrane 综述也得出相似的观点。作者指出腹腔化疗可使患者获益,可延长满意减瘤的Ⅲ期卵巢癌患者的总生存和无进展生存期。但是研究者同时指出腹腔化疗存在导管相关并发症和更高的不良反应发生率,需要在后续的临床研究中探索腹腔化疗的最佳剂量、给药时机、给药机制等问题。目前腹腔化疗仍有争议,一些学者认为截止目前的研究并非纯粹的探索腹腔化疗,而且存在缺陷。这些学者对腹腔化疗的技术问题和较严重的不良反应存在担心[183]。尽管卵巢癌患者的初始治疗需要个体化,但由于满意减瘤的Ⅲ期卵巢癌患者存在总生存方面的优势,应考虑是否所有满意减瘤者都需要腹腔化疗。GOG172 最近更新的生存结果强调了腹腔化疗的价值。腹腔化疗组患者和静脉化疗组患者的中位生存期分别为 61.8 个月(95%CI 55~69.5)和 51.4 个月(95%CI 46~58.2)。腹腔化疗可使患者疾病死亡风险降低 23%(校正 $HR=0.77$,95%CI 0.65~0.90,$P=0.002$),腹腔化疗周期数越多生存期越长[184]。

新辅助化疗

一些学者建议对于术前评估无法满意减瘤的Ⅲ期和Ⅳ期卵巢癌患者可在肿瘤细胞减灭术前给予化疗。耶鲁大学 Schwartz 等学者将一组新辅助化疗+手术+辅助化疗患者和既往在该中心接受肿瘤细胞减灭术+辅助化疗患者的历史数据进行了比较[185]。2~3 周期的新辅助化疗对合并大量胸腹腔积液的患者有益。新辅助化疗可减少浆膜腔积液,改善患者的体力状态,减少术后并发症,尤其是胸部并发症的发生。Bristow 等总结了有关新辅助化疗的系统性综述,经有经验的卵巢癌手术团队评估为无法满意减瘤的患者,新辅助化疗是可行的替代方案[186]。但是目前的数据提示采用新辅助化疗患者的生存仍劣于接受满意的初次减瘤术患者。

1995 年,EORTC 报告了一项关于中间型肿瘤细胞减灭术的前瞻随机研究的结果。初次手术未达到满意减瘤的患者接受 3 周期含铂方案化疗后行中间型肿瘤细胞减灭术。接受中间型肿瘤细胞减灭术组患者较对照组患者生存有获益[187]。经过 10 年的随访,随机至中间型肿瘤细胞减灭术组患者的死亡风险降低超过 40%[188]。可是 GOG 开展的一项关于中间型肿瘤细胞减灭术的前瞻Ⅲ期研究并未证实上述结论[189]:接受中间型肿瘤细胞减灭术的 216 例患者中位生存期为 32 个月,未行中间型肿瘤细胞减灭术的 209 例患者中位生存期为 33 个月。研究者认为两组患者生存无统计差异的原因可能是患者入组前已经由妇科肿瘤医师尽最大努力完成了减瘤手术[190]。

有些学者认为新辅助化疗+中间型肿瘤细胞减灭术适用于体力状态较差的患者[185,191,192]。2010 年,Vergote 等报告了 EORTC-NCIC 一项对比初次肿瘤细胞减灭术和中间型肿瘤细胞减灭术的研究结果[193]。该研究纳入了 670 例ⅢC~Ⅳ期卵巢癌、输卵管癌和原发性腹膜癌患者。所有患者均为肿瘤广泛的ⅢC 期和Ⅳ期患者。超过 60%的患者转移病灶直径超过 10cm,74.5%的患者转移病灶直径超过 5cm。患者被随机分至直接肿瘤细胞减灭术+至少 6 周期含铂化疗组或 3 周期新辅助化疗,如患者肿瘤化疗有效或稳定,则接受中间型肿瘤细胞减灭术,术后接受至少 3 周期含铂化疗。直接手术组和新辅助化疗组患者中位生存期分别为 29 个月和 30 个月。两组患者无进展生存期均为 12 个月,可能和纳入患者本身预后较差有关。接受新辅助化疗组患者的术后并发症率和死亡率低于直接手术组。

在两组患者中，完全切除肿瘤是总生存最重要的独立预后因素。这项研究的结果饱受质疑和批评[194~197]。Du Bois 等发现该研究纳入患者的体力状态比大多数研究中患者的体力状态差，而且肿瘤完全切除率在不同国家之间差异较大，并相对较低[194]。在直接肿瘤细胞减灭术组，仅有约 20%的患者达到了无肉眼残存肿瘤，这一比例远低于有经验的中心的数据。满意减瘤比例在不同国家之间差别较大，从比利时的 62%到荷兰的 3.9%不等，这说明各国家手术能力有差异。该研究的中位总生存仅 30 个月，远低于其他满意减瘤+辅助化疗研究所报道的超过 60 个月，提示该研究纳入了体力状态较差、疾病较晚的患者。

另有两项关于新辅助化疗的随机研究已完成了入组。第一项是在英国开展的研究，设计类似 EORTC 的 CHORUS 研究[198]。最近该研究公布了结果，和 EORTC 的结果非常类似。552 例患者随机分为两组，一组患者接受新辅助化疗+中间期肿瘤细胞减灭术+3 周期化疗，另一组患者接受直接肿瘤细胞减灭术+6 周期含铂方案化疗。直接手术组满意减瘤率仅为 16%，新辅助化疗组满意减瘤率为 40%。两组的中位手术时长均为 120min，对于完成最大限度的减瘤手术来说都不足够。直接手术组患者术后并发症发生率（5.6%）明显高于预期，这可能和入组患者的选择有关。直接手术组和新辅助化疗组的中位 PFS 分别为 10.7 个月和 12 个月，没有显著差异；中位总生存期分别为 22.6 个月和 24.1 个月。死亡的风险比是 0.87，有利于新辅助化疗组，单侧 90%CI 的上限是 0.98（95%CI 0.72~1.05）。直接手术组患者术后 28 天内的严重并发症和死亡发生率更高。作者认为Ⅲ或Ⅳ期卵巢癌患者接受新辅助化疗的生存不劣于接受直接手术，对于部分患者是合理的治疗选择。

对于新辅助化疗的观点仍有分歧。一项调研提示 82%的 SGO 成员认为并没有足够的证据支持新辅助化疗[199]。相反，70%的 ESMO 会员认为已有足够的证据推荐新辅助化疗。基于上述的考虑，在患者的整个治疗过程中尽早实施肿瘤细胞减灭术仍是标准治疗[200]。新辅助化疗适用于体力状态或营养状态较差的患者，新辅助化疗后行中间减瘤术可降低患者术后并发症的发生率。

贝伐珠单抗辅助治疗

抗血管生成药物如贝伐珠单抗在复发卵巢癌中显示出疗效及益处，基于此，开展了两项大规模随机研究，旨在探讨晚期卵巢癌患者中标准卡铂加紫杉醇辅助治疗的基础上加用贝伐珠单抗的作用。已有证据表明在其他类型的肿瘤中，如结肠癌、肺癌，在化疗的基础上加用贝伐珠单抗能够增加有效率、延长无进展生存期及总生存期[201,202]。

两项大规模的Ⅲ期研究（GOG 218 和 ICON 7）探讨了贝伐珠单抗在一线治疗中的作用。GOG 218 是一项三臂的随机研究，共招募了 1 873 位Ⅲ期或Ⅳ期卵巢癌、输卵管癌及腹膜癌患者[203]。Ⅲ期患者要求有肉眼可见的残存病灶。所有患者被随机分入以下三组：①对照组患者进行 6 个周期的紫杉醇+卡铂化疗，第二至第六周期加用安慰剂，随后每 3 周一次单药安慰剂，共 22 个周期；②患者接受 6 个周期的标准方案化疗，第二至第六周期加用贝伐珠单抗（15mg/kg），随后单独使用安慰剂共 22 个周期；③患者进行 6 个周期的标准方案化疗，第二至第六周期加用贝伐珠单抗，然后继续贝伐珠单抗单药治疗共 22 个周期。中位随访时间 17.4 个月，第 2 组化疗期间加用贝伐珠单抗组与对照组相比疾病进展或死亡风险相似（$HR = 0.908$，$P = 0.16$），贝伐珠单抗联合化疗并维持治疗组与对照组相比疾病进展或死亡风险显著降低（$HR = 0.717$，$P < 0.001$）。在进行无进展生存时间（PFS）分析时排除了 CA125 升高的患者，对照组中位 PFS 为 12 个月，贝伐珠单抗维持治疗组为 18 个月（$HR = 0.645$，$P = 0.001$）。最近，对 GOG 218 研究的所有患者进行独立影像学评估，结果也证实了这一观点。迄今为止，总体生存时间（OS）似乎无明显差异，这可能是因为许多病人在复发后接受了多种后续方案的治疗，包括交叉使用贝伐珠单抗或其他抗血管内皮生长因子（VEGF）药物，这些药物可能潜在的影响总体生存时间。

ICON 7 与 GOG 218 研究设计相似，共入组 1 528 例高危型（透明细胞或高级别）患者[204]。除了Ⅲ期和Ⅳ期患者，Ⅰ期和Ⅱ期卵巢癌、输卵管癌或腹膜癌患者也被纳入。入组患者被随机分入 6 周期化疗组或 6 周期化疗加贝伐珠单抗治疗组（7.5mg/kg），之后 12 周期每 3 周一次的贝伐珠单抗维持治疗。中位随访时间 19.4 个月，对照组中位 PFS 为 17.3 个月，贝伐珠单抗组为 19 个月（$HR = 0.81$，$P = 0.004$）。中位随访 28 个月时，贝伐珠单抗组 PFS 的改善仍得以维持。探索性的 OS 分析显示高危亚组（残存肿瘤>1cm 的Ⅲ期和Ⅳ期）患者的生存显著改善（$HR = 0.64$，$P = 0.002$）。最近新发表的生存分析数据也证实了这一观点，高危亚组的中位生存时间从 35 个月延长至 39 个月，改善了 4 个月[205]。然而，ICON 研究总人群中两组间无生存优势。贝伐珠单抗可导致毒性反应增加，包括出血（主要是 1 级的皮肤黏膜出血）、2 级及以上高血压（贝伐珠单抗组 18% vs 标准治疗组 2%）、3 级及以上血栓形成（贝伐珠单抗组 7% vs 标准治疗组 3%）以及胃肠道穿孔（贝伐珠单抗组发生 10 例 vs 标准治疗组发生 3 例）。

与 GOG 218 研究相比，ICON 7 研究包括了晚期肿瘤术后无肉眼残存病灶的患者，同时包括高危型早期肿瘤患者。ICON 7 研究中，使用了较低剂量的贝伐珠单抗（7.5mg/kg vs GOG 218 的 15mg/kg），持续了较短的维持治疗时间（12 周期 vs 16 周期）。两组研究中，停用贝伐珠单抗几个月后 PFS 曲线趋于一致，表明抗血管生成治疗能够延缓，但不能阻止疾病进展。这引发了对高危型患者进行无限期治疗的合理性的话题。这点目前正在进行研究，但对成本效益有显著的影响。目前还没有好的生物标记物能预测哪些的患者最可能从贝伐珠单抗联合一线治疗中获益，最佳剂量也有待明确。

晚期侵袭性卵巢癌的治疗

一次的化疗：卡铂（AUC 5~6）联合紫杉醇（175mg/m^2，滴注超过 3h）（表 104-7）。正如之前讨论的，和加用贝伐珠单抗一样，剂量密集方案或腹腔灌注方案也是基于循证医学的选择。有严重神经病变风险的患者，以糖尿病患者为例，可以采取替代方案即多西他赛（75mg/m^2）和卡铂（AUC 5），可以降低神经毒性。对于无法耐受紫杉烷毒性的患者，单药卡铂（AUC 5~6）化疗也是一种合理的选择。

表 104-7　晚期上皮性卵巢癌、输卵管癌及腹膜癌的化疗：推荐方案

药物	剂量	应用时间/h	间隔	治疗周期数
标准方案				
卡铂紫杉醇	AUC=5~6	3	每3周	6~8个周期
	175mg/m²			
卡铂紫杉醇	AUC=5	3	每3周	6个周期
	80mg/m²		每周	18周
卡铂多西他赛	AUC=5	3	每周	6个周期
	75mg/m²		每3周	
顺铂紫杉醇	75mg/m²	3	每3周	6个周期
	135mg/m²	24		
卡铂（单药）[a]	AUC=4~6	3	每3周	6个周期可耐受时

[a] 年老、体弱或状态不佳的患者。
AUC，卡尔弗特公式的曲线下面积。
摘自 Reproduced from Berek et al.，2015，p. 510[130]。

晚期交界性肿瘤的治疗

化疗对于晚期交界性肿瘤患者的作用是不确定的，而且有争议。GOG 正在评估化疗对于初次手术后复发的晚期交界性肿瘤的作用。在知道这项试验结果前，现有的治疗方案主要是手术。患者应该进行肿瘤细胞减灭术，术后随访观察。交界性肿瘤即使是晚期，也有良好的预后。首次有症状的复发可能发生在诊断后的数年。与晚期侵袭性卵巢上皮癌 20%~25%的生存率相比，Ⅲ期交界性肿瘤患者的生存率超过 60%。因此，再次肿瘤细胞减灭术通常可以创造另一段长期无症状的生存期。化疗疗效不确切并且反应率低，但对于不能进行肿瘤细胞减灭术的患者可行化疗。

临床无肿瘤患者的疗效评估

很多上皮性卵巢癌患者经过理想的肿瘤细胞减灭术和后续的治疗后可能在治疗结束后没有疾病证据。已经证明肿瘤标记物和放射性评估过于不敏感，以至于无法精确除外亚临床病灶的存在[206~208]。二次探查手术是曾用来评估残存病灶的一项技术，由于目前可使用的化疗的作用，二次探查开腹手术并不影响患者的生存，故现已不再常规使用[209,210]。二次探查手术仅在研究的情况下进行，为了评价可能受病灶大小影响的二线或挽救性治疗的作用，如免疫治疗或抗自噬治疗。

维持治疗

辅助化疗后实现临床完全缓解的患者的最佳管理措施仍有待确定。即使是手术明确已经完全缓解的患者也有 30%~50%的复发率。一些研究者推荐进行二次探查开腹手术，以鉴别出可能需要进行腹腔灌注治疗的患者[211]。然而，没有证据能够证明静脉辅助化疗后常规行腹腔灌注能延长生存。

已经开展临床研究来评价维持化疗是否对手术证实临床完全缓解的患者有益。GOG 和 SWOG 进行了一项研究，比较 3 周期和 12 周期每月一次的紫杉醇（135~175mg/m² 静脉滴注超过 3h）巩固化疗在初始紫杉醇和卡铂化疗后临床缓解的患者中的作用[212]。3 周期和 12 周期紫杉醇化疗组无进展间期分别是 21 个月和 28 个月（$P=0.035$）。结果，9 个月的额外化疗增加了 7 个月的无进展生存期。目前为止，两组的总体生存时间没有差异。在欧洲，有两项安慰剂对照的随机临床研究，紫杉醇和卡铂化疗后临床缓解的患者接受 4 个周期的拓扑替康巩固化疗。两项研究中，研究组与安慰剂组相比生存期均没有改善[213,214]。

随访检查

最佳的随访检查频率尚不确定，但是完成化疗并且临床缓解的患者可以在 1~2 年内每 3 个月行一次盆腔和 CA125 检查。CA125 升高可先于出现复发的临床表现或症状近 3~6 个月。GCIG（Gynecologic Cancer Inter Group）为 CA125 进展制定了标准的定义，现已广泛应用于临床研究：治疗前 CA125 升高、随后曾降至正常的患者，必须在间隔一周以上两次随机检测时 CA125 大于或等于正常上限的 2 倍；治疗前 CA125 升高治疗过程中未曾降至正常的患者，必须在间隔一周以上两次随机检测时 CA125 大于或等于谷底值的 2 倍。

CA125 升高可能会促使进行 CT 检查。PET 扫描在这种情况下的作用还不明确。最近一篇综述总结到，PET 检查发现复发卵巢癌的敏感性约 90%，特异性约 85%。对于 CA125 升高而传统影像不能作出判断或检查阴性时，PET 检查对复发的诊断可能尤其有用，但这一作用尚存争议。氟-18 脱氧葡萄糖（^{18}FDG）-PET/CT 设备能同时进行^{18}FDG-PET 摄取和 CT 成像，可能对于检测复发卵巢癌更有价值；这项技术有助于筛选可能受益于再次肿瘤细胞减灭术的复发患者[215]。

初步缓解的患者，在体格检查或 CT 扫描没有变化而仅有 CA125 升高确实是个难题。目前，额外的化疗并不推荐用于仅有 CA125 升高而没有临床症状或影像学复发证据的情况。有时患者可给予他莫昔芬或阿那曲唑治疗，尽管 20%的患者可能出现 CA125 稳定或下降，但这项干预措施的作用并不明确。GOG 比较了他莫昔芬和沙利度胺在 CA125 升高但没有其他复发证据的患者中的作用。研究观察到两者疗效相似，但他莫昔芬的毒性更小。也有一些研究用 CA125 升高评估新型细胞抑制靶向药物的活性。随着更多有效的挽救性治疗可以使用，血清标记物如 CA125 可能会发挥更大的用处。对于从未发现胸腔转移或从未有胸腔积液的患者，不强制进行胸部放射性检查随诊。如果没有 CA125 的升高，化疗后的前三年应该谨慎使用 CT 和 MRI 扫描进行随访。

复发上皮性卵巢癌的治疗

大部分复发的女性会接受进一步的化疗，可能的获益部分取决于初始治疗的反应和反应持续时间。治疗的目标包括缓解疾病相关症状，保持或改善生活质量，推迟疾病进展的时间，

并尽可能延长生存，尤其是对于铂敏感复发的患者。许多有效的化疗药物（铂类、紫杉醇、拓扑替康、多柔比星脂质体、多西他赛、吉西他滨、培美曲塞和依托泊苷）及靶向药物（贝伐珠单抗）可以使用，治疗的选择基于许多因素，包括可能的获益、潜在的毒性和患者的依从性[216,217]。初始治疗后大于6个月复发的女性归为“铂敏感复发”，通常继续接受铂类为基础的化疗，缓解率为27%～65%，中位生存时间为12个月～24个月[218,219]。一线化疗后6个月内复发的患者归为“铂耐药复发”，中位生存时间6个月～9个月，化疗缓解率可能为10%～30%。治疗过程中病情进展的患者属于“铂难治性”。铂难治性卵巢癌患者对化疗的客观缓解率非常低，通常小于10%[216]。

铂敏感复发肿瘤

总体而言，随机研究表明铂类为基础的联合化疗的缓解率、中位无进展生存和总体生存率均优于单药铂类化疗。两项多国Ⅲ期随机研究[220]和一项Ⅱ期随机研究[221]比较了铂类联合紫杉醇化疗和铂类单药化疗的效果。在ICON4和AGO-OVAR-2.2研究报告中，802例在无治疗间隔至少6～12个月的铂敏感复发卵巢癌，随机被分为铂类为基础的化疗组（72%卡铂或顺铂单药；17%环磷酰胺、多柔比星和顺铂；4%卡铂加顺铂；3%顺铂加多柔比星）和紫杉醇加铂类为基础的化疗组（80%紫杉醇加卡铂；10%紫杉醇加顺铂；5%紫杉醇加卡铂和顺铂；4%紫杉醇单药）。AGO-OVAR-2.2研究未达到计划入组人数。在两项研究中，很大比例的患者最初未接受紫杉醇化疗。综合这些研究进行分析，在42个月的中位随访时间内，紫杉醇联合治疗组有显著的生存获益（HR=0.82）。绝对2年生存获益是7%（57% vs 50%），中位生存时间改善了5个月（29个月vs 24个月）。紫杉醇方案的PFS更好（HR=0.76）。1年PFS有10%的差异（50% vs 40%），中位PFS延长了3个月（13个月vs 10个月）。除了紫杉醇组神经毒性和脱发的发生率更高，而不含紫杉醇组骨髓抑制发生率更高外，两组毒性相当。

两项随机试验比较了卡铂单药与卡铂联合吉西他滨或卡铂联合多柔比星脂质体[222,223]。联合治疗组缓解率更高，PFS更长，但研究不足以评价总体生存。其中GCIG研究比较了卡铂联合吉西他滨与卡铂单药，联合组缓解率为47.2%，卡铂组为30.9%，PFS分别为8.6个月和5.8个月。SWOG研究比较了卡铂单药与卡铂联合多柔比星脂质体，因为入组速度慢被提前终止。共入组61例患者，联合治疗组缓解率为67%，卡铂组缓解率为32%。PFS是12个月vs 8个月，有趣的是，总生存期分别是26个月vs 18个月（P=0.02）[224]。法国的一项Ⅱ期研究证实了在铂敏感复发的卵巢癌患者中，卡铂联合多柔比星脂质体化疗的有效率高，为67%。

一项大规模的GCIG研究（CALYPSO）招募了约1 000名患者，对卡铂联合多柔比星脂质体（CD）与卡铂联合紫杉醇（CP）进行比较。中位随访时间为22个月，CD组PFS优于CP组，并有统计学意义（HR=0.821，95%CI 0.72～0.94，P=0.005）；中位PFS分别为11.3个月和9.4个月。总的来说，CP组发生严重的非血液学毒性（36.8% vs 28.4%，P=0.01）导致提早中断治疗（15% vs 6%，P=0.001）的概率更高。可以看到，CP组发生2级及以上脱发（83.6% vs 7%）、过敏反应（18.8% vs 5.6%）、感觉神经病变（26.9% vs 4.9%）的频率更高；CD组发生手足综合征（2～3级12% vs 2.2%）、恶心（35.2% vs 24.2%）和黏膜炎（2～3级13.9% vs 7%）更多。这项研究表明多柔比星脂质体联合卡铂与紫杉醇联合卡铂相比，PFS更优，治疗指数更好。目前这种治疗方案被广泛采用。

一些研究者猜测使用非铂类药物治疗可延长无铂间期，一段时间后能使肿瘤再次变得对铂更敏感[225]。然而，没有数据能够支持非铂类药物的插入延长了距末次铂类化疗的间隔，导致铂敏感性增加这一假说。

研究者对非铂类药物作为二线治疗进行了研究[226,227]，包括一项曲贝替定联合多柔比星脂质体对比单药多柔比星脂质体的大规模Ⅲ期研究[228]。这项研究包括铂敏感复发及铂耐药复发患者。在铂敏感复发患者中，曲贝替定联合多柔比星脂质体治疗的有效率更高（35% vs 23%），中位PFS分别为9.2个月和1.5个月（HR=0.73，95%CI 0.56～0.95，P=0.017 0）[228]。作者没有报道铂敏感或铂耐药患者后续接受含铂化疗后的有效率，也没有报道是否在增加无铂间期后能明显增加肿瘤对铂类的反应性。

OCEANS研究是贝伐珠单抗用于484例铂敏感复发卵巢癌的随机研究。患者距一线含铂治疗≥6个月复发，且有可测量病灶，随机进行卡铂联合吉西他滨加贝伐珠单抗或安慰剂治疗6个周期～10个周期，持续给予贝伐珠单抗或安慰剂直到疾病进展。主要研究终点是PFS，根据RECIST进行疗效评估。贝伐珠单抗组的PFS优于安慰剂组（HR= 0.484，95%CI 0.388～0.605，P<0.000 1）。贝伐珠单抗组PFS为12.4个月，安慰剂组为8.4个月。加用贝伐珠单抗组的客观缓解率（78.5% vs 57.4%，P<0.000 1）及缓解期（10.4个月vs 7.4个月；HR=0.534，95%CI 0.408～0.698）明显改善。未进行生活质量评估，但未观测到新的或不可预测的毒性反应。这项研究的结果支持贝伐珠单抗在部分铂敏感复发卵巢癌患者中的作用。

其他形式的抗血管生成治疗正在通过临床研究进行评估[229]。VEGF捕获剂（阿柏西普）是一种可溶性的诱饵受体，能够在配体与受体相互作用前吸收配体，正在复发卵巢癌患者中进行Ⅱ期研究。也有许多其他的口服药通过抑制酪氨酸激酶靶向抑制血管生成。

铂耐药或难治性复发肿瘤

铂难治患者定义为在治疗中进展的患者，二线化疗的缓解率小于10%（表104-7）。铂耐药患者（即化疗完成后6个月内复发进展）的治疗是复杂的，应该提供机会给这些患者参加临床研究。然而，最近AURELIA研究指出，在化疗基础上联合贝伐珠单抗能够得到额外的获益，这可能会改变标准治疗，因为近期FDA基于AURELIA的结果批准贝伐珠单抗用于铂耐药复发卵巢癌[230]。

所有联合化疗对比单药化疗治疗耐药或难治卵巢癌的随机研究均未显示出联合化疗比单药化疗更有优势。有很多可能有效的单药，最常使用的有紫杉醇、多西他赛、拓扑替康、多柔比星脂质体、吉西他滨、异环磷酰胺、曲贝替定、口服依托泊苷、他莫昔芬、培美曲塞和贝伐珠单抗[226,227,231～234]。

约200例铂耐药复发卵巢癌患者随机接受吉西他滨或多柔比星脂质体化疗。吉西他滨组和多柔比星脂质体组的中位PFS分别是3.6个月和3.1个月，中位总体生存分别是12.7个月和 13.5 个月，总体有效率分别是 6.1%和 8.3%。在有可测量病灶的亚组患者中，总体缓解率分别是 9.2%和 11.7%。治疗组间没有一个有效性终点显示出统计学差异。多柔比星脂质体组有更多的手足综合征和黏膜炎，吉西他滨组有更多的便秘、恶心呕吐、乏力和神经病变[235]。

这些结果和一项大规模的对比帕土匹龙（patupilone）与多柔比星脂质体在 829 例铂耐药/难治卵巢癌患者中疗效的Ⅲ期随机研究相似[236]。帕土匹龙是一种微管稳定剂，当与它的分子靶点 β-微球蛋白结合后，能够诱导细胞周期的停滞和凋亡，据报道在铂难治或铂耐药复发卵巢癌患者中，总体有效率为 16%。研究的主要终点是总生存期。两种治疗的患者结局没有差异。两组的中位 PFS 均为 3.7 个月，帕土匹龙组总生存期是 13.2 个月，多柔比星脂质体组是 12.7 个月，试验组 20%的患者由于毒性反应中断治疗。观察到的所有级别的常见不良反应包括帕土匹龙组的腹泻（85%）和外周神经病变（39%）以及多柔比星脂质体组的口腔炎/黏膜炎（43%）和手足综合征（41.8%）。这项研究中大多数的患者为铂耐药，而不是铂难治复发。而且，几乎所有的患者 WHO 体力状态评分为 0 或 1，因此，这个选择性的人群不一定能代表整体铂耐药/难治卵巢癌。研究结果强调这些患者预后差，并且强调了症状改善及生活质量关怀的重要性。值得讨论的是，这些应该是化疗的主要目标，并且应该与临床研究中 PFS、OS 这样传统的研究终点一起，作为共同的主要研究终点。

多项Ⅱ期临床研究显示单药紫杉醇在铂耐药复发卵巢癌中客观缓解率为 20%~30%[237~242]。主要的毒性是虚弱和外周神经病变。紫杉醇周疗比 3 周疗更有效，毒性更轻。在一项 53 例铂耐药复发卵巢癌参与的研究中，紫杉醇周疗（80mg/m²，>1h）在有可测量病灶的患者中客观缓解率为 25%，无可测量病灶的患者有 27%血 CA125 水平下降了 75%[240]。

多西他赛在铂耐药患者中也有一定的活性[243~245]。GOG 研究了 60 例铂耐药复发卵巢癌或腹膜癌[245]。尽管客观缓解率达 22%，但是中位缓解间期仅仅是 2.5 个月，由于四分之三的患者出现严重的神经病变，加大了治疗难度。

拓扑替康对于铂敏感或耐药复发患者是一种有效的二线治疗[246~259]。在一项研究中，139 例女性每天接受拓扑替康 1.5mg/m²，持续 5 天，铂敏感和铂耐药患者缓解率分别为 19%、13%[246]。拓扑替康的主要毒性是血液学毒性，尤其是中性粒细胞减少。5 天的给药剂量时，70%~80%的患者发生严重的中性粒细胞减少，25%的患者出现粒缺性发热，合并或不合并感染[246,251]。一些研究中，5 天方案比其他较短期的方案有更好的缓解率[246~256]，但在一些其他的研究中，减少剂量为 1mg/(m²·d)持续 3 天，缓解率相似，但毒性更低。在一项 31 例患者的研究中，一半患者为铂难治性[259]，每 21 天给药拓扑替康 2mg/(m²·d)，持续 3 天，缓解率为 32%。在铂难治患者中持续输注拓扑替康（0.4mg/(m²·d)，14~21 天）客观缓解率为 27%~35%[252]。拓扑替康周疗每周给药 4mg/m²，持续 3 周，停药一周，缓解率和 5 天方案相似，但毒性大大减少。因此，这被认为是这种药物可以考虑的选择方案。

多柔比星脂质体（美国商品名 Doxil，欧洲商品名 Caelyx）在铂或紫杉烷难治的患者中有活性。它的主要严重毒性是手足综合征，也叫掌跖感觉丧失性红斑或肢端红斑，发生于 20%的接受 50mg/m²、每 4 周一次的患者[260,261]。多柔比星脂质体不引起神经毒性或脱发。它每 4 周给药，这令它使用起来更方便。较低的剂量 40mg/m² 相对更容易耐受，已被广泛应用。在一项 89 例铂难治患者的研究中，82 例为紫杉醇耐药患者，多柔比星脂质体的缓解率为 17%（1 例完全缓解，14 例部分缓解）。在另一项研究中，客观缓解率为 26%，但在一线治疗中进展的患者没有发生缓解[262]。

有两项随机研究比较了多柔比星脂质体与拓扑替康或紫杉醇。在一项研究中，237 例女性在接受一种含铂方案化疗后复发，其中 117 例（49.4%）为铂难治性复发，多柔比星脂质体 50mg/(m²·d)，>1h，每 4 周一次，与拓扑替康 1.5mg/(m²·d)，连续 5 天，每 3 周一次比较。两种治疗有相似的总体缓解率（20% vs 17%）、至进展时间（22 周 vs 20 周）和中位总体生存期（66 周 vs 56 周）。多柔比星脂质体治疗的患者骨髓抑制显著降低。第二个研究在 214 例既往接受过铂类治疗但之前未使用紫杉烷类的患者中，比较了多柔比星脂质体与单药紫杉醇的作用[263]，多柔比星脂质体和紫杉醇的总体缓解率分别是 18%、22%，中位生存分别是 46 周、56 周，两者之间没有显著的差异。实际上，大部分患者初始治疗剂量为多柔比星脂质体 40mg/m²，每 4 周一次。因为最初使用 50mg/m² 时，减量很常见。

吉西他滨是一类胞嘧啶的核苷类似物，据报道在铂耐药复发患者中缓解率为 10%~20%，在铂难治性患者中为 6%[231~233,264,265]。主要毒性是骨髓抑制和胃肠道反应。

口服依托泊苷的最常见毒性是骨髓抑制、恶心呕吐。可以观察到大约四分之一的患者出现 4 级中性粒细胞减少，10%~15%的患者有严重的恶心呕吐[234]。尽管最初的一项静脉使用依托泊苷的研究报道，在 24 例患者中缓解率仅为 8%[234]，随后的一项延长口服给药依托泊苷时间（每天 50mg/m²，共 21 天，每 4 周一次）的研究在 41 例铂耐药复发患者中的缓解率为 27%，其中 3 例持续完全缓解。在 25 例铂或紫杉烷耐药的患者中，报道了 8 例（32%）客观缓解。口服依托泊苷可以考虑用于紫杉醇及铂耐药的患者。

免疫治疗

在卵巢癌患者中使用免疫检查点抑制剂引起了人们极大的兴趣。抗 PD1 及 PD-L1 抗体在黑色素瘤和肺癌中的结果促进了在卵巢癌中的研究。来自日本京都的 Hamanishi 和他的同事开展了一项使用纳武单抗（抗 PD1 抗体）的Ⅱ期研究，在这项研究中既往接受过多次治疗并且铂耐药者的客观缓解率为 17%，包括 1 例完全缓解的卵巢透明细胞癌患者[266]。其他包括卵巢癌在内的实体瘤的报道也是鼓舞人心[267]。利用基因工程 CAR T 细胞疗法正在逐渐开展，主要作用靶点包括间皮素和 ESO-NY[268]。

激素治疗

上皮性卵巢癌经常有雌激素和雄激素受体表达阳性，尤其是在低级别的肿瘤中。一些上皮性卵巢肿瘤患者对内分泌治疗有反应，但似乎在高级别肿瘤的总体缓解率约 10%~20%。在晚期患者中，孕激素类药物、他莫昔芬、芳香化酶抑制剂和促性腺激素释放激素激动剂可单独或联合细胞毒化疗使用[269~272]。在晚期、主要是高级别上皮性卵巢癌患者的一项研究中，他莫昔芬仅有13%的部分缓解率，但30%的患者推迟了疾病进展。在复发的ER强表达的低级别卵巢癌中使用芳香化酶抑制剂的小型研究报道了较高的缓解率。

靶向治疗和PARP抑制剂

贝伐珠单抗的研究显示其客观缓解率为20%，6个月的无进展生存率为40%，大量单药靶向药（索拉非尼、坦罗莫司、吉非替尼、伊马替尼、米非司酮、enzastaurin、拉帕替尼及伏林司他）在复发上皮性卵巢癌中的客观缓解率不到10%，6个月PFS <25%。当前的研究集中于确定能够发挥协同致死作用的联合用药。

协同致死的概念看似简单，并且解释了PARP抑制剂在同源重组修复功能障碍细胞中的选择性和靶向作用。*BRCA1/2*功能丧失增加了对PARP抑制剂的敏感性，导致增殖细胞中未修复的单链DNA断裂积累，从而导致复制叉的崩溃，引起双链DNA的断裂（DSB）[273]。在同源重组修复缺陷的*BRCA1/2*肿瘤细胞中，DSB未被修复，这引起基因不稳定和细胞死亡。*BRCA1/2*和PARP抑制剂协同致死的相互作用已在体外以及1和2期复发卵巢癌研究中得到了确认[274,275]。奥拉帕利最初的Ⅰ期研究报道在*BRCA*突变的复发卵巢癌中有63%的显著临床获益率[275]。这导致扩大注册队列为50例*BRCA1/2*突变的患者，证实了在既往多次治疗的复发卵巢癌组的活性，临床获益率为46%[276]。可以观察到40%的患者有RECIST影像学缓解或GCIG CA125缓解。对奥拉帕利的反应和铂敏感性有关；铂耐药或难治患者的临床获益率分别为46%和23%，铂敏感患者的临床获益率为69%[276]。这些发现引发了大量的2期随机研究和广泛的兴趣，不仅针对*BRCA*突变的女性，还包括“散发”卵巢癌。高级别散发浆液性卵巢癌的分子异质性现在得到了更好的认识，而且显然至少50%的肿瘤有同源重组修复通路的障碍，并也可能对*PARP1*抑制剂敏感[277]。挑战在于如何更好地识别哪些肿瘤存在同源重组修复损伤，更可能对PARP抑制剂有反应。有大量的医药公司开发了伴随诊断检测来帮助识别最可能从*PARP*抑制剂中获益的患者。

PARP抑制剂维持治疗的研究已经非常令人兴奋。Ledermann等[278]报道了铂敏感复发卵巢癌患者在化疗缓解后，随机进行奥拉帕利维持或安慰剂维持治疗，奥拉帕利组PFS显著延长。BRCA突变的女性获益更高（HR = 0.18，95% CI 0.11，0.31，P<0.000 01；中位PFS为11.2个月 vs 4.3个月）[279]。基于这项研究的结果，已经开展了关于奥拉帕利及其他PARP抑制剂的大规模验证试验。在不远的将来，PARP抑制剂可能将在BRCA相关的卵巢癌或HRD患者的治疗中扮演越来越重要的角色。有一些PARP抑制剂联合化疗或血管生成抑制剂的研究，而且这是一个非常活跃的研究领域，至少五种不同的PARP抑制剂在被不同的医药公司研发之中。Liu等最近报道，与奥拉帕利单药相比奥拉帕利联合西地尼布的缓解率高达79%，PFS显著延长（17.7个月 vs 9个月），这些引发了新的研究，在未来这些新的治疗有望取代化疗[280]。

在一项多中心Ⅲ期随机安慰剂对照的铂敏感复发卵巢癌的研究中，尼拉帕利维持治疗组显示出无进展生存的优势：在携带胚系*BRCA1/2*突变的女性中为21个月 vs 5.5个月，在同源重组缺陷（HRD）的女性中为12.9个月 vs 3.8个月，在BRCA阴性的女性中为9.3个月 vs 3.9个月（均有显著差异P<0.001）。

姑息性放疗

如果患者只有一个主要的有症状的病变局限于某一部位，能够被有限的放疗野安全包裹，放疗作为一种姑息性治疗可能有效。例如，一个固定的盆腔包块侵犯了阴道黏膜引起出血、疼痛，或者肠道或膀胱功能障碍，但没有明显播散症状的腹膜病变。腹膜后淋巴结或腹腔外的局限病灶，如锁骨上或腹股沟淋巴结、骨转移、脑转移，都可能从姑息性放疗中受益，就像肝被膜扩张导致的疼痛性肝肿大。对可利用的化疗药物耐药的复发卵巢癌患者接受放疗后的客观和主观缓解率已有报道。一项Memorial Sloan-kettering癌症中心的研究显示铂难治患者的客观或主观缓解率为70%[281]。尽管用于姑息治疗的最佳剂量尚未确定，但是化疗后复发的卵巢癌患者局部放疗可能取得持久的缓解，即使对于化疗耐药的患者也是如此。对于已经证实脑转移的预期生命只有数周到数月的患者，姑息性全脑放疗是有指征的。

（曾嘉　赵羽西　李一帆　王甜甜 译　李宁 校）

参考文献

The complete reference list can be found on the Wiley Companion Digital Edition of this title (see inside front cover for login instructions).

1 Siegel R, Ma J, Zou Z, et al. Cancer statistics. *CA Cancer J Clin*. 2015;**65**:5–29.

2 SEER Cancer Statistics Factsheets. *Ovary Cancer*. Bethesda, MD: National Cancer Institute; 2005. http://seer.cancer.gov/statfacts/html/ovary.html.

9 Erickson BK, Conner MG, Landen CN. The role of the fallopian tube in the origin of ovarian cancer. *Am J Obstet Gynecol*. 2013;**209**:409–414.

27 Collaborative Group on Epidemiological Studies of Ovarian Cancer, Beral V, Gaitskell K, et al. Menopausal hormone use and ovarian cancer risk: individual participant meta analysis of 52 epidemiological studies. *Lancet*. 2015;**385**:1835–1842.

35 Struewing JP, Hartge P, Wacholder S, et al. The risk of cancer associated with specific mutations of BRCA1 and BRCA2 among Ashkenazi Jews. *N Engl J Med*. 1997;**336**:1401–1408.

47 Moyer VA. U.S. Preventive Services Task Force. Screening for ovarian cancer: U.S. Preventive Services Task Force reaffirmation recommendation statement. *Ann Intern Med*. 2012;**157(12)**:900–904.

55 Rebbeck TR, Lynch HT, Neuhausen SL, et al. Prophylactic oophorectomy in carriers of BRCA1 or BRCA2 mutations. *N Engl J Med*. 2002;**346**:1616–1622.

56 Haber D. Prophylactic oophorectomy to reduce the risk of ovarian and breast cancer in carriers of BRCA mutations. *N Engl J Med*. 2002;**346**:1660–1661.

60 Domchek SM, Friebel TM, Singer CF, et al. Association of risk-reducing surgery in BRCA1 or BRCA2 mutation carriers with cancer risk and mortality. *JAMA*. 2010;**304(9)**:967–975.

63 Genetic Testing for Heritable Mutations in the BRCA1 and BRCA2 Genes EVIQ Guidelines Cancer Institute NSW November 2013. https://www.eviq.org.au

68 Bast RC Jr, Romero I, Mills GB. Molecular pathogenesis of ovarian cancer. In: Mendelsohn J, Howley PM, Israel MA, Gray JW, Thompson CB, eds. *The Molecular Basis of Cancer*, 4th ed. Philadelphia, PA: Elsevier Health; 2015:531–547.

69 Merritt WM, Lin YG, Han LY, et al. Dicer, drosha and outcomes in patients with ovarian cancer. *N Engl J Med*. 2008;**359**:2641–2650.

70 Bast RC Jr, Hennessy B, Mills GB. The biology of ovarian cancer: new opportunities for translation. *Nat Rev Cancer*. 2009;**9**:415.

72 Kurman RJ, Shih IM. Molecular pathogenesis and extraovarian origin of epithelial ovarian cancer – shifting the paradigm. *Hum Pathol*. 2011;**42**:918.

74 Cancer Genome Atlas Research Network. Integrated genomic analyses of ovarian carcinoma. *Nature*. 2011;**474**:609.

82 Bast RC Jr, Klug TL, St. John E, et al. A radioimmunoassay using a monoclonal antibody to monitor the course of epithelial ovarian cancer. *N Engl J Med*. 1983;**309**:883–887.

83 Bast RC Jr, Feeney M, Lazarus H, et al. Reactivity of a monoclonal antibody with

human ovarian carcinoma. *J Clin Invest*. 1981;**68**:1331-1337.

86 Bast RC, Spriggs DR. More than a biomarker: CA125 may contribute to ovarian cancer pathogenesis. *Gynecol Oncol*. 2011;**121**:429-430. PMID: 21601106.

95 Goff BA, Mandel LS, Drescher CW, et al. Development of an ovarian cancer symptom index: possibilities for earlier detection. *Cancer*. 2007;**109**(**2**):221-227.

98 Jacobs I, Oram D, Fairbanks J, Turner J, Frost C, Grudzinskas JG. A risk of malignancy index incorporating CA 125, ultrasound and menopausal status for the accurate preoperative diagnosis of ovarian cancer. *Br J Obstet Gynaecol*. 1990;**97**(**10**):922-929.

99 Ueland FR, Desimone CP, Seamon LG, et al. Effectiveness of a multivariate index assay in the preoperative assessment of ovarian tumors. *Obstet Gynecol*. 2011;**117**:1289-1297.

101 Moore RG, Miller C, Disilvestro P, et al. Evaluation of the diagnostic accuracy of the risk of ovarian malignancy algorithm in women with a pelvic mass. *Obstet Gynecol*. 2011;**118**:280-288.

112 Lu KH, Skates S, Hernandez MA, et al. A two-stage ovarian cancer screening strategy using the risk of ovarian cancer algorithm (ROCA) identifies early stage incident cancers and demonstrates high positive predictive value. *Cancer*. 2013;**119**:3454-3461.

113 Menon U, Gentry-Maharaj A, Hallett R, et al. Sensitivity and specificity of multimodal and ultrasound screening for ovarian cancer, and stage distribution of detected cancers: results of the prevalence screen of the UK Collaborative Trial of Ovarian Cancer Screening (UKCTOCS). *Lancet Oncol*. 2009;**10**:327-340.

114 Menon U, Ryan A, Kalsi J, et al. Risk algorithm using serial biomarker measurements doubles the number of screen-detected cancers compared with a single-threshold rule in the United Kingdom Collaborative Trial of Ovarian Cancer Screening. *J Clin Oncol*. 2015;**33**:2062-2071.

130 Berek JS, Friedlander ML, Hacker NF. Epithelial ovarian, fallopian tube, and peritoneal cancer. In: Berek JS, Hacker NF, eds. *Berek & Hacker's Gynecologic Oncology*, 6th ed. Philadelphia: Lippincott Williams & Wilkins; 2015:464-529.

133 Griffiths CT. Surgical resection of tumor bulk in the primary treatment of ovarian carcinoma. *Natl Cancer Inst Monogr*. 1975;**42**:101-109.

146 McGuire WP, Hoskins WJ, Brady MF, et al. Cyclophosphamide and cisplatin compared with paclitaxel and cisplatin in patients with stage III and stage IV ovarian cancer. *N Engl J Med*. 1996;**334**:1-6.

147 Piccart MJ, Bertelsen K, James K, et al. Randomized intergroup trial of cisplatin-paclitaxel versus cisplatin-cyclophosphamide in women with advanced epithelial ovarian cancer: three year results. *J Natl Cancer Inst*. 2000;**92**:699-708.

148 Muggia F, Braly PS, Brady MF, et al. Phase III randomized study of cisplatin versus paclitaxel versus cisplatin and paclitaxel in patients with suboptimal stage III or IV ovarian cancer: a Gynecologic Oncology Group study. *J Clin Oncol*. 2000;**18**:106-115.

157 Swenerton K, Jeffrey J, Stuart G, et al. Cisplatin-cyclophosphamide versus carboplatin-cyclophosphamide in advanced ovarian cancer: a randomized phase III study of the National Cancer Institute of Canada Clinical Trials Group. *J Clin Oncol*. 1992;**10**:718-726.

158 Ozols RF, Bundy BN, Greer B, et al. Phase III trial of carboplatin and paclitaxel compared with cisplatin and paclitaxel in patients with optimally resected stage III ovarian cancer. *J Clin Oncol*. 2003;**21**:3194-3200.

160 The International Collaborative Ovarian Neoplasm (ICON) Group. Paclitaxel plus carboplatin versus standard chemotherapy with either single agent carboplatin or cyclophosphamide, doxorubicin and cisplatin: in women with ovarian cancer: the ICON3 randomised trial. *Lancet*. 2002;**360**:505-515.

164 Aabo K, Adams M, Adnitt P, et al. Chemotherapy in advanced ovarian cancer: four systematic meta analyses of individual patient data from 37 randomized trials. Advanced Ovarian Cancer Trialists' Group. *Br J Cancer*. 1998;**78**:1479-1487.

169 Vasey PA, Paul J, Birt A, et al. Docetaxel and cisplatin in combination as first-line chemotherapy for advanced epithelial ovarian cancer. Scottish Gynaecological Cancer Trials Group. *J Clin Oncol*. 1999;**17**:2069-2080.

170 Bookman MA, Brady MF, McGuire WP, et al. Evaluation of new platinum-based treatment regimens in advanced-stage ovarian cancer: a Phase III Trial of the Gynecologic Cancer Intergroup (GOG182). *J Clin Oncol*. 2009;**27**:1419-1425.

178 Alberts DS, Liu PY, Hannigan EV, et al. Intraperitoneal cisplatin plus intravenous cyclophosphamide versus intravenous cisplatin plus intravenous cyclophosphamide for stage III ovarian cancer. *N Engl J Med*. 1996;**335**:1950-1955.

179 Markman M, Bundy B, Benda J, et al. Randomized phase III study of intravenous cisplatin/paclitaxel versus moderately high dose intravenous carboplatin followed by intraperitoneal paclitaxel and intraperitoneal cisplatin in optimal residual ovarian cancer: an Intergroup trial (GOG, SWOG, ECOG). *J Clin Oncol*. 2001;**19**:921-923.

180 Armstrong D, Bundy B, Wenzel L, et al. Intraperitoneal cisplatin and paclitaxel in ovarian cancer. *N Engl J Med*. 2006;**354**:34-53.

187 van der Burg MEL, van Lent M, Buyse M, et al. The effect of debulking surgery after induction chemotherapy on the prognosis in advanced epithelial ovarian cancer. *N Engl J Med*. 1995;**332**:629-634.

201 Cohen MH, Gootenberg J, Keegan P, Pazdur R. FDA drug approval summary: bevacizumab (Avastin) plus Carboplatin and paclitaxel as first-line treatment of advanced/metastatic recurrent nonsquamous non-small Cell lung cancer. *Oncologist*. 2007;**12**(**6**):713-718.

203 Burger RA, Brady MF, Bookman MA, et al. Gynecologic Oncol ogy Group. Incorporation of bevacizumab in the primary treatment of ovarian cancer. *N Engl J Med*. 2011;**365**(**26**):2473-2483.

204 Perren TJ, Swart AM, Pfisterer J, et al. A phase 3 trial of bevacizumab in ovarian cancer. *N Engl J Med*. 2011;**365**(**26**):2484-2496.

222 Pfisterer J, Plante M, Vergote I, et al. Gemcitabine plus carboplatin compared with carboplatin in patients with platinum-sensitive recurrent ovarian cancer: an intergroup trial of the AGO-OVAR, the NCIC CTG, and the EORTC GCG. *J Clin Oncol*. 2006;**24**:4699-4707.

223 Alberts DS, Liu PY, Wilczynski SP, et al. Randomized trial of pegylated liposomal doxorubicin (PLD) plus carboplatin versus carboplatin in platinum-sensitive (PS) patients with recurrent epithe- lial ovarian or peritoneal carcinoma after failure of initial platinum- based chemotherapy (Southwest Oncology Group Protocol S0200). *Gynecol Oncol*. 2008;**108**:90-94.

224 Pujade-Lauraine E, Wagner U, Aavall-Lundqvist E, et al. Pegylated liposomal doxorubicin and carboplatin compared with paclitaxel and carboplatin for patients with platinum-sensitive ovarian cancer in late relapse. *J Clin Oncol*. 2010;**28**(**20**):3323-3329.

230 Poveda AM, Selle F, Hilpert F, et al. Bevacixumab combined with weekly paclitaxel, pegylated liposomal doxorubicin, or topotecan in platinum-resistant recurrent ovarian cancer: analysis by chemotherapy cohort of the fandomized phase III AURELIA Trial. *J Clin Oncol*. 2015;**63**:1408.

235 Mutch DG, Orlando M, Goss T, et al. Randomized phase III trial of gemcitabine compared with pegylated liposomal doxorubicin in patients with platinum-resistant ovarian cancer. *J Clin Oncol*. 2007;**25**:2811-2818.

275 Fong PC, Boss DS, Yap TA, et al. Inhibition of poly(ADP-ribose) polymerase in tumors from BRCA mutation carriers. *N Engl J Med*. 2009;**361**(**2**):123-134.

276 Fong PC, Yap TA, Boss DS, et al. Poly(ADP)-ribose polymerase inhibition: frequent durable responses in BRCA carrier ovarian cancer correlating with platinum-free interval. *J Clin Oncol*. 2010;**28**(**15**):2512-2519.

278 Ledermann J, Harter P, Gourley C, et al. Olaparib maintenance therapy in platinum-sensitive relapsed ovarian cancer. *N Engl J Med*. 2012;**366**(**15**): 1382-1392.

281 Mizra MR, Monk BJ, Herrstedt J, et al. Niraparib Maintenance Therapy in Platinum-Sensitive, Recurrent Ovarian Cancer. *NEJM*. DOI: 10.1056/NEJMoa1611310.

第105章　非上皮性卵巢恶性肿瘤

Jonathan S. Berek, MD, MMS, FASCO ■ Michael L. Friedlander, MD, MBChB, PhD ■ Robert C. Bast Jr., MD

概述

与卵巢上皮癌相比，非上皮性卵巢肿瘤并不常见，在所有卵巢恶性肿瘤中占<10%[1,2]。非上皮性卵巢恶性肿瘤包括生殖细胞肿瘤、性索间质肿瘤、卵巢转移性癌以及各种罕见的卵巢恶性肿瘤，包括肉瘤和脂质细胞肿瘤。尽管这些肿瘤患者的症状、诊断和治疗上有很多相似之处，但他们仍有各自的特点，治疗方法不尽相同[1~5]。恶性生殖细胞肿瘤起源于卵巢原始生殖细胞，可以通过组织学类型和肿瘤标记物甲胎蛋白（AFP）、人绒毛膜促性腺激素（hCG）进行鉴别，无性细胞瘤（AFP-hCG-）、胚胎性癌（AFP+hCG+）、未成熟畸胎瘤（AFP-hCG-）、内胚窦（卵黄囊）瘤（AFP+hCG-）以及卵巢绒毛膜癌（AFP-hCG+）。生殖细胞肿瘤常发生于初潮前女孩和年轻女性，生长迅速，可以表现为有症状的盆腔包块。因为保留生育是重要需求，治疗通常选择单侧附件切除，之后辅以铂为基础的化疗。在生殖细胞肿瘤中，无性细胞瘤有10%~15%为双侧发生，有5%的患者性腺发育不全。即使是肿瘤晚期，发生转移的生殖细胞肿瘤对化疗也相当敏感，长期生存率也很高。在有些医院，ⅠA期的生殖细胞肿瘤年轻患者在手术切除后严密随访，只有复发时才给予化疗，结果也很好。性索间质肿瘤包括颗粒细胞瘤、幼年型颗粒细胞瘤和支持间质细胞瘤。颗粒细胞瘤可以发生在任何年龄，并可产生雌激素，使得少部分女孩出现假性性早熟，绝经前女性出现停经，绝经后女性子宫内膜增生。颗粒间质肿瘤生长缓慢，常常局限于一侧卵巢，手术通常可治愈75%以上的Ⅰ期病例。完全切除后通常不再辅助化疗。然而也会出现远期复发。持续或复发肿瘤对铂为基础的化疗和激素治疗敏感，包括孕激素、促黄体激素释放激素拮抗剂以及芳香化酶抑制剂。抑制素B是一个有用的标记物。Sertoli-Leydig细胞瘤常发生于20~40岁的患者，产生雄激素，在70%以上的患者引起男性化。由于很多Sertoli-Leydig细胞瘤处于早期，很少累及双侧，因此经常采用单侧附件切除术，5年生存率达70%~90%。

生殖细胞恶性肿瘤

生殖细胞肿瘤（GCT）来源于卵巢的原始生殖细胞，发病率约为睾丸恶性生殖细胞肿瘤的十分之一。尽管它们也可以出现在性腺外的部位如纵隔和腹膜后，但绝大部分生殖细胞肿瘤发生于性腺，来源于未分化的生殖细胞。这些肿瘤发生位置的变异归结于生殖细胞进入正在发育的性腺性索前从卵黄囊尾侧至背侧肠系膜的胚胎迁移[1,2]。

生殖细胞肿瘤是可被治愈的肿瘤的典范。卵巢生殖细胞肿瘤的治疗很大程度借鉴更常见的男性睾丸生殖细胞肿瘤的治疗经验。睾丸生殖细胞肿瘤的随机试验很多，为治疗的选择提供了强大的证据支持[6,7]。睾丸生殖细胞瘤的治疗结果在有经验的治疗中心比较好，因此可以推测对于相对少见的卵巢生殖细胞肿瘤预后应该也是如此。由于治愈率很高，目前更关注的是如何在保证生存的前提下降低毒副反应。仍有一小部分患者死于该病，有研究正在探讨如何改善这部分高风险、预后差的患者的治疗结局[6,7]。

Murugaesu等[8]报道了一项最大样本的研究，包括113例晚期卵巢生殖细胞肿瘤患者，进行顺铂为基础的化疗，结果表明分期和肿瘤标记物升高是预后差的独立因素。这些发现很重要，明确了卵巢生殖细胞肿瘤与睾丸生殖细胞肿瘤的预后因素相似，与在临床上观察到卵巢及睾丸生殖细胞肿瘤行为相似是一致的。这对卵巢生殖细胞肿瘤的治疗很重要，因为可以有助于明确哪些患者预后差，需要更积极的治疗[8]。

组织学及生物标记物

卵巢生殖细胞肿瘤的组织学分类见表105-1[1,10]。一些生殖细胞肿瘤分泌甲胎蛋白（AFP）及人绒毛膜促性腺激素（hCG）。AFP和β-hCG升高有助于盆腔包块的鉴别诊断以及

表105-1　卵巢生殖细胞瘤的组织学类型[9]

Ⅰ. 无性细胞瘤
Ⅱ. 畸胎瘤
A. 未成熟型
B. 成熟型
1. 实性
2. 囊性
a. 皮样囊肿（成熟囊性畸胎瘤）
b. 皮样囊肿恶变
C. 单胚层及高度特异性
1. 卵巢甲状腺瘤
2. 类癌
3. 卵巢甲状腺瘤和类癌
4. 其他
Ⅲ. 内胚窦瘤
Ⅳ. 胚胎性癌
Ⅴ. 多胚瘤
Ⅵ. 绒毛膜癌
Ⅶ. 混合型

术后随访监测。胎盘碱性磷酸酶（PLAP）和乳酸脱氢酶（LDH）可在 95% 的无性细胞瘤患者中升高，连续监测血清 LDH 水平对随诊该疾病可能有用。PLAP 作为免疫组化标记物比血清标记物更有意义。生殖细胞肿瘤的分类既要根据组织学特点也要参考肿瘤标记物的表达（图 105-1）[12,13]。

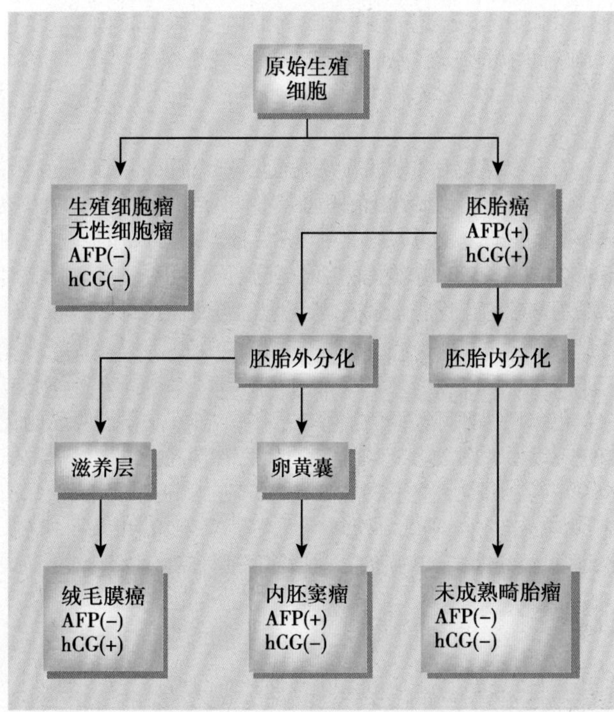

图 105-1 纯恶性 GCT 与其分泌的标志物的关系举例。AFP，甲胎蛋白，hCG，人绒毛膜促性腺激素。摘自 Berek 2015[11]. Reproduced with permission of Wolters Kluwer Health

在此分类中，胚胎癌由未分化细胞组成，可合成 hCG 及 AFP，是其他几种生殖细胞肿瘤的前身[4,13]。分化程度更高的生殖细胞肿瘤，如内胚窦瘤（EST），可分泌 AFP；绒毛膜癌可分泌 hCG，这些肿瘤起源于胚胎外组织；未成熟畸胎瘤源于胚胎组织，不分泌 hCG，但 AFP 可能升高。hCG 可在 3%的无性细胞瘤患者中升高，升高水平往往小于 100 国际单位。单纯无性细胞瘤中未见 AFP 升高[1]。

流行病学

尽管所有卵巢良恶性肿瘤中有 20%～25%来源于生殖细胞，但生殖细胞来源的恶性肿瘤仅占卵巢恶性肿瘤的 5%[1]。在亚洲和黑人群体中，上皮性卵巢癌相对欧美不常见，生殖细胞恶性肿瘤在卵巢恶性肿瘤中可占达 15%。在 20 岁以前，几乎 70%的卵巢肿瘤来源于生殖细胞，这其中有 1/3 是恶性的[1,2]。在这个年龄段生殖细胞肿瘤占卵巢恶性肿瘤的 2/3。生殖细胞恶性肿瘤也会发生在 20～30 岁之间，但在之后就很少见。

症状

与生长相对缓慢的卵巢上皮癌相比，生殖细胞恶性肿瘤生长迅速，常因包膜扩张、出血或坏死引起的亚急性盆腔疼痛为特征。快速增大的盆腔包块可能会使膀胱或直肠产生压迫症状，在月经初期的患者中可能出现月经周期紊乱。一些年轻患者可能会误以为这是怀孕的表现，导致延误诊断。破裂或扭转可能会引起急性症状。这些症状可能会与急性阑尾炎混淆。更晚期的患者可能会出现腹水，表现为腹胀[3]。

体征

对于可触及附件包块的患者，可与如前所述的卵巢上皮癌一样进行评估。部分生殖细胞肿瘤患者可能是初潮前患者。如果超声评估病变主要是实性的，或者是囊实性的，则很可能是肿瘤，并且可能是恶性肿瘤。体格检查还应该注意是否有腹水、胸腔积液和脏器肿大的迹象。

诊断

初潮前女性≥2cm 或绝经前女性≥8cm 的混合性附件包块常常需要手术探查。在年轻患者中，术前血液学检查需要包括血清 hCG、AFP、LDH、CA125 水平，全血细胞计数和肝功能检查。胸部影像学检查很重要，因为生殖细胞肿瘤可以转移到肺或纵隔。因为这些肿瘤倾向于出现在发育异常的性腺，所以对于初潮前女性患者理想情况下术前应进行染色体核型分析，但实践中不一定可行[3,14]。术前 CT 或 MRI 检查可显示腹膜后淋巴结是否有肿大及其位置，或者是否有肝转移。除非有非常广泛的转移，一般还是先行手术。初潮后的患者如果有附件囊性肿物，直径不超过 8cm，可以先观察或尝试激素抑制治疗 2 周期[15]。

无性细胞瘤

无性细胞瘤是最常见的恶性生殖细胞肿瘤，大约占所有生殖细胞来源卵巢恶性肿瘤的 30%～40%[2,12]，占所有卵巢恶性肿瘤 1%～3%，但是在小于 20 岁的卵巢恶性肿瘤中占 5%～10%。75%的无性细胞瘤发生于 10 岁到 30 岁之间，5%出现在 10 岁以前，50 岁以后很少见[1,4]。该病主要发生在年轻女性，20%～30%与妊娠相关的卵巢恶性肿瘤是无性细胞瘤。

与异常卵巢的相关性

约 5%的无性细胞瘤在性腺异常的女性表型患者中发现[1,14]。这种恶性疾病与单纯性腺发育不全（46XY，双侧条索状性腺）、混合性腺发育不全（45X/46XY，单侧条索状性腺，对侧睾丸）或雄激素不敏感综合征（46XY，睾丸女性化）的患者相关。因此合并盆腔肿物的初潮前患者应确定其染色体核型，尤其是怀疑为无性细胞瘤的患者（图 105-2）。

在多数性腺发育不全的患者中，无性细胞瘤常起源自性腺母细胞瘤——由生殖细胞和性索间质组成的良性卵巢肿瘤。若在性腺发育不全患者的性腺内有性腺母细胞瘤，超过 50%会发展成卵巢恶性肿瘤[16]。

大约 65%的无性细胞瘤诊断时为Ⅰ期[1,3,5,17~21]。85%～90%的Ⅰ期肿瘤局限在一侧卵巢，10%～15%侵犯双侧。其他生殖细胞肿瘤很少累及双侧。在保留对侧卵巢的患者中，5%～10%会于 2 年内再发无性细胞瘤[1]。这里面包括未接受全身化疗的患者和合并有性腺发育不全的患者。

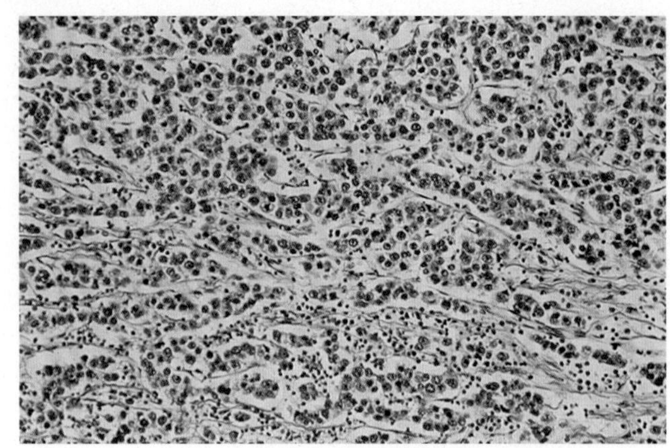

图 105-2 无性细胞瘤

转移途径

在 25%发生转移的该病患者中,肿瘤最常见的是通过淋巴结转移,尤其是转移至更高的腹主动脉旁淋巴结[19]。其次还有血行转移和直接蔓延,即穿透卵巢被膜后肿瘤细胞在腹膜表面的脱落和播散。即使没有其他转移证据时也可能出现肿瘤向对侧卵巢转移的情况。骨转移很少见,多位于脊柱下段椎体。肿瘤很少转移至肺、肝、脑,可见于长期患病或复发的患者。纵隔和锁骨上淋巴结转移是该病的晚期表现[17,18]。

治疗

早期无性细胞瘤主要的治疗方式是手术,包括切除病灶,有限的手术分期—冲洗液、网膜活检、仔细触诊所有的腹膜表面及腹膜后淋巴结,以及对任何怀疑有肿瘤侵犯地方的活检。肿瘤发生转移的患者需行化疗。因为该病主要发生在年轻女性,保留生育功能必须加以考虑[19,22]。一项在 Norwegian Radium 医院的对比研究显示了化疗相对于放疗的优越之处。化疗组的生存率更好,并发症更少[22]。

手术

卵巢无性细胞瘤手术至少切除单侧卵巢[20,23]。如果有生育需求——很多患者有该需求——即使是存在转移的情况,对侧卵巢、输卵管以及子宫也应该原位保留,因为该肿瘤对化疗敏感。如果不要求保留生育功能,对于晚期患者应行全子宫双附件切除[5],尽管这只对于一小部分患者合适。对于染色体核型分析有 Y 染色体的患者,应切除双侧卵巢,但是可以保留子宫,以备将来可能进行胚胎移植。肿瘤细胞减灭术并未证明有益,但是容易切除的大块肿瘤(比如网膜饼)应该在第一次手术时切除。重要的是不要进行容易导致并发症的手术,因为那可能会推迟化疗的开始。

无性细胞瘤患者检查时发现肿瘤局限于卵巢的患者,应进行仔细分期手术以确定是否有隐匿性转移。这些肿瘤经常转移至肾血管周围的腹主动脉旁淋巴结。应取腹腔冲洗液送细胞学,彻底探查所有腹膜表面以及腹膜后淋巴结,发现任何异常都应取活检或切除。应该仔细检查对侧卵巢,因为无性细胞瘤是唯一倾向侵犯双侧卵巢的生殖细胞肿瘤,而且不是所有的双侧病变都会出现明显的卵巢增大。因此,需要对对侧卵巢进行仔细的检查和触诊,并对任何可疑病变进行切除活检[5,20,21,23]。如果对侧卵巢发现小的肿瘤,切除肿瘤并保留部分正常卵巢或许可行。

许多表面上局限于一侧卵巢的无性细胞瘤患者,因仅接受了单侧附件切除术而未行分期术再次就诊。这些患者可选择:①重新进行开腹分期术;②规律的盆腔及腹部 CT 检查;③辅助化疗[19]。因为大部分无性细胞瘤局限于一侧卵巢且生长迅速,作者更倾向于选择规律密切监测这些患者[24,25]。

放疗

失去生育能力和继发恶性肿瘤是放疗重要的远期并发症,因此放疗不再作为无性细胞瘤患者的初始治疗[22]。放疗可被选择性地用于复发患者[5,21,22]。无性细胞瘤对放疗很敏感,剂量在 2 500~3 500cGy 就有效;但是已不再常用,因为该肿瘤对以铂为基础的化疗非常敏感,被治愈的可能性很高。

化疗

化疗是一种可选择的治疗[23,26~35]。与放疗相比明显的优势是可以使大多数病人保留生育能力,并且降低继发肿瘤的风险[23,36~40]。最常用的化疗方案是 BEP 方案(博来霉素、依托泊苷、顺铂)。过去,VBP(长春碱、博来霉素、顺铂)以及 VAC(长春新碱、放线菌素、环磷酰胺)方案很常用,但目前很少使用(表 105-2)[23,26~30]。

表 105-2 卵巢 GCT 联合化疗方案

方案及用药	剂量及计划[a]
BEP	
博来霉素	30IU/周,最长使用 12 周
	15U/(m² · 周)×5;之后在第 4 程第一天给药
依托泊苷	100mg/(m² · d)×5 天,每 3 周
顺铂	20mg/(m² · d)×5 天,或 100mg/(m² · d)×1 天,每 3 周

[a] 以上均为静脉给药。

妇科肿瘤协作组(GOG)研究了三个疗程 EC 方案(依托泊苷联合卡铂):依托泊苷(120mg/m²,第 1、2 和 3 天静脉给药,每 4 周重复),卡铂(400mg/m²,第 1 天静脉给药,每 4 周重复),治疗 39 例完全切除的卵巢无性细胞瘤(ⅠB 期、ⅠC 期、Ⅱ期或Ⅲ期)的效果[33]。试验结果非常好,GOG 报道持续无病生存率为 100%。对于晚期、未完全切除的生殖细胞肿瘤,GOG 进行了两项以顺铂为基础的连续研究[27]。在第一项研究中,患者接受 4 周期的长春碱(12mg/m²,每 3 周 1 次)、博来霉素[20U/(m² · 周)静脉给药,共 12 周]和顺铂[20mg/(m² · d)×5 天,静脉给药,每 3 周 1 次]化疗。二次探查手术发现病灶持续存在或进展的患者给予 6 周期的 VAC 方案。在第二项研究中,患者先接受 3 周期的 BEP 方案化疗,之后用 VAC 方案进行巩固[27]。VAC 方案在 BEP 方案之后使用并没有改善预后,因此不再应用。

两项研究中共有 20 例Ⅲ到Ⅳ期的无性细胞瘤患者接受治疗并可评价疗效,19 例存活,无病生存期 6~68 个月(中位 26 个月)。这些患者中 14 例进行了二次探查术,都没有发现残存肿瘤。一项在 MD Anderson 癌症中心的研究中,14 例有残存肿瘤的患者使用 BEP 方案化疗,所有患者在长期随访中均无瘤生存[30]。在另一项研究中,有 26 例卵巢无性细胞瘤患者接受了 BEP 化疗,这些患者有 54%是ⅢC 或Ⅳ期,经过 3~6 个周期的化疗,25(96%)例患者长期无瘤生存[35]。

这些结果显示对于晚期,未完全切净肿瘤的无性细胞瘤患者使用以顺铂为基础的联合化疗也可以有很好的预后[34~39,41]。依据睾丸肿瘤治疗的数据,最佳方案是 3~4 周期的 BEP 方案化疗,周期数根据肿瘤侵犯程度以及是否有内脏转移决定[40~42]。如果博来霉素因为肺毒性有使用禁忌,应该考虑给 4 周期的顺铂联合依托泊苷而不是 3 周期的 BEP。

对于无性细胞瘤患者没有必要进行二次探查术[43~45]。无性细胞瘤患者化疗后是否需进行手术切除残存病灶尚不明确,因为绝大多数这种患者化疗后只剩下坏死组织或者没有活性的肿瘤组织。一般来说,这些患者应该用影像学和肿瘤标记物密切监测。化疗结束 4 周后仍残存有 3cm 以上肿块的患者应考虑正电子发射断层显像(PET-CT)检查。在这种情况下,PET-CT 可以敏感地检测男性精原细胞瘤的残存肿瘤[46],发现 30%~50%患者中有残存肿瘤。如果 PET-CT 结果阳性或者影像学扫描显示肿瘤进展,最好在进行挽救性治疗之前有组织学证据[47]。

肿瘤复发

无性细胞瘤患者很少出现复发,75%的复发出现在初次治疗后的一年以内[1~4],最常见的部位是腹腔和腹膜后淋巴结。这些患者应根据其初次治疗的情况和复发部位选择放疗或者化疗。仅接受过手术治疗的复发患者应接受化疗。如果已经使用过 BEP 方案,则可以尝试 TIP(紫杉醇、异环磷酰胺和铂类)方案,该方案是睾丸生殖细胞肿瘤常用的挽救性方案[48]。

治疗决策应在多学科合作的基础上包括对生殖细胞肿瘤治疗有经验的内科医师的参与。对于部分患者,可以考虑给予大剂量化疗的同时外周干细胞支持治疗。一些大剂量化疗方案正处在Ⅱ期研究,具体方案的选择应依据前次化疗方案、肿瘤复发时间和既往治疗遗留的毒性反应情况[49,50]。目前还不清楚作为复发患者的一线挽救治疗,大剂量化疗是否优于常规剂量化疗。目前只有一项随机试验,来自欧洲血液和骨髓移植协会(EBMT)-IT-94,3 周期的 VIP 化疗或者长春碱、异环磷酰胺、顺铂(VeIP)化疗后行大剂量化疗,与 4 周期的常规剂量化疗相比,并没有显示出优势。一项国际随机对照研究(TIGER)计划将 390 名复发生殖细胞瘤患者随机分为两组:一组是常规剂量以铂为基础的 TIP 方案 4 周期,另一组是先进行 2 周期的紫杉醇、异环磷酰胺化疗,之后在自体干细胞支持下行 3 周期的大剂量卡铂和依托泊苷化疗(TICE)[50]。

对于部分局部复发的无性细胞瘤患者可以考虑放疗,但是放疗有一个主要的缺点,如果需要对盆腔和腹部照射,则有可能丧失生育能力,并且如果放疗失败还有可能会降低继续给予化疗的可能[22]。

妊娠

因为无性细胞瘤常发生在年轻患者,该病可能发生于妊娠期。ⅠA 期的肿瘤可以被完整切除,继续妊娠。对于更晚期的患者,能否继续妊娠取决于孕周。对于妊娠中期和晚期患者可给予常规剂量化疗而不会对胎儿造成明显损害[36,51]。在妊娠期间应用 BEP 方案化疗的患者很少,有引起胎儿畸形和并发症的报道,必须强调妊娠期间只有确实需要化疗的患者才会给予化疗[52]。

预后

ⅠA 期无性细胞瘤患者行单侧卵巢切除术后 5 年无瘤生存率高达 95%以上[5,21]。容易复发的特征包括肿瘤直径大于 10~15cm、年龄小于 20 岁、显微镜下可见大量的有丝分裂、异型性以及髓质型[1,12]。

Kumar 等从 SEER 数据库中提取了 1988 年到 2004 年恶性卵巢生殖细胞肿瘤的资料。共 1 296 例无性细胞瘤、未成熟畸胎瘤和混合型生殖细胞肿瘤,其中 613(47.3%)例进行了淋巴结清扫术,淋巴结转移见于 28%的无性细胞瘤、8%的未成熟畸胎瘤以及 16%的混合型生殖细胞肿瘤患者中($P<0.05$)。淋巴结阴性的患者 5 年生存率为 95.7%,淋巴结转移的患者 5 年生存率为 82.8%($P<0.001$)。同一个项目组近来更新了结果,1 083 例临床上认为病变局限于卵巢的生殖细胞肿瘤患者进行了手术[54]。其中 590(54.5%)例患者未行淋巴清扫术,493(45.5%)例患者进行了淋巴结清扫术。对于后者,52(10.5%)例患者因为发现淋巴结转移分期为 FIGO ⅢC 期。未行淋巴清扫术的患者 5 年生存率为 96.9%,进行了淋巴结清扫术的为 97.7%,而淋巴清扫术后发现分期为ⅢC 期的患者 5 年生存率为 93.4%。这些生存率没有统计学上的差异,强调了无性细胞瘤患者的预后较好[26~39]。

未成熟畸胎瘤

未成熟畸胎瘤包含未成熟的神经上皮,可以是单纯的未成熟畸胎瘤或者与其他生殖细胞肿瘤并存而称为混合型生殖细胞肿瘤。单纯的未成熟畸胎瘤仅占所有卵巢恶性肿瘤不到 1%,但该病是第二常见的卵巢恶性生殖细胞肿瘤,在不到 20 岁的年轻女性中占所有卵巢恶性肿瘤的 10%~20%[1]。大约 50%的卵巢单纯未成熟畸胎瘤发生在 10~20 岁之间,该病很少在绝经后女性中出现。

神经上皮细胞数目的半定量与卵巢未成熟畸胎瘤的预后相关,也是该病病理分级的基础[55~57]。切片中未成熟神经上皮最多的地方少于一个低倍镜视野(G1)者,生存率在 95%以上,而未成熟神经上皮细胞密度更高(G2、G3)的患者总体生存率较低(约 85%)[57]。这点并不适用于儿童卵巢未成熟畸胎瘤,因为儿童卵巢未成熟畸胎瘤无论其分化程度如何,单纯手术效果很好。这些结果来自于并非所有患者接受以铂为基础的化疗的年代[58,59]。

一些病理学家推荐两级分级系统,建议将未成熟畸胎瘤分为低级别或高级别,因为按照 3 级分级系统,无论一个病理医生重复阅片还是病理医生之间都难以得到一致的结论[55],这也是作者目前的实践情况。

卵巢未成熟畸胎瘤可能与腹膜神经胶质瘤相关，后者如果由完全成熟的组织组成则提示预后良好。最近的报道指出，这些神经胶质"种植成分"不是来源于肿瘤，而是畸胎瘤诱导的腹膜多潜能 Müllerian 干细胞化生而成[58,60,61]。研究者发现卵巢畸胎瘤一个独特之处：畸胎瘤含有一套母系染色体的复制，因此在微卫星多态位点为纯合，而相匹配的正常组织 DNA（脱氧核糖核酸）同时包括来源于母系以及父系的遗传成分，因此相应的微卫星多态位点显示为杂合。

成熟畸胎瘤转化为恶性很少见，鳞状细胞癌是最常见的恶性类型，腺癌、原发性黑色素瘤、类癌也会发生，但很少见（见下面的讨论）[32]。据报道畸胎瘤恶变的风险在 0.5%到 2%之间，常发生在绝经后患者。

诊断

术前评估及鉴别诊断和其他生殖细胞肿瘤相同。某些未成熟畸胎瘤也会像成熟畸胎瘤一样含有钙化，这可以通过腹部 X 线片或超声发现。很少情况下，该病可能会产生类固醇激素，可能会伴有假性性早熟[4]。在一些单纯未成熟畸胎瘤患者中 AFP 可能升高，但 hCG 不升高。

手术

对于肿瘤局限于一侧卵巢的绝经前患者，应行单侧卵巢切除术和有限的分期手术。对于少见的绝经后未成熟畸胎瘤患者，应行全子宫及双附件切除术。对侧卵巢受侵比较少见，因此没有必要将对侧卵巢行常规切除或楔形切除活检[2]。腹膜表面任何可疑病变都应取样送检做组织病理学评估。最常见的转移部位是腹膜，更少见的是腹膜后淋巴结。血行转移至脏器实质如肺、肝或大脑等并不常见。当出现脏器实质转移的时候，患者通常处于晚期或复发，肿瘤通常为高级别[4]。

对转移病灶行减瘤术是否提高对化疗的疗效尚不明确[62,63]。疗效基本上取决于是否能立即开始化疗。任何可能会导致潜在并发症而延误化疗的手术应暂不进行，可以在化疗完成后考虑手术切除残存病灶。

化疗

ⅠA 期 G1 的患者预后很好，不需要行辅助化疗。对于高级别ⅠA 期未成熟畸胎瘤，通常给予辅助化疗，但是这也存在争议，因为有报道指出通过密切随访监测复发后给予治疗也能有好的预后[19,22,28~30,44,59,64~78]。

过去最常用的联合化疗方案是 VAC[72~74]，但是 GOG 一项研究显示对于未完全切除肿瘤的患者无病生存率仅为 75%[74]。过去 20 年，含顺铂联合方案加入该病的一线治疗中，以前 VBP 是最常用的方案，近来 BEP 更常用[67]。

GOG 对完全切除肿瘤的Ⅰ期、Ⅱ期、Ⅲ期卵巢生殖细胞肿瘤患者进行了一项 3 程 BEP 方案化疗的前瞻性研究。总体来讲，毒性是可以耐受的，93 例非无性细胞瘤患者中 91 例（97.8%）可达临床治愈。在非随机性研究中，对于完全切除肿瘤的卵巢非无性细胞瘤的生殖细胞肿瘤患者，BEP 方案优于 VAC 方案。由于部分患者术后会迅速进展，对于需要化疗的患者，术后应尽快开始化疗，最好在 7~10 天内开始。

BEP 替代 VBP 方案的提出来源于睾丸癌的治疗经验，依托泊苷替代长春碱可以有更好的治疗效果（同等的效果和更低的并发症），更少的神经和胃肠道毒性，并提高预后[67,68]。此外，博来霉素的应用在这组患者中也很重要。在一项随机试验中，在 166 例睾丸生殖细胞肿瘤患者中，给予 3 个周期的 EP（依托泊苷+顺铂）或 BEP（依托泊苷+顺铂+博来霉素）方案，BEP 方案无复发生存率为 84%，EP 方案为 69%（$P=0.03$）[40]。

已发生转移的睾丸生殖细胞肿瘤中顺铂优于卡铂。一项研究纳入了 192 例预后好的睾丸生殖细胞肿瘤患者，给予 4 周期的 EP 或 EC 方案化疗。EP 方案化疗的有 3 例复发，EC 方案化疗的有 7 例患者复发[42]。一项德国的研究随机将患者分为：①3 周期标准剂量的 BEP 方案，第 1~5 天；②CEB 方案：卡铂（AUC 5）第 1 天，依托泊苷 120mg/m^2 第 1~3 天，博来霉素 30mg 第 1、8、15 天[79]。给予 4 周期的 CEB 化疗，第 4 周期不使用博来霉素，以便两种方案中依托泊苷和博来霉素的累积剂量相当。54 例患者纳入了该试验。29 例给予了 BEP，25 例给予了 CEB 方案化疗。CEB 方案化疗组复发的患者更多（32% vs 13%）。4 例（16%）患者 CEB 方案化疗后死于疾病进展，而 BEP 组 1 例（3%）患者化疗后死于疾病进展。中期分析后该试验提前终止。另一项由 Horwich 等报道的更大的随机试验也印证了卡铂的劣势[80]。根据这些结果，BEP 方案是更推荐的治疗方案[67,81~83]。BEP 的 3 天方案与 5 天方案疗效相当。BEP 方案包括依托泊苷 500mg/m^2：100mg/m^2 第 1~5 天，或者 165mg/m^2 第 1~3 天，顺铂 100mg/m^2：20mg/m^2 第 1~5 天，或者 50mg/m^2 第 1~2 天，博来霉素 30mg 第 1、8、15 天，第 1~3 周期。

肿瘤复发

复发未成熟畸胎瘤的治疗原则及方案同前面所讨论的复发无性细胞瘤一致。

二次开腹探查术

对于接受辅助化疗的卵巢生殖细胞肿瘤患者，一般不推荐二次剖腹探查术（如ⅠA 期，G2 和 G3）。但是，对于化疗后仍有残存肿瘤的转移性未成熟畸胎瘤应考虑手术，因为这些患者可能存在残存的成熟性畸胎瘤，有发生成熟畸胎瘤综合征的风险，这是未成熟畸胎瘤一种少见的并发症[84~86]。此外，残存的成熟畸胎瘤将来可能恶变，切除残存肿瘤和排除持续性病变很重要，而且可能需要进一步化疗。

手术原则借鉴了较多的男性生殖细胞肿瘤合并未成熟畸胎瘤化疗后仍有残存肿瘤患者的手术经验[87]。Mathew 等[88]报道了他们卵巢生殖细胞肿瘤化疗后残存肿瘤进行开腹探查评估其性质的经验。68 例患者完成了含顺铂的联合方案化疗，其中 35 例影像学显示有残存肿瘤。这 35 例患者中 29 例进行了开腹手术，其中 10 例（34.5%）证实有肿瘤残存，包括 7 例（24.2%）未成熟畸胎瘤。19 例（65.5%）患者没有恶性证据，其中 3 例（10.3%）为成熟畸胎瘤，16 例（55.2%）仅为坏死或纤维组织。没有一例无性细胞瘤和胚胎性癌影像学显示残存肿瘤小于 5cm 的患者残存有活性的肿瘤，然而所有原发肿瘤含有畸胎瘤成分的患者均有残存肿瘤，更强调了转移性未成熟畸胎瘤有任何残存肿瘤需行手术[88,89]。

预后

未成熟畸胎瘤最重要的预后因素是肿瘤的分级[1,55]。此外，初始治疗前肿瘤的分期以及肿瘤大小对预后也有影响[4]。总之，对于所有期别的单纯未成熟畸胎瘤患者 5 年生存率为 70%～80%，手术分期为Ⅰ期的患者 5 年生存率为 90%～95%[11,44,55,64]。

未成熟程度或分级通常可以预测肿瘤的转移倾向及预后。据报道 G1、G2、G3 患者的 5 年生存率分别为 82%、62% 和 30%[55]。但是这些患者中很多发生在尚无合适的化疗手段的年代，这些数据和现在的经验以及最近报道的数据无法匹配[69]。比如，Lai 等[90]报道了 84 例卵巢生殖细胞肿瘤患者的长期结局，包括 29 例未成熟畸胎瘤，5 年生存率为 97.4%。

偶尔，这些肿瘤可能与成熟或低级别神经胶质成分相关，可通过腹膜种植。这些患者有良好的长期生存[4]。成熟的神经胶质成分可以生长，模拟恶性肿瘤的行为，可能需要切除来减轻对周围组织的压迫。

内胚窦瘤

内胚窦瘤也被称为卵黄囊瘤，因为它们来源于原始卵黄囊[1]。该病是第三常见的卵巢恶性生殖细胞肿瘤。内胚窦瘤中位诊断年龄为 18 岁[1~3,91,92]。大约 1/3 的患者发现时为初潮前患者。腹部或盆腔痛的发生率约 75%，而无症状的盆腔包块见于约 10%的患者[11]。大部分内胚窦瘤分泌 AFP，很少情况下也分泌可检测到的 α-1-抗胰蛋白酶（AAT）。肿瘤的严重程度与 AFP 的水平显著相关，尽管也有观察到不一致的情况。血清 AFP 水平可用来监测患者对治疗的反应，以及用于随访[91~98]。

手术

内胚窦瘤的治疗包括手术探查，单侧附件切除，冰冻病理诊断以及有限的分期手术。不应行子宫切除术及对侧附件切除术[4,94,95]。像其他生殖细胞肿瘤一样，保守手术及辅助化疗可以保留生育[23]。对于发生转移的患者，应尽可能切除所有可见的病变。术中所见肿瘤通常为实性，较大，直径在 7～28cm（中位 15cm）。几乎没有双侧发生的内胚窦瘤，只有在腹腔有其他部位转移时，对侧卵巢才可能受侵。大多数患者处于早期：71%Ⅰ期，6%Ⅱ期，23%Ⅲ期[95,99]。

化疗

所有内胚窦瘤患者应该在术后短期内开始化疗。在常规应用联合化疗前，2 年生存率约为 25%。应用 VAC 方案化疗后，生存率提高到了 60%～70%，显示出该病大多数患者对化疗敏感[73,74]。所有患者应该行以顺铂为基础的化疗，比如 BEP，该方案被认为是标准治疗。早期患者的治愈概率将近 100%，更晚期患者至少 75%[95]。

卵巢生殖细胞肿瘤中最佳的化疗周期数尚未确定，但是从更有经验的睾丸生殖细胞肿瘤中可以合理地推测，3 周期的 BEP 方案对于预后好，低风险的患者是最佳的，4 周期对于中危到高危患者是合适的[100]。对于因为毒性不能使用博来霉素的患者，推荐 4 周期的顺铂联合依托泊苷。对于更晚期的博来霉素为禁忌的患者，一个可选择的方案为 VIP（依托泊苷、异环磷酰胺、顺铂）。4 周期的 VIP 与 4 周期的 BEP 疗效相当，但是 VIP 的骨髓毒性更重，需要生长因子的支持[6,7,101]。需要对生殖细胞肿瘤有经验的临床医生来治疗这些患者，因为没有经验的医生会影响患者的疗效。

近来印度的一项 21 例患者的研究显示，新辅助化疗后行保留生育的手术对于无法完成满意减瘤术的晚期卵巢生殖细胞肿瘤也可能是一种合理的选择[102]。

胚胎癌

卵巢胚胎癌非常少见。因为其缺少合体滋养层和细胞滋养层细胞，可以与绒毛膜癌鉴别。患者非常年轻，在两项研究中，患者年龄从 4 到 28 岁不等（中位 14 岁）[103]。也有报道过年纪更大的患者[104]。胚胎癌可能分泌雌激素，导致一些患者会出现假性性早熟或者阴道不规则出血[1]。其他表现与内胚窦瘤相似。原发病灶一般会比较大，发现时大约 2/3 局限于一侧卵巢。这些病变常常分泌 AFP 和 hCG，可以通过这些标记物随访评估患者对治疗的反应[96]。胚胎癌的治疗原则与内胚窦瘤相同[57]。

卵巢绒毛膜癌

单纯卵巢非妊娠绒毛膜癌非常少见。该病患者多小于 20 岁，与转移至卵巢的妊娠相关绒癌的组织学表现相同[105]。hCG 可用来监测患者对治疗的反应。如果 hCG 水平很高，在初潮来临前出现肿瘤的患者大约 50%会出现同性性早熟[106,107]。

仅有少量关于非妊娠相关的绒毛膜癌化疗的报道，但是已有报道显示该病像妊娠相关的滋养细胞疾病一样应用 MAC 方案（甲氨蝶呤、放线菌素 D、环磷酰胺）可完全缓解[105]。该病非常少见所以没有很好的研究数据，其他选择可有 BEP 或 POMB-ACE 方案（表 105-3）。卵巢绒毛膜癌预后较差。大部分初诊时已发生脏器实质转移的患者应按照高危生殖细胞肿瘤进行治疗。

表 105-3　卵巢生殖细胞肿瘤 POMB/ACE 化疗方案

POMB	
第 1 天	长春新碱 $1mg/m^2$ IV，甲氨蝶呤 $300mg/m^2$，12h 输注
第 2 天	博来霉素 15mg，24h 输注，亚叶酸解救在 MTX 开始 24h 后，15mg/12h，共 4 次
第 3 天	博来霉素 15mg，24h 输注
第 4 天	顺铂 $120mg/m^2$，同时给予水化及补充 3mg 硫酸镁
ACE	
第 1～5 天	依托泊苷（VP16）$100mg/m^2$，第 1～5 天
第 3～5 天	放线菌素 D 0.5mg IV，第 3～5 天
第 5 天	环磷酰胺 $500mg/m^2$ IV，第 5 天
OMB	
第 1 天	长春新碱 $1mg/m^2$ IV，甲氨蝶呤 $300mg/m^2$，12h 输注
第 2 天	博来霉素 15mg，24h 输注，亚叶酸解救 24h 后开始
第 3 天	博来霉素 15mg，24h 输注

治疗计划是 2 周期 POMB 后 ACE。POMB 之后与 ACE 交替直至患者通过 hCG、AFP、PLAP、LDH 评估生化缓解。通常 POMB 为 3～5 周期。生化缓解后，ACE 与 OMB 交替直至缓解持续大约 12 周。两程化疗间隔尽量缩小（通常 9～11 天）。如果 ACE 化疗后因为骨髓抑制延误，在接下来的 ACE 化疗中则省去前两天的依托泊苷。

多胚瘤

卵巢多胚瘤是另一种极其少见的肿瘤，由“拟胚体”组成。该肿瘤复制早期胚胎分化的结构（即三个体细胞层：内胚层、中胚层和外胚层）[1,12]。该病发生在非常年轻的初潮前女孩，有假性青春期表现，AFP 和 hCG 水平升高。多胚瘤局限在一侧卵巢的患者术后可以通过连续的肿瘤标记物和诊断性影像学检查随访，免于细胞毒药物化疗。对于需要化疗的患者，常用 BEP 方案[73]。

混合型生殖细胞肿瘤

卵巢混合型生殖细胞恶性肿瘤包含上面提到的两种或更多种成分。在一项研究中，混合型生殖细胞肿瘤中最常见的成分是无性细胞瘤，占 80%，其次是内胚窦瘤，占 70%，未成熟畸胎瘤，占 53%，绒毛膜癌占 20%，胚胎性癌占 16%。最常见的组合是无性细胞瘤合并内胚窦瘤。混合型生殖细胞肿瘤可能分泌 AFP 和/或 hCG，或者两者均无，这取决于肿瘤的组成成分。

该病应该联合化疗，最合适的方案是 BEP。血清肿瘤标记物如果最初是阳性的，化疗后可能转阴，但这可能只反映该其中某一种成分的消退。因此如果化疗后仍有残存肿瘤可能需要二次手术，尤其是初始肿瘤中含有未成熟畸胎瘤成分者。

最重要的预后因素为初始肿瘤的大小和最恶性成分所占的比例[74]。Ⅰ A 期，肿瘤小于 10cm 的患者存活率为 100%。肿瘤成分中内胚窦瘤、绒毛膜癌或 G3 未成熟畸胎瘤占比小于 1/3 的预后也很好，但是当这些成分占肿瘤的大部分时患者预后不佳。

Ⅰ期卵巢生殖细胞肿瘤的随访

对Ⅰ期睾丸生殖细胞肿瘤的年轻患者，术后常规随访监测。大量证据支持术后随访监测，有许多指南推荐如何进行合适的随访[6,7]。虽然多达 20%～30%患者会出现复发，但几乎所有的患者可以通过 BEP 挽救性化疗而治愈，化疗潜在的副作用多数也可以避免。

年轻男性患者常规进行监测随访，但仍未广泛用于女性卵巢生殖细胞肿瘤患者。目前有一些数据支持对一部分肿瘤局限于卵巢的患者进行随访。Cushing 等人[108]报道了一项 44 例儿童卵巢未成熟畸胎瘤的研究，该研究中患者肿瘤均完全切除，随后进行严密的影像学和血清学随访。31 例（70.5%）患者为单纯卵巢未成熟畸胎瘤，其中有 17 例 G1、12 例 G2、2 例 G3。13 例（29.5%）患者为卵巢未成熟畸胎瘤合并镜下卵黄囊瘤。4 年无瘤和总生存率在卵巢未成熟畸胎瘤组和卵巢未成熟畸胎瘤合并卵黄囊瘤组分别为 97.7%（95%CI 84.9%～99.7%）和 100%。未成熟畸胎瘤合并卵黄囊瘤组中仅 1 例患者出现卵黄囊瘤复发，通过化疗进行挽救性治疗[108]。

Charing Cross 小组最先报道了一项前瞻性研究，该研究中 24 例Ⅰ A 期卵巢生殖细胞肿瘤患者也纳入了随访监测。其中包含 9 例（37.5%）无性细胞瘤，9 例（37.5%）单纯未成熟畸胎瘤，6 例（25%）内胚窦瘤（合并或未合并未成熟畸胎瘤）。治疗为手术切除，没有进行辅助化疗，术后监测项目包括临床症状、血清学以及影像学检查。所有患者进行了二次开腹探查术，在中位随访时间 6.8 年时，除 1 例外其余患者都存活且获得缓解。5 年 OS 为 95%，5 年的 DFS 为 68%。8 例患者因为疾病复发或者第二原发生殖细胞肿瘤需要化疗。这其中包括 3 例 G2 未成熟畸胎瘤，3 例无性细胞瘤以及 2 例在 4.5 和 5.2 年后对侧卵巢出现无性细胞瘤的患者。除了 1 例患者死于肺栓塞外，其余患者全部通过化疗挽救成功[109]。

同一研究组更新了他们的经验，报道了其对Ⅰ A 期女性卵巢 GCT 患者术后随访观察的安全性[25]。37 例（中位年龄为 26 岁，范围 14～48 岁）Ⅰ期肿瘤患者从 1981 年到 2003 年进入 Mount Vernon 和 Charing Cross 医院进行治疗。患者进行手术及分期，之后通过定期肿瘤标记物及影像学进行严密随访。中位随访时间为 6 年。Ⅰ A 期非无性细胞瘤的复发率为 36%（8/22），无性细胞瘤为 22%（2/9）。此外，1 例成熟畸胎瘤合并胶质瘤患者同样出现肿瘤复发。这 11 例复发患者中，10 例（91%）通过铂类药物为基础的化疗治愈。1 例因为化疗耐药而死亡。所有的肿瘤复发均出现在手术后 13 个月以内。恶性卵巢 GCT 总疾病特异性生存率为 94%。

接受保留生育功能手术的患者 50%以上能够成功受孕。研究者认为与睾丸肿瘤类似，所有Ⅰ A 期卵巢 GCT 的监测均为安全可行。他们同时对所有非无性细胞瘤患者进行有潜在毒性的辅助化疗提出质疑，因为这些患者即便出现肿瘤复发，也有大于 90%的机会通过化疗挽救。

上述随访监测方案很吸引人，并有更大量儿科文献支持，但在成年人中的经验较少，需要国际合作来进一步研究。如果有研究者拟开展该监测项目，并使用 Charing Cross 小组的方案，应严格执行该方案并让患者知晓该方案在成年人的研究数据有限。

监测方案非常严格，如果术前未行检查，术后应行胸腹盆 CT。如果未行充分的手术分期，术后 12 周应复查腹盆 MRI/CT 或者行二次腹腔镜探查术。如果以上均为阴性，12 个月后复查 MRI/CT。患者第一年每一个月复查一次，第二年每 2 个月复查一次，第三年每 3 个月复查一次，直到第 5 年，之后 5 年每 6 个月复查一次。每间隔一次需要复查盆腔超声及胸片。肿瘤标记物包括 AFP、β-hCG、CA125、LDH 在 6 个月内应该每 2 周复查一次，之后 6 个月每月复查一次，第 2 年每两月复查一次，第 3 年每 3 个月复查一次，直到第 5 年，之后 5 年每 6 个月复查一次[25,109]。

卵巢恶性生殖细胞肿瘤治疗的远期并发症

已有大量数据报道关于以顺铂为基础的化疗在男性睾丸癌治疗中的远期副作用，但针对卵巢生殖细胞肿瘤的文献却很少。BEP 方案化疗毒性在男性患者中记载较清楚，包括会使 5%的患者出现严重肺毒性，1%的患者出现致死性肺毒性，0.2%～1%的患者出现急性髓性白血病或骨髓增生异常综合征，20%～30%会出现神经病变：20%出现雷诺现象，24%出现耳鸣，多达 70%患者会出现高音听力损失。另外还包括对性腺功能的影响，高血压、心血管疾病风险增加，以及在 30%的患者中会出现一定程度的肾脏损伤[110,111]。这些副作用强调了限制化疗周期数的重要性：低风险患者限制在 3 周期，高风险患者限制在 4 周期 BEP 方案，患者寻求有经验医师的必要性[89,112]。

性腺功能

引起卵巢生殖细胞肿瘤患者不孕的一个重要原因是不必要的双侧附件及子宫全切术。尽管以铂为基础的化疗常常会导致暂时的卵巢功能障碍，大部分患者可以恢复正常的卵巢功能，生育能力可以保留[14,21,23,36~40]。在一项纳入了 47 例联合化疗的生殖细胞恶性肿瘤患者的研究中，91.5%的患者恢复了正常的月经，有 14 个健康的婴儿存活，并且没有出生缺陷[23]。一些因素比如开始化疗的年龄较大、累积药物剂量更高、治疗时期更长等因素都会对将来性腺功能产生不利影响[37,89,112~114]。

GOG 近来报道了一项较大的卵巢生殖细胞肿瘤患者进行以铂为基础的化疗后生育及性腺功能的研究，该研究纳入了 132 例存活患者。令人吃惊的是，只有 71 例(53.8%)患者接受了保留生育的手术，在这些患者中，87.3%仍有规律的月经周期。24 例患者接受癌症治疗后育有 37 名子女[82,115]。

继发恶性肿瘤

生殖细胞肿瘤患者化疗后远期发病及死亡的一个重要原因就是继发恶性肿瘤[89]。尤其依托泊苷被认为与治疗相关的白血病相关。

治疗相关白血病的发生率与依托泊苷的使用剂量相关。依托泊苷累积剂量小于 2 000mg/m^2[116] 的患者患白血病的概率为 0.4%～0.5%(概率提高了 30 倍)，而依托泊苷累积剂量大于 2 000mg/m^2[117] 的患者患白血病的概率高达 5%(概率提高了 336 倍)。在标准的 3 或 4 周期 BEP 方案化疗后，患者接受的依托泊苷累积剂量分别为 1 500mg/m^2 和 2 000mg/m^2。

尽管存在继发白血病的风险，但风险-获益分析得出结论：含依托泊苷的化疗方案对于晚期生殖细胞肿瘤有益。与 PVB(顺铂、长春新碱、博来霉素)相比，每 20 名接受 BEP 治疗的患者预计会有 1 例发生治疗相关白血病。对于低风险患者，或者高剂量依托泊苷进行挽救性治疗患者的风险-获益分析尚不清楚[117]。

性索间质肿瘤

卵巢性索间质肿瘤占所有卵巢恶性肿瘤的 5%～8%[1~4,118~123]。该肿瘤来源于性索和卵巢基质或间质，常包含多种不同成分，包括“女性”细胞(颗粒细胞和卵泡膜细胞)、“男性”细胞(支持细胞和间质细胞)，还有一些形态学上属于未分化细胞。该肿瘤的分类见表 105-4[10,124]。

表 105-4　性索间质肿瘤[9]

A. 颗粒间质细胞肿瘤
1. 颗粒细胞瘤
2. 卵泡膜-纤维瘤组
a. 卵泡膜细胞瘤
b. 纤维瘤
c. 未分类
B. 男性母细胞瘤：支持-间质细胞瘤
1. 分化良好
a. 支持细胞瘤
b. 支持-间质细胞瘤
c. 间质细胞瘤；门细胞瘤
2. 中分化
3. 低分化(肉瘤样)
4. 含异源组织成分
C. 两性母细胞瘤
D. 未分类

颗粒间质细胞肿瘤

颗粒间质细胞肿瘤包括颗粒细胞瘤、卵泡膜细胞瘤和纤维瘤。颗粒细胞瘤为低度恶性，卵泡膜细胞瘤和纤维瘤是良性的，很少情况可能会出现恶性形态学表现，一旦出现则称之为纤维肉瘤[1,125]。

颗粒细胞瘤可分泌雌激素，可以发生在任何年龄女性中，分为成人颗粒细胞肿瘤和幼年型颗粒细胞肿瘤。青春期前女性患者占总数的 5%；其他患者分布在整个生育期至绝经后[122,123,126,127]。只有 2%的患者出现双侧病变(图 105-3)。

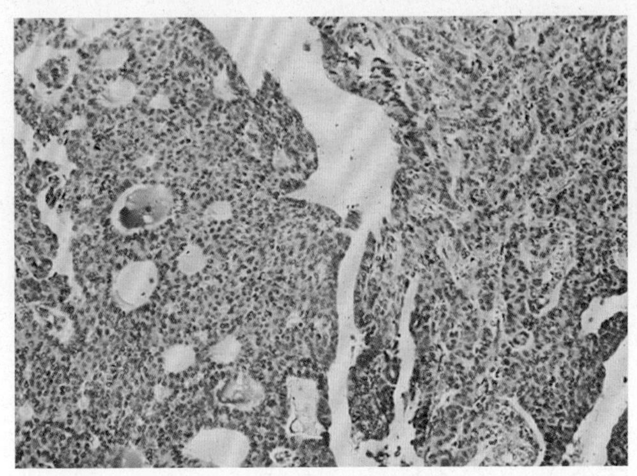

图 105-3　颗粒细胞瘤

而在青春期前发病的患者中，因为分泌雌激素，75%与假性性早熟有关[123]。育龄患者中，多数可出现月经不调或继发闭经。而在绝经后患者中，子宫异常出血是常见的症状。至少5%颗粒细胞瘤与子宫内膜癌发生相关，25%~50%与子宫内膜增生相关[1,120,122,123,126]。极少数情况下，颗粒细胞瘤可能分泌雄激素，引起女性男性化。

颗粒细胞肿瘤的其他一些症状和体征则不特异，与大部分卵巢恶性肿瘤相似。大约10%的患者会出现腹水，很少出现胸腔积液[122,123]。该肿瘤可导致出血，偶尔肿瘤出现破裂，会造成腹腔积血。

颗粒细胞瘤在诊断时多为Ⅰ期，但在初始治疗5~30年后可能复发[121]。肿瘤可通过血行转移，在多年后转移至肺、肝和脑。恶性泡膜细胞瘤很少见，其症状、治疗和预后等情况与颗粒细胞瘤相似[125,127]。

在所有卵巢成人型颗粒细胞肿瘤中发现都存在编码FOXL2基因的体细胞错义突变。FOXL2 402 CG导致功能的增加或改变，被认为是成人颗粒细胞肿瘤的驱动突变。目前正在尝试将其作为治疗靶点[128~130]。

诊断

颗粒细胞瘤会分泌抑制素，可作为诊断和监测的肿瘤标记物[131~135]。它是一种主要由颗粒细胞分泌的多肽激素，抑制垂体分泌FSH。绝经后抑制素的水平下降，检测不出。某些卵巢肿瘤（黏液性卵巢上皮癌、颗粒细胞瘤）分泌抑制素，可以在出现临床复发症状之前该激素水平升高[136~138]。在绝经期前女性，血浆抑制素水平升高合并闭经或不孕症提示颗粒细胞肿瘤。

过去，抑制素的检测方法不能区分抑制素A和B，只能检测总的抑制素的量。但是，现在已经有特有的免疫分析方法分别检测抑制素A和B。颗粒细胞瘤主要分泌的是抑制素B，有报道显示抑制素B比A更能准确地反映疾病状态。检测抑制素B的浓度而不是总的抑制素或抑制素A，可以更好地随访颗粒细胞瘤[134,139]。

抗Müllerian管激素（AMH），也被称作Müllerian管抑制因子（MIS），由颗粒细胞分泌，是这些肿瘤新兴的潜在肿瘤标记物[135]。升高的AMH显示出高特异性。检测方法在商业上可行，AMH在颗粒细胞瘤治疗中的作用正在研究中[140]。升高的雌激素水平不是颗粒细胞瘤敏感的标记物[137]。

卵巢颗粒细胞瘤的标记物（如抑制素、CD99、AMH）进行染色有助于组织学诊断[131,132]。抑制素抗体似乎最有用，但并不特异[128]。在一个报道中，94%的颗粒细胞瘤和10%~20%的卵巢子宫内膜样癌以及转移癌，抑制素染色阳性[135]。后者显示染色强度明显减弱。如果不能确诊，目前可以通过分子检测进行FOXL2突变检测协助诊断[129,130]。

治疗

颗粒细胞瘤的治疗取决于患者的年龄以及病变范围。对于大多数患者，初始治疗仅行手术即可，放疗和化疗可以用于复发或转移的患者[122,123,126,127]。

手术

颗粒细胞瘤在大约2%的患者中累及双侧，因此单侧输卵管-卵巢切除术对于ⅠA期儿童或育龄期女性较为合适[119]。如果开腹手术冰冻切片发现颗粒细胞瘤，应该进行适当的分期手术，包括评估对侧卵巢[141~144]。同恶性生殖细胞肿瘤一样，分期术包括冲洗液、网膜活检、腹膜表面和腹膜后淋巴结的仔细触诊以及对任何可疑病变的活检。如果对侧卵巢增大，应取活检。如果有转移病灶，应尽可能切除干净，因为该肿瘤会缓慢生长而且对化疗不敏感。对于围绝经期及绝经后女性，保留卵巢意义不大，应采取子宫切除和双附件切除术。对于绝经前未行子宫切除的女性，由于可能同时合并子宫内膜腺癌，应行刮宫术。

放疗

尽管盆腔放疗可以治疗孤立的盆腔复发灶，但尚无证据支持颗粒细胞瘤患者进行辅助放疗[121,122,138]。对于持续存在或复发的颗粒细胞瘤，尤其是已进行手术减瘤的患者，放疗可以诱导临床缓解，偶尔可获得长期缓解[138,145,146]。在一项单中心34例患者随访超过40年的回顾性研究中，14例（41.2%）有可测量病灶的患者进行了治疗[145]，3例（21%）在放疗后10~21年存活且无肿瘤进展。

化疗

目前尚无证据对Ⅰ期患者进行辅助化疗能够阻止复发。出现转移的颗粒细胞瘤患者过去数年一直采取多种不同的抗肿瘤药物。虽然已经有报道单药环磷酰胺和美法仑以及联合方案VAC、PAC（顺铂、多柔比星和环磷酰胺）、PVB和BEP化疗达完全缓解的患者，但没有一个持续有效的治疗方案[4,119,147~158]。近年来卡铂和紫杉醇[138]以及贝伐珠单抗[159]显示出一定的疗效。

因为这类肿瘤较罕见，很难对Ⅱ~Ⅳ期患者开展设计合理的随机试验。回顾性研究显示，Ⅲ~Ⅳ期患者术后化疗可以提高PFS[138,149]，但是并没有提高OS[150]。尽管缺乏支持生存受益的数据，但由于疾病进展风险高，并且以铂类为基础的化疗可能会提高存活率，一些专家仍建议Ⅱ~Ⅳ期的患者手术完全切除后进行化疗[138,151~154]。目前可选择的方案包括BEP、EP、PAC以及卡铂和紫杉醇[138]。

对于未满意减瘤的患者，BEP治疗的总体缓解率为58%~83%[138,151,155]。一项38例进展期患者的研究显示，患者完成4个疗程的BEP化疗，行二次手术探查，14例（37%）患者无阳性发现[151]。中位随诊时间为3年的随访中，16例原发晚期肿瘤患者中11例（69%）未出现疾病进展，而41例复发患者中，21例（51%）未出现疾病进展。该方案有严重的毒副作用，并出现两例博来霉素相关的死亡。据报道，卡铂联合依托泊苷[156]、PVB[122,157]、PAC[147,158]也有相当高的缓解率。

对于年长患者，需要寻找新的毒性小、疗效相当的治疗方案。紫杉醇有一定的抗肿瘤活性，有研究报道铂类联合紫杉醇缓解率可达60%，可能是更有效的治疗选择[160~162]。

肿瘤复发

复发的中位时间是诊断后大约4~6年[119,121,142,154]。对于复发肿瘤的治疗没有标准方案。常见的复发部位是盆腔，上腹部也可能累及。如果肿瘤局限，进一步的手术可能是有效的，而弥漫性腹部转移治疗比较困难。化疗和放疗对部分患者可能有效。

约 30%的颗粒细胞瘤患者雌激素受体阳性,100%的患者孕激素受体阳性[163,164]。激素制剂如孕酮、促黄体生成素释放激素(LHRH)拮抗剂等可用于治疗,但相关数据有限[137]。一些小样本量的研究和个案报道显示,13 例患者中 LHRH 拮抗剂缓解率为 50%[164~166]。5 例患者中 4 例(80%)对促孕激素有反应[167]。Freeman 近期报道了两例复发成人型颗粒细胞瘤患者。此两例患者接受了包括化疗在内的多种治疗,并在接受亮丙瑞林治疗时,疾病发生进展。两例患者阿那曲唑治疗后,抑制素 B 水平和临床检查维持正常,两例患者分别维持治疗 14 个月和 18 个月[168]。

因为数量很少,不能得出有效结论,这其中可能存在明显的发表偏倚,报道的更多的是治疗有效的病例[169]。

预后

卵巢颗粒细胞瘤的预后取决于肿瘤的手术分期[121,123,138,170~173]。大多数颗粒细胞瘤是惰性的,诊断时局限于一侧卵巢,Ⅰ期肿瘤的治愈率为 75%~92%[123,144,154,173]。但是,远期复发也并不少见[119,121,123]。在一项纳入了 37 例Ⅰ期患者的研究中,5 年、10 年、20 年的生存率分别为 94%、82%和 62%。Ⅱ~Ⅳ期患者的 5 年和 10 年生存率分别为 55%和 34%。

在成人肿瘤中,细胞异型性、有丝分裂率和缺乏 Call-Exner 小体是早期复发唯一、重要的病理预测因子[153]。肿瘤核型异常和 *P53* 过表达似乎都与预后无关[174]。肿瘤的 DNA 倍体数与生存期相关。Holland 等[148]报道了 37 例原发性颗粒细胞瘤患者中的 13 例(35%)DNA 非整倍体。有残存肿瘤是无进展生存的最重要的预测因子,但 DNA 倍体数是一个独立的预后因素。无残存肿瘤和肿瘤 DNA 为二倍体的患者 10 年无进展生存率为 96%。

幼年型颗粒细胞瘤

卵巢幼年型颗粒细胞瘤很少见,在幼年和青春期卵巢恶性肿瘤中占不到 5%[156]。大约 90%诊断时为Ⅰ期,预后较好。幼年型颗粒细胞瘤的侵袭性弱于成人型颗粒细胞瘤。晚期肿瘤可以通过铂为基础的联合化疗获得很好的治疗效果(比如 BEP)[138]。

支持-间质细胞瘤

支持-间质细胞肿瘤最常发生于 20~40 岁,75%的患者年龄小于 40 岁。这类肿瘤在卵巢恶性肿瘤中的比例不足 0.2%[13]。支持-间质细胞瘤多为低级别恶性肿瘤,但分化差的肿瘤可能更具有侵袭性。

该肿瘤产生雄激素,临床上 70%~85%患者出现女性男性化[175,176]。男性化的表现包括月经稀发甚至闭经、乳腺萎缩、痤疮、多毛、阴蒂增大、声音变粗以及发际线后移。血清雄激素检测提示睾酮、雄烯二酮增高,伴硫酸脱氢表雄酮正常或轻度增高[1]。少数情况下支持-间质细胞瘤与雌激素化表现相关,例如性早熟,不规则出血或绝经后出血[176]。

治疗

由于这类低级别肿瘤仅有不到 1%累及双侧,育龄期女性的治疗通常采取单侧附件切除术,同时评估对侧卵巢[176]。对于年龄较大的患者,应行子宫切除及双附件切除术。

对于病变持续存在者应用化疗的资料有限,但是有报道显示,对于存在可测量的瘤灶的患者,应用顺铂联合多柔比星或异环磷酰胺或联合两者[176],或者应用上述提到的颗粒细胞瘤的化疗方案,能够有一定缓解。因为该病少见,大多数研究都包括颗粒细胞瘤[152]。盆腔放疗也可以用于盆腔复发肿瘤,但效果有限。

预后

5 年生存率为 70%~90%,此后复发并不常见[1,2,176]。大多数死亡病例为分化差的肿瘤患者。

罕见卵巢肿瘤

还有几种少见的卵巢恶性肿瘤,合起来只占卵巢恶性肿瘤的 0.1%。这些病变包括脂质细胞瘤、原发卵巢肉瘤和小细胞卵巢癌。

脂质细胞瘤

脂质细胞瘤被认为来源于靠近卵巢的肾上腺皮质残迹。目前已经报道了超过 100 例脂质细胞瘤,只有少数患者累及双侧[1]。大多数患者为女性男性化,有时伴肥胖、高血压、糖耐量异常,提示有糖皮质激素的分泌。少数患者为雌激素分泌型,可表现为性早熟。

多数脂质细胞瘤为良性和低级别,但约有 20%的患者可发生腹腔转移,极少数发生远处转移。主要的治疗方式是手术,对于放疗和化疗,目前无相关报道。

肉瘤

卵巢恶性中胚叶混合瘤通常是异源的,80%发生在绝经后的女性[177~183]。这类肿瘤生物学行为具有侵袭性,临床表现与大多数卵巢上皮癌类似。

这类患者需接受肿瘤细胞减灭术及术后含铂联合化疗。Silasi 等[184]报道了耶鲁大学 22 例患者的治疗经验,除了 2 例其余全部为晚期肿瘤。全部研究对象的中位生存时间为 38 个月。18 例满意减瘤(<1cm)患者的中位生存时间为 46 个月,4 例未达满意减瘤(>1cm)患者的中位生存期为 27 个月。6 名患者满意减瘤术后进行顺铂、异环磷酰胺化疗,他们的中位无病生存间隔为 13 个月,中位生存时间为 51 个月。4 例患者满意减瘤术后,进行卡铂和紫杉醇联合化疗,他们的中位无病生存间隔为 6 个月,中位生存时间为 38 个月。顺铂联合异环磷酰胺组与卡铂联合紫杉醇组生存时间的差异没有统计学意义($P=0.48$)。一线顺铂和异环磷酰胺或卡铂和紫杉醇化疗可以达到卵巢上皮癌的生存率。

Leiser 等[185]报道了 Memorial Sloan-Kettering 使用铂类联合

紫杉醇治疗 30 例卵巢癌肉瘤的经验。12 例(40%)患者完全缓解,7 例(23%)患者部分缓解,2 例(7%)患者疾病稳定,9 例(30%)患者肿瘤进展。对于缓解患者,中位进展时间为 12 个月,中位随访时间 23 个月,存活者中位生存时间为 43 个月。3 年和 5 年生存率分别为 53%和 30%。

卵巢小细胞癌

这一罕见肿瘤发病的平均年龄为 24 岁(2~46 岁)[186],累及双侧,约有 2/3 的患者伴随副肿瘤性高钙血症。该肿瘤占所有卵巢肿瘤相关高钙血症的一半。约 50%的患者在诊断时已发生卵巢外转移。

治疗方法包括手术及术后以铂类为基础的化疗。部分患者可以考虑放疗。除了肿瘤本身的治疗,控制高钙血症需要充分水化、使用袢利尿剂和双膦酸盐。

在一项妇科肿瘤协作组的合作研究中,收集了来自澳大利亚、加拿大、欧洲的 17 名患者的数据[187],所有患者中位随访时间为 13 个月,存活患者的中位随访时间为 35.5 个月。10 例(58.8%)患者为 FIGO Ⅰ期,6 例(35.3%)为Ⅲ期,1 例分期不详。所有患者均采取手术切除和铂类为基础的辅助化疗。7 例患者进行了辅助盆腔、全腹或者延伸野放疗。Ⅰ期肿瘤患者的中位生存时间未达到,Ⅲ期患者为 6 个月。10 例Ⅰ期患者中 6 例进行了辅助放疗,其中 5 例无瘤存活;4 例未进行辅助放疗的患者,1 例无瘤存活。7 例Ⅲ期和分期不详的患者,只有 1 例存活。唯一长期存活的一例患者进行了铂为基础的化疗(BEP),之后进行了腹主动脉旁及盆腔放疗。盆腔和腹腔复发最为常见。接受放化疗挽救治疗的患者效果不佳。

尽管该肿瘤的最佳治疗方案未知,但通过对这些研究进行回顾,作者主张多种手段综合治疗,包括对所有病灶进行手术切除,进行卡铂联合紫杉醇或顺铂联合依托泊苷化疗,以及序贯或同时进行盆腔照射。也有其他学者提倡在干细胞支持下进行大剂量化疗,并有部分患者长期生存的报道[188,189]。

转移瘤

大约 5%~6%的卵巢肿瘤是由其他器官转移而来,最常见的是来自女性生殖道、乳腺或胃肠道[190~207]。转移途径可以是通过其他盆腔肿瘤直接浸润,通过血行转移、淋巴转移或通过种植播散在腹膜表面。

妇科原发肿瘤

非卵巢的生殖道肿瘤可以通过直接浸润或转移至卵巢[1]。某些情况下,当卵巢和输卵管同时受累时,很难区别哪个是原发肿瘤。前面我们已经讨论过,很多高级别浆液癌我们原来一直以为原发于卵巢,现在被认为实际上是来自输卵管[208]。宫颈癌仅少数情况下会转移至卵巢(<1%),且多数为晚期肿瘤或组织类型为腺癌者。约 5%的子宫内膜腺癌可以转移或直接种植在卵巢表面,但原发卵巢肿瘤合并子宫内膜癌的可能性会更大。在这种情况下,卵巢宫内膜样腺癌往往与子宫内膜腺癌相关[209]。

非妇科原发肿瘤

乳腺癌转移至卵巢的概率根据判断方法不同而有所不同,但乳腺癌转移至卵巢比较常见,尤其是雌激素受体阳性的转移性乳腺癌。乳腺转移癌患者尸检表明 24%的患者卵巢受累,其中 80%为双侧受累[190~196]。与此类似,当绝经前的乳腺转移癌患者行卵巢切除术作为一种治疗时,发现大约 20%~30%患者有卵巢转移,其中 60%为双侧受累。乳腺癌早期卵巢受累相当少见,但无确切数据。在大多数病例中,卵巢转移多表现隐匿,在一些患者中,当其他部位转移灶出现明显症状时可能会发现有盆腔包块。

库肯勃瘤

库肯勃瘤占卵巢转移癌的 30%~40%,特征是卵巢间质中的黏蛋白填充及印戒细胞[200,201]。原发肿瘤最常来源于胃,其次是结肠、乳腺或胆道。少数情况下来自宫颈或膀胱。库肯勃瘤占卵巢恶性肿瘤的 2%,通常累及双侧。库肯勃瘤往往在原发肿瘤晚期时才会被发现,因此大部分患者在一年之内死于该病。在某些患者中,原发肿瘤可能一直没有找到。

其他胃肠道肿瘤

其他来自胃肠道的卵巢转移瘤,没有库肯勃瘤经典的组织学表现,大部分来自结肠,少数为小肠。女性小肠癌患者中约 1%~2%在病程中会转移至卵巢[192,197~199,202,203]。年龄大于 40 岁的附件肿瘤女性患者,如果有任何胃肠道症状,都应在术前先行胃肠镜除外胃肠道原发癌转移至卵巢。

转移性结肠癌的组织学表现可与卵巢黏液性囊腺癌相似,两者在组织学上难以鉴别[202~206]。阑尾癌也常常累及卵巢,与原发卵巢癌混淆,尤其是腹膜假黏液瘤[202,206]。当出现卵巢转移时,行结肠癌手术的同时行双侧附件切除术[197,207]。

黑色素瘤

已报道的恶性黑色素瘤转移至卵巢的病例很少[210],而且必须与另一种罕见的起源自卵巢畸胎瘤的黑色素瘤区分开[211]。在该转移瘤中,黑色素瘤通常已经广泛播散。手术通常用于减轻盆腹腔疼痛、出血或扭转。

类癌

类癌转移占卵巢转移癌的比例不足 2%[212]。相反地,只有 2%的原发类癌有卵巢转移的证据,这些患者中仅有 40%在发现转移时候表现为类癌综合征[213]。因此,对于围绝经期和绝经后肠道类癌患者,切除卵巢预防转移的发生是合理的。此外,发现卵巢类癌应该迅速仔细寻找原发肠道病变。

淋巴瘤和白血病

淋巴瘤和白血病可以累及卵巢。一旦发生通常是双侧受累[214~217]。大约 5%的霍奇金病发生淋巴瘤样卵巢累及,但多发生于晚期肿瘤。而 Burkitt 淋巴瘤卵巢受累很常见。其他类型的淋巴瘤则不常累及卵巢,白血病浸润卵巢也较少见。

有时卵巢可能是腹盆腔脏器内淋巴瘤受累的唯一明显部位,这种情况下可能需要仔细手术探查。如果卵巢实性肿块的冰冻切片显示为淋巴瘤,则应术中咨询血液学-肿瘤学家,以决定是否需继续手术。一般来说,尽管肿大的淋巴结通常会取活检,大部分淋巴瘤患者不需要行广泛分期手术。在某些霍奇金病例中，可能需要进行更广泛的评估。治疗通常涉及对淋巴瘤或白血病原发病的治疗。切除大的卵巢病灶可能会提高患者的舒适度以及提高对后续放化疗的反应[216]。

（王婷婷 译 李宁 校）

参考文献

The complete reference list can be found on the Wiley Companion Digital Edition of this title (see inside front cover for login instructions).

1 Scully RE, Young RH, Clement RB. Tumors of the ovary, maldeveloped gonads, fallopian tube, and broad ligament. In: *Atlas of Tumor Pathology: 3rd series, Fascicle 23*. Washington, DC: Armed Forces Institute of Pathology; 1998:169–498.

2 Chen LM, Berek JS. Ovarian and fallopian tubes. In: Haskell CM, ed. *Cancer Treatment*, 5th ed. Philadelphia, PA: WB Saunders; 2000:900–932.

11 Berek JS, Friedlander ML, Hacker NF. Germ cell and nonepithelial ovarian cancer. In: Berek JS, Hacker NF, eds. *Berek & Hacker's Gynecologic Oncology*, 6th ed. Wolters Kluwer: Philadelphia, PA; 2015:530–559.

19 Lu KH, Gershenson DM. Update on the management of ovarian germ cell tumors. *J Reprod Med*. 2005;**50**:417–425.

29 Williams SD, Blessing JA, Liao S, et al. Adjuvant therapy of ovarian germ cell tumors with cisplatin, etoposide, and bleomycin: a trial of the Gynecologic Oncology Group. *J Clin Oncol*. 1994;**12**:701–706.

30 Gershenson DM, Morris M, Cangir A, et al. Treatment of malignant germ cell tumors of the ovary with bleomycin, etoposide, and cisplatin. *J Clin Oncol*. 1990;**8**:715–720.

54 Mahdi H, Swensen RE, Hanna R, et al. Prognostic impact of lymphadenectomy in clinically early stage malignant germ cell tumour of the ovary. *Br J Cancer*. 2011;**105(4)**:493–497.

66 Mann JR, Raafat F, Robinson K, et al. The United Kingdom Children's Cancer Study Group's second germ cell tumor study: carboplatin, etoposide, and bleomycin are effective treatment for children with malignant extracranial germ cell tumors, with acceptable toxicity. *J Clin Oncol*. 2000;**18**:3809–3818.

95 de La Motte RT, Pautier P, et al. Prognostic factors in women treated for ovarian yolk sac tumour: a retrospective analysis of 84 cases. *Eur J Cancer*. 2011;**47(2)**:175–182.

112 Matei D, Miller AM, Monahan P, et al. Chronic physical effects and health care utilization in long-term ovarian germ cell tumor survivors: a Gynecologic Oncology Group study. *J Clin Oncol*. 2009;**27**:4142–4149.

113 Zhang R, Sun YC, Zhang GY, et al. Treatment of malignant germ cell tumors and preservation of fertility. *Eur J Gynaecol Oncol*. 2012;**33**:489–492.

114 Monahan PO, Champion VL, Zhao Q, et al. Case–control comparison of quality of life in long-term ovarian germ cell tumor survivors: a Gynecologic Oncology Group Study. *J Psychosoc Oncol*. 2008;**26(3)**:19–42. PMID: 19042263.

115 Gershenson DM, Miller AM, Champion VL, et al. Reproductive and sexual function after platinum-based chemotherapy in long-term ovarian germ cell tumor survivors: a Gynecologic Oncology Group Study. *J Clin Oncol*. 2007;**25**:2792–2797.

120 Boyce EA, Costaggini I, Vitonis A, et al. The epidemiology of ovarian granulosa cell tumors: a case control study. *Gynecol Oncol*. 2009;**115**:221–225.

124 Roth LM. Recent advances in the pathology and classification of ovarian sex cord-stromal tumors. *Int J Gynecol Pathol*. 2006;**25**:199–215.

128 Zhao C, Vinh TN, McManus K, et al. Identification of the most sensitive and robust immunohistochemical markers in different categories of ovarian sex cord-stromal tumors. *Am J Surg Pathol*. 2009;**33**:354–366.

129 Shah SP, Köbel M, Senz J, et al. Mutation of FOXL2 in granulosa-cell tumors of the ovary. *N Engl J Med*. 2009;**360**:2719–2729.

130 Köbel M, Gilks CB, Huntsman DG. Adult-type granulosa cell tumors and FOXL2 mutation. *Cancer Res*. 2009;**69**:9160–9162.

131 Lappohn RE, Burger HG, Bouma J, et al. Inhibin as a marker for granulosa-cell tumors. *N Engl J Med*. 1989;**321**:790–793.

138 Schumer ST, Cannistra SA. Granulosa cell tumor of the ovary. *J Clin Oncol*. 2003;**21**:1180–1189.

139 Chang HL, Pahlavan N, Halpern EF, et al. Serum Müllerian Inhibiting Substance/anti-Müllerian hormone levels in patients with adult granulosa cell tumors directly correlate with aggregate tumor mass as determined by pathology or radiology. *Gynecol Oncol*. 2009;**114**:57–60.

140 Geerts I, Vergote I, Neven P, et al. The role of inhibins B and anti-müllerian hormone for diagnosis and follow-up of granulosa cell tumors. *Int J Gynecol Cancer*. 2009;**19(5)**:847–855.

142 Brown J, Sood AK, Deavers MT, et al. Patterns of metastasis in sex cord-stromal tumors of the ovary: can routine staging lymphadenectomy be omitted? *Gynecol Oncol*. 2009;**113**:86–90.

143 Abu-Rustum NR, Restivo A, Ivy J, et al. Retroperitoneal nodal metastasis in primary and recurrent granulosa cell tumors of the ovary. *Gynecol Oncol*. 2006;**103**:31–34.

144 NCCN (2013) *National Comprehensive Cancer Network (NCCN) Guidelines*, www.nccn.org (accessed 15 May 2013).

161 Brown J, Shvartsman HS, Deavers MT, et al. The activity of taxanes in the treatment of sex cord-stromal ovarian tumors. *J Clin Oncol*. 2004;**22**:3517.

169 Sommeijer DW, Sjoquist KM, Friedlander M. Hormonal treatment in recurrent and metastatic gynaecological cancers: a review of the current literature. *Curr Oncol Rep*. 2013;**15(6)**:541–548.

173 Auranen A, Sundström J, Ijäs J, et al. Prognostic factors of ovarian granulosa cell tumor: a study of 35 patients and review of the literature. *Int J Gynecol Cancer*. 2007;**17**:1011–1018.

176 Tomlinson MW, Treadwell MC, Deppe G. Platinum based chemotherapy to treat recurrent Sertoli-Leydig cell ovarian carcinoma during pregnancy. *Eur J Gynaecol Oncol*. 1997;**18**:44–46.

184 Silasi DA, Illuzzi JL, Kelly MG, et al. Carcinosarcoma of the ovary. *Int J Gynecol Cancer*. 2008;**18**:22–29.

185 Leiser AL, Chi DS, Ishill NM, et al. Carcinosarcoma of the ovary treated with platinum and taxane: The Memorial Sloan-Kettering Cancer Center experience. *Gynecol Oncol*. 2007;**105**:657–661.

187 Harrison ML, Hoskins P, du Bois A, et al. Small cell of the ovary, hypercalcemic type—analysis of combined experience and recommendation for management. A GCIG study. *Gynecol Oncol*. 2006;**100**:233–238.

188 Pautier P, Ribrag V, Duvillard P, et al. Results of a prospective dose-intensive regimen in 27 patients with small cell carcinoma of the ovary of the hypercalcemic type. *Ann Oncol*. 2007;**18**:1985–1989.

189 Nelsen LL, Muirhead DM, Bell MC. Ovarian small cell carcinoma, hypercalcemic type exhibiting a response to high-dose chemotherapy. *S D Med*. 2010;**63(11)**:375–377.

193 Moore RG, Chung M, Granai CO, et al. Incidence of metastasis to the ovaries from nongenital tract tumors. *Gynecol Oncol*. 2004;**93**:87–91.

196 Yada-Hashimoto N, Yamamoto T, Kamiura S, et al. Metastatic ovarian tumors: a review of 64 cases. *Gynecol Oncol*. 2003;**89**:314–317.

197 Ayhan A, Guvenal T, Salman MC, et al. The role of cytoreductive surgery in nongenital cancers metastatic to the ovaries. *Gynecol Oncol*. 2005;**98**:235–241.

204 Seidman JD, Kurman RJ, Ronnett BM. Primary and metastatic mucinous adenocarcinomas in the ovaries: incidence in routine practice with a new approach to improve intraoperative diagnosis. *Am J Surg Pathol*. 2003;**27**:985–993.

208 Levanon K, Crum C, Drapkin R. New insights into the pathogenesis of serous ovarian cancer and its clinical impact. *J Clin Oncol*. 2008;**26**:5284–5293.

211 Davis GL. Malignant melanoma arising in mature ovarian cystic teratoma (dermoid cyst): report of two cases and literature analysis. *Int J Gynecol Pathol*. 1996;**15**:356–362.

213 Robbins ML, Sunshine TJ. Metastatic carcinoid diagnosed at laparoscopic excision of pelvic Endometriosis. *J Am Assoc Gynecol Laparosc*. 2000;**7**:251–253.

216 Azizoglu C, Altinok G, Uner A, et al. Ovarian lymphomas: a clinicopathological analysis of 10 cases. *Arch Gynecol Obstet*. 2001;**265**:91–93.

第 106 章　葡萄胎及妊娠滋养细胞肿瘤

Donald P. Goldstein, MD ■ Ross S. Berkowitz, MD ■ Neil S. Horowitz, MD

概述

妊娠滋养细胞瘤(GTN)是几个少见的、即使存在广泛转移仍可被治愈的恶性肿瘤之一。GTN 包括一系列相互关联的肿瘤,包括葡萄胎、侵袭性葡萄胎,绒毛膜癌,胎盘部位滋养细胞瘤(PSTT)和上皮样滋养细胞瘤(ETT),这些肿瘤有不同程度的局部浸润和转移倾向。除了 PSTT 和 ETT 外,所有的 GTN 都来自绒毛表面的细胞滋养细胞和合体细胞,并产生大量的人类绒促性素(hCG)。hCG 水平的测定可作为 GTN 肿瘤诊断、治疗反应监测和复发随访的可靠指标。PSTT 和 ETT 起源于绒毛外滋养细胞的中间滋养细胞,产生的 hCG 较少,因此对于这 2 类肿瘤,hCG 作为肿瘤标记物的可靠性较低。GTN 大多数来源于葡萄胎妊娠,但也可继发于任何形式的妊娠,包括人工或自然流产、异位妊娠或足月妊娠。在 1956 年开展有效化疗之前,大部分局限于子宫的 GTN 患者均采用子宫切除术治愈,但转移性疾病几乎都是致命的。目前,如果能尽早接受规范化治疗,大多数患者可以被治愈并保留生育功能。GTN 患者依据预后评分系统被分为低危组及高危组。低危 GTN 一般对单药治疗有反应,而高危组则需要联合化疗才能达到缓解。尽管接受了化疗,GTN 患者治愈后的妊娠结局与一般人群相似。

葡萄胎妊娠和妊娠滋养细胞肿瘤(GTN)包括一组相互关联的疾病,包括完全性葡萄胎(CHM)和部分葡萄胎(PHM),侵袭性葡萄胎,绒毛膜癌(CCA),胎盘部位滋养细胞肿瘤(PSTT)和上皮样滋养细胞肿瘤(ETT)。葡萄胎妊娠和 GTN 产生一种独特的肿瘤标志物,人类绒促性素(hCG),可用于诊断、治疗效果的监测,并随访疾病是否复发。完全性和部分性葡萄胎是非浸润性的局部肿瘤,由异常受精而导致的增殖过程发展而来。其他滋养细胞肿瘤统称为 GTN,因为存在局部侵袭性及转移而被视为恶性肿瘤。GTN 最常继发于葡萄胎妊娠,但也可继发于任何其他类型的妊娠。虽然这些肿瘤较少见,但对于肿瘤医生来说,了解它们的自然历史和治疗管理是非常重要的,因为尽管此类疾病威胁生育期女性的生命,但如果及时接受规范的治疗,有很高的可能性达到治愈并保留生育功能[1,2]。尽管在过去 60 年中 GTN 的治疗取得了较大的进展,但对于长期延误诊断的患者,尤其是继发于非葡萄胎妊娠的患者,仍然存巨大的肿瘤负担,面临治疗失败和死亡的重大风险。

发生率

世界各地报道的葡萄胎妊娠和 GTN 的发病率各不相同[3]。完全性和部分性葡萄胎妊娠在北美和欧洲的发病率约分别为 1∶1 250 和 1∶650,而亚洲国家的发病率则要高 3~10 倍[4,5]。全世界葡萄胎妊娠发病率的差异可能是由于数据来源是基于医院或者基于人群的。

GTN 的发病率难以确定的原因是大多数国家都没有准确的流行病学数据。大约 50% 的 GTN 病例来自葡萄胎妊娠,25% 来自流产或输卵管妊娠,25% 来自足月妊娠或早产[6]。非葡萄胎相关的 GTN 主要为绒毛膜癌,而 PSTT 和 ETT 很少见。非葡萄胎相关的 GTN 在北美及欧洲的发病率约 2/100 000~7/100 000 次妊娠,而在东南亚和日本,发病率则增加至 50/100 000~200/100 000 例的比例[7,8]。

危险因素

葡萄胎妊娠及 GTN 的两个主要危险因素是极端的妊娠年龄(特别是大于 35 岁和小于 16 岁)以及既往葡萄胎妊娠病史[9~13]。Parazzini 等学者[11]指出,CHM 的风险对于年龄超过 35 岁的女性增加了两倍,而年龄超过 40 岁的女性增加了 7.5 倍。虽然高龄妇女的卵子更容易发生异常受精,但大多数葡萄胎和 GTN 病例发生在 35 岁以下的女性,因为这个年龄组的怀孕次数更多。PHM 的患病风险与母亲年龄无关。

GTN 的组织病理学分类

根据大体形态、组织病理学及染色体核型,葡萄胎可分为完全性葡萄胎和部分性葡萄胎[14,15]。CHM 的特征为绒毛水肿与滋养细胞增生。无可识别的胚胎或胎儿组织。部分性葡萄胎的特征为存在两种类型的绒毛,其中一部分外形正常,另一部分表现为局灶水肿和滋养层增生。通常存在胎儿和胚胎组织。由完全性或部分性葡萄胎发展而来的局部侵袭性或转移性 GTN,既可具有葡萄胎组织学特征也可具有 CCA 的组织学特征。

CCA 不含绒毛结构,但包含大片状退行性发育的细胞滋养细胞和合体滋养细胞。尽管 CCA 大多来源于 CHM,但它也可发生于任何妊娠后。非葡萄胎妊娠后的、持续性 GTN 通常具有 CCA 的组织病理学特征,很少表现为 PSTT 或 ETT。CCA 是一类血管丰富的肿瘤,可通过血行转移,最早扩散到肺。在延误诊断的患者中,远处转移部位,如脑,肝脏,肾脏,胃肠道和脾脏转移通常为病变的晚期表现。

PSTT 和 ETT,几乎完全由单核的中间型滋养细胞构成,不含绒毛结构[16,17]。PSTT 和 ETT 都更容易出现子宫肌层浸润,与 CCA 相反,转移是该疾病的晚期表现。这些肿瘤的临床表现多样,即使手术和化疗也难以控制转移。其特点是 hCG 水平较低,因此在诊断疾病之前可能就已经存在较大的肿瘤负荷。

临床表现及诊断

葡萄胎后的 GTN

完全性葡萄胎患者中有 15%会出现子宫侵犯,4%出现转移[18]。1%~4%的 PHM 患者会发生非转移性持续性肿瘤[19]。葡萄胎排出后,所有患者都必须密切监测,警惕葡萄胎后 GTN 的发生。那些 hCG 水平持续升高,需要化疗和/或手术切除,或有转移证据的患者被定义为葡萄胎后的 GTN。根据国际妇产科联合会(FIGO)的标准,葡萄胎后 GTN 的诊断应该满足下列条件:①血清 hCG 水平处于平台(间隔超过 3 周、至少 4 次测定下降小于 10%);②血清 hCG 水平升高(连续 2 周以上增长超过 10%);③病理诊断为 CCA 或 IM[20]。

另外有一些少见的情况会由于非 GTN 的原因出现血清 hCG 浓度的假阳性升高,hCG 升高的鉴别诊断包括:①妊娠;②卵巢或其他部位的生殖细胞肿瘤;③产生促性腺激素的非滋养细胞肿瘤(如肝细胞瘤);④或因为异嗜性抗体造成的幻觉 hCG[21]。绝经后妇女也有报道可测到脑垂体来源的 hCG,可用激素替代疗法抑制[22]。

非转移性 GTN

非葡萄胎妊娠后的局部浸润性 GTN 很少发生[18]。这些患者可表现为 hCG 水平持续升高,不规则阴道出血,子宫复旧不全或不对称的子宫增大。在没有高水平的 hCG(>100 000mIU/ml)时,很少出现卵巢黄素化囊肿。滋养细胞肿瘤可能侵蚀到子宫血管,导致阴道出血,或者可能穿过子宫肌层,造成腹腔内出血。子宫腔内大量的肿瘤坏死病灶也可造成感染败血症,引发盆腔疼痛和脓性分泌物。

转移性 GTN

大约 4%的患者在完全性葡萄胎后发生病灶转移,其他妊娠后较少发生[18]。当发生转移时,病理通常为绒癌,因为具有早期侵蚀血管和播散的特性。这些患者的症状和体征依据转移部位各异,肺部病变表现为咯血,颅内出血可引起急性神经功能障碍,等等。

最常见的转移部位是肺部,80%的转移性 GTN 患者行胸部 X 线检查或 CT 检查可发现肺转移。由于呼吸系统症状和影像学表现可能很突出,患者在诊断为 GTN 前可被考虑为肺部原发疾病。滋养细胞栓塞造成肺动脉闭塞时,可引起肺动脉高压。随着呼吸功能衰竭的进展,需要插管治疗,预示结局很差[23]。即使患者有广泛转移,妇科症状可能不明显或没有妇科症状。任何生育年龄的妇女出现不明原因的肺部或全身症状时,应考虑 GTN 的诊断。

转移性 GTN 患者中 30%有阴道转移。由于这些病灶血运丰富,活检可引发大量出血[18]。

转移性 GTN 患者中约 10%发生肝转移和脑转移。肝转移和脑转移病灶的组织学类型与绒癌相同,通常发生于非葡萄胎妊娠后。这些患者常常有诊断的延误,肿瘤负荷较大。几乎所有肝转移和脑转移的患者同时伴有肺转移和阴道受累[24,25]。

分期及危险评估

1982 年 FIGO 采用了 GTN 的临床解剖分期。

Ⅰ期:病变局限于子宫

Ⅱ期:病变超出子宫但局限于阴道和盆腔

Ⅲ期:病变转移至肺,存在或不存在子宫或盆腔病灶

Ⅳ期:病变转移至其他部位(脑、肝、肾、胃肠道、脾等)

除临床解剖分期外,世界卫生组织(WHO)采用了预后评分系统(表 106-1),可预测耐药的风险和有助于选择合适的化疗方案[20,27]。预后评分小于 7 分时对单药化疗耐药率较低。当预后评分大于等于 7 分的患者对单药化疗有较高的耐药率,需要联合化疗以获得缓解。Ⅰ期 GTN 患者往往为低危组,Ⅳ期患者通常为高危组。因此,低危和高危的区分主要适用于Ⅱ期和Ⅲ期患者。FIGO 分期由罗马数字表示,改良的 WHO 预后评分以阿拉伯数字表示,中间冒号隔开(如Ⅱ:6)。

表 106-1　妊娠性滋养细胞肿瘤预后评分系统

	计分[b]			
	0	1	2	4
年龄/岁	<39	>39	—	—
末次妊娠	葡萄胎	流产	足月产	—
妊娠中止至化疗开始的间隔/月[a]	<4	4~6	7~12	—
hCG/(IU/L)	$<10^3$	$10^3\sim10^4$	$10^4\sim10^5$	—
肿瘤最大直径,包括子宫肿瘤	—	3~5cm	5cm	—
转移部位	—	脾、肾	胃肠道、肝	脑
转移瘤数目	—	1~4	5~8	>8
既往化疗史	—	—	单药化疗	多药化疗

[a] 妊娠中止至化疗开始的间隔时间以月为单位。
[b] 各项分数加和得到总分,患者评分<7 为低危;≥7 分为高危。
摘自 Matsui et al 2004[26]。

Charing Cross 医院的数据显示,低危患者中 WHO 预后评分为 5~6 分者当中,只有 30%可以通过单药治疗治愈,表明这部分患者在初始治疗时应给予联合化疗治疗。这些患者的特征是治疗前 hCG 水平>100 000mIU/ml 和超声检查肿瘤负荷较大[28]。

GTN 的治疗

治疗前评估和 GTN 分期

GTN 的患者必须进行全面的评估以确定分期和危险分层,从而指导临床医生选择恰当的治疗方案(图 106-1)。体格检查

包括妇科阴道检查，以发现阴道转移灶，它可能会造成出血。影像学评估应包括盆腔超声检查，以此来发现子宫内是否有滋养细胞组织的残留，子宫肌层的侵犯，是否有盆腔局部病灶的播散。同样也必须进行胸片检查，因为肺部是最常见的转移部位。尽管胸部CT扫描检查与胸部X线检查相比，有更高的敏感性，但由于肺部的隐匿病灶并不影响结局，它并未被纳入分期系统。胸部X线阴性的患者经肺CT检查后，约40%可发现肺转移灶[29]。没有肺部和阴道转移的患者，远处转移如脑和肝脏的转移罕见。随着中枢神经系统扫描技术的提高，脑脊液中hCG水平检测不再有指导意义。只要临床影像符合GTN的诊断，转移病灶无须行组织活检来确诊，因为这些种植灶血运丰富，活检有出血的风险。

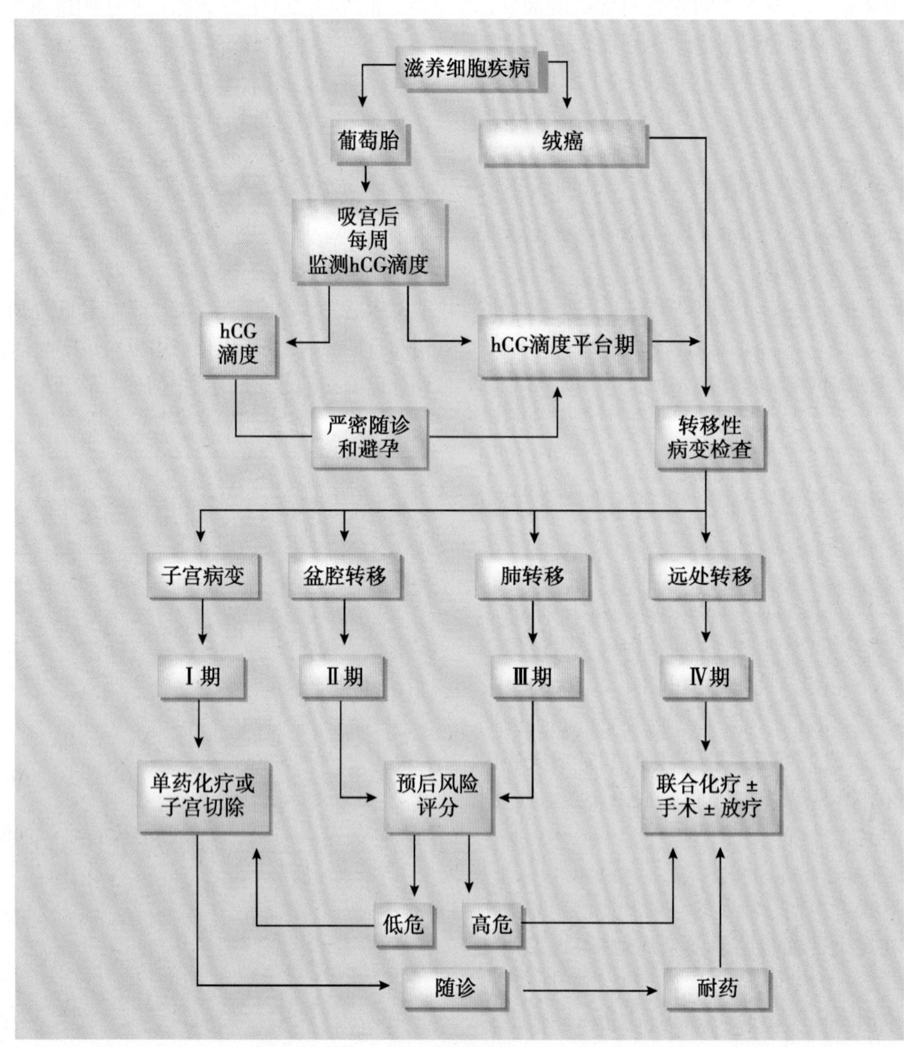

图106-1　妊娠滋养细胞疾病（GTD）治疗流程

低危GTN的治疗

低危GTN初始治疗

低危GTN包括Ⅰ期（非转移性）和Ⅱ/Ⅲ期（转移性）GTN患者中预后评分小于7分者。Ⅰ期GTN患者治疗方案的选择，基于患者是否要求保留生育功能。如果患者已完成了生育，可行全子宫切除[30]。在手术的同时，我们建议同时行辅助性单药化疗一疗程来治疗任何的隐匿转移灶，可以采用甲氨蝶呤（MTX）或放线菌素D（ACTD）。

MTX/ACTD单药序贯化疗适用于那些渴望保留生育功能的Ⅰ期GTN和低危转移GTN患者。MTX联合亚叶酸（MTX-FA）是新英格兰滋养细胞疾病中心（New England Trophoblastic Disease Center，NETDC）首选的单药方案[31]。MTX-FA治疗Ⅰ期GTN患者完全缓解率为90.2%（147/163），Ⅱ期和Ⅲ期低危患者的完全缓解率为68.2%（15/22），这些完全缓解的患者中一程化疗的缓解率为81.5%（132/162）。首选ACTD治疗用于那些肝功能异常的患者，因为应用MTX-FA方案可能加重肝脏毒性，以及序贯用药中提示MTX耐药的患者[32]。

对于非转移性和低危转移的GTT患者，应用单药MTX或ACTD化疗均可获得很好的和类似的缓解率[2,18,32]。一些采用MTX和ACTD的联合化疗方案对GTN有效，但目前尚无前瞻性对照研究比较这些方案（表106-2）[32]。单药化疗方案的实施依据固定的时间间隔。hCG水平下降小于一个对数预示患者对该药物相对耐药，可更换化疗药物。

表 106-2　单药化疗方案

甲氨蝶呤方案
MTX-FA
MTX 1.0mg/kg 肌内注射第 1、3、5、7 天
亚叶酸 0.1mg/kg 肌内注射或 po 第 2、4、6、8 天
5 天 MTX
MTX 0.4mg/(kg·d)静脉注射或肌内注射×5 天
MTX 周疗(脉冲)
MTX 50mg/m^2 肌内注射每周
放线菌素 D 方案
5 天 Act-D
Act-D 12μg/(kg·d)静脉注射×5 天
Act-D 周疗(脉冲)
Act-D 1.25mg/m^2 静脉注射每 2 周 1 次(最大 2mg)

FA,亚叶酸。

低危 GTN 的挽救治疗

低危 GTN 患者单药序贯化疗耐药后采用联合化疗通常可以获得缓解,方案中包括 MTX、ACTD、环磷酰胺、依托泊苷和 Oncovin(EMA/CO)(依托泊苷、甲氨蝶呤、放线菌素 D、环磷酰胺、长春新碱)(表 106-3)[33]。依托泊苷的使用,特别是对于低危 GTN 患者,引发人们的担忧,因为根据 Rustin 等人[34]的报道,它的使用可能导致继发的其他恶性肿瘤。近期,来自同一机构的更大样本量的报道显示该风险有限[35]。如果病变对单药和联合化疗均耐药,可考虑行全子宫切除术或可考虑行局部切除术(若患者渴望保留生育功能)。如果计划行局部病灶切除术,超声检查,MRI 扫描,盆腔动脉显影和/或 PET 扫描有助于明确耐药病灶的部位。在低危疾病患者中,有效治疗后,给予三个疗程的巩固化疗可减少复发的风险[36]。

表 106-3　EMACO 方案

时间方案	
第 1 天	依托泊苷 100mg/m^2 静脉注射(200ml 生理盐水静脉注射超过 30min)
	Act-D 0.5mg 静脉推注
	MTX 100mg/m^2 静脉推注
	MTX 200mg/m^2 静脉注射大于 12h
第 2 天	依托泊苷 100mg/m^2 静脉注射(200ml 生理盐水静脉注射超过 30 分)
	Act-D 0.5mg 静脉推注
	FA 15mg IM 或口服在 MTX 开始后 24h,每 12h 1 次,共 4 次
第 8 天	CTX 600mg/m^2 静脉注射
	长春新碱 1.0mg/m^2 静脉推注

Act-D,放线菌素 D;FA,亚叶酸;MTX,甲氨蝶呤。

高危 GTN、Ⅱ期和Ⅲ期的治疗

初始治疗

FIGO 分期为Ⅱ期和Ⅲ期以及 WHO 评分≥7 分的患者有很高的耐药和复发的风险。这些患者应当首选 EMACO 方案联合化疗,它的完全缓解率为 76%~86%[37~39]。

挽救治疗

对 EMACO 耐药的患者可采用改良方案:EMACE,方案中第 8 天更换为顺铂和依托泊苷化疗[33]。联合化疗间隔时间为 2~3 周,如果化疗毒性可耐受,化疗持续到 hCG 水平连续 3 周检测阴性,在此之后给予至少 3 周期巩固化疗以减少复发风险。

Ⅳ期 GTN 的治疗

Ⅳ期患者包括那些有疾病快速进展和化疗耐药高风险的患者。初始治疗采用联合化疗方案并联合手术及放疗可显著改善患者生存期。在 NETDC,1975 年前,仅有 30%的Ⅳ期患者存活。1975 年后,随着早期大剂量多药联合化疗的出现,80%的Ⅳ期患者可获得持续的完全缓解。

所有Ⅳ期 GTN 患者均可首选 EMA/CO 方案联合化疗。当出现中枢神经系统转移时,MTX 的剂量可增加到 1g/m^2[40]。EMA/CO 耐药的患者可采用 EMA/CE 方案,详见表 106-4。有小的病例队列报道了许多其他有效的挽救方案。依托泊苷联合顺铂和博来霉素(BEP)或长春碱联合顺铂和博来霉素(PVB)的二线化疗方案也已被证明对耐药 GTN 患者有效[41~44]。

表 106-4　EMACE 方案

时间	治疗方案
第 1 天	依托泊苷 100mg/m^2 静脉注射(200ml 生理盐水静脉注射超过 30 分)
	Act-D 0.5mg 静脉推注
	MTX 100mg/m^2 静脉推注
	MTX 1 000mg/m^2 静脉注射超过 12h
第 2 天	依托泊苷 100mg/m^2 静脉注射(200ml 生理盐水静脉注射超过 30 分)
	Act-D 0.5mg 静脉推注
	FA 30mg 肌内注射或口服,在 MTX 治疗开始后 32h,每 12h 1 次,共 6 次
第 8 天	顺铂 60mg/m^2 静脉注射(同时水化),依托泊苷 100mg/m^2 静脉注射(200ml 生理盐水静脉注射超过 30 分)

Act-D,放线菌素 D;FA,亚叶酸;MTX,甲氨蝶呤。
摘自 Bagshawe 1976[1]。经 Wiley 出版社许可转载。

自体骨髓移植或干细胞解救在 GTN 治疗中的作用仍不明确。但是有个案报道在难治性 GTN 患者中,采用大剂量化疗联合自体骨髓移植或干细胞支持,可获完全缓解[45,46]。

尽管已有成熟有效的方案,仍需要努力寻找新的治疗耐药病变的有效药物。异环磷酰胺和紫杉醇已被成功地应用于临床,但是仍需进一步地研究以明确其作为一线或二线治疗的作用[47,48]。Osborne 等报道一种新的包括 3 种药物的二联方案:紫杉醇、依托泊苷和顺铂(TE/TP),治疗 2 例复发高危 GTN 患者,获得完全缓解[49]。Wan 等证实含有氟尿嘧啶(FUDR)药物的方案对耐药患者有效[50]。Matsui 等发现氟尿嘧啶联合 ACTD 可作为有效的挽救治疗方案[26]。

手术的作用

手术可用于治疗相关并发症,以及切除耐药病灶[51]。全子宫切除术可用于控制子宫出血和败血症,或降低肿瘤负荷,从而减少化疗的应用。阴道转移灶的出血可采用填塞、局部扩大切除或下腹动脉栓塞治疗[52]。开胸术可用于切除大剂量化疗后仍持续可见的肺部病灶[53]。但是,在促性腺激素达到完全缓解后,胸片检查可能仍会显示持续存在的模糊的纤维结节。必须进行全面的转移灶检查,以除外其他部位持续存在的肿瘤。PET 扫描有助于确定有活性肿瘤的隐匿部位[54]。尽管血管栓塞也可用于治疗出血,可能仍需行肝切除术以治疗肝转移病灶的出血[55]。开颅手术可用于紧急降颅压,或控制出血,也可用于颅内孤立转移灶的切除[32]。

放射治疗的作用

在 NETDC,当确定发生颅内转移时,迅速进行全脑照射和全身化疗,可降低脑出血的风险。Yordan 等报道脑转移患者单独应用化疗的死亡率为 44%(11/25),但是采用脑部放疗和化疗的 18 例患者中没有死亡[56]。在局部切除的特定病例中也取得了优异的结果,特别是当肿瘤是孤立的且位于周边时[32,40,51]。

单独进行强化化疗的脑转移患者也有非常好的治愈率。Newlands 等报道脑部受累患者仅接受化疗的缓解率极高[40]。35 例脑部病变的患者,接受包括大剂量静脉和鞘内 MTX 的强化联合化疗后,30 例(86%)患者持续缓解。对于有表面孤立性脑转移的患者,在治疗开始时进行开颅手术。

开颅手术也是急性颅内减压或控制出血的必要方法。开颅手术还应解决威胁生命的并发症,从而提供一个化疗控制疾病的机会。偶尔,当脑转移灶对化疗耐药时,可以选择手术切除。Athanassiou 等报道,接受开颅手术治疗急性颅内并发症的 5 例患者中,有 4 例最终得以治愈[57]。幸运的是,大多数脑转移患者达到缓解后没有残留的神经系统缺陷,除非出现过颅内出血。

然而,我们观察到在接受全颅照射的患者中,有极少的患者出现严重痴呆和进行性记忆丧失。尽管关于脑转移瘤最佳治疗方案的争议尚未解决,Neubauer 等报告说,包括化疗、手术和放疗(全脑或立体定向)在内的多种联合治疗方法已将患者总体生存率从 46%提高到 64%[58]。

PSTT 和 ETT 的治疗

因为疾病独特的生物学特性,PSTT 和 ETT 的患者的治疗需要特殊的考虑。我们认为,所有非转移性 PSTT 和 ETT 患者的主要治疗方式应该是子宫切除术,而无须辅助化疗,因为这种绒毛膜癌(CCA)变异体对化疗相对耐药[16,59,60]。如果患者存在深肌层受累,我们的治疗策略是同时行盆腔淋巴结清扫。与绒毛膜癌不同,这些肿瘤在转移之前往往会长期定植在子宫内。一旦发生转移,PSTT 和 ETT 的死亡率都很高。Kingdon 等报道,他们回顾 GTN 的死亡病例,发现 30%的 GTN 死亡患者具有 PSTT 组织学成分[61]。在没有明显转移迹象的情况下,不需要进一步的治疗。

由于 PSTT 和 ETT 患者稀缺,目前还没有普遍认可的关于如何治疗 PSTT 和 ETT 的临床指南,但鉴于其侵袭性的临床行为,将包括外科手术、放射治疗和化学治疗多模式治疗方法结合起来可提患者的生存率。EMA/EP 对 PSTT 转移患者有效[62]。Papadopoulos 等报道,从前次妊娠到临床发病的间隔时间是最重要的预后因素[62]。间隔时间<4 年的所有 27 例患者均存活,而间隔时间超过 4 年的所有 7 例患者均死亡。尽管不适用于大多数患者,但保留生育功能的手术也有成功的个例[63,64]。

治疗结果

Ⅰ期 GTN

1965 年 7 月至 2013 年 12 月,在 NETDC 治疗的 624 例Ⅰ期 GTN 患者均获得了缓解。在 582 例接受单药化疗的患者中,478 例(82%)通过续贯 MTX/ACTD 治疗后缓解。所有 35 例行子宫切除术和辅助单药化疗的患者均获得缓解,无须进一步治疗。7 例高危患者通过联合化疗获得了缓解。其余 104 例耐药的患者通过联合化疗或手术干预均获得缓解。

Ⅱ期和Ⅲ期 GTN

在 NETDC 治疗的所有 37 例Ⅱ期 GTN 患者和 226 例Ⅲ期 GTN 患者中的 225 例获得完全缓解。单药化疗后,21 例Ⅱ期低危患者中的 16 例(76.2%)和 154 例Ⅲ期低危患者中 113 例(73.3%)获得缓解。所有对单药化疗耐药的患者均通过联合化疗获得缓解。Ⅱ期高危组的 16 例患者和 13 例Ⅲ期高危组患者中的 12 例(92.3%)通过联合方案获得了缓解。Ⅲ期高危组有 1 例死亡病例。

Ⅳ期 GTN

1975 年之前,在 NETDC 只有 6/20 例(30%)Ⅳ期 GTN 患者获得缓解。但是,在 1975 年之后,33 例Ⅳ期疾病患者中有 25 例(75.5%)获得缓解。存活率的显著提高是由于在治疗早期使用了大剂量综合治疗疗法。尽管在美国,脑转移瘤通常采用脑照射治疗,但仅接受化学疗法治疗的脑转移瘤患者也有极高的缓解率。最近,Alifrangis 等[65]报道了,使用低剂量依托泊苷和顺铂联合的初始治疗,可提高高危 GTN 和肿瘤负荷大的患者的生存率。

hCG 的随访和复发

所有患有Ⅰ、Ⅱ和Ⅲ期 GTN 患者均需每周监测 hCG 水平,直到连续三周检测结果正常,然后每月一次,直到 12 个月。由于Ⅳ期 GTN 患者的晚期复发风险高,需要每月随访一次至正常水平持续 24 个月。在整个监测期间,建议所有患者使用有效的避孕措施。NETDC 的复发率如下:Ⅰ期,2.9%;Ⅱ期,8.3%;Ⅲ期,4.2%;Ⅳ9.1%。从最后一次 hCG 水平正常至复发的平均时间为 6 个月,这在Ⅰ~Ⅳ期患者之间没有差异[66]。

一旦复发,患者需要重新分期,并更换先前未采用过的化疗方案。Ⅰ、Ⅱ和Ⅲ期的所有复发患者均获得缓解,而两名Ⅳ期的复发患者均死亡。

静止 GTN

持续性(至少 3 个月)低水平 hCG(范围 0.5~200mIU/ml)的一个罕见原因是静止 GTN,最常见于葡萄胎妊娠后。静止 GTN 被认为是由于存在高度分化的非侵袭性合体滋养层细胞。其特征如下:①临床上难以发现病灶;②hCG 水平对治疗无反应,大概是因为这些细胞的生长周期与正常细胞相当。静止 GTN 患者不应接受化疗,但应密切随访,因为 6%~10%的患者最终会发展成需要治疗的活性 GTN。低水平的高糖基化 hCG 的存在表明存在静止 GTN。高糖基化 hCG 水平的升高时提示发展为活性 GTN,需要治疗[21]。

治疗后的妊娠

完全性和部分性葡萄胎患者将来可正常生育[67]。但是,这些患者在以后的妊娠中发生葡萄胎妊娠的风险增加。接受过 GTN 化疗的患者将来也可正常妊娠[68]。重要的是,先天畸形的发生率没有增加。来自 NETDC 和其他 10 个中心的数据报道了化疗后 3 191 例妊娠结果。其中 2 342(73.4%)得到活产婴儿,早产 89 例(4.7%),死产 40 例(1.3%)和自然流产 457 例(14.3%)。尽管死产的发生率似乎有所增加,但只有 46(1.6%)的婴儿存在先天性畸形,这与普通人群一致。Woolas 等人指出[68],单药 MTX 治疗的妇女与接受联合化疗的妇女相比,受孕率或妊娠结局无差异。此外,只有 7%希望怀孕的妇女未怀孕。

由于再次葡萄胎妊娠的风险增加了 10 倍,因此再次妊娠后,在早孕期末应进行产科超声检查,以确认胎儿的发育是否正常。此外,应在妊娠结束后 6 周进行 hCG 检测,以排除隐匿性 GTN。任何自然流产或治疗性流产后,妊娠排除物必须进行病理检查。

(雷呈志　赵羽西　袁华 译　向阳　蒋芳 校)

参考文献

The complete reference list can be found on the Wiley Companion Digital Edition of this title (see inside front cover for login instructions).

1 Bagshawe KD. Risks and prognostic factors in trophoblastic neoplasia. *Cancer*. 1976;**38**:1373–1385.

2 Goldstein DP, Berkowitz RS. *Gestational Trophoblastic Neoplasms: Clinical Principles of Diagnosis and Management*. Philadelphia: WB Saunders; 1982:1–301.

4 Palmer JR. Advances in the epidemiology of gestational trophoblastic disease. *J Reprod Med*. 1994;**39**:155–162.

12 Elias KM, Goldstein DP, Berkowitz RS. Complete hydatitdform mole in women older than age 50. *J Reprod Med*. 2010;**55**:208–212.

13 Elias KM, Shoni M, Bernstein MR, et al. Complete hydatidiform mole in women aged 40-49 years. *J Reprod Med*. 2012;**57**:254–258.

16 Feltmate C, Genest DR, Wise L, et al. Placental site trophoblastic tumor: a 17-year experience at the New England Trophoblastic Disease Center. *Gynecol Oncol*. 2001;**82**:415–419.

19 Berkowitz RS, Goldstein DP. Presentation and management of molar pregnancy. In: Hancock BW, Newlands ES, Berkowitz RS, eds. *Gestational Trophoblastic Disease*. London: Chapman and Hall; 1997:127–142.

20 Kohorn EI. The new FIGO 2000 staging and risk factor scoring system for gestational trophoblastic disease: Description and critical assessment. *Int J Gynaecol Cancer*. 2001;**11**:73–77.

21 Cole LA, Khanlian SA, Giddings A, et al. Gestational trophoblastic diseases: 4. Presentation with persistent low positive human chorionic gonadotropin test results. *Gynecol Oncol*. 2006;**102**:165–169.

23 Bakri YN, Berkowitz RS, Khan J, et al. Pulmonary metastases of gestational trophoblastic tumor: risk factors for early respiratory failure. *J Reprod Med*. 1994;**39**:175–178.

24 Newlands ES, Holden L, Seckl MJ, et al. Management of brain metastases in patients with high risk gestational trophoblastic tumours (GTT). *J Reprod Med*. 2002;**47**:465–471.

25 Bakri YN, Subhi J, Amer M, et al. Liver metastases of gestational trophoblastic tumor. *Gynecol Oncol*. 1993;**48**:110–113.

27 World Health Organization. *Trophoblastic diseases: technical report series 692*. Geneva: WHO; 1983.

28 McGrath S, Short D, Harvey R, et al. The management and outcome of women with post-hydatidiform mole 'low-risk' gestational trophoblastic neoplasia, but hCG levels in excess of 100,000 IU/L. *Br J Cancer*. 2010;**102**:810–814.

29 Garner EIO, Garrett A, Goldstein DP, Berkowitz RS. Significance of chest computed tomography findings in the evaluation and treatment of persistent gestational trophoblastic neoplasia. *J Reprod Med*. 2004;**49**:411–414.

30 Clark RM, Nevadunsky NS, Ghosh S, et al. The evolving role of hysterectomy in gestational trophoblastic neoplasia at the New England Trophoblastic Disease Center. *J Reprod Med*. 2010;**55**:194–198.

31 Berkowitz RS, Goldstein DP, Bernstein MR. Ten years experience with methotrexate and folinic acid as primary therapy for gestational trophoblastic disease. *Gynecol Oncol*. 1986;**23**:111–118.

32 Seckl M, Sebire N, Berkowitz RS. Gestatioanl trophoblastic disease. *Lancet*. 2010;**376**:717–729.

33 Newlands ES, Bower M, Holden L, et al. Management of resistant gestational trophoblastic tumors. *J Reprod Med*. 1998;**43**:111–118.

34 Rustin GJS, Newlands ES, Lutz JM, et al. Combination but not single-agent methotrexate chemotherapy for gestational trophoblastic tumors increases the incidence of second tumors. *J Clin Oncol*. 1996;**14**:2769–2773.

35 Savage PM, Cook R, O'Nions J, et al. The effects of chemotherapy treatment for gestational trophoblastic tumours on second tumour risk and early menopause. XVII World Congress on Gestational Trophoblastic Diseases, 2014;71-2. (Abstract).

36 Lybol C, Sweep FC, Harvey R, et al. Relapse rates after two versus three consolidation courses of methotrexate in the treatment of low-risk gestational trophoblastic neoplasia. *Gynecol Oncol*. 2012;**125**:576–579.

37 Newlands ES, Bagshawe KD, Begent RH, et al. Results with the EMA/CO (etoposide, methotrexate, actinomycin D, cyclophosphamide, vincristine) regimen in high risk gestational trophoblastic tumours, 1979 to 1989. *Br J Obstet Gynaecol*. 1991;**98**:550–556.

40 Newlands ES, Holden L, Seckl MJ, et al. Management of brain metastases in patients with high risk gestational trophoblastic tumor. *J Reprod Med*. 2002;**47**:465.

44 Lurain JR, Schink JC. Importance of salvage therapy in the management of high-risk gestational trophoblastic neoplasia. *J Reprod Med*. 2012;**57**:219–224.

49 Osborne R, Covens A, Merchandani DE, Gerulath AS. Successful salvage of relapsed high-risk gestational Trophoblastic neoplasia patients using a novel paclitaxel-containing doublet. *J Reprod Med*. 2004;**49**:655–658.

51 Lurain JR, Singh DK, Schink JC. Role of surgery in the management of high-risk

gestational troph0blastic neoplasia. *J Reprod Med*. 2006;**51**:773-777.

53 Fleming EL, Garrett L, Growdon WB, et al. The changing role of thoracotomy in gestational trophoblastic neoplasia at the New England Trophoblastic Disease Center. *J Reprod Med*. 2008;**53**:493-498.

54 Dhillon T, Palmieri C, Sebire NJ, et al. Value of whole body 18 FDG-PET to identify the active site of gestational trophoblastic neoplasia. *J Reprod Med*. 2006;**51**:879-883.

57 Athanassiou A, Begent RHJ, Newlands ES, et al. Central nervous system metastases of choriocarcinoma: 23 years' experience at Charing Cross Hospital. *Cancer*. 1983;**52**:1728-1735.

58 Neubauer NL, Latif N, Kalakota K, et al. Brain metastasis in gestational trophoblastic disease: an update. *J Reprod Med*. 2012;**57**:288-292.

59 Palmer JE, Macdonald M, Wells M, et al. Epithelioid trophoblastic tumor: a review of the literature. *J Reprod Med*. 2008;**53**:465-475.

61 Kingdon SJ, Coleman RE, Ellis L, Hancock BW. Deaths from gestational trophoblastic neoplasia. Any lessons to be learned? *J Reprod Med*. 2012;**57**:293-296.

62 Papadopoulos AJ, Foskett M, Seckl MJ, et al. Twenty-five years clinical experience of placental site trophoblastic tumors. *J Reprod Med*. 2002;**47**:460-464.

65 Alifrangis C, Agarwal R, Short D, et al. EMA/CO for high-risk gestational trophoblastic neoplasia:good outcome with induction low-dose etoposide-cisplatin and genetic analysis. *J Clin Oncol*. 2013;**31**:280-286.

66 Goldstein DP, Zanten-Przybysz I, Bernstein MR, Berkowitz RS. Revised FIGO staging system for gestational trophoblastic tumors; recommendations regarding therapy. *J Reprod Med*. 1998;**43**:37-43.

67 Vargas R, Barroilhet L, Esselen K, et al. Subsequent pregnancy outcomes in patients with molar pregnancy and persistent gestational trophoblastic neoplasia: updated results. *J Reprod Med*. 2014;**59**:188-194.

68 Woolas RP, Bower M, Newlands ES, et al. Influence of chemotherapy for gestational trophoblastic disease on subsequent pregnancy outcome. *Br J Obstet Gynecol*. 1998;**105**:1326-1327.

第 107 章　妇科肉瘤

Jamal Rahaman, MD ■ Carmel J. Cohen, MD

概述

妇科肉瘤非常罕见，占妇科恶性肿瘤的不到 1.5%。子宫肉瘤中，癌肉瘤和平滑肌肉瘤各占 35%～40%，子宫内膜间质肉瘤（ESS）占 10%～15%，其他肉瘤包括腺肉瘤占 5%～10%。子宫癌肉瘤应该被归类于转化型子宫内膜癌。大多数腺肉瘤和 ESS 预后较好，且激素治疗有效。未分化子宫内膜肉瘤（UES）和肉瘤成分过度生长的腺肉瘤较为罕见，预后差，需要化疗。ESS 从组织学和临床表现有别于 UES，有不同的基因重排方式。超过 50% 的 I 期平滑肌肉瘤（LMS）和癌肉瘤患者会出现复发。晚期或复发病变需要化疗。对于 LMS，有效的化疗药物为多柔比星、异环磷酰胺、吉西他滨和多西他赛。对于子宫癌肉瘤，可供选择的药物为异环磷酰胺、顺铂/卡铂和紫杉醇。对部分经选择的子宫癌肉瘤患者行放射治疗可提高局部控制率。激素治疗可用于晚期或复发低级别 ESS 和腺肉瘤，包括孕激素、促性腺激素释放激素激动剂和芳香化酶抑制剂。

历史回顾与展望

外阴、阴道、宫颈、子宫和卵巢的肉瘤（包括间质细胞和上皮-间质细胞混合性恶性肿瘤）占这些器官恶性肿瘤的不到 1.5%。

表 107-1　子宫肉瘤的分类美国病理学家协会关于子宫肉瘤的分类

组织学类型（选择所有适用类型）	未分化子宫/子宫内膜肉瘤
子宫平滑肌肉瘤	腺肉瘤
低级别子宫内膜间质肉瘤#	腺肉瘤伴有：
低级别子宫内膜间质肉瘤伴有：	• 横纹肌分化
• 平滑肌分化	• 软骨分化
• 性索成分	• 骨分化
• 腺体成分	• 其他异源性成分（列举）______
其他（列举）_______	腺肉瘤伴有肉瘤样过度生长
高级别子宫内膜间质肉瘤	其他（列举）_______

低级别子宫内膜间质肉瘤与良性的子宫内膜间质结节的区别在于浸润入周围的子宫肌层和/或淋巴血管脉管间隙受侵。子宫内膜间质结节可出现轻微边缘不规则，形成指状突起，但不能超过 3mm。这一方案不适用于子宫内膜间质结节。

摘自 Tavassoli[3] 和 Otis[4]。

这些恶性肿瘤的分类是个难题，直到 1959 年[1] Ober 提出一种分类方法，于 1970 年 Kempson 和 Bari[2] 予以修订，并于 2003 年世界卫生组织（WHO）[3] 和美国病理学家协会[4] 将其重新进行分类（表 107-1）。子宫癌肉瘤不再归类于子宫肉瘤，应该归类于化生型子宫内膜癌[5]，但是在本章中论述。

发病率和流行病学

女性盆腔肉瘤最常见的部位是子宫，但子宫肉瘤仅占子宫恶性肿瘤的 4%～9%，每年的发病率低于 20/100 万[6,7]。黑人女性的总体发病率是白人的二倍，但是接受相同治疗后，生存率没有明显差别[6,7]。癌肉瘤的患病风险随年龄增大而急剧增加。癌肉瘤的年发病率为 8.2/100 万，子宫平滑肌肉瘤（LMS）为 6.4/100 万，子宫内膜间质肉瘤（ESS）为 1.8/100 万，未分类肉瘤为 0.7/100 万[6,7]。据报道癌肉瘤和 LMS 各占子宫肉瘤的 35%～40%，ESS 占 10%～15%，其他肉瘤占 5%[7]。

危险因素

子宫肉瘤的流行病学危险因素尚不甚明确，既往放射治疗[8,9]和他莫昔芬治疗史[10,11]，子宫肉瘤发生的危险性增加。

病理

子宫是妇科肉瘤最常见的部位，ESS 单纯起源于子宫内膜，LMS 单纯起源于子宫肌层，而癌肉瘤的起源则两者都有[1,12]。同源性肿瘤含有癌以及子宫固有组织分化的肉瘤成分，而异源性肿瘤包括癌加上宫外来源组织（骨、软骨、横纹肌）的肉瘤。中肾旁管腺肉瘤是混合性中肾旁管肿瘤，包括恶性的间叶成分和良性的上皮成分[3,13,14]。

子宫内膜间质病变

子宫内膜间质结节（ESN）罕见。其特征是清晰的非浸润性边界，无肌层和脉管侵犯的证据。2/3 病例为子宫肌层的孤立性病变，与子宫内膜无关[3]。

ESS 肿瘤为低级别有转移潜能，与 ESN 类似，它们由大小一致的细胞组成，类似增殖期子宫内膜间质细胞，但是有子宫肌层和/或脉管受侵[3]。组织学上，其特征是密集分布的间质细胞，大小一致，伴有极少量的细胞多形性，轻微的核异型性，核分裂象罕见。值得重视的是，在其他典型的低度 ESS 中，单独发现核分裂数增加并不意味着不良的预后[15]。

诊断 ESS 可能比较棘手，因为其具有不同的形态学特征（表 107-1）[3]。在伴有灶状平滑肌分化的肿瘤中，如果平滑肌成分小于整个肿瘤体积的 30%，肿瘤被分类为 ESS。肿瘤含有更多平滑肌成分组成多被归类于混合性子宫内膜间质和平滑肌肿瘤[3,16]。

未分化子宫内膜肉瘤（UES-以前被称为高级别 ESS）的特征为细胞异型性明显，核多形性，核分裂数高，广泛浸润。另外 UES 常表现为破坏性的子宫肌层受侵[3]。

分子和基因改变

ESS 的分子特征，也可见于 ESN，主要为：大多数免疫组化染色检查雌激素受体（ER）和孕激素受体（PR）阳性。通常 CD10 阳性，连接蛋白和钙调节蛋白阴性，PTEN 杂合子丢失，Wnt 信号转导通路反常[5,17,18]。

UES 表现为与增殖相关的标志物（Ki67、P16 和 P53）染色阳性率增加，而 ER、PR、连接蛋白或平滑肌抗原（SMA）染色常为阴性[5]。UES 也表达酪氨酸激酶受体 CD117（c-KIT）[19]、CyclinD1[20]、人表皮生长因子受体 2（HER2 或 ERPB2），而这些通常在 ESS 上不表达[5]。

至少有 75%的 ESS 患者被证实存在基因重排[21,22]。最常见的细胞遗传学异常是 7 号染色体 t（7;17）的易位导致的 *JAZF1-SUZ12* 基因融合，见于 35%～50%的子宫内膜间质肉瘤患者[22]。其他已知的基因融合有 *JAZF1-PHF1*、*EPC1-PHF1*、单 *JAZF1*、单 *PHF1*[21～25]。

UES 缺乏这些以 *JAZF1* 为基础的基因重排，但却常出现 *YWHAE-FAM22A/B* 基因融合[26～29]，这可能为肿瘤特征性表现，因为在其他 55 种肿瘤类型的 827 例患者中均没有检测到这种基因重排[27]。

扩散的途径

子宫肉瘤可通过淋巴管和血行播散，也可通过局部蔓延和腹膜扩散[30～38]。

Rose 等[30]研究了 73 例子宫肉瘤患者的尸检结果，包括 43 例癌肉瘤，19 例 LMS，9 例 ESS 和 2 例 ESM。腹膜腔和网膜是最常受累的部位（59%），随后是肺（52%），盆腔（41%），腹主动脉旁淋巴结（38%）和肝实质（34%）。值得重视的是，肺转移通常是孤立性的。

成人软组织肉瘤的淋巴结转移率<3%，因组织学亚型不同而有差异[39]。在一项包含 357 例 LMS 患者的研究中，总的淋巴结转移的危险性约为 6.4%[40]。但是，在 57 例接受手术分期的 LMS 患者中，临床诊断淋巴结正常且病变局限于子宫，有 3.5%存在隐匿性淋巴结转移[35]。癌肉瘤总淋巴结转移和隐匿性淋巴结转移率更高，分别为 25%[41]和 18%[35]，而 ESS 则分别为 16%和 6%[42]。深肌层受侵和广泛的淋巴管-血管间隙受侵（LVSI）进一步增加了隐匿性转移的危险[32,43]。腺肉瘤的淋巴结转移率约为 3%[44]。

临床特点

子宫内膜间质肿瘤

子宫内膜间质肿瘤患者常为围绝经期女性，表现为不规则阴道出血。肿瘤组织可由宫颈口突出，即使体积很大也未穿透子宫壁。通常进行子宫内膜取样可以确诊[16,45,46]。

子宫平滑肌肉瘤

LMS 常发生于 40～50 岁女性，在 45 岁时发病率最高，此后直至 80 岁发病率逐渐降低。病变常与良性平滑肌瘤有关，虽然在平滑肌瘤中的恶变率不到 1%[47]。关于肉瘤病变是由良性平滑肌瘤“发展”而来或独立发生有相当多的争论。Ferenczy 等[48]未能证实这种发展的关系，然而 Spiro 和 Koss[49]发现平滑肌瘤中有交界性改变，提出存在恶性转化的概念。LMS 经常在肌瘤剔除术或子宫切除术时被意外发现[47,50]。

癌肉瘤

癌肉瘤的发病率在 50 岁时开始增加，到 75 岁后稳定。特征性的临床表现为阴道出血、阴道分泌物增多和腹痛。与 LMS 相比，癌肉瘤更多通过子宫内膜取样确诊，因为 LMS 常不累及宫腔。

肿瘤生物标志物

Goto 等报道血乳酸脱氢酶（LDH）在少部分 LMS 患者中升高，与动态磁共振联合应用有助于诊断。联合应用的阳性预测值为 91%，与之相比，单独应用 LDH 的 39%，单独应用 MRI 的 71%[51]。

影像学检查

ESS 在超声检查时无特异性表现[52]。ESS 在磁共振弥散加权成像的特征为肿瘤沿着血管或韧带投射导致的蚯蚓状改变[53]。很少有研究描述 UES 的特征性表现[54]。

Kurjak 等[55]评价了经阴道彩色多普勒超声波检查在鉴别子宫肉瘤和平滑肌瘤中的作用。计算机断层扫描（CT）可确定子宫外的扩散，磁共振扫描（MRI）可评估子宫肌层受侵的深度。围术期进行影像学检查可显示子宫肿物的特征，评估是否累及淋巴结及存在其他转移，但是不能可靠地区分子宫肉瘤和其他子宫病变。很少有资料提示影像学检查的最佳选择[54,56]。FDG-PET 比腹部 CT 扫描能更好地发现盆腔外转移病灶[57～59]。

诊断

子宫肉瘤患者 75%～95%可出现异常阴道出血[60,61]。盆腔疼痛、阴道分泌物增加、排出组织常见。绝大多数癌肉瘤患者可通过子宫内膜活检确诊[62]，而 LMS 和 ESS 分别至少有 40%和 20%的病例漏诊[34,63,64]。

TNM 和 FIGO 分期

子宫肉瘤需要手术分期。国际妇产科联盟(International Federation of Gynecology and Obstetrics, FIGO)在 2009 年之前没有专门针肉瘤的特异性分期系统而应用子宫内膜的分期原则。2009 年 FIGO 制订了专门针对 LMS, EES 和 UES 的子宫肉瘤的分期系统,以及针对腺肉瘤的分期系统(表 107-2 和表 107-3)。癌肉瘤的分期采用 2009 年 FIGO 修订的子宫内膜癌分期系统(参见第 103 章)。

表 107-2 分期:子宫平滑肌肉瘤、子宫内膜间质肉瘤和未分化子宫肉瘤

TNM 分类	FIGO 分期	定义
原发肿瘤(T)		
TX		原发肿瘤无法评估
T0		无原发肿瘤的证据
T1	Ⅰ	肿瘤局限于子宫
T1a	ⅠA	肿瘤最大直径小于等于 5cm(≤5cm)
T1b	ⅠB	肿瘤最大直径大于 5cm(>5cm)
T2	Ⅱ	肿瘤扩散超出了子宫,但仍局限于盆腔(肿瘤延伸至子宫外盆腔组织)
T2a	ⅡA	肿瘤累及附件
T2b	ⅡB	肿瘤累及其他盆腔组织
T3	Ⅲ	肿瘤侵犯腹腔组织(并非仅仅突向腹腔)
T3a	ⅢA	一个病灶
T3b	ⅢB	多处病灶
T4	ⅣA	肿瘤侵及膀胱黏膜和/或直肠
区域淋巴结(N)		
NX		区域淋巴结无法评估
N0		无区域淋巴结转移
N1	ⅢC	区域淋巴结转移至盆腔淋巴结
远处转移(M)		
M0		无远处转移
M1	ⅣB	远处转移(除外附件,盆腔和腹腔组织)
		列举部位,如果知道:________

表 107-3 分期-子宫腺肉瘤

TNM 分类	FIGO 分期	定义
原发肿瘤(T)		
TX		原发肿瘤无法评估
T0		无原发肿瘤的证据
T1	Ⅰ	肿瘤局限于子宫
T1a	ⅠA	肿瘤局限于子宫内膜/颈管内膜,无肌层浸润
T1b	ⅠB	肿瘤浸润≤1/2 肌层(≤50%)
T1c	ⅠC	肿瘤浸润>1/2 肌层(>50%)
T2	Ⅱ	肿瘤扩散超出了子宫,但仍局限于盆腔(肿瘤延伸至子宫外盆腔组织)
T2a	ⅡA	肿瘤累及附件
T2b	ⅡB	肿瘤累及其他盆腔组织
T3	Ⅲ	肿瘤侵犯腹腔组织(并非仅仅突向腹腔)
T3a	ⅢA	一个病灶
T3b	ⅢB	多处病灶
T4	ⅣA	肿瘤侵及膀胱黏膜和/或直肠
区域淋巴结(N)		
NX		区域淋巴结无法评估
N0		无区域淋巴结转移
N1	ⅢC	区域淋巴结转移至盆腔淋巴结
远处转移(M)		
M0		无远处转移
M1	ⅣB	远处转移(除外附件,盆腔和腹腔组织)
		列举部位,如果知道:________

预后因素和预后

三种主要类型子宫肉瘤的预后因素各不相同。Major 等报道 GOG 针对临床分期为Ⅰ期和Ⅱ期的子宫肉瘤患者进行的临床病理学研究结果,本研究有 453 例患者符合入组条件,430 例接受包括淋巴结切除术的完整分期手术,这其中包括 59 例 LMS 和 301 例癌肉瘤[35]。同源性癌肉瘤的中位生存时间为 62.6 个月,异源性癌肉瘤为 22.7 个月,LMS 为 20.6 个月。同源性癌肉瘤总的复发率为 56%。

在 LMS 患者中,常伴有淋巴血管间隙受侵和子宫峡部及宫颈受累,但是淋巴结转移、附件转移和腹腔细胞学阳性较为

罕见。核分裂数是唯一与无进展间隔有关的手术病理学因素[2,35,37,65]。3 例核分裂数小于 10 个/10HPF 的患者无复发，61%的核分裂数为 10~20 个/10HPF 的患者和 79%的核分裂数大于 20 个/10HPF 的患者复发。

与 LMS 患者相反，与癌肉瘤患者无进展间隔时间相关的手术病理因素包括附件转移、淋巴结转移、组织学细胞类型（同源性或异源性）以及肉瘤的级别。值得重视的是，癌肉瘤患者淋巴结和附件转移率及腹腔细胞学阳性率较高。盆腔淋巴结转移率为腹主动脉旁淋巴结转移的两倍（15% vs 7.8%），有 5%可同时出现盆腔及腹主动脉旁淋巴结转移[35]。

粉碎术

对怀疑为子宫肉瘤的患者行腹腔镜下子宫切除术时，不宜采用强力粉碎术。Wright（2014）通过研究大型保险数据库的数据发现，36 470 名妇女在接受微创子宫切除术时采用强力粉碎术，子宫恶性肿瘤的发生率为 27/10 000（99 例）[66]。除此以外，发现了 26 例其他妇科恶性肿瘤（发生率为 7/10 000），39 例子宫恶性潜能未定平滑肌瘤（11/10 000）以及 368 例子宫内膜增生（101/10 000）[66]。

子宫平滑肌肉瘤

子宫平滑肌肉瘤患者采用粉碎术与不良预后相关[67]。Park 等[68]等报道了一组接受肿瘤粉碎术后被诊断为子宫平滑肌肉瘤的病例，5 年无瘤生存率（DFS）为 40%，而未接受粉碎术者为 65%（P=0.04）。同样地，粉碎术后患者的 5 年总生存率（OS）为 46%，而未接受粉碎术者为 73%（P=0.04）[68]。

子宫内膜间质肿瘤

在一项研究中，子宫内膜间质肉瘤患者采用肿瘤粉碎术与未行粉碎术患者相比较，5 年无瘤生存率（DFS）较低（分别为 55% vs 84%，OR 风险比为 4.03，95%CI：1.06~15.3）[69]。但是据报道粉碎术对总生存率（OS）无明显影响。

手术治疗

除了胚胎性横纹肌肉瘤外，女性生殖系统肉瘤的初始治疗为手术。子宫肉瘤患者需要行腹式全子宫切除术和仔细地分期，包括盆腔和腹主动脉旁淋巴结取样。通过病理分期证实肿瘤局限于子宫的癌肉瘤患者，腹腔冲洗液细胞学发现恶性细胞为不良预后因素。

绝经前的 LMS 患者应该保留卵巢，因为保留卵巢有可能会改善预后[12,64,70,71]。但是，其他的所有患者必须行双侧输卵管-卵巢切除术，包括低级别 ESS 患者[72,73]，因为这些肿瘤可能为激素依赖性或反应性，有可能扩散至子宫旁组织、阔韧带和附件。

临床分期为Ⅰ期或Ⅱ期的癌肉瘤患者很大一部分在剖腹手术分期后出现分期升高[74,75]；因此对这部分患者进行分期手术是合理的。目前关于淋巴结取样在 LMS 和 ESS 患者中作用的研究有限，但这些肉瘤患者中几乎所有出现淋巴结转移者同时也存在腹腔内转移[47]。

与其他妇科恶性肿瘤不同，开胸手术或电视辅助胸腔镜检查对于子宫肉瘤肺转移患者有作用。Levenback 等回顾分析了 Memorial Sloan-Kettering 癌症中心 45 例因子宫肉瘤肺转移而切除肺部转移灶的患者，其中多数病例为 LMS（84%）[76]。单侧病变患者的平均生存时间（39 个月）明显长于双侧病变的患者（27 个月）。复发或转移的低级别 ESS 患者，其盆腔病变或肺部转移灶同样也应手术切除。

妇科肉瘤的术后治疗

虽然完全手术切除是妇科生殖系统肉瘤患者理想的初始治疗方法，但没有随机研究证实肿瘤细胞减灭手术对晚期或复发患者的总生存率有影响。同样地，淋巴结切除的治疗意义未被证实，但理论上是有益处的。对于子宫或卵巢肉瘤的患者，没有正式的研究评价在全子宫和双输卵管-卵巢切除术的基础上进一步进行淋巴结切除术的价值。

对于子宫肉瘤患者，目前尚无经前瞻性研究得出的确定结论表明任何类型的辅助治疗可改善总体生存率。为了探讨目前已知的放疗和化疗在肉瘤中的作用，将 LMS 从剩余的同源性和异源性癌肉瘤区分开来，因为前者的复发方式与后者稍微有些不同。

放射治疗

LMS 的放射治疗

与其他肉瘤相反，局限于子宫的 LMS 患者复发的主要方式为盆腹腔外复发（65%），少部位患者最初的复发部位局限于腹腔和/或盆腔（28%）[77~79]。因此，在 LMS 中，虽然盆腔复发率不低，但给予盆腔放疗作为术后辅助治疗潜在获益很少，2/3 的患者在首次复发时即存在远处转移。仅保留放疗作为孤立盆腔复发病灶的治疗。

癌肉瘤的放射治疗

历史上，术前或术后盆腔照射被用于癌肉瘤手术的辅助治疗。许多回顾性文献阐明了这种常见的应用[60,75,80~86]。在一些有关癌肉瘤的报道中，盆腔复发率为 56%，而远处转移率为 45%。这表明与 LMS 患者相比，癌肉瘤患者盆腔复发的危险性较高[60,80~82,86]。同样也表明即使对于病变明显局限于子宫的患者，仅行手术治疗对于控制盆腔病变是不够的。有一些研究已表明术后放射治疗的益处[87,88]，尤其在控制局部病变方面，尽管不是所有研究均支持上述结论[60,84,88~93]。应用或未应用辅助性盆腔放疗患者的远处转移率类似，在 35%~45%[60,81,84]。

仅有一项随机临床试验评估Ⅰ期和Ⅱ期子宫肉瘤患者

辅助盆腔放疗的作用。EORTC 在 1998 年至 2001 年招募了 224 例患者(103 例 LMS,91 例癌肉瘤和 28 例 ESS),结果表明放疗可提高癌肉瘤患者的局部控制率(放疗组 24%复发,观察组 47%复发),但不改善总体生存。盆腔放疗对 LMS 的局部控制率没有影响(放疗组 20%复发,观察组 24%复发)[93]。

鉴于子宫肉瘤盆腔复发率较高,因此,应对癌肉瘤患者给予辅助性盆腔放疗以提高局部控制率,尽管尚无放疗的标准化剂量,但至少不应低于 50Gy,分割至少 5 周。

GOG[94]另外进行了一项Ⅲ期研究,将全腹放疗(WAI)与顺铂+异环磷酰胺+美司那(CIM)三周期化疗在 206 例符合条件的Ⅰ~Ⅳ期满意减瘤术的癌肉瘤患者中进行比较,虽然没有明显的统计学优势,但仍然观察到化疗的生存差异,CIM 患者的调整复发率降低了 21%,调整死亡率降低了 29%。此外,WAI 患者的晚期不良事件显著增加[95]。

被认为无法手术的子宫肉瘤患者极少采用初始盆腔放射治疗。文献报道约一半或 2/3 的患者可通过常规分割放疗方案控制盆腔病变,其中小部分患者可达到治愈[60,80~82]。

最后,对于复发或者未控的盆腔肿瘤导致疼痛或出血者,放射治疗可作为有效的姑息性治疗方法。

化疗

子宫肉瘤的两个特征增加了系统治疗的必要性:①即使Ⅰ期病变的患者复发率至少为 50%;②肿瘤易发生远处复发转移。然而由于该病发病率低,探讨系统性治疗价值的研究数量有限。GOG 的研究最早发现癌肉瘤和 LMS 在药物治疗敏感性上存在差异[96]。因为这两种细胞类型对化疗的反应性不同,它们分别被讨论。

单药治疗

部分药物被研究在晚期或复发癌肉瘤和/或 LMS 中的应用价值(表 107-3 和表 107-4),其中包括顺铂[101,100,103,102]、异环磷酰胺[97~99]、多柔比星[96,104]、脂质体多柔比星[105]、依托泊苷[106~108]、米托蒽醌[109]、紫杉醇[110,111]、托泊替康[112]、吉西他滨[113]、三甲曲沙[116]和多西他赛[117,115]。

表 107-4 子宫肉瘤单药化疗疗效

药物	既往化疗	化疗方案	有效,n(%)			参考文献
			CS	LMS	ESS	
异环磷酰胺	无	1.5g/(m²·d)+美司纳,0.3g/(m²·d),第 1~5 天,每 4 周为一周期	9/28(32)	6/35(17)	7/21(33)	97~99
顺铂	无	50mg/m²,每 3 周为一周期	12/63(19)	1/33(3)	—	100
	有	50mg/m²,每 3 周为一周期	5/28(18)	1/19(5)	—	101,102
	无	75~100mg/m²,每 3 周为一周期	5/12(42)	—	—	103
多柔比星	无	60mg/m²,每 3 周为一周期	4/41(10)	7/28(25)	—	96
	无	50~90mg/m²,每 3 周为一周期	0/9(0)	—	—	104
脂质体多柔比星	无	50mg/m²,每 4 周为一周期	—	5/32(16)	—	105
依托泊苷	有	100mg/(m²·d),第 1~3 天,每 4 周为一周期	2/31(6)	3/28(11)	—	106
	有	50mg/(m²·d),第 1~21 天,每 4 周为一周期	—	2/29(7)	—	107
	无	100mg/(m²·d),第 1~3 天,每 3 周为一周期	—	0/28(0)	—	108
米托蒽醌	有	12mg/m²,每 3 周为一周期	0/17(0)	0/12(0)	—	109
紫杉醇	无	175mg/m²,每 3 周为一周期	—	3/34(9)	—	110
紫杉醇	有	170mg/m²,每 3 周为一周期	8/44(18)	—	—	111
托泊替康	无	1.5mg/(m²·d),第 1~5 天,每 3 周为一周期	—	3/36(8)	—	112
吉西他滨	有	1 000mg/m²,第 1,8,15 天,每 4 周为一周期	—	9/44(20.5)	—	113
他比特啶	无	1.5mg/m²,每 3 周为一周期	—	2/20(10)	—	114
多西他赛	无	100mg/m²,每 3 周为一周期	—	0/16(0)	—	115

ESS,子宫内膜间质肉瘤;LMS,子宫平滑肌肉瘤;CS,癌肉瘤。

癌肉瘤

异环磷酰胺是治疗晚期或复发子宫癌肉瘤最有效的单药，对既往未接受过化疗的患者总有效率为 32.2%[97]。紫杉醇[111]和顺铂[100]是另外两个非常有效的单药，总有效率分别为 18.2%和 18%。

子宫平滑肌肉瘤

多柔比星[96]、吉西他滨[113]和异环磷酰胺[98]是 LMS 试验过的单药中（表 107-4）最有效的，有效率分别为 25%、20.5%和 17.2%。

子宫内膜间质肉瘤

妇科文献中有关 ESS 应用化疗的资料有限[34,63,118]，异环磷酰胺[99]被报道在 21 例转移性 ESS 患者中总有效率为 33.3%。

联合化疗

子宫平滑肌肉瘤

最有效的联合化疗方案为吉西他滨（900mg/m² 静脉滴注，第 1 天和第 8 天）联合多西他赛（100mg/m² 静脉滴注，第 8 天），第 9~15 天皮下注射粒细胞集落刺激因子。GOG 进行了两项Ⅱ期研究，分别探讨本方案[吉西他滨固定剂量率为 10mg/（m²·min）]在转移性 LMS 一线和二线治疗中的价值。作为转移性子宫平滑肌肉瘤的初始治疗，42 例患者总有效率为 36%，另外 26%患者疾病稳定[119]。作为二线治疗的 48 例患者中，总有效率为 27%，另外 50%疾病稳定（中位时间为 5.4 个月）[120]。

其他非常有效的联合化疗方案为多柔比星联合异环磷酰胺。GOG[121]报道 33 例患者给予常规剂量异环磷酰胺作为一线治疗，总有效率为 30%。Leyvraz 等[122]对 37 例患者采用了更高剂量强度的方案：异环磷酰胺（10g/m²，连续静脉滴注 5 天）联合多柔比星[（25mg/（m²·d）静脉滴注，第 1~3 天]，总有效率达到 49%。

癌肉瘤

有三个随机临床研究确定了子宫癌肉瘤最优的联合化疗方案。GOG-0108 比较了在晚期、顽固或复发子宫癌肉瘤患者中应用异环磷酰胺-美司那单药或联合顺铂作为一线治疗的疗效。联合用药组的总有效率（54%）明显高于单药组（36%），但是无显著的生存受益。

在 GOG-0161 研究中，子宫癌肉瘤患者接受紫杉醇-异环磷酰胺/美司那-生长因子联合方案化疗，与接受异环磷酰胺单药化疗的患者比较，调整后死亡的危险度减少 31%，调整后肿瘤进展的危险度减少 29%[123]。因此，紫杉醇/异环磷酰胺成为未来 GOG 关于子宫癌肉瘤研究中试验联合化疗的标准方案。

GOGⅡ期研究（GOG-0232B）正式试验了 55 例晚期子宫癌肉瘤患者应用紫杉醇和卡铂（T/C）方案化疗的有效性。结果证实完全缓解和部分缓解率分别为 13%和 41%，使得总有效率达到 54%，中位无进展生存期为 7.0 个月，中位生存期为 14.4 个月[124]。因此，GOG 目前关于子宫癌肉瘤的Ⅲ期研究（GOG 261）设计为非劣性研究，比较 T/C 方案与紫杉醇/异环磷酰胺方案化疗的有效性。此研究已完成入组，预期将证实紫杉醇和卡铂成为治疗子宫癌肉瘤的最好的主要化疗方案。

局限病变的辅助化疗

子宫平滑肌肉瘤

手术完全切除的早期子宫平滑肌肉瘤患者术后辅助化疗的作用仍在研究中，但初步结果令人期待。迄今为止仅有一个随机研究探讨了早期子宫肉瘤辅助化疗价值（GOG 20）。该研究将患者随机分入多柔比星（60mg/m²，每 3 周为一周期，共 8 个周期）化疗组或无治疗组。但因子宫平滑肌肉瘤亚组仅纳入 48 例患者，病例数较少不足以评估复发率或生存率是否存在显著性差异[125]。

肉瘤协作研究联盟进行了一项Ⅱ期多中心研究，47 例病变局限于子宫的平滑肌肉瘤患者，接受 4 个周期的固定剂量率吉西他滨-多西他赛加 4 个周期的多柔比星辅助化疗。虽然 78%的患者 2 年无进展，但随访至 3 年时下降至 50%[126]。一项Ⅲ期多中心随机研究（GOG 277）将吉西他滨-多西他赛化疗后加多柔比星与目前标准的方案化疗后观察相比较，此研究目前正在进行中。

癌肉瘤

GOG 报道了一项研究（GOG 117），探讨在 65 例手术完全切除且术后不补充放疗的Ⅰ或Ⅱ期子宫癌肉瘤患者中应用异环磷酰胺+美司那+顺铂方案辅助化疗。24 个月时无进展生存率和总生存率分别为 69%和 82%，84 个月时无进展生存率和总生存率分别为 54%和 52%。5 年总生存率为 62%[127]。由于超过半数以上的复发病例出现了盆腔复发，因此该研究建议术后放疗联合序贯化疗可能使此类患者获益。

激素和生物治疗

子宫肉瘤患者中存在雌激素和孕激素受体[45,128]。Sutton 等研究 43 例不同类型的子宫肉瘤患者的激素受体表达情况，发现其中 55.5%雌激素受体阳性，55.8%孕激素受体阳性[128]。受体的存在不受分期或分级影响，但是低级别 ESS 的患者受体水平及阳性率均非常高，因此这类肿瘤对孕激素治疗通常反应率较高[45,46,118,129~131]，同时建议停止对此类肿瘤使用雌激素替代治疗和他莫昔芬治疗[45,132]。

最近有报道将芳香化酶抑制剂[59,133]和促性腺激素释放激素激动剂[134]用于治疗 ESS，可显著提高缓解率、延长缓解时间[45,132,135]。在一项 GOGⅢ期研究中，102 例既往未接受过化疗的转移性子宫平滑肌肉瘤患者应用固定剂量率吉西他滨-多西他赛化疗的基础上联合贝伐单抗并未提高总反应率、无进展生存期及或总生存期。

中肾旁管腺肉瘤

“中肾旁管腺肉瘤”这一名词创造于 1974 年，是一种独特的子宫肿瘤，特征为间叶成分为恶性，通常为低级别；腺上皮成分通常为良性、少数为非典型性[13]。大多数腺肉瘤起源于子宫内膜，极少数起源于颈管内膜、子宫下段和子宫肌层[14,136,137]。GOG 一项 1993 年的研究中发现，腺肉瘤占子宫肉瘤的 7%[35]。子宫腺肉瘤可发生于所有年龄的女性，但最常见于绝经后妇女。迄今最大样本量的研究报道发病最高年龄为 80 岁，38%的患者年龄小于 50 岁[136]。最常见的症状是不规则阴道出血，但一些患者以盆腔疼痛、腹部包块或阴道分泌物增加为主诉。

大体上，大多数为单发的息肉状肿物，有小囊腔，其次为肿瘤切面海绵状[14,136]。Clement 和 Scully[136] 在研究了 100 例腺肉瘤患者的镜下组织学表现后于 1990 年提出并发表了本病的组织学诊断标准：应包括以下至少一项：核分裂数≥2/10HPF；明显的间质细胞密集；显著的间质细胞不典型性。当少量病例的肿瘤中超过 25% 由纯肉瘤组成时，被称为“肉瘤样过度生长”，这些病例肉瘤成分一般为高级别，病变具有侵袭性[14,138]。大多数腺肉瘤，无间质过度生长，其肉瘤成分中表达 ER 和 PR，可作为治疗的靶点。但当腺肉瘤出现间质过度生长，肉瘤成分的激素受体表达通常为阴性[14,139,140]。除了间质过度生长，与生存期降低唯一相关的组织病理学特征是子宫肌层受侵[14,44,136,138,140]。

子宫外的中肾旁管腺肉瘤包括卵巢、阴道子宫内膜异位病灶、直肠阴道隔、胃肠道、膀胱、Douglas 窝、腹膜和肝脏[14,137,140~142]。卵巢腺肉瘤的恶性程度较子宫腺肉瘤更高，可能的原因是由于缺乏解剖屏障而导致腹膜种植播散[14,142]。

非子宫妇科肉瘤

外阴

迄今文献报道的外阴肉瘤不足 500 例。最常见的外阴肉瘤为 LMS、横纹肌肉瘤和纤维肉瘤[143]。这些肿瘤的临床表现与它们的级别、核分裂数、组织学类型以及分期有关[143,144]。对于低级别的肿瘤，扩大局部切除已足够。但对于侵袭性较高的肿瘤，应考虑实施根治性外阴切除术加淋巴结切除术，术后给予细胞毒药物辅助化疗，但辅助性化疗的治疗价值尚缺乏相应研究[144]。

阴道

阴道肉瘤占原发性阴道恶性肿瘤的 3%[145]。成年人中最常见的阴道肉瘤是 LMS，在 40 岁以上患者中最常见的症状是阴道出血[146]。虽然这种肿瘤高度恶性，但接受手术治疗（全子宫双附件及阴道切除术）的患者才可能得到生存获益。

胚胎性横纹肌肉瘤（RMS），以前称为葡萄状肉瘤，最常发生于儿童，具有典型的葡萄串状外观。以往该病致死率极高，年幼的女孩子需接受广泛性的除脏手术。目前儿童胚胎性阴道 RMS 最好的是治疗方式为多药联合诱导化疗，如 VAC 方案，随后给予局部切除，术后必要时可给予腔内放疗，而根治性手术仅作为持续性或复发病例的挽救治疗[147]。

卵巢

大多数在阴道、外阴或子宫中常见的肉瘤类型亦可发生于卵巢[148,149]。卵巢癌肉瘤较罕见，且极具侵袭性，预后差，仅占所有卵巢恶性肿瘤的 1%~4%[150]。主要的治疗方法仍然是对转移性病变行最大限度的减瘤术，术后给予以铂类为基础的化疗。早期病变和肿瘤有同源性间质成分的患者预后较好[150]。

输卵管

在女性生殖系统肉瘤中，输卵管原发肉瘤最为少见。最常见的组织学类型是癌肉瘤[151,94,152~154]，治疗与卵巢癌肉瘤相同，对转移性病变行最大限度的减瘤术，术后辅助以铂类为基础的化疗[151]。

（程敏　佐晶 译　程敏 校）

参考文献

The complete reference list can be found on the Wiley Companion Digital Edition of this title (see inside front cover for login instructions).

2 Kempson RL, Bari W. Uterine sarcomas. Classification, diagnosis, and prognosis. *Hum Pathol*. 1970;**1**(**3**):331–349.

3 Tavassoli FA, Devilee P. Tumors of the uterine corpus. In: *World Health Organization Classification of Tumours. Pathology and Genetics of Tumours of the Breast and Female Genital Organs*. Lyons: IARC Press; 2003:217–258.

4 Otis COAC, Nucci MR, McCluggage WG. Protocol for the Examination of Specimens from Patients with Sarcoma of the Uterus. College of American Pathologists 2013 [cited 2015 01/04/2015]; Available from: http://www.cap.org/apps/docs/committees/cancer/cancer_protocols/2013/UterineSarcomaProtocol_3000.pdf.

5 D'Angelo E, Prat J. Uterine sarcomas: a review. *Gynecol Oncol*. 2010;**116**(**1**):131–139. Epub 2009/10/27.

6 Harlow BL, Weiss NS, Lofton S. The epidemiology of sarcomas of the uterus. *J Natl Cancer Inst*. 1986;**76**(**3**):399–402.

13 Clement PB, Scully RE. Mullerian adenosarcoma of the uterus. A clinicopathologic analysis of ten cases of a distinctive type of mullerian mixed tumor. *Cancer*. 1974;**34**(**4**):1138–1149. Epub 1974/10/01.

14 McCluggage WG. Mullerian adenosarcoma of the female genital tract. *Adv Anat Pathol*. 2010;**17**(**2**):122–129. Epub 2010/02/25.

21 Chiang S, Ali R, Melnyk N, et al. Frequency of known gene rearrangements in endometrial stromal tumors. *Am J Surg Pathol*. 2011;**35**(**9**):1364–1372. Epub 2011/08/13.

30 Rose PG, Piver MS, Tsukada Y, Lau T. Patterns of metastasis in uterine sarcoma. An autopsy study. *Cancer*. 1989;**63**(**5**):935–938.

35 Major FJ, Blessing JA, Silverberg SG, et al. Prognostic factors in early-stage uterine sarcoma. A Gynecologic Oncology Group study. *Cancer*. 1993;**71**(**4 Suppl**):1702–1709.

44 Arend R, Bagaria M, Lewin SN, et al. Long-term outcome and natural history of uterine adenosarcomas. *Gynecol Oncol*. 2010;**119**(**2**):305–308. Epub 2010/08/07.

45 Amant F, Floquet A, Friedlander M, et al. Gynecologic Cancer InterGroup (GCIG) consensus review for endometrial stromal sarcoma. *Int J Gynecol Cancer*. 2014;**24**(**9, Suppl. 3**):S67–S72. Epub 2014/07/18.

46 Rauh-Hain JA, del Carmen MG. Endometrial stromal sarcoma: a systematic review. *Obstet Gynecol*. 2013;**122**(**3**):676–683. Epub 2013/08/08.

47 Leibsohn S, d'Ablaing G, Mishell DR Jr, Schlaerth JB. Leiomyosarcoma in a series of hysterectomies performed for presumed uterine leiomyomas. *Am J Obstet Gynecol*. 1990;**162**(**4**):968–974; discussion 74-6.

51 Goto A, Takeuchi S, Sugimura K, Maruo T. Usefulness of Gd-DTPA contrast-enhanced dynamic MRI and serum determination of LDH and its isozymes in the differential diagnosis of leiomyosarcoma from degenerated leiomyoma of the uterus. *Int J Gynecol Cancer*. 2002;**12**(**4**):354–361. Epub 2002/07/30.

65 Gadducci A, Cosio S, Romanini A, Genazzani AR. The management of patients with uterine sarcoma: a debated clinical challenge. *Crit Rev Oncol Hematol*. 2008;**65**(**2**):129–142. Epub 2007/08/21.

66 Wright JD, Tergas AI, Burke WM, et al. Uterine pathology in women undergoing minimally invasive hysterectomy using morcellation. *JAMA*. 2014;**312**(**12**):1253–1255. Epub 2014/07/23.

68 Park JY, Park SK, Kim DY, et al. The impact of tumor morcellation during surgery on the prognosis of patients with apparently early uterine leiomyosarcoma. *Gynecol Oncol*. 2011;**122**(**2**):255–259. Epub 2011/05/14.

69 Park JY, Kim DY, Kim JH, Kim YM, Kim YT, Nam JH. The impact of tumor morcellation during surgery on the outcomes of patients with apparently

early low-grade endometrial stromal sarcoma of the uterus. *Ann Surg Oncol.* 2011;**18(12)**:3453–3461. Epub 2011/05/05.

70 Aaro LA, Symmonds RE, Dockerty MB. Sarcoma of the uterus. A clinical and pathologic study of 177 cases. *Am J Obstet Gynecol.* 1966;**94(1)**:101–109.

71 Garg G, Shah JP, Liu JR, et al. Validation of tumor size as staging variable in the revised International Federation of Gynecology and Obstetrics stage I leiomyosarcoma: a population-based study. *Int J Gynecol Cancer.* 2010;**20(7)**:1201–1206. Epub 2010/10/14.

75 Silverberg SG, Major FJ, Blessing JA, et al. Carcinosarcoma (malignant mixed mesodermal tumor) of the uterus. A Gynecologic Oncology Group pathologic study of 203 cases. *Int J Gynecol Pathol.* 1990;**9(1)**:1–19.

93 Reed NS, Mangioni C, Malmstrom H, et al. Phase III randomised study to evaluate the role of adjuvant pelvic radiotherapy in the treatment of uterine sarcomas stages I and II: an European Organisation for Research and Treatment of Cancer Gynaecological Cancer Group Study (protocol 55874). *Eur J Cancer.* 2008;**44(6)**:808–818. Epub 2008/04/02.

95 Wolfson AH, Brady MF, Rocereto T, et al. A gynecologic oncology group randomized phase III trial of whole abdominal irradiation (WAI) vs. cisplatin-ifosfamide and mesna (CIM) as post-surgical therapy in stage I-IV carcinosarcoma (CS) of the uterus. *Gynecol Oncol.* 2007;**107(2)**:177–185.

96 Omura GA, Major FJ, Blessing JA, et al. A randomized study of adriamycin with and without dimethyl triazenoimidazole carboxamide in advanced uterine sarcomas. *Cancer.* 1983;**52(4)**:626–632.

114 Monk BJ, Blessing JA, Street DG, Muller CY, Burke JJ, Hensley ML. A phase II evaluation of trabectedin in the treatment of advanced, persistent, or recurrent uterine leiomyosarcoma: a Gynecologic Oncology Group study. *Gynecol Oncol.* 2012;**124(1)**:48–52.

119 Hensley ML, Blessing JA, Mannel R, Rose PG. Fixed-dose rate gemcitabine plus docetaxel as first-line therapy for metastatic uterine leiomyosarcoma: a Gynecologic Oncology Group phase II trial. *Gynecol Oncol.* 2008;**109(3)**:329–334. Epub 2008/06/07.

120 Hensley ML, Blessing JA, Degeest K, Abulafia O, Rose PG, Homesley HD. Fixed-dose rate gemcitabine plus docetaxel as second-line therapy for metastatic uterine leiomyosarcoma: a Gynecologic Oncology Group phase II study. *Gynecol Oncol.* 2008;**109(3)**:323–328. Epub 2008/04/09.

122 Leyvraz S, Zweifel M, Jundt G, et al. Long-term results of a multicenter SAKK trial on high-dose ifosfamide and doxorubicin in advanced or metastatic gynecologic sarcomas. *Ann Oncol.* 2006;**17(4)**:646–651. Epub 2006/02/28.

123 Homesley HD, Filiaci V, Markman M, et al. Phase III trial of ifosfamide with or without paclitaxel in advanced uterine carcinosarcoma: a Gynecologic Oncology Group Study. *J Clin Oncol.* 2007;**25(5)**:526–531.

124 Powell MA, Filiaci VL, Rose PG, et al. Phase II evaluation of paclitaxel and carboplatin in the treatment of carcinosarcoma of the uterus: a Gynecologic Oncology Group study. *J Clin Oncol.* 2010;**28(16)**:2727–2731. Epub 2010/04/28.

125 Omura GA, Blessing JA, Major F, et al. A randomized clinical trial of adjuvant adriamycin in uterine sarcomas: a Gynecologic Oncology Group Study. *J Clin Oncol.* 1985;**3(9)**:1240–1245.

126 Hensley ML, Wathen JK, Maki RG, et al. Adjuvant therapy for high-grade, uterus-limited leiomyosarcoma: results of a phase 2 trial (SARC 005). *Cancer.* 2013;**119(8)**:1555–1561. Epub 2013/01/22.

130 Cheng X, Yang G, Schmeler KM, et al. Recurrence patterns and prognosis of endometrial stromal sarcoma and the potential of tyrosine kinase-inhibiting therapy. *Gynecol Oncol.* 2011;**121(2)**:323–327. Epub 2011/02/01.

136 Clement PB, Scully RE. Mullerian adenosarcoma of the uterus: a clinicopathologic analysis of 100 cases with a review of the literature. *Hum Pathol.* 1990;**21(4)**:363–381. Epub 1990/04/01.

142 Eichhorn JH, Young RH, Clement PB, Scully RE. Mesodermal (mullerian) adenosarcoma of the ovary: a clinicopathologic analysis of 40 cases and a review of the literature. *Am J Surg Pathol.* 2002;**26(10)**:1243–1258. Epub 2002/10/03.

144 Curtin JP, Saigo P, Slucher B, Venkatraman ES, Mychalczak B, Hoskins WJ. Soft-tissue sarcoma of the vagina and vulva: a clinicopathologic study. *Obstet Gynecol.* 1995;**86(2)**:269–272. Epub 1995/08/01.

147 Raney RB Jr, Gehan EA, Hays DM, et al. Primary chemotherapy with or without radiation therapy and/or surgery for children with localized sarcoma of the bladder, prostate, vagina, uterus, and cervix. A comparison of the results in Intergroup Rhabdomyosarcoma Studies I and II. *Cancer.* 1990;**66(10)**:2072–2081. Epub 1990/11/15.

148 Oliva E, Egger JF, Young RH. Primary endometrioid stromal sarcoma of the ovary: a clinicopathologic study of 27 cases with morphologic and behavioral features similar to those of uterine low-grade endometrial stromal sarcoma. *Am J Surg Pathol.* 2014;**38(3)**:305–315. Epub 2014/02/15.

149 Lan C, Huang X, Lin S, Cai M, Liu J. Endometrial stromal sarcoma arising from endometriosis: a clinicopathological study and literature review. *Gynecol Obstet Invest.* 2012;**74(4)**:288–297. Epub 2012/09/19.

150 del Carmen MG, Birrer M, Schorge JO. Carcinosarcoma of the ovary: a review of the literature. *Gynecol Oncol.* 2012;**125(1)**:271–277. Epub 2011/12/14.

151 Yokoyama Y, Yokota M, Futagami M, Mizunuma H. Carcinosarcoma of the fallopian tube: report of four cases and review of literature. *Asia Pac J Clin Oncol.* 2012;**8(3)**:303–311. Epub 2012/08/18.

第 108 章　乳腺肿瘤

Hope S. Rugo, MD ■ Melanie Majure, MD ■ Anthony Dragun, MD ■ Meredith Buxton, PhD ■ Laura Esserman, MD, MBA

概述

女性乳腺癌仍然是一个影响公共卫生和社会的重大医疗问题，包括筛查、风险因素、预防、诊断、治疗和预后等问题。目前主要的研究进展显著提高了人们对乳腺癌的生物学和临床特性，以及驱动肿瘤生长和抵抗的生物学途径的认识。这些进展也在治疗方面产生了巨大影响，使乳腺癌死亡率在过去二十年中显著下降，同时这些进展也成为了正在进行的临床研究的基础。分子学研究有助于对乳腺癌亚型异质性的了解；生物学和肿瘤负荷的研究提供了风险和治疗的分层，促进了个体化筛查、预防和治疗的进展。随着新信息的增加，新的管理范式也成为国际指南中的护理标准。我们的挑战是适当有效地应用新的治疗方式，并且了解乳腺癌对其的反应和抵抗情况。本章将着重介绍从分子、生物和病理研究以及临床试验中获得的信息。

流行病学

乳腺癌是北美女性和整个工业化世界中女性最常见的恶性肿瘤。在美国，乳腺癌占所有女性恶性肿瘤的 29%。据美国癌症协会估计，在 2015 年，将有 231 840 名女性诊为乳腺癌[1]。

女性一生中患乳腺癌的风险约为 1/8 或 12%[2]。年龄相关的患乳腺癌的可能性如表 108-1 所示。具有某些危险因素的女性患病风险更高，例如具有很强的家族史或某些已知的基因突变。这些数据还不包括预计的 64 640 例新发的乳腺原位癌。

表 108-1　乳腺癌的终身患病概率（女性，所有种族，2008—2010）

年龄/岁	10 年内患乳腺癌风险(%)	概率
20	0.06	1/1 732
30	0.44	1/228
40	1.45	1/69
50	2.31	1/43
60	3.49	1/29
70	3.84	1/26
终身风险	12.29	1/8

摘自 DeS 抗-s 2014[3] 经 Wiley 许可转载。

此外，将有 2 350 名男性诊为乳腺癌。

西方国家 1980—1990 年末乳腺癌的发病率增加了约 30%，2002—2003 年间明显下降。发病率的增加可以归因于乳腺摄影（mammography）的频繁应用，以及绝经后激素替代疗法（HRT）的使用增加和生殖因素的变化。2002 年妇女健康行动（Women Health Initiative，WHI）的随机对照研究提供了确定性的结论，即接受 HRT 的绝经后妇女患乳腺癌的风险显著增加。这些结果导致 HRT 的使用大幅减少，相应地，在 2002—2003 年期间，乳腺癌发病率下降了 7%，主要范围是 55 岁及以上的白人女性[4,5]。自 2004 年以来，美国乳腺癌的发病率相对稳定[2,3]，不同种族之间有很大差异，如表 108-2 所示。然而，白人和非裔美国妇女的发病率正趋于一致[3]。

表 108-2　按种族或种族划分的乳腺癌发病率：美国，2007—2011 年

	非西班牙裔白人	非裔美国人	西班牙裔拉丁美洲人	美国印第安人/阿拉斯加土著	亚裔/太平洋岛民
发病率/(/10 万人)	127.6	123.0	86	91.7	86.0
死亡率/(/10 万人)	22.2	31.4	14.5	15.2	11.3

摘自 Siegel 2015[1]。经 Wiley 许可转载。

乳腺癌是全世界女性中最常被诊断出的癌症。2012 年，预计 170 万例乳腺癌被确诊，占所有女性癌症病例的 25%[6]。发病率因地理区域而异，约有一半发生在较发达国家，一般北美、澳大利亚/新西兰、北欧和西欧发病率较高。相比之下，中欧和东欧、拉丁美洲、加勒比和西亚的发病率居中，而非洲、南亚和东亚的大部分地区则处于低水平。欠发达地区患乳腺癌的累积风险为 3.3%（直到 74 岁），而较发达地区的风险为 8%。国际发病率的变化可能是由于风险因素的差异以及早期检测方法的实用性不同[7]。亚洲，南美洲和非洲的许多国家的乳腺癌发病率一直在上升，可能是因为生活方式的变化，包括生育模式、饮食、肥胖和体育锻炼[6,8]。

从 1975 年到 1990 年，美国乳腺癌的死亡率缓慢上升了 0.4%，然后从 1990 年到 2010 年下降了 34%[3]。死亡率的降低很可能是早期检测和治疗进步的结果[9]。

50 岁以下的女性降幅最大（每年降低 3.1%，而 50 岁及以上的女性每年减少 1.9%）。在美国，乳腺癌是女性癌症相关死亡的第二大病因（位于肺癌之后），但在年龄介于 20 岁到 59 岁之间的女性中，则是癌症相关死亡的首位病因。美国癌症协会估计，2015 年乳腺癌相关死亡人数为 40 290 人，占美国女性全部癌症相关死亡的 6.8%。尽管发病率低于白人女性，但非裔美国女

性的年均乳腺癌死亡率最高,死亡率因种族和民族而异。这种差异主要是由生物亚型、诊断时疾病的分期造成的,很大程度上也是由于社会经济地位的差异。从2001年到2010年,几乎所有种族群体的死亡率都有所下降,白人的死亡率降低明显多于非裔美国妇女。大多数乳腺癌在早期被诊断出来,61%的乳腺癌新发病例是局限期(淋巴结阴性);32%是区域期,还有6%在初始诊断时就已经出现远处转移。5年生存率取决于肿瘤的发现阶段,局限期的存活率为98.6%,肿瘤扩散到局部淋巴结时的存活率为84.9%,远处扩散时的存活率仅为26%。

危险因素

乳腺癌的发病率随着危险因素的不同而有所变化,有的危险因素已明确。其中,性别和年龄是两个最突出的因素。DNA修复基因的种系突变显著增加了罹患乳腺癌和其他癌症的终身风险,并增加了年轻时患乳腺癌的风险。其他与生活方式相关的因素对风险的影响更小,而改变可改变因素对个体患乳腺癌风险的影响在很大程度上是未知的。与乳腺癌发展相关的危险因素见表108-3。

表108-3 与乳腺癌发生相关的危险因素

明显增加
BRCA1、*BRCA2* 突变,Li-Fraumeni 综合征年龄增长
发达国家
一级亲属中有乳腺癌或卵巢癌家族史
45岁以前患有不典型增生、乳腺小叶原位癌电离辐射暴露史
中度增加
既往诊断为乳腺癌
月经初潮早
月经停经晚
未生产或首次足月妊娠延迟(30岁以上)
社会经济地位高
酒精摄入
45岁以后患有不典型增生、乳腺小叶原位癌
肥胖(仅绝经后女性)
乳腺X线实质分型不佳
儿子或女儿诊断为软组织肉瘤
既往患有子宫癌、卵巢癌或结肠癌
轻度增加
良性乳房增生性疾病(非异型性)
口服避孕药(10年以上)
绝经后雌激素替代疗法
可疑增加(无证据支持)
首次怀孕中断身心因素
高脂饮食
复杂性纤维腺瘤
降低风险
20岁以前足月妊娠多次妊娠
45岁以前行卵巢切除术
规律运动,尤其是在青春期和成年早期母乳喂养
无影响
乳房缩小术

性别

美国女性乳腺癌的年龄调整发病率比男性高出近100倍,这和全世界是一致的。男性乳腺癌在所有男性癌症中所占比例不到1%,在所有乳腺癌中所占比例约为1%。*BRCA1* 和 *BRCA2* 的基因突变是男性乳腺癌的最容易理解的危险因素,其终身风险范围从略高于1%(*BRCA1*)到近7%(*BRCA2*)。在世界范围内,男性的死亡率比女性下降得更少,由于累积发病低,所以迄今为止的临床试验一直不成功。最近,一个国际组织开始了针对男性乳腺癌的合作临床试验。

年龄

美国乳腺癌诊断的中位年龄是64岁,大多数病例的确诊年龄在55~64岁之间。在世界其他平均寿命更短的地区,发生乳腺癌的中位年龄要提前10~15年。而年龄相关死亡率与发病情况平行。

社会经济阶层

乳腺癌在经济阶层和教育地位较高的女性中发现更为频繁[10,11]。这很可能与生活方式因素相关,例如饮食、首次生育年龄、外源性激素的使用以及酒精摄入。然而,乳腺癌的死亡率在贫困阶层女性中更高,这与诊断时肿瘤分期较晚、肿瘤生物学更具侵袭性,以及获得护理的机会减少有关。

种族

如表108-2所示,乳腺癌的发病率和死亡率因种族不同而有很大差异。在美国,从2010年到2012年,白人被诊断出乳腺癌和死于乳腺癌的风险分别为12.64%和2.66%,黑人为11.14%和3.26%,亚洲/太平洋岛屿居民为10.25%和1.74%,拉美裔分别为9.81%和2.08%,美洲印第安人和阿拉斯加人分别为8.15%和1.66%。移民人口的研究显示,当低危群体迁徙至高危地区(如从亚洲至美国)时,其乳腺癌的发病率迅速上升,接近一代或两代以内本土人群的发病率[12]。

家族史/遗传学

家族史是乳腺癌的一个重要风险因素,但是在常规基因检测之前建立的关联使现有数据变得复杂(见下文)[13]。一般来说,一级亲属有乳腺癌病史的女性,与无此家族史女性相比,发生乳腺癌的风险增加一倍。有两个一级亲属的风险是三倍,三个或更多的是四倍。如果一级亲属分别在40岁以下、40~59岁和50~60岁分别诊断乳腺癌,那么早期患病的风险将进一步分别增加约3倍、2倍和1.5倍。除非有多个家庭成员被诊断出患有乳腺癌,否则在老年时被诊断出乳腺癌的风险较小。

那些具有 *BRCA1* 或 *BRCA2* 突变的个体,患卵巢癌和乳腺癌的概率较普通人更高。乳腺癌的终身患病风险为50%~85%,发病时间通常更早[14]。第二原发乳腺癌的风险也在增加,估计为40%~60%。这些突变是通过常染色体显性遗传的,已有2 000多种不同的突变、多态性和变异在17号染色体上的 *BRCA1* 和13号染色体上的 *BRCA2* 上发现[15,16]。在具有相同种族的人群中携带突变的风险更高,例如在德系犹太人中已发现了特征性的 *BRCA1*(185delAG,5382insC)和 *BRCA2*(617delT)突变位点;而这些基因的组合频率在一般人群中超过了2%[17~19]。在比利时、丹麦、芬兰、法国、荷兰、匈牙利、冰岛、挪威、俄罗斯和西非的其他种族社区中,也发现了类似的“建立者”突变(“founder”mutation)[20]。*BRCA* 基因编码的 DNA 修复酶通过同源重组途径在双链 DNA 修复中发挥重要作用。BRCA 活性异常细胞的 DNA 修复缺陷目前已被用于设计特定的治疗方法,如进一步损伤 DNA、导致肿瘤细胞死亡的 PARP 抑制剂(见治疗部分)。

家族性乳腺癌占所有乳腺癌不到 10%,其中 *BRCA1* 和 *BRCA2* 相关的家族性乳腺癌似乎仅占 2/3。其他一些基因也被发现会增加患乳腺癌和其他癌症的风险,包括 TP53(Li-Fraumeni 综合征)、PTEN(考登综合征)、ATM、CHECK2 和 PALB2,以及其他基因[21~25]。在过去十年中,全基因组关联研究(GWAS)发现了大量(>75)更常见的对风险有中度影响的变异(>5%)[26,27],并得到了验证[(*RR*)<1.5][28]。虽然它们单独对乳腺癌的影响不大,但结合起来却会大大增加总体风险。

有趣的是,尽管已经报道了所有的表型,但某些乳腺癌表型与特定的突变密切相关。三阴性乳腺癌在 *BRCA1* 突变的女性中发生得更频繁,HR+乳腺癌在 *BRCA2* 或 *CHEK2* 突变的女性中发生频繁,在 Li-Fraumeni 综合征患者中易发生 HER2/neu 和 HR+[29,30]。重要的是,许多常见的风险等位基因与 HR+乳腺癌的发展密切相关[28,31]。共有 7 个突变基因与更具侵略性的激素受体阴性(HR-)乳腺癌相关[32],其中四个突变位点最近发现[33]。多基因检测现在已经广泛使用,并且可以检测另外 4%的具有遗传咨询价值的潜在有害突变位点[34]。

美国国家癌症中心建议有乳腺癌病史或者符合以下条件的人应做基因检测:*BRCA1* 或 *BRCA2* 有害突变的家族史,45 岁前诊断为乳腺癌,50 岁前患有原发性癌症,任何年龄的有一级亲属乳腺癌,未知或有限的家族史,或 60 岁前确诊三阴性乳腺癌(TNBC)。其他标准包括任何年龄诊断为乳腺癌的患者和 1 名近亲诊断为乳腺癌或卵巢癌的患者,≥2 名近亲诊断为乳腺癌或胰腺癌和/或前列腺癌的患者。有卵巢癌、男性乳腺癌病史的患者,以及其他一些标准也包括在本建议中。一般来说,应首先对受影响的家庭成员进行检测,并对没有癌症诊断的家庭成员进行检测,以备受影响的家庭成员无法进行检测时使用[378]。最近对 200 多名 TNBC 患者进行的一系列研究发现,*BRCA* 突变率为 15.4%;在符合 NCCN 肿瘤临床实践指南(NCCN 指南)筛查的患者中,这一比例上升到 18.3%;比率因年龄、种族和种族而异[35]。

基因筛查的其他标准包括任何年龄的乳腺癌诊断;卵巢癌、胰腺癌或前列腺癌的近亲;或者任何患有乳腺癌的男性亲属。对于突变频率较高的人种,应考虑进行检测。一项试验发现,德系犹太人妇女中约 12%的乳腺癌可归因于 *BRCA1* 或 *BRCA2* 基因突变[17]。

确定患有乳腺癌的妇女和有发生突变危险的妇女是极其重要的。筛查和降低风险的手术可以降低癌症死亡率[36~39]。教育人们这些策略以及识别肿瘤的机制是至关重要的。

内分泌和生殖危险因素

无论亚型如何,暴露于雌激素和孕酮的持续时间和程度明显影响患乳腺癌的风险。排卵期长,月经初潮早,绝经年龄晚,可患乳腺癌的风险每年增加 3%~4%[11]。从 30 岁到 20 岁,首次生育的年龄越小,每年乳腺癌的风险就会降低 3%,而多胎生育的保护作用就越小。在 30 岁后生育第一个孩子的妇女比未生育的妇女患乳腺癌的风险更高,尤其是在分娩后的头 5 年内。这种风险明显增加的可能机制可能是怀孕的刺激作用(以及怀孕时激素环境的改变)对其他上皮细胞的影响。长时间的母乳喂养似乎可以降低风险,而短时间的母乳喂养几乎不会产生什么影响,而且在哺乳年龄较小时可以降低风险[40]。在最近的荟萃分析中,每一次生育都可降低乳腺癌相对危险度(relative risk,*RR*)7%,而每哺乳一年另外还降低相对危险度的 4.3%[41]。

外源性激素

虽然过去的很多年里,人们对外源性激素替代或口服避孕药与乳腺癌风险都有争议,但是妇女健康行动(Women Health Initiative,WHI)的随机对照研究得到了定论。在该项研究中,16 608 名绝经后的健康女性被随机分配口服共轭雌激素加醋酸甲地孕酮或安慰剂[42]。因为健康风险超过了健康获益,雌激素和孕酮联合用药组在随诊 5.2 年后被停止。与 HRT 相关的冠心病风险比(hazard ratio,*HR*)增加 29%,乳腺癌增加 26%,脑卒中增加 41%,肺栓塞增加 13%。同时,在使用激素替代的女性中,结直肠癌的 *HR* 下降 47%,髋骨骨折下降 34%。没有在记忆力下降和其他智力功能的测量方面发现保护性作用。百万妇女研究(Million Women Study)和 HERS Ⅱ 研究(心脏与雌/孕激素替代研究(Heart and Estrogen/Progestin Replacement Study)也获得了相似的结果[43~45]。

美国预防服务特别工作(United States Preventative Services Task Force)组给出结论:雌激素和孕激素在大多数女性中的不良作用超过了其对慢性疾病的预防作用。尽管短期应用 HRT 可能对控制与更年期有关的血管舒缩症状有益,但不推荐长期使用。

长期以来,口服避孕药的使用与乳腺癌风险的轻微增加有关。最近,一项针对美国 20~49 岁女性医疗服务体系的大型研究发现,近期服用高剂量雌激素制剂的女性风险增加,而服用低剂量雌激素避孕药的女性风险则没有增加[46]。停止使用后,风险似乎不会持续。

体育锻炼和肥胖

有证据表明,缺乏身体活动是绝经后乳腺癌的一个风险因素,经常锻炼的女性患乳腺癌的风险相对降低[47,48]。这种益处主要受到体重的影响,肥胖的女人运动过程几乎没有受益。在妇女健康倡议中,35 岁时经常进行剧烈运动的妇女患乳腺癌的风险相对降低了 14%。与久坐不动的女性相比,即使每周 1.25~2.5h 的快走也可使乳腺癌风险相对降低 18%,而那些额外 10h 快走或等效运动的人的风险降低更多[49]。

高体重指数(>25kg/m^2),尤其是绝经后体重增加和腹部肥胖,明显与绝经后乳腺癌风险增加有关[10,50~52]。对于绝经后妇女、体重指数>25 的妇女相对危险度为 1.5,肥胖女性(BMI>30)的相对危险度为 2。在妇女健康行动中,肥胖还与 HR+乳腺癌和更严重的乳腺癌类型患病风险增加有关[53]。绝经前妇女的数据更为复杂,她们的体重和患乳腺癌的风险之间没有明确的关系[54]。

较高强度的体力活动和较低的体重指数与较低的雌二醇

和雌酮水平以及血清胰岛素水平相关,这可能部分解释了运动对乳腺癌风险的影响[55~57]。ACS 已发布指南关于运动和营养可以降低癌症风险[58,59]。乳腺癌风险降低与遵守这些指南有关[54]。

二甲双胍和糖尿病

在妇女健康行动中,糖尿病妇女使用二甲双胍可降低乳腺癌的风险[60]。已知二甲双胍可提高胰岛素敏感性和降低高胰岛素血症,而在临床前模型中,高胰岛素血症与癌症的发生和增殖有关[61]。此外,胰岛素样生长因子受体表达的信号通路与乳腺癌的增殖和治疗耐药有关,二甲双胍可能通过 mTOR 这一靶点抑制下游信号通路[62~65]。在一些研究中,糖尿病与乳腺癌的高风险有关,但在另一些研究中则不然;然而,在乳腺癌诊断后,糖尿病会导致更糟的结果[52,66~69]。目前多中心临床试验正在对二甲双胍在早期乳腺癌(ESBC)患者中进行试验[70,71]。

乳腺密度

乳腺密度是各种族乳腺癌的常见和重要危险因素,与年龄和体重指数呈负相关[72~76]。许多州的法律要求在进行乳房 X 线检查时向妇女报告乳房密度信息[75]。乳腺密度四分位数最高的女性,患病风险似乎明显升高,比乳腺密度最低的女性高出 4.5~5 倍。不同的研究显示,标准乳腺摄影检查所显示的乳腺密度(1、2、3、4 分别表示脂肪性、散在纤维腺体型、不均质型和致密型),与乳腺癌风险有着很强的相关性且结果具可重复性[76]。对于 BCSC5 年或 5 年风险高或非常高且乳房密度非常大的患者,乳腺间期癌病例的危险比为 1.62,而在 70~74 岁的患者中,危险比上升到 3.45。为此,一个结合 BCSC 风险模型和乳腺密度与良性乳腺疾病(BBD)的风险模型已建立,该模型可帮助准确确定需要进行一级预防的高危妇女[70]。Gail 风险模型用于估计乳腺癌的 5 年和终身风险,纳入乳腺密度对乳腺癌风险评估的影响不大[77,78]。此外,这些患者可能需要额外的影像学检查,尽管到目前为止还没有确切的数据表明替代的影像学检查将提供更好的信息、改善癌症检测、提高乳腺癌分期或生存率诊断。

酒精

流行病学研究一致发现,女性饮酒者发生乳腺癌的风险增高。这被认为是由于酒精影响肝功能,使雌二醇的血清和组织浓度增加。在女性健康行动观察研究中,酒精摄入与乳腺癌风险的增加相关,最大限度的增加与最高的每日摄入量有关。这种影响似乎因不同亚型而异[79]。与那些从不饮酒的女性相比,那些每周饮酒量超过 7 杯的女性患浸润性小叶癌的风险几乎增加了两倍(*HR*=1.82,95%*CI*:1.18~2.81),但酒精对浸润性导管癌的风险没有影响,尽管这两种亚型都是 HR+型。

电离辐射

接触电离辐射是乳腺癌已知的危险因素。原子弹的幸存者和使用放射线治疗产后乳腺炎、痤疮、多毛症和关节炎的患者,即使照射的剂量很低或很弱,乳腺癌的发病率也会增高[80,81]。过去用于监测结核的治疗效果而反复进行的胸部 X 线检查也与乳腺癌风险增高有关。乳腺癌的发病率在霍奇金病(Hodgkin disease)患者中有所增加,青春期或年轻时接受了胸部放射治疗,尤其是放射治疗与化疗结合时,患乳腺癌的风险显著增加[82]。从辐射暴露到发生乳腺癌之间的潜伏期很长(中位数 30 年),但是放射治疗与化疗结合时,这个时间会缩短。普通诊断性的放射检查所导致的乳腺癌发生风险是极低的,并且放射技术人员的乳腺癌发病率没有升高[83]。为治疗原发性乳腺癌所实施的放疗,5 年后对侧乳腺癌的发病风险增高(大约 30%)[84]。

乳腺良性病变

大多数其他形式的乳腺良性病变似乎与乳腺癌的风险增加无关。因此,大部分具有乳腺结节或良性乳腺病变的女性,乳腺癌的风险并没有明显增加。

然而,很多研究显示,乳腺良性病变的存在(或既往有该病史)与乳腺癌风险增加相关[85]。其他研究已发现,既往因为良性病变接受过乳腺活检的女性,发病风险也增高。但是,这种联系在很大程度上是局限于经活检证实、组织学显示为异型性或增生性病变者(异型性导管或小叶增生)(表 108-4)[87,88]。与从未接受乳腺活检的女性相比,患有良性乳腺病变且不伴增生的女性,乳腺癌的比值比(odds ratio,*OR*)为 1.5;伴有增生但无异型性的女性 *OR*=1.9;而同时伴有增生和异型性的女性,其 *OR*=2.6~5.3,而对于有异型性和家族史的女性[86,89],这个比值增加到 11。在 Mayo Clinic 的一项最近的研究中,9 807 名患有良性乳腺疾病的女性中,年轻(45 岁以下)且伴有异型性的女性,发生乳腺癌的 *HR*=6.99。确定这一风险因素的重要性在于能够使用激素治疗进行化学预防以及使用基于风险的筛查方法来显著降低风险[87,88]。

表 108-4 浸润性乳腺癌的相对危险度[a]——基于未患癌乳腺组织的组织学检查

风险不增加(无增生性病变)
腺病
顶泌汗腺改变
导管扩张症
常见类型的轻度上皮增生
风险轻度增加(1.5~2 倍)(不伴异型性的增生性病变)
常见类型的中度或旺炽性增生
硬化性腺病
风险中度增加(4~5 倍)(非典型增生或交界性病变)
非典型导管增生
非典型小叶增生
高危(8~10 倍)(原位癌)[b]
小叶原位癌——双侧乳腺
导管原位癌(非粉刺型)——单侧,局部

[a] 每一类型的女性都与未接受过乳腺活检且年龄匹配的女性相比较,以考察在接受乳腺活检后的 10~20 年内发生浸润性导管癌的风险。上述风险并非终身风险。

[b] 在只接受活检后,只有很少例数的非粉刺型导管癌一直被作为风险指标。

其他

双膦酸盐

口服双膦酸盐可以降低侵袭性乳腺癌的风险，尤其是 HR+ 型乳腺癌的发病率[90~92]。骨质疏松症可能是绝经后较低的雌激素水平的一个标志，并与较低的乳腺癌风险相关[93,94]。最近的一项荟萃分析表明，使用双膦酸盐超过 1 年的患者与不使用双膦酸盐的患者相比，乳腺癌的发病率降低 15%，侵袭性疾病的发病率降低 32%[95]。

钙和维生素 D

虽然以前的研究支持维生素 D 和钙在降低乳腺癌发病率方面的作用，但随后的研究未能发现乳腺癌风险之间存在关联[96]。一项大型研究显示，服用补充维生素 D 的年轻女性乳房密度较低，另一项研究则表明服用补充维生素 D 可对乳房密度高的女性乳房密度产生影响[93,94]。

其他饮食饮食

动物脂肪含量高，水果和蔬菜含量低的饮食与患乳腺癌的风险较高有关。然而，这也与运动和体脂等其他因素密切相关。在没有乳腺癌病史的 48 000 多名绝经后妇女中进行了一项初步干预试验[97]，试验组的妇女被分配到总脂肪摄入量低(20%的能量)和 5~6 份蔬菜，水果和谷物的饮食组。进行 8 年的随访，浸润性乳腺癌风险没有降低，但依从性最高组的风险有降低的趋势。鉴于这种饮食也与其他一些并发症的减少有关，并且较长时间的干预可能会产生更大的影响，这似乎是一种合理且可行的生活方式。

乳腺癌风险评估模型

统计学模型可以用于评估女性患乳腺癌的风险。一些模型用于预测包括短期和终身风险在内的乳腺癌发生风险。这些模型高度依赖于对象的年龄；因此，一个年轻女性的很低的短期风险，可能伴随着很高的终身风险。Gail 风险评估模型(Gail risk assessment model)[98~100]和 Claus 模型[101]是预测女性乳腺癌风险最常用的模型[102]。其他模型，例如 BRCA-PRO[103]、Frank[104]和 Couch[105]模型，是预测携带基因突变者的风险或概率的，应用于指导决定是否进行 *BRCA1* 或 *BRCA2* 基因突变的检测。这些模型并不能确定是否会发生乳腺癌。确切地说，它们是依靠遗传易感性的检测结果来预测风险的。检测结果的解释取决于所检测的是否是先证者(患癌的人)和家族中是否存在已知的致癌突变。在过去的 5 年里，出现了新的模型，包括乳腺密度、风险暴露、家族史和单核苷酸多态性，如乳腺癌监测联盟模型已在 100 多万妇女中得到有效验证[106]。

Gail 模型

对于每年都接受筛查的女性，Gail 风险评估模型是最常用的评估乳腺癌患病风险的统计模型。Gail 等利用来自 Breast Cancer Detection Demonstration Project 的 28 个参与中心的 284 780 名女性(以白人女性为主)的数据，建立了这一模型。这是一个基于 *HR*(具有特定危险因素者的患病风险/不具危险因素者的患病风险)的非条件 logistic 回归模型。模型中所使用的危险因素包括年龄、初潮年龄、首次生育的年龄、一级亲属患乳腺癌的人数(仅限于母亲、姐妹或女儿)、接受乳腺活检的次数和乳腺病理为不典型增生。

Gail 模型适用于绝大多数女性。美国的 NASBP 预防试验以 1.67 分(这是 60 岁女性 5 年 Gail 分数的平均值)作为入组的最低风险标准。Gail 风险模型现在广泛用于个体化的临床决策，可用多种方式获得(NCI 网站、手持设备或计算机软件)。这个模型可以很好地预测人群的患病风险，但 1.67 的临界值并没有显示出良好的区分能力[107]。Ozanne 等通过将研究对象的 Gail 风险与其他女性的风险相比较，从而提出了改进方法。这样一来，患病风险的四分位数或十分位数最高的女性辨识度更佳，也更有助于确定真正高危的女性[108]。这个模型的缺陷在于对家族史的处理不够好，无论是父亲一方的乳腺癌家族史还是亲属的发病年龄，均未计算在内。研究者目前正在修订这个模型，以预测非洲裔美国人的乳腺癌风险。改进方法正如上文所提到的那样，可以将乳腺密度与风险相乘，以进一步提高模型的预测能力[74,109]。

遗传模型

在 100 多万名美国女性组成的多种族群体中，BCSC 模型(一种包含 BI-RADS 乳腺密度的类似工具)显示出 Gail 模型更好的风险识别和校准能力。Gail 和 BCSC 都没有纳入基因危险因素的现代知识。添加多基因风险(76 个单核苷酸多态性)改善了 BCSC 模型的性能，包括密度和多基因风险。其他模型也被开发出来，包括多种风险因素，如家族史、更全面的遗传因素和暴露。RO[101]、Frank[102]和 Couch[103]是用于预测携带 *BRCA1* 或 *BRCA2* 基因突变的可能性，是基于常染色体显性遗传模式和高危人群突变率，BRCAPRO 模型还预测患乳腺癌和卵巢癌的风险。该模型基于母亲和父亲癌症史中的多个变量，包括诊断年龄、多种原发性癌症、双侧乳腺癌、德系犹太人血统以及患有乳腺癌的一级、二级和三级亲属人数。BRCAPRO 模型还包括卵巢癌和胰腺癌。这种高风险的情况很少发生。

这些遗传模型临床用于具有乳腺癌阳性家族史的女性，模型经过很好的校准，能够辨识性地预测 *BRCA* 突变的存在。据预测，至多 10%~15%的女性乳腺癌患者存在 *BRCA1* 或 *BRCA2* 的突变。BRCAPRO 不仅可以预测白人家族中的基因突变，还可以预测非裔美国人家族中的基因突变。然而，研究者怀疑，接近 20%的乳腺癌是由于不确定的遗传因素导致的，而剩下的 70%则被认为是散发性或非遗传性疾病。

生物标志物

BRCA1 和 *BRCA2* 的突变可以肯定地预测乳腺癌的终身风险和早期风险，但不能准确的预测短期风险。明确可以作为风险量化指标的生物标志物就显得至关重要。生物标志物在预防中的最佳应用是既能够预测短期风险的增加，又能够预测针对性干预所带来的获益。潜在可变的、且一直显示与乳腺癌风险更高相关的生物标志物包括异形性和乳腺密度。异型性也预示着他莫昔芬(tamoxifen)的使用可以带来更大的获益。在 NSABP P-1 研究中，他莫昔芬的使用降低了高达 89%的乳腺癌风险[110]。许多研究者正在致力于生物标志物的研究，以确定这些标志物是否可作为评价干预效果的可靠的替代指标[111]。如果这些生物标志物用于检测预防性干预效果会如何呢？一

些药物，如针对 ER 阳性乳腺癌发挥作用的选择性雌激素调节剂（selective estrogen modifiers）和芳香化酶抑制剂（aromatase inhibitors），可以用于治疗细胞学检查发现异形性的女性，其干预效果可以通过异形性的减少来衡量。治疗过程中（6~12 个月）还可以对乳腺密度的改变进行评估，并将其作为代替指标来确定那些最有可能从预防性干预中获益的人群。其他可改变的风险包括运动，饮食和体重。沟通和共同决策对于降低风险至关重要[112~114]。

乳腺癌生长的调控

了解乳腺癌的发展及其生长调控方面的基本知识，为我们制订预防和治疗策略奠定了基础。成年女性的乳腺由上皮组织构成的输乳管和泌乳腺泡构成，其中泌乳腺泡位于纤维组织框架和脂肪中，且开口于输乳管末端。正常乳腺的生长和发育是通过许多激素和生长因子之间复杂的相互作用进行调控的，其中一些激素和生长因子是由乳腺细胞自身分泌的，可能具有自分泌功能。雌二醇调控与肽和蛋白相关的一些基因的表达，而这些肽和蛋白参与了乳腺细胞生长的控制机制。这些生长因子与特异性受体结合而发挥作用。多肽激素的受体多是位于细胞膜上的，而类固醇激素家族的受体则主要位于细胞核内[115,116]，但也可位于细胞膜上。生长因子、细胞因子、激素和特异性膜受体之间的相互作用，触发了细胞内生物化学信号的级联反应，导致不同基因的活化或抑制。

研究显示其中的一些激素对乳腺上皮细胞的生长、发育和乳腺的泌乳具有促进作用。由于这些激素及其受体对正常乳腺组织具有调节作用，因此乳腺起源的恶性细胞可能表达其中很多激素的受体，并可能保持一定程度的激素依赖，就不足为奇了。

生长因子信号通路的基因异常（大部分是获得性的）与发育异常和多种包括癌症在内的慢性疾病有着千丝万缕的联系。恶性细胞的产生是遗传事件（genetic events）逐步发展的结果，这些遗传事件包括生长因子或其信号通路成分的表达失去调控[114]。

激素和生长因子对乳腺癌细胞的生长调控图示于图 108-1 中。雌激素的生物作用是通过分子与 ER 高亲和性结合介导的。这些分子属于配体诱导核受体家族。类固醇、甲状腺素和维生素是其已知的配体[117]。最近的研究显示乳腺癌细胞在雌激素的调控下可以合成和分泌自身的生长因子，通过自分泌或旁分泌机制自发性刺激乳腺癌细胞或邻近的间质组织。芳香化酶在许多乳腺癌中大量表达，使恶性细胞能够合成自身重要的生长因子和雌激素。间质组织可能也分泌能够刺激乳腺癌细胞的 IGF-1 和 IGF-2。潜在的自分泌/旁分泌生长因子有 EGF、TGF-α、IGF-2、血小板源性生长因子（platelet-derived growth factor）和成纤维细胞生长因子（fibroblast growth factor）。研究发现培养的乳腺癌细胞和人乳腺癌组织标本都表达和分泌 EGF、TGF-α、IGF-1 和 IGF-2，它们是肿瘤上皮（恶性）成分的潜在有丝分裂原[118]。血小板源性生长因子和成纤维细胞生长因子是由乳腺癌细胞分泌的，可能与许多乳腺癌中的间充质基质成分明显增殖有关。

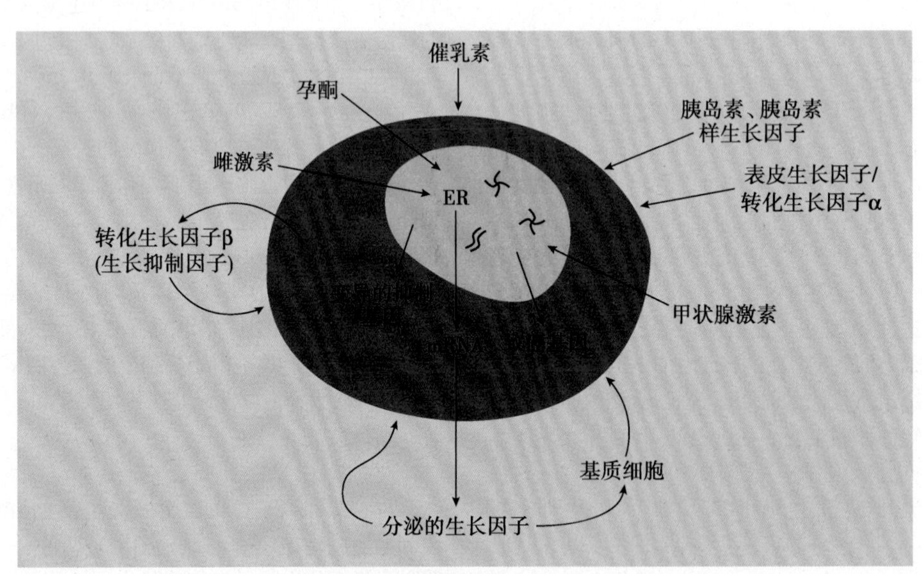

图 108-1　激素和生长因子对乳腺癌生长的调控

人乳腺癌细胞还分泌数种可能具有自分泌抑制活性的肽。TGF-β 是一个生长因子家族，它能够抑制上皮组织的增殖，并促进间质组织的增殖[50]。研究显示 ER 阴性的乳腺癌细胞，比 ER 阳性的细胞对 TGF-β 更为敏感。乳腺癌细胞的恶性潜能，部分程度上取决于肿瘤所产生的生长刺激因子和抑制因子之间的平衡。肿瘤的上皮和/或间质细胞也分泌蛋白酶，如组织蛋白酶（cathepsins）、基质溶解素（stromelysins）、明胶酶（gelatinases）或尿激酶型纤溶酶原激活物（urokinase plasminogen activator）等，这些蛋白酶也参与了肿瘤侵袭和转移的潜能。

在 ER 阳性的乳腺癌细胞中，某些自分泌生长因子的表达和分泌，如 TGF-α、IGF-2 等，是由雌激素刺激、抗雌激素（抗-estrogen)抑制的。在 ER 阴性的乳腺癌细胞中,这些因子的分泌则不是由雌激素调控的。研究者推测,这些分泌的因子的表达,在某种程度上介导了雌激素和抗雌激素的生长效应。雌激素和抗雌激素对于乳腺癌细胞有多种作用。雌激素刺激 RNA、DNA、蛋白质的合成和关键调节酶的活性,而抗雌激素则在大部分组织中具有相反作用。雌激素最终通过细胞周期和有丝分裂调节细胞的运动。

干扰细胞的正常生长控制机制会导致细胞分裂失控和癌的发生。这种细胞转化的发生是通过癌基因(oncogenes)的激活和抑癌基因(tumor suppressor genes)的突变或丢失所导致的。癌基因正常对应的是原癌基因(proto-oncogenes),它在正常细胞中起生长调节作用。原癌基因的改变与动物和人体内肿瘤的发生、发展和/或维持有关。癌基因的产物通常是生长因子、生长因子受体、分子开关或转录因子。人乳腺癌组织中常见的过表达的癌基因包括 *myc* 和 *ras* 家族成员(*c-myc*、*Ha-ras-1*)、*int-2*[参与老鼠(和人,据推测)的乳腺癌的发生]和 EGF 受体(EGFR、erbB)家族成员[包括 erbB-2(也就是 HER2 或 neu)、HER3 和 HER4]。生长因子受体的过表达和突变经常导致这些受体的组成性激活(即受体在缺乏同源配体的情况下发出信号)。生长促进信号被不断的传送给细胞,导致多条信号转导通路的激活和细胞生长失去调控。正常情况下参与细胞周期控制的基因,尤其是 *cyclin D* 和 E 家族成员,也可能作为癌基因发挥功能。这些癌基因的过表达可能有助于恶性表型的启动和维持。研究表明,转基因小鼠乳腺中 *myc*、*ras* 和 *HER2* 基因的组织特异性过表达导致良性和恶性乳腺疾病的发病率升高。这些本来正常的基因表达发生改变,对于乳腺上皮的生长稳态具有深远的影响。最近的研究显示阻断这些生长因子受体或通路具有治疗作用[68]。这些研究表明,不论是在临床前模型还是人乳腺癌中,HER2 的单克隆抗体都具有显著的抗肿瘤作用,并下调 PI3K 信号通路。此外,这些单克隆抗体还和细胞毒药物具有协同作用,如蒽环类(anthracyclines)、铂类似物(platinum analogs)、长春瑞滨(venorelbin)和紫杉类(taxanes)等。肿瘤组织中 EGFR 过表达,意味着患者的预后不佳。然而,EGFR 似乎并不是肿瘤恶性行为的关键驱动者,其单克隆抗体在临床试验中只取得了很小的成功。

研究发现,在乳腺癌标本中对这些癌基因的表达进行量化,为肿瘤的侵袭性、预后和治疗敏感性提供了宝贵的信息[69]。恶性细胞的细胞表面受体下游的信号分子经常被激活或改变。因此,乳腺癌中 PI3 激酶通路和 MAP 激酶通路经常被激活,甚至在没有 EGFR 或 HER2 过表达的情况下亦然。

抑癌基因对于乳腺癌的形成也具有作用。这些基因发生突变或缺失,失去了正常的抑制功能,可能会导致癌症的发生。在人乳腺癌细胞和其他实体瘤中,都明确存在已知抑癌基因的改变,如视网膜母细胞瘤基因(RB1)和人 *TP53* 基因。研究者发现在患有 Li-Fraumeni 综合征的家族中,存在 *TP53* 基因的突变,而这些家族的乳腺癌和其他肿瘤的发病率明显上升。另外,研究显示高达 50% 的乳腺癌中存在 *TP53* 基因的突变。两个与家族性乳腺癌相关的突变基因——*BRCA1* 和 *BRCA2*,也被认为是抑癌基因。这些基因所表达的蛋白的正常功能是控制细胞增殖(RB1 和 TP53)或促进/介导 DNA 的修复(TP53、BRCA1、BRCA2)。基因突变导致蛋白突变,并由此导致细胞周期的调控失常。认识到抑癌基因的突变失活可以早期发现高危家族,并带来新的治疗策略——不论是在实验室还是在早期临床试验中,都可以通过基因疗法导入正常基因的拷贝,或使用正常抑制蛋白本身进行治疗,以逆转恶性表型。

雌激素和孕激素受体

雌激素受体是核激素受体超家族的成员,具有多个功能域,分为 2 个亚型,每个亚型具有多个同型异构体和剪切变异体。ERα(alpha)基因位 6 号染色体长臂(6q24 ~ q27),而 ERβ(beta)基因则位于 14 号染色体的 q22 ~ 24 带。PR 至少有 3 种亚型,其组织分布和功能正在积极的探索中。其他雌激素诱导蛋白调控导致细胞增殖的事件。当受体与抗雌激素(如他莫昔芬等)结合时,生长促进基因的转录被阻断,但其他基因可能会被他莫昔芬激活。

ER 与其配体相结合,所形成的 ER-配体复合物与雌激素反应元件相结合,并启动雌激素驱动基因的转录。位于细胞膜的 ER,与配体结合后,介导非基因效应,这主要是通过与肽生长因子受体(EGFR、HER2)的交互作用而实现的。在抗雌激素耐药方面,ER 的非基因效应增加明显。

ER 检测最重要的应用是选择适合内分泌治疗的患者。有 50% ~ 60% 的 ER 阳性患者从内分泌治疗中获益,其中包括通过内分泌治疗获得客观缓解(部分或完全)和长期稳定(>6 个月)的转移性乳腺癌患者,这两组患者具有相同的生存预期。肿瘤无法检测到 ER 或 PR 的患者无法从内分泌治疗中获益。然而,ER 和/或 PR 含量很低但可检测到的乳腺癌患者,也可对内分泌治疗产生反应,尽管这种情况非常少见。

ER 和 PR 的状态可以随着时间或干预治疗而改变,因此,对于可获取的组织进行重复活检,有助于后续治疗的选择。然而,原发肿瘤的 ER 状态仍然能够对复发后内分泌治疗的疗效进行非常合理的预测。ER 阴性的肿瘤有一个很强的趋势,即化疗有效率更高,因此激素受体状态通常情况下可能有助于预测化疗的疗效。目前还不知道为什么 40% ~ 50% 的 ER 阳性肿瘤尽管存在受体,但却对内分泌治疗无效。显然,一个检测方法如果能够明确真正对内分泌治疗敏感的肿瘤,将会对临床更有帮助。至少有一个多基因检测——21 基因检测(Oncotype Dx),在美国被越来越多地用于显示 ER 阳性女性乳腺癌患者在服用他莫昔芬 5 年后发生远处转移风险的特征[119]。

研究者已经明确乳腺癌组织中存在变异和/或突变的 ER[120]。其中一些是组成性激活的(无雌激素的情况下激活转录),一些是失活的,还有一些则具有优势负性效应(dominant negative activity)。这些变异体及其在激素耐药状态方面的作用(如果存在任何作用的话)所具有的生物重要性有待阐明。

病理

组织学类型

乳腺癌的病理分类对于非乳腺病专家来说往往是难以理解的。表 108-5 列出了各种组织学类型的浸润性乳腺癌。

表 108-5 浸润性乳腺癌组织学类型的发病率

组织学类型	人数	%
腺癌	287 384	97.4
浸润性导管癌	216 104	73.2
小叶癌	26 726	9.1
混合性导管癌和小叶癌	27 371	9.3
炎性乳腺癌	1 003	0.3
黏液癌	5 737	1.9
管状癌	1 850	0.6
乳头状癌	1 754	0.6
佩吉特病	1 259	0.4
其他腺癌	3 336	1.1
腺癌,NOS	2 176	0.7
鳞状细胞癌	145	0
其他特殊类型癌	2 415	0.8
髓样癌	815	0.3
其他	1 600	0.5
非特殊型	3 356	1.1

NOS,非特殊型(not otherwise specified)。来源:Howlader 2015[2]

乳腺上皮性肿瘤

导管上皮产生的肿瘤可以只在来源导管的管腔内发现,也就是说,肿瘤位于导管内,并未穿透基底膜或侵犯周围间质。最常见的情况是这种肿瘤从大的导管中产生,并表现为数种类型。如果肿瘤进入到导管中,并伴有乳头状结构,则被认为是乳头状癌(papillary carcinoma)(图 108-2)。这种病变是罕见的,约占乳腺癌的 1%。在组织学上可以发现极性紊乱的多形性导管上皮细胞,以及它们"堆积"而形成的乳头。乳头状癌和良性非典型性乳头状瘤的鉴别较为困难。

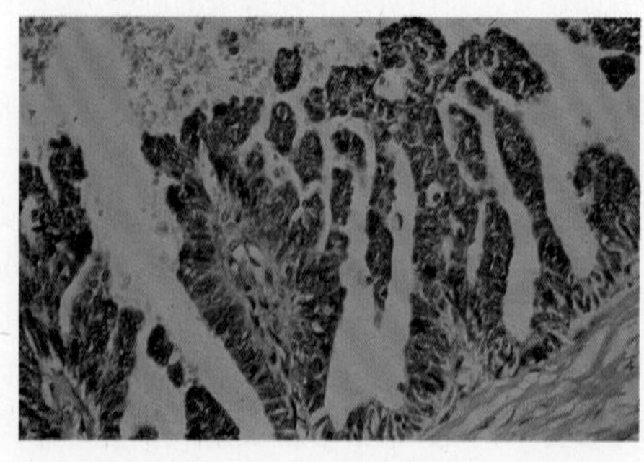

图 108-2 乳腺乳头状癌,少见肿瘤,<1%,极少浸润,预后良好

乳头状癌极少侵犯周围间质,完全切除的预期生存率接近 100%。当侵犯到周围间质时,这种肿瘤的生长非常缓慢,并形成很大的肿物。乳头状癌通常不会累及皮肤和筋膜,腋窝淋巴结转移是其晚期特征。临床发现非浸润性肿瘤是可以切除的,病变边界清楚,质地柔软,与纤维腺瘤的质地不同。

非浸润性导管癌,又称导管内癌(intraductal carcinoma)或导管原位癌(ductal carcinoma in situ,DCIS),其上皮细胞亚群的增殖局限于乳腺导管内,光镜下没有穿过基底膜侵犯到间质的征象。DCIS 的组织学诊断存在一定的问题。区分良性但高度异型性增生与 DCIS 往往是困难的,有时小灶的间质浸润也难以确定。偶尔情况下,DCIS 与小叶原位癌(lobular carcinoma in situ,LCIS)之间难以辨别,这是因为 DCIS 可以延伸到乳腺小叶,而 LCIS 也可以包括小叶外的导管,因此一些病变可能介于两者之间。目前已经认识到 DCIS 存在多种组织学类型,最常见的是粉刺状(comedo)、筛状(cribriform)、实体状(solid)、乳头状(papillary)和微乳头状(micropapillary)(图 108-3)。不同的组织学类型与不同的生物学行为有关。DCIS 的增殖比率依据其组织学特征而不同。粉刺样 DCIS 的增殖比率高,而筛状、乳头状和实体状 DCIS 的增殖比率低。粉刺癌(comedocarcinoma)是一种癌的类型,其特征是导管扩张并被癌细胞充填。这些癌细胞是坏死的,可称为半固体坏死性栓子(semisolid necrotic plugs)。这些组织学类型的肿瘤通常不被视为一个独立的细胞类型,而是代表了导管内癌的不同的描述方式。研究显示粉刺型 DCIS 与其他类型相比,局部复发率更高,进展为浸润性乳腺癌更快(图 108-4)。目前发现人 EGF 受体 2(HER2/neu)的过表达只存在于在实体样和粉刺样 DCIS 中,但不存在于乳头状和筛状 DCIS 中。ER 的检测是评估 DCIS 不可或缺的部分,对于选择最佳治疗干预是必不可少的。

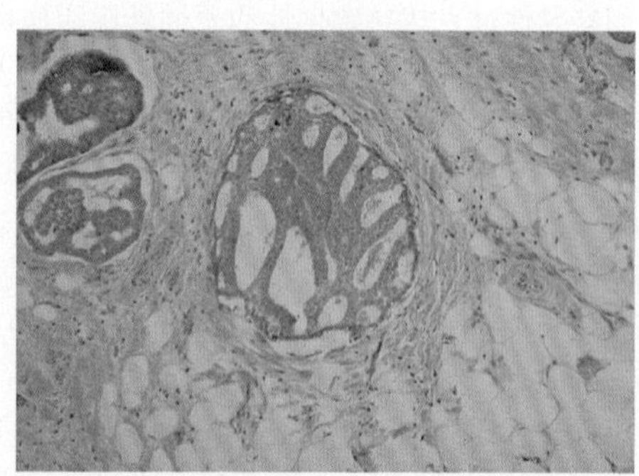

图 108-3 导管原位癌(ductal carcinoma in situ,DCIS)筛状型。导管空间被增殖的导管细胞所填充。导管细胞的细胞核相对一致,细胞排列于背靠背的(筛状)腺体上。腺体的大小和形状完全一致,并呈现刚性内侧缘(所谓的"甜面包切割"样外观)

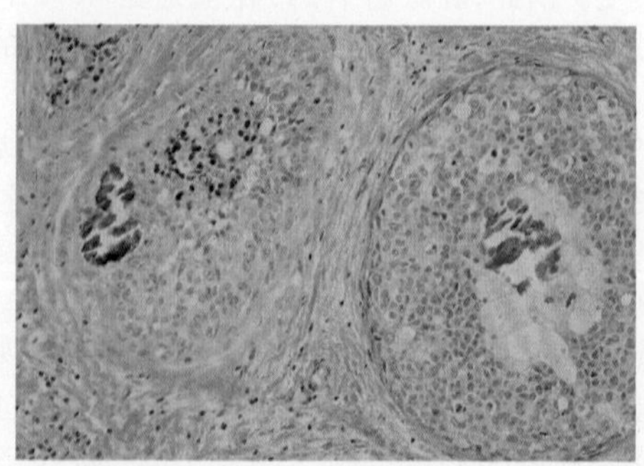

图 108-4 导管原位癌(DCIS),粉刺型。两个导管包含具有高核分裂相、局灶坏死和钙化的肿瘤细胞。高级别的核分裂相和中央坏死是诊断粉刺型导管原位癌的依据

小叶癌(lobular carcinoma)源自乳腺小的末端导管。小叶癌的非浸润性类型,即小叶原位癌的特征是:低核级别的小细胞充填小叶并使之扩张,但没有穿透基底膜(图 108-5)。当病变延伸超过小叶范围或其来源的终末导管,就成为浸润性小叶癌(invasive lobular carcinoma)。小细胞经常在胶原束之间相互交错排列成单行,也就是所谓的"印度列兵样排列"(India file)。其他时候小叶癌可能同常见的浸润性导管癌几乎没有区别(图 108-6)。非浸润性癌几乎占女性所有乳腺肿瘤病变的 22%,其中 LCIS 占 60%,也就是全部乳腺肿瘤的 12%。DCIS 往往伴随着浸润性导管癌,或是其早期形式;LCIS 可以随后出现任何一侧乳腺的浸润性导管或小叶癌,因此 LCIS 更是一个全身疾病的标志,而非局部早期病变。随着乳腺摄影越来越多的应用,检测的非浸润性癌的比例明显升高。

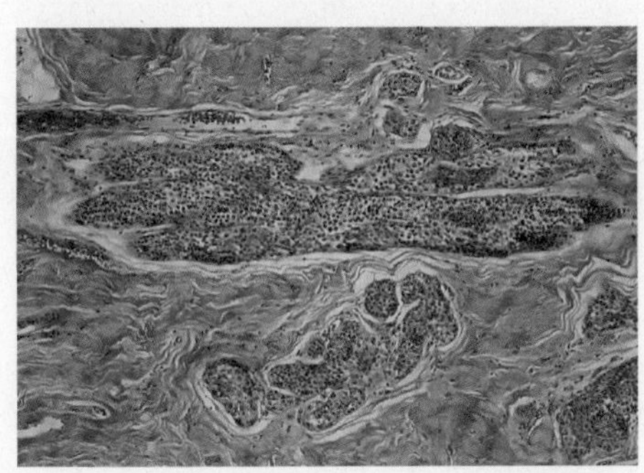

图 108-5 小叶原位癌(lobular carcinoma in situ,LCIS)。大小形状一致的小细胞增殖,完全充满终末导管和腺泡并使之扩张

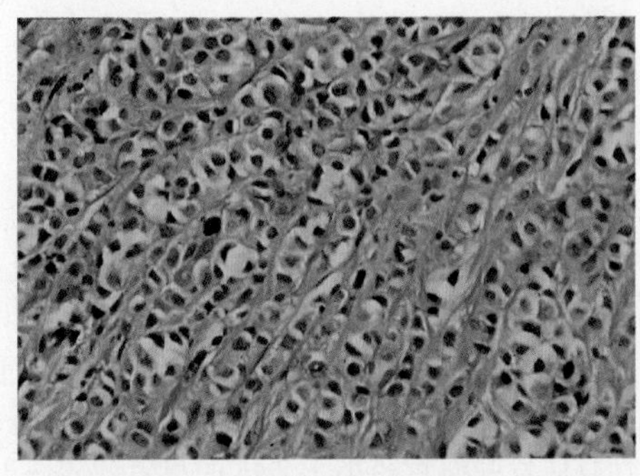

图 108-6 浸润性小叶癌。肿瘤细胞的细胞核相对一致,发生侵袭,细胞呈单行排列或线形排列(所谓的"印度列兵样排列")

我们将没有特殊类型组织学结构的浸润性导管癌规定为"非特殊型"(not otherwise specified,NOS),这是最常见的导管癌,几乎占乳腺癌的 80%(图 108-7)。遇到坚硬的阻力,切面下肿瘤回缩,可发现呈淡黄色、灰白色条纹的坏死灶,组织学上存在不同程度的纤维化反应。浸润性导管癌 NOS 经常转移至腋窝淋巴结,是不同肿瘤类型中预后最差的一种。一半以上(52.6%)的乳腺癌是单纯浸润性导管癌 NOS。

还有几个其他类型的浸润性癌源自大的导管,每一种都有其各自不同的组织学表现。髓样癌(medullary carcinoma),占所有乳腺癌的 3%~6%,体积往往较大(图 108-8),由相对高核级别的细胞形成,肿瘤中通常存在小淋巴细胞的广泛浸润。髓

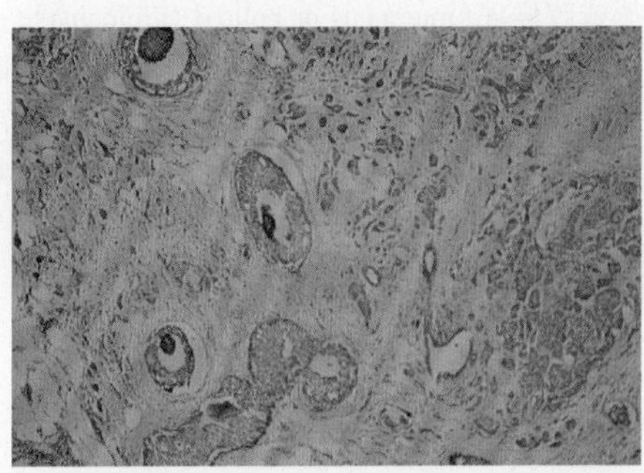

图 108-7 非特殊型乳腺浸润性导管癌(not otherwise specified,NOS)。接近 80% 的乳腺癌组织学呈这种表现,约 1/3 伴有其他类型的分化

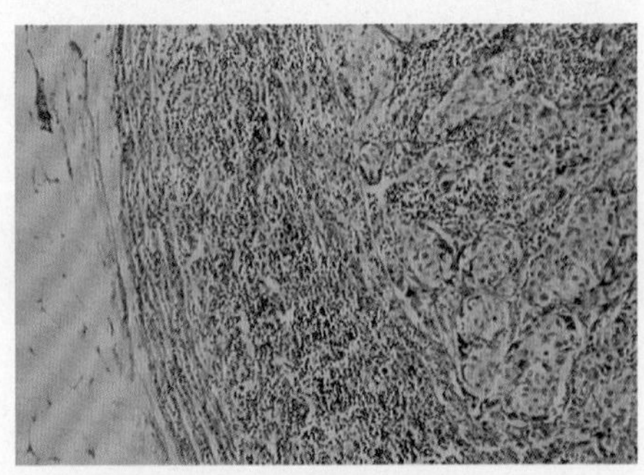

图 108-8 髓样癌大约占乳腺癌的 5%~7%,分化相对较差,预后仍然好于浸润性导管癌

样癌的边界相对清楚,有时被描述为"推挤性"边界("pushing" border),相比之下,NOS 肿瘤中的小的细胞巢倾向于更为广泛地浸润到邻近间质中去。一项关于髓样癌的研究观察了 336 名典型和 273 名不典型髓样癌患者,这些患者来源于多个 National Surgical Adjuvant Breast Project(NASBP)Ⅰ期、Ⅱ期试验中入组的 6 404 名患者。研究发现,典型髓样癌患者的生存优于浸润性导管癌 NOS,非典型髓样癌患者的生存则与 NOS 相似[121]。

管状癌(tubular carcinoma)是一种非浸润性癌,肿瘤中小管形成非常明显。它占乳腺癌的 1%~2%,低核级别,一些细胞具有极性(图 108-9)。管状癌预后良好,当其体积较小时,是可以治愈的。

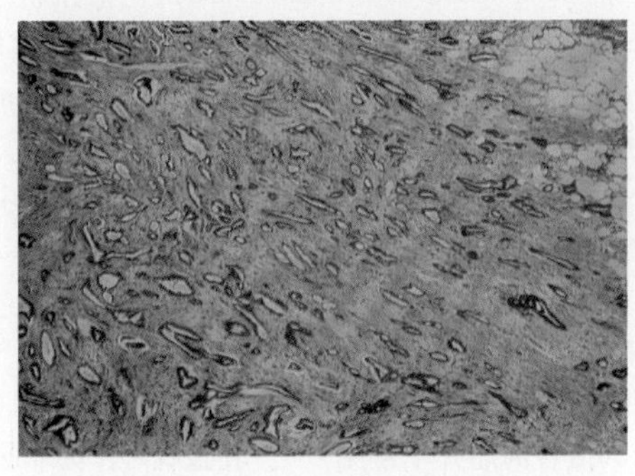

图 108-9 乳腺导管癌。单纯的导管癌罕见,小于 1%,预后好于非特殊型浸润性导管癌(infiltrating duct carcinoma not otherwise specified,NOS)。20% 的浸润性导管癌 NOS 可以见到部分管状分化

黏液癌或胶样癌(mucinous or colloid carcinoma),占所有乳腺肿瘤的1%~2%,其特点是镜下可见上皮,细胞呈巢状或条索状漂浮于黏液间质中。这一类型的肿瘤生长缓慢,可以形成很大的肿物。当肿瘤以黏液为主时,预后较好(图 108-10)。

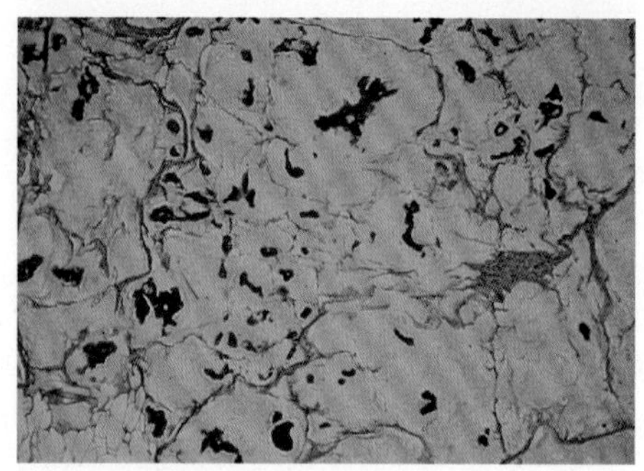

图 108-10　乳腺黏液癌或胶样癌。这一类型少见(约2%),但预后相对较好

还有两种特殊类型的乳腺癌。乳腺佩吉特病(Paget disease)发生于1%~4%的乳腺癌患者。临床上,患者表现为具有相对较长的乳头湿疹。样变病史,并伴有瘙痒、灼热、渗出和/或出血。乳头的改变与乳腺潜在的癌变有关,这种癌变在大约2/3的患者中触诊可及。下方的肿瘤类型上可能是导管内癌,也可能是浸润性导管癌,预后与相应肿瘤的侵袭性和组织学类型相关。组织学上看,乳头上皮包含有癌细胞巢。

炎性乳腺癌(inflammatory breast cancer,IBC),或称乳腺真皮淋巴管性癌病(dermal lymphatic carcinomatosis),其临床特征是皮肤发红、发热、水肿、[橘皮样变(peaud orange)],明显的丹毒样边缘,乳腺下组织硬块,本病进展迅速,从出现首个征象到诊断时间通常小于 3 个月。诊断时必须具有这些表现。红斑区域和周围外观正常的皮肤的活检,经常(但并非总是)提示分化差的癌细胞充满并阻塞皮下淋巴管。炎性细胞是罕见的。患者通常具有晚期乳腺癌的表现,包括可触及的腋窝淋巴结、锁骨上淋巴结和/或远处转移。炎性乳腺癌在美国和西欧占乳腺癌的1%~2%,而报道的北非和中东的发病率则更高。

乳腺癌还有其他一些类型,但十分罕见(<1%),包括腺样囊性癌(adenocystic carcinoma)、癌肉瘤(carcinosarcomas)、单纯鳞状细胞癌(pure squamous cell carcinoma)、化生性癌(metapalstic carcinoma)(肿瘤中存在骨或软骨基质)、基底细胞癌(basal cell carcinoma,BCC)以及所谓的富脂质癌(lipid-rich carcinoma)等,但是由于其罕见性,尚无法确定其与临床的联系。转移癌以前很少见,现在越来越多地被认为是三阴性乳腺癌中一个独特且预后较差的亚型。

乳腺非上皮性肿瘤

乳腺也可出现非上皮性肿瘤。纤维肉瘤、平滑肌肉瘤、横纹肌肉瘤和血管肉瘤并不常见[122]。乳腺既可作为非霍奇金淋巴瘤的原发灶,也可作为全身性疾病的一部分。发生于乳腺的非霍奇金淋巴瘤通常为 B 细胞型,其中一些在组织学上与癌相似,免疫组化往往有助于解决这一问题。只有少数霍奇金病和白血病(leukemia)首发于乳腺。叶状肿瘤(phyllodes tumor)[叶状囊肉瘤(cystosarcoma phyllodes)]是一种双相肿瘤,部分是上皮成分,部分是间质成分(图 108-11)。叶状肉瘤有时体积较大,常常对邻近乳腺组织有所侵犯。最好的治疗方法是局部切除,并需将一部分周围正常乳腺组织包括在内。叶状肿瘤可以分为良性、交界性/行为不确定的或恶性肿瘤。已经知道恶性叶状肿瘤可以发生转移并导致患者死亡。高有丝分裂速率、细胞异型性、间质增生、浸润性边缘、出血和坏死被认为是恶性叶状肿瘤的特征。恶性的组织学和间质增生是转移的预测因素,尽管很难从临床或组织学表现上确定哪些叶状肿瘤具有恶性行为并将发生转移[123]。

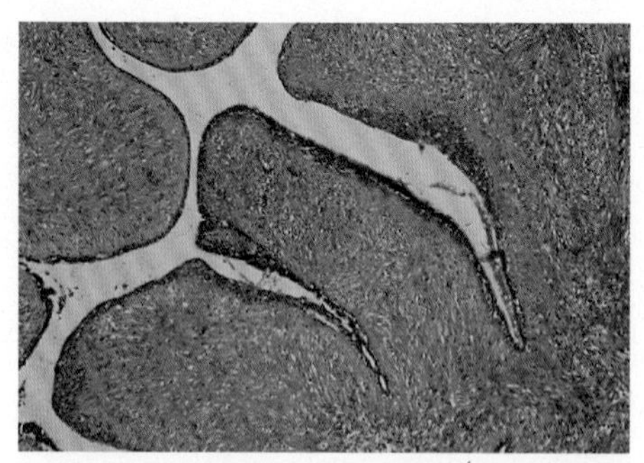

图 108-11　叶状肿瘤(phyllodes tumor)[叶状囊肉瘤(cystosarcoma phyllodes)]。叶状突起,由良性上皮排列形成,间质细胞数目明显增多

预后因素

肿瘤大小

肿瘤的大小不仅可以决定局部治疗的最佳方法,而且对决定其他治疗具有预后意义。随着肿瘤大小的增加,不论是淋巴结阴性还是阳性的肿瘤,复发或转移的风险均会增加。由于淋巴结阳性的乳腺癌患者治疗失败的风险已经很高,肿瘤增大所增加的预后价值相对极小。但是,在淋巴结阴性的乳腺癌中,肿瘤大小常常是主要的预后指标。这一指标在决定淋巴结阴性的乳腺癌患者是否使用辅助性系统治疗方面尤其重要。肿瘤大小仅指侵袭的部分,应该有病理学家在三维上进行确定。淋巴结阴性且原发肿瘤直径小于 2cm 的患者,25%~30%会在随诊的 20 年内出现复发[124]。肿瘤直径 1cm 或 1cm 以下的患者预后极佳,在不接受有效辅助治疗的情况下,10 年的复发率小于 15%。一个最大的数据库,来自监测、流行病学、最终结果(surveillance,epidemiology,and end results,SEER)计划,显示了肿瘤大小、淋巴结状态和乳腺癌生存之间的关系[1]。肿瘤 1cm 以下且淋巴结阴性的患者,5 年内死于乳腺癌的概率小于 2%,10 年内则仅有 4%[125]。考虑到肿瘤很小的这一组患者极佳的预后,以及治疗的费用和毒性,不推荐常规使用化疗。一小部分 T1a、bN0M0 的患者(约 10%)同时具有低核级别和淋巴管浸润,则意味着这部分患者复发风险较高(高达 30%),需要给予全身性辅助治疗[126]。

腋窝淋巴结受累

同侧腋窝淋巴结受累仍然是原发性乳腺癌最可靠且最具

可重复性的预后指标。一般而言，淋巴结阳性的患者 50%～70%出现复发，而淋巴结阴性的患者在只接受局部区域治疗后，只有 15%～45%的患者出现复发。原发性乳腺癌患者的肿瘤复发风险与腋窝阳性淋巴结数目密切相关[127]。每发现一个额外的阳性淋巴结，复发和转移的风险就增加数个百分点。因此，具有 4～10 个阳性淋巴结的患者比 1～3 个的患者复发风险更高，而具有 10 个或 10 个以上阳性淋巴结的患者，复发和转移的可能性在 80%以上。

由于淋巴结状态不能够通过临床方法进行准确的评估，因此进行包括Ⅰ、Ⅱ水平在内的腋窝淋巴结清扫（axillary lymph node dissection，ALND），被认为是标准治疗[128]。临床研究已经表明，只有在清扫和检查的淋巴结至少是 6 个，但最好是 10 个以上时，淋巴结阴性才是可靠的。

淋巴结的宏转移和微转移具有相似的预后意义[128]。最近的数据表明，微转移（N1mic）与大细胞转移（macrometastases）相比，存在中度风险，尽管这仍存在争议[129,130]。相比之下，孤立的肿瘤细胞（ITC，<0. 2mm）似乎没有预后意义[131]。

近年来，原发性乳腺癌已经在早期、主要是局部阶段就得以诊断。经典的腋窝淋巴结清扫并未给淋巴结阴性的患者带来治疗获益，但却可导致明显的短期和长期并发症。前哨淋巴结活检成为这部分患者的替代性的（诊断性）分期方式[132]。这一手术方式明显减少了外科手术在腋窝的操作范围，对于大多数腋窝淋巴结阴性的患者，排除了其接受正式腋窝淋巴结清扫的必要，同时提供了相似（某些情况下更好）的诊断和预后信息。在确定单个（或只有数个）前哨淋巴结状态方面，病理学家可以通过联合使用光镜、IHC 甚至更敏感的分子技术，开展更详细的评估以对微转移进行检测。比较腋窝淋巴结清扫和前哨淋巴结活检的随机试验结果显示后者的并发症明显减少。根据这一结果，在临床上腋窝淋巴结阴性的局部早期乳腺癌患者中，前哨淋巴结活检已经代替相当一部分经典的腋窝淋巴结清扫术。

尽管腋窝淋巴结状态是最强有力的预后指标，但在腋窝淋巴结不存在转移的患者中，仍然有 15%～45%的患者出现复发并死亡。因为这一局限性，研究者已在寻找其他的预后指标以提高预后的准确性，尤其是淋巴结阴性的这一组患者的预后。

基于基因表达的分子检测显示，肿瘤的生物学可能比分期更重要。最近发表的数据显示，在淋巴结阳性的女性乳腺癌患者中，通过 *NKI70* 基因检测确定为低危的患者，无论是否接受化疗，无复发生存率（recurrent-free survival）极好。这与该检测所确定的高危患者的无复发生存率形成对比。肿瘤的分子检测仍将继续是一个重要的研究领域，并可能在将来成为决定治疗的重要工具。

组织学类型

已有报道显示多个组织学因素具有预后意义[120]。导管癌和小叶癌的预后基本相似，可以使用同样的治疗方式。而多个少见肿瘤，包括单纯的管状癌、黏液癌或胶样癌、乳头状癌和所有的非浸润性癌，预后明显更好，尤其是发现时处于淋巴结阴性阶段者[135]。鉴于这些组织学类型的预后更好，不采用辅助性系统治疗是合理的，尤其是对于小肿瘤而言（<3cm）。由于这些特殊类型的肿瘤大多数在诊断时体积较小，且多为淋巴结阴性，局部治疗就是所需的全部治疗。

组织学分级或分化

研究显示肿瘤的分级是一个重要的预后指标。一般而言，表现出高度分化特征的肿瘤预后最好。多个研究显示，高级别与较高的复发转移率和较低的生存率有关，而且这种联系与肿瘤大小和淋巴结受累无关。高级别肿瘤也与激素受体阴性和化疗疗效增加有关，相反，低级别则与激素敏感性和化疗疗效降低有关。各种组织学分化级别的明确定义使人们认识到这些分化级别具有预后价值，且这种预后价值是可以重复的。在核分级上也存在类似的看法，但有些学者发现组织学分级是更为可靠的预后指标，因为它包括了细胞和组织相关的标准。

目前最常使用的分级系统是 Scarf-Bloom-Richardso 系统的 Elston Ellis 修改版。这个系统依据腺管形成的程度、细胞核多形性及每个高倍视野中核分裂象的计数，将浸润性导管癌分为 3 个组织学等级。每项的分数可评为 1～3，1 代表最有利的发现（如明显的腺体形成、细胞多形性少见、低有丝分裂速率），而 3 代表最差的发现。把每一项的分数相加，总分 3～5 分是Ⅰ级（分化好或低级别），6～7 分是Ⅱ级（中分化或中级别），8～9 分是Ⅲ级（低分化或高级别）。

肿瘤坏死

在 NSABP B-04 项目中，1 539 名浸润性乳腺癌患者中有 60%存在不同程度的肿瘤坏死。坏死，尤其是程度明显时，与治疗失败的比率升高呈正相关。尽管坏死与一些据称和乳腺癌不良预后相关的临床病理特征关系密切，但与病理淋巴结状态无关，而且多变量分析显示坏死对治疗失败的影响，在病变最大径小于 5cm 时，是与肿瘤大小无关的。

淋巴和血管侵犯

在许多临床报道中，淋巴和血管侵犯都与不良预后相关。在 NSABP 的患者中，有 1/3 在其大肿物内发现有淋巴管侵犯，另外还有 23%认为存在可疑侵犯（图 108-12）。这一发现与其他不良特征有关。仅有 5%的患者发现血管侵犯。血管侵犯与 4 个或 4 个以上腋窝淋巴结阳性、淋巴管侵犯及其他不利发现有关（图 108-13）。其他研究中报道的血管侵犯为 5%～50%。

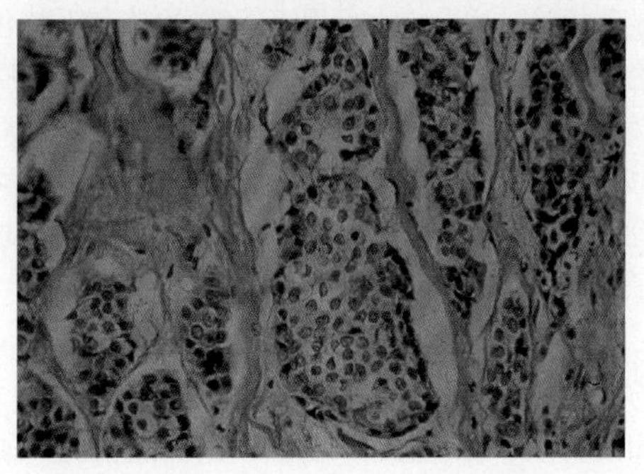

图 108-12　乳腺癌淋巴管侵犯。管壁变薄，内皮细胞沿管壁排列

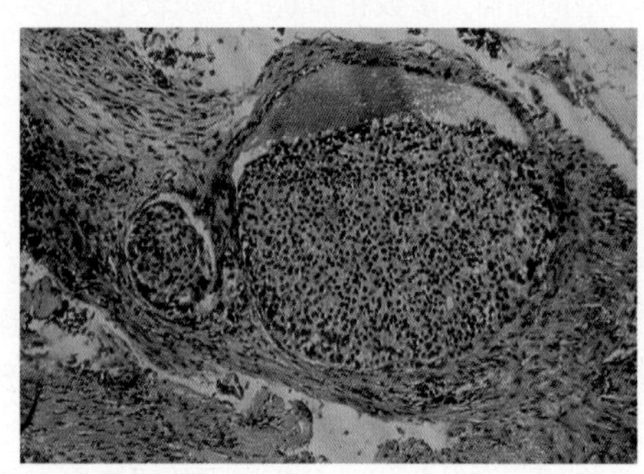

图 108-13 乳腺癌血管侵犯。管壁结构仍可识别，管腔内存在红细胞

多中心性

许多乳腺癌是多中心来源的。研究者对 NSABP 中 904 例患者进行检查，13.4%发现了作为独立病灶存在的浸润性或非浸润性癌。非浸润性和浸润性多中心癌的比例分别为 4.1%和 9.3%。乳腺磁共振成像(magnetic resonance imaging，MRI)来越多地用于病变范围的术前评估，检查显示乳腺癌的多中心性比之前使用乳腺摄影时更为常见。

尽管原发性乳腺癌的女性双侧乳房发生多灶病变的概率较高，但在最初的乳腺中出现两个或两个以上临床明显的原发癌还是少见的。同样，双侧乳腺同时发生肿瘤的情况也很少见，而在未受累乳腺或对侧乳腺出现异时性第二原发肿瘤的十年发生率为 4%～6%，这个数字并未达到通过随机活检、尸检或 MRI 检测到的隐匿性病变而推测出的发生率。

增殖能力标志

恶性组织增殖比率的测量，对包括乳腺癌在内的多种肿瘤具有很强的预后价值。评估恶性细胞的增殖能力可使用多种技术，包括有丝分裂指数、胸腺嘧啶标志指数(thymidine-labeling indices，TLI)和 SPF。有丝分裂指数的确定方法是，将肿瘤标本用苏木精和伊红染色后，在光镜下对其核分裂象进行计数。这种方法已通过单因素和多因素分析得到验证。许多蛋白在细胞周期的控制方面发挥作用，或在细胞周期的某些阶段表达水平升高。Ki-67 和增殖细胞核抗原(proliferating cell nuclear antigen，PCNA)是另外两个恶性肿瘤增殖比率的标志[92,93]。其中 Ki-67 的研究更为广泛，它与 SPF 的结果以及长期预后显著相关。这一技术可用于新鲜、冷冻和石蜡包埋的材料。不论腋窝淋巴结状态如何，Ki-67 数值低说明肿瘤增殖较慢，与复发比率较低有关 Ki-67 分数高与其他不良预后因素显著相关，如组织学和细胞学级别高、非整倍体和类固醇受体阴性状态等。因此，调控增殖的基因部分程度上推动了现有的预测性分子分析方法的进步，就不足为奇了。

免疫因素

肿瘤浸润性淋巴细胞[137]与侵袭性乳腺癌亚型(如 TNBC)的预后改善有关。初步数据显示免疫抑制剂对乳腺癌的疗效，强调需要更好地了解个体的免疫环境。

诊断和筛查

在以前，乳腺癌的首发症状是可触及的肿物，多由患者首先发现。而现在，乳腺摄影越来越多的应用，尤其是在筛查项目中的应用，导致许多乳腺癌在临床前阶段就被发现。简单的讨论乳腺癌的体征和症状，而不考虑这些临床前发现，这样的讨论是不完整的。从某种程度上，这意味着选择哪些被怀疑有乳腺癌的患者来进行活检具有更大的复杂性。具有乳腺癌解剖学和生物学的背景知识——肿瘤如何生长并在局部增大，才能最好地理解临床和乳腺摄影的体征和症状。

病史

病史应该包括标准的流行病学和生育信息以便评估相对风险因素。与肿物、疼痛或任何乳腺改变有关的信息都应该被包括在内，并与体征相联系。尽管乳房疼痛是导致患者就诊的最常见的主诉，但极少是乳腺癌的症状。乳腺癌，尤其是在早期阶段，通常是没有疼痛的。大多数乳腺疼痛与激素刺激和乳腺组织的肿胀有关(尽管这些症状可能将注意力引向肿物并发现肿瘤)。对患者进行仔细的问诊通常会发现疼痛具有周期性，可在排卵和月经来临之间的任何时候开始，并通常在月经前数天疼痛程度最重。疼痛往往在经期的第一天或第二天消失，在下一周期再次出现。50%以上的育龄期女性的周期性疼痛为中等程度，极少数可以出现剧烈疼痛。一些患者叙述，在疼痛程度最重时，甚至无法淋浴。

对此最有效的治疗是解释与安慰，但有些患者疼痛极重并严重影响行动，可能需要激素或激素阻断剂的治疗。偶有文献报道咖啡因限制或低脂饮食有助于病情，但似乎只有个别患者的病情得到缓解，并且这些报道没有得到具有说服力的临床试验的支持。

医师应该对叙述乳房出现肿物或其他任何查体改变的患者给予仔细的关注。病史应该描述肿物特征或大小的任何改变以及肿物是否变软，还应描述疼痛在月经周期中出现的时间。与纤维囊性病有关的肿物可以增大或缩小，这与只会增大的肿瘤明显不同。如果不能确定，应在经期后对患者进行复查。

还应对其他改变进行描述，如皮肤变厚或颜色改变，出现腋窝肿物或乳头溢液等。乳头溢液可以是浆液性、水样或乳汁样，可以质清或表现为黄色或绿色，也可以是浆液血性或直接呈血性。尽管后者可能提示肿瘤，这一症状最常见于导管内乳头状瘤，这是一个良性疾病；所有的血性分泌物都需要进一步检查。

澄清或浆液性分泌物，尤其是累及一个以上开口于乳头的大导管时，有可能是良性的。不能自行分泌而需人为挤压才可排出的非血性分泌物，也可能是良性的。在像乳腺这样的顶浆分泌系统中，经常有一些细胞脱屑和液化，因此导管系统中可有一些液体出现。如果这些液体没有被很好地吸收，就可以通过乳腺集合管到达乳头，从而表现为分泌物。同样地，如酚酞管因纤维化或浓缩的物质发生堵塞，分泌的压力会导致导管扩张和囊肿形成。分泌物细胞学检查的准确性低，不是非常有用。

还应对其他改变进行描述,如皮肤变厚或颜色改变,出现腋窝肿物或乳头溢液等。乳头溢液可以是浆液性、水样或乳汁样,可以质清或表现为黄色或绿色,也可以是浆液血性或直接呈血性。尽管后者可能提示肿瘤,这一症状最常见于导管内乳头状瘤,这是一个良性疾病;所有的血性分泌物都需要进一步检查。

澄清或浆液性分泌物,尤其是累及一个以上开口于乳头的大导管时,有可能是良性的。不能自行分泌而需人为挤压才可排出的非血性分泌物,也可能是良性的。在像乳腺这样的顶浆分泌系统中,经常有一些细胞脱屑和液化,因此导管系统中可有一些液体出现。如果这些液体没有被很好地吸收,就可以通过乳腺集合管到达乳头,从而表现为分泌物。同样地,如酚酞管因纤维化或浓缩的物质发生堵塞,分泌的压力会导致导管扩张和囊肿形成。分泌物细胞学检查的准确性低,不是非常有用。

体格检查

医师应该首先让患者取坐位、然后取仰卧位对其进行体格检查。当患者坐直时,视诊比触诊可以得到更多有用的信息。当患者抬起双臂并向上伸展时,皮肤的轮廓被拉紧,使得医师可以更容易的发现乳房上半部分的轮廓异常。这个体位也使得乳房的酒窝征更加明显,尤其是位于下半部分乳房的酒窝征。由于坐位时大部分乳腺组织聚结在一起,触诊时很难发现真正的肿物,而且很容易与融合的组织相混淆。使患者的手臂放松并内收,对腋窝进行触诊,这在患者取坐位时触诊最佳。

让患者仰卧,手臂抬起,手置于头后,肘部平放于枕上,乳腺组织会分布于胸壁上,以便进行恰当的触诊。患者应该稍微转向对侧以帮助触诊。按照一种方式进行检查是很重要的,不过是按象限触诊还是条状触诊则取决于检查者。皮肤的改变,例如酒窝征、橘皮征(水肿)、红斑或出现固定和溃疡的区域,提示晚期乳腺癌已经侵袭皮肤或接近皮下组织。当患者取坐位抬起双臂或向前倾斜时,皮肤的回缩往往更易于发现。乳头内陷或不对称是另外一个不良征象,除非患者叙述该症状自出生后就一直存在。乳头和乳晕隐隐发红变厚,或表面的上皮出现脱落,可能提示佩吉特病。

在对腋窝、锁骨上和锁骨下淋巴结以及肝脏进行触诊以检查有无肿大之后,查体就可以结束了。尽管可触及的肿大淋巴结提高了转移的可能性,仔细的研究显示临床判断是高度不准确的。在 NSABP 开展的一项研究中,一组被临床医师判断为腋窝淋巴结正常的患者,对其标本进行病理学检查,38%的患者组织学检查证明有淋巴结转移瘤[120]。相反,在表现为淋巴结肿大并被判断为转移癌的患者中,发现有 25%淋巴结是正常的。

最困难的临床决定是对病理性肿物和与纤维腺体(或纤维囊肿)改变有关的生理性改变进行鉴别。许多女性表现为后者,其特征是质韧致密物且边界不清。真正的肿物是有明确边界的,不论其边界是光滑的肉眼可见的囊肿或纤维腺瘤,还是有些不规则(如肿瘤),显示出不连续肿物的则需要进一步检查。浸润性导管癌通常质硬,在乳房中十分明显,相比较而言,多发的质硬的肿物可能是良性乳腺病。小叶癌一般不会如此坚硬,因此更加难以识别。

使用卡尺测量肿物的大小是重要的,这样一来就可以在之后的检查中更加精确地确定肿物大小的任何改变。移动性病变通常被认为是良性的,但这是另外一个临床不能确定的问题。晚期肿瘤可以是固定的,但是早期可触及的病变相对于皮肤或胸壁的筋膜和肌肉一定是可移动的。但是,囊肿或纤维腺瘤的移动性(称为"可移动性"更合适)特征有些细微的不同,两者有包膜,在周围的乳腺组织中移动起来容易得多。另一方面,肿瘤没有包膜,在浸润性结缔组织增生的过程中被包绕起来,往往是随着周围的乳腺组织一起移动,而不是在周围的组织内移动,即使肿瘤没有被像皮肤或肌肉这样的周围结构所固定。即使是最有经验的医师,有时也不能准确区分良性与恶性病变。

影像学

近 30 年来,40 岁以上女性的每年例行乳房 X 线检查已成为降低乳腺癌死亡率的基本措施。我们在乳腺癌生物学的上取得的进展和普查的开展使我们对筛查策略修正和改进[138]。

2009 年,USPSTF 对筛查指南进行了修改,建议将所有 40~75 岁女性的年度乳房 X 线照片替换为 50~75 岁女性的两年一次筛查,40~50 岁之间的筛查应该是考虑患者背景个性化设计的。2015 年更新进一步支持了这些建议(http://www.uspreventiveservicestaskforce.org/)。ACS 于 2015 年 10 月修订了其乳腺 X 线摄影筛查指南[139],仍然强烈建议进行筛查,但修改了其开始时的年龄。建议年龄在 45~54 岁女性进行年度筛查,55 岁的女性可以过渡到每隔一年筛查。ACS 还指出,女性应该有机会进行年度筛查,并且只要她们的预期寿命至少为 10 年或更长,就应该继续筛查。它还建议 40~44 岁之间的妇女应有机会进行年度筛查(表 108-6)。

表 108-6　国际筛选策略

国家	起始年龄/岁	结束年龄/岁	频率
美国	40	—	一年一次
瑞士	40	74	两年一次
英国	50	70	三年一次
荷兰	50	70	两年一次
法国	50	74	两年一次
意大利	50	70	两年一次
德国	50	70	两年一次

有关筛选的建议仍在讨论中,关于年度筛选有效性的意见也大不相同。一方认为,从 40 岁开始的年度乳房 X 线筛查可以减少间隔期癌症发病率,但其他人认为年度筛查会导致更多的假阳性与不必要的治疗,并且更有针对性的方法可以减少假阴性和过度诊断而不增加间隔期癌发病率。对于大多数女性来说,年度乳房 X 线可以在早期可治愈阶段发现癌症的特点可以抵消其带来的不适和不便。遗憾的是,常在晚期发现的或预后更差的癌症常在筛查间歇期发现,或者不太容易通过标准 X 线发现。2009 年 USPSTF 推荐的筛选频率降低旨在平衡利益和危害,更符合大多数其他西方国家的政策。

越来越多的人质疑筛查的有效性。加拿大国家乳腺筛查研究(CNBSS)是早期关键的筛查试验之一,其25年的随访结果于2014年2月发表,当时他们得出结论(证实了他们此前10~15年的随访结果),与简单的临床乳腺检查相比,每年的乳房X线检查并不能减少死亡率[140]。瑞士已经建议彻底停止乳房X线检查,因为没有证据表明这样做的好处大于坏处[141]。期刊上经常出现相反观点[142~144],反映出对筛查指南的广泛分歧。

乳房X线摄影仍是目前的标准筛查方式,其根源在于20世纪80年代的大型随机筛查试验[145]。瑞典试验中乳腺癌死亡率相对降低了21%,其中60多岁的妇女受益最大。在瑞典的试验中,筛查的时间间隔从18个月到33个月不等。自这些初步研究以来,情况发生了很大变化。目前使用的有效的系统疗法大多数在这些筛查试验开始时还未使用,但目前在降低乳腺癌死亡率方面有明确的作用[146]。目前,全身治疗被认为可降低2/3死亡率,乳腺影像学检查大约可降低1/3[9,147]。重要的是,内分泌治疗[148,149]的广泛应用可能会减轻某些癌症晚期才被发现的影响。

乳房X线检查对女性最为熟悉的潜在危害是"假阳性"。每次乳房检查,女性得到假阳性而后续活检的是良性的风险都会增加。经过10年的年度筛查,超过一半的女性得到假阳性结果,7%~9%将进行假阳性活检[150]。一般来说,乳房X线检查的特异性约为90%,表明发生假阳性结果的概率是1/10。然而,只有大约1/5的女性在接受筛查时确实患有乳腺癌,因此大多数异常乳房X线检查都是假阳性[151]。这对女性有多种影响。最近的一项系统评价显示,心理困扰可持续长达3年,从而导致对随后筛查的依从性降低[152]。同样,来自荷兰的一项研究表明,93%的女性在阴性筛查后被召回,但一次假阳性结果后,只有56%的召回率,在两次假阳性结果后,只有44%的召回率。BCSC显示相对于年度筛查,每两年一次筛查[153],假阳性率降低50%,虽然会稍增加晚期癌症发病率,但是统计学意义不明显[154]。

乳房筛查的另一个潜在危害来自"过度诊断"[155]。二十年的研究已经向我们证明,乳腺癌是上皮起源[155]的侵袭性疾病。根据CNBSS的25年随访结果突出显示,筛查本质上更有可能识别缓慢生长的肿瘤[136]。有一半的通过乳腺X线发现的癌症是无法通过常规乳房检查发现的[138]。最近的一项荟萃分析估计,20%的癌症(高达50%是通过筛查检出的)被归于过度诊断的类别[157]。数据表明,女性被过度诊断的可能性大于筛查检出乳腺癌[158]。使用分子标记物诊断超低风险疾病时,也获得了类似的结果[159,160]。

大多数乳腺癌前病变和导管原位癌可能属于过度诊断。导管原位癌在筛查之前很少被诊断出来,但在筛查之后诊断增加了500倍[161]。组成导管原位癌的肿瘤细胞在形态学上与侵袭性肿瘤细胞相似,因此人们认为导管原位癌最终发展为侵袭性肿瘤。由于导管原位癌的常规治疗是乳房切除或肿瘤切除和放疗,因此导管原位癌的自然病史尚不清楚[162,163]。流行病学证据表明,只有一小部分人在一生中会发展成侵袭性疾病[164]。此外,切除宫颈癌癌前病变可引起的子宫颈癌发病率急剧下降,与之不同的是,每年50 000多名妇女切除导管原位癌,经过10年的观察,浸润性乳腺病变的发生率没有下降[162](有一个短期下降,但这是由于妇女健康行动大幅减少荷尔蒙替代疗法的结果)。目前已有4 165个分子标记物可识别出一种低风险的乳腺导管原位癌,其5年罹患乳腺癌的风险与65岁女性的平均风险(2.5%)[166,167]大致相同,但每年2万例乳腺导管原位癌切除术,其中许多是双侧的[168,169]。

改善筛查的研究正在进行中,重点是确定最有可能受益的患者群体,并发现分子标记物,以确定进展风险较低的癌症。筛查和活检异常的回召标准和阈值正在被积极评价改进[156,170,171]。BI-RADS[172]推荐评分为4分的进行活检,有>2%~95%的机会要么是侵袭性癌症或导管原位癌。BI-RADS4A(低度可疑<10%)、4B(中等可疑10%~50%)和4C(中度>50%,但小于95%可疑)分类可以帮助更好地细化活检阈值[173]。

然而,可减少过度诊断和假阳性回召的负担的最好的方法是结合我们对个体乳腺癌风险的更好理解来提升我们的筛查方法。

风险分层筛选最近受到广泛关注[174]。医学研究所提倡在开展乳腺筛查时采用技术一体化、生物学和风险分层。他们指出,个性化——对高危人群进行更频繁的筛查——可以提高筛查试验的阳性预测值,并可能减少不必要的相互干扰[175,176]。由于大多数人的患病风险相对较低,个性化筛查将导致大多数人不那么频繁地接受检查,减少假阳性回召和活检率。这也是USPSTF在对2009年[155]的乳房X线进行全面审查后得出的结论,即筛查的利弊取决于40多岁女性的个体风险因素和74岁以上女性的患病情况。与50多岁的女性相比,40多岁的177名女性从筛查中获得的益处是平均风险的两倍[178]。因此,是否对40多岁的妇女进行筛查应根据个人的危险因素作出决定。USPSTF敦促临床医生根据个人风险与患者讨论筛查的利弊。对于年龄在50~74岁之间的妇女,USPSTF发现,与每年进行一次筛查相比,每隔一年进行一次筛查可以保留益处,并将风险降至最低。

医学界未能就USPSTF指南这个问题达成共识[179~181]。女性也不愿意相信减少筛查会有好处[177]。最后,USPSTF准则没有说明如何将风险评估纳入实践。因此,尽管我们见证了乳腺癌在诊断、预后和治疗方面的重大进展,但自20世纪80年代以来,我们的筛查方法没有发生根本性的改变。当务之急是超越目前的争论,测试乳腺癌筛查的新方法,以最大限度地提高效益,并将对妇女的危害降到最低。显然,这意味着要有可帮助我们在现代辅助治疗的背景下筛查的新的研究,同时它也表明要使用关于乳腺癌自然史的30年知识,以及导致个人患乳腺癌和/或死于乳腺癌的风险的因素。正如我们的治疗方法已经从一刀切发展到更加个性化、以患者为中心、以证据为基础的治疗,我们的筛查方法也必须如此[147]。

在过去十年中,随着我们对疾病机制和分析能力理解的进步,我们有能力以比以往任何时候都更高的精度治疗疾病。在乳腺癌中,这反映在我们如何根据个体疾病的可测量的特征选择特定的治疗方法[117,168,182,183]。与之相反是我们在很大程度上对待乳腺癌筛查的态度是好像每个人都是一样的。作为一种更适应风险的方法是可以使患者、提供者和消费者受益的。作为《平价医疗法案》(*Affordable Care Act*)的一部分而成立的以患者为中心的结果研究所(PCORI)最近资助了一项随机试验,对个性化筛查与年度筛查进行了对比,目的是把重点放在如何让筛查更好地惠及女性及其提供者(wisdomstudy. org)。

这项被提议的实用的试验试图通过每年一次的乳房检查和更新的个体化检查方法来解决这一争议。尽管我们对乳腺癌风险的认识有了很大的提高,但确定女性筛查建议的唯一标准是她的年龄(如果已知 BRCA 状况)。然而,目前已有一些模型将家族史和乳腺密度、内分泌暴露、基因突变和非典型性结合起来评估乳腺癌风险[100,103,184~186]。最近,一些常见的基因变异也被证实是预测因子[187]。乳腺癌生物学、风险评估(基因组学)和成像(密度)方面的进展为我们提供了实现个性化模型所需的所有工具和知识;它提供了何时开始、何时停止以及多久筛查的建议,具体取决于对其个人风险的明确衡量。这项研究是由加州大学雅典娜乳腺健康网络开展的。基于风险的筛查对医疗保健支付者的潜在好处是众多且巨大的。我们目前的乳腺癌筛查费用每年有 80 亿~100 亿美元,每年有 60 万例活检结果是良性的。如果我们将最广泛采用的 40~80 岁女性的年度筛查方法的成本与 USPSTF 的建议进行比较,两者之间的成本差异约为 63 亿美元——比 NCI 的年度预算要高[188,189]。

MRI 检查

MRI 在乳腺癌的治疗中得到越来越多的应用。其优点是能够提供乳腺的三维图像,对致密型乳腺敏感性高,且不使用电离辐射。MRI 也有很明显的缺点,包括成本高、影像学表现的多样性以及中等的特异性,后者与其高度敏感性相结合经常导致不必要的检查[190]。

MRI 不适合作为普通筛查工具。其价格至少是乳腺摄影的 10 倍,这将使美国的筛查成本提高到 1 000 亿美元的范畴。MRI 应该专用于如下情况:发现乳腺癌的先验概率(prior probability)高(高危)且以高灵敏度检查为首选;已知其他更便宜且可靠的筛查工具(如乳腺摄影)较不敏感[156,191],如乳腺癌终身风险为 85%的 *BRCA1* 或 *BRCA2* 突变携带者。虽然平均 35 岁发生乳腺癌的可能性为 1/10 000,但突变携带者的风险介于 1/100~5/100,而 MRI 在这部分人群中较乳腺摄影敏感得多。五年 Gail 风险很高且乳腺组织非常致密的女性也属于此类。密度校正的 Gail 风险评分[58]将风险与乳腺摄影所报告的乳腺密度(BIRADS 密度)相结合,使用这一评分能够确定高危或乳腺摄影具有假阴性风险的女性。密度校正的 Gail 风险的计算方法是,对于 BIRADS 分级为 1、2、3、4 的女性,分别将其 Gail 风险与 0. 59、1. 00、1. 41 或 1. 94 相乘。对于通过密度校正的 Gail 风险计算出的乳腺癌终身风险>50%的女性,推荐其采用 MRI 筛查。该工具计算出的终身风险在 35%~49%的女性,可以考虑 MRI 筛查,但是目前没有证据支持每年都进行 MRI 筛查。

真正衡量一种筛查检测方法,不在于这种方法是否发现了更多的肿瘤,而在于其对肿瘤的发现是否降低了乳腺癌的死亡率和发病率。目前还没有研究发现 MRI 筛查降低了乳腺癌的死亡率。但是,两项大的研究已经显示,使用 MRI 对高危女性进行筛查要敏感得多,这两项研究的结果显著相似[192,193]。如果用肿瘤大小和淋巴结受累代替检查结果,MRI 的确提高了风险最高的这组女性的肿瘤分期。在荷兰研究中,对 1 909 例患者使用乳腺摄影和 MRI 进行筛查,对照组由未接受过 MRI 筛查的突变携带者和高危患者构成,将研究组中所发现的乳腺癌与合适的对照组相比较。在最高风险组中(估算的终身风险为 50%~85%),在由 MRI 筛查发现肿瘤的突变携带者中,63%为淋巴结阴性,与之相比,对照组 47%为淋巴结阴性;在中危组中(估算的终身风险为 15%~30%),研究组只有 12%淋巴结受累,87%为淋巴结阴性(与之相比,对照组 52%~56%具有阳性淋巴结,44%~48%为阴性淋巴结)。因此,MRI 似乎能够在更早的阶段发现乳腺癌。但是,肿瘤的检出率也很重要,当肿瘤检出率高、且比普通筛查组明显增高时,应该使用 MRI。值得注意的是,突变携带者、高危和中危女性,乳腺癌的检出率分别为每 1 000 人每年 26. 5 例、5. 4 例和 7. 8 例,这与年龄介于 50~70 岁的女性中 5/1 000~7/1 000 的检出率形成对比,在后者中,乳腺摄影性价比虚高。发生乳腺癌风险较高的是最高风险组和突变携带者,对于这部分风险最高的女性,我们应该仔细限制 MRI 的使用。

不论在经济上还是心理上,筛查都要付出代价。在荷兰研究中接受 10 年筛查的 1 909 名女性中,进行了 1 200 项额外的检查。在发现 45 例乳腺癌的过程中,MRI 导致的额外检查(420 项)是乳腺摄影的 2 倍(207 项),导致的不必要的活检是乳腺摄影的 3 倍,分别为 24 例和 7 例[190]。MRI 作为筛查工具,应该具有严格的标准,非常审慎地加以应用,这样我们就不会滥用资源,避免因为疏忽导致患者因假阳性而感到苦恼。假阳性更需要追随和解决,但这会十分困难,因为尚不具备 MRI 引导下活检的工具。在影像学发现异常后,通常推荐 3 个月或 6 个月的随诊观察。然而,MR 检查的花费是 1 000~2 000 美元,除非是在发现异常的可能性比一般人群高很多,以及乳腺摄影不可能有效的情况下,否则使用 MR 检查是不合适的。两个关键的要旨是我们需要找到风险分层的方法以合适地调整技术的应用;MRI 筛查应该在有能力对 MRI 发现的异常进行检查的机构中进行,如有必要,可以使用超声和 MRI 引导下活检。2003 年蓝十字会/蓝盾(Blue Cross/Blue Shield)技术评估得出结论,即 MRI 筛查用于具有乳腺癌遗传易感性的女性是合理的。荷兰和加拿大研究[190,194]只是强化了这一结论而已。总体来说,中危和高危女性可能患乳腺癌较少,因为其风险不是那样高,这意味着 MR 必须变得更具特异性且异常情况的随诊变得更为简单,我们才能对中危女性进行广泛筛查。

并不是所有的 MR 检查都相似。技术、序列、读片以及随诊和活检能力具有很大的变化性。尽管乳腺 MRI 的运用增长迅速,仍然没有标准存在。临床医师在申请乳腺 MRI 检查时需要了解这一技术、月经的时间(月经中期,最好是在月经开始后的 4~14 天[190]),还需具备对有意义的结果进行解释的技能。因为相对无法以电子的方式传输和查看影像,所以对不同机构的影像结果进行解释是一个挑战。研究者对 MRI 的每一个领域都在进行积极的探索,进一步的研究和技术改进竟会极大地提高我们的能力,从而将 MRI 很好地整合进乳腺癌的治疗中。

在诊断性检查显示存在异常后,依然可以使用 MRI。在评价乳腺摄影异常表现和可触及肿物的 MRI 表现特征方面,最确定性的研究是由国际乳腺 MRI 协会组织的多机构(International Breast MRI Consortium,IBMC)研究。14 家机构使用 MRI 对 841 名患者进行了评估。所有患者均接受了高分辨率扫描,500 名伴有强化病灶的患者在48h内返回接受动态扫描。研究确定了MRI的高度敏感性和中度特异性，还发现高分辨率技术和动态扫描具有同样的表现特征。高分辨率扫描可以给出更好的解剖学细节，且不需要专门的计算机软件以进行动态分析。这是重要的一点，因为高分辨率扫描对临床医师而言更易于解释，因此有可能够被包括进所有的MRI检查。病变在MRI上的诊断特征正在改进，但还不具备足够的特异性来代替活检。在乳腺摄影诊断显示异常之后进行MRI检查明显提高了假阳性。目前，除非无法对乳腺摄影的可疑发现进行评估或定位，或有其他令人信服的原因需要申请MRI(如患者是突变携带者，或者具有很高的患病风险和非常致密的乳腺组织)，MRI在乳腺癌的诊断上是没有作用的。

或许MRI最重要的作用是对已知的乳腺癌进行分期并检测疗效[190]。MRI能够发现乳腺癌的独特类型，小叶或炎性癌等不同类型肿瘤是最常见的独特类型。最初的影像学特征能够确定疗效可能极差的患者，如体积大的弥漫性肿瘤[195]。

风险和预防

根据USPSTF的建议，如果我们能够降低风险较低者的筛查频率，那些患乳腺癌风险较低的人将被筛选得更少，从而减少假阳性结果。假阳性复查和活检的过程非常紧张，可导致在问题解决后很长时间内持续存在焦虑增加和筛查方式选择的变化[152,193]。个人风险评估可以提高对他们个人乳腺癌的风险的一般理解。目前，只有十分之一的女性对她的个人风险有准确的认知，而十分之四的女性从未与医生讨论过她们的个人乳腺癌风险[196]。她们不知道有些肿瘤在体检间歇期快速出现并生长，所以不管以前的筛查是否正常，都需要引起注意[197]。估计有200万美国女性有高风险，但很多人完全没有意识到自己的风险[198]，因此无法从中受益。有三项Ⅰ级研究证明了内分泌治疗可降低风险。NSABP P-01对超过13 000名Gail风险至少为1.67的女性进行了研究，随机分为他莫昔芬组和安慰剂组，结果显示，患侵袭性乳腺癌或导管内癌的风险可降低50%甚至更多(85%)[199]。这已得到IBIS试验证实[200]，此外，年龄较小的女性(50岁以下)可获得更多益处，并且即使在5年后停止治疗，受益仍持续10年。STAR试验比较了他莫昔芬和雷洛昔芬，并研发了选择性雌激素受体调节剂(SERM)来改善乳腺密度，但在后续研究中注意到它可以降低绝经后妇女的激素阳性乳腺癌和骨折风险[201]。雷洛昔芬不刺激子宫内膜，对子宫内膜有较少的副作用，如出血和子宫内膜癌，虽然降低风险的效果不如他莫昔芬高，但它被认为是绝经后妇女更好的选择[202]。这得到了IBIS-2试验的长期随访的验证[203]，该试验表明服用他莫昔芬的绝经后妇女死于子宫内膜癌的风险增加。最后，使用依西美坦的预防研究(MAP.3)显示，与服用他莫昔芬的女性相比，绝经后女性发生HR+浸润性乳腺癌的风险降低了60%[204]。在美国和世界范围内，人们对内分泌治疗降低乳腺癌的风险的认识不足，这可能是由于未能将风险评估自动化或集成到初级保健中，未能认识到风险降低的好处，未能评估妇女是否获得了特定的好处。例如，胆固醇是一种用来证明降低心脏风险的指标。乳房密度被认为是一种可能的动态风险测量方法，服用他莫昔芬的女性如果表现出乳腺癌密度的降低，就能获得风险降低的好处[205,206]。这是一个重要的研究点，并可能纳入未来的预防研究。此外，我们知道，沟通个人风险可以促进更多的筛查[207]，当女性知道自己风险很高，而且能从中受益时，她们会更积极地使用预防性干预措施。

活检

当一名女性表现出诊断性异常时，应该根据病变为浸润性癌或原位癌的可能性、年龄、基础健康状况以及患者的寿命做出干预决定。考虑到将来治疗的需要，再决定进行哪一种活检其目的是使操作次数(包括最终的肿瘤手术)、不适和恐惧、诊断等待的时间和焦虑减至最低，并使患者能够获得最佳治疗时机。

关于肿物和乳腺摄影异常的诊断，有很多选择可以提供。对于可触及的病变，选择包括细针抽吸活检(fine-needle aspiration，FNA)、空芯针活检和切除活检。微创技术——空芯针活检和FNA，在有经验的医师手里和当使用“三重评估”(triple assessment)时，是非常精确的。三重评估就是仔细考虑影像学、临床和病理学发现。如果存在明显的不一致，则应进行进一步评估。一般而言，切除活检不是最佳的诊断方式。微创活检技术可以在办公室里即刻施行，有助于快速诊断和治疗选择的讨论，并帮助在确定性手术之前对乳腺病变的程度进行充分评估。FNA和空芯针活检也可用于确定可疑的多中心病变，从而避免多次手术，一般情况下允许我们按照最佳顺序进行治疗。

所要进行活检的类型取决于指定机构的专业建议。FNA是高度精确的，在有经验的医师手里其敏感性和特异性分别为98%和99%。在瑞典和英国，FNA是标准的诊断工具，被广泛而成功地用于可触及性和乳腺摄影提示的病变。这一技术要求医师在病变取样(这方面容易出现最大的错误)、切片制备和细胞学检查的解释方面经过训练并具有经验[208]。FNA的优点是可以立即进行操作并在一天内得到结果。当高度怀疑浸润性癌且预计要进行前哨淋巴结切除(sentinel lymph node dissection，SLND)时，不论FNA还是空芯针活检均可作为首选。当采用SLND时，活检的类型会影响SLND的准确性。当其后要进行SLND时，FNA和空芯针活检的假阴性率比较低，在切取活检(incisional biopsy)中，FNA与空芯针活检的假阴性率相较而言分别为8%和14%，而切除活检的假阴性率为15%。在患者肿瘤大而明显的情况下，FNA可以有助于快速确诊并治疗选择的讨论，包括新辅助治疗(neoadjuvant therapy)和临床试验。对于选择外科治疗的患者，不需要做进一步的检查。对于选择新辅助治疗的患者，应进行空芯针活检，获取组织学标本，以对侵袭性疾病进行确认；如果出现病理完全缓解(complete pathologic response)的情况，则可为以后的研究保留标本；空芯针活检还可为可能的临床试验保留标本。在指定机构不具备细胞学专业知识的情况下，医师也能够在办公室中快速施行空芯针活检。

因乳腺摄影异常而召回患者是很常见的，而且通过乳房摄影活检(mammographic biopsy)诊断肿瘤[肿瘤活检率(cancer to biopsy rate)或CBR]的可能性变化很大，各地报道的CBR为10%~40%。低CBR并不是高度敏感性所必需的，事实上，最有经验且训练有素的乳腺摄影医师发现的恶性肿瘤较多，而对良性的肿瘤较少申请活检[116]。在将活检质量提高和操作反馈作为常规的机构中,CBR 随着时间而下降。有数种方法可以避免对非肿瘤组织进行活检。在超过 2 年的时间里保持稳定的局限性肿物病变,很可能是良性的,不需要活检。如果有经验的乳腺摄影医师尚未阅读过该 X 线片,可将请有经验的医师阅片作为第二个选择。

在推荐活检的情况下,非常重要的一点是确定病变是不可触及的。如果是可以触及的病变,尤其是如果怀疑其为肿瘤时,FNA 不仅是确定诊断,而且确定这个可触及的肿物的确是肿瘤,从而避免在乳房肿物切除术时需要进行导丝定位。对于乳腺摄影发现的不可触及的可疑肿物,尝试用超声对其定位,这使得诊断和确定过程在超声引导下进行,对患者而言更为舒适。在病变只能在乳房摄影 X 线片中看到的情况下,可以施行立体定向活检(stereotactic biopsy),使用数字影像定位病变并引导空芯针活检。通过有经验的医师,这一方式的敏感性可以高达 98%[206]。拍摄标本的 X 线片以确定已获得靶病灶(通常是钙化)。如果去除所有钙化存在风险,那么在病变部位留下夹子以便之后对该部位进行定位是至关重要的。

进行操作很重要的一点是要考虑其在患者整体治疗中的价值。如果不存在肿瘤,则应对钙化或病变进行充分的取样。如果存在肿瘤,最小数量的取样用以确诊就足够了。这时候,诊断方式不是决定性的,需要进行广泛切除。一些放射科医师会取得 30 个以上的空芯针活检标本,这是不需要的,而且会引起组织血肿和变形,并使得我们难以评价病变的真正范围。这对患者而言也并不愉快。

一些乳腺摄影病变不能使用立体定向技术进行活检,原因或者是病变距胸壁太近,或者是在放置活检针的方向上乳房压缩到小于 3cm。在这种情况下,必须施行切除活检。放射科医师会放置导丝,让其末端位于钙化或肿物水平上或其下方,以指导外科手术。外科医师将会根据放射科医师所估计的恶性肿瘤的可能性来决定切除范围。对于肿瘤可能性更大的病变,应该切除肿瘤及其周围 1cm 的组织。对于较不可疑的病变,切除的组织可以少一点。为了避免切除不必要的组织,切口应该靠近导丝的末端或病变估计的位置。在导丝插入处开始切除只会导致切掉过多的组织,并导致导丝末端切缘靠近肿瘤。在需要进行额外切除的情况在病变上方进行切开有助于对活检腔进行定位。所有的标本均需要送交乳腺摄影或使用 Faxitron 进行评估,使外科医师能够确定靶病灶已被切除。对任何病变属 BIRADS(breast imaging reporting and data system scale)4 级或以上者,乳腺摄影医师会常规推荐活检。但是,BIRADS 4 级包括的病变属于恶性肿瘤的风险可低至 3%,或高达 75%;病变可以怀疑为原位癌或浸润性癌——BIRADS4 级不提示两者的差别。外科医师应该确定他们不仅了解可疑病变的类型,还了解更具体的风险评估,因为风险评估使得如何评估患者有所不同。一个年级较大的女性,同时患有多种并发症,乳腺摄影分级为 BIRADS 4 级,如果病变有接近 90%的可能性为良性,10%的可能性为 DCIS,则患者可能不需要活检。这是可以通过乳腺摄影追随的病变类型。一般而言,我们推荐使用微创活检来进行确诊,但是如果患者有局限的成簇的线性钙化,高度怀疑为 DCIS,切除活检也可是一种选择方式。在这种情况下,空芯针可能提示 DCIS,而活检阴性则与乳腺摄影不一致,需要进行导丝定位和切除。如果相关的浸润性癌的可能性较低,将不需要进行前哨淋巴结解剖或腋窝淋巴结取样,因此,在开始的时候进行立体定向活检几乎没有价值。

导管原位癌

导管原位癌(ductal carcinoma in situ,DCIS),细胞学检查中发现恶性上皮细胞位于乳腺导管细胞内,没有浸透基底膜到达乳腺间质。图 108-3 显示的是 DCIS 的组织学实例。

DCIS 在乳腺摄影筛查之前是不常见的,约占乳腺癌检出率的 3%。大多数诊断为 DCIS 的患者是无症状的、不可触及的小病变,在乳腺摄影显示局灶区域的多形性钙化之后而得到发现。DCIS 目前约占筛查发现乳腺癌的 20%~25%。在病理和分子水平上,构成 DCIS 的细胞与侵袭性癌症相似,因此可以推断这些病变是癌前病变,早期切除和治疗可以降低癌症的发生率和死亡率。然而,长期流行病学研究充分证明,每年切除 5 万至 6 万个乳腺导管原位癌病灶并没有降低侵袭性乳腺癌的发生率[209]。这与切除结肠息肉和宫颈上皮内瘤变(CIN)病变形成对比,切除癌前病变分别导致结肠癌和宫颈癌的发病率下降[164]。对于低级别 DCIS,SEER 并没有证据表明,无论是否进行干预,女性的生存率都是一样的。在 57 222 名诊断为 DCIS 的女性中,只有 2%(1 169 名)的患者接受了观察。在低级别 DCIS 患者中,手术前后 10 年生存率相同(分别为 98.6%和 98.8%)[210]。

Narod 和同事对 10 万余名确诊为 DCIS 的女性进行了大规模观察研究,结果显示死于乳腺癌的风险极低。在这项为期 20 年的研究中,只有不到 1%的患者死于乳腺癌(与之相比,5%的患者死于其他原因)。使用 Kaplan-Meier 方法,20 年乳腺癌的特异性死亡率为 3.3%,与 ACS 列出的乳腺癌将导致女性死亡的概率(ACS.org)统计数据几乎相同。

关于 DCIS 的治疗,当前的主要的问题是放疗和激素治疗的使用。虽然放疗降低了浸润性乳腺癌发生的概率,并减少了乳腺导管原位癌的复发,但对乳腺导管原位癌进行肿瘤切除后的放疗并不能降低乳腺癌的死亡率。这一点得到大量证明[212]。一些研究发现,切缘>10mm 的只接受手术而不接受放射治疗的低级别 DCIS 有 3%复发。

关于 DCIS 的治疗,当前的主要的问题是放疗和激素治疗的使用。虽然放疗降低了浸润性乳腺癌发生的概率,并减少了乳腺导管原位癌的复发,但对乳腺导管原位癌进行肿瘤切除后的放疗并不能降低乳腺癌的死亡率。这一点得到大量证明[212]。一些研究发现,切缘>10mm 的只接受手术而不接受放射治疗的低级别 DCIS 有 3%复发。Dana-Farber 癌症研究和东部肿瘤协作组(Eastern Cooperative Oncology Group,ECOG)的两项前瞻性研究发现,低、中级导管原位癌的局部复发率分别为 12.5%和 7%。

Silverstein 及其同事支持只用肿块切除术治疗预后良好型 DCIS,他们在 1995 年开发了 Van Nuys 预后指数(Van Nuys Prognostic Index,VNPI)来帮助界定低复发风险患者的选择标准[136]。最初的 VNPI 分类是通过对两家机构在 1979—1995 年收治的 333 名患者进行回顾性分析确定的。患者在 3 个因素中每个可以得到 1~3 分:肿瘤分级和是否存在坏死(合并为同一类)、肿瘤大小及切缘状态。超过 2/3 的患者属于中危 VNPI

（累计分数为5~7），而且，与随机数据相似，放疗减少了这部分患者乳腺癌复发的可能性（32% vs 15%，$P=0.017$）[160]。不足1/3的患者属于较小的低级别病变，手术切缘广泛阴性，在只接受保乳术治疗后乳腺癌复发风险较低（在76例未经放疗的患者中乳腺癌的复发率为3%）。研究小组随后将患者的年龄纳入到预后指数中。在对旧金山地区只使用肿块切除术治疗DCIS的1 036名≥40岁的女性进行了基于人群的队列研究后，报道了相似的数据。这一研究发现总体上复发率相对较高（5年的总复发率和浸润性癌复发率分别为20%和10%）；但是研究还发现，对于由乳腺摄影发现的低级别DCIS且外科治疗达到广泛切缘阴性的这部分亚组患者，在只接受手术治疗后，复发率较低[157]。

Silverstein和其同事扩大了这一原始队列，对其数据进行重新分析，将焦点集中于DCIS患者切缘状态的重要性上。在这一分析中[138]，他们报道93例切缘宽度≥10mm的患者，八年复发率只有3%。当切缘宽度为1~10mm和小于1mm时，肿块切除术治疗后不经放疗8年的局部复发可能性则高出很多，复发率分别为20%和58%。当对研究进行更新和扩大、收入212例切缘宽度≥10mm的患者时，这组患者的乳腺复发率增加到14%[139]。另外，在10mm切缘情况下注意到的低复发率，在Dana-Farber/Harvard Cancer Center所开展的单臂前瞻性试验中并没有得到证实。在该项试验中，157名1级或2级DCIS，肿瘤≤2.5cm的患者，只接受了局部切除且阴性切缘达到≥1cm[142]。因为复发率达到了预先界定的停止条件，这项试验被提前关闭，试验估计的5年局部复发率为12.5%（6%的浸润性癌复发率）。作者的结论是，即使是这组高度选择的患者，仍然存在很高的局部复发率。ECOG也已开展了一项前瞻性研究，711例经过手术治疗的DCIS患者被分为加或不加他莫昔芬两组，两组患者均不接受放疗。研究入组了两类不同的患者：①低级别或中级别DCIS，肿瘤<2.5cm；或②高级别DCIS，肿瘤<1cm。所有患者都要求肿块切除术后乳腺摄影是阴性的且手术阴性切缘≥3mm。低级别或中级别组同侧乳房肿瘤复发（IBTR）的五年风险为7%，而高级别组为14%[141]。我们知道单一手术治疗作为挽救治疗（salvage therapies）是成功的，肿瘤相关死亡率较低，因此，合理的做法是告诉患者现有的数据，让她们参与局部区域治疗的决定。

目前，由于过去十年来乳腺筛查技术的进步，关于现代单纯DCIS的过度诊断和随后的过度治疗一直存在争议。与此同时，NSABP B-17和B-24试验的长期联合随访显示，导管原位癌仅手术治疗的人群术后复发增加了乳腺癌相关死亡率，而放疗将浸润性乳腺癌复发率的风险降低了一半以上（19.4% vs 8.9%）[211]。尽管VNPI和ECOG研究在鉴别DCIS低风险亚群方面提供了指导，但它们并不具有与前瞻性随机试验相同的重要性。

1998年，RTOG开始了一项针对低/中级导管内原位癌，肿瘤最大2.5cm，切缘≤3mm的妇女的试验，最初设计用于1 800名患者[213]。遗憾的是，由于收益不佳，研究于2006年结束；然而，在纳入的636名患者中，放射治疗在7年中将局部失败率从6.7%降低到0.9%（$P<0.001$）。这一临床影响有待讨论，而且必须就辅助放疗的毒性和不便与更高的复发风险（可能是浸润性的）和后续抢救治疗的需要向患者说明，让患者进行权衡。基因组测序是为DCIS患者提供咨询和个性化提供辅助建议的一种新兴临床工具。在对上述Ⅱ期ECOG试验中治疗的300多名患者的组织分析中，根据浸润性复发的风险使用*21*基因测序试验（见辅助治疗部分）对患者进行评分具有可预测性，而且与临床因素无关[165]。与目前的临床应用相比，这种方法是否具有成本效益还有待观察[214]。

放疗的风险很小，但却是实实在在的。考虑到死亡率低的优势，有多种高风险因素的乳腺导管原位癌发生浸润性乳腺癌时，应当考虑保留外束放射治疗用于保乳治疗。许多侵入性病变在绝经后不需要放疗[215~217]，因此，放疗对浸润性乳腺癌没有的好处也就不足为奇了。

关于DCIS的治疗，第二个研究和争论的主要领域是内分泌治疗的使用。在完成B-17试验后，NSABP进行了B-24试验，将1 802名接受肿块切除术和放疗的患者随机分为接受五年他莫昔芬治疗或口服五年安慰剂[218]。这一试验与B-17纳入标准的不同之处在于：该试验包括了手术切缘阳性的患者，在试验结束时这部分患者占试验人群的25%。此外，研究的主要终点不是同侧乳腺复发，而是发生同侧乳腺复发和对侧乳腺癌的可能性。因此，这一试验设计的初衷是研究联合他莫昔芬治疗DCIS的获益，以及他莫昔芬在减少以后的新发乳腺癌方面的化学预防作用。

B-24试验的结果显示，使用他莫昔芬、手术和放疗的患者，非浸润性或浸润性乳腺癌的5年发生率为8.2%，与之相比，只接受手术和放疗的患者为13.4%[142]。显然，这种获益的一部分是他莫昔芬的化学预防作用。在B-24试验中，使用他莫昔芬导致对侧乳腺癌的5年发病率减少41%。这些数据与他莫昔芬辅助试验和NSABP P-1试验中第二原发乳腺癌的减少是一致的——这两个试验发现，对于患病风险增高的女性，他莫昔芬使乳腺癌的发生降低了49%[110]。研究者随后对保存的628例患者（327例服用安慰剂，301例使用他莫昔芬）肿瘤标本的ER表达进行了回顾性分析，发现他莫昔芬的获益局限于482名ER阳性的患者（占研究人数的77%）。在这组患者中，他莫昔芬明显减少了同侧乳腺复发和对侧乳腺癌的发生。ER阴性的患者未能从他莫昔芬中明显获益，而且由于样本量太小，无法发现较小的获益。

关于DCIS患者肿块切除术后放疗和他莫昔芬的相互作用，UK/ANZ提供了其他信息[219]。在这一研究中，对于术后没有接受放疗的患者，他莫昔芬的使用降低了DCIS的复发率，但没有降低浸润性癌的复发率。然而，在肿块切除术后接受放疗的患者中，他莫昔芬没有为同侧乳房事件提供获益。不同于B-24试验，这项试验要求所有患者都要具有阴性的手术切缘，并且研究在评价原发癌的结果时没有把对侧乳腺癌的发生作为事件包括进来。

这些数据显示，对于接受充分的肿块切除术治疗即达到手术切缘阴性）并随后接受放疗的患者，他莫昔芬在降低同侧乳腺复发方面的治疗获益可能是很低的，但对于对侧乳腺具有保护作用。有趣的是，一项最近的调查发现56%的美国医师常规推荐DCIS患者使用他莫昔芬，而只有22%的医师如此[146]。尽管他莫昔芬在DCIS方面的治疗获益缺乏明晰性，对于ER阳性的患者，加用他莫昔芬可能具有化学预防作用，使之后的新发乳腺癌的风险降至最低。NSABPB-35是一项三期试验，比较了

3 104 名诊断为导管原位癌的绝经后妇女使用 5 年他莫昔芬和阿那曲唑的效果[220]。这种差异在 60 岁以下的女性中被放大，绝对差异为 6.7%。与之前的研究一致，总体生存率(OS)没有发现差异；阿那曲唑治疗的患者子宫癌较少，骨质疏松性骨折较多。

在乳腺导管原位癌(DCIS)患者中，乳腺癌特异性死亡率与诊断时的年龄、种族和导管原位癌特征有关，如 ER 状态、分级、大小(>5cm)和坏死情况。尽管它们在多变量分析中具有重要意义，但高风险特征，如 ER-和高等级，往往是重叠的。只有一小部分患者会有一种或多种高危特征。对于有 DCIS 症状的年轻女性(<40 岁)，约占总人口的 5%，我们应该认识到这是一种不同于一般 DCIS 的疾病。此外，非裔美国女性更有可能是 HR-和 HR-/HER2+乳腺癌。总的来说，这些群体可能占患 DCIS 人口的 20%左右。

DCIS 与高风险相关并不常见。当 DCIS 在 35 岁甚至 40 岁之前被诊断出来时，其中一些病变确实会增加乳腺癌特异性死亡率的风险。40 岁以前诊断的乳腺导管原位癌多伴有肿块或乳头溢血等症状，因为 40 岁以前的筛查很少见。

乳腺导管原位癌被认为有局部复发风险，但是长期随访发现 DCIS 同时也具有同侧和对侧浸润性乳腺癌复发风险，分别为 5.9%和 6.2%，这提示 DCIS 可能为癌前病变。DCIS 基因检测提示仅手术切除低风险的病变仍有如同 2.5Gail 的风险。单侧复发的 DCIS 或对侧 DCIS 事件对死亡率没有影响。然而，侵袭性癌症确实如此：单侧为 18 倍，对侧为 13 倍，这表明所有风险都取决于侵袭性癌症发生的概率。对于绝经前妇女，他莫昔芬是 HR+DCIS 的良好选择。对于绝经后的妇女，芳香化酶抑制剂(AI)被证明对降低风险有更高的影响。如果 AI 产生不良副作用，雷洛昔芬是一个很好的替代品。他莫昔芬可能不应该用于绝经后妇女的 DCIS，因为据报道，在较长时间的激素治疗存在风险[203]。

高危病变(如 HER2+、<40 岁、ER-、肿瘤较大)应积极治疗，但 Narod 分析表明，我们目前的手术切除和放疗方法可能不足以治疗导死亡的乳腺癌，需要研究新的方法。在一项研究中，我们发现与复发相关的肿瘤微环境中充满了活化的巨噬细胞，而活化的 T 细胞则很少[221]。

早期乳腺癌治疗

分期和分类

分期的目的是：①计划最适合患者的治疗策略；②使得研究者根据患者的疾病状态得出更多的富于才智的成果；③便于我们对不同治疗方法的疗效进行比较。目前常用的分期方法是临床和病理分期，但包括了生物学评估的更新的方法正处于发展和验证中。不考虑所使用的分期方法，记住分期代表着患者个体的肿瘤状态或生物潜能，是非常重要的。特定分期方法的应用应该根据其在这一任务中的准确性来进行判断。

TNM 分类由国际抗癌联盟(International Union Against Cancer，UICC)制订，并被美国癌症分期联合委员会(American Joint Commission on Cancer Staging)所接受，是一个世界性的标准[222]。TNM 分期的基础是肿瘤的临床特征(T)、区域淋巴结(N)和是否存在远处转移(M)。肿瘤以其大小为特征，因此 T1 是肿瘤小于 2cm，T2 是 2~5cm，T3 是大于 5cm。同样的，N0 代表区域淋巴结阴性或正常等(表 108-7)。

临床分期系统通常低估了疾病的程度。将病理信息包括进来提高了分期的准确性，这是大多数现代临床试验的基础。在所有情况下，我们首要的目标是确定肿瘤的生物活性。Cox 回归统计模型显示淋巴结转移的存在是最重要的因素。而且，受累淋巴结的数目可用于进一步划分预后亚组。一般认为，淋巴结转移穿透包膜并浸润到邻近的结旁组织，会导致预后更差。

回归分析模型发现肿瘤大小与淋巴结受累密切相关[84,223]。在腋窝淋巴结阳性患者组，肿瘤大小不是重要的判断要点，但要除外淋巴结受累 4 个以上者。因此，肿瘤大小可以与时间或生长率密切相关，作用小于淋巴结受累，后者是肿瘤生物侵袭性的更为特异的指标。而且，一些患者的大肿物可能是生长缓慢的肿瘤，多年未予注意，肿物并未发生转移。在对乳腺摄影筛查发现的肿瘤小且具侵袭性的患者进行分类时，也存在类似的问题，这部分患者已经存在远处转移，尽管初期的局部临床特征比较有利，仍可能迅速死亡。而生物学分期可以比 TNM 系统更准确地确定这部分患者。

表 108-7 TNM 分期定义

原发肿瘤(T)	
TX	原发肿瘤无法评估
T0	没有原发肿瘤证据
Tis	原位癌
Tis(DCIS)	导管原位癌
Tis(LCIS)	小叶原位癌
Tis(Paget)	乳头佩吉特病，不伴有肿块
T1	肿瘤最大直径≤2cm
T1mic	微小浸润癌，最大直径≤0.1cm
T1a	肿瘤最大直径>0.1cm，但≤0.5cm

续表

T1b	肿瘤最大直径>0.5cm,但≤1.0cm
T1c	肿瘤最大直径>1.0cm,但≤2.0cm
T2	肿瘤最大直径>2.0cm,但≤5.0cm
T3	肿瘤最大直径≥5.0cm
T4	不论肿瘤大小,直接侵犯胸壁(a)或皮肤(b),如下所述
T4a	侵犯胸壁,不包括胸肌
T4b	患侧乳腺皮肤水肿、溃破或卫星结节
T4c	T4a 与 T4b 并存
T4d	炎性乳腺癌
区域淋巴结(N)	
NX	区域淋巴结无法评估(如曾经切除)
N0	无区域淋巴结转移
N1	同侧腋窝淋巴结转移,可活动
N2	同侧腋窝淋巴结转移,固定或相互融合或缺乏同侧腋窝淋巴结转移的证据,但临床上发现有同侧内淋巴结转移
N3	同侧锁骨下淋巴结转移伴或不伴腋窝淋巴结转移;或有临床上发现同侧内乳淋巴结转移和腋窝淋巴结转移的临床证据;或同侧锁骨上淋巴结转移伴或不伴腋窝或内乳淋巴结转移
病理学分期(pN)	
pNX	区域淋巴结无法评估(如过去已切除,或未进行病理学检查)
pN0	无区域淋巴结转移
pN1	1~3 个腋窝淋巴结转移,和/或通过前哨淋巴结切除发现内乳淋巴结有微笑转移灶,但临床上未发现
pN2	4~9 个腋窝淋巴结转移,或临床上发现内乳淋巴结转移,但腋窝淋巴结无转移
pN3	≥10 个腋窝淋巴结转移,或锁骨下淋巴结转移,或临床上发现同侧内乳淋巴结转移;或有 1 个或更多腋窝淋巴结阳性,临床上未发现内乳淋巴结转移但镜下有微小转移;或同侧锁骨上淋巴结转移
远处转移(M)	
MX	远处转移无法评估
M0	无远处转移
M1	有远处转移
AJCC 分期	
0 期	Tis,N0,M0
Ⅰ期	T1,N1,M0
ⅡA 期	T0,N1,M0 T1,N0,M0 T2,N0,M0
ⅡB 期	T2,N1,M0 T3,N0,M0
ⅢA 期	T0,N2,M0 T1,N2,M0 T2,N2,M0 T3,N1,M0 T3,N2,M0
ⅢB 期	T4,任何 N,M0
ⅢC 期	T4,N1,M0 T4,N2,M0
Ⅳ期	任何 T,任何 N,M1

外科手术

在过去的 30 年里，原发性乳腺癌的局部治疗已经发生了革命性的改变，其结果是乳腺癌根治术和扩大根治术(extended radical mastectomy)已经成为外科历史。一系列随机对照临床试验将乳腺癌根治术(radical mastectomy)与手术范围较小的术式进行了对比，研究结果的发表促使 NIH 发起的共识发展会议(NIH-sponsored consensus development conference)(1990)做出如下推荐：对于乳腺癌Ⅰ期和Ⅱ期的患者，由于保乳术的生存数据与全乳切除加腋窝解剖相当，并同时使患者的乳房得以保存，因此保乳术是更加合适的治疗[224]。

多种来源的信息显示，许多乳腺癌患者在临床确诊时就已经存在肿瘤播散。这并不奇怪，因为 1cm 的乳腺肿瘤其生长经过了理论上 30~40 次倍增，使得肿瘤接近 1kg，这个大小对于患者来说可以是致命的。然而，我们现在知道乳腺癌是一种具有异质性的疾病，一些患者的肿瘤转移扩散潜能较低，而一些患者即使其肿瘤小且局限于乳房，仍然具有很高的转移扩散风险[86,89]。分子谱(molecular profile)可能会很大程度上提高我们区分这些肿瘤并据此调整方案的能力。

对于临床上认为已经"治愈"的乳腺癌，如果根治术后发现腋窝淋巴结转移而未进行化疗，将有 3/4 的患者在 10 年后出现复发转移，对于 4 个以上腋窝淋巴结转移的患者，这一比例将上升至 9/10。这些发现强调一些乳腺癌是全身性质的疾病[144]，并提示广泛的局部和区域手术作为唯一的治疗手段用于转移风险高的患者是不够的。

保乳治疗

保乳的目的是切除肿瘤及其周围的正常组织，同时保持乳房的轮廓和形状。留在切缘上的肿瘤将增加复发风险。Recht 等在一项 533 例患者的研究中显示，复发风险取决于切缘上肿瘤的残留量：肉眼可见的阳性切缘(grossly positive margins)、局灶性阳性切缘(focally positive margins)和肿瘤贴近切缘(close margins)的复发风险分别为 27%、14%与 7%。本研究中所有的患者都接受了放疗，近切缘实质上没有改变复发风险。广泛的导管内癌曾经被认为是保乳手术的禁忌证，现在已经发现如果全部的 DCIS 都被切除，则与更高的局部复发风险无关。在诊断后的头 10 年内，保乳术后所有的乳腺复发，90%位于同一象限，遗传上等同于原发性乳腺癌。然而，保乳手术与乳房切除术(mastectomy)对比的长期随访研究显示，10 年后乳腺存在发生新发肿瘤的持续风险，但经常是发生于其他象限。

随着乳房肿块切除法的出现，我们需要采用二步法(two-stage procedure)进行活检然后行确定性手术。术前空芯针活检，不论是临床进行还是在放射学检查引导下进行，都应该被认为是标准做法，这样外科医师在进行任何手术前就可以得到明确的诊断并更好地设计手术。图 108-14 详细描述了原发性乳腺癌最佳外科治疗决策的制订方法。

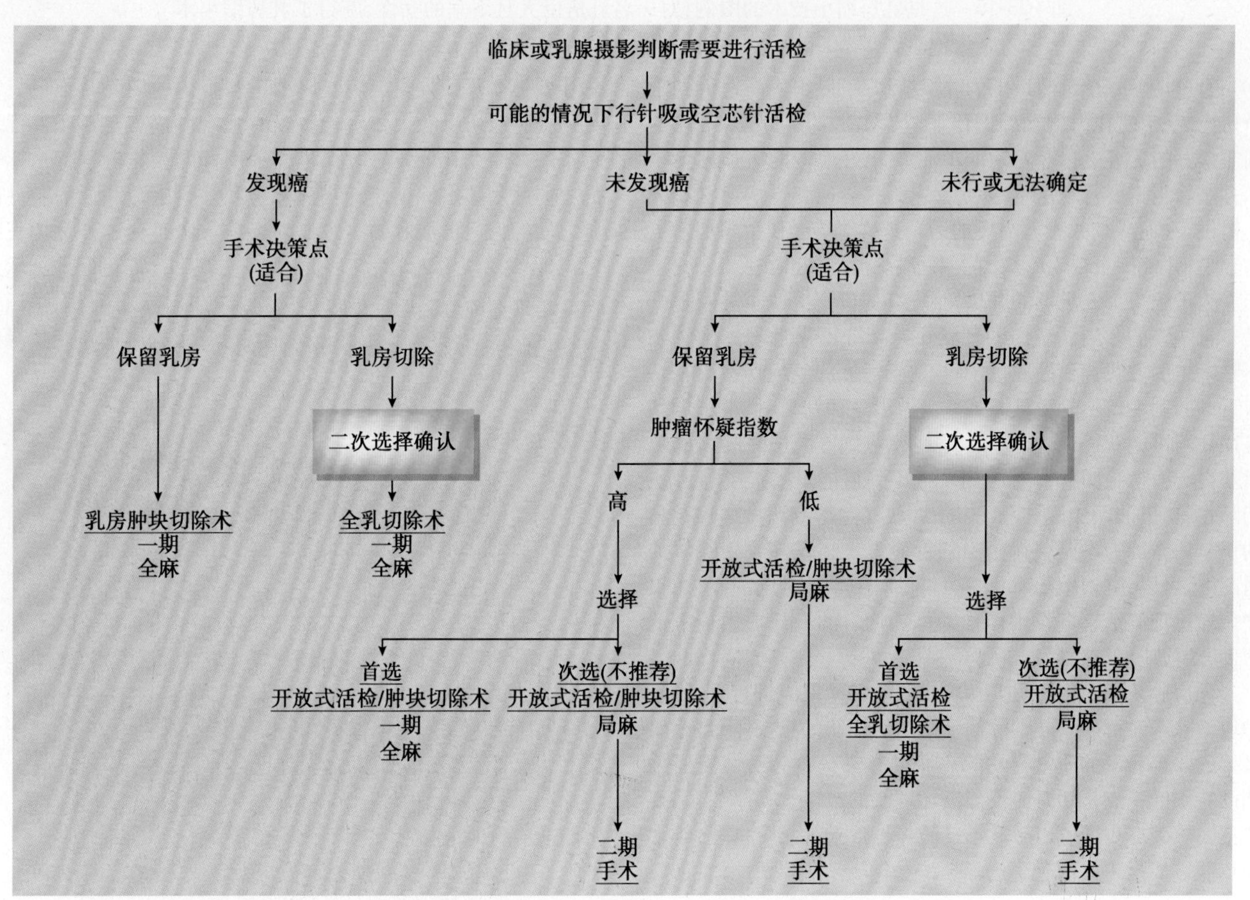

图 108-14　原发性乳腺癌治疗的外科决策推荐

如果必须进行开放式手术活检，则应按照乳腺肿物切除术的方式进行。如果遇到的是恶性肿瘤，手术者必须注意确保切缘没有肿瘤。在所有保乳术可行的情况下，不论腋窝手术是同时还是以后进行，为确诊乳腺病变而施行的手术都变为确定性治疗。大多数乳腺癌手术（活检、肿块切除术、腋窝解剖甚至乳房切除术）都可以在门诊进行，手术并发症的程度非常轻，患者自身和社会可以一样或者更好地适应手术过程。

技术和美容考虑

为了达到最佳美容效果，应该根据肿瘤的范围、位置和乳房本来的形状设计切口。现在需要接受乳房手术的患者有很多选择。可以切除的组织的范围取决于乳房的大小。整形外科技术可为对侧乳房行或不行美容手术，以改善乳房的对称性。一旦乳腺组织被切除，解剖乳腺组织到达筋膜水平，为从内侧向外侧方向闭合乳腺组织提供机会，并因此避免了乳头组织的上下移位。可以对对侧乳房施行乳房固定术（mastopexy）或缩小术以改善对称性。如果乳房下垂（ptosis）的程度非常明显，可以在部分乳房切除术后完成乳房缩小术（breast reduction），由此将提高美容效果与切除乳腺组织的肿瘤手术结合起来（图 108-15）。在乳房缩小术中，可以切除一半以上的乳房，因此这一技术可以用于较大的肿瘤或单个象限上散在分布的原位癌。图 108-15（a）和 15b 显示的是一例因巨大乳房带来极大不适、一直想要接受乳房缩小术的患者。

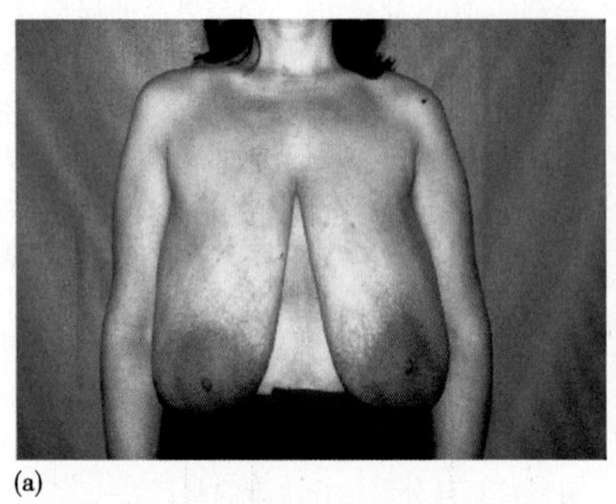
(a)

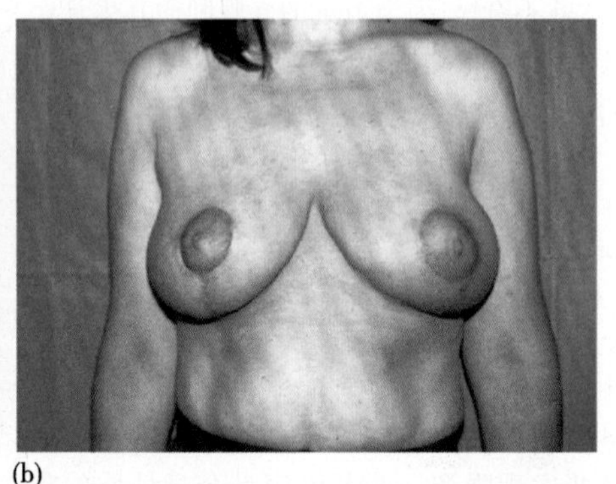
(b)

图 108-15 这是乳房缩小技术的图例：对一名乳房巨大且下垂的女性，施行了乳房缩小术加部分乳房切除术。（a）术前照片；（b）术后照片

通过切除一个象限以上的乳腺组织，可以很容易地得到干净切缘，手术时在内侧和外侧留下至少 1cm 的乳腺瓣，可以达到非常好的美容效果。术前 MRI 能够很好地帮助医师设计手术方法。当需要行乳房手术时，手术为患者改变乳房形状和大小提供了机会（如果患者需要的话），这样可能会使手术切除更加容易，并使一个令人不快的手术过程变得轻松很多。

为了施行令人满意的肿块切除术，切口直接位于肿瘤上方是非常重要的。用乳晕周围环状切口切除不靠近乳晕的肿物不是理想的方式，而且通过皮下隧道穿过乳腺组织切除不在切口下方的病变也不是最佳方式。当做出这种切口时，很难做到且往往不可能获得干净切缘。经这种切口再次切除肿瘤部位以获得干净切缘同样困难。如果考虑到可能最后需要行肿块切除术，切口的做法应该考虑一下肿块切除术应该做哪种类型的切口。在因为不能获得干净切缘而无法施行肿块切除术的情况下，可以将肿块切除术的切口融合到乳房切除术的切口中。通过穿刺活检进行术前诊断可为切口的设计提供很大的帮助，活检应该按照标准进行。

乳房肿块切除术不需要切除皮肤。如果术前进行过活检，肿块切除术时可以一并移除瘢痕周围的皮肤，但这并不是绝对必要的。美容术的质量与切除皮肤的数量呈负相关。需要强调的特别的一点是切开时不能破坏皮肤的边缘，这样就不需要薄皮瓣。破坏皮肤可以导致不佳的美容效果，因此一些时候切除皮肤可能是更好的美容选择。

肿瘤切除与标本切缘检查

切除肿瘤使之被完全封在正常脂肪和/或乳腺组织内。这一步并不需要预先确定病变周围正常组织的切除其数量只需要达到肿瘤切缘的大体观检查没有发现肿瘤就足够了。标示标本的方向尤其重要。医疗机构采用标准操作流程标示标本的方向并用墨水标志，会使病理医师、外科医师和放射肿瘤医师之间的沟通更加通畅。经典的标准方法是标本外侧用长线标志，上缘用短线标志，在后面固定一片 Telfa 以更好地标示方向。这种方法对于需要进行 X 线摄影的标本尤其有用，可以保留标本的形状，提高确定并进一步切除靠近标本的特定切缘的机会（图 108-16）。

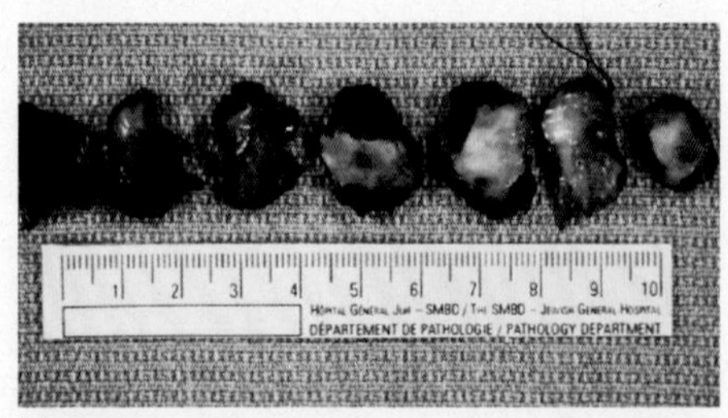

(a)

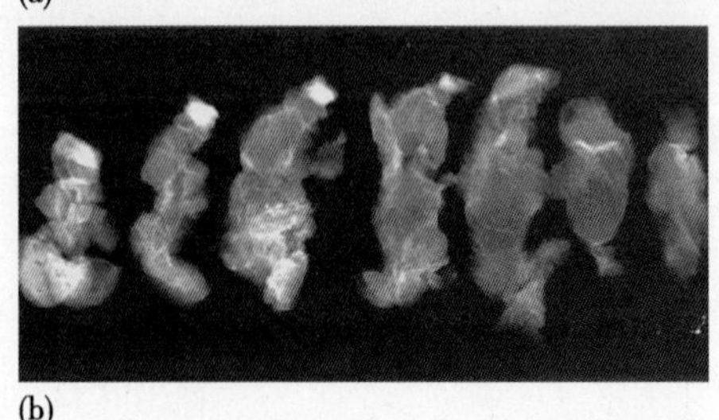
(b)

图 108-16 （a）标本肉眼观（b）标本影像学显示钙化

如果之前进行了切除活检而未评估切缘，则必须在进行淋巴结解剖时再次手术切除以确定切缘没有肿瘤。

标本被立即送交病理学家，或者更加理想的是，病理学家在手术室接收标本并想象标本的方向。病理学家的作用是确认或确定肿瘤的诊断(如果未行针刺活检)，帮助外科医师在术中确定标本切缘在大体检查下是否没有肿瘤，并取走部分标本进行一些专门的研究。

病理学家收到标本并根据外科医师放置的缝线标签确定其方向。在测量后，大体检查未被切开的肿瘤的切缘受累情况。如果有证据显示肿瘤已被切断，病理学家会立即通知外科医师手术边缘残留病灶的准确位置，这样在病理学家完成标本检查时，外科医师可以切除残留部分的其他组织。然后病理学家在标本的整个表面涂上一层墨汁，用吸墨纸吸干，再把肿瘤或标本横向切成两等份。一些病理学家会用多种颜色(如后面、前上半部分、前下部分)以提高准确描述阳性切缘位置的能力。如果在大体检查中发现肿瘤靠近所切除的组织边缘，病理学家会制作冷冻切片(frozen sections)以确定切缘受累。在认为无法确定切缘受累时，任何时候都可以切除其他的乳腺组织以获得新的真正的肿瘤边界。不应该为了确定切缘是否没有肿瘤而制作大量冰冻切片。用精细的方法制作固定切片可以更好地对切缘做出评估。

如果之后在镜下发现二次切除的标本切缘受累，并且没有证据显示肿瘤大体标本已经被切断，可以考虑不切除乳房。在这种情况下，当明确肿瘤大体标本未被切断，放疗加系统治疗可能会达到足够的局部区域肿瘤控制，大部分患者仍将保持无局部复发。波士顿(Boston)的对接中心(Joint Center)更新了关于切缘控制的系列报道，显示阳性切缘的复发率与真正的阴性切缘相同[225]。同样的，当乳腺肿块切除术后肿瘤复发，如果这样的肿瘤体积小，能够切除且标本切缘干净，再次行肿块切除术可能还将获得肿瘤控制。

用于决定肿瘤是否累积标本切缘的病理标准可以不同。许多病理学家使用像肿瘤"非常接近"切缘这样的主观说法来表示切缘受累。病例复阅显示只有 12%的全乳切除术标本因为切缘仅而有残损肿瘤。因此，只有在肿瘤被切断时才认为切线受累是最合适的。对于由乳腺摄影发现的需要 X 线引导的肿瘤，需要在乳腺内放置一根或多跟导丝，以将钙化包括起来或准确标示病变中心或钙化。一旦病变被切除，就需要对标本进行 X 线摄影，确认病变的存在和乳腺摄影异常相对于切缘的位置。对于能够使用超声确定的不可触及的病变，只要有可能，就应该使用超声进行定位，因为这种方式患者可以更好地耐受，且不必像乳腺摄影定位那样需要压紧乳房。一些外科医师正在接受使用超声的训练，这样他们能够在手术室里更好地对实体病变的进行针对性切除。这减少了手术室与放射科交流的需要与时间。然而，这需要外科医师受过专门训练，技术非常熟练，能够确定哪些病变可以准确发现以免在术中遗漏病变。

乳房切除术

接受乳房切除术的患者可以选择是否接受乳房重建。患者是否选择乳房重建，美容考虑是很重要的。设法在胸壁上留出一个平面是很重要的，这样患者可以佩戴义乳并感觉舒适。手术要在腋线处避免皮肤皱褶，可以在腋窝部分做鱼尾形切口(fish tail incisions)，或应用整形外科技术设计腋窝处的切口，从而避免出现多余的皮肤。

当使用合适的多学科综合治疗时，即使是局部晚期病变，即刻重建(immediate reconstruction)也是安全的[226](图 108-17)。因此，任何考虑乳房切除术的患者都应被告知重建的选择，包括即刻重建和延迟重建。重建后的并发症是常见的，不论外科医师还是患者都应该对其有所预料。对结果的预期应该予以恰当地设定，患者应该对采用多种外科手段以达到最佳重建效果的可能性有所准备。

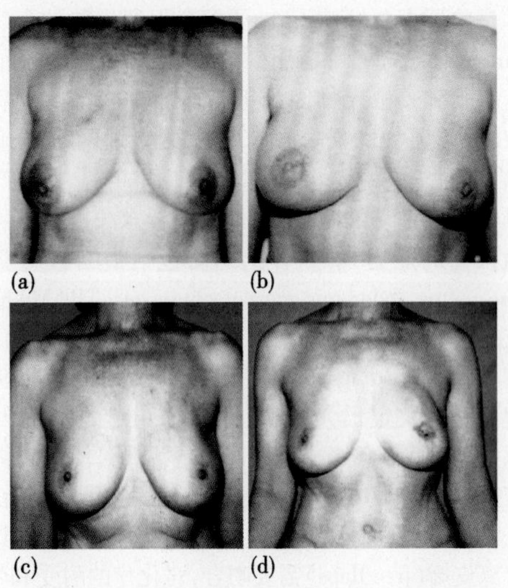

图 108-17 37 岁(a，b)及 65 岁患者护皮乳房切除术后即刻重建 TRAM 皮瓣及延后乳头重建，术后照片分别为 12 周(c)及 8 周(d)，均为乳头重建后 5 天

如果使用化疗这一决定使我们不需要切除额外的组织或对原发肿瘤进行确定性切除，又如果化疗是特定患者多学科综合治疗的一部分，以及如果患者强烈考虑乳房切除术，根据疾病的程度或患者的偏好，应该强烈考虑新辅助化疗(neoadjuvant chemotherapy)。在辅助治疗后进行外科手术和重建使因并发症延迟辅助治疗的风险降至最低，并给患者更多的时间考虑外科手术的选择、调整和适应诊断并更清楚地考虑手术选择。对全身治疗后的手术和重建顺序进行合理安排可以最大限度地降低并发症延迟辅助治疗的风险，并使女性有更多时间针对诊断考虑手术方式的选择。新辅助全身治疗可提高乳房保留率。在最近一项关于卡铂和贝伐单抗(bevacizumab)加入蒽环类和紫杉烷类化疗的研究中，手术前治疗能够使 42%的不能保乳乳腺癌变为可保乳[227]。93%选择保乳手术的患者能成果保乳。然而，在满足保乳条件的患者中大约 30%的女性最终选择了乳房切除术。新辅助化疗允许许多大乳腺肿瘤的患者实现具有临床意义的肿瘤缩小，提示进行保乳的可能性。然而，治疗反应因成像方式和肿瘤亚型而异。在 ISPY-1 试验中，肿瘤体积在 MRI 和手术病理的一致性，在三阴性乳腺癌中较高，但在内分泌受体阳性乳腺癌中较低[228]。

对于对重建感到矛盾的女性，延期重建(delayged reconstruction)可能是最好的。但是，即刻重建的美容效果是最好的，可以使瘢痕做到最小，并根据已选择的重建类型设计切口。在仅仅几天内作出重建的决定是困难的，对正在决定中的女性应该打消其疑虑,额外一周到两周的时间研究手术选择并作出好的决定是不会影响其生存预后的。患者将可能带着其选择的结果生活数十年,因此投入数周的时间(如果需要的)话——来确定她们对于自己的决定不会存在忧虑是重要的。

有两种基本类型的重建可以提供——植入物重建(implant reconstruction)和自体组织重建(autologous tissue reconstruction)。植入物可以放置组织扩张器或永久性植入物。组织扩张器是最常使用的重建形式。将之放置于胸大肌下,扩张袋逐渐扩张直到大于所需的乳房大小。然后扩张器被永久性植入物替代并塑造乳房外形。整个过程可能需要 6~8 周时间。另一种技术是放置永久性植入物,要配合保留皮肤的乳房切除术(skin sparing mastectomy)使用[128]。大部分用于重建的植入物是盐水。尽管硅胶植入物因为担心增加自体免疫疾病的风险而退出市场,几项大的研究并未显示两者之间存在确定性联系。其结果是,硅胶植入物得以再次使用[146]。硅胶产品可能更好的具体实例是有的(如如果即刻放置永久性植入物但又需要扩张植入物的能力)。自体组织瓣包括横断腹直肌肌皮瓣(transverse rectus abdominis musculocutaneous, TRAM)或腹壁下动脉穿支皮瓣(deep inferior epigastric perforator, DIEP),或背阔肌肌皮瓣(latissimus dorsi flaps)(图 108-18 和图 108-19)。

重建类型的决定很大程度上取决于患者的偏好,尽管治疗上的考虑也起到了重要作用。如果需要放疗,使用自体组织的并发症较少。关于 TRAM 皮瓣是否能够耐受化疗是有争议的。已经发表的几篇报道显示放疗对皮瓣具有显著的有害影响。这可能是游离皮瓣(free flaps)需要吻合,对化疗的耐受和带蒂皮瓣(pedicle flaps)相同,或者更有可能的是,使用更高剂量放疗(包括瘤床在内高达 6 500cGy)的机构可能会遇到更多的并发症。一家来自苏格兰 Dundee 的机构最近报道,将胸壁放疗剂量限制在 4 500~5 000cGy,在大量患者中均显示出极佳的效果。

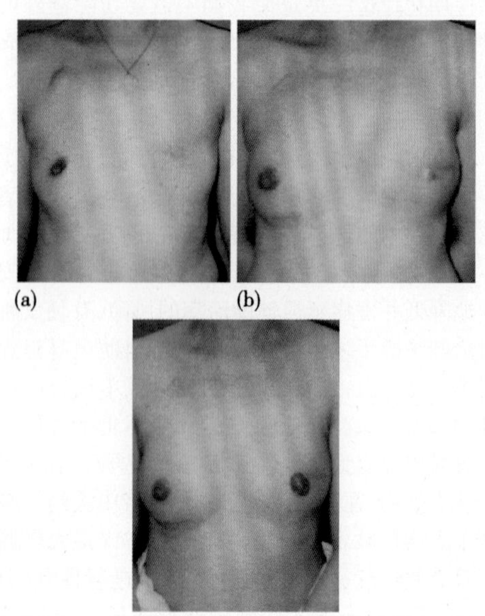

图 108-18 保留全部皮肤的手术配合多种重建技术。(a)立即植入重建,乳房固定术切口及对侧乳房固定术。左侧乳房做了切除,图片是术后 3 周时拍摄。(b)亚厘米级导管原位癌病灶切除后复发的高危险患者双侧乳房切除并立即植入重建。(c)右侧乳房切除术后立即用 TRAM 皮瓣重建

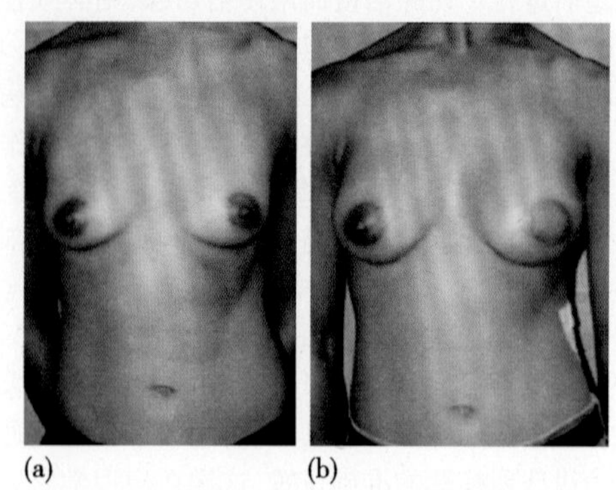

图 108-19 39 岁患者背阔肌双侧重建。术前(a)及(b)术后 12 周图片

保留全部皮肤的乳房切除术(total skin sparing mastectomy)是乳房切除术的一项新技术[229,230]。这一技术去除了包括乳晕和乳头组织在内的全部乳腺组织,但保留覆在上面的真皮。最近的一篇包括 171 例患者的报道显示,随着时间的推移,这项技术已经变得可靠起来,而且可以使用不同切口以达到极佳的效果。这一技术使得 99% 的乳晕和乳头得以保留。尽管随访有限,早期结果显示局部复发率很低(<2%),并且我们预测保留全部皮肤的乳房切除术将不会影响复发风险。这一技术的关键是完成乳管组织的切除(图 108-18 和图 108-19)。除了使用永久性植入体以外,这项技术可以与任何重建技术联合使用,因为术中即时扩张皮肤显著增加皮肤坏死的风险。尽管具有挑战性,这项技术振奋人心的发展是将全部乳腺组织的切除和出色的美容效果相结合,同时安全性好。当对患病风险最高的女性考虑预防性乳房切除术时,使用保留全部皮肤的乳房切除术的时机是尤其重要的,可以使患者对手术的美容效果感到足够满意。

腋窝淋巴结清扫

腋窝淋巴结清扫的目的不在于提高治愈可能性,因为区域淋巴结被认为是肿瘤远处转移的指示信号,而不是促进远处转移。腋窝淋巴结清扫的切口应该与切除乳腺肿瘤的切口分开。可以沿胸大肌后外侧缘做纵向切口,也可以在腋线下方行横向切口。目前的淋巴结解剖包括腋窝Ⅰ、Ⅱ水平的淋巴结。其解剖学边界以背阔肌为外界,腋静脉为上界,胸小肌内侧缘为内界,手术不需要切除胸小肌,并应找到和保留支配前锯肌和背阔肌的神经。找到腋静脉并沿胸小肌下方到达其内侧缘,这是切除的最小范围。切除淋巴结的平均数目大约是 15 个。尽管肿块切除部位不做引流,腋窝应该在术后数天里留置负压引流。

由于前哨淋巴结清扫的引入,腋窝的处理已经发生了很大变化。这种方式大大限制了外科在腋窝的手术范围,对于绝大部分腋窝淋巴结阴性的患者,免除了正规腋窝淋巴结清扫的需要,同时提供相似的(有些情况下更好的)诊断和预后信息。检测单个(或只有几个)前哨淋巴结使得病理学家可以通过分析前哨淋巴结的多水平切片(multiple level sections)作出更为详细的评估。通过将光学显微镜、免疫组化(immunohistochemistry, IHC)以及更加敏感的分子技术相结合,显著提高了微转移

的检测。然而,通过更敏感的技术在组织学阴性的淋巴结中确定孤立的转移细胞,其预后意义尚不确定;因此,目前并不认为其足以构成Ⅱ期病变。大型合作研究小组正在对前哨淋巴结活检和评估进行广泛的评定,其中包括 NSABP 和 ACOSOG。ACOSOGZ-010 试验要求临床医师在其医院内不使用免疫组化分析,这样所有的淋巴结能够在中心实验室染色并对结果采取盲法,以评估淋巴结微转移的预后意义。NSABP B-32 随机将 5 611 名阴性 SLN 的患者分为只接受 SLN 活检或 SLN 活检后进行腋窝淋巴结清扫(axillary lymph node dissection, ALND)两组。发现阳性 SLN 的女性亦接受全 ALND。研究的力度在于它是最大的 SLND 的随机试验,它是参与该研究的全国 80 家中心 232 名外科医师协作的典范。尽管还不知道其远期疗效、区域控制和生存情况,SLN 活检技术的结果是知道的。平均来看,每个患者切除 3 个 SLN;SLN 的确认率是 97.2%,并随着外科医师的经验而提高,26%的患者前哨淋巴结阳性。在只有一个前哨淋巴结阳性的患者中,有 61.5%其他淋巴结是阴性的(38.5%其他淋巴结阳性)。假阴性率(SLN 阴性时腋窝淋巴结受累)是 9.7%,这一点没有随着医师的经验而改变,但明显受到用于诊断的活检类型的影响;对于 FNA/空芯针活检、切开活检和切除活检,假阴性率分别为 8.0%、14.3%和 15.2%。发现的 SLN 的数目也对 SLN 的假阴性率有影响。如果检测到 1 个以上的 SLN,则阴性结果的可信度更高,但对于阳性淋巴结先验概率较高的女性则可信度可能降低。

前哨淋巴结活检

使用放射示踪剂或可视的蓝色染料来定位和切除前哨淋巴结(SLN)(直接引流肿瘤部位的淋巴结),正成为评估腋窝的标准技术。这项技术最先用于黑色素瘤,然后用于乳腺癌的研究。只要术者熟练掌握该技术,就具有高度的准确性。文献报道术者识别前哨淋巴结的能力范围介于 85%~97%。ACOSOG 在招募外科医师参与前哨淋巴结注册试验和确定 SLN 切除后行全腋窝清扫是否具有价值的试验时,要求他们能够识别 90%以上患者的前哨淋巴结且假阴性率在 5%以下。有报道显示 SLND 后淋巴水肿(lymphedema)的比率小于 7%,与 ALND17%~25%的比率形成鲜明对比[231]。研究显示 SLND 在新辅助化疗后具有相似的结果[232],尽管 SLN 的识别可能较少,假阴性率是非常相似的。尽管仍然存在一些争议,新辅助化疗后行 SLND 的潜在益处是使患者在开始化疗前免于其他手术,由于淋巴结的肿瘤可能随着化疗消失,患者可能会避免腋窝清扫术,而且化疗后淋巴结存在肿瘤的信息在预测局部复发率和决定需要放疗方面具有价值[151]。术中冰冻切片在检测淋巴结转移方面始终不如实验室之后所进行的专门检测准确。最近报道印迹细胞学(imprint cytology)具有非常低的假阳性率,但敏感性不如冰冻切片高。在 NSABP B-32 试验中,的确发现印迹细胞的假阳性率低,为 0.4%,但敏感性只有 61.5%。这在术中淋巴结转移检测方面具有价值,因为能够使外科医师在行 SLND 时进行全腋窝淋巴结清扫,由此避免了第二次手术。临床医师应该在自己所在的机构中使用这一技术,做到最低的假阳性率,从而使不必要的额外的手术降到最少。

使用伽马(gamma)同位素标志的胶体进行放射性核素注射并用手持探头扫描的方法正在取代蓝色染料注射法,后者提示淋巴结的方式是可以见到蓝色淋巴管通向蓝色前哨淋巴结。尽管一些作者强烈支持这两种方法中的一种,大部分报道显示将两者的结果相结合后,辨识前哨淋巴结的水平是最高的。NSABP B32 试验中放射性核素比蓝色染料具有更高的 SLN 辨识力。淋巴蓝染料过敏风险很小但的确是存在的,概率小于 1%。NSABP B-12 试验显示严重过敏的风险是 0.2%。使用蓝色染料时,麻醉医师应注意到这一可能性。

腋窝淋巴结清扫的必要性

人们经常问是否所有行肿块切除术的患者都需要腋窝分期。如果系统治疗的必要性和治疗类型能够由患者和肿瘤的特征而非腋窝淋巴结状态所决定,腋窝分期的必要性就变得不那么确定了。而且,如果所有的淋巴结阴性和阳性的患者都给予同样的全身性辅助治疗,正如术前新辅助化疗试验的情况那样,那么似乎就没有理由知道淋巴结状态了,除非是需要预测患者的结果。早期乳腺癌试验协作组(Early Breast Cancer Trialists' Collaborative Group)的回顾性结果显示,辅助化疗为淋巴结阴性和阳性的患者带来益处,两组降低治疗失败的风险是相同的,因此许多肿瘤学家对所有患者都进行化疗,除非患者的风险降低比例太小以至于几乎不能真正获益。研究者设计了决策制订工具,例如 Adjuvantonline.com,这款工具得到过很好的验证,用于预测化疗的绝对获益[233];此外还有提供复发分数的分子工具,例如 Oncotype DX[234]使得能够更好地指导肿瘤学家进行系统治疗。在决定是否给予辅助治疗和使用什么类型的辅助治疗方面,肿瘤的分子特征可能比分期更重要。美国和欧洲所使用的两种分子检测正处于临床试验中以更好的回答这些问题(美国的是 TAILORx 试验,欧洲的是 MINDACT 试验)。当这些数据成熟时,前哨淋巴结清扫和腋窝清扫的作用就会得到明确。在分子时代,有些情况下,对手术为主要治疗手段的患者切除所有可能的局部区域肿瘤非常重要的,如患者的复发预测风险低,或已经接受过新辅助化疗,其残余病灶可能对治疗抗拒。在新辅助化疗后达到病理完全缓解的情况下,有些患者可能不需要手术;临床 N0 的患者在新辅助化疗后,将更多地接受前哨淋巴结清扫,而不考虑治疗前的淋巴结状态,这是根据疗效调整外科手术范围的范例。人们可能尤其会质疑 ER 阳性且计划接受内分泌治疗的老年女性腋窝清扫的必要性。在这种情况下,腋窝淋巴结的状态不太可能改变化疗的使用。但是,在几乎所有临床上腋窝阴性的患者中,前哨淋巴结清扫是分期和外科治疗的标准部分,且能够在大部分女性中成功实施,给患者带来的不良反应也较小。在前哨淋巴结阳性的情况下,Ⅰ、Ⅱ水平的腋窝淋巴结清扫被认为是标准治疗。尽管人们普遍接受腋窝清扫可以提供最佳的腋窝局部控制,一项随机试验将全乳切除术加或不加腋窝清扫进行了对比,结果显示在不进行腋窝清扫的情况下,不是所有的腋窝阳性淋巴结都会发生复发:事实上只有一半会出现复发。

多中心的 ACOSOG Z011 临床研究将接受保乳手术且前哨淋巴结具有 1 个阳性淋巴结的乳腺癌患者随机分为做与不做腋窝淋巴结清扫两组[235]。目标入组 1 900 名患者,实际入组 991 名乳腺癌患者。两组间 5 年腋窝和乳腺复发率无显著差异,更重要的是,两组间无病生存率和总生存率无差异。这个重要结果已经改变了对腋窝淋巴结的治疗规范,也使很多女性免除了腋窝淋巴结清扫带来的并发症。但对于接受乳腺全切的乳腺癌患者一枚前哨淋巴结阳性是否仍需要淋巴结清扫有待进一步研究,除非进行全乳放疗。

自乳房X线筛查的常规使用以来,绝大多数被诊断患有浸润性乳腺癌的患者肿瘤在T1~T2期,适于进行保乳治疗。保乳手术已成为早期乳腺癌的标准治疗方式。这项治疗包含三个重要步骤:切除肿瘤并获得阴性切缘(通常称为乳房肿瘤切除术或乳房区段切除术),腋窝淋巴结处理包括前哨淋巴结活检或Ⅰ/Ⅱ组腋窝淋巴结清扫术,以及乳腺放疗。大部分接受现代保乳治疗的患者都获得了较好结局。结合全身系统治疗,对于适宜人群保乳术后年均复发风险在0.5%以下[236,237]。此外,随着外科和放疗技术的进步,保乳治疗的并发症也非常低。

虽然如此,保乳治疗在美国仍未得到充分应用。在一项比较早期乳腺癌两种内分泌治疗方法的多中心研究中,美国的保乳率仅为49%[238]。相比之下,英国的保乳率为58%,在瑞典,德国或澳大利亚/新西兰观察到甚至更高的比率。既往数据还表明,在美国各地区,乳房保护的使用情况各不相同,南部和中西部地区的妇女乳房保护的可能性低于东部或西部海岸的妇女[239]。影响保乳治疗的因素的多方面的。遗憾的是,一些女性接受乳房切除术是基于一种误解,认为乳房切除术可能会取得更好的结果。因此,至关重要的是,乳腺癌提供者应了解有关乳房保护的数据,以便新诊断的疾病患者可以选择适当的治疗方案。

保乳治疗与乳房切除术比较

保乳术作为代替乳房切除术的局部区域治疗已经被研究了40余年。在一些单机构获得了最初的成功结果后,人们开展了一些3期临床试验,直接比较保乳术患者和乳房切除术患者的疗效[240~242]。其中一个比较重要的试验是NSABP B-06研究[234]。这项试验开始于1976年,入组了1 843名患者。T1或T2、N0或N1、M0、乳腺肿瘤≤4cm的患者被随机分到3个治疗组中:①改良根治术;②肿块切除术加腋窝淋巴结清扫术;或③肿块切除术加腋窝清扫术,随后进行放疗。这项试验随访了20年,结果显示保乳治疗与乳房切除术的生存相当。

保乳治疗的禁忌证

原发肿瘤不能通过肿块切除术成功切除的早期乳腺癌患者不适合保乳治疗。例如,存在弥散的可疑钙化,无法采用美容效果较好的肿块切除术的患者最好接受乳房切除术治疗。与之相似,对于保乳术中反复尝试均无法获得阴性手术切缘的患者,最好也行乳房切除术。然而,越来越多的情况是,Ⅱ期和Ⅲ期的乳腺癌患者可以接受新辅助化疗或激素治疗,并且超过50%的患者其原发肿瘤的收缩足以实现保乳术。患者不适合进行保乳术的第二个原因是其为放疗并发症的高危患者。这类患者具体的例子包括曾经接受过放疗的患者、怀孕女性及某些结缔组织病患者。对于处于怀孕早期的女性,完整乳腺的照射所导致的体内辐射散射(internal radiation scatter)能够达到致死和致畸的剂量水平[243]。某些胶原血管病(collagen vascular diseases),如系统性硬皮病(systemic scleroderma)、多发性肌炎(polymyositis)、皮肌炎(dermatomyositis)、红斑狼疮(lupus erythematosus)及混合性结缔组织病(mixed-connective tissue disorders)都与明显的风险相关,包括乳房纤维化(breast fibrosis)和疼痛、胸壁坏死(chest wall necrosis)和臂丛神经病变(brachial plexopathy)[244]。

放射治疗

一个世纪以来,放射治疗在乳腺癌的有效治疗中起着至关重要的作用。从过去的辅助性放疗到20世纪70年代放射治疗使得保乳术能够革命性的取代根治性,放射肿瘤学家和外科医生组成了第一个"多学科"癌症团队。绝大多数乳腺癌患者会在治疗的某个阶段接受放疗。因此,在乳腺癌诊断时,放射肿瘤学家必须和乳腺外科医生、肿瘤内科医生一起制订患者的个体化治疗方案。目前,放射治疗处于技术高速发展之中,也在循证医学和个性化治疗的平衡方面产生了一些挑战和争议。

浸润性乳腺癌保乳术后放疗的作用

确定放疗在保乳治疗中的作用一直是过去30余年来许多前瞻性随机临床试验的焦点[241,242]。总体而言,这些试验显示保乳术后放疗明显改善了局部控制,使以后的远处复发风险降至最低,并减少乳腺癌死亡率。

NSABP B-06是第一个评估肿瘤切除术后放疗益处的随机研究。这项试验显示,对于接受保乳术治疗的患者,放疗提供了显著的临床获益。20年后,只接受肿块切除术的患者乳腺部位的复发率为40%,与之相比,接受肿块切除术加放疗的患者复发率为14%。复发风险降低了几乎2/3,这与其他类似设计的试验所观察到的下降非常相似[234]。早期乳腺癌试验协作组(EBCTCG)对NSABPB-06和其他前瞻性临床试验(评估放疗对浸润性乳腺癌患者接受保乳术治疗的作用)的数据进行了分析。这项重要的荟萃分析研究了来自7 300名女性的患者个体资料。肿块切除术后进行乳腺放疗使淋巴结阴性患者10年的乳腺内复发率(in-breast recurrence)由29%降低至10%,淋巴结阳性患者的复发率由47%降低至13%。更重要的是,放疗的应用使死于乳腺癌的15年风险明显降低。对于淋巴结阴性的患者,乳腺癌的死亡率由31%减少到26%;对于淋巴结阳性的患者,则由55%减少到48%[242]。

全乳照射后瘤床加量

在WBRT后进一步减少局部复发的策略是通过增加术后对瘤床中风险最高的组织来增加放射剂量来实现的。第一项在5 000cGy WBRT后进行1 000cGy瘤床加量的随机试验在法国里昂进行。瘤床加量使得5年时局部复发率得到了具有统计学差异的小幅降低(3.6%对4.5%,$P=0.04$)[245]。随后,EORTC完成了一项更大规模的试验,随机分组超过5 000例患者为5 000cGy WBRT,有或没有额外的1 600cGy瘤床加量。该试验再次表明,瘤床加量能使10年复发率降低(10.2% vs 6.2%,$P<0.001$)[246]。在亚组分析中,所有年龄段都有这种益处,但在年轻女性中最为明显。

适宜人群的放疗选择

尽管荟萃分析和像NSABP B-06这样的大型试验提供了决定性的数据,即放疗对于大多数接受保乳手术的患者是有益的,但是关于亚组患者是否只接受保乳手术就能取得很好的疗效,人们仍然很感兴趣。因此,一些试验将入选标准限定为疾病特征更为有利的患者。意大利米兰(Milan,Italy)的研究者进行了一项试验,以评估小肿瘤切除且具有广泛阴性切缘之后是否需要放疗。在这项研究中,肿瘤≤2.5cm 的患者被随机分为接受象限切除术(quadrantectomy)加腋窝清扫术和上述手术加乳腺放疗。试验的 10 年结果显示放疗将乳腺复发率由 24%减少到 6%(P<0.001)[247]。Ⅰ期患者代表了潜在有利的另外一组患者。在这些患者中,一项瑞典试验的数据显示放疗使五年乳腺复发率由 18%减少到 2%(P<0.000 1)[248]。芬兰(Finland)的一项相似的随机试验将研究对象限定于Ⅰ期且阴性切缘≥1cm 的患者,也发现放疗将乳腺复发由 14.1%减少到 6.2%,P=0.029[248,249]。

试验数据也已显示系统治疗(化疗或他莫昔芬)的使用不会消除乳腺放疗的必要性。在 NSABP B-06 试验中,淋巴结阳性的患者均接受化疗,当这部分患者未使用放疗时,20 年的乳腺复发率为 44%;而当使用放疗时,复发率则为 9%[234]。苏格兰(Scotland)的一项随机试验要求所有患者都接受系统治疗,589 名入组患者中接近 75%接受他莫昔芬作为唯一的系统治疗。在这项试验中,手术、系统治疗、放疗组的 6 年乳腺复发率为 6%,而在随机分入到手术加系统治疗不行放疗的患者中,复发率则为 25%[250]。

四项更近一些的试验已经进一步界定了选择标准[215,216,251,252]。在所有这 4 项试验中,尽管一些只接受手术治疗的亚组患者复发率相对较低,放疗对于乳腺复发的减少均具有统计学意义。NSABP B-21 试验只入组淋巴结阳性且原发肿瘤≤1cm 的患者。所有的患者都接受了肿块切除术和腋窝淋巴结清扫术,被随机分为单用他莫昔芬、单用放疗或他莫昔芬加放疗[249]。加拿大试验具有非常相似的入选标准和结果。最后,CALGB/Intergroup 研究将焦点集中到年龄超过 70 岁的有利的早期乳腺癌患者。在后 2 项试验中,ER 阳性接受他莫昔芬治疗的患者复发率低。在 CALGB 试验中,单用他莫昔芬和他莫昔芬加放疗的 10 年复发率分别为 10%和 2%[215]。两组间全乳切除术、远处转移和总生存率并无差异。类似设计的 Scottish PRIMEⅡ临床研究入组了 1 300 名 65 岁以上的早期乳腺癌患者,单用他莫昔芬和他莫昔芬加放疗的 5 年复发率分别为 4%和 1%(P=0.000 2)[216]。

总之,几乎所有的临床研究迄今为止都已显示保乳术后乳腺放疗减少局部复发,因此应该被认为是所有早期浸润性乳腺癌患者治疗的标准组成部分。到目前为止,关于早期乳腺癌患者可能不需要放疗的亚组界定,除了年龄大于 70 岁、淋巴结阴性、ER 阳性、适合他莫昔芬治疗的女性,大部分尝试都是失败的。在这组患者中,关于是否使用放疗的决定,应该基于患者的寿命和偏好。

放疗作为淋巴结阳性早期乳腺癌患者腋窝淋巴结清扫的替代品

在钼靶诊断、全身治疗和前哨淋巴结活检等技术的支持下,人们对腋窝淋巴结阴性或者少数前哨淋巴结阳性的患者免除腋窝淋巴结清扫越来越感兴趣。减少腋窝淋巴结清扫尤其对于需要放疗的患者尤为重要,因为腋窝淋巴结清扫手术和放疗联合应用会造成更高的淋巴水肿风险并影响生活质量(quality of life,QOL)。之前的 ACOSOG Z0011 试验证实对于将进行全乳放疗的保乳术患者,1~2 枚前哨淋巴结阳性时,腋窝淋巴结清扫并不能改善患者 5 年无病生存率或总生存率[233]。EORTC 10981-22023(AMAROS)研究分析了一个类似的患者人群,包括有两个以上阳性淋巴结(5%)的患者和接受过乳房切除术的患者(18%)[253]。超过 1 400 名 SNLB 阳性的患者随机接受腋窝淋巴结清扫术或腋窝放疗,随访 6 年两组间腋窝复发无统计学差异。尽管由于事件总数较低,试验的说服力不足,但接受腋窝淋巴结清扫的患者上肢淋巴水肿的发生率明显较高。这两项试验结合在一起,对早期淋巴结阳性患者的局部治疗的指南产生了广泛影响,使得更多患者能够免于乳腺癌根治术。鉴于腋窝复发常见于 2 年内[234,254],这两项研究的长期随访也未必会改变临床实践。

乳腺切除术后放疗

对于经过选择的乳腺癌患者,将放疗和乳房切除术的有利作用结合起来具有很强的理论基础。探索乳腺切除术后放疗的最初的研究开始于 20 世纪 50 年代,并且代表了肿瘤学历史上一些最早的对照临床试验。因此,在经过 50 余年的研究后,关于乳腺切除术后放疗(postmastectomy radiation)的价值和合适的应用选择标准,依然存在很大的争议,这多少有些令人感到吃惊。这种持续的不确定性是由许多因素促使而成的。随着时间的推移,发生的第二个改变是加入了化疗作为常规治疗的组成部分。这一改变是重要的,因为它降低了远处转移的风险,并借此改善了局部区域控制,从而改善了患者的生存。

现代乳腺切除术后放疗的试验

3 项较新的随机试验对乳腺切除术后放疗进行了研究,这 3 项试验所发表的文献均被 EBCTCG 的荟萃分析所采用。EBCTCG 能够从 PMRT 的每项随机前瞻性试验中获得原始数据,包括近 10 000 例在乳房切除术和腋窝清扫后随机接受放疗与观察的病例。对于淋巴结阳性患者,PMRT 将局部复发风险降低到 1/3(从 29%到 8%),导致 15 年乳腺癌死亡率(从 60%到 55%)绝对降低 5%。对于淋巴结阴性的患者,局部区域受益较小(从 8%到 3%),但生存率差异无收益[242]。总体而言,该荟萃分析的数据表明,长期生存获益仅表现在 5 年局部区域控制改善 10%的试验[242]。因此,有明确的迹象表明 PMRT 在清除手术后的镜下肿瘤残留,防止其成为远处转移的来源,避免其最终导致患者死亡。

试验结果为放疗的潜在获益提供了新的见解,但也进一步引起了有关其应用的争议。更重要的是,所有这 3 项试验都使用了更加现代的放疗技术,而且所有的患者都接受了系统治疗。丹麦乳腺癌协作组(Danish Breast Cancer Coopera tive Group,DBCCG)82b 试验或许是这 3 项试验中最重要的一个。1 708 例Ⅱ期或Ⅲ期的绝经前乳腺癌患者随机分为乳腺切除术后进行 9 周期 CMF 化疗,或乳腺切除术、放疗和 8 周期 CMF 化疗两组。放疗范围包括胸壁和引流淋巴管(包括内乳淋巴结),总剂量 50Gy(分 25 次完成),并使用电子线在心脏上方的区域进行照射,以使心血管组织的受量降至最低[255]。大部分入组的患者为 1~3 个阳性淋巴结。但是,这项试验的大部分患者没有接受正规的腋窝Ⅰ、Ⅱ水平淋巴结清扫。切除的腋窝淋巴结的中位数只有7个，只有24%的患者切除了10个或10个以上的淋巴结，有15%的患者只切除了3个或更少的淋巴结。这项试验最显著的发现是随机分入放疗组的患者总生存率提高（10年生存率分别为54%和45%，$P<0.001$）。这种生存优势可能是接受放疗的患者局部区域复发率减少的结果（9% vs 32%，$P<0.001$）。同时，加拿大不列颠哥伦比亚省温哥华（Vancouver，British Columbia）的研究者进行了具有类似设计的小规模试验。试验中318例具有阳性淋巴结的患者被随机分为接受乳房切除术和CMF，或乳房切除术、放疗和CMF256。结果与DBCCG非常相似，放疗的应用与总生存（20年生存率分别为47%和37%，$P=0.03$）和局部区域控制（20年局部区域控制率分别为87%和61%，$P<0.0001$）的提高有关。

最后是DBCCG 82c试验，将1300例绝经后患者随机分为乳腺切除术和他莫昔芬，或乳腺切除术、他莫昔芬和放疗[257]。肿瘤的分期和腋窝手术的范围也与82b试验非常相似。82c试验在总生存和局部控制方面的获益程度与前面的两项研究相似。被随机分入接受放疗的患者十年总生存率更为有利（分别为45%和36%，$P=0.03$），局部控制率也是如此（十年局部控制率分别为92%和65%，$P<0.001$）。DBCCG82b &c的综合数据的18年更新继续显示放疗的应用与局部控制率（86% vs 51%，$P<0.0001$）和无远处转移生存率（distant metastasis-free survival）（47% vs 36%，$P<0.0001$）的继续获益有关[258]。

目前乳房切除术后放疗的适应证

约15年前发表的美国临床肿瘤学会（ASCO）PMRT共识指南推荐治疗Ⅲ期疾病患者（定义为原发肿瘤T3伴淋巴结转移，原发肿瘤T4，或有4个或更多淋巴结）[259]乳房切除术、标准腋窝淋巴结清扫术和化疗，使得这些局部晚期患者获得较大生存获益。然而，这一具有里程碑意义的指南却对于PMRT在Ⅱ期伴1~3个阳性淋巴结的患者中作用尚存争议。其原因在于，尽管丹麦和不列颠哥伦比亚省试验中的大多数患者有1~3个阳性淋巴结，但PMRT的意义外科医生提出异议，在较大规模的丹麦研究中标准治疗组中腋窝研究不足。事实上，丹麦试验中这些没有PMRT治疗的患者的长期局部复发率为41%，而在不列颠哥伦比亚省的试验中接受更完全腋窝清扫的类似患者中为21%[256,260]。值得注意的是，腋窝手术不充分可能导致低估了阳性淋巴结的真实数量，并且许多这些患者可能已经有4个或更多淋巴结并已经接受过更广泛的手术。

丹麦和加拿大研究的结果显著影响了ASCO对PMRT的共识指南（2001年出版），也改变了十多年的临床实践模式。最近，EBCTCG于2014年发表的一项荟萃分析试图阐明PMRT对最具争议的患者，即原发性肿瘤较小但伴有1~3个阳性淋巴结的患者的效用[258]。来自22项随机试验的数据，包括超过3700名腋窝淋巴结清扫至第Ⅱ水平后接受PMRT的患者，分析了10年局部复发和20年生存率的差异。对于接受全身治疗的1~3个阳性淋巴结的患者（$n=1133$），PMRT显著减少超过3/4的局部复发（20%~4%，$P<0.0001$），并改善约8%的乳腺癌特异性死亡率（50%~42%，$P=0.01$）。有趣的是，在四个或更多阳性淋巴结的患者的亚组分析中，局部区域复发（32% vs 13%，$P<0.00001$）和乳腺癌死亡率（80% vs 70，$P=0.04$）受益几乎相同。

因此，对于所有淋巴结阳性且预期寿命超过10年的患者，PMRT的效用毫无疑问。除了阳性淋巴结的数量之外，还应该考虑其他不良病理特征，例如淋巴结转移的体积，淋巴结转移的范围以及转移淋巴结的百分比来指导临床决策。总之，EBCTCG的更新[261]以及上述AMAROS试验[253]表明，在腋窝淋巴结清扫的作用逐渐减弱时，PMRT的应用范围正在扩大。对肿瘤生物学和基因组分析的更全面理解可能会在不远的未来进一步指导临床实践中发挥作用。

乳房切除术后放疗与乳房再造相结合

过去十年的两大趋势是选择乳房切除术后放疗的人和接受乳房再造的人越来越多，这两者可能会存在一定的碰撞[262]。虽然基于植入物或组织瓣的乳房重建对放射治疗提出了一定的挑战，但它不应被视为PMRT的禁忌证。虽然整形外科实践模式的变化很大，而且临床经验比随机临床试验更多，但随着时间的推移，也具有一些共同的原则。通常，在需要PMRT的患者中立即重建，最好用基于组织扩张器（tissue expander，TE）/植入物的技术完成[259]。这是最常用的方式，因为它巩固了外科手术程序，并允许通过长达一个月的辅助化疗过程进行全组织扩张。TE可以在PMRT之前换成永久性植入物[263]，或者在PMRT过程中排空以改善放射剂量测定[264]。另外，自体皮瓣技术是延迟重建的首选，其中带血管组织瓣可以改善伤口愈合和美容效果[262]。乳房切除术后的乳房再造对于许多患者治疗后的QOL来说至关重要，但重要的是患者不要因为担心影响重建效果的而改变他们的肿瘤治疗方法，因为重建的美容效果是可以纠正。

新辅助化疗后放疗

改良根治性术后辅助化疗和PMRT已成为局部晚期如乳腺癌患者经典的标准治疗方法。然而，在过去三十年中，新辅助化疗（术前化疗）的使用在分期较晚的患者中显著增加。该方法首先用于无法切除或无法彻底切除的患者，此类患者的初步临床数据表明新辅助化疗可获得较高的肿瘤反应率。随后，在初诊时肿瘤较大的乳腺癌的患者中也应用了这种方法。

新辅助化疗后的保乳治疗

最早的研究化疗和手术顺序的研究是为了判断原发肿瘤较大的乳腺癌能够通过新辅助化疗实现保乳术。为了研究这一点，NSABP和EORTC独立进行临床试验，比较新辅助化疗和辅助化疗对Ⅱ~Ⅲ期乳腺癌患者的影响。虽然两项试验均发现新辅助化疗组的乳房保留率较高[265,266]，但NSABP研究显示，这一增加主要是由于T3疾病化疗后患者保乳率增加了近三倍（22% vs 8%）[264]。对于晚期疾病患者，保乳治疗的目标是同时实现可接受的美容结果和较低的乳房复发风险。因此，对于具有大的原发灶的患者，切除范围需根据化疗后肿瘤床，而不是原发肿瘤的初始体积。然而，仅切除残余疾病的化疗后体积的一个问题是，一些晚期乳腺癌在新辅助化疗的反应中不会向心性缩小到单独的病灶，而是在原发灶的体积内缩小为多个病灶[193]。在这种情况下，针对初始原发灶核心的切除术可能会面临漏掉很多显微病灶的压力，在理论上会增加局部复发风险。

在 NSABP B-18 试验中,接受新辅助化疗的患者与辅助化疗相比在乳腺癌复发率总体上没有统计学差异(16 年复发率分别为 13%和 10%)[267]。然而,对新辅助化疗后进行保乳手术的患者,原发肿瘤较大的患者乳腺癌复发率较高。在接受新辅助化疗的患者中,8 年乳腺局部复发率为 16%,是初诊即符合保乳条件小肿瘤患者的两倍多[264]。其他多中心研究也显示接受新辅助化疗的患者乳腺局部复发率相对较高[268,269]。

与这些数据相比,一项单中心的研究通过谨慎的筛选患者和深度的多学科合作实现了很好的局部控制率。得克萨斯大学 MD 安德森癌症中心的研究人员最近公布了新辅助化疗后行保乳术的最大规模研究之一[267]。在这项研究中,340 名谨慎选择对化疗有良好反应的患者接受了保乳手术和放疗。尽管该研究中有 72%的患者患有临床ⅡB~Ⅲ期疾病,但 5 年和 10 年的乳腺癌复发率分别仅为 5%和 10%。四种肿瘤相关因素与乳腺癌复发和局部复发有关:淋巴结临床分期 N2 或 N3、淋巴血管区域浸润、残余病灶的多灶分布及直径高于 2cm 的残留疾病[270]。研究者随后制订了相应的预后指数,对于指数为 0 或 1 的患者,保乳术将提供与乳房切除术和放射治疗相似的效果。然而,对于具有 3 个或 3 个以上不良因素的患者乳房切除术联合放射治疗将获取更低的局部复发风险[271]。

新辅助化疗后乳腺切除术后放疗

对接受新辅助治疗的患者在乳腺切除术后进行放疗的指征和疗效进行研究的数据很少。对于首先接受乳腺切除术治疗的患者,主要是根据病变范围决定放疗。这是因为临床和影像对原发肿瘤的大小和淋巴结受累数目的评估是不准确的。显然,新辅助化疗改变了 80%~90%的患者的病理程度,而且有研究发现,乳腺切除术后肿瘤的病理程度与局部区域复发之间的联系,在接受新辅助化疗的患者中和在首先接受手术治疗的患者中是不同的[268]。这些数据提示我们,对于接受新辅助化疗和乳腺切除术的患者,在评估其局部区域复发风险时,不论是术前的临床分期,还是化疗后病理上确定的残余肿瘤的范围,都应该考虑在内。事实上,在对接受新辅助化疗、乳腺切除术而未行放疗的患者的分析中,局部复发预测因素的多变量分析发现,术前和术后因素都与局部区域复发独立相关[272]。对于接受新辅助化疗和乳腺切除术的患者,放疗在减少局部区域复发方面的作用,尚未经过前瞻性随机试验的评估。不过,有一项前瞻性试验对比了 579 例接受新辅助化疗、乳腺切除术和放疗的患者和 136 例只接受新辅助化疗和乳腺切除术的患者[273]。放疗在这部分人群中并不是随机给予的,而且两组的预后因素存在显著的不平衡。总体而言,与不接受放疗的患者相比,接受放疗的患者病变更为广泛,疾病特征较差。除此之外,术后放疗的患者与仅接受新辅助化疗和手术的患者相比,局部复发率显著降低(10 年局部区域复发率分别为 8%和 22%,$P=0.001$)。在临床 T4、ⅢB/C 期的患者及化疗后阳性淋巴结≥4 个的患者亚组中,局部区域复发率的绝对改善为 30%~40%。放疗在同样亚组中的应用能够将总生存和病因特异性生存(cause-specific survival)改善 15%~20%。随后只针对术后放疗组中达到病理完全缓解的患者进行分析,放疗降低了临床Ⅲ期患者的局部区域复发率(33% vs 7%,$P=0.04$)[274]。

对于在化疗后仍然具有阳性淋巴结的临床Ⅱ期患者,是否使用化疗尚不清楚。有研究报道了 132 例临床Ⅱ期的患者,这些患者在新辅助化疗和乳房切除术后均未行放疗,显示临床 T3N0 或具有≥4 个阳性淋巴结的患者局部区域复发率较高[275]。余下的患者中 5 年局部复发率小于 10%。新辅助化疗后具有 1~3 个阳性淋巴结的临床Ⅱ期患者,5 年局部区域复发率为 8%。重要的一点是要认识到这项研究的样本量较小,研究人群容易出现选择偏倚,因为她们只代表治疗医师为其选择不使用放疗的患者。

基于可以获得的数据,推荐在初始诊断时即对临床Ⅲ期的患者在乳腺切除术后进行放疗时合理的。对于化疗后具有≥4 个阳性淋巴结的临床Ⅰ期或Ⅱ期患者,或疾病进展导致原发肿瘤超过 5cm 的患者,假定其局部区域复发的风险较高且应接受放疗,也是合理的。对于新辅助化疗后具有 1~3 个阳性淋巴结的临床Ⅰ期或Ⅱ期患者,目前尚不知道放疗是否能够使之获益[276]。美国两项正在进行的前瞻性随机试验正在对这两个难题进行研究。NSABP B-51 试验通过入组病理证实的淋巴结阳性并在新辅助化疗后转为淋巴结阴性的患者。然后将患者随机分配到 WBRT,有或没有腋窝淋巴结放疗或 PMRT 对比切除术后观察[277]。Alliance A011202 试验入组类似患者,将化疗后淋巴结仍为阳性患者随机分配到腋窝淋巴结清扫术与 PMRT 治疗两组[278]。

放射治疗的细节

乳腺癌治疗野的计划和设计以及放射治疗的实施都是至关重要的,需要现代的设备,并要求注重细节。显然,放射治疗能够导致正常组织的严重损伤,甚至引起危及生命的放射性损伤,而这些都能够通过现代治疗技术得以避免或使之减至最低。我们已经在放射肿瘤学领域取得了许多最新进展,这些进展可以直接为乳腺癌患者带来益处。其中一个重要的进展是使用三维成像技术辅助靶区设计。计算机断层扫描模拟定向[computered tomography(CT)-based simulation]技术允许放射肿瘤学家采集患者治疗部位的 CT 图像,并在其 CT 图像上设计治疗野,因此可以更好地显示靶区和希望避免正常组织,例如心脏。图 108-20 显示的是左侧Ⅰ期乳腺癌在乳房肿块切除术后进行放疗的治疗野设计图例。在这幅图像中,放疗医师在患者本人的 CT 片上对瘤床进行勾画,并进行图像重建。乳腺治疗使用的是内侧切线定向线束,射线在照射野边缘可以深达中线附近,并横向穿过前胸,从腋中线附近穿出。外侧切线线束(lateral tangent beam)与治疗野相对,这样当射线穿过乳腺时,可以调整乳腺内剂量的跌落,并最终形成均匀的剂量分布。其他令人感兴趣的区域,例如腋窝淋巴结、内乳链(internal mammary chain)或锁骨上窝,也可以这样勾画以显示其相对于治疗野边界的解剖位置。图 108-21 显示的内侧切线线束的射野方向观(beam eyeview),内侧切线线束用于治疗乳腺(包括瘤床)、上部内乳淋巴结及Ⅰ水平和部分Ⅱ水平的腋窝。

第二个主要进展是三维剂量计算系统(three dimensional dose calculation systems)的发展,这个系统可以在整个三维治疗区(three dimensional treatment volume)上更精确地计算和显示 CT 图像上的剂量。最后,现代治疗工具也使得我们可以在三维空间上进行剂量调整。这样调整的目的是提供均匀的剂量分布,使正常组织的受量高于处方剂量(prescribed dose)的风

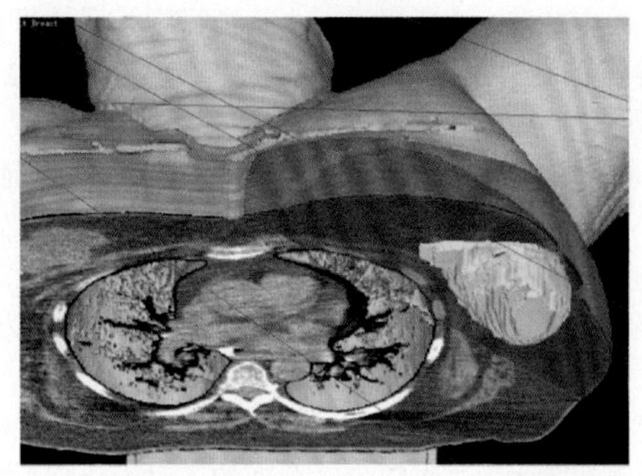

图 108-20　用于左侧浸润性乳腺癌治疗的照射野横断面图像。红色阴影区域代表包含入照射野的区域。黄色实心区域代表瘤床，通过在连续计算机断层扫描片上对这一区域进行勾画实现瘤床重建。使用两个相对的治疗野：内侧切线野——斜向进入乳房内侧并从乳房外侧穿出——与之相对的是外侧切线野。当射线穿过组织时会出现放射剂量的跌落，两野相对以调整剂量的跌落

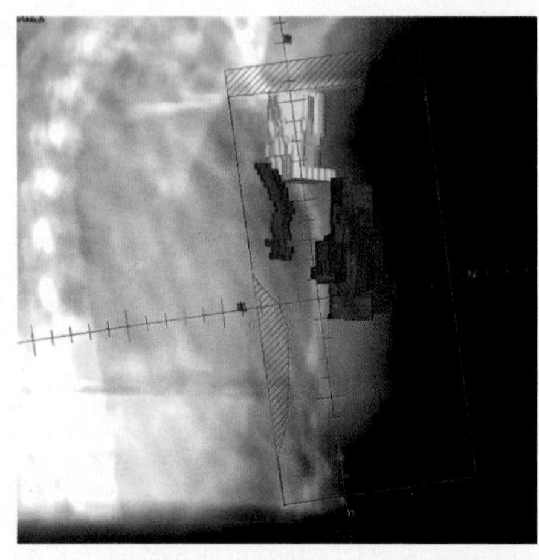

图 108-21　内侧切线野的射野方向观。内侧切线野的设计应该包括乳房、腋窝下部、和内乳淋巴结链的上部。图中显示的是瘤床(红色)、内乳淋巴结区域的上部(蓝色)和腋窝下部(黄色)的重建轮廓

险及靶区受量低于处方剂量的风险降至最低。在乳腺癌的放射治疗中，治疗计划过程是最初至关重要的一步。让患者取仰卧位，手臂置于外展外旋位，固定患者的体位。然后进行 CT 扫描，获得用于治疗计划的图像。在患者乳腺的皮肤上画出定位线(reference mark)。在治疗计划过程中，放疗医师对治疗野进行设计，并使剂量分布达到最佳，这个过程通常需要 2~3 天，不需要患者的参与。在完成计划后，开始进行每日治疗，通常需要每日在治疗室治疗 15min。治疗是没有疼痛的。最常见的疗程需要治疗 25~28 次，乳房或胸壁每日照射 180~200cGy，包括或不包括存在风险的淋巴引流区。上述疗程后通常给予 6~8 次补充治疗，在瘤床区域每日照射 180~200cGy(经常称为瘤床或胸壁推量)。每周治疗 5 天，总共治疗 6~6.5 周。这种在较长时间内每天提供最低生物有效剂量的策略适用于单纯切除术后或乳腺癌切除术后的患者(包括或不包括区域淋巴结清扫)，被称为传统分割放射治疗(CFRT)。

早期乳腺癌的放疗新方法

一些早期乳腺癌患者接受保乳手术治疗，并不接受其后的放射治疗；还有许多非常适合保乳治疗的患者为了避免放疗而选择接受乳房切除手术。导致这两种情况的一个主要原因是考虑到与外照射(external beam radiation)相关的不便和费用。早期乳腺癌的常规外照射治疗通常需要 5~7 周 CFRT。这种安排对于需要在交通上花费数小时才能到达放疗机构的患者而言是尤其沉重的。此外，全世界能为早期乳腺癌患者提供这种治疗方案的机构和设备还太少。

由于这些和其他的原因，人们正在研究许多策略以缩短放疗时间和减轻经济负担。最简单的策略是高分割放射治疗(HFRT)，即增加每次治疗的放射量，使整个治疗过程减少一半左右。随着每部分放射量的增加，所提供的总剂量也相应地向下调整，以提供与 CFRT 剂量相同的放射生物学特性。HFRT 大型随机试验结果见表 108-8。

1986 年，Royal Marsden 医院开展了一项临床试验，其中约 1 500 名患者随机接受 CFRT 治疗，与两种 HFRT 治疗方案中的一种方案进行对比[284]。这一结果导致了英国乳腺放射治疗标准化试验小组的建立，该小组开展了两项随机试验，对大约 4 500 名患有早期乳腺癌的妇女进行 CFRT 和 HFRT 的比较。在 START A 试验的 HFRT 组中，285 名患者在 5 周内接受了 4 160cGy 或 3 900Gy 的 13 个分量的治疗，而在 START B 组中，287 名患者在 3 周内接受了 15 个分量的 4 050cGy 的治疗。长期随访 10 年结果表明，HFRT 是一种安全有效的治疗早期乳腺癌的方法[284,286,288]。在同一时间在加拿大，Whelan 和其同事开展了一项随机试验，在 1 000 名早期乳腺癌且淋巴结阴性的女性行 HFRT，经过 10 年随访，两组的局部控制、生存或乳房美容没有区别[283,287]。

缩短治疗总时间的第二个策略是使照射的乳房体积最小化从而给予更高剂量的照射。这项策略的合理之处在于因原发肿瘤较小而接受肿块切除术的患者，在肿块切除术后或肿瘤在 2cm 以内时，80%的患者是没有肿瘤残存的[289]。部分乳腺照射(partial breast irradiation)的 5 年随访或更长时间的结果数据，大部分是来源于探索以组织间近距离放射治疗(interstitial brachytherapy)作为唯一的放疗剂量给予方式的研究。对于这种治疗方式，医师通常需要以手术的方式为患者放置导管以在瘤床周围形成 2~2.5cm 的空间，然后在导管内暂时放置高剂量率放射粒子(high-dose-rate radioactive seeds)，每日两次，共放置 5 天。到目前为止，在小规模前瞻性和随机化的研究中，采用该方法对具有良好疾病特征的高选择性患者进行 10 年的预后数据非常好[290,291]。然而，其他研究者已经注意到，与常规的乳房外照射相比，这种方法的临床脂肪坏死率更高，疗效更差。使用球囊近距离治疗的结果数据也很好，美国乳腺外科医生协会(ASBS)注册中心对大约 1 500 名患者进行的研究显示，5 年内乳房复发的风险为 4%[294]。由于在单独的外科手术中放置近距离治疗导管有其自身的风险，因此已有其他的 APBI 辐射方法。三维适形外束 APBI 可利用其复杂的非侵入性方法达到和近距离放射同样的良好效果[293]。

表 108-8　比较常规分次放疗(CFRT)与次分次放疗(HFRT)的部分随机临床试验结果

试验	平均随访时间/年	N	剂量/cGy	#分割	IBTR[a]/%	LRR[a]/%	DFS[a]/%	OS[a]/%	美观效果(好和极好)/%	急性毒性反应(3 级以上)
Canada[283]	10	612	5 000	25	6.7	—	—	84	71.3	3.0
		622	4 250	16	6.2	—	—	85	69.8	3.0
Royal Marsden[284]	10	470	5 000	25	12	—	—	—	71	—
		466	4 290	13	9.6	—	—	—	74	—
		474	3 900	13	15	—	—	—	58[b]	—
START A[285,286]	9	749	5 000	25	6.7	7.4	77	80	—	0.3
		750	4 160	13	5.6	6.3	77	82	—	0.0
		737	3 900	13	8.1	8.8	76	80	—	0.0
START B[286,287]	10	1 105	5 000	25	5.2	5.5	78	81	—	1.2
		1 110	4 050	15	3.8	4.3	82[c]	84[c]	—	0.3

N,患者人数;IBTR,乳腺癌内肿瘤复发;LRR,局部复发;DFS,无病生存;OS,总生存期。
[a]除非另有说明,否则所有统计 P 值在 CFRT 与 HFRT 的比较中均无意义。
[b]测量值在统计学上不如 CFRT($P<0.05$)。
[c]测量值在统计学上优于 CFRT($P<0.05$)。

综上所述,这些数据表明,APBI 需要在一个大的随机前瞻性试验中进行补充研究,并严格保证质量,以确保适当的标准化和体积目标覆盖率。为了解决这一问题,NSABP 和 RTOG 在十年前联合赞助了一项Ⅲ期试验(NSABP B-39/RTOG 0413),对 4 000 多名 0、Ⅰ、Ⅱ期乳腺癌患者随机进行 CFRT 或 APBI(近距离治疗或外照射)[21]。本研究在达到预期结果后,于 2013 年结束,这可能是数十年来最有效的乳腺放疗研究。

APBI 的另一种方案已经在三期临床试验中与 CFRT 进行了比较,该方案使用专门的设备在肿瘤切除时将可扩张球囊放置于瘤床腔内,这样就可以在球囊中心插入高剂量率放射源。迄今为止发表的最大的Ⅲ期 APBI 试验(TARGIT-A)随机选择 2 200 多名绝经后早期乳腺癌患者接受 CFRT 或单剂量术中放疗(2 000cGy to The tissue-applicator interface)[296]。4 年后,每组局部复发的风险相同(1%),尽管 15%的手术内患者因术后不良病理发现接受了额外的乳房照射。在这样一项控制良好的大型研究中,对接受术中 APBI 治疗的部分早期患者所看到的良好结果,可能如同 NSABP B-39/RTOG 0413 最终预期结果一样。考虑到这一点,ASTRO 制订了使用 APBI 的共识标准,以帮助选择目前适合这些选择的患者[297]。虽然有待提高,但这些准则只是在 B-39 的结果可用之前提供临床使用指导。

与此同时,研究人员正在开发更多的新技术,如立体定向消融放疗,以扩大 APBI 的范围,使其侵入性更低,甚至更少的治疗[298,299]。随着未来的发展,APBI 作为其多种形式之一,将越来越多地成为对特定的早期乳腺癌进行改良治疗的一种方法。

乳腺癌放射治疗的并发症

乳腺癌的现代放射治疗相对耐受性良好,发生长期并发症的概率低。放疗所引起的并发症包括急性反应(acute effect)或晚期反应(late effect)。急性反应通常是在治疗期间或在治疗后立即发生,大部分具有自限性。与乳腺或乳房切除术后放疗相关的常见急性反应包括治疗相关的疲劳和放射性皮炎。早期乳腺癌患者这些反应通常相对较轻,能够继续工作,进行日常生活和活动。

治疗后的晚期反应相对少见,尤其对于因早期乳腺癌或 DCIS 接受保乳手术的患者。对于这部分患者,最常见的晚期反应是乳腺美容的改变。肿块切除术和乳房放疗之后的美容效果受到技术、患者体型、系统治疗的使用以及手术范围的影响。在接受保乳手术和放疗的患者中,有 70%~85%认为其美容效果良好或极佳[300,301]。

局部区域治疗所导致的其他更为常见的并发症是淋巴水肿。腋窝Ⅰ、Ⅱ水平淋巴结清扫后,对锁骨上窝和腋顶(axillary apex)进行照射会使淋巴水肿的概率加倍,从 8%~10%(只手术)升高到 15%~20%。如果对腋窝Ⅲ水平进行淋巴结清扫,或者锁骨下窝或锁骨上窝存在未切除的受累淋巴结,需要对这一区域进行更高剂量的放疗,在这种情况下,淋巴水肿的概率会进一步升高。其他促使淋巴水肿的患者相关因素包括肥胖和同侧手臂之后受伤或感染。

接受放射治疗的乳腺癌患者理论上也有发展为肺毒性的风险,因为标准切向场掠过一小部分同侧肺组织,因为胸部的自然弯曲和乳房处于仰卧位。人们普遍认为肺组织对辐射很敏感,即使是最小的剂量也超过了耐受范围[302]。因此,通常的策略是使用三维规划、强度调节和/或俯卧位,以尽量减少暴露在处方剂量下的肺的体积。在现代化放疗技术治疗下,放射性肺炎的发展或整个乳房辐射后随之而来的临床显著纤维化是非常罕见的[300,303]。

臂丛损伤是治疗局部晚期乳腺癌时需要局部淋巴结照射而产生的问题。使用 CFRT,臂丛的剂量应保持在理论剂量阈值以下(通常 4 500~5 000cGy),6 000~6 500cGy 辐射 5 年导致损伤风险为 5%。如果患者在锁骨上窝有严重的疾病,剂量增加接近或超过这个阈值是必要的,而且应仔细注意臂丛的位置和剂量。在这种情况下,肿瘤直接侵犯引起的臂丛损伤的风险远远超过医源性损伤。

心血管并发症已经成为与乳腺癌放疗相关的最重要的问题,受到长期关注。显然,如果下方的心血管系统受到高剂量照射,乳腺癌的放射治疗能够导致严重的心血管相关死亡[304]。与早期的放射技术相比,乳腺癌的现代放射治疗与心血管并发症和死亡率减少有关。在丹麦的术后放疗试验中,专门使用电子束技术治疗胸壁以使心脏结构的受量达到最小。在中位随访117个月后,大约1 500名被随机为接受放疗的患者,与1 500名随机为不接受放疗的患者相比,死亡率或心脏相关的住院日数未增加[305]。Vallis等对加拿大研究的分析显示了相似的并发症和死亡率。对接受放疗作为保乳治疗组成部分的2 128例患者进行长期随访,患者的中位随访时间超过10年,作者发现左侧乳腺癌的患者与右侧相比,心血管的并发症并未增加[306]。最近,一篇报道分析了右侧乳腺癌患者SEER的数据,发现在20世纪70年代,对于接受放疗的乳腺癌患者,左侧患病比右侧患病的心血管死亡增加。但是,20世纪80年代和90年代治疗的患者中未见死亡增加[307]。

总之,在乳腺癌放疗中没有真正的"安全"心脏辐射剂量,而且必须评估其风险和与当前治疗相关的全身细胞毒性和心脏毒性风险。现代放射治疗应该是安全而有效的。为了确保使放疗相关的并发症达到最少,治疗的技术和设备是重要的。

早期乳腺癌的系统治疗

乳腺癌是一种复杂的异质性疾病,临床表现和预后各不相同。当患者被诊断为早期乳腺癌(ESBC)后,她应该接受多学科的治疗。遗憾的是,20%~30%被诊断为ESBC的妇女最终会复发并伴有远处转移[308]。

当患者被诊断为ESBC后,治疗会受到临床病理指标的影响。临床因素如年龄、月经状况、肿瘤大小、淋巴结状况,以及病理因素如肿瘤分级、生物标志物和增殖率等,被用来确定癌症的侵袭性并指导选择治疗方案。由免疫组化和原位杂交(ISH)染色法确定的肿瘤生物标志物表达状态,以此将乳腺癌分为三种主要类型,这三种类型可以预测患者预后及对特定治疗的反应。乳腺癌的主要类型为激素受体阳性型、HER2过表达型和三阴性乳腺癌。

HR+乳腺癌阳性表达雌激素受体和孕激素受体,目前的标准检测方法为IHC。ER是一种配体调节的转录因子,通过对细胞增殖的影响,是HR+乳腺癌发生的主要驱动力。ER和PR与雌激素具有高亲和力的相互结合,导致构象改变,进入细胞核。这种激素受体复合物与雌激素特异性反应元件结合,激发或抑制基因表达。当ER或PR与抗雌激素结合时,促生长基因被阻断。ER或PR的存在与内分泌治疗的反应性有关。

免疫组化可以在新鲜或冰冻的组织或细胞学标本上进行。ER和PR表达状态因肿瘤不同而异。ASCO/美国病理学家学院(CAP)指南建议将HR阳性定义为肿瘤细胞中ER或PR的阳性率≥1%,因为肿瘤细胞表达ER或PR的阳性率<1%的患者对内分泌治疗有显著的疗效反应[309]。60%~80%的乳腺癌标本表达ER。

15%~20%的乳腺癌过度表达HER2,这些患者中约50%也同时是HR+。HER2癌基因编码具有细胞内酪氨酸激酶活性的跨膜糖蛋白受体。HER2受体是EGFR受体家族的成员之一,参与激活信号转导通路,调控正常和恶性乳腺上皮细胞的生长和分化。HER2过表达可预测此类患者对特定化疗和HER2靶向治疗反应的预后。

最近的ASCO/CAP指南推荐所有ESBC患者或转移性乳腺癌(MBC)患者都可以通过有效的HER2检测来评估HER2的表达状态[310]。HER2表达状态可通过免疫组化法测定HER2膜蛋白的表达,或用ISH[荧光原位杂交(FISH)、显色性ISH或双原位杂交(DISH)]检测*HER2*基因扩增。FISH既可以用单探针检测HER2,也可以用双探针检测HER2和着丝粒17(CEP17)。

当膜染色状态为3+时,免疫组化法此乳腺癌定义为HER2阳性(≥10%的肿瘤细胞有完整而强烈的膜染色)[308]。IHC(0~1)为HER2阴性(HER2-),IHC(2+)为模棱两可,应进行FISH检测。FISH检测结果中当HER2与CEP17之比为>2.0,或虽然HER2与CEP17之比<2.0,但平均每个细胞中的HER2拷贝数>6.0时,将乳腺癌定义为HER2阳性。HER2与CEP17之比<2和/或平均每个细胞中的HER2拷贝数<4时阴性,HER2与CEP17之比<2和/或平均每个细胞中的HER2拷贝数介于4.0~6.0个时为可疑,应进行免疫组化。如果结果与其他组织病理学发现不一致,应考虑重复检查。

根据定义,TNBC缺乏IHC染色下ER、PR、HER2的表达和FISH检测中HER2的扩增。ASCO/CAP指南将HR-定义为在适当的外部和内部对照染色的情况下,肿瘤细胞的免疫组化染色阳性细胞<1%[311]。ASCO/CAP指南将IHC或FISH检测中非扩增性的HER2定义为HER2 0~1+[308]。

乳腺癌复发的年危险率在初次治疗后的头几年最高,在3~5年达到峰值,并在7或8年后下降到稳定状态。然而,复发模式因乳腺癌亚型而异。HR+ESBC的远处复发率在诊断后的前5年高达50%,但在接下来的15年间,复发率和/或死亡率每年增加0.5%~3%。相比之下,TNBC的ROR在确诊的前3年内最高,但此后风险迅速下降,只有很少的复发发生在5年后。即使考虑到年龄、种族、分期、肿瘤大小、淋巴结状态、种族和治疗方案,TNBC的OS明显差于HR+乳腺癌(HR=2.72,95%CI:2.39~3.10,P<0.000 1)[309]。与HER2-的ESBC相比,HER2+ESBC具有更具侵袭性的临床进程,复发和OS的时间更短。随着HER2靶向单克隆抗体曲妥珠单抗(trastuzumab)的出现,其疾病自然史显著改善,复发率降低了50%,OS增加了约30%。然而,HER2+ESBC的预后也依赖于激素受体的状态,HR+/HER2+ESBC对内分泌治疗的反应降低就证明了这一点。

ESBC的最佳治疗包括局部治疗和全身治疗的结合。全身疗法主要用于降低侵袭性疾病患者远处复发的风险,但内分泌疗法在减少局部复发和对侧原发肿瘤方面都非常有效。HR+疾病的治疗使用以下几种药物之一,包括SERM他莫昔芬、芳香化酶抑制剂以及使用促性腺激素释放激素激动剂(GnRHa)以抑制绝经前妇女的卵巢功能,无论是否进行化疗。化疗是TNBC的主要全身治疗方法,与曲妥珠单抗合用可治疗HER2+乳腺癌。

针对ESBC的靶向生物治疗的研究正在积极开展。总的来说，在 MBC 的治疗中，与标准治疗相比，生物靶向治疗药物与标准治疗药物联合使用显示出更高的疗效。此类药物包括 HER2 靶向单克隆抗体和口服酪氨酸激酶抑制剂、环磷酰胺依赖性激酶 4/6（CDK4/6）抑制剂或结合内分泌治疗的 PI3K 抑制剂，以及逆转肿瘤免疫耐受的免疫治疗。有关这些试验的详细信息可访问 http://www.cancer.gov/abcancer/treatment/clintrials/search。

ESBC 的标准治疗通常适用于基于生物亚型、疾病程度和患者相关因素等的特定的风险组。这些风险组的不同预后表明，表型多样性的基础是分子通路的不同。在过去的 20 年里，生物医学研究和技术的快速发展使得人们对驱动癌症生长的分子信号通路有了更多的了解，这些分子信号通路影响着癌症的预后和治疗反应。目前的技术可以判断患者预后，并有助于预测 HR+乳腺癌化疗的获益，但遗憾的是，无法预测哪种化疗方案或联合化疗方案最有效，这样会导致过度治疗。新的检测方法有助于确定晚期复发风险较高的患者。希望正在进行的研究能够识别出这些生物标志物或基因标记的组合，从而帮助个体化治疗，并为最需要的患者提供新的靶向生物治疗。

乳腺肿瘤的临床实践正在迅速发展，鼓励肿瘤学家通过美国和国际组织提供的治疗指南和共识声明随时了解这些变化。NCCN 指南提供证据证明和共识，并经常更新，可在 NCCN.org 上获得。关于早期乳腺癌治疗的圣加仑国际专家共识近期有所更新，并可在 http://www.oncoconferences.ch/mm//mm001/Ann_Oncol-2015-Coates-annonc_mdv221.pdf 中查阅。ASCO 中的质量研究所已根据专家小组对现有最佳证据的审查制订了治疗指南，并可在 http://www.instituteforquality.org/practice-guidelines 中找到。

预后及预测

研究者为整合预后信息形成标准化的预后指数，已经进行了多次尝试。诺丁汉大学指数以肿瘤分级、腋窝淋巴结受累和激素受体状体为基础[312,313]，已经过独立研究中心的前瞻性验证和确定，但这个指数在确定个体预后方面作用仍然有限。Adjuvantonline 项目（图 108-22）（https://www.adjuvantonline.com/index.jsp）是应用最多的预后指数。这个免费的在线软件包括患者的年龄、伴随疾病、肿瘤大小、分级、腋窝淋巴结阳性数和 ER 状态，软件利用这些信息对患者个体的十年复发率和死亡率进行计算[231]。通过估计的风险水平，程序还可计算患者从辅助他莫昔芬、芳香化酶抑制剂和不同的化疗方案中所获得的绝对益处。加拿大不列颠哥伦比亚省（British Columbia）的研究者最近通过在不到 2%的预测患者中所观察到的结果，对程序进行验证。然而，Adjuvantonline 是在 HER2 作为常规检测前开发的，并且复发包括局部复发和远处复发。因此，化疗的作用可能被不恰当的放大或缩小。

乳腺癌亚型

基因表达谱可以同时检测多个基因的变化，并测量单个乳腺癌细胞内数千个基因的活性，从而提供更准确的肿瘤分类。2000 年，Perou 等[314]使用该技术评估了 189 个乳腺癌样本，其中 122 例样本含有显著的基因簇表达模式。这些基因簇的表达分别代表四种不同的乳腺癌亚型：Luminal A 和 B，HER2 过表达型和基底型。回顾性研究表明，这些亚型与预后和预测治疗结果有关。

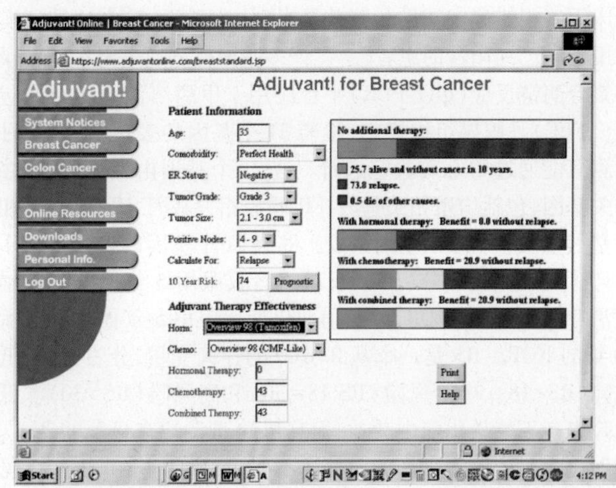

图 108-22　在线预后软件，预测十年的复发率与死亡率，并根据患者个体自身以及肿瘤的特点预测从不同的全身性治疗选择中获益的可能性

乳腺癌的腔内亚型包括与正常乳腺组织腔内上皮细胞相关的基因，与 HR+乳腺癌明显重叠，其中大多数（90%~95%）为腔内亚型[315]。Luminal A 亚型具有最好的预后，大约占乳腺癌的 40%，与雌激素受体相关基因的高表达，HER2 和增殖相关基因簇的低表达有关。相比之下，Luminal B 亚型在所有乳腺癌中占 30%~40%，并且与 *HER2* 基因的低表达以及增殖相关基因簇的高表达有关。无论系统性治疗如何，Luminal B 亚型乳腺癌患者的远期无复发生存率低于 Luminal A 亚型的患者。

HER2 过表达型与 HER2 及增殖相关基因的高表达有关，且比其他乳腺癌有更高的基因组突变频率[313]。有趣的是，一些 HER2-乳腺癌被鉴定为 HER2 过表达型。

基底亚型与增殖相关基因簇如表皮生长因子受体的高表达，和 ER 及 HER2 相关基因的低表达有关，因此一般为 ER、PR 和 HER2 阴性[313]。然而，基底亚型并不等同于三阴性乳腺癌，它与乳腺导管上皮的基底层蛋白的表达相关。基底亚型乳腺癌预后较差，发病后 5 年内乳腺癌复发的风险明显增加，但此后，复发风险则迅速下降。后续研究通过评估新辅助化疗后三阴性乳腺癌的不同预后，又把三阴性乳腺癌分为 7 种亚型：基底细胞 1 型和 2 型、免疫调节型、间充质型、间充质干细胞样型、腔内雄激素受体（AR）型和不稳定型[316,317]。

多基因检测

过去二十年中开发了数种多基因检测方法，包括 Oncotype DX、MammaPrint（MP）、Prosigna、乳腺癌指数（BCI）和 EndoPredict（EP），可以为遗传性乳腺癌患者提供复发风险评估，并在某些情况下预测患者辅助治疗的获益。最重要的是，这些检测通过预测内分泌治疗或预测化疗的获益度，有利于合理的个体化治疗。最常用的支持数据最多的检测方式是 Oncotype DX 和 MP。

Oncotype DX 测定法自 2004 年投入市场以来，最初的目的是作为一种评估淋巴结阴性、激素受体阳性的乳腺癌患者的预后，并预测其化疗获益的工具。对这类患者而言，仅利用传统临床因素很难确定辅助化疗效果[117,181]。最近，该方法被证实可用于淋巴结阳性的患者[134]。该多基因检测通过定量反转录酶聚合酶链反应(qRT-PCR)平台应用于甲醛溶液固定石蜡包埋(FFPE)乳腺癌组织样本，检测 21 个基因的表达[117]。这种检测只能通过中心实验室进行。这 21 个基因由 16 个乳腺癌相关基因，包括增殖相关基因、ER 调控相关基因、HER2 通路相关基因以及 5 个参照基因组成。将这 21 个基因的表达水平用于计算复发风险评分(RS)，反映患者仅服用 5 年他莫昔芬辅助治疗后 10 年的 ROR，以及辅助化疗后服用 5 年他莫昔芬后 10 年的 ROR。RS 是一个从 0～100 的连续变量，分为三类：低风险(RS<18)、中等风险(RS 18～30)和高风险(RS>30)。低风险患者不能从化疗中获益，而高风险患者却有显著的获益。辅助化疗对中风险患者的益处尚不明确，目前正在研究中(见下文；TAILORx 试验)。

Oncotype DX 的开发人员分析从基因组数据库中选定 250 个基因，从几个临床试验的肿瘤样本中测试他们的表达，包括 NSABP B-14 和 NSABP B-20[117]。从这些测试中确定最终 21 个基因的选择，并用于计算每个肿瘤样本的 RS。共获得 668 个样本分析和 RS。按照 10 年远处复发转移率分为三组：6.8%(95%*CI*：4.0～9.6)为低风险组(RS<18)，14.3%(95%*CI*：8.3～20.3)为中风险组(RS 18～30)，和 31%(95%可信区间，23.6～37.4)为高风险组(RS>30)。低 RS 组的 ROR 明显低于高 RS 组($P<0.001$)。

多项研究表明 Oncotype DX 能够预测不同复发风险评分组患者化疗的疗效。Paik 等人检测了 NSABP B-20 试验中部分肿瘤样本的($n=651$)的 RS 值[181]。NSABP B-20 是一项针对 HR+，腋窝淋巴结阴性的绝经后妇女进行研究的临床试验[318]。Paik 等观察到化疗获益与 RS 之间的相关性存在明显的统计学意义($P=0.038$)，RS 高者化疗获益较大[*RR*=0.26，95%*CI*：0.13～0.53]，10 年远处复发率平均下降 27.6%(SE，8.0%)。相比之下，低 RS 组患者化疗后(*RR*1.31，95%*CI*：0.46～3.78)的 10 年远处复发率无明显下降(1.1%；2.2%)。

Albain 等人[134]回顾性的分析了一项三期临床试验 SWOG-8814 中的部分患者，研究其 RS 和无病生存期(DFS)之间的关系。SWOG-8814 研究绝经后女性，激素受体阳性，腋窝淋巴结转移的 ESBC 患者，对比单药他莫昔芬治疗和他莫昔芬+CAF 治疗。在母试验的 927 名患者中，40%的患者接受了 RS 评分。单药他莫昔芬组中，RS 可预测 DFS(*HR*=2.64，95%*CI*：1.3～5.27，$P=0.006$)。低 RS 患者未发现明显的 CAF 获益(log-rank $P=0.97$；*HR*=1.02，0.54～1.93)，而高 RS 组的 DFS 则有统计学意义上的改善(*HR*=0.59，95%*CI*：0.35～1.01；log-rank $P=0.033$)。

辅助化疗对淋巴结阴性，Oncotype DX 检测中复发风险组患者的获益判断不明确，目前两项随机Ⅲ期临床试验正在进行评估。TAILORx(NCT00310180)试验研究的是淋巴结阴性，HR+且 RS 值在 12～30 的乳腺癌患者。这项研究始于 2006 年，共有 10 273 名患者参与其中[319]。RS 值介于 11～25($n=6\,897$)的患者被随机分为两组，一组接受辅助化疗+内分泌治疗，另一组仅接受内分泌治疗。RS 值在 26～30 的患者均接受化疗联合内分泌治疗，RS 值<11 的患者仅接受内分泌治疗。推荐标准的局部治疗。最终数据的收集计划于 2017 年 12 月进行，但低风险组的结果数据于 2015 年发表[320]。共有 1 626 例患者接受治疗，中位年龄 58 岁，中位肿瘤大小 1.5cm；59%的患者为中等组织学分级。超过一半的患者接受人工智能治疗(59%)。5 年无侵袭性疾病生存率(IDFS)为 93.8%，5 年远处无复发率(DRFI)为 99.3%，OS 为 98%。复发风险不受年龄、肿瘤大小或组织学分级的影响。这些数据支持了基因检测在决定低风险乳腺癌患者不需要化疗的临床应用。人们急切地期待着来自中风险人群的结果数据。

RxPONDER1007 临床试验(NCT01272037)是一项前瞻性研究，评估 HR+，HER2-、淋巴结阳性(1～3 个淋巴结)、RS≤25 的接受内分泌治疗和内分泌联合化疗的乳腺癌患者获益[321]。共有 4 000 名患者接受化疗联合内分泌治疗或仅接受内分泌治疗。每位患者的辅助治疗方案将由治疗医师根据标准治疗方案选择。本研究预计完成日期为 2022 年 2 月。

MP*70* 基因检测是为 62 岁以下、淋巴结阴性或阳性(1～3 个淋巴结)、HR+或 HR-、ESBC 原发肿瘤不大于 5cm 的妇女进行的一项预后检测[322]。采用 DNA 芯片技术检测乳腺肿瘤标本中 70 个特异性基因的 mRNA 表达水平。该测试最初是为新鲜冷冻样本设计的，但后来在石蜡标本上得到了验证。70 个基因的表达水平被用来将患者分成低或高风险组。在没有辅助治疗的情况下，低风险组患者在 10 年内发生转移的概率为 13%，而高风险组患者发生转移的概率为 56%。

该检测由荷兰癌症研究所(Netherlands Cancer Institute)开发，使用了 78 名淋巴结阴性乳腺癌患者的肿瘤组织样本，这些患者没有接受系统性辅助治疗，并且有相关结果记录[323]。用微阵列技术对每个肿瘤样本的整个基因组进行评估，以确定与复发风险最相关的基因。选择 70 个最能预测复发的基因进行 MP 检测。后来，通过使用几种不同的组织库，回顾性地验证了该方法在区分低和高复发风险的淋巴结阴性、HR+乳腺癌患者的能力。一项研究对 307 例 HR+，淋巴结阴性的 ESBC 患者的组织样本进行了检测，结果显示，高危组与低危组预后差异显著(*HR*=2.32)[167]。后续的数据也验证了 MP 检测在淋巴结阳性患者中的预后价值[324,325]。

MINDACT 试验是一项前瞻性多中心试验，在乳腺国际组织(BIG)中进行，评估 MP *70* 基因在淋巴结阴性和 1～3 个淋巴结阳性乳腺癌中的表达情况[133]。MINDACT 登记了 6 600 名患者，按 MP 和临床病理风险指标分为高风险组和低风险组，风险判定结果一致。一致判定为高风险组患者接受辅助化疗，一致判定为低风险组患者不接受化疗[326]。风险判定结果不一致的患者随机接受基于 MP 或临床病理风险指标的辅助化疗。接受化疗的患者也被随机分为两种不同的化疗方案，接受内分泌治疗的患者同样的被随机分为两种不同的辅助内分泌治疗方案。第一批疗效结果于 2016 年公布。

Prosigna 评分旨在评估绝经后 HR+乳腺癌患者 10 年远处复发的风险，包括淋巴结阴性(Ⅰ期或Ⅱ期)或淋巴结阳性(仅Ⅱ期)。Prosigna 评分，也被称为 ROR 评分，是用一种专有算法计算的，该算法结合了患者的乳腺癌亚型(由微阵列 50(PAM-50)的预测分析决定)和肿瘤大小。PAM-50 是 Perou 等人在 2000 年定义乳腺癌固有亚型时使用的较大基因集的 50 个基因子集。应用 PAM-50 对 761 例未接受任何系统性治疗的 ESBC 患者的组织标本进行预后评估。PAM-50 和原发肿瘤大小的数据用来计算ROR评分，然后用于将HR+乳腺癌患者分为低、中、高复发风险亚组。选择的50个基因和相关的亚型在包括标准参数的多变量分析评估时仍然显著有意义。

Gnant等人[327]进行了一项独立的回顾性研究，该研究表明，与标准临床预测因子相比，PAM-50派生ROR评分的预后可靠性提高了一级证据。研究队列包括1 478例来自ABCSG-8临床试验患者的组织样本，其中3 091例HR+的ESBC患者未接受辅助化疗，而是接受2年辅助他莫昔芬+3年阿纳曲唑或5年的辅助他莫昔芬治疗。与标准临床预测因子相比，ROR评分增加了具有统计学意义的预后信息（$P<0.000\ 1$）。Luminal A亚组的样本在10年内的ROR评分明显低于Luminal B亚组。

BCI包括一个双基因比（HOXB13∶IL17BR；H/I）和一个五基因分子级别指数（MGI）（BUB1B，CENPA，NEK2、RACGAP1RRM2），被用于针对接受他莫昔芬治疗患者的随机斯德哥尔摩试验且BCI可以提供一个乳腺癌远期复发的连续风险模型[328,329]。BCI已被证明可以显著预测0~10年的ROR，效果超过标准的临床病理因素评价，并预测晚期远处复发[330]。来自扩大辅助内分泌治疗MA.17试验的肿瘤样本的亚组分析表明，H/I可以在5年他莫昔芬组中确定高危组，并发现H/I评分高的人群，5年后接受来曲唑治疗者远处复发的可能性降低[331]。

EP是一种基于RNA的多基因评分，包括8个癌症相关基因和3个参考基因，用于预测早期、ER阳性和HER2阴性，且仅接受辅助内分泌治疗的乳腺癌患者远处复发的可能性[332,333]。EP结合淋巴结状态和肿瘤大小，组成一个综合风险评分，即EPclin。

激素受体阳性乳腺癌的内分泌治疗

雌激素在乳腺癌发生和进展中的作用在一个多世纪前就得到了证实，当时一部分晚期乳腺癌患者接受了卵巢切除手术，从而获得了暂时的疾病控制。在整个20世纪中期，有ESBC切除史的绝经前妇女通过放射治疗或手术进行了卵巢消融术，随后发现这些妇女的复发率有所降低[334]。这样的结果使得研究者进一步评估系统性内分泌治疗对晚期乳腺癌的治疗以及对预防ESBC疾病复发的作用。

直到他莫昔芬于1985年被批准用于绝经后妇女以及于1990年被批准用于绝经前妇女，系统性内分泌治疗才被普遍用于HR+的ESBC患者。作为一种选择性雌激素受体调节剂（SERM），他莫昔芬竞争性地抑制雌激素与雌激素受体结合，随后的拮抗剂作用和激动剂作用则取决于靶组织。虽然尚未完全解释清楚，但这些差异效应可能是由于参与雌激素受体介导的基因调控的辅助激活蛋白和辅助抑制蛋白之间的相互作用不同造成的。

他莫昔芬最初是在他莫昔芬辅助治疗（NATO）的临床试验中作为辅助治疗药物进行评估的，该临床试验始于1977年，随机将1 285名ESBC患者分为两组，一组服用10mg的他莫昔芬bid，为期两年，而另一组则不接受如何进一步治疗。在最长8年的随访中，接受他莫昔芬治疗的患者复发率降低了36%（$\chi^2=17.69$，$P=0.000\ 1$），全因死亡风险降低了29%（$\chi^2=7.48$，$P=0.006\ 2$）[335]。最初5年的辅助他莫昔芬治疗试验显示5年生存率略有提高，但经过较长时间的随访显示，5年后该组患者死亡率明显下降，在诊断后15年，试验组死亡率下降3倍。在第5~9年和第10~14年期间死亡率的下降均相当于第0~4年死亡率的下降。1988年EBCTCG发表的一项荟萃分析了28项他莫昔芬辅助试验，明确证实他莫昔芬可降低所有患者的5年死亡率，但对50岁以上的妇女的影响大于50岁以下的妇女[336]。2011年EBCTCG荟萃分析内分泌治疗的报道称，在5年他莫昔芬对比安慰剂的试验中，平均随访13年发现，他莫昔芬可显著减少乳腺癌15年复发风险（相对危险度0.61，95%可信区间0.57~0.65）和乳腺癌15年死亡风险（相对危险度0.70，95%可信区间0.64~0.75）[337]。辅助他莫昔芬治疗5年可减少乳腺癌的年复发率近40%，死亡率31%，且与年龄、化疗、淋巴结状态和绝经状态无关。遗憾的是，ROR并没有随着时间的推移而降低，超过50%的复发和2/3的死亡发生在诊断后5年内。

虽然他莫昔芬在减少乳腺癌复发和增加总生存率方面有很大的益处，但它并不是没有副作用，包括一些不常见但很严重的不良事件（AE）。对中枢神经系统（CNS）的拮抗作用导致功能失调的热调节，近80%的患者在服用他莫昔芬后出现潮热，这在绝经前妇女中最为显著。子宫组织的兴奋性活动可促进子宫内膜增生，进而发展成肌瘤、息肉和恶性肿瘤。EBCTCG综述分析了他莫昔芬与安慰剂试验中个体患者数据，结果显示子宫内膜癌的发病率增加了2.4倍，但对死亡率没有负面影响[338]。子宫内膜癌的患者几乎全部>50岁。长期随访显示，子宫肉瘤的发生率有较小的增加，通常出现在晚期，在他莫昔芬治疗开始后的2~5年。几项综合分析显示，他莫昔芬可使静脉血栓栓塞事件增加两到三倍，这种效应主要见于55岁以上及体重指数较高的女性。其他副作用包括阴道溢液、性功能障碍、月经紊乱和白内障。

AI最初被批准在绝经后晚期乳腺癌患者中进行评估，后来作为他莫昔芬的替代方案用于绝经后妇女的辅助治疗。芳香化酶将外周组织中的雄激素转化为雌激素。芳香化酶抑制剂通过抑制这种酶的活性从而快速降低循环雌激素水平。它们不能阻止卵巢组织分泌雌激素，因此不适用于卵巢功能正常的绝经前妇女。

第一代和第二代芳香化酶抑制剂毒性太大，无法进一步发展，但第三代芳香化酶抑制剂——依西美坦、阿那曲唑和来曲唑则更安全，耐受性更好。阿那曲唑和来曲唑是非甾体类药物，它们可逆地与芳香化酶结合，而依西美坦是一种甾体类药物，不可逆地与芳香化酶结合。芳香化酶抑制剂的副作用及症状如下：AI与骨质疏松症、骨折、关节僵硬、骨痛、潮热和性功能障碍的风险增加有关。

绝经后妇女的辅助内分泌治疗

第三代芳香化酶抑制剂的发展受到挑战，后来取代他莫昔芬成为绝经后激素受体阳性ESBC患者的主要辅助内分泌治疗药物。20世纪90年代开始了几项重要的Ⅲ期临床试验，以证明AI在降低复发风险和改善绝经后妇女总生存率方面优于他莫昔芬。其他研究验证了辅助内分泌治疗的最佳时间，以优化降低风险，同时限制毒性。临床前试验数据显示，鉴于他莫昔芬在乳腺癌细胞系中的耐药性以及与他莫昔芬长期治疗相关的毒性反应的大型临床试验报道，研究人员在经过2~3年的辅助他莫昔芬治疗（即序贯治疗）之后，会在评估后改为芳香化酶抑制剂治疗。延长辅助内分泌治疗，即使用他莫昔芬治疗 10 年或使用他莫昔芬治疗 5 年，然后使用芳香化酶抑制剂治疗 5 年，可进一步降低激素受体阳性 ESBC 患者的晚期复发风险。

阿那曲唑，他莫昔芬，单药或联合使用(ATAC)研究是第一个证明芳香化酶抑制剂序贯他莫昔芬疗效的临床试验[336,339,340]。所有 9 241 名随机参与者均为绝经后患者，并已完成手术、放疗和/或化疗等基本治疗。未根据激素受体情况排除患者，其中 84%为激素受体阳性。三个研究小组包括：5 年内，每天服用阿那曲唑 1mg，他莫昔芬 20mg，或者两者同时服用。初始分析中位随访时间 33.3 个月，结果显示阿那曲唑组 3 年 DFS 为 89.4%，他莫昔芬组为 87.4%，*HR*=0.83，具有统计学意义(95%*CI*:0.71~0.96，*P*=0.013)。联合用药组与他莫昔芬组比较，两者的 *HR* 值相似，为 1.02(95% *CI*:0.89~1.18，*P*=0.8)。阿那曲唑在子宫内膜癌(*P*=0.02)、阴道出血或分泌物(*P*<0.000 1)、脑血管事件和静脉血栓栓塞事件(*P*=0.000 6)、潮热(*P*<0.000 1)的发生率更低。然而，他莫昔芬组患者关节僵硬和骨折的发生率明显低于阿那曲唑组(*P*<0.000 1)。在 10 年的随访中，与单药他莫昔芬组和联合用药组相比，阿那曲唑在延长无病生存期(*HR*=0.91，95%*CI*:0.83~0.99，*P*=0.04)和延长复发间隔时间方面更加有效。

BIG 1~98 研究是对患有 ESBC 的绝经后妇女进行的Ⅲ期双盲临床试验，旨在对比来曲唑与他莫昔芬 5 年的辅助单药治疗以及利曲唑在他莫昔芬前后的序贯治疗效果[341]。共有 8 010 名手术治疗后患者被随机分为四组术后辅助治疗方案：来曲唑每日 2.5mg，5 年；每日他莫昔芬 20mg，5 年；来曲唑 2 年后序贯他莫昔芬 3 年；他莫昔芬 2 年后序贯来曲唑 3 年。2005 年的一项协议修正案允许从他莫昔芬治疗转为来曲唑治疗，因为其可显著的延长无病生存期。在 8.7 年的中位随访中，无论是从治疗意向评估还是从截尾加权的逆概率(IPCW)评估，来曲唑单药治疗的 DFS 和 OS 均明显优于他莫昔芬单药治疗，这也解释了从他莫昔芬到来曲唑的选择性交叉。在 8 年的中位随访中，两组间的差异无统计学意义。

2011 年发表的一篇荟萃分析研究了来自 ATAC 和 BIG 1~98 试验的 9 856 名患者，随机接受 5 年的 AI(阿那曲唑或来曲唑)或他莫昔芬治疗，结果证实接受 AI 治疗的患者，复发率降低了 2.9%(SE=0.7%)。AI 组的复发率为 9.6%，而他莫昔芬组的复发率为 12.6%(2*P*<0.000 01)，乳腺癌死亡率下降 1.1%(SE=0.0%)。

依西美坦组间研究(IES)随机选取了 4 742 例绝经后激素受体阳性的 ESBC 患者，这些患者在接受了 2~3 年的他莫昔芬治疗后仍然没有出现任何疾病。这些患者要么改用依西美坦，要么继续服用他莫昔芬，共接受了 5 年的辅助内分泌治疗[342]。在 30.6 个月的中位随访中，依西美坦转换组患者的 DFS 显著改善(未经调整的 *HR*=0.68，95%*CI*:0.56~0.82，*P*<0.001)，3 年获益 4.7%。在 91 个月的中位随访中，这一改善没有下降，也未见更多的获益(*HR*=0.94，95%*CI*:0.80~1.10，*P*=0.60)。不过却发现 OS 的明显改善(*HR*=0.86，95%*CI*:0.75~0.99，*P*=0.04)。亚组分析显示，无论孕激素受体状况如何，腋窝淋巴结阳性或阴性的雌激素受体阳性疾病患者都有所获益。骨质疏松症(9.2% vs 7.2%，*P*=0.01)和骨折(7% vs 4.9%，*P*=0.003)发生率的增加与之前预期一致。

2014 年，福布斯等人在 ASCO 上发表了一项最新的荟萃分析，其中包括约 3.7 万名女性，该研究结果进一步支持了绝经后女性中 AI 的使用[344,345]。在比较芳香化酶抑制剂和他莫昔芬的试验中，共有 22 533 名绝经后激素受体阳性的 ESBC 患者，在 0~1 年(*RR*=0.66，95%*CI*:0.54~0.80)和 2~4 年(*RR*=0.75，95%*CI*:0.64~0.88)的复发率显著降低。荟萃分析还报道了序贯辅助治疗组与单药他莫昔芬组相比，乳腺癌相关死亡风险明显减少(*RR*=0.84，95%*CI*:0.73~0.97)。在临床试验中，对比芳香化酶抑制剂以及他莫昔芬序贯芳香化酶抑制剂组的患者(*n*=12 799)，前者在 0~1 年复发率显著降低(*RR*=0.75，95%*CI*:0.75~0.89)，但在 2~4 年，两者复发率类似(*RR*=0.99，95%*CI*:0.85~1.15)。2~4 年复发率的相似性最有可能是由于在这段时间内，序贯组的患者有可能已转化为接受 AI 治疗。

对于绝经后的 ESBC 患者而言，AI 类比他莫昔芬更有效，因此开展更多临床试验来评估延长 AI 治疗。MA.17 是一项Ⅲ期临床试验，随机选取了 5 187 名绝经后的 ESBC 患者，她们既往已服用了 5 年他莫昔芬，随后服用 5 年来曲唑或安慰剂。在 64 个月的中位随访中，DFS(*HR*=0.68，95%*CI*:0.45~0.61)及 OS(*HR*=0.51，95%*CI*:0.42~0.61)均有明显获益。结果导致他莫昔芬序贯来曲唑的辅助治疗被广泛批准。在试验结果公布后，随机分为安慰剂组的患者被允许服用来曲唑，且患者知情。那些选择服用来曲唑的患者的 DFS 仍进一步增加，尽管两次治疗之间的间隔时间较长，平均为 2.8 年。

两项大型跨国临床试验评估了他莫昔芬延长治疗的广泛应用，并得出了类似的结果。辅助他莫昔芬较长时间治疗对比较短时间治疗(ATLAS)的临床试验纳入了 12 894 例 ESBC 患者，在完成了 5 年的他莫昔芬治疗后，部分患者继续服用他莫昔芬至满 10 年，剩余患者则在那个时候就停止服药。超过一半的参与者(53%)已知 ER 阳性，对他们来说，使用他莫昔芬对降低乳腺癌复发率(18%对 21%，*P*=0.002)和总体死亡率(639 例死亡 vs 722 例死亡，*P*=0.01)有显著的益处[346]。随着时间的推移，复发率的降低变得更加显著，5~9 年复发率为 0.9(95%*CI*:0.79~1.02)，后期复发率为 0.75(95% *CI*:0.62~0.90)。在 5~14 年，随机选择继续服用他莫昔芬的患者罹患子宫内膜癌的累积风险为 31%，而对照组为 16%，绝对死亡率上升 0.2%。

提供更多辅助他莫昔芬治疗(aTTom)的临床试验随机选择 6 953 名 ESBC 患者，这些患者在服用不少于 4 年他莫昔芬后，再服用 5 年他莫昔芬或安慰剂[347]。平均随访 4.2 年，延长治疗组复发率明显降低(*RR*=0.94，95% *CI*:0.81~1.09，*P*=0.4)。平均随访 5 年后，继续他莫昔芬治疗组可见明显的时间依存性复发风险的降低[*RR*=0.995~6 年(95% *CI*:0.86~1.15)，*RR*=0.847~9 年(95% *CI*:0.73~0.95)，之后为 0.75(95%*CI*:0.66~0.86)][348]。值得注意的是 61%的患者没有接受激素受体状态检测。服用他莫昔芬 10 年后，子宫内膜癌的发病率翻了一番，但死亡率并没有增加。

EBCTCG 最近发表了一篇关于 AI 和他莫昔芬治疗激素受体阳性的 ESBC 患者的荟萃分析，其中包括 31 920 名绝经后妇女[349]。接受 5 年 AI 治疗的患者与接受 5 年他莫昔芬治疗的患者的复发率在 0~1 年(RR=0.64,95%CI:0.52~0.78)和 2~4 年(RR=0.80,0.68~0.93)有显著性差异,但在随后的几年中不再显著。AI 治疗 10 年的死亡率低于他莫昔芬(RR=0.85,95%CI:0.75~0.96,2P=0.009)。比较 5 年 AI 或 5 年他莫昔芬与 2~3 年他莫昔芬序贯 AI 5 年的研究结果表明,只有在治疗方法不同的时候,AI 的复发率比才更低。然而,无论采用相似或不同的治疗方法,在整个研究过程中,AI 降低了乳腺癌相关死亡率和全因死亡率。AE 结果与预期一致,10 年子宫内膜癌的发生率与他莫昔芬相比有所增加(1.2% vs 0.4%),5 年骨折风险与他莫昔芬相比增加了更多(8.2%与 5.5%)。表 108-9 给出了 2011 年和 2015 年 EBCTCG 荟萃分析评估的各种内分泌治疗的疗效比较。

表 108-9　辅助内分泌治疗的疗效比较[337,349]

	术后 0~4 年复发率	术后 5~9 年复发率	术后 10~14 年复发率	术后 15 年复发率差异	术后 15 年乳腺癌死亡率
TAM[a](5 年) vs 观察组	0.53(2P<0.000 01)	0.68(2P<0.000 01)	0.97	13.2%(RR=0.61,95% CI:0.57 ~ 0.65,2P <0.000 01)	0.70(P<0.000 01)
	术后 0~1 年复发率	**术后 2~4 年复发率**	**术后 5 年及以上年复发率**	**术后 10 年复发率差异**	**术后 10 年乳腺癌死亡率**
AI[b](5 年) vs TAM (5 年)	0.64 (95% CI:0.52~0.78,P <0.000 01)	0.80 (95% CI:0.68~0.93,P <0.000 01)	术后 10 年后无显著差异	3.6%(95%CI:1.7~5.4)	0.85(95% CI:0.75~0.96,2P=0.009)
AI(5 年) vs TAM (2~3 年)至 AI 满 5 年	0.74 (95% CI:0.62~0.89,2P =0.002)	0.99 (95% CI:0.85~1.15)	术后 7 年后无显著差异	无显著差异(2P=0.045)	0.89(95% CI:0.78~1.03,2P=0.11)
TAM(2~3 年)至 AI 满 5 年 vs TAM(5 年)	无显著差异(截至数据收集日期)	0.56 (95% CI:0.46~0.67,P <0.000 1)	术后 10 年后无显著差异	2.0%(95%CI:0.2~3.8)	0.84(95% CI:0.72~0.96,2P=0.015)

[a]TAM,他莫昔芬。
[b]AI,芳香化酶抑制剂。

2014 年 ASCO 临床实践指南重点更新了辅助内分泌治疗,建议绝经后 HR+的 ESBC 患者接受至少 5 年的 AI 或他莫昔芬序贯 AI 治疗[350]。她们应该接受总共 10 年的辅助治疗。2015 年 St. Gallen 关于初级治疗的共识指出,一些绝经后妇女可以用 5 年的他莫昔芬治疗,但高风险患者应该在某个时候接受 AI 治疗[345]。此外,不管月经状况如何,腋窝淋巴结阳性,HR+的 ESBC 患者应接受 10 年内分泌治疗。

绝经前女性的辅助内分泌治疗

绝经前妇女的 HR+乳腺癌发病率在过去二十年中有所增加,这很可能与饮食和生活方式有关。1995 年,他莫昔芬被列为绝经前 HR+乳腺癌妇女的标准辅助内分泌治疗方案。随后在 2001 年进行的 EBCTCG 荟萃分析显示,服用他莫昔芬 5 年,不论年龄大小,复发率降低了 50%,乳腺癌相关死亡率降低了 31%[351]。其他治疗方法如卵巢抑制、化疗或其他内分泌治疗,如 AI 的作用,目前仍不清楚。

INT 0101(E5188)是一项针对绝经前淋巴结阳性、HR+ESBC 患者的Ⅲ期随机临床试验。患者被随机分为只接受 CAF 组,CAF 序贯戈舍瑞林组,及 CAF 联合戈舍瑞林联合他莫昔芬组[352]。在随访 11.5 年后发现,CAF 联合戈舍瑞林联合他莫昔芬治疗与 CAF 序贯戈舍瑞林治疗相比,可显著延长复发时间及无病生存期。回顾过去,年龄小于 40 岁的女性为获益人群,这可能是因为她们最有可能恢复卵巢功能。遗憾的是,该研究设计并没有包括 CAF 序贯他莫昔芬治疗,因为在起初设计研究时,该方案并不被认为是有益的。戈舍瑞林的加入与体重增加、糖尿病的发展和潮热有关。

INT 0101(E5188)是第一个评估 LHRH 激动剂作为绝经前妇女辅助治疗作用的临床试验。Cuzick 等人[353]于 2007 年对 16 项随机临床试验进行了荟萃分析,评估了 LHRH 激动剂作为辅助治疗绝经前 HR+乳腺癌的疗效。纳入的试验仅评估 LHRH、LHRH 联合他莫昔芬、LHRH 联合化疗或 LHRH 联合化疗+他莫昔芬。所有纳入的试验都没有对他莫昔芬联合化疗和 LHRH 联合化疗进行比较。LHRH 试验只显示了无统计学意义的 RR 的降低和死亡率的降低,但缺乏数据支持。主要的发现是,LHRH 联合化疗加上或不加他莫昔芬均对 40 岁的妇女有显著的益处。值得注意的是,荟萃分析在评估许多重要问题方面的能力不足,比如他莫昔芬在绝经前妇女中的作用,此外,没有一种化疗方案是基于紫杉醇的,只有少数是基于蒽环类药物的。

奥地利乳腺癌和结肠直肠癌研究小组 12(ABCSG-12)的临床试验随机选择 1 803 名 HR+的 ESBC 女性患者,她们接受为期 3 年的戈舍瑞林治疗,从而接受阿那曲唑或他莫昔芬治疗,并在 3 年内服用唑来磷酸或不服用唑来磷酸[354]。在 48 个月的中位随访中,随机选择卵巢抑制联合 AI 的妇女并没有发现 DFS 相关获益(HR=1.10,95%CI:0.78~1.53)。

SOFT/TEXT 临床试验已被证实是绝经前 HR+的 ESBC 患者最有效的辅助内分泌治疗。SOFT/TEXT 是由国际乳腺癌研究组织(IBCSG)、BIG 和北美乳腺癌组织在 2003 年发起的Ⅲ期随机临床试验[355]。TEXT 试验是对比他莫昔芬联合依西美坦、他莫昔芬联合卵巢抑制以及依西美坦联合卵巢抑制 5 年后的结果。术后随机抽取 2 672 例患者进行化疗。相比之下,卵巢功能抑制试验(SOFT)仅用了 5 年时间,涉及 3 组患者,比较卵巢抑制联合他莫昔芬、卵巢抑制联合依西美坦和单药他莫昔芬。共有 3 066 名妇女在完成手术和/或化疗后被随机分配到上述组,并要求在试验开始前保持绝经前状态。超过一半的研究参与者(53%)接受了化疗。除非患者骨质减少或骨质疏松,否则两项试验都不允许使用双膦酸盐。

最初针对 SOFT 和 TEXT 的数据分析计划是分别比较各个治疗组之间的 DFS,但因为该相对低风险人群目标事件发生率较低,2011 年试验修正案决定分析 SOFT 联合 TEXT 两项试验,比较依西美坦+卵巢抑制和他莫昔芬+卵巢抑制[356]。TEXT/SOFT 联合分析了 4 960 例患者,截至 2014 年 7 月中位随访时间为 68 个月。其中依西美坦+卵巢抑制组 5 年 DFS 为 91.1%,他莫昔芬+卵巢抑制组 5 年 DFS 为 87.3%,总生存率无差异。AE 发生率与以往绝经后妇女的研究相似,分别为 30.6% 和 29.4%(依西美坦组和他莫昔芬组)。结果表明,HR+的 ESBC 合并高危疾病的患者,卵巢抑制+芳香化酶抑制剂,可大幅度降低远处复发。然而,数据还没有完全成熟,超过 50% 的预期复发事件尚未发生,这表明目前的结论需要谨慎接受。

SOFT 在 2014 年 12 月举办的圣安东尼奥乳腺癌研讨会上发表了关于在卵巢抑制的基础上联合他莫昔芬的研究。经过中位时间 67 个月的随访,卵巢抑制联合他莫昔芬组的 5 年 DFS 为 86.6%,而单药他莫昔芬组的 5 年 DFS 为 84.7%(HR=0.83,95%CI:0.66~1.04,P=0.10)[357]。然而,化疗后接受他莫昔芬联合卵巢抑制的患者与化疗后仅用他莫昔芬的患者相比,前者治疗效果更好(HR=0.78,95%CI:0.60~1.02)。来自 SOFT 和 TEXT 研究的结果如表 108-10 所示。

表 108-10　TEXT 和 SOFT 临床试验结果总结

TEXT 和 SOFT 临床试验中位随访 68 个月(n=4 690)[355]				
	5 年 DFS	**5 年乳腺癌无复发率**	**5 年无远处转移率**	**5 年总生存率**
他莫昔芬/卵巢功能抑制	87.3%	88.8%	92.0%	96.9%
依西美坦/卵巢功能抑制	91.1%	92.8%	93.8%	95.9%
	5 年 DFS(复发,新发肿瘤或死亡的 HR)	5 年乳腺癌无复发率(复发的 HR)	5 年无远处转移率(HR)	5 年总生存率(HR)
他莫昔芬/卵巢功能抑制 vs 依西美坦/卵巢功能抑制	0.72(P<0.001)	0.66(P<0.001)	0.78(P=0.02)	无统计学差异
SOFT 临床试验中位随访 67 个月(n=3 066)[357]				
	5 年 DFS	**5 年乳腺癌无复发率**	**5 年乳腺癌无复发率(化疗后患者)**	**5 年总生存率(化疗后患者)**
依西美坦/卵巢功能抑制	未报告	90.9%	87.8%	未报告
他莫昔芬/卵巢功能抑制	86.6%	88.4%	84.8%	94.5%
他莫昔芬	84.7%	86.4%	83.6%	90.9%
他莫昔芬/卵巢功能抑制 vs 他莫昔芬	0.83(95% CI:0.66~1.04,P=0.10)	0.81(95% CI:0.63~1.03,P=0.09)	0.64(95% CI:0.42~0.96)	
SOFT 试验中年龄<35 岁的患者(n=350),233 例患者被纳入基础研究,其中 4%的患者接受了化疗				
	依西美坦/卵巢功能抑制	**他莫昔芬/卵巢功能抑制**	**他莫昔芬**	
5 年乳腺癌无复发率	83.4%	78.9%	67.7%	

由于试验设计的差异,比较 TEXT/SOFT 和 ABCSG-12 试验的结果是困难的。在 ABCSG-12 研究中,只有 5%的患者接受了化疗,纳入的患者更少,卵巢抑制仅进行了 3 年,而唑来膦酸的加入可能已经抵消了 AI 的作用,研究组间无显著差异。

2014 年 ASCO 临床实践指南重点更新了辅助内分泌治疗,建议 HR+ESBC 绝经前妇女服用 5 年他莫昔芬[350]。该指南指出,如果患者在最初服药 5 年之后仍处于围绝经期或绝经前期,那么他莫昔芬应延长至 10 年。如果一名妇女在服用他莫昔芬 5 年后绝经,她应该继续服用他莫昔芬,或者改用 AI 类药物 5 年。2015 年 St. Gallen 原发性治疗共识建议,对于 HR+ESBC 高危的绝经前妇女,应考虑卵巢抑制联合他莫昔芬或 AI 治疗[345]。高危患者定义为年龄≤35 岁、绝经前、化疗后、多发腋窝淋巴结转移。

HR+/HER2-ESBC 患者的辅助化疗

首次证明乳腺癌的自然史可以通过系统性治疗来改变的是那些随机接受乳腺癌根治术的患者,他们在手术或安慰剂开始时服用了 3 天的噻替帕[358]。与安慰剂相比,1968 年有报道称,至少 4 个腋窝淋巴结转移的绝经前妇女使用噻替帕治疗后,5 年生存率显著提高,这一发现在随访 10 年后仍然存在。20 世纪 60 年代的第二代临床试验进一步证明,通过全身治疗可以延长无病期。NSABP 和 ECOG 联合进行的一项临床试验表明，L-苯丙氨酸芥(L-PAM)口服 24 个月，可延长乳腺癌根治初期淋巴结阳性的 ESBC 患者的无病期[354]。随访超过 20 年后证实，使用这种单药不仅可显著延长 DFS，而且对绝经前患者的 OS 也有显著的延长。最初在绝经后妇女中观察到的相似的趋势并没有持续。

在上述早期临床试验中检验的单药方案表明，全身化疗可以改善预后，并可作为设计多药方案的基础。20 世纪 70 年代的第三期临床试验引入了至今仍在使用的治疗方案。Bonadonna 等人 1976 年发表在 Milan Study 的研究，评估 CMF 方案(环磷酰胺 14 天每天 100mg/m^2，甲氨蝶呤 40mg/m^2 第 1 和第 8 天联合氟尿嘧啶 600mg/m^2 第 1 天和第 8 天)12 个周期对比根治性乳房切除术后淋巴结阳性的女性 ESBC 患者[359]。研究显示所有接受 CMF 治疗的亚组患者均显著减少了治疗的失败率(5.3% vs 24%，$P<10^{-6}$)。2/3 的患者经历了各种各样的毒性反应，包括恶心、呕吐、畏食症、脱发、膀胱炎和口臭。一项中位随访时长 19.4 年的米兰试研究结果表明绝经前妇女可受益，但绝经后妇女没有获益[360]。尽管最初报道 CMF 对绝经后妇女的疗效获益较差，但较长时间的随访表明，年龄较大的妇女更有可能减少药物剂量，当提供相同剂量时，各年龄组的疗效是相似的[361]。

CMF 在 20 世纪 80 年代被广泛用作首选的主要化疗方案，并继续为选定的一组患者提供合理的辅助化疗。然而，在 21 世纪初，含蒽环类药物序贯紫杉烷类药物的化疗方案被明确定义为标准的辅助化疗方案。

1975 年报道指出，多柔比星(doxorubicin)联合环磷酰胺(AC)治疗对 MBC 患者而言是有效和安全的化疗方案[362]。一项大量患者前瞻性试验评估不同组合的蒽环霉素多柔比星和盐酸表柔比星(epirubicin)以确定最优组合以及治疗的频率和时长。

设计 NSABP B-15 用于评估短期化疗的益处，AC(多柔比星 60mg/m^2 和环磷酰胺 600mg/m^2)每 3 周给予 4 个周期，疗效优于时间更密集的 CMF 方案，即每 4 周给予 6 个周期[363]。本研究随机选取 2 194 名淋巴结阳性的他莫昔芬无反应性 ESBC 患者，在她们初次手术治疗后给予 AC 或 CMF 方案化疗。(他莫昔芬无反应性 ESBC 被定义为年龄≤49 岁的所有 ESBC 女性和 50~59 岁患有 PR 疾病的女性)。中位随访 3 年，DFS 和 OS 无明显差异。然而，NSABP B-15 提示，由于 AC 的治疗时间较短，因此优于 CMF。在 NSABP B-16 中也发现了类似的结果，该试验包括对他莫昔芬有反应的 ESBC 患者。对现有随机试验的进一步分析表明，包含三种或三种以上药物(如 FAC、CAF 和 FEC)的含蒽环类药物方案优于 CMF。

HR+/HER2-乳腺癌的辅助化疗已使用紫杉烷类联合蒽环类药物。包括 CALGB 9344、NSABP B-28、BCIRG 001 和 E1199 在内的几项临床试验证明了该组合的有效性。

CALGB 9344 有多个研究目标，其中之一就是评价 AC 联合紫杉醇.[364]共 3 121 例淋巴结阳性的 ESBC 患者随机接受 AC(不同剂量多柔比星，下面详细描述)，联合或不联合每 3 周四个周期的紫杉醇 175mg/m^2。中位随访 5 年，仅接受 AC 的 DFS 为 65%，而 AC 联合紫杉醇的 DFS 为 70%，联合紫杉醇后复发的 *HR*=17%。仅接受 AC 治疗的患者 OS 为 77%，而 AC 联合紫杉醇治疗的 OS 为 80%，联合紫杉醇治疗的患者死亡 *HR*=18%。紫杉醇的加入使 DFS 和 OS 在 5 年内的绝对改善分别为 5%和 3%。这些结果酚酞致 2005 年批准紫杉醇与 AC 联合作为 ESBC 的辅助化疗方案。

NSABP-28 开展于 1995 年，纳入 3 060 例可接受手术的淋巴结阳性乳腺癌女性患者。随机 1∶1分为接受四个周期的标准 AC 序贯每 3 周四个周期紫杉醇 225mg/m^2(AC/T)，或仅接受四个周期标准 AC 方案化疗[365]。所有患者均接受他莫昔芬治疗。经过 64.6 个月的中位随访后，AC/T 组的 DFS 为 76%，而仅 AC 组为 72%，疾病复发的 *RR* 值显著降低(*RR*=0.83，95%*CI*：0.72~0.95，*P*=0.006)。虽然 AC 联合紫杉醇明显改善了 DFS，但两组的 5 年 OS 均为 85%，未见改善。

乳腺癌国际研究组(BCIRG)001 是一项三期临床试验，于 1997 年开展，比较 3 周 6 个周期的 FAC 和 6 个周期的多西他赛 75mg/m^2 联合 AC 方案(TAC)[366]。共有 1 491 名淋巴结阳性的 ESBC 妇女被随机分至两组。在 55 个月的中位随访中，TAC 可降低复发风险(*HR*=0.72，95%*CI*：0.59~0.88，*P*=0.001)和死亡风险(*HR*=0.70，95%*CI*：0.53~0.91，*P*=0.008)。124 个月的中位随访后，复发风险和 OS 的获益依旧维持，*HR*=0.80(95%*CI*：0.68~0.93；log-rank*P*=0.004 3)和 *HR*=0.74(95%*CI*：0.61~0.90；log-rank *P*=0.020)[367]。获益与阳性淋巴结的数量、激素受体状态和 HER2 状态无关。BCIRG 001 清楚地显示了多西他赛在佐剂中的作用。

E1199 临床试验采用 2×2 因子设计，比较紫杉醇与多西他赛，按照每周或每 3 周的时间周期[368]。共有 4 950 名可手术的、淋巴结阳性或高风险的淋巴结阴性 ESBC 患者，随机手术后接受四个周期的 AC 每 3 周序贯以下化疗方案：①紫杉醇每周 80mg/m^2(静脉注射持续 1h)共 12 周；②紫杉醇 175mg/m^2(静脉注射持续 3h)每 3 周 4 次；③多烯紫杉醇每周 35mg/m^2(静脉注射持续 1h)共 12 周；或④多西他赛 100mg/m^2(静脉注射持续 1h)每 3 周 4 次。63.8 个月的中位随访后，紫杉烷类药物和治疗方案的初步比较中没有发现差异。然而，每周使用紫杉醇组与每 3 周给予紫杉醇组相比，前者可显著改善 DFS(*HR*=0.79，*P*=0.006)和 OS(*HR*=0.76，*P*=0.01)。该研究结酚酞致 NCCN 推荐每周紫杉醇联合 AC 作为 ESBC 的首选辅助化疗方案[369]。中位随访时间为 12.1 年后，DFS 仍显著改善(*HR*=0.84，*P*=0.011)，而 OS 仅略有改善(*HR*=0.87，*P*=0.09)[370]。此外，每 3 周给予多西他赛与每 3 周紫杉醇比较，DFS 有显著改善(*HR*=0.79，*P*=0.001)，OS 有微小改善(*HR*=0.86，*P*=0.054)。

研究人员清楚地指出，蒽环类药物和紫杉烷对 ESBC 的治疗都非常有益，他们试图通过评估不同剂量和强度来优化治疗方案，同时降低其毒性。剂量密度可改善预后，但增加多柔比星的剂量并无法改善预后。

CALGB 8541 选择 1 572 例淋巴结阳性乳腺癌患者，随机接受 CAF 化疗方案中不同剂量或频率的环磷酰胺[371]。包括环磷酰胺 400mg/m^2+多柔比星 40mg/m^2+氟尿嘧啶 400mg/m^2 28 天六个周期；环磷酰胺 600mg/m^2+多柔比星 60mg/m^2+氟尿嘧啶 600mg/m^2 每天两次共 28 天四个周期；以及环磷酰胺 300mg/m^2+多柔比星 30mg/m^2+氟尿嘧啶 300mg/m^2 每天两次共 28 天四个周期。前两组的总剂量相同，但第二组的单次剂量更高；第三组的总剂量是前两组的一半，但强度与第一组相同。在 3.4 年的中位随访中，接受较高或中等剂量强度治疗的患者的 DFS 和 OS 在统计学上显著延长，提示存在剂量-反应效应，因此在 ESBC 中选择环磷酰胺 600mg/m^2 作为辅助 AC 化疗的标准剂量。

CALGB 9344(如上所述)的第二个研究目标是评估增加多柔比星剂量是否能提供额外获益[364]。所有纳入 CALGB 9344 的患者随机接受 AC+三种剂量多柔比星之一(60mg/m^2、75mg/m^2、或 90mg/m^2 静脉注射)+标准环磷酰胺(600mg/m^2 静脉注射)每

3周4周期,序贯紫杉醇四周期(如上所述)或没有额外的化疗。接受60mg/m^2、75mg/m^{2}和90mg/m^{2}多柔比星的患者,DFS分别为69%、66%和67%,高剂量多柔比星未发现任何获益。

临床前研究显示,特定剂量的化疗杀死了一定比例的癌细胞,而不是特定数量的乳腺癌,它们以非指数Gompertzian动力学增长,但细胞减少后的再生实际上比指数模型更快[372]。一些研究人员假设,更频繁地给予细胞毒性化疗将比增加剂量更有效的控制疾病。研究这一假设的最初限制是增加骨髓抑制的风险。然而,非格司亭的研发,一种降低中性粒细胞减少的重组人粒细胞集落刺激因子(CSF),为评估剂量强化方案提供了可能[373]。

CALGB 9741是一项关键的临床试验,该试验表明,剂量密度、缩短化疗间隔时间可以改善预后[374]。本研究还评估了序贯或同时给予化疗药物是否会提供更多的益处,假设序贯治疗可达到更高剂量密度的疗效,从而进一步减少化疗毒性。本研究纳入2 005名淋巴结阳性ESBC患者,分别接受以下四种方案:①多柔比星(A)60mg/m^2 4剂量序贯紫杉醇(T)170mg/m^2 4剂,序贯环磷酰胺(C)600mg/m^2 4剂,每3周给予所有剂量;②按上述ACT顺序,每2周给予所有剂量,加非格司亭;③每3周给予4次AC,序贯T 4次,每3周给予所有剂量;④同时给予4个周期AC,4个周期T,每2周给予所有剂量,加非格司亭。所有方案均提供相同剂量的药物。在36个月的中位随访中,剂量密集的方案者(每2周给予所有剂量)DFS明显改善(HR=0.74,P=0.010)和OS(HR=0.69,P=0.013)。4年的DFS在高剂量组为82%,低剂量组为75%。序贯或同时给予化疗药物之间没有差异。与其他方案相比,剂量密集方案的患者中性粒细胞减少的严重程度较轻。

从CALGB 9741、CALGB 9344和BCIRG 001的结果来看,剂量密集的AC+紫杉烷成为治疗淋巴结阳性和高风险淋巴结阴性乳腺癌的标准化疗方案。然而,这样的治疗方案有明显的药物毒性,伴有短期和长期的风险。骨髓抑制最初是一种更为常见的并发症,但随着G-CSF的发展而改善。蒽环类药物与增加心脏毒性有关(OR=5.43,95%CI:2.34~12.62),是一种剂量限制的副作用。因此,研究人员为风险较低的ESBC女性寻求毒性更小、同样有效的治疗方案。美国癌症研究试验9735,一项三期临床试验,随机选取1 016例术后ESBC患者,每3周给予多西他赛75mg/m^2+环磷酰胺600mg/m^{2}静脉注射(TC),共4个周期;或标准AC不跟随G-CSF治疗[375]。16%的参与者年龄在65岁以上,这一人群在ESBC的许多关键试验中都没有得到很好的代表。年龄较大的女性比年轻女性更容易出现淋巴结转移。在平均5.5年的随访时间里,86%的TC组保持无病状态,对比AC组的80%(HR=0.67,95%CI:0.50~0.94,P=0.015)。这一优势在7年的中位随访中仍持续(HR=0.74,95%CI:0.50~0.97,P=0.033)。此外,TC组的OS为87%,对比AC组的82%(HR=0.69,95%CI:0.50~0.97,P=0.032)[376]。DFS和OS的获益与年龄、淋巴结状态或激素受体状态无关。毒性反应因治疗方案的不同而不同,AC组恶心呕吐较重,而TC组肌痛、关节痛、水肿和发热性营养不良更重。发热性中性粒细胞减少在老年患者中并不常见。

CALGB 40101是为了评估单药紫杉醇在治疗低风险淋巴结阳性(一至三个淋巴结转移)或淋巴结阴性ESBC患者时,是否不亚于AC方案[377]。共有3 871名患者随机分配到四组化疗方案。每3周接受标准AC进行4~6次循环,每周接受紫杉醇共进行12~18周。然而,研究进展缓慢,两个较长时间的方案被中止,并随机分配于剩下的两组。由于未能实现4 646名患者的原计划获益目标,该研究于2010年7月初结束。在中位6.1年的随访中,DFS和OS的HR分别为1.26和1.27,支持AC是更佳的治疗方案,且未能提供证据表明,单药紫杉醇不亚于AC。正如预期的那样,紫杉醇组出现更多的神经病变,而AC组出现更多的血液毒性反应;总的来说,认为紫杉醇毒性较小。

考虑到联合化疗(如AC/T、TAC和TC)对ESBC治疗效果的改善,其他最初在MBC中评估的方案也在辅助设置中进行了评估。截至2015年,没有其他辅助化疗方案能进一步改善HR+/HER2-ESBC的疗效。表108-11列出了ESBC的首选和替代辅助(和新辅助)化疗方案。加用卡培他滨或吉西他滨并没有改善预后。

表108-11 不同亚型早期乳腺癌新辅助化疗和辅助化疗的首选和替代方案

新辅助/辅助化疗的首选方案	
HER2-早期乳腺癌	累积剂量多柔比星+环磷酰胺(ddAC)/累积剂量紫杉醇(ddT)
	累积剂量多柔比星+环磷酰胺(ddAC)/每周紫杉醇(T)
	多西他赛+环磷酰胺(TC)
HER2+早期乳腺癌	多柔比星+环磷酰胺(AC)/紫杉醇+曲妥珠单抗(TH)±帕妥珠单抗
	多西他赛+卡铂(TCH)±帕妥珠单抗
新辅助/辅助化疗的替代方案	
HER2-早期乳腺癌	累积剂量多柔比星+环磷酰胺(ddAC)
	多柔比星+环磷酰胺(AC)
	氟尿嘧啶+多柔比星+环磷酰胺(FAC)
	氟尿嘧啶+表柔比星+环磷酰胺(FEC)
	多西他赛+多柔比星+环磷酰胺
HER2+早期乳腺癌	(TAC)环磷酰胺+甲氨蝶呤+氟尿嘧啶(CMF)
	紫杉醇+曲妥珠单抗(TH)
	FEC/紫杉醇+曲妥珠单抗±帕妥珠单抗
	AC/紫杉醇+曲妥珠单抗±帕妥珠单抗

单药卡培他滨是氟尿嘧啶的前药形式，对高达 30%的 MBC 患者有治疗效果。与其他化疗不同的是，卡培他滨是口服的，这对许多患者来说更容易接受。卡培他滨作为 ESBC 治疗的一部分，首次在 CALGB 49907 临床试验中被评估[379]。这项研究主要针对老年患者，因为对他们而言口服治疗的耐受性更好。CALGB 49907 选择 633 名≥65 岁的乳腺癌术后患者，随机接受卡培他滨 14 天，21 天为一个周期；或接受肿瘤学家选择的 CMF 或 AC。在中位 2.4 年的随访中，卡培他滨的复发和死亡比率是标准疗法的两倍，复发 *HR*=2.09(*P*<0.001)。

FINXX 临床试验评估了基于 AC/T 治疗中联合卡培他滨[380]。患者随机接受多西他赛联合卡培他滨治疗 3 个周期，序贯环磷酰胺、表柔比星和卡培他滨（TX/CEX）治疗 3 个周期或 3 个周期的多西他赛联合 CEF 治疗 3 个周期（T/CEF）。中位随访 59 个月，无复发生存率无显著差异，*HR*=0.79(95%*CI*: 0.60~1.04，*P*=0.087)。

鉴于其对 MBC 的疗效，评估吉西他滨是否可作为蒽环类和紫杉烷的联合辅助治疗药物。tAnGo 三期临床试验将高危 ESBC 患者随机分配为每 3 周接受表柔比星 90mg/m^2 静脉注射和环磷酰胺 600mg/m^2 静脉注射（EC），共 4 周期，序贯吉西他滨 1 250mg/m^2 静脉注射（第 1 天和第 8 天）和紫杉醇 175mg/m^2 静脉注射（第一天）（GT）四个周期；或仅接受 EC/T 方案化疗[381]。共纳入 3 152 例患者，其中 55%≤50 岁，77%为淋巴结阳性，41%为 ER+，26%为 HER2+。在 30 个月的预先计划的中期分析中，两组间的 DFS(*HR*=1.0，95%*CI*:0.8~1.2，*P*=0.96)和 OS(*HR*=1.1，95%*CI*:0.9~1.4，*P*=0.35)没有显著差异，表明吉西他滨的加入并没有增加任何获益。

2015 年 St. Gallen 会议成员中，绝大多数人都认为 luminal A 型 ESBC 对化疗的反应一般较差[345]。专家组同意，*21* 基因检测、MP 和 Prosigna 检测中低风险评分的 luminal B 型 ESBC 患者不应接受化疗。luminal 型 ESBC 患者化疗的相对适应证为组织学 3 级、超过 4 个阳性淋巴结、高 Ki-67 以及广泛的脉管浸润。

HER2+ESBC 患者的化疗

对几个关键辅助化疗试验的回顾性分析显示，HER2 过表达的患者亚群获益最大。设计 CALGB 8869 试验以确定分子标记物是否能够预测 CALGB 8541 试验组患者对辅助化疗的反应[382]。从 CALGB 8541 临床试验中随机抽取 442 个肿瘤样本。发现 c-erbB-2 过表达超过 50%的肿瘤患者在接受高剂量 CAF 方案治疗后 DFS 和 OS 明显延长，而没有 HER2 过表达的患者则无获益。

如前所述，CALGB 9344 评估增加多柔比星剂量的影响以及在蒽环类化疗方案基础上添加紫杉醇对淋巴结阳性 ESBC 患者 DFS 和 OS 的影响[364]。海耶斯等[383]对 CALGB 9344 肿瘤样本进行回顾性分析，评估 HER2+ESBC 患者是否存在额外获益。大约 50%的研究参与者是随机选择的，他们的肿瘤样本通过 IHC 和/或 FISH 共同评估 HER2 状态。如其他地方所述，当患者接受多柔比星治疗的剂量超过 60mg/m^2 时，没有发现任何益处；与早期发现一致，在 HER2+肿瘤患者中，高剂量的多柔比星并没有带来任何益处。然而，加用紫杉醇对 HER2+患者有显著的益处，*HR*=0.59(*P*=0.01)。HR+/HER2-ESBC 患者获益甚微。

Hugh 等人评估了以上详细描述的 BCIRG 001[384] 中 90%以上患者的肿瘤亚型对辅助化疗的预后意义和预测反应，对比淋巴结阳性乳腺癌患者术后接受 TAC 和 FAC。使用免疫组化染色法对 ER、PR、HER2 和 Ki-67 状态进行鉴定，从而确定肿瘤亚型。将患者分为三阴性型(14.5%)、HER2 过表达型(8.5%)、luminal B 型(61.1%)和 luminal A 型(15.9%)。以 luminal B 为参照，计算 3 年 DFS 差异的 p 值。ER-/PR-/HER2+患者的 DFS 具有微弱的优势，*HR*=0.50(95%*CI*:0.29~1.83)。

认识到蒽环类药物和紫杉醇类药物对 HER2+ESBC 患者的显著疗效，因此普遍建议 HER2+乳腺癌患者接受辅助化疗。

曲妥珠单抗为基础的治疗

抗 HER2 抗体药物-曲妥珠单抗的研发显著改善了 HER2+乳腺癌患者的预后，显著降低了乳腺癌的复发。曲妥珠单抗是一种人源性单克隆抗体，可抑制 HER2 过表达癌细胞的生长、增殖和存活。抗体针对 HER2 的细胞外区域，防止其与其他 HER2 分子形成二聚体。科学家们提出了几种机制来解释曲妥珠单抗的细胞活性和分子活性。一个令人信服的假设是曲妥珠单抗通过免疫靶向 HER2+肿瘤细胞激活抗体依赖性细胞毒性。体外研究表明，除去曲妥珠单抗的 Fc 部分会破坏曲妥珠单抗的活性，而增强 Fc 受体则会增加小鼠 HER2 肿瘤模型的抗体活性[385,386]。另一种说法是，曲妥珠单抗结合 HER2 后，自然杀伤细胞并促进凋亡。一个被广泛接受的机制是曲妥珠单抗干扰 MAPK 和 PI3K/Akt 细胞通路上的信号因子，而这些通路参与细胞生长和增殖[387]。曲妥珠单抗结合 HER2 可阻止 HER2 形成二聚体，而二聚是 Akt 磷酸化所必需的，从而阻断酪氨酸激酶 Src 信号通路。

曲妥珠单抗的毒性

曲妥珠单抗通常耐受性良好，但心脏毒性是一种少见却严重的副作用。心脏毒性是最初曲妥珠单抗的 MBC 研究中一个意外的发现。曲妥珠单抗引起的心脏功能障碍定义为左心室射血分数(LVEF)降低≤5%，伴有充血性心力衰竭症状，或无症状时 LVEF 降低≤10%[388]。Seidman 等人对曲妥珠单抗临床试验中心脏毒性的荟萃分析报告，使用蒽环类药物联合曲妥珠单抗可引发不可接受的心脏毒性(27%)[389]。仅接受曲妥珠单抗(3%~7%)或曲妥珠单抗+紫杉醇(13%)治疗的患者心脏毒性相对较轻。相比之下，接受蒽环类药物而无曲妥珠单抗治疗的患者，8%出现了心脏毒性反应。大多数曲妥珠单抗治疗后的患者患有可逆的心脏毒性，此时可以恢复曲妥珠单抗治疗。对曲妥珠单抗治疗后患者 LVEF 的最佳监测时间还没有很好的定义，建议每 3~6 个月进行一次。

有历史意义的曲妥珠单抗(B3-1，N9831，BCIRG-006 和 HERA)

曲妥珠单抗在 2006 年被批准作为 Her2 靶向的辅助治疗，在四项大型临床试验的背景下，评估了 13 000 多名妇女，一致报告 3 年复发风险降低了约 50%。四项研究大约在 2000 年开始，且提出了几个设计上略有不同的问题。

NSABP B-31 招募了 2 030 名 HER2+乳腺癌淋巴结阳性的女性，她们都接受了标准 AC 序贯紫杉醇治疗，每 3 周或每周一次[390]。患者随机分配至接受紫杉醇+曲妥珠单抗治疗，共 52 周；或仅接受紫杉醇治疗。另一项研究，北部中央癌症治疗组

(NCCTG)N9831,招募了 3 506 名淋巴结阳性 HER2+ESBC 患者,分配至 NSABP B-31 中的两组以及接受 52 周曲妥珠单抗的第三组,但只有在完成 AC/T(XX)后。综合分析 NSABP B-31 和 NCCTG N9831 的前两组研究,中位随访 2 年,发现曲妥珠单抗组的 DFS 明显延长($HR=0.48$,95% CI:0.39~0.59,$P<0.001$),3 年 DFS 绝对差异为 2%。曲妥珠单抗组较对照组远处复发风险降低 53%(95% CI:0.48~0.93,$P=0.015$),死亡率降低 1/3(95% CI:0.37~0.61,$P<0.0001$)。

BCIRG006 是一项全球性的多中心临床试验,3 222 名女性参与了这项试验,她们被随机分至 3 组:两组类似于 NSABP B-31 和 NCCTG N9831 的研究(标准 AC 序贯多西他赛+曲妥珠单抗(AC/TH)),第三组含有非蒽环类药物,包括多西他赛、卡铂和曲妥珠单抗(TCH)[387]。中位随访 2 年,含曲妥珠单抗组的 DFS 明显改善,AC/TH 组复发风险降低 51%($P<0.0001$),TCH 组复发风险降低 39%($P=0.0002$)。由于研究设计的原因,AC/TH 组和 TCH 组的疗效没有可比性。含曲妥珠单抗的组中,生存获益无统计学意义。

赫赛汀辅助(HERA)Ⅲ期临床试验纳入了 5 090 名 HER2+ESBC 患者,这些患者已完成了四个周期的辅助(或新辅助)化疗和放射治疗(根据需要)。将研究对象分为三组:观察组、1 年曲妥珠单抗组和 2 年曲妥珠单抗组[391]。第一次中期分析报告示,1 年曲妥珠单抗组与观察组相比,2 年 DFS 绝对获益 8.4%。观察组的无事件患者被允许交叉接受曲妥珠单抗治疗[392]。即便如此,1 年曲妥珠单抗组与观察组相比,4 年 DFS 仍有显著延长(78.6% vs 72.2%;$HR=0.76$,95% CI:0.66~0.87,$P<0.0001$)。OS 没有差异。下面讨论 1 年与 2 年曲妥珠单抗相关的结果。

NSABP B-31、NCCTG N9831、BCIRG 006 和 HERA 均提示 HER2+ESBC 患者辅助化疗中加入曲妥珠单抗对 DFS 有显著的获益。2015 年更新的乳腺癌 NCCN 指南规定,原发性肿瘤>0.5cm 或阳性淋巴结的 HER2+ESBC 患者应接受曲妥珠单抗辅助化疗[395]。表 108-11 列出了 HER2+ESBC 的首选和替代辅助(和新辅助)化疗方案。指南指出,曲妥珠单抗对淋巴结阴性的 T1a(≤0.5cm)或 T1b(0.5~1.0cm)患者的疗效尚不确定,必须仔细权衡毒性反应。这个问题最近在 APT 临床试验中得到了解释,下文将对此进行详细描述。

NCCN 指南目前建议,辅助曲妥珠单抗应先与以紫杉醇为基础的化疗药物一起使用,然后作为单药使用,总共 1 年(或 52 周)[393]。NSABP B-31、NCCTG N9831 和 BCIRG 006 只评估了 1 年曲妥珠单抗,而 HERA 评估了 1 年和 2 年曲妥珠单抗。中位随访 8 年,发现接受 1 年或 2 年曲妥珠单抗组的 DFS 无明显差异($HR=0.99$,95% CI:0.85~1.14,$P=0.86$)[394]。此外,接受曲妥珠单抗治疗 2 年的患者发生 3~4 级 AE 和左心室功能障碍的发生率(分别为 20.4% 和 7.2%)高于 1 年者(分别为 16.3% 和 4.1%)。

考虑到曲妥珠单抗的毒性和成本,研究人员研究了缩短曲妥珠单抗疗程(9 周、3 个月或 6 个月),疗效是否不低于推荐的 52 周疗程。迄今为止,短疗程治疗方案还没有被证明与标准的 52 周曲妥珠单抗方案疗效相同。

芬兰赫赛汀(FIN-HER)临床试验评估了短期曲妥珠单抗限制心脏毒性的疗效[392]。该三期临床试验纳入了 1 010 名淋巴结阳性或高危淋巴结阴性乳腺癌患者,她们接受多西他赛三个周期序贯 FEC,或长春瑞滨三个周期,序贯 FEC。共有 232 名 HER2+患者,随机分为在接受多西他赛或长春瑞滨同时,接受或不接受为期 9 周的曲妥珠单抗治疗。曲妥珠单抗组 3 年 DFS 明显改善(复发或死亡 $HR=0.42$,95% CI:0.21~0.83,$P=0.01$)。没有观察到左心室射血分数或心力衰竭事件的减少。

赫赛汀辅助治疗减少暴露方案(PHARE)Ⅲ期临床试验纳入 3 384 例 HER2+ESBC 患者,他们已经完成了初次手术,术后至少接受了四个周期化疗,并使用曲妥珠单抗 6 个月[395]。患者随机分为 2 组;继续使用曲妥珠单抗 6 个月(共 12 个月)或停止使用曲妥珠单抗(共 6 个月),以证明其非劣效性。在 42.5 个月的中位随访中,12 个月组和 6 个月组的 DFS 分别为 87.8% 和 84.9%,OS 分别为 95% 和 93.1%,短期组没有表现出非劣效性。

希腊肿瘤学研究小组最近报道了一项三期临床试验,随机选取了 481 名淋巴结阳性或高危淋巴结阴性 HER2+ESBC 的妇女,进行 12 个月或 6 个月曲妥珠单抗联合辅助化疗[396]。在初次手术后,所有患者均接受剂量密集的 FEC,序贯每 14 天给予多西他赛 75mg/m^2,共 4 个周期,同时给予曲妥珠单抗,然后延长至共 12 个月或 6 个月。12 个月组和 6 个月组的 3 年 DFS 分别为 95.7% 和 93.3%($HR=1.57$,95% CI:0.86~2.10,$P=0.137$),6 个月组并没有表现出非劣效性。

短期 HER2 临床试验(NCT00629278)比较了 3 个月和 12 个月曲妥珠单抗的疗效[397]。该研究将 2 500 名淋巴结阳性或高风险淋巴结阴性 HER2+ESBC 患者,随机接受 4 个周期蒽环类药物为基础的化疗,序贯四个周期的紫杉醇为基础的化疗+18 个周期或 3 个周期的曲妥珠单抗(每三周);或 3 个周期的多西他赛+曲妥珠单抗(每三周),序贯三个周期的 FEC 而无额外的曲妥珠单抗。该研究于 2010 年完成,但截至 2015 年 8 月尚未公布结果。

Synergism or Long Duration(SOLD)研究是由芬兰乳腺癌组赞助的Ⅲ期临床试验(NCT00593697),评估 9 周与 52 周曲妥珠单抗的疗效[398]。共有 2 168 名 HER2+ESBC 患者被随机分为两组,一组为每 3 周多西他赛联合曲妥珠单抗(TH)治疗 3 个周期,序贯 FE75C 治疗 3 个周期;另一组为相同的治疗方案,每 3 周给予曲妥珠单抗治疗,共 52 周。该研究于 2014 年 11 月完成,但截至 2015 年 8 月尚未公布结果。

PersephoneⅢ期临床试验纳入 4 000 例 HER2+EBSC 患者,比较 6 个月与 12 个月标准曲妥珠单抗的疗效。该研究于 2007 年开始,截至 2014 年共 3 166 名患者被随机分组,2016 年首次计划进行非劣效性中期分析[399]。

既往临床试验证明,曲妥珠单抗靶向治疗淋巴结阳性或高危淋巴结阴性 HER2+ESBC 患者的重要性。这些研究未纳入 HER2+ESBC 小淋巴结阴性的妇女,对这类患者适当的治疗方案尚不清楚。分析 NCCN 数据库 520 例 HR-/HER2+ESBC 的患者肿瘤直径≤1cm 的患者信息,5 年 DFS 分别为 94%(T1bN0)、93%(T1aN0)和 94%~96%(T1a~bN0)[400]。辅助紫杉醇联合曲妥珠单抗(APT)临床试验是一项多中心研究人员发起的临床试验,旨在开发一种有效的治疗方案,限制 HER2+ESBC 小淋巴结阴性患者的药物毒性反应,因为此类患者的预后一般较好[401]。所有患者每周接受紫杉醇 80mg/m^2 静脉注射 12 周+12 周曲妥珠单抗治疗共 9 个月。共纳入 410 例患者，其中 87.7%的患者完成治疗。研究表明，紫杉醇联合曲妥珠单抗治疗是更合适的。3 年 DFS 为 98.7%(95%*CI*:97.6~99.8)，优于历史对照。13 例出现 AE，包括 1 例 3 级神经病患者和 13 例无症状射血分数下降的患者，除 2 例患者外，其余均痊愈。

帕妥珠单抗辅助/新辅助化疗研究

帕妥珠单抗是一种人源性单克隆抗体，是 HER 的第一类异质二聚体抑制剂，可与 HER2 二聚体结合，阻止 HER2 与其家族成员发生相互作用。与曲妥珠单抗不同，帕妥珠单抗只阻止 HER2 的同源二聚体，抑制 HER2:HER3 结合，这是最活跃的 HER 复合物[402]。帕妥珠单抗于 2012 年被 FDA 批准用于 MBC 患者，这是基于 CLEOPATRA 临床试验的结果表明，多西他赛、曲妥珠单抗和帕妥珠单抗联合使用优于单纯的多西他赛加曲妥珠单抗。NeoSphere 临床试验评估了帕妥珠单抗联合多西他赛和曲妥珠单抗作为新辅助化疗药物的疗效，并于 2014 年在新辅助药物中获得批准。设计帕妥珠单抗和赫赛汀在乳腺癌辅助化疗(APHINITY)临床试验(NCT01358877)用于确定当帕妥珠单抗与标准辅助化疗药物和曲妥珠单抗联合使用时，是否会提高疗效[403]。共 4 810 例 HER2+ESBC 淋巴结阳性患者，采用双盲法随机 1∶1分为两组。所有患者都根据研究人员的选择，接受了 6~8 个周期的蒽环类药物或紫杉醇方案辅助化疗。研究组同时使用曲妥珠单抗和帕妥珠单抗并延长至 1 年，而比较组则同时使用曲妥珠单抗和安慰剂并延长至 1 年。初步结果将于 2016 年公布。

帕妥珠单抗还没有被批准用于辅助化疗。然而，最新的 NCCN 乳腺癌指南指出，病理分期为 T2N1、HER2+ESBC 的患者，如果没有接受含帕妥珠单抗的新辅助化疗，可以接受含帕妥珠单抗的辅助化疗[395]。

HER2+ESBC 患者新辅助治疗的研究

拉帕替尼(lapatinib)是一种口服小分子双酪氨酸激酶 HER2 和 EGFR 抑制剂。拉帕替尼联合卡培他滨被批准用于 HER2+MBC 合并曲妥珠单抗耐药的患者[404]。虽然拉帕替尼的耐受性一般较好，但它与轻度至中度腹泻、皮疹和轻度、短暂的肝转氨酶升高有关。化疗后的 Tykerb 评估(TEACH)试验评估了拉帕替尼辅助治疗 HER2ESBC 患者的有效性和安全性[405]。该跨国、双盲Ⅲ期临床试验随机选择 3 147 名患者在辅助化疗结束后随时开始接受拉帕替尼或安慰剂。中位随访 47.4 个月的拉帕替尼组和 48.3 个月的安慰剂组后发现，DFS 没有显著差异(13% vs 17%，*HR*=0.83，95%*CI*:0.70~1.00，*P*=0.053)。然而，对 HER2 状态的集中评估显示，只有 79%的参与者是 HER2+，且 DFS 的获益是微不足道的。研究者认为，拉帕替尼可作为 HER2ESBC 患者无法接受曲妥珠单抗辅助化疗的合适备选药物。

辅助拉帕替尼和/或曲妥珠单抗优化治疗(ALTTO)临床试验随机选择 8 381 例 HER2+ESBC 患者，随机接受 1 年的拉帕替尼+曲妥珠单抗(L+T)；或 1 年的曲妥珠单抗；或 1 年的拉帕替尼或曲妥珠单抗单药辅助治疗[406]。ALTTO 是 NEOALTTO 临床试验的一项联合研究(在新辅助治疗部分中有描述)，该研究显示，与单药曲妥珠单抗相比，L+T 的 pCR 率增加了一倍[407]。ALTTO 临床试验的初步结果于 2014 年在 ASCO 会议上公布。与曲妥珠单抗(86%)相比，L+T(88%)组 4 年 DFS 明显改善(*HR*=0.84，97.5%*CI*:0.70~1.02，*P*=0.048)；曲妥珠单抗序贯拉帕替尼组为 87%(*HR*=0.93，97.5%*CI*:0.76~1.13，*P*=0.044)。ALTTO 的初步结果在 NEOALTTO 结果的背景下既令人惊讶又令人失望，这导致研究人员质疑 pCR 的实用性。

奈拉替尼(neratinib)是一种口服多酪氨酸激酶(HER2，HER4，和 EGFR)抑制剂。该新药物最初是在针对 HER2+MBC 患者接受曲妥珠单抗联合紫杉醇的二期临床试验中研究的，该药物可改善无进展生存(PFS)[408]。转移和新辅助治疗的阳性结酚酞致进一步评估奈拉替尼作为 HER2+ESBC 的扩展辅助治疗药物。ExteNET 临床试验是一项双盲、安慰剂对照、Ⅲ期临床试验，评估标准曲妥珠单抗化疗后使用 12 个月奈拉替尼的疗效。本研究选取 2 840 例 HER2+ESBC 患者，他们在完成一期手术，并接受标准的曲妥珠单抗辅助化疗后，随机接受奈拉替尼或安慰剂治疗 1 年。在 2 年的中位随访中，奈拉替尼组与安慰剂组相比，可明显改善 DFS(93.9% vs 91.6%；*HR*=0.67，*P*=0.004 6)。奈拉替尼组最常见的副作用为腹泻，有 40%的患者出现 3 级腹泻。

ATEMPTⅡ期临床试验(NCT01853748)正在评估单药曲妥珠单抗(T-DM1)作为辅助治疗药物的使用情况，其目标是在 APT 研究结果的基础上，避免化疗相关毒性反应，同时降低疾病复发的风险[401]。T-DM1 是一种连接曲妥珠单抗和细胞毒性药物 DM1 的抗体-药物偶联物。根据 EMILIA 临床试验的结果(见 MBC 部分)，T-DM1 于 2013 年被 FDA 批准为 HER2+MBC 的二线治疗药物。ATEMPT 于 2013 年 5 月启动，招募 500 名Ⅰ期 HER2+乳腺癌患者。将患者按照 3∶1的比例随机分为 2 组，每 3 周给予一次 T-DM1，持续 51 周，每周紫杉醇联合曲妥珠单抗治疗，共 12 个周期，再序贯 9 个月的曲妥珠单抗，完成 1 年的曲妥珠单抗治疗。DFS 的最终数据收集于 2017 年 5 月完成。

三阴性乳腺癌

与 HR+和 HER2+ESBC 分别可采用内分泌治疗和 HER2 靶向治疗相比，TNBC 尚无靶向治疗。因此，化疗是 TNBC 患者唯一的辅助治疗方法。在关键的辅助化疗试验中，对肿瘤亚型的回顾性分析大多未能明确 TNBC 的预后。然而，现有的分析清楚地表明，基于紫杉醇的化疗方案对 TNBC 有显著的益处。

上述详细描述的 E1199 临床试验比较了紫杉醇和多西他赛的疗效，以及淋巴结阳性或高风险淋巴结阴性 ESBC 患者术后，在已经历四个周期的标准 AC 化疗后的治疗频率(3 周 vs 每周)[366]。一项前瞻性分析纳入 1 025 例 TNBC 患者，经历 12.1 年的随访后，证实紫杉醇每周给药组与每三周给药组相比，可显著改善 DFS 和 OS(DFS *HR*=0.69，*P*=0.001；OS *HR*=0.69，*P*=0.019)[368]。这些发现表明，TNBC 患者在接受 AC 序贯每周紫杉醇治疗，10 年 DFS 和 OS 可改善 10%。上述详细描述的美国肿瘤临床试验 9735[374] 表明，TNBC 患者接受 4 个周期 TC 化疗的 DFS 和 OS 优于接受 4 个周期的标准 AC 化疗。

贝伐单抗是一种针对血管内皮生长因子(VEGF)的人源性单克隆抗体，它的一些Ⅲ期临床试验表明，联合化疗对转移性 TNBC 患者有一定的益处。贝伐单抗辅助治疗 TNBC(BEA-

TRICE)临床试验随机选择2 591例原发TNBC可手术患者进行化疗，包括或不包括贝伐单抗，每周剂量为5mg/kg，为期1年[410]。在大约32个月的中位随访中，两组患者3年的DFS和OS相似。

一些铂类药物的新辅助化疗临床试验(在其他地方讨论过)表明，*BRCA1* ESBC患者的pCR得到了改善，其中大多数为TNBC。目前还没有研究专门来评估TNBC在辅助治疗中的铂类药物方案。

新辅助化疗：重新排序手术和化疗

乳腺癌的治疗过去是从手术切除开始，然后根据需要进行化疗、放疗和内分泌治疗。然而，越来越多的乳腺癌患者在手术前已接受化疗。术前(或新辅助)化疗最初用于患有炎性或不可手术的乳腺肿瘤的妇女，使之可手术。随后，新辅助化疗作为一种治疗手段，使得肿瘤体积较大的T2或T3乳腺癌患者得以保乳治疗。最近，新辅助化疗甚至已被作为一种治疗选择，以允许早期评估系统治疗的有效性，并测试新药。因此，这些治疗理念使得大多数乳腺癌患者有条件接受新辅助化疗。表108-12回顾了些潜在的好处。

表108-12 乳腺癌新辅助化疗的潜在获益

获益
推进乳腺切除术在无法手术的乳腺癌或炎性乳腺癌患者中的应用
增加患者的保乳手术比率
如果肿瘤对化疗有效，切除的乳腺较少，则能提高保乳手术的美容效果
确定肿瘤是否对于治疗耐药，以便临床医师可以停止无效的化疗方案
减少术后放疗照射范围
肿瘤对新辅助化疗的病理反应是预后因素。因此，这种顺序策略无法对下述情况进行评价：
直接比较两种化疗方案的疗效，或在标准治疗中添加靶向药物的疗效
直接研究影响化疗敏感性/耐药性的生物因素
为新药的临床研究确定患者-尽管这些患者接受了最佳标准方案的治疗，仍然具有很高的复发风险
在等待更大规模的辅助研究完成的同时，允许对已被证明能够改善对标准治疗反应的治疗进行早期监管批准

多年来，已开展多项研究来评估术前化疗对原发性可手术乳腺癌的价值。NSABP B-18是一项随机试验，比较了可手术乳腺癌患者术前和术后给予4个周期的多柔比星和环磷酰胺(AC)[411]，发现术前新辅助化疗组的DFS和OS与术后辅助化疗组无差异。EORTC[365]完成了相似设计的验证性试验，结果与NSABP B-18的结果非常相似。

B-18的问题是在最初的治疗之后是否需要进一步的治疗，这在阿伯丁试验中得到了解决[412]。在这个小型研究中，162名患者接受了4个周期的多柔比星、环磷酰胺、长春新碱和泼尼松龙(CVAP)治疗，有应答者随机继续接受4个周期的CVAP或4个周期的多西他赛(100mg/m^2)治疗，无应答者继续接受4个周期的多西他赛。接受多西他赛治疗的患者中，反应率有所改善，且较长时间后转为无复发率和OS的改善。本研究证实pCR率的提高与无复发生存(RFS)和OS的改善有关。MD Anderson[413]和NSABP B-27[414]研究也证实，与继续使用多柔比星相比，非交叉耐药方案与改善RFS和OS相关。

NSABP B-27也证实了pCR率可预测RFS，并验证了pCR作为长期治疗获益的替代标记物。因此，pCR被认为是用于比较治疗方案的一个有效工具。

新辅助化疗的反应成为评估DFS和生存率的预后指标。因此，术前化疗效果可以作为检测新治疗方案的中间终点，也可以作为检测成熟方案中加入新药物的辅助效果的中间终点，而不必等待数年，直到DFS和死亡才可以进行比较。由于术前化疗与术后化疗在DFS和生存率上的价值是等价的，因此新的化疗方案可以在这种情况下进行测试，而不用担心会使患者处于不利地位。

因此，大量的术前(或新辅助)治疗研究接踵而至，研究了化疗的选择和治疗顺序。与不含紫杉醇的方案相比，同时或序贯给予紫杉醇的基于蒽环类药物的化疗方案在新辅助治疗中表现出更高的治疗效果[364,401~412,415~417]。

新辅助治疗的研究包括化疗、内分泌治疗和生物学治疗(如HER2靶向治疗)。研究表明，特定的化疗方案可以使特定的肿瘤亚型患者受益。

对于TNBC患者，铂类药物已显示出对转移者的益处；因此，卡铂与NACT联合研究表明，卡铂可以提高pCR率[418,419]。卡铂联合PARP抑制剂也有一定希望[420]。

对于HER2+乳腺癌患者，HER2靶向治疗已被证明在提高pCR率和长期预后方面是有益的。曲妥珠单抗的益处已在几项研究中被证实，尤其是NOAH研究[421,422]，这表明，标准新辅助化疗+曲妥珠单抗(术后继续曲妥珠单抗治疗)与没有曲妥珠单抗(19%)相比，可提高pCR(38%)($P=0.001$)；与接受标准化疗患者相比，可显著提高EFS率。在NeoSphere[379]和TRYPHAENA[423]两项研究中，与对照组(NACT+曲妥珠单抗)相比，帕妥珠单抗联合NACT+曲妥珠单抗组均显示出更高的获益。基于这些结果以及辅助试验APHINITY(NCT01358877)已获得收益，FDA加速批准在新辅助治疗中，在化疗和曲妥珠单抗中添加帕妥珠单抗。拉帕替尼还没有取得与帕妥珠单抗类似的成功，有几项研究表明，拉帕替尼代替曲妥珠单抗时，疗效没有增加，且两者联合使用时，疗效有限[404,424,425]。此外一些针对Her2靶向治疗的研究正在开展中，并在Ⅱ期研究中显示出一些初步的希望[426]。

新辅助研究也着眼于反应调整安排，即根据临床对有疗效反应或无疗效反应的评估，在一系列治疗周期之后继续进行相同或非交叉耐药治疗[427]。虽然这些研究没有体现出增加疗效的证据，但这项研究设计是朝着根据早期疗效反应量身订制个性化治疗迈出的重要一步。

表108-13总结了几个关键的新辅助化疗研究的具体细节。

表 108-13　新辅助研究结果总结

乳腺癌亚型	研究	化疗药物	比较	pCR	总结
HER2 阳性 HER2 阴性[422]	NOAH	多柔比星、紫杉醇、环磷酰胺、甲氨蝶呤和氟尿嘧啶	+/-曲妥珠单抗(H)		新辅助化疗与化疗相比,增加了 pCR 和 EFS 的发生率
HER2 阳性[425]	CALGB 40601	紫杉醇(T)	曲妥珠单抗(H) 拉帕替尼(L) H+L	TH:46%(37%~55%) TL:32%(22%~45%) THL:56%(47%~65%)	L 因疗效不佳而提前停用; 在 H 中加入 L 不增加 pCR
HER2 阳性[424]	NSABP B-41	多柔比星+曲妥珠单抗,序贯紫杉醇(T)	曲妥珠单抗(H) 拉帕替尼(L) H+L	H:49. 4. 5%(41. 8%~56. 5%) L:47. 4%(39. 8%~54. 6%) H+L 60. 2%(52. 5%~67. 1%)	L 或 L+H 并没有表现出比 H 单独更高的疗效
HER2 阳性[407]	NeoALTTO	紫杉醇(T)	曲妥珠单抗(H) 拉帕替尼(L) H+L	L(54. 9%),H+L(69. 8%) H 36. 49%(25. 60~48. 49) L 33. 78%(23. 19~45. 72)	L+H 的 pCR 率高于单独的 H 或 L
HER2 阳性[428]	GeparQuinto	盐酸表柔比星和环磷酰胺(EC)其次是多西他赛(D)	曲妥珠单抗(H) 拉帕替尼(L)	L+H 61. 33%(49. 38~72. 36) ECH-DH:30. 3%(25. 2%~35. 8%) ECH-DL:22. 7%(18. 2%~27. 8%)	H 的 pCR 率高于 L,不良事件更少
HER2 阳性[358]	NeoSphere	曲妥珠单抗(H)+多西他赛(D)	A 组:H+D B 组:帕妥珠单抗(P)+H +D C 组: D 组:P+D	A 组(H+D):29. 0%(20. 6%~38. 5%) A 组(P+H+D):45. 8%(36. 1%~55. 7%) C 组(P+H):16. 8%(10. 3~25. 3) D 组(P+D):24. 0%(15. 8%~33. 7%)	P+H+D(B 组)pCR 明显高于 H+D 组
HER2 阳性[423]	TRYPHAENA	氟尿嘧啶、表柔比星和环磷酰胺(FEC),多西他赛(D),卡铂+曲妥珠单抗(H),帕妥珠单抗(P)	A 臂:FEC+H+P×3→D+H +P×3 B 臂:FEC×3→T+H+P×3 C 臂:T 卡铂 H+P×6	A 臂:54. 7%(42. 7%~66. 2%) B 臂:56. 2%(44. 1%~67. 8%) C 臂:63. 6%(51. 9%~74. 3%)	H+P 对蒽环类药物心脏耐受性及疗效的研究。并发蒽环类抗生素耐受性良好,但没有增加 pCR
HER2 阳性及三阴性乳腺癌(TNBC)[418]	GeparSixto; GBG 66	紫杉醇(T)+脂质体 A HER2 阳性:曲妥珠单抗(H)+拉帕替尼(L) TNBC:贝伐单抗	+/-卡铂	不加卡铂:36. 9%(31. 3%~42. 4%) 卡铂:43. 7%(38. 1%~49. 4%)	添加卡铂可提高 TNBC 患者的 pCR 率
TNBC[419]	CALGB 40603	紫杉醇(T)序贯多柔比星/环磷酰胺(AC)	卡铂 贝伐单抗	卡铂:54%(48%~61%) 不加卡铂:41%(35%~48%) Bev:52%(45%~58%) No Bev:44%(38%~51%)	在新辅助化疗中添加卡铂 PCR 率
全部[266]	NSABP B-18	多柔比星/环磷酰胺(AC)	治疗顺序(4 个 AC 周期化疗后手术 vs 手术后 4 个 AC 周期化疗)	术后 AC 与术前 AC 的危险比比较 DFS:0. 99,DDFS:0. 70,OS:0. 83	术前化疗组与术后化疗组 DFS、OS 无差异

续表

乳腺癌亚型	研究	化疗药物	比较	pCR	总结
全部[265]	EORTC 10902	氟尿嘧啶、表柔比星和环磷酰胺(FEC)	治疗顺序(4 个 FEC 周期化疗后手术 vs 手术后 4 个 FEC 周期化疗)	OS(危害比,1.16;PFS(危害比,1.15,$P=0.27$),时间相关 LRR(危害比 1.13,$P=0.61$)	术前化疗组与术后化疗组 OS、PFS、时间相关 LRR 无差异
全部[414]	NSABP B-27	多柔比星/环磷酰胺(AC)序贯多西他赛(D)	第 1 组:术前 AC 方案化疗 4 个周期 第 2 组:术前 4 周期 AC 方案,序贯 4 周期 D 方案 第 3 组:术前 4 周期 AC 方案化疗,术后 4 周期 D 方案化疗	pCR: 第 1 组:12.9% 第 2 组:26.1% 第 3 组:14.5%	术前 4 周期 AC 后加入 4 周期 D,与单纯 AC 相比,可显著提高 pCR 率
全部[427]	GeparTrio	多西他赛(D)+多柔比星/环磷酰胺(AC)2 周期	4 周期 DAC 或 6 周期 DAC(适用于肿瘤减少 50%的 1 390 例患者)	8 个周期(23.5%):6 个周期(21%);AOR1.27(0.90~1.81)	8 个周期的 DAC 的 pCR 率没有高于 6 个周期
HR 阴性或 HR 阳性及临床结节阳性[429]	GeparQuattro	表柔比星、环磷酰胺(EC)、多西他赛(D)	D+卡培他滨(DX)或者 D 序贯 X(D-X)	D:22.3%,DX:19.5%,DX:22.3% pCR+/-D:2.8%~(2.4%~8.0%);EC+DX vEC plus DX:2.8%(-8.0%~2.4%)	同时 D 和 X 方案与 D 序贯 X 方案的乳房保存率或 pCR 无差异
全部[420,426,430]	I-SPY2Trial	紫杉醇(T)和小多柔比星/环磷酰胺(AC)	veliparib 和卡铂(VC)	pCR(95%概率区间):VC 与对照组分别为 51%(35%~69%)及 26%(11%~40%)	在随机分配中进行多臂试验可以有效地确定反应肿瘤亚型。VC 加标准化治疗可以提高 pCR 率
			奈拉替尼(N)	N 与 HER2+/HR=56%(37%~73%) vs 33%(11%~54%)	在 HER2+/HR-乳腺癌中,N 加标准治疗极有可能改善 pCR
			MK-2206+/-曲妥珠单抗(H)	HER2+/HR 的 MK-2206 与对照:67.5% vs 36%; HR-:49.5% vs 26.2%; HER2+:52.6% vs 29.0%	MK-2206 的三个标记(HER2+/HR-,HR-和 HER2+)表明其在 HR-和 HER2+疾病中的活性
			T-DM1(曲妥珠单抗)+帕妥珠单抗(P)	TDM1+P 与对照(TH):HER2+:52% vs 22% HER2+/HR+:64% vs 33%	TDM1+P 在所有 HER2+亚型中(包括 HR+和 HR-亚群)呈逐步递增趋势
			帕妥珠单抗(P)+曲妥珠单抗(H)(迄今为止正在测试的其他 6 种研究试剂)	HER2+:54% vs 22%HER2+/HR-:74% vs 33% HER2+/HR+:44% vs 17%	THP→AC 显著提高了 pCR 率,超过了标准的 TH→AC,并且在所有 HER2+(包括 HR+和 HR-亚群)中呈逐步递增趋势

内分泌治疗的研究比较有限,主要集中在绝经后妇女[431]。绝经后妇女内分泌治疗的作用可能相当于化疗,尽管证据有限,需要更多的研究[432,433]。在绝经后妇女的临床试验中,对不同内分泌治疗方案的研究表明,芳香化酶抑制剂比他莫昔芬更有效,在保乳手术方面也有改善,这与暴露时间有关[434~436]。在接受芳香化酶抑制剂的患者中,临床疗效反应无明显差异[437]。目前正在研究 Ki-67 和一个评价肿瘤残留和增殖的评分系统作为对新辅助激素治疗的早期疗效反应或耐药性的标志物[438,439]。目前已评估在 AI 新辅助内分泌治疗的基础上增加一些靶向治疗效果,这些治疗已显示出在晚期疾病的控制方面的改善[440]。其中包括 PI3K 和 CDK 4/6 抑制剂[441]。mTOR 抑制剂依维莫司首先在新辅助治疗环境中进行研究,然后在二线转移治疗环境中进行注册试验。在最初的研究中无法确定疗效反应和耐药的标志物,而这一目标在新辅助内分泌试验中也是难以捉摸的[442]。

在绝经前和绝经后 HR+乳腺癌队列中研究新辅助内分泌治疗的兴趣越来越浓;然而,pCR 并不是一个很好的疗效反应替代终点。目前,在 HR+乳腺癌中,我们还没有很好的早期疗效反应标志物。因此,新辅助治疗可以为理解不同乳腺癌的生物学特性和疗效反应提供平台,并帮助我们针对性地改善疗效反应和治疗结果。

新辅助治疗作为新药测试终点

I-SPY 2 试验使用一个创新模式(一种自适应设计,允许您根据自己的需要去学习)加速检测和识别新药物治剂与 NACT 结合[443]。该研究的目的是开展新药物的Ⅰ和Ⅰb 期(联合紫杉醇)在原发病高危早期复发患者的安全数据检测,研究对哪种肿瘤亚型最有效,并提高三期试验的成功机会。如果药物制剂可提高一种或多种疾病亚型的 pCR 率(与对照相比),那么它们将从试验中"毕业",并且能够预测,在验证性Ⅲ期试验中成功的可能性为 85%,这样,可以选择最有效的药物来推进三期临床试验,从而提高肿瘤三期临床试验 10%~30% 的成功率[444]。FDA 同意新辅助剂的设置将作为一个提高新药物测试效率的机会[445]。美国食品药品监督管理局(FDA)对 12 项国际试验进行了荟萃分析,通过认可 pCR 作为无事件生存试验(EFS)替代终点的证据基础,表明了它对新辅助临床试验的支持[446]。他们的主要目标包括建立 pCR 与 EFS 和 OS 之间的关系,以确定 pCR 是否与某些亚型的长期生存最相关,以及 pCR 率的增加是否能预测 EFS 和 OS。他们的发现确立了 pCR 的最佳定义。无论是乳腺癌还是淋巴结肿瘤的根除或消失,ypT0ypN0 或 ypT0/is ypN0(仅与乳腺癌相比,ypT0/is)与 EFS 和 OS 的相关性更好[(EFS *HR*:ypT0ypN0:0.44;ypT0/is ypN0:0.48 vs ypT0/is:0.60 和/或 OS *HR*:ypT0ypN0 0.36;ypT0/is ypN0:0.36 vs ypT0/is:OS 0.51)]。他们还发现,pCR 在 TNBC 患者中(EFS:*HR*=0.24,95% *CI*:0.18~0.33;OS:0.16,0.11~0.25),以及在接受曲妥珠单抗治疗的 HER2+/HR-肿瘤患者中(EFS:0.15,0.09~0.27;OS:0.08,0.03,0.22)与长期预后结果的相关性最强。

FDA 随后发布了将病理反应作为加速审批的终点的指南[447]。在 ESBC 中,新药的常规批准通常需要显示出能够改进 DFS 或 OS 的临床试验来体现临床获益。FDA 可以加速批准新药是基于替代终点已被证明取得近似的临床效益,因此 FDA 提出了使用 pCR 率作为 HER2+,三阴性,更具增生特性 HR+疾病的 DFS 和 OS 的代替终点。重要的是,在批准加速审批之前,必须完成 EFS 终点的应计项目(在新辅助试验中或作为单独的辅助试验)[448]。如果验证性试验中没有显示出 DFS 或 OS 改善的迹象,则新辅助适应证的标签将被移除。一项随机试验可以支持这种加速批准,即基于 pCR 率提高,最终通过改进 DFS 和 OS 来证实其临床获益。新辅助治疗为快速设计和测试新的治疗策略以及加速药物开发提供了一个平台。

有人担心,ALTTO[449] 和 NeoALTTO[404] 两项研究产生的不一致结果将使人们对 pCR 作为替代终点产生怀疑。然而观察发现,ALTTO 试验关于拉帕替尼和曲妥珠单抗的研究 *HR*=0.86 被 NeoALTTO 实际预测,但事件的数量并不足以使其统计学意义,NeoALTTO 试验是在术后而非术前给予 AC 化疗,与 NeoALTTO 研究相比,ALTTO 的研究对象处于较低风险(较小的肿瘤和少量淋巴结阳性患者)[450]。这些研究也显示了使用相同研究对象进行 pCR 评估和 EFS 评估的重要性,这是 I-SPY 3 国际试验的目标。一旦结果确定,一项新的关于 Her2 靶向新辅助治疗研究的荟萃分析正在计划开展中。

晚期乳腺癌的治疗

放疗对复发性及转移性乳腺癌的作用

姑息性放疗在有症状的 MBC 患者中已经确立了良好的治疗价值,但它还在继续发展,作为系统性细胞毒性、靶向治疗和内分泌治疗的补充疗法。非负重骨出现的疼痛的骨转移和普通的病理骨折对短期定向放射治疗反应良好。然而,局部放射治疗并不能替代骨内固定。RTOG 的一项Ⅲ期随机试验比较了 800cGy 单次照射与标准的 3 000cGy 分 10 次照射,两者在控制骨转移方面获得了相同的结果[451]。虽然多学科联合治疗可能适用于累及邻近软组织的复杂骨转移,但单一治疗方法可缩短治疗时间,这在大多数临床情况下肯定是更合适的。对于存在广泛骨病的患者,现代静脉药物,如 samarium-153 lexidronam,有非常好的止痛和改善骨功能的效果,且没有像早期药物带来的严重、不可逆的骨髓抑制现象发生[452]。

就脑转移癌的治疗而言,在控制效果较差的全身广泛转移的情况下,放射治疗是相当标准且优于外科治疗的治疗方法。对于多发性病变,尤其是对于广泛颅内转移,常规接受的姑息性全脑疗程为 3 000~3 750cGy,分 10~15 次照射[453]。对于单发或有限的脑转移,尤其是颅外疾病控制良好的患者,最佳治疗方法是从全脑放疗转为立体定向放疗(SRS),以避免神经认知毒性[454]。在这类患者中,与全脑放疗相关的毒性可能存在于那些有多发性脑转移或 SRS 后复发性转移的患者。

对于患有寡转移(三个或更少的癌灶部位)的患者,有新的证据表明,局部放疗可能是全身治疗的重要补充,即使对无症状的患者也是如此[455]。目前一项Ⅱ/Ⅲ期试验正在评估在标准全身治疗的基础上增加立体定向放疗或手术切除有限转移瘤的益处[456]。最后,对于局部复发性疾病患者,即使是那些已经接受过放疗、定向放疗和现代再放疗的患者,同样可以安全地与手术和全身治疗相结合,这对提供长期的局部控制和改善

QOL 至关重要[457,458]。

对转移性乳腺癌的系统治疗

转移性乳腺癌的发生率没有被正式统计过，但据估计，在所有诊断为早期乳腺癌的患者中，约有 1/4 的患者最终会发展为复发性疾病，伴有远处转移。在所有被诊断为乳腺癌的妇女中，发现 5%的人有原发性转移性乳腺癌，其特征是在最初诊断时存在远处转移。一般情况下，早期乳腺癌的复发率在初次治疗后 3~5 年达到高峰，然后在 8 年后下降到稳定状态。尽管 50%的远处复发发生在确诊后的前 5 年内，但 HR+早期乳腺癌妇女仍在长达确诊后的 20 年内存在复发风险。相比之下三阴性乳腺癌的复发一般发生在最初 3 年内，此后风险显著降低。既往，HER2+乳腺癌的预后较差，并沿着类似三阴性乳腺癌的时间轴复发，但如补充部分所述，HER2 靶向治疗显著改善了 ROR 和 OS。

如本章补充部分所述，临床病理因素，如年龄；绝经情况；肿瘤的大小、分级、组织形态学和生物标志物状态；节点状态影响 ROR。然而，完成最佳辅助治疗后淋巴结阴性乳腺癌患者清楚地表明，临床病理因素并不能完全解释风险。无论辅助治疗如何，与 Luminal A 型患者相比，Luminal B 亚型患者在诊断后 5~10 年无复发生存率更差[313]。基底样亚型的患者在诊断后 5 年比腔内 B 亚型的患者病情更严重，但是实际上这些生存曲线在 10 年后交叉。

像复发的时间一样，转移的位置和范围通常与特定的癌症亚型有关。HER2+乳腺癌易发生内脏和中枢神经系统转移。三阴性乳腺癌倾向于在肺或大脑的局部复发，但在骨中复发的概率较低[309]。HR+乳腺癌通常累及骨骼和软组织，病程缓慢，但在某些情况下，累及内脏的表现更为严重。

转移性乳腺癌患者的中位生存期为 2~3 年。长期预后由肿瘤生物学、生长速度、疾病负担、器官定位、治疗反应持续时间、对干预措施的耐药性或敏感性决定。大多数有明显远处转移的患者目前无法治愈。转移性乳腺癌的中位生存期为 2~3 年。皮肤转移、淋巴结转移和骨转移较少的患者，生存期较长，多处脏器受累的患者生存期较短，尤其是对于发生内脏转移（肝脏、脑、肺脏）的患者。与激素受体阴性或对系统治疗无反应的患者相比，ER 阳性以及化疗达到完全缓解的患者生存期较长。

对于大多数转移性乳腺癌患者来说，治疗严格意义上是姑息性治疗，目的是通过减轻疾病和治疗引起的症状，延缓疾病的进展，同时改善生活质量。被诊断为转移癌的患者应该被告知，他们的疾病是无法治愈的，但可以治疗，并鼓励患者可以带瘤生存多年。鉴于转移性乳腺癌具有相当大的异质性，个体化治疗计划应包括但不限于医学、外科和放射专科医师、姑息治疗专家、心理肿瘤学家、肿瘤专科护士、社会工作者和患者导航员在内的多学科小组合作[460]。

当患者有症状或体检结果不确定是否复发时，病史和体格检查应该集中检查胸壁、皮肤、余下的乳腺、区域和远处淋巴结、中轴骨、肺脏、肝脏和中枢神经系统这些部位的转移。实验室评估应该包括全血计数、血小板计数、血钙和肝肾功能检查。如果血清肿瘤标志物 CA15~3、CA27.29 和 CEA 比基线水平升高，则可以每月结合体检和影像学对其进行评估，以跟踪治疗效果。

发现有可疑的复发转移癌，应该强烈考虑诊断性活检[409,458]。活检可以检测组织的 ER、PR、HER2/neu 和其他标志物，有助于治疗决策。这些标志物的表达可能会发生改变，与原发性乳腺癌诊断时的表达情况不同。10%~30%的病例存在 ER 不一致，20%~50%的病例存在 PR 不一致，HER2 不一致的比例更高[461]。在无法获得的肿瘤标本的组织中，患者和肿瘤特征有助于确定肿瘤是否有可能对激素治疗敏感。有 HR+/HER2-早期乳腺癌病史、无病间隔超过 3 年、主要位于软组织和/或骨骼的小体积转移性疾病的老年绝经后患者比具有相反特征的患者更有可能对内分泌治疗产生反应。对于呈惰性临床经过的患者，ER 阴性的检测结果意味着应该进行重复检测，以确保假阴性结果不会使患者错失有可能带来获益的内分泌治疗。

治疗指南的使用与存活率的提高之间存在明显的关联。转移性乳腺癌的管理有几个指导原则。2013 年 11 月，在葡萄牙里斯本举行的第二届晚期乳腺癌国际共识会议（ABC2）上，欧洲肿瘤学会（ESO）和欧洲肿瘤医学会（ESMO）共同制订了指南[458]。ASCO 的临床实践指南提供了基于证据的建议，这些建议是由多学科专家小组通过对Ⅲ期临床试验和临床经验的系统回顾而制订的。关于转移性乳腺癌有几个 ASCO 临床实践指南，可以在 http://www.instituteforquality.org/practice-guidelines 找到[462~465]。

HR+/HER2-早期乳腺癌的系统治疗

大多数新诊断为 HR+/HER2-早期乳腺癌的患者都采用内分泌治疗。化疗应用于那些有终末器官功能障碍风险或已经存在终末器官功能障碍的患者，对他们来说，迅速减轻肿瘤负担至关重要。只有少数临床试验对 HR+/HER2-早期乳腺癌患者的内分泌治疗与化疗进行了比较。2003 年发表的 Cochrane 荟萃分析评估了 10 项相关研究，并报告说，尽管化疗的反应速度更快（$RR=1.25$，95% CI：1.01~1.54，$P=0.04$），OS 无差异（$HR=0.94$，95% CI：0.79~1.12，$P=0.5$）[466]。纳入的试验是几十年前进行的，评估了各种激素疗法，但未能充分评估生活质量。考虑到治疗目标，大多数指南重新修订了 HR+/HER2-早期乳腺癌患者应早期使用激素治疗，除非病情进展迅速[409,458]。

HR+/HER2-乳腺癌患者的内分泌治疗方案包括他莫昔芬、非甾体芳香化酶抑制剂阿那曲唑和来曲唑、甾体依西美坦和氟维司群，以及不太常用的其他药物，如醋酸甲地孕酮和雌二醇。在选择治疗方案时，必须考虑辅助治疗前的内分泌治疗以及辅助治疗和复发之间的间隔时间。药物副作用情况也应在个体化的基础上加以考虑。

大约 50%的患者对一线激素治疗有反应。完成辅助激素治疗并达到长期无病间隔的患者可能对一线激素治疗有反应。内分泌治疗引起大鼠不良反应的时间可能会延长，不应过早放弃治疗。在使用其他治疗前，如果没有发生进展，患者应该进行连续 6~12 周的试验性治疗。无临床反应或经两种激素治疗后病情进展的患者应转用化疗。对激素治疗有反应的患者通常可以继续进行几个连续的激素治疗，直到没有进一步的激素治疗方法可用或发生内脏风险。

事实上，所有 HR+/HER2-早期乳腺癌患者最终都会对激素治疗产生继发性耐药性。在过去的十年中,分子靶向药物已经与一线和二线激素治疗相结合,以克服或预防激素耐药性。其中一些组合已经可提高 PFS,进一步扩大了内分泌治疗的适应证。

绝经前 HR+/HER2-早期乳腺癌的内分泌治疗

对于绝经前激素受体阳性的转移性乳腺癌患者,抗雌激素治疗是首选,除非在辅助抗雌激素治疗的一年内发生转移。LHRH 激动剂戈舍瑞林和亮丙瑞林在 20 世纪 80 年代开始在 MBC 中使用,提供了类似的临床效益,无须手术干预。他莫昔芬最初并不是作为绝经前乳腺癌的单一药物,而是与 LHRH 激动剂联合使用。Klijn 等人[468]于 2001 年发表了一项荟萃分析,对 506 名患有早期乳腺癌患者评估 LHRH 激动剂(包括或不包括他莫昔芬)的四项Ⅱ期临床试验显示,对于绝经前的激素反应性转移性乳腺癌,他莫昔芬和 LHRH 类似物联合用药[299]是内分泌治疗的首选。

ABC2 共识指南和 NCCN 指南都建议,对于 HR+/HER2-早期乳腺癌[409,458]的绝经前妇女,首先应采用卵巢去势或消融联合内分泌治疗。如果证实了对他莫昔芬的耐药,或者患者在使用或不使用 LHRH 激动剂的情况下使用一线他莫昔芬,那么可以遵循绝经后妇女推荐的相同治疗顺序,但要继续使用 LHRH 激动剂。

绝经后 HR+/HER2-乳腺癌的内分泌治疗

1977 年,他莫昔芬被批准用于绝经后乳腺癌患者,并在 20 多年的时间里一直是 HR+乳腺癌的主要治疗药物。早期临床试验比较了他莫昔芬与现有的激素疗法,如二乙基雌酚、炔雌醇、醋酸甲地孕酮和氟氧酮。在许多病例中发现,他莫昔芬对 HR+ MBC 患者的反应率高达 50%,而且副作用更容易耐受[469]。

几个多中心在 2000 年和 2001 年发表的Ⅲ期临床试验表明,第三代非甾体类 AI 作为一线治疗绝经后乳腺癌妇女治疗效果优于或者相当于他莫昔芬 470~472。最大的一项Ⅲ期随机临床试验,纳入 907 名绝经后 HR+(或激素受体状态未知)乳腺癌患者,来曲唑每天 2.5mg 或他莫昔芬每天 20mg[469]。来曲唑组患者临床获益率(CBR)高于对照组(49% vs 38%),与他莫昔芬组相比显著延长肿瘤进展时间(41 周:26 周;HR=0.70,95%CI:0.60~0.82,P=0.001)。Mauriet 等人[473]在 2006 年的一项荟萃分析中评估了 AI 与他莫昔芬和其他激素疗法的疗效对比,并证明了作为一线治疗,第三代 AI 具有显著的生存优势(相对危险率降低 11%(95%CI:1%~19%,P=0.03)。补充部分讨论了与他莫昔芬和 AI 相关的副作用和毒性。类固醇和非类固醇 AI 之间存在不完全的交叉耐药性[474]。研究表明,在一种 AI 上取得进展的患者,可以通过另一种类型的药物获得具有临床意义的益处[475,476]。

氟维司群是纯雌激素拮抗剂,阻断 ER 的两个活性功能域的转录活性,还影响受体的二聚化,促使受体降解,导致细胞中的 ER 受体浓度显著下降,抑制雌激素信号转导。根据三期临床试验结果显示,氟维司群与阿那曲唑有相似的反应率和肿瘤进展时间(TTP),在 2002 年被 FDA 批准可每月肌内注射使用。最初准予每月肌内注射 250mg 氟维司群,但是随后在复发性或转移性乳腺癌试验中的比较(如下所述)表明,每月注射 500mg 氟维司群效果优于前者[478]。

北美试验 0021 是Ⅲ期、双盲、双模拟临床试验,随机选取 400 名绝经后 HR+乳腺癌患者,每月氟维司群 250mg 肌内注射或每日服用阿那曲唑片 1mg[481,479]。大约 96%的患者接受了他莫昔芬作为辅助治疗或转移治疗。中位随访 16.8 个月,TTP、CBR、OR、AE 的差异均无统计学意义(HR=0.92,9.14%CI:0.74~1.15,P=0.42)。

随机、双盲、双模拟Ⅲ期临床试验对比氟维司群和依西美坦在使用非甾体类 AI 治疗后进展或复发的 HR+乳腺癌女性患者的疗效[480]。纳入的 693 名妇女中 60%的患者在这项研究之前接受了至少两种内分泌治疗。氟维司群首日给药量为 500m,第 14、28 天每日 250mg,之后每 4 周 250mg,依西美坦每日给药量为 25mg。与试验 0021 相似,差异无统计学意义。两组患者 TTP 中位数均为 3.7 个月(HR=0.963,95%CI:0.819~1.133,P=0.653 1)。氟维司群与依西美坦相比 ORR 分别为 7.4%、6.7%,P = 0.736,CBR 分别为 32.2%、31.5%;,P = 0.853)。相当大比例的患者可耐受这两种疗法。

Ⅲ期 CONFIRM 试验旨在确定是否如临床前和临床Ⅱ期结果所示,更高剂量的氟维司群方案会提高治疗效果[476]。共有 736 名绝经后 HR+乳腺癌妇女接受氟维司群 500mg 肌内注射(第 0 天、第 14 天、第 28 每日 250mg,此后每 28 天 250mg)。所有参与者都曾在辅助治疗或转移治疗中接受过抗雌激素或 AI 治疗。氟维司群 500m 与 250mg 相比较,PFS 可得到延长(HR=0.80,95%CI:0.68~0.94,P=0.006)。两组注射部位疼痛、恶心、骨痛等不良反应的发生率和严重程度相似。这些结果促使 2010 年 9 月 FDA 批准了氟维司群 500mg。

FIRST 是一项随机、开放、平行设计的多中心Ⅱ期临床研究,旨在比较氟维司群 500mg 与阿那曲唑 1mg 在晚期乳腺癌一线内分泌治疗中的疗效。研究结果显示,对于初诊的绝经后晚期乳腺癌患者,给予氟维司群 500mg 较阿那曲唑能够显著延长无进展生存期(PFS)达 10.3 个月,总生存期(OS)获益长达 54.1 个月。随机选择 205 名 HR+患者接受氟维司群 500mg(第 0 天、第 14 天、第 28 每日 500mg,此后每 28 天 500mg)和阿那曲唑每日 1mg 相比较[477]。晚期患者未接受内分泌治疗,<30%的患者已完成多于 12 个月辅助内分泌治疗。晚期一线治疗中,氟维司群(HD)较阿那曲唑能显著延长 PFS(中位 PFS:23.4 个月对 13.1 个月;HR=0.66,95%CI:0.47~0.92,P=0.01),且耐受性良好[483]。

SoFEAⅢ期临床试验评估了联合内分泌治疗对绝经后 HR+乳腺癌患者的作用[484]。共有 723 名女性随机接受氟维司群联合阿那曲唑、氟维司群联合安慰剂或依西美坦联合安慰剂治疗。在 PFS 方面,氟维司群加阿那曲唑组与氟维司群加安慰剂组没有差异,依西美坦组与氟维司群加安慰剂组也没有差异。然而,该研究使用了 250mg 的氟维司群。

对于激素治疗进展缓慢,但肿瘤负荷低,症状轻微,或对其他药物如炔雌醇和醋酸甲地孕酮缺乏候选药物的患者,还存在其他内分泌疗法。临床研究表明,HR+乳腺癌细胞在长期缺乏雌激素后发生雌二醇诱导的凋亡。Ellis 等人进行了一项Ⅱ期临床试验,随机选择了 66 名 HR+乳腺癌的女性,她们在 AI 治疗上取得疗效,每天服用雌二醇 30mg 或 6mg。两组均显示

485CBR 约为 30%，但低剂量组的严重 AE 较低。醋酸甲地孕酮在 HR+乳腺癌有疗效。

早期研究表明，乳腺癌 . 486 中位 PFS 为 15 个月，对醋酸甲地孕酮的应答率为 25%，剂量为每日 4 次，每次 40mg。值得注意的副作用包括体重增加、体液潴留、阴道出血、静脉血栓栓塞性疾病和生活质量低下。

内分泌疗法研究

一些正在进行的临床试验已经评估了标准激素疗法以及新的抗雌激素疗法的最佳顺序。一项全球范围的Ⅲ期随机、双盲、多中心临床试验 FALCON 研究，头对头地比较了氟维司群 500mg 与阿那曲唑用于绝经后激素受体阳性晚期乳腺癌一线内分泌治疗的疗效。研究纳入 450 例既往未接受过内分泌治疗的 ER 和/或 PR 阳性的局部晚期或转移性乳腺癌患者，在中位随访 25 个月后，与阿那曲唑治疗组相比，氟维司群能够显著改善患者 PFS：16.6 个月对 13.8 个月，$HR=0.797$（95% CI：0.637～0.999），$P=0.0486$。研究结果于 2016 年秋季公布。

FALCON 研究结果揭示，对既往未接受辅助内分泌治疗的乳腺癌患者，氟维司群 500mg 一线治疗绝经后激素受体阳性晚期乳腺癌的疗效优于 AI，奠定了氟维司群 500mg 作为激素受体阳性晚期乳腺癌的一线治疗地位。

其他评估集中在新的激素制剂上，如 ER 降解剂、雄激素拮抗剂和 AR 抑制剂。有关这些试验的详细信息可在 http://www.cancer.gov/abcancer/treatment/clintrials/ 中找到。

内分泌治疗联合靶向药物治疗

内分泌治疗是一种有效的、普遍耐受良好的治疗方案，可以控制病情，同时延迟 HR+/HER2-乳腺癌患者向化疗的过渡。遗憾的是，所有的患者最终都会对内分泌疗法产生抵抗。辅助性内分泌治疗开始后 2 年内复发、内分泌治疗结束后 12 个月内复发、早期乳腺癌开始内分泌治疗后 6 个月以内进展者为继发性或获得性耐药[458]。参与原发性和继发性耐药的分子机制很复杂。临床前研究已经认识到 ER 和各种生长因子受体以及细胞内信号通路之间存在适应性交叉。使乳腺癌细胞逃避内分泌治疗的假定机制包括 *ER* 基因的突变（ESR），通过上调生长因子受体通路增强信号转导，诱导激素非依赖型增长，过敏性低雌激素浓度，细胞周期蛋白 D1 超表达。通过临床前模型对激素抵抗机制的理解的提高促进了临床试验的发展，这些临床试验旨在通过将传统的基于激素的疗法与选择性靶向肿瘤生物学的药物相结合，延缓或逆转内分泌抵抗。表 108-14 列出了许多研究中的治疗方法，它们的作用机制和分子靶点，以及有关的乳腺癌亚型。

表 108-14 正在进行的临床试验中的研究药物、相关分子靶标和乳腺癌亚型

分子靶点	研究药物	作用机制	在单药或联合用药测试下正在研究的乳腺癌亚型
成纤维细胞生长因子（FGF）通路	德立替尼	FGF 受体抑制剂；VEGF 受体抑制剂；PDGF 受体抑制剂	任何 *FGFR* 突变的亚型（用单药）
胰岛素样生长因子（IGF）通路	cixutumumab（IMC-A12）	抗 IGF-1 受体单克隆抗体	任何亚型（用替西罗莫司） HER2+（用细胞毒类药物和拉帕替尼）
JAK/STAT 通路	ruxolitinib（INCB-18424）	JAK1/2 抑制剂	HER2+（用曲妥珠单抗） HER2-（用细胞毒性药物）
MAPK 通路	selumetinib（AZD6244，ARRY-142886）	MEK 抑制剂	HR+（用 EBT）
PI3K/Akt/mTOR 通路	阿哌利西（BYL719） taselisib（GDC-0032）	α 特异性 PI3K 抑制剂	HR+/HER2-（用 EBT） HER2+用 HER2 定向治疗 TNBC（用恩佐鲁胺）
	buparlisib（BKM120） pictilisib（GDC-0941）	1 型 Pan PI3K 抑制剂	HR+/HER2-（用 EBT；瑞博西尼；细胞毒类药物） TNBC（用细胞毒类药物）
	MK-2206	Akt 抑制剂	任何亚型（用细胞毒类药物） HR+/HER2-（用 EBT）
	替西罗莫司	mTOR 抑制剂	HR+/HER2-（用 EBT） TNBC（用细胞毒类药物；贝伐单抗）
	sapanisertib（MLN0128）	mTORC1/2	HR+/HER2-（用 EBT）
细胞周期蛋白依赖性激酶（CDK）	玻玛西林（LY2835219） dinaciclib（SCH727965） 瑞博西尼（LEE-001）	CDK 4/6 抑制剂	HR+/HER2-（用 EBT）

续表

分子靶点	研究药物	作用机制	在单药或联合用药测试下正在研究的乳腺癌亚型
集落刺激因子(CSF)-1	PLX3397	CSF-1R 抑制剂;KIT 抑制剂	TNBC(用细胞毒药物)
受体糖蛋白 NMB(gpNMB)	glembatumumab vedotin (CDX-011)	抗 gpNMB 抗体-药物缀合物	TNBC(单药)
热休克蛋白 90(HSP90)	ganetespib(STA-9090)	HSP90 抑制剂(一种新型小分子抑制剂)	HR+/HER2-(用细胞毒药物) Any subtype(单药)
HER2	奈拉替尼(HKI-272)	HER2/EGFR 双靶点酪氨酸激酶抑制剂	HER2+(单药) HER2+(用细胞毒药物) HER2+(用曲妥珠单抗) HER2equivocal(用细胞毒药物)
	margetuximab	Fc 优化的抗 HER2 单克隆抗体	HER2+(单药;用细胞毒药物)
	MM-302	HER2 靶向脂质体多柔比星(一种新型抗体-药物偶联物)	HER2+(单药)
	ONT-380(ARRY-380)	HER2 特异性抑制剂(一种新型小分子抑制剂)	HER2+(单药)
HER3	patritumab(U3~1287)	抗 HER3 单克隆抗体(新药)	HER2+(用细胞毒药物;曲妥珠单抗)
组蛋白去乙酰化酶(HDAC)	恩替诺特 vorinostat panobinostat	HDAC 抑制剂	HR+/HER2-(用 EBT;免疫治疗) HER2+(用细胞毒药物;曲妥珠单抗) 任何亚型(单药)
PARP	奥拉帕利(olaparib) veliparib(ABT-888)	PARP1/2 抑制剂	TNBC(单药;用细胞毒药物)
	talazoparib(BMN-673)	PARP1/2 抑制剂;PARP1/2 捕集剂	gBRCA(单药)
PD-1 和 PD-L1	帕博利珠单抗(MK-3475)	抗 PD-1 单克隆抗体	TN(用细胞毒类药物) HR+/HER2-(用 HDAC 抑制剂;EBT)
	阿特珠单抗(MPDL3280A)	抗 PD-L1 单克隆抗体	TNBC(单药) HER2+(用细胞毒类药物;曲妥珠单抗)
SRC	Dasatinib	SRC 抑制剂	HER2+(用曲妥珠单抗和细胞毒类药物)
类固醇激素	bazedoxifene	选择性雌激素受体调节剂	HR+(用 CDK 4/6 抑制剂)
	enobosarm(GTx-024)	选择性雄激素受体调节剂	TN/AR+(单药) ER+/AR+(单药)
	bicalutamide	抗雄激素	HR+或 HR-/AR+(用 CDK 4/6 抑制剂)
	恩佐鲁胺	雄激素受体抑制剂	HR+/HER2-(用 EBT) TNBC(单药;用 PI3K 抑制剂)

EBT,内分泌疗法。

基于内分泌的治疗和抗血管生成剂

临床前研究表明,由 HR+乳腺癌细胞分泌的 VEGF 通过新血管生成驱动肿瘤增殖。VEGF 水平升高与早期复发和激素治疗耐药相关。来曲唑/氟维司群和安维汀(LEA)研究是第一个评估激素治疗与抗 VEGF 单克隆抗体贝伐单抗联合作为 HR+/HER2-转移性乳腺癌患者的一线治疗的Ⅲ期临床试验[488]。研究随机分配 380 名接受内分泌治疗(来曲唑或氟维司群)的患者,每 3 周静脉注射贝伐单抗 15mg/kg 或仅接受内分泌治疗。大约一半的研究参与者在辅助治疗中接受了内分泌治疗,其中只有 20%接受了 AI。中位随访时间为 23.7 个月,贝伐单抗组中位 PFS 为 19.3 个月,对照组为 14.4 个月(HR = 0.83,95%

CI:0.65~1.06,*P*=1.26)。治疗失败的时间和 OS 在两组中相似,但含贝伐单抗组的毒性更为显著。

Dickler 等人在 2015 年 ASCO 上报道了 CALGB40503(Alliance)的初步结果,这是一项大型Ⅲ期临床试验,评估了 HR+转移性乳腺癌患者中来曲唑联合贝伐单抗一线治疗的效果[489]。中位随访 39 个月,共观察到 258 例 PFS 事件,联合组的中位 PFS 为 20 个月,而单用来曲唑组仅为 16 个月(*HR*=0.74,95%*CI*:0.58~0.95,*P*=0.016)。ORR(*P*=0.004)和 CBR(*P*=0.005)在含贝伐单抗组中体现出显著优势,但 OS 没有明显差异。但在联合组中毒性反应也明显加强,其中 50%的患者报告了高级别不良事件,而对照组仅有 14%的患者发生。

基于内分泌的疗法和 PI3K/Akt/mTOR 途径抑制剂

PI3K/Akt/mTOR 通路在细胞增殖、代谢和存活中起关键作用。PI3K/Akt/mTOR 途径的过度活化导致下游信号转导增加以及 ER 配体的非依赖性激活。PI3K/Akt/mTOR 通路经常在大约 50%的 HR+MBC 中失调,并且不适当的上调与不良预后和激素疗法的耐药性相关。mTOR 抑制剂联合内分泌治疗的临床前研究证明其可以对 HR+乳腺癌细胞产生协同抑制作用。二线激素疗法依西美坦联合 mTOR 抑制剂依维莫司治疗 MBC 可使患者的 PFS 增加一倍以上,同时 OS 上升但并无统计学差异。这一结果使得在此情况下常规使用依维莫司得到批准[488]。但是毒性反应(如口腔炎)的发生也明显增强[489]。一些评估依维莫司以及其他 PI3K 途径的抑制剂在各种疾病环境中的使用情况的试验正在进行。PI3K-α 特异性亚基抑制剂已经提供了令人鼓舞的早期试验结果,同时具有不同以往且可能更有利的毒性结果。

应用依维莫司治疗乳腺癌(BOLERO-2)临床试验是一项双盲,随机,Ⅲ期研究,该研究评估了在 NSAI 治疗后疾病进展的 HR+/HER2-MBC 患者中联合使用依西美坦加依维莫司(一种 mTOR 抑制剂)的疗效[490]。经过 18 个月的中位随访时间后,依维莫司+依西美坦组的中位 PFS 为 7.8 个月,而安慰剂+依西美坦组只有 3.2 个月[491]。上述结果是 FDA 批准对 NSAI 治疗后疾病进展的乳腺癌患者使用依西美坦联合依维莫司的基础。39 个月后的最终分析显示了联合用药组拥有 4 个月的 OS 获益,差异具有统计学意义(*HR*=0.89,95%*CI*:0.73~1.10,*P*=0.14)[492]。但依维莫司与许多特定类别的 AE 相关,这些 AE 具有剂量限制性,可显著提升口腔炎,皮疹和非感染性肺炎的发病率。一些正在进行的研究已经在新辅助,辅助和转移环境中对依维莫司进行了评估。实验细节详见 http://www.cancer.gov/about-cancer/treatment/clinical-trials/search。

HORIZON 是一项随机,安慰剂对照的Ⅲ期临床试验,随机分配 1 112 名患有 HR+MBC 的绝经后妇女接受一线 mTOR 抑制剂替西罗莫司(temsirolimus)每日 30mg(每 2 周 5 天)+来曲唑每日 2.5mg 或安慰剂+来曲唑[493]。大约 60%的患者在辅助治疗中没有接受内分泌治疗。总人群中(*HR*=0.90,95%*CI*:0.76~1.07,*P*=0.25)或先前接受过辅助内分泌治疗的患者中(*HR*=0.84,95%*CI*:0.66~1.08,*P*=0.17)PFS 均没有明显改善。BOLERO-2 和 HORIZON 结果之间的差异部分归因于药代动力学,给药方案和研究人群的变化。

内分泌治疗和 CDK4/6 抑制剂

CDK 是一类丝/苏氨酸激酶,在细胞复制和分裂的调节中起关键作用。CDK4/6 与细胞周期蛋白 D 形成复合物以使视网膜母细胞瘤蛋白(Rb)失活,从而激活基因转录。CDK 的失调可导致过度的细胞增殖,同时因为肿瘤生长和抗性而变得更复杂。临床前研究表明,CDK4/6 抑制剂可诱导乳腺癌细胞系的细胞生长停滞和凋亡,当 ER+乳腺癌细胞暴露于 CDK4/6 抑制剂和以内分泌为基础的治疗时,会产生协同效应。CDK4/6 抑制剂是口服给药的一类新型小分子治疗剂,主要毒性是自限性的、无并发症的中性粒细胞减少症。研究人员在临床试验中积极研究了几种 CDK4/6 抑制剂,结果令人满意。

帕博西尼(palbociclib)是一种口服 CDK4/6 抑制剂,在Ⅱ期和Ⅲ期试验中均有很好的结果。一项Ⅱ期试验显示,在一线治疗中,来曲唑基础上加用帕博西尼会使 PFS 加倍,但 OS 没有明显改善[495]。这些数据加速了 FDA 批准帕博西尼联合来曲唑作为 HR+转移性乳腺癌的一线治疗方案。最终批准取决于第三阶段试验的结果,该项结果应于 2016 年公布。在二线治疗的环境中,氟维司群加用帕博西尼也使 PFS 增加一倍以上,但 OS 的数据尚不成熟[496]。帕博西尼的主要毒性是自限性、无并发症的中性粒细胞减少症。

PALOMA-1/TRIO-18 是一项国际、随机、开放的Ⅱ期临床试验,评估在一线环境中对来曲唑加用帕博西尼(一种 CDK4/6 抑制剂)在 HR+/HER2-转移性乳腺癌中的疗效[493]。共有 165 名绝经后妇女被随机分配到帕博西尼(125mg/(次·天),每 28 天中服用 21 天)加用来曲唑每日 2.5mg 组或单用来曲唑组。大约 50%的患者是新发的 MBC,因此之前没有接受治疗。单用曲唑组的中位 PFS 为 10.2 个月,而含帕博西尼的组为 20.2 个月(*HR*=0.488,95%*CI*:0.319~0.748;单侧 *P*=0.000 4)。该研究无法评估 OS。在含帕博西尼的组中,54%的患者存在 3~4 级中性粒细胞减少症,而单用来曲唑组仅有 1%。研究期间未发生粒细胞减少性发热或中性粒细胞减少相关感染病例。2015 年 2 月公布的这些结果使得 FDA 加速批准帕博西尼联合来曲唑用于 HR+/HER2-MBC 的初始激素治疗[497]。

PALOMA-2Ⅲ期临床试验是一项持续的确认性研究,其设计与 PALOMA-1 相似(ClinicalTrials.gov 编号:NCT0201740427)。超过 650 名患者随机按 3:1比例分到帕博西尼+来曲唑组或安慰剂+来曲唑组。初步结果预计在 2016 年公布。

PALOMA-3 是一项Ⅲ期临床试验,评估氟维司群与帕博西尼联合用于 HR+/HER2-MBC 患者,这些患者在之前的激素治疗中疾病已经进展或复发[494]。共有 521 名患者被随机按 2:1 的比例分入帕博西尼+氟维司群组或安慰剂+氟维司群组。该研究允许纳入接受过戈舍瑞林卵巢抑制的绝经前妇女。含帕博西尼组的中位 PFS 为 9.2 个月,而安慰剂组为 3.8 个月(进展或死亡的 *HR*=0.42,95%*CI*:0.32~0.56,*P*<0.001)。

帕博西尼是迄今为止唯一被批准的 CDK4/6 抑制剂,但正在进行的临床试验正在研究 CDK4/6 抑制剂瑞博西尼(ribociclib)和玻玛西林(abemaciclib)在转移以及新辅助和辅助环境中的作用。

瑞博西尼和玻玛西林

MONALEESA-1 是一项随机Ⅱ期临床试验，评估瑞博西尼(LEE-001)，一种 CDT4/6 抑制剂，在新辅助治疗中的生物学活性(ClinicalTrials. gov 编号：NCT 01919229)。该研究已经完成，预计初步结果于 2016 年公布。MONALEESA-2 是一项双盲，安慰剂对照的Ⅲ期临床试验，评估每日联合使用 2.5mg 来曲唑和 600mg 瑞博西尼(4 周为一个周期，前 3 周每日 1 次然后停药一周，)在大概 500 名疾病进展且之前未接受过治疗的 HR+/HER2-MBC 患者中的作用(ClinicalTrials. gov 编号：NCT01958021)。2016 年中期的新闻宣布 MONALEESA-2 已达到其疗效终点，数据预计在 2016 年晚些时候发布。

玻玛西林(LY2835219)是一种 CDK4/6 抑制剂，血液学毒性较弱，但比其他类药物胃肠道毒性更强。MONARCH-1 是一项Ⅱ期临床试验，评估单用玻玛西林(LY2835219)在 HR+/HER2-复发的、局部晚期或在转移性环境中激素治疗和化疗均有进展的 MBC 患者中的疗效(ClinicalTrials. gov 编号：NCT02102490)。在 2016 年的 ASCO 会议上，由 Dickler 等人呈现的数据证明了该方案整体有效率为 19.7%，临床受益率为 42.4%。MONARCH-3 是一项随机，双盲Ⅲ期临床试验，招募了大约 450 名患有 HR+/HER2-MBC 的绝经后妇女，在一线环境中接受 NSAI+玻玛西林或 NSAI+安慰剂(ClinicalTrials. gov 编号：NCT02246621)。最终的 PFS 数据收集工作预计于 2017 年 6 月进行。一项Ⅱ期研究正在评估玻玛西林在患有脑转移的 HR+/HER2-乳腺癌患者中的疗效和安全性(ClinicalTrials. gov 编号：NCT02308020)。

基于内分泌的治疗和雄激素受体抑制剂

AR 在乳腺癌亚型中的表达差异很大，84%~95%的 HR+乳腺癌都表达 AR，而仅有 10%~43%HR-乳腺癌也表达 AR[498]。临床前数据表明 AR 参与了抗 AI 的过程。一项多中心，双盲，Ⅱ期临床试验将 247 名患有 HR+/HER2-MBC 的患者随机分到依西美坦+恩佐鲁胺(enzalutamide)160mg/d 或依西美坦+安慰剂两组中。该实验正在进行中(ClinicalTrials. gov 编号：NCT02007512)。

基于内分泌的治疗和 PI3K 抑制剂

一些正在进行中的Ⅱ期和Ⅲ期临床试验旨在评估口服 PI3K 抑制剂，如Ⅰ类 pan-PI3K 抑制剂 buparlisib(BKM120)、α-选择性 PI3K 抑制剂阿哌利西(alpelisib)(BYL719)和 taselisib 作为 MBC 患者的一线和二线治疗方案的疗效。BELLE-2 是一项随机、双盲、安慰剂对照的Ⅲ期临床试验，评估了氟维司群肌注 500mg(第 0,14,28 天给药，此后每 28 天给药 1 次)与 buparlisib 100mg/(次·d)联合用药在 AI 治疗后进展的 HR+/HER2-MBC 的绝经后妇女中的作用(ClinicalTrials. gov 编号：NCT01610284)。在 2015 年的圣安东尼奥乳腺癌会议上，由 Baselga 等人呈现的数据表明了该试验 PFS 获益很小，而毒性反应却很显著。有趣的是，研究人员在一小部分患者中检测了循环 DNA，并证明了 *PIK3CA* 突变的患者有更大的获益。这个有趣的来源于假设的数据是令人鼓舞的，但在 PFS 上的低获益率和毒性反应让 buparlisib 的进一步研发变得不现实。BELLE-3 是唯一正在进行的有关 buparlisib 的试验。它是一项随机，安慰剂对照的Ⅲ期临床试验，评估了氟维司群 500mg 肌内注射(第 0、14、28 天给药，之后每 28 天给药 1 次)与 buparlisib 100mg/d 一次的组合对 mTOR 抑制剂与内分泌治疗联合治疗后疾病进展的 HR+/HER2-MBC 的绝经后妇女的作用(ClinicalTrials. gov 编号：NCT01633060)。该研究将有助于确定在应用 mTOR 抑制剂疾病进展后使用靶向 PI3K/Akt/mTOR 途径的替代药物是否有益。

尽管 buparlisib 的试验结果令人沮丧，但在两个令人振奋的早期研究数据的基础上，两种 PIK3CA-α 靶向药物正处于Ⅲ期试验阶段。这两项试验均在比较氟维司群+靶向药物和氟维司群+安慰剂在 HR+HER2-MBC 的绝经后女性中的效果。其中，SOLAR-1 正在评估阿哌利西(NCT02437318)，SANDPIPER 正在评估 taselisib(NCT02340221)。

内分泌治疗和 PI3K 抑制剂的组合也在新辅助治疗的大背景中进行研究。NEOBELLE，一项随机、双盲Ⅱ期临床试验，针对 HR+HER2-ESBC(early-stagebreastcancer，早期乳腺癌)的绝经后女性比较了来曲唑(每日 2.5mg)+α 特异性 PI3K 抑制剂(阿哌利西)和来曲唑+安慰剂的组合(ClinicalTrials. gov 编号：NCT01923168)。随机分配到实验组的患者每天接受 300mg 的阿哌利西。治疗将持续 24 周，当发生不可接受的毒性反应或疾病进展时治疗停止，此时患者将接受手术。该试验最初还包括 buparlisib，但在 BELLE-2 令人失望的结果之后，相关试验也停止了。

许多正在进行的研究正在评估针对 ESBC 和 MBC 中 PI3K/Akt/mTOR 途径的药物。有关这些试验的详细信息，请访问 http://www. cancer. gov/about-cancer/treatment/clinical-trials/search。

基于内分泌的治疗和 HDAC 抑制剂

恩替诺特(entinostat)是一种新的 1 类组蛋白去乙酰化酶(HDAC)抑制剂。其临床前模型证明了它可以通过下调生长因子信号通路，正常化 ER 水平和升高芳香化酶水平来恢复激素敏感性[499]。ENCORE301 是一项随机Ⅱ期临床试验。该试验随机选择了 130 名 NSAI 治疗后疾病进展的 HR+/HER2-MBC 的绝经后女性接受每日 25mg 依西美坦+每周口服 5mg 恩替诺特或依西美坦+安慰剂的治疗方案[500]。治疗分析结果显示含恩替诺特组 PFS 得到改善，为 4.3 个月，而对照组 PFS 为 2.3 个月(HR=0.73,95% CI:0.50~1.07；单侧 P=0.055)。选择中位 OS 作为试验终点，与对照组(19.8 个月)相比，含有恩替诺特的组 OS(28.1 个月)显著改善(HR=0.59,95% CI:0.36~0.97,P=0.036)。这些结酚酞致恩替诺特于 2013 年被 FDA 定义为突破性疗法。E2112 是一项Ⅲ期临床试验，比较依西美坦联合或不联合恩替诺特的疗效。该试验拟招募 600 名患有 HR+/HER2-MBC 的患者(ClinicalTrials. gov 编号：NCT02115282)。

Pan-HDAC 抑制剂伏立诺他目前正在与免疫检查点抑制剂帕博利珠单抗(pembrolizumab)共同处于研究中，以评估激素治疗耐药型 MBC 对表观遗传免疫启动的反应。下面将对帕博利珠单抗进行详细讨论。这项Ⅱ期临床试验旨在招募 58 名 HR+MBC 患者在转移性环境中进行激素治疗，每日接受他莫昔芬

20mg+伏立诺他 400mg(每周给药 5 天,停药 2 天,21 天 1 个周期),并每 3 周静脉注射 200mg 帕博利珠单抗(ClinicalTrials.gov 编号:NCT02395627)。患者随机在第 2 周期或第 4 周期开始时使用帕博利珠单抗。

HR+/HER2-MBC 治疗指南和建议

ABC2 共识指南指出,对于患有 HR+/HER2-MBC 的绝经后女性,优选的一线内分泌治疗是 AI 或他莫昔芬,具体取决于辅助治疗的类型和持续时间[458]。高剂量的氟维司群也是一线治疗的一种选择。其次,指南规定患有 HR+/HER2-MBC 的患者在接受 NSAI 治疗后若出现疾病进展,应考虑使用依维莫司联合依西美坦进行治疗。NCCN 指南与 ABC2 的建议一致[409]。

MBC 的化疗

在 MBC 中是否应用化疗在很大程度上取决于患者疾病的亚型。化疗是唯一可用于转移性 TNBC 的治疗方法,通常与 HER2+MBC 中的 HER2 靶向药物联合使用。如前所述,HR+/HER2-MBC 的化疗应仅限于快速管理内脏危象,初次治疗产生的激素抵抗,或当患者对基于内分泌的疗法产生不可逆的抵抗时。表 108-15 中包括了 MBC 中常用的单药和联合化疗方案。

表 108-15 HER2-和 HER2+转移性乳腺癌的常用单药和联合化疗方案

HER2-MBC	单药化疗	紫杉醇(每周)
		多西他赛(每三周)
		白蛋白紫杉醇(nab-paclitaxel)
		多柔比星
		聚乙二醇脂质体多柔比星
		表柔比星
		卡培他滨
		艾日布林
		伊沙匹隆
		长春瑞滨
		吉西他滨
		卡铂
		顺铂
	联合化疗	多西他赛+卡培他滨
		吉西他滨+紫杉醇(或多西他赛)
		吉西他滨+卡铂(或顺铂)
HER2+MBC	紫杉醇(或多西他赛)+曲妥珠单抗+帕妥珠单抗	
	T-DM1	
	拉帕替尼+卡培他滨	
	紫杉醇+曲妥珠单抗	
	长春瑞滨+曲妥珠单抗	

摘自 2015 年网络 NCCN。经 NCCN 肿瘤学临床实践指南(NCCN 指南®)批准,适用于乳腺癌 V.3.2015。National Comprehensive Cancer Network,Inc 2015。保留所有权利。[2015 年 9 月 15 日]访问。要查看指南的最新和完整版本,请在线访问 NCCN.org。美国综合癌症网络®,NCCN®,NCCNGUIDELINES®和所有其他 NCCN 内容是 National Comprehensive Cancer Network,Inc 拥有的商标。

化疗既可以选择单一药剂,也可以选择两种及以上药物的更强化方案。从历史上看,联合化疗方案优于单药化疗,因为联合方案中增加的 *RR* 和 TTP 被认为同时也改善了 OS。Carrick 等人在 2009 年进行的一项荟萃分析中通过评估了涉及 9 742 名患者的 43 项 MBC 化疗试验,对单药与联合化疗相关的结果进行了评估[501]。本项分析中有 55%的参与者接受了一线治疗。联合治疗方案在 *RR*、PFS 和 OS 方面优于单药治疗(OS 的 $HR=0.88$,95%CI:0.83~0.94,$P<0.0001$),但同时毒性反应也增强了,差异具有统计学意义[502]。随后 Dear 等人在 2013 年进行的荟萃分析中通过评估 12 项试验,其中包括 9 项不同治疗方案的比较,以评估联合化疗与按顺序使用相同药物的疗效差异。荟萃分析显示组合和按顺序使用化疗药物之间 OS 无差异($HR=1.04$,95%CI:0.93~1.15,$P=0.45$)。但是与顺序单药化疗相比,联合化疗组的肿瘤反应增强(RR:1.16,95%CI:1.06~1.28,$P=0.001$),并且肿瘤进展风险降低($HR=1.11$,95%CI:0.99~1.25,$P=0.08$)。

维持化疗是在达到最佳疗效之后的治疗的延续。2011年，Gennari等人报告了一项随机临床试验的荟萃分析，该试验比较了化疗作为预先设定疗程内的一线治疗或作为维持治疗的疗效差异[503]。这项荟萃分析纳入了11项试验，2 269名患者，结果表明维持性化疗与OS（$HR=0.91$，95%CI：0.84~0.99，$P=0.046$）和PFS（$HR=0.64$，95%CI：0.55~0.76，$P<0.001$）的改善有关。最近在韩国的一项多中心Ⅲ期临床试验中评估了维持化疗的作用[504]。共有324名患有MBC的患者入组并在一线环境中接受了六个周期的紫杉醇+吉西他滨化疗。然后将231名疾病得到控制的患者随机分配至紫杉醇+吉西他滨维持组或持续观察组（停止任何治疗）。维持组的中位PFS显著长于观察组（分别为7.5个月和3.8个月，$P=0.026$）。此外，维持治疗组的中位OS也显著长于观察组（分别为32.3个月和23.5个月，$P=0.047$）。不出所料，维持化疗与骨髓抑制和神经病变增加有关。该研究包括转移性TNBC和HR+MBC患者。观察组HR+MBC患者没有接受维持性的激素治疗，其中只有20%先前接受过内分泌治疗。亚组分析表明，PFS的益处主要体现在TN亚型患者身上。在诱导化疗达到最佳反应后维持内分泌治疗方案尚未在临床试验中进行过研究，但是一项合理的选择[458]。

大多数患者对一线治疗有反应。尚没有临床试验证明在MBC的一线治疗中使用特定化学疗法比另一种更能提高OS。一般来说，蒽环类和紫杉醇类药物被认为是最有效的乳腺癌化疗药，并且是一线治疗中常用的治疗方法。当然，治疗方案的选择应当个性化，综合考虑先前的辅助化疗方案、复发时间、总寿命、蒽环类暴露情况和并发症。

单药化疗

紫杉醇类化合物如紫杉醇（paclitaxel）和多西他赛（docetaxel）通过稳定微管从而诱导细胞周期停滞，是治疗乳腺癌最有效和最耐受的化学疗法之一。FDA最初于1994年批准单药使用紫杉醇，剂量为175mg/m^2，每3周静脉注射一次，给药时间为1~3h。CALGB9840是一项Ⅲ期临床试验，随机分配585名MBC患者，静脉给予80mg/m^{2}紫杉醇（每月给药3周），或静脉给予紫杉醇175mg/m^2（每3周1次）作为一线或二线化疗方案[505]。在CALGB9342研究中的一项联合分析中，有158名患者每3周接受1次紫杉醇175mg/m^{2}治疗，结果表明每周给药组的OS（24个月）较每3周组的OS（12个月）明显改善（$HR=1.28$，$P=0.0092$），RR（42% vs 29%）和中位TTP（9个月vs 5个月）也显著增加。与每3周给药组相比，3级神经病变在每周给药组更常见（24% vs 12%，$P=0.0003$），而每3周给药组的骨髓抑制和感染并发症的发生率更高。

多西他赛通常以每3周75~100mg/m^{2}的剂量静脉注射1h使用。几项小型Ⅱ期和Ⅲ期临床试验比较了多西他赛每周35~40mg/m^{2}与每3周75~100mg/m^{2}静脉注射的疗效，同时在2010年Mauri等人进行的荟萃分析证明了多西他赛各种使用方案之间的ORR，PFS或OS没有显著差异[506~509]。然而，每周给药的方案中出现了较少的骨髓抑制和神经病变，但出现了更频繁的指甲改变和溢泪。

一项Ⅲ期临床试验在含有蒽环类药物治疗后进展的MBC患者中比较了多西他赛每3周100mg/m^{2}静脉注射与紫杉醇每3周175mg/m^{2}静脉注射的疗效。在372例随机分组的患者中，与紫杉醇组相比，多西他赛组的TTP更长（5.7个月vs 3.6个月；$HR=1.64$，95%CI：1.33~2.02，$P<0.0001$）同时OS也较长（15.4个月vs 12.7个月；$HR=1.41$，95%CI：1.15~1.73，$P=0.03$）[510]。然而，优选治疗方案中，每周一次紫杉醇和每3周1次多西他赛没有在平行对照研究中进行过比较。多西他赛和紫杉醇并不是完全交叉耐药的，有许多患者在对其中一种药物产生抗药性后使用另一种紫杉醇类药物治疗仍可在临床获益[511,512]。

研发纳米颗粒白蛋白紫杉醇（nab-paclitaxel）是为了避免与紫杉醇和多西他赛，聚氧乙烯蓖麻油（cremophor EL）和聚山梨酯80（polysorbate 80）一起使用而出现溶剂相关输液反应。2005年，FDA批准了白蛋白紫杉醇的应用，因其在Ⅲ期临床试验中与每3周紫杉醇方案相比具有卓越的疗效[513]。特别的是，有454名MBC女性被随机分配接受白蛋白紫杉醇260mg/m^{2}每3周静脉注射一次或紫杉醇175mg/m^2。大约40%的参与者在转移性的治疗方案中未接受过化疗。与紫杉醇组相比，白蛋白紫杉醇组患者的ORR显著提高（33% vs 19%，$P=0.001$），TTP也显著延长（23.0周vs 16.9周；$HR=0.75$，$P=0.006$）。白蛋白紫杉醇组的4级中性粒细胞减少症发生率比紫杉醇组低（9% vs 22%，$P<0.001$），但3级感觉神经病变更常见（10% vs 2%，$P<0.001$），但大多数并发症可通过中断治疗和减少剂量而消退。在白蛋白紫杉醇组中没有使用糖皮质激素或抗组胺药，并且没有发生过敏反应。尚没有研究比较每周白蛋白紫杉醇方案与优选的每周紫杉醇方案的疗效差异。

一项Ⅱ期临床随机试验比较了白蛋白紫杉醇的几种不同方案和每3周多西他赛的疗效差异[514]。在这项研究中，300例初次诊治的MBC患者随机分为紫杉醇静脉注射300mg/m^{2}每3周一次、100mg/m^{2}每4周的前3周各1次、150mg/m^{2}每4周的前3周各1次或多西他赛100mg/m^{2}每3周一次。在白蛋白紫杉醇150mg/m^{2}每4周的前3周各1次方案下出现了最高的RR、PFS和OS[515]。白蛋白紫杉醇引起的周围神经病变率与紫杉醇和多西他赛相当，但是中性粒细胞减少的发生率更低。

蒽环类药物是MBC合理的一线化疗药，但评估患者的心脏危险因素和终身蒽环类药物暴露剂量（多柔比星450~550mg/m^{2}和表柔比星900mg/m^2）对降低心脏毒性风险至关重要。多柔比星通常以每3周60~75mg/m^{2}或每周20mg/m^{2}的剂量给予。表柔比星可以每3周75~100mg/m^{2}或每周20~30mg/m^{2}的剂量给予。聚乙二醇脂质体多柔比星（pegylated liposomal doxorubicin，PLD）是多柔比星的增强形式，其被包封在脂质体中以最小化不良影响，同时保持治疗功效。比较PLD和多柔比星的几项Ⅲ期临床试验已经证明两者具有相同的疗效，但PLD的心脏毒性风险显著降低，同时允许患者转移性的治疗方案中进行蒽环类药物的再治疗[516~518]。应用PLD同时会减少脱发和恶心的发生，但会增加手足综合征和黏膜炎发生频率。

一项随机对照试验通过比较一线多柔比星与紫杉醇（每3周一次，疾病进展时允许交叉使用），发现一线多柔比星的RR和PFS更高，但两者的OS没有统计学差异[519]。多柔比星会导致更多的毒性，但能更好控制肿瘤相关症状。相比之下，在E1193临床试验中，每3周使用1次单药多柔比星或紫杉醇显示出相当的 RR 治疗失败时间，OS 和 QOL[520]。一项包含三个临床试验的荟萃分析中，纳入了 919 名随机分组的患者单药使用蒽环类药物或每 3 周使用紫杉醇类药物，结果两组表现出相似的 *RR*（33%和 38%，*P*=0.08）和 OS（*HR*=1.01，95%*CI*：0.88～1.16，*P*=0.90），但含蒽环类药物组 PFS 显著增加（*HR*=1.19，95%*CI*：1.04～1.36，*P*=0.011）[521]。但尚没有临床试验在一线治疗中比较蒽环类药物与每周使用紫杉醇的疗效差异。

卡培他滨（capecitabine）是口服给药的第三代氟嘧啶氨基甲酸酯，在胸苷磷酸化酶的作用下优先在肿瘤组织中转化为其活性代谢产物氟尿嘧啶，从而允许更具选择性的细胞毒性，同时具有更少的毒副作用。一些Ⅱ期临床试验表明，单药卡培他滨对之前接触蒽环类和紫杉醇类药物的 MBC 患者有效，*RR* 为 15%～29%，OS 为 10.1～15.2 个月[522～525]。1998 年 FDA 批准卡培他滨用于 MBC 患者，作为蒽环类和紫杉醇类药物难治性 MBC 患者的单药治疗，并于 2001 年与多西他赛联合使用，如下所述。FDA 和卡培他滨说明书均建议卡培他滨初始剂量为 1 250mg/m^2，每日 2 次，持续 2 周，然后停药 7 天。然而，较低的起始剂量 1 000mg/m^2 每日 2 次，持续 2 周，然后停药 1 周的效果与上述相似，但手足综合征和腹泻发生较少[526]。

艾日布林（eribulin），一种新型微管蛋白聚合抑制剂，在 EMBRACE 研究结果显著的背景下，在 2010 年被 FDA 批准用于在转移性的治疗方案中接受过 2 次化疗后的 MBC 患者。该研究是一项重度预处理 MBC 患者的Ⅲ期临床试验[527]。在这项开放性研究中，762 名患者以 2∶1的比例随机分组，在 21 天为一周期的第 1 天和第 8 天静脉注射艾日布林 1.4mg/m^2 或按医生的选择进行化疗。与医生选择的化疗组相比（10.6 个月，95%*CI*：9.3～12.5；*HR*=0.81，95%*CI*：0.66～0.99，*P*=0.041），艾日布林组的中位 OS 显著改善（13.1 个月，95%*CI*：11.8～14.3）。但有 5%的患者因外周神经病变停用艾日布林。在Ⅲ期临床试验中比较了艾日布林和卡培他滨对 OS 和 PFS 的影响，试图确定用于 MBC 患者的标准疗法，该疗法适用于对蒽环类和紫杉醇类治疗后疾病进展的患者[528]。共有 1 102 名患有 MBC 的女性被随机分配接受艾日布林或卡培他滨作为其一线，二线或三线化疗。在 OS（15.9 个月 vs 14.5 个月；*HR*=0.88，95%*CI*：0.77～1.00，*P*=0.56）或 PFS（4.1 个月 vs 4.2 个月；*HR*=1.08，95%*CI*：0.93～1.25，*P*=0.30）上，艾日布林并不优于卡培他滨。同时观察到客观 *RR* 没有差异，艾日布林为 11.0%，卡培他滨为 11.5%。QOL 评分也相似，大多数 AE 为 1 或 2 级。

伊沙匹隆（ixabepilone）是一种埃坡霉素，用于克服紫杉醇类和蒽环类耐药的新型抗微管剂。Ⅱ期研究显示在重度预处理的 MBC 患者中，每 3 周静脉注射伊沙匹隆 40mg/m^2 的客观 *RR* 约为 12%，40%～50%的患者病情稳定[529,530]。短暂性周围神经病变、骨髓抑制、脱发和疲劳是这些研究中的常见毒性反应。2007 年 FDA 的批准是基于评估伊沙匹隆和卡培他滨联合的Ⅲ期临床试验，但标注允许作为单药治疗。伊沙匹隆目前仅在美国有售。

长春瑞滨（vinorelbine）是一种半合成长春花生物碱，已被用于广泛评估治疗 MBC 并在临床实践中使用了几十年，但从未获得 FDA 的监管批准。Ⅱ期临床试验已经证实，在 21 天周期的第 1 天和第 8 天以 30mg/m^2 剂量单药给予长春瑞滨治疗，一线治疗的 MBC 患者的 *RR* 为 40%～50%，二线治疗的 MBC 患者为 20%～35%[531,532]。长春瑞滨耐受性良好，主要副作用为骨髓抑制。

在 MBC 患者中应用的一些化疗药物已经被批准作为单药化疗方案，但联合化疗方案更常用，如下所述。吉西他滨（gemcitabine）是一种嘧啶类抗代谢物，通过独特的作用机制抑制 DNA 合成。研究人员已对其作为 MBC 患者的一线，二线和三线治疗方案进行了研究，平均 *RR* 分别为 37%，26% 和 13%[533～535]。鉴于其有限的毒性和独特的作用机制，通常将其与其他化疗药物联合使用，如紫杉醇类和铂类。2004 年，美国 FDA 批准吉西他滨联合紫杉醇用于在先前的蒽环类药物治疗中疾病进展的 MBC 患者。顺铂和卡铂是 DNA 交联剂，在先前未进行治疗的 MBC 中具有相似的活性，客观反应率在 8% 和 35%之间[536～538]。

根据 NCCN 指南用于复发性 MBC 的优选的单药化学疗法，有多柔比星、PLD、紫杉醇、卡培他滨、吉西他滨、长春瑞滨和艾日布林[409]。

联合化疗方案

当需要快速的肿瘤反应来改善癌症相关症状或在危及生命的内脏危象的情况下，可以采用几种联合化疗方案。然而，这些方案通常毒性更大，使用前应仔细评估患者情况。一些批准用于佐剂或新辅助治疗的联合用药也被证明在转移性环境中有效，如蒽环类加环磷酰胺（伴或不伴氟尿嘧啶），以及 CMF 方案。不含蒽环类的紫杉醇类化疗方案包括紫杉醇/多西他赛+吉西他滨、多西他赛+卡培他滨或紫杉醇+顺铂/卡铂。对于蒽环类和紫杉醇类药物治疗后肿瘤进展的患者，可用的组合方案有吉西他滨+卡铂。建议的联合化疗方案可在 NCCN 乳腺癌指南中找到（NCCN.org）[395,409]。

Ⅲ期 Intergroup E1193 随机临床试验比较了单药多柔比星、单药紫杉醇和多柔比星+紫杉醇在 MBC 患者上的疗效，患者在疾病进展后允许单药交叉[518]。联合化疗组的反应率（47%）和 TTP（8 个月）在统计学上均优于两个单药组（单药多柔比星组为 36%和 5.8 个月；单药紫杉醇组为 34%和 6.0 个月）。然而，与顺序单药治疗相比，在联合用药组中没有观察到 OS 明显获益。此外，所有组的 QOL 结果相似。

联合化疗方案通常是在两种具有不同机制药物之间具有协同作用的临床前证据的基础上形成的。紫杉醇通过上调胸苷磷酸化酶来增强卡培他滨的活性，早期Ⅰ期研究清楚地证明了多西他赛和卡培他滨之间的协同作用[539]。O'Shaughnessy 等人在 2002 年报告的一项Ⅲ期临床试验中随机分组了 511 例蒽环类耐药的 MBC 患者在第 1～14 天每天 2 次接受口服卡培他滨 1 250mg/m^2，并在每个周期第 1 天（21 天为 1 个周期）给予静脉注射多西他赛 75mg/m^2 或者每周期 1 次静脉注射多西他赛 100mg/m^2。联合组的 ORR（42% vs 30%，*P*=0.006）、中位 TTP（6.1 个月 vs 4.2 个月；*HR*=0.652，95%*CI*：0.545～0.780，*P*=0.001）和 OS（14.5 个月 vs 11.5 个月；*HR*=0.75，95%*CI*：0.634～0.947，*P*=0.0126）均显著增加。这个临床试验第一次证明了含多西他赛的联合化疗方案可改善患者的 OS。然而，试验完成后，与单药治疗组相比，联合治疗组接受单药序贯多西他赛治疗的比例更大（20% vs 7%），使 OS 的解释变得更加复杂。

一项Ⅲ期临床试验随机分配170名患者在21天为1个周期的第1天和第8天静脉注射吉西他滨1 000mg/m²,同时第8天静脉注射多西他赛75mg/m²或每3周静脉注射多西他赛175mg/m²,结果证明与单药化疗组相比,联合化疗组TTP增加(*HR*=0.77,95% *CI*:0.59~1.01;log-rank=0.06),但*RR*或OS没有差异[540]。然而,参加本研究的患者很少接受二线或三线治疗。一项全球范围开展的Ⅲ期临床试验随机分配529例接受蒽环类药物治疗的患者在第1天和第8天静脉注射吉西他滨1 250mg/m²,每21天的第1天静脉注射紫杉醇175mg/m²,或者仅服用紫杉醇[541]。与单药化疗组相比,联合用药组的TTP较长(6.14个月 vs 3.98个月;log-rank *P*=0.000 2)并且*RR*增加(41.4% vs 26.2%,*P*=0.000 2)。然而,该试验没有使用紫杉醇的每周最佳方案。这些结果使得FDA在2004年批准了吉西他滨联合紫杉醇作为MBC患者的一线治疗方案。一项Ⅲ期临床试验评估了每3周1次或每周1次吉西他滨联合紫杉醇或多西他赛的方案[542]。这项纳入了240名患者的研究表明,各组之间的TTP和OS相似。虽然联合不同的紫杉醇类药物得到的ORR相似,但每周1次方案优于每3周1次方案。此外,多西他赛联合吉西他滨或卡培他滨方案已在几项Ⅲ期临床试验中进行了比较。汇总的结果分析显示不同组间的OS,PFS和ORR没有差异[543]。

临床前研究证明了吉西他滨和铂类药物之间的协同作用,随后的临床试验证明,这种联合用药方案在先前接触蒽环类和紫杉醇类药物的患者中具有中等活性。一项多中心Ⅱ期临床试验,对39例重度预处理的MBC患者第1天和第8天静脉注射吉西他滨1 000mg/m²,每3周第1天注射卡铂AUC4,其ORR为31%(95% *CI*:17%~48%),中位TTP为5.3个月(95% *CI*:2.6~6.7个月)[544]。一项多中心Ⅱ期临床试验对33例重度预处理的MBC患者在21天周期的第1天和第8天静脉注射吉西他滨1 000mg/m²,顺铂30mg/m²,最终ORR为25.8%(95% *CI*:17%~48%),中位TTP为4个月(95% *CI*:2.15~5.85个月)[545]。

抗血管生成剂联合化疗在MBC中的应用

如辅助治疗章节中所述,新血管生成在乳腺癌的发展中起着重要作用,并且研究人员已经在转移性环境中评估了几种抗血管生成剂的作用。2008年,FDA批准将单克隆抗体贝伐单抗与化疗联合用于MBC的一线治疗。该批准是在Ⅲ期E2100临床试验结果的基础上通过的。该试验将722名患有MBC的患者随机分配至每周1次接受紫杉醇化疗(使用或不使用贝伐单抗,按10mg/kg的剂量每2周静脉注射1次)[546]。与对照组的PFS相比(5.9个月;*HR*=0.6),含有贝伐单抗的组在PFS(11.8个月)中具有显著益处,但在OS中没有明显差异(*P*=1)。贝伐单抗与一线化疗相结合的后续Ⅲ期研究表明,患者的PFS改善程度较低,且对OS无影响,导致2011年FDA撤回对贝伐单抗治疗MBC的批准。

Ⅲ期AVastin和DOcetaxel(AVADO)临床试验将736例MBC患者随机分配接受静脉注射多西他赛100mg/m²联合静脉注射贝伐单抗7.5mg/kg或15mg/kg或多西他赛加安慰剂,每3周给药1次[547]。中位随访时间为25个月,PFS在含贝伐单抗的两组中均占优势。PFS获益最显著的是贝伐单抗15mg/kg组,为10.1个月,而对照组为8.2个月。Ⅲ期RIBBON-1临床试验将1 237名HER2-MBC的患者随机分配至研究者选择的一线化疗方案(含或不含贝伐单抗15mg/kg),并且发现当贝伐单抗联合卡培他滨、紫杉醇类或蒽环类药物时,中位PFS改善最显著。Rossari等人于2012年发表的关于E2100,AVADO和RIBBON-1的荟萃分析显示,含贝伐单抗组的1年OS改善最显著,但中位OS无差异(*HR*=0.97,95% *CI*:0.86~1.08,*P*=0.056)[548]。

许多Ⅱ期和Ⅲ期临床试验已经评估了在一线,二线和多线化学疗法中添加贝伐单抗的疗效。Ⅲ期RIBBON-2临床试验评估了贝伐单抗与研究者选择的二线化疗的组合,发现贝伐单抗联合卡培他滨、紫杉醇类药物、吉西他滨或长春瑞滨后患者的中位PFS从5.1个月提升到7.2个月,差异具有统计学意义[549]。与其他研究相似,OS没有显著变化。除了没有生存获益外,贝伐单抗联合化疗还可能增加3~4级高血压(4.4%),血栓栓塞性疾病(3.2%),蛋白尿(1.7%)和出血(1.4%)的风险[550]。正在进行的全球双盲Ⅲ期MERiDiAN临床试验正在评估HER2-MBC患者中含或不含贝伐单抗的一线每周一次紫杉醇方案[551]。该研究将评估所有患者以及用VEGF-A高浓度作为治疗获益的预测标志物的亚组患者的PFS。

同时研究人员也已经评估了用于治疗MBC的其他类型的抗血管生成剂。舒尼替尼(sunitinib)是一种抑制VEGF受体的小分子多靶点TKI,在Ⅲ期临床试验中研究了其与卡培他滨联合治疗蒽环类和紫杉醇类药物耐药的MBC患者的疗效[552]。该研究随机分配了442名先前最多接受过两个疗程治疗的MBC患者接受卡培他滨2 000mg/m²,每天口服或不服用舒尼替尼37.5mg。结果表明两组间的ORR,PFS和OS是相似的。

雷莫芦单抗(ramucirumab)是一种抗人VEGF受体-2的人源化单克隆抗体,在第三阶段ROSE/TRIO-12临床试验中研究人员对其与多西他赛联合用药进行了研究[553]。这项双盲研究将1 144例HER2-MBC患者随机分组接受一线多西他赛75mg,然后分别静脉注射雷莫芦单抗或安慰剂10mg/kg,每3周1次。检测结果表明各组间的中位PFS(*HR*=0.88,*P*=0.077)或OS(*HR*=1.01,*P*=0.915)无明显统计学差异,而含雷莫芦单抗组的疲劳程度,高血压,手足综合征和口腔炎等毒性明显提高。截至2015年,尚未有任何抗血管生成剂批准用于治疗MBC,但许多药物正在评估中,相关信息可在www.clinicaltrials.gov上找到。

HER2+MBC的全身治疗

在缺乏HER2-靶向治疗的情况下,由于肿瘤侵袭性行为而缩短了HER2+乳腺癌患者的OS[554]。1998年批准了曲妥珠单抗联合紫杉醇作为治疗HER2+MBC的一线方案,接着2006年批准其作为治疗ESBC的一线方案,这些显著改善了这些患者的预后。遗憾的是,15%的HER2+ESBC患者在完成1年曲妥珠单抗辅助治疗后会出现无法治愈的转移性疾病,30%~50%的患者在转移性环境下接受曲妥珠单抗治疗1年内疾病将会进展。三种额外的HER2定向疗法拉帕替尼,帕妥珠单抗和T-DM1的进一步研发以及FDA的批准进一步改善了HER2+MBC患者的存活率。许多新的HER2定向疗法目前正在评估中并将在下面描述。

曲妥珠单抗在 HER2+MBC 中的关键试验

在用曲妥珠单抗治疗 HER2+MBC 患者的早期临床试验中，研究人员评估了一线和二线曲妥珠单抗单药治疗和曲妥珠单抗联合化疗的疗效。一项针对 114 名 HER2+MBC 女性的一线曲妥珠单抗单药治疗的单臂研究显示，*RR* 为 26%，CBR 为 38%[555]。相比之下，一项有关曲妥珠单抗单药治疗 222 例在 1 个或 2 个化疗方案治疗后进展的 HER2+MBC 患者的比较研究中，患者的 ORR 为 15%，中位反应持续时间为 9.1 个月[556]。

FDA 批准曲妥珠单抗是在 Slamon 等人的关键性Ⅲ期试验的结果的基础上进行的，该试验将 469 名 HER2+MBC 女性随机分配至标准化疗（蒽环类加环磷酰胺或紫杉醇）加曲妥珠单抗组或仅在一线治疗中进行化疗组[557]。静脉注射给予曲妥珠单抗负荷剂量 4mg/kg，然后每周静脉注射 2mg/kg。与单独化疗相比，联合曲妥珠单抗的患者可以获得更长的 TTP（7.4 个月 vs 4.6 个月，$P<0.001$），较高的 ORR（50% vs 32%，$P<0.001$），更长的反应时间（9.1 个月 vs 6.1 个月）和更长的 OS（25.1 个月 vs 20.3 个月，$P=0.046$）。与曲妥珠单抗相关的主要毒性是 LVEF 降低，这在接受蒽环类和环磷酰胺联合曲妥珠单抗的患者中最为突出（27%），其次为接受紫杉醇联合曲妥珠单抗的患者（13%），仅接受蒽环类和环磷酰胺的患者（8%）或仅接受紫杉醇的患者（1%）。这种毒性的增强导致一般建议在转移性环境中蒽环类抗生素不与曲妥珠单抗联合使用[409,464]。

在一线环境中单药化疗加曲妥珠单抗的其他几个Ⅱ期和Ⅲ期临床试验已经开展。在 Marty 等人于 2005 年报道的多国Ⅱ期临床试验中，186 名患有 HER2+的 MBC 患者随机接受多西他赛 100mg/m^2 静脉注射，每 3 周一次，伴或不伴曲妥珠单抗，随访至疾病进展[558]。与对照组相比，多西他赛中加入曲妥珠单抗与患者中位 TTP（11.7 个月 vs 6.1 个月，$P=0.0001$）、ORR（61% vs 34%，$P=0.0002$）和 OS（31.2 个月 vs 22.7 个月，$P=0.0325$）增加相关。对照组患者在疾病进展时变为单药曲妥珠单抗治疗方案与多西他赛联合曲妥珠单抗治疗方案的 OS 相似（30.3 个月 vs 31.2 个月），清楚地证明了曲妥珠单抗在二线治疗的有效性。

几项单臂Ⅱ期临床试验报道，HER2+MBC 患者使用长春瑞滨联合曲妥珠单抗治疗的 ORR 为 63%~78%，这种治疗方案通常对原发性不良事件如中性粒细胞减少症和神经病变的耐受良好[559~561]。基本上所有联合曲妥珠单抗和化疗的其他研究已证实安全性和有效性，尽管大多数是单臂试验。在许多国家，无论使用何种化学疗法及其疗效如何，曲妥珠单抗联合化疗已成为 HER2+MBC 患者的标准治疗方法[562]。

临床前研究证明了铂类药物，紫杉醇类和曲妥珠单抗之间具有协同作用，随后的临床试验试图通过合并这些药物来进一步提高临床获益[563]。一项多中心Ⅲ期临床试验随机分配了 196 例 HER2+MBC 并且未在转移性治疗方案中进行治疗的女性每 3 周 1 次静脉注射曲妥珠单抗和紫杉醇 175mg/m^2，伴或不伴静脉注射卡铂 AUC6，然后每周维持曲妥珠单抗治疗[564]。含卡铂组的患者的 ORR（52% vs 36%，$P=0.04$）和 PFS（10.7 个月 vs 7.1 个月；*HR*=0.66，95%*CI*：0.59~0.73，$P=0.03$）以及 4 级中性粒细胞减少的发生均增加。其中一项预先指定的亚组分析显示，在上述治疗中，HER2+，IHC3+的患者（与 2+相比）有更高的 ORR（57% vs 36%，$P=0.03$）和 PFS（13.8 个月 vs 7.6 个月；*HR*=0.55，95%*CI*：0.46~0.64，$P=0.005$）。但分析中没有观察到 OS 的改善。

BCIRG007 是一项多中心Ⅲ期临床试验，评估在一线治疗中向多西他赛和曲妥珠单抗中加入卡铂的效果[565]。将未曾接受治疗的 263 名女性 HER2+MBC 患者随机分配接受 8 个周期的曲妥珠单抗+多西他赛 100mg/m^2 每 3 周 1 次静脉注射，或接受曲妥珠单抗+卡铂 AUC6+多西他赛 75mg/m^2 静脉注射每 3 周一次，其后用曲妥珠单抗维持治疗。与 Robert 等人的上述研究相比，在 TTP，*RR*、OS 或毒性方面没有显著差异。认为加入卡铂并没显示出任何益处是因为在对照组中使用了更高剂量的多西他赛。向紫杉醇类和曲妥珠单抗中加入卡铂尚未成为标准的一线或二线方案很大程度上是由 HER2-定向剂的开发造成的，因为该方案可以改善患者的 PFS 和 OS，如下所述。

很少有研究比较曲妥珠单抗单药治疗与曲妥珠单抗联合化疗。一项Ⅲ期研究比较了一线曲妥珠单抗联合多西他赛与曲妥珠单抗单药治疗（疾病进展时改用曲妥珠单抗联合多西他赛）的疗效，结果显示联合组患者的中位 PFS（*HR*=4.24，$P<0.01$）和 OS（*HR*=2.72，$P=0.04$）显著改善[566]。这项研究中的 112 名患者中的大多数有内脏转移和多个转移灶。一项对 101 名患者进行的类Ⅱ期研究比较了一线多西他赛加曲妥珠单抗与单药曲妥珠单抗方案的疗效，（疾病进展时改为单药多西他赛治疗）[567]。两组患者的 PFS 相似，但联合组的 *RR* 改善，OS 升高但无统计学差异。该试验设计未反映当前临床实践中疾病进展后继续应用曲妥珠单抗联合化疗方案的效果（该方法在德国乳腺组（GBG）26/BIG03~05 临床试验中被证实可改善患者预后）如下所述。

在 FDA 批准拉帕替尼和 T-DM1 之前，对一线紫杉醇类药物加曲妥珠单抗治疗进展的患者的最佳二线治疗方案尚不清楚。一些研究人员认为进展是由化疗耐药性造成的，因此曲妥珠单抗应该在疾病进展时继续使用[568,569]。GBG26/BIG03~05 研究是一项Ⅲ期临床试验，将一线紫杉醇类加曲妥珠单抗治疗进展的 HER2+MBC 患者随机分组接受二线卡培他滨+持续曲妥珠单抗治疗或仅接受卡培他滨治疗[570]。GBG26/BIG03~05 仅在完成目标的 1/3 后就早早结束，部分原因是拉帕替尼联合卡培他滨已经得到批准用于二线治疗。尽管如此，持续应用曲妥珠单抗联合卡培他滨与单独应用卡培他滨相比，ORR（48.1% vs 27.0%，$P=0.0115$）和 TTP（8.2 个月 vs 5.6 个月，$P=0.0338$）显著改善。由于研究动力不足，尽管 OS 在数值上有改善，但无统计学差异（24.9 个月 vs 20.6 个月，$P=0.73$）。尽管仍有其他研究尝试证明在进展后持续使用曲妥珠单抗的有效性，但 GBG26/BIG03~05 是唯一一项证明其有效性的前瞻性研究。

曲妥珠单抗的给药剂量可以为 4mg/kg 静脉注射 1 次，接着每周静脉注射 2mg/kg，也可以为负荷剂量 8mg/kg 静脉注射 1 次，接着每 3 周静脉注射 6mg/kg[409]。最近开发的曲妥珠单抗皮下制剂是标准静脉注射制剂的一种有效替代方法[571]。新辅助赫赛汀（neoadjuvant herceptin，HannaH）加强疗法，一项多国、开放、随机的Ⅲ期临床试验最近证明，曲妥珠单抗 600mg 每 3 周皮下给药 1 次在新辅助治疗中的 PCR 率并不优于标准曲妥珠单抗静脉给药疗法[572]。而皮下组的患者感染更频繁。曲妥珠单抗固定剂量的皮下制剂最近在欧盟被批准作为患者优选的替代品，因为其给药时间更短且不适感更轻。正在进行的Ⅲ期临床试验，优先考虑赫赛汀皮下注射或静脉注射给药（PrefHER），同时评估患者和医生的偏好以及皮下制剂带来的成本节约（ClinicalTrials. gov 编号：NCT01401166）。

曲妥珠单抗之外的疗法：附加的 HER2 定向疗法

30%～50%的单纯曲妥珠单抗治疗的 HER2+MBC 的患者在一线治疗中没有达到曲妥珠单抗加化疗的客观反应率，随后还经历了较短的 TTP（7～17 个月）和 OS（22～38 个月）[557,560]。此外，最终在所有患者中都将发展为对曲妥珠单抗的获得性耐药。人们设想的曲妥珠单抗原发性耐药和获得性耐药的机制包括 HER2 的内在分子变化，平行代偿信号通路的上调，抗体依赖性细胞毒性的缺陷和细胞凋亡的改变[573,574]。在通过阻断 HER2 途径下游效应作为替代方法的发展下，已使患者预后得到明显改善，如下所述。

拉帕替尼治疗 HER2+乳腺癌

拉帕替尼是一种口服小分子 TKI，靶向调控细胞内 HER2 激酶结构域，对曲妥珠单抗耐药的 HER2 过表达乳腺癌细胞具有活性。2007 年 FDA 批准拉帕替尼联合卡培他滨用于对含有紫杉醇类药物加曲妥珠单抗治疗方案进展的患者进行Ⅲ期临床试验。共有 324 名 HER2+MBC 患者被随机分配至拉帕替尼 1 250mg/d 口服，加卡培他滨 2 500mg/m^2 每日口服（21 天 1 周期，第 1～14 天给药）或仅服用卡培他滨[402]。与对照组相比，在含拉帕替尼的组上观察到独立评估的 PFS 得到显著改善（8.4 个月 vs 4.4 个月；HR = 0.49，95% CI：0.34～0.71，P < 0.001）。最终分析显示，与卡培他滨组相比，含拉帕替尼组的患者具有生存优势（75.0 周 vs 64.7 周）[575]。试验中未观察到 LVEF 下降或心肌病的情况。腹泻在联合组比对照组更常见（60% vs 39%，P<0.001），但大多数为 1 级或 2 级，3 级腹泻的发生率相似（12% vs 11%）。在含拉帕替尼的组中观察到 CNS 转移的病例较少（4 例患者 vs 11 例患者），但这一发现无统计学意义[402]。从 2007 年至 2012 年，拉帕替尼加卡培他滨被认为是 HER2+MBC 在紫杉醇类药物加曲妥珠单抗治疗进展后恰当的二线治疗方案[576]。

临床前研究证明了拉帕替尼和曲妥珠单抗之间的协同作用及其不含交叉耐药性。EGF104900 是一项Ⅱ期临床试验，将 296 名重度预处理的 HER2+MBC 患者随机分配至拉帕替尼加曲妥珠单抗组或单用拉帕替尼组[577]。参与者平均已经接受过 3 种含曲妥珠单抗的方案。拉帕替尼联合曲妥珠单抗的组合的 PFS（HR = 0.74，95% CI：0.58～0.94，P = 0.011）、CBR 和 OS（14.5 个月 vs 9.5 个月；HR = 0.74，95% CI：0.57～0.97，P = 0.026）均优于单用拉帕替尼组[578]。联合组腹泻率高于拉帕替尼组（60% vs 48%，P = 0.03），但 3 级腹泻率相同（7%）。

NCIC-CTG-MA-31 是一项国际性的开放性Ⅲ期临床试验，随机分配了 652 名未接受治疗的 HER2+MBC 女性接受 24 周紫杉醇类联合拉帕替尼或曲妥珠单抗治疗，然后进行相同的 HER2 定向单药治疗[579]。与曲妥珠单抗联合紫杉醇类组相比，拉帕替尼联合紫杉醇类药物组在 PFS（9.1 个月 vs 13.6 个月，P<0.001）和 OS 方面均较差，从而表明曲妥珠单抗在一线治疗中优于拉帕替尼。

HER2+乳腺癌有发展为 CNS 的倾向。遗憾的是，曲妥珠单抗不能透过血脑屏障。尽管控制了全身性疾病，估计有 10%～15%的 HER2+MBC 患者在用曲妥珠单抗治疗后会发生脑转移。高频率的 CNS 转移可能是由多种因素造成的，但曲妥珠单抗通过控制全身疾病延长寿命可能会增加临床上 CNS 转移的可能性。如前所述，Geyer 等人报道了与单用卡培他滨方案相比，拉帕替尼联合卡培他滨治疗后 CNS 转移病例出现较少，但差异不具有统计学意义[402]。几项研究随后评估了拉帕替尼预防或治疗 CNS 转移的能力。

接受了放射治疗的进展性脑转移瘤患者再接受单药拉帕替尼治疗的 ORR 仅为 6%，但与卡培他滨组合使用时 ORR 更为显著，为 21%～31.8%[580～582]。Ⅱ期 LANDSCAPE 临床试验对未经治疗的 HER2+脑转移患者使用拉帕替尼联合卡培他滨方案，CNS 患者的 ORR 为 65.9%，TTP 为 5.5 个月，OS 为 17.0 个月[583]。

CEREBEL 是一项多中心，开放的Ⅲ期临床试验，旨在评估拉帕替尼联合卡培他滨对 CNS 转移作为最初进展部位的患者的影响[584]。共有 540 名 HER2+MBC 患者被随机分配至每日拉帕替尼 1 250mg/m^2 加每日两次卡培他滨 2 000mg/m^2（21 天周期的第 1～14 天）或曲妥珠单抗加卡培他滨 2 500mg/m^2 每日两次（21 天为 1 周期，第 1～14 天给药）。该研究提前终止，因为含有拉帕替尼组（3%）和含有曲妥珠单抗组（5%）以 CNS 作为初始复发部位的转移率没有差异。此外，含曲妥珠单抗组的患者表现出较高的 PFS（HR = 1.30，95% CI：1.04～1.64）和 OS（HR = 1.34，95% CI：0.95～1.64）。

帕妥珠单抗在 HER2+MBC 中的运用

帕妥珠单抗（pertuzumab），如辅助部分所述，是一种人源化单克隆抗体，通过结合不同于曲妥珠单抗的表位来阻止 HER2 二聚化[585,586]。帕妥珠单抗和曲妥珠单抗联合使用会得到更全面的 HER2 信号通路阻断。在临床前研究中，与单药活性相比，联合用药大大增强了抗肿瘤活性[587]。一项Ⅱ期临床试验比较了单药帕妥珠单抗与帕妥珠单抗联合曲妥珠单抗用于曲妥珠单抗联合化疗后进展的 HER2+MBC 患者的疗效[588]。帕妥珠单抗仅表现出最小的抗肿瘤活性，联合治疗下患者的 CBR 为 50%，ORR 为 24.2%，PFS 为 5.5 个月，且具有最小的额外毒性。

帕妥珠单抗和曲妥珠单抗的临床评估研究（CLEOPATRA）是一项国际性多中心临床试验，该试验促使 FDA 于 2012 年批准帕妥珠单抗联合多西他赛和曲妥珠单抗的方案[589]。该研究随机分组了 808 名 HER2+MBC 患者，并且不曾在转移性环境中接受过治疗。患者每 3 周静脉注射曲妥珠单抗加多西他赛 75mg/m^2 之后每三周使用帕妥珠单抗或安慰剂。给予帕妥珠单抗的负荷剂量为 840mg，然后每 3 周使用 420mg。曲妥珠单抗联合帕妥珠单抗或安慰剂在患者停止化疗后继续进行，直至肿瘤进展或死亡。不到 50%的参与者接受了辅助治疗，约 10%的患者接受了曲妥珠单抗辅助治疗。

CLEOPATRA 研究表明，与对照组相比，加用帕妥珠单抗会使研究者评估的 PFS 得到 6.3 个月的改善（18.7 个月 vs 12.4 个月；HR = 0.68，95% CI：0.51～0.75，P<0.001），同时使 OS 得到 15.7 个月的改善（56.5 个月 vs 40.8 个月；HR = 0.68，95%

CI:0.58~0.80,*P*<0.001)[590]。ORR 在帕妥珠单抗组中为 80.2%,在对照组中为 69.3%[591]。在对照组(1~41 个周期)和帕妥珠单抗组(1~35 个周期)中,每位患者接受的多西他赛周期中位数为 8。添加帕妥珠单抗不会导致心功能不全的发生率增加,但与对照组相比,腹泻(66.8% vs 46.3%)和皮疹(33.7% vs 24.2%)的发生率更高。

以 CNS 转移为疾病进展第一部位的发生率在帕妥珠单抗组和对照组之间相似(13.7% vs 12.66%)[589]。然而,与对照组(11.9 个月)相比,帕妥珠单抗组(15.0 个月)CNS 转移发生的中位时间延长(*HR*=0.58,95%*CI*:0.39~0.85,*P*=0.004 9)。以 CNS 转移作为疾病进展第一部位的患者的 OS 在帕妥珠单抗组显示出一定优势,但无统计学差异(34.4 个月 vs 26.4 个月)。

在 CLEOPATRA 临床试验中,有几种具有预测性的生物标志物得到了认可。升高的血清 HER2 蛋白、血清 HER2 和 HER3mRNA 水平以及降低的血清 HER2 细胞外结构域(sHER2)水平与较好的预后相关(*P*<0.05)[592]。与 PIK3A 发生突变的对照组(13.8 个月 vs 8.6 个月)和帕妥珠单抗组(21.8 个月 vs 12.5 个月)相比,野生型 PIK3CA 患者的中位 PFS 均较长。

一些正在进行的临床试验已经评估了曲妥珠单抗和帕妥珠单抗联合各种化学疗法在 ESBC 和 MBC 两种环境中的效果。有关这些试验的详细信息,请访问:http://www.cancer.gov/about-cancer/treatment/clinical-trials/search。

T-DM1 在 HER2+MBC 中的应用

新型抗体药物缀合物 T-DM1 可以将高效抗微管细胞毒性药物 emtansine 直接递送至 HER2+乳腺癌细胞。在辅助治疗部分讨论了 T-DM1,但对其最初的研究是在转移性环境中进行的。2013 年,FDA 批准 T-DM1 用于治疗在转移的情况下接受含有曲妥珠单抗的紫杉醇方案后疾病有进展的 HER2+MBC 患者。T-DM1 得到批准是基于 EMILIA 研究,这是一项国际,多中心,开放的Ⅲ期临床试验,将 991 例 HER2+MBC 患者随机分配至 T-DM1 组或拉帕替尼联合卡培他滨组,后者是当时在曲妥珠单抗治疗后疾病进展患者的标准选择[593]。纳入的患者在曲妥珠单抗和紫杉醇方案治疗后疾病进展。与拉帕替尼联合卡培他滨相比,T-DM1 组的患者中位 PFS(9.6 个月 vs 6.4 个月;*HR*=0.65,95%*CI*:0.55~0.75,*P*<0.001)和中位 OS(30.9 个月 vs 25.1 个月;*HR*=0.68,95%*CI*:0.55~0.85,*P*<0.001)均得到显著改善。此外,T-DM1 耐受性更好,总体毒性更低,最常见的 3~4 级不良反应是血小板减少症(12.9%)和转氨酶升高(2.9%~4.3%)。

有关 T-DM1 疗效的其他证据呈现在 TH3RESA 试验中。这是一项国际、随机、开放的Ⅲ期临床试验,评估 T-DM1 在经两种或多种 HER2 靶向治疗后进展的 HER2+MBC 患者身上的疗效[594]。研究人员对这项研究的参与者进行了大量预处理,其中大约 50%的患者接受过 4 次 MBC 化疗。共有 602 名患者以 2∶1的比例随机分配至 T-DM1 组或医生选择的治疗方案组。与对照组相比,T-DM1 组患者的中位 PFS 增加 2.9 个月(6.2 个月 vs 3.3 个月;*HR*=0.528,*P*<0.001),中期中位数增加(*HR*=0.552,*P*=0.003 4,功效停止边界未交叉),安全性结果与 EMILIA 相似。

第三阶段 MARIANNE 临床试验比较了单药 T-DM1、T-DM1 联合帕妥珠单抗和曲妥珠单抗联合化疗在 HER2+MBC 一线治疗中的作用[595,596]。该研究是在帕妥珠单抗加曲妥珠单抗联合多西他赛方案得到批准之前设计的,因此不包括目前 HER2+MBC 的一线治疗标准。大约 31%的患者接受了新辅助或辅助 HER2 定向治疗,而 37%原发性 HER2+MBC 的患者下接受了初始治疗。初步结果在 ASCO 2015 上发表,虽然与曲妥珠单抗联合化疗相比,含有 TDM-1 组在 PFS(*HR*=0.91,97.5%*CI*:0.73~1.13,*P*=0.31)中并非劣势,但它们也未能表现出优势。

HER2+MBC 的治疗建议

所有已知的 HER2 定向疗法中的最佳方案尚不清楚。表 108-15 列出了可用于 HER2+MBC 的 HER2 定向疗法的常见化疗方案。CLEOPATRA,EMILIA 和 TH3RESA 的结果被用来制订最近在 ABC2,ASCO 和 NCCN 上发布的最新指南[409,458,464]。一般而言,曲妥珠单抗,帕妥珠单抗和紫杉醇的组合是 HER2+MBC 的首选一线治疗方案。一种常见且恰当的临床实践是停用紫杉醇类药物,同时在完成该一线方案的八个周期后继续生物治疗。T-DM1 是首选的二线治疗方案(与拉帕替尼加卡培他滨相比),如果未在二线治疗中提供,在之后的治疗中也要优先选择使用(与医生选择的其他治疗相比)。不支持在一线治疗中使用帕妥珠单抗(除了其与曲妥珠单抗和化学疗法联合使用)。但是,如果患者没有接受过帕妥珠单抗,可以在一线以外的治疗中使用它。

与 HR-/HER2+患者不同的是,几乎 50%的 HER2+乳腺癌患者也患有 HR+疾病,这与其对内分泌治疗会产生一定耐药性的生理特征相关。患有 HR+/HER2+疾病的患者通常被归类为管腔 B 内在亚型组[313]。临床前和临床试验表明,HER2 定向治疗可部分治疗对激素疗法的耐药性,这表明 ER 与 HER2 之间存在交叉对话。患有非内脏,惰性疾病和化疗受限的并发症的患者是激素治疗联合 HER2 靶向药物治疗的合适候选者[458]。

曲妥珠单抗和阿那曲唑针对 ER+HER2+乳腺癌的Ⅲ期临床试验(TAnDEM)随机分配了 207 名患有 HR+/HER2+MBC 的绝经后女性,接受阿那曲唑伴或不伴曲妥珠单抗的方案[597]。与单用阿那曲唑组相比,含曲妥珠单抗组的患者 PFS 显著改善(4.8 个月 vs 2.4 个月;*HR*=0.63,95%*CI*:0.47~0.84,*P*=0.001 6),但 OS 没有区别。一项国际、开放的Ⅲ期临床试验 eLEcTRA 将患有 HR+/HER2+MBC 的绝经后女性随机分为在一线治疗中使用来曲唑组或来曲唑联合曲妥珠单抗组[598]。因为获益较差,在计划招募的 370 名患者中仅招募到 57 名患者,所以该研究被迫提前结束。与联合用药组相比,单用来曲唑组的中位 TTP 更短(3.3 个月 vs 14.1 个月;*HR*=0.67,*P*=0.23),CBR 降低(39% vs 65%,95%*CI*:1.01~8.84)。虽然差异无统计学意义,但这些发现与 TAnDEM 临床试验中的结果相似。虽然大多数 HR+/HER2+MBC 的患者通常选择接受 HER2 靶向药物联合化疗,但是那些接受内分泌治疗而非化疗的患者应该同时联合使用 HER2 靶向药物,因为 TAnDEM 临床试验显示该方案有使 PFS 获益的效果[458]。

HER2-乳腺癌中 HER2 的体细胞突变

癌基因组测序研究表明,HER2-乳腺癌患者存在 HER2 体细胞突变。Bose 等人的一项研究评估了 25 名类似的患者,确定了13种激活突变,并推测这些突变会驱动癌基因转化[599]。用奈拉替尼治疗这些含激活突变的乳腺癌细胞可有效抑制肿瘤细胞。正在进行的多中心Ⅱ期临床试验目前正在评估奈拉替尼在实体瘤和HER2体细胞突变患者中的应用(ClinicalTrials.gov编号:NCT01953926)。第二项正在进行的Ⅱ期临床试验评估了奈拉替尼伴或不伴氟维司群在HER2-MBC和HER2体细胞突变患者上的疗效(ClinicalTrials.gov编号:NCT01670877)。

HER2定向治疗与靶向药物联合使用

如前所述,研究人员已经对贝伐单抗联合激素疗法以逆转HR+MBC中的激素抵抗,并与化疗相结合的方案进行了评估,但应用该方案治疗乳腺癌在美国尚未获得批准。VEGF在HER2过表达的乳腺癌细胞中上调,并且抗血管生成剂在HER2+MBC中也具有重要意义。在小型Ⅱ期临床试验中,应用贝伐单抗、曲妥珠单抗和卡培他滨的组合患者的ORR为73%,PFS为14.4个月。Ⅲ期AVEREL临床试验将424例HER2+MBC患者随机分为在一线治疗中使用多西他赛伴或不伴曲妥珠单抗组[600]。独立评估显示,加用贝伐单抗治疗后,临床获益变化无统计学差异,PFS未达到方案规定的主要终点(对照组vs含贝伐单抗组:13.9个月vs 16.5个月;HR=0.016 2)。曲妥珠单抗和贝伐单抗联合使用时未发生意外不良事件。有趣的是,较高浓度的血浆VEGF-A不仅与较差的预后相关,还与较好的贝伐单抗治疗效果相关。

曲妥珠单抗耐药与肿瘤抑制基因PTEN的缺失,PI3K途径的改变和mTOR活化的增加有关[601,602]。几项Ⅲ期临床试验研究了mTOR抑制剂依维莫司联合化疗在HER2+MBC患者身上的应用,但未能证明该方案有益。在BOLERO-3临床试验中,569名患有HER2+MBC的女性被随机分配接受依维莫司5mg/d或安慰剂,同时所有参与者每周接受长春瑞滨加曲妥珠单抗治疗[603]。在曲妥珠单抗辅助治疗期间在12个月以内复发或在MBC环境中曲妥珠单抗治疗4周内进展被认为出现了曲妥珠单抗耐药。依维莫司组的PFS稍稍延长(7个月),而对照组为5.78个月(HR=0.78,95%CI:0.65~0.95,P=0.006 7),OS的比较情况尚未报道。亚组分析显示依维莫司在<65岁和非内脏HR-/HER2+MBC患者身上获益更多。但同时,正如在其他试验和临床实践中所经历的那样,依维莫司与更明显的毒性反应相关。对保存的肿瘤组织进行探索性分析显示,与PTEN浓度较高的患者相比,在PTEN浓度低的患者中(HR=0.40,95%CI:0.20~0.82,P=0.01);与pS6浓度低的患者相比,pS6浓度高的患者加入依维莫司可获得更显著的益处(HR=0.48,95%CI:0.24~0.96,P=0.04)。*PIK3CA*突变似乎没有预测出益处(HR=0.65,95%CI:0.21~1.45,P=0.32)。

在Ⅲ期BOLERO-1临床试验中,依维莫司还被评估为HER2+MBC的一线治疗药物,该试验以2:1的比例将719名初治患者随机分配至多西他赛联合曲妥珠单抗治疗伴依维莫司10mg/d组或安慰剂组[604]。初步结果由Hurvitz等人发表在SABCS2014上,显示PFS没有改善(14.95个月vs 14.49个月;HR=0.89,95% CI:0.73~1.08,P=0.116 6)。依维莫司组HR-/HER2+参与者的PFS值得注意,但未达到方案制订的显著标准。安全性结果与BOLERO-3试验和其他基于依维莫司的试验报告相似。结合BOLERO-3和-1的数据,依维莫司在HER2+MBC的治疗中没有起到任何治疗作用。

HER2+MBC中的新型靶向药物

MM-302是一种聚乙二醇化脂质体抗体——一种药物偶联物,可特异性地向HER2+乳腺癌细胞递送多柔比星,从而限制健康组织在化疗中的暴露。Ⅰ期临床试验证明了MM-302联合曲妥珠单抗在HER2+MBC中的安全性和抗肿瘤活性[605]。HERMIONE是一项正在进行的国际性、多元化、开放、随机的Ⅱ期临床试验,评估比较了每3周静脉注射30mg/m^{2}MM-302加曲妥珠单抗方案与医生选择的化疗方案(如长春瑞滨、卡培他滨或吉西他滨)加曲妥珠单抗方案治疗帕妥珠单抗和T-DM1治疗后进展的蒽环类幼稚HER2+MBC患者的有效性(ClinicalTrials.gov编号:NCT02213744)[606]。margetuximab是一种类似于曲妥珠单抗的嵌合单克隆抗体,其Fc片段经过工程改造以促进与CD16A的结合,并在随后保持了曲妥珠单抗的抗肿瘤增殖作用。临床前研究表明margetuximab优于曲妥珠单抗,Ⅰ期试验显示margetuximab耐受性良好。一项正在进行的Ⅱ期试验评估了margetuximab在HER2经IHC检测可疑,而FISH检测为阴性的MBC患者上的疗效(ClinicalTrials.gov编号:NCT01838021)。计划进行的Ⅲ期临床试验SOPHIA旨在随机分配528例HER2+MBC患者接受margetuximab或曲妥珠单抗化疗,这些患者均曾在曲妥珠单抗,帕妥珠单抗和T-DM1治疗后进展(ClinicalTrials.gov编号:NCT02492711)。这些和其他研究性HER2定向治疗的药物被列于表108-14中。

ONT-380,以前被称为ARRY-380,是一种口服,可逆的选择性的小分子HER2抑制剂。在HER2+MBC患者中,ONT-380正在进行两项Ⅰb期临床试验。第一项试验旨在评估ONT-380联合T-DM1在先前用紫杉醇类和曲妥珠单抗治疗的患者中的疗效(ClinicalTrials.gov编号:NCT01983501)。第二项试验旨在评估ONT-380联合卡培他滨和/或曲妥珠单抗在先前接受过曲妥珠单抗和T-DM1治疗的患者中的疗效(ClinicalTrials.gov编号:NCT02025192)。两项研究的中期分析表明,ONT-380耐受性良好,具有临床益处[607,608]。

许多小分子TKI已经在MBC环境中进行了评估。奈拉替尼,如辅助部分所述,是一种HER1、2和4的强效不可逆TKI,在临床前研究中克服了HER2+乳腺癌细胞对曲妥珠单抗的耐药性。一项Ⅰ期临床试验评估了奈拉替尼联合每周紫杉醇和曲妥珠单抗方案治疗先前接受过HER2定向治疗和紫杉醇类治疗的HER2+MBC患者的疗效,结果显示ORR为38%,CBR为52%,PFS为3.7个月[405]。一项Ⅱ期临床试验未能证明奈拉替尼单药方案在治疗至少接受过两种含曲妥珠单抗方案的HER2+MBC患者方面优于拉帕替尼联合卡培他滨方案[609]。一项多国、开放的Ⅰ/Ⅱ期临床试验评估了曲妥珠单抗预处理的HER2+MBC患者使用奈拉替尼联合卡培他滨方案的安全性和有效性[610]。首次拉帕替尼治疗患者的ORR为64%,曾经接触过拉帕替尼的患者的ORR为57%,中位PFS分别为40.3周和35.9周。最常见的毒性是腹泻(88%)和手足综合征(48%)。一项正在进行的Ⅱ期NEfERTT临床试验将479名HER2+MBC患者随机分配到一线紫杉醇联合奈拉替尼组或曲妥珠单抗组(ClinicalTrials.gov编号:NCT00915018)。2014年

11月的一份新闻稿报道了两个治疗组之间具有相似的PFS,但接受奈拉替尼治疗的患者与曲妥珠单抗相比脑转移发生率较低(7.4% vs 15.6%,$P=0.006$)[611]。但奈拉替尼组毒性增加,接受奈拉替尼和曲妥珠单抗治疗的患者3级腹泻发生率分别为30%和4%。NEfERTT临床试验未使用预防性止泻治疗,一些试验报告使用预防措施可显著减少腹泻。正在进行的Ⅲ期NALA研究旨在随机分配600名在转移性环境中接受过2种HER2定向治疗后进展的HER2+MBC患者至奈拉替尼+卡培他滨组或拉帕替尼+卡培他滨组(ClinicalTrials.gov编号:NCT01808573)。

一项Ⅰ期临床试验评估了α-选择性PI3K抑制剂阿哌利西(BYL719)与T-DM1联合治疗之前接受曲妥珠单抗和紫杉醇为基础的治疗后疾病进展的HER2+MBC患者的疗效(ClinicalTrials.gov编号:NCT02038010)。Ⅰb期临床试验目前正在评估PI3K抑制剂taselisib(GDC-0032)与几种目前批准的HER2定向疗法的组合(ClinicalTrials.gov编号:NCT02390427)。在一项Ⅰ/Ⅱ期临床试验中,Ⅰ类pan-PI3K抑制剂pilaralisib(SAR245408)将与曲妥珠单抗和紫杉醇联合用于曲妥珠单抗难治性HER2+MBC患者中[612]。

三阴性乳腺癌的全身治疗

MBC化疗仍然是各阶段TNBC的主要治疗方法。正如新辅助部分所述,TNBC对蒽环类和紫杉醇类药物非常敏感。几项评估新辅助环境中在标准化疗方案中加入卡铂的临床试验显示,TNBC的PCR率为22%~53%[416,613]。PFS和OS的长期结果尚不明确,但铂类药物不是早期TNBC的标准治疗方案。

铂类药物也已在转移性TNBC的环境中得到了评估,初步结果来自第一阶段Ⅲ期临床试验,在2014年SABCS的报告中比较了一线卡铂与多西他赛的疗效差异[614]。多中心TNT研究将376名未治疗的转移性TNBC女性随机分配至卡铂AUC 6每3周静脉注射1次,或多西他赛100mg/m^{2}每3周静脉注射1次,并当疾病进展时允许方案交叉。中位随访11个月,两组的ORR和PFS率相似。一项预先指定的纳入了43名*BRCA1/2*家族突变的试验参与者的亚组分析显示,与多西他赛组相比,卡铂组中患者的ORR显著增加,差异具有统计学意义(68% vs 33%,$P=0.03$)。

来自TNT研究参与者的原发性肿瘤样品接受了由Myriad Genetics开发的同源重组缺陷(HRD)测定法的HRD分析[615]。具有家族或体细胞*BRCA*突变的患者倾向于具有高HRD评分。在HRD评分较高或较低的患者中,两个治疗组之间未观察到PFS或OS的显著差异。

与*BRCA1/2*相关的乳腺癌大约分别有75%和50%为三阴性。*BRCA1/2*是肿瘤抑制基因,其产物在通过同源重组修复双链DNA断裂中起关键作用。当肿瘤前体细胞中剩余的野生型BRCA等位基因在家族*BRCA1/2*突变的患者中丢失时,由于HR效率降低而导致基因组不稳定。如TNT试验所示,这种受损的DNA修复机制被认为可以赋予铂类药物更高的敏感性。

多腺苷二磷酸核糖聚合酶(PARP)通过碱基切除修复识别和修复单链DNA断裂。PARP抑制剂阻止单链DNA的修复,并且对*BRCA*突变体肿瘤细胞具有高度选择性。虽然单个突变基因产物可能与细胞活力相容,但相关基因中的其他多个突变很可能导致细胞死亡。这种合成致死性的概念是一个关键的遗传概念,它指导了PARP抑制剂用于治疗BRCA相关和BRCA样TNBC的评估。

在一项国际多中心Ⅱ期临床试验中证实了PARP在BRCA相关肿瘤中的活性,该试验治疗了54名患有BRCA相关的先前至少使用一种单药奥拉帕利(olaparib)化疗过的MBC女性[616]。当参与者每日2次接受奥拉帕利400mg/次时,患者的*RR*为41%,中位PFS达到5.7个月。一项Ⅰ期临床试验目前正在评估奥拉帕利与buparlisib(BKM120,一种新型Ⅰ类pan-PI3K抑制剂)或阿哌利西(BYL719,一种新型α-选择性PI3K抑制剂)在TNMBC患者中联合使用的疗效(ClinicalTrials.gov编号:NCT01623349)。

其他几种PARP抑制剂正在作为单一疗法或与其他靶向疗法或化疗联合进行研究,包括veliparib(ABT-888)、talazoparib(BMN-673)、iniparib、尼拉帕尼(niraparib)和鲁卡帕尼(rucaparib)。一项关于PARP抑制剂veliparib(ABT-888)与卡铂联合用于转移性TNBC或*BRCA1/2*家族突变的HER2-MBC患者中的Ⅰ期剂量递增研究正在进行中(ClinicalTrials.gov编号:NCT01251874)。一项卡铂加紫杉醇联合veliparib(ABT-888)或安慰剂治疗BRCA相关HER2-MBC患者的Ⅲ期临床试验正在进行(ClinicalTrials.gov Identifier NCT 02163694)。该研究旨在招募270名患者,估计最初于2017年1月完成。

talazoparib的临床前研究表明,这种PARP抑制剂具有比其他类成员高得多的效力[613]。第二阶段ABRAZO临床试验对talazoparib在*BRCA1/2*突变和MBC患者身上进行了评估。其中,MBC患者要么在最后铂剂治疗后进展时间超过8周,要么曾在转移性环境中接受两种以上但不含铂剂的方案(ClinicalTrials.gov编号:NCT020234916)。一项国际多中心、Ⅲ期EMBRACA临床试验对家族性*BRCA*突变且局部晚期或MBC的患者进行了单药talazoparib的评估[617]。计划将先前在转移性环境中接受不超过两种化疗方案的429名患者以2:1的比例随机分配至talazoparib每日1.0mg(21天1周期)组或医生选择治疗(卡培他滨、艾日布林、吉西他滨或长春瑞滨)组,将PFS作为主要的终点。talazoparib Beyond BRCA(TBB)是一项单臂Ⅱ期临床试验,评估talazoparib治疗野生型*BRCA1/2*突变的转移性TNBC患者,但HRD由Myriad®研发的HRD酶检测确定(ClinicalTrials.gov编号:NCT02401347)。

有关转移性TNBC最近的临床试验

10%~32%的TNBC患者表达AR,阻断AR信号转导的药物正在MBC环境中进行积极的研究[314]。在一项针对AR阳性患者的Ⅱ期临床试验中研究人员评估了在AR+/HR-MBC患者中使用非甾体抗雄激素Bicalu-tamide的单药疗法的效果[618]。在筛选出HR-MBC的424名患者中,通过IHC的检测,发现12%的患者肿瘤AR+程度>10%。患者6个月的CBR为19%(95%*CI*:7~39),中位PFS为12周(95%*CI*:11~22),这清楚地证明了原理的正确性。Traina等人在2015年的ASCO中报告了一项开放的Ⅱ期临床试验的结果,该试验评估了单药恩佐鲁胺(一种有效的AR抑制剂)在AR+转移性TNBC患者中的作用[619]。在IHC筛查AR+的404名患者中,79%的患者AR>0%并且55%的人AR达10%。共有118名患者每天用160mg

恩佐鲁胺治疗。基因谱分析用于开发雄激素相关的基因标记，具有标记的患者的中位 PFS 优于无标记的患者（32 周 vs 9 周）。正在进行的Ⅰb/Ⅱ期临床试验正在评估 PI3K 抑制剂 taselisib（GDC-0032）与恩佐鲁胺联合治疗转移性 AR+TNBC 患者的效果（ClinicalTrials. gov 编号：NCT02457910）。这些和其他的研究性药物列于表 108-14 中。

通过免疫疗法逆转 MBC 中的免疫耐受性最近引起了关注。肿瘤细胞的免疫耐受可以通过肿瘤表面配体（如程序性细胞死亡配体 1（PD-L1））与抗肿瘤 T 细胞的抑制性受体（如程序性细胞死亡蛋白 1（PD-1）和 B7）的结合而发生[620,621]。PD-L1 在大约 20%的 TNBC 中表达，显著高于其他类型的乳腺癌[622]。针对 PD-L1 和 PD-1 的单克隆抗体的临床前研究表明肿瘤特异性 T 细胞免疫可以得到恢复，特别是在转移性 TNBC 环境中。2014 年的 SABCS 中报告了抗 PD-1 和抗 PD-L1 抗体的两个Ⅰb 期扩增研究的初步结果。研究人员应用高度选择性抗 PD-1 抗体帕博利珠单抗（MK-3475）对 32 例重度预治疗的 TNMBC 女性进行单药治疗的方案进行了评估，其中 58%表达 PD-L1[623]，25. 9%的患者疾病稳定，18. 5%的患者疾病出现了反应。在 21 名重度预治疗的 PD-L1 阳性转移性 TNBC 的患者中评估了抗 PD-L1 抗体阿特珠单抗（atezolizumab）（MPDL3280A）的效果，其中 ORR 为 19%，包括 2 例完全应答和 2 例部分应答。24 周的 PFS 为 27%（95%*CI*：7～47）[624]。

许多新型药物正在研究转移性 TNBC，包括巨噬细胞抑制剂，生物制剂和 FGFR 抑制剂（表 108-14）。PLX3397 是一种新型口服酪氨酸激酶抑制剂，能有效抑制 CSF-1 受体激酶，后者在调节肿瘤相关巨噬细胞中起关键作用。一项 PLX3397 联合艾日布林的Ⅰb/Ⅱ期临床试验正在患有转移性 TNBC 的患者中进行（ClinicalTrials. gov 编号：NCT01596751）。CDX-011（glembatumumab vedotin）是与糖蛋白（gp）NMB 结合的抗体-药物偶联物。第二阶段 METRIC 临床试验旨在将 300 名 gpNMB 过表达的 TNMBC 患者随机分配接受 CDX-011 或卡培他滨，以评估 CDX-011 的安全性和有效性（ClinicalTrials. gov 编号：NCT01997333）。大约 25%的乳腺癌表现出异常的 FGF 信号[625]。德立替尼（lucitanib）是一种新型的成纤维细胞 FGF 受体 1、2 和 VEGFR1～3 的口服抑制剂，在临床前研究中具有抗乳腺癌细胞的活性。在一项Ⅰ期临床试验中，应用德立替尼单药治疗的 FGF 异常的 MBC 患者的 ORR 为 50%。一项具有相似实验设计思路的Ⅱ期临床剂量测定试验目前正在 FGF 异常的 MBC 患者中（包括那些 TNBC 患者）进行[626]。

MBC 中 CNS 转移的处理

总体而言，CNS 转移仅发生在一小部分 MBC 患者中，但在转移性 TNBC 和 HER2+MBC 中，CNS 发生率在 30%～45%[627～630]。脑实质转移瘤的管理通常需要神经外科医生、放疗医生和肿瘤内科医生之间的合作。单个或数量较少的潜在可切除的脑转移瘤患者应接受手术或放疗。软脑膜癌病是 MBC 的一个严重且复杂的并发症，常常预示着患者的肿瘤已到晚期。软脑膜癌病的治疗可包括鞘内化疗，放疗和支持治疗。如前所述，在过去的二十年中，用曲妥珠单抗治疗的 HER2+乳腺癌患者脑转移的发生率有所增加。这种趋势很可能是由曲妥珠单抗治疗患者的 OS 得到总体改善以及曲妥珠单抗不能穿透 CNS 造成的[651]。如前所述，拉帕替尼显示出使 CNS 转移减少的趋势，但统计学意义不明显。目前正在评估拉帕替尼、奈拉替尼和其他靶向治疗 CNS 转移的疗法。

MBC 中针对肝转移的靶向治疗

目前尚缺乏关于肝脏病变病灶管理的前瞻性随机临床试验数据（如 PFS 和 OS）。然而，存在着许多局部治疗手段。只有在与多学科肿瘤委员会进行充分讨论后，才能在高度选择的患者中尝试局部治疗肝脏转移[458]。

MBC 中针对骨转移的靶向治疗

骨是最常见的转移部位，高达 80%的 MBC 患者在临床过程中发生骨转移。骨转移是与乳腺癌相关的伴有疼痛，骨折，脊髓压迫和高钙血症的并发症最常见的发病和致残来源。骨转移靶向药物与抗肿瘤治疗相结合是全身治疗的一个重要方面，而局部放疗或手术治疗可作为对即将发生的或活动性骨折的更精确的处理方案。建议对主要负重部位（如髋部，股骨，肱骨和肩部）的转移性病变进行骨科的评估，以防止致残或致死的病理性骨折。对负重骨中骨转移的疼痛部位或即将发生的骨折部位的放疗通常与全身治疗联合使用。

骨修饰疗法应该从发现溶骨性骨转移的第一个证据开始。双膦酸盐是破骨细胞活化的有效抑制剂。在几项Ⅲ期临床试验中，发现与帕米磷酸盐（pamidronate）和安慰剂相比，双膦酸盐唑来磷酸可降低骨骼相关事件（SRE）的风险、SRE 的平均时间和年度骨骼发病率[631,632]。一项大型Ⅲ期试验发现与唑来磷酸相比，地诺单抗（denosumab）显著延迟了首次和之后 SRE 出现的时间，而在 OS、DFS 和严重的 AE 方面两者没有明显差异[633]。地诺单抗会引起更频繁的低钙血症并且成本更高，但同时其给药时间更快，急性期反应和肾脏副作用更少。两类药物具有相似的下颌骨坏死率。

特殊话题

对侧预防性乳房切除术

接受乳房切除术治疗的单侧乳腺癌患者通常考虑进行对侧预防性乳房切除术以降低对侧乳腺癌的风险。在美国进行乳腺癌切除术治疗单侧乳腺癌患者的几项大型机构和相关地理研究显示，在过去的二十年中，对侧预防性乳房切除术的数量增加了[374,634～636]。但这与乳腺癌死亡率降低无关。然而，对于对侧乳腺癌高风险的患者，例如 *BRCA1/2* 突变的患者，对侧预防性乳腺切除术可提高长期生存率并具有成本效益[677～639]。低龄和家族史与对侧乳腺癌的高风险相关，并且新出现的数据表明这可能是由多基因引起的[640]。

与对侧预防性乳房切除术相关的因素包括患者年龄<50 岁，高加索人种，乳腺癌家族史，*BRCA* 突变检测，组织学特征为浸润性小叶癌，术前 MRI，乳房重建和在 NCI 指定的癌症中心治疗[634,641～643]。在过去的 15 年中，随着对侧预防性乳房切除术的增加，乳房切除术的技术可以保留乳头-乳晕复合体（NAC）的皮肤，保留乳头的乳房切除术（NSM）和需要立即进行乳房重建的 TSSM 已经越来越多地开始被使用了[229,644～648]。

许多研究表明，*BRCA1/2* 突变的患者发生乳腺癌的风险增加，而对侧预防性乳房切除术可改善这些患者的长期生存率[637,638,642,649,650]。在一项比较 *BRCA1/2* 阴性家系和阳性家系的研究中发现，*BRCA1* 突变 25 年内患对侧乳腺癌的风险为 44.1%，*BRCA2* 突变患对侧乳腺癌的风险为 33.5%，未发现突变为 17.2%[651]。

最近一项评估在接受 TSSM 和立即乳房再造的患者中进行对侧预防性乳房切除术的研究显示，2006—2013 年期间接受对侧预防性乳房切除术的患者比例增加，这与之前的报告一致[374,634,635,642]。在这项研究中，50%的患者接受了对侧预防性乳房切除术：这其中 45%的患者没有已知的有害突变，100%的患者存在有害突变。这些比例明显高于此前报道的数据[374,635,642]。这可能是由以下固有选择偏倚造成的：患者主要是高加索人，相对年轻，并且在 NCI 指定的癌症中心有机会接受外科医生伴立即乳房重建的 TSSM 治疗[642,643]。

基因突变检测呈阴性但仍进行对侧预防性乳房切除术（选择乳房切除术的女性）的患者范围为 27%～58%[642,652,653]。在该组中，对侧预防性乳房切除术有增加的趋势，这可能与患者年龄相对较小、患有乳腺癌或卵巢癌的亲属的年龄较小以及患有乳腺癌或卵巢癌的家庭成员的数量增加有关。之前的研究报道，乳腺癌亲属数量的增加与 *BRCA1/2* 阳性家族中对侧预防性乳房切除术的风险增加相关[654]。在 *BRCA1/2* 阴性家族的患者中，对那些在初次诊断乳腺癌时年龄小于 40 岁的患者来说，对侧乳腺癌的 25 年风险为 28.4%，而在 *BRCA2* 突变的患者中接近 33.5%[649]。这些研究结果表明，年龄较小或有较强家族史的患者患对侧乳腺癌的风险可能会有所增加，但具体风险无法测量。有证据表明，多基因风险评分可以评估对侧乳腺癌的遗传风险，并鉴别出有对侧乳腺癌风险的患者，相当于 BRCA 携带者[640]。对侧预防性乳房切除术在那些存在对侧乳腺癌危险因素的患者和那些病理分期较低的肿瘤患者中被更频繁地选择[651]，这表明与担心对侧乳腺癌发生相比，病理分期较高的女性可能更会担心同侧复发的风险。对预防性乳房切除术标本的病理学检查显示，仅有 2.2%～4.7%的患者表现出病理异常，包括 DCIS，LCIS 和黏液性癌[661,655,656]。

然而，女性应该知道额外的对侧预防性乳房切除术可能会导致患者术后并发症的风险增加，虽然风险较小。对侧预防性乳房切除术会使浅表乳头坏死和植入物暴露的风险增加一倍。这也与伤口破裂和需要口服抗生素抗感染的风险增加有关，但这些 *RR* 估计值<2。对侧预防性乳房切除术不会导致植入式乳房重建患者植入物丢失的风险增加。其他研究发现，与单侧乳房切除术相比，对侧预防性乳房切除术可使并发症增加 1.5～2.1 倍[657~660]，与上述研究结果一致。

一些研究表明，患者认为对侧预防性乳房切除术带来的获益，比如对侧乳腺癌风险降低，筛查次数减少以及重建后更好的美学效果，可能已经超过了对侧预防性乳房切除术后并发症风险的增加。即使在没有任何数据证明该方案会降低死亡率。那些选择对侧预防性乳房切除术的人表达了对乳腺癌家族史、罹患癌症的主观恐惧，同时希望保持或改善乳房的美观[661~666]。患者的主观脆弱感可能远高于其对侧乳腺癌的实际风险[666]。一些欧洲作者认为，对癌症恐惧的增加和整形手术的可接受性已导致美国对侧预防性乳房切除术的使用频率增加[677]。来自患者报告的结果研究表明，接受对侧预防性乳房切除术的患者对乳房和整体重建结果的满意度高于未进行对侧预防性乳房切除术的患者[668]。

孤立性局部复发的处理

如果检测到孤立的胸壁或区域淋巴结复发，建议进行组织活检和手术切除。如果不进行早期照射，则需要对胸壁进行放射治疗，放疗范围应涉及局部淋巴结区域，并应对 HR+疾病进行激素治疗。一项开放试验（CALOR 试验）随机分配了手术切除的局部区域复发患者（无论是否进行了化疗）[455]。HR+疾病的患者接受了辅助内分泌治疗，显微镜下手术切缘需进行放射治疗。该试验仅纳入 162 例患者，但中位随访时间为 4.9 年。接受化疗的患者与未接受化疗的患者相比，DFS 事件的发生频率显著降低（28% vs 44%）。对于患有 HR-疾病的患者，化疗明显更加有效，但数量太小而无法得出明确的结论。

根据这些数据，局部复发患者应在疾病亚型和既往治疗的基础上选择合适的治疗方法，包括放射治疗、激素治疗和化疗。

孕期乳腺癌

有 1%～2%的乳腺癌女性在妊娠时确诊，平均年龄为 35 岁。在相同疾病阶段内，妊娠与非妊娠乳腺癌患者的预后相似。遗憾的是，由于妊娠期间相关体格检查的变化，妊娠患者的诊断通常会延迟，并且由于诊断时疾病阶段较晚，她们的预后往往更差[669]。

一般而言，只有在结果可能会改变疾病治疗方案的时候才应进行放射学评估(670)。超声检查通常是对孕妇进行的初步影像学检查[671]。钼靶检查并非禁忌，胎儿受到的辐射照射也很小，但仍建议进行腹部屏蔽。然而，由于妊娠期间乳房密度增加，孕期或哺乳期患者的钼靶照片检查的敏感性降低。对比磁共振成像是禁忌的，因为尚不存在其对胎儿影响的数据[672]。

妊娠期间乳腺癌管理的治疗建议必须基于外科医生，肿瘤内科医生和产科医生之间的详细讨论。此外，必须考虑患者的信念和价值体系。在妊娠期间乳腺癌患者的治疗选择与非妊娠患者的选择相似。然而，治疗的时间和顺序取决于确诊时的妊娠时长以及疾病是否发展为局部晚期[670]。虽然很少有必要，但应考虑终止妊娠，特别是在妊娠早期诊断时。如果在妊娠晚期诊断为低风险乳腺癌，通常可以适当延迟治疗直至分娩后。在妊娠期间的任何时候乳房切除术都是适当的，且对胎儿的风险最小，而放射治疗明显禁忌并且应延迟到分娩后进行[673~675]。

化疗可引起胎儿畸形，必须在妊娠早期避免。一项前瞻性和几项回顾性临床试验评估了妊娠期化疗的使用，并且一致认为基于多柔比星的疗法适用于妊娠中期和晚期，对母体、胎儿或新生儿毒性最小[676~679]。一项 2012 年的回顾性研究证明了在接受每 3 周多柔比星加环磷酰胺（AC）或接受剂量密集的 AC 加培非格司亭（pegfilgrastim）的患者中，新生儿出生体重、妊娠异常率或中性粒细胞减少率没有显著差异[680]。其他研究也证实了类似的发现。其他化学疗法或生物制剂的数据不足以支持其使用，而他莫昔芬明显与流产和先天性畸形有关。

男性乳腺癌

男性乳腺癌最常见的症状包括乳房肿块，乳头溢液，乳头内陷，腋窝肿块和局部或远处疼痛。由于缺乏诊断的认识，男性患者通常表现出更晚期的疾病。对男性乳腺癌的评估和诊断与女性相似。大多数患有早期乳腺癌的男性都接受了简单的乳房切除术和 SLND 治疗,那些患有局部晚期疾病的患者应首先接受新辅助治疗。辅助放射遵循与女性相同的模式。

由于男性乳腺癌十分罕见,没有针对乳腺癌男性特异性全身治疗的随机临床试验。男性乳腺癌的辅助治疗选择与女性相似。Giordano 等人 2005 年的回顾性研究报告了 156 名乳腺癌患者在单一机构接受治疗的结果[681]。其中 135 名男性患有 ESBC,85%的患者患有 HR+疾病。接受激素治疗的患者 OS 显著升高(HR=0.45,P=0.01)。同时发现他莫昔芬优于 AI。一项对 257 名接受了激素治疗的 ESBC 男性的回顾性分析表明,患者接受 AI 比他莫昔芬的死亡风险更高(HR=1.55,95%CI:1.13~2.13,P=0.007)。男性患者应用他莫昔芬的依从性普遍较差,并且与高依从性相比,低依从性组患者的 10 年 DFS 率(42% vs 80%,P=0.007)和 OS(50% vs 80%,P=0.008)明显更差[682]。

许多回顾性研究表明,男性 HR+乳腺癌患者的反应率高达 80%。其他基于激素的疗法以及新的靶向疗法的经验非常有限。一般而言,化疗在男性中具有与 MBC 的女性相似的效果。

炎性乳腺癌

炎性乳腺癌(inflammatory breast cancer,IBC)是一种侵袭性,局部晚期的乳腺癌,占美国新诊断乳腺癌的 2%。IBC 患者的预后较差,在全身化疗出现之前,最佳局部区域治疗后的 5 年生存率<5%[683]。虽然多学科方法改善了预后,但使用 2004—2007 年间的 SEER 数据进行了基于人群的研究证实,IBC 患者患乳腺癌的 HR 局部晚期非 IBC 患者增加 43%(HR=1.43,95%CI:1.10~1.86,P=0.008)[684]。

IBC 是一种临床诊断,其特征为体表检查发现至少占乳房皮肤的 1/3 红斑和水肿(peaud'orange)并且存在时间不超过 6 个月[685]。皮肤淋巴受累不是支持诊断的必备条件,乳房的核心活检通常能提供明确的诊断。因为经常无法触及基础肿块,IBC 经常被误认为是乳腺炎,并对患者使用抗生素进行治疗。

IBC 的标准疗法是新辅助化疗,建议使用含有蒽环类和紫杉醇类药物的方案[409,683]。HER2+IBC 患者应采用与 HER2+非 IBC 对应部分相同的新辅助治疗方案。大多数 IBC 病例对化疗有显著反应,并且>90%的患者通常没有局部区域疾病。新辅助化疗后的局部治疗应包括乳房切除术和放射治疗。一些治疗中心在新辅助化疗出现完全反应后采取了保乳手术,但国际共识委员会并未建议采用这种方式。此外,SSM 在 IBC 中是禁忌的[683]。

老年患者的治疗

美国增长最快的人口是 65 岁左右的群体。目前,该群体占全美人口的 12%,但 50%的乳腺癌发生在该群体中。由于美国女性的预期寿命为 80 岁,而且因为今天的老年人更健康,大多数乳腺癌患者的预期寿命也超过了 10 年。目前很少可以看到有关老年女性乳腺癌患者治疗的临床研究[686,687]。"老年"的定义可能是在实际年龄、生理年龄或预期寿命的基础上形成的。在这个群体中的治疗决策要越来越多地基于患者的综合身体条件,这些条件通常会比乳腺癌本身更能限制预期寿命。不同年龄组患者的治疗方法不应有所不同。同时存在的其他疾病改变了患者的预期寿命,从而也改变了我们对乳腺癌的所有干预措施的预期效益。老年 ESBC 患者的标准治疗方法应为乳房肿瘤切除术,SLNB 和放疗,并根据预后因素 ER,PR 和 HER2 的情况确定是否进行全身辅助治疗。预示肿瘤生物学行为的分子分型越来越多地帮助我们调整患者的治疗方案。最近在《Adjuvant! Online》上发表的一项关于 MP 对>60 岁中度风险女性的影响的研究结果在通过临床数据预测的方法之外为我们提供了额外的信息[688]。我们将在未来使用分子测试来定义一群患者,并在其身上测试较少人为干预的影响。

目前,AI 或他莫昔芬的应用已经成为任何年龄下 HR+乳腺癌女性的标准疗法。HR-乳腺癌患者不适用内分泌治疗。值得注意的是,在 CALGB9343 研究中,70 岁以上接受他莫昔芬或他莫昔芬+放射治疗的 ER+的乳腺癌女性更容易死于其他疾病。在随访第八年时,乳腺癌相关死亡率为 3%,而其他原因造成的死亡率为 21%。

一旦患者肿瘤复发风险高到必须接受化疗,同时化疗的获益大于其相关风险,我们就应该给予老年患者足量化疗[689]。小于标准足量的化疗通常是无效的,且给患者带来了不必要的治疗相关毒性。但是在 CALGB 研究中,当 HER2/neu 测定结果为阴性的情况下,在 CAF 方案中接受每 4 周 4 次注射 40mg/m^2 多柔比星的女性与那些接受 4 次 60mg/m^2 或 6 次 40mg/m^2 的女性预后相似。当然,我们需要前瞻性研究来验证这些结果。最近,人们很有兴趣设计方案来评估可能对这些患者产生更小毒性的新药。一项Ⅲ期临床试验比较了单药口服卡培他滨与经典 CMF 或 AC 方案在 65 岁以上患者的辅助治疗中的疗效。卡培他滨组的 DFS 明显不如标准方案,同时标准化疗耐受性良好[690]。

症状监控和幸存者

据 ACS 估计,截至 2014 年 1 月,乳腺癌幸存者超过 300 万[1],大约 72%的乳腺癌幸存者(>200 万女性)年龄为 60 岁;不足 10%的患者年龄<50 岁。了解年轻和老年幸存者面临的问题对于支持其生活质量、适当降低风险和症状的监控至关重要。

ESBC 幸存者的治疗后标准随访护理应包括监测癌症复发或新的原发灶和预防继发性癌症,同时应对患者进行晚期心理社会和身体状况的评估,并对治疗带来的不良后果(如新的医疗问题,症状和心理困扰)进行干预。最后,初级保健提供者和癌症专家应共同对患者的生存状况进行管理和关怀。

在完成原发性乳腺癌联合治疗后的前 3 年内,患者应每 3~6 个月就诊一次,并且每次就诊都需要仔细进行完整的体格检查[409]。随后的 2 年内,患者应每 6~12 个月就诊 1 次,之后每年一次。接受保乳手术的患者应在完成放射治疗后 6 个月,即初次钼靶检查后 1 年进行乳房检查,之后每年进行一次。只有在出现症状或体检结果异常的情况下才应进行影像学检查。由于 MBC 的早期检测不能使 OS 获益,因此不建议在缺乏临床症状或体检结果无异常的情况下进行全血细胞计数、综合代谢组学、肿瘤标志物和影像学的检查。目前较活跃的研究领域包括监测循环 DNA 作为疾病复发的早期标志。

对于许多患者而言,从接受强效的治疗过渡到频率较低的随访观察可能很困难,特别是在资源贫乏,中低收入的环境中。应教育患者识别疾病复发的体征和症状,管理短期和长期的身体和社会心理状况，以及认识到通过适当的体力活动保持健康体重是一种重要的健康生活方式[692,693]。此时，一般建议癌症幸存者每周达到150min的中等强度活动。此外患者的生存问题还包括生育能力、疲劳和抑郁、认知功能障碍、疼痛、淋巴水肿、性功能障碍、睡眠障碍、骨骼健康、心脏毒性和健康的生活方式选择。其中一些问题在NCCN生存指南1.2016.691版本中进行了详细说明[691]。

乳腺癌中的肥胖和糖尿病

Patterson等人[692]评估了综合身体状况对2 542例ESBC女性乳腺癌结局的影响，中位随访时间为7.3年。最值得注意的是，糖尿病患者的ROR（*HR*=2.1，95%*CI*：1.3~3.4）和死亡率（*HR*=2.5，95%*CI*：1.4~4.4）超过非糖尿病患者两倍。Sparano等人在2012年发表的荟萃分析表明，在HR+乳腺癌患者中，肥胖患者与较差的DFS（*HR*=1.24，95%*CI*：1.06~1.46，*P*=0.000 8）和OS（*HR*=1.37，95%*CI*：1.13~1.67，*P*=0.002）相关，但在其他亚型中没有得到体现[694]。

一些临床试验已经评估了旨在改善预后的各种减肥和营养干预措施。WINS研究是1994年开始的一项Ⅲ期临床试验，该研究将2 437名ESBC患者按60∶40的比例随机分组，接受注册营养师指导的低脂饮食计划。在SABCS2014中提出了长期分析[42]。在中位随访5年时，干预组的患者脂肪卡路里减少了9.2%，体重增加了2.7kg（6磅）。在平均60个月的随访中，干预组的复发率降低了24%。该干预的最大益处是使HR-ESBC女性的死亡率降低了54%，而HR+ESBC女性没有获益。然而，妇女健康饮食和生活（WHEL）随机临床试验比较了蔬菜和水果含量高的低脂饮食在3 088名妇女中的作用，随访7.3年后，发现对乳腺癌事件或死亡率没有影响[695]。

生育管理

全世界浸润性乳腺癌中，育龄女性占15%[459]。这些女性在接受化疗后经常会出现卵巢早衰或不育，这可能会损害卵巢储备[696]。ASCO癌症患者生育能力保留的临床实践指南建议如果不孕症是一种潜在的风险，那么开始治疗前应对所有育龄患者的生育能力保留问题进行讨论[697]。处在希望保留生育能力矛盾之中的患者应该转诊给生殖专家。胚胎和卵母细胞冷冻保存是唯一成熟的保存方法。新出现的数据表明，HR-ESBC患者在辅助化疗期间使用戈舍瑞林（goserelin）可降低卵巢功能衰竭的风险[698]。

一项预防更年期的早期研究（POEMS）/S0230临床试验是一项Ⅲ期临床试验，评估了绝经前HR-ESBC女性接受化疗加戈舍瑞林治疗后卵巢功能衰竭的发生情况。遗憾的是，由于资金不足，该研究未能达到招募416名患者的目标而提前关闭。共有257名女性随机接受含或不含戈舍瑞林的标准环磷酰胺化疗。中位随访时间为4.1年，仅218名女性的研究结果可用。戈舍瑞林组8%的患者发生卵巢功能衰竭，相比之下，对照组为22%（*OR*=0.30，95%*CI*：0.9~0.97；双侧*P*=0.04）。戈舍瑞林组女性的妊娠率高于对照组（21% vs 11%，*P*=0.03）。虽然数据缺失，但研究人员据此得出结论，戈舍瑞林与HR-ESBC妇女联合化疗时，似乎可以降低早期绝经的风险，并提高生育能力。

由于绝经前HR+ESBC患者接受了几年的辅助内分泌治疗，所以她们推迟了分娩。这些患者通常在开始治疗前考虑胚胎或卵母细胞冷冻保存，但理论上卵巢刺激和雌激素水平增加会导致肿瘤生长的风险增加。Oktay等[696]最近描述了HR+ESBC患者的卵巢刺激方案，该方案使用来曲唑与促卵泡生成激素相结合来限制雌激素水平的增加。在该研究中，131名ESBC女性在化疗和卵细胞冷冻保存前接受卵巢刺激的同时进行了5mg/d的来曲唑治疗。研究人群中每次胚胎移植率的成功率为51.5%，与未患癌症的美国全国女性的平均值相似。

脱发

化疗引起的脱发对许多乳腺癌患者造成了情感创伤，并且通常被列为治疗中最可怕的副作用。几十年来，促进头皮冷却和预防化疗导致的脱发的装置已经在欧洲和加拿大投入研究并广泛使用，最近在美国的研究证明了其对接受常用化学治疗方案的ESBC患者的疗效。荷兰头皮冷却登记处对化疗期间接受头皮降温治疗的近1 500名妇女进行调查，结果发现该方案对50%患者有效，并且在5年的随访中未发现头皮转移病例[699]。过去几年中使用较新的设备（如Penguin冰帽，Digni帽和PAXMANOrbis头皮冷却器）的几项小型临床试验已经报道了更高的疗效，在65%~75%的使用者中脱发率为25%。美国正在进行的临床试验正在继续评估这些设备的安全性和有效性（NCT01831024、NCT01986140）。

淋巴水肿

手臂淋巴水肿的特点是局部肿胀，因为体内组织中富含蛋白质的液体积聚，影响美观，同时伴有运动功能下降[700]。淋巴水肿影响大约21%的乳腺癌幸存者，其发病率取决于患者的手术类型。除了功能下降外，患者还会出现感觉异常，疼痛和心理困扰，导致QOL降低。早期的生理治疗包括手动淋巴引流、瘢痕组织按摩和肩部运动。手术后若尽早开始治疗，淋巴水肿的发生率较低。淋巴水肿的治疗方案包括理疗以增加患肢的活动范围，穿弹力服进行渐进阻力训练，减重并适当配合弹力服的穿着[691]。患者应条件允许时转诊至淋巴水肿专科医生。手术疗法被认为是最后的选择，并仍处在研究中。

潮热

65%~80%的ESBC幸存者部分布位会出现潮热，可能是化疗或抗雌激素治疗引起的卵巢抑制。几项随机对照试验表明，文拉法辛、加巴喷丁或可乐定（SSRI）的药物干预比安慰剂更有效地降低了潮热的频率[701]。但是包括针灸和认知行为疗法在内的非药物干预措施的有效性尚不清楚，部分原因是对照干预无法实施。

骨骼健康

雌激素含量下降会导致骨吸收，骨质快速丢失。因此，接受AI治疗的女性骨密度减少和随后出现的不良骨骼事件的风险增加。AI患者应进行骨折风险评估，双能X线吸收测定法

(DEXA)测定骨密度以及临床因素(如年龄、骨折史、低体重指数、烟草和酒精滥用情况)的评估。骨密度应每 1~2 年重复测量一次。此外,应鼓励患者服用钙和维生素 D。在 AI 治疗期间出现骨质减少或骨质疏松症的患者应考虑使用双膦酸盐或地诺单抗。

几十年来,研究人员已经评估了用于降低 ESBC 女性远程复发风险的辅助双膦酸盐治疗,结果各不相同。EBCTCG 最近发表了接受双膦酸盐辅助治疗的个体患者的随机研究的荟萃分析[702]。共有 18 766 名女性参加了 2~5 年的双膦酸盐治疗试验。骨复发率显著减少(HR=0. 83,95%CI:0. 87~1. 01;双侧 P=0. 004)。在绝经后患者中观察到复发,远处复发,骨复发和乳腺癌死亡率明显减少。

(刘嘉琦　张梦璐　孟祥志　冯轲昕 译
王翔　王昕 校)

参考文献

The complete reference list can be found on the Wiley Companion Digital Edition of this title (see inside front cover for login instructions).

1 Siegel RL, Miller KD, Jemal A. Cancer statistics, 2015. *CA Cancer J Clin*. 2015;**65**:5-29.

14 Mavaddat N, Peock S, Frost D, et al. Cancer risks for BRCA1 and BRCA2 mutation carriers: results from prospective analysis of EMBRACE. *J Natl Cancer Inst*. 2013;**105**:812-822.

42 Chlebowski RT, Rohan TE, Manson JE, et al. Breast cancer after use of estrogen plus progestin and estrogen alone: analyses of data from 2 Women's Health Initiative randomized clinical trials. *JAMA Oncol*. 2015;**1**:296-305.

98 Gail MH. Twenty-five years of breast cancer risk models and their applications. *J Natl Cancer Inst*. 2015;**107**.

119 Paik S, Shak S, Tang G, et al. A multigene assay to predict recurrence of tamoxifen-treated, node-negative breast cancer. *N Engl J Med*. 2004;**351**:2817-2826.

138 Esserman LJ, Thompson IM, Reid B, et al. Addressing overdiagnosis and overtreatment in cancer: a prescription for change. *Lancet Oncol*. 2014;**15**:e234-e242.

139 Oeffinger KC, Fontham ET, Etzioni R, et al. Breast cancer screening for women at average risk: 2015 guideline update from the American Cancer Society. *JAMA*. 2015;**314**:1599-1614.

146 Early Breast Cancer Trialists' Collaborative Group (EBCTCG). Effects of chemotherapy and hormonal therapy for early breast cancer on recurrence and 15-year survival: an overview of the randomised trials. *Lancet*. 2005;**365**:1687-1717.

148 Dowsett M, Cuzick J, Ingle J, et al. Meta-analysis of breast cancer outcomes in adjuvant trials of aromatase inhibitors versus tamoxifen. *J Clin Oncol*. 2010;**28**:509-518.

199 Fisher B, Costantino JP, Wickerham DL, et al. Tamoxifen for the prevention of breast cancer: current status of the National Surgical Adjuvant Breast and Bowel Project P-1 study. *J Natl Cancer Inst*. 2005;**97**:1652-1662.

204 Goss PE, Ingle JN, Ales-Martinez JE, et al. Exemestane for breast-cancer prevention in postmenopausal women. *N Engl J Med*. 2011;**364**:2381-2391.

235 Giuliano AE, Hunt KK, Ballman KV, et al. Axillary dissection vs no axillary dissection in women with invasive breast cancer and sentinel node metastasis: a randomized clinical trial. *JAMA*. 2011;**305**:569-575.

241 Morris AD, Morris RD, Wilson JF, et al. Breast-conserving therapy vs mastectomy in early-stage breast cancer: a meta-analysis of 10-year survival. *Cancer J Sci Am*. 1997;3:6-12.

242 Early Breast Cancer Trialists' Collaborative Group. Favourable and unfavourable effects on long-term survival of radiotherapy for early breast cancer: an overview of the randomised trials. Early Breast Cancer Trialists' Collaborative Group. *Lancet*. 2000;**355**:1757-1770.

267 Rastogi P, Anderson SJ, Bear HD, et al. Preoperative chemotherapy: updates of National Surgical Adjuvant Breast and Bowel Project Protocols B-18 and B-27. *J Clin Oncol*. 2008;**26**:778-785.

337 Early Breast Cancer Trialists' Collaborative Group, Davies C, Godwin J, et al. Relevance of breast cancer hormone receptors and other factors to the efficacy of adjuvant tamoxifen: patient-level meta-analysis of randomised trials. *Lancet*. 2011;**378**:771-784.

342 Coombes RC, Hall E, Gibson LJ, et al. A randomized trial of exemestane after two to three years of tamoxifen therapy in postmenopausal women with primary breast cancer. *N Engl J Med*. 2004;**350**:1081-1092.

345 Coates AS, Winer EP, Goldhirsch A, et al. Tailoring therapies-improving the management of early breast cancer: St Gallen International Expert Consensus on the Primary Therapy of Early Breast Cancer 2015. *Ann Oncol*. 2015;**26**:1533-1546.

350 Burstein HJ, Temin S, Anderson H, et al. Adjuvant endocrine therapy for women with hormone receptor-positive breast cancer: American Society of Clinical Oncology clinical practice guideline focused update. *J Clin Oncol*. 2014;**32**:2255-2269.

364 Henderson IC, Berry DA, Demetri GD, et al. Improved outcomes from adding sequential Paclitaxel but not from escalating Doxorubicin dose in an adjuvant chemotherapy regimen for patients with node-positive primary breast cancer. *J Clin Oncol*. 2003;**21**:976-983.

365 Mamounas EP, Bryant J, Lembersky B, et al. Paclitaxel after doxorubicin plus cyclophosphamide as adjuvant chemotherapy for node-positive breast cancer: results from NSABP B-28. *J Clin Oncol*. 2005;**23**:3686-3696.

366 Martin M, Pienkowski T, Mackey J, et al. Adjuvant docetaxel for node-positive breast cancer. *N Engl J Med*. 2005;**352**:2302-2313.

367 Mackey JR, Martin M, Pienkowski T, et al. Adjuvant docetaxel, doxorubicin, and cyclophosphamide in node-positive breast cancer: 10-year follow-up of the phase 3 randomised BCIRG 001 trial. *Lancet Oncol*. 2013;**14**:72-80.

371 Wood WC, Budman DR, Korzun AH, et al. Dose and dose intensity of adjuvant chemotherapy for stage II, node-positive breast carcinoma. *N Engl J Med*. 1994;**330**:1253-1259.

374 Citron ML, Berry DA, Cirrincione C, et al. Randomized trial of dose-dense versus conventionally scheduled and sequential versus concurrent combination chemotherapy as postoperative adjuvant treatment of node-positive primary breast cancer: first report of Intergroup Trial C9741/Cancer and Leukemia Group B Trial 9741. *J Clin Oncol*. 2003;**21**:1431-1439.

404 Geyer CE, Forster J, Lindquist D, et al. Lapatinib plus capecitabine for HER2-positive advanced breast cancer. *N Engl J Med*. 2006;**355**:2733-2743.

405 Goss PE, Smith IE, O'Shaughnessy J, et al. Adjuvant lapatinib for women with early-stage HER2-positive breast cancer: a randomised, controlled, phase 3 trial. *Lancet Oncol*. 2013;**14**:88-96.

457 Aebi S, Gelber S, Anderson SJ, et al. Chemotherapy for isolated locoregional recurrence of breast cancer (CALOR): a randomised trial. *Lancet Oncol*. 2014;**15**:156-163.

460 Cardoso F, Costa A, Norton L, et al. ESO-ESMO 2nd international consensus guidelines for advanced breast cancer (ABC2). *Breast*. 2014;**23**:489-502.

466 Wilcken N, Hornbuckle J, Ghersi D. Chemotherapy alone versus endocrine therapy alone for metastatic breast cancer. *Cochrane Database Syst Rev*. 2003;**2**:CD002747.

471 Mouridsen H, Gershanovich M, Sun Y, et al. Superior efficacy of letrozole versus tamoxifen as first-line therapy for postmenopausal women with advanced breast cancer: results of a phase III study of the International Letrozole Breast Cancer Group. *J Clin Oncol*. 2001;**19**:2596-2606.

479 Osborne CK, Pippen J, Jones SE, et al. Double-blind, randomized trial comparing the efficacy and tolerability of fulvestrant versus anastrozole in postmenopausal women with advanced breast cancer progressing on prior endocrine therapy: results of a North American trial. *J Clin Oncol*. 2002;**20**:3386-3395.

490 Baselga J, Campone M, Piccart M, et al. Everolimus in postmenopausal hormone-receptor-positive advanced breast cancer. *N Engl J Med*. 2012;**366**:520-529.

495 Finn RS, Crown JP, Lang I, et al. The cyclin-dependent kinase 4/6 inhibitor palbociclib in combination with letrozole versus letrozole alone as first-line treatment of oestrogen receptor-positive, HER2-negative, advanced breast cancer (PALOMA-1/TRIO-18): a randomised phase 2 study. *Lancet Oncol*. 2015;**16**:25-35.

496 Turner NC, Ro J, Andre F, et al. Palbociclib in hormone-receptor-positive advanced breast cancer. *N Engl J Med*. 2015;**373**:209-219.

502 Dear RF, McGeechan K, Jenkins MC, et al. Combination versus sequential single agent chemotherapy for metastatic breast cancer. *Cochrane Database Syst Rev*. 2013;**12**:CD008792.

503 Gennari A, Stockler M, Puntoni M, et al. Duration of chemotherapy for metastatic breast cancer: a systematic review and meta-analysis of randomized clinical trials. *J Clin Oncol*. 2011;**29**:2144-2149.

504 Park YH, Jung KH, Im SA, et al. Phase III, multicenter, randomized trial of maintenance chemotherapy versus observation in patients with metastatic breast cancer after achieving disease control with six cycles of gemcitabine plus paclitaxel as first-line chemotherapy: KCSG-BR07-02. *J Clin Oncol*. 2013;**31**:1732-1739.

520 Sledge GW, Neuberg D, Bernardo P, et al. Phase III trial of doxorubicin, paclitaxel, and the combination of doxorubicin and paclitaxel as front-line chemotherapy for metastatic breast cancer: an intergroup trial (E1193). *J Clin Oncol*. 2003;**21**:588-592.

557 Slamon DJ, Leyland-Jones B, Shak S, et al. Use of chemotherapy plus a monoclonal

antibody against HER2 for metastatic breast cancer that overexpresses HER2. *N Engl J Med*. 2001;**344**:783–792.

565 Valero V, Forbes J, Pegram MD, et al. Multicenter phase III randomized trial comparing docetaxel and trastuzumab with docetaxel, carboplatin, and trastuzumab as first-line chemotherapy for patients with HER2-gene-amplified metastatic breast cancer (BCIRG 007 study): two highly active therapeutic regimens. *J Clin Oncol*. 2011;**29**:149–156.

589 Baselga J, Cortes J, Kim SB, et al. Pertuzumab plus trastuzumab plus docetaxel for metastatic breast cancer. *N Engl J Med*. 2012;**366**:109–119.

593 Verma S, Miles D, Gianni L, et al. Trastuzumab emtansine for HER2-positive advanced breast cancer. *N Engl J Med*. 2012;**367**:1783–1791.

631 Rosen LS, Gordon D, Kaminski M, et al. Long-term efficacy and safety of zoledronic acid compared with pamidronate disodium in the treatment of skeletal complications in patients with advanced multiple myeloma or breast carcinoma: a randomized, double-blind, multicenter, comparative trial. *Cancer*. 2003;**98**:1735–1744.

633 Stopeck AT, Lipton A, Body JJ, et al. Denosumab compared with zoledronic acid for the treatment of bone metastases in patients with advanced breast cancer: a randomized, double-blind study. *J Clin Oncol*. 2010;**28**:5132–5139.

681 Giordano SH, Perkins GH, Broglio K, et al. Adjuvant systemic therapy for male breast carcinoma. *Cancer*. 2005;**104**:2359–2364.

第 109 章　恶性黑色素瘤

Justin M. Ko, MD, MBA, FAAD ■ Susan M. Swetter, MD ■ Jonathan S. Zager, MD ■ Vernon K. Sondak, MD ■ Scott E. Woodman, MD, PhD ■ Kim A. Margolin, MD

概述

恶性黑色素瘤是起源于各类包括皮肤、黏膜和眼内的色素细胞的恶性肿瘤。尽管这些肿瘤都被归类为黑色素瘤，具有共同的色素沉着的分子生物学特征，且共同起源于神经嵴，但重要的区别在于各自具有不同的分子学特征、暴露于紫外线辐射是否作为致癌的高危因素等，这决定了其不同的自然病程，包括对于治疗的临床疗效。虽然多数的黑色素瘤都在早期被确诊，可通过极小的手术达到治愈，但黑色素瘤在早期便可能通过淋巴管和血行途径转移。外科手术是治疗原发、局限性以及部分单发或寡转移性黑色素瘤的主要方法，但是系统性全身治疗已显著改善了转移性黑色素瘤的预后，尤其是可增强现有机体细胞免疫功能的免疫治疗。新的分子靶点的迅速发现、免疫治疗的联合应用（包括放射治疗的应用）以及对治疗抵抗机制的理解均有望在不久的将来使黑色素瘤患者的预后得到更大的改善。

黑色素瘤的皮肤学原理

流行病学与病因学

全球黑色素瘤的发病率和死亡率持续升高，这是由于紫外线辐射（自然光源和人工光源）的增加，且不同的年龄和性别其预后有所差异。在美国，2016 年有 76 380 例新确诊的侵袭性皮肤黑色素瘤病例，其中大约 10 130 例死亡[1]。在过去的 30 年里，发病率一直持续上升，自 2004 年以来，白种人的发病率每年增加 3%，几乎比其他所有癌症的发病率都要快[2]。紫外线辐射（UVR）增加导致西部各州发病率更高[3]。年轻女性（15~39 岁）的发病率上升了两倍以上，而中年和老年男性的发病率则更是急剧上升[3,4]。

黑色素瘤发病率的增加可归因于以下因素：白种人间歇性紫外线照射的增加、皮肤活检率的增高，从而检测到了更薄、更早期的病变，以及组织学上将早期病变从原来的定义成非典型黑色素细胞增生或严重发育不良逐渐变化为定义成原位黑色素瘤[5,6]。然而，较厚的肿瘤的发病率持续上升，包括社会经济地位较低的人群的发病率急剧上升，这表明潜在致命病例的发病率确实上升，并且缺乏筛查是解释最近黑色素瘤发病趋势的一个关键因素[7]。

危险因素

环境因素

黑色素瘤的致病风险与急性、强烈的和间歇性的紫外线照射有关，但紫外线照射并非黑色素损伤的直接致病因素。黑色素瘤经常发生在衣服遮盖的地方，室内工作人员在阳光照射的地方黑色素瘤的发病率更高，这些观察结果均支持黑色素瘤是通过不同的分子途径致病的观点[8,9]。暴露在阳光下和暴露较少的身体区域的黑色素瘤发病率也有不同的年龄高峰[10]，在间歇性暴露部位（如躯干和肢体近端）的黑色素瘤发病率约为 55 岁，这可能反映出生命早期易受紫外线辐射影响，逐渐发展至完全黑色素损伤，致使生命晚期的黑色素瘤发病率下降，应该归因于这些机制[11]。相反，长期暴露的部位如面部和肢体远端的黑色素瘤会随着年龄的增长而持续增长。紫外线诱导的标志性 *DNA* 突变通常出现在黑色素瘤中识别的驱动突变中[12]，但不像非黑色素瘤皮肤癌中那样与长期日光照射直接相关，因此可能存在其他的突变源。然而，澳大利亚的一项随机研究表明，每日持续使用抵挡 UVA 和 UVB 的广谱防晒霜（与不规律使用或不使用相比）可降低黑色素瘤的发病率[13]。室内晒黑已被证实是年轻女性皮肤黑色素瘤发病率增加的主要原因，其发病风险与晒黑的方式剂量成正比，包括增加室内晒黑的年限、小时数和疗程[14,15]。令人担忧的是，在白种人皮肤的受试者中，76%的黑色素瘤与年轻时日光浴频繁相关。与此同时，研究证实日光浴喜好与药物成瘾有很强的相关性，提示成瘾的基因介导机制[16]，这与动物研究显示出的结果，即阿片类相关物质通过内啡肽受体诱导个体寻求日光照射的行为相一致[17]。

自身因素

虽然正常黑色素细胞转化为黑色素瘤细胞的过程并未被完全了解，但进行性遗传突变可能改变了细胞的增殖、分化和死亡，并影响了细胞对紫外线辐射致癌作用的敏感性。

黑色素瘤在很大程度上是白色人种易患的疾病，包括那些红色或金色头发，易被灼伤或有严重晒伤病史，或不易被晒黑的人[18]。痣数量增多或易长雀斑的白种人也有更高的风险发展成黑色素瘤[19]。通过对黑色素痣表型的综合分析，即使在不同的纬度，也证实了在体表常见/典型痣、大痣和/或临床不典型痣（CAN）的数量增加，增加了皮肤黑色素瘤的患病风险[20]。既往病史和家族史都是黑色素瘤发病的重要危险因素[21]。与普通人群相比，实体器官移植人群患鳞状细胞癌的风险更大，而且黑色素瘤的发生率也更高[22]。

遗传易感性与家族性黑色素瘤

大多数黑色素瘤都是散发性的,只有5%~10%的病例具有确定的家族倾向[23]。家族性黑色素瘤的特征表现为黑色素瘤的发病风险增高,多发性原发黑色素瘤的发病率更高,一般发病年龄更早[24]。家族性黑色素瘤的发病机制与特异性遗传改变有关。染色体 9p21 上 *CDKN2A* 位点的突变,编码肿瘤抑制因子 *p16* 和 *p14/ARF*,约占家族病例的 1/3。另外,黑色素瘤发病风险还发生在表达黑素肾上腺皮质激素受体基因 *MCR1* 变体的 *CDKN2A* 突变携带者身上,这与红色头发、白色皮肤和雀斑相关。由于这两种基因的突变只存在于家族性黑色素瘤家族的一个亚组中,因此可能存在着其他黑色素瘤易感性基因。对于有 3 个或更多侵袭性黑色素瘤或癌症"事件"个人史或家族史(即患者本人或家族中有 2 个侵袭性黑色素瘤和 1 个胰腺癌)的患者,*p16* 基因突变的检测已被正式列入诊疗建议,因为这意味着个人患病的风险提高 20%[25]。然而,由于即使在高危人群中突变的频率仍然很低,且对皮肤学监测筛查缺乏指导意义,因此一般不建议进行除研究目的以外的遗传检测。

非典型痣综合征/表型

大量的临床不典型痣(CAN),也被称为"混合痣",是黑色素瘤最重要的临床危险因素。与普通人群相比,患有临床不典型痣的患者患上黑色素瘤的风险高出 2~15 倍,并且风险随着 CAN 数量和/或黑色素瘤个人或家族史的增加而增加[26]。不典型痣表型的特征是多发性普通痣(数量>100)及多发大痣(一般数量>5 个,大小>8mm),颜色不均,边缘不规则,形状不对称。黑色素瘤很少来源于先前已存在的不典型痣,在体表存在各种类型的黑色素痣(典型、不典型或先天性)的黑色素瘤患者中,超过 70%的黑色素瘤是新生的,尽管具有严重的组织学发育异常的非典型痣可能是真正的黑色素瘤前体[27]。与不典型/混合痣相关的黑色素瘤通常是薄的表浅扩散型,可能是由于对易感人群皮肤监测的增加所致。

先天性黑色素痣(CMN)

先天性黑色素痣(CMN)仅见于 1%~6%的新生儿,很少转变为黑色素瘤[28]。患有"大或巨大"先天性痣(成人病变直径大于 20cm,婴儿躯体病变直径大于 6cm,或婴儿头部病变直径大于 9cm)的患者,其黑色素瘤的发病风险小于 5%[29~32],约一半发生在生命的前几年[33]。在小尺寸(<1.5cm)和中等尺寸的 CMN 中出现黑色素瘤的风险较低,几乎不发生在青春期前[34]。CMN 的管理取决于多种可变因素,包括监测的便宜性和外科手术带来的潜在的社会心理方面的获益及损害。

黑色素瘤风险评估

一些风险评估工具已被用于针对黑色素瘤高危人群,特别是 65 岁以上的白种人和社会经济地位较低的人群,这两类人群的黑色素瘤死亡率最高。

目前的风险评估工具来源于一项对 718 名非西班牙裔白人患者和 945 名对照者的大型病例对照研究,其中涉及对背部可疑痣的检查,并询问了两个关于肤色和阳光照射史的问题[35]。轻度雀斑和浅肤色被证明是男性和女性的危险因素。此外,男性大于 17 个小痣和大于 2 个大痣或女性背部大于 12 个小痣也是显著的危险因素。黑色素瘤风险评估工具的这些数据可从美国癌症研究所获得(http://www. cancer. gov/melanoma risk tool/)。该工具计算了年龄高达 70 岁的患者未来 5 年发生黑色素瘤的绝对风险。

预后因素

许多临床因素影响患者的预后,包括年龄、性别和原发肿瘤的解剖位置。一般来说,男性、老年人以及头颈部有黑色素瘤的患者预后更差。2004—2008 年在法国进行的一项基于人群的研究表明,男性患者的肿瘤更厚,且肿瘤更常发生溃疡。老年患者的肿瘤更厚、更晚期,更常发生在头颈部[36]。

虽然黑色素瘤最新的分类发放表明其具有独特的分子、遗传、解剖部位和紫外线暴露等相关特征,但某些组织学亚型的生长动力学似乎也在预后中起到作用。快速生长的黑色素瘤结节亚型仅凭临床特征往往无法及早发现。结节性黑色素瘤(NM)占美国和澳大利亚黑色素瘤亚型病例的不足 15%,但与其他组织学亚型相比,较厚的肿瘤(>2mm)和黑色素瘤死亡人数更多。

最新的分子技术,如基因表达谱分析,可能很快有助于识别具有更积极行为的黑色素瘤[37]。

临床表现

皮肤黑色素瘤可以发生在任何部位,但最常见于女性下肢和背部以及男性躯干。从临床角度来看,新的或不断变化的"痣"或皮肤损伤是黑色素瘤最常见的警示。Rigel[38]等人首先提出了所谓"ABCDE"的早期诊断,它是一种简单的记忆方法,可以提高对黑色素瘤典型早期症状的认识(表 109-1)。为了进一步简化,Weinstock[39]简洁地集中了信息,强调最重要的警示是新发的或有变化的皮损。"丑小鸭"警示是指看起来与其他病变不同的色素沉着或临床无色素病变,这可有助于鉴别缺乏经典 ABCD 标准的黑色素瘤(如结节性、无色素性或去纤维增生亚型)[40,41]。

表 109-1　ABCDE:黑色素瘤临床表现

A	不对称性	病变的两半不对称
B	边界不规则	可能出现粗糙、缺口或扇形
C	颜色多样	颜色不均匀或病变可能有多种颜色,呈褐色、棕色或黑色阴影,特别是白色、红色或蓝灰色渐变色
D	直径	通常大于 6mm(大约是一块铅笔橡皮的直径),但黑色素瘤的直径也可能更小;痣的任何生长都需要评估
E	病变变化	大小或颜色的变化;特殊的结节性或无色素性黑色素瘤可能不符合上述 ABCD 标准

由于原发性黑色素瘤的组织学特征对黑色素瘤的分期和预后至关重要,对可疑病变进行适当的初次活检至关重要。为了提供准确的诊断和组织学显微标记,最好是在色素病变的周围,超过正常皮肤窄小切缘(1~3mm)的范围内进行切除活检。这一规则的一个重要例外是雀斑样恶性黑色素瘤原位癌亚型,如果病变只行少量或部分活检的话,误诊风险很高。在这种情况下,最好的诊断活检技术通常是广泛的刮除活检,至少延伸到乳头状真皮,排除微浸润黑色素瘤的机会,并允许对肿瘤进行最佳的组织病理学解释。

病理特点

除结节性黑色素瘤外，其他临床病理亚型的生长模式特征是首先处在原位（辐射状生长）阶段，缺乏转移的生物学潜力，可能持续数月至数年，然后进入皮肤浸润（垂直生长）阶段。

真皮浸润的黑色素瘤具有转移的可能性，最大的风险发生在垂直生长（致瘤）阶段[42]。免疫组化谱系［S-100，人黑色素瘤黑 45（HMB-45），黑色素 A/Mart-1］或增殖指数（Ki-67）在某些情况下可能有助于鉴别黑色素瘤与其类似病变（如黑色素瘤痣、斯皮茨痣、细胞蓝痣、透明细胞肉瘤或周围神经鞘恶性肿瘤）的组织学差异[43]。一项生物标志物在黑色素瘤进展中表达的研究中揭示了痣、原发性黑色素瘤和转移瘤之间生物标志物的不同表达[44]。结合 Ki-67/Anti-Mart-1（Melan-A）和 HMB-45/MITF 免疫染色的方法也被证明给黑色素瘤的诊断带来了希望[45]。

黑色素瘤的病理报告应包括细胞形态和结构，以及肿瘤厚度（Breslow 深度）、是否存在溃疡、皮肤有丝分裂率（以每平方毫米的数目测量）、微卫星和淋巴血管侵犯（如果存在）。解剖层面的浸润（Clark 分级）预后意义较小，现在作为病理报告的可选项。

儿童和青少年的非典型黑色素细胞病变可能难以与真正的黑色素瘤区分开来，包括非典型 Spitz 肿瘤和具有不确定恶性潜能的 Spitz 或黑色素细胞肿瘤（STUMP 或者 MelTUMP）。因此，比较基因组杂交（GGH）和荧光原位杂交（FISH）等分子技术已被用来协助确定病变的恶性和良性生物学行为[46~49]。新的基因表达谱分析技术可能对非典型黑色素细胞肿瘤的分子检测有进一步的诊断价值，并有助于预后和风险分层[50~53]，其中一些发现可能对未来黑色素瘤的分期系统有极大的预测意义。

临床病理学亚型

原发性皮肤黑色素瘤的四个主要经典的“组织遗传学”黑色素瘤亚型是基于组织病理学发现、解剖部位和晒伤程度分型的。分别包括浅表扩散型黑色素瘤、结节性恶性黑色素瘤、恶性雀斑样痣黑色素瘤、肢端雀斑痣样黑色素瘤。此外，还有其他更罕见的病种（<5%的黑色素瘤），包括：①成纤维/神经性黑色素瘤；②黏膜（雀斑样）黑色素瘤[53]；③蓝痣样黑色素瘤；④巨大先天性痣发生的黑色素瘤；⑤软组织黑色素瘤（透明细胞肉瘤）。

浅表扩散型黑色素瘤

在皮肤黑色素瘤中，浅表扩散型黑色素瘤约占 70%，通常表现为 ABCDE 征，是 30~50 岁非典型/发育异常痣患者最常见的亚型。它最常见于男性和女性的躯干和女性的腿部。

结节性黑色素瘤

结节性黑色素瘤是次常见的黑色素瘤亚型，占黑色素瘤患者的 15%~30%，男性和女性最常见于腿部和躯干。典型表现为深褐色至黑色丘疹或穹顶状结节，数周至数月快速生长，轻微创伤后可溃疡出血。大多数厚黑色素瘤被诊断为这种亚型[54,55]。

恶性雀斑样痣黑色素瘤

恶性雀斑样痣黑色素瘤的发病率在美国正在上升[56]。它通常发生于皮肤白皙的老年人（平均年龄 65 岁）的皮肤（头部、颈部和手臂）长期受到阳光照射而受损，经过几年到几十年的缓慢生长而形成。恶性雀斑样痣黑色素瘤的原位前体病变通常是一个长期存在的大于 1~3cm 的大的（黄斑）病变，表现为从深褐色到黑色的色素沉着，其内常见白色或色素不足的区域。皮肤浸润表明恶性雀斑样痣黑色素瘤的进展，其特征是在原位病变内出现凸起的棕黑色结节。

肢端黑色素瘤

肢端黑色素瘤是白种人中最不常见的黑色素瘤亚型（占黑色素瘤病例的 2%~8%），但却是肤色较深的人种（即非洲裔美国人、亚裔和西班牙裔人）中最常见的黑色素瘤亚型，占这些人群中黑色素瘤病例的 29%~72%。由于诊断的延误，可能导致预后的恶化[57,58]。肢端雀斑样黑色素瘤发生在手掌、脚底或指甲下方（甲下黑色素瘤），可能表现为指甲变色或手指或脚趾指甲内的纵向色素带（黑甲）。近端或外侧指甲皱褶的色素扩散称为 Hutchinson 征，这是甲下黑色素瘤的标志。

不常见的亚型

成纤维黑色素瘤是一种不常见但重要的黑色素瘤亚型，由于其好发于老年人，临床特征类似于非黑色素瘤（角蛋白细胞）皮肤癌，广泛切除后辅助放射治疗的潜在指征取决于肿瘤的厚度、神经侵犯和切缘状态。无色素黑色素瘤（<5%的黑色素瘤）可以发生在任何的亚型，常与基底细胞或鳞状细胞癌、皮肤纤维瘤或毛囊破裂相似。它最常见于结节性或成纤维亚型或皮肤转移性黑色素瘤，可能是因为这些分化差的癌细胞无法合成黑色素。

遗传学与分子病理学

临床和组织病理学表现、起源细胞（上皮细胞相关与非上皮细胞相关）、与紫外线辐射的因果关系、发病年龄、体细胞突变和种系遗传易感性等均存在显著的复杂性。黑色素瘤不是一种疾病，而是由生物学上不同的亚型组成，其表型是由潜在的遗传改变驱动的[59]。

与黑色素瘤相关的一种生长因子途径是 RAS-RAF-MAPK-ERK（丝裂原相关蛋白激酶，MAPK）信号级联备受关注。MAPK 通路中丝氨酸三胺激酶 *BRAF* 基因 1799 位点的突变发生在约一半的皮肤黑色素瘤中，导致 600 位的谷氨酰胺（约 75%~80%的病例）或赖氨酸替代缬氨酸（大部分其余病例），这种致癌突变导致细胞过度增殖和对凋亡的抵抗[60]。依赖 *BRAF* 突变的细胞中黑色素瘤的生物学也受到共存突变或其他连锁途径中基因表达的改变的影响，特别是 PTEN/AKT/PI3K/MTOR 途径对代谢传感器和癌症/微环境营养素的控制至关重要。激活 *NRAS* 的突变，以及较不常见的癌基因，如 *c-kit*（见下文），会导致这两种途径的下游激活。

大多数 *BRAF* 突变的黑色素瘤出现在间歇性暴露于阳光下的皮肤中，而长期暴露于阳光下区域的黑色素瘤 *BRAF* 突变的发生率较低，偶尔携带 *c-kit* 突变或扩增，c-kit 是一种受体酪氨酸激酶[61,62]，在 15%~20%的肢端和黏膜黑色素瘤[61~63]。激活 c-kit 可刺激 MAPK 和 PI3K-AKT 通路，使癌细胞获得增殖和生存优势[64]。

Bastian 等发现，良性黑色素细胞痣[65]中发现的 *BRAF* 突变通常发生在青春期早期，其发生频率与非 CSD 黑色素瘤相同，他们认为获得性痣和非 CSD 黑色素瘤患者可能有特殊的易感性，在相对低剂量的紫外线照射下发展成 *BRAF* 突变的黑色素细胞肿瘤。这一概念在随后的研究中得到了支持，该研究证明了促黑素（melanocortin）受体 1（MC1R）的种系变异对这种易感性有显著影响[66,67]。更具体地说，*MC1R* 的变异被证明能显著增加 *BRAF* 突变的非 CSD 黑色素瘤的风险。

在黑色素瘤中鉴定的癌基因或肿瘤抑制基因中，没有一个被认为是黑色素瘤发病的唯一原因，而且由于下游功能重叠，一些似乎相互排斥。例如，如上所述，NRAS 激活 RAF 激酶以响应生长因子受体激活，并在 15%~20%的黑色素瘤中存在激活突变，但几乎从未发生 *BRAF* 突变[67]。p16 肿瘤抑制因子的缺失是黑色素瘤的一个相对常见的事件，与 *BRAF* 突变有明显的重叠[68]。*PTEN* 突变和缺失已在少数黑色素瘤中被描述，并且似乎与 *BRAF* 突变一致（图 109-1）[69]。

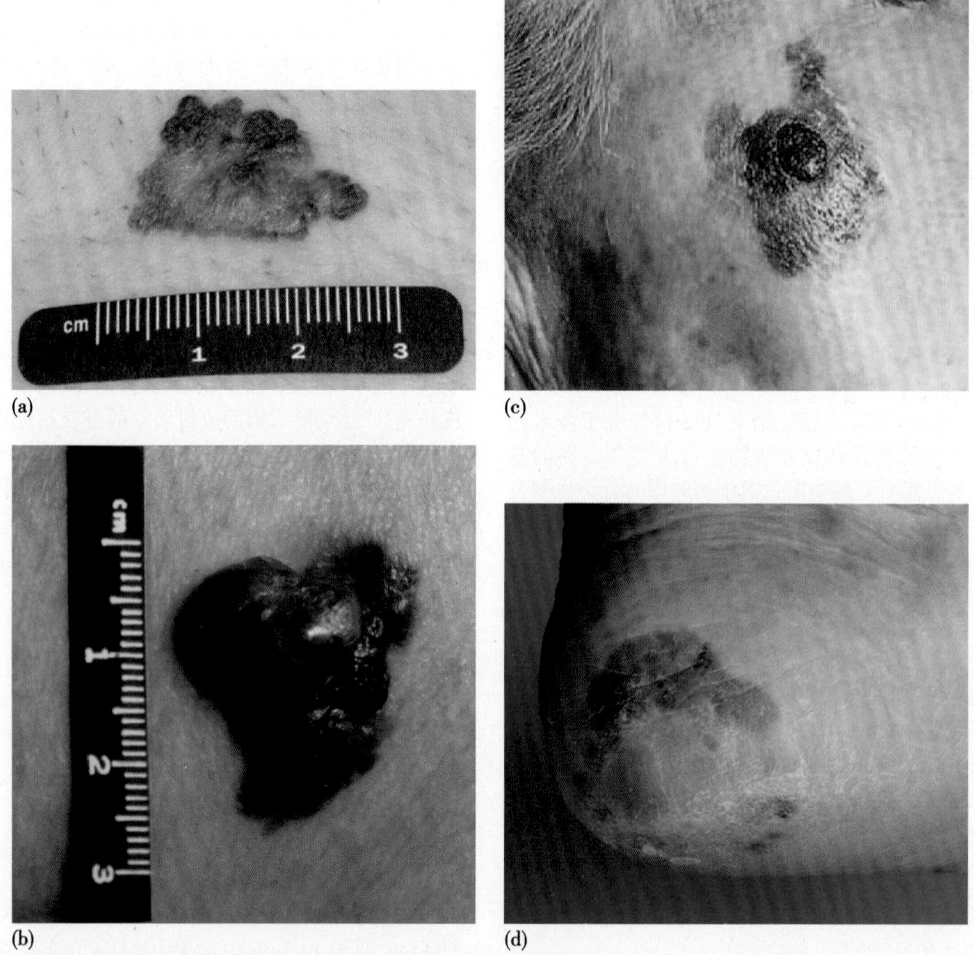

图 109-1 （a）浅表扩散型黑色素瘤。边界不规则，各种颜色不均，直径大于 6mm。（b）结节性黑色素瘤。（c）恶性雀斑样痣黑色素瘤具有快速生长的结节区。（d）足跟的肢端雀斑样黑色素瘤（承蒙 Jeffrey E. Gershenwald，MD 惠赠）

黑色素瘤的外科治疗

原发性皮肤黑色素瘤的治疗

外科手术仍然是治疗原发性皮肤黑色素瘤的主要手段，过去十年来具体的手术方式没有明显改变。原发性黑色素瘤采用广泛切除术，并有明确的切除范围。切除的边缘取决于肿瘤的深度和原发部位。手术时从活检瘢痕或残余色素的边缘测量宽度；不等同于切除标本的组织病理学的测量。然而，组织学上的阴性边缘一直是切除原发肿瘤的目标。目前关于侵袭性黑色素瘤切除宽度的建议（表 109-2）得到了随机试验的验证，总结在表 109-3 中[71~74]。对于原位黑色素瘤，建议边缘为 0.5~1cm[75]。对于深度小于 1mm 的侵袭性黑色素瘤，建议切缘为 1cm，这与局部复发率低相关。对于 1~2mm 的黑色素瘤，考虑到美观或功能性预后，建议 1~2cm 的边缘。对于大于 2mm 的黑色素瘤，只要可行，建议边缘为 2cm[75]。一项荟萃分析发现，哪怕是深度更厚的原发黑色素瘤的边缘均不需要>2cm，而且对于任何的侵袭性黑色素瘤，边缘都不应小于 1cm[76]。

表 109-2　根据原发性肿瘤的厚度和位置，推荐皮肤黑色素瘤广泛切除的切缘

厚度	原发部位	推荐广泛切除切缘(cm)
原位癌	任何部位皮肤	0.5~1
0.01~1.00mm	任何部位皮肤	1
1.01~2.00mm	头颈部，肢体远端[a]	1
	躯干，肢体近端[b]	2
>2.00mm	头颈部，肢体远端[a]	1
	躯干，肢体近端	2

[a] 甲下原发性肿瘤可能需要远端截指。

[b] 如果需要皮肤移植重建切除缺损，可接受 1cm 的切缘。

局部解剖限制和特定的患者因素可能会导致与标准推荐边缘的微小偏差。

摘自 Sondak and Gibney 2014[70]。

表 109-3　ASCO-SSO 对黑色素瘤前哨淋巴结活检的建议总结

- SLNB 建议用于任何解剖部位的厚度为 1~4mm 皮肤黑色素瘤
- SLNB 可被推荐用于分期，并有利于厚度大于 4mm 的黑色素瘤患者的区域疾病控制
- 没有足够的证据支持黑色素瘤厚度小于 1mm 的患者进行常规的 SLNB 治疗，但在某些高危患者中可被考虑
- 所有 SLNB 阳性患者建议进行完整的淋巴结清扫

SLNB，前哨淋巴结活检。

摘自 Wong et al，2012[85]。

区域淋巴结的治疗

前哨淋巴结活检的作用

临床阴性淋巴结内隐匿性肿瘤转移(AJCC 分期系统将其定义为“显微镜下”疾病)是临床Ⅰ期和Ⅱ期黑色素瘤预后的关键预测因子[77]，有证据表明即使是微小的淋巴结微转移也具有临床相关性[78,79]。区域淋巴结中的黑色素瘤微转移不能通过任何影像方式(包括 PET/CT[80,81]或超声检查[82,83])被可靠地检测到。前哨淋巴结活检(SLNB)可识别低发病率的微转移瘤[84]。2012 年，ASCO 和外科肿瘤学会(SSO)联合发布了黑色素瘤 SLNB 适应证的循证医学评估(表 109-4)[85]。

根据前瞻性随机多中心选择性淋巴结切除试验Ⅰ(MSLT-1)的中期结果[77]，最有力的证据支持中等厚度黑色素瘤患者的 SLNB。表 109-3 总结了主要的 ASCO-SSO SLNB 建议。MSLT-1(表 109-5)[86]和回顾性机构系列的成熟结果也支持临床结阴性厚黑色素瘤(>4mm)患者的 SLNB[89~92]。对于在 MSLT-1 研究中没有充分评估，也没有纳入前瞻性但非随机的日光浴黑色素瘤试验的薄黑色素瘤(<1mm)患者中使用前哨淋巴结活检仍存在争议[93~95]。

目前，大多数新诊断的皮肤黑色素瘤是 T1 病变(厚度不超过 1mm)，淋巴结转移或黑色素瘤死亡的总风险较低[96]。建议所有 T1 黑色素瘤患者进行前哨淋巴结活检并不具有成本效益[95]。ASCO-SSO 建议在具有“高风险”特征的特定病例中考虑针对薄黑色素瘤的 SLNB(表 109-6)[85]。

根据大量回顾性收集登记数据，SLNB 似乎对许多 0.76~1.00mm 的黑色素瘤患者是合理的，但对大多数厚度小于 0.76mm 的黑色素瘤患者则并不合理[96]。此外，关于 SNLB 的决策需要考虑到患者的年龄、需求和并发症。

表 109-4　多中心选择性淋巴结清扫术试验 1(MSLT-1)的最终结果总结

	结果	注释
可行性	99.5%接受 SLNB 的患者中至少发现一个前哨淋巴结	SLNB 在全球范围内具有高度可行性
得出假阴性率	黑色素瘤≥1.2mm 患者中 19%的前哨淋巴结呈阳性：黑色素瘤 1.2~3.5mm 患者为 16%，黑色素瘤>3.5mm 患者为 33%	SLNB 是一种有效的假阴性率可被接受的分级方法
	阴性前哨淋巴结患者的淋巴结复发率为 5.9%：1.2~3.5mm 的黑色素瘤为 4.8，大于 3.5mm 的黑色素瘤为 10.3%	
预后意义	阳性前哨淋巴结与 1.2~3.5mm 黑色素瘤的疾病复发和死亡增加 2.5 倍有关；阴性前哨淋巴结的黑色素瘤患者 10 年肿瘤特异性生存率为 85%，而阳性前哨淋巴结的患者为 62%	前哨淋巴结状态是已知最明显的临床淋巴结阴性的中-厚黑色素瘤的预后指标
SLNB 的生存影响	与观察相比，随机接受 SLNB 治疗的中-厚黑色素瘤患者的 10 年黑色素瘤特异性生存率增加 3%，无显著性差异	SLNB 对接受手术的所有患者的生存率没有显著影响
无复发生存的影响	与观察相比，随机接受 SLNB 治疗的患者无复发生存率有统计学上的显著改善	SLNB 显著降低中-厚黑色素瘤的复发率，主要是通过减少之后的淋巴结复发
对淋巴结阳性患者的影响	随机接受 SLNB 治疗的中厚黑色素瘤以及阳性淋巴结患者(完成淋巴结清扫术)与临床未行区域淋巴结干预的观察组相比，在统计学上显著改善了远处无转移生存率和黑色素瘤特异性生存率；SLNB 组和观察组的厚黑色素瘤患者和阳性淋巴结患者没有显著差异	根治性淋巴结清扫术早期治疗中-厚淋巴结阳性黑色素瘤显著改善预后；淋巴结阳性的厚黑色素瘤患者可能有很高的远处转移疾病风险，因此淋巴结切除的时机并不重要

SLNB，前哨淋巴结活检。

摘自 Sondak and Gibney 2014[70]。Original data from Morton。

表 109-5 选择前哨淋巴结活检的 T1 黑色素瘤的高危特征

高风险标准	对发现阳性淋巴结可能性的影响	注释
厚度 0.76~0.99mm	在一个 1 250 名黑色素瘤≤1mm 患者的登记系列中，根据各种标准选择接受 SLNB 治疗，891 例≥0.76mm 黑色素瘤中 6.3%的患者发现转移瘤，而 359 例≤0.75mm 黑色素瘤中只有 2.5%的患者发现转移瘤。<0.5mm 黑色素瘤患者前哨淋巴结未发现转移[87]。在一个大型的单中心的试验中，SLNB 通常提供给大于 0.76mm 的黑色素瘤患者，而不需要任何其他高风险特征，8.4%的患者有一个阳性前哨淋巴结[86]	大多数薄黑色素瘤且前哨淋巴结阳性的患者都出现在 T1 厚度谱的上端；极少数黑色素瘤<0.76mm 的未经选择的患者有足够的淋巴结转移风险来证明 SLNB 的合理性
溃疡	18.3%的注册试验[87]患者和 23.5%的单中心试验[88]伴有溃疡的 T1 黑色素瘤的前哨淋巴结呈阳性	在 T1 黑色素瘤中的前哨淋巴结阳性相当罕见（在<10%的病例中出现），但溃疡可能是薄黑色素瘤中前哨淋巴结阳性的最高危险因素
有丝分裂计数	有丝分裂计数≥1/mm^2 不能预测注册试验[87]中的淋巴结转移，但可以预测单中心试验[88]中的转移	在目前的 AJCC 分期系统中，T1 黑色素瘤中即使有一个真皮有丝分裂，也会使肿瘤从 T1a 升级到 T1b。目前尚不清楚皮肤有丝分裂是否足以证明 SLNB，特别是在小于 0.76mm 的黑色素瘤中
患者年龄	—	年轻患者在所有肿瘤厚度类别中均具有较高的前哨淋巴结阳性风险，且淋巴结复发风险更大
Clark 分级	Clark 分级是一个重要的预测前哨淋巴结状态的注册试验[87]，而不是一个单中心试验[88]	Clark Ⅳ级的黑色素瘤更可能在较厚的（≥0.76~1.00mm）T1 患者中出现淋巴结转移。Clark Ⅳ级黑色素瘤小于 0.76mm 时 SLNB 的价值尚未被证实

SLNB，前哨淋巴结活检。

摘自 Han 2012[87] and Han 2013[88]。

表 109-6 各国和国际组织对完全切除的黑色素瘤患者的随访指南总结
（这些指导方针尚未经过前瞻性验证，因此应仅作为建议予以考虑）

分期	体格检查	影像学
Ⅰ期	每 3~12 个月×5 年，每年随访超过 5 年	除非有临床指征，否则无须影像学检查
Ⅱ期	每 3~6 个月×2 年，然后每 3~12 个月再进行 3 年的随访，每年随访超过 5 年[a]	高危患者可考虑行 CT 和/或 PET/CT，以筛查复发性疾病。每年考虑一次头颅磁共振检查[b]
Ⅲ-Ⅳ期	每 3~6 个月×2 年，然后每 3~12 个月再进行 3 年的随访，每年随访超过 5 年[c]	对于高危患者，必须行 CT 和/或 PET/CT，以筛查复发性疾病。每年考虑一次头颅磁共振检查[b]

[a] 考虑对原发性肿瘤较厚和/或溃疡的高危Ⅱ期患者进行更频繁和更长的随访。

[b] 超声检查可以用来评价区域淋巴结情况。

[c] 考虑对高危ⅢB/C 期患者进行更频繁和更长的随访。

CT，计算机断层扫描；PET/CT，正电子发射断层扫描/计算机断层扫描。

摘自 Fields and Coit 2011[145]。

还有一些需要考虑的与采用 SLNB 有关的临床情况。一般而言，成纤维性黑色素瘤的淋巴结转移风险较低[97,98]，一些研究者主张放弃这种组织学类型的 SLNB[99]。在最近的一系列研究中，淋巴结转移的风险已经被证明是足够高的，足以证明所有厚度大于或等于 1mm 的成纤维性黑色素瘤患者常规考虑 SLNB 的合理性。儿童黑色素瘤患者淋巴结转移的发生率更高，但与成人相比，其总体预后明显更好，而且 SLNB 在这些患者中的作用仍存在争议，尤其是对于儿童期所谓的非典型黑色素细胞增生[100~103]。

前哨淋巴结阳性疾病的完全性淋巴结清扫术

NCCN 指南[75]，在数十年的临床经验的有力支持下，呼吁对所有临床阳性淋巴结且无远处转移的影像学证据的黑色素瘤患者进行淋巴结清扫术的常规治疗[104]。尽管在缺乏临床试验参与的情况下，ASCO/SSO 指南建议将其作为标准治疗，但在 SLNB 阳性后常规使用完成淋巴结清扫术仍存在争议[85]。MSLT-1 试验表明，中厚度黑色素瘤患者行完全淋巴结清扫术的结果优于那些在区域淋巴结内复发的患者[86]，但根据试验性质，完全淋巴结清扫术对肿瘤治疗的贡献是否优于前哨淋巴结切除则还无法评估。非前哨淋巴结仅在少数病例中有肿瘤累及[107]，而且至少一些前哨淋巴结阳性的患者即使没有完成淋巴结清扫术也能在较长时间内预后良好[86]。淋巴结清扫术后，特别是严重淋巴水肿的发病率，在 SLNB 阳性的情况下进行的淋巴结清扫术后的并发症发病率低于淋巴结复发后的治疗性淋巴结清扫术的[109]。一项前瞻性随机试验，比较前哨淋巴结阳性患者（MSLT-2）对区域淋巴结超声监测及即刻完成淋巴结清扫术之间的疗效，最近完成了病例收集等待试验结果（clinicaltrials. gov NCT 00297895）。

肉眼淋巴结转移的根治性淋巴结清扫术

与 SLNB 鉴别出的显微镜下疾病不同，治疗性根治性淋巴结清扫几乎总是指临床上明显的、可切除的淋巴结转移；全身治疗和/或放射治疗不足以替代临床区域淋巴结阳性患者的手术治疗[75]。

移行转移及局部复发性黑色素瘤的治疗

广泛切除适用于被活检证实的没有远处转移的局部复发、卫星灶或移行转移。在对复发肿瘤进行治疗性切除之前，应进行完整的影像学分期(使用 PET/CT 或 CT 以及脑部 MRI 或 CT)。

动脉内局部灌注疗法

高温隔离肢体灌注(HILP)和隔离肢体灌注(ILI)是治疗肢端不可切除的局部复发或移行转移黑色素瘤的方法，它可将有病灶的肢端从全身循环中隔离出来，并在动脉内进行高剂量的化疗，同时限制了全身对化疗的暴露。HILP 是通过直接解剖和插管四肢的主要血管和通过心肺转流机循环化疗来完成的，该机允许温度升高和充氧灌注液。在肢体温度达到 39~41℃的情况下，HILP 在肢体内的浓度可达到全身系统耐受浓度的 15~25 倍。由于热疗的浓度增加和潜在的协同效应，如果全身用药，极少或几乎将没有活性，因此如美法仑等药物就成为高效的区域性药物[110,111]。报道的反应率在 80%~90%，完全缓解(complete remission，CR)率高达 60%~70%[111~114]。美法仑是美国最常用的药物，而美法仑联合肿瘤坏死因子 α (TNF-α)则在欧洲使用[115]。TNF-α 的价值尚未被明确证实。在一项大型多中心随机试验中，在总生存或 CR 率方面均未发现统计学上的显著差异，并且联合 TNF-α 与显著较高的区域毒性相关[114]。

在 HILP 期间隔离肢体可大大降低大剂量化疗的全身毒性风险；然而，仍可能发生严重的并发症。最常见的是淋巴水肿，据报道有 12%~36%的患者发生。严重的区域毒性，包括高达 5%的病例发生室间隔综合征，以及高达 3.3%的病例可发生肢体坏死功能丧失[115,116]。

ILI 的侵袭性比 HILP 更小，是一种通过低流量输液，在轻度高温、酸中毒和低氧环境中进行的治疗。导管经皮置入未受累肢体的动脉和静脉中，并在病变部位近端进入受累肢体的血管中，避免了开放性外科插管的需要及其并发症的发生率。人工循环化疗 30min[117]。ILI 后局部 CR 率在 23%~44%，部分缓解率在 27%~56%[117,118]。尽管这些结果低于 HILP 报告的结果，但在临床试验中，这两种技术还没有被前瞻性地以头对头的方式进行比较。在最近对 HILP 和 ILI 的回顾性比较中(ILI = 94，ILP = 109)，ILI 的总有效率为 53%，ILP 的总有效率为 80%(P>0.001)。ILI 的中位总生存期(OS)为 46 个月，而 ILP 为 40 个月(P=0.31)。两组之间的年龄、性别或 N 分期无差异；然而，ILI 组的 BOD 较高(58%比 44%，P=0.04)[119]。重要的是，如有必要 ILI 可以很容易地重复进行，并且似乎比 HILP 的区域毒性更小(皮肤红斑和水肿是最常见的副作用之一，组织损失小于 1%的时间)，实际上没有全身毒性[116~119]。

关于 ILI 或 HILP 是否应首选用于治疗移行转移的黑色素瘤存在一些争论，这一决定部分是基于存在需要进行淋巴结清扫的淋巴结或肿瘤负荷高的肢体，这两种情况都可以更好地用 HILP 来解决，尽管如此仍缺乏数据支持这一理论。考虑到相对的发病率和有效性，HILP 通常被保留作为一种补救措施，用于那些在 ILI 后进展迅速而无远处转移迹象的患者。对于对 ILI 有良好初始反应但最终进展的患者，可以尝试重复 ILI。

病灶内和局部治疗

黑色素瘤的病变内治疗比区域性或系统性治疗有几个优势。当地药品管理局允许输送浓度增加的药剂，减少区域和系统接触，潜在地提高疗效和降低毒性。此外，肿瘤微环境的改变可能是免疫原性的，并引起局部免疫反应，导致“旁观者效应”，其中未注射的远处病变表现出反应，有多种不同类型的病变内治疗被报道过。

Bacille Calmette-Guèrin(BCG)是治疗移行转移的最早治疗方法之一。在最初的标志性试验中，90%的注射皮肤病变复发，17%的患者也有未注射病变的复发。一些患者在完成卡介苗注射后几年内保持无病状态[120]。重组人白介素-2(IL-2)也被用于黑色素瘤的病灶内注射，其毒性明显优于卡介苗。存在着局部治疗的风险，注射后的流感样症状最常见(85%)[121]。用 IL-2 进行病变内治疗相对昂贵。pv-10 是一种 10%的玫瑰红孟加拉溶液，这是一种水溶性黄嘌呤染料，数十年来用作静脉内诊断剂，眼科医生局部使用来评估肝功能，使其成为一种潜在的低成本治疗方法，在“重新调整用途”时用于病灶内给药显示出一定的疗效[122]。已有报道对既往系统性伊普利单抗、抗 PD1 和维莫非尼(vemurafenib)不敏感的患者有反应，有证据表明在未注射的病变中有旁观者效应[123]。

Talimogene Laherparepvec(TVEC，以前称为 OncoVEX)是一种基因修饰的溶瘤疱疹病毒，包含人类粒细胞-巨噬细胞集落刺激因子(GM-CSF)的编码序列。溶瘤病毒被设计成选择性地在肿瘤中复制，从而感染和破坏癌细胞，并诱导针对癌细胞的免疫反应。*GM-CSF* 基因(*GM-CSF*)在肿瘤细胞中的表达可聚集并激活抗原递呈细胞和免疫抑制因子，从而介导有效的抗肿瘤 T 细胞毒性。这种方式的肿瘤破坏也可以诱导 T 细胞在附近和远处的未被注射的转移灶中循环并发挥抗肿瘤作用。Ⅲ期 OPTiM 研究入组 436 名患者，分别以 2∶1的方式随机分为病变内 TVEC 组和皮下 GM-CSF 组。TVEC 组有 26.4%的客观缓解率，而 GM-CSF 组有 5.7%的客观缓解率(P<0.001)。长期缓解率(DRR)作为主要终点事件在统计学意义上有显著升高，即 PR 或 CR 的时间持续 6 个月或更长时间。TVEC 和 GM-CSF 的 DRR 分别为 16.3%和 2.1%(P<0.001)。总生存的结果也更倾向于 TVEC，尽管没有统计学意义[126]。这种有预期的病毒介导免疫基因疗法目前正在与免疫检查点阻滞剂和其他免疫调节干预措施结合进行测试，其他有或无转基因的溶瘤病毒也在黑色素瘤和其他恶性肿瘤中被研究[124]。

咪喹莫特和二苯莎莫酮(DPCP)是局部外用，而不是通过皮内注射。这种方法特别适用于多发性皮肤小结节的患者。局部应用咪喹莫特，加上或不加其他药剂，如局部 5-氟脲类药物，可使得治疗后的面部病变减少 90%[125,126]。DPCP 是一种引起接触过敏的接触致敏剂；在 50 名接受 DPCP 治疗的患者中，23 名患者(46%)达到 CR，另外 19 名患者(38%)达到 PR。DPCP 的副作用是可耐受的，包括最常见的皮肤副作用如起疱和刺激[127]。

放射治疗

对于移行转移或区域性复发的患者，放射治疗可能获益。治疗方案尚不明确，但可能对症状的控制使得放射治疗可以作为不可切除局部黑色素瘤患者[128]的一种选择，目前正在作为免疫调节剂被进行积极的研究,详见本章下文。

Ⅳ期黑色素瘤的外科转移灶切除术

孤立的、可切除的远处转移性黑色素瘤患者可作为外科治疗的候选者,目的是清除所有已知的病变部位。确定哪些患者能从转移灶切除中获益需要良好的临床判断和彻底的术前分期,包括全身的 PET/CT 和头颅的 MRI,以排除隐蔽的转移灶部位[129]。

西南肿瘤学组开展的 S9430 试验,对Ⅳ期黑色素瘤患者进行了仅有的一项前瞻性(尽管非随机)手术评估[130]。Ⅳ期黑色素瘤患者在接受正式手术之前,即在确定了潜在可切除性时就被纳入研究。这使得研究者可以评估切除率,确定完全切除后的无复发生存率和总生存率。在 77 名试验患者中,3 名患者在切除标本中没有发现黑色素瘤的证据(怀疑转移性病灶是第二原发恶性肿瘤或良性病变),2 名患者仅是Ⅲ期病变。另外 8 名患者不能全部切除病灶。因此,64 名患者(88.9%)实际上被切除至无瘤状态。中位随访 5 年后,除 6 例(9.4%)外,其余均复发,中位无复发生存期(RFS)约为 5 个月。中位总生存期为 21 个月,可评估的 12 个月生存率为 75%,4 年生存率为 31%[130]。尽管这是一个很小的前瞻性研究,而且存在着其他未入组的患者,但 S9430 报告的可切除率和生存率是比较外科和非外科方法治疗Ⅳ黑色素瘤最具代表性的数据。如果是现在进行这项研究,可以使用目前更敏感的影像学方法来发现可切除的单一或少转移的病灶可能会获得更佳的研究结果。然而,对于转移性黑色素瘤的新的全身系统治疗方法目前被发现其有效率在逐渐升高,因此可能应该适当的重新考虑手术作为一线治疗的作用,而且重要的是从分子水平上研究新辅助治疗的潜力。分子靶向药和新的免疫疗法,特别是 pd-1 抑制剂,作用相对较快,可能使以前无法切除的病变更易于手术切除。

辅助治疗在Ⅱ期和Ⅲ期黑色素瘤中的作用

免疫治疗

免疫治疗是黑色素瘤最广泛被研究评价的辅助治疗方法,其中最广泛被评价的辅助免疫治疗是干扰素-α(IFN-α),有多种剂量、用药时间和方案。大剂量 IFN-α 是一种为期 1 年的辅助治疗方案,包括两个部分:首先是 1 个月的“诱导”阶段,静脉注射 2 000 万单位 IFN-α_{2b}/m^2(体表面积)/d,5 日/周,持续 4 周,随后是 11 个月的“维持”阶段,持续皮下注射 1 000 万单位。3 次/周。三项随机试验表明,高剂量的 IFN-α 可改善 RFS,两项试验也显示了可改善 OS[131,132]。在美国,大剂量 IFN-α 被批准用于厚的、淋巴结转移阴性和淋巴结转移阳性黑色素瘤的辅助治疗。迄今为止,还没有关于大剂量 IFN-α 的研究明确定义对治疗有较好或较差反应的亚组患者。诱导和维持阶段的相对重要性尚未得到充分定义,但仅应用 4 周诱导阶段的治疗似乎并不充分[133]。

还对较低剂量的 IFN-α(300 万~1 000 万单位/次,3 次/周,未根据体表面积进行剂量调整,且非静脉给药)的辅助 IFN-α 方案进行了研究评估。在一些欧洲国家,低剂量的 IFN-α 被批准用于辅助治疗,并被提倡用于中等厚度的淋巴结转移阴性的黑色素瘤患者[134]。在缺乏高剂量和低剂量 IFN-α 方案之间的直接比较的情况下,对其进行了荟萃分析,以评估辅助 IFN-α 疗法的总体和相对疗效。荟萃分析结果清楚地显示 IFN-α 治疗可延迟复发时间,在最新的分析中,总的 RFS 改善了 17%(复发风险比 0.83),但没有明确区分高剂量和低剂量方案的疗效差异。荟萃分析结果也显示辅助性 IFN-α 的 OS 在统计学上显著改善,有 9%(生存风险比 0.91)的改善[135]。

根据一项随机试验的结果,聚乙二醇 IFN-α 在 2011 年在美国被批准作为Ⅲ期黑色素瘤的替代辅助治疗[136]。这项试验表明,与标准 IFN-α 试验一致,在统计学上 RFS 有显著改善,但没有显示出 OS 的获益。然而,一项有趣的观察表明,伴有溃疡的原发性前哨淋巴结阳性亚组黑色素瘤患者接受聚乙二醇 IFN-α 治疗后,生存获益显著提高(41%)。尽管其他一些 IFN-α 试验在这一亚组中也有类似的获益[137,138],但最好认为这是一个还未经证实但具有可观性的发现,有待最终的验证。聚乙二醇 IFN-α 与大剂量的 IFN-α 没有直接的比较,但从药理学特性角度看,其严重的副作用似乎更少,这可能使其成为更适合维持阶段的药物。与高剂量的 IFN-α 不同,聚乙二醇 IFN-α 拟皮下注射 5 年[3μg/(kg·周)],静脉注射 1 个月的诱导期替换为高剂量[6μg/(kg·周)]的 2 个月的皮下注射诱导期。

正在研究中的其他辅助系统治疗

在不可切除的转移性黑色素瘤中,新药物的有效性和生存获益结果激励了一些药物在辅助治疗中的试验研究。在已无病灶或可能治愈的患者中,这些药物是否比现有的 IFN-α 方案效果相同或更优,以及这些新药的毒性是否可耐受,还有待观察。尽管如此,对黑色素瘤生物学和抗肿瘤免疫反应调节器的了解及进展,已经深刻地改变了Ⅳ期黑色素瘤患者的治疗方法,可能最终会转化为新的、更有效的、预期毒性更小的预防黑色素瘤复发的辅助治疗方法。

在一项随机试验中,将由 IFN-α、重组人白介素-2、达卡巴嗪(dacarbazine)、长春新碱和顺铂组成的多药生物化学治疗方案与大剂量 IFN-α 进行比较,结果显示,在统计学上具有显著的 RFS 优势,但在 OS 中没有差异[139]。尽管这是第一个随机试验,显示了其统计学上明显优于大剂量 IFN-α,但该方案的毒性限制了其使用,并且缺乏 OS 优势,这表明它不能成为黑色素瘤辅助治疗的新标准。

伊匹木单抗(ipilumimab)已被证明能提高Ⅳ期黑色素瘤的生存率(本章后面将详细介绍),其毒性低于生物化学治疗,因此在辅助治疗中评估它是一个合理可选择的治疗方法。比较 10mg/kg 伊匹木单抗(剂量高于批准用于治疗不可切除转移性黑色素瘤的剂量)与安慰剂的随机试验的初步数据显示,伊匹木单抗组的 RFS 在统计学上有显著改善[140]。遗憾的是,该方案的毒性出乎意料地严重。关于这种伊匹木单抗辅助治疗方案对 OS 的改善的数据尚待公布。重要的是,目前还不清楚伊匹木单抗与 IFN-α 相比对辅助治疗的效果。鉴于伊匹木单抗辅助治疗的毒性为 10mg/kg 剂量组的,还需要评估相对于标准 3mg/kg 伊匹木单抗剂量组的风险效益比。与大剂量 IFN-α(E1609,NCT 01274338)相比,目前已经进行了一项随机试验,以评估伊匹木单抗在 10mg/kg 和 3mg/kg 剂量下的疗效。这项试验已经完成了病例累积,结果令人期待。抗 PD1 抗体的安全性和耐受性似乎优于 IFN-α 和伊匹木单抗,这使得这些抗体成为评价辅助治疗的理想候选。伊匹木单抗与纳武单抗(nivolumab)(Checkmate 238,NCT 02833906)和帕博利珠单抗(pembrolizumab)与安慰剂(EORTC Keynote 054,NCT 02362594)的随机试验已完成但结果尚未成熟,它们可能会重新定义未来的辅助系统治疗的建议。

研究辅助治疗 BRAF 抑制剂单独或联合 MEK 抑制剂活性的其他试验已完成病例累积并等待结果数据。人们对这些药物在辅助治疗中的耐受性提出了合理的担忧,特别是考虑到服用这些药物的患者可能快速出现耐药性和继发其他恶性肿瘤,并且不建议在辅助治疗中常规使用这些药物[141]。

可切除的区域淋巴结的辅助放疗

根治性淋巴结切除术后区域淋巴结复发风险高的患者的确定标准包括多发性(≥4)或融合的肿瘤累及淋巴结,至少一个淋巴结有淋巴结外受累,任何一个淋巴结尺寸较大(≥3cm)。在一项前瞻性试验中,217 名符合这些标准的患者在淋巴结清扫术后随机接受了观察或术后区域淋巴结放射治疗[108]。中位随访 40 个月后,观察组 108 例患者中 34 例(31.5%)出现淋巴结复发,证实了这些患者区域复发的高风险。与观察组相比,辅助放射治疗组的淋巴结复发率明显降低,但当所有复发部位都包括在内时,RFS 和 OS 无差异[108]。这证实了高复发风险患者术后放疗能显著降低淋巴结区域复发的可能性,对于选择的高危病例应考虑放疗。在高危黑色素瘤的辅助治疗中,研究局部辅助放射治疗与免疫检查点阻断的相互作用也具有重要意义。

高危黑色素瘤患者的观察随访

关于手术治疗后黑色素瘤患者随访评估的频率和内容,已经提出了各种方案[142~144]。迄今为止,还没有研究表明,通过任何影像学或实验室检查(包括胸部 X 线、PET/CT 或 MRI 扫描)对黑色素瘤手术治疗后的患者进行监测具有成本效益。一项评估Ⅲ期黑色素瘤患者术后随访结果的研究发现,一半的复发是由患者自己检测到的,"无论是更广泛检查的随访还是更频繁的随访,都与发现可切除的首次复发无关"[142]。尽管大多数建议的随访方案在术后最初几年会更频繁地随访,但在术后的第一个十年内,Ⅰ期和Ⅱ期黑色素瘤复发的条件概率实际上相当稳定[144]。教育是关键,应该关注患者和家庭,以及初级保健医生、皮肤科医生和外科医生,黑色素瘤中心可能希望能集中培训甚至"认证"。患者应愿意返回黑色素瘤中心评估可疑的复发,因为正确诊断复发(如通过针吸细胞学记录病变复发,而不是通过开放活检)对成功治疗很重要。重要的是,我们需要对随访进行个性化制订,确定哪些患者最适合在黑色素瘤中心外进行大部分监测,哪些患者应该更频繁地返回。

表 109-6 总结了各国和国际组织对完全切除黑色素瘤患者的随访指南。这些指导方案尚未经过前瞻性验证,因此应仅作为建议考虑[142]。

葡萄膜黑色素瘤和罕见的眼部黑色素瘤

葡萄膜黑色素瘤(UM)是成人最常见的眼内原发性肿瘤,占所有黑色素瘤的 5%。术语"UM"用于出现在葡萄膜内的黑色素瘤(即虹膜、纤毛体或脉络膜),而更广泛的术语"眼"黑色素瘤包括结膜和眼睑等表现类似于皮肤黑色素瘤的部位。葡萄膜黑色素瘤进一步被指定为前(虹膜)或后(睫状体和/或脉络膜)腔肿瘤。前房 UM 较少见(<10%的 UMS),且不易转移,而大约一半诊断为后房 UM 的患者会发生转移。

UM 的局部治疗采用放射性斑块、质子治疗或原发性 UM 肿瘤的摘除。在一项比较Ⅰ型斑块近距离放射治疗与去核术的随机研究中[128],85%接受放射治疗的患者保留了眼睛,37%接受放射治疗的患者在治疗后 5 年内视力超过 20/200。放射性斑块组和去核组之间没有生存差异[145]。因此,放射治疗方法已成为原发性 UM 治疗的首选策略,保留了小于 10%的不可能进行放射治疗的病例(如体积大的疾病、技术困难的肿瘤位置、患者偏好)的摘除术。由于大多数患者没有进行摘除,针吸活检技术现在被用来获得病理和分子诊断信息,这对预后至关重要。

UM 转移是血行性的,因为葡萄膜道似乎不包含淋巴结引流的透明淋巴管。肝脏最终参与了 95%的转移瘤病例,并且是大约 50%患者转移瘤的唯一部位。最常见的其他转移灶是肺(24%)、骨(16%)和皮肤(11%)。与皮肤黑色素瘤不同,很少转移到淋巴结或大脑。UM 患者的临床病程高度依赖于肝脏疾病进展。肝转移患者诊断后的中位生存期为 4~6 个月,1 年生存率为 10%~15%。局限于肝外部位的转移患者的中位生存期为 19~28 个月,1 年生存率约为 76%。因此,肝病与单纯肝外疾病可能代表不同的生物学实体[146]。

大约 90%的 UM 在 G 蛋白 αq(GNAQ)或 11(GNA11)亚单位基因中具有激活性、互斥性、复发性突变。几乎所有的 *GNAQ/11* 基因突变都定位于外显子 5(Q209)的一个热点,尽管少数基因定位于外显子 4(R183)。*GNAQ/11* 基因突变是早期的致瘤事件,不足以引发转移性疾病,但由于额外的分子畸变(如蛋白激酶 C 等)而引起的 UM 中的一些下游通路可能是研究性药物的靶向发展[147]。*SF3B1*(大多数情况下改变 R625 氨基酸位置)或 *EIF1AX*(外显子 1 或 2)基因的额外复发错义突变在大约 40%的 UM 肿瘤中以相同比例出现,并且基本上相互排斥。染色体 3p21.1 上的核泛素羧基末端水解酶 *BAP1* 基因存在短义和非短义突变。*BAP1* 基因畸变往往与单体 3 同时发生,导致 *BAP1* 杂合子丢失。*BAP1* 基因突变和单体 3 均不易与 *SF3B1* 或 *EIF1AX* 基因突变同时发生,前者与发生转移瘤的高风险有关[148]。与 *BAP1* 突变导致肿瘤抑制功能丧失一致的是,在家族中有许多种系 *BAP1* 突变的报道,导致了 UM 的高发病率[149]。在 UM 中观察到的另一个复发性染色体畸变是 8q 拷贝数增加(通常伴有 8p 丢失),这往往伴随着单体 3,并且与较短的复发时间有关。相反,6p 拷贝数增加(通常 6q 丢失)通常出现在缺乏单体 3 或 8q 拷贝数增加的肿瘤中,并且与转移的低风险相关。还描述了较不常见的染色体畸变,如 1p 和/或 16q 缺失。除 *BAP1* 外,还不太清楚功能上与这些染色体畸变相关的特异基因[150]。

原发肿瘤的多个解剖、组织学和分子特征与预后不良有关:①纤毛体位置(较差)>脉络膜>>虹膜(很少转移);②肿瘤大小较大;③巩膜外侵犯;④上皮样细胞>梭形细胞组织学;⑤有丝分裂率增多;⑥存在单体 3±CHR 为 8q 增益;⑦2 类≫

1b 类≫1a 类基因表达谱(精确预测结果且不需要染色体分析的 15 个基因表达谱)。然而,转移的最大危险因素是拷贝数谱(如单体 3/CHR 为 8q 增益和/或)1b/2 类基因表达谱[151,152]。

转移性 UM 已被证明基本上对传统化疗和免疫治疗方法是抵抗耐药的。鉴于目前无法针对上述的分子畸变特性进行治疗,目前主要集中在针对与这些基因改变相关的"影响因子"分子。迄今为止,最成功的系统性治疗方法是针对明显由 *GNAQ/11* 突变激活的 MEK-MAPK 途径。一项Ⅱ期随机临床试验表明,单一药物司美替尼(selumetinib)(一种小分子 MEK 抑制剂)治疗转移性 UM 患者可导致 50%的肿瘤退缩,15%的患者出现 RECIST 应答。与达卡巴嗪(7 周)相比,司美替尼(15.9 周)治疗后中位无进展生存率有显著差异,尽管总体生存率没有改善[153]。突变型 *BAP1*/单体 3 的靶向作用仍在研究中。回顾性分析多中心接受伊匹木单抗治疗的转移性 UM 患者表明,在亚组(约 5%)中观察到长期肿瘤反应,在稍大的晚期疾病患者亚组中观察到长期稳定疾病(SD)[154]。最近,一个多机构回顾性试验报道了用抗体阻断剂 PD-1 或 PD-L1 治疗转移性葡萄膜黑色素瘤的方法,并显示出非常低的活性[155],进一步的证据表明,成功治疗这种黑色素瘤的特异性策略需要关注免疫肿瘤微环境中的分子生物学及其靶点。

对于单纯肝转移或主要为肝转移的患者,已经探索了针对肝脏的多种治疗方法:单独或经皮肝灌注化疗、经动脉化疗栓塞(TACE)、放射性栓塞或冷冻栓塞或选择性内放射治疗(SIRT)。肝导向治疗研究的患者数量往往较低,但总的来说,在接受治疗的患者中,肿瘤反应率相对较高,进展时间间隔相对较长,和/或生存率相对较高。9 项研究(共 209 名患者)使用 TACE(主要是以顺铂为基础)显示,总体 CR 率为 2%,PR 率为 24%,SD 率为 33%。八项综合研究(共 277 名患者)显示肝动脉内化疗(主要采用福莫司汀或美法仑方案)对该方法有 9%的 CR、22%的 PR 和 29%的 SD 率。最后,四项研究(共 59 例)显示肝动脉灌注有 8%的 CR、44%的 PR 和 10%的 SD 发生率(参考文献 156 中进行了综述)。

如果有一个相对稳定和安全的可切除的孤立性病变,对转移瘤的外科切除可能是有效的。在一项 61 名患者除接受化疗外还接受了手术切除的研究中,在有疗效的患者中观察到 22 个月的总中位生存期,而在没有疗效的患者中观察到 10 个月的总中位生存期。在所有这些结果中,患者转诊和选择标准的变化是重要因素,必须通过进行良好控制的前瞻性随机试验加以验证。

目前应用最具预测性的分子标记来预测转移发生的风险,原发性肿瘤具有明确的基因驱动因素,以及广泛的临床治疗方法(分子抑制剂、免疫疗法、放射治疗和外科手术)现在可用。这种治疗方法无论在辅助治疗还是在进展期治疗实践中都是有效的治疗 UM 的方法。

眼结膜表面的黑色素瘤是罕见的,可能使原发性获得性黑色素病复杂化。最近的报告显示,在 78 例结膜黑色素瘤试验中,29%的患者存在典型的激活性 *BRAF* 突变,18%的患者存在 *NRAS* 突变,进一步证明了该部位黑色素瘤与皮肤黑色素瘤之间的密切关系,并有病例报告表明,维莫非尼对黑色素瘤有临床疗效,并证实了 BRAF 作为结膜黑色素瘤致癌因子的重要性[157,158]。

晚期黑色素瘤的生物学和治疗

转移性黑色素瘤的诊断可由有黑色素瘤病史的患者(大约一半的表现)的新症状或体征发现,也可是根据初始诊断时的分期、复发的时间依赖性风险在进行随访复查时由影像学发现的新的但无症状的病灶,将改变疾病自然病程。与内脏部位相比,皮肤和软组织是最常见的初始转移性疾病部位,少数患者有继发于血源性传播的广泛转移性疾病,如黏膜黑色素瘤。

不常见的是,即使在中枢神经系统中,晚期黑色素瘤也可能以孤立或多发性转移的形式出现,虽然没有已知的病史或同时出现新的原发性黑色素瘤的证据。据推测,免疫介导的控制或由局部免疫反应控制的原发性缺失的回归解释了这一现象,与已知原发性缺失的病例相比,后者的预后稍好[159]。黑色素瘤广泛转移的器官或部位很少,但对大脑有特殊的亲和力,通常是出血和水肿作为直接或主要原因导致死亡。其他癌症罕见的黑色素瘤转移部位包括小肠和大肠,甚至心脏。原发性黑色素瘤对转移的特定部位的倾向正在被研究中。例如,CCL25 和 CCR9 趋化因子:趋化因子受体相互作用在肠道转移中有报道[160],磷酸酶和紧张素同系物(PTEN)相关途径的活性增加与最终转移到大脑的比率较高有关(参考文献 161 中进行了综述)。许多其他的分子改变,最近的一种变化是 CD44V6 分子的表达,它是一种透明质酸的受体,在大脑中高度表达[162],已经被报道影响已确定的脑转移的风险和/或生物学行为(参考文献 163 中进行了综述)。

黑色素瘤的分子靶向治疗

转移性黑色素瘤根据生存曲线被分为三个亚分期:M1a,局限于皮肤和软组织;M1b,肺,有/没有皮肤/软组织转移;和 M1c,转移到任何内脏器官和/或血清乳酸脱氢酶(LDH)较正常高限升高[94]。如巴斯蒂安小组所详细描述的那样,随着对不同黑色素瘤分子基础的理解的快速增长,这些亚组之间的差异正在逐渐消失[61]。然而,除了一些值得注意的例子,如具有可操作的致癌驱动基因突变(BRAF、C-KIT、NRAS)和 UM 的黑色素瘤,这通常被排除在免疫治疗的大多数临床试验之外,晚期黑色素瘤的临床试验包括未经选择的患者,这些患者具有如 LDH 和性能状态等已知的预测变量。

在所有人类恶性肿瘤中,黑色素瘤和肺癌的每个细胞突变的频率最高,这主要归因于太阳紫外线照射引起的频繁 C→T 的转变[12]。少数突变导致"驱动"癌基因(如激活 *BRAFv600*^{E} 或 *v600*^{K} 突变或 G12、G13 或 Q61 处的 *NRAS* 突变和/或)在肿瘤发生中不同程度协作的重要"乘客"改变(如 PTEN 功能丧失,至少在 20%~30%的黑色素瘤中发生)。通常与 *BRAF* 突变有关的黑色素瘤[164],以及许多其他肿瘤,如 TP53 和 p16INK4a 和 p14ARF[12])。未经 BRAF 抑制剂治疗的原发性黑色素瘤中很少发现 BRAF 和 NRAS 同时突变。通过大量的途径激活机制,包括 PTEN 启动子的高甲基化和 AKT 或 PI3kinase 等的罕见突变,阐明了 PTEN 途径及其下游具有多种增殖、代谢和抗凋亡功能的介质的重要性(综述见参考文献 165)。

目前治疗黑色素瘤的靶向药物的分子驱动因素仅限于 *BRAF* 激活突变,该突变通过基于 PCR 或基因测序方法检测编

码 *BRAF* $V600^E$ 的突变或残基 600 处较不常见的布拉夫丝氨酸-苏氨酸激酶的激活突变之一[166]。*BRAF* $V600^E$ 从缬氨酸转变为谷氨酸（V→E），约占 75%，其次是缬氨酸转变为赖氨酸（V→K），约占 17%。其他氨基酸被取代占少数剩余的病例[167]。携带 $V600^K$ 的肿瘤与更高的发病年龄、慢性日光损伤、尽管应用 BRAF 抑制剂但预后不良等相关[168]。有许多可用于下一代基因组测序的分析可检测具有治疗意义的其他变化，例如，在约 20%的黏膜和 15%的肢端黑色素瘤中激活 *c-kit* 突变，偶尔对伊马替尼[170~172]及相关酪氨酸激酶抑制剂有反应，*NRAS* 突变即 MEK 和细胞周期蛋白依赖激酶（CDK）4/6 抑制剂有反应，尽管不如 *BRAF* 突变的黑色素瘤敏感[172]。这些分析对于发现新的耐药机制也很有价值，尤其是在治疗前和治疗中对活检进行连续检查时。最近在 Spitzoid 痣中观察到 *BRAF* 基因与其他几种分子融合，这为已经在试验中的几种药物提供了独特的靶点[173]。

大多数接受单药 BRAF 或 MEK 抑制剂治疗的患者会出现肿瘤缩小（表 109-7），且可以通过联合使用抑制剂来改善病情，这表明联合用药比单剂 BRAF 抑制剂具有更好的生存获益。由于 BRAF 抑制剂的一些毒性是通过事与愿违地增强上游途径的信号来发生的，同时也激活了 MEK[174]，因此在联合治疗过程中，这些作用并不明显；此外，继发性低级别皮肤增生（角化棘皮瘤和鳞状癌）在治疗过程中也会发生。在联合治疗期间，给予突变的 HRAS 活化的 MEK[175]上游也会减少。联合用药有更高的反应率和更高的肿瘤退缩，如个体受试者最大退缩的"瀑布"图所示。据报道，相较于单药治疗组，联合治疗组的无进展生存期更长，总生存期更长[176~179]。使用 BRAF 或 MEK 抑制剂进行单剂治疗的毒性通常是可以耐受的，但联合用药可能需要减少剂量、缩短用药间隔或更换药物。表 109-7 对其进行了简要总结，但从最近的经验中可以获得进一步的治疗指南[181,182]，而且毫无疑问，由于这些药物的应用获批已使其能更广泛地使用，因此也将产生更多的临床经验。

表 109-7　分子靶向药物的抗肿瘤活性和毒性[a]

药物（参考文献）	威罗非尼[178]	威罗非尼[177]	达拉非尼[176]	曲美替尼[179]	达拉非尼+曲美替尼[176]	达拉非尼+曲美替尼[177]	威罗非尼+克比替尼[b,178]
病例数	239	352	212	214	211	352	254
客观有效率/%	45	51	51	22	67	64	68
CR/%	4	8	9	2	10	13	10
无进展生存率（中位数，月）	6.2	7.3	8.8	4.8	9.3	11.4	9.9
毒性[c]							
所有 3 级/%	49	57	34	3 或 4 级	32	48	49
所有 4 级/%	9	1.4	3	8	3	1	13
发热	22	21	28	—	51	53	26
疲劳	31	—	35	26	35	—	32
头痛	—	—	29	—	30	—	—
恶心或呕吐	24	15	26	18	30	29	10
寒战	—	8	16	—	30	31	—
关节痛	40	51	27	—	24	24	32
腹泻	28	38	14	43	24	32	17
皮疹	35	43	22	57	23	22	17
高血压	—	—	14	15	22	—	—
外周水肿	—	—	5	26	14	—	—
转氨酶升高	18	—	5	—	11	—	18
光过敏	15	22	—	—	—	4	28
表皮角化病	29	25	32	—	9	4	10
棘皮瘤	20	KA 或 SCC	21	—	—	KA 或	1
鳞癌	11	18	9	—	—	SCC 1	3
脱发	—	26	26	17	—		2
手足综合征	—	25	27	—	5	4	—
左室射血分数降低	—	—	2	—	4	8	—

[a] 来自临床试验。

[b] 30%的患者有无症状的 1~2 级肌酐磷酸激酶升高。

[c] 可逆性短暂性药物性视网膜病变，很少报道。

对单一 MAPK 抑制剂的获得性耐药发生在中位数为 6 个月后，而与 MAPK 抑制剂联合用药后获得性耐药发生在中位数为 8~11 个月，尽管部分患者可能得到长期稳定控制[183]。许多临床试验表明，在治疗前、治疗过程中或进展时，耐药机制和耐药保护机制都是显而易见的。多数获得性 MAPK 抑制剂耐药的情况下，通过 BRAF（基因扩增或截断突变）的改变，MEK 信号重新激活；NRAS 中的二次突变，其下游结果是 CRAF 异二聚体增加，阻断突变 BRAF 重新激活。下游信号转导；罕见的 *MEK* 突变或相关（COT1）激活；以及一些也激活 PI3kinase/AKT 途径的受体激酶改变（图 109-2）[182,183]。Kugel 和 Aplin 称为"适应性"的一种早期治疗耐药形式涉及代谢或受体酪氨酸激酶信号转导的改变，该信号传递生长优势或细胞凋亡的耐药，也可能以小分子抑制剂或抗体为靶点，但已被认为是抗凋亡的药物，目前比获得性机制正被更广泛地研究[184]。延迟或预防耐药性出现的治疗试验至关重要，因为任何形式的靶向治疗都难以克服既定的耐药性。例如，在 BRAF 抑制失败（只有 15% 的反应率，PFS<4 个月[185]）后，MEK 和 BRAF 抑制剂联合是可行的，目前的研究重点是通过改进前线治疗和分子分型来预防或延迟耐药性。基于大量临床前数据[188]和临床经验，间歇给药的使用也在研究中（clinicaltrials. gov NCT 02196181）。

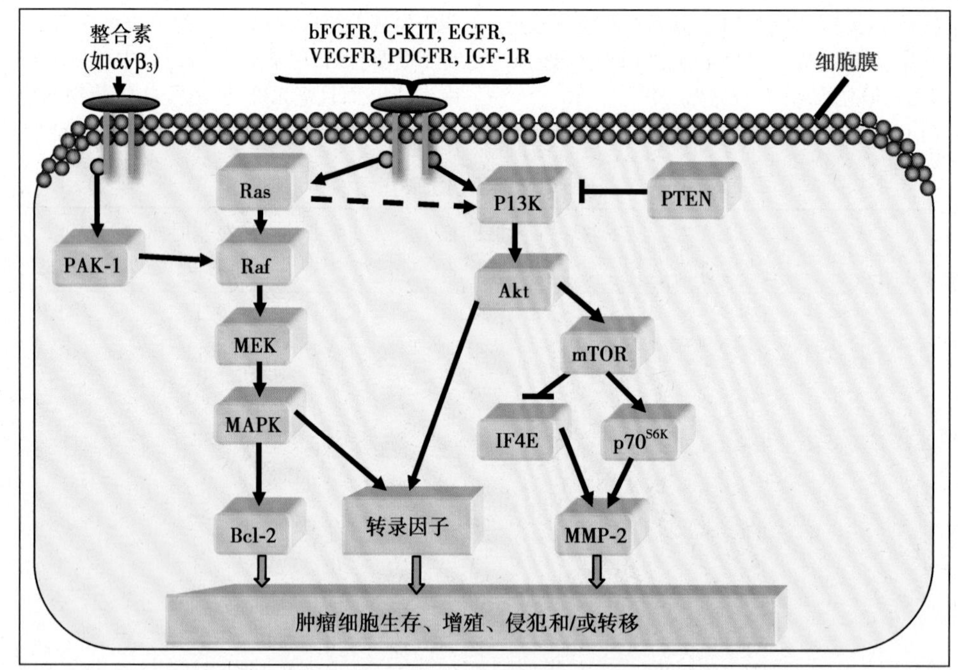

图 109-2　多种分子通路能够促进黑色素瘤增殖和生存。已经发现有许多通路，比如 RAF/MEK/MAPK 通路和 PI3K/AKT 通路，能够促进黑色素瘤增殖和生存。对这些通路的理解将有助于黑色素瘤靶向治疗的发展

对于 BRAF 活化突变的黑色素瘤，选择免疫治疗还是靶向药物作为一线方案目前仍不明确，因为两者的起效机制迥异。MAPK 抑制剂可快速起效，数天到数周内症状即缓解，而免疫治疗则需要数周到数月，尤其是伊匹木单抗，治疗反应可呈多种表现，包括客观进展后治疗反应延迟，以及尚未总体客观缓解即已出现新的病灶[189]。计划性药物序贯试验的完成（见下述）为此问题提供了答案，总体推荐 *BRAF* 突变型黑色素瘤快速进展期、症状型或肿瘤负荷很高的患者早期联合 MAPK 抑制剂治疗。美国一项大型多团队协作临床试验（NCT 02224781）针对该问题做了研究，BRAF 活化突变的黑色素瘤进展期患者随机分配为 2 组，一组予以初始治疗（达拉非尼联合曲美替尼），另一组予以伊匹木单抗联合纳武单抗。在肿瘤进展期，两组患者的治疗方式互换。这个临床试验界定了患者的最佳初始治疗和后续治疗方式，以及每种治疗方法获益的重要预后因素（包括常规临床检验如血清 LDH、复杂的血液或肿瘤免疫学指标）。其他亟待解决的问题包括：对于需要姑息性放疗的患者，是否及如何继续靶向治疗（可能相互增加皮肤和肝毒性）。如果其他病灶已获控制、仅单发病灶有症状性进展，是否及如何进行外科治疗。

进展期黑色素瘤的免疫治疗

重组人白介素-2 和其他细胞因子

重组人白介素-2（interleukin-2，IL-2）IL-2 是一种免疫调节细胞因子，在大剂量应用时，可通过多种机制作用于免疫效应细胞而治疗黑色素瘤。最新的数据表明，其具有 15%~25% 的客观缓解率，无复发生存率可稳定在 20%[190]。目前，大剂量 IL-2 应用的临床安全性标准、专家团队以及相关的支持治疗都被用以选择接受此类治疗的患者；尽管已经有很多关于剂量、应用时机和毒性反应的研究，但原始治疗方案的改进仍然起效甚微。大剂量 IL-2 的毒性是由于由小分子血管活性物质如氧化亚氮介导的广泛的血管渗漏所致，其可能导致伴有多器官功能损伤的可逆性全身炎性反应，可能也与 IL-2 介导产生的炎性介质，如肿瘤坏死因子和 IFN-γ 有关。目前关于 IL-2 疗效预测的免疫或遗传因素研究（clinicaltrials. gov NCT 01288963）正在进行中，参加研究的患者将有更多的治疗选择，其他免疫治疗药物（见下文）可作为单药应用，更多见的是作为联合或序贯治

疗的药物之一。还有其他的临床试验检测了IL-2与免疫检查点阻断剂联合或序贯应用的治疗效果以及新的细胞因子的可能作用，尤其是可刺激细胞毒性T细胞的细胞因子，但与IL-2不同，它们也不刺激调节性T细胞或激活诱导的细胞死亡。在治疗前或治疗中以及其他任何时候，血液和肿瘤组织中的生物标志物对于阐释疗效和耐药性（以及可能的毒性）都很重要，也决定了一线和其他治疗方案的选择标准。

进展期黑色素瘤的免疫检查点抑制剂

伊匹木单抗是CTLA4的完全人源化抗体，这种分子可通过与肿瘤或树突细胞中的B7.1配体结合并将其从活化的CD28受体中分离而激活效应T细胞，从而提供"免疫检查点"。CTLA4抗体的存在使活化被修复，本已存在但无效的抗肿瘤免疫反应也被增强。CTLA4阻滞剂也促进效应T细胞向肿瘤的归巢，并消除Treg细胞[190,191]。应用伊匹木单抗3mg/kg，每隔3周用4次，10%～15%的患者可客观缓解，而在另外10%～15%的患者中，呈现出小部分的逆转或疾病稳定[192]。存活率在2.5年左右达到平稳期约20%，因此这些患者可以通过持久和有效的免疫反应获得治愈（参考文献193综述）。可能还存在其他机制，阻断CTLA4的治疗方式并不典型，且有所延迟，因而很难把握进展期患者转为二线治疗的时机。然而，随着新的检查点阻断剂的出现，特别是阻断PD-L1/PD-1相互作用的抗体（表109-8）[194～197]，越来越多的学者推荐应用单药伊匹木单抗。对于黑色素瘤和其他一些恶性肿瘤，CTLA4和PD-1或PD-L1抑制剂联合或最佳序贯方式的作用方式目前是最关键的临床问题。其余问题包括辅助伊匹木单抗的生存受益和应用的安全性/耐受性（见前文）以及CTLA4抑制剂的更高剂量和更长时间给药方案的治疗效果以及与其他免疫调节剂的新联合方案（图109-3）。例如，最近的研究显示，每3周×4次，然后每12周给予10mg/kg剂量的伊匹木单抗，同时给予GM-CSF（每3周给药2周，每日给药），以提高生存率并减少伊匹木单抗的毒性[192]，研究结果很有意义，有助于进一步研究晚期黑色素瘤及其辅助治疗。尽管*BRAF*突变与较高复发率及较强侵袭性的转移瘤相关[199]，但它与黑色素瘤对伊匹木单抗的反应似乎没有太大关系[200]。

大分割放疗或其他放疗方式通过增强抗原和MHC的表达、减少抑制细胞和分子、促进树突状细胞炎症物质的诱导功能等多种机制，增强肿瘤抗原特异性反应。从而改善伊匹木单抗和其他免疫治疗药物的耐药性。大量的临床试验已经开始研究上述作用机制在黑色素瘤和其他肿瘤中的作用[201～203]。这些药物之间重要的相互作用见图109-3。

伊匹木单抗的毒性以免疫反应为主，包括瘙痒、皮疹、疲劳和腹泻（约1/3至半数患者），而需要干预的结肠炎较少见（7%～10%），但可能引起出血甚至肠穿孔（<1%）。垂体炎可能导致肾上腺、甲状腺和生殖激素缺乏，需要激素替代治疗，有时还需要短期应用糖皮质激素治疗局部炎症，尤其是垂体炎引起的视交叉受压而致的视力障碍。免疫相关性肝炎及较为罕见的其他器官受累，如神经病变也有报道。针对大多数免疫相关不良反应的一线治疗方案通常是短期应用糖皮质激素，必要时使用抗肿瘤坏死因子抗体（对于罕见激素抵抗性肝炎，推荐使用吗替麦考酚酯）[204]。对于CTLA-4抗体治疗，有研究报道了自身免疫反应和肿瘤消退之间的关系[205]，而且治疗期间，血液淋巴细胞数更高也与治疗反应相关，但证据级别仍不高，不能作为在治疗前预测疗效或毒副作用发生可能性的指标。但最近有一项研究详细报道了黑色素在治疗前进行活检，并检测肿瘤组织

表109-8 选择性CTLA4和PD-1阻断性抗体对进展期黑色素瘤的疗效和毒性（数据来源于Ⅲ期临床试验结果）

药物（参考文献）	纳武单抗[194]		帕博利珠单抗[195],a		伊匹木单抗[195]		伊匹木单抗[196]		纳武单抗+伊匹木单抗[196]		纳武单抗[196]		帕博利珠单抗[197],b	
例数	206		277		256		315		314		316		178	
ORR/%	40		33		12		19		58		44		38	
总生存率	1年	79%	1年	74%	1年	58%	NR		NR		NR		NR	
毒性/%[c]，级别	全部	3～4	全部	3～4	全部	3～4	全部	3～4	全部	3～4	全部	3～4	全部	3～4
疲劳	20	0	21	0	15	1	28	1	35	4	34	1	21	1
结肠炎/腹泻	16	1	17	2.5	23	3	33	6	44	9	19	2	8	0
皮炎/瘙痒/皮疹	17	0.5	15	0	25	1	35	2	40	5	26	0.6	21	0
垂体炎/内分泌疾病[c]	NR	NR	0.4	0.4	1	2	4	0	15	0.3	9	0	5	0
肝炎	NR	NR	1	1	1	0.4	4	0.6	18	8	4	1	NR	NR
肺炎	NR	NR	0.4	0	0	0	NR	NR	NR	NR	NR	NR	NR	NR
肾病	NR	NR	0	0	0.4	0.4	NR	NR	NR	NR	NR	NR	NR	NR
发热	NR	NR	NR	NR	NR	NR	7	0.3	18	0.6	6	0	NR	NR
关节痛	6	0	9	6	5	0.8	6	1	10	0.3	8	0	7	1
恶心	16	0	10	0	9	0.4	16	0.6	26	2	13	0.6	4	0

[a] 帕博利珠单抗每3周10mg/kg。

[b] 帕博利珠单抗每2周2mg/kg。

[c] NR，未报道。

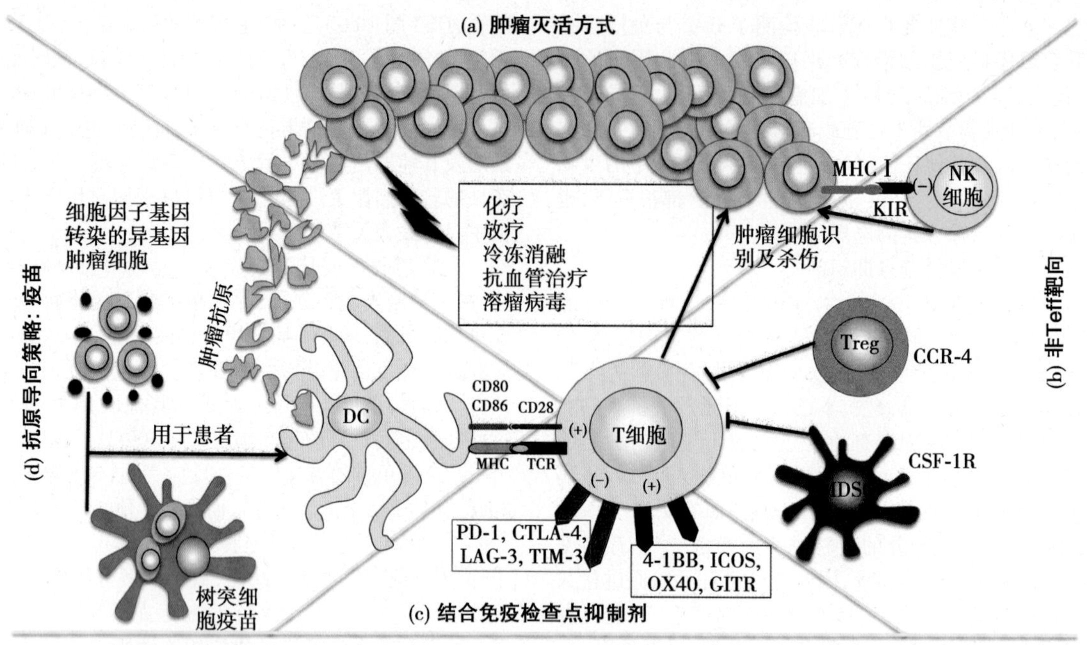

图 109-3 细胞毒性 T 淋巴细胞相关抗原 4(CTLA-4)抑制剂的联合治疗。(a)常规和新型疗法可以有效地破坏肿瘤并释放肿瘤相关抗原(TAA),从而增强抗原呈递和肿瘤特异性适应性免疫;(b)新型靶向药物可抑制调节性 T 细胞(Treg)和髓源性抑制细胞(MDSC)的抑制作用,或通过自然杀伤(NK)细胞杀伤免疫球蛋白样受体(KIR)活性而增强先天免疫;(c)免疫检查点和共刺激受体可与 CTLA-4 联合靶向以增强 T 细胞功能;(d)通过使用肽、全蛋白、全细胞、DNA 或基于病毒载体的疫苗等方法可增强对已知 TAA 的适应性免疫。CSF-1R,集落刺激因子 1 受体;DC,树突状细胞;GITR,糖皮质激素诱导的肿瘤坏死因子受体(TNF)受体相关蛋白;ICOS,诱导型 T 细胞共刺激分子;LAG-3,淋巴细胞活化基因 3;MHC,主要组织相容性复合体;PD-1,程序性细胞死亡 1;TCR,T 细胞受体;Teff,效应 T 细胞;TIM-3,T 细胞免疫球蛋白和含黏蛋白的结构域 3。摘自 Funt 等,2014[198]。转载经 UBM Medica 许可

中的常见外显子突变序列,为使用 CTLA-4 阻断剂获益的患者提供新的免疫原性 MHC Ⅰ类肿瘤相关位点[206]。该报道还针对使用伊匹木单抗获益的患者进行了研究,证实了此类患者与黑色素瘤抗原特异性免疫应答相关的治疗效果[207],为免疫检查点抑制剂的抗肿瘤免疫应答提供概念性的支持,目前多认为这是肿瘤特异性突变,可能源自肿瘤发生过程中某些重要致癌物所诱导的损伤[208]。因此,其与其他免疫调节剂联用可协同起效,并减少肿瘤微环境中的负信号转导,或增强抗原递呈细胞的功能,目前这些相关研究正在进行中。在治疗前和治疗后,肿瘤组织和血液中细胞变化及其基因表达和作用机制等进一步研究也不断有新的进展,这为患者的个体化初始治疗提供了更好的选择标准。

PD-1(程序性死亡)具有两个重要的配体,PD-L1(在多种细胞上表达,且在肿瘤中常由浸润的淋巴细胞产生的细胞因子广泛诱导)和 PD-L2(主要在造血细胞中表达)。PD-1 的配体结合触发了效应 T 细胞中的负信号转导,使其对下游的抗原刺激和最终凋亡不产生反应,这种级联效应可能是表达 PD-L1 的肿瘤细胞摆脱免疫控制的机制之一。这个机制在“适应性耐药”中尤其重要,“适应性耐药”是指浸润性 CD8 淋巴细胞产生 IFN-γ 诱导肿瘤细胞产生 PD-L1,这可为 PD-1 或 PD-L1 抑制剂的有效免疫治疗奠定基础[209~211]。近期,一些研究将这些完全人源化或广泛人源化抗体应用于晚期黑色素瘤和其他几种恶性肿瘤的治疗,结果显示,应用伊匹木单抗的患者中有 25%~30%有客观缓解,如果存在 *BRAF* 突变,还可联合应用 BRAF 抑制剂;因而,在 2014 年年末,帕博利珠单抗和纳武单抗被批准用于治疗进展期黑色素瘤。但有随机试验首次对未经治疗的 BRAF 野生型患者进行了研究,证实了纳武单抗对比达卡巴嗪在无进展生存和总生存方面的显著优势(死亡风险比为 0.42,1 年生存率为 73%相比于 42%)[194,214](图 109-4);即使对于 *BRAF* 突变型黑色素瘤,这些抗体也作为常规一线治疗被快速而广泛地应用。

PD-1 抑制剂的毒性数据证实了相对于伊匹木单抗单药治疗,前者具有更好的疗效,而后者具有较少的获益和较多的免疫相关毒副作用(表 109-8)。PD-1 抑制剂的大多数毒性作用与伊匹木单抗的免疫相关毒副作用类似,有相同的靶向组织,但发生率更低,程度也更轻;在部分 PD-1 通路抑制的病例中,已报道可见肺炎、肾炎和神经炎等具特征性的副作用,还有其他一些罕见的病例表现为检查点抑制剂所致的其他不良反应,可能与免疫抗性缺失相关。通过表 109-8 可见,虽然 CTLA4 联合 PD-1 抑制剂与伊匹木单抗单药相比,具有更高的反应率和无进展存活率(见下文),但联用的毒副作用发生率更高,程度更为严重,而且出现了分别单药应用时均没有出现过的新的并发症。但联合方案的优势很明显,值得进一步研究。正如这项开创性试验的亚群回顾性分析结果所示,对于 PD-L1 高表达的肿瘤,纳武单抗单药治疗的患者获益等同于联合治疗,而对于 PD-L1 无表达的肿瘤,联合方案仍然是最佳的治疗方式。据推测,阻断 PD-L1(而非阻断 PD-1)会产生完全的免疫耐受,这是由 PD-L2 与 PD-1 的相互作用所决定的。目前,两种 PD-L1 抗体[阿特珠单抗(atezolizumab)和度伐单抗]用于黑色素瘤和其他恶性肿瘤的研究已初见效果,并可与其他黑色素瘤药物联用,包括贝伐单抗(抗血管内皮因子,具有免疫增强活性)、MAPK 抑制剂以及其他免疫调节剂,共同刺激产生细胞毒性或抑制肿瘤微环境中的细胞或分子。

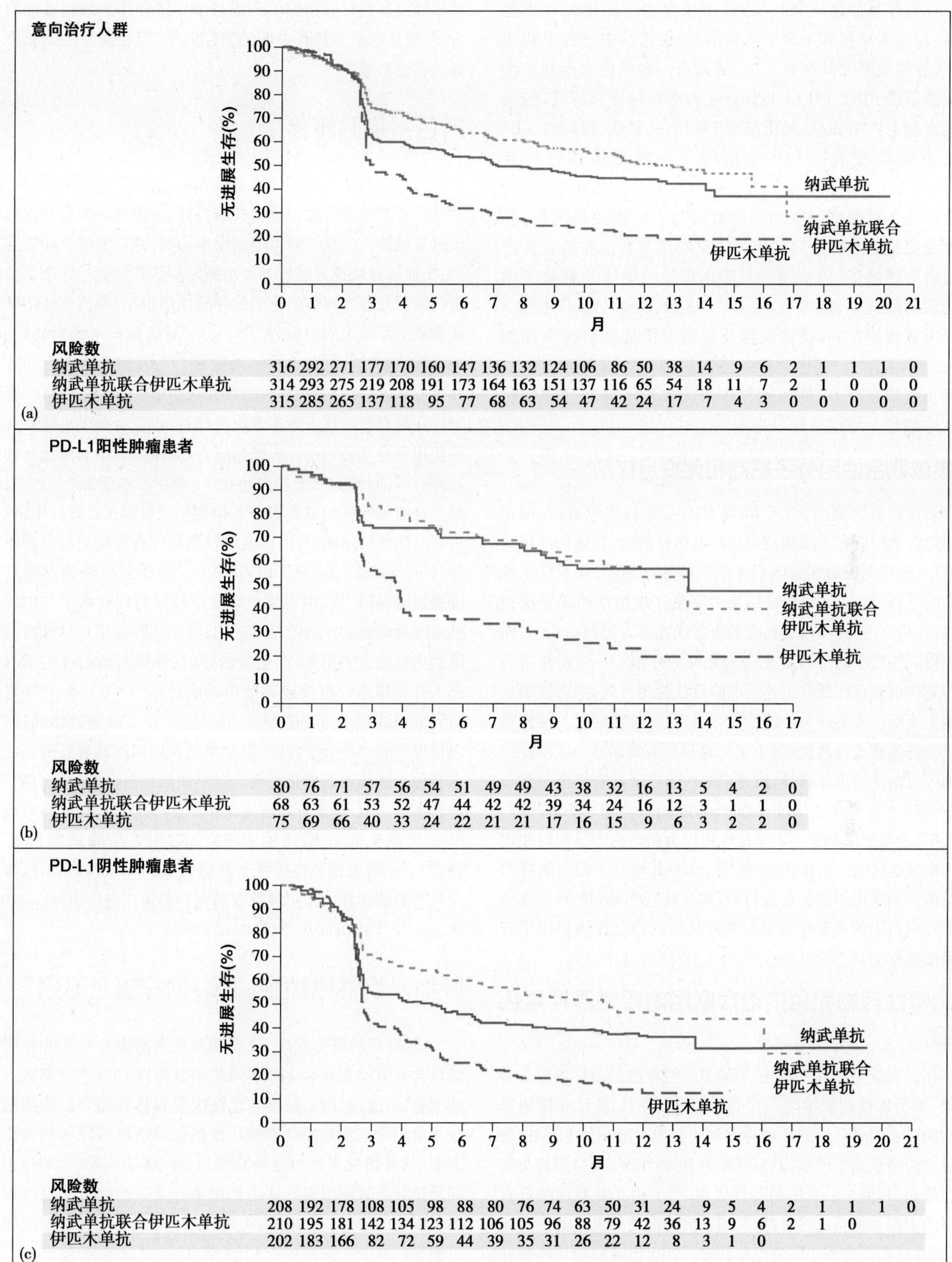

图 109-4　PFS,纳武单抗联合伊匹木单抗与单药相比。(a)意向治疗人群无进展生存的 Kaplan-Meier 曲线。纳武单抗组的中位无进展生存期为 6.9 个月(95%*CI*:4.3~9.5),纳武单抗-伊匹木单抗组为 11.5 个月(95%*CI*:8.9~16.7),伊匹木单抗组为 2.9 个月(95%*CI*:2.8~3.4)。对于纳武单抗联合伊匹木单抗,观察到的 PFS 明显长于伊匹木单抗(死亡或疾病进展的风险比,0.42;99.5%*CI*:0.31~0.57;*P*<0.001),纳武单抗对比伊匹木单抗(风险比,0.57;99.5%*CI*:0.43~0.76;*P*<0.001)。(b)PD-L1 阳性肿瘤患者的 PFS,及(c)PD-L1 阴性肿瘤患者的 PFS。摘自 Larkin 等,2015[196]。经《新英格兰医学杂志》许可转载

一项Ⅲ期临床研究证实：对于未经治疗的进展期黑色素瘤，伊匹木单抗和纳武单抗联用，与仅用其中一种单药相比，抗肿瘤效果尤具优势[197]。近期有一些黑色素瘤和非小细胞肺癌因 PD-1/PD-L1 抗体获益的潜在标记物研究，包括黑色素瘤中肿瘤和/或间质细胞 PD-L1 的表达、浸润性 CD8 淋巴细胞及浸润性 CD8 细胞中 T 细胞受体的寡核苷酸[215,216]，临床中越来越多地对这些药物的应用进行评估，定会有利于对预测因素和药物有效与否的相关机制研究。其他免疫检查点抑制剂和相关的免疫调节剂也在黑色素瘤中具有应用前景，包括通过与活化相关的配体共刺激 T 细胞的激动性抗体（激动性 CD137、OX40、CD40、CD27 抗体）和树突状细胞（Toll 受体配体及肿瘤疫苗抗原与树突细胞靶向抗体结合）。其他治疗方法包括抑制肿瘤微环境中的其他免疫抑制信号，例如吲哚胺双加氧酶或抑制性肿瘤相关巨噬细胞上的信号转导受体。

序贯或联合使用分子靶向和免疫治疗剂

回顾性研究显示，对于 *BRAF* 突变型恶性黑色素瘤，最初使用靶向治疗后在进展期接受伊匹木单抗治疗，与最初使用免疫治疗、而在免疫治疗失败后采用靶向治疗相比，前者会出现更多的不良反应[217,218]。该结果由完全序贯治疗的研究所得出，且在研究中，肿瘤侵袭性强的患者优先进入靶向治疗组，而肿瘤侵袭性较小的患者优先进入免疫治疗组。一项正在进行中的随机试验正在探究上述情况的最佳给药方式，将恶性黑色素瘤主流治疗方案作为一线治疗方案，与在进展期引入使用替代疗法的患者进行对比（见下文），这项研究将回答一线治疗方案和序贯治疗的更优选择，研究中纳入的进展期恶性黑色素瘤患者大约一半发生在皮肤（clinicaltrials. gov NCT 02224781）。经证实，维莫非尼和伊匹木单抗联用作为初始治疗且同时使用 MAPK 抑制剂的毒副作用超量[219]，许多其他分子靶向治疗与免疫治疗的联用研究正在进行中，部分研究为 *BRAF* 突变在免疫治疗耐药中的重要性及其对免疫反应的抑制作用提供了有前景的数据支持[220]。

细胞毒性药物和免疫治疗联用治疗进展期黑色素瘤

在大剂量 IL-2 出现以前，转移性黑色素瘤的治疗效果非常有限，细胞毒性药物单药治疗的客观缓解率低，IL-2 和细胞毒性药物或者两者联用的缓解持续时间有限。唯一经 FDA 批准的标准药物是达卡巴嗪，其反应率为 10%~12%，与口服替莫唑胺疗效相似，但是后者的耐受性更高[221]。由于替莫唑胺具有很好的中枢神经系统渗透性，其用于治疗脑转移患者的期望值很高，并且广泛应用于原发性脑肿瘤。达卡巴嗪和替莫唑胺在黑色素瘤中应用比较少，现在主要用于上述药物治疗失败或无法耐受的患者。尽管报道多药联合作为替代方案可获得较高的反应率，但其毒性更大，且并无证据证实患者获益更多，特别是与至少 3 种细胞毒性药物和 2 种免疫治疗联用的“生化疗法”组合，通常是 IL-2 和 IFN-α[222]。纳米颗粒-白蛋白结合的紫杉醇或非紫杉醇作为单药或与卡铂组合作为细胞毒性治疗方案，对黑色素瘤具有中度的治疗效果，但在前瞻性试验中未显示存活获益[223]。

黑色素瘤脑转移

黑色素瘤是成人实体瘤中最容易血行转移至脑部的肿瘤，并且由于其嗜血管和快速生长的特性，对患者的生存和健康造成严重威胁。一旦诊断可能需手术切除，并且常需立即缓解水肿、出血以及快速进展性神经功能障碍等并发症。标准剂量或替代剂量及分次照射的全脑放疗的作用很小，与简单使用糖皮质激素治疗并无明显差异[224]。尽管缺乏随机对照对比研究，但立体定向放疗（SRS）的结果最好[225]，且对病变大小和数量并无要求，可灵活变化各种治疗方法（伽玛刀或射波刀）。全脑放疗在姑息性治疗方面患者也可获益，包括合并多出转移或之前使用全身性药物治疗失败的患者，如逐步证实对黑色素瘤脑转移有效的药物（分子靶向药物[226]与伊匹木单抗[227]）。对于黑色素瘤脑转移的双重 MAPK 抑制研究目前正在进行中，包括可切除病变的术前治疗，以及对转移治疗有无反应的分析研究等（clinicaltrials. gov NCT 01978236）。尽管这些药物不能直接渗透血脑屏障[228]，但对黑色素瘤脑转移的疗效水平与中枢神经系统外病变的疗效的是相近的，可能与肿瘤生长导致血脑屏障的完整性丧失相关，在免疫治疗时，外周激活的淋巴细胞可进入并迁移至中枢神经系统中的病灶处[229,230]。为了寻找预防和治疗脑转移的最佳方法，需要进一步了解脑转移的过程，包括原发病灶的分子特征，以及黑色素瘤细胞转移至脑部之前在其他转移灶处的变化过程。对早期黑色素瘤的研究有限，且结论不尽一致，但最近的研究证实了肿瘤细胞自身或与邻近星形胶质细胞相互作用的 PTEN/AKT/PI3 激酶通路的重要性[163]。研究其他免疫检查点抑制剂如 PD-1 和 PD-L1 抗体对黑色素瘤脑转移的作用等重要研究目前正在进行中（clinicaltrials. gov NCT 02085070，NCT 02320058）。

肿瘤浸润淋巴细胞（TIL）治疗黑色素瘤

近 20 年的研究发现，进展期黑色素瘤患者切除的肿瘤组织以含有 IL-2 的培养基培养可扩增获得以 CD8 淋巴细胞为主的细胞，可通过分离、扩增和输注大量自体肿瘤来源的细胞毒性 T 淋巴细胞治疗黑色素瘤。使用包括淋巴清除大剂量化疗方案、某些情况下进行全身辐照以稳定细胞因子、大剂量 IL-2 刺激抗肿瘤效应细胞的体内扩增和存活等治疗方法也可用于黑色素瘤的治疗。据报道，约 20%的患者使用足量肿瘤浸润淋巴细胞（TIL）生长并足疗程治疗，其完全缓解率为 50%[231]。进一步的前期治疗包括 BRAF 抑制剂、“幼稚”TIL 细胞和免疫检查点抑制剂的使用，这些方案中对 HDIL-2 的需求可能会被更多的可耐受因素所取代，以扩增和维持输注的细胞毒性细胞产物。最近关于黑色素瘤中 TIL 细胞免疫生物学的研究发现，与 PD-1 检查点抑制剂的免疫治疗效果一致，包括存在多个免疫检查点(PD-1、LAG3、TIM3)和共刺激分子(4-1BB、ICOS)对CD8效应T细胞和CD8细胞上的T细胞受体β基因序列的寡核苷酸具有肿瘤特异性突变的抗原特异性[232]。

最近出现的多种新的靶向药物和免疫检查点抑制剂将为研究TIL细胞治疗的作用提供更有利的条件,这些治疗方案既可用于目前药物治疗失败的患者,也可作为部分进展期黑色素瘤患者的联合用药选择。虽然进展期黑色素瘤对部分患者来说仍致命,但分子靶向药物和免疫治疗的迅速出现和可观的治疗效果为治疗黑色素瘤提供了更多机会,并将成为黑色素瘤治疗方法的新领域。

小结

黑色素瘤的发病率和死亡率呈上升趋势,这也反映了(自然光和人造光)紫外线的暴露和其他不明致癌物的作用。家族性风险因素包括细胞周期蛋白激酶基因的罕见突变和更常见的基因多态性,如控制皮肤和毛发色素沉着的促黑素受体等。其他风险因素包括大量的痣和非典型色素痣。在临床病理学亚型中,结节性黑色素瘤因生长较快、无早期非侵袭性辐射状生长阶段、且倾向于无色素病变而导致诊断困难,使得其预后最差。手术切除标准包括在病变周围有足够的外科边缘,以减少局部复发的可能性;在局部广泛切除时,可行由淋巴示踪显影剂引导的前哨淋巴结活检;对于一个或多个前哨淋巴结阳性的患者则行淋巴结清扫术。根据Breslow厚度、溃疡、有丝分裂率以及淋巴结转移的数量和大小,使用2009年美国癌症联合委员会(American Joint Committee on Cancer,AJCC)分期,可预估远期预后及风险。血源性转移主要发生在葡萄膜和黏膜黑色素瘤以及一些皮肤黑色素瘤,而淋巴结转移也常见于皮肤黑色素瘤。转移性黑色素瘤的外科治疗取决于转移的数量和位置,但可能与无复发生存期延长相关。转移性黑色素瘤按照预后分为仅皮肤/软组织、肺和内脏转移和/或血清乳酸脱氢酶升高。尽管立体定向放疗、新型分子靶向治疗和免疫治疗已显示在脑转移中具有良好效果,但相比其他恶性肿瘤,黑色素瘤更易发生脑转移,且预后差。黑色素瘤是一种免疫原性肿瘤,已成功采用大剂量重组人白介素-2、体外扩增的肿瘤浸润淋巴细胞和阻断CTLA4和PD-1/PD-L1免疫检查点的抗体进行治疗。结合放疗通过多重调节肿瘤免疫微环境中的抑制因子,也显示出其治疗前景。分子靶向药物,特别是抑制BRAF致癌活化突变的黑色素瘤中丝裂原活化蛋白激酶下游通路的药物,也提高了黑色素瘤患者的存活率,而且预防或治疗耐药性和靶向其他分子驱动因子的新的靶向药物正在研究中。黑色素瘤似乎起源于那些具有易在脑中运输和繁殖的分子特征的细胞。尽管靶向治疗和免疫治疗在脑转移中有一定疗效,但脑转移仍是黑色素瘤死亡的重要原因,应该进行更深入的研究。

(刘婷 张鑫鑫 译 李晓阳 于胜吉 校)

参考文献

The complete reference list can be found on the Wiley Companion Digital Edition of this title (see inside front cover for login instructions).

12 Hodis E, Watson IR, Kryukov GV, et al. A landscape of driver mutations in melanoma. *Cell*. 2012;**150**:251–263.

26 Choi JN, Hanlon A, Leffell D. Melanoma and nevi: detection and diagnosis. *Curr Probl Cancer*. 2011;**35**:138–161.

28 Price HN, Schaffer JV. Congenital melanocytic nevi-when to worry and how to treat: Facts and controversies. *Clin Dermatol*. 2010;**28**:293–302.

37 Abbas O, Miller DD, Bhawan J. Cutaneous malignant melanoma: update on diagnostic and prognostic biomarkers. *Am J Dermatopathol*. 2014;**36**:363–379.

55 Demierre MF, Chung C, Miller DR, Geller AC. Early detection of thick melanomas in the United States: beware of the nodular subtype. *Arch Dermatol*. 2005;**141**:745–750.

61 Curtin JA, Fridlyand J, Kageshita T, et al. Distinct sets of genetic alterations in melanoma. *N Engl J Med*. 2005;**353**:2135–2147.

84 Valsecchi ME, Silbermins D, de Rosa N, et al. Lymphatic mapping and sentinel lymph node biopsy in patients with melanoma: a meta-analysis. *J Clin Oncol*. 2011;**29**:1479–1487.

85 Wong SL, Balch CM, Hurley P, et al. Sentinel lymph node biopsy for melanoma: American Society of Clinical Oncology and Society of Surgical Oncology joint clinical practice guideline. *J Clin Oncol*. 2012;**30**:2912–2918.

86 Morton DL, Thompson JF, Cochran AJ, et al. Sentinel node biopsy or nodal observation in melanoma: final trial report. *N Engl J Med*. 2014;**370**:599–609.

88 Han D, Zager JS, Shyr Y, et al. Clinicopathologic predictors of sentinel lymph node metástasis in thin melanoma. *J Clin Oncol*. 2013;**31**:4387–93.

94 Balch CM, Gershenwald JE, Soong S-j, et al. Final version of 2009 AJCC melanoma staging and classification. *J Clin Oncol*. 2009;**27**:6199–6206.

106 Wong SL, Morton DL, Thompson JF, et al. Melanoma patients with positive sentinel nodes who did not undergo completion lymphadenectomy: a multi-institutional study. *Ann Surg Oncol*. 2006;**13**:809–816.

108 Burmeister BH, Henderson MA, Ainslie J, et al. Adjuvant radiotherapy versus observation alone for patients at risk of lymph-node field relapse after therapeutic lymphadenectomy for melanoma: a randomised trial. *Lancet Oncol*. 2012;**13**:589–597.

114 Cornett WR, McCall LM, Petersen RP, et al. Randomized multicenter trial of hyperthermic isolated limb perfusion with melphalan alone compared with melphalan plus tumor necrosis factor: American College of Surgeons Oncology Group Trial Z0020. *J Clin Oncol*. 2006;**24**:4196–4201.

119 Dossett LA, Ben-Shabat I, Olofsson Bagge R, Zager JS. Clinical Response and Regional Toxicity Following Isolated Limb Infusion Compared with Isolated Limb Perfusion for In-Transit Melanoma. *Ann Surg Oncol*. 2016;**23**:2330–5.

124 Andtbacka RH, Kaufman HL, Collichio F, et al. Talimogene laherparepvec Improves durable response rate in patients with advanced melanoma. *J Clin Oncol*. 2015;**33**:2780–2788.

130 Sosman JA, Moon J, Tuthill RJ, et al. A phase II trial of complete resection for stage IV melanoma: results of Southwest Oncology Group (SWOG) clinical trial S9430. *Cancer*. 2011;**117**:4740–4746.

136 Eggermont AM, Suciu S, Testori A, et al. Long-term results of the randomized phase III trial EORTC 18991 of adjuvant therapy with pegylated interferon alfa-2b versus observation in resected stage III melanoma. *J Clin Oncol*. 2012;**30**:3810–3818.

140 Eggermont AM, Chiarion-Sileni V, Grob JJ, et al. Adjuvant ipilimumab versus placebo after complete resection of high-risk stage III melanoma (EORTC 18071): a randomised, double-blind, phase 3 trial. *Lancet Oncol*. 2015;**16**:522–530.

143 Romano E, Scordo M, Dusza SW, et al. Site and timing of first relapse in stage III melanoma patients: implications for follow-up guidelines. *J Clin Oncol*. 2010;**28**:3042–3047.

151 Harbour JW. A prognostic test to predict the risk of metastasis in uveal melanoma based on a 15-gene expression profile. *Methods Mol Biol*. 2014;**1102**:427–440.

174 Solit DB, Rosen N. Towards a unified model of RAF inhibitor resistance. *Lancet Oncol*. 2014;**15**:323–332.

176 Long GV, Stroyakovskiy D, Gogas H, et al. Combined BRAF and MEK inhibition versus BRAF inhibition alone in melanoma. *N Engl J Med*. 2014;**371**:1877–88.

177 Robert C, Karaszewska B, Schachter J, et al. Improved overall survival in melanoma with combined dabrafenib and trametinib. *N Engl J Med*. 2015;**372**:30–39.

178 Larkin J, Ascierto PA, Dréno B, et al. Combined vemurafenib and cobimetinib in BRAF-mutated melanoma. *N Engl J Med*. 2014;**371**:1867–1876.

188 Payne R, Glenn L, Hoen H, et al. Durable responses and reversible toxicity of high-dose interleukin-2 treatment of melanoma and renal cancer in a Community Hospital Biotherapy Program. *J Immunother Cancer*. 2014:**14**:13.

194 Robert C, Long GV, Brady B, et al. Nivolumab in previously untreated melanoma without BRAF mutation. *N Engl J Med*. 2015:**372**:320–330.

196 Larkin J, Chiarion-Sileni V, Gonzalez R, et al. Combined nivolumab and ipilimumab or monotherapy in untreated melanoma. *N Engl J Med*. 2015;**373**:23–34.

202 Demaria S, Pilones KA, Vanpouille-Box C, et al. The optimal partnership of radiation and immunotherapy: from preclinical studies to clinical translation. *Radiat Res*. 2014;**182**:170–81.

212 Topalian SL, Sznol M, McDermott DF, et al. Survival, durable tumor remission, and long-term safety in patients with advanced melanoma receiving nivolumab. *J Clin Oncol*. 2014;**32**:1020–1030.

第110章　其他类型皮肤癌症

William G. Stebbins, MD ■ Eric A. Millican, MD ■ Victor A. Neel, MD, PhD

概述

本章论述了几种较为常见的非黑色素瘤皮肤癌，主要对病因和目前的治疗方案进行介绍。

皮肤是一个异质性器官，由来源于外胚层、中胚层和内胚层的多种成分组成。这种多样的组成导致多种良性或恶性肿瘤的形成。其中许多肿瘤极为罕见，在这一章节中不作探讨。表110-1列举了最常见的恶性肿瘤及癌前病变，并在本章中详细介绍。这些肿瘤与肿瘤学家密切相关，因为它们具有转移的能力，并导致严重的机体损伤。我们还将简单介绍几种罕见的良性皮肤肿瘤可能导致的肿瘤综合征，以促使临床医师发现这些综合征后能进一步发现潜在的疾病，包括黑色素瘤、卡波西肉瘤（Kaposi sarcoma，KS）、恶性组织细胞增多症及皮肤淋巴瘤，皮肤淋巴瘤将在本书中的其他章节进行介绍。

表110-1　常见的皮肤恶性肿瘤和癌前病变

	癌前病变	恶性肿瘤
表皮	光化性角化病	角化棘皮瘤
	砷角化病	基底细胞癌
	HPV致癌前丘疹样病变（表皮增生，鲍温样丘疹病）	梅克尔细胞癌
	黏膜白斑病	鳞状细胞癌
真皮		皮肤纤维肉瘤突起
		恶性组织细胞瘤
		血管肉瘤
		皮脂腺癌
		乳房外佩吉特病
附件	皮脂腺痣	
与癌症综合征相关的良性皮肤肿瘤		
	毛膜瘤→考登病（乳腺/内脏肿瘤）	
	皮脂腺瘤→Muir-Torre综合征（GI/GU肿瘤）	
	黏膜神经瘤→MEN Ⅱ B型（甲状腺癌/嗜铬细胞瘤）	

GI，胃肠道；GU，泌尿系；HPV，人乳头状病毒；MEN，多发性内分泌瘤。

非恶性黑色素瘤皮肤癌（nonmelanoma skin cancer，NMSC），包括鳞状细胞癌（squamous cell carcinoma，SCC）和基底细胞癌（basal cell carcinoma，BCC）的发生率一直在上升（表110-2）。1983年美国有480 000人被确诊为NMSC[1]。到2008年，报道的病例数超过100万[2]，到2014年则估算超过350万[3]。在美国、澳大利亚和英国的白种人中，基底细胞癌和鳞状细胞癌的比例为4∶1[1,4,5]。这两种肿瘤约占所有皮肤肿瘤的90%。近年来，日光在这些常见皮肤肿瘤形成中的作用日益受到重视[6]。

表110-2　非黑色素瘤皮肤肿瘤统计（U. S. 2014）

	基底细胞癌和鳞状细胞癌	梅克尔细胞癌
病例的数量/每年	>3 500 000的新发病例	1 000~1 500新患者
疾病的严重程度/每年	2%的患者死于SCC	300~500的死亡数
	毁容	发生率增加
	残疾	

摘自http://www.skincancer.org/skin-cancer-information/skin-cancer-facts，accessed September 2，2014。

紫外线辐射在皮肤肿瘤发病中的作用

在过去的几十年中，由于人们逐渐意识到平流层臭氧层的缺失导致地球表面紫外线B（UVB）辐射的增加可能造成严重的后果，因而对日光和皮肤癌相关性的研究也越来越多。目前对于日光在NMSC发病机制中的作用已达成广泛的共识[7,8]。Chuang等[9]研究发现生活在考艾岛、夏威夷的日裔人非恶性黑色素瘤皮肤癌的发生率较日本本土居民高45倍。另一项研究显示生活在美国马里兰的高加索渔民，其鳞状细胞癌而非基底细胞癌的发生率与日光暴露量直接相关[10]。还有一项接近12 000例患者的大样本研究显示鳞状细胞癌和慢性累积性日光暴露密切相关[11]。从地理学上看，白种人居住区越接近赤道则皮肤癌的发生率越高，进一步证实了日光在肿瘤发病中的作用。

UVB对其损伤的DNA进行了特殊的标志，细胞的自行修复则导致CC>TT的突变或C→T的转换。UVA也可以诱导这些突变，尽管其更可能的机制是间接通过产生活性氧物质[12,13]。在SCC的癌前病变（亦被称作光化性角化病）中，肿瘤抑制物的失活突变或*P53*携带有这些UV诱导的错误[14]。因为*P53*与DNA修复基因、细胞周期调控基因的转录调节以及细胞死亡的诱导相关，UV辐射对这一重要的调控因子的损伤则可导致受损细胞的过度增殖。

除了自然光照射外，室内晒黑越来越被认为是致癌因素。据一项荟萃分析报道，曾使用晒黑床的患者发生 SCC 的风险增加 67%，BCC 风险增加 29%[15]。另两项独立的病例对照研究也发现超过 60% 的 BCC 早期发病（50 岁以下）的风险增加[16,17]。总体而言，美国超过 419 000 例皮肤癌病例可归因于每年的室内晒黑[18]。这些类似的发现使得国际癌症研究总署将紫外线晒黑设备归类Ⅰ类致癌物[19]。近期，美国 FDA 将该类设备重新归类为Ⅱ类（中高风险）设备，并且几个州已通过立法限制其在青少年中使用。UVB 和 UVA（320~400nm）还通过直接和间接作用影响皮肤免疫系统，降低细胞介导的免疫并诱导抑制性 T 细胞的增生[20]。组织免疫的缺失被认为是影响肿瘤形成的另一因素。

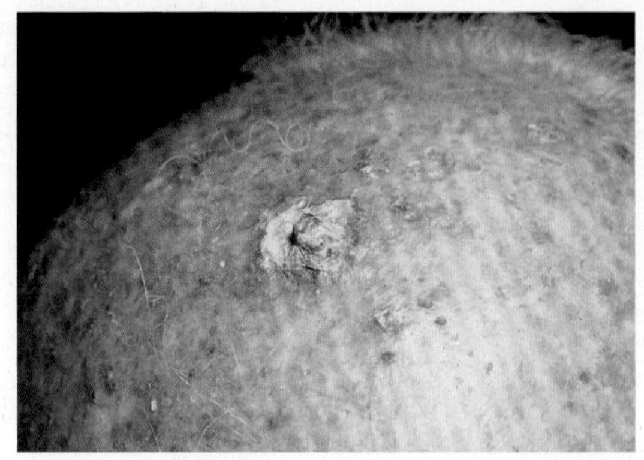

图 110-1　光化性角化病。头皮的多发性非连续性病变。这些病变触诊呈“沙砾样”。图片中央最大的病变即为肥大性的变种。必须与原位鳞状细胞癌相鉴别

表皮来源的肿瘤

光化性角化病

定义

光化性角化病（actinic keratoses，AK），亦被称作日光性角化病，是一种非常常见的皮肤损伤，多发生于易感人群接受长时间和反复的日光暴露之后。紫外线辐射导致角质细胞的损伤并产生单处或多处的、散在的、干燥的、粗糙的、附有鳞屑的病变。这种癌前病变可能最终会演变成鳞状细胞癌。

流行病学

光化性角化病主要发生于浅肤色人群身上日光暴露的部分。在某些人群的老年白种人中发生率接近 100%[1]。光化性角化病亦可见于从事户外职业的更年轻（小于 30 岁）的易感人群，如农民、牧民、海员，或者长期进行户外运动和娱乐的人群。这种病变在移植受体[21]和白化病患者[22]中更为常见。这种病变在有色人种中罕见，几乎从不发生于黑人、东印度人和其他亚洲人群中。

临床特征

光化性角化病通常起病隐匿，往往不易被发现。典型的皮损较为粗糙，触诊呈沙砾样，感觉如同粗糙的砂纸。病变多为皮肤颜色或黄棕色，稍有发红，表现为圆形至椭圆形皮损，直径通常小于 1.0cm。有的病变较平坦，也有的表现为结节性，为光化性角化病的肥大性变种（图 110-1）。多为单发或多个散在分布的病变，主要局限于日光暴露的区域。有一种色素沉着的光化性角化病，称为播散色素性光化性角化病，是一种棕色的缓慢生长并伴有少量鳞屑的皮损，多发生在面部，直径可大于 1.5cm，往往与恶性雀斑样痣难以鉴别。

诊断

光化性角化病的诊断通常只需通过临床检查即可确诊。肥大性的变种有时则容易与早期 SCC 相混淆。Suchniak 等[23]发现有 50%的原位或浸润性 SCC 被临床诊断为肥大性光化性角化病。

治疗

扁平光化性角化病多采用冷冻治疗[24]。对大多数病例简单地采用棉签拭子或喷枪蘸取液氮涂于患处即可。对较顽固的病变可能还需反复治疗。无须对起疱的病变进行冷冻。刮除术和电干燥对病变同样有效，但造成瘢痕和色素沉着的风险更大。而肥大性病变最好行活检诊断以除外浸润性 SCC。

当病变累及范围较大时，可采用氟尿嘧啶（5-FU）制剂涂于患处，每日 2 次，不超过 4 周。这将会导致治疗区域刺激性反应，从发红、疼痛和渗液到浅溃疡并结痂（图 110-2）。这些反应在停用细胞毒性软膏后会逐渐消退。现有新型的含 0.5%氟尿嘧啶的制剂，每日 1 次连用 4 周可能对皮肤的刺激性更小[25]。

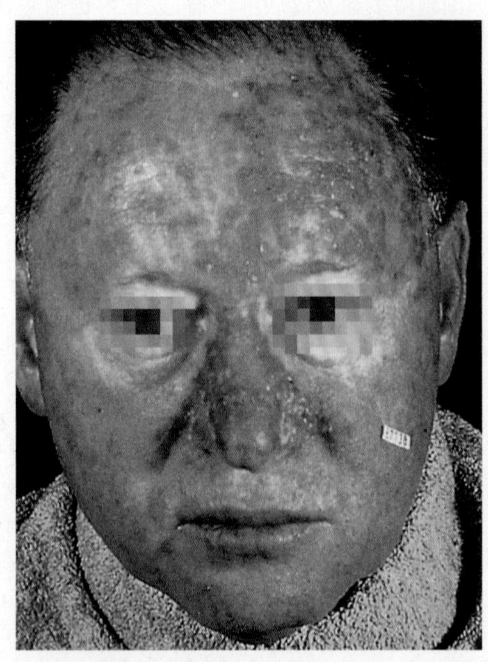

图 110-2　光化性角化病。颜面的弥漫性光化性角化病。注意右侧为对照，左侧的前额和鼻部已接受 5%氟尿嘧啶治疗 14 日

此外还有其他多种有效的治疗方法。最广泛使用的是 5% 咪喹莫特软膏，每周两次，连用 16 周，主要针对免疫功能健全的患者位于头面部的非肥大性光化性角化病[18]。副反应包括发红、瘙痒和/或局部的烧灼感，亦可见局部的过度色素沉着。咪喹莫特通过刺激 toll 样受体 7（TLR7）上调炎症性细胞因子发挥作用。有报道称 3%的双氯芬酸或钠盐凝胶局部应用对光化性角化病亦有效[26]。每周使用两次，应用 60~90 日。完全

缓解的发生率似乎较氟尿嘧啶和咪喹莫特低，且治疗可引起皮肤刺激。FDA 最近批准了另一种外用药物：巨大戟醇甲基丁烯酸酯，它通过直接诱导细胞死亡以及非特异性炎症起作用。已证实该药与其他局部治疗具有等同的结果，其优点疗程较短，仅需 2~3 日[27]。

最后，光动力学疗法（photodynamic therapy，PDT），采用光敏剂氨基乙酰丙酸局部应用，可被癌前病变的细胞优先摄取，暴露于蓝光或红光激活可出现光活化。在患有面部和头皮的广泛光化性角化病的患者中，PDT 可清除 90% 的光化性角化病[28]。在轻度暴露后可发生治疗区域皮肤的刺痛。治疗后会发生类似于日晒后的反应。

病程和预后

光化性角化病的皮损有可能自发地消失，但多数情况下如不治疗则会长期存在。光化性角化病一生中有轻度的风险（<10%）转化成 SCC。Marks 等[29]报道有 60% 的 SCC 来源于先前存在的日光性角化病。

角化棘皮瘤

定义

角化棘皮瘤是一种常见的，生长迅速的良性肿瘤，即使不治疗也可能自行消退。目前认为其来源于毛囊。

流行病学

关于角化棘皮瘤发生率的研究较少[30]。Chuang 等[31]报道在考艾岛、夏威夷的小样本人群中，其发生率为每 10 万人中 103.6 发病。该疾病在 60~65 岁高发，而在小于 20 岁的人群中罕见。与鳞状细胞癌和基底细胞癌不同，角化棘皮瘤的发病率在老年人中并无增高的趋势。其在黑人和日本人中少见，男性的发病率是女性的 2~3 倍。大多数患者为单发病变。

目前认为日光暴露和化学致癌剂的暴露如焦油为致病因素。可能还存在病毒性的致病因素，但目前尚在探讨中。DNA 杂交和聚合酶链反应研究发现了 HPV 的存在[32]。还有人提出遗传缺陷的可能性，因为这种肿瘤在 Muir-Torre 综合征患者中较普通人群更为常见。

临床特征

角化棘皮瘤主要来源于具有毛发的皮肤。最常见的发病区域为颜面的中央区：面颊、鼻部、耳朵、嘴唇、眼睑以及前额。手、腕部和前臂的背侧也是好发的部位。躯干和头皮较为少见。典型的病变表现为单发的，迅速生长的硬质圆顶形肉色至浅粉色病变，其顶部中央区的凹陷还可见角质栓（图 110-3）。进展期的病变通常在 2~4 周内直径可增至 2cm。成熟的病变数月后可自行消退，并遗留瘢痕。从生长到自发性消退的整个周期为 4~6 个月[33]。亦可见多发或复发的病变，尤其在焦油暴露相关的情况下。多发性病变可能与细胞介导的免疫缺陷和体内多发恶性肿瘤以及皮脂腺瘤相关，被认为是 Muir-Torre 综合征的临床表现之一。尚无证据证明单发型病变与体内的恶性病变有关。

诊断

角化棘皮瘤最主要的鉴别诊断为 SCC。病变迅速地进展，自发性消失，典型的圆顶状形态以及角化的中央栓，患者相对年轻，均为诊断的线索。多数情况下有必要进行楔形活检以除外浸润性 SCC。

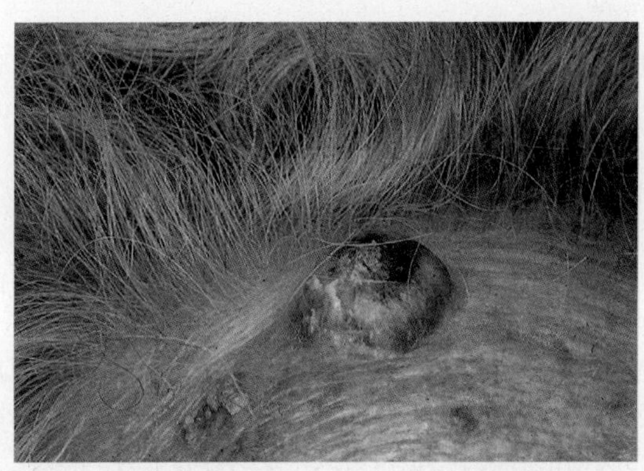

图 110-3　角化棘皮瘤。一种粉色、圆顶样病变，中央附有角质栓。这种迅速增长的病变位于前额中部（承蒙 P. I. McCarthy，MD 惠赠）

治疗

角化棘皮瘤有可能自行消退，伴有瘢痕的残留。外科手术切除既能保证美容的效果又能提供病理诊断的组织。放疗[34]被成功地用于不能除外 SCC 的病变中，亦被称为巨型进展性角化棘皮瘤[35,36]。放疗的剂量为 4 000~6 000cGy，与用于 SCC 的根治性剂量相同。在治疗前对病变进行活检以谨慎排除 SCC。

病程和预后

角化棘皮瘤是一种预后极好的良性肿瘤。有关恶性转化和转移病变的报道极有可能实为误诊的 SCC。

鳞状细胞癌

定义

鳞状细胞癌（squamous cell carcinoma，SCC）是一种来源于表皮或附属器角质细胞或鳞状黏膜上皮细胞的恶性肿瘤。患者通常有外源性致癌剂损伤的病史，如阳光、电离辐射、局部刺激、砷摄入等。肿瘤细胞有形成角质的趋势。鲍恩病（Bowen disease）是一种原位 SCC。疣状癌是一种临床病理学表现为疣状的低级别 SCC。巨大型尖锐湿疣（Buschke-Loewenstein 瘤）是发生于生殖器的疣状癌的一种亚型；口腔乳头状瘤病侵及口腔；跖部疣状癌侵及足底皮肤。

流行病学

皮肤 SCC 的发生率由于地域、人种、生活习惯、职业的不同在世界各地大相径庭。1983 年报道每 10 万人中发患者数为 41.4 人[1]，且发生率还在增加[2]。在过去三十年中，美国的 SCC 发病率增加了 200% 以上，每年确诊在 70 万例以上[37]。

如前所述，在许多 SCC 中已发现了 *P53* 抑癌基因的突变[38]。采用光动力疗法治疗皮肤病的患者，如银屑病、蕈样肉芽肿（mycosis fungoides，MF）（皮肤 T 细胞淋巴瘤），因接受 UVB 或补骨脂素和紫外线 A（psoralen plus ultraviolet A，PUVA），其发生 SCC 的风险更高[39,40]。众所周知，SCC 的发生率在免疫抑制的患者中更高，对这类患者应密切随访。许多皮肤病学中心现已为免疫抑制或移植后的患者设立专门的门诊[41]。根据免疫抑制剂的药物剂量和既往的日光暴露量，移植患者发生 SCC 的概率最高可达普通人的 65 倍[42]。SCC/BCC 的比值在普通人群中为 0.25∶1，而在移植患者中则逆转为 1.5∶1~3∶1。这类患者中肿瘤的临床生物学行为更具侵袭性[39,43]。

皮肤疣状癌是一种罕见的肿瘤，报道的例数约 100 多例[44]。80%~90%的患者为男性，中位年龄 52~60 岁。Buschke-Loewenstein 瘤被认为是生殖器黏膜的疣状癌。阴茎的 Buschke-Loewenstein 瘤最为常见，占全体阴茎癌的 5%~24%。阴道、宫颈、肛周、直肠周围的 Buschke-Loewenstein 瘤较阴茎病变略少见。这些肿瘤的发病机制与 HPV 相关，尤其是 HPV6 和 HPV11[44]。

鲍恩病的发生率尚无大规模的研究报道。据报道，明尼苏达州罗彻斯特市的人群中每 10 万的发患者数为 14 人[45]；在夏威夷考艾岛的居民中，每 10 万人中发病患者数为 142 人[46]。

对于 NMSC 的遗传危险因素的研究已取得进展[47]。促黑素-1 受体的基因多态性与黑色素瘤的发生相关，而与 SCC 和 BCC 的发生无关。

临床特点

SCC 通常来源于受损皮肤或受到慢性刺激的皮肤。因此肿瘤附近的皮肤可能表现出日光性损伤的特征，如光化性角化病、皱纹和干燥、毛细血管扩张以及不规则的色素沉着。或者可见既往放疗后的放射性皮炎[48]，深部的骨髓炎相关的窦道，或是烧伤后的瘢痕[马乔林溃疡(Marjolin ulcer)][49]。下肢的慢性静脉溃疡与鳞状细胞癌发生风险相关[50]。慢性溃疡表现出超过正常肉芽形成范围的过度的增殖时，应警惕有恶性转化的可能。

SCC 通常较 BCC 发展迅速，但较角化棘皮瘤缓慢。早期病变即所谓的表皮内 SCC 或原位癌，主要表现为日光暴露部位的附有鳞屑的红斑。病变通常有锐利的分界线，但边缘不规则(图 110-4)。鲍恩病在临床上等同于原位 SCC。龟头的鲍恩病亦被称作 Queyrat 增殖性红斑。

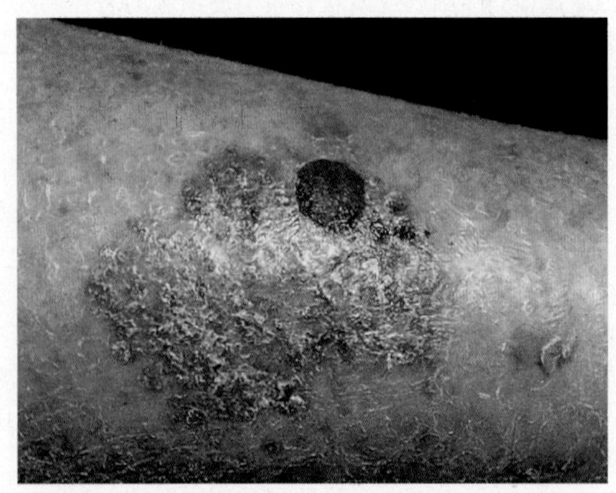

图 110-4　鳞状细胞癌(SCC)：来源于原位的 SCC。下肢的浸润性 SCC 结节起源于分界清楚的红斑样并附有鳞屑的原位 SCC

浸润性 SCC(图 110-5)几乎均来源于既往存在的癌前病变或原位癌，尽管也有新生鳞状细胞癌的报道[51]。病变通常表现为发红的、硬质丘疹、斑块或结节。病变的形状可为多角形、椭圆形、圆形或疣状(图 110-6，图 110-7)。肿瘤一般会随着时间增高增大。SCC 的一个标志为触诊时质地较硬。晚期的病变通常被侵蚀，伴结痂和溃疡，边缘有硬结。溃疡常被脓性渗出物覆盖，易出血(图 110-7)。早期的溃疡往往是不典型病变的标志。局部的淋巴结肿大可能是对溃疡的炎性反应，也可能是由转移造成的。后者往往呈橡皮样或更加不规则，可能有周围组织粘连固定。

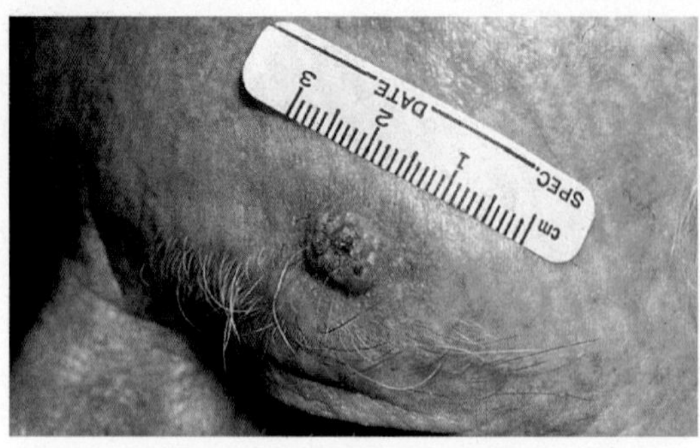

图 110-5　浸润性鳞状细胞癌。类似于角化棘皮瘤(图 110-3)位于前额的红斑样、过度角化结节。有必要行切开或切除活检来鉴别这两种疾病

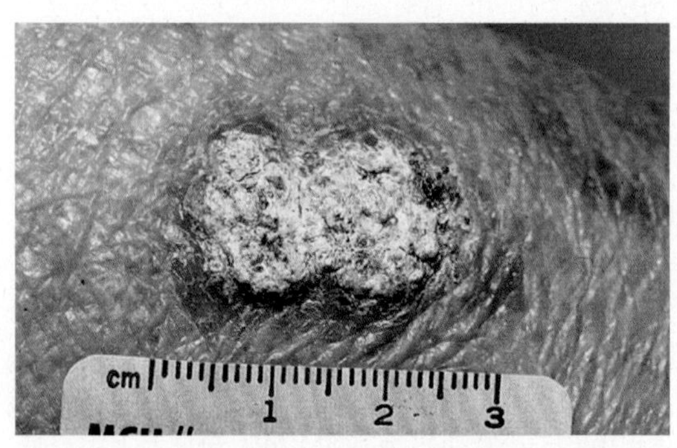

图 110-6　浸润性鳞状细胞癌。前臂的过度角化、带痂斑块。注意周围皮肤的日光损伤：皱纹、擦伤样、缺乏光泽的表现

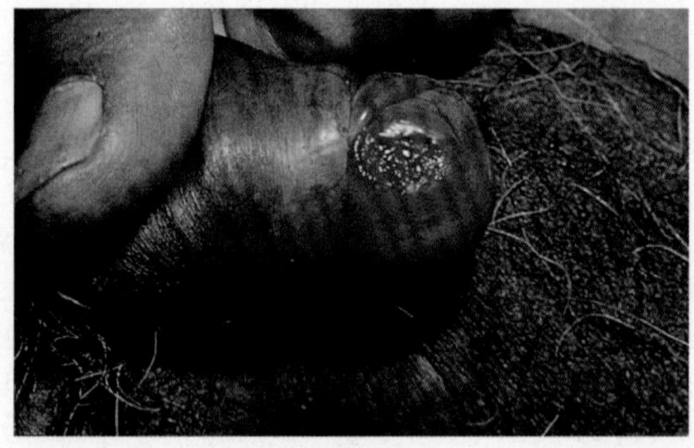

图 110-7　浸润性鳞状细胞癌。龟头的破溃病变，伴有边缘的硬结。溃疡通常较易出血

疣状癌最好发于男性的足底[44]。其典型表现为缓慢增大的菜花样肿物。该疾病具有局部侵袭性，可形成巨块。超过 50%的患者足底形成球状物。其他的病变部位包括面部、臀部、口腔、躯干以及四肢。肿瘤质地柔软甚至“腐烂”，可能形成恶臭。如果不治疗，肿瘤将穿透下方的软组织和骨，但转移却极少见。

Buschke-Loewenstein 瘤好发于龟头以及未行割礼的男性的包皮，表现为冠状沟上菜花样、真菌样的恶臭肿瘤。女性则发

生于阴道、宫颈或阴阜。Buschke-Loewenstein 瘤易向深部浸润，导致下方软组织的损伤。

嘴唇的 SCC 可来源于黏膜白斑或光化性唇炎的病变区域，大部分发生于下唇。这种肿瘤较无毛发皮肤来源的肿瘤更具有侵袭性，以及更高的转移率。

来源于晚期放射性皮炎的恶性肿瘤往往不典型，并极具侵袭性。此种肿瘤的转移率较高[52]。

治疗

治疗手段的选择取决于肿瘤的分化程度以及有无转移。还应考虑肿瘤的大小、形状及易感因素。如果为局限性的高分化肿瘤，且无转移的证据，治疗的目标应是病变的完整切除。如为低分化的复发肿瘤，或已存在淋巴结转移，完整切除不可能的情况下，则建议行姑息性治疗。现有的多种治疗手段包括电干燥法刮除术(ED&C)、手术切除、Mohs 手术、冷冻治疗、电切术，以及放射治疗[34,53~55]。

电干燥法刮除术

电干燥法刮除术(ED&C)可用于原位 SCC，尤其是躯干部位的病变。主要不足是肿瘤边缘缺乏明确的组织学证据，但在符合适应证的患者中，复发率与切除手术相近[56]。侵袭性 SCC 和具有高风险特征的肿瘤均具有较高的复发风险，但是，对于这些肿瘤，最佳的治疗方法应能允许进行适当的边缘评估。ED&C 残留的大的圆形瘢痕也成为某些患者的顾虑之一。

切除手术

针对较小且边界清楚的病变，可采用外科手术一期缝合或植皮。应保证 3~5mm 的充足的切缘，将复发的风险降至最低。Brodland 和 Zitelli[57]报道 4mm 的切缘可达到 95%的肿瘤清除率。对于浸润性或较大的病变(直径>2cm)，或高危的区域，如头皮、耳朵、鼻部、眼睑或嘴唇，Mohs 手术是最好的治疗方式。

由于淋巴结转移的发生率较低，不推荐进行预防性淋巴结清扫。对于高危肿瘤，前哨淋巴结活检成为一种治疗选择，但具体指征仍然不明确。已经转移到区域淋巴结的肿瘤最好通过切除、淋巴结清扫和放化疗来治疗。

Mohs 手术

少数医生用 Mohs 显微外科手术切除肿瘤，并获得了 100%切除的外科切缘。该技术在所有治疗方式中具有最低的局部复发率，同时还可最大限度地保护周围的正常组织，从而获得最佳的美容效果[57]。它是美容敏感区域或功能敏感区域以及复发肿瘤的首选治疗方法。它还适用于免疫功能低下的患者、之前已放疗的皮肤肿瘤，或具有高危特征的肿瘤，包括分化差、厚度≥2mm、直径≥2cm 或周围神经受侵。Mohs 手术的应用标准已经发表[57,58]。

冷冻治疗

液氮冷冻治疗 SCC 最好仅用于非美容敏感区的原位癌。如果运用得当，其简便易行、治愈率高的优势显而易见[54,59]。

放射治疗

对于不能耐受其他有创性治疗方式的患者，放射治疗是一种选择。治疗方案由肿瘤的治疗方式、大小、深度和部位，以及专门的时间-剂量-分次方案所决定。分次照射可获得最佳的治愈率和最低的不良反应，方案从 5~30 个次不等[34]。美国大多数皮肤癌的放射治疗是使用电子束或表层 X 线治疗，总剂量在 4 000~6 000cGy 之间。对于原发性和复发性 SCC，报道的 5 年控制率分别为 89%和 68%[60]。虽然治疗合理，但显著低于切除或 Mohs 显微手术的 5 年治愈率。近年来，高剂量率电子近距离放射治疗越来越普遍，但缺乏 5 年的对照数据[61]。术后放射治疗也可作为某些高危肿瘤的辅助治疗，包括神经受侵或其他高风险特征(AJCC 高风险特征参见下述)。

患者和肿瘤部位的选择对于所有放射治疗都至关重要。经过仔细甄选，一些鼻子、嘴唇、眼睑和眼角的小病灶，可以获得良好的美容效果，尽管这些病灶可能会随着时间而恶化。由于存在放射性坏死的风险，手背上的病变以及骨、软骨结构上的病变不应使用放射治疗。由于存在放疗后恶变的风险，应谨慎治疗较年轻的患者。在慢性放射性皮炎区域出现的肿瘤不应使用更多的放射治疗。

化疗

维 A 酸作为预防性化疗药物口服使用时，可降低 SCC 的发生率。但如长期使用，需权衡获益与毒副作用，包括高脂血症、关节痛、黏膜皮肤干燥症和脱发等。在接收器官移植的患者中，皮肤癌发生率和 SCC 病死率增高，则可考虑长期使用维 A 酸类药物[62]。

病程和预后

与局部复发和转移率相关的危险因素包括治疗手段、既往治疗、部位、大小、深度、分化程度、神经受侵的组织学证据，还有非紫外线的诱发因素，以及宿主免疫抑制。皮肤鳞状细胞癌的总体转移率为 3%~6%[63]。来源于阳光损伤性皮肤的肿瘤发生转移的概率较低，而来源于慢性骨髓炎窦道、刺激部位以及烧伤瘢痕的肿瘤发生转移的概率则明显升高(分别为 31%、20%和 18%)。位于下唇的肿瘤虽然多是日光造成的，但转移的发生率达 15%。发生于龟头(图 110-7)、阴阜以及口腔黏膜的肿瘤也有较高的转移率。2012 年估计死于 SCC 的患者多达 8 800 例[37]。

第 7 版美国癌症联合委员会(AJCC)SCC 分期系统于 2010 年发布，包括肿瘤直径≥2cm、肿瘤厚度>2mm 或 Clark 分级≥Ⅳ、分化差、周围神经受侵、颅骨受侵、发生于耳或唇部等高危特征[64]。虽然相对第 6 版分期系统已做了改进，但更有学者提出了可以更准确地将高危肿瘤分组分层为不同预后人群的替代分期系统[65]。(《AJCC 癌症分期指南》第 8 版中文版于 2021 年 4 月出版)

如接受正规的治疗，总体的 5 年转移率为 90%，包括唇部的 SCC[63]。Frankel 等[66]建议 SCC 治疗后第一年每 3 个月随访，之后每半年随访至少 4 年。

基底细胞癌

定义

基底细胞癌(basal cell carcinoma，BCC)是一种转移罕见的恶性肿瘤。由来源于上皮和类似表皮基底层的附件的细胞组成，并具有典型的基质。该疾病生长缓慢，并形成局部浸润长达数年，最终导致溃疡，因此也被称作“侵蚀性溃疡”。

流行病学

在美国，BCC 占每年确诊的非恶性黑色素瘤皮肤癌的 75%[67,68]。BCC 的发生率从夏威夷考艾岛的每 10 万人中的 422 人[30]到明尼苏达州罗彻斯特市的每 10 万人中的 146 人不等[69]。它是白种人中最常见的皮肤肿瘤[1]，在有色人种中较少见。最好发于40岁以上。男性所占比例稍高。其他的危险因素包括日照强度高的地理位置、无机三价砷的电离辐射、免疫抑制等。某些皮肤病患者，如接受UVB或PUVA治疗的银屑病或蕈样肉芽肿患者，也属于高危人群[39]。近期已有多项研究证实BCC和间歇性（娱乐性）的日光暴露有关[70,71]。这与过去认为BCC是终身累积性日光暴露造成的理论是相悖的。基因研究显示肿瘤抑制基因片功能失能突变，或平滑基因的获能突变，导致了散发性基底细胞癌的形成[72,73]。这些基因的种系突变可导致Gorlin或基底细胞痣综合征。

临床表现

BCC往往缓慢生长数月至数年。早期症状通常不典型，溃疡形成之后则伴有出血。最常发生于日光暴露的区域如面部和上肢，手掌和足底罕见。

早期的病变表现为圆形或椭圆形的丘疹或结节，中央的脐形凹陷多为溃疡。颜色呈粉色或红色，半透明或珍珠样质地（图110-8）。BCC触诊质地较硬，如果不治疗，病变缓慢增大，并对周围结构产生破坏性的侵袭。长期存在的病变必然会发生溃疡（图110-9）。周围的皮肤多伴有毛细血管扩张，以及其他日光损伤的证据，如光化性角化病、肥大、皱纹、干燥以及不规则的色素沉着。某些BCC呈现出泛蓝的色调[74]。这种情况可能与恶性黑色素瘤相混淆（图110-10）。这种所谓的浅表性BCC多位于躯干，表现为不规则的肥大斑块，边缘轻微隆起（图110-11）。平坦型的BCC较难诊断。通常为乳白色，形态上与局限性硬皮病相似，因此被称为局限性硬皮病样BCC。这种类型的病变通常发生于面部，具有更强的侵袭性[75]。

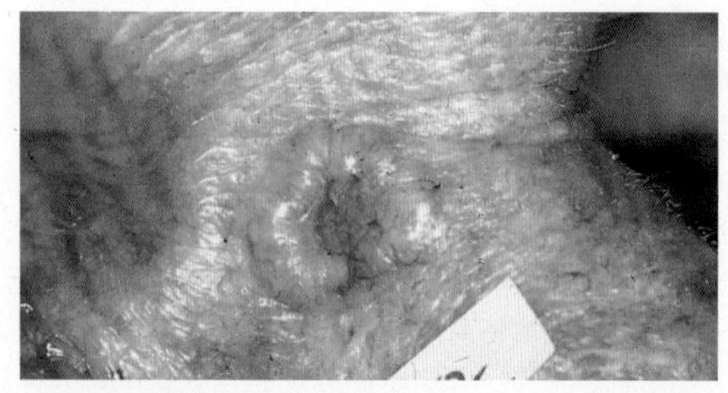

图110-8 基底细胞癌。带有脐形凹陷的珍珠样小结节，中央破溃并伴有毛细血管扩张

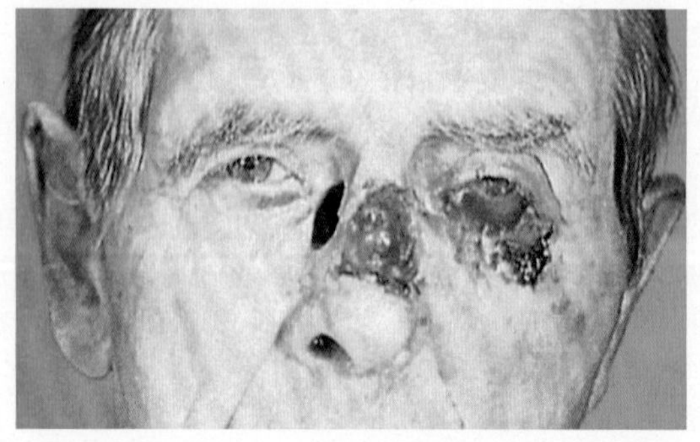

图110-9 基底细胞癌。注意这种长期存在病变的腐蚀性质

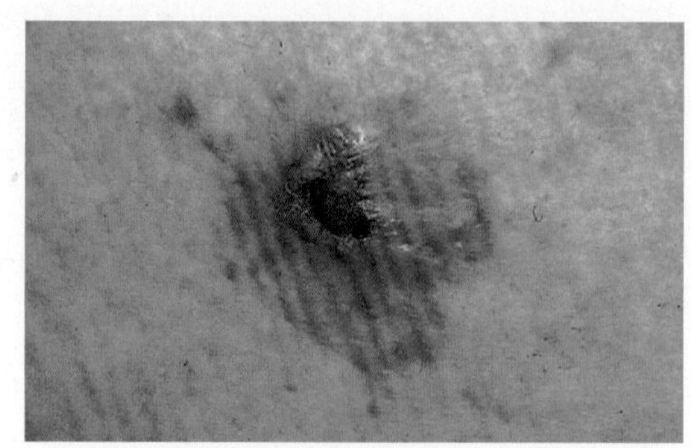

图110-10 色素沉着基底细胞癌。粉色且边缘不规则斑块，中央呈深蓝色至黑色的色素沉着，类似于浅表扩散型黑色素瘤。斑块具有光泽是诊断线索之一

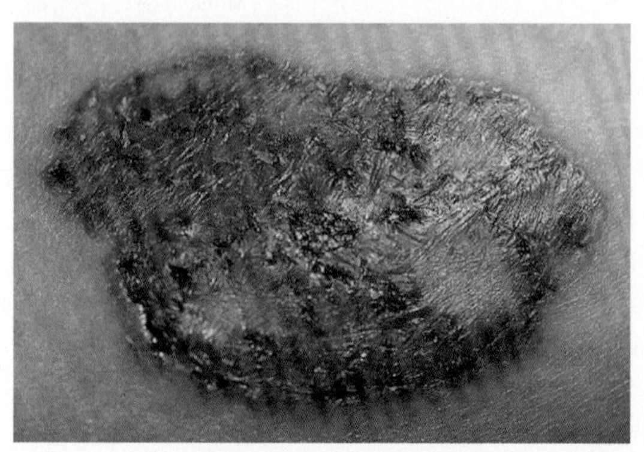

图110-11 浅表性基底细胞癌。腹部的5cm大型病变。串珠样边缘是临床诊断的线索

治疗

治疗的选择取决于病变的类型和大小、部位、患者的大体状况、美容要求，尤其是术者的经验和技术[67]。局限性硬皮病样的BCC通常具有清晰的边缘，而导致对肿瘤病变程度的低估，进而导致治疗的不足。位于鼻唇沟、眼周及耳后的病变往往浸润较深，远超出了其临床表现出的边界（图110-12）。早期出现溃疡的病变更具有侵袭性。在进行治疗的选择时，对BCC不同临床和病理类型的生物学行为的了解至关重要。治愈仍是BCC治疗的首选目标。治疗不足将会导致复发和更深的浸润。

电干燥法和刮除术

ED&C适合位于低危险区域、直径小于1cm、低侵袭性组织类型的肿瘤。如治疗病例选择恰当，其复发率与手术切除相似；如选择不当，复发率将超过20%[76]。该治疗方法的主要劣势包括缺少组织学证据以及治疗后在外观上留有圆形低色素瘢痕。

手术切除

切缘4mm、切除肿瘤后一期缝合可获得良好的美容效果，同时还能让病理学家检查手术切缘以判断切除边缘是否足够[77]。如侧切缘残存肿瘤，可能导致切缘处的复发，这往往发现早，容易再次手术切除。如果是切缘深度不够导致的复发，往往发现晚，并伴有深部结构的浸润。位于躯干和肢体的非侵袭性组织类型的肿瘤，其复发率小于5%[77]。

Mohs手术

Mohs显微手术是所有治疗方法中复发率最低的治疗手

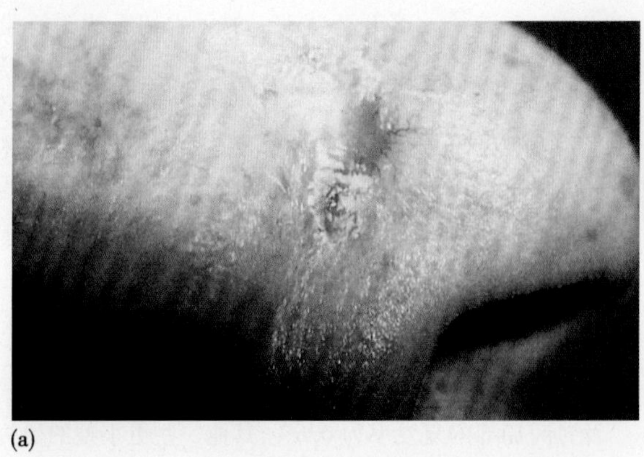
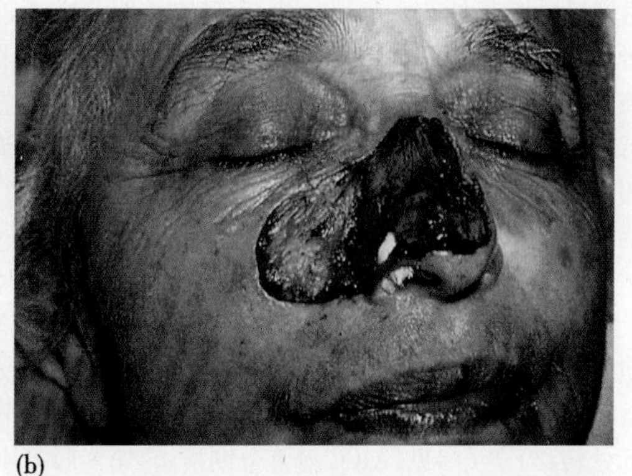

(a)　(b)

图 110-12　(a)基底细胞癌肉眼所见病变较为局限。(b)同一患者接受手术后，说明潜在的扩散远超过临床所见的边界

段，它同时最大限度地保留了周围的正常组织(图 110-12)。依据 2012 年发布的适用标准，Mohs 手术适用于侵袭性组织类型的肿瘤，包括硬斑病样、浸润性、变异性和微结节型。它还适用于几乎所有的复发肿瘤，位于头颈、生殖器、胫前、手足以及躯干部位大于 2cm 的结节型肿瘤[58]。该治疗方法的优势在于肿瘤切缘的全面评估和最大限度的组织保留。其劣势包括费用高，某些地区接受 Mohs 手术培训的外科医生有限[78]。

放疗

有些患者可以选择电离辐射进行治疗，特别适合于不能耐受侵入性操作的老年或体弱的患者。电子线和浅层 X 线治疗原发性和复发性 BCC，其 5 年控制率分别为 95%、86%[60]。已经初步成功地使用电子线近距离放射治疗 BCC，但研究项目少，而且缺少长期数据资料[61]。大于 5cm 的病变其复发率高于较小的病变[79]。治疗的日程需根据肿瘤的类型、位置、大小、深度，以及放疗的总剂量和分割次数来决定。将总剂量 4 000~6 000cGy 分割成多次小剂量治疗数周，可将肥厚、坏死和痂皮的反应减至最低。为方便患者，推荐使用 5~8 次的大分割放疗，特别是高剂量近距离照射。但是，相对于常规放疗 20~30 次，大分割放疗副作用更大，美观效果更差[80]。

化疗

每日两次局部涂抹 5%氟尿嘧啶软膏，使用数周，最适合于小而表浅的病变，尤其是不能耐受其他局部更具侵袭性治疗手段的老年人。但目前认为复发率较高。针对结节性的病变亦有尝试瘤内注射氟尿嘧啶[81,82]。对于免疫功能正常的患者，5%咪喹莫特软膏，每周五次，连用 6 周，可用于经活检证实的浅表性 BCC。大于 2.0cm 或非位于躯干、颈部或肢体(手足除外)的病变不是 FDA 批准的适应证。

2012 年 FDA 批准维莫德吉(vismodegib)用于治疗转移性或“局部晚期”BCC。维莫德吉抑制跨膜蛋白平整，阻断 hedgehog 信号转导通路。在关键的非随机二期临床实验中，30%转移患者、43%局部晚期(不能手术)患者显示至少部分缓解。中位缓解时间 7.6 个月[83]。不良反应普遍存在，包括肌肉痉挛、味觉障碍、脱发、腹泻和闭经[84]。

病程和预后

基底细胞癌均呈缓慢生长。但如果不治疗，可逐渐增至较大体积，造成严重的组织损伤。一项针对原发性 BCC 复发率的回顾性研究显示，不同治疗手段的结果高度一致[78]。多数研究报道的治愈率达 95%或更高[76,85]。有报道称 Mohs 手术的 5 年复发率较其他常用的治疗手段低。尽管转移很少见，但在较大和长期的病变中仍可能发生[86]。在这种情况下，预后往往欠佳，1 年生存率不足 20%，5 年生存率约为 10%。普遍而言，BCC 患者 5 年内发生再次发生 BCC 的概率高达 45%[87]。

梅克尔细胞癌

定义

梅克尔细胞(Merkel cell)于 1875 年由 Merkel 首次提出。这是一种非树突状，非角化细胞的表皮透明细胞，常见于哺乳动物和人类的表皮和真皮。梅克尔细胞癌在 1972 年由 Toker 提出。被认为是来源于皮肤的梅克尔细胞。它是一种高级别的恶性肿瘤，具有较高的局部复发和转移率。3 年死亡率达 33%，甚至超过了皮肤恶性黑色素瘤。

流行病学

梅克尔细胞癌是一种较为罕见的肿瘤。来自 SEER 的数据显示从 1996 年到 2001 年发病率翻了两倍(每 10 万人的年发病率由 0.15 升至 0.6)[88,89]。这部分归因于诸如细胞角蛋白 20(CK20)等免疫标记物的出现，诊断准确性得到提高。据估计 2007 年 1 500 例新病例被确诊，而且普遍认为近几年其发病率居高不下。中位的确诊年龄为 69 岁。90%以上的梅克尔细胞癌患者超过了 50 岁。并具有轻度的男性多发趋势。在患 HIV，CLL 或实体器官移植的患者中梅克尔细胞癌的发病率更高。一种既往未知的多瘤病毒近期被证实在 80%的 MCC 肿瘤中存在[90]。

临床表现

最常见的发病部位为头颈(49%)，肢体(38%)，且下肢较上肢更为常见，以及躯干(13%)，主要为下背部和臀部。病变表现为丘疹或结节，粉色、红色或紫色，表面常伴有毛细血管扩张。肿瘤通常小于 2cm。梅克尔细胞癌可根据 AEIOU 原则协助诊断(无症状/无触痛，增长迅速，免疫抑制，大于 50 岁，肤色白皙的患者的紫外线暴露部位)[88]。细胞角蛋白 20 免疫染色(核周型)与梅克尔细胞癌的诊断显著相关。

治疗

局部扩大切除是标准的治疗手段[91]。此外，根据冷冻切片病理进行的显微切除也是有一定价值的[92]。研究表明前哨淋巴结活检对淋巴结侵犯有预测作用[93]。前哨淋巴结阴性患者是否行术后辅助放疗仍然存在争议。然而，研究表明前哨淋巴结阳性患者接受术后辅助放疗能够改善复发的局部控制以及淋巴结局部控制，对于淋巴结转移负荷大以及多发淋巴结转移患者推荐术后辅助放疗[89]。放疗对于控制局部复发或淋巴结清扫后的局部控制均有效[94]。尚无证据证实化疗可延长生存。

病程和预后

梅克尔细胞癌患者的3年总生存约为33%。疗效取决于原发肿瘤的大小和分期。前哨淋巴结活检对确定患者的淋巴结病变具有一定的价值（Ⅲ期）。2010年AJCC将梅克尔细胞癌分为4期（Ⅰ期，肿瘤小于2cm；Ⅱ期，肿瘤≥2cm；Ⅲ期，淋巴结转移；Ⅳ期，远处转移）[89]（参见《AJCC癌症分期指南》第8版第46章）。与免疫健全患者相比，免疫抑制患者有更高的发病率[95]。

来源于真皮的肿瘤

隆突性皮肤纤维肉瘤

定义

隆突性皮肤纤维肉瘤（dermatofibrosarcoma protuberans，DFSP）是一种来源于真皮的局部恶性、缓慢生长的肿瘤。肿瘤细胞与成纤维细胞类似，但异型程度不同。

流行病学

这是一种好发于青年到中年的罕见肿瘤。在儿童中鲜有报道。男性的患病率为女性的4倍。黑种人较白种人常见。有报道称该疾病与砷剂暴露、烧伤或外科瘢痕、黑棘皮病有关，孕期增长迅速。

临床特点

DFSP最常见于躯干和肢体远端。往往表现为单发的，缓慢增长的不规则结节[96]。早期病变与皮肤纤维瘤，瘢痕疙瘩，或鳞状细胞癌相似（图110-13）。病变触诊坚硬，呈肉色、红色或黄色。中心可能伴有溃疡。如无治疗肿瘤可长至较大的体积，并形成卫星灶。特征性的不规则表面及质硬斑块样基地可提示该病的诊断。活检可确诊。手术时的平均体积为5cm。

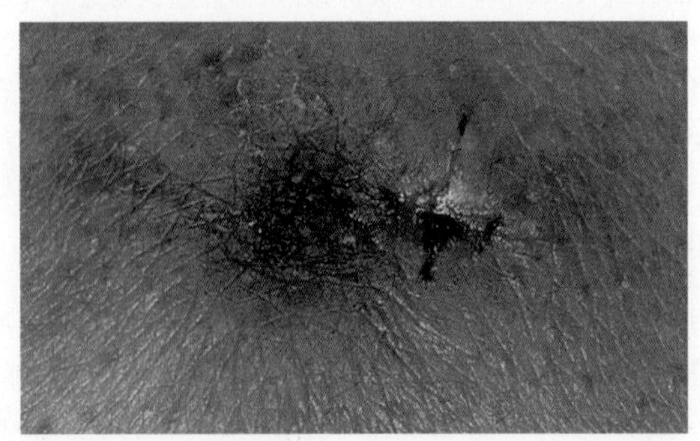

图110-13　颈背部的隆突性皮肤纤维肉瘤。类似于皮肤样纤维瘤的质硬结节

最近，DFSP被证实含有染色体易位，为胶原Ⅰ型*alpha*基因和血小板衍生生长因子*B*基因的融合[97]。这种特殊的t(17;22)易位可协助疑难病例确诊为DFSP。

治疗

传统的外科切除之后，DFSP有较高的复发率，范围为30%~50%[98]。旁开至少3cm的手术切缘达深筋膜为当前推荐的常规治疗。在一项大型研究中，这一治疗手段获得的复发率约为10%。由于手术可能造成皮肤缺损，亦可推荐在显微镜下控制手术切缘的Mohs手术。这种术式可以在手术时标志亚临床边缘，并更精准地确定手术切缘。由于初始的转移风险低，不推荐进行预防性淋巴结切除。近来酪氨酸激酶受体抑制剂伊马替尼已被成功地用于多发的复发和转移性DFSP患者[99]。

病程和预后

在一项136例的回顾性研究中，DFSP患者接受Mohs手术治疗，局部的复发率为6.6%，其他一些更小型的研究报道的复发率更低[100]。Mohs术者的经验在预防复发方面是至关重要的。组织学上，晚期复发常见，因此建议长期随访。

皮肤血管肉瘤

定义

皮肤血管肉瘤（angiosarcoma，AS）是内皮细胞的一种侵袭性恶性肿瘤，来源于慢性淋巴水肿，慢性放射性皮炎或是老年人的颜面和头皮。

流行病学

皮肤AS累及老年人，男性多于女性。日光并非重要的影响因素，因为肿瘤往往发生于毛发下方[101]。来源于慢性淋巴水肿的AS（所谓的Stewart-Treves综合征）是一种罕见的术后并发症，可见于乳房切除术后、黑色素瘤腋窝淋巴结清扫术后，亦可继发于丝虫感染的淋巴水肿以及慢性特发性淋巴水肿。遗憾的是，约0.5%的女性在乳房切除术和淋巴结清扫术后的1~30年内发生AS。放疗引起的AS是发生于照射区以及邻近的一种罕见的医源性并发症。在某些病例中潜伏期可达40年。

临床特征

在所有三种表现中，临床特点相似。外形呈挫伤样斑点、丘疹以及结节样，往往增长迅速。溃疡可见于晚期的病变。在面部，颜面水肿为临床表现。在所有的患者中，病变实际都超出临床所见。

治疗

AS的治疗并不乐观。临床医师面临的问题是到疾病确诊时，肿瘤已超出临床可见边界好几厘米。颜面和头皮的AS在诊断时很少低于10cm。扩大切除序贯放疗为主要的治疗手段。一项24例头面部AS患者的研究中，局部控制率为57%。但在这些患者中，47%发生远处转移[102]。对于外科不能切除的肿瘤，放疗、重组IL-2和IFN-α_{2b}[103]或者脂质体多柔比星[104]瘤内注射辅助治疗，可能延长某些患者的寿命。诸如甲磺酸伊马替尼和贝伐单抗等生物靶向治疗也在研究中[105]。

病程和预后

5年生存率约12%[101]。

来源于附属器的肿瘤

皮脂腺癌

定义

通常发生于眼睑，皮脂腺癌是一种附属器的恶性肿瘤。

流行病学

皮脂腺癌是仅次于 BCC 的最常见的眼睑恶性肿瘤。

临床表现

皮脂腺癌往往易于被误诊。肿瘤通常表现为位于上下眼睑的无痛、肉色丘疹或结节，易被误诊为睑板腺囊肿或慢性睑炎。多数患者因发生溃疡而引起临床怀疑并进行活检。局灶的睫毛脱失或黄染是辅助诊断的线索。皮脂腺癌通常与 Muir-Torre 综合征相关，后者将在本章中进行介绍。

治疗

在最近的一项针对眼睑恶性肿瘤处理的循证医学研究中，根据冰冻切片指导切除肿瘤的 Mohs 显微手术是优于其他治疗手段的，包括放疗[106]。

病程和预后在一项 Mohs 手术治疗 18 例皮脂腺癌的研究中，Spencer 等报道平均随访 37 个月之后，复发率为 11%[107]。一名患者发生了转移(5.6%)。这一结果优于其他研究报道的复发率和转移率，分别高达 30%和 22%。

乳房外佩吉特病

定义

乳房外佩吉特病(extramammary Paget disease，EMPD)是一种顶浆分泌腺的恶性肿瘤，临床表现与乳房佩吉特病相似，但发生于富含顶浆分泌腺的部位，包括会阴和腋窝。

流行病学

在妇女和白人中更常见，EMPD 通常在 50 岁后发生。

临床表现

EMPD 是一种附有鳞屑、边缘锐利的斑块，最常见于阴阜。由于最常见的症状是瘙痒和烧灼感，常被误诊为擦烂红斑或局部湿疹，从而导致误诊。颜面部接受激素或抗真菌治疗处理后的进行性增大的斑块提示 EMPD 可能。

治疗

明确有无潜在的肿瘤是十分重要的。对原发性 EMPD 建议行外科切除。尽管传统的手术复发率高达 40%，但是显微控制的手术(Mohs 手术)在尽可能保存组织的情况下可获得同样的结果。一项小样本研究显示高剂量放疗(4 000cGy)引起局部病变的退化。二氧化碳激光消融治疗是姑息性的，且复发率较高。最近，有报道单独局部使用 5%咪喹莫特软膏或同时联合其他方法治疗 EPD，获得一定的成功[108]。

病程和预后

当 EMPD 与腺癌相关时，预后较差。即使原发性 EMPD 最终将形成溃疡，导致局部浸润并转移至淋巴结，但其浸润深度 >1mm 仍是重要的预后因素。即使进行了扩大切除，局部复发率仍达 25%。

与癌症综合征相关的良性皮肤肿瘤

毛膜瘤(考登病)

定义

毛膜瘤是一种具有毛发外根鞘特性的肿瘤。在考登病中，多发性毛膜瘤与多发外胚层、中胚层或内胚层来源的错构样新生物有关。在考登病中，多发性毛膜瘤同时伴发多种错构瘤和其他脏器的肿瘤；其中最重要的包括纤维囊性病和乳腺癌，甲状腺腺癌和甲状腺滤泡癌，胃肠道息肉，以及脂肪瘤[109]。

流行病学

毛膜瘤是一种罕见伴有表现变异性的常染色体显性疾病。迄今为止的报道还不到 100 例。在这些报道的病例中男性略多于女性。既往报道的患者中仅有一例日本人和两例黑人，其余患者均为白种人。年龄范围为 4~75 岁，中位年龄 39 岁。

临床特征

毛膜瘤表现为小的苔藓样、皮肤颜色或黄褐色的丘疹，表面光滑。病变多集中于面部，尤其在口部和耳部。类似的丘疹可能出现在肢体，包括掌跖部，以及口腔，尤其是在齿龈和舌(图 110-14 和图 110-15)。这些丘疹的症状往往早于乳腺癌的症状出现，因此可作为相关肿瘤的标志物。

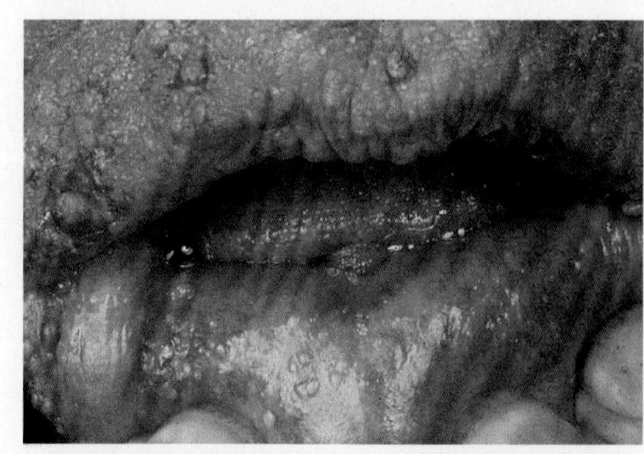

图 110-14　考登病。上唇的多发性毛膜瘤。类似的结节亦可见于下唇的黏膜面

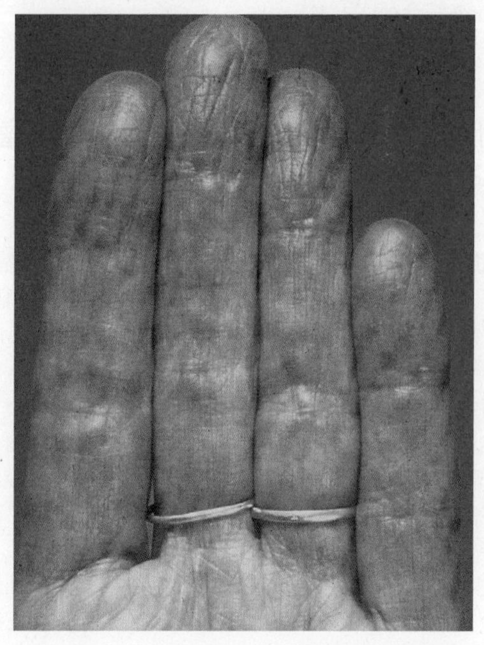

图 110-15　考登病。掌面半透明的角化性丘疹

遗传学

蛋白酪氨酸磷酸酶 PTEN 的种系突变与多个考登病家族相关[110]。

治疗

治疗的目的是获得良好的美容效果以及根据指征治疗多

种相关的良恶性肿瘤。考虑到女性患者中乳腺癌的高发生率，最高达50%，应根据情况经常进行乳腺检查和乳房造影。

皮脂腺腺瘤（Muir-Torre 综合征）

定义

皮脂腺腺瘤（Muir-Torre 综合征）是一种罕见的良性肿瘤，由真皮内不完全分化的皮脂腺小叶构成。在 Muir-Torre 综合征中，多发的皮脂腺腺瘤和癌与多发内脏恶性肿瘤相关。在 Muir-Torre 综合征中，多发的皮脂腺腺瘤，包括腺瘤和癌，以及角化棘皮瘤，与多发的脏器肿瘤相关，最常见的为结肠癌和 Vater 壶腹癌。这些皮脂腺肿瘤极为罕见，因此当一个正常人发现单个病变时应进一步检查以除外内脏肿瘤。

流行病学

单发性皮脂腺腺瘤较为罕见，可发生在老年患者中，男女性均有发生。而与 Muir-Torre 综合征相关的多发性皮脂腺瘤则是家族性的，报道的超过50%的患者有直系亲属患体内肿瘤的病史，最常见的是结肠[111]。

临床特征

皮脂腺腺瘤的典型表现为质硬，肉色或蜡黄色丘疹或带蒂的病变，大小通常小于1cm。表面可能光滑或呈疣状。长期的病变可能呈斑块样或伴溃疡。病变多位于面部或头皮，增长缓慢。

遗传学

DNA 错配修复基因 HMSH2 是 Muir-Torre 综合征患者异常表现的基因之一[112]。作为筛选检查手段，尽管其敏感性和特异性不高，皮脂腺腺瘤的错配基因免疫组化检测仍有助于诊断 Muir-Torre 综合征[113]。

治疗

治疗的手段为外科切除。肿瘤对放疗也敏感。

多发性黏膜神经瘤（多发性内分泌腺瘤 2B，MEN2B）

定义

黏膜神经瘤表现为小的、不连续的、部分融合的无痛结节，通常侵犯嘴唇，并可影响舌的边缘。多发性黏膜神经瘤、甲状腺髓样癌以及嗜铬细胞瘤的三联征已被确证为家族性的综合征。

流行病学

非连续性的黏膜神经瘤较为常见，通常是由直接的外伤引起的，例如典型的咬伤后神经瘤。文献中报道的与内分泌瘤相关的多发性神经瘤已超过150例[114]。

临床特征

在 MEN2B 中，嘴唇的弥漫性肿大是一个早期特征。在病程将近十年时，舌部会出现弥漫性及对称性的肉色丘疹和结节。全身的黏膜都可能受累。患者通常伴有马方综合征体质。最重要的是，在青年人中就可能发生甲状腺髓样癌。这些肿瘤产生降钙素，并可刺激甲状旁腺增大。嗜铬细胞瘤也较为常见。

遗传学

迄今发现的所有病例中，已发现了一种受体酪氨酸激酶 RET 的原癌基因的突变[115]。

病程和预后

甲状腺髓样癌通常是死亡的原因。采用超声常规筛查这类肿瘤，监测血清降钙素有助于早期诊断，但目前推荐是 *RET* 突变的患者进行预防性甲状腺切除术[116]。

转移到皮肤的肿瘤

内脏肿瘤罕见皮肤转移。在一项7 316例非黑色素瘤皮肤肿瘤的研究中[117]，仅1%的患者在诊断时发现了皮肤的转移。而另一项研究表明2 298例死于内脏恶性肿瘤的患者中，仅2.7%有皮肤转移的证据[118]。一项更近的研究发现，4 020名转移性恶性肿瘤和黑色素瘤的患者中，10%发生皮肤转移。总之，各种肿瘤转移至皮肤的概率与特定原发肿瘤的发生率相关[119]。

肿瘤的转移谱在两种性别间有轻微的差别[119]。有研究发现，男性中最易转移至皮肤的原发恶性肿瘤包括恶性黑色素瘤（32%），肺癌（12%）、大肠癌（11%）、口腔癌（9%）、喉癌（5.5%）以及肾癌（5%）。在女性中，乳腺是目前最常见的皮肤转移来源（70%），其次为黑色素瘤（3%），其他包括卵巢、大肠及口腔，占所有病例的1.3%～2.3%[119]。近年来，女性肺癌的发生率显著升高，导致肺癌皮肤转移的发生率在女性中也相应地升高。其他转移至皮肤的肿瘤包括甲状腺、胰腺、肝脏、胆囊、膀胱、子宫内膜、前列腺以及睾丸。但上述肿瘤发生皮肤转移的概率极低。

转移性的皮肤肿瘤通常表现为多发性、质硬、非溃疡的结节。当这种结节单发时，可能被误诊为原发性皮肤肿瘤。类似蜂窝织炎的皮肤转移可能发生于10%的乳腺癌患者。皮肤转移最好发的部位是胸部和腹部，其次为头颈部，肢体的转移较为罕见。位于头皮的转移灶可能导致秃顶（“肿瘤学脱发”）。肿瘤扩散可能经血液或淋巴道进行。乳腺和口腔的肿瘤往往经淋巴道转移，而其他肿瘤则多经血行转移。淋巴道扩散可以解释为什么皮肤转移多发生于原发肿瘤的附近：肺癌转移至胸部，胃癌转移至腹壁，而肾癌则转移至后背部。

发生皮肤转移的患者预后通常较差。Lookingbill 等的研究发现，各种原发肿瘤从确诊皮肤转移到死亡的时间为1～34个月[119]。在过去的几十年中，预后的变化可能是肿瘤治疗进展的结果。那些仅有皮肤转移的恶性黑色素瘤患者，可能获得更长的无疾病生存时间。

（张鑫鑫 赵振国 译 李晓阳 于胜吉 校）

参考文献

The complete reference list can be found on the Wiley Companion Digital Edition of this title (see inside front cover for login instructions).

2 Cancer Facts & Figures. *In: Society AC, editor*. Atlanta: American Cancer Society; 2008:2008.

7 Weinstock MA. Death from skin cancer among the elderly: epidemiological patterns. *Arch Dermatol*. 1997;**133(10)**:1207–1209.

9 Chuang TY, Reizner GT, Elpern DJ, Stone JL, Farmer ER. Nonmelanoma skin cancer in Japanese ethnic Hawaiians in Kauai, Hawaii: an incidence report. *J Am Acad Dermatol*. 1995;**33(3)**:422–426.

11 Franceschi S, Levi F, Randimbison L, La Vecchia C. Site distribution of different types of skin cancer: new aetiological clues. *Int J Cancer*. 1996;**67(1)**:24–28.

20 Clydesdale GJ, Dandie GW, Muller HK. Ultraviolet light induced injury: immunological and inflammatory effects. *Immunol Cell Biol*. 2001;**79(6)**:547–568.

21 Ramsay HM, Fryer AA, Hawley CM, Smith AG, Harden PN. Non-melanoma skin cancer risk in the Queensland renal transplant population. *Br J Dermatol.* 2002;**147(5)**:950–956.

22 Lookingbill DP, Lookingbill GL, Leppard B. Actinic damage and skin cancer in albinos in northern Tanzania: findings in 164 patients enrolled in an outreach skin care program. *J Am Acad Dermatol.* 1995;**32(4)**:653–658.

23 Suchniak JM, Baer S, Goldberg LH. High rate of malignant transformation in hyperkeratotic actinic keratoses. *J Am Acad Dermatol.* 1997;**37(3 Pt 1)**:392–394.

24 Drake LA, Ceilley RI, Cornelison RL, et al. Guidelines of care for actinic keratoses. Committee on Guidelines of Care. *J Am Acad Dermatol.* 1995;**32(1)**:95–98.

25 Gupta AK, Weiss JS, Jorizzo JL. 5-fluorouracil 0.5% cream for multiple actinic or solar keratoses of the face and anterior scalp. *Skin Therapy Lett.* 2001;**6(9)**:1–4.

26 Jarvis B, Figgitt DP. Topical 3% diclofenac in 2.5% hyaluronic acid gel: a review of its use in patients with actinic keratoses. *Am J Clin Dermatol.* 2003;**4(3)**:203–213.

32 Hsi ED, Svoboda-Newman SM, Stern RA, Nickoloff BJ, Frank TS. Detection of human papillomavirus DNA in keratoacanthomas by polymerase chain reaction. *Am J Dermatopathol.* 1997;**19(1)**:10–15.

39 Katz KA, Marcil I, Stern RS. Incidence and risk factors associated with a second squamous cell carcinoma or basal cell carcinoma in psoralen + ultraviolet a light-treated psoriasis patients. *J Invest Dermatol.* 2002;**118(6)**:1038–1043.

40 Nijsten TEC, Stern RS. The increased risk of skin cancer is persistent after discontinuation of psoralen+ultraviolet A: a cohort study. *J Invest Dermatol.* 2003;**121(2)**:252–258.

41 Christenson LJ, Geusau A, Ferrandiz C, et al. Specialty clinics for the dermatologic care of solid-organ transplant recipients. *Dermatol Surg.* 2004;**30(4 Pt 2)**:598–603.

42 Jensen P, Hansen S, Möller B, et al. Skin cancer in kidney and heart transplant recipients and different long-term immunosuppressive therapy regimens. *J Am Acad Dermatol.* 1999;**40(2 Pt 1)**:177–186.

43 Martinez J-C, Otley CC, Stasko T, et al. Defining the clinical course of metastatic skin cancer in organ transplant recipients: a multicenter collaborative study. *Arch Dermatol.* 2003;**139(3)**:301–306.

44 Schwartz RA. Verrucous carcinoma of the skin and mucosa. *J Am Acad Dermatol.* 1995;**32(1)**:1–21.

46 Reizner GT, Chuang TY, Elpern DJ, Stone JL, Farmer ER. Bowen's disease (squamous cell carcinoma in situ) in Kauai, Hawaii. A population-based incidence report. *J Am Acad Dermatol.* 1994;**31(4)**:596–600.

51 Lebwohl M. Actinic keratosis: epidemiology and progression to squamous cell carcinoma. *Br J Dermatol.* 2003;**149(Suppl 66)**:31–33.

52 Maalej M, Frikha H, Kochbati L, et al. Radio-induced malignancies of the scalp about 98 patients with 150 lesions and literature review. *Cancer Radiother.* 2004;**8(2)**:81–87.

62 De Graaf YG, Euvrard S, Bouwes Bavinck JN. Systemic and topical retinoids in the management of skin cancer in organ transplant recipients. *Dermatol Surg.* 2004;**30(4 Pt 2)**:656–661.

63 Cherpelis BS, Marcusen C, Lang PG. Prognostic factors for metastasis in squamous cell carcinoma of the skin. *Dermatol Surg.* 2002;**28(3)**:268–273.

68 Hoy WE. Nonmelanoma skin carcinoma in Albuquerque, New Mexico: experience of a major health care provider. *Cancer.* 1996;**77(12)**:2489–2495.

70 Kricker A, Armstrong BK, English DR. Sun exposure and non-melanocytic skin cancer. *Cancer Causes Control.* 1994;**5(4)**:367–392.

72 Johnson RL, Rothman AL, Xie J, et al. Human homolog of patched, a candidate gene for the basal cell nevus syndrome. *Science.* 1996;**272(5268)**:1668–1671.

73 Lam CW, Xie J, To KF, et al. A frequent activated smoothened mutation in sporadic basal cell carcinomas. *Oncogene.* 1999;**18(3)**:833–836.

81 Newman MD, Weinberg JM. Topical therapy in the treatment of actinic keratosis and basal cell carcinoma. *Cutis.* 2007;**79(4 Suppl)**:18–28.

88 Heath M, Jaimes N, Lemos B, et al. Clinical characteristics of Merkel cell carcinoma at diagnosis in 195 patients: the AEIOU features. *J Am Acad Dermatol.* 2008;**58(3)**:375–381.

90 Feng H, Shuda M, Chang Y, Moore PS. Clonal integration of a polyomavirus in human Merkel cell carcinoma. *Science.* 2008;**319(5866)**:1096–1100.

91 Allen PJ, Zhang ZF, Coit DG. Surgical management of Merkel cell carcinoma. *Ann Surg.* 1999;**229(1)**:97–105.

92 O'Connor WJ, Roenigk RK, Brodland DG. Merkel cell carcinoma. Comparison of Mohs micrographic surgery and wide excision in eighty-six patients. *Dermatol Surg.* 1997;**23(10)**:929–933.

93 Messina JL, Reintgen DS, Cruse CW, et al. Selective lymphadenectomy in patients with Merkel cell (cutaneous neuroendocrine) carcinoma. *Ann Surg Oncol.* 1997;**4(5)**:389–395.

95 Skelton HG, Smith KJ, Hitchcock CL, McCarthy WF, Lupton GP, Graham JH. Merkel cell carcinoma: analysis of clinical, histologic, and immunohistologic features of 132 cases with relation to survival. *J Am Acad Dermatol.* 1997;**37(5 Pt 1)**:734–739.

97 Wang J, Hisaoka M, Shimajiri S, Morimitsu Y, Hashimoto H. Detection of COL1A1-PDGFB fusion transcripts in dermatofibrosarcoma protuberans by reverse transcription-polymerase chain reaction using archival formalin-fixed, paraffin-embedded tissues. *Diagn Mol Pathol.* 1999;**8(3)**:113–119.

98 Parker TL, Zitelli JA. Surgical margins for excision of dermatofibrosarcoma protuberans. *J Am Acad Dermatol.* 1995;**32(2 Pt 1)**:233–236.

99 Maki RG, Awan RA, Dixon RH, Jhanwar S, Antonescu CR. Differential sensitivity to imatinib of 2 patients with metastatic sarcoma arising from dermatofibrosarcoma protuberans. *Int J Cancer.* 2002;**100(6)**:623–626.

100 Snow SN, Gordon EM, Larson PO, Bagheri MM, Bentz ML, Sable DB. Dermatofibrosarcoma protuberans: a report on 29 patients treated by Mohs micrographic surgery with long-term follow-up and review of the literature. *Cancer.* 2004;**101(1)**:28–38.

102 Sasaki R, Soejima T, Kishi K, et al. Angiosarcoma treated with radiotherapy: impact of tumor type and size on outcome. *Int J Radiat Oncol Biol Phys.* 2002;**52(4)**:1032–1040.

103 Ulrich L, Krause M, Brachmann A, Franke I, Gollnick H. Successful treatment of angiosarcoma of the scalp by intralesional cytokine therapy and surface irradiation. *J Eur Acad Dermatol Venereol.* 2000;**14(5)**:412–415.

104 Wollina U, Füller J, Graefe T, Kaatz M, Lopatta E. Angiosarcoma of the scalp: treatment with liposomal doxorubicin and radiotherapy. *J Cancer Res Clin Oncol.* 2001;**127(6)**:396–399.

107 Spencer JM, Nossa R, Tse DT, Sequeira M. Sebaceous carcinoma of the eyelid treated with Mohs micrographic surgery. *J Am Acad Dermatol.* 2001;**44(6)**:1004–1009.

109 Gustafson S, Zbuk KM, Scacheri C, Eng C. Cowden syndrome. *Semin Oncol.* 2007;**34(5)**:428–434.

110 Liaw D, Marsh DJ, Li J, et al. Germline mutations of the PTEN gene in Cowden disease, an inherited breast and thyroid cancer syndrome. *Nat Genet.* 1997;**16(1)**:64–67.

111 Pettey AA, Walsh JS. Muir-Torre syndrome: a case report and review of the literature. *Cutis.* 2005;**75(3)**:149–155.

115 Santoro M, Carlomagno F, Romano A, et al. Activation of RET as a dominant transforming gene by germline mutations of MEN2A and MEN2B. *Science.* 1995;**267(5196)**:381–383.

116 Sanso GE, Domene HM, Garcia R, Pusiol E. de M, Roque M, et al. Very early detection of RET proto-oncogene mutation is crucial for preventive thyroidectomy in multiple endocrine neoplasia type 2 children: presence of C-cell malignant disease in asymptomatic carriers. *Cancer.* 2002;**94(2)**:323–330.

第 111 章　骨肿瘤

Timothy A. Damron, MD, FACS

概述

骨肿瘤是少见疾病，可发生于各个年龄阶段，能累及全身任何一块骨骼。骨病损可以是良性肿瘤、反应性病变、原发骨的肉瘤、骨转移癌、骨髓瘤和淋巴瘤等。良性骨病损主要发生于儿童和青少年，其生物学行为可为静止的、活跃的和侵袭的，侵袭性病损可类似恶性骨肿瘤。原发骨的肉瘤发病年龄呈双峰分布，转移性骨肿瘤、骨髓瘤和淋巴瘤主要发生于成人。尽管骨肿瘤种类繁多，但是每种骨肿瘤具有独特的临床和影像学表现、特殊的好发部位，这些特征可以缩小鉴别诊断，选择合适的治疗方案。

骨的肉瘤占所有癌症不足 0.2%。2014 年间新诊断 3 020 例原发骨的肉瘤，1 460 例死亡。前三位最常见的骨的肉瘤是骨肉瘤、软骨肉瘤和尤因肉瘤。然而，最常见的原发于骨的恶性肿瘤是骨髓瘤，最常见累及骨的恶性肿瘤是转移癌。

骨肿瘤的病理学分类不断进展。分类方法仍然主要依据细胞起源或组织类型。原发骨肿瘤来源于软骨细胞、骨细胞、血管细胞或其他，但一些肿瘤来源不明。目前最常用的病理学分类系统是 WHO 骨肿瘤分类法。

前言

骨肿瘤属少见肿瘤。它起源于骨骼系统的各类细胞，可发生于任何年龄段的患者，见于全身各处的骨组织。其中包括良性骨肿瘤、原发骨骼系统肉瘤、骨转移癌、骨髓瘤及淋巴瘤。良性骨肿瘤可表现为静息的、活跃的或侵袭性的。尽管骨肿瘤种类繁多，但每一种都有其自身不同的临床表现及 X 线特点，比如特异的好发部位，可以缩小鉴别诊断的范围，进而选择合适的治疗方法。

骨骼系统肉瘤发病率仅占全部肿瘤发病率的 0.2% 或更小[1]。在 2014 年，约有 3 020 例原发骨骼系统肉瘤的新发病例，约 1 460 例死亡病例。3 种最常见的骨骼系统肉瘤分别为骨肉瘤（45%）、软骨肉瘤（36%）、尤因肉瘤（18%）[2]。但最常见的原发于骨骼系统的恶性肿瘤是骨髓瘤，最常见的侵及骨骼的恶性病变是转移癌。骨的恶性肿瘤仅占少数，绝大多数的骨肿瘤为良性。

骨肿瘤的病理学分类不断进展。分类方法仍然主要依据细胞起源或组织类型。原发的骨肿瘤可起源于软骨细胞——成软骨细胞（内生软骨瘤、骨膜软骨瘤、软骨母细胞瘤、软骨黏液样纤维瘤、软骨肉瘤）、骨细胞——成骨细胞（骨瘤、骨样骨瘤、骨母细胞瘤、骨肉瘤）和血管细胞（血管瘤、血管肉瘤），但其中一些肿瘤的细胞来源并不清楚。目前最为广泛认可的是 WHO 病理分类，本章中会沿用其中大部分分类，但像良性纤维瘤等一些肿瘤的分组有所不同[3]。在本文上一版之后骨肿瘤 WHO 分类法有所更新（表 111-1）。

表 111-1　WHO 第 4 版骨与软组织肿瘤分类中骨肿瘤分类[3]

软骨性肿瘤
骨软骨瘤
软骨瘤：内生软骨瘤，骨膜软骨瘤
软骨黏液样纤维瘤
骨软骨黏液瘤
甲下外生骨疣和奇异性骨旁骨软骨瘤样增生
滑膜软骨瘤病
软骨母细胞瘤
软骨肉瘤（1~3 级）包括原发、继发和骨膜软骨肉
去分化型软骨肉瘤
间叶型软骨肉瘤
透明细胞型软骨肉瘤
骨源性肿瘤
骨瘤
骨样骨瘤
骨母细胞瘤
低级别中心性骨肉瘤
传统型骨肉瘤
毛细血管扩张型骨肉瘤
小细胞型骨肉瘤
骨膜型骨肉瘤
骨旁型骨肉瘤
高级别表面骨肉瘤
纤维源性肿瘤
骨的促结缔组织增生性纤维瘤
骨的纤维肉瘤
纤维组织细胞性肿瘤
非骨化性纤维瘤和骨的良性纤维组织细胞瘤
尤因肉瘤
造血系统肿瘤
浆细胞骨髓瘤
骨的孤立性浆细胞瘤
骨的原发性非霍奇金淋巴瘤
富含骨巨细胞的肿瘤

续表

小骨的巨细胞病变
骨巨细胞瘤
脊索组织肿瘤
良性脊索组织肿瘤
脊索瘤
血管源性肿瘤
血管瘤
上皮样血管瘤
上皮样血管内皮瘤
血管肉瘤
肌源性、脂肪源性、上皮性肿瘤
平滑肌肉瘤
脂肪瘤
脂肪肉瘤
成釉细胞瘤
未明确肿瘤性质的肿瘤
动脉瘤样骨囊肿
单纯性骨囊肿
纤维结构不良
骨性纤维结构不良
朗格汉斯细胞组织细胞增生症
Erdheim-Chester 病
软骨间叶性错构瘤
Rosai-Dorfman 病

本章的前言部分主要涉及治疗前阶段（评估、分期及活检），中间部分涉及手术治疗（重建的选择和手术切缘）、放射治疗、药物治疗，最后部分讨论特殊的良性和恶性骨肿瘤以及与骨肿瘤相关的先天性综合征。

评估

评估骨肿瘤的重要信息来自病史、查体及 X 线特点。骨肿瘤的评价目的是达到缩小鉴别诊断的范围，指导随后的治疗。某些情况可以借助特异性诊断，依据诊断，后续可进行观察（如非骨化性纤维瘤、内生软骨瘤）、活检（如动脉瘤样骨囊肿、软骨母细胞瘤、骨巨细胞瘤、骨肉瘤）、冲洗或清创（如骨髓炎）、针吸或注射（如单腔骨囊肿）、射频消融术（如骨样骨瘤）、切除（如骨软骨瘤）、预防性固定（如骨转移癌、骨髓瘤）。而某些肿瘤根据生物学行为分为静息、活跃或侵袭性。静息的骨肿瘤可进行观察，活跃的骨肿瘤通常需要活检并刮除或植骨。侵袭性骨肿瘤几乎都需要在治疗前行活检确认，其中包括良性侵袭性病变（如动脉瘤样骨囊肿、软骨母细胞瘤、骨巨细胞瘤）和恶性肿瘤（如原发骨肉瘤、骨转移癌、骨髓瘤、淋巴瘤）。

患者的年龄及通过何种途径发现的骨肿瘤都是重要的病史特征。如果是小于 5 岁的患者，那么年龄分层非常有利于诊断，因为转移性神经母细胞瘤几乎特异性发生在这个年龄段。如果患者大于 40 岁，那么就会做出不同的诊断，依次见于转移癌、骨髓瘤、淋巴瘤、原发骨的肉瘤，如软骨肉瘤、骨的恶性纤维组织细胞瘤及纤维肉瘤。

发现骨肿瘤的途径多种多样。由于其他原因检查时无意中发现的骨肿瘤，通常为静止的病损，仅需要定期观察。在成年患者中，最常在无意中发现的骨肿瘤是内生软骨瘤；在儿科患者中，则是非骨化性纤维瘤。无痛的骨性肿物通常是骨软骨瘤，但其他的骨表面肿瘤也可有类似的表现。包括范围最广的还是痛性骨肿瘤，其中包括多种活跃及侵袭性的骨肿瘤。病理性骨折前伴发疼痛的，通常为活跃或者侵袭性骨肿瘤；不伴发疼痛的，则更倾向于静息性肿瘤。病理性骨折前伴发疼痛者通常需要活检，而不伴有疼痛者往往需观察至少骨折愈合，当然存在例外的情况。

影像学评估骨肿瘤的标准是通过 X 线平片。可就 4 个方面进行评估：肿瘤的解剖部位（骺端、干骺端、骨干、表面或是皮质内）、边缘骨质破坏的特征（1 型（地图形）、2 型（虫蚀样）或是 3 型（渗透浸润））、骨的反应（骨膜反应）、骨质矿化状况（钙化、骨化、磨玻璃样）（表 111-2）。1 型骨质破坏的边缘又能分为三个亚型[5]。1A 型的特点是厚的硬化边缘，通常提示良性病变。1B 型边缘清晰，但无硬化边，提示病损潜在快速生长可能，特殊病例可能为低度恶性。1C 型开始出现虫噬样改变，提示侵袭性增大，包括骨皮质破坏[6]。普遍而言良性肿瘤具有硬化边缘，透明软骨肿瘤是个例外，大部分内生软骨瘤没有 1A 型边缘。结合平片特征及临床表现通常就可缩小鉴别诊断的范围。

表 111-2 骨肿瘤边缘破坏、骨反应及骨质矿化状况的典型 X 线表现

X 线平片类别	表现类型	典型病种[a]
边缘破坏的特征	地图形（边缘清晰）	1A 非骨化性纤维瘤
		单发骨囊肿
		1B 动脉瘤样骨囊肿
		软骨母细胞瘤
		1C 骨巨细胞瘤
		淋巴瘤
	虫蚀样（模糊不清）	转移癌
		骨髓瘤
		骨髓炎
	渗透浸润（边缘不清）	骨肉瘤
		尤因肉瘤
		转移癌
		淋巴瘤
骨反应	边缘硬化	非骨化性纤维瘤

续表

X 线平片类别	表现类型	典型病种[a]
		纤维异常增殖症
	皮质增厚	骨样骨瘤
		骨髓炎
	薄层骨膜反应	应力性骨折
	骨内膜膨胀呈扇贝样	低级或中级软骨肉瘤
	骨包壳	动脉瘤样骨囊肿
		骨巨细胞瘤
	Codman 三角	骨肉瘤
	葱皮样骨膜反应	尤因肉瘤
骨质矿化状况	弧形或环形点状钙化	透明软骨肿瘤(内生软骨瘤/软骨肉瘤)
	磨玻璃样	纤维异常增殖症
	成骨样	骨样骨瘤
		骨母细胞瘤
		骨肉瘤
		转移癌(前列腺,乳腺)
		淋巴瘤

[a] 此表中的影像学表现并不特异,其中有很多交叉,因此表中涉及的肿瘤特征可能较典型,但并不是唯一的特征。

摘自 Damron 2008[4]. Reproduced with permission of Wolters Kluwer Health。

骨扫描是通过判断病变是否摄取放射性核素^{99m}Tc,来提示肿瘤为活跃性还是侵袭性,是单发还是多发。但骨髓瘤是个例外,它在骨扫描中显示为冷点。某些像肾转移癌的侵袭性病变,如果肿瘤破坏超过了受累骨的成骨能力,那么在骨扫描时也可能不显示为热点。

正电子发射断层扫描(PET)在骨肿瘤评估和分期的作用与日俱增[6]。大体而言,PET 更适合恶性骨肿瘤。但是,有研究表明 18F-FDG PET 对恶性肿瘤缺乏特异性,尽管许多良性肿瘤,包括骨化纤维瘤和骨样骨瘤等,有更大的变异型,但 PET 检查仍缺乏特异性。PET 扫描在恶性骨肿瘤分期的作用越来越重要,但对诊断肺转移而言,与常规胸部 CT 相比,PET 敏感性更低。

骨肿瘤的磁共振成像(MRI)一般在 X 线平片诊断证据不足时应用,它可以判断骨肉瘤的局部侵犯范围。一些特殊的骨肿瘤可能需要 MRI 来确认,如骨囊肿(囊性病变的边缘强化)、动脉瘤样骨囊肿(由多个充满血液的分隔组成)。骨肉瘤病变周围水肿常见,但也可见于某些特定的良性病变,如骨髓炎、骨样骨瘤、软骨母细胞瘤、朗格汉斯细胞组织细胞增生症(LCH)、软骨黏液样纤维瘤等。计算机断层扫描(CT)可显示在骨样骨瘤的周围出现反应性的透光区,对于软骨肿瘤,可通过骨内膜是否存在扇贝样变来鉴别内生软骨瘤和软骨肉瘤,病变区可发现形态不清晰的矿化,还可以辅助评估 MRI 难以显示的解剖部位,如骶骨、骨盆、肩胛骨等。

分期

骨骼系统肉瘤的分期可同时评估原发病灶及远处转移。为了评估原发病灶,那么应该进行包括全身骨骼的 X 线及 MRI 检查来明确有无"跳跃性"的病变。骨骼系统的肉瘤最易发生远处转移的部位是肺,其次是骨。因此,严格的分期应通过胸片、胸部 CT 来评估肺部情况,全身骨扫描或 PET 来评价其余的骨骼。

骨骼肌肉系统的肉瘤分期系统通常应用的是由 William Enneking 提出的,它后来被美国骨骼肌肉系统肿瘤协会(Musculoskeletal Tumor Society, MSTS)所采用(表 111-3)。MSTS 分期系统包括有无转移、级别(高或低)、肿瘤的局部侵犯(骨内或软组织侵犯)。典型的软骨肉瘤是低级别、间室内(局限在骨)的,因而通常是ⅠA 期。传统高级别骨肉瘤通常侵犯周围软组织,且 80% 当前无远处转移证据的通常分期为ⅡB 期。在该分期系统中,若有转移证据则为Ⅲ期。

表 111-3 骨骼肌肉肿瘤协会分期系统

分期	级别	局部侵犯	转移
Ⅰ	低	A-间室内	无
		B-间室外	
Ⅱ	高	A-间室内	
		B-间室外	
Ⅲ	任何	任何	有

摘自 Enneking 1980[7]. Reproduced with permission from the Association of Bone and Joint Surgeons。

目前最为广泛应用于骨骼系统肉瘤的分期系统来自 American Joint Commission on Cancer(AJCC)[8](表 111-4)。该系统具有更充分的依据指导预后(图 111-1)。AJCC 系统包含有无转移(区别于远处转移的多个非连续的骨肿瘤)、级别(分级 1、2 或是 3、4)、大小(≤8cm 或是>8cm)。该系统在根据不同级别区分Ⅰ、Ⅱ期时与 MSTS 分期相似,但在界定 A、B 时依据的是肿瘤大小。对于骨肉瘤和尤因肉瘤的患者,ⅡB 比ⅡA 期的转移发生率要高。存在"跳跃性"病变(同一骨骼上的非连续性病变)的患者分到Ⅲ期。发生远处转移的为Ⅳ期,但是肺外转移(如骨转移)的预后较单一肺转移的预后要差,因此又单独分为两组(ⅣA 和ⅣB)。因此,对于<8cm 的低级别软骨肉瘤,典型的分期为ⅠA 期。无非连续性病变或远处转移、>8cm 的高级别骨肉瘤,典型的分期为ⅡB 期。AJCC 分期系统在 2002—2012 年未做更改[10]。

表 111-4 AJCC 骨肿瘤分期系统

原发肿瘤[T]				
Tx	原发肿瘤无法评估			
T0	无原发肿瘤证据			
T1	肿瘤最大径≤8cm			
T2	肿瘤最大径>8cm			
T3	原发骨存在不连续的肿瘤			
区域淋巴结[N]				
Nx*	区域淋巴结无法评估			
N0	无区域淋巴结转移			
N1	区域淋巴结转移			
远处转移[M]				
Mx	远处转移无法评估			
M0	无远处转移			
M1	远处转移			
M1a	肺转移			
M1b	其他远处转移灶			
组织学分级[G]				
Gx	分级无法评估			
G1	分化好-低级别			
G2	中度分化-低级别			
G3	分化差-高级别			
G4	未分化-高级别			
分期	**肿瘤[T]**	**淋巴结[N]**	**转移[M]**	**级别[G]**
ⅠA	T1	N0	M0	G1,2 低级别
ⅠB	T2	N0	M0	G1,2 低级别
ⅡA	T1	N0	M0	G3,4 高级别
ⅡB	T2	N0	M0	G3,4 高级别
Ⅲ	T3	N0	M0	任何 G
ⅣA	任何 T	N0	M1a	任何 G
ⅣB	任何 T	N1	任何 M	任何 G
	任何 T	任何 N	M1b	任何 G

* 因为肉瘤中淋巴结受累较少见，Nx 定义并不适合，且如临床证据不足，可视为 N0。尤因肉瘤分作 G4。

摘自 Edge 2010[9]，Reproduced with permission from Springer。

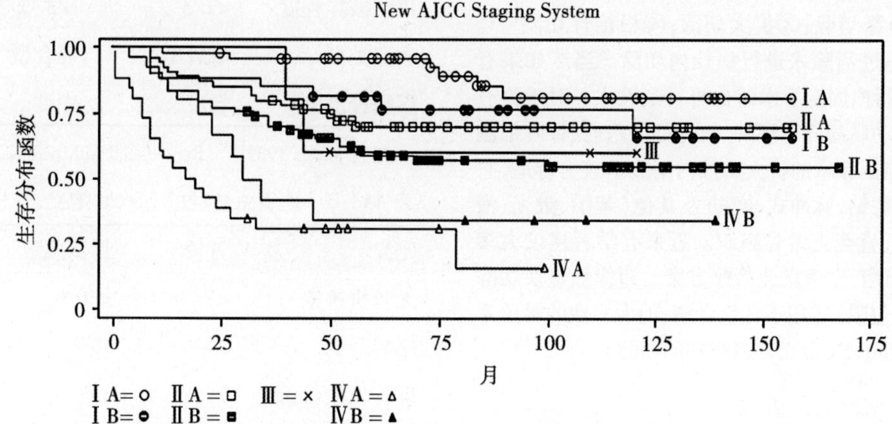

图 111-1 根据新的 AJCC 骨肿瘤分期系统的不同分期的生存率。摘自 ACS 2014[1]。Reproduced with permission of The American Cancer Society

活检

当仅通过影像学评估后仍不能明确诊断肿瘤为良性时，就应当进行活检。当静息性肿瘤，如非骨化性纤维瘤、单发骨囊肿、内生软骨瘤等，可通过临床影像学诊断的话，一般不需要活检。某些活跃性的肿瘤，如骨纤维结构发育不良、骨内脂肪瘤、骨软骨瘤，如果通过影像学可以诊断的话，也并不一定需要活检。但对于大多数的活跃性肿瘤及所有的侵袭性肿瘤，均需要活检来明确诊断。如果怀疑为高级别肉瘤，则应该新辅助治疗前就进行活检。

因为骨转移癌的治疗与原发骨肿瘤的治疗截然不同，所以当怀疑为转移癌时需要更为慎重。因此，即使明确有易发生骨转移的癌症病史（如乳腺、前列腺、肺、肾、甲状腺癌），首发的骨转移一般也需要通过活检确诊，除非临床资料提示为晚期（已有其他部位的广泛转移）。对怀疑为骨转移癌的患者需要进行活检，但钻孔取得活检标本的方法并不是最好的，因为一旦因穿透病变而使髓内屏障被破坏，所有邻近的相关骨和软组织都有潜在被肿瘤污染的可能。如果病理结果提示为肉瘤，而非转移癌，那么先前未受累的组织也发生了不必要的污染。

有 4 种适用于骨肿瘤的活检技术：①细针活检；②粗针活检；③切开活检；④切除活检。细针活检（FNA）仅可提供细胞进行细胞学检验，通常在影像学引导下完成。FNA 应用在骨肿瘤时，针对 2 种临床情况：①强烈怀疑为骨肿瘤时（骨转移癌、复发的肉瘤）；②取出病变较为困难的部位（脊椎、骨盆、肩胛骨）。粗针活检有助于解释除了细胞学细节外组织结构的异常。对于骨及软组织的肿瘤，粗针活检的应用范围与 FNA 相似。切开活检则可提供足够多的组织进行组织学鉴定，但若进行切开活检需要考虑到的是，无论最终诊断如何，切开活检应由将来施行根治性切除术的同一名医生来完成[11,12]。切除活检通常只用于如骨软骨瘤这样的骨肿瘤，因为它可通过影像学诊断，切除的并发症很小，且位置表浅，较易切除。

手术切缘

根据不同的骨肿瘤类型应选择更恰当的手术切除方式。选用不同的术式就会有不同的手术切缘。共有 4 种切除方式：①病灶内切除；②边缘切除；③扩大切除；④根治性切除[13]。多数良性骨肿瘤可通过刮除术进行病灶内切除。当然如果有必要，骨转移瘤在进行内固定手术时也可行刮除术。对于具有侵袭性的良性肿瘤（动脉瘤样骨囊肿、软骨母细胞瘤、骨巨细胞瘤），选择有别于单纯刮除术的扩大病灶内刮除术较为合适，它利用了机械性（高速磨钻、脉冲式冲洗）及其他（苯酚、激光、液氮）技术来扩大切缘，直至正常骨组织。近来有学者建议大多数肢端低级别软骨肉瘤，也考虑此治疗方案。边缘性整块切除（包括肿瘤周围的假包膜）适用于骨软骨瘤，但大多数的骨骼系统肉瘤应采用扩大切除术（带正常组织袖的切除）。

保肢术与截肢术

在保肢与截肢之间选择时必须要考虑 2 个方面：肿瘤学安全性与肢体功能。首先，如果选择行保肢术，从肿瘤学的角度来说，患者预期的生存期不应低于行截肢术的生存期。前瞻性提出此问题，在选择适当患者时，保肢患者预期生存时间不应少于截肢患者[14,15]。但是对于患者个体，治疗方案的决定仍需谨慎。肿瘤学安全性需考虑 2 个因素：化疗的敏感性（如果可行）及手术切缘。化疗的敏感性越差，局部复发的可能性就越大，与采用何种切缘无关。因此，对于化疗敏感性差的患者（肿瘤进展），就相对不适于保肢。骨骼系统肉瘤手术的目标是扩大切除，并不是全部进行保肢手术，详尽的术前计划确定适宜的截肢水平同样能达到手术目的。如果肉瘤侵犯的周围软组织中存在重要的结构（主要的血管及神经），此时为了切除肿瘤，不得不同时切除其中重要的结构，那么此时对于保肢术则为禁忌证，选择截肢术就更为合适。

就肿瘤学安全性来说，如果选择了保肢术，那么重建后的预期功能应至少与相应水平截肢术后的功能相仿。对于下肢胫骨远端病变，膝下平面截肢术后的下肢功能总体上要优于胫骨远端重建术，因而此时相对较适于行截肢术。针对上肢，如果能保留 3 支主要神经（桡神经、尺神经、正中神经）其中的 2 支，即可选择保肢术。如果上肢主要神经中一支以上的神经和/或腋窝及肱动静脉被肿瘤包绕，则是截肢术的适应证。

转移癌、骨髓瘤及淋巴瘤的手术治疗

转移癌、骨髓瘤及淋巴瘤的骨病变有 4 种情况可能需要手术治疗：①活检病理确诊；②对即将发生的病理性骨折进行预防性内固定；③手术固定病理性骨折；④整块切除孤立的病灶。先前已经讨论过活检，但未充分强调的是：需在手术治疗前明确诊断。对发生骨折的风险预测手段正在不断发展。现今对骨折的预测基于临床及影像学标准。Mirels 设计了由 4 个因素组成的等级评定系统[16]（表 111-5 和表 111-6）。Mirels 评分系统经验上可行，但其特异性较低，大约只有 33%[17]。基于 CT 生物力学分析的评估研究正在进行中[18]。

表 111-5 骨转移癌病理性骨折风险预测 Mirels 评分系统

	1分	2分	3分
解剖部位	上肢	下肢	转子周围
皮质破坏程度	<1/3	1/3~2/3	>2/3
病变类型	成骨型	混合型	溶骨型
疼痛程度	轻度	中度	影响功能

摘自 Mirels 1989[16]. Reproduced with permission from Wiley。

表 111-6 基于总分数的 Mirels 定义、骨折风险及治疗建议

定义	分数	骨折风险	建议
无骨折迹象	<7	<10%	观察
临界骨折	8	15%	考虑固定
即将发生骨折	9	33%	预防性固定
即将发生骨折	>10	>50%	预防性固定

摘自 Mirels 1989[16]. Reproduced with permission from Wiley。

当广泛播散的恶性肿瘤患者发生病理性骨折时，尽管这些患者的生存期有限，但是通常为了改善功能而进行内固定手术。而无法耐受手术的垂死或临终前患者，发生病理性骨折通常采用非手术治疗。为了患者能从手术治疗中获益，预期生存时间应长于治疗后恢复时间。

在这种情况下，手术固定原则与标准骨折固定的原则不同。因为晚期的病变还会在骨的其他部位发展，所以使用髓内钉固定，而不是钢板/螺钉固定，从而可以保护其他骨骼，尤其在长骨中是更好的选择。众所周知，转移癌及骨髓瘤病例，骨折愈合非常缓慢，因此制订术前计划时，不妨假设骨折可能将不愈合。因此常见以骨水泥进行即时固定，目的在于缩短患者功能受损后的恢复时间。已经证实，术后放疗有助于功能的恢复，并降低再手术的概率[19]。

重建方案的选择

良性骨肿瘤

良性骨肿瘤行刮除术后的骨缺损可用自体骨、人工骨、合成骨或骨水泥来填充[20]。骨水泥常应用于骨巨细胞瘤行扩大病灶内刮除术后骨缺损的填充。骨水泥能够即刻提供充分承重的固定，且在凝固过程中的产热可以扩大外科边界，并形成清晰的影像学边界，如发生局部复发则便于后期诊断。在某些情况下，当体积较大的病灶被刮除后，可用髓内针或钢板/螺钉行预防性固定来避免骨折的发生。

原发骨骼系统肉瘤

骨骼系统肉瘤切除术后，大范围骨与周围软组织缺损的重建可有多种选择方案。对于患者个体，选择恰当的重建方式需要考虑到患者的年龄、预期效果、预后、辅助治疗、手术类型及解剖部位等因素。一般来讲，重建技术包括人工关节假体置换、结构性异体骨移植、同种异体骨-假体复合物、血管化骨移植等。随着时间的推移，人工关节假体置换、同种异体骨-假体复合物的使用逐渐增多，而结构性异体骨移植的使用逐渐减少。除了同种异体骨-假体复合物，结构性异体骨移植的主要作用是重建骨干的缺损（缺损上下方的关节均可保留时）。最常见的切除肉瘤的类型是关节内切除术（切除包括关节面的骨骼），需要重建关节表面，常行关节的置换。如肿瘤侵入关节，则应用关节外切除术（从关节的两侧截除），这时使用同种异体骨行关节融合往往是更好的重建方案。

患者的年龄是需要考虑的主要因素，因为骨骼未成熟的患者可能发展成为双侧肢体不等长，但如果行重建术时考虑到了这一点，对术侧骨骼生长停滞造成的长度缺失进行代偿，则可避免双侧肢体不等长的发生。对于 8 岁以下的患者，很有可能发生肢体不等长，致使标准的重建方案根本无济于事，这种情况处理起来较为棘手，可考虑截肢、旋转成形术、保留骨骺的带血管蒂腓骨瓣移植等[21~27]。下肢的旋转成形术是在膝关节周围的肿瘤切除术后，将足及踝从正常旋转至 180 度重建，这样足跟可向前运动，踝部活动与患者膝部相协调。在这种情况下，患者肢体功能类似膝下截肢，而不必一定要接受膝上截肢术。8 岁以上的患者，能够使用可延长假体进行重建[28~32]。近些年来，这种非侵入性可延长假体的临床应用引人注目[31]，但其并发症的发生率较高，并且患者骨骼成熟后其耐久性也是个问题[33]。

上肢

在肩部骨的恶性肿瘤切除术后进行重建，其功能取决于肿瘤切除时是否保留三角肌[34,35]。如果肱骨近端的肿瘤侵犯三角肌，必须要切除三角肌才可以实现扩大的切缘，无论采用何种重建方式，肩关节功能都会很差。如果保留三角肌，多采用同种异体骨-假体复合物进行功能重建[36]。这种重建方法可以将保留的肩袖肌腱与同种异体肌腱缝合，以求改进其功能。如果选择骨关节的异体骨移植重建，术后并发症风险增加，包括同种异体移植骨连接处不愈合、骨折、软骨下塌陷等。肩胛骨及肱骨所有的部分可通过假体来重建。上肢远端是骨骼系统肉瘤发生的少见部位。

下肢

保留肢体的骨盆肉瘤切除术（内半骨盆切除术），如能保留髋关节（如前方耻骨支/坐骨支的切除和髋臼以上的髂骨切除），则无须进行重建，一些外科医生甚至将累及髋臼的肿瘤切除后都不予重建。内半骨盆切除术后的髋臼和髋关节有多种重建方法，但也有很多并发症[37,38]。股骨近端的重建可采用半关节成形术（置换股骨头，而不处理髋臼），也可采用同种异体骨-假体复合物重建[39~41]，将臀部外展肌与同种异体肌腱缝合进行重建，有利于增加稳定性和保持正常步态。

大多数股骨远端的重建采用股骨远端人工假体行全膝关节重建。胫骨近端肿瘤切除后需要重建伸膝装置，通过将髌韧带缝合至胫骨粗隆来实现，此时可采用胫骨近端假体进行全膝关节重建或同种异体骨-假体复合物重建。无论采取何种重建方式，都可用腓肠肌内侧头覆盖同种异体移植物和/或假体同时重建伸膝装置。用同种异体骨-假体复合物重建胫骨近端时，患者剩余的髌韧带可与同种异体肌腱缝合，以进一步完善伸膝装置的重建。

并发症

骨骼系统肉瘤重建和修复后的并发症非常多，且较常见。所有的重建术后都担心感染，特别是术后大死腔的形成、辅助治疗后的伤口延迟愈合、化疗诱导的中性粒细胞减少。然而，某些并发症的发生与特定的解剖位置和重建的类型相关。胫骨近端因局部缺乏软组织覆盖而特别容易感染。肩关节与髋关节行定制人工假体重建时，常可发生关节不稳，甚至完全脱位。所有人工假体都存在松动的可能，但假体的寿命尚可接受（近端股骨-90%，远端股骨-60%，近端胫骨-50%）[42]。值得关注的是，与以往常用的关节成形术不同的新的内固定术式已经出现，目前正在进行密切随访[43]。据报道在膝关节周围使用这种方法，显示 10 年生存率达 80%[44]。同种异体骨与宿主骨的连接处不易愈合，当仅使用同种异体骨重建时尤可发生，进而引起骨折。

骨肿瘤的放射治疗

放射治疗在治疗原发性骨肿瘤中作用有限，它主要应用于骨转移癌、骨髓瘤和淋巴瘤等骨病损的局部治疗。放射治疗一般不用于良性骨肿瘤的治疗，但对发生于脊柱、症状明显的顽固性组织细胞增多症,低剂量放疗一直是其有效的治疗方案[45]。骨骼系统的肉瘤中,放疗可用于尤因肉瘤的治疗,但却不是骨肉瘤或软骨肉瘤的标准治疗方法。

骨辐射的潜在并发症包括放射后肉瘤、自发和脆性骨折、骨坏死、小儿生长停滞或成角畸形等。放射后肉瘤通常发生在放射暴露至少 3 年后,接受的平均剂量约为 50Gy[46]。放射后骨折的危险因素包括骨膜剥离、新辅助化疗、病变发生于股骨、高剂量辐射、圆周照射等[47]。因其难于治疗、治疗时间长及较高的骨折不愈合率(45%~67%),所以需要多次手术治疗或彻底的骨切除/重建术和/或截肢术,因而放射后骨折受到越来越多的关注[47]。

骨肿瘤的药物治疗

骨肿瘤药物治疗的地位逐步提升。一般而言,对于高级别骨骼系统肉瘤,化疗可以系统性消灭肉眼不可见的病变。骨骼系统肉瘤的化疗通常首先在手术前进行(新辅助化疗),在手术或者放疗后继续完成。因此,治疗典型的高级别骨肉瘤和尤因肉瘤时,均先进行新辅助化疗。但化疗应用于低级别的软骨肉瘤则没有明确的意义。

使用二磷酸盐抑制破骨细胞介导的骨破坏已成为治疗骨髓瘤和多数骨转移癌的标准方法,其中包括乳腺癌、前列腺癌和肺癌[48]。最近,二磷酸盐药物也用于适应证之外的某些良性骨病变,包括纤维发育不良和骨巨细胞瘤,但其疗效尚未确定。值得关注的是,应用二磷酸盐有发生下颌骨坏死和非典型性股骨近端转子下骨折的风险[48,49]。

常见的良性骨肿瘤

软骨源性肿瘤

软骨源性肿瘤可以分为成熟的透明软骨源性肿瘤(软骨瘤和骨软骨瘤)和未成熟软骨源性肿瘤(软骨母细胞瘤和软骨黏液样纤维瘤)。

软骨瘤

在 WHO 分类中"软骨瘤"标题下包括内生软骨瘤和骨膜软骨瘤。内生软骨瘤是位于髓内的良性透明软骨肿瘤,骨膜软骨瘤是生长于骨表面的软骨肿瘤。内生软骨瘤病(多发性内生软骨瘤/Ollier 病和 Maffucci 综合征)则在先天性综合征部分来进行讨论。Maffucci 综合征表现为多发内生软骨瘤同时伴血管瘤。

内生软骨瘤在原发骨肿瘤中相对常见,约占总数的 17%。这类肿瘤很可能来源于未成熟骨的透明软骨生长板。这类病变绝大多数无症状,或由于其他原因引起疼痛行 X 线检查而偶然发现的[50]。内生软骨瘤是发生于手足短管状骨的最常见骨病变。在长管状骨中,好发于股骨(常因髋部或膝部疼痛而行 X 线检查时发现)和肱骨(常因肩部疼痛而行影像学评估时发现)。单发的内生软骨瘤位于扁平骨者少见,但发生在该部位的软骨病变需要考虑软骨肉瘤的可能。因为透明软骨的影像学特点很典型,所以最需要与内生软骨瘤鉴别的疾病是软骨肉瘤。

内生软骨瘤随着自然病程的进展逐渐钙化。因此,成人中发生的内生软骨瘤常常显示出弧形或环形的特征性点状钙化灶,其特征性的改变使医生单纯通过影像学检查而不需要活检即可确诊该病(图 111-2)。病变处骨内膜常呈扇贝样改变。然而,当这些病变出现骨膜反应,超出骨皮质之外,广泛骨皮质破坏,软组织肿物形成时,就一定要考虑软骨肉瘤。内生软骨瘤典型的 MRI 表现为分叶状,在 T1 加权像上呈低信号,T2 加权像上呈高信号。骨扫描显像呈摄取增加是内生软骨瘤的典型表现,但它不能作为恶性的标志,因其很可能是周围骨持续重塑所造成的。

在显微镜下,内生软骨瘤是由良性、稀疏的透明软骨构成,但是细胞结构和异型性的程度是可以变化的。在手指和其他小骨等特定部位的内生软骨瘤,尽管其呈良性行为,但其组织学特征却呈现出更强的侵袭性。

绝大多数内生软骨瘤,尤其是无症状性病变且具有典型影像学表现者,可仅行观察以确保病变不再进展。然而,无论是影像学改变还是所引起的疼痛使诊断不确定时,病变部位均应行彻底的刮除术和全面的组织学检查以区别软骨肉瘤。软骨性病变在刮除术后很少复发。

相反,骨膜软骨瘤是完全不同的良性透明软骨病变。常因手指、足趾的肿块或其他部位的轻度疼痛而发现。X 线片上在

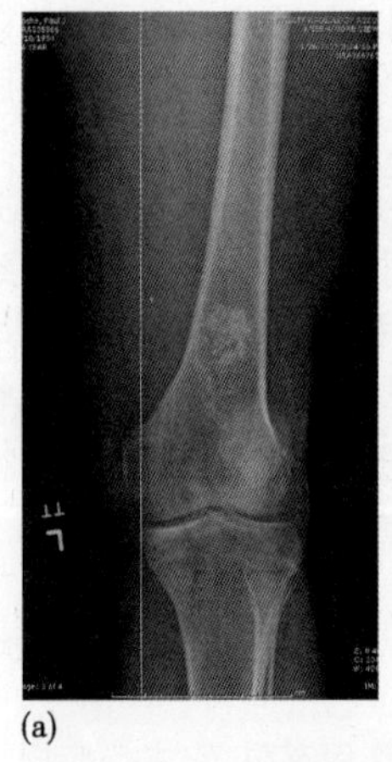
(a)

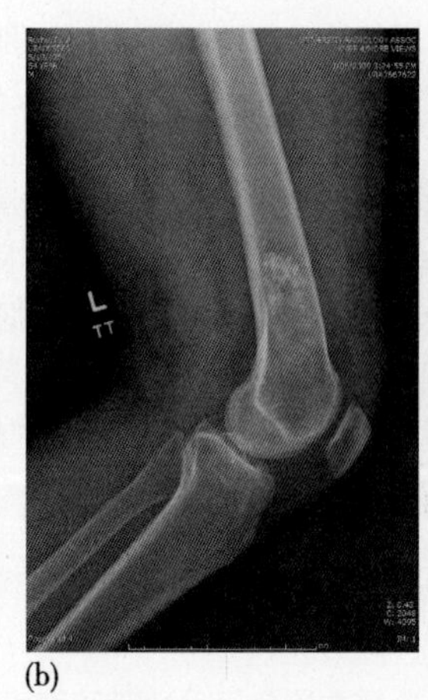
(b)

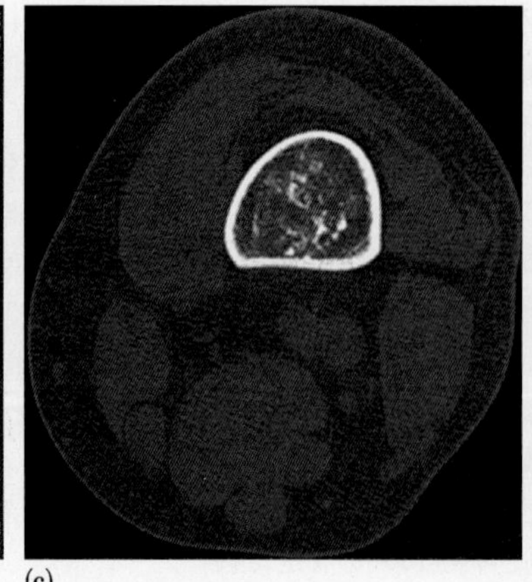
(c)

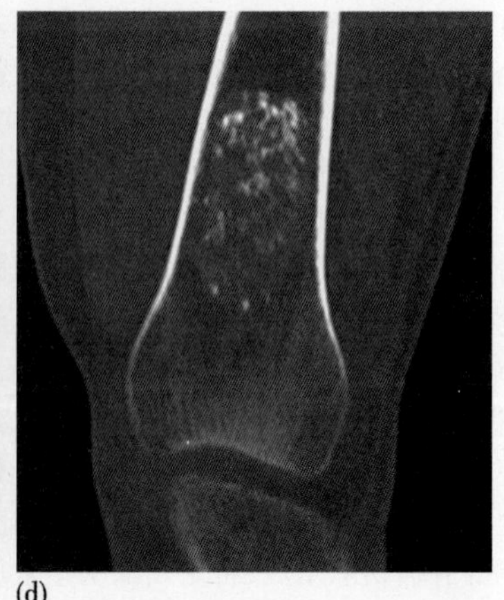
(d)

图 111-2 股骨远端 X 线正位像(a)侧位像(b)及其横切面(c)冠状面(d)CT 扫描显示特征性的弧形或环形的点状透明软骨,没有提示病变为软骨肉瘤的明显的骨内膜扇贝样改变和皮质破坏

病变表面呈典型的蝶形凹陷。骨膜软骨瘤需要与皮质旁软骨肉瘤相鉴别。较小的病变(小于 7cm)常是骨膜软骨瘤。根据肿瘤位置,骨膜软骨瘤可通过刮除术或整块切除来治疗。

软骨母细胞瘤

这种未成熟的软骨来源的肿瘤是一种不常见的良性病变,以关节疼痛为典型特征,诊断较困难,好发于长骨骨骺[51]。绝大多数病例发生在未成熟骨,表现为关节疼痛(由于位于长骨骨端),类似常见病的症状。由于病变初期只有微小的影像学改变,使疾病在很长一段时间难以诊断。该病可以累及多处骨骼,但最常见的部位是肱骨近端、股骨远端和胫骨近端。

由于未成熟软骨通常难以出现透明软骨病变中的特征性钙化,因而其在 X 线上的表现常不明显。另外,软骨母细胞瘤在骺端圆形的射线透亮区常没有明显的硬化边包绕。在 MRI 上更易看出,软骨母细胞瘤在 T1 加权像上呈低信号,T2 加权像上呈高信号,而且表现出广泛的病变周围的水肿。骨扫描可见病灶的核素浓聚。

组织学上,软骨母细胞瘤以"鹅卵石"样排列的圆形细胞为主,清晰可见的胞核内凹呈"咖啡豆"样。还可见到巨细胞和软骨基质。

软骨母细胞瘤虽然常常只表现为活跃的病变,但它也可表现出侵袭性,治疗的时候必须考虑到这一点。扩大的瘤内刮除术仍是软骨母细胞瘤的经典治疗手段,但是近期采用 RFA 治疗入选病例获得相当成功的结果[52]。当 RFA 治疗位于负重软骨面下体积大的病灶时,必须考虑到塌陷的风险[52]。软骨母细胞瘤是具有肺转移潜能的两种良性骨病变之一(另一种是骨巨细胞瘤)。因此术前和术后随访一定要注意肺部的情况。

软骨黏液样纤维瘤

软骨黏液样纤维瘤与软骨母细胞瘤一样,也是一种未成熟软骨来源的良性肿瘤[53]。不同的是,它好发于长骨干骺端,与骺板毗邻。软骨黏液样纤维瘤是一种罕见肿瘤,只占骨肿瘤总数的百分之一。最常累及的长骨是胫骨。这类肿瘤有 1/3 发生在扁平骨。疼痛是软骨黏液样纤维瘤的主要症状。

软骨黏液样纤维瘤的影像学特征包括病变常位于干骺端,偏心,分叶状的溶骨改变,无基质矿化的皂泡样改变,以及相应的骨皮质变薄。在某些情况下,由于伴有骨皮质的破坏甚至软组织的侵犯,外观看起来像侵袭性肿瘤(图 111-3)。在显微镜下,肿瘤呈小叶状排列,更多的细胞聚集在肿瘤外围,黏液样中心只聚有少量散在的细胞。典型的细胞呈"星形"。

治疗主要是刮除植骨术。局部复发率在 15%~25%。软骨黏液样纤维瘤不发生转移。

骨软骨瘤

骨软骨瘤是最常见的骨肿瘤,它是生长软骨在远离骺板

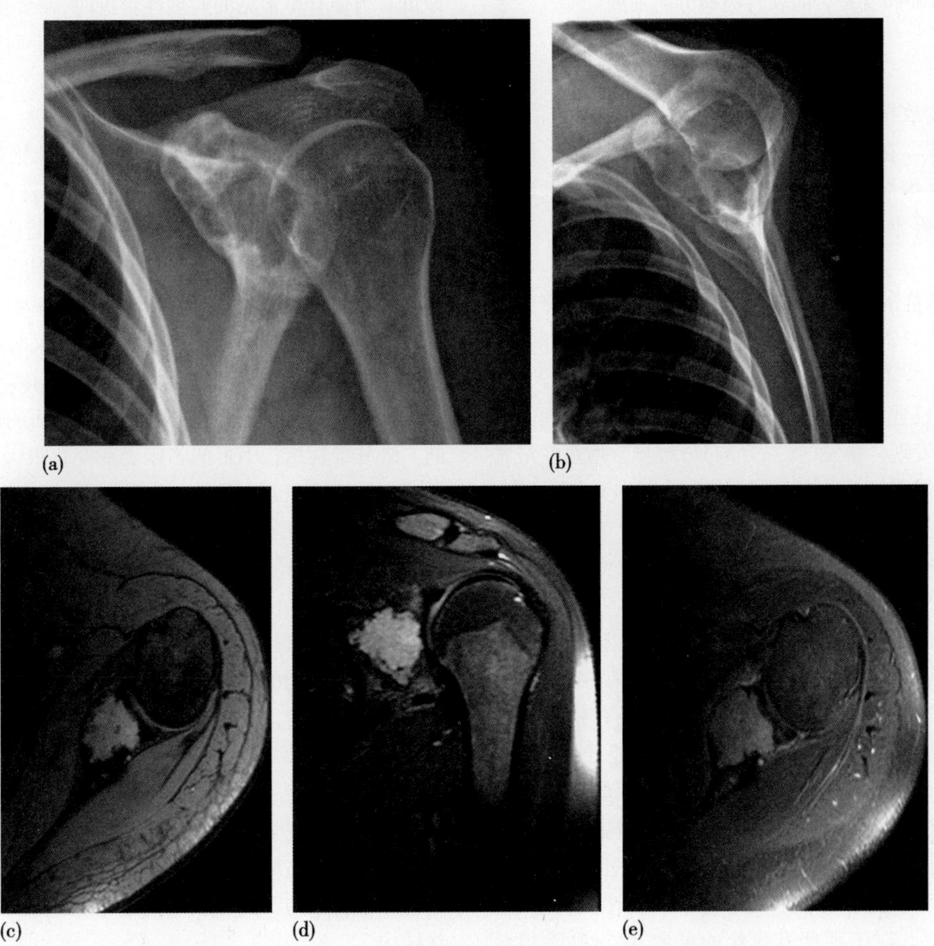

图 111-3　软骨黏液样纤维瘤。肩部正位像(a)、肩胛 Y 位(b)、T2 加权像横断面(c)、冠状面(d)、质子密度横断面(e)MR 显示了软骨黏液样纤维瘤的征象,这一例病变发生在扁骨——肩胛骨。皮质变薄,病灶的皮质破坏是侵袭性行为的特征,易与软骨肉瘤混淆

和关节的部位发生外生型生长所形成的肿瘤，且与长骨生长的某一阶段有关联[54]。伴随着软骨的生长，遗留下来有或无蒂的骨突起。这类肿瘤在骨骼未成熟时期形成和生长，在骨骼成熟时期停止生长，如果不将其切除，肿瘤将伴随终身。它可以表现为疼痛或无痛的肿块。疼痛常是由于肿瘤表面覆盖的软组织的刺激或滑囊炎，但也可由肿瘤蒂部的骨折或恶性变引起。恶性变在孤立的骨软骨瘤很少见，但在具有家族史的患者中较常见，即多发性遗传性外生性骨疣（见先天性综合征部分）。

骨软骨瘤的X线平片即可确诊。肿瘤常表现为干骺端的外生型突起，其特点是骨皮质和骨髓的连续性。当肿瘤有蒂时，骨软骨瘤的软骨帽常指向远离邻近关节的一端。MRI有时用来评估软骨帽的厚度，其厚度在儿童时期有时可达到3cm。然而，成人的软骨帽多在1.5cm以下，较厚的软骨帽应该怀疑由骨软骨瘤起源的软骨肉瘤。在显微镜下，骨软骨瘤可见一良性的透明软骨帽覆盖在正常骨小梁上。

骨软骨瘤的治疗基于患者的症状和临床体征。当患者没有症状时可以考虑观察。当儿童患骨软骨瘤伴有疼痛时，可以考虑切除。儿童的年龄越大，病变距骺板越远，复发的可能性越小。在成人，任何有症状的或有增长的骨软骨瘤应该进一步行MRI检查，以明确病变是否向软骨肉瘤方向发展[54]。

纤维性肿瘤

以下三种病变放在一起讨论是因为其组织学相似性，它们均由纤维组织构成。在最近的WHO骨病变分类系统中，纤维异常增殖症和骨纤维性结构不良都被列为“未明确肿瘤性质的肿瘤”。非骨化性纤维瘤被列为纤维组织细胞性肿瘤[3]。

纤维异常增殖症

纤维异常增殖症的病因被证实为*GNAS*基因突变，突变使骨形成过程中出现异常。它是一种相对常见的骨形成疾病，可在儿童时期发病，亦可在成年时得出诊断。临床表现基于年龄、病变的数目和位置而呈多样化。患者常因疼痛或病理性骨折就诊，也可偶然发现。单发的（孤立的）纤维异常增殖症最常见于颅骨，其次是股骨、胫骨和肋骨。多发性纤维异常增殖症（相对于单发者少见）最常累及股骨、骨盆和胫骨。多发性纤维异常增殖症也称McCune-Albright综合征（见先天性综合征部分）和Mazabraud综合征（相关的肌内黏液瘤）。

X线上，纤维性结构不良通常表现为地图型溶骨性病变。在长骨，这类病变常常被描述为“长骨中的长病变”。它们可以影响骨的任何一部分（骺、干骺端和骨干），而且有特征性的“毛玻璃”样改变。在股骨近端，广泛的受累可能导致“牧羊拐”样畸形。在Tc99骨扫描上摄取增高。在显微镜下，未成熟的编织样骨被描述为“汉字样”，缺少骨纤维结构不良中可见的成骨细胞环绕，周围可见稀疏的成纤维细胞。

治疗基于年龄、位置和症状。当影像学表现比较典型，且无症状时可以观察。对于那些有症状的患者，可行刮除植骨术，但是结构性植骨更可取，因为颗粒性植骨通常被吸收。在股骨近端的纤维性结构不良常要考虑预防性固定，此处病变的小梁骨杂乱无序，易于发生应力性骨折，并反复重塑。对于有症状的多发性纤维异常增殖症，二磷酸盐治疗有一定的效果[55,56]。

非骨化性纤维瘤和纤维皮质缺损

非骨化性纤维瘤和纤维皮质缺损属于未成熟骨发育异常的不同表现形式[57]。纤维皮质缺损相对较小，多局限在皮质，然而非骨化性纤维瘤相对较大，可延伸至骨髓腔。它们如此多见以至于被认为是正常的变异体。因膝关节受伤急诊医治的儿童，1/3的都可发现一处或多处这类病变。它们常无任何症状，检查时被偶然发现。少数病例是在骨折之后被发现的，其特点是骨折之前无疼痛史。无疼痛说明了这类病变属于静止型，没有活跃的特征。长骨干骺端是这类病变最常见的部位，尤其是膝关节周围。

几乎所有的这类病变可以在X线片上得以确诊。其特征性的表现有至少一部分位于皮质内，常发生在干骺端，偏心，皂泡样溶骨性改变，边界呈地图形，病变周围存在薄层硬化边。如有必要可行磁共振成像，其特征是在T1和T2加权像上均呈低信号。无骨折发生时病变周围无水肿。极少数情况下，需要行活检来确诊，此类情况下其病理学特征为席纹状、旋涡状成纤维细胞的背景下伴有散在的巨细胞。

对于绝大多数纤维皮质缺损和非骨化性纤维瘤仅行观察即可。当伴有不常见的病理性骨折时，需要根据骨折部位和类型决定治疗方案，当需要行手术内固定时应同时行刮除植骨术。

骨纤维性结构不良

过去，骨纤维性结构不良又称为骨化性纤维瘤或Campanacci病[57]。在纤维性肿瘤中，骨纤维性结构不良具有独特性，在于它的发病部位（几乎均发生在胫骨前面）和组织学特点（骨岛被成骨细胞包绕，从而与纤维性结构分开）。该病基本上属于儿童时期发生的肿瘤，绝大多数在8岁以前发病，且多发生于在相对表浅的骨骼内（胫骨、腓骨、尺骨、桡骨），可以双侧发病或在同一骨内存在多发病灶。它应该与造釉细胞瘤相鉴别，造釉细胞瘤也是一种好发于胫骨前面的肿瘤，但它是恶性的。骨纤维性结构不良的临床表现变化很大，一些患者因胫骨无痛性肿块而发现，还有一些患者因应力性骨折而发生间歇痛，少数患者发展为胫骨弓形弯曲。

影像学上，绝大多数骨纤维性结构不良呈现为胫骨中上1/3的溶骨性病灶，偏心、皂泡样或锯齿样外观。对于老年患者，其影像学表现与造釉细胞瘤类似，需要进一步的鉴别。与造釉细胞瘤不同的是，骨纤维性结构不良在MRI上没有软组织侵犯。作为一种活跃的病变，骨纤维性结构不良在骨扫描上摄取增高。在显微镜下需要与骨纤维性结构不良鉴别的疾病有纤维异常增殖症和造釉细胞瘤。骨纤维性结构不良与纤维异常增殖症均表现为在良性纤维组织背景中有编织状骨岛，不同的是前者的骨岛周围存在成骨细胞环。与造釉细胞瘤鉴别点是骨纤维性结构不良不表现为恶性程度更高的上皮细胞样岛状结构。

骨纤维性结构不良的治疗基于年龄、症状和影像学表现。在骺板闭合之前，无临床症状、影像学典型表现的病变，仅需观察即可。当发生应力性骨折时，应该考虑支具治疗。若影像学表现不典型,应行活检进一步诊断。外科切除±植骨术仅适用于有进行性畸形或骨骼成熟后有症状的患者。由于刮除植骨后复发率高,有学者建议对所有患者行骨膜外切除[58]。

巨细胞肿瘤

骨巨细胞瘤是一种相对常见(占所有骨肿瘤的 5%~10%)的良性骨肿瘤,以其独特的组织学和生物学行为特征[59]。在最新的 WHO 分类系统中,它分为一种"富于巨细胞的破骨细胞肿瘤"。它是具有潜在侵袭性表现的四种良性骨肿瘤之一(同动脉瘤样骨囊肿、软骨母细胞瘤和骨母细胞瘤一起)。除此之外,同软骨母细胞瘤一样,它虽然是良性肿瘤,但却有肺转移的潜能。由于巨细胞瘤具有典型的生长活跃和侵袭性强的行为特点,其临床表现常为疼痛、肿胀、邻近关节功能障碍和病理性骨折。骨巨细胞瘤多发生于成人,高峰年龄为 20~40 岁。罕见发生于未成熟骨骼患者。最好发于膝关节(股骨远端和胫骨近端)、腕关节(桡骨远端)、骶骨和肩关节(肱骨近端)周围。

在影像学上,骨巨细胞瘤多位于长骨干骺端,常常延及骺板,呈偏心、透亮的病灶,并有虫蚀状边缘,呈 1C 型,常延及邻近关节的软骨下骨。但在骨骼未成熟的患者,病变常位于干骺端。骨巨细胞瘤呈纯溶骨性病变,无基质钙化,影像学上可见到皮质破坏和软组织浸润的侵袭性表现。尽管在组织学上骨巨细胞瘤的主要特征是多核巨细胞,但是真正的肿瘤细胞是作为背景的细胞核均匀一致为特征的基质细胞。

骨巨细胞瘤的局部治疗取决于病变部位。在可以弃置的部位,如腓骨近端和尺骨远端,适合选择整块切除。然而,对于大多数部位,推荐的治疗方法是彻底的病灶内刮除术加植骨术或骨水泥填充术。彻底的刮除术包括机械刮除(刮匙)和高速磨钻外,还有其他残腔边缘的处理方法(如苯酚、液氮或激光)。骨巨细胞瘤在仅行病灶内刮除术时局部复发率为 30%~47%,但彻底的刮除术后局部复发率仅为 25%[59]。对骨巨细胞瘤患者的全程治疗包括潜在肺转移的评估及局部复发的早期诊断。术后 20 年还有复发的报道[59]。对"不能手术切除的"骨巨细胞瘤,治疗的选择包括:放疗、栓塞治疗或地诺单抗(denosumab)。地诺单抗是一种 RANK 配体抑制剂,具有抑制骨巨细胞瘤中基质细胞聚集形成巨细胞的能力[60]。尽管使用地诺单抗早期效果令人鼓舞,但长期使用的疗效以及其副作用仍然有待进一步研究[61]。

骨血管瘤

骨血管瘤是脊柱最常见的骨良性肿瘤,它源于血管的增殖,在其他部位很少见。绝大多数的骨血管瘤,尤其是脊柱的血管瘤都是无症状的,因而常是偶然情况下发现的。如有任何临床症状,都要在除外血管瘤的情况下究其原因。极少数情况下,它会引起骨的膨胀性改变或病理性骨折。在脊柱,这些情况可能累及神经系统。

在脊柱,骨血管瘤的影像学表现很典型,因此大多数情况下不需要活检来确诊。在 X 线片上病变呈栅栏样纵条纹改变。CT 和 MRI 扫描横切面上病变呈"波尔卡圆点状"改变。在 MRI T2 加权像上骨血管瘤呈高信号,加入造影剂后,病变显示得更清楚强化明显。当影像学不典型时,活检可显示大小不一的良性血管,表现为多种组织学亚型。在脊柱以外的部位,影像学表现多样,常常需要行活检。

由于多数血管瘤都是无症状的,因此仅需观察即可。对于少见的真正有症状的、"非典型"或"侵袭性"病灶,可以考虑切除、放疗、栓塞术和硬化治疗[62]。

成骨性肿瘤

内生骨疣

内生骨疣,又叫骨岛,是髓腔内松质骨出现的局灶致密层状骨[63]。内生骨疣是良性潜在型病变,无任何症状,多由其他原因行影像学检查时被偶然发现。当发生在成人时,常被考虑为常染色体显性遗传的脆弱性骨硬化的一部分。当出现多发性病变时,则需要与成骨性转移瘤相鉴别。

在平片和 CT 扫描上,内生骨疣是出现在松质骨内的密集硬化区,但它没有中心瘤巢(可在骨样骨瘤中见到),病灶边缘可见放射样针状骨,在骨扫描上无摄取(除了巨大的内生骨疣)(图 111-4)。通常不需要活检,但在显微镜下可见到成熟的层状骨。

通常不需要治疗。在确诊后仅行观察即可。

骨样骨瘤

骨样骨瘤是一良性成骨性肿瘤,其典型表现为独特的疼

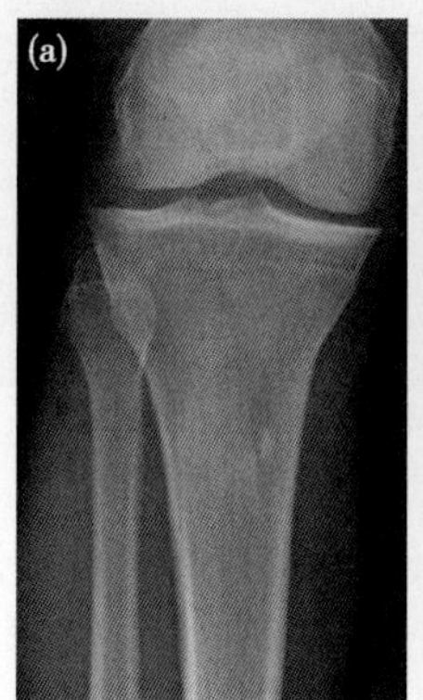

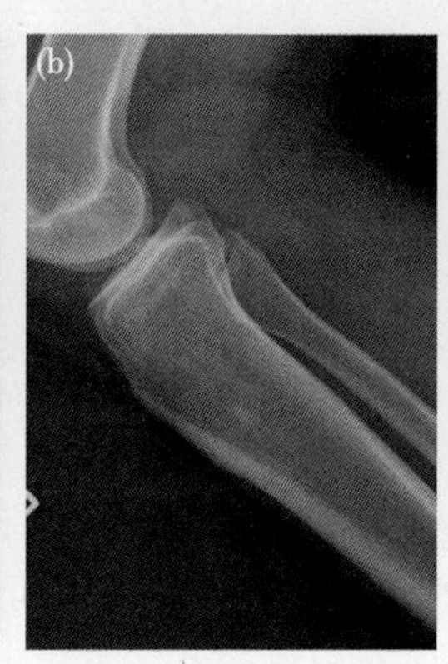

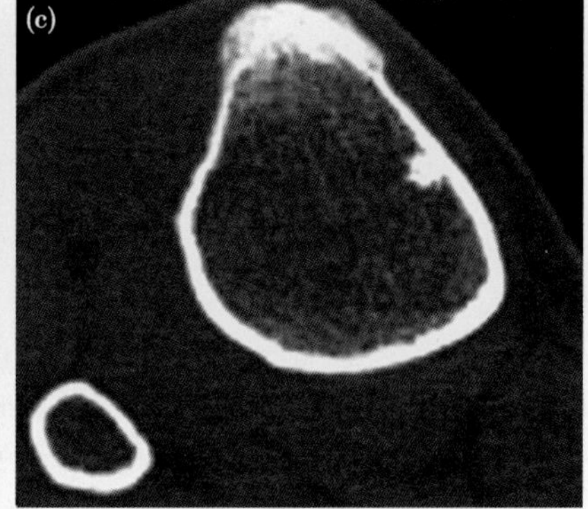

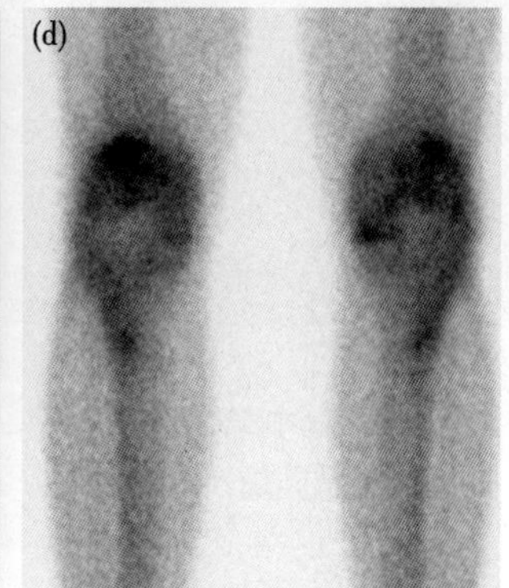

图 111-4　内生骨疣(骨岛)。正位片(a)、侧位片(b)膝关节 X 线片显示了偶然发现的小块不透光的骨病变。CT 横断面(c)显示了特征性的硬化骨边缘周围的放射样骨针,并且与周围骨小梁相互交叉。(d)骨扫描上通常无摄取增加

痛方式，最常见于青少年和年轻的成年人。疼痛特点是夜间痛，而且大多数患者（70%的患者）在服用非甾体抗炎药后的一段时间内（20~30min）疼痛明显减轻或完全消失。据推测非甾体抗炎药的镇痛机制是降低骨样骨瘤病灶内的前列腺素浓度。骨样骨瘤最常发生于股骨和胫骨，它还是椎体附件区最常见的三类肿瘤之一（与骨母细胞瘤和动脉瘤样骨囊肿一同）。在脊柱，骨样骨瘤能引起痛性脊柱侧凸，病变位于侧凸的凹面。当病变位于近关节处时，可能引起渗出性的关节病和滑膜炎。

骨样骨瘤在X线上常表现为直径小于2cm的透亮瘤巢，周围可见致密的硬化的反应骨包绕。病变常位于皮质内，偏心性，反应骨可侵入髓腔或引起骨膨胀。由于反应骨可能很致密，因此只有在CT和MRI上可见到瘤巢。在MRI上，骨样骨瘤的典型表现为病灶周围广泛的水肿带。骨扫描上骨样骨瘤呈高摄取。组织学上，骨样骨瘤瘤巢的特征为不规则排列的矿化类骨质周围被混有成骨细胞和破骨细胞的血管纤维基质包绕。

骨样骨瘤的治疗在不断地完善。现在最主要的手术治疗方式是射频消融（RFA）[65]。首次射频消融治疗后90%的患者症状消失。当RFA不可行时（脊柱病变邻近神经根、近关节处或病变难以定位时），外科切除病灶就会使疼痛症状消失。虽然已经有多种技术来定位瘤巢，但有时术中难以准确定位病灶位置。第三种选择是服用非甾体抗炎药，但是疼痛症状消失的平均治疗期是2.5年。

骨母细胞瘤

骨母细胞瘤与骨样骨瘤有很多共同点，其最主要的区别是瘤巢的体积更大[64]。相同点包括它们潜在的组织学，都好发于青少年和年轻的成年人，多发生于脊柱附件区。不同点包括没有骨样骨瘤典型的疼痛特点，具有潜在的侵袭性及直径大于2cm的瘤巢。除此之外，大部分骨母细胞瘤（70%）发生于脊柱，而发生于长骨者相对少见。

骨母细胞瘤在影像学上除了可见到更大的伴有钙化的瘤巢外，其他影像学表现与骨样骨瘤很相似。显微镜下与骨样骨瘤很相似，可见不规则排列的矿化类骨质周围被混有成骨细胞和破骨细胞的血管纤维基质包绕。

由于其相比较骨样骨瘤有更大的体积和侵袭性，骨母细胞瘤的治疗为彻底的囊内刮除术。术后复发率为10%~30%。在脊柱等手术较为困难的部位复发后可以考虑放疗。

囊肿和其他肿瘤

动脉瘤样骨囊肿

动脉瘤样骨囊肿可以是原发性或继发性病变[66]。原发性动脉瘤样骨囊肿是由致癌基因USP6和启动子*CDH11*的基因重排为特点的瘤性增殖[67,68]。继发性动脉瘤样骨囊肿与其他的原发性骨病变有关，而没有染色体的异[68]。与软骨母细胞瘤、骨巨细胞瘤和骨母细胞瘤一样，动脉瘤样骨囊肿是四种具有侵袭性表现的良性肿瘤之一。其高峰发病年龄为1~20岁，典型的临床表现为疼痛，有时伴有肿胀和/或病理性骨折。动脉瘤样骨囊肿的好发部位是长骨，尤其是股骨和胫骨，但它也是脊柱附件最常见的三种肿瘤之一（与骨样骨瘤和骨母细胞瘤一起）。

X线上，典型的动脉瘤样骨囊肿呈偏心、溶骨性、“吹气球样”外观，周围包绕“蛋壳样”薄层反应骨。然而，并不是在所有的病例都有这样的改变，在平片上，其成像与骨囊肿、非骨化性纤维瘤和纤维异常增殖症等良性病变有相似之处（图111-5）。动脉瘤样骨囊肿的MRI表现为病变被分割成小腔，其内充满血液，有的可见液-液平面。然而，典型的影像学表现并不足以确诊，还需要进一步明确潜在的原发病变。因此，确诊需行活检，以此来区别在影像学上与其相像的毛细血管扩张性骨肉瘤。显微镜下，动脉瘤样骨囊肿内可见充满血液的多个血湖，稀疏的成纤维细胞组成的隔膜将血湖隔开，并可见含铁血黄素沉积和散在的巨细胞。

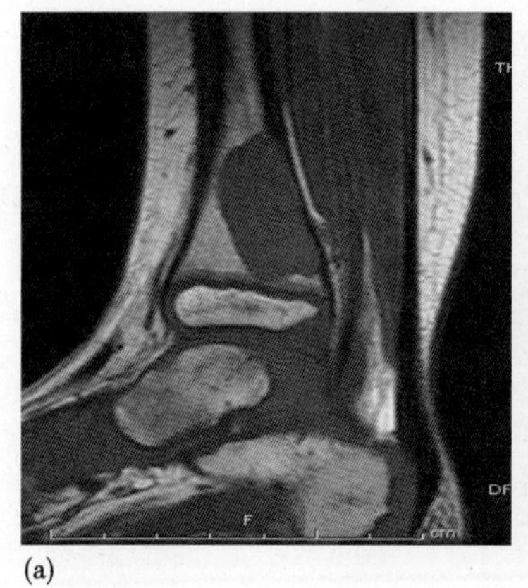
(a)

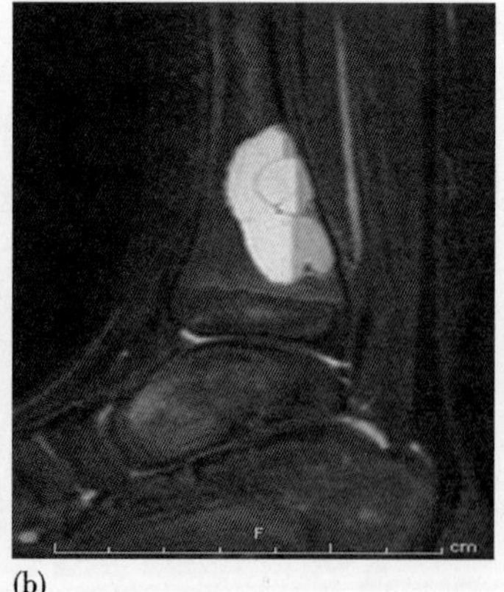
(b)

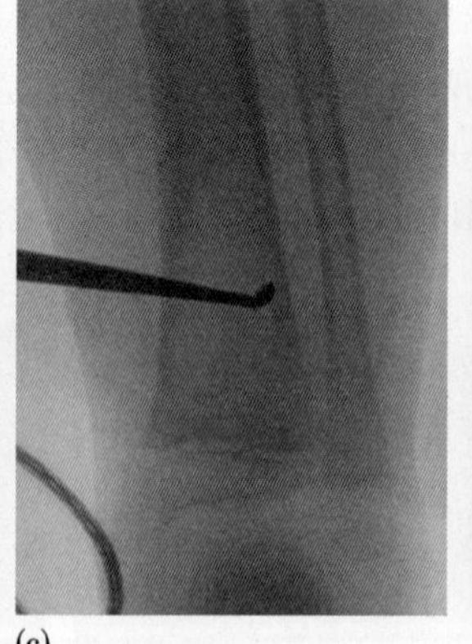
(c)

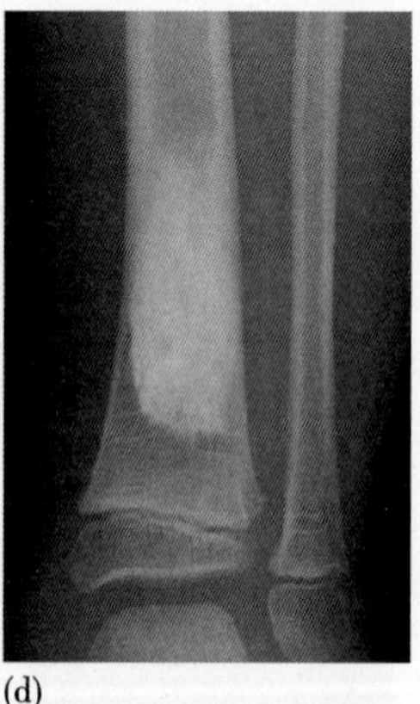
(d)

图111-5 动脉瘤样骨囊肿。4岁患儿，伴有疼痛，MRI显示为透亮的骨病变，病变为典型的液体信号，T1加权矢状位像（a），但是动脉瘤样骨囊肿的分隔和液-液平面的特点在T2加权像上显示的最清楚（b），术中荧光成像（c），这个病变并没有显示出动脉瘤样骨囊肿的侵袭性（气球样皮质）。这个病变用刮匙彻底刮除并用合成的移植物填充（d）

由于动脉瘤样骨囊肿的潜在侵袭性和富含血管组织，它的治疗面临挑战，而且其自然病程有时很难预测[69]。在大多数情况下，常选择彻底的刮除术，进而行全面的组织学检查以发现潜在的原发病变，并与毛细血管扩张型骨肉瘤相鉴别。在刮除术前，应考虑行术前栓塞术，尤其是位于不能用止血带控制出血的部位。术中的大出血可能是致命性的。一些学者建议行栓塞术或抽吸/注射作为治疗方案，但这些方法不能行全面的组织学检查[70]。局部复发并不总以侵袭的方式进展，但必须密切观察。当局部病变未完全切除，病变侵袭性进展，或在手术困难的部位复发时应考虑低剂量放疗。

单纯性骨囊肿

与动脉瘤样骨囊肿相比，单纯性骨囊肿常是不活跃的病变，最坏的情况是活跃性病变。在没有骨折前，它是充满浆液性或血性液体的独立的骨腔。大多数单纯性骨囊肿在儿童时期诊断，常位于肱骨近端、股骨近端和跟骨。在年轻的成人中，更常见于跟骨和髂骨。单纯性骨囊肿在骨折之前常无症状，多数病理性骨折发生在轻微的外伤之后。

X线上，单纯性骨囊肿常位于长骨干骺端或骨干干骺端，呈中心性，在骨折前是完全溶骨性病灶，边缘无明显硬化，有时周围皮质轻度膨胀，但很少能见到骨折后具有诊断意义的“碎片陷落征”。碎片陷落征（落叶征）是骨折的薄片皮质骨垂到囊肿远端。在MRI上，单纯性骨囊肿病变与液体信号是相同的，均为T1加权像上低信号，T2加权像上高信号。病灶边缘强化而中心无强化。在骨折之后的一些病例，血性成分混有浆液性液体可能会产生液-液平面。但是缺少分隔和多种液性成分可用来与单纯性骨囊肿相鉴别。在没发生骨折时，可抽出清亮的浆液性液体，若有骨折，则可能为血性的液体。行刮除术后，组织学检查可发现只有纤维薄膜和散在的组织细胞。

单纯性骨囊肿的治疗基于发病部位、年龄和临床症状。在肱骨近端，应先等待病理性骨折愈合。大约1/7的单纯性骨囊肿发生骨折后会治愈（图111-6）。假如骨折后囊肿仍然存在，那就需要行抽吸术或注射的方法来治疗。常用的注射剂有甲泼尼龙、脱钙骨基质、骨髓或联合应用。一项一级证据的临床研究比较注射骨髓和类固醇的疗效，通过影像学骨愈合标准显示注射类固醇效果更好[71]。在股骨近端的骨囊肿发生骨折的风险更高，骨折后果更严重，因此应考虑行刮除植骨术预防骨折。当位于股骨近端的单纯性骨囊肿发生病理性骨折时，应在切开复位内固定的同时行刮除植骨术。在跟骨和髂骨等部位发生单纯性骨囊肿时，如果无临床症状可行观察，因为这些部位并不常发生骨折。不论哪种治疗方案，大约60%的病变会治愈。另有30%病变会部分痊愈，但有10%的病变会持续存在或复发。单纯性骨囊肿的自然病程必须铭刻在心，在典型部位发生的单纯性骨囊肿随着骨骼的发育成熟会自愈。因此，患者的骨骼越接近成熟，病变的侵袭性越小。

朗格汉斯细胞组织细胞增生症

朗格汉斯细胞组织细胞增生症起源于朗格汉斯细胞组织细胞，它是网状内皮系统的组成成分，参与吞噬外来碎片的，起源于骨髓[45]。朗格汉斯细胞组织细胞增生症包括孤立的嗜酸性肉芽肿、Hand-Christian-Schüller病（包括多发性骨病变、眼球突出和尿崩症）和莱特勒-西韦病（Letterer-Siwe disease）（病变弥散，且常致命）。患者越年轻，越可能是播散性的疾病。大多数播散性疾病的患者都是2岁以下儿童，而嗜酸性肉芽肿的患者最常见于5~20岁。目前LCH的分类包含

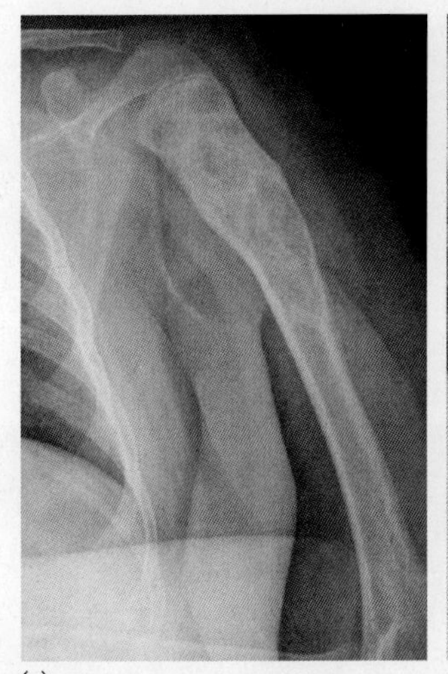
(a)

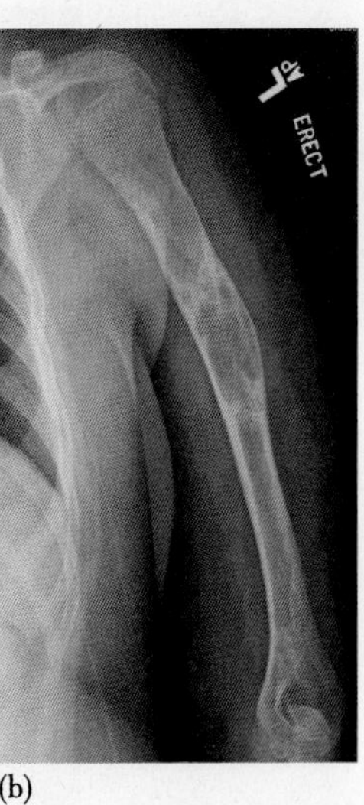

(b)

图111-6 单纯性骨囊肿。9岁儿童，左肱骨正位片（a），肱骨近端处受轻微外伤后导致2次骨折，X线片上可见在肱骨近端邻近骺板处呈溶骨性病变，而且病变正在愈合。单纯性骨囊肿发生骨折后约1/7的患者会自愈。然而，2年后（b）病变复发，肱骨中段透射性增强，肱骨近端骺板距骨囊肿渐远。这类病变在骨骼未成熟时活跃

“非危险”器官（骨、皮肤和淋巴结），“危险”器官（肝脏、脾、肺和骨髓），“中枢神经系统危险”区域（眼眶、乳突、颞骨），后者有形成尿崩症、其他内分泌异常和脑病变的危险。单发非危险部位受累通常认为是一良性疾病[72]。单发的嗜酸性肉芽肿最好发的部位是颅骨、骨盆、肋骨和椎体等扁骨。发生于长骨者则多位于骨干和干骺端。多发病变时，最常累及颅骨、颚骨和手足骨。

朗格汉斯细胞组织细胞增生症的临床表现取决于疾病的阶段。单发病变或多发病变中较孤立的病变常引起局部疼痛或因影响下肢而造成跛行，但也可无症状，因意外发现病变。该病的全身表现包括尿崩症、眼球突出、发热、感染、肝脾肿大、淋巴结病和皮疹等。

X线上，朗格汉斯细胞组织细胞增生症的表现是多种多样的，因此常与其他疾病相混淆（与骨髓炎一样）。由于其侵袭性表现，与骨肉瘤较难鉴别（图111-7）。该病常表现为溶骨性，可见穿凿样边界和软组织侵犯。也常被误认为尤因肉瘤。发生在椎体上的病变常表现为扁平椎。MRI可显示病变周围的水肿带。骨扫描有30%的假阴性率，因此任何类型的朗格汉斯细胞组织细胞增生症都要骨骼的全面检查。由于临床表现与尤因肉瘤和淋巴瘤类似，为明确诊断常常需要活检。在高倍镜下可见病变以朗格汉斯细胞为主（核大、嗜碱、呈咖啡豆样），伴有许多嗜酸细胞。

由病理证实的朗格汉斯细胞组织细胞增生症的治疗取决于疾病的阶段、症状、部位、大小和病变的数目。累及危险器官的全身受累需要化疗。当椎体病变有塌陷的风险时可以考虑低剂量放疗。外科治疗包括单纯刮除术、刮除植骨术、预防性内固定和抽吸/类固醇注射术。单发的朗格汉斯细胞组织细胞增生症较易缓解，在某些情况下仅行活检就能治愈。发病年龄越小、病变累及范围越广，患者预后越差。

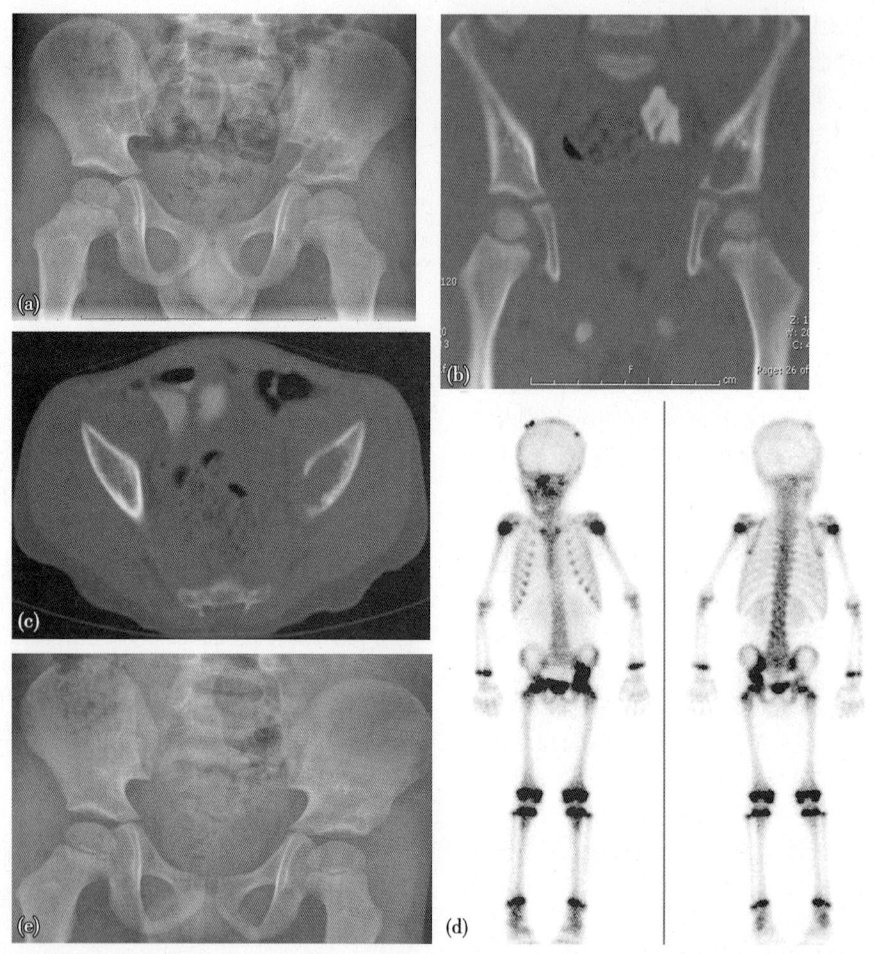

图 111-7　朗格汉斯细胞组织细胞增生症(嗜酸性肉芽肿)骨盆正位片(a),4 岁男性患者,左侧髋臼上缘溶骨性病变,边缘呈虫蛀样。CT 冠状位(b)和横断位(c)可见骨皮质破坏,需要鉴别转移性神经母细胞瘤和尤因肉瘤,但是活检见到层状的朗格汉斯细胞及散在的嗜酸细胞。(d)骨扫描可见病变处摄取增高,但还需要全面检查来排除其他在骨扫描呈阴性的病变。该病例只有一处单发病变,没有涉及其他脏器。(e)活检和刮除术后 1 年,病变在 X 线上不易看出,患者无症状

原发性恶性骨肿瘤

成釉细胞瘤

成釉细胞瘤是上皮性肿瘤,一种罕见的低度恶性的原发性恶性骨肿瘤,被认为是来源于异位的上皮细胞[73]。大概占所有骨肿瘤的 0.4%。最常见于年龄较大的儿童和年轻的成年人。95%的病变发生于胫骨,尤其是胫骨前面,或同时发生在胫骨和腓骨。最常见的临床表现是进行性疼痛和小腿中段的肿胀。

X 线上,成釉细胞瘤为偏心性溶骨性病灶,常造成胫骨中段前侧的皮质破坏,局部软组织肿物形成。在骨髓质部分常可见到透光病灶周围有硬化性的反应骨。病变在 MRI T1 加权像上呈低信号,在 T2 加权像上呈高信号,常有软组织侵犯,有时可见到多发病灶。显微镜下可见上皮组织细胞呈腺样排列,周围被纤维组织包绕。

成釉细胞瘤的治疗是手术,包括广泛切除受累的骨与软组织至正常组织。虽然 85%患者可治愈,仍需要长期随访,因为其可能在数年后复发或转移。

软骨肉瘤

软骨肉瘤来源于对骨的发生与生长很重要的软骨细胞[74~77]。软骨肉瘤属于相对多见的骨肿瘤,发生率仅次于骨肉瘤,是第二常见的骨的肉瘤。绝大部分的软骨肉瘤为低度恶性,可发生于成人的多个部位,最常见于骨盆,其次为股骨、肋骨、肱骨、肩胛骨及胫骨。患者常因疼痛就诊。由于软骨源性肿瘤发生率高,且良性、恶性在临床特点、影像学表现、甚至组织学特征方面具有相似性,所以诊断最大的难点在于内生软骨瘤与软骨肉瘤的鉴别。

软骨肉瘤除了以恶性程度划分之外,还有其他分类标准。后面分别讨论不同于经典性低级别软骨肉瘤的特殊组织学亚型(透明细胞软骨肉瘤、去分化型软骨肉瘤、间质细胞软骨肉瘤)。经典性低级别软骨肉瘤最初可能以“原发型软骨肉瘤”出现,或以继发于既有的良性软骨病变(内生软骨瘤与骨软骨瘤)“继发性软骨肉瘤”(图 111-8)。此外,软骨肉瘤可发生于髓腔,为“中央型”;也可发生于骨表面(发生于既有的骨软骨瘤中的骨膜旁/皮质旁软骨肉瘤或继发型软骨肉瘤),为“周围型”。

经典性软骨肉瘤的 X 线平片可观察到与内生软骨瘤相似

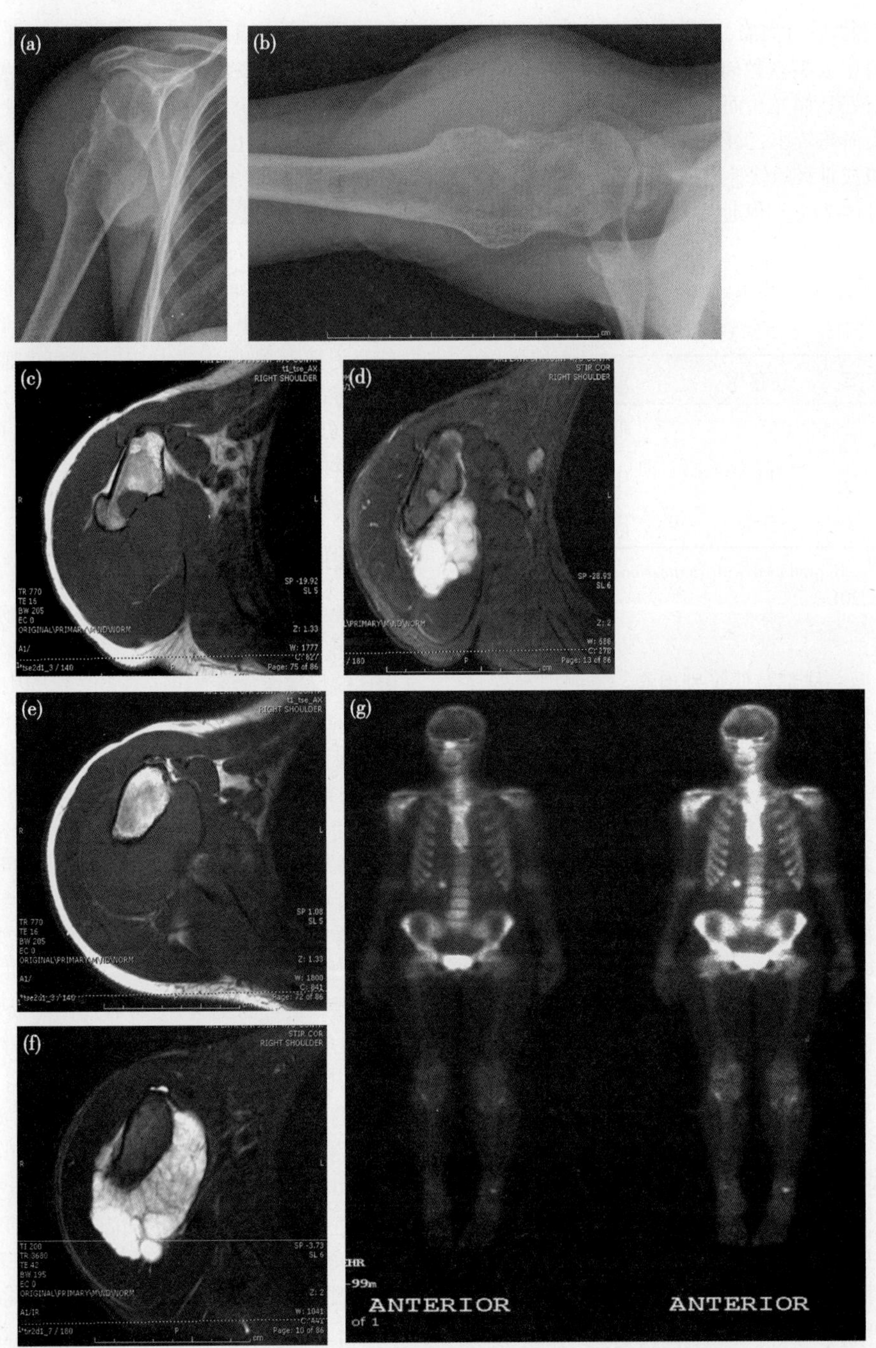

图 111-8　继发性周围型软骨肉瘤。女性，26 岁，多发性骨软骨瘤病，出现右肩关节疼痛、肿胀。右肩关节正位片（a）与侧位片（b）可见右肱骨近端干骺端多发性骨软骨瘤，骨周围可见巨大软组织影。此外，尤其在侧位片可见骨皮质受侵。MRI T1 加权像（c，e）与 T2 加权像（d，f）可见厚度约 2cm 的软骨帽形成，提示原有骨软骨瘤发生软骨肉瘤改变，且原有骨质受侵。（g）骨扫描可见右肱骨近端摄取增高。该患者接受了肱骨近端肿瘤切除、假体置换术

的弧形或环形软骨钙化。此外，还可观察到很多恶性特征，如骨皮质破坏并软组织肿块形成、肿瘤进行性增大、骨皮质膨胀、超过半数的骨膜内出现虫蚀样“扇贝征”、膨胀区域 X 线透过性增加及骨膜反应。虽然 MRI 可以更清晰地显示软组织肿块及病变周围水肿，但是良恶性均表现为 T1 加权像低信号、T2 加权像高信号。CT 能更好地显示“扇贝征”和骨皮质破坏的程度。在骨扫描上，任何性质的软骨肿瘤均显示为病变区域放射性浓聚，因而骨扫描不能作为鉴别良恶性软骨肿瘤的手段。组织学上，内生软骨瘤与软骨肉瘤的典型不同在于，内生软骨瘤的病变呈“包壳”样变（孤立的分叶状软骨周围被反应骨包绕），而软骨肉瘤的病变呈“浸润”性改变（软骨肉瘤向周围的骨小梁浸润）。此外，细胞构成丰富、细胞异型性、双核细胞，均提示软骨肉瘤。肿瘤的发生部位也应考虑在内。发生于手部或 Ollier 病好发部位的内生软骨瘤组织学表现为恶性，但病程为良性。总体来讲，软骨肿瘤的良性与低度恶性很难通过组织病理学进行鉴别，还需要考虑临床表现和影像学特征。软骨肿瘤的确切诊断，更依赖于临床表现和影像学特征。

由于肿瘤为大量基质，细胞相对较少，目前的治疗仅限于

手术。对于多数低度恶性软骨肉瘤,放疗或化疗的作用尚不明显。近年来,对于Ⅰ级中央型软骨肉瘤,建议囊内彻底刮除并局部辅助治疗(苯酚、液氮、激光),而不是以往常用的肿瘤广泛切除[78~80]。这种术式损伤较小,仅限于没有软组织受侵的软骨肉瘤,不适用于Ⅱ级或Ⅲ级的软骨肉瘤。软骨肉瘤的预后与其分级密切相关(表 111-7)。与其他多数低度恶性肿瘤一样,建议进行长期随访。

表 111-7 按照肿瘤分级,软骨肉瘤的生存率、转移率及局部复发率

分级	5 年生存率	转移率	局部复发率
Ⅰ级	90%	0	低
Ⅱ级	81%	10%~15%	中
Ⅲ级	29%	>50%	高

摘自 Damron 2008[81]. Reproduced with permission from Wolters Kluwer Health(table 6.3-4,p.201)。

透明细胞软骨肉瘤

与经典型软骨肉瘤一样都是低级别肉瘤。透明细胞软骨肉瘤的发病部位(长骨干骺端)和组织学表现(细胞体积大,胞质丰富、透亮,分布于软骨基质中)均有特异性。透明细胞软骨肉瘤较为少见,常发生于股骨、胫骨或肱骨的近端干骺端。高发年龄是 20~40 岁。主要症状是疼痛。

如果患者年龄不大,发生于干骺端的透明细胞软骨肉瘤需要与软骨母细胞瘤鉴别(因为大部分软骨母细胞瘤均发生于骨骼尚未发育成熟的人群)。X 线平片可见透明细胞软骨肉瘤病变呈放射性透亮区,病变范围延伸至软骨下骨,与骨巨细胞瘤相似。镜下可见具有特征性的大的透明细胞,向周围侵犯,具备恶性特征。

广泛性整块切除是治疗透明细胞软骨肉瘤的标准方法。治疗得当,预后很好。总的复发率约为 15%。

去分化软骨肉瘤

软骨肉瘤中,去分化的侵袭性最强,预后最差。依照定义,去分化型软骨肉瘤是低级别软骨肉瘤中出现高级别肉瘤成分,通常为骨肉瘤。最常见于股骨、骨盆、肱骨、肋骨及肩胛骨。影像学上,在典型的软骨肉瘤中存在进展性溶骨病变,则提示去分化软骨肉瘤。软骨肉瘤的治疗应针对其高级别成分,化疗的效果仍不明确,预后较差,5 年生存率 10%~15%[74,82,83]。一项新近研究指出,与不含异环磷酰胺的标准化疗相比,手术联合异环磷酰胺为基础的化疗,可以提高生存率[82]。

间质细胞软骨肉瘤

骨的软骨肉瘤中最为少见的一类,具有高度侵袭性,主要发生于青少年与相对年轻的成年人。多见于中轴骨,肿瘤多呈偏心性生长。镜下表现为血管间隙周围环绕着结节状细胞软骨样组织。与多数软骨肉瘤相同,虽然新近研究不断在探讨化疗的潜在疗效,手术仍是主要治疗方法[75]。5 年生存率报道不一,从小于 30%到 52%[2]。

脊索瘤

脊索瘤是起源于胚胎残留脊索组织的低度恶性肿瘤。依照残留脊索组织的分布,脊索瘤可发生于骶尾部、蝶枕部及脊柱各部位。脊索瘤多发生于成年人,骶骨为最常见发病部位。非裔美国人很少发病。年轻患者多见于颅骨。脊索瘤仅占所有原发骨肿瘤的 3%~4%。临床症状因发病部位而异,常见症状是疼痛。如发生于骶骨,可出现排尿、排便及性功能障碍。如发生于颅骨,可出现脑神经功能障碍。如发生于脊柱,可出现背痛或下肢痛等症状。

因解剖结构复杂,溶骨性破坏较轻微,X 线平片较难发现脊索瘤。只有 CT 或 MRI 可以显示肿瘤前方的软组织肿块,多伴有骨破坏。镜下观察,脊索瘤组织中包含有灶状或条索状分布的空泡细胞,细胞胞体大,内含空泡状胞质,较具特征性。

可能的话,脊索瘤的治疗应当是广泛切除的手术治疗。但是,放疗可以提高边缘切除或切缘不净的脊索瘤患者的无瘤时间[84]。对于此种低度恶性肿瘤,化疗没有作用。局部复发常见(高达 70%)。5 年生存率 75%~85%,10 年生存率 40%~50%。

尤因肉瘤

总体来讲,尤因肉瘤仅次于骨肉瘤与软骨肉瘤,位居骨恶性肿瘤的第 3 位[2]。5~30 岁(尤因肉瘤的高发年龄)的患者群中,尤因肉瘤仅次于骨肉瘤位居第 2 位。尤因肉瘤来源于原始的间质细胞,恶性、分化差、体积小、圆形、蓝染,与尤因肉瘤家族中的其他类型相似[85]。尤因肿瘤家族包括尤因肉瘤、原始神经外胚瘤(PNET)、Askin 瘤,均有 22 号染色体的 *EWS* 基因易位。常见部位是股骨和骨盆,其次为椎体及肋骨。主要症状为疼痛、肿胀,约 20%伴有发热和不适感。10%的患者在初诊时即出现病理性骨折。辅助检查可见血沉增快,部分存在贫血及白细胞增多。

影像学特征因发病部位的不同而表现各异。发生于长骨的尤因肉瘤可见骨干受累,骨皮质呈"葱皮样"改变(肿瘤周围存在多层反应性新生骨,随着肿瘤的不断增大,反应骨层层增多所致)多见,肿瘤边缘不清,呈虫蚀状,骨皮质破坏明显,常伴有软组织肿块。影像学表现几乎多为溶骨性。镜下观察,尤因肉瘤的瘤细胞体积小、圆形、蓝染,与其他实体瘤(如淋巴瘤、神经母细胞瘤骨转移)较难鉴别,研究较少。95% 的免疫组化 CD99(MIC2 蛋白)呈阳性。荧光原位杂交(FISH)检测发现 t(11;22)(q24;q12)或近似易位(t(21;22))可确诊。这些易位导致相关蛋白融合是 EWS-FLI1 与 EWS-ERG。

尤因肉瘤的治疗包括多药物新辅助化疗的全身治疗、扩大切除手术和局部放疗[85]。尤因肉瘤的有效化疗药物包括多柔比星、长春新碱、环磷酰胺、放线菌素 D。化疗可以明显提高生存率。新的趋势是对可以接受放疗的部位进行手术治疗。以往认为,尤因肉瘤是放疗敏感的肿瘤。对于中轴部位难以切除(如骨盆、骶骨、脊柱、颅骨)或转移的尤因肉瘤,放疗是有效的。对于手术切缘阳性的尤因肉瘤,放疗是手术的辅助治疗。手术切除最初仅适用于非承重骨(如髂骨翼、肋骨、腓骨、桡骨近端、尺骨远端等),目前更多地应用于可以重建的骨(股骨、胫骨、肱骨)。虽然手术应用越来越多、疗效可以接受,骨盆尤因肉瘤的局部治疗仍有争议[86]。目前,尚无随机研究比较放疗与手术的疗效,而回顾性分析又存在选择性偏差,因为放疗多应用于难以切除的躯干部位肿瘤。目前,很多临床试验表明,尤因肉瘤预后较好,5 年生存率为 65%~70%。但是,基于美国国家癌症中心的数据,一项包含 3 225 例尤因肉瘤的 5 年以上随访显示,尤因肉瘤的 5 年存活率仅为 50.6%[2]。

骨肉瘤

作为最常见的骨的肉瘤，骨肉瘤包含有很多种类的亚型，多数是高度恶性，但有 3 种是低度恶性或中度恶性（表 111-8）。它们的共同点是起源于成骨细胞，是成骨性肿瘤[87,88]。90%的骨肉瘤是传统型高度恶性。发病年龄呈双峰形，第一高峰为 10~30 岁。第二高峰为老年患者，多为佩吉特病（Paget 样骨肉瘤）或放疗后患者（放射性骨肉瘤）。临床表现常为进行性疼痛，有时合并肿胀。最常见于骨骼未成熟患者的生长活跃部位，依次为股骨远端、胫骨近端、肱骨近端。男女比约为 1.5∶1。

影像学上，骨肉瘤表现为成骨性，多位于干骺端，边界不清，伴有软组织肿块，表现为"积云样"成骨（图 111-9）。部分组织学亚型，尤其是成纤维细胞型骨肉瘤与毛细血管扩张型骨肉瘤，瘤体呈放射线透亮，没有典型的成骨。毛细血管扩张型骨肉瘤充满血窦，影像上与良性的动脉瘤样骨囊肿（ABC）表现相近，需行鉴别诊断。MRI 上，典型骨肉瘤是 T1 加权像呈低信号，T2 加权像呈不均匀高信号，常显示软组织肿块，髓腔内可见跳跃性病变。骨扫描可见放射性摄取增高。镜下表现各异，特别是低度恶性与高度恶性，但关键部分都是恶性类骨质形成。最常见的组织亚型为成骨细胞型，其次为成软骨细胞型、成纤维细胞型，毛细血管扩张型骨肉瘤最为少见。

表 111-8　骨肉瘤分级与类型

低度恶性	中度恶性	高度恶性
低度恶性中心型骨肉瘤	骨膜骨肉瘤	普通型骨肉瘤
骨旁骨肉瘤		高度恶性表面骨肉瘤
		继发性
		Paget 样
		放射性
		小细胞性骨肉瘤

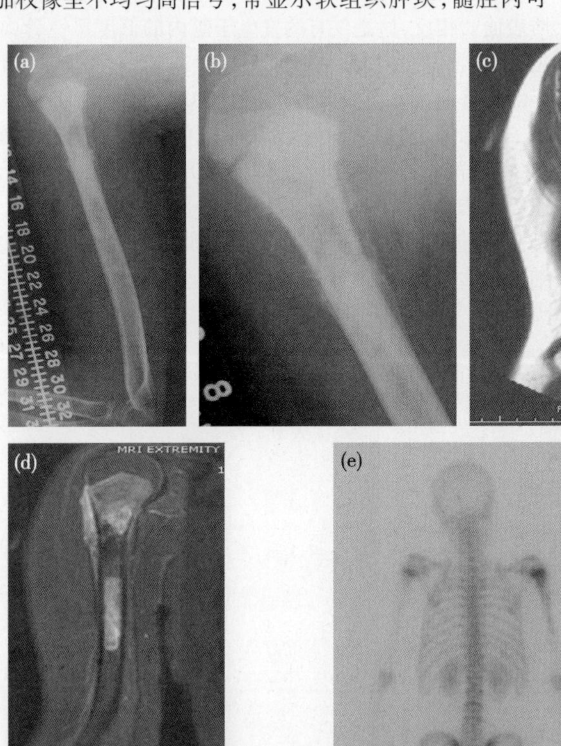

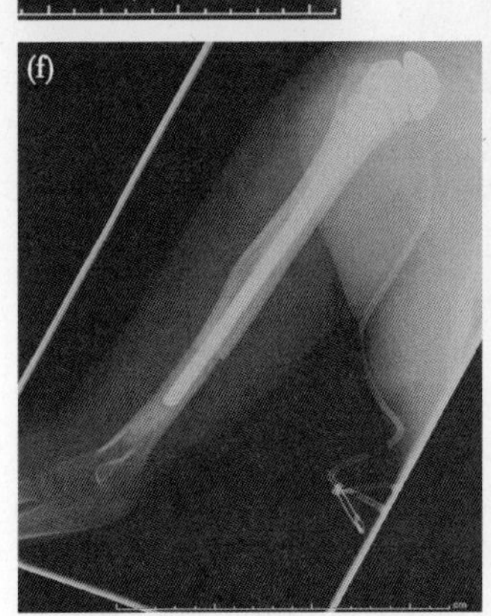

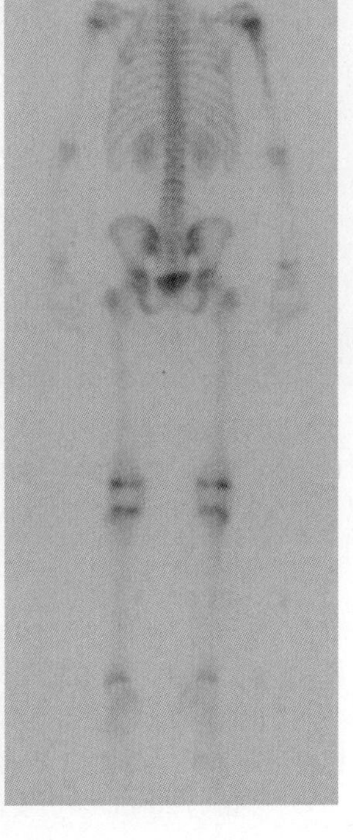

图 111-9　普通型骨肉瘤。13 岁女性患者，右肩关节疼痛、肿胀，X 线片检查（a~b）发现肱骨近端干骺端高密度病变，边界不清，Codman 三角样骨膜反应及软组织肿块。MRI 冠状位 T1 加权像（c）与 T2 加权像（d）显示软组织肿块和肿瘤在髓腔内的边界。骨扫描（e）显示肱骨近端放射性摄取增高。对于年轻患者，这些特征几乎可以确诊为骨肉瘤。活检证实为高度恶性骨肉瘤。进行新辅助化疗后，患者接受扩大切除并肱骨近端同种异体骨复合人工假体重建（f）

治疗取决于肿瘤恶性程度与侵犯范围。对于高度恶性骨肉瘤，新辅助多药联合化疗是关键，包括多柔比星、异环磷酰胺、顺铂和甲氨蝶呤[89]。新辅助化疗可致肿瘤明显坏死、软组织肿块缩小，有利于手术操作。肿瘤坏死率大于95%，多提示较长的无瘤生存和总生存时间。p-糖蛋白膜泵（*MDR-1* 基因编码）与耐药相关，它可将化疗药物的大分子泵出细胞外。局部病变可以行广泛手术切除。放疗不是骨肉瘤的标准治疗。低度恶性中心型及骨旁骨肉瘤（低级别亚型）的治疗仅为广泛切除，无须化疗或放疗。

骨肉瘤各临床病理亚型的特征分述如下。

普通型骨肉瘤

影像上，作为典型的骨肉瘤，普通型高度恶性骨肉瘤多发生于干骺端，好发部位依次是股骨远端、胫骨近端、肱骨近端。X线平片上常表现为“积云样”成骨，边界不清，骨皮质受累，可见软组织肿块与Codman三角（肿瘤增大突破骨皮质及骨膜，形成反应性新生骨所致）（图111-9）。

组织学上，可见骨肉瘤细胞呈多形性，核分裂象多见，可见花边样粉红色类骨质形成。普通型骨肉瘤呈典型的成骨性（成骨细胞型），也可见大量的软骨基质（成软骨细胞型）与纤维组织（成纤维细胞型），或血窦的存在（毛细血管扩张型）。成软骨细胞型骨肉瘤与软骨肉瘤和成纤维细胞型骨肉瘤的鉴别主要依赖于是否有恶性类骨质的存在。

多药联合化疗使得骨肉瘤的预后明显提高。临床研究表明，无转移骨肉瘤的5年生存率为75%~80%。美国国家癌症数据库的美国外科医师学会的数据显示，对于包括转移病例在内的所有年龄的患者，骨肉瘤的预后仍不尽如人意[2]。一项自1985—1998年对8 104例骨肉瘤随访至少5年的研究显示，高度恶性骨肉瘤的相对5年生存率为52.6%。30岁以下的相对5年生存率为60%，30~49岁的相对5年生存率为50%，50岁及以上的仅为30%。大约20%的骨肉瘤患者发生转移，进一步治疗后的5年生存率为30%~40%。再次发生转移的患者，5年生存率仅为15%~20%。

高度恶性表面型骨肉瘤

这里所说的表面型骨肉瘤不同于另外两类表面骨肉瘤（骨旁骨肉瘤与骨膜骨肉瘤），后者均为低度恶性或中度恶性。高度恶性表面型骨肉瘤无论在影像学特征、组织学表现，还是临床行为方面，均表现为高度恶性。此外，其临床表现、发生人群、病理学特征及治疗方法都与经典性高级别骨肉瘤有所差别。

低度恶性中心型骨肉瘤

与骨旁骨肉瘤相似，低度恶性中心型骨肉瘤是另一种低度恶性骨肉瘤。但是，与骨旁骨肉瘤和骨膜骨肉瘤这两种低度或中度恶性的骨肉瘤相比，低度恶性中心型骨肉瘤并不存在于骨质表面。相反，这是仅有的发生于髓内的低度恶性骨肉瘤。少见，仅占骨肉瘤的1%~2%。临床表现多为疼痛。典型患者的年龄比普通型骨肉瘤更大，多见于20~30岁。

影像学上，髓内存在界限清晰的低度恶性高密度影，易与纤维异常增殖症混淆（图111-10）。镜下表现与高级别普通型骨肉瘤明显不同。类似于骨旁骨肉瘤，低度恶性中心型骨肉瘤可见有骨小梁存在的条带状类骨质，其中穿梭有细胞较少的成纤维性基质，细胞异型性不明显，核分裂象少见。

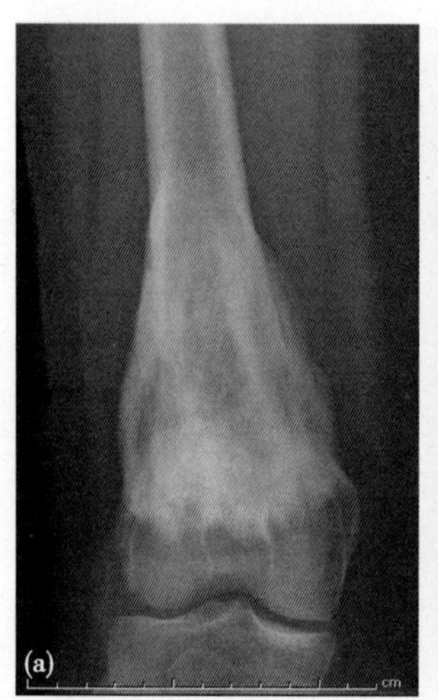

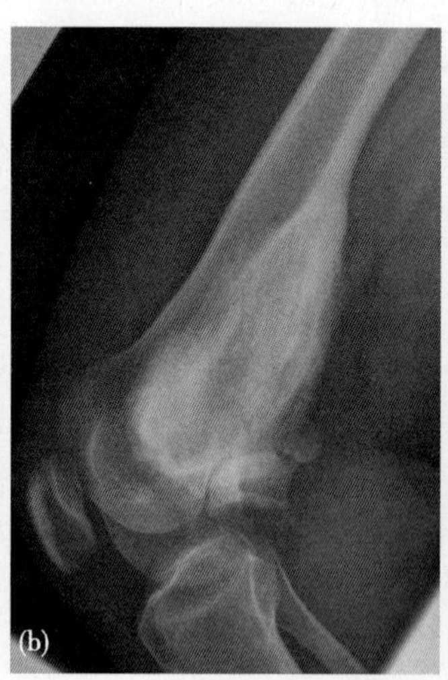

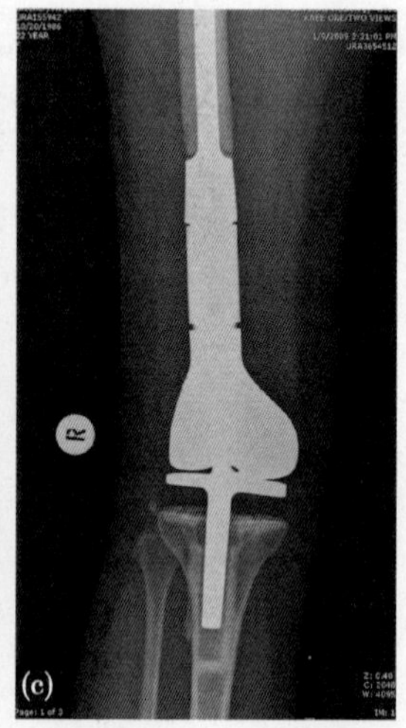

图111-10 低度恶性中心型骨肉瘤。26岁女性患者，疼痛、肿胀持续数年，诊断为低级别中心型骨肉瘤。X线正位片（a）与侧位片（b）显示股骨远端干骺端髓内钙化病灶。活检显示，条索状类骨质中可见稀疏的纤维组织。病变扩大切除后，以股骨远端全膝人工关节假体置换术进行功能重建（c）

与另外两种低度恶性骨肉瘤一样，低度恶性中心型骨肉瘤的治疗采用广泛性切除，无须化疗或放疗。总体来讲，预后很好。经过得当的外科治疗，局部复发率仅约为5%，5年生存率为90%，10年生存率可达85%。极少数病例发生去分化，在相邻组织中出现高度恶性肉瘤成分。

骨旁骨肉瘤

骨旁骨肉瘤是生长于骨表面的低度恶性骨肉瘤，其临床表现、影像学特征及组织学特点都具有明显的特征性，占骨肉瘤的5%。与发生于髓内的骨肉瘤相似，骨旁骨肉瘤的发病高峰年龄为20~30岁。女性较男性多见（男女比例为1∶2）。骨旁骨肉瘤最常发生于股骨远端后侧(占 80%);胫骨近端与肱骨近端是相对常见部位。多表现为大腿远端后侧的无痛性肿块,膝关节活动受限。

影像学上,骨旁骨肉瘤常表现为分叶状、密度均一的成骨性肿块,基底"附着"于骨皮质。少数病例可见肿瘤环绕骨骼生长,被覆盖的骨皮质可见骨膜反应。镜下表现类似于低度恶性中心型骨肉瘤,细胞基质较少,可见成熟的带状类骨质。

骨旁骨肉瘤的治疗是单纯切除手术,化疗或放疗均不明确。极少数病例可能出现去分化成分。总体的 5 年生存率为 86%[2]。

骨膜骨肉瘤

骨膜骨肉瘤为另一种生长于骨表面的肿瘤,仅占骨肉瘤的 1%~2%。临床表现、发病年龄与普通型骨肉瘤相同,但是多见于胫骨骨干与股骨骨干。影像学上,除生长于骨干表面外,还可多见钙化,可出现"日光征"骨膜反应或斑片状钙化,反映了其组织学的成软骨化。镜下所见与普通型骨肉瘤相似,但是表现为中度恶性和部分成软骨化。治疗采用常规的新辅助化疗联合扩大切除手术。预后介于骨旁骨肉瘤与普通型骨肉瘤之间。

继发性骨肉瘤

继发性骨肉瘤多见于老年患者,是所有骨肉瘤中预后最差的一类,且与外界相关因素关系密切,如骨的佩吉特病(Paget disease)及接受的放射剂量。在软骨肉瘤章节中,我们讨论了去分化软骨肉瘤中出现的高度恶性骨肉瘤成分。

Pagetoid 骨肉瘤

佩吉特病继发 Pagetoid 肉瘤样变的发生率为 1%~15%,这种代谢性骨病的特点是骨转换迅速。高峰年龄为 55~85 岁。临床表现为与之前性质不同的疼痛,伴或不伴有软组织肿块或肿胀。由于佩吉特病多见于扁平骨,因而 Pagetoid 骨肉瘤多见于肩胛骨、骨盆、肋骨。影像学上,Pagetoid 骨中出现侵袭性成骨性或溶骨性病变。治疗包括化疗(如果患者能够耐受)及扩大切除手术。化疗的效果尚无定论。预后较差,5 年生存率为 5%~18%[2]。

放射性骨肉瘤

诊断标准为发生于先前接受过照射部位的骨肉瘤,之前并无肉瘤成分,自初次接受放疗及病变进展至肿瘤发生至少经过 3~4 年。放射性骨肉瘤发生于之前曾接受过照射的骨骼,并且占所有放射后骨的肉瘤的 70%,其他还包括恶性纤维组织细胞瘤或纤维肉瘤。临床表现为先前接受照射的部位发生肿胀、疼痛。影像学上,放射性骨肉瘤表现为发病部位的侵袭性骨病变。镜下的组织学特征与高度恶性普通型骨肉瘤、恶性纤维组织细胞瘤或纤维肉瘤相似。治疗包括手术切除和辅助化疗(如患者可耐受),但化疗的效果尚无定论[90]。预后极差,5 年生存率为 5%~30%。

小细胞性骨肉瘤

除了组织学特征以外,小细胞性骨肉瘤与高级别普通型骨肉瘤相似。镜下,可见大量的小圆形蓝染细胞,胞质模糊;与尤因肉瘤相区分的唯一特征是小细胞性骨肉瘤中可见类骨质,有时甚至活检都难以鉴别。治疗与预后同普通型骨肉瘤。

骨血管性肉瘤

依据最新的 WHO 分类系统,骨的血管性肉瘤分为两种亚型,上皮样血管内皮瘤和血管肉瘤[91~93]。最新 WHO 分类中,将以前囊括入内的血管外皮瘤定义为纤维性实体瘤[94]。此类肿瘤代表了一系列肿瘤,其中血管内皮瘤的侵袭性最小,而血管肉瘤的侵袭性最强。该类肿瘤较少见,还不及骨的肉瘤的 1%。临床上,发病年龄范围广,多见于中年和老年成人。与大部分骨恶性肿瘤一样,临床表现主要为疼痛与肿胀。很少发生病理性骨折,多见于血管肉瘤。骨血管性肉瘤中,大约 1/3 的患者为多灶性病变,表现为单侧肢体的超关节"跳跃性"病变或波及全身的弥散性病变。任何骨都可能发生,长骨多见。

影像学上,表现为典型的溶骨性骨破坏,但可见溶骨与成骨共存。软组织肿块不常见。镜下,每类肿瘤均可见到原始的血管样通道,较具特征性。骨血管性肉瘤的治疗包括扩大切除手术或放疗。血管内皮瘤对放射线特别敏感,可首先进行放疗。化疗效果不确定。对于弥漫性或多灶性病变,放疗也是有效的。

转移性骨肿瘤

骨转移癌是侵及骨骼最常见的恶性病变。发病率高于骨的肉瘤或骨髓瘤。最常见的"亲骨性"肿瘤多原发于乳腺、前列腺、肺、肾及甲状腺。乳腺癌与前列腺癌在发生骨转移时,原发病灶多已经过治疗。肺癌患者常常以骨转移为首先症状。肾癌与甲状腺癌的骨转移可以与原发肿瘤同时发生,也可延迟发生。对于原发灶不明的骨转移患者,最为常见的是肺癌或肾癌。骨转移癌患者多为 40 岁以上。5 岁以下儿童中,转移性神经母细胞瘤多见。年龄更大一些的儿童中,原发病多为横纹肌肉瘤。临床表现为疼痛、肿胀,或可出现病理性骨折。但也有骨病变发病隐匿、在常规复查时发现的。发生于脊柱的转移瘤,可出现神经症状,甚至截瘫。常见的部位为脊柱、股骨近端、骨盆、肋骨、胸骨、肱骨近端及颅骨。转移至肘关节和膝关节以远的较少见,如果确有发生,多为肺癌骨转移。

疑似肿瘤骨转移的评估需要结合体格检查、实验室检查,以及影像学表现。由于成人骨髓瘤与骨转移癌难以区分,可做血清蛋白与尿蛋白电泳加以鉴别。淋巴瘤中会出现乳酸脱氢酶升高,并非特异性指标。前列腺癌可出现特异性抗原升高。肾癌可出现血尿。标准影像学评估应当包括检查全身骨的全身骨扫描和胸腹盆 CT。PET/CT 的应用也越来越多。

骨转移癌的影像学表现各种各样。某些肿瘤,如前列腺癌骨转移,是典型的成骨性改变,乳腺癌骨转移常表现为溶骨性与成骨性并存。肺癌、肾癌、甲状腺癌骨转移多为单纯溶骨性改变。骨扫描可显示多部位摄取增高。孤立性骨转移不少见,但是,某些高度侵袭性肿瘤(如肾癌或甲状腺癌)骨转移在骨扫描上可能不显示摄取增高。病理上通常是大类的描述,如腺癌、鳞癌、低分化癌等。此时,免疫组化指标对于鉴别其原发灶是相当重要的(表 111-9)。某些肿瘤具有特异性的组织病理学特征,如肾透明细胞癌、甲状腺高分化滤泡状癌、转移性皮肤恶性黑色素瘤。

表 111-9 骨转移癌的部分免疫组化标志

免疫组化标志	原发肿瘤
前列腺特异性抗原(PSA)	前列腺癌
甲状腺转录因子(TTF-1)	肺癌
白细胞共同抗原(LCA)	淋巴瘤

骨转移癌的治疗分为全身与局部治疗。全身治疗包括针对原发肿瘤(本书其他章节有论述)和针对骨破坏(调控破骨细胞)的治疗。双膦酸盐广泛应用于骨转移的治疗,它可抑制破骨细胞对骨质的进一步破坏。转移癌、骨髓瘤及淋巴瘤的手术治疗已在之前的章节论述。如果确诊为骨转移,预后较差,生存率与原发病的种类相关(表 111-10)。

表 111-10 易发生骨转移的常见原发肿瘤:骨转移发生率与转移发生后的生存率

原发肿瘤	转移发生率/%	临床骨转移发生率/%	诊断为转移后的中位生存期/月	5 年生存率均数/%
乳腺癌	65~75		24	20
前列腺癌	65~75	30~40	40	25
肺癌	30~40	20~40	<6	<5
肾癌	20~25	15~25	6	10
甲状腺癌	60	20~40	48	40

摘自 Damron 2008[95]. Reproduced with permission from Wolters Kluwer Health。

骨髓瘤

骨髓瘤是骨骼系统常见的原发恶性肿瘤。由于其他章节已介绍,这里仅介绍与骨相关的问题。骨髓瘤多见于50~80岁老年患者,黑人多见,与高加索人的比例约为2∶1。临床表现包括疼痛、病理性骨折、骨髓损害(表现为贫血所致的乏力、易疲劳,血小板减少所致的出血,中性粒细胞减少所致的感染)、肾损害及高钙血症。骨单发性浆细胞瘤与骨髓瘤的诊断不甚一致。骨髓瘤的诊断标准为骨髓中浆细胞的比例为10%以上,血清(血清蛋白电泳单克隆 γ-球蛋白)或尿液(尿蛋白电泳本周蛋白)中单克隆抗体阳性,终末器官损害(高钙血症、肾损害、贫血、骨质病变)。

骨髓瘤的影像学表现包括单发或多发"穿凿样"小灶状溶骨性改变,可相互融合成范围较大的病变。80%骨髓瘤的骨扫描并不显示高摄取,因而在初诊时需要考虑到是否存在骨骼病变。镜下可见大片的浆细胞,体积大、圆形、深染、核圆、偏心、核仁清晰。

骨髓瘤的骨病变对放疗很敏感。但是,范围较大的病变或伴发病理性骨折,可考虑手术固定。骨髓瘤骨病变的手术治疗见前述章节。

骨淋巴瘤

骨的原发性淋巴瘤最初称为"网状细胞肉瘤",是骨内恶性淋巴瘤的浸润,不伴有淋巴结或内脏侵犯。任何年龄均可发病,最常发生于股骨、髂骨、肋骨。临床表现为疼痛、软组织肿块或病理性骨折。与弥漫性淋巴瘤不同的是,此类患者很少有全身症状。

影像学上,骨淋巴瘤 X 线平片表现为骨干或干骺端出现浸润性、边界不清的病变。多数为溶骨性病变,少数为成骨性,类似于骨肉瘤。镜下,骨的原发性淋巴瘤显示为小圆形蓝染的肿瘤细胞,需要做免疫组化将其与尤因肉瘤相鉴别。90%原发骨淋巴瘤为大 B 细胞淋巴瘤。免疫组化 B 细胞的标志物包括 CD19 与 CD20。

骨原发性淋巴瘤的治疗需要多学科综合治疗。化疗为主要治疗方法,手术应用于活检、骨折固定及对濒临骨折的预防性固定。化疗药物通常包括环磷酰胺、阿柔比星、长春新碱、泼尼松(CHOP 方案)与利妥昔单抗(rituximab)(CD20 单克隆抗体)。

先天性综合征

很多先天性综合征常累及骨骼,或易于发生骨恶变。本章介绍其中一部分。

多发内生软骨瘤病

多发内生软骨瘤病可以表现为单纯的多发性内生软骨瘤(Ollier 病)或伴有多发软组织血管瘤的多发性内生软骨瘤(Maffucci 综合征)。这两类疾病发病均散在,且原因不明。临床不常见,典型病例在儿童时即已确诊。影像学上,内生软骨瘤单个病灶的影像学表现与单发性内生软骨瘤并无差别。这两种综合征的最重要差别在于恶变的发生率。

Ollier 病

多发性内生软骨瘤病有 20%~30%的风险转变为单个或多个软骨肉瘤。因而此类患者每年都应该复查或随访。Ollier 病发生软骨肉瘤的常见部位为骨盆、股骨近端、肱骨近端。

Maffucci 综合征

Maffucci 综合征有可能恶变为软骨肉瘤,也可能转变为其他恶性肿瘤。实际上,Maffucci 综合征的恶变率几乎是 100%。主要有急性淋巴细胞白血病、星形细胞瘤、胃肠道恶性肿瘤等。此类肿瘤在确诊早期就需要严密观察。

家族性腺瘤性息肉病

多发性结直肠息肉为结肠腺瘤性息肉病基因(*APC* 基因)

突变所致常染色体显性遗传病。家族性腺瘤性息肉病伴发骨病变(以及相关的 Gardner 综合征)仅表现为骨瘤。骨病变无须特殊治疗,也不会出现恶变。家族性腺瘤性息肉病伴发的唯一恶性病变为结肠癌。

多发性骨纤维异常增殖症(McCune-Albright 综合征、Mazabraud 综合征)

大部分骨纤维异常增殖症为单发(单骨性),部分为多骨性(多发性纤维异常增殖症)。此外,30%~50%的多发性纤维异常增殖症患者伴有明显的皮肤色素沉着,且色素沉着的边界不规则,呈"缅因州海岸线"状,且伴有性早熟及内分泌紊乱,称为 McCune-Albright 综合征(或 Albright 综合征)。少数纤维异常增殖症伴有软组织黏液瘤(Mazabraud 综合征),其发病机制为 *GNAS1* 基因的突变。依据骨骼病变的临床表现(疼痛、跛行、肿胀、成角畸形、肢体不等长、颅面部异常)与特征性的皮肤病变、性早熟,以及内分泌相关性症状(甲状旁腺功能亢进、甲状腺功能亢进、库欣综合征、肢端肥大症、糖尿病、佝偻病、骨软化症、高催乳素血症),此类患者在儿童期或青春期即可确诊。

如前所述,多发性骨纤维异常增殖症的单个病灶与单发性骨纤维异常增殖症的影像学和组织学表现相同。治疗应该兼顾伴随症(尤其内分泌相关性疾病)与骨病变。由于多发性骨纤维异常增殖症多伴有进行性骨畸形的发生,尤其是股骨近端,因而需要行预防性治疗(包括手术干预及双膦酸盐治疗)。该类疾病很少恶变,且多在放疗后发生。

多发性骨软骨瘤病

多发性骨软骨瘤病(遗传性多发性外生骨疣)为 *EXT1* 或 *EXT2* 基因突变所致的常染色体显性遗传病,与最为常见的良性骨肿瘤,即单发性骨软骨瘤相比,此病少见。确诊常在 2~10 岁儿童期。典型表现为近关节处的"多节状"骨隆起、身材矮小、肢体较短、髋关节外翻、桡骨头脱位及疼痛。影像学可见多处骨软骨瘤,每处病变与单发性骨软骨瘤相同。治疗与单发性骨软骨瘤一样,可手术切除有症状的肿瘤。恶变发生率为 3%~10%,多为低度恶性软骨肉瘤(图 111-11)。

视网膜母细胞瘤综合征

rb1 基因突变患者易于发病,不仅易发生视网膜母细胞瘤,而且通过"二次打击"突变为其他恶性肿瘤,多为骨肉瘤。因而,此类疾病又被称为"视网膜母细胞瘤/成骨性肉瘤综合征"。视网膜母细胞瘤多在 3 岁前确诊,骨肉瘤高发年龄为青少年。影像学表现、组织学表现及治疗与普通型高度恶性骨肉瘤相同,见前述。

Rothmund-Thomson 综合征

Rothmund-Thomson 综合征虽然少见,但在骨肿瘤中不应忽视,因为它可能进展为骨肉瘤。Rothmund-Thomson 综合征为常染色体隐性遗传病,为 8 号染色体的 RECQL4 解旋酶基因突变所致。通过特征性的光敏性红色斑疹及最终形成的色素沉着或色素缺失性皮肤异色等临床表现,Rothmund-Thomson 综合征

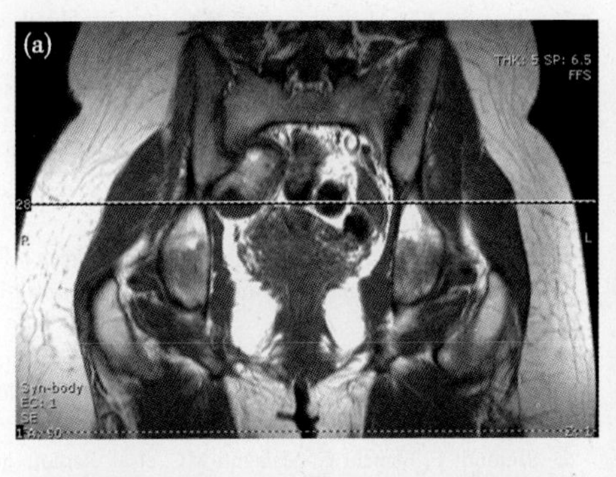

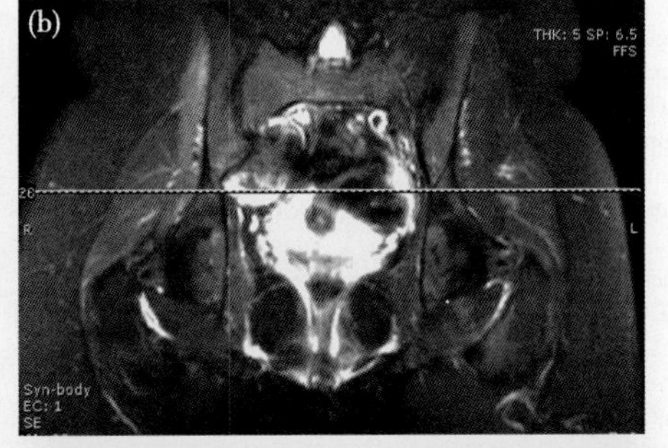

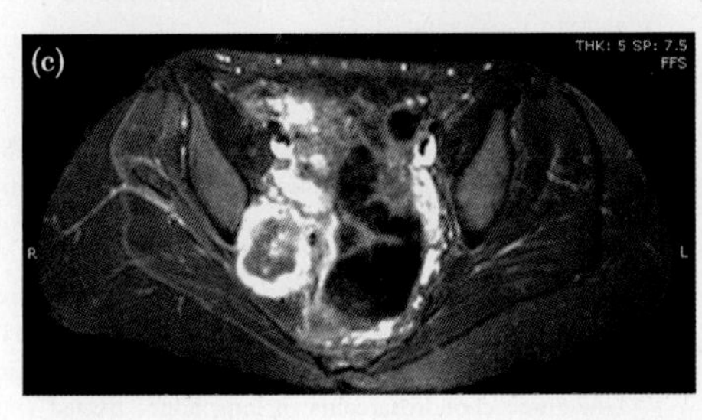

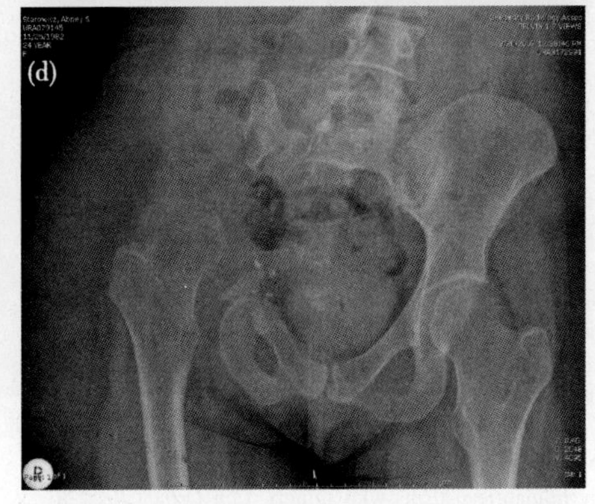

图 111-11　多发性骨软骨瘤病继发软骨肉瘤。23 岁女性患者,曾诊断为遗传性多发性外生骨疣,出现骨盆疼痛。X 线片未发现、但 MRI(a~c)可见,肿块起源于骨盆内壁体积较小的骨软骨瘤,平骶髂关节,延伸至坐骨切迹。活检证实为低度恶性软骨肉瘤。患者接受内侧半盆切除并旷置术(d)。骨盆是骨软骨瘤病继发软骨肉瘤的最常见部位,建议定期检查

常在出生 6 个月内确诊。基因检测证实了大量病例，但需排除相关疾病，如 Werner 综合征及布卢姆综合征（Bloom syndrome）。其他需要排除的骨相关病变，包括骨质疏松、锁骨发育不全、并指（趾）畸形、膝关节发育不良、膝关节外翻和良性骨病变。该病尚无特异性治疗方法。需要高度警惕肌肉骨骼系统恶变的发生，如骨肉瘤。

Werner 综合征

Werner 综合征（成人早衰症），与 Rothmund-Thomson 综合征的发病基因具有同源性，且部分临床症状也相似。它是由 8 号染色体上的 *WRN* 基因突变所致的常染色体隐性遗传病。RECQ 解旋酶合成缺陷导致发生广泛的恶变（如骨肉瘤），但是，软组织肉瘤、甲状腺癌、黑色素瘤更为常见。临床表现早期就会出现（硬皮病、过早白发或秃发、非老年性白内障、心脏瓣膜钙沉积、动脉粥样硬化、糖尿病、性功能障碍），患者成年后可以通过基因检测与尿液玻璃酸酶含量确诊。伴发的其他肌肉骨骼系统病变包括骨质疏松、肌肉萎缩、钙沉积、扁平足。对于确诊 Werner 综合征的患者，需要警惕早期出现恶变。

（赵振国 许宋锋 译 王鲁强 于胜吉 校）

参考文献

The complete reference list can be found on the Wiley Companion Digital Edition of this title (see inside front cover for login instructions).

1 American Cancer Society. *American Cancer Society: Cancer Facts and Figures 2014*. Atlanta: American Cancer Society, http://www.cancer.org/acs/groups/content/@research/documents/webcontent/acspc-042151.pdf; 2014.

2 Damron TA, Ward WG, Stewart A. Osteosarcoma, chondrosarcoma, and Ewing's sarcoma: National Cancer Data Base Report. *Clin Orthop Relat Res*. 2007;**459**:40–47.

3 Fletcher CDM, Bridge JA, Hogendoorn P, Mertens F (eds). *WHO Classification of Tumours of Soft Tissue and Bone*, 4th ed. Lyon, France: WHO Press; 2013.

4 Damron TA (ed.). *Orthopaedic Surgery Essentials: Oncology and Basic Science*. Philadelphia, PA: Lippincott, Williams and Wilkins; 2008.

5 Davies AM, Sundaram M, James SJ (eds). *Imaging of Bone Tumors and Tumor-Like Lesions: Techniques and Applications*. Berlin: Springer Science & Business Media; 2009.

7 Enneking WF, Spanier SS, Goodman MA. A system for the surgical staging of musculoskeletal sarcoma. *Clin Orthop Relat Res*. 1980;**153**:106–120.

10 AJCC. Bone sarcoma. In: *AJCC Cancer Staging Manual*, 7th ed. New York, NY: Springer; 2010.

12 Mankin HJ, Mankin CJ, Simon MA. The hazards of the biopsy, revisited. Members of the Musculoskeletal Tumor Society. *J Bone Joint Surg Am*. 1996;**78**:656–663.

16 Mirels H. Metastatic disease in long bones. *Clin Orthop Relat Res*. 1989;**249**:256–264.

17 Damron TA, Morgan H, Prakash D, Grant W, Aronowitz J, Heiner J. Critical evaluation of Mirel's rating system for impending pathologic fractures. *Clin Orthop Relat Res*. 2003;**415S**:S201–S207.

18 Snyder BD, Hauser-Kara DA, Hipp JA, Zurakowski D, Hecht AC, Gebhardt MC. Predicting fracture through benign skeletal lesions with quantitative computed tomography. *J Bone Joint Surg Am*. 2006;**88**:55–70.

19 Townsend PW, Smalley SR, Cozad SC, Rosenthal HG, Hassanein RE. Role of postoperative radiation therapy after stabilization of fractures caused by metastatic disease. *Int J Radiat Oncol Biol Phys*. 1995;**31(1)**:43–49.

22 Hanlon M, Krajbich JI. Rotationplasty in skeletally immature patients. Long-term follow-up results. *Clin Orthop Relat Res*. 1999;**1(358)**:75–82.

29 Eckardt JJ, Kabo JM, Kelley CM, et al. Expandable endoprosthesis reconstruction in skeletally immature patients with tumors. *Clin Orthop Relat Res*. 2000;**1(373)**:51–61.

32 Hoffman C, Hillmann A, Krakau H, et al. Functional results and quality of life measurements in patients with multimodal treatment of a primary bone tumor located in the distal femur. Rotationplasty versus endoprosthetic replacement. *Med Pediatr Oncol*. 1998;**31**:202–203.

33 Cipriano CA, Gruzinova IS, Frank RM, Gitelis S, Virkus WW. Frequent complications and severe bone loss associated with the repiphysis expandable distal femoral prosthesis. *Clin Orthop Relat Res*. 2014;**473(3)**:831–838.

35 Damron TA, Rock MG, O'Connor MI, et al. Functional laboratory assessment after oncologic shoulder joint resections. *Clin Orthop Relat Res*. 1998;**348**:124–134.

36 O'Connor MI, Sim FH, Chao EY. Limb salvage for neoplasms of the shoulder girdle. Intermediate reconstructive and functional results. *J Bone Joint Surg Am*. 1996;**78(12)**:1872–1888.

37 O'Connor MI, Sim FH. Salvage of the limb in the treatment of malignant pelvic tumors. *J Bone Joint Surg*. 1989;**71A**:481–494.

42 Malawer MM, Chou LB. Prosthetic survival and clinical results with use of large-segment replacements in the treatment of high-grade bone sarcomas. *J Bone Joint Surg Am*. 1995;**77**:1154–1165.

44 Healey JH, Morris CD, Athanasian EA, Boland PJ. Compress knee arthroplasty has 80% 10-year survivorship and novel forms of bone failure. *Clin Orthop Relat Res*. 2013;**471(3)**:774–783. doi: 10.1007/s11999-012-2635-6.

45 Azouz EM, Saigal G, Rodriguez MM, et al. Langerhans' cell histiocytosis: pathology, imaging and treatment of skeletal involvement. *Pediatr Radiol*. 2005;**35**:103–115.

46 Sheppard DG, Libshitz HI. Post-radiation sarcomas: a review of the clinical and imaging features in 63 cases. *Clin Radiol*. 2001;**56(1)**:22–29.

47 Cannon CP, Lin PP, Lewis VO, Yasko AW. Management of radiation-associated fractures. *J Am Acad Orthop Surg*. 2008;**16(9)**:541–549.

48 Body JJ. Bisphosphonates for malignancy-related bone disease: current status, future developments. *Support Care Cancer*. 2006;**14(5)**:408–418.

49 Shane E, Burr D, Abrahamsen B, et al. Atypical subtrochanteric and diaphyseal femoral fractures: second report of a task force of the American Society for Bone and Mineral Research. *J Bone Miner Res*. 2014;**29(1)**:1–23. doi: 10.1002/jbmr.1998. Epub 2013 Oct 1.

50 Levy JC, Temple HT, Mollabashy A, et al. The causes of pain in benign solitary enchondromas of the proximal humerus. *Clin Orthop Relat Res*. 2005;**431**:181–186.

51 Springfield DS, Capanna R, Gherlinzoni F, et al. Chondroblastoma: A review of seventy cases. *J Bone Joint Surg Am*. 1985;**67**:748–755.

53 Wu CT, Inwards CY, O'Laughlin S, et al. Chondromyxoid fibroma of bone: a clinicopathologic review of 278 cases. *Hum Pathol*. 1998;**29**:438–446.

56 Chapurlat RD. Medical therapy in adults with fibrous dysplasia of bone. *J Bone Miner Res*. 2006;**21(Suppl 2)**:P114–P119.

58 Lee RS, Weitzel S, Eastwood DM, et al. Osteofibrous dysplasia of the tibia. Is there a need for a radical surgical approach? *J Bone Joint Surg (Br)*. 2006;**88(5)**:658–664.

59 O'Donnell RJ, Springfield DS, Morwani HK, et al. Recurrence of giant cell tumors of the long bones after curettage and packing with cement. *J Bone Joint Surg Am*. 1994;**76(12)**:1827–1833.

61 Xu SF, Adams B, Yu XC, Xu M. Denosumab and giant cell tumour of bone-a review and future management considerations. *Curr Oncol*. 2013;**20(5)**:e442–e447. doi: 10.3747/co.20.1497.

64 Greenspan A. Benign bone-forming lesions: osteoma, osteoid osteoma, and osteoblastoma. Clinical, imaging, pathologic, and differential considerations. *Skeletal Radiol*. 1993;**22**:485–500.

65 Rimondi E, Bianchi G, Malaguti MC, et al. Radiofrequency thermoablation of primary non-spinal osteoid osteoma: optimization of the procedure. *Eur Radiol*. 2005;**15**:1393–1399.

66 Ramirez AR, Stanton RP. Aneurysmal bone cyst in 29 children. *J Pediatr Orthop*. 2002;**22(4)**:533–539.

71 Wright JG, Yandow S, Donaldson S, Marley L, Simple Bone Cyst Trial Group. A randomized clinical trial comparing intralesional bone marrow and steroid injections for simple bone cysts. *J Bone Joint Surg Am*. 2008;**90(4)**:722–730.

72 Allen CE, McClain KL. Langerhans cell histiocytosis: a review of past, current and future therapies. *Drugs Today (Barc)*. 2007;**43(9)**:627–643.

78 Verdegaal SH, Brouwers HF, van Zwet EW, Hogendoorn PC, Taminiau AH. Low-grade chondrosarcoma of long bones treated with intralesional curettage followed by application of phenol, ethanol, and bone-grafting. *J Bone Joint Surg Am*. 2012;**94(13)**:1201–1207. doi: 10.2106/JBJS.J.01498.

85 Weber KL. Current concepts in the treatment of Ewing's sarcoma. *Expert Rev Anticancer Ther*. 2002;**2(6)**:687–694.

第 112 章　软组织肉瘤

Robert G. Maki, MD, PhD, FACP ■ Chandrajit P. Raut, MD, MSc, FACS ■
Brian O' Sullivan, MD, FRCPI, FRCPC

概述

软组织肉瘤的治疗是由原发性肉瘤的解剖部位和组织学决定的，并且越来越多地受到肉瘤特殊遗传学的影响。在本章中，我们将重点介绍这组 50 多种亚型肿瘤的治疗原则，强调手术的解剖结构限制、辅助放疗的特殊性、针对不同组织学类型选择系统治疗方案。

在本章中，我们将讨论软组织肉瘤患者的病因、表现、诊断、分期和多学科治疗。合适时机下，放射治疗可以用于较大的肿瘤。本章重点介绍了越来越复杂的辐射技术的发展。关于系统疗法，本章针对软组织肉瘤一线治疗可能改变的情况，提出了辅助疗法的一些未知的新问题。我们试图将特异性组织学或分子变化与治疗方案联系起来，期待新的药物将取代现有药物。但在过去几年中，除了胃肠道间质肿瘤（gastrointestinal stromal tumor, GIST）外，几乎对其他肿瘤没有实质性影响。

非骨组织的肉瘤，即传统意义上的软组织肉瘤（soft tissue sarcoma, STS），是一类相对罕见的恶性肿瘤。它们分布于各种解剖部位，有多种组织病理学特征。这类肿瘤有共同的胚胎学起源——中胚层。例外的是被认为起源于外胚层的神经组织来源的肉瘤［如恶性外周神经鞘瘤（MPNST）］和尤因肉瘤/原始神经外胚层肿瘤（primitive neuroectodermal tumor, PNET）家族，以及起源于内胚层的血管肉瘤。尽管身体中非骨性组织占体重达 75%之多，但这些结缔组织的原发肿瘤相对罕见，大约只占成人恶性肿瘤的 1%、儿童恶性肿瘤的 15%。在美国，每年大约有 12 000 例新确诊的软组织肉瘤，其中每年有 5 000 例死亡[1]。了解这类肿瘤是十分重要的，如果初始治疗方法不得当，患者的预后会受到影响。此外，肉瘤的生物学研究为检测、治疗和预防更常见的恶性肿瘤提供了新的策略。

本章综述了目前对于非骨组织的肉瘤在诊断、分级和综合治疗上的观点。同时，还综述了不同分化程度和临床行为的软组织肉瘤的分子生物学发展和基础研究进展。组织病理学对肉瘤的分类很重要，但原发病灶的解剖学部位仍然是重要的分类标准之一，因为这是确定治疗方法和判断预后的基础。肢体的肉瘤占全部肉瘤的 50%，是本章“治疗”部分关注的重点。腹膜后肉瘤（retroperitoneal sarcoma, RPS）、胃肠道间质肿瘤（gastrointestinal stromal tumor, GIST）、隆突性皮肤纤维肉瘤（dermatofibrosarcoma protuberans, DFSP）将在本章单独论述。其他解剖部位的肉瘤由于罕见，本章没有涉及。本章重点是阐明现有确切证据证实我们已经知道的和还需要进一步研究的问题。

病因

多数肉瘤是自发形成的。对于多数癌症来说，这越来越容易理解[2]。通过对软组织肉瘤患者及其家属的肉瘤和正常组织的分子学分析，逐渐发现，软组织肉瘤是由间充质干细胞恶变而来的。遗传和环境因素在软组织向肉瘤的转化上起到一定作用[3]。

30 多年前，我们就认识到肉瘤有一定的遗传倾向。最早的关于家族性肿瘤（如恶性肿瘤的基因遗传倾向）的研究之一，是研究某些家族中肉瘤和其他类型肿瘤（如乳腺癌）的发生[4]。这种常染色体显性遗传倾向现在称为 Li-Fraumeni 综合征，在分子水平上是生殖细胞系中的 *TP53* 基因突变导致的。此时，它可能是一个有缺陷的抑癌基因[5,6]。

某些基因缺陷也会增加特定肉瘤的发病风险。最典型的例子，就是神经纤维瘤病更容易发展为恶性外周神经鞘瘤（malignant peripheral nerve sheath tumors, MPNST），也被称为神经纤维肉瘤或恶性施万细胞瘤[7,8]。Ⅰ型神经纤维瘤病（von Recklinghausen 病）是一个常染色体显性遗传病，其位于染色体 17q11.2 上的 *NF1* 基因的功能受到破坏。*NF1* 基因产物——神经纤维瘤蛋白的内在功能尚不清楚，但该基因通过激活三磷酸鸟苷表现为抑癌基因。*NF1* 基因的常见突变形式是基因截断，NF1 功能缺失导致对 ras 途径的信号失控，从而影响治疗方案[9,10]。NF1 缺失可能是促使神经纤维瘤患者经过一段时间发展成恶性外周神经鞘瘤的基本过程。Ⅰ型神经纤维瘤病患者一生中有 10%的风险发展成肉瘤（通常是恶性外周神经鞘瘤）；考虑到 ras 激活的蛋白质效应，恶变风险却不高，这一点尚不清楚；其他因素，如 PRC2 复合体表观遗传调控因子的失活，也可能出现肿瘤表型[11~13]。

研究发现，儿童视网膜母细胞瘤的生存者在晚期出现肉瘤的风险较高[14,15]。这提供了另一个功能失调或缺失抑癌基因（即染色体 13q14 上的 *Rb* 基因产物）的例子。视网膜母细胞瘤患者及其家族出现软组织肉瘤的风险升高，出现其他类型肿瘤的风险也升高，如骨肉瘤、乳腺癌和肺癌。*Rb* 突变患者会出现哪一种恶性肿瘤还没有令人信服的证据，这也是今后肿瘤转化机制研究中有待解决的重要问题。

Gardner 综合征是上皮细胞和间充质细胞功能失调之间的重要遗传联系。Gardner 综合征是肠道（通常是结肠）的家族性腺瘤样息肉病中的一种亚型。患有这一综合征的人同时还有肠外表现，如表皮样囊肿和骨瘤。其分子水平的异常为位于染色体 5q21 上的结肠腺瘤样息肉基因（adenomatous polyposis coli, APC）的缺陷。Gardner 综合征的患者患肠系膜和腹膜内硬纤维瘤的风险更高[16,17]。硬纤维瘤是一种间充质细胞以侵袭性纤维瘤方式生长的肿瘤，特征性细胞为温和细胞（组织学上是良性的)，但表现出不受控制的增长和向机体侵袭的恶性特征。自发性硬纤维瘤常出现 β-连环蛋白基因 CTNNB1，与 APC 的信号通路相同[18,19]。有些 Gardner 综合征患者会发展为硬纤维瘤而另一些则不会，这一点还不清楚。但 Gardner 综合征患者一生中发展成硬纤维瘤的风险为 10%~20%，比普通人群的风险高近 1 000 倍。

特定环境的暴露也与肉瘤的发生有关。最重要的因素之一就是电离辐射。辐射相关肉瘤通常是放疗治疗其他疾病(常是以前的恶性肿瘤)的晚期效应。放疗治疗乳腺癌、霍奇金淋巴瘤、非霍奇金淋巴瘤和其他肿瘤之后可以出现肉瘤[20]。辐射剂量似乎与放疗后肉瘤发生有关，接受 10Gy 以下的辐射发生肉瘤的风险非常低。其分子机制可能很复杂，因为从临床观察上来看，肉瘤多发生在之前辐射区域的边缘。这表明，诱变效应可能在之前辐射的边缘区域最大，在此区域内辐射既达到了足够诱发突变的剂量又不至于使突变细胞死亡。传统上我们认为，辐射相关肉瘤是在接受辐射平均 9 年后发生的，也有研究表明早期就有发生。辐射相关肉瘤主要是恶性外周神经鞘瘤、血管肉瘤和未分化多形性肉瘤(undifferentiated pleomorphic sarcoma，UPS)。尽管它们是侵袭性的，但这些放疗相关肉瘤并没真正表现出和其他高度恶性肉瘤不同的行为。与原组织学类型相比，辐射相关肉瘤患者的临床预后更差。辐射相关肉瘤应作为新的原发性疾病进行治疗，以得到最好的疗效。

特定化学暴露与肉瘤发生的相关性较弱，虽然化学物质诱导肉瘤发生的动物模型是较广泛应用于各实验室研究肿瘤转化的模型。肝血管肉瘤与许多种化学物质的暴露有关，如聚氯乙烯和砷化物[21]。其他化合物暴露和肉瘤发生的关系还不清楚，包括二噁英(如落叶剂和其他苯氧醋酸类除草剂)和用于保存木材的氯酚类[22]。

组织的慢性刺激或炎症是引起肉瘤的一个有争议的潜在原因。可以肯定的是，在女性接受根治性乳房切除术后的淋巴水肿上肢中，发生肉瘤的风险较高，通常与以往放疗引发的复杂变化有关(称为 Stewart-Treves 综合征)[23,24]。有限的数据(个案报道)提示，其他来源的慢性组织刺激和炎症可能与肉瘤的发生有关[25]。虽然软组织肉瘤患者常有外伤史，但外伤对肉瘤发生的影响是不确定的。

实体器官移植后的严重、慢性免疫抑制是肉瘤发生的另一个危险因素。实体器官移植患者的肉瘤发生比例较高(10%)，其中卡波西肉瘤占大多数[26,27]。

筛查

考虑到普通人群中肉瘤的罕见性，常规体检没有对肉瘤进行筛查。但是，医生们应当知道遗传倾向和环境暴露可能增加肉瘤发生的风险，这一点很重要。一个完整的家族史可能提供肉瘤遗传倾向的线索，如息肉、神经纤维瘤病、视网膜母细胞瘤、一级亲属年轻时患的任何癌症或肉瘤的家族史。遗传咨询应当讨论与这些遗传倾向相关的问题，尤其要考虑到缺乏典型 *TP53* 突变的 Li-Fraumeni 样家族[28]。对于肉瘤风险较高的患者，可能需要借助更多检查进行更详细的临床评估，而不是普通检查。对于神经纤维瘤病患者，如果发现快速生长的肿块，尤其是有临床症状的，应该考虑手术切除，以排除神经纤维瘤发生肉瘤转化的可能。同样，对于之前接受过放疗的患者，如果发现皮肤或软组织的任何浅表或深部的异常，都应该进行彻底检查。

临床表现、分类和诊断

原发部位

非骨组织肉瘤几乎出现在任何解剖部位。图 112-1 标明了安德森癌症研究中心(University of Texas MD Anderson Cancer Center)5 113 例肉瘤的解剖学部位分布及部位特异性的组织学亚型。大约 1/3~1/2 的非骨组织肉瘤发生在下肢，传统上最常见的组织学亚型是脂肪肉瘤和未分化多形性肉瘤(以往称为恶性纤维组织细胞瘤，MFH)。随着病理学进行肉瘤分类技术的进展(如免疫组化、DNA 和 RNA 分析)，逐渐认识到未分化多形性肉瘤可能具有一些与低分化脂肪肉瘤或平滑肌肉瘤以及其他组织学亚型相同的特征[29]。腹膜后肉瘤占所有软组织肉瘤的 15%~20%，其中脂肪肉瘤和平滑肌肉瘤为主要组织学亚型。内脏肉瘤占另外的 24%，头颈部肉瘤占全部肉瘤约 4%。

临床表现

大多数非骨组织肉瘤的患者表现为无痛的肿块，其中 1/3 有疼痛表现[30]。肉瘤的诊断延误很常见，最常见的误诊是四肢和躯干的血肿或“脂肪瘤”。腹膜后肉瘤的诊断延误尤为常见，因为这个区域的肿瘤往往长到很大体积之后才会引起症状(如腹胀或腰大肌刺激症状，伴有背部或腹股沟区的不适)或功能异常，如输尿管梗阻引起的肾积水。

查体应该评估肿物的大小和活动度，注意肿物和筋膜(浅筋膜和深筋膜)及周围神经血管、骨的关系。还应该进行部位特异性的神经血管检查和局部淋巴结情况的评估。肉瘤很少转移到淋巴结，仅限于一些特定的组织学亚型。出现真正的淋巴结转移时，临床医生应当考虑肉瘤的诊断是否正确。

组织学分类

分类方法

广义上，肉瘤可以分为骨来源的肉瘤和非骨或骨周围软组织来源的肉瘤。非骨组织的肉瘤进一步可分为脏器(如胃肠或女性生殖器官)来源和非脏器软组织来源的肉瘤，如肌肉、肌腱、脂肪组织、胸膜、滑膜和其他结缔组织。

最普遍使用的软组织肉瘤分类基于组织来源，如最新的世界卫生组织(World Health Organization，WHO)肉瘤分类系统[31]。这一分类系统在病理医生间是可重复的，以便更好地鉴别肿瘤。然而，随着组织学分化程度的降低，细胞学起源的确定变得越来越困难。例如，病理医生在诊断未分化多形性肉瘤与低分化平滑肌肉瘤的标准上可能有所不同；使用特定 DNA 检测和免疫组化标记的增加已经提高了诊断的一致性。尽管如此，总体缺少对肉瘤的熟悉，使得 20% 以上的会诊病例存在误诊。

由于临床研究人员没有足够的数据把组织学亚型直接与生物学行为或特定的治疗措施联系起来，因此确定软组织肉瘤的特定细胞起源的困难有时还在于其临床的重要性有限。但

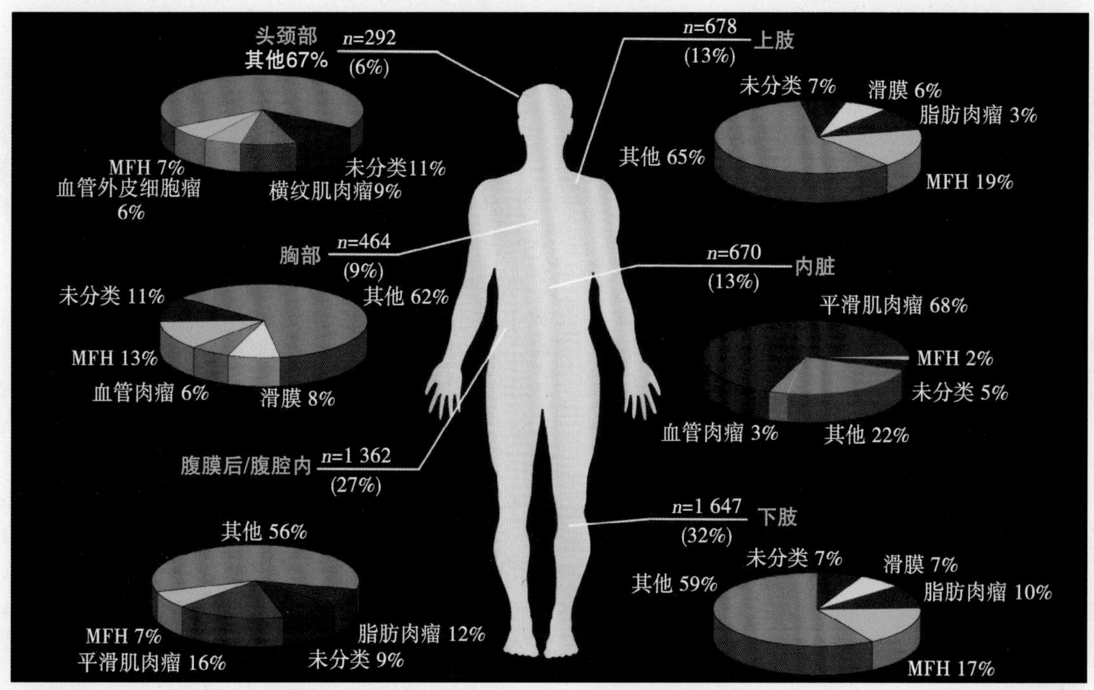

图 112-1　得克萨斯大学安德森癌症研究中心(University of Texas MD Anderson Cancer Center)肉瘤中心的连续的 5 113 例 STS 的解剖学部位分布和部位特异性组织学亚型(MDACC 肉瘤数据,1996 年 6 月至 2005 年 6 月)

也有例外,包括上皮样肉瘤、透明细胞肉瘤、血管肉瘤和胚胎横纹肌肉瘤,它们都有更大的局部淋巴结转移的风险[32,33]。一项单中心研究表明,患者就诊时的区域淋巴结转移率只有 2.7%,而某些组织学亚型肉瘤的淋巴结转移率要高很多,如血管肉瘤(13.5%),胚胎型横纹肌肉瘤(13.6%)和上皮样肉瘤(16.7%)。因此,治疗策略可能有所不同。对于其他亚型,生物学行为更多是由组织学分级而不是组织学亚型来决定的。但是,随着对肿瘤恶性转化的基础生物学和分子机制的研究深入,更准确的分类可能会有重要的临床意义。目前,在分子水平上诊断肉瘤或进行亚型分类的工具,已经越来越多地应用于肉瘤亚型,如胃肠间质瘤、滑膜肉瘤、脂肪肉瘤、尤因肉瘤/原始神经外胚瘤和横纹肌肉瘤(表 112-1)。未来的临床试验应当以比过去 30 年的研究更复杂的方式考虑组织学和分子特性,而过去并没有这么多标记物。

表 112-1　非骨组织肉瘤的细胞遗传学畸变

组织学亚型	细胞遗传学改变	基因
黏液性脂肪肉瘤	t(12;16)	*FUS-DDIT3*
高分化脂肪肉瘤	环状和巨大标志	扩大 12q13~15 *HMG1C* *CDK4* *HDM2*
脂肪瘤(微小非典型)	12q 异常	扩大 12q13~15
脂肪瘤	12q14~15 异常 6p 异常	
滑膜肉瘤	t(X;18)	*SS18-SSX1*,*SSX2* 或 *SSX4*
尤因肉瘤家族/PNET	t(11;22)及其他	*EWSR1-FLI1*(及其他)
横纹肌肉瘤	t(2;13)或 t(1;13)	*PAX3*(或 7)-*FOXO1*(腺泡状)
透明细胞肉瘤	t(12;22)	*EWSR1-ATF1*
骨外黏液样软骨肉瘤	t(9;22)	*EWSR1-NR4A3*
	t(9;17)	*TAF15-NR4A3*
隆突性皮肤纤维肉瘤	t(17;22)	*COL1A1-PDGFB*
子宫内膜间质肉瘤(低恶)	t(7;17)	*JAZF1-SUZ12*
促纤维组织增生性小圆细胞瘤	t(11;22)	*EWSR1-WT1*
软组织腺泡状肉瘤	t(X;17)	*ASPSCR1-TFE3*

PNET,原始神经外胚层肿瘤

组织学分级

生物学侵袭性常依据肉瘤的组织学分级来预测[34]。不同组织学亚型之间的分级是不同的(图 112-2)。多因素比较分析表明,组织学分级是评估远处转移和肿瘤相关死亡风险最重要的预后因素[34,36]。虽然有许多分级系统,但是软组织肉瘤分级时是否应当采用细胞形态标准,仍未达成共识。

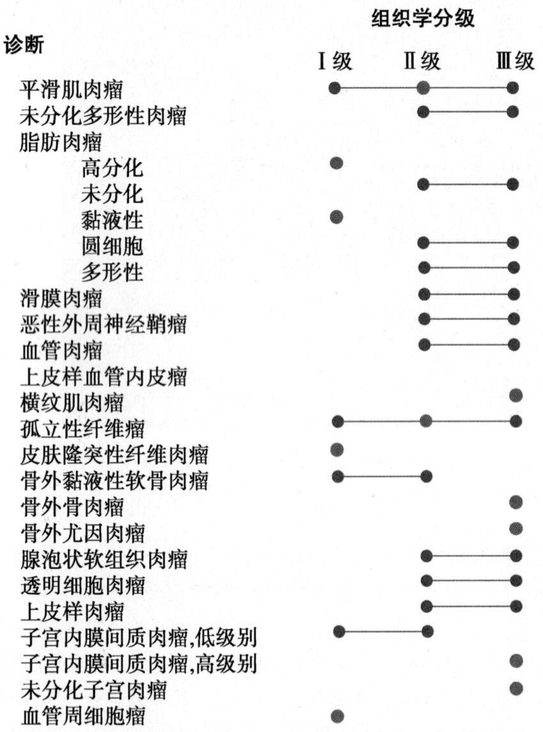

图 112-2　软组织肉瘤不同组织学亚型的恶性程度分级。摘自参考文献 35,Enzinger FN and Weiss SW, editors. Soft tissue tumors. 5th ed. Mosby-Year Book Inc;2008

最常用的两个分级系统是由 Costa 等提出的美国国立癌症研究所(US National Cancer Institute,NCI)系统和美国抗癌联盟(Federation Nationale des Centres de Lutte Contre le Cancer,FNCLCC)肉瘤组提出的系统,都是首次发表于 1984 年[29,30,37]。NCI 系统根据肿瘤的组织学亚型、部位和坏死量进行分级,但在某些情况下也考虑肿瘤细胞丰度、细胞核多形性和有丝分裂数量。FNCLCC 系统采用三种参数进行分级:肿瘤分化程度、有丝分裂细胞比例和肿瘤细胞坏死量。一项比较这两个系统的回顾性研究,对 410 例无转移的成年软组织肉瘤患者做单因素和多因素分析,表明 FNCLCC 系统在预测患者远处转移和肿瘤相关死亡方面要稍好一些[38]。1/3 的病例在特定分级上存在显著差异。利用 FNCLCC 系统会使得Ⅲ级的病例数量增多,Ⅱ级的病例数量减少,与总生存率和无转移生存率的相关性更好。FNCLCC 系统是目前最好的分级系统,是美国癌症联合委员会(American Joint Committee on Cancer, AJCC)/国际抗癌联盟(Union for International Cancer Control, UICC)软组织肉瘤分级系统的一部分。但需要注意的是,自 1984 年以来,已经确定了几个新的诊断类别,其组织学分级不受 FNCLCC 标准的限制。

在讨论分级时,要注意清楚描述肉瘤的特征。首先,单个肉瘤存在很大的异质性。因此,凭借非常少的肿瘤标本进行诊断可能是不准确的,如仅凭细针抽吸活检(fine-needle aspiration,FNA)的标本进行诊断。这种异质性在去分化脂肪肉瘤中表现尤为明显,一部分肿瘤可能相对来说是低到中度恶性表现,而同一肿瘤的另一部分却可能是更明显的高度恶性部分。任何关于分级的临床相关性的讨论都必须考虑诊断过程中固有的变异性,这会导致某种特定分级肉瘤的临床结果发生变化。

其次,肿瘤的分级会随时间而改变。此过程很好地体现在同一患者的高分化脂肪肉瘤演变为去分化脂肪肉瘤的过程。其他的例子包括由以前的黏液性脂肪肉瘤和纤维肉瘤变性为圆形细胞脂肪肉瘤,偶尔伴发于多发性复发型皮肤隆突性纤维肉瘤。

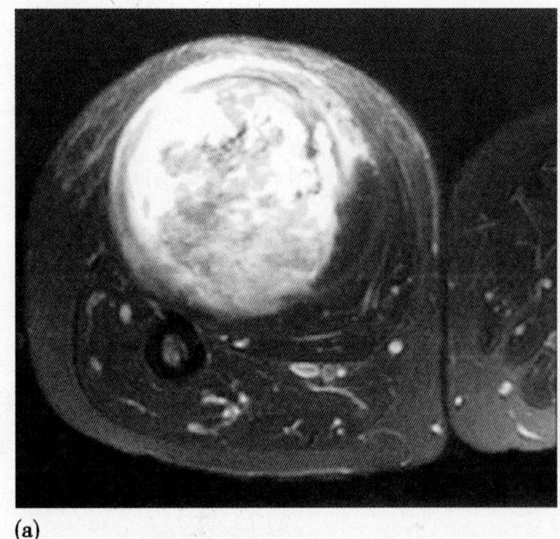

(a)

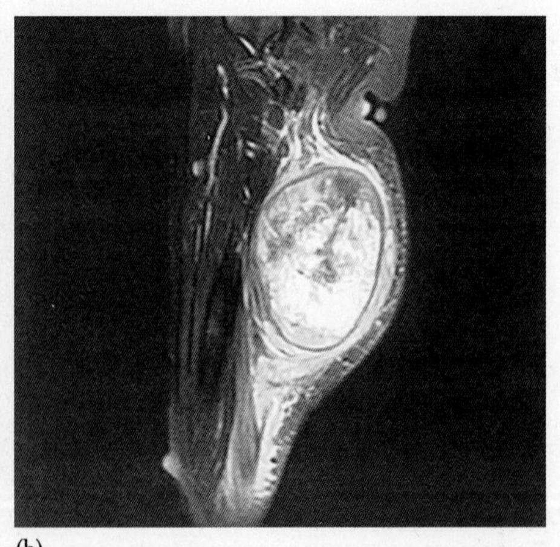

(b)

图 112-3　(a)55 岁女性患者大腿后侧的 TNM T2b 高度恶性肉瘤的 MRI T2 加权压脂相。肿瘤位于大腿后侧肌肉内,被皮下的浅筋膜所限制,其周围有“条纹形”水肿。肿瘤前方与股骨界限清晰,但肿瘤的边缘没有其浅表部分那么分界明显,可能是由于肿瘤向肌肉的浸润。(b)同一患者矢状面 MRI 显示,主要病变边界清晰。但是,上图显示肿瘤上方的水肿区域向近端股骨头发展。肿瘤远端水肿更加明显,呈增强的三角形并指向远端。无法确定水肿区域是否存在显微镜下微小病灶,这种不确定性将影响精确切除肿瘤的计划(见正文)

影像学

肿瘤所在部位决定了原发性肿瘤最佳影像检查方法。对于肢体、躯干及头颈的软组织肿物，磁共振成像（MRI）通常是最佳选择（图 112-3 和图 112-4），因为 MRI 可增强肿瘤和肌肉之间、肿瘤和邻近血管之间的对比度，并提供了病变的多平面信息[39]。但是，肿瘤放射诊断协作组（Radiation Diagnostic Oncology Group）的一项研究，对恶性骨肿瘤（$n=183$）和恶性软组织肿瘤（$n=133$）的 MRI 和 CT 进行比较，结果表明 MRI 并不比 CT 强[40]。尽管这两种检查在诊断方面没有差别，但是手术和放疗计划需要 MRI 提供的多平面图像信息以及进行 MRI/CT 图像融合[41,42]。对于盆腔病变或特定固定器官（如直肠或肝脏）的评估，MRI 的多平面成像功能可提供优越的单模式成像（图 112-4）。然而，对于腹膜后和腹部，CT 通常会提供满意的解剖学位置。有时，MRI 的梯度序列成像可以很好地表现出肿瘤和血管结构的关系，特别是下腔静脉和主动脉（图 112-5）。

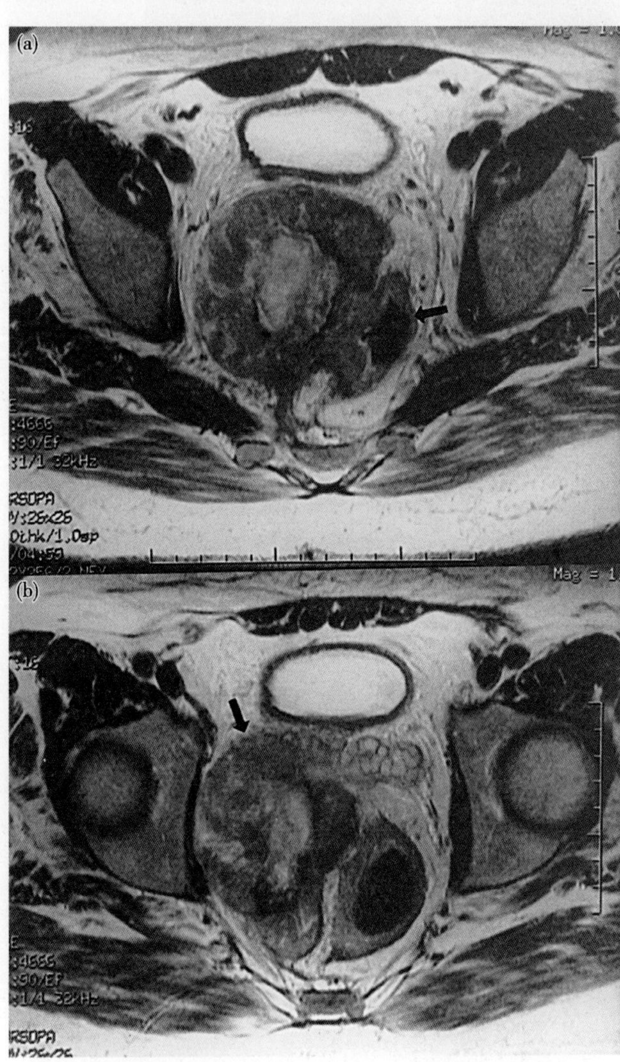

图 112-4　57 岁男性患者的 T2 期盆腔平滑肌肉瘤。（a）轴位 MRI 快速自旋回波 T2 加权相，显示累及直肠的不均质肿块（箭头：直肠内空气）。（b）注意肿物紧邻右侧精囊（箭头）

有创性检查如血管造影或腔静脉造影，在软组织肉瘤的评估中很少使用。

选择用来排除远处转移的最经济的影像学检查，应考虑原发肿瘤的大小、分级和解剖学部位。一般情况下，低度、中度或者是直径 5cm 以下的高度恶性肿瘤仅需要清晰的胸片就可达到满意的胸部评估，因为这些患者出现肺转移的风险相对较低[43,44]。但是，直径大于 5cm（T2）的高度恶性肿瘤患者应该接受胸部 CT 检查，因为这些患者的转移风险更高[44,45]。腹膜后肉瘤和腹腔内脏器肉瘤患者应该进行肝脏检查来排除同步肝转移的可能性。肝脏是这些病变首次转移的更常见部位。通常，CT 检查肝脏已足够，但如果在 CT 上有任何可疑的发现，敏感度更高的 MRI 会很有价值。

正电子发射断层扫描（PET）可以选择性地用来检查肿瘤的程度，特别是诊断不清的病变，这可能是其他影像检查发现的可能的转移。但是，PET 并没有常规用于软组织肉瘤的分期。

活检

对大多数出现软组织肿块的患者来说，原发肿瘤的活检是必不可少的。总的来说，任何成人逐渐增大（即使没有症状）的软组织肿物、大于 5cm 的肿物或是持续超过 4～6 周的肿物都需要进行活检。首选活检方法是损伤尽可能小又能提供明确的组织学诊断和分级的方法。在绝大多数医疗中心，芯针活检可以获得足够的组织进行诊断，并且比切开活检更经济[46,47]。但是，对于大体积的肿瘤来说，芯针活检不能获得足够的组织进行诊断时，考虑到肉瘤的异质性，应当采用切开活检以获得足够的组织进行组织病理评估，同时还能提供足够组织进行详细的分子学和细胞遗传学分析。直接触诊能用于引导大多数浅表病变的针刺活检，但不易触及的肉瘤通常需要影像学引导，以便对肿块最可疑的部位进行安全的经皮穿刺。经皮活检针道部位的肿瘤复发是很少见的，但是也有报道，这使得一些医生建议在活检部位做标志以利于以后的切除。细针抽吸活检（fine-needle aspiration，FNA）通常不能为初步诊断提供足够的组织，但可用于确认复发或转移。这种想法也有例外：内镜超声引导下的内脏肉瘤（如 GIST）FNA 可以提供足够的组织用于诊断，同时最大限度地降低肿瘤破裂的风险，但无法评估有丝分裂率。最后，在 FNA 基础上使用芯针活检的主要理由，是需要足够的组织来进行更深入的分子检测。与芯针活检相比，FNA 的另一个主要局限是没有保存组织结构的外观来评估组织特征（如坏死率）。

图 112-6 概述了针对原发肢体软组织肿物患者的实用的活检和分期方法。肢体的较小（<5cm）的浅表病灶（如远离关节、肌腱及血管神经束等可影响外科切出边界的结构），切除活检后复发风险较低，可行切除活检，并在显微镜下评估切缘。肢体病变切除活检的切口应沿肢体长轴纵向定位。对 T2 期、深筋膜下的 T1 期以及邻近关节肌腱血管神经的浅表 T1 期的病变，最好进行经皮针芯穿刺活检。

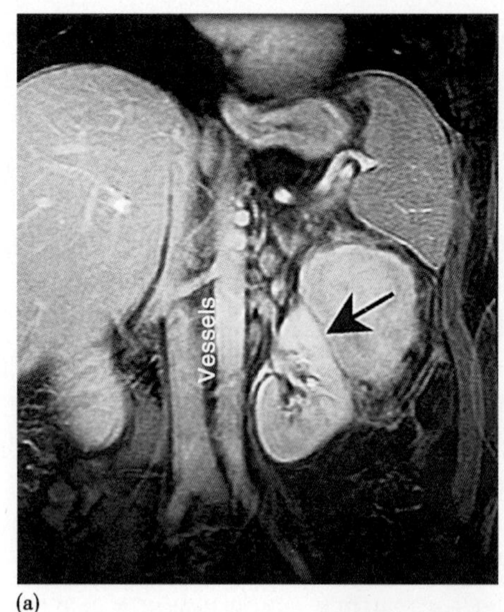

(a)

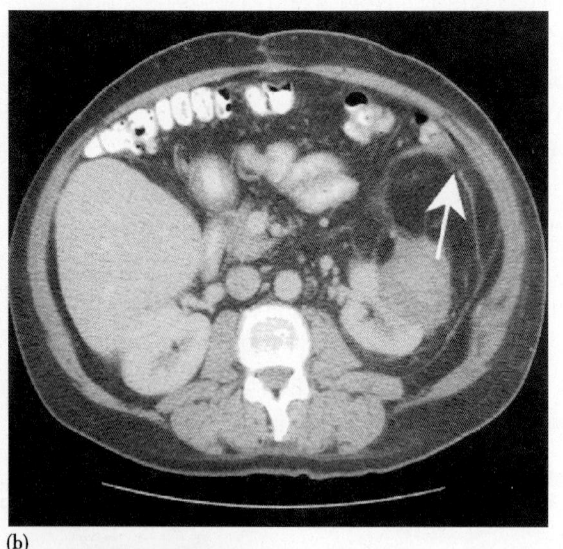

(b)

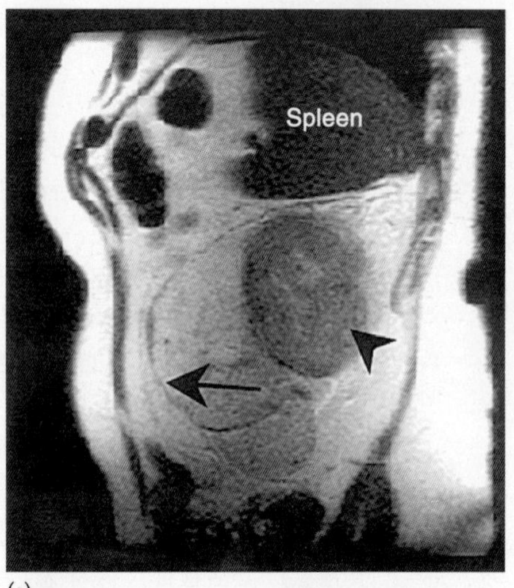

(c)

图 112-5 (a)冠状位压脂钆增强 MRI 显示一个实性脂肪肉瘤,大小 8.3cm×6.6cm,靠近并压迫左肾上极。这个肿物位于脾下方,与肾脏不相连(有分界线,箭头所示),是一个更大的脂肪性肿物的一部分。中线血管显示得很清楚。(b)同一病变的 CT 表现。同之前的 MRI 表现一样,可以看到肿物靠近肾脏。另有一个信号减低的脂肪性肿物,其前方被一个环形的灰色区域围绕,可能是水肿、炎症或细胞增生(箭头)。这个肿物有异常脂肪的表现,制订治疗计划时应予考虑。注意含有造影剂的肠道。(c)同一病变矢状位 MRI 平扫图像。此 MRI 图像的优点在于它能将腹膜后肉瘤的前缘(长箭头所示)与普通脂肪分开。实性区域(箭头)同样可以在脾下看到。此外,这些图像可以数字化输出到三维的放疗计划工作站或 CT 模拟器工作站,使 MRI 图像和 CT 分层融合。这可以为选定病例提供比单独 CT 图像更精确的肿瘤整体体积显示和临床靶目标。这在 CT 和 MRI 没有显示肿瘤的情况下特别有用

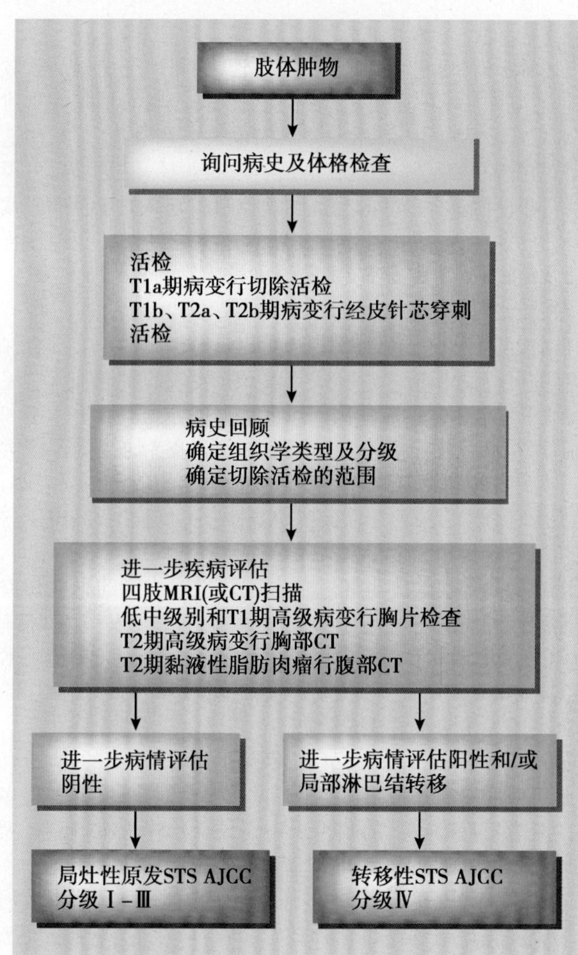

图 112-6　原发肢体软组织肿瘤患者治疗前评估和分级方法。AJCC，美国癌症联合会。摘自 Pisters 1998[48]

分期及预后影响因素

分期

软组织肉瘤相对罕见、所在解剖部位各异、不同级别肿瘤的组织亚型多达 50 余种，这些使得建立一个适用于各种肉瘤分期的完善的分期系统是非常困难的。AJCC/UICC 的第 7 版分期系统是目前最广泛应用于软组织肉瘤的分期系统（表 112-2）[49]。该系统不仅适用于肢体肿瘤，还可应用于躯干、头颈部以及腹膜后肿瘤；对于胃肠道间质瘤有单独的分期系统。

目前分期系统的一个主要局限性是它没有考虑 STS 的解剖部位，这被认为是影响预后的重要因素[50,51]。因此，尽管目前分期系统没有将解剖部位考虑在内，但在可能的情况下，预后分析应当结合解剖部位进行。此外，分期系统也没有包括组织学这项预后的关键因素。

常规预后因素

制订 STS 患者的治疗计划时，深入了解影响疗效的临床病理因素至关重要。已经开展了对局部肉瘤患者预后因素的多变量分析研究[52~54]。但是，除了少数以外，多数研究的病例数量少于 300 例。

大规模的临床研究确定了肢体软组织肉瘤公认的高危因素，包括：体积大（直径≥5cm），高度恶性，部位深在。此外，未被重视的预后因素包括特定的组织学亚型（如 MPNST）、切缘阳性或局部复发导致的风险增加。显微镜下切缘阳性的类型也很重要。低级别脂肪肉瘤的局部复发（LR）风险较低，还有为了保护重要结构术前计划了切缘阳性并术后放疗可清除残余的。但是，两类切缘阳性可导致局部复发风险升高，非计划

表 112-2　美国癌症联合委员会（AJCC）软组织肉瘤分期系统（第七次修订）

TX	无法评估原发肿瘤					
T0	无原发肿瘤证据					
T1	肿瘤最大径小于 5cm					
T1a	浅表肿瘤					
T1b	深在肿瘤					
T2	肿瘤最大径大于 5cm					
T2a	浅表肿瘤					
T2b	深在肿瘤					
N1	局部淋巴结转移					
G1	分化好					
G2	中度分化					
G3	分化不良					
G4	低分化或未分化（仅当四分类时）					
Ⅰ期	T1a，1b，2a，2b	N0	M0	G1～2	G1	低
Ⅱ期	T1a，1b，2a	N0	M0	G3～4	G2～3	高
Ⅲ期	T2b	N0	M0	G3～4	G2～3	高
Ⅳ期	任一 T	N1	M0	任一 G	任一 G	高或者低
	任一 T	N0	M1	任一 G	任一 G	高或者低

摘自 Edge et al，2010[49]。

手术且扩大切除后仍为切缘阳性、按术前计划手术后出现预想不到的切缘阳性[55]。"非计划手术"的定义是，在没有充分的术前分期或考虑切除肿瘤周围正常组织的必要性的情况下进行的切除活检或切除手术。

与其他实体瘤不同，软组织肉瘤局部复发的不良因素不同于预测肿瘤远处转移和患者死亡的危险因素[52]。换言之，患者具备局部复发的不良因素，并不意味着增加远处转移和患者死亡的风险。因此，用于评估肿瘤远处转移和肿瘤相关死亡的分期系统并不适用于预测肿瘤局部复发。

纽约纪念医院斯隆-凯特林癌症研究中心（Memorial Sloan-Kettering Cancer Center，MSKCC）的 Kattan 等耗时 12 年利用一个包含 2 000 余例软组织肉瘤病例的随访数据库，前瞻性研究肉瘤相关死亡的可能性[51]。其研究结果构建并内部验证了一个预测肉瘤相关死亡的量表（图 112-6）。这一量表已经在多种临床情况下得以验证，如腹膜后肉瘤（RPS），或针对特定肿瘤（如脂肪肉瘤），或针对个体患者[56~59]。此量表可用于患者咨询、制订随访计划以及确定临床试验合理性。

可能的分子水平预后因素

一些特异性的分子标志物已经被应用于评估软组织肉瘤的预后，如 *TP53* 突变、MDM2 扩增、Ki-67 指数、*RB* 基因在高级别肉瘤中的异常表达、组织分级。但不包括 SS18-SSX 融合，这似乎是滑膜肉瘤患者的一个重要预后因素[60]。关于肉瘤分子预后因素的详细文献讨论超出了本章的范围。读者可以参考更详细的评论[61,62]。

即使是最常见的公认的标记物也很难作为预后因素，例如 Ki-67，一种在细胞周期的大部分阶段都会表达的抗原。Ki-67 被用作细胞分裂的评价指数。初步研究表明，不同来源的成人软组织肉瘤 Ki-67 核染色与组织学分级有关，但在考虑组织学分级时，Ki-67 并不是独立的预后影响因素[63]。相反，对更多患者的进一步研究表明，Ki-67 指数是临床疗效的独立预后因素[64]。只有在关于 Ki-67 免疫组化本质及其解释的共识指导方针的制订之后，我们才能期望在肉瘤疗效中看到对这种生物标志物的更仔细、准确的评估[65]。从 Ki-67 数据的不一致性可以看出，使用越来越多的遗传标记来确定疗效的难度。尽管特异性蛋白、DNA 和 RNA 指标已被确定具有独立的预后意义，但目前还没有关于这些预后因素如何应用于临床实践的共识。

肢体局部原发软组织肉瘤的治疗

手术

概述

手术依然是原发局部软组织肉瘤治疗的基础。以下内容主要涉及最常见的肢体软组织肉瘤，其原则亦适用于其他部位。

随着 20 世纪 70~80 年代保肢技术的进展，以往作为原发肢体软组织肉瘤主要治疗方式的截肢手术已经大大减少。当今，多学科综合治疗策略的广泛应用，意味着绝大多数肢体局部 STS 患者都会接受保肢治疗，通常是保功能；现在仅有不到 10%的患者行截肢手术[66,67]。对于某些患者，单纯手术切除即可达到保肢的目的。

截肢

大多数外科医生认为，重要的血管、骨和神经受累是截肢的相对适应证。术中连同受累骨、血管及神经整块切除并重建的手术方式虽然可行，但相关并发症也很多。因此，对某些这种情况的患者（如足部），截肢仍是唯一的选择，但是术后可很快康复，并且可获得良好的局部肿瘤控制和较高的生存率。截肢的其他适应证包括肿瘤伴有皮肤真菌感染或伴有病理性骨折，难以保肢。

综合保肢治疗

目前，至少 90%肢体局部肉瘤可以进行保肢治疗。综合保肢治疗的可行性来自一项 1982 年由 NCI 发表的Ⅲ期临床试验证据，适于保肢手术的肢体肉瘤患者被随机分到截肢手术组和保肢手术并术后放疗组[68]。术后，这两组患者均接受了多柔比星、环磷酰胺和甲氨蝶呤化疗。超过 9 年的随访结果表明，保肢手术联合术后放化疗在保留功能性肢体的同时，获得了与截肢相当的疾病相关生存率。

满意的局部切除应当经过包含正常组织边缘的纵向切口切除原发性肿瘤。紧贴肿瘤假包膜切除的局部复发率为 1/3~2/3。反之，正如评价术后放疗的随机试验的对照组（单纯手术组）和其他单机构研究所述，包含正常组织边缘的广泛性切除的局部复发率为 10%~31%[69]。

如今，谈及保肢治疗就必须提及辅助治疗，常见的是放疗。许多随机对照研究都强调辅助治疗的重要性，并且制订了很多重要的具有里程碑意义的软组织肉瘤局部治疗方案。除一项研究外，多数研究关注于四肢肉瘤以及手术和辅助放疗。

Yang 等将 91 例高度恶性肢体软组织肉瘤保肢手术患者随机分为辅助化疗组和序贯化疗放疗组[70]。另外 50 例低度恶性软组织肉瘤保肢手术患者随机分为辅助放疗组和无后续治疗组。局部控制率在接受放疗的患者中达到 99%，而未接受放疗的在 70%左右，两者有显著性差异（$P=0.000\ 1$）。高度恶性组和低度恶性组的结果类似（表 112-3）。

1982—1987 年，126 例患者被随机分组评估术后辅助放疗的作用（表 112-3）[69]。术后行短距离放疗（brachytherapy，BRT），方法为术后植入铱-192，4~6 日内释放 42~45Gy。5 年随访表明，高度恶性肉瘤行术后 BRT 组的局部控制率为 91%，而单纯手术组为 70%（$P=0.04$）。值得注意的是，低度恶性肉瘤的 BRT 并未改善局部控制率（单纯手术组为 74%，术后 BRT 组为 64%）。肿瘤恶性程度不同对 BRT 反应不同的原因尚未明确。有一种说法提出低度恶性肉瘤细胞周期较长，在相对较短的 BRT 期间，细胞尚未进入放疗敏感的周期。在"放射治疗方法"一节中，对 BRT 与体外放射治疗（EBRT）的优缺点进行了进一步讨论。

满意的外科切缘可能无须放疗

尚无随机试验证据来定义满意的肉瘤大体标本的外科切缘到底是多少。一般来讲，应尽力达到扩大的外科边界（通常主观的选择肿瘤外 2cm），除非肿瘤毗邻重要血管神经；且其未受肿瘤累及时，可紧贴血管神经切除肿瘤。肢体软组织肉瘤的外科切除技巧不在本节讨论范围之内，可参见其他研究[71]。无论如何，手术原则仍是在与肿瘤距离足够的情况下切除肿瘤及有可能受累的组织（至少 2cm 距离），或将肿瘤连同限制其延伸的天然屏障整块切除。对于这些病例，即使存在一些预后不良的危险因素如体积较大、高度恶性等，术后放疗往往也是非必需的。但在例外的情况下，如术前"非计划"切除、周围组

表 112-3　躯干及肢体肉瘤依据级别不同关于辅助放疗的Ⅲ期临床试验

组织学分级	第一作者/单位（参考文献）	治疗组	放疗剂量	患者数量	局部复发/%	无复发生存率/%	总生存率/%
高级别	Pisters/MSKCC[69]	手术+近距离照射	42~45	56	5(9)	89	27
		手术	—	63	19(30)	66	67
	Yang/NCI[70]	手术+体外放疗	45+18(瘤床加量)	47	0(0)	100	75
		手术	—	44	9(20)	78	74
低级别	Pisters/MSKCC[69]	手术+近距离照射	42~45	22	8(36)	73	96
		手术	—	23	6(26)	73	95
	Yang/NCI[70]	手术+体外放疗	45+18(瘤床加量)	26	1(4)	96	NR
		手术	—	24	8(33)	63	NR

MSKCC,纽约纪念医院斯隆-凯特林癌症研究中心(Memorial Sloan-Kettering Cancer Center);NCI,国家癌症研究中心(National Cancer Institute);NR,无报道。

织被肿瘤明显污染、肿瘤的确切边界无法明确时,可行术后放疗。根据组织学,当合适的生物屏障(如肌肉筋膜)形成边缘时,小于 2cm 的切缘是可行的。组织学具有浸润边界的肿瘤(如黏液纤维肉瘤),可能需要更大的切缘或彻底切除。另一方面,预后良好的肿瘤(如分化良好的脂肪肉瘤/非典型脂肪肉瘤),可通过边缘切除进行治疗。

区域淋巴结的处理

成人肉瘤的淋巴结转移率较低(2%~3%),多数患者没有必要常规接受区域淋巴结清扫[32]。但是,对于血管肉瘤、胚胎/腺泡状横纹肌肉瘤或上皮样肉瘤,淋巴转移的概率相对较高,需要进行详细的区域淋巴结检查排除其转移的可能性。包含区域淋巴结的术后辅助放疗可能对这些患者有益。

对于软组织肉瘤的患者来说,淋巴结转移被认为是特别的预后不良因素,等同于 TNM 分期中的远处转移。区域淋巴结清扫的患者生存率升至 34%,因此,淋巴结受累而无结外病变的患者应行治疗性淋巴结清扫术[32]。以前,孤立性淋巴转移(与同时性远处转移截然不同)被 TNM 分级系统归类为预后不良和远处转移。最新的研究表明,如果积极治疗,其预后与Ⅲ期肿瘤(如高度恶性、深在、大于 5cm 的肿瘤)相似。孤立性淋巴结转移使得 AJCC/UICC 分级系统将单纯 N1 归为Ⅲ期[49]。随访结果对于将 N1 归为Ⅲ期的有效性提出了质疑,因为与 AJCC 分级系统中淋巴结阴性的Ⅲ期相比,N1 患者的生存率更接近于Ⅳ期[72]。

放疗

手术联合放疗的基本理论

两项Ⅲ期临床试验支持手术联合放疗治疗软组织肉瘤(表 112-3)。基于两个前提:肿瘤切除术后的显微镜下肿瘤细胞微残留可以被放疗消灭;当手术和放疗联合时,可避免进行破坏正常组织很大的根治性手术[69,70]。尽管传统观念认为软组织肉瘤对于放疗不敏感,但体外肉瘤细胞放疗敏感性试验表明软组织肉瘤对于放疗的敏感性与其他恶性肿瘤相似,这支持第一个前提[73,74]。第二个前提强调通过放疗减少切除范围以保留肢体、躯干、乳房以及头颈部肉瘤的患者的局部外观和功能[75~77]。类似的原则也适用于在容易出现问题部位的肉瘤,如腹膜后肉瘤、头颈部伴有颅底侵犯的高风险肉瘤或椎旁病变侵犯椎管的肉瘤。虽然通过前瞻性随机临床试验证实了放疗治疗肢体肉瘤的有效性,但其他部位尚未得到证实。目前,有一个评估原发性腹膜后肉瘤的术前放疗的Ⅲ期试验正在进行中。

内脏器官肉瘤常规不做放疗,主要因为胸腔、腹腔、盆腔内器官位置不固定,所以此类肿瘤行手术切除后可能肿瘤残留部位的放疗定位比较困难。被污染的肠管及其系膜在术后可能移至离手术野较远的部位。胸腔病灶切除后可能发生胸膜污染或纵隔移位。盆腔内位置固定的肿瘤或与躯干体壁连接紧密的肿瘤较适合做术前或者术后放疗。然而巨大的放射野需覆盖整个体腔,加上体腔内器官可接受的安全放射剂量有限,另外,这些部位的肿瘤远处转移风险远远大于局部复发等因素,限制了辅助放疗的实施。

体外放射计划需考虑的重要要素

肿瘤的精确定位是放疗计划制订的首要要素。由于经济原因,最主要应用的是 CT,但 MRI 可提供更为准确的肿瘤范围,并可通过电脑工作站进行图像融合后模拟出肿瘤形象[41,42]。肿瘤病理报告和手术记录可提供进一步信息,术中留置金属夹亦可帮助肿瘤定位。

应有效固定患处以减少放疗区域设置的误差以及治疗中发生移动。舒适的肢体位置或定制的支具有助于固定患肢,从而使每次治疗放疗区域设置一致。通过合适的组织学材料的应用,也可对浅表组织包括手术瘢痕进行放疗,但有可能导致组织纤维化、萎缩以及毛细血管扩张等。对于不规则的放疗区域,可应用光束分割、剂量补偿及滤光片等来优化调整放疗剂量。然而,这在很大程度上已经被强度调节放射治疗(IMRT)所取代,解决了包括目标的大小、形状和位置,以及周围正常组织的性质(包括轮廓和宽度)等问题。IMRT 特别适用于靶区接近关键正常组织(如颅底或腹部)的情况。整个肢体、关节以及软组织条件不佳的部位如(肘部、足跟部等)应避免全剂量放疗,否则将可影响肢体功能并造成肢端水肿。

如果放疗可能导致对称器官之一丧失功能(如眼、肾脏等)时,应在放疗前评估其功能,确定对称能否有效代偿,这点非常重要。这种情况在腹膜后肉瘤的治疗中经常遇到。如果肿瘤偏右侧或体积巨大,腹膜后肉瘤可侵及肝脏包膜或被肝脏覆盖,使得确定肿瘤周围的放疗区域变得十分困难。所以这个区域放疗最适合采用 IMRT 方法,原因在于这种方法可精确模拟肿瘤的外形,尽量将肝组织及其他重要的正常组织排除在放疗区域之外[78,79]。幸运的是,尽管整个肝脏的放疗耐受性很低,但如果仅有部分肝组织受到较高剂量的放疗,还是比较安全的。通过剂量-体积直方图可更好地利用"体积效应"以及更加迅捷、安全地制订治疗方案。当腹膜后肉瘤可能粘连或侵及肝脏被膜需切除部分肝脏时,外科医师及放疗科医师应详细讨论治疗方案以确定经过手术及放疗仍有足够的正常肝组织保留。

剂量分配问题

术后放疗的剂量依据软组织肉瘤的分级及外科切缘来确定[70,80,81]。对于低度恶性肿瘤常规剂量为 60Gy,高度恶性为 66Gy。如果进行术前放疗,大多数医院多采用 50Gy 左右,并以每日 1 次的方式 5 周内完成[81,82]。但有关剂量反应的研究数据非常有限,且大多数为说服力较低的回顾性研究。目前数据表明,术后放疗往往应用较大剂量(同术前放疗相比),但仍需寻求术后较低剂量放疗可行性数据的研究。下面将讨论使用的剂量和使用不同剂量对潜在发病率的影响。

单次分割剂量通常从 1.8~2.1Gy 不等[81,83]。单次分割剂量越小,期望后期并发症越少,这对于重要组织的放疗十分重要。目前已有一些不同的分割方案诸如超分割、低分割以及加速方案等[84~87]开始应用。最近,评估了一项 272 名肢体和躯干软组织肉瘤患者参与的术前低分割放疗研究。术前放疗连续 5 日,每次 5Gy。低分割治疗组的复发率(19%)高于同期的常规治疗组[88]。需要进行更长时间的后续研究。大剂量及低剂量分割方法在近期无法取代常规的放射治疗,包括一系列原因,小规模的非随机研究、需要一些规范协议、有效性和毒性及现代靶向治疗技术辅以 IMRT 可以抵消一部分改变分割剂量所产生的潜在优势等。

放疗剂量和靶区

近期,关于放疗靶区技术设计的新的指南已经发布。对于这一内容将会在下面详细介绍[89]。

很多软组织肉瘤受限于肢体轴向平面上的天然屏障,如骨、骨间膜或主要的筋膜平面,因此肢体软组织肉瘤倾向于在肢体特定肌群内沿肢体长轴蔓延。因此,放射区域在肿瘤的头尾方向上必须足够大。在横截面上,可安全地确定非放疗区域,特别是被完整屏障所隔开的组织。骨、骨间膜、筋膜被认为是肿瘤在轴向扩散的重要屏障,因此,放疗边界的勾画主要取决于头尾方向。对于非肢体病变,肿瘤蔓延的方向同样是沿着受累的肌肉组织,但此时应尤其关注筋膜平面并应包括在放射靶区域内。

本章中前文总结了肉瘤蔓延的解剖平面以及易于向哪个方向转移的原理。这些信息有助于设计放疗靶区。制订放疗计划的基本要素首先是确定肉眼肿瘤区(gross tumor volume, GTV),然后在肿瘤周围设定边界以包含所有可能存在镜下残留肿瘤风险的区域(临床肿瘤区,clinical tumor volume,CTV)(图 112-7a-c 和图 112-8)[90]。一般来说,放疗可分期实施,初始剂量(总剂量 40~50Gy,每次 1.8 或 2.0Gy)消除高危区域内所有镜下肿瘤细胞(第一期)。当进行术后放疗时,通常至少有一个区域可以使更高的放射剂量集中于最高危区域(第二期)。这时的放射剂量通常是 15~16Gy,但存在肉眼残留病变时这个剂量还可以增加。对于第一期的放疗靶区,外放至手术区域外 1.5cm,在头尾方向达 4cm,以期包括周围组织的微小病变;缩野"强化"放疗范围原发肿瘤外 1.5cm,在头尾方向达 2cm。对于术前放疗,历史上也是目前流行的做法是,GTV 50Gy/25f,4~6 周后再进行手术。通常,CTV 包括 GTV,外放至原发肿瘤外 1.5~2.0cm,在头尾方向达 4.0cm。CTV 也应该包括肿瘤外水肿带(可能隐藏有距 GTV 有一定距离的肿瘤细胞)[91]。术

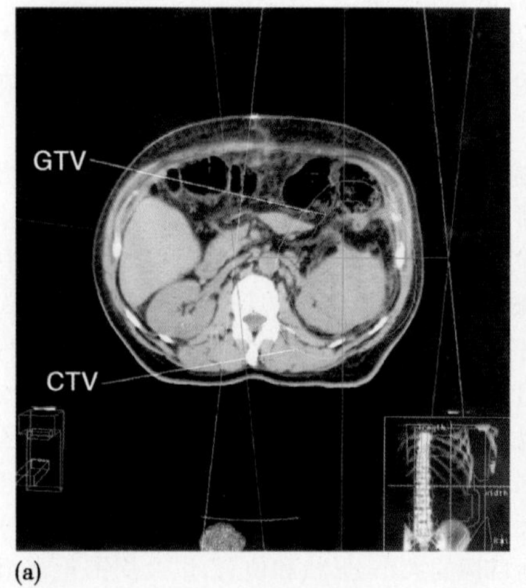

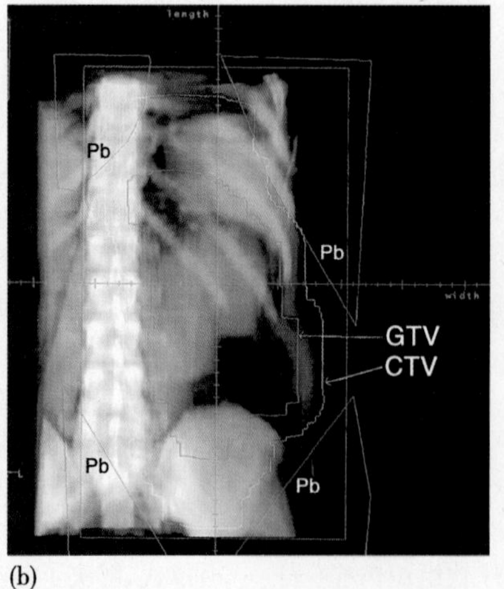

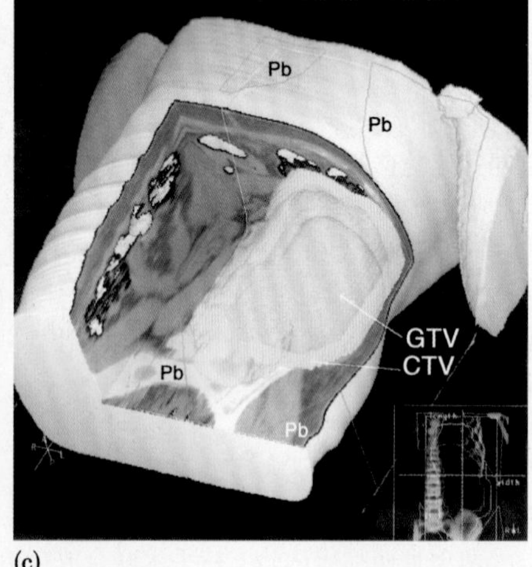

图 112-7 (a)GTV 在 CT 模拟工作站中被绘制出来(红色边框区域)。这包括前文述及的肿瘤前方异常脂肪像(图 112-5b 和 c)。这一处理由许多薄层 CT 断层片组成,以使三维治疗规划中的图像重建得以实现。CTV 在图中被黄色边框勾勒出来,代表着超出 GTV 范围的可能的镜下肿瘤扩散范围。此外图中尚有一些边界,这些边界是在考虑个体差异以及器官移动所造成的偏差而设计出的。注意被肿瘤推挤移位的肠管。图中直线表示常规的前后对穿照射野的照射方向。(b)在射束方向视图(beam eye view,BEV)中显示的 GTV 和 CTV 的轮廓。这是应用 CT 模拟器对 X 线片进行数码重建后得出的图像。一旦在 BEV 中发现靶区域内的射线线路,屏蔽(Pb)即可设定。(c)该图显示了三维重建的 GTV、CTV 以及屏蔽区域(Pb),并将腹壁以及前方的组织结构略去。总的来说,这种"剖开立体图"在需要显示危险解剖结构旁的靶区域边界时有重要作用,因为这些解剖结构往往需要保护,而它们与放射靶区域之间的空间关系往往在常规的影像学检查中不能被很好地界定

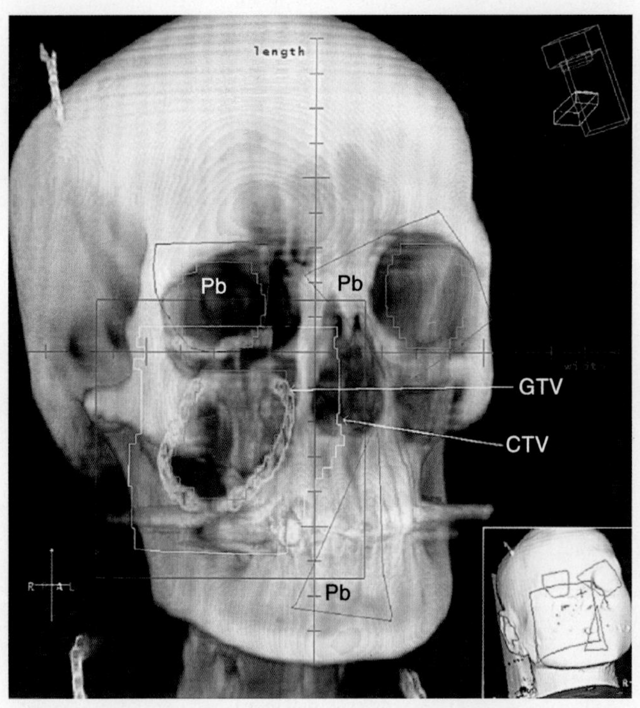

图 112-8　一位患右颊部 STS 年轻女性的头颈部数码重建 X 线片。由于照射区域接近右眼，术前放疗被选用于该患者的治疗，这是因为术前放疗能够最大地将 CTV 限制于肿瘤局部环境中。与图 112-6 中所述相同的应用 CT 模拟器的图像处理方法也在此处被用到。图中颊部 GTV 在 CTV 包围下，屏蔽(Pb)区域也是清晰可见的。患者在进行 CT 检查时所佩戴的发夹可以在右顶部见到，同时也可以看到她所戴的项链。右下角的小图显示的是患者在应用可能的照射之后的三维重建图像

前放疗后，术后“强化”放疗通常只用于手术切缘阳性的患者。这是因为，即便不进行术后“强化”放疗，切缘阴性患者的局控率也超过 90%[81,92,93]。当标本的边缘出现染色，则说明肿瘤细胞达到切缘，为切缘阳性；反之，则无论肿瘤多么接近切缘，仍为切缘阴性[81]。

在 216 例肢体软组织肉瘤的回顾性研究中，52 例患者只接受术前放疗(50Gy)，41 例接受术前放疗，并接受术后放疗(通常 16Gy)。术前放疗和手术后切缘阳性的患者是否需要术后“强化”放疗目前遭到怀疑。一部分未接受放疗或接受术后放疗的患者被排除在外(123/216)。术后“强化”放疗组的 5 年局控率更低(74%相比于只接受术前放疗组的 90%)[94]。类似的研究(n=67)也得到一样的结论[95]。这些结果提示：在软组织肉瘤的治疗中，术前放疗和手术后进行术后“强化”放疗有待于探讨，而且由于放射剂量的增加从而增加放射治疗的远期风险和挑战(如放疗导致的骨折)，这些都是需要考虑的。

加拿大肉瘤研究组关于肢体软组织肉瘤精确体外放疗靶区的随机临床研究的预期结果有待于以后进一步讨论[96]。但是，最近已经完成的英国术后随机Ⅲ期临床“VORTEX”研究(NCT NCT00423618)，比较长轴上 5cm 和经典的 GTV 2cm，结果值得期待[97]。已经完成的 RTOG-0630 试验(NCT NCT00589121)发现，IMRT 可以有更小的术前放疗靶区(长轴 3cm)，尽管这个结果可能被解释为是非随机研究[98]。综上所述，放疗靶区在长轴上不能小于 4cm。当然，为了更好地保护感兴趣的正常组织，减少放疗靶区，更多的研究需要进一步进行。

尽管放疗靶区有所差异，手术结合放疗治疗肢体软组织肉瘤的局部控制率都接近 90%，这些结果提示镜下累及的区域可能小于我们以前的认识。近来外科技术的提高，可能更加降低肿瘤的术中播散，因此照射所有外科处理区域、瘢痕、引流区域，可能并非必需。这似乎与外科手术是否在有良好肉瘤处理经验的肿瘤中心进行很有关系。也必须考虑病例的选择，以解释近距离放疗和体外放疗的差异。

放疗和手术的先后顺序

体外放疗的 2 种常用方式是术前放疗和术后放疗。术前放疗在肿瘤未受任何干扰、肿瘤细胞氧合状况可能较好的状况下实施，这也就解释了为何低剂量术前放疗确实不会对局部肿瘤控制造成负面影响[99]。Nielsen 等[100]对接受过术前放疗以及手术的患者重新设计放疗方案后发现，接受术前放疗的患者的放射区域和被动放疗的关节数量均显著少于仅接受术后进行放疗的患者。术前放疗的另一个优势是它可以促进外科肿瘤医师与放射肿瘤医师之间的合作，并易于在其他治疗开始前先制订一套整体的、互相协调的诊疗计划。

加拿大肉瘤研究组进行的临床试验(SR2)对于术前以及术后放疗进行了前瞻性随机对照研究[96]。与预期的一样，这个试验发现术前放疗导致急性伤口并发症的增加。另一方面，也和预期的一样，试验发现术后放疗也增加了肢体纤维化、水肿、关节僵硬和骨折。

加拿大肉瘤研究组 NCIC 试验(SR2)的长期随访发现，在可评估晚期毒性的 129 例患者中，术后放疗组中 48%相比于术前放疗组中 32%发生 2 级或更高级别的纤维化(P=0.07)[101]。水肿更常见于术后放疗组(23%相比于 16%)，关节僵硬也类似(23%相比于 18%)。有这些并发症的患者，不管在多伦多肢体救助评分还是肌肉骨骼肿瘤社会分级评分中，功能评分均更差(p 值均 < 0.01)。照射野大小可预测更多的纤维化(P=0.002)、关节僵硬(P=0.006)和周围水肿(P=0.06)。与术后放疗组相比，术前放疗组的急性伤口愈合并发症通常可达 2 倍。这些增加的风险几乎完全局限于下肢(术前放疗组 43%相比于术后放疗组 21%；P=0.01)。有意思的是，另外的一些报道，包括来自得克萨斯大学的安德森癌症研究中心，使用和加拿大 NCI 试验一样的急性伤口愈合并发症评级系统，几乎发现同样的结果[66]。

术前体外放疗与手术的间隔时间对于肢体软组织肉瘤急性伤口愈合并发症的影响，也进行了研究。尽管间隔时间影响很小，研究数据仍然建议降低急性伤口愈合并发症的最佳时间为 4~5 周[67]。

在最初的中位随访年限为 3.3 年的 SR2 报告中，术前放疗组患者的总生存率显著提高(P=0.048 1)，这可能与术后放疗组中非肉瘤原因死亡数增多有关[96]。两组的局部肿瘤未控制率相同(7%)(图 112-9)。但是，最近公布的结果中，最初的生存率差异已经消失了[101]。术前放疗和术后放疗在 5 年时的结果对比如下：局部控制率，93%相比于 92%；无转移率，67%相比于 69%；无复发生存率，58%相比于 59%；总生存率，73%相比于 67%(P=0.48)；病因特异性生存率，78%相比于 73%(P=0.64)。Cox 模型显示只有切缘是局部肿瘤控制的显著影响因素，肿瘤大

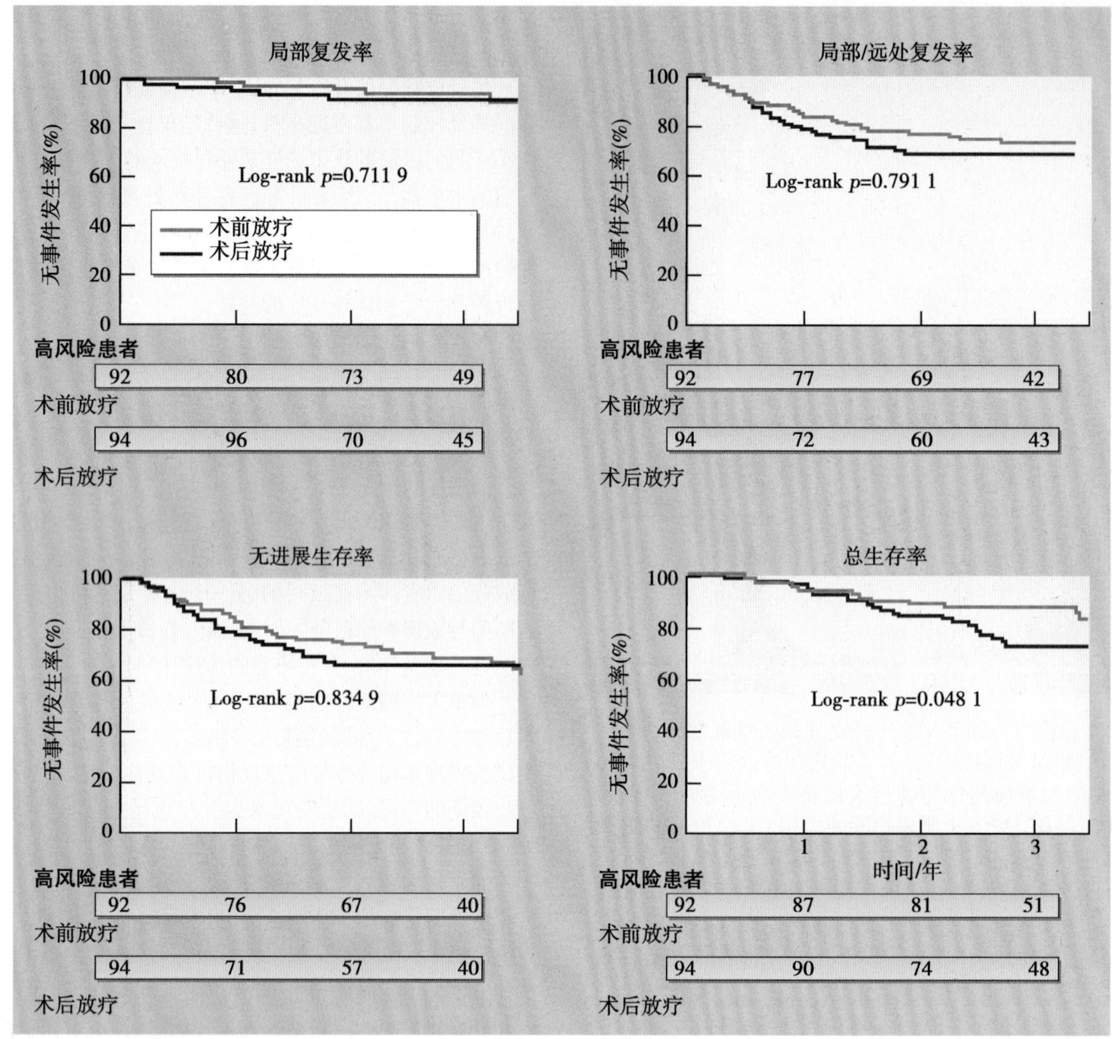

图 112-9 应用 Kaplan-Meier 方法对属于加拿大 NCI 临床试验组的加拿大肉瘤研究组进行的随机试验的局部复发率、转移率(局部和区域性复发)、无进展生存率和总生存率进行比较。这一临床试验以比较术前放疗和术后放疗效果为目的。摘自 O'Sullivan 等 2002[96]。Elsevier 公司授权复制

小以及分期是转移/复发、总生存率以及病因特异性生存率的显著影响因素,肿瘤分期是无复发生存率的唯一预测因素。

现阶段,对于术前、术后放疗的选择应当个性化,并综合考虑肿瘤位置、肿瘤大小、放疗靶区、并发症以及危险因素。总之,术前放疗相较术后放疗来说有更多的优势,但是会显著提高患者术后伤口并发症的发生风险。表 112-4 总结了选择术前放疗的相对适应证。另外,尽管很多关于术前放疗的讨论都集中于肢体病变,腹膜后肉瘤术前放疗的耐受性优于术后放疗。这是由于肿瘤作为组织扩展器将肠管推出放疗靶区(图 112-7a-c)。这将在"腹膜后肉瘤"章节详细讨论。

表 112-4 不考虑伤口并发症术前放疗的相对适应证

治疗环境/肿瘤部位	焦点问题	评论
头颈部		
鼻窦	接近视觉结构(眼、眶视交叉)	视觉功能损伤可被降至最低
颅底	接近脊髓、脑干	因其剂量和照射区域体积均较小,"较少"发生的损伤(牙齿,口腔黏膜损伤)的发生率也很小
颊部与面部	见较早的研究资料	见较早的研究资料
中厚皮瓣重建(特别是下肢)	皮瓣裂开以及继发感染	数月或数年后可能发生肢体活动或就业损害(罕见)
较大的涵盖体腔的 GTV 或 CTV	见较早的研究资料	见较早的研究资料

续表

治疗环境/肿瘤部位	焦点问题	评论
腹膜后	接近肠、肝、肾	重要器官可以被肿瘤推离原位或者不固定或者与其他组织粘连,这一情况与术后放疗中类似;可在肿瘤污染体腔前治疗全部肿瘤
一些小肠病变	接近重要解剖结构,特别是在小肠侧壁粘连时	腹腔污染使术后放疗无法进行
胸壁/胸膜	接近肺或心	肺可被胸壁或胸膜肿瘤推离原位,这一点可被术前放疗所避免。或者在手术前先行对 GTV 的治疗
腹壁,盆侧壁	接近肾、肠、肝、卵巢	避免 CTV 涉及较为脆弱的解剖结构 GTV 与剂量依赖性重要解剖结构相邻
胸廓入口/上胸部	接近臂丛	重要解剖结构剂量限制,采取胸壁和下颈部放疗。考虑额外增加剂量
大腿内侧(年轻男性)	接近睾丸	可避免永久性不育症
肢体中央肿瘤	接近其他间室	能够减少肿瘤周围的组织的照射,这在术后放疗中是不能做到的

CTV,临床靶区;GTV,肉眼肿瘤区。

摘自 O'Sullivan 等,1999[77]。Elsevier 公司授权复制。

放疗实施方法

一般而言,最常用的放疗方式包括体外放疗和近距离放疗。体外放疗,也包括关于体外放疗的时间顺序(术前放疗相比于术后放疗)的争论,已经在前面讨论。通常而言,也需要关注适形调强放疗的潜在作用,这也在前面提到过。至今尚无随机试验对体外放疗和近距离放疗直接进行比较,但这两种放疗方式都已经单独与手术进行了比较。除了 2 个前瞻性Ⅱ期临床试验正在等待研究结果,也没有重点关注适形调强放疗的随机试验。

适形调强放疗

对于肢体软组织肉瘤而言,适形调强放疗对于靶区覆盖和正常组织高剂量区的保护优于传统技术[102]。近期,一项非同时期的回顾性研究比较了手术联合适形调强放疗($n=165$)和常规体外放疗($n=154$)。考虑到已知的由于不同时期治疗所导致的研究缺陷,适形调强放疗显著降低肢体原发软组织肉瘤的局部复发率(局部复发率:适形调强放疗 7.6%相比于常规放疗 15.1%,$P=0.02$)[103]。

2 项前瞻性Ⅱ期临床试验(来自 Princess Margaret(NCT 00188175)和放射治疗肿瘤研究组(RTOG 0630;NCT 00589121))研究了术前影像引导放疗(IGRT)(采用适形放疗/适形调强放疗)是否可以降低放疗相关并发症[98,104]。Princess Margaret(PMH)试验和 RTOG 0630 试验在一些试验设计上并不相同:特别是 PMH 排除了上肢病变,RTOG 0630 试验术前放疗后进行了"强化"补量放疗,RTOG 0630 试验也允许化疗,一些靶区覆盖的选择(将在后续提及)。两项研究的原始观察终点也不相同。

PMH 试验发现:与加拿大肉瘤研究组 SR2 试验只采用 2D 和 3D 放疗相比,PMH 试验降低伤口愈合相关并发症(31%相比于 43%)[96],也降低了需要组织修复、放疗慢性并发症以及导致再次手术的严重伤口愈合相关并发症,同样也保全了好的肢体功能,增加局部控制率(93%)。RTOG 0630 试验报道:与 NCIC-SR2 试验相比,显著降低了晚期并发症(11%相比于 SR2 的 37%)。这个结果与 IGRT PMH 试验类似。重要的是,PMH 试验和 RTOG 0630 试验定义的 CTV 并不相同(RTOG 0630 试验:高级别病变:大体肿瘤外长轴边缘 3cm,低级别病变:2cm;PMH 试验:长轴边缘 4cm)。降低 CTV 至这种程度可以解释在同等的局部控制率基础上获得更好的肢体功能,尽管另一种选择是在各个方向降低靶区周围正常组织的剂量,这在上述 2 项试验中分享过。最后,与传统的适形技术相比,适形调强放疗能够更好地适形所需要照射的靶区。

适形调强放疗可能的最大优势是,不但可以增加局部控制率,而且也可以通过避免骨骼照射以减少骨骼毒性和迟发骨折,这经常在讨论肢体软组织肉瘤联合治疗时被忽视。近期的一项 230 例患者(176 例下肢和 54 例上肢)参与的、中位随访时间 41.2 个月的研究重点讨论了适形调强放疗避免骨损伤的循证医学剂量[105]。总的骨折风险是 2%(4/230),这与以前报道的 6%相比,比较不错,从而建议:避免骨骼照射的努力是恰当的。

近距离放疗

相对于外照射放疗,BRT 具有更多的优势,主要包括较短的总治疗时间(4~6 日相比于 5~6.5 周),以及术后在克隆源性细胞数目处于最小值时更早地开始放疗。由于 BRT 较为简单,比外照射放疗更容易被整合到包括系统化疗的治疗方案中,因为外照射治疗相对滞后。BRT 的放射剂量相对较小,这也有助于促进功能恢复。BRT 在正常组织对放疗耐受不良时也具有优势。当手术后需要对手术区域进行强化放疗时,对于已行术前放疗的患者可以采用上述的放疗方案。对已行照射过的组织行 BRT 是达到保肢目的的另一种途径[106,107]。如前所述,对于低级别的病变来说,BRT没有明显的优势,体外照射更加有效(表112-3)[69,70,108]。BRT也可以通过术中情况勾画靶区。美国近距离放疗社会指南将BRT和体外放疗做了区分,也提出BRT作为一种单独的治疗模式有以下的禁忌证:①由于内置物几何外形原因,CTV无法充分包括;②邻近的关键解剖结构,例如神经血管,可能被必需的放射所干扰;③外科切缘阳性;④肿瘤累及皮肤[109,110]。

BRT在一些内置物几何外形无法优化的位置,例如上肢或肢体近段区域,似乎作用有限[111]。这些BRT随机临床试验的结果已经在前面讨论过。另外,在一项134例高级别肢体软组织肉瘤参与的回顾性研究中发现,BRT相对于适形调强放疗也得出相似的不利结果[112]。适形调强放疗的5年局部控制率为92%,BRT为81%($P=0.04$)。遗憾的是,BRT,包括严格控制适应证,仍发现效果低于体外放疗,但是并没有随机临床试验去比较这些似乎有效的局部治疗手段。

传统上,BRT研究,包括前面提到的那些,用的是低剂量技术。高剂量BRT在理论上有潜在的优势,包括更低的放射职业暴露、门诊操作、通过改变停延时间优化剂量分布等。但是,当放置导管邻近神经血管等位置时,在肉瘤治疗中可能发生伤口愈合相关并发症,也推荐注意。至今,仍没有大宗病例研究去评估软组织肉瘤的高剂量BRT,也没有直接和低剂量BRT比较,部分是由于技术的差异。

其他放疗手段

除了外照射放疗、BRT以及IMRT,还有许多其他放疗方法,包括粒子束放疗(电子、质子、π介子或者中子)、术中放疗(intraoperative radiotherapy,IORT),即应用外照射或者BRT方式结合其他技术(如热疗)。IORT最常用于腹膜后肉瘤的治疗中,将于下文详细讨论。一些研究还描述了IORT治疗肢体肉瘤[113,114]。正式的临床试验并没有对这些方法的相关优点进行比较,选择哪一种治疗方法是根据某一治疗中心是否拥有该种这类方法,并且认为该方法有效。以质子束放疗为例,它作用于目标区域的精确性使它在对十分接近重要组织结构的肿瘤的治疗具备优势[115,116]。一般来说,虽然有许多应用这些方法的报道,但是需要考虑到治疗方法选择中存在倾向性的问题,因为实际上这些治疗方法并不是被随机选择的[117,118]。

化疗

化疗药物,包括传统的细胞毒性药物和新的小分子口服激酶抑制剂(SMOKI),被广泛应用于有转移的软组织肉瘤患者。化疗作为在STS的辅助治疗的作用目前仍有争议。但是,如果化疗在肉瘤的治疗中能有与放疗以及手术同等的地位的话,必将会有有效的药物被研发出来,有效地改善原发肿瘤患者以及不可见的镜下转移患者的治愈率。这一章节将主要回顾化疗在辅助治疗以及肿瘤转移中的应用,同时也包括对化疗联合放疗的简单讨论。

手术切除后化疗

虽然局部复发或局部区域复发是一小部分患者初期治疗后的一个问题,但威胁肉瘤患者生命的主要危险因素仍是无法控制的全身性转移。尽管系统治疗可以使高级别肉瘤缩小(尽管效果常常并不理想),但问题是早期应用系统治疗是否会对镜下转移病灶产生影响并真正改善肿瘤总生存率以及无病生存率(disease-free survival,DFS)。

当然,对于尤因肉瘤/PNET、横纹肌肉瘤以及成骨肉瘤来说,辅助化疗或新辅助化疗是恰当的标准治疗方式[119~122]。但是,对于更多常见的软组织肉瘤,如平滑肌肉瘤、脂肪肉瘤以及高级别未分化多形性肉瘤(曾被称为恶性纤维组织细胞瘤),来说,化疗的收益即使有也很小[123]。虽然辅助化疗已经被许多医师应用于收益相对较小的疾病(如Ⅰ期乳腺癌以及Ⅱ期结肠癌)中,但是在肉瘤治疗中,化疗这一很小的潜在优势需要个体化讨论。当然目前缺乏对转移性肉瘤有效的药物妨碍了这一领域的发展,但是伊马替尼对GIST治疗有效给予了人们希望,新的药物有望达到系统治疗的最终治愈目标,提高了新发患者的治愈率。

目前已有许多以蒽环类药物为基础的辅助化疗方案应用于软组织肉瘤治疗中的研究,最早的应用与多柔比星的出现几乎同时开始[124,125]。由于以蒽环类抗药物/异环磷酰胺为基础的治疗已成为一种辅助化疗标准方案,并且之前只有一项在1992年完成的研究中提及了应用异环磷酰胺,因此这些研究将不会再本文中回顾。

在目前最大的联合化疗临床研究中,意大利肉瘤研究组(Italian sarcoma Study Group,ISSG)对一组肢体或肢体带的,可切除的,原发或复发的,经放疗或未经放疗的软组织肉瘤病例进行了研究[126,127]。104位患者被随机地分为无化疗组和化疗组。化疗组接受异环磷酰胺(1 800mg/(m^2·d)加用美斯纳,连续5日),表柔比星(60mg/m^2,连续2日),加用非格司亭(filgrastim)支持治疗。在1996年的中期分析结果得出了一项早期结论,因为试验达到了一个主要终点——无瘤生存率提高。在中位随访时间为36个月的随访结果中,化疗组的总生存率对无化疗组总生存率为72%相比于55%($P=0.002$)。但是,在长期随访过程中,应用意向性分析(intention-to-treat)得到的总生存率差异已无统计显著性[126]。这项研究是文献中对于辅助化疗效果的最强论据。虽然如此,在研究进行到4年时观察到的相同的远处和局部复发率并无很好的解释。

相反,在一项EORTC的Ⅲ期化疗组(每周期多柔比星75mg/m^2,异环磷酰胺5g/m^2,共5周期,非格司亭支持治疗)对比观察组的临床研究中并没有看到生存获益[128]。1995—2003年一共纳入351例患者,80%(130/163)的患者完成了全部5周期化疗。总生存率并没有统计学差异(治疗组的$HR=0.94$,95%CI:0.68~1.31,$P=0.72$),无复发生存率也没有显著性差异($HR=0.91$,CI 0.67~1.22,$P=0.51$)。治疗组的5年总生存率为67%,对照组为68%。这一研究和ISG研究的主要区别是,ISG研究的异环磷酰胺剂量更低,ISG研究应用的是表柔比星。但是并不清楚,病变的转移是否与这些差异有关。

最近的关于肢体软组织肉瘤辅助化疗的综合性分析是2008年包括18项研究所有解剖位置肉瘤的荟萃分析[129]。在这项研究中,一共考察了93项潜在的研究,最终选择了18项研究,包括1 953例肢体或非肢体的软组织肉瘤。病理并没有集中复阅。荟萃分析的结果,包括精确的概率结果、危险比等,在图112-10和表112-5中总结。

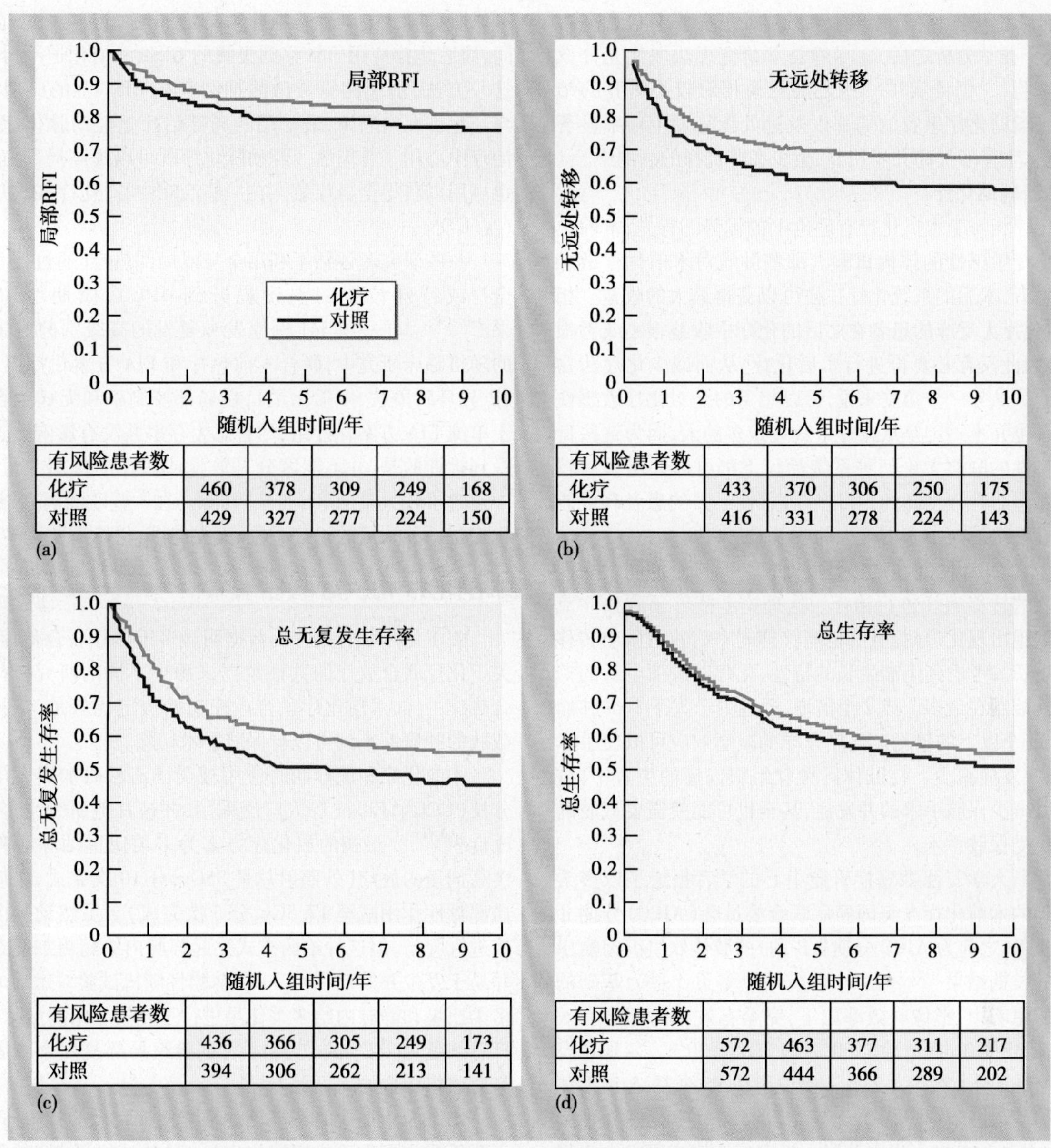

图 112-10　针对单个患者所得数据进行荟萃分析（继后分析）的统计曲线：(a)无局部复发期（RFI）；(b)无远处转移期；(c)总无复发生存率；(d)总生存率。摘自 O'Bryan 等，1977[130]。Wiley 公司授权复制

表 112-5　辅助化疗的临床结果：风险比和 95%*CI*（2008 年荟萃分析）

	多柔比星	多柔比星-异环磷酰胺	联合
无局部复发期	0.75(0.56~1.01)	0.66(0.39~1.12)	0.73(0.56~0.94)
无远处转移期	0.69(0.56~0.86)	0.61(0.41~0.92)	0.67(0.56~0.82)
总无复发生存率	0.69(0.56~0.86)	0.61(0.41~0.92)	0.67(0.56~0.82)
总生存率	0.84(0.68~1.03)	0.56(0.36~0.85)	0.77(0.64~0.93)

摘自 Pervaiz 等，2008[129]。Wiley 公司授权复制。

18 项临床试验的研究数据都被综合起来，但并没有对每个病例的数据进行检查。结合所有的数据，化疗的局部复发风险、远处转移风险、总复发风险和总生存率被优先考虑。对于总生存率而言，化疗的死亡相对风险是 0.77（95% *CI*：0.64~0.93），$P=0.01$；相对复发风险是 0.67（95% *CI*：0.56~0.82），$P=0.0001$。各种复发的绝对风险降低 10%，总生存率的绝对风险降低 6%。但是，正如在这项荟萃分析的评论中所说，这些数据必须被慎重接受[131]，这是因为：①每个病例的数据并没有被复阅和询问；②在更早的分析中，18%的病例并没有病历可以复阅，无法通过专业中心的复阅以了解病理的错误率；③较

高的不适合入组患者比例；④最大的独立研究并没有包含在内（发表于这个荟萃分析之后）。尽管荟萃研究无法取代充分设计的随机试验，它仍证实了一些之前规模相对较小研究的结论——接受辅助化疗患者的局部以及远处无复发生存率显著提高了，但总生存率提高并不明显，至少在非选择的病例中。

术前化疗(新辅助化疗)

术前化疗相对于术后化疗有理论上的优势。首先，术前化疗提供了化疗敏感性的体内试验。那些肿瘤对术前化疗敏感性较高的患者，术后的系统化疗往往可以获得最大的收益。相反，对术前化疗无反应的患者在之后的化疗中收益很小或者根本无收益，因此没有必要再进行术后化疗，从而减少化疗药物的毒性反应。从另一个角度来说，可以想象的是对化疗敏感性较高的患者也并不一定是从化疗中获益最多的人，因为这些良好生物学特性的肿瘤无论何种系统治疗下都可以注定预后较好，相反，那些恶性程度高的，对化疗敏感性不强的患者有可能在新的高效系统治疗中获得最大的收益。

其次，术前化疗的潜在优势是可以在肿瘤诊断的同时立即开始对隐匿的转移病灶进行治疗。这理论上能够预防独立克隆的转移细胞出现化疗耐药性，也能够抑制术后残留微小转移灶的快速生长。考虑到肉瘤生长的特性，化疗对肿瘤生长的控制可以使其控制在最多 1 或 2 个倍增，远远少于大于 1cm 肿瘤所需要的 35 个以上的倍增。化疗介导的减瘤效应可以使手术范围缩小、并发症减少。在肢体巨大软组织肉瘤的患者中，减瘤效应可以减少保肢手术的并发症，甚至也可能使需要截肢的患者得以接受保肢手术。

得克萨斯大学安德森癌症研究中心的学者报道了以多柔比星为基础的术前化疗在美国癌症联合委员会（AJCC）分期Ⅱ C 期以及Ⅲ期（之前为 AJCC 分期ⅢB 期）的肢体软组织肉瘤患者中应用的长期结果[132]。在 76 名应用以多柔比星为基础的术前化疗的患者中，影像有效率如下：完全有效 9%；部分有效 19%；效果轻微 13%；病情稳定 30%；病变发展 30%。客观总有效率（完全和部分有效）为 27%。中位随访 85 个月，5 年无复发生存率、无远处转移生存率、无瘤生存率和总生存率分别为 83%、52%、46%和 59%。得克萨斯大学安德森癌症研究中心报道的无事件发生率与Ⅲ期术后化疗临床试验中所得到的结果类似。此外，有效患者（完全有效者和部分有效者）与无效患者的无事件发生率并无显著性差异。相反，在一项美国 MSKCC 的小型研究中，接受了 2 个周期以多柔比星为基础的化疗后，只有 1/29 的患者出现符合 WHO 定义的肿瘤缩小[133]。

包含异环磷酰胺的联合用药方案已经应用于术前治疗中。选择病例使用以异环磷酰胺为基础的激进的化疗方案，肿瘤出现良好的反应。初步结果提示这一方案的效率要高于历史对照中应用无异环磷酰胺化疗方案[134]。然而，正如前文所提到的，应用多柔比星和异环磷酰胺的新辅助化疗Ⅱ期临床试验在治疗组中并未显示出更好的疗效，尽管这一研究并不是针对确定生存率是否提高而设计的[135]。

化疗的局部应用

理论上，辅助化疗的抗肿瘤作用可以通过改良与药物转运相关的影响因素而提高。其中一种改良方法是进行局部化疗而不是全身给药。腹腔化疗最早应用于卵巢癌或阑尾癌——那些位于比较表浅、容易接受腹膜化疗的位置；相比那些容易形成明显肿块的其他恶性肿瘤，腹腔化疗难以穿透。在一段时间，腹腔化疗应用于转移到腹膜的 GIST 和消化道平滑肌肉瘤。这一方法，由于酪氨酸激酶抑制剂在 GIST 上的应用，而被放弃。也许在肉瘤中，最常用的局部治疗是经动脉化疗，在一些治疗中心用于骨肉瘤。经动脉化疗既可以提高局部血药浓度，也可用以获得全身疗效。在一些治疗中心，化疗在放疗后应用（见下文）。

一些研究者评估了利用全身或局部热疗（通过技术手段将全身或特殊位置的温度提升到 41℃），以期增加化疗效果[136~138]。在一项 341 例原发和复发的高级别肉瘤患者参与的随机临床研究中，联合术前热疗和 EIA 方案化疗组（依托泊苷、异环磷酰胺、多柔比星），在局部控制率和无病生存率上优于单纯 EIA 方案化疗组，尽管总生存率并没有影响。这项研究受到批评的是，并不能区分是放疗或热疗的作用，而且在研究中包含了较大量的 R1 和 R2 切除。在一些欧洲国家，热疗联合化疗是一种认可的治疗手段，而在美国，仍然需要更多的研究。

术前化疗和放疗联合

关于化疗联合放疗的数据明显多于热疗联合化疗，大部分关于化疗联合放疗的共性数据来源于不同的研究机构。和联合热疗一样，术前化疗联合放疗初始假定优势是，使只能采取截肢的肿瘤缩小到可以行保肢手术切除。

术前化疗和放疗同时应用被美国洛杉矶加州大学洛杉矶分校（UCLA）Eilber 等人广泛采用，并被其他研究组多次检验、改良[139,140]。最初的放化疗方案为多柔比星动脉给药联合每次高剂量的放疗（外照射总量 35Gy，分 10 次完成，之后为减少局部毒性作用减至 17.5Gy，分 5 次完成）。虽然动脉内给药直接进入肿瘤，但这种给药方式比起静脉内给药更加复杂、昂贵，并易于发生并发症[141]。一项前瞻性随机试验对术前动脉内给多柔比星和静脉内给多柔比星进行了比较。给药后都进行了 8 日总剂量为 28Gy 的放疗，术后试验组局部复发率或者生存率与对照组相比均无显著差异[140]。

迄今为止最大的直接针对系统化疗联合放疗进行的研究，主要检测应用和不应用雷佐生（一种放疗增敏剂）的随机对照临床试验，病例选择为可切除的或不可切除的软组织肉瘤[142]。试验组雷佐生出现急性皮肤反应，但迟发毒性反应较对照组并没有明显的增加。即使两组中病例存在一定的不平衡，但 130 例可评价病例中的 82 例相比于仅用外照射放疗的患者仍表现出了升高的有效率（74%相比于 49%）以及改善了的局部控制率（64%相比于 30%，$P<0.05$）。外照射放疗中位剂量为 56~58Gy，雷佐生放疗期间每日口服剂量为 150mg/m^2。

在尤因肉瘤和横纹肌肉瘤的治疗中，不管是异环磷酰胺还是环磷酰胺已被常规地与放疗联合作为其固定治疗方案的一部分，在最大限度局部控制肿瘤的同时进行全身系统化治疗[119]。总的来说，该治疗方案的毒性反应并不比仅用放疗时高。但是，联合治疗的皮肤反应要高于仅用放疗时[143]。

另一种化疗和放疗序贯治疗方案在局限的、高级别的、大的（>8cm）肢体软组织肉瘤进行验证[144~146]。这一治疗方案包括 3 周期多柔比星、异环磷酰胺、美斯纳、达卡巴嗪（dacarbazine）联合化疗以及两次 22Gy 剂量的放疗（每次分 11 次完成），也就是术前进行总剂量为 44Gy 的放疗，而后进行手术治疗,术后对切缘进行仔细显微镜下评估。对于镜下阳性手术边界者给予 16Gy 的术后强化放疗(8 次完成)。经该方案治疗的 48 名患者预后显著好于匹配的历史对照[144]。相对于 MAID 化疗方案组和对照组患者,该方案组五年局部控制率、无远处转移生存率、无瘤生存率和总生存率分别为 92%相比于 86%(P=0.115 5),75%相比于 44%(P=0.001 6),70%相比于 42%(P=0.000 2),以及 87%相比于 58%(P=0.000 3)。中性粒细胞减少症发热的并发症发生率为 25%。14 名(29%)接受化疗和放疗序贯治疗的患者出现伤口愈合并发症。1 名接受了化疗的患者发生了迟发型致死性骨髓异常增生综合征。鉴于该研究与历史对照相比的良好结果,肿瘤放射治疗协作组(Radiation Therapy Oncology Group)已开始组织一项多中心试验,改良化疗方案从而更好地处理局部毒性问题。这项研究结果建议,联合治疗可以在各个机构成功进行,尽管有一些毒性。这一结果和以往的单中心研究结果一致[145,146]。目前问题是,肢体高风险软组织肉瘤在密集新辅助化放疗和手术治疗后,是否可以生存获益,这还需要长期随访研究。

尽管在之前的研究中发现了明显的毒性反应,但局部控制率得到明显提高,从而向人们提出了安全应用化放疗联合治疗以降低局部肿瘤控制风险的可能。Pisters 等[132]将多柔比星和放疗联合应用于 27 名患有肢体软组织肉瘤患者的新辅助化疗中。术前外照射 25 次,每次 2Gy;多柔比星每周 4 日持续输注,每日剂量均较前一天增加一支。在化放疗后 4~7 周进行影像学检查以对肿瘤进行重新分期,之后无转移患者行手术切除肿瘤。联合标准术前放疗时,术前持续输注多柔比星最大耐受剂量为每周 17.5mg/m^2;23 位患者中 7 人(30%)出现了三级皮肤毒性反应。全部 26 名接受手术的患者均完整切除了肿瘤(R0 或 R1)。在 22 名接受了最大耐受剂量多柔比星治疗后手术的患者中,11 位患者(50%)化疗坏死率达 90%以上,其中 2 名患者为 100%。这一方案正在和放射增敏剂(如吉西他滨)同时应用进行临床试验[147]。对于联合治疗更进一步的研究将在之后的"腹膜后肉瘤"章节中详细讨论。

其他关于软组织肉瘤辅助化疗的多中心临床试验

众所周知,不同的肉瘤亚型具有不同的化疗敏感性,例如:恶性外周神经鞘瘤)对多柔比星耐药;平滑肌肉瘤对异环磷酰胺敏感性较其他类型的肉瘤低;转移的滑膜肉瘤和黏液型/圆细胞型脂肪肉瘤比其他类型的肉瘤对化疗更敏感,并且是对蒽环类抗生素和异环磷酰胺敏感的两种肉瘤亚型[61]。这提示辅助化疗应当在肉瘤亚型特异性的基础上进行选择。整合 UCLA 和 MSKCC 的非随机资料显示应用于滑膜肉瘤和黏液型/圆细胞型脂肪肉瘤的辅助化疗确实有效,同时也支持根据 MSKCC 和 Dana-Farber 癌症研究所的数据得出的所有软组织肉瘤都应当进行新辅助化疗的结论[148~150]。有趣的是,在安德森癌症研究中心和 MSKCC 所有接受或没接受过化疗的患者的资料显示,无论患者接受的是辅助化疗还是新辅助化疗,接受化疗组和未接受化疗组患者的总生存率并无统计学差异[151]。然而,这些数据存在一定的偏倚,原因在于被选择接受化疗往往是年轻、健康、肿瘤较大、肿瘤分期较高的患者。然而即便如此,在肉瘤较大的患者中,尤其是脂肪肉瘤患者倾向于采取辅助化疗,这可能是选择偏倚的原因,但同时也可以使这些本来预后较差的患者有了与预后较好患者形成相同概率的机会。

总的来说,对于 AJCC 分期Ⅲ期的软组织肉瘤患者来说,即便辅助化疗有益处,益处也比较有限。在不同的治疗中心和不同的实施者之间,对于准备化疗患者的实践操作并不相同。鉴于这种情况,笔者会权衡系统治疗的收益与风险,并根据具体临床情况制订个体化治疗计划。50 岁以下的患者可以得到最大的收益。当然,在 35%或更多的、有特定的基因易位或突变的软组织肉瘤患者,与伊马替尼对于 GIST 的治疗一样,在肢体和躯干软组织肉瘤的辅助治疗(传统细胞毒性化疗联合新的治疗方法)中提供希望。

"小儿"肉瘤与辅助治疗

几乎所有针对于小儿肉瘤患者的标准化治疗方案均包括化疗,其对于成骨肉瘤、尤因肉瘤、横纹肌肉瘤患者均有明确的疗效。以下为一些简略的针对该类化疗敏感肿瘤的讨论。

新辅助化疗方案是成骨肉瘤初始治疗的标准方案[121]。在化疗应用之前的时代,即便对于原发肿瘤行截肢术,治愈率仅约为 15%。化疗的应用,生存率提高到了 65%~70%。然而 30%~35%的复发患者仍是一个临床非常棘手的问题,尽管加用新药,治愈的概率也是微乎其微。这一新药在美国的随机临床研究中并没有证实可以得到获益[120]。新辅助化疗的效果(化疗后肿瘤坏死率)与疾病的预后直接相关,这也为那些初始化疗效果不佳的患者提供了更换化疗方案的机会。标准化的辅助化疗方案是以顺铂和多柔比星为核心的,在大部分的小儿和部分成人应用甲氨蝶呤。1997 年的一篇文章对甲氨蝶呤作为辅助治疗的一部分提出质疑,他们指出单纯应用多柔比星和顺铂可以达到和包括毒性强的高剂量甲氨蝶呤的方案(类似于 Rosen 的 T10 方案)相同的效果[152]。然而,在其他一些研究中,甲氨蝶呤是新辅助治疗的重要组成部分,是骨肉瘤联合治疗中不可分割的一部分[153]。非特异性免疫系统刺激剂胞壁三肽(muramyl tripeptide,MTP)的益处并没有遭到特别多的疑问。胞壁三肽在一个大型小儿临床试验中,作为辅助性治疗,提高了总生存率;然而,加入异环磷酰胺至甲氨蝶呤-多柔比星-顺铂(MAP)为基石的治疗中,并没有看到生存获益[120]。

纵观一系列国际临床研究,横纹肌肉瘤的辅助化疗方案首先进行诱导化疗,而后进行放化疗联合治疗,最后再进行化疗以满足全疗程化疗的要求。这一治疗方案在患儿中一般耗时约 48 周。标准化疗方案包括长春新碱、放线菌素 D 和环磷酰胺,这一方案与 VAI、VIE 方案效果相当但毒性更小[119]。在此方案中加入多柔比星对于该方案总生存率并没有明显的提高,因此在横纹肌肉瘤的治疗中常不采用[154]。与儿童患者相比,成人对长春新碱的耐受性差,成人患者必须调整剂量或缩短化疗疗程。在大多数研究中,也在日常临床实践中,儿童患者预后往往好于相同分期的成人患者[155,156]。

对于尤因肉瘤的患者来说,与横纹肌肉瘤的治疗不同,在长春新碱、多柔比星和环磷酰胺为基础的化疗方案中再加入额外的化疗药物(异环磷酰胺和依托泊苷)能够改善未转移肿瘤的预后,2 周方案优于 3 周方案[122];然而,并没有数据(超过 18 岁的患者可以从 2 周方案获益)发表。这种五药联合化疗方案是对于新诊断尤因肉瘤患者的一种良好的标准化方案。对于成人 14 周期化疗往往十分困难,因而缩短辅助化疗方案势在必行。全部14周期化疗是否可以获得更好的疗效,目前也并不十分明确。与横纹肌肉瘤一样,其他条件一样的情况下,尤因肉瘤儿童患者的预后好于成人患者[157~159]。

对于局部晚期肿瘤的治疗

隔离肢体热灌注化疗、隔离肢体热输注化疗和局部热疗

作为一项在美国正处于研究中的技术(虽然在世界上部分国家已被监管部门许可应用),隔离热灌注化疗技术(hyperthermic isolated limb perfusion,HILP)在晚期,无法手术切除的软组织肉瘤治疗中的应用受到了越来越多的关注。ILP包括在高温条件下局部灌注高剂量化疗药(最常用是美法仑),如果可以,也包括肿瘤坏死因子。ILP通过动脉和静脉插管以及旁路泵,建立一条氧合回路,并通过近端放置止血带,以最小化全身血药浓度。

在两种情况下考虑HILP:①对于只能行截肢治疗的晚期恶性肿瘤,尝试保肢者;②对于已伴肺有转移的、预期生存时间较短的局部晚期恶性肿瘤,(Ⅳ期病变),尝试改善患肢功能者。

一项多中心Ⅱ期临床试验评估了影像学确认无法手术切除的55名肢体软组织肉瘤进行HILP(灌注大剂量IFN-α和美法仑,部分患者只用IFN-α)[160]。大部分看到肿瘤反应,超过80%的患者保留肢体。局部毒性反应有限,全身毒性反应为低至中度。无治疗相关的死亡病例。尽管ILP获得较高的CR率(15%~30%)和保肢率(>80%),并没有随机临床试验比较软组织肉瘤的ILP和侵袭性保肢手术联合放疗。因此,对于一些患者而言,当其他治疗受限或无法实现时,ILP被认为是一种潜在的治疗手段。合适的患者可以被推荐至有治疗条件的治疗中心。

肢体软组织肉瘤的隔离肢体热输注化疗(isolated limb infusion,ILI)被研究得比较有限,经动脉化疗也差不多。和ILP一样,ILI依赖于隔离肢体循环的高剂量化疗药物。与ILP不同的是,ILI可以经皮放置导管,并在乏氧的条件下进行。然而,肢体软组织肉瘤ILI治疗的经验尚比较有限。与ILP一样,并没有随机临床试验直接比较ILI和侵袭性保肢手术联合体外放疗。但是,准备ILP和ILI的患者在初次评估时,通常不再考虑手术联合体外放疗,因此在一些患者,ILP和ILI被认为是一种潜在的治疗手段。

为了局部控制的精准放疗

除了对放疗十分敏感的肉瘤亚型的患者,大多数把放疗作为唯一的治疗方式的患者被认为是局部晚期,无法手术切除的病变。单纯放疗是一种罕见的治疗选择,应当仅在对治疗肉瘤十分专业的治疗中心中应用。身体健康,具有肉眼"无法切除",但无全身转移的肉瘤患者应该到专科治疗中心,接受多学科联合的综合治疗方案,包括手术、放疗以及可能的化疗。比如,腹股沟或腋窝的肿瘤可能会包绕肢体主要的血管,肿瘤连同主要的动静脉切除后,进行血管重建,也通常应用术后辅助放疗。在罕见的情况下,患者具有真正无法切除的局部晚期肿瘤可能仅行放疗,如光子束或粒子束(质子、中子或介子)[161~163]。没有正式的临床试验对这些方案进行互相比较,仅在上述不良临床预后情况下采用单纯放疗。局部控制率可达到40%~70%。

转移性病变的治疗

转移的临床问题

软组织肿瘤患者诊断复发或转移,通常令人心碎。患者和医师都很明白,一般来说,这一诊断是致命的。多学科肉瘤治疗协作组在治疗转移性肉瘤患者中发挥的作用是:寻找机会使综合治疗仍能改善一些重要的预后因素,比如生存率或生活质量。在某些患者手术和全身化疗仍能在提高患者的治疗效果发挥重要作用。总的来说,很重要的是意识到对于无法手术切除的转移性软组织肉瘤(罕见例外病例),最终都是致命的,但姑息性化疗,仍有可能达到延长生命和改善生活质量。

最常见的肢体软组织肉瘤转移部位是肺。的确,无论原发肢体还是躯干软组织肉瘤发生转移,80%都在肺,且肺是唯一的转移部位[61]。原发内脏、胃肠道肉瘤通常转移到肝和肺。肺外转移作为肢体肉瘤的首发转移并不常见,它往往作为肉瘤广泛播散的晚期表现。远处转移发生后中位生存时间为12个月(图112-11)[165],尽管,对于接受细胞毒性化疗的非选择的同时期患者的中位生存时间目前为15~18个月。对转移性软组织肉瘤合理的治疗需要充分了解肿瘤的自然发展过程,并根据患者因素、疾病因素以及既往治疗情况为患者制订个体化治疗方案。

随着时间的推移,对于晚期或转移性肉瘤的治疗方法也在不断发生变化。我们认识到临床试验必须进行合理、正确的分组才能获得有价值的数据。对于"肉瘤"不考虑分组的研究就如同对于"癌"不考虑其来源的研究一样天真。虽然皆为间叶组织来源,且均在"肉瘤"的名下,但去生物学行为却大不相同,对它们的研究应当认真考虑进行合理分组。如要进行临床研究,需要获得足够的病例数和进行可信的统计学分析,因此需要国内或国际水平的合作。这种合作组织目前已经在欧洲国家中建成(EORTC的软组织与骨的肉瘤协作组),以及在斯堪的纳维亚半岛、意大利和加拿大中心。同时,新的合作组织也在美国外科医师学会肿瘤组(ACOSOG)的赞助下在美国启动。在这些合作组织的共同努力下,相信进一步的研究会迅速地将研究成果转化成为新的治疗方式,这也是肉瘤患者所迫切需要的。

转移病灶的切除

许多研究者报道了成人软组织肉瘤肺转移灶切除的经验[166,167]。开胸肺转移灶切除术后3年生存率为23%~54%。由于能否完全切除所有转移病灶是疾病预后的重要判断指标,上述报道的各机构转移灶切除术后生存率的差异可能是在统计生存率时,有的选取了所有接受开胸手术的患者,有的仅选取了能完全切除所有转移灶的患者进行统计。

预测哪一位肺转移的肉瘤患者能从肺切除术中受益是十分困难的。单因素分析确定的临床标准包括无转移间歇期、转移结节数量以及肿瘤倍增时间。NCI和Roswell Par癌症中心进行的多因素分析证实较短的无转移间歇期和肺部转移灶切除不完全是肺转移患者的不良预后因素[166~169]。另外,MDACC

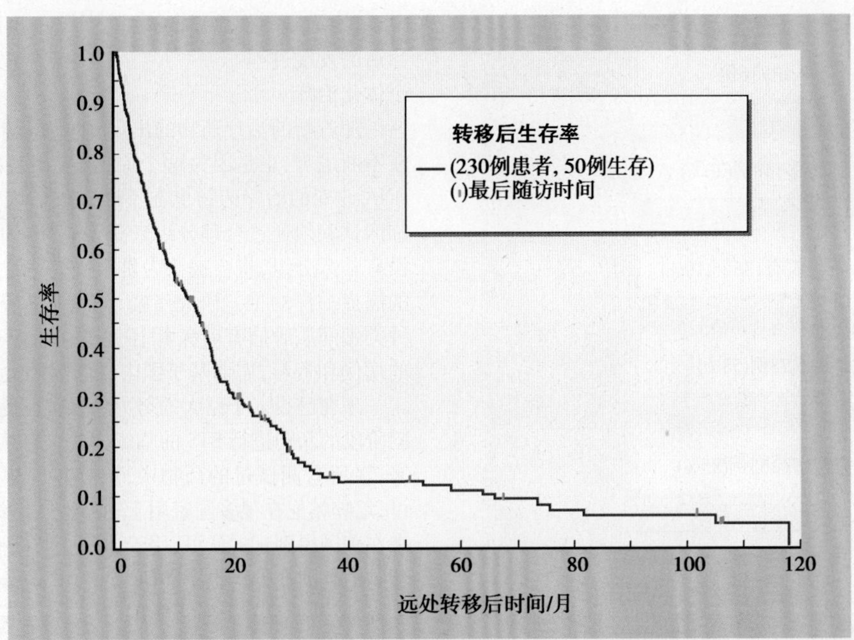

图 112-11　230 位肢体 STS 的患者的转移后生存率(在确诊为 M1 期后)。中位转移后生存时间为 11.6 个月。摘自 Slater 等 1986[164]。Elsevier 公司授权复制

的一项多因素分析认为术前胸部 CT 中肺转移结节多于 3 个也是一项不良预后因素。不过,影响患者生存率的最重要的预后因素仍是能否完全切除所有的转移病灶。MSKCC 的 Billingsley 等对于转移灶切除术患者生存率的回顾分析中,经彻底转移病灶切除的患者中位生存时间为 20 个月,而无法彻底切除转移病灶的患者中位生存时间为 10 个月(图 112-12)[165]。总之,能否达到彻底切除转移病灶以及肺部结节数量为预测术后预后的重要可靠因素。

遗憾的是,转移病灶切除术仅对肺转移患者中的少部分(<15%)有帮助。MSKCC 的资料可以很好地支持这一观点(图 112-13)[170]。在资料中共有 716 名原发肢体肉瘤患者入组,其中 148 名患者(21%)继发肺转移。在 148 名患者中仅发生肺转移的为 135 例(91%),其中 78 例(58%)有手术指征。在这 78 例中有 65 例(83%)能够对全部肺部转移灶进行完全切除。也就是说,44%的患者能够接受彻底的转移病灶切除术。彻底切除转移病灶后中位生存时间为 19 个月,3 年生存率为 23%。所有未行开胸手术的患者均在 3 年内死亡。对于全部 135 例仅发生肺转移的患者来说,3 年生存率仅有 11%。

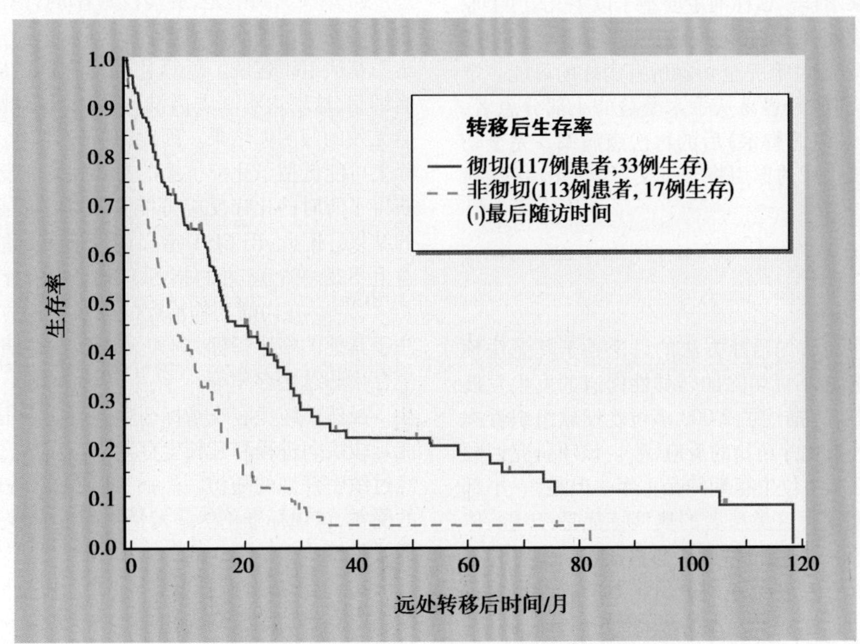

图 112-12　转移灶被切除后的患者生存率。彻底切除肺部转移病灶的患者中位生存时间为 20 个月。摘自 Slater 等 1986[164]。Elsevier 公司授权复制

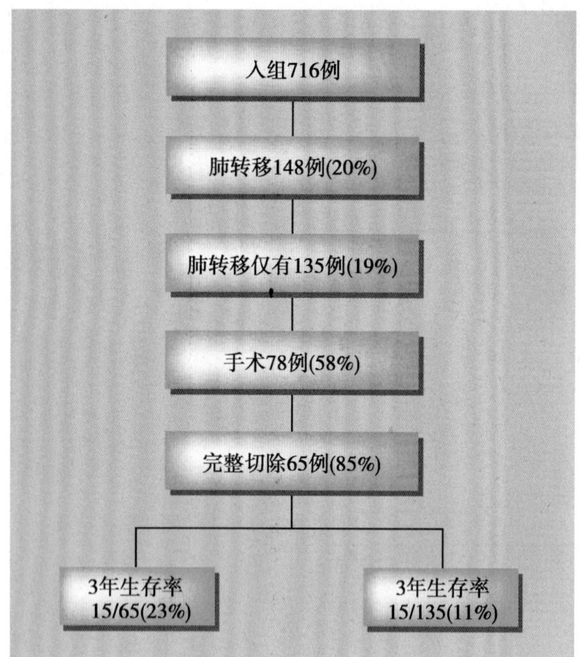

图 112-13 716 例原发或局部复发的肢体 STS 患者的肺转移风险评估及后续治疗。摘自 Brennan 等 1996[170]。Elsevier 公司授权复制。

一些关于反复开胸肺转移病灶切除的研究也被发表。在 NCI 进行上述治疗的 43 名患者中,72%的患者接受二次开胸手术消除了所有肺转移灶,二次开胸手术后中位生存时间为 25 个月[171]。MDACC 的 39 例患者接受了二次开胸转移病灶切除术,他们发现二次开胸术后长期生存率的预测因素仍为是否为单发转移灶以及能否进行彻底的切除术[172]。二次孤立性转移患者的预后明显好于可切除的多发病变患者。

之所以转移性肺叶切除的筛选指征严格,是因为有转移病灶患者的总体治疗效果不佳。该标准主要基于以下几点:①原发肿瘤已被控制或可控制;②没有胸外疾病;③患者有开胸术或肺叶切除术的临床指征;④有完全切除所有病灶的可能。严格筛选切肺的患者,使那些最容易从手术受益的小部分患者,控制其在开胸术(或者反复开胸术)后的再次患病率。完全切除转移性病灶后的系统化疗的作用将于下文“个体化治疗”章节进一步讨论。

转移性疾病的化疗

肿瘤转移的自然病程

不可切除的转移性肉瘤的治疗方法的讨论始于其无法预料的病程。EORTC 为描述不可切除的转移性肉瘤的发生发展过程作出了突出的贡献,它描述了 2 000 多位晚期软组织骨肉瘤的预后特征及对蒽环类化疗药物的反应[173]。该项研究回顾了 20 多年来的病例,总的中位生存期约是 1 年。但是,一小部分患者有更长的生存期限。这类患者的典型特征是:年轻、体质好、骨肉瘤分化级别低、没有肝转移,从初次发病到发生转移经历了很长的时间。重要的是,这项研究所提示的改善预后的因素,与预测化疗反应的指标不同(后者包括例如高分化肿瘤、脂肪肉瘤等等)。因此,专家认为对转移性骨肉瘤预后影响最大的是肿瘤本身的生物学特性及某些患者的临床特征,例如年龄和并发症等。过去在收治这些患者时,临床资料的收集非常重要,因为新药或治疗的选择,需基于疾病的自然发生或者治疗后的发展过程。

个体化治疗

随着新的治疗药物的出现,晚期或转移性肉瘤的治疗方法在不断进步,正是因为这个原因,应用直接作用于特殊组织或 DNA 改变的治疗药物也在不断进展。人们越来越多地认识到临床试验须通过合理分组来获得有用的信息。“肉瘤”的研究没有临床分组,将会被认为是跟研究“癌症”而不区分哪种类型的癌症一样幼稚。研究者需考虑到在“STS”称谓下的多于 50 种类别间质肿瘤有着大相径庭的生物学行为。为了获得足够的病例和资料,需要基于国内或国际的大规模合作。

现在已投入了巨大的努力将多种已商业化的药物和处于试验阶段的新药进行 STS 的临床试验。自从环磷酰胺普遍应用以来,在所有测试过的药物中,只有曲贝替定在欧洲得到正式认可;培唑帕尼在很多国家用于转移性软组织肉瘤;艾日布林也近来在美国得到正式认可,用于治疗脂肪肉瘤;此后其他一些经典药物的新的变异体也正在研究,例如 aldoxorubicin。对于特殊的诊断,伊马替尼和其他 SMOKI 用于肉瘤具有一定的活性,但并还没有得到特殊的正式认可,除了伊马替尼治疗隆突性皮肤纤维肉瘤。即便如此,在一些随机研究中,吉西他滨不管与多西他赛还是 DTIC 联合,在无进展生存率和总生存率上优于吉西他滨单药。这些数据的出彩之处将在下面章节介绍。

阿柔比星和异环磷酰胺

虽然不同类型的肉瘤对不同的化疗药物敏感度不一,多柔比星和异环磷酰胺仍然是转移性肉瘤最有效的两种药物,RECIST 确定这两种药物的反应率在 10%~20%[174]。如果按照过去的研究中敏感和不敏感 STS 的亚型的比率来计算化疗的反应率,那么反应率应该更高。例如:滑膜肉瘤和黏液样/小圆细胞脂肪肉瘤相对于异环磷酰胺(和阿柔比星)敏感,但是,GIST、肺泡软组织肉瘤和血管外皮细胞瘤/孤立纤维瘤明显对以上两种药物耐药。

需要认识到的是,肿瘤反应率的计算越来越被质疑,因为它不能反映出肿瘤患者真正的临床获益。很多肉瘤有致密的透明基质组织包绕。就算化疗药在体内成功地杀死了大量肿瘤细胞,这层透明基质仍没有变化,导致影像学上化疗药对肿瘤无效的假阴性结果。因此,基于影像学表现的客观反应率实际上可能低估了化疗抗癌的有效性。相反,肿瘤的简单皱缩并获得了暂时的化疗反应可能并不能说明是多药联合强效化疗的结果。因此,RECIST 定义的反应率可能在反映肉瘤治疗效益上不是一个理想的指标,GIST 的治疗就是一个典型的例子[175,176]。在肉瘤药物治疗的效益反应方面,越来越多的人关注于其他的临床指标,例如无进展生存期、给定时间范围内的生存率和总生存率等。

虽然单纯凭客观指标药物的反应率很低,有些药物仍有可能延缓疾病进程和延长生存期限。当然,这样结论的得出必须经过缜密仔细的随访。然而,即使 RECIST 标准容易低估患者的受益,该项标准仍然是衡量临床反应率的标尺。

量效关系

20 世纪 70 年代早期,第一次研究证实了肉瘤对阿柔比星敏感[124]。紧接着,阿柔比星在肉瘤治疗过程中的研究应用证实存在量效反应关系,每周期 50mg/m^2 的药量远不及每周期 60mg/m^2 的大剂量药物的抗癌效果好。但虽然存在这种量效关系,还需认识到其他变量可能影响抗癌效果,例如上述肉瘤的组织病理学亚型等。既然其他对化疗敏感的实体瘤,尤其是乳腺癌,在阿柔比星的使用上有最佳用药剂量:在每周期 60mg/m^2 以上,那么治疗肉瘤的阿柔比星使用剂量也类似。临床证实给予高于常量每周期 60~75mg/m^2 的阿柔比星未见肿瘤反应率的提高。

关于异环磷酰胺已有大量有关剂量和化疗方案的研究。已证实大剂量的异环磷酰胺的抗癌效果更好[134,177]。通过每周期高剂量的环磷酰胺(>10 000mg/m^2)作用于过去的低剂量(如<6 000mg/m^2)治疗失败的患者有很好的疗效。但是,鉴于这种药物高剂量使用时的潜在毒副作用,高剂量环磷酰胺最好用于对于该药非常敏感并可获得很好疗效的小部分患者(如计划手术切除转移灶前)。

单药和联合化疗

一个持续争论的焦点是晚期肉瘤患者的最佳治疗途径是联合化疗还是序贯单药化疗。最负盛名的有关联合化疗的随机临床试验是,美国的一项关于是否联合应用异环磷酰胺与阿柔比星和达卡巴嗪化疗转移性或晚期初治的 STS 的试验。结果显示虽然联合异环磷酰胺与阿柔比星、达卡巴嗪组在客观反应率明显提高,但是长期生存率并未得到改善[178,179]。统计学研究显示在异环磷酰胺给予后化疗药物的毒副作用明显增加使联合化疗的地位受到质疑。虽然通过小而显著的反应率证实了抗癌作用的提高,但是加用第三种药物并没有生存受益。

类似的方式,多柔比星(每周期 75mg/m^2)加入更高剂量的环磷酰胺(每周期 10g/m^2),可以获得满意的、显著增加的 RECIST 反应率(26%相比于 14%),中位无进展生存时间(7.4 个月相比于 6.4 个月),更高的毒性和可能的生存获益(14.3 个月相比于 12.8 个月,$P=0.076$)[180]。从这些数据中,并不清楚,这两种药物的续贯使用是否可以和联合使用一样,得出相似的结果。特别是生存数据,作为我们判断转移性肉瘤治疗成功的试金石。这两项随机临床试验数据支持,对于有症状、需要得到治疗反应的患者,进行化疗药物的联合使用;同样的原因,对于症状不明显或无症状、只需要维护治疗的患者,使用单药,以降低药物毒性,也并非不合理。

增加化疗效果的策略

利用干细胞增加药物剂量

经检验在血液恶性肿瘤、乳腺癌和其他恶性肿瘤中,提高化疗反应率的另一个有效策略是增加药物剂量的同时添加干细胞支持。最初,这种尝试应用于自体骨髓移植的支持治疗,而在过去十年里,通过造血细胞因子改善机体对化疗药骨髓抑制的耐受已让患者有显著的获益。随着对肉瘤标准化疗的进行,以确定粒细胞集落刺激因子可使外周血祖细胞活动并产生血液细胞[181]。含剂量阿霉素、异环磷酰胺、顺铂以及干细胞支持对于骨肉瘤的治疗效果并不优于标准剂量,验证了剂量密集化疗的局限性[182]。就算在化疗敏感的尤因肉瘤使用了剂量密集化疗加上自体干细胞支持治疗,生存率似乎并未改善,可能与肿瘤细胞污染了干细胞群有关。因此对肉瘤,是否进行剂量密集化疗加上干细胞及细胞因子支持治疗仍然需进一步研究。

包被的蒽环类化疗药

另一种增加疗效的治疗策略是利用脂质载体包被蒽环类化疗药。目前至少有三种蒽环类药物的脂质胶囊被测试,都证实对肉瘤有显著疗效。值得注意的是,目前最广泛运用的药剂相比于旧的载有多柔比星的大脂质体更能减少心脏毒性。聚乙二醇化的脂质体多柔比星(Doxil/Caelyx)是一种利用聚乙二醇固定在脂质双层膜上的小的脂质体,类似用亲水性外衣来降低循环中脂质体的半衰期和阻止体内网状内皮组织系统降解药物。这种制备相比于未包被的多柔比星,化疗药物剂量更小,更容易为机体耐受,因而患者更少出现骨髓抑制、心脏毒性、脱发以及未知的该药物首次使用引起的特殊反应,但手足综合征可能更重;但是,当剂量更低时,它可以有很长的循环半衰期(30~70h),导致曲线下面积达 50mg/m^2,这是多柔比星自身的 300 倍。在Ⅰ期随机研究第二阶段,聚乙二醇包被的脂质体多柔比星与原多柔比星一样有效(在 GIST 被认为是另一种类型的肉瘤之前,反应率为 9%相比于 10%),虽然形式上的非劣效性或等价性尚未确定,但聚乙二醇脂质体多柔比星的毒性明显小于多柔比星[183]。这种毒性更小的蒽环类药物的制备方式让身体状态更差的患者有了系统治疗的机会,是一种治疗缓慢进展的结缔组织疾病,例如黏液样脂肪肉瘤或者硬纤维瘤的新方法。

非蒽环类和环磷酰胺药物

几乎没有其他药物可以超越蒽环类和异环磷酰胺,在软组织肉瘤中证实活性。但是,这是一个需要更多组织学特异性数据进行治疗决策的时代性概括。目前公认的是,达卡巴嗪在软组织肉瘤中有轻微活性,研究证实,平滑肌肉瘤和较少的孤立性纤维性肿瘤这两种病理诊断,对达卡巴嗪和其口服类似物替莫唑胺有很强的活性[184~186]。吉西他滨和多西他赛联合应用,在绝对令人失望的吉西他滨单药Ⅱ期临床试验后,首次在子宫平滑肌肉瘤中展示活性,提示这两种药物有协同作用[187,188]。随机临床试验显示,吉西他滨和多西他赛联合应用,在一组非选择的肉瘤中,在 PFS 和 OS 上均优于吉西他滨单药[189]。UPS 和多形性脂肪肉瘤的治疗反应最为明显,明显强于平滑肌肉瘤。有一项随机临床试验发现,吉西他滨和达卡巴嗪在 PFS 和 OS 上优于达卡巴嗪单药,其次,吉西他滨联合用药在影像学和临床结果上均优于单药[190]。贝伐单抗加入吉西他滨-多西他赛中并不能改变化疗的基础,PFS 在数值上,尽管并没有在统计学上,不如这两种化疗药物单独使用[191]。因此,不管吉西他滨-多西他赛还是吉西他滨-达卡巴嗪联合应用,在多柔比星和/或异环磷酰胺治疗失败后,是一种很好的选择。的确,对于吉西他滨为基础治疗的毒性反应和多柔比星为基础治疗的毒性反应的对比认识,导致多柔比星为基础治疗在美国转移性软组织肉瘤治疗中被接受为一线治疗[192]。作者通常用吉西他滨-达卡巴嗪治疗平滑肌肉瘤,吉西他滨-多西他赛治疗 UPS 和多形性脂肪肉瘤,多形性脂肪肉瘤在断断续续的试验中可以看到反应。

新药

肉瘤为药物的发展提供了肥沃的土壤。多柔比星被发现对肉瘤有效后,就迅速发展成为最广泛使用的抗癌制剂。伊马替尼以及其在化疗抵抗患者中的惊人结果,为人们提供了一个原理证据,因此,在其他实体肿瘤中,证实了 EGFR 抑制剂、BRAF 抑制剂以及类似的药物。一些更新的药物以及其在肉瘤中的应用,将在后续详细阐述。这一章节的下一个版本无疑将会包含更多的新药和新的靶向药物针对肉瘤的特殊组织类型或分子特征亚型,很多通过肿瘤内科学发生。

曲贝替定

曲贝替定(ET-743,trabectidin)是一种产自海洋被囊动物海鞘螺的物质。它能共价结合到 DNA 的浅凹槽中,在 S 晚期及 G2 期阻止细胞周期的进行,通过拮抗转录因子 NF-Y 的受体影响转录的进行,进而减少包含多种耐药基因在内的大量基因的表达。经过初始Ⅰ期试验的有效性验证,进行了多项Ⅱ期临床试验,最为成功的一项(一项Ⅱ期随机临床试验关于药物的两种使用时刻表)直接导致药物在欧洲批准用于难治性软组织肉瘤[193,194]。随机临床试验的随访研究发现,曲贝替定的活性明显高于达卡巴嗪[195]。

一项曲贝替定治疗转移性平滑肌肉瘤和脂肪肉瘤的Ⅱ期随机临床试验,比较了药物以周为单位的24h灌输方案[193]。在这270名患者参与的研究中,超过3次的每周灌输方案的中位进展时间为3.7个月相比于3次每周灌输方案的2.3个月,$P=0.03$;OS在数值上长于3次每周灌输方案,13.9个月相比于11.8个月,$P=0.19$。在黏液状圆细胞脂肪肉瘤中发现独特的药物活性,尽管在其他组织类型中也发现了药物活性。

类似的方式,微管靶向药物艾日布林(eribulin)在一项Ⅱ期临床试验中展示了活性[196],这一试验导致上面提及的曲贝替定类似试验的进行。在一项治疗平滑肌肉瘤和脂肪肉瘤的Ⅲ期临床试验中,比较了曲贝替定和达卡巴嗪。Ⅲ期临床试验证实了前面Ⅱ期临床试验所看到的活性。在这项研究中,曲贝替定和达卡巴嗪的OS并没有显著性差异(12.4个月相比于12.9个月),曲贝替定的PFS显著高于达卡巴嗪(4.2个月相比于1.5个月)。

至今为止,除了细胞毒性药物,最为重要的结果包含SMO-KI培唑帕尼。在一项Ⅱ期临床试验展示活性后[197],进行了Ⅲ期临床试验PALETTE,包含369名标准治疗后进展的软组织肉瘤患者。通过培唑帕尼和安慰剂2∶1随机配比,培唑帕尼组展示出令人满意的PFS优势。通过独立的影像学家评估,培唑帕尼组的中位PFS为4.6个月,安慰剂组为1.6个月,配对$HR=0.35$($P<0.001$)。在最终分析后,安慰剂组的中位OS为10.7个月,培唑帕尼组的为12.6个月,$HR=0.87$,$P=0.26$[198]。这些数据使培唑帕尼用于标准治疗后失败的转移性软组织肉瘤,在国际上得到广泛认可。

一些特殊肉瘤的分子特征越来越多地指导治疗选择。基于肿瘤DNA改变(基因丢失、移位或突变),mTOR抑制剂,例如西罗莫司,在血管周上皮细胞瘤(PEComas)显示活性[199];伊马替尼和其他PDGF受体、CSF1受体抑制剂在DSFS[200]和腱鞘巨细胞瘤(TGCT)[201,202]显示活性。克唑替尼(crizotinib),一种ALK抑制剂,在ALK易位的炎性肌成纤维细胞肿瘤(IMT)显示活性。越来越多的靶向其他(不只是激酶)的这类药物,显示活性,进入治疗的焦点,可能包括高频*IDH1*和*IDH2*突变的软骨肉瘤,滑膜肉瘤、尤因肉瘤、MPNST(分别可能具有表观遗传调节剂*PRC1*、*LSD*、*BRD*突变,都有可能很快成为靶点,类似其他表观遗传调节剂,例如EZH2。

局部复发的治疗

若有孤立的局灶复发,治疗目标和原发肿瘤一样,名义上,需在尽可能多地维持功能和美观的基础上行最理想的局部控制[107]。早期发现局部复发可增加成功救治的机会,并像初治的患者一样,需在专业的多学科的肉瘤治疗中心得到良好的评估和治疗。局部复发的STS评估、治疗流程在图112-14中总结。初始的评估必须包含既往病史的全面回顾,因为这对治疗方案的选择有影响。因此,所有既往手术及病理资料、既往放化疗方案,尤其是照射范围、剂量以及照射强度均需详细地回

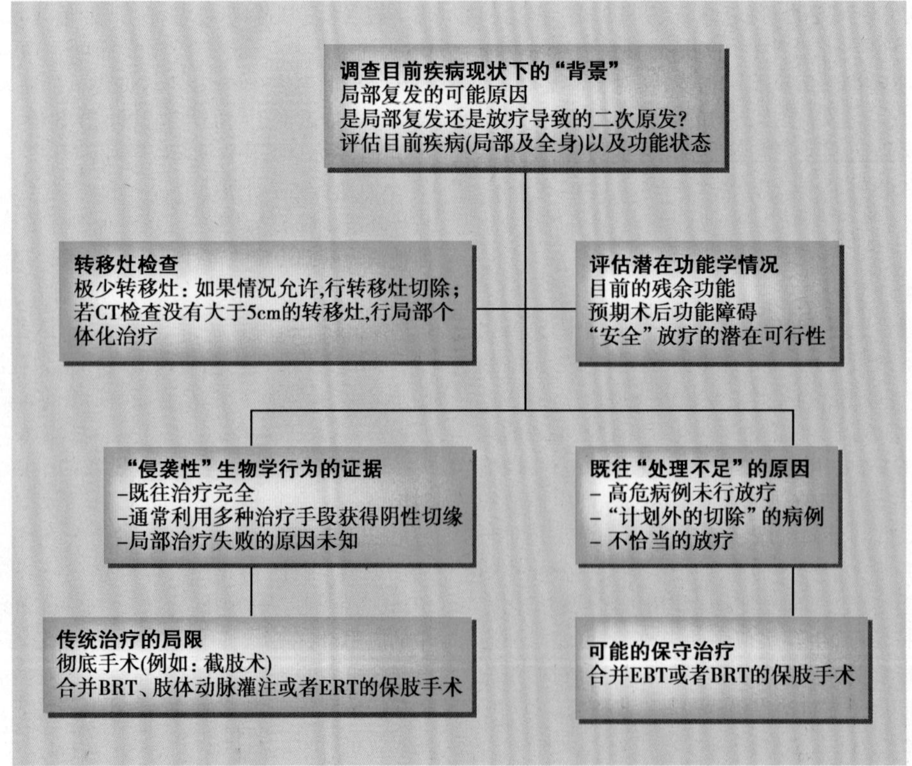

图112-14 局部复发的STS患者的治疗流程。该图专为肢体病灶设计,但是对于其他部位的病灶一样使用(如头部、颈部及腹膜后)。简写:BRT,短距离放射治疗;ERT,外粒子放疗。摘自Catton等1999[107]。Elsevier公司授权复制

顾和分析。

局部复发需像新发肿瘤一样进行分期。邻近原发病灶的区域及被既往手术干预过的潜在“被污染”的区域需仔细检查。这些区域及邻近复发的组织，包括潜在肿瘤延伸的部位，都被认为是高危区，需要被切除和/或被列为放疗区域。

“局部复发”疾病标志下的几项典型分组包括：①先前治疗不含放疗的病例；②既往放疗过的病例；③出现远处转移的病例；④难以区分局部复发和放疗导致的再发肿瘤的病例。虽然在局部复发的病例中可选择的治疗方案更为有限，治疗的挑战更大，但有一部分患者仍可以获得痊愈。给这些局部复发的疾病选择最佳的治疗方案需要更多的临床经验。

胃肠道间质瘤

肉瘤中的一种特殊亚型胃肠道间质瘤(GIST)改变人们对于实体肉瘤认识。认识到 KIT 是可以作为区分 GIST 与其他肉瘤的标志，以及 KIT 或者 PDGFRA 活化突变可能激化了 KIT 的分子构成[203]，临床研究迅速地，和这些分子的生物学研究平行地探究了 GIST 的生物学特性。值得注意的是，免疫组织化学标记的存在不一定对肿瘤有作用，因为这是由声称这是事实的公司提出的。尤因肉瘤标志的 KIT 也阳性但 KIT 在该瘤中并不突变，因而尤因肉瘤对伊马替尼不敏感。

原发性 GIST 的外科处理原则不同于其他肉瘤和内脏腺癌。通常，手术切除只需要很小的安全边缘，不像其他肉瘤和内脏腺癌需要广泛切缘。不像胃癌，GIST 通常不转移到局部-区域淋巴结(除了一些小儿 GIST)，在大部分患者中淋巴结清扫并非必需。因此，胃 GIST 通常只需要楔形切除，极少需要胃大部切除(通常由于解剖结构限制)。同样的，起源于小肠、结肠和直肠的 GIST 也可以很小的安全边缘手术切除。而且，肉眼切除干净的、但镜下切缘阳性的 GIST 患者，与那些切缘阴性的相比，并不增加 LR 风险[204]。

认识到伊马替尼在体内对 GIST 细胞系的作用[203]，转移性疾病的治疗手段迅速进步，从Ⅰ、Ⅱ期到Ⅲ期临床试验发展到转移性疾病的治疗试验[205~209]，结果是始终如一的惊人。伊马替尼至少比其他任何用来治疗 GIST(以前被称为胃肠道平滑肌肉瘤)的药物有用 10 倍。该肿瘤对于伊马替尼的反应率约为 50%，30%～50%疾病稳定，约 15%在治疗过程中显著进展。美国的Ⅲ期临床试验的数据提示 400mg 和 800mg 产生同等的时间-进展曲线，但是欧洲/澳大利亚的Ⅲ期临床试验研究显示时间-进展曲线在高剂量组(每日 800mg)得到改善[206]。显然，患者的 *KIT* 基因型的突变决定了他们的反应率(图 112-15)[210]。*KIT* 外显子 *11* 突变的患者有 80%～90%的反应率，而外显子 *9* 突变的患者只有 1/3～1/2 有反应。没有 *KIT* 或 *PDGFRA* 基因突变的患者反应率更低，但是仍然比其他化疗药物观察到的反应率高。目前，不考虑基因突变的因素，伊马替尼是转移性 GIST 的标准治疗用药。对大多数患者每日 400mg 的剂量是一个合理的用药起点，若有疾病进展或外显子 *9* 基因突变的证据，可将药量调至 800mg[211]。若在肝脏发现显著的新发低密度灶，伊马替尼的治疗不能中止；它们可能在一开始就有隐性转移，和影像学和临床经验证实的那样[176]。

伊马替尼作用于转移性 GIST 的中位时间接近 2 年。低剂量伊马替尼治疗的患者若疾病进展，可对高剂量的该药再次起反应。伊马替尼的Ⅰ期临床试验提示，每日的最大耐受剂量为

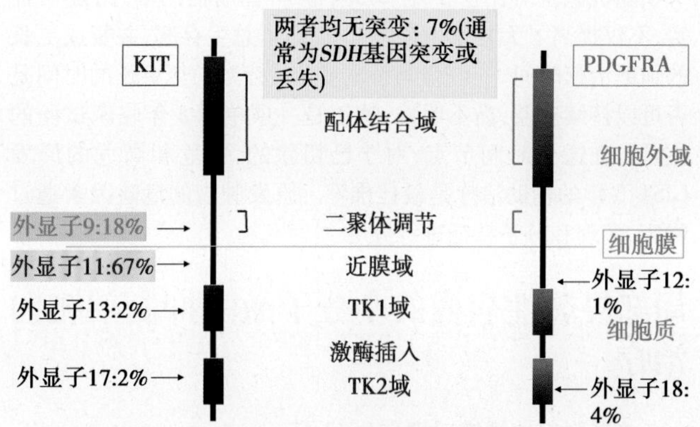

图 112-15 胃肠道间质肿瘤的突变情况和 KIT 或 PDGFRA 蛋白的定位

800mg(口服 400mg，一天二次)。患者疾病进展方式有不同寻常，所谓的“肿瘤中的肿瘤”，代表 *KIT* 发生了二次突变[160]。有些病例的再次生长肿瘤灶中可见明显的坏死，而在另外一些病例，与大多数晚期 GIST 患者出现多发转移灶不同的是，只能看到单个转移灶残留。因而，有些患者通过谨慎筹备的手术切除单一转移病灶达到治疗的目的。

通过伊马替尼疾病控制稳定的转移性 GIST 行转移灶切除的原因为：通过伊马替尼达到病理学完全缓解非常少(<5%)，许多(可能大多数)患者会因第二次基因突变而最终对伊马替尼二次耐药。大规模的临床试验中心报道谨慎挑选伊马替尼治疗的患者，行病灶切除术可有很好的无疾病进展生存率。该结果的得出是由于病例选择偏倚还是由于手术真实有效，还不清楚[212,213]。美国、欧洲和中国进行了随机对照试验，评估对疾病稳定或伊马替尼治疗有效的患者行转移病灶切除术的效果。获益不佳导致欧洲和中国临床试验的终止，美国的试验并因此没有启动。

伊马替尼在转移性 GIST 的应用，衍生了新的 SMOKI，部分通过Ⅲ期临床试验，并得到后续管理部门的批准。转移性病变出现伊马替尼耐药，加入 mTOR 抑制剂依维莫司(everolimus)至伊马替尼，可以出现轻微的活性[214]。然而，其他靶向 KIT 的 SMOKI 已经观察到更强的活性。舒尼替尼在伊马替尼耐药的 GIST 可以展示活性，与安慰剂相比，显著提高 PFS 和 OS[215]。随着索拉非尼(sorafenib)在 GIST 展示活性[216,217]，瑞格拉非尼(一种氟化的索拉非尼)在Ⅲ期试验(更多的关注在安慰剂组)中，与安慰剂相比，展示了活性；在这个 GRID 试验中，安慰剂组的患者很快横跨到包含舒尼替尼的研究中，可能由于 GRID 试验缺乏 OS 获益[218]。在其他药物治疗失败后，一些形式的 SMOKI 似乎适合于进一步的治疗[219]。

鉴于其在转移性肿瘤中的卓越活性，并不令人惊奇，伊马替尼也在辅助治疗中进行了尝试。0 相比于 1 年、0 相比于 2 年和 1 年相比于 3 年伊马替尼的研究数据发现，均持续地证实更长时间的治疗的持续获益。伊马替尼的辅助治疗作用，最初在美国通过 ACOSOG Z9001 试验证实，在其中，对于>3cm 的 GIST 完全切除后，1 年伊马替尼治疗(400mg/d)相比于安慰剂。结果由于 762 例患者在中期随访发现伊马替尼组患者的无疾病进展率远高于对照组(97%相比于 83%)而中止[220]。

一项随机试验对比了 1 年和 3 年伊马替尼辅助治疗,随后证实,不仅提高了无复发生存率,也提高了总生存率,并赞成更长的辅助治疗时间[221]。伊马替尼辅助治疗延长至更长的时间是否可以持续获益,尚不明确,这正是一项单臂 5 年临床试验的主题。在这个时间节点,对于已切除的、中危和高危的原发 GIST,3 年的辅助治疗是最佳推荐。原发肿瘤的危险因素通过临床、病理和分子特征进行分层[222~224]。

局部侵袭性病变的小分子激酶抑制剂靶向治疗

皮肤隆突性纤维肉瘤(dermatofibrosarcoma protuberans,DFSP)是源于表皮的结节的"外突"病灶,有持续多年特征性的缓慢生长史。虽然它在组织学上呈现为低级别或交界性恶性肿瘤,DFSP 在单纯切除后容易局部复发。染色体异位 t(17;22)和基因融合的产物(表 112-1)促进 *COL1A1-PDGFB* 基因融合蛋白的表达,进而促使 PDGF-B 的成熟,让 DFSP 细胞表面的 PDGF-B 受体与自分泌或旁分泌的 PDGF-B 相互作用。尤其是,伊马替尼抑制 PDGF 酪蛋白激酶受体,以类似的方法,其在慢性髓细胞性白血病中抑制 BCR-ABL 酪蛋白激酶受体,在 GIST 中抑制 KIT 酪蛋白激酶受体。在复发性 DFSP,伊马替尼具有活性,从而证实,在实体瘤中,激酶可以是一个很好的靶点,甚至在罕见的肿瘤,只要肿瘤的基因组学有所提示[200,225~227]。

同样的原因,腱鞘巨细胞瘤(以前曾命名为色素沉着绒毛结节性滑膜炎)的 t(1;2)COL6A3-CSF1 产生融合蛋白,其负责侵略性炎症浸润。伊马替尼可以拮抗 CSF1R(FMS,CD115)的活性,使复发病变缩小[201]。更特异性 SMOKI 和拮抗 CD115 的单抗,也可以使复发性 TGCT 缩小。最后,PEComa,在遗传性综合征结节性硬化患者中发现,其相关病变淋巴管肌瘤病不仅缺乏 TSC1,也缺乏 TSC2(抑癌基因)。TOR(西罗莫司的靶点)在 TSC1 和 TSC2 失活后,被激活,因此,并不令人惊奇的是,SMOKI 西罗莫司和结构相关复合物,在这种情况下被激活,作为进一步原理证据——封闭实体瘤的"启动"激酶可以获得影像学和临床获益[199]。

腹膜后肉瘤

腹膜后肉瘤(retroperitoneal sarcoma,RPS)约占 STS 的 15%。不易早期发现,往往位于手术和放疗照射难以到达的区域(如邻近小肠和肝脏的区域)。因此,通过联合治疗对 RPS 的局部控制率不如肢体 STS[54,228~232]。在玛格丽特公主医院的 102 名 RPS 患者中,仅有 45 例患者获得完全切除,29 例残存肉眼病灶,28 例术后活检镜下残留病灶[232]。总的 5 年和 10 年的局部无复发率分别为 28%和 9%。放疗,尤其是高剂量的放疗,对总生存率无改善,但似乎显著延长复发的时限。只有肿瘤完全切除可增加远期生存率、减少局部复发和远处转移,同前面提到的其他病例研究类似。RPS 患者应在治疗之前行多学科临床评估以获得专家治疗意见和建设性的治疗方案。

来自欧洲有争议的报告探索了定义为间室切除的扩大手术对改善 RPS 患者局部病灶控制的价值[233,234]。这些分别来自法国和意大利的回顾性的研究资料提示切除病灶邻近区域脏器,例如肾脏和结肠,可增强对病灶的局部控制。这些研究结果的解读有明显的选择偏倚,且复杂,正如报告附件上编者所指[235],这些数据没有给予特殊的治疗意见。目前,没有临床试验证实通过联合邻近脏器的根治性切除可以改进病灶的局部控制。

术前及术后放疗方法

各种辅助放疗已运用于 RPS。一项在随机前瞻性临床试验进行一次性术中照射(in-operation radiotherapy,IORT,20Gy),加术后外照射(35~40Gy),与传统的术后放疗(50~55Gy)比较。在这项 35 人的试验中,局部复发率降低,但未发现生存率的改善[236]。IORT 导致周围神经病变的发生率较高,原因在于剂量大,有时相互重叠的放疗区域,使骶神经丛承受过大的放射剂量。然而,在对照组,由于高剂量的射线照射到肠道,胃肠道并发症更常见。

其他研究者探索了术前放疗的策略。来自麻省总医院的 Gieschen 等报告 37 例患者术前放疗后手术切除病灶,随后对一部分患者行 IORT[237]。完全切除率为 83%,五年总生存率、无瘤生存率、局部控制率和无远处转移率分别为 50%、38%、59%和 54%。该研究的早期报告描述完全切除率为 70%,4 年局部控制率为 81%。更新的研究显示肿瘤完全切除和 IORT 治疗组相比,无 IORT 组(30%相比于 61%)改善了总生存率和局部控制率(74%相比于 83%)。但是,该研究为非随机的,可能选择了更适用于 IORT 照射的病灶。目前在 Mayo 临床中心的 Petersen 等发现利用类似的治疗手段对原发肿瘤也可改善局部控制[238]。

多伦多大学肉瘤研究组描述了超乎寻常的可喜结果,尤其对原发肿瘤,他们前瞻性非对照研究了术前放疗(25 例,平均剂量为 45Gy),术后选择病例行 BRT[239]。有趣的是,在他们的试验中,患者术前放疗的毒副反应与其他试验报道的毒副反应不同。虽然中位照射体积达到 7L,但患者术前外照射的胃肠道毒性评分极低。没有患者因为急性毒副作用住院,也没有因为急性毒副作用而干预或停止治疗。术前放疗的显著低毒性与肠道不在照射区域内有关。而选择性使用术后 BRT 的患者胃肠道毒副作用大,况且没有证据证明 BRT 对控制肿瘤有益。

得克萨斯大学安德森癌症研究中心与玛格丽特公主医院工作组将他们的Ⅱ期试验和小样本的初期试验数据进行整合,荟萃分析发现术前放疗合并手术切除病灶可很好地提高患者总生存率[240]。但是,我们仍应该非常小心诠释这个结果,因为这些患者都是被推荐在大的专业机构病灶接受高水平的肿瘤切除技术,存在病例的选择偏倚。同样地,人们仍不清楚是 BRT 还是 IORT 为最佳放疗方式,这依赖方案的制订和病例的选择。但是,术前放疗在 PMH 研究的长期随访中持续展示良好的局部控制率和 OS。

以上 3 份研究报告对 RPS 患者的术前放疗肯定了以下几点优势:①在高剂量放射区,由于肿瘤将小肠推挤移位,使治疗更安全、毒副作用更小;②术前放疗没有手术造成肠管粘连固定的问题,可以安全地在肿瘤区域实施高剂量放疗;③肿瘤定位明确,使照射区域更为准确;④肿瘤被完整腹膜限制,使肿瘤扩散转移有物理屏障;⑤手术时腹膜内肿瘤扩散的风险可因术前放疗的生物学影响而减少;⑥根据肉瘤传统放疗的原则,术前状态下的较低剂量的放疗可达到有效的生物学效应。虽然 RPS 术前放疗计划复杂,但适形或调强保证邻近器官免受高剂量放射性照射。当术前有大块肝脏被照射时，必须让手术和放疗医师都集中在手术室评估残存肝脏的体积。我们不能过分强调放射剂量的精确调节，需确定在手术时有足够未照射体积的肝脏残留[241]。

目前公认的 RPS 治疗原则是尽可能地完整切除病灶。上述辅助放疗的多种放疗方式还处于试验阶段，需进一步评估。目前，正为 RPS 的治疗实施设计一个更为科学合理的临床试验，计划通过随机对照试验探索外粒子束的放疗作用[174]。欧洲癌症研究与治疗组织（EORTC）目前正在进行一项关于术前放疗加手术和单纯手术的Ⅲ期随机临床研究（NCT 01344018），即将顺利完成[242]。

化-放疗方法

虽然单纯化疗已证明对 RPS 没有显著效果，但正如其他实体瘤，化-放疗也逐渐成为 RPS 治疗的一个选择。该种治疗方法对预后更差的高级别 RPS 尤其适用。

初步试验性研究发现，在可接受毒性范围内，对有巨大肿瘤的患者，术前利用碘脱氧嘧啶核苷和多柔比星化疗联合外粒子照射治疗后，术后切缘阴性的患者的局部病灶可得到很好的控制[141,243]。这些研究说明化疗联合放疗是可行的。Ⅱ期后续试验需说明有关反应率和毒副反应的情况，以决定联合放化疗的治疗方式是否能进入Ⅲ期试验。肿瘤放疗协会（Radiation Therapy Oncology Group，RTOG）完成了Ⅱ期术前多柔比星和异环磷酰胺化疗和术前放疗，切除肿瘤后对中到高级别的 RPS 行术中或术后高剂量照射的试验。结果发现这些患者出现了显著的毒性反应，而无瘤生存改善有限[144,146]。

STS 治疗的其他问题

功能结果和治疗后遗症

肢体肉瘤治疗后的功能情况在结果评估中占有重要的地位。评价功能情况较困难，因为它需要有效且可重复的指标。在发展和使用这些方法方面，很多研究中心也缺乏经验，且大多文献中患者情况有很大的不同。

因此到目前为止，与功能差相关的因素包括：肿瘤体积大、放疗剂量高和范围广、神经损伤、术后骨折和伤口愈合并发症等[244,245]。为了评估和比较功能结果，必须具有统一的评价功能学的指标。三个疾病特异性评分标准被报道在评估功能方面有用[246]。Davis 已将这方面详细讨论，他发现在文献中“功能”有许多含义[246]。损伤（impairment）、残疾（disability）和活动障碍（handicap）的概念常被误解和误用。Davis 注意到损伤是结构或功能的紊乱；而残疾是被限制或缺乏正常活动的能力。损伤和残疾导致了活动障碍，它使人不能作为一个正常的个人在社会上担任对应的角色。对于肉瘤患者，损伤可被表现为软组织纤维化、关节不能活动和肌力降低；残疾可表现为活动受限、难以自理和日常活动；而活动障碍则是在家庭、社会及工作领域的能力限制。

损伤最常见在肢体 STS 保肢手术后的后遗症，超过 50%的患者出现显著的损伤性改变[246]。残疾较少发生，尽管各报道自相矛盾。似乎很多肉瘤患者学会去适应损伤性改变。而在文献中很少注意到活动障碍。但是，有限资料显示超过 50%的患者可能在肢体 STS 治疗后经历了在他们就业和社会角色方面的改变。肉瘤治疗的持续性挑战是确定肢体肉瘤患者的治愈比率。尤其是多学科联合治疗的目的将是在维持或改进目前疾病控制情况的同时，尽可能减少创伤，进而降低治疗的致残率和改善患者生活质量。

伤口并发症

文献报告伤口并发症的发生率差异非常大。有肢体肉瘤手术后大于 40%的伤口并发症的报道[85,247~249]。伤口并发症的定义不同可能是报道发生率不同的原因。回顾性研究数据显示与伤口愈合不良相关的因素包括：高龄、营养不良、肿瘤位于肢体末梢、肿瘤体积大、术前辅助治疗尤其是放疗[247,248,250]。特别高的并发症发生在术前放疗和术中热疗的患者中[117]。虽然很多学者报告伤口并发症与术前放疗有关，但是也存在未行放、化疗的患者术后并发症发生率很高的情况[251]。最常见肢体远端肿瘤扩大切除后可能出现高的伤口并发症的风险。利用带血管蒂的组织转移覆盖伤口，可减少多数伤口并发症的发生，并使更多扩大切除肿瘤的保肢手术成为可能[250,252,253]。SR2 临床研究以前瞻性的方式较早注意到术前放疗对伤口愈合的负面影响，但这基于术者个人是否倾向于行转移性皮瓣填补创面组织[96]。

基于分子及病理生物学方面的肉瘤治疗

肉瘤的治疗越来越被疾病本身的特殊性质所影响，最重要的是其病理亚型。正如 Pasteur 和 Koch 的研究成为我们认识和定义病原微生物的基础，如今许多实验室对肉瘤的分子生物学和细胞生物学的研究重新确定了肉瘤的科研领域。其中的一个例子就是认识到尤因肉瘤/PNET 家族肿瘤是骨外 STS 而不是骨的肉瘤。这些肿瘤应从联合化疗开始，用激进的多种综合治疗来达到治愈的目的。如果手术已切除了可见的病灶，辅助化疗必须进行。如果手术切缘可能残余病灶，需考虑术后辅助放疗。PNET 及 Askin 肿瘤采用尤因肉瘤类似的治疗方案，治疗效果已明显改善。这个家族肿瘤的分子水平变化的类似性使我们认为它们具有相同的疾病发生分子机制，只是肿瘤形态和临床病理学的表型变异[254,255]。

随着对易位基因产物分子生物学越来越多的了解，表明表观遗传学事件在肉瘤的形成过程中非常重要，影像化疗的效果。尤因肉瘤和滑膜肉瘤是有化疗反应的软组织肉瘤亚型。虽然 *TP53* 可能是这些肉瘤化疗敏感的原因，*TP53* 状态并不是提示化疗敏感的唯一因素，因为其他 *TP53* 野生型肉瘤的化疗敏感性明显减低，例如骨外黏液样软骨肉瘤和腺泡状软组织肉瘤。表观遗传学 mSW1/SNF（BAF）复合物的惊人研究结果以及其在滑膜肉瘤中的作用，将阐明提高滑膜肉瘤生存率的一些机械方面的基础——为了更好地使肿瘤细胞死亡[256,257]。

作为最后的例子，对脂肪肉瘤的多种组织病理亚型的研究和认识越来越深入，关于一些其所获得的、特有的 DNA 信号的机制也逐渐了解[258]。黏液和圆细胞脂肪肉瘤表现出特征性的染色体重排 T（12;16）（q13;p11）FUS-DDIT3。这类脂肪肉瘤倾向于多柔比星为基础的化疗方案敏感，曲贝替定对这一特殊类型突显出最强活性。曲贝替定似乎可以抑制 FUS-DDIT3 融合蛋白和DNA结合，从而导致脂肪肉瘤细胞的死亡或分化[259,260]。更为罕见的多形性脂肪肉瘤亚型与其他脂肪肉瘤亚型相比，和未分化多形性肉瘤更为相同。最后，分化好的脂肪肉瘤在细胞遗传学分析呈现出环状和巨大的标志性染色体以及其表观遗传学的异常，经常包含染色体12q的大量扩增，同样也贯穿去分化脂肪肉瘤。在高分化-去分化脂肪肉瘤中，解除CDK24和HDM2位点和扩增数百倍的染色体12q结合，可能可以提供思路——怎么更好地攻击这些化疗相对不敏感的肉瘤[261~263]。

STS的免疫治疗

值此本书出版之时，检查免疫系统作为肉瘤的治疗手段，甚至还没有开始考虑，尚处于婴儿期，或宁可说是产前状态。免疫治疗，在一些国家，已经被认可用于治疗骨源性肿瘤，通过使用非特异性免疫辅助药物米伐木肽(MTP-PE)，作为辅助治疗的一部分，提高治愈率[120]。虽然，Robbins等演示了在NY-ESO-1阳性的肉瘤，例如滑膜肉瘤，应用T细胞治疗的原理证据[264,265]，但是，免疫检查点阻滞剂的潜在益处仍然非常不清楚，直到2015年还没有研究在肉瘤上进行。按照假设，有越多的*DNA*突变和改变的肿瘤，越有可能对免疫治疗有反应，因此，我们期望看到未分化多形性肉瘤、平滑肌肉瘤和骨肉瘤在这些最佳反应者中，在易位相关肉瘤活性不佳。相反，CAR-T治疗可能更容易靶向易位相关肉瘤，假如适当的靶向抗原被识别。

总结

显然，STS的治疗在过去的十年有了长足的进步。在不到三十年内，在各个肿瘤中心治疗的标准方法均向多途径联合治疗发展，增加保肢手术及改善患者生活质量的目标努力。明智地联合使用多种激进的治疗方法可减少患者的复发率和改善生存率。肿瘤的基因组学和免疫学革命进一步更新了对这些罕见病的基本认识；提供了崭新的诊断技术，这有助于我们放弃既往无根据的奇想和缺乏治疗的连贯性；也提供了选择新的靶向药物的资源。新的治疗主动权在一些特定亚型的软组织肉瘤，开始攻击肉瘤细胞形成的基本机制，有希望的是，这些主动权不同于目前的必需治疗，可以通过降低发病率，提高患者的预后。大规模的合作研究将极大推进此项工作的深入。

(许宋锋 徐立斌 译 王鲁强 于胜吉 校)

参考文献

The complete reference list can be found on the Wiley Companion Digital Edition of this title (see inside front cover for login instructions).

3 Thomas DM, Ballinger ML. Etiologic, environmental and inherited risk factors in sarcomas. *J Surg Oncol*. 2015;**111**:490–495.

4 Li FP, Fraumeni JF Jr. Soft-tissue sarcomas, breast cancer, and other neoplasms. A familial syndrome? *Ann Intern Med*. 1969;**71**:747–752.

6 McBride KA, Ballinger ML, Killick E, et al. Li-Fraumeni syndrome: cancer risk assessment and clinical management. *Nat Rev Clin Oncol*. 2014;**11**:260–271.

7 Kolberg M, Holand M, Agesen TH, et al. Survival meta-analyses for >1800 malignant peripheral nerve sheath tumor patients with and without neurofibromatosis type 1. *Neuro Oncol*. 2013;**15**:135–147.

14 MacCarthy A, Bayne AM, Brownbill PA, et al. Second and subsequent tumours among 1927 retinoblastoma patients diagnosed in Britain 1951-2004. *Br J Cancer*. 2013;**108**:2455–2463.

20 Gladdy RA, Qin LX, Moraco N, et al. Do radiation-associated soft tissue sarcomas have the same prognosis as sporadic soft tissue sarcomas? *J Clin Oncol*. 2010;**28**:2064–2069.

28 Mitchell G, Ballinger ML, Wong S, et al. High frequency of germline TP53 mutations in a prospective adult-onset sarcoma cohort. *PLoS One*. 2013;**8**:e69026.

31 WHO. *Classification of Tumours of Soft Tissue and Bone*. Lyon: International Agency for Research on Cancer; 2013.

32 Fong Y, Coit DG, Woodruff JM, Brennan MF. Lymph node metastasis from soft tissue sarcoma in adults. Analysis of data from a prospective database of 1772 sarcoma patients. *Ann Surg*. 1993;**217**:72–77.

34 Brennan MF, Antonescu CR, Moraco N, Singer S. Lessons learned from the study of 10,000 patients with soft tissue sarcoma. *Ann Surg*. 2014;**260**:416–421; discussion 421-412.

36 Lahat G, Tuvin D, Wei C, et al. New perspectives for staging and prognosis in soft tissue sarcoma. *Ann Surg Oncol*. 2008;**15**:2739–2748.

38 Guillou L, Coindre JM, Bonichon F, et al. Comparative study of the National Cancer Institute and French Federation of Cancer Centers Sarcoma Group grading systems in a population of 410 adult patients with soft tissue sarcoma. *J Clin Oncol*. 1997;**15**:350–362.

44 von Mehren M, Randall RL, Benjamin RS, et al. (2015) *NCCN Clinical Practice Guidelines in Oncology: Soft Tissue Sarcoma* (accessed March 01 2015).

49 Edge SB, Byrd DR, Compton CC, Fritz AG, Greene FL, Trotti A III (eds). Soft tissue sarcoma. In: *AJCC Cancer Staging Manual*. New York: Springer; 2010:291–298.

51 Kattan MW, Leung DH, Brennan MF. Postoperative nomogram for 12-year sarcoma-specific death. *J Clin Oncol*. 2002;**20**:791–796.

52 Pisters PW, Leung DH, Woodruff J, Shi W, Brennan MF. Analysis of prognostic factors in 1,041 patients with localized soft tissue sarcomas of the extremities. *J Clin Oncol*. 1996;**14**:1679–1689.

54 Gronchi A, Miceli R, Shurell E, et al. Outcome prediction in primary resected retroperitoneal soft tissue sarcoma: histology-specific overall survival and disease-free survival nomograms built on major sarcoma center data sets. *J Clin Oncol*. 2013;**31**:1649–1655.

61 Brennan MF, Antonescu CR, Maki RG. *Management of Soft Tissue Sarcoma*. New York: Springer; 2013.

62 Dei Tos AP. A current perspective on the role for molecular studies in soft tissue tumor pathology. *Semin Diagn Pathol*. 2013;**30**:375–381.

69 Pisters PW, Harrison LB, Leung DH, Woodruff JM, Casper ES, Brennan MF. Long-term results of a prospective randomized trial of adjuvant brachytherapy in soft tissue sarcoma. *J Clin Oncol*. 1996;**14**:859–868.

70 Yang JC, Chang AE, Baker AR, et al. Randomized prospective study of the benefit of adjuvant radiation therapy in the treatment of soft tissue sarcomas of the extremity. *J Clin Oncol*. 1998;**16**:197–203.

72 Maki RG, Moraco N, Antonescu CR, et al. Toward better soft tissue sarcoma staging: building on american joint committee on cancer staging systems versions 6 and 7. *Ann Surg Oncol*. 2013;**20**:3377–3383.

77 O'Sullivan B, Wylie J, Catton C, et al. The local management of soft tissue sarcoma. *Semin Radiat Oncol*. 1999;**9**:328–348.

78 O'Sullivan B, Ward I, Haycocks T, Sharpe M. Techniques to modulate radiotherapy toxicity and outcome in soft tissue sarcoma. *Curr Treat Options Oncol*. 2003;**4**:453–464.

89 Haas RL, Delaney TF, O'Sullivan B, et al. Radiotherapy for management of extremity soft tissue sarcomas: why, when, and where? *Int J Radiat Oncol Biol Phys*. 2012;**84**:572–580.

96 O'Sullivan B, Davis AM, Turcotte R, et al. Preoperative versus postoperative radiotherapy in soft-tissue sarcoma of the limbs: a randomised trial. *Lancet*. 2002;**359**:2235–2241.

100 Nielsen OS, Cummings B, O'Sullivan B, Catton C, Bell RS, Fornasier VL. Preoperative and postoperative irradiation of soft tissue sarcomas: effect of radiation field size. *Int J Radiat Oncol Biol Phys*. 1991;**21**:1595–1599.

101 Davis AM, O'Sullivan B, Turcotte R, et al. Late radiation morbidity following randomization to preoperative versus postoperative radiotherapy in extremity soft tissue sarcoma. *Radiother Oncol*. 2005;**75**:48–53.

102 Hong L, Alektiar KM, Hunt M, Venkatraman E, Leibel SA. Intensity-modulated radiotherapy for soft tissue sarcoma of the thigh. *Int J Radiat Oncol Biol Phys*. 2004;**59**:752–759.

104 O'Sullivan B, Griffin AM, Dickie CI, et al. Phase 2 study of preoperative image-guided intensity-modulated radiation therapy to reduce wound and combined modality morbidities in lower extremity soft tissue sarcoma. *Cancer*. 2013;**119**:1878–1884.

107 Catton CN, Swallow CJ, O'Sullivan B. Approaches to local salvage of soft tissue sarcoma after primary site failure. *Semin Radiat Oncol*. 1999;**9**:378–388.

112 Alektiar KM, Brennan MF, Singer S. Local control comparison of adjuvant brachytherapy to intensity-modulated radiotherapy in primary high-grade sarcoma of the extremity. *Cancer*. 2011;**117**:3229–3234.

119 Crist WM, Anderson JR, Meza JL, et al. Intergroup rhabdomyosarcoma study-IV: results for patients with nonmetastatic disease. *J Clin Oncol*. 2001;**19**:3091–3102.

120 Meyers PA, Schwartz CL, Krailo MD, et al. Osteosarcoma: the addition of muramyl tripeptide to chemotherapy improves overall survival–a report from the Children's Oncology Group. *J Clin Oncol*. 2008;**26**:633–638.

121 Whelan JS, Bielack SS, Marina N, et al. EURAMOS-1, an international randomised study for osteosarcoma: results from pre-randomisation treatment. *Ann Oncol*. 2015;**26**:407–414.

122 Womer RB, West DC, Krailo MD, et al. Randomized controlled trial of interval-compressed chemotherapy for the treatment of localized Ewing sarcoma: a report from the Children's Oncology Group. *J Clin Oncol*. 2012;**30**:4148–4154.

126 Frustaci S, De Paoli A, Bidoli E, et al. Ifosfamide in the adjuvant therapy of soft tissue sarcomas. *Oncology*. 2003;**65(Suppl 2)**:80–84.

127 Frustaci S, Gherlinzoni F, De Paoli A, et al. Adjuvant chemotherapy for adult soft tissue sarcomas of the extremities and girdles: results of the Italian randomized cooperative trial. *J Clin Oncol*. 2001;**19**:1238–1247.

128 Woll PJ, Reichardt P, Le Cesne A, et al. Adjuvant chemotherapy with doxorubicin, ifosfamide, and lenograstim for resected soft-tissue sarcoma (EORTC 62931): a multicentre randomised controlled trial. *Lancet Oncol*. 2012;**13**:1045–1054.

129 Pervaiz N, Colterjohn N, Farrokhyar F, Tozer R, Figueredo A, Ghert M. A systematic meta-analysis of randomized controlled trials of adjuvant chemotherapy for localized resectable soft-tissue sarcoma. *Cancer*. 2008;**113**:573–581.

141 Eilber F, Eckardt J, Rosen G, Forscher C, Selch M, Fu YS. Preoperative therapy for soft tissue sarcoma. *Hematol Oncol Clin North Am*. 1995;**9**:817–823.

144 DeLaney TF, Spiro IJ, Suit HD, et al. Neoadjuvant chemotherapy and radiotherapy for large extremity soft-tissue sarcomas. *Int J Radiat Oncol Biol Phys*. 2003;**56**:1117–1127.

145 Kraybill WG, Harris J, Spiro IJ, et al. Long-term results of a phase 2 study of neoadjuvant chemotherapy and radiotherapy in the management of high-risk, high-grade, soft tissue sarcomas of the extremities and body wall: Radiation Therapy Oncology Group Trial 9514. *Cancer*. 2010;**116**:4613–4621.

151 Cormier JN, Huang X, Xing Y, et al. Cohort analysis of patients with localized, high-risk, extremity soft tissue sarcoma treated at two cancer centers: chemotherapy-associated outcomes. *J Clin Oncol*. 2004;**22**:4567–4574.

160 Wardelmann E, Merkelbach-Bruse S, Pauls K, et al. Polyclonal evolution of multiple secondary KIT mutations in gastrointestinal stromal tumors under treatment with imatinib mesylate. *Clin Cancer Res*. 2006;**12**:1743–1749.

165 Billingsley KG, Lewis JJ, Leung DH, Casper ES, Woodruff JM, Brennan MF. Multifactorial analysis of the survival of patients with distant metastasis arising from primary extremity sarcoma. *Cancer*. 1999;**85**:389–395.

166 Billingsley KG, Burt ME, Jara E, et al. Pulmonary metastases from soft tissue sarcoma: analysis of patterns of diseases and postmetastasis survival. *Ann Surg*. 1999;**229**:602–610; discussion 610–602.

167 van Geel AN, Pastorino U, Jauch KW, et al. Surgical treatment of lung metastases: The European Organization for Research and Treatment of Cancer-Soft Tissue and Bone Sarcoma Group study of 255 patients. *Cancer*. 1996;**77**:675–682.

173 Van Glabbeke M, van Oosterom AT, Oosterhuis JW, et al. Prognostic factors for the outcome of chemotherapy in advanced soft tissue sarcoma: an analysis of 2,185 patients treated with anthracycline-containing first-line regimens–a European Organization for Research and Treatment of Cancer Soft Tissue and Bone Sarcoma Group Study. *J Clin Oncol*. 1999;**17**:150–157.

176 Choi H, Charnsangavej C, Faria SC, et al. Correlation of computed tomography and positron emission tomography in patients with metastatic gastrointestinal stromal tumor treated at a single institution with imatinib mesylate: proposal of new computed tomography response criteria. *J Clin Oncol*. 2007;**25**:1753–1759.

177 Patel SR, Vadhan-Raj S, Burgess MA, et al. Results of two consecutive trials of dose-intensive chemotherapy with doxorubicin and ifosfamide in patients with sarcomas. *Am J Clin Oncol*. 1998;**21**:317–321.

178 Antman K, Crowley J, Balcerzak SP, et al. An intergroup phase III randomized study of doxorubicin and dacarbazine with or without ifosfamide and mesna in advanced soft tissue and bone sarcomas. *J Clin Oncol*. 1993;**11**:1276–1285.

180 Judson I, Verweij J, Gelderblom H, et al. Doxorubicin alone versus intensified doxorubicin plus ifosfamide for first-line treatment of advanced or metastatic soft-tissue sarcoma: a randomised controlled phase 3 trial. *Lancet Oncol*. 2014;**15**:415–423.

183 Judson I, Radford JA, Harris M, et al. Randomised phase II trial of pegylated liposomal doxorubicin (DOXIL/CAELYX) versus doxorubicin in the treatment of advanced or metastatic soft tissue sarcoma: a study by the EORTC Soft Tissue and Bone Sarcoma Group. *Eur J Cancer*. 2001;**37**:870–877.

187 Hensley ML, Maki R, Venkatraman E, et al. Gemcitabine and docetaxel in patients with unresectable leiomyosarcoma: results of a phase II trial. *J Clin Oncol*. 2002;**20**:2824–2831.

189 Maki RG, Wathen JK, Patel SR, et al. Randomized phase II study of gemcitabine and docetaxel compared with gemcitabine alone in patients with metastatic soft tissue sarcomas: results of sarcoma alliance for research through collaboration study 002 [corrected]. *J Clin Oncol*. 2007;**25**:2755–2763.

190 Garcia-Del-Muro X, Lopez-Pousa A, Maurel J, et al. Randomized phase II study comparing gemcitabine plus dacarbazine versus dacarbazine alone in patients with previously treated soft tissue sarcoma: a Spanish Group for Research on Sarcomas study. *J Clin Oncol*. 2011;**29**:2528–2533.

191 Hensley ML, Miller A, O'Malley DM, et al. Randomized phase III trial of gemcitabine plus docetaxel plus bevacizumab or placebo as first-line treatment for metastatic uterine leiomyosarcoma: an NRG Oncology/Gynecologic Oncology Group Study. *J Clin Oncol*. 2015;**33**:1180–1185.

193 Demetri GD, Chawla SP, von Mehren M, et al. Efficacy and safety of trabectedin in patients with advanced or metastatic liposarcoma or leiomyosarcoma after failure of prior anthracyclines and ifosfamide: results of a randomized phase II study of two different schedules. *J Clin Oncol*. 2009;**27**:4188–4196.

195 Demetri G, Schoffski P, Placeholder P (2015) Trabectedin vs Dacarbazine in L-sarcomas.

196 Schoffski P, Ray-Coquard IL, Cioffi A, et al. Activity of eribulin mesylate in patients with soft-tissue sarcoma: a phase 2 study in four independent histological subtypes. *Lancet Oncol*. 2011;**12**:1045–1052.

198 van der Graaf WT, Blay JY, Chawla SP, et al. Pazopanib for metastatic soft-tissue sarcoma (PALETTE): a randomised, double-blind, placebo-controlled phase 3 trial. *Lancet*. 2012;**379**:1879–1886.

206 Verweij J, Casali PG, Zalcberg J, et al. Progression-free survival in gastrointestinal stromal tumours with high-dose imatinib: randomised trial. *Lancet*. 2004;**364**:1127–1134.

207 Demetri GD, von Mehren M, Blanke CD, et al. Efficacy and safety of imatinib mesylate in advanced gastrointestinal stromal tumors. *N Engl J Med*. 2002;**347**:472–480.

211 Debiec-Rychter M, Sciot R, Le Cesne A, et al. KIT mutations and dose selection for imatinib in patients with advanced gastrointestinal stromal tumours. *Eur J Cancer*. 2006;**42**:1093–1103.

214 Schoffski P, Reichardt P, Blay JY, et al. A phase I-II study of everolimus (RAD001) in combination with imatinib in patients with imatinib-resistant gastrointestinal stromal tumors. *Ann Oncol*. 2010;**21**:1990–1998.

215 Demetri GD, van Oosterom AT, Garrett CR, et al. Efficacy and safety of sunitinib in patients with advanced gastrointestinal stromal tumour after failure of imatinib: a randomised controlled trial. *Lancet*. 2006;**368**:1329–1338.

218 Demetri GD, Reichardt P, Kang YK, et al. Efficacy and safety of regorafenib for advanced gastrointestinal stromal tumours after failure of imatinib and sunitinib (GRID): an international, multicentre, randomised, placebo-controlled, phase 3 trial. *Lancet*. 2013;**381**:295–302.

221 Joensuu H, Eriksson M, Sundby Hall K, et al. One vs three years of adjuvant imatinib for operable gastrointestinal stromal tumor: a randomized trial. *JAMA*. 2012;**307**:1265–1272.

222 Joensuu H, Vehtari A, Riihimaki J, et al. Risk of recurrence of gastrointestinal stromal tumour after surgery: an analysis of pooled population-based cohorts. *Lancet Oncol*. 2012;**13**:265–274.

224 Joensuu H, Rutkowski P, Nishida T, et al. KIT and PDGFRA mutations and the risk of GI stromal tumor recurrence. *J Clin Oncol*. 2015;**33**:634–642.

225 Heinrich MC, Joensuu H, Demetri GD, et al. Phase II, open-label study evaluating the activity of imatinib in treating life-threatening malignancies known to be associated with imatinib-sensitive tyrosine kinases. *Clin Cancer Res*. 2008;**14**:2717–2725.

228 Gronchi A, Miceli R, Allard MA, et al. Personalizing the approach to retroperitoneal soft tissue sarcoma: histology-specific patterns of failure and postrelapse outcome after primary extended resection. *Ann Surg Oncol*. 2015;**22**:1447–1454.

231 Singer S, Antonescu CR, Riedel E, Brennan MF. Histologic subtype and margin of resection predict pattern of recurrence and survival for retroperitoneal liposarcoma. *Ann Surg*. 2003;**238**:358–370; discussion 370–351.

235 Pisters PW. Resection of some–but not all–clinically uninvolved adjacent viscera as part of surgery for retroperitoneal soft tissue sarcomas. *J Clin Oncol*. 2009;**27**:6–8.

238 Petersen IA, Haddock MG, Donohue JH, et al. Use of intraoperative electron beam radiotherapy in the management of retroperitoneal soft tissue sarcomas. *Int J Radiat Oncol Biol Phys*. 2002;**52**:469–475.

245 Stinson SF, DeLaney TF, Greenberg J, et al. Acute and long-term effects on limb function of combined modality limb sparing therapy for extremity soft tissue sarcoma. *Int J Radiat Oncol Biol Phys*. 1991;**21**:1493–1499.

246 Davis AM. Functional outcome in extremity soft tissue sarcoma. *Semin Radiat Oncol*. 1999;**9**:360–368.

254 Antonescu C. Round cell sarcomas beyond Ewing: emerging entities. *Histopathology*. 2014;**64**:26–37.

255 Antonescu CR, Dal CP. Promiscuous genes involved in recurrent chromosomal translocations in soft tissue tumours. *Pathology*. 2014;**46**:105–112.

256 Kadoch C, Crabtree GR. Reversible disruption of mSWI/SNF (BAF) complexes by the SS18-SSX oncogenic fusion in synovial sarcoma. *Cell*. 2013;**153**:71–85.
257 Su L, Sampaio AV, Jones KB, et al. Deconstruction of the SS18-SSX fusion oncoprotein complex: insights into disease etiology and therapeutics. *Cancer Cell*. 2012;**21**:333–347.
258 Garsed DW, Marshall OJ, Corbin VD, et al. The architecture and evolution of cancer neochromosomes. *Cancer Cell*. 2014;**26**:653–667.
259 Di Giandomenico S, Frapolli R, Bello E, et al. Mode of action of trabectedin in myxoid liposarcomas. *Oncogene*. 2014;**33**:5201–5210.
261 Crago AM, Socci ND, DeCarolis P, et al. Copy number losses define subgroups of dedifferentiated liposarcoma with poor prognosis and genomic instability. *Clin Cancer Res*. 2012;**18**:1334–1340.
263 Dickson MA, Tap WD, Keohan ML, et al. Phase II trial of the CDK4 inhibitor PD0332991 in patients with advanced CDK4-amplified well-differentiated or dedifferentiated liposarcoma. *J Clin Oncol*. 2013;**31**:2024–2028.
264 Robbins PF, Morgan RA, Feldman SA, et al. Tumor regression in patients with metastatic synovial cell sarcoma and melanoma using genetically engineered lymphocytes reactive with NY-ESO-1. *J Clin Oncol*. 2011;**29**:917–924.
265 Robbins PF, Kassim SH, Tran TL, et al. A pilot trial using lymphocytes genetically engineered with an NY-ESO-1-reactive T-cell receptor: long-term follow-up and correlates with response. *Clin Cancer Res*. 2015;**21**:1019–1027.

第 113 章　骨髓增生异常综合征

Lewis R. Silverman, MD

概述

20 世纪初期人们就发现存在一类以贫血和发育异常为特点的造血系统疾病，其发生于急性髓细胞性白血病(acute myeloid leukemia, AML)之前。这类综合征最初被称为白血病前期，其定义未明确，只能通过回顾性分析确定。然而这一术语本身信息传递具有不确定性，临床转归并不一定会发生白血病。1976 年法美英协作组(FAB)采用了更准确的描述和更恰当的命名——骨髓增生异常综合征(myelodysplastic syndrome, MDS)。FAB 分型有助于发现患有这类异质性克隆性疾病的患者。

MDS 起源于多能造血干细胞，临床特点为骨髓增生活跃、无效造血，并伴有一系或多系外周血细胞减少。多数患者骨髓衰竭后因出血和感染而死亡，而高达 40% 的患者转化为急性白血病。疾病的发展过程符合肿瘤发生的多次打击致病理论，因此可以作为深入理解肿瘤转化过程的重要模型。

伴随这一系列的发现，问题随之而来：MDS 究竟是明确的肿瘤状态，还是仅仅是转化中的癌前病变。该综合征似乎代表了一种疾病过程：初始的基因组损伤(虽然临床上难以发现)，随后更多的获得性基因和表观遗传学损伤，到最后明确的瘤变状态。

将这种疾病命名为 MDS 而非白血病前期，可以将其区别于其他已知与急性白血病发生有关的疾病。后者包括经典的骨髓增殖综合征(真性红细胞增多症、慢性髓细胞性白血病、原因未明的髓样化生、原发性血小板增多症)、再生障碍性贫血、阵发性睡眠性血红蛋白尿症(paroxysmal nocturnal hemoglobinuria, PNH)，以及范科尼综合征、布卢姆综合征和唐氏综合征。这些特殊的“白血病前期状态”不在本章讨论范围内。

MDS 可进一步分为原发性和继发性综合征。前者是原发性的，病因不明；而后者有明确的环境、职业或医源性诱因。

MDS 的发病率是 AML 发病率(美国每年约有 14 000 例新发病例)的 1~2 倍。SEER 数据库目前正在追踪该疾病，将来会有更精确的数据。根据医疗保险索赔估计，2009—2011 年期间共有 10.7 万例病例。普遍认为发病率升高的原因很多，包括认知度的提高、诊断更精准以及人口老龄化。

历史

Luzzatto 首次描述了一例骨髓红系增生活跃的慢性贫血，他称为“假性再生障碍性贫血”[1]。然而直到 Rhoads 和 Bomford 描述了这种疾病，疾病的名称“难治性贫血(refractory anemia, RA)”才被广泛接受[2,3]。

20 世纪 50 年代初发现部分难治性贫血患者确实会进展为白血病，因而有了“白血病前期”这一术语[4,5]。然而由于许多患者因骨髓衰竭死亡，并没有进展为白血病，“白血病前期”这一命名似乎常是错误的。1976 年 FAB 制订了 MDS 的诊断标准以便于对潜在患者作出诊断[6]。

MDS 的发病率是 AML 发病率(美国每年约有 14 000 例新发病例)的 1~2 倍[7,8]。SEER 数据库目前正在追踪该疾病，将来会有更精确的数据。根据医疗保险索赔估计，2009—2011 年期间共有 10.7 万例病例[8]。

分型

根据骨髓细胞学[9]，将该综合征分为 3 个亚型：获得性铁粒幼细胞性贫血、难治性贫血伴原始细胞增多(RAEB)和慢性粒-单核细胞白血病(CMML)。1982 年 FAB 协作组修订了 MDS 分型体系，根据形态学特征和骨髓及外周血原始细胞比例将 MDS 分为 5 型[6]。这 5 个亚型包括：①难治性贫血(refractory anemia, RA)；②难治性贫血伴环形铁粒幼细胞(refractory anemia with ringed sideroblasts, RARS)；③难治性贫血伴原始细胞增多(refractory anemia with excess blasts, RAEB)(5%<原始细胞<20%)；④慢性粒-单核细胞白血病(chronic myelomonocytic leukemia, CMML)；⑤难治性贫血伴原始细胞增多转化型(RAEB in transformation, RAEB-T)(20%≤原始细胞<30%)。考虑到该分型方案可能导致急性髓细胞性白血病 M6 型(红白血病)的误诊，1985 年又进行了进一步的修订和完善[10]。

CMML 的归类仍存在一些争议：CMML 究竟真的是 MDS 的一种亚型，还是归为骨髓增殖性疾病(myeloproliferative disorders, MPD)的一个亚型更为恰当。部分 CMML 患者既有 MDS 的特点，也有 MPD 的特点，是一种兼具两种疾病特征的重叠综合征[9]。其生物学行为似乎与骨髓原始细胞百分比密切相关[11~13]。

国际预后积分系统(IPSS)是根据骨髓原始细胞百分比，细胞遗传学和血细胞减少程度制订的[14]。IPSS 对生存和急性白血病转化的风险具有预测价值(表 113-1)。

修订后的 IPSS(IPSS-R)将患者分为 5 个亚组，具有更高的预测价值，并对外周血细胞计数加以区分利用[16]。细胞遗传学亚组也根据进一步的风险评估进行了修订。与原版 IPSS 的 816 例病例相比，此次修订对 7 012 名患者进行了分析。IPSS-R 能够更好地对患者进行危险分组，不仅能够动态地预测新诊断患者的预后，而且在患者病程中能随时判断其预后。这种分组方法已经得到验证，并与世界卫生组织(WHO)分型[17]一起成为标准的分类方法(表 113-2 和表 113-3)。然而如果无法获得细胞遗传学数据，IPSS 的预测能力会显著降低。

表 113-1 IPSS 积分系统

预后变量	积分				
	0	0.5	1.0	1.5	2.0
骨髓原始细胞/%	<5	5~10	—	11~20	21~29
染色体核型	良好	中等	差	—	—
血细胞减少	0/1	2/3	—	—	—
积分	**细胞遗传学**				
低危:0 分	预后良好:	正常核型			
中危-1:0.5~1.0 分		-y			
中危-2:1.5~2.0 分		del(5q)			
高危:>2.5 分		del(20q)			
	预后差:	7 号染色体异常			
		≥3 种复杂核型异常			
	预后中等:	其他			

改编自 Nazha 2013[15]。

表 113-2 修订的国际预后积分系统(IPSS-R)根据预后危险度分组进行 MDS 分类

国际预后评分系统(IPSS)	急性髓细胞性白血病转化的风险(25%患者转化的时间)/年	中位生存/年
极低危	未达到	8.8
低危	10.8	5.3
中危-1	3.2	3.0
高危	1.4	1.6
极高危	0.73	0.8

改编自 Greenberg 2012[16]。

表 113-3 世界卫生组织(WHO)分型

难治性贫血(RA)
• 伴环形铁粒幼细胞
• 不伴环形铁粒幼细胞
难治性血细胞减少伴多系发育异常(RCMD)
• 伴环形铁粒幼细胞
• 不伴环形铁粒幼细胞
难治性贫血伴原始细胞增多
• RAEB-Ⅰ(原始细胞 6%~10%)
• RAEB-Ⅱ(原始细胞 11%~19%)
5q-综合征
CMML(MDS/MPD)
骨髓增生异常综合征,不能分类

改编自 Fenaux 2009[18]。

1999 年,WHO 工作组发布了另一个分型系统,不仅沿用了 FAB 系统的常规形态学标准,还考虑了细胞遗传学标记(表 113-3)。根据 1 600 名原发 MDS 患者的数据评估结果,在 FAB 系统基础上增加了两类,共计 7 类,均与预后密切相关。将 WBC>13×10^9/L 的 CMML 从 WHO 分型的 MDS 中剔除,归入 MPN,将 WBC<13×10^9/L 的 CMML 归为 MDS/MPN。将 RA 分为单纯的难治性贫血(pure refractory anemia,PRA)和难治性血细胞减少伴多系发育异常(refractory cytopenia with multilineage dysplasia,RCMD)。之前被归为 RARS 的部分病例现被列入单纯铁粒幼细胞性贫血组[19],而伴有其他系发育异常的患者以及不伴环形铁粒幼细胞的 RA 被归入 RCMD。RAEB 根据骨髓和外周血原始细胞计数分为 RAEB-Ⅰ和 RAEB-Ⅱ。RAEB-T 则纳入 AML 中。

此外,将有 5q 相关核型异常的 MDS 作为一种独立的分型,当骨髓原始细胞比例小于 5%时,其预后相对较好。如表 113-3 所示,WHO 分型已进行了一些更新修订。

病因

虽然大多数 MDS 患者的致病因素不能明确,但部分患者发病可能与暴露于电离辐射、化学物质、药物或其他环境因素有关。

电离辐射暴露与干细胞畸变有明确的相关性[20]。此外，原子弹爆炸幸存者在发生白血病前通常会经历白血病前期状态[21]。原子弹爆炸幸存者在暴露于射线后很长一段时间内，基因不稳定的发生率持续性增高，这种不稳定性包括染色体结构和数目的异常，这种异常可能导致 MDS 和 AML 的发生[22]。

化学因素对骨髓的损伤已经是公认的现象，在暴露于石油化工产品（特别是苯）和橡胶工业的工人中，白血病的发生风险增加[23]。许多苯诱导的白血病患者在早期都有白血病前期综合征的表现。人类细胞系暴露于氢醌（苯的代谢物）后，可发生 5 号、7 号和 8 号染色体的畸变，在一定程度上导致与化学物质暴露相关的 DNA 损伤[24]。在伴或不伴有环形铁粒幼细胞的患者中，接触柴油汽体（$P<0.01$）、柴油液体（$P<0.01$）或氨水（$P<0.05$）都与 MDS 发生有关[25]。仔细询问患者环境和职业危害暴露史是接诊 MDS 患者的重要组成部分。其他环境因素可能包括使用染发剂和吸烟[26]。

放化疗后出现的治疗相关 MDS 和白血病，最初是在治疗后的霍奇金病患者中观察到的[27]。自霍奇金病治疗后发生 MDS 的报道后，陆续报道了乳腺癌、肺癌、卵巢癌和胃肠道肿瘤、非霍奇金淋巴瘤、精原细胞瘤、多发性骨髓瘤、真性红细胞增多症、慢性淋巴细胞白血病（chronic lymphocytic leukemia，CLL）以及非恶性疾病治疗后出现了治疗相关 MDS[28~30]。烷化剂、亚硝基脲类和丙卡巴肼（procarbazine）的致白血病作用最强。接触这些特殊药物的致病风险得到了证实，这些患者中 5 号和 7 号染色体异常的发生率较接受蒽环类药物或抗代谢药物治疗的患者增高，尽管蒽环类药物也有风险[30]。在接受美法仑或苯丁酸氮芥（chlorambucil）治疗的卵巢癌患者中观察到，致白血病作用似乎与药物暴露的剂量和时间有关。在生殖细胞肿瘤患者中，接受依托泊苷联合顺铂或其他烷化剂治疗与 MDS 或 AML 风险的增加有关[31]。依托泊苷或替尼泊苷的累积剂量与 MDS 或治疗相关 AML 的发生之间的关系仍有待确定[32]。17 号染色体短臂（17p）部分缺失与 *TP53* 基因突变或过表达相关，目前认为也与既往的化疗有关[19]。这一结果在使用烷化剂治疗的淋巴系统肿瘤患者以及使用羟基脲或 p 治疗的 MPN 患者中均得到了证实。最近有报道治疗相关 MDS 与氟达拉滨和克拉屈滨（cladribine）有关[20]。

长期以来一直存在争论，白血病发生风险的增加是辐射和/或化疗暴露的直接结果，还是仅仅反映了与疾病本质相关的自然倾向。据报道，有些肿瘤的 MDS 和/或异时性白血病的发病风险增加，如多发性骨髓瘤、淋巴瘤、肺癌和 CLL[33,34]。而真性红细胞增多症或霍奇金病经不同治疗方法治疗后，白血病发生率存在差异，这表明治疗是最关键的致病因素。在真性红细胞增多症患者中，与单用放血治疗的患者相比用苯丁酸氮芥治疗的患者发生白血病的风险显著升高[35]。同样，与 MOPP 方案（氮芥、长春新碱、丙卡巴肼和泼尼松）相比，ABVD 方案（多柔比星、博来霉素、长春新碱和达卡巴嗪）治疗的霍奇金病患者治疗相关白血病的发生率要低得多[36]。认识到这些潜在风险有助于开发疗效相同但较少致白血病的治疗方案，尤其是对于有可能长期存活的疾病。在一项非格司亭（filgrastim）治疗的慢性中性粒细胞减少症患者的回顾登记中，9%的先天性中性粒细胞减少症患者出现 MDS 和/或白血病，而周期性或特发性中性粒细胞减少症患者没有病例出现 MDS 和/或白血病[37]。在这些患者中非格司亭的应用与 MDS 的发生之间的关系尚不明确。

大剂量化疗后干细胞支持作为根治性疗法用于治疗多种恶性肿瘤，如非霍奇金淋巴瘤。如前所述，已发现淋巴瘤相关 MDS 或异时性白血病的发病风险增加。目前认为 MDS 是大剂量化疗方案治疗的晚期并发症[38]，尽管经标准剂量化疗的非霍奇金淋巴瘤患者中也出现了治疗相关 MDS。保险统计报告的 6 年风险在 6.4%~18%[39]。目前正在研究的策略是预后差的患者在病程早期使用大剂量清髓治疗，因此了解这一问题的严重性愈发重要。研究表明 MDS 患者存在多个异常造血克隆，这些克隆共存并可产生亚克隆[40]。在转化为 AML 的患者中这些克隆可以产生白血病克隆[41]。

病理生物学

克隆起源

大量证据集中在 MDS 的克隆起源上。在 30%~70%的 MDS 患者中可检测到非随机染色体异常，证实这可能是一种克隆性疾病[42~47]。疾病起源于多能造血干细胞，其证据来源于 MDS 进展为双表型和淋巴系统白血病的病例报道[42,48]。

X 连锁的多态酶如葡萄糖-6-磷酸脱氢酶（G-6-PD）的灭活模式分析是分析肿瘤克隆起源的有用工具。Raskind 等人[49]证实，在 24 个 EB 病毒（Epstein-Barr virus）转染的 B 淋巴细胞系中，21 个细胞系表达单一轻链免疫球蛋白，而且仅含一种 G-6-PD 同工酶。相反，T 细胞同时表达 G-6-PD-A 和-B 同工酶。MDS 发生淋巴系异常克隆的频率差异较大。B 淋巴细胞发生异常克隆较 T 细胞更常见[50~53]。其他研究发现只有髓系定向干细胞参与 MDS 克隆，而淋巴细胞是多克隆起源的[50~53]。用荧光原位杂交（FISH）或聚合酶链反应（PCR）分析杂合子的缺失，证实了早期干细胞的受累，这些干细胞能够分化为 CD34+ 细胞，也能分化为红系、巨核细胞系和髓单核细胞系细胞，但不分化为淋巴细胞[54]。随后，在一项免疫分型联合 FISH 的研究中发现，B 淋巴细胞与 5q-综合征有关[55]。对 T 细胞克隆性进行分子和流式细胞学分析，也表明 T 细胞参与了部分患者的 MDS 克隆。结果矛盾的原因尚不清楚，但也反映了疾病的异质性和患者间的变异较大。分子学研究表明，MDS 患者中存在多种克隆：一种起始克隆，以及携带重现性基因突变和新基因通路突变的多种亚克隆[41]。

体外前体细胞生长特点

对各种类型 MDS 患者的骨髓和外周血的克隆分析表明，造血前体细胞的生长存在一系列异常[56]，但均未证明对临床反应有指导意义。

骨髓微环境

骨髓活检的组织学检查表明微环境存在异常[57]。他们发现不成熟的前体细胞在骨髓的骨小梁间区中央呈簇状分布，而不是沿着骨内膜表面分布，他们将此作为不成熟前体细胞异常定位（abnormal localization of immature precursors，ALIP）的证据。在一项 40 例患者的研究中，ALIP 的存在与生存期缩短显著相关,并与AML转化风险增高有关。这些结果与FAB亚型无关,甚至在难治性贫血患者中也能发现。但是必须注意鉴别真正的ALIP和伪ALIP。伪ALIP中成簇细胞为红系或巨核细胞系来源,与ALIP髓系来源的前体细胞相比,并不具有相同的预后价值。通过免疫组化方法检测不成熟前体细胞表型有助于鉴别ALIP的真伪。然而ALIP并不是MDS患者所特有的,不能作为诊断依据[58]。

最近的小鼠模型数据表明在骨髓微环境中成骨细胞对白血病细胞有调节作用[58]。成骨细胞的减少与白血病进展和生存期缩短有关[59]。成骨细胞数量有可能成为调节MDS/AML进展的药物靶点。

信号转导

尚不确定导致成熟和功能异常的早期病理生理缺陷是造血前体细胞所固有的,还是造血前体细胞与辅助细胞和其他微环境因素的相互作用造成的,或是两者皆有。造血细胞缺陷可能不仅与前体细胞的数量异常有关,对增殖和分化途径中的细胞因子或其他调节分子的应答也出现信号转导异常。由于细胞因子受体的数量或功能异常,或是结合后信号转导功能失调,MDS患者的造血细胞对许多细胞因子的反应受损,无法对外源信号产生应答。

造血前体细胞对细胞因子刺激的反应异常,CFU-GM、CFU-GEMM和BFU-E克隆数量减少[60]。MDS患者纯化后的原始细胞在粒细胞集落刺激因子(G-CSF)和粒细胞-巨噬细胞集落刺激因子(GM-CSF)的作用下可以增殖但不分化成熟。MDS患者纯化的CD34+细胞也出现对G-CSF的反应受损[61]。MDS中受体异常并不常见[62~64],部分患者存在受体数量减少或结构异常。在促红细胞生成素受体缺陷的患者中,缺少促红细胞生成素的作用,前体细胞分化受阻,细胞发生凋亡[65]。另一方面,信号转导缺陷似乎在造血前体细胞对调节分子的反应异常中发挥巨大作用[63,64,66]。这涉及细胞因子信号转导途径和调节凋亡的因子[63,64,66]。MDS患者STAT5不能被促红细胞生成素激活,但可以被IL-3激活,提示促红细胞生成素信号通路存在缺陷。虽然功能受损,但增加细胞因子浓度可部分纠正这种缺陷[67,68]。导致转录沉默的表观遗传学改变是影响细胞因子信号转导的另一可能机制。有证据表明,31%的MDS患者*SOCS-1*基因异常高甲基化与JAK/STAT通路活性增强有关[69]。在MDS患者骨髓中发现DNA甲基转移酶1和3A过表达,这也许能部分解释其他基因中发生的高甲基化,如*p15*基因[70]。

多数MDS患者骨髓细胞增生活跃,各系细胞明显增生。这种现象可解释为骨髓对外周血细胞减少的反馈信号的代偿性反应。然而,这种反应并不能产生有效的造血;提示凋亡增加起了作用[71~73]。细胞因子的缺乏或相对抵抗可以解释这种无效造血现象。在一些研究中显示,MDS患者骨髓细胞中Fas和Fas配体的表达增加。在骨髓培养中,阻断肿瘤坏死因子(TNF)介导的信号,如应用抗TNF-α抗体,造血细胞集落数量比对照组显著增多。其他研究认为Fas通路和TNF-α功能失调可以导致无效造血[71~73]。部分患者TGF-β过表达,抑制TGF-β信号通路可恢复造血,提示TGF-β具有负性调节作用。

通过检测膜联蛋白V、线粒体膜电位和细胞溶解产物胱天蛋白酶3活性,发现与初治AML患者相比,MDS患者成熟细胞和不成熟CD34+细胞的凋亡均增加。这些结果表明所有FAB亚型的MDS患者细胞凋亡增加,包括RAEB-T亚型,这有别于AML患者[74]。

细胞遗传学

30%~70%的MDS患者中发现与AML患者类似的染色体异常,主要为染色体的完全或部分缺失,最常受累的是染色体5(-5,5q-)、7(-7,7q-)和8(8+)[75,76]。与核心结合因子重排有关的核型异常,例如急性早幼粒细胞白血病(M3)中的t(15;17),AML(M2)中的t(8;21)和AML(M4)中的inv16,在MDS中非常罕见。这些AML亚型患者预后良好,有治愈的可能,因此这部分患者应按AML对待给予相应治疗。此外,涉及20号染色体长臂部分缺失(20q-)的核型异常,在MDS尤其是RARS、真性红细胞增多症和骨髓增生综合征中较常见,初治AML患者通常不出现。染色体异常最常见于高危患者。与AML不同,虽发现了特异的染色体异常,但没有FAB亚型特异性异常。除显带染色技术外,FISH技术能检测出患者的其他染色体异常,可以作为标准技术的补充[77]。

多项研究表明,核型异常是一个独立的预后因素。与单个克隆异常或正常核型相比,复杂核型异常的生存期缩短。某些特殊的克隆亚型对生存和白血病转化风险具有不同的预后意义。7号染色体单体、5号染色体单体和7q与生存期缩短有关,而孤立的20号染色体长臂缺失(20q-)、孤立的5号染色体长臂缺失(5q-综合征)及孤立的Y染色体缺失[78]与生存延长有关。在IPSS评分中细胞遗传学结果是一个独立的预后变量,据其将患者分为预后良好、预后中等、预后差3个亚组。进一步的研究加深了我们对MDS中细胞遗传学危险度分组的认识。对German-Austrian和MD Anderson数据库的病例分析表明,IPSS评分低估了细胞遗传学作为危险因素的权重,预后差的细胞遗传学异常是与原始细胞>20%一样差的危险因素[75]。因此对IPSS细胞遗传学分组进行了修订。在2 900多名患者中发现了19种不同的细胞遗传学类型。这些类型被归为预后非常好、良好、中等、差和非常差5个亚组,并已被纳入修订的IPSS积分系统(表113-4)[16]。

相当大比例的患者具有遗传不稳定性,克隆演变可以证实。20%~35%的患者病程中经历了克隆演变,与初始的核型状态无关。克隆演变对白血病转化和生存的意义最初并不明确。在部分研究中克隆演变与预后不良有关,但并不增加白血病转化的风险。相反,Glenn等在临床稳定患者中发现了核型变化[79]。一项纳入31例从MDS进展为AML患者的研究表明,涉及染色体1、7、8、11和17的其他异常可能参与转化过程[80]。亚克隆演变提示基因组不稳定。在部分MDS患者尤其是治疗相关疾病患者中发现了微卫星不稳定性,与DNA错配修复系统缺陷有关[81]。骨髓中的克隆结构评估表明,MDS患者存在一个正常克隆和多个伴有获得性突变的继发克隆,导致了克隆演变[41]。

5号染色体长臂部分缺失(5q-)特别值得注意。如前所述,5q-综合征表现为难治性大细胞性贫血,血小板计数正常或增高,巨血小板,红系病态造血,巨核细胞分叶减少,多为女性,生存期长以及白血病转化率低。将5q-综合征与5q-伴其他染色体异常或FAB分型不是RA的病例区分开非常重要,后者临床病程更具侵袭性,生存期更短。目前发现5q-患者RPS14核糖体RNA缺陷是导致这些患者骨髓衰竭的遗传缺陷(见"基因突变和失调"一节)[82]。

表 113-4　细胞遗传学：修订的细胞遗传学 IPSS-R 分组

危险度分组	细胞遗传学分组	双重	复合	中位总生存/月
极低危	Del 11q	—	—	60.8
	-Y			
低危	正常	包括 del(5q)	—	48.6
	del(5q)			
	del(12p)			
	del(20q)			
中危	del 7q	任何其他	—	26
	+8			
	i(17p)			
	+19			
	任何其他独立克隆			
高危	inv(3)/t(3q)/del(3q)	包括-7/del(7q)	3	15.8
	-7			
极高危	—	—	>3	5.9

改编自 Schanz 2012[76]。

致突变剂或致癌剂暴露所继发的 MDS 患者，染色体异常的核型和临床意义也是类似的。应用表鬼臼毒素（依托泊苷和替尼泊苷）治疗的患者可以发生 11q23 断裂点的特殊易位。这导致混合白血病（mixed lineage leukemia，MLL）融合蛋白的转录。

已开发出新的技术用于检测正常中期细胞遗传学（MC）无法分辨的基因组异常[83]。单核苷酸多态性分析（SNP-A）的基因异常检出率比 MC 高。

基因突变和失调

在细胞基因组中原癌基因调控和表达的改变会导致细胞增殖和分化异常，被认为是参与肿瘤转化的分子基础[84]。*ras* 癌基因家族的点突变与人类多种肿瘤有关，包括肺癌、胰腺癌、结肠肠癌及造血系统肿瘤[85]。在 20%～30% 的 AML 患者和 9%～48%的 MDS 患者中发现了 12、13 和 61 密码子的特殊点突变，这些突变与 *ras* 基因激活有关。这些发现提示，*ras* 基因激活可能不仅与 MDS 的发展有关，还可能参与受损干细胞的转化过程。仅有少数病例涉及 Ki-ras 和 H-ras。CMML 是与 *ras* 基因突变有关的最常见的 FAB 亚型。40%的患者存在 *ras* 突变[86~88]。

最近发现在 MDS 患者中，许多基因伴有重现性体细胞突变，涉及许多不同的途径，与表观遗传学调控、RNA 剪接、信号激活和转录因子（表 113-5）有关。其中有许多突变是致癌的，并且部分突变之间存在关联或互斥的关系。这些突变并非 MDS 所特有的，亦见于包括 AML 和 MPN 在内的髓系疾病[89,90]。部分研究数据表明，有些突变出现在 MDS 病程早期，而另一些突变是后期出现的。有些突变具有预后意义，尤其是 *EZH2*、*TP53*、*Runx1*、*DNAMT3A* 以及 *ASLX1*[91]。其中一些突变可能导致亚克隆演变倾向增加，而且突变数量的增加似乎与预后更差和 AML 转化率更高有关。*TET2*、*IDH1*、*IDH2* 等突变的功能失调导致羟甲基化异常，但这些异常对信号通路的主要影响尚不清楚。这些重现性突变有助于深入理解疾病发病机制和预后信息，并提供潜在的治疗靶点（图 113-1）。

表 113-5　MDS 中的基因突变

候选基因	染色体	在 MDS 中的频率/%	假定的功能意义
表观遗传学途径			
ASXL1 * 612990	20q	11～15	未知
IDH1/IDH2 * 147700/ * 147650	2q/15q	4～11	生存缩短
DNMT3A * 602769	2p	8	生存缩短
EZH2 * 601573	7q	2～6	生存缩短
TET2 * 612839	4q	11～26	未知
SETBP1	18	—	未知
信号通路	—	—	—
JAK2 * 147796	9p	2	未知
N/KRAS * 164790/ * 190070	1p/12p	3～6	增加 AML 转化的风险
CBL * 165360	11q	1	未知
FLT3ITD * 136351	13q	0～2	生存缩短

续表

候选基因	染色体	在 MDS 中的频率/%	假定的功能意义
转录因子			
RUNX1[*] 151385	21q	4~14	生存缩短;治疗相关 MDS 中更常见
其他			
TP53[*] 191170	17p	10~18	生存缩短且增加 AML 转化的风险
NPM1[*] 164040	5q	2	未知
RNA 剪接			
SF3B1	—	14	蛋白质剪接异常
SRSF2	—	12	蛋白质剪接异常
U2AF1	—	7	蛋白质剪接异常
ZRSR2	—	3	蛋白质剪接异常

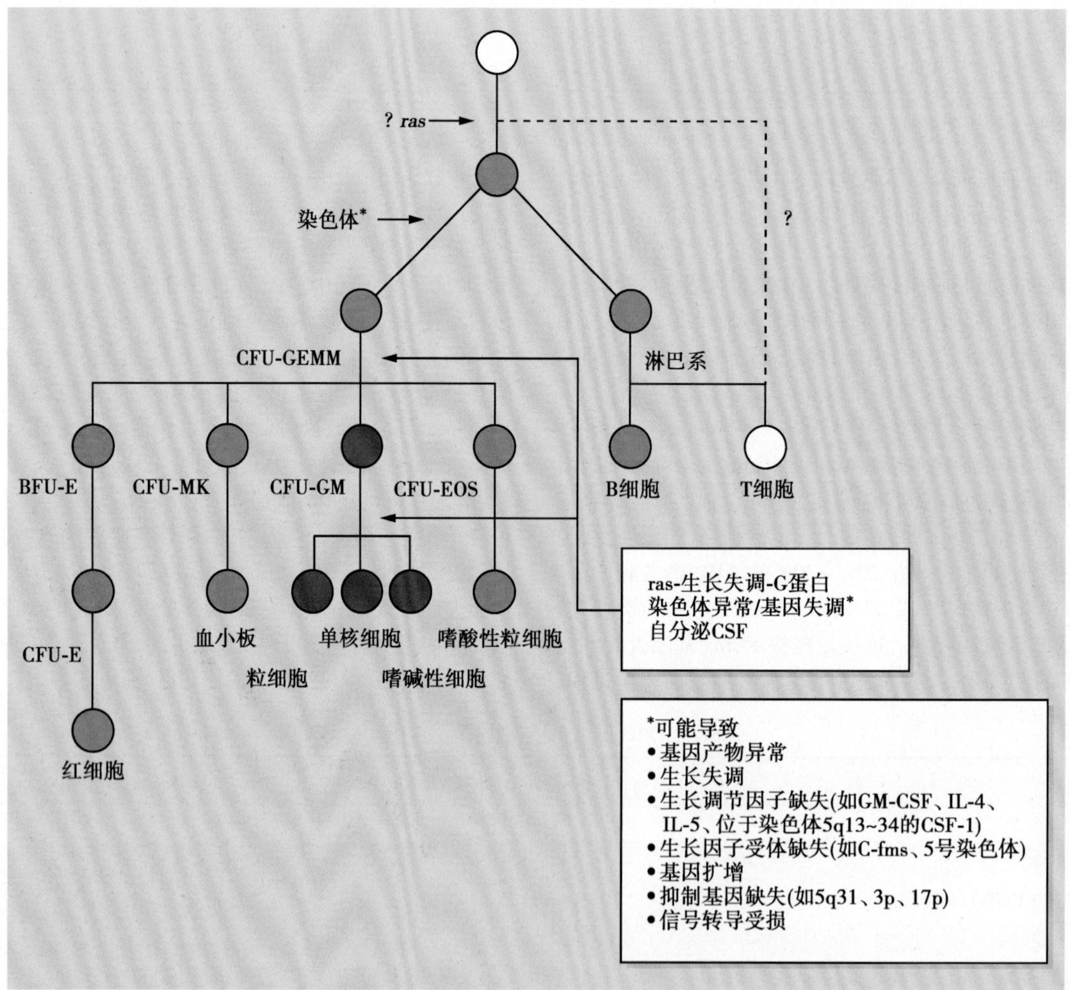

图 113-1 在 MDS 发病机制中影响多能造血干细胞的多个步骤(白色圈)。染色体畸变和 *ras* 突变可以发生在疾病发病的早期或晚期。年轻患者疾病起源于定向干细胞,似乎沿着固定系别途径进展(红色圈),与部分初发 AML 患者的干细胞起源类似。在大多数 MDS 患者中,疾病起源于多能干细胞,影响多个造血系列(淡橘色圈和红色圈)。[*]可能导致基因产物异常、生长失调、生长调节因子缺失(如 GM-CSF、IL-3、IL-4、IL-5、位于染色体 5q13~34 的 CSF-1 等)、生长因子受体缺失(如 cfms、5 号染色体)、基因扩增、抑制基因缺失(如 5q31、3p、17p)、信号转导异常。IL 白介素;CSF 集落刺激因子

已经发现修饰后表达 *N-ras* 突变的 CD34+前体细胞对促红细胞生成素的反应存在分化缺陷。表现为增殖减少，倍增时间延长，S/G2M 期细胞数量减少，导致中晚幼红阶段细胞分化受阻。这些细胞趋向于加速凋亡，提示 *N-ras* 突变的表达可能是 MDS 的部分病理生理学基础[92]。

在大量原发或继发性 MDS 患者中，5 号染色体的完全或部分缺失引发了肿瘤抑制基因假说，该基因位于 5 号染色体长臂 5q21～5q34 的狭窄区带内。该区域是深入研究的焦点，已经发现了缺失或失调的候选基因，研究范围逐渐缩小。干扰素调节因子-1（IRF-1）是一种 DNA 结合调节因子，通过与启动子结合而部分调控干扰素和干扰素诱导基因的表达。作为激动子，具有抗增殖和拮抗癌基因活性的作用，并可以逆转表型的转化。*IRF-1* 基因就位于 5q31 区域。已发现在伴有 del 5q 的 MDS 或 AML 患者中可出现一个或两个 IRF 等位基因的缺失。体外研究表明，*IRF-1* 基因的缺失与表型转化和/或放化疗诱导的细胞凋亡有关。尽管这些数据提示了 *IRF-1* 基因可能的作用，但尚无研究证实这些观察结果[93,94]。最近的一项研究表明，*IRF-1* 过表达可能导致 Toll 样受体上调，从而激活凋亡途径。由于没有发现疾病相关的明确的肿瘤抑制基因，因此需要其他方法研究潜在机制。Ebert 等用 RNA 干扰（RNAi）来鉴别可能相关的基因。他们发现核糖体亚单位蛋白 *RSP14* 基因功能部分缺失，该基因与 5q-患者的前体细胞向红系分化受阻有关。利用体外 RNAi 技术可以构建 5q-患者的细胞表型。del 5q 患者的细胞中 *RSP14* 基因过表达能够纠正表型并恢复正常的红系造血，提示该基因与 del 5q-患者造血相关。*RSP14* 功能缺失导致 18s 前体 rRNA 的加工减少。这与先天性骨髓衰竭 Diamond-Blackfan 贫血的发病机制类似[82]。

据报道，8%的 MDS 患者存在 *TP53* 抑癌基因的点突变[95]。在一项研究发现，继发性 MDS（sMDS）或治疗相关 AML（tAML）患者白血病细胞 *TP53* 基因突变率高于预期，但不包括生殖组织。在之后的随访中发现，在转化为 AML 时 *TP53* 突变增高[96]。发现微卫星不稳定性，且与突变表型一致，提示这些患者发生治疗相关 MDS/AML 的风险更高。17p-综合征以粒细胞发育异常为特点，中性粒细胞有假性 Pelger-Huët 核异常，胞质内有小空泡。在一项研究中，16 名 17p-患者中有 15 名存在 *TP53* 相关的缺失，提示肿瘤抑制基因的缺失可能对 17p-综合征的形态学、细胞遗传学和分子表型有影响。最近发现部分 MDS 患者中存在其他几种基因的表达失调，包括 *E Ⅵ-1*、*c-mpl*、*PDGF*、*MLL* 和 *CSF-1* 受体[97]。位于 3 号染色体的 *E Ⅵ-1* 基因在髓系和红系分化中发挥作用。基因表达失调与骨髓系和红系成熟受阻有关[97]。

V617F JAK2 突变见于 MPD、真性红细胞增多症、骨髓纤维化和原发性血小板增多症的患者。少部分 MDS 患者也带有此突变。这些患者通常血小板计数增高，可能出现铁粒幼细胞性贫血。有些人将这部分患者称为 RARS-T 亚型（T＝血小板增多）。

临床和实验室特征

MDS 患者的临床和实验室特征主要是由多功能造血干细胞的缺陷决定的。MDS 主要发生于 60 岁以上的成人，儿童和青少年偶有发生。大多数报告中，中位年龄在 65 岁以上，以男性为主。临床表现无特异性。症状主要与细胞减少有关，贫血所致症状最常见。贫血症状包括疲劳、虚弱、面色苍白、呼吸困难、心绞痛和心力衰竭。其他少见的症状和体征有容易擦伤、瘀斑、鼻出血、牙龈出血、瘀点和细菌感染，尤其是呼吸道和皮肤的感染。查体无特异性体征。据报道 10%～40%的患者出现肝脏和/或脾脏肿大，最常见于 CMML。淋巴结肿大和皮肤浸润并不常见。有报道称非治疗相关 MDS 与其他肿瘤有关，包括淋巴增殖性疾病、浆细胞疾病及上皮来源的肿瘤。

血液学特点包括外周血一系或多系血细胞减少，与病态造血和功能异常有关，详见表 113-6。多数患者骨髓增生活跃，部分或全部前体细胞有病态造血。红细胞酶、表面抗原、血红蛋白合成和铁代谢的异常都有报道。部分酶活性的改变会影响红细胞的生存，例如丙酮酸激酶。转移酶 A 和 H 以及半乳糖基转移酶活性异常将导致血型的改变。血红蛋白的合成受胎儿血红蛋白（HbF）增加、珠蛋白链合成异常和铁代谢异常的影响。

表 113-6 MDS 细胞形态和功能的异常

红细胞
形态
红细胞大小不一
异形红细胞
椭圆形大红细胞
小红细胞
嗜碱性点彩
Howell-Jolly 小体
外周血出现有核红细胞
巨幼样变
多核前体细胞
核出芽
核破裂
血红蛋白合成异常
环形铁粒幼细胞
可染铁增多
酶学
己糖激酶增高
丙酮酸激酶减少
2,3-二磷酸甘油酸变位酶减少
磷酸果糖激酶减少
腺苷脱氨酶增高
丙酮酸激酶增高
血型抗原表达降低或缺失
胎儿血红蛋白增加
珠蛋白链合成异常
铁代谢异常
白细胞
形态
假性 Pelger-Huët 细胞

续表

异常染色质凝集
异常核间桥
单核细胞增多
颗粒形成缺陷(颗粒减少)
巨幼样变
Auer 小体
LAP 升高
髓过氧化物酶减少
胞壁酸酶减少(CMML)
颗粒膜糖蛋白缺失
表面抗原不适宜表达
系别特异性缺失
黏附降低
趋化缺陷
吞噬缺陷
吞噬作用降低
巨核细胞
形态
小巨核细胞
核分叶减少
大单圆核巨核细胞
外周血出现巨核细胞碎片
巨血小板
血小板聚集缺陷
血栓素 A2 缺乏
Bernard-Soulier 样缺陷
免疫缺陷
T 细胞 IL-2 受体减少
IL-2 分泌减少
NK 细胞活性降低
NK 细胞对 γ 干扰素反应降低
对丝裂霉素反应降低
T4 细胞减少
免疫球蛋白异常
自身抗体
自身免疫现象
自我识别功能受损

髓系通常表现为白细胞减少,幼稚细胞增多,大型不染色细胞(large unstained cell,LUC)增加。相较 RA 和 RARS 患者,RAEB 和 RAEB-T 患者中性粒细胞减少更常见[27]。白细胞增多常见于 CMML,根据定义,诊断时要求单核细胞绝对计数增多(>1×10^9/L)。单核细胞增多也见于其他 MDS 亚型。胞质异常导致细胞颗粒形成减少或缺乏,出现 Aure 小体或异常的嗜天青颗粒。组化研究表明,白细胞碱性磷酸酶水平升高或降低,髓过氧化物酶染色减弱,颗粒膜糖蛋白丢失。表面抗原分析显示,系别特异性抗原缺失,不适宜抗原持续表达或表达增加,系别间区别不明显。部分患者的异常抗原持续表达,或者表达这些抗原的细胞比例增高,这些都与白血病转化风险增高和生存缩短有关。单核细胞活化表面表型的异常表达见于所有 FAB 亚型患者,而粒细胞活化表面抗原几乎仅见于幼稚细胞增多的患者。粒细胞功能受损包括呼吸暴发异常、趋化缺陷、超氧化物释放以及中性粒细胞刺激信号的异常[98,99]。核的表型及功能异常见表 113-6。

巨核细胞可减少,常有形态异常(表 113-6)。RAEB 和 RAEB-T 患者更易出现血小板减少、巨核细胞减少、巨核细胞的病态造血更明显。外周血可出现巨核细胞碎片和巨血小板。这些患者的出血症状可能不仅仅是血小板减少造成的,也与血小板功能异常有关。血小板聚集缺陷、血栓素 A2 活性缺乏或 Bernard-Soulier 型血小板缺陷可导致血小板功能异常。后一种缺陷是由血小板膜糖蛋白 GP Ib-IX 复合物缺陷引起的。

少部分患者表现为骨髓增生减低和血细胞减少,形态学上与再生障碍性贫血难以区分[100]。细胞遗传学分析联合或不联合间期 FISH 有助于 MDS 的诊断。

MDS 与免疫系统异常的关系特别令人感兴趣,因为曾经报道过很多免疫方面的异常。T 细胞白介素-2(IL-2)受体数量和 IL-2 的分泌量都减少。后者部分是由于免疫调节 B 细胞衰竭导致的。NK 细胞活性和对 α 干扰素的反应性降低,α 干扰素分泌减少,而 NK 细胞的总数变化很大。T 细胞数量减少,对有丝分裂原刺激的反应性降低,总细胞数减少,T4/T8 细胞比例下降。后者主要是由 T4 细胞总数减少所致。

免疫球蛋白异常较常见,表现为出现自身抗体或直接库姆斯试验(Coombs test)阳性。MDS 与免疫紊乱的关系还不清楚。患者的免疫系统失调很普遍。与此一致的是 MDS 患者存在自身反应性 IgM 和 IgG,提示自我识别机制存在异常。目前尚不清楚一些异常是否部分与红细胞输注有关,经有效治疗是否可逆。如果多能干细胞多向分化的潜能存在缺陷,T 细胞和 B 细胞的失调就不足为奇了。

诊断的建立

在大多数患者中,通过标准化检查可以很容易确立诊断,这些检查包括病史和体检、全血计数和外周血涂片镜检。血细胞减少应该除外生化、维生素缺乏、出血、毒素/药物或感染原因,然后进行骨髓穿刺和活检。此外必须进行常规细胞遗传学检查。MDS 的诊断首先要根据形态学标准,外周血及骨髓前体细胞有明确的形态异常特征(表 113-6)。虽然部分分类系统包含了细胞遗传学信息(IPSS、IPSS-R 和 WHO),但主要还是依赖骨髓和外周血的形态。用流式细胞术进行骨髓细胞群分析已经成为急性白血病患者诊断和分型的标准,它也更常规地应用于 MDS 的诊断。可以发现异常细胞群和偏移的抗原表达。然而,目前尚未进行骨髓形态学与流式细胞术结果的对比研究,单独使用流式细胞检测结果建立 MDS 的诊断和分类并不可靠。根据 FAB、IPSS、IPSS-R 或 WHO 标准进行精确的分类时,必须或至少部分地以骨髓形态学为基础。因此,流式细胞分析应被视为一个补充检查,但不足以建立诊断和分类。高达 70% 的患者细胞遗传学存在异常,这些异常虽然不足以诊断,但可能提示诊断。骨髓疾病中常见突变基因的基因突变分析正在商业化,可用于支持MDS的诊断。然而,非血液恶性肿瘤的普通患者中可发现基因突变,该突变的意义尚不确定[101]。因此,仅靠基因突变是不足以建立诊断的。

诊断的难点

部分MDS患者也可表现出MPN的特征,也就是"重叠综合征"[102]。在这些患者中,血细胞减少可与白细胞或血小板的增多同时存在。部分患者中,白细胞计数的升高可能同时伴有单核细胞增多。根据现有的分类系统,一部分患者可以明确诊断为MPN,而另一部分患者仍然归类为MDS,主要取决于分类系统中设定的白细胞的上限。还有一些患者有骨髓纤维化,伴或不伴明显脾脏肿大和外周血细胞减少,如果有病态造血特征,也提示MDS。这些患者的分类就更困难。有骨髓纤维化、脾脏明显肿大、外周血涂片提示典型的红白血病样改变的患者更容易被归入骨髓纤维化伴髓样化生,而没有明显脾脏肿大和/或外周血出现红白血病样改变的患者就有可能被考虑为MDS伴骨髓纤维化。除了RARS-T患者外,存在*JAK2V617F*突变更倾向于诊断为MPN而非MDS。

低增生MDS通常很难与再生障碍性贫血区分,具有很多相同的特点[103,104]。这些患者HLA-DR15的表达增加,并有PNH的表型(CD59的表达降低),无论是MDS还是再生障碍性贫血都对免疫调节治疗有反应。如果存在MDS中常见的染色体异常等细胞遗传学异常,可支持MDS的诊断,但不能完全除外再生障碍性贫血。在这些患者中,在没有其他标准的情况下,治疗方案可能决定着诊断方向。

最后,还有一部分患者表现为严重全血细胞减少,但骨髓检查没有阳性发现(没有任何病态造血表现,没有髓系原始细胞增高),也没有任何细胞遗传学异常。这些患者中的一部分可能有MDS,只有持续的观察与检测才能明确诊断。基因突变也可能提示MDS。其他患者可能有骨髓损伤接触史(毒素、感染因素等),但可能永远不会被发现,血细胞可以在数月或数年后最终完全或部分恢复。后面这种情况,如果没有明确的诊断依据,就应耐心观察,支持治疗(supportive care,SC)通常是确诊前最合适的治疗选择。这些患者还应该考虑免疫介导的造血干细胞损伤。鉴别诊断还应包括大颗粒淋巴细胞(large granular lymphocytic,LGL)白血病,T细胞受体、免疫球蛋白基因重排以及T细胞亚群可能能提供信息[105]。

发病机制及与白血病转化的关系

影响多能干细胞的病变的发生发展可能与多种因素有关,包括化学损伤、射线或感染,都可以造成基因表达的改变。由于大多数患者都在50~80岁,细胞衰老可能也起了作用。一旦发生畸变,经过多个致癌步骤造成克隆损伤,导致40%患者向急性白血病转化。疾病的进展很可能需要多个事件的发生,最终出现优势的细胞克隆[106,107]。根据对大量已经发生的病变的认识,可以推测这些导致发病的事件之间的可能的关系。*ras*癌基因的突变可以发生疾病发展的早期,也可以发生在晚期,可能参与肿瘤发生的某一过程。在*ras*突变的一个模型中发现,*ras*突变导致生长和分化异常,对促红细胞生成素反应发生异常,凋亡增加,这些都与体内表型的反应相似。这些突变可能造成了突变后细胞的生长优势,导致侵袭性增殖。作为迟发事件,选择性生长优势足以触发白血病转化。但是,如果在早期发生*ras*基因改变,就不足以触发疾病进一步进展,还需要其他因素的辅助,例如伴随染色体异常和基因失调。随着识别更多涉及不同途径的体细胞突变,包括涉及表观遗传调控、信号、转录因子和RNA的剪接,表明发病机制更为复杂。能够研究这些突变作用的模型将是至关重要的[108]。

造血前体细胞的异常反应提示存在潜在的信号转导异常。细胞因子受体的突变可以导致信号静默或过表达。已经发现FLT3和G-CSF受体突变与MDS患者的AML转化有关。但多数研究都没有发现细胞因子受体的异常,这提示在配体-受体反应的下游也存在异常[109,110]。骨髓细胞凋亡增加,TNF-α和TGF-β明显失调,进一步提示细胞因子失调。在没有专有存活因子存在时,对细胞因子信号反应异常的造血前体细胞加速细胞凋亡。如果发生能够触发增殖优势和AML转化的基因的或生长调节的其他改变,那么这类表型就会占优势。在患有严重先天性中性粒细胞减少的患者中,进展到MDS或急性白血病时通常伴有获得性G-CSF受体的突变[111]。G-CSF受体基因的点突变导致受体胞质区的C端断裂。受损细胞就不能在G-CSF作用下成熟为粒细胞。在大鼠模型中,G-CSF受体突变导致G-CSF受体反应性前体细胞的增殖。用G-CSF治疗可以增加中性粒细胞,转录因子激活增加,由于内化异常,细胞表面的表达时间延长。克隆扩增中发生的更多的基因突变造成白血病发生。

79%的MDS患者有核型异常,晚期更常见。这提示,从多能干细胞分化下来的克隆更容易发现核型异常,骨髓原始细胞增多的患者核型异常的发生率更高。在部分研究中,复杂核型的白血病转化风险更高也提示这些异常能造成克隆的优势生长,也反映了基因不稳定性。这种不稳定性表现为获得附加染色体异常的克隆演变,也与疾病进展、恶性转化或直接转为AML有关。最后,多数核型异常与染色体全部或部分缺失有关,提示基因缺失也许在发病机制中起作用。5号染色体长臂的关键区域q13-q34区域,含有编码大量重要蛋白的基因,包括*GM-CSF*、*IL-3*、*IL-4*、*IL-5*、*CSF-1*和癌基因*cfms*(编码CSF-1受体)。这一关键区域的变化导致产生异常基因产物或发生点突变。染色体的缺失导致本来可以表达的等位基因突变而造成半合子细胞,或造成抑癌基因的缺失。MDS患者常见的染色体缺失包括1q-、5q-、17p-和3p-,这些缺失区域可能包含抑癌基因,这些基因的缺失可能在转化过程中起作用。

细胞周期的失调可能与白血病转化有关。在MDS患者的研究中发现,超过50%的患者的周期素依赖的激酶抑制因子(CDKI)基因p15INK4B的CpG岛甲基化异常。与低危MDS相比,高危MDS患者甲基化的频率更高。另外,在疾病进展时甲基化更明显。

治疗

多年来,由于患者的年龄偏大、常继发骨髓衰竭、合并症多,而且缺乏有效的治疗手段,MDS 患者的处理是令人失望和棘手的。主要的治疗是支持治疗(SC),包括输血和抗感染来减轻症状,但对疾病的最终结果没有影响。治疗效果受疾病的异质性影响,每个患者的预后都不同。其他混杂因素包括缺乏大宗的随机研究,也没有统一的疗效标准,这都造成治疗结果很难解释。近 10 年来,MDS 的治疗引起了更多人的兴趣,出现了新的有效治疗药物。

分化诱导剂和新作用机制的药物

自从 Charlotte Friend 等首次证实二甲基亚砜(DMSO)能在体外诱导小鼠红白血病细胞分化并改变恶性表型以后,人们就对分化治疗抗肿瘤的模式产生了极大的兴趣[112]。虽然已经在体外观察到了这种现象,但在临床上获得证实非常困难。有些药物能在体外有效诱导分化,但在 MDS 治疗中没有获得成功[例如顺式和反式维 A 酸、维生素 D_3、酪酸盐和六亚甲基二乙酰胺(HMBA)]。

低甲基化药物(HMA)阿扎胞苷(AzaC)已经产生了良好的疗效(表 113-7)[113~116]。基因启动子区域的失表达通常与 CpG 岛的过多甲基化有关。异常的获得性甲基化改变或表观遗传学事件影响基因间区和内含子区,导致基因静默,对细胞周期和分化过程中的基因调控有重要影响。Christman、Acs、Talyor 和 Jones 等建立了一种生化模式对 AzaC 的分化诱导作用进行解释:AzaC 通过影响 DNA 甲基化而诱导分化[117~119]。AzaC 一旦与 DNA 结合,可以与 DNA 甲基转移酶共价结合,这种酶在哺乳动物细胞内负责新合成 DNA 的甲基化。结合后导致结合点的 DNA 远端去甲基化,原来甲基化的静默基因可以转录。在 β 珠蛋白生成障碍性贫血患者中[120],用 AzaC 治疗可以增加胎儿血红蛋白合成,而这与 γ 球蛋白基因区域的去甲基化有关。根据这个模型,癌症白血病协助组 B(CALGB)进行了两项 AzaC 治疗 MDS 的疗效观察,结果显示,高危 MDS 患者的反应率为 50%[115,121]。据此 CALGB 进行了比较 AzaC 与 SC 疗效的Ⅲ期试验。根据试验设计,SC 组的患者在最少观察 4 个月后,有疾病进展的患者可以交叉进入治疗组。AzaC 组反应率达 60%(7%CR、16%PR、37%改善),而 SC 组只有 5%(改善)($P<0.0001$)。AzaC 组的白血病转化或死亡的中位时间明显延迟(21 个月 vs SC 组 13 个月,$P=0.007$)。AzaC 组的首次 AML 转化事件的概率(15%)低于 SC 组[116]($P=0.001$)。通过几种检查方法,AzaC 组患者的生活质量(quality of life,QOL)都明显优于对照组。他们的生活质量随之显著提高。随着时间的推移,AzaC 组患者在疲劳、生理功能、呼吸困难、心理压力和积极情绪方面的改善明显大于 SC 组。交叉进入 AzaC 治疗组的患者,在疲劳、生理功能、呼吸困难和总体健康方面有显著改善[122]。AzaC 组和 SC 组的中位生存期(不管交叉情况如何,均通过意向性治疗进行分析)分别为 20 个月和 14 个月($P=0.1$)。AzaC 组 24 个月生存率为 41%,sc 组为 25%($P=0.03$)。为了消除 49 名交叉患者在生存分析中的混杂效应,进行了 3 个亚组的 6 个月生存节点比较分析。这些亚组包括从未交叉或仅在 6 个月后交叉的 SC 患者,6 个月内交叉的 SC 患者,以及最初随机分成的 AzaC 组。节点分析前死亡的 36 名患者已被剔除。这三组的额外中位生存期(在 6 个月节点之后)分别为 11、14 和 18 个月。AzaC 组与晚交叉或未交叉的 SC 亚组相比有显著性差异($P=0.03$)。早期交叉的 SC 亚组(第 2 亚组)患者的中位生存时间高于晚交叉或从未交叉的患者(第 1 亚组),但差异没有统计学意义($P=0.11$)。结果表明,与 SC 组相比,AzaC 治疗组患者有更高的缓解率,生活质量提高、进展时间延迟,提高了 24 个月生存率,延迟白血病转化或死亡时间,以及显著降低转化为 AML 的风险。在交叉接受 AzaC 治疗时,根据相同的系列随访对相同的个体进行生活质量评估,他们的生活质量显著提高。与 SC 组患者相比,AzaC 组患者在疲劳(EORTC,$P=0.001$)、生理功能(EORTC,$P=0.002$)、呼吸困难(EORTC,$P=0.0014$)、心理压力(MHI,$P=0.015$)和积极情绪(MHI,$P=0.0077$)等方面都有明显的改善。治疗后红细胞输注的差异持续存在。交叉之前 SC 组的生活质量是稳定或者日益恶化的。交叉到 AzaC 组后,患者在疲劳(EORTC,$P=0.0001$)、生理功能(EORTC,$P=0.004$)、呼吸困难(EORTC,$P=0.0002$)和总体状态(MHI,$P=0.016$)方面都得到了改善。详细的分析表明,安慰剂或 Hawthorne 效应不能解释 AzaC 对 QOL 的改善。其他研究也证实,AzaC 使 45%的患者脱离输血,对符合 WHO AML 分类(原始细胞>20%)的患者也有效,中位生存达 19.3 个月,提示这类患者也能潜在获益[123]。因此,AzaC 是除了异基因骨髓移植(bone marrow transplantation,BMT)外唯一能改变 MDS 自然病程的有效药物。而且,AzaC 没有骨髓移植那样存在年龄限制。第二个随机对照试验也确证了,并在扩大观察范围后发现,与传统治疗方案(医师指导下选择最佳 SC、低剂量阿糖胞苷或蒽环类药物联合阿糖胞苷的诱导化疗)组相比,AzaC 治疗组患者有明显的生存优势,AzaC 治疗组的中位总生存期(OS)为 24.4 个月,而传统治疗组只有 15 个月[18]。AzaC 治疗组在进展到 AML 或死亡的时间明显延迟。AzaC 治疗组中 45%的患者脱离输血,需要静脉应用抗生素的感染的发生率下降了 33%。所有 AzaC 研究结果一致发现,初始反应时间较慢,需要每月重复的周期用药才能看到反应,中位反应时间为三个周期。其他分析提示 AzaC 维持治疗也可获益[124]。

AzaC 通过多种机制发挥作用。它可以作为细胞毒药物,但体外实验数据显示,它还可以作为生物反应调节剂影响细胞因子的信号转导途径而发挥作用[125]。另一个去甲基化药物地西他滨(2-deoxy-5-AzaC)也被评估试验[126~129]。虽然疗效反应标准不同,地西他滨与 AzaC 一样都有疗效。在北美进行的一项地西他滨与 SC 随机对照研究中,地西他滨的缓解率优于 SC,CR+PR 达 17%,而 SC 组为 0。但次要研究终点——进展至 AML 或死亡时间方面,两组之间没有差异[129]。在欧洲 EORTC 进行的第二个地西他滨和 SC 治疗中危-2 或高危组患者的随机试验中,在进展到 AML 或死亡以及生存时间方面,两组之间都没有差异[126]。采用一种改良方案($20mg/(m^2 \cdot d) \times 5d$,每 4 周一次)后,治疗缓解率相当,但骨髓抑制减轻[130,131]。但这不是对照试验,对疾病结局的影响还不能肯定[132]。

表 113-7　MDS 患者中的随机对照研究：药物对比支持治疗(SC)±安慰剂

药物	治疗反应	生活质量	AML 转化率	进展时间	转化 AML 或死亡的时间	24 个月的生存
顺式维 A 酸	NSSD	—	—	—	—	NSSD
小剂量阿糖胞苷	阿糖胞苷	—	NSSD	NSSD	NSSD	NSSD
G-CSF	G-CSF	—	NSSD	NSSD	SC[a]	SC[a]
GM-CSF	GM-CSF	—	NSSD	—	—	NSSD
阿扎胞苷	阿扎胞苷[b]	阿扎胞苷[c]	阿扎胞苷[b]	阿扎胞苷[d]	阿扎胞苷[e]	阿扎胞苷[f]
地西他滨	地西他滨	地西他滨	NSSD	NSSD	NSSD	NR

[a] RAEB 患者有差异。对 RAEB-T 患者，在 G-CSF 和 SC 之间 NSSD。
[b] $P<0.001$。
[c] 疲劳($P=0.001$)；体力($P=0.002$)；呼吸困难($P=0.0014$)；精神健康指数($P=0.0077$)。
[d] $P<0.0001$。
[e] $P=0.004$。
[f] $P=0.03$。
NSSD，在试验药物和安慰剂或支持治疗(SC)之间没有统计学差异；-，试验中终点未评价；NR，没有报道。

表观遗传组合

单剂 HMA 对半数接受治疗的患者有反应但是不能治愈。人们已探索用去甲基化药物 HMA 和多种组蛋白去乙酰化酶抑制剂(HDAC)进行表观遗传学联合治疗的方法[132]。在体外研究，联合 HMA 和 HDAC 有协同作用，使表观遗传学沉默基因重新表达。该作用依赖于序贯用药，需要在 HDAC 之前施用 HMA 以观察作用，且该观察引领一系列联合转化试验。在一项随机试验中，比较了 AzaC 联合恩替诺特组与单药 AzaC 组，结果示联合治疗组与单用 AzaC 治疗组在缓解或总生存方面没有差异。对两组患者甲基化差异的分析表明，联合治疗组和单药治疗组之间存在负相互作用，联合治疗组的低甲基化程度降低[133]。在 AzaC 与伏林司他(vorinostat)联合应用的Ⅰ-Ⅱ期研究表明，AzaC($75mg/(m^2 \cdot d)$，第 1～第 7 日)联合伏林司他(200mg，每日两次，第 3～第 9 日)的队列中，缓解率高达 75%，并且进展至 AML 或死亡的时间及总生存均增加[134]。很多联合治疗组患者在研究过程中出现与胃肠道毒性相关的恶心、呕吐及疲劳。这些毒性可以被一些患者耐受，但可能会阻碍患者的长期耐受性，并可能导致患者无法维持治疗以获得完整的疗效。AzaC 联合 mocetinostat 也显示阳性的临床反应；然而，因出现心包炎症而此研究被停止。

信号抑制剂：多激酶抑制剂

rigosertib 是一种具有多激酶抑制活性的 ras 模拟分子。它是一种 PI3 激酶/Akt 途径的广泛抑制剂，已单独或联合应用于 MDS 研究中[135]。rigosertib 单药应用时，在大多数 HMA 治疗失败的患者中，其静脉注射能改善外周血计数和降低骨髓幼稚细胞百分比[135]。在一项随机三期研究中，患者被随机分为 rigosertib 或 BSC 治疗组(可能包括小剂量阿糖胞苷)，OS 是 HMA 治疗失败患者的主要终点。研究中的趋势提示 rigosertib 效果更好，8.2 个月对 5.9 个月[$P=0.33$，$HR=0.87$(95% CI：0.67～1.14)]。虽然该试验未达到主要终点，但有几个亚组证明了生存获益[136]。rigosertib 正在一项新的Ⅲ期研究中进行试验。rigosertib 与 AzaC 联合治疗的体外研究也在进行中。体外研究表明，两种药物之间存在协同作用，可以促进细胞凋亡。联合用药的Ⅰ期研究的数据显示，该方案耐受性良好，并在 MDS 和 AML 患者中产生效果，包括那些之前使用 HMA 治疗失败的患者[137]。

在体外试验中，维 A 酸及其衍生物是很有效的分化诱导剂，但在几个临床试验中的疗效很差，令人失望[138]。

抗 TNF 和 IMID 免疫调节剂

由于在 MDS 发病机制中观察到 TNF 发挥了作用(见前文“信号转导”部分)，所以在一些小型探索研究中进行了 TNF 的疗效观察。依那西普是一种抗 TNF 的融合蛋白，在一项试验中发现，在 30%的患者中观察到红系有反应，而其他系细胞的反应很低[139]。沙利度胺(thalidomide)具有抗 TNF 活性，但也可以用它对血管内皮生长因子(VEGF)的影响来解释，主要对红系有影响，反应率在 10%～19%[140]。嗜睡和神经病变导致患者停药。来那度胺(lenalidomide)是沙利度胺的类似物，但没有嗜睡或神经病变的副作用，在体外的抗 TNF 活性和抗 VEGF 活性更强，已经进行了Ⅱ期临床试验。在 148 例有 5q-(单独或伴有其他细胞遗传学异常)的低危和中危-1 组患者中，67%的患者脱离了输血[141]。脱离输血的中位时间为 115 周[141]。这些数据在第二个研究中得到证实，其中 10mg/d 应为初始剂量。随后进行了无 5q-的低危和中危-1 组患者的观察，26%的患者脱离输血，中位时间为 41 周。来那度胺与 AzaC 联合治疗，总有效率为 67%[142]。联合治疗耐受性良好，但需要更多的试验来确定是否优于单独使用两种药物。

在低危的红细胞输注依赖性 MDS 患者中，具有对活化素 2 型受体的配体捕获活性的 TGFβ 超配体家族正在临床开发中。在早期试验中，一些药物如索他特西普(sotatercept)和拉斯帕西普(luspatercept)，能减少一些患者的输血需求，并消除了低输血负担低风险患者输注红细胞的需求[143]。这些药物正在进行进一步的临床试验。

激素

虽然部分再生障碍性贫血患者能从非特异性红系刺激药物治疗中获益，但并未证实雄激素对 MDS 有效。早期的观察结果显示，雄激素治疗会加速疾病的进展，与白血病转化相关，但没有被后续的研究证实,但也没有观察到疗效[144,145]。

糖皮质激素治疗的总反应率在9%~24%,但无效患者的副作用也很明显。

有报告称达那唑能改善 MDS 患者的血小板减少和贫血。对那些存在免疫介导细胞破坏情况的患者,达那唑是有帮助的。

化疗

单独或联合应用化疗药物都被用于治疗 MDS 患者。这些药物用于一系列治疗方案,从长程小剂量方案[99]到常规用于抗白血病的骨髓毒性方案。也被用来治疗所有疾病阶段的患者。抗白血病类治疗并没有改变多数患者的最终结果,而多数患者的毒副作用明显。在一项对化疗诱导与 HMA 比较的回顾性分析中,其趋势表明 HMA 是获益的[15]。

氟达拉滨和阿糖胞苷在药理学上的相互作用可以增加细胞内的 ara-CTP 浓度,多用于治疗复发 AML 患者并有一定疗效。随后,与 G-CSF 联合(FLAG)或不联合(FA)的方案用于治疗 MDS 和初发 AML 患者[146]。这两种方案的完全缓解(complete remission,CR)率相当,分别为 60%和 55%,在原始细胞增多的 MDS 患者中的缓解率更高。在全部患者中(MDS 和 AML),有 27%在诱导阶段死亡。FA 组的预计的中位生存期为 29 周,而 FLAG 组为 39 周,差异没有统计学意义。在有 5 号或 7 号染色体缺失的患者中,FLAG 方案的缓解率为 64%,而 FA 组只有 36%。但作者将缓解率的差异归功于其他因素,而与治疗无关。加用 G-CSF 与中性粒细胞恢复加速有关,但这并不能降低感染率或感染相关死亡。总体而言,MDS 患者的治疗结果与 AML 相比没有差异。

阿糖胞苷已经过广泛的检验。在文献综述中有报道称,170 名患者应用低剂量阿糖胞苷后,CR 为 16%[147,148]。CR 的中位持续时间为 10.5 个月,但获得缓解似乎对总生存几乎没有影响。在东部合作肿瘤组(ECOG)和西南肿瘤组(SWOG)进行的一项随机试验中,MDS 患者接受低剂量阿糖胞苷或 SC 治疗。进展的 SC 患者可以交叉接受阿糖胞苷治疗。阿糖胞苷和 SC 组在总生存、进展时间或 AML 转化率方面没有显著差异(表 113-7)。在最近一项随机试验的亚组分析中,与传统治疗方案相比,AzaC 明显优于低剂量阿糖胞苷,显著提高了中危-2 型和高危 MDS 患者的生存[18]。

氯法拉滨在 15~40mg/m^2 的不同剂量下每日静脉注射×5 日,在未接受治疗和 HMA 治疗失败的患者中,有 25%~50%的患者有反应,反应持续时间不同。氯法拉滨在 MDS 治疗中的作用和效果仍有待确定[149]。

总之,早期的研究结果显示,MDS 患者或 MDS 转化的 AML 患者的疗效比初发 AML 患者差。年龄似乎影响了缓解率和缓解持续时间,年轻患者比老年患者更容易获得 CR,缓解的时间也更长。与没有获得 CR 的 MDS 患者相比,获得 CR 的患者的生存提高,但缓解持续时间比获得 CR 的初发 AML 患者短。在转化为 AML 之前进行治疗与缓解率更高有关,从诊断 MDS 到转化为 AML 的间期更短的患者的缓解率也比较高。但采用积极的抗白血病方案治疗与死亡率升高和并发症增加有关,约 30%的患者死于药物相关的并发症。

铁螯合 对于红细胞输血依赖的低危患者来说,铁的积累导致铁过载和血色病导致的最终组织损伤是一个长期的问题。对于已接受了≥25 个单位的输注红细胞或血清铁蛋白>2 000ng/ml 的患者,推荐使用螯合疗法(NCCN 指南 2.2014 版)。使用地拉罗司已被证明可以降低血清铁蛋白和不稳定血浆铁[150]。一些研究表明其对生存有影响,但还没有相关的随机试验,其他因素包括患者选择偏倚也可能起作用。然而,螯合剂应该是红细胞输血依赖性低危患者管理策略的一部分。对于高危患者,螯合剂的作用尚不确定。在患者对初级治疗有血液学反应之前或除非患者对初级治疗有血液学反应,否则在这种患者群体在缺乏有效的应用中螯合剂可能是不合理的。

骨髓移植

异基因和同基因骨髓移植治疗 MDS 患者的小型研究结果显示,35%~40%的患者能够获得长期无病生存[151]。两个大型单中心研究证实了这一结果。在一个大宗病例的研究中,评价了 1981—1996 年中的 251 例患者。Appelbaum 等报道,预计的(Kaplan-Meier)5 年无病生存率(DFS)为 40%。年轻患者、病程较短、女性和初发 MDS 都是 DFS 较好的预后指标。20 岁以下患者的 DFS 为 60%,而 20~50 岁组和大于 50 岁组患者的 DFS 分别为 40%和 20%。低危 MDS 患者的 6 年 DFS 为 55%,而高危 MDS 患者只有 30%[152,153]。这一差异与疾病进展患者的复发率更高有关。在 IPSS 评分为低危和中危-1 组患者中,几乎都没有复发。低危和中危-1 组患者的 5 年 DFS 为 60%,而中危-2 组为 36%,高危组只有 28%。接受配型相合非血缘供者(match unrelated donor,MUD)骨髓移植患者的疗效非常差。在美国骨髓供者计划的结果分析中,在最初 4 年(1986—1990)的登记资料中,接受 MUD 的患者的疗效令人失望,2 年 DFS 只有 18%,2 年的总生存只有 24%。有研究发现原发 MDS 患者的生存优于继发 MDS 患者(56% vs 27%)。

骨髓移植的确切疗效和时机以及最佳预处理方案都还不清楚。近期对低危患者的分析表明,除非有疾病进展的证据,观察等待比立即移植的生存时间长。对高危患者,诊断后尽快进行移植,生存时间更长[154]。这些数据最近针对 60~70 岁的患者进行了更新,移植对于高危患者是有利的,他们的预期寿命有所增加,而非移植方法则更适合于低危患者[155]。对 40 岁及以下的年轻患者,如果有合适的同胞供者,建议进行移植,因为除此之外没有根治的办法。但是哪些 50 岁以下的患者适合移植还没有答案。有年轻的低危 MDS 患者单用 SC 的中位生存期超过 15 年[156]。超过 40 岁的患者进行移植的很少,但这部分用同胞供者进行移植患者的有限资料显示,无病生存率达 30%。考虑到上述结果,无同胞供者患者的移植选择就更为困难。考虑到大多数 MDS 患者的年龄和有合适供者的比例,未来移植的价值可能非常有限,只有 5%~10%的 MDS 患者可以受益[151]。

因为大多数 MDS 患者的年龄较大,全剂量清髓性移植预处理方案的毒性又很大,改用减低剂量预处理方案进行造血干细胞移植的吸引力逐渐增加。这些治疗常采用氟达拉滨为主的预处理方案,耐受性较好,不会完全清除患者的骨髓。形成同胞或非血缘供者和患者的嵌合体。最近的报告证实,这种方法可以用于 60 岁以上的患者,死亡率在 0~21%。83%的患者能够形成嵌合体。与清髓移植相似,缓解和复发的时间取决于 IPSS 分类。因此,这种方法更容易应用到老年患者身上,但还需要进一步的研究证实其治疗的潜在作用[151,155]。

在同种异基因移植之前，AzaC 被认为是异基因移植前的一个桥接，在移植后，也被用于一种维持治疗策略[157,158]。移植前和移植后的治疗都有良好的耐受性，但需要随机试验来评估移植前或移植后的 AzaC 是否对疾病结果产生积极影响。

大剂量化疗加自体骨髓或外周血干细胞移植曾经在小范围内流行。欧洲组报告了 79 例患者采用强化治疗，在第一次 CR 期进行自体骨髓移植。79 例中有 55 例患者明确处于第一次 CR 期，与 110 例初发 AML 患者进行配对比较研究。所有 79 例患者的 2 年生存率为 39%，55 例 MDS/sAML 患者的 2 年 DFS 为 28%，而初发 AML 患者的二年 DFS 为 51%。MDS/sAML 组的复发率为 69%，初发 AML 的复发率为 40%（$P=0.007$）[159,160]。采用 PBSC 注的问题较多，因为只有不到一半的 MDS 患者能够采集到足够的细胞。

生长因子　造血生长因子是控制骨髓干细胞增殖和分化的调节性糖蛋白[161]。有几项研究探讨了在 MDS 中应用 GM-CSF 的疗效[162]。在一项对照研究中，患者被随机分为观察组和 rhGM-CSF 治疗组。与不用细胞因子治疗的观察组相比，治疗组患者的中性粒细胞、嗜酸性粒细胞、单核细胞和淋巴细胞明显升高，而感染率下降。血小板计数、血红蛋白或输血需求在两组间没有差异。骨髓原始细胞大于 15% 的患者白血病转化风险最高，对白血病转化而言这是一个关键数值。

已经评价了非格司亭（G-CSF）的疗效。在随机对照研究中，102 例 RAEB 或 RAEB-T 患者采用 G-CSF 或 SC 治疗[161]。两组在进展到 AML 的时间上没有差异。在 RAEB-T 患者中的生存也没有差异。但在 RAEB 患者中，治疗组患者的生存明显短于对照组，因此试验提前中止。

促红细胞生长素也被用于治疗 MDS，试验组的红细胞反应率为 20%～25%[77,163,164]。疗效仅限于红系。荟萃分析显示，骨髓衰竭加重时疗效降低。血清促红细胞生长素水平低、输血需求少的患者更容易获得疗效。对用 G-CSF 治疗获得疗效的患者进行体外红系造血观察，因此引发了两个促红细胞生长素和 G-CSF 联合治疗的临床试验。治疗反应率在 35%～40%，并可以增强促红细胞生长素的活性。与其他试验结果相似，这些试验中的血清促红细胞生长素水平具有预后价值，血清促红细胞生长素水平高于 500U/L 的患者疗效不佳。在另一个报告中，G-CSF 的增强效应并不持久。在一个 191 例联合治疗的研究中，总反应率为 39%。低危组患者的反应率较高，获得 CR 的患者的缓解时间更长。根据输血需求和血清促红细胞生长素水平制订的治疗策略也许对患者的选择更有指导意义。促红细胞生长素治疗对生存的影响表明不输血对生存有益[78]。

以骨髓增生极度低下和全血细胞重度减少为特点的 MDS 患者的临床表现类似于重症再生障碍性贫血（低增生 MDS），在一项 25 例 MDS 患者用抗胸腺球蛋白治疗的研究中，有 11 例患者获得反应（14 例 RA 中 9 例，6 例 RAEB 中 2 例）[79,80]。主要疗效是脱离输血，25 例患者中有 3 例患者的血常规恢复正常。但骨髓增生程度或病态造血的特点并没有变化。在一项已经完成的试验中，61 例患者进行了治疗，21 例（34%）有反应。在有反应的患者中有 76% 的患者输血需求减少，所有患者中有 25% 的患者输血需求减少。疗效可能部分是由免疫抑制剂减轻了 T 细胞对造血前体细胞的抑制带来的。部分年轻患者有多系细胞减少，红细胞输注依赖时间缩短，HLA-DRB1-15 阳性，这些患者更有可能获得疗效。

临床处理

MDS 患者如何选择治疗方案非常困难（图 113-2）。对 RA 或 RARS、低危或中危-1 患者，预后相对较好，疾病主要表现为无症状贫血，观察和 SC 是主要的选择。对那些需要红细胞输注的患者，这本身就是一个不良的预后因素，无论是否联合 G-CSF，应用促红细胞生长素都是合理的[81]。可考虑在 ESA 治疗失败或患有严重白细胞减少症或血小板减少症的患者中使用来那度胺或 AzaC 治疗。对于那些核型异常的患者（不包括 5q-综合征和预后良好的细胞遗传学风险），预后相对较差。这些患者应该密切随访，并准备进入临床试验，特别是骨髓原始细胞比例增高或外周血有明显的中性粒细胞减少和血小板减少时。对促红细胞生长素（无论是否联合 G-CSF）治疗贫血反应不好或有其他系严重细胞减少的低危组患者，应该考虑 AzaC 的治疗，已经证实 AzaC 对低危组患者治疗有效，能减轻其症状。单药来那度胺或 HMA 可导致 25%（来那度胺）和 50%（AzaC）患者脱离输血。对于进展中的低危患者，如果来那度胺和/或 HMA 治疗失败，并且有相合供体，应考虑采用同种异基因骨髓移植，因为这是迄今为止唯一能实现治愈的疗法[154,155]。

有高危因素的患者（中危-2 或高危；高危和极高危-IPSS-R）预后很差，都应该用 HMA 进行治疗。没有其他高危因素（如异常核型、严重的血小板减少或严重的中性粒细胞减少）的 RAEB-1（原始细胞 5%～10%）患者应该密切观察并判断疾病的稳定程度。有病情进展证据的患者应该立即进行治疗。

较高风险组的患者可以从 AzaC 治疗中受益，AzaC 应该被认为是这些患者的标准一线治疗。AzaC 治疗明确优于 SC，可以诱导缓解，减少输血需要，延长生存期，提高生活质量[116,122]。这种疗法有可能成为治疗标准。这些高危患者也可以参加临床试验。干细胞移植是高危患者治愈疾病的重要治疗策略，如果有合适的供者，且患者的年龄合适并且其危险分层需要，在诊断后进行评估的早期就应该考虑干细胞移植的问题。但是，由于复发率很高，许多中心并不把这些患者作为移植治疗的对象。在移植前达到诱导缓解可能是有效的策略[154,155,165]。

对于已经转化为白血病的患者，可以进行积极的抗白血病化疗，或者考虑对老年患者进行 HMA 治疗。抗白血病化疗的 CR 率在 30%～60%，但与治疗相关的发病率和死亡率较高。大多数患者复发。HMA 已用于这些患者并可提高生存率[166]。低增生 MDS 患者，尤其是年轻患者，可受益于抗胸腺细胞免疫球蛋白，无论是否联合环孢素或其他免疫调节治疗。一线或二线 HMA 治疗方案失败的患者预后不良，应考虑使用试验药物[167]。

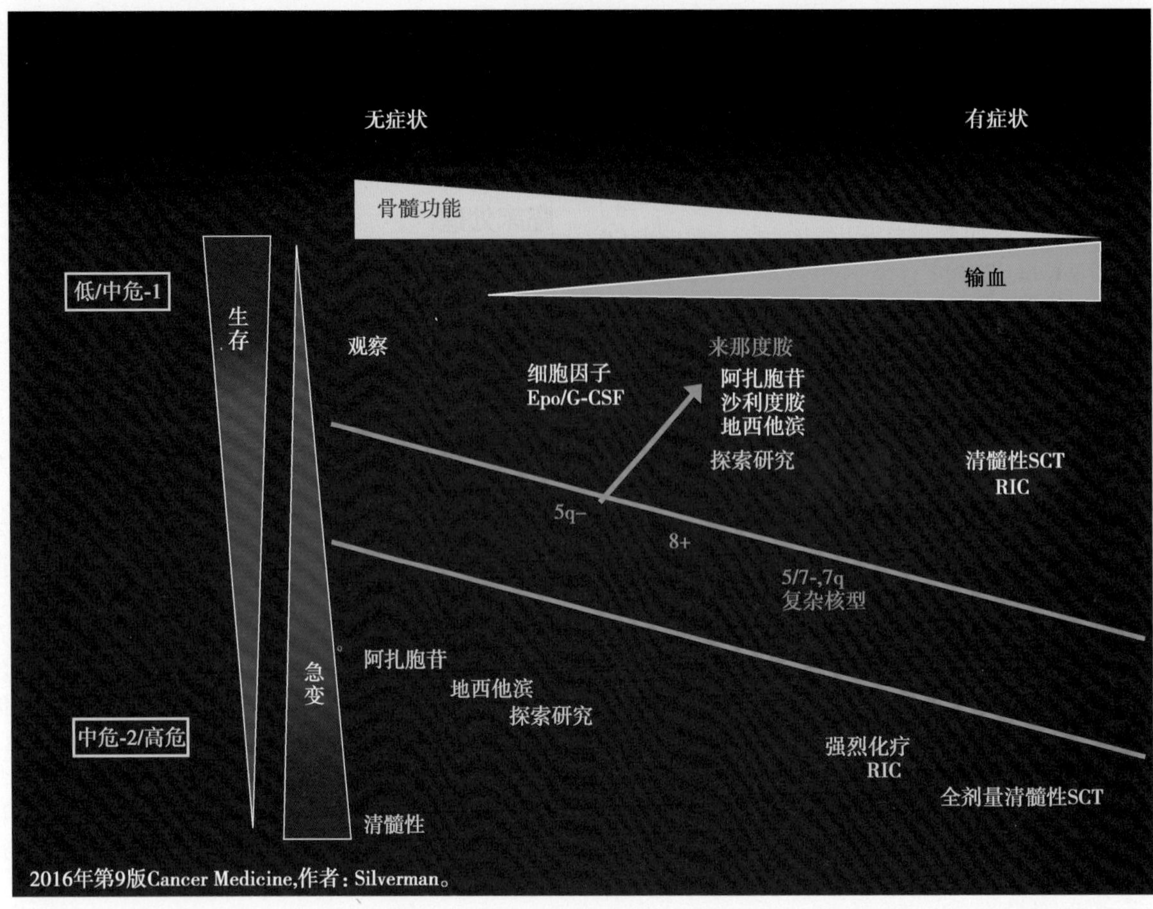

图 113-2 MDS 患者的治疗策略

未来的方向

MDS 治疗与预防的进展依赖于对导致这种疾病的生化和分子缺陷的了解程度。基因突变和表观基因组的鉴定提供的信息有助于个体化治疗的决策。关键是要进行使用明确的生物学终点、设计严谨的临床试验。生存是最终目标，但作为唯一的治疗标准又太宽泛。生活质量评估在检验治疗效果是否获益中是有用的手段。Ⅱ期和Ⅲ期临床试验应该常规包括这些评估指标，在姑息治疗中也同样重要。费用分析也是另一个重要的治疗效益指标。在未来的Ⅲ期临床研究中，也应该涵盖药物经济学内容。

在以细胞成熟与增殖的不平衡逐渐加重为特征的疾病中，诱导分化是有吸引力的治疗方法。在全反式维 A 酸治疗急性早幼粒细胞白血病的过程中已经证实了诱导分化是非常有效的策略。AzaC 可能作为一种生物反应调节剂，作用于表观基因组和基因信号的传导，而发挥部分作用，与 HDAC 等其他药物合用更有优势[132]。干扰或阻断异常信号转导的药物（如酪氨酸和多激酶抑制剂）可能有效[135]。能刺激自体或异基因 T 细胞的肿瘤疫苗及免疫调节策略的应用，将和 PD-1/PDL-1 检测点抑制剂一样成为未来探索的热点。

（白元松 顾桂颖 朱镇星 译 白元松 顾桂颖 朱镇星 赵亚男 顾柱颖 校）

参考文献

The complete reference list can be found on the Wiley Companion Digital Edition of this title (see inside front cover for login instructions).

3 Bomford PR, Rhoads CP. Refractory anaemia. I. Clinical and pathological aspects. *Q J Med*. 1941;**10**:175.

4 Block M, Jacobson LO, Bethard WF. Preleukemic acute human leukemia. *J Am Med Assoc*. 1953;**152**:1018.

6 Bennett JM, Catovsky D, Daniel MT, et al. Proposals for the classification of the acute leukaemias. French-American-British (FAB) co-operative group. *Br J Haematol*. 1976;**33**:451–458.

7 Aul C, Gattermann N, Schneider W. Age-related incidence and other epidemiological aspects of myelodysplastic syndrome. *Br J Haematol*. 1992;**82**:358.

10 Bennett JM, Catovsky D, Daniel M-T, et al. Proposed revised criteria for the classification of acute myeloid leukemia. A Report of the French-American-British Cooperative Group. *Ann Intern Med*. 1985;**103**:620–625.

16 Greenberg PL, Tuechler H, Schanz J, et al. Revised international prognostic scoring system for myelodysplastic syndromes. *Blood*. 2012;**120(12)**:2454–2465.

17 Harris N, Jaffe E, Diehold J, et al. World Health Organization classification of neoplastic diseases of the hematopoietic and lymphoid tissues: report of the Clinical Advisory Committee Meeting — Airlie House, Virginia, November 1997. *J Clin Oncol*. 1999;**17**:3835–3849.

21 Kamada N, Uchins H. Preleukemic states in atomic bomb survivors. *Blood Cells*. 1976;**2**:57.

25 Farrow A, Jacobs A, West RR. Myelodysplasia, chemical exposure, and other environmental factors. *Leukemia*. 1989;**3**:33.

30 Kantarjian HM, Keating MJ. Therapy-related leukemia and myelodysplastic syndrome. *Semin Oncol*. 1987;**14**:435.

35 Berk PD, Goldberg JD, Silverstein MN, et al. Increased incidence of acute leukemia in polycythemia vera associated with chlorambucil therapy. *N Engl J Med*. 1981;**304**:441.

116 Silverman LR, Demakos EP, Peterson BL, et al. Randomized controlled trial of azacitidine in patients with the myelodysplastic syndrome: a study of the cancer

and leukemia group B. *J Clin Oncol.* 2002;**20**:2429–2440.

122 Kornblith AB, Herndon JE 2nd, Silverman LR, et al. Impact of azacytidine on the quality of life of patients with myelodysplastic syndrome treated in a randomized phase III trial: a Cancer and Leukemia Group B study. *J Clin Oncol.* 2002;**20**:2441–2452.

123 Silverman LR, McKenzie DR, Peterson BL, et al. Further analysis of trials with azacitidine in patients with myelodysplastic syndrome: studies 8421, 8921, and 9221 by the Cancer and Leukemia Group B. *J Clin Oncol.* 2006;**24**:3895–3903.

124 Silverman LR, Fenaux P, Mufti GJ, et al. Continued azacitidine therapy beyond time of first response improves quality of response in patients with higher-risk myelodysplastic syndromes. *Cancer.* 2011;**117**:2697–2702.

126 Lübbert M, Suciu S, Baila L, et al. Low-dose decitabine versus best supportive care in elderly patients with intermediate- or high-risk myelodysplastic syndrome (MDS) ineligible for intensive chemotherapy: final results of the randomized Phase III Study of the European Organisation for Research and Treatment of Cancer Leukemia Group and the German MDS Study Group. *J Clin Oncol.* 2011;**29**:1987–1996.

127 Wijermans P, Lubbert M, Verhoef G, et al. Low-dose 5-aza-2′-deoxycytidine, a DNA hypomethylating agent, for the treatment of high-risk myelodysplastic syndrome: a multicenter phase II study in elderly patients. *J Clin Oncol.* 2000;**18**:956–962.

130 Kantarjian H, Oki Y, Garcia-Manero G, et al. Results of a randomized study of 3 schedules of low-dose decitabine in higher-risk myelodysplastic syndrome and chronic myelomonocytic leukemia. *Blood.* 2007;**109**:52–57.

131 Steensma DP, Baer MR, Slack JL, et al. Multicenter study of decitabine administered daily for 5 days every 4 weeks to adults with myelodysplastic syndromes: the alternative dosing for outpatient treatment (ADOPT) trial. *J Clin Oncol.* 2009;**27**:3842–3848.

132 Navada SC, Steinmann J, Lubbert M, et al. Clinical development of demethylating agents in hematology. *J Clin Invest.* 2014;**124**:40–46.

133 Prebet T, Sun Z, Figueroa ME, et al. Prolonged administration of azacitidine with or without entinostat for myelodysplastic syndrome and acute myeloid leukemia with myelodysplasia-related changes: results of the US Leukemia Intergroup Trial E1905. *J Clin Oncol.* 2014;**32**:1242–1248.

134 Silverman LR, Verma A, Odchimar-Reissig R, et al. A phase II trial of epigenetic modulators vorinostat in combination with azacitidine (azac) in patients with the myelodysplastic syndrome (MDS): initial results of study 6898 of the New York Cancer Consortium. *Blood.* 2013;**122(21)**:386.

135 Silverman LR, Greenberg P, Raza A, et al. Clinical activity and safety of the dual pathway inhibitor rigosertib for higher risk myelodysplastic syndromes following DNA methyltransferase inhibitor therapy. *Hematol Oncol.* 2015;**33(2)**:57–66.

136 Garcia-Manero G, Fenaux P, Al-Kali A, et al. Overall survival and subgroup analysis from a randomized phase III study of intravenous rigosertib versus best supportive care (BSC) in patients (pts) with higher-risk myelodysplastic syndrome (HR-MDS) after failure of hypomethylating agents (HMAs). *Blood.* 2014;**163**: abstract.

137 Navada SC, Garcia-Manero G, Wilhelm F, et al. A phase I/II study of the combination of oral rigosertib and azacitidine in patients with myelodysplastic syndrome (MDS) or acute myeloid leukemia (AML). *Blood.* 2014;**124**: abstract 3252.

166 Kantarjian HM, Thomas XG, Dmoszynska A, et al. Multicenter, randomized, open-label, phase iii trial of decitabine versus patient choice, with physician advice, of either supportive care or low-dose cytarabine for the treatment of older patients with newly diagnosed acute myeloid leukemia. *J Clin Oncol.* 2012;**30**:2670–2677.

167 Prébet T, Gore SD, Esterni B, et al. Outcome of high-risk myelodysplastic syndrome after azacitidine treatment failure. *J Clin Oncol.* 2011;**29**:3322–3327.

第 114 章　成人急性髓细胞性白血病：肥大细胞白血病和其他肥大细胞肿瘤

Richard M. Stone, MD ■ Charles A. Schiffer, MD

概述

急性髓细胞性白血病（acute myeloid leukemia, AML）是成人急性白血病中最常见的类型，约占 20 岁以上急性白血病的 80%左右。随着输血医学、感染治疗的进步、强效止吐药的发展、化疗方法的改进以及更安全的同种异体移植的增多，至少在年轻患者中改善了白血病的预后。而且，对病理生理学，特别是基因组学领域更深入的理解，AML 患者可以采取毒性低、个体化和更有效的治疗方法。目前，大约 80%的年轻（年龄<60 岁）成人和 30%～50%的老年患者能够达到完全缓解（complete remission, CR），CR 定义为骨髓形态学正常，中性粒细胞和血小板计数正常，无髓外病变证据。患者年龄和其他生物学因素不同，CR 比例也不同，CR 患者中有 10%～70%可能实现长期生存，其中大多数患者存在治愈可能。然而，大多数 AML 本质上是一种耐药性疾病，老年患者的预后几乎没有改变，化疗方法仍然有待进步。

简介

AML 可发生于所有年龄段的成年人，但在老年人中尤其常见。AML 患者的中位年龄大约是 70 岁（图 114-1）。AML 可表现为发病即为白血病而没有明显的先前疾病；而另一些 AML 患者从其他骨髓疾病进展而来，这些疾病包括骨髓增生异常、骨髓增殖性肿瘤、再生障碍性贫血、范科尼贫血（Fanconi anemia）等，或是在治疗其他类型的癌症或非恶性疾病之后发生[1~4]。没有骨髓疾病史或没有抗肿瘤治疗经历的 AML 称为原发性 AML，而其他类型 AML 称为继发性 AML。由于突变谱更能反映 AML 的生物学异质性，因此突变谱可能比这种分类方法能更好地预测治疗反应和长期预后[5]。对 AML 患者的恰当治疗是一项多学科的工作，这项工作会从团队协作中获益。治疗 AML 不仅需要多方面的专业知识，包括输血医学、感染性疾病、留置导管的放置和护理、营养和抗肿瘤药物药理学等，还需要先进精密的实验诊断设备和为患者及其家属提供所需的社会心理咨询。最理想的是能够进行异基因干细胞移植，目前主要用于 75 岁以下的 AML 患者。这些学科的内容在本书的其他章节也有描述，但它们在白血病患者治疗中的关键作用不能被高估。

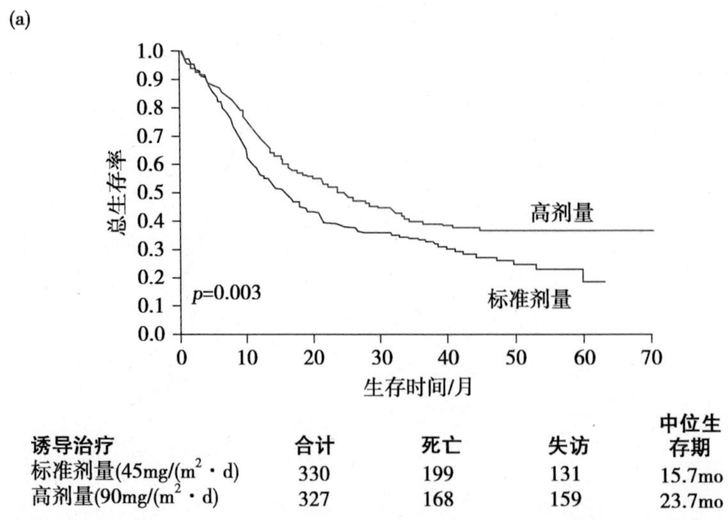

诱导治疗	合计	死亡	失访	中位生存期
标准剂量(45mg/(m^2·d)	330	199	131	15.7mo
高剂量(90mg/(m^2·d)	327	168	159	23.7mo

图 114-1　来自 ECOG 的数据表明，年龄小于 60 岁的 AML 患者的总生存率接近 40%，根据细胞遗传学风险和柔红霉素（daunorubicin）剂量不同总生存率有所变化。摘自 Fernandez 2009[4]，经 NEJM 许可转载

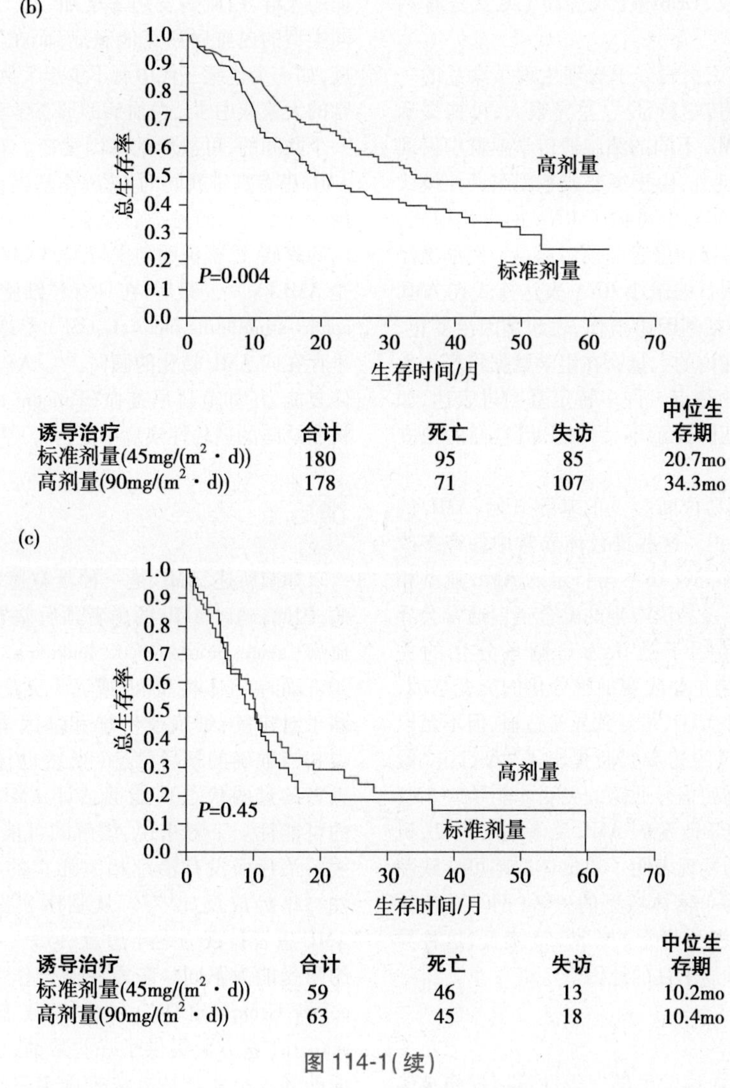

图 114-1(续)

发病机制和病因

病理生理学

造血干细胞的获得性遗传学变化可以部分解释 AML 的病理生理过程，这些遗传学变化既促进自我更新，又损害正常的造血干细胞分化，最终导致不成熟细胞的积累。最近对原发性 AML 的遗传学特征进行了阐述[6]。每个患者的白血病细胞中平均存在 5 个突变，"只有"30 个突变是重现性的（在 3%以上的患者中能够观察到）。在 30 个重现性突变中，有一些是相对常见的，这其中就包括功能获得性突变，针对这些突变的靶向治疗正在积极研发中。FLT3 是一种跨膜酪氨酸激酶，在大约 30%的 AML 患者中发生 *FLT3* 突变[7]。这些突变中大约 3/4 是长度或内部串联重复（internal tandem duplication，ITD）突变，FLT3 蛋白的膜旁区域被 3 到多于 100 个以上的氨基酸拉长。由于 *FLT3* 突变患者的复发率高，因此这种突变与不良预后有关。*ITD* 突变和不常见的酪氨酸激酶域点突变（通常为 D835Y）都会导致配体非依赖的受体结构活化。目前有几种 FLT3 抑制剂正在积极研制中，在 *FLT3* 突变患者中既可作为单药使用，也可与化疗联合使用。第二个常见的突变是 NPM1 穿梭蛋白的点突变[8]。这种突变，特别是在没有 *FLT3* 突变的正常核型患者中发生，提示预后良好[9]。Ras 鸟嘌呤核苷酸结合蛋白的突变与过度增殖有关，发生在大约 20% 的 AML 患者中[10]。翻译后修饰是 Ras 活化所需的步骤，但抑制翻译后修饰在 AML 治疗中几乎没有取得成功[11]。应用 MEK 抑制剂（在黑色素瘤和其他实体肿瘤中有效）阻断 Ras 通路提供了希望[12]。异构橼酸脱氢酶基因 *IDH1* 和 *IDH2* 突变发生在大约 20%的 AML 患者（每种突变的病例~10%）[13]。虽然这些突变的预后意义尚不清楚，但它们导致了新形态 2-羟葡萄糖酸盐（2-hydroxy gluterate，2HG）的生成，而不是通常的反应产物 α-酮葡萄糖酸盐。而且 2HG 水平可能与疾病活性有关[14]。应用小分子抑制 *IDH1* 或 *IDH2* 可能成为一种有效的治疗手段。在 AML 中经常见到具有表观活性（即 DNA 的翻译后修饰）的转录复合物和酶发生突变，这些突变可能会对基因表达有明显影响[6]。*DNMT3* 突变发生在大约 20%的 AML 患者，该突变可能与诱导治疗期间剂量强化的柔红霉素（daunorubicin）治疗有关[15]，提示预后不良[16]。这些被称为表观遗传修饰酶，如 ASXL1、EZH2 和 TET2 的存在，通常与骨髓增生异常综合征（myelodysplastic syndrome，MDS）发展而来的 AML 有关。*TP53*

突变提示预后不良[17]。相反，CEBPα（双等位）突变是有利突变[18]。

AML的遗传学复杂性是该疾病分子病理生理学紊乱的一个重要特征。AML的表观遗传学特征[19]差异很大，可能提示存在特异的治疗方法。在AML不同的细胞遗传学亚群中发现了特异的表观遗传学特征。此外，由于突变或基因组调控模式的改变，所以信使RNA[20]和实际上是微小RNA的表达模式，提供了AML病理生理学的解释和患者的预后信息。例如已经发现，尤其是部分控制免疫调节的微小RNA表达模式在AML中发挥重要作用[21]。整合包括基因组损伤、表观基因组变化、RNA和微小RNA表达模式在内的大量潜在组学数据将产生大量信息，并将成为未来研究的热点。许多特定基因过表达，如BAALC[22]或WT1[23]，已被证明提示不良预后，但它们的独立意义仍有待证实。

从识别细胞遗传学平衡易位断裂点的基因开始，AML的遗传学变化开始被大家所认识。这些染色体异常中的许多改变，例如t(8;21)、t(15;17)和inv(16)，与特定的AML亚型相关，并具有重要的预后意义。由易位产生的融合蛋白通常会导致转录因子的紊乱，而转录因子被认为是髓系分化的关键[24~27]。小鼠实验表明，转染主要改变细胞分化的突变基因，如t(8;21)易位产生的AML1/ETO，可导致异常造血，但不足以直接导致AML[27]。基于小鼠的初步实验提出了"双打击"假说，即需要同时影响分化和增殖信号通路的突变才能导致AML发生[28]。具有复杂细胞遗传学改变的AML患者预后不良，机制仍有待阐明。5q-MDS中的发现表明了单倍体缺陷可导致髓系恶性肿瘤[29]。许多被称为单倍体核型的患者（两个单倍体或一个单倍体合并一种骨髓基质异常）携带*p53*突变，这种异常可能解释了这一类AML预后不良的原因[17]。

暴露和风险

虽然越来越多的导致白血病发生的获得性基因损伤被确定，但有确切原因造成DNA损伤致AML发生的患者仅占AML的一小部分。暴露于核弹[30]或治疗性辐射[31]后，以及应用某些化疗药物后[32,33]，或严重持续的职业暴露于苯或石油化学产品后[34,35]，白血病发生的频率增加。与化疗相关的白血病有两种类型：①典型烷化剂诱导型AML，该型白血病常常继发于有克隆异常的骨髓增生异常，常伴有5号染色体和/或7号染色体的缺失[33]；②表鬼臼毒素/拓扑异构酶Ⅱ抑制剂相关型AML，该型潜伏期比典型烷化剂诱导型AML短（中位潜伏期是2年对比5年），该型常伴有粒单核细胞或单核细胞分化和11q23区域异常[33]。关于治疗相关白血病起源的一些观点受到了最近一些研究的挑战：①部分曾接受化疗的患者存在基因[5]或细胞遗传学损伤[36]，其临床表现与原发AML无明显区别；②由于突变的"正常"随机积累，业已存在*p53*突变的造血干细胞克隆在接受基因毒性治疗后，为了生存，*p53*突变可能被保留，从而有利于AML的发展[37]。

家族性AML

AML通常不是一种家族性疾病或遗传性疾病，这是一个值得被相关家庭关注的事实。在确诊后的头6个月内，同卵双胞胎患AML的发病率似乎有所增加[38]。一些具有家族综合征的人群，白血病发病率增加[39~41]。在这些家族中发现了不同类型的白血病和其他癌症，而在其他潜在信息量更大的家族，如一个连续三代中有不少于7例的红白血病或骨髓增生异常的大家族中[41]，白血病的形态学和临床特征相似，提示存在一个共同的、可遗传的基因突变。有报道在一个家族中，三名AML患者携带共同的*CEBPA*基因（该基因参与粒细胞分化）遗传突变[42]；而另一个有家族性血小板异常伴有AML转化倾向的家族，已被证明与携带编码CBF-α的基因突变有关（以前是AML1）[43]。最后，在具有粒细胞集落刺激因子（granulocyte colony-stimulating factor，G-CSF）受体遗传多态性的个体中，似乎存在向AML转化的倾向[44]。AML在某些不具有DNA损伤修复能力［如范科尼贫血（Fanconi anemia）］[45]或存在端粒酶机制缺陷的遗传性疾病中更为常见[46]。

预后

如前所述，AML是一种具有遗传学和生物学异质性的疾病，因此，确诊AML的患者预后差异很大；急性早幼粒细胞白血病（acute promyelocytic leukemia，APL）的治愈率为80%～90%，而单倍体核型和/或*p53*突变患者的治愈率几乎为零。基于对年龄、细胞遗传学和基因学等三方面的了解可以获得相当准确的预后信息（当然也包括明显的并发症和老年患者的衰弱状态），能够估计AML患者获得长期良好预后的可能性。一般来说，缓解的可能性，即顺利接受标准诱导缓解治疗而没有治疗相关死亡的概率，以及不复发的可能性与年龄成反比[47]。从临床实践考虑，55～65岁以上的AML患者被视为老年患者；但是，不同个体对细胞毒性化疗的耐受能力不同。东方肿瘤合作组（Eastern Cooperative Oncology Group，ECOG）的一般状态量表（performance status scale）在这方面提供了一些帮助，但有倾向应用更详细和全面的老年患者评估方法来确定患者是否能够耐受化疗[48]。除了随着年龄的增长发生并发症的可能性随之增加以外，其他的考虑包括老年人干细胞储备有限[49]以及不可避免的肝肾功能下降。此外，老年人白血病在生物学上更具侵袭性，其骨髓不良染色体异常的比例增加[50]，并且骨髓增生异常相关的遗传学异常的可能性增加，以及先前的骨髓干细胞疾病，这些因素都与较差的预后相关。对于有明显不良预后的老年AML患者通常采用不同的治疗方法。

在过去的40年中，我们已经在根据AML诊断时染色体的特征来判断预后，并且在某些情况下指导治疗。许多研究已经将新诊断的年轻成人AML患者分为三个预后类别[51,52]。大约15%的患者存在预后良好的异常改变（不包括APL），包括核心结合因子易位，如t(8;21)和染色体16的臂间倒位，这些患者的完全缓解率较高而复发率相对较低；其中至少有2/3的患者因携带C-kit酪氨酸激酶基因相关突变而增加了不良预后的可能性[53]。约15%的患者有预后不良的染色体异常[50]，包括复杂核型（通常大于3个，但在某些分类中界定为5种不同的染色体异常）或单倍体核型（2个单倍体或1个单倍体加1个结构异常）[54]。不良预后分类中的患者约有15%的长期无病生存可能性，但是那些单倍体核型的患者预后会更差[55]。该亚组中*TP53*基因突变的高发生率可能部分解释了预后差的原因[17]。约 70%的患者被认为是中等预后,长期生存率约为 40%。其中一些患者有很明显的特征性染色体异常,如+8 或涉及 11q23(*MLL* 基因)的易位。

然而,绝大多数中等预后组由正常核型的患者组成。在过去的 10~20 年里,人们做出了巨大的努力将核型正常的患者进行预后分组。目前,人们普遍使用以下三个基因的信息来指导分类:*CEBPα*,*NPM1* 和 *FLT3*。白血病细胞中存在双等位基因 *CEBPα* 突变的患者无病生存率往往高达 80%;然而,只有少数患者有这种异常[18]。*FLT3ITD*(*ITD*)突变导致跨膜酪氨酸激酶长度的变化,被认为是不利突变,而 NPM1 核穿梭蛋白的突变是有利的。当考虑到这两种突变可能同时存在,只有 *NPM1* 突变的而不伴有 *FLT3ITD* 突变的患者会表现出较高的生存率[9]。这是染色体中等预后类别中唯一的患者亚组,推荐在缓解后仅进行以化疗为基础的治疗[9]。最近的一项研究表明,只有那些具有 *NPM1* 突变和 *FLT3ITD* 野生型遗传学模式,以及 *IDH1/IDH2* 突变的患者具有较高的总体存活率[16],但这一点仍有待于其他研究的证实。*DNMTA3* 突变也意味着不良预后[15,56],预后与伴有 *EZH2* 和 *ASXL1* 突变等 MDS 相关异常改变的 AML 患者类似[57]。

在老年患者中,复杂或不利的细胞遗传学改变发生率较高。然而,少数老年人具有良好的核型,如果他们的其他医学指标允许,应采用常规诱导和巩固治疗方案[50]。此外,在具有正常核型的老年患者中,如果有 *NPM1* 突变而没有 *FLT3ITD* 突变,可能这部分患者的生存率高于没有这种遗传学模式改变的老年人[58]。

表 114-1 描述了改良的欧洲白血病网(European Leukemia Net,ELN)分类方案[59],显示了年轻成人各种细胞遗传学和基因改变的频率和一般预后。随着时间的推移,其他遗传学异常的引入,这个列表可能会有变化。

表 114-1　细胞遗传学和基因为基础的危险度分层

危险分组	特征	近似四年生存率/%	近似患病率/%
极高危	单体核型(两条单体或一个染色体加平衡易位)	10	6
高危	复杂核型(>3 个异常)或不利的(-7,7q-,-5,5q-,3q 或 t(6;9))细胞遗传学	20	12
中等	正常细胞遗传学(伴 *FLT3* 突变或 *FLT3-ITD* 不存在/*NPM1* 野生型/*CEBPα* 野生型)或其他核型	35	25
	16 号染色体倒位或 t(8;21)伴 *c-KIT* 突变	40	5
	正常细胞遗传学(*FLT3-ITD* 不存在/*NPM1* 突变)	50	25
良好	正常细胞遗传学(具有 *CEBPα* 双等位基因突变)	60	5
	t(8;21)或 16 号染色体倒位(伴 *c-KIT* 野生型)	65	10
非常好	t(15;17)	85	12

摘自 Stone2013[59]。经美国临床肿瘤学学会许可转载。

形态学分类与临床和实验室相关

AML 的诊断有赖于对取材良好的外周血和骨髓标本的检测。应同时评估骨髓穿刺和骨髓活检。虽然活检通常对识别单个细胞没有帮助,但它提供了细胞结构的最佳评估,偶尔可以识别在骨髓穿刺液中未发现的聚集的白血病细胞,而且活检对于评估骨髓纤维化是必要的。1976 年,来自法国、美国和英国的形态学家提出了一个分类系统,旨在对临床和生物学上不同亚型的 AML 和急性淋巴细胞白血病(acute lymphoblastic leukemia, ALL)进行标准定义[60]。这种法国,美国和英国(French,American,and British,FAB)分类方法已经进行了系列的修改,最初是在 2002 年[61],在 2016 年[62]由世界卫生组织(World Health Organization,WHO)发起采纳,这代表了为提高不同研究者之间一致性所做的努力,也整合了免疫学、细胞遗传学和分子研究的新发现。

AML 的诊断通常在 Wright 或 Wright-Giemsa 染色涂片上评估,要求原始粒细胞占骨髓细胞或外周血白细胞(white blood cells,WBC)的 20%及以上。FAB 分类要求>30%的原始细胞以区分 AML 和骨髓增生异常。虽然这一变化是基于一项研究,该研究表明 AML 预后可能仅基于原始细胞计数[63],但目前尚不清楚这在生物学上是否有充分根据。在比较过去的 AML 试验与最近的研究时,这种资格标准的差异是需要考虑的。肿瘤性的早幼粒细胞、原始单核细胞或幼稚单核细胞、原始巨核细胞包括在该百分比中,并且它们的存在定义了下面讲述的各种形态学亚型。各种组织化学染色被用于辅助亚型分类和 AML 与 ALL 的鉴别诊断。应用针对仅存在于髓系分化细胞抗原[称为簇标志(cluster designations,CD)]的单克隆抗体,有助于进行鉴别诊断。最常用的抗体包括的抗 CD11b、CD13、CD14、CD33 和 C117 抗体[64]。这些抗原存在于正常的造血干细胞上,不是白血病特有的,也不是某些 AMLFAB 亚型所特有的。一般而言,这些抗原与预后无关,其中 CD34 抗原可能是个例外[65],CD34 可在未分化的造血祖细胞上检测到,并且可以在 AML 或 ALL 患者的原始细胞中检测到。原始细胞 CD34 强表达的 AML 患者,尤其是同时形态学分化较差、髓系相关抗原表达不太强的患者对化疗耐药,因此预后不良[66]。

FAB 和 WHO 根据最相似的正常骨髓成分对 AML 的亚型进行分类命名。然而,这并不表明白血病仅涉及在形态上表现最有特征的细胞系。直到最近,其他造血谱系的参与也只能通过这些其他细胞系中突出的形态学异常的存在来推断。在患有骨髓增生异常或红白血病的患者中,通常存在三系增生异常的形态学证据,由此推断恶性转化的初始细胞是具有多系成熟能力的造血干细胞前体[67]。Fialkow 等[68]对女性患者的葡萄糖-6-磷酸脱氢酶的 X 染色体连锁多态性进行研究,证明在一些 AML 患者中,髓系细胞而不是红系或巨核细胞的祖细胞参与 AML 发生。这项首次观察证明是有预见性的;但是目前我们认为大多数造血细胞来自紊乱的干细胞,多系受累非常普遍。此外,AML 应被视为寡克隆,而不是单克隆;诊断时存在克隆异质性;考虑到化疗的选择压力,主导性克隆可以随时间变化。例如,有证据表明在缓解期或复发时存在某种亚克隆,这些亚克隆已经获得"进展"突变(或者这些突变在诊断时存在于非常小的亚克隆中)[5],并且在诊断时存在的一个小克隆可能是导致复发的原因。

AML 的不同亚型的代表性病例展示在图 114-2~图 114-11 中。表 114-2 回顾了这些形态学亚型的免疫学,细胞遗传学和临床相关性(如果存在)。

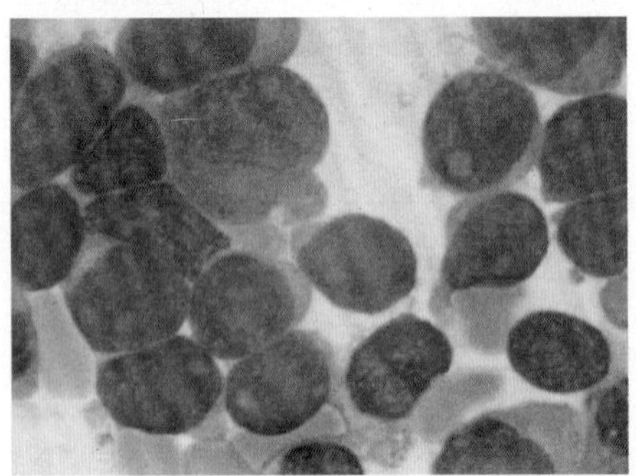

图 114-2　M0。未分化类型的急性髓细胞性白血病(acute myeloid leukemia,AML)患者的骨髓原始细胞质量不等、无颗粒。过氧化物酶和苏丹黑染色阴性,可与 FABM7 或 FABL2 混淆。通过使用针对髓系抗原的抗体进行免疫表型分析和/或使用透射电子显微镜观察过氧化物酶阳性颗粒的超微结构,可以证实为髓系细胞

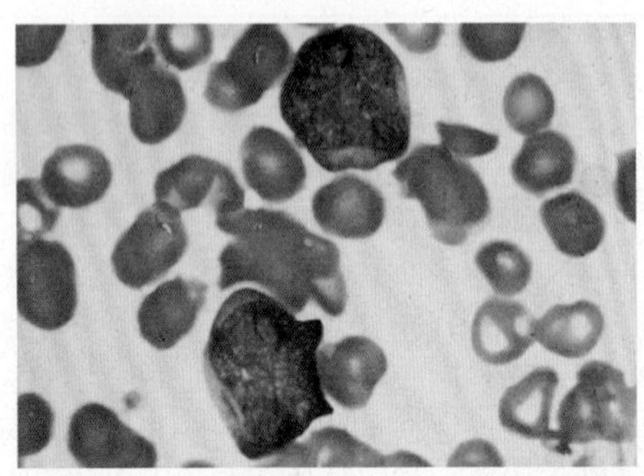

图 114-3　来自一例 M1 急性髓细胞性白血病患者的一个原始细胞,可见明显的 Auer 小体

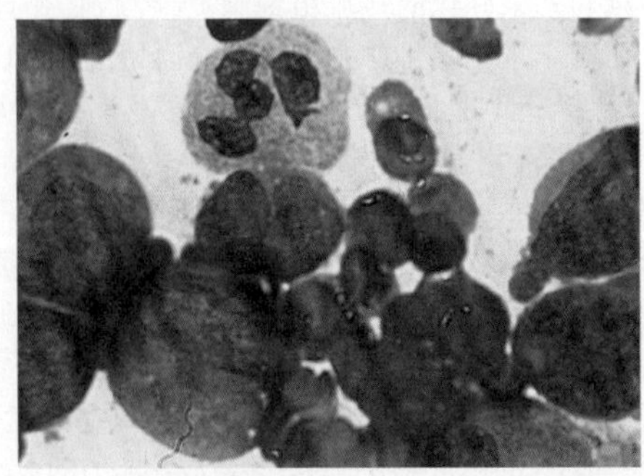

图 114-4　M2 白血病的特征是骨髓髓系细胞部分分化和更成熟的髓系细胞存在

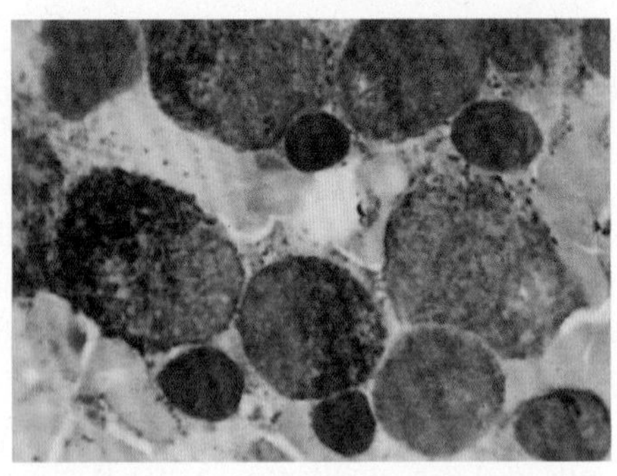

图 114-5　M3 早幼粒细胞白血病细胞通常具有不规则的细胞核,胞质可见大量颗粒。常有细胞外浆,且常见具有多个 Auer 小体(未示出)的原始细胞。这种白血病具有典型的 t(15;17)染色体易位和弥散性血管内凝血的特征性临床表现

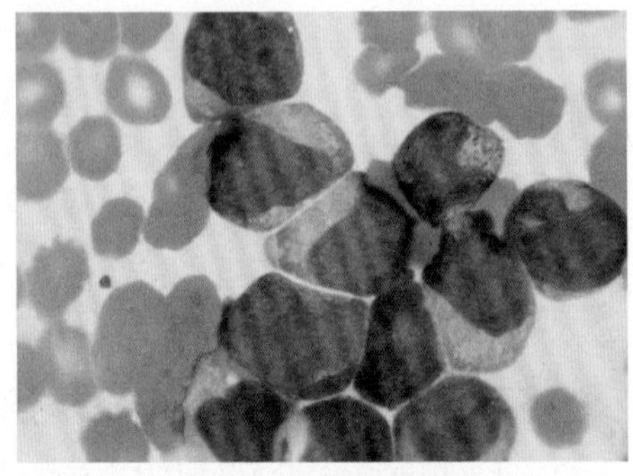

图 114-6　M4,急性粒单核细胞白血病的原始细胞具有髓系和单核细胞样外观(原始细胞包括粒系和单核系的原始细胞)

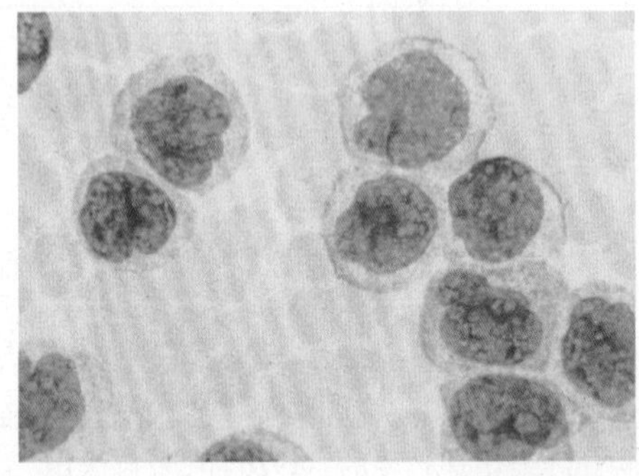

图 114-7　M5,单核细胞白血病。一些细胞可见明显的核仁、少量颗粒、胞质嗜碱性,使这些细胞具有早幼粒细胞样外观

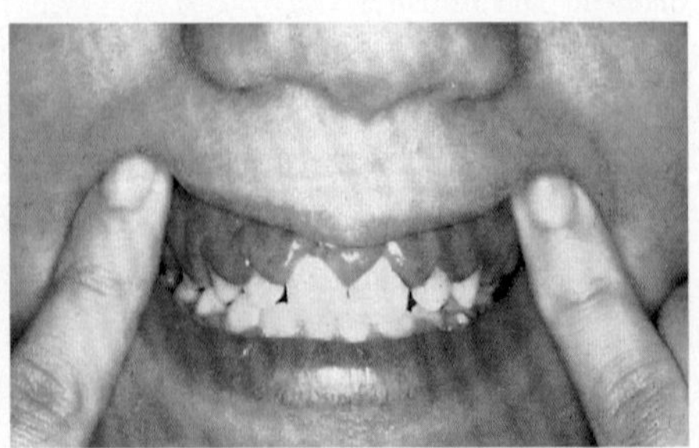

图 114-8　M5,单核细胞白血病,由于白血病细胞浸润导致的牙龈肥大

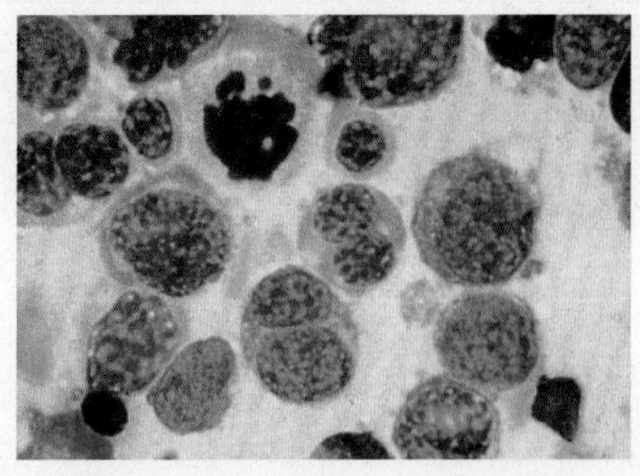
图 114-9 M6,红白血病的特征是存在异常的较早阶段的巨幼红细胞和多核红细胞。在一些细胞中可见到核分裂象。FABM6 和伴有过量原始细胞转化的骨髓增生异常综合征之间的区别主要是髓系原始细胞的比例不同

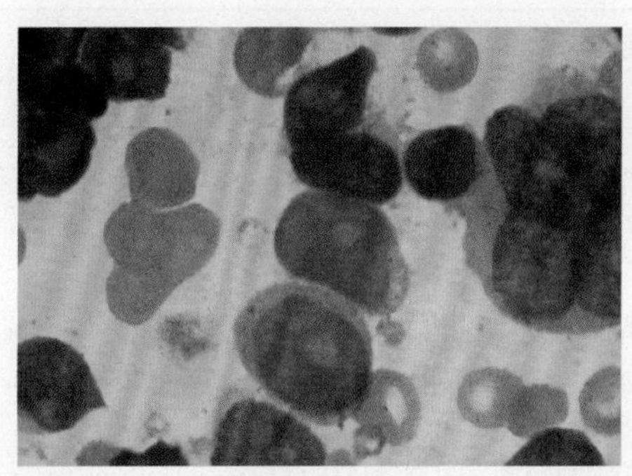
图 114-10 M7,巨核细胞白血病。此型白血病的原始细胞通常在形态上是未分化的。多核细胞,发育异常的小巨核细胞和胞质出芽有助于诊断。该诊断可通过免疫表型分析或超微结构检查证实

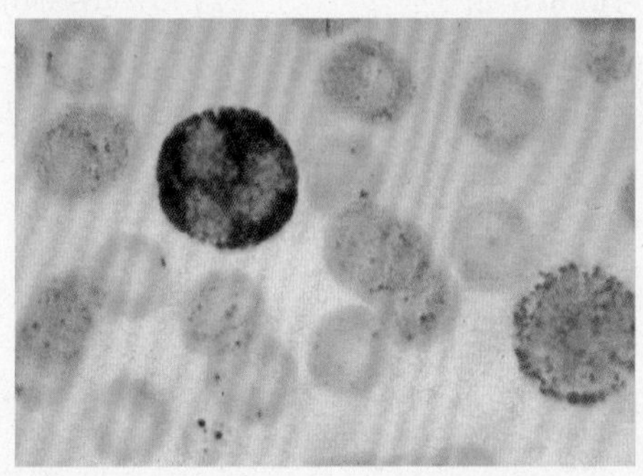
图 114-11 FABM1AML 患者原始细胞和中性粒细胞的典型苏丹黑 B 染色

表 114-2 AML 中的重现性核型和分子异常

细胞遗传学异常	FAB 分型	累及基因	中位年龄	在原发 AML 中发病率	预后价值	评价
t(8;21)	M2	*AML1/ETO*	30 岁	5%~7%	好	常见 Auer 小体
t(15;17)	M3	*PML-RARa*	40	5%~8%	ATRA 为基础治疗治愈率高	DIC
t(11;17)	与 M3 相似	*PLZF/RARa*	?	<1%	对 ATRA 反应差	
abn16q22	M4 伴嗜酸细胞增多	*CBFA/MYH11*	35~40	5%	好	复发后再诱导缓解率高
Abn11q23	M5	*MLL*+多种伙伴基因	>50	3%	差,除了 t(9;11)	高白细胞、髓外侵犯
+8	不定		>60	5%~10%	差	
del5, del7, 5q-, 7q-或混合存在	不定,常见 FABM6		>60	15%~20%	差	在继发 AML 或 MDS 病史者常见
Inv3	异常巨核细胞	*Ribophorin/EVI 1*	?	<1%	差	血小板数多,其他异常常见(del5,del7)
+13	不定,有些是未分化型		可能>60	1%~2%	差	常见混合特征
t(6;9)(p2;q34)	M2/M4 嗜碱性粒细胞增多	*DEK/CAN*	?	<1%	差	嗜碱性粒细胞明显增多

续表

细胞遗传学异常	FAB 分型	累及基因	中位年龄	在原发 AML 中发病率	预后价值	评价
t(9;22)	常见于 M1	*BCR-ABL*	可能>50	约 1%	差	脾大
t(1;22)	常见于 M7	*MOZ/CBP*	婴儿	<1%	差	脏器肿大
t(8;16)	M4,5		?	<1%	差	嗜血现象
分子异常						
FLT3 突变[8]	不定,常见 CN-AML,可见于 t(6;9);t(15;17)	*ITD* 或点突变	?	约 30%CN-AML	差	
(NPM1)突变(5q35)[47]	不定	NPM,常伴其他突变	?	约 35%AML 约 50%CN-AML	好(除了伴有其他突变)	
CEBPα[48]	不定	减少 CEBPα 水平	?	约 15%CN-AML	好(除了伴有其他突变)	
过表达 BAALC(脑和急性白血病胞质)蛋白	不定	过表达 BAALC	?	主要在 CN-AML 中研究	差,需进一步研究	
MLL 部分串联重复[57]	不定	影响 *HOX* 基因功能	?	约 8% CN-AML	不清楚,需进一步研究	
IDH1,*IDH2*	不定	异构橡酸脱氢酶	?	*IDH1*10%, *IDH2*18%	不定	临床试验中的特异性抑制剂
TET2	不定(常见于 MDS)	DNA 甲基化	>60%	15%	不良	与年龄正相关
DNMT3A	不定	DNA 甲基化	>60%	20%	不良	与年龄正相关
ASXL1	不定	表观调控	?	6%	不良	与其他突变相关

AML,急性髓细胞性白血病;ATRA,维 A 酸;DIC,弥散性血管内凝血;FAB,法国、美国、英国;MDS,骨髓增生异常综合征。

外周血

大多数 AML 患者存在贫血(中位血红蛋白 8g/dl),血小板减少症(中位血小板计数 40 000~50 000/μl)和白细胞增多(中位数 WBC 计数 10 000~20 000/μl)。红细胞形态通常相对正常。可以观察到体积偏大、颗粒减少的血小板,血小板功能缺陷可以导致出血。大多数患者中性粒细胞减少,并伴有形态学异常(核分叶多、颗粒减少、Pelger-Huet 畸形)。大多数患者仔细检查可以检测到外周血的原始细胞,但当外周血细胞数量较少时很难区分白血病亚型(或偶尔可明确诊断急性白血病)。少数白细胞明显减少(称为低白细胞性白血病)的患者可能较难诊断,最终需进行骨髓检查确诊。

AML 伴重现性遗传学异常

临床发现 t(8;21)、inv(16)和 t(15;17)已有几十年,我们在 M2、M4 伴嗜酸性粒细胞增多和 M3(APL)章节中有所描述。具有 t(8;21)和 inv(16)的 AML 被称为"核结合因子"(core binding factor,CBF)白血病,因为这些易位导致转录的分子异常。在大约 25% 的 CBFAML 患者中发现 C-KIT 酪氨酸激酶受体的突变,其导致增殖信号持续激活,数据表明这种附加突变的患者以及相应蛋白过表达的患者预后较差[53]。

2008 年 WHO 分类在这一类白血病中增加了 inv3(q21;q26.2)、t(3;3)(q21;26.2)、(1;22)(p13;q13)[RBM15-MLK1](常见于婴儿,见章节 M7)和 t(6;9)(p23;q23)[DEK-NUP214]。t(6;9)易位并不常见,可能在年轻患者中更多一些,并且可以与多种 AML 形态相关,这类患者通常嗜碱性细胞显著增多[69]。*FLT3ITD* 突变在大约 2/3 的 t(6;9)患者中存在[70],化疗效果差,应尽可能进行同种异体造血干细胞移植。

AML 与 MDS 相关的变化

增加这一类别表明很多 AML,特别是老年患者,是从先前的骨髓增生异常疾病发展而来。这类患者包括既往有 MDS 病史,至少有两系病态造血>50%和伴有"MDS 细胞遗传学"改变的患者,包括-5、-7、i(17)/t(17p)、-13、del11q、del(12p)、del9q 和复杂核型以及具有标志染色体改变[67]。这些白血病似乎起源于非常早期的造血干细胞,这些患者倾向于低的缓解率和较短的持续缓解时间。似乎仅基于形态学异常的这类患者,可能会呈现基于突变谱的多种致癌途径,因此可能不会有一致的不良预后[5]。

治疗相关 AML

此类别包括因其他疾病接受化疗和/或放射治疗后发病的 AML。形态学和核型同 MDS 相似,另外也包括一组之前接受过拓扑异构酶Ⅱ抑制剂治疗、有 11q23 异常的患者,这类患者常在短期内发生 AML[32,33]。治疗相关的 AML 往往对化疗耐药性更强,达到缓解的患者应考虑同种异体造血干细胞移植。值得注意的是,一些与治疗相关的 AML 患者可能具有 inv(16),t(8;21)和 t(15;17)(APL)或原发 AML 典型遗传学改变,尽管可能与具有这些核型的原发性 AML 不同,但这些亚型患者对标准方案反应良好[5,36]。

髓外 AML(又称髓样肉瘤)

偶尔有患者初诊时通过组化染色证实在髓外病变组织存在髓系原始细胞,而骨髓没有明显的受累。肿物可能累及皮肤、胃肠道、卵巢、中枢神经系统(CNS),以及几乎每个身体器官。该病如果不治疗患者最终全身复发的风险极高[71],但对这类患者治疗的系统性研究报道很少。多数医师在初次诊断后就开始考虑对适合患者给予诱导、巩固治疗。尽管这种"早期"治疗复发率很高,而干细胞移植的作用尚不清楚,但考虑移植以维持病情缓解是合理的。某些患者具有 t(8;21)染色体易位,但可能并没有像更典型的 t(8;21) AML 一样具有有利的预后[72]。

非特殊型 AML

这一类别包括大量未划分于以上分组的 AML。

FAB 分型

虽然目前不再使用旧版 FAB 分类,但可以讨论其临床病理相关性。Wright-Giemsa 染色的外周血或骨髓穿刺涂片可以更好地区分 AML 而不是 ALL。一般来说,AML 患者的原始细胞较大、胞质较丰富、核仁较明显且可见多个核仁。然而,最终的诊断取决于 Auer 小体的存在,Auer 小体是胞质内线性排列的髓系颗粒。细胞化学染色,如髓过氧化物酶,存在于 73%的原始细胞中,可以帮助诊断 AML。

M0:微分化 AML

如图 114-2 所示,一些患者的原始细胞类似于髓系原始细胞,但在用髓过氧化物酶、苏丹黑 B 或其他组织化学染色检查时,在光学显微镜下是阴性的。但是这些白血病的髓系性质可以通过免疫方法或通过电镜观察过氧化物酶染色预处理的标本发现。电镜可见到过氧化物酶颗粒的超微结构。电子显微镜能够显示超微结构的过氧化物酶阳性颗粒,免疫分型可以发现白血病细胞表达髓系抗原而不表达淋系抗原[73,74]。这些细胞通常表达 CD34。一般来说,末端脱氧核苷酸转移酶(terminal deoxynucleotidyl transferase,TdT)不表达,但有时可以在少数原始细胞中被检测到。

大约 7%的初治 AML 患者属于微分化 AML(M0AML),对药物相对耐药[75]。这种未分化的白血病很容易与 ALL 混淆,因此获得原始细胞免疫表型对形态学未分化白血病的患者至关重要。除了对化疗耐药外,M0 在临床表现上无特殊性。许多 M0 患者具有复杂的异常核型[75]。除 13 号染色体三倍体外,没有发现明显的细胞遗传学特征,这种特征在一些形态学分化差的白血病患者中也有报道[76]。

M1:髓细胞性白血病未成熟型

M1 型患者的原始细胞核圆形、胞质量中等、颗粒少,可见 Auer 小体(图 114-3)。与 M2 不同,几乎没有髓系成熟的证据,早幼粒细胞以下阶段的髓系细胞比例<10%。在年龄、性别、临床特征、细胞遗传学异常方面无特殊性。

M2:髓细胞性白血病成熟型

与 M1 不同,M2 型表现为髓系连续分化成熟,有早幼粒细胞、中幼粒细胞和更成熟阶段的粒细胞。细胞的颗粒性更加明显,Auer 小体常较明显(图 114-4)。20%~25%的 M2 患者具有特征性易位[t(8;21)(q22;22)];该染色体易位主要见于有 Auer 小体的 M2。此类患者的中位年龄(30 岁)较低,初始完全缓解率非常高(大多数患者>85%),复发率较低,长期无病生存期长,特别是接受大剂量阿糖胞苷为基础的巩固化疗的患者[77],但是如果同时存在 *c-kit* 突变或其他预后不良基因时其预后变差[78]。髓外粒细胞性肉瘤的发生率在 t(8;21)M2 患者中可能增加,其细胞表面表达黏附分子 CD56。有时表现为散在肿块,有时发生在脊柱旁,预后差,和单核细胞白血病的牙龈和皮肤累及不同[71]。

M3:急性早幼粒细胞白血病

APL 是 AML 最独特的亚型之一,主要体现在形态学、临床特征、细胞遗传学以及对诱导分化治疗药物,如维 A 酸(ATRA)和砷剂的反应敏感等方面[79]。在大多数患者中,形态学诊断更直接,骨髓可见大量多颗粒的异常早幼粒细胞。细胞核呈圆形,核仁明显,胞质充满大量的嗜天青颗粒(图 114-5)。Auer 小体常见,常见多个 Auer 小体(被称为柴束状细胞),少数患者的白血病细胞颗粒少,有时只有通过电镜才能看到颗粒[80]。这类少颗粒型 APL 的细胞表现为双分叶核或多分叶核,有时会与 AML 的单核细胞白血病相混淆。与 APL 的典型白细胞减少表现相反,少颗粒型患者的白细胞计数偏高。在这两类 APL 中,苏丹黑 B 或髓过氧化物酶染色是强阳性的。HLA-DR 在所有造血前体细胞上表达,但是 APL 细胞不表达 HLA-DR。这一发现的原因和生物学意义尚不清楚。相反,CD33 始终强表达[81]。

APL 可见于所有年龄阶段,但大部分患者一般较年轻,中位年龄为 30~40 岁。APL 约占 AML 的 10%,可能在拉丁人[82]和肥胖人群中更为普遍[83]。APL 几乎都表现为低纤维蛋白原血症、其他凝血因子的消耗、纤维蛋白降解产物增多、内源性和输注的血小板破坏增加。颗粒中含有强效的促凝血成分,化疗导致细胞裂解后通常会增加弥散性血管内凝血(diffuse intravascular coagulation,DIC)的概率[84],通常伴有出血增加,而使用 ATRA 可以迅速改善[85]。对于某些患者,有研究表明纤溶亢进可能是引发凝血功能障碍的主要原因[86]。APL 与极高的出血性并发症和死亡率相关,死亡通常与颅内出血有关,因此初次考虑 APL 时即应用 ATRA 治疗是极为重要的[87]。在 ATRA 控制 DIC 之前,严重的低纤维蛋白原血症(<100mg/dl)可能需要补充冷沉淀,并且应该通过积极使用血小板输注来纠正血小板减少。

几乎所有 APL 患者都有涉特征性染色体易位[t(15;17)

(q22;q12)][88],同时可能伴有其他细胞遗传学异常,如8号染色体三倍体[89]。反转录聚合酶链反应(RT-PCR)可用于检测融合转录产物,可用于评估微小残留病(minimal residual disease,MRD)[90],也可以对临床特征和形态学上典型的APL和正常核型的患者进行正确分类。17号染色体上的断裂点位于视黄酸受体α基因的内含子中。这个基因已经命名为*PML*基因,该基因具有DNA结合能力,从15号染色体易位形成融合蛋白,其功能以显性方式阻断RAR-α控制的基因转录,导致RAR-α控制的基因转录受阻,可能通过招募核共抑制因子发挥作用。维A酸治疗解除了共抑制物的活性[91,92],允许参与分化的基因发生转录[93]。另一种有趣的方法是在APL患者中使用组蛋白去乙酰化酶抑制剂以增强基因表达[94]。可以检测到大约1/3的APL患者存在*FLT3ITD*突变,这与较高的白细胞计数和M3变异形态有关。但与非APL的AML情况不同,并不总是有不良的预后[95,96],与APL在形态上相似但具有交替易位如t(11;17)(q23;q21)的白血病已被报道。尽管具有RAR-α重排,但这些患者对ATRA无反应。这类患者不是15号染色体的*PML*基因,而是11号染色体上的新型锌指基因PZLF易位至RAR-α,产生一种融合蛋白,其抑制了ATRA介导的转录共抑制活性[97]。

从历史角度看,用蒽环类化疗药治疗APL患者的缓解率非常高。最初的耐药性非常罕见,大多数治疗失败与出血或感染性死亡有关。APL对单药蒽环类药物治疗具有独特的敏感性,CR率可以>80%[98]。与其他类型的AML相比,APL化疗可以获得缓解而不会产生骨髓抑制[99]。治疗后的骨髓常常残存异常的早幼粒细胞,无须进一步化疗,这些细胞也会逐渐消失,恢复正常造血。尽管形态异常的细胞持续存在,但DIC不会再次发生。毫无疑问,APL的这一独特特征与对具有分化和非细胞毒性作用机制的药物的敏感性有关(见“急性早幼粒细胞白血病(APL)的治疗”一节)。目前至少有80%的患者在使用ATRA和三氧化二砷联合化疗的情况下得到治愈[100]。

M4:粒单核细胞白血病

粒单核细胞白血病的形态学特征为粒细胞系和单核细胞系成分共存,约占新诊断AML患者的15%~20%。根据FAB标准,该亚型在形态上单核细胞系的原始细胞占白血病细胞的比例需>20%,以此与FABM1型,特别M2型相区分。单核细胞系的白血病细胞通常与部分分化的单核细胞类似,颗粒较少,胞质浅灰,细胞核呈折叠状,这在外周血中很常见(图114-6)。单核系白血病细胞可以通过用非特异性酯酶如α-醋酸萘酯和α-萘基丁酸酯染色来确认。

该亚型没有特异的临床特征,可能因为形态学入选标准宽泛导致此分类纳入了各种类型的患者。M4中位发病年龄略微偏大,高白细胞和髓外侵犯的发生率可能升高(也常见于单核细胞白血病)。M4没有特殊的染色体异常,而且其短期及长期生存亦难以准确预测。

M4EO:粒单核细胞白血病伴嗜酸性粒细胞升高

大约5%的原发性AML患者具有典型粒单核细胞白血病的形态学特征,且同时存在处于不同成熟阶段的异常增生的嗜酸性粒细胞。这种独特的嗜酸性粒细胞通常仅占骨髓细胞的5%~10%[101]。一般来说,除典型的嗜酸性成分外,这些细胞还含有大的嗜碱性颗粒。M2型伴嗜酸性粒细胞增多也偶有报道。

M4E0发病年龄较小(中位年龄35~40岁),预后非常好[102]。CR率高(通常大于85%),原发性耐药很少。有些研究报道这类AML的预后最好。最近发现C-KIT突变在部分CBF AML患者中存在,是一个预后不良的指标[53,78]。除了CR1的持续时间很长,复发后获得的CR2持续时间也很长[103]。早期文献报道骨髓中嗜酸性粒细胞增多的患者出现中枢神经系统(CNS)复发率高。应用大剂量阿糖胞苷(ara-C)为主的强烈化疗后,AML患者很少发生CNS复发,因此FAB M4E0患者不需要进行CNS治疗。

所有FAB M4E0的患者均存在16号染色体长臂22带(16q22)细胞遗传学异常。尽管也存在同时伴有16q22同源缺失的两条16号染色体之间的易位[104],大多数患者为16号染色体中心倒位(inv16)。该断裂点涉及CBF-β链基因与平滑肌肌球蛋白重链基因的融合。由此产生的融合蛋白可能具有核共抑制因子活性(以组蛋白去乙酰化酶的形式),并以类似于t(8;21)M2AML中的CBF-α/ETO融合的方式抑制髓系分化所需基因的转录[105]。虽然inv(16)白血病患者对高强度化疗反应非常好[接受HiDAC(HiDAC)的患者3年DFS率>60%~70%][102],但其具体原因仍不清楚。

M5:单核细胞白血病

单核细胞白血病具有两种亚型(M5a,M5b);两者大于80%的原始细胞都来自单核细胞系。M5a不太常见,其原始单核细胞具有球形核和少量呈嗜碱性的细胞质,没有形态分化的迹象。M5b伴有形态学分化的特征,至少20%的原始细胞与幼稚单核细胞类似,细胞核折叠,胞质丰富且颗粒较少,通常没有Auer小体。核折叠在核染色质稀疏的情况下非常明显(图114-7)。骨髓涂片中经常可以看到这些细胞对其他造血细胞的吞噬作用。这些单核细胞成分可以被非特异性酯酶明显染色,并可被氟化物抑制。

虽然单核细胞白血病见于各个年龄段,但老年人更常见。FAB M5患者在诊断时原始细胞计数更高,由高白细胞淤滞带来的问题比较常见(参见“并发症”部分[106]),此外,M5髓外白血病的发生率最高,特别是伴有形态学分化的患者[107]。例如,患者因齿龈增生就诊牙科的情况较常见(图114-8)。皮肤浸润在诊断和复发时都很常见,且皮肤通常为初始复发部位,即使有时骨髓形态仍正常。其他不常见的髓外侵犯部位包括胃肠道,结膜和中枢神经系统。髓外浸润很可能与幼稚单核细胞向这些部位的活跃迁移有关。这些部分分化的细胞在体内能够迁移到皮肤窗口,在体外可以胞吞微生物,黏附于尼龙纤维[108]。

大多数AML患者的血清溶菌酶水平升高,但单核细胞白血病患者的溶血酶水平通常要高得多[109]。溶菌酶可影响肾小管功能,导致FAB M4和M5白血病患者出现严重的症状性低钾血症。该问题通常随着细胞减少而缓解,但呕吐和腹泻也可加重低钾血症。

除了因白细胞增多并发症引起的初始问题外,单核细胞白血病患者往往因耐药问题导致CR率低。虽然既往研究表明单核细胞白血病CR持续时间往往较短,长期无病生存率很低,但对ECOG治疗的大量患者的分析表明,当考虑到其他危险因素时,它与其他AML形态学亚型的结局相似[110]。单核细胞白血病存在着各种各样的细胞遗传学异常,其中最常涉及 11 号染色体 q23 频带。这个被称为混合谱系白血病(MLL)基因的断裂点参与髓系或淋巴来源的白血病的发生,以及表皮鞘毒素和其他针对拓扑异构酶Ⅱ的药物治疗后的白血病[111]。*MLL* 基因,也称为 All-1 或 HRX,可以与平衡易位中的至少 16 种不同基因组合[112]。MLL 与果蝇发育中重要的基因同源,并且包括 DNA 结合元件。涉及 *MLL* 基因的 t(9;11)易位相对常见,其预后比预料中要好,初始 CR 率高[113,114]。M5b 伴有明显的噬血现象和 t(8;16)(p11;p13)有相关性,该易位累及 CBP 类转录因子,CBP 类转录因子促进髓系分化[115]。

M6:红白血病

红白血病,以前常被称为 Di Guglielmo 综合征,是 AML 的一种亚型,其中红系形态学异常最为突出[116]。纯红白血病的病例很少见,其主要的恶性细胞为原始红细胞。相反,这是三系造血明显异常的骨髓干细胞疾病。除了髓系原始细胞增多外,红白血病中红系还存在形态学异常,包括明显的巨幼红细胞增多,多核,核破裂,有丝分裂增加,以及高碘酸-Schiff(PAS)染色团块状阳性(图 114-9)。铁储存一般增多,同时经常伴有环状铁幼粒细胞增多。这些与骨髓增生异常综合征患者的形态学改变类似,并且许多观察者认为大多数红白血病从生物学上与伴原始细胞的难治性贫血相似。两组患者疗效非常差,易发生于老年人,以及存在类似的细胞遗传学异常(复杂核型,5 号染色体和/或 7 号染色体部分或全部缺失,以及标记染色体)[116]。尽管如此,为了使临床试验方案的准入和报告保持一致,FAB 和 WHO 通过对原始红细胞和原始粒细胞数量的量化,多少有些武断地区分了 M6、骨髓增生异常(RAEB)和其他具有大量原始红细胞的 FAB 亚型。在最近的 WHO 更新中,大多数这些患者现在属于"AML 伴 MDS 相关变化"。M6 定义为大于 50%的骨髓有核细胞是红系,且原始细胞在非红系中的比例超过 30%。Gly2A 是红系特异的,但是很少需要免疫表型来鉴定这些形态学亚型。

M7:巨核细胞白血病

巨核细胞生成的形态学异常,通常以单核或双核小巨核细胞的存在为特征,这在许多 AML 亚型中很常见,在 M6 或骨髓增生异常综合征中尤为突出。这些患者中有少数有血小板增多和 3 号染色体异常[inv(3)(q21;q26)]。这种细胞遗传学异常通常与其他染色体缺失有关,见于多种原发形态(M1,M2,M4),及有 MDS 先驱病史的患者[117]。这些患者对初始治疗的反应较差且整体生存(OS)短。血小板增多不仅存在于 inv(3)核型的患者中,也存在于其他初诊的 AML 患者中[118]。染色体 3q21 断点处的基因与 EⅥ1 转录因子的激活有关[119]。

FABM7 的白血病细胞主要来自巨核细胞系[120],在一些患者中,存在巨核细胞异常增生或多核细胞,表明巨核细胞显著受累(图 114-10),而在其他情况下,白血病细胞形态上未分化,具有数量不等的无颗粒细胞质,有时与 M1 或 ALL 混淆。苏丹黑 B(图 114-11),髓过氧化物酶和 α-萘基丁酸盐染色阴性,而 PAS 和酸性磷酸酶可能是阳性的,通常是弥漫的斑点状图案。然而,组织化学染色是非诊断性的,确诊需通过超微结构技术或多种表达在原始细胞表面的血小板抗原(通常是糖蛋白Ⅱb/Ⅲa[CD41]或 von Willebrand 因子)来检测血小板特异性过氧化物酶[121]。因为大多数患者的骨髓网状蛋白增加,使骨髓纤维化和骨穿干抽,诊断有时很难确定。这些患者需要仔细评估外周血细胞。大多数急性骨髓硬化患者实际上可能即为急性巨核细胞白血病,但不应该与原发性骨髓纤维化的晚期相混淆;事实上,显著的脾肿大不是 M7 的临床特征。虽然它是 AML 的一种罕见亚型,大多数研究表明其预后非常差。M7 诱导化疗后骨髓抑制时间往往较长,而且由于骨髓纤维化,通常难以通过重复骨髓穿刺来跟踪治疗结果。对该亚型的细胞遗传学评估相对较少,除了 inv(3)核型和在婴儿中发现的 t(1;22)(p13;q13)[RBM15/*MKL1* 基因融合]的病例外,没有发现其他一致的细胞遗传学异常[122]。

急性全骨髓增生伴骨髓纤维化

这是一种非常罕见的来源于造血干细胞的 AML 亚型,其骨髓表现为网状纤维明显增加,三系造血形态异常,不同数量的具有未成熟髓系免疫表型的原始细胞[123,124]。患者通常出现全血细胞减少症和全身症状。有时全骨髓增生伴骨髓纤维化,与急性巨核细胞白血病伴骨髓纤维化(APMF)或 MDS 伴骨髓纤维化很难区分。APMF 对标准化疗反应不佳。

混合表型白血病

相当数量的急性白血病无法轻易分类,因为白血病细胞可能同时具有淋巴系和髓系的特征。WHO 2008 年统一使用关于造血和淋巴组织分类的专业使用术语"混合表型急性白血病"(MPAL)来涵盖这些异质性肿瘤。MPAL 的白血病细胞在细胞化学或免疫表型上同时具有髓系和淋巴系的特征(双表型),或者存在两种不同的白血病细胞群:髓系和淋巴系(双系列)。双表型和双系列之间的差异通常不会改变诊断治疗方法。尽管之前使用了诸如 EGIL(欧洲急性白血病免疫学表征组)之类的系统[125],但最近的分类基于 2008 年 WHO 白血病专题[126]。这些疾病往往具有急性 B 淋巴细胞白血病(B-ALL)与急性髓细胞性白血病(AML)的特征,或急性 T 淋巴细胞白血病(T-ALL)与急性髓细胞性白血病(AML)的特征,因此分别被命名为 B-髓系疾病或 T-髓系疾病。如果存在已知的重现性遗传病变,例如费城染色体阳性白血病,MLL 重排白血病或 AML 定义性的平衡易位如 t(8;21),则具有来自两系的证据的白血病需特殊指明。从技术上讲,MPAL 还排除了继发性白血病,伴有 *FGFR1* 突变的白血病,和急变期的 CML[127]。

MPAL 的基本特征是某些谱系定义性标记在两个类别中的特定表达。尽管该方式稍微复杂,但 CD3 表达是 T 淋巴细胞来源的证据,CD19 与一个或两个其他标记共同提示 B 淋巴细胞来源。髓系来源可以通过一组单核细胞免疫表型标记或最常见的髓过氧化物酶表达来确定。ALL 中具有特征性的表现 TdT;然而,25%的 AML 患者也表达 TdT,所以并不能认为它是谱系定义性的异常。值得一提的是,许多 AML 可以通过流式细胞术检测到淋巴系抗原,但不符合双表型白血病的诊断标准,此类病例应在 AML 预后和治疗评价中予以考虑[127]。

MPAL 的治疗没有清晰一致的指南。比较特殊的是 *BCR-ABL* 阳性白血病,其应通过化疗和酪氨酸激酶抑制剂联合治疗。大多数其他 MPAL 应该应用 ALL 治疗方案,而对于显著表达髓过氧化物酶或甚至存在 Auer 小体的患者则存在争议。联合 AML 和 ALL 的治疗方案也是可行的,但可能比更典型的 ALL 方案毒性更大。鉴于 MPAL 的相对原发耐药的特性,异体造血干细胞移植可作为缓解后的巩固治疗。

临床症状和体征

AML 患者通常表现出与全血细胞减少有关的症状,包括虚弱,易疲劳,不同程度的感染,出血,如齿龈出血、瘀斑、鼻衄或月经过多等。少数患者出现明显的髓外症状,表现为皮肤或牙龈浸润。成年 AML 患者很少发生骨痛,但部分患者会感觉胸骨不适或压痛,偶尔伴有长骨,尤其是下肢骨痛。AML 的起病时间难以确切判断,因为个体就医的症状阈值不同。大多数患者在诊断之前数周,甚至数月内即出现不易察觉的白血病证状。

体格检查表现多种多样,且没有特异性状。如果有发热症状,须积极寻找感染部位,并使用广谱抗生素进行经验性治疗。大部分患者发热仅与白血病疾病本身有关,且随着白血病治疗而好转。皮肤查体可发现苍白、浸润性结节,可能是原发性或栓塞性的皮肤感染,或最常见的与血小板减少和/或凝血功能障碍有关的瘀点或瘀斑。眼底检查发现大多数患者存在出血和/或渗出(参见"眼科并发症"的部分)。根据贫血的严重程度,结膜可表现为不同程度的苍白。由于白血病浸润的概率很低,因此仔细检查口咽和牙齿尤为重要。AML 患者很少有可触及的淋巴结,并且明显的淋巴结肿大更为罕见。同样,肝脾肿大并不常见,如果出现,可能提示急性淋巴细胞白血病或慢性髓细胞性白血病急变期。以上发现都不是诊断依据,最终的诊断和分类取决于外周血和骨髓的检查。

成功治疗 AML 需要严格的化疗,应特别注意可能使患者治疗复杂化的其他医学问题。充血性心力衰竭或其他心脏病的病史可能会影响蒽环类药物的应用,而且因为诱导治疗导致的全血细胞减少会持续 3~4 周,期间需要大量静脉输液,包括抗生素,红细胞和血小板输注,肾毒性抗菌药物时水化,以及肠外营养,这时必须密切监测患者情况。既往的输血史或多次妊娠可以导致血小板输注困难或红细胞或血小板输血反应。对可能的药物过敏进行仔细评估,因为几乎每个患者都需要抗生素治疗。单纯疱疹病毒感染史(抗体滴度升高)的患者需预防性应用阿昔洛韦[128]。绝经前妇女需使用 GNRH 激动剂或雌激素和/或孕激素化合物抑制月经,直至血小板减少恢复为止。应与有需求的患者讨论保留生育能力的事宜。尽管许多患者在诊断时是低精子症或无精子症。渴望有家庭的男性应该考虑精子冻存,通过在化疗期间抑制垂体-卵巢轴,GNRH 拮抗治疗可以保留具有生育潜力的女性的生育能力[129]。

一旦确诊(表 114-3),医护人员必须向患者及其家属介绍治疗目标和副作用。这种讨论可以强化几乎所有患者对治疗的短期和长期的潜在获益的认识。患者住院期间与其重复此讨论和咨询是合适和必要的。一般而言,对于年轻患者,适合诱导治疗随后强化化疗和/或同种异体移植进行缓解后治疗。对于年龄较大的患者(>60~65 岁),可能会从标准的,更激进的方法中获益,但必须与患者及家属讨论去甲基化药物的治疗。

表 114-3 初始诊断评级

病史和体格检查要全面,重点放在以下方面:
• 症状持续时间
• 月经史
• 以前妊娠史,输血反应史
• 药物过敏(抗生素)
• 感染部位:直肠、阴道、口咽部、牙龈、皮肤
• 出现体征
• 髓外白血病体征——皮肤、牙龈
• 牙齿情况
骨穿和骨髓活检
• 形态学
• 细胞化学
• 免疫分型
• 细胞遗传学
• TdT
• 基因组研究
血生化
• 血尿素氮、肌酐、电解质,尿酸
• 转氨酶,碱性磷酸酶,胆红素,LDH,钙,磷
凝血
• PT,APTT,纤维蛋白原、纤维蛋白降解产物
胸片,ECG,左室射血分数(必要时)
HLA 配型(患者和家属);淋巴细胞毒(抗-HLA)抗体筛查
单纯疱疹病毒和巨细胞病毒血清学检测
腰锥穿刺(仅在有症状时做)

HLA,人类白细胞抗原。

治疗:概述

传统上,AML 的治疗分为以下阶段:诱导,缓解后治疗以及后复发治疗。初诊的 AML 诱导治疗的目标是获得 CR,然后给予旨在最大化多数患者的无病生存和治愈率的后续治疗。完全缓解的定义主要根据形态学标准,包括:原始细胞的骨髓小于 5%,无髓外白血病,中性粒细胞(>1 500/μl)和血小板(>150 000/μl)。即使骨髓原始细胞<5%,但可见到白血病的典型形态学特征,例如 Auer 小体,这种情况不能定义为 CR。血红蛋白没有恢复正常以及存在与白血病无关的症状不能作为判断 CR 依据,因为它们通常与治疗相关,并且会逐渐恢复正常。

目前假说认为,细胞毒性化疗显著减少了白血病克隆的细胞数量,进而残存的正常造血祖细胞重建增殖受抑的骨髓,最终骨髓达到 CR。观察结果也证实了这一解释,即在缓解的患者中无法检测到原始白血病细胞中存在的细胞遗传学异常。然而,在一些患者中,强化化疗似乎解除了分化阻滞,使得 CR 期间在骨髓和外周血中看到的似乎正常的细胞实际上是白血病克隆产生的后代[130,131]。X 染色体连锁多态性(葡萄糖-6-磷酸脱氢酶同工酶或限制性片段长度多态性)或在 CR 期间正常细胞仍存在疾病特异性的突变证明了这一点[132]。这种"克隆性 CR"的发生频率、可能与特定 AML 亚型相关性、缓解时间、生物学机制等重要的检测技术问题需要进一步研究确定。

诱导治疗：一般原则

诱导治疗目的是快速清除外周血中的白血病细胞，进而导致骨髓抑制。但是急性早幼粒细胞白血病患者（FAB M3）比较特殊，尽管白血病细胞形态学上持续 2~3 周后仍能实现缓解[133]，因此，特别是考虑到基于维 A 酸/亚砷酸的应用，急性早幼粒细胞白血病不需要多次骨髓穿刺。标准诱导治疗（所谓的"3+7"；3 日多蒽环类药物，通常是柔红霉素和 7 日连续输注阿糖胞苷）后大约 1 周（通常在治疗开始后 2 周），需进行骨髓穿刺和活检以评估细胞杀伤的程度。如果骨髓增生明显减低，则需要等待细胞计数恢复。如果骨髓增生并不减低，且第 14 日的骨髓中仅见到白血病细胞，则通常实施第二疗程的化疗。如果使用基于 HiDAC 的方案作为诱导化疗，则不建议进行多次骨髓穿刺。

有时，特别是"第 14 日"骨髓是低增生性的，则可能难以区分残存的白血病细胞和正常的未分化的造血祖细胞。在这种情况下，建议延迟再化疗并在几天内复查骨髓穿刺。如果没有进一步成熟的证据，则提示进行第二疗程的化疗。如果出现红系前体细胞，幼稚巨核细胞或外周血血小板或中性粒细胞计数增加，需延迟第二疗程，因为这是骨髓再生正在进行。应用标准治疗方案，大约 30% 的 AML 患者需要两个疗程才能获得缓解。尽管如此，进行第二疗程化疗的指征，仍然存在相当大的多变性和不确定性。

大多数试验以 CR 或无反应来判断疗效。然而，将预后因素研究或评估不同方案的细胞毒活性的失败原因严格分类，对提高缓解率很有益处。比如将无反应者分为以下几种情况：明显的化疗耐药的白血病，因患者死亡时骨髓增生仍低下以致无法确定对化疗的反应，以及那些早期死亡，死亡前未能获得足够的骨髓标本，而无法确定白血病是否持续存在。耐药白血病患者包括治疗中存活下来的患者和那些在骨髓或外周血中有白血病形态学证据但已死亡的患者。尽管获得 CR 的中位时间通常在治疗开始后的 30~35 日，患者达到足够水平的外周血中性粒细胞（>500/μl）且不再需要血小板输注（计数为 10~20 000/μl）一般至少提前 7~10 日，这可能有利于筛选新型和/或非细胞毒药物。其他类型的缓解包括部分缓解（骨髓原始细胞减少 50% 且正常细胞计数恢复），CRp（与 CR 相同，但血小板未完全恢复），CRi（与 CR 相同，但中性粒细胞计数低）和无形态学白血病状态（<5% 骨髓原始细胞，但正常细胞计数未恢复）。这种分类在大多数患者中相对简单，可以有助于区分由于耐药和支持治疗不足引起的失败[2,133]。

在大型协作组研究中，标准化疗的 CR 率约为 65%。患者年龄和细胞遗传学是最关键的临床变量，年轻患者的 CR 率为 75%~80%，60 岁以上约为 50%。治疗失败的原因根据患者年龄而异。随着支持治疗的提高，50 岁以下的患者死于化疗并发症的情况并不常见，大约 25% 的诱导失败率是白血病细胞耐药所致。相比之下，在>60 岁的患者中，诱导治疗失败是由于白血病细胞耐药和终末器官耐受性降低导致骨髓抑制期死亡，两者整体发生率分别为 40% 和 10%。

尽管在过去的 25 年中，全世界年轻的 AML 患者的 CR 率逐渐提高，这主要归功于更好的支持治疗而不是治疗方案的改变。除了急性早幼粒细胞白血病应用维 A 酸和亚砷酸外（见下文），自从开始柔红霉素和阿糖胞苷联合诱导治疗方案（即所谓的"7 和 3"方案）应用以来，急性髓细胞性白血病治疗方法的改变相对较少[134]。这种双药组合来自对两者单药活性的观察。柔红霉素通常以 45~90mg/(m^2·d) 的剂量静脉输注，应用 3 日；阿糖胞苷以 100~200mg/(m^2·d) 的剂量连续输注 7 日（表 114-4）。癌症和白血病协作组 B（CALGB）的一系列随机研究显示[134~140]：

表 114-4　急性髓细胞性白血病的代表性化疗方案

	剂量	给药方式	天数
诱导			
阿糖胞苷	100~200mg/m^2	持续 IV	1~7
柔红霉素	45~60mg/m^2	IV	1~3
或 伊达比星	12mg/m^2	IV	1~3
或 米托蒽醌	12mg/m^2	IV	1~3
缓解后			
阿糖胞苷	3g/m^2q12h(>3h)	IV(6 次)	1,3,5
或 阿糖胞苷	1.5 ~ 2g/m^2q12h(>1h)	IV(8 次)	1~4(12 次)
或 阿糖胞苷	100mg/m^2	持续 IV	1~5

有关不同方案的课程数量和患者选择的详细信息，请参阅文本。

1. 7 和 3 方案的临床结果优于 5 日阿糖胞苷和 2 日柔红霉素。

2. 在 7 和 3 方案中加入口服 6-硫鸟嘌呤（DAT 方案）并未增加 CR 率。

3. 与柔红霉素联合使用时，持续输注阿糖胞苷的效果略好于每日两次短期静脉输注。

4. 与 7 日相比，阿糖胞苷持续输注 10 日并未改善治疗效果。

5. 多柔比星替代柔红霉素几乎达到相同的 CR 率，但多柔比星的黏膜毒性更高。

6. 将阿糖胞苷的剂量从 100mg/(m^2·d) 增加到 200mg/(m^2·d) 没有整体获益。

7 和 3 方案的其他调整

大多数改善 3+7 诱导方案的尝试都没有增加总体生存率。一些临床试验应用了其他蒽环类药物如米托蒽醌（mitoxantrone）、佐柔比星（rubidazone）、阿柔比星（aclacinomycin）、安吖啶（amsacrine）和伊达比星（idarubicin）[141~145]。这些研究均未证实这些不同药物能提高生存或 DFS 优势，可能是因为这些药物在结构和作用机制方面相对类似，因此易受相同的耐药机制的影响。伊达比星的临床试验规模是迄今为止最大的，其中三项初步试验显示伊达比星诱导治疗达到了至少与柔红霉素和阿糖胞苷相当的结果[142,144]。一项重要的随机试验表明，与柔红霉素相比，伊达比星在老年患者中没有显示出优势[146]。此外，伊达比星组的骨髓抑制持续时间更长，这使人质疑两组细胞毒性相同的结论。因此，这些替代性的药物不能提高 AML 患者的长期无病生存率。

一项澳大利亚试验在 3+7 方案中联合了依托泊苷[147]。接受依托泊苷治疗的老年患者的 CR 率与柔红霉素和阿糖胞苷组相似，仅轻度延长了年轻患者 CR 的持续时间。这是一项规模相对较小的研究，在诱导和缓解后治疗期间接受依托泊苷治疗的患者的整体无病生存率与其他大型研究中仅使用柔红霉素和阿糖胞苷的疗效相似[148]。

CALGB 的大型Ⅰ期研究表明，依托泊苷联合 3+7 方案的临床结果，与仅使用两种药物的疗效相似。

由于 HiDAC 在缓解后治疗中具有优势（见下文），一些研究小组已经在年轻患者的诱导治疗期间加用 HiDAC。研究比较了标准 3+7 方案与柔红霉素联合中或高剂量阿糖胞苷（2~3g/m^2，8~12 个剂量）进行了比较[149~151]。尽管一项研究记录了随机分配到 HiDAC 组的患者的 CR 持续时间更长（但总生存没有变化），但这些研究未能证实 HiDAC 组的 CR 率的提高[149]。也有研究比较了诱导治疗期间在标准柔红霉素/阿糖胞苷基础上联合 HiDAC。一项小型试验显示，60 岁以下患者的缓解率为 87%[152]，但是一项协作性研究未能证实该结果[153]。临床试验结果表明，HiDAC 在诱导治疗和在巩固治疗中应用疗效相似[154]。

新的诱导治疗策略

虽然 3+7 的策略仍然是标准治疗方案，但新的数据表明，许多患者（可能所有 65 岁以下的患者）柔红霉素的剂量应该超过既往使用的 45mg/m^2。ECOG1900 研究将患者随机分配至 45mg/(m^2·d)或 90mg/(m^2·d)的柔红霉素共 3 日，结果发现高剂量组延长了大多数亚组（甚至是高白细胞或随访时间较长的 FLT3ITD 患者）的生存期[155]。一项针对欧洲老年人的类似设计的研究也表明，至少在 60~65 岁之间的患者，每日 90mg/m^2 的剂量优于 45mg/m^2[156]。英国的一项研究报告指出 60mg/m^2 与 90mg/m^2 同样有效[157]。如上所述，在 3+7 基础上联用其他药物或用 HiDAC 替代 3+7 标准连续输注阿糖胞苷的研究并未增加总生存。然而，波兰急性白血病研究小组研究显示，克拉屈滨（cladribine）联合蒽环类/阿糖胞苷优于 3+7 方案[158]；然而，该研究中年轻成人的对照组的 CR 率低于预期，这些结果需要其他研究证实。MD 安德森教授癌症中心的非随机 2 期研究应用持续输注 HiDAC 和伊达比星方案，取得了较好的结果[159]。一项法国试验中老年人可从 CCNU 联合 3+7 方案中获益[160]。FLAGIDA 方案虽然用药密集且毒副作用大，但是却有高 CR 率和无病生存率[161]。另一种可能与 3+7 基础方案联合的药物是吉姆单抗/奥佐米星（gemtuzumab ozogamicin，GO），它是一种针对表达于大多数 AML 原始细胞上的 CD33 抗原的抗体毒素偶联物；它最初被批准作为复发性老年 AML[162] 的单药治疗，然后在随机试验中比较标准诱导治疗联合或不联合 GO 显示出了边际效益和/或模棱两可的结果，因此撤市[163]。然而，法国[164] 和英国[165] 的试验表明，标准化疗联合相对小剂量的 GO 可能使 70 岁以下的 AML 获益。直到撰写本文时，该药仍未重新进入市场；虽然具有预后良好的染色体异常的患者从中获益较多，但仍需要在北美进行验证性试验，以证明常规使用这种药物是有益的[166]。

老年患者和其他不良预后亚组的治疗方法

对于几乎没有机会获得长期益处的患者，应用 3+7 诱导方法进行细胞毒性化疗是否值得？对于 60~65 岁以上的老年患者，以及一些诊断时已知，预后较差的单倍体核型[54] 或 *p53* 突变[17] 的年轻患者的治疗，仍是一个主要的讨论和争议的话题。具有已知不良预后特征的年轻成人，目前似乎很少采用 3+7 或类似方案诱导治疗，随后缓解后治疗，进而进行同种异体造血干细胞移植。如果没有兄弟姐妹供体、相合的非亲缘供体或“有利的”部分不相合的非亲缘供体，那么这些情况应首先考虑单倍体相同或脐带血干细胞移植（SCT）。在这种情况下，化疗耐药程度是非常严重的，即使异体移植的结果仍然相对较差，但比基于化疗的缓解后治疗方法略好[17]。

与标准 3+7 方案相比，应用低剂量化疗初始治疗可能会使一些老年人获益更多。多数患者的标准化疗中柔红霉素剂量应≥60mg/m^2。相反，特别是当存在不良预后因素时，可以考虑应用诸如去甲基化药物-阿扎胞苷或地西他滨的低剂量化疗，或在临床试验中合理应用毒性稍高的单药治疗氯法拉滨。虽然老年人有许多预后评估方法，但通常认为从 3+7 为基础的化疗获益可能性较低的特征是在氯法拉滨Ⅱ期临床试验[167] 中应用的一些因素，包括年龄>70 岁，既往血液学异常，合并疾病，不良细胞遗传学。一项 2 期试验应用 30mg/m^2 的氯法拉滨共 5 日，达到了 35%的 CR 率，并有 10%的毒性相关死亡。部分是因为“不适合强化治疗”的患者难以定义，该试验未获得美国食品药品管理局（FDA）的批准。一项 ECOG 主导的大型Ⅲ期试验中正在评估氯法拉滨在这个年龄段与 3+7 方案相比的疗效。

在欧洲，对于被认为不适合或至少“不适合”标准诱导化疗的患者，低剂量阿糖胞苷是另一种常用的选择。低剂量阿糖胞苷似乎比羟基脲效果略好[168]，但美国很少使用。两项重要的试验比较了去甲基化药物与老年 AML 患者常用的其他疗法。一项此类试验比较了地西他滨与低剂量阿糖胞苷或支持治疗，CR 率达到 25%[169]。虽然欧洲批准了地西他滨用于老年 AML 患者的初始治疗，但其在美国尚未获得批准，主要是因为关键性试验并没有达到延长总生存的主要研究终点。一项试验初步结果表明，对于白细胞计数小于 15 000/μl 的 AML 患者，5-阿扎胞苷与常规治疗方案相比，虽然并未达到主要研究终点，但是，5-阿扎胞苷仍是低剂量阿糖胞苷或支持治疗的可行替代方案[170]。然而，应该强调的是，应用去甲基化药物和低剂量阿糖胞苷的 CR 率远低于标准化疗，并且较低强度的治疗方法仅在低增生的 AML 患者中得到评估。如果这些治疗方法用于高外周血原始细胞计数或高骨髓原始细胞浸润的患者，结果可能比上述结果的更差。因此，理想情况下，在临床试验的背景下，3+7 的诱导方案应该是 75 岁以下相对适合的老年人的默认化疗方案。

应用去甲基化剂药物治疗的患者应该与接受此类药物的 MDS 相同的方式进行管理。患者应每 4~6 周持续接受去甲基化剂药物的治疗,直至出现细胞毒性反应或明显进展。当然,长期使用这些药物有利于实现相对良好的长期效果。如果患者取得了非常好的结果,例如应用去甲基化药物后达到 CR,那么 75 岁以下的老年人,则可以考虑进行非清髓性的异基因造血干细胞移植[171]。这种情况通常只应用于选择或正在接受强化疗方案的人群,但接受较低强度化疗方案的患者也应该考虑[172]。

缓解后治疗

CR 的形态学评估是主观的,且相对不敏感。更好地定量 CR 时仍存在的白血病细胞[微小残留病(minimal resisual desease,MRD)]可以将患者分成不同的预后亚组。据估计,具有明显形态学 CR 的患者中仍可残留多达 10^9 个白血病细胞。只有少数患者的 CR 状态可以在没有进一步治疗的情况下持续 1~2 年,但普遍认为获得 CR 后仍需要某种形式的治疗才能实现长期无病生存。在德国白血病协作组进行的一项试验中,37 名患者由于各种协议和医学原因未接受缓解后治疗,这些患者后来均全部复发[173]。ECOG 报告了一项随机研究,其中达到 CR 的患者被随机分为无治疗组,低剂量维持治疗组或缓解后高强度方案[174]。无治疗组的所有患者均迅速复发,中位 CR 持续时间为 4 个月,导致该试验组提前终止。Embury 等报告的一项较小的随机研究中也证实了类似的结果[175]。如果在诱导后早期恢复阶段,患者接受额外化疗,即使不接受缓解后化疗也可以延长缓解的持续时间[176,177],但这种治疗方案更类似于巩固治疗。因此,常规方案达到缓解后应用化疗(有或没有后续造血干细胞移植)仍然是标准治疗方案。

年轻的成年人通常接受以治愈为目标的治疗,应接受缓解后化疗,包括强化(或骨髓抑制性的)"巩固"化疗和/或造血干细胞移植。"维持治疗"通常指间歇性给予数月至数年的低剂量门诊治疗,与儿童 ALL 成功使用的模式相似,但这种方法尚未明确证实对 AML 患者适用。

多种药物已经用于缓解后治疗,包括在初始诱导中成功施用的药物,特别是作为巩固治疗的 HiDAC,以及不同类别的化合物,其中一些已经证实在 AML 中有效,而其他药物则疗效有限。因为各种预后因素显著影响最终结果,且与应用的治疗方案无关,小的非随机研究中的良好结果可能反映了患者选择偏倚,所以最终必须通过多中心研究证实。

总体而言,接受某种形式的缓解后强化化疗后,成人 AML 患者的中位 CR 持续时间为 12~18 个月,其中 20%~25%的 CR 患者可达到长期无病生存(图 114-10)。对已达到 CR 的 CALGB 患者进行的大量回顾性研究显示,CR 后的前 6 个月,每月复发率相对恒定为 4.7%。在随后的 6 个月间隔中复发率出现下降趋势(第 7~12 个月每月 3.5%,第 13~16 个月每月 2.4%),CR 3 年后曲线达到平台期[178]。一般情况下,与晚期复发的患者相比,早期复发的患者的白血病细胞更加耐药[179]。CALGB 早期进行的缓解后治疗的随机试验:①隔月治疗与每月维持治疗方案相比;②3 年相对低剂量的维持治疗与 8 个月相比(实际上,8 个月后停止治疗的患者存在一定程度的生存优势);③维持治疗期间阿糖胞苷的剂量从 100mg/m² 加倍至 200mg/m²;④维持治疗联合甲醇可提取的结肠杆菌(MER)残留物形式的非特异性免疫疗法。发现以上变化对长期疗效无影响。有关维持化疗的作用,较早的 ECOG 研究表明,DAT(柔红霉素、阿糖胞苷、硫鸟嘌呤)两个疗程后,继续 2 年的维持治疗并无获益[180]。德国 Buchner 等人报道的研究[181,182]显示,虽然对长期存活率的影响仍是未知数,但是在缓解后一个疗程 DAT 后,长期维持治疗一定程度延长了 CR 持续时间。后续研究显示在维持之前使用了更强烈的缓解后巩固治疗,这时维持治疗的效果较弱[181,182]。

两项重要的随机试验表明,年轻患者缓解后应用 HiDAC 优于低剂量[183]。ECOG 研究中,与接受 2 年低剂量维持治疗的患者相比,随机接受一次高强度的缓解后 HiDAC 巩固治疗的患者,缓解的中位持续时间更长[183]。CALGB 研究中,596 例 CR 的 AML 患者均接受四个疗程的阿糖胞苷治疗,并随机分为以下三种不同的剂量水平:100mg/m² 连续静脉输注(CIV)5 日,400mg/m² 静脉输注 5 日,3g/m² 静脉注射 3h,在第 1、3 和 5 日每 12h 一次(总共六个剂量/疗程)。年龄>60 岁的患者未显示从高剂量组获益,CR 的中位持续时间约为 13 个月,长期无病生存率仅为 10%~12%[184]。此外,老年患者中枢神经系统毒性的发生率较高,主要表现为小脑功能障碍。其他研究也未能证实老年患者可以从较高剂量的阿糖胞苷获益[185]。相比之下,小于 60 岁的患者在无复发生存和总生存方面均从 HiDAC 方案中获益匪浅。小于 40 岁的患者的长期效应与接受自体或异体骨髓移植(BMT)者相似。

这些研究强烈支持年轻的 AML 患者使用 HiDAC 的巩固治疗。目前尚不清楚 HiDAC 的疗程数,最佳剂量和安排,以及联合其他药物能否改善这些结果。结合到 DNA 中的阿糖胞苷可能的最大剂量为 1~1.5g/m²。最近完成的英国随机研究表明,1.5g/m² 的剂量与最初 CALGB 应用的 3g/m² 相比总生存相同[186]。在另一项随机研究中,应用其他潜在非交叉耐药的药物方案替代 HiDAC,结果并不优于三个周期的 HiDAC 治疗[187]。英国医学研究委员会(MRC)的研究证实,多个疗程的缓解后治疗使用各种不同的药物,其总体结果与 HiDAC 类似[188,189]。CALGB 数据表明,在预后良好的细胞遗传学患者中[t(8;21)和 inv(16)]HiDAC 的获益最为明显,而在通常与耐药有关的核型不良的患者中效果则要小得多[77]。如果化疗可行,大多数临床医生应尝试应用至少三个疗程基于 HiDAC 的缓解后治疗方案。由于异体造血干细胞移植目前正变得越来越普遍,基于 HiDAC 的缓解后治疗最适于年轻的 inv16,t(8;21)的患者或具有正常细胞遗传学且 *NPM1* 突变但没有 *FLT3ITD* 突变的患者[9]。

关于缓解后使用何种治疗类型必须考虑患者的医疗状况,诱导期间可能发生获得性持续感染(特别是真菌感染),以及提供足够的血小板输血治疗,以尽量平衡强化后缓解治疗的优势与风险。根据巩固方案的强度,尽管巩固治疗后使用髓系生长因子可明显缩短严重中性粒细胞减少的持续时间,并可能使这种疗法更安全[190,191],预计 CR 后的死亡率为 5%,这点必须仔细向患者解释。

在 AML 中替代高剂量化疗的方法是自体造血干细胞移植。冷冻保存的自体骨髓可以迅速重建接受清髓治疗患者的骨髓,尽管与异基因造血干细胞移植相比,骨髓恢复时间可能会延迟[192]。与骨髓相比,应用细胞因子动员的外周血干细胞(PBSC)的中性粒细胞减少,以及血小板减少的持续时间缩短[193]。自体移植耐受性良好,可以很容易地用于65岁甚至年龄更大的患者。其主要缺点包括无移植物抗白血病效应,以及仍具活性的白血病祖细胞将与自体干细胞同时植入患者体内。目前已应用了大量新涌现的技术,包括针对髓系原始细胞的单克隆抗体,以及将骨髓与高浓度细胞毒性药物一起孵育[192],最大限度保留造血祖细胞(尽管骨髓延迟重建并不罕见)[193]。目前还不清楚这些体外处理是否有益。回顾性比较表明,在高剂量巩固治疗后仍未清髓情况下富集自体造血干细胞,其复发率并未增加。许多中心和小组报道了首次CR时自体造血干细胞移植无复发生存率>40%[194,195,196]。历史上,自体干细胞移植经验显示复发率约为50%,这可能是最好的自体移植结果。该方法的其他潜在证据来自AML患者[192]第二次和第三次移植的治愈率为20%的报告[192]。

异基因造血干细胞移植是年轻患者缓解后治疗的主要替代治疗选择,并且在高度选择的老年患者中越来越多地应用非清髓性造血干细胞移植。同卵双胞胎作为供者的同源造血干细胞移植[197],以及HLA相合的同胞作为供者的异基因造血干细胞移植[198],首先在晚期难治性AML患者中评估使用。在证实该难治性患者的长期无病生存率约为10%,并且首次缓解后接受同源移植的患者的无病生存率达到40%~50%后,AML患者首次缓解后异基因造血干细胞移植的研究陆续开展[199]。早期的小规模研究证明异基因造血干细胞移植复发率低,大部分死亡与急性和慢性移植物抗宿主病(GVHD)的并发症有关。随着目前支持治疗的进步,特别是新型GVHD预防性及治疗性的策略的应用,异基因造血干细胞移植更安全,更常用[200,201]。

20世纪90年代,一些大型前瞻性试验"遗传地"将具有HLA相合同胞的患者分配到异体造血干细胞移植(通常仅在≤45岁的患者中),同时将其他患者随机分配至自体造血干细胞移植或化疗[188,202]。这些试验中的第一个纳入了422例<45岁患者(中位年龄33岁),异基因造血干细胞移植(预计4年为55%)和自体造血干细胞移植(48%)患者的无病生存率相似,且优于接受第二次中剂量阿糖胞苷和胺苯吖啶巩固化疗组(30%)[202]。总生存期是相似的,因为许多化疗后复发的患者可以成功再次诱导,然后在第二次CR中接受造血干细胞移植。许多患者没有接受随机治疗,也没有提供关于不同细胞遗传学风险组中三种治疗的反应的信息。

在法国进行的另一项类似设计的试验显示任何类型的造血干细胞移植并不优于接受强化缓解后化疗的患者[203]。在德国进行的一项大型研究显示作为巩固治疗组成部分的自体移植没有益处。在英国进行的MRC10试验[188]显示自体造血干细胞移植是有益的。未接受异基因造血干细胞移植的患者接受三个周期的CR后化疗,然后随机分为非清髓自体造血干细胞移植或观察组。自体造血干细胞移植延长了CR持续时间,但两组之间的总生存没显著差异。异基因造血干细胞移植并不显著优于自体造血干细胞移植;在不同的细胞遗传学风险组中,没有一种方式明显优于另一种方式。更新了的MRC试验意向性分析了有或无匹配的同胞供者的患者的结果[189]。同样,对于有供者并进行移植的患者,移植与化疗相比无明显的生存获益,并且有供者的患者移植与否之间亦无优劣之分。

组织实施的试验[204]意向性分析发现,化疗至少与自体或异基因造血干细胞移植具有同样的治愈效果。与所有其他研究一样,许多分配到造血干细胞移植模式的患者由于各种原因未接受这种治疗。关于异基因造血干细胞移植在首次CR患者AML治疗中的作用,可以得出一些一般性结论:

1. 该技术的适用性在某种程度上受到患者的年龄限制。GVHD的死亡率以每十年计逐渐增高。随着支持治疗的进步,以及应用非清髓预处理方案的减低强度的移植和外周血干细胞移植的逐年增加,老年人移植的应用越来越多。非清髓方法显著降低早期副作用,并且在大多数老年患者中可行[205]。一项系统的前瞻性研究表明,由于临床、管理和供体可获得性的问题,只有一小部分首次CR的老年患者能够进行移植[206]。尽管如此,由于老年人接受化疗效果较差,且减低强度的异基因造血干细胞移植效果较好(至少对那些成功进行移植的患者(35%的无病生存)),因此一般认为75岁以下的成年人接受异基因造血干细胞移植是可行的。

2. 有合适的HLA相合的家庭供者的潜在受者不到1/3。替代方案包括使用相合的无关供者,部分不相合的家庭供者,半相合供者或脐带血。尽管世界范围内有数百万HLA型捐献者,但确定合适供者仍然存在监管方面的延误[207]。对于具有不常见HLA类型的少数族裔患者尤其如此,并且在无关供者移植的报道中存在相当大的选择偏倚,因为一些高风险的患者在等待供者时复发。尽管如此,通过使用分子组织相容性分型,非亲缘异基因移植与同胞相合移植的疗效相当。这一技术扩大了异基因造血干细胞移植的应用范围,可以让更多的AML患者在首次缓解时移植[208,209]。脐带血可能是没有相合的同胞或无关供者患者的干细胞替代来源。即使许多移植来自不相合的供者,脐带血移植后GVHD的发生率要低得多。然而,尽管使用双脐带移植有助于解决成年接受者剂量的问题[210,211],但移植仍然会因此延迟。目前,来自部分匹配的同胞,父母或孩子的半相合移植复发率虽然可能高于全相合供者,但几乎所有受者都可以得到合适的供者[212]。

3. 虽然异基因造血干细胞移植可以治愈一些化疗耐药的患者,但复发仍客观存在。一些化疗后耐药和复发的因素也适用于造血干细胞移植患者[213,214]。

4. 由于移植物的抗白血病效应,造血干细胞移植后的抗白血病作用与GVHD的发生和严重程度相关。通过各种免疫抑制方法减弱GVHD减少了GVHD的发生,但也增加了疾病复发风险[215]。相关研究正在评估选择性T细胞耗竭方法和移植物的其他免疫操作方法,以使造血干细胞移植更安全且不增加复发风险[216,217]。

5. 由于慢性GVHD,多达10%~20%的幸存患者可能有明显的症状和体力状态受损。长期存活者中继发性肿瘤的发生率也略有增加[218]。

CBF细胞遗传学异常患者应用基于大剂量阿糖胞苷的缓解后治疗方案,根据诊断时的分子或核型确定的预后不良的患者采用异基因造血干细胞移植,这种方法的适用性目前已达成共识。然而,中度风险特别是染色体正常的患者的治疗仍然存在争议。荟萃分析表明,一般所有存在不良细胞遗传学的患者应用造血干细胞移植的方法疗效稍好一些[219~221]。中等预后组中唯一不明确的亚组是具有正常细胞遗传学和*NPM1*突变,

但没有 *FLT3ITD* 突变的亚组。这些患者化疗的存活率更高，并且对于这些患者以及存在预后良好易位的患者，可以在第二次缓解时应用造血干细胞移植。

AML 复发和难治性 AML 的治疗

许多药物单独或联合应用对复发或难治性 AML 有明显活性，包括安吖啶、米托蒽醌、亚胺醌（diaziquone）、伊达比星、氟达拉滨（fludarabine）、2-氯脱氧腺苷（2-chlorodeoxy-adenosine）、依托泊苷、高三尖杉酯碱（homoharringtonine）、托泊替康、卡铂和氯法拉滨。复发患者存在较大的异质性，除了药物外还有许多因素影响疗效[222~224]。诸如：①原发耐药患者普遍疗效较差，尤其是首次 CR 持续时间短、治疗过程中复发的患者；②既往血液病基础上转化的白血病、预后不良核型者容易出现耐药；③二次或多次复发者比首次复发者预后更差、缓解持续时间逐渐缩短。

英国 MRC 的结果，前瞻性地跟踪所有进入诱导性 AML 试验的患者，都支持以上结论[244]。在另一项研究中，首次缓解期大于 18 个月的患者比小于 18 个月的患者再诱导缓解率高，分别为 64%（37/58）和 29%（80/278）。此外，第二次 CR 持续时间前者高于后者，分别为 8 个月和 3 个月。患者年龄和细胞遗传学结果也是重要的预后因素，强调根据Ⅱ期临床研究结果重视患者选择。在没有对照组的临床研究中，疗效差异可能史尤其患者选择而非特定治疗方案的优越性。

复发患者的治疗方案和时机选择应个体化。对初始治疗反应差并伴有并发症的患者，再诱导的强化疗可能使生存期更短。这些患者中有些人经过支持治疗（输注红细胞及血小板、口服羟基脲控制高白和骨痛）可以维持基本的生活质量长达数月之久。但是不能延长生存期。相反，具有初治较长缓解期的年轻患者可以从强化疗后序贯异基因干细胞移植中获益。

白血病复发时患者通常无症状、血象正常，只在骨髓中发现原始细胞增多。除非为了后续骨髓移植做准备，否则没有证据证实理论上认为的应该在肿瘤负荷低的复发早期开始治疗。早期治疗的弊端是再诱导治疗疗效差并且导致并发症和早期死亡率增加，但是如果目标是长期存活（如同种异体干细胞移植），则没有理由延迟治疗。

基本上没有对照试验来指导药物选择，通常是选择既往有效的药物进行再诱导，与某些试验性的新药作比较。如果患者在接受化疗时复发，使用原来的药物进行再次诱导是没有意义的。但是如果最近接受传统剂量阿糖胞苷治疗复发的患者可以选用大剂量阿糖胞苷进行再诱导治疗（2～3g/m² 每 12h 一次，8～12 次），患者可以获得短期缓解，是否长期获益尚不清楚。没有证据证实在实现第二次或第三次缓解的患者进行缓解后治疗是有益的。相反可以使原本没有症状在家的患者接受没有长期益处的化疗。

目前尚不清楚是否应在首次复发时就进行 SCT，还是再诱导达到第二次缓解后再移植。遗憾的是，多数患者无法达到再次缓解，即使缓解也因为出现并发症而无法进行移植。来自西雅图的报告显示：第一次复发进行移植比第二次或多次复发再移植的疗效相似或更好[225]。识别早期复发患者并及时将此类患者转到移植中心常常是一个实际问题。尽管如此，如果有合适的供体，特别是在年轻患者中，最好考虑对早期复发的患者进行同种异体移植。同样的，异基因移植可以使用一些原发性难治性白血病患者的长期存活，因此有必要在诊断时进行患者和亲属的 HLA 配型。但是由于组织分型，捐赠者的鉴定和干细胞采集导致的延迟，对于此类患者进行无关供者移植难度较大。目前，大多数移植中心已建议更多复发的患者首先接受诱导化疗，因为 SCT 作为此类患者的主要治疗效果不佳。由于许多 75 岁以下的患者在 CR1 中进行了同种异体移植，许多出现了复发。同种异体 SCT 后复发特别明显，2 年生存率仅为 7%[226]。一般来说，可以耐受化疗的 BMT 复发患者可以从供体淋巴细胞输注[226]或第二次 BMT[227]中获益。SCT 后复发者可以从诸如针对治疗 AML[228,229] *FLT3ITD* 突变的索拉非尼（sorafenib）或免疫检查点抑制剂[230]中获益。

对于 CR2 的患者进行异基因移植可以增加长期存活概率。因此，对于准备进行异基因移植的复发患者进行再诱导期间需要进行供者查询。对再诱导化疗有反应的患者会对化疗有一定程度的敏感性，预示着能够从异基因移植中获益。

急性早幼粒细胞白血病的治疗

急性早幼粒细胞白血病（APL）的治疗有别于其他类型 AML，因此需要单独论述。从理论上讲，如果白血病祖细胞能够在体外诱导分化，白血病细胞克隆将会失去自我更新的能力而被消除，这种诱导方法比强烈的细胞毒化学疗法副作用更少。除了 HL-60 细胞系和从 APL 患者获得的原代细胞外，其他细胞在体外很难重复诱导体外分化。

进行“分化治疗”的临床试验（如维生素 D 和小剂量阿糖胞苷）很少且结果不甚满意，偶尔 APL 患者接受顺式维 A 酸治疗后出现短期疗效[231]。然而，中国报道的口服维 A 酸 30～90 日分化治疗模式的疗效显著，获得了成功[232]。难治性和初诊的 APL 患者 CR 率超过 80%，且诱导过程中未出现骨髓抑制，通过定期骨髓涂片证实异常早幼粒细胞分化成熟[233,234]。ATRA 治疗后 DIC 快速纠正，血小板输注需求大幅减少。虽然出血性并发症减少，但 20%～30%的患者单独接受维 A 酸治疗时会出现明显的副作用，包括发烧，快速肺功能衰竭，心包和胸腔积液。该综合征可以不伴有白细胞增多且可能致命。最佳治疗是在“ATRA”综合征的最初征兆时及时给予糖皮质激素[235,236]治疗。复发患者可以出现对 ATRA 的耐药，单独应用 ATRA 的患者都会复发。可能的药代动力学机制包括快速诱导的 ATRA 代谢、诱导正常组织中的细胞质中维 A 酸结合蛋白和 ATRA 的结合，使得药物对 APL 细胞的作用减弱[237]。

一经认可 ATRA 在 APL 中的疗效，许多研究开始来确定使用该药的最佳用药方案。在大西洋两岸进行的试验表明，在诱导和缓解后治疗期间，维 A 酸与蒽环类的联合化疗组合优于单独的任何一种药物[85,238]。基于初诊是血小板和白细胞计数的风险评分就来自这些试验的结果，特别是来自西班牙（PETHEMA）的持续研究，表明白细胞计数>10 000/μl 具有最差的长期预后。而白细胞计数<10 000/μl，血小板计数>40 000/μl 具有最佳长期预后[239]。在引入三氧化二砷之前，标准治疗可归纳为蒽环类加 ATRA 的诱导，序贯 2～3 周期的维 A 酸+蒽环类作为巩固。在完成强化化疗后，继续口服抗代谢物和 ATRA 维持

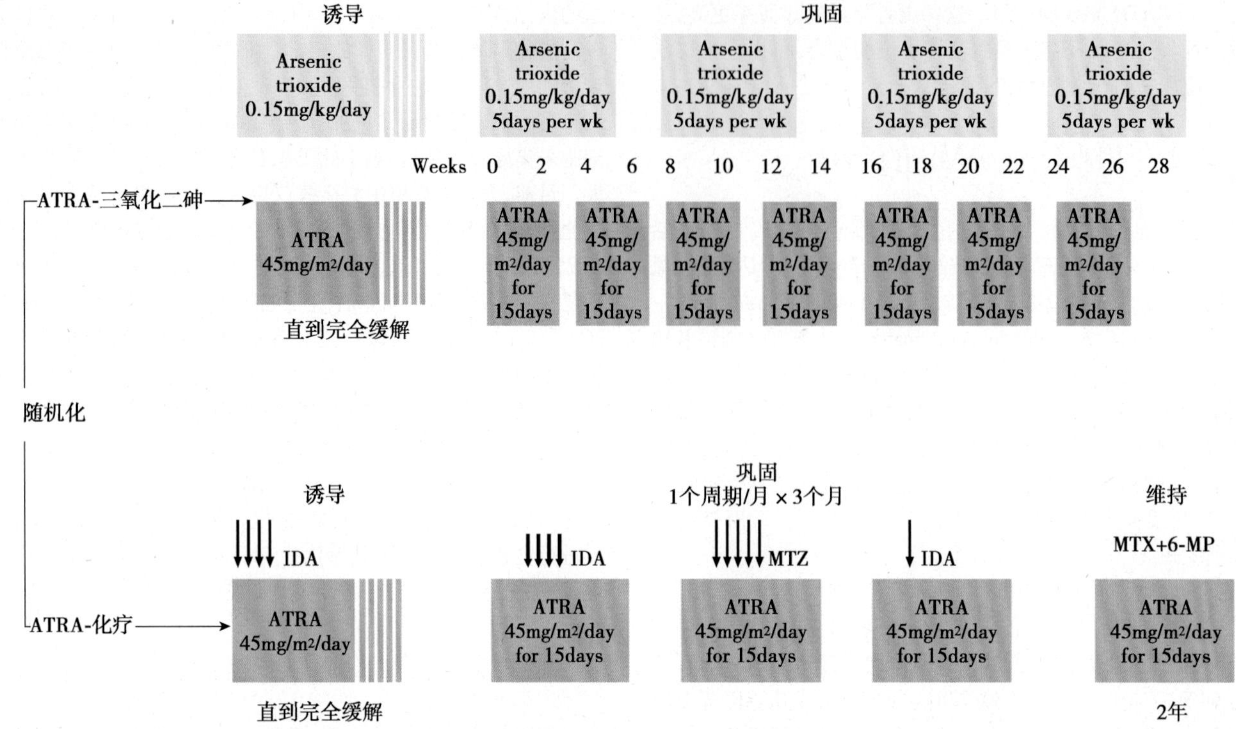

图 114-12 治疗组。在维 A 酸(ATRA)-化疗组中,化疗方案如下:伊达比星(IDA),在第 2,4,6 和 8 日每日 12mg/m^2 体表面积的剂量。诱导期;在第一轮巩固治疗的第 1~4 日,剂量为 5mg/(m^2·d)的 IDA;在第二轮巩固治疗的第 1~5 日,米托蒽醌(MTZ)剂量为 10mg/(m^2·d);在第三周期巩固治疗的第 1 日,IDA 剂量为 12mg/(m^2·d);剂量为 15mg/m^2/周的肌注或口服甲氨蝶呤(MTX)和口服巯嘌呤(6-MP),剂量为 50mg/(m^2·d),与 ATRA 交替,剂量为 45mg/(m^2·d),每 3 个月 15 日,为期 2 年。诱导治疗箱中的垂直线表示缓解诱导治疗持续时间的变化。箭头表示不同化学治疗剂的大致时间和剂量。摘自 Lo-Coco2013[100]。经 NEJM 许可转载

治疗约 1 年,可以增加无病生存和 OS 获益[238]更高剂量的 Ara-C 被认为对白细胞计数>10 000/μl 的高风险人群有益[240]。此外,疾病复发可以在形态学复发之前通过 PCR 测量分子学证据(PML-RARα)来预测[90]。需要通过额外治疗使分子学转阴的患者可以行自体移植挽救治疗,而分子学阳性患者则可以通过异基因移植获益[241]。一些晚期复发是在中枢神经系统[242],所以常规应用预防性鞘内注射,尤其是诊断时白细胞计数高的患者和凝血异常、血小板减少控制后复发的患者。还有一些问题,例如这种强化化疗是否会导致 MDS 和/或继发性白血病[243]。

APL 治疗的新进展又是在中国出现,静脉应用三氧化二砷即使在晚期复发的患者中也会有较高的 CR 率[244],这是对 APL 治疗方法的重大改变。尽管三氧化二砷治疗 APL 确切的特异性作用机制仍待阐明,但可以肯定的是其可以加速 APL 细胞凋亡[245]。近年来,四硫化四砷也被证实对初诊和复发 APL 患者有效,并且具有口服优势[246]。虽然三氧化二砷成为复发性 APL 的标准疗法,但目前常规用于 APL 的诱导和/或缓解后治疗。中国学者证实 ATRA 和三氧化二砷联合诱导治疗可以获得较高的缓解率[247],而来自印度[248]和伊朗[249]的研究报告显示仅在使用三氧化二砷时呈现高分子缓解率。得克萨斯大学安德森癌症医学中心研究组证实,对于不适合联合蒽环类药物为主的双诱导方案中,对于高白细胞和疗效不理想的患者加入 CD33 单抗可以提高无病生存。尽管随访的时间相对较短,其疗效与多个中心研究应用的标准治疗疗效相似[250,251]。

北美洲国际组评估了两个疗程的砷作为缓解后的巩固治疗,显示与没有砷的标准治疗相比显示出生存获益[252]。高危患者(WBC>10 000)这种治疗效果较好。澳大利亚研究者也肯定了化学/ATRA/砷联合治疗的价值[253]。

我们治疗 APL 的方式中最显著的变化之一是来自意大利成人血液病组(GIMEMA)的试验,该试验比较了无化疗方法(ATRA 和三氧化二砷一起作为诱导)和使用蒽环霉素和维 A 酸对上述 PETHEMA 方法进行前缓解治疗(图 114-12)[100]。该试验被设计为非劣效性研究,仅限于<70 岁,诊断时白细胞计数<10 000/μl 的患者。分配到 ATRA/砷组的患者有 93%的无病生存和 95%的 OS,这在统计学上优于分配到含化疗组患者的结果。因此,诊断时白细胞计数<10 000/μl 的新治疗标准是 GIMEMA 试验中使用的 ATRA 和砷的治疗方案。白细胞计数>10 000/μl 的患者的治疗标准尚未出现,但在这些患者中使用 CALGB9710[252]或 EORTC 试验[240]方法是合理的,因为这些方案在该亚组中已获得获益结果。未来对于 APL 治疗涉及细胞毒性药物剂量的最低使用,很快就可以通过口服药物治愈绝大多数 APL 的患者,因为三氧化二砷的口服制剂可能能够取代频繁且相对麻烦的静脉砷剂输注。

治疗 APL 的主要问题是预防出血性死亡,这通常是诊断延迟和 ATRA 治疗导致的。对于出现出血性症状并伴有凝血异常(包括低纤维蛋白原血症),伴有凝血酶原时间延长和纤维蛋白溶解加快证据的患者,应怀疑 APL。ATRA 应该在这些患者中凭经验启动治疗,然后在细胞遗传学或分子学研究未能证

实 APL 的诊断时停止。

其他支持疗法和治疗方法

造血生长因子

由于骨髓抑制相关毒性和死亡率较高，特别是在患有 AML 的老年人中，造血生长因子（HGF）有利于减轻这种副作用。HGF 包括粒细胞-巨噬细胞集落刺激因子（GM-CSF），G-CSF 和白介素（IL）-3 以及血小板生成因子，巨核细胞生长和发育因子（MGDF），IL-11 和新的血小板生成剂［罗米司亭（romiplostim）和艾曲波帕（eltrombopag）］。AML 中这些药物的使用落后于实体肿瘤，因为担心会导致原始细胞增殖和临床结果不佳。尽管尚未证实该临床问题的不利影响，但由于其他原因，HGF 尚未达到预期效果。

多项随机研究已经在老年患者中完成，初始诱导治疗后随机接受 HGF 和安慰剂，目的是通过缩短严重骨髓抑制持续时间，从而减少感染并发症来提高 CR 率[254~259]。所有试验均指出到中性粒细胞减少<500/μl 的天数减少 2~5 日，有时可以使住院时间缩短 1~2 日。但是 ECOG 报道的一个较小的试验[254]的研究结果是严重感染的发生率、感染死亡率、完全缓解率或生存率没有显著差异。一项针对老年 AML 患者诱导治疗后使用 G-CSF 的随机试验显示，G-CSF 能提高 CR 率[258]。令人意外的是，两组患者的感染死亡率是相似的，但是完全缓解率增加的原因目前还不清楚。且总生存期没有区别。

总之，HGF 最好在诱导治疗完成后应用[260]。相比之下，巩固强化治疗后应用 G-CSF 明显缩短了中性粒细胞减少的持续时间，尽管完全缓解持续时间或生存期没有改善[190]。为了缩短住院时间，可以在巩固治疗后应用 HGF。使用聚乙二醇化血小板生成素的较小研究未能显示在 AML 的诱导或巩固治疗期间血小板输注的需求减少[261]。血小板生成素激动剂罗米司亭和艾曲波帕，均在难治性 ITP 中被批准，已用于 MDS 的临床试验[262,263]，但有证据表明能够刺激白血病细胞故不能应用于 AML 和 MDS。

尽管体外证据表明 HGF 可以增加细胞进入 S 期从而增强 Ara-C 的细胞毒性作用[264,265]，但这种预激策略的临床疗效却不理想。MD 安德森研究小组的一项早期研究表明，化疗前和化疗期间给予 GM-CSF 的反应率和生存率低于仅接受化疗的历史对照组[266]。之后的多数随机对照研究均没能证实诱导前、诱导中或诱导后应用 GM-CSF/G-CSF 的优势[267~269]。其中一些研究使用了 HIDAC，而其他研究评估了更常规的连续输注方案。其中一项声称显示出优势的研究[270]无法在后续调查中得到证实。

免疫调节

异基因 SCT 的疗效关键是存在移植物抗白血病效应。虽然这是一个复杂的多因素效应，进一步的研究可以考虑应用淋巴因子来刺激特定细胞进行免疫治疗。

血液循环中的 NK 细胞在体外对白血病细胞具有细胞毒性，可以在自体和同种异体移植后检测到，但在化疗后检测中未能检测到[271]。尽管低剂量 IL-2 可以通过扩增 T-reg 细胞来改善 GVHD[272]，但 NK 细胞的数量可以通过移植后应用 IL-2 来扩增[273]。标准或高 IL-2 对 AML 复发患者有一定的抗白血病作用[274,275]。有小样本试验证实了化疗后给予 IL-2 的可行性，可惜在大样本随机试验中未能证实[276]。年轻成人的类似试验中发现 IL-2 能提高 LFS 和 OS，但许多患者拒绝随机接受 IL-2 治疗[277]。另一项随机试验显示在晚期缓解后治疗时应用组胺和 IL-2 有益[278]，但由于随机前化疗方案的不同而受到质疑。目前正在开发应用树突状细胞来递呈白血病相关抗原（如 WT1 和 PR1、工程化 T 细胞或转染 AML 细胞）以刺激免疫应答[279~282]。

规避耐药性

耐药性可能是由一小群能够有效自我更新的白血病细胞决定的[283,284]。研究这些白血病“干细胞”非常困难，因为在单个患者身上很难重复克隆出白血病细胞来进行系列研究。此外，存在潜在的取样偏差，因为体外结果仅反映了在人工环境中可以生长的单个时间点获得的细胞的特征。尽管如此，人们对研发白血病“干细胞”的靶向药物非常感兴趣[285]。

多药耐药性（MDR）表型在大多数情况下与膜糖蛋白（p-170）的量增加相关，膜糖蛋白用作加速多种药物外流的泵，包括蒽环类抗生素，长春新碱，紫杉烷类和米托蒽醌[286]。p-170 的水平可以通过单个 AML 细胞的流式细胞术、Westernblots、mRNA 表达水平和基因表达来检测，并且在化疗耐药的患者中水平增加[287,288]。MDR 表型最常见于复发、难治、老年和其他有不良预后因素的患者[289,290]。

在体外与多种化合物一起培养，包括钙通道阻滞剂维拉帕米，奎宁和环孢素，可以逆转 p-170 的作用[290]。在产生这种效应所需的维拉帕米剂量下会发生心脏毒性。环孢素可以在药物水平上体外逆转 MDR 表型，在毒性方面是临床上可接受的。对于复发性 AML 患者，阿糖胞苷加连续输注柔红霉素方案中加入环孢素的随机试验表明，实验组成人总生存期有益[291]。PSC-833 是一种更有效的非免疫抑制性环孢素类似物，已在随机试验中作为标准疗法的辅助手段进行评估。可惜没有提高 CR 率，还有一些试验显示 PSC833 受体的毒性增加[292,293]。由于它们对正常组织如肝脏和肾脏的影响，并且这些调节剂也影响抗肿瘤药物的药代动力学，所以如果给予 MDR 调节剂，蒽环类或依托泊苷的剂量通常必须减量[294]。其他 MDR 调节剂也同样令人失望[295]。

微小残留病（MRD）

许多技术可以检测形态学完全缓解患者的残留白血病细胞，包括（以灵敏度的近似降序排列）传统细胞遗传学[296]，已知基因重排的 Southern 印迹，荧光原位杂交（FISH），多参数流式细胞仪和 RT-PCR[297,298]。MRD 的定期监测是 APL、慢性髓细胞性白血病和儿童 ALL 的治疗的重要组成部分，但是尚无充分标准在 AML 患者中常规使用[299]。技术问题比比皆是，包括应用分子技术时对已知且已克隆异常的要求，以及使用免疫监测时抗原表达随时间变化的可能性。关于这个主题只进行了很少的大型前瞻性研究。尽管理论上如果持续检测到残留病的存在，疾病最终会复发，但是假阳性和假阴性问题是由存在，可能误导下一步治疗。连续检测比较费时，希望今后的研究能够明确哪些特定的监测点最有预后价值。对于不同的 AML 类型需要检测的标本也可能不同。一个关键的临床问题是:如果严重复发之前给予进一步治疗或异基因 SCT 的干预是否有意义。然而尚无前瞻性数据去解决这一问题,但回顾性研究显示,具有可检测 MRD 的同种异体移植受者的复发率远高于预期。由于残留的存在,自体移植和大剂量化疗可能效果不佳。

小分子抑制剂和其他新方法

虽然多年来没有任何新批准的非 APL/AML 药物(不包括经批准然后撤销的 GO),但是许多药物都正在研发中。对所有药物进行全面讨论超出了本章的范围;然而,值得强调的是酪氨酸激酶抑制剂治疗的进展以及其他一些有趣的药物研发。

伊马替尼和其他 BCR-ABL 抑制剂在 CML 治疗中的成功促使人们在 AML 中寻找类似的功能获得性突变,这种抑制可能创造治疗益处。

大约 30%的新发 AML 患者发生 FLT3 跨膜酪氨酸激酶的功能获得性突变,最常见的是 *ITD* 突变,其使近膜区域延长 3~100 个氨基酸;少数患者在酪氨酸激酶结构域中具有活化点突变[7]。两种类型的突变均可导致配体非依赖性激活[300]和鼠模型中的骨髓增生性疾病[301]。几种 FLT3 抑制剂正在开发中,尚未获得 FDA 批准。使用米哚妥林(midostaurin)[302]、来他替尼(lestaurtinib)[303]和索拉非尼[304]的单药试验均显示晚期突变型 FLT3AML 患者有反应。索拉非尼被公认为晚期肾癌和肝细胞癌患者血管内皮生长因子受体抑制剂。米哚妥林可以抑制酪氨酸激酶结构域突变细胞的生长,而大多数其他药物(除了克雷诺兰尼(crenolanib)[305])不能并且仅在具有 *ITD* 突变的 FLT3 群体中开发。奎扎替尼(quizartinib)是一种有效且相对特异的 FLT3ITD 抑制剂,作为单一药物已显示出相对较高的反应率[306],并且正在与 *AML* 复发中的突变 FLT3ITD 患者的化学疗法进行比较;然而,一个重要的抗性机制是具有 *FLT3TKD* 突变的克隆的生长[307]。

鉴于相对罕见的 CR 和单药 FLT3 抑制剂治疗的短暂反应持续时间,与化疗联合开发这些药物已成为主要推动力。一项在复发突变 FLT3ITD 患者中加入来他替尼治疗的试验,其试验结果为阴性[308],其他几个与加入或不加入 FLT3 抑制剂的化疗作比较的临床试验正在进行中。此外,FLT3 抑制剂,特别是索拉非尼,似乎对一些异基因干细胞移植后复发的 *FLT3AML* 突变患者有效[228,229]。

鉴于有相当数量的具有良好染色体的 AML 患者(所谓的 CBF 易位)具有 c-kit 过量和/或 c-kit 酪氨酸激酶的突变,c-kit 抑制剂达沙替尼(dasatinib)已被添加到 AML 患者的细胞遗传学亚组的化疗中。初步结果是令人鼓舞的,并且随机试验也正在进行中[309]。大约 20%的 AML 患者发现的另一种功能获得性突变发生在 *IDH1* 或 *IDH2* 基因中,其产物催化 2-羟基葡萄糖酸盐的新形态产生,并以前白血病的方式外成地影响基因表达[310]。*IDH1* 和 IHD2 抑制剂的初步结果令人鼓舞[311]。具有活化的 *RAS* 癌基因突变的患者[12]对 MEK 途径抑制剂也有反应。

除了这些基因疗法外,还有许多其他药物正在开发中,它们利用了 AML 细胞和正常干细胞之间潜在的生物学差异。骨髓生态位中的 AML 细胞通过骨髓基质中内皮细胞和其他细胞所合成的因子促进其生存[312]。CXCR4 抑制剂普乐沙福等药物可能破坏生存信号,使 AML 细胞更容易被细胞毒性剂杀死[313]。ABT199 是一种 BCL2 抑制剂,在 CLL 治疗中具有显著优势[314],可单独使用或与化学疗法联合使用以促进 AML 细胞的凋亡。另一种在开发中的药物是 KPT330,是一种核输出蛋白抑制剂,主要通过阻止肿瘤抑制基因从癌细胞核中排出,特别是在 AML 细胞中[315]。有几种针对 CD123 的抗体和免疫复合物[316]被认为在白血病干细胞上有特异性表达。AML 中任何药物的发展途径都有点令人生畏,因为必须确定它是否可用作晚期患者的单一药物,以及是否需要在患者的疾病早期阶段中加入化疗。在后一种情况下,鉴于患者对化学疗法的初始反应率相对较高,需要进行大型试验或具有新颖设计的试验。

并发症

高白细胞血症

由于细胞表面黏附分子的表达,白血病母细胞比成熟粒细胞更不易变形[317],并且比淋巴母细胞"更黏"。随着外周血白血病母细胞计数的增加,通常在髓系白血病中>$10^5/\mu l$ 的水平,微循环中的血流可能受到这些更黏且不易变形的细胞形成的栓塞所阻碍。局部低氧血症可能因分裂中的白血病母细胞的高代谢活动、内皮损伤和出血而加剧。红细胞输注可能会进一步增加血液黏度并使情况变得更糟,应该停止给药或缓慢给药,直至 WBC 减少。凝血异常包括 DIC,进一步增加了局部出血的风险。建议大量血小板输注,特别是当血液涂片中存在血小板碎片时,血小板计数经常被高估,因为自动血细胞计数器会将白血病细胞破坏产物错误地计为血小板[318]。

尽管在具有极高白血病母细胞计数的患者的大多数器官中都可以发现白细胞停滞的病理学证据,但临床症状通常与中枢神经系统和肺部受累有关[319,320]。有时在治疗中出现白血病细胞溶解,可能会出现低氧血症恶化的呼吸困难。在凝血期间由于钾从白细胞中释放,可能发生血清钾的假性升高,因此有时有必要用肝素抗凝血浆测定血钾水平。类似地,由于白细胞的代谢活性增强,即使在运输到实验室期间将样本适当地放置在冰上,PO_2 也会出现假性降低。在这种情况下,脉搏血氧仪可以准确评估血氧饱和度。高白细胞血症常见于粒单核细胞白血病或单核细胞白血病,可能是白血病性幼稚单核细胞容易迁移到组织中并进一步增殖所致。

有症状的高白细胞血症患者的早期死亡率很高[320]。即使这种患者诱导期间存活,缓解率也较低并且 CR 持续时间较短。有症状的高白细胞血症(ALL 患者很少)是一种医学急症,需要积极快速降低白细胞计数。大多数患者可以通过化疗实现快速细胞减少,方案有标准诱导方案或大剂量羟基脲($3g/(m^2 \cdot d)$)。一些中心还提倡低剂量颅内照射以防止中枢神经系统白血病细胞的增殖,因为这些药物理论上难以通过血脑屏障。虽然没有比较性研究来确定结果是否优于化疗,但这种治疗耐受性良好。

一些患者因为存在肾功能不全、代谢性问题（未及时给予别嘌醇治疗来预防高尿酸血症）而导致不能立即开始化疗。这时可以紧急进行白细胞去除术来降低或稳定白细胞计数[321,322]。尽管通过白细胞单采（手术时间通常持续数小时）可以改善肺部和中枢神经系统症状，但在理论上和实际操作中有些困难。例如，白细胞单采很难祛除已有的血管内血栓，特别是如果已经发生了血管侵犯。在这种情况下，虽然理论上白细胞单采可以减少这些部位白细胞的进一步积累，但是化疗仍是主要的解决方法。此外，当治疗过程中白细胞增长过快时，应用细胞周期特异性化疗药物最可能快速起效。当细胞毒性药物化疗过程中出现肺部问题时，白细胞单采也可能有好处，因为在此类患者中，有一部分症状与白细胞溶解后的局部炎症反应有关[323]。

中枢神经系统白血病

AML 患者的中枢神经系统（CNS）受累程度远低于成人和小孩的 ALL 患者。大多数临床医生感觉近年来发病率进一步下降，可能是因为使用了大剂量阿糖胞苷，可以透过血脑屏障进入 CNS。近年来大样本 AML 临床试验中，CNS 白血病的发生率<5%[324]。因此，初诊时在没有中枢神经系统症状的情况下，并不做常规诊断性腰椎穿刺，化疗方案也不包括 CNS 预防。CNSL 最常见的症状是颅内压增高，通常包括持续性头痛，嗜睡或其他精神变化。AML[325] 脑神经体征（最常见的是第Ⅲ或Ⅵ对脑神经），继发于神经根受累，偶尔还有周围神经表现并可伴有头痛或单独发生[325]。

通过腰椎穿刺后检查脑脊液（CSF）的细胞离心涂片可确认诊断。细胞计数可以从 5/μl 到>1 000/μl 变化。大多数患者的 CSF 蛋白中度升高，葡萄糖水平降低。对于 CNSL 治疗包括注射化疗药物，对于反应不佳者、脑神经受累者可以加以颅脑放疗（常用剂量 2 400cGy）[325]。初始治疗的鞘注药物包括甲氨蝶呤（15mg/次）、阿糖胞苷（50mg/次），在出现不适或复发时与其他药物交叉使用。经典治疗方案是鞘注 2~3 次/周，直到脑脊液清亮为止，改为每周一次（共两次），然后每月一次直到 1 年。由于难以进行重复的腰椎穿刺或担心某些个体的 CSF 流量不能从腰椎间隙向整个 CNS 输送足够量的药物，因此经常需要脑室内给药的 Omaya 留置管[326]。此外还报道了使用系统性药物穿透中枢神经系统的成功治疗方法，如亚胺醌（AZQ）、大剂量甲氨蝶呤或 HIDAC[327]。阿糖胞苷的缓释（depo）制剂可能是另一种选择[328]。遗憾的是，复发率很高，也可与骨髓复发同时发生，或者是独立发生，即使在最初的成功治疗后，也会发生这样的结果。

目前认为 FAB M4E0 中枢白血病的发病率较高，在单核细胞白血病和循环中高白血病母细胞计数的患者中中枢白血病的发病率可能较高[329]。使用更现代的治疗方案可能就不再是这种情况了，且预防性治疗在这些人的观点中并没有说明。如上所述，CNS 受累易发生在具有高白细胞计数的 APL 患者中。有些医师对 CR_2 的 APL 患者进行预防性鞘注。

眼部并发症

基本上每个眼部结构都可被白血病累及，在没有化疗的时代这是一个重要的临床问题[330]。白血病细胞浸润结膜和泪腺，局部形成明显的肿块，需要放射治疗。然而，脉络膜和视网膜受累是最常见的。一项前瞻性研究对 53 名新诊断的 AML 成人进行了分析，其中 64% 的患者出现视网膜或视神经异常[331]。出血和棉絮斑（神经纤维缺血的后果）是最常见，这些事件的发生与患者年龄、FAB 类型、白细胞计数或血细胞比容无关。视网膜病变患者的初始血小板计数较低。共有 10 名患者视力下降，其中 5 名患有黄斑出血。据认为，许多棉絮斑点是贫血所引起的缺血的结果或这种情况加剧的表现。明确的视网膜白血病浸润无法被确定。所有患者均接受了积极的化疗和血小板输注支持；没有患者接受颅内或眼部照射。在达到完全缓解的患者中所有眼部发现都得到了解决，并且都没有残留的视力缺陷。眼部感染似乎并不常见，可能是因为及时经验性的使用抗细菌和抗真菌药物降低了眼部血源性感染的发生。

怀孕

AML 偶尔会在怀孕时被诊断出来，常是因为出现临床症状或体检查血常规时发现异常。如果在妊娠早期发现，建议终止妊娠并给予化疗。妊娠后期诊断的患者（如在妊娠中期晚期）的治疗比较复杂。如果白血病进展相对缓慢，有时可以通过白细胞单采和/或输血等保守治疗，并尽快引产和分娩[332]。也有关于妊娠后期的患者接受化疗的报道[333,334]。这些患者中的大多数没有流产，新生儿没有发生白血病，其他异常风险也没有增加。

代谢异常

接受 AML 治疗的患者可能会出现各种代谢问题，如呕吐、腹泻、营养不良或肾功能不全，通常是因为抗生素，特别是两性霉素 B 的副作用。一些代谢紊乱与白血病本身有关。高尿酸血症偶尔伴有尿酸性肾病和肾功能不全，是 AML 最常见的代谢并发症。所有患者一旦确诊急性白血病，应立即服用别嘌醇（≥300mg/d 或更大剂量），以便在情况允许时立即进行化疗。通过大量水化和碱化可以使多数患者的尿酸性肾病避免或减轻。别嘌醇通常可在化疗完成后 1 或 2 日内停药。偶尔患者出现尿酸水平显著升高，可以应用重组尿酸氧化酶，数几小时内使尿酸水平迅速下降[335]。一般一次剂量就足够了，通过连续监测尿酸水平再决定后续治疗剂量[336]。

ALL 患者更容易发生肿瘤细胞溶解综合征，一些 AML 患者体内大量白血病细胞破坏，表现为高磷血症，低钙血症，高钾血症和肾功能不全。原因是白血病细胞破坏释放大量磷酸盐，其与肾脏中的钙形成沉淀，导致低钙血症，有时导致少尿型肾功能不全。高尿酸血症使病情进一步恶化，通过正确水化可以改善，并且常有自限性。

尽管 AML 患者中有明显的大量细胞损伤，但高血钙症并不常见。严重的低钾血症比较常见，特别是在单核细胞白血病时。可能由于这些患者溶菌酶水平升高导致肾小管损伤而引起肾脏钾丢失增多。这时及时静脉补钾非常必要，在化疗后白血病细胞下降后症状随之好转。乳酸酸中毒可以在初诊和复发时出现，不过这种情况非常少见，机制不清，推测可能与白血病在局部瘀积后无氧代谢有关[337]。

小结

由于支持治疗和并发症处理水平的提高,60 岁以上 AML 患者的总体疗效在全球范围内得到了改善。但是疗效已经进入一个平台期,需要开展新的方法使更多的白血病患者得到根治。分子遗传学的快速发展为实现这一目标带来了希望,对白血病生物学和小分子,单克隆抗体,细胞因子和具有潜在临床效用的 HGF 的产生有了更多的了解。进一步揭示药物耐药机制以及提高现有药物有效性的可能性也是一个令人兴奋和可实现的前景。以上策略以及评估开展干细胞移植和新的化疗药物的临床试验可以减少经验治疗,为 AML 治疗的成功提供了希望。

肥大细胞白血病和其他肥大细胞肿瘤

肥大细胞疾病被列为髓系增生性疾病,临床表现多样,可以表现为皮肤受累的反应性良性综合征,也可以表现为肥大细胞浸润多个器官(包括骨髓)的恶性肿瘤[338,339]。

反应性肥大细胞增生

肥大细胞增生经常表现为受累组织(如过敏性鼻炎的鼻黏膜)的速发性或迟发型超敏反应。许多恶性疾病均可出现骨髓中肥大细胞数量的增加,如淋巴细胞增生性疾病[340],毛细胞白血病[341]和髓系肿瘤[342,343]。这类患者的肥大细胞增多似乎是反应性的,而不是来自恶性克隆。

肿瘤性肥大细胞病

色素性荨麻疹是迄今为止肿瘤性肥大细胞增殖最常见的临床表现[344]。典型的荨麻疹色素性暴发由多个分散的色素沉着过度的结节性病变组成,呈良性临床过程,尤其是儿童患者。皮肤表现包括机械损伤反应(Darier 征)、瘙痒或间歇性潮红导致的肥大细胞脱颗形引起的典型荨麻疹风疹皮肤肥大细胞增多症(CM)[345]与系统性肥大细胞病(SMCD)不容易区分,后者是一种惰性疾病,其肥大细胞可在皮肤以外的部位发现。SMCD 中的血清类胰蛋白酶水平高于 CM[346]。全身肥大细胞增多症可以表现为全身症状和/或胃肠道症状,这与肥大细胞因子大量释放有关。这些症状在色素性荨麻疹患者中不常见,包括鼻炎、哮喘、恶心、呕吐、腹泻、晕厥、胸痛、骨痛和直肠不适[347]。骨骼,胃肠道和脾脏也可以是肥大细胞浸润的部位。

恶性肥大细胞增多症是 SCMD 的一个更具侵袭性的类型,临床预后不佳[347]。惰性全身性肥大细胞增多症不影响寿命,但是恶性肥大细胞增多症后诊断后存活期很少超过 1~2 年。常累及骨髓,并存在嗜酸粒细胞增多和全血细胞减少,腺体病变和/或器官肿大也较常见[348]。在 20 世纪 90 年代早期,人们认识到全身性肥大细胞增生患者的肥大细胞能够独立于 C-KIT 配体(肥大细胞生长的关键因子)的刺激而生长[349]。通过细胞系和患者样本证明,这种生长独立的基础是 C-KIT 的自身活化[350,351],最常与激酶结构域中 816 位点的突变相关,跨膜区域突变也可出现[352]。在患者的 B 细胞和单核细胞中均检测到 *ASP-816 VAL* 突变,表明全身性肥大细胞增多症是一种从早期造血干细胞进化而来的克隆性疾病[352]。相反,来自肥大细胞白血病的患者的原始细胞没有这种突变,提示可能还有其他原因[353]。

肥大细胞白血病是一种罕见的侵袭性恶性肥大细胞增生亚型,其特征是外周血中存在大量非典型肥大细胞[354~356]。肥大细胞白血病患者的中位生存期<6 个月,与非白血病型恶性肥大细胞增多症患者相比,后者往往存活较长时间。大多数报道的肥大细胞白血病病例常见于已有恶性肥大细胞病的患者。肥大细胞白血病的诊断标准是:①外周血白细胞分类中肥大细胞比例≥10%;②白血病肥大细胞应表现出形态异型性;③细胞组化证实细胞为肥大细胞来源(氯醋酸酯酶染色出现异染颗粒,过氧化物酶染色阴性)[355]。

尽管肥大细胞白血病骨髓中不典型肥大细胞浸润明显,但是初诊时血液学指标变化较大。贫血常为轻到中度;初始白细胞计数范围可以正常也可以>50 000/μl[355]。虽然外周血非典型肥大细胞(具有碎片,胞浆伪足和多个细胞核的低度颗粒化的同色染色细胞)的百分比可能相对较低(但>10%),但几乎总是随着病程数量大幅增加。肥大细胞白血病患者的染色体核型基本正常,核分裂像少影响核型分析。全身性肥大细胞增多症的患者的骨髓细胞常存在细胞遗传学异常,如+8、-7/7q-,20q-,和骨髓增生性疾病相似[355,356]。如果患者同时存在嗜酸性粒细胞增多,需要检测细胞遗传学以排除血小板衍生生长因子受体(PDGFR,涉及染色体 5q31-32)的异常,因为这类患者对伊马替尼敏感。

治疗

肥大细胞肿瘤的治疗基于疾病类型和临床表现。CM 患者通常不需要治疗。然而,SMCD 具有多种多样的临床表现。例如,那些患有血液学异常的人可能需要支持治疗,其中可能包括输血或经验性使用 HGF。避免麻醉、酒精、阿司匹林和吗啡等肥大细胞刺激物可以减少潮红、瘙痒、腹泻和可能与组胺有关的症状[357~359]。H_1 和 H_2 抗组胺药或色甘酸二钠可以减轻症状,放射治疗可以控制局部症状而不引起组胺释放[360]。

典型的 *ASP-816 VAL* 突变对 C-KIT 抑制剂甲磺酸伊马替尼[351,361,362]和尼洛替尼(nilotinib)[363]都不敏感,虽然体外研究表明这种突变的 C-KIT 可能对达沙替尼(dasatinib)[364]敏感。前期数据表明多靶点激酶抑制剂 PKC412(米哚妥林)也可能抑制这种激活突变的产物,并且早期的报道提示有潜在的临床应用前景[365,366]。克拉屈滨和 α 干扰素可以使全身性肥大细胞增多症患者的细胞减少,对于有全身症状的患者可以考虑应用[367,368]。恶性肥大细胞增多症或肥大细胞白血病(不伴 *c-kit* 突变)对治疗的反应通常是短暂的,尚无标准治疗方案。可以选择蒽环类药物与阿糖胞苷联合进行诱导化疗,然后进行大剂量阿糖胞苷巩固治疗。异基因造血干细胞移植在合适患者可以考虑进行,但是这方面的经验较少。

(白元松 孟令俊 赵亚男 丛丹 译 白元松 孟令俊 赵亚男 丛丹 韩冷 毕林涛 校)

参考文献

The complete reference list can be found on the Wiley Companion Digital Edition of this title (see inside front cover for login instructions).

1 Leukemia SSFSAM, 2013, www.seer.cancer.gov/statfacts/html/amyl.html (accessed 2 Apr 2016).

2 Cheson BD, Bennett JM, Kopecky KJ, et al. Revised recommendations of the International Working Group for Diagnosis, Standardization of Response Criteria, Treatment Outcomes, and Reporting Standards for Therapeutic Trials in Acute Myeloid Leukemia. *J Clin Oncol*. 2003;**21**:4642–4649.

3 Rowe JM, Tallman MS. How I treat acute myeloid leukemia. *Blood*. 2010;**116**: 3147–3156.

5 Lindsley RC, Mar BG, Mazzola E, et al. Acute myeloid leukemia ontogeny is defined by distinct somatic mutations. *Blood*. 2015;**125(9)**:1367–1376.

6 Network TCaGAR. Genomic and epigenomic landscapes of adult de novo acute myeloid leukemia. *N Engl J Med*. 2013;**368**:2059–2074.

7 Kindler T, Lipka DB, Fischer T. FLT3 as a therapeutic target in AML: still challenging after all these years. *Blood*. 2010;**116**:5089–5102.

8 Marcucci G, Haferlach T, Döhner H. Molecular genetics of adult acute myeloid leukemia: prognostic and therapeutic implications. *J Clin Oncol*. 2011;**29**:475–486.

9 Schlenk RF, Dohner K, Krauter J, et al. Mutations and treatment outcome in cytogenetically normal acute myeloid leukemia. *N Engl J Med*. 2008;**358**:1909–1918.

16 Patel JP, Gönen M, Figueroa ME, et al. Prognostic relevance of integrated genetic profiling in acute myeloid leukemia. *N Engl J Med*. 2012;**366**:1079–1089.

17 Rucker FG, Schlenk RF, Bullinger L, et al. TP53 alterations in acute myeloid leukemia with complex karyotype correlate with specific copy number alterations, monosomal karyotype, and dismal outcome. *Blood*. 2012;**119**:2114–2121.

47 Ossenkoppele G, Lowenberg B. How I treat the older patient with acute myeloid leukemia. *Blood*. 2015;**125**:767–774.

48 Hurria A, Lachs MS, Cohen HJ, et al. Geriatric assessment for oncologists: rationale and future directions. *Crit Rev Oncol Hematol*. 2006;**59**:211–217.

50 Frohling S, Schlenk RF, Kayser S, et al. Cytogenetics and age are major determinants of outcome in intensively treated acute myeloid leukemia patients older than 60 years: results from AMLSG trial AML HD98-B. *Blood*. 2006;**108**: 3280–3288.

51 Grimwade D, Hills RK, Moorman AV, et al. Refinement of cytogenetic classification in acute myeloid leukemia: determination of prognostic significance of rare recurring chromosomal abnormalities among 5876 younger adult patients treated in the United Kingdom Medical Research Council trials. *Blood*. 2010;**116**:354–365.

54 Slovak ML, Kopecky KJ, Cassileth PA, et al. Karyotypic analysis predicts outcome of preremission and postremission therapy in adult acute myeloid leukemia: a Southwest Oncology Group/Eastern Cooperative Oncology Group Study. *Blood*. 2000;**96**:4075–4083.

62 Vardiman JW, Thiele J, Arber DA, et al. The 2016 revision of the World Health Organization (WHO) classification of myeloid neoplasms and acute leukemia: rationale and important changes. *Blood*. 2009;**114**:937–951.

78 Cairoli R, Beghini A, Grillo G, et al. Prognostic impact of c-KIT mutations in core binding factor leukemias: an Italian retrospective study. *Blood*. 2006;**107**:3463–3468.

100 Lo-Coco F, Avvisati G, Vignetti M, et al. Retinoic acid and arsenic trioxide for acute promyelocytic leukemia. *N Engl J Med*. 2013;**369**:111–121.

133 Dohner H, Estey EH, Amadori S, et al. Diagnosis and management of acute myeloid leukemia in adults: recommendations from an international expert panel, on behalf of the European LeukemiaNet. *Blood*. 2010;**115**:453–474.

157 Burnett AK, Russell N, Hills RK, et al. A randomised comparison of daunorubicin 90 mg/m^2 Vs 60 mg/m^2 in AML induction: results from the UK NCRI AML17 trial in 1206 patients. *Blood*. 2014;**124**:7.

158 Holowiecki J, Grosicki S, Giebel S, et al. Cladribine, but not fludarabine, added to daunorubicin and cytarabine during induction prolongs survival of patients with acute myeloid leukemia: a multicenter, Randomized Phase III Study. *J Clin Oncol*. 2012;**30**:2441–2448.

161 Burnett AK, Russell NH, Hills RK, et al. Optimization of chemotherapy for younger patients with acute myeloid leukemia: results of the medical research council AML15 trial. *J Clin Oncol*. 2013;**31**:3360–3368.

164 Castaigne S, Pautas C, Terré C, et al. Effect of gemtuzumab ozogamicin on survival of adult patients with de-novo acute myeloid leukaemia (ALFA-0701): a randomised, open-label, phase 3 study. *Lancet*. 2012;**379**:1508–1516.

165 Burnett AK, Russell NH, Hills RK, et al. Addition of gemtuzumab ozogamicin to induction chemotherapy improves survival in older patients with acute myeloid leukemia. *J Clin Oncol*. 2012;**30**:3924–3931.

166 Rowe JM, Lowenberg B. Gemtuzumab ozogamicin in acute myeloid leukemia: a remarkable saga about an active drug. *Blood*. 2013;**121**:4838–4841.

179 Breems DA, Van Putten WL, Huijgens PC, et al. Prognostic index for adult patients with acute myeloid leukemia in first relapse. *J Clin Oncol*. 2005;**23**:1969–1978.

183 Cassileth PA, Lynch E, Hines J, et al. Varying intensity of postremission therapy in acute myeloid leukemia. *Blood*. 1992;**79**:1924–1930.

184 Mayer RJ, Davis RB, Schiffer CA, et al. Intensive postremission chemotherapy in adults with acute myeloid leukemia. Cancer and Leukemia Group B. *N Engl J Med*. 1994;**331**:896–903.

202 Zittoun RA, Mandelli F, Willemze R, et al. Autologous or allogeneic bone marrow transplantation compared with intensive chemotherapy in acute myelogenous leukemia. European Organization for Research and Treatment of Cancer (EORTC) and the Gruppo Italiano Malattie Ematologiche Maligne dell'Adulto (GIMEMA) Leukemia Cooperative Groups. *N Engl J Med*. 1995;**332**:217–223.

206 Estey E, de Lima M, Tibes R, et al. Prospective feasibility analysis of reduced-intensity conditioning (RIC) regimens for hematopoietic stem cell transplantation (HSCT) in elderly patients with acute myeloid leukemia (AML) and high-risk myelodysplastic syndrome (MDS). *Blood*. 2007;**109**:1395–1400.

219 Koreth J, Schlenk R, Kopecky KJ, et al. Allogeneic stem cell transplantation for acute myeloid leukemia in first complete remission: systematic review and meta-analysis of prospective clinical trials. *JAMA*. 2009;**301**:2349–2361.

221 Stelljes M, Krug U, Beelen DW, et al. Allogeneic transplantation versus chemotherapy as postremission therapy for acute myeloid leukemia: a prospective matched pairs analysis. *J Clin Oncol*. 2014;**32**:288–296.

226 Schmid C, Labopin M, Nagler A, et al. Donor lymphocyte infusion in the treatment of first hematological relapse after allogeneic stem-cell transplantation in adults with acute myeloid leukemia: a retrospective risk factors analysis and comparison with other strategies by the EBMT Acute Leukemia Working Party. *J Clin Oncol*. 2007;**25**:4938–4945.

240 Ades L, Sanz MA, Chevret S, et al. Treatment of newly diagnosed acute promyelocytic leukemia (APL): a comparison of French-Belgian-Swiss and PETHEMA results. *Blood*. 2008;**111**:1078–1084.

252 Powell BL, Moser B, Stock W, et al. Arsenic trioxide improves event-free and overall survival for adults with acute promyelocytic leukemia: North American Leukemia Intergroup Study C9710. *Blood*. 2010;**116**:3751–3757.

260 Schiffer CA. Hematopoietic growth factors as adjuncts to the treatment of acute myeloid leukemia. *Blood*. 1996;**88**:3675–3685.

289 Leith CP, Kopecky KJ, Godwin J, et al. Acute myeloid leukemia in the elderly: assessment of multidrug resistance (MDR1) and cytogenetics distinguishes biologic subgroups with remarkably distinct responses to standard chemotherapy. A Southwest Oncology Group study. *Blood*. 1997;**89**:3323–3329.

316 Mardiros A, Dos Santos C, McDonald T, et al. T cells expressing CD123-specific chimeric antigen receptors exhibit specific cytolytic effector functions and antitumor effects against human acute myeloid leukemia. *Blood*. 2013;**122**:3138–3148.

322 Röllig C, Ehninger G. How I treat hyperleukocytosis in acute myeloid leukemia. *Blood*. 2015;**125**:3246–3252.

354 Bain BJ. Systemic mastocytosis and other mast cell neoplasms. *Br J Haematol*. 1999;**106**:9–17.

365 Gotlib J, Berube C, Growney JD, et al. Activity of the tyrosine kinase inhibitor PKC412 in a patient with mast cell leukemia with the D816V KIT mutation. *Blood*. 2005;**106**:2865–2870.

第 115 章　慢性髓细胞白血病

Jorge Cortes, MD ■ Richard T. Silver, MD ■ Hagop M. Kantarjian, MD

概述

慢性髓细胞白血病(chronic myeloid leukemia, CML)是第一个被发现与一种独特的染色体异常,即费城染色体相关的恶性血液病。这种异常的分子生理改变也得到进一步阐明,即形成 *BCR-ABL* 融合基因并能够翻译成为具有酪氨酸激酶活性的融合蛋白;这一发现促进了特异性酪氨酸激酶抑制剂的开发。使用此类药物作为初始治疗已经导致该疾病自然历程发生巨大变化,得到恰当的治疗患者的预期寿命有望与总人口平均寿命相似。而且,已有多种治疗药物可用于对初始治疗没有最佳反应的患者。目前的研究集中在使更多患者成功治愈并停止治疗的方法上。

慢性髓细胞白血病是一种多能干细胞克隆的异常增生,涉及骨髓的粒系、红系、巨核细胞、B 或 T 淋巴细胞,但不涉及骨髓成纤维细胞。CML 的特征是存在独特的染色体异常,即费城染色体(Philadelphia chromosome, Ph)。

历史背景

1960 年,CML 患者中发现了一条微小的染色体片段,这一异常后来被确定为 9 号和 22 号染色体的平衡易位[1,2]。随后的研究表明,这种易位导致 *BCR-ABL* 融合基因的产生,当这种基因被转染到小鼠体内时会诱发 CML[3]。该嵌合基因会翻译产生具有酪氨酸激酶活性结构的融合蛋白[4]。IFN-α 是第一种诱导费城染色体消失的疗法,治疗反应的金标准是获得完全的细胞遗传学反应(complete cytogenetic responses, CCyR)[5]。对酪氨酸激酶活性的认识促进了酪氨酸激酶抑制剂(tyrosine kinase inhibitors, TKI)的发展,由一代伊马替尼[6],到第二代和第三代药物,从根本上改变了疾病的自然历程(图 115-1)[7]。目前,被诊断为 CML 的患者,如果治疗得当,他们的预期寿命与总人口平均寿命相似。

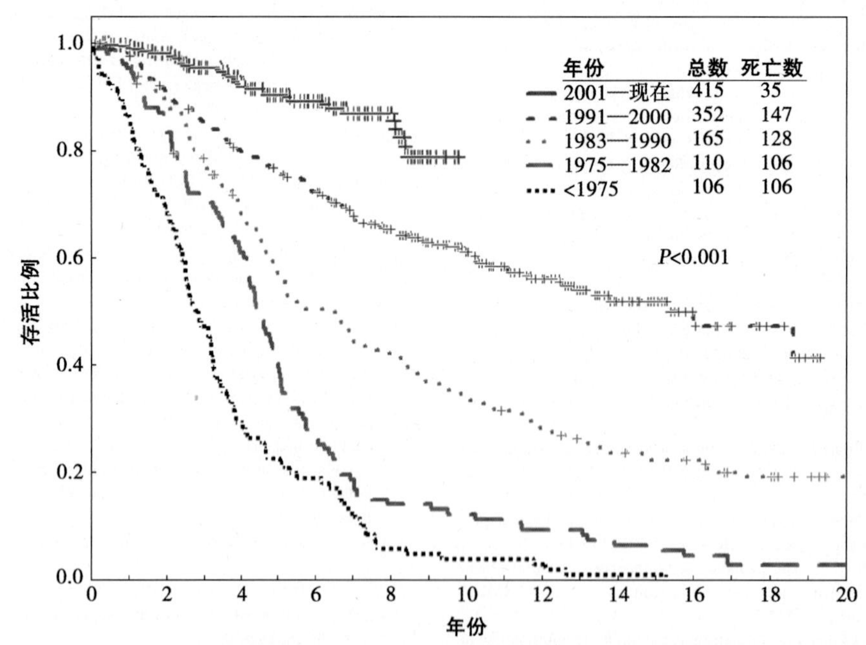

图 115-1　MD 安德森癌症中心新诊断慢性期 CML 患者的生存率(n = 1 148;1965—2010)。摘自 Kan-tarjian 等,2012[7]。这项研究最初发表在《血液》杂志上。© 美国血液病学会

发病率与流行病学

CML 占所有白血病发生的 15%[1,2]。CML 发病的中位年龄是 55~65 岁,发病率随着年龄增长而增加,男性比例略高(比例为 1.8∶1)[8]。据估计,2014 年在美国有 5 980 例 CML 新诊断病例,并有 810 名患者死于 CML[9]。美国 CML 的发病率一直保持在大约 1.81∶10 万。使用伊马替尼治疗后,每年的死亡率已经从 15%~20%下降到 2%,预计平均存活期可能超过 20 年。因此,在美国 CML 患者在未来三十年可能超过 20 万例[10]。

危险因素

对于多数 CML 患者，尚无确定的致病因素。尽管电离辐射可以导致白血病，但辐射所致的最常见的白血病是急性髓细胞性白血病（acute myeloid leukemia，AML）。在 1945 年日本原子弹爆炸后就有 CML 发病的报道，而且在早期研究中发现放射科医师和接受放射线治疗的强直性脊柱炎患者亦有发病[3,4,11,12]。目前还没有发现其他已知的危险因素。

病理学

典型的 CML 病程表现为两期或三期，即慢性期、中间期或加速期、终末期或急变期[13]。白细胞增多常见，白细胞计数常常高于 100×10^9/L，从回顾性数据来看，慢性期患者的中位生存期为 3～6 年，在慢性期患者中，2 年内，急变转化率为每年 5%～10%，之后每年有 15%～20%的风险。CML 加速期的特点是成熟障碍的细胞增多。加速期的定义有不同的标准。常见的一种分类定义为加速期存在下列任何情况：原始细胞≥15%，原始粒细胞加早幼粒细胞≥30%，嗜碱性粒细胞≥20%，出现与治疗无关的血小板下降并且<100×10^9/L，或细胞遗传学出现克隆演变[14]。也有其他标准被提出，如世界卫生组织（World Health Organization，WHO）的建议，但其中的一些分类标准[7,15]还没有得到临床验证[16]。加速期患者的中位生存期为 1～2 年[8,17]，但使用 TKI 会显著提高生存期[18]。急变期定义为外周血或骨髓中原始细胞≥30%，或有不成熟细胞的髓外疾病存在[19]。WHO 建议将其更改为原始细胞≥20%，但此项建议未被证实[10,16]。急变期可根据免疫表型分为髓系、淋巴系，双表型或混合表型（淋巴和粒细胞系）。20%～30%的患者发生急淋变，急髓变占 50%，还有 25%不能分型[11,20]。急变期 CML 的平均生存期为 3～6 个月。急淋变患者有较好的预后，采用 TKI 联合化疗，缓解率（response rate，RR）≥90%，中位生存期为>18 个月[21]。

慢性期的实验室特征包括白细胞增多和核左移（图 115-2），并常常伴有嗜碱性粒细胞和嗜酸性粒细胞增多。血小板增多常见，但并不容易见到血栓现象。一定程度的贫血也比较常见。白细胞碱性磷酸酶（ALP）的活性减低，而血清中维生素 B_{12} 水平显著升高。

骨髓细胞增殖活跃。在慢性期，存在各个分化阶段的细胞，中性粒细胞为主，原粒和早幼粒细胞比例小于 10%（图 115-3 和图 115-4）。巨核细胞数可能会增加，还可能存在网状纤维的增加，且骨髓纤维化可能随着疾病的进展而加重，但 TKI 治疗可以逆转这一过程[22]。

在急变期，急淋变细胞中含有末端脱氧核酸转移酶（terminal deoxynucleotidyl transferase，TDT），淋巴母细胞通常表达 CD10、CD19、CD22 以及其他的 B 细胞标志[20]。T 淋巴细胞急变很少发生。慢粒急髓变与急性髓细胞性白血病相似。原始粒细胞髓过氧化物酶染色阳性并且表达包括 CD13、CD33 和 CD117 的髓系标志。

较少的患者不经过慢性期而直接表现为急淋变或急粒变。

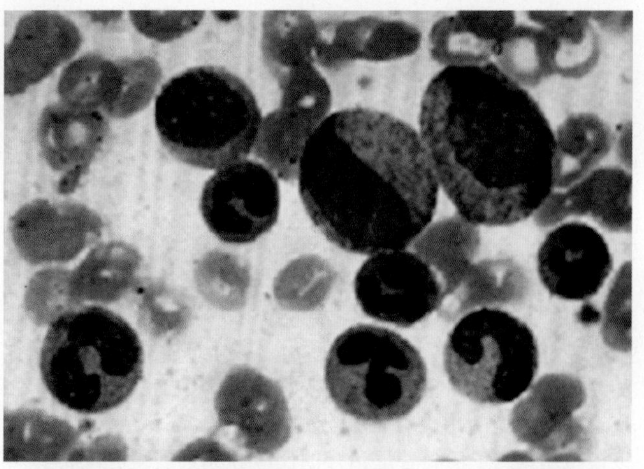

图 115-2　慢性骨髓细胞性白血病。包括中幼粒细胞，晚幼粒细胞，杆状核细胞，多形核粒细胞的白细胞增多是疾病慢性期外周血的特点

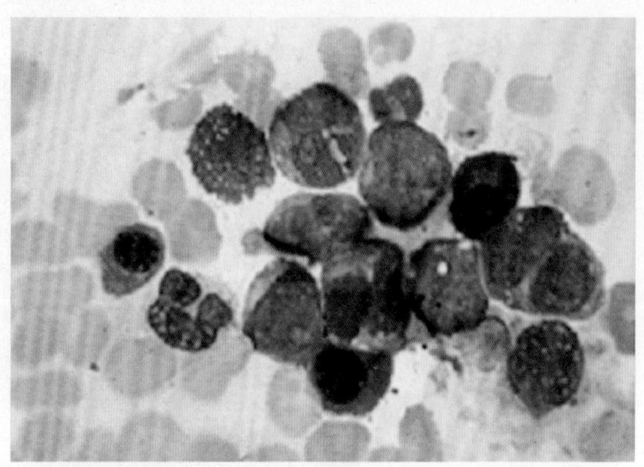

图 115-3　CML，急粒变时。骨髓穿刺的涂片显示原始粒细胞占优势

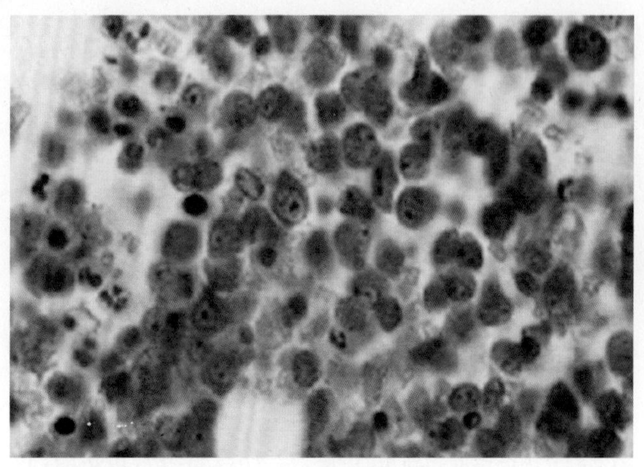

图 115-4　CML，急变期。骨髓穿刺涂片显示 75%的骨髓细胞为有核仁的原始细胞

这种情况区分慢粒急变与 Ph 阳性的急性淋巴细胞白血病(acute lymphoblastic leukemia, ALL)或急性髓细胞性白血病(acute myeloid leukemia, AML)是很困难的但这种区分只是语义的区别,而治疗和预后是一样的。很少出现巨核细胞白血病、红白血病和嗜碱性细胞白血病转化。

预后分类

CML 预后是多种的。已提出对患者进行危险度分层协助治疗决策的选择。Sokal 模型是最常用的[23],它定义了三个危险组,即低危组(40%~50%的患者),中危组(约 30%的患者)和高危组(10%~20%的患者),按此分类使用白消安(busulfan)或羟基脲治疗的中位存活期分别为 4.5 年、3.5 年和 2.5 年。该模型还预测了伊马替尼治疗的反应和无进展生存期,当然,三组的疗效比过去都好。其他的分类包括,Harford 评分(更适用于干扰素治疗的患者)[24]、简单但未得到普遍验证的 EUTOS 评分(仅基于嗜碱性细胞百分比和脾脏大小)[25~27],或用于干细胞移植(stem cell transplant, SCT)的 Gratwohl 评分[20,28]。TKI 治疗已降低或消除了几个预后因素的价值(如年龄,骨髓纤维化,Del9q,及复杂 Ph 染色体)[21~23,29~32]。值得注意的是,青少年和年轻人可能会有更差的预后,这可能是因为他们对治疗的依从性较差[33]。

发病机制

CML 的主要生物学缺陷是干细胞无节制的扩增,成熟不协调,细胞凋亡减少,与骨髓基质的黏附不良[34~36]。

细胞遗传学

CML 的特征性改变是 Ph 染色体。它是由于第 9 号染色体上 q34.1 的 3′端的 *ABL* 基因片段和 22 号染色体 q11.21 的 5′端的 *BCR* 基因片段相互易位后形成的 t(9;22)(q34.1;q11.21)[2]。这一染色体异常将产生 *BCR-ABL* 融合基因(图 115-5)。

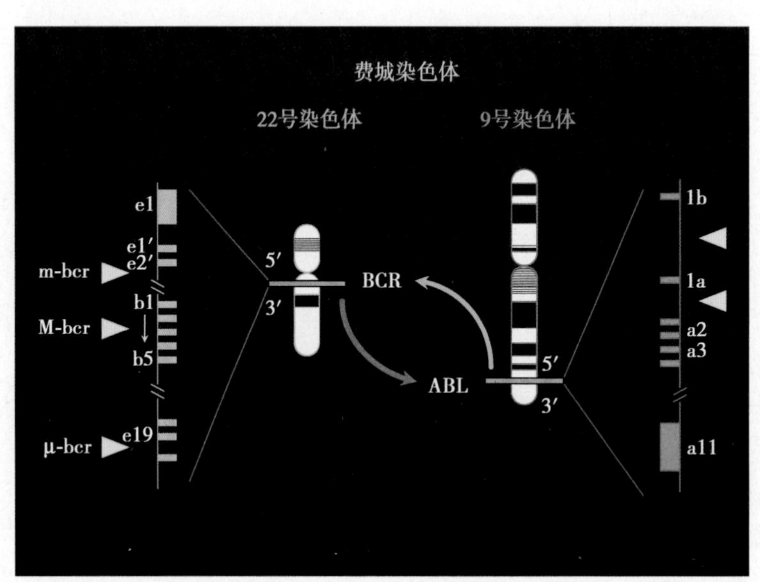

图 115-5　9;22 染色体易位的示意图

在大约 95%的 CML 患者中能发现 Ph 染色体。Ph 染色体在 5%的儿童和 15%~30%成人急性淋巴细胞白血病以及 2%的初诊急性髓细胞性白血病患者中也可以观察到[37]。有些患者会出现变异易位,易位可能是简单易位(涉及 22 号染色体和 9 号染色体以外的另一条染色体)或复杂易位(涉及 22 号染色体,9 号染色体,及至少一个其他染色体)[38]。这些患者以往的治疗效果较差,但接受伊马替尼治疗后,其预后与经典的 Ph 染色体阳性患者类似[31,32]。

CML 的疾病进展往往伴随着其他的细胞遗传学异常。最常见的异常包括+Ph,17 号等臂染色体(i(17q)),+8,+19,20q 缺失[39]。这些细胞遗传学异常导致的分子后果尚不清楚。肿瘤抑制基因的突变和缺失,比如 *p16*、*TP53* 和 *ABL*、*BCR*、*p15* 以及 *cadherin-13* 的甲基化可能在转化过程中起作用[40~44]。JAK-STAT 通路活化可能是白血病干细胞存活的原因[45,46]。在急变期,粒-巨噬细胞祖细胞是候选干细胞,β-catenin 活化可能增强这些细胞的自我更新活性[47]。

TKI 成功治疗后,在 10%~15%的患者中发现,Ph 染色体阴性细胞中存在染色体异常,最常见是+8,单体 7 或 5,20q 缺失[48]。这些异常可能会自行恢复,但在极少数情况下(<1%)可能会发展为骨髓增生异常综合征或 AML[40~42,49~51]。

分子生物学

9 号和 22 号染色体易位产生一种 *BCR-ABL* 融合基因,该基因可编码一个具有改变酪氨酸激酶活性的 *BCR-ABL* 蛋白[46,52]。

发生于 9 号和 22 号染色体的断裂点具有某些程度的异质性。在 9 号染色体上,断裂点可能发生在 200kb 或以上,导致大部分 *c-abl* 基因被易位[46]。*ABL* 基因的断点可发生在最上游外显子Ⅰb 区,也可发生于下游外显子Ⅰa 区,或最常见的外显子Ⅰb 和Ⅰa 之间的区域。BCR 的断裂点常常出现在主要断裂点簇区域,包括 *e12-e16* 外显子(以前称为 *b1-b5*),导致 *b2a2* (*e13a2*)或 *b3a2*(*e14b2*)的融合转录,它们都产生一种 210kDa 的融合蛋白($p210^{BCR-ABL1}$)。在少数新诊断 CML 的患者(但常见于 Ph 阳性的 ALL),断裂点可能会出现在次要的断裂点簇区,产生成一个 *e1a2* 融合(翻译成 190-kDa 的蛋白质)[53]。一些较少见的断点可能发生在其他不同的区域,如 μ-bcr 发生在更远端断点区域。

Bcr-Abl 融合基因转录成为嵌合的 Bcr-Abl mRNA,根据的 *BCR* 基因断裂点的位置不同而翻译出三种分子量不同的融合蛋白 $p190^{Bcr-Abl}$,$p210^{Bcr-Abl}$,和 $p230^{Bcr-Abl}$(图 115-6)。所有这些融合蛋白在结构上都具有不受调节的酪氨酸激酶活性,可激活细胞内信号通路,如 STAT、RAS、RAF、JUN 激酶、MYC、AKT 和 BCL-2 等通路,这就使得 CML 具有了恶性表型[52]。

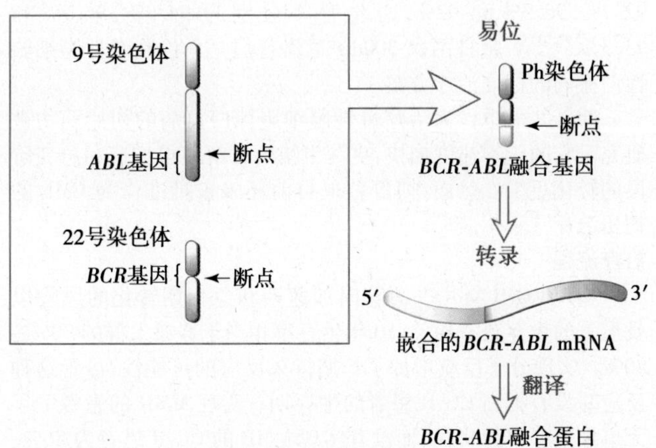

图 115-6　Ph 染色体的细胞遗传学和分子生物学的变化

大多数典型的 CML 患者慢性期为 *b2a2*(*e13a2*)或 *b3a2*(*e14b2*)重排。两者的临床特征,对药物的治疗反应及预后是相似的。Ph 阳性的急性淋巴细胞白血病患者既可以表达 $p210^{Bcr-Abl}$(30%~50%)也可以表达 $p190^{Bcr-Abl}$(50%~70%)。极少数慢性期 CML 患者表达 *e1a2*($p190^{Bcr-Abl}$)蛋白,预后较差[53,54]。表达 $p230^{Bcr-Abl}$ 蛋白与更惰性的 CML 相关,并且其表现更类似于慢性中性粒细胞白血病。

在 5%~10%具有典型形态学表现的 CML 病例中,并未发现 Ph 染色体存在。其中的 1/3 患者,存在 *BCR-ABL* 的基因重排,这些患者具有与 Ph 阳性 CML 患者相似的临床特征、治疗反应和预后[16,55]。其他 2/3 患者不伴有 *BCR-ABL* 重排(在 WHO 分类中称为“非典型 CML”),有着不同的临床特征和血液学特征,包括疾病初期较低的白细胞和血小板计数,以进行性血细胞减少和器官肿大为疾病进展特征,而不是急性白血病转化,中位生存期为 18~24 个月[17,56,57]。这种类型的白血病不在这个章节讨论。反转录酶链式反应(RT-PCR)检测 *BCR-ABL* 转录本的敏感性是 10^{-5}[48,58]。应用 RT-PCR(敏感性是 10^{-8})能够检测出的高达 25%~30%的正常成年人中存在 *BCR-ABL* 重排,大约比临床应用的 RT-PCR 的敏感性高 3 个对数级[59]。这说明克隆性疾病的发生需要逃避免疫监视和/或第二致癌事件。

一部分接受 TKI 治疗的患者会发展为 TKI 耐药。几种耐药机制已被阐明;最常见的是 *BCR-ABL* 激酶域(kinase domain,KD)突变。目前已报道超过 50 种不同的突变,涉及 *BCR-ABL* 结构中的许多域,包括 P-环(ATP 结合区)、活化环、催化域及伊马替尼与 BCR-ABL 结合的氨基酸位点[60]。不同激酶突变的 CML 对不同的 TKI 敏感性不同。某些位点突变可以用比抑制野生型稍高的 TKI 浓度就可以;而其他位点的突变则对 TKI 完全不敏感[61,62]。突变分析有助于帮助 TKI 耐药患者,根据突变对应的不同 TKI 药物的 IC50 值,选择其可能敏感的 TKI。例如,*F317L* 和 *V299L* 突变对达沙替尼(dasatinib)不敏感,*V299L* 突变对博舒替尼(bosutinib)不敏感,F359V 和 E255K/V 对尼洛替尼(nilotinib)不敏感,而 T315I 只对帕纳替尼(ponatinib)敏感(第三代 TKI 对所有突变都有效)[63~65]。

诊断

大约 90%的患者诊断时为慢性期,通常无症状。症状的发展通常是隐匿性的,并且通常由脾肿大(疼痛、腹胀、早期饱腹感)或贫血症状(疲劳)表现出来[13]。临床不常见的症状是出现痛风、厌食、体重减轻、不明原因的发烧或血小板功能障碍(如瘀斑或出血)。WBC 非常高的患者可表现为高黏滞血症的症状(阴茎异常勃起、脑血管意外、耳鸣、精神错乱、视网膜出血)。加速期的症状包括发烧、盗汗、体重减轻或与血小板减少相关的出血。偶尔,常规随诊的患者中并没有加速期的症状,但血液和骨髓的变化已预视加速期的转化。CML 的急变期症状包括相关的全身症状(盗汗、体重减轻、发烧、骨痛)、贫血、感染风险增加和/或出血。

当怀疑为慢性髓细胞性白血病诊断时,必须进行骨髓穿刺。虽然 CML 可以通过检测外周血进行诊断,但只有通过对骨髓和外周血的全面评估,才能识别疾病的所有特征和进行正确的分期。骨髓穿刺应包括以下内容:①细胞分化以进行适当的分期;②评估纤维化和其他特征;③通过 G 显带进行细胞遗传学分析,以确认存在 PH 染色体和可能的额外染色体异常;至少需要 20 个处于分裂中期的细胞来正确判断核型和评估治疗反应。此外,在诊断时推荐 RT-PCR。虽然 *BCR-ABL* 转录的数量与预后无关(基线使用 *ABL* 作为对照基因不可靠),但它允许对标准 PCR 检测不到的异常转录(如 *e19a2*、*b2a3*、*b3a3*)进行检测。

在治疗过程中,每 6 个月进行一次骨髓穿刺以行细胞遗传学分析,直到确认有 CCyR。因此,在大多数患者中,并不需要频繁的骨髓穿刺,或者根本不需要。在 ph 阴性有明确的染色体异常的患者中需要继续进行核型分析。FISH 可用于评估细胞遗传学治疗反应的情况,可用外周血进行检测,但它不提供 ph 阳性细胞(即克隆进化)或 ph 染色体阴性细胞中是否存在额外染色体异常的信息。所有外周血计数有不明原因变化的患者或失去主要分子反应(MMR)(如果国际范围内的水平接近 1%)的患者都应进行骨髓穿刺检查。在治疗期间,还应在治疗开始后 3 个月、6 个月和 12 个月以及之后每 6 个月对患者进行 RT-PCR 监测。

在慢性期患者的诊断时,不需要对突变进行评估,因为在这种情况下,使用标准方法尚未发现突变。当 CCyR 不能持续时,应进行突变的检测。根据欧洲白血病网(ELN)建议,在给定时间内未达到建议的反应标准的患者可以进行突变分析,但比起那些有初始抵抗力的人(即没有达到最佳反应),突变更常见于继发性耐药(即丧失细胞遗传学反应)的患者中。

分期和预后因素

CML有三个阶段:慢性期、加速期和急变期。在前面的"病理"一节中对定义每个阶段的特征进行了描述,对于已经处于慢性期的患者提出了风险分类,其中包括Sokal[23]、Hasford(欧洲)[24]和EUTOS分类[25]。这些分类主要用于预测预后;治疗建议通常同样适用于所有风险组。Sokal评分是最常用的,通过公式得到:exp(0.011 6×(年龄[岁]-43.4))+(0.034 5×(脾脏大小[cm]-7.51)+(0.188×(血小板[10^9/L]/700)^2-0.563))+(0.088 7×(细胞[%]-2.10))。根据评分确定三个风险组:低危(得分<0.8)、中危(得分0.8~1.2)和高危(>1.2)。在美国,只有10%~15%的患者在诊断时具有高风险评分,而在世界其他地区,这些患者可能占所有患者的1/3。

治疗

所有CML患者的初始治疗均采用TKI。甲磺酸伊马替尼是20世纪90年代推出的一种选择性Bcr-Abl TKI,它改变了CML的自然历史[6,66-70],使用TKI治疗的慢性期患者的预期寿命与一般人群相当[71]。

甲磺酸伊马替尼

伊马替尼是一种有效的Bcr-Abl和少数其他酪氨酸激酶,如c-kit和PDGF的抑制剂[6,72]。它最初使用在INF-2治疗失败或不能耐受的CML[73,74]。共有454例患者接受治疗,伊马替尼每日口服400mg,CCyR为57%。预计5年生存率为76%[73]。

对于初治患者,伊马替尼的疗效是通过一个比较伊马替尼和IFN-α联合小剂量阿糖胞苷[卒中后胰岛素耐受干预试验(insulin resistance intervention after stroke,IRIS)]的多中心随机临床试验来证实的[75,76]。随访8年,83%的患者实现了CCyR,无事件生存率81%,无转化生存率92%,总生存率85%[77]。在慢性期,伊马替尼标准的起始剂量为每日400mg。更高剂量的伊马替尼(每日600~800mg)治疗可改善反应率,并可能会更早取得疗效[78,79]。高剂量是否能改善患者的长期预后尚存争议[65,80-82]。到目前为止,每日400mg仍然是标准的初始剂量。若使用伊马替尼每日400mg治疗的慢性期患者出现疾病进展,提高伊马替尼剂量到每日600~800mg可使一些患者重新获得完全细胞遗传学缓解[83,84]。

第二代酪氨酸激酶抑制剂

达沙替尼和尼洛替尼是第二代TKI,分别比伊马替尼强效约300倍[85]和30倍[86]。它们最早被研究并批准用于治疗对伊马替尼产生耐药性或不耐受的患者。随后的试验表明,这两种药物都可以产生比伊马替尼更强大、更快速的反应[87-89]。与伊马替尼相比,其转化为加速阶段和急变阶段的速率更低。因此,这两种药物都被批准并作为慢性CML患者的初始标准治疗。

在达沙替尼与伊马替尼的随机试验中,12个月时达到CCyR的比例达沙替尼为77%,伊马替尼为66%,36个月时MMR累积率分别为69%和55%。3个月时,接受达沙替尼治疗的患者中,84%的患者的*BCR-ABL/ABL*转录水平<10%,而伊马替尼治疗的患者为64%。转化为加速期或急变期的比例分别为3%和5%。在至少4年的随访中,无事件生存率或总生存率无差异[90,91]。达沙替尼治疗新诊断CML慢性期患者的标准起始剂量为每日100mg。

类似的随机试验研究了尼洛替尼两种不同的剂量(每日两次300mg和每日两次400mg)并与伊马替尼对比。第12个月时,尼洛替尼组(400mg每日2次)CCyR率为80%,尼洛替尼组(300mg每日2次)CCyR率为78%,伊马替尼组CCyR率为65%。到第3年,MMR的发生率分别为73%、70%和53%。若以*BCR-ABL/ABL*水平<10%为标准,其中尼洛替尼300mg每日2次达标率为91%,尼洛替尼400mg每日2次达标率为89%,伊马替尼达标率为67%;第4年未进展到加速或急变阶段的分别为96.7%、97.8%和93.1%。4年无进展生存率分别为92.7%、96.3%和92%,总生存率分别为94.3%、96.7%和93.3%[92,93]。每日两次300mg尼洛替尼是新诊断慢性髓细胞性白血病的标准治疗方案。

博舒替尼也作为治疗慢性髓细胞性白血病的初始药物被研究。它的应答速度加快,更深更快的缓解使得加速和急变阶段的转化更少。然而,博舒替尼目前还未被批准作为CML的初始治疗[94]。

治疗流程

实现CCyR与几乎消除向加速期和急变期转化的风险以及显著的生存获益相关,10年生存率相当于普通人群的70%~80%。实现分子反应增加了长期持久反应的可能性,尽管这种反应并没有提高CCyR患者的生存期。实现MMR的患者7年无事件生存率为95%,而没有实现MMR的CCyR患者为86%。无加速期或急变期转化的生存率和总生存率没有差异。更深层次的反应考虑停止治疗的可能性,而这在今天是只能通过临床试验来考虑的观点。

除了反应的深度,反应的时间对改善长期结果也很重要。治疗开始后3个月*BCR-ABL/ABL*<10%的患者与>10%患者相比,EFS的发生率显著提高(分别为90%和80%)[95-98]。总体存活率也有显著但较小的差异。这决定了被认为是最佳治疗反应的建议,包括在第3个月用RT-PCR分型的*BCR-ABL/ABL*<10%和/或用标准核型分型的Ph<35%,在第6个月的*BCR-ABL/ABL*<1%和/或Ph0%,和在第12个月的*BCR-ABL/ABL*<0.1%。以上级别定义失败(表115-1)[99]。

获得最佳治疗的患者可以不加改变地继续治疗。目前的治疗流程包括无限期地继续治疗,尽管目前正在进行一些研究以确定是否可以停止某些患者的治疗。符合警告定义的患者可以继续治疗,但应评估依从性,优化治疗,并每3个月严格监测患者,如果发现治疗失败,应考虑治疗变化。一旦符合失败的定义,就应该实施治疗的更改[99]。

改变治疗方法的另一个原因可能是不耐受。尽管TKI的总体耐受性很好,但它们都有不良事件,需要监测和适当的管理。适当的管理[100]可能包括短暂的治疗中断、剂量调整、不良事件的医疗管理和支持性护理,按经验来说大多数患者可以继续治疗和充分应答。一般情况下,患者不应根据首次发生的不良事件而改用不同的TKI,除非这是危及生命的情况(如Stevens-Johnson综合征、心肌梗死、卒中)。只有大约5%的患者对TKI是有真正的不耐受。对最常见不良事件的管理建议见表115-2。

表 115-1　伊马替尼常见相关不良事件的管理建议

不良事件	处理	不良事件	处理
恶心/呕吐	与食物、液体同服	关节痛，骨痛	非甾体抗炎药
	止吐药	转氨酶升高(罕见)	中断治疗并密切观测
腹泻	洛哌丁胺		缓解后减剂量
	复方地芬诺酯	骨髓抑制	暂停治疗/减低剂量一般不选择
外周水肿	利尿剂	贫血	考虑使用促红细胞生成素或促红细胞生成刺激蛋白[a]
眶周水肿	含激素的乳膏		
皮疹	避免暴露于阳光	中性粒细胞减少症	3 级以上(如 ANC<1×10^9/L)则中断治疗，复发/症状持续或出现败血症时考虑非格司亭
	局部使用激素		
	系统性使用激素(早期处理很重要)	血小板减少症	3 级以上(如血小板<50×10^9/L)则中断治疗，考虑予 IL-11[a] 10μg/kg 每周用 3~7 日
肌肉痉挛	奎宁水或奎宁		
	必要时用电解质替代治疗		
	葡萄糖酸钙		

[a] 促红细胞生成素、促红细胞生成刺激蛋白、非格司亭、IL-11 的使用并非标准用法，需要根据情况考虑使用

表 115-2　根据欧洲白血病网的反应标准

时间/月	反应		
	失败	警告	最优的
3	无 CHR 和/或 Ph+>95%	*BCR-ABL*>10%和/或 Ph+>36%~95%	*BCR-ABL*≤10%和/或 Ph+≤35%
6	*BCR-ABL*>10%和/或 Ph+>35%	*BCR-ABL* 1%~10%和/或 Ph+>1%~35%	*BCR-ABL*<1%和/或 Ph+0
12	*BCR-ABL*>1%和/或 Ph+>0	*BCR-ABL*>0.1%~1%	*BCR-ABL*<0.1%
任意	CHR 缺失，CCyR 缺失，证实 MMR 缺失 CCA/Ph+突变	CCA/Ph-(-7,或者 7q-)	*BCR-ABL*<0.1%

CHR，完全血液学缓解；Ph+，存在费城染色体的中期细胞的百分比(完全评估至少需要 20 个)；CCyR，完全细胞变异反应；MMR，主要分子反应；CCA/Ph+，费城染色体的细胞克隆染色体异常。

改编自 Quintas-Cardama 等，2009。这项研究最初发表在《血液》杂志上。© 美国血液病学会。

早期 TKI 失败后的治疗方案

有几种 TKI 可用于治疗耐药(如 ELN[99] 所定义)或对早期 TKI 不耐受的患者。这些药物包括达沙替尼、尼洛替尼、博舒替尼和泼那替尼(ponatinib)。此外，高三尖杉酯碱是一种蛋白质合成抑制剂(不是 TKI)，也被批准用于接受过至少两次 TKI 治疗的患者。

在以前仅接受伊马替尼作为早期 TKI 治疗并经历了耐药或不耐受的患者中，每日服用一次剂量为 100mg 的达沙替尼可诱导 44%的耐药患者和 67%的不耐药患者发生 CCyR。MMR 发生在 37%的耐药或不耐受患者中，6 年无进展生存率为 49%，总生存率为 71%[101,102]。同样，在每日两次 400mg 剂量(二线治疗的标准剂量)尼洛替尼能够诱导 41%的伊马替尼耐药患者和 51%的耐药患者发生 CCyR，4 年无进展生存率为 57%，总生存率为 78%[103]。博舒替尼也是第二代 TKI，具有抗 Src 和 Abl 的活性，是伊马替尼抗 Abl 活性的 30~50 倍，但与用于 CML 的其他 TKI 相比，对 c-kit 或 PDGF-R 的抑制作用最小。博舒替尼也有效地诱导了 48%的耐药患者和 52%的对伊马替尼不耐受患者发生 CCyR，CCyR 患者中分别有 64%和 65%的患者实现了 MMR。这导致无进展生存率分别为 73%和 95%[104]。这些药物在 *T315I* 突变患者中均不起作用。

博舒替尼和泼那替尼在已接受两种或两种以上 TKI 治疗的患者中进行了研究。每日服用一次博舒替尼 500mg，118 名接受伊马替尼治疗的患者中有 30%~35%的患者产生了主要的细胞遗传学反应，这些患者已经对达沙替尼产生了耐药性或不耐受，或对尼洛替尼产生了耐药性。相应的 CCyR 率分别为 14%、28%和 27%，预计 2 年无进展生存率分别为 65%、81%和 77%[105]。泼那替尼是一种有效的 Abl 酪氨酸激酶活性抑制剂以及包括 c-kit、FLT3 和 VEGFR 在内的其他激酶的有效抑制剂。重要的是，它对未突变的 *BCR-ABL* 或任何经过检测的 *KD* 突变，包括多重耐药的 T315I，都具有强大的抑制活性[106]。泼

那替尼每日剂量为45mg,在267例患者中93%至少接受过2次TKI治疗(60%至少接受过3次TKI治疗),56%(46%完全)获得了主要的细胞遗传学反应,34%获得了MMR。91%患者的主要细胞遗传学反应至少持续了12个月,12个月的总生存率为94%。对于T315I患者,应答率分别为70%、66%和56%,应答的持久性和总体生存率相似[107,108]。使用高三尖杉酯碱,20%的慢性期患者在对至少两种TKI产生耐药性后,获得了主要的细胞遗传学反应,平均总生存期为33.9个月[109]。包括T315I患者在内无论突变状态如何,均可看到应答[110]。对TKI有耐药性的患者也应考虑异基因SCT。

干细胞移植

异基因SCT在40%~80%的患者中可能是有效的,这些患者接受的移植来自HLA相合同胞或不相关的捐赠者[111]。在首次慢性期移植的患者中,来自匹配相关的同胞的3 514例和来自不相关的捐赠者的1 052例,5年生存率分别为63%和55%,无白血病生存率分别为55%和50%。5年复发的累积发生率为12%~14%[111]。然而,对于在持续完全缓解≥5年存活的患者,接收同胞供者细胞的15年的存活率是88%,而接受那些不相关的捐赠者是87%,复发的累积发病率分别为8%和2%,移植后18年有复发记录[112]。接受干细胞移植治疗的患者在移植后的前14年的死亡率高于年龄、性别和种族相近的一般人群[112]。近年来,由于使用脐带血或单倍体相合供体进行移植取得越来越成功的结果,供者的可获得性有所改善,并且通过使用非清髓性条件治疗方案,供体的可获得性已扩展到更高年龄组。此外,通过改善支持治疗和GVHD(移植物抗宿主病)预防和管理,早期死亡率已经下降。然而,随着TKI的应用,SCT的作用发生了重大变化。一些报道证实,尽管从诊断到SCT的时间仍然是影响移植后预后的重要因素,既往暴露于TKI对SCT后的预后没有不良影响[113,114]。同样,慢性期移植患者的预后明显好于晚期移植患者[111]。在泼那替尼和高三尖杉酯碱出现之前,SCT是治疗*T315I*突变的唯一有效方法,慢性期移植的患者的2年生存率为59%[115,116]。

加速期或急变期移植患者的预后明显较差,加速期5年生存率为40%,急变期为10%~15%。在第2个慢性期后进行急变期移植的患者可能具有与加速期移植患者相似的长期结果[28,117,118]。

2015年的CML治疗建议

迄今为止,伊马替尼的疗效非常好且持久,随着随访时间的缩短,达沙替尼和尼洛替尼的疗效在早期和较深的反应以及较低的转化率方面似乎更好,尽管这些结果没有在无事件或整体生存中转化为显著的差异。TKI治疗患者的预期寿命与普通人群相似,尤其是达到CCyR的患者。基于此TKI是所有慢性期CML患者的标准初始治疗。由于与伊马替尼相比,达沙替尼或尼洛替尼在随机试验中的疗效有所提高,因此在许多情况下首选这些药物[90~93]。然而,伊马替尼可能仍然是全世界大部分(可能是主体)患者的首选治疗方法。应当强调的是,伊马替尼也是适当的治疗方法。为患者提供最佳长期结果的最重要方面是对患者的适当管理。这包括发现和管理不良事件的密切随访。所有TKI都有与之相关的不良事件,但大多数都可以通过短暂的治疗中断、剂量调整和/或医疗干预来控制。很少有患者(约5%)对某种药物真的不耐受。在有后续研究表明早期改变治疗方案的长期益处之前,在3个月内没有主要细胞遗传学反应(或没有BCR-ABL/ABL转录物<10%)的患者可以继续不改变治疗方案,但需要在第6个月后再次检查[99]。对于在治疗6个月后仍未达到主要细胞遗传学反应(或仍有BCR-ABL/ABL转录物>10%)的患者,可以考虑改变治疗方案,尽管也没有研究表明,在这种情况下改变治疗方案会改变长期预后。患者需要至少每6个月进行一次详细的监测。当达到失败的标准时(如ELN所定义的),明显需要治疗方法的改变。随机试验表明在这些情况下(比如失败),与伊马替尼剂量的增加相比,从伊马替尼换到第二代TKI的治疗改变改善了结局[119]。在符合失败标准的情况下,通常需要进行突变分析,并且还需要进行骨髓穿刺,以确定患者在改变治疗前的细胞遗传学和所处阶段。如果确定了突变,这可以指导预期诱导应答的TKI是哪一种(如果确定了*F317L*或*V299L*,考虑尼洛替尼或泼那替尼;如果确定了F359V,考虑博沙替尼、达沙替尼或泼那替尼;对于T315I,可能考虑泼那替尼或高三尖杉酯碱)[61,62]。如果没有突变,或者有一个没有可用的信息的突变或不同的TKI没有有意义的差异的突变,那么其他的考虑因素可能有助于决定使用什么药物,例如使用一种或另一种药物可能使患者更多地暴露于不良事件的并发症,对于特定的患者可能更容易接受的不良事件谱,以及患者发现更方便或更容易接受的剂量,从而来优化依从性。对至少两种TKI有耐药性的患者可以考虑进行SCT。在长期治疗可能不理想或不可行的其他情况下(如出于成本考虑),也可以考虑SCT。

在诊断时具有加速期特征的患者可以用TKI治疗,特别是达沙替尼或尼洛替尼,在这种情况下他们的预后与慢性期患者几乎相同[120]。除非没有足够的反应,否则这些患者不需要SCT。对于在接受TKI治疗时进展到加速期的慢性期患者,应接受一种不同的TKI并考虑进行SCT。急变期CML患者应接受TKI治疗,通常合并化疗并且应该强烈考虑SCT。尽管在这种情况下,SCT的效果最好,残留疾病最少,但一旦患者达到血液学完全缓解,就可以继续进行移植,因为进一步的化疗可能会导致并发症,这可能会使SCT不能进行或有更大的风险并且反应可能不会进一步改善。

生存和随访

CML患者应持续治疗,并进行密切的无限期随访。这不仅包括监测疾病状态(每6个月用PCR检测一次外周血),还包括注意并发症和可能的副作用。需要持续进行评估从而对不良事件的认识有所提高。这些包括动脉血栓性事件,如缺血性心脏病(包括心绞痛和心肌梗死)、缺血性脑病(包括短暂的缺血性发作和卒中)和外周动脉闭塞性疾病等动脉血栓事件,尤其是泼那替尼和尼洛替尼。应注意监测和管理危险因素,如高血压(经常由泼那替尼引起或加重)、糖尿病(经常由尼洛替尼引起或加重)、高脂血症(也与TKI治疗相关)等。最近的分析也表明TKI可能会损害肾功能,尤其是伊马替尼。使用达沙替尼有呼吸道症状的患者应评估胸腔积液或肺动脉高压。尽管大多数不良事件发生在病程的早期,但对于某些(如胸腔积液或动脉血栓事件)来说,其发生率是恒定的,并且第一次事件可能会发生在治疗的几年后。

正在进行的研究在探索对合适的患者中止治疗[124,125]。在至少 2 年内持续检测不到转录本(PCR 敏感性至少为 4.5log)的患者中,经过 3~4 年的随访约 40%的患者中止治疗后病情得到持续缓解。目前这种方法只应在临床试验中考虑,患者应继续密切监测,前 6 个月至少每月监测一次,2 年内每 2~3 个月监测一次,然后持续每 6 个月监测一次。

结论

自从 TKI 问世,CML 患者的预后有了显著的改善。预计现今确诊的慢性髓细胞性白血病患者的预期寿命可能与普通人群相似。要使患者获得如此良好的结果,充分的管理是很重要的,包括合适的剂量优化、合适的不良事件管理、持续的定期疾病反应监测、如有指征及时的干预以及在患者的整个生命周期中持续的支持。通过这种方式,进展期转化不常见,并且死于 CML 的患者将越来越少。

总结

慢性髓细胞性白血病(CML)的特征是存在费城染色体。这导致了 *BCR-ABL* 融合基因的产生,而 *BCR-ABL* 融合基因进而转化为具有结构激酶活性的酪氨酸激酶。该病分为三个阶段:慢性期、加速期和急变期。大多数患者在慢性期被诊断并且诊断时没有症状。使用 TKI 治疗改变了该疾病的自然病史,其预期寿命与普通人群相似。伊马替尼是第一个应用的 TKI,仍然是一线治疗的标准和有效疗法。大多数患者将达到一个完全细胞遗传学反应(CCyR),使其转化为加速期和急变期的情况非常罕见。更高剂量的伊马替尼可以达到更高的应答率,包括更深的分子应答。达沙替尼和尼洛替尼也是一线治疗的批准治疗方案,可以提高完全细胞遗传学和主要分子(以及更深的分子)应答的速率,并且很少转化到加速期和急变期,但在随机试验中与伊马替尼相比,没有改善无事件生存率或总生存率。对于对一种 TKI 产生耐药性或不耐受的患者,可以更换其他抑制剂。在这种情况下,博舒替尼和泼那替尼是额外的选择。总的来说,大约 40%对初始治疗有耐药性或不耐受的患者可能在随后的 TKI 治疗中实现 CCyR。最常见的耐药机制是 *KD* 突变的出现。不同的突变可能对不同的抑制剂有不同的敏感性,当存在这种突变时,可以选择最合适的治疗方案。尽管一般耐受良好的 TKI 可能导致不良事件,其中一些可能是严重的并且需要适当的识别和管理;这可能包括在某些情况下改变治疗方案。对于那些对各线治疗方案都没有实现充分反应的患者,SCT 仍然是一种有用的和潜在的治疗方法。在充足的治疗方法和适当的管理下,诊断为 CML 的患者应该能够获得正常的预期寿命。

(白元松　周迪 译　白元松　周迪　李军　丛丹 校)

参考文献

The complete reference list can be found on the Wiley Companion Digital Edition of this title (see inside front cover for login instructions).

1 Nowell PC, Hungerford DA. A minute chromosome in human chronic granulocytic leukemia. *Science*. 1960;**132**:1497–1501.

7 Kantarjian H, O'Brien S, Jabbour E, et al. Improved survival in chronic myeloid leukemia since the introduction of imatinib therapy: a single-institution historical experience. *Blood*. 2012;**119(9)**:1981–1987.

14 Kantarjian HM, Dixon D, Keating MJ, et al. Characteristics of accelerated disease in chronic myelogenous leukemia. *Cancer*. 1988;**61(7)**:1441–1446.

23 Sokal JE, Cox EB, Baccarani M, et al. Prognostic discrimination in "good-risk" chronic granulocytic leukemia. *Blood*. 1984;**63(4)**:789–799.

31 Quintas-Cardama A, Kantarjian H, Talpaz M, et al. Imatinib mesylate therapy may overcome the poor prognostic significance of deletions of derivative chromosome 9 in patients with chronic myelogenous leukemia. *Blood*. 2005;**105(6)**:2281–2286.

33 Pemmaraju N, Kantarjian H, Shan J, et al. Analysis of outcomes in adolescents and young adults with chronic myelogenous leukemia treated with upfront tyrosine kinase inhibitor therapy. *Haematologica*. 2012;**97(7)**:1029–1035.

47 Jamieson CH, Ailles LE, Dylla SJ, et al. Granulocyte-macrophage progenitors as candidate leukemic stem cells in blast-crisis CML. *N Engl J Med*. 2004;**351(7)**:657–667.

48 Medina J, Kantarjian H, Talpaz M, et al. Chromosomal abnormalities in Philadelphia chromosome-negative metaphases appearing during imatinib mesylate therapy in patients with Philadelphia chromosome-positive chronic myelogenous leukemia in chronic phase. *Cancer*. 2003;**98(9)**:1905–1911.

52 Quintas-Cardama A, Cortes J. Molecular biology of bcr-abl1-positive chronic myeloid leukemia. *Blood*. 2009;**113(8)**:1619–1630.

58 Hughes T, Deininger M, Hochhaus A, et al. Monitoring CML patients responding to treatment with tyrosine kinase inhibitors: review and recommendations for harmonizing current methodology for detecting BCR-ABL transcripts and kinase domain mutations and for expressing results. *Blood*. 2006;**108(1)**:28–37.

62 Redaelli S, Piazza R, Rostagno R, et al. Activity of bosutinib, dasatinib, and nilotinib against 18 imatinib-resistant BCR/ABL mutants. *J Clin Oncol*. 2009;**27(3)**:469–471.

63 Kantarjian H, Schiffer C, Jones D, Cortes J. Monitoring the response and course of chronic myeloid leukemia in the modern era of BCR-ABL tyrosine kinase inhibitors: practical advice on the use and interpretation of monitoring methods. *Blood*. 2008;**111(4)**:1774–1780.

69 Druker BJ, Talpaz M, Resta DJ, et al. Efficacy and safety of a specific inhibitor of the BCR-ABL tyrosine kinase in chronic myeloid leukemia. *N Engl J Med*. 2001;**344(14)**:1031–1037.

74 Kantarjian H, Sawyers C, Hochhaus A, et al. Hematologic and cytogenetic responses to imatinib mesylate in chronic myelogenous leukemia. *N Engl J Med*. 2002;**346(9)**:645–652.

75 Druker BJ, Guilhot F, O'Brien SG, et al. Five-year follow-up of patients receiving imatinib for chronic myeloid leukemia. *N Engl J Med*. 2006;**355(23)**:2408–2417.

79 Kantarjian H, Talpaz M, O'Brien S, et al. High-dose imatinib mesylate therapy in newly diagnosed Philadelphia chromosome-positive chronic phase chronic myeloid leukemia. *Blood*. 2004;**103(8)**:2873–2878.

82 Hehlmann R, Lauseker M, Jung-Munkwitz S, et al. Tolerability-adapted imatinib 800 mg/d versus 400 mg/d versus 400 mg/d plus interferon-alpha in newly diagnosed chronic myeloid leukemia. *J Clin Oncol*. 2011;**29(12)**:1634–1642.

88 Cortes JE, Jones D, O'Brien S, et al. Results of dasatinib therapy in patients with early chronic-phase chronic myeloid leukemia. *J Clin Oncol*. 2010;**28(3)**:398–404.

91 Kantarjian HM, Shah NP, Cortes JE, et al. Dasatinib or imatinib in newly diagnosed chronic-phase chronic myeloid leukemia: 2-year follow-up from a randomized phase 3 trial (DASISION). *Blood*. 2012;**119(5)**:1123–1129.

92 Kantarjian HM, Hochhaus A, Saglio G, et al. Nilotinib versus imatinib for the treatment of patients with newly diagnosed chronic phase, Philadelphia chromosome-positive, chronic myeloid leukaemia: 24-month minimum follow-up of the phase 3 randomised ENESTnd trial. *Lancet Oncol*. 2011;**12(9)**:841–851.

94 Gambacorti-Passerini C, Cortes JE, Lipton JH, et al. Safety of bosutinib versus imatinib in the phase 3 BELA trial in newly diagnosed chronic phase chronic myeloid leukemia. *Am J Hematol*. 2014;**89(10)**:947–953.

95 Jain P, Kantarjian H, Nazha A, et al. Early responses predict better outcomes in patients with newly diagnosed chronic myeloid leukemia: results with four tyrosine kinase inhibitor modalities. *Blood*. 2013;**121(24)**:4867–4874.

99 Baccarani M, Deininger MW, Rosti G, et al. European Leukemia Net recommendations for the management of chronic myeloid leukemia: 2013. *Blood*. 2013;**122(6)**:872–884.

102 Shah NP, Guilhot F, Cortes JE, et al. Long-term outcome with dasatinib after ima-

tinib failure in chronic-phase chronic myeloid leukemia: follow-up of a phase 3 study. *Blood*. 2014;**123(15)**:2317–2324.

103 Giles FJ, le Coutre PD, Pinilla-Ibarz J, et al. Nilotinib in imatinib-resistant or imatinib-intolerant patients with chronic myeloid leukemia in chronic phase: 48-month follow-up results of a phase II study. *Leukemia*. 2013;**27(1)**:107–112.

104 Gambacorti-Passerini C, Brummendorf TH, Kim DW, et al. Bosutinib efficacy and safety in chronic phase chronic myeloid leukemia after imatinib resistance or intolerance: minimum 24-month follow-up. *Am J Hematol*. 2014;**89(7)**:732–742.

107 Cortes JE, Kim DW, Pinilla-Ibarz J, et al. A phase 2 trial of ponatinib in Philadelphia chromosome-positive leukemias. *N Engl J Med*. 2013;**369(19)**:1783–1796.

109 Cortes JE, Nicolini FE, Wetzler M, et al. Subcutaneous omacetaxine mepesuccinate in patients with chronic-phase chronic myeloid leukemia previously treated with 2 or more tyrosine kinase inhibitors including imatinib. *Clin Lymphoma Myeloma Leuk*. 2013;**13(5)**:584–591.

111 Arora M, Weisdorf DJ, Spellman SR, et al. HLA-identical sibling compared with 8/8 matched and mismatched unrelated donor bone marrow transplant for chronic phase chronic myeloid leukemia. *J Clin Oncol*. 2009;**27(10)**:1644–1652.

112 Goldman JM, Majhail NS, Klein JP, et al. Relapse and late mortality in 5-year survivors of myeloablative allogeneic hematopoietic cell transplantation for chronic myeloid leukemia in first chronic phase. *J Clin Oncol*. 2010;**28(11)**:1888–1895.

120 Ohanian M, Kantarjian HM, Quintas-Cardama A, et al. Tyrosine kinase inhibitors as initial therapy for patients with chronic myeloid leukemia in accelerated phase. *Clin Lymphoma Myeloma Leuk*. 2014;**14(2)**:155–162.

124 Mahon FX, Rea D, Guilhot J, et al. Discontinuation of imatinib in patients with chronic myeloid leukaemia who have maintained complete molecular remission for at least 2 years: the prospective, multicentre Stop Imatinib (STIM) trial. *Lancet Oncol*. 2010;**11(11)**:1029–1035.

125 Ross DM, Branford S, Seymour JF, et al. Safety and efficacy of imatinib cessation for CML patients with stable undetectable minimal residual disease: results from the TWISTER Study. *Blood*. 2013.

第 116 章　急性淋巴细胞白血病

Nitin Jain, MD, MSPH ■ Stefan Faderl, MD ■ Hagop M. Kantarjian, MD ■ Susan O' Brien, MD

概述

成人急性淋巴细胞白血病(acute lymphoblastic leukemia, ALL)预后不良。近年来在 ALL 的生物学行为、预后和治疗方面取得了很大进步。治疗方面的进步包括单克隆抗体、抗体药物偶联物(antibody-drug conjugates, ADC)、酪氨酸激酶抑制剂(tyrosine kinase inhibitors, TKI)等药物的进展，以及最新的嵌合抗原受体 T 细胞治疗(chimericantigen receptor T-cell therapy, CAR-T)。这些治疗方法正在逐步改善 ALL 患者的生存。

引言

急性淋巴细胞白血病是一种异质性疾病。ALL 细胞遗传学-分子生物学特征的识别使 ALL 亚型分类更加准确，并促进按照预后风险进行分层治疗和新药研发。更为重要的是，短短几十年中 ALL 的治疗进展已经使大多数儿童 ALL 得以治愈。将儿童 ALL 的成功治疗策略应用于成人明显提高了疗效，但长期无病生存率(disease-free survival, DFS)仅 40%左右。但是，不断进步的 ALL 分子生物学危险度分层、改良的联合化疗方案、新型靶向药物的研发、对微小残留病的理解，以及对药物基因组学特征和耐药机制认识的不断深入，将有望于提高成人 ALL 患者的预后。

流行病学和病因学

ALL 好发于儿童，占全部儿童白血病的 80%，占全部儿童肿瘤的 25%，高发年龄为 2~5 岁，发病率为 3.5/10 万~4/10 万。与之相反，ALL 在成人肿瘤中的比例低于 1%。在美国，ALL 年龄标准化发病率约为 1.7/10 万，每年大约有 6 000 例新诊断的 ALL 患者[1]。

ALL 常见于高加索人种，发病率存在地理差异，生活在西班牙和拉丁美洲的西班牙裔 ALL 发病率较高[2]。在儿童 ALL 中男性的发病率略高于女性，而在大于 20 岁的患者中男性 ALL 的发病率显著高于女性(1.3∶1)。此外，在工业化和城市化地区 ALL 的发病率高，使得人们推测社会经济学因素很可能也参与了 ALL 发病[3]。

大多数患者无明确的致病因素。在儿童中，仅有少数患者(<5%)与遗传因素有关(如 Down 综合征、布卢姆综合征(Bloom syndrome)、运动失调性毛细血管扩张症、Nijmege 断裂综合征)[4]。增加儿童 ALL 风险的因素包括父母的职业，母亲的生产史，父母的吸烟或饮酒史，母亲的饮食状况，出生前的维生素使用情况，杀虫剂或有机溶剂的暴露史，居住地高水平的供电线相关磁场暴露史(>0.3μT 或 0.4μT)，但这些危险因素存在争议[5,6]。研究还关注药物代谢的遗传变异，DNA 修复，可能与环境相互作用的细胞周期检查点，饮食，母系遗传以及其他可能影响白血病发生的外部因素。全基因组相关性研究已经明确了几个增加 ALL 发生风险的基因(如 ARID5B、IKZF1、CDKN2A、TP63、GATA3)[7~12]。

儿童 ALL 的高发年龄为 2~5 岁，鉴于 ALL 与工业化及城市化的相关性，及偶发的儿童 ALL 聚集现象(特别是在新建城市)，由此产生了两个假说：①人口混合假说；②延迟感染假说[13~15]。第一个假说认为，儿童 ALL 聚集发生是由于非病原学感染的易感者(非免疫的)混入携带者人群[13,14]。第二个假说建立在二次打击学说基础上，认为一些出生前获得前白血病克隆的易感者由于生活水平较高，年轻时无或仅有轻度的常见感染[15]，未经历感染使这些人的免疫系统更易于对常见感染产生异常或病理反应，病原体感染的时间与患者淋巴细胞快速增殖的年龄相一致。实际上，对新生儿血迹和单卵双生子的回顾性研究已经证实存在白血病前克隆，并支持出生后获得性的转化事件是完成白血病转化的必要条件[16~19]。

临床表现

ALL 患者的临床症状和体征的差异很大。疾病可能在诊断前潜伏发展并持续数月，但是大多数患者都是急性发病，临床症状与骨髓中白血病细胞增殖并向外周血、淋巴结、肝脏、脾脏和中枢神经系统(central nervous system, CNS)等髓外组织浸润相关。常见临床症状包括：乏力、全身症状(发热、盗汗和体重减轻)、容易淤青或出血、呼吸困难。儿童患者尤其是婴幼儿，可能仅出现四肢和关节疼痛。T-ALL 可因纵隔肿物导致喘鸣和哮鸣，心包积液和上腔静脉压迫综合征。睾丸浸润发生率低，主要见于婴儿期和青少年期的男性患者。尽管 CNS 白血病更常见于成熟 B-ALL(Burkitt 白血病/淋巴瘤)患者，但是确诊时仅有不到 10%的患者具有 CNS 浸润。脑神经麻痹(特别是第Ⅲ、Ⅳ、Ⅵ和Ⅶ对脑神经)可导致复视、眼球运动异常、面部感觉迟钝和面部肌肉下垂。恶心、呕吐、头痛或视乳头水肿提示可能存在脑膜侵犯和高颅压。中枢神经受累所致的颏麻木，由于症状较轻，若患者无主诉很容易漏诊。可通过脑脊液(CSF)涂片确诊 CNS 浸润。尽管以往指南中 CNS 浸润的诊断指标为脑脊液中>5 个白细胞/μl，并可见原始淋巴细胞，但对于脑脊液中可见原始淋巴细胞，但<5 个白细胞/μl 的患者 CNS 浸润的诊断尚存争议[20]。最新明确了以下三种 CNS 状态：①脑脊液中无原始淋巴细胞(CNS1)；②<5 个白细胞/μl，可见原始淋巴细胞(CNS2)；③>5 个白细胞/μl，可见原始淋巴细胞或者出现脑神经麻痹(CNS3)[21]。体格检查可以有苍白、瘀点、瘀斑、全身淋巴结肿大和肝脾肿大。肿瘤溶解综合征常见于成熟 B-ALL 患者，但是也可见于具有高白细胞计数的其他类型的白血病患者。弥散性血管内凝血(diffuse intravascular coagulation, DIC)以实验室检查异常多见,很少具有明显的DIC临床特征。表116-1总结了就诊于三级转诊中心的接受初始治疗为hyper-CVAD方案的成人ALL患者的临床和实验室特征[22]。

表116-1 接受hyper-CVAD化疗作为初始治疗的成人急性淋巴细胞白血病的特征(n=204)

特征	变量
中位年龄(岁)	39.5
范围	16~79
≥60岁/%	22
ECOG身体状况评分>2/%	7
器官受累(%)	1
淋巴结肿大	32
脾大	25
肝大	16
中位白细胞计数($\times10^9$)	7.7
白细胞计数>30×10^9	26
生化检查异常/%	—
乳酸脱氢酶增高	59
肌苷≥1.3mg/dl	16
胆红素≥1.3mg/dl	13
免疫表型/%	—
前B细胞型	67
成熟B细胞型	9
T细胞型	12
其他(未分化,双表型)	12
髓系标记阳性/%	54
核型/%	—
二倍体	22
Ph染色体阳性	16
t(8;14);t(8;2);t(8;22)	4
超二倍体	4
亚二倍体	5
危险度分层/%	—
标危	22
高危	78

ALL的诊断

根据外周血、骨髓或组织切片检测到白血病细胞来确定ALL的诊断。临床工作中对ALL患者的白血病细胞进行细胞形态学、细胞化学和免疫表型的彻底评估非常重要。明确细胞遗传学和分子生物学异常能更准确地将白血病细胞分类,有助于更加准确的判断患者预后。目前正在进行的全基因组分析能够重新定义ALL的亚型并且能够将预后不同及需要特殊治疗的患者进行分组,而以目前的手段仅能部分区分患者[23,24]。

形态学和细胞化学

ALL白血病细胞是大小和形状不同的异质性群体,最初就是依据ALL原始细胞的形态学特征进行ALL分型诊断。法国-美国-英国(FAB)协作组据此将ALL分为三型:L1型白血病细胞体积小,核浆比大,核仁不清楚,细胞质疏松,嗜碱性不一。L2型白血病细胞以大细胞为主,大小不一,比较丰富的细胞质,核浆比较小,核仁更加清楚。L1型中儿童患者多见,而L2型更多见于成人患者。L3型白血病细胞大小较均一,中等大小,染色质分散,核仁清楚,细胞质呈典型的深蓝色嗜碱性,空泡明显。L3型多见于成熟B-ALL和Burkitt淋巴瘤。成熟B-ALL以细胞更新快为特征,在骨髓活检切片中表现为"满天星"的细胞形态学特征。除L3型与成熟B-ALL相关外,其余分型因不具有预后或治疗相关性已基本失用。

尽管尚无具有确诊意义的细胞化学染色方法,诊断ALL的细胞化学染色的关键特征包括:髓过氧化物酶(MPO)阴性,非特异性酯酶(NSE)阴性,MPO低阳性率(3%~5%)见于急淋变期的慢性髓细胞性白血病患者和其他的罕见病例[25,26]。苏丹黑染色与MPO非常相似,但特异性低,并且MPO染色的简便易行性限制了苏丹黑染色的应用。末端脱氧核苷酰转移酶(TdT)是鉴别反应性和恶性淋巴细胞增多非常有价值的指标,通常见于≥40%的白血病细胞。L3型ALL以TdT阴性为特征[27]。

免疫分型

以流式细胞仪进行免疫分型检测是确诊ALL的重要步骤,能够鉴别诊断并进一步明确亚型。尽管目前尚无公认的诊断ALL的抗体谱,图116-1所列出的常见抗体组合通常足以使>95%的ALL患者确诊,并明确来源。

大部分的(70%~85%)ALL均为B细胞来源。按照B细胞的分化阶段,可将B-ALL分为:(i)早期前B-ALL(pro-B-ALL);(ii)普通型B-ALL(commonB-ALL);(iii)前B-ALL(pre-B-ALL)以及(iv)成熟B-ALL(matureB-ALL)。在可辨别的最早期阶段,早期前B-ALL白血病细胞表现为CD19阳性、CD79a阳性或CD22阳性,但不具有其他B细胞分化抗原。免疫表型特征为CD19阳性、CD10阴性、胞质免疫球蛋白阴性且伴有髓系抗原共表达的B-ALL好发于婴幼儿期,通常与t(4;11)异位及*MLL*基因重排相关,预后差。普通型ALL(cALL,早期前B-ALL)代表白血病细胞发育的中间阶段,是儿童和成人患者中最常见的免疫表型。其免疫表型特征为CD10(普通ALL抗原,CALLA)阳性,常见于Ph染色体阳性ALL(Ph^+-ALL)。处于更为成熟阶段的前B-ALL白血病细胞表达TDT、HLA-DR、CD19、CD79a和胞质免疫球蛋白。在前B-ALL中具有t(1;19)异位的患者比例较高。成熟B-ALL(Burkitt白血病)白血病细胞表达膜表面免疫球蛋白(sIg,通常为IgM),为κ或λ轻链克隆,TDT阴性。成熟B-ALL普遍表达CD20,而在其他类型的ALL中仅有40%~50%的患者CD20阳性。

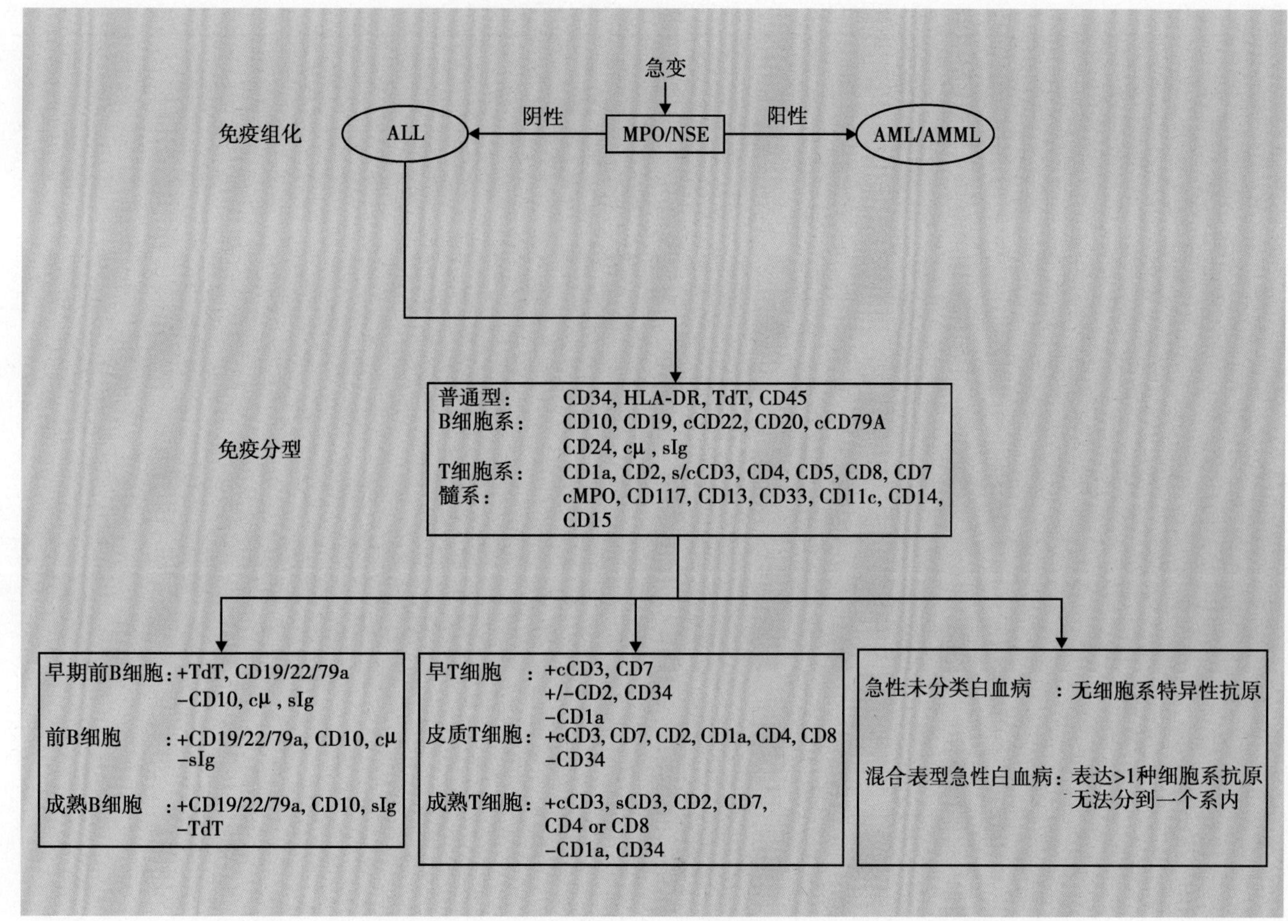

图 116-1　ALL 的诊断方法。MPO，髓过氧化物酶；NSE，非特异性酶；c，细胞质；s，表面

T-ALL 仅 ALL 的占 20%～25%，与 B-ALL 相似可进一步根据胸腺内抗原分化的不同阶段分为不同亚型。T-ALL 表达不同水平的 CD1a、CD2、CD3、CD4、CD5、CD7 和 CD8，其中 CD7 最敏感，但由于 CD7 也可表达于部分 AML 和 NK 细胞白血病，因此其特异性差。目前认为胞质 CD3(cCD3)是最特异的 T 细胞系列分化抗原。成熟 T-ALL 共表达膜表面 CD3(sCD3)和胞质 CD3(cCD3)，CD2，CD4 或 CD8(仅表达其一)。处于更早期分化阶段的 T-ALL 表达 cCD3，但 sCD3 阴性。皮质(胸腺)T 细胞 ALL 以表达 CD1a、双表达 CD4 和 CD8 为特征，并被认为具有良好的预后[28]。最近发现的早期前体 T 细胞 ALL(ETP-ALL)为 T-ALL 的高危亚型，其特征是 CD1a 阴性、CD8 阴性、不表达或弱表达 CD5 以及存在一种及以上的髓系标记(CD117、CD34、HLA-DR、CD13、CD33、CD11b 及 CD65)[29]。ETP-ALL 髓系抗原共表达常见(占成人 ALL 的 15%～50%；占儿童 ALL 的 5%～35%)，但是并不代表具有双系潜能[30]。髓系抗原表达在具有 t(9;22)，t(4;11)，t(12;21)异位的 ALL 中更为常见，而罕见于成熟 B-ALL 中。尽管髓系抗原的表达无预后评估价值[31]，但是可借此来鉴别白血病细胞和正常前体细胞，因而可用于微小残留病(minimal resisual desease，MRD)监测。

细胞遗传学和分子生物学异常

ALL 患者常具有细胞遗传学和分子生物学异常(表 116-2)[4,32]。细胞遗传学和分子生物学检测是非常重要的，不但能够提供病理生物学信息及作为药物靶点，而且可以提供预后信息及危险度分层信息，并指导调整治疗方案[32]。常规的核型分析仍然是识别染色体异常的基础。除此之外，荧光原位杂交(FISH)，以及 mRNA 的实时定量聚合酶链反应(RT-PCR)均已应用于微小残留病检测，监测病情发展。

染色体数量异常

染色体的数量及核型异常严重影响 ALL 患者的预后。少于 44 条染色体的核型即为亚二倍体，发生率<5%但预后较差[33～36]。最近一项基因组分析中，研究>120 个二倍体 ALL，明确两种亚型：①有 24～31 条染色体的近单倍体 ALL，多数存在目标酪氨酸激酶受体信号通路和 RAS 信号通路的改变；②有 32～39 条染色体的低二倍体，90%以上的病例 *TP53* 发生改变[36]。

多于 46 条染色体的核型即为超二倍体。儿童患者超二倍体的发生率高于成人(约 25%比 5%)。最常增多的染色体为 4，8，10 和 21 号，其次为 5，6，14 和 17 号染色体，但并非随机增多。儿童患者的基因表达谱分析显示，归于该组的异常基因中 70%属于 X 染色体或 21 号染色体，而与 X 或 21 号染色体数量是否增加无关[23]。已经证实 ALL 患者的超二倍体白血病细胞蓄积更多的甲氨蝶呤多谷氨酸盐，因而对巯嘌呤，硫鸟嘌呤，阿糖胞苷和门冬酰胺酶等药物更为敏感[37,38]。

染色体结构异常

t(9;22)异位

9 号和 22 号染色体长臂异位形成了 t(9;22)(q34;q11)。Ph 染色体是成人 ALL 中最为常见的染色体异常(占 15%～30%)，但在儿童患者中少见(<5%)[39]。尽管 $p210^{BCR\text{-}ABL}$ 是

表 116-2 ALL 的细胞遗传学和分子生物学异常

细胞遗传学特征	受累基因	频率/%	
		成人	儿童
t(1;14)(p32;q11)	*TAL-1*	10~15	5~10
del(5)(q35)	*HOX11L2*	<2	<2
t(5;14)(q35;q32)	*HOX11L2*	1	2~3
del(6q),t(6;12)	?	5	<5
del(7p)	?	5~10	<5
+8	—	10~12	2
t(8;14),t(8;22),t(2;8)	*c-MYC*	5	2~5
t(9;22)(q34;q11)	*BCR-ABL*	15~25	2~6
del(9)(p21~22)	*CDKN2A* 和 *CDKN2B*	6~30	20
del(9)(q32)	*TAL-2*	<1	<1
附加染色体 9q	*NUP214/ABL*	<5	?
t(10;14)(q24;q11)	*HOX11*	5~10	<5
del(11)(q22)	*ATM*	25~30[a]	15[a]
del(11)(q23)	*MLL/AF4*	5~10	<5
del(12p) or t(12p)	*ETV6-AML1*	<1[b]	20~25[b]
del(13)(q14)	*miR15/miR16*	<5	<5
t(14q11-q13)	*TCRα and δ*	20~25[c]	20~25[c]
t(14q32)	IGH,*BCL11B*	5	?
t(1;19),t(17;19)	*E2A-PBX1*,*E2A-HLF*	<5	4~5
超二倍体	—	2~15	10~26
亚二倍体	—	5~10	5~10

[a] 通过 LOH(杂合子丢失)评估。
[b]通过 PCR(聚合酶链反应)评估。
[c]在 T-ALL,总发生率<10%。
IgM,免疫球蛋白 M;Igκ,免疫球蛋白 κ;Igλ,免疫球蛋白 λ;TdT,末端脱氧核糖核酸转移酶。

CML 中最常见的原癌蛋白,但 Ph$^+$-ALL 患者最常见的是 p190$^{BCR-ABL}$。老年 ALL 患者常具有 t(9;22),表现为初诊时高白细胞(WBC)数和高原始细胞数、表达前 B 细胞的免疫表型,并经常伴有髓系抗原共表达[40]。尽管 Ph$^+$-ALL 曾是长期无病生存率最差的亚型之一,但是目前酪氨酸激酶抑制剂(TKI,见下文)以及多药联合化疗的应用改善了该类患者的预后。

t(12;21)异位和 del(12p)

12 号染色体短臂异常涉及的 ETV6(TEL),是转录因子 Ets 家族的转录调节基因。ETV6 与 21q22 位点上的 RUNX1(AML1,CBFA2)融合形成 t(12;21)异位[41]。该融合蛋白为组蛋白去乙酰化酶的新成员,使染色质结构更为紧凑并抑制转录,从而降低自我更新能力和分化潜能。利用分子生物学的方法在近 30%的 ALL 儿童中检测到 t(12;21)异位,使其成为儿童前 B-ALL 中最为常见的细胞遗传学-分子生物学异常,但是该异位在成人 ALL 患者中较为少见[42]。尽管可能会发生延迟复发,ETV6-RUNX1 阳性的 ALL 儿童患者预后较好[4]。ETV6-RUNX1 阳性的白血病细胞被证实能够抑制多药耐药-1(*MDR-1*)基因,降低新的嘌呤合成并抑制调控嘌呤代谢的基因[43]。

9p21 缺失

9p21 缺失在 ALL 患者中的发生率接近 15%[44],这些患者有较高的复发率和较短的生存期,预后较差。其与预后的相关性在儿童患者中较成人患者更为显著[45,46]。del(9p21)通常累及的基因包括 cyclin-依赖的激酶抑制基因 CDKN2A(MTS1、p16INK4a)和 CDKN2B(MTS2、p15INK4b)。利用 FISH 或 PCR 技术,接近 80%的儿童 T-ALL 和 20%的前 B-ALL 中可检测到 CDKN2A 的杂合子和/或纯合子缺失。

***MLL* 基因重排(11q23)**

11q23 异常通常涉及混合细胞系白血病基因 MLL(ALL-1、HRX、HTRX1)。MLL 编码一种维持 HOX 家族特定成员表达的核蛋白,并经常与位于染色体 4q21、9p22、19p13、1p32 和许多其他染色体上的基因进行重排[47]。85%婴幼儿 ALL 患者检测到位于 4q21 位点上的 *MLL-AF4* 融合基因,但在成人 ALL 中仅占 3%～8%[48]。具有 *MLL* 基因的成人 ALL 的临床特征包括：高龄、WBC 计数较高、肝脾大、不易受侵的中枢神经系统常常受累。CD10 阴性，胞质免疫球蛋白阳性的前 B-ALL 中 *MLL* 基因重排的发生率较高[49]。髓系抗原共表达常见。携带 *MLL* 基因的婴儿和成人 ALL 白血病患者预后差，而大于一岁的儿童患者则预后中等[50]。

E2A 基因重排(19p13)

19p13 位点上已知的两个 *E2A* 基因重排包括 t(1;19)(q23;p13)和 t(17;19)(q21;p13)。t(1;19)异位与胞质免疫球蛋白阳性的前 B-ALL 密切相关。E2A 与其并列的同源 *PBX1* 基因发生异位形成 E2A-PBX1，具有潜在的转录启动子活性，在体外可使多种类型细胞包括成纤维细胞，髓系祖细胞和淋巴样祖细胞发生转化。E2A-PBX1 阳性的 ALL 对于标准剂量或小剂量化疗的疗效差，但是大剂量化疗可以提高疗效[51]。

8q24 基因重排

位于 8q24 位点的 *c-MYC* 基因参与以下三种易位形成并可与成熟 B-ALL 的 κ 或 λ 免疫球蛋白轻链位点结合：①t(8;14)(q24;q32)发生率为 80%，是最为常见的异位[52]。该异位由 *c-MYC* 基因与免疫球蛋白的重链(*IgH*)基因在 14q32 位点处并列形成；②t(8;22)(q24;q11)占 B-ALL 患者的 15%，累及 22q11 上的 *Igλ* 基因位点；③t(2;8)(p12;q24)异位的发生率最低，累及 2p12 位点上的 *Igκ* 基因位点。

其他的分子生物学异常

超过 60% 的 T-ALL 患者存在 NOTCH1 的活化突变，*NOTCH1* 基因通过编码跨膜受体调控正常 T 细胞[53]。确切地说，*NOTCH1* 突变激活可能启动大多数 T-ALL。存在 *NOTCH1* 突变的 T-ALL 患者预后较好[54,55]。大约 2% 的儿童 ALL 患者存在 21 号染色体内的扩增，这些患者常具有前 B 细胞的免疫表型，临床上具有高龄，低白细胞计数，复发风险较高的特征[56]。

基因表达谱芯片分析

利用基因芯片技术进行基因表达谱分析，可用来进一步划分 ALL 亚型，按照危险度及疗效反应将患者进行分层，识别与药物敏感性和耐药通路相关的基因标记，从而对 ALL 的发病机制和生物学特征确定新认识。基于基因表达谱分析，明确了 B-ALL 中一种新的高危亚型，Ph 样 ALL(见下文)[57,58]。

ALL 的治疗

联合化疗已成为儿童和成人 ALL 治疗的主要手段[59]。设计联合用药原则基于将全部有抗 ALL 活性的药物以序贯或扩展方式应用。联合化疗的目的是防止出现耐药的白血病亚克隆，以及尽快恢复正常造血功能。通过借鉴儿童 ALL 的化疗方案，成人 ALL 已经形成了固定的治疗模式。尽管与儿童方案相比，成人 ALL 的各种联合化疗方案在用药顺序和药物种类的选择上均存在一定的差异，但是两者均遵循共同基本原则：诱导治疗、早期强化治疗、巩固治疗、维持治疗、中枢神经系统白血病的防治[60,61]。鉴于这些化疗方案已取得了较高的缓解率，目前 ALL 的治疗方案更加关注于延长缓解期、提高成人 ALL 患者的生存期，以及改善儿童 ALL 患者的生活质量。所以验证亚型特异性预后模型、完善危险度分层和靶向治疗，已经成为目前临床试验的主要目的。

初诊患者的治疗

ALL 的治疗方案非常复杂并且许多治疗的细节可以改变，图 116-2 是目前普遍接受且便于操作的工作框架图。由于 ALL 的治疗变得越来越个体化，且越来越依赖于合理的预后风险分层，因此我们在制订化疗方案前需明确预后因素。

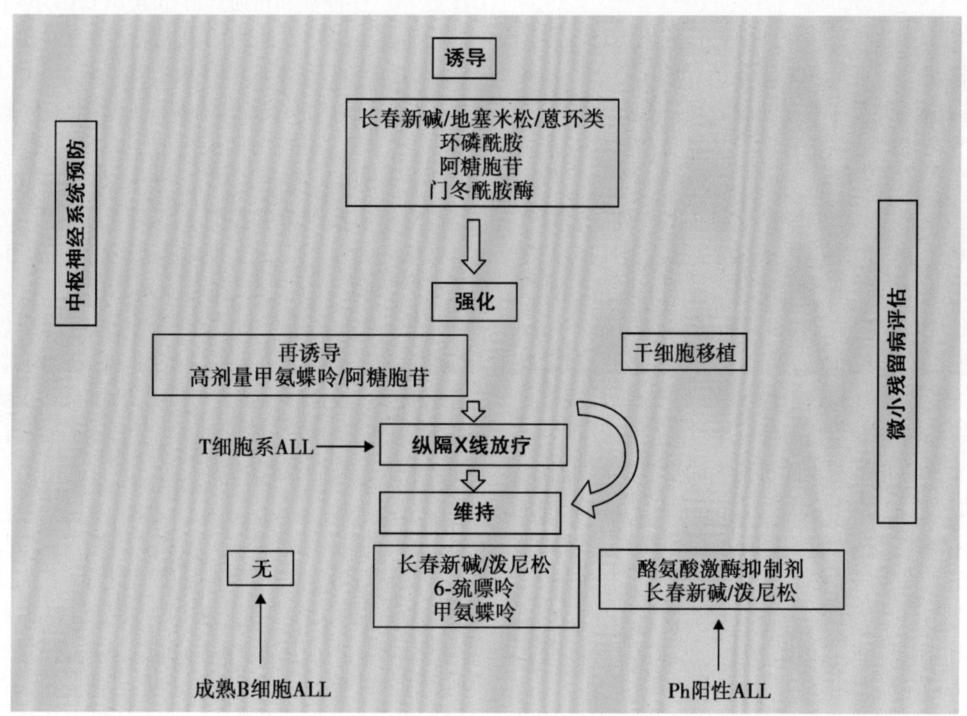

图 116-2　ALL 治疗方案框架图

预后因素

ALL 预后风险分层工作可追溯到 20 世纪 80 年代，并且因临床试验积累经验的增多而不断得到改进。尽管目前的诱导化疗药物已经取得了较高的缓解率，预后模型对于根据预后分层指导缓解后治疗仍然是有意义的，其不但在成人和儿童高危 ALL 患者中提高了无病生存期率，而且避免预后良好 ALL 患者的过度治疗。值得注意的是，治疗方案的改进已经克服了许多临床、实验室和生物学变量对预后的影响。例如，曾经被认为预后不良的 T-ALL，通过应用目前包括环磷酰胺和阿糖胞苷的化疗方案已经使得成人 T-ALL 的长期 DFS 率大于 50%，而儿童 DFS 率大于 80%[59]。成熟 B-ALL 通过接受短期强化的化疗方案，成人患者的完全缓解（complete remission，CR）率已达到 90%，DFS 率>50%，而儿童患者的 DFS 率>80%。细胞形态学、免疫分型、染色体核型分析、分子遗传学以及微小残留病（minimal resisual desease，MRD）检测均有助于对患者进行更为精确的危险度分层。已确定的不良危险因素包括年龄>60 岁，诊断时白细胞计数升高［B 细胞>30 000/μl，T 细胞>10^5/μl］，早期前 B 细胞或早期 T 细胞免疫表型，存在 T(4;11)(q21;q23) 和其他 MLL 重排，以及低二倍体或复杂核型[39]。

诱导治疗后及巩固化疗期间 MRD 监测已经成为预测复发的敏感指标之一，特别是有利于对标危患者进行预后分层[62]。德国成人 ALL 多中心研究协作组（GMALL）前瞻性地对 196 例标危 ALL 患者在开始治疗后的第一年中分别在 9 个时间点通过定量 PCR 的方法检测 MRD[63]。MRD 有助于复发预测，根据 MRD 转阴的速度或 MRD 阳性的持续时间，可将 ALL 患者按照复发风险分为三组，3 年复发风险分别波动于 0（低危组）到 94%（高危组）之间。

诱导治疗

长春新碱、糖皮质激素联合第三种药物（成人为蒽环类药物，儿童为门冬酰胺酶）一直是 ALL 诱导治疗的基石[4]。尚无证据表明应用不同蒽环类药物治疗的患者预后存在差异及在诱导过程中蒽环类药物剂量强化有助于提高目前已经较高的 CR 率和 DFS[64,65]。

另一些药物已经成为 ALL 诱导治疗和强化治疗的一部分。这些药物包括阿糖胞苷、甲氨蝶呤、环磷酰胺、左旋-门冬酰胺酶，以及较少应用的依托泊苷、替尼泊苷、m-安吖啶或其他药物。由于 CR 率已经在 90%左右，很难再进一步提高 CR 率。但是，数据表明强化的诱导治疗能够延长缓解期及生存期，特别是在某些亚型尤为显著。环磷酰胺和阿糖胞苷已经提高了 T-ALL 患者的缓解率和 DFS[39]。另外一个重要的药物是左旋-门冬酰胺酶。儿童 ALL 的大样本随机临床试验结果表明，在整个缓解期和/或缓解后治疗期间持续应用左旋-门冬酰胺酶能够提高患者的生存率[66~68]。左旋-门冬酰胺酶是一种细菌酶能够有效清除血清天冬酰胺。白血病细胞合成蛋白的过程中需要天冬酰胺的参与，但是与正常细胞不同，因其自身不能合成天冬酰胺，所以依赖更高浓度的血清天冬酰胺水平来维持细胞生存。最常用的门冬酰胺酶来源于大肠埃希菌，其缺点是成人比儿童患者更容易出现耐药和不耐受。PEG 天冬酰胺酶是大肠埃希菌来源门冬酰胺酶的一种修饰体，具有更长的血清半衰期，并且降低了耐药的风险，已经有成人 ALL 患者应用 PEG 天冬酰胺酶的报道[68,69]。

单克隆抗体已经被纳入成人 ALL 患者的诱导化疗方案中。目前抗 CD20 抗体利妥昔单抗［其他单克隆抗体，包括抗体-药物偶联物（ADC）的详情见下文］的应用积累了大量的经验。已经证实表达 CD20 的成人前 B-ALL 患者的复发率高[70]，多个临床试验均显示化疗联合利妥昔单抗改善了临床预后，特别在成熟 B-ALL 患者中疗效更为显著[70,71]。来自安德森癌症研究中心一个研究小组关于最新的改良方案 hyper-CVAD（环磷酰胺、长春新碱、多柔比星和地塞米松）的数据表明，联合利妥昔单抗使年轻 ALL 患者（<60 岁）3 年总生存率（OS）从 47%提高到 75%（P=0.003）[70]。

糖皮质激素是 ALL 标准诱导方案中的重要药物，泼尼松或泼尼松龙是最常用的糖皮质激素，特别在维持治疗期。地塞米松比泼尼松和泼尼松龙具有更强的体外抗白血病作用，并且在脑脊液中能够达到更高的药物浓度。儿童肿瘤协作组和英国医学研究委员会的随机临床试验结果证实，在整个化疗期间应用 6mg/m^2 或 6.5mg/m^2 地塞米松降低了孤立的中枢神经系统复发并且明显延长了无事件生存期[72,73]。然而，来自东京儿童癌症研究协作组的一项纳入 231 例标危和中危儿童 ALL 患者的较小样本量的临床研究结果表明，地塞米松（诱导化疗期间 8mg/m^2，强化治疗期间 6mg/m^2）与泼尼松龙（诱导化疗期间 60mg/m^2，强化治疗期间 40mg/m^2）对临床预后的影响并无差异[74]。

鉴于诱导化疗的强度，支持治疗已经成为 ALL 治疗中的重要组成部分。造血细胞生长因子可以通过缩短骨髓抑制期来降低感染并发症。此外，化疗后骨髓功能的快速恢复将有利于及时进行下一个疗程的强化治疗。ALL 的随机临床研究证实了应用粒细胞集落刺激因子（G-CSF）等造血细胞生长因子的优势[75~77]。癌症和白血病协作组 B（CALGB）开展一随机双盲的临床试验 9111，与仅接受支持治疗的 102 例患者相比，G-CSF 治疗组（n=96）患者的中性粒细胞恢复至>1×10^9/L 的时间和血小板恢复时间明显缩短（16 日 vs 22 日，P<0.001；16 日 vs 19 日，P=0.003），住院时间缩短（P=0.02），缓解率提高（87% vs 71%，P=0.01），死亡率下降（5% vs 11%，P=0.04）[77]。

对于成人 ALL 患者而言，诱导化疗期间至少在中性粒细胞计数恢复到>1 000/μl 之前均需要预防性应用抗生素，包括抗细菌药物（左氧氟沙星、环丙沙星、甲氧苄啶/磺胺甲噁唑等），抗真菌药物（氟康唑、伏立康唑、泊沙康唑等）以及抗病毒药物（阿昔洛韦等）。具有高白细胞的 ALL 患者应警惕肿瘤溶解综合征及弥散性血管内溶血（DIC）的发生，并应该及时给予恰当处理。大剂量糖皮质激素的应用可能会导致器官功能障碍（如 ALL 相关的高胆红素血症）。

缓解后治疗

缓解后治疗包括巩固强化和维持治疗，对于某些患者还需要进行造血干细胞移植（SCT）。通过借鉴儿童 ALL 的治疗经验，巩固强化治疗已经提高了成人 ALL 患者的预后，对于高危的成人 ALL 患者尤为显著。但是目前关于最佳的巩固治疗方案及其治疗时间尚无定论。经典的巩固治疗方案包括重复诱导治疗方案，或者与其他化疗方案轮流使用，巩固治疗可能使某些特定的 ALL 亚型患者受益。有关细胞生长抑制药物应用的剂量、顺序和联合方案各临床研究之间的差异很大，因此目前仍很难评估不同化疗方案中单个化疗药物的作用。

举例来说，表 116-3 详细阐述了 hyper-CVAD 方案。在 hyper-CVAD 方案期间，不同剂量的环磷酰胺联合大剂量阿糖胞苷和甲氨蝶呤应用 8 个疗程，大体相当于缓解后强化治疗 6 个月[22]。与早期剂量较小的 VAD 方案相比，hyper-CVAD 方案的 CR 率更高（91% 比 75%），生存期更长。在 CALGB8811 研究中，ALL 患者在 5 药联合的诱导化疗后需要接受共 8 种药物的早期和晚期强化治疗[60]。维持治疗至少到确诊后 2 年。中位缓解期为 29 个月，中位生存期为 36 个月，结果明显优于早期无强化治疗的临床试验。

表 116-3　用于急性淋巴细胞白血病的 hyper-CVAD 化疗方案

成分	药物	亚型				
		非特异	CD20-阳性	成熟 B 细胞	T-系	Ph-阳性
诱导与巩固治疗						
Hyper-CVAD（1，3，5，7 周期）	环磷酰胺	√	√	√	√	√
	多柔比星	√	√	√	√	√
	长春新碱	√	√	√	√	√
	地塞米松	√	√	√	√	√
	抗-CD20 抗体（如利妥昔单抗）	—	√[a]	√	—	√[a,b]
	TKI（如达沙替尼）	—	—	—	—	√[c]
甲氨蝶呤＋大剂量阿糖胞苷（2，4，6，8 周期）	甲氨蝶呤	√	√	√	√	√
	阿糖胞苷	√	√	√	√	√
	抗-CD20 抗体（如利妥昔单抗）	—	√[a]	√	—	√[a,b]
	TKI（如达沙替尼）	—	—	—	—	√[c]
CNS 预防						
鞘内注射治疗[d]	鞘注甲氨蝶呤[e]	√	√	√	√	√
	鞘注阿糖胞苷	√	√	√	√	√
维持前治疗						
纵隔放疗	—	—	—	—	√[f]	—
奈拉滨	奈拉滨	—	—	—	√[g]	—
维持治疗						
POMP	巯嘌呤	√[h]	√[h]	—	√[h]	—
	口服甲氨蝶呤	√[h]	√[h]	—	√[h]	—
	泼尼松	√[h]	√[h]	—	√[h]	√[i]
	长春新碱	√[h]	√[h]	—	√[h]	√[i]
强化	口服甲氨蝶呤/L-门冬酰胺酶（第 6 和 18 个月）	√	√	—	√	√
	高-CVAD（第 7 和 19 个月）	√	√	—	√	√
TKI（如达沙替尼）	TKI（如达沙替尼）	—	—	—	—	√[j]

[a] 在第 1～4 周期期间。

[b] 若 CD20-阳性。

[c] On 在开始第一个周期的第 1～14 日；每日 1 次持续到开始第二循环。

[d] 根据发生中枢神经系统白血病的风险来决定鞘注次数（低危者 4 次，中危 8 次，高危及成熟 B 细胞型 16 次鞘注）每个诱导剂强化巩固治疗需进行 2 次鞘注

[e] 若通过蛛网膜下腔进行鞘注则甲氨蝶呤的剂量应减少。

[f] 若巨大的纵隔淋巴结肿大（≥7cm）。

[g] 两个疗程分别为 28，35 日。

[h] 总疗程 30 个月。

[i] 总疗程 24 个月。

[j] 维持治疗后仍持续给药。

大部分的维持治疗包括 6-巯嘌呤、甲氨蝶呤，每月应用长春新碱和泼尼松，持续 2~3 年。维持治疗期间进一步的强化治疗目前正在研究中，但是尚处于调查研究阶段。维持治疗的疗效具有亚型特异性的特点：由于成熟 B-ALL 患者复发多在 CR 后一年内，因此对于该亚型的 ALL 患者维持治疗作用不大；TKI 已经成为 Ph^+-ALL 治疗方案中必不可少的药物；其他的如 T 细胞特异性的药物奈拉滨（nelarabine）在 T-ALL 治疗中的作用正在研究中。

SCT 改善了处于第一次 CR 期（CR1）的高危 ALL 患者的预后[78~83]。尽管目前不提倡对处于 CR1 期的标危 ALL 患者进行 SCT，但近期一些研究显示某些标危 ALL 患者可能在 SCT 中获益，标危 ALL 患者是否接受 SCT 可根据 MRD 水平或目前尚未明确意义的其他标记综合判断[79~81]。一些研究比较了处于 CR1 的 ALL 患者接受异基因 SCT，自体 SCT、化疗的疗效。受到种种因素的限制，目前对各种治疗方案进行无偏倚的比较仍然比较困难。大部分患者缺乏配型相合的同胞供者，因此不能在第一时间接受异基因 SCT。并且，移植预处理方案，干细胞来源（外周血，骨髓），T 细胞去除的效果，以及预后标记的一致性等方面均存在较大的异质性[82,83]。

在一项法国的多中心临床试验（LALA87）中，具有同胞相合供者、年龄小于 40 岁并处于 CR 期的 ALL 患者接受异基因 SCT（$n=116$），若年龄>40 岁或无同胞相合供者的 ALL 患者被随机分组接受化疗（$n=96$）或者自体 SCT（$n=95$）[84]。除高危 ALL 患者（Ph^+-ALL，未分化 ALL，年龄>35 岁，白细胞计数>30×10^9/L，达到 CR 时间>4 周）以外，两组患者 5 年生存率无明显差异（48%比 35%，$P=0.08$）。而对于高危 ALL 患者，异基因 SCT 组具有更好的 5 年生存率（44%比 22%，$P=0.03$）和无病生存率（39%比 14%，$P=0.01$）。LALA87 最新随访数据表明对于高危 ALL 患者，异基因 SCT 组的 10 年总体生存率为 44%，明显优于化疗组的 11%（$P=0.009$），而对于标危 ALL 患者异基因 SCT 和化疗组的 OS 分别为 49%和 39%（$P=0.6$）[85]。

LALA-94 研究关注根据危险度分层调整缓解后治疗策略及异基因 SCT[86]。共 922 例患者被分为标危、高危、Ph+以及 CNS 浸润组。全部患者均接受标准的 4 周诱导治疗，之后标危组患者继续接受化疗，具有 HLA 相合同胞供者的非标危组患者接受异基因 SCT；无供者的患者接受自体 SCT，若这些患者无 Ph 染色体及 CNS 浸润也可被随机分组接受自体 SCT 或化疗。该研究证实对于高危 ALL 患者在 CR1 期进行异基因 SCT 可获得更好的无病生存。另一方面，该研究结果并未表明自体 SCT 比化疗更具优势。

法国 GOELAMS 协作组研究比较了高危 ALL 患者在 CR1 期进行异基因 SCT 与无 HLA 相合供者或者年龄>50 岁的患者延迟进行自体 SCT 的疗效差异[87]。在一项 50 岁以下患者的研究结果表明，异基因 SCT 患者的 6 年总体生存率明显优于自体 SCT（75%比 40%，$P=0.002\,7$）。

MRCUKALLXⅡ/ECOGE2993 临床试验是一项旨在探讨异基因 SCT 是否能够使全部具有移植适应证的成年 ALL 患者受益的多中心研究；同时还探讨单纯进行自体 SCT 能否和缓解后化疗一样有效[79]。该项研究包括了年龄在 15~59 岁的 1 929 例患者。具有 HLA 相合同胞供者的患者均进行异基因 SCT，而无 HLA 相合同胞供者或者年龄>55 岁的患者随机进行自体 SCT 或化疗。随机分组前均进行诱导化疗及大剂量甲氨蝶呤强化治疗。高危患者定义：年龄>35 岁、高白细胞（B-ALL 白细胞≥30×10^9/L，T-ALL 白细胞≥100×10^9/L）和 Ph^+-ALL。全部患者的 CR 率为 90%，5 年生存率为 43%。结果如下：①具有 HLA 相合供者和无供者 Ph^--ALL 患者的 5 年生存率分别为 53%和 45%（$P=0.02$）；②具有 HLA 相合供者和无供者的标危 Ph^--ALL 患者的 5 年生存率为 62%比 52%（$P=0.02$）；③具有 HLA 相合供者和无供者的高危患者的 5 年生存率无明显差异（41%比 35%，$P=0.2$）。该组患者中，考虑移植相关毒性降低了异基因 *SG* 更好疗效的取得，同时抵消了移植降低复发率的作用；④缓解后化疗组患者的无事件生存率和总体生存率均优于自体 SCT 组（分别为 $P=0.02$ 和 $P=0.03$）。

尽管对 ALL 患者在 CR1 期进行异基因 SCT 已经得到了越来越多的认可，但是最佳的移植时机尚不明确。新的治疗药物（如 TKI 在 Ph^+-ALL 患者中的应用）可能会影响预后，因此需要在某些高危患者中重新明确异基因 SCT 的适应证。非清髓 SCT 已成功应用于老年患者[83,88,89]。仅有不到 30%的患者具有 HLA 相合的同胞供者，这仍是影响 SCT 应用的主要障碍。为了提高 SCT 的数量，近年来在部分相合的同胞供者，相合的无关供者以及脐带血方面进行了大量工作[82,83,90,91]。

中枢神经系统白血病的预防

初诊时 ALL 患者的中枢神经系统浸润少见（儿童患者<5%，成人患者<10%）[60,92~94]。但是如果不进行 CNS 白血病预防，40%~50%的患者会出现中枢神经系统白血病，并且严重影响 ALL 患者治愈[95]。中枢神经系统复发可表现为孤立的中枢神经系统白血病，可发生于骨髓复发后或伴随骨髓复发或睾丸复发，或者三个部位同时复发。CNS 复发导致患者预后差，因此有效的中枢神经系统白血病的预防极其重要[21]。已经证实延迟进行中枢神经系统白血病的预防将增加发生中枢神经系统白血病的风险，因此应在诱导治疗的早期即开始中枢神经系统白血病的预防治疗，而且应在整个诱导治疗期和早期强化治疗期间持续进行预防性治疗。

发生中枢神经系统浸润的危险因素包括：低龄、T-ALL 和成熟 B-ALL、初诊时高白细胞计数及 CSF 中检测到 WBC[21]。研究证实 CD7、CD56 和白介素-15 的表达可预测 ALL 患者髓外复发[96,97]。血清乳酸脱氢酶（LDH）升高和增殖指数高（S+G2M>14%）是发生中枢神经系统白血病的敏感预测指标[98]。

中枢神经系统白血病的预防性治疗包括鞘注（IT）化疗药物（甲氨蝶呤、阿糖胞苷、糖皮质激素），大剂量全身化疗（甲氨蝶呤、阿糖胞苷、门冬酰胺酶、地塞米松、巯嘌呤）和全颅脊髓放疗（XRT）。尽管三药联合较单药甲氨蝶呤鞘注更为有效，但是一项随机临床试验结果证实三药联合鞘注的患者发生治疗相关中枢神经系统并发症的风险更大，且骨髓及睾丸复发风险更高[99]。对于这种矛盾现象的解释之一是孤立的 CNS 复发实际上可能是全面复发的一种早期征象，早期更好地控制中枢神经系统白血病有利于延缓之后其他部位白血病的复发。一些儿童和成人 ALL 的临床研究表明鞘注与全颅脊髓放疗的疗效相当，因此目前对全颅脊髓放疗的作用尚存争议[21]。XRT 的副作用是严重的致残性的，例如可以导致癫痫发作、痴呆、智力障碍及复杂的内分泌病等其他并发症。单独应用大剂量化疗对中枢神经系统白血病预防疗效不佳。选择性颅底照射可能使脑神经根受累的患者获益。

微小残留病

目前认为残存的白血病细胞是儿童和成人 ALL 患者复发的原因，白血病细胞在获得形态学和细胞遗传学缓解后仍持续存在，但是通过显微镜和细胞化学染色等常规的方法检测不到。目前已研发了包括多参数流式细胞术和 PCR 技术在内的多种敏感的检测方法。不管采用哪种检测方法，均需要通过识别特异性的白血病细胞标记来检测残存的白血病细胞。对于流式细胞术而言，可监测细胞表面多种抗原的异常表达。而对于 PCR 来讲，白血病细胞特异性的融合基因（如 *BCR-ABL*、*MLL-AF4*、*ETV6-RUNX1*）或者特异性重组免疫球蛋白或 T 细胞受体基因结合区域的检测是很好的 MRD 检测标记[62]。

关于儿童和成人 ALL 的大量研究已经证实 MRD 监测能够准确地预测复发[62,100~105]。通过儿童 ALL 研究已经达成共识：诱导治疗之后，整个巩固治疗和维持治疗期间 MRD 水平均较高或任意时点检测的 MRD 水平持续增高，这些患者具有较高的复发风险[106]。尽管在诱导治疗结束时，更多的成人患者 MRD 水平较儿童患者高，但即便 MRD 水平比儿童患者低，复发率也高于儿童。已经证实在不同的时间点对 MRD 水平进行持续监测同样能够有效预测成人 ALL 患者的复发[101,102]。

目前 MRD 水平监测已被纳入多个临床研究以便指导缓解后化疗强度。但是尚存在以下问题：①何为与临床相关的 MRD 水平阈值，高于该阈值是否需要进行临床干预治疗；②在诱导治疗后，最准确的 MRD 监测时间点包括哪些？对于接受特异性治疗的患者如何调整 MRD 监测时间；③根据分子生物学复发进行干预治疗是否能够提高临床疗效？如果可以，目前所采用的缓解标准是否应该包括分子生物学反应；④不同的实验室之间 MRD 监测结果的可重复性如何？除了可作为根据危险度分层调整治疗策略的有利工具之外，MRD 研究将有望用于更好地揭示 ALL 自身的生物学特性。

青少年及年轻成人 ALL（AYA）

AYA 组（临床研究大多定义为 16~39 岁）患者可采用类儿童化疗方案或成人 ALL 方案。通常儿童的化疗方案更为强化，包括非骨髓抑制药物如类固醇、长春新碱、天冬酰胺酶，并且通常采用更强化的 CNS 预防。几个回顾性和前瞻性研究表明，与成人方案相比，应用儿童方案治疗的患者预后更好。安德森癌症研究中心最近公布了相似的结果[107]。与使用 hyper-CVAD 方案治疗的患者相比，使用儿童方案（强化的 BFM 方案）治疗的 AYA 患者预后较好[108]。最近在 AYA-ALL 患者中明确 Ph 样基因（见下文）及其与较差预后的相关性，以及随着年龄增加 Ph 样基因的发生率增加使 AYA 患者人群管理更加复杂[24,109]。

挽救治疗

复发的成人 ALL 患者的预后仍然很差。复发后治疗仅使 30%~40% 的患者达到 CR2，5 年 OS 仅为 10% 左右。在 MRCUKALL12/ECOG2993 研究中，复发的成人 ALL 患者的 5 年总生存率仅为 7%[110]。预后较好（指 5 年总生存率为 11%~12%）的因素包括：年龄小于 20 岁并且缓解期超过 2 年。尽管尚无标准的挽救治疗方案，目前普遍认为异基因 SCT 应作为挽救治疗的首选。对于大部分患者而言，SCT 并不是无合适供者、合并发症（如感染、PS 评分高）或伴有其他无法控制疾病的患者的首选治疗。与一线治疗方案相似，非 SCT 的挽救治疗方案已基本确定，包括：①联合应用长春新碱、糖皮质激素和蒽环类药物；②联合应用门冬酰胺酶和甲氨蝶呤；③大剂量阿糖胞苷。由于患者特性、之前药物的接触史和敏感性、挽救方案的疗程数量、化疗药物应用的剂量和顺序等均存在较大差异，并且由于总体生存率较差，一些患者接受 SCT 作为巩固治疗，这些均导致直接比较各方案的疗效比较困难。所以为 ALL 患者研发新的治疗办法势在必行。

疾病亚型

Ph^+-ALL

Ph^+-ALL 曾经是标准化疗下生存率最低的一个亚型，多见于成人患者且与成人 ALL 患者预后差有一定的相关[111]。

伊马替尼及新一代 TKI 药物的上市使 Ph^+-ALL 未来出现更多的治疗办法变为可能。伊马替尼通过竞争结合 BCR-ABL 的 ATP 位点抑制癌蛋白的自动激活及下游细胞内蛋白的磷酸化。Ph^+-ALL 患者单独使用伊马替尼的血液学缓解率在 20%~30%，但缓解期较短[112]。激酶抑制剂联合低剂量化疗（长春新碱和糖皮质激素）在不适宜接受更为积极治疗的老年和衰弱患者中显著获益[113]。

多个研究已成功将伊马替尼和强化化疗方案联合应用[114~116]。MDACC 研究小组采用伊马替尼联合 hyper-CVAD 方案[114]。伊马替尼 600mg/d，共 14 日，联合诱导治疗，之后持续应用至剂量增至 800mg/d 作为维持治疗。54 例研究对象的中位年龄为 51 岁（17~84 岁），93%的患者获得了完全缓解，其获得 CR 的中位时间为 21 日。通过巢式 PCR 检测其分子学缓解率为 52%。从开始治疗后的 5 个月（中位时间）内 16 例患者接受了异基因 SCT，接受 SCT 患者的 3 年生存率较未移植患者无明显提高（63%比 56%）。联合伊马替尼的疗效明显优于单用 hyper-CVAD；3 年 OS 率分别为 55%和 15%（$P<0.001$）。目前普遍认为在诱导治疗的早期即开始使用伊马替尼，且在诱导治疗和巩固治疗期间持续应用的疗效要比伊马替尼与化疗交替应用的疗效更好[117]。

达沙替尼（dasatinib）和尼洛替尼是两种二代 TKI 药物，在体外实验中已多次证实其疗效优于伊马替尼，包括对大多数伊马替尼耐药的激酶突变有效。这两种药物均对伊马替尼耐药的 Ph^+-ALL 有效。MD 安德森癌症中心的研究人员对 63 名新诊断的 Ph^+-ALL 患者进行达沙替尼联合 hyper-CVAD 治疗[118,119]。93%的患者达到主要分子学缓解，65%的患者达到完全分子学缓解。DFS 和 OS 的中位时间分别为 31 个月和 44 个月。另一些研究同样得到了上述结果，目前早期应用 TKI 药物是 Ph^+-ALL 的标准治疗方案[39,120~124]。Ph^+-ALL 患者还可以应用尼洛替尼联合多药化疗[125]。泼那替尼（ponatinib）是第三代 TKI 药物，目前正在研究其联合 hyper-CVAD 化疗作为

ALL 患者的一线治疗[126]。

成熟 B-ALL(Burkitt 白血病)

成熟 B-ALL 是 ALL 中的罕见亚型，主要见于儿童患者。该疾病的遗传学基础是 8q24 位点的 *MYC* 易位至 14 号染色体上的免疫球蛋白重链区，也可少见地易位于 λ(22q11)或 κ(2p12)位点。快速诊断并明确分型对于 Burkitt 白血病最佳治疗结局至关重要。由于该病发生肿瘤溶解综合征的风险很高，所以给予水化并应用别嘌醇和/或拉布立酶非常重要。强化的化学免疫疗法是成熟 B-ALL 患者的标准治疗方法[71,127]。Thomas 等采用 hyper-CVAD 联合利妥昔单抗治疗 31 例成熟 B-ALL 或淋巴瘤的初治患者，中位年龄为 46 岁(29%患者>60 岁)[127]。总体 CR 率为 86%。3 年 OS 率和 DFS 率分别为 89%和 88%，老年患者的疗效与之相似。年轻患者及利妥昔单抗治疗是独立的预后较好的因素。最近，德国 ALL 研究组公布了令人惊喜的结果，对 363 例 Burkitt 白血病/淋巴瘤患者采用化学免疫方案联合利妥昔单抗[71]，CR 率、5 年 PFS 和 5 年 OS 分别为 88%、71%、80%。

Ph 样 ALL

2009 年，在 ALL 儿童患者中发现新的 B-ALL 亚组，其基因表达谱与 Ph^+-ALL 相似，但无 Ph 染色体[57,58]。这些被称为"Ph 样 ALL"的患者占儿童 B-ALL 的 15%，占 AYAALL 的 20%~25%[24,128]。Ph 样 ALL 患者的疾病复发率较高，总生存率较低[24,128~131]。

大约 50%的 Ph 样 ALL 患者有 CRLF2 重排，位于 Xp22.3/Yp11.3 的假常染色体区，CRLF2 可以在 14q32.33 位点与免疫球蛋白重链增强区形成(IGH-CRLF2)易位，或者近 CRLF2 处的局灶性缺失导致 P2RY8-CRLF2 融合基因表达[109,129,132~135]。

大约 50%的 CRLF2 重排患者有 *JAK* 基因突变(*JAK2*，最常见的是 *JAK2R683* 和 *JAK1*)[24]。据报道，非 CRLF2 重排患者可有以下几种基因融合，包括 *ABL1*、*ABL2*、*JAK2*、*EPOR* 和 *PDGFRB*。这些不同的遗传改变激活了信号通路，特别是 *ABL1*、*PDGFRB*(两者都可以被 TKI 药物抑制，例如达沙替尼)和 JAK-STAT 信号通路，其可以被 JAK 抑制剂如芦可替尼(ruxolitinib)抑制[109,136]。

Harvey 等人对 207 名"高危"B-ALL 的儿童进行了评估，发现 14%的儿童 CRLF2 过度表达[129]。令人感兴趣的是，西班牙裔患者更容易有 CRLF2 过度表达(35%比 7%，$P<0.001$)。

早期前体 T-ALL(ETP-ALL)

具有髓系表达特征的 T 细胞被明确为高风险 T 细胞亚组，这些幼稚 T 淋巴细胞来源于早期前体 T 细胞(ETP)，其处于造血干细胞向 T 系分化的原始阶段并具有多系分化潜能[29]。10%~15%的儿童 T-ALL 和 7%~10%的成人 T-ALL 都具有 ETP 表型[29,137]。ETP-ALL 的特异性免疫表型包括：①CD1a 阴性；②CD8 阴性；③CD5 弱或缺失；④存在一种或多种髓系/干细胞标记如 CD117、CD34、HLA-DR、CD13、CD33、CD11b 和 CD65[29]。ETP-ALL 患者的预后显著低于 T-ALL 患者(StJude 的儿科数据-10 年 OS，ETP-ALL 为 19%，非 ETPT-ALL 为 84%，$P\leqslant 0.0001$；10 年复发率，ETP-ALL 为 72%，非 ETPT-ALL 为 10%，$P\leqslant 0.0001$)[29,138]。德国 ALL 研究组报道，ETP-ALL 占成人 T-ALL 的 7.4%[137,139,140]，ETP-ALL 患者中 *FLT-3* 突变发生率为 35%，DNMT3A 发生率为 14%。

新的治疗策略

对疾病生物学的深入理解为 ALL 患者带来了新的治疗方法(表 116-4)。治疗白血病的有效药物多为核苷类似物。氯法拉滨是以氟达拉滨和克拉德里滨为模型的新一代嘌呤核苷，但具有不同的作用机制和活性谱[141]。在 61 例复发或难治性 ALL(R/R-ALL)儿童中进行氯法拉滨Ⅱ期临床试验，反应率达到 30%[142]。氯法拉滨已被美国食品药品管理局(FDA)批准用于 R/R-ALL 儿童。Kantarjian 等报道[143]，对于 R/R-ALL 患者，单药氯法拉滨的反应率为 17%。西南肿瘤学研究组进行了一项Ⅱ期临床试验，即氯法拉滨和阿糖胞苷联合用于 R/R-ALL，反应率为 17%[144]。奈拉宾为 9-β-D-阿糖呋喃糖鸟嘌呤(ara-G)的水溶性前体药物，在复发的 T 淋巴恶性肿瘤中取得较显著的疗效，并被 FDA 批准用于此适应证[145~149]。121 名儿童和 39 名成人复发 T 白血病/淋巴瘤组的反应率分别为 33%和 41%。神经毒性是奈拉滨的主要不良事件，呈剂量和时间依

表 116-4 急性淋巴细胞白血病的新药

分类	举例
核苷类似物	氯法拉滨
	奈拉滨
脂质体和聚乙二醇化合物	脂质体长春新碱(Marqibo)
	脂质体多柔比星
	聚乙二醇门冬酰胺酶
单克隆抗体	
非结合的	利妥昔单抗(CD20)
	奥法木单抗(CD20)
	依帕珠单抗(CD22)
	阿伦珠单抗(CD52)
抗体药物/毒素结合物	奥英妥珠单抗(CD22/卡阿奇霉素)
	SAR3419(CD19/美登木碱)
	莫西托莫单抗(CD22/铜绿假单胞菌毒素)
双特异性抗体	博利那单抗(CD19/CD3)
酪氨酸激酶抑制剂	伊马替尼
	达沙替尼
	尼洛替尼
	泼那替尼
	芦可替尼
T 细胞免疫治疗	嵌合抗原受体 T 细胞

赖性。MD 安德森研究组报告了 40 例新诊断的 T-ALL 或 T 细胞淋巴母细胞淋巴瘤患者，应用奈拉滨联合 hyper-CVAD 方案化疗[149]。患者在维持治疗的早期(4 或 5 疗程 CVAD 后)和晚期(代替维持治疗的第 6 和 7 疗程)接受 2 周期奈拉滨静点($650mg/m^2$,5 日)。总反应率(ORR)和 CR 率分别为 97%、91%。3 年的 DFS 和 OS 分别为 61%、63%。长春新碱是治疗 ALL 的重要药物。脂质体长春新碱可以提高长春新碱用量，并更易于富集在肿瘤组织。O'Brien 等人评估脂质体长春新碱单药治疗复发及多次复发的成人 Ph-ALL 患者[150]。65 例接受脂质体长春新碱的患者 CR/CRi 率为 20%,ORR 率为 35%。基于这项研究，脂质体长春新碱已被 FDA 批准用于这类患者。

靶细胞表面受体

利妥昔单抗是一种针对细胞表面 CD20 的嵌合单克隆抗体，在 B-ALL 中具有明确的作用(见前文)[70]。奥法木单抗(ofatumumab)作用于不同的 CD20 表位，在体外比利妥昔单抗有更强的促进补体依赖的细胞毒(CDC)效应。目前正在 ALL 患者中进行研究[151,152]。

CD19 在 B-ALL 中一致表达。博利那单抗(blinatumomab)是一种新型抗体(双特异性 T 细胞结合抗体)，靶向结合患者的 T 细胞并作用于表达 CD19 的肿瘤细胞，引起细胞毒性 T 细胞效应[153]。博利那单抗已被证实可以在绝大多数 ALL 患者中清除 MRD[154,155]。德国 ALL 研究组对 R/R B-ALL 患者进行了博利那单抗Ⅱ期临床试验[156]。博利那单抗连续静脉滴注 28 日，间歇 14 日。有疗效的患者可以继续治疗 3 周期或骨髓移植。在 36 名接受治疗的患者中，25 名患者(69%)获得 CR/CRi。中位 OS 为 9.8 个月，中位无复发生存期为 7.6 个月。在一项国际多中心Ⅱ期研究中，189 名 R/R ALL 患者接受了博利那单抗治疗[157]。该研究包括特别高危的患者群体[原发难治或复发 ALL(首次缓解后 12 个月内复发，同种异体 SCT 后 12 个月内复发，或首次挽救治疗无效及治疗后复发)]。43%的患者在用博利那单抗治疗的两个周期内达到 CR/CRi。中位总生存期为 6.1 个月。基于这些数据，博利那单抗已在美国被批准用于治疗 R/R B-ALL 患者。

SAR3419 是针对 CD19 的抗体药物偶联物(ADC)。ADC 是抑制微管蛋白聚合和组装的有效药物，可通过 IgG1 抗体 huB4 与美登木素生物碱 DM4 的结合产生。在一项Ⅰ期研究中，复发的 B 细胞淋巴瘤患者每 3 周应用一次 SAR3419[158]。最常见的药物相关毒性是眼毒性，发生率高达 44%。在可评估疗效的 35 名患者中，26 名(74%)患者的肿瘤体积缩小。第二阶段的研究旨在评估一周一次的 SAR3419 的疗效和副作用[159]。结果显示眼部副作用发生率明显降低，55%的患者发现肿瘤缩小。

90%以上 ALL 患者表达 CD22。奥英妥珠单抗(inotuzumab ozogamicin)是 CD22 单克隆抗体，与卡雷霉素(calecheamicin，一种毒素)结合，单药治疗 R/R ALL 表现出有效性[160]。在一项Ⅱ期研究中，49 名患者接受了每 3~4 周静脉注射一次奥英妥珠单抗($1.8mg/m^2$)。总反应率(ORR)为 57%(CR 18%，骨髓 CR 39%)。体外试验结果显示，缩短用药间隔产生更高的疗效，给予每周用药方案(第 1 日为 $0.8mg/m^2$，第 8 日和第 15 日为 $0.5mg/m^2$，每 3~4 周 1 次)[161]。每周方案 ORR 为 53%，并减少了毒副作用。已在 R/R NHL 患者中，对奥英妥珠单抗联合利妥昔单抗(rituximab)进行评估[162]。奥英妥珠单抗联合利妥昔单抗方案中，奥英妥珠单抗的最大耐受剂量(MTD)为每 4 周 $1.8mg/m^2$。最常见的 3~4 级不良事件是血小板减少(31%)和中性粒细胞减少(22%)。在最大耐受剂量下，复发的滤泡淋巴瘤(FL)和弥漫大 B 细胞淋巴瘤(DLBCL)的客观缓解率分别为 87%和 74%。

依帕珠单抗(epratuzumab)，一种靶向 CD22 的非结合单克隆抗体，已在 ALL 中进行研究。Advani 等人[163]在成人 R/R B-All 中应用依帕珠单抗联合氯法拉滨和阿糖胞苷方案(西南肿瘤学组研究 S0910)。结果显示，CR/CRi 率为 52%，显著高于反应率仅为 17%的氯法拉滨联合阿糖胞苷的临床试验结果。依帕珠单抗联合长春新碱和类固醇治疗老年 R/R-ALL 患者，CR/CRi 率均为 20%[164]。

莫西托莫单抗(moxetumomab)是一种重组免疫毒素，由假单胞菌毒素融合抗 CD22 单克隆抗体的 Fv 片段组成[165]。在复发/难治性 CD22+B-ALL 的儿童患者的Ⅰ期研究中，莫西托莫单抗给予的剂量范围为 5~40μg/kg，隔日一次，共 6 次[166]。21 名患者接受了治疗。最常见的治疗相关不良事件是体重增加、转氨酶增高和低蛋白血症。ORR 为 29%。成人 R/R-ALL 患者莫西托单抗Ⅰ/Ⅱ期试验目前正在招募患者(NCT01891981)。

几乎所有正常和恶性 B 淋巴细胞、T 淋巴细胞、单核细胞和巨噬细胞都表达 CD52[167]。阿伦珠单抗(alemtuzumab)是一种直接抗 CD52 的非结合单克隆抗体。在Ⅰ/Ⅱ期 CALGB 研究中，阿伦珠单抗用于治疗 24 例处于 CR1 期的患者，目的是清除 MRD[168]。对 11 例患者进行 MRD 连续评估，其中 8 例患者的 MRD 中位数下降 1 个对数。但阿伦珠单抗单药治疗复发/难治性儿童和成人 ALL 患者疗效有限[169,170]。

嵌合抗原受体(CAR)治疗

目前嵌合抗原受体(CAR)的免疫治疗是研究热点。CAR 是合成受体，由融合到跨膜域的抗原结合域和一个或多个胞质信号域组成。合成的受体在自体或同种异体 T 细胞上表达。在 R/R B-ALL 患者中，CD19-CARs 治疗取得显著疗效，CR 率大于 80%[171~174]。Davila 等人[171]报告 16 例 R/R B-ALL 患者，应用 CD19 CAR-T 细胞治疗，CR 率为 88%。Maude 等人报告 30 例儿童和成人 R/R ALL 患者用 CD19 CAR-T 细胞治疗[174]。27 名患者 CR 率达到 90%。6 个月的无事件生存率(EFS)为 67%，OS 为 78%。CAR-T 细胞输注后，细胞因子释放综合征常见。将 CD19 作为治疗靶点也可导致 B 细胞发育不良，患者需要定期免疫球蛋白替代治疗。

T-ALL

与 B-ALL 一些治疗靶点正在临床研究不同，目前只有有限的几个针对 T-ALL 的药物/靶点正在研究。

Notch 抑制剂在 T-ALL 的研究

Notch 信号是进化高度保守的信号通路，在干细胞分化成 T 细胞的过程中起到重要的调节作用[175,176]。Ellisen 等描述易位 t(7;9)(q34;q34.3)时，首先报道了 Notch 通路参与 T-ALL[177]。Weng 等人报道，在 56%的 T-ALL 患者中有激活的 *NOTCH1* 突变[53]。Asnafi 等人报道，成人 T-ALL 患者中

NOTCH1 和 *FBXW7* 突变的发生率为 72%[55]。NOTCH1/*FBXW7* 突变与更好的临床预后相关[55,178]。在 R/R-T-ALL 患者Ⅰ期试验中口服 γ-分泌酶抑制剂 MK-0752 取得一定的临床疗效，但具有显著的胃肠道毒性[179]。胃肠道毒性是一种靶向毒性效应，特异性的作用于小肠上皮细胞的杯状细胞，而不是肠上皮细胞[180]。目前正在进行一项为期一周的 γ-分泌酶抑制剂 BMS-906024 的Ⅰ期试验（NCT01363817）。

总结

随着对 ALL 生物学特性的深入理解以及预后评估体系的不断完善，使得 ALL 治疗越来越复杂。成熟 B-ALL 患者最好接受短期强化治疗，而 T-ALL 患者疗效的提高得益于化疗方案中增加了环磷酰胺和阿糖胞苷。目前普遍认为 Ph^+-ALL 治疗方案中应该包括 TKI，诱导治疗初始即开始应用并维持治疗数年。随着更为完善和更具预测性的危险度分层体系的应用，造血干细胞移植的适应证已经有所调整。无移植禁忌证的高危患者应在 CR1 期进行移植，而处于第二次或更多次缓解期的患者均应进行移植。移植是否应该推广至标危 ALL 患者尚无定论，但不应作为常规治疗。对于任何其他类型的恶性肿瘤，深入进行更为精确的 ALL 亚型分类是提高 ALL 患者，特别是成人 ALL 患者预后的关键。Ph 样 ALL 和 ETP-ALL 是最新被定义的两种高危 ALL 亚型，TKI 靶向治疗可能有效。ALL 的治疗方案是复杂的并会一直如此。新药研发如 ADC 和 CAR-T 是非常有前景的。将这些新的药物纳入目前已建立的治疗方案仍然是一个持续的挑战。

（白元松　杨杨　王世宝 译　白元松　杨杨　王世宝 校）

参考文献

The complete reference list can be found on the Wiley Companion Digital Edition of this title (see inside front cover for login instructions).

9 Mulligan CG, Goorha S, Radtke I, et al. Genome-wide analysis of genetic alterations in acute lymphoblastic leukaemia. *Nature*. 2007;**446(7137)**:758–764.

22 Kantarjian H, Thomas D, O'Brien S, et al. Long-term follow-up results of hyperfractionated cyclophosphamide, vincristine, doxorubicin, and dexamethasone (Hyper-CVAD), a dose-intensive regimen, in adult acute lymphocytic leukemia. *Cancer*. 2004;**101(12)**:2788–2801.

24 Roberts KG, Li Y, Payne-Turner D, et al. Targetable kinase-activating lesions in Ph-like acute lymphoblastic leukemia. *N Engl J Med*. 2014;**371(11)**:1005–1015.

28 Marks DI, Paietta EM, Moorman AV, et al. T-cell acute lymphoblastic leukemia in adults: clinical features, immunophenotype, cytogenetics, and outcome from the large randomized prospective trial (UKALL XII/ECOG 2993). *Blood*. 2009;**114(25)**:5136–5145.

29 Coustan-Smith E, Mullighan CG, Onciu M, et al. Early T-cell precursor leukaemia: a subtype of very high-risk acute lymphoblastic leukaemia. *Lancet Oncol*. 2009;**10(2)**:147–156.

36 Holmfeldt L, Wei L, Diaz-Flores E, et al. The genomic landscape of hypodiploid acute lymphoblastic leukemia. *Nat Genet*. 2013;**45(3)**:242–252.

53 Weng AP, Ferrando AA, Lee W, et al. Activating mutations of NOTCH1 in human T cell acute lymphoblastic leukemia. *Science*. 2004;**306(5694)**:269–271.

55 Asnafi V, Buzyn A, Le Noir S, et al. NOTCH1/FBXW7 mutation identifies a large subgroup with favorable outcome in adult T-cell acute lymphoblastic leukemia (T-ALL): a Group for Research on Adult Acute Lymphoblastic Leukemia (GRAALL) study. *Blood*. 2009;**113(17)**:3918–3924.

57 Den Boer ML, van Slegtenhorst M, De Menezes RX, et al. A subtype of childhood acute lymphoblastic leukaemia with poor treatment outcome: a genome-wide classification study. *Lancet Oncol*. 2009;**10(2)**:125–134.

58 Mullighan CG, Su X, Zhang J, et al. Deletion of IKZF1 and prognosis in acute lymphoblastic leukemia. *N Engl J Med*. 2009;**360(5)**:470–480.

60 Larson RA, Dodge RK, Burns CP, et al. A five-drug remission induction regimen with intensive consolidation for adults with acute lymphoblastic leukemia: cancer and leukemia group B study 8811. *Blood*. 1995;**85(8)**:2025–2037.

61 Kantarjian HM, Cortes JE, O'Brien S, et al. Long-term survival benefit and improved complete cytogenetic and molecular response rates with imatinib mesylate in Philadelphia chromosome-positive chronic-phase chronic myeloid leukemia after failure of interferon-alpha. *Blood*. 2004;**104(7)**:1979–1988.

63 Bruggemann M, Raff T, Flohr T, et al. Clinical significance of minimal residual disease quantification in adult patients with standard-risk acute lymphoblastic leukemia. *Blood*. 2006;**107(3)**:1116–1123.

70 Thomas DA, O'Brien S, Faderl S, et al. Chemoimmunotherapy with a modified hyper-CVAD and rituximab regimen improves outcome in de novo Philadelphia chromosome-negative precursor B-lineage acute lymphoblastic leukemia. *J Clin Oncol*. 2010;**28(24)**:3880–3889.

71 Hoelzer D, Walewski J, Dohner H, et al. Improved outcome of adult Burkitt lymphoma/leukemia with rituximab and chemotherapy: report of a large prospective multicenter trial. *Blood*. 2014;**124(26)**:3870–3879.

79 Goldstone AH, Richards SM, Lazarus HM, et al. In adults with standard-risk acute lymphoblastic leukemia, the greatest benefit is achieved from a matched sibling allogeneic transplantation in first complete remission, and an autologous transplantation is less effective than conventional consolidation/maintenance chemotherapy in all patients: final results of the International ALL Trial (MRC UKALL XII/ECOG E2993). *Blood*. 2008;**111(4)**:1827–1833.

80 Cornelissen JJ, van der Holt B, Verhoef GE, et al. Myeloablative allogeneic versus autologous stem cell transplantation in adult patients with acute lymphoblastic leukemia in first remission: a prospective sibling donor versus no-donor comparison. *Blood*. 2009;**113(6)**:1375–1382.

86 Thomas X, Boiron JM, Huguet F, et al. Outcome of treatment in adults with acute lymphoblastic leukemia: analysis of the LALA-94 trial. *J Clin Oncol*. 2004;**22(20)**:4075–4086.

92 Lazarus HM, Richards SM, Chopra R, et al. Central nervous system involvement in adult acute lymphoblastic leukemia at diagnosis: results from the international ALL trial MRC UKALL XII/ECOG E2993. *Blood*. 2006;**108(2)**:465–472.

107 Stock W. Adolescents and young adults with acute lymphoblastic leukemia. *Hematol Am Soc Hematol Educ Program*. 2010;**2010**:21–29.

108 Rytting ME, Thomas DA, O'Brien SM, et al. Augmented Berlin-Frankfurt-Munster therapy in adolescents and young adults (AYAs) with acute lymphoblastic leukemia (ALL). *Cancer*. 2014;**120(23)**:3660–3668.

109 Roberts KG, Morin RD, Zhang J, et al. Genetic alterations activating kinase and cytokine receptor signaling in high-risk acute lymphoblastic leukemia. *Cancer Cell*. 2012;**22(2)**:153–166.

114 Thomas DA, Faderl S, Cortes J, et al. Treatment of Philadelphia chromosome-positive acute lymphocytic leukemia with hyper-CVAD and imatinib mesylate. *Blood*. 2004;**103(12)**:4396–4407.

116 Fielding AK, Rowe JM, Buck G, et al. UKALLXII/ECOG2993: addition of imatinib to a standard treatment regimen enhances long-term outcomes in Philadelphia positive acute lymphoblastic leukemia. *Blood*. 2014;**123(6)**:843–850.

118 Ravandi F, O'Brien S, Thomas D, et al. First report of phase 2 study of dasatinib with hyper-CVAD for the frontline treatment of patients with Philadelphia chromosome-positive (Ph+) acute lymphoblastic leukemia. *Blood*. 2010;**116(12)**:2070–2077.

120 Bassan R, Rossi G, Pogliani EM, et al. Chemotherapy-phased imatinib pulses improve long-term outcome of adult patients with Philadelphia chromosome-positive acute lymphoblastic leukemia: Northern Italy Leukemia Group protocol 09/00. *J Clin Oncol*. 2010;**28(22)**:3644–3652.

126 Jabbour E, Kantarjian H, Thomas DA, et al. Phase II study of combination of hyper-CVAD with ponatinib in front line therapy of patients (pts) with Philadelphia Chromosome (Ph) positive acute lymphoblastic leukemia (ALL). *Blood* (ASH Annual Meeting Abstracts). 2013;**122**:2663a.

127 Thomas DA, Faderl S, O'Brien S, et al. Chemoimmunotherapy with hyper-CVAD plus rituximab for the treatment of adult Burkitt and Burkitt-type lymphoma or acute lymphoblastic leukemia. *Cancer*. 2006;**106(7)**:1569–1580.

129 Harvey RC, Mullighan CG, Chen IM, et al. Rearrangement of CRLF2 is associated with mutation of JAK kinases, alteration of IKZF1, Hispanic/Latino ethnicity, and a poor outcome in pediatric B-progenitor acute lymphoblastic leukemia. *Blood*. 2010;**115(26)**:5312–5321.

130 Harvey RC, Mullighan CG, Wang X, et al. Identification of novel cluster groups in pediatric high-risk B-precursor acute lymphoblastic leukemia with gene expression profiling: correlation with genome-wide DNA copy number alterations, clinical characteristics, and outcome. *Blood*. 2010;**116(23)**:4874–4884.

138 Zhang J, Ding L, Holmfeldt L, et al. The genetic basis of early T-cell precursor acute lymphoblastic leukaemia. *Nature*. 2012;**481(7380)**:157–163.

143 Kantarjian H, Gandhi V, Cortes J, et al. Phase 2 clinical and pharmacologic study of clofarabine in patients with refractory or relapsed acute leukemia. *Blood*.

2003;**102**(**7**):2379–2386.

150 O'Brien S, Schiller G, Lister J, et al. High-dose vincristine sulfate liposome injection for advanced, relapsed, and refractory adult Philadelphia chromosome-negative acute lymphoblastic leukemia. *J Clin Oncol*. 2013;**31**(**6**): 676–683.

154 Topp MS, Kufer P, Gokbuget N, et al. Targeted therapy with the T-cell-engaging antibody blinatumomab of chemotherapy-refractory minimal residual disease in B-lineage acute lymphoblastic leukemia patients results in high response rate and prolonged leukemia-free survival. *J Clin Oncol*. 2011;**29**(**18**):2493–2498.

155 Topp MS, Gokbuget N, Zugmaier G, et al. Long-term follow-up of hematologic relapse-free survival in a phase 2 study of blinatumomab in patients with MRD in B-lineage ALL. *Blood*. 2012;**120**(**26**):5185–5187.

156 Topp MS, Gokbuget N, Zugmaier G, et al. Phase II Trial of the anti-CD19 bispecific T cell-engager blinatumomab shows hematologic and molecular remissions in patients with relapsed or refractory B-precursor acute lymphoblastic leukemia. *J Clin Oncol*. 2014;**32**(**36**):4134–4140.

160 Kantarjian H, Thomas D, Jorgensen J, et al. Inotuzumab ozogamicin, an anti-CD22-calecheamicin conjugate, for refractory and relapsed acute lymphocytic leukaemia: a phase 2 study. *Lancet Oncol*. 2012;**13**(**4**):403–411.

172 Brentjens RJ, Davila ML, Riviere I, et al. CD19-targeted T cells rapidly induce molecular remissions in adults with chemotherapy-refractory acute lymphoblastic leukemia. *Sci Transl Med*. 2013;**5**(**177**):177ra38.

173 Grupp SA, Kalos M, Barrett D, et al. Chimeric antigen receptor-modified T cells for acute lymphoid leukemia. *N Engl J Med*. 2013;**368**(**16**):1509–1518.

174 Maude SL, Frey N, Shaw PA, et al. Chimeric antigen receptor T cells for sustained remissions in leukemia. *N Engl J Med*. 2014;**371**(**16**):1507–1517.

第117章 慢性淋巴细胞白血病

Kanti R. Rai, MD ■ Jacqueline C. Barrientos, MD

概述

慢性淋巴细胞白血病(chronic lymphocytic leukemia, CLL)是一种以无功能的小淋巴细胞在外周血,骨髓和淋巴组织中聚集为特征的惰性B细胞肿瘤。由于病情进展缓慢,仅当全身症状出现时才开始治疗。慢性淋巴细胞白血病主要发生在有明显的临床伴随疾病的老年人。鉴于化疗方案的已知毒性,传统免疫化疗限于耐受性良好的患者。近年来,新靶向药物应用于具有不良预后标记和高危险患者展现了前所未有的疗效,也促成了CLL患者管理的重大转变:基于CLL患者的临床和生物学特性新药联合以期获得最优化的治疗策略。

慢性髓细胞性白血病

CLL生物学:历史进程

CLL是CD5+单克隆B细胞淋巴组织增殖性肿瘤,因免疫球蛋白(Ig)V基因突变的水平不同而在临床上呈现较大的异质性[1]。表117-1总结了以往和现在对CLL认识的一些重要区别。染色体核型分析和基因突变检测技术进步,有助于判定临床表现的异质性并预测疾病预后,这些使CLL研究在过去十年中取得了突破性的进展。值得注意的是,骨髓微环境的作用以及信号转导通路异常在CLL发病机制中具有同样重要的临床意义[2~5]。对疾病的深入理解,有助于靶向肿瘤细胞增殖、生存通路的药物研发。最近研究发现,新药可以使复发难治CLL患者的长期生存预期显著改善。尽管CLL研究进展迅速,大多数初始治疗达到缓解的患者最终会复发。目前,研究的重点在于阐明新型靶向药物的耐药机制。

表117-1 过去与现在对B细胞慢性淋巴细胞白血病的认知

过去	现在
• 一种同类细胞来源的临床异质性疾病	• 一种来源于B淋巴细胞的异质性疾病,这些细胞主要在细胞的激活及成熟状态或细胞亚群上不同
• 来源于B淋巴细胞的疾病	• 因免疫球蛋白(Ig)*V*基因突变的水平不同而在临床上表现为一种源于抗原经历的B淋巴细胞来源的异质性疾病
• 因先天凋亡缺陷导致的白血病细胞堆积发生,进而形成白血病细胞肿块	• 白血病细胞堆积形成的肿块是由于先天凋亡缺陷所致,而非最初就已存在。细胞累积的发生是因通过一些受体(如B细胞受体(BCR),趋化因子及细胞因子受体等)和它们绑定的/可溶性配体将源于外界环境的生存信号传递给了白血病细胞
• 一种累积性疾病	• 一种累积性疾病,其增殖水平超越以往的预期
• 在低危/A期及中危/B期患者中,用一些预后指标将异质性患者进行Ral分期(低/中/高危或Binet分期(A/B/C期)(与临床预后比对)	• 更新的分子及蛋白标记将不同临床经过的低危/A期及中危/B期患者进一步分层
• 治疗上主要依靠临床观察以及试错法	• 以上已知的新发现将为研发出根据假说而来的有效治疗药物提供线索,找到靶点

发病率和流行病学

在西方成年人群中CLL是最常见的白血病,在美国的发病率约占所有白血病的30%。2014年美国约有15 720例新诊断的CLL,有4 600例CLL患者死亡[6]。CLL男女的发病比例为1.5∶1,以老年患者居多,中位诊断年龄为71岁[6,7]。与亚洲、非洲或其他较不发达国家相比,CLL在欧洲、澳大利亚和北美更为常见[8]。

CLL的诊断

世界卫生组织(WHO)对造血系统肿瘤的分类中,将CLL定义为白血病样的淋巴细胞淋巴瘤,其有别于小淋巴细胞淋巴瘤(SLL)之处在于白血病表现[9]。在该分类中,CLL均为B细胞来源,而以前的所谓T-CLL现在被称为T-幼淋巴细胞淋巴瘤

(T-PLL)[10]。国际 CLL 研讨会(IWCLL)确定 CLL 的最低诊断标准要求经流式细胞术证实外周血单克隆 B 细胞计数≥5×10^9/L(5 000/μl)[11]。外周血涂片特征性的表现为小的而形态成熟、胞质较少的淋巴细胞显著增多(图 117-1)。此类细胞胞质较少,核染色质紧密,核仁不明显,染色质部分聚集,外周血淋巴细胞中大的或不典型淋巴细胞、分裂细胞及前体淋巴细胞比例超过 55%。此外,涂抹细胞在 CLL 较为常见(实质为细胞碎片)[12]。

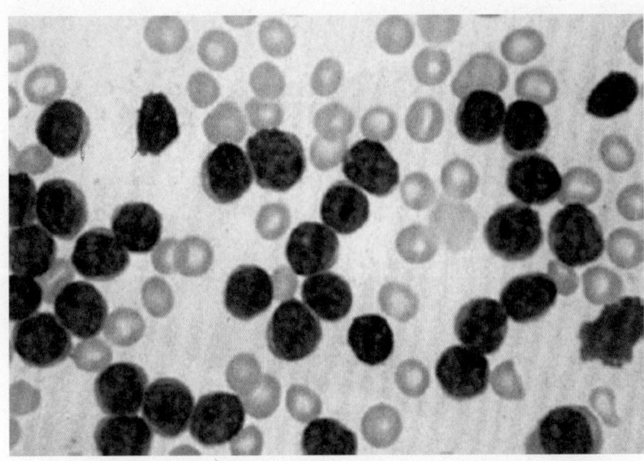

图 117-1　外周血涂片中 CLL 的形态。白细胞计数 100×10^9/L。绝大多数淋巴细胞呈成熟的形态,血小板在这个伴血小板减少的患者中缺如(Wright-Giemsa 染色;放大 100 倍)

病因和发病机制

单克隆 B 细胞淋巴细胞增多症和家族性 CLL

单克隆 B 淋巴细胞增多症(MBL)是指健康个体外周血中存在低水平的单克隆 B 淋巴细胞。诊断标准:①B 细胞克隆性异常;②外周血 B 淋巴细胞<5×10^9/L 且无 B 症状;③无肝、脾、淋巴结肿大;④无贫血及血小板减少[13]。Rawstron 等[14]发现 CLL 患者一级亲属中发生 MBL 概率约为 13.5%。这个数据已经远高于 Rawstron 等所报道的 3.5%[15]。此外,在 CLL 患者的家庭成员中,CLL 的发病率增加[17,16]。未来的研究需要进一步阐明 CLL 可能的易感基因或者可能的 CLL 携带状态。与 Kyle 统计 MGUS 进展为多发性骨髓瘤的数据相似[18],MBL 者每年进展为需要治疗的 CLL 比例为 1.1%[19]。

CLL 细胞的免疫生物学和免疫表型

在形态学上,CLL 淋巴细胞类似于正常外周血中成熟的淋巴细胞,共同表达 T 细胞抗原 CD5,B 细胞表面抗原 CD19, CD20 和 CD23。与正常 B 细胞相比,膜免疫球蛋白 CD20 和 CD79b 的表达水平极低[20],限制性表达 κ 或 λ 免疫球蛋白轻链中的一种。其他几种成熟淋巴细胞恶性肿瘤的临床特征与 CLL 相似(表 117-2),因此,通过流式细胞术有助于鉴别(表 117-3)[21~23]。

表 117-2　成熟 B 淋巴细胞的恶性肿瘤

慢性淋巴细胞白血病/小细胞淋巴瘤(CLL/SLL)
B-幼淋巴细胞白血病(B-PLL)
毛细胞白血病(HCL)
滤泡细胞淋巴瘤的白血病期(FL-L)
套细胞淋巴瘤的白血病期(MCL-L)
伴绒毛淋巴细胞的脾淋巴瘤(SLVL)
淋巴浆细胞样淋巴瘤

表 117-3　淋巴增生性疾病的表型

疾病	典型表型
慢性淋巴细胞白血病	CD20(d), CD19+, CD22(d), sIg(d), CD23+, FMC-7-, CD5+, CD10-, CD38+/-
套细胞淋巴瘤	CD20(i), sIg(i), CD23+/-, FMC-7+/-, CD5+, CD10-, cyclin-D1+
幼淋巴细胞白血病	CD20(+i), sIg(+i), FMC-7+/-, CD5+/-, CD10-
边缘区 B-细胞淋巴瘤	CD23-, CD11c+/-, CD103+/-, CD5+/-, CD10-, CD138(b)
淋巴浆细胞淋巴瘤	CD23(-/d), sIg+/-, cIg+, CD5+/-
滤泡性淋巴瘤	CD20(+i), CD5-, CD10+, bcl-2+, CD43-
弥漫大 B 细胞淋巴瘤	CD20(+i), CD5-, CD10+, bcl-2+/-, CD43+/-, CD5+/-
Buekitt 淋巴瘤	Bcl-2-, CD10(+b), CD43+, CD5-
毛细胞白血病	CD22(b), CD11c(b), CD25+, CD103+, sIg(i), CD123+, CD5-

+. 阳性;-,阴性;±,可能为阳性或阴性;d,低表达;i,中度表达;b,强表达;sIg,表面免疫球蛋白;cIg,胞质免疫球蛋白。

临床方面

患者不常出现全身症状。典型症状被称为"B 组"症状:体重骤降 10%或以上,发热高于 38℃或夜间盗汗超过 1 个月,没有感染征象。也有文献报道 CLL 可出现乏力症状。

外周血淋巴细胞绝对值

根据 IWCLL 标准,外周血单克隆 B 淋巴细胞计数至少为 5×10^9/L,且该群淋巴细胞免疫表型须为 CD19+、CD20+、CD23+和 CD5+,用以鉴别感染以及其他淋巴增殖性肿瘤(如淋巴瘤白血病,毛细胞白血病(HCL),图 117-2 所示的幼淋巴细胞白血病(PLL)和大颗粒细胞白血病)。

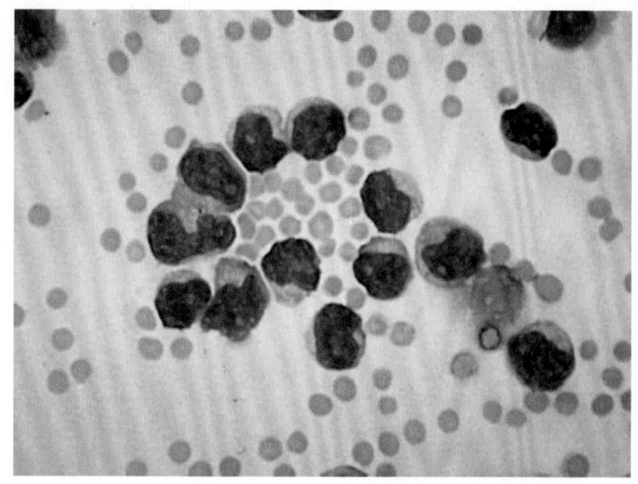

图 117-2 幼淋细胞白血病。外周血涂片显示明显的细胞核和丰富的胞质(Wright-Giemsa 染色;放大 1 000 倍)

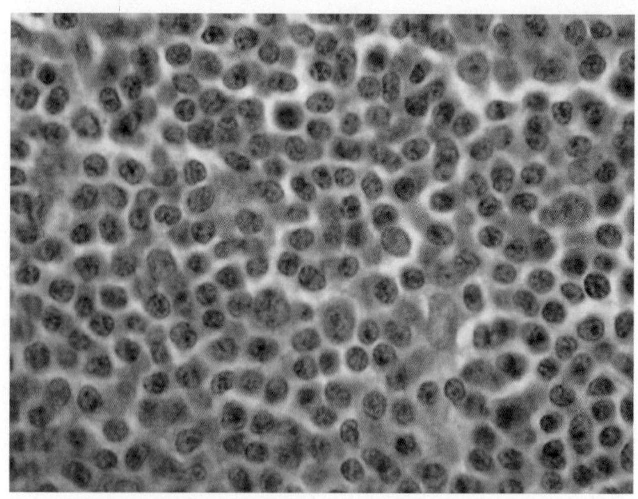

图 117-3 CLL 骨髓活检示弥漫浸润的 CLL 细胞(HE 染色:放大 600 倍)

临床表现

CLL 的淋巴结具有圆形、质韧、分散、无触痛且触诊可自由滑动的特点。体格检查中最常发现是淋巴结肿大,部分可存在脾大或肝大。淋巴结肿大范围既可广泛也可局限,肿大程度也不尽相同,引起邻近器官压迫症状。除了可触及的浅表淋巴结、肝和脾外,初诊时其他淋巴组织也可增大,如 Waldeyer 环或扁桃体。此外,CLL 细胞浸润可发生于任何器官或组织。与其他类型非霍奇金淋巴瘤相比,胃肠黏膜浸润及脑膜侵犯少见。

影像学表现

影像学检查在初诊和随访评估病情时既非必要也不是必须。CT 扫描或胸片经常会找到体格检查不能发现的淋巴结病变,但这些发现并不能改变临床 Rai 或 Binet 分期。除非出现新临床症状或发生其他特殊临床情况,否则不建议上述检查。美国血液学会提倡早期无症状患者通过实验室检查而非 CT 扫描来进行临床分期。对于临床试验的方案设计,具体问题具体分析。

实验室检查异常

虽然 CLL 诊断要求外周血淋巴细胞绝对值的下限是 $5\times10^9/L$,多数患者的计数会远高于该值,甚至超过 $100\times10^9/L$。外周血涂片分类见白细胞增多,以成熟的小淋巴细胞为主,比例在 50%~100%不等。

除骨髓细胞学检查见成熟淋巴细胞比例增加之外,还可以通过骨髓病理学检查见到三种淋巴细胞的浸润方式(图 117-3):结节型,间质型以及弥散型。研究发现伴有弥散浸润型的患者通常处于疾病进展阶段,且预后相对较差。从预后的角度看,结节型和间质型由于预后相对良好,可以将它们一并归为"非弥散组"[24~26]。

症状性贫血和血小板减少也可见于初诊阶段,但一般程度相对较轻。直接抗人球蛋白阳性者不超过 25%,但典型的自身免疫性溶血性贫血并不常见。在缺乏可信的血小板抗体检测试验的情况下,自身免疫性血小板减少的诊断依赖于骨髓中的巨核细胞数量及外周血中的血小板计数。

初诊时可出现高 γ 球蛋白血症,但多数病例仅见于疾病的晚期阶段。三种类型免疫球蛋白(IgG、IgA 和 IgM)常常低于正常,部分患者仅出现一至两种球蛋白降低。低球蛋白血症和粒细胞减少增大了 CLL 患者发生细菌、病毒以及机会性感染的概率。由于 B 细胞比例明显增加,淋巴细胞亚群分析常常提示 T 细胞与 B 细胞的比例改变了(正常是 2:1)。由于患者免疫功能不健全,应该避免接种任何活疫苗(水痘、麻疹、卡介苗等)。在这类免疫缺陷的群体中,接种后病毒复制增加,活疫苗实际上能诱发活动性感染[27,28]。

CLL 在血生化检查上没有特征性的异常,有时可见乳酸脱氢酶、尿酸、转氨酶(谷丙转氨酶(AST)或谷草转氨酶(ALT))升高,血钙升高较为罕见。极度白细胞增多症患者偶尔会发生假性高钾血症。

自然病程和终点事件

CLL 通常被认为是一种相对惰性的疾病,病程较长,最终的死因多为与 CLL 无关的并发症。然而,这种现象仅见于少于 30%的病例中。CLL 的自然病程异质性很大。多数患者一直处于初级阶段并可生存 5~10 年,病情进展相对缓慢,一旦发展为终末期,通常仅可维持 1~2 年。在没有症状的疾病初期,患者可保持原有的生活规律,但在疾病终末期,体力状态迅速恶化。进展期患者的死因多与原发病或治疗并发症直接相关。其中感染致死率较高,占所有死亡原因的 30%~50%。

转化为高级别疾病的特征是对常用的化疗药物复发耐药[29]。高达 10%的 CLL 患者最终会转化为弥漫大 B 细胞淋巴瘤[30](Richter 转化或 Richter 综合征,图 117-4)。Richter 综合征病程进展迅速,对目前多种化疗药物耐药,总生存期(OS)较差[31,32]。诊断 Richter 综合征需要完整淋巴结的组织病理检查,常见增殖指数(Ki-67)较高的大 B 细胞。此外,少数患者存在"幼淋巴细胞样转化",其外周血可见混合形态的小成熟淋巴细胞和幼淋巴细胞,这与典型的 B 幼淋巴细胞白血病(B-

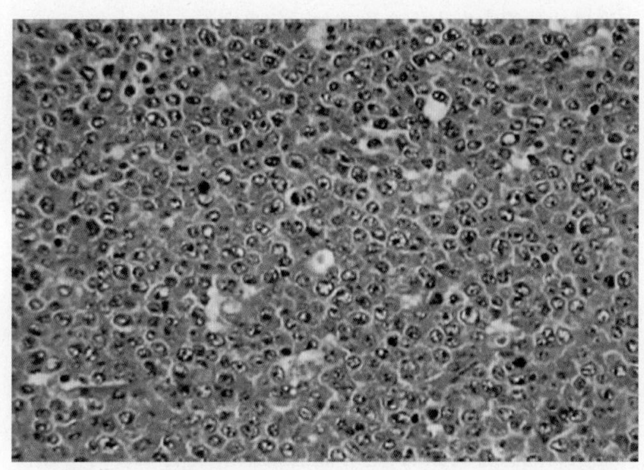

图 117-4　慢性淋巴细胞白血病，Richter 综合征。表现为淋巴母细胞增生的淋巴结切片，细胞较大，核仁明显（HE 染色：放大 600 倍）

prolymphocytic Leukemia，B-PLL）不同，B-PLL 外周血的幼淋巴细胞形态一致。幼淋巴细胞样转化与 Richter 转化相似，临床经过具有侵袭性。

急性白血病仅见于极少数的 CLL 患者终末期。一旦发生，通常是髓系来源（粒细胞的，粒单细胞的或急性红白血病）。由于只对很少一部分之前未接受过烷化剂治疗的患者进行了随访，烷化剂导致急性白血病的观点尚未被认可。对于转变为急性白血病的患者可采用相应的治疗方案处理，但通常预后不良。

CLL 继发第二肿瘤的风险高于正常人群的两倍。皮肤癌和其他实体瘤一样，在 CLL 中的发生率增加。因此推荐所有 CLL 患者（包括不需治疗的患者）遵守适龄者的癌症筛查指南。

临床分期和其他预后因素

由于简单（依靠简单的体检和实验室检查）并可精准判定预后，Rai[34] 和 Binet[38] 这两种分期系统广泛应用于临床。

Rai 和其同事的分期系统

Rai 系统是基于这样一种概念：CLL 是一种克隆性淋巴细胞增殖导致肿瘤负荷在体内不断增加最终出现临床症状的疾病。这些临床表现首先从血液开始，逐渐累及淋巴结、脾和肝，最终抑制骨髓功能。最早期为单克隆淋巴细胞增多症（临床 0 期），晚期（如贫血和血小板减少，除 AIHA 和 ITP 之外）被视为疾病进展，CLL 细胞浸润骨髓所致。

接近 25%的初诊患者处于疾病的最早期（0 期），少于 25%的患者处于进展期（Ⅲ～Ⅳ期），剩余 50%患者在Ⅰ期或Ⅱ期。表 117-4 提示各个中心的 CLL 各期患者所占比例基本一致。Rai 和他同事的研究发现，0 期患者从诊断开始的中位生存时间是 150 个月，Ⅰ期为 101 个月，Ⅱ期为 71 个月，Ⅲ期和Ⅳ期均为 19 个月[34]。尽管 Rai 和其同事在 1975 年发表的文章中对生存情况只作了三组数据分析（0 期，Ⅰ期和Ⅱ期合并，Ⅲ期和Ⅳ期合并），但他们仍建议应保留 5 期分期系统以便前瞻性地观察在Ⅰ与Ⅱ期、Ⅲ与Ⅳ期之间是否存在生物学和临床上的差异。到了 1987 年，分期系统调整为三组：低危（Rai 分期 0 期），中危（Rai 分期Ⅰ和Ⅱ期合并）以及高危组（Rai 分期Ⅲ和Ⅳ期合并）[39]。20 世纪 90 年代，一项具有里程碑意义的研究评价了经改良的 Rai 分期系统进行危险分层 CLL 患者一线接受苯丁酸氮芥（chlorambucil）与氟达拉滨的疗效，进而确立了氟达拉滨的优势[40]。氟达拉滨和嘌呤类似物现在可作为没有严重并发症 CLL 的一线治疗选择[41,42]。

表 117-4　来自不同研究组的根据 Rai 分期的病例分布情况

研究组	病例（n）	系列/年	分期/%				
			0	Ⅰ	Ⅱ	Ⅲ	Ⅳ
Rai et al.[34]	125	18	23	31	17	11	14
Geisler and Hansen (1981)[35]	102	20	36	19	17	8	31
Baccarani et al. (1982)[36]	188	26.5	26.5	21	9	17	9
Skinnider (1982)[37]	745	19	21	31	16	13	31
MRC CLL-1a (1989)	660	28	18	29	10	15	31

在英国 CLL 医学研究委员会上Ⅲ期血红蛋白的标准是<110g/L。

Binet 和其同事的分期系统

Binet 将所有贫血、血小板减少（贫血定义为 HGB 小于 100g/L，血小板减少定义为低于 100×10^9/L）或两者均有的患者定义为 C 期[38]。所有剩余的患者（非 C 期）再根据少于三个区域（A 期）或三个及以上区域（B 期）可触及的淋巴结肿大情况分为两组。这种分期顾及 5 个部位：颈部、腋下、腹股沟（单侧/双侧，每个区域算一个部位）以及肝脏和脾脏的情况。该体系被证实对预测患者预后有很大帮助，A、B、C 三期患者的生存曲线分别与 Rai 分期中的低、中、高危组对应。

预测低、中危险组疾病进程的标准

实际上所有处于高危组的患者（Ⅲ、Ⅳ期）都呈现相对迅速的临床进程和较短的生存期。其他危险组的疾病进程并不尽相同。低危/中危组患者（分别是 0 期、Ⅰ期和Ⅱ期）可能由于进展缓慢而表现为相对良性的临床经过，获得长达几年甚至是几十年的生存时间。同样，低危/中危组患者也可能出现迅速进展，生存期较短。区分疾病异质性的主要预后标志物包括染色体畸变，*IGHV* 突变状态，CD38 和 Zap-70 表达（表 117-5）。其他预后因子包括年龄、性别、并发症、复杂的染色体核型[43]、分子遗传学标记[44]以及 β_2-微球蛋白等被证实对于 CLL 病程预测有一定帮助。

表 117-5　预测慢性淋巴细胞白血病（CLL）的分子学和遗传学标记

	标记	
	良好预后	不良预后
IgVH 突变状况	突变	未突变
ZAP-70	阴性	阳性
CD38	阴性	阳性
FISH 遗传学	13q 缺失	11q 缺失，17p 缺失

主要的预后标记物

IGHV 突变

白血病 B 细胞表达的 *IGHV* 基因是否存在突变将 CLL 分为两个预后亚组。*IGHV* 基因突变的患者有相对缓慢的疾病进程和更长的无病进展期和总体生存期[46,47]。可能部分原因是未突变的 CLL 病例的 B 细胞受体（BCR）刺激性下游转导通路信号的能力大于突变细胞[1,48]。有或没有 *IGHV* 突变的患者可根据其他重要预后指标进一步细化，如是否存在 *TP53*[49]，NOTCH1[50] 和 *SF3B1*[44] 突变，是否表达 ZAP-70[51] 和 CD38[46]，这些都被证实对该病的临床进程有影响。

细胞遗传学

CLL 的细胞遗传学的预后价值是有限的，因为利用传统的显带分析很难将白血病细胞诱导进入分裂中期。应用荧光原位杂交（FISH）技术可以在 82% 的病例中检测到染色体畸变[52]。Döhner 等人的一项开创性研究发现 CLL 患者存在以下常见突变及其所占比例如下：13q14 缺失患者占 55%，11q 缺失占 18%，12 三体占 16%，17p 缺失占 7%，6q 缺失占 7%。该研究中，正常核型占 CLL 患者 18%。在上述突变中，13q、11q 及 17p 缺失意义最大。伴有单一 13q 缺失患者的中位生存期为 133 个月，11q 或 17p 缺失者预后不良，中位生存期分别为 79 和 32 个月。11q 和 17p 的缺失被认为分别涉及了编码毛细血管共济失调基因突变和肿瘤抑制基因 p53 的失活。这些高风险突变与疾病的侵袭性和对化疗耐药相关[53,54]。正常核型与 +12 患者生存时间相近，分别为 111 个月和 114 个月。

Zap-70 表达

Zap-70 是一种参与激活信号的胞内蛋白。它通常存在于 T 淋巴细胞和自然杀伤细胞上，很少表达于正常 B 细胞[55]。尽管通过流式细胞术可检测 ZAP-70 的表达，这些检测的可重复性和方法学都需要再进一步标准化。研究表明其在白血病 B 淋巴细胞上的异常表达与无突变的 *IGHV* 基因有关（U-CLL）[51,56]。数据显示 Zap-70 阳性可作为 CLL 进展和不良预后的独立预测因素[55,57]。ZAP-70 的表达在预测治疗时间上优于突变状态[58,59]。

分子遗传学

一系列的基因突变对 CLL 具有预后价值。抑癌基因 *TP53* 突变是多种人类肿瘤中最频发的改变之一，该突变常与不良预后相关。德国 CLL 研究小组（GCLLSG）发现，8.5%既往未治疗的 CLL 患者有 *p53* 突变，其中一些甚至没有 17p 缺失[49]。无论 17p 是否缺失，*p53* 突变的预后都很差，并且与治疗反应差、无进展生存期（PFS）和生存期较短有关。此外，在多变量分析中，*TP53* 突变分析的预后价值远远超过本章前面提及的公认不良遗传因素[60]。

在 CLL 中具有预后意义的其他突变包括 NOTCH1[61] 和 *SF3B1*[44] 突变。关于这些异常的详细研究结果使得一些专家提出了风险算法，该算法将包含有关基因突变、染色体异常和克隆进化过程中发生的变化的预后信息[62,63]。

治疗

早期干预被认为是治疗大多数恶性疾病的关键，但并不适用于 CLL。没有证据表明 CLL 接受现有的治疗手段后能够治愈[64]，因此“观察与等待”是多数初诊患者最适合的治疗策略。也就是说，每 3~4 个月进行一次包括病史采集，体格检查和全血细胞计数的随访（如果有迹象表明有侵袭性疾病，则需要缩短随访周期）。

如果临床试验结果表明应用嘌呤类似物，单克隆抗体以及近期针对 BCR 信号通路的小分子靶向药物早期干预可以改善无症状高危患者的预后，这可能会在未来改变 CLL 的治疗模式。目前，除临床试验之外并不推荐早期药物干预。

CLL 一线和挽救治疗的方案选择分别见表 117-6 和表 117-7。

表 117-6　慢性淋巴细胞白血病的一线治疗

患者人群	治疗方案
患者年龄<70 岁或者没有重大并发症及不伴 17p 缺失年龄更大的患者	• 氟达拉滨+环磷酰胺+利妥昔单抗
	• 苯达莫司汀±利妥昔单抗
	• 氟达拉滨+利妥昔单抗
	• 喷司他丁（pentostatin）+环磷酰胺+利妥昔单抗
	• 奥妥珠单抗+苯丁酸氮芥
	• 奥法木单抗+苯丁酸氮芥
	• 伊布替尼
患者年龄>70 岁或者合并重大并发症及不伴 17p 缺失的年龄更小的患者	• 奥妥珠单抗+苯丁酸氮芥
	• 奥法木单抗+苯丁酸氮芥
	• 伊布替尼
	• 苯达莫司汀±利妥昔单抗
	• 环磷酰胺±利妥昔单抗±糖皮质激素
	• 氟达拉滨±利妥昔单抗
	• 减少剂量的氟达拉滨+环磷酰胺+利妥昔单抗
	• 苯丁酸氮芥
合并重大并发症不能耐受嘌呤类似物	• 奥妥珠单抗+苯丁酸氮芥
	• 奥法木单抗+苯丁酸氮芥
	• 苯丁酸氮芥
伴 17p 缺失的患者	• 伊布替尼
	• idelalisib+利妥昔单抗
	• 阿伦珠单抗（alemtuzumab）
	• 临床试验

表 117-7 复发慢性淋巴细胞白血病的挽救治疗

患者人群	治疗方案
年龄<70 岁的对初始治疗缓解时间短或者没有重大并发症及不伴 17p 缺失的>70 岁的患者	• 伊布替尼
	• idelalisib+利妥昔单抗
	• 氟达拉滨+环磷酰胺+利妥昔单抗
	• 喷司他丁+环磷酰胺+利妥昔单抗
	• 苯达莫司汀±利妥昔单抗
	• 氟达拉滨+阿伦珠单抗
	• 奥法木单抗
	• 来那度胺±利妥昔单抗
	• 阿伦珠单抗±利妥昔单抗
	• 大剂量甲泼尼龙+利妥昔单抗
	• R-CHOP
	• OFAR
	• 临床试验
年龄≥70 岁及不伴 17p 缺失的对初始治疗缓解时间短的患者	• 伊布替尼
	• idelalisib+利妥昔单抗
	• 苯达莫司汀±利妥昔单抗
	• 奥法木单抗
	• 大剂量甲泼尼龙+利妥昔单抗
	• 阿伦珠单抗±利妥昔单抗
	• 临床试验
伴 17p 缺失的患者	• 伊布替尼
	• 文尼克拉
	• 艾代拉里斯+利妥昔单抗
	• 阿伦珠单抗±利妥昔单抗
	• 临床试验

国际 CLL 工作组初始治疗指征

①Rai 分期Ⅰ或Ⅱ(Binet 分期 B)伴有疾病相关症状者；

②Rai 分期Ⅲ或Ⅳ期(Binet 分期 C)；

③巨大或快速增长的有症状的淋巴结病变或脾肿大；

④淋巴细胞倍增时间小于 6 个月；

⑤糖皮质激素治疗反应差的 AIHA 或血小板减少(或两者均有)。

淋巴结增大和/或淋巴细胞倍增的时间短暂，需要谨慎评估。没有证据表明淋巴细胞计数达到特定阈值需要治疗。部分证据表明，在少数患者中，高白细胞血症可能会导致高黏滞血症。因此，在有风险的特定患者中，可考虑进行治疗。

治疗的目标

最佳的个体化治疗方案选择取决于患者年龄，身体状态和遗传学改变。以往，CLL 的治疗需持续到症状消失或有临床表现的淋巴结病变得到控制。随着抗 CD20 单克隆抗体(mAb)利妥昔单抗(在化疗基础上联合使用)的出现，微小残留病变(MRD)阴性与更好的 PFS 和 OS 相关[65]。因此，定义完全缓解(complete remission，CR)和 MRD 阴性的标准进一步提高了[11]。

然而，考虑到疾病的异质性和 CLL 并发症的发生率，很难为 CLL 治疗制订精准的目标。尽管 CR 和 MRD 阴性是终极理想目标，但是在某些情况下，由于药物毒性使其并非适合于所有患者。临床医生需将患者的个体情况同现有疗法相匹配，并设定个体化的治疗目标。

以 BCR 信号转导和微环境的小分子靶向药物的临床应用，需要更新先前的疗效评价标准[66]。BCR 抑制剂动员骨髓和淋巴结中 CLL 细胞进入外周血，可引起淋巴细胞增多症，容易被误认为是疾病进展(PD)或缺乏反应。

治疗反应的标准

完全缓解意味着临床症状消失，体格检查未见异常，淋巴细胞计数小于 4×10^9/L，中性粒细胞≥1.5×10^9/L，血小板≥100×10^9/L，并且血红蛋白≥110g/L。血浆免疫球蛋白正常并非完全缓解的必要条件。对于参加临床试验的患者，骨髓穿刺和活检至少要在停止治疗后的 2 个月内进行，要求形态学正常，淋巴细胞在有核细胞中的比例小于 30%，才被认定达到完全缓解(CR)。骨髓中仍有 CLL 的被定义为部分缓解(PR)。在接受治疗后，骨髓中有淋巴样结节的称为结节性 PR。指南推荐应对这些结节行免疫组化染色以确定是否为 CLL 细胞。治疗后伴有持续性血细胞减少而无 CLL 的证据被认为是达到 CR 而骨髓未完全恢复(CRi)。

其他严格意义上的 PR 标准包括之前升高的淋巴细胞计数减少，增大的淋巴结、脾或肝缩小比例大于等于 50%。外周血至少有以下一种表现：中性粒细胞计数≥1.5×10^9/L，血小板≥100×10^9/L，血红蛋白≥110g/L(或上述指标较治疗前改善≥50%)。这些反应须持续至少 2 个月[11]。

“淋巴细胞部分反应增生”(PRL)的新概念要求满足除外周淋巴细胞计数外所有 PR 标准。在缺乏其他 PD 的客观证据的前提下，仅仅淋巴细胞增多不被视为 PD 的指标。淋巴细胞增多症患者在没有 PD 的其他证据时，需要继续治疗，直至出现明确的 PD 征象[66]。

MRD 阴性要求无论四色流式细胞学检测还是等位特异性寡核苷酸 PCR 的方法均查不到白血病细胞。MRD 检测需要在临床试验性治疗结束后的至少 3 个月后[11]。尽管 MRD 阴性预示预后更佳，但它作为一种评价治疗目标的意义尚不明确。

苯丁酸氮芥单药治疗

尽管现有证据表明与其他可用的药物相比，苯丁酸氮芥

(chlorambucil)单药治疗具有较低的反应率和较短的缓解期,由于便于使用、耐受性良好,苯丁酸氮芥仍然被广泛用于体弱和老年患者。研究表明,苯丁酸氮芥具有剂量依赖性和时间依赖性[67,68]。一项 CALGB 的研究发现苯丁酸氮芥每日给药和间歇给药的疗效相当[69]。苯丁酸氮芥通常是给药治疗一段时间直至获得最大临床反应,维持治疗并不常见。最近的数据表明,与靶向 CD20 的单克隆抗体联合可以获得更好的疗效且具有良好的耐受性。单药治疗的地位可能在未来发生变化。

糖皮质激素

泼尼松曾被单独用于 CLL 患者的治疗,通常的初始剂量为 20~60mg,之后逐渐减量[67,70]。外周血淋巴细胞计数通常在接受治疗后 1~2 个月出现一过性升高,随后降低,这是由于淋巴细胞从淋巴结和骨髓释放入外周血所致。大约 2/3 患者的贫血和血小板减少会得到改善。不良事件主要为慢性糖皮质激素治疗相关的副作用及感染。目前,泼尼松的主要适应证为自身抗体诱发的贫血和血小板减少症。

氟达拉滨-环磷酰胺-利妥昔单抗(FCR)

FCR 仍然是 CLL 患者早期治疗的金标准。一项单中心单臂研究中,应用氟达拉滨、环磷酰胺及利妥昔单抗(FCR)成功治疗了 224 例既往未接受过治疗的患者[40,71]。总体反应率为 95%,72%的患者获得了 CR,多数 MRD 阴性。许多患者无病生存时间达到十年以上。该研究中,出现了 3~4 级中性粒细胞减少的患者比例高于 50%。

在德国 CLL 研究组的一项设计周密的 3 期临床试验中,纳入了 817 例既往未接受过治疗的患者,旨在评价 FC 方案中加入利妥昔单抗的获益[41]。该研究中位随访 47 个月,发现 FCR 组患者具有较高的 PFS(两组分别为 57.9 和 32.9 个月,$P<0.001$)[72]。FCR 组发生中性粒细胞减少的患者较多,但出现 3~4 度感染的患者不多。与其他嘌呤类似物联合烷化剂及利妥昔单抗方案一样,使用 FCR 方案期间应给予抗生素预防肺孢子虫、水痘-带状疱疹病毒及念珠菌感染。最近,将 FCR 与毒性较低的 BR(苯达莫司汀和利妥昔单抗)方案进行了比较,发现 FCR 优于对照组 BR(参见标题为"苯达莫司汀"的部分)。一项大规模正在进行的临床试验(E1912)目前正在招募患者评估 FCR 与利妥昔单抗联合伊布替尼在一线 17p 缺失的年轻 CLL 患者中的疗效。该研究的主要终点比较组间 PFS 及生活质量的改善情况。

苯达莫司汀

基于一项比较既往未接受过治疗的 CLL 中苯达莫司汀(bendamustine)和苯丁酸氮芥疗效的临床试验结果,苯达莫司汀在 2008 年获 FDA 批准使用[73]。在该研究中,苯达莫司汀静脉每 4 周给药一次,100mg/m² 使用 2 日,总体反应率及无疾病进展生存期均优于苯丁酸氮芥。鉴于苯达莫司汀联合利妥昔单抗在一线和复发 CLL 患者的疗效和耐受性[74,75],该方案可作为 FCR 方案出现早期和晚期毒性后的选择。

一项名为 CLL10 的Ⅲ期临床试验比较了一线治疗方案 BR 与 FCR 的差异,该研究将 del17p 的高危者排除在外。虽然两个组的 ORR 相同(97.8%),但 FCR 组治疗的患者中 CR 率更高,并且有更长的 PFS,两组患者 OS 的差异无统计学意义。与 BR 组患者相比,FCR 组严重的中性粒细胞减少、骨髓抑制和感染等 3/4 级不良事件发生率明显更高。由于 BR 的毒性较轻,该方案可用于一般状态欠佳 CLL 患者的前期治疗[76]。

奥法木单抗

奥法木单抗(Ofatumumab)是一种由转基因小鼠产生的完全人源化的抗 CD20 单克隆抗体(mAb),与利妥昔单抗相比,它可结合于 CD20 的不同表位。它属于Ⅰ型 mAb,在 CLL 细胞系中显示出比利妥昔单抗更强的补体依赖性细胞毒性,由此被获批单药治疗复发的 CLL[77,78]。近期,奥法木单抗被批准与苯丁酸氮芥联合用于一线治疗[79]。

奥妥珠单抗

奥妥珠单抗(obinutuzumab)是一种人源 CD20 单克隆抗体,与苯丁酸氮芥联合用于未经治疗的 CLL 患者。未经治疗的 CLL 患者被随机分配到苯丁酸氮芥组、苯丁酸氮芥联合利妥昔单抗组与苯丁酸氮芥联合奥妥珠单抗组[80]。Goede 等人发现,与利妥昔单抗联合苯丁酸氮芥相比,奥妥珠单抗与苯丁酸氮芥联合可使多重衰弱的 CLL 患者(中位年龄 73 岁)PFS 延长,CR 增加,MRD 阴性率增加。此外,与苯丁酸氮芥单药相比,联合奥妥珠单抗可取得显著的 OS 获益。这表明,即使体弱的患者也可取得更深的缓解并转化为生存优势。将该药与新型 BCR 抑制剂联合的试验在研中。

伊布替尼

伊布替尼(ibrutinib)是一种口服生物利用度高,小分子不可逆的 BTK 抑制剂,已被证明可诱导 CLL 患者迅速出现淋巴结缩小。与其他激酶抑制剂一样,伊布替尼抑制包括 BCR、Toll 样受体、BAFF 和 CD40 在内的多种信号通路,并可以干扰基质细胞的保护作用[3]。在早期Ⅰb/Ⅱ期临床试验中,伊布替尼单药被用于治疗复发/难治性 CLL 患者。所有受试患者组(包括高龄患者和高危患者)的总体有效率(ORR)高达 71%,并获得持久缓解(26 个月 PFS 为 75%)[81]。为期三年的随访显示了伊布替尼的持久反应[82]。RESONATEⅢ期临床研究中,比较了伊布替尼与奥法木单抗于复发/难治性 CLL/SLL 患者的疗效[83],两组患者的 ORR 分别为 42.6%和 4.1%。该研究结果与 17p 状态无关,甚至在嘌呤类似物难治的患者也有疗效,且毒性微小。

在 17p 缺失高危患者的大规模前瞻性研究中,伊布替尼显著改善了 ORR 和 PFS,具有良好的风险获益比[84]。中位随访 13 个月时,在 12 个月中疾病无进展生存的患者占 79.3%,与早期研究结果一致[81]。该研究中,复发难治患者的 PFS 优于初治接受 FCR 的 17p 缺失患者[42],后者的中位 PFS 仅为 11 个月。这些结果支持伊布替尼可作为 17p 缺失的 CLL/SLL 患者的有效药物。

idelalisib

idelalisib 是一种靶向的,高选择性的口服磷酸肌醇 3-激酶 δ(PI3K)抑制剂。PI3K 仅存在于白细胞中,可促进恶性 B 细胞的生存和增殖。一项随机双盲安慰剂对照的Ⅲ期临床试验中,利妥昔单抗联合 idelalisib 和利妥昔单抗联合安慰剂的患者的 ORR 分别为 81% 和 13%，由于两组疗效差异悬殊而被独立数据和安全管理委员会提前叫停[85,86]。亚组分析表明，无论是否存在 *17p*、*TP53* 或 *IGHV* 突变，idelalisib 联合利妥昔单抗均有效[87]。小样本的Ⅱ期临床试验表明，艾代拉里斯联合利妥昔单抗一线治疗 *17p* 缺失患者也有效[88]。

维奈克拉

BCL-2 蛋白家族是调节内源性细胞凋亡的重要因子。它们通常在 CLL 细胞中过度表达，并有助于肿瘤细胞的存活和耐药。维奈克拉（venetoclax）是第一代选择性 BCL2 抑制剂。由于可以迅速降低包括复发性 del（17p）在内 CLL 患者外周血、淋巴结和骨髓中的肿瘤负荷，从而产生较高的总体反应率，该药最近获得了美国 FDA 的批准。维奈克拉（与利妥昔单抗合用）用于复发或难治性 CLL 患者的适应证仍待评估获批。

干细胞移植

尽管造血干细胞移植（HSCT）是治疗多种侵袭性血液系统恶性肿瘤的选择，但在 CLL 中的作用尚存争议。自体干细胞移植（stem cell transplant，SCT）并没有为 CLL 带来明显获益[89]。鉴于该方法较高的治疗相关死亡率，HSCT 仅用于非常特殊的病例。

CLL 的社会心理方面

被诊断为白血病对患者来讲是一种很大的精神挑战。初诊时详细解释 CLL 的自然发展病程，强调一些患者不需要治疗，早期治疗并不能获益。患者需要知道当疾病进展或出现症状时会有很多有效的疗法。要告知患者许多早期的 CLL 患者的生存期与相同年龄、性别的正常人群是相似的。也应该告诉患者需要关注一些新的预后因素。良好的预后标记进一步确证观察是可取的方法，但多数存在高危标记的患者难于接受这种初始治疗的方式。要拉近与患者的关系，特别是那些处于疾病早期的患者，对患者所提出的问题应予详细的解答，同时为患者及家属提供精神及心理上的安慰。当前治疗的选择迅速增多，尤其是年轻患者，在需要治疗时可以抱着更乐观的态度。

未满足的需求和未来的方向

目前的目标是根据患者临床表现制订个体化治疗策略。如本章前面所述，开始治疗的确切时间取决于几个因素。如果患者有 CLL 引起的症状，治疗是必要的。高危标记的存在不是治疗的指征。通常 CLL 还有一个灰色区域，即无明显的症状学表现，细胞减少也呈良性过程。如果患者愿意，可以继续观察，至细胞计数下降至预期水平之下再治疗。

以嘌呤类似物为基础的方案，如 FCR，仍然是没有并发症的年轻 CLL 患者的一线标准方案。对 Coombs 试验阳性或有 AIHA 病史者应避免使用嘌呤类似物。对于存在并发症的年老体弱者，如果没有 17p 缺失，强烈推荐奥妥珠单抗联合苯丁酸氮芥，BR，奥法木单抗和苯丁酸氮芥或伊布替尼的一线治疗；如果存在复杂情况，禁止使用这些方案中的任一种。

新型靶向药物单药或联合细胞毒药物化疗将对 CLL 患者的临床预后产生重大影响。这是目前开展大型Ⅲ期临床试验的原因，这些试验比较了一线免疫化疗与有可能改变当前标准治疗的靶向药物疗效。在未来，一些患者（包括年轻健康的患者）可能会接受不包含细胞毒性化疗药物的治疗方案。还可以预想到，将新药与免疫化疗方案联合用于一线治疗可以产生更深的治疗反应率和更长的缓解时间且不增加治疗相关毒性。

最具挑战性的治疗决策是有症状的 17p 缺失的初治患者。专家对这组患者的最佳治疗没有明确的共识。尽管添加了单克隆抗体，但细胞毒性化疗方案的效果仍然欠佳。使用伊布替尼单药或联合利妥昔单抗的小样本Ⅰ-Ⅱ期试验数据令人鼓舞[90~92]，因此应该明确考虑使用伊布替尼。伊布替尼和维奈克拉是美国为数不多获批用于治疗 17p 缺失 CLL 的药物。如果无法耐受伊布替尼或维奈克拉，idelalisib 将是合理的选择，因为它已被证实于 17p 缺失者具有临床获益[87,88]。值得一提的是，对于一般状态较好的年轻高危患者（17p 缺失，新药治疗失败，初始治疗获得较短 PFS）需进行干细胞移植评估。

然而，CLL 治疗的目标和持续时间仍不明确。免疫化学治疗方案的高 CR 率和 MRD 阴性率在十年前已取得了很大的进步，但这些成功的长期获益仍未在使用 BCR 抑制剂患者中得到证实。因此，MRD 阴性仅作为临床试验设计的治疗目标。

在过去几年取得了一场突破性的革命，包括 B 细胞信号转导抑制剂的发展，CLL 微环境的免疫调节剂和单克隆抗体[93]。CLL 的靶向治疗时代已经明确到来，并可预见这种进展将持续下去。我们希望新疗法和新治疗模式将改变今天 CLL 管理的方式。

致谢

Jacqueline Barrientos 的工作得到了 NIH/NCATS 基金# UL1TR00457 和 2015 年美国血液学会-哈罗德阿莫斯医学院发展计划（ASH-AMFDP）奖学金的部分支持。

（白元松　张文龙 译　白元松　张文龙　周迪 校）

参考文献

The complete reference list can be found on the Wiley Companion Digital Edition of this title (see inside front cover for login instructions).

1 Chiorazzi N, Rai KR, Ferrarini M. Mechanism of disease: chronic lymphocytic leukemia. *N Engl J Med*. 2005;**352**:804–815.

3 Wiestner A. Emerging role of kinase-targeted strategies in chronic lymphocytic leukemia. *Blood*. 2012;**120**:4684–4691.

9 Jaffe ES, Harris NL, Stein H, et al. Chronic lymphocytic leukemia/small lymphocytic lymphoma. In: Jaffe ES, Harris NL, Stein H, Vardiman JW, eds. *World Health Organization Classification of Tumours: Pathology and Genetics of Tumours of Haematopoietic and Lymphoid Tissues*. Lyon, France: IARC Press; 2001:127–130.

11 Hallek M, Cheson BD, Catovsky D, et al. Guidelines for the diagnosis and treatment of chronic lymphocytic leukemia: a report from the International Workshop on Chronic Lymphocytic Leukemia updating the National Cancer Institute–Working Group 1996 guidelines. *Blood*. 2008;**111**:5446–5456.

18 Rawstron AC, Bennett FL, O'Connor SJ, et al. Monoclonal B-cell lymphocytosis and chronic lymphocytic leukemia. *N Engl J Med*. 2008;**359**:575–583.

31 Apostolia-Maria T, Sijin W, Peter M, et al. Other malignancies in chronic lymphocytic leukemia/small lymphocytic lymphoma. *J Clin Oncol*. 2008. doi: JCO.2008.17.5398.

34 Rai KR, Sawitsky A, Cronkite EP, et al. Clinical staging of chronic lymphocytic leukemia. *Blood*. 1975;**46**:219-234.

38 Binet JL, Auquier A, Dighiero G, et al. A new prognostic classification of chronic lymphocytic leukemia derived from a multivariate survival analysis. *Cancer*. 1981;**48**:198-206.

40 Rai KR, Peterson BL, Appelbaum FR, et al. Fludarabine compared with chlorambucil as primary therapy for chronic lymphocytic leukemia. *N Engl J Med*. 2000;**343**:1750-1757.

41 Keating MJ, O'Brien S, Albitar M, et al. Early results of a chemoimmunotherapy regimen of fludarabine, cyclophosphamide, and rituximab as initial therapy for chronic lymphocytic leukemia. *J Clin Oncol*. 2005;**23**:4079-4088.

42 Hallek M, Fischer K, Fingerle-Rowson G, et al. Addition of rituximab to fludarabine and cyclophosphamide in patients with chronic lymphocytic leukaemia: a randomised, open-label, phase 3 trial. *Lancet*. 2010;**376(9747)**:1164-1174.

44 Wang L, Lawrence MS, Wan Y, et al. SF3B1 and other novel cancer genes in chronic lymphocytic leukemia. *N Engl J Med*. 2011;**365**:2497-2506.

46 Damle RN, Wasil T, Fais F, et al. Immunoglobulin V gene mutation status and CD38 expression as novel prognostic indicators in chronic lymphocytic leukemia. *Blood*. 1999;**94**:1840-1847.

47 Hamblin TJ, Davis Z, Gardiner A, et al. Unmutated IgVH genes are associated with a more aggressive form of chronic lymphocytic leukemia. *Blood*. 1999;**94**:1848-1854.

52 Döhner H, Stilgenbauer S, Benner A, et al. Genomic aberrations and survival in chronic lymphocytic leukemia. *N Engl J Med*. 2000;**343**:1910-1916.

58 Rassenti LZ, Huynh L, Toy TZ, et al. ZAP-70 compared with immunoglobulin heavy-chain gene mutation status as a predictor of disease progression in CLL. *N Engl J Med*. 2004;**351**:893-901.

60 Gonzalez D, Martinez P, Wade R, et al. Mutational status of the TP53 gene as a predictor of response and survival in patients with chronic lymphocytic leukemia: results from the LRF CLL4 trial. *J Clin Oncol*. 2011;**29**:2223-2229.

62 Rossi D, Rasi S, Spina V, et al. Integrated mutational and cytogenetic analysis identifies new prognostic subgroups in chronic lymphocytic leukemia. *Blood*. 2013;**121**:1403-1412.

63 Pflug N, Bahlo J, Shanafelt TD, et al. Development of a comprehensive prognostic index for patients with chronic lymphocytic leukemia. *Blood*. 2014;**124(1)**:49-62.

65 Böttcher S, Ritgen M, Fischer K, et al. Minimal residual disease quantification is an independent predictor of progression-free and overall survival in chronic lymphocytic leukemia: a multivariate analysis from the randomized GCLLSG CLL8 trial. *J Clin Oncol*. 2012;**30(9)**:980-988.

66 Cheson BD, Byrd JC, Rai KR, et al. Novel targeted agents and the need to refine clinical end points in chronic lymphocytic leukemia. *J Clin Oncol*. 2012;**30(23)**:2820-2822.

74 Fischer K, Cramer P, Busch R, et al. Bendamustine in combination with rituximab for previously untreated patients with chronic lymphocytic leukemia: a multicenter phase II trial of the German Chronic Lymphocytic Leukemia Study Group. *J Clin Oncol*. 2012;**30**:3209-3216.

75 Fischer K, Cramer P, Busch R, et al. Bendamustine combined with rituximab in patients with relapsed and/or refractory chronic lymphocytic leukemia: a multicenter phase II trial of the German Chronic Lymphocytic Leukemia Study Group. *J Clin Oncol*. 2011;**29**:3559-3566.

76 Eichhorst B, Fink AM, Busch R, et al. Frontline chemoimmunotherapy with fludarabine (F), cyclophosphamide (C), and rituximab (R) (FCR) shows superior efficacy in comparison to bendamustine (B) and rituximab (BR) in previously untreated and physically fit patients (pts) with advanced chronic lymphocytic leukemia (CLL): final analysis of an international, randomized study of the German CLL Study Group (GCLLSG) (CLL10 study). *Blood*. 2014;**124(21)**:19.

78 Wierda WG, Padmanabhan S, Chan GW, Gupta IV, Lisby S, Österborg A. Hx-CD20-406 Study Investigators. Ofatumumab is active in patients with fludarabine-refractory CLL irrespective of prior rituximab: results from the phase 2 international study. *Blood*. 2011;**118**:5126-5129.

80 Goede V, Fischer K, Busch R, et al. Obinutuzumab plus chlorambucil in patients with CLL and coexisting conditions. *N Engl J Med*. 2014;**370**:1101-1110.

81 Byrd JC, Furman RR, Coutre SE, et al. Targeting BTK with ibrutinib in relapsed chronic lymphocytic leukemia. *N Engl J Med*. 2013;**369**:32-42.

82 O'Brien SM, Furman RR, Coutre SE, et al. Independent evaluation of ibrutinib efficacy 3 years post-initiation of monotherapy in patients with chronic lymphocytic leukemia/small lymphocytic leukemia including deletion 17p disease. *J Clin Oncol*. 2014 (suppl; abstr 7014);**32**:5s.

83 Byrd JC, Brown JR, O'Brien S, et al. Ibrutinib versus ofatumumab in previously treated chronic lymphoid leukemia. *N Engl J Med*. 2014;**371**:213-223.

84 O'Brien S, Jones JA, Coutre S. Efficacy and safety of ibrutinib in patients with relapsed or refractory chronic lymphocytic leukemia or small lymphocytic leukemia with 17p deletion: results from the phase II RESONATE™-17 trial. *Blood*. 2014;**124**:327.

85 Furman RR, Sharman JP, Coutre SE, et al. Idelalisib and rituximab in relapsed chronic lymphocytic leukemia. *N Engl J Med*. 2014;**370**:997-1007.

88 O'Brien S, Lamanna N, Kipps TJ. Update on a phase 2 study of idelalisib in combination with rituximab in treatment-naïve patients ≥65 years with chronic lymphocytic leukemia (CLL) or small lymphocytic lymphoma (SLL). *Blood*. 2014;**124(21)**:1994.

89 Esteve J, Villamor N, Colomer D, et al. Stem cell transplantation for chronic lymphocytic leukemia: different outcome after autologous and allogeneic transplantation and correlation with minimal residual disease status. *Leukemia*. 2001;**15**:445-451.

90 O'Brien S, Furman RR, Coutre SE, et al. Ibrutinib as initial therapy for elderly patients with chronic lymphocytic leukaemia or small lymphocytic lymphoma: an open-label, multicentre, phase 1b/2 trial. *Lancet Oncol*. 2014;**15(1)**:48-58.

91 Farooqui MZ, Valdez J, Martyr S, et al. Ibrutinib for previously untreated and relapsed or refractory chronic lymphocytic leukaemia with TP53 aberrations: a phase 2, single-arm trial. *Lancet Oncol*. 2015;**16(2)**:169-176.

第118章　霍奇金淋巴瘤

Carol S. Portlock, MD ■ Anita Kumar, MD ■ James Armitage, MD

概述

本章将回顾过去几十年中在放疗和化疗领域使霍奇金淋巴瘤(HL)成为可治愈性疾病的具有里程碑意义的进展。我们将介绍HL典型特征和新的流行病学,生物学,病理特点。重点介绍HL在分期、影像检查和先进的治疗方法,这一章将着重介绍当前对HL日常管理方法,例如:精准的危险分层,PET影像检查的应用和如何缩小放疗野和降低放疗剂量,寻找治疗的长期毒性有限而又具有良好治愈率的药物。最后作者还介绍了发展新的生物靶向治疗是如何改进复发耐药HL的治疗现状的。

引言

经典的霍奇金淋巴瘤(cHL)至少有80%的患者是潜在可以治愈的。这与有明确的诊断标准,预后因素,影像学检查的改进,尤其是先系统治疗和后续选择限制性治疗野的巩固放疗相关。

对于生存期内提高治愈率/生活质量需求的增加已经成为尽可能在不损害治愈率的情况下减少初始治疗强度的重要目标。化疗和放疗剂量/放疗野的改变也导致长期毒性比如不孕,心肺毒性和继发恶性肿瘤的减少。

历史

1832年Thomas霍奇金向伦敦的医学外科学会提交了一篇具有历史意义的论文[1],题为"外分泌腺和脾脏的一些病态表现",文中描述了他在伦敦Guy医院对一些患者的研究,包括临床病史和尸检所见的巨大的淋巴结和脾脏明显肿大[1]。霍奇金意识到这些患者罹患了一种起源于颈部、胸部和腹部大血管周围淋巴结的疾病。Samuel Wilks和后来的W. S. Greenfield描述了这些淋巴结的微观特征。Carl Sternberg和Dorothy在1898年和1902年对霍奇金淋巴瘤首次进行了详细的微观描述[2,3]。19世纪末Roentgen发现X线后、Becquerel发现放射活性以及Curies夫妇发现镭后不久,1901年即开始了天然射线早期治疗霍奇金淋巴瘤。之前的血清及其他生物制剂、砷、碘及外科手术治疗对霍奇金淋巴瘤都无效。因此第一个关于X线治疗可使肿大的淋巴结明显缩小的报道曾令人兴奋一时甚至预言霍奇金淋巴瘤可以治愈[4,5]。

现代放疗技术始于20世纪20年代Gilbert的研究。Gilbert是第一个提出科预测霍奇金淋巴瘤特定临床模式的医生之一。Gilbert提倡除了治疗受累的淋巴结外,对于没有明显受累但存在可疑显微镜下病灶的邻近受累的淋巴结也需要治疗[6]。

在1950年,Vera Peters进一步扩展了这种方法,报告了用这种方法治疗1期患者5年和10年的生存率分别为88%和79%[7]。然而应用RT可以治愈早期霍奇金淋巴瘤的观点没有很快被接受。Henry Kaplan研制出直线加速器并且成功用这种方法治cHL。他确定了放疗范围和剂量,改进了诊断分期的方法,开发将实验室成果转化为临床实践的模型,在美国他和Saul Rosenberg推进了早期的随机对照临床研究[8~10]。

在联合化疗出现之前,晚期cHL一直是致命的肿瘤。在20世纪40年代,发现氮芥是有效的药物,20世纪60年代中期Vincent DeVita及其团队首先用MOPP方案,一种有效的四药方案(氮芥、长春新碱、丙卡巴肼和泼尼松)治疗患者[11]。MOPP方案有较高的完全缓解率和显著延长生存,使cHL成为可以治愈的疾病[12]。

像放射治疗一样,随机对照研究也在联合化疗的发展中发挥关键作用。研究显示维持化疗并没有获益,明确相对短的化疗疗程就能治愈淋巴瘤,最后显示ABVD方案(多柔比星、博来霉素、长春新碱和达卡巴嗪)能够降低毒性,同时与MOPP方案(或者含有MOPP的方案)疗效相当,因此确认了ABVD作为标准治疗方案[13,14]。

流行病学和病因学

2014年,美国预计有9 190例新发cHL病例。cHL的发病率是每年2.7/10万,在20年间发病率保持稳定。在美国,新发病例的中位发病年龄是39岁,31%的患者年龄在20~34岁之间。男性略多于女性(3.1/10万~2.4/10万)[15],尽管以前在经济发达国家cHL的发病呈现双峰分布,第二峰不明显但持续,发现这些病例是更好病理类型的非霍奇金淋巴瘤。

霍奇金淋巴瘤的病因仍然不清楚。流行病学数据提示感染和遗传改变是两个主要因素[16,17]。病毒病因学提示在年轻患者中的霍奇金淋巴瘤患者与儿童时期在经济发达国家增加产妇教育,兄弟姊妹和玩伴少,兄弟姊妹中排行靠前,居住在独家住宅这些因素暴露减少相关[18,19]。这种相关性也使研究者提出,霍奇金淋巴瘤似乎类似一种病毒性疾病,是年龄相关的宿主对感染的应答(如在脊髓灰质炎和传染性单核细胞增多症中见到的),支持这一理论的依据是,经济发达国家10岁以下的儿童中霍奇金淋巴瘤罕有发生。

EB病毒(Epstein-Barr virus,EBV)是霍奇金淋巴瘤中首要的疑似病原[16,20,21]。EBV是非洲Burkitt淋巴瘤的病原体,且文献记载在免疫缺陷疾病和器官移植后的患者中发现了EBV相关淋巴瘤。既往有单核细胞增多症的患者,cHL的发病率增加2~3倍。另外,后来发展为cHL的患者对EBV抗原应答模式发生了改变。

最近细胞和分子生物学数据为EBV和cHL的相关性提供

了额外的证据支持。通过使用灵敏的分子探针，30%～50%的霍奇金淋巴瘤的标本发现在诊断性 Reed-Sternberg（R-S）细胞中含有 *EBV* 的基因组片段[22]。在研究中发现，初次活检和复发时 *EBV* 基因组状态保持稳定。*EBV* 基因组阳性的里-施细胞代表所谓的Ⅱ型潜伏谱，即表达潜伏感染膜蛋白（LMP）-1，LMP-2a，EBNA-1 和 EBV 编码核糖核酸（EBER）。LMP-1 在转录中发挥至关重要的作用，在转染研究中发现 LMP-1 发挥致癌基因的作用，而 EBNA-1 在游离病毒基因组复制中是必需的。

在一些研究中发现同卵双生子间，父母-子女间，这些一级亲属中存在遗传易感性，发病率明显增加，而配偶间并非如此。另外，cHL 与特定的人类白细胞抗原（HLA）相关，而 HLA 和 EBV 感染相关；基因组相关性研究已经鉴别出 non-HLA 易感性基因，但还没有证实[17]。

患者的免疫异常

cHL 以治疗前即存在的细胞免疫功能缺陷和 T 细胞介导的免疫应答功能缺陷为特征。这些缺陷在已治愈的患者中持续存在[23]，包括迟发性皮肤超敏损害，T 细胞丝裂原刺激所致的增殖反应受抑，免疫球蛋白生成增强，和自然杀伤细胞的细胞毒性作用降低。这些免疫异常提示是由于细胞因子的慢性过度刺激导致的继发性免疫抑制。在活动性 cHL 患者中，这些发现与里-施细胞释放细胞因子增加一致。然而在已经治愈的患者中持续存在免疫异常的现象却难以解释。

治疗后这种治疗所致的免疫抑制逐渐恢复正常，但似乎在治疗后的头几年内免疫抑制效应最明显[23]。例如发生过多的带状疱疹感染，超过 75%的患者在第 1 年内发生，少数患者在第 3 年后发生（6%）。带状疱疹的风险随治疗强度的增加而增加[24]。

与迟发性超敏反应存在的缺陷不同，多数 cHL 的患者在诊断时 B 细胞的数目和功能相对正常，B 细胞功能会受到治疗的不利影响[23]，因此鼓励患者保持接种疫苗。

病理学

霍奇金淋巴瘤以其组织学上的多样性区别于其他类型的淋巴瘤[25]。受累淋巴结有不同程度的反应性细胞和炎细胞浸润和纤维化，同时存在散在分布的、特征性的恶性肿瘤细胞，即里-施细胞（Reed-Sternberg cell）和单个核肿瘤细胞。典型的里-施细胞有丰富的胞质，2～3 个胞核，每个核都有单个的、明显的核仁，与背景中周围体积较小的细胞形成鲜明对比。单个核肿瘤细胞是其变异型，它具有里-施细胞的胞核和胞质特征，但仅有单个胞核。在没有里-施细胞存在时，通常很少诊断霍奇金淋巴瘤，然而，仅存在这些细胞也不足以做出霍奇金淋巴瘤的诊断。R-S 样的细胞在传染性单核细胞增多症，非霍奇金淋巴瘤和某些癌症和肉瘤中也存在。因此 cHL 的诊断标准包括存在里-施细胞和同时存在包括正常淋巴细胞质细胞，嗜酸性粒细胞的特征性背景。

cHL 的病理分类包括：结节硬化型（NSHL）、混合细胞型（MCHL）、淋巴细胞富集型（LRHL）消减型（LDHL），还有结节性淋巴细胞为主型霍奇金淋巴瘤（NLPHL）。cHL 的亚型不影响临床管理，预后或治疗。然而，不同霍奇金淋巴瘤的组织学亚型在发病部位、自然病程和预后上都表现不同，在 NLPHL 中表现更明显。

霍奇金淋巴瘤的亚型

NSHL 的两个组织学特点有助于与其他的 cHL 亚型进行区分：胶原纤维条索状增生，并把淋巴组织分隔成小结节状；这些结节含有一种变异的里-施细胞，称为陷窝细胞。在甲醛溶液固定的组织中，细胞丰富的胞质经甲醛溶液固定液处理后胞质收缩形成空白的胞质，造成细胞位于陷窝中的假象（图 118-1～图 118-3）。分子谱研究显示 NSHL 与原发纵隔大 B 细胞淋巴瘤密切相关。NSHL 是罕见的存在灰色区域的肿瘤，它兼具着两种肿瘤的特点[26～28]。

结节硬化型病变是唯一的一种男女发生率大致相当的霍奇金淋巴瘤类型，好发于青少年和青壮年，在 50 岁后不常见。显著倾向累及下颈部、锁骨上和纵隔淋巴结，通常按顺序播散[29]。在发达国家占 cHL 的 60%～70%，而在发展中国家通常少见。

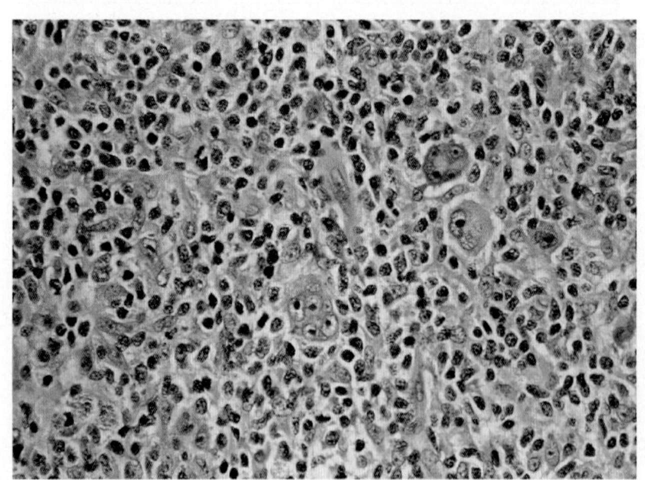

图 118-1　结节硬化型霍奇金淋巴瘤里-施细胞和变体，大的多核或者多分叶的细胞，少数具有大核仁的单核细胞可与细胞成分明显区分

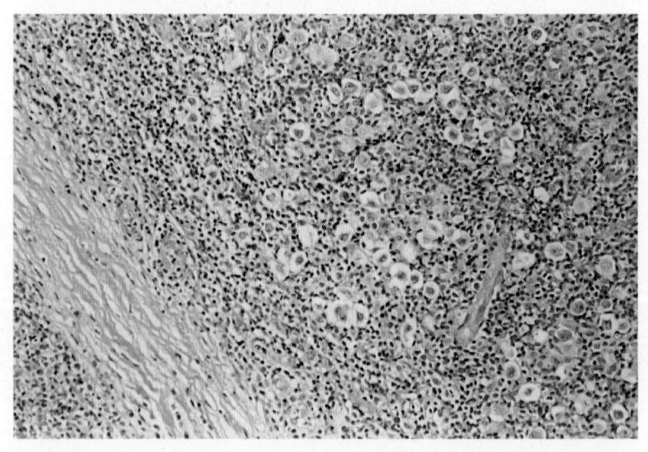

图 118-2　霍奇金病，结节硬化。在这个视野的左下方有一个纤维条索，肿瘤腔隙细胞有丰富的清晰的细胞质，与周围的淋巴细胞明显区分开来

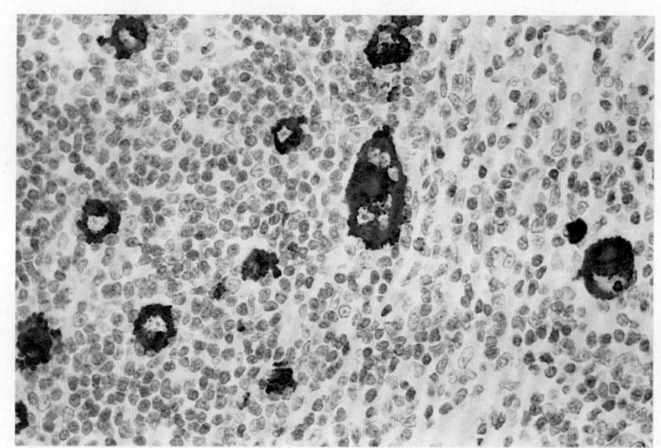

图 118-3　在霍奇金病结节硬化型中 CD15 的免疫标记。肿瘤里-施细胞和单核霍奇金细胞呈现免疫反应阳性

MCHL 在高倍镜下表现为炎症性背景中含有丰富的正常细胞,还有 5~15 个里-施细胞和变体(图 118-4 和图 118-5)。患者一般年龄较大,常存在 B 症状,患者常常存在腹部受累或者为晚期疾病。在美国大约 25%的 cHL 是 MCHL,在不发达国家这种类型更为常见。MCHL 可能与周围 T 细胞淋巴瘤混淆,PAX5 抗原作为一种 B 细胞标志物在鉴别上可能尤其有帮助。

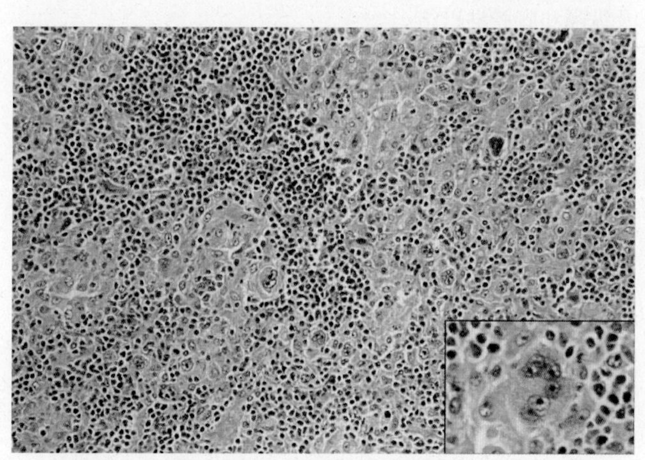

图 118-4　霍奇金病,混合细胞型。里-施细胞存在于背景中富含组织细胞中。插图:高倍镜下多核里-施细胞

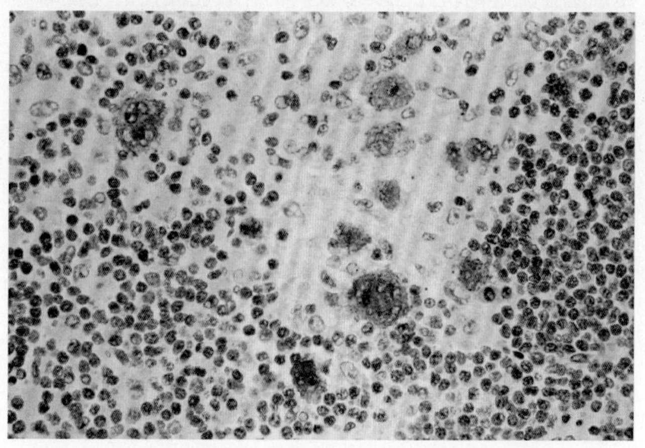

图 118-5　霍奇金病,混合细胞型膜蛋白 EB 病毒免疫标记(与图 118-4 相同的标本)

LRHL 代表了另外一种组织学亚型,可能是结节状的或者弥散的,里-施细胞相对少见(图 118-6 和图 118-7),通常以成熟的小淋巴细胞为主。嗜酸性粒细胞和中性粒细胞通常仅存在于血管内。

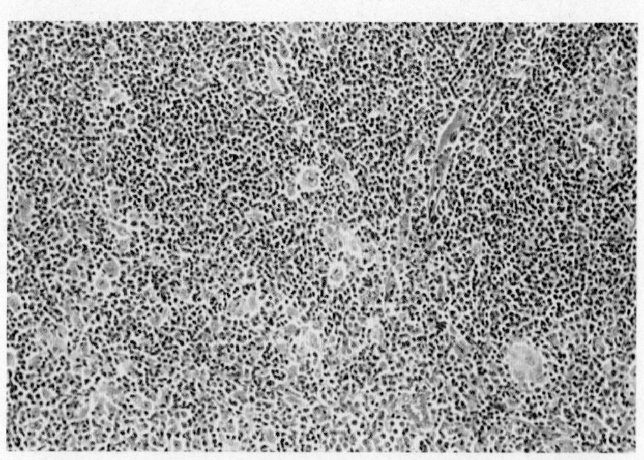

图 118-6　经典霍奇金病淋巴细胞富集型。在增殖的小淋巴细胞和组织细胞的背景中里-施细胞和单核霍奇金细胞罕见

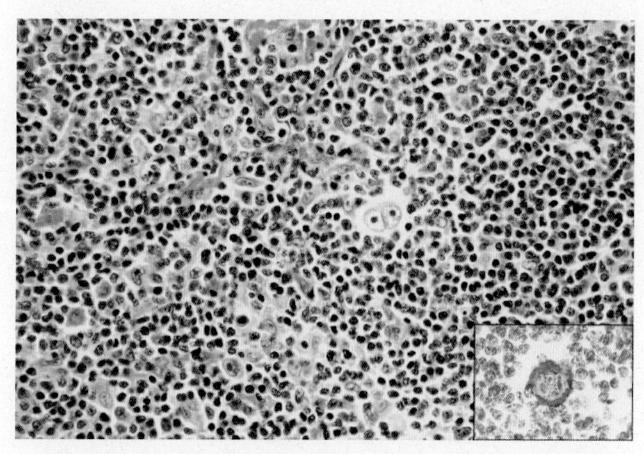

图 118-7　经典霍奇金病淋巴细胞富集型。在中央视野中见到双核里-施细胞,里-施细胞 CD15 免疫染色是阳性的

LDHL 已经很少被诊断,在经济发达国家所占比例不足霍奇金淋巴瘤的 1%。通常为晚期患者,存在 B 型症状。里-施细胞和多形性变异细胞常见,多数患者只有稀疏的正常淋巴细胞。

在 NLPHL 亚型中,尽管残留某些正常的结节结构,淋巴结结构已经消失,见不到诊断性的里-施细胞,但是变异淋巴细胞(LP 细胞)是非常典型的(图 118-8 和图 118-9)。这些细胞通常多数有分叶状核,由于形态上与爆米花相似,故称为"爆米花细胞"。纤维化不常见。LP 或者"爆米花"样 R-S 变体细胞存在于多克隆 B 淋巴细胞的背景中(图 118-9)[30,31]。通常 LP 细胞代表 B 细胞的标志物 CD20 是阳性的,但 cHL 的标志物 CD15 和 CD30 是阴性的(图 118-10 和图 118-11)[31,32]。在 NLPHL 中很少检测到 EBV[33]。生发中心进行性转化这种良性的异常改变通与 NLPHL 相关。这种病变中

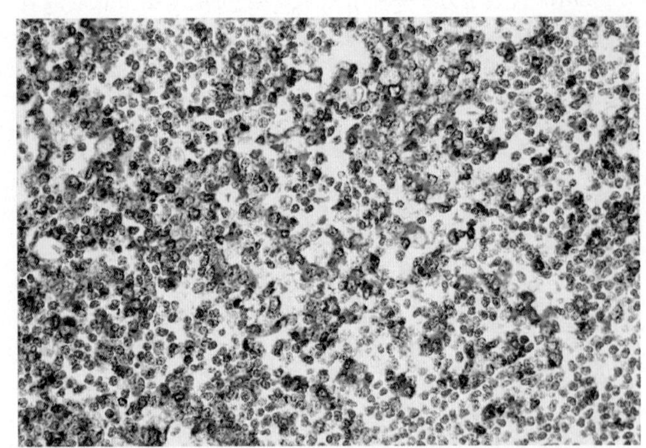

图 118-8 淋巴细胞为主型霍奇金淋巴瘤(图 118-9~图 118-11 是同一个标本)CD57 染色阳性提示免疫反应细胞显著增加,存在非免疫反应细胞的周围

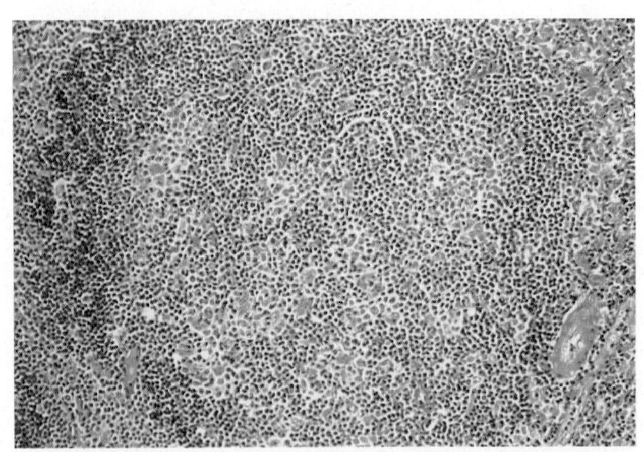

图 118-9 淋巴细胞为主型霍奇金淋巴瘤。淋巴结的结构隐约可见

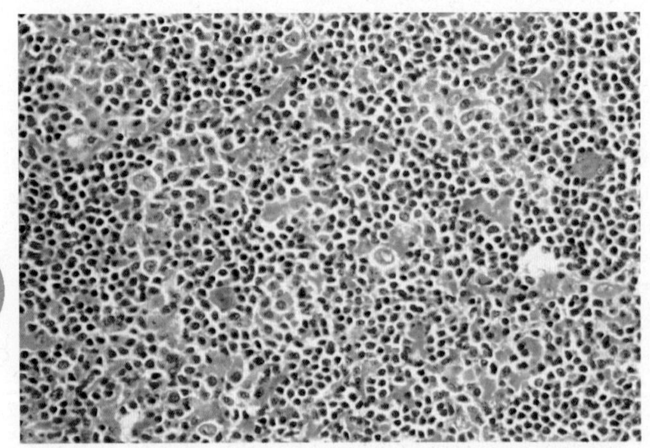

图 118-10 高倍镜视野下的淋巴细胞为主型霍奇金淋巴瘤(与图 118-9 为同一标本)。在淋巴细胞和组织细胞的背景下分散存在一些大的具有染色质、核仁相对较小的,稀疏的细胞质的分裂细胞,也称为 L 或 H 细胞

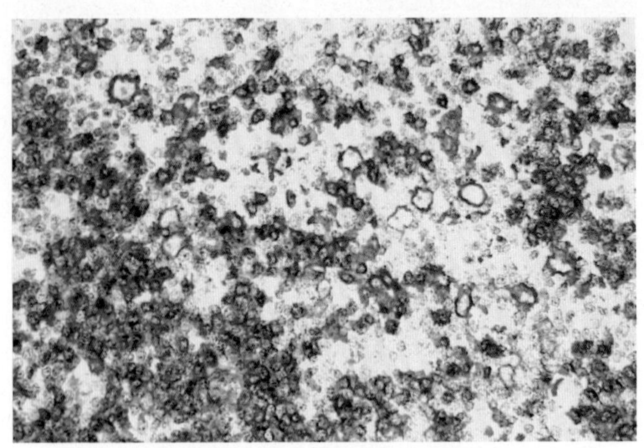

图 118-11 淋巴细胞为主型霍奇金淋巴瘤(与图 118-9 和图 118-10 为同一标本)CD20 染色阳性的 L 或 H 细胞还有淋巴结内高比例的淋巴细胞

没有里-施细胞和 LP 变体。生发中心进行性转化可以与 NLPH 存在于同一个病灶或者邻近的结节[32]。在美国,NLPH 占所有 HL 的 5%~10%。这种病变局限于一组周围淋巴结(上颈部、下颌部、肘部、腹股沟及腋窝淋巴结),很少累及纵隔和腹腔淋巴结。

免疫表型和生物学特征

里-施细胞是 B 淋巴细胞来源的[25]。这些细胞可表达静息的或者活化的淋巴细细胞抗原,通常是 B 细胞抗原:PAX5 通常是阳性的,CD20 或 CD79a 很少阳性,T 细胞表面抗原(CD3,CD4,和 CD8)阳性罕见。NLPHL 亚型中的 LP 细胞一致性表达 B 细胞抗原。在 cHL,CD30 和 CD15 表面抗原存在于多数的里-施细胞,几乎所有的病例 CD30 都是阳性的,大约 80%的患者 CD15 是阳性的,而 CD45(白细胞常见抗原)通常是阴性的。相反,NLPHL 中的 LP 细胞 CD15 和 CD30 是阴性的,CD45 是阳性的[33]。

尽管这些细胞免疫球蛋白基因表达异常缺少,单个里-施细胞显微解剖研究证实多数病例存在克隆性的免疫球电白基因重排,证实了细胞的克隆形成和 B 细胞组系的建立[34,35]。而且里-施细胞拥有体细胞 *V* 基因突变,提示是生发中心或后生发中心起源。突变的模式也许可以解释缺乏免疫球蛋白表达。另一可能的解释包括肿瘤基因转录的表观遗传学沉默或者 Notch1 和 STAT5 的组成型表达[25]。正常生发中心的 B 细胞缺少功能性的免疫球蛋白受体,通过凋亡机制从生发中心清除。因此里-施细胞对通常的凋亡机制表现为耐药。FAS/CD95 介导的凋亡途径被 c-FLIP(里-施细胞组成型表达)抑制[36]。目前有几种假设解释这种现象,包括 NF-κB 途径的活化,普遍的家族性乱交,EBV 感染。来自霍奇金淋巴瘤的细胞系都始终表达 NF-κB,这支持 NF-κB 在霍奇金细胞存活和生长过程中的作用。在 HL 衍生的细胞系中观察到 NF-κB 途径的组成型表达的证据,在联合免疫缺陷鼠模型和细胞系中，发现 NF-κB 的抑制影响肿瘤的生长[37]，表观遗传学研究也显示规律应用阿司匹林与减少 HL 发生相关，可能是与抑制 NF-κB 的转录有关[38]，NF-κB 组成型活化也与诱导 *REL* 基因扩增，NF-κB 抑制性突变和体细胞 *TNFA1P3* 突变有关[25]，在 EBV 感染相关的病例，LMP-2a 表达可以替代 B 细胞受体的功能。

LP 细胞显微微切割研究也证实存在克隆性免疫球蛋白基因的重排，再次确认了单克隆和 B 细胞祖系[34]。另外也证明 *V* 基因体细胞突变，克隆内测序的多样性也可以检测到，这些提供了 NLPHL 是生发中心起源的证据。cHL 与之相反，这些突变与功能抗原受体相容。

细胞遗传学异常在里-施细胞非常常见。然而，没有一致的描述。罕见的 t(14∶18)易位通常在滤泡 B 细胞淋巴瘤可以检测到。比较基因组杂交研究也证实在染色体 2p 上 *NF-κB*、*REL* 和 *BCL11a* 基因所在位点，9p(*JAK2* 位点)和 12q(MDM2 位点)的反复获得和 4p16、4q23～q24、9p23～p24(与 PD-L1 蛋白高表达相关)区域的获得。在大多数 cHL 利用全基因组扫描技术已经证实了这种反复的失衡[39]。

肿瘤微环境在 HL 的发病机制、相关的表现及预后中起着重要作用[40,41]。据推测，细胞因子与 cHL 存在显著的炎症成分、纤维化、多种组织学类型以及与发热，体重减轻，盗汗的临床症状有关[42～44]。许多病例与肿瘤坏死因子受体(TNFR)和配体家族成员，Th2 和少量的 Th1 细胞因子，以及其他趋化因子上调有关。坏死因子受体(NFR)成员可导致 NF-κB 组成型活化，NF-κB 是 B 淋巴细胞增殖和存活的重要因子。优先表达 Th2 细胞因子和趋化因子可以解释嗜酸性粒细胞和成纤维细胞的频繁存在，还有细胞免疫的局部抑制。EBV 可能有助于细胞因子的产生，例如，由 LMP-1-诱导的 NF-κB 激活和刺激白介素(IL)-10 的产生，IL-10 是一种有效的细胞免疫抑制剂。在一些病例中，特殊的细胞因子可能与特殊的组织学特点相关。例如，转化生长因子(TGF)，已知能刺激纤维增殖和胶原形成，与 NSHL 相关[45]，和 TARC(CCL27)是一种霍奇金淋巴瘤细胞分泌的淋巴细胞诱导 CC 趋化因子，与 CD4+T 细胞浸润有关[46]。组织嗜酸性粒细胞增多症可能是由于 IL-5、IL-9、CCL11 和 CCL28 的表达，IL-13 可能在里-施细胞自分泌中发挥作用[47]。

分期

大多数 cHL 都有淋巴结受累的核心模式(颈部、纵隔和主动脉旁)，其中>80%的最初出现在膈肌上方，相反，某些淋巴结受累(肠系膜、胃下、骶前、表核和腘窝)少见。脾脏受累与膈下淋巴结病变和系统症状有关，孤立的肝脏病变少见，骨和骨髓受累通常是局限的。最近 Lugano 分类更新了分期，Lugano 分类合并了原来的 Ann Arbor 分期和后来的 Cotswolds 修订(表 118-1)[48] PET 影像现在被认为是鉴别所有 cHL 受累部位的最准确方法，不再推荐常规骨髓活检，治疗前评价见表 118-2。

表 118-1　Lugano 分期 48

Ⅰ期	侵犯单个淋巴结或者一组邻近的淋巴结区
	ⅠE 期：侵犯单个结外部位
	扁桃体、韦氏环和脾脏被认为是淋巴组织
Ⅱ期	侵及横膈同侧两个或两个以上的淋巴结区
	ⅡE 期：侵犯Ⅰ期或者Ⅱ期淋巴结，累及横膈同侧有限的结外器官
Ⅲ期	累及横膈两侧淋巴结
Ⅳ期	累及非邻近的结外器官伴有或不伴有淋巴结受累
以下分组适用于各期	
A	无症状
B	发热[体温>38℃(100.4℉)]，盗汗，诊断前 6 个月内无法解释的体重减轻超过平时体重的 10%
X	巨块(CT 测量单个淋巴结肿块的最大直径>10cm)

表 118-2　推荐的分期程序

充分的外科活检，并由有经验的血液病理学家阅片(首选手术切除标本；一些病例空心针穿刺也是足够的；针吸活检不能提供充足的标本)
病史需要注明是否存在全身症状
仔细的体格检查，强调淋巴结链、肝脾大小和韦氏环的检查
实验室检查：全血细胞计数和分类、血沉和包括肝功能在内的完整的代谢功能检查；HIV，乙型肝炎和丙型肝炎血清学检查
PET 扫描
如果需要进行放射治疗，选择颈部、胸部、腹部、盆腔的 CT 检查
除非 PET 扫描可疑不推荐进展骨髓活检，活检的结果将改变治疗
含多柔比星方案的需要评估射血分数
含博来霉素方案需要进行肺功能评估
咨询：生育保护

经典霍奇金淋巴瘤的治疗原则

cHL 初始治疗是由分期和临床预后分类决定的，总的来说，分为有独特治疗的三组：早期，预后良好；早期，预后不良和晚期。

放疗

早年，仅使用放疗进行治疗，而且应用的是大剂量/大照射野，随后放疗的范围被显著缩小。几项随机对照研究证实，联合治疗模式(CMT，化疗+放疗)受累野放疗与扩大野放疗对疾病的控制是等同的，对生存的影响是相似的[49,50]。巩固放疗限于最初累及的范围,放疗剂量也减少[51]。这样的降低剂量和放疗范围的治疗预期可减轻放疗的延迟影响[52]。目前,放射野包括受累的淋巴结,INRT(化疗前病变体积小,需要良好的化疗前成像),或者受累区域,ISRT(最初累及的组织体积,但需要更多的临床判断来规划边界,由于治疗前的影像是次优的)。许多组织采用ISRT作为cHL的标准放疗野[53]。INRT和ISRT比受累野放疗明显要小。

化疗

联合化疗的引入促使放疗剂量和放射野的减少,目前化疗是cHL治疗的基石。之前与不孕和继发性白血病相关的有毒的化疗方案MOPP已经被等效的,低毒的方案ABVD所取替[13]。ABVD方案是美国的标准治疗方案。已经研发了许多方案进一步改善疗效。剂量密集的改良的BEACOPP(博来霉素、依托泊苷、多柔比星、环磷酰胺、长春新碱、丙卡巴肼和泼尼松)能够改善FFTF,但是却增加了急性和慢性毒性,而且没有生存获益[54~56]。

风险适应性中期PET评估

为了改善预后降低毒性,中期FDG-PET(PET)扫描经常用来评估应答,PET是在完成治疗之前进行的,通常是第二和第四个周期化疗后进行。2周期ABVD治疗后,中期PET检查预测治疗应答和临床结果[57~59],由此引出了"应答适应疗法"的概念,因此,治疗强度可能随着良好的早期反应而降低,如果早期反应不足则可升高[60]。

cHL的PET应答标准采用"五点量表"(PFS)或Deauville标准:基线和中期PET扫描是根据初始淋巴瘤部位的摄取情况进行评分的:①无摄取;②摄取=纵隔血池;③摄取=肝脏;④摄取>肝脏中度增加;或⑤摄取显著增加>肝脏及/或新病变[61]。1~3分通常被解释为没有淋巴瘤,而4或5分为被认为阳性。在临床试验中,阴性被严格的定义为1~2分,中期PET阴性的患者治疗随后被减少。

早期cHL

早期患者被定义为有利的风险组和不利的风险组[62~65]。通常不利的特征包括:巨大的纵隔肿块,B组症状,ESR升高,累及多组淋巴结。巨大肿块有多种定义:>1/3纵隔肿块比(MMR,肿块的最大径除以最大胸腔直径),>纵隔胸廓比值的1/3(MTR,肿块的最大直径除以T5~T6水平胸腔直径)或者任何超过10cm的肿块。三个风险系统对早期cHL进行4个周期ABVD+IFRT进行了回顾性分析,其主要特征是肿瘤负荷(巨大的肿块或者较多的肿瘤数目)[66]。

预后良好患者

早期预后良好的cHL的许多研究在不损害治疗的前提下减少迟发作用。GHSG HD10研究纳入1 131例没有危险因素的ⅠA~ⅡB期患者[67]。随机分为4个治疗组:ABVD×2周期+30Gy IFRT;ABVD×2周期+20Gy IFRT;ABVD×4周期+30Gy IFRT;ABVD×4周期+20Gy IFRT。ABVD治疗2周期组5年的无治疗失败率(FFTF)分别为91.1%和93%,与之相似的是两种放疗方案20Gy和30Gy治疗组的FFTF分别为92.9%和93.4%,也没有差异。不良反应和急性毒性在ABVD×4周期+30Gy IFRT治疗组更为常见。对于预后良好的早期患者作者推荐ABVD×2周期+20Gy IFRT。

在选择性的早期cHL患者去除放疗作为一种新的治疗标准正在兴起。在2004年,MSKCC报告了一项纳入152例没有大肿块的Ⅰ、ⅡAⅡB、ⅢA期的cHL患者,随机接受6周期ABVD+RT或者单独6周期ABVD治疗[68]。ABVD+RT和ABVD治疗组在5年的FFS分别为86% vs 81%($P=0.61$)和5年的OS率分别为97% vs 90%($P=0.08$)。NCIC和ECOG HD.6选择ⅠA或ⅡA没有大肿块的cHL随机接受ABVD单独治疗或者ABVD+次全淋巴结放疗(sTLI)[69]。在RT组预后因素好的患者仅接受sTLI,然而有不良预后因素的患者(年龄≥39岁,ESR≥50mm/h,混合细胞型或者淋巴细胞消减型,≥4个病灶)接受2周期的ABVD治疗联合sTLI。只接受4~6个周期ABVD治疗的患者是根据中期CT评估确定。ABVD组12年的OS率显著获益为94%,ABVD+sTLI组12年OS率为87%($P=0.04$),CMT组有过多的继发恶性肿瘤。考虑到sTLI已经过时,这项研究一直受到批评,然而这项研究也证实ABVD单独治疗的价值,也强调了对CMT的关注。

通过中期PET评估的ABCD单独治疗也开始进行研究[70,71]。英国的RAPID研究是一项纳入602例没有大肿块的ⅠA或ⅡA期cHL患者随机非劣效研究,纳入的患者包括有不良预后因素和无不良预后因素的患者。所有患者接受3周期ABVD治疗后进行PET影像检查。如果是阴性(Deauville1~2分)的患者,患者不接受进一步治疗或者1周期ABVD+30Gy IFRT;如果PET检查为阳性,所有患者接受1周期ABVD+30Gy IFRT治疗。中位随访60个月,CMT和仅接受3周期化疗的患者3年的PFS率分别为94.6%和90.8%,绝对风险相差3.8%。EORTC/LYSA/FIL H10研究是一项随机非劣效研究,纳入有不良预后因素和无不良预后因素的早期cHL患者采用ABVD方案治疗,2周期后PET评估,经过事先计划的中期无用性分析,得出结论,与CMT相比,单纯化疗组应该终止,而ABVD组1年的PFS率也是极好的,大约为95%,也提出是否过早得出结论这样的问题。正在进行的PET适应性研究的长期结果将进一步阐释是否单独ABVD是对选择性的早期的cHL患者有效的治疗策略。

有不良预后因素的患者

对于早期有不良预后因素的cHL标准的治疗选择为联合治疗,5年的PFS率是80%~85%[50,72]。一些有巨大肿块的有不良预后因素的患者,早~中期PET评估为阴性也有较好的预后,这些患者也是单纯化疗的候选人群[70]。有巨大肿块的患者增加放疗是尤其重要的,忽略放疗的PET适应性研究通常将这些患者排除在外[73]。

在早期,有不良预后因素的cHL中几项随机对照研究已经评价了联合治疗的剂量和顺序[50,72,74~76]。GHSG HD11研究在1 570例患者中评估了CMT方案:4ABVD+20GyIFRT,4ABVD+30GyIFRT,4BEACOPP+20GyIFRT,vs 4BEACOPP+30GyIFRT。在这项研究中ⅡB期患者被认为是晚期患者而排除在外,5年的FFTF率分别为:81%(4ABVD+20Gy),85%(4ABVD+30Gy),87%(4BEA-COPP+20Gy),和87%(4BEACOPP+30Gy)[72]。当

联合 20Gy IFRT,结果倾向于 BEACOPP,然而联合 30Gy 时,ABVD+RT 具有较低的毒性。作者推荐 4ABVD+30GyIFRT 是早期有不良预后因素 cHL 患者的治疗选择。

GHSGHD14 研究比较了 4 周期 ABVD+30GyIFRT vs 2 周期改良 BEACOPP+2 周期 ABVD(2+2)+30GyIFRT[76]。“2+2”组的 5 年 FFTF 率是 94.8%,4ABVD+IFRT 组为 87.7%($P=<0.001$),然而在“2+2”组急性毒性显著增加。在中位随访 43 个月时,治疗相关的死亡和继发恶性肿瘤没有显著不同。

组间试验 E2496 比较了 6~8ABVD+36GyIFRT 和 Stanford V[77]。对于有巨大肿块(巨大肿块的定义为 MMR≥1/3 胸部 X 线片或者在 CT 上≥10cm)的Ⅰ或Ⅱ期患者,ABVD+IFRT 和 Stanford V 治疗 5 年的 FFS 率分别为 85%和 79%($HR=0.68$;95%CI:0.37~1.25),这两种方法间没有显著的不同。更多的患者接受 Stanford V+IFRT(巨大肿块定义为>5cm),更多的 ABVD 患者接受长疗程化疗[75]。基于这样的结果,ABVD 后巩固放疗仍然是巨大肿块型早期 cHL 的标准治疗。

晚期 cHL

在晚期 cHL 中,国际预后评分(IPS)确定了 7 个独立的、与病程进展和总生存率相关的预后因素:血清白蛋白<4g/dl;血红蛋白<10.5g/dl;男性;Ⅳ期疾病;年龄≥45 岁;白细胞计数≥15 000/mm[3];淋巴细胞计数<600/mm[3]或少于白细胞总数的 8%[78]。最高风险组(≥5 个风险因子)5 年的 FFS 率为 42%,而没有风险因子的患者 5 年的 FFS 率是 80%。分析了 1990 年以前的 IPS 数据,促使了一项新的评估。这项研究包括不列颠哥伦比亚癌症机构(BCCA)数据库中 740 例接受 ABVD 和 ABVD 样方案治疗的患者[79]。发现 IPS 仍然是对预后影响最显著的,但是差异缩小了:>4 个 IPS 风险因素的患者 5 年的 FFS 率为 70%,没有不良预后因素的患者 5 年的 FFS 为 88%,两者 5 年的 OS 率分别为 73%和 98%。这些结果表明,由于使用统一的含有蒽环类药物化疗(ABVD),生长因子的支持,分期更加精准以及更加精准的病理诊断改善了预后。

治疗

晚期 cHL 的标准治疗方案是 6 周期的 ABVD 方案。剂量密集型的化疗方案也被研究。尽管在Ⅱ期研究提示 Stanford V 方案较 ABVD 方案可能有更好的疗效,而在晚期 cHL 患者的组间研究中 FFS 却没有不同:5 年的 FFS 率 ABVD 方案是 74%,Stanford V 方案是 71%[80~82]。而且 Stanford V 组与更高的淋巴细胞减少和神经系统疾病发生相关。

GHSG 改良的 BEACOPP 方案在欧洲广泛应用,但由于过度的毒性和没有明确的生存获益,在美国并没有获得普遍使用。GHSG 的三项Ⅲ期研究 HD9、HD12 和 HD15 已经检验了 BEACOPP 方案[55,56,83]。

在 HD9 研究中,1 196 例患者随机接受:COPP-ABVD;标准剂量的 BEACOPP;高剂量的 BEACOPP[55]。原发灶≥5cm 的患者都接受 8 周期化疗+RT。研究显示 escBEACOPP 比 COPP-ABVD 和标准剂量的 BEACOPP 方案有更好的 5 年(82%、70%和 64%)和 10 年的 FFTF 和 OS(86%、80%和 75%)

escBEACOPP 对于 IPS 评分 4~7 分的患者有更高的临床获益,但是有较高的骨髓抑制,不孕,继发性脊髓发育不良/急性白血病。

HD12 研究比较了 esc BEACOPP 和 4 周期 escBEACOPP+4 周期 BEACOPP(4+4)[83]。患者然后随机接受不进一步治疗和 30Gy RT 的巩固治疗。escBEACOPP 和 4+4,方案 5 年 FFTF 分别为 86.4%和 84.8%,5 年的 OS 率分别为 92%和 90.3%。尽管 OS 没有显著改善,RT 组在 FFTF 方面更具优势。

HD15 研究包括了 2 182 例患者 8 周期 escBEACOPP,6 周期 escBEACOPP,标准剂量、时间密集型 BEACOPP[56]。RT(30Gy)限于 PET 阳性残留病灶的患者(≥2.5cm)。5 年的 FFTF 率分别为 4.4%,89.3%,5 年的 OS 率分别为 91.9%,95.3%,94.5%。作者推荐有更好的结果的,更少的治疗相关死亡率,更少的继发肿瘤的 6 周期的 escBEACOPP 方案治疗。

里-施细胞表达 B 细胞抗原 CD20+的 cHL 亚型患者。Ⅱ期研究报告了用 ABVD 联合利妥昔单抗每周一次共 6 周[84,85]。在一项研究中,5 年的 EFS 和 OS 率分别为 83%和 96%,对于这个组织学亚群似乎很有希望[84]。

风险适应性中期 PET 影像也应用在晚期 cHL。一项来自以色列的Ⅰ期研究提示风险和应答适应治疗可能是有效的。在这项研究中 45 例低危(IPS≥3)患者接受 2 个周期的 escBEACOPP,然后进行 PET 扫描。如果 PET 是阴性的,患者后续接受 4 周期 ABVD 方案治疗。31 例早期-中期 PET 评估获得阴性的患者,4 年 PFS 率是 87%[60]。来自 SWOG S0816 和英国 RATHL 研究的早期结果显示应用中期 PET 评估应答适应性治疗策略也是充满希望的[86]。

复发性、难治性霍奇金淋巴瘤的治疗

复发耐药的 Chl(r/r-cHL)的标准治疗方法是通过挽救性化疗以达到缓解状态,随后给予清髓性化疗和自体干细胞移植(ASCT)。不同的组织已经研究出能够预测 r/r-cHL 完成 ASCT 结局的模型[87~91]。不利的预后因素包括:存在结外疾病,一线治疗后缓解时间短(通常≤1 年;存在 B 症状)。另外一个强的独立的预后因素是移植前的功能影像状态[92,93]。在一项中位随访时间是 51 个月的研究中,移植前 PET 扫描阴性的患者有更好的生存,无事件生存>80%,而 PET 扫描阳性的患者为 29%[92]。

r/rcHL 挽救性治疗的方案包括:ICE(异环磷酰胺,卡铂,依托泊苷)DHAP(地塞米松,高剂量阿糖胞苷和顺铂),ESHAP(依托泊苷、甲泼尼龙、大剂量阿糖胞苷和顺铂),IGEV(异环磷酰胺,吉西他滨和长春瑞滨),GVD(吉西他滨,长春瑞滨和聚乙二醇脂质体多柔比星)[88,94~97]尽管这些方案没有前瞻性的进行疗效比较,但在Ⅱ期研究中有相似的疗效。

由于移植前有持续性疾病的患者预后极差,因此挽救性治疗的目的就是在巩固性 ASCT 之前获得 PET 阴性缓解。这一目标可以通过一个或多个含有或者没有放疗的挽救性方案来实现。在 r/r-cHL 中 ASCT 潜在的治疗作用和生存获益已经通过两项大的比较单独化疗和化疗后 ASCT 确立[98,99]。

HL 治疗新药

大约有 15%的 HL 患者会在一线、二线治疗中失败,需要新的治疗。2012 年 FDA 批准了 brentuximab vedotin(BV)用于治疗 ASCT 失败或那些至少两种多药方案不是 ASCT 候选的患者[100,101]。其他认为有效的药物包括组蛋白去乙酰化酶抑制剂、PI3K/Akt/mTOR 抑制剂、来那度胺(lenalidomide)、苯达莫司汀[102]。最近,针对程序性死亡-1(PD1)-PD1 配体通路的免疫检查点抑制剂在 cHL 中显示出良好的前景。PD-1/PD-L1 途径损害免疫应答,抑制这一途径能够使宿主的抗肿瘤免疫应答增强。早期的数据显示两种这类药物帕博利珠单抗和纳武单抗治疗 cHL 的总的 ORR 在 50%~89%[103,104]。

brentuximab vedotin(BV),是一种偶联药物(ADC),含有嵌合型抗体 CD30 的单克隆抗体的抗体 cAC10,与单甲基金葡菌素 E(MMAE)形成化学共轭[105,106]。MMAE 内化进入里-施细胞,是导致细胞周期停滞和凋亡的微管蛋白抑制剂[107]。在最初的Ⅰ期研究中,纳入了 45 例 CD30 阳性的复发难治的血液恶性肿瘤,每 3 周静脉注射一次 BV,剂量从 0.1mg/kg 到 3.6mg/kg 不等,剂量限制性毒性包括:3~4 级的血小板减少,3 级的高血糖和粒缺性发热,最大耐受剂量(MTD)是 1.8mg/kg,每 3 周期 1 次,研究看到了充满前景的应答,在 2 期研究中 102 例 ASCT 的 r/r cHL 进一步证实这一结果。101 例患者每 3 周接受 1.8mg/kg BV,持续 16 个周期。总的 ORR 是 75%,CR 为 33%(34/102),中位 PFS 和 OS 分别为 5.6 个月和 40.5 个月,而且 14 例患者 BV 后持续缓解,其中 9 例没再进行其他治疗,5 例已开始巩固同种异体 SCT[108]。

目前正在研究 BV 与 AVD 联合初始治疗 cHL 的方法:一项国际Ⅲ期研究比较了 BV+AVD 和 ABVD 治疗晚期 cHL。相似的 BV 联合方案也正在早期 cHL 和老年 cHL 进行研究。另外的策略是 ASCT 之前应用 BV,以代替或补充标准的挽救治疗,如 ICE[109]。

Post-ASCT,是一项在高危 cHL 患者中进行的,BV 与安慰剂比较的维持治疗的Ⅲ研究,BV 维持的中位 PFS 显著改善(42.9 个月 vs 24.1 个月)[110]。

特殊人群

NLPHL

淋巴瘤的罕见亚型(参看病理诊断部分)现在被认为是高度可治疗的,但可能无法用 cHL 的标准治疗方法治愈[111~113]。管理的措施包括早期患者的单纯的切除 INRT 或者 CMT,监测,利妥昔单抗单药或者联合化疗,复发/晚期的患者采用姑息性的 INRT。最重要的是,生存仍然很好,但先前治疗晚期副作用可能有一些不良的影响。因此在这种患者,需要注意年轻患者,治疗的强度,有限的治疗可能取得良好的结果。像无痛性淋巴瘤,NLPHL 与晚期发生组织学转化有关(T 细胞富集型 B 细胞淋巴瘤,DLBCL 的亚型,或者 DLBCL)。这种转化最终可能发展成威胁生命的疾病,而需要含有多个药物的方案化疗来治疗 DLBCL。

老年患者

在老年患者中,尽管治疗方法由于耐受性可能需要进行改变,获得疗效的 cHL 治疗仍然是可以现实的。尽管博来霉素可能对肺毒性更大,ABVD 仍是标准的治疗方案,其他方案也经常被考虑(不含多柔比星或博来霉素)。brentuximab vedotin 可能是 ABVD 中博来霉素的替代(见前文)。复发/难治性 cHL 患者中年龄小于 70 岁的选择性患者中采用挽救性化疗/ASCT 治疗,一般患者的生理年龄在 70 岁或以下。没有二线 ASCT 治疗时,大多数患者没有治疗选择,可以参加Ⅰ~Ⅱ期临床研究,姑息化疗,或者 RT。

孕妇

cHL 可能发生在年轻的女性,非常罕见的也发生在孕妇。这些患者的管理的细节在其他地方进行讨论。最重要的是,cHL 通常是一种进展缓慢的淋巴瘤,治疗往往可以推迟直到分娩,或 ABVD 可以在第二和/或第三个月期间安全使用。妊娠期应尽量减少 MRI,不应行 PET 检查。

HIV

cHL 也可能与 HIV 相关,在这种情况下,病理更可能是混合细胞或淋巴细胞减少的组织学亚型,和分期更晚的发生在不寻常的位置,如皮肤。治疗方案与没有 HIV 的患者是相同的。CD4 细胞计数超过 200 的患者接受同步的 cART 治疗,有指证的患者接受预防抗感染治疗。存在过度免疫治疗的患者出现感染性并发症的可能性更多,需要更加选择的治疗方案[114]。

治疗后的随访

PET 成像有能力预测持续缓解和治愈。这就提出了一个重要的问题:什么时候、怎样的频率、多久应该进行 PET 影像检查。一致的意见认为在监测中,PET 过于敏感,出现过多的假阳性。CT 或 MRI 可以在需要时作为替代。由于大多数复发发生在治疗后的头两年,因此不建议在此时间段后进行常规影像学检查[115]。

(程颖 张爽 译 程颖 校)

参考文献

The complete reference list can be found on the Wiley Companion Digital Edition of this title (see inside front cover for login instructions).

1 Hodgkin's T. On some morbid appearances of the absorbent glands and spleen. *Medico-Chirurgical Trans.* 1832;**17**:68–97.

7 Peters M. A study of survivals in Hodgkin's disease treated radiologically. *Am J Roentgenol.* 1950;**63**:299–311.

8 Kaplan H. The radical radiotherapy of regionally localized Hodgkin's disease. *Radiology.* 1962;**78**:553–561.

9 Kaplan HS. Role of intensive radiotherapy in the management of Hodgkin's disease. *Cancer.* 1966;**19**:356.

10 Jacobs C. *Henry Kaplan and the Story of Hodgkin's Disease.* Stanford, CA: *Stanford University Press*; 2010:456. http://www.sup.org/books/title/?id=16764(accessed 9 Jan 2015).

12 DeVita VJ, Simon R, Habbard S, et al. Curability of advanced Hodgkin's disease with chemotherapy: longterm follow up of MOPP-treated patients at the National Cancer Institute. *Ann Intern Med.* 1980;**92**:587–595.

13 Canellos GP, Anderson JR, Propert KJ, et al. Chemotherapy of advanced Hodgkin's disease with MOPP, ABVD, or MOPP alternating with ABVD [see comments]. *N Engl J Med.* 1992;**327**:1478–1484.

14 Bonadonna G, Zucali R, Monfardini S, et al. Combination chemotherapy of Hodgkin's disease with Adriamycin, bleomycin, vinblastine, and imidazole carboxamide versus MOPP. *Cancer.* 1975;**36**:252–259.

16 Vockerodt M, Yap LF, Shannon-Lowe C, et al. The Epstein-Barr virus and the pathogenesis of lymphoma. *J Pathol.* 2015;**235**(2):312–322. doi: 10.1002/path.4459.

17 Kushekhar K, van den Berg A, Nolte I, Hepkema B, Visser L, Diepstra A.

Genetic associations in classical Hodgkin lymphoma: a systematic review and insights into susceptibility mechanisms. *Cancer Epidemiol Biomarkers Prev.* 2014;**23**(**12**):2737-2747.

25 King RL, Howard MT, Bagg A. Hodgkin lymphoma: pathology, pathogenesis, and a plethora of potential prognostic predictors. *Adv Anat Pathol.* 2014 Jan;**21**(**1**):12-25. doi: 10.1097/PAP.0000000000000002.

29 Mauch PM, Kalish L, Kadin M, et al. Patterns of presentation of Hodgkin's disease. *Cancer.* 1993;**71**:2062-2071.

40 Steidl C, Connors JM, Gascoyne RD. Molecular pathogenesis of Hodgkin's lymphoma: increasing evidence of the importance of the microenvironment. *J Clin Oncol.* 2011 May 10;**29**(**14**):1812-1826.

41 Steidl C, Lee T, Shah SP, et al. Tumor-associated macrophages and survival in classic Hodgkin's lymphoma. *N Engl J Med.* 2010;**362**(**10**):875-885.

48 Cheson BD, Fisher RI, Barrington SF, et al. Recommendations for initial evaluation, staging, and response assessment of Hodgkin and non-Hodgkin lymphoma: the Lugano classification. *J Clin Oncol.* 2014 Sep 20;**32**(**27**):3059-3068.

52 Ng AK, Travis LB. Acute and long-term complications of radiotherapy in Hodgkin lymphoma. In: Specht L, Yahalom J, eds. *Radiotherapy for Hodgkin Lymphoma.* Heidelberg: Springer; 2011:183-196.

53 Specht L, Yahalom J, Illidge T, et al. Modern radiation therapy for Hodgkin lymphoma: field and dose guidelines from the international lymphoma radiation oncology group (ILROG). *Int J Radiat Oncol Biol Phys.* 2014;**89**:854-862.

54 Diehl V, Franklin J, Pfreundschuh M, et al. Standard and increased-dose BEACOPP chemotherapy compared with COPP-ABVD for advanced Hodgkin's disease. *N Engl J Med.* 2003;**348**:2386-2395.

55 Engert A, Diehl V, Franklin J, et al. Escalated-dose BEACOPP in the treatment of patients with advanced-stage Hodgkin's lymphoma: 10 years of follow-up of the GHSG HD9 study. *J Clin Oncol.* 2009;**27**:4548-4554.

57 Gallamini A, Rigacci L, Merli F, et al. The predictive value of positron emission tomography scanning performed after two courses of standard therapy on treatment outcome in advanced stage Hodgkin's disease. *Haematologica.* 2006;**91**:475-481.

61 Gallamini A, Barrington SF, Biggi A, et al. The predictive role of interim positron emission tomography for Hodgkin lymphoma treatment outcome is confirmed using the interpretation criteria of the Deauville five-point scale. *Haematologica.* 2014;**99**(**6**):1107-1113.

64 Meyer RM, Gospodarowicz MK, Connors JM, et al. Randomized comparison of ABVD chemotherapy with a strategy that includes radiation therapy in patients with limited-stage Hodgkin's lymphoma: National Cancer Institute of Canada Clinical Trials Group and the Eastern Cooperative Oncology Group. *J Clin Oncol.* 2005;**23**:4634-4642.

66 Klimm B, Goergen H, Fuchs M, et al. Impact of risk factors on outcomes in early-stage Hodgkin's lymphoma: an analysis of international staging definitions. *Ann Oncol.* 2013;**24**:3070-3076.

67 Engert A, Plutschow A, Eich HT, et al. Reduced treatment intensity in patients with early-stage Hodgkin's lymphoma. *N Engl J Med.* 2010;**363**:640-652.

68 Straus DJ, Portlock CS, Qin J, et al. Results of a prospective randomized clinical trial of doxorubicin, bleomycin, vinblastine, and dacarbazine (ABVD) followed by radiation therapy (RT) versus ABVD alone for stages I, II, and IIIA nonbulky Hodgkin disease. *Blood.* 2004;**104**:3483-3489.

69 Meyer RM, Gospodarowicz MK, Connors JM, et al. ABVD alone versus radiation-based therapy in limited-stage Hodgkin's lymphoma. *N Engl J Med.* 2012;**366**:399-408.

70 Radford J, Illidge T, Counsell N, et al. Results of a trial of PET-directed therapy for early-stage Hodgkin's lymphoma. *N Engl J Med.* 2015;**372**:1598-1607.

72 Eich HT, Diehl V, Gorgen H, et al. Intensified chemotherapy and dose-reduced involved-field radiotherapy in patients with early unfavorable Hodgkin's lymphoma: final analysis of the German Hodgkin Study Group HD11 trial. *J Clin Oncol.* 2010;**28**:4199-4206.

77 Advani RH, Hong F, Fisher RI, et al. Randomized phase III trial comparing ABVD plus radiotherapy with the Stanford V regimen in patients with stages I or II locally extensive, bulky mediastinal Hodgkin lymphoma: a subset analysis of the North American intergroup E2496 trial. *J Clin Oncol.* 2015;**33**:1936-1942.

78 Hasenclever D, Diehl V. A prognostic score for advanced Hodgkin's disease. International prognostic factors project on advanced Hodgkin's disease. *N Engl J Med.* 1998;**339**:1506-1514.

79 Moccia AA, Donaldson J, Chhanabhai M, et al. International Prognostic Score in advanced-stage Hodgkin's lymphoma: altered utility in the modern era. *J Clin Oncol.* 2012;**30**:3383-3388.

86 Johnson P, McKenzie H. How I treat advanced classical Hodgkin lymphoma. *Blood.* 2015;**125**:1717-1723.

89 Moskowitz CH, Yahalom J, Zelenetz AD, et al. High-dose chemo-radiotherapy for relapsed or refractory Hodgkin lymphoma and the significance of pre-transplant functional imaging. *Br J Haematol.* 2010;**148**:890-897.

92 Moskowitz CH, Matasar MJ, Zelenetz AD, et al. Normalization of pre-ASCT, FDG-PET imaging with second-line, non-cross-resistant, chemotherapy programs improves event-free survival in patients with Hodgkin lymphoma. *Blood.* 2012;**119**:1665-1670.

100 Younes A, Bartlett NL, Leonard JP, et al. Brentuximab vedotin (SGN-35) for relapsed CD30-positive lymphomas. *N Engl J Med.* 2010;**363**:1812-1821.

102 Moskowitz AJ. Novel agents in Hodgkin lymphoma. *Curr Oncol Rep.* 2012;**14**:419-423.

104 Ansell SM, Lesokhin AM, Borrello I, et al. PD-1 Blockade with Nivolumab in relapsed or refractory Hodgkin's lymphoma. *N Engl J Med.* 2015;**372**:311-319.

108 Gopal AK, Chen R, Smith SE, et al. Three-year follow-up data and characterization of long-term remissions from an ongoing phase 2 study of brentuximab vedotin in patients with relapsed or refractory Hodgkin lymphoma. *Blood ASH Annual Meeting Abstracts.* 2013;**122**(**21**):4382.

109 Moskowitz AJ, Schoder H, Yahalom J, et al. PET-adapted sequential salvage therapy with brentuximab vedotin followed by augmented ifosamide, carboplatin, and etoposide for patients with relapsed and refractory Hodgkin's lymphoma: a non-randomised, open-label, single-centre, phase 2 study. *Lancet Oncol.* 2015;**16**:284-292.

110 Moskowitz CH, Nademanee A, Masszi T, et al. Brentuximab vedotin as consolidation therapy after autologous stem-cell transplantation in patients with Hodgkin's lymphoma at risk of relapse or progression (AETHERA): a randomised, double-blind, placebo-controlled, phase 3 trial. *Lancet.* 2015;**385**: 1853-1362.

113 Shankar A, Daw S. Nodular lymphocyte predominant Hodgkin lymphoma in children and adolescents — a comprehensive review of biology, clinical course and treatment options. *Br J Haematol.* 2012;**159**:288-298.

114 Uldrick TS, Little RF. How we treat classical Hodgkin lymphoma in patients infected with human immunodeficiency virus. *Blood.* 2014 **125**:1226-1235 . pii: blood-2014-08-551598..

115 Ng AK. Current survivorship recommendations for patients with Hodgkin lymphoma: focus on late effects. *Blood.* 2014;**124**(**23**):3373-3379. doi: 10.1182/blood-2014-05-579193.

第 119 章　非霍奇金淋巴瘤

Arnold S. Freedman, MD ■ Ann S. LaCasce, MD

概述

恶性淋巴瘤主要是由淋巴组织内的细胞转化形成的肿瘤。虽然霍奇金淋巴瘤(HL)和非霍奇金淋巴瘤(NHL)均侵犯淋巴造血组织,但它们的生物学特征和临床行为仍存在区别,其肿瘤细胞起源、发生部位、特殊症状和对治疗的反应均有所不同。虽然两者都是对放疗和化疗最敏感的恶性肿瘤之一,但治愈率有着显著差异,采用传统和解救治疗策略,有接近 80%的霍奇金淋巴瘤患者被治愈,而非霍奇金淋巴瘤治愈率则不到 50%。

流行病学和病因学

发病率和死亡率

2014 年美国新诊断非霍奇金淋巴瘤 70 890 例,预计死亡 18 990 例[1]。发病随着年龄的增长而稳步增加,男性发病率略高于女性,高加索人群的发病率高于非裔美国人。尽管自 20 世纪 90 年代中期以来,发病率的增长速度有所放缓,但仍在以每年 1.5%~2%的速度增长。

非霍奇金淋巴瘤各病理类型的发生率随年龄变化而有显著差异。在儿童中,以 Burkitt 淋巴瘤(BL)、淋巴母细胞淋巴瘤(LBL)和弥漫性大 B 细胞淋巴瘤(DLBCL)为主。随着年龄的增长,滤泡性淋巴瘤(FL)和其他侵袭性淋巴瘤的发生率持续增高,小淋巴细胞淋巴瘤和滤泡性淋巴瘤是 60 岁以上患者最常见的诊断类型。

增加 NHL 发病风险的相关因素和疾病

感染是某些 NHL 的致病因素(表 119-1),EB 病毒与 Burkitt 淋巴瘤、自然杀伤细胞淋巴瘤和人类免疫缺陷病毒(HIV-1)相关淋巴瘤的发生密切相关[2,3],45%~70%的 HIV 相关淋巴瘤与 EB 病毒有关,HIV 感染者的原发中枢神经系统淋巴瘤几乎 100%与 EB 病毒有关。人类 T 细胞白血病病毒-1(HTLV-1)与高发于加勒比海及日本南部的成人 T 细胞白血病/淋巴瘤有关[4];胃边缘带淋巴瘤(MZL)与幽门螺杆菌感染有关[5];脾边缘带淋巴瘤与丙型肝炎感染有关[6];慢性乙型肝炎感染也增加 NHL 的风险[7]。在欧洲,眼附件的边缘带淋巴瘤与鹦鹉热衣原体感染有关[8],伯氏包柔氏螺旋体感染与边缘带淋巴瘤侵犯皮肤有关,免疫增殖性的小肠疾病(地中海淋巴瘤,α 重链病)与空肠弯曲菌感染有关[9],原发渗出性淋巴瘤与卡波西肉瘤相关疱疹病毒即人类疱疹病毒-8(HHV-8)有关[10,11]。

表 119-1　淋巴瘤发生的风险因素

遗传性免疫缺陷疾病	获得性免疫缺陷疾病	自身免疫性和炎症性疾病	感染因子(除了 HIV)	化学因素和药物
自身免疫性淋巴细胞增殖性疾病	HIV-1 感染	类风湿关节炎	EB 病毒	除草剂,杀虫剂,有机溶剂
共济失调毛细血管扩张综合征	医源性疾病	系统性红斑狼疮	HTLV-1	电离辐射
白细胞异常色素减退综合征(Chediak-Higashi syndrome)	肿瘤坏死因子激动剂	干燥综合征	HHV-8	化疗,放疗
常见变异型免疫缺陷病		乳糜泻	幽门螺旋杆菌	
WAS		桥本甲状腺炎	空肠弯曲杆菌	
X 连锁淋巴组织增殖性疾病		炎症性肠病	鹦鹉热衣原体	
			伯氏疏螺旋体	
			HCV	

WAS,威斯科特-奥尔德里奇综合征(Wiskott-Aldrich syndrome);HCV,丙肝病毒;HHV-8,人疱疹病毒-8 型;HIV-1,人类免疫缺陷病毒 1 型;HTLV-1,人嗜 T-淋巴病毒 1 型。

NHL 发病风险增加与许多因素和/或疾病状态有关，与某些化学物质的接触，包括除草剂苯氧醋酸、砷、杀虫剂、杀菌剂、氯酚、有机溶剂、卤甲烷、铅、氯乙烯或石棉等会增加患 NHL 的风险，但其证据仍存在争议[12~14]，增加患病风险的职业性暴露包括农业工作、焊接、木材行业[15,16]。

遗传性和获得性免疫缺陷病以及自身免疫性疾病与淋巴瘤的发病增加有关[17,18]。免疫抑制与诱发 NHL 之间的关系值得关注，因为随着免疫抑制的消退，有一部分淋巴瘤可以发生自发消退[19]。做过器官移植而需要长期服用免疫抑制药物的患者，其 NHL 的发病风险增加近 100 倍，且发病最常发生在移植后的第一年，弥漫性大 B 细胞淋巴瘤（DLBCL）是这种情况下最常见的 NHL，其常与 EB 病毒感染相关[20]。罕见的遗传性免疫缺陷病，如 X 连锁淋巴细胞增殖综合征、威斯科特-奥尔德里奇综合征（Wiskott-Aldrich syndrome）、白细胞异常色素减退综合征（Chediak-Higashi syndrome）、共济失调毛细血管扩张综合征和普通变异免疫缺陷症，因发生高侵袭性淋巴瘤而更加复杂。在 NHL、HL 和慢性淋巴细胞白血病（CLL）的一级亲属中可观察到 NHL 发病风险增加[21]。

非霍奇金淋巴瘤病理学、免疫生物学和自然病程

WHO 发表了淋巴造血系统肿瘤的新分类（表 119-2），其策略是整合形态学、免疫分型和遗传学特征以及临床表现进行综合分类[22]。在这里，将把这个分类的众多病种分别以“惰性”“侵袭性”和“高度侵袭性”范畴分组介绍（表 119-2）。

表 119-2　2008 年 WHO 淋巴瘤分类：B 细胞和 T 细胞肿瘤

前体 B、T 细胞肿瘤	前体 B-淋巴母细胞白血病/淋巴瘤
	前体 T-淋巴母细胞白血病/淋巴瘤
成熟 B 细胞肿瘤	慢性淋巴细胞白血病/小淋巴细胞性淋巴瘤
	B 细胞前淋巴细胞白血病
	淋巴浆细胞性淋巴瘤
	脾边缘带淋巴瘤
	毛细胞白血病
	脾 B 细胞淋巴瘤，无法分类
	浆细胞肿瘤
	结外边缘带淋巴瘤
	结内边缘带淋巴瘤
	滤泡性淋巴瘤
	原发皮肤滤泡中心性淋巴瘤
	套细胞淋巴瘤
	弥漫大 B 细胞淋巴瘤
	T 细胞/组织细胞丰富的大 B 细胞淋巴瘤
	原发中枢神经系统 DLBCL
	原发皮肤 DLBCL，腿型
	老年性 EBV 阳性 DLBCL
	慢性炎症相关弥漫大 B 细胞淋巴瘤
	淋巴瘤样肉芽肿病
	原发纵隔大 B 细胞淋巴瘤
	血管内大 B 细胞淋巴瘤
	ALK 阳性大 B 细胞淋巴瘤
	浆母细胞淋巴瘤
	伯基特淋巴瘤
	不能分类的 B 细胞淋巴瘤，特征介于 DLBCL 和 Burkitt 淋巴瘤之间
	不能分类的 B 细胞淋巴瘤，特征介于 DLBCL 和霍奇金淋巴瘤之间
成熟 T 细胞肿瘤	T 细胞前淋巴细胞白血病
	T 细胞大颗粒淋巴细胞白血病
	成人 T 细胞白血病/淋巴瘤
	结外 NK/T 细胞淋巴瘤，鼻型
	肠病型 T 细胞淋巴瘤
	肝脾 T 细胞淋巴瘤
	皮下脂膜炎样 T 细胞淋巴瘤
	蕈样真菌病
	Sézary 综合征
	原发皮肤 CD30+T 细胞增殖性疾病
	原发皮肤外周 T 细胞淋巴瘤，罕见型
	外周 T 细胞淋巴瘤，非特指型
	血管免疫母细胞 T 细胞淋巴瘤
	ALK 阳性间变性大细胞淋巴瘤
	ALK 阴性间变性大细胞淋巴瘤

ALK，间变性淋巴瘤激酶；DLBCL，弥漫性大 B 细胞淋巴瘤；EBV，EB 病毒；NK，自然杀伤细胞。

染色体易位和癌基因重排

免疫球蛋白(Ig)和T细胞受体(TCR)在正常淋巴细胞中存在基因重排,淋巴瘤常可发现染色体易位,这些染色体易位涉及癌基因的激活或抑癌基因的失活。其中癌基因的激活更为常见,即原癌基因受到构成性活性启动子的控制,导致癌基因及其蛋白产物的过表达,例如BL中(8;14)(q24;q32)的易位涉及*MYC*原癌基因和*IgH*基因;FL中(14;18)(q32;q32)的易位涉及*BCL2*原癌基因和*IgH*基因;套细胞淋巴瘤(MCL)中(11;14)(q13;q32)的易位涉及编码*cyclinD1*(*CCDN1*)基因和*IgH*基因。而染色体易位产生编码嵌合致癌蛋白的融合基因是不常见的,包括间变性大细胞淋巴瘤(ALCL)中(2;5)(p23;q35)涉及ALK和*NPM1*基因的易位,以及在MZL淋巴瘤中涉及API2和*MLT*基因的t(11;18)易位。这些易位和重排可以通过跨越染色体断点的探针聚合酶链反应(PCR)检测,反转录酶聚合酶链反应(RT-PCR)检测融合基因的RNA产物,或使用探针到特定染色体片段的荧光原位杂交(FISH)检测。利用免疫组织化学技术可检测易位导致一部分正常淋巴细胞中从未表达(如ALK激酶)的蛋白。

惰性淋巴瘤

惰性NHL通常以年为单位计算患者的存活率,即使不治疗这种患者也能存活相当长时间,但通常传统疗法无法治愈。在西方国家诊断的NHL中,惰性淋巴瘤占35%~40%,其中最常见的3种类型是滤泡性淋巴瘤(FL)、小淋巴细胞性淋巴瘤和边缘带淋巴瘤(MZL),分别占所有NHL病变的22%、6%和5%。相比之下,淋巴浆细胞性淋巴瘤、蕈样真菌病/塞扎里综合征(Sézary syndrome,SS)及脾脏MZL都属于少见类型,仅占所有NHL的1%以下或者更少。

滤泡性淋巴瘤(follicular lymphoma,FL)是最常见的惰性NHL,形态上类似于次级淋巴滤泡的生发中心(图119-1)。WHO依据每高倍视野中大细胞的数目将FL分为三级:1级,0~5/10倍高倍视野(HPF)(图119-2);2级,6~15/10HPF;3级,>15/10HPF,3级又细分为3A级(以有丝细胞为主)和3B级(以成丝细胞片为主)。1级和2级FL以及许多3A级FL处理方法类似,3B级FL是一种侵袭性疾病,与DLBCL分类合并。

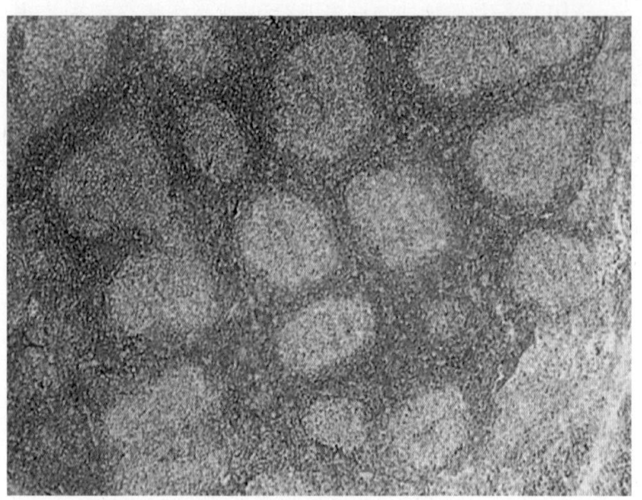

图119-1 滤泡性淋巴瘤Ⅰ级(低倍镜视野)

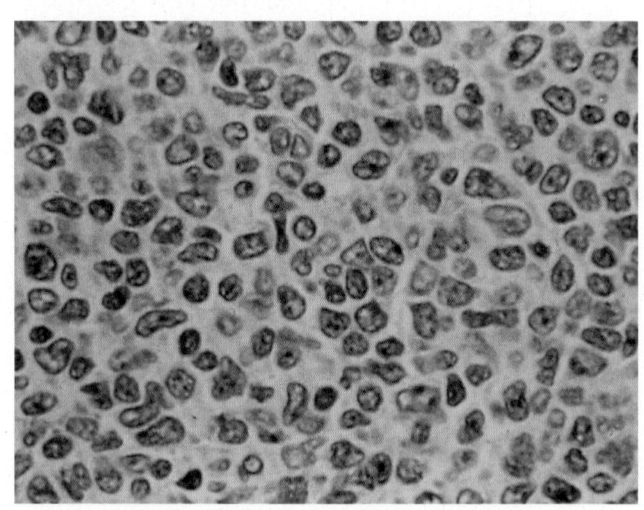

图119-2 滤泡性淋巴瘤Ⅰ级(高倍镜视野)

FL和正常卵泡中心B细胞表达细胞表面抗原,包括单克隆免疫球蛋白和B细胞抗原CD19、CD20、CD10、CD79a,但缺乏CD5。bcl-2蛋白过表达基本上存在于所有的1级和2级病变,bcl-6核阳性至少见于部分肿瘤细胞。t(14;18)是最常见的细胞遗传学异常,这种改变导致bcl-2蛋白在超过85%的病变中过表达(参见第8章)。最近的测序研究发现,FL(90%的肿瘤)最常见的突变与MLL2有关,这是一种编码组蛋白H3甲基化酶的基因。其他不常见的复发性突变包括涉及表观遗传修饰基因的其他基因,如*EZH2*、*CREBBP*和*EP300*[23,24]。

FL占NHL的22%[25],40岁以前不常见,诊断时的中位年龄约为60岁,少见于亚裔与黑人。患者经常存在颈部、腋窝、腹股沟、股部淋巴结区等外周淋巴结无痛性增大。通常淋巴结增大在诊断前已存在一段时间,且时长时消。肺门及纵隔淋巴结常常受累,但纵隔大肿块罕见。一些患者存在无症状性腹腔大肿物。分期研究证实晚期病变存在脾脏、肝脏、骨髓受累的概率分别为40%、50%、70%。FL骨髓受累为单一模式的骨小梁旁浸润。极少患者存在髓外受累,仅有约20%患者存在B症状或乳酸脱氢酶(LDH)增高,仅有肠道受侵的患者预后良好[26]。尽管外周神经的压迫及硬膜外肿物造成的脊索压迫可能形成受累,但中枢神经系统受累并不常见。

3级FL以前被称为滤泡性大细胞淋巴瘤,在3B级病例中*BCL6*重排的比例很高。大多数研究都包括3A和3B级FL,这影响了对结果的解释。临床3B级FL更接近DLBCL[22,27],相比之下,许多3A级的FL患者具有更惰性的病程。

FL的自然进程多种多样,一些患者观察5年肿物时长时消,没有必要治疗[28]。另外一些存在播散性病变,快速增长,由于脏器肿大、淋巴管阻塞、脏器梗阻从而需要治疗。

高达60%的FL在疾病进展过程中发生组织学转化,通常转化为DLBCL,临床上表现为淋巴结病进展加快、结外部位受累、出现B症状和LDH水平升高。发生组织学转化的患者预后较差[29,30]。

小淋巴细胞性淋巴瘤

在WHO分类中,小淋巴细胞性淋巴瘤和B细胞慢性淋巴细胞白血病被视为同一个疾病类型。尽管绝大部分肿瘤细胞看起来像正常的小淋巴细胞,淋巴结病变中还是可以看到一些体积较大的细胞,位于所谓生长中心(proliferation centers),形态上类似于前体淋巴细胞白血病细胞(图 119-3、图 116-2 和图 116-3)。小淋巴细胞性淋巴瘤在表型上与 B 细胞慢性淋巴细胞白血病几乎完全相同,表达 HLA-DR 及 B 细胞抗原 CD19、CD20 和 CD23,低水平表达表面免疫球蛋白和 CD5。细胞遗传学改变包括染色体 12 三体以及 13q、11q 和 17p 异常,检出率分别为 40%、45%~55%、17%~20%和 7%~10%。携带有 13q 缺失的患者预后最好,而 11q 或者 17p 异常的患者预后最差[31]。

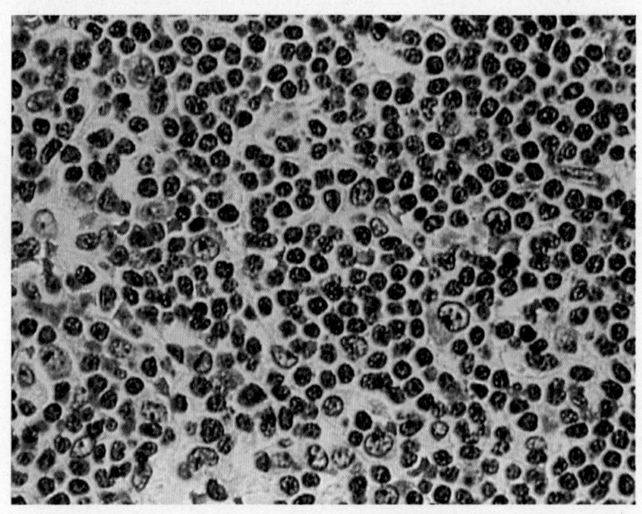

图 119-3　小淋巴细胞性淋巴瘤

最近的研究提示,这种病变中 30%~50%携带有非突变性的免疫球蛋白可变区基因,这种表现型所对应的是初始型 B 细胞(naïve Bcells)。这些病变常常表达 CD38 和酪氨酸激酶 ZAP-70,预后较差[32]。其余的 50%~70%病变携带有已突变的免疫球蛋白可变区基因,来源于生发中心或者生发中心后 B 细胞[33],预后良好[34]。对慢性淋巴细胞白血病的深入测序研究发现了一些复发性突变,包括 *NOTCH1*、*MYD88* 和 *SF3B1* 基因[35]。

小淋巴细胞淋巴瘤占所有非霍奇金淋巴瘤的 6%[25],临床表现与 FL 类似。与 B 细胞慢性淋巴细胞白血病不同,70%~90%的患者骨髓呈阳性,但外周血淋巴细胞可能正常或仅有轻度增多。约 20%患者存在血清副蛋白,约 40%患者存在低丙球蛋白血症。小淋巴细胞淋巴瘤与 B 细胞慢性淋巴细胞白血病均能转化为 DLBCL 或更少见的 HL(Richter 综合征,图 119-4)[36]。

淋巴浆细胞性淋巴瘤

淋巴浆细胞性淋巴瘤是一种由弥漫增生的小淋巴细胞构成的惰性淋巴瘤,肿瘤细胞表现出向浆细胞方向分化成熟[37]。通过特殊染色可以证明免疫球蛋白存在,包含体的出现也说明了这一点。肿瘤细胞表达 B 细胞抗原 CD19、CD20 和表面免疫球蛋白 M 同种型分子,一般不表达 CD5、CD10 和 CD23。40%~60%的淋巴浆细胞性淋巴瘤存在 6q21 缺失,这种综合征与 Waldenström 巨球蛋白血症相关。参与 Ig 受体下游信号通路的 MYD88 蛋白几乎在 100%的病例中存在活化突变[38]。

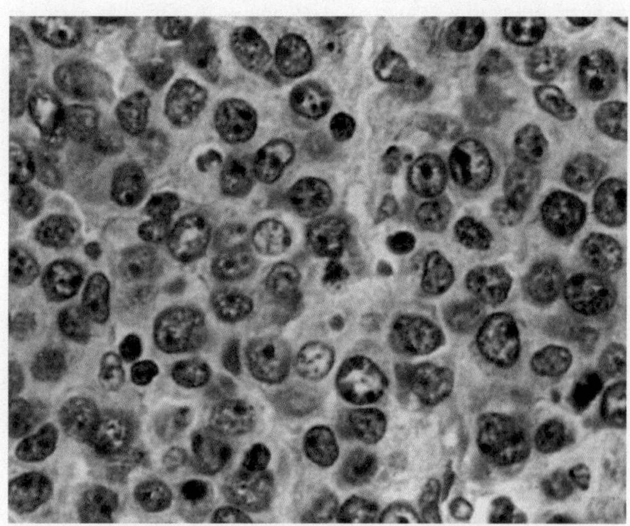

图 119-4　弥漫性大 B 细胞性淋巴瘤

淋巴浆细胞性淋巴瘤约占所有 NHL 的 1%,临床表现类似于小淋巴细胞淋巴瘤。中位发病年龄 60 多岁,几乎所有患者均因骨髓受累而进入Ⅳ期,淋巴结和脾脏受累较常见。B 症状和血清 LDH 升高是罕见的,血清 M 成分是常见的。与 B-CLL 一样,副蛋白可能具有自身抗体或冷球蛋白活性,然而大多数情况下混合冷沉球蛋白血症已被证明与并发丙型肝炎病毒(HCV)感染[39]和针对丙型肝炎治疗的疗效有关,在 WHO 临床研究中,5 年总生存期(OS)(58%)和无病生存(25%)与小淋巴细胞性淋巴瘤相同。

边缘带淋巴瘤

边缘带淋巴瘤(MZL)是一组疾病,包括结内型、结外型和脾脏型 MZL,其中结外型病变又被称为黏膜相关淋巴样组织淋巴瘤(MALTs)[40,41]。结内型 MZL 肿瘤细胞形态上似于正常"单核样"B 细胞,常累及淋巴窦。免疫表型上,这种肿瘤表达表面免疫球蛋白 M 及 B 细胞抗原(CD19 和 CD20)。与其他惰性淋巴瘤相似,MZL 能够转化为高级别淋巴瘤。结内型 MZL 占所有 NHL 的 1%,超过 70%的患者就诊时疾病已经进入Ⅲ/Ⅳ期,多数患者没有症状。与绝大多数其他惰性淋巴瘤相比,骨髓累及比较少见,5 年生存率为 55%~79%。

结外型 MZL 肿瘤细胞与单核细胞样 B 细胞相似,表达 CD19、CD20 和表面免疫球蛋白 M,被认为起源于记忆 B 细胞。淋巴上皮病变可能与着丝粒细胞有关,这肿瘤细胞本身并不形成滤泡,但却排列在反应性滤泡周围。当结外型 MZL 播散到淋巴结时,肿瘤细胞首先累及边缘带。染色体 3 三体和 t(11;18)是最常见的细胞遗传学异常,其发生率高达 60%(胃的结外型 MZL)和 25%~40%[42]。

结外型 MZL 约占所有 NHL 的 5%,约占所有胃淋巴瘤的 50%。B 症状不常见,大部分患者为Ⅰ期或Ⅱ期。没有明显的年龄分布倾向,最常侵犯胃肠道(胃最常见)、肺、硬脑膜、泪腺、唾液腺、皮肤、甲状腺、乳腺。MZL 与自身免疫性疾病和幽门螺杆菌、伯氏疏螺旋体、鹦鹉热衣原体和 HCV 感染有关[43~46]。少于 25%的患者有淋巴结和骨髓受侵,患者可表现为消化性溃疡、腹痛、干燥综合征,或受侵部位的肿块。这些淋巴瘤能够播散到其他黏膜相关淋巴组织，大约30%的患者有骨髓受侵，典型的出现在病程的晚期，这在非胃边缘带淋巴瘤中更常见[47]。这些肿瘤完全缓解率高，可能长期生存，10年以上的生存率高达80%[48]。与所有惰性NHL一样，可以转化为DLBCL。

脾脏MZL占全部NHL的2%以下，中位年龄65岁，50岁以前少见[25]，可见脾内边缘带的扩增，也能侵犯骨髓和外周血（被称为伴绒毛淋巴细胞脾淋巴瘤）。脾边缘带淋巴瘤中有39%病例出现3号染色体三体，患者的10年生存率超过70%。测序研究表明复发体细胞突变基因参与NOTCH，NF-κB，和B细胞受体途径以及*TP53*突变[49]。

侵袭性淋巴瘤

套细胞性淋巴瘤

一般情况下，套细胞性淋巴瘤（MCL）表现出侵袭性行为[50,51]，这种肿瘤相当于套区的初始B细胞。形态上，MCL可表现为弥漫性生长，亦可以呈模糊地小结节样外观，偶尔表现为次级滤泡的套区扩张。细胞学表型上，肿瘤细胞体积中等，有一个不规则的胞核。有的MCL病变主要由母细胞化的肿瘤细胞组成，有丝分裂指数高。肿瘤细胞表达B细胞抗原和表面免疫球蛋白M（伴有或者不伴有表面免疫球蛋白D）、CD5和CD43表达，但缺乏CD10和CD23表达，过表达细胞周期素D1。t(11;14)(q13;q32)存在于大约70%的MCL，这种改变造成*bcl-1*基因（编码细胞周期素D1）重排。大约8%的MCL呈细胞周期素D1阴性，这些病变具有细胞周期素D2、4或者细胞周期素D3过表达，但不携带染色体重排[52]，临床上与细胞周期素D1阳性的病例表现相似[53]。深度测序[54]已经在少数病例中发现*NOTCH1*突变，这可能与预后不良有关，SOX11过表达也与预后较差有关[52,55]。

套细胞淋巴瘤大约占全部NHL的7%，约75%为男性，中位年龄63岁，大约70%的患者为Ⅳ期，近1/3有B症状。典型受累部位是淋巴结、脾、肝、韦氏环和骨髓，25%~50%的患者就诊时出现外周血受侵。套细胞淋巴瘤能够侵犯胃肠道的任何区域，偶尔表现为小肠多发息肉。套细胞淋巴瘤的中位生存期3~6年，诊断时为母细胞型套细胞淋巴瘤患者的中位生存仅有18个月。母细胞转化发生在35%的患者中，4年的发病风险为42%，一旦发生转化则中位生存仅为3.8个月[56]，*p53*的突变和缺失也与预后较差有关[57]。

弥漫性大B细胞性淋巴瘤

弥漫性大B细胞淋巴瘤（DLBCL）由弥漫增生的大细胞构成，核分裂指数高。肿瘤细胞有中等量的胞质，有裂或无裂的胞核，常常有几个核仁，这类肿瘤的形态可以变化很大（图119-4）。DLBCL代表许多不同的疾病类型[22]，（表119-2）已经对DLBCL进行了基因表达谱分析，据此把DLBCL分成不同的遗传学类型[58~61]。有证据表明，DLBCL病变具有生发中心B细胞或者活化B细胞的表现型。一般情况下，肿瘤细胞表达B细胞抗原（CD19和CD20）和单克隆性表面免疫球蛋白M，偶尔也表达其他重链亚型。CD5阳性不常见，这样的患者可能预后较差[62]。CD10和BCL-6阳性支持生发中心起源，而MUM1表达支持非生发中心起源。大约70%的病变表达BCL-6蛋白，与生发中心起源一致[63]。

DLBCL存在多种染色体异常，BCL-6与3q27的染色体重排有关[64]。基因重排发生在20%~40%的弥漫性侵袭性淋巴瘤中，大约30%的DLBCL患者中观察到t(14;18)，其中一些患者可能由FL的组织学转变为DLBCL。通过基因表达谱（GEP）发现生发中心B细胞（GCB）类型通常与2号染色体上的t(14;18)和REL癌基因的扩增有关。相比之下，活化的B细胞（ABC）类型与6q21的缺失、三体3、3q和18q21~22的增加以及*EZH2*的突变有关[65,66]。活化的B细胞类型也有较高水平NF-κB的激活[67]。10%的DLBCL发生*MYC*重排，其中伴随基因占60%，替代基因占40%。约20%的*MYC*重排同时伴有*BCL2*或*BCL6*重排，这一组合被称为“双打击淋巴瘤”[68]。*MYC*的扩增和/或过表达独立于*MYC*重排，扩增也与预后不良有关[69,70]。

DLBCL占所有NHL的31%，是最常见的组织学亚型，发病人群一般为中年或老年（中位年龄64岁），患者均有淋巴结肿大或结外疾病。大约20%的DLBCL为局部发病（Ⅰ期或ⅠE期），30%~40%的患者会出现Ⅰ期或Ⅱ期疾病，大约40%的患者出现Ⅳ期疾病。30%的患者出现B症状，与大多数NHL不同，半数以上患者LDH升高。在疾病的过程中，可能涉及肝脏、肾脏、肺、骨骼和周围神经，骨髓受累最初见于10%~20%的患者，结外疾病、特别是睾丸、骨髓、鼻窦、多个结外部位和LDH升高是中枢神经系统传播的其他风险[71]。DLBCL的罕见病例表现为弥散性的血管内大淋巴细胞增殖，累及小血管，但没有明显的瘤块[72~74]，最常累及中枢神经系统、肾脏、肺和皮肤。

DLBCL中有一个独特的临床类型，称为原发性纵隔大B细胞淋巴瘤（PMLBCL）（占所有DLBCL病例的7%）[75]，PMLBCL组织学上细胞浸润是不均匀的，常存在硬化。免疫表型包括B细胞抗原（CD19、CD20），但表面和胞质免疫球蛋白呈阴性。GEP表明这种亚型不同于DLBCL的生发中心或ABC类型。最近的研究表明，PMLBCL的GEP模式与HL的里-施细胞（Reed-Sternberg cell）非常相似[76,77]，在含有*JAK2*基因的染色体9p区域和程序性细胞死亡配体1和2（PDL1和PDL2）以及具有抑制T细胞功能的程序性细胞死亡受体1（PD-1）的配体上，常见拷贝数的增加，类似于经典HD[76]。PMLBCL以女性为主，中位年龄为40岁，超过70%的患者表现为累及纵隔大肿块的Ⅰ/Ⅱ期疾病，大约1/3的患者可见胸腔和心包积液，上腔静脉综合征很常见。与DLBCL相似，大多数情况下存在LDH升高，而骨髓受累并不常见，PMLBCL患者的预后与DLBCL患者相似。

外周T细胞性淋巴瘤

外周T细胞性淋巴瘤（PTCL）包括一组疾病类型，占成年人所有NHL的15%[78]。依据发病率高低依次是PTCL、未指定的类型（not otherwise specified，NOS）、间变性大细胞性淋巴瘤（ALCL）、血管免疫母细胞性T细胞性淋巴瘤（AITL）、鼻型结外NK/T细胞性淋巴瘤以及其他少见类型，包括脂膜炎样T细胞性淋巴瘤、肠病型T细胞性淋巴瘤以及肝脾型γ/δT细胞性淋巴瘤。

PTCL可发生于淋巴结，也可位于结外，肿瘤细胞呈弥漫浸润生长，细胞形态变化较大。部分病变中由小细胞和大细胞混合组成；也可以由多形性肿瘤细胞和Reed-Sternberg样细胞构成，背景细胞包括上皮样组织细胞、浆细胞和嗜酸性粒细胞；还有部分病变主要由大细胞构成。与B细胞性淋巴瘤不同，

PTCL 中 T 细胞表面抗原的表达方式变化非常大，多数肿瘤表达 CD2、CD3 和 CD4，一部分还表达 CD8[79]。在多数病变中，存在一种或者一种以上的所谓"成熟"T 细胞抗原丢失，如 CD5 和 CD7。许多 PTCL 病变呈 EBV 阳性，尤其是鼻型结外 NK/T 细胞性淋巴瘤[80]，EBV 阳性与预后不良有关。

90%的 T 细胞性淋巴瘤具有有丝分裂中期异常改变，外周 T 细胞性淋巴瘤中最常见的染色体转位是 t(7;14)、t(11;14)、inv(14)和 t(14;14)，AITL 与三倍体 3 和/或 5 有关[81]，这些转位都累及位于 14q11、7q34~35 和 7p15 的 T 细胞受体(TCR)基因。发生于年轻人的 ALCL 大部分携带有 t(2;5)，少部分携带 t(1;2)[82]；发生于成年人的病变一般缺乏 t(2;5)，肝脾型 γ/δT 细胞性淋巴瘤与染色体 7q 等臂和 8 三体改变有关[83]。

PTCL 发病的中位年龄与 DLBCL 相似，与 DLBCL 相比，80%的 PTCL 为Ⅲ/Ⅳ期疾病，B 症状更常见，包括肝脾肿大和结外疾病如皮肤病变，PTCL 的预后一般比 DLBCL 差[84,85]。许多不常见的 PTCL 亚型具有独特的组织学特征。AITL 除了多形性的、不同种类的浸润细胞外，还存在丰富的高内皮小静脉。这个亚型的病变约 10%显示出 Ig 重链基因重排；大部分病变中能够检测到 *EBV* 基因组序列，既可以在 B 细胞中，也可以在 T 细胞中[86]。AITL 主要影响老年人，表现为急性全身淋巴肿大、肝脾肿大、皮疹和 B 型症状[86]。免疫异常多见，包括浆细胞增多症，多克隆高人免疫球蛋白血症和 Coombs 检测阳性，中位存活时间为 30 个月，感染是最常见的死亡原因，其次是 T 细胞淋巴瘤或发展为 EBV 阳性 DLBCL。

ALCL 是一种 T 细胞 NHL，可表现为原发性全身 ALCL，ALK 阳性；原发性全身 ALCL，ALK 阴性；原发性皮肤 ALCL。当累及淋巴结时，表现为淋巴窦内有怪异的大细胞。这种病变的肿瘤细胞通常具有活化成熟 T 细胞的表型，表达 HLA-DR、CD30 和 CD25。应用 ALK1 的单克隆抗体可以在 40%~60%的 ALCL 病变中检测到 ALK 表达，在携带 t(2;5)的病例中表现为胞核和胞质阳性[87]。由此产生的融合基因编码具有组成酪氨酸激酶活性的嵌合 NPM-ALK 融合蛋白。ALK 阳性病例在儿童和年轻人较常见，其预后好于 ALK 阴性病例[88]。

ALCL 占成人 NHL 的 2%，是第二常见的 T 细胞淋巴瘤，发病中位年龄 34 岁，以男性为主。该病呈双峰分布，高峰出现在儿童、青年和成年后期。在成人中，B 症状、外周淋巴结肿大和腹膜淋巴结肿大常见，皮肤是结外病变常见部位(约 25%的患者)，骨髓受侵不常见。ALCL 有一种不寻常的表现形式，发病在乳房内，这与乳房植入物有关[89]。全身性 ALCL ALK 阳性患者与 DLBCL 预后相似[90]，在 ALCL、PTCL NOS 和 AITL 三者中，ALCL 的 OS 最高，而 AITL 最低[91]。

灰区淋巴瘤

灰色区淋巴瘤包括无法分类的 B 细胞淋巴瘤，其特征介于 BL 与 DLBCL 之间(B-UNC/BL/DLBCL)和 DLBCL 与经典 HL 之间(B-UNC/cHL/DLBCL)[22]。

特征介于 BL 和 DLBCL 之间(B-UNC/BL/DLBCL)的无法分类的 B 细胞淋巴瘤，具有中至大的肿瘤细胞大小，可能有很高的 Ki67 指数和 CD10(+)，细胞的大小比 BL 变化更大，通常是 BCL2 阳性，BCL6 可能是阴性，Ki67 指数可能低于 100%，GEP 已经证明这些具有异质性[92]。30%~45%的患者有染色体易位，包括 *c-myc* 和 BCL-2，被称为"双打击"淋巴瘤[68]。B-UNC/BL/DLBCL 常伴有高 IPI 的结外病变，预后较差。组织学上表现为双打击淋巴瘤的患者预后很差，中位 OS 为 4 个月[93]。

特征介于 DLBCL 与经典 HL 之间(B-UNC/cHL/DLBCL)的无法分类的 B 细胞淋巴瘤，特征介于 PMBCL 与经典 HL 之间，或 B-UNC/cHL/DLBCL。这种罕见的疾病常见于纵隔肿块的男性。组织学上与经典 HL 的里-施细胞相似，与 DLBCL 或 PML-BCL 的大细胞相似，可见纤维间质和炎性浸润。恶性细胞表达 CD45、CD20、CD79a 和 CD30，但通常 CD15(-)；其他 B 细胞标志物如 PAX5、OCT-2 和 BOB1 通常呈阳性，这些患者的预后均差于经典 HL 和 PMLBCL，尚未证实其最佳治疗方法[94]。

高度侵袭性淋巴瘤

前体 T 细胞性或者 B 淋巴母细胞性白血病/淋巴瘤

淋巴母细胞性淋巴瘤(LBL)与急性淋巴母细胞性白血病(ALL)(参见第 116 章)是同一疾病的两种表现，LBL 的定义是骨髓受累小于 25%，肿瘤细胞核/浆比高，胞质少，细胞核染色质细，有多个小核仁，核分裂指数高，胞核可以折叠或者扭曲。一般情况下，受累淋巴结结构消失，代之以恶性细胞(图 119-5)。

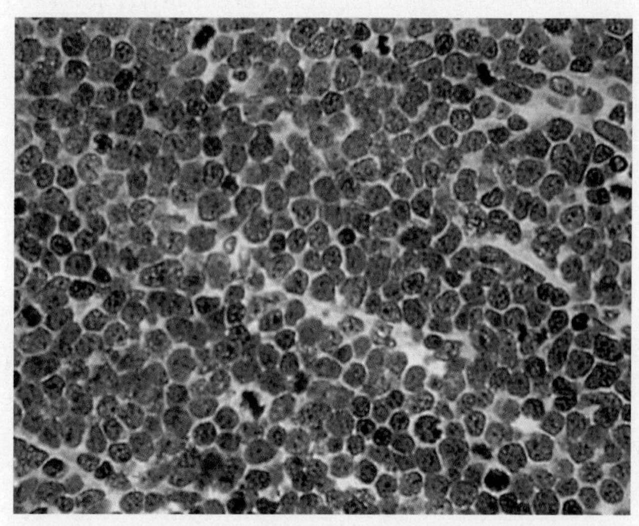

图 119-5　T-淋巴母细胞性淋巴瘤

绝大多数 LBL 来源于 T 细胞。几项研究已经表明大多数 T 细胞性 LBL 相当于胸腺细胞分化的不同阶段(参见第 116 章)。

虽然 LBL 是儿童 NHL 的一个主要亚群，但在成人中并不常见(占成人 NHL 的 2%)。患者通常为 20~30 岁男性，表现为颈部、锁骨上、腋窝淋巴结肿大(50%)或纵隔肿块(50%~75%)，这与上腔静脉综合征、气管阻塞和心包积液有关。一小部分患者表现为结外疾病(如皮肤、睾丸或骨骼受侵)。超过 80%的患者为晚期疾病，近 50%有 B 症状，大多数患者 LDH 升高。虽然初始骨髓通常是正常的，但几乎所有的患者都会发展为骨髓浸润和随后的白血病阶段。骨髓受侵的患者发生中枢神经系统浸润概率也很高。B 细胞 LBL 是一种非常罕见的变异,患者的中位年龄为 39 岁[95],B 细胞 LBL 无纵隔肿块出现,但会累及淋巴结和结外部位。

Burkitt 淋巴瘤

Burkitt 淋巴瘤(BL)细胞与正常次级滤泡生发中心的小无裂细胞相似。由于核分裂速度快,分裂象很常见。与正常生发中心类似,可见吞噬小体巨噬细胞,呈经典的“满天星”(starry sky)表现。一般来讲,Ki-67 抗原标记指数(增殖细胞所占比例)应该为 99%或者更高[22]。

Burkitt 淋巴瘤是一种 B 细胞肿瘤,表达 B 细胞限制性抗原,包括 CD19、CD20、表面 IgM、CD10 和 BCL-6 核蛋白[96]。地方性 Burkitt 淋巴瘤呈 EBV 阳性,而大部分非地方性 Burkitt 淋巴瘤 EBV 阴性,Burkitt 淋巴瘤缺乏 BCL-2 蛋白。

95%的 Burkitt 淋巴瘤携带 8q24 与 14、2 或者 22 之间的染色体转位[22]。在基因表达谱方面,经病理诊断检出的 Burkitt 淋巴瘤以及非典型 Burkitt 淋巴瘤表现为 *myc* 靶基因过表达、正常生发中心基因不同程度地表达以及 MHC Ⅰ和 NF-κB 的靶基因表达减低,这些研究有助于一些难分类病例的组织学诊断[92,97,98]。

一般来说,BL 是一种儿童肿瘤,有三种主要的临床表现地区性、散发性和免疫缺陷相关。地区性(非洲)表现为颌面部骨肿瘤,可扩散到结外部位包括卵巢、睾丸、肾脏、乳房,尤其是骨髓和脑膜。散发性表现为腹部肿块、腹水、肾脏、睾丸和卵巢受累,而且与地区性一样,也会扩散到骨髓和中枢神经系统。与免疫缺陷相关的患者常涉及淋巴结和外周血。BL 以男性为主,多在 35 岁以下发病,这些肿瘤很容易侵犯骨髓和中枢神经系统。

成人 T 细胞白血病/淋巴瘤

ATLL 是一种罕见的疾病,发病全部与 HTLV-1 感染有关[99-101],在日本南部、加勒比海流域、非洲和美国东南部流行。正常肿瘤细胞对应的是活化的 CD4+T 细胞,表达 CD2、CD3、CD5 和 CD25。发病中位年龄为 60 岁[102],该病可表现为四种变异型:急性(最常见和高度侵袭性)、淋巴瘤性、慢性和冒烟性,这些变异型的中位生存期分别为 6 个月、10 个月、24 个月和“未达到”[103]。该病浸润骨髓和外周血,高白细胞计数、血钙过多(由于 PTH-相关蛋白质、TGF-β 和等级配体),溶骨性病变,淋巴结肿大,肝脾肿大,皮肤病变、间质性肺浸润。

鉴别诊断和肿瘤侵犯部位

超过 2/3 的非霍奇金淋巴瘤患者表现为持续的无痛性外周淋巴结肿大,就诊时与普通淋巴结病变的鉴别诊断必须排除感染性病因。一般认为较硬的大于 1.5cm×1.5cm 的淋巴结,与已确定的感染无关,持续 4~6 周以上,并且进展增大,应该考虑做活检。然而,某些病理类型的非霍奇金淋巴瘤经常表现为有时增大有时缩小。对于青少年人,应该在鉴别诊断时首先考虑传染性单核细胞增多症和霍奇金淋巴瘤。与霍奇金淋巴瘤相比,非霍奇金淋巴瘤患者韦氏环、滑车上和肠系膜淋巴结受侵更常见。不像霍奇金淋巴瘤患者常常伴有消瘦、发热、盗汗症状,只有大约 40%的非霍奇金淋巴瘤患者伴有全身症状。在侵袭性病理类型的患者中 B 症状更常见,接近 50%。发生率低于 20%的少见症状包括疲劳、乏力和皮肤瘙痒。

非霍奇金淋巴瘤也会出现胸部、腹部和/或结外部位的症状。虽然比霍奇金淋巴瘤少见,但将近 20%的非霍奇金淋巴瘤患者具有纵隔淋巴结病变。这些患者最常出现持续性咳嗽、胸部不适,或者虽然无临床症状,但有胸部影像学的异常。偶尔会出现上腔静脉压迫综合征。纵隔病变的鉴别诊断包括感染(如组织胞浆菌病、结核、传染性单核细胞增多症)、结节病、霍奇金淋巴瘤,以及其他肿瘤。腹膜后、肠系膜、盆腔淋巴结受侵常见于大多数非霍奇金淋巴瘤病理类型中。除非有巨大肿块或引起梗阻,这些部位的淋巴结增大通常不引起症状。相反,腹部肿块、显著的脾肿大,或原发胃肠道淋巴瘤患者的症状与那些其他腹部占位病变引起的症状相似。这包括慢性疼痛、腹胀、与内脏梗阻有关的早饱症状,甚或急性穿孔和胃肠道出血,少见的患者出现不可解释的贫血症状。那些侵袭性非霍奇金淋巴瘤可以出现原发皮肤病灶、睾丸肿块、急性脊髓压迫、孤立的骨病灶和罕见的淋巴瘤脑膜炎。原发中枢神经系统淋巴瘤的症状包括头痛、昏睡、局灶性神经系统症状、癫痫发作、瘫痪。

当非霍奇金淋巴瘤侵犯结外部位时,鉴别诊断就更为困难。非霍奇金淋巴瘤不常侵犯肺,表现为支气管血管束、淋巴管炎、结节、肺泡受侵[104]。虽然很少表现为肝内大肿块,25%~50%的非霍奇金淋巴瘤会出现肝浸润。晚期惰性淋巴瘤中,近 75%的患者在就诊时可有镜下肝浸润。相反,原发肝的淋巴瘤罕见,且几乎总是侵袭性的病理类型。另一结外受侵部位是原发骨的淋巴瘤,发生于不到 5%的患者,表现为局部骨痛。最常见的表现是在标准 X 线片下可见溶骨性病灶。原发骨淋巴瘤的最常见部位是股骨、骨盆、椎骨。将近 5%的非霍奇金淋巴瘤是原发胃肠道的淋巴瘤。这些患者表现为出血、疼痛或梗阻,胃是最常受侵的部位,其次分别是小肠和结肠。大多数胃肠道淋巴瘤属于弥漫性侵袭性病理类型,特别是弥漫性大 B 细胞淋巴瘤、套细胞淋巴瘤和小肠 T 细胞淋巴瘤。结外边缘带淋巴瘤最常见的侵犯部位是胃。套细胞淋巴瘤的一个亚群表现为多发小肠息肉,可侵犯胃肠道的任何部位。肾浸润不常见(2%~14%),前列腺、睾丸、卵巢的局部浸润更少见,这些部位的典型病理学类型是 DLBCL 和 Burkitt 淋巴瘤,原发于其他罕见部位的淋巴瘤包括眼眶、心、乳腺、唾液腺、甲状腺、肾上腺。

分期和检测

1971 年开始用于霍奇金淋巴瘤的 Ann Arbor 分期系统,也被用于非霍奇金淋巴瘤的分期[105]。这个分期系统着重于肿瘤侵犯区域(结内和结外)的数量、部位和有无全身症状。表 119-3 总结了 Ann Arbor 分期的基本特点。因为非霍奇金淋巴瘤通常是经血行播散,这个分期系统对 NHL 作用远不如 HL。

全身“B”症状(发热、盗汗和体重减轻)不再包括在 NHL 分期系统中,因为这些症状不是患者的独立预后因素。

对于非霍奇金淋巴瘤,分期的意义比在霍奇金淋巴瘤中小很多。多个研究显示,相比于就诊时的分期,非霍奇金淋巴瘤的预后更多地依赖于组织学和临床参数。对非霍奇金淋巴瘤进行分期的目的是识别出少量能采用局部治疗或联合治疗模式的患者,以及在不同病理类型内再分层,以决定预后和评价治疗的影响。

表 119-3 非霍奇金淋巴瘤修订分期系统

分期	受累部位	结外病变(E)
局限期		
Ⅰ期	侵及单一淋巴结区	单个结外器官或组织受侵,没有淋巴结受累
Ⅱ期	侵及横膈同侧两个或多个淋巴结区	横膈同侧的单一结外器官或部位的局限受侵伴有区域淋巴结受侵
Ⅱ期(巨块型)*	巨块型Ⅱ期疾病	不适用
进展期		
Ⅲ期	横膈两侧的淋巴结区受侵;横膈上方淋巴结区受有脾脏受侵	不适用
Ⅳ期	弥漫性或播散性侵犯一个或更多结外部位	不适用

* Ⅱ期巨块型疾病按局限期还是进展期治疗,取决于组织学类型和预后因素。

诊断和初步评估

分期检查必须结合病理类型来进行。在最初活检之后,应完成血液学检查,包括全血细胞计数、常规生化、肝功能,以及血清蛋白电泳以确定血液循环中是否存在单克隆副蛋白。应进行 HIV、乙肝(可能通过淋巴瘤治疗重新激活)和丙肝血清学检查。血清 β_2-微球水平在惰性淋巴瘤中可代表肿瘤负荷,在非霍奇金淋巴瘤中血清 LDH 的浓度是重要的独立预测生存指标。孤立的韦氏环受侵与小肠受侵相关,约出现在 20% 的患者,因此应考虑进行内镜检查。要精确分期必须进行胸、腹、盆腔 CT 检查评价淋巴结病变。应行单侧骨髓活检,因为淋巴瘤侵犯骨髓的可能性还是相对较高的,特别是对于大多数惰性淋巴瘤,大部分患者会发生骨髓受侵。近年来骨髓活检在 DLBCL 中的作用受到质疑,在近期 PET/CT 对 DLBCL 患者进行初步分期的分析中,PET 扫描对骨髓受累的敏感性和特异性分别为 89% 和 99% 以上,PET 扫描阴性的患者仍应行骨髓活检,但 PET 扫描阳性显示骨髓受累的患者的活检价值有限[106]。对于有骨髓受侵、鼻旁窦受侵、椎旁肿块、睾丸受侵或有临床指征的侵袭性淋巴瘤,应进行腰穿检查脑脊液(CSF)。PET 使用[18]氟脱氧葡萄糖是一种高灵敏度和特异性的扫描模式,用于检测淋巴结和结外部位的 NHL,对 DLBCL、MCL 和 FL 非常有用,推荐在这些类型在初始分期中进行 PET 扫描。PET 扫描对 SLL 和 MZL 不敏感[107]。

International Harmonization Project 关于 PET 扫描提出一致的建议,包括建议 PET 用于弥漫性大 B 细胞淋巴瘤和霍奇金淋巴瘤;治疗期间的 PET 扫描仍然只是临床研究的一部分。全部治疗完成后的 PET 扫描至少应在化疗后 3 周再做,但推荐在化疗后 6~8 周进行,在放疗后或放化疗后 8~12 周进行,没有证据在长期随访时采用 PET 扫描[108],评价脑和脊髓时 MRI 是最有价值的。

免疫和分子研究

生物学研究包括细胞表面标志、细胞遗传学、用于诊断和分期的分子技术、微小肿瘤检测。针对淋巴样细胞表达的表面抗原的单抗,确定免疫球蛋白和 T 细胞受体基因重排的分子技术都是评估肿瘤细胞浸润的敏感工具。免疫表型和细胞遗传学研究能够帮助确定淋巴瘤的病理类型。对于那些具有已知的染色体易位的非霍奇金淋巴瘤,采用 FISH、细胞遗传学、PCR 方法进行检测,有可能鉴定出特有的染色体断点,微小肿瘤的检测研究可提供重要的预后信息。

影响预后及疗效评判的疾病参数

非霍奇金淋巴瘤的预后因素

侵袭性非霍奇金淋巴瘤

目前已经为许多 NHL 亚型建立了临床预后模型,基于一项包括 2 031 例罹患侵袭性弥漫性非霍奇金淋巴瘤且接受含蒽环类药物治疗的患者的大型临床研究分析,确立了著名的国际预后指数(international prognostic index,IPI)来对于预后情况进行预测(表 119-4)[109]。在众多可能影响的因素中,年龄(≤60 岁 vs >60 岁)、血清乳酸脱氢酶(LDH)水平(在正常上限内 vs 超出正常上限)、一般状况(ECOG 评分 0~1 vs 2~4)、分期(Ⅰ/Ⅱ期 vs Ⅲ/Ⅳ期),以及淋巴结外受侵(≤1 处 vs >1 处)均是总生存的独立预后因素。资料显示,依据危险评分可分成 4 组:低危-0~1 分,低中危-2 分,中高危-3 分,高危-4~5 分;5 年总生存率(OS)分别为 73%(0~1 分)、51%(2 分)、43%(3 分)和 26%(4~5 分)。IPI 评分也适用于评价接受 R-CHOP 方案治疗的弥漫大 B 细胞淋巴瘤,一项研究显示,对于评分为 0~1、2 及≥3 分的患者,其 4 年肿瘤无进展生存(PFS)分别为 94%、80% 和 53%[110]。

表 119-4 国际预后指数(IPI 评分)

国际预后指数(IPI)				
年龄>60 岁				
LDH>正常值上限				
ECOG PS 评分≥2 分				
Ann Arbor 分期:Ⅲ期或Ⅳ期				
结外病变受侵部位数>1				
危险因子	预后分组	3 年 EFS/%	3 年 PFS/%	3 年 OS/%
0~1	低危	81	87	91
2	低中危	69	75	81
3	高中危	53	59	65
4~5	高危	50	50	59

采用标准来源(Ziepert M,Hasenclever D,Kuhnt E,et al,Standard In-ter-national Prognostic Index remains avalid predictor of outcome for patients with aggressive CD20+B-cell lymphoma in the rituximab era. J Clin Oncol 2010;28:2373)。

ECOG,东部肿瘤协作组;EFS,无病生存期;LDH,乳酸脱氢酶;OS,总生存期;PFS,无进展生存期。

滤泡性非霍奇金淋巴瘤

基于对超过4 000例滤泡淋巴瘤患者生存的观察,确立的滤泡淋巴瘤国际预后指数(FLIPI),具有如下预后不良因子:年龄>60岁、Ⅲ/Ⅳ期、具有4个以上的受侵淋巴结区域、血清LDH增高及血红蛋白低于12g/dl。10年的总生存率对于不同评分的患者分别为:0~1分(低危)-71%,2分(中危)-51%和3分以上(高危)-36%(表119-5)[111]。同弥漫大B细胞淋巴瘤相似,利妥昔单抗显著改善了滤泡淋巴瘤的预后生存,而FLIPI评分对于预后的判断依然有效[112]。对于其他类型NHL,已经从统一治疗的患者人群中开发出预后模型。套细胞淋巴瘤国际预后指数(MIPI),包括年龄、PS、LDH和WBC作为预后因素[113]。单一的增殖指数以及增殖指数合并入MIPI时可以提供额外的预后效用[114]。已有多种预测PTCL NOS的模型报道,但总体上IPI提供了一个合理的结果分层,低风险患者2年OS为55%,高风险患者2年OS<15%[115]。

表119-5 滤泡淋巴瘤国际预后指数(FLIPI)

年龄>60岁			
LDH>正常值上限			
Hgb<12g/dl			
Ann Arbor分期:Ⅲ期或Ⅳ期			
受累淋巴结区的数目>4			
危险因子	预后分组	5年OS/%	10年OS/%
0~1	低危	91	71
2	中危	78	51
3~5	高危	52	36

采用标准来源(Solal-Celigny P, Roy P, Colombat P, et al, Follicular lymphoma international prognostic index. Blood 2004;104:1258)。

Hgb,血红蛋白;LDH,乳酸脱氢酶;OS,总生存期。

基因表达谱作为预后因素

通过基因芯片技术,基因表达谱可以将弥漫大B细胞淋巴瘤患者分成不同的预后[58~60,116]。基于基因表达的不同,弥漫大B细胞淋巴瘤可分为生发中心型或活化B细胞型两种不同的亚型;生发中心型弥漫大B细胞淋巴瘤总生存明显好于后者。基于来自基因表达谱的发现,利用组织芯片的免疫组化技术,可通过有限的基因产物来作为标志物以判断预后[116]。生发中心型或非生发中心型B细胞可以通过CD10、BCL-6和MUM1的表达来加以区分。应用组织芯片区分,弥漫大B细胞淋巴瘤中,42%为生发中心型,58%为非生发中心型。

在滤泡淋巴瘤,基因表达谱显示根据非肿瘤细胞浸润相关的基因可以将患者分为预后良好和预后不良亚组,具有Ⅰ类免疫应答标志(与某些T细胞和巨噬细胞标志物相关的基因表达)预后良好,Ⅱ类免疫应答标志(在巨噬细胞中高表达的基因)预后不良[117]。套细胞淋巴瘤患者的基因表达谱显示,细胞周期蛋白D1的增殖信号和高表达与预后不良有关[114]。

根据WHO分类的治疗手段

惰性淋巴瘤

早期惰性淋巴瘤的治疗

10%~20%的惰性淋巴瘤患者分期为Ⅰ/Ⅱ期,所有的组织学亚型均应行根治性局部放疗。一项来自Stanford的研究对177名患者(44%Ⅰ期和56%Ⅱ期)进行分析,其中大多数患者接受了扩大范围的放疗[118],该项研究中患者的10年、15年、20年生存率分别为64%、44%、35%,无复发生存率为44%、40%、37%。在最近的一项报告中超过6 000例Ⅰ期或Ⅱ期滤泡性淋巴瘤患者,最初接受放疗的34%的患者有更高的疾病特异性生存期(disease-specific survival),5年、10年、15年、20年的生存率分别为90% vs 81%,79% vs 66%,68% vs 57%,63% vs 51%[119]。最近的一项回顾性分析表明,与单纯放疗相比,化疗免疫疗法或全身疗法联合放疗可改善PFS,但对OS无影响[120]。在一项小规模的回顾性研究中,报道了观察即没有立即治疗可成为一种替代方案,特别是对Ⅱ期患者[121],中位OS为19年,中位随访7年,63%的患者不需要治疗。

淋巴结外的边缘带淋巴瘤(MZL)常为局限性疾病,常侵犯胃肠道、唾液腺、甲状腺、眼眶、眼结膜、乳腺和肺。在幽门螺杆菌相关的胃MZL患者中,使用抗生素和质子泵抑制剂治疗可诱导80%以上的患者疾病消退,长期疾病控制良好,并有少数患者长期生存[122~124]。BCL-10核表达和/或t(11;18)有助于前瞻性识别那些不能从抗HP中获益的胃边缘带淋巴瘤[125]。眼的MZL有使用多西环素抗衣原体治疗报道了不同的结果[8],单药利妥昔单抗对初诊患者的总有效率(RR)为87%[130]。

对于经抗HP治疗进展或HP阴性的局限期胃MZL,行受累野放疗±手术治疗10年无病生存率超过90%[126,127]。其他的结外MZL,由于其长期处于局限期,手术是非常有效的治疗手段,术后考虑受累野放疗。一项回顾性研究中,ⅠE及ⅡE期MZL行单独放疗,5年无病生存率及总生存率分别为76%与96%,发病部位在胃与发病部位在甲状腺与其他部位相比,5年无病生存率分别为93%与69%($P=0.006$)[128]。MZL患者使用烷化剂、氟达拉滨或单用利妥昔单抗治疗的有效率高[129,130]。

晚期惰性淋巴瘤的治疗

无症状瘤负荷小的患者可密切监测而无须积极治疗,惰性淋巴瘤的自然病程很长,一些患者在诊断时缺乏症状,这些患者中有很多把密切观察作为首要手段。在Stanford和British National Lymphoma Investigation的研究中[131],将无症状的患者随机分为两组,一组接受初始治疗,另一组推迟治疗,直到出现症状(通常进展为体积较大肿瘤),两者总生存无差异。在Stanford研究中,到需要治疗的中位时间为3年[132]。在利妥昔单抗时代,已经研究过"观察等待"与"观察"之间的疗效比较。一项前瞻性研究比较观察组、利妥昔单抗单药组或利妥昔单抗维持治疗组对未经治疗滤泡性淋巴瘤的疗效,观察等待的患者到下一次治疗的中位时间为34个月,但利妥昔单抗治疗组中位时间没有达到,患者进行观察、利妥昔单抗单药治疗、利妥昔单抗维持治疗的3年PFS率分别为33%、80%、90%,三组中3年OS率均为95%[133]。

利妥昔单抗的应用改变了晚期FL的治疗模式,三期随机试验显示利妥昔单抗联合化疗方案可以显著改善疗效[134~138]。所有这些研究都表明含利妥昔单抗组可以改善缓解率、至疾病进展时间和总生存时间。

有研究用其他治疗方案与利妥昔单抗加环磷酰胺、多柔比星、长春新碱、泼尼松(R-CHOP)方案比较,以提高疗效和减少毒性。一项Ⅲ期试验比较苯达莫司汀-利妥昔单抗(BR)与R-CHOP方案疗效,主要包括滤泡性淋巴瘤、套细胞淋巴瘤和边缘带淋巴瘤[139],在45个月时中位PFS R-CHOP方案优于BR方案(69.5个月 vs 31.2个月),两组OS无差异。此外BR组具有更低的毒性,包括3/4级中性粒细胞降低和白细胞降低的发生率更低。几项Ⅱ期试验采用利妥昔单抗单药作为懒惰性淋巴瘤的初始治疗,总缓解率为54%~73%[140~142]。其中一项试验的中位随访时间为30个月,中位PFS为34个月。此外,与观察相比,利妥昔单抗延长治疗可增加2倍的无事件生存率(EFS)。对于初始治疗的患者使用短期的利妥昔单抗维持治疗,8年的无进展生存率是45%[143]。初治的滤泡性淋巴瘤应用放射免疫疗法,^{90}Y-替伊莫单抗(ibritumomab-tiuxetan)和^{131}I-托西莫单抗(不再可用)在Ⅱ期研究中取得了优异的结果[144,145],但与利妥昔单抗相比是否获益尚未评估。在一项随机试验中,比较R-CHOP方案和CHOP方案化疗后应用^{131}I-托西莫单抗治疗的疗效,两组PFS无差异[146]。

一个大型Ⅲ期试验研究化疗免疫治疗后应用利妥昔单抗维持治疗[147],与观察相比,利妥昔单抗维持治疗改善了PFS,但到目前为止,化疗免疫治疗[R-CVP、R-CHOP或氟达拉滨、环磷酰胺、米托蒽醌和利妥昔单抗(FCM-R)]后缓解的初治滤泡性淋巴瘤患者,利妥昔单抗维持治疗对OS没有影响。

其他惰性淋巴瘤的治疗

除FL外的其他惰性NHL包括结内型和结外型MZL,通常与FL治疗相似。SLL患者采用慢性淋巴细胞白血病的化学免疫治疗方案治疗(参见第117章),MZL应用R-CHOP方案和BR方案治疗,PFS无明显差异。对于淋巴浆细胞性淋巴瘤,治疗方案包括地塞米松、利妥昔单抗、环磷酰胺[148]、BR、硼替佐米和利妥昔单抗±地塞米松[149]。地塞米松、利妥昔单抗和环磷酰胺方案总缓解率和完全缓解率分别为83和7%,2年OS和PFS率分别为81%和67%。脾脏MZL常从脾脏切除中获益,且症状得到良好控制,血细胞减少也得到改善[150]。单药利妥昔单抗和免疫化疗的缓解率和5年PFS率均超过90%[130]。

高剂量治疗和自体干细胞移植(ASCT)已用于FL患者首次缓解时[151~156],这会增加了患者患有包括MDS/AML和实体瘤在内的第二种恶性肿瘤的风险,大多数随机试验在使用利妥昔单抗之前进行,研究显示PFS有显著改善,但OS没有获益[157]。

复发的惰性淋巴瘤仍然对利妥昔单抗单药和利妥昔单抗联合化疗等药物敏感;但是化疗免疫疗法的中位无复发生存时间随着每次复发而逐渐降低。利妥昔单抗单药治疗复发性FL的最新进展来自随机的SAKK试验,Martinelli等人发现35%的应答者在8年后仍处于缓解状态。然而利妥昔单抗单药作为诱导治疗方案,其疗效是否会与未接受利妥昔单抗的化疗患者一样好或持久,目前仍不确定。

一项Ⅱ期试验显示利妥昔单抗治疗复发的惰性NHL总缓解率为40%[158],其中11%患者完全缓解,预计中位PFS为18个月。利妥昔单抗与其他药物联合治疗复发/耐药患者,取得不错的疗效。一项Ⅲ期研究[159]对之前没有接受过蒽环类药物或利妥昔单抗治疗的复发的滤泡性淋巴瘤患者,随机分配至CHOP和R-CHOP组,产生应答的患者接受第二次随机分组,给予利妥昔单抗最多2年的维持治疗(375mg/m^{2}静脉注射,每3个月一次),或给予观察。总缓解率(85% vs 72%)、完全缓解率(30% vs 16%)和PFS(33个月 vs 20个月),在R-CHOP组中均显著升高。无论采用何种诱导方案,第二次随机化时接受利妥昔单抗维持治疗的患者中位PFS更长(52个月 vs 15个月)。此外,与观察组结果相比,利妥昔单抗维持治疗也显著改善了3年OS率(85% vs 77%)。许多Ⅱ期试验应用其他药物联合利妥昔单抗治疗与高的缓解率相关,其中BR方案的缓解率为90%,中位PFS为2年[160,161]。

放射免疫耦合剂被美国食品药品管理局(FDA)批准用于治疗复发FL,^{90}Y-替伊莫单抗治疗复发患者的缓解率为82%,完全缓解率为26%,中位缓解持续时间>12个月[162]。在一项Ⅲ期临床研究中,143例复发难治的低度恶性淋巴瘤、FL和转化型非霍奇金淋巴瘤患者,利妥昔单抗或利妥昔单抗联合^{90}Y-替伊莫单抗治疗的总缓解率分别为56%和80%[163],放射免疫疗法在惰性淋巴瘤治疗模式中的作用仍不确定。PI3Kδ亚型特异性抑制剂艾代拉里斯(idelalisib)最近被批准用于复发滤泡性和小淋巴细胞性淋巴瘤,总缓解率为57%,中位缓解持续时间为12.5个月[164]。

FL对低剂量(如总剂量为4Gy,连续2日给予2Gy量)放射治疗敏感,可用于单个部位的姑息治疗,完全缓解率为57%,总缓解率为82%,且耐受性良好[165]。

复发惰性淋巴瘤的自体造血干细胞移植

长期随访的Ⅱ期临床研究提示化疗敏感的复发FL亚组经过自体造血干细胞支持下的大剂量化疗预后好,12年无病生存率为48%[71,144,166]。在欧洲CUP临床试验中[167],89例复发进展的FL患者接受3周期CHOP方案,获得缓解且骨髓受累少于20%者随机接受3周期以上CHOP方案或自体造血干细胞支持下的大剂量化疗,进行或不进行抗B细胞单抗的净化。中位随访69个月,所有入组患者的5年生存率为50%,自体造血干细胞移植组的中位生存还未达到,无病生存与总生存均有利于自体移植组,但与有无净化并无差异。

同种异体干细胞移植治疗复发性FL

对于复发的FL患者,采用了清髓和降低强度预处理(RIC)两种方法,清髓性移植治疗相关的死亡率高达40%,然而复发率<20%[168]。相比之下,RIC alloSCT具有较低的治疗相关死亡率[169~171],但有报道表明其复发率可能高于传统的清髓性移植。alloSCT与ASCT对FL的疗效比较尚不清楚,最近一项NCCN数据库的回顾性分析发现,ASCT的3年OS明显高于alloSCT(87% vs 61%)[172]。对于经过选择的患者,alloSCT仍是复发性FL的潜在治疗方案。

组织转化

惰性淋巴瘤发生组织转化后预后很差,尤其是以前治疗过的患者[173]，大宗报道显示FL发生组织转化后中位生存仅11个月[174]。在Stanford研究的一项报道中，获得完全缓解者5年实际生存率75%，除此以外中位生存期仅有22个月[175]。几项研究报道了FL组织学转化后患者ASCT的疗效，DFS为40%~50%，DLBCL和FL的患者均可复发[176~179]。针对经选择的化疗敏感的患者进行自体移植强化治疗是可行的选择。

侵袭性淋巴瘤

恶性淋巴瘤WHO分类中，侵袭性淋巴瘤包括弥漫大B细胞淋巴瘤（DLBCL）、套细胞淋巴瘤（MCL）、外周T细胞淋巴瘤（PTCL）非特指或特指型、间变大细胞淋巴瘤（ALCL）（表119-2）。

早期侵袭性淋巴瘤的治疗

DLBCL中真正为局限期的患者少于20%，除外临床研究，局限期DLBCL推荐治疗为短疗程化疗联合受累野放疗（involved field radiotherapy，IFRT），或者进行单纯化疗。SWOG的随机研究对8个周期CHOP方案单纯化疗或3周期CHOP化疗联合IFRT治疗局限期DLBCL患者进行了比较，结果显示短疗程化疗联合IFRT优于单纯化疗，具有更好的5年无进展生存率（PFS）和总生存率（OS），分别为77% vs 64%和82% vs 72%[180]，年龄超过60岁的患者通过短疗程化疗联合IFRT获益更大。另一项随机研究比较了8个周期CHOP方案加或不加IFRT治疗初治Ⅰ期具有巨块或结外受累及Ⅱ期弥漫大细胞淋巴瘤患者的疗效，尽管10年OS（68% vs 65%）两组相似，但对于获得完全缓解（complete remission，CR）患者加放疗的无疾病生存率（DFS）更好（73% vs 56%）[181]，放疗对部分Ⅰ/Ⅱ期患者的价值仍不明确。对于年龄≤60岁的低危患者，高强化方案ACVBP单纯化疗的疗效优于CHOP方案联合RT[182]。同样有研究显示，对于年龄>60岁的患者，相比4周期CHOP方案单纯化疗，CHOP方案联合IFRT未能提高DFS和OS[183]。这些研究提出了早期DLBCL放疗必要性的问题，对至少有一个危险因素的早期DLBCL患者（年龄>60岁；血清LDH增高；Ⅱ期疾病；或PS≥1）采用R-CHOP三个周期再进行累及野放射治疗[184]，2年、4年的PFS和OS分别为93%、88%和95%、92%。一项Ⅲ期研究评估≤60岁、IPI评分为0或1分的患者，均为体积较大的肿瘤（肿块>7.5cm）或结外部位接受了累及野放疗，比较CHOP和R-CHOP方案6个周期的治疗效果，对于IPI评分为0分，无大肿块病变，包括早期患者，R-CHOP方案的5年EFS约为90%，提示单纯化疗免疫治疗是早期疾病的一种选择。然而具有大肿块的患者（定义为肿块>7.5cm）预后较差。在比较CHOP与R-CHOP的疗效的MiNT试验中，所有>7.5cm肿块的患者（IPI 0或IPI 1）都接受了30~40Gy累及野的放疗，那些IPI为0和大肿块患者的PFS比没有大肿块者低10%~15%[185]。在对类似群体进行的UNFOLDER试验中，早期数据表明化疗后放疗有获益。目前，对早期DLBCL合并大肿块病变者的最适当治疗仍存在争议。

PMLBCL患者常表现为早期疾病，从历史上看，患者都接受过联合治疗模式。在MInT试验中，87例PMLBCL患者接受了6个周期的R-CHOP方案治疗，其中75%的患者还接受了放疗，接受放射治疗的患者中，只有7%的人后来病情进展或复发[186]。最近的一项研究对51名接受剂量调整的EPOCH联合利妥昔单抗（DA-EPOCH-R）且未接受RT治疗的患者进行评估，结果显示PFS（93%）和OS（100%）表现突出[187]。就是否需要放射治疗而言，最近的一项研究报告表明，在没有放疗的情况下，治疗结束时PET/CT扫描阴性者有较好的疗效[188]。

结外NK/T细胞淋巴瘤早期病变占97%，ⅠE期患者的5年OS和PFS分别为78%和63%，ⅡE期患者的OS和PFS分别为46%和40%，联合治疗模式与单纯放疗疗效无差异[189]。对于ⅠE/ⅡE期患者，早期应用RT（50~55Gy）至关重要，而初始化疗后应用RT效果较差。最近的研究表明联合治疗可能产生更好的结果，几项Ⅱ期试验给予同步放疗联合顺铂（每周给药），随后给予依托泊苷、异环磷酰胺、顺铂和地塞米松方案，总体RR为83%，3年PFS和OS分别为85%和86%[190,191]。

晚期侵袭性淋巴瘤的治疗

如果不能参加临床研究，目前对于晚期DLBCL或PTCL，分别推荐采用R-CHOP或CHOP联合化疗方案。最近临床试验研究的主要问题是化疗的周期数以及周期的间隔时间。对于年龄60~80岁的老年DLBCL患者，GELA的研究显示，无论是PFS、DFS还是OS，8个周期的R-CHOP方案优于单用CHOP方案[192,193]。一项美国60岁以上人群的分组研究[194]，患者先随机接受CHOP方案或R-CHOP方案治疗，有效者再随机分为利妥昔单抗维持治疗组和观察组，加上利妥昔单抗的R-CHOP方案化疗，同样能够带来无事件生存（EFS）和OS的获益，但对已经接受过利妥昔单抗诱导治疗的患者，使用维持治疗并不提高疗效。同样，对于60岁以下的中低危患者（IPI为0或1分），R-CHOP较CHOP能够改善TTF（到治疗失败时间）和OS，特别是IPI为1分的患者获益更大[185]。

在RICOVER研究中，对于60岁以上的患者，6个或8个周期的R-CHOP方案优于CHOP方案（70% vs 57%），8个周期的R-CHOP方案并未优于6个周期的R-CHOP方案[195]。在另一项研究中，给予每21日一次的R-CHOP方案8个周期，与每14日一次的R-CHOP 6个周期进行比较，PFS或OS无差异[196]，这支持给予每21日一次的R-CHOP方案6个周期作为标准治疗。R-CHOP的替代方案已在Ⅲ期试验中得到验证，在60岁以下IPI评分为1分的患者中，应用强化的R-ACVBP方案诱导治疗后与给予甲氨蝶呤联合亮氨酸巩固治疗[197]，与R-CHOP联合鞘内甲氨蝶呤治疗进行比较，在非生发中心亚组中，R-ACVBP加甲氨蝶呤和亮氨酸方案有更高的PFS和OS[198]。

睾丸弥漫大B细胞淋巴瘤

从历史数据上看，原发性睾丸DLBCL的长期治疗结果比通过国际预测指数（IPI）预测的结果要差[199,200]。在一项研究中对53例未经治疗的Ⅰ期或Ⅱ期原发性睾丸淋巴瘤患者给予每21日一次的6~8个周期R-CHOP方案，并鞘内注射每周一次的4个周期甲氨蝶呤（12mg），所有患者行对侧睾丸放疗（30Gy），Ⅱ期患者给予区域淋巴结放疗（30~36Gy），中位随访65个月，5年OS和PFS分别为85%和74%。

使用药物预防DLBCL中枢神经系统浸润存在很大争议[201]，在前利妥昔单抗时代，中枢神经系统受累的风险为2.8%，其中实质内和椎管内疾病发生率为66%，孤立性脑膜转移发生率为26%[202]。危险因素包括疾病部位（睾丸、卵巢、骨髓、乳房、硬膜外间隙、肾脏、肾上腺和鼻旁窦）；IPI评分高；多个结外部位受侵和细胞遗传学的“双打击”。由于脑实质复发数量较多,仅鞘内化疗可能不足以预防,因此高剂量甲氨蝶呤可能是一种更有效的治疗方法。然而,没有足够的证据表明高剂量甲氨蝶呤优于鞘内注射治疗。

新的 WHO 分类亚型 B-UNC/BL/DLBCL 的治疗方法尚不确定[203,204],有回顾性研究表明,改良的 CODOX-M/IVAC(环磷酰胺、长春新碱、多柔比星、高剂量甲氨蝶呤联合异环磷酰胺、阿糖胞苷、依托泊苷和鞘内甲氨蝶呤)、HyperCVAD 和 DA-EPOCH-R 等强化治疗方案的疗效优于 R-CHOP 方案(ORR 86% vs 57%,4 年 PFS 50%~65% vs 0~30%)[205],发生 *c-myc* 易位的患者预后很差。National Cancer Institute 进行的一项应用 DA-EPOCH-R 方案治疗 *myc* 易位阳性的 DLBCL 的Ⅱ期研究颇具前景[206]。目前正在进行一项多中心研究,旨在进一步探索该方案在 BL 和 *MYC* 易位阳性的 DLBCL 的疗效。B-UNC/BL/DLBCL 亚型具有异质性,B-UNC/BL/DLBCL 的亚型中很多是双打击淋巴瘤,这些病变使用 R-CHOP 方案并不能满足临床需要。

对于局限期和晚期 PTCL 患者,采取与 DLBCL 类似的治疗方法。当患者按 IPI 分层时,PTCL 患者的 PFS 和 OS 均普遍低于 DLBCL 患者,目前还没有明确的证据支持其他不同方案治疗 PTCL 的优越性[207]。一项Ⅲ期研究回顾性的亚组分析比较 CHOP 方案和 CHOP+依托泊苷方案的疗效,发现年龄小于 60 岁、诊断时 LDH 正常的 PTCL 患者 EFS 明显改善,但 OS 无差异。ALCL 在 T 细胞淋巴瘤中预后最好,尤其是 ALK 蛋白表达的患者预后更好,5 年 OS 为 79%[88]。抗 CD30 单克隆偶联药物布妥昔单抗(brentuximab)在复发的 CD30+ALCL 中具有很强的活性,目前正在验证其在 ALCL 初始治疗中的疗效。

自体造血干细胞移植治疗首次缓解的侵袭性非霍奇金淋巴瘤

多个研究探讨了高剂量治疗和自体造血干细胞移植(ASCT)对首次获得缓解(CR/PR)的侵袭性淋巴瘤患者的价值,然而并未得出明确结论[208,209]。在 15 项随机试验中,在前利妥昔单抗时代对 3 079 例治疗的患者进行了荟萃分析,对于首次获得 CR 的患者,接受传统疗法或 ASCT 治疗在 EFS、OS 或治疗相关死亡率等方面均无明显差异[210]。

由于 PTCL 患者普遍预后较差,在几项Ⅱ期研究中对首次缓解的 PTCL 患者进 ASCT,结果令人鼓舞[211,212]。

套细胞淋巴瘤

随着化学免疫疗法的出现,现在 MCL 患者的中位生存期是 3~6 年[213]。R-CHOP 一直是 MCL 的首选方案,一项比较 R-CHOP 与苯达莫司汀联合利妥昔单抗(BR)的随机试验,R-CHOP 方案具有更长的 PFS(35 个月 vs 22 个月)且毒性更小[139]。另一项研究比较 R-CHOP 与 FCR 方案(氟达拉滨、环磷酰胺、利妥昔单抗)[214]在 60 岁以上患者的疗效,两组患者的 CR 率相似,但 R-CHOP 方案毒性更小,4 年的 OS 率是 62% 和 47%,R-CHOP 方案更优[214]。另一个随机研究针对接受 R-CHOP 治疗的患者,给予 IFN-α 或利妥昔单抗维持治疗,观察到给予利妥昔单抗维持治疗的患者具有生存获益(4 年的 OS 率为 87% vs 63%)。

自体移植对小于 65 岁、首次治疗 CR 或 PR 的患者,与 IFN-α 维持治疗相比,可以改善 PFS,但 OS 提高无显著的统计学差异[215]。多个Ⅱ期研究在 ASCT 前强化诱导治疗,其中联合高剂量阿糖胞苷治疗效果良好[216],中位 OS 和缓解持续时间超过 10 年,中位 EFS 为 7.4 年。

HyperCVAD 是一种强化治疗方案,使用高剂量环磷酰胺、高剂量甲氨蝶呤和阿糖胞苷。对于初次缓解的患者,它是 ASCT 的替代方案,可以延长 MCL 的缓解时间。一项 MD Anderson 报告提示在 8 年时中位 OS 仍没有达到,而中位至治疗失败时间是 4.6 年[217]。两个多中心试验报告 R-HyperCVAD 方案疾病控制良好,但有很大比例的患者由于毒性不能完成规定的治疗[218,219]。

绝大多数 MCL 患者会复发,三种药物被 FDA 批准用于复发的 MCL:硼替佐米、来那度胺(lenalidomide)和伊布替尼(ibrutinib)。硼替佐米总 RR 为 29%(CR 5%),中位缓解时间为 7 个月[220];来那度胺被批准用于硼替佐米治疗失败的患者,RR 为 26%(CR 7%)和 17 个月的中位缓解时间[221];伊布替尼 RR 为 68%(CR 21%),中位缓解持续时间为 17.5 个月[222];艾代拉里斯 RR 为 40%[223]。ASCT 对复发的 MCL 患者的疗效有限,经过选择的复发患者可以考虑非清髓性异位干细胞移植,3 年期的 PFS 和 OS 分别为 30%和 40%[224]。

高级别淋巴瘤

淋巴母细胞和 Burkitt 淋巴瘤

淋巴母细胞淋巴瘤的治疗详见第 117 章。

针对儿童群体设计的 CODOX-M/IVAC 治疗 BL,低风险患者 2 年 OS 为 82%,高风险患者为 70%[225,226];Hyper-CVAD 方案得到类似的结果[227]。一项 DA-EPOCH-R 的研究报告了良好的结果,中位随访 86 个月,PFS 为 95%,OS 为 100%[228]。目前无证据显示成人患者在初次缓解时应用自体造血干细胞移植可提高疗效[229]。

成人 T 细胞白血病/淋巴瘤

目前采用强化的多药联合方案化疗治疗 ATLL[230],对于冒烟型、慢性亚型可首先考虑给予齐多夫定和 IFN-α 抗病毒治疗[230,231]。对于急性白血病淋巴瘤类型,一项Ⅲ期随机试验报告强化治疗方案(VCAP-AMP-VECP)的 3 年 OS 为 24%,而 CHOP 方案仅为 13%[232]。由于化疗效果欠佳,在 ATLL 中应用了清髓性和低强度的 alloSCT 治疗,但治疗效果有限[233,234]。

复发侵袭性 NHL 的治疗

侵袭性 NHL 大多在化疗免疫疗法治疗结束后 2 年内复发[235],复发后约 60%的患者仍然对传统治疗敏感,但只有不到 10%的侵袭性 NHL 患者使用二线治疗方案可以延长无病生存期。目前治疗复发性 NHL 的有效方法包括高剂量化疗和干细胞移植。

传统解救治疗

绝大多数复发或难治性 DLBCL 患者从传统的解救治疗中获益有限,其缓解持续时间和 OS 约为 6 个月。在随机试验中比较了几种联合化疗方案疗效,获得了较为一致的结果。具体来说,利妥昔单抗+异环磷酰胺、卡铂、依托泊苷方案与利妥昔单抗+地塞米松、阿糖胞苷、铂类方案及利妥昔单抗+吉西他滨、地塞米松、铂类的方案疗效相当[236~239]。解救治疗的目的是明确最有可能从高剂量治疗和 ASCT 获益的化疗敏感的患者。

复发性 PTCL 预后很差,中位 OS 为 6.7 个月[240],吉西他滨和其他常规化疗的疗效有限[241]。治疗复发 PTCL 的新药包括抗叶酸药物普拉曲沙(pralatrexate),HDAC组蛋白去乙酰化酶罗米地辛(romidepsin)和贝利司他(belinostat),有效率均在25%~30%左右,缓解持续时间<18个月[242,243],高选择性非清髓性异位干细胞移植的5年OS和PFS分别为50%和40%[244]。

复发侵袭性NHL的自体干细胞移植

ASCT时的疾病敏感性仍然是预测治疗结果最重要的预后变量,几项大型研究表明,初次诱导治疗耐药的患者行ASCT后,无病生存率低于10%。复发后对化疗仍然敏感的患者长期无病生存率为30%~60%,而耐药患者的长期生存率仅为10%~15%。

对于复发侵袭性NHL,在PARMA试验中ASCT与传统的抢救治疗方法进行比较[245],患者(多为DLBCL)接受2个周期化疗后(顺铂、阿糖胞苷和甲泼尼龙联合方案),将缓解者随机分为两组,一组继续接受4个疗程的化疗,一组接受高剂量化疗联合自体骨髓移植,中位随访时间超过5年,随机至高剂量化疗组的患者无事件生存率(46% vs 12%)和总生存率(53% vs 32%)更优。

迄今为止,研究人员在移植后使用利妥昔单抗[246],抗CD19免疫毒素,口服激酶抑制剂恩扎妥林(enzastaurin)进行维持治疗或加入放射免疫治疗[247],均未能改善结果。对于复发或难治性DLBCL患者,高剂量化疗联合ASCT仍是化疗敏感性患者的治疗选择。如果复发是局部的,在高剂量化疗和ASCT治疗前或治疗后辅助放疗对疾病控制可能是有益的,但可能不会影响OS。对于化疗不敏感的患者,应考虑临床试验或姑息性治疗,但不考虑干细胞移植。一些新的药物包括伊布替尼(特别在ABC亚型中)以及来那度胺和依维莫司(everolimus)已经在复发的DLBCL患者中展现了希望。

NHL的异基因干细胞移植

异基因干细胞移植已经用于复发性和难治性NHL,几乎所有病例均为复发患者,其中许多对传统剂量的治疗耐药。根据European Bone Marrow Transplant登记的资料,侵袭性NHL行异基因移植后的复发率比自体移植的低,但是OS并无差异,因为异基因移植的移植相关死亡率更高,5年EFS和OS为43%,1年治疗相关死亡率为25%。对于PS评分良好且对化疗敏感的ASCT后复发的患者,可考虑alloSCT(通常为RIC alloSCT),几项研究报告结果显示PFS为40%~60%,但RIC alloSCT治疗相关的死亡率为20%,清髓性移植治疗的死亡率高达40%[248,249]。

NHL新的治疗手段

NHL的治疗已经取得了显著进步,其中主要是改善了B细胞淋巴瘤的疗效,然而许多疾病亚型如PTCL和复发及难治性DLBCL的治疗进展较少。目前有大量新的、合理的靶向药物正在研究中,包括抗体偶联物、激酶抑制剂和增强T细胞毒性的免疫疗法(嵌合抗原受体T细胞和检查点抑制剂)。最重要的进展是我们对淋巴瘤生成过程中遗传事件和异常通路的理解,这推动了针对新靶点的药物研发,从而限制了对正常细胞的毒性。

(程颖 张良 译 程颖 校)

参考文献

The complete reference list can be found on the Wiley Companion Digital Edition of this title (see inside front cover for login instructions).

22 Swerdlow SH, Campo E, Harris NL, et al. *WHO Classification of Tumours of Haematopoietic and Lymphoid Tissues*. Lyon, France: IARC Press; 2008.

25 Armitage JO, Weisenburger DD. New approach to classifying non-Hodgkin's lymphomas: clinical features of the major histologic subtypes. Non-Hodgkin's Lymphoma Classification Project. *J Clin Oncol*. 1998;**16(8)**:2780–2795.

29 Montoto S, Fitzgibbon J. Transformation of indolent B-cell lymphomas. *J Clin Oncol*. 2011;**29**:1827–1834.

31 Grever MR, Lucas DM, Dewald GW, et al. Comprehensive assessment of genetic and molecular features predicting outcome in patients with chronic lymphocytic leukemia: results from the US Intergroup Phase III Trial E2997. *J Clin Oncol*. 2007;**25(7)**:799–804.

58 Rosenwald A, Wright G, Chan WC, et al. The use of molecular profiling to predict survival after chemotherapy for diffuse large-B-cell lymphoma. *N Engl J Med*. 2002;**346(25)**:1937–1947.

59 Alizadeh AA, Eisen MB, Davis RE, et al. Distinct types of diffuse large B-cell lymphoma identified by gene expression profiling. *Nature*. 2000;**403(6769)**:503–511.

60 Monti S, Savage KJ, Kutok JL, et al. Molecular profiling of diffuse large B-cell lymphoma identifies robust subtypes including one characterized by host inflammatory response. *Blood*. 2005;**105(5)**:1851–1861.

61 Shipp MA, Ross KN, Tamayo P, et al. Diffuse large B-cell lymphoma outcome prediction by gene-expression profiling and supervised machine learning. *Nat Med*. 2002;**8(1)**:68–74.

68 Aukema SM, Siebert R, Schuuring E, et al. Double-hit B-cell lymphomas. *Blood*. 2011;**117(8)**:2319–2331.

71 Montoto S, Corradini P, Dreyling M, et al. Indications for hematopoietic stem cell transplantation in patients with follicular lymphoma: a consensus project of the EBMT-Lymphoma Working Party. *Haematologica*. 2013;**98(7)**:1014–1021.

78 Rizvi MA, Evens AM, Tallman MS, Nelson BP, Rosen ST. T-cell non-Hodgkin lymphoma. *Blood*. 2006;**107(4)**:1255–1264.

91 Sonnen R, Schmidt WP, Muller-Hermelink HK, Schmitz N. The International Prognostic Index determines the outcome of patients with nodal mature T-cell lymphomas. *Br J Haematol*. 2005;**129(3)**:366–372.

105 Cheson BD, Fisher RI, Barrington SF, et al. Recommendations for initial evaluation, staging, and response assessment of Hodgkin and non-Hodgkin lymphoma: the Lugano classification. *J Clin Oncol*. 2014;**32(27)**:3059–3068.

109 A predictive model for aggressive non-Hodgkin's lymphoma. The International Non-Hodgkin's Lymphoma Prognostic Factors Project. *N Engl J Med*. 1993;**329(14)**:987–994.

111 Solal-Celigny P, Roy P, Colombat P, et al. Follicular lymphoma international prognostic index. *Blood*. 2004;**104(5)**:1258–1265.

115 Schmitz N, Trumper L, Ziepert M, et al. Treatment and prognosis of mature T-cell and NK-cell lymphoma: an analysis of patients with T-cell lymphoma treated in studies of the German High-Grade Non-Hodgkin Lymphoma Study Group. *Blood*. 2010;**116(18)**:3418–3425.

116 Hans CP, Weisenburger DD, Greiner TC, et al. Confirmation of the molecular classification of diffuse large B-cell lymphoma by immunohistochemistry using a tissue microarray. *Blood*. 2004;**103(1)**:275–282.

131 Ardeshna KM, Smith P, Norton A, et al. Long-term effect of a watch and wait policy versus immediate systemic treatment for asymptomatic advanced-stage non-Hodgkin lymphoma: a randomised controlled trial. *Lancet*. 2003;**362(9383)**:516–522.

133 Ardeshna KM, Qian W, Smith P, et al. Rituximab versus a watch-and-wait approach in patients with advanced-stage, asymptomatic, non-bulky follicular lymphoma: an open-label randomised phase 3 trial. *Lancet Oncol*. 2014;**15(4)**:424–435.

136 Marcus R, Imrie K, Belch A, et al. CVP chemotherapy plus rituximab compared with CVP as first-line treatment for advanced follicular lymphoma. *Blood*. 2005;**105(4)**:1417–1423.

139 Rummel MJ, Niederle N, Maschmeyer G, et al. Bendamustine plus rituximab versus CHOP plus rituximab as first-line treatment for patients with indolent and mantle-cell lymphomas: an open-label, multicentre, randomised, phase 3 non-inferiority trial. *Lancet*. 2013;**381(9873)**:1203–1210.

143 Martinelli G, Schmitz SF, Utiger U, et al. Long-term follow-up of patients with follicular lymphoma receiving single-agent rituximab at two different schedules in trial SAKK 35/98. *J Clin Oncol*. 2010;**28(29)**:4480–4484.

147 Salles G, Seymour JF, Offner F, et al. Rituximab maintenance for 2 years in patients with high tumour burden follicular lymphoma responding to rituximab plus chemotherapy (PRIMA): a phase 3, randomised controlled trial. *Lancet*. 2011;**377(9759)**:42–51.

164 Gopal AK, Kahl BS, de Vos S, et al. PI3Kdelta inhibition by idelalisib in patients

with relapsed indolent lymphoma. *N Engl J Med*. 2014;**370**(**11**):1008–1018.

167 Schouten HC, Qian W, Kvaloy S, et al. High-dose therapy improves progression-free survival and survival in relapsed follicular non-Hodgkin's lymphoma: results from the randomized European CUP trial. *J Clin Oncol*. 2003;**21**(**21**): 3918–3927.

169 Khouri IF, McLaughlin P, Saliba RM, et al. Eight-year experience with allogeneic stem cell transplantation for relapsed follicular lymphoma after nonmyeloablative conditioning with fludarabine, cyclophosphamide, and rituximab. *Blood*. 2008;**111**(**12**):5530–5536.

180 Miller TP, Dahlberg S, Cassady JR, et al. Chemotherapy alone compared with chemotherapy plus radiotherapy for localized intermediate- and high-grade non-Hodgkin's lymphoma. *N Engl J Med*. 1998;**339**(**1**):21–26.

184 Persky DO, Unger JM, Spier CM, et al. Phase II study of rituximab plus three cycles of CHOP and involved-field radiotherapy for patients with limited-stage aggressive B-cell lymphoma: Southwest Oncology Group study 0014. *J Clin Oncol*. 2008;**26**(**14**):2258–2263.

185 Pfreundschuh M, Trumper L, Osterborg A, et al. CHOP-like chemotherapy plus rituximab versus CHOP-like chemotherapy alone in young patients with good-prognosis diffuse large-B-cell lymphoma: a randomised controlled trial by the MabThera International Trial (MInT) Group. *Lancet Oncol*. 2006;**7**(**5**):379–391.

187 Dunleavy K, Pittaluga S, Maeda LS, et al. Dose-adjusted EPOCH-rituximab therapy in primary mediastinal B-cell lymphoma. *N Engl J Med*. 2013;**368**(**15**): 1408–1416.

192 Coiffier B, Lepage E, Briere J, et al. CHOP chemotherapy plus rituximab compared with CHOP alone in elderly patients with diffuse large-B-cell lymphoma. *N Engl J Med*. 2002;**346**(**4**):235–242.

194 Habermann TM, Weller EA, Morrison VA, et al. Rituximab-CHOP versus CHOP alone or with maintenance rituximab in older patients with diffuse large B-cell lymphoma. *J Clin Oncol*. 2006;**24**(**19**):3121–3127.

195 Pfreundschuh M, Schubert J, Ziepert M, et al. Six versus eight cycles of bi-weekly CHOP-14 with or without rituximab in elderly patients with aggressive CD20+ B-cell lymphomas: a randomised controlled trial (RICOVER-60). *Lancet Oncol*. 2008;**9**(**2**):105–116.

201 McMillan A, Ardeshna KM, Cwynarski K, Lyttelton M, McKay P, Montoto S. Guideline on the prevention of secondary central nervous system lymphoma: British Committee for Standards in Haematology. *Br J Haematol*. 2013;**163**(**2**):168–181.

209 Stiff PJ, Unger JM, Cook JR, et al. Autologous transplantation as consolidation for aggressive non-Hodgkin's lymphoma. *N Engl J Med*. 2013;**369**(**18**):1681–1690.

214 Kluin-Nelemans HC, Hoster E, Hermine O, et al. Treatment of older patients with mantle-cell lymphoma. *N Engl J Med*. 2012;**367**(**6**):520–531.

217 Romaguera JE, Fayad LE, Feng L, et al. Ten-year follow-up after intense chemoimmunotherapy with Rituximab-HyperCVAD alternating with Rituximab-high dose methotrexate/cytarabine (R-MA) and without stem cell transplantation in patients with untreated aggressive mantle cell lymphoma. *Br J Haematol*. 2010;**150**(**2**):200–208.

222 Wang ML, Rule S, Martin P, et al. Targeting BTK with ibrutinib in relapsed or refractory mantle-cell lymphoma. *N Engl J Med*. 2013;**369**(**6**):507–516.

223 Kahl BS, Spurgeon SE, Furman RR, et al. A phase 1 study of the PI3Kdelta inhibitor idelalisib in patients with relapsed/refractory mantle cell lymphoma (MCL). *Blood*. 2014;**123**(**22**):3398–3405.

224 Fenske TS, Zhang MJ, Carreras J, et al. Autologous or reduced-intensity conditioning allogeneic hematopoietic cell transplantation for chemotherapy-sensitive mantle-cell lymphoma: analysis of transplantation timing and modality. *J Clin Oncol*. 2014;**32**(**4**):273–281.

228 Dunleavy K, Pittaluga S, Shovlin M, et al. Low-intensity therapy in adults with Burkitt's lymphoma. *N Engl J Med*. 2013;**369**(**20**):1915–1925.

245 Philip T, Guglielmi C, Hagenbeek A, et al. Autologous bone marrow transplantation as compared with salvage chemotherapy in relapses of chemotherapy-sensitive non-Hodgkin's lymphoma. *N Engl J Med*. 1995;**333**(**23**): 1540–1545.

第 120 章 蕈样肉芽肿和塞扎里综合征

Richard T. Hoppe, MD ■ Youn H. Kim, MD ■ Ranjana H. Advani, MD

概述

蕈样肉芽肿(mycosis fungoides,MF)/塞扎里综合征(Sézary syndrome,SS)是最常见的皮肤T细胞淋巴瘤。它起源于皮肤,其表现可以是很小的斑块,也可以是广泛的皮肤肿瘤。在累及外周血液时,通常还伴有红皮病,被称为SS。小斑块型疾病的自然病程很长,对各种局部治疗有良好反应,甚至与同龄对照人群有着相似的生存率,而发生皮肤肿瘤或皮肤外疾病的MF/SS则进展极为迅速。对局限型MF/SS的治疗主要是局部治疗,包括局部化疗(氮芥)、放疗和光疗。而当疾病发生进展时,虽然仍需要经常性的局部治疗,但全身治疗则成为关键。常规化疗(单一用药或药物组合)通常无效。而系统生物制剂如组蛋白去乙酰化酶抑制剂、干扰素、光疗、阿伦珠单抗和布妥昔单抗(brentuximab)可能会可能有一定效果。最近,造血干细胞移植,尤其是不做清髓的造血干细胞移植,在一项队列实验中对晚期MF或SS表现出良好疗效。

历史观点

MF最初由法国皮肤科医生Alibert发现。MF/SS是最常见的皮肤T细胞淋巴瘤(CTCL)。SS是MF的红皮、白血病型变体[1]。

发病率和流行病学

美国每年病例数小于1 000[2]。中位年龄55~66岁;但更年青的个体也可能发病[3]。男性患病率约为女性的2倍,发病率无种族间差异。发病原因不明[4]。没有证据显示MF/SS与化学品接触或任何病毒有关[5,6]。

病理

异常的单核"脑质样"细胞单独或成簇浸润表皮和上真皮(Pautrier微脓肿)。他们表现出辅助T细胞的特征(CD4+)[7]。少量病例是CD8+(细胞毒性/抑制性T细胞表型)。研究表明,皮肤、淋巴结和外周血中T细胞受体发生了单克隆重排[8]。根据非典型细胞的浸润程度,淋巴结被分类为LN-0至LN-4[9]。即使在仅有皮肤病变的淋巴结中,也可能观察到克隆细胞的潜在参与[10]。

发病机制和自然病史

MF可能首先出现在肉芽肿期,表现为非特异性、轻微扩张的皮肤损伤。之后,可能会出现斑块、肿瘤或全身性红皮病。该疾病常常分布于下腰和大腿,瘙痒是其常见症状。发生浸润的斑块最终可能发展为溃疡或蕈样肿瘤。受到感染的肿瘤可能导致败血症和死亡。

红皮病患者会有强烈的瘙痒症状。包括红皮病、淋巴结病和血液循环中异常细胞的综合征称为SS[11]。其他表现包括亲毛囊性MF[12]、Paget样网状细胞增生症[13]、肉芽肿[14]和色素减退[15]。

MF通常是惰性的[16,17],但15%~20%的病例会发展为皮肤外疾病,最常见的是皮肤肿瘤或红皮病[18]。局部结节是皮肤外最常见的受累部位,而MF可能影响脾脏、肝脏、肺脏和其他器官[19]。

诊断

可基于常规组织学检查做免疫表型识别。可以通过Southern印迹分析[20,21]或聚合酶链反应(PCR)扩增的方法检测T细胞受体基因重排[8,22]。血液的流式细胞术检查可显示CD4+CD7-细胞群体扩增,这是非典型塞扎里型淋巴细胞的特征[23]。PCR方法可以帮助确定血液[24]或淋巴结受累[10]。

局限型疾病的患者需要接受高质量的体检,做仔细的皮损评估、全血细胞计数、塞扎里细胞检测、化学指标筛查和胸部X线片。如果它们都在正常范围内,则不需要进行额外的检查。全身性疾病患者应进行CT(计算机断层扫描)或PET/CT(正电子发射断层扫描和计算机断层扫描成像)[25]。应对肿大的淋巴结进行组织活检,但骨髓取样需要视情况而定。

TNMB 分期

MF/SS的TNMB(肿瘤、淋巴结、转移瘤、血液)分期系统总结于表120-1和表120-2中[26]。

表 120-1 肿瘤、淋巴结转移、MF 的血液分类

T(皮肤)	
T1	局限的斑片、丘疹或斑块覆盖皮肤表面的<10%
T2	斑块、丘疹和/或斑块覆盖≥10%的皮肤表面
T3	一个或多个肿瘤(直径>1cm)
T4	融合性红斑>80%体表面积
N(淋巴结)	
N0	无临床可扪及的异常外周淋巴结;无须活检
N1	临床扪及异常外周淋巴结;组织病理学 Dutch Gr 1or NCI LN0~2
N2	临床扪及异常外周淋巴结;组织病理学 Dutch Gr 2or NCI LN3
N3	临床扪及异常外周淋巴结;组织病理学 Dutch Gr 3~4 or NCI LN4
NX	临床扪及异常外周淋巴结;无组织病理学证据
M(内脏)	
M0	无内脏器官受累

续表

M1	内脏器官受累(必须有病理学证实,受累器官需详细说明)
B(血液)	
B0	无明显血液受累:<5%的外周血淋巴细胞(PBL)为典型细胞(塞扎里细胞)
B1	低血液瘤细胞负荷:>5%的 PBL 为非典型细胞(塞扎里细胞),但未达到 B2 标准
B2	高血液瘤细胞负荷:>1 000/mcl 塞扎里细胞阳性克隆

摘自 Olsen 等人[26],经美国血液学学会许可使用。

表 120-2　MF/SS 临床分期系统

	T	N	M	B
ⅠA	1	0	0	0,1
ⅠB	2	0	0	0,1
Ⅱ	1~2	1,2	0	0,1
ⅡB	3	0~2	0	0,1
Ⅲ	4	0~2	0	0,1
ⅢA	4	0~2	0	0
ⅢB	4	0~2	0	1
ⅣA1	1~4	0~2	0	2
ⅣA2	1~4	3	0	0~2
ⅣB	1~4	0~3	1	0~2

预后因素和生物标志物

T 分期和皮肤外疾病是生存率的最重要预测因子(图 120-1)[18]。局限性斑块(T1;ⅠA 期)患者的生存率很高,与年龄、性别、种族相匹配的对照人群相当[16]。中位生存期超过 33 年,只有不到 10%的患者会发生恶化。

广泛性斑块且伴有皮肤外受累(T2;ⅠB、ⅡA 期)患者的中位生存时间超过 11 年[17]。约 24%的患者发展为进展性疾病,约 20%会死于 MF。发生皮肤肿瘤(T3;ⅡB 期)或全身性红皮病(T4;Ⅲ期)但无皮肤外受累的患者的中位生存期为 3~5 年,其中大多数患者都将死于 MF[27]。

皮肤外淋巴结受累(ⅣA 期)或内脏受累(ⅣB 期)患者的中位生存期小于 1.5 年[28]。外周血中塞扎里细胞的存在,通常提示更高级的 T 分期(通常是 T4)和皮肤外疾病[29]。

患者可能发生皮肤肿瘤,其皮肤浸润细胞中,非典型淋巴细胞占比超过 25%[30,31]。这被称为大细胞转化。这些细胞可能表达 CD30,增殖速度快,并且与之前存在的 MF 有共同的克隆起源[30,32]。这些大细胞可能丢失一种或多种 T 细胞相关抗原[30,31]。这些患者可能有更快的疾病进展,需要更强化的治疗[33]。

多学科治疗

美国国家综合癌症网络(NCCN)已经建立了治疗 MF 和 SS 的共识指南[34]。常见的皮肤疗法包括糖皮质激素、补骨素加紫外线 A(PUVA)、局部化疗、维 A 酸类和辐射。一些患者(10%~20%)需要治疗全身性疾病。治疗方案选择应基于临床分期(图 120-2)。

外用化疗

外用氮芥(mechlorethamine,HN2)是一种有效的治疗方法,尤其适用于 T1~2 期疾病[35]。其作用机制可能与烷化作用、免疫机制及表皮细胞-朗格汉斯细胞-T 细胞轴的相互作用有关。HN2 可以施用于局部或整个皮肤。它可以是水溶液,但最常见的是凝胶或软膏制剂。在清除阶段,每日至少局部施用一次 HN2。皮肤清除可能需要 6 个月或更长时间,然后需要维持治疗。市售的凝胶制剂浓度为 0.02%(Valchlor)[36]。

如果疗效特别慢,则可以增加 HN2 软膏的浓度或者施用频率。T1~T2 期疾病的完全反应率(CRR)约为 15%,部分反应率(PRR)约为 50%[36]。皮肤清除的中位时间为 6~8 个月,反应可维持超过 10 个月。治疗的耐受性良好。原发性急性并发症包括皮肤过敏[36]、接触性皮炎、皮肤刺激和红斑。没有系统吸收,所以即使对儿童也是安全的[35]。

外用维 A 酸

贝沙罗汀(targretin)是一种 RXR 选择性合成维 A 酸,为浓度 1%的凝胶,可薄薄地涂在斑块上,每日两次。该药物有刺激作用,所以仅适于局部使用。大多数ⅠA~ⅠB 期疾病患者对其有疗效[37]。最常见的毒性反应是局部刺激,大多数患者都会出现这种反应。可能有必要在治疗数周后停止使用,评估疾病状态。贝沙罗汀凝胶被批准用于疑难症状或不能耐受其他疗法的ⅠA~ⅠB 期疾病患者。

光疗

光疗包括 UVA 或 UVB 波长的紫外(UV)辐射。长波 UVA 相对于 UVB 的优势在于更大的穿透深度。对于局限性疾病,单独使用 UVB[38]或家庭 UV 光疗(UVA+UVB[38,39]即可能取得良好效果。起始时,每日或每周三次 UVB 治疗,剂量逐渐增加。在维持期,治疗频率逐渐降低。窄频 UVB(nb-UVB)光疗与宽频 UVB 相比具有较低的毒性,并且在ⅠA~ⅡA 期疾病患者中达到 68%的 CRR[37]。nb-UVB 的临床疗效可能优于宽频 UVB[40]。

UVA 可与光敏剂、补骨素、PUVA 一起使用,这种联合疗法被称为光化学疗法。在 UVA 作用下,补骨素可嵌入 DNA,形成单功能和双功能加合物,抑制 DNA 合成。这导致细胞毒性和抗增殖作用以及潜在的免疫调节作用。使用此疗法时,患者先摄入补骨素(8-甲氧基补骨素),然后 1~2h 后在受控条件下暴露于 UVA。通常只对眼睛做遮盖,但可以遮盖其他选定区域,以尽量减少不必要的光损伤。"阴影"区域,如头皮、会阴、腋窝和其他皮肤皱褶可能不能获得足够的暴露。

PUVA 治疗开始时每周三次,直至皮肤病变被清除,然后降低治疗频率。维持治疗应在一年内停止,以最大限度地降低皮肤癌发生的风险。皮肤清除时间为 2~6 个月。ⅠA~ⅡA 期疾病的 CRR 为 62%,PRR 为 25%[37]。疗效持续时间平均为约 12 个月。PUVA 是ⅠA-ⅡA 期疾病的一线疗法之一,或作用其他治疗失败后的二线疗法。对于 SS 患者,可在 *PUVA* 的基础上辅以全身性 IFN-α[41]或全身性维 A 酸治疗[42]。

PUVA 的主要急性并发症是光毒性反应,伴有红皮病和水疱,发生率约为 20%[37]。摄入补骨素后,患者应在至少 24h 内避免皮肤和眼睛暴露于光照。PUVA 潜在长期并发症包括白内障和恶性皮肤肿瘤[40]。

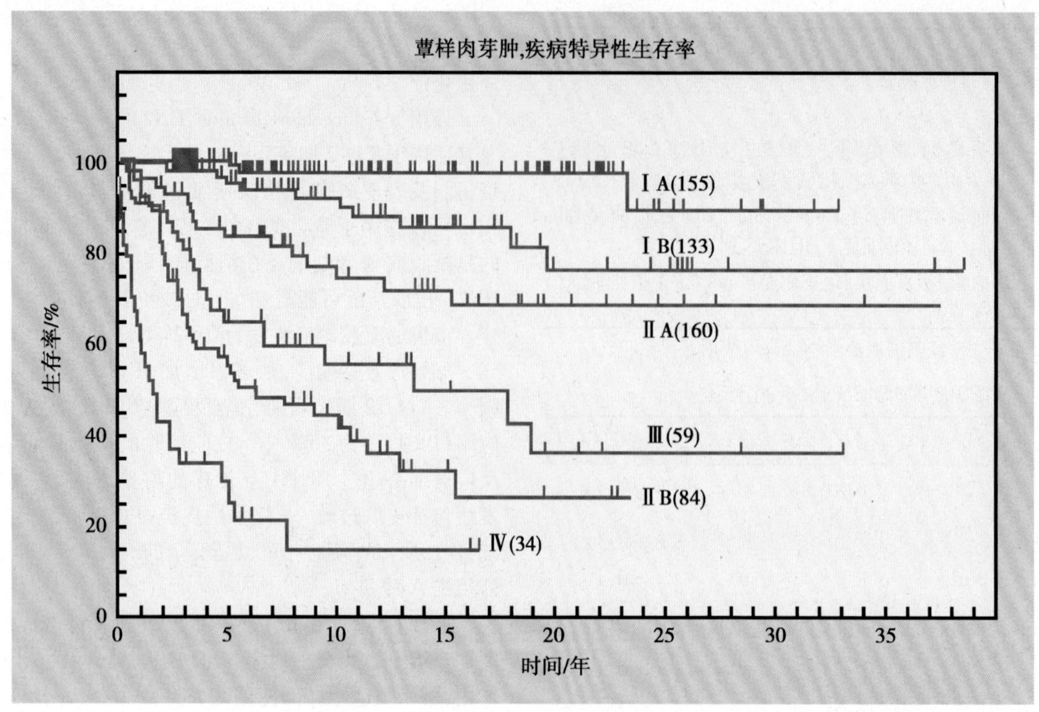

图 120-1　在斯坦福大学接受治疗的 525 名 MF 患者在疾病初始阶段之后的疾病特异性存活率

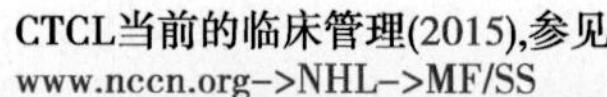

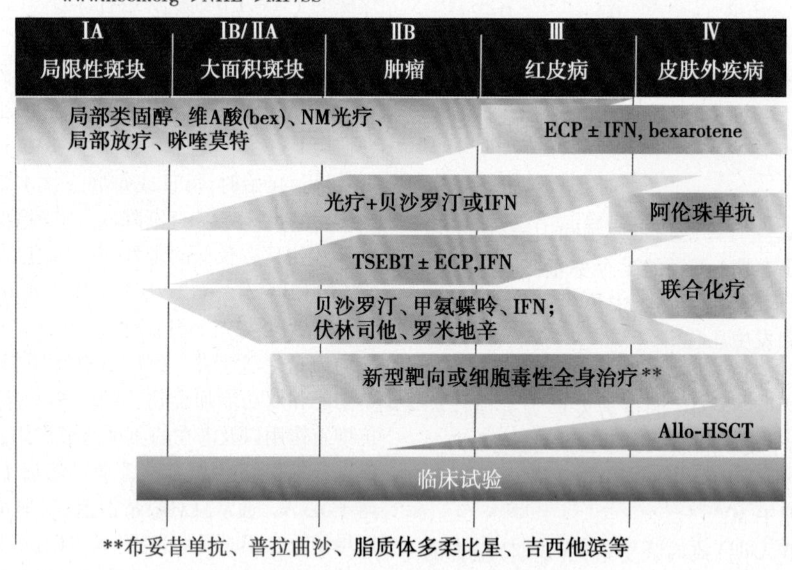

图 120-2　MF/SS 患者的治疗预案

放疗

MF 具有极高的放射敏感性。可以使用 8Gy 的剂量治疗斑块或肿瘤,有约 95%的机会达到局部控制[43]。利用电子束治疗整个皮肤的技术已经面世(全皮肤电子束治疗[TSEBT])[44]。患者在远距离多个位置站立,接受治疗。患者在 9~10 周内接受 30~36Gy 剂量的照射后,总体响应率(ORR)接近 100%,因皮肤受累程度的不同,完全响应率(CRR)为 40%~98%[44,45]。TSEBT 对ⅠB~ⅡB 疾病患者的效果最好。为减少治疗的毒性和持续时间,并能重复使用 TSEBT,引入了低剂量(12Gy)TSEBT 方案,其 ORR 达到 88%,CRR 为 27%[46]。临床获益的持续时间超过 16 个月。

高剂量 TSEBT 的并发症包括红斑、脱屑和暂时性脱毛。患者还会经历指甲和趾甲的暂时丧失,以及长达 12 个月的出汗功能受损。高剂量 TSEBT 还会导致继发性皮肤恶性肿瘤的风险增加。接受 12Gy TSEBT 治疗的患者会出现暂时性脱毛,但一般不会丧失指甲和趾甲,而且其他皮肤不良反应也远低于高剂量 TSEBT。

对于有淋巴结受累的患者,可以在 3~4 周内 30Gy *TSEBT* 的基础上,辅以传统的兆伏(4~15MeV)光子照射,以实现局部控制[44]。

全身化疗

全身化疗适用于患有皮肤外、晚期或疑难疾病的患者。几乎所有对其他淋巴瘤有效的药物都已被尝试用于治疗 MF/SS。遗憾的是,它们通常只会产生短暂的姑息性反应。对 198 例接受全身治疗的 MF/SS 患者的回顾性研究显示,更换治疗药物的时间仅为 3.9 个月,并且耐久性缓解极少[47]。根据 NCCN 发布的指南,预计只有少数 MF 患者(10%～20%)需要全身化疗[48]。

单药化疗试验报告的 526 名患者中,缓解率仅为 20%～80%,缓解的中位持续时间为 3～22 个月[49]。单一用药包括抗甲酸盐甲氨蝶呤[50~53]、普拉曲沙[54]、苯丁酸氮芥[55]、嘌呤类似物[56~63]、喷司他丁、2-CDA、氟达拉滨、吉西他滨[64~67]、聚乙二醇脂质体多柔比星[68~71]、替莫唑胺[72,73]和硼替佐米[74,75]。

目前最大的临床试验使用了环磷酰胺、长春新碱、泼尼松的组合,外加或不外加多柔比星[76,77]。CRR 约为 25%,缓解时间为 3～20 个月[49]。更激进的治疗方案包括依托泊苷、伊达比星、环磷酰胺、长春新碱、泼尼松和博来霉素(ⅥCOP-B)联合化疗[78]和 ESHAP(依托泊苷、高剂量阿糖胞苷和甲泼尼龙)[79]。

联合化疗和 TSEBT 曾被认为是首选治疗方案[80~82]。然而,NCI 的前瞻性随机试验显示,其效果并不优于传统保守治疗[83,84]。

造血干细胞移植(HSCT)

尽管自体移植已成功用于许多淋巴瘤,但它并不适用于 MF/SS[85~87]。患者的缓解时间非常短,中位进展时间不到 3 个月[85]。即便经过 T 细胞分离以充分除去污染的淋巴瘤细胞,也未能改善其疗效[88]。

同种异体移植更具吸引力,因为同种异体移植物抗肿瘤效应可帮助控制恶性 T 细胞。适用标准和准备方案各不相同。早期报道显示,那些经骨髓清除后接受 HLA 匹配亲属的同种异体移植的患者,可以实现完全和持续的缓解,而且轻度的移植物抗宿主(GVHD)反应可能有抗淋巴瘤效应[89,90]。

这些同种异体移植的结果令人鼓舞,但由于移植相关的发病率和死亡率,其适用性有限,特别是对老年患者而言。最新的非清髓方法和低强度预处理方案比清髓方案有效且毒性更低[85]。国际登记处报告的无进展生存率(PFS)在 5 年时高达 32%,7 年时高达 30%[91~95]。

一种新方法是联合使用 TSEBT、全淋巴照射和兔抗人胸腺细胞免疫球蛋白,作为非清髓性准备方案[96]。研究表明,这种方案的 GVHD 风险较低。在斯坦福大学的 29 例ⅡB 或Ⅳ期 MF/SS 患者中,移植后Ⅱ～Ⅳ级 GVHD 的发生率为仅 21%[97]。2 年期 PFS 为 50%,OS 为 76%。

似乎同种异体造血干细胞移植(HSCT)(特别是低强度预处理方案后的移植)可能获得持久的缓解。还需要更大规模的前瞻性研究来确定最佳的移植时机和最佳的预处理方案。由于许多生物制剂显示出良好的活性和耐受性,维持治疗也可能是有效的。

体外光照

体外光照(ECP)是一种体外技术对全身做 PUVA 的方法[98]。该技术中,通过白细胞分离术收集患者的白细胞,将其暴露于光活化药物(8-甲氧基补骨素,Uvadex),然后用 UVA 照射。然后通过静脉将经照射的细胞回输到患者体内。光照治疗的作用机制尚不清楚,但它可能诱导循环肿瘤细胞(塞扎里细胞)的凋亡。凋亡细胞释放的肿瘤抗原被外周树突细胞处理,增强全身抗肿瘤反应[99]。该治疗对红皮病患者最有效(T4)[100]。如果配合生物制剂(如干扰素或维 A 酸[101,104]或皮肤定向疗法(如局部类固醇、局部氮芥或 TSEBT),反应率可能更高[48,102]。ECP 的不良副作用很小。一些患者可能会出现恶心,主要是因为摄入的补骨素,有些患者在治疗后会出现短暂的低烧或轻度不适。没有显著器官损伤,或骨髓/免疫抑制的报道[103]。

全身生物疗法

IFN-α 可以单独使用,但更多的时候是与其他局部或全身治疗同时使用。单用时的 ORR 为 53%～74%,CRR 为 21%～35%[41,104,105]。与光疗法联合使用时,反应率和持续时间似乎更理想[41]。

使用贝沙罗汀做全身性治疗可能是有效的[106]。它可以与 PUVA(Re-PUVA)、IFN-α 或 TSEBT 联合使用。缓解率为 45%～55%(CR 率为 10%～20%)[42,104~111]。最常见的并发症包括光过敏、干燥症、肌痛、关节痛、头痛、高脂血症和中枢性甲状腺功能减退,此外还有可能的致畸作用。停止治疗后,大多数毒性疾病都是可逆的。

两种组蛋白去乙酰化酶(HDAC)抑制剂,伏林司他(辛二酰苯胺异羟肟酸)和罗米地辛(romidepsin),也表现出一定的效果。伏林司他是一种口服药物,其 ORR 率为 24%～30%,但很少有 CR[112,113]。治疗到出现反应的中位时间为 12 周,反应持续的中位时间为 15～26 周。一般能缓解瘙痒。最常见的副作用包括疲劳、腹泻、恶心、厌食、味觉障碍和血小板减少症。

罗米地辛(缩酚酸肽)是一种静脉给药的 HDAC 抑制剂,其 ORR 为 34%[114,115]。主要不良反应包括恶心、呕吐、疲劳、血小板减少和粒细胞减少。

阿伦珠单抗(Campath-1H)是一种靶向 CD52 的人源化单克隆抗体,其 CRR 和 PRR 分别达到 32%和 23%,治疗失效的中位时间为 12 个月[116]。严重感染是其风险之一,需要对这些患者采取抗菌和抗病毒预防措施。已经引入了改良的剂量方案,其毒性有所降低[117,118]。阿伦珠单抗对减少 SS 患者外周血塞扎里细胞计数特别有效。

布妥昔单抗(BV)是一种抗 CD30 单克隆抗体与一甲基澳瑞他汀 E(一种抗微管药物)的缀合物,对 CD30 阳性的恶性肿瘤有强力的选择杀伤作用[119]。MF 即表达不同水平的 CD30,BV 对 MF 的疗效已经得到证实[120]。在 73%的患者中观察到客观整体反应。最常见的 BV 相关不良反应是周围神经病变、疲劳、恶心、脱发和中性粒细胞减少症。

来那度胺(lenalidomide)是一种口服免疫调节药物[121]。ORR 为 28%。主要并发症包括疲劳、感染和白细胞减少症。

结论

MF/SS 是一种具有挑战性的疾病。其临床表现各异,虽然其病程一般较为缓慢,但在许多患者中,表现出恶性行为。局部治疗和全身生物治疗对它有一定疗效,但化疗对其的作用较小。同种异体干细胞移植可能成为部分患者的治愈性治疗。

(程颖　李佩东 译　程颖 校)

参考文献

The complete reference list can be found on the Wiley Companion Digital Edition of this title (see inside front cover for login instructions).

1 Kim YH, Hoppe RT. Mycosis fungoides and the Sézary syndrome. *Semin Oncol.* 1999;**26**:276–289.

11 Willemze R, Jaffe ES, Burg G, et al. WHO-EORTC classification for cutaneous lymphomas. *Blood*. 2005;**105**:3768–3785.

18 Kim YH, Liu HL, Mraz-Gernhard S, et al. Long-term outcome of 525 patients with mycosis fungoides and Sézary syndrome at Stanford: clinical prognostic factors and risks of disease progression and second cancer. *Arch Dermatol.* 2003;**139**:857–866.

26 Olsen E, Vonderheid E, Pimpinelli N, et al. Revisions to the staging and classification of mycosis fungoides and Sézary syndrome: a proposal of the International Society for Cutaneous Lymphomas (ISCL) and the cutaneous lymphoma task force of the European Organization of Research and Treatment of Cancer (EORTC). *Blood*. 2007;**110**:1713–1722.

29 Sausville EA, Eddy JL, Makuch RW, et al. Histopathologic staging at initial diagnosis of mycosis fungoides and the Sézary syndrome. Definition of three distinctive prognostic groups. *Ann Intern Med.* 1988;**109**:372–382.

36 Lessin SR, Duvic M, Guitart S, et al. Topical chemotherapy in cutaneous T-cell lymphoma. Positive results of a randomized, controlled, multicenter trial testing the efficacy and safety of a novel mechlorethamine, 0.02%, gel in mycosis fungoides. *JAMA Dermatol.* 2013;**149**:25–32.

37 Heald P, Mehlmauer M, Martin AG, et al. Topical bexarotene therapy for patients with refractory or persistent early-stage cutaneous T-cell lymphoma: results of the phase III clinical trial. *J Am Acad Dermatol.* 2003;**49**:801.

38 Ponte P, Serrao V, Apetato M. Efficacy of narrowband UVB vs. PUVA in patients with early-stage mycosis fungoides. *J Eur Acad Dermatol Venereol.* 2010;**24**:716–721.

43 Thomas TO, Agrawal P, Guitart J, et al. Outcome of patients treat with a single-fraction dose of palliative radiation for cutaneous T-cell lymphoma. *Int J Radiat Oncol Biol Phys.* 2013;**85**:747–753.

44 Hoppe R. Mycosis fungoides: radiation therapy. *Dermatol Ther*. 2003;**16**:347–354.

46 Hoppe RT, Harrison C, Tavallaee M, et al. Low-dose total skin electron beam therapy as an effective modality to reduce disease burden inpatients with mycosis fungoides: Results of a pooled analysis from 3 phase-II clinical trials. *J Am Acad Dermatol.* 2015;**72**:288–292.

47 Hughes CFM, Khot A, McCormack C, et al. Lack of durable disease control with chemotherapy for mycosis fungoides and Sézary syndrome: a comparative study of systemic therapy. *Blood*. 2015;**125**:71–81.

53 Zackheim HS, Kashani-Sabet M, McMillan AK. Low dose methotrexate to treat mycosis fungoides: a retrospective study in 69 patients. *J Am Acad Dermatol.* 2003;**49**:873–878.

54 Horwitz SM, Kim YH, Foss F, et al. Identification of an active, well-tolerated dose of pralatrexate in patients with relapsed or refractory cutaneous T-cell lymphoma. *Blood*. 2012;**119**:4115–4122.

57 Tsimberidon AM, Giles F, Duvic M, et al. Phase II study of pentostatin in advanced T-cell lymphoid malignancies: update of an M.D. Anderson Cancer Center series. *Cancer*. 2004;**100**:342–349.

71 Dummer R, Quaglino P, Becker JC, et al. Prospective international multicenter phase II trial of intravenous pegylated liposomal doxorubicin monochemotherapy in patients with stage IIB, IVA, or IVB advanced mycosis fungoides: final results from EORTC 21012. *J Clin Oncol.* 2012;**30**:4091–4097.

73 Querfeld C, Rosen ST, Guitart J, et al. Multicenter phase II tri of temozolamide in mycosis fungoides/Sézary syndrome: correlation with O^6-methylguanine-DNA methyltransferase and mismatch repair proteins. *Clin Cancer Res.* 2011;**17**: 5748–5754.

92 Duarte RF, Boumendil A, Onida F, et al. Long-term outcome of allogeneic hematopoietic cell transplantation for patients with mycosis fungoides and Sézary syndrome: a European Society for Blood and Marrow Transplantation Lymphoma Working Party Extended Analysis. *J Clin Oncol.* 2014;**32**:3347–3348.

97 Weng WK, Armstrong R, Arai S, et al. Non-myeloablative allogeneic transplantation resulting in clinical and molecular remission with low non-relapse mortality (NRM) in patients with advanced stage mycosis fungoides (MF) and Sézary syndrome (SS). *Blood*. 2014:2544.

100 Zic JA. The treatment of cutaneous T-cell lymphoma with photopheresis. *Dermatol Ther*. 2003;**16**:337–346.

105 Olsen EA. Interferon in the treatment of cutaneous T-cell lymphoma. *Dermatol Ther*. 2003;**16**:311–321.

106 Apisarnthanarax N, Ha CS, Duvic M. Mycosis fungoides with follicular mucinosis displaying aggressive tumor-stage transformation, successful treatment using radiation therapy plus oral bexarotene combination therapy. *Am J Clin Dermatol.* 2003;**4**:429–433.

107 Duvic M, Martin AG, Kim Y, et al. Phase 2 and 3 clinical trial of oral bexarotene (Targretin capsules) for the treatment of refractory or persistent early-stage cutaneous T-cell lymphoma. *Arch Dermatol.* 2001;**137**:581–593.

113 Olsen EA, Kim YH, Kuzel TM, et al. Phase IIB multicenter trial of vorinostat in patients with persistent, progressive, or treatment refractory cutaneous T-cell lymphoma. *J Clin Oncol.* 2007;**25**:3109–3115.

115 Whitaker SJ, Demierre M-F, Kim EJ, et al. Final results from a multicenter, international, pivotal study of romidepsin in refractory cutaneous T-cell lymphoma. *J Clin Oncol.* 2010;**28**:4485–4491.

118 Querfeld C, Mehta N, Rosen ST, et al. Alemtuzumab for relapsed and refractory erythrodermic cutaneous T-cell lymphoma: a single institution experience from the Robert H. Lurie Comprehensive Cancer Center. *Leuk Lymphoma.* 2009;**50**:1969–1976.

120 Kim Y, Tavallaee M, Sundram U et al. Phase II investigator-initiated study of brentuximab vedotin in mycosis fungoides and Sézary syndrome with variable CD30 expression level: a Multi-Institution Collaborative Project. *J Clin Oncol.* 2015;**33**:3750–3758.

第 121 章　浆细胞肿瘤

Noopur Raje, MD ■ Teru Hideshima, MD, PhD ■ Andrew J. Yee, MD ■ Kenneth C. Anderson, MD

概述

浆细胞肿瘤是指浆细胞发生单克隆增殖，分泌异常的单克隆免疫球蛋白的一类肿瘤。这类疾病包括从具有惰性生物学行为的意义不明的单克隆丙种球蛋白血症到恶性肿瘤，如多发性骨髓瘤，是以高钙血症、贫血、肾功能障碍和/或溶解性骨破坏为主要特征。随着对骨髓瘤分子基础的不断深入研究导致其治疗出现了显著进展。大剂量美法仑联合自体干细胞移植是过去主要的治疗手段。现在，高效和耐受性良好的药物，如蛋白酶体抑制剂（如硼替佐米和卡非佐米）和免疫调节剂［如来那度胺（lenalidomide）和泊马度胺（pomalidomide）］已经迅速转化为骨髓瘤的主要治疗手段，明显提高了总生存率。越来越多治疗策略的出现延长了生存期，如维持治疗和新药的出现如浆细胞特异性单克隆抗体进一步改善预后。

多发性骨髓瘤

多发性骨髓瘤（multiple myeloma, MM）是指骨髓（bone marrow, BM）中浆细胞和类浆细胞样细胞恶性增殖，其特征是在血浆和/或尿液中出现单克隆免疫球蛋白（monoclonal immunoglobulin, Ig）或 Ig 片段的一种疾病[1]。这种疾病于 1845 年第一次被发现，当时第一个患者表现为骨痛和尿液中出现热溶性"动物有机物质"[2,3]。MM 这种疾病是 1873 年正式确认命名，反映不同的 BM 浸润部位。早在 1890 年就发现了浆细胞，此后不久，即 1900 年，发现了 MM 与浆细胞增多有关。1939 年的电泳和 1953 年的免疫电泳技术的应用使得单克隆免疫球蛋白成为 MM 诊断的特有物质[4,5]。

诊断标准

活动性 MM 临床和病理诊断的标准是血清和/或尿中存在单克隆免疫球蛋白，骨髓中浆细胞≥10%，伴有高钙血症、肾功能不全、贫血和/或骨损伤（也称为"CRAB"标准，图 121-1），与 MM 相关（表 121-1）[7,8]。活动性 MM 必须与其他单克隆免疫球蛋白疾病区分开来，包括恶性和其他良性疾病，尤其是意义不明的单克隆丙种球蛋白血症（monoclonal gammopathy of undetermined significance, MGUS）和冒烟型 MM。以及其他单克隆蛋白相关的疾病包括华氏巨球蛋白血症、非霍奇金淋巴瘤、原发性淀粉样变性、特发性冷凝集素病、原发性冷球蛋白血症和重链病。冒烟型 MM 的定义是单克隆蛋白>3g/dl 和/或骨髓中浆细胞≥10%，且无终末器官受累（即"CRAB"标准：高钙血症、肾功能不全、贫血或骨损伤）。国际骨髓瘤工作组（International Myeloma Working Group, IMWG）最近更新了有症状骨髓瘤的定义，纳入了以下生物标志物作为诊断标准，如骨髓克隆性浆细胞比例≥60%，受累血清游离轻链与未受累血清游离轻链（free light-chain, FLC）比值≥100，或 MRI 检查发现局灶性病变部位>1 处[6]。

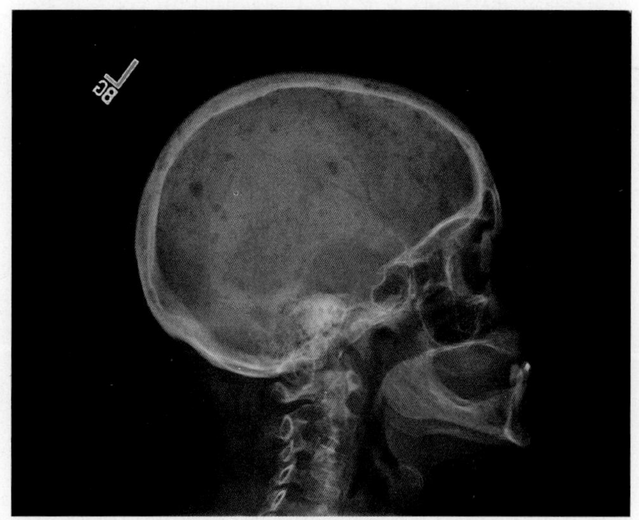

图 121-1　多发性骨髓瘤特征性溶骨性病变

表 121-1　单克隆免疫球蛋白的分类

意义不明的单克隆丙种球蛋白血症
M-蛋白峰值<3g/dl
骨髓中克隆性浆细胞<10%
缺少 CRAB[a] 症状
无症状（冒烟）骨髓瘤
M-蛋白水平≥3g/dl 或骨髓中克隆性浆细胞 10%~60%
缺少 CRAB 症状
活动性骨髓瘤
骨髓中克隆性浆细胞≥10%或活组织检查证实为浆细胞瘤和出现任何一个 CRAB 症状或没有 CRAB 症状需要具有以下条件：MRI 检查示>1 处病灶，骨髓克隆性浆细胞≥60%，受累与未受累血清游离轻链比值（FLC）≥100

[a]CRAB 标准是由浆细胞异常所致的终末器官损害：血钙升高（>1mg/d 升高于正常上限或>11mg/dl）；肾功能不全（肌酐清除率<40ml/min 或肌酐>2mg/dl）；贫血（血红蛋白>2g/dl 低于正常或血红蛋白<10g/dl 下限）；或骨损伤（骨骼 X 线摄片、CT 或 PET CT 上的一个或多个溶骨性病变）。

摘自 *Rajkumar* et al, *2014. 6Reproduced with permission of Elsevier*。

意义不明的单克隆丙种球蛋白血症

MGUS 在 50 岁或 50 岁以上的人群中的发生率为 3. 2%,在 70 岁或 70 岁以上的人群中的发生率为 5. 3%[9]。其诊断标准为血浆中 M 蛋白水平<3g/dl,骨髓中单克隆浆细胞比例<10%,无骨破坏、贫血、高钙血症、肾功能不全(CRAB 标准)[8]。来自梅奥诊所诊断的 1 384 名患者的大型数据,其中 115 名患者进展为 MM、IgM 淋巴瘤、原发性淀粉样变性、巨球蛋白血症、慢性淋巴细胞病白血病或浆细胞肿瘤的相对进展风险分别为 25. 0、2. 4、8. 4、46. 0、0. 9 和 8. 5[10]。MGUS 发展为 MM 或相关疾病的风险约为每年 1%,血清单克隆蛋白的初始浓度是 20 年时病情进展的重要预测因子。Cesana 等人也发表了类似的结果[11]。MGUS 向 MM 转化相关的独立预后因素包括:①骨髓中浆细胞增多>5%;②尿本周蛋白;③多克隆血清免疫球蛋白下降;④红细胞沉降率升高[11]。最近,进展的危险因素包括异常的血清 κ∶λ FLC 比值,血清单克隆蛋白水平≥1. 5g/dl,非 Ig 型单克隆蛋白[12]。从无症状型进展为症状型 MM 相关风险为诊断时骨髓中浆细胞比例、血清单克隆蛋白水平[13]以及血清 FLC 比值异常[14]。在某些情况下,MGUS 是否需要治疗可能与症状有关。例如,血浆置换在 IgG 或 IgA 型 MGUS 有相关的神经症状时似乎是有效的[15]。

流行病学

除了 MGUS 外,MM 发生的潜在危险因素还包括暴露于辐射或石油产品中。与白血病不同,苯暴露不会增加 MM 的风险[16]。据报道,在两个或两个以上受影响的个体家庭可能中存在遗传易感性[17]。MM 在农民、造纸商、家具制造商和木材工人中的发病率也较高(但不到两倍)。

关于 MM 有两个主要的误解。首先,MM 被误认为是一种罕见的疾病。MM 是第二常见的血液恶性肿瘤,2014 年美国新增 24 050 例癌症病例,约占癌症相关死亡人数的 2%[18]。据报道,非裔美国人和太平洋岛民的发病率最高。而欧洲和北美的白人则处于中间水平,生活在亚洲和美国的亚洲人患病概率普遍较低[19]。虽然有人认为 MM 的发病率正在增加,但来自明尼苏达州奥姆斯特德县的研究数据表明,在过去的 46 年里,MM 的发病率并没有发生显著的变化[20]。第二个误解是 MM 只是老年人的一种疾病。来自梅奥诊所的一个大型数据,MM 的中位年龄是 66 岁[21,22]。虽然 98%的患者年龄在 40 岁以上,但是 30%的患者年龄小于 60 岁。事实上有相当大一部分人的年龄低于 70 岁,因此可以采取更积极的治疗方法来影响潜在的治疗策略。

临床特征

通过在表 121-2 中总结的 1985—1998 年 1 027 例新诊断 MM 的临床特征[21]。骨痛和贫血仍然是最常见的临床症状。

表 121-2　多发性骨髓瘤的特征

特征表现	
贫血(血红蛋白≤12g/dl)	73%
血钙≥11mg/dl	13%
肌酐≥2g/dl	19%
X 线异常(平片)[a]	79%
骨痛	58%
乏力	32%
体重下降	24%

[a]67%的患者有溶骨性骨损伤。

摘自 *Kyle et al,2003. 21Reproduced with permission of Elsevier*。

实验室检查

在大多数病例中,实验室检查发现血清和/或尿液中有单克隆 Ig 和骨的 X 线表现异常。其中,50%~60%的 MM 患者血清和尿中同时具有单克隆蛋白;20%~30%的患者仅血清中有,尿中无单克隆蛋白;15%~20%的患者仅尿中有单克隆蛋白;只有 1%~2%的患者在血液和/或尿液中无单克隆蛋白分泌[23];IgG 或 IgA 型单克隆蛋白最为常见,IgD 或 IgE 型较为少见。双克隆现象比以前更为常见,通常只能通过免疫固定电泳技术检测到。IgG 和 IgA 型占 33%;IgM 和 IgG 型占 24%;双克隆和 IgD 型患者的预后与单克隆疾病患者相似[24]。密切观察对于 MGUS 和冒烟型 MM 患者是一个恰当的选择,然而,多发性骨髓瘤的治疗已采用多种方案。MM 的自然病程是随着肿瘤生长逐年增加,M 蛋白倍增时间是衡量 MM 生长速度的一种指标,随着每次复发而缩短。最终,骨髓衰竭发展为缺铁性贫血、白细胞减少症和血小板减少症,从骨髓衰竭到死亡的中位时间间隔为 3 个月(1 个月~9 个月)[25]。感染和肾衰竭分别占 MM 患者死亡的 52%和 21%,急性髓系白血病在一小部分患者中发生,但超出了预期的基线发生率[25]。

生物学

细胞表面表型

B 细胞限制性抗原和相关抗原(antigens,Ag)被用来描述正常和恶性 B 细胞分化的阶段[27]。此外,抗原谱不仅对鉴别恶性 B 细胞分化的阶段很有用,而且对 B 细胞肿瘤的分类也很有用。MM 细胞具有某些 Ag 的细胞表面表达,如 CD38 和 PCA-1(前列腺癌抗原-1),这些细胞表面表达也存在于正常的浆细胞中,提示 MM 的正常细胞对应物是正常的浆细胞。然而,到目前为止,已经有许多其他的 Ag 被发现在 MM 的表面,在某些情况下,一些细胞在分化阶段比浆细胞更早与 B 细胞发生反应,也与非 B 细胞发生反应[28~33]。Harada 等人已经证明正常的浆细胞表达 CD19+CD56-,而 MM 细胞没有这种表型[34]。MUC-1 抗原的核心蛋白在 MM 细胞上表达[35],其抑制作用可导致 MM 细胞死亡[36]。黏附分子在 MM 细胞上的表达和功能将在下面部分描述。这种细胞表面表型的异质性引起了对 MM 细胞起源的争论。

MM 细胞起源

众所周知，MM 患者骨髓中积聚着大量的浆细胞或类浆细胞形态样细胞。然而，自 20 世纪 70 年代以来，基于使用特异性型抗体的研究，人们已经知道，通过特异性抗体可以通过外周血淋巴细胞的克隆来识别巨球蛋白血症、MM、MGUS 和慢性淋巴细胞白血病[37]。特异性决定因子的存在对 MM 中骨髓的细胞质中前体 B 细胞提供了进一步的证据，致癌事件可能发生在前体 B 细胞阶段。研究发现，B 细胞和 T 细胞具有相同的特异性决定因素，这表明致癌转化的靶细胞可能是 B 细胞和 T 细胞克隆的前体细胞[38]。异倍体骨髓 MM 细胞可表达髓系、红系和血小板系细胞表面蛋白的 mRNA，也支持恶性克隆可以从早期分化进展得到观点[39]。此外，MM 患者外周血单克隆 B 细胞系（CD19 和 CD20 低表达，CALLA 和 PCA-1 中等表达，具有较强的 CD45RO 抗原表达）为晚期 B 细胞，不断向浆细胞期发展[31]。然而，目前还不清楚恶性克隆中的哪个细胞是“克隆的”，并且能够自我更新。一些证据表明，前 B 细胞和幼稚 B 细胞从骨髓迁移到淋巴结（lymph node，LN），在那里发生抗原识别、选择和体细胞超突变。记忆 B 细胞被认为是包含 MM 的细胞质 μ-阳性前体细胞，然后在淋巴结中进行 Ig 类转换[40]。Ig 变量（VH）基因序列分析显示 MM 肿瘤细胞是滤泡后的，突变的均质克隆序列表明没有持续暴露于体细胞超突变机制[41]。IgM MM 的 *VH* 基因分析表明其起源于经历同型开关事件的记忆细胞[42]。MGUS 中突变的异质性序列表明，肿瘤细胞仍受突变体的影响，在 MM 中（*IgH* 位置）14q 异常最为常见，由于原癌基因在滤泡性淋巴瘤、伯基特淋巴瘤、慢性淋巴细胞白血病等 B 细胞恶性肿瘤中易位并过度表达，它们也可能在 MM 的肿瘤发生中发挥作用。此外，涉及开关区域的易位表明 MM 中最终的致癌分子事件发生在 B 细胞个体发育的晚期[43]。最近，具有记忆 B 细胞表型的 CD138 细胞被认为是克隆 MM“干细胞”，尽管这一概念需要进一步验证[44]。

黏附分子、细胞因子和基质细胞在 MM 中的作用

黏附分子介导肿瘤细胞对细胞外基质（ECM）蛋白或骨髓基质细胞（BMSC）的同型和异型黏附（图 121-2）[45]。此外，它们在疾病进展的发病机制中起着关键作用。在淋巴结转换之后，黏附分子如 CD44、VLA-4（非常晚的抗原-4）、VLA-5、LFA-1（白细胞功能相关的抗原-1）、CD56、syndecan-1（CD138）和 MPC-1 介导 MM 细胞向骨髓归巢[45~49]。随后，MM 细胞与骨髓间充质干细胞结合，例如通过 VLA-4 与 VCAM-1（血管细胞黏附分子-1）和 ECM 结合，以及通过蛋白多糖与Ⅰ型胶原以及 VLA-4 与纤连蛋白结合。这种结合不仅使肿瘤细胞在骨髓微环境中定位，而且刺激骨髓间充质干细胞的白介素-6（IL-6）转录和分泌，并伴有相关的 MM 细胞旁分泌[50~52]。此外，通过肿瘤细胞上发现的 CD40 触发 IL-6 转录和分泌，并伴有相关的 MM 自分泌细胞生长（图 121-3）[53]。TNF-α 上调对 MM 细胞黏附分子和骨髓间充质干细胞，从而增加黏合物和细胞黏附介导耐药（CAM-DR）[54]。syndecan-1 是 MM 细胞生长、存活和细胞分化的多功能调节剂，血清 syndecan-1 升高与肿瘤细胞负荷增加、金属蛋白酶-9 活性降低和预后不良有关[55~57]。它还能调节破骨细胞的降解和成骨细胞的分化[55]。黏附还可以引起基质金属蛋白酶-1，有利于骨吸收和肿瘤侵袭[58]。随着疾病

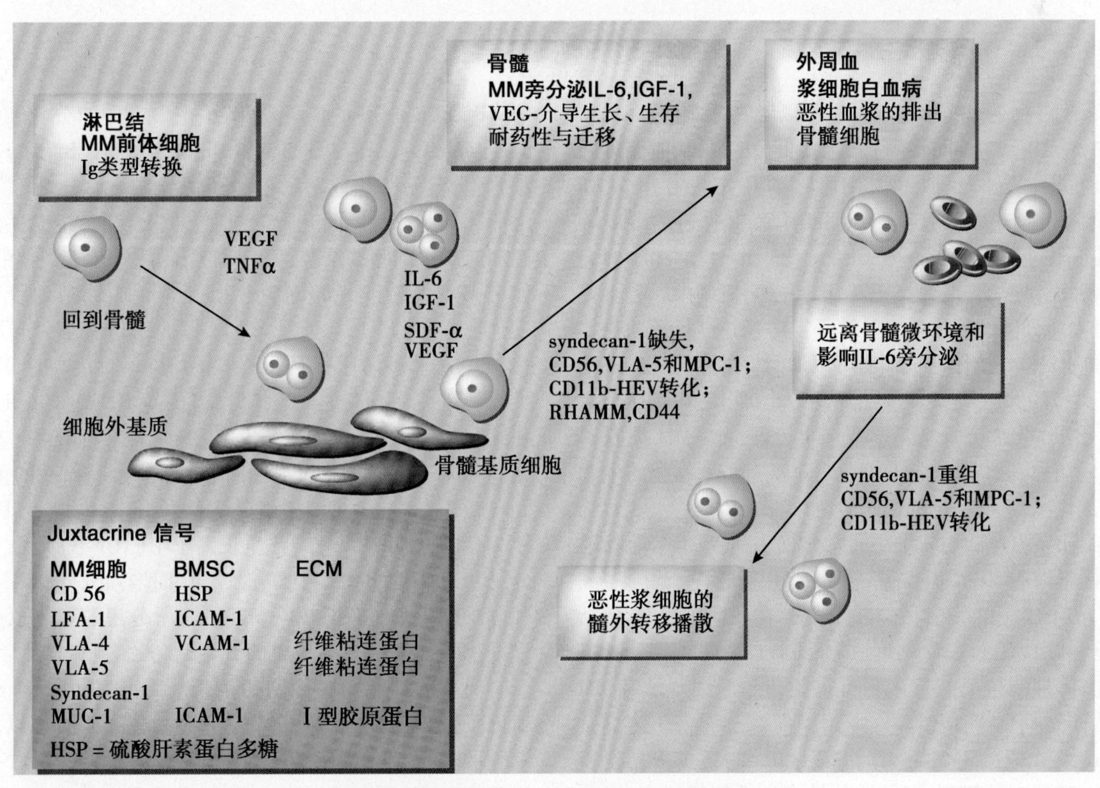

图 121-2　黏附分子在骨髓瘤中的发病过程

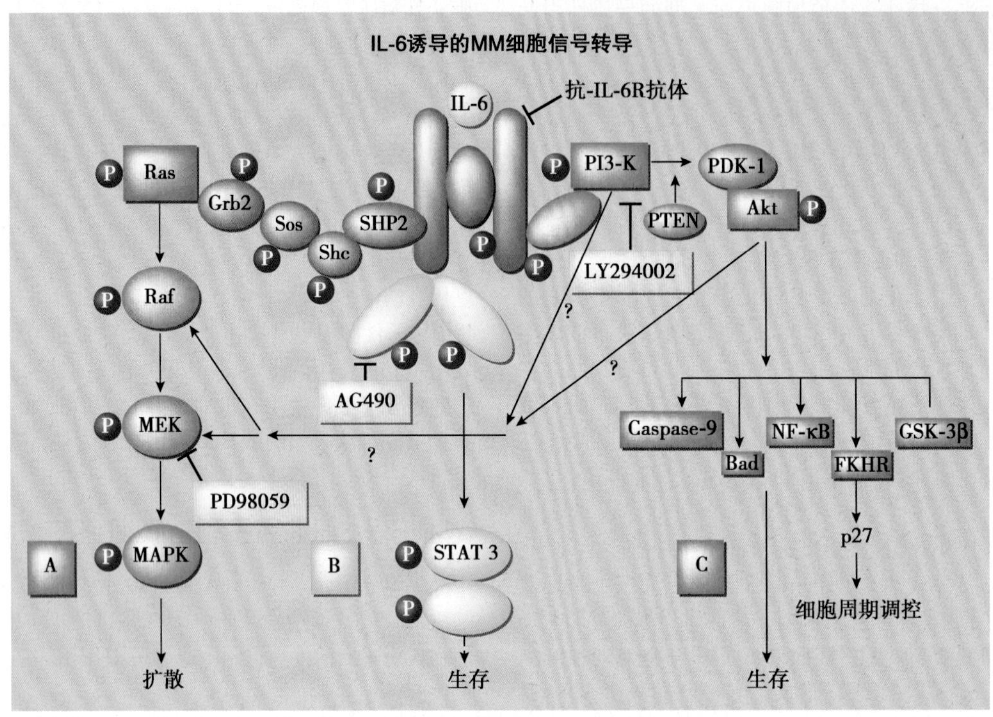

图 121-3　interleukin-6 信号级联

的进展，浆细胞白血病（PCL）的发展以某些黏附分子（如 CD56、VLA-5、MPC-1、syndecan-1）表达减少为特征，从而促进肿瘤细胞的动员。此外，获取 PCL 细胞上的其他黏附分子，如 CD11b、CD44 和 RHAMM，有助于从 BM 中流出时通过内皮细胞。MM 髓外细胞的增殖是由于 CD56、VLA-5、MPC-1 和 syndecan-1 的出现而促进的。黏附分子在 MM 发病机制中起着重要作用，针对黏附分子的治疗策略已被研发出来并进行了动物实验；例如，抗 ICAM-1 抗体已被证明可以抑制重度联合免疫缺陷病（SCID）小鼠的肿瘤发展[59]。此外，在人胎骨移植 SCID 小鼠（SCID-hu 小鼠）中建立的 MM 模型首次为评价人 MM 细胞对人 BM ECM 蛋白和 BMSC 的归巢提供了体内模型，结合的生物学后遗症，以及基于这一过程中断的新疗法的试验[60,61]。对美法仑和多柔比星耐药的 MM 细胞通常过度表达 VLA-4，而黏附于纤维连接蛋白等 ECM 蛋白可诱导 CAM-DR，并上调肿瘤细胞中 p27Kip1 的表达[62]。我们将在接下来的段落中讨论，包括免疫调节药物（IMiD），如沙利度胺（thalidomide）和来那度胺，以及蛋白酶体抑制剂硼替佐米都可以靶向肿瘤细胞及其 BM 微环境，从而克服 CAM-DR[63~67]。

我们已经描述了 MM 细胞作为宿主 BM 的宿主并黏附于 BMSC 和 ECM 蛋白的机制，以及这种结合的功能后遗症，以确定新的治疗靶点。重要的是，我们过去的研究已经确定了那些介导 MM 细胞与纤连蛋白和骨髓间充质干细胞结合的黏附分子，以及这种结合带来的 MM 细胞生长和生存优势[45,52,68~70]。

我们的研究表明，骨髓间充质干细胞分泌细胞因子，如 IL-6[71]、胰岛素样生长因子-1（IGF-1）[72]、血管内皮生长因子（VEGF）[73,74]、基质细胞衍生生长因子（SDF-1α）[75]和 B 细胞激活因子（BAFF）[76,77]，从而增加 MM 在 BM 环境中细胞的生长、生存、耐药性和迁移（图 121-4）。除了在 BM 微环境中定位肿瘤细胞，我们的研究表明，MM 细胞黏附 BMSC 也触发的旁分泌 NF-κB-dependent 转录和 IL-6 在 BMSC 的分泌，通过激活 p42/44MAPK、*JAK2*/STAT3 和 PI3K/AKT 信号级联，介导 MM 细胞生长、存活和地塞米松耐药诱导凋亡[50,52,72,78~89]。VEGF 由 MM 细胞和骨髓间充质干细胞共同分泌，通过 MM 细胞与骨髓间充质干细胞的结合，VEGF 的分泌水平也有类似的上调；它促进 MM 细胞生长和 BM 新生血管的形成，尽管血管生成的病理生理意义尚不明确[90,91]。VEGF 通过 PKC 信号转导诱导迁移[74]。虽然肿瘤坏死因子 α（TNFα）并不直接改变 MM 细胞的生长和生存，我们的研究表明，它诱发 NF-κB-dependent 上调在细胞表面黏附分子的表达（ICAM-1 和 VCAM-1）在 MM 细胞和 bmsc，导致增加细胞黏附和相关诱导 bmsc 的 IL-6 转录和分泌[54]。重组 IL-1β 刺激 MM 细胞产生 IL-6，因此增强 MM 细胞的扩散[92]。转移生长因子-β（TGF-β）是由 MM 细胞分泌和 IL-6 在 BMSC 中分泌[93]，从而增强旁分泌 IL-6 介导的肿瘤细胞生长。TGF-β 由 MM 细胞所分泌的可能也会导致免疫缺陷特征表达下调 MM 的 B 细胞，T 细胞和自然杀伤细胞，没有类似的抑制 MM 细胞的生长。IL-10 是人 MM 细胞的增殖因子，但不是分化因子[94]。IGF-1 已被证明可以增强 MM 细胞的生长、生存和耐药性[72]。巨噬细胞炎性蛋白-1α（MIP-1α）对于 MM 是一个破骨细胞刺激因子[95,96]。BAFF 是由骨髓间充质干细胞，尤其是破骨细胞产生的。它通过多个受体发出信号，包括 BAFF-R、跨膜激活剂、钙调节剂、环亲素配体相互作用体（TACI）和 B 细胞成熟 Ag（BCMA）[76,77]。MM 细胞中 *TACI* 基因表达水平与微环境依赖性有关[97]。这种信号级联对 MM 细胞具有延长生存的作用。由 IL-15[98] 和最近的 IL-21[99] 介导的自分泌生长已在 MM 细胞系和患者细胞中得到证实。

Wnt 信号调控多种疾病发生发展过程，进而导致恶性肿瘤的形成，近年来已在 MM 中研究证实。Wnt 是一类与七次跨膜

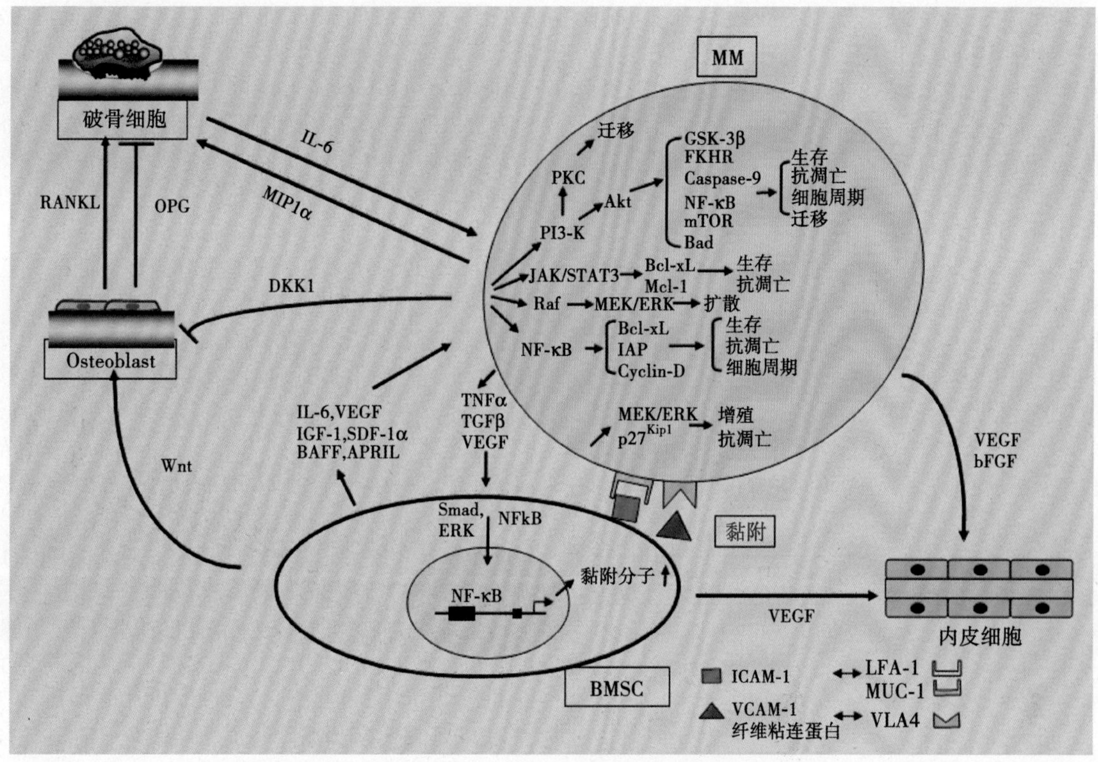

图 121-4　微环境中上下信号级联

受体结合的分泌型糖蛋白。Wnt 信号途径能引起胞内 β-连锁蛋白（β-catenin）积累，在 MM，规范 Wnt 信号通路被激活 Wnt-3a 治疗后，与 β-catenin 积累有关。Wnt-3a 处理进一步导致 MM 细胞发生明显的形态学改变，并伴有肌动蛋白细胞骨架的重新排列[100]。Derksen 等[101]报道 MM 细胞过表达 β-catenin，包括其氨基端磷酸化形式，符合活跃 β-catenin/T 细胞因子转录媒介。进一步积累和 β-catenin 核定位，和/或增加细胞增殖，是通过刺激与 Wnt-3a Wnt 信号，LiCl 或 β-catenin 的持续活跃的突变体。Wnt 信号通路也被认为是间充质干细胞成骨细胞分化的重要调控通路。有趣的是，在 BM 活检标本中 MM 细胞标本中检测到 Dickkopf1（DKK1），是 Wnt 信号级联反应中的负面调节因子和 β-catenin/TCF 通路的靶点[102]。此外，MM 患者骨髓血浆和外周血中 DKK1 水平升高与 *DKK1* 基因表达模式相关，并与局灶性骨病损的存在相关[103]。

最重要的是，MM 细胞与骨髓间充质干细胞的黏附引起基因谱的改变：即肿瘤细胞生长、生存和耐药基因的上调；MM 细胞和骨髓间充质干细胞黏附分子的上调；以及人骨髓间充质干细胞在小鼠体内和体外模型中细胞因子的变化[104~106]。MM 细胞与 BMSC 的相互作用激活 Notch 信号，诱导美法仑耐药[107]。当 MM 细胞与骨髓间充质干细胞结合时，蛋白酶体活性的诱导可能使其对治疗敏感。

我们已经证明亚胺类药物（如来那度胺）可以抑制 VEGF 和 IL-6，而 VEGF 和 IL-6 在 MM 中下调树突状细胞的抗原递呈功能[108]。此外，来那度胺直接激活 T 细胞上的 CD28，从而刺激 IL-2 的转录和分泌，从而上调 T 细胞和 NK 细胞的抗 MM 活性[108,109]。来那度胺可上调抗体依赖性细胞毒性（antibody-dependent cellular cytotoxicity，ADCC）[110]。免疫调节剂还会影响效应细胞与 MM 细胞和骨髓间充质干细胞相互作用所激发的细胞因子信号，这是通过调控细胞因子信号抑制因子（SOCS）基因的 SOCS1 来实现的[111]。

MM 的分子发病机制

MM 内的恶性浆细胞位于骨髓中，与骨髓间充质干细胞密切相关。恶性浆细胞是一种生存期很长的细胞，其标记指数（labeling index，LI）很低（1%~2%），这为恶性 BMPC 的增殖率提供了一个衡量指标，预测了新诊断的 MM 患者的生存率。*Ig* 基因重排以与抗原选择相容的方式广泛地发生体细胞超突变，没有证据表明超突变过程正在持续[41]。然而，MM 细胞的 Ig 分泌率明显低于正常浆细胞。因此，看来 MM 细胞中的关键致癌事件要么发生在长期存活浆细胞的正常分化过程之后，要么不影响大多数正常分化过程。

基因表达谱最近被用来描述从正常浆细胞到 MGUS 再到 MM 的过程中相关的变化[112~114]。MGUS 和 MM 的 mRNA 表达谱相似，且与正常浆细胞有明显差异[114]。这些研究不仅可以提高对基础病理生理学的认识，而且可以确定新的治疗靶点。

通过常规分析，在 MM 的大型研究中，MM 中检测到核型异常发生率占 30%~50%（表 121-3）[115~117]。核型异常的发生率和程度与治疗的分期、预后和对治疗反应有关。例如，大约 20%的Ⅰ期患者出现异常，60%的Ⅲ期患者出现异常，>80%的髓外肿瘤出现异常。这种分析依赖于获得可靠的中间准备工作，并且大大低估了这些不常分裂的细胞群中 DNA 改变的程度。通过荧光原位杂交（fluorescence in situ hybridization，FISH）技术分析，两项研究报告显示，分别有 96%或 89%的 MM 肿瘤样本中至少有一条染色体是三体的[118,119]。虽然传统的核型并没有在 MGUS 常规报道，但似乎有相当一部分的 MGUS 浆细胞也是非整倍体。通过 FISH 分析，两项对 MGUS 细胞的研究中，至少一条染色体的三体发生率分别为43%和53%；在前者中，通过图像分析，61%的细胞含有非整倍体DNA[118,120]。特征性的数值异常为染色体3、5、7、9、11、15和19的13号染色体单体和三分体。非随机结构异常最常涉及1号染色体，无明显的位点特异性；14q32（*IgH*）位点占20%～40%；11q13（bcl-1位点）约占20%，但主要易位于14q32；13q14间质缺失占15%；8q24占10%左右，其中大约一半与易位有关。重要的是，最近的一份报告记录了MGUS和MM中类似的易位，包括t（4；14）（p16.3；q32）和t（14；16）（q32；q23），但没有任何明显的临床或生物学相关性[121]。

许多B淋巴细胞肿瘤的遗传性病变由于涉及*IgH*基因位点（14q32.3）的易位而导致癌基因失调；不太常见的是，变异易位涉及一个IgL位点（2p12，κ或22q11，λ）（表121-3和表121-4）。常规核型分析，约20%～40%MM的异常核型是14q32的

表121-3　骨髓瘤染色体改变

遗传病变	发生率/%
超二倍体	60
t（11；14）	20
t（4；14）	15
MAF 易位	5
Del（13q）/单体13	50～60
Del（1p）	7～40
Chr 1q21 扩增	40
细胞周期素1失调	80
RAS 突变	30～50
FAM46C，DIS3	10～21
NF-κB 激活突变和基因拷贝数异变	15～20
IgH MYC 基因重排	15
UTX 缺失和突变	30
TP53 激活（突变+缺失（17p））	10～20
p18和/或Rb失活	<5
p14启动子甲基化	<5
PTEN丢失	<2

表121-4　异常重组的非免疫球蛋白位点

染色体	基因	功能
11q13	*Cyclin D1*	促进增长
4p16	*FGFR3*，*MMSET*	生长因子
8q24	*MYC*	增长/凋亡
16q23	*c-maf*	转录因子
6p25	*IRF4*	转录因子

摘自*Kuel and Bergsagel 2002*[122]。*Reproduced with permission of Nature Publishing Group*。

易位[123]。在疾病的髓外期和细胞系中，这些易位的发生率明显较高，在更多的检查中被发现。约30%的这些易位，配偶染色体位点为11q13（bcl-1，cyclin D1），但在大多数情况下，配偶没有被识别（14q32+）。细胞周期蛋白D1的转录激活最近在一些原发性肿瘤中得到证实，细胞周期蛋白D3的激活与t（6；14）（p21；q32）易位相关[121,124,125]。其他复发性配偶基因点很少被发现，包括<5%的8q24（*c-myc*）、18q21（bcl-2）、11q23（ml-1）和6p21.1。通过将传统的核型分析与检测*IgH*开关区域易位的Southern blot综合分析相结合，我们发现大多数MM细胞系和一个原发肿瘤都存在*IgH*易位，且主要涉及*IgH*开关区域[43,126]。最近的FISH研究也表明，73%的MM患者存在*IGH*基因重排[127]。由t（4；14）调控的表观癌基因是成纤维细胞生长因子受体3（fibroblast growth factor receptor 3，*FGFR3*）基因，可能由于t（4；14）调控的*FGFR3*表达失调，在骨髓微环境中从基质细胞产生的FGF中接收*FGFR3*介导的信号[128]。除了*FGFR3*，MM中的t（4；14）易位还调控一种新的基因MMSET，导致*IgH/MMSET*杂交转录[129]。*FGFR3*的异位表达促进MM细胞增殖，阻止细胞凋亡，其致癌潜能已在小鼠模型中测试，证实其转化造血细胞的能力[130,131]。最后，有证据表明，在MM中，*c-myc*的表达升高和一个*c-myc*等位基因的选择性表达可能频繁发生，尽管只有10%～20%的肿瘤发现了*c-myc*附近的结构基因变化。

大约39%的新诊断的MM患者发生*Ras*突变，并且*Ras*突变的频率随着疾病的进展而增加。N-和*K-ras*突变很少在孤立的浆细胞瘤和MGUS中检测到，但在MM（9%～30%）和大多数终末期疾病或PCL患者（63%～70%）中更常见[132,133]。激活癌基因突变也可能导致生长因子独立性和抑制凋亡素。在MM中激活*ras*癌基因突变也可能导致细胞生长因子独立性和凋亡抑制。

虽然易位（14；18）在MM中仅有0～15%的发生率，但在大多数MM患者和MM细胞系中均可见过表达Bcl-2[134,135]。高水平的Bcl-2蛋白可能介导MM细胞对IL-6、星孢菌素或其他药物诱导的凋亡的抵抗[136]。在小鼠MM细胞系中，Bcl-XL在环己酰亚胺治疗或IL-6停药后，在抑制细胞凋亡方面发挥了重要作用[137]。同样，过表达Bcl-2或Bcl-XL也可抑制IL-6在B-9IL-6依赖细胞系中的阻止细胞凋亡[138]。在MM细胞中，Mcl-1过表达，IL-6上调，介导细胞对凋亡的抵抗，而Mcl-1下调则触发细胞凋亡（图121-5）[140]。

超过50%的MM存在13号染色体缺失，且与预后不良相关[121,141～143]。然而，这些缺失也与MGUS相关，因此它们在转化为MM中的作用目前还不明确[121,144,145]。

最近对MM的分子发病机制的了解导致了一个新的MM分类[146,147]。大多数MM肿瘤有染色体异常，可广泛分为高二倍体（HRD）或非高二倍体（NHRD）肿瘤。近一半的MM肿瘤是HRD，其余被归为NHRD，包括亚二倍体、假二倍体或亚四倍体肿瘤。这些NHRD肿瘤的预后较差。在MM中发现5例复发性*IgH*易位发生率为40%，包括*MMSET*和*FGFR3*（15%）、*cyclin D3*（3%）、*cyclin D1*（15%）、*c-maf*（5%）和*MAFB*（2%）。最近的证据表明，这五种易位中有三种在NHRD肿瘤中占主导地位。

涉及*TP53*基因组位点的17p染色体缺失在新诊断的骨髓

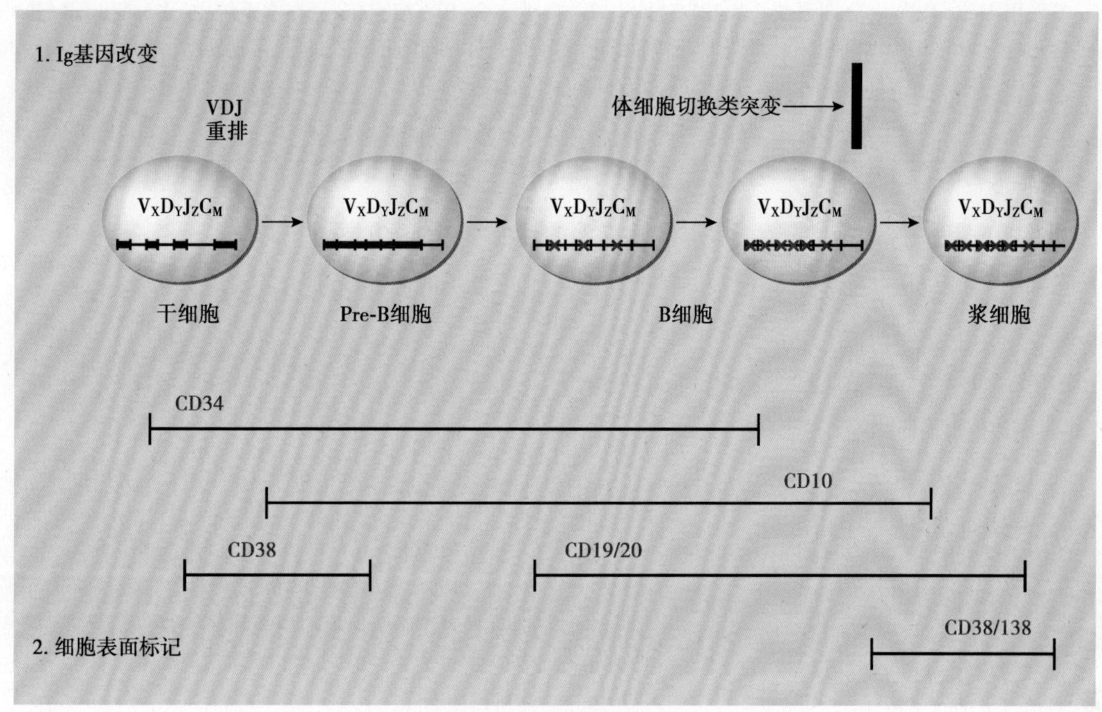

图121-5 凋亡信号通路

瘤中很少见(5%~10%),但在复发和难治性病例中更为常见(20%~40%),且与不良预后相关[148,149]。然而,含硼替佐米的方案可以克服这种不良预后,如HOVON-65/GMMG-HD4试验所示[150]。约40%的新诊断骨髓瘤和70%的复发骨髓瘤可通过FISH检测到1q21扩增。它会对总体生存(OS)产生负面影响。可能的下游靶基因包括 *CKS1B*、*PSMD4*、*MCL1* 和 *BCL9*。CKS1B是一种调节细胞周期蛋白依赖性蛋白激酶的蛋白,PSMD4是一种蛋白酶体亚单位调节对硼替佐米治疗的反应[151~153]。此外,在7%~40%的患者中存在1p缺失,这与自体干细胞移植后PFS(无进展生存期)和OS的降低有关[154~156]。*FAM46C* 缺失或 *FAM46C* 突变(在15%的患者中很明显)尤其与生存时间缩短相关(中位OS 25.7个月 vs 51.3个月,$P=0.004$)[156,157]。FAM46C的生物学功能尚不清楚,但可能与mRNA的稳定有关。其他异常包括 *MYC* 重排,包括染色体8p24上的不平衡易位和插入、小重复、扩增和倒置[158~161];11q22位点纯合缺失导致 *YAP1*、*BIRC3*、*birc2* 基因组区域缺失[162~164];4号染色体、14号染色体和16号染色体畸变,破坏 *FGFR3*、*WWOX* 和 *cyld*;6号染色体缺失或扩增,Xp11.2位点纯合缺失[165,166],包括UTX,一组蛋白H3赖氨酸27(H3K27)去甲基酶突变,发生在10%的骨髓瘤中[157,167]。

随着cDNA技术的出现,一种快速、全面的基因表达谱可能更好地确定疾病生物学,预后因素,并确定潜在新药的治疗靶点[124,168]。这些研究还可能确定对传统和新型MM疗法的敏感性和耐药性的机制[169,170]。已知的靶抗原可能只是冰山一角。最近,微阵列比较基因组杂交(aCGH)已与基因谱分析相关联,分别用于识别染色体扩增和转录过表达[165]。经典的过表达和敲除实验可能首先在癌症模型中进行,然后在MM模型中进行,以确定单克隆抗体(细胞表面)或小分子抑制剂(细胞内)治疗的潜在新靶点。

体细胞突变和克隆间多样性

多发性骨髓瘤通常发生在MGUS或冒烟型骨髓瘤转化为症状性骨髓瘤之前[171,172],其特征是突变的积累,这些突变赋予生长优势(驱动突变)或功能无关突变(乘客突变)。迄今为止,已有300多个骨髓瘤患者的DNA样本采用全基因组测序或全外显子组测序方法进行测序[157,173,174]。经常发生突变的基因包括 *KRAS*、*NRAS*、*FAM46C*、*DIS3* 和 *TP53*。其他重要基因包括 *BRAF*(占4%的患者)、*TRAF3*、*CYLD*、*RBL*、*PRDM1* 和 *ACTG1*。*TRAF3* 和 *CYLD* 突变,加上纯合子缺失在 *BIRC2/BIRC3*、*NIK* 过表达和其他基因的突变(*CARD11* 和 *MYD88*)有助于持续激活NF-κB通路。参与蛋白稳态、未折叠蛋白反应或淋巴/浆细胞发育的基因,如参与浆细胞分化的 *PRDM1* 以及 *XBP1*、*IRF4*、*LRRK2*、*SP140* 和 *LTB* 形成骨髓瘤突变基因簇。其他周期性突变基因 *ROBO1*,参与β-catenin和MET信号跨膜受体,EGR1转录因子,FAT3,属于钙黏蛋白家族的一种跨膜蛋白,组蛋白修饰酶基因(*MLL*、*MLL2*、*MLL3*、*WHSC1/MMSET*、*WHSC1L1* 和 *UTX* 等)。PCL患者往往有不同类型的异常,如 *p14ARF* 启动子甲基化、*PTEN* 缺失、*RBL* 突变以及更高的 *TP53* 突变和缺失率[175]。

最近的数据支持骨髓瘤瘤内异质性的概念,在不同的进化机制(包括线性、分支、平行或趋同进化)下,不同的亚克隆可能出现并成为主导[173,176]。克隆多样性类似于达尔文式的选择,有利于癌症的进展和对治疗的适应。下一代测序分析表明,大多数患者在诊断时具有亚克隆结构,其中一个克隆占主导地位,其他几个克隆可在疾病进化或治疗后的不同阶段重新出现[173,177,178]。

预后因素

已有多种明确的临床和实验室参数具有预后指导意

义[7,179~181]。多采用 Durie-Salmon 分期系统（表 121-5）[7]。Ⅰ期患者肿瘤细胞数较少<0.6×10^{12} 细胞/m^2，Ⅱ期患者肿瘤细胞数介于 0.6~1.2×10^{12} 细胞/m^2 之间，Ⅲ期患者肿瘤细胞数较高，为 1.2×10^{12} 细胞/m^2。在本系统中，ⅠA 期、ⅠB+ⅡA+ⅡB 期、ⅢA 期、ⅢB 期患者的生存期分别为 61.2、54.5、30.1、14.7 个月。

表 121-5 Durie-Salmon（DS）分期标准和国际分期标准（ISS）

分期	Durie-Salmon 分期	ISS 分期	ISS 分期总生存期
Ⅰ期	具有所有以下条件：	血清 β_2-微球蛋白<3.5mg/L	62 个月
	• 血红蛋白>10g/dl	血清白蛋白≥3.5g/dl	
	• 血钙正常或≤12mg/dl		
	• 骨 X 线片，0~1 处病灶或孤立性骨浆细胞瘤		
	• M-蛋白产生水平低		
	○ IgG<5g/dl		
	○ IgA<3g/dl		
	○ 尿中轻链 M-蛋白<4g/24h		
Ⅱ期	非Ⅰ期，非Ⅲ期	血清 β_2-微球蛋白<3.5mg/L，但血清白蛋白 3.5<g/dl 或血清 β_2-微球蛋白 3.5~5.5mg/L，不包含血清白蛋白	44 个月
Ⅲ期	具有一项以上的以下条件：	血清 β_2-微球蛋白≥5.5mg/L	29 个月
	• 血红蛋白<8.5g/dl		
	• 血钙>12mg/dl		
	• 严重溶骨性骨破坏（≥3 处）		
	• M-蛋白产生水平高		
	○ IgG>7g/dl		
	○ IgA>5g/dl		
	○ 尿中轻链 M-蛋白>12g/24h		

许多额外的单一参数已被作为有价值的预后因素。在具有浆细胞形态患者中报道了其具有高的标记指数，血清 IL-6 受体水平，*ras* 突变高，疾病侵袭性强和生存期短的特征[182]。血清 β_2-微球蛋白轻链（serum β_2 microglobulin，β_2M）代表的主要组织相容性复合体的细胞膜，并增加血清 β_2M 结果释放肿瘤增长分数和细胞流动率高。MM 患者肾功能正常，血清 β_2M 增高预测进展[183]。LI 是测量 MM 细胞 DNA 合成的一种方法，它预测了存活率。通常在诊断时低（<1%），复发时高，在 MGUS 和惰性 MM 表达低[184]。超过 50%的 MM 存在 13 号染色体缺失，且与不良预后有关[141~143]；然而，这些缺失也与 MGUS 相关[121,144,145]，因此它们在转换为 MM 中的作用目前还没有确定。HRD MM 预后改善，临床特征明显，13 号染色体缺失无不良影响[185]。此外，它不能预测对硼替佐米的反应，这强调了预后因素对特定治疗的重要性[186]。基因表达谱不仅可以确定疾病的发病机制，还可以确定新的预后因素和潜在的治疗靶点[124,130]。这些研究还将确定对传统和新型 MM 疗法的敏感性和耐药性的机制。细胞周期蛋白 D 失调已被确定为 MM 的早期和统一事件。利用基因表达谱鉴定 5 个复发易位、特定三体和周期蛋白 *D2* 基因的表达，MM 可预测分为 8 组 TC（易位/周期蛋白 D）[187]。还提出了其他的分子分类[188]，高风险骨髓瘤的定义是染色体 1 的基因表达失调[189]。最近，第一个基于 DNA 的分类方案被提出来用于预测高剂量治疗的疗效[165]。

一些研究指出血清 IL-6 水平与疾病分期及生存有关，IL-6 刺激肝细胞产生如 C 反应蛋白类的急性期蛋白[190,191]，C 反应蛋白能够反应 IL-6 水平及骨髓浆细胞增殖状态。事实上，意义未明的单克隆 γ 球蛋白血症（MGUS）患者的 C 反应蛋白水平明显低于多发性骨髓瘤患者，且血清 C 反应蛋白水平与生存有关。血清可溶性白介素-6 受体（sIL-6R）[192]、肝细胞生长因子[193]、syndecan-1[194]水平升高以及血清透明质酸水平降低均可作为预后不良的独立预后因子[195,196]。外周血中循环浆细胞的百分比及其标记指数均可作为评估经过常规治疗及高剂量化疗后的骨髓瘤患者生存的独立预后因子，循环内皮细胞亦与疾病的病程及对沙利度胺的反应性存在相关性[197,198]。最后，循环蛋白酶体水平是生存的独立预后因素[199,200]。

因为多数因子间的相互作用使得其独立价值很有限。一些团队经过多因素分析发现血清 β_2M 及浆细胞增殖活性是预测转归的最佳变量组合，β_2-微球蛋白可反应肿瘤负荷及肾功能，浆细胞增殖活性可通过 LI 或 S 期的肿瘤细胞数目评估。年龄及体力状态亦可改善预后评估[201,202]。

国际分期系统（ISS）基于血清 β_2M 及白蛋白水平制订了

一项三期 ISS(表 121-5),目前该分期系统最为常用且应用于临床研究中[181]。

并发症

多发性骨髓瘤的并发症包括骨质破坏、高钙血症、高黏滞综合征、反复感染、肾衰竭以及心功能异常。

骨质破坏及高钙血症

多发性骨髓瘤的显著特征为溶骨性病变、骨痛、病理性骨折风险增高以及广泛的骨质疏松。骨髓瘤骨病表现为成骨细胞及破骨细胞活性的失衡[203],成骨细胞骨形成功能受抑同时与破骨细胞不成比例激活(图 121-6)。RANKL 与 RANK 受体偶联后刺激破骨细胞的分化[204,205]、形成及存活[206],骨髓瘤细胞可通过直接黏附、信号转导或生成 IL-7 等途径产生 RANKL 并且上调骨髓间充质干细胞及成骨细胞中 RANKL 的表达[207~209]。此外,RANKL 与 RANK 受体偶联后抑制骨保护素(OPG)的形成,OPG 为一种通过可溶性因子[210~212]、$\alpha_4\beta_1$-VCAM1 整联蛋白、DKK1 产物抑制 RANK-RANKL 交互作用的诱导受体[214],通过 syndecan 介导的交互作用失活为骨髓瘤细胞[215]。有趣的是,骨髓瘤患者血清 OPG 水平低于正常且与溶骨性病变的发生相关[216,217],RANKL/OPG 比增高提示预后不良。OPG 重组[218]、RANK、OPG 肽[211,213,219]以及最近研发的一种抗 RANKL 抗体地诺单抗(denosumab)[220]可以调整 RANKL/OPG 轴并降低骨髓瘤患者破骨细胞活性。骨髓瘤细胞产生巨噬细胞抑制蛋白(MIP-1α)或细胞因子 C-C motif 配体并促进前体细胞成熟为破骨细胞,MIP-1α 通过 CCR1 及 CCR5 向破骨细胞发送信号并促进上调间质细胞的 RANKL 水平,骨髓瘤患者中 MIP-1α 水平升高[96,221,222],在体外研究及动物模型中 MIP-1α 失活或阻断 CCR1 可减少骨病的发生[223]。IL-6[96]、PTHrP[224]、膜联蛋白Ⅱ[225,226]以及 ephrinB2/EphB4 轴[227]也会促进骨质吸收[228]。骨髓瘤骨病的发展中另一主要原因为成骨细胞受抑,WNT 信号转导途径(包括 DKK1、FRP-2 以及[229] SOST)干扰成骨细胞的成熟[230]。DKK1 由骨髓瘤细胞表达,可上调成骨细胞 RANKL 的水平并提高破骨细胞活性[103,231],骨髓瘤患者血清 DKK1 水平升高,动物实验中已经检测出抗 DKK1 抗体[232~235],目前相关临床研究正在进行。最后,作为 TGF-β 家族成员的激活蛋白 A、IL-3 以及 IL-7 水平升高可通过阻断 RUNX2/CBFA1 抑制骨形成并促进骨的重吸收。此外,骨的活动范围本身会支持骨髓瘤细胞存活并阻止 TNF-α 介导的细胞凋亡[236]。

治疗

双膦酸盐不仅可以阻断破骨细胞和调节成骨细胞,同时可以减小肿瘤负荷[237],在多发性骨髓瘤的支持治疗中发挥关键作用,在体内异种移植模型中发现 OPG 与 RANKL 的重组片段存在与双膦酸盐相似的作用。双膦酸盐尤其是唑来膦酸,目前在临床不仅用于减少骨病的发生[238],同时通过最近的荟萃分析发现,相对于安慰剂,双膦酸盐与患者 OS 延长存在相关性[239,240]。骨吸收及骨形成的标志物与溶骨性病变范围相关[241]。相比于健康对照组,多发性骨髓瘤患者尿液中尿嘧啶吡啶啉(PYD)和脱氧吡啶-诺林(DPD)交联物,以及血清抗酒石酸酸性磷酸酶异构体 5b(Tracp-5b),包括Ⅰ型胶原 N-末端交联肽(NTX)在内的胶原降解产物水平升高[242],仅由活化的破骨细胞产生的骨吸收标志物,并可预示多发性骨髓瘤骨病的早

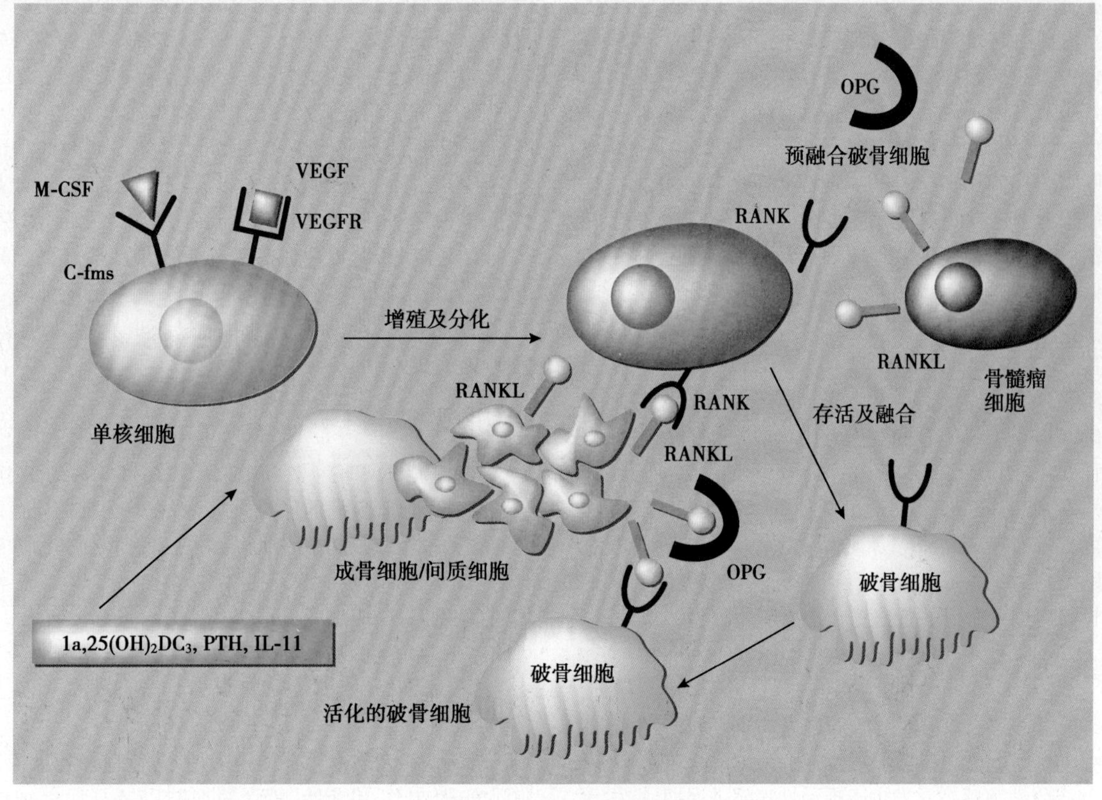

图 121-6 破骨细胞形成

期进展，相反，该人群中如骨碱性磷酸酶及骨钙素等骨形成标志物则相应减少。另一项随机对照研究证实口服氯磷酸盐可减慢骨病及骨不良事件的进展，但其对生存期无影响[242]。一项前瞻性随机对照试验显示在 Durie-Salmon 分期为Ⅲ期且溶骨性病变≥1 处的骨髓瘤患者中，帕米膦酸二钠可减少如病理性骨折、骨放疗以及脊髓压迫症等骨不良事件的发生，该作用可持续 21 个月，其摘要已在 ASCO 提前报告，建议所有的骨髓瘤患者不论化疗效果如何均应持续静脉应用双膦酸盐，因其可能减少骨不良事件及骨痛的发生[243]。有趣的是该研究中的患者即使一线化疗失败其生存期依旧得到延长，这也提示双膦酸盐存在抗骨髓瘤细胞活性的作用[244,245]。目前证据支持的观点为双膦酸盐可减少骨髓基质细胞产生 IL-6 并诱导破骨细胞及肿瘤细胞凋亡[246]。对惰性骨髓瘤的研究中发现，帕米膦酸二钠可以降低骨转换，但并未表现出确切的抗肿瘤活性[247,248]。相比之下，唑来膦酸在作用更强的同时在缩短起效时间方面存在优势，同时对骨不良事件的预防作用与帕米膦酸二钠相似[249]。最近，MRC 骨髓瘤 IX 研究（MRC Myeloma IX trial）证实，与口服双膦酸盐相比，骨髓瘤患者应用唑来膦酸可以得到更长的 OS[250]。但同时需警惕双膦酸盐治疗后出现下颌骨坏死的案例[251]，这种仅在少数患者中新发的并发症导致 ASCO 指南的更新，指南推荐治疗后达到 very good 部分缓解（VGPR）或更好的患者应用双膦酸盐 2 年后停药，而治疗后仅为部分缓解（PR）或更差的患者则需继续应用[252~254]。对于病变局限的患者进行例如椎体成形术或后凸成形术等支持治疗可以保持脊柱的稳定性并缓解疼痛[255~257]。

高钙血症的治疗需在骨髓瘤进行基础治疗的基础上同时应用糖皮质激素、降钙素以及双膦酸盐抑制破骨细胞导致的骨吸收。糖皮质激素可以减少新的破骨细胞形成，降钙素及糖皮质激素可在短期内起效，并且可用于肾功能不全患者，双膦酸盐结合于骨表面并抑制破骨细胞的活性则为治疗的基础。因此骨髓瘤骨病及高钙血症的治疗需包括针对骨髓瘤的基本的细胞毒治疗、水化治疗以及双膦酸盐治疗，而对于一线治疗耐药的患者则需应用降钙素治疗。一项在 287 例存在高钙血症的恶性肿瘤患者中进行的随机对照试验发现，唑来膦酸优于帕米膦酸二钠[257]，由于骨痛或其他原因导致患者活动受限可能加重高钙血症[258]。

高黏滞综合征

高黏滞综合征在临床上通常表现为神经系统自发性出血及视力障碍，238 例 IgG 型骨髓瘤患者中高黏滞综合征发生率为 4.2%，而在 46 例血清 IgG M 蛋白>5.0g/dl 的患者中高黏滞综合征的发生率高达 22%。相对于其他 IgG 亚类，IgG 3 亚类骨髓瘤患者更易出现高黏滞综合征[259]，该综合征的严重程度与血清黏度无直接关系[260]，血浆置换术可改善患者的临床症状并降低骨髓瘤患者血清的蛋白复合物浓度及血清黏度。

反复感染

骨髓瘤患者的感染概率是心脏病患者的 15 倍。肺炎链球菌感染及嗜血杆菌感染通常发生于化疗疾病早期及化疗中[261]，革兰氏阴性菌感染常发生于难治性疾病进展期、抗生素治疗后、有创操作后、固定术、院内菌落定植以及氮质血症。院内感染通常是致命性的，因此对于骨髓瘤患者应尽量减少如留置导管等异物的应用。菌血症（革兰氏阴性或革兰氏阳性）与化疗后粒缺性发热并无确切联系。骨髓瘤患者中真菌、疱疹、分枝杆菌感染以及肺囊虫病较为少见。感染是导致骨髓瘤患者死亡的最主要原因（占发病者的 20%~50%），骨髓瘤患者感染概率增加使得预防措施不断发展，尽管骨髓瘤患者在肺炎球菌疫苗接种后抗体滴度呈正相关增加，但预先免疫滴度则显著减少。因此免疫后滴度水平低且不能起到保护作用[262]。尽管如此，由于此种治疗价格较低且可能对一些患者有效，仍然推荐患者进行肺炎球菌疫苗接种。一项对于骨髓瘤患者进行人免疫球蛋白预防治疗的双盲随机对照试验表明，尽管此种方法对于平稳期患者可能有效[263]，但人免疫球蛋白预防治疗并不能降低感染的发生率，目前，人免疫球蛋白仅应用于存在反复或危及生命的感染患者以及低人免疫球蛋白血症患者[264]。

肾衰竭

骨髓瘤患者出现肾衰竭预示预后不良。一项研究发现 22%的患者在诊断时血清肌酐水平≥2mg/dl，在血清肌酐水平<4mg/dl 的患者中有 48%经过治疗后肾功能可恢复正常[265]。导致骨髓瘤患者出现肾衰竭的因素通常较多，其中包括高钙血症、巨细胞围绕白蛋白、IgG 以及 κ 和 λ 轻链形成的大量层板状管型堵塞近曲小管及远曲小管形成的骨髓瘤肾、高尿酸血症、造影剂肾毒性、脱水、浆细胞浸润、肾盂肾炎以及淀粉样变性。最重要的易感因素则是脱水，积极水化对避免不可逆性肾功能不全至关重要。另外，应积极治疗潜在疾病，应避免静脉应用造影剂（造影剂）。蛋白尿的类型及定量可以鉴别以下疾病：骨髓瘤肾，表现为大量轻链及少量白蛋白；轻链沉积病，特征为尿中轻链及白蛋白水平均较低；淀粉样变性，表现为尿中存在大量白蛋白而轻链较少[266]。与 MM 单克隆轻链产物、轻链沉积病和淀粉样变性相关的肾脏表现是由于本周蛋白（BJP）分别以管型、基底膜沉淀或纤维沉积等形式沉积所致。由于未知原因，肾脏表现的严重程度因人而异[267~269]。将 40 位患者的 BJP 注射到小鼠体内，26 例（65%）以管型、基底膜沉淀或晶体的形式沉积在小鼠肾脏中，其模式与在患者中观察到的模式相似。该实验模型对于肾毒性或淀粉样蛋白形成轻链的鉴别和分化可能存在价值[269]。在 IL-6 转基因小鼠中已经证实了肾损害的进展和 MM 肾的发生，这使我们进一步了解 IL-6 在 MM 发病机制中的作用[270]。

心功能衰竭

MM 患者的平均年龄和中位年龄约为 60 岁，此类患者同时经常存在心血管疾病的风险。然而，由于心肌中淀粉样蛋白浸润导致扩张型或限制性心肌病、高黏血症和/或贫血，患者尤其容易发生心肌缺血和/或充血性心力衰竭（CHF）。广泛性骨破坏的多发性骨髓瘤患者也常合并高输出量心力衰竭，上述情况可归因于骨病变的动静脉分流[271~273]。

贫血

骨髓瘤患者贫血可能是由多种因素引起的，包括骨髓瘤细胞浸润、肾损伤、化疗后的骨髓抑制以及与促红细胞生成素（EPO）水平下降。初步研究已经证实了外源性 EPO 的应用对多发性骨髓瘤的疗效。Osterborg 等人进行了一项随机研究，应用由 2 000U/d 开始爬坡至出现应答的滴定剂量 10 000U/d 的 EPO 对比 24 周内不应用 EPO，出现应答定义为在不输血的情况下 HB 增加>2g/dl[274~277]。60%的 EPO 治疗组患者有效，治疗组中 72%的患者 EPO 水平低于正常，只有 20%的患者 EPO 在正常水平。虽然 40 000 单位 SC 每周一次是目前常用的方法，但 10 000 单位 SC 每周三次是最佳的起始剂量。然而，红细胞生成刺激剂，如 EPO 和达依泊汀，在风险评估和缓解策略（REMS）计划下受到限制，因为有几项试验显示使用这些药物会增加血栓风险，并对生存产生不利影响（尽管 MM 患者中这种风险并没有像实体肿瘤一样得到很好的证明）[278,279]。

神经病变

许多恶性和副蛋白血症性病变与神经性病变有关。在 MM 中，对称性、远端感觉或感觉运动性神经病最常见，考虑与轴突变性有关，有或没有淀粉样蛋白沉积，对于此种病变无特殊治疗方法[280]。在某些情况下，这与抑制周围神经髓鞘的单克隆抗体有关[281]。

伴随疾病

MM 表现均涉及血液学疾病以及实体肿瘤。急性白血病由致白血病物质诱导，如辐射和烷化剂，或者是 MM 自然病程的一部分。从诊断 MM 到急性白血病发病的平均时间为 60（17~147）个月。未经治疗的多发骨髓瘤患者发生急性白血病表明白血病可能是多发骨髓瘤自然病程的一部分。此外，125 例接受烷基化剂治疗的 MM 患者中有 6 例（4.8%）出现急性白血病，其发病率明显高于接受辐照和烷基化剂治疗的卵巢癌患者[282]。据报道，在开始治疗 50 个月后，使用美法仑联合泼尼松（MP）或美法仑、环磷酰胺、卡莫司汀（carmustine）和泼尼松联合治疗的 MM 患者患白血病的风险高达 17.4%[25]。Gonzalez 等人研究发现 476 例 MM 患者中 11 例发展为髓细胞性白血病或成铁粒幼细胞性贫血[282,283]。这些患者均接受了平均为期 3 年的美法仑联合泼尼松治疗，出现了严重的细胞遗传学异常。这项研究表明白血病的发生主要与治疗有关。最后，在 628 例 MM 患者中，实体肿瘤的发生率和多样性与在同年龄健康人相仿[284]。

治疗

MM 一直以来都被认为是一种不可治愈的肿瘤，但即使是老年患者，其对治疗的耐受性敏感性良好。大剂量的美法仑化疗治疗、自体干细胞移植，以及新药免疫调节剂（IMiD）（如来那度胺）和蛋白酶体抑制剂（如硼替佐米）的应用，使得 MM 患者生存期明显延长。一项回顾性研究比较了 1997 年以后及 1997 年以前确诊的 MM 患者，发现其 OS 显著改善，分别为 44.8 个月和 29.9 个月[285]。

对于 MM 患者何时开始治疗是目前研究的热点。目前共识推荐根据癌症研究和生物统计学（CRAB）标准，至少符合一条根据终末器官受累的活动期 MM 需进行治疗。对于无症状的冒烟型 MM 患者，目前共识推荐密切观察[6]。然而，目前已有研究表明，因骨髓瘤治疗具有良好的耐受性和有效性，可以在症状出现之前尽早开始治疗。最近，西班牙骨髓瘤团队进行了一项对比来那度胺联合地塞米松对比密切观察治疗高危冒烟型 MM 患者的随机对照试验。高风险被定义为同时存在骨髓浸润以及血清单克隆蛋白或流式细胞检测标准升高或免疫球蛋白水平降低（免疫低下）[286]。研究发现，积极治疗组中 3 年的 OS 较好优于观察组，OS 分别为 94%和 80%，这是首次在冒烟型 MM 相关研究中发现治疗获益。这些结果表明，早期开始治疗可能是有帮助的，这些发现的普遍性等待进一步试验确认，以及确定最有可能从早期治疗中受益的特定患者。冒烟型 MM 的其他治疗策略包括疫苗，例如用 PVX-410，一种设计用来激发对 MM 细胞的免疫反应的多肽疫苗。这种疫苗以 Xbp1、CD138 和 CS1 为靶点，Xbp1、CD138 和 CS1 为在 MM 细胞中高表达并参与 MM 病理发生的蛋白质。目前，PVX-410 正在进行一期临床试验，并与来那度胺联合使用以增强免疫反应（NCT01718899）[287,288]。

接受 MM 治疗的患者应进行临床和实验室评估以确保治疗的安全性和有效性。应通过免疫电泳和更灵敏的免疫固定技术以及血清游离轻链检测法（FLC）来测定血清和/或尿液中的单克隆蛋白。血清 FLC 检测可用于诊断和评估既往患有寡分泌型或不分泌型骨髓瘤的患者。应每年进行一次骨骼调查及骨髓细胞检查，以供诊断和监测后续临床状态、单克隆免疫球蛋白或血象改变的时间[289]。重要的是，作为肿瘤应答的客观证据，血清或尿 M 蛋减少可以反映蛋白质分解代谢增加，或蛋白质产量下降，或两者同时存在。此外，治疗过程中可能出现非 M 蛋白分泌型 MM 克隆，因此单克隆免疫球蛋白显著减少并不意味着肿瘤负荷减少。

评估移植后疗效的 Blade 标准是由欧洲血液和骨髓移植学会（EBMT）、国际骨髓移植登记处（IBMTR）和自体血液及骨髓移植登记处（ABMTR）制订的。这些标准包括对完全反应（CR）更敏感和严格的定义，包括免疫固定法检测的副蛋白缺失（不包括短暂反应）[290]。最近，血清游离轻链检测已纳入疗效判定标准[291~293]，目前 IMWG 反应标准目则被广泛使用（表 121-6）。对完全缓解的更严格定义导致了严格完全缓解范畴的纳入，此类患者无法通过免疫组织化学或免疫荧光法在骨髓中检测到单克隆浆细胞同时游离轻链比在正常范围。以前使用的接近完全缓解（仅血清单克隆免疫球蛋白免疫固定电泳阳性）现在被列入新的范畴-VGPR，并且先前使用的轻微反应类别被取消。新标准的局限性在于需通过单克隆免疫球蛋白及骨髓评估来确定反应应答。可以通过现代成像技术（如 MRI 和 FDG-PET CT）轻易识别的骨骼事件的动态变化不包括在疗效评估中。

目前，以测序为基准的平台、定量 PCR（聚合酶链反应）和多参数流式细胞技术正用于检测初始治疗后至少达到 VGPR 的患者的最小残余病（MRD），这对于评估预后存在重要作用。Martinez-Lopez 等人最近报道了基于测序的骨髓评估结果，对 113 名经初始治疗后疗效至少达到 VGPR 的患者进行了评估。在达到 CR 的患者中，MRD 阴性患者的 TTP（进展时间）为 131 个月，而 MRD 阳性患者的 TTP（进展时间）为 35 个月。当按 MRD 水平分层时，相应的 TTP 平均数为 27 个月（MRD $\geq 10^{-3}$）、48 个月（$10^{-5} \leq$ MRD $< 10^{-3}$）及 80 个月（MRD $< 10^{-5}$）（$P = 0.003 \sim 0.0001$）。尽管 MRD 目前不是一个检测指标，但未来 MRD 在评估疾病的反应方面可能起到重要作用[295]。

表 121-6 国际骨髓瘤工作组的统一反应标准

反应子范畴[a]	反应标准
CR	血清和尿液免疫荧光检测隐形，同时软组织浆细胞瘤消失以及骨髓中浆细胞数小于 5%[b]
sCR	满足 CR 如上定义，同时游离轻链比正常且免疫组织化学或免疫荧光分析[c] 显示骨髓[b] 中无克隆细胞
VGPR	血清和尿液 M 蛋白可通过免疫固定法检测出，但电泳检测阴性，或血清 M 蛋白减少至少 90%同时尿 M 蛋白<100mg/24h
PR	血清 M-蛋白减少 50%以上，24h 尿蛋白减少至少 90%或小于 200mg/24h
	如果血清和尿液中 M 蛋白无法测量，则需受累 FLC 及未受累 FLC 水平的差异≥50%来代替 M 蛋白标准
	如果血清和尿 M 蛋白均不可测量，且游离轻链也不可测量，则在基线骨髓浆细胞百分比≥30%的情况下，需要血浆细胞减少≥50%来替代 M 蛋白标准
	除上述标准外，如果在基线时出现软组织浆细胞瘤，则需浆细胞瘤缩小至少 50%
SD	不符合 CR、VGPR、PR 或进展性疾病的标准

CR，完全缓解；FLC，游离轻链；PR，部分缓解；sCR，严格的完整缓解；SD，病情稳定；VGPR，非常好的部分缓解；M 蛋白，单克隆蛋白。

[a]所有的反应类别都需要在任何新治疗开始前的任何时候进行两次连续评估；CR、PR 和 SD 类别也不需要已知的证据来证明进行性或新的骨损伤(如果进行了放射检查)。放射研究不需要满足这些反应要求。

[b]不需要重复骨髓活检确认。

[c]克隆细胞的存在/缺失是基于大于4∶1或小于1∶2的 κ/λ。免疫组化和/或免疫荧光显示的异常 κ/λ 比需要至少 100 个血浆细胞进行分析。

不建议使用 SD 作为反应指标；疾病的稳定性最好通过提供进展时间估计来描述。

摘自 Rajkumar 等人 2011[294]。

初始治疗

一直期以来，口服 MP 被认为是一种标准的治疗方式，对 50%～60%的患者客观有效。多个较早的研究已经检验了单纯 MP 方案与 MP 联合化疗(CCT)一样有效(通常与长春新碱和环磷酰胺等较老的药物一起使用)[296,297]。为了确定哪些患者(如果有的话)在更积极的治疗中效果更好，Gregory 等人研究了 18 个随机对照试验的发表报告，比较了 3 814 名患者的初始治疗中 MP 和 CCT 的疗效[298]。总体结果表明，这些治疗方式的疗效没有差异。研究显示高剂量 MP 化疗 2 年生存率高于 MP 方案化疗，但与 CCT 方案治疗的 2 年生存率之间无明显差异。这些结果表明，MP 与 CCT 之间并没有什么区别，MP 对于预后较好的患者应为首选，对于预后不良的患者则次之。

免疫调节药物

沙利度胺是一种免疫调节剂，它的引入是对 MP 方案的首次改进。在 65 岁以上新诊断的骨髓瘤患者中，沙利度胺与 MP(MPT：美法仑、泼尼松、沙利度胺)联合使用达到 76%的 CR 或 PR 率，而 MP 组该比率为 47%[299]。这使得 2 年无事件生存率(EFS)翻了一番，从 27%到 54%。根据这些数据，MPT 是不适合移植患者的标准治疗。然而，所有研究显示 MPT 组的不良事件随之增加，包括感染、神经病变和血栓栓塞，这表明需要进行预防血栓及预防感染的治疗。美法仑、泼尼松和来那度胺联合(MPR)是针对该人群的另一种有效的治疗方案[300]。Palumbo 等人随后评估了在初治的不适合移植的 MM 患者中进行 MPR 诱导治疗后联合来那度胺维持治疗(MPR-R)的疗效和安全性，并与未经维持治疗的 MPR 或 MP 治疗进行对比。中位随访时间为 30 个月，MPR-R 患者的中位 PFS 为 31 个月，MPR 患者为 14 个月，MP 患者为 13 个月。在 65～75 岁的患者中同样观察到这种益处。含来那度胺的治疗方法的有效率在 MPR-R 组为 77%，MPR 组为 68%，而在 MP 组为 5%[301]。

使用其他新药如硼替佐米联合 MP 的随机试验也证明了其有益效果。例如，VISTA 试验比较了不适合自体干细胞移植的患者应用硼替佐米、美法仑和泼尼松(VMP)以及 MP 方案。与 MP 组相比，VMP 组的 OS 显著改善[302]，其 3 年 OS 分别为 68. 5%(VMP)和 54%(MP)[303]。

最近，一项随机Ⅲ期试验 FIRST 试验，对三种治疗方案进行对比，分别为连续使用来那度胺联合低剂量地塞米松(Rd)和使用 18 周期来那度胺与低剂量地塞米松方案(Rd18)以及使用 12 周期 MPT 方案。连续 Rd 方案的中位 PFS 为 25. 5 个月，Rd18 为 20. 7 个月，MPT 为 21. 2 个月。Rd 的 4 年 OS 为 59. 4%，Rd18 为 55. 7%，MPT 为 51. 4%[304]。在连续使用 Rd 组中，ORR 为 75. 1%(15. 1% CR，28. 4% VGPR)，而 Rd18 组中 ORR 为 73. 4(CR 为 14. 2%，VGPR 为 28. 5%)，MPT 组中 ORR 位 32. 3%(CR 9. 3%，VGPR 18. 8%)。连续使用 Rd 组的安全性是可控的，因为血液学和非血液学不良事件与 Rd 和 MPT 组相仿。值得注意的是，连续使用 Rd 的血液系统第二原发性恶性肿瘤的发生率低于 MPT 组。在新诊断的不适合移植的患者中，FIRST 试验确认了连续使用 Rd 方案成为新的标准治疗。目前对硼替佐米、来那度胺和地塞米松三种药物小剂量联合应用以及三种药物剂量进行递减模式治疗的临床研究正在进行(表 121-7)。

在符合移植条件的患者中，两项研究应用沙利度胺联合地塞米松作为 MM 的初始治疗方法，并在 2/3 的患者中的达到了快速反应，从而成功地收集了用于移植的外周血干细胞(PBSC)。在收集自体干细胞和移植前，作为患者的初步治疗，我们将沙利度胺联合地塞米松、VAD 方案(长春新碱、多柔比星、地塞米松)以及地塞米松进行比较[308,309]。Cavo 等人通过一项病例对照分析得出[310]，沙利度胺联合地塞米松获得了较高的总体反应率，而一项随机三期(EGOG)试验显示沙利度胺联合地塞米松的反应率明显高于地塞米松治疗组，其差异存在显著统计学意义。这项研究为 FDA(美国食品药品管理局)批准该方案治疗 MM 提供了依据[311]。

表 121-7　初治的不适合移植患者的新型药物介绍

研究	治疗方案	患者数	中位随访时间/月	中位 OS	中位 PFS
IFM99-06[305]	MP	196	51.5	33.2	17.8
	MPT	125		51.6	27.5
	MEL100	126		38.3	19.4
IFM 01/01[306]	MPT	113	47.5	44	24.1
	MP	116		29.1	18.5
MM-015[305]	MPR-R	152	30	45.2	31
	MPR	153		NR	14
	MP	154		NR	13
VISTA[307]	VMP	344	60	56.4	N/A
	MP	338		43.1	N/A
FIRST[304]	Rd	536	37	59.4%[a]	25.5
	Rd18	541		55.7%	20.7
	MPT	547		51.4%	21.2

MP,美法仑、泼尼松;MPT,美法仑、泼尼松、沙利度胺;MEL 100,美法仑 100mg/m²;MPR,美法仑、泼尼松、来那度胺;MPR-R,美法仑、泼尼松、来那度胺诱导,然后使用来那度胺维持治疗;VMP,硼替佐米、美法仑、泼尼松;Rd,来那度胺、低剂量地塞米松持续治疗;Rd18,来那度胺、低剂量地塞米松 18 个周期;OS,总生存;PFS,无进展生存期;NR,没达到。

[a]4 年 OS。

此外,早期研究显示患者对来那度胺联合地塞米松治疗有效率为 91%,其中 CR 6%、VGPR 32%。基于这些有希望的结果,一项由 ECOG 领导的美国Ⅲ期试验研究了来那度胺联合地塞米松在新诊断 MM 中的作用[312]。研究设计允许所有患者只进行四个周期治疗进行疗效评估,此后患者可以停止研究进行干细胞移植。本试验的安全性数据发现,联合使用来那度胺和低剂量地塞米松方案比联合使用来那度胺和高剂量地塞米松方案更可取,在试验的两个治疗组中,低剂量地塞米松组出现 3 级及以上的非血液学不良事件减少(48%对比 65%),包括血栓栓塞(12%对比 26%)和感染(9%对比 16%)。低剂量地塞米松治疗的确增加了 3 级及以上中性粒细胞减少的发生率(20%对比 12%)[313,314]。重要的是,低剂量地塞米松联合治疗的生存率高于高剂量地塞米松组,其 1 年 OS 分别为 96%和 87%。当患者接受来那度胺治疗时,需要预防性应用阿司匹林、华法林或皮下注射低分子肝素抗凝治疗[313~316]。

蛋白酶体抑制剂

Richardson 等人测试了硼替佐米单药和 Jagan-Nath 等人测试了硼替佐米联合地塞米松作为初始治疗方案[317,318];这两种情况均注意到了高度的反应频率及程度。Richardson 等人通过一项Ⅰ/Ⅱ期试验证实了来那度胺、硼替佐米和地塞米松(RVD)联合用药的安全性和有效性,该研究显示了前所未有的 100%的全面有效率[319]。在这项工作的基础上,RVD 联合方案作为一线治疗的好处同样体现在两项Ⅱ期试验:IFM 2008 试验和 Evo-Lution 试验的结果中。在 IFM 试验中诱导治疗后的 ORR 为 97%(13%sCR,16%CR 和 54%≥VGPR)[320,321]。EVOLUTION 试验旨在将 RVD 与 CyBorD(环磷酰胺,硼替佐米和地塞米松)在随机,多中心环境中进行比较。初次治疗后使用硼替佐米维持 4 个 6 周周期的 RVD 组的 ORR 为 85%(24%CR,51%≥VGPR)。

卡非佐米(carfilzomib)是一种环氧酶素类第二代蛋白酶抑制剂,以高度选择性和不可逆转的方式与 20S 蛋白酶体结合。鉴于其被批准用于复发性疾病的治疗,目前正在对前期背景进行研究。Jakubowiak 等人通过其进行的剂量递增研究对卡非佐米、来那度胺和地塞米松(CRD)联合用药进行评估[322,323],其中患者接受了卡非佐米(20、27 或 36mg/m²,第 1、2、8、9、15 和 16 日,8 个周期,此后第 1、2、15 和 16 日),来那度胺 25mg 第 1~21 日,地塞米松第 1~4 周期每周 40mg,第 5~8 周期每周 20mg,28 日为 1 周期,在 8 个周期后,患者每隔一周进行该用药方案,持续 8 个周期。经过 24 个周期后,推荐使用来那度胺进行维持治疗。平均 12 个周期后,62%的患者达到接近 CR 或更好的疗效,42%的患者达到 sCR。24 个月的 PFS 为 92%。毒性曲线是可接受的,并且值得注意的是,周围神经病变发生较少。

如上文所述,与移植方案相比,新药物联合地塞米松的双联疗法,尤其是三联疗法,可诱导完全缓解率。使用中的现代方案的实例包括来那度胺联合地塞米松、硼替佐米联合地塞米松的双重组合,以及 RVD、cybord 和 CRD 的三重组合(表 121-8)[310,324]。

表 121-8　初治适合移植患者的新型药物介绍

研究	治疗方案	患者数	Cr/nCR/%	ORR/%	结果
Rajkumar 等人[313]	RD	223	18	79	OS:87%at 1year
	Rd	222	14	68	OS:96%at 1year
Harousseau 等人[325]	VAD	121	6.4	62.8	PFS 30months
	Bd	121	14.8	78.5	PFS:36months
Reeder 等人[326]	CyBorD	33	39	88	N/A
Richardson 等人[319]	RVD	66	39	100	OS 97% at 18-months
Jakubowiak 等人[323]	CRD	53	62	98	PFS 92% 24-months

RD,来那度胺、大剂量地塞米松;Rd,来那度胺、低剂量地塞米松;VAD,长春新碱、多柔比星、地塞米松;Bd,硼替佐米、低剂量地塞米松;CyBorD,环磷酰胺、硼替佐米、地塞米松;RVD,来那度胺、硼替佐米(万珂)、地塞米松;CRD,卡非佐米、来那度胺、地塞米松;OS,整体生存期;PFS,无进展生存期;N/A,不适用。

对于计划进行干细胞采集的患者,应避免使用包括烷基化剂如美法仑的组合,因为可能会对正常的造血干细胞造成损害,这可能导致无法收集用于自体造血干细胞移植的干细胞。尽管使用生长因子和化疗的干细胞动员可以克服来那度胺的骨髓抑制作用,来那度胺仍然可能阻碍干细胞的收集。治疗周期数,特别是含有来那度胺的方案,应限制在大约四个周期,因为额外的周期可能会影响干细胞收集的能力[327~331]。

与自体造血干细胞移植相比,新药物联合治疗获得的完全缓解率引导了一项正在进行的临床研究,该研究对新药治疗后立即给予自体造血干细胞移植以及新药物治疗后在疾病复发后给予自体干细胞移植进行对比。新药可能压制一些细胞生成的不良预后因子,如 del 13,t(4;14)和 del 17p。现在放弃自体造血干细胞移植为时尚早，因为新药的临床试验随访期太短，无法确定增加的完全缓解率能否转化为持久缓解以及 EFS 和 OS 是否会增加。

完全缓解率作为最终结果的替代指标证明是不充分的。DETERMINATION 试验(NCT01208662)是一项正在进行的Ⅲ期多中心随机试验，该试验是在 65 岁及以下骨髓瘤患者中早期应用高剂量美法仑联合自体干细胞移植对比疾病复发时进行移植中应用自体干细胞移植，所有患者均接受 RVD 诱导治疗。这项试验旨在新药物的背景下，明确无论是在复发前还是复发时自体干细胞移植的角色。自体移植很可能会增加新药带来的好处。

放射治疗

放射治疗多用于治疗局部病变，包括浆细胞瘤或脊髓压迫综合征，并经常用于缓解症状。半体照射作为诱导 CCT 后的巩固治疗或化疗耐药的 MM 的补救治疗是有一定作用的。全身照射(TBI)已被用作造血干细胞移植前治疗的一个组成部分，但由于高剂量美法仑具有相同的功效和较低的毒性，因此很少使用[332~334]。

高剂量治疗方法

在有或没有 TBI 的情况下，以高于常规剂量给予烷化剂(美法仑、环磷酰胺和白消安)，然后移植同源，同种异体和自体骨髓或外周血祖细胞(PBPC)的原理如下：浆细胞病仍然是致命的；多个研究记录了 MM 细胞对化疗和放疗的敏感性；并且用 HDT 可以获得 CR。

自体干细胞移植

高剂量化疗后自体 BM 或 PBPC 移植也获得了高 CR 率(40%)，但遗憾的是，这些反应的中位持续时间只有 24~36 个月。敏感疾病患者和较少接受重大预处理的患者的预后最好[335,336]。最重要的是，法国的一项全国性试验，纳入 200 名接受了两个疗程的 VMCP 治疗后交替使用 VBAP 的 MM 患者，随机接受常规化疗(另外 8VMCP/VBAP 疗程)或 HDT(美法仑和 TBI)，此后进行自体骨髓移植，与接受常规治疗的患者相比，高剂量治疗患者有效率，EFS 和 OS 显著提高。MM 的另一项随机试验检测了 HDT 在早期和晚期作为常规治疗后复发的挽救治疗的相对优劣性[337]。两组患者的 OS 均为 64 个月，但无症状和无毒性(Q-Twist)的质量调整时间对早期移植组患者有很强的支持作用[338]。美国团体之间的试验支持这一观点。IFM 进行了一项随机试验，比较了 200mg/m^2 的高剂量美法仑与 140mg/m^2 的美法仑加上 TBI 作为消融疗法的疗效[339]。尽管反应率和 EFS 具有可比性，但单独使用高剂量美法仑治疗组的毒性较低且 OS 更长，这表明 TBI 不应该被视为消融方案的一部分[334]。一项斯堪的纳维亚人群研究表明，与接受常规治疗的历史对照组相比，接受强化治疗的<60 岁 MM 患者的生存期延长。另一项随机 MRC 试验证实，与传统疗法相比，接受高剂量治疗的患者生存期可延长 12 个月[340]。虽然这些研究令人鼓舞，但患者不太可能在单次高剂量和自体干细胞移植治疗后治愈[341]。在所有研究中，中位 EFS 均延长，所有五项研究中，四项研究提示移植可以得到更高的 CR 率，三项研究的 OS 得到延长(表 121-9)。

表 121-9 自体移植对比常规化疗治疗初治骨髓瘤

作者	治疗方法	患者数	CR/%	中位 EFS/月	中位 OS/月
Barlogie 等人[342]	常规化疗[a]	116	–	22	48
	HDT	123	40	49	62
Lenhoff 等人[340]	常规化疗[a]	274	–	–	46%at 48
	HDT	274	34	27	61%at 48
Attal 等人[337]	常规化疗	100	5	18	37
	HDT	100	22	27	52%at 60
Fermand 等人[338]	常规化疗	96	–	18.7	50.4
	HDT	94	–	24.3	55.3
Blade 等人[343]	常规化疗	83	11	34.3	66
	HDT	81	30	42.5	61
Child 等人[341]	常规化疗	200	8.5	19.6	42.3
	HDT	201	44	31.6	54.1

CR，完全缓解；EFS，无事件生存；HDT，高剂量治疗；OS，总生存率。
[a]历史对照。

提高自体移植的效果

使用自体 BM 或 PBPC 达到使肿瘤细胞衰竭的作用或者通过 CD34 的表达来选择正常的造血祖细胞的自体移植目前被尝试用于改善 HDT 的效果[344~346]。但事实上其并没有改善预后[347,348]。Barlogie 等人正在进行多种大剂量疗法和干细胞移植[349,350]。与以往匹配的对照组相比，其有效率更高，但对长期无病生存率(DFS)的影响需要进一步随访。最近一项比较是否联合沙利度胺的串联移植的研究结果显示 OS 并无明显差异。一项法国随机对照试验对单次及双次的 HDT 及干细胞移植进行比较，两组 CR 率没有显著差异，EFS 和 OS 曲线仅在 3 年后分离[351]。这表明只有一部分患者可能受益，实际上只有那些在第一次移植中没有获得 CR 的患者才从第二次移植中受益[352]。Bologna 96 研究还表明，双重自体移植主要是能让未达到接近 CR 的患者受益[353]。目前正在进行的一项单次自体移植联合或不联合巩固治疗对比双次自体移植联合来那度胺维持治疗的Ⅲ期多中心临床试验(BMT CTN 0702)正在观察串联移植的作用[354]。

Giralt 等人报告了使用环孢素诱导自体移植后移植物抗宿主病(GVHD)以产生相关的自体移植物抗 MM 效应。该效应可能刺激针对骨髓瘤的自身免疫反应并治疗移植后微小残余病从而改善预后[355]。既往曾有学者尝试在体外培养特异性抗 MM 自体 T 细胞，用于患者自体移植后微小残余病(MRD)的过继免疫疗法。现在可以克隆患者特异性独特型蛋白的基因，鉴定肽类基因序列编码预测患者 HLA 类型的Ⅰ类 HLA 沟内呈现的肽的基因序列，并在体外扩增肽特异性 T 细胞 56 类似的策略可用于扩增针对在 MM 细胞上过表达的共有抗原内的肽的 T 细胞，例如端粒酶催化亚基(hTERT)，MUC-1 或细胞色素 CYP1B1[356]。用以增强整个肿瘤细胞的免疫原性的免疫反应测试正在进行中[35,357,358]。我们已经证明了 MM 细胞可以融合到 DC 中，并且 MM DC 融合体作为抗原递呈细胞可以将整个 MM 细胞呈现为异物。在同基因小鼠 MM 模型中，用 MM DC 融合细胞进行疫苗接种，证明了其保护和治疗效果。最重要的是，我们已经证明，患者 MM 细胞可以融合到自体 DC 中，其融合细胞很容易从患者 BM 或外周血中分离出来，并且自体 MM DC 融合细胞可以在体外触发特定的细胞溶解自体 T 细胞反应[359]。我们正在将这些发现转化为 MM-DC 融合疫苗的临床试验，以评估体内 MM 特异性 T 细胞和 B 细胞反应以及临床疗效[360~362]。

维持治疗

目前已提出维持治疗方案以延长自体干细胞移植后完全缓解的持续时间。新的抗骨髓瘤药物耐受性和有效性的提高增加了这种方法的可行性以及关注度；既往尝试应用传统化疗药物如美法仑或干扰素作为维持治疗的方案均没有好的疗效[363]。

一项荟萃分析对诱导化疗后沙利度胺维持治疗与其他治疗方案进行比较的随机对照试验进行了研究，其中包括来自 6 项试验的 2 786 名患者，证明接受沙利度胺维持治疗的患者的 OS 略有改善（$HR=0.83$，$P=0.07$）。接受沙利度胺和糖皮质激素联合治疗的患者 OS 改善最为显著（$HR=0.70$，$P=0.02$）。沙利度胺可改善 PFS（$HR=0.65$，$P<0.01$），但存在较高的血栓的风险（风险差异 0.024，$P<0.05$）及周围神经病变的风险增加（风险差异 0.072，$P<0.01$）[364]。

三项随机试验探讨了来那度胺作为维持治疗的应用，其中两项试验是在自体干细胞移植后进行的，另一项试验是在不符合高剂量治疗要求的患者中进行 9 个月以美法仑为基础的治疗后进行的[365,366]。在所有三个试验中，例如，CALGB1100104 研究，使用来那度胺维持治疗组的 PFS 几乎翻了一番，从 27 个月到 46 个月[301]。此外，CALGB 研究显示，来那度胺组 OS 亦获益：来那度胺组患者有 15%死亡，安慰剂组为 23%（$P<0.03$）；来那度胺组 3 年 OS 为 88%，安慰剂组为 80%[366]。

使用来那度胺维持治疗的一个重要问题是继发性恶性肿瘤的风险。维持治疗组（7%~7.7%）发生第二种原发性癌症的风险大约是应用安慰剂对照组（2.6%~3%）的两倍。观察到的继发性癌症包括血液学恶性肿瘤，如急性髓细胞性白血病和实体瘤。当来那度胺与口服美法仑联合使用时，继发性血液系统恶性肿瘤的风险似乎最大（$HR=4.86$，$P<0.0001$）。在开始维持治疗前应考虑并与患者讨论继发性恶性肿瘤的风险增加和维持治疗的风险效益比[367]。

硼替佐米也被及和 CR 率从 31%提高到 49%。在表 121-10 中总结了最近的维持治疗试验[368]。

表 121-10　维持治疗方案

研究	治疗方案	患者数	转归
IFM 2005-02[366]	一次或两次 ASCT 后应用来那度胺对比安慰剂维持	614	PFS 41 个月对比 23 个月
CALGB 100104[366]	ASCT 后应用来那度胺对比安慰剂维持治疗	460	TTP 46 个月对比 27 个月
HOVON-65/GMMG-HD4[368]	VAD 对比 PAD 治疗后行 ASCT，此后行沙利度胺或硼替佐米维持	827	PFS 28 个月对比 35 个月

ASCT，自体干细胞移植；CR，完全缓解；PAD，硼替佐米、多柔比星，地塞米松；VAD，长春新碱，多柔比星，地塞米松；PFS，无进展生存；TTP，疾病进展时间。

巩固治疗

于自体干细胞移植治疗后给予短程巩固治疗可以提高 CR 率及降低复发风险。Ladetto 等[369]报道称自体干细胞移植后给予硼替佐米、沙利度胺、地塞米松联合巩固治疗，可能使 22% VGPR 率达到 100%，以及持续的分子反应（PCR 阴性）。据报道，自体干细胞移植后给予硼替佐米和来那度胺单药治疗均可提高 10%~30%CR 率[370,371]，在 IFM 2008 研究中，对移植后 2 周期 RVD 方案维持治疗的安全性及有效性进行评估，研究显示其安全、有效、耐受性良好，巩固治疗后严格完全缓解率由 27%提高至 40%[372]。

维持治疗

基于现有数据，维持治疗对于适合移植及不适合移植患者而言均可改善疾病控制率[373,374]。多项临床研究均证实应用沙利度胺、来那度胺及硼替佐米可使适合移植的多发性骨髓瘤患者临床获益。

迄今为止，关于来那度胺的临床研究结果是最有说服力的。IFM 2005-02 和 CALGB 100104 研究均使得 PFS 加倍[365,366]，尽管只有 CALGB 研究获得 OS 获益。来那度胺作为口服制剂，耐受性良好，很好地满足了骨髓瘤维持治疗的需求。最近，FIRST 研究，比较了 Rd 维持治疗与 18 周期 Rd 以及 MPT 治疗，应用 Rd 维持治疗组中位 PFS 25.5 个月，Rd 18 周期为 20.7 个月，MPT 组 21.2 个月[304]。然而，虽然罹患第二原发恶性肿瘤的风险较低，给予维持治疗时仍需对该种可能性给予充分注意。

同种异体干细胞移植

虽然多发性骨髓瘤较少进行同系骨髓移植，但据西雅图[375]与欧洲骨髓移植协作组（EBMT[376]）报道，部分移植后患者获得较长的无疾病进展时间。据 EBMT 报道[377~379]，72 名（44%）移植后患者最短 4 年总生存率为 32%，7 年总生存率 28%。然而，6 年的总体 PFS 率为 34%，部分患者于移植后获得大于 4 年的持续 CR。女性、IgA 型 MM、低血清 β_2-微球蛋白水平、Ⅰ期、一线治疗后骨髓移植前获得 CR 均为良性预后因素。尤其值得关注的是，由于选择了更为适合的患者、早期移植以及减少移植前治疗，移植相关死亡率（TRM，50%发生于男性）由此前的 41%[380]降至 20%[379]。在西雅图，骨髓移植患者 4.5 年达到 CR 的 OS 及 PFS 率分别为 50%及 43%[381]。不良预后因素包括：诊断后超过 1 年行骨髓移植、移植时血清 β_2-微球蛋白水平大于>2.5mg/dl、女性患者移植男性供体骨髓、移植前接受大于 8 周期化疗、Durie-Salmon 分期Ⅲ期。Again toxicity 较为常见，35 例患者（44%）于移植后 100 日内死于移植相关因素[381,382]。为降低多发性骨髓瘤同种异体移植相关死亡率，我们对 61 例对常规化疗仍敏感的患者应用组织相容同级供体移植进行了去 T（CD6）细胞骨髓移植[346,383~386]。获得了 17 例 CR（28%），34 例（57%）PR，2 例（3%）NR（未达到），仅有 3 例（5%）移植相关死亡。骨髓移植后 DFS 为 1 年，仅有 20%患者无病生存大于等于 4 年。

同种异体移植后分子豁免自体移植更为常见[387~390]，供体淋巴细胞输注（DLI）可用于治疗 MM 移植后复发[391~393]，显示了较好的治疗移植物抗 MM（GVM）效应。在该中心，通过长期观察发现,移植相关毒副反应较高的患者将获得较低的复发风险[394]。为了减轻毒性反应,加强 GVM 效果,在 CD6T 细胞骨髓移植后 6 个月后给予 CD4+DLI[386]。尽管预防性的 DLI 显著提升了 GVM,但是,仅有 58% 的骨髓移植患者进行了该项治疗。

使用非剥离性骨髓移植是保护 GVM 效果的另一种策略,同时避免了同种异体移植的毒性[395]。在高危 MM 患者中,使用 100mg/m² 的美法仑与 DLI 联合[396],虽然一些患者已达到控制疾病的目的,但在这一组患者中仍可注意到明显的 GVHD。几位研究者在非清髓移植前进行了自体移植,验证了该方法的可行性,从而增强抗肿瘤活性及提高抗 MM 免疫能力[397,398]。例如,Maloney 等人[398]报告的总体应答率为 83%,CRS 为 57%,但是移植相关毒性、慢性 GVHD 以及肿瘤复发仍是一个问题。在高危 MM 患者中进行的一项随机试验表明,自体干细胞移植和剂量减少异基因移植(IFM 99-03)的结合并不优于串联自体移植计划。(IFM 99-04)[399],但另一项随机试验显示,接受自体移植的患者存活率更高,然后是异基因移植[400,401]。同种异体移植的 OS 中位数为 80 个月,双自体移植的 OS 中位数为 54 个月。同种异体移植后的 CR 率为 55%,而双侧自体移植后的 CR 率为 26%。相比之下,在高危 MM 患者中进行的随机试验表明,自体干细胞移植和剂量减少异基因移植(IFM 99-03)的结合并不优于串联自体(IFM 99-04)[399]。BMT CTN 0102 也评估了自体 SCT 续贯二次移植对照非清髓性异基因 SCT。

在标准和高危患者中,自体 HSCT 后的非髓性同种异体 HSCT 并不比串联自体 HSCT 更有效[402]。Bjork-strand 等发表一项前瞻性临床研究,比较了单次或串联自体骨髓移植与自体异种 HLA-相同同胞相匹配供体移植的患者。对 357 例接受自体骨髓移植(单次或双次)以及自体异种 HLA-相同同胞相匹配供体的患者进行长期随访发现,PFS 率为 35% 及 18% ($P=0.001$),后者 PFS 为 60 个月。术后未复发死亡率为 12%,而自体组为 3%($P<0.001$),广泛性 GVHD 的发生率分别为 31% 和 23%[403]。

采用异基因移植作为挽救疗法,虽然可行,但在经过大量预处理的人群中不太可能有显著的益处。EBMT 报道了 229 例接受低强度的异基因 SCT 患者的预后。1 年 TRM 为 22%,3 年 OS 为 41%,PFS 为 21%。25% 的患者患有广泛的慢性 GVHD[404]。在缓解期和病程早期接受移植的患者的疗效最佳。影响 OS 的不利因素包括耐受性疾病、多次移植以及女性供体的男性患者。

同种异体移植只应在临床试验的背景下进行,这些试验的目的是减少慢性 GVHD,将 GVM 与 GVHD 分离,并扩大 GVM 效应以提高 Amelio 评级毒物的疗效。使免疫效应细胞的抗髓鞘效应达到最大化。

复发性疾病

几乎所有最初对化疗有反应的 MM 患者最终都会复发。为了克服对现有治疗方法的耐药性以及改善患者预后,需要新的基于生物学的治疗方案,其目标是作用于 BM 中的 MM 细胞,抑制其增殖及存活[405]。为了实现这一目标,我们开发了研究 MM 细胞生长、存活和药物耐药机制的系统。重要的是,我们还开发了体外系统和动物模型,以描述 MM 细胞向 BM 归巢的机制,以及各种促进 MM 细胞在 BM 微环境中的生长、存活、耐药性和迁移的因素(MM 细胞-BMSC 相互作用、细胞因子和血管生成)[73,80,85~87,406~408]。这些模型系统允许开发几种有前景的基于生物学的治疗方法,这些疗法可以针对 MM 细胞及其 BM 微环境,其治疗靶点仅针对 MM 细胞或者仅针对微环境。(图 121-7)。

免疫调节药物

针对 MM 细胞及其 BM 环境从而在体外克服经典耐药性的药物包括 IMiD,比如沙利度胺、来那度胺、泊马度胺[64]以及蛋白酶抑制剂硼替佐米[66]、卡非佐米(carfilzomib)。IMiD 药物来那度胺由实验室转化到临床应用的速度是非常快的。它在 2000 年通过体外及体内试验均证实同时针对 MM 细胞及 BM 微环境[64,409];2001 年结束一期试验明确了其最大耐受剂量、低毒以及显著的抗多发性骨髓瘤活性[410]。二期试验完成于 2002 年[411]。

两项大型的Ⅲ期临床试验,来那度胺/地塞米松对比地塞米松/安慰剂,因为来那度胺/地塞米松治疗组有统计学上显著的更高的应答率以及显著延长 TTP 及 OS,使得上述试验均被提前终止,进一步也使得 FDA 批准来那度胺/地塞米松方案用于治疗一线治疗后复发的 MM[412,413]。泊马度胺也显示出了强大的抗骨髓瘤作用。有几项研究在复发性人群中联合使用了泊马度胺和小剂量地塞米松,第 1~21 日口服泊马度胺 4mg,28 日为 1 周期,直到进展。一项Ⅱ期随机、开放临床研究,比较泊马度胺联合低剂量地塞米松与泊马度胺单药治疗复发、难治性多发骨髓瘤。联合组中位 PFS 为 4.2 个月,单药治疗组 2.7 个月,($HR=0.68$,$P=0.003$),联合治疗组 ORR 为 33%,单药治疗组为 18%,中位 OS 分别为 16.5 个月和 13.6 个月。而对来那度胺和硼替佐米的耐药不影响泊马度胺和地塞米松的疗效[414]。欧洲一项Ⅲ期临床研究比较泊马度胺联合低剂量地塞米松对比单药高剂量地塞米松,联合治疗组 PFS 4 个月,单药治疗组 1.9 个月($HR=0.48$,$P<0.0001$),最常见的治疗副反应为骨髓抑制和感染[415]。

近年来,当人们首次认识到 IMiD 药物可与脑脊液(CBN)[416]结合,其在 MM 中的作用机制(及其致畸性)得到了较好的阐明。IMiD 药物与脑脊液结合后可防止 CBN 的自泛素化,促进转录因子 IKZF 1(Ikaros)和 IKZF 3(Aiolos)的 CBN 依赖性蛋白酶体降解,这对 MM 增殖非常重要[417~419]。

蛋白酶体抑制剂

硼酸蛋白酶体抑制剂硼替佐米的临床转化和随后的 FDA 批准也非常迅速。在 MM 中使用硼替佐米的最初原理是阻断 NF-κB 的活性,因为在 MM 中,NF-κB 被确定为治疗靶点,具有抗药性,调节 MM 细胞和骨髓基质细胞上的黏附分子表达,调节组成和 MM 结合诱导细胞因子的转录和分泌[50]。在多发性骨髓瘤细胞中,硼替佐米可导致未折叠蛋白和内质网应激的积累,随后激活未折叠蛋白反应并阻止细胞周期[420]。Ⅰ期试验显示耐受性和抗-MM 活性的早期证据[421]。Ⅱ期 SUMMIT 试

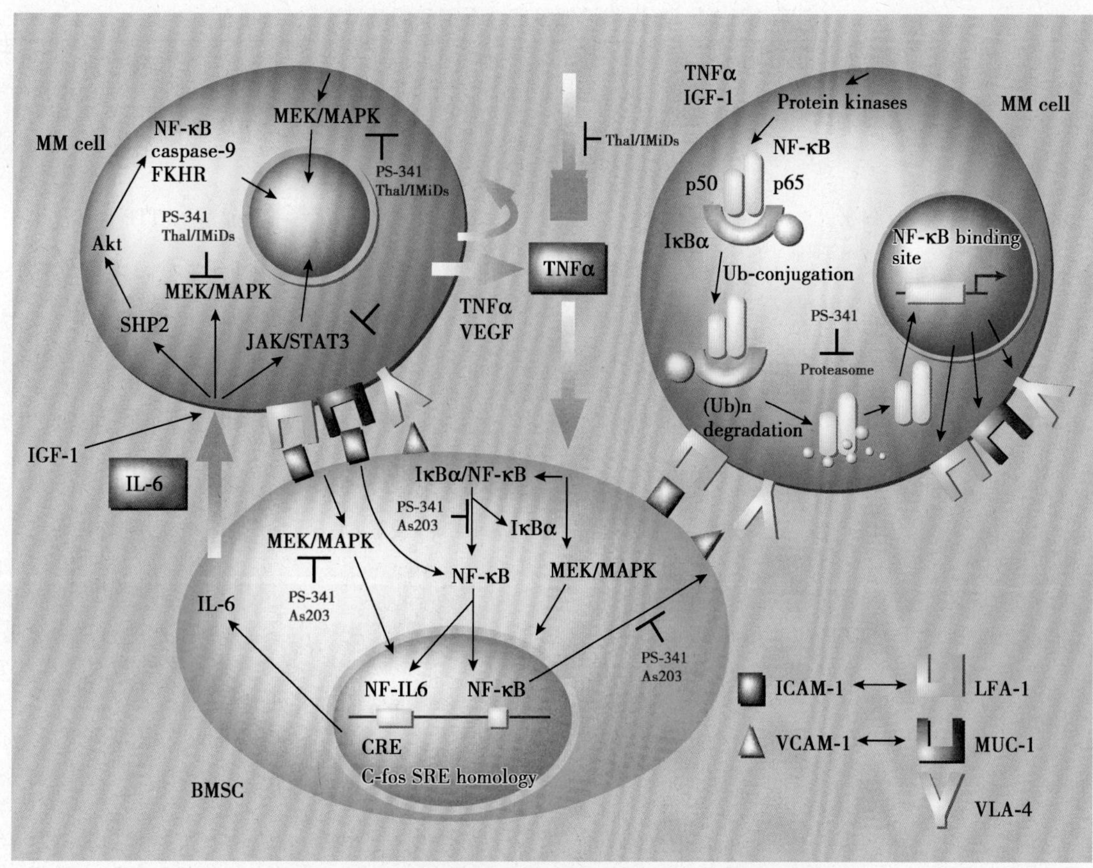

图 121-7 新型治疗剂对多发性骨髓瘤信号通路的抑制作用

验证实了反应,包括 CR、TTP 延长和存活率以及相关的临床效益,为 FDA 加速批准治疗复发难治性 MM 奠定了基础[422]。APEX 试验比较了地塞米松和硼替佐米治疗复发性 MM 的疗效,由于硼替佐米治疗组 TTP 的稳定显著延长,因此未进行盲法检查,这为其 FDA 批准扩展到复发性 MM 奠定了基础[317]。通过随访,TTP 和 OS 明显改善,并且神经并发症可以控制[423]。它的哪种活性导致了 MM 细胞毒性尚不清楚。

下一代环氧酮蛋白酶体抑制剂卡非佐米作为单一药物获得 FDA 的快速批准,用于治疗至少接受过两线治疗的患者,根据单药卡非佐米二期治疗结果,每周两次给药治疗既往接受中位数为五线治疗后的患者的 ORR 为 23.7%。中位反应持续时间为 7.8 个月,中位 OS 为 15.6 个月。该药物耐受性良好。最常见的副作用是疲劳,贫血,恶心和血小板减少,13.9%报道周围神经病变(大多数患者有基础周围神经病变)[424]。7.2%的患者出现心力衰竭事件,如肺水肿。ASPIRE 试验最近报道了卡非佐米与来那度胺和地塞米松联合应用对比来那度胺、地塞米松治疗复发性 MM 患者的研究结果[425]。这种联合治疗耐受性良好,PFS 改善了近 9 个月,强调了即使在复发情况下三药联合治疗的益处。

口服蛋白酶体抑制剂伊沙佐米(ixazomib)和 oprozomib 目前正在临床试验中,可能会获得批准。伊沙佐米已经在复发难治性人群的第一阶段试验中证明了其安全性和有效性。在 60 名接受过包括硼替佐米在内的 6 种先前治疗方案的患者中(83%),有 41 名可评估的患者。有响应的患者包括 1 个 VGPR、5 个 PR、1 个 MR 和 15 个 SD。只有 10%的患者有与药物相关的周围神经病变,没有一个≥3 级[426,427]。在一项Ⅰ/Ⅱ期试验中,对伊沙佐米周疗联合标准剂量来那度胺和地塞米松治疗新诊断的骨髓瘤患者进行评估。58 名可评估反应的患者的初步结果显示,总体反应率为 93%,67%的受试者达到或优于 VGPR,包括 24%的 CR 率[426,428]。基于这些结果,正在进行两项大型的国际三期临床试验对伊沙佐米正在联合来那度胺和地塞米松方案进行评估:复发性、难治性多发性骨髓瘤患者使用 TOURMALINE MM1,新诊断患者使用 TOURMALINE MM2。另一种口服蛋白酶体抑制剂 oprozomib 也正在研究治疗多发性硬化症[429]。这些药物可能会显著影响多发性骨髓瘤的治疗,从而使患者能够完全接受口服药物治疗,从而完全接受门诊治疗。这对患者,尤其是老年人群,具有可测量的生活质量效益,并可能为结合蛋白酶体抑制剂为基础的维持策略提供一种方便的方法。表 121-11 总结了一些用于复发疾病的治疗方法。

组蛋白脱乙酰基酶(HDAC)

组蛋白脱乙酰基酶(HDAC)抑制剂是另一类药物,与硼替佐米联合使用后,在复发难治性骨髓瘤中表现出活性。一项随机对照的Ⅲ期试验 VANTAGE 088,表明非选择性 HDAC 抑制剂伏林司他和硼替佐米的组合是有效的和耐受性良好的。与单用硼替佐米组比较,伏林司他和硼替佐米组的 ORR 分别为 56.2%和 40.6%(P<0.000 1),同样,PFS 分别为 7.63 个月和 6.83 个月(P=0.01)[431]。最近,另一种非选择性 HDAC 抑制剂帕比司他(panobinostat)与硼替佐米和地塞米松联合进行了Ⅱ期研究[436],而 PANORAMA-1 研究是比较了帕

表 121-11 复发难治性多发性骨髓瘤的新疗法

试验	阶段	代理	样本数	ORR/%	OS/月	结果/月
Richardson et al[317]	Ph3	硼替佐米	669	38	29.8	TTP 6.2 vs 3.5
		地塞米松		18	23.7	
Orlowski et al[430]	Ph3	bort/PLD	646	44	76%[a]	TTP 9.3 vs 6.5
		硼替佐米		41	65%[a]	
Weber et al[412]	Ph3	来那度胺	353	61	29.6	TTP 11.1 vs 4.7
		地塞米松		20	20.2	
Dimopoulos et al[413]	Ph3	来那度胺	351	60	NR	TTP 11.3 vs 4.7
		地塞米松		24	20.6	
Richardson et al[319]	Ph2	RVD	64	64	26	中位 TTP 9.5
Siegel et al[322]	Ph2	卡非佐米	266	24	15.6	中位 PFS 3.7
San Miguel et al[415]	Ph3	pom/lo-dex	302	31	11.9	中位 PFS 4.0 vs 1.9
		hi-dex		10	7.8	
Dimopoulos et al[431]	Ph3	vor/bort	637	56	NR	中位 PFS 7.6 vs 6.8
		bort		41	28.1	
San Miguel et al[432]	Ph3	pan/bort/地塞米松	768	61	NR	中位 PFS 12 vs 8.1
		bort/地塞米松		55		
Lokhorst et al[433]	Ph1/2	达雷木单抗	32	42[b]	NR	中位 PFS NR
Lonial et al[434]	Ph2	elo/len/dex	73	92[c]	NR	中位 PFS NR[c]
Lentzsch et al[435]	Ph2	benda/len/dex	29	52	NR	中位 PFS 6.1

benda,苯达莫司汀;bort,硼替佐米;dex,地塞米松;elo,厄罗珠单抗;hi,高剂量;lo,低剂量;NR,未报告/接触;pan,泛铌酸盐;PLD,聚乙二醇脂质体多柔比星;pom,泊马度胺;RVD,来那度胺、硼替佐米、地塞米松;vor,弗瑞斯特。

[a] 15 个月。

[b] 接受剂量≥4mg/kg 的患者。

[c] 在 20.8 个月时接受剂量为 10mg/kg 的患者。

比司他、硼替佐米和地塞米松单独治疗复发难治性人群的Ⅲ期研究[432]。三联疗法治疗的患者的 PFS 为 12 个月 vs 8.1 个月($P<0.0001$)。ORR 为 61% vs 55%,反应持续时间为 13.1 个月 vs 10.9 个月。OS 数据尚不成熟。常见的副作用包括骨髓抑制和腹泻[436]。基于这些发现,帕比司他于 2015 年获得了 FDA 的批准,是第一个适应证为一线治疗 MM 获批的 HDAC 抑制剂[432]。瑞考司他(ricolinostat)(ACY-1215)是一种选择性的 HDAC6 抑制剂,目前正在进行联合来那度胺或硼替佐米联合地塞米松研究[437~439]。与来那度胺、地塞米松配伍,ORR 为 69%。16 例患者中有 13 例曾使用过来那度胺,3/6 患者对来那度胺无反应[440]。联合应用硼替佐米和地塞米松,ORR 为 44%[441]。

单克隆抗体

一些单克隆抗体在骨髓瘤中被研究和证实具有活性。具体来说,针对 CD38、CS1 和 BAFF 的新药正在进行临床试验[427,442]。达拉木单抗(daratumumab)是一种单克隆 CD38 抗体,根据一项Ⅰ/Ⅱ期试验的结果,由 FDA 授予其快速审批和突破性疗法,该试验证明达拉木单抗单药可以抑制复发难治性骨髓瘤细胞的活性。在≥4mg/kg 组($n=12$),观察到 5 个 PRs 和 3 个 MRs。中位 PFS 为 3.8 个月。达拉木单抗联合来那度胺和地塞米松治疗复发难治性疾病目前正在研究中。另一种 CD38 抑制剂 SAR650984 在 MTD 的 RR 患者的剂量递增研究中具有 30.8%的 ORR[443]。达拉木单抗也被用于治疗冒烟型 MM(NCT02316106)。

厄罗珠单抗(elotuzumab),一种针对人 CS1(也被称为 CD2 亚群-1、SLAMF7、CRAC 和 CD319)的人源化单克隆抗体,是一种在 MM 细胞和正常血浆细胞上高度表达的细胞表面抗原糖蛋白,也被 FDA 授予突破性治疗的指定药物。在Ⅰ期研究中,没有观察到客观反应,尽管根据 EBMT 骨髓瘤反应标准,有 26.5%的患者有疾病稳定(SD)[444]。联合应用来那度胺和地塞米松,82%(28 例中有 23 例)的患者获得了客观缓解。在中位数为 16.4 个月的随访后，20mg/kg 队列中接受治疗直至疾病进展的患者的 TTP 中位数为 NR[445]。平均随访 20.8 个月后，10mg/kg 剂量的 ORR 为 92%，平均 PFS 为 NR，这是正在进行的Ⅲ期试验 ELOQUENT-2 中使用的剂量[434]。Ⅰ期试验中厄罗珠单抗联合硼替佐米和地塞米松的疗效也很好，27 例复发难治性疾病可评估患者中 48%的患者疗效为 PR 或更好[446]。厄罗珠单抗与来那度胺以及地塞米松的联合应用也在高风险冒烟型 MM 中进行研究（NCT02279394）。

tabalumab 是一种完全人源化的单克隆抗体，具有针对膜结合和可溶性 BAFF 的活性，并在Ⅰ期研究中与硼替佐米和地塞米松联合使用。在本研究中，ORR 为 45.8%[447]。该组合的Ⅱ期试验已经完成，结果即将公布。

其他治疗

苯达莫司汀作为单一药物或联合来那度胺和地塞米松是复发难治性骨髓瘤患者的另一个选择。在Ⅰ/Ⅱ期试验中评价了苯达莫司汀、来那度胺和地塞米松的联合用药。平均 PFS 为 6.1 个月，PR 率为 52%，VGPR 率为 24%[435]。与先前使用 100mg/m² 的研究相比，苯达莫司汀的 MTD 为 75mg/m²。毒性主要是血液学方面的争论，推荐低剂量，特别是考虑到治疗对象为既往经过多线治疗后患者。

其他的治疗方案也已被探索，硼替佐米和聚乙二醇脂质体多柔比星（多柔比星）和苯达莫司汀与泼尼松和沙利度胺[430,448]。

目前有许多针对新的途径的新药正在开发中[449,450]。例如，filanesib，一种激肽纺锤体蛋白抑制剂，可诱导异常有丝分裂停止和快速细胞死亡并优先作用于包括骨髓瘤细胞在内的 MCL-1 依赖性细胞，与来那度胺和硼替佐米联合显示出治疗活性。目前正在研究其他几种新型药物，包括溴域抑制剂、细胞周期蛋白依赖激酶抑制剂和泛素途径抑制剂。从这些早期研究中获得的数据将更好地理解这些数据将如何被纳入骨髓瘤的治疗选择[451~453]。

另一个值得关注和发展的领域是阻断肿瘤细胞和免疫细胞之间的相互作用。PD-1 和 PD-L1 是两个研究较多的目标。PD-1 是一种存在于 T 细胞上的受体，与肿瘤细胞表达的 PD-L1 相互作用。持续性 MRD 和复发患者的 PD-L1 和 PD-1 表达上调[454]。目前正在进行的临床试验探索将 PD-1 阻断与树突状细胞/骨髓瘤融合疫苗[362,455]结合使用，例如与帕博利珠单抗、来那度胺和地塞米松联合使用（NCT02036502）。复发或难治性患者的治疗选择取决于许多因素，包括自上一次治疗以来的时间、既往是否使用新型药物、单独或联合用药以及既往治疗是否存在并发症，例如神经病变、肾功能障碍和患者生理功能的丧失。在过去的十年中，RR 骨髓瘤患者可接受的治疗方法数量急剧增加。这是肿瘤学中一个非常活跃的领域，随着越来越多的新疗法进入试验并获得批准，这一领域将继续发展。

未来方向

多发性骨髓瘤新治疗模式的演变

我们的体外研究和动物模型研究已经证明了 BM 在促进多发性骨髓瘤细胞生长、存活、耐药性和在 BM 微环境中迁移方面的重要性，并且已经获得了基于在 BM 环境中靶向多发性骨髓瘤细胞的非常有希望的治疗方法。这些研究为多发性骨髓瘤发现新的治疗模式提供了框架，因此，迫切需要针对肿瘤细胞及其微环境的治疗方法，尽管已经有可用的治疗方法，但多发性骨髓瘤仍然无法治愈。

新型靶向多发性骨髓瘤的识别与验证

重要的是，在我们使用传统地塞米松[169]和硼替佐米[170]疗法进行的体外基因队列研究中，从接受这些方案治疗的患者身上获得的样本一方面有助于确定新药物作用的体内靶点和机制，另一方面也有助于确定耐药机制，以及帮助确定这些新疗法的体内靶点是否与其体外抗-MM 活性相关。令人兴奋的是，临床前研究表明，当这些新药物与传统药物结合或相互结合时，活性增强。这些研究建立了一种新的治疗模式，针对骨髓微环境中的骨髓基质细胞，进一步阐明骨髓基质细胞的发病机制，克服耐药性，改善患者预后。

新的抑制剂包括新的蛋白酶体抑制剂 marizomib（NPI-0052）、FGFR3 抑制剂[456,457]、MEK 抑制剂、AZD6244[458]和 HSP90 抑制剂[459]。marizomib[460]是一种新一代蛋白酶体抑制剂，在临床前模型中对硼替佐米耐药型 MM 具有治疗作用并且无毒性，并且已经在进行针对复发的多发性骨髓瘤的临床试验。FGFR3 抑制剂专门针对 15%～20%的 T(4∶14)易位患者。单纯用热休克蛋白 90 抑制剂治疗复发难治性多发性骨髓瘤有较好的疗效。

基因和蛋白表达谱也可以为新的靶向治疗的临床方案提供临床前基础。例如我们的研究表明，硼替佐米在体外治疗多发性骨髓瘤细胞可诱导死亡信号转导，下调生存信号转导，并上调泛素/蛋白酶体和应激反应基因转录物[170]。特别是硼替佐米上调了热休克蛋白 90，热休克蛋白 90 不仅是一种应激反应蛋白，而且在蛋白酶体降解蛋白质前所需的蛋白质展开中起主要作用。我们在生物体外进行的研究表明，HSP90 抑制剂 17-AAG（KOS953）可以阻断硼替佐米诱导的 HSP90 应激反应，从而增加 MM 细胞凋亡。因此，这些基因微队列研究为临床试验提供了框架，将这些药物与多发性骨髓瘤结合，表明 Hsp90 抑制剂 KOS953 可以增敏甚至克服对硼替佐米的耐药性[461]，并且硼替佐米对照硼替佐米联合 KOS953 治疗复发多发性骨髓瘤的Ⅲ期临床试验正在进行中。

蛋白质组学研究也可以为新型靶向治疗的临床前应用提供基础。例如，我们的体外研究表明，MM 细胞暴露于硼替佐米可诱导 DNA 修复激酶，如 DNA PKC，以剂量和时间依赖性方式分裂[462]。这一观察首次表明，硼替佐米抑制 DNA 修复。随后的体外研究表明，将硼替佐米与 DNA 破坏剂（烷化剂和蒽环类）结合，可以提高耐药 MM 细胞对这些药物的敏感性，甚至恢复对这些药物的敏感性[463]。硼替佐米联合脂质体多柔比星[464]或者美法仑[463]的临床方案已显示出良好的临床效果。具体地说，一项针对复发性多发性骨髓瘤患者的，应用脂质体多柔比星联合硼替佐米对照硼替佐米的大型随机试验显示，接受联合治疗的患者的 OR、EFS 和 OS 显著改善，为 2007 年 6 月的 FDA 批准奠定了基础[430]。

为了在合理的临床试验中为这些新型药物的耦合提供框

架，我们还对传统药物和这些新型药物在多发性骨髓瘤细胞中触发的凋亡信号级联进行了分析[70]。例如，应用免疫调节剂和肿瘤坏死因子相关凋亡诱导配体双重触发细胞凋亡蛋白酶8凋亡信号，而使用诸如来那度胺和硼替佐米的免疫调节剂可同时触发细胞凋亡蛋白酶8和细胞凋亡蛋白酶9介导的多发性骨髓瘤细胞死亡。来那度胺和硼替佐米联合应用已显示出显著的活性，即使对两种药物单独耐药的患者也是如此[465]。

mTOR抑制剂西罗莫司使MM细胞对传统和新疗法均敏感[466,467]，西罗莫司酯化物在异种移植模型中具有抗MM活性[468]。口服mTOR抑制剂依维莫司与来那度胺联合治疗复发/难治性骨髓瘤的Ⅰ期试验耐受性良好，在既往经多线治疗的人群中有反应[469]。硼替佐米抑制生长(MEK/ERT)和生存(Jak/STAT)信号转导，但激活AKT为硼替佐米与AKT抑制剂哌立福辛结合提供临床前基础[470]。

我们最近的信号学研究已经确定了侵袭性蛋白在MM中降解泛素化蛋白的作用，并专门使用HDAC6抑制剂tubacin来抑制其向侵袭性蛋白的转运以进行降解。用管肽阻断侵袭性可诱导蛋白酶体的代偿性上调；相反，用硼替佐米阻断蛋白酶体可触发对侵袭性的代偿性上调。重要的是，分别用硼替佐米和tubacin阻断蛋白酶体和聚集体，会产生协同毒性[471]。HDAC6抑制剂瑞考司他(ACY-1215)目前正与来那度胺、泊马度胺或硼替佐米联合进行临床试验[440,441]。

也可以将单克隆抗体与新药物结合。例如，来那度胺能显著增强MM患者中的抗CD40诱导的ADCC[110]。最后，相关临床研究中的基因表达谱将确定药物敏感性与耐药性，并允许预测哪些患者最有可能对传统和新的靶向治疗作出反应。例如，患者肿瘤样本的基因表达谱显示，对硼替佐米有反应的患者与没有反应的患者相比基因表达上调。HSP27上调与固有或获得性硼替佐米耐药相关。临床前研究表明，p38MAPK抑制下调了耐药MM细胞系和患者样本中HSP27的表达，并恢复了硼替佐米的敏感性[472]，为这两种药物结合的试验提供了基础。

其他浆细胞失调

浆细胞瘤

临床特点

浆细胞瘤是来源于骨骼(孤立性骨浆细胞瘤，SOP)或软组织(髓外浆细胞瘤，EMP)的单克隆浆细胞的集合。占血浆细胞比例<10%。在进行SOP或EMP诊断之前，必须排除MM。MRI可用于显示与多发性骨髓瘤一致的其他骨髓异常[473]。SOP或EMP发病的中位年龄约为50岁，比MM发病的中位年龄小近10岁[474~476]。尽管SOP和EMP患者都可以进展到MM，但大多数情况下SOP患者将发展为MM，而EMP患者只有50%最终发展为多发性骨髓瘤。SOP和EMP患者的中位生存期分别为86.4和100.8个月，两者相似；然而，PFS明显不同，SOP患者为16%，EMP患者为71%。在原发性浆细胞瘤治疗后，血清和/或尿液中稳定的单克隆Ig的持续存在不需要额外的治疗，因为它不影响生存或DFS[474]。相反，在有SOP或EMP病史的患者中，单克隆免疫球蛋白水平的升高可能出现复发性浆细胞瘤或MM。有人建议，对于MM来说，血清β_2M在SOP患者中具有预后价值。19例血清β_2M升高的患者中，17例转化为MM，存活时间(31个月)较正常血清β_2M水平高[477]。

治疗

SOP和EMP的治疗是局部治疗，主要是根据解剖学部位进行放射治疗或者手术治疗[474~476]。单独应用化疗或者与放疗以及手术联合应用，均未被证实可作为SOP或EMP的主要治疗。此外，给予辅助化疗以预防复发性疾病和/或进展为MM的益处也未确定。放射野外放疗后的蛋白质缺失可预测长期DFS和可能的治愈率[478]。

免疫球蛋白M单克隆免疫球蛋白病

血清中过量的单克隆IgM可在多种疾病中发生。在Mayo临床系列的430名患者中，有一种单克隆的IgM蛋白被鉴定出来，242名患者(56%)有MGUS，71名患者(17%)有巨球蛋白血症，28名患者(7%)有淋巴瘤，21名患者(5%)有慢性淋巴细胞白血病，6名患者(1%)有淀粉样变性，62名患者(14%)有其他恶性淋巴细胞增生性疾病[479]。从M蛋白识别到恶性淋巴细胞疾病发展的时间为4~9年，这表明对此类患者进行长期随访是必要的。

巨球蛋白血症

巨球蛋白血症(WM)的诊断是基于存在一种IgM单克隆蛋白和10%或更多的BM活检，显示与具有淋巴浆细胞特征的小淋巴细胞和淋巴浆细胞淋巴瘤的免疫表型特征有关(见下文讨论)[480]。巨球蛋白血症与世界卫生组织(世卫组织)淋巴肿瘤分类[修订版欧洲-美洲(real)淋巴瘤分类的LPL/免疫细胞瘤]中的淋巴浆细胞淋巴瘤(LPA)最为接近。巨球蛋白血症约占所有血液恶性肿瘤的2%，男性比女性更常见。它的发病率随着年龄的增长而增加，在白人中比在非洲裔美国人中更常见[481,482]。虽然巨球蛋白血症的病因尚不清楚，遗传因素可能与该病的发生有关，因为有报道称巨球蛋白血症家族与其他淋巴细胞增生和免疫疾病有关[483]。细胞遗传学异常发生在15%~90%的病例中，但没有一例是巨球蛋白血症特有的[484,485]。巨球蛋白血症B-细胞克隆衍生物可将具有大量表面免疫球蛋白的小淋巴细胞的克隆分化为含有胞质内免疫球蛋白的淋巴细胞质细胞和成熟浆细胞。这种形态异质性通过表型标志物的可变表达来反映。所有的巨球蛋白血症细胞都表达单克隆IgM，大多数细胞CD19、CD20、CD22和FMC7阳性。在PCA-1抗原强度不同的情况下，检测到高密度的CD38。可以预见，CD45亚型的表达是异质的，可能反映了正在进行的单克隆B细胞分化。在大约20%的病例中，有CD5和CD23的表达，但它们的共存并不常见[486]。巨球蛋白血症中循环克隆B细胞在治疗无效或进展的患者中增加[487]。最近的研究表明，巨球蛋白血症起源于生发后中心B细胞，该细胞在淋巴滤泡中有欠发达的体细胞突变和抗原选择，具有携带IgM记忆B细胞的特征[488~490]。

巨球蛋白血症发病的中位年龄为61岁。症状特征不明显和非特异性，最常见的是虚弱、厌食和体重减轻。由周围神经病变和雷诺现象引起的症状可能先于更严重的症状。淋巴结肿大、脾大和/或肝大在30%~40%的病例中存在,骨髓中通常存在至少20%~25%的淋巴浆细胞样细胞。小肠和周围神经受累可导致吸收不良和神经病变的临床后遗症。出血并发症可能是由于出血时间异常、血小板黏附性降低或IgM蛋白直接干扰血小板因子3和凝血因子的释放。鉴别诊断的一个重要部分是排除不常见的IgM型多发性骨髓瘤,其特征是溶骨性疾病和无器官肿大和/或淋巴细胞受累;巨球蛋白血症本身很少进展为IgM型多发性骨髓瘤[491]。淀粉样变在巨球蛋白血症中很少发生[492]。高黏度证候群,先前描述为一种罕见的多发性硬化症并发症,通常发生在过量IgM,其特征是黏膜出血和神经、眼部和心血管异常[259]。血浆置换治疗对于清除过量的IgM比在过量的IgG单克隆蛋白和相关的多发性骨髓瘤高黏性的情况下更有用。

治疗

中位生存期约为50个月,与文献记载最好的系列多发性骨髓瘤患者没有太大差异。然而,与患有多发性骨髓瘤的患者相比,许多患有巨球蛋白血症的人长期无须治疗,其生存期可超过20年。尽管高剂量的自体干细胞移植疗法已被证明对许多发性骨髓瘤患者或低度恶性淋巴瘤患者有效,但相对较少的巨球蛋白血症患者接受了移植。尽管如此,初步数据表明高剂量治疗与高CR率和可接受的毒性有关,因此该方法值得进一步研究,尤其是对预后不良的年轻患者[493]。据报道,脾切除术对化疗耐药的巨球蛋白血症患者有效,并导致单克隆蛋白浓度显著降低,且持续缓解[494,495]。用利妥昔单抗(一种嵌合的抗CD20单克隆抗体)治疗的单克隆抗体在治疗和未治疗的低度恶性淋巴瘤患者中均能产生疗效。鉴于CD20抗原通常存在于巨球蛋白血症中,在早期研究中,已将利妥昔单抗给予患者,且在先前治疗过的患者中,约1/3的患者出现临床反应[496,497]。越来越多的方案使用了利妥昔单抗与环磷酰胺[498]或硼替佐米[499]的组合。利妥昔单抗在巨球蛋白血症中的疗效可能与血清黏度增加及IgM的显著增加有关[500]。

最近的证据表明大多数巨球蛋白血症患者存在*MYD88L265P*突变[501]。此外,CXCR4途径的突变可能影响疾病的表现[502]。Bruton酪氨酸激酶(BTK)是MYD88的下游靶点,MYD88是一种Toll样受体的衔接分子[503]。伊布替尼是一种口服的BTK抑制剂,63例以前接受过治疗的巨球蛋白血症患者的伊布替尼Ⅱ期试验表明,73%的患者的单克隆蛋白减少50%或更好,平均时间为8周[504]。这些发现使FDA批准伊布替尼用于巨球蛋白血症治疗。

重链疾病

因为Franklin等人[505]的原始描述,在血清和尿液中含有大量IgG Fc片段的原发性恶性淋巴瘤患者中,γ重链疾病(γ-HCD)的临床和免疫范围已扩大。这些疾病的特征是一部分患者的Ig重链存在于血清或尿液中,或两者兼而有之。确诊时的中位年龄与多发性骨髓瘤相似,约60岁[506]。临床和实验室特征可能是异质的。最常见的症状是虚弱、疲劳和发热,与淋巴结肿大和肝脾肿大有关。除了血清或尿液中的Ig重链外,大多数病例都有淋巴浆细胞浸润。临床病程可能是暴发性的和快速进行的;或者,单克隆重链在其他无症状的患者中可以持续数年。因此存活率是可变的,但中位数只有12个月。活动性疾病患者的治疗方案与淋巴瘤或多发性骨髓瘤患者的治疗方案相似,而惰性疾病患者的治疗应在无须治疗的情况下按期随访。α-HCD、μ-HCD和δ-HCD的病例也有过描述。HCD通常与胃肠道的非霍奇金淋巴瘤有关,首先是血浆细胞在肠道内产生重链和聚集物,然后转变为免疫母细胞型的恶性非霍奇金淋巴瘤,可能是由较成熟的血浆细胞[507]。由于其稀有性,重链疾病的理想治疗方法尚不清楚,但强化化疗包括静脉注射环磷酰胺、多柔比星、长春新碱和口服泼尼松,似乎能使一些患者的症状获得长期缓解[522]。

淀粉样变

淀粉样变作为一种临床上有意义的疾病是相对罕见的。它被分为五类,包括:①原发性,有或无浆细胞和淋巴细胞的肿瘤;②继发性,与慢性感染或自身免疫性疾病有关;③遗传性,与家族性地中海热、葡萄牙下肢神经病等有关;④淀粉样变,与衰老有关;⑤内分泌腺类淀粉样变,伴有甲状腺髓样癌和多发性内分泌肿瘤2型[492,508]。淀粉样变性的大多数病例中发现的淀粉样变可分为两种类型,根据纤维是否主要由Ig轻链的可变区域组成(AL,原发性淀粉样变)或由蛋白质A(AA,继发性淀粉样变)组成。蛋白质A分子量为8 500Da,由76个氨基酸组成,与任何已知的免疫球蛋白无关。确定正确的诊断方法是关键,因为单克隆免疫球蛋白病的意义不明是常见的,在一系列350例疑似淀粉样变的患者中,9.7%的患者实际上在纤维蛋白原Aα链或转甲状腺素中有突变[509]。淀粉样蛋白P的直接分类通过激光显微解剖和质谱法分析蛋白质有助于提高淀粉样变的诊断准确性[510]。

在淀粉样变中,淀粉样蛋白主要涉及心脏、舌头、胃肠道和/或皮肤,而原发性淀粉样变主要导致肝脏、肾脏和脾脏中的纤维沉积。一项对229例原发性淀粉样变患者的回顾性研究显示,47例(21%)患者中有多发性骨髓瘤[508]。最初出现的症状是疲劳和体重减轻,疼痛在同样患有多发性骨髓瘤的患者中更为常见。高达1/3的原发性淀粉样变患者出现肝大和巨舌;一半患者出现肾功能不全,82%的患者出现蛋白尿(定义为免疫球蛋白尿,仅见于多发性骨髓瘤)。肾病综合征、CHF、直立性低血压、腕管综合征和周围神经病变在无多发性骨髓瘤患者(30%~70%的研究患者)中的发生率均高于多发性骨髓瘤患者(<20%)。总的生存期中位数为12个月,多发性骨髓瘤的患者为5个月,而没有多发性骨髓瘤的患者为13个月。虽然已经很难监测疾病的分布和发展,但已经证明放射性标记的血清淀粉样蛋白P组分对淀粉样纤维具有特异性结合亲和力,可以静脉注射,并快速且特异地定位于淀粉样蛋白沉积[511,512]。因此,这种技术可能有助于诊断和监测系统性淀粉样变的程度,包括治疗干预的效果。

治疗

原发性淀粉样变的治疗正在取得进展。早期研究着眼于秋水仙碱或MP或这三种药物,应答率均较低[513]。最初的经验是，使用具有自体干细胞支持[514,515]的剂量密集型美法仑可以达到CR，随着器官特异性疾病的表现状态和临床缓解的改善，指南已经制订，便于患者选择最大限度地提高效益，最大限度地减少相关死亡率[516~518]。在多发性骨髓瘤中，具备资格接受高剂量治疗的患者在化疗中也可能表现良好[519]。为了解决这一问题，一项随机试验将高剂量的美法仑和自体干细胞移植，与标准的美法仑和地塞米松进行比较，本研究未发现高剂量强化治疗的益处[520]。这项试验的一个显著局限性是强化组的高死亡率，在其他研究中没有发现，这表明该试验可能不具有普遍性。

试图改善有症状和晚期多系统疾病患者的预后，可能需要器官和干细胞移植，以及使用低强度的调节疗法。例如，心脏受累的患者在自体干细胞动员和移植过程中具有异常高的TRM，这些患者可以通过心脏移植和自体干细胞移植相结合的方式进行治疗[521]。现在新药用于多发性骨髓瘤的常规治疗，在对原发性淀粉样变患者治疗上也有增加，如CyBorD联合治疗，具有持久的疗效[522]。

（程颖 陈艳 王莹 辛影 译 程颖 校）

参考文献

The complete reference list can be found on the Wiley Companion Digital Edition of this title (see inside front cover for login instructions).

6 Rajkumar SV, Dimopoulos MA, Palumbo A, et al. International Myeloma Working Group updated criteria for the diagnosis of multiple myeloma. *Lancet Oncol*. 2014;**15**:e538–e548.

7 Durie BGM, Salmon SE. A clinical staging system for multiple myeloma. Correlation of measured cell mass with presenting clinical features, response to treatment and survival. *Cancer*. 1975;**36**:842–854.

9 Kyle RA, Therneau TM, Rajkumar SV, et al. Prevalence of monoclonal gammopathy of undetermined significance. *N Engl J Med*. 2006;**354**:1362–1369.

12 Rajkumar SV, Kyle RA, Therneau TM, et al. Serum free light chain ratio is an independent risk factor for progression in monoclonal gammopathy of undetermined significance. *Blood*. 2005;**106**:812–817.

13 Kyle RA, Remstein ED, Therneau TM, et al. Clinical course and prognosis of smoldering (asymptomatic) multiple myeloma. *N Engl J Med*. 2007;**356**:2582–2590.

21 Kyle RA, Gertz MA, Witzig TE, et al. Review of 1027 patients with newly diagnosed multiple myeloma. *Mayo Clin Proc*. 2003;**78**:21–33.

43 Bergsagel PL, Chesi M, Nardini E, Brents LA, Kirby SL, Kuehl WM. Promiscuous translocations into immunoglobulin heavy chain switch regions in multiple myeloma. *Proc Natl Acad Sci U S A*. 1996;**93**:13931–13936.

45 Teoh G, Anderson KC. Interaction of tumor and host cells with adhesion and extracellular matrix molecules in the development of multiple myeloma. *Hematol Oncol Clin North Am*. 1997;**11**:27–42.

64 Hideshima T, Chauhan D, Shima Y, et al. Thalidomide and its analogues overcome drug resistance of human multiple myeloma cells to conventional therapy. *Blood*. 2000;**96**:2943–2950.

70 Hideshima T, Anderson KC. Molecular mechanisms of novel therapeutic approaches for multiple myeloma. *Nat Rev Cancer*. 2002;**2**:927–937.

90 Singhal S, Mehta J, Desikan R, et al. Antitumor activity of thalidomide in refractory multiple myeloma. *N Engl J Med*. 1999;**341**:1565–1571.

146 Bergsagel PL, Kuehl WM. Molecular pathogenesis and a consequent classification of multiple myeloma. *J Clin Oncol*. 2005;**23**:6333–6338.

150 Neben K, Lokhorst HM, Jauch A, et al. Administration of bortezomib before and after autologous stem cell transplantation improves outcome in multiple myeloma patients with deletion 17p. *Blood*. 2012;**119**:940–948.

157 Chapman MA, Lawrence MS, Keats JJ, et al. Initial genome sequencing and analysis of multiple myeloma. *Nature*. 2011;**471**:467–472.

171 Weiss BM, Abadie J, Verma P, Howard RS, Kuehl WM. A monoclonal gammopathy precedes multiple myeloma in most patients. *Blood*. 2009;**113**:5418–5422.

172 Landgren O, Kyle RA, Pfeiffer RM, et al. Monoclonal gammopathy of undetermined significance (MGUS) consistently precedes multiple myeloma: a prospective study. *Blood*. 2009;**113**:5412–5417.

181 Greipp PR, San Miguel J, Durie BG, et al. International staging system for multiple myeloma. *J Clin Oncol*. 2005;**23**:3412–3420.

188 Zhan F, Huang Y, Colla S, et al. The molecular classification of multiple myeloma. *Blood*. 2006;**108**:2020–2028.

243 Berenson J, Lichtenstein A, Porter L, et al. Pamidronate disodium reduces the occurrence of skeletal events in patients with advanced multiple myeloma. *N Engl J Med*. 1996;**334**:488–493.

251 Morgan GJ, Child JA, Gregory WM, et al. Effects of zoledronic acid versus clodronic acid on skeletal morbidity in patients with newly diagnosed multiple myeloma (MRC Myeloma IX): secondary outcomes from a randomised controlled trial. *Lancet Oncol*. 2011;**12**:743–752.

253 Raje N, Woo SB, Hande K, et al. Clinical, radiographic, and biochemical characterization of multiple myeloma patients with osteonecrosis of the jaw. *Clin Cancer Res*. 2008;**14**:2387–2395.

285 Kumar SK, Rajkumar SV, Dispenzieri A, et al. Improved survival in multiple myeloma and the impact of novel therapies. *Blood*. 2008;**111**:2516–2520.

293 Durie BG, Harousseau JL, Miguel JS, et al. International uniform response criteria for multiple myeloma. *Leukemia*. 2006;**20**:1467–1473.

294 Rajkumar SV, Harousseau JL, Durie B, et al. Consensus recommendations for the uniform reporting of clinical trials: report of the International Myeloma Workshop Consensus Panel 1. *Blood*. 2011;**117**:4691–4695.

295 Martinez-Lopez J, Lahuerta JJ, Pepin F, et al. Prognostic value of deep sequencing method for minimal residual disease detection in multiple myeloma. *Blood*. 2014;**123**:3073–3079.

302 San Miguel JF, Schlag R, Khuageva NK, et al. Bortezomib plus melphalan and prednisone for initial treatment of multiple myeloma. *N Engl J Med*. 2008;**359**:906–917.

304 Benboubker L, Dimopoulos MA, Dispenzieri A, et al. Lenalidomide and dexamethasone in transplant-ineligible patients with myeloma. *N Engl J Med*. 2014;**371**:906–917.

313 Rajkumar SV, Jacobus S, Callander NS, et al. Lenalidomide plus high-dose dexamethasone versus lenalidomide plus low-dose dexamethasone as initial therapy for newly diagnosed multiple myeloma: an open-label randomised controlled trial. *Lancet Oncol*. 2010;**11**:29–37.

317 Richardson PG, Sonneveld P, Schuster MW, et al. Bortezomib or high-dose dexamethasone for relapsed multiple myeloma. *N Engl J Med*. 2005;**352**:2487–2498.

341 Child JA, Morgan GJ, Davies FE, et al. High-dose chemotherapy with hematopoietic stem-cell rescue for multiple myeloma. *N Engl J Med*. 2003;**348**:1875–1883.

366 McCarthy PL, Owzar K, Hofmeister CC, et al. Lenalidomide after stem-cell transplantation for multiple myeloma. *N Engl J Med*. 2012;**366**:1770–1781.

381 Bensinger WI, Buckner CD, Anasetti C, et al. Allogeneic marrow transplantation for multiple myeloma: an analysis of risk factors on outcome. *Blood*. 1996;**88**:2787–2793.

394 Alyea E, Weller E, Schlossman R, et al. Outcome after autologous and allogeneic stem cell transplantation for patients with multiple myeloma: impact of graft-versus-myeloma effect. *Bone Marrow Transplant*. 2003;**32**:1145–1151.

398 Maloney DG, Molina AJ, Sahebi F, et al. Allografting with nonmyeloablative conditioning following cytoreductive autografts for the treatment of patients with multiple myeloma. *Blood*. 2003;**102**:3447–3454.

412 Weber DM, Chen C, Niesvizky R, et al. Lenalidomide plus dexamethasone for relapsed multiple myeloma in North America. *N Engl J Med*. 2007;**357**:2133–2142.

415 San Miguel J, Weisel K, Moreau P, et al. Pomalidomide plus low-dose dexamethasone versus high-dose dexamethasone alone for patients with relapsed and refractory multiple myeloma (MM-003): a randomised, open-label, phase 3 trial. *Lancet Oncol*. 2013;**14**:1055–1066.

425 Stewart AK, Rajkumar SV, Dimopoulos MA, et al. Carfilzomib, lenalidomide, and dexamethasone for relapsed multiple myeloma. *N Engl J Med*. 2015;**372**:142–152.

433 Lokhorst HM, Plesner T, Gimsing P, et al. Phase I/II dose-escalation study of daratumumab in patients with relapsed or refractory multiple myeloma. *ASCO Meeting Abstracts*. 2013;**31**:8512.

434 Lonial S, Jagannath S, Moreau P, et al. Phase (Ph) I/II study of elotuzumab (Elo) plus lenalidomide/dexamethasone (Len/dex) in relapsed/refractory multiple myeloma (RR MM): updated Ph II results and Ph I/II long-term safety. *ASCO Meeting Abstracts*. 2013;**31**:8542.

504 Treon SP, Tripsas CK, Meid K, et al. Ibrutinib in Previously Treated Waldenstrom's Macroglobulinemia. *N Engl J Med*. 2015;**372**:1430–1440.

第 122 章　骨髓增殖性肿瘤：原发性血小板增多症，原发性骨髓纤维化，真性红细胞增多症

Ayalew Tefferi，MD

概述

慢性髓系肿瘤（chronic myeloid neoplasm）是一组起源于异常转化的多能造血干细胞的恶性骨髓增殖性疾病。这群异质性疾病均为惰性起病，演变为急性白血病风险的概率不同。即便不转化为白血病，这些疾病特征性的细胞过度增殖或缺乏经常困扰患者甚至致命；这类疾病的并发症包括血栓形成，出血，显著的肝脾肿大，明显的全身症状或恶病质。

依据 2008 年世界卫生组织（World Health Organization，WHO）分类系统修定版，慢性髓系肿瘤包括骨髓增生异常综合征（myelodysplastic syndrome，MDS）（参见第 113 章），骨髓增殖性肿瘤（myeloproliferative neoplasm，MPN）、"骨髓增生异常综合征/骨髓增殖性肿瘤重叠"以及伴血小板衍生生长因子受体（platelet-derived growth factor receptor，PDGFR）（PDGFRα 或 PDFFRβ）或成纤维细胞生长因子受体 1（fibroblast growth factor receptor1，FGFR1）突变和显著嗜酸性粒细胞增多这一类疾病[1,2]。2008 年世界卫生组织对于 MPN 分类包括 4 种经典的"骨髓增殖性疾病"：慢性髓细胞性白血病（chronic myeloid leukemia，CML）、真性红细胞增多症（polycythemia vera，PV）、原发性血小板增多症（essential thrombocythemia，ET）、原发性骨髓纤维化（primary myelofibrosis，PMF），也包括慢性中性粒细胞白血病（chronic neutrophilic leukemia，CNL）、慢性嗜酸性粒细胞白血病非特殊型（chronic eosinophilic leukemia not otherwise specified，CEL-NOS）、肥大细胞增多症（mastocytosis）及无法分类的 MPN（MPN，unclassifiable，MPN-U）。"MDS/MPN"这一类同时具备 MDS（红系或粒系的病态造血）和 MPN（外周血粒细胞增多、单核细胞增多、嗜酸性粒细胞增多或血小板增多）的特征[3]。这一类包括"慢性粒-单核细胞白血病"（chronic myelomonocytic leukemia，CMML），"青少年粒单核细胞白血病"（juvenile myelomonocytic leukemia，JMML），"BCR-ABL 阴性不典型 CML"（aCML）以及"MDS/MPN，未分类"（MDS/MPN unclassifiable）[2]。"MDS/MPN，未分类"包括世界卫生组织暂定类"环形铁粒幼红细胞性难治性贫血伴相关血小板增多"（ring sideroblasts associated with marked thrombocytosis，RARS-T）[3]。

Epstein 和 Goedel（Vienna，1934 年）、Vaquez（Paris，1892 年）和 Heuck（Heidelberg，1879 年）分别最早对 ET、PV 和 PMF 做出描述，而清楚的描述这类疾病距今时间不长[4]。自从 1960 年，CML 被定义为存在费城染色体（Philadelphia chromosome，Ph），即 t(9;22)(q34;q11)[5]。在 20 世纪 80 年代，与费城染色体等效的分子标志 *BCR-ABL* 基因易位被发现，该基因用于诊断 CML 并能够在鼠模型中致病。现在 CML 是 Dameshek 分类的原发 MPD 分类中定义最明确、分子特征最明显的疾病[6]。本章主要讨论三种 *BCR-ABL* 基因阴性的经典 MPN（即 PV、ET 和 PMF）。

原发性血小板增多症

流行病学

ET 并不常见；根据年龄和性别调整的年发病率为 0.2/10 万~2.5/10 万人[7~9]。相对年轻人群中（30~50 岁），女性似乎更常见，但这种性别差异在其他年龄组并不明显。迄今为止尚未发现明确的致病因素。ET 的发病率（同时还有 PV 和 PMF）在犹太人群中似乎呈增长趋势[10]。三种 MPN 的初诊中位年龄约为 60 岁。家族聚集性的 ET 虽然被报道过但非常罕见；一些家族性病例是由于促血小板生成素（thrombopoietin，TPO）基因突变有关，这会使 Tpo 产物增加（一种巨核细胞生长因子）会导致巨核细胞过度刺激[11,12]。

诊断

ET 确诊最大的挑战是鉴别真正的原发血小板增多和"继发性"或"反应性"血小板增多（reactive thrombocytosis，RT）。多达 80%的血小板增多的常规病例中，血小板计数的升高呈多克隆性且由于非骨髓疾病导致[13,14]。与炎症、感染和恶性疾病相关的血小板增多被认为与巨核细胞相关刺激因子，如白介素-6（interleukin-6，IL-6）相关；而缺铁时偶尔并发的血小板增多机制尚不明确，可能由于促红细胞生成素（erythropoietin，Epo）对血小板生成的前体细胞有交叉刺激作用[15]。

临床上鉴别诊断 ET 和 RT 非常重要，因为 ET 并发血栓和出血风险较继发性血小板增多高很多[13]。如果 RT 证据不明显，血清铁蛋白（serum ferritin）和 C 反应蛋白（C-reactive Protein，CRP，一种 IL-6 水平的替代标志物）可能在分别排除缺铁和感染方面有诊断价值[15]。CRP 升高提示 RT，并应更彻底的寻找反应性细胞因子的来源。当然 CRP 升高并不能严格排除 ET，因为患者可能同时存在 ET 和炎症反应，但这种情况非常少见[15]。解读铁蛋白水平同样需慎重：虽然低水平铁蛋白提示缺铁而高水平提示 RT，但与 CRP 类似，同样不能完全排除 ET 的诊断。

从患者病史中较易获得外科手术引起的脾功能减退信息，但是由于淀粉样变性、乳糜泻或其他原因所致的脾功能低下可能并不明显[16]。因此对于每一个慢性血小板增多的患者，初诊时均应进行血涂片检查并寻找特异性的 Howell-Jolly 小体。

完成上述步骤如果尚无 RT 和脾功能低下的证据，则 ET 的可能性较大，而外周血 JAK2、*CALR* 和 *MPL* 突变的筛查可能

有助于诊断潜在的 MPN，而无须区分 ET 与 PV 或 PMF。ET 也应该与其他髓系疾病相鉴别，因为这些疾病有不同的预后和不同的治疗方案。与 ET 相似的髓系肿瘤包括以下疾病的部分病例，如 MDS、CML 及其他两种非 ET 的经典 MPN（如 PV 和 PMF，包括有可能混淆的 PMF“细胞期或纤维化前期”）。如一名疑似 ET 的患者常规细胞遗传学分析中没有显示费城染色体（Philadelphia chromosome），应至少 1 次通过外周血或骨髓的荧光原位杂交（fluorescence in situ hybridization，FISH）检测以排除核型隐匿性 CML 的可能性。

鉴别 ET 和 PMF 通常不难，但仍存在例外。如 15% 的 ET 病例存在轻度（1 或 2 级）的网状纤维[17]。同时细胞器期的 PMF 特点为骨髓细胞过量伴巨核细胞不典型增生，骨髓纤维化并不重，其表现可以与 ET 类似，需进行细致的形态学检查进行鉴别[18]。所有 BCR-ABL 阴性的原发性骨髓纤维化（分为 3 级）的骨髓活检特征是存在异常的巨核细胞簇。初诊患者中不到 10%存在细胞遗传学异常[19]。

发病机制

如上所述，通过 X 染色体链锁 DNA（X-chromosome-linked DNA）或基因产物分析，大部分女性 ET 患者均涉及巨核系、有时是髓系的克隆性骨髓增殖（甚至存在于白细胞计数和血细胞比容均正常的一些病例中）[20,21]。

2005 年发现在大部分 ET 以及 PMF 和 PV 患者中存在 *JAK2* 功能获得性基因突变（*JAK2V617F*）[22~25]。另有非常少的一部分 ET 患者（约 5%）携带 *MPL* 突变[26~29]。最近，在 2013 年，约半数 *JAK2* 未突变的 ET 或 PMF 患者中又发现了钙网蛋白基因（*CALR*）突变[30]，而该突变的精确致病机制尚不清楚。

ET 中的巨核细胞增生和血小板生成呈显著的自发性，正常调控途径存在明显缺陷。大部分病例机制尚不明确。ET 患者来源的巨核细胞不能被关键的生长和分化细胞因子抗体所抑制，这些细胞因子包括 IL-3、IL-6，粒细胞-巨噬细胞集落刺激因子（granulocyte-monocyte colony-stimulating factor，GM-CSF）以及 Tpo 等[31,32]。虽然 Tpo 和它的受体 c-Mpl 是控制巨核细胞生长发育反馈调节环的主要组成部分，但在 ET 和相关疾病中，Tpo 和 c-Mpl 的动力学特征似乎较复杂。ET 患者中尽管存在增多的巨核细胞团，但 Tpo 水平通常为正常或升高，且正常骨髓和 ET 或 RT 之间的差别不具重复性。而 ET 中 c-Mpl 表达（尽管不总是如此）经常明显降低（图 122-1）。而且 c-Mpl 在其他 MPN 中也存在表达下调，所以 c-Mpl 作为 ET 的诊断作用有限[33,34]。ET 中促使巨核细胞增殖的特异性细胞因子目前尚不明确，但该病患者中巨核系祖细胞对于 IL-3 和 Tpo 存在不能解释的高度敏感性[35,36]。

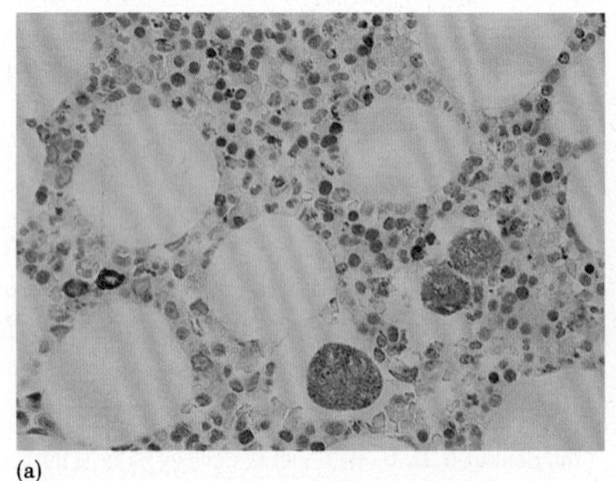
(a)

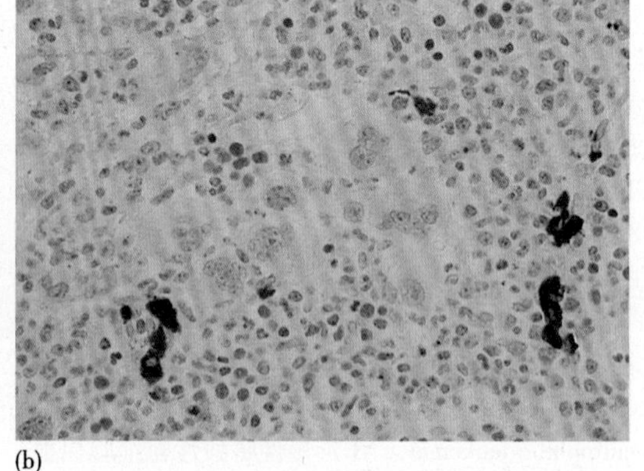
(b)

图 122-1 （a）正常巨核细胞 c-Mpl 免疫组化染色和（b）骨髓增生性疾病中的巨核细胞 c-Mpl 染色减少。摘自 Tefferi2001。经 Elsevier 许可转载

临床表现

至少半数 ET 患者初诊时无特殊症状，通过合理治疗后相当比例的患者能在病程中仍保持无症状，但在整个病程中其预期寿命明显短于性别和年龄匹配的对照组人口[37~39]。25%~50%ET 发病时有微血管和血管舒缩症状。初诊时和随访时分别有 11%~25%和 10%~22%的患者伴广泛血栓，而广泛出血比例分别 2%~5%和 1%~7%[9,38,40,41]。使用阿司匹林（aspirin，ASA）和其他具有抑制血小板功能的非甾体抗炎药（non-steroidal anti-inflammatory drugs，NSAID）会加重出血。与其他 MPN 普遍脾大不同，不到 25% 的 ET 患者起病时脾大可触及[37]。

血管舒缩障碍（如头疼、头晕目眩、视物模糊和盲点等视力症状、心悸、胸痛、红斑性肢痛病及四肢远端感觉异常）使患者感到痛苦但基本无致命危险。这些症状原因尚不清楚，推测与血小板-微脉管系统内皮之间作用：这种作用与局部炎症和一过性血栓血管栓塞相关[42]。许多血小板产物如血栓素 A2 具有血管活性，可能在致病过程中起到相应作用。红斑性肢痛病是最严重的血管症状，以红斑，皮肤发热，和四肢末端疼痛为特征，这个症状较罕见且对 ET 具有特征性[43]。微血管舒缩障碍并不能很明确预测出血或大血管血栓形成。

ET 致命性的并发症包括：大血管血栓（动脉和静脉），出血，疾病转变为 PMF 类似的纤维化期或者急性髓系白血病（acute myeloid leukemia，AML）。动脉血栓可以导致脑血管事件、心血管缺血，器官梗死以及肢端坏疽。ET 的静脉血栓不仅易发于其他血栓性疾病常见发病部位（如肺栓塞和下肢深静脉血栓），还易发于一些罕见部位（如脑静脉窦血栓，视网膜静脉血栓，以及肝和门静脉血栓）[38]。

ET 最常见及影响患者的出血问题见于皮肤黏膜出血（鼻出血、牙龈出血、瘀斑、瘀点）[44]。因为鼻出血和容易擦伤在普

通人群中非常常见,因此评估这些相应症状就是 ET 对受累患者的影响比较困难。如果仔细调控血小板计数可以控制黏膜出血症状,则有理由推测血小板增多对症状有重要作用。ET 的严重出血并发症最常见于肠道,并可因应用 ASA 或 NSAID 加重[45]。中枢神经系统(central nervous system,CNS)和视网膜也可发生出血,幸运的是相对罕见。比较矛盾的是,血小板极度增多的患者可能有特别的出血风险,部分原因可能与血小板吸附大量血管性假血友病因子(von Willebrand factor,vWF)多聚体所造成的获得性 vWF 缺乏相关。这种现象可见于任何原因造成的极度血小板增多[46]。

在初诊 10 年时间内,ET 纤维化或白血病演化属于罕见事件(发生率小于 5%)[37,38]。

治疗和预后

治疗 ET 要注意两点:①ET 一般属于惰性疾病,至少在最初 10 年内预期寿命与年龄、性别匹配的对照健康人群相仿;②迄今为止尚未有治疗手段证明可以影响总生存率[37,47],因此必须谨记不伤害原则。ET 的初始治疗通常是为了减轻微血管症状或预防组织血栓形成以及出血等并发症。小剂量应用 ASA 可以减轻血管舒缩障碍,每日 81mg 通常即有效。当应用 ASA 不能减轻症状时,增加降血小板药物用量通常有效。

因为只有极少数随机对照试验用来评估降低 ET 患者的血栓风险,因此临床决策通常必须建立于前瞻性队列研究和大型回顾性分析基础之上。治疗策略应该基于个性化评估血栓风险。两项临床参数对于临床判断至关重要:血栓病史和年龄超过 60 岁[41,48]。可以根据是否存在这两项危险因素将 ET 患者分为低危组,高危组和中危组并给予相应分层治疗(表 122-1 和 122-2)[49]。该分类方法完善了在 ET 中 *JAK2* 突变和心血管危险因素等是动脉血栓形成独立的危险因素[50]。因此,"低风险",而非"非常低风险",定义为年龄<60 岁且无血栓形成史,但有 *JAK2* 突变或心血管危险因素。无 *JAK2* 突变或心血管危险因素的患者被列为"非常低风险"组。对高风险疾病的定义保持不变,包括患者年龄≥60 岁或存在血栓形成史。*JAK2V617F* 突变等位基因负荷与 ET 患者预后关系不大。

表 122-1　真红细胞增多症和 ET 危险度分级

低危	年龄小于 60 岁,无血栓病史,血小板计数小于 $1\times10^6/\mu l$
中危	年龄大于 60 岁,且无血栓病史,血小板计数大于 $1\times10^6/\mu l$
高危	年龄≥60 岁或有血栓病史

表 122-2　ET 症危险度分层治疗建议

危险度分级	细胞抑制治疗	阿司匹林治疗	可能怀孕
低危	不	是	小剂量阿司匹林
高危	是	是	小剂量阿司匹林和 IFN-α
中危	有时	是(除外获得性 von Willebrand 病)	小剂量阿司匹林(除外获得性 von Willebrand 病)

血小板治疗的获益可知,针对低危、高危组的 ET 症患者每日应用 81~235mg ASA 同样可以降低血栓风险似乎是有道理的[51,52]。然而,如前所述,极低危组的患者可能无须 ASA 抗血小板治疗。对高危患者更常用的策略为降低血小板到正常水平。一项重要的随机对照研究证实,应用羟基脲(hydroxyurea,HU)可以降低 ET 高危组患者 20% 绝对血栓事件风险(3.6)[53]。其他减少血细胞药物尚未在随机研究中证实降低血栓事件。目前尚不明确高危组患者精确的降血小板目标,这是因为即便血小板计数正常也有可能发生血栓事件,但回顾性研究支持血小板小于 4 000 000/μl 即为合理的控制目标[54,55]。低危和中危组患者血栓事件相对少见,目前尚不明确应用降血小板药物能否获益。

基于高质量的循证医学证据,HU 应该列为 ET 一线治疗选择。HU 曾被担心具有致白血病作用,但最近两项应用 HU 治疗 ET 的研究中分别追踪了 5~14 年和 2~12 年,尚未发现继发白血病[56,57]。IFN-α_{2a}(INFα)以及最近的长效聚乙二醇干扰素在 HU 不耐受或难治性病例中可以作为替代治疗方案,但干扰素广为人知的药物毒性限制了它作为一线治疗的应用,特别是高危组 ET 患者多为老人,不易耐受所需的剂量[58~60]。IFN-α_{2a} 适合需要降低血小板的怀孕 ET 患者(参见下文)。

仅有不到 10% 的 ET 症患者出现广泛出血(即大量失血导致血红蛋白降低或导致重要器官出血,如 CNS)[37,38]。极度血小板增多(血小板计数超过 $1\times10^6/\mu l$)似乎是出血的危险因素,部分原因是因为上文描述的获得性 vWF 因子缺乏。降低血小板数量以间接提高 vWF 因子水平的治疗可能间接提示 vWF 多聚体的减少。在急诊情况下单采血小板是最快降低血小板水平的方法,但其效用仍有待证明。

特别考虑

ET 怀孕患者与怀孕前 3 个月自发流产风险升高(约 35%)相关[61]。但产后血栓风险并未升高[62]。自发流产和血小板增生的程度之间并没有明确的联系,同样也没有证据表明预防性单采血小板可以使患者获益[61]。高危 ET 孕妇(如之前有血栓病史的女性)与其他高危患者一样需要降血小板治疗。有单臂试验证明了孕期应用 IFNα 的安全性,但缺乏对照组数据。HU 和哌泊溴烷(pipobroman)存在致畸作用(FDA 孕妇用药安全分级 D),阿那格雷(anagrelide)可以通过胎盘但对胎儿发育作用未知(FDA 孕妇用药安全分级 C)。但是胎儿早期偶然暴露于 HU 并没有严重到必须进行选择性流产[63]。

原发性骨髓纤维化

流行病学

在三种经典的 MPN 中,PMF 侵袭性最强。幸运的是 PMF 是一种罕见病,年发病率仅 0.4/10 万~1.5/10 万人,中位诊断年龄超过 60 岁,男性稍多[7,8]。PMF 与电离辐射(如广岛幸存者)、严重暴露于石油衍生物、二氧化钍造影剂(thorotrast)具有相关性,但绝大部分 PMF 病例无类似暴露史[64,65]。

发病机制

与其他 MPN 疾病类似,通过分析 X 染色体连锁基因和基因产物可证明 PMF 中髓系来源细胞为单克隆性[66]。与此不同,PMF 中骨髓成纤维细胞为多克隆性[66,67]。特征性的 PMF 骨髓间质反应包括成纤维细胞过度增生,细胞外基质蛋白如胶原(大部分为Ⅰ型和Ⅲ型)明显增多,血管增生明显,骨合成和成骨细胞功能活跃[68,69]。骨髓微环境的变化是由于克隆性髓细胞来源的细胞因子风暴介导。事实上已经可以在 PMF 检测到骨髓细胞内外多种细胞因子水平的提高,可以促进纤维产生、血管生成和/或促进成骨,从而支持了前述假设[70]。

在多种小鼠模型中观察到骨髓纤维化伴或不伴髓外造血(extramedullary hematopoiesis,EMH)。强制高表达 TPO 的小鼠会发生骨髓纤维化和骨质硬化,这可能是由于抑制破骨的骨保护素过度分泌[71,72]。转录因子 GATA-1 在造血细胞的发育和分化中起着重要作用,低表达 GATA-1 的小鼠巨核细胞分化受损伴血小板生成减少,最终进展为 EMH 和骨髓纤维化[73]。但是目前尚不清楚此种胚系突变小鼠模型多大程度上模拟人类的疾病状况,我们期望在人类疾病模型中这些突变仅限于造血细胞。但在人类 PMF 中 TPO 或者它的受体 C-Mpl 以及 GATA-1 并没有发现突变或者表达变化,同样 GATA-1 主要的辅因子 FOG-1 也未发现突变[74]。

PMF 潜在的分子功能障碍正逐渐明确。最值得注意的是 2005 年在大部分 PMF,ET 和 PV 患者中发现 *JAK2* 功能获得性突变 *JAK2V617F*[22~25]。在 2006—2007 年间,*JAK2V617F* 阴性病例中发现其他 *JAK2* 突变(PV 中)和 *MPL* 突变(ET 和 PMF 中)[26~29]。最近在 2013 年,在大约 25% 的 PMF 患者中发现 MPN 相关的钙网蛋白基因(*CALR*)的又一个驱动突变,并且与 *JAK2* 或 *MPL* 突变相互排斥[75]。但是,这些突变精确的致病机制尚不清楚。PMF 重现性染色体异常包括 del(13q)、del(20q)、+8、+9、del(12p)以及 1 号和 7 号染色体异常;这些异常亦可见于其他慢性髓系疾病,对 PMF 而言缺乏特异性[76]。大约一半 PMF 患者初诊时存在细胞遗传学异常,但是没有占优势的类型,每一种细胞遗传学异常都只影响不超过 15%~20%患者。

诊断

PMF 典型特征包括骨髓细胞增生伴纤维化;以脾大为典型特征的 EMH;贫血;被称为骨髓增生异常的外周血象[70]。单独的骨髓纤维化和骨髓痨外周血形态并不能确诊 PMF,因为骨髓纤维化和多种疾病状态相关,包括转移癌,其他造血系统异常,风湿病和肉芽肿类疾病(表 122-3)。外周血骨髓痨形态包括:成红细胞显著大小不一,异型红细胞,泪滴状红细胞,以及粒细胞核左移,但形成机制尚不明确。甚至 EMH 也不完全为 PMF 特异性改变,因为也可见于其他疾病,比如转移癌造成的骨髓被替代,或者珠蛋白生成障碍性贫血造成的骨髓造血不充分[77,78]。

表 122-3 骨髓纤维化病因

骨髓异常	非血液系统疾病	其他血液系统疾病
骨髓纤维化伴髓样化生	转移癌	毛白血病
慢性髓细胞性白血病	结缔组织病(如狼疮或系统性硬化)	多发性骨髓瘤
原发性血小板增多症	感染(如肉芽肿,结核,利士曼原虫感染)	淋巴组织增生性疾病
不典型慢性骨髓异常	维生素 D 缺乏(佝偻病)	灰色血小板综合征
高嗜酸性粒细胞综合征	肾性骨病	
真性红细胞增多症	佩吉特病	
骨髓增生异常综合征伴纤维化	甲状旁腺功能亢进	
恶性组织细胞增多症		
系统性肥大细胞增多症		
急性骨髓纤维化		
急性巨核细胞白血病(AML-M7)		
其他急性髓系白血病		

因为细胞过度增生和纤维化，PMF 患者骨穿检查时骨髓非常难以抽取造成“干抽”。骨髓活检主要可见重度胶原纤维化，骨质硬化，窦内造血，以及不典型巨核细胞增殖。标准的苏木素和伊红染色不适用于观察骨髓纤维化，而最好用一些特殊方法，如用于网硬蛋白的染色（一种使基质细胞生成的糖蛋白染色的银浸渍技术）或胶原三色染色。许多 PMF 病例在“细胞期”的诊断较难，因为初始的骨髓纤维化极少，即便已经发展了纤维化分级方案，其临床功用也相当有限[79]。

PMF 的骨髓形态学特征难以与伴纤维化的 MDS（MDS-f）以及“急性骨髓纤维化”相鉴别。后者与巨核细胞白血病（AML-M7）存在重叠[79]。多数 PMF 病例常见巨核细胞一系发育异常，而出现其他细胞系发育异常则倾向诊断为 MDS-f[79]。如果持续症状较重且疾病进展快（病程数周），脾不大则提示急性骨髓纤维化（也称为恶性骨髓硬化或急性骨髓硬化）。针对原始巨核细胞的特异性染色（如 CD61 或 vWF）可以鉴别出其他方式无法识别的细胞群体。尽管很多时候临床医师和病理学家已经尽力，患者诊断仍不能明确且患者必须接受预期治疗。

临床表现

约 25%的 PMF 患者在诊断时无症状，而大多数患者初诊存在贫血和不同程度的脾大。PMF 患者贫血是多因素造成的。致病原因包括纤维化组织替代正常造血骨髓，剩余骨髓组织无效造血，以及脾功能亢进。PMF 患者往往出现巨脾且质地坚硬（图 122-6），肝脾大往往继发于 EMH，并且与高代谢症状（明显的疲劳、体重下降、盗汗、低热），外周水肿（源于静脉压迫），腹泻，早饱（胃部压迫）以及偶发的门脉高压等症状群密切相关。

PMF 患者巨脾可能并发脾梗死，先驱症状为可放射至左肩的中到重度疼痛，经常需要阿片类麻醉药物进行镇痛[80]。脾的 CT 影像学特征可能不明显，或仅有楔形或圆形低密度影。EMH 可以发生于全身各处，常见部位除肝脾外还有淋巴结、皮肤、胸膜、腹膜、肺以及脊柱和硬脑膜外空隙。后两者可能导致脊髓和/或神经根压迫等急症，需要应用糖皮质激素降低水肿并立即进行放射治疗[81]。幸运的是局灶性的 EMH 对低剂量伽马射线辐射（100~150cGy）反应迅速。

PMF 患者普遍依赖输注红细胞支持治疗。患者血清 LDH 水平常升高，反映无效造血和 EMH 造成的肝损伤。高尿酸血症和继发痛风发作也较常见，该症状反映了无效造血伴发的较高细胞更新率。PMF 可见骨痛，与骨髓替代和骨膜炎等多因素相关。PMF 有时可伴发 Sweet 综合征（嗜中性白细胞皮肤病），因治疗方式不同尚须与皮肤的 EMH 相鉴别[82]。

PMF 致死有多种途径，其中严重的感染或转变为耐药的髓系白血病较为常见。在病程最初 10 年中约有 20%的患者转变为白血病[83]。相对少见的死因包括血栓性出血事件和继发于肺动脉高压的心力衰竭。

预后

PMF 目前的预后风险分层是基于构成动态国际预后评分系统（dynamic international prognostic scoring system，DIPSS）plus 的 8 个临床参数[84]。这 8 个参数包括不利的核型（包括+8、-7/7q-、i（17q）、inv（3）、-5/5q-、12p-或 11q23 重组的一种或 2 种异常或包含复杂核型）[85,86]，需要输注红细胞[87,88]血小板计数<100×10^9/L，年龄>65 岁，血红蛋白<10g/dl，白细胞计数>25×10^9/L，循环原始细胞≥1%，以及存在全身症状[89]。基于上述 8 个风险因素建立的四个 DIPSS-plus 风险分层分别为低（无风险因素）、中间 1（一个风险因素）、中间 2（两个或三个风险因素）和高（四个或更多风险因素），对应的中位生存期分别为 15.4、6.5、2.9 和 1.3 年[84]。

自从 DIPSS-plus 发表以来，已经发表了几项研究，表明有更多的预后信息。例如，单体核型、inv（3）/i（17q）异常或包含以下任意两项：循环原始细胞>9%、白细胞≥40×10^9/L[90]或其他不利的核型，预测 PMF 的 2 年死亡率>80%。同样，PMF 中较低的存活率与 *JAK2* 46/1 单倍型[91]、低 *JAK2V617F* 等位基因负荷[92,93]或存在 IDH[94]、EZH2[95]、SRSF2[96]、ASXL1[97]的突变有关。

最近，Tefferi 等人研究了 254 例 PMF 患者，报道了 *JAK2*、*CALR*、*MPL* 的突变频率分别为 58%、25%、8%，9%为三种突变均为野生型（即三阴性）[98]。在 *JAK2/MPL* 未突变的病例中，*CALR* 突变频率为 74%。*CALR* 突变与年龄较小、较高的血小板计数和较低的 DIPSS-plus 评分有关。*CALR* 突变的患者出现贫血、需要输血或显示白细胞增多的可能性不大。剪接体突变在 *CALR* 突变患者中罕见。在随后对 570 名患者进行的一项国际研究中[99]，作者们报告了在 CALR+ASXL1-患者中生存时间最长（中位数为 10.4 年），而在 CALR-ASXL1+患者中生存时间最短（中位数为 2.3 年）。CALR+ASXL1+和 CALR-ASXL1-患者的生存期相似，并被归为中间风险分层（中位生存期 5.8 年）。Guglielmelli 等人[100]随后证明了预后不利突变数量的额外价值。

治疗

传统的 PMF 治疗多为姑息治疗，没有证据表明可以改善总体生存。患者应该考虑参加任何可行的新治疗策略的临床试验。治疗贫血的原有策略包括雄激素（如每日口服氟甲睾酮 10mg 两次或达那唑 400~600mg 一次），但典型的 PMF 老年男性患者应在治疗前排除隐匿性的前列腺癌[101]。同时在这个治疗策略下应用糖皮质激素可以短期获益（口服泼尼松起始剂量每日 30~40mg，持续一月后逐渐减量），遗憾的是雄激素和类固醇激素有效率并不高，仅对 1/3 的 PMF 患者在短期内有效。对于内源性促红细胞生成素（Epo）水平低于 100mIU/ml 的患者，短期内可以考虑促红细胞生成药物（erythropoiesis stimulating agents，ESA）[102]。但是这种治疗会加重 PMF 相关的脾大，对依赖输血的患者无效，还增加其向白血病转化的风险[103]。羟基脲是脾大症状明显的 PMF 患者首选药物[104]。HU 起始剂量 500mg 一天三次，一般在 1~2 周内起效，然后可以根据优化目标调整 HU 剂量。

沙利度胺（thalidomide）可以改善 PMF 患者血细胞减少并缩小脾脏[105]。文献报道，对贫血其的反应率为 20%~62%，对血小板减少症有效率 25%~80%，对脾大有效率 7%~30%[105,106]。常规剂量与治疗多发性骨髓瘤类似（每日 200mg 或更高），在这个剂量下，沙利度胺与严重的骨髓增殖反应相关，如可以加速 EMH[107]。低剂量的沙利度胺（每日 50mg）更容易耐受且反应持久[106,108]。治疗中增加泼尼松可以降低沙利度胺剂量，改善患者耐受并加强该药促红细胞生成活性[106,108]。

已经在 PMF,PV/ET 后 MF 和其他相关 MPN 中评估了几种新药,包括其他免疫调节剂和抑制剂[109]。泊马度胺(pomalidomide)是一种免疫调节药物,当单独使用(2mg/d)或与泼尼松(0.5 或 2mg/d)联合使用时,25%的患者得到贫血改善[110]。在另一个Ⅱ期临床研究中,仅在 *JAK2V617F* 突变的病例中观察到贫血反应(24%对 0%)[111]。58%的患者出现血小板反应,但对脾脏大小影响不大。很少观察到药物相关的神经病变或骨髓抑制。使用>2mg/d 的剂量未能增加活性,但确实产生更大的骨髓抑制[112]。比较泊马度胺与安慰剂的 3 期研究未显示贫血反应的显著差异,但用泊马度胺能显著改善血小板反应[113]。

已经在 MPN 患者中评估了许多 JAK 抑制剂 ATP 模拟物,包括芦可替尼(INCB018424)、菲卓替尼(fedratinib)(SAR302503)、momelotinib(CYT387)、来他替尼(CEP-701)、pacritinib(SB1518)、AZD1480、BMS911543、LY2784544 和 XL019(clinicaltrials.gov)。芦可替尼是一种 *JAK1/JAK2* 抑制剂,最初在 153 例 PMF 或 PV/ET 后 MF 患者的Ⅰ/Ⅱ期研究中进行了评估[114]。毒性包括血小板减少症,贫血和停药后的"细胞因子反弹反应",并伴有急性症状复发和脾肿大[115]。大多数患者的全身症状和体重增加均有改善,44%的患者脾脏大小明显下降≥50%。28 例输血依赖患者中有 4 例(14%)实现了输血非依赖。检测到促炎细胞因子(如 IL-1RA、IL-6、TNF-a 和 MIP-1b)大量减少与全身症状的改善相关。

两项随机研究比较了芦可替尼与安慰剂或最佳支持治疗的疗效[116,117]。在 COMFORT-1 试验中,与安慰剂相比($n=309$)[75],芦可替尼不仅显著改善了脾脏反应(42%对<1%)和全身症状(46%),还能够改善严重的贫血(31%对 13.9%)和血小板减少(34.2%对 9.3%)。在 COMFORT-2 试验中,与"最佳有效治疗"($n=219$)相比 117,芦可替尼改善了脾脏反应(28.5%对 0),但也加重了血小板减少(44.5%对 9.6%)、贫血(40.4%对 12.3%)和腹泻(24.0%对 11.0%)。对 MF 患者的长期随访表明,在中位时间达到 9.2 个月后,相当高比例的患者停用了该药物。停药后出现严重的停药症状:症状急性复发、脾肿大加速、细胞减少加重、偶有血流动力学失代偿(包括感染性休克样综合征)。在 COMFORT-2 中,55%的患者在 3 年内停用了该药物。尽管双臂交叉,存活率在统计学上仍有轻微的提高。最近的报道表明芦可替尼与严重机会性感染相关[118]。

菲卓替尼是一种选择性 *JAK2* 抑制剂,在一项Ⅰ/Ⅱ期研究中对 59 例 PMF 患者或后 PV/ET、MF[119] 患者进行了初步评估。大多数患者的症状得到了持久的缓解。副作用包括恶心(3%)、呕吐(3%)、腹泻(10%)、无症状性血清淀粉酶/脂肪酶轻度升高(27%)、转氨酶升高(27%)或肌酐升高(24%)、血小板减少(24%)和贫血(35%)。一般来说,*JAK2V617F* 的存在与反应无关。一项Ⅲ期研究($n=289$)将菲卓替尼两种不同剂量(500 或 400mg/d)和安慰剂比较,证实了该药物在缓解症状和减少脾脏大小方面的功效(分别为 49%,47%和 1%),但与药物使用相关脑病的相关报道导致其停药未能进一步研究[120]。

momelotinib(MMB、GS-0387 和 CYT387)是一种 *JAK1* 和 *JAK2* 抑制剂,在一项Ⅰ~Ⅱ期研究中,分别在 59%和 48%的参与者观察到了贫血和脾脏大小的改善。33 例患者中,有 70%的患者在入组前一个月内接受了红细胞输注,能维持至少 12 周(4.7 至>18.3 个月),输血需求下降[121]。大多数患者的全身症状有所改善。3/4 级不良反应包括血小板减少(32%)、高脂血症(5%)、肝转氨酶升高(3%)和头痛(3%)。22%的患者出现治疗相关的新发周围神经病变(感觉症状,1 级)。随后,研究扩大到 166 例患者,每日 1 次 150 或 300mg,或每日 150mg 两次,连续 9 个月,结果相似[122]。目前正在对该药与芦可替尼进行Ⅲ期的比较研究。

pacritinib(SB1518)是一种 *JAK2*/FLT3 抑制剂,其产生 MRI 脾反应率有 32%,并伴有症状改善,但在Ⅱ期研究中[123],34 名参与者中仅有 6%出现贫血改善。最常见的治疗相关不良事件是胃肠道反应,尤其是腹泻。

对于患有顽固性脾脏疼痛、体质障碍症状、症状性门静脉高压症和/或需要频繁的红细胞输注的患者,可考虑进行脾切除术。在一组 223 例接受脾切除术的 PMF 患者中,67%、23%、50%和 0%的患者在全身症状、输血依赖性贫血、门脉高压和严重血小板减少方面得到了持久缓解[124]。然而,即使在经验丰富的中心,PMF 脾切除术围术期死亡率可能也高达 9%,总体生存率可能不受影响;脾切除术后中位存活期约为 2 年。即使在没有明显弥散性血管内凝血的情况下,升高的 D-二聚体也可预测更高的手术风险。高达 25%的手术幸存者会出现明显的肝大或极度血小板增多症[124]。脾切除术前血小板减少症与脾切除术后白血病转化的风险相关的原因不明。脾切除术后血小板增多症与围术期血栓形成密切相关。HU 可用于预防脾切除术后血小板计数升高。对于有症状性脾肿大的较差的手术候选患者,脾脏照射的姑息性使用是合理的,但成功是不确定和短暂的[125]。

因为担心骨髓纤维化可能造成干细胞植入失败,异基因造血干细胞移植(allo-HSCT)治疗 PMF 最初比较受限,但并没有证据支持这种推测。移植术后血小板恢复会因骨髓纤维化延后三日,并需稍微增加术后血小板输注支持,但其与植入失败和其他移植相关问题的相关性并不清楚[126]。异基因造血干细胞移植治疗 PMF 目前有增长趋势,但如何选择移植患者和移植时机仍充满争议。虽然植入已经问题不大,但即便采用非清髓的减低预处理强度方案,移植药物毒性问题依然较大[127]。在一项异基因造血干细胞移植治疗骨髓纤维化的研究中,年龄超过 44 岁的患者 5 年生存率仅 14%,另一项研究显示其 2 年生存率仅 41%[128,129]。同时研究报道该病移植术后的慢性移植物抗宿主病比率高达 59%[130]。年轻患者移植术后预后稍好,其生存率可以超过 60%。但必须经过慎重考虑才能移植,且作为挽救治疗手段,应选择预期寿命不佳的患者[128,130]。

真性红细胞增多症

流行病学

真性红细胞增多症(polycythemia vera,PV)的年发病率为每年 0.8/10 万~2.6/10 万人,大部分研究的发病率数据多偏向这个区间较高的一边,并且一直稳定[131,132]。和其他 MPN 一样,PV 的发病率随年龄增长。初诊中位年龄约为 60 岁;但亦可见于年轻人，7%的患者诊断时年龄小于 40 岁[133,134]。该病男性稍多（男女患者比例 1.2∶1），在犹太族裔尤其是德国犹太族发病率较高[10,135]。少数 PV 病例成家族聚集性，但是家族性红细胞增多症经常证明是由于高氧亲和力血红蛋白或生活环境的自然暴露（如定居高海拔区域或者钴中毒）[136,137]。

发病机制

1976 年首先证明通过 X 染色体连锁（G-6-PD）酶分析证明了 PV 造血细胞克隆的特征[138]。2005 年发现大部分 PV 患者存在 *JAK2* 基因的功能获得性突变（*JAK2V617F*）[22~25]。2007 年在 *JAK2V617F* 阴性的病例中发现其他 *JAK2* 基因突变[28]。*JAK2V617F* 为该基因 14 号外显子鸟嘌呤到胸腺嘧啶的点突变。而这个 *JAK2* 基因座 1 849 位的突变也使 JAK2 蛋白 617 位的缬氨酸变为苯丙氨酸。*JAK2V617F* 突变常见于 PV、ET、PMF[22~25]，并可见于其他髓系肿瘤[139,140]。截至目前尚未在淋巴系统疾病[141~144]、实体瘤[145~147]和继发性骨髓增生[148,149]中发现 *JAK2V617F* 突变。总体上来说 *JAK2V617F* 突变可见于 95%的 PV 病例，50%的 ET 或 PMF，在其他骨髓增殖性疾病中，如难治性贫血伴环形铁粒幼细胞和血小板增多（refractory anemia with ringed sideroblasts and thrombocytosis，RARS-T）不超过 20%，在 AML 和 MDS 中不超过 5%[150~153]。

在小鼠移植模型中，*JAK2V617F* 突变可以诱导类似 PV 的症状[24,154,155]。ET 患者中的等位基因突变较 PV 或 PMF 少[156~160]。PV 中通过有丝分裂和基因重组形成 *JAK2V617F* 纯合子，所以等位基因负荷较高[22,23,25]。人类 *JAK2V617F* 突变出现于原始干细胞水平，在血细胞分化过程中属于早期事件[161~163]。部分但不是所有[164]研究提示 *JAK2V617F* 克隆累及 NK[165]、T[166]、B[166]淋巴细胞。另有证据表明 *JAK2V617F* 突变并不见于 PV 或者其他 MPN 最初形成的疾病克隆，而且这个突变对内源性克隆的形成并非必需的[167~169]。最新研究发现 *JAK2V617F* 阴性的白血病克隆起源于 *JAK2V617F* 阳性的 MPN 患者，则进一步阐释了两者独立性[170,171]。

2007 年在一群以红细胞增多为主要特征的 *JAK2V617F* 阴性 PV 患者中存在一系列 *JAK2* 基因 12 号外显子区域的突变[172]。尽管这些患者血中促红细胞生成素水平总是低于参考值，且每例均存在内源性红细胞生成（EEC），根据其临床特征，部分患者还是被诊断为"特发性红细胞增多症"。原报道中 10/11 的大部分病例[172]中存在下列四种 *JAK2* 第 12 号外显子突变中的一种：N542-E543del 4 例，F537-K539delinsL 3 例，K539L 2 例，H538QK539L 1 例。四种 12 号外显子等位基因突变在表达 EPO 受体的细胞系中均会引起非细胞因子依赖的过度增殖，以及 JAK-STAT 信号途径的持续激活[172]。另外，*JAK2*K539L 在小鼠移植模型中诱导产生了 PV 的临床表现。其他研究确证了前述研究的系列结果[28,173~177]，大部分[28,173,174]但非全部研究[175,177]提示 12 号外显子突变实际存在于所有 *JAK2V617F* 阴性的 PV 病例中（全部 PV 病例的 3%）。此外，后续研究也发现了更多的 12 号外显子突变：R541-E543delinsK、I540-E-543delinsMK、V536-I546dup11、F537-I546dup10+547L 和 E543-D544del[174~176]。

PV 患者红系集落形成祖细胞（红系集落形成单位 BFU-E 或爆式集落形成单位 BFU-E）（BFU-E 或 BFU-E）对正常的生长和分化信号如促红细胞生成素（Epo）、粒细胞-巨噬细胞集落刺激因子（GM-CSF）、干细胞因子、白介素-3（IL-3）非常敏感或者完全不依赖[178,179]。尽管这是 PV 的典型特征，但亦可见于 ET 和 PMF，从而缺乏特异性。PV 患者血中 Epo 水平总体来说非常低或者与红细胞增生情况不成比例。并且过量的非 Epo 依赖性的 BFU-E 或 BFU-E 可导致大量红细胞团（red cell mass，RCM）[180,181]。与 ET 病例中 Tpo 类似，难治性 PV 的家族存在 Epo 受体突变。虽经细致研究目前尚未找到非家族性 PV Epo 受体任何结构变化[182,183]。有研究发现 PV 病例中 Epo 受体表达存在异常（如缺乏正常的高亲和力的 Epo 受体），但这项发现并不一致[184]。因为 IGF-1 结合蛋白的改变，包括 IGF-1 受体基础磷酸化水平提高，PV 患者来源的细胞对胰岛素样生长因子 1（IGF-1）非常敏感[185]。另在部分患者中发现 SHP-1 磷酸酶活性降低（与 EPO、SCF、IL-3 受体密切相关，属于受体配体结合产生的负向调节信号），STAT-3 持续激活，抗-凋亡蛋白比如 Bcl-XL 水平升高以及其他生化异常；这些变化的病理生物学机制和关系尚不清楚[186~188]。

未治疗患者 10%～20%存在染色体核型异常[189,190]。这些异常包括典型慢性髓系异常如 8 号染色体三体、9 号染色体三体、20q 缺失、13q 缺失，男性患者缺失 Y、5 号和 7 号染色体异常，但对 PV 而言缺乏特异性[190]。

临床特征

PV 相关的常见症状和体征列于表 122-4 中。许多 PV 的

表 122-4　真红细胞增多症相关临床和实验室特征

症状和体征	发生概率/%
收缩压高	72
脾大	70
多血质面容	67
结膜充血	59
头疼	48
虚弱	47
视网膜静脉充血	46
瘙痒	43
眩晕	43
肝大	40
出汗	33
舒张压高	32
视力受损	31
体重减轻	29
感觉异常	29
呼吸困难	26
关节症状	26
上腹不适	24

摘自 1975 年柏林[191]。经 Elsevier 许可转载。

临床特征都是由于红细胞团(RCM)增加直接造成,这是各种原因红细胞增生的共性特点,但瘙痒和脾大强烈提示 PV。红细胞团增多可导致血液黏滞,从而呈现各种多血质症状和体征。PV 患者常有头疼,同时可有视物模糊,听力改变,黏膜出血,气短,全身不适。高血压同样可能为红细胞团增多所致。至少 2/3PV 患者脾大,因此同时出现红细胞增生和脾大强烈提示 PV 可能性较大[191]。40%患者出现血栓症,常见动脉血栓,每年有 3.9%的患者出现栓塞[133]。动脉血栓较静脉血栓更容易致命。和 ET 一样,PV 的静脉血栓可并发于罕见位置,如肠系膜静脉或肝静脉。PV 可见出血,特别是胃肠道出血,但较血栓少见[133]。瘙痒较常见,且可被温热水激惹(水源性),属于经典 PV 相关不适,其发病机制尚不清楚[192,193]。红斑性肢痛病和其他血管舒缩症状、感觉异常和头疼(在前文 ET 部分描述)亦可见于 PV 患者;大约半数 PV 患者有白细胞和血小板增多。

诊断

诊断 PV 最主要的困难是需要与其他原因引起的红细胞增多相鉴别(表 122-5)。

1975 年,真红细胞增多症协作组(Polycythemia Vera Study Group)制订其诊断标准[191],在当时属于重要进展,但目前只有历史参考价值[194,195]。这些标准包括直接测量红细胞团数目等,但此方法步骤过于烦琐,目前多数病例已经不需该项检查。新诊断方法的进展以及对血细胞比容和 RCM 紧密联系的了解,都极大地降低了红细胞团测量在 PV 诊断中的地位。

因为多达 95%以上的 PV 患者都携带 *JAK2V617F* 突变,怀疑 PV 的患者可先行外周血 *JAK2V617F* 突变筛查。为了尽量减少假阳性和假阴性结果,以及能够识别少数 *JAK2V617F* 阴性的 PV 病例,作者建议同时检查血中 EPO 水平,超 90%的 PV 患者 EPO 异常偏低[196]。如果 *JAK2V617F* 突变和 EPO 检验均支持 PV(即突变阳性且血清 EPO 偏低),则建议行骨髓穿刺,但骨穿并非诊断 PV 所必要条件。如果 *JAK2V617F* 突变和 EPO 检验均不支持 PV 诊断(突变阴性且血 EPO 正常/偏高),则除非有其他明确的临床指征,一般不建议做进一步检查。如果分子突变检查和血清 EPO 结果不一致,则应该首先重复两项检查,在结果不变的情况下应予以骨穿。从这方面来说,血 EPO 较低的 *JAK2V617* 患者可考虑检测 *JAK2* 的 12 号外显子突变。

如果怀疑先天性红细胞增多症,初诊实验室检查需检测血红蛋白氧饱和度为 50%时的氧分压(P50)。如果 P50 降低,即氧解离曲线左移提示常染色体显性遗传病(常染色体显性遗传)[197];氧血红蛋白亲和力异常血红蛋白病,或者常染色体阴性遗传病;双膦酸甘油酸盐变位酶突变所致的 2,3-双膦酸甘油酸盐(2,3-bisphosphoglycerate,2,3-BPG)缺乏[198]。如果 P50 值正常,应该首先考虑先天性红细胞增多症最常见的突变:*VHL* 基因突变,有此突变的俄罗斯族裔应该考虑 Chuvash 红细胞增多症,此症特征为血 EPO 水平升高[199]。目前关于 HIF-1α 脯氨酰羟化酶基因突变[200]资料较少,与正常血清 EPO 水平联系紧密。另外,Epo 受体(EPOR)突变在诊断伴正常或较低血清 Epo 的先天性红细胞增多症时应予以考虑[201]。

表 122-5 红细胞增多症分类

分类
一、相对红细胞增多症
1. 体液浓缩所致相对红细胞增多
2. 极高数值
二、真性的红细胞增多
1. 真性红细胞增多症
2. 继发性红细胞增多症
a. 促红细胞生成素介导
(1)低氧所致
(a)中枢性缺氧
①慢性肺病
②右向左心血管分流
③高原定居
④一氧化碳中毒和吸烟者红细胞增多
⑤包括睡眠呼吸暂停在内的低通气
(b)外周性缺氧
①局限性
肾动脉狭窄
②弥漫
高氧亲和力血红蛋白病(常染色体显性遗传病)
2,3-二磷酸甘油酸变异酶缺乏症(常染色体隐性遗传病)
(2)非缺氧依赖性(病理性促红细胞生成素产生)
(a)恶性肿瘤
①肝癌
②肾癌
③脑成血管细胞瘤
④甲状旁腺肿瘤
(b)非恶性肿瘤疾病
①子宫平滑肌瘤
②多囊肾
③嗜铬细胞瘤
④脑膜瘤
(c)遗传性促红细胞生成素分泌增多
(d)Chuvash 红细胞增多症(遗传,异常的氧内稳态)
(3)EPO 兴奋剂
b. 促红细胞生成素受体介导
(1)促红细胞生成素受体主动突变
(2)常染色体显性遗传红细胞增多症
c. 药物相关
(1)雄激素治疗
(2)持续红细胞生成受体激动剂(CERA)
d. 不明机制
(1)大多数病例为常染色体显性遗传红细胞增多症
(2)少数病例为常染色体阴性遗传性红细胞增多症
(3)肾移植术后红细胞增生

疾病预后

诊断为 PV 患者的中位预期寿命超过 10 年,但仍低于同性别和同年龄段健康对照人群[47]。血栓出血并发症和转变为 AML 是降低生存的主要因素。同 ET 一样,年龄超过 60 岁是发生血栓症的危险因素[203]。除高龄和血栓病史外,目前尚不明确其他预后因素。15%~20%的 PV 患者会最终进入与 PMF 类似的“骨髓衰竭期”,这种转变的特征包括贫血加重、白细胞数上升和脾大。

治疗

与 ET 一样，可以应用小剂量阿司匹林改善 PV 相关的血管舒缩症状。PV 相关的瘙痒可以使用选择性血清素重摄取抑制剂如帕罗西汀（paroxetine）治疗[192]，而抗组胺药如羟嗪和苯海拉明则效果欠佳。

PV 治疗的主要目标是预防严重的血栓性疾病，但不增加出血等其他致命疾患，也不增加转化为骨髓纤维化或急性白血病的风险。治疗性静脉放血是达到治疗目标的主要方法。作为成功治疗方案的组成部分，必须强调规律静脉放血的重要性；骨髓抑制性药物仅能起到辅助作用。在 PV 定义后的最初几十年，在未形成标准的静脉放血治疗前，PV 患者中位生存期约为 2 年，大多数患者因为血栓类似事件致命[204,205]。目前大多数 PV 相关死亡仍是因为血栓症，但单用静脉放血治疗的患者中位生存期即超过 15 年[133]。

研究表明血细胞比容小于 45%的患者其脑血管血流明显改善，并使血液黏稠度正常化，血栓症也将减少。因此 PV 患者采用静脉放血为基础的治疗方案的目的即为降低并保持血细胞比容在此区间内[206,207]。同时因为女性正常血红蛋白范围稍低，目前普遍建议女性患者血细胞比容应该降至低于 42%，但此项建议未经过严格证实，而且全血黏滞度应与性别无关。

一直以来医师都对引入其他治疗方法来降低血栓相关风险非常感兴趣。但仅是何时在静脉放血基础上加入药物治疗尚有争议。虽然 PV 患者血小板升高并非一个主要的血栓风险因素，但和 ET 一样，PV 患者血小板明显升高（即升至 1×10^6/μl）是出血的危险因素[208]。因此，针对无血栓病史且血小板计数接近正常的年轻患者，单独采用静脉放血治疗应该安全性较高。

最近的大规模安慰剂-随机对照临床试验结果显示小剂量阿司匹林（每日 100mg，在美国不能实现的剂量）可以很大程度上降低血栓事件（但未改善总体生存）。因此有学说认为无阿司匹林禁忌证的 PV 患者都应常规采用此药治疗[51]。在这项试验中，联合事件终点包括非致命性心肌梗死，非致命脑卒中，或心血管系统病因所致死亡、联合事件终点的风险包括非致命心肌梗死，非致命脑卒中，肺栓塞，大血管血栓和心血管系统病因所致死亡；试验表明阿司匹林组较安慰剂组降低了事件发生概率和风险（相对风险度分别为 0.41，0.40）。该种剂量下实验组较安慰剂组出血风险稍有提高（相对风险度 1.6）[51]。

多年以来 PV 中骨髓抑制药物的应用都广受关注，并且不断涌现优化治疗方案。在一项 20 世纪 60 年代标志性的三臂随机试验中，分别发现两种特异性药物：在静脉放血治疗基础上，口服的苯丁酸氮芥和静脉给药的放射磷（同位素^{32}P）可以降低血栓症风险[202]。但在总体生存方面，加用这两种药物的实验组都较单用静脉放血治疗组差，其原因可能为实验组的白血病的发病率升高。13～19 年单用静脉放血，分别加用^{32}P 和苯丁酸氮芥的实验组白血病发病率分别为 1.5%，9.6%，13.2%，相应的中位生存期分别为 12.6 年，9.1 年，10.9 年[202]。采用苯丁酸氮芥治疗的实验组出现多例淋巴瘤，胃肠道和皮肤肿瘤发病率也相应提高。

多种其他药物可以像^{32}P 和烷化剂一样降低血栓发病率但没有类似的白血病风险，例如 HU 可以降低血栓风险并作为静脉放血的有效补充治疗，同时其白血病致病率远低于^{32}P 和苯丁酸氮芥。在一项真红细胞增多症协作组（PVSG）的研究中，比较初诊 2 年内应用 HU 与历史队列研究中采用静脉放血的患者，HU 的血栓风险较小（6.6%比 14%），且中位随访时间 8.6 年内仅有 5.9%患者转变为白血病[209]。因为 HU 实际致白血病的风险未知，它仅用于高血栓风险的患者作为静脉放血的补充，如老年患者和先前有血栓病史的患者（表 122-6）。

表 122-6　真红细胞增多症患者建议治疗方案

危险度分级[a]	年龄小于 60 岁	年龄大于 60 岁	育龄妇女
低危	静脉放血+小剂量阿司匹林	分级不适用	静脉放血+小剂量阿司匹林
中危	静脉放血+小剂量阿司匹林（除外 aVWD）	分级不适用	静脉放血+小剂量阿司匹（除外 aVWD）
高危	静脉放血+小剂量阿司匹林+HU/IFN-α	静脉放血+HU+小剂量阿司匹林	静脉放血+小剂量阿司匹林+IFN-α

HU，羟基脲；IFNα，干扰素-α_{2a}；aVWD，获得性 von Willebrand 病。[a] 有关风险分层算法，请参见第 113 章。

IFN-α_{2a} 对 PV 患者健康有益，同时由于有报告描述了用药后良好的母婴状态，干扰素还作为不耐受 HU 或有意愿怀孕患者的治疗选择。干扰素可以控制约 80%可耐受患者的红细胞增度，所需治疗剂量每周 450～2 700 万单位不等（常用的起始剂量为 300 万单位皮下注射每周三次），同时 IFN-α_{2a} 对治疗血小板增多有良好疗效[58,210,211]。干扰素可以减少脾大并可缓解难治性皮肤瘙痒。但是至少有 20%的患者因为副作用中断治疗，其中包括疲劳，全身不适，发热，精神症状，肌肉痛，关节痛[211]。同时 IFN-α_{2a} 比 HU 价格更贵。除了适宜用于可能怀孕的女性患者，对于需要缓解难治性皮肤瘙痒的高危患者和担心 HU 潜在致白血病风险的患者，IFN-α_{2a} 可以作为静脉放血的有效补充治疗。

如前所述，基于对照研究的证据，目前推荐高危（年龄≥60 岁或有血栓病史）PV 患者采用细胞减灭疗法预防血栓形成[4,5]。在这方面，HU 是基于循证选择的一线治疗，而非对照的研究支持使用 IFN-α 和白消安作为二线药物的选择[1]。尽管最近 FDA 批准了在 HU 难治性病例中使用芦可替尼[20]，但我们不在 PV 中使用它，除非足够剂量的 HU、IFN-α 或白消安对此无效时出现严重的瘙痒或症状性脾肿大。

（白元松　韩冷　胡南均 译　白元松　韩冷　胡南均 校）

参考文献

The complete reference list can be found on the Wiley Companion Digital Edition of this title (see inside front cover for login instructions).

2 Tefferi A, Vardiman JW. Classification and diagnosis of myeloproliferative neoplasms: the 2008 World Health Organization criteria and point-of-care diagnostic algorithms. *Leukemia*. 2008;**22**(**1**):14–22.

7 Mesa RA, Silverstein MN, Jacobsen SJ, Wollan PC, Tefferi A. Population-based incidence and survival figures in essential thrombocythemia and agnogenic myeloid metaplasia: An Olmsted County study, 1976–1995. *Am J Hematol*. 1999;**61**(**1**):10–15.

8 Kutti J, Ridell B. Epidemiology of the myeloproliferative disorders: essential thrombocythaemia, polycythaemia vera and idiopathic myelofibrosis. *Pathol Biol (Paris)*. 2001;**49**(**2**):164–166.

9 Jensen MK, de Nully BP, Nielsen OJ, Hasselbalch HC. Incidence, clinical features and outcome of essential thrombocythaemia in a well defined geographical area. *Eur J Haematol*. 2000;**65**(**2**):132–139.

11 Kondo T, Okabe M, Sanada M, et al. Familial essential thrombocythemia associated with one-base deletion in the 5′-untranslated region of the thrombopoietin gene. *Blood*. 1998;**92**(**4**):1091–1096.

20 Elkassar N, Hetet G, Briere J, Grandchamp B. Clonality analysis of hematopoiesis in essential thrombocythemia – advantages of studying T lymphocytes and platelets. *Blood*. 1997;**89**(**1**):128–134.

21 Fialkow PJ, Faguet GB, Jacobson RJ, Vaidya K, Murphy S. Evidence that essential thrombocythemia is a clonal disorder with origin in a multipotent stem cell. *Blood*. 1981;**58**(**5**):916–919.

22 Baxter EJ, Scott LM, Campbell PJ, et al. Acquired mutation of the tyrosine kinase JAK2 in human myeloproliferative disorders. *Lancet*. 2005;**365**(**9464**):1054–1061.

23 Kralovics R, Passamonti F, Buser AS, et al. A gain-of-function mutation of JAK2 in myeloproliferative disorders. *N Engl J Med*. 2005;**352**(**17**):1779–1790.

29 Scott LM, Tong W, Levine RL, et al. JAK2 exon 12 mutations in polycythemia vera and idiopathic erythrocytosis. *N Engl J Med*. 2007;**356**(**5**):459–468.

32 Taksin AL, Couedic JPL, Dusanter-Fourt I, et al. Autonomous megakaryocyte growth in essential thrombocythemia and idiopathic myelofibrosis is not related to a c-mpl mutation or to an autocrine stimulation by Mpl-L. *Blood*. 1999;**93**(**1**):125–139.

39 Tefferi A, Guglielmelli P, Larson DR, et al. Long-term survival and blast transformation in molecularly annotated essential thrombocythemia, polycythemia vera, and myelofibrosis. *Blood*. 2014;**124**(**16**):2507–2513; quiz 2615. Prepublished on 20 July 2014 as DOI: 10.1182/blood-2014-05-579136.

40 Besses C, Cervantes F, Pereira A, et al. Major vascular complications in essential thrombocythemia: a study of the predictive factors in a series of 148 patients. *Leukemia*. 1999;**13**(**2**):150–154.

41 Cortelazzo S, Viero P, Finazzi G, D'Emilio A, Rodeghiero F, Barbui T. Incidence and risk factors for thrombotic complications in a historical cohort of 100 patients with essential thrombocythemia. *J Clin Oncol*. 1990;**8**(**3**):556–562.

43 van Genderen PJ, Michiels JJ. Erythromelalgia: a pathognomonic microvascular thrombotic complication in essential thrombocythemia and polycythemia vera. [Review] [23 refs]. *Semin Thromb Hemost*. 1997;**23**(**4**):357–363.

50 Tefferi A, Barbui T. New and treatment-relevant risk stratification for thrombosis in essential thrombocythemia and polycythemia vera. *Am J Hematol*. 2015. Prepublished on 16 April 2015 as DOI 10.1002/ajh.24037.

51 Landolfi R, Marchioli R, Kutti J, et al. Efficacy and safety of low-dose aspirin in polycythemia vera. *N Engl J Med*. 2004;**350**(**2**):114–124.

84 Gangat N, Caramazza D, Vaidya R, et al. DIPSS plus: a refined Dynamic International Prognostic Scoring System for primary myelofibrosis that incorporates prognostic information from karyotype, platelet count, and transfusion status. *J Clin Oncol*. 2011;**29**(**4**):392–397. Prepublished on 15 Dec 2010 as DOI: 10.1200/JCO.2010.32.2446.

91 Tefferi A, Lasho TL, Patnaik MM, et al. JAK2 germline genetic variation affects disease susceptibility in primary myelofibrosis regardless of V617F mutational status: nullizygosity for the JAK2 46/1 haplotype is associated with inferior survival. *Leukemia*. 2010;**24**(**1**):105–109.

100 Guglielmelli P, Lasho TL, Rotunno G, et al. The number of prognostically detrimental mutations and prognosis in primary myelofibrosis: an international study of 797 patients. *Leukemia*. 2014;**28**(**9**):1804–1810. Prepublished on 20 Feb 2014 as DOI 10.1038/leu.2014.76.

110 Tefferi A, Verstovsek S, Barosi G, et al. Pomalidomide is active in the treatment of anemia associated with myelofibrosis. *J Clin Oncol*. 2009;**27**:4563–4569.

113 Tefferi A, Passamonti F, Barbui T, et al. Phase 3 study of pomalidomide in myeloproliferative neoplasm (MPN)-associated myelofibrosis with RBC-transfusion-dependence. *Blood*. 2013;**122**:394.

114 Verstovsek S, Kantarjian H, Mesa RA, et al. Safety and efficacy of INCB018424, a JAK1 and JAK2 inhibitor, in myelofibrosis. *N Engl J Med*. 2010;**363**:1117–1127.

116 Verstovsek S, Mesa RA, Gotlib J, et al. A double-blind, placebo-controlled trial of ruxolitinib for myelofibrosis. *N Engl J Med*. 2012;**366**:799–807. Prepublished on 2 Mar 2012 as DOI 10.1056/NEJMoa1110557.

117 Harrison C, Kiladjian JJ, Al-Ali HK, et al. JAK inhibition with ruxolitinib versus best available therapy for myelofibrosis. *N Engl J Med*. 2012;**366**:787–798. Prepublished on 2 Mar 2012 as DOI 10.1056/NEJMoa1110556.

119 Pardanani A, Gotlib JR, Jamieson C, et al. Safety and efficacy of TG101348, a selective JAK2 inhibitor, in myelofibrosis. *J Clin Oncol*. 2011;**29**:789–796. Prepublished on 12 Jan 2011 as DOI 10.1200/JCO.2010.32.8021.

120 Pardanani A, Harrison CN, Cortes JE, et al. Results of a randomized, double-blind, placebo-controlled phase III study (JAKARTA) of the JAK2-selective inhibitor fedratinib (SAR302503) in patients with myelofibrosis (MF). *Blood*. 2013;**122**:393.

122 Pardanani A, Gotlib J, Gupta V, et al. Update on the long-term efficacy and safety of momelotinib, a JAK1 and JAK2 inhibitor, for the treatment of myelofibrosis. *Blood*. 2013;**122**:108.

141 Melzner I, Weniger MA, Menz CK, Moller P. Absence of the JAK2 V617F activating mutation in classical Hodgkin lymphoma and primary mediastinal B-cell lymphoma. *Leukemia*. 2006;**20**(**1**):157–158.

142 Lee JW, Soung YH, Kim SY, et al. JAK2 V617F mutation is uncommon in non-Hodgkin lymphomas. *Leuk Lymphoma*. 2006;**47**(**2**):313–314.

143 Sulong S, Case M, Minto L, Wilkins B, Hall A, Irving J. The V617F mutation in Jak2 is not found in childhood acute lymphoblastic leukaemia. *Br J Haematol*. 2005;**130**(**6**):964–965.

144 Levine RL, Loriaux M, Huntly BJ, et al. The JAK2V617F activating mutation occurs in chronic myelomonocytic leukemia and acute myeloid leukemia, but not in acute lymphoblastic leukemia or chronic lymphocytic leukemia. *Blood*. 2005;**106**(**10**):3377–3379.

150 Steensma DP, McClure RF, Karp JE, et al. JAK2 V617F is a rare finding in de novo acute myeloid leukemia, but STAT3 activation is common and remains unexplained. *Leukemia*. 2006;**20**(**6**):971–978.

151 Renneville A, Quesnel B, Charpentier A, et al. High occurrence of JAK2 V617 mutation in refractory anemia with ringed sideroblasts associated with marked thrombocytosis. *Leukemia*. 2006;**20**(**11**):2067–2070.

152 Verstovsek S, Silver RT, Cross NC, Tefferi A. JAK2V617F mutational frequency in polycythemia vera: 100%, >90%, less? *Leukemia*. 2006;**20**(**11**):2067.

163 Delhommeau F, Dupont S, Tonetti C, et al. Evidence that the JAK2 G1849T (V617F) mutation occurs in a lymphomyeloid progenitor in polycythemia vera and idiopathic myelofibrosis. *Blood*. 2007;**109**(**1**):71–77.

164 Lasho TL, Mesa R, Gilliland DG, Tefferi A. Mutation studies in CD3+, CD19+ and CD34+ cell fractions in myeloproliferative disorders with homozygous JAK2(V617F) in granulocytes. *Br J Haematol*. 2005;**130**(**5**):797–799.

171 Campbell PJ, Baxter EJ, Beer PA, et al. Mutation of JAK2 in the myeloproliferative disorders: timing, clonality studies, cytogenetic associations, and role in leukemic transformation. *Blood*. 2006;**108**(**10**):3548–3555.

172 Scott LM, Tong W, Levine R, et al. Somatic mutations of JAK2 exon 12 in polycythemia vera and idiopathic erythrocytosis. *N Engl J Med*. 2007;**365**:459–468.

178 Casadevall N, Vainchenker W, Lacombe C, et al. Erythroid progenitors in polycythemia vera: demonstration of their hypersensitivity to erythropoietin using serum free cultures. *Blood*. 1982;**59**(**2**):447–451.

179 Dai CH, Krantz SB, Dessypris EN, Means RT Jr, Horn ST, Gilbert HS. Polycythemia vera. II. Hypersensitivity of bone marrow erythroid, granulocyte-macrophage, and megakaryocyte progenitor cells to interleukin-3 and granulocyte-macrophage colony-stimulating factor. *Blood*. 1992;**80**(**4**):891–899.

第十二篇

肿瘤并发症治疗

第 123 章　未明原发灶肿瘤

John D. Hainsworth, MD ■ F. Anthony Greco, MD

概述

未明原发灶肿瘤（CUP）是一种临床综合征，是在完整的病理学评估和标准的临床评估之后仍未发现原发灶的一组疾病，占所有恶性肿瘤诊断时的 2%～3%。目前，由于可以对转移病灶进行活检，现在大多数患者可以使用改进的免疫过氧化物酶染色和分子基因表达谱来准确预测组织来源。本章节中，在完成临床和病理评估之后，可以明确约 20% CUP 的原发部位，并且可以提供对应的治疗方案。然而，仍有将近 80% 的患者应用经验性的联合化疗。目前，随着研究的不断进展，实体瘤的治疗多以部位为特异性，经验性化疗可能不会提供最佳的治疗方案。部位特异性的治疗，即以组织起源为指导，可以通过分子分析或免疫过氧化物酶染色等方法来进行预测。部位特异性治疗的新数据也将在以下的文章中进行阐述。

未明原发灶肿瘤（CUP）是临床上常见的一种情况，占所有恶性肿瘤诊断时的 2%～3%[1,2]，诊断 CUP 的患者在临床特征、病理学、治疗反应和预后等方面异质性明显。典型的患者可出现转移部位的相关症状，而在经过常规的病史、物理检查、影像学和实验室检测均未能发现原发部位。虽然大部分患者活检病理结果为癌，但是，组织学检测尚不足以描述这类肿瘤的特征。

近年来，在 CUP 的主要进展是在这群异质性的人群中确定了多个可治疗的亚组。为了鉴别出这类患者，需基于特定的临床和/或病理特征，以及特异性的一线治疗是否可获得最佳的治疗效果。此外，对于其他 CUP 患者（约 80%），经验性广谱化疗方案的治疗疗效仍十分有限。然而，随着治疗水平的发展，不同类型实体瘤的治疗方法愈发特异性，以单一化疗方案为一组异质性明显的 CUP 患者提供治疗的方法愈发赶不上时代的步伐。

近年来，随着诊断技术的进步，包括更加精密的免疫组化（IHC）染色和肿瘤分子基因表达情况（GEP），即使解剖学上的原发部位无法证明，仍可以精确的预测很多 CUP 的原发部位。并且，依据现有的研究结果，与经验性化疗相比，基于肿瘤起源部位预测的部位特异性治疗可以明显改善患者的治疗结局。

病理评估

肿瘤组织的光学显微镜检查是病理学评估的关键一步，可为后续的评估进行系统分类。几乎所有的 CUP 都含有癌的成分，而经过光学显微镜的评估可以将它们分为 5 类：①低分化肿瘤；②低分化癌；③腺癌；④鳞癌；⑤神经内分泌癌。偶尔在初始检查时也可见到黑色素瘤和肉瘤。

由于单纯的组织学检查很难确定肿瘤的原发部位，因此，对每一名 CUP 患者进行额外的病理学评估显得尤为重要。在最初的活检时应计划获得足够的病理组织，以用于所有的病理学检查，而细针活检所获得的组织是不够的。此外，肿瘤学家和病理学家的密切沟通十分必要，以确保获得到的组织可以用于确定更多的争议性的结果。

低分化肿瘤

组织学特点导致病理学家不能区分的介于癌和其他恶性肿瘤之间的肿瘤即可归为低分化肿瘤，如肉瘤、黑色素瘤和血液系统肿瘤。这类人群在 CUP 患者组织学诊断后约占 5%，但在特异性的检查（IHC 染色、GEP）后占比较少。对这组患者来说，良好治疗效果的肿瘤如非霍奇金淋巴瘤等非常常见，因此精准诊断显得尤为重要[3~5]。

低分化癌

低分化癌占到 CUP 患者的 20%左右；此外，另有 10%的诊断为低分化腺癌的患者，常规单独的光学显微镜检查尚不足以诊断为低分化癌。在一组 87 名低分化癌患者中，16 名患者（18%）在 IHC 检查后被确定为其他诊断[6]。而联合应用 IHC 染色和 GEP 可以使更多的患者明确诊断。

腺癌

腺癌是应用光学显微镜最常诊断的病理类型，占 CUP 患者的比例达到 70%。由于不同的腺癌具有不同的组织学特点，因此，原发灶的部位常不能确定。而那些确定的组织学特点常与特定的肿瘤类型相关（“乳头状”对应卵巢和甲状腺癌，“印戒细胞”对应胃癌）；然而，这些结果仍不足以用于最后确定肿瘤的原发部位。

近年来，精准预测腺癌患者原发部位的能力逐年提高。应用 IHC 染色方法鉴定细胞特异性蛋白可以精准预测 35%～55%患者的原发部位[7,8]。需根据临床特点进行 IHC 染色项目的选取（如性别，转移部位）。此外，GEP 也能预测包括那些应用 IHC 染色不能确定的患者在内的大部分原发灶不明患者的原发部位。因此，对原发灶不明腺癌的评估需要这些特异性的病理学方法。

鳞癌

鳞癌占 CUP 患者的比例约为 5%。这些患者中大多数患者会出现特异性的症状，并且可以获得有效的治疗。组织学检查是鳞癌的最佳诊断方法。

神经内分泌癌

由于病理诊断水平的提高，大部分的神经内分泌肿瘤可以被确诊。而在 CUP 患者中 3%可诊断为神经内分泌癌。依据各自的特点可以将它们分为三组，低分化肿瘤（类癌/胰岛细胞型），高分化神经内分泌肿瘤（小细胞癌、非典型类癌、大细胞神经内分泌癌）和低分化癌（专门的病理检测中显示出神经内分泌特点）。而低分化和高分化癌的区分对治疗的选择至关重要。

免疫组化染色

IHC染色在肿瘤分类中广泛使用。特异性的肿瘤染色可以区分不良分化肿瘤的谱系来源（表123-1）[7,9~11]。例如以癌和淋巴瘤的区分，不良分化的神经内分泌癌，偶然鉴别出的黑色素瘤和肉瘤[5,7,12~14]。

当应用IHC评估CUP时，会极大地提高组织来源的鉴别准确率。表123-2列举出了一些恶性肿瘤的典型染色形式。这些结果必须要结合临床和组织学特点来解读，由于染色形式存在重叠，很少有IHC染色是完全特异性的。前列腺特异性抗原（PSA）染色是一个排他性且特异表达于前列腺癌[11]。对于其他癌来说，IHC染色的panels可以提高特异性；这些IHC的panels可以鉴别出大约2/3转移灶的原发部位[15~18]。少量经典的染色模式可以被用于诊断（如CK7+/CK20−/TTF-1+用于肺腺癌，CK7−/CK20+/CDX2+用于结直肠腺癌）。4种染色模式（CK7，CK20，CDX2，TTF-1）适合大部分CUP患者诊断时的初始评估。

表123-1　低分化肿瘤：IHC染色在鉴别诊断中的使用

肿瘤类型	细胞角蛋白	上皮细胞膜抗原	白细胞共同抗原	S-100蛋白，HMB45，Melan-A	波形蛋白	肌间线蛋白	凝血因子Ⅷ抗原	染色颗粒素/突触囊泡蛋白
癌	+	+[a]	−	−	−	−	±	
淋巴瘤	−	±[b]	+	−	−	−	−	−
黑色素瘤	−	−	−	+	+	−	−	−
肉瘤	−	±[c]	−	−	+	+[d]	+[e]	−
神经内分泌肿瘤	+	+	−	−	−	−	−	+

[a] 腺癌；[b] 间变性大细胞淋巴瘤（Ki-1或CD30阳性淋巴瘤）；[c] 上皮样肉瘤，滑膜肉瘤；[d] 平滑肌肉瘤，横纹肌肉瘤；[e] 血管肉瘤。

表123-2　原发灶不明癌：用于组织来源鉴定时IHC染色模式

肿瘤类型	IHC染色
膀胱癌（移行细胞）	CK20（+），CK5/6（+），p63（+），GATA3（+），urothelin（+）
乳腺癌	CK7（+），ER（+），PR（+），GCDFP-15（+），Her2/neu（+），mammaglobin（+），GATA3（+）
结直肠癌	CK20（+），CK7（−），CDX2（+）
生殖细胞肿瘤	PLAP（+），OCT4（+）
肝癌	hepar1（+），CD10（+）
肺：腺癌	TTF1（+），CK7（+），CK20（−），P63（+），CK5/6（+）
肺：神经内分泌癌（小细胞/大细胞）	TTF1（+），chromogranin（+），synaptophysin（+）
肺：鳞癌	CK7（+），CK20（−），P63（+），CK5/6（+）
卵巢癌	CK7（+），ER（+），WT1（+），PAX8（+），mesothelin（+）
胰腺癌	CK7（+），CA19~9（+），mesothelin（+）
前列腺癌	PSA（+），CK7（−），CK20（−）
肾癌	RCC（+），PAX8（+），CD10（+），pan-cytokeratin AE 1/3（+）
甲状腺癌（滤泡/乳头）	thyroglobulin（+），TTF1（+），PAX8（+）

电子显微镜

通过电子显微镜对特定超微结构特征的识别，可以对一些分化较差的肿瘤做出明确的诊断。因为这种方法尚未广泛普及，且活检时需要特殊的组织固定方法，并且相当昂贵，因此，只有当常规光学显微镜、IHC染色和GEP不能确定时，才考虑应用电子显微镜来进行肿瘤的谱系研究。

肿瘤特异性染色体畸形

多种肿瘤特异性的染色体畸形在CUP诊断中扮演重要角色。在很多B细胞及T细胞非霍奇金淋巴瘤中可探测到免疫球蛋白肿瘤特异性的重排或是检测到T细胞抗原受体基因[19]。在一些罕见病例中，免疫过氧化物酶染色或流式细胞免疫表型检测不能明确诊断淋巴瘤时，如果检测到这些特殊基因的重排可协助最终诊断。实体瘤特异的畸形包括染色体异位（相互异位[11：22][q24；q12]），在所有的外周性神经上皮瘤和多数尤因肉瘤中存在[20,21]。t（15：19）在儿童或年轻中线结构受侵肿瘤或组织起源未明肿瘤中存在[22]，12号染色体短臂的等臂染色体（i12p）在多数男性睾丸和非性腺的生殖细胞肿瘤中出现[23]。性腺外胚胎细胞肿瘤常存在i（12p）异常，常常对铂类为基础的化疗敏感[23]。大部分恶性肿瘤可以用染色体异常来识别，而现在却可以用更广泛的方法来识别，包括IHC染色和GEP。

基因表达谱

基于起源部位的特异性基因表达谱目前已经被识别出

来，也反映出了他们与正常组织表达谱之间的差异[24]。通过检测关键部位基因表达的差异，这样的方法适用于多种类型的肿瘤，因此，是一种评估 CUP 的潜在的重要诊断工具。

在过去的 15 年间，开展了一些研究方法用于预测 CUP 患者的组织起源。早期的试验仅检测了少量的基因表达标志物，诊断了相关的少量的肿瘤类型[25~28]。近来，反转录-聚合酶链反应（RT-PCR）或基因芯片技术的应用，以及生物信息学的进展，目前已经开发应用于超过 40 种肿瘤类型/亚型的检测[29~37]。最近的大多数研究，1/3 的商业公司可获得并且使用以下检测方法：CancerTYPE ID（bioTheranostics，Inc.）[34,35]，Cancer Origin Test（Rosetta Genomics）[36,37]或者 Tissue of Origin Test（Pathwork，Inc.）[32,33]。

在验证性研究中，应用晚期肿瘤患者（原发灶已知）的活组织进行盲态检测；通过商业可获得的检测方法可以预测 85%～90%患者的组织来源[33,35,37]。无论活检部位（原发 vs 转移）和组织学分级（高分化 vs 低分化），准确率均很高。

精准的 GEP 预测 CUP 组织来源

精准的 GEP 来评估 CUP 其实有很多的困难，很多患者的组织学原发部位不明确。然后，几项强有力的研究证实 CUP 的准确性与先前使用已知原发部位的晚期肿瘤患者进行的验证研究中所证明的相似。最直接的证据来自一项对患有 CUP 患者应用 GEP 的研究，这些患者在病程中最终确认了原发部位（从初始评估后 9～314 周）[8,38]。在 24 名患者中，有 18 名（75%）患者应用初治活检标本 GEP 正确预测了肿瘤的组织学原发部位。尽管人们对 CUP 独特的生物学特性表示担忧，但这些癌症中的大多数似乎都保留了其原始组织的基因表达谱，足以用目前的检测方法进行识别。

GEP 还可以用于标准评估（包括中位数为 18 的 IHC 染色）后仍然原发灶不明低分化肿瘤的评估[39]。30 名患者中，25 名患者分子肿瘤图谱可以进行谱性预测（癌症 10 名，黑色素瘤 5 名，肉瘤 8 名，造血系统肿瘤 2 名），并且，可以预测所有 10 名癌症患者的组织来源。额外的研究和/或治疗的反应可以支持大多数患者的分子谱预测结果。

对比 IHC vs GEP

应用 IHC 染色 vs GEP 鉴别转移性肿瘤原发部位准确性的大型研究共有两项[40,41]。在这两项研究中，提供给病理学家甲醛溶液固定的组织玻片；并且，临床信息仅提供患者性别和活检部位。这两种方法在已知肿瘤原发部位的患者中均显示出了较高的准确性。并且，GEP 比免疫组化染色更能提供正确的诊断（分别为 79% vs 69%；89% vs 83%），而组织学分化差的患者免疫组化染色的准确性下降[41]。

在 CUP 患者中进行类似的对比研究是不可能的，因为他们的原发部位仍不清楚。在一项研究中，IHC 染色可以鉴别 52/149（35%）名患者的单部位来源[8]。在这 52 名患者中，与 GEP 预测的组织来源一致率达到 77%。然而，当 IHC 不能预测单部位组织来源时，IHC 和 GEP 预测的相关性也较差。这项研究的主要结果将在图 123-1 中列举。

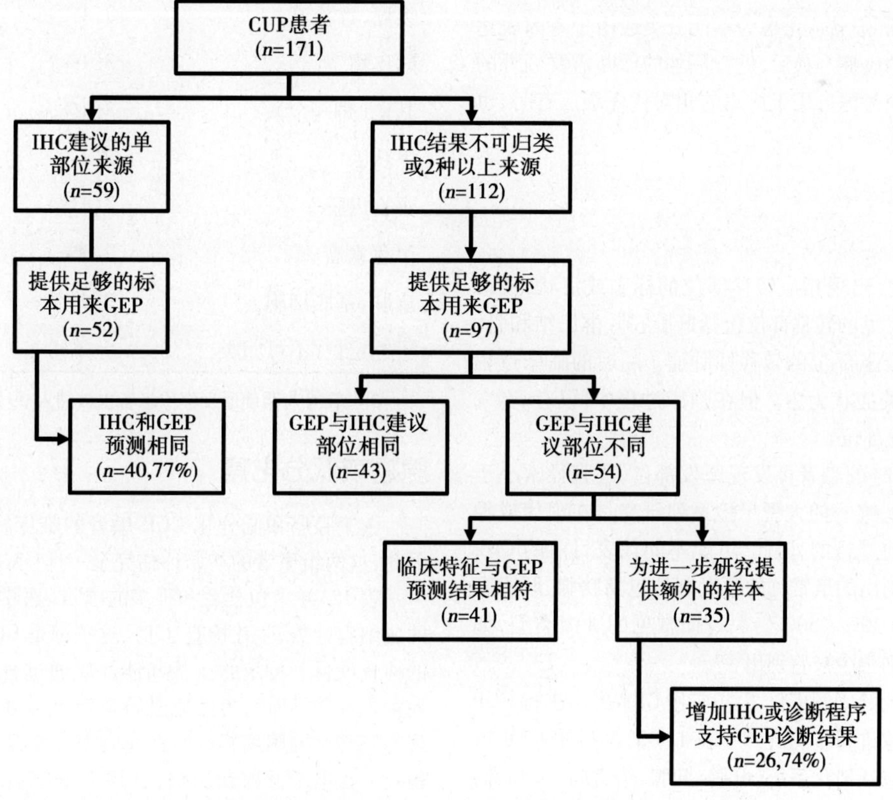

图 123-1　对比 IHC 和 GEP 进行 CUP 患者的组织起源预测

4 项小型研究证明在单一应用 IHC 诊断时 IHC 与 GEP 有较好的相关性[42~45]。总体上看,这 5 个临床研究纳入的 117 名患者,78%的患者单组织来源的预测与临床诊断相符。当然,在所有的研究中,IHC 染色单一诊断的符合率<55%。

总结和结论

虽然在 CUP 患者中很难验证诊断测试的准确性,但目前各大研究的数据基本一致,且最近已经做过详细的评估[46]。依据数据可得出以下结论:

1. GEP 使用商业上可获得的检测方法,可以预测>90% CUP 患者的组织来源。这些预测的准确性在 75%左右。

2. IHC 染色可以预测 35%~55% CUP 患者的单部位组织来源,IHC 和 GEP 的结果一致性较高(78%的病例)。而肿瘤学家往往不愿根据 IHC 预测结果来进行治疗;然而,往往有这样一组患者,GEP 尚不必要,仅需根据 IHC 的检测结果进行部位特异性治疗即可。

3. 除非单个组织来源可以预测,否则 IHC 染色结果对于诊断是没有帮助的。在余下的患者中,GEP 大大增加了预测组织起源的准确性。

由于 GEP 被纳入针对 CUP 患者的诊断评价中,必须考虑几个潜在的问题。第一,即使是在已知肿瘤原发部位的确认性研究中,GEP 的诊断也并不是 100%准确。这些诊断应与临床特征和其他病理研究结果一并考虑。第二,多种肿瘤的基因表达谱存在重叠,而这种情况会导致误诊的可能(如乳腺、唾液腺和皮肤附属器肿瘤的基因表达谱存在重叠)。第三,不包含在正在使用的特定的 GEP 试验中的肿瘤类型不能被诊断。当这种情况发生时,这种肿瘤就应考虑为不能分类或由于基因表达谱重叠而可能误诊的癌症。最后,进行额外的诊断需要额外的活检材料。应该仔细考虑可用于检测的相对优先级。有时,也可以考虑进行二次活检。

临床评价

多数 CUP 患者会出现相应转移部位的标志或症状,被诊断时为晚期癌症。常见的转移部位包括肝脏、肺、淋巴结和骨;多数患者存在一个以上部位的转移性肿瘤。随后的临床过程多以转移部位的相关症状为主。但在临床过程中,仅有 5%~10%的患者显现原发部位。

尸检时,大约 70%的患者可发现原发部位,且直径常小于 2cm。令人遗憾的是,唯一的大型尸检系列研究是在现代成像技术的常规应用之前进行的,因此,可能不能代表目前的 CUP 人群。历史尸检鉴别出的最常见的原发部位包括胰腺、肝胆管和肺,占所有病例的 40%~50%[47,48]。而常见的肿瘤类型,如乳腺和前列腺腺癌则很少被鉴别出[48]。

我们将尸检发现的原发部位[48]与应用 GEP 方法进行 CUP 患者评估的原发部位进行了对比[49](表 123-3)。应用 GEP 方法预测的原发部位包括消化系统(肝脏、胰腺、结直肠)和肺部,与尸检的结果一致。然而,尿道上皮癌、乳腺癌和卵巢癌常与尸检结果不一致。由于卵巢癌和乳腺癌的治疗效果均相对较好,因此这些结果有着重要的实际意义。

表 123-3 起源部位-历史尸检结果与分子肿瘤预测结果的对比

原发部位	分子肿瘤预测结果[49](n=252)	尸检结果[a][48](n=133)
胆管	52(21%)	0
尿道上皮	31(12%)	0
肺	28(11%)	29(22%)
结/直肠	28(11%)	6(2%)
胰腺	12(5%)	28(22%)
乳腺	12(5%)	1(1%)
卵巢	11(4%)	4(3%)
胃/胃食管	10(4%)	8(6%)
肾	9(4%)	8(6%)
肝	8(3%)	16(12%)
肉瘤	6(2%)	0
宫颈	6(2%)	0
神经内分泌	5(2%)	0
前列腺	4(2%)	4(3%)
皮肤	4(2%)	0
生殖细胞	4(2%)	0
类癌,胃肠道	3(1%)	0
间皮瘤	3(1%)	0
其他(每一个)	3(1%)	6(6%)
甲状腺	2(1%)	1(1%)
子宫内膜	2(1%)	0
黑色素瘤	2(1%)	0
皮肤,基底细胞	2(1%)	0
不能定位/不可归类	5(2%)	23(17%)

[a]3 名临终前明确原发部位患者也被纳入

腺癌或低分化癌

由于腺癌和低分化 CUP 患者的临床特点存在很多重叠,因此,这两组患者的初始评估完全一样(表 123-4)。

表 123-4 中包含着和很多的项目(医学史、体格检查、完整的血细胞计数、生化检查、CT),这些都是 CUP 患者诊断过程中的检查项目。特定的症状和体征应通过直接的放射学或内镜检查来评估。所有男性应进行血清 PSA 水平的检测。临床表现与转移性乳腺癌相符的女性应进行乳腺 X 线和乳腺 MRI 的检查。正电子发射断层扫描(PET)的作用存在争议。虽然一些研究推荐 PET 扫描可以用来鉴别至少 30%患者的原发部位[50],但单个的前瞻性研究表明 PET 扫描与 CT 扫描相比并没有明显优势[51]。

表 123-4　推荐初步临床评估

- 完整的病史-包括详细的系统回顾
- 完整的体格检查-包括骨盆检查和便潜血
- 实验室评估-全血细胞计数,综合的代谢结果,乳酸脱氢酶,尿液分析
- CT-胸部,腹部和盆部
- 乳腺 X 线摄影(女性)
- 血清 PSA(男性)
- 选择人群的 PET 扫描
- 病理学评估-包括初始的 IHC 评估(CK7,CK20,TTF-1,CDX2)

初步评估的特殊特征,包括临床和病理学结果,可用于指导更进一步的重点评估。多个常见的患者组,在表 123-5 中列出了初步的临床和病理评价,并提出了进一步评估的建议。

表 123-5　首次评估确定的特定患者的附加评估

患者组	临床评估	病理评估
女性存在乳腺癌特征(骨,肺,肝转移;CK7+)	乳腺 MRI	IHC:ER,GCDFP-15,GATA 3 FISH:HER2
女性存在卵巢癌特征(盆腔/腹膜转移;CK7+)	盆腔/阴道超声	IHC:WT-1,PAX8 GEP(如果需要)
肺癌特征(肺门/纵隔腺病;TTF-1+)	支气管镜	IHC:Napsin A FISH:ALK/ROS-1 突变:EGFR GEP(如果需要)
结肠癌特征(肝/腹膜转移;CK20+/CK7-,CDX2)	结肠镜	突变:KRAS GEP(如果需要)
纵隔/腹膜后肿块	睾丸超声 血清 HCG,AFP	IHC:OCT4,PLAP FISH:i(12p) GEP(如果需要)
低分化癌,存在或不存在清晰细胞特征	-	IHC:CGA,syn,RCC,Hepar-1,HMB-45,Melan-A,血清 AFP(如果 Hepar-1+),奥曲肽(如果神经内分泌染色+) 突变:BRAF(如果黑色素瘤染色+) GEP

鳞状细胞癌

原发灶不明的鳞状细胞癌通常在颈部或腹股沟出现孤立的转移性淋巴结。这些患者的有效治疗较多,因此,最初的评估至关重要:①确定原发部位区域;②确定局部肿瘤受累程度。

颈部淋巴结是最常见的原发灶不明鳞癌的转移部位。患者常为中年或更老一些,多数患者有吸烟或饮酒史。最佳的评估应包括口咽、下咽、鼻咽、喉和上段食管的内镜检查,并在可疑部位进行活检。颈部 CT 检查可以帮助确认疾病的严重程度和原发灶的部位。在标准评估后仍未明确诊断的患者,当应用 PET 检查时,可以鉴别出 25%患者的原发部位[52]。当涉及下颈部或锁骨上淋巴结时,应怀疑原发性肺癌的可能。如果 CT 和头/颈部评估均为阴性结果,应进行支气管镜检查。

如果在上述评估后原发部位仍未确定,则建议采用同侧或双侧扁桃体切除术[53]。在一系列研究中,扁桃体切除后 87 名患者中有 23 名(26%)确定扁桃体为原发部位[54]。

大部分腹股沟淋巴结鳞状细胞癌患者的原发部位多位于生殖系统或肛门直肠区域。在女性患者中,应重点检查外阴、阴道和宫颈,并在可疑区域进行活检检查。男性患者应接受阴茎的检查。为了排除直肠肛管区域的病变,无论男女均应进行详细的内镜检查。对于这些患者来说鉴别出原发部位非常重要,因为无论对于外阴、阴道、宫颈或肛管部位的癌症,即使出现区域淋巴结转移,也可能存在非常有效的治疗方法。

除了颈部和腹股沟淋巴结外的转移性鳞癌通常可能是原发性肺癌的转移。如果其他临床特点怀疑为肺癌应进行胸部 CT 和纤维支气管镜的检查。

神经内分泌癌

神经内分泌癌患者的初始临床评估与表 123-4 中描述一致;但是,在确定治疗方法时应进行特殊的考虑。

低级别神经内分泌癌,有时会在转移灶发现转移性类癌或胰岛细胞瘤而没有明显原发灶提示。在这种情况下,转移灶几乎均会累及肝脏。由于肿瘤分泌生物活性物质,患者会表现出某些临床综合征。对这些患者的其他临床评估应包括对这些物质的血清或尿液筛查。应进行奥曲肽扫描和上、下消化道内镜检查。

高级别神经内分泌癌包括典型的小细胞癌和大细胞神经内分泌癌,以及 IHC 染色或 GEP 检测后考虑为神经内分泌癌的低分化癌。高级别神经内分泌癌诊断时常存在多发转移,很少有分泌生物活性肽导致的相关症状。合并吸烟史的患者应怀疑肺部原发的可能,并需进行支气管镜检查。甲状腺转录因子-1(TTF-1)免疫组化染色的患者也应考虑支气管镜检查。在临床评估中,肺外的小细胞癌可以存在不同的起源部位(唾液腺、食管、胰腺、膀胱、前列腺、结直肠、子宫、宫颈)。CDX2IHC 染色的患者应考虑进行结肠镜检查。

这些高级别神经内分泌癌的起源目前仍不十分清楚。部分小细胞肺癌患者原发部位隐匿。由于很多这样的患者并没有吸烟史,且肺部并未受累,因此,相当一部分人并不会做出这

样的诊断。曾经认为,高级别神经内分泌癌与低级别神经内分泌癌起源相同,但表现出的是肿瘤生物学"光谱"的两端。然而,目前看来,高级别神经内分泌癌有着不同的起源;小细胞肺癌患者中存在常见的染色体异常(3p、5q、10q 和 17p 的缺失),而这些分子异常并没有在类癌中出现[55,56]。

治疗

依据初始诊断评估,患者可被分为几组。在一些患者中,这些评估可以鉴别出组织学的原发部位;这些患者不再是CUP,并且可以根据肿瘤类型进行合适的治疗。第二组患者(约 20%)即使解剖原发部位不能确定,也可以依据临床和/或病理特点分为多个亚组(表 123-6)。每一个亚组的处理方法也将详细介绍。最后,最大的一部分(约 80%)患者并不能区分出合适的亚组。这些患者在近年来一直应用经验性化疗并且进行短期评估。然而,越来越多的证据均支持 IHC 和 GEP 预测组织来源后,可应用部位特异性治疗来治疗这些患者。这些新的数据也将进行阐述。

表 123-6 有利治疗亚组总结

亚组	组织学类型	治疗
女性,孤立腋窝 LN	腺癌	按照Ⅱ期乳腺癌治疗
女性,腋窝 LV+其他转移	腺癌	按照转移性乳腺癌治疗
女性,腹膜转移	腺癌(常浆液性)或低分化癌	按照Ⅲ期卵巢癌治疗
男性,成骨性转移或血清 PSA 升高或 PSA 肿瘤着色	腺癌	按照转移性前列腺癌治疗
结肠癌表现(腹腔内转移+典型组织学/IHC)	腺癌	按照转移性结肠癌治疗
单个转移部位	腺癌或低分化癌	明确的局部治疗(外科切除和/或放疗)
孤立颈部 LN	鳞癌	按照局部晚期头/颈部肿瘤治疗
孤立腹股沟 LN	鳞癌	明确局部治疗(包括外科切除和/或放疗)±化疗
性腺外生殖细胞综合征	低分化癌	按照预后差生殖细胞肿瘤治疗
神经内分泌癌,低级别	类癌/岛细胞特点	按照晚期类癌治疗
神经内分泌癌,侵袭性	小细胞或低分化癌	按照小细胞肺癌治疗

有利的亚组

存在腹膜转移癌的女性患者

在女性患者中,腺癌导致的弥漫的腹膜转移偶见于来自胃肠道肿瘤或乳腺癌,但绝大多数来源于卵巢。此外,腹膜转移癌也可能发生在无卵巢肿瘤且无腹腔内其他原发肿瘤的女性中。这种情况经常会发生在家族性高发卵巢癌风险的女性身上,甚至是在这些患者预防性切除了卵巢以后也可能发生[57]。并且随着 *BRCA1* 基因变异程度的增加,发病的风险也会增加[58]。大部分患者有卵巢癌的组织学特性,例如乳头状癌或砂样癌,临床特征也类似于晚期卵巢癌,转移癌局限在腹膜表面,并且血清中 CA125 水平为阳性结果。如果组织特性提示为卵巢癌,以上症状被称为"多灶性卵巢外浆液性癌"或"腹膜乳头状浆液性癌"。在极少的情况下,男性腹膜转移性癌,乳头状腺癌及血清 CA125 阳性也曾有报道[59]。符合上述特征的患者通常对晚期卵巢癌有效的化疗方案也会有较高的反应率。多项调查研究显示一线治疗反应率为 39%~66%,治愈率为 15%~20%[60~65]。以卵巢癌为例,化疗前给予减瘤术能使患者获得最长的缓解期。理想的治疗包括初始最大限度的减瘤术,后续继续应用紫杉醇/顺铂化疗。

存在腋窝淋巴结转移癌的女性患者

女性患者存在腋窝淋巴结转移性腺癌首先应怀疑转移性乳腺癌[66]。对乳腺钼靶 X 线检查阴性的乳腺癌患者,MRI 和 PET 扫描检查能够发现乳腺上的原发灶,因此,这两项检查是非常必要的[67,68]。淋巴结活检后需要进行雌激素受体和孕激素受体的测定,以及 HER-2 的检测,还需检测其他乳腺 IHC 标志物(表 123-2)。如果结果为阳性,这些检查可以作为诊断乳腺癌的有力证据。

在完善了常规分期检查后,只有孤立性腋窝淋巴结转移的患者通常是可治疗的,而且治疗应依据Ⅱ期乳腺癌的治疗指南。首先要进行改良根治术或乳腺放疗后的腋窝淋巴结切除术[69~71]。即使是在体格检查和其他乳腺辅助检查都是阴性的情况下,乳腺切除术后也可以确诊 44%~82%的乳腺癌[70]。这些原发肿瘤直径常小于 2cm;偶然情况下,也可在乳腺内发现原位癌的存在[72]。术后辅助治疗的选择也应按照淋巴结阳性乳腺癌的治疗指南进行。

女性患者存在腋窝淋巴结以外的转移时也有可能是转移性乳腺癌所致。这部分患者应按照转移性乳腺癌的治疗指南要求接受系统的治疗,尤其是 IHC 染色和 GEP 也支持乳腺癌诊断的患者。激素受体状态和 HER-2 的表达情况也可以指导这些类似于转移性乳腺癌患者的治疗。

男性骨转移

所有男性 CUP 患者均需检测血清 PSA 水平。即使可能临床特点不典型,血清 PSA 水平升高(或肿瘤 PSA 染色阳性)的男性患者需按照转移性前列腺癌治疗进行治疗[73,74]。即使没有发现 *PSA* 的变化,成骨性骨转移也应该按照前列腺癌进行试验治疗。

结直肠癌表现

在过去的 20 年间,越来越多治疗有效的细胞毒药物和靶向治疗药物相继出现,使晚期结直肠癌患者的中位生存期从 8 个月延长到 24 个月[75]。由于针对结直肠癌患者的标准治疗并不能在 CUP 患者经验化疗时使用,因此,在 CUP 患者中鉴别出这样的患者就显得尤为重要。

近来,已经定义了结肠癌的"轮廓",允许 CUP 患者根据相应的特征预测结直肠为可能的原发部位[76,77]。结肠癌的"轮廓"包括:①典型的临床特征(肝、腹膜转移);②组织学类型类似下消化道腺癌;③典型的 IHC 染色(CK20+/CK7-或 CDX2+)。在一组 68 名这样的患者中,根据转移性结直肠癌指南进行治疗的患者中位生存期达到了 28 个月[77]。我们重点要注意的是,结肠镜检查并没有在这些患者中发现任何原发部位的可能。虽然这种治疗不能直接与 CUP 患者的经验治疗相对比,良好的中位生存期(对比经验性化疗中位生存期 8~10 个月)强有力的证明了这种治疗策略的可行性。

表现为单发转移灶的癌

有的情况下,在进行了全面的评估之后,只能确诊为单发转移病灶。这一单发的病灶可以位于不同的部位,包括淋巴结、脑、肺、肾上腺、肝脏、骨及皮肤。当然不排除一些罕见的原发肿瘤看起来像单一转移癌(如原发性皮肤顶泌汗腺癌,小汗腺癌,皮脂腺癌等),所以应充分考虑,其实鉴别起来并不复杂,通常可以通过简单的临床及病理特点鉴别开来。

大多数患者在很短的时间就会出现其他部位的转移。但是,针对原发灶的治疗往往能延长无病生存时间,甚至改善总生存[78]。在开始进行原发灶治疗之前,首先做一次 PET 检查对于明确体内其他转移情况非常有意义[79]。如果并未发现其他转移,在技术允许的情况下,应当先对实体病灶进行切除。有些情况下(如切除了脑内单发病灶),对原发部位再进行放疗也是可行的,目的是达到对原发部位最大限度的控制。系统性化疗对于原发灶控制方面的作用尚未明确;然而,如果 IHC 染色或 GEP 考虑为敏感的肿瘤类型应进行辅助或新辅助化疗。

性腺外生殖细胞肿瘤综合征

一小部分未知原发部位的低分化癌且按照标准组织学检测无法诊断的患者可考虑为性腺外生殖细胞肿瘤[23,80,81]。这类患者通常为青年男性,肿瘤多位于纵隔或腹膜后。部分患者血清肿瘤标志物 HCG 或 AFP 水平显著升高。而大部分这样的患者,可以通过 IHC、GEP 进行诊断[39],或是可通过检测染色体 i(12p)异常确诊生殖细胞肿瘤[23]。

这些性腺外生殖细胞肿瘤患者应接受铂类为基础的化疗 4 个周期,之后对残余肿瘤进行最大限度的切除。治疗效果与典型性腺外生殖细胞肿瘤的治疗效果类似[23,80]。

颈部或锁骨上淋巴结鳞状细胞癌

原发灶不明鳞癌最常见的表现为单侧颈部淋巴结受累。推荐的临床评估方法(前文中已阐述)可以鉴别出 85%原发部位位于头颈部的患者[82]。

当不能明确原发部位时,患者需根据局部晚期头颈部鳞癌的治疗指南进行治疗;约 50%的患者可获得长期的无病生存[83~88]。对于已知原发部位为头颈部的患者,颈部淋巴结广泛受累和肿瘤组织分化不良是不良的预后因素[84,89]。

下颈部或锁骨上淋巴结转移的患者最大的可能是原发性肺癌,治疗效果较差。然而,对于锁骨以下未发现疾病的患者,应采用与颈部高位淋巴结转移患者相同的治疗方案,部分患者可能获得长期生存。

腹股沟淋巴结鳞癌

大部分累及腹股沟淋巴结的鳞癌患者原发灶多位于肛门区域。少部分患者虽然原发灶未明,但对局部腹股沟淋巴结进行手术或放疗有时也能获得长期生存[90]。由于联合化疗也可以改善这个区域(如宫颈、肛门)鳞状细胞癌患者的生存,因此对于原发灶未明患者也可考虑给予额外的化疗。

低级别神经内分泌癌

原发灶不明的类癌或胰岛细胞肿瘤通常表现为惰性生物学行为,对于已知原发部位的这些类型的肿瘤,治疗应当遵循目前的指南。长效奥曲肽(LAR)治疗可以延缓肿瘤的进展并且毒性较低[91]。根据临床情况,适当的治疗也包括局部治疗(孤立病灶的切除,射频消融,冷冻疗法或肝动脉栓塞化疗)。多种细胞毒药物(氟尿嘧啶、链佐星、卡培他滨、替莫唑胺)也有一定的疗效,靶向治疗药物(舒尼替尼、依维莫司)也有一定的希望。

高级别神经内分泌癌

这组患者包括小细胞癌和大细胞神经内分泌癌(组织学诊断),还有一部分患者是低分化神经内分泌癌,IHC 染色可鉴别出神经内分泌癌成分。这类患者应接受小细胞肺癌那样的联合治疗;据报告,这组患者治疗反应率高,但长期生存比例低(10%~15%)[92~95]。

低分化癌

原发部位不明低分化癌患者是一大类异质性明显的肿瘤。20 世纪 70 年代,在一群化疗高度敏感的肿瘤患者中第一次发现[80,81,96]。目前的检测方法可以鉴别出这类人群中疗效较好的患者。其余的低分化 CUP 患者预后与未知原发部位的腺癌患者预后相似。这些患者也需要应用腺癌的推荐治疗方法,特别注意需要使用 IHC 染色和/或 GEP 来确定组织来源。

CUP 的经验化疗

大部分(80%)原发灶未明的腺癌患者不属于以上任何一个特异性临床亚组。多年来,如果组织来源不能确定,经验性化疗是大部分这类患者的治疗选择。在设计经验性化疗方案时,许多类型的实体肿瘤治疗效果不佳。此外,类似的细胞毒药物和方案被用于多种肿瘤的治疗。因此,设计对最敏感肿瘤具有合理活性的"广谱"治疗方案是可能的。

含有大多数常用细胞毒性药物的联合治疗方案(紫杉类、吉西他滨、拓扑异构酶 I 抑制剂、蒽环类、长春碱类)被用于 CUP 患者的经验性化疗。紫杉类和铂类药物的联用是被广泛研究且常用的治疗方案[97~103]。多种其他的方案(吉西他滨/铂类,吉西他滨/紫杉醇)也有类似的活性[104~106]。多个随机2期临床研究对比了不同的两药联合治疗结果类似[105,107~111]。而增加第3种药物并不能提高有效率[109,112~115]。虽然治疗的反应率不同,但大部分的试验报告中位生存期8~11个月,2年生存率14%~24%。在较大型的实验中(大于100个患者),中位生存期则为9个月[107,112,114,116,117]。

少量2期临床研究评估了经验性二线治疗的疗效。单药吉西他滨和联合治疗方案,如吉西他滨/伊立替康,卡培他滨/奥沙利铂和贝伐单抗/厄洛替尼等均有一定的有效率[118~121]。

虽然没有最佳的研究直接对比经验化疗和最佳支持治疗生存期的差异,几项大型注册研究提示目前的治疗可以延长患者的生存[122~129]。瑞典癌症登记处的数据显示,CUP患者的中位生存期是有延长的2001—2008年(6个月)vs 1987—1993年(4个月)[130]。

尽管取得了这些微小的进步,但作者相信,CUP的经验性化疗时代即将结束。精准识别组织来源可以为大部分的CUP患者提供更合理的框架性治疗建议。

组织来源预测指导部位特异性治疗

大部分CUP患者均可精确的预测组织来源。尽管我们可以合理地假设,基于预测组织来源的特异性治疗可能优于经验性化疗,但支持这一假设的临床数据最近才积累起来,而且还不完整。但对这个部位特异性治疗持怀疑态度的原因主要是CUP患者独特的生物学特征(主要部位不明显的事实证明了这一点)。依据临床特点的不同可以推测肿瘤对系统化疗的反应情况也会存在差异。然而,越来越多的证据也证明大部分肿瘤保存了与原发部位肿瘤相同的特点。

多个生物学和临床观察均支持这些相似。首先,CUP患者的基因表达情况与晚期肿瘤相同组织来源类似。其次,目前还没有发现与CUP相同的独立的分子特征。再次,在临床上公认的几个有利的CUP亚群中,对患者的成功治疗是基于假设他们具有特定的癌症类型(如女性腋窝淋巴结转移按照乳腺癌治疗、腹膜转移癌按照卵巢癌治疗)。最后,包含CUP患者的回顾性分析发现,IHC染色或分子特征支持结直肠原发部位的患者应用结直肠癌的标准方案治疗,中为生存期>20个月,与转移性结肠癌患者的生存期类似[131,132]。

最强有力的支持部位特异性治疗的证据来自一项最近的大型、前瞻性临床研究,纳入的是既往未经治疗的CUP患者,所有患者均进行GEP检测(RT-PCR检测92-基因[35])。在这项研究中,可以预测242/253名(98%)患者的组织来源。诊断出26名不同组织的来源(表123-3)。根据GEP预测结果应用部位特异性治疗的患者中位生存期12.5个月[49]。

在这一大组患者中,41%的预测组织来源的患者对相关的标准治疗耐药,因此,不管用什么治疗获益均非常小。像预计的那样,这组患者预后较差,中位生存期仅为7.6个月。然而,余下的患者(59%)应用根据肿瘤类型的部位特异性治疗是有反应的,中位生存期13.4个月($P=0.04$)。尽管个体癌症患者的数量很小,但是这组患者的中位生存期与预测肿瘤类型的那些患者相似(中位生存:卵巢30个月,乳腺28个月,NSCLC 16个月,结直肠13个月,胰腺8个月,胆管7个月)。

除了这项前瞻性研究结果,多项小型的回顾性研究和个案报告均提示预测组织来源的部位特异性治疗是存在获益的[133,134]。但并不是所有的结果均一致,67名初始评估时已经确认组织学原发部位的CUP患者,使用早期的分子谱预测原发部位正确率仅为35%[135]。

筛选CUP“可操作的”分子异常

许多新的肿瘤治疗方法利用肿瘤特异性的分子生物学特性,这些特性对癌细胞的生长和转移至关重要。因此,为这些药物确定合适的患者群体不仅取决于肿瘤类型,还取决于特异性靶向分子异常的存在。对特定肿瘤类型的患者进行靶向分子异常筛查已经成为临床实践的标准,而对更广泛的潜在“可操作”异常进行筛查正变得越来越常见。

目前,CUP患者分子异常的流行病学资料有限。CUP患者异质性明显,一些潜在的“可操作”异常很可能被重新提出。先前的研究和个案报道均证明存在特定的分子生物学异常(EGFR;PI3KCA,MET,和其他)[136~140]。进一步描述这些异常及其频率是很重要的,并可能为一些CUP患者增加额外的治疗选择。

CUP患者组织来源的鉴定也可以导致对特异性分子异常的直接评估。例如,预测CUP为非小细胞肺癌需要进一步评估EGFR活化突变和ALK和ROS-1重排。在一小群这样的患者,研究鉴别了ALK重排,应用克唑替尼(crizotinib)的治疗导致患者明显获益[141]。联合使用GEP进行诊断和额外的分子检测以确定“可操作”分子异常是CUP治疗未来可能的方向。

目前CUP患者的处理-新的治疗模式出现

图123-2所示为建议的CUP患者管理示意图。在初始的临床和病理评估后(包括IHC染色),组织学原发部位已经确认的患者需要考虑相应的治疗,良好治疗亚组的患者需要接受恰当的治疗。应用IHC预测单个组织来源的患者需要接受部位特异性治疗;GEP可能帮助验证IHC结果。当初始的IHC评估不能确定单一组织来源时,需进行GEP检查,根据治疗结果进行部位特异性治疗。在完成诊断评估后,如患者的组织来源不明,可采用经验性化疗。

临床数据已经支持将分子诊断学整合到CUP的管理中,但仍有必要继续研究以完善管理建议。CUP患者治疗水平的提高也依赖于其他癌症类型治疗的进展,并且与对这些肿瘤的精确治疗数量的增加有关。及时地将新药物整合到CUP患者的治疗中,需要持续不断的努力,将关键的分子异常定义为每个患者治疗计划的一部分。

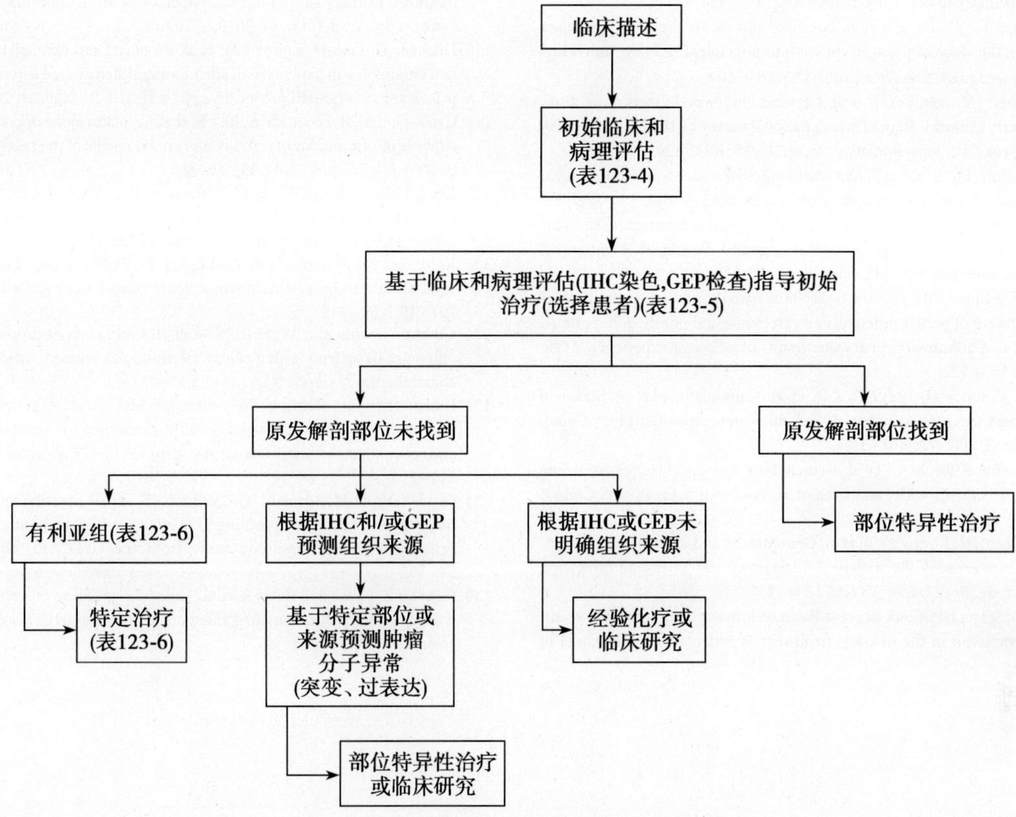

图 123-2　未明原发灶肿瘤患者的处理概览

（程颖　杨长良 译　程颖 校）

参考文献

The complete reference list can be found on the Wiley Companion Digital Edition of this title (see inside front cover for login instructions).

5 Horning SJ, Carrier EK, Rouse RV, et al. Lymphomas presenting as histologically unclassified neoplasms: characteristics and response to treatment. *J Clin Oncol*. 1989;**7**:1281–1287.

7 Oien KA, Dennis JL. Diagnostic work-up of carcinoma of unknown primary: from immunohistochemistry to molecular profiling. *Ann Oncol*. 2012;**23(Suppl 10)**:271–277.

8 Greco FA, Lennington WJ, Spigel DR, Hainsworth JD. Molecular profiling diagnosis in unknown primary cancer: accuracy and ability to complement standard pathology. *J Natl Cancer Inst*. 2013;**105**:782–790.

11 Oien K. Pathologic evaluation of unknown primary cancer. *Semin Oncol*. 2009;**36**:8–37.

16 Dennis JL, Hvidsten TR, Wit EC, et al. Markers of adenocarcinoma characteristic of the site of origin: development of a diagnostic algorithm. *Clin Cancer Res*. 2005;**11**:3766–3772.

17 Park SY, Kim BH, Kim JH, et al. Panels of immunohistochemical markers help determine primary sites of metastatic adenocarcinoma. *Arch Pathol Lab Med*. 2007;**131**:1561–1567.

18 Anderson GG, Weiss LM. Determining tissue of origin for metastatic cancers: meta-analysis and literature review of immunohistochemistry performance. *Appl Immunohistochem Mol Morphol*. 2010;**18**:3–8.

23 Motzer RJ, Rodriguez E, Reuter VE, et al. Molecular and cytogenetic studies in the diagnosis of patients with poorly differentiated carcinomas of unknown primary site. *J Clin Oncol*. 1995;**13**:274–282.

24 Su AI, Welsh JB, Sapinoso LM, et al. Molecular classification of human carcinomas by use of gene expression signatures. *Cancer Res*. 2001;**61**:7388–7393.

33 Pillai R, Deeter R, Rigl CT, et al. Validation and reproducibility of a microarray-based gene expression test for tumor identification in formalin-fixed, paraffin-embedded specimens. *J Mol Diagn*. 2011;**13**:48–56.

35 Erlander MG, Ma XJ, Kesty NC, et al. Performance and clinical evaluation of the 92-gene real-time PCR assay for tumor classification. *J Mol Diagn*. 2011;**13**:493–503.

37 Meiri E, Mueller WC, Rosenwald S, et al. A second-generation microRNA-based assay for diagnosing tumor tissue origin. *Oncologist*. 2012;**17**:801–812.

38 Greco FA, Spigel DR, Yardley DA, et al. Molecular profiling in unknown primary cancer: accuracy of tissue of origin prediction. *Oncologist*. 2010;**15**:500–506.

40 Weiss LM, Chu P, Schroeder BE, et al. Blinded comparator study of immunohistochemical analysis versus a 92-gene cancer classifier in the diagnosis of the primary site in metastatic tumors. *J Mol Diagn*. 2013;**15**:263–269.

46 Hainsworth JD, Greco FA. Gene expression profiling in patients with carcinoma of unknown primary site: from translational research to standard of care. *Virchows Arch*. 2014;**464**:393–402.

48 Nystrom JS, Weiner JM, Heffelfinger-Juttner J, et al. Metastatic and histologic presentations in unknown primary cancer. *Semin Oncol*. 1977;**4**:53–58.

49 Hainsworth JD, Rubin MS, Spigel DR, et al. Molecular gene expression profiling to predict the tissue of origin and direct site-specific therapy in patients with carcinoma of unknown primary site: a prospective trial of the Sarah Cannon research institute. *J Clin Oncol*. 2013;**31**:217–223.

51 Moller AK, Loft A, Berthelsen AK, et al. A prospective comparison of 18 F-FDG PET/CT and CT as diagnostic tools to identify the primary tumor site in patients with extracervical carcinoma of unknown primary site. *Oncologist*. 2012;**17**:1146–1154.

52 Rusthoven KE, Koshy M, Paulino AC. The role of fluorodeoxyglucose positron emission tomography in cervical lymph node metastases from an unknown primary tumor. *Cancer*. 2004;**101**:2641–2649.

65 Piver MS, Eltabbakh GH, Hempling RE, et al. Two sequential studies for primary peritoneal carcinoma: induction with weekly cisplatin followed by either cisplatin-doxorubicin-cyclophosphamide or paclitaxel-cisplatin. *Gynecol Oncol*. 1997;**67**:141–146.

66 Pentheroudakis G, Lazaridis G, Pavlidis N. Axillary nodal metastases from carcinoma of unknown primary (CUPAx): a systematic review of published evidence. *Breast Cancer Res Treat*. 2010;**119**:1–11.

77 Varadhachary GR, Karanth S, Qiao W, et al. Carcinoma of unknown primary with gastrointestinal profile: immunohistochemistry and survival data for this favorable subset. *Int J Clin Oncol*. 2014;**19**:479–484.

78 Nguyen LN, Maor MH, Oswald MJ. Brain metastases as the only manifestation of

an undetected primary tumor. *Cancer*. 1998;**83**:2181－2184.

79 Rades D, Kuhnel G, Wildfang I, et al. Localised disease in cancer of unknown primary (CUP): the value of positron emission tomography (PET) for individual therapeutic management. *Ann Oncol*. 2001;**12**:1605－1609.

84 Grau C, Johansen LV, Jakobsen J, et al. Cervical lymph node metastases from unknown primary tumours. Results from a national survey by the Danish Society for Head and Neck Oncology. *Radiother Oncol*. 2000;**55**:121－129.

90 Guarischi A, Keane TJ, Elhakim T. Metastatic inguinal nodes from an unknown primary neoplasm. A review of 56 cases. *Cancer*. 1987;**59**:572－577.

92 Hainsworth JD, Johnson DH, Greco FA. Poorly differentiated neuroendocrine carcinoma of unknown primary site. A newly recognized clinicopathologic entity. *Ann Intern Med*. 1988;**109**:364－371.

96 Hainsworth JD, Johnson DH, Greco FA. Cisplatin-based combination chemotherapy in the treatment of poorly differentiated carcinoma and poorly differentiated adenocarcinoma of unknown primary site: results of a 12-year experience. *J Clin Oncol*. 1992;**10**:912－922.

97 Briasoulis E, Kalofonos H, Bafaloukos D, et al. Carboplatin plus paclitaxel in unknown primary carcinoma: a phase II Hellenic Cooperative Oncology Group Study. *J Clin Oncol*. 2000;**18**:3101－3107.

104 Pouessel D, Culine S, Becht C, et al. Gemcitabine and docetaxel as front-line chemotherapy in patients with carcinoma of an unknown primary site. *Cancer*. 2004;**100**:1257－1261.

106 Pittman KB, Olver IN, Koczwara B, et al. Gemcitabine and carboplatin in carcinoma of unknown primary site: a phase 2 Adelaide Cancer Trials and Education Collaborative study. *Br J Cancer*. 2006;**95**:1309－1313.

107 Hainsworth JD, Spigel DR, Clark BL, et al. Paclitaxel/carboplatin/etoposide versus gemcitabine/irinotecan in the first-line treatment of patients with carcinoma of unknown primary site: a randomized, phase Ⅲ Sarah Cannon Oncology Research Consortium Trial. *Cancer J*. 2010;**16**:70－75.

110 Huebner G, Link H, Kohne CH, et al. Paclitaxel and carboplatin vs gemcitabine and vinorelbine in patients with adeno- or undifferentiated carcinoma of unknown primary: a randomised prospective phase II trial. *Br J Cancer*. 2009;**100**:44－49.

111 Gross-Goupil M, Fourcade A, Blot E, et al. Cisplatin alone or combined with gemcitabine in carcinomas of unknown primary: results of the randomised GEFCAPI 02 trial. *Eur J Cancer*. 2012;**48**:721－727.

117 Lee J, Hahn S, Kim DW, et al. Evaluation of survival benefits by platinums and taxanes for an unfavourable subset of carcinoma of unknown primary: a systematic review and meta-analysis. *Br J Cancer*. 2013;**108**:39－48.

130 Riihimaki M, Hemminki A, Sundquist K, Hemminki K. Time trends in survival from cancer of unknown primary: small steps forward. *Eur J Cancer*. 2013;**49**:2403－2410.

131 Greco F, Lennington W, Spigel DR, et al. Carcinoma of unknown primary site: outcomes in patients with a colorectal molecular profile treated with site-specific chemotherapy. *J Cancer Ther*. 2012;**3**:37－43.

132 Hainsworth JD, Schnabel CA, Erlander MG, et al. A retrospective study of treatment outcomes in patients with carcinoma of unknown primary site and a colorectal cancer molecular profile. *Clin Colorectal Cancer*. 2012;**11**: 112－118.

133 Gross-Goupil M, Massard C, Lesimple T, et al. Identifying the primary site using gene expression profiling in patients with carcinoma of an unknown primary (CUP): a feasibility study from the GEFCAPI. *Onkologie*. 2012;**35**: 54－55.

140 Gatalica Z, Millis S, Bender R, et al. Molecular profiling cancers of unknown primary: paradigm shift in management of CUP. European Cancer Conference 2013, abstract #LBA39; 2013.

第 124 章　厌食与恶病质

Takao Ohnuma, MD, PhD

概述

癌症恶病质是一种消耗性综合征，表现为骨骼肌质量的大量减少，伴有或不伴有脂肪组织萎缩。可以通过与简单的饥饿作比较，饥饿时脂肪替代葡萄糖成为优选的原料为身体供能。癌症恶病质的起因是由于代谢的变化，而非仅是能量的缺乏，它无法通过强制营养支持逆转。癌症相关恶病质形成的原因是多方面的，包括促恶病质细胞因子及代谢紊乱。欧洲癌症协会致力于开发癌症恶病质的新定义和分类。近期研究发现，阿拉莫林（anamorelin），一种口服胃促生长素（ghrelin）类似物，可以作为治疗癌症恶病质的新药。

简介

恶病质是一种消耗综合征，可伴随多种疾病，包括癌症、慢性阻塞性肺疾病、艾滋病及类风湿关节炎。它与中枢性及系统性促炎因子增加相关，伴有生活质量的下降、对药物治疗反应变差及生存期的缩短[1,2]。

恶病质引起的骨骼肌大量丢失，伴有或不伴有脂肪组织萎缩，可以通过与简单的饥饿做对比，饥饿发生时，脂肪替代葡萄糖成为身体供能的优选能量来源。癌症恶病质的起因是由于代谢的变化，而非仅是能量的缺乏，它无法通过强制营养支持来逆转[3,4]。

恶病质的患者对手术、化疗及放射治疗的耐受性差[5~8]。在接受手术治疗的患者中，第四腰椎水平的横断面图像显示，随着瘦体重的减少，协变量调整后的死亡率显著增加[7~9]。

由于普遍接受的定义、诊断标准及分类方法的缺乏，大大阻碍了临床试验和临床实践的进展。表 124-1 和表 124-2 展示了 2010 年癌症恶病质的定义与分类方法的发展情况[10]。

人们一致认为，治疗的重点应是在抗癌治疗全程对患者进行营养支持及功能状态的改善，而不是关注于终末期的消耗。当恶病质伴随有全身性炎症反应或代谢改变时，则需要包括新药治疗在内的多模式治疗方法。以下三种支持治疗方式是至关重要的：确保足够的能量及蛋白质的摄入、坚持身体锻炼保持肌肉质量及减少（如果存在的话）全身炎症反应。一些基于新的药物治疗靶点（包括细胞因子、胃促生长素受体、雄激素受体及肌肉生长抑素）的Ⅱ/Ⅲ期临床研究结果预计在 2016 年公布。如果出现有效的治疗方法，早期发现营养不良和恶病质将变得越来越重要[11]。

表 124-1　癌症恶病质的诊断

评估项目	量化指标	注释
体重减轻	>5%	在过去的 6 个月内（没有简单饥饿）
或		
体重指数	<20	如果体重减轻>2%
或		
四肢骨骼肌指数		与肌肉减少症一致
双能 X 线	男性<7.26kg/m^2	如果体重减轻>2%
	女性<5.45kg/m^2	
骨密度	男性<32cm^2	上臂
	女性<18cm^2	
人体测量学	男性<55cm^2	腰椎 CT 成像
	女性<39cm^2	
生物电阻抗	男性<14.6kg/m^2	如果肥胖或水肿，则不可靠
	女性<11.4kg/m^2	

摘自 Fearon 等，2011[10]，经 Elsevier 许可转载。

表 124-2　癌症恶病质分期

恶病质前期
厌食，代谢变化，体重减轻<5%
恶病质期
过去 6 个月内体重减轻>5%（除外饥饿状态）
或体重指数<20 及体重减轻>2%
或
厌食和全身炎症改变和肌肉减少症以及体重减轻>2%
难治性恶病质期
癌症患者分解代谢活跃，对抗癌治疗反应不佳；体能状态评分低，以及预计生存期<3 个月

摘自 Fearon 等，2011[10]。经 Elsevier 许可转载。

病因及发病机制

癌症相关恶病质形成的原因是多方面的，大致可以分为相互关联的三大类：厌食与早饱、消化道机械性梗阻以及代谢紊乱。

癌症患者的厌食可以分为疾病相关、治疗相关及情绪困扰相关。厌食可能由早饱、恶心、味觉障碍和口味变化引起。表124-3列出了厌食与早饱的可能病因。癌症患者已被证实对特定的食物香味的味觉及嗅觉发生了异常[48]。

表124-3 癌症厌食的可能原因

名称	特征
细胞因子	TNFα[12~14]
	IL-1[14~16]
	IL-6[14,17~32]
神经肽	大脑神经肽环路失调[33]
5-羟色胺	血清及中枢神经系统(CNS)水平升高[34,35]
血清乳酸	肿瘤分泌产物[36,37]
高血糖素及高血糖素样多肽[38,39]	
满足素(satietins)	一种从人血浆分离出的蛋白质[40,41]
高钙血症	偶尔的副肿瘤发现[42]
铃蟾肽(铃蟾肽)	来自小细胞肺癌的神经肽[43,44]
毒激素-L	从肝癌患者的腹水中纯化的脂肪分解因子[45,46]
抗癌剂(致吐性)	顺铂、多柔比星、氮芥等[47]

细胞因子

TNF-α、IL-1、IL-6[及其亚家族细胞因子如睫状神经营养因子(ciliary neurotrophic factor,CNTF)和白血病抑制因子(leukemia inhibitory factor,LIF)]以及宿主免疫细胞和/或肿瘤细胞产生的IFN-γ均被认为是癌症恶病质的相关介质[49~51]。这些细胞因子被称为原核因子,在动物体内的特征是引起厌食、体重减轻、急性期蛋白质反应、蛋白质和脂肪分解、皮质醇水平上升和高血糖素和胰岛素水平下降,胰岛素抵抗,贫血,发烧,能量消耗增加。这些细胞因子与瘦素、神经肽或血清素之间的直接相互作用被认为是诱导癌症厌食的发生机制。抗恶病质因子,如IL-4,IL-10,IL-12,IL-15,IFN-α以及胰岛素样生长因子I(insulin-like growth factor I,IGF-I)发挥着与促恶病质因子相反作用。

促恶病质细胞因子由宿主免疫细胞产生,包括辅助T细胞1、巨噬细胞及骨髓衍生的抑制细胞,这些细胞也是持续性炎症反应的一部分。蛋白水解诱导因子(proteolysis inducing factor,PIF)仅由肿瘤产生。PIF与TNF-α通过相似的通路,即激活肌肉中的核因子-κB(NF-κB)转录因子来诱导恶病质的发生[52,53]。

肾上腺素能升高的状态在各种肿瘤类型中相似,导致能量消耗率升高[54,55]。瘦体重消耗的主要部位是骨骼肌,这是由于蛋白质转运增加的过程中没有相应的蛋白质合成[54]。现有的数据展示了肌球蛋白重链(myosin heavy chain,MyHC)的缺失及纤维大小的减少[54,56]。调节蛋白质分解的腺苷三磷酸-泛素依赖性途径在某些癌症恶病质病例中被上调[54,57]。

IL-6是一种多功能细胞因子,参与多种宿主防御和病理过程[17]。分泌IL-6的细胞可以诱导肌肉和脂肪储存的消耗并最终导致死亡[18,19]。在大多数恶病质实验模型中血清IL-6水平升高。IL-6被证实是多种肿瘤导致体重减轻的敏感预测因子,包括晚期小细胞肺癌[20]和结肠癌[21,22]。升高的IL-6水平与多种癌症类型的存活率降低有关[23]。除IL-6本身外,其他IL-6家族细胞因子也与肌肉萎缩有关,包括CNTF[24,25]及LIF[26,27]IL-6和相关配体通过与膜结合或可溶形式的配体特异性α肾上腺素受体(IL-6受体-α,也称为gp80)结合而激活信号转导[28]。这些配体受体复合物诱导三种主要通路的激活:信号转导和转录激活因子1和3(STAT1/3),ERK及磷脂酰肌醇3-激酶/Akt途径[29]。这些途径与下游激酶相互作用以影响基因表达[30]。

IL-6家族配体强力激活的一种通路是JAK/STAT3通路。STAT3活化被证明是肌肉萎缩的共同特征,该途径可以在体内和体外通过IL-6在肌肉中激活,也可以通过不同类型的癌症和无菌败血症激活。此外,STAT3活化证明其对于肌肉萎缩是必要和充分的。相反,用JAK或STAT3抑制剂在药理学上抑制STAT3通路,可以减少了IL-6下游的肌肉萎缩。这些结果表明STAT3是癌症恶病质和高IL-6家族信号转导的其他条件下发生肌肉萎缩的主要介质[31,32]。

虽然癌症中恶病质状态下肌肉减少的潜在机制与肌营养不良的机制不重叠,但功能失调的肌营养不良糖蛋白复合物(DGC)是这两种疾病状态之间的共同机制[58~60]。

肿瘤引起的DGC改变是恶病质早期的一个关键事件。DGC是通过肌肉活检检查明确[59]。与健康对照组相比,在60%的胃肠道癌症患者中,肌营养不良蛋白显著减少,这与DGC蛋白的高糖基化有关[59]。

虽然TNF-α诱导IL-1,这两种细胞因子可作用于大脑以及直接作用于胃肠道发挥厌食效应,例如,使胃排空减缓[12,15]。致癌物诱导肿瘤的老鼠模型中,尽管在其他组织中存在变化,IL-1β及其受体mRNA是在大脑中唯一上调的因子,考虑癌症相关的厌食中发挥重要作用[16]。

在肿瘤患者中,血清中的循环TNF-α,IL-1、IL-6和IFN-γ水平与厌食/体重减轻综合征之间无明显相关性[13,14]。恶病质的核心作用机制涉及多种细胞因子,包括IL-1、IL-6、IL-8、TNF-α、IFN-α及其他趋化因子;还与5-羟色胺和神经肽能回路功能障碍相关[34]。此外,癌症患者血浆游离色氨酸水平升高与厌食密切相关。血液中色氨酸的增加会导致脑脊液中色氨酸水平升高,导致血清素合成增加,血清素是癌症厌食的主要介质[35]。

在癌症患者中,蛋白酶体的活性所致恶病质并不常见[54,61]。一些研究结果表明,自噬溶酶体蛋白水解系统和组织蛋白酶B在癌症恶病质的发展过程中发挥作用[61,62]。

胰岛素与胃促生长素

由胰腺分泌的胰岛素和主要由脂肪细胞产生的瘦素均以与体脂含量成比例的进入血液循环,而他们进入中枢神经系统

(central nervous system, CNS)的比例与其在血浆的水平成正比。随着体重增加，胰岛素的分泌在基础状态及餐后均增加。胰岛素促进脂肪细胞中的脂肪储存和瘦素合成。相比胰岛素，瘦素在中枢神经系统控制能量稳态的方面发挥着更为重要的作用，例如，尽管胰岛素水平始终保持较高的状态，瘦素缺乏仍会导致肥胖，提示肥胖并不是由胰岛素缺乏引起的[63,64]。

神经肽网络对食欲的内源性控制可归类为促进食欲和食欲缺乏(表 124-4)。在具有恶病质的荷瘤动物中，已经显示出了较低的瘦素循环水平和降低的脂肪组织瘦素 mRNA 含量[65]。与其相类似的，患有晚期肺癌和结肠癌的患者的血清瘦素水平降低[66,67]。血浆瘦素水平显示出性别相关性，女性恶病质患者血浆瘦素水平明显低于男性恶病质患者[68]。

表 124-4 参与促进食欲(合成代谢)与抑制食欲(分解代谢)的神经肽

促进食欲分子
神经肽 Y(NPY)
刺鼠色蛋白相关蛋白(AGRP)
黑色素聚集色素(MCH)
下丘脑分泌素 1 和 2(食欲肽 A 与食欲肽 B)
加兰肽
去甲肾上腺素
阿片类
胃促生长素
抑制食欲分子
α-促黑激素(α-MSH)
促肾上腺皮质激素释放激素(CRH)
促甲状腺素释放(TRH)
可卡因及安非他命转录产物(CART)
阿黑皮素原(POMC)
胰岛素
IL-1β
尿皮质素
高血糖素样肽 1(GLP-1)
缩宫素
神经降压肽
5-羟色胺
多巴胺
组胺
胆囊收缩素
铃蟾肽
降钙素基因相关肽
垂体腺苷酸环化酶激活多肽瘦素

摘自参考文献[33,63]。

胃促生长素(ghrelin)，作为一种"胃促生长素"由胃肠道中的胃促生长素细胞分泌，在中枢神经系统中挥发神经肽的作用。胃排空时，胃促生长素被分泌；胃充盈时，分泌停止。胃促生长素作用于下丘脑细胞，既增加饥饿感，又增加胃酸分泌和胃肠动力，为食物摄取做准备。胃促生长素与瘦素作用相反，而胃促生长素和瘦素的受体同时存在于相同的脑细胞中。胃促生长素还通过与多巴胺和乙酰胆碱的相互作用，在调节腹侧被盖区(一个在处理性欲和成瘾方面发挥作用的部位)的感知中枢方面起着重要作用。

胃促生长素由 *GHRL* 基因编码，由前肽胃促生长素/肥胖抑制素(obestatin)切割生成。全长前胃促生长素原(preproghrelin)与前胃动素同源，两者均为胃动素家族成员。

胃促生长素结构独特，它由 28 个氨基酸组成，其中一个独立的脂肪酸在 ser 3 上被辛酰化，不仅可以结合生长激素(growth hormone, GH)促分泌素受体，还可以赋予分子对不同代谢途径的多种多效性[69]。血清中可检测到源自相同前体的两种不同形式的胃促生长素：未乙酰化的胃促生长素(unacylated ghrelin, UnAG)和较低浓度的乙酰化胃促生长素。胃促生长素的乙酰化主要在胃内通过细胞内胃促生长素-O-酰基转移酶进行，这种酶仅在 2008 年被发现。乙酰化的胃促生长素，但不是未乙酰化的胃促生长素，可以结合生长激素促分泌素受体-1a (growth hormone secretagogue receptor-1a, GHSR-1a)，广泛表达在下丘脑和垂体区域，介导 GH 释放，能够增强食欲和增加脂肪组织沉积。

在多种高亲和力结合位点中，未乙酰化和乙酰化的胃促生长素共同作用，调节下游介质的释放。此外，已经鉴定出未乙酰化胃促生长素在脑、肠、脂肪和肌肉中的新型受体，其可能促进细胞增殖、分化和存活[70]。

胃促生长素的生理功能包括食欲调节、GH 释放增强、能量稳态、葡萄糖稳态、抗炎作用、对心血管系统的影响、胃肠道运动的调节、性功能和成骨作用。GHSR 广泛表达在控制体重、情绪反应、记忆和学习的大脑区域。

据报道，在患有肌肉萎缩和癌症恶病质的患者中，胃促生长素的循环水平增加。胃促生长素在动物系统中反作用于肿瘤诱导的厌食，其给药增加了食物摄入和体重增加[71~73]。

调节癌症厌食-恶病质综合征的主要分子机制包括脑神经化学的改变。特别是，下丘脑促黑素(melanocortin)系统似乎对外周输入没有适当的反应，其活性主要转向促进分解代谢刺激的活化，促进外周组织中碳水化合物、脂质和蛋白质的代谢，导致胰岛素抵抗、脂肪分解增加、并加速肌肉蛋白水解[74]。促炎细胞因子(TNF-α 和 IL-1β)和下丘脑 5-羟色胺能神经元与下丘脑黑皮素系统的功能障碍有关[33]。特别是两种肽系统似乎在控制摄食行为方面具有强烈影响：这两种肽系统是促食欲神经肽 Y(neuropeptide Y, NPY)和厌食阿黑皮素原(proopiomelanocortin, POMC)系统[75]。许多这些介质通过改变 NPY/POMC 系统发挥作用。两者都起源于下丘脑弓状核(ARC)并在脑中广泛延伸[75]。细胞因子在癌症厌食中的作用可能取决于 NPY 和 POMC 两个系统。研究发现，下丘脑 IL-1mRNA 在甲基胆蒽诱导的携带肉瘤的大鼠中显著增加。这些大鼠的脑脊液中 IL-1

的水平也增加[76,77]。向下丘脑注射IL-1β会导致骨骼肌基因表达在数小时内发生显著变化,包括泛素蛋白酶体途径的上调。这清楚地证明了肌肉蛋白质合成和降解的神经控制潜力[78]。但在癌症恶病质患者中尚未得到完全探索[54]。

消化道功能障碍

癌症患者出现味觉和嗅觉感知异常的情况已有人描述过。口腔、口咽、食管、胃、胰腺、肝脏和腹膜的肿瘤可能通过机械干扰损害口腔的摄入功能。肠梗阻是癌症的常见并发症。吸收不良通常发生在胰腺癌中酶的缺乏或继发于肠或肠系膜的淋巴瘤之后[79,80]。

胃排空延迟和蠕动减慢是导致早饱的致病机制[81]。早饱在上消化道蠕动减少的患者中很常见[82,83]。

生化和代谢紊乱

产生乳酸的葡萄糖高利用率是肿瘤细胞的特征性改变(Warburg效应)。在小鼠体内,移植肿瘤的葡萄糖利用率仅次于大脑[84]。己糖激酶,作为催化糖酵解途径的第一步,通常在肿瘤细胞中高度过表达,是该过程的主要参与者。

肿瘤己糖激酶与外部线粒体膜的结合使酶优先获得线粒体中产生的ATP并增加酶的活性和稳定性[85]。己糖激酶反应的最终产物,葡萄糖-6-磷酸,不仅通过糖酵解产生ATP,而且还是细胞生长和增殖所必需的代谢过程中的关键中间体。通过葡萄糖代谢产生的乳酸可以被其他组织用于供能,或者可以被运输到肝脏以再合成葡萄糖。这种循环代谢途径,也被称为Cori循环,此循环中葡萄糖在肿瘤组织中通过糖酵解转化为乳酸,然后再在肝脏中转化为葡萄糖。癌细胞中葡萄糖转化为乳酸产生2个ATP,而肝脏中乳酸转化为葡萄糖却需要消耗6个ATP。因此,全身能量丢失或无效的基质循环,涉及肿瘤糖酵解和宿主糖异生的相互作用,可能是癌症恶病质的重要原因[86]。假设产生的所有乳酸都被能再次转换成葡萄糖,那么癌细胞就像一个能量的寄生体。然而,也可以计算一下,如果85%的乳酸通过糖异生途径转化,而15%被氧化,那么宿主对肿瘤产生的乳酸的处理则可以认为是能量中立的。研究表明,Cori循环的增加在能量消耗方面是微不足道的,并且增加的葡萄糖分解代谢本身是体重减轻和恶病质发展的原因[87]。

无效循环的另一个机制是棕色脂肪组织(brown adipose tissues,UCP1)中和骨骼肌(UCP2和3)中的解偶联蛋白(uncoupling proteins,UCP)的活化[88~91]。

与6例体重稳定的胃肠道腺癌患者及6例对照组研究对象相比,6例体重明显减轻的胃肠道腺癌患者的肌肉中UCP-3mRNA水平更高。但UCP-2mRNA水平在各组之间没有显著差异[90]。肌肉UCP-3活性的升高可能会增加能量消耗,而这又可能导致组织的分解代谢。导致肌肉萎缩的其他机制也被证实存在,例如线粒体功能障碍和PPARγ共激活因子-1的活化[92~95]。

近期,对Warburg效应的重新审视正在广泛进行[96]。与大多数正常细胞不同,许多癌细胞从有氧糖酵解中获得大量的能量,即使在氧气存在下也能将大部分摄入的葡萄糖转化为乳酸。尽管通过糖酵解生成的ATP比通过氧化磷酸化生成ATP快,但就每单位葡萄糖消耗所生成的ATP而言,其效率要低得多。因此,这种转变要求肿瘤细胞实现异常高的葡萄糖摄取率以满足其对能量、生物合成和氧化还原的需要。有氧糖酵解为肿瘤细胞提供了生物合成优势,这是因为糖酵解的高通量底物能够有效地将碳分流至关键的辅助生物合成途径。由于癌症代谢改变而产生的关键分子是降低的烟酰胺维生素 B_4 二核苷酸磷酸盐(nicotinamide adenine dinu-cleotide phosphate,NADPH),它作为一种辅助因子,在许多大分子生物合成过程中,为至关重要的酶促反应中提供还原能力。NADPH也是一种抗氧化剂,也是对抗快速增殖过程中所产生的活性氧自由基(ROS)活性的组成成分。高浓度的ROS可以破坏大分子,诱导衰老和凋亡。谷胱甘肽(GSH)和硫氧还蛋白(TRX)也同样是抗氧化剂,它们在NADPH的作用下维持还原形式。除了改变肿瘤细胞代谢的遗传变化之外,微环境因素如缺氧、pH和低葡萄糖浓度等,也在确定肿瘤细胞的代谢表型中起主要作用。研究表明癌细胞能分泌过氧化氢。因此可以得出结论,癌症相关成纤维细胞中的氧化应激可以驱动自噬、线粒体自噬和有氧糖酵解。

这种"寄生"代谢偶联将基质转化为"工厂",用于局部再循环和高能量营养素(如L-乳酸)的生成,以促进癌细胞中的氧化线粒体代谢。基质Cavolin-1(Cav-1)的缺失已被证实为缺氧、氧化应激、自噬和"反向Warburg效应"的新的生物标志,它可以导致早期肿瘤复发和不良临床结果[97,98]。

活性氧自由基及氧化应激

在癌症恶病质过程中会发生中远端脂肪组织和肌肉的代谢重编程。脂肪酸被癌细胞摄取和分解以产生ATP并促进肿瘤生长。癌细胞经常侵入脂肪组织,诱导邻近脂肪细胞释放游离脂肪酸,这种释放作用会促进肿瘤生长。

血浆中高水平的游离脂肪酸是癌症恶病质和癌症晚期的关键特征。脂肪酸是用于筛选癌症恶病质的优选血浆分解代谢物,它是通过比较 ^{14}C 标记的棕榈酸酯和葡萄糖的消失并测量 ^{14}C 标记的 CO_2 的产生量来测量。在肿瘤细胞中,游离脂肪酸被分解代谢产生乙酰-CoA,酮体和ATP。总之,癌细胞对远端脂肪细胞和肌细胞产生的分解代谢作用类似于癌细胞对与癌细毗邻的成纤维细胞或肿瘤相关成纤维细胞施加的分解代谢作用。

脂肪组织甘油三酯水解酶(ATGL)和激素敏感性脂肪酶(HSL)是脂肪细胞产生游离脂肪酸并最终身成酮的关键酶。高ATGL和HSL活性与癌症恶病质,肌细胞凋亡和肌肉减少相关。在癌症恶病质中通过自噬和溶酶体降解诱导肌肉萎缩。ATGL和HSL敲除研究表明它们介导肌肉降解过程。这提示了代谢,自噬和恶病质之间显著的相互作用[99]。

MicroRNA,激素水平异常,肿瘤寄生及信号通路

在人恶病质模型中,基因表达的调节与miR-378有关[100,101]。有报道显示,晚期肿瘤患者睾酮水平降低[102,103],血浆皮质醇含量升高[104,105]。这些发现可能与恶病质癌症患者骨骼肌和其他器官蛋白质分解代谢增加有关。

参与癌症恶病质的信号转导途径示于表124-5中。

涉及肌肉萎缩的信号通路是相互依赖的。单一途径的激活或抑制可能对肌肉蛋白质平衡具有级联效应。没有任何一条通路可以单独调控这一过程[132]。

表 124-5　肿瘤恶病质相关信号通路

信号		表达功能	参考文献
NF-κB 依赖的信号途径（IL-1 /TNFα/ TWEAK（和 PIF）↑→TRAF6→NF-κB/ JNK / p38 / ERK→半胱氨酸蛋白酶→MyoD mRNA）（TWEAK→NF-κB ↑→MuRF1 ↑→MyHC 丢失）	↑	凋亡增加 促进蛋白质降解	12,15,106-108,109-113
泛素 - 蛋白酶体途径（UPP）（肌肉特异性泛素连接酶 MAFbx / atrogin-1 ↑和 MuRF1 ↑→肌原纤维蛋白降解）	↑	促进肌原纤维蛋白的降解	58,61a,62a,114a,115-119a,120a,121-123
肌肉生长抑制素/激活素途径（肌肉生长抑制素/ ActRIIB→SMAD2,3→UPP,→AKT,→MAFbx 及 MuRF1）	↑	负向调节肌原纤维蛋白	60,124-126
自噬 - 溶酶体途径（FOXO3A→自噬→组织蛋白酶 B / L）	↑	促进蛋白质降解	61,62,127
IL-6,JAK / STAT 途径（IL-6→gp130→JAK→STAT3→pSTAT3）	↑	促进蛋白质降解（肌原纤维和肌节蛋白）	17-32
抗肌萎缩蛋白糖蛋白复合物（DGC）（肌纤维外膜缺陷和细胞外基质蛋白改变→MAFbx / atrogin-1 ↑和 MuRF1 ↑）	↑	肌肉膜损伤和肌肉萎缩	59
钙依赖性蛋白水解系统（IL-1 /TNFα→p38 / JAK→catepsin→钙蛋白酶和 caspase-3→细胞凋亡）	↑	降低肌肉蛋白质（癌症恶病质中没有报道确切的肌肉位置）	61,120,128
IGF-1 途径（IGF-1 ↓→PI3K→AKT→的 mTOR→↓蛋白质合成）	↓	促进蛋白质降解和增加细胞凋亡	129
丝裂原活化蛋白激酶（MAPKs）,PGC-1α 和 caspase 途径（p38 MAPKs→PGC-1α→ERK1 / 2→JAK→Caspase 8）	↑	拮抗 MAFbx 和 MuRF1,抑制产热作用,抑制骨骼肌	94
聚（ADP-核糖）聚合酶（PARP ↑→细胞凋亡↑→MyoD 的蛋白↓）	↑	肌肉 DNA 片段化胞凋亡,MyoD 下调	130,131a

PIF,蛋白水解诱导因子；MyHC,肌球蛋白重链；PGC-1α,PPARγ 辅激活物-1α；PARP,聚（ADP-核糖）聚合酶。
动物数据不一定可以在患者中重现。参考文献报告了阴性临床数。

治疗

癌症恶病质的根本治疗方法是去除致病肿瘤。在没有实现这一目标的情况下,尽管可采取以下各种措施,但成效有限。

支持治疗

对恶病质发之前早期干预会有帮助。早期营养干预可以改善营养状况并减少炎症反应[133]。化疗期间体重稳定与化疗毒性减低和总体生存期延长有关[5]。

运动在预防癌症方面是有效的[134],在癌症治疗期间是安全的[135],对于癌症患者来说是有利健康的[136],运动可以改善骨骼健康、肌肉力量、生活质量、疲劳、心理社会困扰、抑郁,提升自尊[137]。发生并发症的风险在癌症幸存者中较频繁,可以通过增加身体活动来显著减少。此外,运动与整体死亡率降低相关[138]。体力活动可通过调节肌肉代谢,胰岛素敏感性和炎症来减轻恶病质的作用[137~139]。运动已被证明通过上调抗骨骼肌和脂肪组织中的炎症细胞因子从而达到抗炎作用。应该建议在癌症治疗的最早阶段运动[139],最好在运动期间有一位护理人员或运动专业人员的帮助。

药物治疗

奥氮平是一种选择性单胺能拮抗剂,对 5-羟色胺和多巴胺受体具有很强的亲和性。低剂量的奥氮平具有良好的耐受性,对癌症恶病质的体重、营养和功能恢复具有良好的临床作用[140]。

胃促生长素及其类似物阿拉莫林、BIM-28131、BIM-28125 和 RC-1291。

2010 年,17 名体重减轻的患有实体胃肠道肿瘤的癌症患者开始长期服用胃促生长素[141]。在高剂量或低剂量胃促生长素的随机研究中,高剂量组可改善食欲并减少全身脂肪损失（$P<0.04$）,降低血清 GH（$P<0.05$）。没有观察到不良反应。这些数据使研究人员测试了许多合成的胃促生长素类似物的功效,包括阿拉莫林,BIM-28125,BIM-28131（RM-131）,L163255 和 RC-1291。

阿拉莫林（ONO-7643）（Helsinn Healthcare S. A. Switzerland）是一种新型口服胃促生长素受体激动剂。

在一项缓解癌症患者恶病质的药物和安慰剂短暂交叉临床研究中发现,IGF-1 会使食欲和体重显著增加[142]。

在设计相同的Ⅲ期临床研究 ROMANA 1 和 2 中,将 484 例和 495 例无法手术的Ⅲ期和Ⅳ期非小细胞肺癌,合并恶病质,预期寿命>4 个月的患者,以 2∶1的比例随机分配接受阿拉莫林 100mg/d 或安慰剂 12 周。大多数患者接受化疗,八分之一接受放射治疗。恶病质定义为过去 6 个月内体重减轻超过 5%或体重指数低于 20kg/m^2。两项研究均发现,在 12 周的研究期间,随机分配到安慰剂组的患者体重继续减轻,瘦体重减轻,而分配给阿拉莫林的患者则瘦体重增加。两组体重之间的差异在第 3 周、第 6 周、第 9 周和第 12 周时非常显著,两个实验瘦体重的中位数中分别为 1.10kg 和 0.75kg,而安慰剂组为负 0.44kg 和 0.96kg。阿拉莫林组的体重平均增加 2.2kg 和 0.95kg,而安慰剂组的体重增加 0.14kg 和 0.57kg。在研究过程中发现两组的握力均下降。通过厌食/恶病质治疗功能评估表(FAACT)来评估生活质量也显示出有利于阿拉莫林的显著差异。最常见的不良事件是可控制的恶心和高血糖(预期作为作用机制的一部分)[143]。

BIM-28125是另一种合成胃促生长素类似物,在癌症恶病质的实验模型中具有相似的作用[144],临床试验尚未见报道。最近有报告综述了胃促生长素及其类似物对癌症恶病质的影响[145,146]。

运动员使用同化雄性类固醇类药物来促进肌肉生长和力量。为了证实补充诺龙癸酸是否能够影响非小细胞肺癌患者化疗的效果[147,148],进行了相关随机对照临床试验。

该研究显示,尽管治疗组显示更少的体重下降,两组化疗反应率和生存期却无明显差异。另有一项三臂的Ⅲ期随机对照临床实验表明,氟甲睾酮,合成类固醇的一种,在治疗肿瘤相关恶病质方面,与孕激素甲地孕酮和糖皮质激素地塞米松相比,刺激食欲的作用显著降低,同时减轻毒性方面也未显示出明显优势[149]。

enobosarm(GTx-024)是一种雄激素受体调节剂(SARM),在肌肉和骨骼中具有组织选择性合成代谢作用。在159名癌症患者中(按癌症类型分层),每日1次口服enobosarm或安慰剂给药长达113日。发现总瘦体重显著增加。数据表明enobosarm可能导致瘦体重的改善,而没有与雄激素和孕激素相关的毒性作用[150]。

醋酸甲地孕酮和醋酸甲羟孕酮

在醋酸甲地孕酮治疗的癌症患者中观察到血清IL-1a、IL-1b、IL-2、IL-6和TNF-α水平显著降低,这可能与改善食欲和体重增加的机制有关[151]。

在对包括2 000多名患者在内的15项随机临床试验进行的综述中,高剂量孕激素在改善食欲和增加体重方面具有统计学意义[152]。醋酸甲地孕酮产生的体重增加主要来自增加身体脂肪而不是瘦肉组织[153,154]。有人认为,醋酸甲地孕酮治疗过程中主要增加脂肪组织虽然这一情况不是最理想的,但不应该被贬低,因为体内脂肪的消耗通常是癌症的不良后果。

醋酸甲地孕酮禁用于小儿恶病质患者,因为这类患者中有相当一部分患有肾上腺皮质功能不全[155]。老年癌症患者也应谨慎使用醋酸甲地孕酮因为卧床和血清纤维蛋白原增加而容易发生深静脉血栓形成。

醋酸甲羟孕酮是一种更广泛使用的合成孕激素。甲羟孕酮减少了细胞因子和血清素的产生[156]。已经报道了两项安慰剂对照随机研究[157,158]。尽管食欲增加,但两项研究均未产生体重增加。

在胃排空延迟或胃轻瘫的晚期癌症患者中,口服给予促运动剂,甲氧氯普胺,口服每次10mg,三餐前和睡前共4次,可有效刺激食欲,缓解与厌食相关的其他消化不良症状[159,160]。即使没有证实胃肠道存在异常,控释制剂似乎比立即释放药物更有效,因为它控制了与晚期癌症相关的恶心[161]。

在癌症患者中进行了屈大麻酚的研究[162,163]。所有患者均表示食欲有所改善,但所有患者均继续出现体重减轻。最近,一项随机研究比较了屈大麻酚、醋酸甲地孕酮及两者组合对缓解癌症相关厌食的作用[164]。与单用屈大麻酚相比,醋酸甲地孕酮对晚期癌症患者的厌食缓解更胜一筹,甲地孕酮和屈大麻酚的组合似乎没有带来额外的获益。

大麻粉和烟含有许多不同的大麻类物质,据报道比合成的屈大麻酚更好。科学实验还没有完成,但随着广泛的合法化现在是可能的。

癌症恶病质不等同于简单的饥饿,无论是肠内还是肠外营养支持,仅具有有限的作用。

全肠外营养被证实对于接受化疗和或放疗的患者在治疗耐受性,治疗反应或总生存方面没有显著益处[165,166]。此外,还有其他作者报道全肠外营养治疗是有害的,与肠外营养治疗相关的争议还有待进一步确证[167~169]。

从上述讨论中可以推测单一疗法可能不能成功地治疗恶病质。不同组合的治疗方案可能更有益处[170]。

未来方向与小结

目前人们已经认识到对癌症恶病质的诊断经常太晚,从而不能通过营养补充来逆转。这使得恶病质的早期识别和干预很重要。现在看来,在恶病质前期的早期营养干预是有效的,恶病质前期的概念更有意义。随着对恶病质前期的认识以及各种抗癌药物的出现,我们正处于完成恶病质的有效治疗阶段。

体育锻炼应该是任何抗恶病质治疗方案的一部分。一些潜在的有希望的线索需要进行精心设计的临床试验加以验证。需要更多临床研究的药物包括生长激素/胰岛素[171],生长激素释放肽2(growth hormone releasing peptide 2,GHRP-2)[172,173]和生长激素释放激素表达质粒[174]。

最有希望的抗恶病质药物是胃促生长素类似物,如阿拉莫林[143]。可能用于补充的其他抗恶病质药包括醋酸甲羟孕酮[156~158]、塞来昔布(celecoxib)[175,176]、抗氧化剂[177,178]、奥氮平[140]、天然大麻和β-羟基-β-甲基丁酸酯/L-精氨酸/L-谷氨酰胺[179~183]。

具有潜在益处的研究药物包括胃促生长素模拟物,例如BIM-28131[144],BIM-28125[144],L163255[184]和RC-1291[185];雄激素受体调节剂enobosarm(GTx-024)[150];合成代谢分解代谢转化剂MT-102和espindrol[186,187];抗IL-1α抗体MABp1[188,189];抗IL-1受体拮抗剂IP-1510[189];抗IL-6抗体ALD518[189~191];肌肉生长抑制素抑制剂如bimagrumab(BYM338)[189]和REGN1033[189]以及一种广谱肽-核酸免疫调节剂OHR/AVR118[189]。

恶病质一直以来未引起足够重视,并且目前临床治疗方案并不能满足治疗要求,重新定义癌症恶病质,在恶病质前期早期干预治疗应该彻底改变这种复杂疾病的治疗方法,对所有类型的癌症治疗都有重大益处。

(崔久嵬 李玲玉 译)

参考文献

The complete reference list can be found on the Wiley Companion Digital Edition of this title (see inside front cover for login instructions).

1 Fearon KCH, Glass DJ, Guttridge DC. Cancer Cachexia: mediators, signaling, and metabolic pathways. *Cell Metab*. 2012;**16**:153–166.

2 von Haehling S, Anker SD. Cachexia as a major underestimated and unmet medical need: facts and numbers. *J Cachexia Sarcopenia Muscle*. 2010;1:1–5.

7 Englesbe MJ, Lee JS, He K, et al. Analytic morphomics, core muscle size, and surgical outcomes. *Ann Surg*. 2012;**256**:255–261.

10 Fearon K, Strasser F, Anker SD, et al. Definition and classification of cancer cachexia: an international consensus. *Lancet Oncol*. 2011;**12**:489–495.

11 Aapro M, Arends J, Bozzetti F, et al. Early recognition of malnutrition and cachexia in the cancer patient: a position paper of a European School of Oncology Task Force. *Ann Oncol*. 2014;**25**:1492–1499.

33 Inui A. Cancer anorexia-cachexia syndrome: are neuropeptides the key? *Cancer Res*. 1999;**59**:4493–4501.

54 Johns NA, Stephens KCH, Fearon KC. Muscle wasting in cancer. *Int J Biochem Cell*

Biol. 2013;**45**:2215–2229.

59 Acharyya S, Butchbach ME, Sahenk Z, et al. Dystrophin glycoprotein complex dysfunction: a regulatory link between muscular dystrophy and cancer cachexia. *Cancer Cell.* 2005;**8**:421–432.

61 Jagoe RT, Redfern CP, Roberts RG, et al. Skeletal muscle mRNA levels for cathepsin B, but not components of the ubiquitin-proteasome pathway, are increased in patients with lung cancer referred for thoracotomy. *Clin Sci (Lond).* 2002;**102**:353–361.

62 Tardif N, Klaude M, Lundell L, et al. Autophagic-lysosomal patway is the main proteolytic system modified in the skeletal muscle of esophageal cancer patients. *Am J Clin Nutr.* 2013;**98**:1485–1492.

63 Schwartz MW, Woods SC, Porte D Jr, et al. Central nervous system control of food intake. *Nature.* 2000;**404**:661–671.

69 Molfino A, Gioia G, Muscaritoli M. The hunger hormone ghrelin in cachexia. *Expert Opin Biol Ther.* 2013;**13**:465–468.

86 Mathupala SP, Rempel A, Pedersen PL. Glucose catabolism in cancer cells: identification and characterization of a marked activation response of the type II hexokinase gene to hypoxic conditions. *J Biol Chem.* 2001;**276**:43407–43412.

90 Collins P, McCulloch P, Williams G. Muscle UCP-3 mRNA levels are elevated in weight loss associated with gastrointestinal adenocarcinoma in humans. *Br J Cancer.* 2002;**86**:372–375.

94 Puigserver P, Rhee J, Lin J, et al. Cytokine stimulation of energy expenditure through p38 MAP kinase activation of PPARγ coactivator-1. *Mol Cell.* 2001;**8**:971–982.

96 Cainns RA, Harris IS, Mak TW. Regulation of cancer cell metabolism. *Nat Rev Cancer.* 2011;**11**:85–95.

99 Martinez-Outschoorn UE, Lisanti MP, Sotgia F. Catabolic cancer-associated fibroblasts transfer energy and biomass to anabolic cancer cells, fueling tumor growth. *Semin Cancer Biol.* 2014;**25**:47–60.

106 Guttridge DC, Mayo MW, Madrid LV, et al. NF-kappaB-induced loss of MyoD messenger RNA: possible role in muscle decay and cachexia. *Science.* 2000;**289**:2363–2366.

113 Kumar A, Bhatnagar S, Paul PK. TWEAK TRAF6 regulate skeletal muscle atrophy. *Curr Opin Clin Nutr Metab Care.* 2012;**15**:233–239.

114 Op den Kamp CM, Langen RC, Minnaard R, et al. Pre-cachexia in patients with stages I-III non-small cell lung cancer: systemic inflammation and functional impairment without activation of skeletal muscle ubiquitin proteasome system. *Lung Cancer.* 2012;**76**:112–117.

115 Gomes MD, Lecker SH, Jagoe RT, et al. Atrogin-1, a muscle-specific F-box protein highly expressed during muscle atrophy. *Proc Natl Acad Sci U S A.* 2001;**98**:14440–14445.

116 Bodine SC, Latres E, Baumhueter S, et al. Identification of ubiquitin ligases required for skeletal muscle atrophy. *Science.* 2001;**294**:1704–1708.

120 Smith IJ, Aversa Z, Hasselgren P-O, et al. Calpain activity is increased in skeletal muscle from gastric cancer patients with no or minimal weight loss. *Muscle Nerve.* 2011;**43**:410–414.

131 Bossola M, Mirabella M, Ricci E, et al. Skeletal muscle apoptosis is not increased in gastric cancer patients with mild–moderate weight loss. *Int J Biochem Cell Biol.* 2006;**38**:1561–1570.

134 Thompson R. Preventing cancer: the role of food, nutrition and physical activity. *J Fam Health Care.* 2010;**20**:100–102.

136 Rock CL, Doyle C, Demark-Wahnefried W, et al. Nutrition and physical activity guidelines for cancer survivors. *CA Cancer J Clin.* 2012;**62**:243–274.

140 Braiteh F, Dalal S, Khuwaja A, et al. Phase I pilot study of the safety and tolerability of olanzapine (OZA) for the treatment of cachexia in patients with advanced cancer. *J Clin Oncol.* 2008;**26**:196–203.

142 Garcia JM, Friend J, Allen S. Therapeutic potential of anamorelin, a novel, oral ghrelin mimetic, in patients with cancer-related cachexia: a multicenter, randomized, double-blind, crossover, pilot study. *Support Care Cancer.* 2013;**21**:129–137.

143 Temel J, Currow D, Fearon K, et al. Anamorelin for the treatment of cancer anorexia-cachexia in NSCLC: Results from the phase 3 studies ROMANA 1 and 2. ESMO Congress, Barcelona, Spain. Abst 14830-PR. Presented September 27, 2014.

145 Molfino A, Formiconi A, Rossi Fanelli F, et al. Ghrelin: from discovery to cancer cachexia therapy. *Curr Opin Clin Nutr Metab Care.* 2014;**17**:471–476.

146 Argiles JM, Stemmler B. The potential of ghrelin in the treatment of cancer cachexia. *Expert Opin Biol Ther.* 2013;**13**:67–76.

150 Dobs AS, Boccia RV, Croot CC, et al. Effects of enobosarm on muscle wasting and physical function in patients with cancer: a double-blind, randomised controlled phase 2 trial. *Lancet Oncol.* 2013;**14**:335–345.

152 Pascual Lopez A, Roque i Figuls M, Urrutia Cuchi G, et al. Systematic review of megestrol acetate in the treatment of anorexia-cachexia syndrome. *J Pain Symptom Manag.* 2004;**27**:360–369.

153 Loprinzi CL, Schaid DJ, Dose AM, et al. Body-composition changes in patients who gain weight while receiving megestrol acetate. *J Clin Oncol.* 1993;**11**:152–154.

170 Argiles JM, Lopez-Soriano J, Busquets S. Novel approaches to the treatment of cachexia. *Drug Discov Today.* 2008;**13**:73–78.

176 Mantovani G, Macciò A, Madeddu C, et al. Phase II nonrandomized study of the efficacy and safety of COX-2 inhibitor celecoxib on patients with cancer cachexia. *J Mol Med (Berl).* 2010;**88**:85–92.

188 Ma JD, Heavey SF, Revta C, Roeland EJ. Novel investigational biologics for the treatment of cancer cachexia. *Expert Opin Biol Ther.* 2014;**14**:1113–1120.

190 Clarke SJ, Gebbie C, Sweeney C, et al. A phase I, pharmacokinetic (PK), and preliminary efficacy assessment of ALD518, a humanized anti-IL-6 antibody, in patients with advanced cancer. *J Cachexia Sarcopenia Muscle.* 2010;**1**:98.

第 125 章　止吐治疗

Patrick M. Forde，MD，MBBCh ■ David S. Ettinger，MD，FACP，FCCP

概述

自从 20 世纪 90 年代早期应用的 5-HT_3 受体拮抗剂和 2003 年应用的 NK-1 受体拮抗剂阿瑞匹坦（aprepitant）以来，在预防和治疗化疗导致的呕吐方面已经取得了巨大的进展。最近的调查表明了对于化疗引起的急性呕吐的认识有待进一步提高，特别是关于延迟性恶心和呕吐的频率及严重程度。幸运的是，新药的研发进一步增强止吐药的药效。同时针灸和身心干预等补充疗法也似乎有望能控制化疗导致的恶心，其作用也正在进一步探索。根据预防性止吐治疗的指南来适当地使用特定的化疗药物将减少肿瘤患者出现这些最令人痛苦的化疗副作用。

概述

尽管近年来药物治疗取得了很大的进展，对很多癌症患者而言，化疗导致的恶心和呕吐（chemotherapy-induced nausea and vomiting，CINV）仍然是很严重的问题[1]。除了对机体产生一些不良后果（包括脱水、营养不良、代谢紊乱等）之外，CINV 对患者的生活质量也会产生很大的影响[2]。尽管有关预防性止吐治疗的指南已经颁布，一些患者仍然未能接受理想的预防性抗 CINV 的措施。与化疗前就用合适的药物预防恶心呕吐相比，化疗后产生的恶心呕吐更难控制。此外，如果既往所接受的止吐治疗不够有效，患者可能会对恶心和呕吐产生畏惧心理。因此，对 CINV 的理想控制是控制癌症患者症状的一个非常关键的方面。

在过去，所有接受化疗的癌症患者中，70%～80%会发生呕吐[3]。所幸的是，自从引入有效的止吐治疗后，对呕吐的控制有了明显的进步[1]。过去的 20 年中，很多研究尝试量化化疗副反应对癌症患者的影响。而恶心和呕吐被反复提到是“主要的躯体反应”[4]和“最麻烦和最令人不愉快”的化疗相关副反应[5]。近年来我们在药物预防 CINV 方面取得了进步，但 de Boer-dennert 等在 1997 年发起的一项研究显示，尽管在引入了 5-HT_3 拮抗剂后，恶心和呕吐的总发生率及严重程度有了下降，但它们仍然分别排在最令人感到难受的化疗相关副反应的第一和第三位[6]。Grunberg 等在 2001—2002 年间对患者、肿瘤内科医师以及肿瘤科护士进行调研，以评价 CINV 发生的频率以及医疗实施者对 CINV 的认识[1]。尽管在预防急性恶心和呕吐方面有了提高（急性恶心约 35%，急性呕吐约 13%），延迟性症状的发生频率仍然很高（依据化疗方案的不同，延迟性恶心的发生率在 50%～60%，延迟性呕吐的发生率在 30%～50%）。令人震惊的是，超过 75%的医生和护士低估了延迟性恶性呕吐的发生率。只有更加关注目前存在的问题并更好地使用现有的医疗措施，我们才能在减轻 CINV 的症状方面取得进步。

本章的重点包括 CINV 的病理生理学机制，常见化疗药物的致吐潜能，包括支持治疗在内的止吐措施的分级，以及预防和迅速控制 CINV 的指南。

恶心及呕吐的病理生理学机制

呕吐是由中枢神经系统通过各种传入神经和神经递质组成的复杂通路控制的。在 20 世纪 50 年代，Borison 及 Wang 的研究明确了脑干中与恶心和呕吐相关的两个区域：化学感受器触发区（chemoreceptor trigger zone，CTZ）和催吐中枢[7]。CTZ 位于第四脑室底部的延髓后极区。由于 CTZ 位于血-脑脊液屏障的外部，它对于血流中的诸如化疗药物及其代谢产物等致吐性刺激非常敏感[8]。在 CTZ 上有毒蕈碱、多巴胺 D_2、羟色胺（5-HT_3）、神经激肽 1（NK-1）以及组胺 H_1 的受体。来自 CTZ 的冲动可以传导到催吐中枢，除此之外，来自胃肠道和咽部的传入冲动也可通过迷走神经和内脏神经传导到催吐中枢并在此协调整合[9]。尤其是在预期性呕吐中，来自大脑皮质的冲动也会参与。催吐中枢能够接受传入冲动并协调流涎中枢、腹部肌肉、呼吸中枢以及自主神经的传出活动，最终形成呕吐。催吐中枢位于脑干的孤束核，由这些弥散的受体及效应核组成[8]。

在这些传入及传出通路中最重要的神经递质有羟色胺（5-HT_3）、多巴胺以及 P 物质。其他还包括乙酰胆碱、类固醇、组胺、大麻、阿片和氨酪酸（GABA）[10]。各种止吐药物的药理机制就是阻断以上这些神经递质与其受体的结合。20 世纪 90 年代初，5-HT_3 受体拮抗剂的问世是止吐治疗历史上最重大的进步[6]。与 NK-1 受体结合的 P 物质是近来止吐治疗中的一个新靶点[11]，阿瑞匹坦是一个已获得美国食品药品监督局（FDA）批准的 NK-1 受体阻滞剂，该药已经在止吐治疗中显示出较好的临床疗效[12～14]。诸如甲哌氯奥沙普秦，氟哌利多以及甲氧氯普胺等药物都是通过抑制多巴胺发挥其止吐作用的。然而，目前仍不清楚化疗药物及其代谢产物是在呕吐神经通路的什么部位以及是通过何种机制产生催吐作用的。化疗代谢产物能够直接刺激 CTZ。羟色胺和其他神经递质可能是从被化疗破坏的肠道细胞释放出来的。感受神经元可以释放 P 物质，在 CTZ 和孤束核中已经发现大量的 NK-1 受体。尽管对中枢神经系统以及控制呕吐的神经通路的认识越来越多，但目前还没有发现有一条共同的通路，因此用单药完全预防化疗所致的呕吐仍不现实。

呕吐的分类

化疗所致的呕吐一般分为三类:急性、延迟性和预期性呕吐。

急性呕吐定义为化疗开始后 24h 内发生的恶心和呕吐。如果不进行充足的预防,急性呕吐在化疗后 1~2h 即可发生,在化疗后 4~6h 达到高峰。

延迟性呕吐是指在化疗开始 24h 后发生的恶心和呕吐。比较典型的延迟性呕吐一般在化疗开始后 48~72h 达到高峰,并能够持续 6~7 日。尽管延迟性呕吐的发生率及严重程度可能不如急性呕吐,但它也不如急性呕吐容易控制。与延迟性呕吐最相关的化疗药物是顺铂,此外,卡铂、环磷酰胺和蒽环类药物也可导致延迟性呕吐。预期性呕吐发生在此前曾经历过严重恶心呕吐的患者,这些患者在化疗开始之前就会产生条件反射般的恶心呕吐。

预期性呕吐可由与化疗相关的视觉或活动(如前往治疗中心)而激发。由于预期性呕吐是一种条件反射,它主要是由大脑皮质介导的。随着对 CINV 更好的控制,预期性呕吐的发生率已经明显下降[15]。

暴发性呕吐是指即使进行了预防性治疗但仍出现的呕吐,还需要进行解救性治疗。这是一个难以处理的临床问题,几乎没有临床试验数据来指导这种情况下的止吐药物的选择[16,17]。包括氟哌利多、奥氮平和氯氮平在内的集中药物已经进行了经验性用药[16,17]。

难治性呕吐是指在以往化疗周期中预防性和/或解救性治疗失败,而在接下来的化疗周期中仍然出现的呕吐症状。

除化疗外,其他可导致癌症患者恶心呕吐的潜在因素还包括:不完全或完全性肠梗阻、脑转移、血尿、电解质紊乱(如高血糖、高钙血症、低钠血症)以及胃麻痹。一些癌症患者经常处方用的药物,如阿片类药物,也可能导致呕吐。

致吐性化疗

CINV 的严重性及频率因患者及化疗药物的不同而异。预测 CINV 高发的患者相关性因素包括:有化疗史、有 CINV 史、女性、年纪较轻者、有晕车史以及无饮酒史。化疗相关性因素包括化疗的给药途径、化疗药物的强度。最具有预测意义的因素是所用的化疗药物[18]。

目前并没有一个被大家广泛认可的对化疗药物致呕吐潜能进行分级的系统(表 125-1)。由 Hesketh 等所制定的同时也是最为大家接受的分级系统依据在不进行预防性止吐的情况下患者发生恶心呕吐的概率将化疗药物的催吐能力分为五个级别。具体为:第一级,少于 10% 的患者呕吐;第二级,10%~30%;第三级,30%~60%;第四级,60%~90%;第五级,超过 90% 的患者在不进行预防性止吐处理时会发生呕吐[19]。最近的一项改良将化疗药物的催吐风险分为四个级别[20]。

表 125-1 单个化疗药物的致吐潜能

致吐水平	药物
高危,5 级(不预防情况下预期发生呕吐概率>90%)	卡莫司汀>250mg/m^2
	顺铂≥50mg/m^2
	环磷酰胺>1 500mg/m^2
	达卡巴嗪
	氮芥
	链佐星(streptozocin)
中危,4 级(不预防情况下预期发生呕吐概率在 60%~90%)	氨磷汀>500mg/m^2
	白消安>4mg/d
	卡铂
	顺铂<50mg/m^2
	环磷酰胺>750mg/m^2 且≤1 500mg/m^2
	阿糖胞苷>1g/m^2
	放线菌素 D
	多柔比星>60mg/m^2
	表柔比星>90mg/m^2
	美法仑>50mg/m^2
	甲氨蝶呤>1 000mg/m^2
	丙卡巴肼(procarbazine)(口服)
中危,3 级(不预防情况下预期发生呕吐概率在 30%~60%)	氨磷汀>300mg/m^2 且≤500mg/m^2
	三氧化二砷
	苯达莫司汀
	环磷酰胺≤750mg/m^2
	环磷酰胺(口服)
	多柔比星 20~60mg/m^2
	表柔比星≤90mg/m^2
	异环磷酰胺
	IL-2>1 200 万~1 500 万单位/m^2
	伊立替康
	洛莫司汀
	甲氨蝶呤 250~1 000mg/m^2
	米托蒽醌<15mg/m^2
	奥沙利铂>75mg/m^2
低危,2 级(不预防情况下预期发生呕吐概率在 10%~30%)	氨磷汀≤300mg/m^2
	贝沙罗汀
	阿糖胞苷 100~200mg/m^2
	卡培他滨
	多西他赛
	多柔比星(脂质体剂型)
	依托泊苷

续表

致吐水平	药物
	氟尿嘧啶<1 000mg/m^2
	吉西他滨
	甲氨蝶呤 50~250mg/m^2
	丝裂霉素
	米托蒽醌
	紫杉醇
	培美曲塞
	替莫唑胺
	托泊替康
极低危，1 级（不预防情况下预期发生呕吐概率<10%）	阿伦珠单抗
	天门冬酰胺酶
	贝伐单抗
	α 干扰素
	博来霉素
	硼替佐米
	西妥昔单抗（cetuximab）
	苯丁酸氮芥（口服）
	克拉屈滨（cladribine）
	达沙替尼
	右丙亚胺（dexrazoxane）
	地尼重组人白介素-2
	厄洛替尼
	氟达拉滨（fludarabine）
	吉非替尼（gefitinib）
	吉姆单抗
	羟基脲
	甲磺酸伊马替尼
	美法仑（低剂量，口服剂型）
	甲氨蝶呤≤50mg/m^2
	喷司他丁（pentostatin）
	利妥昔单抗
	索拉非尼（sorafenib）
	舒尼替尼
	巯鸟嘌呤（口服）
	曲妥珠单抗（trastuzumab）
	戊柔比星
	长春碱
	长春新碱
	长春瑞滨

高风险（第五级）：超过 90%

中等风险（第三级和第四级）：30%~90%

低风险（第二级）：10%~30%

极低风险（第一级）：少于 10%

须要注意的是这些分级系统均是按照急性呕吐来划分的。而近期的资料显示延迟性呕吐的发生率及严重程度往往被低估，因此对很多患者而言，这还是一个很大的问题[1]。根据预期症状发生的持续天数，应该给予相应足够的预防性止吐处理。

止吐药物的分类

对调节呕吐反应的中枢神经系统通路中已知神经递质的认识，我们确定了抗呕吐治疗的靶点（表 125-2）。反过来，这些药物在临床中的成功应用也证实了以上神经递质及其受体在呕吐通路中的重要性。控制呕吐的神经受体包括毒蕈碱（M1，乙酰胆碱受体部位），多巴胺（D_2，多巴胺受体部位），组胺（H_1，组胺受体部位），5-HT_3（羟色胺受体部位），NK-1（P 物质受体部位）以及 GABA（苯二氮䓬类受体部位）[21,22]。最有效及最常用的止吐药物有 5-HT_3 受体拮抗剂，多巴胺拮抗剂以及类固醇药物。NK-1 受体拮抗剂作为一类新的药物，进一步扩大了止吐药物的种类。

表 125-2　常见止吐药物的分类及推荐剂量

药物	分类	使用途径	剂量
昂丹司琼	5-HT_3 受体拮抗剂	IV	8~12mg
		PO	12~24mg
格拉司琼		IV	1mg 或 0.01mg/kg
		PO	2mg
多拉司琼		IV	100mg 或 1.8mg/kg
		PO	100mg
帕洛诺司琼		IV	0.25mg
阿瑞匹坦	NK-1 受体拮抗剂	PO	第一天 125mg 第二、三天 80mg
地塞米松	类固醇	IV	8~20mg
		PO	8~20mg
甲哌氯奥沙普秦	多巴胺受体拮抗剂	IV	10mg
		PO	10mg
		直肠栓剂	25mg
甲氧氯普胺	多巴胺受体拮抗剂	IV	1~2mg/kg
		PO	20~40mg
氟哌利多	多巴胺受体拮抗剂	IV	1~3mg
		PO	1~2mg
屈大麻酚	大麻酚	PO	5~10mg

IV，静脉注射；5-HT_3，羟色胺；NK，神经激肽；PO，口服。

羟色胺/5-HT$_3$ 受体拮抗剂

在 20 世纪 90 年代的早期，美国批准了四个 5-HT$_3$ 受体拮抗剂：昂丹司琼，格拉司琼，多拉司琼（dolasetron）以及最近批准的帕洛诺司琼（palonosetron）。这些药物革新了高度及中度致吐性化疗的预防性止吐措施。研究发现单用 5-HT$_3$ 受体拮抗剂与单用高剂量甲氧氯普胺相比有更好的疗效[23]，与高剂量甲氧氯普胺联合地塞米松相比疗效相似，而后者是这类患者之前的标准治疗[24]。然而，经过验证联合应用 5-HT$_3$ 受体拮抗剂与地塞米松是最为有效的[25]。5-HT$_3$ 受体拮抗剂仍然是预防高度及中度致吐性化疗的基石。在 2003 年之前，FDA 批准了三个 5-HT$_3$ 受体拮抗剂：昂丹司琼、格拉司琼、多拉司琼。尽管这三个药物在临床前研究中显示了不同的效果，很多临床研究都显示它们的临床疗效相似[26~31]。化疗前给予单剂量的效果与给予多剂量的效果相似[32~34]。此外，这些药物口服与静脉应用的效果也没有明显差别[35,36]。在 2003 年 7 月，一个新的 5-HT$_3$ 受体拮抗剂，帕洛诺司琼，被 FDA 批准用于预防性止吐。与其他羟色胺拮抗剂相比该药的优点在于它与 5-HT$_3$ 受体具有更高的亲和力并且半衰期更长。两个Ⅲ期临床研究显示帕洛诺司琼效果优于昂丹司琼和多拉司琼，尤其在预防延迟性恶心和呕吐方面更优[37,38]。在第一个研究中，592 例患者在中度致吐性化疗前 30min 随机接受帕洛诺司琼 0.25mg 或者 0.75mg 或者多拉司琼 100mg。少于 5%的患者同时接受了类固醇激素的治疗。在帕洛诺司琼 0.25mg 剂量组和多拉司琼组之间完全缓解（complete remission，CR）率具有明显的差别。CR 的定义为在化疗开始后的第一个 24h 中没有呕吐并且没有进行解救性止吐。帕洛诺司琼 0.25mg 组的 CR 率为 63%，而多拉司琼组的 CR 率为 52.9%（P=0.049），帕洛诺司琼 0.75mg 组的 CR 率为 57%（P=0.412）。就对延迟性恶心呕吐（24～120h）的完全控制（定义为无呕吐，无须解救性止吐，除轻度恶心外没有其他症状）率而言，帕洛诺司琼 0.25mg 组与 0.75mg 组较多拉司琼 100mg 组有明显的提高（帕洛诺司琼 0.25mg 组为 48.1%，多拉司琼组为 36.1%，P=0.027；帕洛诺司琼 0.75mg 组为 51.9%，P=0.016）。各组之间头疼、便秘和疲乏等副反应的发生率没有明显差别[37]。在第二项研究中，帕洛诺司琼是与昂丹司琼 32mg 进行比较的。570 例接受中度致吐性化疗的患者在化疗的第一天随机进入帕洛诺司琼的两个剂量组（0.25mg 或者 0.75mg）或昂丹司琼 32mg 组。没有患者接受类固醇激素。帕洛诺司琼 0.25mg 组在急性和延迟性呕吐方面的 CR 率均较昂丹司琼组明显高（81%比 68.6%，P=0.009；74.1%比 55.1%，P<0.001）。尽管帕洛诺司琼 0.75mg 组较昂丹司琼组缓解率为高，但是该结果没有统计学意义。各组包括头疼、腹泻、便秘和疲乏等副反应的发生率均相似[38]。尽管帕洛诺司琼可能较其他 5-HT$_3$ 受体拮抗剂尤其在预防延迟性症状方面具有优势，我们还需要研究来进一步评价该结果。所有 5-HT$_3$ 受体拮抗剂的耐受性均较好，最常见的副反应是头疼，发生在 15%～20%的患者。其次常见的副反应包括便秘和头晕。最近，格拉司琼被用在透皮系统（Sancuso）以预防 CINV。在Ⅲ期临床研究中比较了透皮的格拉司琼贴剂与口服格拉司琼在控制 CINV 方面的功效。这种贴剂含有 34.3mg 的格拉司琼，其中的活性成分将在 7 日内缓慢释放。一项包含了 641 例接受高度或中度止吐性化疗的患者的多中心研究显示，格拉司琼贴剂不比多剂量口服格拉司琼的效果差[39]。

多巴胺受体拮抗剂

三类多巴胺受体拮抗剂可有效预防和治疗恶心及呕吐：吩噻嗪类，丁酰苯类和苯甲酰胺类。在 20 世纪 60 年代，吩噻嗪类药物首先被证明可以有效预防 CINV。甲哌氯奥沙普秦是这类药物中最常用的，该药可预防除高致吐性化疗外的所有类型化疗所致的呕吐[40]。可能发生包括肌张力异常在内的锥体外系反应。用苯海拉明或者停用甲哌氯奥沙普秦可用于治疗锥体外系反应。而丁酰苯类药物，包括氟哌利多，较少用于预防 CINV，其副作用与吩噻嗪类药物相似。它们可能在治疗暴发性恶心及呕吐方面具有一定的疗效。

在苯甲酰胺类药物中，甲氧氯普胺（胃复安）是研究最透彻并且在 CINV 的治疗中应用最多的一个药物。该药在低剂量时可以阻断中枢及外周的多巴胺（D_2）受体，在高剂量时可产生弱的 5-HT$_3$ 抑制作用。此外，它可以促进胃排空，并在胃食管交界处收缩贲门括约肌。在 5-HT$_3$ 拮抗剂出现之前，静脉联合应用高剂量的甲氧氯普胺和地塞米松是对高致吐性化疗最有效的预防止吐措施[41]。由于能够通过血-脑脊液屏障，甲氧氯普胺可产生肌张力异常和迟发性运动障碍的副作用，尤其是在高剂量应用或是在老年人中应用时。苯海拉明常常作为联合方案中的一部分用以预防这些副作用。这些预防性止吐方案目前已被含有 5-HT$_3$ 受体拮抗剂的方案所取代，因为后者在疗效和安全性方面均占有优势[23~25]。

糖皮质激素类

糖皮质激素类在单独或联合应用于预防各级致吐性化疗的恶心及呕吐方面均有效，其中地塞米松最常用。地塞米松联合 5-HT$_3$ 受体拮抗剂±NK-1 受体拮抗剂可用于中至重度致吐性化疗。一项包含了 32 项随机临床实验的荟萃分析，共纳入 1984—1998 年期间 5 613 例患者，发现地塞米松无论是单独应用或是与其他药物联合应用均对中至重度致吐性化疗有效[42]。随后的研究显示，在高致吐性化疗中，5-HT$_3$ 受体拮抗剂与地塞米松的联合应用效果优于任何一个药物的单独应用[43]。糖皮质激素在呕吐反射通路上的作用位点目前仍不清楚。此类药物可能出现失眠、体重增加以及情绪障碍的副作用。

NK-1 受体拮抗剂

NK-1 受体位于孤束核与延髓后极区，并可以被 P 物质激活[11]。NK-1 受体抑制剂已显示出具有抗呕吐的效应，NK-1 受体已成为一个新的抗呕吐治疗的靶点。阿瑞匹坦是该类药物中第一个被批准的药物，不仅能够预防高度致吐性化疗所致的急性呕吐，还能够预防延迟性呕吐[13,14]。

在前期研究结果基础上，随后的两个Ⅲ期随机临床研究进一步证实了阿瑞匹坦在预防急性及延迟性恶心呕吐方面的疗效。523 例接受高致吐性化疗（顺铂>70mg/m^2）的患者被随机分成两组，一组接受阿瑞匹坦+5-HT$_3$ 受体拮抗剂+地塞米松预防性治疗（第 1 日：阿瑞匹坦 125mg 口服，昂丹司琼 32mg 静推，地塞米松 12mg 口服；第 2～3 日：阿瑞匹坦 80mg 口服，地塞米松 8mg 口服；第 4 日：地塞米松 8mg 口服）；另一组仅接受 5-

HT_3 受体拮抗剂+地塞米松治疗(第 1 日:昂丹司琼 32mg 静推,地塞米松 20mg 口服;第 2~4 日:地塞米松 8mg 一天两次口服)。在第一项研究中,阿瑞匹坦组总体 CR(第一个 24h 内无呕吐并且无须解救止吐)率为 62.7%,而标准治疗组总体 CR 率仅为 43.3%($P<0.001$)。阿瑞匹坦组无论在急性呕吐还是延迟性呕吐的控制方面均较标准对照组有优势,急性呕吐的 CR 率分别为 82.8%和 68.4%($P<0.001$),延迟性呕吐的 CR 率分别为 67.7%和 46.8%($P<0.001$)[13]。第二项研究在 521 例接受含高剂量顺铂化疗方案的患者中证实了以上研究结果。在阿瑞匹坦组总体 CR 率为 72.7%,标准治疗组为 52.3%($P<0.001$)。无论在急性呕吐还是延迟性呕吐的 CR 率方面,阿瑞匹坦组均优于标准治疗组(89.2%比 78.1%,$P<0.001$;75.4%比 55.8%,$P<0.001$)[14]。基于以上研究结果,FDA 在 2003 年批准阿瑞匹坦用于临床。

福沙匹坦(fosaprepitant)是阿瑞匹坦的水溶性磷酸化前体。FDA 已批准福沙匹坦 150mg 可用于替代口服阿瑞匹坦三药联合方案[44]。

阿瑞匹坦是细胞色素 P-450 酶 3A4(CYP3A4)的底物,同时也是其中度诱导剂及抑制剂[45]。化疗药物及其他许多药物都是经该酶代谢,因此使用以下经 CYP3A4 代谢的化疗药物的患者在使用阿瑞匹坦时必须谨慎:多西他赛、紫杉醇、依托泊苷、伊立替康、异环磷酰胺、伊马替尼、长春瑞滨、长春地辛和长春新碱。尽管在临床研究中接受以上化疗药物患者的阿瑞匹坦给药剂量在未经调整的情况下,也并未观察到有副作用及对疗效的影响,但我们仍需对此保持警惕。此外,阿瑞匹坦可能还与一些非化疗药物相互作用。它可以诱导华法林的代谢,使其血药浓度降低,似乎还能增加口服地塞米松和甲泼尼龙的活性,因此,当地塞米松与阿瑞匹坦一起用于预防性止吐时,推荐将地塞米松的剂量进行下调。其他和阿瑞匹坦有相互作用的药物还包括口服避孕药、咪达唑仑、酮康唑、红霉素、卡马西平、利福平以及苯妥英。

奈妥匹坦(netupitant)是一种新型的 NK-1 受体拮抗剂,具有亲和力高和半衰期长(90h)的特性[46]。近期一项Ⅲ期研究中,纳入了 1 455 例接受中毒致吐性化疗(AC 或 EC)的患者,按 1∶1的比例随机分为两组:一组为 NEPA 组,单次固定剂量的奈妥匹坦和帕洛诺司琼口服,联合标准的地塞米松口服;另一组为帕洛诺司琼口服,联合标准的地塞米松口服[47]。有效性终点包括急性(0~24h)、延迟性(25~120h)和总体(0~120h)CR 率,CR 定义为无呕吐并且无须解救药物治疗。结果显示奈妥匹坦与帕洛诺司琼的联合治疗在所有研究终点中均具有优势,在接受 4 个及以上周期的化疗患者中,CR 率从 67%~75%提高到 74%~84%,绝对值增加了 7%~14%,并且组间不良事件的发生率没有显著差异。

其他类型的止吐药物

其他可用于止吐的药物类型还有苯二氮䓬类、抗胆碱药物以及大麻类药物。最常用的苯二氮䓬类的药物是劳拉西泮和阿普唑仑,它们能够阻断 GABA 受体,尤其是大脑皮质中的 GABA 受体,在治疗预期性呕吐以及减轻患者化疗相关的焦虑方面具有最佳的效果[46]。

鉴于美国多个地区的医用大麻合法化,大麻类药物可能会成为越来越受关注的焦点。但应该注意的是,虽然有证据支持合成大麻可用于棘手病例的治疗,但应该将其用于难治性病例,在普通病例中的治疗应用仍需进一步研究[48,49]。

奥氮平,一种硫代苯二氮䓬类药物,被发现在预防急性及延迟性呕吐治疗中有效[17,50]。奥氮平已纳入 NCCN 指南,用于治疗高度及中度致吐性化疗引起的呕吐[17]。

抗胆碱类药物如异奥沙普秦以及苯海拉明常用于治疗暴发性的 CINV,而东莨菪碱透皮贴剂较为少用。尽管目前有一些不确切的证据支持在对常规止吐药物治疗无效的患者中使用大麻类药物如大麻或其合成药物大麻酚或屈大麻酚,然而推荐应用这类药物的随机临床研究非常少[46]。

补充和替代药物疗法

在过去的几十年,人们十分关注补充和替代疗法(complementary and alternative medicine,CAM),尤其是对肿瘤患者的治疗。人们曾尝试用各种各样的 CAM 治疗如针灸、催眠、推拿、音乐及草药辅助药物如生姜等来控制呕吐。其中,针灸及一些身心疗法似乎比较有效[47],但在推荐作为常规应用之前我们还需要对其进行进一步的研究。

在中国,针灸作为一种传统治疗方法,可以用来控制包括呕吐在内的各种不适。最近有一项纳入了 11 项随机研究($n=1\,247$)的荟萃分析评价了针灸在控制中至重度致吐性化疗所致 CINV 方面的作用[48]。该研究发现接受针灸治疗的患者急性呕吐的发生率明显低于对照组(22%比 31%,$P=0.04$),然而延迟性呕吐患者却并未从中获益。值得注意的是,所有这些研究均是在阿瑞匹坦获得批准之前进行的,因此目前针灸的价值并不明确。

据报道,身心疗法如催眠、图像引导、渐进性肌肉放松疗法(progressive muscle relaxation therapy,PMRT)能够显著减少 CINV[49~52]。在中国香港特别行政区进行的一项随机临床研究中,71 例接受甲氧氯普胺+地塞米松止吐治疗的乳腺癌患者随机进入渐进性肌肉放松训练以及图像引导组(化疗前 1h 一次,以后每日 1 次,连续 5 日),另外设置无干预组。与无干预组相比,干预组的患者 CINV 的持续时间短($P=0.05$),发生率低($P=0.07$)。然而,这些患者没有接受包括 $5\text{-}HT_3$ 拮抗剂或者 NK-1 拮抗剂在内的标准预防性止吐措施,因此限制了该研究的临床应用。

一些包括约 30 例患者的小型临床研究发现,其他放松治疗如音乐和推拿也是有效的辅助抗呕吐治疗方法[53,54]。这些放松治疗能够影响大脑皮质,因此对减少呕吐的感知以及控制预期性呕吐尤其有效。

两项评价生姜治疗 CINV 疗效的临床研究均为阴性结果[55,56]。目前许多评估各种 CAM 治疗方法的临床研究正在进行中,这些研究将为我们进一步提供有关 CAM 治疗疗效(或无效)的有用信息,从而有利于将传统临床肿瘤学中的治疗方法优化整合(整合肿瘤学)[47]。

预防及治疗化疗所致呕吐的指南

止吐治疗的目标是完全预防 CINV(表 125-3)。对于接受中至高度致吐性化疗的患者而言,发生恶心呕吐的危险期在化疗后还将持续至少 4 日，因此止吐治疗需覆盖这个时期。对预防性止吐药物的选择取决于如下列出的不同化疗药物的致吐程度[18]。

表 125-3 依据致吐风险预防患者急性及延迟性恶心呕吐的指南

致吐风险	急性	延迟性
高度(>90%)	阿瑞匹坦+$5\text{-}HT_3$ 拮抗剂+地塞米松	阿瑞匹坦+地塞米松
中度(30%~90%)	$5\text{-}HT_3$ 拮抗剂+地塞米松	地塞米松
低度(10%~30%)	地塞米松或吩噻嗪类或甲氧氯普胺	无
极低(<10%)	无	无

$5\text{-}HT_3$，羟色胺。

高度致吐性化疗

顺铂和环磷酰胺是最常用的高度致吐性化疗药物。如果没有充分的预防措施，恶心和呕吐是几乎必然发生的。在 NK-1 受体拮抗剂阿瑞匹坦获得批准之前的指南推荐采用 $5\text{-}HT_3$ 受体拮抗剂联合地塞米松治疗。现在对于所有接受高致吐性化疗的患者推荐治疗方法是：第 1 日：$5\text{-}HT_3$ 受体拮抗剂+阿瑞匹坦(125mg 口服)或者福沙匹坦(115mg 静脉注射)+地塞米松(12mg 口服或静脉注射)，第 2~4 日：阿瑞匹坦(80mg 口服)+地塞米松(8mg 口服或静脉注射)，或者福沙匹坦+地塞米松(第 2 日 8mg 口服，第 3~4 日 8mg/d 两次口服)。所有预防性止吐药物都应该在化疗开始前应用。

中度致吐性化疗

对于所有接受中度致吐性化疗的患者，推荐采用 $5\text{-}HT_3$ 受体拮抗剂+地塞米松的联合方案。最近的临床研究结果表明，帕洛诺司琼在控制延迟性呕吐方面更具有优势，因此更倾向推荐帕洛诺司琼(0. 25mg 仅第 1 日)作为 $5\text{-}HT_3$ 受体拮抗剂。如果应用其他 $5\text{-}HT_3$ 受体拮抗剂，应该在第 1 日化疗开始前应用，并要在第 2~3 日每日 1 次重复应用。地塞米松第一天为 12mg 口服或者静脉注射，在第 2~3 日每日 8mg(8mg/d 一次或者 4mg/d 两次)。在特定的患者中(尽管已经接受足够的预防措施仍然发生暴发性恶心呕吐的患者和有高危因素的患者)，应该考虑使用阿瑞匹坦(第 1 日 125mg 口服或者福沙匹坦 150mg 静脉注射，第 2~3 日 80m 口服)。奈妥匹坦和帕洛诺司琼最近的数据令人鼓舞，但奈妥匹坦尚未获得美国 FDA 的批准。

低度致吐性化疗

对于接受低度致吐性化疗的患者，预防性止吐药物可选地塞米松(12mg 口服或者静脉注射)，或甲哌氯奥沙普秦(每 4~6h 10mg 口服或静脉注射)，或甲氧氯普胺(每 4~6h 20~40mg 口服，或每 3~4h 1~2mg/kg 静脉注射同时应用苯海拉明预防锥体外系反应)。所有预防药物均应在化疗前开始应用。

极低度致吐性化疗

不推荐常规进行预防性止吐。如果确实发生了恶心或者呕吐，推荐应用地塞米松、甲哌氯奥沙普秦或者甲氧氯普胺，并且在下个疗程化疗开始前应该考虑预防性应用这些药物。

特殊情况

暴发性恶心及呕吐

理想情况下，对暴发性恶心呕吐的最佳治疗是预防其发生。有时，虽然进行了积极的预防，仍旧会出现症状。对暴发性症状最好是加用另一类止吐药物。此外，可能需要应用除口服以外的其他给药途径，如经静脉或直肠给药。如果按计划而非按需用药，这些措施的效果可能会更好。当暴发性恶心呕吐已经发生，我们需要重新评价预防性止吐方案，并在下一疗程化疗开始之前对其进行加强。

预期性恶心呕吐

预防预期性恶心呕吐的关键是防止每次化疗恶心呕吐症状的发生。一旦症状产生，应当在预防性止吐方案中加用苯二氮䓬类药物[57]。上文所提及的一些身心治疗手段如行为疗法、系统性脱敏疗法、催眠术等也证实是有效的[49~53]。

多日化疗引起的恶心和呕吐

很多恶性肿瘤患者需接受多日化疗，如生殖细胞肿瘤、淋巴瘤、多发性骨髓瘤和干细胞移植等，这类发生患者急性和延迟性恶心呕吐的风险均有。尽管 NCCN 指南中专门列出了“管理多日致吐性化疗方案的原则”的章节，但仅提示应根据高度致吐性化疗相应方案选择止吐疗法。延迟性恶心呕吐的风险取决于所应用的化疗药物和最后所使用的化疗药物的致吐程度。

有研究评估了帕洛诺司琼重复给药对于多日化疗的效果，但没有明确的结论，仍需进一步的研究来回答是否需要帕洛诺司琼的重复给药[1,2]。

阿瑞匹坦在多药化疗止吐治疗中的作用已经很明确[3~5]，可再多日化疗中应用，但很难针对每日多种致吐性化疗药物来推荐特定的止吐药物。

NCCN 的止吐指南概述了多日化疗止吐治疗的一般原则，提出可应用糖皮质激素(地塞米松)、5-羟色胺拮抗剂(帕罗诺司琼)和神经激肽拮抗剂(阿瑞匹坦)来治疗。

放疗诱导的恶心呕吐

几乎所有在骨髓移植前接受全身照射的患者以及超过 80%的接受上腹部放疗的患者会产生放疗诱导的恶心呕吐(Radiation-induced nausea and vomiting，RINV)[58]。研究已显示无论是与安慰剂的比较[59]还是与甲氧氯普胺和甲哌氯奥沙普秦的联合方案比较[60,61]，预防性应用 $5\text{-}HT_3$ 受体拮抗剂均可显示出其优越性。推荐所有进行上腹部照射或者全身照射的患者接受口服 $5\text{-}HT_3$ 受体拮抗剂 2~每日 3 次，加或者不加地塞米松作为预防[62]。

结论

近年来，我们在预防和治疗化疗所致的恶心和呕吐方面已经取得了显著的进步。近期的调查显示，我们仍需提高对化疗所致急性尤其是延迟性恶心呕吐的频率和严重性的认识。所幸的是，我们又有了加强预防性止吐效果的新武器。支持治疗在控制恶心方面似乎也较有希望，目前正在对此进行进一步探索。正确应用指南，基于所使用的特定化疗药物选择适当的预防措施，将有助于确保更少的患者经受这些令人痛苦的副作用。

（崔久嵬　李玲玉　刘蒙蒙 译）

参考文献

The complete reference list can be found on the Wiley Companion Digital Edition of this title (see inside front cover for login instructions).

1 Grunberg SM, Deuson RR, Mavros P, et al. Incidence of chemotherapy-induced nausea and emesis after modern antiemetics. *Cancer*. 2004;**100**:2261–2268.

2 Mitchell EP. Gastrointestinal toxicity of chemotherapeutic agents. *Semin Oncol*. 1992;**19**:566–579.

6 de Boer-Dennert M, de Wit R, Schmitz PI, et al. Patient perceptions of the side-effects of chemotherapy: the influence of 5HT3 antagonists. *Br J Cancer*. 1997;**76**:1055–1061.

9 Carpenter DO. Neural mechanisms of emesis. *Can J Physiol Pharmacol*. 1990;**68**:230–236.

14 Hesketh PJ, Grunberg SM, Gralla RJ, et al. The oral neurokinin-1 antagonist aprepitant for the prevention of chemotherapy-induced nausea and vomiting: a multinational, randomized, double-blind, placebo-controlled trial in patients receiving high-dose cisplatin—the Aprepitant Protocol 052 Study Group. *J Clin Oncol*. 2003;**21**:4112–4119.

15 Moher D, Arthur AZ, Pater JL. Anticipatory nausea and/or vomiting. *Cancer Treat Rev*. 1984;**11**:257–264.

16 Roila F, Herrstedt J, Aapro M, et al. Group EMGW. Guideline update for MASCC and ESMO in the prevention of chemotherapy- and radiotherapy-induced nausea and vomiting: results of the Perugia consensus conference. *Ann Oncol*. 2010;**21**(**Suppl 5**):v232–v243.

17 National Comprehensive Cancer Network (2014) *Antiemesis Version 1.2016*, www.nccn.org (accessed 02 May, 2016).

19 Hesketh PJ, Kris MG, Grunberg SM, et al. Proposal for classifying the acute emetogenicity of cancer chemotherapy. *J Clin Oncol*. 1997;**15**:103–109.

20 Koeller JM, Aapro MS, Gralla RJ, et al. A. Antiemetic guidelines: creating a more practical treatment approach. *Support Care Cancer*. 2002;**10**:519–522.

21 Mitchelson F. Pharmacological agents affecting emesis. A review (part I). *Drugs*. 1992;**43**:295–315.

22 Bountra C, Gale JD, Gardner CJ, et al. Towards understanding the aetiology and pathophysiology of the emetic reflex: novel approaches to antiemetic drugs. *Oncology*. 1996;**53**(**Suppl 1**):102–109.

23 Chevallier B, Cappelaere P, Splinter T, et al. A double-blind, multicentre comparison of intravenous dolasetron mesilate and metoclopramide in the prevention of nausea and vomiting in cancer patients receiving high-dose cisplatin chemotherapy. *Support Care Cancer*. 1997;**5**:22–30.

24 Warr D, Wilan A, Venner P, et al. A randomised, double-blind comparison of granisetron with high-dose metoclopramide, dexamethasone and diphenhydramine for cisplatin-induced emesis. An NCI Canada Clinical Trials Group phase III trial. *Eur J Cancer*. 1992;**29A**:33–36.

25 Heron JF, Goedhals L, Jordaan JP, et al. Oral granisetron alone and in combination with dexamethasone: a double-blind randomized comparison against high-dose metoclopramide plus dexamethasone in prevention of cisplatin-induced emesis. The Granisetron Study Group. *Ann Oncol*. 1994;**5**:579–584.

28 Martoni A, Angelelli B, Guaraldi M, et al. An open randomised cross-over study on granisetron versus ondansetron in the prevention of acute emesis induced by moderate dose cisplatin-containing regimens. *Eur J Cancer*. 1996;**32A**:82–85.

29 Hesketh P, Navari R, Grote T, et al. Double-blind, randomized comparison of the antiemetic efficacy of intravenous dolasetron mesylate and intravenous ondansetron in the prevention of acute cisplatin-induced emesis in patients with cancer. Dolasetron Comparative Chemotherapy Induced Emesis Prevention Group. *J Clin Oncol*. 1996;**14**:2242–2249.

30 Audhuy B, Cappelaere P, Martin M, et al. A double-blind, randomised comparison of the anti-emetic efficacy of two intravenous doses of dolasetron mesilate and granisetron in patients receiving high dose cisplatin chemotherapy. *Eur J Cancer*. 1996;**32A**:807–813.

46 Spinelli T, Calcagnile S, Giuliano C, et al. Netupitant PET imaging and ADME studies in humans. *J Clin Pharmacol*. 2014;**54**(**1**):97–108.

47 Aapro M, Karthaus, M, Schwartzberg L, et al. (2014) Phase 3 study of NEPA, a fixed-dose combination of netupitant and palonosetron, for prevention of chemotherapy-induced nausea and vomiting during moderately emetogenic chemotherapy cycles. Paper presented at 50th Annual Meeting of the American Society of Clinical Oncology; May 30; Chicago, Il.

48 Hill KP. Medical marijuana: more questions than answers. *J Psychiatr Pract*. 2014;**20**(**5**):389–391.

49 Einhorn LH, Brames MJ, Dreicer R, et al. Palonosetron plus dexamethasone for prevention of chemotherapy-induced nausea and vomiting in patients receiving multiple-day chemotherapy for germ cell cancer. *Support Care Cancer*. 2007;**15**:1293–1300.

50 Giralt SA, Mangan KF, Maziarz RT, et al. Three palonosetron regimens to prevent CINV in myeloma patients receiving multiple-day high-dose melphalan and hematopoietic stem cell transplantation. *Ann Oncol*. 2011;**22**:939–946.

51 Jordan K, Kinitz I, Voigt W, et al. Safety and efficacy of a triple antiemetic combination with NK-1 antagonist aprepitant in highly and moderately emetogenic multiple day chemotherapy. *Eur J Cancer*. 2009;**45**:1184–1187.

52 Olver IN, Grimison P, Chatfield M, et al. Results of a 7-day aprepitant schedule for the prevention of nausea and vomiting in 5-day cisplatin-based germ cell tumor chemotherapy. *Support Care Cancer*. 2013;**21**:1561–1568.

53 Albany C, Brames MJ, Fausel C, et al. Randomized, double-blind placebo-controlled, phase III cross-over study evaluating the oral neurokinin-1 antagonist aprepitant in combination with a 5HT3 receptor antagonist and dexamethasone in patients with germ cell tumors receiving 5-day cisplatin combination chemotherapy regimens: a Hoosier Oncology Group study. *J Clin Oncol*. 2012;**30**:3998–4003.

54 Sharkey KA, Darmani NA. Parker LA regulation of nausea and vomiting by cannabinoids and the endocannabinoid system. *Eur J Pharmacol*. 2014;**722**:134–146. doi: 10.1016/j.ejphar.2013.09.068.

55 Navani RM, Gray SE, Keir AC, et al. Olanzapine versus aprepitant for the prevention of chemotherapy-induced nausea and vomiting: a randomized phase II trial. *J Support Oncol*. 2011;**9**:188–195.

第 126 章　癌症的神经系统并发症

Lisa M. DeAngelis, MD, FAAN

概述

由于癌症患者全身治疗预后较好、生存期延长，神经系统的相关并发症越来越常见。恶性肿瘤可转移至脑组织、硬膜、蛛网膜下腔、脊髓、神经根、神经丛。化学治疗的异环磷酰胺脑病等急性毒性反应会直接影响到有效抗肿瘤治疗周期的完成。除此以外，放射治疗以及化学治疗的远期并发症如放射性脊髓损伤和外周神经病将严重影响患者的生活质量。积极预防、早发现和早治疗将降低恶性肿瘤患者神经系统并发症的发生率。

癌症的神经系统并发症可以由转移引起，也可由非转移引起（表 126-1）。转移病灶可通过以下途径影响神经系统：直接侵犯（如臂丛神经转移）；压迫（如硬膜外脊髓压迫）；影响血供（如颅骨转移引起的矢状窦阻塞）。脑转移性病变将在第 77 章讨论。尽管绝大多数肿瘤都可发生神经系统转移，但某些肿瘤更倾向于导致特定的中枢或外周神经系统疾病（如白血病易转移至软脑膜，但很少转移到脑实质）。前列腺癌易发生椎体转移，而软脑膜和脑实质累及较少，因此常引起硬膜外脊髓压迫[1,2]。

表 126-1　癌症的神经系统并发症

转移性
颅内（常转移至脑，参见第 70 章）
脊柱脊髓（硬膜外）
软脑膜（颅底和马尾）
脑神经（颅底病变）
外周神经（臂丛和腰骶丛）
肌肉（罕见）
非转移性
治疗相关并发症（放疗、化疗）
血管性疾病（出血、梗死）
代谢、营养功能障碍
副瘤综合征
感染

非转移性神经系统并发症通常是肿瘤特异性的。代谢紊乱更常见于肿瘤广泛转移至重要器官时，如肠癌肝转移；或者体液和电解质失衡，如乳腺癌致高钙血症或小细胞肺癌致抗利尿激素分泌异常。中枢神经系统感染更常继发于癌症导致的免疫抑制，如霍奇金病。与实体瘤相比，血管并发症更常见于血液系统恶性肿瘤[7]。影响中枢神经系统的副瘤综合征更常见于特定的肿瘤如小细胞肺癌和卵巢癌[3]。通过患者症状体征准确发现判断神经系统异常将有利于疾病诊断（表 126-2）。

表 126-2　按部位分类的癌症患者神经系统并发症

部位	常见原因	典型症状和体征
脑部	转移	头痛
	软膜转移	意识不清
	代谢性/中毒性脑病	偏瘫
	感染（脑膜炎，脑脓肿）	癫痫
	放射性脑病	共济失调
	脑出血或脑梗死	
	副肿瘤脑病（边缘系统脑病）	
脊髓和马尾	硬膜外转移	背痛
	软膜转移	截瘫
	髓内转移	感觉障碍平面
	硬膜外脓肿或血肿	大小便失禁
	放射性脊髓病	
	鞘内化疗后脊髓病	
	副肿瘤脊髓病	
脑神经和外周神经	肿瘤等外源性压迫（血肿）	局部疼痛
	肿瘤直接侵犯	感觉障碍
	药物毒性	运动障碍
	水痘带状疱疹感染	神经分布区（局部病变）或四肢远端（多神经丛病变）腱反射减弱
	放射性神经丛病	
	副肿瘤性神经病	
神经肌肉连接处	药物（氨基糖苷类抗生素）	不伴感觉障碍的肢体力弱
	副肿瘤性疾病（Lambert-Eaton 肌无力综合征，重症肌无力）	呼吸功能不全
肌肉	转移	近端肢体无力
	类固醇性肌病	不伴感觉障碍的肢体力弱
	恶病质性肌病	
	副肿瘤性多发性肌炎或皮肌炎	

脊柱转移较常见，但由于双膦酸盐的应用，包括脊髓压迫等骨损伤并发症发生率明显下降[6]。椎体转移病灶向椎管蔓延，或椎旁肿瘤通过椎间孔侵犯硬膜外空间均可导致脊髓压迫（图 126-1）。淋巴瘤通过神经孔侵犯椎管而不破坏骨质。肠癌、肾癌、前列腺癌、头颈部恶性肿瘤直接侵犯椎体结构也可导致硬膜外占位。转移癌可致椎体压缩破坏，继之骨质、肿瘤、韧带等受累组织可能凸入椎管压迫脊髓。

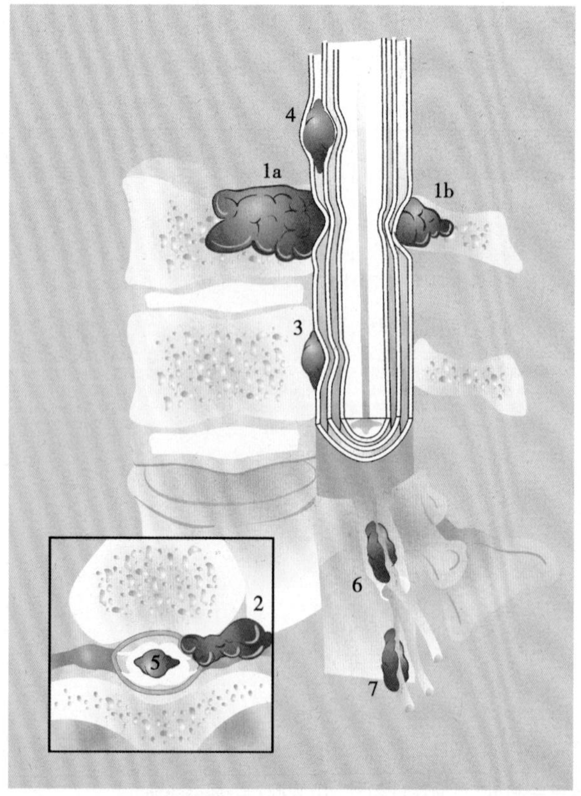

图 126-1　骨转移直接侵犯椎体（1a）或后弓（1b）、椎旁肿瘤通过椎间孔蔓延（2）或直接转移至硬膜外（3）导致硬膜外脊髓压迫。硬膜下转移（4）、髓内生长（5）、椎旁转移侵犯根血管（6）和神经根（7）罕见

转移性并发症

脊柱转移

除了脑转移以外，压迫脊髓和马尾的转移病灶是转移性肿瘤引起的最常见的神经系统并发症状[1,2,4]。脊髓在 L1 或 L2 椎体水平结束，但该水平以下的马尾压迫也被认为是脊髓压迫，因为其诊断和治疗是一样的[1]。脊髓压迫可导致疼痛，如果不治疗会引起瘫痪和尿便失禁。癌症导致瘫痪的患者通常在数月内死亡。然而，临床研究显示，早期诊断及治疗可维持患者独立行走能力并延长生存期。

大约 5%死于癌症的患者在尸检时发现有脊髓压迫。每年美国有 18 000~20 000 的新发脊髓压迫病例[1,5]。引起脊髓压迫转移癌的最常见原发肿瘤为乳腺癌、肺癌、前列腺癌和淋巴瘤（表 126-3）。脊髓压迫通常发生于恶性肿瘤转移的晚期阶段，但是高达 20%的脊髓压迫患者在神经系统症状出现前并未发现原发恶性肿瘤。

表 126-3　MSKCC 583 例有脊髓压迫症状患者的原发肿瘤

原发肿瘤	患者数量/%
乳腺癌	127(22)
肺癌	90(15)
前列腺癌	58(10)
淋巴网状内皮细胞肿瘤	56(10)
肉瘤	52(9)
肾癌	39(7)
胃肠道肿瘤	29(5)
黑色素瘤	23(4)
原发灶不明	21(4)
头颈部肿瘤	19(3)
多部位	69(12)
合计	583

MSKCC，纽约纪念医院斯隆-凯特林癌症研究中心（Memorial Sloan-Kettering Cancer Center）。

引起脊髓压迫最常见的部位是胸椎，其次是腰骶椎和颈椎，发生比例大约为 4∶2∶1。约 25%的脊髓压迫患者有两个或更多的连续性椎体转移。但与感染不同的是，椎间盘可保持正常。多达 32%的脊髓压迫患者除了临床可疑的节段外还有其他节段的脊髓压迫，提示对可疑硬脊膜外占位患者行全椎管影像学检查是非常必要的。

脊髓压迫的病理生理学

近一半患者的硬脊膜外肿瘤可同时累及脊髓的前侧和后侧。约 20%的患者肿瘤为环绕侵犯脊髓。组织学研究显示，最常见的病理改变包括载脂巨噬细胞浸润引起的脱髓鞘、间质水肿和局灶性轴索肿胀。但即使在突发瘫痪的患者中脊髓梗死也很罕见。硬膜外静脉丛压迫（可能造成脊髓水肿）可在脊髓压迫早期发生，而脊髓血流量降低则出现较晚。因此，脊髓压迫之所以成为神经急症是因为难以预测的脊髓静脉梗死常引起急性瘫痪。受压神经组织释放的潜在神经毒性物质如前列腺素和 5-羟色胺可能会导致神经功能障碍。

临床表现和诊断

脊髓压迫的症状和体征取决于受压脊髓的水平（如颈段和胸段）。背痛实际上是脊髓压迫患者的首发症状（表 126-4）[5]。疼痛可为局限性（位于受累椎体）、根性（放射至手臂、躯干或腿部）或两者共存。局限性疼痛为钝痛酸痛，可逐渐进展，常常局限于受累脊柱。活动后局限性疼痛加重提示脊椎不稳定。在颈及腰骶椎，神经根痛往往是单侧的。而在躯干部则往往是双背痛（束带状），这充分提示硬脊膜外占位。患者仰卧时脊髓压迫引起的疼痛通常会加重有助于鉴别椎间盘突出，后者在患者仰卧时疼痛会改善。咳嗽、用力或 Valsalva 呼吸时引起疼痛加重。在胸腹部计算机断层扫描（CT）或磁共振成像（MRI）评估原发肿瘤时会偶然发现脊髓压迫，但患者常无疼痛表现。

表 126-4　MSKCC 213 例脊髓压迫患者的症状和体征

	首发症状		明确诊断后出现症状	
	病例数	比例/%	病例数	比例/%
疼痛	201	94	207	97
肢体无力	7	3	157	74
自主神经功能紊乱	0	0	111	52
感觉障碍	1	0.5	112	53
共济失调	2	0.9	8	4

MSKCC，纽约纪念医院斯隆-凯特林癌症研究中心（Memorial Sloan-Kettering Cancer Center）。

硬膜外脊髓压迫的第二常见特征是无力，通常在出现疼痛后数周至数月内发生，多见于腿部近端肌肉。下肢肌张力常增加，腱反射亢进，并出现足底伸肌反应。如果脊髓压迫发生在脊髓以下的马尾水平，腱反射常减弱或消失。如果因为疼痛不能准确检查肌力，应在使用止痛剂后完成全面查体。

肛门和膀胱功能异常大多发生在脊髓压迫后期。然而当脊髓圆锥受压时（T10 至 L1 椎体病变），膀胱功能障碍可能是首发和唯一症状。由于膀胱感觉功能不全，患者可能意识不到尿潴留。腹部触诊往往提示膀胱膨胀，且排空后超声检查显示尿潴留。通常肛门括约肌松弛。感觉症状包括始于脚趾并向近端蔓延的麻木和感觉异常。除圆锥压迫外，如果出现躯干感觉异常平面，一般不会是骶段受累所致。尽管背痛先于共济失调出现，但部分患者类似小脑疾病的步态或躯干共济失调可能是唯一的神经系统体征。水痘带状疱疹可能是发生于硬膜外转移的皮肤表现。如果该表现的出现早于脊柱转移有可能延误脊髓压迫的诊断。

硬脊膜外脊髓压迫的临床症状和体征都是非特异性的（表 126-5）。椎间盘突出或椎管狭窄可以引起类似的脊髓压迫症状，可能会影响癌症患者病情的判断。其他疾病如硬膜外血肿和脓肿可能与癌症或其治疗直接相关。

表 126-5　硬膜外脊髓压迫的鉴别诊断

诊断	定性分析	诊断方法
髓内肿瘤	胶质瘤	增强 MRI
	转移瘤	
髓外硬膜下肿瘤	脑膜瘤	增强 MRI
	神经纤维瘤	
软膜肿瘤	转移瘤	增强 MRI，CSF 细胞学
	原发淋巴瘤	
放射性脊髓病	脊柱放疗	增强 MRI
动静脉畸形	放疗后海绵状血管瘤	增强 MRI，脊髓血管造影
横贯性脊髓病	感染后脊髓病，多发性硬化	增强 MRI
硬膜外血肿	血小板减少（腰椎穿刺史）	MRI 或 CT
硬膜外脓肿	败血症，硬膜外置管	增强 MRI，细菌培养
脊柱退行性疾病	椎间盘突出，椎管狭窄	MRI
骨质疏松症	脊柱压缩性骨折	MRI，组织活检

CSF，脑脊液；CT，计算机断层成像；MRI，磁共振成像。
摘自参考文献 1，牛津大学出版社。

出现背痛的癌症患者在排除其他诊断后才能判断为脊髓压迫。因为，脊髓明显受压后可能出现超急性损伤和严重的神经功能障碍，应立即进行体检评估。磁共振成像是恶性肿瘤引起脊椎占位唯一重要的诊断方法（图 126-2），应对脊椎全长进行扫描成像。观察脊柱转移或硬膜外肿瘤不需要行增强扫描，但要鉴别髓内转移或软脑膜种植时必须行增强扫描。无法行磁共振检查的患者（如安装心脏起搏器）应行 CT 脊髓造影术，通过三维重建成像提供最佳的脊椎多维图像。

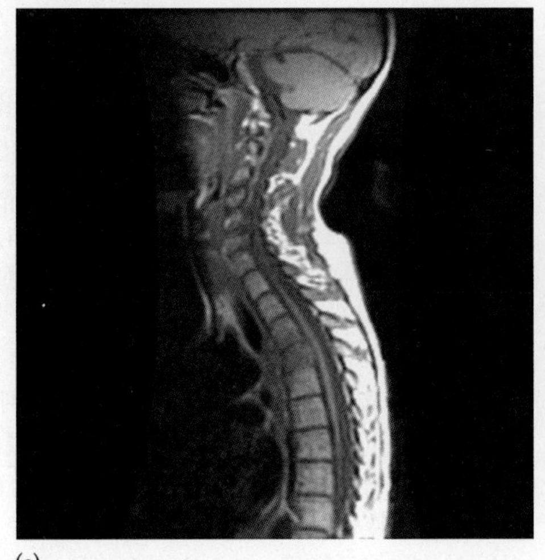

(a)

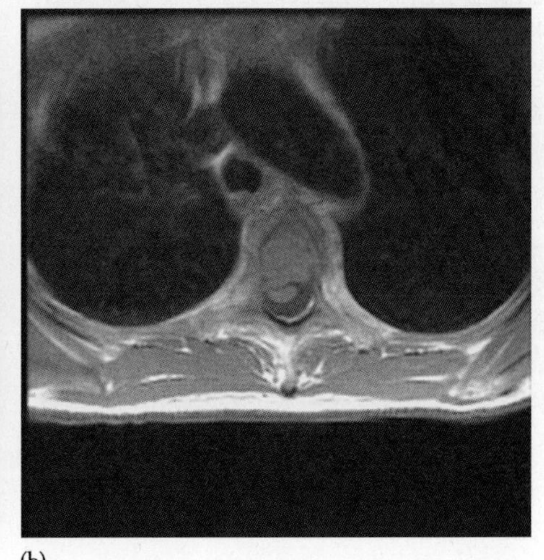

(b)

图 126-2　磁共振显示转移性乳腺癌致脊髓压迫。（a）椎体肿瘤压迫脊髓前部。（b）相同水平轴位图显示脊髓前方和侧方受压变形

治疗

脊髓压迫需要紧急治疗，目的是减压和抑制肿瘤再生长[1,4]。放射治疗是大多数患者的主要治疗手段，但手术和化疗对特定患者也十分重要。所有患者的初始治疗应采用类固醇激素。类固醇激素通过溶瘤效应使肿瘤体积缩小从而缓解脊髓压迫，尤其在淋巴瘤的治疗中效果显著。但在大多数情况下，激素通过减轻脊髓水肿来发挥治疗作用。由于同时应用多种治疗方法，糖皮质激素的作用很难评估，最佳治疗剂量还不明确。

对于仅有疼痛症状的患者，初始治疗可给予地塞米松（每24h 16mg）。若疼痛持续或出现新的症状可增加剂量。对于重度疼痛或有明确脊髓转移的患者，应静脉推注100mg地塞米松，之后每24h分次给予100mg。当患者接受疗效更确切的治疗方法后，该药物可缓慢减量。糖皮质激素可引起一系列副作用，其中部分在脊髓压迫患者中可能更为突出。1%的患者可能出现胃肠道穿孔。便秘是脊髓压迫常见的并发症，有增加胃肠道穿孔的危险。因此，在使用糖皮质激素治疗过程中，特别是初始剂量很大时尽早减量尤为必要。

放疗是脊髓压迫患者最常规的治疗方法。接受放疗的患者多因肿瘤进展或多发椎体转移失去手术指征[1,5]。放疗照射的范围包括受压部位和上下一至两个椎体，照射的单次剂量为300cGy，照射10次，总剂量为3 000cGy。对于初治有效而复发的患者，多程放疗可能有益且风险较小[7]。三维适形调强放疗安全有效，对已经照射过的部位或代替标准的外放射治疗结果满意[8~10]。

手术对于脊髓压迫的治疗意义越来越重要。一般而言，手术只限于下列患者：①已照射过的部位出现脊髓压迫；②患者出现脊髓压迫时未确诊为癌症；③椎体移位或椎间盘碎片引起硬膜外损伤；④骨质破坏引起脊柱不稳；⑤肿瘤对放疗不敏感（如肾癌）。然而，前瞻性Ⅲ期研究结果显示，手术联合放疗治疗脊髓压迫的效果比单纯放疗好[11,12]。肿瘤及受侵椎体切除预后更好，可长期显著改善神经功能，多数患者能恢复行走和括约肌功能。虽然两组间生存时间的长短无显著差异，但手术患者有生存期延长的趋势（129日 vs 100日，$P=0.08$）。上述数据提示脊髓压迫患者应考虑手术治疗。然而，该研究纳入的患者是有选择性的，是不是所有脊髓压迫的手术治疗患者都能获得较好的预后仍不明确。最新报道，椎体成形术和后凸成形术可有效治疗脊髓压迫，特别是对严重疼痛和脊柱压缩性骨折效果较好[13]。

化疗，同步或不同步放疗，对部分敏感性肿瘤尤其是淋巴瘤及少部分实体瘤有效[14]。化疗可有效治疗敏感肿瘤导致的脊髓压迫，但仅适用于那些神经系统症状轻微的患者。如果出现脊髓转移，首要治疗必须是放疗或手术。不论应用何种治疗方法，绝大多数患者在治疗前后均能保证良好的肢体活动。部分瘫痪患者通过治疗能再次行走，少部分患者仅恢复基本功能。

软脑膜转移

软脑膜转移发生率低于脑实质转移和椎旁转移，但在小细胞肺癌、乳腺癌和卵巢癌患者中发生率呈上升趋势。软脑膜转移可严重影像患者的生活质量和生存时间，只有不到一半的患者可从现有的治疗方法中获益。

目前很难准确估计软脑膜转移的发病率，约5%罹患转移性癌症患者可能会发生软脑膜转移。鲜有软脑膜转移的研究能给出明确的发病率数字，其诊断很大程度上取决于仔细的观察和遵循的标准。由于这些局限性，不同恶性肿瘤发生软脑膜转移的比例各不相同（表126-6）。

表126-6　各种恶性肿瘤软膜转移的发生率

恶性肿瘤	软膜转移发生率/%	特点
癌		
乳腺癌	5	发生率可能增加，浸润性小叶癌多见
SCLC	9~25	发生率逐渐增加，风险随生存期延长而增加
NSCLC	?	较乳腺癌少见
黑色素瘤	23	尸检时发生率50%
白血病		
AML	<5	未预防时为10%；表现为白细胞增加、LDH升高，伴髓外占位，呈单核细胞表型
ALL	11	未预防时为30%；呈T细胞表型，表现为Burkitt形态、白细胞增加
CLL	罕见	可能发生于暴发危象
淋巴瘤		
NHL	4~10	表现为弥漫大B细胞和淋巴细胞组织，伴骨髓侵犯
HD	罕见	
总体发生	8.6	MSKCC 649例脑组织尸检患者中56例发生软膜转移

SCLC，小细胞肺癌；NSCLC，非小细胞肺癌；AML，急性粒细胞白血病；LDH，乳酸脱氢酶；ALL，急性淋巴细胞白血病；CLL，慢性淋巴细胞白血病；NHL，非霍奇金淋巴瘤；HD，霍奇金病；MSKCC，纽约纪念医院斯隆-凯特林癌症研究中心（Memorial Sloan-Kettering Cancer Center）。

病理生理学

恶性肿瘤细胞可通过多种途径进入蛛网膜下腔（图126-3）。蛛网膜下侵犯是通过静脉壁和骨小梁浸润来实现的。恶性肿瘤细胞黏附于软脑膜毛细血管壁从而直接进入蛛网膜下腔。脑实质转移瘤会侵蚀脑室或蛛网膜下腔，或因手术播散，从而导致软脑膜转移。40%的小脑转移瘤患者手术切除后出现软脑膜播散，但仅2%~3%的幕上转移瘤患者手术切除肿瘤后发生软脑膜转移。通过脉络丛播散的病例罕见。恶性肿瘤细胞可沿神经根直接侵犯或经神经周围淋巴管进入蛛网膜下腔。

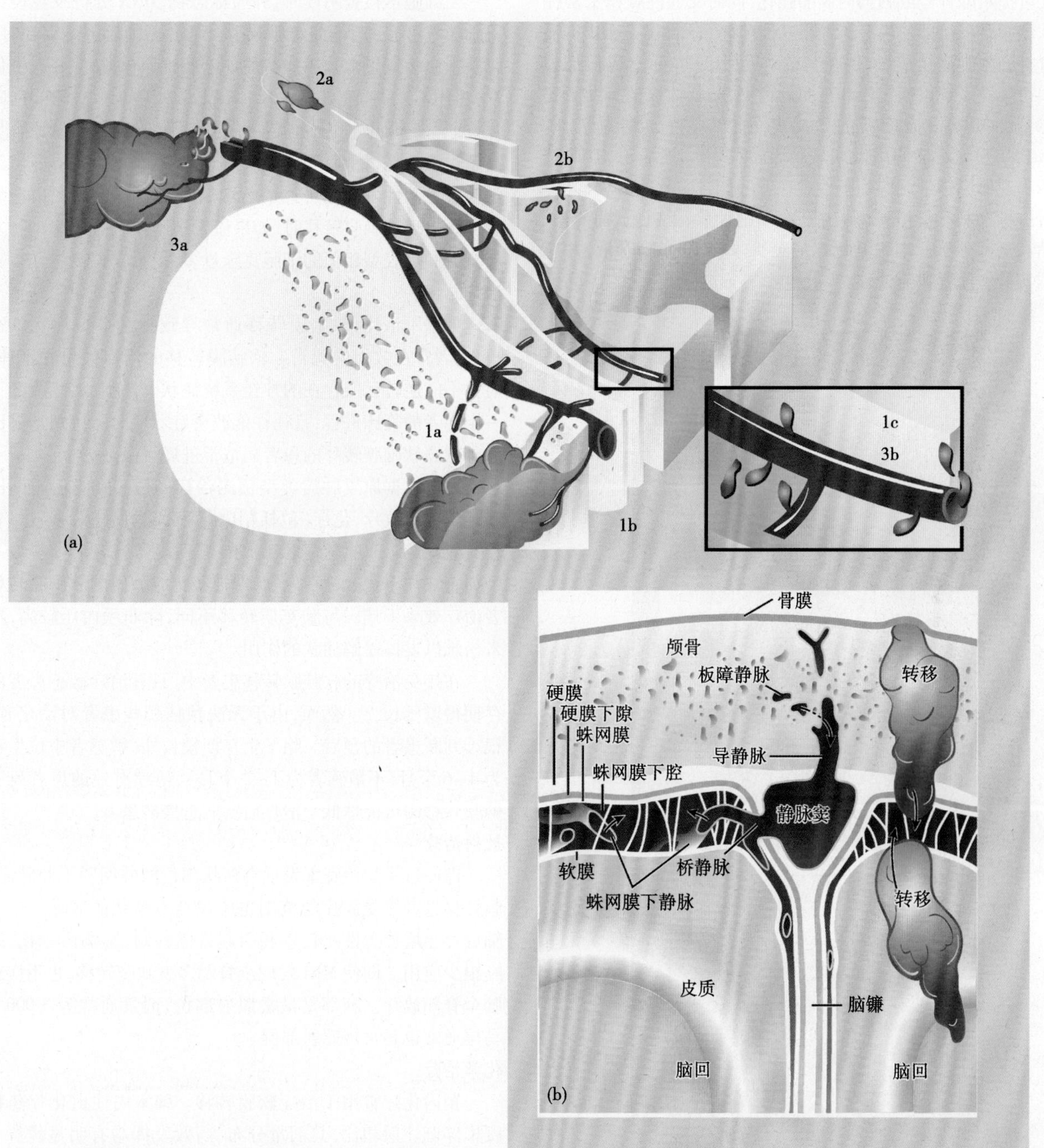

图 126-3　软膜转移的病理生理机制。(a)肿瘤细胞进入脊髓蛛网膜下腔机制。肿瘤侵犯椎体(1a)并沿椎旁静脉丛(1b)进入蛛网膜下腔(1c)。肿瘤还可侵犯椎管外的外周神经或神经根(2a)并沿神经鞘膜侵入椎管向软膜种植(2b)。肿瘤可侵犯中枢神经系统外血管(3a)并沿蛛网膜下腔静脉向蛛网膜下腔播散(3b)。见参考文献 1。(b)肿瘤侵入脑蛛网膜下腔机制。肿瘤可转移至颅骨或脑组织,经颅骨板障静脉或直接经蛛网膜下腔静脉向颅内蛛网膜下腔播散。脉络丛(未显示)也是脑膜转移的偶发部位

软脑膜转移通过多种机制引起神经系统功能异常[1]:①恶性肿瘤细胞直接侵犯脑、脊髓、脑神经和脊神经根;②影响脑脊液释放和吸收从而导致伴或不伴脑积水的颅内压增高;③肿瘤沿 Virchow-Robin 间隙浸润,可能会减少大脑血流灌注从而引起继发脑梗死。

症状和体征

不同部位多发的神经系统异常表现强烈提示软脑膜转移,包括[1,2]:①头痛,尤其是未发现脑转移证据时的晨起或体位性头痛;②脑神经麻痹,尤其是复视或面瘫;③无明确颈椎转移时出现颈部疼痛;④上肢或下肢的根性疼痛,尤其是伴有无局部椎旁痛的肌无力;⑤原因不明的便秘、阳痿、尿失禁或尿潴留;⑥非对称性下肢无力,不伴疼痛或感觉异常的腱反射减退;⑦意识不清、记忆力减退或其他认知障碍。

诊断

软脑膜转移诊断的金标准是在脑脊液中找到恶性肿瘤细胞。然而,影像学检查是目前较常用的诊断方法[15]。头颅

MRI 可提示脑神经或脑沟内肿瘤强化,同时交通性脑积水常提示软脑膜转移。即使没有神经根功能障碍,脊椎增强 MRI 可显示脊神经根肿瘤结节,特别在马尾附近(图 126-4)。应扫描整个中枢神经系统以确定疾病侵犯的范围,特征性改变有助于建立诊断。MRI 扫描诊断的敏感度为 76%,特异度为 77%。FDG-PET 显像可能偶然发现软脑膜转移[16]。然而,具有典型临床表现而影像学无明确阳性发现者不能排除软膜转移诊断。应行腰椎穿刺,进行开放压力测定、细胞计数、蛋白质、葡萄糖、细菌和真菌分析。细胞学标本应至少采样 10ml 脑脊液,并应根据实验室流程快速处理。

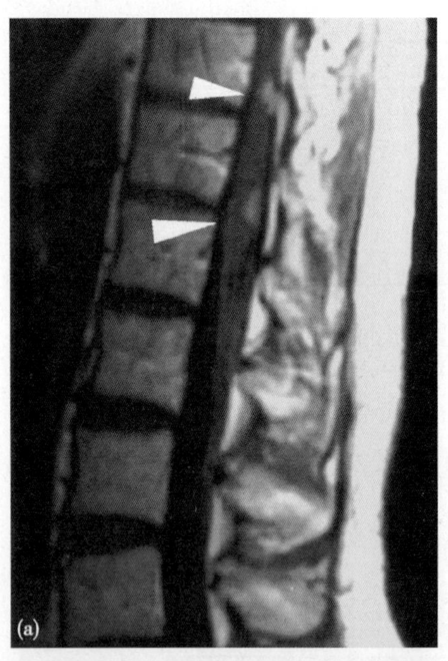

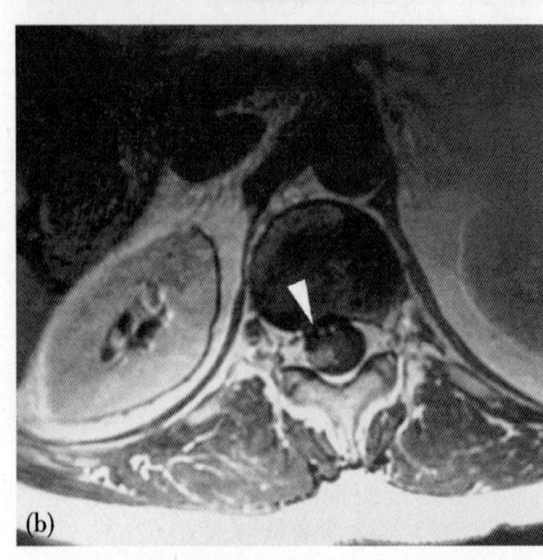

图 126-4 磁共振增强扫描显示肺癌软膜转移。矢状位(a)和轴位图(b)显示硬膜囊内强化结节。该患者脑脊液细胞学检查发现恶性肿瘤细胞

50%~60%的软脑膜转移患者首次脑脊液样本中可找到恶性肿瘤细胞[1]。细胞学检查敏感性为 75%,但特异性几乎为 100%。加送样本可增加阳性检出率。少数腰椎穿刺脑脊液无明确发现的患者脑池脑脊液可能找到阳性细胞。同时,脑室脑脊液细胞学检查可有阳性检出,而腰穿脑脊液检测可能为阴性,反之亦然。细胞捕获技术可较传统细胞学检查更能有效检出恶性肿瘤细胞[17]。

当细胞学检查阴性时,肿瘤标志物、DNA 分析及免疫细胞化学技术可有助于诊断软膜转移。当正常血脑屏障存在时(脑脊液蛋白含量正常),肿瘤抗原如癌胚抗原(CEA)、β 人绒促性素(β-HCG)、癌抗原(CA)125、CA27. 29、CA19~9 和前列腺特异抗原(PSA)的水平不应超过血清水平的 1%。当抗原含量升高超过该水平,特别是当脑脊液含量高于血清水平,即使细胞学检查无阳性发现也可诊断软膜转移。当淋巴瘤或白血病患者怀疑出现软脑膜转移时,如果流式细胞仪或分子标记物发现与全身肿瘤表型相似的细胞克隆过多,提示软膜转移。

治疗

如果不治疗,软脑膜转移通常导致神经系统症状急剧加重,患者常在数周内死亡。软脑膜转移的治疗效果并不理想,通常不能逆转已经存在的神经系统症状。然而,治疗改变了约一半患者的临床进程,且往往能改善症状[1,18]。特别是淋巴瘤和乳腺癌软脑膜转移的患者病情常进展缓慢。

可以根据原发肿瘤类型预测治疗的敏感性。由于淋巴瘤和乳腺癌对放疗、化疗(包括鞘内化疗)相对敏感,多数患者治疗有效。约 1/3 的肺癌和 1/5 的黑色素瘤患者治疗有效。神经损害往往不可逆,所以有严重神经功能障碍的软脑膜转移患者治疗效果不佳。与脑实质转移不同,除非颅内压较高,地塞米松难以发挥缓解症状的作用。

在接受治疗的软脑膜转移患者中,只有治疗敏感患者的生存期得以延长[1]。然而,由于无法预估哪些患者对治疗有效,很难判断患者的预后。除了生存期较长外(敏感者中位生存期为 4~6 个月,不敏感者为 1~2 个月),治疗有效的患者死于软脑膜转移的可能性低于治疗后疾病进展的患者。

放射治疗

即使影像学检查未发现有症状部位的蛛网膜下腔肿瘤,软膜转移患者接受放疗的范围也应包括有症状的区域。全神经轴放疗会增加急性死亡率和引起骨髓抑制,影响后续化疗,已经很少应用。即使 MRI 发现全脊髓多发软膜转移,也不应行全脑全脊髓放疗。脑部是最常照射部位,剂量通常为 3 000cGy,马尾通常也是常规照射部位。

化学治疗

鞘内化疗常用于治疗软膜转移。脑室内注射化疗药物与腰椎穿刺注射相比,其剂量分布、药效发挥均有明显优势。最常使用的药物是甲氨蝶呤(MTX),对乳腺癌、淋巴瘤和白血病均有效,但对其他常见肿瘤导致的软膜转移疗效欠佳。Ommaya 囊可通过手术置于右侧侧脑室。成人鞘内注射 MTX 的剂量是 12~15mg(以不含防腐剂的生理盐水稀释)。在该剂量下,脑脊液中 MTX 浓度在 36~48h 内可维持略超过 10^{-6}M 的治疗浓度。

应用^{111}In-DPTA(二乙烯三胺五溴醋酸)脑池造影评估脑脊液流体动力学发现,大量软膜转移患者脑脊液流动受阻。^{111}In 研究可预测脑脊液 MTX 分布浓度。除非存在完全阻塞,该药物可分布于整个蛛网膜下腔[19]。脑脊液流动受阻的患者脑白质病发生率增加,总体预后较差。若患者出现伴或不伴脑积水的颅内压增高,应首先考虑行脑室腹腔分流。即使存在可临时关闭的分流阀,脑积水或者行分流术后的患者也不应

采用鞘内化疗。Ommaya 囊脑室导管穿刺路径周围出现局灶性脑白质病的软膜转移患者应高度怀疑 CSF 流动受阻（见 MTX）。

鞘内注射后 MTX 可长时间存在于血浆内，易引起骨髓抑制和口腔炎。MTX 注射 12h 后开始口服亚叶酸钙可防止上述并发症发生。脑脊液中并不含亚叶酸钙，但可检测出其活性代谢产物 5-甲基四氢叶酸（5-甲基 THFA）。然而，口服亚叶酸钙后脑脊液中 5-甲基 THFA 水平很低，不会削弱对脑脊液中肿瘤细胞的杀伤效果。

有两项研究显示，鞘内注射 MTX 单药与鞘内注射多药化疗疗效相似，并显著减少全身毒性反应。和接受单独治疗的患者相比，MTX 联合放疗者往往能获得更高的缓解率。对于淋巴瘤、白血病或乳腺癌脑膜转移患者来说，阿糖胞苷（胞嘧啶阿糖胞苷[ara-C]）和噻替哌也可能有效。阿糖胞苷脂质体在脑脊液中半衰期较长，可以间隔 14 日给药。有报道指出，实体瘤软膜转移通常对阿糖胞苷不敏感，而阿糖胞苷脂质体可能有效[20]。但阿糖胞苷脂质体可引起严重的化学性脑膜炎，患者在给药前一天必须服用预防性类固醇激素并持续使用至用药后两天。鞘内注射利妥昔单抗、曲妥珠单抗（trastuzumab）可分别治疗淋巴瘤和 HER2 阳性的乳腺癌软膜转移[21]。对于临床进展稳定的患者以及经过 6 个月治疗后脑脊液无肿瘤细胞的患者，其后续治疗周期方案鲜有相关报道。鞘内注射药物可能会引起神经毒性，这将在本章后进行讨论。

由于软膜转移破坏了血脑屏障，大剂量的全身化疗可能也有一定的治疗效果。大剂量静脉注射 MTX（$3\sim8g/m^2$）并于用药 24h 后保护性应用亚叶酸钙可能会导致脑脊液 MTX 水平超过 10^{-6}M。这可以作为鞘内给药的替代途径，特别是在脑脊液循环受阻时。当鞘内注射药物渗入肿瘤结节剂量不足时，全身给药也可治疗多发脑膜转移。其他可进入脑脊液或对脑膜转移有效的药物包括治疗血液系统恶性肿瘤应用的大剂量阿糖胞苷和治疗乳腺癌的卡培他滨[22]。包括酪氨酸酶抑制剂和贝伐单抗在内的新药对个别患者有效，应根据敏感性选择使用[23,24]。

脑神经及外周神经转移

脑神经及外周神经的疾病常引起严重疼痛，所致的神经功能障碍程度取决于受累神经范围。恶性肿瘤转移灶所致颅内及外周神经功能障碍的发生率目前尚不明确，目前仅对部分特定肿瘤有少量报道。例如，面神经麻痹在恶性腮腺肿瘤的发生率为 5%～25%，其中在腺泡状细胞癌中发生率较低，而在未分化癌中发生率较高。原发肺癌患者约 3% 为肺上沟癌，其中大量患者表现为臂丛神经受侵的疼痛（Pancoast 综合征）。肿瘤可压迫侵犯单个或多组神经（多神经炎）。

发病机制

肿瘤压迫和侵犯神经鞘膜，从而损伤脑神经和外周神经。转移至锁骨上淋巴结的肺上沟瘤（Pancoast tumor）和乳腺癌可压迫但不常直接侵犯臂丛，而面部的鳞状细胞癌、黑色素瘤及前列腺癌可能具有神经源性，显微镜下可见其沿神经走行到达椎管甚至脑干[25]。类似于血脑脊液屏障的血神经屏障可将水溶性化疗药从神经中清除，从而为肿瘤细胞生长提供温床。

症状

脑神经及外周神经功能障碍的特异性症状及体征取决于受累神经和受累机制。疼痛常为首发症状，在受压局部或受累感觉神经或神经丛远端分布区出现。疼痛及神经功能障碍常同时出现在神经受侵部位。总体而言，当混合神经受累时，不论神经受累的机制如何，运动功能受损通常较感觉缺失严重。MRI 检查可以发现压迫神经的病灶（图 126-5）[1,25]。若病灶浸润性生长，影像学检查可无阳性发现，而仅能通过临床症状或活检确诊。增强 MRI 或 PET 检查可以发现向神经丛或神经根浸润性生长的肿瘤。

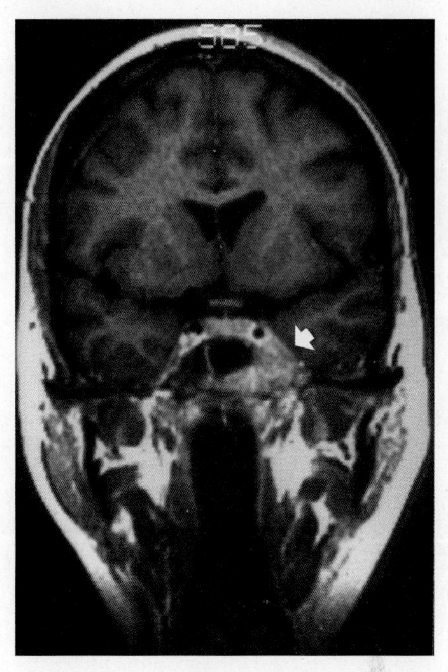

图 126-5　冠状位增强磁共振显示乳腺癌左侧海绵窦转移（箭头）。患者眶后痛，伴部分Ⅲ、Ⅵ、Ⅴ1 脑神经麻痹

脑神经及外周神经病变可能是放疗或化疗的副反应或副肿瘤综合征。鉴别非转移性和转移性外周神经病变比较困难。但总体而言，前者不常引起疼痛，后者通常痛感较重。此外，大部分副肿瘤综合征及药物诱发的神经病变多为双侧对称性，而转移性神经病变则是单侧不对称的。

脑神经病变

肿瘤可转移至从脑干至其投射的终末器官任何部位的脑神经（表 126-7）。脑干转移可能导致特发性脑神经功能障碍，但其他脑干体征常提示病灶的核心位置。软膜转移是脑神经病变通常多发的常见原因。颅底转移常引起特征性脑神经功能障碍，易于病灶定位[1,2]。脑神经最终可能在穿出颅孔后遭到破坏。

增强 MRI 扫描可显示受累脑神经及其全程走行。由于有可能同时发生软膜转移，即使明确诊断颅底转移，也应行腰椎穿刺。恶性肿瘤患者非转移性脑神经病变也很常见（表 126-8）。颅底和眼眶转移通常采用放射治疗。在合适的情况下可使用化疗。

表 126-7　恶性肿瘤转移致脑神经病变

转移部位	临床表现	特点评估
眼	视力下降,视网膜脱落	脉络膜病变较视网膜病变多见;疼痛、突眼、复视少见;原发病灶多来自乳腺和肺
眶	疼痛,突眼,复视,Ⅴ1 感觉障碍,约 1/3 患者出现迟发性视敏度下降	脉络膜转移常见;乳腺癌、前列腺癌、淋巴瘤为常见原发肿瘤
鞍旁	单侧额部痛,眼球活动障碍(Ⅲ Ⅳ Ⅵ),Ⅴ1 感觉异常	很少影像视觉,无眼球突出;多为淋巴瘤转移
鞍区	尿崩	垂体前叶功能不全和视觉障碍少见;上述症状提示原发性垂体肿瘤可能;多为乳腺癌转移
中颅底	面部麻木(Ⅴ2、Ⅴ3),部分患者展神经麻痹	肿瘤压迫致闪电样面痛(三叉神经痛)少见
颈静脉孔	声音嘶哑、吞咽困难、咽痛(Ⅸ Ⅹ),胸锁乳突肌无力(Ⅺ),偶见舌肌无力(Ⅻ)	优势半球的颈内静脉受压可能导致视乳头水肿;舌咽神经痛罕见
枕髁	单侧枕部痛和颈强直,单侧舌肌麻痹(Ⅻ)	疼痛常发射至前额
下颌	单侧下颌和牙龈麻木(“精神性神经病变”)	脑膜或颅底转移;多为乳腺癌、淋巴瘤转移
颈动脉窦或舌咽神经	晕厥,吞咽时颈咽痛	心脏抑制,血管减压性晕厥;头颈部恶性肿瘤,症状出现提示肿瘤复发,可危及生命
左上纵隔	声音嘶哑,喉麻痹	肺癌、乳腺癌、头颈部恶性肿瘤转移

表 126-8　癌症患者脑神经病变的非转移性病因

脑神经症状	病因
Ⅱ(单侧视物模糊)	镓,IFN-α,放疗,颞动脉炎,视网膜出血等疾病
Ⅲ(复视,上睑下垂)	糖尿病(瞳孔常正常),动脉瘤,颅内压增高(颞叶钩回疝),重症肌无力和格雷夫斯病(Graves disease)[a]
Ⅳ(下颌痛,面痛)	长春新碱,三叉神经痛(暴发无感觉障碍的闪电样痛)
Ⅵ(复视)	长春新碱,颅内压增高,头部外伤,糖尿病,药物毒性(毒品、抗惊厥药),斜视
Ⅶ(面瘫)	Bell 麻痹(特发性),水痘单状疱疹病毒感染[Ramsay 亨特综合征(Hunt syndrome)],糖尿病
Ⅷ(听力下降,平衡失调)	顺铂,氨基糖苷类药物,脑退行性变,听神经瘤,放疗诱发浆液性中耳炎
Ⅹ(构音障碍,喉麻痹)	长春新碱

[a] 复视的常见原因,但并非脑神经疾病。

臂丛神经病变

恶性肿瘤患者的臂丛神经病变通常由腋窝、颈淋巴结或局部骨质(锁骨)的转移癌破坏侵袭引起,部分肺上沟肿瘤也可导致臂丛神经病变[1,2]。由于多数转移癌从下方压迫臂丛,患者初发症状通常为肩后部疼痛,或上肢、腕部及前臂内侧放射至第四、五指的疼痛(沿 C8 或 T1 分布)。肌力减弱通常从手部开始出现,而感觉缺失往往始发于第四、五指。上述症状可逐渐进展至整个上肢,且有助于鉴别肿瘤和颈椎间盘突出症,后者的疼痛症状通常影响上肢外侧及前臂背侧,伴有肱三头肌及腕伸肌力弱(C7 神经根病变)。肿瘤可在腋窝及锁骨上区触及。同侧霍纳综合征(Horner syndrome)(上睑下垂、瞳孔缩小及无汗)常提示肿瘤累及椎旁区域星状神经节,此时颈部 MRI 扫描可发现硬膜外占位。

臂丛病变的鉴别诊断包括放疗诱发的神经丛病变、创伤(术中体位或中心静脉置管后)、特发性神经丛病或放疗诱发的恶性外周神经鞘瘤。转移癌导致的臂丛病变往往易与放疗诱发的神经丛病变混淆。对鉴别两者有帮助的临床特征包括:①转移性神经丛病变的首发症状常为疼痛,放疗诱导的神经丛病变常出现感觉异常;②霍纳综合征多见于转移性神经丛病变;③转移性疾病的症状及体征进展更快;④锁骨上窝肿大多见于转移性疾病;⑤淋巴水肿则多提示放疗诱导的神经病变。CT 或 MRI 可发现神经丛内占位(转移性神经丛病变)或由于纤维化而缺失的软组织界面(放疗诱导的神经丛病变)。PET 扫描可能有助于疑难杂症的确诊。

放疗是转移性臂丛神经病变的最佳选择方案。化疗对于部分先前接受放疗的患者可能有效(乳腺癌或淋巴瘤患者)。对于放疗诱发的神经丛损伤目前尚无满意的治疗方案。外科手术松解神经周围纤维组织目前对治疗无益,全身及局部皮质激素治疗、高压氧治疗、贝伐单抗注射等也无明显效果。卡马西平、阿片类制剂、加巴喷丁、普瑞巴林等药物及神经毁损手术可用于疼痛的治疗。

腰骶丛神经病变

腰骶神经丛由 L2 至 S5 的神经根组成。上腰段神经(L2~4)出骨盆延续为闭孔神经(支配内收肌)和股神经(支配股四头肌),而腿部其余部分则由坐骨神经支配(L5~S1)。膀胱、直肠及肛门由 S3、S4、S5 的神经根支配。虽然约 25%的患者是双侧受累,但转移性腰骶丛神经病变的主要症状是一侧下肢无力和麻木。双侧失神经支配会出现尿失禁,因此尿失禁往往提示中枢性(马尾)或骶骨受累。鉴别诊断需要增强脊椎 MRI 及脑脊液分析。盆腔和腹腔恶性肿瘤的局部侵犯是转移性腰骶丛病变的首要原因。需要鉴别的疾病包括:腰椎间盘突出症、马尾水平的硬膜外及硬膜下转移、放疗诱导的神经丛病变(常由盆腔肿瘤大剂量放疗引起)、术中损伤、血肿、脓肿、糖尿病性或特发性腰骶丛病变。转移性与放疗诱导的腰骶神经丛病变间鉴别要点与臂丛病变相似。转移性病变 CT 或 MRI 常显示腰骶丛肿块影。若有脓肿形成或怀疑继发性肿瘤可行活检。放疗是转移性腰骶丛病变最常用的治疗手段。若肿瘤转移累及脊柱,可出现硬膜外受压症状,因此上述区域必须包含在放射野内。

外周神经病变

转移性肿瘤可侵袭单束外周神经,也可沿神经广泛播散,导致单神经元复合体或弥漫性多神经丛病变,从而加重淋巴瘤或者白血病患者的病情。肢体的 PET 扫描有助于诊断[26]。然而,恶性肿瘤患者发生弥漫型多神经丛病变,常有毒物接触史,或伴副肿瘤综合征,后两种情况将在后续部分介绍。

癌症治疗中非转移性并发症

多数癌症治疗可出现神经毒性(表 126-9)。一些药物(如长春新碱)甚至可以在低剂量时引起神经毒性,而其他药物(如阿糖胞苷)只有在大剂量治疗才引起神经毒性。神经毒性已成为癌症治疗(如放疗)的剂量限制因素。患者在治疗中表现出的毒性反应往往超过癌症本身[1,2,27]。以下将介绍癌症治疗常见神经毒性。

化学治疗

长春花生物碱类

长春碱类药物可通过结合周围神经内的微管蛋白,干扰介导快速轴突运输的微管形成而导致神经损害。神经毒性是所有长春碱类药物的剂量限制性副反应,尤其是长春新碱。长春瑞滨也可引起周围神经毒性,尤其在联合或序贯与其他神经毒性药物合用时。其中枢毒性较为罕见,因为长春新碱不能透过血脑屏障。长春新碱不能用于鞘内注射。

表 126-9 癌症患者常用的有神经毒性反应的药物

急性脑病(谵妄)	非脑膜炎性头痛
糖皮质激素	维 A 酸
甲氨蝶呤(大剂量 IV,IT)	甲基苄啶-磺胺甲噁唑
顺铂	糖皮质激素
长春新碱	他莫昔芬
天冬酰胺酶	昂丹司琼
丙卡巴肼	癫痫
氟尿嘧啶(±左旋咪唑)	甲氨蝶呤
阿糖胞苷(大剂量 IV,IT)	依托泊苷(大剂量)
亚硝基脲类(大剂量或动脉注射)	顺铂
异环磷酰胺/美司钠(mesna)	长春新碱
干扰素	天冬酰胺酶
慢性脑病(痴呆)	氮芥
甲氨蝶呤	卡莫司汀
卡莫司汀	达卡巴嗪(动脉注射或大剂量)
阿糖胞苷	白消安(大剂量)
氟达拉滨	脊髓病变(鞘内给药)
视觉障碍	甲氨蝶呤
他莫昔芬	阿糖胞苷
顺铂	噻替哌
IFN-α	外周神经病变
小脑功能障碍/共济失调	长春花生物碱
阿糖胞苷	顺铂
苯妥英钠	奥沙利铂
丙卡巴肼	依托泊苷
无菌性脑膜炎	替尼泊苷
甲基苄啶-磺胺甲噁唑	紫杉醇
IVIg	苏拉明
NSAID	多西他赛
单克隆抗体	硼替佐米
硼替佐米	
卡马西平	
阿糖胞苷(IT)	
甲氨蝶呤(IT)	
糖皮质激素(IT)	

IV,静脉注射;IVIg,静脉人免疫球蛋白注射;IT,鞘内给药;NSAID,非甾体抗炎药。

摘自参考文献 1。

长春碱类药物神经毒性是年龄(成人更严重)及剂量依赖性的,存在肝损伤及在接受其他潜在神经毒性药物治疗的患者中更加严重。几乎所有接受长春新碱治疗的患者指尖都会出现刺痛的异常感觉,且通常在脚趾,而针对感觉功能的临床检查却往往是阴性。踝关节伸展反射缺失是早期普遍发生的征象。随着治疗进行,所有反射可能都减退或者消失,还有可能出现乏力。乏力主要有两种类型:①广泛性远端轴突神经病变更加常见,当乏力较轻时,患者丧失脚跟走路能力及腕伸肌的肌力;乏力严重者可出现走路时足下垂或两脚碰撞。当乏力严重到一定程度时,患者将无法行动或卧床不起,但在出现显著乏力症状前就应及时停药,若既往患有周围神经疾病,尤其是腓骨肌萎缩性神经病及其他可能的神经病变(如糖尿病性多神经病),则可增加长春新碱神经毒性的严重程度。②患者出现局限性乏力(单侧足下垂或脑神经麻痹,例如上睑下垂或眼外肌、面肌或咽肌麻痹),尽管全身毒性在停药后通常可以逆转,显著乏力在患者中可持续存在,自主神经功能紊乱,尤其是腹部绞痛及便秘,通常在每次给药后几小时或几天内发生,麻痹性肠梗阻也会出现且威胁生命,所有患者都必须预防胃肠道并发症的发生,阳痿的发生也有报道。

长春新碱给药的罕见并发症包括:骨痛、下颌及喉部尖锐刺痛,或已有疼痛加剧。这些症状通常在给药几小时内发生,在几天后逐渐缓解。症状往往在初次或二次给药时出现,很少在后续治疗中再次出现。抗利尿激素分泌不当引起的低钠血症在给药后数天内发生,并可能伴随后续给药而反复出现。

甲氨蝶呤

MTX 的毒性有不同的临床表现形式[1,2]。假性脑膜炎、神志不清、发热及脑脊液细胞异常增多等急性反应通常在鞘内注射后 4~6h 出现,并在几天后缓解。该综合征往往易与感染性脑膜炎混淆,但在注射后症状发生往往较细菌感染更加快速。如果革兰氏染色或培养显示没有微生物存在,则不需要使用抗生素治疗。地塞米松可缓解或预防部分症状发生。轻度急性毒性在患者的发生率为 10%,但持续鞘内注射 MTX 时通常较为安全。

截瘫通常会在腰穿滴注 MTX 或阿糖胞苷后出现,表现为腿部乏力及感觉缺失,经过数天后逐渐发展为横断性脊髓病。部分患者可恢复,但多数患者出现持续截瘫。尸检可发现脊髓广泛坏死。目前其发病机制不明,可能是特质性的,而与剂量无关。

鞘内高浓度注射 MTX 后出现的早期迟发反应在接受这一治疗患者中的发生率约为 4%。该反应通常在第三、四次治疗后的 7~10 日出现,表现为麻木或昏迷,并通常伴随偏侧性神经体征并在数小时内不停变化。MRI 弥散序列的高信号可能提示缺血改变。多数患者均可完全恢复且该反应通常不会在 MTX 再次滴注时重复出现。MTX 脑白质病变通常在接受鞘内或静脉 MTX 治疗累积剂量较高或接受 MTX 联合颅内放疗的患者中发生。治疗后存活超过 6 个月的成年患者可发生进行性认知水平下降而不伴有偏身运动感觉障碍。脑白质病变通常在这些患者的神经系统影像学检查中可见,但对于无症状患者则很少可在 MRI 或活检中发现病变。神经病理改变包括白质中多灶区域的凝固性坏死且常伴有广泛钙化,通常在脑室旁区域较明显。不同于脑放射性坏死,这种改变没有血管的纤维蛋白样坏死。

此外,局灶性脑白质病变可围绕导管的行走轨迹发生。当用力将 MTX 注入脑室时,药物沿着导管外壁扩散,产生类似肿块病灶的局灶性脑白质病变。MRI 可见低信号强化肿块(图 126-6)。该病灶可自行吸收或需要移除导管后消退。

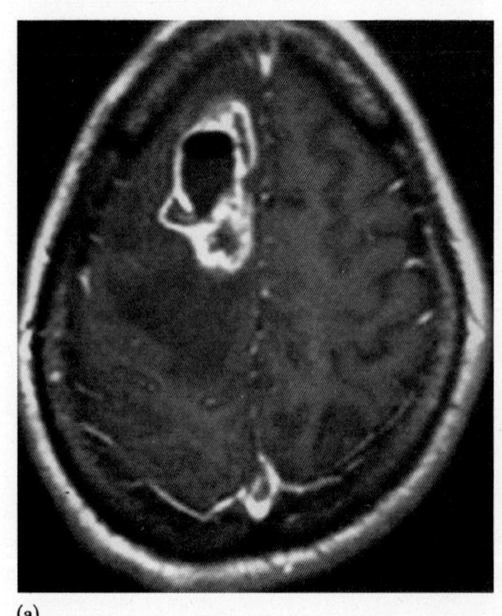
(a)

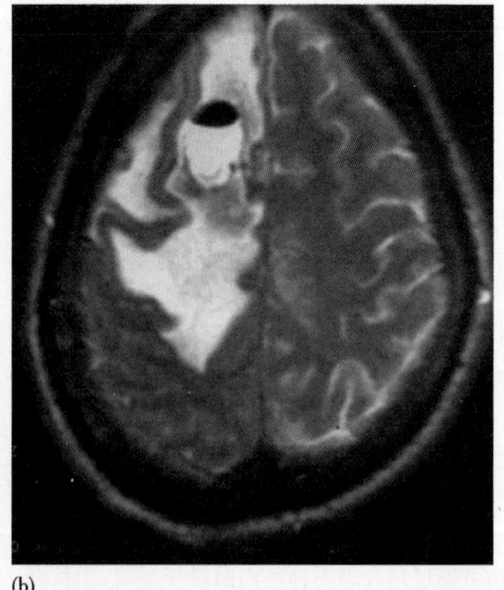
(b)

图 126-6　T1 加权增强 MRI(a)和 T2 加权(b)显示局灶性脑白质病变患者脑内功能异常的 Ommaya 储液囊。储液囊堵塞却未被发现。该患者接受甲氨蝶呤经多程鞘内灌注化疗。药物经导管注入弥散至额叶,造成区域性坏死伴周围脑组织明显水肿。最近一次灌注化疗后可见占位中心气体平面。该患者出现癫痫发作和左侧肢体偏瘫,经激素治疗后好转

铂类

周围神经病变是某些铂类药物的剂量限制性毒性反应，尤其是顺铂及奥沙利铂[1,28]。神经病变的症状一开始表现为手指及脚趾麻木感，也可出现伸展反射丧失、振动及位置觉减弱。疼痛、温度觉及肌力不受影响。可能出现严重的失感觉性共济失调。症状通常在治疗完成后出现，并在数月内进展并继而稳定。随后可出现逐渐缓解，但有些患者可能出现永久性的功能丧失。莱尔米特征（Lhermitte sign）是在颈部前屈时出现的手臂、后背或腿部过电样感觉，通常是铂类较少见的神经毒性。奥沙利铂可能在输液中或输液后短期内引起寒冷诱导的感觉异常[28]。镁剂不能治疗奥沙利铂的神经毒性[29]。

顺铂引起的耳毒性是螺旋器损伤的结果。严重到影响言语感知的毒性并不常见，但听力减退则有可能无法消除。癫痫发作和脑病已在接受顺铂治疗的患者中有所报道，顺铂诱导肾脏过度代谢镁和钙。可产生神经系统症状的血管疾病已被报道是以顺铂为基础化疗的迟发效应。许多产生该不良反应的患者后续出现雷诺现象，部分患者出现短暂脑缺血发作或脑梗死。其他铂类药物的神经毒性较弱。

紫杉烷类药物

紫杉醇和多烯紫杉醇都可与微管蛋白结合，稳定并促进微管的聚集。两者均可导致感觉障碍的周围神经病变，最初表现为足趾的感觉异常，继而扩展到手指[1,30]。严重的感觉缺失及反射消失随用药时间延长而逐渐加剧。撤药后症状常可缓解。乏力较为少见，但通常多在近端出现，类似肌病，但不同的是这可能继发于神经病变。由于紫杉醇通常被同步使用或序贯用于其他神经毒性药物如顺铂，患者在最初几次使用时可出现显著症状。紫杉烷与白蛋白纳米粒结合形成的白蛋白结合型紫杉醇较标准药物神经毒性轻。

氟尿嘧啶

广泛性脑白质病变在治疗中与严重的全身毒性相关，且提示存在遗传性二氢嘧啶脱氢酶缺陷，该酶负责进行嘧啶代谢[31]。口服卡培他滨（双重酯化氟尿嘧啶）较静脉输注氟尿嘧啶神经毒性轻。

阿糖胞苷

鞘内注射阿糖胞苷可引起急性化学性脑膜炎，伴有意识障碍、发热及脑脊液细胞增多。几乎每个接受脂质体治疗（DepoCyt）[20]的患者中均可发生。每次注射 DepoCyt 前和注射后均应该使用地塞米松。

静脉高剂量阿糖胞苷（$3g/m^2$，q12h，6 次）可导致 10%～25%的患者出现神经毒性。年长及肾功能不全患者上述风险增加。有报道指出，神经毒性发生的最小蓄积剂量为 $18g/m^2$，剂量越高（$30\sim40g/m^2$）发生率越高毒性越严重。通常毒性反应表现为全脑功能障碍，在初始治疗数天后出现，并在数天后加剧。一般在发病后两周患者可逐渐恢复，但有约 20%的患者并不能完全恢复，尤其是神经系统障碍严重的患者。包括小脑浦肯野细胞及小脑深部核团的神经元缺失都是可能出现的病理变化。在小脑中毒的情况下可能发生脑白质病变及癫痫发作。神经系统体征可能随再次治疗而出现。

其他药物

其他有神经毒性的药物包括硼替佐米[32]、苏拉明及丙卡巴肼（procarbazine）。这些药物均可导致周围神经病变，尽管使用丙卡巴肼很少出现这一问题。硼替佐米引起的神经病变可表现为剧烈疼痛，易导致压迫性神经病变和弥漫性神经病变。二代蛋白酶体抑制剂卡非佐米一般不会引起严重的外周神经病变。沙利度胺可致外周神经病，但来那度胺和泊马度胺（pomalidomide）神经毒性较小。高剂量白消安治疗过去常用于为患者骨髓移植做准备，它可导致癫痫发作。在标准剂量应用时该药物并不导致神经毒性。吉西他滨在联合腹部放疗时可导致肌炎并伴有急性肌痛及肌紧张，该症状可应用类固醇治疗[1,33]。MEK 抑制剂司美替尼可导致局灶性颈部伸肌力弱，表现为点头征[34]。

抗体介导的神经毒性

伊匹木单抗（ipilumimab）可导致下丘脑垂体炎，在 MRI 上表现为下丘脑增强信号。长期慢性应用利妥昔单抗可导致持续的免疫抑制，由于脑内 JC 病毒的激活，从而引起进展性多中心脑白质病（PML）[35]。上述并发症可能引起偏瘫、意识障碍、甚至危及生命疾病，其唯一有效的治疗方法是重建免疫功能。MRI 可见多发不强化的白质占位。

贝伐单抗以及其他抗血管内皮生长因子（VEGF）药物可引起高血压病和以癫痫、意识障碍为主要表现的可逆性后部脑部综合征（PRES）[36]。PRES 在 MRI 特别是 FLAIR 序列上表现为脑白质占位。PRES 患者需要密切监测并积极控制血压。其他药物如异体干细胞移植后应用的他克莫司、环孢素、吗替麦考酚酯以及许多传统的化疗药物如铂类和吉西他滨也可引起 PRES。博利那单抗是双特异性 T 细胞受体连接抗体（BITE），可用于治疗 B 细胞急性淋巴细胞白血病（ALL）。约 20%的患者可出现中枢神经毒性，导致脑白质病，表现为癫痫和共济失调[35]。

brentuximab vedotin 是 CD30 抗体药物的共轭化合物，可导致感觉性神经元病，停药后症状可以缓解，缓解后可再次用药[35]。brentuximab vedotin 也可导致肌肉痛。

放射治疗

虽然中枢神经系统对放射线不敏感，但是脑、脊髓以及外周神经都可能受到放射线的损害，该损害所产生的症状往往会在放射治疗完成数月甚至数年后出现（表 126-10）[2]。患者在治疗后存活时间越长，放疗对中枢神经系统的影响就越大。

脑损伤

放疗的急性反应多发生于放疗后数小时内。提前使用地塞米松[1]的患者很少出现急性反应。但是病灶较大、患有多病灶肿瘤或者有脑水肿的患者，特别是有颅压增高症状的患者，出现这些副作用的可能性更大。急性放射治疗损伤的症状包括局灶性症状的恶化、头痛、恶心、呕吐、意识障碍等。这些症状往往短暂，且对皮质醇治疗有效。病理学上可归结为放疗引起血脑屏障破坏继而形成的脑水肿。有时通过磁共振能发现更严重的病灶周围水肿。

早期延迟性脑病一般发生在放射治疗后数周到数月间。患者出现单侧病灶症状的恶化或原有意识障碍程度加重。症状往往持续数天到数周，并且在使用糖皮质激素后通常会得到缓解，一般最后会完全消失。早期延迟性脑病常和脑部肿瘤病灶进展或癌细胞转移混淆，因此也被称为假性进展。在磁共振上均表现为强化病灶，与肿瘤进展难以鉴别。PET 或灌注 MRI 检查可有所帮助。然而，症状逐渐加重明确提示病情恶化。

表 126-10　中枢神经系统放射治疗的神经相关并发症

并发症	潜伏期	症状体征	备注
脑			
急性	数小时	神经功能缺陷加重，头痛、恶心、呕吐、意识障碍、乏力	短暂性，糖皮质激素有效
早期性	数周至数月	神经功能缺陷加重，癫痫频发，嗜睡	数天至数周缓解，糖皮质激素有效
迟发性			
a. 放射性坏死	6个月至数年	局部占位效应	激素和手术治疗，可能与肿瘤共存
b. 痴呆	1年	认知水平下降	可能难以发现
c. 内分泌	数年	甲状腺功能减退，闭经/溢乳，性欲改变，生长受限	原发于下丘脑和垂体
d. 继发肿瘤	10~40年，儿童可能提前出现	脑肿瘤症状	脑膜瘤，肉瘤，恶性胶质瘤
e. 卒中	数年	突发神经功能障碍	主干或分支血管
脊髓			
早期性	数周至数月	颈部活动时休克（Lhermitte 综合征）	常为短暂性
延迟性			
a. 脊髓病变	数周至数年	感觉异常为首发症状的脊髓功能进行性障碍	致死率高
b. 下运动神经元综合征	数月至数年	局灶性肌无力和肌萎缩	可自然转归

晚期延迟性脑损伤是脑放射治疗后最为严重的并发症，治疗后数周到数年出现的脑放射性坏死是其最常见的表现[1,2,37]。研究表明，在接受了 4 500cGy 的放射治疗后，6%的患者会出现脑组织放射性坏死[37]。放射总剂量是放射性脑坏死的最主要因素。6 000cGY 是一个界限，超过这个剂量，非常容易发生放射性脑坏死。然而，超分割照射风险较大，放射性坏死特别常见于立体定向放疗治疗脑转移瘤后。头痛、局灶功能缺损以及癫痫都是常见症状。CT/MRI 上显示强化的病灶与周围水肿的占位效应，很难和中枢神经系统肿瘤区分开。PET 和灌注 MRI 可鉴别代谢旺盛的肿瘤和代谢减低的坏死。分辨肿瘤和放射性坏死常比较困难，可能需要活组织检查。使用地塞米松后，患者症状明显好转，有的患者在停用类固醇药物后依然可以保持良好状态。一般来说，需要手术切除坏死组织。而文献报告的抗凝剂及高压氧缓释症状还有待商榷[38]。

放疗还可引起痴呆，但并不能作为脑组织坏死的证据[1,2]。MRI 一般只能发现脑室扩张脑萎缩，以及白质信号增强。部分患者对脑室分流短暂有效或不完全有效[1]。在接受大剂量放疗后，颈动脉或颅内动脉可能闭塞而引起脑梗死[39]。血管畸形和脑出血可能是放疗后远期并发症。SMART 综合征（放疗后卒中样偏头痛）是指颅脑照射后复杂性偏头痛样发作[40]。放疗还可损伤下丘脑或垂体从而导致内分泌功能障碍。成人接受颅脑放疗后，可能在十年或数十年后会出现脑瘤，但同样情况对于儿童来说则出现更早（平均 6 年左右）。放疗可引起的肿瘤包括脑膜瘤、肉瘤以及恶性胶质瘤。

脊髓损伤

由放疗引起的脊髓损伤并不多见。在接受放疗数周或数月后，患者在颈部弯曲时可能会有短暂的触电感（Lhermitte 现象），这种现象也会出现在颈部放疗，包括对霍奇金病的斗篷式放疗之后[1]。治疗原则一般是等其自行消退。但从另一方面来说，这种放射脊髓病，特别是数月到数年（中期位为 20 个月）内疾病进展可能危及生命。放射脊髓病的产生，与放疗中接受的总剂量，以及每次分割的剂量都有关。我们估计，ED5（也就是使 5%的患者出现该病症）的总量在 5 700~6 100cGy，且每次不超过 200cGY。放射脊髓病的患者最初出现腿脚感觉异常，进而表现为感觉缺失、肌无力及括约肌功能障碍。脊髓受损还可能引起疼痛，同时受损处下方则表现为痛觉迟钝。与硬膜外压迫不同的是，在症状进展时，感觉和运动障碍的表现在一开始时往往是非对称的，并且经常会出现 Brown-Sequard 综合征。MRI 表现为正常的、增大的和萎缩的脊髓之间的对比非常明显，但没有实质性的压迫（图 126-7）。激素治疗效果较差。有报道称抗凝血剂和高压氧对这些症状非常有效，但未被严格证明。脊髓病通常是永久性的[1]。

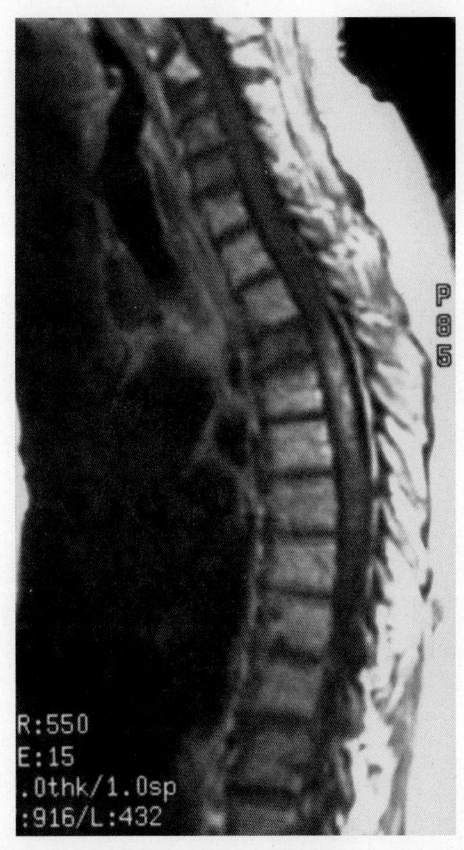

图 126-7 磁共振显示放射性脊髓病变。乳腺癌胸椎转移患者接受放射治疗，照射部位为低信号胸椎椎体。数月后，该患者出现脊髓病变，脊髓强化部位考虑为放射性损伤

癌症的脑血管并发症

有肿瘤转移的癌症患者尸体解剖及神经病理学研究发现，脑血管损伤是第二常见并发症。任何肿瘤转移都可能导致脑出血[41]。最多见的是肺癌。但按并发症出现例数与患者人数的比例来说，在黑色素瘤、肾肿瘤、甲状腺瘤及生殖细胞瘤转移中更常见。与转移无关的脑内出血则常见于白血病、血小板减少病及凝血功能障碍患者人群中[1]。硬膜下出血可能伴随硬膜转移或凝血障碍疾病[42]。出血量较大的患者可能会突然发生头痛、恶心、嗜睡和局灶性功能缺损。怀疑脑出血患者应行脑部影像学检查。对于由血小板减少症和凝血病引起出血的患者来说，应该注意观察，以便处理潜在的问题。脑转移相关的硬膜血肿和脑出血可能需要手术介入。

脑梗死和脑出血同样常见[43,44]。动脉的加速硬化引起的脑梗死一般在放疗后出现，这种放疗往往将颈动脉和脑血管包括在辐射野之中。头部和颈部的放疗容易导致颈动脉狭窄，以及脑血管狭窄，这些都是放射后脑梗死的主要原因。败血症性脑梗死经常与曲霉菌、假丝酵母和毛霉菌感染有关。这些条件致病菌会引起血管炎，其所导致的脑梗死一般为多处且易并发出血。曲霉菌是最常见的致病菌，且常伴有肺部感染，肺部感染灶的发现往往是诊断的线索。抗真菌治疗疗效差，病死率高。

脑静脉血栓形成（如上矢状窦血栓）可由于肿瘤转移对血管造成的压迫或侵入引起，也可由凝血性疾病引起[1,12]。临床上表现为头痛、局灶性功能缺损或癫痫。可通过磁共振静脉造影进行诊断。腰椎穿刺可发现颅压升高，以及脑脊液中红细胞增多。一般来说，如果不是硬脑膜转移（在这种情况中需要采用放疗）引起的，都可自行好转。

癌症患者发生脑卒中的情况中，大约一半是由于脑栓塞引起的[43,44]。这可能是由于心脏问题或非细菌性心内膜炎（NBTE）。肺癌和胃肠道肿瘤是最常见的与 NBTE 相关的原发癌。患有 NBTE 的患者发生栓塞时往往是多病灶的，还常伴随出血。弥漫性脑病和局灶性功能缺损通常伴随出现。在大约 1/3 的 NBTE 患者中，可找到弥散性血管内凝血的实验室证据。二维超声心动图诊断意义不大，但食管超声心动图却可证明瓣膜赘生物。脑血管造影显示多个动脉分支闭塞。在这种情况下，可考虑抗凝剂和肝素配合使用。有证据表明华法林作用不大。富含凝血酶或Ⅹa 因子抑制剂药物是否具有相似疗效还无法证实。DIC 可能导致脑血栓形成。初发神经症状通常表现为突发弥散性脑病和局灶性功能缺损。尽管在 DWI 序列上可以发现小的缺血灶，增强 MRI 的结果通常是阴性的。抗凝剂和肝素配合使用通常可以抑制神经系统功能障碍的发展。

神经系统副肿瘤综合征

副肿瘤综合征是指病因不明并且在癌症患者中发生频率越来越高的一系列生理功能紊乱（表 126-11）[3]。相对于其他已知的癌症并发症，副肿瘤综合征在癌症患者中并不多见，发病率约 1%左右。因为 2/3 的副肿瘤综合征在癌症确诊前就会出现，所以具有一定的积极意义，可以帮助诊断和早期治疗肿瘤。这些功能紊乱往往比恶性肿瘤对患者的影响更大。但其中一些病症有助于成功治疗癌症。

该综合征的发病机制不清，但其中多数可能与自身免疫基础有关。最有利的证据是由免疫系统紊乱引起的 Lambert-Eaton 肌无力（LEM）。该疾病是由于自身抗体抑制了神经肌肉接头的突触前钙通道，从而导致患者肌无力。检查表明，在反复的肌肉收缩后会使肌肉力量增强（与重症肌无力相反）和深部腱反射消失。这些症状与患者自己描述的感到口干、阳痿、大腿异常感都说明存在神经异常。有些症状与特异性抗体的出现有关，包括亚急性感觉神经病变、边缘叶脑炎、亚急性小脑变性和人免疫球蛋白相关性神经病变。这些抗体不仅是副肿瘤综合征的标志，也是可能存在肿瘤的证据[3]。

很多以免疫调节为主的治疗手段，包括血浆置换术、糖皮质激素和免疫蛋白的静脉注射，对由副肿瘤综合征引起的神经功能障碍治疗效果都不佳。LEM 是个例外，免疫抑制治疗对它有良好的效果。当对恶性肿瘤进行有效的治疗后，部分患者副肿瘤综合征的症状有明显改善。因此，应首先对恶性肿瘤积极治疗。

表 126-11 神经系统副肿瘤综合征

综合征	相关肿瘤[a]	临床特点
脑		
边缘系统病变[b]	SCLC	抑郁,记忆力丧失,意识障碍,脑脊液异常
脑干病变[b]	SCLC	共济失调,脑神经功能障碍,皮质脊髓束功能障碍,脑脊液异常
亚急性小脑退行性变	乳腺癌、卵巢癌,SCLC,霍奇金淋巴瘤	共济失调,构音障碍,眼球震颤,脑脊液正常
斜视性眼肌痉挛,肌痉挛	肺癌	眼球和骨骼肌急剧异常活动
视神经炎,视网膜变性	SCLC	无痛性视野缺失,短暂性视物模糊
NMDA 受体脑炎	畸胎瘤	癫痫,精神异常,节律活动,认知水平下降
脊髓		
坏死性脊髓病变	SCLC、淋巴瘤、白血病	脊髓病变加重
亚急性运动神经元病	霍奇金及非霍奇金淋巴瘤	部分性肌无力、肌萎缩、肌束颤动
背根神经		
亚急性感觉神经元病[b]	SCLC	感觉迟钝,感觉性共济失调,腱反射消失
外周神经		
人免疫球蛋白相关性神经元病	骨髓瘤	感觉功能丧失,肌无力,腱反射消失
急性多发神经炎(Guillain-Barré)	淋巴瘤	脑脊液中无细胞、高蛋白
神经肌肉接头		
LEMS	SCLC	近端肌无力,腱反射减弱,眼肌正常
重症肌无力	胸腺瘤	肌无力,眼肌受累
肌肉		
皮肌炎,多肌炎	肺癌、乳腺癌、卵巢癌、GI	肌无力,CPK 升高

[a] 最常见肿瘤。
[b] 常同时发生。
CPK,肌酸激酶;GI,胃肠道肿瘤;LEMS,Lambert-Eaton 肌无力综合征;NMDA,氮甲基-D-天冬氨酸;SCLC,小细胞肺癌。

(左赋兴 译 万经海 校)

参考文献

1 DeAngelis LM, Posner JB. *Neurologic Complications of Cancer*. New York: Oxford University Press; 2008.
2 Schiff D, Kesari S, Wen PY. *Cancer Neurology in Clinical Practice. Neurologic Complications of Cancer and Its Treatment*. Totowa, New Jersey: Humana Press; 2007.
3 Darnell RB, Posner JB. Paraneoplastic syndromes affecting the nervous system. *Semin Oncol*. 2006;**33**:270-298.
4 Liu JK, Laufer I, Bilsky MH. Update on management of vertebral column tumors. *CNS Oncol*. 2014;3:137-147.
5 Cole JS, Patchell RA. Metastatic epidural spinal cord compression. *Lancet Neurol*. 2008;**7**:459-466.
6 Lipton A. Efficacy and safety of intravenous bisphosphonates in patients with bone metastases caused by metastatic breast cancer. *Clin Breast Cancer*. 2007;7(**Suppl 1**):S14-20.
7 Rades D, Evers JN, Bajrovic A, Veninga T, Schild SE. Re-irradiation of spinal cord compression due to metastasis in elderly patients. *Anticancer Res*. 2014;**34**:2555-2558.
8 Sahgal A, Bilsky M, Chang EL, et al. Stereotactic body radiotherapy for spinal metastases: current status, with a focus on its application in the postoperative patient. *J Neurosurg Spine*. 2011;**14**:151-166.
9 Katsoulakis E, Riaz N, Cox B, et al. Delivering a third course of radiation to spine metastases using image-guided, intensity-modulated radiation therapy. *J Neurosurg Spine*. 2013;**18**:63-68.
10 Bydon M, De la Garza-Ramos R, Bettagowda C, Gokasian ZL, Sciubba DM. The use of stereotactic radiosurgery for the treatment of spinal axis tumors: a review. *Clin Neurol Neurosurg*: 2014.
11 Patchell RA, Tibbs PA, Regine WF, et al. Direct decompressive surgical resection in the treatment of spinal cord compression caused by metastatic cancer: a randomised trial. *Lancet*. 2005;**366**:643-648.
12 Bilsky M, Smith M. Surgical approach to epidural spinal cord compression. *Hematol Oncol Clin North Am*. 2006;**20**:1307-1317.
13 Kwok Y, Tibbs PA, Patchell RA. Clinical approach to metastatic epidural spinal cord compression. *Hematol Oncol Clin North Am*. 2006;**20**:1297-1305.
14 Grommes C, Bosl GJ, DeAngelis LM. Treatment of epidural spinal cord involvement from germ cell tumors with chemotherapy. *Cancer*. 2011;**117**:1911-1916.
15 Clarke JL, Perez HR, Jacks LM, Panageas KS, Deangelis LM. Leptomeningeal metastases in the MRI era. *Neurology*. 2010;**74**:1449-1454.
16 Shah S, Rangarajan V, Purandare N, Luthra K, Medhi S. 18F-FDG uptakes in leptomeningeal metastases from carcinoma of the breast on a positron emission tomography/computerized tomography study. *Indian J Cancer*. 2007;**44**:115-118.
17 Nayak L, Fleisher M, Gonzalez-Espinoza R, et al. Rare cell capture technology for the diagnosis of leptomeningeal metastasis in solid tumors. *Neurology*. 2013;**80**:1598-1605.
18 Taillibert S, Laigle-Donadey F, Chodkiewicz C, Sanson M, Hoang-Xuan K, Delattre JY. Leptomeningeal metastases from solid malignancy: a review. *J Neurooncol*. 2005;**75**:85-99.

19 Mason WP, Yeh SD, DeAngelis LM. 111Indium-diethylenetriamine pentaacetic acid cerebrospinal fluid flow studies predict distribution of intrathecally administered chemotherapy and outcome in patients with leptomeningeal metastases. *Neurology*. 1998;**50**:438–444.

20 Glantz MJ, LaFollette S, Jaeckle KA, et al. Randomized trial of a slow-release versus a standard formulation of cytarabine for the intrathecal treatment of lymphomatous meningitis. *J Clin Oncol*. 1999;**17**:3110–3116.

21 Zagouri F, Sergentanis TN, Bartsch R, et al. Intrathecal administration of trastuzumab for the treatment of meningeal carcinomatosis in HER2-positive metastatic breast cancer: a systematic review and pooled analysis. *Breast Cancer Res Treat*. 2013;**139**:13–22.

22 Ekenel M, Hormigo AM, Peak S, Deangelis LM, Abrey LE. Capecitabine therapy of central nervous system metastases from breast cancer. *J Neurooncol*. 2007;**85**:223–227.

23 Ranze O, Hofmann E, Distelrath A, Hoeffkes HG. Renal cell cancer presented with leptomeningeal carcinomatosis effectively treated with sorafenib. *Onkologie*. 2007;**30**:450–451.

24 Vincent A, Lesser G, Brown D, et al. Prolonged regression of metastatic leptomeningeal breast cancer that has failed conventional therapy: a case report and review of the literature. *J Breast Cancer*. 2013;**16**:122–126.

25 Ladha SS, Spinner RJ, Suarez GA, Amrami KK, Dyck PJ. Neoplastic lumbosacral radiculoplexopathy in prostate cancer by direct perineural spread: an unusual entity. *Muscle Nerve*. 2006;**34**:659–665.

26 Zhou WL, Wu HB, Weng CS, et al. Usefulness of 18F-FDG PET/CT in the detection of neurolymphomatosis. *Nucl Med Commun*. 2014;**35**:1107–1111.

27 Kaley TJ, Deangelis LM. Therapy of chemotherapy-induced peripheral neuropathy. *Br J Haematol*. 2009;**145**:3–14.

28 Joseph EK, Chen X, Bogen O, Levine JD. Oxaliplatin acts on IB4-positive nociceptors to induce an oxidative stress-dependent acute painful peripheral neuropathy. *J Pain*. 2008;**9**:463–472.

29 Loprinzi CL, Qin R, Dakhil SR, et al. Phase III randomized, placebo-controlled, double-blind study of intravenous calcium and magnesium to prevent oxaliplatin-induced sensory neurotoxicity (N08CB/Alliance). *J Clin Oncol*. 2014;**32**:997–1005.

30 Argyriou AA, Koltzenburg M, Polychronopoulos P, Papapetropoulos S, Kalofonos HP. Peripheral nerve damage associated with administration of taxanes in patients with cancer. *Crit Rev Oncol Hematol*. 2008;**66**:218–228.

31 Johnson MR, Hageboutros A, Wang K, High L, Smith JB, Diasio RB. Life-threatening toxicity in a dihydropyrimidine dehydrogenase-deficient patient after treatment with topical 5-fluorouracil. *Clin Cancer Res*. 1999;**5**:2006–2011.

32 O'Connor OA, Wright J, Moskowitz C, et al. Phase II clinical experience with the novel proteasome inhibitor bortezomib in patients with indolent non-Hodgkin's lymphoma and mantle cell lymphoma. *J Clin Oncol*. 2005;**23**:676–684.

33 Pentsova E, Liu A, Rosenblum M, O'Reilly E, Chen X, Hormigo A. Gemcitabine induced myositis in patients with pancreatic cancer: case reports and topic review. *J Neurooncol*. 2012;**106**:15–21.

34 Chen X, Schwartz GK, DeAngelis LM, Kaley T, Carvajal RD. Dropped head syndrome: report of three cases during treatment with a MEK inhibitor. *Neurology*. 2012;**79**:1929–1931.

35 Magge R, DeAngelis LM. The double-edged sword: neurotoxicity of chemotherapy. *Blood Rev*. 2014;**29**:93–100.

36 Tlemsani C, Mir O, Boudou-Rouquette P, et al. Posterior reversible encephalopathy syndrome induced by anti-VEGF agents. *Target Oncol*. 2011;**6**:253–258.

37 Ruben JD, Dally M, Bailey M, Smith R, McLean CA, Fedele P. Cerebral radiation necrosis: incidence, outcomes, and risk factors with emphasis on radiation parameters and chemotherapy. *Int J Radiat Oncol Biol Phys*. 2006;**65**:499–508.

38 Boothe D, Young R, Yamada Y, Prager A, Chan T, Beal K. Bevacizumab as a treatment for radiation necrosis of brain metastases post stereotactic radiosurgery. *Neuro Oncol*. 2013;**15**:1257–1263.

39 O'Connor MM, Mayberg MR. Effects of radiation on cerebral vasculature: a review. *Neurosurgery*. 2000;**46**:138–149; discussion 131–150.

40 Black DF, Morris JM, Lindell EP, et al. Stroke-like migraine attacks after radiation therapy (SMART) syndrome is not always completely reversible: a case series. *AJNR Am J Neuroradiol*. 2013;**34**:2298–2303.

41 Navi BB, Reichman JS, Berlin D, et al. Intracerebral and subarachnoid hemorrhage in patients with cancer. *Neurology*. 2010;**74**:494–501.

42 Reichman J, Singer S, Navi B, et al. Subdural hematoma in patients with cancer. *Neurosurgery*. 2012;**71**:74–79.

43 Cestari DM, Weine DM, Panageas KS, Segal AZ, DeAngelis LM. Stroke in patients with cancer: incidence and etiology. *Neurology*. 2004;**62**:2025–2030.

44 Navi BB, Singer S, Merkler AE, et al. Recurrent thromboembolic events after ischemic stroke in patients with cancer. *Neurology*. 2014;**83**:26–33.

第 127 章　肿瘤化学药物治疗的皮肤毒性反应

Anisha B. Patel, MD ■ Madeleine M. Duvic, MD

概述

随着新型靶向抗肿瘤药物的不断研发，肿瘤化疗的皮肤毒性反应日益突出。肿瘤化疗中皮肤黏膜并发症的发生率与受影响组织的高增殖特性有关，如黏膜、皮肤、头发、指甲等，其易于受到化疗药物的作用。本章讨论了与靶向治疗相关的特殊副作用和细胞毒性化学治疗的常见副作用。

肿瘤患者皮肤反应的诊断往往错综复杂，需考虑恶性肿瘤本身，伴随疾病，服用多种药物及免疫抑制。随着骨髓移植技术的进步，并发症如移植物抗宿主病（graft versus host disease，GVHD）、机会性感染和恶性肿瘤也越来越多地出现，并且由于其和化疗诱发反应的相似性造成后者诊断的复杂化。在本章中我们将讨论肿瘤化疗的各种皮肤反应（表 127-1）。这些反应在不同化疗药物中发生的频率和严重程度各不相同（表 127-2）。虽然皮肤毒性反应很少致命，但对潜在皮肤反应的识别十分重要，因为它们可能导致皮肤毒性反应发生率增高、化疗中止或剂量减少、容貌受损和心理困扰。正确处理这些潜在的剂量限制性皮肤毒性可能有利于计划化疗方案实施及疗效的优化。

表 127-1　与化疗相关的主要皮肤反应

药物过敏反应（麻疹、多形红斑、Stevens-Johnsons 综合征、中毒性表皮坏死松解症）
黏膜反应（口腔炎、阿弗他溃疡）
指甲反应（色素沉着、甲剥离、甲沟炎）
外渗反应（刺激性、糜烂性）
色素沉着改变（色素沉着、白癜风）
放射相关反应（放射增强反应、放疗后回忆反应，光敏反应）
脱发（生长期脱发、瘢痕性脱发）
肢端反应（化疗所致的骶部红斑/中毒性红斑、手足皮肤反应）
中性粒细胞皮肤病（Sweet 综合征、结节性红斑）
淋巴细胞恢复性皮肤赘生物（角化病、鳞状细胞癌、雀斑样痣、黑色素瘤）

表 127-2　主要化疗药物类别的常见皮肤黏膜反应

烷化剂类	抗生素类	长春碱类	抗代谢类
色素沉着	脱发	脱发	肢端红斑
超敏反应	口腔炎	化学蜂窝织炎	脱发
	化学蜂窝织炎	炎症性角化病	色素沉着
	色素沉着	嗜中性小汗腺炎	放射相关反应
	放射相关反应		

药物过敏反应

"传统"药物反应可分为免疫反应、非免疫或毒性反应。在免疫药物反应中，按免疫反应分型可分为Ⅰ-Ⅳ亚型（表 127-3）。最常见的反应是 T 细胞介导的延迟型药物反应，包括麻疹或发疹性药疹。临床表现为躯干上的红斑和薄丘疹，向四肢蔓延，通常无症状。当皮疹疼痛时，鉴别诊断包括多形红斑（erythema multiforme，EM）、Stevens-Johnsons 综合征（Stevens-Johnsons syndrome，SJS）和中毒性表皮坏死松解症（toxic epidermal necrolysis，TEN）。EM 的特征常以四肢的靶形红斑丘疹或丘疹起病，可累及手掌和脚掌，进展时可形成中央大疱并累及至口腔和生殖器黏膜。而 SJS 和 TEN 常以集中分布的暗色丘疹和斑块起病，这些丘疹和斑块合并形成囊泡，并伴有严重的黏膜受累。SJS 皮损通常占体表面积比例<10%，而 TEN>30%。SJS 的死亡率为 1%~5%，TEN 是 25%~35%[1]。

表 127-3　免疫介导的药物过敏反应

IgE 依赖的药物反应（原Ⅰ型）	L-天冬酰胺酶、紫杉醇、多西他赛、替尼泊苷、顺铂（膀胱内用药）	荨麻疹、血管性水肿、速发型过敏反应
细胞毒性药物引起的反应（针对固定抗原的抗体；原Ⅱ型）		继发于药物引起血小板减少的瘀点
免疫复合物依赖的药物反应（原Ⅲ型）		血管炎、血清病、荨麻疹（某些类型）
迟发型细胞介导的药物反应（原Ⅳ型）与未定义的类型	丙卡巴肼、半胱氨酸、核苷类似物（也可以有 IgE 依赖和免疫复合物介导的药物反应）	发疹样/麻疹样疹、固定型药疹、苔藓样药物反应、SJS/TEN、AGEP、DRESS
未观察到免疫介导反应	亚硝基、长春碱、阿尔维他明、达汀霉素	

伴嗜酸性粒细胞增多和系统症状的药疹（drug reaction with eosinophilia and systemic，DRESS）和急性全身发疹性脓疱病（acute generalized exanthematous pustulosis，AGEP）的发病机制尚不清楚。DRESS 的皮损并不特异，但以周围水肿、淋巴结病和肝转氨酶升高为特征。AGEP 表现为突然出现成片的皮肤脓疱。通常开始于面部或易摩擦的区域，可能伴有灼烧和瘙痒。可伴有发热、中性粒细胞增多和嗜酸性粒细胞增多[2]。90%的病例是药物引起的，主要是用抗生素如 β-内酰胺类、头孢菌素、氟康唑、制霉菌素（nystatin）、特比萘芬（terbinafine）[1]。其他已报道的诱因包括组蛋白脱乙酰酶抑制剂苔藓抑素（bryostatin）[3]、伊马替尼、汞、铊、碘己醇、斑贴试验、伪麻黄碱、地尔硫䓬、呋塞米和病毒感染[4]。这两种反应不如发疹性皮损常见，但更为严重。

肿瘤靶向治疗

靶向药物在 20 世纪 90 年代中期开始出现，其副作用一直备受关注。虽然全身毒性降低了，但许多靶向药物的信号通路也影响上皮细胞，使其副作用比以往的化疗皮肤反应更为特异。这一变化甚至反映在临床试验的文献中，在临床试验中的不良事件以往被描述为“皮疹”或“病变”，现在描述变得更加具体，更易于对其进行预测和监测。

目前有许多靶向治疗，但只有那些发生率较高特定的皮肤反应在本章节讨论。

表皮生长因子受体抑制剂

近年来，EGFR 已被公认为是肿瘤细胞增殖、凋亡、血管生成和转移的重要调节因子。配体与受体结合使受体形成二聚体，从而激活了细胞内酪氨酸激酶结构域[5]。EGFR 对于维持正常皮肤稳态也起到重要作用[6]。表皮角质形成细胞 EGFR 的激活起到促进细胞周期、分化、迁移的作用，是正常皮肤功能维持和伤口愈合的关键[7]。EGFR 抑制剂常见的皮肤不良反应包括痤疮样皮疹、甲沟炎、干燥病、湿疹及地图舌。痤疮毛囊炎一般在治疗后 8~10 日出现在面部和躯干上部。在Ⅰ期临床试验中，厄洛替尼最大耐受剂量组约有 50%的病例在治疗第二周出现脓疱样痤疮样药疹[8]。皮疹可因异常瘙痒导致超过 75%的患者 EGFR 抑制剂剂量的调整[9]。痤疮毛囊炎的发生和严重程度与肿瘤缓解和生存有关[10]。该皮肤反应在西妥昔单抗（cetuximab）、帕尼单抗（panitumumab）、尼妥珠单抗（nimotuzumab）、厄洛替尼和吉非替尼（gefitinib）中均有报道[11~13]。口服四环素联合局部类固醇是标准治疗。维 A 酸和局部抗生素的有效性仍未得到证实，由于引起皮肤反应的病因是上皮细胞功能失调，并非滤泡堵塞和破裂[11]。葡萄球菌定植会加重皮疹，如果病变为脓疱或结痂，则建议行微生物培养和使用抗生素（图 127-1）。

人类表皮生长因子受体（human epidermal growth factor receptor，HER）1/2 阻滞剂具有与 EGFR 抑制剂相同的副作用，但更为温和。曲妥珠单抗（trastuzumab）、拉帕替尼、达可米替尼（dacomitinib）和阿法替尼都报道过痤疮暴发[14~17]。此外，血管内皮生长因子（vascular endothelial growth factor，VEGF）抑制剂可发生黏膜炎和地图舌，多激酶抑制剂可发生手足皮肤反应（hand-foot skin reaction，HFSR）[18]。

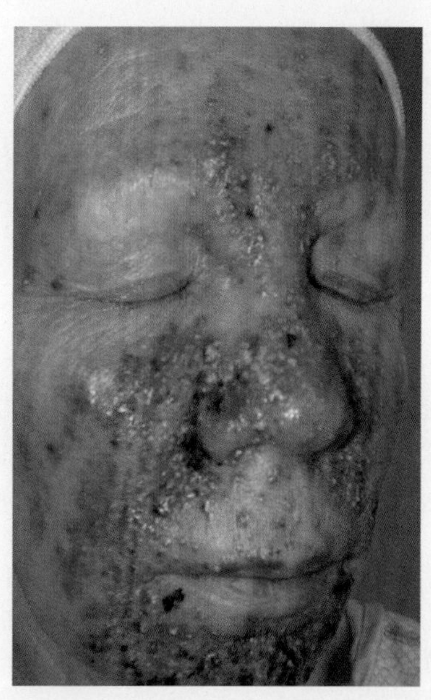

图 127-1　西妥昔单抗治疗相关的脸部严重痤疮样皮疹

BCR-ABL 酪氨酸激酶抑制剂

甲磺酸伊马替尼靶向 *BCR-ABL* 基因，已用于慢性髓细胞性白血病和急性淋巴细胞白血病的治疗。伊马替尼常引起剂量依赖性皮肤反应，包括面部水肿，麻疹样皮疹，荨麻疹，湿疹性皮炎和 AGEP[19,20]。一位患者出现了具有蕈样肉芽肿（mycosis fungoides，MF）组织学特征的湿疹[21]。

第二代和第三代 BCR-ABL 特异性酪氨酸激酶抑制剂如达沙替尼（dasatinib）、尼洛替尼和泼那替尼与手掌、面部和身体的滤泡性苔藓样病变有关，这些疾病会引起瘙痒并导致瘢痕性脱发[22]。这种脱发即使停药也不可逆转。

多激酶抑制剂

舒尼替尼和索拉非尼（sorafenib）是针对 VEGF 受体、血小板衍生生长因子受体（platelet-derived growth factor receptor，PDGFR）、c-Kit 和 FLT-3 的多激酶抑制剂。索拉非尼也抑制 RAF 激酶。它们是为晚期肾细胞癌研发，也被用于肝癌、胃癌和甲状腺癌的治疗。它们与 HFSR、黏膜炎、脱发、干燥症和口干症密切相关。然而，由于它们与多种靶向治疗有重叠，也有 BRAF 抑制剂导致皮肤鳞状细胞癌（squamous cell carcinoma，SCC）和 VEGF 抑制剂导致痤疮样皮疹的报道[23]。

HFSR 发生的高峰期在开始治疗后的 2~4 周内，发生率在 1/5~1/3 之间，索拉非尼的发生率略高。患者在摩擦和压力点形成局灶性角质层，可形成囊泡，最终导致疼痛的水疱（图 127-2）。发生 HSFR 的风险取决于患者使用的药物和正在治疗的癌症类型。最初提出的可能机制是这些药物的 VEGFR 阻断导致患者对压力和创伤的反应能力减弱[24,25]。最近，通过使用抗 Fas 配体抗体阻断反应，Fas/Fas 配体反应被证实与该皮肤反应有关，这也可能参与 Stevens-Johnsons 综合征和 TEN 的发生[26]。

虽然在索拉非尼和舒尼替尼等多激酶抑制剂中更为常见，但有报道称这些病变与 BRAF 抑制剂有关[27]。这些与细胞毒性化疗中常见的手足综合征/肢端红斑（acral erythema，AE）/毒

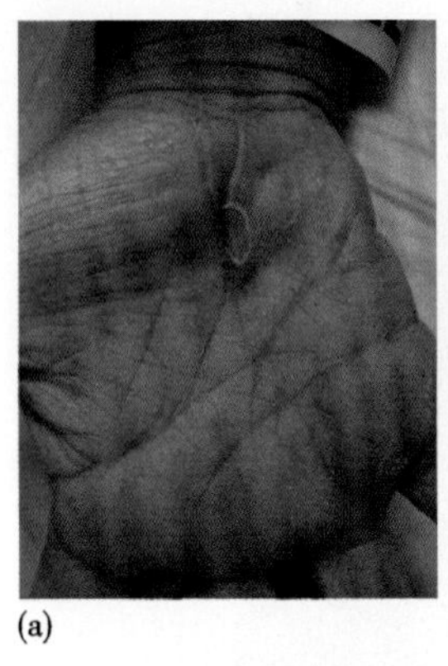

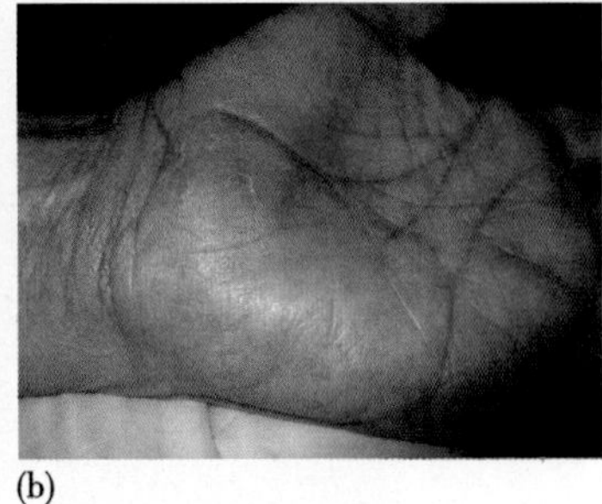

(a) (b)

图 127-2 索拉非尼治疗相关的手足皮肤反应

性红斑不同。HFSR 与手足综合征的区别在于后者伴有弥漫性红斑和水肿，且潜伏期较长（2～4 周）。HFSR 通常在继续使用多激酶抑制剂治疗的过程中自行消退[28]。

mTOR 抑制剂

与 EGFR 信号通路重叠的是 PI3K/AKT 信号通路，后者可激活哺乳动物的西罗莫司靶点（mammalian target of rapamycin，mTOR）。该信号通路与细胞生长和血管生成有关，西罗莫司或西罗莫司是这类的原始药物代表，此外还有依维莫司（everolimus）和坦罗莫司（temsirolimus）。这些药物都与 EGFR 抑制剂导致的丘疹脓疱疮有关，在最新开发的药物坦罗莫司中，这种皮肤反应的发生率为 45.8%。他们也可诱发比较典型的麻疹型药疹和口腔黏膜炎。与细胞毒性化疗相反，类似于口腔溃疡的较深口腔溃疡的案例也有报道。此外，依维莫司和坦罗莫司也可导致湿疹性皮炎[29]。

BRAF 抑制剂

BRAF 抑制剂最早用于转移性黑色素瘤的治疗，具有显著的皮肤副作用如炎症、滤疱疹和肿瘤。这些副作用导致小于 10%的患者停止或减少剂量[30]。在炎性皮肤毒性中，中性粒细胞皮肤病，包括急性发热性中性粒细胞皮肤病（Sweet 综合征）和中性粒细胞脂膜炎，被认为与使用 BRAF 抑制剂有关[30～36]。

已有 2 例躯干和四肢 Sweet 综合征所致红斑性假泡样丘疹和丘疹，伴系统性症状如发热和关节疼痛[36,37]。中性粒细胞性脂膜炎的患者表现为腿部柔软红斑结节，偶尔也出现在手臂，组织学与中性粒细胞小叶脂膜炎一致[31～34]。白癜风[38]，皮肤结节病[39]，Grover 病[40]和化脓性汗腺炎[41]的报道较少。

BRAF 抑制剂治疗的患者对紫外线（ultraviolet，UV）以及放射治疗的辐射敏感性增强，从而导致更快发生、更严重的晒伤和急性放射性皮炎[42,43]。此外，放疗后回忆反应性皮炎的病例也有报道[44,45]。

表皮和毛囊的调节失调在 BRAF 抑制剂皮肤反应中起到关键作用。掌跖角化过度或角化病是一种非炎症性表皮增厚，表现为手掌和脚掌的黄色厚斑块，类似于大的胼胝组织。最常见的是脚部的角质层呈压力点状，不伴有水疱[46]。毛囊表面角化性堵塞可导致角化病的毛状疹，这是常见于躯干和四肢，通常无症状。在 2 期和 3 期临床研究中[47,48]，5%～9%的患者没有注意到该皮肤反应，这个数据仍可能被低估了。

肿瘤病变是这些皮肤反应中发病率最高的。光化性角化病（actinic keratoses，AK）是一种典型的上皮组织癌前病变，与慢性日光损伤有关。维莫非尼治疗的患者中 AK 的发生率为 6%～16%[47～49]，而达拉菲尼治疗的患者为 5%[46,51～53]。疣状角化病是一种乳头状的、高度角化的、界限清楚的丘疹，在 BRAF 抑制剂治疗过程中经常发生。它们在治疗后 3～4 个月出现[53]。这些病变并不是真正的疣，人类乳头瘤病毒检测多呈阴性[54,55]。对于这两种类型的病变，都应及时采用冷冻疗法、光动力疗法、刮除术和局部氟尿嘧啶帮助预防 SCC 的发生（图 127-3）。

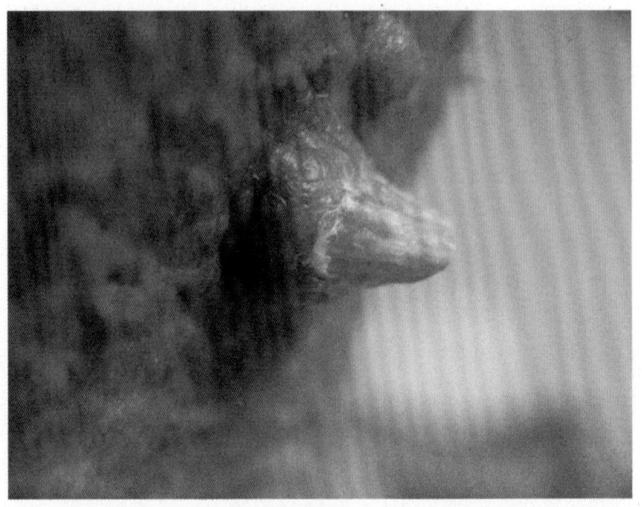

图 127-3 维莫非尼治疗相关的鳞状细胞癌

SCC 患者常表现为球形、界限清楚、角化过度、红斑丘疹和结节。它们生长迅速，在患有慢性太阳损伤的老年患者中发病率更高[46]。

维莫非尼治疗的患者中 SCC 的发生率为 4%～31%[47,48,56]，而达拉菲尼治疗的患者发病率为 6%～11%[51,52,57,58]。Sosman 等人的研究表明，它们主要是分化良好的或角化棘皮瘤型鳞状细胞癌，比普通的太阳诱导的鳞状细胞癌的侵袭性小。SCC 发生的中位时间为 8 周。在部分 BRAF 诱导的部分 SCC 案例中发现 HRAS 的上调与 MAP 激酶通路的反常上调有关[47]。

据报道，患者有色素痣的退化，新出现的色素痣及色素痣变黑的情况发生。新的色素痣通常在 8～14 周出现，表现为 BRAF 野生型，无 *V600E* 突变[59]。这些病变活检被认为是普通痣、发育不良痣和新的原发性皮肤黑色素瘤。在使用维莫非尼治疗的 2 期和 3 期临床研究的 464 名患者中，有 5 名患者出现了新的黑色素瘤[60]。

MEK 抑制剂

司美替尼（selumetinib）和曲美替尼（trametinib）是两种新型 MEK 抑制剂，其靶点位于 BRAF 下游，其副作用与 EGFR 抑制剂相似[61]。有趣的是，在 BRAF 抑制剂中加入 MEK 抑制剂后，与单独使用 BRAF 抑制剂相比，鳞状细胞增殖速度降低，这可能也同时解决了 *HRAS* 突变的问题。

免疫调制剂

随着生物技术的进步，针对肿瘤细胞水平的细胞因子和免疫治疗药物的开发也越来越多。这类药物的特异性略逊色于靶向治疗，主要通过增强机体对转移性和血液系统肿瘤的抗肿瘤免疫反应发挥作用。其皮肤的副作用也常缺乏特异性，常包括反应性炎症过程。

免疫检查点抑制剂

用于治疗黑色素瘤的免疫调节剂包括伊匹木单抗（ipilumimab）和纳武单抗（nivolumab）或帕博利珠单抗（帕博利珠单抗）。伊匹木单抗是一种靶向 CTLA4 的单克隆抗体，可抑制共刺激分子 CD28 的结合。阻断 CTLA4 可使激活细胞毒性 T 细胞活性，增强对转移性黑色素瘤的免疫应答。主要的副作用是麻疹或湿疹[62]。同样，帕博利珠单抗阻断 PD-1，当 PD-1 与配体结合时，可降低 T 细胞的细胞毒性作用。这种分子在肿瘤细胞中上调，被认为是比 CTLA4 更具有特异性。除了具有与伊匹木单抗类似的皮肤副作用外，还可导致白癜风[63]。

细胞因子

重组人白介素-2（interleukin 2，IL-2）已经作为晚期转移性黑色素瘤和肾细胞癌的替代治疗，干扰素-α（interferon-α，IFN-α）已经成为慢性髓細胞性白血病、毛细胞白血病、皮肤 T 细胞淋巴瘤、黑色素瘤及卡波西肉瘤（Kaposi sarcoma，KS）的标准治疗。据报道，除了显著毒性（表 127-4）如毛细血管渗漏综合征外，IL-2 发生皮肤反应的概率大约为 72%[64]。一种瘙痒的弥漫性红皮病通常在用药后 1~3 日出现，在停止治疗 2 日后消退伴有脱屑（图 127-4）[64]。这种皮肤反应临床表现类似于中毒性休克综合征，在一些患者中已证实和金黄色葡萄球菌败血症有关。IL-2 动脉内用药也可导致多达 30% 的患者对含碘的造影剂过敏[65]。重要的是，一项 IL-2 治疗转移性黑色素瘤的研究表明白癜风的发生可能与较好的预后相关[66]。虽然 IFN-α 的毒性比 IL-2 小，文献中也有一些皮肤反应报道。大约 1/3 的患者会发生局部注射部位的反应。在一项对 1 000 名接受 IFN-α 治疗的患者的研究表明，脱发和唇疱疹加重较为常见，发生率分别为 10% 和 5%[65,67]。类似于非修饰的重组 IFN-α，聚乙二醇 IFNα 已被证明会引起皮下注射部位的局部皮肤溃疡[68]。IFN-α 和 IL-2 也可诱发和/或加重脂溢性皮炎和牛皮癣[65]。

表 127-4 细胞因子反应

其他 IFN-α 反应	其他 IL-2
嗜酸性筋膜炎	手术瘢痕的侵蚀
疱疹口唇加重	对碘造影剂过敏
增加睫毛生长	线性 IgA 大疱性皮肤病
坏死性血管炎	寻常性天疱疮（新发，复发性）
副肿瘤性天疱疮	皮肌炎恶化
银屑病（新发，恶化）	牛皮癣恶化
甲状腺炎	葡萄球菌感染
	TEN 样大疱性剥脱性白癜风

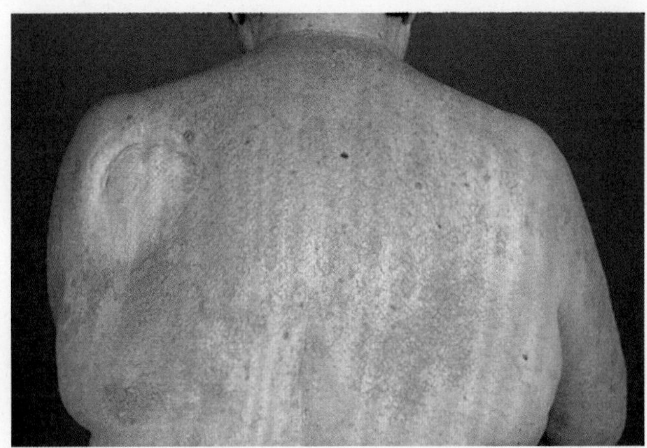

图 127-4 黑色素瘤患者出现与 IL-2 治疗相关的红斑皮疹

脱发

脱发是化疗引起的最常见皮肤毒性反应。大多数药物引起的脱发是诱导正常的头发过早进入休止期而导致休止期脱发，而生长期脱发是除 IL-2 和 IFN-α 之外化疗药物引起的最常见脱发类型（表 127-5）。生长期脱发是由于化疗引起头发基质细胞在毛囊毛发生长期的高有丝分裂活动突然中止所致[70]。生长期脱发从化疗开始 1~2 周内始出现，在化疗 1~2 个月后最为明显[71]。头发再生通常在化疗结束 5 个月后，然后头发的颜色和质感可能会改变[69]。有报道显示白消安/环磷酰胺可引起永久性脱发[72]。

表 127-5 化疗药物相关的脱发

常见或严重		罕见或轻微	
博来霉素	异环磷酰胺	安吖啶	美法仑
顺铂	IFN-α	白消安	巯嘌呤
环磷酰胺	伊立替康	卡铂	甲氨蝶呤
阿糖胞苷	氮芥	卡莫司汀	丝裂霉素
达卡巴嗪	亚硝基脲类	苯丁酸氮芥 表柔比星	丙卡巴肼
放线菌素 D	紫杉醇	吉西他滨	替尼泊苷
柔红霉素	噻替哌	羟基脲	长春瑞滨
多西他赛	托泊替康		
多柔比星	长春碱		
依托泊苷	长春新碱		
氟尿嘧啶	长春地辛		
伊达比星			

脱发往往影响患者接受化疗的情绪。遗憾的是，尽管头皮低温治疗，米诺地尔、维生素 D_3、环孢素和局部多柔比星单克隆抗体被广泛研究。目前尚没有广泛认可的预防和治疗脱发的方法[73,74]。

口腔炎

肿瘤化疗引起的口腔炎和其他口腔并发症在第 135 章和第 136 章中讨论。

指甲反应

色素沉着是接受化疗的患者尤其是深色皮肤患者中最常见的指甲反应[75]。化疗诱导黑色素细胞激活引起的色素沉着应区别于黄甲综合征(yellow nail syndrome,YNS)。YNS 表现为指甲横断面曲率增加、弧影缺失及角质层缺乏。已知的病因学包括副肿瘤反应、获得性免疫缺陷综合征(acquired immune deficiency syndrome,AIDS)相关和药物诱发(图 127-5)[76]。

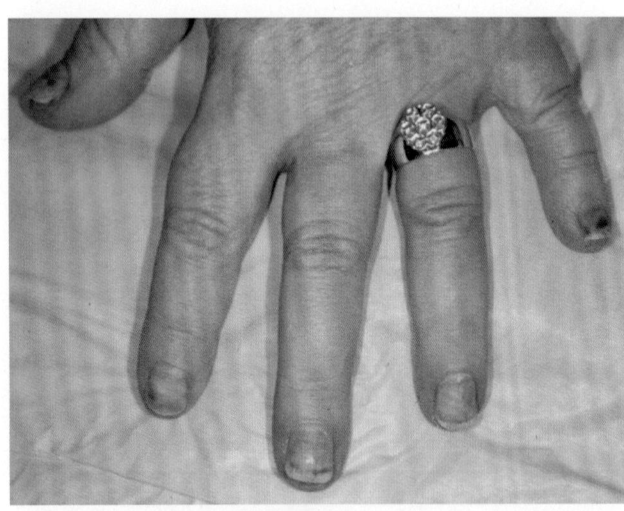

图 127-5 多西他赛导致的指甲色素沉着和甲营养不良

其他常见指甲异常表现包括称为博氏线的甲板横向凹陷(图 127-6),称为 Mees 线的整个甲板宽度的白色变,称为白甲病的部分甲床的横向白色变,甲剥离和甲营养不良。文献中已有报道博来霉素与甲剥离,羟基脲与脆甲症,依托泊苷和甲床色素沉着存在相关性[75,77]。随着 EGFR 抑制剂使用的增多,甲沟炎、甲皱的发炎更为常见并且非常痛苦。金黄色葡萄球菌和白色念珠菌的二重感染也非常常见。表 127-6 总结了其他指甲病变及其相关的化疗药物。这些指甲变化通常是良性的,并且病变在停用相关药物后随着指甲生长而恢复。然而,被化疗损伤的指甲更容易受到酵母菌、皮肤真菌和假单胞菌的感染,可能会对甲床造成不可逆的永久性损伤。

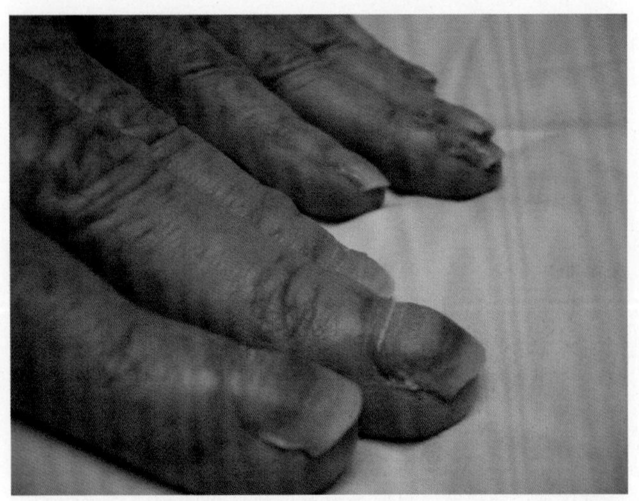

图 127-6 色素沉着和博氏线

表 127-6 指甲异常和相关化疗药物小结

甲病	相关的化疗药物
博氏线	紫杉烷类,博来霉素,顺铂,多柔比星,美法仑,长春新碱
横向指甲白纹	多柔比星
马尔克线	多柔比星,环磷酰胺,长春新碱,甲酰四氢叶酸,左旋咪唑,甲氨蝶呤
甲剥离	紫杉烷类,多柔比星,氟尿嘧啶,米托蒽醌,博来霉素
甲缺失,无甲,脱甲	紫杉烷类,博来霉素,氟尿嘧啶,巯嘌呤,米托蒽醌
缺血改变	博来霉素,紫杉烷类,多柔比星,甲氨蝶呤,氮芥,依托泊苷,环磷酰胺,白消安,美法仑
黑甲	博来霉素,环磷酰胺,柔红霉素,多柔比星,氟尿嘧啶,羟基脲,氨鲁米特,白消安,顺铂,达卡巴嗪,多西他赛,伊达比星,异环磷酰胺,美法仑
非黑色素色素沉着	氟尿嘧啶
急性甲沟炎	甲氨蝶呤,紫杉烷类
脓性肉芽肿	西妥昔单抗(C225),吉非替尼(易瑞沙)

外渗反应

外渗损伤是众所周知的药物不良反应事件,指药物从静脉或者静脉导管进入皮下组织。接受静脉化疗的患者中药物意外外渗的发生率为 0.1%~6%(表 127-7)[78]。外渗的皮肤表现可以从轻微不适和轻度红斑到严重而疼痛的皮肤坏死、溃疡和深部组织结构的破坏。

细胞毒性药物外渗通常引起两类局部皮肤反应:刺激性反应和发泡剂反应。刺激物引起短暂而具有自限性的静脉炎及沿着静脉走行或静脉给药部位局部的热痛红斑反应。蒽环类药物的局部刺激反应表现为红斑和荨麻疹样超敏反应。发泡剂最初引起类似的反应,但是刺激有恶化的可能,取决于外渗药物的量,导致神经和肌腱损伤以及随后的神经功能缺损、肌肉挛缩和关节僵硬。组织损伤的程度在很大程度上取决于渗出物的浓度、体积和囊泡性质[78,79]。

表 127-7 化疗药物相关的化学蜂窝织炎

常见		罕见	
放线菌素 D	安吖啶	伊索比星	普卡霉素
柔红霉素	比生群	依托泊苷	吡唑呋喃菌素
多柔比星	博来霉素	氟尿嘧啶	链佐星
丝裂霉素	卡莫司汀 氯乙链佐星 顺铂 达卡巴嗪 表柔比星	伊达比星 美法仑 氮芥 米托蒽醌 紫杉醇	长春碱 长春新碱 长春地辛 长春瑞滨

紫杉醇可诱导外渗回忆性反应，即一个部位的药物外渗可引起原先药物外渗部位出现红斑，甚至溃疡样的皮肤反应[80]。中心静脉导管移位或者静脉穿孔可诱发潜在的灾难性后果，包括纵隔炎、发热、胸膜剧烈疼痛、上肢和颈部肿胀及纵隔增大。

发泡剂损伤有时也被称为化学蜂窝织炎，表现为愈合不良，通常会持续恶化，需要手术干预。发泡剂可延迟成纤维细胞性伤口收缩，并具有与 DNA 结合的能力，使他们有可能被循环作用，停留在组织中造成较长时间的损害[79]。据估计大约有 1/3 的发泡剂外渗将会发生溃疡，对药物外渗的重视和处理对于限制组织损伤具有重要作用[81]。一旦怀疑药物外渗，推荐立即停止输液，而后吸出残留药物并拔除输液管。通常应用局部冷敷和抬高患肢以减轻反应[80]。单纯应用间歇性局部冷敷可以成功预防 89.1%的溃疡发生[82]。对于长春花生物碱类药物外渗推荐采用热敷，因为冷敷可能诱发溃疡发生[81]。

解毒剂的使用具有争议，有些解毒剂如碳酸氢钠可能有害或诱发溃疡。硫代硫酸钠（氮芥）、玻璃酸酶（长春花生物碱）、粒细胞巨噬细胞集落刺激因子（多柔比星）、吡哆醇（丝裂霉素）已分别被推荐作为局部注射的解毒剂[83~85]。局部注射糖皮质激素的效果也不确切，因为很少有炎症细胞参与外渗反映[85]。有时难以界定局部解毒剂是具有特异作用还是作为稀释剂。已经证实局部注射生理盐水有助于外渗反应消退及防止溃疡发生[86]。虽然保守治疗可适用于大多数发泡剂的外渗反应，但是有时早期手术切除更有利，尤其是涉及最强作用的发泡剂[86,87]。如果溃疡显著或者外渗损伤部位对治疗无效，局部广泛切除和皮瓣重建的手术就很有必要。自由基清除剂二甲基亚砜（DMSO）取得了局部治疗的成功。在 1995 年，对来自多项研究的包括 96 例患者的分析表明，DMSO 使得 98.3%的外渗病例免于发生溃疡[88]。

色素沉着

色素沉着是一种常见的皮肤表现，是患者关心的容貌改变。皮肤、黏膜、毛发、牙齿和指甲可能都会受到影响，可能发生弥漫性或局限性反应。应用烷化剂、抗肿瘤抗生素和吉西他滨常出现色素沉着（表 127-8）[77]。在抗代谢药物中，甲氨蝶呤可能会产生特征性的头发“标志符号”：浅色头发患者出现横向色素沉着带和正常头发颜色交替[77]。接受替加氟治疗的患者中约有 1/3 可出现手掌、脚掌、指甲及龟头的色素沉着。接受博来霉素治疗的患者中有 8%~20%的患者在创伤区域可出现鞭毛虫样带状色素沉着（图 127-7）。白消安的色素沉着与 addison 病类似，会有乏力、体重减轻及腹泻的症状，但是血清促黑素细胞激素和促肾上腺皮质激素水平正常[69]。化疗诱发色素沉着的机制目前尚不清楚，可能与直接毒性、黑素细胞刺激及炎症后改变有关。虽然这些反应有时可能是永久的，但是在大多数情况下，化疗终止后变色反应将会逐渐消退。

表 127-8 化疗药物相关的色素沉着

烷化剂	抗生素类	核算类似物抗代谢药	联合化疗方案
白消安	博来霉素	氟尿嘧啶	博来霉素/多柔比星/长春新碱
顺铂	放线菌素 D	甲氨蝶呤	白消安/环磷酰胺
环磷酰胺	柔红霉素	替加氟	环磷酰胺/多柔比星/长春新碱/泼尼松
福莫司汀	多柔比星	布喹那钠	环磷酰胺/依托泊苷/卡铂
异环磷酰胺	米托蒽醌	多西他赛	多柔比星/博来霉素/长春碱/达卡巴嗪
噻替哌	普卡霉素	羟基脲	异环磷酰胺/卡铂/依托泊苷
局部用卡莫司汀	吉西他滨	丙卡巴肼	甲氨蝶呤/阿糖胞苷/L-门冬酰胺酶/柔红霉素/巯嘌呤/环磷酰胺
局部用氮芥	曲沙他滨	长春瑞滨	

源自参考文献[69]

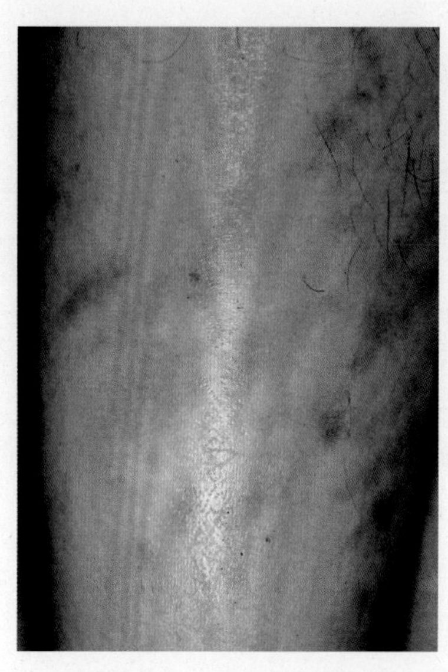

图 127-7 博来霉素引起的皮肤鞭毛样色素沉着

白癜风，一种黑色素细胞完全缺失导致的皮肤褪色性疾病，被认为可作为有针对性的药物疗法，特别是治疗转移性黑色素瘤（表 127-9）[38,62,63]。白癜风存在无症状的、脱色的、常呈对称分布的、无特定位置的皮肤斑块。尽管许多猜测这与疾病反应相关，但还没有被进一步证明。

表 127-9 化疗药物相关的脱色/白癜风

维莫非尼	吉非替尼
达拉非尼（dabrafenib）	干扰素
帕博利珠单抗（pembrolizumab）	重组人白介素-2
伊马替尼	

放射相关反应

放射包括暴露于紫外线以及放射治疗的暴露。三种放射相关的皮肤反应类型已被很好的描述：放射增强反应、放射治疗回忆反应以及光敏性反应（表 127-10 和表 127-11）。

表 127-10 与放射反应相关的化疗药物

放射增强反应	反射治疗回忆反应	
博来霉素	博来霉素	洛莫司汀
喜树碱	阿糖胞苷	美法仑
苯丁酸氮芥	放线菌素 D	甲氨蝶呤
顺铂[a]	柔红霉素	奥沙利铂
环磷酰胺[a]	多西他赛	紫杉醇
放线菌素 D	依达曲沙	他莫昔芬
多柔比星	依托泊苷	三嗪苯酰胺
氟尿嘧啶	氟尿嘧啶	曲美沙特
羟基脲	吉西他滨	维莫非尼
干扰素	羟基脲	长春碱
巯嘌呤	伊达比星	
甲氨蝶呤		
三嗪苯酰胺		
维莫非尼		
长春新碱[a]		

[a] 只在联合用药方案中有报道[69]。

表 127-11 具有光毒性的化疗药物

布喹那钠	甲氨蝶呤
达卡巴嗪	丝裂霉素 C
放线菌素 D	卟啉类
多柔比星	丙卡巴肼
氟尿嘧啶	替加氟
氟他胺	硫鸟嘌呤
羟基脲	长春碱

放射增强反应

放射增强反应一般出现在放化疗开始后的一周内。虽然其他器官也会受到这一增强作用的影响，但是皮肤是这一毒性反应发生的最常见部位。这种反应可能表现为干燥或潮湿脱皮或红斑及水肿。当出现大疱、糜烂、溃疡伴有红斑时，通常是因为发生了葡萄球菌感染[89]。增加放射损伤的程度与给予药物与放射的时间间隔呈负相关。化疗与放疗的时间间隔越短暂，放射增强作用越大[90]。增强作用也取决于药物的剂量及药理机制[75]。

放射治疗回忆反应

放射治疗回忆反应是在原先照射过的区域出现红斑样的炎性反应。严重的放射性皮炎作为一种 ID 反应甚至可以累及照射范围以外的区域。放射治疗回忆反应可在放射治疗后 8 日到 15 年出现，也可能发生于其他器官[77]。回忆反应的发生率及严重程度分别取决于放疗的剂量及放化疗之间的间隔时间[91]。紫外线的回忆反应的发生一般在苏拉明（35%的发生率）、甲氨蝶呤、维莫非尼、依托泊苷/环磷酰胺药物治疗后 1 周内出现皮肤晒伤[92]。

光化性角化病的炎症被称为光化性角化病的回忆反应（表 127-12）。苏拉明和阿糖胞苷诱导的脂溢性角化病的炎症反应以及氟达拉滨诱导的鳞状细胞癌的案例也有报道。全身性氟尿嘧啶和临床亚临床的光化性角化病之间的联系是众所周知的，局部应用氟尿嘧啶也可产生类似的效果。光化性角化病的回忆反应通常出现在给药的 1 周后，并在治疗结束后的 1~4 周消退，当然在治疗的过程中也能消退[93]。这种回忆反应可能与光化性角化病辐射的回忆反应或与 DNA 合成的增加相关，因此存在更多的化学药剂的吸收[93,94]。虽然这些病变都是自限性的，但是存在发生表面溃疡和葡萄球菌定植的风险，因此需要使用抗生素活皮脂类固醇来预防。并且这种反应在接下来的药物治疗中可能还会发生，但也可能不会再发生。与在光化性角化病中局部应用氟尿嘧啶类似，全身性应用氟尿嘧啶也可以消退炎症反应，治疗光化性角化病[95]。

表 127-12 炎性光线性角化相关的化疗药物

放线菌素 D/长春新碱/达卡巴嗪
多西他赛
多柔比星
多柔比星/阿糖胞苷/硫鸟嘌呤
多柔比星/长春新碱
氟尿嘧啶
氟尿嘧啶/顺铂
喷司他丁（pentostatin）

放射治疗回忆反应的机制目前尚不清楚，尽管有理论认为是因为干细胞储备不足或者放疗后存活的细胞发生突变以致影响损伤组织修复[96]。

一般而言，对于放射相关反应给予对症治疗，以努力避免或用合适的抗生素治疗继发感染。严重的溃疡和坏死性反应可能需要清创。局部外用莫匹罗星（mupirocin）和全身应用糖皮质激素是放射治疗回忆反应的主要治疗，甚至可以允许继续使用该药而不再出现回忆反应[96]。

光敏性反应

最后，虽然化疗和紫外线照射相关性皮肤反应报道相对较少，但其相关性还是有据可查的（表 127-11）。一般来说这些皮肤反应大多数涉及外源的光毒性，而这些药剂只是起到了显色的作用。临床和组织学检查显示，这些光毒性反应表现为较为夸张的晒伤。指甲的光毒性反应可表现为巯嘌呤引起的光甲剥离，通常很敏感，常累及指甲末端 1/3。

另外一种光敏反应的形式是氟他胺和替加氟的光变态反应，当再次使用相关药物时皮肤反应会再次出现[97]。

光敏反应的治疗采用局部外用糖皮质激素和止痒药。严重者需要全身应用类固醇。氯喹和 β 胡萝卜素被用于预防光过敏，但是在对照研究中却无效果[98]。此外，由于药物可能在患者的皮肤中留存数周，应建议患者采用防晒措施。

肢端反应

肢端红斑（acral erythema，AE）和手足皮肤反应（hand-foot skin reaction，HFSR）是两种典型的与靶向治疗相关的肢端反应。肢端红斑还有很多别名，包括手足综合征和化疗毒性红斑（表 127-13，表 127-14）。

表 127-13　炎症性肢端红斑相关的化疗药物

常见		罕见	
卡培他滨	顺铂	伊达比星	紫杉醇
阿糖胞苷	环磷酰胺	洛莫司汀	聚乙二醇聚乙二醇脂质体多柔比星
多柔比星	柔红霉素	美法仑	氟尿苷
氟尿嘧啶	多西他赛	巯嘌呤	舒拉明
	去氧氟尿苷	甲氨蝶呤	曲沙他滨（troxacitabine）
	依托泊苷	丝裂霉素	替加氟
	羟基脲	米托坦	长春新碱

源自参考文献[69]

表 127-14　与化疗有关的各种反应

大疱类天疱疮	结节性红斑	潮红（持续的）	多毛症（持续的）
放线菌素 D/MTX	白消安	普卡霉素	氟甲睾酮
微血管炎	己烯雌酚	丙卡巴肼	他莫昔芬
氨鲁米特	IL-2	苏拉明	非黑色素瘤皮肤癌
皮肤粘连，获得性	顽固性药疹	他莫昔芬	氮芥（局部）
多柔比星/酮康唑	达卡巴嗪	替尼泊苷	BRAF 抑制剂
皮肤溃疡	羟基脲	曲美沙特	卟啉症
羟基脲	紫杉醇（天疱疮）	毛囊炎	顺铂
IFN-α，聚乙二醇 IFN-α	丙卡巴肼	放线菌素 D	晚期皮肤卟啉症
IL-2	潮红	柔红霉素	白消安
甲氨蝶呤	左旋天冬酰胺	氟尿嘧啶	环磷酰胺
疱疹样皮炎，恶化	博来霉素	甲氨蝶呤	己烯雌酚
环磷酰胺/多柔比星/长春新碱	卡铂	EGFR 抑制剂	甲氨蝶呤
博来霉素	卡莫司汀（卡莫司汀）	疥疮病	急性间歇性卟啉病
顺铂	顺铂	氟甲睾酮	苯丁酸氮芥
长春新碱	环磷酰胺	甲氨蝶呤	环磷酰胺
皮肌炎样反应	达卡巴嗪	放线菌素 D	脓疱性银屑病
羟基脲	膜海鞘素	甲羟孕酮	氨鲁米特
他莫昔芬	己烯雌酚	丙卡巴肼	脂质体多柔比星
替加氟	多西他赛	长春新碱	脂溢性皮炎，恶化

续表

博来霉素	多柔比星	发色改变	氟尿嘧啶
多烯紫杉醇	依托泊苷	博来霉素	IL-2
药物引起的 SLE	氟尿嘧啶	顺铂	IFN-α
氨鲁米特	氟他米特	环磷酰胺	毛细血管扩张
己烯雌酚	IL-2	甲氨蝶呤	卡莫司汀(卡莫司汀)
羟基脲	亮丙瑞林	他莫昔芬	氟尿嘧啶(局部用药)
亮丙瑞林	洛莫司汀	多毛症	羟基脲
替加氟	紫杉醇	己烯雌酚	IFN-α
IFN-α			

EGFR,表皮生长因子;IFN-α,干扰素-α;IL-2,重组人白介素-2;MTX,甲氨蝶呤;SLE,系统性红斑狼疮。

1974 年 Zuehlke 首次报道肢端红斑与化疗相关[99]。也称作掌跖红肿疼痛、掌跖红斑手足综合征、特殊 AE 和 Burgdorf 反应。有手掌和脚掌感觉迟钝的前驱症状,包括疼痛、麻木,对称性,边界清楚的肿胀及红斑(图 127-8),而后进入脱屑期进而恢复。红斑和肿胀通常出现在大小鱼际隆起处、手指侧面和远端指骨垫。手比足更易受累。在其各种表现中,AE 可表现为交替出现的红斑带,也可能伴随着轻微的红斑或躯干、颈部、胸部、头皮及四肢部位麻疹样暴发[100]。据报道甲氨蝶呤和阿糖胞苷可以诱发大疱样变异的 AE,在恢复之前可能会进展为全层表皮坏死[101]。

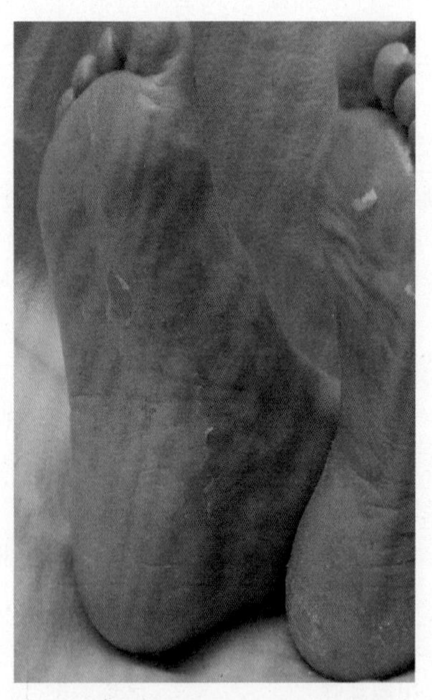

图 127-8 化疗诱导的脚掌肢端红斑

AE 在不同年龄组有 6%~42% 发病率,在成人中更常见[102]。AE 表现为峰值水平和总累积剂量的剂量依赖性,因为与持续低剂量给药(2~10 个月)相比在静脉推注后它发生更早且更严重(24h 到 3 周)[100,103]。AE 随着化疗的进一步应用趋于持久并会加重,可能有剂量限制,因为相关的疼痛可能会加重而导致身体和功能受限。AE 可在停用致病药物 1~2 周内恢复,伴有脱屑和上皮再形成(图 127-9)。再次给药时 AE 不一定再次发生。对于 AE 采取对症治疗,旨在提高耐受性以使化疗可以继续进行。糖皮质激素取得了不同程度的疗效。支持治疗包括局部伤口护理、抬高患肢和止痛药。与治疗脱发的头皮低温概念相似,手与足的降温也利于预防 AE[103]。一项回顾性研究结果表明,环氧化酶 2(COX-2 的)抑制剂塞来昔布可降低 67 例服用卡培他滨的转移性结直肠癌患者 AE 发生率[104]。与单用卡培他滨相比,塞来昔布同时可以减轻卡培他滨引起的腹泻,提高肿瘤疗效,延长肿瘤至中位进展时间。维生素 B_6 也可减轻感觉迟钝和疼痛以使治疗得以继续[105]。

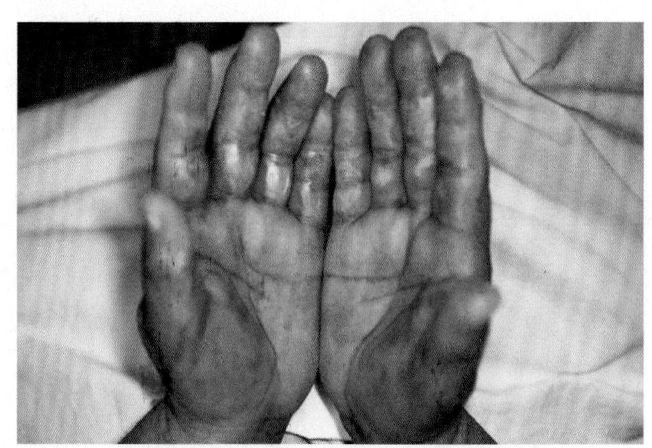

图 127-9 手足综合症脱屑期,卡培他滨二次用药

AE 发病机制目前尚不清楚,可能是多方面的。AE 的病理活检没有组织特异性但是和毒性反应相一致[103]。化疗时,诊断 AE 相对容易。但是对于骨髓移植(BMT)的患者,很难将之与急性移植物抗宿主病(GVHD)鉴别。BMT 患者中 AE 有 35%的发病率,这可能和使用大剂量的化疗及全身照射有关[106]。在最初 3 周,AE 的病理和临床表现均和急性 GVHD 相似:如 AE 一样,急性 GVHD 时手掌受累常见,但是随着疾病进展,身体其他部位也会受累。急性 GVHD 的早期活检与 AE 相似,间隔 3~5 日的系列活检有助于明确疾病进展的模式而支持急性 GVHD 的诊断[106]。区分 AE 和急性 GVHD 很重要,因为后者需要进一步的免疫抑制治疗,如果不治疗,疾病通常进展,可能会致命。

HFSR 常见于多重激酶抑制剂、索拉非尼、舒尼替尼的不良反应,MEK 抑制剂也有报道。它与 AE 的区别主要是自然角化，厚茧以及起泡倾向。

淋巴细胞恢复时的皮疹

淋巴细胞恢复时的皮疹（cutaneous eruption of lymphocyte recovery，ELR）可能在接受清髓性的密集化疗的患者中出现[107]。同 ESS 一样，在多种化疗药物使用中观察到 ELR 现象但是不与特定药物相关。ELR 的临床表现为多样分布的红斑样瘙痒的斑疹、丘疹及斑块，其可能融合成红皮病外观，并且通常伴随数日的发热。在化疗时，这一反应通常发生在化疗所致白细胞计数最低值后的 6~21 日，与外周淋巴细胞的最初恢复时间相关。ELR 可能是高度同种反应性免疫淋巴细胞进入外周循环和皮肤的反应[107]。ELR 呈自限性，在数天的脱屑和轻度色素沉着后可恢复。鉴于 ELR 临床表现的非特异性，需要和引起红斑疹的其他原因相鉴别，尤其是急性 GVHD、败血症、病毒疹、白血病、皮肤淋巴瘤、ESS 及药物过敏。在这些出疹类型中，骨髓移植时急性 GVHD 的出现时间与 ELR 相似，尤其是自体 GVHD 与 ELR 非常相似，两者都存在组织相容性涉及淋巴细胞的恢复。然而，无法可靠地通过皮肤活检将急性自体 GVHD 与 ELR 区分开[108]。Horn 认为 GVHD 可能代表了 ELR 的一种形式[109]。

（崔久嵬　李玲玉　译）

参考文献

The complete reference list can be found on the Wiley Companion Digital Edition of this title (see inside front cover for login instructions).

1 Revuz J, Valeyrie-Allanore L. Drug reactions. In: Bolognia J, Jorizzo J, Schaffer J, et al., eds. *Dermatology*, 3rd ed. Philadephia: Elsevier Saunders; 2012, Chapter 21.

2 Sidoroff A, Halevy S, Bavinck JB, et al. Acute generalized exanthematous pustulosis (AGEP)óa clinical reaction pattern. *J Cutan Pathol*. 2001;**28**:113 - 119.

6 Busam KJ, Capodieci P, Motzer R, et al. Cutaneous side-effects in cancer patients treated with the antiepidermal growth factor receptor antibody C225. *Br J Dermatol*. 2001;**144**(**6**):1169 - 1176.

9 Boone SL, Rademaker A, Liu D, Pfeiffer C, Mauro DJ, Lacouture ME. Impact and management of skin toxicity associated with anti-epidermal growth factor receptor therapy: survey results. *Oncology*. 2007;**72**(**3-4**):152 - 159.

10 Saltz LB, Meropol NJ, Loehrer PJ, Needle MN, Kopit J, Mayer RJ. Phase II trial of cetuximab in patients with refractory colorectal cancer that expresses the epidermal growth factor receptor. *J Clin Oncol*. 2004;**22**:1201 - 1208.

11 Lacouture ME. Mechanisms of cutaneous toxicities to EGFR inhibitors. *Nat Rev Cancer*. 2006;**6**(**10**):803 - 812.

18 Drucker AM, Wu S, Dang CT, Lacouture ME. Risk of rash with the anti-HER2 dimerization antibody pertuzumab: a meta-analysis. *Breast Cancer Res Treat*. 2012;**135**(**2**):347 - 354.

22 Amitay-laish I, Stemmer SM, Lacouture ME. Adverse cutaneous reactions secondary to tyrosine kinase inhibitors including imatinib mesylate, nilotinib, and dasatinib. *Dermatol Ther*. 2011;**24**(**4**):386 - 395.

23 Balagula Y, Lacouture ME, Cotliar JA. Dermatologic toxicities of targeted anticancer therapies. *J Support Oncol*. 2010;**8**(**4**):149 - 161.

24 Chu D, Lacouture ME, Fillos T, Wu S. Risk of hand-foot skin reaction with sorafenib: a systematic review and meta-analysis. *Acta Oncol*. 2008;**47**(**2**):176 - 186.

25 Chu D, Lacouture ME, Weiner E, Wu S. Risk of hand-foot skin reaction with the multitargeted kinase inhibitor sunitinib in patients with renal cell and non-renal cell carcinoma: a meta-analysis. *Clin Genitourin Cancer*. 2009;**7**(**1**):11 - 19.

27 Boyd KP, Vincent B, Andea A, Conry RM, Hughey LC. Nonmalignant cutaneous findings associated with vemurafenib use in patients with metastatic melanoma. *J Am Acad Dermatol*. 2012;**67**(**6**):1375 - 1379.

29 Balagula Y, Rosen A, Tan BH, et al. Clinical and histopathologic characteristics of rash in cancer patients treated with mammalian target of rapamycin inhibitors. *Cancer*. 2012;**118**(**20**):5078 - 5083.

30 Lacouture ME, Duvic M, Hauschild A, et al. Analysis of dermatologic events in vemurafenib-treated patients with melanoma. *Oncologist*. 2013;**18**(**3**):314 - 322.

31 Infante J, Falchook G, Lawrence D, et al. Phase I/II study to assess safety, pharmacokinetics, and efficacy of the oral MEK 1/2 inhibitor GSK1120212 (GSK 212) dosed in combination with the oral BRAF inhibitor GSK2118436 (GSK436) [abstract 8503]. *J Clin Oncol*. 2011;**29**(**suppl**):CRA8503.

32 Zimmer L, Livingstone E, Hillen U, Dömkes S, Becker A, Schadendorf D. Panniculitis with arthralgia in patients with melanoma treated with selective BRAF inhibitors and its management. *Arch Dermatol*. 2012;**148**(**3**):357 - 361.

42 Pulvirenti T, Hong A, Clements A, et al. Acute Radiation Skin Toxicity Associated With BRAF Inhibitors. *J Clin Oncol*. 2014.

46 Anforth R, Fernandez-peñas P, Long GV. Cutaneous toxicities of RAF inhibitors. *Lancet Oncol*. 2013;**14**(**1**):e11 - e18.

49 Huang V, Hepper D, Anadkat M, Cornelius L. Cutaneous toxic effects associated with vemurafenib and inhibition of the BRAF pathway. *Arch Dermatol*. 2012;**148**(**5**):628 - 633.

57 Trefzer U, Minor D, Ribas A, et al. BREAK-2: a phase IIA trial of the selective BRAF kinase inhibitor GSK2118436 in patients with BRAF (V660E/K) -positive metastatic melanoma. *Pigment Cell Melanoma Res*. 2012;**25**:E2.

58 Hauschild A, Grob J-J, Demidov LV, et al. Dabrafenib in BRAF-mutated metastatic melanoma: a multicentre, open-label, phase 3 randomised controlled trial. *Lancet*. 2012;**380**:358 - 365.

59 Cohen PR, Bedikian AY, Kim KB. Appearance of New Vemurafenib-associated Melanocytic Nevi on Normal-appearing Skin: Case Series and a Review of Changing or New Pigmented Lesions in Patients with Metastatic Malignant Melanoma After Initiating Treatment with Vemurafenib. *J Clin Aesthet Dermatol*. 2013;**6**(**5**):27 - 37.

61 Curry JL, Torres-cabala CA, Kim KB, et al. Dermatologic toxicities to targeted cancer therapy: shared clinical and histologic adverse skin reactions. *Int J Dermatol*. 2014;**53**(**3**):376 - 384.

62 Lacouture ME, Wolchok JD, Yosipovitch G, Kähler KC, Busam KJ, Hauschild A. Ipilimumab in patients with cancer and the management of dermatologic adverse events. *J Am Acad Dermatol*. 2014;**71**(**1**):161 - 169.

63 Hamid O, Robert C, Daud A, et al. Safety and tumor responses with lambrolizumab (anti-PD-1) in melanoma. *N Engl J Med*. 2013;**369**(**2**):134 - 144.

64 Wolkenstein P, Chosidow O, Wechsler J, et al. Cutaneous side effects associated with interleukin-2 administration for metastatic melanoma. *J Am Acad Dermatol*. 1993;**28**:66 - 70.

69 DeSpain JD. Dermatologic toxicity of chemotherapy. *Semin Oncol*. 1992;**19**: 501 - 507.

71 Hood AF. Dermatologic toxicity. In: Perry MC, ed. *The chemotherapy source book*, 2nd ed. Baltimore: Williams & Wilkins; 1996:595 - 606.

74 Dmytriw AA, Morzycki W, Green PJ. Prevention of alopecia in medical and interventional chemotherapy patients. *J Cutan Med Surg*. 2014;**18**:1 - 6.

77 Susser WS, Whitaker-Worth DL, Grant-Kels JM. Mucocutaneous reactions to chemotherapy. *J Am Acad Dermatol*. 1999;**40**:367 - 398.

79 Rudolph R, Larson DL. Etiology and treatment of chemotherapeutic agent extravasation injuries: a review. *J Clin Oncol*. 1987;**5**:1116 - 1126.

89 Hill A, Hanson M, Bogle MA, Duvic M. Severe radiation dermatitis is related to *Staphylococcus aureus*. *Am J Clin Oncol*. 2004;**27**:362 - 363.

90 Houtee PV, Danhier S, Mornex F. Toxicity of combined radiation and chemotherapy in non-small cell lung cancer. *Lung Cancer*. 1994;**10**:S271 - S280.

93 Johnson T, Rapini R, Duvic M. Inflammation of actinic keratoses from systemic chemotherapy. *J Am Acad Dermatol*. 1987;**17**:192 - 197.

97 Fava P, Quaglino P, Fierro MT, Novelli M, Bernengo MG. Therapeutic hotline. A rare vandetanib-induced photo-allergic drug eruption. *Dermatol Ther*. 2010;**23**(**5**):553 - 555.

103 Baack BR, Burgdorf WHC. Chemotherapy-induced acral erythema. *J Am Acad Dermatol*. 1991;**24**:457 - 461.

107 Horn TD, Redd JV, Karp JE, et al. Cutaneous eruptions of lymphocyte recovery. *Arch Dermatol*. 1989;**215**:1512 - 1517.

108 Bauer DJ, Hood AF, Horn TD. Histologic comparison of autologous graft-vs-host reaction and cutaneous eruption of lymphocyte recovery. *Arch Dermatol*. 1993;**129**:855 - 858.

第 128 章 骨并发症

Michael A. Via, MD ■ Ilya Iofifin, MD ■ Jeffrey I. Mechanick, MD

概述

由于恶性肿瘤的全身反应、分泌效应以及常用癌症疗法的影响,代谢性骨病在癌症患者中非常普遍。对于急性病理骨折,手术治疗可以极大改善患者生活质量。应用骨吸收抑制剂可以预防骨折的发生,并减少骨转移瘤患者的骨痛症状。

前言

癌症一直是重大的公共健康问题,44%的美国男性及 38%的女性在其一生中都曾患过癌症。据估计,2015 年美国将有 1 658 370 例新发癌症病例[1]。随着癌症治疗的进展和癌症患者生存率持续提高,癌症的骨并发症越来越普遍。这些骨相关并发症包括骨转移引发的疼痛,骨折和恶性肿瘤的高钙血症。骨是最常见的癌转移部位,尸检发现死于癌症的患者中 70%存在骨转移,其中大部分病例具有临床症状且需要治疗(参见第 111 章,表 111-8)[2]。一旦发生骨转移,将无法彻底治愈,患者和医师必须明确治疗的目标是缓解症状而不是治愈[2]。最常发生骨转移的五种癌症类型分别是乳腺癌、前列腺癌、肺癌、肾癌和甲状腺癌。事实上,几乎所有的癌症类型都可以转移到骨。作为最常见的起源于骨的恶性肿瘤,多发性骨髓瘤也可导致严重的骨并发症。与转移癌相同,治愈多发性骨髓瘤的可能性也不大,但可以进行有效的全身控制。随着新疗法的发展,患者的生存时间也在不断改善。总而言之,癌症骨转移的治疗需要一个包括肿瘤内科医师、骨科医师和放射科医师的多学科团队共同参与。

骨病变患者的评估

对患者进行评估,首先要仔细的询问病史和体格检查。治疗方案的制订需要医师了解患者疼痛的部位,加重及缓解因素,既往肿瘤病史及既往治疗措施。除了骨转移瘤之外,关节炎和其他骨科疾病同样可能导致患者疼痛,而骨转移灶的发现可能纯属偶然。对于发生骨转移的骨骼,首先应行整个骨骼的平片检查,因为骨转移可能是多灶性的(图 128-1)。骨病变可以是单纯溶骨性的(仅见骨质破坏,如典型的淋巴瘤,多发性骨髓瘤,肺癌,肾癌和甲状腺癌转移),成骨性的(可见异常骨沉积,前列腺癌转移常见),或混合性的(通常见于乳腺癌转移)。虽然放射性核素锝骨扫描和 MRI 对于检测转移病灶非常敏感,但是普通 CT 扫描在评估骨的完整性方面具有优势,在评估是否需要行手术治疗时往往需要该项检查。同样,应扫描整个病变的骨骼,以便准确评估骨折风险并指导手术治疗。

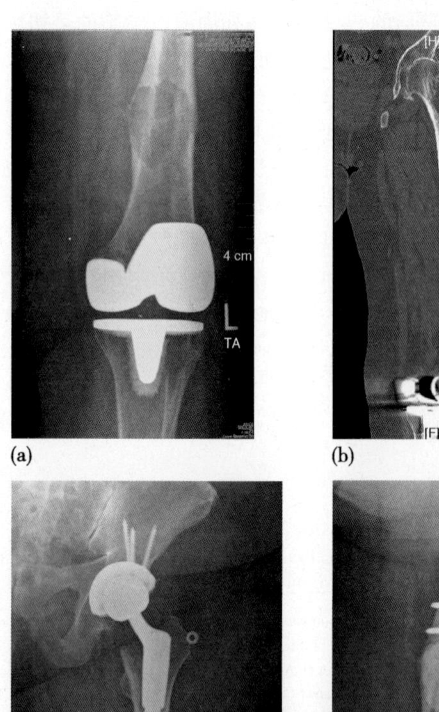

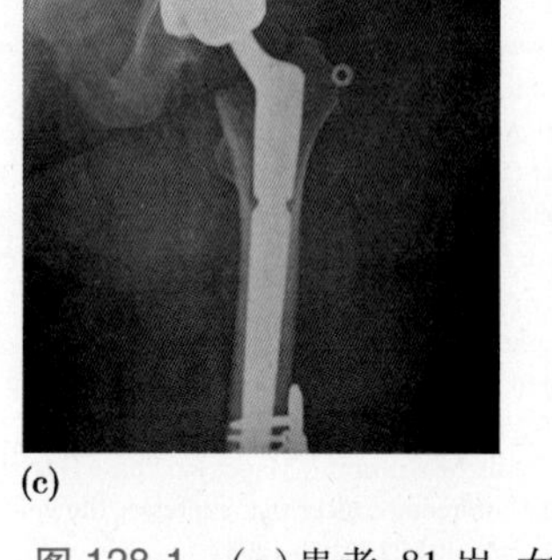

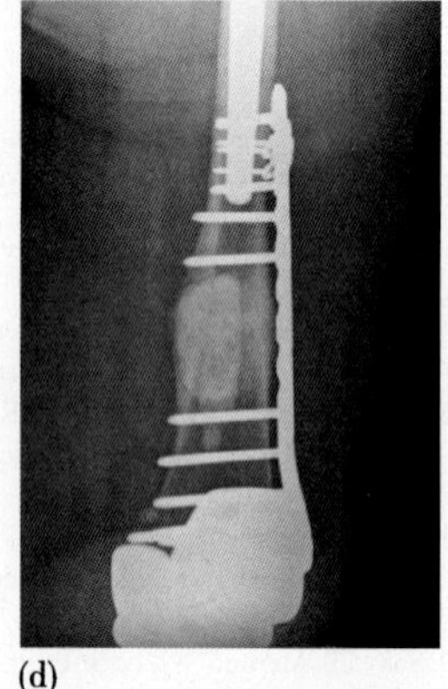

(a) (b) (c) (d)

图 128-1 (a)患者,81 岁,女性,转移性乳腺癌。主诉膝部疼痛,需要注意病变位于固定良好的全膝关节假体上方的股骨远段干骺端。(b)股骨全长的非增强 CT 扫描显示股骨颈的骨质破坏病灶。尽管并无临床症状,但有发生移位性病理骨折的风险。髋关节可见严重退行性病变。(c、d)股骨远端病变行病灶内刮除,锁定钢板固定及骨水泥填充。压配合长柄髋关节置换用于治疗股骨近端病变及骨关节炎。两种内植物重叠可以减少假体骨折的风险,并对整个股骨起到保护作用

骨单发病变

患有孤立性骨病变,但没有活检证实为转移性疾病的患者需要特别注意。有既往癌症病史,那么新发现的骨病变很可能是转移灶,但不是绝对的,因此在进行干预之前需要进行

彻底的评估。最严重的错误之一是认为患者患有转移性疾病,却未能发现有治愈可能的原发恶性骨肿瘤。恶性肿瘤虽然多发生于青少年和年轻人,但在所有年龄组都可能发病,其治疗与转移癌,多发性骨髓瘤和淋巴瘤完全不同。骨原发恶性肿瘤通常需要手术广泛切除,以达到治愈的目的,而大多数转移性病变采用病灶内手术治疗,以姑息治疗为目的。髓内钉植入是治疗转移性疾病最常见的骨科手术方式之一。如果是原发恶性骨肿瘤,髓内钉穿过肿瘤,将会污染整个骨和周围软组织,本来可以进行保肢的患者,将不得不接受更广范围的手术切除,甚至需要半骨盆截肢等截肢手术。此外,扩髓促使肿瘤细胞进入体循环和肺部,增大转移和死亡的风险[3]。即使原发恶性骨肿瘤部位发生病理性骨折,大多数情况下,通过化疗以及不污染周围组织的石膏固定或微创固定等外科手术,保肢也是可以实现的[4]。正确的诊断对于指导治疗是必要的。

因此,当患者被诊断为癌症时,除了评估受影响的骨骼之外,还应进行进一步的分期研究。应行胸部、腹部和骨盆的CT扫描,并通过口服和静脉注射造影剂进行强化,以检查内脏是否有转移以及潜在的原发肿瘤。可通过全身骨扫描检测其他骨骼转移灶,免疫固定或蛋白电泳在血清和/或尿液中检测到单克隆峰可帮助多发性骨髓瘤的诊断[5]。放射性核素骨显像可以检测到由于肿瘤活动,创伤,或退行性关节疾病导致的新骨沉积反应。在大多数情况下它是检测骨转移的敏感方式,但多发性骨髓瘤、转移性肾细胞癌和甲状腺癌通常是纯溶骨性的,很少有骨沉积,这些肿瘤的病变在行骨显像时可能无法发现。当怀疑是其中某一诊断时,应进行骨骼检查(包括长骨、胸部和骨盆的正位X线片以及脊柱和颅骨的侧位X线片)。正电子发射断层扫描(PET)是另一种评估分期的敏感方法,但其确切的适应证仍未确定。所有的受累骨骼应进一步评估发生骨折的风险。转移性前列腺癌患者中通常前列腺特异性抗原(PSA)水平升高,应对怀疑有此诊断的男性进行检查。

这种系统的评估可以区分怀疑为转移性疾病、多发性骨髓瘤或淋巴瘤导致的多发性骨和内脏病变的患者,以及较为少见的高度怀疑为原发恶性骨肿瘤的单发骨病变患者。这种评估方法还有其他优势。可以找到最容易进行活检的部位,这可能与患者最初主诉的部位不同。众所周知转移性肾细胞癌和甲状腺癌血运丰富,在活检时可能大量出血。了解这些知识很重要,术前可以进行肿瘤栓塞和相应的准备工作。

初步诊断通常基于影像学评估,但需通过组织活检确认。如果医生在术前通过影像学、既往转移癌病史或多发性骨髓瘤病史以及实验室检查结果做出诊断,并对诊断有信心,则可以使用术中冰冻切片来确认诊断。但需注意的是,冰冻切片结果并非百分之百准确,骨病变中准确率有86%~94%[6]。如果怀疑是肉瘤,那么应在确定组织学诊断后进行治疗。此外,冰冻切片的可靠性取决于病理学家的经验,而大多数病理学家对原发性骨肿瘤的经验有限。需要特别注意活检通道被肿瘤细胞污染并需要一并切除,特别是在开放活检的情况下。虽然这对转移性疾病或多发性骨髓瘤几乎没有影响,但对肉瘤患者来说,活检位置不当显著影响患者预后,甚至导致4.5%的病例不得不接受截肢手术[7]。因此,活检应在三级转诊中心进行,或至少与接受过培训并具有骨恶性肿瘤治疗专业知识的外科医生合作进行。

骨病变的治疗方案选择

对于骨病变有一系列的治疗方案:对于无症状、无病理性骨折风险的病变可以观察,发生移位及潜在病理性骨折的病变行手术干预。除了癌症的全身治疗外,应用二磷酸盐及地诺单抗药物治疗已被证实可以减少骨骼事件的发生,例如椎体的压缩性骨折,以及骨转移瘤和多发性骨髓瘤患者的手术或放疗需求[8]。70%的接受放疗的患者疼痛症状得到缓解,存在多种治疗方案:8Gy单剂量照射具有与传统的、时间更长的30Gy剂量10日疗程相似的疗效。偶尔会出现癌症疼痛症状复发,需要再次治疗,单剂量照射更容易执行。不同组织学类型的肿瘤对放射的敏感性不同。多发性骨髓瘤、淋巴瘤、前列腺癌和乳腺癌对放射敏感,而肾细胞癌则对放射不敏感[9]。对患有骨骼病变的患者选择最合适的治疗方法时,肿瘤对系统治疗和放射治疗的敏感性是需要考虑的众多因素之一。对于没有明显骨折风险的病变,放射治疗是最合适的。在大多数情况下,骨盆,脊柱,肋骨和肩胛骨是放射治疗的合适部位,而长骨的病变,特别是下肢骨的病变,存在较高的骨折风险,应评估是否可行外科手术干预。

对于结构改变不明显的小病变,放疗并不能缓解疼痛症状,射频消融(RFA)和冷冻消融是有效的微创治疗选择。在CT引导下,将探针放入病灶内进行局部治疗。在RFA时,针头探头向周围组织输送高频交流电,导致热坏死。可以将聚甲基丙烯酸甲酯(PMMA骨水泥)注射到肿瘤留下的空腔中,以维持结构稳定,并起到止痛效果[10]。从概念上讲低温消融是一种类似于RFA的热技术,在这种技术中,肿瘤细胞不是通过加热被破坏,而是通过放置在病灶内的探针释放加压氩气,形成快速冷冻循环破坏肿瘤细胞,然后缓慢解冻,与RFA不同,在CT上可以看到热坏死区[11]。这两种方式都可以与经皮聚甲基丙烯酸甲酯注射相结合。这种图像引导的热消融技术最适合应用于骨折风险低的病变,如椎体、骶骨和髂骨病变,以及许多髋臼病变。一旦发生骨折或骨骼由于结构完整性丧失而具有显著的骨折风险,通常需要手术。在患者情况不支持行手术干预时,特别是在椎体转移时,PMMA稳定可以减轻疼痛,恢复患者的活动能力。

病理性骨折的治疗原则

病理性骨折治疗的目的是改善功能和减轻疼痛。患者及其家属必须知晓,并了解治疗的目的是姑息性的,并不是治愈。必须仔细权衡并发症的风险和潜在的获益。虽然癌症患者的生存时间难以预测，但应超过预期的手术恢复时间。病理性骨折往往不能愈合，即使能愈合，过程也很缓慢。在一个系列研究中，123 名患者共发生 129 例病理性骨折，整体骨折愈合率仅为 35%。在存活超过 6 个月的患者中，该比率上升至 74%[12]。同时病理性骨折患者往往存在多种系统性并发症，在选择最佳治疗方案时，必须牢记这些。常规的非肿瘤导致的骨折，在相对较短的限制性负重期后会愈合，而病理性骨折不同，无法实现这种预期。固定必须足够持久，允许即刻的不受限制的负重，并持续患者的整个寿命。尽量避免多次手术。化疗具有细胞毒性，为使手术伤口愈合常需暂停化疗。由于全身性疾病可在全身治疗中断期间发展，因此应尽量减少手术次数，以减少治疗中断的时间和次数。

肿瘤导致的骨结构完整性破坏，是导致骨折的首要因素。肿瘤的病灶内切除，常需 PMMA 骨水泥固定以提供稳定固定，从而获得更好的肿瘤局部控制。已经证明内固定合并骨水泥植入相比单纯内固定术[13]，可以有效缓解疼痛，并可提供更稳定的生物力学结构[14]。骨移植不能用于正在接受化疗和放疗的患者，因此不能用于转移性疾病或多发性骨髓瘤的治疗。PMMA 骨水泥提供即时稳定性，便宜且易于使用，优于骨移植。在骨水泥存在情况下骨折也可愈合（图 128-3）。除了肿瘤刮除术以及高速磨钻处理腔壁以降低复发风险之外，冷冻手术可作为对放射不敏感肿瘤的治疗方式，可能延长患者存活时间，例如寡转移性肾细胞癌[15]。

病理性骨折的治疗方法包括髓内钉、钢板和螺钉固定、假体置换和不重建的骨切除。治疗方法的选择取决于肿瘤生物学、位置和周围骨骼的完整性。例如，多发性骨髓瘤导致的锁骨病理性骨折通常可以采取非手术治疗，而转移性肾细胞癌导致的锁骨骨折最好的治疗方法是锁骨切除。放射治疗是骨病变手术治疗的重要辅助手段，因为它可以抑制肿瘤进展，避免再次手术，并改善功能。一个系列研究证实，术后放疗将再次手术率从单独接受手术组的 15%减少到仅 3%[16]。

髓内钉

髓内钉有诸多优点，是治疗四肢骨转移瘤最常用的手术方法。整个骨骼得到髓内钉的支撑保护，因此如果在同一骨内发生其他病变，则可能不需要再次手术。手术可以微创的方式进行，恢复更快，并降低手术风险。然而在某些情况下，需要根据骨折特征和肿瘤对化疗和放射的敏感性，可以采用开放式方法和 PMMA 骨水泥填充。对放疗不敏感的肿瘤可能需要采取开放的方法，以降低局部肿瘤进展导致并发症的风险，例如转移性肾细胞癌。骨水泥可沿整个髓腔注入，髓内钉嵌入其中，以增强结构的稳定性（图 128-2），或者骨水泥可以包裹髓内钉填充到肿瘤留下的缺损中（图 128-3）。

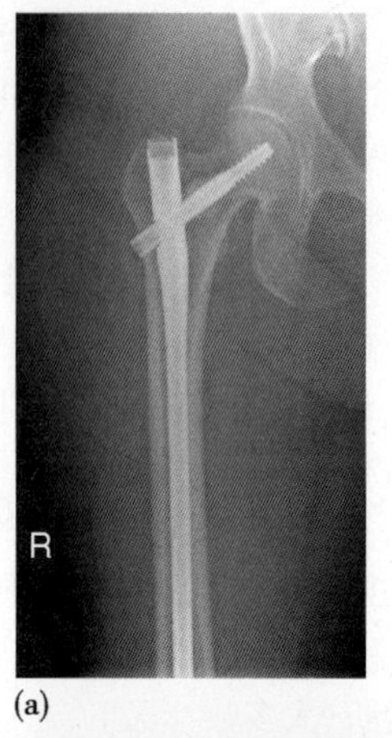

(a)

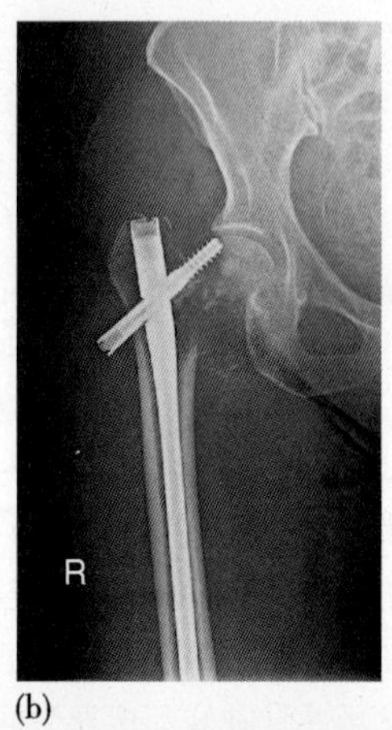

(b)

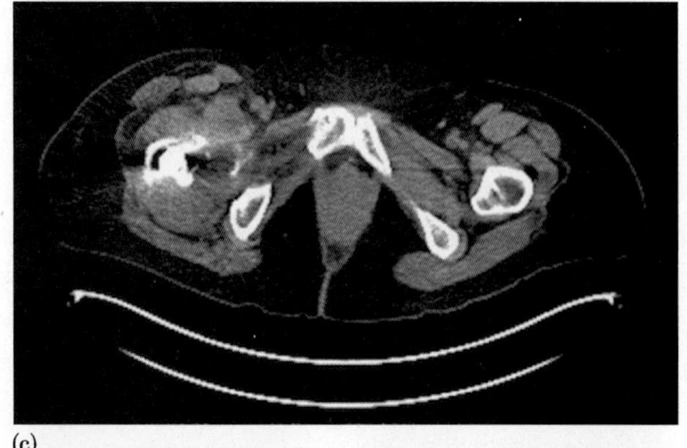
(c)

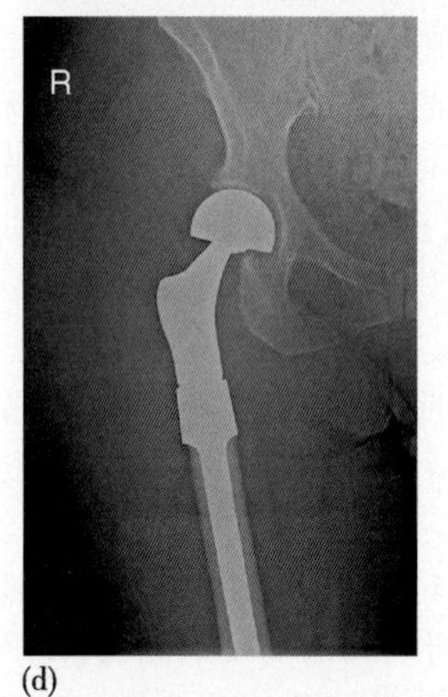

(d)

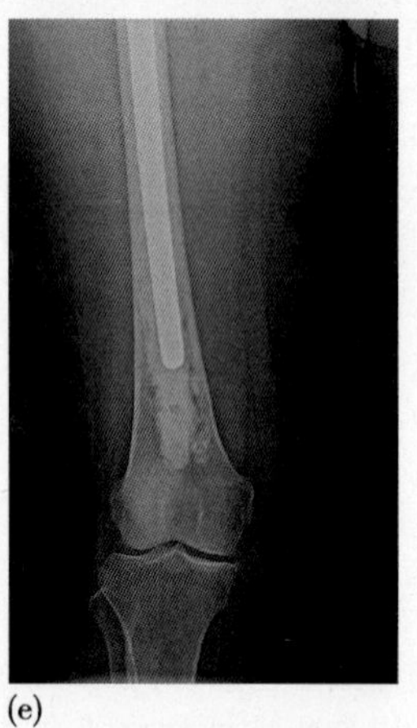
(e)

图 128-2　（a）患者，67 岁，女性，右股骨颈病变。伴疼痛症状，于外院进行了髓内钉治疗。没有进行术前分期。病理证实为转移性肾细胞癌。注意骨质破坏范围很小。手术时沿拉力螺钉注入少量骨水泥。（b）术后 6 周 X 线显示肿瘤进展迅速，股骨颈和大转子大部分破坏，内固定失效。（c）骨盆 CT 显示股骨近端巨大肿块。（d、e）患者接受肿瘤切除，内固定移除和组配股骨近端假体置换。本病例强调了对骨病变患者行术前评估分期的重要性。如果在第一次手术时明确了肾细胞癌的诊断，那么就可以采用广泛肿瘤切除以及半关节置换术，使患者免于再次手术

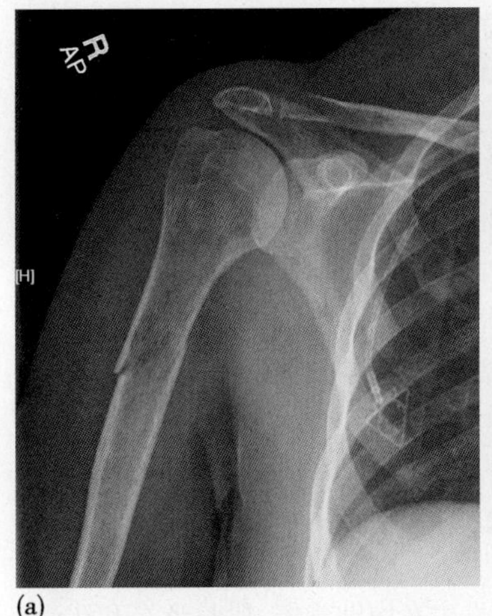

(a)

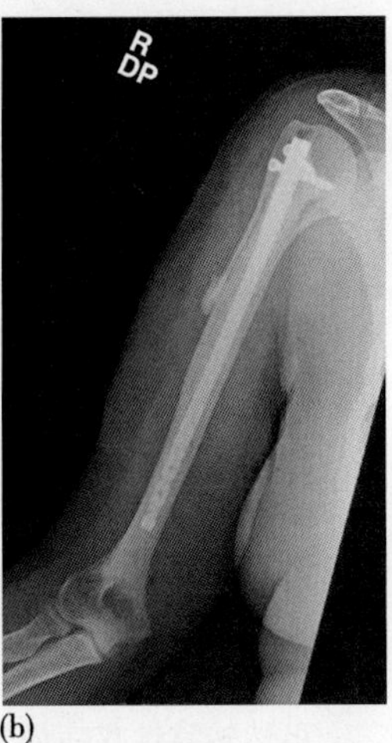

(b)

图 128-3 (a)患者,49 岁,女性,多发性骨髓瘤。右侧肱骨近端病变。(b)骨折距肱骨头使用骨水泥髓内钉。注意骨水泥填充直至近端骨干。未使用远端互锁螺钉,因为整个钉由骨水泥支撑

股骨最常采取髓内钉治疗。头髓钉较常采用,因为拉力螺钉可以固定股骨颈,而股骨颈易受转移性疾病或多发性骨髓瘤的影响。骨骺和骨干肱骨病变也可行髓内钉固定。胫骨很少受转移性疾病或多发性骨髓瘤的影响,但如果发生也可以行髓内钉固定。更少见的是前臂长骨病变;然而,在某些特定的病例中,病理性前臂骨折也可以使用髓内钉固定,安全有效,而不使用部该位常规采用的钢板和螺钉固定。

长骨的近端和远端必须有足够的骨,以使髓内钉有足够的固定和生物力学稳定性。虽然髓内钉最适合于骨干病变,但是在干骺端位置也可以使用髓内钉,但需距关节有足够的距离以允许良好的固定。股骨颈病变最适合采用关节置换术,肱骨头病变可用关节置换术或钢板螺钉固定辅以骨水泥增强来治疗。

钢板和螺钉固定

锁定板技术已经彻底改变了骨折固定,并且已经成为治疗病理性骨折的重要工具。与依赖于钢板与骨骼摩擦的传统钢板技术相比,锁定板有固定角度,每个螺钉的头部固定到板中。因此,所有的螺丝需要一起失效,才会导致固定失效,而这需要巨大的受力。传统的钢板,螺钉可以顺序失效,较小的力就可使整个结构失效。锁定钢板已被证明是治疗关节附近骨折的最佳选择,而传统的固定方法无法提供更佳的结果[17]。锁定钢板结合 PMMA 骨水泥的使用应优先于传统钢板,最适用于关节附近,例如股骨近端,胫骨近端,肱骨近端和肱骨远端,这些部位髓内钉无法充分固定。该方法优于关节成形术,有利于功能恢复[18]。此外,当有其他植入物(如全关节置换术或先前的骨折固定术会干扰髓内固定装置的放置)时,可以使用这种固定方法(图 128-1)。

关节置换术

关节置换术是针对离关节非常近的病变,无论是髓内钉还是钢板螺钉固定都不能提供可靠稳定的固定,最常用于股骨头及股骨颈的病变,因为该部位移位骨折愈合率很低。对于转子间及转子下病变采用关节置换术优于内固定术,而采用肿瘤切除、内固定辅以 PMMA 骨水泥增强优于单独进行内固定[19]。在肿瘤已累及互锁螺钉进钉点的骨干骨折中,使用关节置换术优于髓内钉,因为肿瘤导致骨质破坏,互锁螺钉不能提供足够的支撑而容易脱出(图 128-4)。在预期寿命有限的肿瘤患者中髋臼磨损引起的疼痛不是主要问题,因此不易采用有更高的脱位风险和更长的手术时间的全髋关节置换术,半关节置换术是较好的选择,除非伴有严重的关节炎或需要外科手术干预的髋臼病变(图 128-1)。半关节置换术也可用于肱骨近端病变,那里没有足够的骨量以固定植入物。

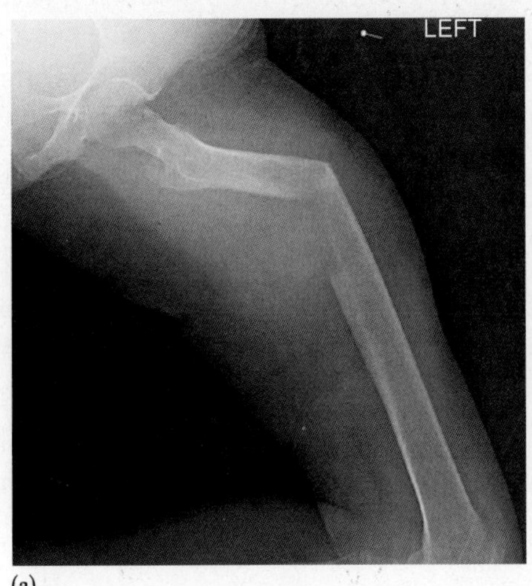

(a)

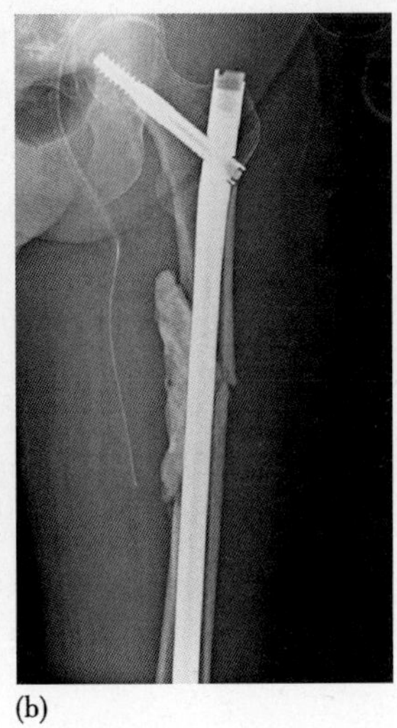

(b)

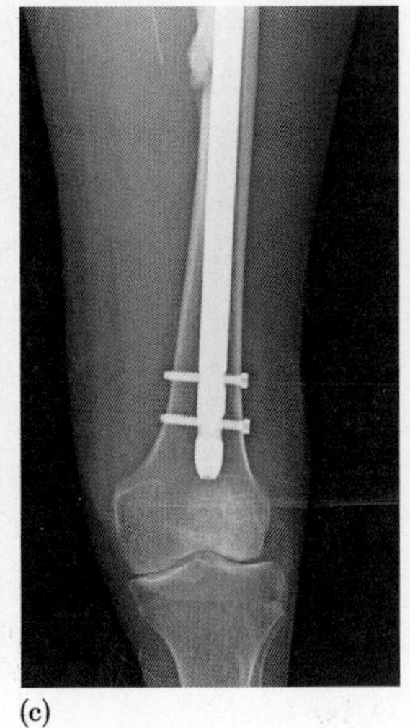

(c)

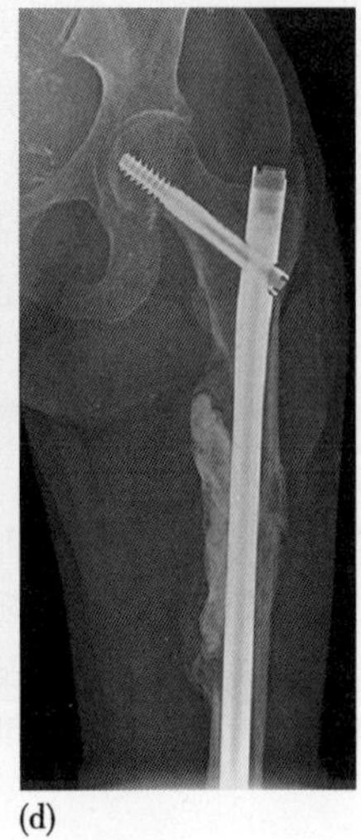

(d)

图 128-4 (a)患者,57 岁,女性,骨转移癌。左股骨中段骨干骨折。(b、c)患者行肿瘤刮除,髓内钉固定,PMMA 骨水泥填充假体周围,以填充肿瘤造成的骨缺损。(d)4 个月后,外侧皮质上的骨折线已消失,并且可见骨痂,表明骨折愈合。注意在骨水泥的内侧有骨痂形成

对于股骨头和股骨颈的孤立病变，一些外科医生使用传统的关节成形术，而另一些医生使用骨水泥型长柄假体半髋置换术，以保护股骨免于疾病进展的影响。在病变累及股骨近端大部分股的情况下，需要长柄半髋置换术（图 128-4）。该手术术中发生心搏骤停风险约为 2%，使用加压骨水泥导致的术中或术后早期死亡风险约为 1%。为降低这种不良事件的风险，在术前及术中必须与麻醉团队进行充分沟通。在骨水泥注入之前于股骨远端放置通气孔可以降低髓内压力，但没有数据表明这可以降低术中心搏骤停的临床风险[20]。从理论上讲，通气孔可以导致应力提高，从而导致假体远端骨折。

大型假体

虽然大型肿瘤假体通常用于修复骨肉瘤切除后留下的巨大缺损，但在转移性疾病和多发性骨髓瘤的治疗中偶尔也可使用，其适应证主要有三个：一是当肿瘤广泛切除而骨量不足以安装骨合成装置和关节置换假体。二是由于肿瘤进展或骨不连导致的内固定失败。三是罕见的单发转移病灶，切除病灶可提高长期生存率。虽然在某些特定的病例中，大型假体是一个合适的选择，但手术时间较长、有较高的并发症发生率（如感染和脱位）以及较长的恢复时间。病变部位同样重要，股骨远端及近端置换术后功能较好，而胫骨近端和肱骨近端置换功能较差。在有较大的骨干缺损的情况下，可以用节段型人工假体代替髓内钉，该假体比骨水泥增强的髓内钉更具生物力学稳定性[21]，假体两侧的髓腔至少长 5cm，以保证假体柄的置入。

髋臼周围病变的治疗

髋臼周围病变的手术治疗可能发生严重畸形、并发症及术中大出血。幸运的是，有很多非手术治疗效果也很好，如限制负重及放疗。对放射不敏感的小病变可以用骨水泥成形术治疗，并可以结合消融技术，如冷冻手术或射频消融。但是，对于非手术治疗失败且预期寿命足够长的患者，仍需进行手术治疗。在骨储备充足且软骨下板保存完好的情况下，可行病灶内刮除和 PMMA 骨水泥充填。对于发生移位的病理性髋臼骨折或影响内侧壁和/或软骨下板的大病变，需要进行复杂的全髋关节置换术。重建的目的是将来自髋臼的力分配到不受疾病影响的骨盆部分，例如髂骨和坐骨。常用的治疗方法有内半骨盆髋臼加强环、植入髂骨的斯坦曼针以及肿瘤缺损填充骨水泥等。在极少数情况下，骨质破坏非常严重，甚至用臼笼重建也不能提供足够的机械支撑，可以考虑使用半骨盆假体置换，但有较高的术后并发症发生率。治疗髋臼周围病变还有一种手术方式是髋臼病灶切除后股骨头旷置术。这种手术方式没有进行重建，因此会造成肢体短缩约 5cm 左右，导致肢体运动功能下降，但患者术后可行走。该手术方式具有并发症发生率低、手术时间短、相对简单的优点，最适合应用于无法行大范围病灶清除及重建或对术后肢体功能要求不高的患者[22]。髋臼周围肿瘤，尤其是多发性骨髓瘤、肾细胞癌、甲状腺癌可能血运丰富，需要作好输血及术前肿瘤栓塞准备。

不重建的手术切除

虽然转移性疾病最常发生在中轴骨骼、股骨近端和肱骨，但也可发生在锁骨、桡骨近端、尺骨远端和腓骨近端等较小骨骼。这些骨骼非常细小，即使用骨水泥增强固定，内植物失败风险仍很高。幸运的是，只切除这些部位的骨病变而不重建，仍可以获得良好的功能。切除已发生骨折的骨段或整个骨，可以极大限度地缓解疼痛症状。这种方法可以减少手术时间并降低并发症的风险，同时提供与骨折固定相同（如果不是更好）的结果。如前所述，对于疼痛明显的严重髋臼周围病变患者，如果其力线很差，或者无法行有广泛髋臼周围切除重建术，股骨头和髋关节切除而不重建的手术方式也是一种很好的选择。

脊柱病变

脊柱是最常见的转移部位，但大部分的脊柱转移病变并不需要手术治疗。通常在行骨扫描、胸腹盆 CT 时偶然发现。脊柱的机械完整性通常不受损害，因此通过放疗治疗轴向性背痛通常是有效的。在没有神经功能损害的压缩性骨折病例中，超过 90% 的患者可以通过后凸成形术联合放疗减轻疼痛[23]。椎体后凸成形术是在影像引导下，经椎弓根将球囊插入椎体，充气以恢复椎体高度，然后将聚甲基丙烯酸甲酯（PMMA）骨水泥注入所形成的空隙中以维持椎体高度。手术减压和融合术适用于神经受压导致的严重的和进行性的神经损害患者（图 128-5）。在脊髓或尾静脉受压的情况下，外科手术干预比单独的放疗起到更好的止痛效果，并且更有可能保持甚至恢复患者的活动能力[24]。在不可逆的神经损伤之前及时进行手术减压至关重要。对于因多发性骨髓瘤、淋巴瘤等放疗敏感性病变导致神经功能损害的病例，急诊放疗是首选的治疗方式。在进行治疗时，应使用糖皮质激素以减轻脊髓周围的水肿，并尽可能地保持神经功能[24]（译者注）。

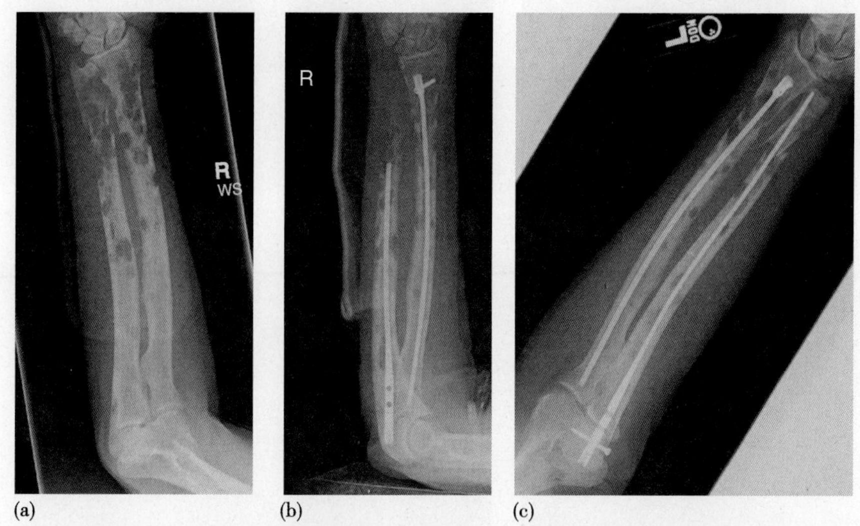

(a)　(b)　(c)

图 128-5　(a)患者,69 岁,男性,多发性骨髓瘤。双侧尺骨及桡骨的多发透光病灶导致病理性骨折。(b、c)双侧尺骨及桡骨行髓内钉固定,右侧尺骨远端没有足够的骨量行固定,因此行手术切除,对功能影响小。髓内钉是以微创的方式进行的,优于钢板和螺钉固定,因该患者全身情况较差,钢板和螺钉需要暴露整个桡骨和尺骨

疼痛性转移病灶及潜在病理骨折的治疗

手术的适应证,除了包括已有移位的病理性骨折,还包括即将发生的病理性骨折和对放疗或其他非手术治疗无效的疼痛性病变。与发生骨折后进行治疗相比,预防性手术的恢复更快、术后功能更好[25,26]。目前已有数个评估系统用来评估病理性骨折风险,最常用的一种由 Mirels 在 1989 年提出,通过四个类别对病变进行评分(参见第 111 章,表 111-4)[27],每个类别的得分为 1~3 分,再计总分(图 128-6 至图 128-10)。各参数如下：

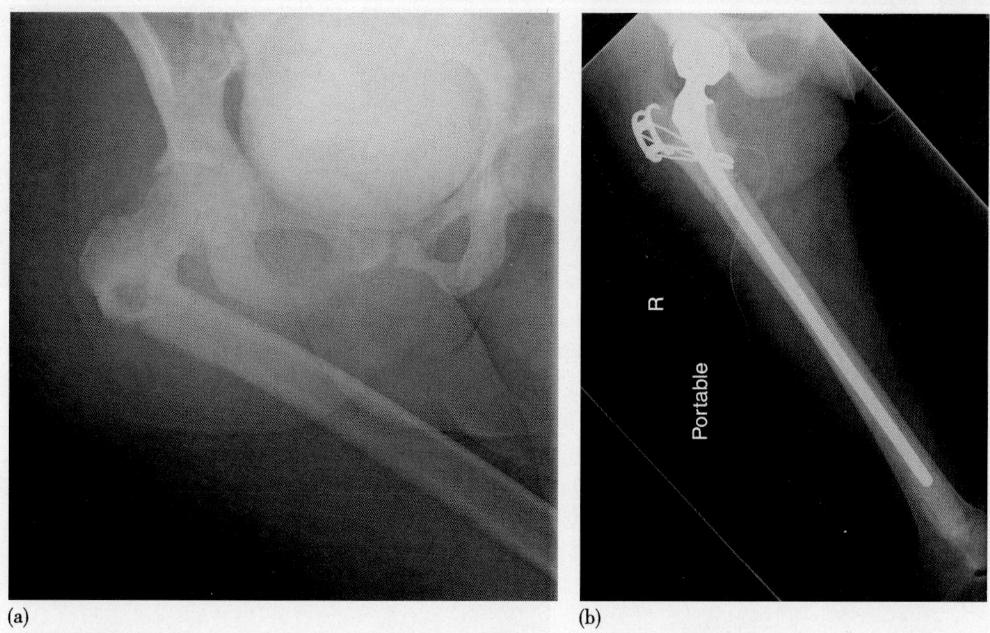

(a)　(b)

图 128-6　(a)患者,40 岁,女性,乳腺癌骨转移。右侧股骨转子间骨折。股骨头及大部分骨盆骨的溶骨性及成骨性改变。(b)行长柄骨水泥型假体半髋关节置换术。对于此病例,股骨髓内钉固定并不是理想的手术方式。这是由于股骨头已经被转移性肿瘤破坏,如果行髓内钉固定,拉力螺钉脱出的风险会非常高。关节置换假体柄具有与髓内钉相同的固定骨折功能,同时受损的股骨头则被假体头替代

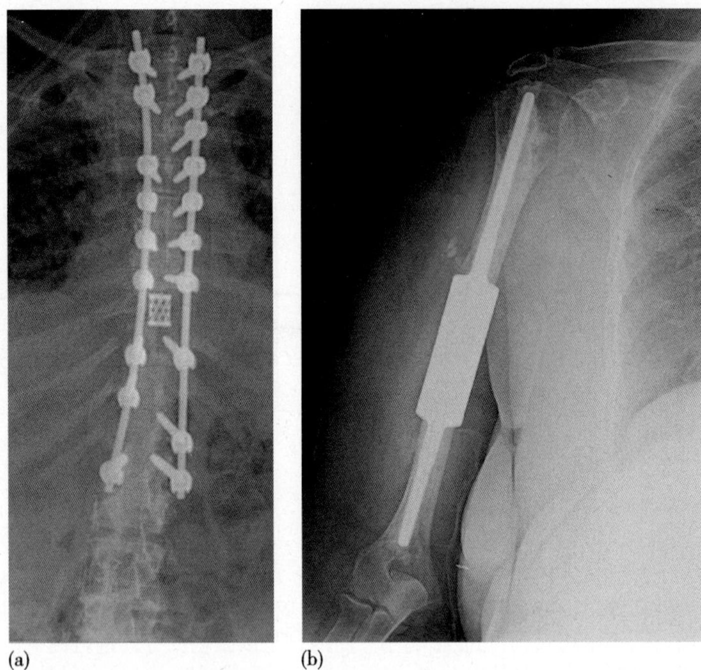

图 128-7 (a)患者,71 岁,女性,肾癌骨转移。肱骨干大范围骨折破坏并病理性骨折。(b)对于髓内钉固定或钢板及螺钉固定没有足够的骨量支撑,因此使用节段型人工假体置换来重建缺损。利用骨水泥将假体固定于骨干远端和近端,使得构造类似于骨水泥型髓内钉

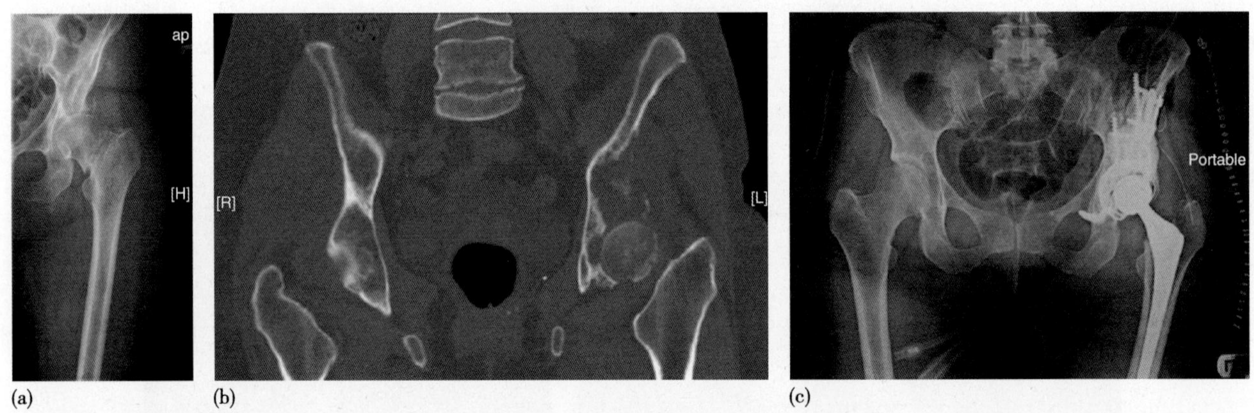

图 128-8 (a)患者,60 岁,女性,外伤致移位性股骨颈骨折。注意髋臼外侧缘有细微的皮质不规则。(b)冠状位 CT 显示髋臼上区域有大的破坏性病变,软骨下板破坏。活检显示转移性乳腺癌。股骨颈骨折与患者的癌症无关。(c)患者接受肿瘤刮除术并用髋臼笼进行全髋关节置换术重建缺损。肿瘤留下的空腔填充 PMMA 骨水泥

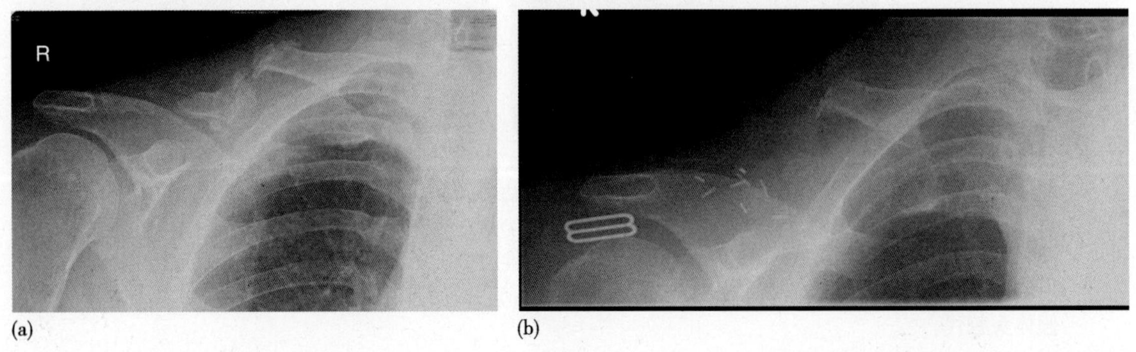

图 128-9 (a)患者,60 岁,女性,右锁骨透光性病变导致病理性骨折。曾患有创伤性锁骨骨折,后来发展成无症状的骨不连。(b)切除包括病理性骨折部位在内的锁骨外侧,患者在手术后 2 周内恢复到基线状态

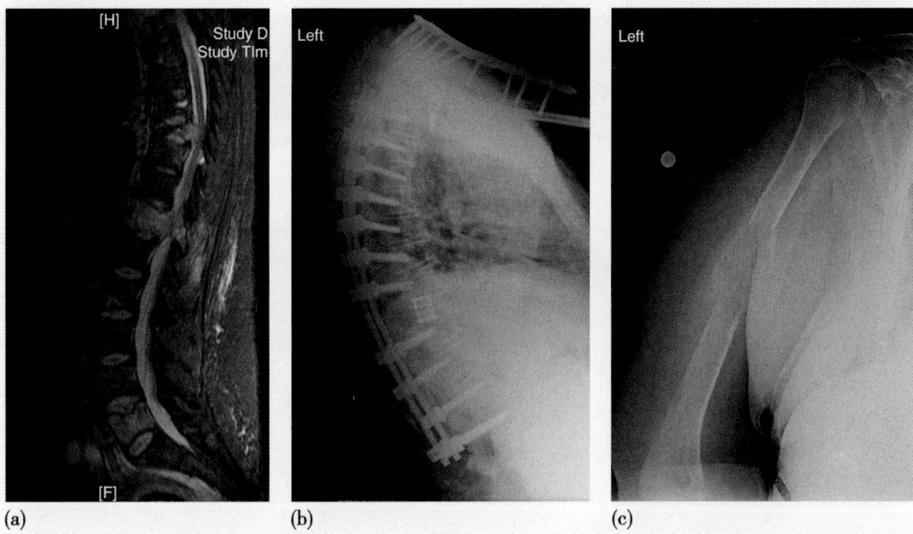

(a) (b) (c)

图 128-10　(a)患者,56 岁,女性,子宫内膜癌骨转移。T9 椎体病理性骨折引起脊髓压迫而出现明显的下肢无力。其他椎体中可见转移性成骨。(b、c)患者行 T9 椎体切除,椎间融合器植入,后路 T8-T10 半椎板切除术,T1-L1 固定融合

1. 病变部位。股骨转子间受力最大,评分为 3 分,而上肢无负重,评分为 1 分。

2. 疼痛程度。活动后疼痛加重评分最高,因为这表明病变部位结构不稳定。在 Mirels 的研究中,所有活动后疼痛加重的患者都发生了骨折,而无功能性疼痛的患者只有 10% 发生骨折。

3. 病变类型。溶骨性病变最容易骨折,因为骨质被肿瘤破坏,所以计 3 分。成骨性病变形成异常的肿瘤骨,其强度比正常骨降低,但较溶骨性病变的骨强度稍高,因此计 1 分。

4. 病变大小。较大的病灶有较高的骨折风险,因此得分较高。

将四个类别的分数相加,得到总分 4～12 分。评分为 9 分的患者有 33% 的骨折风险,因此建议 9 分及以上的患者进行手术,7 分及以下的患者建议进行放射治疗。评分为 8 分的患者骨折风险为 15%,因此必须考虑患者的活动情况、体重、预期寿命以及肿瘤对化疗和放疗的敏感性等因素(参见第 111 章,表 111-4B)。Mirels 系统灵敏度为 91%,其特异性仅为 35%[28],因此需要特异性更高的基于 CT 的评价系统[29]。

(王鲁强 译　李晓阳　于胜吉 校)

参考文献

1 American Cancer Society. *Cancer Facts & Figures 2015*. Atlanta: American Cancer Society; 2015.

2 Coleman RE. Clinical features of metastatic bone disease and risk of skeletal morbidity. *Clin Cancer Res*. 2006;**12**(**20**):6243s–6249s.

3 Gaston CL, Nakamura T, Reddy K, et al. Is limb salvage surgery safe for bone sarcomas identified after a previous surgical procedure? *Bone Joint J*. 2014;**96**(**5**):665–672.

4 Abudu A, Sferopoulos NK, Tillman RM, et al. The surgical treatment and outcome of pathological fractures in localised osteosarcoma. *J Bone Joint Surg Br*. 1996;**78**(**5**):694–698.

5 Rougraff BT, Kneisl JS, Simon MA. Skeletal metastases of unknown origin. A prospective study of. *J Bone Joint Surg Am*. 1993;**75**:1276–1281.

6 Bui MM, Smith P, Agresta SV, et al. Practical issues of intraoperative frozen section diagnosis of bone and soft tissue lesions. *Cancer Control*. 2008;**15**(**1**):7–12.

7 Mankin HJ, Lange TA, Spanier SS. The hazards of biopsy in patients with malignant primary bone and soft tissue tumors. *J Bone Joint Surg*. 1982;**64A**:1121–7.

8 Henry DH, Costa L, Goldwasser F, Hirsh V, et al. Randomized, double-blind study of denosumab versus zoledronic acid in the treatment of bone metastases in patients with advanced cancer (excluding breast and prostate cancer) or multiple myeloma. *J Clin Oncol*. 2011;**29**(**9**):1125–1132.

9 Schocker JD, Brady LW. Radiation therapy for bone metastases. *Clin Orthop*. 1982;**169**:38–43.

10 Toyota N, Naito A, Kakizawa H, et al. Radiofrequency ablation therapy combined with cementoplasty for painful bone metastases: initial experience. *Cardiovasc Intervent Radiol*. 2005;**28**(**5**):578–583.

11 Callstrom MR, Charboneau JW, Goetz MP, et al. Image-guided ablation of painful metastatic bone tumors: a new and effective approach to a difficult problem. *Skeletal Radiol*. 2006;**35**(**1**):1–15.

12 Gainor BJ, Buchert P. Fracture healing in metastatic bone disease. *Clin Orthop Relat Res*. 1983;**178**:297–302.

13 Laitinen M, Nieminen J, Pakarinen TK. Treatment of pathological humerus shaft fractures with intramedullary nails with or without cement fixation. *Arch Orthop Trauma Surg*. 2011;**131**(**4**):503–508.

14 Pugh J, Sherry HS, Futterman B, Frankel VH. Biomechanics of pathologic fractures. *Clin Orthop Relat Res*. 1982;**169**:109–114.

15 Kollender Y, Bickels J, Price WM, et al. Metastatic renal cell carcinoma of bone: indications and technique of surgical intervention. *J Urol*. 2000;**164**(**5**):1505–1508.

16 Townsend PW, Rosenthal HG, Smalley SR, et al. Impact of postoperative radiation therapy and other perioperative factors on outcome after orthopedic stabilization of impending or pathologic fractures due to metastatic disease. *J Clin Oncol*. 1994;**12**(**11**):2345–2350.

17 Friess DM, Attia A. Locking plate fixation for proximal humerus fractures: a comparison with other fixation techniques. *Orthopedics*. 2008;**31**:1183.

18 Siegel HJ, Lopez-Ben R, Mann JP, Ponce BA. Pathological fractures of the proximal humerus treated with a proximal humeral locking plate and bone cement. *J Bone Joint Surg Br*. 2010;**92**(**5**):707–712.

19 Wedin R, Bauer HC. Surgical treatment of skeletal metastatic lesions of the proximal femur: endoprosthesis or reconstruction nail? *J Bone Joint Surg Br*. 2005;**87**(**12**):1653–1657.

20 Patterson BM, Healey JH, Cornell CN, Sharrock NE. Cardiac arrest during hip arthroplasty with a cemented long-stem component. A report of seven cases. *J Bone Joint Surg Am*. 1991;**73**(**2**):271–277.

21 Henry JC, Damron TA, Weiner MM, et al. Biomechanical analysis of humeral dia-

physeal segmental defect fixation. *Clin Orthop Relat Res*. 2002;**396**:231–239.

22 Issack PS, Kotwal SY, Lane JM. Management of metastatic bone disease of the acetabulum. *J Am Acad Orthop Surg*. 2013;**21(11)**:685–695.

23 Gerszten PC, Germanwala A, Burton SA, et al. Combination kyphoplasty and spinal radiosurgery: a new treatment paradigm for pathological fractures. *J Neurosurg Spine*. 2005;**3(4)**:296–301.

24 Patchell RA, Tibbs PA, Regine WF, et al. Direct decompressive surgical resection in the treatment of spinal cord compression caused by metastatic cancer: a randomised trial. *Lancet*. 2005;**366(9486)**:643–648.

25 Katzer A, Meenen NM, Grabbe F, Rueger JM. Surgery of skeletal metastases. *Arch Orthop Trauma Surg*. 2002;**122**:251–258.

26 Ward WG, Holsenbeck S, Dorey FJ, Spang J, Howe D. Metastatic disease of the femur: surgical treatment. *Clin Orthop*. 2003;**415**:230–244.

27 Mirels H. Metastatic disease in long bones. *Clin Orthop*. 1989;**249**:256–64.

28 Damron TA, Morgan H, Prakash D, Grant W, Aronowitz J, Heiner J. Critical evaluation of Mirel's rating system for impending pathologic fractures. *Clin Orthop Relat Res*. 2003;**415S**:S201–S207.

29 Snyder BD, Hauser-Kara DA, Hipp JA, Zurakowski D, Hecht AC, Gebhardt MC. Predicting fracture through benign skeletal lesions with quantitative computed tomography. *J Bone Joint Surg Am*. 2006;**88**:55–70.

第 129 章　血液学并发症和血库支持

Richard M. Kaufman, MD ■ Kenneth C. Anderson, MD

概述

许多用于治疗癌症的基本方法(化疗和干细胞移植)都会破坏骨髓正常的造血功能。因此,癌症患者输血治疗是一种必不可少的支持治疗方法。本章主要关注"经典"血液成分支持:如何收集红细胞、血浆、血小板和粒细胞,并对其进行检测、存储和管理,以解决癌症患者的特定缺陷。特别关注了预防性血小板输注的研究,在过去几十年里,血小板输注在骨髓抑制治疗应用于各种恶性疾病时发挥了关键作用。同时也综述了目前血液制品的感染风险。

癌症患者经常发生血液并发症,和原发疾病或癌症治疗相关[1,2]。红细胞(RBC)、白细胞(WBC),以及血小板数量和功能异常需要输血医学专家提供适当的血液成分支持[3,4]。的确,迄今为止如果没有治疗技术的同步发展以支持患者渡过治疗所致的血液系统并发症,采用高剂量联合化疗方案所取得的治疗进展是不可能的。

全血细胞减少的原因

癌症及其治疗可能通过对造血干细胞直接作用或通过抑制造血生长因子的产生和对造血生长因子的反应而改变正常的造血功能(表 129-1)。

表 129-1　癌症患者贫血、血小板减少和白细胞减少的原因

原发肿瘤替代正常骨髓(如白血病)
转移性肿瘤累及骨髓(如乳腺癌和前列腺癌)
正常生理紊乱
• 营养性(如叶酸、铁和负氮平衡)
• 异常反馈(如造血作用的刺激/抑制)
• 骨髓反应(如纤维化)
• 外周血破坏(如免疫性溶血,弥散性血管内凝血,脾肿大)
• 失血
化疗或放疗对骨髓的抑制作用

疾病相关

骨髓造血细胞可以被来自骨髓细胞的原发肿瘤所替代,或被来自其他器官的肿瘤转移到骨髓所替代。霍奇金淋巴瘤和非霍奇金淋巴瘤(NHL)、恶性黑色素瘤、神经母细胞瘤以及乳腺、前列腺、肺、肾上腺、甲状腺和肾的肿瘤都常常表现为骨髓受累。最终,骨髓弥漫性受累可导致骨髓纤维化或坏死,可能与脾肿大、血小板减少和外周血中所有谱系的未成熟细胞有关[5]。

化疗相关

治疗在骨髓损伤和恢复中的作用因所用药物和不同血液学谱系细胞的正常周转率而异。几种药物对骨髓的特征性作用如表 129-2 所示。骨髓有一个储备池能够在干细胞池停止功能后 8~10 日内向外周血供应成熟细胞。因此,外周血中的事件比骨髓中的晚一周。在初治患者中,治疗后第 9 日或第 10 日出现白细胞减少和血小板减少,第 14 日和第 18 日为计数最低点。计数在第 21 日明显恢复,第 28 日完成。细胞毒性剂量-反应关系通常与 WBC 和血小板计数的最低点有关,而与血细胞减少的持续时间无关。这是由于正常骨髓的干细胞处于休眠状态以保护它们免受伤害。

表 129-2　药物和治疗对骨髓的特征性作用

治疗	血液系统并发症
大多数化疗药物	第 9~10 日白细胞减少和血小板减少;第 14~18 日为最低点;第 21~28 日恢复
亚硝基脲	4~6 周时骨髓抑制
长春新碱,1-天冬酰胺酶,博来霉素,含亮氨酸的骨髓抑制甲氨蝶呤	无骨髓抑制
伽马辐射	慢性淋巴细胞减少
全身辐射	严重抑制体液和细胞免疫反应

伽马辐射相关

辐射损伤的细胞可在所有子代细胞无法增殖前分裂一次或多次;因此,受辐射的细胞在分裂之前不会出现损伤[6]。在放射后第一次分裂时,细胞可能死亡,分裂异常并产生不寻常的形态,无法分裂并保持生理功能,或无法产生一代或多代后代,直至细胞不能增殖。由于骨髓干细胞修复亚致死辐射损伤的能力非常低,多个较小的辐射分割可能保护其他正常组织(如肺和肠),但不会保护骨髓。

相关流程

在癌症病程和/或治疗过程中可能发生正常生理紊乱而导致全血细胞减少,对这些紊乱的认识至关重要。这些包括营养因素,如叶酸、铁或维生素缺乏。造血过程中可能存在异常的

反馈环,如再生障碍性贫血中细胞介导的造血抑制或抗体介导的血小板破坏中血小板生成的刺激[7]。纤维化可能是病程的一部分,也可能是治疗的反应,从而破坏骨髓储备。免疫介导的细胞破坏和其他因素,如脾肿大可导致细胞减少。此外,隐匿性出血一直被认为是造成持续性贫血和难治性血小板减少症的原因。这些临床实例强调了在将血液并发症的病因归因于肿瘤之前,应仔细对癌症患者进行评估。

红细胞异常和红细胞支持

贫血

癌症患者的贫血可能是轻重不一和多病因的。早期癌症患者的造血可能是正常的。另一方面,肿瘤替代骨髓细胞对贫血的发生并不重要,即使是转移性癌症患者。最常见的是随着病情的发展癌症患者贫血的发生率和程度增加。只有当骨髓细胞形态接近正常、血清铁和铁结合能力较低、骨髓铁含量正常或增加、血清铁蛋白升高时才可诊断为慢性贫血[8]。低血铁水平和充足的铁储存同时存在有助于鉴别慢性疾病贫血和缺铁性贫血。此外,必须排除贫血的其他原因,例如明显的溶血、出血、营养不良或骨髓置换。在某些患者中,如霍奇金病(HD),噬红细胞作用或脾功能亢进可能是导致红细胞存活率下降的原因,但在其他患者中病因尚不清楚。

红细胞输注

红细胞输注可增加贫血患者的携氧能力,而正常的生理机制不能充分弥补。当血容量充足时,7g/dl 血红蛋白(约 21%的血细胞比容)的携氧能力可满足维持心肺功能[9]。在危重症患者的多中心随机试验中,证明限制性输血策略(将血红蛋白水平维持在 7~9g/dl 之间)至少与更随意的输血策略一样安全,但急性心肌梗死或不稳定心绞痛患者可能除外[10]。随后的随机试验比较了接受髋关节手术[11]或心脏手术[12~14]的心血管疾病患者、败血症患者[15]、上消化道出血患者[16]中限制性输血策略与自由输血策略的差异。对绝大多数住院患者而言,限制性输血策略(血红蛋白输血阈值为 7~8g/dl)是安全和合适的。然而,目前仍需等待高质量的临床试验数据来指导恶性肿瘤患者的 RBC 输注。总的来说,没有一种血红蛋白水平可以普遍用于"输血指征"。在决定是否给特定患者输血时,医生应考虑患者的年龄、贫血程度、血容量以及是否同时存在心脏、肺或血管疾病[17]。为了满足氧需要,一些患者可能需要更高血红蛋白水平的 RBC 输注。特别是在癌症及其治疗中,血红蛋白水平通常维持在 8g/dl 的水平。平均体重为 70kg 的成年人,输注一单位 RBC 通常会使血红蛋白增加 1g/dl,血细胞比容增加 2%~3%。

红细胞悬液(PRBC)是由全血(WB)通过血浆去除法或红细胞除去法制备而成的。采用过滤法使白细胞减少,从而制备出去白红细胞(LRBC)。白细胞减少可有效预防输血者出现发热性非溶血性输血反应和巨细胞病毒(CMV)感染[18]。在美国和国际上,有普遍输注去白红细胞成分的趋势,以避免白细胞的多种不良后遗症。洗涤 RBC 通过从 PRBC 中进一步去除血浆制备而成。这些血液制品有时用来预防对血浆蛋白的过敏反应[19]。目前 PRBC 在 4℃时可储存 42 日。回顾性研究表明,输注储存时间较长的 PRBC 可能与输血者的不良后果有关[20]。然而在多中心随机对照试验中,并未证实陈旧 RBC 会比新鲜 RBC 增加发病率或死亡率[21~23]。

白细胞减少和白细胞支持

白细胞减少

白细胞减少可能与癌症及其治疗相关。1965 年,Hersh 等总结了在美国国立癌症研究所治疗的急性白血病患者死亡的原因,发现输注血小板明显减少了致命性出血的发生,但单纯感染所致的死亡随之增加[24]。在白血病患者中循环白细胞和感染之间有显著相关性;特别是发生感染的可能性与白细胞减少的严重程度和持续时间成正比[25]。

粒细胞输注

近 30 年前,治疗性粒细胞首次被用于伴有白细胞减少和严重感染的白血病患者。最早的试验证明了粒细胞输血的潜在价值,利用从慢性髓细胞性白血病患者身上采集的粒细胞,并达到了正常供者无法达到的细胞剂量[26]。剂量的重要性被定义为:小于 10^{10} 个粒细胞为无效,大于 10^{11} 个粒细胞为有效。事实上,在一个不发热、未感染的男性体内,循环中粒细胞的半衰期为 6.7h(4~10h),每日更新率为 230%。在犬模型中进行的平行研究也表明,故意采用辐射使狗的白细胞减少,通过粒细胞输血可以成功治疗革兰氏阴性菌血症和肺炎[27]。

已有 6 项预防性白细胞输血的前瞻性随机临床研究,旨在预防白细胞减少患者的感染[28,29]。然而,因为同种异体免疫、输血反应、CMV 感染及肺浸润在输血组更常发生,以上研究并未能改善生存。由于供-受者匹配不足及粒细胞输血剂量不足,这些研究受到了质疑。一项已经完成的大型随机试验应用 G-CSF 和地塞米松动员供者造血,收集高剂量粒细胞[29]。目前,粒细胞输血的作用仍存在争议。当使用粒细胞输血时,产品必须经过放射线照射,以预防免疫缺陷的宿主输血后出现移植物抗宿主病(GVHD)。

血小板减少和血小板支持

血小板减少

癌症患者的血小板减少通常是由化疗和放疗引起的。由于巨核细胞减少或缺乏而导致血小板生成受损是癌症患者血小板减少最常见的原因(表 129-3)。然而,血小板减少也可能是由于患者原发肿瘤进程中出现脾肿大导致的脾隔离症所致。在这种情况下,巨核细胞数量明显增加,除非存在广泛的骨髓浸润。免疫介导的血小板减少也可能与抗人类白细胞抗原(anti-human leukocyteantigen,anti-HLA)或抗血小板特异性的同种抗体有关。最后,血小板减少可能与弥散性血管内凝血(diffuse intravascular coagulation,DIC)有关,特别是在急性髓细胞性白血病(acute myeloid leukemia,AML)、淋巴瘤、肺癌、乳腺癌、胃肠道肿瘤或泌尿系肿瘤患者中。因为早幼粒细胞亚细胞成分中同时存在促凝血物质和纤溶蛋白酶，所以 DIC 常并发于急性早幼粒细胞白血病[30]。

表 129-3 血小板减少的原因

增加导致的急性血小板减少
• 血小板消耗（使用、隔离或破坏）
• 大量血液替换
• 心脏手术
• 脾肿大
血小板免疫破坏
• 自限性的特发性血小板减少性紫癜（ITP）
• 输血后紫癜
• 药物性紫癜
• 慢性特发性血小板减少性紫癜
• 消耗性血小板减少症
遗传缺陷
血小板生成减少引起的血小板减少症
• 再生障碍性贫血
• 急性白血病
特发性巨核细胞发育不全
骨髓浸润
• 恶性浸润
• 非恶性浸润-戈谢病，肉芽肿性疾病
放射或骨髓抑制药物治疗后
特异性抑制血小板产生的药物（如噻嗪类利尿剂、酒精和雌激素）
营养缺乏-巨幼红细胞性贫血，严重的缺铁性贫血（少见）
病毒感染
阵发性睡眠性血红蛋白尿症

血小板功能异常

几种慢性骨髓增生性疾病可能出现血小板功能异常。尽管大多数急性髓细胞性白血病（acute myeloid leukemia，AML）患者的出血与血小板减少有关，但已有报道提示其与血小板功能内在异常有关，包括血小板促凝活性降低、聚集降低和对 ADP、肾上腺素或胶原蛋白的血清素释放反应降低[31]。血小板功能障碍在部分 IgA 骨髓瘤或华氏巨球蛋白血症，多发性骨髓瘤和单克隆人免疫球蛋白病患者中明显，但意义不明[32]。

血小板输注

1910 年，首次给血小板减少患者输注新鲜 WB，结果血小板计数增加、止血效果和出血时间缩短都很显著[33]。在 20 世纪 50 年代，血小板首次用于接受联合化疗后出现的血小板减少的白血病患者[34]。美国国家癌症研究所 20 世纪 60 年代初的数据明确表明，白血病患者在化疗诱导缓解期间死于出血，并确定了血小板计数与出血之间的定量关系[35]。结果表明，血小板治疗可以改变儿童和成人的出血过程，唯一的区别是所需的剂量。最近有两项随机试验比较了预防性血小板输注与治疗性血小板输注对增殖性血小板减少症患者的影响。两项研究都证明了预防性血小板治疗的益处，尽管有限，但均表明与接受自体干细胞移植的患者相比，预防性输注血小板对接受化疗的白血病患者的出血风险有更大的影响[36]。

单供体和多供体血小板

在美国，一个单位浓缩血小板是从一个单位的 WB 经离心分离得到，并含有约 5.5×10^{10} 血小板/单位［这种制备血小板的方法被称为“富含血小板血浆法（platelet-rich plasma，PRP）”。在其他国家，浓缩血小板是通过交替“白膜层”法从 WB 制备而成］。来自多个（4~6 个）供者的浓缩血小板汇集在一起成为一个输血成分。机采血小板技术可以在一个供者一次捐献过程中采集相当于几个单位的浓缩血小板。单个供者血小板单位通常包含至少 3×10^{11} 血小板/单位。单供血小板的使用正在增加；它们通常被用于恶性肿瘤患者的血小板输注[37]。同种免疫患者对随机供者的血小板治疗无效，所以采用 HLA-匹配供者的单供体血小板采集。在美国，血小板在室温下可保存 5 日。

治疗性和预防性血小板输注的适应证

肿瘤患者经常需要输注血小板。大多数为预防性血小板输注以防止出血，而不是治疗活动性出血的治疗性输注[38]。血小板输注的适应证已经成为最近 AABB 临床实践指南的主题[39]。目前，一个剂量的机采血小板（或等同于随机供体浓缩血小板）常规用于血小板小于 10 000/mm^3 肿瘤患者的输注以降低出血风险。来自 Gmur 等的研究数据证明预防性血小板输注的阈值在无发热或无出血的急性白血病患者可以安全地设定在 5×10^9/L，如果发热或出血均无则设定在 10×10^9/L [40]。前瞻性临床试验显示，急性白血病患者血小板输注阈值无论设定在 10×10^9/L 或 20×10^9/L，大出血的风险是相似的，而较低的阈值减少了血小板的使用[41~43]。

在不同的临床情况中，特定血小板计数下出血的风险可能不同。例如，AML 患者在血小板低于 10 000/mm^3 时出血风险增加，而相比之下，急性淋巴细胞白血病（acute lymphoblastic leukemia，ALL）患者在血小板低于 20 000/mm^3 时才有相似的出血风险[44]。由于血小板生成降低引起的慢性血小板减少症（如骨髓增生异常）患者可能需要输血，而相比之下，血小板破坏加速、但生成正常的患者（如特发性血小板减少性紫癜），可能不需要常规输注血小板。此外，慢性血小板减少症患者可能会耐受较低的绝对血小板计数而不需要输血。在血小板功能异常的患者，重要的不是血小板的绝对数量，而是功能性血小板的数量。因此，很难为所有患者界定输注血小板的绝对阈值，预防性血小板输血的时机和剂量必须基于临床考虑[39,45~47]。

多中心随机 PLADO(PLAtelet DOsing)研究证实,与标准剂量预防相比,低剂量的预防性血小板输注不增加 2 级或更高级别的出血。尽管血小板总量要求降低了,但患者接受了更频繁的低剂量预防性血小板输注[48]。

血小板输注有效性的临床和实验室评估

血小板输注的疗效可以通过实验室参数(输注后 1h 或 10~15min 的血小板计数增加)和输注后的观察到的临床效果进行评估[49-52]。校正后的计数增加定义为:从输注前到输注后血小板计数的增加量,该增加量根据输注单位数和受者体表面积进行了校正。新鲜的、适当储存的血小板被输注后,通常在 18~24h 时 CCI 为 15 000~20 000/mm^3[52]。

由于脾隔离,特别是在脾肿大的情况下,输血后血小板计数的增加可能低于预期[50]。已经证明药物诱导的血小板抗体可介导血小板的免疫破坏。如果受者拥有对抗供者 HLA-A 基因位点抗原、ABO 系统或血小板同种抗原的抗体,则输注的血小板的存活也可能受到损害。对造血干细胞移植受者血小板输注疗效也进行了专门研究。

同种异体免疫

血小板含有 HLA-A 和-B 抗原,但缺乏 HLA-C 和-DR 的抗原,并且受者淋巴细胞毒素类抗 HLA 抗体与对随机供者的血小板产生抵抗有显著相关性[53]。目前,使用 HLA 抗原包被珠的流式细胞术可非常容易检测到患者血清中的抗 HLA 抗体。

Yankee 等首先证明,从 HLA-相同的兄弟姐妹或在 HLA-A 和-B 位点(分级 A 或 B 匹配)匹配的非亲属供者获得的血小板,可能使对随机供者的血小板抵抗的同种异体免疫受者获得满意的血小板输注后增量[54]。随后,Duquesnoy 等发现,供者的 HLA 抗原与患者相同(B 匹配)或与患者的抗原交叉反应(BX 匹配)是相当的[55]。

由于认识到抗-HLA 抗体的抵抗性,人们试图通过修饰输注的血小板来避免或延迟同种异体免疫。由于 HLA 抗原在白细胞上表达,而血小板本身免疫原性差,研究人员已经尝试过:①从血小板中去除白细胞,或采用紫外线(UV)照射血小板以去除白细胞的抗原递呈功能;②使用单个而不是多个供者的血小板以减少暴露 HLA 的机会;③输注只有 HLA-匹配或去白细胞的 HLA-匹配的血小板。降低血小板同种异体免疫(trial to reduce alloimmunization to platelets,TRAP)的多中心、前瞻性研究证实,与接受不过滤随机供者浓缩血小板相比,接受过滤或者紫外线处理的随机供者浓缩血小板,或者过滤的单个供者的血小板,单独的抗 HLA 和血小板特异性抗体的发生率及血小板抵抗相关抗体发生率,在白血病受者中是降低的[56]。只有 13%的患者发生和淋巴细胞毒抗体相关的血小板抵抗,这表明大多数输血小板无应答是和其他因素相关的。当敏感受者仍然对 HLA-匹配血小板抵抗,有些时候会提供交叉-匹配的血小板。处理 HLA 免疫耐受性的第三种方法是提供抗原阴性的血小板,类似于为 RBC 同种抗体的患者提供抗原阴性 RBC。

ABO 血型决定因素是血小板膜固有的[57]。与 RBC 输注不同,供者和受者 ABO 血型不匹配并不是血小板输血的绝对禁忌。就是说,ABO 血型相同的血小板输血优先。输注 ABO 血型不相容的血小板(如供者 A 型和受者 O 型)的恢复率比输注 ABO 血型相同的血小板低 1/3 左右[58,59]。

此外,被动输注存在于浓缩血小板的血浆中的高滴度同族血凝素(如供者 O 型,受者 A 型),有时会引起严重溶血。值得注意的是,英国已经常规检测抗 A/B 血小板单位来防止该问题的发生。但包括美国在内的其他国家,都没有采取统一的策略来阻止类似问题的发生[59]。

其他治疗方法

新鲜冰冻血浆的输注

新鲜血浆是一个单位(450ml)WB 在-18℃及以下的温度下通过离心、分离和冷冻而成。它含有生理水平的凝血因子。新鲜冰冻血浆用于纠正凝血因子缺乏;逆转华法林的作用;治疗血栓性血小板减少性紫癜、弥散性血管内凝血、肝病所致凝血障碍、溶栓剂过量、蛋白 C 或 S 缺乏[60,61]。除了从供者的 WB 的血浆中获得外,应用血浆置换法可以获得一些血制品:凝血因子(Ⅷ因子和Ⅸ因子),免疫球蛋白和白蛋白制剂。

输血对免疫系统的影响

同种异体免疫

输血最可靠的效果是刺激受者体内产生对抗输血成分中抗原的抗体。输注血液中的细胞抗原和血浆抗原都使受者暴露于数百种已知的同种抗原中。

超过了 400 种红细胞抗原已被确定,但我们通常只是确保其中三个抗原的相容性:A,B 和 D。已经确定了超过 100 种 HLA 抗原和粒细胞及血小板特异性抗原。等位基因导致全部血浆中蛋白的结构和抗原性不同,导致受者对供者的免疫球蛋白产生同种抗体。大多数同种异型抗原由于其抗原性较弱在输血治疗中被忽略。然而,研究表明受血者对输血中的抗原产生的抗体不仅同输血的次数有关还和时机相关。特别是不同个体接受相同次数的输血,较长时间内重复输血较短期内重复输血更容易产生抗体。一些癌症患者由于长期接受反复输血,更有可能产生同种异型免疫。RBC 的同种抗体可导致受者发病和红细胞存活时间缩短;白细胞抗体与发热性输血反应有关,可削弱输注粒细胞的有效性和存活率[62]。抗 HLA-A 和抗 HLA-B 的抗体和血小板特异性同种抗体一样会削弱输注的血小板的存活时间。最后,抗 IgA 抗体有时会在 IgA 缺乏的受者中产生过敏反应,但是抗 IgG、抗 IgM 和抗脂蛋白的抗体不会产生明显的临床副作用[63]。

输血相关 GVHD

历史观点

GVHD 通常在发生在同种异体骨髓移植(bone marrow transplantation,BMT)后,但很少发生在输血或其他器官移植后。输血相关的(TA)-GVHD 通常发生在免疫抑制的受者(如

BMT 接受者)，但在单方面 HLA 不匹配的情况下，也可发生在免疫功能强的受者中[64]。临床表现包括发热、皮疹、厌食、恶心、呕吐和水样或血性腹泻伴或不伴肝酶升高和胆红素升高。由于 GVHD 没有特定的诊断性特征，这种综合征有时候难以同病毒感染或药疹相鉴别。TA-GVHD 通常比较严重，但与同种异体 BMT 的情况不同，它经常导致继发于骨髓再生障碍的全血细胞减少。大多数报告的 TA-GVHD 病例对免疫抑制治疗无效而且往往是致命的。

风险人群的定义

1986 年，美国国立卫生研究院共识发展会议将接受 BMT 的患者或其他免疫缺陷的患者定义为需要输注接受照射的浓缩血小板以避免出现 GVHD 的适应人群。白血病或其他肿瘤患者由于化疗和/或放疗出现的继发免疫抑制或原来的免疫功能失调(如 HD)而可能存在 TA-GVHD 风险。在 HD 患者中，原来认为联合放化疗是 TA-GVHD 的必要易感因素，但最近报道了一些仅接受化疗的 HD 患者发生 TA-GVHD 的情况。大剂量化疗后接受自体干细胞移植的患者同样也有 TA-GVHD 风险[65]。最后，与 HLA 纯合子供者共享 HLA 单倍型的免疫健全患者似乎也有患 TA-GVHD 的风险[66,67]。HLA 纯合性更容易出现在一级家庭成员之间(如父母、子女和兄弟姐妹)。因此，目前推荐来自上述供者的血细胞成分都需要在输注前接受 25Gy 的照射处理。的确，由于有输注来自二级亲属的血液引起 TA-GVHD 的报道，所以直接来自所有家庭成员的血液都需要辐照处理[68]。接受从纯合子献血者向杂合子的非血亲输血后，都有 TA-GVHD 发生的报道，表明伽马射线照射处理的指征需要放得更宽[69,70]。在日本，从 HLA 纯合献血者向不相关的 HLA 杂合患者输血的风险为 1/874，在美国，这一风险为 1/7 174 [71]。最终，报道证实所有 HLA 匹配的细胞成分都应该进行照射[69~72]。

预防策略

目前唯一预防 TA-GVHD 的有效方法是输注血制品前进行伽马照射处理。研究表明与未照射的对照组相比，15~20Gy 的照射能够使有丝分裂原反应淋巴细胞降低 5~6 个指数级别[71]。美国血库学会(American Association of Blood Banks, AABB)和 FDA 的标准是血液和细胞成分需要接受中位至少 25Gy 的照射处理[72]。目前的研究表明，照射不会对血小板的储存产生影响，但照射后钾释放对经照射红细胞储存的临床意义尚未明确，输血后受照射单位的红细胞的恢复可能会降低[73,74]。

输血相关的感染性疾病

B 型肝炎

虽然以前认为乙型肝炎(HB)是常见的输血相关性感染，但目前应用几代对 HB 表面抗原检测法来筛选潜在供者，以及使用志愿者而不使用商业供血者能明显减少经输血传播的 HB 发生[75]。现在也经常使用核酸检测(nucleic acid testing, NAT)技术来检测 HB。目前估计每一单位血制品发生 HB 的风险大约是 1/200 000(表 129-4)[76]。

表 129-4　输血风险

并发症	频率(发生:单位)
反应	
发热性非溶血反应	1∶100~4∶100
变态反应	1∶100~4∶100
输血相关急性肺损伤	1∶10 000
急性溶血	1∶250 000
迟发性溶血	1∶1 000
过敏反应	1∶150 000
感染	
丙肝	1∶2 000 000
乙肝	1∶200 000
HIV-1	1∶2 000 000
HIV-2	未报道
HTLV-Ⅰ和Ⅱ	1∶250 000~1∶2 000 000
疟疾	1∶4 000 000
红细胞细菌感染	1∶500 000
血小板细菌感染	1∶75 000
其他并发症	
RBC 同种致敏	1∶100
HLA 致敏	1∶10
移植物抗宿主病	罕见

HIV，人类免疫缺陷病毒。
HLA，人类白细胞抗原。
HTLV，人类 T 细胞白血病/淋巴瘤病毒。
RBC，红细胞。

C 型肝炎

在确认了甲型肝炎和乙型肝炎病毒之后，人们很快认识到这两种病毒都不是大多数输血后肝炎病例的罪魁祸首。因此，引入了非 A 型非 B 型肝炎(NANBH)这一术语。20 世纪 80 年代中期，对供体进行了谷丙转氨酶(ALT)和抗 HBc 的筛查；这些指标也被作为具有 20%机会传播 NANBH 的个体的“替代”标志物[77,78]。

通过克隆感染 NANBH 的黑猩猩的病毒 cDNA 片段，最终发现了 NANBH 的致病因子[79]。随后，现在所谓的丙型肝炎病毒(hepatitis C virus, HCV)的整个基因组被克隆出来。建立了血源性 NANBH 的特异性检测方法，其中重组 HCV 多肽用于捕获病毒抗体[80]。随后的多抗原 HCV 酶检测证实，几乎所有输血后 NANBH 病例都是由 HCV 引起的。1990 年开始对献血者进行抗 HCV 抗体的统一筛查。NAT 现在被用来提高检测感染的敏感性[81]。与艾滋病毒(下文讨论)一样，美国所有的献血者都要经过 HCV 筛查。通过将血清前转化窗口期从大约 75 日缩短到少于 30 日，使用 NAT 使每单位 HCV 的风险降低到了大约 1/2 000 000 [76]。

巨细胞病毒

从 CMV 血清阳性供者向 CMV 血清阴性移植受者和新生儿输注细胞血液成分可引起 CMV 血清转化和感染。尽管同等数量的自体和异体 BMT 受者要么血清转化为 CMV,要么分泌 CMV,但自体 BMT 受者很少出现临床后遗症。传统的 CMV 血清阴性血液制品是从 CMV 血清阴性献血者中提取的红细胞和血小板。LRBC 和血小板已被证明可减少婴儿、急性白血病患者以及自体和异体 BMT 受者的输血获得性巨细胞病毒感染[82~85]。一项多中心随机试验比较了接受自体 BMT 的 CMV-血清阴性患者和接受 CMV 血清阴性献血者同种异体移植的血清阴性患者中的血清阴性和过滤细胞血液成分[82]。CMV 血清转化率和感染率在血清阴性和输注过滤成分的患者中是相同的,但只有接受过滤的和未筛选成分的患者才会出现明显的临床后遗症。这些结果表明,过滤处理能显著降低 CMV 传播,过滤成分现在被认为是"CMV 安全"的;不过,断定过滤处理和血清学阴性血制品是相同的结论可能还为时过早。

西尼罗病毒

西尼罗病毒(West Nile virus,WNV)是一种蚊媒黄病毒,可经输血传播。绝大多数的 WNV 感染是由蚊虫叮咬引起的。大约 80%感染 WNV 的人无症状。20%有症状的患者中,绝大多数表现轻微(WNV 发热)。低于 1%的感染者发展为严重脑膜脑炎,高龄是最强的危险因素[86]。1999 年 WNV 首次在美国出现。在 2002 年报道了超过 4 000 例有明显临床症状的 WNV 感染病例,其中 23 例确定和输血相关。2003 年,按照 FDA 试验性新药(investigational new drug,IND)方案,在全国范围内开展血液制品的 NAT。这项检测已经排除了大多数输血传播 WNV 的风险。

败血症

在 4℃储存的 WB 中细菌很少存活。与此相反,血小板储存在室温的搅拌器上是细菌污染的潜在来源,可能导致输血相关的败血症[87]。AABB 现在要求美国的血液采集设备既要检测又要限制血小板的细菌污染[76]。目前正在使用各种筛选技术来处理血小板内的细菌污染,例如自动培养系统[88,89]。

人类免疫缺陷病毒(HIV)

自 1985 年以来,美国所有的献血者均使用 ELISA 法筛选抗 HIV 抗体。经输血传播艾滋病毒现在是非常罕见的;少数发生的病例几乎完全是由于血清阴性窗口期献血所致。在最初实施 HIV 抗体筛查之后,HIV-1 和 HIV-2 ELISA 敏感性的改善将血清阴性窗口期限制在大约 22 日左右[90]。在美国,所有捐赠的单位都要经过微量混合 NAT 检测。NAT[输血介导的扩增(TMA)或聚合酶链反应(PCR)]测试是在 16~24 个样品池中进行;这项技术从暴露时间起将窗口期缩短到大约 10 或 11 日。据估计,目前剩余的每单位 HIV 传播的风险低于 1/2 000 000[76]。

人类 T 细胞淋巴病毒 1 型

人类 T 细胞淋巴病毒 1 型(human T-cell lymphotrophic virus type,HTLV-1)与成人 T 细胞白血病/淋巴瘤(ATL)和热带痉挛性轻截瘫(tropical spastic paresis,TSP)/HTLV-1 相关的脊髓病(HAM)相关,存在流行地区地理集群分布,如日本部分地区和加勒比地区。在美国,ATL 的发病率同加勒比地区类似,因为在美国的病例都发生在非裔美国人或在美国以外地区出生的患者中[91]。

1988 年,开始对所有献血者在每次献血前进行 HTLV-1 检测,一旦确认血清学阳性,将永久延迟献血。美国的研究证明 HTLV-1 是通过输血传播的,并证明了筛查的有效性。每单位的输血风险在 1/250 000~1/2 000 000 之间[76]。

寄生虫病

由于没有对疟疾进行实际的实验室筛查试验,排除旅游到过疫区或从流行地区移民来的捐献者是防止输血相关的感染唯一有效的措施。其他寄生虫病,如巴贝虫病或莱姆病,可通过被蜱咬伤的无症状捐献者传染,这对免疫功能低下或无脾脏患者可能特别重要。输血传播的巴贝虫病是一种区域性疾病。目前,美国有 7 个流行登革热的州:马萨诸塞州、康涅狄格州、罗德岛州、纽约州、新泽西州、威斯康星州和明尼苏达州[92]。虽然通过输血传播梅毒是可能的,但它要求在相当短的螺旋体病期间抽取血液,而且在输血时螺旋体保持活性才能传播。尽管对梅毒进行血清学检测并不能预防梅毒的传播,因为这种检测直到短暂的感染期之后才会呈阳性,但美国联邦法规确实要求将其用作潜在捐赠者的筛查检测。

另一个公认的输血相关感染是南美锥虫病[93]。在大多数情况下会自发好转,患者进入终身携带的、低级别寄生虫血症,具有抗寄生虫抗原抗体,不表现症状。在不确定的 10%~30%的患者出现症状。然而,在免疫功能低下的患者,这种疾病可能会出现更暴发性的病程。寄生虫的血液涂片可用来诊断急性感染,慢性感染则可以通过检测血清抗体诊断。

克-雅病

有家族痴呆症病史、曾接受过角膜或脑外科手术的血液制品的潜在捐献者被拒绝献血[94~97]。由于在 1996 年确诊一个变异型克-雅病(variant Creutzfeldt-Jakob disease,vCJD),这可能与牛海绵状脑病(bovine spongiform encephalopathy,BSE)或"疯牛病"相关,1980—1996 年在英国居住 3 个月的潜在捐献者是被拒绝献血的。从 1980 年起在欧洲居住累计 5 年的捐献者也被拒绝献血。这些旅行限制,以减少美国 5%献血者为代价估计可以消除每日 90%的人接触到 vCJD 的病原体。英国已报道少数的人类输血传播的 vCJD 病例。基于发现 B 淋巴细胞是 vCJD 传播载体的这一事实,许多国家正在建议普遍使用去白细胞成分输血。

移植后血液成分支持

BMT 后,有一段全血细胞减少的时期,患者需要多次 RBC 和血小板输注。在捐献者-接受者 ABO 不相容的情况下(大约 1/3 的同种异体移植),必须特别注意血液制备。在这种情况下,要选择捐献者和接受者 ABO 相容的血液制品。

骨髓捐献者和接受者之间 ABO 血型不相容可能是主要的，接受者中有抗捐献者 RBC 抗原的血凝素，也可能是次要的，捐献者中有抗接受者红细胞抗原的血凝素。主要 ABO 血型不相容有严重溶血反应、移植排斥反应或移植延迟的潜在风险[98~100]。试图克服 ABO 血型不相容的方法包括在 BMT 前从骨髓移植中去除红细胞和/或通过大容量血浆交换或免疫吸附从接受者中去除血凝素，但这些并不是常规操作[101,102]。尽管研究表明，与 ABO 血型匹配的移植相比，ABO 血型不相容 HLA-匹配的移植并不增加患者的死亡率，排异发生率，重建延迟或 GVHD，但一些报告表明，在这种情况下，红细胞重建可以延迟[98,103]。在主要 ABO 血型不相容的非骨髓性干细胞移植中，红细胞的移植可能会特别延迟，因为宿主抗供者血凝素水平的下降往往比骨髓性 BMT 慢[104]。

骨髓捐献者与接受者 ABO 血型不相容的潜在不良后果包括：输注捐赠骨髓时由于被动输注了骨髓血浆中的同种血凝素造成的快速免疫溶血或由捐献者淋巴细胞生产的抗红细胞抗体引起的延迟性免疫性溶血[105]。次要 ABO 血型不相容不会影响到移植物的排异、GVHD 的发生率和严重程度或患者的生存。虽然 BMT 前用移植捐献者的红细胞交叉输血被用来防止被动输注的骨髓同种血凝素造成的溶血，但这是很少有临床意义的问题，并且可以通过在移植前从骨髓去除血浆更容易地避免。由于捐献者骨髓淋巴细胞在移植后早期（1~3 周）产生抗 A 和/或抗 B 抗体，特别是在接受环孢素治疗的患者或接受 T 细胞减少的同种异体移植的患者中，轻微的 ABO 血型不相容可导致不良反应[106,107]。在这种情况下，使用 O 组或捐献者组的红细胞的输血来稀释接受者红细胞；在某些情况下，由于捐献者淋巴细胞的快速移植和抗 RBC 抗体的产生，需要进行换血处理。

结论

如果没有血液成分支持的同步发展，迄今为止癌症新疗法的发展和实施是不可能实现的。在未来，血液成分实验室将提供专门的细胞成分，以促进目前无法治愈的患者使用新的、有前景的移植和细胞疗法。

（程颖　柳菁菁 译　程颖 校）

参考文献

The complete reference list can be found on the Wiley Companion Digital Edition of this title (see inside front cover for login instructions).

10 Hebert PC, Wells G, Blajchman MA, et al. A multicenter randomized, controlled clinical trial of transfusion requirements in critical care. Transfusion Requirements in Critical Care Investigators, Canadian Critical Care Trials Group. *N Engl J Med*. 1999;**340**:409–417.

11 Carson JL, Terrin ML, Noveck H, et al. Liberal or restrictive transfusion in high-risk patients after hip surgery. *N Engl J Med*. 2011;**365**:2453–2462.

14 Murphy GJ, Pike K, Rogers CA, et al. Liberal or restrictive transfusion after cardiac surgery. *N Engl J Med*. 2015;**372**:997–1008.

15 Holst LB, Haase N, Wetterslev J, et al. Lower versus higher hemoglobin threshold for transfusion in septic shock. *N Engl J Med*. 2014;**371**:1381–1391.

16 Villanueva C, Colomo A, Bosch A, et al. Transfusion strategies for acute upper gastrointestinal bleeding. *N Engl J Med*. 2013;**368**:11–21.

21 Fergusson DA, Hebert P, Hogan DL, et al. Effect of fresh red blood cell transfusions on clinical outcomes in premature, very low-birth-weight infants: the ARIPI randomized trial. *JAMA*. 2012;**308**:1443–1451.

22 Steiner ME, Ness PM, Assmann SF, et al. Effects of red-cell storage duration on patients undergoing cardiac surgery. *N Engl J Med*. 2015;**372**:1419–1429.

23 Lacroix J, Hebert PC, Fergusson DA, et al. Age of transfused blood in critically ill adults. *N Engl J Med*. 2015;**372**:1410–1418.

35 Gaydos LA, Freireich EJ, Mantel N, et al. The quantitative relation between platelet count and hemorrhage in patients with acute leukemia. *N Engl J Med*. 1962;**266**:905–909.

36 Wandt H, Schaefer-Eckart K, Wendelin K, et al. Therapeutic platelet transfusion versus routine prophylactic transfusion in patients with haematological malignancies: an open-label, multicentre, randomised study. *Lancet*. 2012;**380(9850)**:1309–1316. doi:10.1016/S0140-6736(12)60689-8. Epub 2012 Aug 8. PMID: 22877506.

39 Kaufman RM, Djulbegovic B, Gernsheimer T, et al. Platelet transfusion: a clinical practice guideline from the AABB. *Ann Intern Med*. 2015;**162**:205–213.

40 Gmur J, Burger J, Schanz U, et al. A safety of stringent prophylactic platelet transfusion policy for patients with acute leukemia. *Lancet*. 1991;**338**:1223–1226.

41 Rebulla P, Finazzi G, Marangoni F, et al. The threshold for prophylactic platelet transfusions in adults with acute myeloid leukemia. *N Engl J Med*. 1997;**337**:1870–1875.

42 Wandt H, Frank M, Ehninger G, et al. Safety and cost effectiveness of a 10×10^9/L trigger for prophylactic platelet transfusions compared with the traditional 20×10^9/L trigger. A prospective comparative trial in 105 patients with acute myeloid leukemia. *Blood*. 1998;**91**:3601–3606.

48 Slichter SJ, Kaufman RM, Assmann SF, et al. Dose of prophylactic platelet transfusions and prevention of hemorrhage. *N Engl J Med*. 2010;**362(7)**:600–613.

51 O'Connell B, Lee EJ, Schiffer CA. The value of 10-minute posttransfusion platelet count. *Transfusion*. 1988;**28**:66–67.

54 Yankee RA, Graff KS, Dowling R, Henderson ES. Selection of unrelated compatible platelet donors by lymphocyte HLA matching. *N Engl J Med*. 1973;**288**:760–764.

56 Slichter SJ. Leukocyte reduction and ultraviolet B irradiation of platelets to prevent alloimmunization and refractoriness to platelet transfusions. *N Engl J Med*. 1997;**337**:1861–1869.

58 Julmy F, Ammann RA, Mansouri T, et al. Transfusion efficacy of ABO major-mismatched platelets (PLTs) in children is inferior to that of ABO-identical PLTs. *Transfusion*. 2009;**49**:21–33.

76 Stramer SL. Current risks of transfusion-transmitted agents: a review. *Arch Pathol Lab Med*. 2007;**131**:702–707.

81 Stramer SL, Caglioti S, Strong DM. NAT of the United States and Canadian blood supply. *Transfusion*. 2000;**40**:1165–1168.

82 Bowden RA, Slichter SJ, Sayers M, et al. A comparison of filtered leukocyte-reduced and cytomegalovirus (CMV) seronegative blood products for the prevention of transfusion-associated CMV infection after marrow transplant. *Blood*. 1995;**86**:3598–3603.

89 Kaufman RM. Platelets: testing, dosing and the storage lesion. *Hematology Am Soc Hematol Educ Program*. 2006:492–496.

第 130 章　肿瘤患者的凝血障碍并发症

Maria T. De Sancho, MD, MSc ■ Jacob H. Rand, MD

概述

出血和血栓性疾病在肿瘤患者中十分常见。出血性疾病通常由血小板异常或凝血因子缺乏引起，需要相应的血液或凝血因子替代治疗。血栓栓塞事件包括深静脉栓塞和肺栓塞，此类疾病常见并且伴有严重的并发症。新的生物标志物、诊断性成像方法和抗凝治疗显著改善了这些患者的预后。随着对各种止血障碍的了解、新的治疗手段的应用及在肿瘤患者中应用适当的血栓预防策略，将进一步降低这类疾病的发病率和提高患者的生存期。

出血及血栓性疾病仍然是导致肿瘤患者致残或致死的重要原因。随着肿瘤治疗的进步，这些疾病的发生近年来明显增加。白血病患者通常容易发生出血，尤其是急性早幼粒细胞白血病（acute promyelocytic leukemia，APL）患者，然而，由于靶向治疗的改进，在临床试验研究中早期失血性死亡已下降到5%～10%，但在近期基于人群的登记信息中，这一结果在临床实践中未能重现[1]。总体来说，出血性疾病在实体瘤患者中相对少见，除了黑色素瘤、生殖细胞瘤、大肠癌和前列腺癌[2]，而肾、膀胱、子宫内膜和子宫颈的癌症可能以出血为首发症状。特别是以吉西他滨和贝伐单抗为基础的治疗，与增加实体瘤患者发生高级别出血的风险相关[3,4]。肿瘤介导的高凝状态是癌细胞直接激活促凝通路的结果。在新近诊断的静脉血栓事件（venous thrombosis event）中，肿瘤患者约占20%，在尸检研究中占高达50%[5]。本章回顾了正常止血的生理过程，并探讨了凝血系统与肿瘤的关系，以及肿瘤患者出血和血栓形成的病理生理学机制。然后介绍了肿瘤患者常见的出血及血栓性疾病的诊断和治疗方法。最后，还介绍了新一代口服直接抗凝药物（direct oralanti coagulants，DOAC），如抗Ⅹa因子和抗Ⅱa因子的抑制剂。

正常止血的生理学

阻止因血管损伤而引起的出血的生理机制，依赖于细胞成分和可溶性血浆蛋白参与的止血过程。血液循环中的血小板在血管损伤处黏附和聚集。血小板的黏附依赖于血管性假性血友病因子（von Willebrand factor，vWF）及随即发生的聚集反应。血小板的激活导致了胞质膜内外极性的翻转，进而暴露了带负电荷的磷脂类物质，并成为凝血酶原复合物聚集的平台。当血液暴露于组织因子（tissue factor，TF）时，外源性凝血通路就被激活了，组织因子是一种跨膜蛋白，在血管壁的深部表达，也可能存在于被激活的内皮细胞中。血栓的形成始于血液内生成并激活的TF进入形成中的血凝块[6]。TF与被激活的Ⅶ因子（Ⅶa因子）结合，随后这一复合物激活了Ⅹ因子和Ⅸ因子。被激活的Ⅸ因子（Ⅸa因子）与Ⅷa因子结合，这成为了激活Ⅹ因子的另一途径。Ⅹa因子复合物与Ⅴa因子及凝血酶原形成凝血活酶，后者是止血过程中的关键酶，可将凝血酶原裂解为凝血酶。在凝血级联反应的终末步骤，凝血酶剪切纤维蛋白原，形成纤维蛋白单体，继而形成纤维蛋白多聚体。纤维蛋白多聚体与ⅩⅢa因子（凝血酶剪切ⅩⅢ因子而形成）共价交联，形成在化学上稳定的凝血块。凝血酶还可反馈性激活辅因子Ⅴ、Ⅷ及Ⅺ，从而放大了凝血级联反应[7]。

纤维蛋白的降解受到内源性抗凝系统限制。抗凝血酶是一种血浆蛋白，属于丝氨酸蛋白酶抑制剂家族的一员，可以抑制所有被激活的凝血因子的活性，特别是Ⅱa和Ⅹa因子。C蛋白是一种维生素K依赖性蛋白，可以蛋白水解Ⅴa及Ⅷa因子，使之形成无活性片段。C蛋白与内皮细胞C蛋白受体（endothelial cell protein receptor，EPCR）结合[8]，并可被结合于血栓调节蛋白的凝血酶激活，血栓调节蛋白是另一种内皮细胞膜蛋白，该反应可被辅因子S蛋白所调节。TF通路抑制物是一种血浆蛋白，可以和TF，Ⅶa因子，Ⅹa因子形成四合物，从而抑制外源性凝血通路。

越来越多引起人们关注的证据表明，除了止血作用外，Ⅺ因子在静脉血栓形成中也发挥作用。最近的一项临床试验支持这一观点，该试验把Ⅺ因子反义寡核苷酸应用在因膝关节置换手术而DVT风险增加的患者中，该策略显著降低了静脉血栓形成。这种抗凝策略有可能为肿瘤患者带来重要的临床获益，而且似乎不需要将Ⅺ因子水平降低到20%的稳态水平以下，即可获得预防效果。因此，这种策略可能在不显著增加出血风险的情况下降低血栓形成率[9]。然而，这种可能性需要在设计良好的临床试验中验证。

纤维蛋白溶解过程包括一系列导致纤维蛋白降解和血栓溶解的丝氨酸蛋白酶级联反应。这一过程的终末步骤是将循环中的纤溶酶原转化为其活性形式的纤溶酶。在循环中，这主要是通过阿替普酶（tissue-type plasminogen activator，t-PA）实现的。这种催化作用高度依赖于纤维蛋白的存在，因为不论是纤溶酶原还是t-PA，在与纤维蛋白结合后可使纤溶酶的产生增加两个数量级以上。在结构上，纤溶酶原与纤维蛋白暴露的赖氨酸残基结合，这些结合位点在纤维蛋白分解过程中数量增加，从而使更多纤溶酶原发生结合，该过程不断放大，产生更多的纤溶酶。天然存在于血浆中的纤溶酶抑制剂（α_2-抗纤溶酶，纤溶酶原激活物抑制物（plasminogen activator inhibitor，PAI）-1和PAI-2）也能限制循环中纤溶酶的活性和生成。其中最有效的是α_2-抗纤溶酶，纤溶酶与纤维蛋白结合后在很大程度阻止了纤溶酶与α_2-抗纤溶酶的结合，进而使纤维蛋白发生裂解。其他关键的调控步骤发生在t-PA的水平，因为t-PA和尿激酶型纤溶酶原激活物（urokinase-type plasminogen activator，u-PA）的活性，都是受到 PAI-1 和 PAI-2 调控的，u-PA 是又一重要的内源性纤溶酶原激活物。

最近发现的限制纤溶系统的机制是通过"凝血酶激活的纤溶抑制剂"。该蛋白称为凝血酶激活的纤溶抑制剂（thrombin activa 表 fibrinolysis inhibitor，TAFI）是一种羧肽酶，可特异性地清除纤维蛋白中暴露的赖氨酸残基，从而去除纤溶酶原和 t-PA 与纤维蛋白赖氨酸结合位点结合的能力。TAFI 需要凝血酶的激活，因此凝血会直接导致 TAFI 参与稳定和保护血凝块不被纤溶系统过早清除[10]。

凝血系统、炎症和肿瘤的关系

凝血与肿瘤的关系最早见于 19 世纪下半叶的医学文献，Trousseau 报告了游走性血栓性静脉炎与胃癌的关系[11]。1878 年，Billroth 证实了血栓中含有肿瘤细胞，并提出肿瘤细胞是通过血栓栓塞扩散的[12]。凝血与肿瘤血管形成及生长之间的相互关系涉及多种凝血因子，尤其是 TF 和凝血酶在肿瘤新生血管形成、生长和扩散中发挥着作用。在此期间，肿瘤细胞或宿主细胞引起了局部或全身性的炎性刺激，使血管内皮成为易形成血栓的表面[13]。血管内皮的损伤使内皮下 vWF 因子和 TF 暴露。vWF 可引起血小板和肿瘤细胞黏附，继而导致血小板的激活和聚集。TF 在凝血级联反应中发挥着关键作用。TF 在激活的血管内皮细胞、单核细胞及肿瘤细胞表面的表达异常增加[14]。有证据显示 TF 在肿瘤等病理状态下的内皮中表达上调，例如发现 TF 及交联纤维蛋白在人类肿瘤内的新生血管内皮中表达增加[15]。

微粒

细胞来源的囊泡，特别是细胞外囊泡（extracellular vesicles，EV），如微粒（microparticles，MP）和微泡，也包括外泌体，作为一种新颖独特的疾病检测方法，正受到越来越多的关注[16]。MP 通常定义为大小 0.1～1μm 的膜粒子，它们暴露出带负电荷的磷脂磷脂酰丝氨酸以及代表细胞起源的膜抗原。血小板衍生微粒（platelet-derived microparticles，PMP）有最丰富的 MP 亚型。它们的存在反映了血小板活性、生理病理状态和肿瘤患者的血栓状态。由于血小板在肿瘤进展和转移中起到关键作用，PMP 也可能在肿瘤细胞增殖、肿瘤细胞间的相互作用、转移和进展、血管生成和炎症中发挥重要作用[17]。

虽然这是一个很有研究价值和诊断潜力的方法，但还没有在临床常规应用中充分标准化的 MP 分析方法。最近，一个共识研讨会的发起者们得出结论，即使应用共同的检测方案，实验室之间也存在显著的变异性[18]。

出血性疾病

肿瘤可引起血小板数量及质量的变化[19]。近 60%的肿瘤患者可发生反应性血小板增多，而近 11%未经治疗的恶性肿瘤患者可以发生血小板减少（表 130-1）。

表 130-1　肿瘤患者的止血异常

异常	机制
血小板	
血小板减少	肿瘤骨髓浸润
	化疗反应
	生物效应修饰剂
	单克隆抗体和免疫毒素
	蛋白酶体抑制剂（硼替佐米）
	弥散性血管内凝血
	脾功能亢进
	免疫介导（自身免疫，同种免疫）
	血栓性微血管病（TMA）
血小板增多	产生增多
	反应性
	原发性
	骨髓增殖性疾病
血小板功能异常	尿毒症
	获得性 von Willebrand 综合征
	骨髓增殖性疾病
凝血因子和临床可获得的凝血活化标记物异常	
低纤维蛋白原血症	门冬酰胺酶，DIC
异常纤维蛋白原血症	肝细胞癌
X因子（减少）	淀粉样变性
凝血因子减少	肝合成受损，DIC，维生素 K 缺乏
D-二聚体和纤维蛋白降解产物增多	炎症，血栓，纤维蛋白降解，DIC，肾功能不全，肝衰竭
凝血酶原片段 1+2 升高	肿瘤播散，DIC
纤溶	
纤溶酶原激活物分泌增加	急性早幼粒细胞白血病（APL）
链接素Ⅱ过表达	APL
纤溶酶原激活物的抑制物水平降低	增加的纤维蛋白（原）降解产物和 D-二聚体增加
获得性血栓形成倾向	
抗凝血酶缺乏	肝脏合成抗凝血蛋白受损，DIC，L-门冬酰胺酶，普通肝素，低分子量肝素
蛋白 C 缺乏	肝脏合成受损，DIC，维生素 K 拮抗剂（VKA）
蛋白 S 缺乏	肝脏合成受损，DIC，VKA
组织因子通路抑制剂缺乏（TFPI）	肝脏合成受损，DIC
细胞因子与止血	
促炎症细胞因子（IL-1，IL-6，TNF）	单核细胞和内皮细胞组织因子表达的关键作用

微粒的增多与肿瘤环境下血栓形成相关；然而，这些检验尚没有充分标准化而可供应用。

DIC，弥散性血管内凝血；TMA，血栓性微血管病；IL，白介素；TNF，肿瘤坏死因子最主要的出血常由于肿瘤侵犯血管及邻近器官，或治疗引起的并发症，以及维生素K缺乏导致。肿瘤患者的出血，可以表现为肿瘤侵犯引起的局部出血，或者由于血小板缺乏、血小板病、特异的凝血因子缺乏、弥散性血管内凝血(diffuse intravascular coagulation，DIC)或纤溶亢进(DIC)引起的全身性出血倾向[19]。对肿瘤患者出血的适当处理取决于能否解决引起出血的潜在疾病。

血小板减少症

血小板减少是肿瘤患者最常见的止血异常疾病，发生于约10%的患者，甚至在化疗之前也可发生。发生快速血小板减少的患者，往往是由于化疗和/或放疗后继发的血小板生成减少或者由于骨髓浸润、脾脏内血小板聚集或者外周性血小板破坏增多，比如脓毒血症、DIC和血栓性微血管病(thrombotic microangiopathy，TMA)[20](表130-2)。硼替佐米(bortezomib)是一种蛋白酶体抑制剂，用于初治或复发的多发性骨髓瘤的治疗，可引起短暂性、周期性和可逆性的血小板减少[20]。由骨髓浸润引起的血小板常见于小细胞肺癌、乳腺癌和前列腺癌患者，以及急性白血病患者。此外，继发于脾脏破坏的血小板减少常见于骨髓增殖性疾病(myeloproliferative disorders，MPD)，但在淋巴瘤及慢性淋巴细胞白血病中相对不常见。当血小板减少是由巨核细胞减少而不是由免疫破坏引起时，临床上更容易发生明显的出血。

表130-2 肿瘤患者血小板减少症的鉴别诊断

血小板生成减少
肿瘤骨转移
急性及慢性白血病
淋巴瘤
浆细胞疾病
药物，包括细胞毒性化疗药物和靶向药物
放射治疗
血小板破坏
药物
免疫介导
细菌性败血症
病毒，真菌及原虫感染
DIC
肝素诱导的血小板减少
血栓性微血管病(TMA)
脾脏内破坏
骨髓增生性疾病
淋巴瘤
慢性淋巴细胞白血病
上述因素的综合作用

DIC，弥散性血管内凝血。

肝功能不全可能是血小板减少的病因之一，因为促血小板生成素合成减少。

血小板减少引起的出血，临床上表现为皮肤、黏膜出血。可以表现为瘀点、瘀斑、鼻出血、口腔、胃肠道及泌尿道出血。一般自发性出血极少发生，除非血小板计数小于5 000~10 000/mm^3。但是，在脓毒血症、尿毒症、外伤或手术等情况下，血小板计数较高时也可发生出血并发症，包括中枢神经系统出血。

确定血小板减少的诊断时必须回顾临床病史、体格检查、药物史以及既往化疗、免疫治疗或放射治疗的时间安排。此外，检查外周血涂片在血小板减少症的诊断工作中也是至关重要的。必须排除外周血涂片上的血小板聚集或血小板卫星现象(血小板在多形核白细胞周围)所表现的假性血小板减少症。

治疗血小板减少相关性出血通常是经验性的，也包括无法明确原因的血小板减少。表130-3列出在不同条件下的临界血小板计数，以及血小板输注的一般性指南。对于无出血症状的患者，不推荐预防性输注血小板，除非血小板计数低于5 000/mm^3。但是，对于接受化疗以及白血病患者，当血小板计数低于10 000/mm^{3}时，预防性血小板输注可减少出血的风险[21,22]。对于接受大手术或侵入性操作的肿瘤患者，如中心静脉置管，支气管或内镜下活检，腰穿，胸腔穿刺术，胸廓造口导管置入，腹腔穿刺术，一般推荐输注血小板至血小板计数达到50 000/mm^{3}以上。对于小型的侵入性操作，如动脉穿刺或套管插入术，如果血小板计数不低于20 000/mm^3，则无须预防性输注血小板，只需在穿刺部位加压即可达到止血的效果[23]。当发生镜下或可见出血，如大便隐血阳性或皮肤黏膜出血时，往往需输注血小板使血小板计数维持于50 000/mm^{3}以上。一般来说，发生中枢神经系统出血的风险较小，而且出血依赖于以下几个因素，如同时的抗凝治疗，血小板减少的病因，凝血异常，肾或肝功能受损，严重脓毒症、外伤和机械通气的使用。接受造血干细胞移植的白血病患者[25,26]发生硬膜下和颅内血肿的概率分别为2.5%~5%[24]和2%。比较性研究发现，来源于单个或多个供者的血小板，输注后的效益相似，止血作用及不良反应也均相似。

表130-3 肿瘤患者推荐血小板输注时的临界血小板计数[a]

血小板计数临界值	
皮肤黏膜或消化道出血	>50 000
白血病	
诱导前化疗	>20 000
急性早幼粒细胞白血病	>5 000~10 000
预防性	
无症状	>5 000
大手术	>50 000
创伤性操作	
大型	>50 000
小型	>20 000

[a] 这些数值只是作为常规指南，实际治疗依赖于特殊情况而变化

血小板性疾病

肿瘤除了可引起血小板量的变化，还可以引起血小板质的异常。主要的异常从以下几个方面介绍。

获得性 von Willebrand 综合征

据文献报告，有几种类型的肿瘤与获得性 von Willebrand 综合征（acquired von Willebrand syndrome，aVWS）相关。在淋巴结增殖性疾病中，意义未明的单克隆丙种球蛋白血症（monoclonal gammopathy of undetermined significance，MGUS）是最常见的与 aVWS 相关的疾病，此外，aVWS 还与多种疾病相关，如多发性骨髓瘤，华氏巨球蛋白血症，慢性淋巴细胞白血病，毛细胞白血病和非霍奇金淋巴瘤。在这些骨髓增殖性疾病中，真性血小板增多症（essential thrombocythemia，ET）是最常见的，而真性红细胞增多症（polycythemia vera，PV）和慢性髓细胞性白血病相对少见。实体瘤中包括肾母细胞瘤（Wilms tumor）和腺瘤也常与 aVWS 相关[27]。

aVWS 的临床表现和遗传性 VWS 的患者相似，只是 aVWS 患者不存在明显的家族史或伴随终身的出血史。aVWS 可表现为自发性皮肤黏膜出血及胃肠道出血，也可表现为术后出血。实验室检查通常可表现为活化部分凝血酶时间（activated partial thromboplastin time，aPTT）延长，出血时间正常或接近延长的临界值，或采用 PFA-100 体外检测暴露时间延长。治疗包括针对潜在恶性肿瘤的治疗及支持治疗，如皮质激素，脱氨基-8-精氨酸升压素（deamino-8-D-arginie vasopressin，DDAVP）（醋酸去氨加压素），Ⅷ/vWF 因子浓缩物，以及输注免疫球蛋白[27,28]。

获得性血友病（Ⅷ因子自身抗体）

实体瘤、浆细胞疾病及淋巴增殖性疾病的患者可以发生获得性血友病，因为这类患者产生针对Ⅷ因子的抗体，被称为“获得性抑制物”。这些抑制物几乎都是 IgG 型免疫球蛋白。最常见的症状是无出血体质的患者出现皮肤和肌肉出血。最典型的实验室表现是血浆凝血酶原时间（prothrombin time，PT）正常情况下 aPTT 延长，血浆混合实验可发现 aPTT 在 37℃温育 1~2h 后仍然延长；与之相反，凝血因子缺乏的患者，血浆混合实验 aPTT 正常。肝素污染血样，往往是由于维持静脉输液管道通畅时滴注肝素造成的结果，这将人为延长 aPTT 并影响血浆混合实验。已混入血样的肝素可以用肝素酶或树脂吸附去除，然后重新进行检测。处理急性出血时，如果抑制物的滴度较低［<5BU（Bethesda units，BU）］，可用醋酸去氨加压素、人或猪型的Ⅷ因子治疗。当抑制物滴度呈中-高度时（>5BU），可用Ⅷ因子替代物，如重组人Ⅶa 因子，或者活化的凝血酶原复合物治疗。除了治疗潜在的肿瘤外，可以联合免疫抑制治疗，包括肾上腺皮质激素、长春新碱、环磷酰胺、环孢素和静脉输注免疫球蛋白（intravenous immunoglobulin，IVIg）。利妥昔单抗可用于一线治疗耐药或者不能耐受标准免疫抑制治疗的患者[29]。

尿毒症

血小板功能异常在患有慢性肾功能不全的肿瘤患者中常见，并可引起明显的出血。尿毒症出血的病理生理学是多因素的，包括 vWF 功能异常、循环中的单磷酸腺苷增多、血小板产生的氧化亚氮水平升高、尿毒症毒素的增高及贫血，以上因素导致血小板从血管内皮移走，降低了因内皮损伤而引起的血小板黏附和聚集的能力[25]。对于有活动性出血或接受有创性操作的患者，如血液透析，推荐给予治疗。患者通常对血液透析及静脉给予 0.3mg/kg 的 DDAVP 反应良好；有时也需要输注冷沉淀（静脉滴注 10 袋，30min 以上）和给予结合雌激素（0.6mg/（kg・d），30~40min 输注，连续 5 日）。促红细胞生成药物，如促红细胞生成素和达依泊汀（darbepoietin），对于尿毒症患者有预防及减少出血的作用，其作用效果比 DDAVP 或结合雌激素更持久[30]。

骨髓增殖性疾病

在骨髓增殖性疾病（myeloproliferative disorders，MPD）中，真性红细胞增多（PV）和真性血小板增多（ET）最可能引起出血及血栓性疾病。12%~39%的 ET 和 PV 患者的首要症状表现为血栓形成[28]。高龄（>65 岁）和既往血栓史是血栓形成的主要危险因素[31]。分别有将近 97%的 PV 患者和 50%的 ET 患者发现有 *JAK2*（Janus kinase2）的假激酶域的获得性点突变（*JAK2*（V617F））。

其他潜在的血栓形成因素还包括心血管系统的危险因素。白细胞增多是与 PV 和 ET 患者血栓形成及生存相关的独立危险因素[32,33]。所有的 PV 患者可采用静脉放血治疗并口服低剂量阿司匹林。治疗的推荐目标是 HCT 低于 45%。对于有大血管并发症风险的低危 ET 患者可观察而不予治疗。对于存在微血管症状的患者可给予低剂量的阿司匹林。伴随的心血管危险因素应给予认真纠正。在高危患者中，羟基脲（hydroxyurea，HU）仍然是大部分需要行去细胞治疗的 PV 和 ET 患者的首选药物，这是目前被证实唯一有效的可降低致命血栓栓塞的治疗方法[34,35]。年轻患者或对 HU 耐药或不能耐受的患者可应用 IFN-α 和阿那格雷（anagrelide），孕妇可应用 IFN-α。*JAK2* 抑制剂副反应较少，可考虑用于需要治疗的 PV 和/或 ET 患者[36]。

凝血因子缺乏

肿瘤患者可能会发生因营养不良、腹泻、肝脏疾病、胆道梗阻、口服抗凝药物及抗生素治疗而引起的维生素 K 缺乏，从而引起各种不同的凝血因子异常。与肝硬化患者相似，原发或转移性肝细胞癌的患者可能发生维生素 K 依赖的凝血因子缺乏（Ⅱ、Ⅶ、Ⅸ、Ⅹ因子、蛋白 C 及蛋白 S）。这些患者往往有纤维蛋白原的升高，而肝硬化或急性肝功能衰竭的患者，其纤维蛋白原水平降低。获得性凝血因子抑制物常见于多发性骨髓瘤及其他浆细胞疾病患者。

除了肿瘤本身的治疗以外，肿瘤患者凝血因子缺乏的处理一般是支持性治疗，包括给予维生素 K、新鲜冰冻血浆和冷沉淀。也可选择口服维生素 K 治疗。冷沉淀采用静脉输注，一般采用 1U/5kg 的剂量[37]。

淀粉样变性

止血障碍在淀粉样变性的患者中常见。实验室检测异常包括PT和aPTT的延长。此外,还包括与肝脏淀粉样物质浸润有关凝血酶时间(thrombin time,TT)的延长,以及蛇毒凝血酶时间(reptilase time,RT)延长。PT而非TT可在临床上预测出血倾向[38]。

药物的作用(门冬酰胺酶)

门冬酰胺酶与其他药物联用,可以用于急性淋巴细胞白血病的诱导治疗。门冬酰胺酶可引起许多凝血因子的消耗,进而引起血栓形成及出血风险。治疗期间,如果排除DIC,t-PA和PAI增加的同时,交联的纤维蛋白降解的产物可在正常范围内[39]。

急性早幼粒细胞白血病

急性早幼粒细胞白血病(acute promyelocytic leukemia,APL)相关的凝血功能障碍至少是因为两种完全不同的机制,包括白血病细胞释放促凝活性物质及纤溶酶原激活。T15-17易位可引起TF过度表达并导致患者处于高凝状态。纤溶酶依赖的原发性纤溶亢进似乎是APL患者低纤维蛋白原水平的主要原因。维A酸的体内诱导分化治疗,可引起纤溶酶活性的快速下降,以及纤维蛋白原水平的正常化,这与*TF*基因在骨髓细胞中的表达显著下降相关[40]。肝素目前已经不再应用于包含ATRA的APL治疗策略中。肝素曾被认为能通过抑制血管内纤维蛋白聚集和减少凝血因子和血小板的消耗,来控制凝血异常,进而减轻出血倾向。

血栓性并发症

肿瘤患者发生血栓栓塞的病因是多方面的。除了常见的容易引起血栓的原因,如运动减少、静脉淤滞、高龄、既往有血栓疾病史,脓毒血症和中心静脉置管以外,肿瘤细胞具有独特的易引发血栓的特性。转化的恶性细胞可以导致血小板异常、凝血级联反应的异常激活、肝脏合成的抗凝及促凝蛋白的下降、纤维蛋白溶解异常、获得性血栓形成倾向及炎症和促血管生成因子的表达(表130-1)。多种生物标志物与肿瘤相关血栓形成有关。化疗前血小板和白细胞计数升高、血红蛋白水平偏低是目前证据等级最高的因素。D-二聚体也可以预测肿瘤相关的VTE。许多肿瘤患者在没有明显血栓形成的情况下,D-二聚体水平已经升高,但对于预测肿瘤相关血栓形成的D-二聚体阈值没有达成共识。TF是止血的生理性诱发因子,在多种肿瘤中广泛表达。TF以MP的形式释放到循环中,在肿瘤患者中可以检测到其水平。然而,目前还没有一致的"标准"TF检测方法。最初的报告显示TF升高与随后的VTE有显著的关联。这些数据大部分来自特定肿瘤患者,尤其是胰腺癌患者。

多种因素可导致肿瘤患者出血和血栓性疾病的风险增加(表130-4)。肿瘤患者血栓形成可能表现为以下几种形式:游走性血栓性静脉炎或Trousseau综合征、静脉血栓栓塞(venous thromboembolism,VTE)、血栓性微血管病(thrombotic microangiopathy,TMA)、动脉栓塞和DIC。

表130-4 肿瘤患者发生出血及血栓并发症的危险因素

导管置入	血栓形成
系统性炎症反应综合征(SIRS)	血栓形成
败血症	血栓形成和出血
既往接受过化疗及放疗	出血为主,也可有血栓形成
选择性雌激素受体调节药物(SERM):他莫昔芬、雷洛昔芬	
同时采用激素替代治疗或口服避孕药	血栓形成
抗血管生成药物(沙利度胺、来那度胺、贝伐单抗[a]、舒尼替尼、索拉非尼)	血栓形成
促红细胞生成药物	血栓形成
肝和/或骨转移性肿瘤	出血为主
维生素K缺乏	出血为主
急性消化道溃疡	出血
近期手术后缝线脱落	出血

[a] 也可导致出血。

游走性血栓性静脉炎(Trousseau综合征)

Trousseau综合征是一种好发于上肢及胸部浅表静脉以复发性和游走性为特点的静脉血栓形成的变异形式[11]。这种综合征强烈提示某种隐匿的恶性肿瘤,尤其是当患者的复发性、游走性静脉血栓出现在某些少见部位,如锁骨下静脉或上肢、腋窝、颈部静脉等。Trousseau综合征与产生黏蛋白的腺癌高度相关[41]。癌症患者的临床特点还包括与微血管病相关的慢性DIC,非细菌性心内膜炎,以及动脉栓塞。另外,游走性血栓性静脉炎的发生还与生长抑素或奥曲肽在恶性类癌综合征中的应用有关。

静脉血栓栓塞

静脉血栓栓塞,包括深静脉血栓(deep vein thrombosis,DVT)和肺栓塞(pulmonary embolism,PE),可发生于4%~20%的肿瘤患者,是导致肿瘤患者死亡的主要原因之一。一些尸检研究表明,肿瘤相关的静脉血栓栓塞的发生率高达50%。初发的特发性VTE患者有并发肿瘤的高风险,尤其是在诊断为血栓栓塞症后的一年内。VTE风险最大的肿瘤患者包括分泌黏蛋白的肿瘤(如胰腺和胃肠道恶性肿瘤)、肺癌、脑瘤、前列腺癌、乳腺癌、卵巢癌以及APL和骨髓增殖性疾病,尤其是PV和ET患者。VTE常常使在大手术后的癌症患者以及接受化疗和/或激素治疗的患者的护理变得复杂[5]。

肿瘤患者血栓进展的风险受到患者的年龄和激素状态的影响。绝经后的进展期乳腺癌患者如果在接受辅助化疗的基础上加用他莫昔芬治疗,其发生血栓形成的风险要高于绝经前的同类患者[42]。在使用过血管生成抑制剂(如沙利度胺,来那度胺和贝伐单抗）的患者中也有发生血栓栓塞事件的报道[15,43]。沙利度胺相关的血栓栓塞事件的致病机制认为是与获得性活化蛋白 C 抵抗程度以及血栓调节蛋白水平下调有关[15,44]。沙利度胺联合化疗造成的内皮损伤以及后续的内皮细胞 PAR-1 表达恢复可能是促使血栓形成的可能因素[45]。肿瘤患者接受促红细胞生成药物治疗贫血也导致血栓并发症风险增加[46]。

在诊断 VTE（不仅包括癌症相关 VTE）方面的主要进展是发展和验证了一个用以预测 VTE 发生概率的标准化临床模型（表 130-5）[47]和血浆 D-二聚体的检测。这两方面进展的结合使得诊断方法更为安全，从而减少了一系列的有创性检查[48]。一项针对肿瘤患者的研究表明 D-二聚体对 PE 具有很高的阴性预测价值和敏感性，如果 D-二聚体为阴性，可以排除 PE 诊断[49]。

表 130-5　肺栓塞的 Wells 标准

变量	得分
既往 DVT 或 PE	1.5
心率≥100/分	1.5
4 周内接受手术或制动	1.5
咯血	1
活动性肿瘤	1
DVT 的临床征象	3
除 PE 外无其他可能的诊断	3

0~1 分：临床可能性低；2~6 分：临床可能性中等；>7 分：PE 临床可能性强（摘自 Wells 等，1997[47]，经 Elsevier 许可转载）。

与其他患者一样，肿瘤患者的 DVT 多数起源于髂静脉系统。DVT 的影像诊断方法包括逆行静脉增强造影、加压超声以及磁共振血管造影。虽然逆行静脉增强造影目前仍然是诊断深静脉血栓的金标准，但它属于有创性操作，需要造影剂，可能引起和导致并发症。血栓被造影剂包绕形成的腔内充盈缺损表现对 DVT 具有诊断意义。加压超声测得的下肢近端静脉的不可压缩率对于深静脉血栓诊断的敏感性为 97%，特异性为 94%[50]。虽然加压超声检测对于诊断近端 DVT 具有高度敏感性，但它对于孤立的远端 DVT 的诊断还不够准确。磁共振血管造影诊断近端 DVT 的敏感性 92%、特异性 95%[51]，可用于诊断盆腔静脉的 DVT，尤其是对于加压超声诊断困难的孤立性髂静脉血栓更有诊断意义。

一些在疑似 DVT 的肿瘤患者中进行的研究显示，满足两种以下情况能够可靠地排除 DVT 并减少创伤性检查：检查前预测概率低，D-二聚体水平正常，以及加压超声显像正常[47]。

非肿瘤的 VTE 患者的标准抗凝治疗包括初始给予皮下或静脉注射治疗剂量的普通肝素（unfractionated heparin，UFH）、皮下注射治疗剂量的低分子量肝素（low-molecular-weight heparin，LMWH）或磺达肝素（fondaparinux，间接Ⅹa 抑制剂），以及后续至少 3 个月的口服华法林治疗，并以国际标准化比值（international normalized ratio，INR）控制在 2.0~3.0 为治疗目标[52]。而对于活动性肿瘤患者，推荐在首次发现 VTE 之后持续给予抗凝治疗[52]。静脉注射肝素以 80U/kg 的初始剂量开始，之后以 18U/kg/h 的剂量静脉维持，保持 aPTT 为 1.5~2.5 倍正常值并据此调整剂量。LMWH 剂量可根据体重调整，每日 1~2 次皮下给药，给药剂量无须实验室监测。华法林治疗于肝素治疗后 24h 内开始。肝素治疗持续至少 5 日，直到 INR 值连续两天维持在治疗范围内。然而，对于大的髂静脉血栓形成或大面积 PE 患者，专家建议将肝素治疗延长到 7~10 日。

回顾性与前瞻性研究均已表明，在明确诊断有血栓形成的肿瘤患者中使用 LMWH 能够带来生存获益[53,54]。与普通肝素相比，LMWH 有以下优点：几乎不需要实验室监测，仅需皮下注射，出血、肝素诱导的血小板减少症（heparin-induced thrombocytopenia，HIT）[55]及骨质疏松症[56]的发生率均较低。目前，有两个临床研究对急性 VTE 的肿瘤患者长期使用 LMWH 替代华法林的治疗做了分析。CANTHANOX 试验在患有 VTE 和/或 PE 的肿瘤人群中，对 3 个月的华法林和依诺肝素（enoxaparin）抗凝治疗的疗效做了比较。虽然依诺肝素组的 VTE 风险相对较低，但两组结果无统计学差异。华法林与高出血风险相关[57]。在 CLOT 试验中，6 个月的 VTE 累积复发风险在口服抗凝血剂组为 17%，而在 LMWH 组为 9%，两者具有统计学差异[58]。总体上，两组之间的出血发生率无显著性差异。目前指南推荐，对于发生 VTE 的肿瘤患者，在初始 3~6 个月给予 LMWH 作为长期治疗[52]。肿瘤合并复发性 VTE 的患者生存期短。对按照体重调整剂量的 LMWH 或者维生素 K 拮抗剂（VKA）耐药的患者，提高 LMWH 的剂量可能是无效的[59]。

全身性溶栓药，如 tPA，存在与溶栓相关的高出血风险，因此其应用应限于大的髂静脉 DVT 或大面积 PE 及血流动力学不稳定的患者[52]。而且，尽管溶栓药物在改变 PE 患者的放射学和血流动力学异常方面已有肯定的疗效，但迄今为止并没有证据表明其能给血栓形成的患者带来生存获益。使用导管内溶栓作为 VTE 初始治疗的适应证仅局限于需要保留肢体的患者。在一般情况下，对于存在脑转移合并 VTE 的肿瘤患者，溶栓治疗由于其可能导致颅内出血的高风险而被列为禁忌[60]。外科进行血栓栓子切除术仅限于溶栓治疗无效或者有禁忌的大面积 PE 患者[52]。对于那些存在抗凝治疗禁忌或者已经使用抗凝治疗的复发性 VTE 肿瘤患者，都建议放置一个可回收的或者永久性的下腔静脉（inferior vena cava，IVC）滤器。然而，下腔静脉滤器也存在一些非预期的副作用，如由滤器相关血栓形成引起的下肢水肿症状[61]。最近的一项研究报告肯定了 IVC 滤器使用的安全性并且认为它能够很有效地预防合并 VTE 的肿瘤患者发生 PE 相关死亡[62]。然而，对于那些既往有 DVT 和出血史或者疾病处于转移性或播散阶段的患者，其置入 IVC 滤器后的生存期是最短的。

肿瘤患者 VTE 治疗的主要关注点在于其出血和 VTE 复发比非肿瘤患者风险高。一项前瞻性队列研究表明，12 个月累积 VTE 复发率在肿瘤患者和非肿瘤患者分别为 20.7%和 6.8%，两组大出血的发生率分别为 12.4%和 4.9%[63]。复发和出血均与肿瘤的严重程度相关，并且主要发生在抗凝治疗的第一个月，但这些都不能用抗凝治疗不足或过度来解释。肿瘤患者 VTE 复发和大出血的风险分别是非肿瘤患者的 2~3 倍和 3~6 倍[58]。

对中心静脉置管的患者不推荐行常规的预防性抗凝治疗[64]。重组 tPA 对于疏通被血栓阻塞的置管是有效的[65]。围术期肿瘤患者,尤其是那些正在接受化疗或者选择性雌激素受体调节剂治疗的乳腺癌患者,以及有 VTE 高风险的癌症患者,如脑肿瘤、结直肠癌、胰腺癌、肺癌、肾癌、卵巢腺癌等,均应采取间歇性充气加压装置或压缩性弹力袜,以及应用 LMWH 来预防性抗血栓治疗。推荐的剂量为达肝素钠(dalteparin)皮下注射 5 000U/d,或依诺肝素皮下注射 40mg/d,或磺达肝素皮下注射 2.5mg,术后 8~12h 开始[64,65]。两个研究报道了在肿瘤患者出院后 3 个星期内持续使用 LMWH 预防治疗,能够将迟发静脉造影 DVT 的发生率降低 60%。最后,对于那些长期卧床或者因急症活动受限或卧床的肿瘤患者,也应接受低剂量 UFH 或 LMWH 的预防性抗血栓治疗。然而,能走动的肿瘤患者不需要行 VTE 的预防性治疗。正在接受化疗或激素治疗的肿瘤患者也不需要行常规的预防性抗血栓治疗[66]。此外,阿司匹林、华法林或 LMWH 等药物也被临床广泛应用在接受沙利度胺或来那度胺联合化疗或大剂量激素治疗的多发性骨髓瘤患者,用于预防性抗血栓治疗[67,68]。

一般预防及治疗

最近的一份 ASCO 临床实践指南描述了对肿瘤患者 VTE 进行预防和治疗的建议,基于文献的系统回顾,建议大多数肿瘤住院患者在住院期间需要血栓预防。门诊肿瘤患者不推荐常规的血栓预防,考虑选择性地用于高风险患者。多发性骨髓瘤患者在接受抗血管生成药物联合化疗和/或地塞米松的治疗时,应使用 LMWH 或低剂量阿司匹林进行血栓预防。接受大型肿瘤手术的患者应从手术前开始接受血栓预防,并持续至少 7~10 日。高危人群应考虑将预防治疗延长至 4 周。LMWH 被推荐用于治疗深静脉血栓和 PE 的初始 5~10 日,以及长期(6 个月)的二级预防。目前不建议恶性肿瘤和 VTE 患者使用新型口服抗凝药物[66]。

抗凝治疗的抗肿瘤作用

实验和间接临床证据都显示抗凝药物尤其是 LMWH 可能具有抗肿瘤效应。有报道认为抗凝剂会干扰肿瘤血管生成和肿瘤细胞增殖潜能,作用于免疫系统会增强肿瘤坏死因子和 NK 细胞介导的干扰素的抗肿瘤活性[69]。抗凝药物还可能干扰各阶段的肿瘤转移级联过程。

肝素诱导的血小板减少症(heparin-induced thrombocytopenia,HIT)

HIT 是一种免疫介导的血小板减少症,发生于 1%~5% 的接受肝素治疗的患者[89]。患者的血小板计数下降通常发生于肝素治疗开始后的 5~10 日,但如果在此之前三个月接受过肝素治疗,那么血小板计数下降可发生于 24h 之内。血小板计数下降偶尔也会仅发生于停止肝素治疗后(称为迟发性 HIT)。HIT 发生的频率随着肝素种类(牛肝素>猪肝素>低分子肝素)、暴露人群(术后患者>内科患者>孕妇)、性别(女性>男性)的不同而有所变化[70]。HIT 的发生由能识别与肝素结合的血小板因子(platelet factor 4,PF4)的肝素依赖性血小板活化抗体所介导。由此产生的血小板活化与凝血酶生成增加有关。这种现象在静脉或动脉血栓形成包括 DVT、PE、肢体动脉血栓形成、血栓性脑卒中、心肌梗死中都会发生。一个临床预测概率的评分系统 4T(血小板减少的程度、血小板减少的时间、其他血小板减少的相关病因、血栓形成)在临床实践中非常有用。如果评分为中度或者高度概率者应考虑 HIT 的诊断,并且立即开始相关治疗[71]。在临床实践中,HIT 的实验室诊断主要通过阳性的 PF4 依赖性免疫检测来完成。治疗包括停止使用所有形式的肝素,应用与 HIT 抗体无交叉反应的直接凝血酶抑制剂,如来匹卢定(lepirudin)或阿加曲班(argatroban)。对于正在应用华法林的 HIT 患者,推荐使用维生素 K 来逆转华法林的抗凝作用。

血栓性微血管病

血栓性微血管病(thrombotic microangiopathy,TMA)包括溶血性贫血、血小板减少症、神经症状、肾功能不全和发热。其中大多数病例报告为腺癌患者,尤其是胃癌;然而,TMA 也发生在乳腺癌和肺癌患者,以及霍奇金淋巴瘤和非霍奇金淋巴瘤患者中[72]。血栓性血小板减少性紫癜/溶血性尿毒症综合征的发生也与肿瘤化疗,特别是丝裂霉素 C、博来霉素、顺铂,以及他莫昔芬[73]、环孢素[74]和干扰素[75]的使用,造血干细胞移植后[76]以及马来酸舒尼替尼的使用(一个批准用于转移性肾细胞癌的口服多靶点酪氨酸激酶抑制剂)[77]有关。

肿瘤相关 TMA 的病理生理学与一般原发性 TMA 相似,是由于缺乏一种 vWF 裂解蛋白酶(ADAMTS-13)引起血小板聚集,导致超大 vWF 多聚体的释放,进而导致血管内皮的损伤[78,79]。

典型的微血管病性溶血性贫血和血小板减少是十分严重的,通常伴有网织红细胞增多,乳酸脱氢酶水平升高,反映了血管内溶血的发生。外周血涂片显示大量的裂体细胞。肾衰竭、神经功能障碍和肺功能障碍是常见的。TTP 标准治疗方法是血浆置换。其他可用于难治性病例的治疗方法包括长春新碱、静脉输注人免疫球蛋白、利妥昔单抗和脾切除术[80~82]。血小板输注通常是禁忌的,因为输注血小板可能会加重微血管血栓形成的严重程度和范围。无论接受何种治疗,TMA 患者的预后普遍较差。

动脉血栓形成和非细菌性血栓性心内膜炎

癌症和动脉血栓形成之间的关系目前尚不明确,一些个案报道认为化疗可能是个诱因[83]。选择性雌激素受体调节剂他莫昔芬和雷洛昔芬(raloxifene)增加了脑卒中的风险[84],特别是在冠脉事件风险增加的绝经后妇女以及当前吸烟的患者中尤为明显[85]。值得注意的是,急性缺血性脑卒中伴有活动性肿瘤(特别是腺癌)的患者,其短期内缺血性脑卒中复发和其他血栓栓塞形成的风险显著增高[86]。

非细菌性血栓性心内膜炎(non-bacterial thrombotic endocarditis,NBTE)是一种消耗性凝血病,在肺腺癌和胰腺腺癌中最为常见。对于任何一个发生缺血性栓塞事件的癌症患者都需要考虑到 NBTE 的可能。超声心动图对于寻找心脏瓣膜上的无菌性血栓性赘生物具有诊断价值。除了瓣膜赘生物,18% 合并 NBTE 的癌症患者还存在由无症状的冠脉栓塞所致的心室室壁运动异常。其处理基本上以支持治疗为主，还包括原发肿瘤治疗和普通肝素或低分子肝素的抗凝治疗。

弥散性血管内凝血

弥散性血管内凝血（diffuse intravascular coagulation，DIC）是一个导致癌症患者病情恶化的临床病理综合征。实体瘤（前列腺癌，胰腺癌，肺癌，胃癌，结肠癌和乳腺癌）和白血病患者，尤其是 APL 患者，并发 DIC 时可能以出血为首发症状。恶性血液病患者常常处于慢性 DIC 状态，缺乏活动性血栓形成和/或出血症状。通常认为 APL 患者的出血是 APL 细胞上的连接素 A2 的异常高表达，继而使纤溶酶增多，导致不可控的纤维蛋白溶解而引起。连接素 A2 是一种内皮细胞表面的磷脂结合蛋白，主要结合纤溶酶原及其激活物 tPA。APL 细胞的 t15～17 易位，导致白血病细胞的 TF 高表达，从而将肿瘤的发生与高凝状态的形成联系起来[87]。

血浆微粒相关 TF 的促凝血活性可能在不同类型恶性肿瘤的 DIC 演变过程中起到了重要的致病作用[88]。

与 DIC 相关的血栓性疾病包括复发性静脉血栓形成、外周动脉血栓形成，脑血管血栓形成、伴随器官功能衰竭的弥散性动脉疾病、外周肢体缺血和坏疽。慢性 DIC 的特点是没有明显的临床表现，但存在细微的、持续的实验室检查异常。转移性肿瘤是慢性 DIC 的一个常见原因。随着时间的推移，大约 25%的转移性肿瘤患者会出现血栓事件。在肿瘤患者中，DIC 的诊断需要结合临床和一系列的实验室检查异常来证实（表 130-6）[89]。单一的实验室检测结果不能明确或排除 DIC 的诊断。在大多数情况下，需要结合检验结果和 DIC 相关的临床症状，才能够合理而明确的诊断 DIC。当存在与 DIC 相关的基础疾病时，有 50%～60%的 DIC 患者会出现初始血小板计数低于 $10^5/mm^3$ 或血小板计数迅速下降，PT 和 aPTT 延长，以及血浆中出现纤维蛋白（原）降解产物和 D-二聚体。由于急性期反应物纤维蛋白原合成的增加，纤维蛋白原水平在面临消耗时仍然可维持在正常范围内。低纤维蛋白原血症仅仅在非常严重的 DIC 病例中具有诊断意义。外周血液涂片可能发现红细胞碎片或裂体细胞的存在，但很少超过 10%。仅在血管内生成的可溶性纤维蛋白单体（soluble fibrin monomer，SF）检测对于 DIC 诊断具有一定灵敏度，但特异度不高[90]。天然抗凝蛋白 C 和/或抗凝血酶（AT）的检测似乎没有更多意义[91]。国际血栓与止血学会（ISTH）下属的 DIC 科学与标准化委员会（SCC）推荐使用显性 DIC 评分系统[91]。ISTH 显性 DIC 评分系统的灵敏度和特异度分别为 91%和 97%[92]。基于 DIC 的实验室结果和临床特征，重复检测对于动态监测疾病变化十分重要。

表 130-6　患有 DIC 的肿瘤患者的异常表现

血小板减少症
PT 和 aPTT 延长
低纤维蛋白原血症[a]
凝血因子Ⅴ和Ⅷ水平下降[b]
出现纤维蛋白（原）的降解产物和 D-二聚体[c] 并与纤维蛋白多聚物和血小板聚集产生二级反应
外周血涂片出现裂体细胞或红细胞碎片，提示微血管病理性溶血

[a] 因为生成增加，纤维蛋白原在消耗后仍可能在正常范围内：低纤维蛋白原血症仅在严重的 DIC 患者具有诊断意义。

[b] 某些早期 DIC 患者的凝血因子Ⅷ可能上升，是由于凝血酶激活因子Ⅷ。

[c] 当内源性纤溶系统降解纤维蛋白时，血浆 D-二聚体由特异性交叉纤维蛋白诱导产生。

一般来说，DIC 的治疗主要是针对潜在肿瘤进行治疗，同时也需要对出血或血栓相关的症状进行支持治疗。正在出血或者有出血高风险的 DIC 肿瘤患者（如接受手术或有创性操作的患者）应接受血小板输注，以保证血小板计数大于 50 000/μl，如果存在 PT 或 aPTT 延长，应输注新鲜冷冻血浆（虽然 30ml/kg 的剂量能够更完全地纠正凝血因子水平，但目前推荐的初始剂量仍为 15ml/kg）。一般不推荐输注纯化凝血因子浓缩物，除非患者体液超负荷，无法接受新鲜冷冻血浆输注。凝血因子浓缩物仅含有一些特定的凝血因子，而 DIC 通常面临凝血因子的全面缺乏。如果条件允许，严重的低纤维蛋白原血症（<1g/L）需要用冷沉淀或纤维蛋白原浓缩物治疗。3g 的纤维蛋白原浓缩物剂量可以将血浆纤维蛋白原水平提高 1g/L，这相当于给予两组冷沉淀物（10 单位）。这些输注性支持治疗的效果需要临床观察和实验室检查的监测[89]。维 A 酸治疗急性早幼粒细胞性白血病的 DIC 出血通常效果显著[86]。

虽然目前没有随机对照临床研究证明在 DIC 患者中使用肝素可以改善临床预后，但对于正在接受抗肿瘤治疗的肿瘤患者，如果存在 DIC 相关血栓形成，仍可静脉注射肝素以稳定血栓，除非该患者出现了中度到重度的血小板减少或出血。肝素的推荐剂量为 10U/（kg・h）持续静脉滴注，不需要负荷剂量。虽然监测 aPTT 可能烦琐，但对于监测出血征象非常重要。对于危重的、非出血性的 DIC 患者推荐使用普通肝素或低分子量肝素进行药物血栓预防[89]。一般来说，DIC 患者不宜使用抗纤溶药物。然而，对于原发性纤溶出血的 DIC 患者（如前列腺癌），可以使用纤溶抑制剂氨基己酸，初始静脉负荷剂量为 4～6g（输注时间大于 1h），然后以 1g/h 的剂量静脉输注，同时监测临床疗效。氨基己酸推荐的口服剂量为 50～60mg/kg 每 4～6h[93]。然而，对于那些存在原发性血栓和继发性纤溶的患者，应避免使用纤溶抑制剂，除非血栓形成的过程得到控制[89]。

治疗出血和血栓性疾病的药物

重组Ⅶa 因子

重组凝血因子Ⅶa（rFⅦa）被 FDA 批准用于已产生因子Ⅷ和Ⅸ的抑制因子的血友病 A 或 B 的出血患者[94]，以及应用于遗传性因子Ⅶ缺乏的患者。它也被证实在控制血小板减少、血小板疾病、获得性凝血因子缺乏所致的出血和肿瘤手术患者中有效。越来越多的证据支持在恶性造血系统疾病和造血干细胞移植相关的大出血患者中使用 rFⅦa[95]。

促血小板生成素受体激动剂

促血小板生成素受体激动剂(TPO-RA):罗米司亭和艾曲波帕(eltrombopag),被 FDA 批准用于增加慢性免疫性血小板减少性紫癜(ITP)患者的血小板计数。脾切除和非脾切除的患者均能获益。TPO-RA 也被批准用于治疗丙型病毒性肝炎和肝硬化背景下的血小板减少,最近又被批准用于治疗再生障碍性贫血。这两种药物对治疗 MDS 和非清髓性化疗虽然尚未获批,但也有效果。短期的有效性和安全性已十分明确,而长期的有效性和安全性正逐步完善。潜在的风险包括血栓形成、骨髓纤维化、恶性造血系统疾病以及艾曲波帕导致的肝毒性[96]。

口服抗凝药(DOAC)

口服Ⅹa 因子抑制物如利伐沙班(rivaroxaban)、阿哌沙班(apixaban)和依度沙班(edoxaban)以及口服凝血酶抑制剂如达比加群(dabigatran),被用于预防非瓣膜性心房纤颤的脑卒中和全身性血栓以及预防 VTE 的临床研究。对具有肿瘤背景的患者,目前临床实践指南全部推荐应用治疗剂量的 LMWH 进行肿瘤相关血栓形成的初始和长期治疗。如果 LMWH 不可获得时,也可应用维生素 K 拮抗剂(vitamin K antagonists, VKA)。对于长期治疗 VTE 的肿瘤患者,LMWH 相比于 VKA 能减少静脉血栓栓塞事件发生,但不能减少死亡率。肿瘤 VTE 患者究竟选择长期 LMWH 还是口服新型抗凝药物,应该平衡获益和风险,综合考虑患者的价值观和对临床结果及治疗策略的选择权。

在 VTE 的紧急治疗中,DOAC 和传统治疗方法相比疗效相当,但在肿瘤患者中的有效性和安全性尚不明确。DOAC 的应用无法获得支持,除非获得了与 LMWH 相比较的对照研究[97,98]。

总结

出血和血栓性并发症常见于肿瘤患者中。近年来,有关肿瘤、凝血和肿瘤血管生成之间关系的认识取得了重大进展。出血并发症通常由血小板异常或凝血因子缺乏所导致,需要特定的血液或凝血因子替代治疗。血栓栓塞事件包括 DVT 和 PE,是肿瘤患者中常见并且严重的并发症。新分子标志物、诊断性影像学的进步以及新型抗凝药物的面世极大地促进了这类患者的治疗。正在进行的关于止血过程的各种紊乱机制的理解、新颖治疗模式的应用及肿瘤患者进行适当血栓预防的研究,能够最终降低患者发病率并改善生存率。

(白元松 丛丹 译 白元松 丛丹 代恩勇 刁建东 校)

参考文献

The complete reference list can be found on the Wiley Companion Digital Edition of this title (see inside front cover for login instructions).

1 Choudhry A, DeLoughery TG. Bleeding and thrombosis in acute promyelocytic leukemia. *Am J Hematol*. 2012;**87**(**6**):596–603.

5 Donnellan E, Kevane B, Healey Bird BR, Ni Ainle F. Cancer and venous thromboembolic disease: from molecular mechanisms to clinical management. *Curr Oncol*. 2014;**21**(**3**):134–143.

21 Estcourt L, Stanworth S, Doree C, et al. Prophylactic platelet transfusion for prevention of bleeding in patients with haematological disorders after chemotherapy and stem cell transplantation. *Cochrane Database Syst Rev*. 2012;**16**:5.

23 Slichter SJ. Evidence-based platelet transfusion guidelines. *Hematology Am Soc Hematol Educ Program*. 2007;**2007**:172–178.

27 Sucker C, Michiels JJ, Zotz RB. Causes, etiology and diagnosis of acquired von Willebrand disease: a prospective diagnostic workup to establish the most effective therapeutic strategies. *Acta Haematol*. 2009;**121**(**2-3**):177–182.

34 Marchioli R, Finazzi G, Specchia G, et al. Cardiovascular events and intensity of treatment in polycythemia vera. *N Engl J Med*. 2013;**368**(**1**):22–33.

35 Kiladjian JJ. The spectrum of JAK2-positive myeloproliferative neoplasms. *Hematology Am Soc Hematol Educ Program*. 2012;**2012**:561–566.

37 O'Shaughnessy DF, Atterbury C, Bolton Maggs P, et al. Guidelines for the use of fresh-frozen plasma, cryoprecipitate and cryosupernatant. *Br J Haematol*. 2004;**126**(**1**):11–28.

38 Mumford AD, O'Donnell J, Gillmore JD, Manning RA, Hawkins PN, Laffan M. Bleeding symptoms and coagulation abnormalities in 337 patients with AL-amyloidosis. *Br J Haematol*. 2000;**110**(**2**):454–460.

41 Varki A. Trousseau's syndrome: multiple definitions and multiple mechanisms. *Blood*. 2007;**110**(**6**):1723–1729.

46 Bennett CL, Silver SM, Djulbegovic B, et al. Venous thromboembolism and mortality associated with recombinant erythropoietin and darbepoetin administration for the treatment of cancer-associated anemia. *JAMA*. 2008;**299**(**8**):914–924.

47 Wells PS, Anderson DR, Bormanis J, et al. Value of assessment of pretest probability of deep-vein thrombosis in clinical management [see comments]. *Lancet*. 1997;**350**(**9094**):1795–1798.

49 King V, Vaze AA, Moskowitz CS, Smith LJ, Ginsberg MS. D-dimer assay to exclude pulmonary embolism in high-risk oncologic population: correlation with CT pulmonary angiography in an urgent care setting. *Radiology*. 2008;**247**(**3**):854–861.

51 Huisman MV, Klok FA. Diagnostic management of acute deep vein thrombosis and pulmonary embolism. *J Thromb Haemost*. 2013;**11**(**3**):412–422.

52 Kearon C, Akl EA, Comerota AJ, et al. Antithrombotic therapy for VTE disease: antithrombotic therapy and prevention of thrombosis, 9th ed: American College of Chest Physicians Evidence-Based Clinical Practice Guidelines. *Chest*. 2012;**141**(**2 Suppl**):e419S–e494S.

53 Siragusa S. Low molecular weight heparins as antineoplastic agents. *Recent Pat Anticancer Drug Discov*. 2008;**3**(**3**):159–161.

58 Lee AY, Levine MN, Baker RI, et al. Low-molecular-weight heparin versus a coumarin for the prevention of recurrent venous thromboembolism in patients with cancer. *N Engl J Med*. 2003;**349**(**2**):146–153.

60 Goldhaber SZ. Thrombolysis for pulmonary embolism. *N Engl J Med*. 2002;**347**(**15**):1131–1132.

62 Wallace MJ, Jean JL, Gupta S, et al. Use of inferior vena caval filters and survival in patients with malignancy. *Cancer*. 2004;**101**(**8**):1902–1907.

64 Holbrook A, Schulman S, Witt DM, et al. Evidence-based management of anticoagulant therapy: antithrombotic therapy and prevention of thrombosis, 9th ed: American College of Chest Physicians Evidence-Based Clinical Practice Guidelines. *Chest*. 2012;**141**(**2 Suppl**):e152S–e184S.

66 Lyman GH, Bohlke K, Khorana AA, et al. Venous thromboembolism prophylaxis and treatment in patients with cancer: American Society of Clinical Oncology clinical practice guideline update. *J Clin Oncol*. 2015;**33**(**6**):654–656.

70 Linkins LA, Dans AL, Moores LK, et al. Treatment and prevention of heparin-induced thrombocytopenia: antithrombotic therapy and prevention of thrombosis, 9th ed: American College of Chest Physicians Evidence-Based Clinical Practice Guidelines. *Chest*. 2012;**141**(**2 Suppl**):e495S–530S.

71 Lo GK, Juhl D, Warkentin TE, Sigouin CS, Eichler P, Greinacher A. Evaluation of pretest clinical score (4 T's) for the diagnosis of heparin-induced thrombocytopenia in two clinical settings. *J Thromb Haemost*. 2006;**4**(**4**):759–765.

76 Tsakiris DA, Tichelli A. Thrombotic complications after haematopoietic stem cell transplantation: early and late effects. *Best Pract Res Clin Haematol*. 2009;**22**(**1**):137–145.

82 Riedl M, Orth-Höller D, Würzner R. An update on the thrombotic microan-

giopathies hemolytic uremic syndrome (HUS) and thrombotic thrombocytopenic purpura (TTP). *Semin Thromb Hemost*. 2014;**40(4)**:413–415.
83 Javid M, Magee TR, Galland RB. Arterial thrombosis associated with malignant disease. *Eur J Vasc Endovasc Surg*. 2008;**35(1)**:84–87.
85 Mosca L, Grady D, Barrett-Connor E, et al. Effect of raloxifene on stroke and venous thromboembolism according to subgroups in postmenopausal women at increased risk of coronary heart disease. *Stroke*. 2009;**40(1)**:147–155.
89 Levi M, Toh CH, Thachil J, Watson HG. Guidelines for the diagnosis and management of disseminated intravascular coagulation. *Br J Haematol*. 2009;**145(1)**:24–33.
91 Toh CH, Hoots WK, SSC. on Disseminated Intravascular Coagulation of the ISTH. The scoring system of the scientific and standardisation committee on disseminated intravascular coagulation of the international society on thrombosis and haemostasis: a 5-year overview. *J Thromb Haemost*. 2007;**5(3)**:604–606.
93 Mannucci PM, Levi M. Prevention and treatment of major blood loss. *N Engl J Med*. 2007;**356(22)**:2301–2311.
96 Mitchell WB, Bussel JB. Thrombopoietin receptor agonists: a critical review. *Semin Hematol*. 2015;**52(1)**:46–52.
97 Carrier M, Cameron C, Delluc A, Castellucci L, Khorana AA, Lee AY. Efficacy and safety of anticoagulant therapy for the treatment of acute cancer-associated thrombosis: a systematic review and meta-analysis. *Thromb Res*. 2014;**134(6)**:1214–1219.
98 Akl EA, Kahale L, Barba M, et al. Anticoagulation for the long-term treatment of venous thromboembolism in patients with cancer. *Cochrane Database Syst Rev*. 2014;7:CD006650.

第 131 章　泌尿系统并发症

Rachel A. Sanford, MD ■ Ala Abudayyeh, MD ■ Christopher J. Logothetis, MD ■
Nizar M. Tannir, MD, FACP

概述

在癌症患者的临床管理中需要对相关泌尿系统并发症的发生有所预期并能及时干预，包括尿路梗阻、膀胱炎、肾炎和化疗药物相关的肾毒性反应。针对接受治愈性治疗的局限期癌症患者，专业的泌尿系统并发症处理对于完成足剂量的化疗至关重要，并可避免剂量减少所致的治愈性降低的风险。在转移性患者中，针对泌尿系统并发症（如尿路梗阻）的专业处理可显著缓解相关症状。本章节探讨了发生在输尿管，膀胱和尿道等部位尿路梗阻的相关诊断和处理。阐述了化疗性、放射性膀胱炎和肾炎的机制及其处理方法。最后，重点概述了常见的潜在肾毒性药物相关的诊断、治疗与预防。除细胞毒性化疗外，本章还讨论了靶向药物治疗引起的肾毒性反应，并概述了可能影响肾功能的免疫相关不良事件（irAE）的新见解。

前言

预防性和及时地干预癌症相关的泌尿系统并发症，有助于局限期患者的治疗，也为转移性患者提供更多治疗的机会。尿路梗阻的处理，药物相关肾毒性损害的及时监测，以及在不过度减量的情况下处理毒性损害，对于癌症患者取得成功治疗至关重要。基于患者肾功能水平的药物剂量调整以及针对具有肾毒性潜在肾损害的多种药物的临床监测是必需的，也是肿瘤学实践的必要组成部分，并且泌尿系统并发症的处理需要多学科的协调管理。本章总结了常见的泌尿系统并发症及其处理。

尿路梗阻

肿瘤的直接浸润，压迫或侵袭输尿管、膀胱或尿道等多个部位均可导致尿路梗阻。梗阻性尿路疾病的自然病史和处理取决于梗阻的位置，时间（急性与慢性）以及针对恶性肿瘤所致梗阻治疗的预期反应。在可治愈性肿瘤的治疗方案中，往往包括一些具有肾毒性的药物的应用［顺铂，异环磷酰胺和甲氨蝶呤（MTX）］，梗阻性尿路疾病的及时逆转对于实现这些药物的足量化疗至关重要。晚期泌尿系统肿瘤患者合并的尿路梗阻或严重的泌尿系统尿路症状威胁着患者的生活质量，而尿流改道是一种重要的姑息性手术，旨在缓解疼痛、延长生存期和提高生活质量。在上述两种情况下，由泌尿科医生或介入科医生进行的一系列微创干预措施（包括支架置入和尿路外引流）可实现早期干预并降低实施大型手术的风险。

梗阻性尿路疾病首先表现为肌酐升高，尤其是无痛的输尿管梗阻。膀胱出口或尿道梗阻导致的膀胱膨隆可在查体时触及。由于肾素-血管紧张素系统的激活，急性单侧肾积水可能引起血压升高[1]；而这种高血压可通过缓解尿路梗阻实现可逆。尿常规可能没有特异性异常，也可能出现有镜下血尿[2]。主要依靠影像学诊断，包括超声和增强 CT。通常首选 B 超以避免造影剂引起的潜在肾毒性反应和放射暴露。增强 MRI 可获得详细的解剖信息，但由于担心肾源性纤维化（NSF），也限制了其在 GFR<30ml/min 患者中的应用。

无论尿路梗阻的位置高低，随着梗阻时间延长，均会导致肾盂压力增加，肾积水和肾小管萎缩。如果任其进展，可能发生不可逆肾损害[3]。尿路梗阻也可能诱发感染。急性和慢性阻塞的情况下肾脏的影像学改变是明显的，前者表现为正常或增厚肾皮质的肾脏增大，后者表现为肾皮质变薄的肾萎缩。尿路梗阻的缓解可能难以明显改善慢性梗阻导致的肾功能不全，并且超声提示肾皮质变薄的肾萎缩也难以恢复。

随着急性梗阻的解除，肾功能的恢复期有可能很长，但一般 7~10 日可恢复至正常[4]。在梗阻缓解后的一段时间内，由于肾小管的重吸收功能异常，可能导致一段时间的去梗阻后多尿。这种情况最常见于高位的急性尿路梗阻。

输尿管梗阻

输尿管位于腹膜后腔隙，病理性腹膜后淋巴结肿大或腹膜后纤维化压迫输尿管特别容易导致机械性梗阻。这种梗阻性尿路疾病最常见于原发性淋巴结肿大（淋巴瘤）或泌尿系肿瘤所致的主动脉周围淋巴结转移，尤其是前列腺癌和生殖细胞肿瘤。处理化疗高度敏感的恶性肿瘤所引起的腹膜后病变压迫输尿管时，尤其是生殖细胞肿瘤或侵袭性淋巴瘤，及时有效的化疗可让临床医生避免梗阻的紧急干预，特别是单侧或不完全输尿管梗阻。在根治性化疗中使用潜在肾毒性药物（如顺铂）时，即便是针对化疗的正常反应，可能也需要预先解除输尿管梗阻。对治疗反应预期的速度与程度，肾功能的代偿程度以及单一细胞毒性化疗药物缓解梗阻的可靠性，共同决定了患者经皮肾造瘘的必要性。

当需要解除输尿管梗阻时，可选择输尿管支架或经皮肾造瘘治疗。输尿管多部位梗阻、闭塞段长或输尿管扭曲的患者可能均需要直接行经皮肾造瘘治疗[5]。虽然单侧经皮肾造瘘术可以保留充足的肾功能以保证姑息性治疗，但长期无疾病生存且依赖于肾毒性药物治疗的患者，需要最大限度地保留肾功能，此时经常需要行双侧肾造瘘术。尽管肾造瘘是保证治疗顺利的关键，但其并没有风险，因存在潜在的感染风险，可能会使治疗计划复杂化、延迟甚至需要重新更改[6,7]。肾造瘘的位置及护理细节也应值得重视，包括选择最佳放管位置以减轻术后疼痛，导管的更换频率以及造口部位的护理等。

放置肾造瘘管时，可利用超声和/或透视下实现肾内集合系统成像以选择穿刺通路。对于经验丰富的医师，98%的病例可以成功留置肾造瘘管，主要并发症发生率约占 4%[5]，主要包括血肿、出血、血管损伤、败血症、肠道或肺损伤和死亡。放置肾造瘘管缓解梗阻及改善肾盂内压后，部分患者可以通过造瘘口顺行放置输尿管 D-J 管。对于初期无法接受治疗的患者，经皮肾造瘘或支架管置入术后可以实行治愈性的治疗。而对于无法治疗的晚期肿瘤患者，两种治疗方案的风险效益可能有所不同。最近研究表明，尿路梗阻的干预治疗显著增加了转移性癌症患者的住院概率[7,8]，并且长期以来人们认为肾衰竭引起的进行性尿毒症可为症状严重的终末期患者带来平缓的死亡结局。因此针对合并非梗阻性重度疼痛且预期寿命很短的患者，不建议对尿路梗阻进行干预，而以缓解症状为主。但这种困难的决策需要医生、患者及家属间的仔细沟通。

膀胱出口和尿道梗阻

恶性疾病导致膀胱出口和尿道梗阻最常见于前列腺癌或膀胱癌患者，也可见于卵巢癌，宫颈癌和子宫内膜癌患者。虽然输尿管梗阻通常无明显症状，但膀胱出口和尿道梗阻的患者经常困扰于膀胱刺激和膨胀所致的不适。这些可能会严重影响患者的生活质量[9,10]。紧邻尿道前列腺部的前列腺癌在体积较小时便可引起显著的梗阻症状。由于充溢性尿失禁，尿量可能会出现波动并伴有相对少尿期和多尿期。

前列腺癌所致尿路梗阻的处理取决于前列腺癌分期。初诊前列腺癌可能对激素非常敏感，通过在留置尿管期间给予雄激素剥夺疗法（ADT），可顺利拔除尿管并缓解梗阻。相反，去势抵抗性前列腺癌接受 ADT 和二线内分泌或化疗后短期内病情仍会进展，不会对上述治疗表现出快速反应，而需要长期的肾造瘘或耻骨上造瘘以缓解梗阻。此外，大体积的前列腺癌或膀胱癌，无论其对预期治疗的反应如何，都可能需要直接经皮肾穿刺造瘘[3]。膀胱出口或尿道梗阻可通过耻骨上膀胱造瘘得到缓解。通常情况下，耻骨上穿刺造瘘可缓解症状，但因其改变了尿路的正常解剖结构，故不推荐应用于有治愈性可能的肿瘤患者。

尿道梗阻患者的症状往往难以缓解。尽管经皮肾造瘘或耻骨上膀胱造瘘可分流尿液，但仍不能完全缓解尿频、尿急、排尿困难和血尿等症状。经尿道前列腺切除术可能有助于缓解晚期癌症患者的症状，对这些晚期肿瘤的症状处理仍是临床医师面临的挑战。

膀胱炎和肾炎

对于肿瘤患者，血尿是一件令人害怕的事件。血尿可起源于尿路的任何部位，肉眼血尿可能需要治疗以防失血过多。血尿的特点可提示尿路出血的部位：长条蚯蚓状血块提示上尿路出血，无血块的新鲜出血常提示下尿路出血。恶性肿瘤治疗后再次血尿可能提示尿路系统内肿瘤复发。

处理血尿的重点在于控制出血，防止血块滞留堵塞引起尿路梗阻和肾功能损害。下尿路出血最常见的初步处理是生理盐水持续膀胱冲洗。膀胱镜下清除血块可能有助于缓解症状。在某些特定患者中，放疗可控制肿瘤出血[11]。环磷酰胺、异环磷酰胺等药物引起的化学性膀胱炎或放射治疗引起的放射性膀胱炎而导致的出血的相关处理是一个具有挑战性的临床难题。膀胱介入栓塞或类固醇注射治疗偶尔可缓解出血，但疗效并不满意。可利用稀释的甲醛使黏膜表层组织变性并固定达到止血效果。急诊膀胱切除手术可避免患者过度失血。其他治疗包括静脉水化[12]，膀胱冲洗，口服或膀胱内注射氨基己酸（仅用于下尿路出血）[13]，膀胱内注射明矾[14]或前列腺素[15,16]。试验性的治疗方法包括氩激光凝固[17]、氨磷汀治疗[18]、高压氧[19]和共轭雌激素治疗等[20]。

化学性膀胱炎

环磷酰胺和异环磷酰胺是最常用的恶唑磷酰胺类化疗药物。其他可引起肉眼血尿的膀胱内灌注治疗药物包括多柔比星、丝裂霉素和卡介苗[21]。环磷酰胺和异环磷酰胺均可代谢成丙烯醛，为一种尿路上皮毒性代谢物[22]。其次化疗引起的血小板减少症也可能会加重出血。据报道，高达 20%接受高剂量环磷酰胺治疗的患者以及 8%异环磷酰胺治疗的患者可出现无菌性出血性膀胱炎[23]。使用常规剂量的环磷酰胺化疗时，可通过大量饮水以预防膀胱炎。在使用异环磷酰胺时，可通过静脉水化或利用美司钠（mesna）尿路保护剂缓解膀胱炎。在异环磷酰胺给药前 15min，给药后 4h 和 8h，静脉注射相当于异环磷酰胺剂量 20%的美司钠（美司钠的总剂量应相当于异环磷酰胺剂量的 60%）。也可以按照异环磷酰胺等同剂量持续静脉滴注美司钠。异环磷酰胺输注后应连续输注美司钠 4~8h。环磷酰胺联合美司钠主要用于骨髓移植行高剂量化疗时的处理，美司钠剂量约为环磷酰胺总剂量的 60%~160%，并分 3~5 等份静脉注射或持续静脉滴注[21,24]。

在不含环磷酰胺的化疗方案中，化疗所致的血小板减少也会引起出血性膀胱炎，另外恶性尿路系统肿瘤也可成为出血灶。骨髓移植中化学性出血性膀胱炎必须与腺病毒[25]或人类 BK 多瘤病毒[26]感染所引起的感染性血尿相鉴别。

放射性膀胱炎

放射性膀胱炎虽然相对少见，外放射或近距离放射治疗盆腔肿瘤后仍可能会引起出血性膀胱炎。相关病理生理学机制涉及血管内皮损伤及动脉内膜炎，导致膀胱进行性缺血，炎症，肌肉萎缩，最终组织坏死[27]。放射性膀胱炎可在结束放疗后半年至数十年内发生。一项研究表明，6.5%的患者接受盆腔放疗后出现放射性膀胱炎[28]。骨髓移植时全身放疗所引起的出血性膀胱炎占 10%~17%[14,29]。出血风险最高的患者是同时使用环磷酰胺或曾接受泌尿外科手术者。放射性膀胱炎可在放射治疗后数十年出现，但由于这种情况也可能意味肿瘤复发，因此在将血尿归因于放射性膀胱炎之前应仔细检查。

放射性肾炎

肾区放疗通常可以控制放射敏感性肿瘤的淋巴结转移（如淋巴瘤和精原细胞瘤）。放射性肾炎可能因肾区辐射而致，与辐射剂量和范围有关[30]。然而现代屏蔽技术大大降低了该并发症的发生率。成人肾脏的耐受剂量（TD5/5）约为 20Gy，15Gy

时肾小球功能开始下降，25～30Gy 时肾功能几乎丧失。顺铂、卡莫司汀（BCNU）和放线菌素 D 等放射增敏剂会降低正常组织的放射耐受性。放疗后 6 个月内肾炎症状并不明显，放疗后 6～12 个月，可能会出现相关症状和阳性体征，包括高血压、水肿、白蛋白尿、尿沉渣增多以及 BUN 和血肌酐升高。高血压是慢性期（大于 12 个月）最常见症状，患者将出现肾脏瘢痕形成，肾皮质小管萎缩和肾小球硬化相关的高肾素性高血压。极少数情况下，患者肾功能逐渐恶化而需要血液透析或肾移植治疗[31]。避免此类并发症是现代实施先进放疗技术的一个重要方面和保障。

骨髓移植中的全身照射与剂量依赖的远期肾毒性相关，包括高血压、贫血、肾小球滤过率（GFR）降低、血尿和蛋白尿。病理改变包括血管坏死和基底膜内皮细胞及上皮细胞破碎[32]。一项综述分析表明，接受 14Gy 全身放疗的骨髓移植患者中，肾病的发病率随着肾屏蔽的范围扩大而降低：未接受肾屏蔽保护的患者中出现肾病者占 30%，接受 30%肾区屏蔽的患者无肾病发生[33]。

癌症治疗药物相关肾毒性的诊断、治疗与预防

常用的化疗药物多数都具有潜在肾毒性（表 131-1）。相关不良反应包括肿瘤溶解综合征，副肿瘤性肾小球肾炎，梗阻性尿路疾病和导致肾衰竭的直接肾毒性反应以及电解质紊乱。这些更常见于多药联合治疗的或伴有并发症的老年人群。由于高剂量化疗、多药联合治疗及全身放疗，这些药物的肾毒性作用在骨髓移植中更常见。下文中我们阐述了几种常见的导致严重肾毒性的药物。表 131-2 列出了可能导致肾毒性的其他药物。表 131-3 列出了几种药物的肾损伤机制。药物的相互作用是潜在肾毒性药物使用的另一个重要参考因素；表 131-4 总结了一些药物的相互作用。这些表中内容并不全面，仔细审查所有处方药和非处方药对于预防癌症患者肾毒性并发症至关重要。表 131-5 总结了几种常见化疗药物的剂量调整。

表 131-1　与肾毒性相关的治疗药物

类型	药物
烷化剂	AZQ（亚胺醌）、卡铂、顺铂、环磷酰胺、异环磷酰胺、亚硝基脲（链佐星、卡莫司汀、洛莫司汀）、奥沙利铂
抗肿瘤抗生素	丝裂霉素 C、普卡霉素
抗代谢药物	5-氮杂胞苷、氯法拉滨、吉西他滨、大剂量甲氨蝶呤
叶酸拮抗剂	培美曲塞
靶向治疗	VEGF 抑制剂（贝伐单抗、舒尼替尼、索拉非尼、培唑帕尼、阿昔替尼、卡博替尼）、mTOR 抑制剂（依维莫司、坦罗莫司）
生物制剂	注射用重组人白介素-2（IL-2）、干扰素
免疫疗法	伊匹木单抗
其他	天冬酰胺酶、环孢素、硝酸镓、吉非替尼（gefitinib）、伊马替尼、喷司他丁（pentostatin）、他克莫司

表 131-2　化疗相关肾毒性的临床特点及病理特点

药物	损伤类型	临床特征	尿液分析	毒性起始时间	治疗/结果	预防
5-氮杂胞苷	急性肾小管损伤	肾小管酸中毒	无特征或治疗相关性低渗	治疗后 7～10 日多尿及肌酐升高	置换 HCO_3、PO_4、Mg；完全恢复	每日监测肌酐、BUN 和电解质
贝伐单抗	肾小球病	蛋白尿	蛋白尿	随累积剂量加重	出现肾病综合征时停药；单纯尿蛋白阳性继续治疗	定期监测
卡铂	肾小管损伤	低镁血症	无特征	治疗 5～10 日后肌酐上升	停药，必要时透析；通常恢复欠佳	避免使用其他肾毒性药物，以前使用顺铂治疗的患者补充 Mg
顺铂	急性肾小管损伤	低镁血症	无特征	随累积剂量肌酐上升	停药，必要时透析；通常恢复欠佳	充分水化，利尿、甘露醇利尿、使用硫代硫酸钠、避免使用氨基糖苷类药物

续表

药物	损伤类型	临床特征	尿液分析	毒性起始时间	治疗/结果	预防
环孢素	肾小管损伤和入球小动脉血管收缩	高钾血症和低镁血症、肾小管酸中毒、高血压	蛋白尿	治疗后肌酐从几日到几月内上升	停药,必要时透析;通常完全恢复	周期性给药、监测肌酐、BUN和电解质
AZQ(亚胺醌)	肾小管及肾小球损伤	无尿、蛋白尿和肾小管酸中毒	蛋白尿	治疗后5~10日肌酐上升	停药,必要时透析;通常完全恢复	避免药物剂量>245mg/m²
硝酸镓	肾小球病	蛋白尿和氮质血症	蛋白尿	治疗期间及治疗后几天内出现蛋白尿所致肌酐升高	停药;通常完全恢复	每日尿量>2L,连续7日药物剂量不能>300mg/(m²·d)
异环磷酰胺	急性肾小球损伤	少尿	无特征	治疗后1~2日内肌酐升高	支持透析;通常完全恢复	既往使用顺铂的患者易少尿,使用美司钠保护剂
白介素2	肾前性氮质血症	少尿和低血压	蛋白尿和血尿	治疗期间肌酐升高	当肌酐≥4.5mg/dl或>4mg/dl伴有酸中毒、水中毒,钾升高时停药;通常1~2周内恢复	给予肾负荷量的多巴胺及充分水化
伊匹木单抗	间质性肾炎	肌酐上升	蛋白尿、含少量红细胞、含少量白细胞	数周	停药;类固醇可能有效	仔细监测血肌酐
甲氨蝶呤	急性肾小管损伤	少尿	无特征	给药1~2日内剂量肌酐升高	根据甲氨蝶呤水平使用大剂量四氢叶酸,大量碱性尿排出;完全恢复	充分水化并碱化尿液,减少治疗肾功能不全的药物剂量,避免氨基糖苷类和非甾体抗炎药
普卡霉素	急性肾小管损伤	突然肾衰竭	轻度蛋白尿	给药期间肌酐升高	停药;如能完全恢复可重新治疗	隔天给药,每日监测肌酐和BUN
丝裂霉素C	肾血管损伤	高血压、贫血	血尿、蛋白尿	两次或多次给药后肌酐升高(12~40周后开始)	永久停药;SPA免疫治疗和透析;很难恢复	累积剂量到60mg时停药
mTOR抑制剂	急性肾小管损伤、局灶性结节性肾小球硬化(FSGS)	肌酐上升	蛋白尿	数周或数月	停药;能完全恢复或带有并发症	定期监测
亚硝基脲	间质性纤维化、肾小球硬化	迟发性并发症	无特征	治疗数月或数年后肌酐升高	支持透析;通常能完全恢复	累计剂量>1 200mg/m²时停止使用该药

续表

药物	损伤类型	临床特征	尿液分析	毒性起始时间	治疗/结果	预防
链霉素	肾小管损伤	间歇性蛋白尿加重	蛋白尿、氨基酸尿	治疗期间出现蛋白尿所致肌酐升高	停药;通常能完全恢复	发现蛋白尿时立即停药,水化不能阻止损伤
VEGF 抑制剂	肾小管损伤、微血管损伤	蛋白尿、高血压	蛋白尿、肾病可能	数周或数月	高血压:积极降压管理 蛋白尿:治疗过程应保持中度蛋白尿以下,出现肾性蛋白尿应永久停止使用此类药物	定期监测

表 131-3 化疗药物所致肾损伤的类型

病理结果	致病药物	病理结果	致病药物
急性肾小球肾炎	无报道	梗阻性尿路病变	甲氨蝶呤
急性肾小管坏死	普卡霉素、mTOR 抑制剂、顺铂	肾小管酸中毒	5-氮杂胞苷
间质性肾炎	亚硝基脲、伊匹木单抗	肾血管炎	丝裂霉素 C
膜性肾小球肾炎(蛋白丢失)	AZQ(亚胺醌)、贝伐单抗		

表 131-4 提高抗肿瘤药物血清浓度或加重肾毒性的药物

阿昔替尼	CYP3A4/5 抑制剂	重组人白介素-2	任何肾毒性药物
卡博替尼	CYP3A4 抑制剂	美法仑	丁硫酸铵
卡培他滨	甲酰四氢叶酸	甲氨蝶呤	有机酸、青霉素、顺铂、NSAID、胺碘酮、阿司匹林、环丙沙星、复方磺胺甲噁唑、环孢素、多西环素、巯基嘌呤、丙磺舒、丙卡巴肼
卡铂	环磷酰胺、氨基糖苷、托泊替康	巯基嘌呤	别嘌醇、甲氨蝶呤、TPMT 抑制剂
顺铂	任何肾毒性药物,美法仑(melphalan)、紫杉醇(paclitaxel)、利妥昔单抗、托泊替康	丝裂霉素	氟尿嘧啶相关溶血性尿毒症综合征
克拉屈滨	环磷酰胺(高剂量)	培唑帕尼	CYP3A4 抑制剂和诱导剂
环磷酰胺	别嘌醇(allopurinol)	链佐星	任何肾毒性药物
环孢素	任何肾毒性药物、万古霉素、美法仑、西咪替丁、保钾利尿剂、萘普生(naproxen)、舒林酸(sulindac)、双氯芬酸(diclofenac)、别嘌醇、细胞色素 P-450 抑制剂、甲氨蝶呤	舒尼替尼	CYP3A4 抑制剂和诱导剂
		坦罗莫司	CYP3A4 抑制剂和诱导剂、许多抗病毒药物、地塞米松
依托泊苷	阿瑞匹坦、环孢素、缬司波达(valspodar)		
依维莫司	选用强 CYP3A4 抑制剂、多种抗病毒药物、酮康唑	他克莫司	任何肾毒性药物、环孢素、顺铂、代谢通过细胞色素 P-450 3A 的药物抑制剂
吉非替尼	细胞色素 P-450 3A4 抑制剂	硫鸟嘌呤	TPMP 抑制剂
吉西他滨	氟尿嘧啶	托泊替康	顺铂、卡铂
异环磷酰胺	细胞色素 P-450 抑制剂、阿瑞匹坦	曲美沙特	西咪替丁、细胞色素 P-450 抑制剂

表 131-5　基于肾功能不全的抗肿瘤药物剂量调整

药物	剂量调整
氮杂胞苷	无法解释的肌酐或 BUN 升高；延长推迟直到恢复正常；减量 50%
博来霉素	肌酐清除率 10～50ml/min：减量 25%
	肌酐清除率<10ml/min：减量 50%
卡培他滨	肌酐清除率 30～50ml/min：减量 25%
	肌酐清除率<30ml/min：不建议继续给药
卡铂	根据 Calvert 公式计算剂量：总剂量(mg)= 目标 AUCx(GFR+25)
卡莫司汀	肌酐清除率<60ml/min：小剂量
顺铂	肌酐清除率 10～50ml/min：减量 25%
	肌酐清除率<10ml/min：减量 50%
氯法拉滨	谨慎使用
环磷酰胺	肌酐清除率 10～50ml/min：减量 25%
	肌酐清除率<10ml/min：减量 50%
阿糖胞苷	肌酐清除率<60ml/min：谨慎使用；减量或改变治疗方案
柔红霉素	肌酐>3mg/dl：减量 50%
依托泊苷	肌酐清除率 15～50ml/min：减量 25%
	肌酐清除率<15ml/min：减量 50%
氟达拉滨	肌酐清除率 30～70ml/min：减量 20%～50%
	肌酐清除率<30ml/min：不建议继续给药
吉非替尼	使用时注意严重的肾功能损害
吉西他滨	使用时注意严重的肾功能损害
羟基脲	肌酐清除率<10ml/min：减量 80%
异环磷酰胺	肌酐清除率 46～60ml/min：减量 20%
	肌酐清除率 31～45ml/min：减量 25%
异环磷酰胺	肌酐清除率≤30ml/min：减量 30%
洛莫司汀	肌酐清除率<60ml/min：小剂量
美法仑	减量是必要的；IV：BUN > 30mg/dl 或肌酐 > 1.5mg/dl：减量 50%
巯嘌呤	减量或延长间隔时间
甲氨蝶呤	肌酐清除率 10～50ml/min：减量 25%
	肌酐清除率<10～30ml/min：停药
丝裂霉素 C	肌酐清除率<10～60ml/min：减量 25%
	肌酐清除率<10mml/min：减量 50%
奥沙利铂	使用时小心中重度肾功能损伤
培美曲塞	肌酐清除率<45ml/min 暂停用药：3/4 级不良反应；非血液系统毒性时需减量 25%
喷司他丁	肌酐清除率<30～60ml/min：可能需要减量
普卡霉素	肌酐清除率 10～50ml/min：减量 25%
	肌酐清除率<10ml/min：减量 50%～70%
丙卡巴肼	肌酐清除率<30ml/min：小剂量
雷替曲塞	肌酐清除率<25～30ml/min：减量 50%
	肌酐清除率<25ml/min：小剂量
链佐星	谨慎使用
噻替哌	必要时减量
替尼泊苷	必要时减量
托泊替康	肌酐清除率 20～39ml/min：减量至 0.75mg/m^2
	肌酐清除率<20ml/min：证据不足
维 A 酸	最大量为 25mg/m^2
曲美沙特	肌酐>2.5mg/dl 时暂停治疗；必要时调整剂量

顺铂

顺铂的临床应用揭示了化疗药物相关肾毒性的潜在危害[34]。顺铂相关肾毒性的有效预防和处理对于该药的临床使用至关重要，并且铂类似物的药物研发部分依赖于如何减轻铂类的肾毒性。顺铂的研究，给药方式的改变以及对肾毒性的预期和监测为肾毒性药物的研究提供了范例。顺铂主要由肾排泄，然而在治疗最初几天内，只能在尿液中检测出微小剂量[35]。大部分药物与蛋白质呈不可逆结合，但在超滤血浆成分中发现了水合二氨基衍生物及其母体的活性代谢产物。该血浆成分的清除是三相的，几乎所有药物在 4h 内消除，但终末半衰期大于 24h。顺铂相关肾毒性是由于肾近曲小管坏死所致，其严重程度可通过充分水化而缓解。由于顺铂是一种高度致吐的药物，快速静脉输液和积极止吐可有效避免患者脱水所致的肾毒性加重[36,37]。

临床上顺铂导致的肾毒性反应可表现为血清肌酐升高和 GFR 下降。其他表现可包括肾小管功能不全所致的低镁血症和中度蛋白尿[38]。当顺铂联合博来霉素时容易出现溶血性尿毒症综合征(HUS)[39]。建议定期监测 GFR 以及钙、镁和磷等电解质。同时也建议顺铂给药间隔至少 7 日，因为最大肾毒性通常不会在 7 日内出现。肌酐清除率显著下降时应延缓治疗。

通过水化预防肾毒性反应至关重要。生理盐水提供了丰富氯离子，通过质量作用减少了铂类水合分子的形成，从而减轻肾毒性。关于甘露醇[40]和呋塞米(Lasix)[41]于顺铂水化中的作用在既往报道中存在争议。与其他潜在肾毒性药物(包括异环磷酰胺和甲氨蝶呤)联合给药可加重肾脏损害，此时给予充分水化至关重要。据报道，同时使用顺铂和氨基糖苷类抗生素会显著损伤肾功能[42]。尽可能地密切关注检验结果、充分水化及避免药物相互作用，对减轻肾功能损害至关重要。

甲氨蝶呤

甲氨蝶呤(MTX)主要经肾排泄。MTX 引起的肾毒性反应可能特别严重,且长期接触会显著增加骨髓毒性和黏膜炎症。MTX 的肾毒性属于剂量依赖性反应,肾衰竭所致死亡与使用该药物有关[43]。由于 MTX 与蛋白质高度结合,在药物过量的情况下透析治疗难以将其清除[39]。MTX 的肾毒性主要表现在肾小管的广泛坏死,该病变称为结晶性肾积水,由 MTX 沉积所致。MTX 及其在肾小管中溶解度较低的主要代谢产物 7-羟基-TTX 在肾区小管沉积,导致肾小球前血管压力改变及肾小球滤过率显著降低。

通过选择肾功能良好的患者,确保充足的水化,并将尿液碱化至 pH=7 或更高,可以避免 MTX 的肾毒性反应。MTX 可能会积聚在液体环境中,因此,需要在给药前引流胸腔积液或腹水。给予 MTX 前,应确保良好的肾功能(正常血清肌酐,最低尿量为 100ml/h)。其他保护措施包括在开始治疗后 24~36h 内给予亚叶酸,并持续至血浆 MTX 水平<0. 1umol/L。监测潜在的药物相互作用至关重要:弱有机酸如水杨酸盐等可通过血浆蛋白结合位点的分子交换而增加 MTX 浓度。此外,丙磺舒和水杨酸盐可降低肾小管运输功能。因此在使用 MTX 期间应避免使用上述药物。

亚硝基脲

各种亚硝基脲(洛莫司汀[CCNU],甲基-洛莫司汀和卡莫司汀)都会引起显著的肾毒性反应[44,45],且已被Ⅲ期临床试验证实[46,47]。与 MTX 和顺铂不同,亚硝基脲会引起间质性肾炎。水化似乎并不能防止亚硝基脲引起的肾毒性反应,而限制累积剂量是预防肾毒性反应的主要方法。

丝裂霉素 C

丝裂霉素 C 是从链真菌中提取的抗生素。虽然已经在多瘤种中显示出显著的抗肿瘤活性,但由于持续血小板减少症等副作用,限制了其临床应用。丝裂霉素 C 也与溶血性尿毒症综合征(HUS)有关,药物暴露与 HUS 发病间的时间间隔差异很大[48]。接受丝裂霉素 C 治疗的患者应密切监测 HUS 的早期症状或体征(如肌酐或 LDH 升高,贫血等)。总剂量小于 30mg/m^2 很少发生 HUS,大多数发生于剂量>60mg 的患者[49]。虽然类固醇可以降低该药物的肺毒性,但并没有明显的肾脏保护作用。

靶向治疗

西罗莫司(mTOR)抑制剂如依维莫司(everolimus)和坦罗莫司可导致蛋白尿和急性肾损伤(AKI)[50],其机制主要为活检已证实的局灶性节段性肾小球硬化[51]以及急性肾小管坏死[52]。已有关于需要透析的不可逆肾损伤病例的报道。mTOR 抑制剂引起 AKI 时应即刻停药,且缺乏再次用药的指南证据。同时,对于合并有低蛋白血症,高血压或既往慢性肾病(CKD)的 65 岁以上患者发生不可逆肾损伤的可能性较高,因此不应再使用 mTOR 抑制剂[51]。

通过 VEGF 途径抑制血管生成的靶向药物(贝伐单抗、舒尼替尼、索拉非尼、培唑帕尼、阿昔替尼和卡博替尼)可能由于影响肾功能而产生蛋白尿和高血压。VEGF 表达于肾小球足细胞或毛细血管细胞,通过减少足细胞紧密连接而导致蛋白尿。这些副作用是剂量依赖的,并且停药后症状可逆。使用 VEGF 抑制剂的患者应定期监测血压,如果血压升高,应立即开始使用降压药物。利用 2~3 种药物控制血压的情况并不罕见,然而通过积极的血压管理可允许 VEGF 抑制剂的持续治疗。发生高血压和蛋白尿时建议使用 ACE 抑制剂作为一线抗高血压治疗。依照每种 VEGF 抑制剂的说明书治疗不同程度的蛋白尿。一般而言,中度蛋白尿应暂停治疗,如果蛋白尿达到肾病范围,则应永久停止治疗[53]。

免疫制剂

重组人白介素-2 可通过毛细血管渗漏性的肾前性氮质血症而引起肾功能不全。通过停药,静脉水化,必要时使用加压剂和肾功能所耐受剂量的多巴胺,可恢复肾功能[43]。环孢素可使肾入球小动脉收缩,引起动脉压升高以及肾素介导的肾功能不全[54]。急性肾毒性反应可通过调整剂量而恢复正常。相反,长期用药可能导致肾小管硬化继而发生不可逆的肾衰竭[55]。

近几年免疫检查点抑制剂已成为晚期癌症治疗的重要策略之一。伊匹木单抗:一种完全人类 IgG1 单克隆抗体,可阻断细胞毒性 T 淋巴细胞相关抗原 4(CTLA-4);纳武单抗:一种完全人 IgG4 抗体,可阻断程序性死亡受体-1(PD-1);帕博利珠单抗:一种人源化单克隆抗体针对 PD-1 的 IgG4-κ 同型抗体,都已成为抗癌的新型武器。这些抗体通过活化 T 细胞、恢复 T 细胞活性,从而增强免疫应答以达到显著的肿瘤杀伤效果[56]。但伊匹木单抗的副反应与患者多种自身免疫疾病相关,包括结肠炎,肺炎和极少数肾炎[57]。上述炎症与高度活化的 CD4 和 CD8 T 细胞的浸润和炎症细胞因子水平升高有关[58]。肾损伤的机制通常为间质性肾炎,而肾病综合征者报道较少[59,60]。停药后肾功能可恢复正常;类固醇或许也有所帮助[61]。纳武单抗与帕博利珠单抗的毒性反应均与人体免疫功能相关,但其副作用轻于伊匹木单抗。其原因可能是 PD-1/PD-L1 检查点相互作用于肿瘤细胞,而 CTLA4/B7 相互作用主要发生在淋巴器官,后者具有全身免疫反应进而影响肾功能[62]。基于上述药物作为单药治疗的疗效,以及 PD-1 和 CTLA-4 阻断效果的潜在协同作用,显然下一步探讨的便是这两种免疫途径相关药物的联合治疗。一项关于晚期黑色素瘤患者的Ⅰ期研究中联合使用了伊匹木单抗和纳武单抗,客观反应率达到 53%,80%以上的患者肿瘤缩小[56]。3/4 级不良事件(AE)发生率在既往多药治疗研究中达到最高(53%),高于单药治疗。与治疗相关的严重 AE 包括肝脏事件(15%),胃肠道事件(9%)和肾脏事件(6%)[56]。

其他药物

其他具有潜在肾毒性的药物见表 131-2。

药物相关肾毒性的临床监测

采用何种监测方式应参考预期的肾损伤机制。例如,由顺铂肾毒性引起的肾小管损伤可能不会立即反映在 GFR 下降,而高镁尿症和低镁血症是顺铂肾毒性的特征。使用可引起间质性肾炎(亚硝基脲)的药物时,需定期常规的检测尿液以评估肾毒性反应，而可能引起 HUS 的药物（丝裂霉素 C 和吉西他滨）应密切监测相关实验室数据。镜下血尿提示临床医师应进一步探索药物引起的肾损伤。

由细胞毒性药物引起的最常见肾功能异常表现为 GFR 下降，提示可能需要调整剂量或改变治疗方案。应特别注意根据体重所计算的准确肾功能。根据 Cockcroft-Gault 公式（表 131-6）计算的肌酐清除率对于一般正常体质的患者是准确的，但在偏瘦或超重人群中结果可能存在预测偏差。在接受肿瘤相关治疗时，患者的体重会出现大幅波动，需要规律监测体重并在每次化疗前计算 GFR。

表 131-6 Cockcroft-Gault 公式

$$\text{肌酐清除率}=\frac{(140-\text{年龄})\times\text{体重(kg)}}{72\times\text{血清肌酐(mg/dl)}}$$

（曹传振 寿建忠 译 邢念增 校）

参考文献

The complete reference list can be found on the Wiley Companion Digital Edition of this title (see inside front cover for login instructions).

2 Gutmann FD, Boxer RJ. Pathophysiology and management of urinary tract obstruction. In: Rieselbach RE, Garnick MB, eds. *Cancer and the Kidney*. Philadelphia: Lea & Febiger; 1982:594–624.

6 Bahu R, Chaftari AM, Hachem RY, et al. Nephrostomy tube related pyelonephritis in patients with cancer: epidemiology, infection rate and risk factors. *J Urol*. 2013;**189(1)**:130–135.

7 Misra S, Coker C, Richenberg J. Percutaneous nephrostomy for ureteric obstruction due to advanced pelvic malignancy: have we got the balance right? *Int Urol Nephrol*. 2013;**45(3)**:627–632.

8 Little B, Ho KJ, Gawley S, Young M. Use of nephrostomy tubes in ureteric obstruction from incurable malignancy. *Int J Clin Pract*. 2003;**57(3)**:180–181.

12 Trotman J, Nivison-Smith I, Dodds A. Haemorrhagic cystitis: incidence and risk factors in a transplant population using hyperhydration. *Bone Marrow Transplant*. 1999;**23(8)**:797–801.

14 Kohno A, Takeyama K, Narabajashi M, et al. Hemorrhagic cystitis associated with allogeneic and autologous bone marrow transplantation for malignant neoplasm in adults. *Jpn J Clin Oncol*. 1993;**23**:46–52.

16 Abt D, Bywater M, Engeler DS, Schmid HP. Therapeutic options for intractable hematuria in advanced bladder cancer. *Int J Urol*. 2013;**20(7)**:651–660.

18 Srivastava A, Nair SC, Srivastava VM, et al. Evaluation of uroprotective efficacy of amifostine against cyclophosphamide induced hemorrhagic cystitis. *Bone Marrow Transplant*. 1999;**23**:463–467.

21 Drake MJ, Nixon PM, Crew J. Drug-induced bladder and urinary disorders. Incidence, prevention and management. *Drug Saf*. 1998;**19**:45–55.

22 Brade WP, Herdrich K, Varani M. Ifosfamide—pharmacology, safety and therapeutic potential. *Cancer Treat Rep*. 1985;**12**:1–47.

24 Abudayyeh A, Abdelrahim M. Current strategies for prevention and management of stem cell transplant-related urinary tract and voiding dysfunction. *Curr Bladder Dysfunct Rep*. 2015;**10(2)**:109–117.

27 West NJ. Prevention and treatment of hemorrhagic cystitis. *Curr Opin Support Palliat Care*. 2014;**8(3)**:235–240.

28 Levenback C, Eifel PJ, Burke TW, Morris M, Gershenson DM. Hemorrhagic cystitis following radiotherapy for stage Ib cancer of the cervix. *Gynecol Oncol*. 1994;**55(2)**:206–210.

30 Krochak RJ, Baker DG. Radiation nephritis. Clinical manifestations and pathophysiologic mechanisms. *Urology*. 1986;**27(5)**:389–393.

31 Perez C, Brady L. *Principles and Practice of Radiation Oncology*, 3rd ed. Philadelphia: Lippincott-Raven; 1998.

32 Kapur S, Chandra R, Antonovych T. Acute radiation nephritis. Light and electron microscopic observations. *Arch Pathol Lab Med*. 1977;**101(9)**:469–473.

33 Lawton CA, Cohen EP, Murray KJ, et al. Long-term results of selective renal shielding in patients undergoing total-body irradiation in preparation for bone marrow transplantation. *Bone Marrow Transplant*. 1997;**20**:1069–1074.

34 Walker EM, Gale GR. Methods of reduction of cisplatin nephrotoxicity. *Ann Clin Lab Sci*. 1981;**11**:397–410.

35 Speer RJ, Ridgway H, Hall LM. Coordination complexes of platinum as antitumor agents. *Cancer Chemother Rep*. 1979;**59**:629–641.

36 Ozols RF, Cordon BJ, Jacobs J, et al. High-dose cisplatin in hypertonic saline. *Ann Intern Med*. 1984;**100**:19–24.

37 Gonzales-Vitale JC, Hayes DM, Cvitkovic E, Sternberg SS. The renal pathology in clinical trial of cisplatinum (II) diamminodichloride. *Cancer*. 1977;**39**:1362–1371.

38 Buamah PK, Howell A, Whitby H, et al. Assessment of renal function during high-dose cisplatin therapy in patients with ovarian carcinoma. *Cancer Chemother Pharmacol*. 1982;**8**:281–284.

39 Berns J, Ford P. Renal toxicities of antineoplastic drugs and bone marrow transplantation. *Semin Nephrol*. 1997;**17**:54–66.

41 Santoso JT, Lucci JA 3rd, Coleman RL, Schafer I, Hannigan EV. Saline, mannitol, and furosemide hydration in acute cisplatin nephrotoxicity: a randomized trial. *Cancer Chemother Pharmacol*. 2003;**52(1)**:13–18.

42 Gonzales-Vitale JC, Hayes DM, Cvitkovic E, Sternberg SS. Acute renal failure after cis-dichlorodiammineplatinum (II) and gentamicin-cephalothin therapies. *Cancer Treat Rep*. 1978;**62**:693–698.

43 Jariwala P, Kumar V, Kothari K, Thakkar S, Umrigar DD. Acute methotrexate toxicity: a fatal condition in two cases of psoriasis. *Case Rep Dermatol Med*. 2014;**2014**:946716.

44 Denine EP, Harrison SD, Pechkam JC. Qualitative and quantitative toxicity of sublethal doses of methyl-CCNU in BDF1 mice. *Cancer Treat Rep*. 1977;**61**:409–417.

45 Carter SK, Broder L, Friedman M. Streptozotocin and metastatic insulinoma. *Ann Intern Med*. 1971;**74**:445–446.

46 Harmon WE, Cohen HJ, Schneeberger EE, Grupe WE. Chronic renal failure in children treated with methyl CCNU. *N Engl J Med*. 1979;**300**:1200–1203.

47 Ellis ME, Weiss RB, Kuperminc M. Nephrotoxicity of lomustine. *Cancer Chemother Pharmacol*. 1985;**15**:174–175.

48 Medina PJ, Sipols JM, George JN. Drug-associated thrombotic thrombocytopenic purpura-hemolytic uremic syndrome. *Curr Opin Hematol*. 2001;**8(5)**:286–293.

49 El-Ghazal R, Podoltsev N, Marks P, Chu E, Saif MW. Mitomycin-C-induced thrombotic thrombocytopenic purpura/hemolytic uremic syndrome: cumulative toxicity of an old drug in a new era. *Clin Colorectal Cancer*. 2011;**10(2)**:142–145.

50 Hudes G, Carducci M, Tomczak P, et al. Temsirolimus, interferon alfa, or both for advanced renal-cell carcinoma. *N Engl J Med*. 2007;**356(22)**:2271–2281.

51 Izzedine H, Boostandoot E, Spano JP, Bardier A, Khayat D. Temsirolimus-induced glomerulopathy. *Oncology*. 2009;**76(3)**:170–172.

52 Izzedine H, Escudier B, Rouvier P, et al. Acute tubular necrosis associated with mTOR inhibitor therapy: a real entity biopsy-proven. *Ann Oncol*. 2013;**24(9)**:2421–2425.

53 Izzedine H, Rixe O, Billemont B, Baumelou A, Deray G. Angiogenesis inhibitor therapies: focus on kidney toxicity and hypertension. *Am J Kidney Dis*. 2007;**50(2)**:203–218.

56 Wolchok JD, Kluger H, Callahan MK, et al. Nivolumab plus ipilimumab in advanced melanoma. *N Engl J Med*. 2013;**369**:122.

57 Voskens CJ, Goldinger SM, Loquai C, et al. The price of tumor control: an analysis of rare side effects of anti-CTLA-4 therapy in metastatic melanoma from the ipilimumab network. *PLoS One*. 2013;**8(1)**:e53745.

58 Kaehler KC, Piel S, Livingstone E, Schilling B, Hauschild A, Schadendorf D. Update on immunologic therapy with anti-CTLA-4 antibodies in melanoma: Identification of clinical and biological response patterns, immune-related adverse events, and their management. *Semin Oncol*. 2010;**37**:485–498.

59 Fadel F, El Karoui K, Knebelmann B. Anti-CTLA4 antibody-induced lupus nephritis. *N Engl J Med*. 2009;**361(2)**:211–212.

60 Forde PM, Rock K, Wilson G, O'Byrne KJ. Ipilimumab-induced immune-related renal failure—a case report. *Anticancer Res*. 2012;**32(10)**:4607–4608.

61 Izzedine H, Gueutin V, Gharbi C, Mateus C, Robert C, et al. Kidney injuries related to ipilimumab. *Invest New Drugs*. 2014;**32(4)**:769–773.

62 Robert C, Soria JC, Eggermont AM. Drug of the year: Programmed death-1 receptor/programmed death-1 ligand-1 receptor monoclonal antibodies. *Eur J Cancer*. 2013;**49**:2968–2971.

第 132 章　心脏并发症

Michael S. Ewer, MD, MPH, JD, LLM, MBA ■ Steven M. Ewer, MD ■ Thomas Suter, MD

概述

恶性肿瘤患者通常会伴有心血管方面的问题，或者面临恶性肿瘤本身所致的严重心血管并发症。这些疾病可能由于动脉粥样硬化、高血压、瓣膜异常等潜在的原因所致，或者直接由肿瘤及其治疗所致（表 132-1）。此外，在非肿瘤患者中少见的心血管疾病可能在肿瘤患者中更常见且有时不易被考虑到。同时在非肿瘤患者中常见的心血管疾病在肿瘤患者中更不能忽略，在肿瘤患者中，这些心血管疾病的表现可能不典型，难以诊断。对于这类易感人群来说，需要更加仔细的临床观察。由于肿瘤、肿瘤相关治疗及心血管系统的相互作用，导致大量临床问题难以用单一因素进行解释，影响其中一个疾病通常也会改变另一个疾病的表现和病程。本章将着眼介绍肿瘤及其治疗相关的常见心血管并发症，并阐述一些肿瘤患者伴有心脏方面问题是所面临的棘手的临床问题。

癌症患者的心血管系统评估

癌症患者的心血管系统评估首先要进行详细的病史采集和完整的体格检查。在肿瘤患者中，常见有提示心力衰竭、心律不齐、心肌缺血和心包疾病的症状及体征，通常需要进行更严格的心血管系统评估[1]。针对个体的检测需要包括表 132-1 中列举的临床情况。如果临床评估结果预示患者可能合并心血管疾病，须进一步评估心电图、胸部 X 线检查及超声心动图。部分特殊的患者可能需要额外的影像学检查及诸如冠脉造影、心电生理检查等侵入性检查。心脏超声，或超声心动图在癌症患者中的应用最为广泛，在评估心脏收缩功能及心脏结构的完整性方面具有重要的作用[2]。完整的超声心动检查包括几项互补的检查，每一项检查都从不同的视角提供心脏异常的信息。经胸二维超声心动图显示了心脏的大部分结构，在部分切面中，可以观察到所有四个心腔以及肌壁的异常运动，从而评估节段性或弥漫性功能异常。使用二维超声心动图可以发现局限性或者包裹性心包积液以及原发或者转移性肿瘤，其他的影像学方法可以提供额外信息[3]。在一些超声图像结果显示不理想的情况，声学造影剂可以用来改善超声心动图图像结果，而这些造影剂也都已被认为安全可行并被广泛应用[4]。

作为心脏超声常规评估的一个部分，频谱与彩色血流多普勒超声可以显示血液在心腔及跨瓣膜时的方向及流速，这部分信息通常以图像的形式叠加在二维超声心动图上。多普勒超声最合适用来评估瓣膜血流动力学、心内分流、血流动力学紊乱以及血流方向异常。多普勒超声也用来评估心脏舒张功能，而心脏舒张功能作为心脏生理的组成部分，目前在临床工作中

表 132-1　癌症的重要心血管并发症

原发心脏肿瘤
• 恶性肿瘤
■ 心脏肿瘤
■ 心包肿瘤
转移瘤
• 心包转移
■ 心包积液
■ 心脏压塞
• 心肌转移
■ 心肌病
■ 心律失常
○ 快速心律失常
○ 心脏传导系统疾病
肿瘤治疗的并发症
• 冠脉痉挛
■ 心肌梗死
• 心律失常
■ 室上性
■ 室性
○ QT 间期延长
• 心肌病
■ Ⅰ型心肌功能异常（不可逆）
○ 慢性充血性心力衰竭
○ 心源性猝死
■ Ⅱ型心肌功能异常（可逆）
■ 舒张期充盈功能异常
• 高血压
• 放疗作用
其他病变
• 心肌淀粉样变
• 类癌性心脏病
• 血栓栓塞事件
• 肺动脉高压

占有越来越重要的作用。应变超声心动图(strain echocardiograph)可以辨别心肌细胞的主动及被动收缩。这些新技术的发展提高了超声检测技术的预测价值[5]。相比于经胸超声检查,经食管超声心动图可以提高某些特殊心脏结构的分辨率。尽管经食管超声心动图是半侵入性的,但是一般认为诊断敏感度的提高可以抵消这个缺点。经食管超声检查在检测赘生物等瓣膜病变或肿瘤的心肌受累具有很大优势,而这些病变在经胸超声中非常难以评估(图 132-1)。由于超声探头位置的原因,经食管超声检查科作为重要的辅助工具用来评估后壁心包积液(如术后)以及发现及监测心内的肿物或者血栓(图 132-2)[6]。术中经食管超声心动图有助于记录下腔静脉肿瘤累及范围及相关肿瘤切除后的结果(图 132-2)[5]。三维心脏超声现在已经开始应用于部分医学中心,可提供心脏内结构(如心脏瓣膜)的空间位置关系。这种技术可以允许二维的图像在一个选定的轴上旋转,可提供特殊方向上的图像[6]。

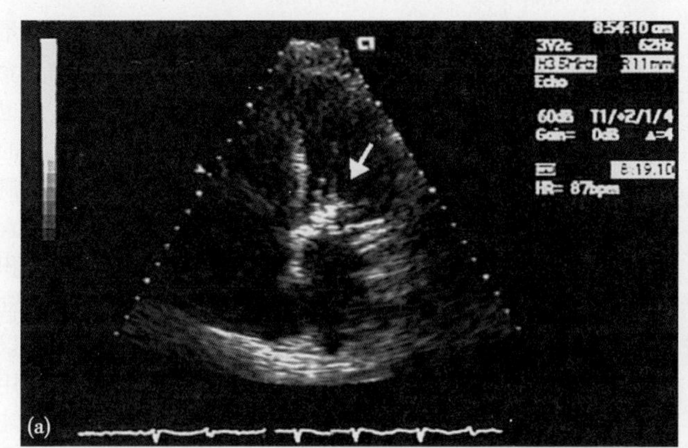

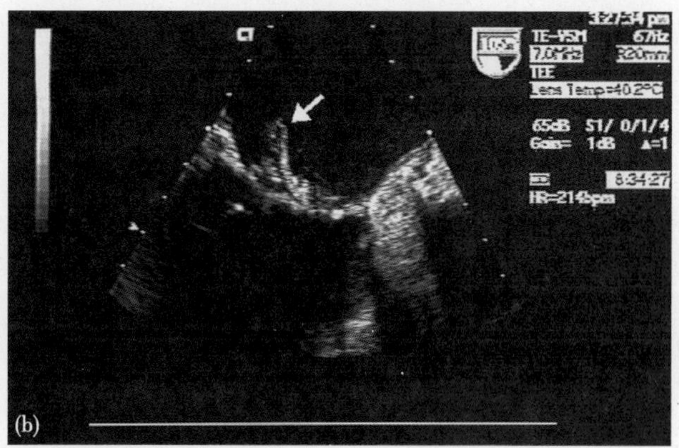

图 132-1 一名感染性心内膜炎累及二尖瓣患者的超声心动图。(a)患者可疑感染性心内膜炎累及主动脉瓣,经胸超声心动图五腔心切面显示主动脉瓣尖明显增厚。(b)同一天相同患者的经食管超声心动图能更清晰地显示主动脉瓣上的巨大赘生物

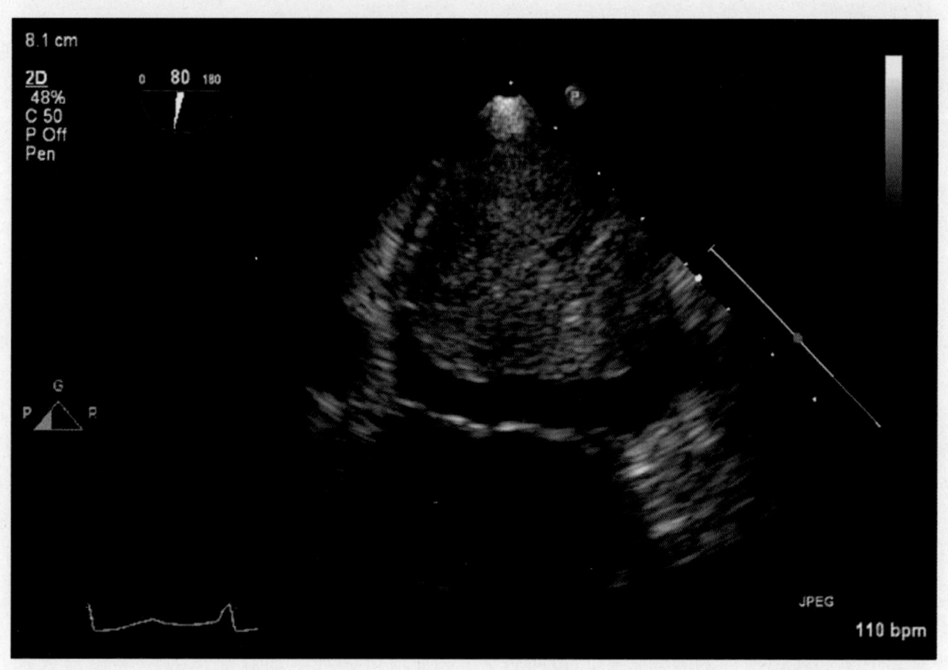

图 132-2 经食管超声心动图显示心绞痛患者左侧动脉的巨大肿物。超声心动表现符合肿瘤,病理显示为多形性黏液样肉瘤

核素显像技术可以同时提供心脏功能以及缺血性心脏病的评估。在患者接受已知或潜在具有心毒性药物治疗时,多重门控的心脏血池扫描仍是评估用药后左心室射血分数的常见手段。相比于超声心动图,核素显像技术的观察者内部差异及观察者间差异较小。这项技术需要心电图门控技术,因此在心律失常的患者中可能会出现问题。此外,多重门控扫描需数分钟进行数据采集,此时需要患者保持不动。一旦图像数据采集完毕,心脏放射性核素扫描可提供估算的射血分数、室壁运动异常的评估及心脏舒张功能的参数。尽管心脏放射性核素扫描过去常常用在大型肿瘤临床研究中用来评估心脏功能,但是由于心脏超声技术的进步以及对放射性暴露的担心,使得超声在临床研究内外都逐渐获得更多应用。无论应用哪种检测方

法,需要强调的是心功能可以被大量非心源性的因素影响,对于患者的心功能改变不能掉以轻心[7]。此外,需要注意的是,左室功能的轻微变化(左心室射血分数改变小于10%)通常与肿瘤以及其相关治疗无关,而更多的是与心脏功能的生理性改变相关,如患者的代谢状态、贫血程度或其他状态。

磁共振成像(magnetic resonance imaging,MRI)可以描述心内、心包及大血管的解剖关系,也可以显示心内及心包内的肿物[8]。尽管目前还未替代心脏超声,快速成像MRI、MR血管造影、增强MRI等技术在肿瘤患者的常规评估中具有越来越广泛的作用[9,10]。在某种程度上,MRI目前已经可以作为定量评估心室容积、心脏功能及肿瘤的金标准[11]。MRI的花费较大,同时其采集时间过长也是部分患者需要难以解决的难题。当患者无法接受其他评估方式评估射血分数时,越来越多的患者选择使用MRI进行评估。心脏计算机断层扫描(computerized tomography,CT)目前的应用也愈发广泛,与MRI类似,心脏CT可以清晰地显示心包及附近的心外结构。正电子发射断层显像(positron emission tomography,PET)其成像原理相较于传统的影像学技术具有优势,目前逐渐应用于肿瘤患者心肌活性评估[12]。

转移累及心脏结构

有8%~10%的肿瘤患者会出现累及心脏结构的转移瘤,而在老年患者中这一比例会降低[13]。这类转移通常由尸检时意外发现或者是肿瘤首发的灾难性表现。原发肿瘤的部位和类型各异,但新的影像学技术能更早地辨认出心脏受累,通常发现时能采取有效治疗措施。肿瘤侵及心脏结构可以通过直接侵犯(如肺癌及食管癌),逆行性淋巴转移(如肺癌及乳腺癌),或者通过血行播散(如黑色素瘤、白血病或淋巴瘤)。鉴于肺癌及乳腺癌相对高发,两者是最常累及心脏的肿瘤类型。

恶性黑色素瘤一旦转移多累及心脏结构[14]。其中以累及心包结构最为多见,其余可能被累及的部位包括心肌及心内膜。因此,对于霍奇金/非霍奇金淋巴瘤、白血病、消化道及妇产科肿瘤、多发性骨髓瘤及肉瘤的患者寻找转移灶时需要常规评估心脏(图132-2)[15]。此外,肾细胞癌可以通过下腔静脉累及右心房及右心室,而这些多可通过手术切除。

心包转移

心包积液

肿瘤患者的心包积液的性质可以是恶性或非恶性的,可能与肿瘤或其相关治疗相关,或者与合并的心脏或系统性疾病相关。恶性心包积液通常定义为病理确证的肿瘤侵犯心包所致的积液,尽管有时心包积液的常规细胞学检查无法获得恶性细胞的证据。在放疗、抗癌治疗、淋巴管阻塞、心包积液、体液分布的变化以及感染都可以导致心包积液。由于积液的量不同以及其施加于心包及心腔上的压力不同,不同心包积液的表现具有极大差异。液体聚集的速度以及心包腔的扩张性决定了心包积液对血流动力学的影响及相应的症状[16]。对心包上具有瘢痕或者心包壁层因受浸润而失去扩张性的患者而言,即使100ml的少量心包积液也会引起明显症状;而当心包腔弹性好,心包积液聚集缓慢的情况下,即使是1L的大量心包积液也不会引起明显的症状。恶性心包积液的出现通常提示预后不良[17]。

一般来说,心包积液并不是静态的,而是与其他体液处于流动平衡的状态。当心包腔内液体生成速度大于吸收速度时,异常的液体聚集便会出现,这种不平衡可能由于输出淋巴管阻塞或是隆突下淋巴结转移阻塞影响有效引流所致。恶性心包积液通常为血性浆液或血性液,常伴有细胞学可辨认的肿瘤细胞。当恶性积液为乳糜性时,其病因多为淋巴瘤,也有报道指出妇科肿瘤放疗后可造成乳糜性积液[18]。

伴有恶性心包积液的患者的可能没有明显的症状。大量具有大量心包积液的患者完全没有症状,他们通常通过胸片发现心影增大从而怀疑伴有心包积液。心电图QRS电压减低也预示着心包积液,但是在癌症患者中其他可导致电压减低的病因十分普遍,因此这个征象特异性低。新发的电压下降需要警惕心包积液的发生。心包积液通常为超声、放射性核素检查以及其他心脏影像学检查时偶然发现的,这些液体多积聚于分隔心脏与肝/肺血管的惰性区域。心脏在积液内摆动预示着血流动力学不稳定(心脏压塞)。胸部CT图像也可以显示心包积液,但是对定量提供不了显著帮助。胸部CT常用来评估胸部及纵隔的累及情况,可以同时提供有关心包积液的第一手信息。一旦怀疑患者出现心包积液,超声心动图可以用来明确诊断,其后积液的进展或吸收也可以通过超声心动图随访[19~21]。

心脏压塞

心包积液的积聚会导致心包内压整体性或局限性增高,影响心排出量(压塞)[22]。症状主要包括呼吸困难及活动耐量减低,体征包括低血压、心动过速、颈静脉扩张、肝大、心源性休克。心脏听诊多表现为心音遥远,难以听诊,有时可以闻及心包摩擦音。患者常有定位困难的胸闷及胸部不适。心包内压力显著增高的患者常伴有吸气时脉压显著下降;正常吸气时收缩压下降10mmHg以上称为奇脉。心脏压塞的典型表现还包括电交替,即指心电图的QRS波群电压呈高低交替性改变。这种现象是由心脏跳动时在含液体的心包腔内来回摆动,时而靠近电极时而远离电极所致。尽管电交替现象在心脏压塞内并不常见,但敏感性较高。心脏压塞通常可以通过体格检查及无创性的方法诊断。超声心动图可以用于心包积液的诊断以及判断心包积液的范围及位置。收缩时右心房塌陷是一种敏感但不特异的表现,当右心塌陷持续时间大于心动周期的1/3时这一征象的特异度显著提高。舒张期的右心室壁塌陷预示血流动力学不稳定,因此是一个更具特异性的表现。心脏压塞普遍表现为下腔静脉扩张,不可压缩。多普勒血流可显示主动脉流出及二尖瓣流入速度受呼吸影响极大。目前不推荐使用心导管明确心脏压塞的诊断,但可以用来显示奇脉的压力图,可发现随着心脏压塞的进展,心腔内舒张压将逐渐提升并重新达到平衡。心脏压塞时,患者吸气时的脉搏将变弱或消失,表现为心排出量减低的心源性休克。如果心脏压塞无法迅速缓解,会导致患者出现严重的心动过缓,甚至死亡。

对恶性心包积液及心脏压塞的治疗

对恶性心包积液的治疗取决于以下几点,包括肿瘤对局部(手术、放疗以及腔内治疗)或系统性抗癌治疗的效果,心包积液的范围以及所致症状以及患者的预期生存期[23,24]。对系统性治疗效果好的肿瘤患者应继续他们目前的治疗方案，恶性胸水可仅因抗癌治疗而消失。但是对于对治疗反应差的患者则需要局部干预。对于肿瘤预后好，身体一般情况好可以耐受全麻手术的肿瘤患者而言，可以选择心包开窗术。尽管经胸或者经剑突下入路效果类似，但是经剑突下入路住院期间死亡率要显著更高[25,26]。无论通过何种入路，形成的交通都能保持通畅，更大的胸膜面积重吸收液体的效率更高。对于大量心包积液或进展为心脏压塞的患者，为保证术前的稳定，心包腔穿刺引流有时很有必要。在积液清除后，患者的症状可以显著消失，此时的患者可以再次从事一些之前无法进行的体力活动。

目前穿刺引流通常在超声心动图引导下进行或者使用透视确认引流管位置，目前更小的穿刺设备以及更新的影像学技术显著减低了心包穿刺的风险[27]。部分患者在心脏压塞缓解后会出现一过性左室功能异常，因此需要进行一定时间的监护[28]。目前相较于经皮心包穿刺术，心包开窗未显示出明确的优势，部分研究显示由于心包开窗具有更大的创伤，其优势并不明确。对于大量心包积液但未发展为心脏压塞的患者来说，是否选择引流仍然存在争议。Merce 等指出该种方法诊断阳性率低，治疗效果差[29]。因此临床上对于类似患者的治疗需要综合他们的功能状态、肿瘤预后以及治疗中心的临床经验。

心包穿刺后可考虑硬化治疗，但是目前硬化治疗的应用已较前减少，这可能部分由于经过硬化治疗后患者会出现与操作相关的不适。已经经过研究报道使用的硬化剂包括：高渗葡萄糖、放射性金、博来霉素、无菌滑石粉、多西环素以及噻替哌(triethylenethiophosphoramide；thio-TEPA®)[30,31]。其中多西环素 250~500mg 可以达到有效的硬化效果[32]。许多患者在没有接受硬化治疗的情况下，每日引流至残留的心包积液量<50ml 可有效防止液体的再聚集[33]。球囊心包切开术(balloon pericardiotomy)目前正逐渐被外科心包切开术所取代，因为后者可在较小创伤下完成[34]。

恶性转移累及心肌

随着影像学技术的广泛应用，恶性肿瘤侵犯心肌逐渐被人们认识，在此之前心肌累及多是尸检时发现。大量生前确诊心肌受累的患者同时也伴有心包的受累。

心肌受累最典型的表现为突发的心律失常[35,36]。心源性猝死并不常见，而心脏穿孔及冠脉受侵蚀导致的出血或心肌梗死出现概率极低。一般而言，心肌受累的患者受有功能的心肌减少的影响，表现为进行性呼吸困难、运动耐量减低，检查可见心脏射血分数的减低。心电图表现为电位减低，其与冠脉阻塞导致的心肌梗死难以鉴别(图 132-3)。即使冠脉造影结果正常，这些患者仍可能出现 ST 段抬高，T 波倒置以及 Q 波等心电图表现[37]。

心肌受累的诊断难以确立。当高度怀疑患者合并心肌受累时，需行特殊的影像学检查进行明确，MRI 可以用来协助确定是否有心肌受累以及受累范围。尽管对于心肌转移的治疗通常为支持治疗，较大病灶或可导致瓣膜阻塞的病灶需要考虑行手术切除[38,39]。

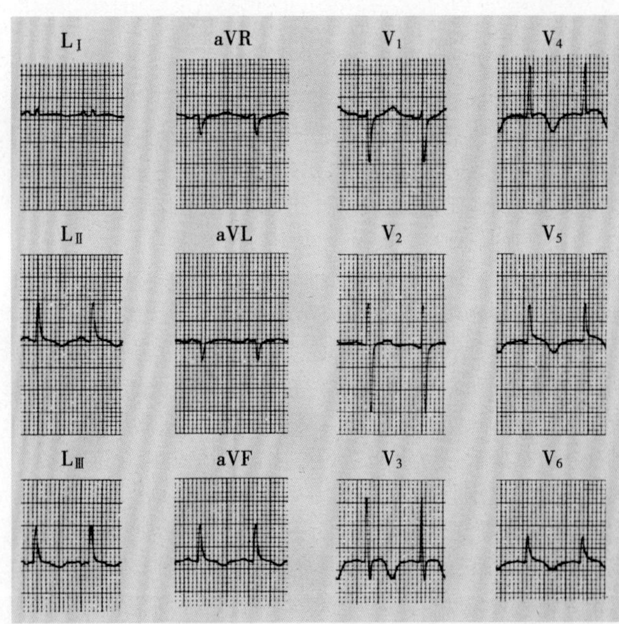

图 132-3 21 岁男性伴有经 MRI 证实的心肌受累，既往无心电图异常的病史，此次表现为心肌缺血。注意其下壁导联(2，3 与 AVF)及心前导联(V_4~V_6)显示的 T 波导致

肿瘤患者细胞介质释放、高输出状态以及浸润性病变对心脏功能的影响

代谢活跃的细胞介质通常与部分肿瘤性疾病相关，也可以导致很多肿瘤患者症状及体征[40]。细胞介质导致的疾病，即副肿瘤综合征，对心血管系统有直接及间接的影响。

类癌性心脏病

类癌起源于肠道嗜铬细胞来源的神经内分泌组织，多发生在肠道或者肺中，关于这类肿瘤的特点在本书其他章节有提及。肿瘤释放的大量具有生物活性的细胞介质使心脏产生特征性的纤维斑块并且破坏了心脏瓣膜的完整性，从而导致类癌性心脏病[41~46]。类癌性心脏病最常出现在肝转移的回盲部类癌患者中。而在支气管及卵巢类癌患者中也可能出现类癌性心脏病，此外如果来源于门脉系统以外，即使在没有肝转移的患者中也会出现类癌性心脏病。斑块形成及心肌损伤的原理还未阐明，但是一些可能的细胞介质包括激肽、血清素、五羟色胺、组胺及前列腺素可能参与相关途径，但仍有其他未明确的成分或组合可能也参与相关过程[47]。

细胞介质从肝脏转移瘤中释放进入肝静脉，从而使右心系统更易受损。此外，由于这些细胞介质在肺被清除，除非心脏存在右向左分流，否则左心系统多不受累及。这些病变多出现在大静脉、右心房及冠状窦的内膜。三尖瓣瓣叶边缘及远端(心室或其下游)通常增厚，而且通常累及腱索。肺动脉瓣可能会出现增厚、短缩。这些损伤会随着血流动力学紊乱而加剧，而这也解释了这些损伤的位置特点。当原发或者转移瘤位于肺的时候，细胞介质会直接释放进入肺静脉血管床，绕过肺组织的灭活作用，此时，左心瓣膜的损伤才会出现[48]。左心瓣膜损伤出现频率小于右心瓣膜损伤，但是更容易导致血流动力学异常。一项关于手术切除的瓣膜的回顾性分析显示不同瓣膜的组织学表现差异非常明显[49~51]。

类癌性斑块最明显的结果是瓣膜的增厚及纤维化,导致瓣膜及瓣环的扭曲变形。三尖瓣关闭不全及肺动脉瓣狭窄是其典型表现,而当病变进展,也会出现三尖瓣僵硬导致同时出现狭窄及反流的血流动力学异常。明显的肺动脉瓣反流是罕见的。右心房的僵硬可导致颈静脉扩张,颈静脉扩张是类肿瘤综合征患者中常见体征。同时也可能导致高输出状态,这同样可能是由于细胞介质的释放所致[52]。

类癌性心脏病的临床表现差异极大。部分患者对由瓣膜病导致的血流动力学问题耐受较好,但是有部分患者症状出现较早,特别是那些老年或者有心脏基础疾病的患者[53]。早期的症状包括疲乏、劳力性呼吸困难,以及高输出状态和/或心律失常所致的心悸。后期的症状主要为右心充血性心力衰竭所致的症状,主要包括水肿、肝大、腹水。心脏杂音通常早于症状出现,三尖瓣反流的杂音通常是早期表现。这种心脏杂音通常为沿左下胸骨缘分布的高调、全收缩期吹风样杂音,吸气时杂音增强。肺动脉狭窄的杂音难以与三尖瓣反流杂音相鉴别,两者常同时存在,其中肺动脉瓣杂音更加粗糙,其分布主要位于左侧第二肋间。

胸片可显示右心室扩大。与类癌性心脏病不同,先天性肺动脉狭窄通常包括继发于狭窄后的肺动脉干的扩张。心电图可显示右心容积及压力负荷的变化,伴或不伴右心房畸形、右心室增生、右束支传导阻滞、电轴右偏,同时也可以显示肢体导联的低电压。

超声心动图是类癌性心脏病的最有效的非侵入性诊断方法(图 132-4)。它不仅可以诊断瓣膜异常,当与多普勒超声检查结合时,它可以同时提供血流动力学数据用来评估瓣膜受累的程度[54]。随着三尖瓣瓣叶的增厚及活动度下降,舒张期跨三尖瓣的血流流速上升。右心房收缩期也常可见看到反流。此外,右心房及右心室的增大为此阶段特征性表现,而超声心动图也可以定量测量右心房及右心室的大小。当大小足够大时,超声心动图在诊断转移性类癌累及心脏方面非常有帮助[55]。

对于类癌性心脏病的治疗通常十分困难而且需要进行个体化考虑。尽管类癌斑块通常不可逆,但是控制及清除致病的细胞介质可延迟斑块进展。在这个方面来说,对原发及转移肿瘤的治疗是十分重要的。当类癌性心脏病诊断明确时,患者首先接受利尿剂、减低后负荷以及限盐的治疗。β 肾上腺素能拮抗剂的效果尚未被证实。手术干预如瓣膜成形术或者瓣膜替换术因为其能改善患者的预后,因此目前的应用愈加频繁,而且也有学者提出应早期干预治疗[44]。

高输出状态以及高输出性心力衰竭

在很多癌症患者中会出现心排出量增高,主要原因包括贫血、甲状腺功能亢进、抗利尿激素分泌异常或血液向肿瘤的分流。在多发性骨髓瘤的患者中高输出状态较为普遍[56]。此外,肝脏疾病(营养不良性肝硬化及感染性肝炎)、发热、情绪激动、低氧血症同样也是导致心排出量增加及高动力状态的常见原因。高输出状态也常出现在一些生物反应调节剂治疗后,包括干扰素(可能由于发热及流感样反应)以及白介素,而这些反应多持续时间较短。

高输出状态通常伴有心率上升(通常 85~110 次/min,但有时更高)及心脏每搏输出量上升。由于右心压力未上升,因此体格检查颈静脉通常未见明显异常。外周脉搏通常波动性强,通常伴有快速的上升及下降,一般收缩期血压提高但是舒张期血压通常降低。听诊显示第四心音。肺瘀血在高充血状态下并不常见。

超声心动图以及放射性核素显象对于诊断非常具有帮助。二维超声检查可以在所有切面下显示室壁运动增强。在某些特殊患者中,可以看到收缩期右心室近乎完全消失,射血分数升高。多普勒超声显示在四个瓣膜区均有血流上升。心脏放射性核素扫描可以提供左心室射血分数及心脏输出量的信息。使用右心导管测量心排出量可以明确诊断,但是临床上应用较少。需要注意的是不要将其与临床上更常见的低输出量的充血性心力衰竭的临床影像相混淆。对于高输出状态需要针对病因治疗,对于肿瘤患者而言,转移瘤是最常见的病因,可伴或不伴有分流、甲状腺功能亢进、低氧血症、贫血以及感染。因此输血、利尿剂、吸氧以及退热药可治疗高输出状态。在某些特殊病例中,β 肾上腺素受体拮抗药也可以提供一定的帮助。但是除非患者有症状,高输出状态并不需要特殊的对症治疗,而需要直接对潜在病因进行治疗。

心脏淀粉样变

淀粉样变指淀粉样蛋白质的异常沉积,可由多种病理性过程产生,出现在心脏等多种器官之中[57]。淀粉样蛋白是由反向平行的 β 折叠的原纤维构成,常沉积在间质中难以被蛋白水解酶水解。它们由多种前体蛋白组成[57,58]。临床上大量肿瘤相关性淀粉样变的患者为多发性骨髓瘤患者,其中少量为霍奇金淋巴瘤患者。与这些疾病相关的淀粉样蛋白为 AL 型淀粉样蛋白,它们是由免疫球蛋白轻链片段(Igλ 及 Igκ)沉积导致。AL 型淀粉样蛋白沉积在心房及心室的心肌中,可导致限制性心肌病或扩张性心肌病。也有报道指出心内膜下淀粉样蛋白沉积会导致瓣膜异常。

心脏淀粉样变的患者易疲劳,并表现出心排出量减低的症状。呼吸困难以及水肿为其常见表现,有时也会伴有厌食、体重减低以及晕厥。除了心力衰竭以外,也有报道指出会发生房性或者室性心律失常以及心脏栓塞事件。会出现的体征包括颈静脉压升高、水肿、肝瘀血、腹水、低血压、巨舌、眶周紫癜。传导异常可以出现在心脏淀粉样变患者中,当其合并心率减低或者低输出状态时可出现症状。急性应激性的晕厥可能是心源性猝死的前兆[59,60]。心脏淀粉样变可同时导致心脏舒张及收缩功能受损。临床上限制性心肌病与缩窄性心包炎难以鉴别,即使右心导管也难以得到确诊。胸片显示心影正常或略微增大。当心力衰竭出现时,肺瘀血及胸腔积液都可能出现。心电图表现包括电压下降、假性心肌梗死表现、传导系统异常以及房性心律失常[61]。超声心动图对于诊断心脏淀粉样变十分有帮助(图 132-5)。超声虽然显示左心室心腔体积未见明显异常,但是会显示室间隔及后壁的增厚。此外,超声心动图中常可显示颗粒状强回声,心包积液较少见。即使没有房性心律失常,心肌淀粉样变患者仍可出现心房通常增大,机械功能减低。超声心动图上显示的左心室增厚与心电图上电压减低的相悖

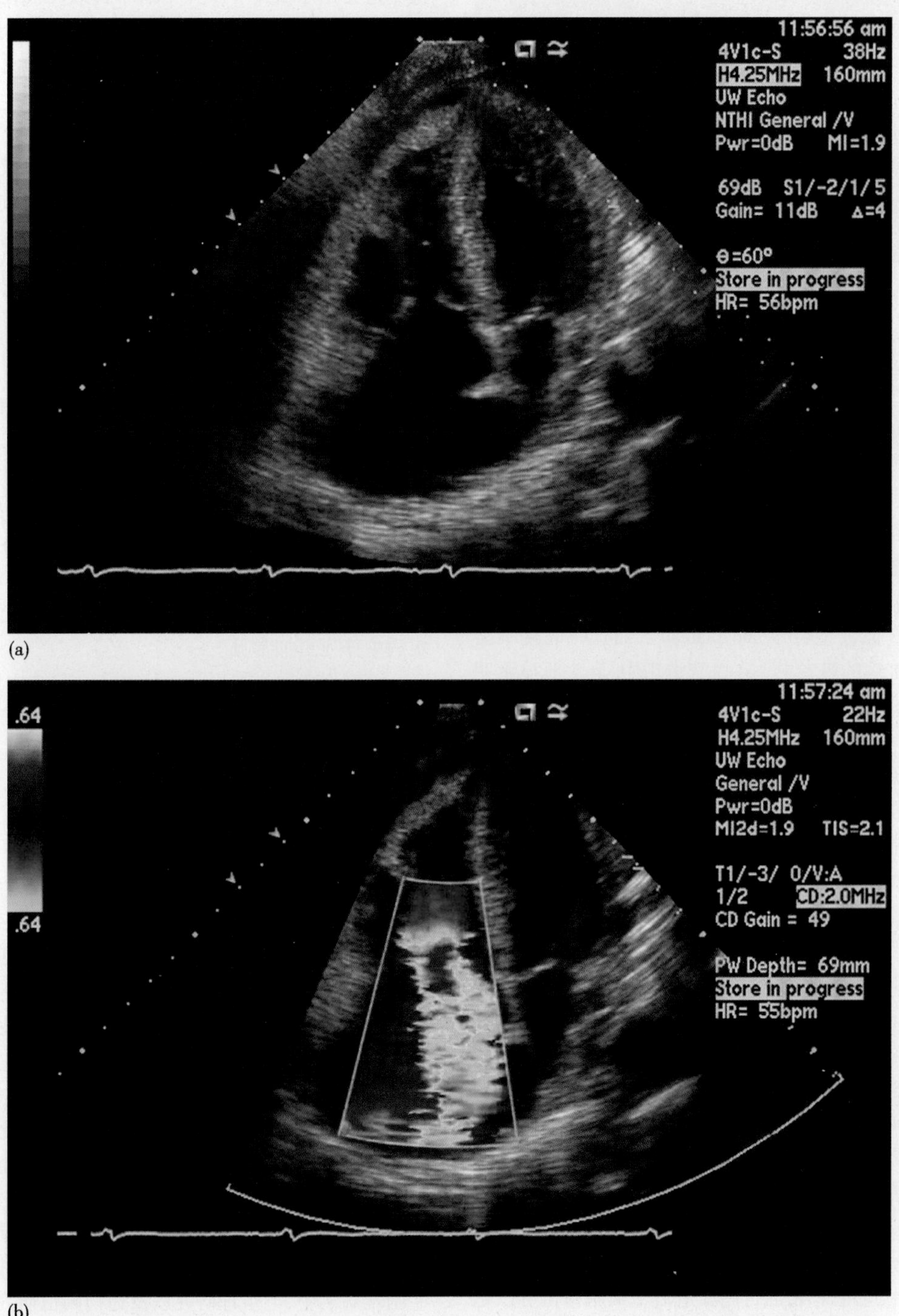

图 132-4　类癌性心脏病:(a)二维四腔心切面显示三尖瓣瓣叶的增厚及粘连。(b)相同的四腔心切面联合彩色多普勒超声显示严重的三尖瓣反流。同样的证据显示右心房、右心室的增大以及少量心包积液

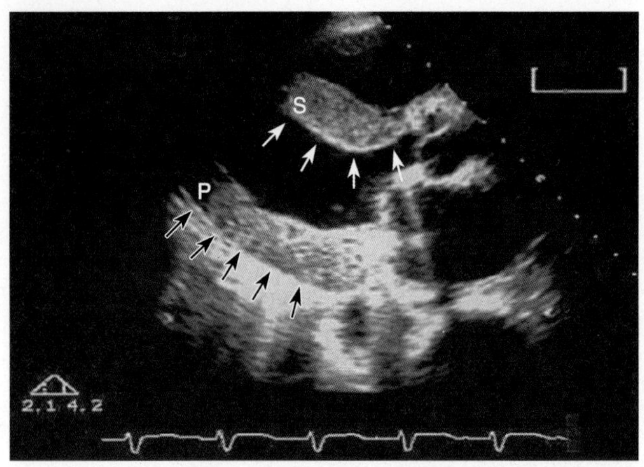

图 132-5　心脏淀粉样变患者的超声心动图长轴观。注意增厚的室间隔及后壁伴有颗粒样回声增强

提示心脏淀粉样变[62]。有报道指出在抗肌球蛋白闪烁显现(anti-myosin scintigraphy)中出现左心室增厚以及弥漫性心肌抗肌球蛋白高摄取预示淀粉样心脏病。心脏 MRI 对诊断淀粉样变心肌浸润十分有帮助,其延迟增强的特点有助于鉴别淀粉样心脏病以及其他心肌病[63]。

心导管显示全心腔压力增高,其中左室压力通常升高至少10mmHg。缩窄性心包炎患者中常见的舒张期心室压力曲线呈现早期下陷晚期高原波型(dip and plateau),而这一表现不会出现在淀粉样心脏病的患者中。在血管造影中,乳头肌显示明显。刚果红染色的心内膜心肌活检组织对于明确诊断十分有帮助[64]。

目前缺乏对于心脏淀粉样变的治疗手段。袢利尿剂是内科治疗的基础。强心苷类药物由于致心律失常作用,对于淀粉样心脏病患者非常危险,有报道称在淀粉样心脏病患者使用强心苷类药物后出现猝死[65]。β 肾上腺素受体抑制剂以及非二氢吡啶钙通道阻滞剂可进一步减低心排出量,血管紧张素转化酶抑制药可引起严重的低血压。临床上使用植入式除颤器治疗恶性心律失常,但是目前没有证据支持其在淀粉样变心脏病患者中的使用[66]。患者临床状况的改善与患者淀粉样变的控制是平行的,对于黑色素瘤的系统性治疗可延迟或减轻患者的黑色素瘤相关心脏淀粉样变的症状[67]。心内血栓是心肌淀粉样变患者的显著风险。在一项尸体解剖的序列研究中显示心内血栓的发生率为 33%。因此临床上建议心脏淀粉样变的患者接受抗凝治疗。目前临床治疗方案包括美法仑、环磷酰胺、卡莫司汀以及长春新碱等抗肿瘤药物以及造血干细胞移植[58]。极少数由于轻链沉积导致的限制型心肌病可以逆转。在某些特定人群中,心脏移植后行同源造血干细胞移植可以达到治疗效果[68]。

肿瘤患者的心律失常

在肿瘤患者中心律失常十分普遍。节律异常可能是由于肿瘤导致的,但是其更普遍的原因包括抗肿瘤治疗、代谢异常以及患者合并的心脏疾病导致患者更易发生心律失常。肿瘤患者的节律分布在形态及功能上与非肿瘤患者的一致。在某些情况下,我们需要积极地抑制心律失常,但在其他情况下,心律失常可能是由于体内稳态变化导致的临时变化,多仅需稍加干预或无须进行干预。大量抗肿瘤药与短暂性心律失常相关,这一心律失常多无明显症状,因此这一现象目前尚未被足够重视。这类化疗相关节律异常通常持续时间短、临床意义不大,但是其可能为心肌受累的表现,其后可能就会出现明显症状。因此,与抗肿瘤治疗相关的心律失常并不能作为替换肿瘤药物的绝对指征。

临床上需要面临许多问题,包括哪部分患者需要进行治疗,何时开始他们的治疗,治疗进行多久以及该进行何种形式的治疗(药物治疗或者行电刺激)。多种的抗心律失常药没有简化这些临床问题。其中有助于判断该如何进行治疗的方法即为判断心律失常的原因,判断其是源于毒性物质或其他代谢异常所致抑或是由心脏结构异常所致[36]。

心律失常的分类:原发性(结构性)或继发性(代谢性)

心脏结构的异常包括一大类可导致心脏异常的心脏疾病。此类疾病包括缺血性心脏病、心肌肥大、瓣膜疾病以及浸润性疾病。在肿瘤患者中,肿瘤侵犯、化疗过程中的细胞丢失、药物所致的缺血以及放疗导致的纤维化也包括在这类疾病中。无论是室上性还是室性的严重心律失常可无任何前兆,而迅速导致血流动力学不稳定以及心源性猝死。在淀粉样变等浸润性疾病中猝死更加常见。

癌症患者的心律失常也可由非心脏结构异常的病因所致。最常见的原因包括容量变化、电解质紊乱、药物作用以及激素水平变化,其他可影响心脏起搏器以及传导组织的代谢因素也应包括在此类中。

对心律失常的治疗

对于由于代谢异常导致的未威胁生命的心律失常可行保守治疗,此时治疗原发病时行密切观察即可。当心律失常导致血流动力学异常,心律失常进展至威胁生命或者持续的心律失常导致血栓栓塞事件发生率上升时需要进行积极治疗。室性心律更为常见,其中包括室性期前收缩、良性加速性室性自主心律以及恶性室性心律失常以及心室纤颤。发热、乏力等伴随症状可增加组织缺血情况,使患者出现室性心律失常,这种情况在贫血患者中更严重。肿瘤患者的意外死亡多由于心律失常。无论病因如何,当出现血流动力学不稳定时就需要考虑结合高级心脏生命支持的医学急救。

一旦决定对心律失常患者进行治疗,需结合指南选择药物治疗以及植入起搏器、除颤仪或消融治疗等非药物治疗。在某些困难病例中,电生理研究以及药物阈值研究可有帮助。在肿瘤患者中,植入性设备的使用比例逐渐增高,恶性疾病不应成为植入性设备使用的禁忌,但是使用时需考虑患者的预后情况。

目前有越来越多的药物涉及尖端扭转型室速这一特殊的室性心律失常。这种多形性的心律失常(图 132-6)出现之前多有 QT 间期延长。QT 间期的测量从 QRS 波群开始至 T 波结束为止,并且需要依据心率校准。这种心律失常与一些因素相关,包括部分抗生素(红霉素、克拉霉素及喷他脒)、抗精

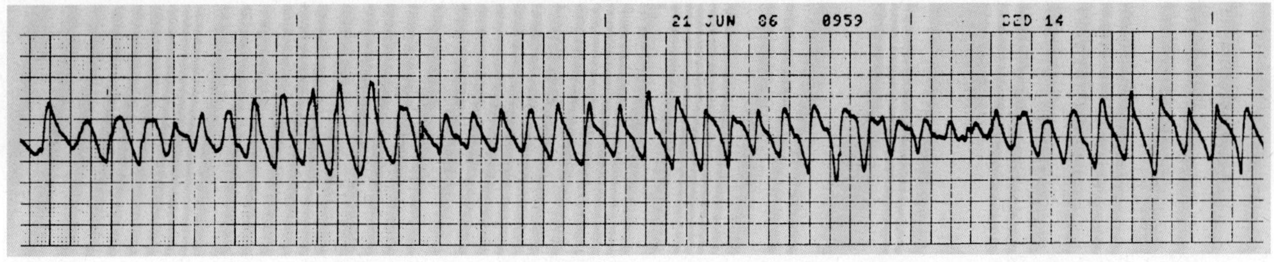

图 132-6　尖端扭转型室速患者的心率记录。之前的心律记录(未显示)显示 QT 间期延长

神病药(氟哌利多)、止吐药、部分高剂量化疗方式以及骨髓移植[69~71]。作为治疗急性早幼粒细胞白血病药物的三氧化二砷也可致 QT 间期延长,因此患者治疗期间因密切关注是否有 QT 间期延长[72,73]。及时识别这种潜在的恶性心律失常并且停用致病药物可能为其最合适的治疗方式。有部分消息指出,尖端扭转型室速更易出现在非裔美国人中。QT 延长在男性及低血钾患者中发生率更高。推荐对高危患者进行 QT 间期的检测[74]。表 132-2 列出了与 QT 延长相关的最重要的药物。

表 132-2　与 QT 间期延长以及已知可致尖端扭转型室速的药物

胺碘酮(amiodarone)	盐酸卤泛群(halofantrine,氯氟菲醇)
阿那格雷(anagrelide)	氟哌利多(haloperidol)
三氧化二砷(arsenic trioxide)	伊布利特(ibutilide)
阿司咪唑(astemizole)	左氧氟沙星(levofloxacin)
阿奇霉素(azithromycin)	levomethadyl
苄普地尔(bepridil)	美索达嗪(mesoridazine)
氯喹(chloroquine)	美沙酮(methadone)
氯奥沙普秦(chlorpromazine)	莫西沙星(moxifloxacin)
环丙沙星(ciprofloxacin)	昂丹司琼(ondansetron)
西沙必利(cisapride)	喷他脒(pentamidine)
西酞普兰(citalopram)	匹莫齐特(pimozide)
克拉霉素(clarithromycin)	普罗布考(probucol)
可卡因(cocaine)	普鲁卡因(procainamide)
丙吡胺(disopyramide)	丙泊酚(propofol)
多非利特(dofetilide)	奎尼丁(quinidine)
多潘立酮(domperidone)	七氟烷(sevoflurane)
决奈达隆(dronedarone)	索他洛尔(sotalol)
氟哌利多(droperidol)	司帕沙星(sparfloxacin)
红霉素(erythromycin)	舒必利(sulpiride)
艾司西酞普兰(escitalopram)	特非那定(terfenadine)
氟卡尼(flecainide)	硫利达嗪(thioridazine)
氟康唑(fluconazole)	凡德他尼(vandetanib)
格帕沙星(grepafloxacin)	

摘录自亚利桑那州治疗教育和研究中心。参考文献:https://crediblemeds.org/(访问时间 2015 年 5 月 1 日)。

对于尖端扭转型室速急救是通过非同步电除颤。一线内科治疗方案包括静脉内注射硫酸镁,无论患者血清镁浓度如何。注射异丙肾上腺素以及超速起搏可以通过增加心率缩短 QT 间期以抑制尖端扭转型室速。利多卡因及苯妥英钠是另外的治疗选择[75,76]。维持钾和镁稳态对于预防这种心律失常复发至关重要。影响 QT 间期的药物需要被鉴别出来并停用,另外避免使用其他可以导致 QT 延长的药物。

癌症治疗的心脏并发症

癌症非手术治疗方式可在多方面影响心脏。这些治疗包括多种药物、生物制剂以及诸如电离辐射等物理治疗(表 132-3)。多种不同方法及其组合可以有各自独立作用、累加作用或者协同作用,蒽环类药物联合心脏放疗可产生累加作用及协同作用的毒性。癌症治疗的损伤可影响心包、心肌、脉管、传导系统及心脏瓣膜。在某些治疗方式中,心脏可发生亚临床损伤,之后的损伤以及一系列应激变化可导致心功能不全的临床表现[77]。

具有心脏毒性的抗癌药物

具有心脏毒性的抗癌药物可导致永久或临时的收缩功能障碍、心肌缺血、心律失常以及血压波动。接下来将按照下述分类对这些具有心脏毒性的抗癌药物进行讨论。

导致左心室功能异常的药物

蒽环类药物以及其相关蒽醌类药物是最常被研究的影响收缩功能异常的药物,其他药物可能通过其他途径影响心脏功能。常基于药物的基础功能及其他性质将抗肿瘤药物分为两种类型,Ⅰ型及Ⅱ型[78]。Ⅰ型药物为原发性,通常直接导致心肌细胞损伤及细胞死亡。一旦心脏损伤达到阈值导致细胞死亡就会导致永久损伤。Ⅰ型药物导致的损伤通常可累积,具有剂量效应,心内膜心肌活检可有典型的改变。Ⅱ型药物导致的心脏功能异常可导致心肌冬眠或晕厥等可逆的心肌功能异常,此外这些药物可通过增加前负荷及液体潴留导致室壁应力上升继而损伤脆弱的心肌细胞。Ⅱ型药物的毒性未显示可累积及剂量效应,并且与蒽环类药物导致损伤不同,这些药物不导致典型的心内膜心肌损伤[77]。这些区别总结在表 132-4 中。

Ⅰ型抗肿瘤治疗相关药物:蒽环类及其相关药物

蒽环类药物的作用是目前所有具有心脏毒性药物中研究最普遍的,此次使用多柔比星的心脏毒性模型作为理解蒽环类药物相关的Ⅰ型心肌病变的模型。

表 132-3　心脏毒性相关抗肿瘤药物

Ⅰ. 与Ⅰ型心肌抑制相关药物	IFN-α
蒽环类药物	Ⅳ. 缺血相关抗肿瘤药物
多柔比星	氟尿嘧啶
吡柔比星	卡培他滨
伊达比星	长春碱
表柔比星	长春新碱
柔红霉素	博来霉素
蒽醌类药物	顺铂
米托蒽醌	生物反应调节剂
潜在的毒性增强剂	Ⅴ. 与低血压相关的抗肿瘤药物
环磷酰胺	重组人白介素-2
异环磷酰胺	高三尖杉酯碱
丝裂霉素 C	Ⅵ. 与高血压相关的抗肿瘤药物
依托泊苷	贝伐单抗
美法仑	舒尼替尼
长春新碱	Ⅶ. 与肺动脉高压相关抗肿瘤药物
博来霉素	达沙替尼(dasatinib)
紫杉醇	Ⅷ. 已知或潜在具有其他心脏毒性作用的药物
毒性抑制剂	紫杉醇(心动过缓)
右丙亚胺	三氧化二砷(延长 QT 间期/尖端扭转型室速)
Ⅱ. Ⅱ型心肌抑制相关药物	博来霉素
曲妥珠单抗	放线菌素 D
拉帕替尼	丝裂霉素 C
舒尼替尼	烷化剂
格列卫	环磷酰胺
其他单克隆抗体或酪氨酸激酶抑制剂	异环磷酰胺
Ⅲ. 其他心脏抑制作用药物	Ⅸ. 放疗(剂量依赖性,可以影响所有心脏结构)
环磷酰胺(高剂量)	

表 132-4　Ⅰ型与Ⅱ型治疗相关心脏功能异常

Ⅰ型(如多柔比星)	Ⅱ型(如曲妥珠单抗)
细胞死亡	细胞功能异常
首次使用即可造成损失	
活检改变(蒽环类典型改变)	无典型蒽环类活检改变
剂量累积效应	无剂量累积效应
永久性损伤(心肌细胞死亡,预后差)	大多数可逆改变(心肌细胞功能异常,预后好)
危险因素:	危险因素:
联合化疗[译者注:原文为 CT 检查(computed tomographic,CT),应为化疗 CT (chemotherapy)]	既往或同时使用蒽环类药物或者紫杉醇治疗
既往或者同期联合放疗	
年龄	年龄
既往心脏疾病	既往心脏疾病
高血压	肥胖(BMI>25kg/m^2)

多柔比星的心脏毒性可见于治疗的早期或晚期，也可以在治疗结束后数月或数年出现。心脏毒性的早期表现包括心电图异常以及心肌心包炎。以目前的药物剂量而言，早期显著的心脏功能异常较为少见，但是也有报道指出首次用药几周内出现心力衰竭[79,80]。早期的心脏毒性更多出现在老年以及接受单次大剂量药物治疗的患者中，也有报道指出使用柔红霉素的患者心脏毒性的发生率高于使用多柔比星的患者。也有极少报告指出使用多柔比星后患者出现猝死。当使用多柔比星时会出现室性及室上性心律失常，但是极少危及生命。目前有证据指出这些现象与多柔比星导致的细胞损伤及细胞死亡有关，而这也被用药后肌钙蛋白 T 等心脏损伤的标志物升高所证实[81,82]。因此早期临床表现可能比之前的认识更重要，用药后肌钙蛋白的释放是早期细胞死亡的重要标志物。这种初始的损伤标志着心肌损伤的开始，但是由于心脏对于心肌损失的巨大代偿能力，这种变化一般难以识别，虽然目前常使用射血分数来评估心肌损伤，但是临床上尚缺乏评估心肌储备的微小变化的手段[83]。

多柔比星的累积剂量与心力衰竭的发生率相关。当累积剂量低于 400mg/m^2 时，患者明显的临床症状并不普遍，但是当多柔比星快速输入累积剂量达到 450mg/m^2 时患者发生明显临床症状的风险显著提高[84]。当合并其他心脏毒性药物时，多柔比星所致心肌病可能在低剂量时出现（详见之后的讨论）。多柔比星导致的心肌损伤在不同患者间差异显著而且难以解释，其原因可能为之前的心脏损伤、其他可提高心肌损伤易感性的情况，基因可能在其中发挥一定的作用，这也是近年来研究的热点。当患者在早期，即最后一次使用多柔比星 4 周内出现心脏功能失代偿，预示患者预后不良，甚至有生命危险。早期出现毒性反应的患者可能具有更严重的初始损伤以及更少的基线心脏功能储备。多柔比星心肌病的症状可能在接近或达到临床最大推荐剂量的常规化疗的几个月或者几年后出现。这种延迟的心肌病可能包括额外的损伤以及应激反应[77]。一系列的应激反应及损伤可能可以解释在部分病例中出现的延迟心肌病。多柔比星进入临床应用已四十余年，对罹患白血病、淋巴瘤、肉瘤及乳腺癌的患者具有治疗作用，但是治疗期间可能会出现亚临床心脏损伤，此类患者在遇到额外的心脏损伤事件时更易出现有症状的心力衰竭。目前还没有证据证实多柔比星对于冠脉疾病、缺血性心肌病等年龄相关的心脏损伤的作用。但是在既往的回顾分析中，在 43 名多柔比星所致的心肌病患者中，有 12 名因进行性心脏功能不全而死亡[85]。

蒽环类药物相关心脏毒性的机制

蒽环类药物所致心脏损伤的机制尚未被完全阐明，但是自由基的形成被认识是其中的重要因素。自由基会损伤心肌细胞的脂质结构，而脂质结构的过氧化反应会损伤内质网及线粒体的功能。在退行性变之前，心肌细胞会因为缺乏过氧化氢酶及过氧化物歧化酶而导致其处理自由基的功能弱于其他细胞[86]。细胞死亡是这种损伤的最终结果。有证据指出心脏毒性药物的原理与肿瘤疗效并不一致，因此对于心脏的保护是可行的。氧自由基的产生与心脏毒性相关，目前越来越多证据指出拓扑异构酶Ⅱβ 也在其中起重要作用，可能可以通过使用右旋丙亚胺对拓扑异构酶的抑制从而起到心脏保护作用[87,88]。目前认为在部分出现多柔比星相关心脏毒性的患者中，其心房钠尿肽水平会增高，这一表现相比于收缩功能与舒张功能更加相关[89]。

蒽环类药物相关心脏毒性的临床表现

蒽环类药物相关心肌病的临床表现与其他充血性心力衰竭的症状难以鉴别。在早期患者多无症状或仅表现轻微的心脏功能异常。在大多数患者中，最早出现的症状为运动后短时间内无法恢复到基线心率。患者也可能出现休息时心动过速以及失去心率的呼吸变异。当心力衰竭进展时，患者呼吸困难会加重，出现静息时呼吸困难时预后不良的标志。

已进展为心肌病的患者通常表现为 S3 奔马律、心脏浊音界增大、轻微运动后心率显著升高以及当肺瘀血时出现弥漫性啰音。胸片显示心影增大以及脉管系统充血的非特异性表现。有时可发现胸腔积液。心电图表现为非特异性的复极化改变。作为容量过剩以及高心室充盈压的标志，B 型钠尿肽通常增高，增高的比例与心力衰竭的程度相匹配[90,91]。对于接受蒽环类或者相关药物治疗的患者来说，左室射血分数仍是最常见的监测心功能的指标。

心肌活检显示心肌的结构改变可提供证明多柔比星及其相关物质所致心脏毒性的重要信息[92~94]。在一些高选择性的患者中，心肌活检可以在安全的前提下提供必要的信息[95]。心脏活检可以通过电镜评估病变的程度以及范围，并决定最终的分级。但是就目前使用的蒽环类方案而言，已不再采用心脏活检。

目前已经证实了在某些患者中即使接受相对低累积剂量的多柔比星，也有较高的心功能不全风险。这些患者包括老年患者、儿童患者以及既往有心血管疾病以及基线射血分数低的患者[96]。现在一般认为如果患者心功能储备低以及氧化应激水平高会增加多柔比星心脏毒性的风险[81]。尽管有些报道与此相反，认为多柔比星与冠脉痉挛以及原发性心肌缺血没有关联[97]。对于高风险的患者而言，应该考虑加强监护，在治疗方案可行的情况下，应用非蒽环类的无心脏毒性的药物。大量证据指出，包含心脏的放疗是心肌病的危险因素，因此，对于拟行同步或者序贯心脏放疗的患者应给予心脏保护以及额外的监护[98,99]。

大量抗肿瘤药可增加多柔比星的心肌毒性。环磷酰胺（下文将进一步进行讨论）会增加多柔比星的心脏毒性作用，而且由于在化疗方案中这两种药物经常联用，因此这个问题在临床上十分重要[100]。据报道，放线菌素 D、普卡霉素、达卡巴嗪以及丝裂霉素 C 均可增加多柔比星的心脏毒性，但是前三种的作用尚未被完全证实[100]。即使在多柔比星治疗结束后，使用丝裂霉素 C 也会增加多柔比星的心脏毒性[101]。也有报道指出紫杉醇也可增加多柔比星的心脏毒性。然而一项研究显示，在联合用药的情况下，患者接受多柔比星的累积浓度低于 340～380mg/m^2 并不会表现出累加效应[102]。当两种药物在短时间内应用可导致心脏毒性发生率的提高，这可能与紫杉醇影响多柔比星的药代动力学从而导致多柔比星以及其代谢产物多柔比星醇的全身浓度增高有关[103]。另一种解释是，这种明显的毒性增加可能仅是在频繁监测心功能的患者中，采用不完善的检测手段以及检测次数增加所致。其他蒽环类及相关药物，如米托蒽醌（蒽醌类），本身的心脏毒性具有累加效应，调整为不同的蒽环类药物并不能提供心脏保护作用[104,105]。

降低多柔比星的心脏毒性有多种策略。临床观察显示当累积剂量<300mg/m^2 时，心脏毒性的发生一般不普遍，但是当累积剂量达到 400mg/m^2，心脏毒性的发生率可以达到5%[84]，因此降低累积剂量是策略之一。在没有危险因素的患者中限制多柔比星的累积剂量可以保证心脏毒性的发生率保持在一个可接受的范围。限制用量也可因减少心脏毒性的可能性从而减少心电监护的需求。而因假阳性的检测结果而过早停止有效治疗的风险可能超过了这些检查的益处。对于接受限制剂量的化疗药物并且治疗有效的患者而言，无须考虑剂量限值。即使合并其他危险因素，大多数患者均可耐受300mg/m^2 的多柔比星以及与其等量心脏毒性的其他蒽环类药物[96]。

将多柔比星制成脂质体可有效减低严重心脏毒性的发生率[106~108]。聚乙二醇及非聚乙二醇的制备方法均有相关研究，在美国聚乙二醇包被的聚乙二醇脂质体多柔比星已被批准用于治疗卡波西肉瘤、卵巢癌以及多发骨髓瘤。聚乙二醇包被的聚乙二醇脂质体多柔比星对于治疗乳腺癌及卵巢癌也很有效，聚乙二醇脂质体多柔比星与传统多柔比星相比具有确证的心脏保护作用，且抗肿瘤效果相当[109,110]。在蒽环类药物敏感的肿瘤亚组中，聚乙二醇包被的聚乙二醇脂质体多柔比星与其母体化合物疗效相当[111]。无论是否使用聚乙二醇包被的聚乙二醇脂质体多柔比星均具有心脏保护作用[112,113]。其中聚乙二醇包被的聚乙二醇脂质体多柔比星的心脏保护作用已被心肌活检以及非侵入性研究所证实[110]。心脏保护的程度难以定量，但是研究显示，在相同程度的心脏毒性时，聚乙二醇脂质体多柔比星的治疗周期是无保护的母药的至少两倍（表 132-5）。脂质体包埋的多柔比星抗癌谱较原先略有差别，但是其口炎及手足综合征的发生率稍高[114]。

表 132-5 蒽环类药物相关毒性：不同心脏毒性药物及剂量方案的相对毒性比较

药物	给药方案	相对于多柔比星标准方案的骨髓抑制能力	相关心脏毒性[a]	与多柔比星标准方案相比的心脏毒性指数[b]	推荐的最大剂量(mg/m^2)[c]
多柔比星	快速输注(20min)	1	1	1	400
多柔比星	每周	1	0.73	0.73	550
多柔比星	24h 输注	1	0.73	0.73	550
多柔比星	48h 输注	1	0.62	0.62	650[d]
多柔比星	96h 输注	1	0.5	0.5	800~1 000[d]
	快速输注	1	(基础值)		
聚乙二醇包被的聚乙二醇脂质体多柔比星	快速输注	1	不确定，可能<0.7	不确定，可能<0.7	不确定
表柔比星	快速输注	0.67	0.66	0.44	900
米托蒽醌	快速输注	5	0.5	2.5	160
柔红霉素	快速输注	0.67	0.75[e]	0.5[e]	800[e]
伊达比星	快速输注	5	0.53	2.67	150
吡柔比星	快速输注	1	0.62	0.62	650[e]
多柔比星+右丙亚胺	快速输注	1[e]	0.5	0.5[e]	800~1 000[e]
多柔比星，300mg/m^2+右丙亚胺	快速输注	1[e]	0.73[e]	0.73[e]	550[e]

[a] 这个因素是用来进行当给予导致同样水平骨髓移植水平的剂量时，其他药物、组合以及给药方案的累积剂量所致心脏毒性与快速输注多柔比星累积剂量所致心脏毒性的比较。

[b] 多柔比星快速输注最大推荐剂量为 400mg/m^2，以此为基础计算其他方案的最大推荐剂量。心脏毒性指数是指当药物累积剂量乘以心脏毒性指数时，其预期所致的心脏毒性与快速输注多柔比星所致心脏毒性一致。例如，当米托蒽醌累积剂量达到 120mg/m^2，患者预期出现的心脏损伤与快速输注 300mg/m^2 多柔比星一致（120×2.5=300）。这个值在调换心脏毒性药物的使用时非常有用。当所用用药的累积剂量与心脏毒性指数的综合超过 400 时，患者发生具有临床显著的心脏毒性事件的比率超过 5%。

[c] 在 5%患者出现具有明显症状的剂量所致充血性心力衰竭。

[d] 心内膜心肌活检显示心脏毒性更低。

[e] 数据不足。

对给药方案进行调整已经被证实可以减少蒽环类药物的心脏毒性。目前已开展了一系列研究，通过心内膜心肌活检检测持续灌注多柔比星 24~96h 后的心脏毒性[115,116]。尽管接受了更高累积剂量的多柔比星，持续灌注多柔比星的患者其高级别心内膜心肌病变的发生率较低。尽管其疗效相当，但是灌注时间大于 96h 会导致黏膜炎及手足综合征发生率显著上升，从而限制这种方案的应用[117]。在儿科患者中灌注化疗的心脏保护作用仍有争议[118,119]。不同多柔比星给药方案的相对心脏保护作用均列在表 132-5 中。尽管持续灌注有心脏保护的明确证据，但所需的便携性输液泵以及留置导管不方便，以及多柔比星累积剂量相对较低，大量临床医师不愿使用这类方案。

现在大量具有可能的心脏保护特性的复合物已被研究。目前唯一批准的心脏保护剂为铁螯合剂右丙亚胺（dexrazoxane）。一项研究将 92 名患者随机分类到两组，其中一组接受含多柔比星的治疗方案（每 21 日一次 50mg/m^2 多柔比星联合 500mg/m^2 环磷酰胺以及 500mg/m^2 氟尿嘧啶的联合方案），另一组接受联合右丙亚胺的相同方案，结果显示通过使用射血分数、心肌活检以及心功能不全的体征及症状来评估，联合右丙亚胺组其心脏毒性显著减低[120]。同时其他毒性作用以及抗肿瘤作用并未受到明显影响。但是，之后的一项研究显示右丙亚胺在保护心脏的同时其抗肿瘤作用明显减低[121]。在患者接受 300mg/m^2 多柔比星后使用右丙亚胺并不减低其抗肿瘤作用[122]。其他研究也未显示右丙亚胺可降低蒽环类药物的抗肿瘤能力。也有研究报道了右丙亚胺联合表柔比星以及米托蒽醌[123,124]。这些研究均显示右丙亚胺也可以减少除多柔比星以外其他心脏毒性药物的毒性。右丙亚胺也被用于需要特别灌注晚期毒性的儿童患者[125]。最近的研究显示右丙亚胺可抑制拓扑异构酶Ⅱ复合物，这可能可以解释为什么是右丙亚胺而非其他抗氧化剂具有心脏保护作用[126]。

患者接受多柔比星治疗过程中的心电监护

即便是老年患者或者那些具有已知心脏疾病的患者，大部分经历肿瘤治疗的患者可以耐受一定量的多柔比星[96]。但是需除外具有显著扩张性心肌病的患者以及既往因使用蒽环类或者相关药物而出现心脏毒性的患者。对于既往因心肌梗死导致射血分数减低的患者而言，只要多柔比星累积剂量低于 300~400mg/m^2，并采取相应的心脏保护措施，大部分患者均可耐受多柔比星。对于这些患者而言，需谨慎提高监测频率。当患者考虑进行多柔比星治疗时，首先需要进行心脏功能评估，其中包括射血分数的测定以及标准（12 导联）心电图，这些检查为未来的比较提供基线数据[127~130]。

无论伴或不伴心脏损伤的症状及体征，对于没有危险因素的患者而言，标准给药方案的多柔比星累积剂量达到 300~350mg/m^2 之前或者与其相当的其他药物以及其他给药方案时无须再次评估（表 132-5）。此后，推荐每 2 个周期的治疗便需要再次进行品评估。当累积剂量超过表 132-5 中所示时，应进行额外详细的检查。无论在哪种剂量水平，具有导致早期心脏毒性高危险因素的患者需要更密切的检测。当患者未合并其他心脏危险因素时，患者接受表 132-5 的推荐剂量治疗时其心力衰竭的发生率接近 5%。

患者射血分数低于 50% 时心脏风险较高。当射血分数未改变时，患者接受多柔比星治疗的剂量不应超过 300mg/m^2，并且需要进行密切检测。对于射血分数降低 15% 以上或者射血分数低于 45% 的患者，强烈建议停止多柔比星并采用非心脏毒性药物的替代治疗方案。

其他蒽环类及其相关（Ⅰ型）药物

临床上，柔红霉素、伊达比星、表柔比星、吡柔比星（pirarubicin）以及米托蒽醌的心脏毒性与多柔比星基本一致。在不同药物间，其肿瘤疗效以及以 mg/m^2 为单位的累积剂量不一致导致心脏毒性不一致。这些药物的心脏毒性尚未与多柔比星一样被充分研究。但是，目前也有数据记录了相同抗肿瘤剂量下患者的射血分数以及心肌活检结果。相比于多柔比星，快速注射表柔比星心脏毒性发生率较低（表 132-5）[131,132]。表柔比星在乳腺癌患者的治疗中使用比例逐渐增高，其心脏保护作用提高了药物的安全性，这对于具有较高心脏风险的患者而言十分重要，但是一项 Cochrane 评论指出其心脏保护作用并不如之前认为的那么有效[133]。一些研究显示相比于多柔比星联合紫杉醇，表柔比星联合紫杉醇心脏毒性较小，并归因于紫杉醇对表柔比星的代谢影响更小[134,135]。目前的数据显示，对于未接受过蒽环类药物的患者而言，150mg/m^2 累积剂量的伊达比星是安全的[136]。作为在日本及法国广泛使用的多柔比星类似物，吡柔比星（THP 多柔比星）目前尚未被批准在美国使用，目前有研究显示在标准用药方案下，吡柔比星相较于多柔比星的心脏毒性显著减低[137]。米托蒽醌是一种蒽醌类药物，与多柔比星相比，在达到同样骨髓抑制水平的情况下，米托蒽醌的心脏毒性较低[104,138]。药物的替换并不能提供心脏保护，因此当既往曾接受过Ⅰ型心脏毒性药物治疗的患者需要接受另一种心脏毒性药物治疗时，临床医生需要进行谨慎考虑。

Ⅱ型抗肿瘤治疗相关药物

Ⅱ型抗肿瘤药物并未显示出与累积剂量相关的毒性反应，因此其心脏毒性表现难以预测。目前这些药物中研究最全面的药物为曲妥珠单抗（trastuzumab），但是其他药物也应在此类型药物中。曲妥珠单抗是一种抗 HER2 的人源化单克隆抗体，对过表达 HER2 的乳腺癌及其他肿瘤（20%~25% 的乳腺癌）的治疗十分有效。早期临床研究发现曲妥珠单抗所致心肌病在体征及症状上与蒽环类药物所致心肌病类似。这种心脏毒性的担忧促使开展了大量多中心、涉及超过 10 000 名使用曲妥珠单抗的患者的临床研究。这些临床研究及其各治疗组方案均列在表 132-6 中[139~141]。目前已得出一些重要的结论，对于心脏毒性最重要的几点如下：①蒽环类药物序贯曲妥珠单抗治疗组的心脏功能异常发生率高于单纯蒽环类药物治疗组，尽管组间的差别<4%，但临床上仍受到关注；②心脏毒性大多是可逆的；③心源性死亡发生率极低；④之前未接受过蒽环类药物治疗的患者在接受包含曲妥珠单抗的治疗方案时其心脏功能异常的发生率更低；⑤曲妥珠单抗相关心脏毒性与多柔比星不同，但心脏放射性核素扫描以及超声心动图均表现为收缩功能减低，难以从临床上进行鉴别。这些研究也指出蒽环类药物以及曲妥珠单抗之间的治疗间期长短至关重要[129,142]。

尽管曲妥珠单抗所致心肌病的原理尚未被阐明，但是其始发事件被认为是曲妥珠单抗与 HER2 的特异性结合，之后影响了心脏中 ErbB-2 信号通路。ErbB-2（HER2/neu）通路属于具有受体酪氨酸激酶活性的表皮生长因子受体（epidermal growth factor receptor，EGFR）家族，该家族有四位成员，包括 EGFR、HER2/neu、HER3 以及 HER4。分布在心脏上的 EGF、调蛋白以及神经调节蛋白这些 EGF 家族的配体可激活 EGFR 家族受体。这些 EGF 配体与 EGFR、HER3 以及 HER4 结合会导致其与 HER2 的异源二聚体产生，引起受体的磷酸化并且起始下游的信号通路。下游被激活的通路包括 Ras/Raf，PI3K/Akt，JNK 以

表 132-6 曲妥珠单抗治疗的辅助研究中心脏毒性的总结

研究	患者数	入选标准	分组	心脏事件/%	可逆性改变	随访时间/年
NSABP B-31	2043	淋巴结+	①AC-T ②AC-TH	①0.8 ②4.1	是	7
BCIRG 006	3222	淋巴结+或者高风险淋巴结	①AC-T ②AC-TH ③TPH	①0.4 ②1.9 ③0.4	不适用	3
NCCTG N9831	1944	淋巴结+或高风险淋巴结	①AC-T ②AC-T-H ③AC-TH	①0.3 ②2.8 ③3.3	是	3
HERA	3386	淋巴结+或高风险淋巴结	①Std ②Std-H	①3.6 ②0.6	是	8
FinHer	232	淋巴结+或高风险淋巴结 年龄<66	①V/T-FAC ②V/T(H)-FAC	①3.4 ②0	不适用	5

A，蒽环类药物；C，环磷酰胺；T，紫杉烷；H，曲妥珠单抗；Std，标准（新）辅助治疗（94%包括蒽环类药物）；V/T，长春瑞滨或紫杉醇；F，氟尿嘧啶。随访时间反映了最近报道的数据。

及 MAPK 这些影响心肌细胞转录的重要调节因子。这些通路涉及心脏的发育、正常心脏功能的维持、对应激的反应、心肌肥大以及对凋亡的调节。在小鼠模型中对 *HER2* 基因进行选择性敲除显示这一受体在调节应激状态下心肌细胞的生长、修复以及生存这些过程中发挥了重要的作用[143]。曲妥珠单抗对 HER2 信号通路的暂时影响会引起对心肌应激的不充分甚至不恰当反应，会导致收缩功能异常以及充血性心力衰竭[144]。曲妥珠单抗对心肌细胞的修复的影响也可以解释为何患者既往接受过蒽环类药物治疗后更易受曲妥珠单抗毒性的影响。

曲妥珠单抗所致心脏功能异常多为可逆的[7,139~142,145]。但是当器官损伤包括之前使用蒽环类药物所致的损伤时，能在多大程度上恢复功能仍然是一个问题。是否以及何时停药，是临时停药抑或是永久停药，如何评估功能恢复后再次用药的风险以及如何进行后续的检测都是需要考虑的问题。一些组织提出了相关指南，但是所有指南都仅基于专家共识而非前瞻性临床研究数据结果[129,146]。

其他Ⅱ型药物

除了曲妥珠单抗，拉帕替尼、舒尼替尼、伊马替尼以及其他药物可能的心脏毒性也逐渐被关注。这些药物的潜在副作用具体包括心功能不全、QT 间期延长以及心肌缺血。目前的数据显示这些药物所致心脏毒性的心肌活检显示线粒体结构改变，尚未发现蒽环类药物所致的心肌活检典型表现。有趣的是，这些药物所致毒性尚未显示出累积效应，对于大量患者而言即使出现心脏毒性仍可以延长给药时间。此外考虑到心脏抑制所致继发效应，使用舒尼替尼可能会出现显著的高血压，当使用伊马替尼时，液体潴留是关键性因素[142,147~149]。

使用这些药物时会出现不同程度的 QT 间期延长，但是严重的 QT 间期延长导致需要暂停或终止用药的情况以及心肌缺血事件十分罕见[70]。报道显示拉帕替尼所致心脏功能异常在接受过蒽环类药物治疗的患者中的发生率为 2.2%，在之前未接受过心脏毒性药物的患者中的发生率为 1.5%，大多数患者（88%）的心脏毒性在不同程度上是可逆的[147]。

其他可导致心脏功能减低的药物

一些无法分类到Ⅰ型及Ⅱ型的药物有时也会导致心肌功能的显著减低。在极少数情况下，α 干扰素可导致射血分数的显著减低[149]。其原理仍未知，可能涉及炎性反应以及高代谢需求。如患者可渡过初次病程后通常可逐渐恢复心功能[150]。高剂量的环磷酰胺会导致特殊的心脏功能异常。严重时心脏损伤表现为出血性心肌炎[151]。这个过程通常急性发作，其发生原因可能与单次高剂量相关（通常大于 4.5g/m^2），而非与累积剂量相关。这一过程通常表现为低射血分数以及低 QRS 电压。尽管严重的出血性心肌炎可致死，但是轻中度出血性心肌炎可以无症状并且是其病理性改变是可逆的。

治疗相关心力衰竭或心脏功能异常的患者的治疗方法

对于蒽环类药物相关心脏功能异常患者最重要的治疗方法是避免再次使用蒽环类药物。一旦诊断明确，蒽环类药物相关心脏功能不全与其他类型的心肌病差别不大，因此它们的治疗方法相似。美国心脏学会以及美国心脏学会公布了成人慢性心力衰竭诊断及治疗的指南[152]。接受蒽环类药物但是没有心脏功能异常的患者在合并其他使心脏功能恶化的情况下需要进行积极治疗。推荐进行高血压的控制及生活方式的改变。当患者射血分数低于 45%～50%时需要考虑进行药物治疗。一些证据支持早期进行药物治疗时最有效的，因此当左室功能异常时就应开始进行药物治疗[153]。血管紧张素转化酶抑制药（ACEI）以及 β 肾上腺能阻滞剂适用于左室功能异常的患者。有症状的心力衰竭患者需加入限盐以及利尿剂治疗。洋地黄可减轻症状，在房颤患者中可协助控制患者的心室反应，但是并不能改善患者的生存。当患者出现房颤时，需行抗凝治疗。目前尚缺乏对于蒽环类药物相关心肌病的特异性治疗方案。恶性肿瘤不应该成为心力衰竭积极治疗的禁忌证，对于肿瘤情况稳定或者肿瘤已治愈的患者而言，也可以考虑机械辅助装置以及心脏移植[154]。Ⅱ型药物所致的心力衰竭多可自行恢复，之后再次给药也是可以考虑的。

与心肌缺血及血栓栓塞事件相关的药物

大量的药物可导致心肌缺血,伴有或不伴有心肌梗死。研究最全面的药物为氟尿嘧啶,特别是当其与顺铂联合使用时[155]。卡培他滨作为氟尿嘧啶氨基甲酸酯类抗肿瘤药,目前常用于治疗胃肠道及乳腺恶性肿瘤,它是一种口服的前药,可在酶的作用下转换为氟尿嘧啶。两种药物中均报道出现了心肌梗死以及心律失常[156,157]。冠脉血管弹性或痉挛会导致缺血。也有报道指出,使用长春碱、长春新碱、博来霉素、顺铂以及生物反应调节剂可导致心肌缺血。广谱的缺血反应提示抗癌治疗同时出现的心肌缺血比一般情况下更普遍。在接近一半接受氟尿嘧啶治疗的患者中会出现非特异性心电图改变,此外16%的患者表现出ST段压低或者抬高以及心肌梗死等缺血相关的心电图表现(图132-7)。大多数受影响的患者均具有基础的冠脉病变,预示着冠脉病变可增大氟尿嘧啶及其相关疾病

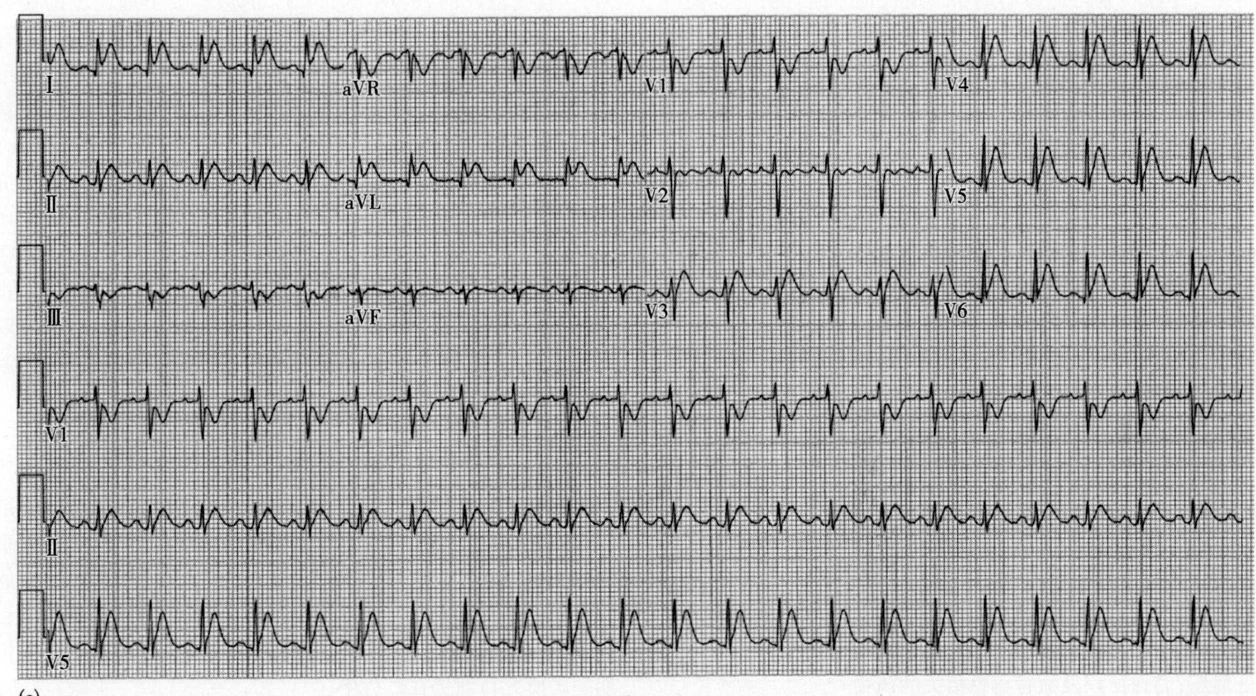

(a)

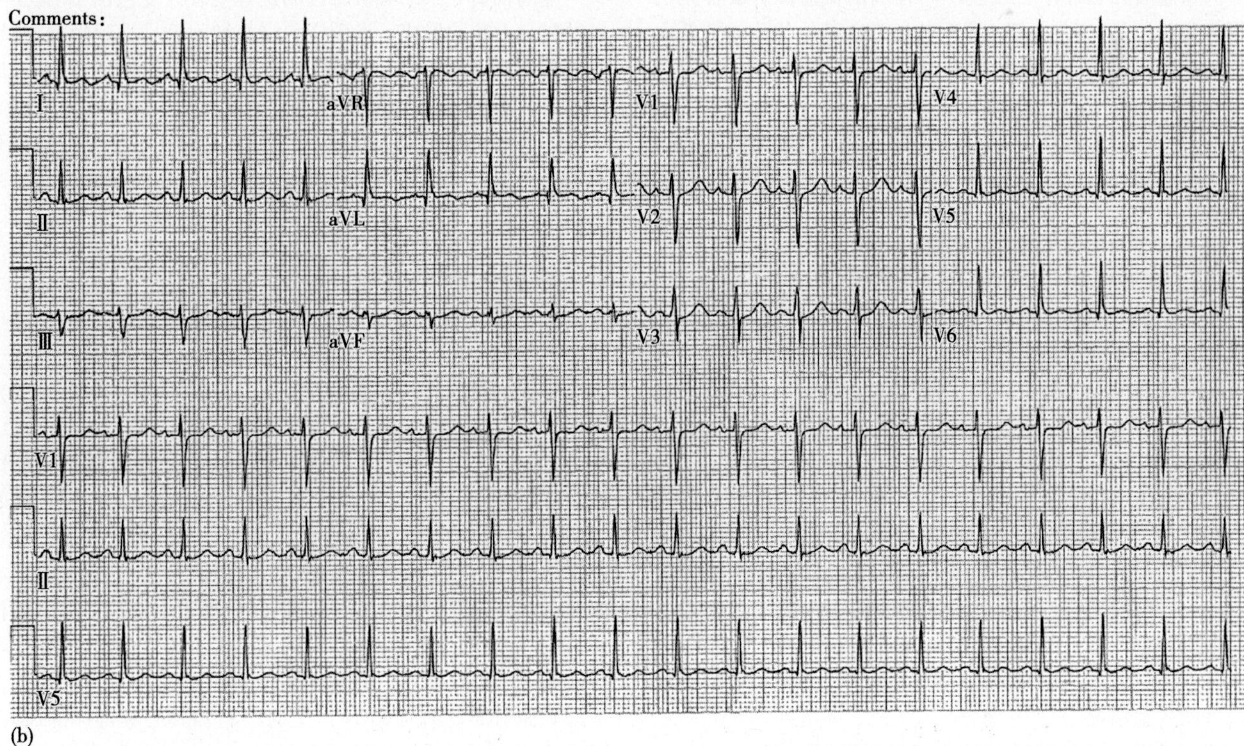

(b)

图132-7 接受氟尿嘧啶治疗后的44岁女性胸痛期间的心电图。(a)冠脉痉挛导致急性前壁ST段抬高。(b)应用硝酸甘油后症状缓解,心电图恢复正常

的缺血风险。有报道指出钙通道阻滞药的使用可预防缺血事件的发生[158]。在部分接受氟尿嘧啶的患者中静脉注射硝酸甘油可预防心肌缺血或心肌梗死事件的发生。当心脏缺血事件可以被控制时,治疗可以继续,但应更加谨慎并增强监护。

当伴有动脉粥样硬化的患者中出现了治疗相关高输出状态时将会导致心肌缺血,其原因为粥样硬化斑块导致血管不能扩张,无法增加血液供应,这一现象称为"冠状动脉窃血"。在这种模式下干扰素可能参与起始缺血反应。通常由生物反应调节剂导致的发热以及甲状腺功能亢进可能会引起缺血。肿瘤坏死因子与高凝状态相关,这可能会导致血管阻塞,这可能可以解释使用细胞因子以及其他生物反应调节剂时出现的缺血。贫血可因携氧能力减低而导致缺血恶化,因此是重要的共存因素。

当患者出现任何原因导致的心肌缺血时均需要密切观察,防止心律失常,尽管观察及治疗需基于总体预后考虑。患者合并冠脉疾病时可以使用 β 肾上腺素能阻滞剂以及长效硝酸酯类药物治疗,有助于减低缺血事件的发生率。已控制的缺血以及与特定治疗相关的缺血不应成为相关药物的治疗绝对禁忌。伴有冠心病的癌症患者通常需要行血管再通,这有助于改善患者耐受治疗的能力以及生存质量。

在大量绝经后乳腺癌人群中进行了激素治疗相关心脏事件的研究。他莫昔芬会导致胆固醇水平减低,而这能提供一定程度的心脏保护作用,但是他莫昔芬与血栓栓塞风险升高相关。芳香酶抑制药阿那曲唑、来曲唑以及依西美坦与胆固醇增多相关,与他莫昔芬相比,芳香酶抑制药所致心血管疾病的风险较高,这可能与他莫昔芬的心脏保护作用相关[159]。

与低血压、高血压以及血管毒性相关的药物

大量患者在化疗中会出现不同程度的低血压。最常见的原因为容量不足,通常由恶心及呕吐所致。其他化疗导致低血压的可能原因包括心排出量减低、血管张力减低、小血管以及毛细血管渗透性增高(毛细血管渗漏)。大部分化疗后出现低血压的患者多为一过性的,可以通过密切监测、补液以及使用血管加压药进行治疗。仅有少量报道指出会出现严重及威胁生命的低血压。

白介素 2 的使用与显著的低血压相关,但是通常为一过性的,经常需要升压药治疗[160,161]。毛细血管渗漏也与其相关。白介素 2 相关心肌缺血可能与低血压相关,但不能除外其直接毒性作用。白介素 2 也可导致室上性心律失常以及心肌炎的发生率上升[162]。白介素 2 导致的舒血管作用可能与其介导了氧化亚氮的释放相关。NG-单甲基-L-精氨酸(NG-monomethyl-L-arginine)作为氧化亚氮合成酶的抑制剂,可以逆转白介素 2 导致的低血压,这既可以支持氧化亚氮在低血压产生中的作用,也预示着 NG-单甲基-L-精氨酸的潜在治疗效果[163]。

高三尖杉酯碱(omacetaxine mepesuccinate,曾用名 homoharringtonine)现在已证实可用于治疗难治性慢性髓细胞性白血病。当静脉输注这种药物时很快出现剂量相关性的低血压,有时十分严重[164]。在这种情况下静脉注射肾上腺素可以帮助稳定患者的一般情况。

研究者对于紫杉醇潜在的心脏毒性作用也十分感兴趣。在一项研究中,在接受可耐受的最大剂量紫杉醇时,有 29% 的患者会出现无症状的心动过缓。更严重的节律异常也有报道,但是通常出现在既往有心脏基础病以及现有电解质紊乱的患者中[165]。紫杉醇所致严重的心脏疾病发生率低,但是大多数患者在治疗期间无须特殊检测[166]。同时也需警惕超敏反应的发生[167]。

顺铂作为常用于治疗泌尿生殖系统、头颈部的恶性肿瘤以及非小细胞肺癌,可导致高血压。沙利度胺以及紫杉醇可导致低血压。贝伐单抗作为抗血管内皮生长因子的单克隆抗体,在接受治疗的患者中超过 25% 的患者会出现血压的显著提高。高达 14% 的患者会发展为严重甚至永久高血压,罕有患者会发生高血压危象。既往有高血压的患者在接受贝伐单抗治疗时出现高血压的风险更高,因此在治疗期间需要注意检测[168]。对于血压难以控制的患者需要行降压治疗,同时需考虑调整治疗方案。包括舒尼替尼(sunitinib)、阿伦珠单抗(alemtuzumab)、吉姆单抗(gemtuzumab)、英夫利西单抗(infliximab)、muromanoa-CD3、利妥昔单抗、索拉非尼(sorafenib)在内的所有抗血管形成的药物均可增加高血压风险,一般当中止或终止给药时血压可恢复正常。一旦高血压被控制以后,可以再次给药,大量患者可在心脏风险可控的情况下继续之前的治疗方案。

放疗所致心脏并发症

对胸部恶性肿瘤的放疗以及随后的心脏疾病之间的关系已经研究得比较明确。包括心脏组织的照射野可以导致一系列疾病,一般通常出现在照射后 10 余年。在这几年对这些危险因素的认识极大提高了放疗技术,但是改良的放疗技术对心脏损伤的减低程度仍未明确,对使用现代技术放疗的患者的长期随访研究目前仍在进行中。

电离辐射导致的心脏毒性的病理生理改变包括 DNA 损伤以及氧自由基的形成。增殖能力强的细胞更易受到影响,特别是血管内皮细胞。小血管损伤将导致心肌组织的炎性反应,最终形成纤维化。心脏各层都受累,加速冠脉疾病进程以及引起急慢性心包疾病、心肌病、瓣膜疾病以及传导系统异常。也有报道指出放疗可导致继发的心脏恶性肿瘤[169]。随时间发展,放疗对心脏的影响表现为迟发性及慢性进行性心脏功能减低,损伤与放疗率呈直接关系。动物模型显示放射剂量相关的伴有心肌微血管病变的慢性充血性心力衰竭,病理学检查显示毛细血管密度显著减低,心肌退行性变、凋亡并伴有间质纤维化[170,171]。细胞动力学研究照射后 30~100 日时内皮细胞增生能力增强。在动物研究中显示这一形态变化与心排出量以及左室射血分数减低情况平行。

放疗对心脏功能的人体研究大多来源于霍奇金淋巴瘤以及乳腺癌患者,这些患者既接受了相当剂量的心脏放射,同时也适合长期随访研究。与之相反,肺癌患者的生存较差因此难以进展出现明显的心脏并发症。危险因素包括总照射剂量、心脏照射剂量以及使用的特殊技术,其他因素也发挥了一定的作用,诸如放疗时患者年龄(年轻患者风险更高)、治疗过程中联合使用蒽环类化疗药以及传统的心脏危险因素。传统观点认为心脏照射剂量达到 35Gy 以上时会增加其心脏毒性的风险,但是目前的研究显示在更低剂量时也会如此。儿童癌症幸存者研究(Childhood Cancer Survivor Study)显示当照射剂量达到 15~35Gy 时,患者心力衰竭、心肌梗死、心包疾病以及瓣膜病的风险提高了两倍以上[172]。其他稍小的研究显示当心脏照射剂量达到 5~15Gy 时,患者心源性猝死的相对危险度为 12.5,当>15Gy 时,心源性猝死的相对危险度为 25[173]。

由于纵隔淋巴结离心脏近、确诊时患者更年轻以及患者预后较好、可长期生存的特点,霍奇金淋巴瘤的放疗的患者出现心脏并发症的风险更高。研究显示包含放疗的治疗方案后发生致死性心脏事件的相对危险度可达 7.2[174]。放疗相关心脏病多需要数年或者数十年才会出现临床症状,一些主要并发症仅在晚期随访评估时才会被发现。最重要的并发症包括瓣膜疾病(反流为主)以及心肌梗死,也会出现限制性心肌病、心律失常以及自主神经功能障碍(图 132-8)。由于更好的心脏遮挡以及其他技术的进步,心包疾病的发生率已减低[175]。

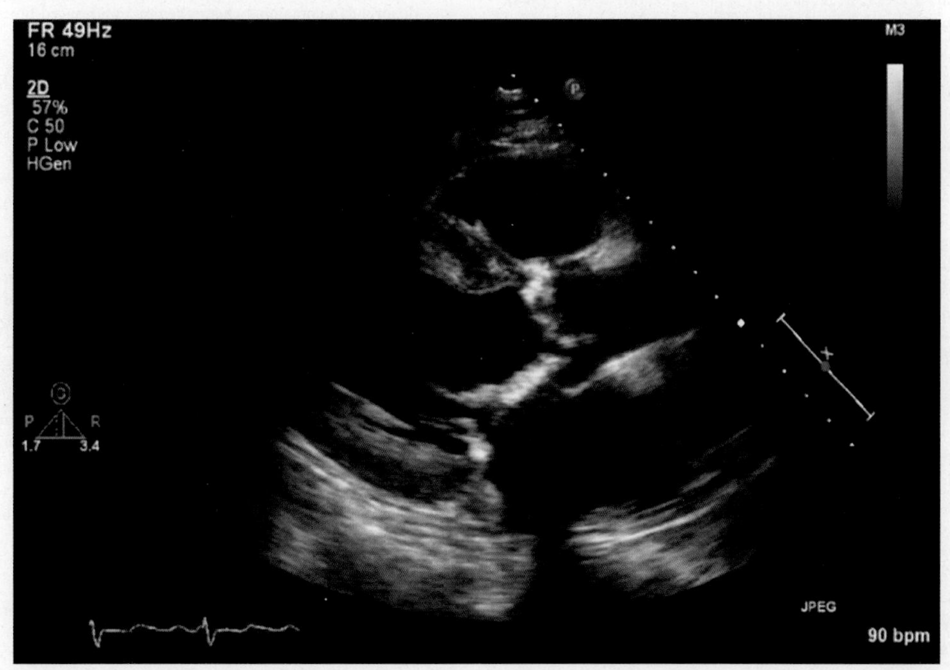

图 132-8　40 岁接受超声心动图胸骨旁长轴观,该患者 20 年前接受淋巴瘤斗篷野照射。注意主动脉瓣及二尖瓣的严重增厚及钙化。这名患者同样伴有严重的冠脉疾病,心肌炎以及异常的心包增厚,可能均与之前的肿瘤治疗相关

得益于总体疾病发生率以及左右对比的优势,乳腺肿瘤患者队列为研究放疗的心脏作用提供了最多证据。一些研究用这一天然的对照组来鉴别化疗的系统性反应以及放疗的局部作用。在早期的随机性试验中证实了放疗与心血管事件的死亡率显著相关[176]。包括心脏遮蔽、切向场、呼吸门控等新技术切实减少或延缓了心脏相关并发症的发生率及死亡率,但是目前特别是对于左侧乳腺癌而言仍然存在显著的危险因素。包括双侧内乳淋巴链的照射野可显著增加后续心血管并发症的发生。与霍奇金淋巴结的数据结果相似,放疗后心脏事件的发生风险随着随诊时间的延长、蒽环类药物的使用以及传统心血管危险的存在而提高。

放疗后心脏毒性反应的临床表现十分广泛。急性心包炎可以在放疗时发生,同时伴有急性或亚急性心包积液,但有时也可以表现为慢性心包积液。这种胸腔积液与恶性心包积液难以鉴别,有时需要行积液细胞学检查已明确诊断。心脏压塞罕有发生。慢性炎症反应可以表现为限制性心包炎,这通常难以诊断,除非患者身体情况可以耐受心包切除术,否则患者预后不佳。

放疗后冠脉疾病可表现为心绞痛、心肌梗死以及猝死,这随着时间延长风险逐渐增加。至少以下两个机制与大血管病变相关。首先,放疗导致的内膜及外膜的增生继发动脉壁的增厚,会导致管腔狭窄。其次,放疗可加速动脉粥样硬化的病程,可同步加速胆固醇沉积以及腔内溃疡的发生[177]。因此,如前所述,诸如抽烟以及血脂异常等传统的心脏危险因素也在此病理过程中发挥了重要的协同因素。由于解剖位置的原因,左前降支是最常被影响的血管。

对放射相关血管损伤的治疗与对缺血性心脏病的传统治疗基本是一致的,硝酸盐、β 肾上腺素能阻滞剂、抗血小板治疗以及钙通道阻滞剂是药物治疗的基础。针对缺血性心脏病的有创治疗通常也对放射相关血管损伤有帮助,但是与缺血性心脏病并不完全一致,使用球囊血管成形术治疗放射相关血管损伤时,球囊压力通常要更高以及球囊释放时间通常需要更长。与治疗缺血性心脏病相比,使用旁路手术治疗放射相关血管损伤更加困难,其原因为血管管腔更小以及术者需要在之前放射治疗后的区域内手术。但是,旁路手术仍然是这些患者的重要治疗手段。

放疗所致心肌病包括舒张功能异常、收缩功能异常以及限制性心肌病。病理显示小血管缺血事件以及纤维化为最主要的改变,伴随随后可能的心室重构。限制性心肌病与心包缩窄难以鉴别,特别是当两者同时出现在同一名患者中。有时在心包切开术之前行心内膜下心肌活检以明确是否共存心肌病变,合并心肌病变会导致极高的手术死亡率。

尽管瓣膜受累更加常见,但是通常并不严重。尽管如此,瓣膜损伤是进行性的,在放射所致心脏病患者中发病率很高。

所致最常见的疾病包括三尖瓣反流、二尖瓣反流以及主动脉反流，但是主动脉狭窄发病率不高[178,179]。组织学上，这些瓣膜变现为心内膜增厚以及心内膜弹力纤维增生[180]。

心脏传导系统的放疗损伤也有报道，一般是通过心电图发现异常。通常可以发现PR间期延长，这是由于房室结上以及结下的房室传导阻滞所致。偶见完全性房室传导阻滞，这类患者植入心脏起搏器可以挽救生命。自主神经功能障碍可以表现为不适当的窦性心动过速、心动过缓以及运动时心率反应异常。

（龚涛 桑铭辰 译 李肖 校）

参考文献

1 Ewer MS, Benjamin RS, Yeh ET. Cardiac complications. In: Holland J, Frei E, eds. *Cancer Medicine*, 6th ed. Hamilton, Ontario: BC Decker; 2003.

5 Plana JC, Galderisi M, Barac A, et al. Expert consensus for multimodality imaging evaluation of adult patients during and after cancer therapy: a report from the American Society of Echocardiography and the European Association of Cardiovascular Imaging. *J Am Soc Echocardiogr*. 2014;**27(9)**:911–939.

7 Ewer M, Gibbs H, Swafford J, Benjamin R. Cardiotoxicity in patients receiving trastuzumab (Herceptin): primary toxicity, synergistic or sequential stress, or surveillance artifact? *Semin Oncol*. 1999;**26(suppl 12)**:96–101.

21 Klein AL, Abbara S, Agler DA, et al. American Society of Echocardiography clinical recommendations for multimodality cardiovascular imaging of patients with pericardial disease: endorsed by the Society for Cardiovascular Magnetic Resonance and Society of Cardiovascular Computed Tomography. *J Am Soc Echocardiogr*. 2013;**26**:965–1012.

22 Spodick D. Current concepts: acute cardiac tamponade. *N Engl J Med*. 2003;**349**:684–690.

36 Ewer SM, Yusuf SW. Arrhythmia in the cancer patient. In: Ewer MS, Yeh ETH, eds. *Cancer and the Heart*, 2nd ed. Shelton, CT: Medical Publishing House-USA; 2013:190–209.

51 Strickman N, Rossi P, Massumi A, Hall R. Carcinoid heart disease: a clinical, pathologic and therapeutic update. *Curr Prob Cardiol*. 1982;**6(11)**:1–41.

66 Kristen AV, Dengler TJ, Hegenbart U, et al. Prophylactic implantation of cardioverter-defibrillator in patients with severe cardiac amyloidosis and high risk for sudden cardiac death. *Heart Rhythm*. 2008;**5**:235.

70 Kim PY, Ewer MS. Chemotherapy and QT prolongation: overview with clinical perspective. *Curr Treat Options Cardiovasc Med*. 2014;**16**:303–308.

78 Ewer MS, Lippman S. Type II chemotherapy-related cardiac dysfunction: time to recognize a new entity. *J Clin Oncol*. 2005;**23(13)**:2900–2902.

82 Cardinale D, Sandri MT, Colombo A, et al. Prognostic value of troponin I in cardiac risk stratification of cancer patients undergoing high-dose chemotherapy. *Circulation*. 2004;**109(22)**:2749–2754.

84 Swain S, Whaley F, Ewer M. Congestive heart failure in patients treated with doxorubicin: A retrospective analysis of three trials. *Cancer*. 2003;**97**:2869–2879.

87 Zhang S, Liu X, Bawa-Khalfe T, et al. Identification of the molecular basis of doxorubicin-induced cardiotoxicity. *Nat Med*. 2012;**18**:1639–1642.

92 Ewer MS, Ali MK, Mackay B, et al. A comparison of resting and exercise ejection fractions with cardiac biopsy grades in patients receiving adriamycin. *J Clin Oncol*. 1984;**2**:112–117.

99 Von Hoff D, Layard M, Basa P, et al. Risk factors for doxorubicin-induced congestive heart failure. *Ann Intern Med*. 1979;**91**:710–717.

114 O'Brian M, Wigler N, Inbar M, et al. Reduced cardiotoxicity and comparable efficacy in a phase III trial of pegylated liposomal doxorubicin HCL (CAELYX/Doxil) versus conventional doxorubicin for first-line treatment of metastatic breast cancer. *Ann Oncol*. 2004;**15**:440–449.

116 Hortobagyi G, Frye D, Buzdar A, et al. Decreased cardiac toxicity of doxorubicin administered by continuous intravenous infusion in combination chemotherapy for metastatic breast carcinoma. *Cancer*. 1989;**63**:37–45.

119 Lipshultz SE, Miller TL, Lipsitz SR, et al. Continuous versus bolus infusion of doxorubicin in children with ALL: long-term cardiac outcomes. *Pediatrics*. 2012;**130**:1003–1011.

121 Swain S, Whaley F, Gerber M, et al. Cardioprotection with dexrazoxane for doxorubicin-containing chemotherapy in advanced breast cancer. *J Clin Oncol*. 1997;**15(4)**:1318–1332.

125 Lipshultz SE, Scully RE, Lipsitz SR, et al. Assessment of dexrazoxane as a cardioprotectant in doxorubicin-treated children with high-risk acute lymphoblastic leukaemia: long-term follow-up of a prospective, randomised, multicentre trial. *Lancet Oncol*. 2010;**2010**:950–961.

133 van Dalen EC, Michiels EMC, Caron HN, Kremer LCM. Different anthracycline derivates for reducing cardiotoxicity in cancer patients. *Cochrane Database of Systematic Reviews*. 2010;(5. Art. No.: D005006). doi: 10.1002/14651858.CD005006.pub4.

134 Gennari A, Salvadori B, Donati S, et al. Cardiotoxicity of epirubicin/paclitaxel-containing regimens: role of cardiac risk factors. *J Clin Oncol*. 1999;**17**:3596–3602.

139 Tan-Chiu E, Yothers G, Romond E, et al. Assessment of cardiac dysfunction in a randomized trial comparing doxorubicin and cyclophosphamide followed by paclitaxel, with or without trastuzumab as adjuvant therapy in node-positive, human epidermal growth factor receptor 2-overexpressing breast cancer: NSABP B31. *J Clin Oncol*. 2005;**23**:7811–7819.

140 Suter T, Procter M, Van Veldhuisen D, et al. Trastuzumab-associated cardiac adverse effects in the Herceptin Adjuvant Trial. *J Clin Oncol*. 2007;**25**:3859–3865.

141 Joensuu H, Bono P, Kataja V, et al. Fluorouracil, epirubicin and cyclophosphamide with either docetaxel or vioorelbine, with or without trastuzumab as adjuvant treatment of breast cancer. Final results of the FinHer Trial. *J Clin Oncol*. 2009;**27**:5685–5692.

142 Ewer MS, Ewer SM. Cardiotoxicity of anticancer treatment. *Nat Rev Cardiol*. 2015;**12(9)**:547–558.

144 Crone S, Zhao Y, Fan L, et al. ErbB2 is essential in the prevention of dilated cardiomyopathy. *Nature Med*. 2002;**8**:459–465.

145 Ewer MS, Vooletich M, Durand J, et al. Reversibility of trastuzumab-related cardiotoxicity: new insights based on clinical course and response to medical treatment. *J Clin Oncol*. 2005;**23**:7820–7827.

147 Perez EA, Koeler M, Byrne J, Preston AJ, Rappold E, Ewer MS. Cardiac safety of lapatinib: pooled analysis of 3689 patients enrolled in clinical trials. *Mayo Clin Proc*. 2008;**83**:679–686.

148 Ewer MS, Suter TM, Lenihan DJ, et al. Cardiovaxcular events among 1090 cancer patients treated with sunitinib, interferon or placebo: a comprehensive adjudicated database analysis demonstrating clinically meaningful reversibility of cardiac events. *Eur J Cancer*. 2014;**50**:2162–2170.

159 Forbes JF, Cuzick J, Buzdar AU, Howell A, Tobias JS, Baum M. Effect of anastrozole and tamoxifen as adjuvant treatment for early-stage breast cancer: 100-month analysis of the ATAC trial. *Lancet Oncol*. 2008;**9**:45–53.

168 Zhong J, Ali AN, Voloschin AD, et al. Bevacizumab-induced hypertension is a predictive marker for improved outcomes in patients with recurrent glioblastoma treated with bevacizumab. *Cancer*. 2015;**121(9)**:1456–1462. doi: 10.1002/cncr.29234.

172 Mulrooney DA, Yeazel MW, Kawashima T, et al. Cardiac outcomes in a cohort of adult survivors of childhood and adolescent cancer: retrospective analysis of the Childhood Cancer Survivor Study cohort. *BMJ*. 2009;**339**:b4606.

173 Tukenova M, Guibout C, Oberlin O, et al. Role of cancer treatment in long-term overall and cardiovascular mortality after childhood cancer. *J Clin Oncol*. 2010;**28**:1308–1315.

第 133 章　呼吸系统并发症

Vickie R. Shannon, MD ■ George A. Eapen, MD ■ Carlos A. Jimenez, MD ■ Horiana B. Grosu, MD ■ Rodolfo C. Morice, MD ■ Lara Bashoura, MD ■ Scott E. Evans, MD ■ Roberto Adachi, MD ■ Michael Kroll, MD ■ Saadia A. Faiz, MD ■ Diwakar D. Balachandran, MD ■ Selvaraj E. Pravinkumar, MD, FRCP ■ Burton F. Dickey, MD

引言

呼吸系统很容易遭受肿瘤及肿瘤治疗并发症影响，这种易感性来源于气体交换的严格结构要求、呼吸道对外部环境持续的暴露，以及伴随呼吸道损害所产生的严重症状。气体交换要求特定的气道，肺泡毛细血管膜，有效的肌肉骨骼通气泵，和足够的肺循环血流。在肿瘤患者中，胸部的原发和转移肿瘤会危害主要的气道；肿瘤的恶性胸腔积液从外部压迫肺部同时影响膈肌功能；肿瘤种植、血液或淋巴道的转移会取代有功能的肺实质；切除性的外科手术减少了肺实质的容积，而非切除性的外科手术可导致肺功能暂时性受损。放射治疗、化疗、干细胞治疗和感染会损害肺的毛细血管膜；肿瘤也可以直接或间接的损害肌肉骨骼泵；静脉血栓和肺血管病变会阻碍肺血流。

正常人的呼吸系统具有大量的生理储备，甚至能够耐受手术切除一侧肺叶。但是在肿瘤患者中，对呼吸系统多个组分的损伤会导致生理储备的丢失和渐进的呼吸困难。呼吸困难、咳嗽、喘息、喘鸣、胸痛和咯血是癌症患者肺部并发症的常见症状。

在这一章节，我们将探讨肿瘤和肿瘤治疗所导致的主要呼吸道并发症的病理生理学、诊断和治疗。我们以肿瘤及肿瘤治疗对肺部的直接影响开始，然后回顾肿瘤对肺部的主要间接影响，最后以肿瘤患者的呼吸衰竭结束。

恶性气道阻塞

恶性的呼吸系统疾病可以是中央的或外周的，局限的或弥散的，腔内的或腔外的或两者共存。病变的范围和部位决定了与病程相关的主要的症状，同时也决定了治疗方案的选择。

常见的肿瘤类型和临床表现

恶性气道阻塞最常见的原因是邻近部位肿瘤的直接侵犯，特别是支气管癌。食管癌和甲状腺癌同样也经常直接累及气道。原发于大气道的肿瘤相对少见，最常见的病理类型包为鳞癌、囊腺癌和类癌[1,2]。肾癌和乳腺癌或胸内淋巴瘤的转移瘤也会引起气道阻塞。管腔内的病变和外周压迫都会严重缩小气道管腔的直径。管径的减少和结构的扭曲共同影响了气流的通畅和黏膜的清除能力，导致了呼吸费力和呼吸困难[3]。气管和支气管主干的管径狭窄导致了典型的症状：包括咳嗽、呼吸困难、喘息、喘鸣和肺不张。支气管主干以上的气道阻塞通常导致肺不张、阻塞性肺炎、咳嗽和呼吸困难。根据气道阻塞严重程度，患者可以表现为无症状至不同程度的呼吸衰竭[4]。当管径小于 8mm 时会产生典型的劳力性呼吸困难，当管径继续减小至 5mm 时，会产生静息性呼吸困难[5]。慢性阻塞性肺疾病（COPD）加重或黏膜水肿，合并肺炎产生的过多分泌物都可以促进呼吸衰竭的产生，即使这些患者只有中度的肿瘤相关气流受限。因此针对感染或 COPD 恶化的治疗可以改善呼吸道症状。

鉴别诊断

虽然诊断明显的呼吸道阻塞并不困难，但临界点以下的气道阻塞产生的症状可能并不容易鉴别。喘鸣是明显气道阻塞的诊断性症状。其他的一些临床表现，包括呼吸困难和哮鸣音可以非常显著，但是并不特异。一些并发症如充血性心力衰竭、胸膜腔积液和肺栓塞，可以产生类似症状，从而影响诊断。

诊断评估

诊断性检查的目的是建立明确的诊断，量化气流受限程度，描述解剖范围，以便优化治疗策略。肺功能测试中肺容量特征性地降低，往往是气道阻塞最早的征象。但这是一个相对不敏感的检测手段，只有在气道直径低于 10mm 时才能检测出阳性结果[6]。肺活量测定可能诱发严重气道阻塞患者的呼吸衰竭，因此对这类患者应谨慎应用。在极少数的情况下，胸部平片上可以见到气管的偏离和压迫。胸部平片在明确肿瘤解剖范围和治疗选择上意义有限。标准的胸部 CT 以及最新的低剂量多层扫描和先进的气管成像技术使多维和三维重建成为可能，提供了关于肿瘤区域范围和优化治疗策略的有价值的附加信息[7]。支气管镜，不管是软式的还是硬式的，始终是气道阻塞诊断的金标准，同时可以获得组织学恶性的证据。另外，支气管镜使病灶可视化，使得我们可以准确地描述血管分布和阻塞范围，以及管腔及管外病灶对阻塞的贡献大小。最近的研究同样肯定了支气管超声内镜在治疗计划制订中的辅助作用[8]。

恶性气道阻塞的治疗策略

肿瘤的特性，包括病理类型、分期、部位、患者的情况比如症状的缓急、PS 评分，决定了治疗策略。治疗策略根据肿瘤和阻塞的部位、当地的医生和医疗机构资源的不同而变化。手术切除为疾病的长期控制提供了最好的前景，应该作为所有初诊患者的首选治疗方法。如果可行，对于小气道和肺实质的局部病灶，手术是最好的治疗手段。但在很多情况下，外照射治疗或全身化疗可能是唯一的选择。中央型气道阻塞的患者常常不能耐受手术或病灶无法手术切除。虽然对肺癌多种治疗手段的全面综述不在本章的讨论范围之内，但是一些基本的原则已经在图 133-1 中进行了概述。在紧急的情况下，硬式纤支镜可以用来机械性地挖出肿瘤或扩张气道，达到姑息治疗缓解症状的目的。在此紧急情况下，可以应用软式纤支镜和气囊支气管成形术[9]。电烧灼术、氩离子束凝固术、激光治疗、冷冻疗法、近距离放射疗法、光动力疗法都是针对管腔内为主的病灶的合理治疗手段（图 133-2）。

管腔外为主的病变最好使用外照射放射治疗和支气管内支架置入术治疗（图 133-3）。因为大多数病变为腔内和腔外混合病变，多种治疗手段相结合的综合治疗很常见，如使用支气管镜激光治疗物理性减瘤术后置入支架，随后外照射巩固治疗。姑息减症治疗可降低护理难度，大多数情况下可以通过合理使用内镜技术得以实现[10]。患者应该尽早转诊到经验丰富的、能为患者提供各种个体化治疗方法的支气管镜检查医师，然后进行仔细评估。

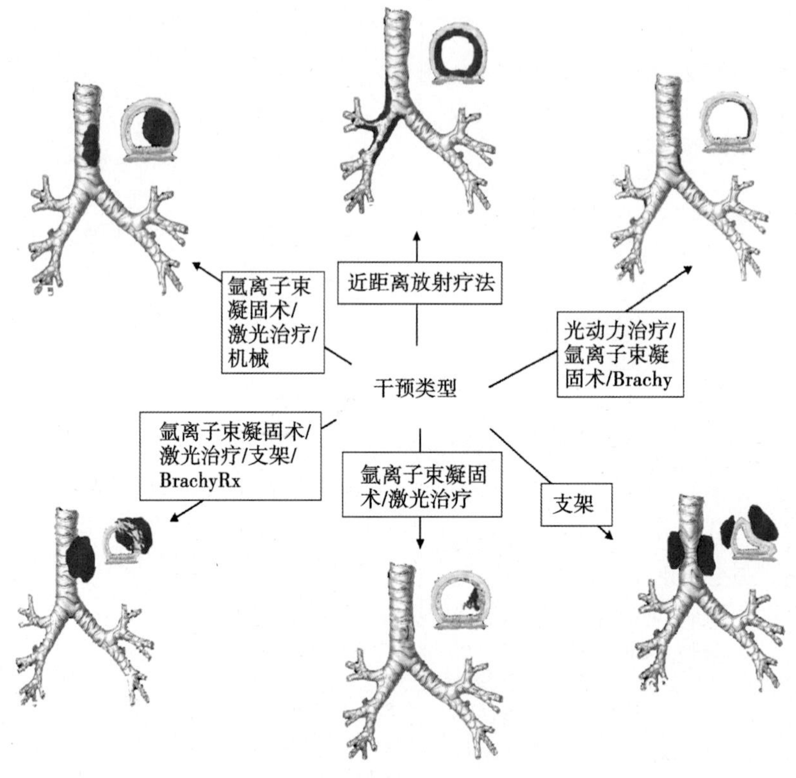

图 133-1　使用支气管镜干预治疗气道阻塞的方法

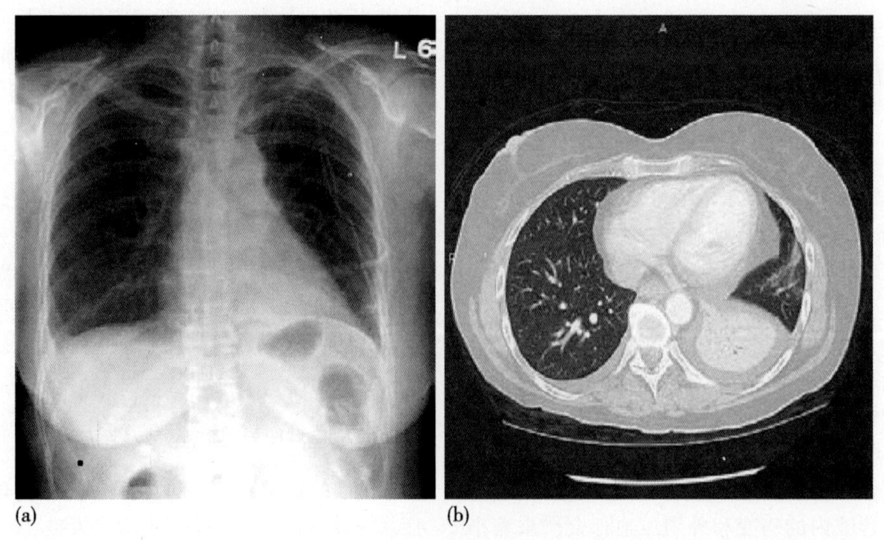

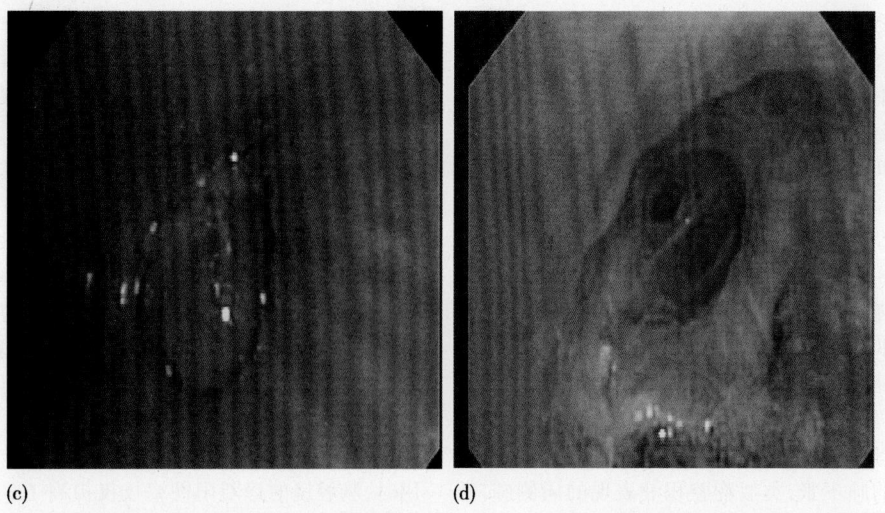

图 133-2　转移性肉瘤所致的左下肺叶塌陷(a 和 b)。支气管镜检查发现由于大的梗阻性肿块导致 LLL 基底部完全性阻塞(c),使用圈断器手术钳和氩离子凝固切除肿块,显露出畅通的远端气道(d)

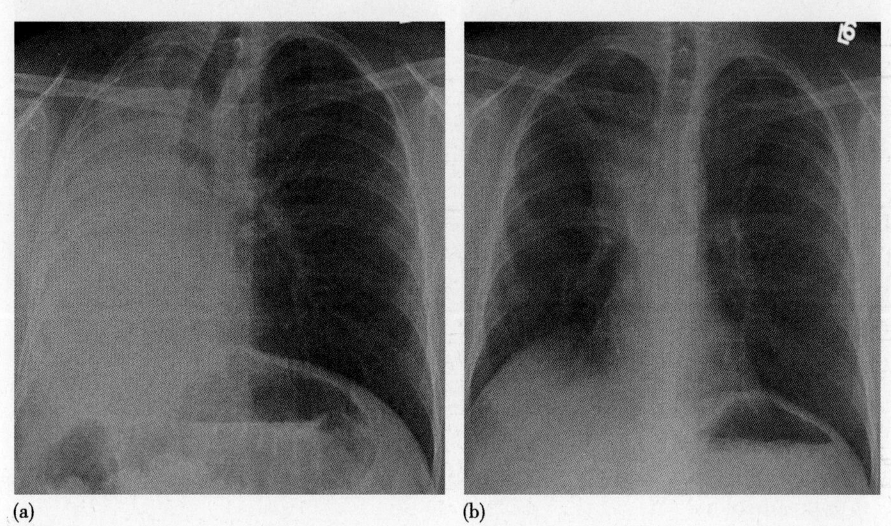

图 133-3　腔外为主的大肿块堵塞右主支气管所致的右肺完全不张(a)。金属支架置入中间支气管(b),使右肺部分复张

恶性胸腔积液

胸水中出现肿瘤细胞是恶性肿瘤常见的临床问题,昭示着肿瘤的远处转移,因此被认为是晚期疾病。恶性胸腔积液有很大的诊断和治疗上的意义。在美国每年有接近 150 000 的恶性胸腔积液病例[11]。在肿瘤胸膜转移的患者中,有高达 45%不会出现胸腔积液[12]。在原发恶性胸膜疾病如恶性间皮瘤中,胸腔积液也可以不出现。几乎所有类型的肿瘤都可以影响胸膜。在所有引起恶性胸腔积液的疾病中,肺癌占据一半的比例,其次是乳腺癌和淋巴瘤。恶性胸腔积液也可以继发于急慢性白血病及骨髓异常增生综合征。白血病患者的胸腔积液往往是感染所致,然后才是白血病胸膜浸润[13]。5%～10%的恶性胸腔积液患者原发灶不明[14,15]。大多数的胸膜恶性肿瘤产生于脏层胸膜的癌栓,壁层胸膜的肿物可能继发于脏层胸膜的播散种植。肺部、胸壁、纵隔组织肿瘤的直接侵犯或肿瘤血行转移至壁层胸膜,是恶性胸水产生的其他机制[16]。除了肿瘤性病因,壁层胸膜与纵隔淋巴结之间任何部位的淋巴回流受阻都可以导致恶性胸水[17]。局部血管内皮生长因子(VGEF)水平的升高在恶性胸水产生中也发挥重要作用,因为 VEGF 具有很强的介导血管通透性升高的作用[18]。VEGF 同源物中,VEGF-D 在恶性胸腔积液的阳性率为 92.6%,使其可以成为一个重要的诊断标志物[19]。肿瘤患者中 17%的胸腔积液是“副恶性”的,这个术语是指积液并不是由胸膜范围内的恶性肿瘤侵犯所直接产生的[16]。这种积液的产生是由于肿瘤的局部或全身效应、肿瘤治疗的并发症或者合并的非肿瘤性疾病所致[20]。淋巴阻塞与副恶性及恶性胸水都有关联、并且是副恶性胸水的最常见病因。其他的常见病因包括支气管阻塞、肺萎陷以及肺栓塞。

临床表现、影像学及诊断

患者最常见的症状是渐进性的劳力性呼吸困难,大量胸水时可以出现严重的咳嗽。全身性症状的出现是疾病进展的常见信号,因此,随着PS评分的降低,周身不适、体重下降、食欲差的主诉反复出现并越来越频繁。胸痛和咯血是提示支气管内肿物和胸壁肿瘤性侵犯的次常见症状。

常规胸部平片和双侧卧位胸片可以为第一步诊断提供重要信息,包括积液量、纵隔和膈肌的位置、有无分隔、气液线的位置以及肺实质的情况。确定纵隔的位置在制订治疗方案中是必不可少的。在导致整个半侧胸腔模糊不清的大量积液评估中,侧卧位投影没有太多的意义。大量胸腔积液伴随纵隔对侧移位通常需要立即进行胸腔穿刺,然而伴随纵隔同侧移位或中心位置的情况,胸腔穿刺则应谨慎施行(图133-4,图133-5)。除了胸腔积液,其他可以导致纵隔同侧移位或纵隔中心位伴胸片模糊影的疾病有:淋巴瘤或间皮瘤相关的冰冻纵隔,同侧中央气道阻塞导致的肺不张,类似胸腔积液表现的同侧肺广泛浸润[20]。CT在鉴别诊断和确定分隔性胸腔积液中特别有价值:CT能够提供更多的关于胸壁、脏层、壁层胸膜、肺实质、纵隔结构的解剖信息[21]。超声可以很方便地用于分析和提供胸腔穿刺的最佳位置,在局限性胸腔积液中尤其有帮助。通过组织运动超声确定内陷的肺,可以在胸腔穿刺前行变形分析[22,23]。PET-CT及MRI对于胸膜外疾病的诊断都有帮助[21]。PET对于诊断恶性间皮瘤有帮助,但是PET扫描对诊断其他恶性胸膜疾病的价值还有待证明。生化分析显示大部分胸水的性质是渗出液,只有5%的恶性胸水为漏出液[20]。恶性胸水诊断的金标准是在胸水中找到癌细胞。62%的患者胸水中癌细胞学检查阳性[24]。流式细胞仪肿瘤标记物检测可以使细胞学阴性的胸水提高33%的敏感性,当怀疑白血病、淋巴瘤、多发性骨髓瘤时,这项检查尤其有价值[25,26]。流式细胞检测在间皮瘤中的价值还存在争议[27]。胸腔镜下胸膜活检诊断胸膜肿瘤的敏感性为95%。当与胸水细胞学检查联用时,胸腔镜的诊断阳性率仅仅提高1%。相反,当与胸水细胞学检查联用时,闭式胸膜活检的阳性率可以从44%提高到77%[24]。

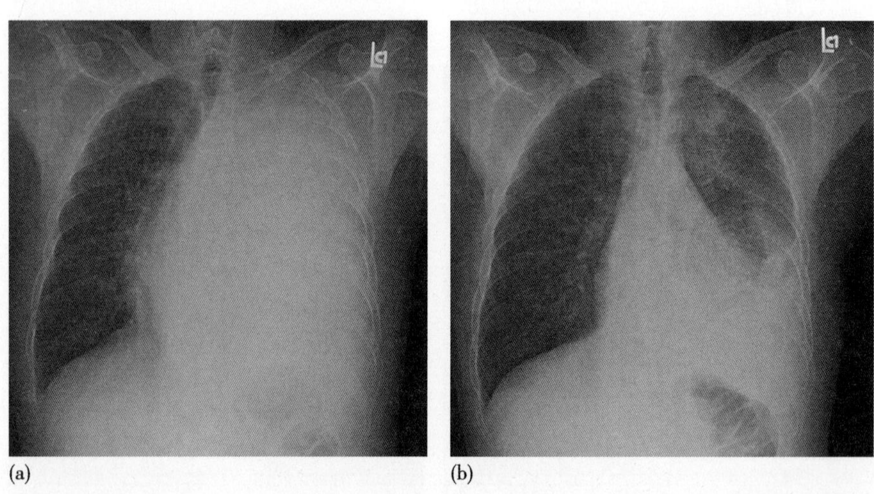

图133-4 左侧大量胸腔积液,造成左边半胸混浊,和对侧纵隔偏移(a)。经胸腔穿刺引流后,纵隔移回中线(b)

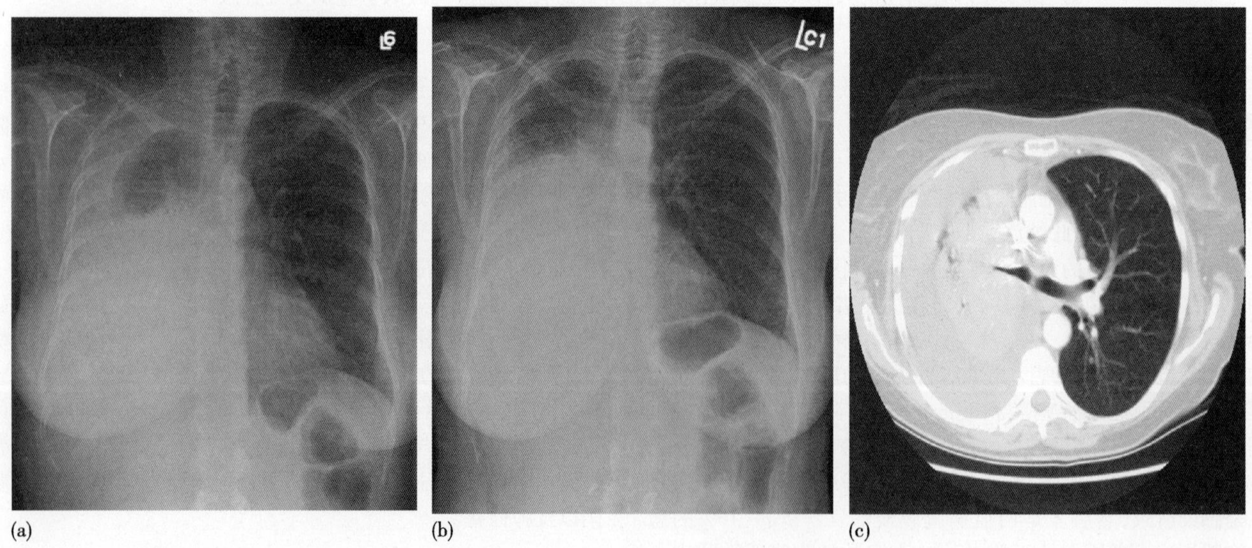

图133-5 右侧大量胸腔积液(a)同侧纵隔以下胸腔移位(b)肺不张或肿块引起肺容积减少。胸部CT扫描(c)可见一个大肿块压迫右主支气管

恶性胸腔积液的治疗

因为恶性胸腔积液往往预示着疾病的晚期和不可治愈，治疗一般都倾向于姑息的手段。因此，注意选择合适的治疗手段以满足患者的个体化需求是非常重要的。患者的 PS 状态以及之前的胸腔穿刺信息，包括抽出的积液的量、是否达到症状的缓解和肺的重新扩张，再次胸腔穿刺的时间间隔都是对制订后续治疗方案有价值的重要因素。对于反复胸腔积液的患者，PS 评分是评价预后的最佳指标[28]。胸壁局部畸形的存在、未来的肿瘤治疗计划、家庭的支持、个人的意愿等因素都会影响患者的治疗。在等待确定治疗方案起效时，胸腔穿刺这一简单的姑息手段对初诊的放化疗敏感肿瘤是合理的，例如淋巴瘤、乳腺癌、小细胞肺癌、生殖细胞肿瘤、卵巢癌、前列腺癌和甲状腺癌等。在初始的临床和影像学评估后，推荐控制症状的治疗性胸穿。最近美国胸科学会和欧洲呼吸协会发表联合声明，推荐每次缓慢引流不超过 1.0~1.5L 的胸水，当患者产生胸部不适、咳嗽、呼吸困难的症状时，应立刻停止引流[11]。根据经验，对于影像学证实的有对侧纵隔移位的大量胸腔积液患者，只要不发生引流相关的胸部不适、咳嗽、呼吸困难等症状，可以安全耐受 2.0~2.5L 一次性胸水引流。但是，一次性大量引流胸水应谨慎进行，尤其是当影像学检查提示有纵隔居中或同侧纵隔移位时。排放大量胸水时测定胸腔压力，可以减少胸腔引流术相关的并发症[29]。就减轻症状的引流术的安全性而言，胸腔压力测量不是必需的，其作用仍需要进一步研究。胸腔穿刺术后肺复张可以通过胸部后前位、侧位片检查来评估。间隔 1~2 日再重复胸腔穿刺术对恰当评估大量胸腔积液的肺复张可能是必要的[30]。在恶性胸腔积液的患者中，97%会在 1 个月内复发，大多数在引流后的 1~3 日内再次出现[31]。对于那些预期寿命有限（<30 日）、PS 评分不佳或者胸水增长缓慢的患者，最好给予反复胸腔穿刺治疗。对那些化疗和/或放疗预期有效的恶性肿瘤患者，反复胸腔穿刺也是一种合理的治疗方法。然而，频繁胸腔穿刺可能引起局部细胞因子和纤维蛋白的产生，导致包裹性胸腔积液，这不仅使得胸腔穿刺变得更复杂，也使后续的姑息模式受到限制[32]。在过去几年，留置胸腔导管，作为有反复恶性胸腔积液的患者姑息治疗的替代选择，正越来越多地被接受。这种姑息治疗适合的人群为预期寿命超过 30 日并且既往胸腔穿刺引流可以有效缓解症状的患者。胸腔导管植入术在这组患者中是有效的，无论胸腔穿刺后是否有肺复张。留置胸腔导管可在门诊进行。在证实导管的位置恰当之后，患者、经过培训的家庭成员或护理人员可以在家里间歇性地引流积液。建议在最初的时候每日进行胸腔引流。每一个环节通常持续不到 15min，引流应直到患者出现咳嗽、胸部不适或液体流出自然停止，可能是因为胸膜腔空间已经被排空。在我们研究所中，92%进行留置导管的患者呼吸困难明显缓解，52%进行了有效的胸膜固定术。从导管置入到导管拔除的平均时间为 32 日。观察到的导管相关并发症的发生率仅占 4%，包括 1 例患者合并脓胸，2 例患者在插管部位出现持续性疼痛。只有 6%的患者在拔除导管后需要再次进行胸腔引流[33]。胸腔置管后接受放化疗的患者和在基线状态呼吸短促的患者能够获得最大限度的改善[34]。在一项亚组分析中，符合胸膜固定术标准的患者在留置胸腔导管后 70%取得有效的胸膜固定[35]。

传统上化学性胸膜固定术是使用最广泛的控制复发性恶性胸腔积液的方法。遗憾的是，由于缺乏前瞻性研究，我们无法对现有化学粘连剂与胸膜粘连术进行有效性、安全性和成本效益的进行比较分析。现有文献的研究结果表明，非化疗药物的粘连剂更有效，是最符合成本效益的硬化剂[11]。不含石棉的无菌滑石粉是首选的胸膜粘连剂。并发症因滑石粒子的剂量，大小和表面特性而异。小于 5mm 的滑石粉颗粒的使用与肺损伤有关，其中包括与成人呼吸窘迫综合征（ARDS）有关的急性肺炎和呼吸衰竭。应该注意避免这些肺损伤[36]。大颗粒滑石粉胸膜固定术的安全性，最近在欧洲的一项大规模多中心试验中获得证实，认为与 ARDS 没有关联[37]。作为一种致组织硬化治疗方法，胸腔镜滑石粉喷洒对于滑石粉浆的优势存在着争议。据报道，这两种技术的成功率均>90%，总体并发症或疾病复发率无显著性差异[11]。已公布的最大前瞻性随机试验纳入 501 例 PS 评分为 1 或 2 的患者，比较了胸腔镜滑石粉喷洒和滑石粉浆的疗效。结果表明：胸导管滑石粉浆和胸腔镜滑石粉喷洒的胸膜固定术的 30 日存活率以及成功率没有差异，但是在两个研究组中均报道了超出预期的高发病率和死亡率。亚组分析表明，胸腔镜滑石粉喷洒可能在肺癌或乳腺癌患者中更有优势[38]。根据现有资料，本研究组认为对所有具有良好的 PS 状态（ECOG 评分 0，1 或 2），且初次引流胸水后达到缓解症状和肺复张的患者，留置胸腔导管或者胸腔镜滑石粉喷洒胸膜固定术作为首选的姑息治疗方式。

在少数情况下，胸腹分流和壁层胸膜部分切除术等替代方式可以用于治疗胸膜固定术失败后的复发性和有症状的胸腔积液或与肺萎陷相关的胸腔积液。与恶性肿瘤相关的乳糜胸通过治疗原发肿瘤可以得到控制。这些富含蛋白质、脂肪和淋巴细胞为主的乳糜液的长期丢失，可能会导致淋巴细胞减少，严重营养消耗，及水、电解质的丢失。乳糜胸引起的死亡率可以高达 50%。在这些症状反复的乳糜胸和癌症复发或疾病进展的患者中，除了给予适当治疗外，肠外营养和滑石粉胸膜固定术[39]或留置胸腔导管仍是合理的治疗选择[40]。胸腹分流装置是一个很好的选择，因为乳糜不会丢失，而是从胸膜腔调动到腹膜腔，在腹膜被重吸收，从而减轻营养不良和免疫抑制的风险。遗憾的是，胸腹分流泵的排量一次只有 1.5~2.5ml，这使得其使用很烦琐。此外，泵堵塞的发生率很高。理论上还可以通过引流泵引起腹腔肿瘤播散，但这并没有被明确证实。胸导管栓塞是复发性乳糜胸的一个治疗选择，这种方法的耐受性很好，但还没有确切证据证实其在癌症人群中的有效性。壁层胸膜部分切除术，胸膜纤维板剥脱术或胸膜全肺切除术与高死亡率有关，并没有比其他姑息治疗更好地控制症状[11]。利用化合物单独或与其他姑息治疗方式相结合以阻止血管内皮生长因子（VEGF）的方法很有前景。从理论上说，使用 VEGF 阻断减少胸腔积液的产生，然后引流胸腔积液并注入化学粘连剂以获得胸膜粘连，可加速胸膜固定，减少住院时间[41]。遗憾的是，在一项 VEGF 受体抑制剂凡德他尼（vandetanib）联合留置胸腔导管治疗复发性恶性胸腔积液非小细胞肺患者的单臂Ⅱ期临床研究中，这一方法并未显著降低胸膜固定术的时间[42]。

总之，在预期寿命有限的患者中，有最佳缓解症状可能，最低手术相关发病率和死亡率，以及最短住院时间的治疗方式就是合理的复发性恶性胸腔积液的治疗方法。一个涉及肿瘤学、肺内科学、介入放射学和胸外科的多学科治疗方法（图 133-6），提供了实现这些目标的最好的机会。

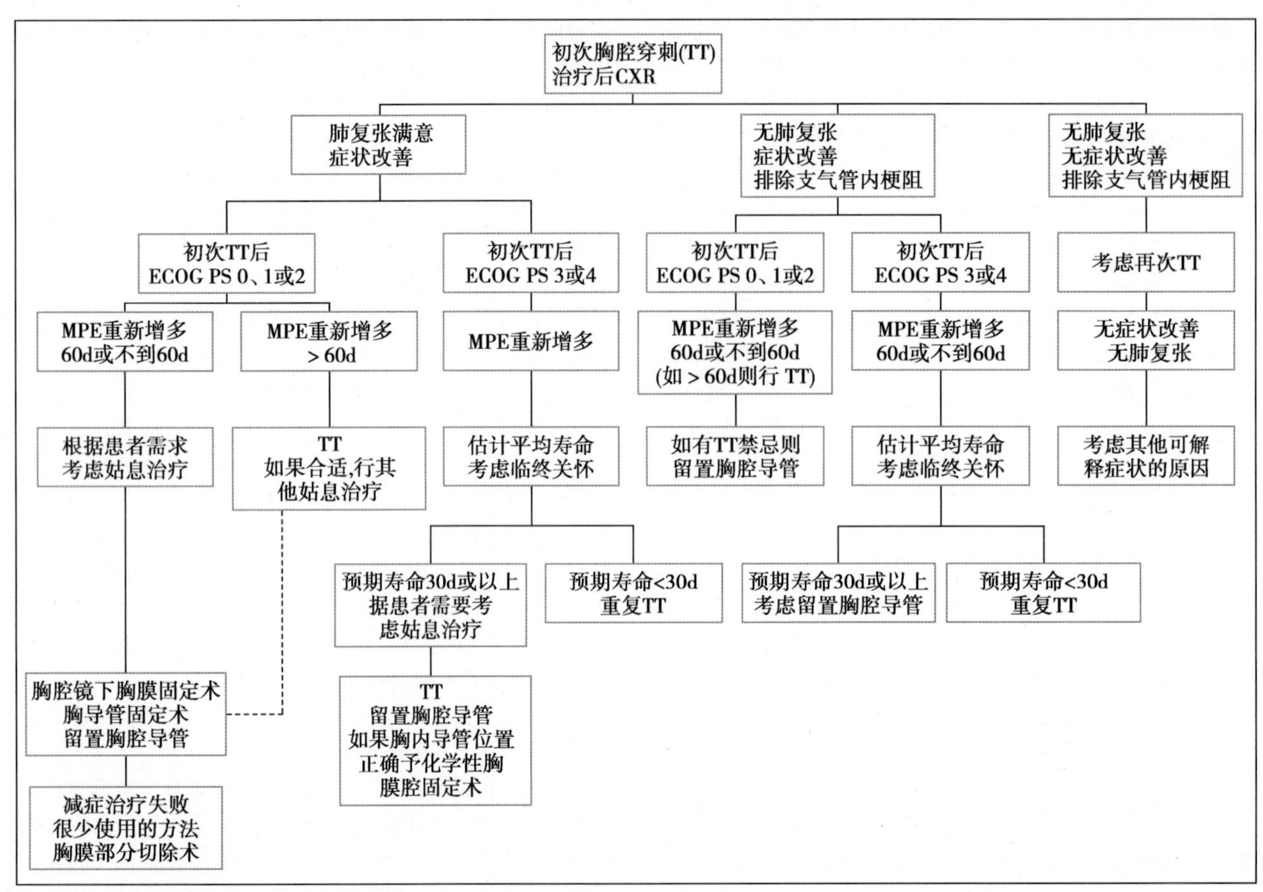

图 133-6 恶性胸腔积液（MPE）的治疗。化疗或放疗初始治疗敏感的肿瘤患者（淋巴瘤，乳腺癌，小细胞肺癌，生殖细胞，卵巢癌，前列腺癌和甲状腺肿瘤）适宜做进行胸腔穿刺术，同时等待全身治疗结果

术后呼吸功能不全

诊断评估

对于解剖上可切除肿瘤的患者的初步评估方法包括，确定患者的器官功能耐受手术的可能性和预测肺切除后的远期肺功能障碍。这可以通过特异性的肺部检查以及其他常规检查来发现同时存在的系统性疾病。肺的评估包括三个序贯的步骤：①肺功能基线测定；②放射性核素定量肺通气/灌注分析计算术后肺功能；③前两个步骤结果不满意的患者进行运动负荷试验[43]。在用于术后预后的预测的肺功能检测试验中，其中一秒钟用力呼气容积（FEV_1）和一氧化碳肺弥散量（DLCO）的减少值的可重复性最高，也最常用于预测肺切除术后并发症[44]。对于决策，考虑到患者的身高，性别和种族的变异，FEV_1 的报告值中百分预测值优于绝对单位（L）值。在我们的实验室中，超过一半 FEV_1 为预测值 60%~80%的患者，通过放射性核素研究得出估计的肺切除术后 FEV_1，这个 FEV_1 值低于安全切除术的可接受值（<40%预计值）。因此，我们建议，只有那些患者基线 FEV_1 和 DLCO≥80%预测值且没有对侧肺疾病临床证据的患者，可不需进一步测试考虑肺切除术。所有其他的患者应进行“拆分功能”的评价，即区域性肺通气和灌注的放射性核素的定量评估。在这项研究中，每侧肺的放射性离子摄入通过吸入 ^{133}Xe 和静脉注射溶解在生理盐水的 ^{133}Xe 或 ^{99}Tc 浓聚测定。在实践中，仅估计肺灌注是最简单和最常见的测量方法。每侧肺贡献的放射性百分比与该侧肺整体功能贡献有关。术后 FEV_1 预测值（FEV_1ppo），和术后 DLCO 预测值（DLCOp-po）通过总百分摄入值减去切除肺区域的百分功能摄入值。许多研究者已经证实了拆分功能对并发症风险以及肺切除后肺功能损失的预测的价值[45,46]。在这些研究中，术前预测值接近于全肺切除术和超过三个肺段的肺段切除术的术后测量值[47]。全肺切除术后肺功能保持相对稳定。这种预测对于切除范围小的手术如肺叶切除是不可靠的，因为早期损失不成比例，之后随着时间推移功能可显著改善[48]。Kearney 等也认为 FEV_1ppo 是并发症唯一显著的独立预测因素[49]。其他可变因素，包括年龄≥60 岁，男性，吸烟史，肺切除术史，高碳酸血症史，（二氧化碳分压≥45mmHg），运动中血氧测定法去饱和（血氧饱和度≤90%），术前 FEV_1≤1L，是无法预测并发症的。Markos 等[50]报道了，DLCOppo<40%的预测值是与较高的发病率和死亡率有关，并且是术后呼吸衰竭最好的预测值。

总之，拆分功能研究中 FEV_1ppo 和 DLCOppo≥40%预测值是肺切除术包括全肺切除术的判断标准。要求进行较小的手术如肺叶切除术但不符合这些标准的患者应在可以进行手术之前进行运动试验进一步评估。

在这些高危患者中使用运动试验的原理基于两个概念：①肺功能不是性能的唯一决定因素，②肺叶切除或更少切除的损耗随着时间的推移而改善，这往往被放射肺量测定研究过高估计[43]。运动试验还显现了单组研究中应激状态下检查心肺和肌肉相互作用的优势。运动试验的最具验证效力的形式是通过增加症状-限制最大值（$VO_{2最大值}$）的工作负荷进行周期性肌力测试。Smith 等人使用这种方法发现，$VO_{2最大值}$>20ml/（kg·min）患者中，1/10 术后出现并发症，而所有 $VO_{2最大值}$<15ml/（kg·min）的患者都出现并发症[51]。我们对由于 FEV_1≤40%、预计术后 FEV_1≤33%和/或动脉血 PCO_2≥45mmHg 而被认为手术不能治愈的患者进行了两项研究。$VO_{2最大值}$≥15ml/（kg·min）的患者接受手术治疗；其他患者进行放疗和/或化疗。所有手术治疗的患者在 24h 内拔管，出院的中位时间是 8 日。无在院死亡者，但是可逆的术后并发症的发生占这类患者的 40%。此外，观察到了这些进行手术的高危患者的生存获益[52,53]。最近，我们确定了 $VO_{2最大值}$作为百分预测值更准确地估计了手术风险，并最大限度地增加了可安全进行肺切除的患者人数。我们的结论是运动中 $VO_{2最大值}$≥60%预测值的高危患者在肺切除术后取得了可接受的预后，即使 $VO_{2最大值}$<15ml/（kg·min）[33]。我们对肺切除术的术前评估方法进行了总结，如图 133-7。除了手术风险和术后功能的评估之外，术前评估的目标还包括方案的完善，以降低风险和使可从手术治疗中获益的患者人数最大化。最后，必须牢记的是，没有任何一个试验能预测所有并发症，患者和医生应该对手术治疗的风险效益作出最后的判定。

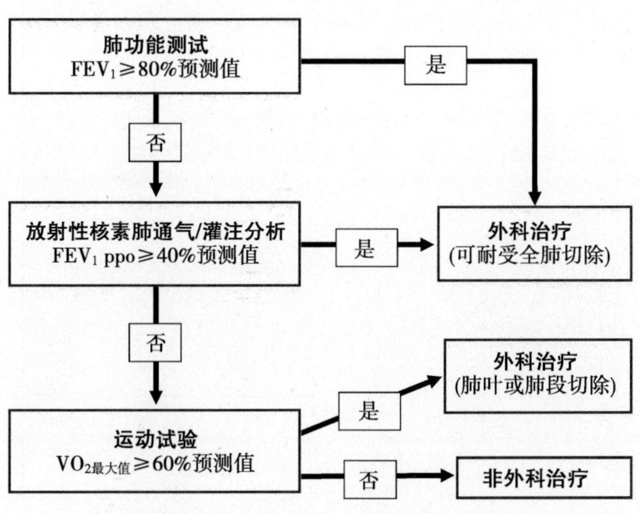

图 133-7　肺切除术术前评估的方法

化疗引起的肺损伤

传统的化疗，以及越来越多的分子靶向抗肿瘤药物，常常会涉及肺损伤。不同类型抗肿瘤药物的肺毒性可能是特殊的、不可预测的或者可变的。另外，统一类抗肿瘤药物的不同剂型可以引起相同类型的肺损伤，但是其发生频率可能不同。比如在靶向 EGFR 的小分子酪氨酸激酶抑制剂（TKI）中，吉非替尼（gefitinib）与厄洛替尼有时会与致命性的间质性肺炎相关；而 EGFR-HER2 双靶点的 TKI 拉帕替尼的肺毒性则比较少见[54]。同样，细胞毒性烷基化剂白消安和环磷酰胺给药后致死的肺损伤是众所周知的，而烷基化剂氯霉素对肺的损伤是非常罕见的，而且仅限于罕见的病例报告[55-57]。

传统化疗相关肺损伤

化疗相关肺损伤的发病机制尚不清楚。可能的机制包括对Ⅱ型肺细胞和/或肺泡壁内皮细胞的直接细胞毒性、导致内皮功能障碍和毛细血管渗漏综合征的细胞因子释放、与释放自由基相关的氧化损伤和/或细胞介导的肺损伤[58~60]。

个别药物毒性可能局限于肺间质、肺泡、胸膜、肺循环或气道，或者可能涉及多个胸腔内结构。肺对药物性损伤（DLI）的反应非常有限，引起固定的病理损伤模式或综合征。主要的间质和肺泡损伤类型最常见，包括各种类型的间质性肺炎，如非特异性间质性肺炎（NSIP）、脱屑性间质性肺炎（DIP）、超敏性肺炎（HP）、机化性肺炎（OP）和嗜酸性粒细胞肺炎（EP）。非心源性肺水肿（NCPE）、弥漫性肺泡损伤（DAD）、急性呼吸窘迫综合征（ARDS）和弥漫性肺泡出血（DAH）是药物性肺损伤的另外形式。除了直接的肺损伤，化疗引起的免疫抑制可能使患者更容易发生危及生命的感染，其中肺炎是最常见的。药物引起的肉芽肿病和淋巴结病也有报道。传统的化疗方案以及分子靶向和免疫调节剂治疗引起的肺损伤模式也有报道。表 133-1 和表 133-2 分别描述了与常规和分子靶向癌症治疗相关的肺损伤模式。

由于经常同步或续贯使用复杂的多药和多学科方案，使个体药物引起的肺损伤发生率的估计变得困难。年龄，累积剂量，同步或序贯放疗，氧疗，既往肺损伤和使用多药方案等诱发因素因个体药物而异，并可能影响发病率以及药物暴露到临床症状出现之间的潜伏期。心源性或非心源性肺水肿、感染、肿瘤复发或放疗引起的肺损伤在临床、影像及病理表现上是有交叉的，这使得这些肺损伤在临床上很难区别，也使得药物性肺损伤的估计变得困难。其他可能与药物性肺损伤相似的情况包括吸入性肺炎，心源性肺水肿，急性肺损伤（ALI）和 ARDS[61,62]。临床症状从低烧伴干咳和呼吸困难到可迅速发展为呼吸衰竭和 ARDS 的暴发性疾病。出现皮疹、潮红和支气管痉挛时，可能提示超敏反应或非 IgE 介导的假过敏反应。这些症状可能在治疗后几分钟到几小时内出现。最近的一项研究发现，使用阳离子药物直接激活肥大细胞是引起假过敏反应的原因[63]。过敏反应通常需要一个过敏期，症状出现在第二个或随后的治疗周期。假过敏反应正好相反，可能发生在第一个化疗周期后的几分钟内。其他形式的药物性肺损伤的临床表现，包括间质性肺炎，通常发生在早期，在开始治疗后的几周到几个月内[59,60]。延迟性肺纤维化，发生在暴露于博来霉素、白消安、环磷酰胺、吉西他滨和亚硝酸钠后数月至数年，是药物性肺损伤的一种晚期表现[64~67]。

全身炎症标志物，如白细胞增多、血沉和 c 反应蛋白升高，是常见但非特异性的表现。PET 在评估药物相关肺损伤的程度时特异性和重要性都不高。DLCO 作为评估肺癌化疗相关肺损伤的反应最敏感的参数，获得了普遍接受，但是其早期变化检测的预测潜力一直是变化的[68~73]。随着疾病进展，限制性

表 133-1 化疗引起的肺损伤的主要临床症状和组织学类型

药物类型	药物	DAD，ARDS，DAH	咯血（非DAH相关）	NCPE	IP	EP	肉芽肿形成	支气管痉挛/IR	BOOP	PHTN（PVOD，PAH）	VTE/PE	胸膜疾病	机会性感染	高血红蛋白	放射记忆性肺炎
烷化剂	白消安	✓			✓	✓			✓						
	环磷酰胺	✓			✓	✓		✓	✓			✓		✓	
	异环磷酰胺	✓		✓	✓			✓	✓					✓	
	替莫唑胺	✓			✓								✓		
	奥沙利铂	✓		✓	✓	✓	✓	✓	✓						
	卡铂							✓							
	顺铂							✓							
	美法仑	✓			✓										
抗代谢药	甲氨蝶呤	✓		✓	✓	✓	✓	✓	✓			✓	✓		
	硫唑嘌呤	✓		✓	✓										
	阿糖孢苷	✓		✓	✓	✓									
	氟达拉滨	✓		✓	✓	✓							✓		
	azacitabine				✓										
	吉西他滨	✓		✓	✓	✓		✓				✓			✓
	喷司他丁			✓		✓									
	培美曲塞	✓						✓							
	净司他丁	✓								✓					
细胞毒药物	博来霉素	✓			✓	✓		✓	✓	✓					
	丝裂霉素 C	✓		✓	✓			✓		✓					
	氨柔比星				✓										✓

续表

药物类型	药物	DAD，ARDS，DAH	咯血（非DAH相关）	NCPE	IP	EP	肉芽肿形成	支气管痉挛/IR	BOOP	PHTN（PVOD，PAH）	VTE/PE	胸膜疾病	机会性感染	高血红蛋白	放射记忆性肺炎
	聚乙二醇脂质体多柔比星				✓			✓							✓
拓扑异构酶抑制剂	伊立替康				✓										
	托泊替康	✓			✓				✓						
鬼臼毒素	依托泊苷	✓				✓		✓							
	替尼泊苷							✓							
亚硝基脲类	BCNU					✓		✓	✓	✓					
	CCNU					✓									
紫杉类	紫杉醇	✓			✓	✓		✓				✓			✓
	多西他赛	✓		✓	✓	✓									✓
	长春新碱	✓						✓							
	长春碱	✓						✓							
	长春地辛	✓						✓							
	长春瑞滨	✓						✓				✓			
	伊沙匹隆														
其他	ATRA	✓			✓			✓			✓	✓			
	三氧化二砷	✓			✓			✓				✓			
	丙卡巴肼				✓	✓	✓					✓			
	左旋天冬酰胺酶							✓	✓						

表 133-2 分子靶向治疗引起的肺损伤的主要临床症状和组织学类型

药物类型	药物	DAD，ARDS，DAH	咯血（非DAH相关）	NCPE	IP	EP	肉芽肿形成	支气管痉挛/IR	BOOP	PHTN（PVOD，PAH）	VTE/PE	胸膜疾病	机会性感染	高血红蛋白	放射记忆性肺炎
单克隆抗体	西妥昔单抗	✓			✓			✓	✓						
	帕尼单抗	✓			✓			✓	✓			✓			✓
	贝伐单抗		✓					✓			✓				
	阿伦珠单抗	✓	✓		✓			✓							
	利妥昔单抗	✓	✓	✓	✓			✓							
	奥妥珠单抗							✓							
	奥法木单抗	✓						✓					✓		
	替伊莫单抗	✓						✓					✓		
	曲妥珠单抗							✓							
	帕妥珠单抗	✓						✓							
	吉姆单抗			✓				✓							
	伊匹木单抗						✓	✓							
酪氨酸激酶抑制剂	吉非替尼	✓			✓										
	厄罗替尼	✓			✓										✓
	伊马替尼	✓		✓	✓							✓			
	达沙替尼				✓						✓	✓			
	博舒替尼											✓			
	泼那替尼										✓				

续表

药物类型	药物	DAD，ARDS，DAH	咯血（非DAH相关）	NCPE	IP	EP	肉芽肿形成	支气管痉挛/IR	BOOP	PHTN（PVOD，PAH）	VTE/PE	胸膜疾病	机会性感染	高血红蛋白	放射记忆性肺炎
	索拉非尼	✓	✓	✓	✓										
	舒尼替尼		✓		✓										
	培唑帕尼		✓								✓				
	凡德他尼	✓			✓										
	艾代拉里斯				✓								✓		
	曲美替尼				✓										
	克唑替尼	✓			✓						✓				
	维莫非尼														✓
	芦可替尼	✓											✓		
西罗莫司抑制剂	依维莫司	✓			✓		✓						✓		
	坦罗莫司	✓			✓										
	硼替佐米	✓			✓				✓	✓					
	卡非佐米				✓					✓					
免疫调节剂	沙利度胺			✓	✓	✓			✓		✓				
	来那度胺				✓										
	pomalidmine														
	IL-2		✓	✓		✓				✓		✓			
	TNF		✓												
	IFN-g		✓				✓		✓	✓		✓			

通气功能障碍会逐渐显现[65,74]。在某些形式的化疗引起的肺损伤后，肺功能在暴露后2年内几乎完全恢复正常是常见的[73]。影像学包括高分辨率计算机断层扫描（HRCT），是评估疑似药物性肺损伤的重要工具，尽管这些发现并不具有特异性。CT上最常见的影像学表现是肺间质和混合性肺泡-间质异常，表现为位于外周和下肺的磨玻璃密度影。上肺阴影在药物过敏反应后比较可以见到。结节性病变可能与潜在的恶性肿瘤相似，可以观察到网状线、间隔增厚和镶嵌样图像。随着病情恶化，影像学主要表现为肺间质纤维化（牵拉性支气管扩张，蜂窝状改变）。基于博来霉素、依托泊苷和利妥昔单抗的治疗后，在PET/CT成像上18F-FDG的弥漫性摄取增高提示肺炎可能。类似的发现也可以在肿瘤的淋巴结转移中看到[75,76]。

支气管肺泡灌洗（BAL）伴或不伴肺活检可能有助于排除感染或基础疾病的诊断。研究表明，其对肺部感染的诊断率高达70%~90%，淋巴瘤和肺癌的淋巴结转移的诊断率高达35%~70%[77,78]。药物性肺损伤BAL的为典型的高细胞性伴中性粒细胞或淋巴细胞数量增加。BAL液CD4/CD8比值下降也可以提供支持诊断的证据，但是比例变化很大，不能充分区分药物诱导还是其他原因引起的ILD[79]。药物诱导的HP表现为BAL液淋巴细胞升高超过50%伴CD4/CD8比值较低。BAL液嗜酸性粒细胞升高超过25%支持药物诱导的EP。连续取样发现进行性加重的血性BAL，和/或BAL液中含铁血黄素的巨噬细胞数目增加的细胞学证据，支持DAH诊断。经支气管和外科肺活检可能有助于诊断IP、DAD、EP和OP，并同血管炎、感染和潜在的恶性肿瘤等进行鉴别。虽然在20%的组织活检中可以看到DLI的病理表现，但DLI的组织病理学标准尚未建立，也没有特征性的发现。尽管如此，肺活检在鉴别诊断和描述肺损伤的组织病理学模式方面是有意义的。这些信息不仅对DLI的诊断有意义，而且对指导治疗方案也很有用。DLI的诊断通常基于药物暴露与肺损伤发生之间的时间关联；整合兼容的临床、影像学和实验室检查结果；排除相互矛盾的诊断。

化疗相关DLI的治疗仍然是基于经验，而不是基于证据。在大多数情况下，停用相关药物是主要的治疗手段。多数患者在停药后症状会得到改善，尽管即使停药后也可能发生疾病进展。一般来说，一旦有足够的临床证据怀疑该药物与肺毒性有关，就应停止使用该药物。这也有明显例外，如采用维A酸（ATRA）或三氧化二砷治疗急性早幼粒细胞白血病后出现分化综合征[80]，需全身类固醇治疗并降低药物剂量，而不是停药，这可以与成功解决轻至中度形式的分化综合征毒性。

如果有临床表现，应开始全身糖皮质激素和支持治疗（包括吸入支气管扩张剂、吸氧和机械通气）。糖皮质激素已被证明可以在某些类固醇反应性肺损伤模式中消除DLI的症状，如HP、EP和阻塞性细支气管炎并机化性肺炎（BOOP）。其他情况包括肺纤维化，肺血管疾病，和闭塞性细支气管炎（BO），糖皮质激素没有确切的作用。目前的专家意见，主张对无症状的ILD进行高分辨率CT扫描密切监测，并在不调整剂量的情况下继续治疗。对于有症状的患者，应使用肺毒性级别来指导临床决策，包括剂量调整或停药，是否使用糖皮质激素治疗[81]。对于中度（2级或以上）IP患者，建议停用化疗药物并开始糖皮质激素治疗，剂量为0.75~1mg/(kg·d)的泼尼松或同等剂量。类固醇通常维持在较高的剂量，直到症状得到改善。然后在1~3个月的时间内根据治疗反应逐渐减少。建议使用支气管镜肺泡灌洗术来排除感染和/或肺泡出血[82]。除非特殊情况，如ATRA和砷相关的分化综合征，一般不建议重新给予同样的化疗药[80,83]。随着间质性肺炎的发展，再次使用致病的同类药物，应根据具体情况，并应根据不同药物、反应的严重程度和替代疗法的可行性综合来做决定。

分子靶向治疗及免疫治疗相关肺损伤

恶性肿瘤细胞中异常表达的蛋白（过表达或表达下调），会导致肿瘤细胞的快速生长。分子靶向抗肿瘤药物，由于抗肿瘤谱比较特异，最初被认为造成正常器官毒性较小，不像传统的化疗药物。靶向治疗的毒性谱（皮肤、血管、凝血、眼、肺）与传统的细胞毒性药物的毒性谱（骨髓抑制、黏膜炎、脱发、严重恶心、呕吐、肺）不尽相同，但是这两种治疗方法的毒性的频率和强度是相近的。ILD、输液反应（IR）、血管病变、胸腔积液是靶向治疗的常见并发症。与靶向治疗相关的肺损伤可能发生于靶点（抑制预期目标）或非靶点（抑制非预期目标）机制。由于多种信号通路的相互作用，也可能发生重叠毒性。

在治疗后2个月就可以影像学上发现ILD，临床肺炎通常发生在靶向治疗的前6个月。最常见的症状是干咳、呼吸困难和发烧。暴发性呼吸衰竭很少见，但在利妥昔单抗治疗后以及西罗莫司（mTOR）和EGFR抑制剂靶向治疗后都有报道（图133-8）。

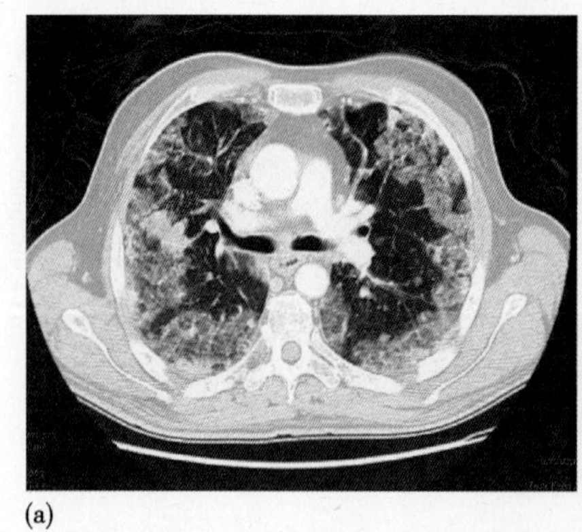
(a)

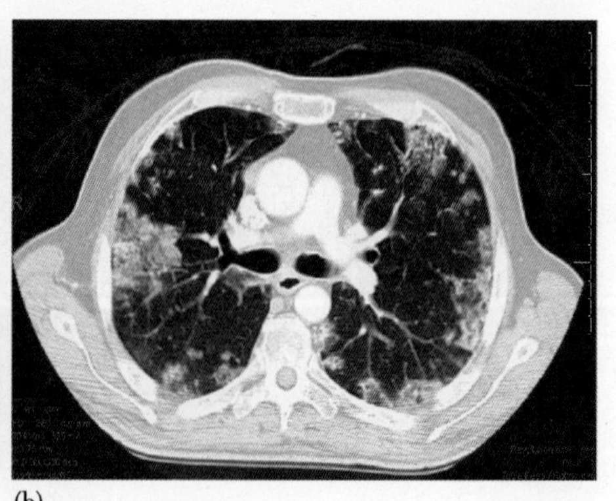
(b)

图133-8　60岁男性，因晚期胰腺癌接受厄洛替尼治疗12周后出现斑疹性丘疹，进行性干咳伴呼吸急促。肺部广泛的磨玻璃影和结节状胸膜浸润（a）；在系统性类固醇治疗2周后明显改善（b）

药物介导的肺部综合征

肺间质疾病(ILD)

非特异性间质性肺炎(NSIP)是药物性肺损伤的 ILD 最常见的形态学类型。隐匿性发展的干咳和呼吸困难是损伤的信号,通常发生于药物暴露后数周到数月内。影像学改变通常比临床症状滞后数天到数周。间质和肺泡间质混合异常是最常见的肺部影像学表现,通常局限于外周或下肺区域。还观察到结节性病变、网状线、间隔增厚、镶嵌样图像和磨玻璃样改变。ILD 的危险因素随各个药物不同,但一般包括高龄、同步放疗或药物联合治疗、既存的肺部疾病、高氧吸入的需求。与 ILD 相关的早期病理变化包括上皮和血管内皮细胞的损害,导致肺泡间质水肿。肺泡水肿和 DAD 是进展期 ILD 的常见特征,尽管停药并予糖皮质激素治疗,仍可能进展至终末期肺纤维化。

高达 20%的博来霉素治疗过的患者发展成为博来霉素诱导的肺炎(BIP),其发生率表现为剂量相关性,总积累剂量超过 400U 时更易发生。BIP 的发生率和严重程度在以下因素存在时增加:年龄超过 70 岁、尿毒症、大剂量给药方案、多种药物治疗、综合治疗或序贯放疗、高通量吸氧[58,84,85]。有证据表明,高流量吸氧可能引发或加剧博来霉素诱导的肺毒性,但是证据级别不高。吸入氧气流量或氧疗时间增加肺损伤的风险尚未确定。此外,博来霉素治疗后降低高氧相关博来霉素毒性风险的时间间隔尚不清楚。尽管如此,我们建议谨慎地提高氧流量,以达到或高于 89%~92%的氧饱和度。干咳、劳力性呼吸困难这些 BIP 相关的临床症状往往在使用博来霉素 1~6 个月之后出现,但是这些表现经常被描述成博来霉素的晚期(>6 个月)毒性(图 133-9)。博来霉素引起 DLCO 预测值下降,最初被认为是早期肺损伤的标志和停药的指征。然而,基于 DLCO 下降的停药阈值尚未确定。此外,只有一小部分接触博来霉素的 DLCO 发生变化的患者会产生临床毒性[86]。在我们的实践中,化疗前存在肺部疾病和/或肺功能受损的患者,需使用系列 PFT 监测 DLCO。当累积剂量接近 400U 或出现提示博来霉素毒性的临床症状时,也需对 DLCO 进行连续监测。糖皮质激素治疗的最佳剂量尚不明确。泼尼松或其等效药物的起始剂量为 0.75~1mg/kg(基于理想体重),在前 4~6 周每日推荐最大剂量为 100mg/kg。泼尼松的减量通常要根据患者的病情和临床治疗反应,需在几个月内逐渐完成。BIP 的消退通常是随着时间的推移而发生的,大多数患者在 15 个月或更长时间内肺功能和肺部影像学均有改善。延迟诊断、持续使用博来霉素或纤维化的发展预示着预后更差。

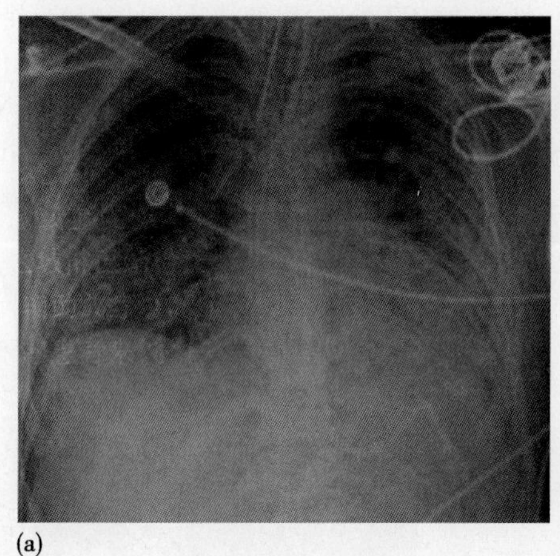

(a)

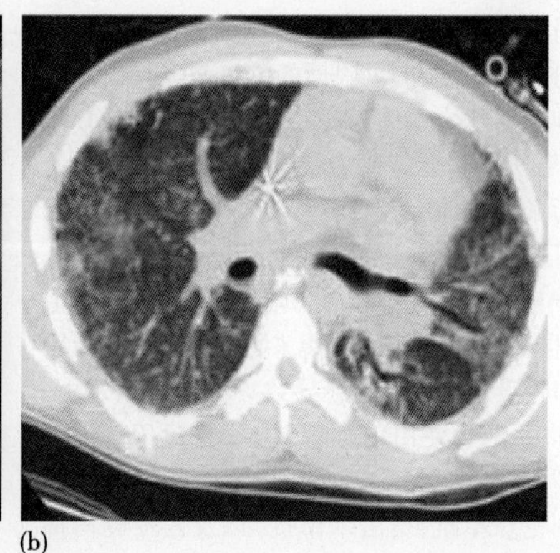

(b)

图 133-9　24 岁女性,在完成以博来霉素为基础的霍奇金淋巴瘤治疗 3 个月后,因无关疾病腹部手术后出现呼吸窘迫。CXR(a)和 CT(b)显示双侧斑片状网状结节和气道病变。检查结果与博来霉素毒性相关的 ARDS 一致,可能是手术期间高氧引起的

BCNU(氮芥)同样也可以引起剂量依赖肺毒性,在累积剂量超过 1 500mg/m^2 的患者中,发生率高达 50%。与其他药物诱导的 IP 不同,BCNU 诱导的间质性肺炎多发于中叶或上叶的特点使之容易被鉴别。上肺叶难治性纤维化及气胸可能发生于结束治疗后几年。白消安和环磷酰胺方案后的迟发型肺炎也有过报道。紫杉醇和多西他赛等紫杉醇类药物治疗后数小时或数周内,可以发生急性和亚急性 IP,这也有确切报道[87]。紫杉醇相关 IP 的发生率和严重程度,受剂量和给药计划的影响。化疗前的肺纤维化,以及合并使用其他增强肺毒性的药物(如吉西他滨)和同步放疗会增加紫杉醇 IP 的发生率。

多种靶向药都会诱导 IP,包括 mTOR 抑制剂(依维莫司、坦罗莫司)、EGFR 抑制剂(吉非替尼、厄罗替尼(erlotinib)、西妥昔单抗、帕尼单抗),多激酶血管生成抑制剂(索拉非尼、舒尼替尼),HER2 抑制剂(曲妥珠单抗),多激酶 Bcr-Abl 抑制剂(伊马替尼、达沙替尼、尼洛替尼、博舒替尼)、蛋白酶体抑制剂(硼替佐米、卡非佐米),ALK 抑制剂(克唑替尼),c-Met 抑制剂(tivantinib),免疫调节剂(沙利度胺、来那度胺、泊马度胺)。ILD 在 mTOR 治疗后最为常见,在接受 mTOR 治疗的实体瘤患者中发生率高达 39%[81,88-90]。大多数患者并无症状;然而,暴发性呼吸衰竭已被报道。最近的研究表明,mTOR 抑制剂诱导的肾癌患者的 ILD 可能与抗肿瘤活性有关[81]。如果这一结果得到证实,将有助于指导伴 mTOR 相关 IP 影像表现且无症状患者的治疗策略。达沙替尼、依维莫司和坦罗莫司诱导 IP 之后,都成功地进行了再挑战[81,91]。

超敏性肺炎(HP)

HP 样反应的典型特征是反复暴露于化疗药后出现发热、呼吸困难、干咳、头痛、疲劳、皮疹和淋巴细胞增多。在最初药物暴露之后的三到四星期内出现的间质性肺炎,并且即使在治

疗未调整的情况下也可能时好时坏。边界不清的非干酪样肉芽肿和单核细胞浸润是亚急性、慢性 HP 的典型组织学表现。肺门腺病和胸腔积液在高达 10%的患者中发生。组织学证实的边界不清的肉芽肿，皮疹以及肺门腺病或胸腔积液的影像学表现可能有助于区别甲氨蝶呤诱导性肺损伤和其他类型药物诱导 HP。影像学改变包括常聚集在外周和上肺叶的均匀斑片状影，特别多见于慢性病程的患者。甲氨蝶呤诱导的 HP 已经有大量的研究，肺损伤在口服、静脉注射、鞘内注射、肌注等给药途径治疗中都有报道。总的来说，化疗诱导的 HP 的患者预后是非常良好的。类固醇治疗之后，处于疾病早期的患者的临床症状和影像学改变通常可以完全缓解。

肺泡病变

非心源性肺水肿、弥漫性肺泡损害以及成人呼吸窘迫综合征

非心源性肺水肿（noncardiogenic pulmonary edema，NCPE）是由于肺泡毛细血管膜损伤，导致毛细血管渗漏和非心源性（渗透性）肺水肿。随着疾病的进展，其病生理表现与成人呼吸窘迫综合征（adult respiratory distress syndrome，ARDS）及其组织学特征相一致，弥漫性肺泡损害（diffuse alveolar damage，DAD）可能随之而来。药物诱导的 NCPE 通常是特异性的反应，与治疗的药物剂量、持续时间无关。患者的典型表现是急性呼吸困难、缺氧、肺泡浸润同时不伴有心力衰竭。尽管偶尔发展为致命的 ARDS，但大部分反应是温和、自限性的。停药、给氧、谨慎使用利尿剂通常可迅速康复。除了 ATRA-和砷诱导的 NCPE 外，再次使用该致病药物通常会导致症状复发，因此不推荐使用。促使病情发展为 ARDS 的因素包括多药方案和同步或续贯放疗或氧疗，特别是在使用博来霉素或白消安治疗后[92,93]。一旦发生，ARDS 对早期停药和并开始皮质醇治疗的反应有很大差异。一些药物（白消安，环磷酰胺，博来霉素）尽管停药后仍然会出现进行性的呼吸系统损害最终导致呼吸困难和死亡。在分子靶向药物中，以下药物使用后可能引起 ARDS：EGFR 抑制剂（吉非替尼，厄罗替尼，西妥昔单抗，）；抗淋巴细胞单克隆抗体（利妥昔单抗，阿伦珠单抗，奥法木单抗）以及西罗莫司抑制剂（依维莫司，坦罗莫司）。*JAK2* 抑制剂芦可替尼的快速停药与细胞因子反弹反应导致的 ARDS 的发生有关。建议优先使用糖皮质激素，同时辅以支持治疗和该药物缓慢减量，以缓解这一潜在问题[94,95]。

弥漫性肺泡出血及其他出血问题

药物诱导弥漫性肺泡出血（DAH）的发生经常与肺泡毛细血管损伤有关，偶尔是不伴肺结构紊乱的轻微型肺泡出血的结果。不伴 DAD 的 DAH 比较罕见，与利妥昔单抗[96]及阿伦珠单抗[97]相关。在使用贝伐单抗治疗中央气道肿瘤的过程中，肿瘤中央坏死空化有时可引起致命的大出血[96]。

嗜酸性肺炎

嗜酸性肺炎（EP）的特征是发热、呼吸困难、缺氧和均匀的磨玻璃密度影，这种磨玻璃影常见于肺的外周和上叶。肺泡和外周血嗜酸性粒细胞增高是常见的特征，BAL 显示嗜酸性粒细胞比例>20%的白细胞。“反向式肺水肿”是典型的影像学特征，但仅在 33%的患者中可见。越来越多的药物与 EP 的发生相关，包括博来霉素、白消安、甲氨蝶呤、丙卡巴肼、氟达拉滨，以及最近基于奥沙利铂和紫杉醇的方案。停用药物和使用高剂量类固醇，患者一般预后良好[61,98~101]。

胸膜疾病

胸腔积液和纤维化

药物引导的胸膜病变通常是整体胸膜病变的一个组成部分，但也可以作为一个孤立事件发生[102]。孤立性胸腔积液可见于甲氨蝶呤、达沙替尼、博舒替尼、多西他赛、ATRA 和粒细胞集落刺激因子（GCSF）治疗后[103,104]。以淋巴细胞为主的渗出液为典型，可为单侧或双侧，体积小至中等。药物引起的胸腔积液的最佳治疗方法尚未明确，胸腔穿刺、利尿剂和类固醇疗法都有报道，但成功率各不相同。在某些情况下，停药后胸腔积液可自行消退。胸膜增厚伴肺纤维化是环磷酰胺、BCNU、博来霉素的迟发性毒性。

肺血管紊乱（PVD）

血栓栓塞性疾病、肺动脉高血压、肺静脉闭塞性疾病（PVOD）

化疗药物对肺血管的副作用可能导致血栓形成、肺性高血压或 PVOD。诊断 PVD 的依据是孤立性的弥散功能（DLCO）或在肺功能检测项目中相对其他肺功能参数，DLCO 不成比例地下降。他莫昔芬的促进血栓形成作用似乎和药物相关的蛋白-C 和抗凝血酶Ⅲ水平下降有关[105]。他莫昔芬和其他化疗药物结合，如环磷酰胺、甲氨蝶呤、氟尿嘧啶，使血栓栓塞现象的风险增加了三倍[106,107]。据报道血栓栓塞事件，在接受以沙利度胺为基础的化疗，与固醇、多西他赛或 BCNU 相结合化疗的患者中发生率为 14%~43%[108~111]。VEGF 阻滞剂：贝伐单抗、舒尼替尼、索拉非尼（sorafenib），与血栓栓塞事件同样有关（图 133-10）[2,96,112,113]。肺动脉高压（PAH）是一种罕见的抗肿瘤药物并发症，提示可能与个体易感性相关。有报道 Bcr-Abl 酪氨

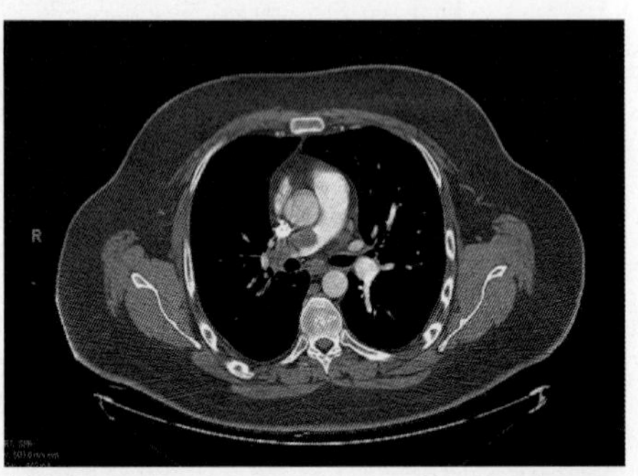

(a)

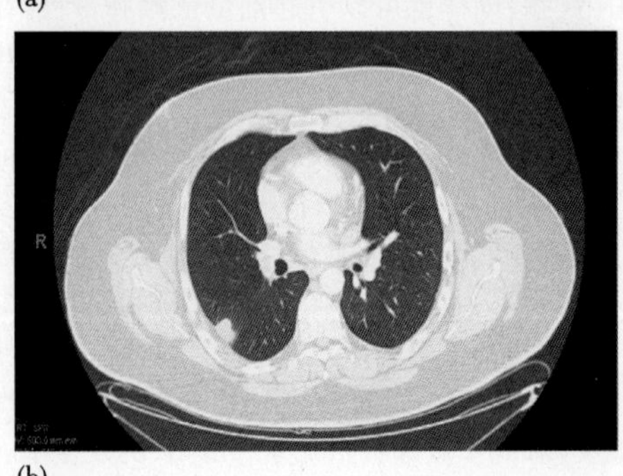

(b)

图 133-10 CT 血管造影显示，接受以贝伐单抗为主的胆道癌化疗的患者中存在大的中央栓子（a）。右肺中叶外侧段呈楔形胸膜下密度，提示合并肺梗死（b）

酸激酶抑制剂达沙替尼会引起严重的 PAH,但是大多数情况下,在停药后仅能部分恢复[114~117]。有假说认为这是多激酶抑制剂脱靶所导致的,目前尚未发现高选择性 Bcr-Abl 酪氨酸激酶抑制剂引起 PAH。实际上在使用达沙替尼引起 PAH 后改用高选择性的 Bcr-Abl 酪氨酸激酶抑制剂如尼洛替尼或伊马替尼目前已经有报道[115,118]。一旦怀疑是达沙替尼引起的 PAH,应立即停药,而且不建议再次考虑使用达沙替尼[119]。干扰素治疗后的 PAH 被认为可能是干扰素诱导的内皮功能障碍[120,121]。抗肿瘤抗生素净司他丁,可引起肺血管壁肥厚,导致肺动脉高压,可能是由于对肺动脉内皮细胞的直接毒性引起的[122]。还有,化疗相关肺动脉高压作为 PVOD 的结果发生,这一过程的特点是肺静脉和小肺静脉纤维化闭塞(见“肿瘤患者肺动脉高压”)。尽管许多药物涉及 PVOD 的发生,博来霉素和 BCNU 与之相关性的数据最为确切[123,124]。

药物诱导的气道疾病

支气管痉挛

支气管痉挛合并呼吸困难、喘息和缺氧是一种常见的、有时致命的化疗相关急性输液反应。事实上,所有化疗药物都可能引发输液反应,其定义为与药物输注相关的暂时性不良反应,其症状和体征与药物已知毒性不一致。急性输液反应往往在药物输注后几分钟内发生,虽然也有报道在药物输注后 10~12h 发生的迟发性输液反应。这种反应通常是 IgE 介导的对外来蛋白的超敏反应(Ⅰ型超敏反应)或非 IgE 介导的假超敏反应。后者是由某些阳离子药物引起的,这些药物可能触发肥大细胞的活化和随后的细胞因子释放(过敏反应)[63]。使用某些药物,如卡铂、奥沙利铂和 L-天冬酰胺酶后,可以产生 IgE 抗体并与肥大细胞和嗜碱性细胞结合。随后再次接触该药物可能会减少血管活性介质(组胺、白三烯和前列腺素)从嗜碱性细胞和肥大细胞的爆炸性释放,引发Ⅰ型超敏反应和过敏反应。Ⅰ型超敏反应通常发生在输液后几分钟内。相关的呼吸症状包括咳嗽、呼吸困难、喘息和胸闷。由于咽喉水肿引起的喉鸣也可能发生。随着病情的进展,双侧肺浸润伴渗透性肺水肿,可发展为 ARDS。有时,这些反应可能严重到足以导致呼吸衰竭、休克和死亡[125]。

紫杉醇类(紫杉醇,多西他赛)引起的输液反应在临床上与 IgE 介导的Ⅰ型超敏反应相似;然而,紫杉醇类药物引起输液反应的潜在机制可能不同。紫杉醇溶于一种聚氧乙烯基蓖麻油溶剂,聚氧乙烯蓖麻油(cremophor EL),它具有高度致敏性,可能触发肥大细胞/嗜碱性细胞的激活及随后的过敏反应。聚山梨酯 80(polysorbate 80)是多西他赛的合成载体,可能通过类似的机制诱导输液反应[126]。紫杉醇诱导的输液反应,归因于紫杉醇的组分及这些溶剂。因此,对于有紫杉醇引起输液反应病史的患者,不推荐使用溶于聚氧乙烯蓖麻油(cyclosporine, teniposide, ixabepilone)及聚山梨酯 80(依托泊苷)的抗肿瘤药物[127]。典型的紫杉醇相关的输液反应在第一次或第二次输注时较早发生。使用组胺受体拮抗剂和类固醇的标准预防已将紫杉醇引起的支气管痉挛的发生率从 30%降低到 2%[128]。最近的研究表明,BRCA1/2 突变是乳腺癌或卵巢癌患者接受卡铂类化疗发生输液反应的独立危险因素。在这种情况下,输液反应往往在药物累积值较低时即可发生[129]。

大多数单克隆抗体的输注可能会引发细胞因子释放综合征,这是一种以呼吸困难、喘息和“流感样症状”为特征的免疫反应,通常发生在用药后的最初几小时内[130]。症状通常比较轻微,少数患者会出现致命反应。小鼠蛋白的百分比被认为与免疫原性反应有关,包括输液反应。最早的单克隆抗体是鼠源性的,在人类中具有高度的免疫原性。降低单克隆抗体免疫原性的一种策略是开发嵌合小鼠-人(西妥昔单抗、利妥昔单抗、布妥昔单抗),部分人源化(贝伐单抗、曲妥珠单抗、阿伦珠单抗、吉姆单抗、奥妥珠单抗)和完全人源化[伊匹木单抗、ofatumumab、帕尼单抗(panitumumab)、雷莫芦单抗(ramucirumab)]的抗体。在最近的一项研究中,基于单抗小鼠免疫原性的降低,帕尼单抗治疗后 IR 的严重程度(0.5%)较西妥昔单抗治疗后(2%)下降了 3/4[131]。单克隆抗体诱发输液反应的危险因素包括药物过敏史、给药途径和给药速度、药物形式和多药治疗。注射前的测试剂量不能准确地预测随后的输液反应。单克隆抗体治疗后诱发的温和的输液反应,需要支持治疗(吸氧、抗组胺药、类固醇和吸入 β 肾上腺素受体激动剂),同时根据具体情况决定是否停用单克隆抗体。抗组胺、糖皮质激素和解热镇痛药通常推荐用于嵌合小鼠-人单克隆抗体治疗前使用,如利妥昔单抗和西妥昔单抗。在几种人源化单克隆抗体(阿伦珠单抗、曲妥珠单抗)和完全人源单克隆抗体(雷莫芦单抗、奥法木单抗)中,输液反应的风险也足够高,值得预防性用药。一般来说,决定是否要预防性用药以及停药后再挑战,需基于过敏反应的严重程度,并在个案的基础上作出决定[132]。尽管有预防措施,输液反应仍可能发生。因此,建议在药物输注期间和输注后立即密切监测。

一类与支气管痉挛有关的药物包括植物碱。尽管长春瑞滨和其他植物碱几乎与肺毒性无关,但也有报道这些药物与丝裂霉素同时或序贯联合化疗时出现以咳嗽、支气管痉挛、呼吸困难、腹痛、低血压为特点的急性反应[133,134]。

其他临床病理综合征

肉芽肿病

非干酪性肉芽肿是一种罕见的药物诱导的肺损伤表现。最常见于甲氨蝶呤和干扰素治疗后[135,136]。甲氨蝶呤和干扰素诱导的肉芽肿淋巴结病很难与结节病鉴别。除了甲氨蝶呤和干扰素,除了甲氨蝶呤和干扰素外,丙卡巴肼(procarbazine)、伊匹木单抗和西罗莫司也可能诱发肉芽肿性肺炎。停药可能会使疾病缓解。

胸部放疗的肺并发症:放射性肺炎和纤维化

放疗的诸多挑战之一是精确地使辐射剂量到达靶器官,同时保护周围正常组织的关键部位不受辐射。在胸部肿瘤中,治疗过程中的解剖变化和肿瘤运动随呼吸变化是常见的现象。胸部放疗后出现明显临床表现的肺部毒性的发生率为 5%~20%。事实上,放射导致的肺损伤(radiation-induced lung injury, RILI)是胸部放疗和放化疗的最常见的剂量限制性并发症。放射技术、成像和传输系统的最新进展,如质子治疗、三维适形放射治疗(CRT)、调强放射治疗(IMRT)和立体定向体放射治疗(SBRT),有可能实现靶区更高的目标剂量,同时减轻对邻近正常组织的辐射。然而，在较新的放射治疗策略中也确实有放射损伤，与之相关的放疗模式和 RILI 的严重程度可能与常规放射治疗引起的肺损伤不同。辐射总剂量、单位剂量、受照射肺体积、射线特征及排列等因素均影响放射性肺炎（RP）的发生发展。先前存在的肺部疾病、潜在的肺功能储备不足、先前的放射治疗和快速停用类固醇也会影响肺损伤的临床表现和严重程度[137]。将放疗与丝裂霉素、环磷酰胺、长春新碱、多柔比星、博来霉素、吉西他滨、紫杉醇、放线菌素 D 等化疗药物联合应用，不仅加重了肺的放疗副反应，还缩短了射线暴露后的潜伏期[138]。尽管关于能够使肺损伤缓和的最佳剂量分割和剂量体积关系的数据仍然在更新，但有种观点还是被普遍认同的，即使用超分割的放射疗程和最小的肺照射体积能够使肺毒性发生可能性最低。影像学上明显的肺损伤是常见的总辐射剂量超过 40Gy。在剂量为>70Gy 时，可能出现了严重的肺部并发症，包括支气管狭窄、支气管软化、纵隔纤维化和喉返神经损伤。在 20Gy 以下的放疗剂量下，肺损伤是罕见的[139]。

放射性肺炎（RP）和放射性肺纤维化（RF）分别代表了 RILI 的急性期和晚期，并且是放射性毒性的最常见形式。急性 RP 的早期症状包括发热、呼吸困难、干咳，通常在治疗后最初的 1~3 个月为隐匿性的，然后发展为影像学可见的肺炎。3~4 个月达到高峰。最早在放射治疗后 3~4 周，可观察到肺部影像学改变，其特征为散在的磨玻璃影，界限不清的斑片影，或合并支气管充气征和在辐射范围内的肺体积损失。在轻微的急性 RP 病例中，这些变化可能在 6 个月内消失，留下线性瘢痕。几乎所有患者都有局部瘢痕，包括那些没有临床症状的人。PET 的可测量的变化，包括肺容量和扩散能力的减少，可以在放射治疗后 2~3 个月观察到。早期 RP 的组织病理学特征包括肺间质水肿、出血和伴有反应性Ⅱ型肺细胞的纤维性渗出物。随着损伤加重，可以发展为 RF。RF 以出现边界清晰的区域，其肺容积下降、线样密度影、支气管扩张、肺实质回缩、膈膜上抬以及同侧胸膜增厚为特征。与常规放疗后的 RP 一样，这些变化通常发生在照射野内。RF 通常在治疗后 6~12 个月发生，在放疗结束后 1~2 年内稳定。PET 可以定量分析 RP，表现为 FDG 摄取增加。PET/CT 影像上的高 SUV 与有症状的 RP 的风险增加相关[140,141]。目前正在研究这种成像方式在识别有症状的 RP 高风险人群中的应用。

另外一种较少见和散发的 RP 也有报道[116]。散发性局限性肺炎在少数（5%）患者中发生，被认为代表了一种过敏性肺炎的类型，其特点是散在的包括双肺野的 CD4+T 淋巴细胞肺泡炎。因此，影像学研究的放射性改变应该延伸至放射野以外。患者在胸部放疗后 1~3 个月出现与肺照射容积不成比例的呼吸困难、干咳症状。这类肺炎和与之有关的症状基本上在 6~8 周内减轻，不伴有任何长期后遗症[116,142,143]。

放射回忆性肺炎是一种罕见但研究较深入的炎症性反应，在使用某些药物后发生于既往放射野的肺组织中。放射回忆性肺炎最常发生于在紫杉醇和蒽环类药物治疗后。吉西他滨、依托泊苷、长春瑞滨、曲妥珠单抗和厄洛替尼也被认为是引发这种疾病的诱因（表 133-1 和表 133-2）[144,145]。患者通常表现在最初和随后几个疗程中出现干咳，低烧和呼吸困难。回忆性肺炎的肺损伤通常在完成放疗后几周到几月内使用促发的抗肿瘤药物治疗后立刻发生。影像学上，可以看到与放射性肺炎一样的磨玻璃影或实变影。停药、使用糖皮质激素以及支持治疗通常预后良好。关于成功治疗这些烦人的药物所致放射回忆性肺炎有过几例报道[146]。

与放疗相关的胸腔积液可作为放射性胸膜炎的早期并发症（6 个月内）发生，也可作为纵隔辐射的晚期后遗症（1~5 年）发生，伴有纵隔纤维化、全身 PH 或淋巴管阻塞。这些渗出通常是小范围的，同侧的，无症状的。患者偶尔可能会出现呼吸急促或胸痛。胸水细胞学无肿瘤细胞，反应性间皮细胞在胸水中常见。PVOD 也被认为是一种罕见的放射性肺毒性并发症。最近有关于乳腺癌放疗后在非放射区域出现 OP 和 EP 的研究报道[147,148]。放疗诱导的 OP 被认为是一种免疫介导的、以淋巴细胞为主的超敏反应。EP 和 OP 均可在胸片上产生迁移性肺斑片状影，一般在放疗后 1~3 个月出现。血液或组织嗜酸性粒细胞的存在，加上既往哮喘或特应性病史，有利于 EP 的诊断。糖皮质激素治疗与放疗诱导的 OP 和 EP 的迅速恢复有关，停用类固醇后很少会复发。放疗的另一个胸内并发症包括肺瘀血，这可能是辐射引起的心肌和/或瓣膜功能障碍的后遗症。

原发肿瘤的位置、类型、范围等因素以及放射线的物理特征和入口直接影响放射性肺损伤的形态和分布。较新的放射治疗和影像学模式如 3D-CRT 和 IMRT，所导致的 RILD，可能不会出现典型的直边浸润，而是呈现肿块样或螺旋状外观，或者表现为边缘较模糊的不规则结节。因此，更新的放射技术造成的肺损伤可能非常难以与其他疾病（如感染或潜在恶性肿瘤的复发）区分开来[149]。这些新的放疗模式后也会出现肺体积损失、支气管扩张等，但其损伤程度较传统放疗轻[150]。质子治疗在达到肿瘤靶区之前，以更少的弥散改善了肿瘤的放射剂量传递。这一结果可能使辐射剂量安全上升到杀死肿瘤的水平，同时不损伤关键的正常肺组织[151,152]。在一项小型研究中，接受质子治疗的非小细胞肺癌患者比接受常规放疗的患者耐受更高剂量的辐射，肺炎发生率更低[151]。当然仍需要进一步研究这些放疗模式及其减少 RP 风险的真正影响。

RILI 主要与感染、药物毒性和复发性肿瘤鉴别。与放射治疗计划的相关性、RILI 的预期模式以及与放射治疗的时间相关性对放射损伤的诊断具有重要意义。在放射治疗完成前出现的肺阴影应考虑另一种诊断。肺纤维化区域内的空洞可能是由于重叠的感染如结核病或曲霉菌所致，或者肿瘤复发或肿瘤坏死所致。由肿瘤或感染引起的支气管扩张的消失也是合并疾病的重要影像学表现。

RILI 代表由炎症性肺炎引发的一系列变化，这些变化发展为纤维化，尽管肺炎和纤维化是一个连续还是单独的病还没有明确答案。遗憾的是，还没有明确的药物可以程度成功预防和治疗 RILI。RP 可能对类固醇治疗有反应。虽然没有基于证据的推荐剂量，但一般来说，每日 40~60mg 泼尼松持续数周，随后数周逐渐减少，可以缓解大多数患者的症状。没有确凿的证据表明，成功地治疗急性肺炎可以减轻 RF 的后期发展。没有证据表明，类固醇在治疗这种放疗的晚期并发症方面有益处。

造血干细胞移植的肺部并发症

对许多复发和高危造血系统恶性肿瘤患者来说，造血干细胞移植（HSCT）是唯一根治性的治疗选择。尽管治疗方案和支持治疗在不断进步，仍有高达 60%的接受 HSCT 患者发生肺部并发症，占发病率和死亡率的相当一部分比重[153~155]。正如大多数移植，肺部并发症也可以分为早期(移植最初的 100 日内)发生和晚期(超过移植后 100 日)发生的(表 133-3)。这些并发症主要是由于移植治疗方案的直接毒性作用，延迟性骨髓再生、持续性免疫抑制治疗，以及移植物抗宿主反应(GVHD)所引起。由于 GVHD 的高发生率和持续性免疫抑制疗法，感染性并发症最常发生于异体 HSCT 后。由于成功的预防治疗能够有效地减少感染性肺部并发症的发生率，非感染性肺部并发症就成为导致 HSCT 后死亡的主要原因。

表 133-3　造血干细胞移植后的非感染性肺部并发症

早期(100 日内)	晚期(100 日后)
• 肺水肿	• 阻塞性细支气管炎
• 特发性肺炎综合征	• 隐源性机化性肺炎
• 弥漫性肺泡出血	• 移植后淋巴增生性疾病
• 围移植期呼吸窘迫综合征	• 淋巴细胞间质性肺炎(少见)
• Ⅱ型肺泡蛋白沉积(少见)	
• 肺静脉闭塞性疾病(少见)	

移植相关早发性非感染性肺部并发症

肺水肿及胸腔积液

弥漫性肺水肿是移植后最常见的早期并发症。病因包括体液潴留导致的毛细血管流体静力压增大相关的体液容积的增加以及心脏功能障碍。与基础疾病相关的肺部毛细血管渗透性增加导致的非心源性肺水肿也可发生[155,156]。流体静力学和渗透性两方面的病因可以在移植后肺水肿中同时存在，并与其他早期出现的肺部并发症相重叠。迅速出现的呼吸困难、缺氧和双肺浸润，同时在诊断评价中未发现感染的迹象支持本病的诊断。肺部水肿可以伴随胸腔积液。胸腔积液伴体重增加可保守治疗而无须胸腔穿刺引流。

围移植期呼吸窘迫综合征(PERDS)

PERDS 发生于 HSCT 后中性粒细胞恢复早期，典型表现为发热、非心源性肺水肿，红斑性皮疹和低氧血症。根据美国国立卫生研究院(NIH)启动的造血干细胞移植临床研究协作组将 PERDS 归入特发性肺炎综合征(IPS)，鉴于本病对糖皮质激素治疗有效且死亡率较低，可能将其单独考虑更有助于治疗本病[156]。由于报道之间对疾病的定义和研究人群不同，发病率的报道差异很大，但是在自体干细胞移植患者中应用严格的诊断标准时，其发病率通常为 5%~10%[157,158]。尽管其病理生理还未完全明确，但似乎与植入期释放的前炎性细胞因子和预处理造成血管内皮细胞损伤有关。危险因素包括生长因子的使用、输入的单核细胞或 CD34(+)细胞的数目、中性粒细胞恢复速度、预处理的方案、潜在疾病和外周血来源的干细胞。一些研究表明糖皮质激素可以改善病情[158,159]。

特发性肺炎综合征(IPS)

1993 年，由 NIH 召集的委员会提出了一个 IPS 的宽泛的工作定义，即 X 线摄影下广泛的非叶性浸润灶而无充血性心力衰竭和下呼吸道感染的证据[160]。IPS 在造血干细胞移植受体的发生率约 10%，通常在移植后 14~90 日发生。其死亡率 50%~70%[161~163]。其危险因素包括：为治疗非白血病的恶性肿瘤进行移植、高龄、接受的总放射剂量、移植前化疗方案类型、高级别的移植物抗宿主病(GVHD)、巨细胞病毒阳性供体、白细胞抗原差异和 PS 评分较低[162]。IPS 可能的病因包括：预处理放化疗方案的直接毒性，隐匿性感染和炎性细胞因子的释放。但是异基因骨髓移植后 IPS 与急性 GVHD 之间的联系提示同种异体 T 细胞损伤也是发病的重要因素[162,163]。临床表现无特异性，如急性呼吸困难、干咳、发热，伴胸部放射影像学检查弥漫性肺浸润表现。IPS 的诊断在很大程度上依赖于排除感染和无心脏、肾脏或医源性水钠潴留。治疗手段包括大剂量糖皮质激素、支持治疗如吸氧和使用广谱抗生素。最近的临床前和临床数据表明肿瘤坏死因子-α(TNF-α)对 IPS 有潜在的致病作用。但是最新的随机对照临床研究结果表明，IPS 对糖皮质激素前具有较高的反应率，但是加用依那西普(肿瘤坏死因子受体融合蛋白)治疗后为显著增加有效性[164]。

弥漫性肺泡出血(DAH)

移植后 DAH 的特征是在同种异体和自体干细胞移植后非感染前提下双侧弥漫性肺部浸润和损伤[165~169]。血液和骨髓移植临床试验网络在 IPS 的定义中包括 DAH。DAH 也已在三分之一的围移植期患者中被描述[157,170]。其支气管肺泡灌洗发现至少 3 个不同的支气管亚段有进行性加重的血性液体或是 20%以上灌洗液的细胞为含铁血黄素的巨噬细胞。因此，血性的 BAL 液体对 DAH 的诊断既不敏感也不特异，其仅仅可以简单地代表肺泡损伤的严重程度和伴随凝血功能障碍而不是单独的综合征[171]。DAH 的发生与凝血功能障碍或血小板减少之间没有任何关联。此外，输注血小板不会改善呼吸状态。DAH 的治疗包括高剂量静脉内皮质类固醇和支持性护理，如氧疗、机械通气和血小板输注。重组人凝血因子Ⅶa(rFⅦa)曾经被用于改善凝血，但最近的回顾性分析显示，在高剂量皮质类固醇治疗基础上添加 rFⅦa 并无生存获益[172]。

肺静脉闭塞性疾病(PVOD)

肺静脉闭塞性疾病是在干细胞移植后的一种罕见并发症。它是肺静脉闭塞和内膜增生纤维化导致的肺动脉高压[173]。大剂量化疗和感染是可能发生的诱因。通常发生在移植后数周，发病隐匿，进行性呼吸困难、乏力[124,174,175]。PVOD 目前的治疗选择有限，2 年内死亡率高达 100%。

移植相关迟发性非感染性肺部并发症

移植后阻塞性支气管炎综合征(BOS)是 HSCT 后长期存活患者中最常见的并发症，它是一种 GVHD 的晚期表现，导致为进行性呼吸功能不全，部分会导致死亡。BOS 几乎从来不会在没有 GVHD 的情况下出现，因此只会影响异基因骨髓移植的患者[154,176,177]。由于缺乏规范的诊断标准，其发病率从 5%~26%不等[178]。BOS 影响小气道，导致慢性炎症、黏膜上皮化生、黏膜下瘢痕、平滑肌肥大和同心性支气管纤维化。已知的最常见的危险因素包括慢性 GVHD、高龄、移植后一百天内出现的病毒感染、移植前出现气流受限、血清 IgG 浓度偏低和在预处理方案中使用甲氨蝶呤或白消安[157,179]。BOS在早期可能无症状，这将导致诊断延迟。随着气道阻塞的进展，呼吸困难、咳嗽和喘息等临床表现在晚期更为常见[180,181]。胸片通常没有异常但是高分辨率CT可能显示一些气道圈闭、小气道的增厚或扩张、“马赛克”衰减的证据。支气管镜及支气管肺泡灌洗和经纤支镜肺部活检通常对诊断本病没有太多帮助。肺功能检查(pulmonary function tests, PFT)是诊断和随访的最基本手段。气道受阻的证据1s用力呼气容积(FEV_1)和用力肺活量(FVC)的下降支持PFT的诊断。NIH对于诊断BOS的指南共识如下：①肺功能检测第1s用力呼气量/肺活量(FEV_1/FVC)<0.7及FEV_1<75%的预测值，残气量>预测值的120%；②高分辨肺部CT显示有气道圈闭、小气道增厚或支气管扩张，或病理证实的限制性细支气管炎；③影像学、实验室和临床试验没有任何感染的迹象[179]。这些诊断标准通常与严重的气道阻塞和纤维化有关，是PTCB的晚期表现，并通常对治疗干预抗拒。最新的文献建议修订这些标准，以便在早期阶段对BOS进行诊断[178]。

BOS的治疗方案尚未在前瞻性试验中评估。加强使用全身的免疫抑制剂糖皮质激素和钙依赖磷酸酶抑制剂是主要的治疗手段[163]。然而，最近两个回顾性分析中表明吸入高剂量糖皮质激素可稳定FEV_1并能显著的改善症状[182,183]。一项肺移植的观察性的研究显示阿奇霉素也有一定的帮助，可能是由于其抗炎作用，因此在一些选择性的患者中使用[184]。最近的一项回顾性研究表明，使用一种毒性较低的组合药物(氟替卡松、阿奇霉素和孟鲁司特)有助于在较短的时间内缓解症状，并减少全身免疫抑制治疗[185]。对一些患者来说，肺移植是一种选择。慢性GVHD仍是引起HSCT长期生存者的主要发病因素和死亡原因，BOS则是其中一个重要的因素。临床过程和疾病进展是波动的，但是持续性气流受阻与死亡率的明显升高有关[176]。早期诊断和合理BOS管理的前瞻性临床研究对提高生存率至关重要。

隐源性机化性肺炎(COP)

COP也被称为特发性闭塞性细支气管炎伴机化性肺炎(bronchiolitis obliterans organizing pneumonia, BOOP)，COP多发生在有GVHD的异体干细胞移植患者或巨细胞肺炎之后[186,194]。COP是一个不同的疾病，不应该与BOS混淆[177,186~188]。与BOS相比相对少见，在长期生存者中发生率1%~2%。干咳、呼吸困难，胸片和CT影像上肺斑片状浸润灶是最主要的临床表现。肺组织活检可以确诊。COP通常对糖皮质激素治疗反应较好；但是目前尚无标准的治疗指南[156]。

移植后淋巴增生性疾病(PTLD)

PTLD是供体来源的EB病毒感染的B淋巴细胞对不充分的细胞毒T淋巴细胞功能产生免疫应答，导致不受控制的扩增性疾病[154,189]。在HSCT患者中发生率约1%，通常发生在移植后的4~12个月，只有20%患者肺组织在此期间受累，常表现为边界不清的结节性浸润灶。治疗方法包括抗CD20单克隆抗体(利妥昔单抗)，抗病毒药物，以及注射EB病毒特异性细胞毒性T淋巴细胞。

肺炎

肺部感染使肿瘤病情及其治疗复杂化[190,191]。提示下呼吸道感染存在的经典征象有：肺实质的浸润、白细胞增多、发热和咳脓痰等。但是由于免疫抑制，这些症状体征可能不会出现在患有肺炎的肿瘤患者中，因此需要对本病提高警惕，防止漏诊。此外，肿瘤患者如出现不能解释的临床病情恶化或在常规影像学检查中出现新的浸润灶提示尽早进行放射影像学检查，通常包括CT的检查。

肺炎确诊要依据病原学(如血液、尿液和胸水)或者在呼吸道分泌物中找到非共生生物体。尽管痰液对于肺炎的诊断价值存在争议，细胞学证实的下呼吸道样本对于诊断似乎有帮助。纤支镜和肺泡灌洗可以作为一种诊断方法来获取下呼吸道样本。这一方法对大多数肿瘤患者是安全的[192]，而且传统方法有效培养出真正病原菌的比例仅25%~51%[193~196]。如果早期使用纤支镜，特别在抗生素使用之前进行检查，BAL对临床带来的帮助会更大。经支气管肺活检可发现血管浸润的共生微生物(如曲霉菌等)，但活检材料培养并未证明其诊断有效性高于肺泡灌洗，且需排除具有凝血功能障碍和/或血小板减少的患者。肺泡灌洗液培养或组织学培养的结果可能会由于定植于上呼吸道的非致病微生物的影响导致其结果难以解释。相反，培养阴性并不能排除感染，特别是在近期使用了广谱抗生素的情况下。分子生物学技术，如对病原体基因组或抗原检测(如血清半乳甘露聚糖、尿液组织胞浆菌抗原)的聚合酶链反应(polymerase chain reaction, PCR)试验可为诊断提供补充。

早期和准确的诊断是成功治疗和良好预后的关键，尽管不应该因为正在进行诊断检查而延误治疗。抗菌药物的选择应基于对病原体的认识(如果能够找到的话)，基础免疫状态以及并发症[197,198](参见第“肿瘤患者感染”章)。延误正确使用抗菌的时机会增加继发的并发症和感染相关死亡的风险，尤其是对那些严重免疫抑制的患者。因此常规的临床实践是一旦高度怀疑感染即开始经验性和/或预防性使用抗生素治疗。但是，应当注意除了感染性肺炎外，肿瘤患者容易受多种原因的影响导致发热和肺部浸润，包括治疗的毒性、与肺外感染有关的全身炎症反应、心力衰竭、实质性肿瘤侵犯或肺出血。

静脉栓塞

肺栓塞(PE)和深静脉血栓(DVT)是静脉栓塞(VTE)的两种表现。在所有的静脉血栓中，约20%与肿瘤有关，肿瘤使静脉栓塞发生率提高4~6倍。肿瘤的治疗，包括手术、化疗、激素、生长因子、血管生成抑制剂、促红细胞生成剂和中心静脉置管的使用又进一步增加血栓生成的风险[199]。VTE的治可能会延迟、中断或影响多种癌症治疗方式[200,201]。癌症相关VTE与总体死亡率显著升高有关，但它是一种罕见的死亡原因[202]。一项研究发现3.5%的癌症患者死于静脉血栓栓塞[203]。

VTE的临床表现多数为非特异性。结合D-二聚体检测评估DVT和PE的评分系统可用于排除癌症患者的VTE；然而，在癌症患者中发现正常D-二聚体水平的可能性不到30%。此外，D-二聚体升高在癌症患者中没有显著的阳性预测价值[204]。多普勒超声是诊断DVT的首选方法，而在一些特殊的情况下可能需要MRI和CT，如髂静脉或下腔静脉血栓。HRCT或CT血管造影是诊断PE的最佳方法，其优点是提供了更多关于胸部病理的信息，这些信息的不足可能会混淆诊断[205]。对于怀疑大量PE的不稳定患者,急诊床旁超声心动图可进行诊断和危险分层[206]。

在所有的肿瘤患者中都应该考虑VTE的预防[207]。接受腹部或盆腔手术的肿瘤患者应预防性使用低分子肝素至少4周[208]。化疗患者不常规推荐预防使用LMWH,仅推荐化疗并联合应用沙利度胺或来那度胺的多发性骨髓瘤患者预防性用药[208]。没有证据表明抗凝能预防导管相关性血栓形成,指南建议不使用抗凝剂[207]。

常规VTE诱导治疗用于癌症患者。在这种情况下,低分子肝素是VTE初始治疗的首选药物。单纯肝素应用于肾功能受损的患者。目前还没有系统地研究溶栓药物在癌症患者中的应用,对于大的PE进行溶栓治疗,当有明确的抗血栓治疗的禁忌时放置IVC[207,209]。基于有限的证据,偶然发现的VTE应作为有症状的VTE进行管理[210]。用于维持治疗,低分子肝素优于维生素K拮抗剂(VKA),因为低分子肝素在预防复发方面更好[199]。如果耐受,维持治疗可以一直用于癌症患者[202~204]。一般不鼓励在癌症患者中使用新型口服抗凝剂,因为很少有癌症患者被纳入这些抗凝药的主要试验,而且没有对这些药物进行监测的既定程序[205]。

肿瘤患者的肺动脉高压

肺血管高压(PH)是指静息时平均肺动脉压(MPAP)≥25mmHg,本病在肿瘤这一特殊情况下的表现还正在进一步的认识之中。经胸超声心电图(TTE)用来评估肺动脉收缩压(PASP)并可以作为肺血管高压的非侵入性筛查工具。肺动脉高压(PAH)指肺末楔压≤15mmHg且肺血管阻力为>3Woods单位的肺毛细血管前PH亚群[207],确诊则需要右心导管插入术(RHC)[208]。RHC可评估血流动力学损伤和肺循环的血管反应活性,同时指导后续的分类和管理。急性PH诊断,必须排除继发性原因,如急性血栓栓塞性疾病、低氧性呼吸功能不全或心功能障碍。

PH可能出现在癌症诊断之前,也可能发生在癌症治疗连续过程中的任何时间点。还可以在癌症治疗完成后发生。癌症相关PH的估计因特定癌症、相关癌症治疗和检测方法的不同而存在很大差异。在疾病的早期仅表现为劳力性呼吸困难、乏力,故使得本病的诊断非常困难,并延误治疗。成功的治疗需要对本病有高度的警觉性,因为以晕厥、心绞痛、血管神经性水肿、腹胀、血流动力学不稳定为标志的进展期患者往往对治疗抗拒。急性PH诊断,必须排除继发性原因,如急性血栓栓塞性疾病、低氧性呼吸功能不全、气管狭窄或心功能障碍。

在2013年世界卫生组织修订的临床分类方案中,PH被分为五组,它们具有相似的病因、血流动力学特征和治疗方法。其中包括PAH(1组)、左心疾病引起的PH(2组)、肺疾病和/或缺氧引起的PH(3组)、慢性血栓性肺动脉高压(CTEPH,4组)和多因素机制不明的PH(5组)[209]。肿瘤相关事件对各亚型均有影响,导致PH的发生。例如,TKI,dasatanib,现在被认为是PAH的一个危险因素,并被纳入1组[209]。该药物可导致中到重度毛细管PH,在停药后可改善或完全消除[115]。PVOD是一种罕见的引起PH的原因,其特征是肺静脉闭塞或狭窄,它代表了1型PH的一个亚组。感染、紫杉醇类药物、胸部放疗和干细胞移植都是PVOD的假定危险因素,但尚未建立明确的因果关系[101,174,211]。PVOD预后差,虽然有些患者可能耐受动脉血管扩张剂,但肺血管扩张剂治疗引起的致命肺水肿也有报道。

慢性骨髓增生性疾病(MPD)是一种罕见的PAH病因。MPD相关的PH的几个潜在机制包括:高心排出量、脾切除、肺动脉直接阻塞、慢性血栓栓塞、门静脉高压和充血性心力衰竭[209,212]。涉及肺血管系统的其他癌症和癌症治疗方法也可能导致PH。包括腺病、肿瘤或纵隔纤维化对肺的大静脉的外压和/或闭塞。霍奇金淋巴瘤和生殖细胞肿瘤引起PH的主要病因基础是纵隔压迫。辐射和感染(如真菌、结核分枝杆菌、芽孢菌、毛霉菌、隐球菌等)造成的纤维化纵隔炎也有报道[213~215]。涉及肺血管的原发性恶性肿瘤主要是肉瘤。这些罕见而往往致命的肿瘤通常来源于肺动脉主干,尽管来源于肺静脉的肉瘤也有报道[216]。肺动脉肉瘤患者常表现有类似慢性栓塞性肺动脉高压(CTEPH)的症状和体征(呼吸困难、胸痛、咳嗽、咯血)。但是,同时出现不能解释的发热、消瘦、杵状指、贫血和血沉增快的表现应高度怀疑恶性肿瘤。继发的肿瘤侵犯血管床者可表现为大血管中央性癌栓或较小的肿瘤细胞团堵塞小血管。后者可能伴或不伴淋巴道扩散。绒毛膜癌和起源于乳腺、肺、胃肠道和肾脏的黏液性肿瘤发生肿瘤栓塞率是最高的[217]。癌栓栓塞的临床症状包括从突发起病,呼吸困难,胸痛和心血管性虚脱,到咳嗽、劳力性呼吸困难和不明原因的肺动脉高压相关的运动不耐受等亚急性症状。肺肿瘤血栓性微血管病(PTTM)是恶性肿瘤相关性肺动脉高压的一个罕见原因,多见于腺癌,尤其是胃腺癌[218]。患者表现为严重的、难治性肺性高血压,可迅速发展导致突发的循环衰竭和死亡。肺微血管细胞学的发现具有诊断价值;然而,PTTM的诊断仅最常用于尸检。到目前为止,对PTTM没有明确的治疗方法。尽管在绝大多数较大的医疗中心,在评价血栓栓塞性事件时,CT血管成像已经取代了通气与血流扫描。在怀疑肿瘤血栓形成的情况下,通气-灌注扫描(ventilation-perfusion,V/Q)可能比胸部CT的诊断价值更高。V/Q闪烁显像中多个亚段的不匹配缺损支持本病的诊断。多个亚段不匹配的V/Q显像缺陷支持结论在RHC时从楔形肺动脉导管中获取的肺微血管细胞学标本可以提供更多支持癌栓形成的证据[217]。

在肺微血管中的白血病性隔离和白细胞血栓形成是粒细胞性和淋巴细胞白血病相关的高白细胞血症(WBC>50 000/dl)和原始细胞危象的罕见并发症。患者通常表现为间质浸润相关的呼吸困难、干咳、低氧血症,和肺动脉高压、肺心病体征。大血管癌栓栓塞的临床表现类似于急性肺血栓栓塞性疾病。然而,微血管癌栓栓塞通常表现为隐匿的呼吸困难,干咳,低氧血症和严重的肺动脉高压症状。肺心病和弥漫性间质性浸润是常见的表现,提示本病已经淋巴道播散,使得不良预后更加恶化。急性非淋巴细胞白血病化疗开始后的急性低氧性呼吸衰竭也有报道。这种综合征,被称为白血病细胞裂解性肺病,通常发生在治疗最初的48h,被认为是由化疗所致的肺白细胞淤滞症和血管周围出血引起的。在无肺部受累的高白细胞白血病患者,由于动脉血气注射器内的白细胞氧代谢,测定的PaO_2可能会人为降低。在这种情况下,由脉搏血氧测量法测得的氧饱和度是正常的。将动脉血气标本保存在冰上或在动脉血气注射器中加入氰化物并进行快速分析解决了这个问题。

在过去二十年中,基于循证医学的治疗策略导致了PAH

治疗指南的演变，这些策略改善了患者的生存，并显著提高了患者的生活质量[219]。应评估所有患者是否需要支持性治疗，包括吸氧、利尿剂、抗凝治疗和锻炼。更进一步的治疗方法是针对PAH本身，应该根据进一步的研究结果和治疗指南。目前和新兴的PAH靶点是内皮素、氧化亚氮和前列腺素通路。具体的治疗策略可能包括单一治疗或更常见的联合治疗[220]。遗憾的是，目前还没有治愈这种疾病的方法。将PAH治疗指南外推到其他形式的PH时需要谨慎。目前还没有研究表明肺血管扩张剂在治疗与癌症相关的PH方面的有效性。多巴酚丁胺、米力农、静脉依前列醇、吸入血管扩张剂和体外生命支持在一般人群中是公认的血流动力学失代偿的PH治疗方法[221]。对于PH和相关血流动力学恶化的危重癌症患者，指南中尚未阐明血管升压素治疗的最佳使用方案。

肿瘤患者睡眠障碍

睡眠障碍和时间生物学在癌症患者的整体护理中有重要意义，可影响癌症的预防、治疗和生存。

癌症的预防

延长睡眠时间和睡眠不规律与癌症风险增加有关。日本一项队列研究收集了超过10万例患者的数据，在每晚睡眠5h或超过9h的患者中发现癌症患病率更高[222]。轮班和夜间倒班工作，也可能增加癌症患病风险。一项研究发现在轮班工作大于30年的护士中患乳腺癌的相对危险度增加。褪黑素，是一种有抗癌潜力的天然激素，受夜间灯光照射抑制，可能会增加慢性睡眠障碍患者的癌症风险[223~225]。睡眠中断和昼夜节律异常与免疫系统介导的肿瘤监测功能受损有关，这也可能增加癌症风险[226,227]。阻塞性睡眠呼吸暂停(OSA)似乎会增加患癌症的风险，导致夜间严重缺氧[228-230]。这些发现表明睡眠障碍和癌症之间存在联系，并强调良好的睡眠卫生和睡眠障碍的治疗是预防癌症的重要目标。

癌症的治疗

白天嗜睡和疲劳，与血浆细胞因子增加有关，如IL-6。良好的夜间睡眠可以降低这种细胞因子的水平。特定癌症的干预或癌症本身所产生的炎症介质可能加剧睡眠中断。例如，治疗乳腺癌的化疗方案可能诱导与睡眠中断有关的血管内皮生长因子(VEGF)表达上升[231]。睡眠剥夺，尤其是损失快速眼动(REM)睡眠，已知会引起痛觉过敏。因此，常见于许多癌症患者的睡眠质量下降包括REM的睡眠剥夺被认为会增加疼痛的敏感性[232]。

原发性睡眠障碍，不宁腿综合征和周期性下肢运动障碍常常伴有失眠和白天嗜睡。这些障碍在某些癌症的亚群比较常见，这可能归因于化疗导致的贫血和周围神经病[233]。OSA综合征可能同样更常见于某些癌症。在对56例头颈部肿瘤患者的研究中，84%符合OSA的临床标准(图133-11)[234]。阿片类药物会加重中枢性睡眠呼吸暂停的症状。这种形式的睡眠呼吸紊乱可能是癌症患者的特定问题，因为许多患者使用阿片类药物以减轻癌痛[235]。

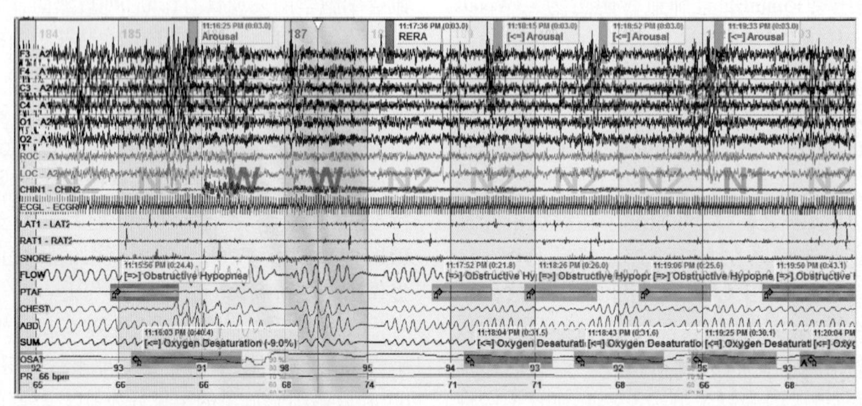

图133-11　76岁男性，扁桃体鳞状细胞癌放化疗9年后，出现鼾声，呼吸暂停，白天嗜睡。发病时BMI为22kg/m²。重度阻塞性睡眠呼吸暂停-低通气综合征，多导睡眠图显示呼吸暂停-低通气指数为32次/小时，氧饱和度最低点为72%(5min图)

通过利用肿瘤细胞周期与宿主组织的昼夜节律的差异，时间生物学和生物钟疗法可以优化癌症治疗的效果而最大限度地减少毒性。人类和动物研究已经表明，这种疗法不仅降低了毒性和提高治疗效果，而且可以增加剂量强度[236,237]。

癌症生存

多达51%的癌症幸存者可能会出现睡眠紊乱、疲劳和失眠[238]。认知和行为疗法(cognitive and behavioral therapy，CBT)被认为是这种疾病的首选治疗。CBT的已被证实可改善失眠，降低镇静催眠药物的使用，并提高生活质量。CBT也可以通过提高IL-1β和IFN-γ水平来影响免疫功能，这被认为可提高睡眠质量[239]。

肺部康复

肺部康复(pulmonary rehabilitation，PR)代表了一个多学科策略，这种策略将慢性呼吸困难和疲劳患者的运动训练，患者及其家属的教育，心理和行为干预和预后评估结合在一起。在

COPD 患者肺部康复的循证医学证据，使得这一治疗策略在本组患者管理中作为标准方案得以实施。与癌症相关的全身症状与疾病，特别是疲劳、呼吸困难、贫血、骨骼肌损伤、肌肉萎缩、缺乏运动耐力、抑郁、去适应和焦虑，大大加重了疾病的负担。PR 针对这些症状，从而减少呼吸困难和疲劳，提高锻炼耐力和生活质量。运动耐受性差会导致肺切除后的预后不佳，并限制了患者耐受化疗潜在毒性的能力[240,241]。因此，为癌症患者提供 PR 的理由是非常充分的，特别是在 COPD 和肿瘤经常共存的肺癌患者中。最近的一些小的研究表明，PR 可能通过改善各种有临床意义的结果，如 PS 评分、化疗相关的疲劳、耗氧量、运动耐受性和健康相关的生活质量，对肺癌的治疗产生积极的影响[242]。Bobbio 等在一项研究中发现，在经过 4 周的术前肺部康复训练后，劳动率以及最大耗氧量（VO_2max）得到提高，使得那些原来术前 VO_2max 被认为不可手术的患者能够成功地接受肺切除手术[243]。在其他研究中，术后 6~8 周 PR 患者的运动耐力、肌肉力量和呼吸困难评分的改善，导致肺癌患者住院时间减少，生活质量提高[243~248]。在非手术患者中，一些小的研究表明，PR 可以解决化疗相关性疲劳，改善行为状态和减少癌症患者住院的长度/频率[249~252]。

急性呼吸衰竭

急性呼吸衰竭（ARF）是成人癌症患者入住 ICU 最常见的原因。可以将癌症患者急性和慢性呼吸功能不全的易感条件分为两类：引起“肺”衰竭或“泵”衰竭的因素。肺衰竭通常与通气/灌注异常，分流，或肺泡毛细血管弥散的改变有关，至少在其早期阶段主要导致缺氧。肺衰竭的典型例子是 ARDS。本章其他章节讨论了癌症 ARDS 多种多样的原因，包括手术，感染，化疗，放疗，以及造血干细胞移植相关的并发症。在无 ARDS 的情况下，肺衰竭也可发生于肺炎，肺不张或肺栓塞有关的通气/灌注比例失调，或肺水肿相关的分流。肺衰竭的其他常见原因列举于表 133-4。相比之下，泵衰竭，主要起源于肺泡

表 133-4　急性呼吸衰竭的肺衰竭和泵衰竭：特征和内因

	肺衰竭	泵衰竭
特征	低氧血症	严重的高碳酸血症和酸中毒：轻度低氧血症
发病机制	通气/灌注比例失调 分流 肺泡毛细血管膜的改变	通气泵耗竭（CNS，PNS 或呼吸肌）
内因	急性肺损伤/急性呼吸窘迫综合征 肺炎 肺不张 肺栓塞/癌栓 肿瘤淋巴管扩散 化疗/放疗 肺白细胞停滞 输血相关的急性肺损伤 术后呼吸功能不全	慢性阻塞性肺疾病或 OSA 并存 内源性或外源性气道压缩 头颈恶性肿瘤引起的阻塞性睡眠呼吸暂停

CNS，中枢神经系统；PNS，周围神经系统。

通气量衰竭，并导致严重呼吸过度和仅轻度低氧血症的酸中毒。ARF 的多种因素，如严重 COPD 急性发作合并肺炎，可导致肺衰竭和泵衰竭。这种混合性情况时癌症患者呼吸衰竭常见的原因，这需要一个系统的方法，针对每个呼吸衰竭的组成部分原因，以便于合理地制订治疗策略。

通气泵的主要组成部分包括位于中枢神经系统（CNS）驱动呼吸的呼吸控制器，胸壁（包括呼吸肌），连接中央控制器与呼吸肌（脊髓和周围神经）的通路。肺泡通气量原发性衰竭，也简称为Ⅱ型呼吸衰竭或通气泵功能不全，任何通气泵组成部分产生足够危害时都可发生。在癌症中，多种原因造成的神经和肌肉功能障碍是泵衰竭频繁发生的基础。肺部康复已越来越多地用于泵衰竭相关的慢性呼吸功能不全患者的治疗。

泵衰竭病因

中枢神经系统疾病：受损驱动器

孤立的呼吸驱动器的抑制是一种少见的泵衰竭原因，可能起源于中枢神经系统损害，如延髓肿瘤或梗死，或镇静、麻醉药物。获得性中枢性低通气/通气不足可发生于脑干肿瘤外科手术之后，特别是接近第四脑室底部者。颅底放射可能有类似的不利影响。隐匿性甲状腺功能减退，尤其是中老年妇女和头颈部肿瘤治疗后，也可能造成中枢性低通气和呼吸衰竭。更多的时候，中央驱动器受抑制引起的呼吸衰竭以附加的损害发生，叠加于慢性呼吸功能不全之上。在这种情况下，小剂量的麻醉或镇静药物可能对肺泡通气量产生重要的影响。呼吸肌疲劳，也可能导致中枢性低通气，这是通过发送抑制信号到 CNS 呼吸中枢以减少驱动实现的，从而保护了肌肉免受损伤和进一步减轻肌肉疲劳。

周围神经系统疾病：神经肌肉能力不足

从 CNS 到呼吸肌的信号传输是通过脊髓和周围神经发生的。因此，导致神经肌肉功能障碍的疾病，如原发性神经系统疾病，脊髓病变，神经肌肉阻断药和肌无力，可导致呼吸衰竭。全身麻醉剂，造成明显的神经肌肉阻滞和通气抑制。其他药物，包括镇静剂，抗焦虑药，安眠药，和氨基糖苷类药物，通常只有在已经存在神经肌肉疾病情况下产生严重的呼吸抑制，如重症肌无力和重症肌无力伴癌综合征或大量的药物过量后。这个原则的一个例外是美沙酮，长期用药可能会导致通气功能不全。肌肉疲劳是癌症中普遍存在的问题，是呼吸衰竭发生的关键。许多原因会加重癌症相关性肌肉疲劳，包括低灌注状态（心源性、感染性或失血性休克），过多的乳酸或氢离子产生，严重贫血，由此引起呼吸衰竭。营养不良和恶病质是晚期癌症的常见并发症。相关性最大的癌症恶病质表现之一是肌肉丢失，这引起了骨骼肌的力量和耐力明显减低，包括膈肌[253]。与慢性阻塞性肺疾病有关的胸部膨胀过度和横膈变平，是肺癌常见的并发症，进一步引起呼吸肌功能损害和呼吸衰竭。电解质紊乱，如低磷血症，低钾血症和低镁血症，常使化疗变得复杂化，并可能会引起癌症患者严重肌肉无力。此外，许多用于呼吸衰竭治疗的药物，包括 β 肾上腺素受体激动剂，利尿剂，糖皮质激素可能会加剧低磷血症和加重肌肉无力。用于癌症患者治疗的化疗药物和其他药物也可能对神经肌肉系统造成有害影响。虽然糖皮质激素引起的肌病已经有很多报道，这些药物加强呼吸肌功能障碍的作用最近才得以认识[254,255]。在化疗药物中，

长春碱,顺铂和紫杉烷类的外周神经毒性最常见。在没有神经肌肉异常之类的诱因存在的情况下,这些药物对肺功能的临床表现可能比较微弱。除了中枢神经系统的影响,麻醉剂的使用可能通过减少膈肌收缩引起呼吸抑制,尤其是氟烷、丙泊酚、氧化亚氮[256,257]。头颈癌手术或前纵隔、食管或肺部手术后膈神经损伤可能会导致持久性的膈肌功能不全和呼吸衰竭。肿瘤直接浸润膈神经致膈肌功能丧失也有发生,尤其见于淋巴瘤、肺癌或头颈癌患者。副肿瘤综合征导致的弥漫性神经功能障碍是癌症呼吸衰竭的另一个原因。Lambert-Eaton 肌无力综合征影响约 3%小细胞肺癌患者,重症肌无力发生于 10%～15%胸腺瘤患者,脱髓鞘性周围神经病变发生于 50%的骨硬化性骨髓瘤患者,这三者是副肿瘤综合征中周围神经系统疾病中最常见的类型。这些疾病通常有一个可能会导致呼吸衰竭的亚急性和衰竭的过程。

呼吸做功增加:呼吸系统负荷增加和胸壁异常

多种癌症相关因素可能会导致急性或慢性呼吸道系统负荷增加。呼吸道阻力负荷增加,表现为气道阻力异常和顺应性增加的生理特点,是 COPD,呼吸道炎症,气道水肿,或黏液、血液或肿瘤机械性阻塞的最重要的特征。气管狭窄引起的上呼吸道梗阻与前插管和头颈部放射有关,并以小气管内管(<7.5mm 内径)进行插管,也是气流阻力和呼吸阻力沉淀剂增加的重要原因。肿瘤、放疗或手术引起的胸壁和胸椎异常可能会导致胸壁弹性负荷增加,呼吸做功增加和呼吸衰竭。

肺衰竭(肺水肿,急性呼吸窘迫综合征,急性肺损伤)

肺水肿/急性呼吸窘迫综合征/急性肺损伤

癌症肺水肿的好发于很多原因造成的肺损伤,这些肺损伤可根据基础的微循环通透特性、有或无弥漫性肺泡病理性损伤进行分类。在正常通透性的肺水肿中,Starling 力不平衡造成的静水压增加导致流体被滤过进入肺部。心源性肺水肿和神经源性肺水肿,以及肺复张,淋巴管阻塞引起的肺水肿,和上呼吸道梗阻解除引起的肺水肿通常微血管的通透性正常。

微血管通透性增加的组织病理学标志是肺泡毛细血管膜完整性的破坏导致肺泡、间质内蛋白质液的沉积。通透性增加的肺水肿发生在无弥漫性肺泡损害的情况时,被称为毛细血管渗漏综合征。在癌症中,这种类型肺水肿可以发生在使用细胞因子之后,如干扰素,重组人白介素-2(IL-2)和 TNF,这些细胞因子可以破坏毛细血管内皮完整性,也可能直接导致心肌毒性,引起与通透性正常和通透性增加病因有关的混合或重叠型的肺水肿。神经源性及复张性肺水肿,是混合型肺水肿的另外两个病因,常见于癌症患者。频繁输注血液制品(红细胞、血小板和粒细胞)使癌症患者易患输血相关的肺损伤综合征(syndrome of transfusion-related lung injury,TRALI),这是非心源性肺水肿的另一种表现形式。左心室舒张末期压力正常的肺动脉高压也是该综合征的重要特征。其治疗为对症支持治疗。临床症状和影像学改变的消退通常始于在症状出现后 2～3 日内,而无肺部永久后遗症,但 20%患者的症状和影像学变化可能会持续一个星期,并与急性肺损伤(ALI/ARDS,见下文)有关[258,259]。

急性肺损伤(acute lung injury,ALI)和急性呼吸窘迫综合征(acute respiratory distress syndrome,ARDS)是指伴有弥漫性肺泡组织病理损伤的不同严重程度的肺水肿。ARDS 特指有双侧肺浸润和严重低氧血症[定义为动脉血氧分压与吸入氧浓度比值(PaO_2/FiO_2)<200]而无左心房高压临床依据的严重肺损伤[260]。ALI 的肺损伤较轻,其 PaO_2/FiO_2 比值在 200 和 300 之间。与 ARDS 有关的癌症相关促发条件很多。病因二分类法为 ARDS 提供了简单的方法,该方法将 ARDS 病因分为造成直接肺损伤的病因(肺炎、胃抽吸术)和全身性疾病相关的促进间接肺损伤(败血症,输血相关的急性肺损伤)的病因,但由于激发事件通常是多方面或未知的,病因常常被混淆。在临床上,患者可表现为急性呼吸衰竭和激发事件 24～48h 内相关的低氧血症。即使没有感染存在,肺损伤炎症反应导致的发热和白细胞升高仍可能是主要结局。虽然急性呼吸窘迫综合征的影像学变化不明显,胸部 X 线检查在鉴别诊断如排除气胸,感染和充血性心脏衰竭中的作用仍然很重要。早期可以看见肺部受累的片状区域呈磨玻璃状,之后可能进展为弥漫性实变区。影像学检查提示心源性肺水肿,如 Kerley B 线,心脏增大,通常无心尖血管再分布。常常会进展到纤维增生期,导致持续性低氧血症与肺顺应性差、死腔增加、通气灌注失调和肺血管高压。

呼吸衰竭的治疗

内科治疗

呼吸衰竭的危重癌症患者的治疗,应包括积极的支持治疗,及针对病因的治疗策略。标准的支持治疗策略,包括吸氧,吸入型支气管扩张剂,营养支持,胸部理疗和肺部清洁,谨慎地使用利尿剂,升压药,必要时使用抗生素。虽然液体负荷增强了耗氧量和组织氧输送,但注意液体动态平衡是必要的,因为持续的液体正平衡与预后不良有关[261,262]。更具体的干预措施,如使用氦氧混合物可暂时缓解近端气道阻塞相关的急性呼吸窘迫,发挥通往进一步治疗的桥梁作用。DAH 患者可从早期使用高剂量类固醇、DDAVP 和积极输血和血液制品支持治疗中获益[263]。一些研究已经证实,重组因子Ⅶ(rFⅦa)和抗纤溶药物如氨基己酸已被用于治疗与移植相关的 DAH,尽管没有令人信服的证据支持这一做法[264～266]。应用活化蛋白 C 治疗在降低败血症相关性 ARDS 死亡率的效果是令人振奋的[284,285],但是,在亚组分析中得到的矛盾结果和严重出血的问题限制了这种药物的使用[267～269]。

在过去十年里,支持治疗的进步以及早期诊断和诱因治疗及减轻呼吸机相关肺损伤,显著增加了 ARDS 的生存率[270]。过去几个试验均未能证实在早期 ARDS 使用大剂量糖皮质激素取得生存获益。一些小型研究表明在 ARDS 的纤维增生期给予大剂量糖皮质激素起到有益的作用,尽管在一个大型多中心由美国国立卫生研究院(ARDS-Net)支持的试验中并未得到证实[271～274]。

机械通气

无创通气(NIV)

内科保守治疗无效的 ARF 患者通常需要辅助通气治疗。机械通气的新模式以及无创通气(NIV)的使用已显示出很有前途的结果,并在癌症患者呼吸衰竭的治疗中获得广泛接受。在几个治疗泵衰竭的随机对照研究[275,276]以及选择性的肺衰竭[275]病例中，NIV 的有效性已经得到明确证实。最近一项关于癌症患者因 ARF 转至 ICU 预后的回顾性研究表明，使用 NIV 明显改善患者的生存[277]。此外，在低氧性急性肾衰竭早期（PaO_2/FiO_2 比值<250）间歇使用 NIV 与常规机械通气显著的减少、ICU 期间和 ICU 之后住院死亡率的下降有关[278~280]。来自一些小的临床研究的证据支持对免疫功能缺陷的急性肾衰竭患者早期使用 NPPV 有利于降低气管插管使用率，缩短 ICU 监护时间和 ICU 死亡率[278,281,282]。免疫功能缺陷的需要机械通气的呼吸衰竭患者预后非常之差，估计机械通气的肺炎风险每日增加 1%[283]。因此，在这种情况下，NIV 在癌症患者的呼吸衰竭治疗中被迅速地广泛接受。

有创机械通气（IMV）

IMV 仍然是急性 ARF 以及 NIV 治疗失败后的标准方案。常规机械通气潮气量高时发生的吸气末肺部过度膨胀和呼气末肺部重复塌陷，可能会引发更严重的肺损伤。这一观察推动了肺保护性呼吸机的发展，它可减轻肺泡过度膨胀和增加肺不张的肺泡补充量，从而减少呼吸机相关性肺损伤的发病率。肺保护性机械通气方法，可通过传统通气模式如辅助控制和压力控制得以实现，可有或没有反比通气或替代方法，如双相气道正压通气（BIPAP），气道压力释放通气（APRV），喷射式和高频振荡通气，和差异性肺通气。这些通气模式还没有任何一种被证实是优于传统通气方式的。美国国立卫生研究院 ARDS-Net 试验得出令人信服的、支持使用保护性呼吸机策略的依据。在该试验中，相比给患者使用更高的潮气量和膨压力的机械通气，较低的潮气量（6ml/kg 预测体重）和有限的静态吸气压（<30cmH_2O）使得生存率提高了 22%[284,285]。目前已经提出了 ARF 患者呼吸机管理的其他辅助治疗，包括体外膜肺氧合（ECMO）和部分液体通气（PLV），俯卧位和表面活性剂滴注。但是，这些疗法相对于传统治疗策略的优点尚未得到明确证实。早期气管切开也许能改善危重患者的预后。基于近 20 年来对机械通气 21 日后考虑气管切开的共识，操作指南提到在适当的时机对需要长期机械通气患者进行气管切开术。虽然这些建议仅仅是以专家的意见为根据，但在当今实践却受到广泛遵循。最近的一项荟萃分析发现，接受早期行气管切开术患者（有创机械通气开始 7 日之内）与气管切开相对较晚的患者相比，总机械通气天数减少了 8.5 日，在 ICU 住院天数明显减少，但死亡率没有显著改变[286]。

呼吸衰竭预后

呼吸衰竭的危重癌症患者的死亡率至少比无呼吸衰竭者高 3 倍[287~289]。危重癌症患者的常见情况，如心脏，肾或肝功能不全，弥散性血管内凝血，血流动力学不稳定，和需要进行机械通气，都是预示预后不良的独立预测因素[287,288,290]。早期报道显示因 ARF 进行机械通气的癌症患者死亡率超过 90%，尤其是恶性血液病患者和接受造血器官移植的患者[291~294]。最近一些调查研究报道死亡率为 69%～84%[288,289,295,296]，提供了一个较好的前景。生存获益可能归因于较好的感染预防措施、移植技术的改善、预防措施的规范使用以减轻吸气困难，移植后更积极使用造血生长因子支持治疗，和使用外周血干细胞移植而非骨髓作为供体干细胞来源的趋势。此外，更新的通气方法，包括 NIV 和肺保护性呼吸机方法，可能起到改善生存的作用[289]。最后，医院普通病房的病情恶化患者的早期诊断和早期治疗方案的实施，和 ICU 住院和分流标准的改善，不仅有助于整体改善 ICU 生存，而且有助于合理利用医院资源[297,298]。

（王镇 译　赵峻 校）

参考文献

The complete reference list can be found on the Wiley Companion Digital Edition of this title (see inside front cover for login instructions).

2 Keefea D, Bowena J, Gibsonb R, Tanc T, Okerac M, Stringer A. Noncardiac vascular toxicities of vascular endothelial growth factor inhibitors in advanced cancer: a review. *Oncologist*. 2011;**16**:432–444.

13 Faiz SA, Sahay S, Jimenez CA. Pleural effusions in acute and chronic leukemia and myelodysplastic syndrome. *Curr Opin Pulm Med*. 2014;**20(4)**:340–346.

34 Ost D, Jimenez CA, Lei X, et al. Quality-adjusted survival following treatment of malignant pleural effusions with indwelling pleural catheters. *Chest*. 2014;**145**:1347–1356.

37 Janssen JP, Collier G, Astoul P, et al. Safety of pleurodesis with talc poudrage in malignant pleural effusion: a prospective cohort study. *Lancet*. 2007;**369(9572)**: 1535–1539.

40 Jimenez C, Mhatre A, Martinez C, et al. Use of an indwelling pleural catheter for the management of recurrent chylothorax in patients with cancer. *Chest*. 2007;**132**:1584–1590.

44 Datta D, Lahiri B. Preoperative evaluation of patients undergoing lung resection surgery. *Chest*. 2003;**123(6)**:2096–2103.

52 Morice RC, Peters EJ, Ryan MB, Putnam JB, Ali MK, Roth JA. Exercise testing in the evaluation of patients at high risk for complications from lung resection. *Chest*. 1992;**101(2)**:356–361.

53 Walsh GL, Morice RC, Putnam JB Jr, et al. Resection of lung cancer is justified in high-risk patients selected by exercise oxygen consumption. *Ann Thorac Surg*. 1994;**58(3)**:704–710; discussion 711.

58 Sleijfer S. Bleomycin-induced pneumonitis. *Chest*. 2001;**120(2)**:617–624.

78 Shannon V, Andersson B, Lei X, Champlin R, Kontoyiannis DP. Utility of early versus late fiberoptic bronchoscopy in the evaluation of new pulmonary infiltrates following hematopoietic stem cell transplantation. *Bone Marrow Transplant*. 2010;**45(4)**:647–655.

80 Rogers J, Yang D. Differentiation syndrome in patients with acute promyelocytic leukemia. *J Oncol Pharm Pract*. 2012;**18(1)**:109–114.

82 Dy G, Adjei A. Understanding, recognizing, and managing toxicities of targeted anticancer therapies. *CA Cancer J Clin*. 2013;**63(4)**:249–279.

87 Nagata S, Ueda N, Yoshida Y, Matsuda H, Maehara Y. Severe interstitial pneumonitis associated with the administration of taxanes. *J Infect Chemother*. 2010;**16(5)**:340–344.

88 Duran I, Goebell PJ, Papazisis K, et al. Drug-induced pneumonitis in cancer patients treated with mTOR inhibitors: management and insights into possible mechanisms. *Expert Opin Drug Saf*. 2014;**13(3)**:361–372.

93 Shannon V, Price K. Pulmonary complications of cancer therapy. *Anesthesiol Clin North Am*. 1998;**16(3)**:563–585.

95 Beauverd Y, Samii K. Acute respiratory distress syndrome in a patient with primary myelofibrosis after ruxolitinib treatment discontinuation. *Int J Hematol*. 2014;**100(5)**:498–501.

114 Godinas L, Guignabert C, Seferian A, et al. Tyrosine kinase inhibitors in pulmonary arterial hypertension: a double-edge sword? *Semin Respir Crit Care Med*. 2013;**34(5)**:714–724.

115 Montani D, Bergot E, Gunther S, et al. Pulmonary arterial hypertension in patients treated by dasatinib. *Circulation*. 2012;**125**:2128–2137.

129 Moon D, Lee JM, Noonan AM, et al. Deleterious BRCA1/2 mutation is an independent risk factor for carboplatin hypersensitivity reactions. *Br J Cancer*. 2013;**109(4)**:1072–1078.

140 Castillo R, Pham N, Ansari S, et al. Pre-radiotherapy FDG PET predicts radiation pneumonitis in lung cancer. *Radiat Oncol*. 2014;**9(74)**:1–10.

146 Ding K, Ji W, Li J, Zhang X, Wang L. Radiation recall pneumonitis induced by chemotherapy after thoracic radiotherapy for lung cancer. *Radiat Oncol*. 2011;**6(24)**:1–6.

153 Diab KJ, Yu Z, Wood KL, et al. Comparison of pulmonary complications after nonmyeloablative and conventional allogeneic hematopoietic cell transplant. *Biol Blood Marrow Transplant*. 2012;**18(12)**:1827–1834.

164 Yanik GA, Horowitz MM, Weisdorf DJ, et al. Randomized, double-blind, placebo-controlled trial of soluble tumor necrosis factor receptor: enbrel (etanercept) for the treatment of idiopathic pneumonia syndrome after allogeneic stem cell transplantation: blood and marrow transplant clinical trials network protocol. *Biol Blood Marrow Transplant*. 2014;**20(6)**:858–864.

172 Elinoff JM, Bagci U, Moriyama B, et al. Recombinant human factor VIIa for alveo-

lar hemorrhage following allogeneic stem cell transplantation. *Biol Blood Marrow Transplant*. 2014;**20(7)**:969–978.

178 Chien J, Duncan S, Williams KM, Pavletic SZ. Bronchiolitis obliterans syndrome after allogeneic hematopoietic stem cell transplantation-an increasingly recognized manifestation of chronic graft-versus-host disease. *Biol Blood Marrow Transplant*. 2010;**16(1 Suppl)**:S106–S114.

185 Norman BC, Jacobsohn DA, Williams KM, et al. Fluticasone, azithromycin and montelukast therapy in reducing corticosteroid exposure in bronchiolitis obliterans syndrome after allogeneic hematopoietic SCT: a case series of eight patients. *Bone Marrow Transplant*. 2011;**46(10)**:1369–1373.

187 Nakasone H, Onizuka M, Suzuki N, et al. Pre-transplant risk factors for cryptogenic organizing pneumonia/bronchiolitis obliterans organizing pneumonia after hematopoietic cell transplantation. *Bone Marrow Transplant*. 2013;**48(10)**:1317–1323.

189 Rasche L, Kapp M, Einsele H, Mielke S. EBV-induced post transplant lymphoproliferative disorders: a persisting challenge in allogeneic hematopoetic SCT. *Bone Marrow Transplant*. 2014;**49(2)**:163–167.

199 Lee AY, Peterson EA. Treatment of cancer-associated thrombosis. *Blood*. 2013;**122(14)**:2310–2317.

203 Lyman GH, Khorana AA, Kuderer NM, et al. Venous thromboembolism prophylaxis and treatment in patients with cancer: American Society of Clinical Oncology clinical practice guideline update. *J Clin Oncol*. 2013;**31(17)**:2189–2204.

204 Carrier M, Khorana AA, Zwicker JI, Noble S, Lee AY, Subcommittee on Haemostasis and Malignancy for the SSC of the ISTH. Management of challenging cases of patients with cancer-associated thrombosis including recurrent thrombosis and bleeding: guidance from the SSC of the ISTH: a reply to a rebuttal. *J Thromb Haemost*. 2014;**12(1)**:116–117.

205 Yeh CH, Gross PL, Weitz JI. Evolving use of new oral anticoagulants for treatment of venous thromboembolism. *Blood*. 2014;**124(7)**:1020–1028.

209 Simonneau G, Gatzoulis MA, Adatia I, et al. Updated clinical classification of pulmonary hypertension. *J Am Coll Cardiol*. 2013;**62**:D34–D41.

230 Nieto FJ, Peppard PE, Young T, Finn L, Hla KM, Farre R. Sleep-disordered breathing and cancer mortality: results from the wisconsin sleep cohort study. *Am J Resp Crit Care Med*. 2012;**186**:190–194.

234 Faiz SA, Balachandran D, Hessel AC, et al. Sleep-related breathing disorders in patients with tumors in the head and neck region. *Oncologist*. 2014;**19**:1200–1206.

242 Mujovic NMN, Subotic D, Marinkovic M, et al. Preoperative pulmonary rehabilitation in patients with non-small cell lung cancer and chronic obstructive pulmonary disease. *Arch Med Sci*. 2014;**10(1)**:68–75.

245 Granger CLCC, McDonald CF, Berney S, Denehy L. Safety and feasibility of an exercise intervention for patients following lung resection: a pilot randomized controlled trial. *Integr Cancer Ther*. 2013;**12(3)**:213–224.

274 Steinberg K, Hudson LD, Goodman RB, et al. Efficacy and safety of corticosteroids for persistent acute respiratory distress syndrome. *N Engl J Med*. 2006;**354(16)**:1671–1684.

282 Caples S, Gay PC. Noninvasive positive pressure ventilation in the intensive care unit: a concise review. *Crit Care Med*. 2005;**33(11)**:2651–2658.

296 Kew A, Couban S, Patrick W, Thompson K, White D. Outcome of hematopoietic stem cell transplant recipients admitted to the intensive care unit. *Biol Blood Marrow Transplant*. 2006;**12(3)**:301–305.

第 134 章　癌症患者的胃肠道和肝脏并发症

Robert S. Bresalier, MD ■ H. Franklin Herlong, MD ■ Boris Blechacz, MD, PhD

概述

胃肠道和肝脏并发症代表了一些最重要的与治疗相关的常见和可能危及生命的疾病,癌症患者治疗选择的增加也伴随着一系列后果,直接地和间接地影响胃肠道细胞的快速分裂。细胞毒性,免疫学和感染性损伤通常会增加毒性。认识这些并发症,并进行适当的评估和干预,是使这些患者保持健康的关键。

随着越来越多的治疗方法被应用于治疗癌症。化疗、放疗和包括免疫疗法在内的分子靶向疗法会在多个器官中导致一系类不良反应,其中就包括胃肠(GI)道的系统。GI 并发症在接受癌症治疗的患者中非常常见。其中一些并发症可能危及生命并要求及时和适当的诊断和治疗。本章介绍了由癌症治疗引发的常见胃肠道并发症,重点是对这些并发症的评估和干预。

食管疾病

食管炎

食管炎可以由化疗或放疗的细胞毒性反应或肿瘤治疗引起的免疫抑制而导致的感染引起(表 134-1)。细胞死亡导致了黏膜萎缩,溃疡和炎症反应的发生。活性氧、促炎症细胞因子和定殖生物的代谢副产物也起到了放大组织损伤的作用[1,2]。化疗和放疗之间的协同作用可能会增加联合治疗方案导致的食管炎的严重程度。药物诱导的损伤,酸性反流疾病以及发生在造血干细胞移植受体的移植物抗宿主反应也可能引起食管炎。当怀疑食管炎时,特别是对于那些免疫功能受损的患者,应立即进行内镜活检和/或刷检以迅速评估并指导早期诊断和治疗。

表 134-1　接受肿瘤治疗的患者患食管炎的主要原因

感染原因/损伤	内镜表现	治疗
白色念珠菌	食管黏膜白斑样病变,周围有红斑	用氟康唑、伊曲康唑、伏立康唑或棘白菌素进行全身抗真菌治疗
单纯疱疹病毒	小水疱,合并形成溃疡	阿昔洛韦和膦甲酸钠
巨细胞病毒	线性或丝状溃疡	阿昔洛韦,膦甲酸钠和缬更昔洛韦
口腔菌群	在活组织检查样本中,细菌与坏死的上皮细胞混合	广谱抗生素
放化疗导致的损伤	易碎黏膜伴红斑水肿	盐酸利多卡因,麻醉性镇痛药,质子泵抑制剂,内镜扩张/支架

放射性食管炎

放射性食管炎常发生于肺癌、头颈肿瘤、食管癌的治疗过程中。急性放射性食管炎主要是由于基底上皮质快速分裂细胞的损伤,导致食管黏膜变薄和剥脱。食管炎的严重程度随着放疗剂量的增加以及某些化疗药物(如顺铂)的使用而增加[3~5]。患者通常主诉为吞咽疼痛、吞咽困难和胸痛。内镜检查可发现红疹、水肿易碎的食管黏膜以及溃疡或伴狭窄的形成。急性食管炎的治疗包括使用局麻药,如口服盐酸利多卡因凝胶,全身性麻醉镇痛药和质子泵抑制剂。一些患者的症状严重到需要接受临时经皮胃造口术(PEG)。术前放置 PEG 可能有助于部分接受头颈部扩大手术和同步放化疗预防术后严重症状。最近癌症支持护理多国协会(MASCC)和国际口腔肿瘤学会(ISOO)发布共识建议使用静脉注射氨磷汀预防化疗和化疗治疗非小细胞肺癌过程中诱发的食管炎,通过内镜扩张治疗狭窄。在发生气管-食管瘘的食管癌患者中,覆膜支架(自膨式金属或塑料支架)是首选的治疗方法,可以使 70%~100%瘘管闭合[6]。

真菌感染

食管念珠菌病在免疫缺陷患者中很常见,白色念珠菌是导致食管和口咽念珠菌病(OPC)最常见的致病微生物。患者以吞咽痛和/或吞咽困难为主诉。内镜检查中,可以看到白色斑样病灶及其周围包绕的红斑覆盖在食管壁上。食管活检或刷检可证实酵母菌或菌丝侵入黏膜细胞。伴有吞咽痛和/或吞咽困难的患者推荐接受全身性抗真菌治疗。如果症状 72h 无改善,应进行内镜检查。抗真菌药的一般持续时间治疗是 14~21 日。免疫功能低下患者出现念珠菌性食管炎需要全身抗真菌治疗,局部用药治疗无效[7~10]。患者无法耐受口服药物治疗时需要静脉给药。治疗食管念珠菌病的药物包括唑类、棘白菌素(echinocandins)或两性霉素 B[7~15]。唑类通过抑制霉菌细胞膜的主要成分麦角固醇的合成来阻止细胞膜的形成。氟康唑属于唑类,其治疗效率高、易于使用且成本低,是推荐的一线药物。对于氟康唑难治性食管念珠菌病的患者如果能耐受口服治疗,可使用新型唑类(伏立康唑和泊沙康唑)。已发现伊曲康唑与氟康唑用于治疗食管念珠菌病一样有效,由于它可能会产生严重的恶心及抑制细胞色素 p 450 酶而发生药物相互作用，所以它的使用受到了限制。

需要静脉治疗的患者应使用氟康唑治疗或一种棘白菌素（卡泊芬净，米卡芬净或阿尼芬净），而不是两性霉素 B，因为它们毒性更低。棘白菌素抑制霉菌细胞壁的重要组成部分 β(1,3)-D-葡聚糖的合成。哺乳动物细胞不需要 β(1,3)-D-葡聚糖，从而限制了潜在的毒性。与唑类相比，棘白菌素的复发率更高，通常作为唑类治疗失败时的二线治疗。两性霉素 B 用于患有食管念珠菌病的孕妇和患有耐药性念珠菌病的个体。OPC 是一种局部感染，其风险因素包括接受放射，化疗，抗生素和类固醇治疗。治疗方法包括局部应用制霉菌素或克霉唑锭剂。有发生 OPC 风险的患者可给予抗真菌预防。外用抗真菌药，如克霉唑或咪康唑可有效预防[16]。

病毒感染

病毒感染性食管炎是由单纯疱疹病毒（HSV）、巨细胞病毒（CMV）及极少数由带状疱疹病毒（VZV）感染引起[8,17]。患者常表现为吞咽疼痛和吞咽困难，相对少见的症状包括恶心、呕吐、胃灼热、上腹痛以及发热。在 HSV 食管炎中，有些患者合并口唇疱疹或口咽溃疡[30]。诊断可通过内镜检查和活检确立（图 134-1）。在早期，HSV 病变可表现为小水疱，尽管他们极少被发现。这些小水疱最终融合为大的溃疡，而这种溃疡通常直径小于 2cm。这些溃疡都被表面正常的、插入的黏膜很好的包绕[31]。CMV 引起的溃疡呈线性或匍行，比 HSV 相关溃疡深，也会出现渗液[31]。从 HSV 相关溃疡边缘取的活检组织可见细胞核内包含体和多核巨细胞。使用针对 HSV 的单克隆抗体的免疫组化方法也可以检测到核内包含体[31]。病毒分离培养有助于识别出对阿昔洛韦不敏感患者的耐药菌株。在患带状疱疹的成人中，VZV 也可以引发食管炎，但通常是在播散性感染的情况下。在内镜下，VZV 引起的溃疡表现与 HSV 溃疡相似。在活检标本中，与 HSV 的鉴别需要借助于免疫组化或培养。

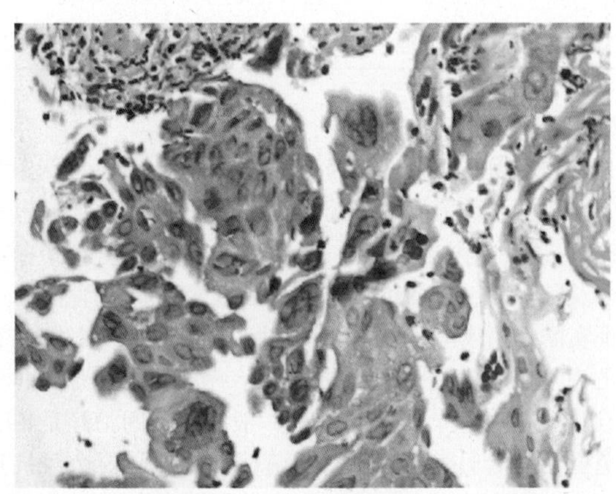

图 134-1 单纯疱疹病毒（HSV）食管炎。高倍镜视野食管黏膜鳞状细胞伴磨玻璃样核病毒中性粒细胞背景下的包含体和多核巨细胞渗出液

CMV 感染内皮细胞和成纤维细胞，但是与 HSV 和 VZV 不同，它不能感染上皮细胞。CMV 感染患者的常规活检可见成纤维细胞和上皮细胞的核内容物。使用抗 CMV 抗体的免疫组化同样有助于诊断。

对于 HSV 食管炎的患者，阿昔洛韦（400mg 5 次/d 口服持续 14～21 日或 5mg/kg 每 8h 静脉注射 7～14 日）是治疗首选[8,9,18,19]。阿昔洛韦耐药 HSV 由与 HSV 胸苷激酶（*TK*）基因突变引起。具有 *TK* 突变的病毒通常具有伐昔洛韦交叉抗性，但仍然容易受可影响 DNA 聚合酶药剂的直接作用，如膦甲酸（2～3 次分开注射 80～120mg/（kg · d），直至临床有效）。严重地持续性阿昔洛韦耐药的 HSV 感染病例几乎全部发生在存在免疫受损的宿主。泛昔洛韦或伐昔洛韦可以用于能够耐受口服治疗的患者，尽管将这些药物应用于治疗 HSV 相关性食管炎的临床经验有限。因为 VZV 食管炎静脉患者通常有传染性，最初通过注射阿昔洛韦治疗。待临床症状改善后，可以改为使用用于 HSV 食管炎的口服药物治疗。治疗 CMV 食管炎需静脉注射更昔洛韦（5mg/（kg · d）两次）或膦甲酸钠（每 8h 静脉输注 68mg/kg 或每 12h 输注 90mg/kg）持续 3～6 周[8,20-22]。一旦患者能够吸收和耐受口服治疗，可以改用缬更昔洛韦（每 12h 900mg）。缬更昔洛韦是更昔洛韦的口服前体。剂量为 900mg/d，缬更昔洛韦产生的全身药物当量相当于更昔洛韦 5mg/kg 静脉注射。感染清除后的维持治疗的作用并不确定。

细菌感染

免疫缺陷患者可发生细菌性食管炎，并常为来源于口腔菌丛的多重微生物感染。其诊断依靠内镜下活检，使用广谱抗生素进行治疗。

药物性食管炎

口服药物诱发的食管炎可发生于那些睡前服药但是饮用的液体不足时或平卧体位的患者。和这一疾病有关的最常见的药物包括：氯化钾、四环素、阿司匹林、非甾体抗炎药、奎尼丁、铁剂和阿仑膦酸钠。损伤是由于食管黏膜接触药物的腐蚀性成分的时间延长所致。患者常表现为突然发生的吞咽痛，这种痛甚至可能会严重到吞咽唾液困难和疼痛。内镜检查有助于明确诊断；但更重要的是需要排除其他诊断，如感染性食管炎或恶性肿瘤。内镜下常见位于近端食管分散的、单个的溃疡。有时损伤可表现为提示肿瘤或狭窄的结节状、息肉状病灶（图 134-2）。食

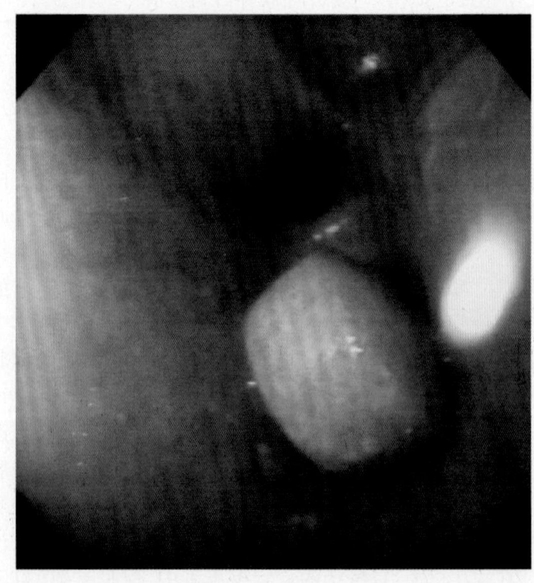

图 134-2 药物介导的食管损伤。在食管狭窄上方的内镜检查中可以看到一片药丸

管活检表现为非特异性改变或者仅仅为急性炎症反应的表现。这种疾病没有特异性的治疗方法，因为它不需要任何干预可以几天内自愈。食管狭窄则需要食管扩张治疗。

恶性吞咽困难

食管癌患者会在进展性、不可治愈的阶段表现这一症状。对那些不是放化疗或手术适应证的患者，还有那些治疗后出现反复吞咽困难的患者，已经有多种内镜技术被用于改善食管腔的开放。

食管扩张可以通过经内镜气囊、水银橡胶探条、线导管聚乙烯探条（Savary-Gilliard 扩张器）进行。在明确的治疗开始前，扩张器可以安全暂时地缓解吞咽困难症状[1,2]。要达到成功的扩张，必须每几星期重复一次。自膨式金属支架（self-expanding metal stents，SEMS）作为一种有效的非手术治疗手段正越来越多地被用于梗阻的、进展性食管肿瘤的姑息治疗[23~27]。SEMS 由多种合金制成，并有不同的形状和型号以适应恶性肿瘤组织的长度和位置。此外，已批准的支架款式包括无覆膜，部分覆膜的和完全覆膜 3 型。此外，它们的材质（镍钛合金、外科钢、塑料）和功能（全能型和"抗反流"型）也各不相同。SEMS 通过内镜引导置入可行或不进行透视检查（图 134-3）。全新设计的双层镍钛合金（Niti-S）支架与以前的设计相比患者的生存时间更长，并发症更少。一旦金属支架展开后，便不能再移动。目前已经有许多随机临床试验比较不同支架在恶性狭窄的中的应用效果，SEMS 的优势有：置入物相对舒适、支架口径较大、穿孔的风险低及彻底消除了额外进行食管扩张的需要。其缺点则包括：花费高、支架移位、膨胀不良、气道梗阻以及出血。随着聚氨酯涂层覆盖的支架的引入，肿瘤向内生长的发生率现已降低，这种被包覆的支架也可用于治疗气管食管瘘的患者。最近，由于自膨式塑料支架（self-expanding plastic stents，SEPS）的发展，使食管癌的姑息治疗又多了一种新的选择。据报道，SEPS 在某些情况下，支架的放置失败率和迁移率较高，不太容易出现狭窄。支架在缓解放化疗后食管恶性肿瘤患者症状方面也很有效。并发症如食管呼吸瘘的风险的增加与辐射剂量相关。目前正在研发可以随着时间的推移逐渐溶解的可降解生物支架。支架也被提议作为一种接受新辅助治疗的人接受手术前的过渡治疗。

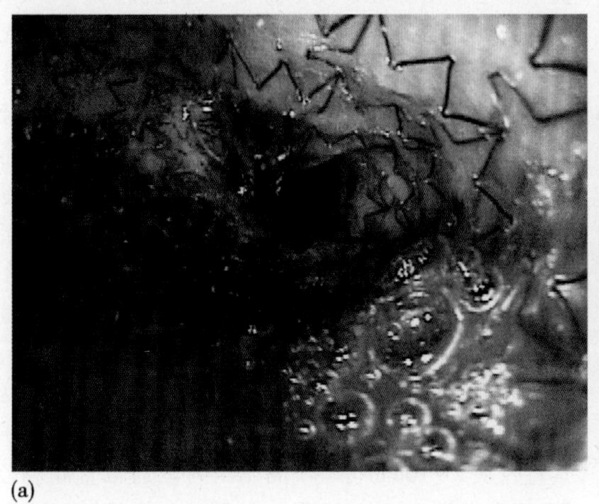
(a)

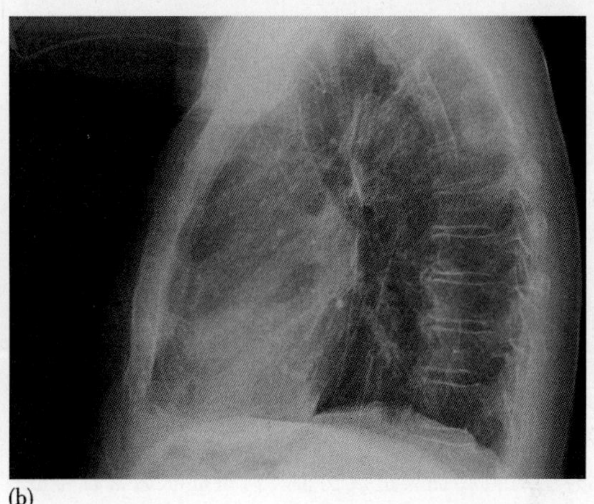
(b)

图 134-3　自膨胀食管（a）食管内自扩张支架用于治疗食管狭窄的内镜视图。（b）胸片显示食管内有支架

射频消融技术，比如激光，光动力疗法（PDT）和大剂量近距离放射治疗等，已成功应用于恶性食管梗阻的缓解，但大部分已被 SEMS 取代。激光能量来自钕：钇铝石榴石晶体，或 Nd：YAG，这一技术是使用石英纤维通过内镜的活检通道引导控制射线的能量，过去被广泛用于缓解食管癌症状。这个方法可能需要事先进行食管扩张才能通过内镜。主要并发症包括食管穿孔，气管-食管瘘，出血和菌血症。Nd：YAG 射线治疗的缺点包括：对于长的、弯曲的病灶或病灶位于近端食管时治疗困难，需要许多治疗阶段以及费用较高。PDT 是使用一种光敏剂和低能量射线来达到肿瘤坏死和管道再通的作用。卟吩姆钠（光卟啉）是唯一被美国食品药品管理局批准用于治疗食管癌的光敏剂。光卟啉静脉注射后，选择性的在肿瘤组织中保持较高浓度。注射后约 48h，通过内镜辅助通道放置的、附在石英光纤终端的圆柱形扩散器使患者暴露于 630nm 的单色激光下引发光化学反应组织导致氧自由基的形成，缺血和肿瘤坏死。

最近 Cochrane 协作分析对 53 项关于食管癌吞咽困难的干预性研究进行了广泛深入的分析[28]。该分析得出结论，与其他方式相比 SEMS 能够安全、有效并更为快速地缓解吞咽困难，但那高剂量腔内近距离放射治疗是一种合适的替代疗法可以提供额外的生存益处和更好的生活质量。近距离放射治疗和 SEMS 的组合可以减少再次介入的需要。刚性塑料支架插入，单独扩张或与其他方式相结合因为并发症发生率较高和复发性吞咽困难单独化疗不建议用于缓解因吞咽困难。

腹泻

放化疗引起的腹泻

腹泻是细胞毒治疗的常见并发症，最常发生于氟尿嘧啶类（特别是氟尿嘧啶）、伊立替康、甲氨蝶呤以及顺铂药物（表 134-2）[29~31]。腹泻也常见于接受小分子表皮生长因子受体酪氨酸激酶抑制剂（厄洛替尼和索拉非尼）的患者。腹泻可导致严重虚弱，并且在一些严重的病例中可导致治疗延误，生活质量下降，依从性下降。腹泻是剂量限制性因素并且是含嘧啶和/或伊立替康化疗方案的主要毒性表现。化疗所致的腹泻其严重程度通常是按照美国国立癌症研究所共同毒性标准（National Cancer Institute Common Toxicity Criteria, NCICTC）来描述的，对于以研究为目的的临床实践更是如此。分级则是根据每日腹泻次数、夜间腹泻表现以及是否需要肠外营养支持或重病特别护理来决定。

表 134-2 癌症与造血细胞移植患者腹泻的鉴别诊断

化疗相关（氟吡嘧啶、伊立替康、甲氨蝶呤、顺铂、小分子表皮生长因子受体酪氨酸激酶抑制剂：厄洛替尼和索拉非尼）及其他因素
继发性结肠炎的免疫调节剂（伊匹木单抗，纳武单抗，lambrizumab）及其他因素
放射治疗
预处理方案
移植物抗宿主病
感染
艰难梭菌
病毒（包括巨细胞病毒）

亚叶酸钙与氟尿嘧啶联用会加重腹泻严重程度，此外，快速推注氟尿嘧啶会加重腹泻，而静脉持续灌注则会减轻。伊立替康可引起早发性腹泻，同时伴有腹绞痛、流泪、流涎增多及其他的类胆碱能综合征表现。伊立替康相关的迟发型腹泻无法预测，且与剂量无关。目前观察到三周方案的发生率低于每周方案。已有文献报道，与氟尿嘧啶联合亚叶酸钙方案相比，伊立替康、氟尿嘧啶联合亚叶酸钙方案腹泻程度更重。据报道，1~2 级腹泻接受厄洛替尼治疗的患者占 56%，服用索拉非尼的患者占 34%[32,33]。

放射治疗会对胃肠黏膜造成伤害。典型症状通常发生在分次放疗的第三周。盆腔或腹部放射可导致急性肠炎，大约 50%的患者以腹部绞痛和腹泻为特征。同步化疗时这些症状变得更为的严重。

阿片受体激动剂是治疗的基础药物[34]。洛哌丁胺和地芬诺酯都被广泛应用于治疗此类腹泻，并获得了美国食品药品管理局批准（FDA）批准。洛哌丁胺更为有效。对于轻中度腹泻，洛哌丁胺的初始剂量为 4mg，然后每 4h 或每次便后 2mg。对于重度或伊立替康诱发的腹泻来说，则需要更强的剂量，洛哌丁胺的初始剂量为 4mg，然后每 2h 2mg 或每 4h 4mg，直到腹泻控制 12h 后停止。奥曲肽是一种合成的长效生长抑素类似物，已被用作阿片类药耐药物患者的二线治疗药物。奥曲肽的推荐初始剂量为 100~150μg，皮下注射，一日 3 次，或 25~50μg/h 静脉点滴。对于无反应者奥曲肽的剂量可调大为 500~2 500μg，每日 3 次。

对于化疗诱发的轻中度腹泻，其他用于轻至中度腹泻的辅助治疗的药物，包括收敛剂如白岭土和活性炭、阿片酊、阿片樟脑酊及可卡因。

由于对伊立替康相关的腹泻风险的充分认识，最近的一些研究已经研究出来预防化疗引起的腹泻的方案。奥曲肽（奥曲肽 LAR）的长效缓释制剂可以每月肌注一次。一旦已达到稳态水平，通过显著降低奥曲肽波峰和波谷浓度的波动，每 4 周一次肌注剂量为 20mg 奥曲肽 LAR 所产生相同的药理学效果相当于 150μg 奥曲肽每日 3 次。另外，奥曲肽 LAR（起始剂量为 20mg）能够有效控制与类癌综合征相关的腹泻[31]，目前正在研究每月 20~30mg 的剂量治疗和预防化疗引起的腹泻。

对于接受造血干细胞移植的患者（HCT），腹泻可能是由于预处理方案引起（全身照射和/或高剂量化疗）。移植前预处理方案可损伤胃肠黏膜，引起黏膜恢复后可治愈的分泌性腹泻。第 20 日后，急性 GVHD 是这些患者腹泻的最常见原因。GVHD 将单独讨论。

艰难梭菌相关性腹泻

如果腹泻不是化疗或放疗的直接结果，特别对于住院患者发生的腹泻，应该考虑艰难梭菌感染，因为这是住院患者感染性腹泻最常见的原因。虽然艰难梭菌感染所致的腹泻或结肠炎通常与使用抗生素治疗相关，但其风险因素还包括肠道手术，免疫缺陷状态和使用包括抗真菌药物及化疗药物等可能抑制肠道正常菌群的治疗。接受化疗的癌症患者即使没有使用抗生素也易出现艰难梭菌感染引起的腹泻。一项关于这类患者的研究表明，甲氨蝶呤、多柔比星和环磷酰胺是最常引起艰难梭菌感染的药物。其临床表现可以有很大的差别，从不合并结肠炎的轻度腹泻，合并全身症状的结肠炎，伴或不伴有蛋白丢失性肠病的伪膜性肠炎至发展为中毒性巨结肠症的暴发性结肠炎。诊断艰难梭菌的方法已有了明显进步，过去通过酶免疫测定法（EIA）检测毒素 A 或毒素 B 是应用最广泛的诊断方法。这些测试的灵敏度为 75%~95%，特异性为 83%~98%。艰难梭菌实验室诊断的两个主要进展是使用谷氨酸脱氢酶（GDH；一种由艰难梭菌产生的酶），在粪便中检测（75%~>90%的敏感性，阴性预测值接近 100%）和毒素基因的核酸扩增试验（PCR）。在内镜检查中，假膜呈现为黏附的黄色斑块，其直径从 2~10mm 不等（图 134-4）。通常直肠和乙状结肠受累，但在大约 10%的病例中，结肠炎仅存在于近端结肠中并且在乙状结肠镜检查时被漏掉。

感染的严重程度不同，艰难梭菌感染的治疗策略也不同，艰难梭菌感染所致腹泻标准治疗方法是口服甲硝唑或万古霉素。甲硝唑 500mg/d 分 3 次口服或静脉注射 10~14 日，同万古霉素 125mg，每日 4 次口服疗效相当。轻度至中度的情况下，较低剂量的万古霉素 125mg 每日 4 次与每日 4 次 250mg 的高剂量一样有效，并且便宜得多。甲硝唑与万古霉素相比具有很多优势，费用低并能抑制对万古霉素选择性耐药的粪肠球菌。因此甲硝唑时治疗轻中度的艰难梭菌感染引起的腹泻的初始治疗方法。如果 3 日内症状没有改善，应开始用万古霉素治疗。对于严重感染并有全身毒性表现的患者，专家推荐的初始治疗为万古霉素 125mg，每日 4 次口服，若患者病情未见好转，则在 48h 中将剂量提高至 500mg/d 分 4 次口服。当口服万古霉素无法起效时，应当考虑给予联用甲硝唑 500mg，静点，每 8h 一次或万古霉素保留灌肠（0.5~1g 的万古霉素溶解在 1~2L 的生理盐水中每 4~12h 一次）。

不建议使用抗蠕动剂，因为它们可能会掩盖症状，并且有证据表明，运输时间的减少会导致并发症并延长疾病的持续时间。CDI 的复发很常见，在所有 CDI 患者中发生率高达 10%~25%。复发通常发生在初期治疗结束 1~3 周内，可能是由于细

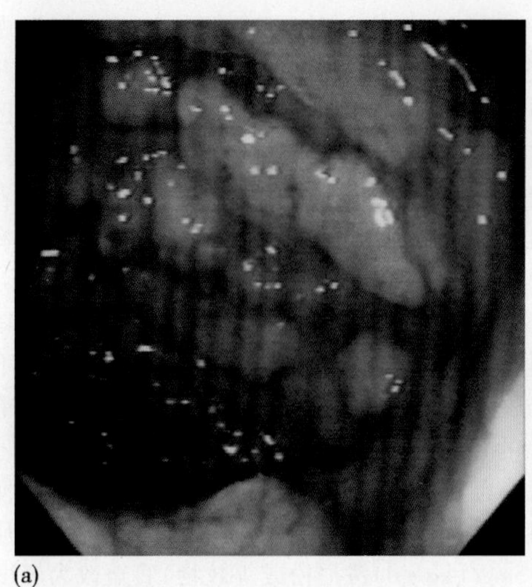
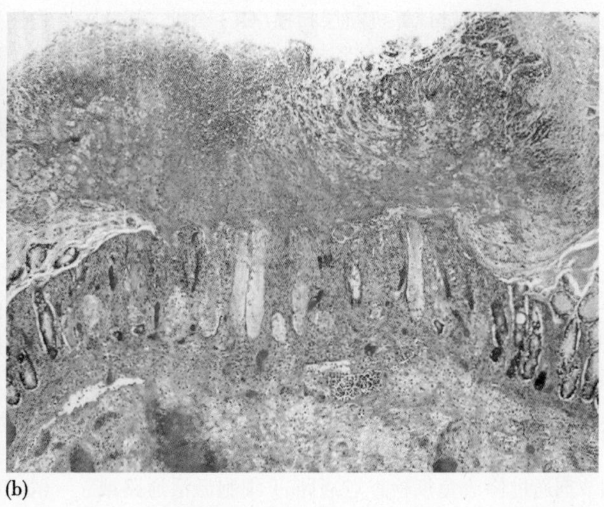

(a)　(b)

图 134-4　伪膜性结肠炎。(a)结肠镜下结肠黏膜上的假膜。(b)结肠黏膜低倍镜显示典型的火山状(蘑菇状)外观,可见腔内炎性渗出物

菌没有得到根除。初次复发处理为再次给予 10~14 日的口服甲硝唑或万古霉素,对于接受第二程抗生素治疗后仍复发的患者,建议治疗方案包括给予窄谱抗生素冲击治疗及阴离子结合树脂如考来烯胺或考来替泊单药或联合万古霉素治疗。非达米星(fidaxomicin)是治疗 CDI 初始复发的替代药物。用于治疗初期 CDI 复发,非达米星和万古霉素治疗的初始效果相当,但非达米星治疗后续复发的可能性低于万古霉素(20% vs 36%)。如果第三次复发,应考虑粪便微生物群移植。在小样本病例中,2 周的万古霉素随后 2 周的利福昔明(rifaximin)已经证明可成功控制复发性感染。最近的一项研究使用了两种中性人单克隆抗体对抗毒素 A(CDA1)和 B(CDB1),治疗 101 名使用甲硝唑或万古霉素有症状的艰难梭菌患者,用单克隆抗体治疗的患者中,艰难梭菌感染的复发率显著降低。

其他感染引起的腹泻

造血干细胞移植后患者的感染性腹泻相当少见。病毒是发现的最常见的生物体(星状病毒,腺病毒,巨细胞病毒和轮状病毒),其次是院内获得性感染(艰难梭菌和产气单胞菌)。巨细胞病毒特别值得一提,因为它可以造成黏膜溃疡而引起腹泻和出血。巨细胞病毒是通过内镜活检来诊断(图 134-5),活组织标本应该被送检免疫组化和病毒培养。感染性腹泻有关的沙门菌、志贺菌、空肠弯曲物种在住院的移植患者中是非常罕见的。寄生虫(隐孢子虫、贾第鞭毛虫、阿米巴)有关的腹泻也是罕见的腹泻原因,这些患者大多数是移植前就已感染。

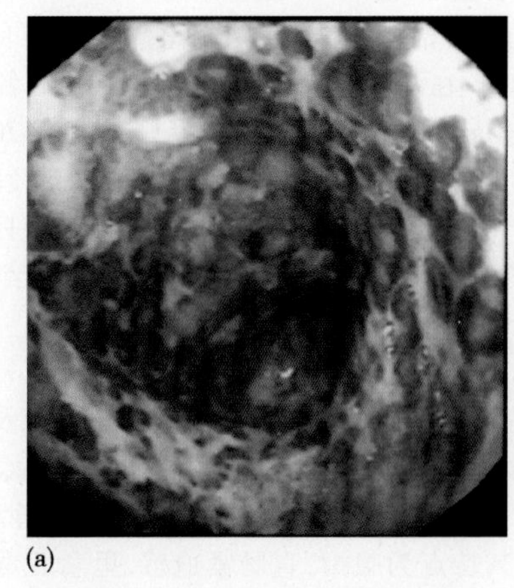
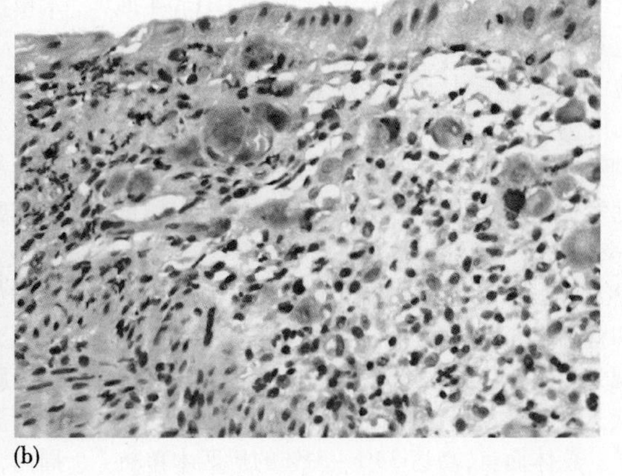

(a)　(b)

图 134-5　巨细胞病毒(CMV)结肠炎。(a)内镜下 CMV 结肠炎。(b)结肠黏膜炎症高倍镜显示间质细胞内存在多种病毒包含体

结肠炎

中性粒细胞减少性小肠结肠炎

中性粒细胞减少性小肠结肠炎或盲肠炎是发生于中性粒细胞减少患者的临床综合征,其特点为发热和右下腹痛。可出现在患有血液系统恶性肿瘤,再生障碍性贫血及治疗实体恶性肿瘤之后骨髓抑制的儿童和成人中[37~42]。来自中性粒细胞减少性小肠结肠炎患者的活检样本的组织学检查的特征是肠壁增厚,水肿,黏膜溃疡,局灶性出血和黏膜或透壁坏死。在手术标本和腹水的标本中已经鉴别出多种病原微生物,中性粒细胞

减少性小肠结肠炎通常通过计算机断层扫描(CT)诊断。超声和CT成像的异常表现包括积液、盲肠扩张、右下腹部炎性包块、盲肠周围积液或是盲肠周围软组织炎性改变,治疗包括肠道休息,静脉输液和应用广谱抗生素。因为中性粒细胞减少症促进了此类疾病的发生,同时凝血功能障碍可能与黏膜出血失血有关,所以应该首先纠正肿瘤治疗相关的血细胞减少和凝血功能障碍。可以使用重组粒细胞集落刺激因子(G-CSF)促进白细胞恢复,这有助于白细胞恢复治疗中性粒细胞减少性小肠结肠炎。手术已被推荐对于已经纠正了血细胞减少症和凝血功能障碍,但仍有持续胃肠道出血的患者,以及穿孔或药物治疗后临床恶化的患者。

免疫调节剂和抗肿瘤药引起的结肠炎

免疫调节剂通过修改免疫检查点通路、T细胞激活通路或过继细胞疗法来增强肿瘤定向免疫应答[43]。然而,这种方法也会引起肠道副反应,特别是与免疫检查点的靶向治疗相关,(如细胞毒性T淋巴细胞抗原-4(CTLA-4)和PD-1)。CTLA-4是一种关键的负向调节因子负责调节免疫应答中的T细胞活化。瞬时的、抗体介导的CTLA-4抑制剂能够增强T细胞应答。伊匹木单抗和替西利姆单抗(tremelimumab)是完全人源的针对CTLA-4的单克隆IgG1抗体。替西利姆单抗与伊匹木单抗的GI不良反应相似,最近的一项随机对照Ⅲ期临床试验中,替西利姆单抗对黑色素瘤化疗没有生存获益[44]。CTLA-4抑制剂主要用于黑色素瘤,尽管它们也已经在其他实体恶性肿瘤如胰腺癌、前列腺癌、肾癌、卵巢癌和小细胞肺癌中进行了评估[45,46]。鉴于抑制剂的调节作用,作为CTLA-4和PD-1在适应性免疫反应中,它们具有广泛的免疫介导的不良事件(imAE),包括小肠结肠炎、肝炎、皮炎、垂体炎、葡萄膜炎和肾炎;小肠结肠炎是最常见的不良反应,在诱导和再诱导期间观察到大多数免疫相关不良事件。

尽管它们也已经在其他实体恶性肿瘤中进行了测试,如胰腺癌,前列腺癌,肾细胞,卵巢和小细胞肺癌,但目前CTLA-4抑制剂主要用于黑色素瘤[45,46]。鉴于CTLA-4和PD-1等抑制剂在适应性免疫反应中的调节作用,它们会产生广泛的免疫介导的不良事件(imAE),包括小肠结肠炎、肝炎、皮炎、垂体炎、葡萄膜炎和肾炎;小肠结肠炎是最常见的不良反应[47]。大多数免疫相关不良事件发生在诱导期和再诱导期[46]。伊匹木单抗相关性小肠结肠炎的发展与周期数无关,但似乎与剂量有关[47,48]。有证据表明小肠结肠炎的发展可能是用伊匹木单抗治疗的黑色素瘤和肾细胞癌患者肿瘤有效的预测因子[47]。小肠结肠炎最常表现为腹泻,但也有腹痛、恶心/呕吐、发烧、肛门疼痛和便秘等症状。大多数小肠结肠炎发生在患者最后一次给药后21日内[47]。总体而言,高达33%~51%的伊匹木单抗治疗患者出现腹泻,其中16%为3级和<1%的4级[44~46,48]。在腔内,高达8%的患者发展为结肠炎,包括4%~5%3级和0~1%的4级结肠炎[45,46]。腹泻通常是白细胞很少,很少有血液阳性水样便。在放射学上,伊匹木单抗相关结肠炎的特征在于肠系膜血管充血,结肠壁增厚,黏膜增强和充满液体的结肠扩张。结肠炎可以表现为弥漫性,也可以表现为与憩室炎(SCAD)相关的节段性结肠炎。虽然小肠炎已有报道,但结肠是最常见的受累区域[49,50]。伊匹木单抗相关性结肠炎的内镜表现是非特异性和严重依赖于肉眼可见的发现,如黏膜红斑、脆性、水肿和溃疡[47]。在大多数患者中,组织学发现包括伴有隐睾炎的中性粒细胞炎症和偶尔的隐窝脓肿,或中性粒细胞-淋巴细胞混合的炎症图像。在少数患者中,可见淋巴细胞为主的炎症,伴随隐窝中CD8+T细胞数量增加和固有层CD4+细胞数量增加[47,49]。0.7%~6.6%的伊匹木单抗治疗患者会出现结肠穿孔或需要结肠切除术[5]。患有继发于伊匹木单抗治疗的小肠结肠炎的患者的死亡率据报道高达5%[47]。伊匹木单抗相关不良事件的治疗以严重程度为指导(表134-3),但需要排除其他病因[51]。轻度胃肠道症状可以对症治疗而不停用伊匹木单抗;然而,需要持续性地反复评估来确定更严重症状或危及生命的并发症。在中度小肠结肠炎的情况下,应停用伊匹木单抗并在症状显著地改善或解决后7日重新开始使用。如果中度症状在7日后仍然存在,则建议开始使用糖皮质激素治疗(如0.5mg/(kg·d)泼尼松或等效物)直至改为轻度症状或症状消退。一旦症状是变为轻度和糖皮质激素剂量已逐渐减少至≤7.5mg/d,可以恢复使用伊匹木单抗。严重的小肠结肠炎和危及生命的并发症需要永久停药伊匹木单抗。在这些情况下,当肠穿孔被排除时,应该应用全身性糖皮质激素(如1~2mg/(kg·d)泼尼松或等同物[51])。有限的报道中,英夫利西单抗的成功应用于糖皮质激素难治性病例中[47,52,53]。和伊匹木单抗一起预防性应用布地奈德并未显著降低腹泻或结肠炎[54,55]。程序性细胞死亡蛋白-1(PD-1)是一类在T细胞上表达的受体,在其配体PD-L1(B7-H_1)和PD-L2结合后(B7-DC)减弱T细胞活化。虽然PD-L2通常由APC表达,但在肿瘤中观察到PD-L1的过度表达[43,56]。纳武单抗和lambrizumab是PD-1靶向的人源化单克隆IgG4抗体,目前正在进行或计划随机的Ⅱ期和Ⅲ期临床试验评估[43]。在最近的非随机对照试验,用纳武单抗治疗的患者中最常见的胃肠道不良事件为腹泻,发病率为18%,3~4级腹泻为2%。其他GI不良事件包括恶心,呕吐,腹痛和口干发生率为5%~8%[15]。纳武单抗/伊匹木单抗联合治疗与单一疗法相比,胃肠道不良事件的发生率并不高[57]。在两项临床试验中分别包括173名和135名患者,观察到与lambrizumab相关的腹泻只有1%~20%[56,58]。考虑到这些药物的新颖性,目前在优化使用方面经验不足,但有人提出在严格的指导下,可以使用类似于治疗伊匹木单抗诱导的小肠结肠炎保守治疗方法[43]。

放射性直肠炎和结肠炎

为治疗妇科、泌尿生殖系、胃肠道系统及其他恶性肿瘤而接受腹部及骨盆放射治疗的患者,会有发生急慢性肠道损伤的风险。在直肠和远端结肠,急性放射损伤通常发生在治疗后6周内,其特点为腹泻,直肠紧迫感,里急后重,偶尔直肠出血。这些症状通常在治疗结束后6个月内自行好转,慢性结肠直肠炎通常发生更晚,平均在放疗后1年或更晚时间出现。慢性损伤是由于上皮萎缩和纤维化所致的闭塞性动脉内膜炎和慢性黏膜缺血。其最终的结果是缺血肠管易形成狭窄和出血。患者可能会主诉腹泻、排便困难、出血、里急后重、直肠紧迫感,少数情况下会出现大便失禁。

结肠镜或乙状结肠镜检查可作出诊断。镜下所见包括黏膜水肿、红斑、易碎和毛细血管扩张。严重病例可见黏膜溃疡伴或不伴有出血和狭窄。

表 134-3　伊匹木单抗导致的回结肠炎的处理

严重性	定义	治疗	进一步治疗
轻度		• 继续使用伊匹木单抗	如果症状严重程度进展：见下文
中度	• 4~6 次排便/d • 腹痛 • 黏液脓血便	• 暂停用伊匹木单抗 • 对症治疗 • 内镜评估	如果 7 日后没有解决： • 全身糖皮质激素(0.5mg/(kg·d)或当量) • 一旦症状改善到轻度加糖皮质激素≤7.5mg/d，立即恢复伊匹木单抗 如果进展到严重症状：见下文
严重	• 大于 7 次排便/d • 腹膜炎 • 肠梗阻 • 发热	• 永久停用伊匹木单抗 • 内镜评估 • 全身应用糖皮质激素(1~2mg/(kg·d)或当量)	持续的症状： • 持续评估穿孔或腹膜炎 • 考虑重复内镜检查 • 考虑替代免疫抑制剂治疗(如英夫利西单抗)

放射性直肠炎的治疗取决于症状，在一些研究中，蔗糖素灌肠已被用于治疗放射引起的慢性直肠炎，但可能增加直肠的出血风险，在一些些小样本的临床试验中其他治疗方法包括高压氧和短链脂肪酸灌肠也显示出益处。包括氩等离子体凝固(APC)等各种热内镜治疗也成功治疗放射线直肠炎出血。手术治疗被应用于有顽固性症状如狭窄、疼痛或出血的患者。关于内镜的详细讨论和放射性直肠炎的外科治疗超出了这一章节的范围。放射性直肠炎的治疗应根据症状的类型和严重程度以及当地的经验选择适当的治疗方案。为了预防接受放射治疗的患者发生放射性直肠炎，推荐静脉注射氨磷汀的剂量为>340mg/m^2[1]。

移植物抗宿主疾病的肠道表现

同种异体造血细胞移植(HCT)的使用和适应证在过去几十年中显著增加，每年约 25 000 次手术[59]。HCT 的主要并发症是 GVHD，其中 54%的患者有胃肠道受累[60,61]。移植物抗宿主疾病(GVHD)是供体 T 细胞对基因特定的受体细胞表面蛋白的反应。人类白细胞抗原(HLA)包括一类 HLA(A、B、C)和二类(DR、DQ、DP)蛋白。前者由所有有核细胞表达，而后者主要由造血细胞表达；然而，HLA Ⅱ类蛋白也可以在炎症和损伤的情况下被其他细胞表达。HLA Ⅰ类和Ⅱ类错配与急性 GVHD 的发生频率呈正相关[62,63]，然而，由于个体差异，在普遍表达的小组织相容性抗原(即 HY 和 HA-1)[64~66] HLA 匹配的患者仍然可能发展成 GVHD。有趣的是，脐带来源的 HCT 错配后发生急性 GVHD 的发生率与骨髓来源的 HCT 相似，但外周血干细胞移植后发生慢性 GVHD 的发生率较高，分别为 53%和 41%[67,68]，自体 GVHD 是自体干细胞移植后发生的自身免疫性 GVHD 样综合征，与环孢素和阿伦珠单抗等药物有关[69,70]。

根据发病时间，移植物抗宿主病分为急性(移植后≤100 日)或慢性(移植后>100 日)。后一种形式可以是急性 GVHD 的延伸，成功治疗的急性形式的复发，或者可能是原发的。然而，由于病情方案的改变，这种分类被发现并不准确，导致急性 GVHD 和重叠综合征的晚期发作[59,71]。因此，专家小组建议对 GVHD 进行新的分类(表 134-4)[73]。

表 134-4　急性和慢性移植物抗宿主病(GVHD)的改良分类[72]

分类	造血干细胞移植后出现症状的时间	存在急性 GVHD 特征	存在慢性 GVHD 特征
急性 GVHD：			
经典急性 GVHD	≤100 日	是	否
持续性、复发性或迟发性急性 GVHD	>100 日	是	否
慢性 GVHD：			
经典慢性 GVHD	无时间限制	否	是
重叠综合征	无时间限制	是	是

急性移植物抗宿主疾病

急性 GVHD 的最常见表现是大量、分泌性腹泻。胃肠道出血与预后不良有关，在 GVHD 的背景下，提示黏膜溃疡，但同时必须考虑其他原因[74,75]。GVHD 相关腹泻被描述为一种渗出性、蛋白大量丢失的肠道疾病；然而，粪便 α_1-antitrypsin 诊断 2~3 期 GI-GVHD 的敏感性和特异性的分别只有 79%和 62%[76]。有时，GI-GVHD 也会导致胰腺供血不足，从而可能导致腹泻。其他常见的 GVHD 相关症状包括厌食、恶心、呕吐、腹痛和肠梗阻。考虑到积极的调节方案、多药联用以及 HCT 后严重中性粒细胞减少导致感染的易感性，这些症状的鉴别诊断在 HCT 患者中很宽泛，没有这些症状并不能排除 GVHD 的存在，因此，需要高度怀疑 GVHD。体格检查时，应评估 GVHD 的后遗症及并发症，如皮肤 GVHD、脱水、体重减轻、发育不良等。偶尔，患者会出现腹水。口咽 GVHD 的表现包括牙龈炎、黏膜炎和红斑[72]。肠 GVHD 的影像学特征包括肠壁增厚、肠扩张、黏膜增强和胃壁增厚。弥漫性小肠壁增厚与较差的预后相关，CT 显示任何一部分结肠受累与 GVHD 严重程度相关[77,78]。急性和迟发性 GVHD 的影像学表现无显著差异[79]，GVHD 的内镜表现包括从轻度红斑到黏膜水肿和弥漫性黏膜丢失，特别是黏膜脱落诊断 GVHD 具有高度特异性[80]。虽然内镜已被证明对 GVHD 的诊断具有很高的预测性，但在经组织学证实的 GVHD 患者中，约有 1/5 的患者在内镜评估中没有明显的肉眼表现[81]，因此，急性 GVHD 的诊断通常需要组织诊断。典型的组织学表现包括隐窝上皮细胞凋亡、隐窝破坏（"破裂的隐窝细胞"），以及上皮细胞和固有层的多种淋巴细胞浸润（图 134-6）。重要的是，在移植前治疗继发的暂时性移植后反应期间，即使没有发生 GVHD 的情况下也可以观察到类似的表现。然而，非 GVHD 相关的组织学改变通常在移植后 20 日就会消失[24]，其他需要鉴别诊断排除的类 GVHD 症状和组织学表现包括感染原（如 CMV 和隐孢子虫）和药物副反应（如吗替麦考酚酯和质子泵抑制剂）。组织学上，消化道 GVHD 历来根据严重程度被分类为 1～4 级[71]，内镜评估的争议包括内镜评估的程度，据报道，高达 45%的 GI-GVHD 患者近端小肠活检和直肠活检之间存在不一致。症状不能预测受累部位，虽然一些研究表明直肠活检是足够的，但其他研究报道胃活组织检查在诊断 GI-GVHD 方面提供了更高的收益。远端结肠评估通常是足够的并且与结肠镜检查相比具有较低的并发症发生率[82]。降低治疗方案强度在减少组织损伤方面是有效的，并被证明可以将急性 GVHD 的发病延迟 100 日以上，但也与一些患者的复发率更高有关[83,84]。GVHD 预防的主要方法是药理学上抑制钙调神经磷酸酶（如钙调神经磷酸酶、环孢素、他克莫司或西罗莫司）与其他免疫抑制剂（如 MTX 或吗替麦考酚酯）在移植后早期阶段使用[85,86]；然而，最近的 Cochrane 数据库分析表明，需要高质量的随机对照试验来证实最佳的 GVHD 预防策略[87]。通常，急性 GVHD 的患者需要在移植后的第二个月使用钙调神经素抑制剂来预防。任何形式的内脏 GVHD 都需要高剂量的糖皮质激素治疗，其结果是急性 GVHD 的发生率高达 60%[1,2,31]。糖皮质激素类难治性 GVHD 病例，治疗策略如体外光照射和抗-TNFα 药物（如 etanercept）但还需要进一步的研究[59]。除了免疫抑制治疗外，还需要诸如感染预防、补液和营养补充等支持性治疗。

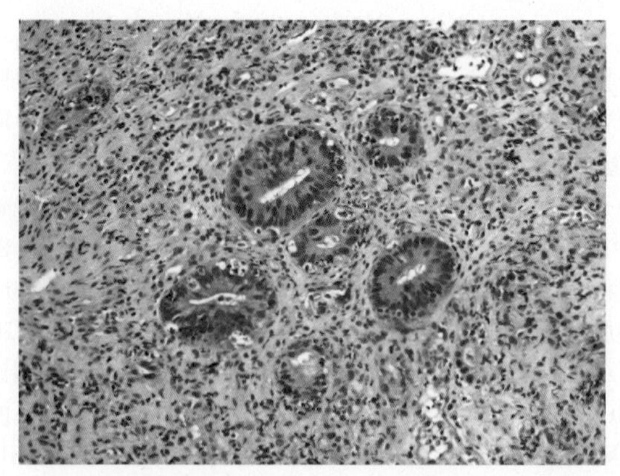

图 134-6　结肠移植物抗宿主病。肠黏膜显示明显的隐窝细胞凋亡和局部隐窝的脱落肉芽组织

慢性移植物抗宿主疾病

慢性 GVHD 在 HCT 长期存活者中的发生率>50%，这是导致 HCT 患者晚期非复发性死亡的主要原因[59]。与疾病进展有关的风险因素包括年龄，急性 GVHD 病史，从移植到慢性 GVHD 的时间，供体类型，移植时疾病状况，GVHD 预防和性别不匹配[88]。遗憾的是，病理机制、诊断标准和最佳治疗目前尚不清楚。最近，美国国家卫生研究院（NIH）制订了若干关于慢性 GVHD 的临床试验标准的专家共识[72]。在本章中，诊断是根据慢性 GVHD 的诊断症状，或独特的症状（定义为急性 GVHD 的不典型症状但不经进一步检查无法诊断为慢性 GVHD）同时经活组织检查、实验室检查或放射学证实。与急性 GVHD 相似，慢性 GVHD 可表现为厌食，恶心、呕吐、腹泻、体重减轻和发育不良，慢性 GVHD 的口咽表现包括地衣扁平样改变，角化过度斑块，口干，黏膜萎缩，黏膜，假膜和溃疡。食管发现包括食管网、狭窄和同心环。其他表现包括黏膜红斑、水肿和糜烂。组织学评价也可显示上皮细胞凋亡和隐窝细胞丢失，但这些变化并不是特异性的，因此也不考虑诊断为慢性 GVHD。支持性护理是慢性 GVHD 治疗的关键因素之一。患者需要监测感染并发症。移植后 3 年口咽发生病变的 HCT 患者应注意评估鳞状细胞癌和其他继发性恶性肿瘤。同样，吞咽困难和吞咽痛的患者需要评估其他病因，如口服避孕药或放疗食管炎和病毒性食管炎等。由狭窄引起的吞咽困难可以经内镜扩张；遗憾的是，穿孔率方面的研究较少。腹泻患者需要评估感染原因，吸收不良，胰腺营养不足。43%的慢性 GVHD 患者营养不良，严重营养不良比例为 14%；因此，应该提供营养评估和营养支持[89,90]。免疫抑制是治疗慢性 GVHD 的关键因素。可局部应用糖皮质激素（如布地奈德（budesonide）和倍氯米松（beclomethasone）GVHD[91,92]。然而，中重度慢性 GVHD 和不能口服的 GVHD 需要全身糖皮质激素通常剂量为 1mg/（kg・d），持续 2 周，然后 6～8 次/周；患者应在 3 个月后彻底复查决定是否进一步减量，还是维持或二线治疗[93]。

癌症治疗的肝脏并发症

化疗相关的肝损伤是治疗许多癌症治疗的不幸后果。因此，在治疗前和治疗期间仔细评估肝功能很重要（表 134-5 和表 134-6）。

肝脏疾病对癌症治疗的影响

先前存在的肝脏疾病不仅会影响治疗方案的选择，而且对于需通过肝脏进行代谢的药物，需要进行剂量调整。肝酶的检测，通常称为"肝功能检测"，不能评估肝脏的功能。肝酶是急性肝损伤的敏感指标，但不能衡量肝脏代谢药物或合成重要蛋白质的能力。白蛋白和胆红素浓度是肝脏合成和进行生物转化潜力的替代标志物，但由于外部因素的影响限制了其敏感性和特异性。因此，对肝功能的可靠评估不应基于检测的几项实验室检测，而应基于临床，实验室和影像学数据的综合评定。此外，经常使用的肝脏实验室检测都不能准确评估肝纤维化。常见的肝脏疾病，例如非酒精性脂肪肝疾病，可以在转氨酶和胆红素正常或极低的情况下隐匿地进展为肝硬化。慢性肝病的唯一证据可能是体检中发现门脉压升高或影像学发现肝结节形成。

对于某些药物，已发布的指南根据现有的肝脏血清学检测说明了其使用限制和剂量。然而，对于许多治疗药物，临床医生必须使用主观数据来设计治疗方案。许多治疗方案需要根

表 134-5　癌症患者肝脏异常的原因

先前存在的肝脏疾病
病毒性肝炎
非酒精性脂肪肝
酒精性肝病
血红蛋白沉着病
自身免疫性肝炎
肝豆状核变性
乳糜泻
α_1-抗胰蛋白酶不足
肿瘤的直接影响
肝转移
门静脉血栓形成
胆道梗阻
肿瘤的间接影响
副瘤综合征
癌症治疗中引起肝病的原因
药物引起的肝脏疾病
移植物抗宿主病(急性和慢性)
肝窦阻塞综合征
病毒性肝炎
败血症诱导的胆汁瘀积
缺血性肝损伤
全胃肠外营养(TPN)
受癌症治疗影响的肝脏疾病
乙型肝炎
非酒精性脂肪肝
自身免疫性肝炎

表 134-6　与癌症治疗相关的肝脏生化检查异常的鉴别诊断

	AST/ALT	碱性磷酸酶	胆红素
药物性肝损伤	正常上限 2~10 倍	正常上限 2~10 倍	正常上限 2~20 倍
病毒性肝炎	正常上限 2~10 倍	正常上限 2~3 倍	正常上限 2~10 倍
肝窦阻塞综合征	正常上限 2~5 倍	正常上限 2~3 倍	正常上限 2~10 倍
移植物抗宿主病	正常上限 2~5 倍	正常上限 2~10 倍	正常上限 2~20 倍

简称：AST：门冬氨酸氨基转移酶；ALT：氨酸转氨酶。

据胆红素浓度进行剂量调整，但仅依靠胆红素浓度可能会产生误导。吉尔伯特综合征(Gilbert syndrome)是一种良性的胆红素代谢紊乱，可以虚假地提高总胆红素浓度，会导致不当地调整治疗方案。

接受癌症治疗的患者中有多达 30%有先前存在肝病的证据，非酒精性脂肪肝最常见。许多药物会加剧肝脏中的脂肪沉积。最常见的是用于治疗乳腺癌和前列腺癌的激素疗法。接受他莫昔芬治疗的女性多达 1/3 会出现肝脏脂肪变性，但通常无症状且与进行性肝病无关[94]。前列腺癌的抗原治疗可加剧代谢综合征的成分，导致肝脏脂肪变性加速[95]。

化疗或放化疗可导致潜在的乙型肝炎的重新激活，这是由于免疫抑制疗法撤退时对乙型肝炎病毒(HBV)的免疫反应增强所致。虽然 HBV 的再活化可以发生在任何化疗方案中，但抗 CD20 单克隆抗体(利妥昔单抗和奥法木单抗)的风险最高[96]。没有可检测的表面抗原(HBsAg)，仅有核心抗体(抗-HBc)阳性伴有不明显的乙型肝炎感染的患者可能会发生再激活。在一份报告中，接受利妥昔单抗治疗的 21 例 HBsAg 阴性/抗 HBc 阳性患者中有 5 例发生了再激活[97]。几个主要学组已经发布了评估和治疗接受癌症治疗的患者 HBV 感染的指南[98~100]。大多数建议在癌症治疗开始时和治疗结束后至少 6 个月进行预防性抗病毒治疗。拉米夫定可用于 HBV DNA 检测不出来且免疫抑制时间短(<12 个月)的患者[101]。由于潜在的病毒耐药性，当检测到 HBV DNA 或预期治疗超过 1 年时，应使用替诺福韦(tenofovir)或恩替卡韦(entecavir)[102]。

与乙型肝炎患者相比，潜在丙型肝炎患者对化疗的反应似乎不同[103]。约有一半 HCV 病毒感染的患者转氨酶和 HCV RNA 水平出现中度升高，但严重肝炎暴发很少见。因此，通常不提示修改剂量。用于治疗不需要干扰素的 HCV 的有效口服抗病毒方案表明，更多正在接受癌症治疗的 HCV 感染患者将成为抗病毒治疗的候选者。

癌症治疗引起的肝毒性

药物不良反应通常发生在接受癌症治疗的患者身上。由于癌症患者经常使用多种药物，并且可能存在许多肝脏异常的潜在原因，包括肿瘤进展，全身感染或肠胃外营养，因此认识到肝毒性是具有挑战性的。

大多数肝毒性反应是特异性的，由代谢紊乱或对药物或其代谢物之一的免疫反应引起[104]。通常这些反应发生在没有潜在肝病的患者中，停药后这些反应消失，而没有明显纤维化或合成功能受损。由于更严重的药物毒性，往往表现为血清胆红素升高，即使在治疗方案可能有限的情况下，也必须停止使用该致敏剂。

通常用于癌症治疗的抗代谢物包括阿糖胞苷(cytosine arabinoside，Ara-C)、氟尿嘧啶、巯嘌呤(6-MP)、硫唑嘌呤、6-硫鸟嘌呤和 MTX。肝脏代谢在这些药物的加工中起着重要作用，肝功能障碍患者通常需要减少剂量。用于治疗急性髓细胞性白血病(AML)的 Ara-C 在极少数情况下与胆汁瘀积有关，一般是可逆的[105]。动脉使用氟尿嘧啶代谢物氟尿苷(氟脱氧尿嘧啶[FudR])与两种类型的毒性有关：第一种是肝细胞损伤，第二种是硬化性胆管炎，肝内胆管狭窄，碱性磷酸酶和胆红素升高[106~108]。

在肝转移瘤切除术之前，氟尿嘧啶和奥沙利铂或伊立替康的组合用于结肠直肠癌患者的新辅助治疗。这些新辅助治疗方案，特别是那些含有奥沙利铂的方案，与肝脏血管系统的脂肪变性和损伤有关，会导致慢性鼻窦阻塞综合征（SOS）相关性疾病[109~112]。

6-MP 通常用于急性淋巴细胞白血病（ALL）的维持治疗。相关的两种毒性已经报道：肝细胞损伤和胆汁瘀积[113]。当日剂量超过 2mg/kg 时，毒性更常见。硫唑嘌呤是 6-MP 的硝基咪唑衍生物。与 6-MP 相比，其毒性较低且剂量依赖性较小。有三种不同的毒性模式：过敏反应，胆汁瘀积反应和内皮细胞损伤伴门静脉压力升高，SOS 和肝脏损伤[114]。

大剂量 MTX 治疗与转氨酶的可逆性有关[115]。接受慢性低剂量 MTX 治疗银屑病或类风湿关节炎的患者有发生肝纤维化和肝硬化的风险。接受累积剂量低于 1.5g MTX 的患者风险较低[116]。

烷化剂引起的肝毒性十分罕见。除环磷酰胺和异环磷酰胺外，接受烷化剂的患者不需要减少剂量。替莫唑胺是一种用于治疗脑肿瘤的烷化剂，会引起严重的肝毒性，因此 FDA 建议在整个治疗过程中监测肝酶[117]。

其他烷化剂（包括美法仑，氯霉素，氮芥和白消安）不依赖肝脏代谢，也通常与肝毒性不相关。

抗肿瘤抗生素包括多柔比星和柔红霉素。多柔比星可引起肝细胞损伤和脂肪变性。胆汁瘀积患者建议减少剂量，以避免更大的毒性[118]。柔红霉素遵循类似的原则。

天冬酰胺酶，用于治疗急性淋巴细胞白血病，会导致一种形式的线粒体损伤的肝脏，特别是那些潜在的脂肪肝疾病。一些天冬酰胺酶肝损伤患者对肉碱有反应[119]。天冬酰胺的分解也能引起高氨血症[120]。

许多分子靶向激酶抑制剂在肝脏中发生代谢紊乱，需要对潜在肝病患者进行剂量调整。拉帕替尼是人类表皮生长因子受体 2 和表皮生长因子受体 EGFR 的双重抑制剂，在接受该药物治疗的患者中，大约有一半的患者有肝毒性，并有几篇潜在的致命反应的报道[121]。某些 HLA 等位基因的存在与肝毒性风险的增加有关[122]。培唑帕尼针对多种酪氨酸激酶，在大约 20%的患者中引起重型肝炎[123]。在吉尔伯特综合征的患者中，它也与一种更为良性的高胆红素血症有关[124]。

检查点抑制剂是针对细胞毒性 T 淋巴细胞相关抗原 4（伊匹木单抗和曲美替尼）和程序性细胞死亡-1 受体（纳武单抗和帕博利珠单抗）的免疫调节抗体。通过增强对肿瘤抗原的免疫反应，这些药物提高了晚期黑色素瘤患者的存活率。在接受两种检查点抑制剂治疗的患者中，只有不到 10%的患者出现转氨酶升高[56,125,126]，这种升高在治疗开始后约 8 周出现。由于肝毒性反应具有自身免疫性肝病的临床和组织学特征，一旦排除了其他潜在的肝损伤来源，应立即开始使用糖皮质激素进行免疫抑制[126]。

肝窦阻塞综合征

SOS，以前称为静脉闭塞性疾病（VOD），通常发生在 HCT 后，但也可能是由于暴露于毒素（Senecio 生物碱）、非移植化疗药物、对肝脏的高剂量放疗或肝移植后[127,128]。临床表现为肝大、黄疸、腹水伴体重增加。SOS 的患病率在已发表的研究中差异很大，但据估计在 20% 左右。SOS 的临床表现类似于巴德-基亚里综合征（Budd-Chiari syndrome），肝静脉阻塞导致窦后门静脉高压。然而，在 SOS 中，是靶向的肝窦内侧细胞，而不是肝静脉[129,130]。内皮细胞受损后，凝血级联激活并形成凝块。纤维蛋白栓，细胞内液体截留和细胞碎片逐渐阻塞血窦，引起肝内窦状隙高压（图 134-7）。

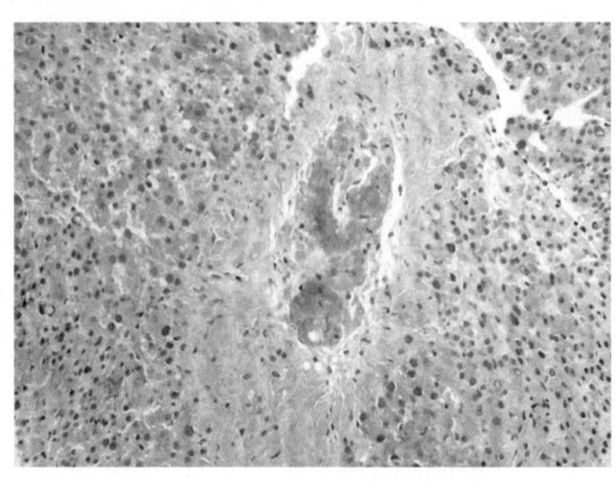

图 134-7 肝窦阻塞综合征（静脉闭塞性疾病）。肝小静脉纤维性闭塞，纤维蛋白沉积。静脉周围肝细胞可见明显的窦性充血

SOS 发展的移植前风险因素包括年龄较大的移植受者年龄，女性，功能差状态，供体-受体 HLA 差异，晚期恶性肿瘤，既往腹部放射，第二次清髓移植，肺扩散能力（DLCO）降低和既往肝脏疾病[131~134]。

移植方案的类型和强度是发生严重 SOS 的最大风险因素。随着全身照射剂量的增加，以及某些药物的使用，如 6 巯基嘌呤（6-mp）、6-硫鸟嘌呤、放射线霉素 D、硫唑嘌呤、白消安（busulfan）、阿糖胞苷（cytosine arabinoside，Ara-C）、环磷酰胺、达卡巴嗪、吉姆单抗/奥佐米星（gemtuzumab ozogamicin，GO）、美法仑、奥沙利铂和尿烷（urethane）等，风险会随之增加[130,131]。

SOS 通常在移植后的第一周内以无法解释的体重增加和肝大为首发症状。大约 25%的患者会出现腹水。转氨酶中度升高，伴有直接高胆红素血症，随后出现峰值胆红素水平低于 20mg/dl[135]。

在排除病毒感染、GVHD、全身感染和肿瘤浸润等其他情况后，可根据典型的体征和症状作出诊断。两种诊断 SOS 的系统，巴尔的摩和西雅图标准已经发表，但这些标准的准确性尚未确定[135,136]。肝活检很少用于 SOS 诊断，典型表现为窦状扩张伴 3 区出血坏死。纤维蛋白沉积伴充血见于窦状和小叶中央静脉。随着时间的推移，胶原蛋白沉积在窦腔和静脉腔内，并阻塞终末肝静脉。如果诊断需要活检，经颈静脉入路是最安全的途径，可以同时测量肝静脉梯度（HVPG）[137]。评估 HVPG 可以区分 GVHD 和 SOS，因为后者的 HPVG 更大。

预防 SOS 应成为所有 HCT 的一个目标。减少潜在的肝毒性药物的使用和降低强度的调节方案可以潜在地限制 SOS 的严重程度。许多移植中心经常使用药物预防。对于同种异体 HCT，在方案之前开始使用熊去氧胆酸，持续 3 个月，与安慰剂相比，将会导致 SOS 发生率降低。一些中心在自体 HCT 中使用低剂量肝素的持续输注。轻度至中度 SOS 可以通过支持疗法治疗,包括用于右上腹疼痛缓解的镇痛药和用于控制血管外液积聚的利尿剂。严重 SOS 患者很少单独使用支持疗法。由于严重 SOS 患者肝静脉中微血栓形成和纤维蛋白沉积的组织学,已经使用了在有或没有抗凝的情况下促进纤维蛋白溶解的治疗。这些治疗策略包括单独使用阿替普酶(重组组织型纤溶酶原激活剂或 tPA)或与肝素和去纤维蛋白多核苷酸联合使用。阿替普酶和肝素治疗后的反应率约为 30%,但与危及生命的出血风险显著相关,特别是多器官衰竭患者[138~140]。去纤维蛋白多核苷酸是一种具有抗血栓形成作用的多脱氧核糖核苷酸-不会引起明显的抗凝。静脉注射去纤维蛋白多核苷酸,剂量范围为每日 5~60mg/kg,至少 14 日,导致 42%~55%的患者出现反应,无明显的治疗相关毒性[141]。使用去纤维蛋白多核苷酸治疗的生存预测因素包括年龄较小,自体干细胞移植和门静脉血流异常,而对于白消安和脑病的方案预测治疗结果更差[142]。经颈静脉肝内门体分流术(TIPS)的插入在少数严重 SOS 患者曾有报道。TIPS 可有效改善门静脉压力梯度;在一些患者中,它与肝和肾症状的临床改善有关。尽管如此,这些影响可能是短暂的,并且可能无法提高整体生存率[143~145]。据报道原位肝移植(OLT)当没有任何药物治疗反应时可作为干细胞移植后 SOS 患者的救治疗法,然而,由于存在恶性肿瘤和/或多器官衰竭,大多数严重 SOS 患者不适合 OLT[146,147]。

肝脏移植物抗宿主病

肝脏是急性 GVHD 中第二大最常见的累及器官,约有 50% 的患者受此影响。没有其他器官参与的严重肝 GVHD 是罕见的。最早的生化发现是结合胆红素和碱性磷酸酶浓度的升高,反映了潜伏的病理损伤。典型的是广泛的胆管损伤,胆管上皮变性和异型性,细胞脱落,小胆管混合细胞浸润导致胆汁淤积[148]。虽然临床和实验室数据可能高度提示肝 GVHD,但可能需要肝活检才能作出明确诊断,并排除 SOS、感染或药物毒性等混淆诊断。在某些情况下,由于造血细胞移植后不久血小板减少导致出血的风险,经皮肝活检可能不可行。在这些情况下,如果肝活检被认为是必要的诊断,经颈静脉途径可能是首选。对于急性 GVHD,首选也是最有效的治疗选择是单独使用糖皮质激素或与他克莫司联合使用。如果这种组合在控制肝 GVHD 方面不成功,二线治疗包括兔抗人胸腺细胞免疫球蛋白和吗替麦考酚酯[149~150]。慢性肝移植物抗宿主病可在既往无急性移植物抗宿主病病史,曾有急性移植物抗宿主病或新发移植物抗宿主病后发生。大约 50%的慢性 GVHD 患者的肝脏受累,最常见的是胆红素和碱性磷酸酶浓度无症状升高[151]。慢性肝 GVHD 的组织学表现类似于另一种免疫介导的肝病——原发性胆汁性肝硬化,伴有慢性炎症细胞对小叶和间隔胆管的损伤[148,152]。慢性肝移植物抗宿主病的初期治疗与急性肝移植物抗宿主病相同,均采用糖皮质激素和他克莫司。难治性慢性肝 GVHD 患者可能对沙利度胺有反应[153]。

其他胃肠道并发症

便秘

便秘是癌症患者治疗中的一个常见问题。在这种情况下,便秘通常是由于经口进食不足,体力活动减少,以及昂丹司琼和阿片类镇痛药等止吐剂导致的。便秘是阿片类药物引起的最常见的不良反应之一[154],阿片类药物的效果是减缓肠道蠕动时间。服用长春新碱类药物的患者也有便秘的报道,特别是长春新碱和沙利度胺。梗阻、肠梗阻、结肠假性梗阻在开始药物治疗便秘前必须解除。在癌症患者中便秘是可以预测的,应采取措施避免这种并发症。电解质异常和其他可逆原因应该被纠正。如果可能的话,引起便秘的药物应该停止使用。在便秘的初期治疗可使用泻药,包括或不包括大便软化剂。双氯联苯和塞纳等刺激性泻药会改变肠道黏膜电解质转运和增加肠道运动活性。如果这些药物无效,高渗药物,如乳果糖或山梨醇可以有效改善大便频率和持续性。聚乙烯乙二醇溶液以粉末的形式存在,并且已经被证实可有效改善慢性便秘。使用药物改善结肠运输的效果一直令人失望。甲氧氯普胺似乎是无效的,而替加色罗(tegaserod)(5-羟色胺受体激动剂)对心血管有明显的副反应,在美国不常规使用,只有在 FDA 的新药(IND)紧急调查流程之后才能使用。鲁比前列酮(lubiprostone),一种氯通道激活剂,是 FDA 批准的治疗慢性特发性便秘的一种双环酸,作用于小肠的顶端,有助于增加细胞内液体和肠道蠕动。对于化疗引起的、症状随阿片类药物的使用时间增加而加重便秘患者,它可能是有效的。它是 FDA 批准用于治疗非癌性疼痛相关阿片类药物引起的便秘。甲基纳曲酮是一种微阿片受体拮抗剂,用于治疗晚期疾病的阿片类药物引起的便秘,已获准在美国使用。该药物是纳曲酮的衍生物,可选择性地拮抗胃肠道内的外周微感受器,对中枢神经系统无影响。在临床试验中,阿片类药物引起便秘后在初次皮下给药甲基纳曲酮后,50%~60%的患者可逆转[155]。在大多数情况下,有效的缓解发生在给药 1h 内,不影响阿片类镇痛药效果或也不会诱发阿片类药物戒断症状。神经胃肠病学方面的最新进展正引领着新的药物研发,这可能有助于治疗严重便秘[156]。外周的活性 μ 阿片受体拮抗剂(帕莫拉)可保留这些药物的中枢镇痛作用,同时对抗胃肠道的周围效应。纳洛昔醇(naloxegol)和 TD-1211 是这个类药物的原型药物。纳洛昔醇是一种口服聚乙二醇化纳洛酮偶联物。纳洛西格最近获批用于治疗无癌症疼痛成人阿片诱导的腹泻[157]。

恶心和呕吐

恶心和呕吐经常发生在使用化疗药物之后。化疗后出现恶心和呕吐的可能性取决于多种因素包括化疗剂量和药物本身的致呕作用[158]。静脉注射抗肿瘤药的致呕作用可以分为五个级别,风险范围从最小或小于 10%(如贝伐单抗)到高或大于 90%的风险(如顺铂)。呕吐可能是急性的(即发生在接受化疗的 24h 内)或延迟的。

现在可以使用各种止吐药来预防和治疗化疗引起的恶心和呕吐。这些药物包括具有高治疗指数的药物如 5-羟色胺 3($5\text{-}HT_3$)受体拮抗剂(如昂丹司琼、格拉司琼、多拉司琼、托烷司琼(tropisetron)和帕洛诺司琼),神经激肽 1 受体拮抗剂(如阿瑞匹坦),以及糖皮质激素(通常与其他药物联用)。也使用治疗指数低的药物,例如盐酸甲氧氯普胺、丁苯酮、吩噻嗪、大麻素和奥氮平。首选药物和治疗方案取决于既定化疗药物的致呕级别。对于呕吐风险低的化疗药物,仅在化疗之前给予止吐药，而对于那些化疗药物呕吐风险(级别 3 或更高)之前和之后都给予止吐药。

胃肠道穿孔，瘘管形成，动脉血栓形成和出血

胃肠穿孔，瘘管形成，动脉血栓形成和出血已经报道了可见于使用贝伐单抗的患者，贝伐单抗是一种抗血管生成因子的单克隆抗体。据报道使用贝伐单抗治疗转移性结直肠癌患者肠道穿孔的发生率为 1%～2%[159,160]。与穿孔相关的危险因素包括完整的原发肿瘤，预照射，急性憩室炎，腹腔内脓肿和胃肠道梗阻。

急性胰腺炎

患有急性胰腺炎的癌症或接受过造血干细胞移植的患者能够被包括结石和酒精摄入等一般人群原因引起。但是，在治疗癌症患者的胰腺炎时应考虑其他病因，包括药物和化疗药。药物性胰腺炎没有明显的临床特征，因此，请仔细询问药物史并排除其他病因对诊断至关重要。一些已知引起急性胰腺炎的最常见药物包括甲硝唑、磺胺类、四环素、呋塞米、噻嗪类、雌激素和他莫昔芬。在化疗过程中，据报道、使用硫唑嘌呤、泼尼松阿糖胞苷和各种组合方案化疗包括长春新碱、MTX、丝裂霉素、氟尿嘧啶、环磷酰胺、顺铂和博来霉素可导致胰腺炎。相关疾病和多药方案常常使确定病因与效果的关系变得困难[161]。

口腔黏膜炎或口咽溃疡

口腔黏膜炎或黏膜内膜的溃疡性溃疡口咽经常发生在接受放射治疗和化疗治疗实体恶性肿瘤的个体中。它发生在 20%～40%接受常规化疗的患者中，80%接受大剂量化疗的患者中，及高达 98%的接受造血干细胞移植治疗的人。基于循证医学的预防建议口腔黏膜炎的治疗和治疗最近已经发表 134-[1]。帕利夫明，一种重组人角质形成细胞生长因子-1，降低正在接受化疗的血液系统恶性肿瘤和需要干细胞移植治疗的患者的口腔黏膜炎的发生率和持续时间，已经获得 FDA 批准。新指南建议该药物可用于预防血液系统恶性肿瘤患者接受大剂量化疗和全身照射自体干细胞移植后导致的口腔黏膜炎[1]。还建议使用口服冷冻疗法来预防接受氟尿嘧啶化疗的口服黏膜炎患者。建议使用低强度激光疗法以预防口腔人干细胞移植联用大剂量化疗患者的黏膜炎。苯达明漱口水(但不能使用其他抗菌漱口水或锭剂)用于预防头颈部接受中等剂量放疗但不伴化疗的患者的口腔黏膜炎。锌补充剂可能有益于预防接受放射或化学疗法治疗的口腔癌患者的黏膜炎。对于接受化疗或放疗的头颈癌患者，不建议使用苏铁漱口水来预防或治疗黏膜炎，因为苏铁漱口水的效果不佳。

(刘昊 译 田艳涛 校)

参考文献

The complete reference list can be found on the Wiley Companion Digital Edition of this title (see inside front cover for login instructions).

1 Lalla RV, Bowen J, Barasch A, et al. MASCC/ISOO clinical practice guidelines for the management of mucositis secondary to cancer therapy. *Cancer*. 2014;**120**:1453–1461.

3 Konig CC, Wouterse SJ, Daams JG, et al. Toxicity of concurrent radiochemotherapy for locally advanced non-small-cell lung cancer: A systematic review of the literature. *Clin Lung Cancer*. 2013;**14**:481–487.

8 Masur H, Brooks JT, Benson CA, et al. Prevention and treatment of opportunistic infections in HIV-infected adults and adolescents: updated guidelines from the Centers for Disease Control and Prevention, national Institutes of Health, and HIV Medicine Association of the Infectious Diseases Society of America. *Clin Infectious Dis*. 2014;**58**:1308–1311. (see also http://aidsinfo.nih.gov/guidelines/html/4/adult-and-adolescent-oi-prevention-and-treatment-guidelines/0).

15 Villanueva A, Gotuzzo E, Arathoon EG, et al. A randomized double-blind study of caspofungin versus fluconazole for the treatment of esophageal candidiasis. *Am J Med*. 2002;**113**(**4**):294–299.

24 Didden P, Spaander MCW, Kuipers EJ. Esophageal stents in malignant and benign disorders. *Curr Gastroenterol Rep*. 2013;**4**:319–328.

28 Dai Y, Lee C, Xie Y, et al. Interventions for dysphagia in oesophageal cancer (review). *Cochrane Database Syst Rev*. 2014;(**10**.Art. No. CD005048.). doi: 10.1002/14651858.CD005048.pub4.

35 Surawicz CM, Brandt LJ, Binion DG, et al. Guidelines for diagnosis, treatment and prevention of *Clostridium difficile* infections. *Am J Gastroenterol*. 2013;**108**:478–498.

36 Lowy I, Molrine DC, Leav BA, et al. Treatment with monoclonal antibodies against Clostridium difficile toxins. *N Engl J Med*. 2010;**362**(**3**):197–205.

37 Nesher L, Rolston KV. Neutropenic enterocolitis, a growing concern in the era of widespread use of aggressive chemotherapy. *Clin Infect Dis*. 2013;**56**:711–717.

38 Ebert EC, Hagspiel KD. Gastrointestinal manifestations of leukemia. *J Gastroenterol Hepatol*. 2012;**27**:458–463.

43 Gangadhar TC, Vonderheide RH. Mitigating the toxic effects of anticancer immunotherapy. *Nat Rev Clin Oncol*. 2014;**11**:91–99.

50 Kim KW, Ramaiya NH, Krajewski KM, et al. Ipilimumab-associated colitis: CT findings. *AJR Am J Roentgenol*. 2013;**200**:W468–W474.

51 Squibb B-M. *YERVOY™ (ipilimumab): Immune-mediated Adverse Reaction Management Guide* [online], 2011; www.hcp.yervoy.com/pdf/rems-management-guide.pdf (accessed 12 August 2015).

56 Hamid O, Robert C, Daud A, et al. Safety and tumor responses with lambrolizumab (anti-PD-1) in melanoma. *N Engl J Med*. 2013;**369**:134–144.

58 Robert C, Ribas A, Wolchok JD, et al. Anti-programmed-death-receptor-1 treatment with pembrolizumab in ipilimumab-refractory advanced melanoma: a randomised dose-comparison cohort of a phase 1 trial. *Lancet*. 2014;**384**:1109–1117.

59 Ferrara JL, Levine JE, Reddy P, Holler E. Graft-versus-host disease. *Lancet*. 2009;**373**:1550–1561.

62 Fernandez-Vina MA, Klein JP, Haagenson M, et al. Multiple mismatches at the low expression HLA loci DP, DQ, and DRB3/4/5 associate with adverse outcomes in hematopoietic stem cell transplantation. *Blood*. 2013;**121**:4603–4610.

67 Anasetti C, Logan BR, Lee SJ, et al. Peripheral-blood stem cells versus bone marrow from unrelated donors. *N Engl J Med*. 2012;**367**:1487–1496.

71 Washington K, Jagasia M. Pathology of graft-versus-host disease in the gastrointestinal tract. *Hum Pathol*. 2009;**40**:909–917.

72 Filipovich AH, Weisdorf D, Pavletic S, et al. National Institutes of Health consensus development project on criteria for clinical trials in chronic graft-versus-host disease: I. Diagnosis and staging working group report. *Biol Blood Marrow Transplant*. 2005;**11**:945–956.

76 Rodriguez-Otero P, Porcher R, Peffault de Latour R, et al. Fecal calprotectin and alpha-1 antitrypsin predict severity and response to corticosteroids in gastrointestinal graft-versus-host disease. *Blood*. 2012;**119**:5909–5917.

85 Cutler C, Logan B, Nakamura R, et al. Tacrolimus/sirolimus vs tacrolimus/methotrexate as GVHD prophylaxis after matched, related donor allogeneic HCT. *Blood*. 2014;**124**:1372–1377.

87 Kharfan-Dabaja M, Mhaskar R, Reljic T, et al. Mycophenolate mofetil versus methotrexate for prevention of graft-versus-host disease in people receiving allogeneic hematopoietic stem cell transplantation. *Cochrane Database Syst Rev*. 2014;7:CD010280.

88 Arora M, Klein JP, Weisdorf DJ, et al. Chronic GVHD risk score: a Center for International Blood and Marrow Transplant Research analysis. *Blood*. 2011;**117**:6714–6720.

93 Wolff D, Gerbitz A, Ayuk F, et al. Consensus conference on clinical practice in chronic graft-versus-host disease (GVHD): first-line and topical treatment of chronic GVHD. *Biol Blood Marrow Transplant*. 2010;**16**:1611–1628.

96 Mitka M. Increased HBV reactivation risk with of atumumab or rituximab. *JAMA*. 2013;**310**:1664.

99 Artz AS, Somerfield MR, Feld JJ, et al. American Society of Clinical Oncology provisional clinical opinion: chronic hepatitis B virus infection screening in patients receiving cytotoxic chemotherapy for treatment of malignant diseases. *J Clin Oncol*. 2010;**28**:3199.

101 Loomba R, Rowley A, Wesley R, et al. A systematic review: the effect of preventive lamivudine on hepatitis B reactivation during chemotherapy. *Ann Intern Med*. 2008;**148**:519.

103 Torres HA, Davila M. Reactivation of hepatitis B virus and hepatitis C virus in patients with cancer. *Nat Rev Clin Oncol*. 2012;**9**:156.

121 Azim HA, Agbor-Tarh D, Bradbury I, et al. Pattern of rash, diarrhea, and hepatic toxicities secondary to lapatinib and their association with age and response to

neoadjuvant therapy: analysis from NEoALTTO trial. *J Clin Oncol*. 2013;**31**:4504.

123 Shibata SI, Chung V, Synold TW, et al. Phase 1 study of pazopanib in patients with advanced solid tumors and hepatic dysfunction: a National Cancer Institute Organ Dysfunction Working Group study. *Clin Cancer Res*. 2013;**19**:3631.

149 Martin PJ, Rizzo JH, Wingard JR, et al. First- and second-line systemic treatment of acute graft-versus-host disease: recommendations of the American Society of Blood and Marrow Transplantation. *Biol Blood Marrow Transplant*. 2012;**18**:1150.

150 Wolff D, Ayuk F, Elmaagacli A, et al. Current practice in diagnosis and treatment of acute graft-versus-host disease: results from a survey among German-Austrian-Swiss hematopoietic stem cell transplant centers. *Biol Blood Marrow Transplant*. 2013;**19**:767.

154 Siemens W, Gaertner J, Becker G. Advances in pharmacotherapy for opioid-induced constipation-a systematic review. *Expert Opin Pharmacother*. 2014;**16**:515–532. Dec 24, epub ahead of print.

156 Camilleri M. Novel therapeutic agents in neurogastroenterology: advances in the past year. *Neurogastrowenterol Motil*. 2014;**26**:1070–1078.

157 Corsetti M, Tack J. Naloxegol, a new drug for the treatment of opioid-induced constipation. *Expert Opin Pharmacother*. 2015;**16**:399–406.

158 Hesketh PJ. Chemotherpay-induced nausea and vomiting. *N Engl J Med*. 2008;**358**:2482–2494.

160 Scott LJ, Chakravarthy U, reeves BC, Rogers CA. Systemic affect of anti-VEGF drugs: a commentary. *Expert Opin Drug Saf*. 2014;**14**:379–388. Dec 9; epub ahead of print.

161 Morgan C, Tillet T, Braybrooke J, et al. Management of uncommon chemotherapy-induced emergencies. *Lancet Oncol*. 2011;**12**:806–814.

第 135 章　肿瘤的口腔并发症及治疗

Stephen T. Sonis, DMD, DMSc ■ Anna Yuan, DMD

概述

口腔是癌症治疗中直接和间接不良副作用的常见部位。在骨髓抑制的患者中，口腔中多样的微生物群使得其既是局部感染的部位又是菌血症和败血症的潜在来源。虽然接受化疗或放射治疗的所有患者中约有一半会出现某种形式的口腔毒性或感染，但几乎每位接受过积极的清髓治疗方案或局部头颈放疗的患者都会出现急性和慢性口腔毒性。在口腔内或周围的组织多样性——角化和非角化黏膜、骨、唾液腺和牙齿——加剧了方案相关的口腔并发症的易感性范围，敏锐度和临床意义。在几乎所有情况下，在癌症治疗前消除或控制现有口腔疾病或癌症治疗期间积极管理口腔健康对预后是有利的。

口腔是癌症治疗的急性和慢性不良副作用的常见部位。这些并发症的性质，发病率，严重程度和病程各不相同，但都会对患者的生活质量，耐受治疗的能力，治疗的总体成本，局部和全身感染的风险以及康复产生不利影响。癌症治疗中的口腔并发症在一些人群中被认为是常见的，例如头颈癌（HNC）患者，但在其他人群中相对罕见。这种观念的形成在很大程度上是由患者报告不足导致的，他们会担心在治疗期间由于提及口腔毒性症状导致治疗剂量降低，从而使最佳的抗癌治疗有所妥协。虽然这种现象并非口腔并发症所独有，但仍有大量的口腔毒性相关数据被低估。另外，随着多种的治疗药物如西妥昔单抗、双膦酸盐和 mTOR 抑制剂的涌现，与其相关的口腔副作用也被逐步报道。目前越来越清楚的是口腔并发症很少孤立地发生。可能由于其共同的生物学基础，他们常常可预见其与其他药物相关的毒性伴随发生[1]。

总体而言，大约 40%的非头颈癌患者在接受治疗中会出现某种形式的口腔相关问题，包括口腔干燥症和黏膜炎[2]。对于接受治疗的 HNC 患者，发生移植物抗宿主病（GVHD）以及接受积极清髓治疗的患者，发生率可上升至 75%以上。口腔并发症的症状性和功能性后果包括：止痛药和抗生素的使用增加，住院时间延长，因疼痛和体液管理而入院、护理资源的利用、诊断性治疗与肠外营养。对费用和成本的影响是巨大的。在一项针对 HNC 和非小细胞肺癌患者的研究中，单独因口腔黏膜炎而增加的成本达 17 244 美元[3]。在过去，口腔并发症很大程度上被认为是不可避免的，常常不是在早期被发现，而且其治疗往往是采用回顾性而非前瞻性或预防性的方式进行治疗。在过去十年，由于对口腔并发症的生物学和流行病学的了解取得了显著进展，已经开发出针对发病机制的干预措施，同时对高危人群也有了更多的了解。

治疗前评估

通过在抗癌治疗前消除存在的牙齿疾病，可以成功地减少多种影响口腔的副作用风险[4~6]。强烈建议在抗癌治疗前到口腔科就诊，因为它可以实现一系列的目标。首先，它提供了一个在患者耐受性最好并且出现治疗后不良后遗症风险最低时，发现和消除活动性及慢性的牙齿或牙周感染来源，如感染或坏死的机会。其次，可以发现原发性癌症的口腔表现。再次，它为患者提供了关于癌症及其治疗对短期和长期口腔健康影响的教育和讨论的机会。最后，对于即将对口腔周围的肿瘤进行外科手术的患者，预处理评估对于优化假体的制造是至关重要的。在放射治疗开始之前制作防护用具可能会降低治疗导致的散射性损伤的影响。

不出意外，在筛查癌症患者时报告的牙科疾病或错误假体或恢复的频率反映了一般人群中这些病症的发生率。虽然在干细胞移植（HSCT）之前评估的 2/3 患者中报告了口腔健康低于理想情况，但只有约 1/3 的筛查患者病理严重到需要干预[7]。类似的，对于在放射治疗前进行筛查的头颈部癌症患者，半数到 2/3 的患者需要拔牙，这主要与牙周病相关[8,9]。虽然在化疗前清除可能的口腔和牙齿感染对局部感染和败血症的发病率具有显著的有利的影响[4]，确切的数据证明需要预照射根除口腔感染的病灶，从而有效地改善预后[10]。在癌症治疗开始前进行有效的牙科筛查与合适的治疗，可以通过减少粒细胞减少期间的感染发生率来显著地节省成本[11]。

牙科评估和治疗的时机

如果在邻近癌症治疗前才开始口腔筛检会使得这个处理失去价值。牙科治疗结束尤其是拔牙后，与放射治疗开始之间的理想间隔一直存在很多争论。然而，考虑到口腔伤口的愈合率，尤其是拔牙的部位，似乎至少 2 周才可以接受，3 周更为理想[12]。而对于即将接受化疗的患者，要求在完成牙科治疗和患者预期的最低粒细胞值之间（<500 细胞/ml）有足量的时间。在通常情况下，如果患者有明显的血小板减少（<10^5 血小板/ml），非紧急的牙科治疗不应该在普通门诊设施中执行[13]。

由于一些恶性血液病起病较急，需要立即化疗，在这种高危人群进行治疗前，口腔筛检和牙齿预治疗可能不太现实。在这种情况下，应在尽可能接近治疗开始的时间进行口腔评估，主要有两个原因：第一，该检查提供了口腔健康情况的重要基线；第二，在这种高度骨髓清除性的群体中，发现和消除活动性口腔感染对于其整个疾病的进程都非常重要。消除已查明的牙源性感染源不应再拖延，因为有重要的数据支持这一结论：在处理得很好的前提下，对这种人群进行拔牙手术也可以很安全，当然最好是在医院中进行处理[10]。有恶性血液病的患者拔牙并发症的发生率据报道为 13%，对住院时间或死亡率没有影响。最常见的并发症包括疼痛和出血。重要的是要注意,没有证据表明积极地拔除无症状的牙齿对预防全身性感染有任何好处。

预处理的评估包括:基线数据,如内科和牙科的病史;实验室数据,如关于1型单纯疱疹病毒抗体水平以及一份包括有除口腔检查外的头颈部检查、口腔内软组织检查、牙周疾病筛查和牙科评价的临床评估。放射学评估应包括那些对确诊牙周疾病、龋齿、根尖周病理、阻生牙必要的X线片。同样重要的是评估患者对牙齿护理的了解和动机。已经被证明存在有未经处理的根尖周病理、进展性龋齿或牙周疾病的牙齿都应被拔除。

有可活动义齿的患者应鼓励他们在癌症治疗时尽量减少使用或不使用,因为哪怕是细微的黏膜创伤可加速黏膜炎的风险和发病。同样,化疗开始前去除矫正牙齿环是预防对萎缩性黏膜造成损伤的重要一环[14]。

放射治疗的口腔并发症

放射治疗的口腔并发症主要由急性和慢性局部组织损伤所致。此外,辐射引起的口腔干燥症可能导致在牙齿和牙周产生继发效应。辐射的剂量率、总剂量、同步化疗的使用以及照射野的大小和结构是口腔毒性的主要决定因素。因此,患口腔、口咽部、舌、鼻咽和唾液腺肿瘤治疗的患者的风险最高。患下咽或喉部肿瘤的患者也常常受到影响,尽管发生率略低。近距离放射治疗比外照射更容易出现口腔毒性。虽然调强放疗(IMRT)(参见第83章)可能保护了部分组织,但其对口腔黏膜的影响仍然非常明显。受辐射直接影响的口腔组织包括黏膜(上皮细胞和固有层组织)、唾液腺、骨骼和肌肉。在儿童中,包括了颌骨的放射治疗将会对颅面和牙科发育产生不良影响[15]。

黏膜炎

作为治疗的毒副反应之一,放疗和化疗都可以对口腔黏膜产生明显的毒性。当描述抗肿瘤治疗引起的黏膜损伤时,黏膜炎这个术语(ICD9代码528.1)比口腔炎更加常用,因为后者是一个通用术语,它可与一系列与化放疗无关的感染或创伤有关。放射诱发口腔黏膜炎的严重程度和动力学与靶向口腔黏膜的剂量率和总剂量有关。局部黏膜的刺激、继发感染、口干这些因素可使辐射对组织的破坏性被放大。

过去5年关于黏膜炎的讨论可概括为三个主题:第一,对黏膜炎的病理描述更加全面;第二,黏膜损伤发生机制具有共性,适用于消化道的所有部分;第三,黏膜炎很少作为一个孤立的毒副作用发生[16]。除此以外,基因组对包括黏膜炎在内的毒性风险的影响,也正被描述的更为全面。

历史上,黏膜炎被视为放疗或化疗直接介导的对位于口腔黏膜基底层的干细胞损伤的结果。有观点认为这些迅速分裂的细胞被不加选择地破坏造成萎缩和之后的溃疡。同时,结缔组织损伤被认为会导致血管通透性增加和组织水肿。然而,基础研究显示黏膜炎发生的过程在生物学上要复杂得多。虽然上皮干细胞是黏膜损伤的最终介导,但是现在已很清楚,它们的死亡既有直接的也有间接机制[17,18]。事实上,这些直接克隆源的细胞死亡是不足以产生临床上所观察到的那些典型程度的损伤。相反,固有层细胞产生的活性物质会在内皮细胞、结缔组织、细胞外基质触发一系列级联事件和炎症浸润。这一系列事件几乎在黏膜最初暴露于射线后即已开始,使一系列的调节和信号分子渗透到上皮细胞并导致损伤、细胞凋亡和坏死。

放射导致的口腔黏膜炎通常在治疗开始后的2周之内出现,累积剂量在10~20Gy。虽然临床改变在这些剂量下才观察到,但是产生这些变化的细胞和组织事件几乎在(见下文)照射开始后立即触发。黏膜红斑、轻度上皮脱落、角化岛的形成是黏膜炎早期的特征性改变。这些改变伴随着一些相对轻的症状。这症状特点是烧灼样疼痛,类似于热奶酪引起的食物烫伤。患者往往难以忍受辛辣食物。除了舌头背面、硬腭和牙龈,任何口腔黏膜表面都是易感部位。最常受影响的地方是颊黏膜(脸颊),舌的腹侧面及双侧面,口底(图135-1)。软腭和口咽也常常受累,这是导致吞咽疼痛的原因。因此,患者可能在他们的治疗早期会主诉喉咙痛。

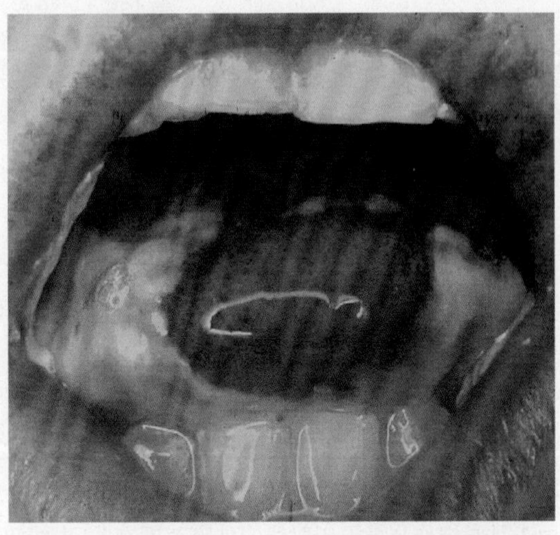

图 135-1　位于舌的腹侧面、双侧及颊黏膜的严重的口腔黏膜炎伴溃疡和伪膜形成,由造血干细胞移植前清髓性化疗所致

在累积剂量约30Gy时,黏膜的完整性被破坏,出现溃疡。在开始时溃疡通常是孤立性的,但随后融合成大的、无间隔的黏膜断裂,往往覆盖含大量死细胞和细菌的伪膜。在严重的情况下,病变可出血(图135-2)。患溃疡性黏膜炎极其痛苦,溃疡

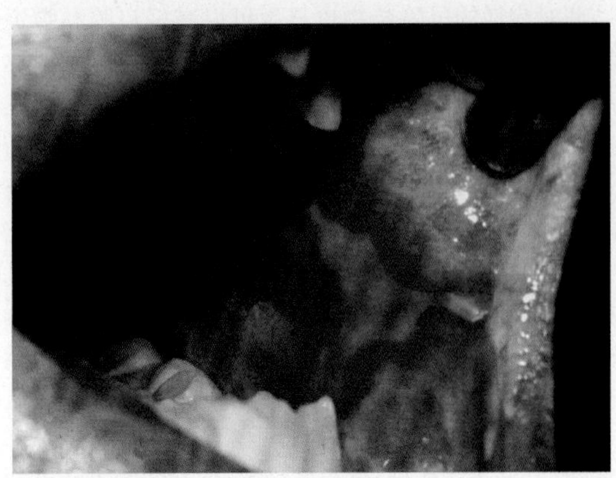

图 135-2　位于左颊黏膜的严重口腔黏膜炎伴有溃疡,红斑和伪膜形成,由治疗口腔癌的放射治疗所致

不仅覆盖了大面积黏膜表面区域，而且也很深。在接受放射线治疗并发生黏膜炎患者的描述中，该并发症往往是他们治疗中最重要的并发症[19]。许多情况下，黏膜炎导致了放射治疗的中断，以及因液体支持或处理疼痛、肠外营养而需要的住院治疗[20]。在这一群体中，因口腔黏膜炎而增加的经济成本非常显著[3]。重要的是，对于即将开始治疗的患者，使他们对可能会面对的黏膜炎的严重性有所了解是很重要的。而在治疗前通常用来描述黏膜炎的“口疮”一词似乎弱化了它们对患者的重要性，一个更实际的描述和处理计划可能会更有帮助。对大多数患者，溃疡性黏膜炎是自限性的，在放射治疗结束后4～6周自发缓解。

黏膜炎的评估

因为缺少一个普遍接受的评分系统，对治疗方案口腔毒性的比较和黏膜炎干预措施的疗效评估存在障碍。目前，最常用于描述口腔黏膜毒性的分级系统是世界卫生组织（WHO）和美国癌症研究所不良事件通用术语标准（NCI-CTCAE）量表。WHO量表结合了红斑和溃疡的客观发现与患者进食固体、液体食物或经口进食的能力（表135-1）。在其最新的版本中（第4版），CTCAE量表消除了对黏膜健康的客观评估，并完全依赖于症状和功能（口服摄入）终点。虽然这种方法最大限度地减少了临床医生评估黏膜炎的工作，但由于依赖患者对功能和症状的反馈，会由于镇痛剂使用、个体疼痛感知和非黏膜炎相关因素（如牙龈炎，恶心等）而变得复杂。

预防和治疗

目前在美国还没有已经被批准的针对放射引起黏膜炎的有效预防或治疗手段。现有的共识认为，改善口腔状况可能会降低黏膜炎的发生风险或严重程度。治疗期间维持高水平的口腔卫生被认为是有帮助的。

表135-1 治疗相关颌骨坏死的分期和处理[21]

分期	临床表现	处理
有风险	无暴露骨	患者教育
0	无坏死骨的临床证据，但有非特异临床发现、影像学改变、症状	系统处理，包括使用止痛药、抗生素
1	无症状的暴露和坏死骨，或骨骼瘘管没有感染迹象	患者教育；抗菌漱口水；密切随访
2	暴露和坏死骨，或骨骼瘘管有感染迹象（如暴露区域骨骼的疼痛、红斑，伴或不伴脓液引流）	患者教育；抗菌漱口水；抗生素；止痛；骨表面清创去除松散的碎片并使粗糙的表面变光滑；密切随访
3	暴露骨有疼痛，通常有相关软组织发炎或感染；可见溶骨延伸至下颌骨下边界或病理性骨折；有时可见口外瘘	患者教育；抗菌漱口水；抗生素；姑息性手术，密切随访

摘自Ruggiero等，2014年[21]。已获得Elsevier的重印许可。

由于黏膜损伤与暴露于射线的黏膜范围有关，中线辐射挡板的使用[22]和三维立体放射治疗[23]可能会减少口腔毒性的范围。

盐酸苄达明是一种非甾体类漱口剂，具有消炎镇痛、麻醉的特性，已经在加拿大，澳大利亚和欧洲被批准用于预防和治疗放射导致的黏膜炎。多项研究的结果显示其对该适应证有效[24,25]。MASCC委员会建议在接受中等剂量的放疗治疗的患者中使用盐酸苄达明[26]。尚无数据支持该药物在接受同步化疗的患者中使用。

一些对症性的屏障药物也显示可以减轻口腔黏膜炎相关的症状。Gelclair是被美国FDA作为一种装置批准，据称它可以在受伤的黏膜上形成一个屏障[27]。硫糖铝，被广泛应用于胃溃疡治疗的药物，可以在溃疡黏膜部位形成一种蛋白药物复合体。已经有一些将它作为漱口剂用于治疗口腔黏膜炎的报道，虽然其疗效似乎并不一致[28,29]。在MASCC指南中它被特别提及不推荐使用。MuGard是一种水凝胶，在一项多机构随机安慰剂对照试验中表现出显著的缓解作用[30]。

还有各种外用制剂用于处理黏膜炎引起的疼痛，包括黏性利多卡因，苯佐卡因口内胶，苯海拉明果胶悬浮制剂或氧化镁乳剂。Caphosol是最初被开发用于口干症患者的牙齿再矿化冲洗剂，是一种含磷酸钠、氯化钙、氯化钠和蒸馏水的电解质溶液，据称可以润滑黏膜，从而减轻黏膜炎。该溶液被作为方案批准，但其临床试验的结果并不一致[31-33]。口服芦荟作为一种舒缓剂被应用已经有一段时间。然而，它在一项双盲、随机、安慰对照的Ⅱ期临床研究中未能证明疗效[34]。表面舒缓漱口水通常只对轻度黏膜炎有效。根据WHO疼痛阶梯系统性地处理疼痛往往是必要的。此外，冷的食物，如冰激淋或冰棒，可舒缓症状。应指导患者取出假牙。

微生物对放射导致的黏膜炎严重程度和病程的作用目前还不清楚[35]。采用黏膜消毒作为黏膜炎的干预措施产生了矛盾的结果。葡萄糖酸氯己定漱口水似乎在黏膜炎的预防或治疗没有作用，事实上还可能会导致病情恶化[36]。已经有一些使用黏菌素、妥布霉素和两性霉素含片的研究，似乎仅有临界的治疗作用，而不推荐使用[37]。

鉴于其重要的需求尚未满足，目前有许多不同种类的可能用于放疗所致黏膜炎的干预措施正处于不同的研发阶段。目前针对氧化应激，先天免疫反应和促炎因子的药物的临床试验正在进行[38]。低水平激光治疗也正在研究其作为口腔黏膜炎干预的潜在用途。虽然临床试验的结果令人鼓舞，但问题是目前仍然缺乏其与肿瘤反应相关的生物学效应的实质性研究。目前确定的是需要更多的研究，以确保其对癌前和癌组织的影响是良性的[39]。

口干症

口干症（xerostomia）将唾液腺包括在照射野内的放疗所引起的持续时间最长、最令人困扰的副作用之一[40]，并且可能因同步化疗而加重。放疗对唾液流量的影响变化不定，口干症状可能与观察到的唾液流量不一致。口干症是由于放疗作用于腺泡细胞所引起的，特别是浆液腺（腮腺）。因此，腺体实质出现炎症、变性和纤维化。范围、持续时间和恢复的程度与剂量率、总剂量、放疗部位密切相关。在放疗开始 1 周后（累积剂量 10Gy），口干症发生就可能被注意到[41]。因为浆液性功能减退但仍有黏液产生，所以唾液变得稠厚。耳部和颈部照射累积剂量达 60Gy 的患者常常发生不可逆转的口干症，伴有唾液腺 80%功能损失[42]。持续 12 个月或以上的口干症不太可能自行恢复[43]。但是对于小剂量的辐射，腺体组织的炎症和水肿通常在治疗结束后一年内自行消退[44]。

除口干症引起的如吞咽困难和味觉改变等功能变化，唾液减少也与口腔清除能力下降、唾液免疫球蛋白 A（IgA）水平和唾液抗菌酶的减少有关。因此，口干症患者容易发生口腔局部感染，包括龋齿、牙周病和口腔念珠菌病。积极的口腔卫生以减少牙支抗的细菌负荷，对降低牙科疾病的风险至关重要。

放疗引起的龋齿在口干症患者中很常见[42]。唾液成分的变化、缓冲能力下降，唾液清洁作用的丧失引起了细菌累积，增加局部致龋菌群和牙齿脱钙进而发生龋齿[45,46]。通常情况下，放射性龋齿表现在牙颈部边缘，然后迅速进展。此外还可以看到牙齿切缘脱钙（白色、白垩的牙釉质）。对于那些存在放射性骨坏死（ORN）风险的患者，除牙齿脱落外，不控制龋齿的主要后果是可能会形成脓肿。

预防和治疗口干症应该考虑四个目标。保护唾液腺功能是至关重要的。只要有可能，就应使用组织保护技术，目的在于最大限度地减少直接辐射暴露的涎腺组织数量。双侧野照射可能会引起唾液流量减少 80%，斗篷野放射通常只减少 30%~40%。应用三维适形放疗或调强放疗技术保护腮腺，使腺体获得最大修复[47]。XRT 的同时应刺激唾液流量，还应预防龋齿以保护齿列。一旦需要即应开始对分泌物减少进行替代治疗。

刺激唾液流量可以通过局部或全身性的方法来实现。可用无蔗糖柠檬汁或无糖口香糖。应避免肉桂、薄荷糖或薄荷味口香糖，因为它们可能会刺激黏膜。

药物疗法也可能有助于刺激腮腺流量[48]。在胆碱能药物中，毛果芸香碱的研究最充分。其可刺激腮腺功能，但对刺激干燥综合征和放疗引起口干症患者的下颌下腺或舌下腺功能无效[49,50]。其他药物，如溴已新、茴三硫、胆碱盐酸、碘化钾、新斯的明和利血平，已用于刺激唾液腺，但证实这些药物效用的数据仍不足。相反，有大量数据支持使用盐酸毛果芸香碱片可以刺激因放疗导致的口干症患者的唾液流量[51]。在放疗结束后有症状而使用毛果芸香碱的病例中，至少需保留部分唾液腺功能。且患者需要注意，在治疗开始后 3 个月内可能都无法实现临床上唾液流量的显著改善。或选择与放疗同时开始毛果芸香碱治疗。无论哪种情况，常规剂量为 5mg，每日 3 次，滴注，但是其剂量用法应根据患者的治疗反应和不良反应进行滴定。

氨磷汀（amifostine），是一种非蛋白类自由基清除剂，已获批为唾液腺细胞保护剂以预防放疗引起口干症[52]。氨磷汀的推荐剂量是 $200mg/m^2$，每日 1 次，3min 滴注，在常规分割放射治疗前 15~30min 开始用药。静脉滴注的要求、给药频率、成本和潜在副作用限制了氨磷汀的应用。此外，最近一项荟萃分析的结果表明，在接受放射治疗同时给予化疗的患者中，氨磷汀的作用是温和的[53]。

唾液替代可以通过使用唾液替代品或人工唾液实现[54]。这些物质大都含有羧甲基纤维素，并可能使黏膜干燥症状获得短暂缓解。唾液替代品，可作为非处方漱口水或喷雾剂提供，在饭前和睡前使用是最有效的。已有许多牙膏和口香糖开发专门供口干症患者使用。

最近报道了令人兴奋的恢复唾液腺功能新的再生方法，但仍限于临床前研究[55]。

毫无疑问，对放疗引起的龋齿最有效的保护是积极使用外用氟化物[56]。外用氟化物补充剂应在放疗开始时使用。放疗后接续使用氟化物是至关重要的，尤其在口干症患者中。牙科使用的氟化物有 3 种：漱口液，通过牙刷或定制的托盘使用的凝胶，以及通过适合患者牙齿的托盘使用的氟滴剂。预期会发生口干症的患者应在放疗开始前制作氟托盘。氟凝胶或氟滴剂应放置在托盘中供患者每日使用。使用托盘可辅以使用酸性氟漱口液；通常早上使用漱口液，睡觉前使用托盘是最简单有效的方法。酸性氟化物效果可能最好，但是酸性物质对口腔黏膜可能有刺激性，或对烤瓷牙产生酸蚀，故中性氟化物漱口液对口腔黏膜炎患者，或对做烤瓷牙患者较为适用。也可以考虑补充使用再矿化牙膏[57]。积极的口腔卫生是值得鼓励的，患者应经常去牙科就诊。定期接受牙齿检查对确保早期发现和治疗龋齿和牙周疾病是至关重要的。

对于因为压迫或黏膜炎不能忍受托盘的患者，可通过牙刷使用氟凝胶，可以用 1.1%氟化钠或 0.4%氟化亚锡。后者似乎更有效。应指导患者避免食用蔗糖。

味觉丧失是暂时的，但也是令人困扰的头颈部放疗后遗症[58]。放疗剂量达 30Gy 剂量时，味觉丧失的严重程度迅速加重，但通常之后就达到了平台期。接受 30Gy 或以上剂量的患者可能会失去分辨咸或甜的味觉能力。幸运的是，味觉减退通常是暂时的，治疗结束后 1~2 个月内味觉开始恢复。完全恢复可能需要长达一年。如果放疗后味觉没有改善，应排除念珠菌感染。

放射性骨坏死

放射性骨坏死（ORN）是头颈部放射治疗最重要的口腔并发症之一[59]。放射性骨坏死最早于 1927 年被描述，其导致软组织剥脱、骨暴露和坏死[60,61]。尽管 ORN 并不局限于颌部，但最常见发生于该区域。ORN 造成一个极其疼痛的、慢性的、恶臭的开放性伤口，往往给患者造成了很大的困扰。大多数病例最终以保守治疗治愈，但这个过程大多漫长。ORN 曾被认为是创伤（通常是拔牙）、放疗和感染的三者综合的结果[62]。然而，随后的研究表明，ORN 表现为伤口愈合缺陷而不是一个真正意义上的骨髓炎[63]。病因似乎与 XRT 引起的血管减少有关[64]。动脉和小动脉壁增厚的组织学改变证实了这一假说。细菌培养结果是否阳性提示有无感染性因素参与[65]。

关于骨坏死的总体发病率还没有共识。虽然有报道其范围为 4% ~ 44%，但绝大多数的经验表明发病率在 15%左右[59,63]。一项最近的荟萃分析报道 HNC 患者的风险仅为 2%[66]。下颌骨比上颌骨更常受累，这可能反映了两者之间的供血和血管差异。XRT 后 ORN 的发生时间是有争议的。一些学者报道,ORN 可以在早至 XRT 后 2 周出现,而其他学者报道,ORN 是晚期病变。大多数病例发生在 XRT 后第一个三年以内(74%)。同样有争议的是 XRT 完成后 ORN 的风险随时间的推移而减少的速率,虽然风险从未达到零[67]。

ORN 的许多危险因素已经明确[68]。据报道,男性发生 ORN 的风险比女性高 3 倍[61]。缺齿患者发生 ORN 的风险可能是有齿患者的 2 倍。此外,ORN 的发病率在患活动性牙科疾病(如牙周病、龋齿、根尖周病、不合适的义齿)的患者中急剧增加[59]。50%病例似乎与放疗后拔牙有关。这些发现有力地支持 XRT 前需行牙科评估、积极修复和去除病变的牙齿。XRT 放射野范围大小、剂量率和总剂量对 ORN 发病率有显著影响。接受下颚或上颚照射累积剂量 65Gy 或以上的患者发生 ORN 的可能性比接受较低剂量的患者更大。三维适形放射治疗技术的使用使得 ORN 的风险略有减少[69]。肿瘤与骨相邻或相连的患者也存在更高的 ORN 风险。这可能是因为骨被包括在放射野内,而暴露于 XRT 的骨量直接影响 ORN 的风险。营养和免疫状态不良患者也易患此病。ORN 的诊断通常基于临床表现。在诊断不能明确的病例中,磁共振成像可能有诊断价值[70]。

ORN 的治疗是以其病情严重程度和长期性为依据的[71]。幸运的是,大多数病变(60%),经过约 6 个月保守治疗包括局部清创、唾液冲洗、口服抗生素可最终治愈[72]。利用己酮可可碱(pentoxifylline)抗 TNF 活性的研究,其评估结果并不一致[73,74]。

没有改善或证实有进展的病变需要更积极的治疗。对于这些病例,可进行清创手术、高压氧(hyperbaric oxygen,HBO)治疗[75,76]。对病变广泛的病例,涉及邻近微血管重建的根治性骨切除术已成功地用于很多保守治疗失败(包括 HBO)的患者[77]。最近报道了成功治疗在常规方法无效的患者中联合使用自体骨髓抽吸浓缩物、同种异体牙髓干细胞和富含血小板的血浆的结果[78]。

因为大多数口腔内 ORN 病例与牙科疾病及 XRT 后拔牙有关,所以放疗开始前消除潜在牙源性病理部位是预防 ORN 的基础。有侵犯牙髓、牙骨质断裂或根尖周病风险的牙周疾病、严重龋齿应在 XRT 开始前拔牙。相邻或累及潜在的手术切除部位(因肿瘤切除的需要)的牙齿也应拔除。鉴于 ORN 的后果,甚至可疑患病的牙齿,尤其是在放射野内的牙齿,也应该拔除。将接受 XRT 治疗患者拔牙的时机是众多研究分析、讨论和争议的主题;无论如何,共识是应在 XRT 前拔牙[13]。理想的情况下,期望最少有 21 日的愈合期,但是根据不同情况下可能制订了更短的时间。在任何一种情况下,XRT 前拔牙比治疗开始后拔牙更理想。因为多项研究表明,无论在 XRT 后多长时间拔牙,都有显著的 ORN 风险。在任何情况下,拔牙术应尽可能防止损伤,需特别注意保护软组织,尽可能Ⅰ期闭合和术后伤口行有效的局部治疗。围术期使用抗生素也是推荐的。

从 XRT 一开始,积极的口腔卫生、使用氟化物、牙科保健是预防牙科疾病发生的重要组成部分。如果 XRT 后发生牙科疾病且是可恢复的,根管治疗比拔牙更可取。但有时拔除放射野内的牙齿是不可避免的[79]。据报道,这些病例发生 ORN 的风险是可以接受的(5.6%),甚至不需要使用 HBO。在这些病例中 HBO 疗效还不确定。一项研究发现,放疗后第一年拔牙的患者,98.5%的术前和术后 HBO 治疗的拔牙部位者愈合且不出现并发症。然而,据报道,拔除的牙齿离放射野越远,HBO 的疗效越差[80]。HBO 的使用,就其成本和多重就诊而言,有必要进一步研究[81]。

化疗口腔并发症

癌症化疗的口腔并发症是由药物作用于口腔黏膜(直接或主要的口腔毒性)、骨髓抑制期间患者对局部较小的口腔病变(间接或次要的口腔毒性)无法进行修复所致,或者两种情况都有。

危险因素

并非所有的接受癌症化疗患者的口腔并发症风险都相同。这一点对于口腔黏膜炎尤为明显。虽然已经知道一些对口腔并发症的发病率和严重程度有影响的一些变量,但总体而言,他们的预测值还有待明确界定。危险因素可分为与患者相关的因素和与治疗方案相关的因素[82]。

与患者相关的危险因素包括肿瘤的诊断、年龄、性别、体重、遗传因素、癌症治疗前的口腔状况、治疗期间口腔护理的水平、治疗基线是否患口干症、基线的中性粒细胞计数。血液系统恶性肿瘤(即白血病和淋巴瘤)患者发生口腔并发症风险比非头颈部实体肿瘤患者更高。例如,超过 66%的白血病和 33%的非霍奇金淋巴瘤患者会出现口腔问题。肿瘤相关骨髓抑制可能至少在一定程度上是此现象的基础[83]。而几乎所有接受局部治疗的头颈肿瘤患者在治疗后会出现口腔问题。

年龄作为黏膜炎的危险因素的作用目前还不清楚,因为很少有研究比较同一诊断而年龄不同的患者口腔黏膜炎的发病率。在儿童中,已观察到中性粒细胞计数的最低点、低体重、更高的肌酐峰值与黏膜炎高发率有关[84]。而在使用氟尿嘧啶治疗实体肿瘤的成年患者中,似乎较年长的患者黏膜炎更加严重、持续时间更长。

性别可能对口腔并发症风险有影响。有报道表明,女性比男性更有可能出现与氟尿嘧啶相关的毒性[85]。这种趋势在接受高剂量化疗(BEAM)或大剂量美法仑(melphalan)化疗之后进行自体造血干细胞移植(HSCT)的患者中也已有报道[86]。造成这一现象的机制目前仍有待明确。遗传因素可能至少通过两种途径影响黏膜炎的风险[87]。有影响药物代谢的遗传缺陷的患者,发生黏膜炎的风险增加[88,89]。例如,在用甲氨蝶呤治疗慢性髓细胞性白血病的患者中,观察到亚甲基四氢叶酸还原酶活性较低(*TT* 基因型)的患者的毒性增加(包括黏膜炎)。同样的,二氢嘧啶脱氢酶(DPD)缺乏的患者易出现氟尿嘧啶引起的毒性。另外,遗传可能会影响和调节一些机制,而这些机制是化疗引起黏膜损伤的生物学基础。例如,炎性细胞因子产物在不同人群中是不同的,且由遗传控制。这些细胞因子对非血液系统毒性的发生发挥一定作用,并且密切相关。因此,这类蛋白容易高表达的患者患黏膜炎和其他毒性的风险有可能增加。例如,在异体造血干细胞移植 HSCT 受者的队列研究中,存在特异性肿瘤坏死因子基因多态性者发生严重不良反应的相对危险度(RR)超过 17 倍[90]。最近的一项关于儿科各种恶性肿瘤的队列研究结果报告了其与 ABO 血型之间的关联性。O 型血患者发生口咽黏膜炎的 RR 为 2.86，而 A 型血患者 RR 为 0.47，B 型血患者 RR 为 0.59[91]。需要进一步的研究以彻底地阐明功能基因对黏膜损伤的影响，但这将对明确基于发病机制的干预的风险性，和预测反应性有重要作用[92]。一般认为，口腔预处理不佳的患者发生某些口腔并发症的风险比较大，而不是所有口腔并发症[93]。不适合的义齿引起的慢性刺激或有缺陷的修复术使患者易患溃疡性黏膜炎。患者存在严重牙周病、牙髓病或轻度软组织感染如第三磨牙（即第三磨牙）部分萌出相关的感染时，一旦出现骨髓抑制发生口源性败血症的风险就会增加。然而，感染风险的增加与放射影像学证实而无症状的根尖病进行根管治疗无关[94]。

治疗期间的口腔护理水平对口腔并发症和感染的预后有重要影响[95]。患者及其医疗服务提供者减少口腔菌群负荷的能力对降低局部和全身感染的风险可产生正面影响[96]。包括牙齿和软组织机械性清创的侵入性技术和抗菌漱口液对口腔保健是有效的。

化疗前和化疗期间口干症可能与口腔黏膜炎风险增加有关[97]。研究证实干燥的口腔黏膜的健康状态改变和口腔定植菌群的增加会加大黏膜炎的可能性。有些研究评估了旨在增加唾液和口腔水分的治疗方案，并得出了非常不一致的研究结论。有一项研究报道了毛果芸香碱对化疗引起的口腔黏膜炎有有利的影响，但未能在类似的试验[98]或自体造血干细胞移植（HSCT）受者中重复[99]。

黏膜炎程度与中性粒细胞计数呈负相关。中性粒细胞计数基线低于 4 000 与较高的黏膜炎发病率相关[97]。在某种程度上，这一研究结果可能解释了恶性血液病患者黏膜炎发病率更高的现象。

并发症的风险也与化疗方式、顺序和剂量有关[16]。同步放疗，包括 TBI，也增加了口腔问题的风险。例如，已有报道在降低强度的干细胞移植受者中口腔黏膜炎的发病率（30.9%）远低于接受传统预处理方案治疗者（90.2%）[97]。化疗药物口腔毒性程度分级有显著性差异[16]。含蒽环类、紫杉烷类、铂和氟尿嘧啶的药物或方案常常有口腔毒性。TBI 的预处理方案也有高比例的黏膜炎发病率。有 17 个明确的口腔黏膜炎率（3~4 级）在患者中占相当大比例（>25%）的药物或联合方案：

- 多西他赛/氟尿嘧啶
- 多西他赛+XRT
- 紫杉醇+XRT
- 多西他赛+氟尿嘧啶
- 紫杉醇/氟尿嘧啶+XRT
- 多西他赛/铂类+XRT
- 紫杉醇/铂类+XRT
- 多西他赛/铂类/氟尿嘧啶
- 紫杉醇/铂类/氟尿嘧啶
- 奥沙利铂+XRT
- 铂类/紫杉类+XRT
- 铂类/甲氨蝶呤/亚叶酸钙
- 氟尿嘧啶/铂类
- 氟尿嘧啶/亚叶酸钙/紫杉类
- 依立替康/氟尿嘧啶 CI+XRT
- 阿糖胞苷/伊达比星/氟达拉滨
- 甲氨蝶呤
- 异环磷酰胺/依托泊苷
- 美法仑

就上表而言，重要的是要记住口腔并发症的发病率，特别是黏膜炎，其发生率和严重程度往往被大大低估。在当前医疗设备条件下，实际上几乎每个化疗药物都有引起口腔毒性反应的潜在可能，至少在部分经治患者中有此可能。

低剂量、重复方案的毒性往往比同一药物单次剂量方案低。放疗继发的毒性依赖于累积剂量；脉冲治疗的应用并不能显著减少口腔的变化。

溃疡性黏膜炎通常发生在化疗后 5~8 日，持续 7~14 日。病变自行愈合且无瘢痕形成。化疗引起的黏膜炎局限于可活动的口腔黏膜：颊黏膜，舌的侧面和腹面，口唇内侧，口底和软腭。与放疗引起的黏膜炎不同，化疗引起的黏膜炎不影响硬腭或牙龈。舌背表面也不会受到影响。这种现象很可能是由于各种黏膜表面的上皮特点不同引起的。口腔各个部位中，以颊黏膜、舌的侧面和腹面、口底最常受累。在接受多个周期化疗的患者中，病变往往会重复出现在相同的部位。许多研究已经证实，黏膜炎并非起源于感染（特别是病毒）。

化疗引起口腔黏膜炎的生物学机制，是当前的重点研究主题[18,100]。如上所述，黏膜炎被视为化疗对口腔基底快速分裂上皮细胞的非特异性毒性的结果。尽管有数据支持这一假设，但药物能通过使上皮细胞几乎或完全失去活性而改变黏膜炎发展过程，这一观察提示其有更广泛的病因学基础。这样看来，口腔黏膜炎这个临床结局是由于局部组织的毒性（内皮细胞，结缔组织和上皮）、骨髓抑制的水平和局部环境间复杂的相互作用的结果。自由基启动的结缔组织和血管内皮细胞的破坏，可能会激活一系列转录因子，并使许多能刺激炎性细胞因子生成和组织损伤的基因的表达增加。同时激活其他信号通路和酶的活性，从而使直接和间接上皮损伤的神经酰胺、蛋白水解酶和其他调节剂增加。因此，除了由直接 DNA 损伤引起的基底细胞克隆死亡，二级途径也产生一连串引起细胞凋亡或坏死的机制。最终，由于再生停止，上皮首先出现萎缩，并完全分解形成溃疡。值得注意的是，在一些患者中，基底上皮细胞累积损伤的程度没有达到溃疡发生所需的阈值。在这些患者中，变薄的黏膜表现为轻度至中度症状（1 级口腔黏膜炎）。当溃疡发生时，口腔中的细菌（包括革兰阳性和革兰阴性菌）发生二次定植。这些细菌的细胞壁产物使其进入下方的结缔组织，并在那里有效地刺激浸润的巨噬细胞产生其他促炎细胞因子。

更好地了解口腔黏膜炎的病理是发展基于发病机制干预措施的基础[38]。这些药物中第一个获得批准的是帕利夫明（角化细胞生长因子 1，Kepivance，Amgen 公司），用于预处理方案为 HSCT 做准备治疗的血液恶性肿瘤患者预防和治疗口腔黏膜炎。在Ⅲ期试验阶段，212 名 HSCT 受者接受了一种口腔毒性预处理方案——帕利夫明，在移植前和移植后多剂量给药明显有效地降低了口腔黏膜炎的持续时间、发病率和严重程度。对研究中患者的生活质量，减少阿片类药物使用和发热的时间有积极的作用[101]。帕利夫明的作用效果不仅是因为它能刺激上皮细胞增殖的结果，还因为它能通过增加调节转录因子的表达而介导细胞保护的作用。在美国，每年 45 万例患者出现黏膜炎，其中进行 HSCT 患者只占 5%。因此，将这些药物和其他药物延伸到其他肿瘤人群是一个重大目标。

低能量（氦氖）激光（λ=632.8nm）疗法（LLLT）已经被证实在减少口腔黏膜炎严重程度和症状的部分有效[102]。在需要进一步研究证实其价值的同时，LLLT 的成本和后勤工作可能会限制其总体效用。随着对 LLLT 影响与肿瘤进展和生长相关的广泛细胞和分子通路的能力有了更多的了解，研究表明其缺乏活性影响肿瘤反应。

许多细胞保护治疗方案和药物已被推荐可作为黏膜炎的干预治疗。口腔冷冻疗法便宜且没有风险，在氟尿嘧啶、依达曲沙（edatrexate）或美法仑注药前 5min 开始，共使用 30min，其使用可能有助于降低黏膜炎的严重程度[26]。许多研究已对己酮可可碱进行研究，研究结果好坏参半。据报告，在结直肠癌和 HNC 患者中，Trefoil 局部用药是有益的[38,103]。维生素 E 和 β-胡萝卜素的抗氧化治疗得出了不一致的结果。生物制剂、基因转移和其他针对特定生物途径的疗法的开发也在研究之中[38]。

由于口腔微生物的存在被认为不利于口腔黏膜炎的病程，抗菌治疗作为一个干预的手段已被广泛研究[36]。从总体上看，有关数据表明通过药物治疗使口腔细菌负荷减少对黏膜炎的发病率或严重程度没有意义。在随机双盲试验中，外用抗菌药物的使用如氯已定葡萄糖酸，一直未能改善黏膜炎发病率和疾病过程[104,105]。

减轻症状是使用最广泛的治疗黏膜炎的方法。生理盐水已使用多年，并且比过氧化氢溶液更有效，犹如“神奇的漱口水”[106]。屏障型缓冲液，如硫糖铝悬液和 Gelclair 也可以使用，虽然其益处尚未得到令人信服的证实。局部应用加入利多卡因或苯海拉明的白陶土和果胶制剂或氧化镁乳剂可能会得到一些局部缓解，但往往不能完全抵消注射药物镇痛的需要。

靶向治疗的影响

mTOR 抑制剂相关的溃疡

哺乳动物西罗莫司靶蛋白（mTOR）抑制剂对晚期恶性肿瘤的疗效已经在临床试验中取得令人鼓舞的结果。口腔溃疡是与这些药物相关的最重要剂量限制性毒性之一[107]，一般上报为黏膜炎。然而，mTOR 抑制剂引起的口腔溃疡的临床过程、生物学行为、症状和可能的发病机制强烈提示这是一种明显不同于由放射治疗或细胞毒性药物化疗引起的黏膜炎[108]。

与化疗引起的典型黏膜炎不同，口疮性病变表现为分散的卵圆形的浅表溃疡，周围有特征性边缘红斑（图 135-3）。给药后病变进展迅速，且通常在一个极其痛苦的过程后自发消退。虽然尚无随机研究，但常见口疮性口腔炎治疗方法可能有效。

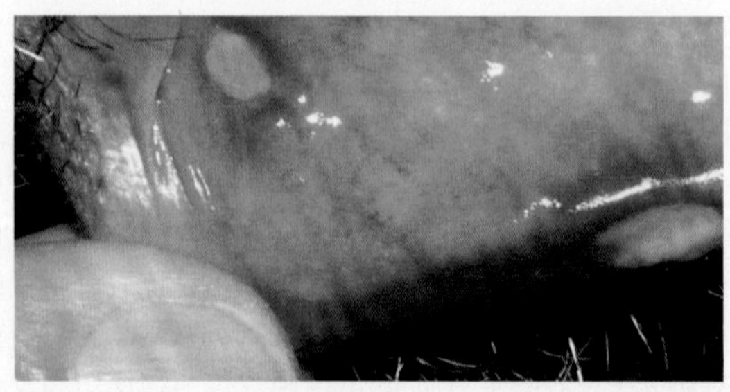

图 135-3 mTOR 抑制剂治疗相关的口腔黏膜溃疡。病变很容易辨认，呈椭圆形，有中央坏死区，和易让人联想到口疮性口腔炎的边缘红斑

与 mTKI 药物相关的感觉异常

多靶点酪氨酸激酶抑制剂（mTKI）为越来越多的恶性肿瘤提供了特异性的癌症治疗方法。这些小分子抑制剂与口腔不适有关，但常无阳性体征。感觉异常这个术语更精确，更具描述性；通常说的口腔炎是非特异性的，但在以前的研究中常使用。这些感觉异常可表现为黏膜过度敏感，灼热，味觉障碍或味觉减退，口腔干燥（有足够的唾液流动），以及其他的感觉异常，如刺痛和麻木。这些症状可能发生在 mTKI 治疗的高达 60%的患者中，并且可能与治疗的其他副作用相关，包括手掌-足底红斑感觉异常[109]。

钙调神经磷酸酶诱导的炎性纤维血管增生

用于免疫抑制的钙调神经磷酸酶抑制剂可以在口腔中诱导炎性纤维血管增生。环孢素与牙龈组织广泛的致密纤维化相关，而他克莫司诱导的化脓性肉芽肿更常见于舌和颊黏膜，表现为局部的纤维性息肉[110]。

骨坏死

化疗同时给予双膦酸盐或 RANK-L 抑制剂地诺单抗已被作为减少骨转移的治疗策略。在接受这类治疗的患者中，颌骨坏死的发病率增加，特别是下颌骨坏死（是上颌骨的 2 倍）[111]。据报道其发病率为 3%~8.5%[112]。较新的报道包括使用舒尼替尼和贝伐单抗等血管生成抑制剂的病例，并出现了一个新的术语，称为药物相关的颌骨坏死（MRONJ）[21]。这类患者中骨坏死的表现因症状而异。虽然有些患者会感到疼痛，但其他患者却没有。大多数病例似乎与牙齿操作、例如拔牙有关，或与软组织创伤有关。这种病理学现象背后的机制尚不清楚，其自然病程也不清楚。保守治疗似乎是最合适的（表 135-1）。目前，最明智的策略是在开始治疗之前确保积极的牙科筛查和治疗，以便尽可能减少以后牙科治疗的需求。

感染

口腔上皮不断脱落的同时，由于骨髓抑制的原因，患者清除丰富的口腔菌群的能力下降。因此，在粒细胞减少的癌症患者中，口腔变成菌血症和败血症的重要感染来源，也是局部继发性感染的来源。这些间接口腔毒性的表现与骨髓状态成正比；因此，患者粒细胞水平到最低点时，口腔毒性最大或即将达到最大。口腔草绿色链球菌的全身感染尤为常见。其中轻型链球菌感染后果最严重。

真菌感染

在骨髓抑制患者中引起口腔局部感染，按发病率由高到低依次为真菌、病毒和细菌。念珠菌感染是最常见的口腔感染，特点表现为白色凝乳状，或红斑、黄斑病变[113]。它最常发生于上腭、舌头和口角。控制不良的口腔念珠菌病可以增加肺部误吸、引发念珠菌性食管炎或真菌血症的风险。此外，曲霉菌和毛霉菌病在骨髓抑制患者中并不罕见；这些病变可表现为侵袭性口腔溃疡，伴有疼痛并可能累及骨质。

由于全身性念珠菌病有很高的发病率和死亡率[114]，对预期长期存在中性粒细胞减少的患者预防性使用抗真菌药是合理的，例如 HSCT 或有接受有口腔毒性的、清髓性化疗患者。

一般来说,外用药物对此类患者是无效的。治疗药物可选氟康唑(fluconazole)、卡泊芬净(caspofungin)、米卡芬净(micafungin)[115]。

对接受头颈部放疗、有口干症和使用类固醇引起免疫抑制的患者,外用抗真菌药物预防性抗白念珠菌可能有好处。多烯类抗真菌剂(如制霉菌素)或咪唑剂,克霉唑同样有效。制霉菌素剂型是黏稠的樱桃味的混悬液,因化疗导致恶心的患者不一定喜欢这种口味。克霉唑剂型是片剂。对于儿童患者,药物加水放入冰块托盘制成的制霉菌素冰棒更受欢迎。其他两种咪唑类药物也可供选择:酮康唑和氟康唑,用于预防和治疗均有效。酮康唑需在酸性环境下起效,这限制了它用于进食困难患者。唑类药物耐药性可能与真菌感染的治疗有相关性。有些念珠菌对唑类抗真菌药物天然不敏感,如光滑念珠菌和克柔念珠菌[116]。

氯己定葡萄糖漱口液作为一种外用抗真菌剂的功效并不明确[117]。但体内研究数据表明氯己定降低了制霉菌素的活性[118]。因此,建议不要与用制霉菌素同时使用。

早已已证实通过真菌培养预测真菌感染或病程没有什么价值,但聚合酶链反应(PCR)在口腔念珠菌感染的快速诊断和鉴别中可能有一定作用[119]。

病毒感染

1 型单纯疱疹病毒(HSV-1)是接受化疗和头颈部放疗患者最常见的口腔病毒感染,抗体检测是风险评估的重要部分。口腔 HSV-1 感染可以是原发性病毒感染,或者既往暴露的宿主体内潜伏病毒的激活[120]。在接受治疗的癌症患者中以后者常见。既往暴露 HSV-1 的患者中,病毒血清反应阳性者比血清反应阴性者感染风险更大。HSV-1 感染最常见的表现是口腔溃疡。虽然其临床表现可能与其他的黏膜炎类似,但通常在其病程和分布范围不同。

接受化疗或 HSCT 的患者 HSV-1 感染的时机通常是相当一致的[121]。一般在治疗开始后约 18 日出现病变。这种时间关系很重要,可用于鉴别病变可能由 HSV-1 感染引起还是化疗的直接口腔毒性引起,化疗的直接口腔毒性通常在治疗开始后 5~7 日出现。并与继发性表面感染(通常是细菌感染)相鉴别。继发性表面感染出现在患者骨髓抑制最严重时(即粒细胞降到最低点),这大约发生在第 12~14 日。病变可以出现在任何黏膜表面,包括硬腭和牙龈这些角化最明显的组织。病毒培养是诊断 HSV-1 感染最明确的方法,建议积极地进行培养,尤其是在病毒血清反应阳性患者。阿昔洛韦(acyclovir)全身用药仍是 HSV 感染的预防和治疗首选[121]。

在进行治疗的癌症患者中,带状疱疹也可表现为口腔病变[115]。这些病变往往成片出现。它们开始呈水疱状,但很快破裂,形成疼性小溃疡。与 HSV-1 形成的病变不同,这些病变常常位于一侧,条带状,沿第五脑神经的分支之一分布。

细菌感染

在骨髓抑制的癌症患者中,口腔可能是局部和全身细菌感染常见来源,粒细胞减少的癌症患者链球菌感染发病率增加可以为证[115]。细菌感染可能是来源于软组织或牙龈或齿源性的感染。接受治疗的癌症患者往往由于口腔卫生下降和口干症导致口腔微生物数量增加。同时,口腔菌群的组成由以革兰阳性菌为主转变为以革兰阴性菌为主。

大多数情况下,龋齿后细菌入侵导致牙髓退化和感染,进而引起牙源性感染。因为患者无法启动炎症反应,所以没有常见的牙齿感染的迹象(如脓肿形成或肿胀),患者主诉有局部齿痛。临床上有叩痛或对热敏感,和/或放射学证据是龋齿进展到牙髓的诊断依据。接受生物碱类药物治疗的患者的神经毒性可能会导致牙齿疼痛,这种疼痛类似牙源性感染。牙源性感染主要来源于厌氧菌,这些厌氧菌与牙菌斑的菌种相似。治疗应包括消除感染源,多数情况下需要拔牙。许多研究者报道过骨髓抑制时拔牙的安全性问题[122]。这些研究指出,拔牙同时应该使用抗生素,必要时输注血小板,重视组织的处理和良好的缝合。不建议用明胶海绵之类的止血材料填塞牙槽,因为它们可能成为感染源。一般来说,在血小板计数大于 50 000 个/ml 的时候,不需要输注血小板。抗生素的全身用药应直到伤口愈合为止。

牙龈感染在接受骨髓抑制治疗的患者中比较常见。有些是局限性的,如第三磨牙萌出不全(即第三磨牙)有关的感染,而其他往往是弥漫性的。有慢性牙龈炎或牙周病的患者,急性牙龈和牙周感染更重。

发生在粒细胞减少期的急性牙龈感染,其临床表现类似急性坏死性溃疡性牙龈炎。特点是疼痛和牙龈退缩,特别是齿间乳突的坏死。这些病变往往是混合性细菌感染,包括各种病原体,如表皮葡萄球菌、铜绿假单胞菌、与牙周疾病有关的细菌如拟杆菌和韦荣球菌。

治疗包括局部清创和全身应用抗生素。病变局部培养可能比血培养更有意义,因为不一定有细菌入血。没有培养结果时建议进行经验性治疗。

在骨髓抑制患者中,黏膜感染往往发生在因口腔毒性导致的溃疡区。溃疡可以表现为穿透性的,形成圆形边界和黄白色坏死中心。由于缺乏炎症反应,通常没有红色边界。如果是创伤引起溃疡,血小板减少症患者可能会出现继发性血肿。革兰阴性菌往往是软组织感染的病因,但必须排除 HSV-1。治疗应包括清创、对症治疗和抗生素。同时应进行细菌和病毒培养。

口腔感染的预防措施包括去除黏膜刺激来源和减少局部口腔菌群数量[6]。此外,在化疗开始前,先处理轻度的无症状的感染可以最大限度降低骨髓抑制后的急性感染风险。减少口腔菌群可以通过物理或化学的方法。可以用普通牙刷进行牙齿局部清洁,而且应使用软刷毛。根据常识,血小板减少症并不是物理清洁的禁忌证。在有明显出血时应该停止刷牙。也可以考虑用棉签或毛巾包裹手指来清洁牙齿。牙线是用于清洁的好工具,但对不熟悉其使用的患者来说有一定困难。未达到重度血小板减少的患者都可以使用牙线。基本上,可用于清除牙垢和微生物的任何东西都将是有益的。棉签,海绵和橡胶都可以用。

漱口液对保持口腔卫生有不同程度的帮助。任何冲洗口腔的液体,包括水,都会有一定的帮助。常用的有盐水和稀释的过氧化物。通常不建议使用酒精作为活性物质的漱口液,因为酒精可灼伤萎缩的黏膜。氯己定葡萄糖酸盐的效果报道不一。如果使用氯己定漱口液,应避免与制霉菌素同时使用,因为后者可以被氯己定灭活。同样,聚维酮碘漱口液也被证实能减少口腔常驻菌群。其他药物也已被尝试用于预防性用药,氟化物漱口液可降低口腔细菌附着于牙齿的能力。所以它们也可能会有所帮助。

应告知有活动义齿的患者在骨髓抑制期间将它们取出。骨髓抑制期间口腔出血大多来源于齿龈。当血小板计数大于20 000个/ml时，自发性牙龈出血很少发生。血小板减少时可能出现缓慢渗血，尤其在有牙周疾病的位置。牙龈出血的局部治疗包括清创、不扰动已形成的血栓、局部应用凝血酶压迫止血。牙龈出血通常被认为是血小板计数已低到足以出现其他更致命的出血的征象。

血肿形成常发生在创伤区域，尤其是口腔黏膜、牙槽黏膜或缺齿区。黏膜下出血的地方形成蓝色水疱样区域，然后变成黄白色、由纤维素形成的瘤样肿物。肿物下方开始上皮化。如果出血发生在完全愈合前，局部治疗应包括凝血酶、微纤维胶原蛋白或其他止血凝胶。完全愈合前，微生物会在血凝块处生长。应每日检查血凝块，上皮一旦完全愈合应立即清除血凝块。未发现的舌下出血，可能会引起舌上抬致呼吸困难。

HSCT相关口腔并发症

黏膜炎

HSCT患者患黏膜炎的风险主要取决于HSCT预处理方案的强度，而发病率差异很大，可高达76%[123]。接受全身放射会影响黏膜炎发生的风险[16]。与其他化疗引起的黏膜炎一样，病变位于在可活动的口腔黏膜，常见于口底、舌系带、唇和颊黏膜（图135-1）。在自体或异体HSCT受者中，无论是移植后黏膜炎的出现时间，还是黏膜炎的持续时间，都没有显著性差异。Woo等[124]报道了自体HSCT受者移植后黏膜炎发病的平均时间为5日，而异体移植受者为6日。两组黏膜炎平均持续时间都大约为6日，消退时间为10~12日。在另一项研究中，接受环磷酰胺和TBI的患者进行了自体HSCT，WHO分级3/4级的黏膜炎持续时间更长。黏膜炎几乎都是在移植后3周消退，这是患者下一步发展为GVHD的一个重要的诊断性标志。中性粒细胞绝对计数（ANC）与黏膜炎消退有相关性。除非患者有十分严重的病灶，否则ANC大于500个/ml时，黏膜炎一般都会自行消退。不过，似乎使用GCSF或GM-CSF并不能预防黏膜炎的发生或减轻黏膜炎的发展。

本章其他地方对黏膜炎诱发机制进行了讨论。值得指出的是，黏膜炎的发生独立于病毒或真菌感染。如上所述，帕利夫明最近已获得批准用于自体HSCT受者的口腔黏膜炎的预防和治疗（见前文）。

感染

口腔感染是HSCT受者出现并发症的一个主要发病原因。尤其重要的是，在这类患者中，口腔是全身感染或远处感染的感染源[125]。HSCT受者链球菌感染率急剧上升。因此，在治疗前必须对HSCT受者进行筛查，以发现和消除无症状、处于休眠状态或潜在的牙齿感染或刺激。

除了细菌感染，HSCT受者在粒细胞减少期还存在口腔病毒和真菌感染的风险。与其他骨髓抑制的患者相似，在BMT人群中这些感染的临床表现，通常不同于这类感染的典型临床表现。因此，必须尽早和积极地进行病原体培养。病毒感染大多由疱疹病毒类所致；单纯疱疹、水痘和带状疱疹都与HSCT患者口腔感染有关。但是，阿昔洛韦预防性用药这一常规基本已经停止了。此外，在HSCT患者中已有关于耐阿昔洛韦的皮肤黏膜单纯疱疹病毒感染的报道。念珠菌病是最常见的真菌感染，但毛霉菌病和曲霉菌病感染也有报道。深部真菌感染的病变一般表现为难愈性牙龈溃疡。活检是首选的诊断方法。

移植物抗宿主病（GVHD）

口腔是急性和慢性GVHD的常见的表现部位[126,127]。急性GVHD的口腔症状报道相对较少，但三种口腔病变的临床模式已见报道，并最早在移植3周后和皮肤病变出现接近1周后可出现口腔症状（图135-4）。起初，可活动黏膜区出现多个白色乳头状小病变。这些病变进展为白色花边样角化病变，临床上类似扁平苔藓，而实际上也被描述为苔藓样。接下来，可能会出现脱屑性病变，这也类似于糜烂或大疱性扁平苔藓病变。与其他两种类型不同，这些表现往往是有症状的，而且需要治疗干预。

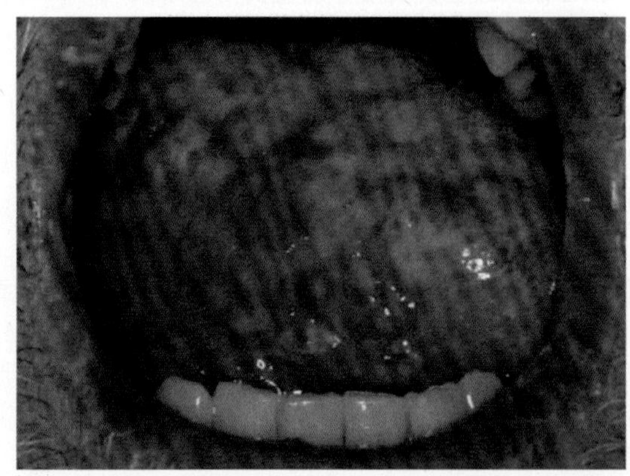

图135-4 移植物抗宿主病口腔表现的特点是以黏膜起疱和苔藓样改变（蒙Nathaniel Treister博士提供）

慢性GVHD的临床表现中，口腔症状仅次于皮肤。慢性GVHD的口腔病变出现在移植约3个月或3个月后。约70% GVHD患者会出现口腔病变，其中最典型者表现为苔藓样病变。有症状的病变一般表现为口腔黏膜的糜烂性、水疱性病变，边缘有角化条纹。此外，在慢性GVHD患者常有口干症。黏膜和唾液腺的变化都是淋巴细胞浸润引起的；由此产生的组织变化类似于其他口腔自身免疫性改变。

为确诊慢性GVHD，唇部小涎腺活检是准确、灵敏的方法，比颊黏膜或腮腺活检更具有预测性。技术上，小涎腺活检只需少许组织，很容易在局麻下在诊室内完成。组织学上，可见腺泡萎缩和/或淋巴细胞浸润下的组织破坏，富含CD3+T细胞。

局部或全身性类固醇治疗一般对苔藓样病变有效。据报道，紫外线A光疗法有助于治疗严重的难治性病变。在本章前面部分讨论了口干症的治疗。和其他口干症患者一样，GVHD患者患龋齿的风险增加，应进行相应的治疗。

另外，HSCT及GVHD的迟发性反应也影响到口腔。在这一人群中，口腔是继发恶性肿瘤最常见的发生部位。因此，患者应常规接受全面的口腔检查，以筛查鳞状细胞癌。据报道，小儿HSCT也有明显的远期口腔及颅面部并发症。建议早期转诊和由小儿牙科专家积极随访治疗。

（王朝阳 金立超 朱一鸣 译 刘绍严 校）

参考文献

The complete reference list can be found on the Wiley Companion Digital Edition of this title (see inside front cover for login instructions).

2 Epstein JB, Guneri P, Barasch A. Appropriate and necessary oral care for people with cancer: guidance to obtain the right oral and dental care at the right time. *Support Care Cancer*. 2014;**22**:1981-1988.

6 Elad S, Raber-Durlacher JE, Brennan MT, et al. Basic oral care for hematology-oncology patients and hematopoietic stem cell transplantation recipients: a position paper from the joint task force for the Multinational Association of Supportive Care in Cancer/International Society of Oral Oncology (MASCC/ISOO) and the European Society for Blood and Marrow Transplantation (EBMT). *Support Care Cancer*. 2015;**23**:223-236.

8 Jham BC, Reis PM, Miranda EL, et al. Oral health status of 207 head and neck cancer patients before, during and after radiotherapy. *Clin Oral Investig*. 2008;**12**(**1**):19-24.

15 Jawad H, Hodson NA, Nixon PJ. A review of dental treatment of head and neck cancer patients, before, during, and after radiotherapy: part 1. *Brit Dent J*. 2015;**218**:65-68.

16 Sonis ST, Elting LS, Keefe D, et al. Perspectives on cancer therapy-induced mucosal injury: pathogenesis, measurement, epidemiology and consequences for patients. *Cancer*. 2004;**100**(**9 Supp**):1995.

17 Russi EG, Raber-Durlacher JE, Sonis ST. Local and systemic pathogenesis and consequences of regimen-induced inflammatory responses in patients with head and neck cancer receiving chemoradiation. *Mediators Inflamm*. 2014:1-14, Article ID 518261.

18 Sonis ST. The pathobiology of mucositis. *Nat Rev Cancer*. 2004;**4**:277.

21 Ruggiero SL, Dodson TB, Fantasia J, et al. American Association of Oral and Maxillofacial Surgeons position paper on medication-related osteonecrosis of the jaw — 2014 update. *J Oral Maxillofac Surg*. 2014;**72**:1938-1956.

26 Lalla RV, Bowen J, Barasch A, et al. MASCC/ISOO clinical practice guidelines for the management of mucositis secondary to cancer therapy. *Cancer*. 2014;**120**:1453-1461.

38 Yuan A, Sonis S. Emerging therapies for the prevention and treatment of oral mucositis. *Expert Opin Emerg Drugs*. 2014;**19**:343-351.

42 Agular GP, Jham BC, Magalhaes CS, et al. A review of the biological and clinical aspects of radiation caries. *J Contemp Dent Pract*. 2009;**10**:83-89.

51 Saleh J, Figueiredo MA, Cherubini K, et al. Salivary hypofunction: an update on aetiology, diagnosis and therapeutics. *Arch Oral Biol*. 2015;**60**:242-255.

53 Gu J, Zhu S, Li X, et al. Effect of amifostine in head and neck cancer patients treated with radiotherapy: a systematic review and meta-analysis based on randomized controlled trials. *PLoS*. 2014;**9**:e95968.

54 Villa A, Connell CL, Abati S. Diagnosis and management of xerostomia and hyposalivation. *Ther Clin Risk Manag*. 2015;**11**:45-51.

56 Hong CH, Napenas JJ, Hodgson BD, et al. A systematic review of dental disease in patients undergoing cancer therapy. *Support Care Cancer*. 2009;**2010**(**18**):1007-1021.

58 Hong JH, Omur-Ozbek P, Stanek BT, et al. Taste and odor abnormalities in cancer patients. *J Support Oncol*. 2009;**7**:58-65.

59 Reuther T, Schuster T, Mende U, Kubler A. Osteoradionecrosis of the jaws as a side effect of radiotherapy of head and neck tumour patients—a report of a thirty year retrospective review. *Int J Oral Maxillofac Surg*. 2003;**32**:289-295.

62 Lee IJ, Koom WS, Lee CG, et al. Risk factors and dose-effect relationship for mandibular osteoradionecrosis in oral and oropharyngeal cancer. *Int J Radiat Oncol Biol Phys*. 2009;**75**:1084-1091.

63 Jacobson AS, Buchbinder D, Hu K, et al. Paradigm shifts in the management of osteoradionecrosis of the mandible. *Oral Oncol*. 2010;**46**:795-801.

66 Nabil S, Samman N. Risk factors for osteoradionecrosis after head and neck radiation: a systematic review. *Oral Surg Oral Pathol Oral Med Oral Radiol*. 2012;**113**:54-69.

71 Rice N, Polyzois I, Ekanayake K, et al. The management of osteoradionecrosis of the jaws — A review. *Surgeon*. 2015;**13**:101-109.

72 McCaul JA. Pharmacologic modalities in the treatment of osteoradionecrosis of the jaw. *Oral Maxillofac Surg Clin North Am*. 2014;**26**:247-252.

75 Fritz GW, Gunsolley JC, Aubaker O, et al. Efficacy of pre- and postirradiation hyperbaric oxygen therapy in the prevention of postextraction osteoradionecrosis: a systematic review. *J Oral Maxillofac Surg*. 2010;**68**:2653-2660.

79 Koga DH, Salvajol JV, Alves FA, et al. Dental extractions and radiotherapy in head and neck oncology: review of the literature. *Oral Dis*. 2008;**14**: 40-44.

81 Chuang SK. Limited evidence to demonstrate that the use of hyperbaric oxygen (HBO) therapy reduces the incidence of osteoradionecrosis in irradiated patients requiring tooth extraction. *J Evid Based Dent Pract*. 2012;**12**(**3 Suppl**): 248-250.

82 Peterson DE, Keefe DM, Sonis ST. New frontiers in mucositis. *Am Soc Clin Oncol Educ Book*. 2012;**2012**:545-551.

89 Schwab M, Zanger UM, Marx C, et al. Role of genetic and nongenetic factors for fluorouracil treatment-related severe toxicity: a prospective clinical trial by the German 5-FU Toxicity Study Group. *J Clin Oncol*. 2008;**26**:2131-2138.

92 Sonis S, Antin J, Tedaldi M, et al. SNP-based Bayesian networks can predict oral mucositis risk in autologous stem cell transplant recipients. *Oral Dis*. 2013;**19**:721-727.

102 Oberol S, Zamperlini-Netto G, Beyene J, et al. Effect of low level laser therapy on oral mucositis: a systematic review and meta-analysis. *PLoS One*. 2014;**9**(**9**):e107418.

105 McGuire DB, Fulton JS, Park J, et al. Systematic review of basic oral care for the management of oral mucositis in cancer patients. *Support Care Cancer*. 2013;**21**:3165-3177.

108 Sonis S, Treister N, Chawla S, et al. Preliminary characterization of oral lesions associated with inhibitors of mammalian target of rapamycin in cancer patients. *Cancer*. 2010;**116**:210-215.

109 Boers-Doets CB, Epstein JB, Raber-Durlacher JE, et al. Oral adverse events associated with tyrosine kinase and mammalian target of rapamycin inhibitors in renal cell carcinoma: a structured literature review. *Oncologist*. 2012;**17**: 135-144.

113 Worthington HV, Clarkson JE, Eden OB. Interventions for treatment of oral candidiasis for patients with cancer receiving treatment. *Cochrane Database Syst Rev*. 2007;**18**:CDOO1972.

115 Lerman MA, Laudenbach J, Marty FM, et al. Management of oral infections in cancer patients. *Dent Clin N Am*. 2008;**52**:129-153.

120 Djuric M, Jankovic L, Jankovic T, et al. Prevalence of oral herpes simplex virus reactivation in cancer patients: a comparison of different techniques of viral detection. *J Oral Pathol Med*. 2009;**38**:167-173.

121 Glenny AM, Fernandez MLM, Pavitt S, et al. Interventions for the prevention and treatment of herpes simplex virus in patients being treated for cancer. *Cochrane Database Syst Rev*. 2009;**21**:CD006706.

122 Filmore WJ, Leavitt BD, Arce K. Dental extraction in the thrombocytopenic patient is safe and complications are easily managed. *J Oral Maxillofac Surg*. 2013;**71**:1647-1652.

125 Herbers AHE, de Haan AFJ, van der Velden WJFM, et al. Mucositis not neutropenia determines bacteremia among hematopoietic stem cell transplant recipients. *Tansplant Infect Dis*. 2014;**16**:279-285.

126 Imanguli MM, Alevizos I, Brown R, et al. Oral graft-versus-host disease. *Oral Dis*. 2008;**14**:396-412.

第 136 章　生殖腺并发症

Vignesh Narayanan, MD ■ Catherine E. Klein, MD

概述

过去的 50 年来，癌症治疗最引人注目的进步是儿童肉瘤、儿童白血病、年轻成人的高级别淋巴瘤、霍奇金淋巴瘤和睾丸肿瘤等肿瘤患者的生存时间获得了空前的改善。越来越多的患乳腺癌的绝经前妇女在接受辅助化疗后生存期显著延长，使得更多的人开始关心长期生育健康的问题。许多新的治疗方法使得大批的患者能够活到成年期，但同时也带来了现代化疗最常见的重要副作用之一：暂时或永久的性腺功能改变。癌症幸存的妇女面临性腺功能早衰的症状，包括绝经、不孕、骨质疏松加速和早期心脏疾病的可能性。男性则面临无精症导致的生育能力低下和亚临床的间质细胞功能障碍，这些可能导致长时间的"男性更年期"表现，包括骨密度下降、肌肉体积减小、性功能下降和冠心病风险增加。

随着对这些并发症的认识，对他们的发生频率和严重程度的记录更加完善，对患者的咨询更加有效，同时改进治疗方法来减轻或预防这些毒性。这些干预措施包括激素治疗，替代治疗，治疗前的生殖细胞预冻存，但是这些方法需要治疗前进行，遗憾的是，许多患者仍然说他们并未被告知这些潜在的灾难性的后果或者关于生育能力丧失的可替代方法。随着癌症治疗的持续发展，存活下来的年轻肿瘤患者的数量正在增加，通过及时的、善解人意的方式来处理这些问题对于肿瘤学家来说极为重要。

过去 50 年癌症治疗的进步使得儿童肉瘤和白血病幸存者以及年轻的高分化淋巴瘤、霍奇金病（HD）和睾丸肿瘤患者可能会存活到成年，但有些人要长期忍受这些治疗带来的痛苦。性腺功能改变是现代癌症治疗中常见的令人痛苦的副作用。女性面临卵巢功能早衰（POF）的症状，包括绝经、不孕、可能加速骨质疏松或早期心脏病。男性有精子减少症以及亚临床间质细胞功能障碍，导致不孕和"雄激素暂停"的长期作用，包括骨密度降低、肌肉萎缩、性欲降低，并增加冠状动脉疾病的风险。

随着文献对这些并发症的频率和严重程度的认识提高，对患者更有效的咨询和创新的方法用来降低性腺毒性。这包括激素干预、选择替代处理、胚胎或生殖细胞的低温保存等，但这些措施必须在治疗前提供，患者仍保留有未明显受损的生育能力或选择保护生育能力。随着癌症治疗的进步癌症幸存者的数量也在增加，肿瘤学家必须及时敏感地应对这些问题。

历史背景

一个世纪前人们就意识到放射线和化疗对性腺功能的影响。1903 年出现了测试放射敏感性的有关报道，并且在后来的 50 年里也有大量的文献集中在这一主题上。原子能委员会于 20 世纪 60 年代完成的对正常男性的研究证实，精原细胞对放射性额外敏感，小到 10cGy 的放射量，相当于引起老鼠产生相应损伤所需剂量的 1/3 就会对其产生损伤[1]。卵母细胞对辐射的耐受稍强，但仍然是一种可再生的剂量依赖的放疗敏感性，这可导致随年龄增长而不孕的发生率和绝经期的提前的发生率增加。1939 年的数据显示，500cGy 的放射剂量照射人类卵巢与停经相关，停经可持续长达 18 个月。所有超过 40 岁的妇女都永久不孕[2]。

最初提出化疗可损害人的生殖功能的报道被一个病理的研究所证实，该研究的结果从 20 世纪 40 年代时接受过氮芥治疗的 30 位男性检测中获得。其中 27 位男性表现出明显的睾丸萎缩和精子发生异常[3]。

最早可信的提出妇女的月经不规则与癌症的治疗方法相关的报道出现在 1956 年[4]。四个年轻的女性在接受白消安治疗慢性髓细胞性白血病时，在治疗开始的 3 个月内出现停经。卵巢和子宫内膜的组织学检查均一致表现为原发性卵巢衰竭。随之多个药物的生殖毒性也被发现，可能损害睾丸或卵巢的化疗药物的名单还在持续增长（表 136-1）。

表 136-1　常用抗癌药物引起性腺功能下降的概率

下降频率	男性	女性
常见	环磷酰胺	环磷酰胺
	氮芥	氮芥
	丙卡巴肼	丙卡巴肼
	亚硝基脲	亚硝基脲
		白消安
		美法仑
		沙利度胺
可能	长春碱	长春碱
	依托泊苷	依托泊苷
	顺铂	顺铂
	卡铂	卡铂
	类固醇	苯丁酸氮芥
	异环磷酰胺	羟基脲
	干扰素	放线菌素 D
	阿糖胞苷	他莫昔芬
	伊马替尼	伊马替尼

续表

下降频率	男性	女性
可能	硫鸟嘌呤	紫杉醇
		硫鸟嘌呤
		干扰素
		阿糖胞苷
很少	长春新碱	甲氨蝶呤
	多柔比星	多柔比星
	博来霉素	博来霉素
	甲氨蝶呤	长春新碱
	氟尿嘧啶	氟尿嘧啶
	硫唑嘌呤	达卡巴嗪
证据不足	长春瑞滨	长春瑞滨
	紫杉醇	依托泊苷
	吉西他滨	吉西他滨
	白介素	培美曲塞
	吉非替尼	异环磷酰胺
	阿伦珠单抗	贝伐单抗
	培美曲塞	吉非替尼
		阿伦珠单抗

生殖毒性治疗后性腺功能的评估

男性的评估

精液分析一直是评估男性性腺功能的基石，在儿童和青春期前男孩中使用促性腺激素（FSH，LH），抗 Millerian 激素（AMH）和抑制素-B 水平的测量。

AMH 由 sertoli 细胞产生，通过引起 Millerian 导管的消退影响男性的性分化[5]。在 9 岁后，AMH 水平下降表明雄激素对 sertoli 细胞和早期精子发生的影响[6]。在 9 岁以上的青春期前的男孩中，抑制素-B 和基础睾酮水平具有更大的相关性。间质细胞比生殖细胞对化疗的影响更具抵抗力，因此，患有癌症的儿童幸存者尽管是无精症，但可能有正常的睾酮[6]。

精液量，精子浓度，流动性和形态学是成年男性睾丸功能的标志。精子发生的标志物，如 FSH 和抑制素-B 水平波动很大，不能预测生殖结果。低或正常的睾酮水平以及伴随 LH 水平升高通常见于成年癌症幸存者[7]，但也受个体间变异差异性的影响，并且缺乏对微小但很重要的睾丸功能变化的检测敏感性。新的生物标志物，包括精子 mRNA，micro-RNA，组蛋白修饰和 DNA 甲基化模式正在开发中[7]。使用荧光原位杂交（FISH）和 DNA 片段化对精子进行遗传测试，鉴别性染色体中的染色体非整倍体，并评估性腺毒性治疗后 DNA 损伤的程度。在接受 BEP 化疗治疗睾丸癌和 ABVD 方案治疗霍奇金淋巴瘤的男性中，发现精子非整倍体的发生率较高[8,9]。非整倍体在几个月内可恢复到基准值，但一些患者在治疗后持续长达 2 年的异常。这些检测方法的未来影响将是耐人寻味的。

女性的评估

卵母细胞数量在出生时是固定的，不会再生[10]。年龄的增长和抗肿瘤治疗可以定量和定性地减少卵母细胞数并对生育能力产生不利影响。在保留生育功能之前评估卵巢储备很重要，尤其对于 35 岁以上女性。测量 FSH，抑制素 B，氯米芬枸橼酸盐激发试验，窦卵泡计数（AFC）和 AMH 评估卵巢储备并通过辅助生殖技术预测卵母细胞产量。月经周期早期卵泡期 FSH 升高（>20mIU/ml）表明卵巢储备受损并预测辅助受孕失败[11]。但是，FSH 水平在月经周期期间波动较大，且在青春期前的女孩中，FSH 和抑制素 B 水平都不可靠。可以通过经阴道超声来量化 AFC 以评估卵巢储备，但是对于测定卵母细胞质量或 IVF 预测妊娠结局没有帮助[12]。

卵巢窦卵泡的颗粒细胞产生 AMH，其血清水平是发育中卵巢卵泡数量的替代指标。AMH 水平随年龄增长逐渐下降直至更年期。和 FSH，抑制素 B 不同，血清 AMH 水平在月经周期内不会波动，并且在儿童中可靠[10]。

低血清 AMH 水平首先见于描述既往儿童期患有癌症的女性，她们仍然有规律的月经指示低卵巢储备[13]。高质量研究发现，乳腺癌和儿童 HD 幸存者的 AMH 水平较低，化疗周期数与血清 AMH 水平之间存在明显的剂量-反应关系[14,15]。使用烷化剂和骨盆/全身照射的治疗通常导致 AMH 水平较低甚或不可检测[16]。治疗前 AMH 水平低的乳腺癌患者在化疗后更容易发生闭经[17]。结合年龄和 AMH 水平的 Nomograms 已经建立，以预测新诊断的乳腺癌患者的化疗后卵巢恢复，并准确地评估对生育保留技术的需求。AMH 水平不能预测自然怀孕或妊娠结局。

化疗对性腺的影响

对男孩的影响

早期有关治疗的报道指出，对于青春前期和青春期的男孩，欠成熟的睾丸似乎对化疗引起的副作用有一定的抵抗力。然而，在不同的研究中，显著睾丸功能障碍的发生频率差异很大。三个主要因素决定了青春期前接受细胞毒性化疗的青春期前男孩睾丸损伤的程度：特定药物，药物的累积剂量和青春期。绝大多数男孩可正常通过青春期发育而不需要额外补充雄激素[18,19]。但是睾丸的体积可能会减小，而 LH 水平的升高也提示间质细胞有一定程度上的功能障碍[6]。

在小的不同患者人群的研究报道，单药环磷酰胺治疗后，甚至治疗几年后的患者能达到正常成年人精子数目的比率范围从 0~100% 不等[20,21]。一篇综述报道口服环磷酰胺的累积剂量为 0.7~52g 时，63 名受试的青春前期的男孩性腺损伤比例为 16%，而青春期受试男孩的性腺损伤比例可高达 67%[22]。应用苯丁酸氮芥单药或联合泼尼松、硫唑嘌呤治疗 6~15 岁的肾病患者，21 名患者中有 17 名在治疗终止后长达 11 年没有精子产生[23]。

大多数可用的数据与多药化疗有关。MOPP 化疗方案对患有霍奇金病的男孩青春期精子产生功能具有显著的损伤，这种损伤将会持续多年[19,24]。

一项关于对包括 456 名接受环磷酰胺治疗肾病、霍奇金病或白血病患者的 30 项研究进行的荟萃分析发现，在接受环磷酰胺剂量低于 400mg/kg（总剂量）的青春期前男孩中，只有不到 10%的人有性腺功能障碍，而在超过 400mg/kg 的青春期前男孩中，有 30%的人有性腺功能障碍[25]。在青春前期男孩中性功能障碍的发生率为 0～24%，但是性成熟的男生却上升到了 68%～95%。最近对 214 名接受烷化剂治疗的成年男性癌症幸存者的分析发现，少精子症和无精子症的发生率分别为 28%和 25%[26]。当累积环磷酰胺当量剂量（CED）小于 4 000mg/m^2 时，精子发生不太可能受损。CED 与无精子症和少精子症的风险与每 1 000mg/m^2 的增加而存在着显著的相关[26]。遗憾的是，对这些总趋势的了解不足和缺乏对任何特定患者的可靠预测都是有问题的。在青春期前的儿童中，即使是小剂量的烷基化药物也可能导致永久性的不孕症。

青春期男性睾丸间质细胞的功能是否受化疗的影响尚不清楚。据报道，在接受 MOPP 治疗的青春期男孩中出现了 FSH 和 LH 升高的男性乳房[19]。其他研究发现正常的基础和刺激的促性腺激素试验[18]，和异常的睾酮对人绒促性素（HCG）的反应是不常见的。最近的一项针对童年时期接受过霍奇金病治疗的 40 名男性的调查发现，32 名患者中有 29 名人促性腺激素分泌正常；28 名患者中有 26 名促性腺激素水平升高，但血清睾酮和第二性征正常。13 例经过测试的患者中有 11 例精子缺乏，并且这些改变在化疗后持续长达 17 年[27]。对 17 名儿童期患肉瘤并存活下来的成年人进行随访发现，其中 58%有精子缺乏，另外 30%精子减少，94%睾酮水平正常。然而，在睾酮水平正常的患者中有 40%促黄体素升高，所有患者中 92%促黄体素升高，提示不同程度的睾丸间质细胞功能不全[6]。虽然青春期前男孩化疗后的 LH，FSH 和血清睾酮水平可能是正常的，但急性淋巴细胞白血病或霍奇金病联合化疗后的睾丸活检通常显示生精小管损伤和间质纤维化。

对成年男性的影响

烷化剂单药应用时，可对输精管上皮产生永久性损伤。环磷酰胺总量达 9g 时可导致普遍的精子缺乏。总剂量达到 18g 时，这种精子缺乏通常是不可逆的[28]。霍奇金病患者接受联合治疗的多项研究，使用或不使用丙卡巴肼（procarbazine）的化疗，表明该药物具有独特的性腺毒性。在一项研究中，所有被研究的 19 例病例接受环磷酰胺、长春新碱（Oncovin）、丙卡巴肼及泼尼松（COPP）方案联合化疗，在化疗后 11 年仍然精子缺乏，而采用去除丙卡巴肼的 COPP 方案治疗的 10 例患者中，有 7 例患者在 3 年内精子生成恢复正常[29,30]。

甲氨蝶呤产生的长期生殖毒性最低。可用于评估长春新碱或长春碱的潜在危害的信息有限，但从 MOPP 化疗方案导致不育的发生率比联合氮芥、长春碱、丙卡巴肼、泼尼松（MVPP）方案略低可以推断，长春新碱的毒性比长春碱略低。尽管也没有单独应用柔红霉素的研究，但似乎柔红霉素与不包含环磷酰胺的方案联合时长期的毒副作用最小。而当与环磷酰胺联合用，柔红霉素可增强对性腺的毒性。长期应用硫唑嘌呤似乎并不影响精子质量。

随着治愈性联合化疗的出现，多个报道显示幸存者，尤其是幸存于霍奇金病和非精原细胞睾丸癌的患者会出现永久性不育。有观察显示，即使在化疗前已有多达 30%患霍奇金病和 50%患生殖细胞瘤的青年患者精子缺乏，精子活力和形态不正常者更多[31～33]，这一现象使得对现有研究的解释更加复杂。一项多变量分析的研究发现，红细胞沉降率升高和处于进展期是预测霍奇金患者化疗前不育的两个最好指标[34]。治疗前的 FSH 水平可为患生殖细胞肿瘤的年轻男性随后的精子产生情况提供一项有用的预测血清指标[35]。MOPP 或 MOPP 类的方案用于治疗霍奇金病在治疗过程中可导致所有的男性不育，并且治疗后能恢复的比例也很低（表 136-2）。在一项前瞻性研究中，37 例男性接受 MVPP 联合方案治疗，12 例在开始治疗前就有精子数量减少，治疗结束后的头 12 个月，所有接受 2 周期化疗后的患者的精子仍然缺乏[38]。更长时间的随访发现仅有 5%～15%的男性曾恢复精子产生。比较 MOPP 化疗方案与多柔比星、博来霉素、长春碱和达卡巴嗪（ABVD）化疗方案治疗霍奇金病的研究提供了令人信服的证据证实 ABVD 方案导致的性腺损伤更小[22,36]。

对于晚期霍奇金淋巴瘤患者，BEACOPP（博来霉素，依托泊苷，多柔比星，环磷酰胺，长春新碱，丙卡巴肼和泼尼松）被越来越多地使用。德国霍奇金研究小组（GHSG）发现无精子症的发生率在接受 8 个周期或 4 个周期的 BEACOPP 治疗的患者中明显较高比较了两个周期的 COPP/ABVD（分别为 93%、91%和 56%）[45]。近期有研究报道 13 例接受更新的 Stanford V 方案（包括长春碱、多柔比星、长春新碱、博来霉素、氮芥、依托泊苷和泼尼松）治疗后存活的 13 名男性患者共生育 19 次[43]。

尽管治疗非霍奇金淋巴瘤的相关数据非常少，但仍然有一些证据显示环磷酰胺、长春碱、泼尼松方案的毒性要小于 MOPP 方案[30]。近期的一项研究分析了 14 例男性患者接受长春新碱、多柔比星、泼尼松、依托泊苷、环磷酰胺和博来霉素联合治疗，结果显示这个方案是治疗非霍奇金淋巴瘤有效且相对无毒性的方案[47]。尽管白血病患者接受自体或异体骨髓移植可显著增加长期不育的风险，白血病治疗似乎毒性较小[71]。Kreuser 等发现 10 例年龄为 14～38 岁接受联合化疗的急性白血病的患者在维持治疗的第二年就已经 100%的恢复了[39,52]。

大多数男性睾丸肿瘤是少精子症。在一组前瞻性的研究中，Dradga 等报道 41 例患者中 77%的患者为少精症，17%的患者为无精症，仅有 6%的患者精子数足够可考虑冻存[48]。至少精子活动异常是常见的。在使用顺铂、长春碱和博来霉素治疗 2 个月后，无论是否使用多柔比星，Drasga 研究中 94%的男性为无精子症患者。

睾丸癌化疗后恢复精子产生是常见的。大多数的研究均显示精子产生的恢复呈时间依赖性，接近 50%的患者 2 年后可恢复部分产生精子的功能（表 136-2）[50,51]。更长期的随访结果没有发现不育或性功能减退的并发症发生[51]。生殖功能的恢复可能与顺铂的累积剂量有关。男性接受顺铂剂量超过 400mg/m^2 就有可能产生永久的不育。部分数据显示，在相同的情况下异环磷酰胺导致的不可逆转的不育要少于环磷酰胺[70,72]。

表 136-2　联合化疗对于性腺的作用

病种	治疗方案	病例数	精子缺乏/闭经/%
男性			
霍奇金病	MOPP(成人)[25,30,36]	150	73~95
	MOPP(青春期前)[25]	18	78
	MOPP(儿童)[25,37]	27	14~80
	ABVD[25]	13	0
	ChIVPP[27]	13	87
	MVPP[32,33,38~40]	210	84~100
	PACEBOM[41]	12	0
	NOVP[42]	21	5
	Stanford V[43,44]	79	<80
非霍奇金淋巴瘤	BEACOPP[45]	15	93
	COPP[46]	7	66~100
	VAPEC-B[30]	14	14
	MACOP-B[47]	15	0
睾丸癌	PVB[48,49]	112	15~28
	PVB+Dox[50,51]	36	17~39
	PEB[42]	42	12
急性白血病	标准剂量[52]	48	3~75
	大剂量[52,53]	104	14~32
肉瘤	Dox/MTX(rt)[54,55]	222	6~90
女性			
卵巢癌	P+其他[56~58]	66	0~8
乳腺癌	L-PAM+FU[59,60]	98	21~72
	CMF[61,62]	549	54~96
	丝裂霉素[63]	15	26
霍奇金病	MOPP(成人)[38,64]	95	55~71
	MOPP(青春期前)[25]	15	7
	MVPP[19]	72	36
	ABVD[27,36]	24	0
	PACEBOM[65]	15	0
	Stanford V[43,44]	63	<60
急性白血病	各种方案[66]	47	15
非霍奇金淋巴瘤	各种方案[67,68]	36	44
	大剂量[40,49,69,70]	怀孕的病例	

ABVD,多柔比星、博来霉素、长春碱、达卡巴嗪;ChIVPP,苯丁酸氮芥、长春碱、泼尼松、丙卡巴肼;CMF,环磷酰胺、甲氨蝶呤、氟尿嘧啶;COPP,环磷酰胺、长春新碱、泼尼松、丙卡巴肼;FU,氟尿嘧啶;MACOP-B,甲氨蝶呤、多柔比星、环磷酰胺、长春新碱、泼尼松、博来霉素;MOPP,氮芥、长春新碱、泼尼松、丙卡巴肼;MVPP,氮芥、长春新碱、泼尼松、丙卡巴肼;NOVP,米托蒽醌、长春碱、长春新碱、泼尼松;PACEBOM,多柔比星、环磷酰胺、依托泊苷、博来霉素、长春新碱、甲氨蝶呤、泼尼松;PEB,顺铂、依托泊苷、博来霉素;L-PAM,L-美法仑;PVB,顺铂、长春碱、伯劳霉素;PVB+Dox,顺铂、长春碱、博来霉素、多柔比星;VAPEC-B,长春新碱、多柔比星、泼尼松、依托泊苷、环磷酰胺、博来霉素。

男孩的睾丸间质细胞功能的抵抗力更强,且通常也有很好的代偿,所以尽管在这些男性中促性腺激素的水平升高很常见,但很少有人需要雄激素替代治疗[24,30]。临床不典型的睾丸间质细胞功能障碍可能存在未被充分验证的后遗症,包括心血管疾病过多,高胆固醇血症和肥胖,以及睾酮降低和 LH/FSH 升高[73]。

对青春前期女孩的影响

化疗对青春前期的女孩卵巢的影响是多变的,取决于治疗所用的药物,药物的剂量以及化疗持续的时间。单药环磷酰胺用于治疗非恶性疾病时,很少会导致青春期的延迟或永久的不孕[74]。接受丙卡巴肼和亚硝基胺治疗脑瘤的大多数女孩的生化检测显示原发性卵巢功能障碍,但是基本上所有的女孩均可正常进入和度过青春期。大多数的女性几年后卵巢功能可恢复正常,并且升高的促性腺激素水平回到正常基准。80%接受急性淋巴细胞白血病联合化疗的幸存者都顺利通过了青春期[75]。在一项大规模的针对童年时期癌症幸存者的随访调查中,出现提前闭经的风险是其姐妹的 13 倍,累积发生率在 40 岁前达到 8%[76]。这种风险增加与烷化剂剂量的升高、对卵巢进行放疗及诊断为霍奇金淋巴瘤相关。在尤因肉瘤患者中,67%的幸存者发生 POF,发生的中位时间为 5.7 年。所有接受盆腔放疗的患者均发生 POF[77]。

然而,在组织学上可看到肿瘤化疗对青春前期卵巢的损伤显著。在单药环磷酰胺或以阿糖胞苷为基础的抗白血病化疗后出现滤泡成熟受阻,基质纤维化,卵细胞数目减少都有报道。

对成年女性的影响

抗肿瘤药物对女性性腺功能的影响主要通过闭经,促性腺激素水平和长期生育率和生育结果来判断。接受抗急性白血病治疗的患者的尸检报告显示,初级卵泡数目没有区别,但次级卵泡显著减少[51]。临床上,接受这些药物化疗的女性出现 POF:如阴道干燥,性交困难,子宫内膜发育不全,性欲下降,潮热,月经减少甚至闭经,血清雌激素水平下降,代偿性血清卵泡刺激素和促黄体素水平升高[33,78]。

出现永久性闭经和不孕的概率取决于采用的药物及总剂量,是否合并放疗以及患者接受治疗时的年龄。在单药治疗的研究中,烷化剂是与 POF 关联最大的药物。小样本研究的报道显示,50%~75%的接受环磷酰胺治疗的女性在开始化疗一个月内出现闭经,但这一现象存在显著的年龄相关的敏感性。在一项研究中,出现闭经前给予的环磷酰胺总剂量,40 岁以上的女性是 5.2g,30~39 岁的女性是 9.3g,20~29 岁的女性是 20.4g。40 岁以下的女性有 50%月经恢复[63]。对于 40 岁以下的女性,月经恢复似乎与月经停止后应用的环磷酰胺量有紧密关联。

过去有研究显示,乳腺癌患者接受美法仑辅助化疗的患者出现显著的年龄相关的 POF;73%的 40~49 岁的女性患者在治疗过程中进展到绝经,但是 39 岁以下的女性患者绝经的只有 22%[59]。白消安或苯丁酸氮芥单药治疗相关的卵巢毒性也被证明和年龄、剂量相关[79,80]。

接受高剂量甲氨蝶呤辅助化疗的肉瘤患者相关的闭经现象不常见,而且血清促性腺激素水平在化疗中和化疗后都保持正常[54]。给予妊娠期患滋养细胞肿瘤的女性低剂量的甲氨蝶呤并没有出现显著的毒性。但英国的一项调查发现,接受化疗的女性闭经发生的时间比未接受化疗的女性早3年[81]。单药氟尿嘧啶、柔红霉素和博来霉素的耐受性也可能很好。

关于依托泊苷的数据较少,但是有报道称,一些女性接受该药治疗妊娠期肿瘤时可出现卵巢功能障碍[82]。

他莫昔芬具有轻微的类雌激素效应,可降低绝经前、后的乳腺癌患者促性腺激素的水平。月经不调很普遍,但持续性闭经的发病率不清楚。长期使用干扰素治疗各种良、恶性疾病的妇女,均有成功怀孕的报道[65]。

大部分关于化疗对性腺功能影响的信息都与联合化疗相关。在接受MOPP、MVPP或COPP治疗的女性霍奇金淋巴瘤患者中,闭经的发生率为15%~80%(表136-2)[29,35,44,83~85]。2/3的患者在化疗期间即出现闭经。目前尚未建立一个明确的剂量-反应关系模型。至少在一项研究中,接受MOPP方案治疗三个周期与六个周期的女性似乎没有差异[86]。开始治疗时的年龄已被证明是影响永久闭经发生率和闭经开始时间的一个重要因素。一般来说,25岁以上的女性患者在治疗期间,60%~100%出现永久闭经。25岁以下的女性患者中5%~30%在开始治疗的同时出现卵巢早衰,更多的女性在未来数月将出现闭经。更年轻的女性患者预计超过50%在5~10年的治疗中可能出现过早绝经[87]。初步报告表明,ABVD或多柔比星、环磷酰胺、依托泊苷、博来霉素、长春新碱、甲氨蝶呤和类固醇等治疗霍奇金病的替代方案延迟闭经的概率可能较低[38,56]。Horning等报告了19名接受Stanford V方案五的女性患者在治疗中怀孕24人次[43]。在一些小型的研究中,接受甲氨蝶呤、多柔比星、环磷酰胺、长春新碱、泼尼松、博来霉素治疗的侵袭性淋巴瘤女性患者仍能保持生育能力[41]。接受Mega-CHOP治疗4个疗程的NHL女性患者,有12人恢复了卵巢功能[88],这些患者中8人自然受孕。另一项对象为40岁以下接受CHOP方案治疗的非霍奇金淋巴瘤女性患者的研究中,36名患者中只有2人出现POF[89]。这些患者中有50%在首次疾病缓解期内怀孕。

接受包含顺铂方案治疗的生殖细胞肿瘤的女性患者,通常在治疗过程中会出现闭经,但90%以上的患者治疗结束后几个月内会恢复月经周期[57,90~92]。患有乳腺癌的妇女本身可能有与年龄有关的生育能力的下降,80%接受环磷酰胺,甲氨蝶呤氟尿嘧啶(CMF方案)治疗的患者在疗程的前10个月内会出现绝经[61,62]。接受CMF联合治疗的患者中出现绝经的平均比例,报道的范围为20%~100%[93]。接受多柔吡星和环磷酰胺的患者通常3个月内进入无排卵期,之后很快进入围绝经期。30岁以下,接受含多柔比星方案治疗的患者中只有少数有绝经现象,30~40岁之间约有1/3,而几乎所有40岁以上的患者会出现绝经。含表柔比星的治疗方案与之类似。多西他赛联合多柔比星和环磷酰胺的辅助化疗方案可导致平均年龄为49岁的患者中绝经的发生率为61%[94]。

高剂量化疗后的生育力

随着越来越多的年轻患者经受大剂量、骨髓抑制的化疗,个案报道和小样本研究显示只有极少数患者可恢复生育力。一项针对超过37 000名经历了一次自体或异体造血干细胞移植(SCT)的患者的回顾性调查示,仅有0.6%的患者后来成功怀孕[95]。随访187名先前接受过骨髓移植治疗的再生障碍性贫血或白血病年轻女性患者,发现了预期的环磷酰胺对卵巢功能的年龄依赖效应[53]。57%的女性患者在SCT后2.3年出现生育能力受损。144例患者中仅7%的患者恢复了生育能力,女性恢复生育能力的时间要比男性长。一项纵向研究,纳入217例儿童时期接受异体SCT的患者,经过2.6年中位随访时间,56%的男性生育能力受损,FSH/LH升高,低睾酮水平。15例患者中14例有无精症。SCT后3.4年,仅3%恢复生育能力[96]。因再生障碍性贫血行骨髓移植的患者整体较好,尤其是25岁以下患者。

放疗对性腺功能的影响

对男性的影响

对患有急性白血病的男孩的进行放射治疗是预防睾丸复发的标准疗法。低于1 200cGy的剂量不足以控制疾病,大多数诊疗规范建议对两个睾丸使用2 400cGy的剂量。在这个剂量下,大多数患者的睾丸间质细胞发生永久性损害,青春期延迟,睾酮水平经常明显降低,促性腺激素水平增加[97]。

在成人中,单次剂量400~600cGy的睾丸放疗可能会产生5年或更长时间的无精症[1]。对骨盆或下肢的分次放疗产生的散射也可能影响睾丸。Berthelsen评价了接受预防性放疗的精原细胞瘤患者,结果发现2/3产生了无精症,估计这些患者接受的散射剂量为20~130cGy[98]。Shapiro等已经证明即使接受低至27cGy的放疗,少精/无精症可持续长达24个月[99]。当辐射剂量超过2 000~3 000cGy时,成人睾丸间质细胞即发生功能障碍,同时伴有LH值升高,这可能需要激素替代治疗。大多数患者睾丸功能可以恢复,一系列的研究报道了希望生育的男子其伴侣怀孕成功率为37%~66%[100]。

骨髓移植后的全身放疗通常与永久无精症相关。继发不育与针对下丘脑或垂体的同期放化疗治疗颅内肿瘤有关[101]。对于接受辐射的男性幸存的生殖细胞是否会有永久性的影响仍存在争议,但大多数研究都不能证明子代恶性肿瘤的增加[102]。

对女性的影响

人类卵巢放射敏感性并没有像男性睾丸一样被准确地定义。原始的小卵母细胞被认为比大卵泡细胞敏感。卵巢的放射敏感性也呈剂量依赖性和年龄依赖性。在成年女性中,单次剂量500cGy能导致所有年龄的妇女月经紊乱。对于40岁以上的妇女,600cGy即可诱发绝经。如果分次照射超过6周,年龄20~30岁的女性可以耐受高达3 000cGy的剂量[103]。童年时子宫放疗增加了不孕、自发性流产、胎儿宫内生长迟缓的危险,所以即使保留卵巢功能仍无法保证生育能力。一项回顾性纳入162例Ⅱ~Ⅲ期结直肠癌患者,研究发现直肠癌患者闭经的发生率高于结肠癌患者,可能与直肠癌的盆腔放疗有关[104]。

靶向治疗对于性腺功能的影响

在分子靶向治疗的时代,一些新的药物类别已经进入临床使用,但是关于它们对生育能力影响的数据很少。此外,此类药物通常联合细胞毒性剂同时使用,尚未研究联合治疗对性腺功能的影响。

TKI 的影响

伊马替尼抑制对于 Leydig 细胞功能至关重要的 c-KIT,同时抑制对于生殖细胞迁移必需的血小板衍生生长因子受体(PDGFR)。c-KIT 和 PDGFR 也在卵母细胞中表达,并在卵泡生成和雌性生育中起重要作用。有报道显示在青春期前的男性中出现少精症,男子女性型乳房和睾丸衰竭[105]。有病例报告显示有男性出现少精症,但大多数男性可生育正常的后代[106]。接受伊马替尼治疗的妇女似乎可正常怀孕,但可能会增加先天性畸形的风险,因此建议在怀孕前停止治疗[107]。

在用克唑替尼治疗的男性中已经描述了性腺功能减退症和低睾酮的快速发作[108]。一项随访研究记录了低睾酮水平、性激素结合球蛋白、LH、FSH 和游离睾酮减少,表明中枢性腺功能减退症[109]。达沙替尼和舒尼替尼与男性乳房发育相关,但它们对生育能力的影响尚不清楚。

M-TOR 抑制剂的影响

西罗莫司和依维莫司(everolimus)也抑制 c-KIT。从器官移植患者推断出 m-TOR 抑制剂的生殖系统副作用。接受西罗莫司和依维莫司治疗的男性睾丸激素低,出现少精症,FSH 和 LH 升高,停止治疗后可恢复[110]。在用西罗莫司体外处理人卵巢皮质时发现颗粒细胞破坏卵母细胞,但既往有报道示 m-TOR 抑制剂介导的细胞凋亡是丧失卵母细胞的机制[111]。

单克隆抗体和免疫疗法的影响

阿伦珠单抗是一种针对 CD52 的单克隆抗体,可引起精子的固定和凝集,因为 CD52 也在精子表面表达[112]。伊匹木单抗阻断细胞毒性 T 淋巴细胞相关抗原 4(CTLA-4)和程序性细胞死亡-1(PD-1)受体阻断剂用于治疗黑色素瘤可引起垂体下垂和垂体功能低下。在伊匹木单抗在黑色素瘤的前期试验中,严重垂体功能低下的发生率低至 1.8%[113]。CTLA-4 和 PD-1 阻断的生殖毒性的发生率尚不清楚。

保护措施

男性的保护

长期以来,人们一直推测,通过激素调控来阻止精子生成可能会改善睾丸损伤,因为大多数化疗药物对分裂细胞有选择性毒性。在接受霍奇金淋巴瘤化疗的男性的临床试验中,两次使用 GnRH 类似物的尝试均未成功[114,115]。对于晚期霍奇金淋巴瘤合并化疗后希望生育的男性,ABVD 明显优于 MOPP38。使用 GnRH 类似物并不会缩短精子形成的恢复时间。Masala 等人记录了使用睾酮对环磷酰胺治疗的患者的一些保护作用。ASCO 指南表明,该程序是实验性的。

预期癌症治疗的男性应考虑精液冷冻保存。与非癌症对照相比,精子冷冻过程对癌症患者精子质量的危害并不更大[116]。由于治疗前患者经常存在精子质量异常,很多患者被认为并不适合做精子保存,但目前人工授精技术的改进使得很少的精子数量或很低的精子活力也能成功受孕[117]。在细致的生殖技术辅助下,这样受孕的成功率可达到 45%。而且,体外受精和随后的受精卵植入在更低的精子数量和活力[118]的情况下也取得了成功[101]。随着胞质内精子注射技术的进展,受孕的概率即使在精子数量极低的情况下也能大大提高。Garcia 比较了接受相同辅助生殖程序的恶性肿瘤患者和非癌症患者的胞质内精子注射的情况,结果发现癌症患者的累积妊娠率和累积活产率分别为 69% 和 62%,与非癌症患者相当[119]。据报道,在几个无精子症睾丸癌存活者中,使用睾丸活检获取的精子和在睾丸切除术时从输精管中提取的精子进行受精[120]。然而,许多中心报告说,选择保存精液的男性的总体成功率可能有限,并且可能受到精液质量以外的其他因素的影响。纽约纪念医院斯隆-凯特林癌症研究中心(Memorial Sloan-Kettering Cancer Center, MSKCC)的一个系列报告指出,69 名男性中有 48 名储存了精子,但治疗后 27 个月的中位数只有 11 人试图使用他们的精子进行人工授精。在这些人中,只有 3 人成功怀孕[117,121]。

对于青春期的男性,可采取阴茎震动取精和电激取精法[122]。有关睾丸循环隔离技术的初步研究显示,这种技术手段在小鼠模型中具有保护作用,并有可能用于人类的临床试验[123]。

据报道,睾丸精液取出术可使 55%~85% 各种原因引起的非梗阻性精子缺乏症男性精子恢复。Damani 等报道了一组化疗后的精子缺乏症患者,65% 的患者发现有存活的精子,其中 12 对患者夫妇总共进行了 26 次的胞质内精子注入,受孕率为 65%,目前为止所有新生儿都符合正常的检查标准[124]。

睾丸组织活检和精液冻存还处于试验阶段,正如从睾丸组织中分离生殖细胞储存技术一样。性腺屏蔽仍然是目前放射治疗防护的主要手段,尚没有令人信服的证据表明阴囊低温有保护作用。

女性的保护

和男性保护的假设相似,也有人提出使用口服避孕药或 GnRH 类似物抑制卵巢功能,为即将接受对卵巢有损伤作用的放疗或化疗的女性患者提供保护,一些动物模型证实了这一设想,无论是用于保护放疗还是化疗产生的卵巢损害[125]。然而类似的人类研究结果还存在争议,研究的病例数还相对较少。这些研究当中最有希望的是 Chapman 和 Sutcliffe 的报道,他们对计划接受 MVPP 方案治疗霍奇金淋巴瘤的女性患者应用口服避孕药,平均随访时间达 26 个月时,6 例患者中有 5 例恢复了月经[126]。

Pacheco 等给 12 例年龄在 15~20 岁之间,预计要接受抗淋巴瘤治疗的患者予醋酸亮丙瑞林治[127],具体为通过连续皮下注射缓释剂型来实施治疗前抑制,以克服卵巢功能抑制的推迟,注射每月一次直至化疗停止后一个月,结果所有 12 例患者均在 6 个月内恢复了正常的月经周期,其中有 3 人成功受孕,而没有接受醋酸亮丙瑞林抑制治疗的 4 例患者无一恢复月经周期。一项纳入了 6 项随机对照试验（RCT）的荟萃分析，主要研究 HD，卵巢癌和乳腺癌女性的生殖系统情况，化疗时使用 GnRH 类似物与恢复自然月经周期和排卵显著相关（OR 分别为 3.46、5.70）[128]。随后对仅包含乳腺癌患者的 RCT 进行的荟萃分析在预防 POF 和使用 GnRH 激动剂恢复自然月经周期方面得出了矛盾的结果[129~131]。一项评价淋巴结阳性绝经前女性乳腺癌患者辅助化疗疗效的大型研究发现（NSABP-B-30 研究），闭经期较长的患者有更好的无病生存率和总体生存率[132]。因此，乳腺癌患者通过卵巢抑制对于保留生育能力存在争议。

促排卵和胚胎冻存活产率最高，对于有稳定婚姻关系的女性是目前的最佳选择。受精前需要超数排卵，时间控制或人工控制激素水平均可以接受。移植率在 8%～30%。总的受孕率超过 60%[133]。

卵巢组织保存仍处试验阶段，但对于急需抗肿瘤治疗的患者可考虑尝试。卵巢皮质组织也具有包含大量卵泡的优势，因此增加了将来成功受孕的可能。卵巢组织最终可重新植回患者体内以恢复生殖能力，据报道植入的卵巢组织可以使患者恢复正常的月经周期[134]，甚至在残存卵巢皮质原位移植后有活产的报道。比利时一项研究，纳入 114 例接受冻卵的恶性肿瘤患者，33 例患者中共 49 次自然受孕，2 次人工受孕，中位随访时间 50 个月[135]。这种技术最终可能为年轻女孩以及性成熟的年轻女性提供选择。

近来用于筛选性腺毒性治疗后 POF 高风险患者的爱丁堡选择标准的有效性得到验证，可以用于筛选患者进行干预[136]。这些技术的医疗和伦理问题仍然有争议[137]。

对于要进行盆腔放疗的患者，可考虑行卵巢移位固定术，一般是在行探查术或开腹分期手术时把卵巢移到子宫底的后面或向侧方移出放射野以外，这样可使卵巢的照射剂量降低 90%，激素功能可保存 55%～99%。然而，生殖功能仍会受到损伤，可能是由于卵巢输卵管解剖学变异和散射线所致。一个小型研究显示，腹腔镜下骶前卵巢固定术可更好地保护卵巢的功能[138]。在这种情况下，可选择将其中一个卵巢移位而另一个卵巢切下冻存[139]。特殊的卵巢屏蔽装置在某些患者中可能有效。

儿童的保护

当前尚无被证实有效的可用于保护儿童将来生殖功能的方法，一些中心提供实验性的卵巢组织和睾丸组织冻存技术，但这个领域的研究面临许多伦理问题。目前可查到很多关于保留生殖功能的技术和伦理问题的优秀综述（表 136-3）[127,135]。

表 136-3 肿瘤患者保留生殖能力的选择

	男性	状态	女性	状态
儿童	睾丸组织冻存	未证实	卵巢组织冻存	未证实
成人	GnRH 类似物	未证实	GnRH 类似物	有效?
			口服避孕药	未证实
	精子冻存	被接受	卵细胞冻存	试验阶段
	睾丸取精术	试验阶段	卵巢组织冻存	可选用
			胚胎冻存	可选用
			卵巢组织移植	试验阶段

GnRH 类似物，促性腺激素释放激素。

妊娠结局

化学治疗

个别案例显示即使用最强烈的化疗方案后也有成功妊娠和生育的例子，无论是男性还是女性在肿瘤化疗后都不能肯定永久失去生育能力。几项回顾性的研究评估了在儿童或青少年时期完成化疗后怀孕女性的妊娠结局。

一项大的研究评估了儿童时期接受针对各种肿瘤化疗的患者的后代情况，发现总共 286 例之后怀孕生产的胎儿中，先天性异常的发生没有增加，对其中 24 例婴儿进行的染色体分析中 23 例是正常的[140]。先前患胚胎滋养层肿瘤并接受过化疗的女性，其妊娠也没有显示先天性胎儿异常、自然流产或新生儿死亡的风险有所增加[141]。

Holmes 评估了治疗霍奇金淋巴瘤的女性患者，并把 93 例接受化疗患者的妊娠和 288 例同胞对照组的妊娠相比较，总体而言，两组没有差异，但是在对同时接受放疗和化疗的患者进行分层分析时，发现似乎联合治疗更多地导致男性患者的妻子自发性流产，而接受联合治疗的女性患者后代发育异常似乎比对照组稍微多一些[142]。

大样本研究显示，男性患者化疗后的子女似乎正常，近 1 400 个这样的婴儿发生先天性异常的概率是 4%，和普通人群没有差别。这些异常大部分都是普通的，而非基因导致的异常[142]。

进一步的随访显示这些孩子的发育，成长以及学校表现都是正常的。一项美国国家癌症研究所的研究显示，与同胞匹配的对照组后代相比，经过化疗的患者其后代肿瘤发病率有轻微的升高但无统计学意义（0.3% vs 0.23%），这一数据和普通人群没有差别。但当根据年龄和性别来分析时，似乎患病年龄在

5 岁以下的男性肿瘤患者的后代肿瘤发病率高一些[143]。

化疗对子宫内胎儿的危险性取决于妊娠年龄、药物种类和剂量。叶酸拮抗剂不应在妊娠前三个月使用。其他抗代谢药物很少和先天畸形有关。妊娠前三个月暴露于氟尿嘧啶、环磷酰胺、白消安、苯丁酸氮芥与婴儿出生低体重或其他一些少见的先天异常有关[144]。有报道母亲使用蒽环类药物后婴儿出现心肌坏死[145]。伊马替尼被证实可导致动物的胎儿畸形,但是也有女性接受伊马替尼治疗时受孕并成功生育的个案报告。一孕妇无意中使用美罗华治疗后顺利生产一健康的婴儿[146]。在少数女性患者中,妊娠期间给予 IFN-α 治疗也被报道是安全的[147]。

化疗药物联合应用是否增加对胎儿的毒性尚没有定论。个案报道和小规模的研究显示在妊娠中晚期暴露于化疗药物会轻微增加胎儿畸形的风险性,但这些后代的长期发育是正常的[148,149]。化疗的非致畸作用(包括低出生体重、宫内生长迟缓,以及更多细微的发育异常)还有待明确。在子宫内暴露于己烯雌酚的女性婴儿生殖细胞透明细胞瘤的发生率增高,但子宫内化疗暴露对其他肿瘤的致癌作用还缺乏明确的文献报道,对这些儿童生殖潜能的影响也仍不清楚。

放射治疗

放射治疗对于基因的影响大部分数据都来源于原子弹爆炸的幸存者,尽管已经累积了大量他们的后代的数据,但对这些数据的解释要结合很多因素,特别要计算性腺实际的接受量。不过,估计接受量在 0.001 82 性腺雷姆(人类等量伦琴射线),即相当于 1 拉德(cGy)电离辐射产生的生物效应时,很明显胎儿异常(主要的先天性异常,死产、出生后一周内死亡)增加的比率较小。有报道称这些婴儿头围偏小[140],但在妊娠期间接受放疗的女性患者后代中这一异常发生率并非始终如一。

在接受横膈以下放射治疗的女性患者中,早产发生率高达 20%,另外低体重婴儿也有增加。这些不良事件主要发生在治疗后的一年内,提示也许是由于子宫局部或激素的因素而不是基因的缺陷所造成[46,150]。

在妊娠第二周到第八周器官形成期的婴儿接受照射发生畸形的风险最大,最主要的畸形包括生长迟缓、眼睛疾病以及小头畸形。安全剂量还没有确定,但是通常在妊娠的头 3 个月子宫的治疗剂量达到 10cGY 时建议进行流产。横膈上的放射治疗由于射线的散射仍可对胎儿造成影响,但大部分可通过腹部防护来防止,而在妊娠的头 3 个月接受颈部和腋窝的局部放射治疗可能是安全的[144]。

社会心理问题

社会心理问题,包括容貌变化,生育能力丧失,对下一代出生缺陷的担心,性功能减低以及肿瘤的复发,都会对单身患者面临约会和伴侣选择以及已婚患者如何维持稳定的夫妻关系产生重要影响,这些患者的离婚率是普通人的 4 倍[46,149,150]。细节内容超出了本问的范畴,有兴趣的读者可以找到很多这方面的优秀综述[42,149,151~155]。

对于性功能的生理评估,Andersen 提出了一个供评估者实施的模型,可以帮助预防一些问题的出现[42]。

总结

- 性腺功能异常和药物剂量以及年龄相关
- 年轻患者更易保留生育功能
- 烷化剂对各年龄组均有伤害
- 儿童接受化疗后无论性别,均正常进入青春期
- 传统内分泌水平的检测对于性腺毒性的判断不敏感
- 烷化剂毒性最高,尤其是丙卡巴肼
- 很多细胞毒性药物缺乏详细的研究数据
- 年轻 HD 患者最好接受 ABVD,取代 MOPP
- 围绝经期乳腺癌患者化疗后较易进入绝经状态
- 新药具有理论风险,但尚未得到充分研究
- 生育风险应该是化疗同意中讨论的一部分
- 经证实的保护男性生育能力的选择仅限于精液冷冻保存
- 许多患有 HD 或睾丸肿瘤的男性存在少精症
- 少精症亦可行低温保存
- 新的有效保留女性生育能力的方法有待进一步发展
- 孕三月之后暴露于大多数化疗药对于胎儿是安全的
- 孕期行化疗结局乐观
- 儿童时期化疗对于之后的怀孕影响一般
- 胎儿早期应避免暴露于叶酸拮抗剂

(杨晰 译 安菊生 校)

参考文献

The complete reference list can be found on the Wiley Companion Digital Edition of this title (see inside front cover for login instructions).

3 Gilman A. The initial clinical trial of nitrogen mustard. *Am J Surg*. 1963;**105**:574.

5 Josso N, Cate RL, Picard JY, et al. Anti-Müllerian hormone: the Jost factor. *Recent Prog Horm Res*. 1993;**48**:1–59.

7 Dere E, Anderson LM, Hwang K, Boekelheide K, et al. Biomarkers of chemotherapy-induced testicular damage. *Fertil Steril*. 2013;**100**:1192–1202.

10 Dewailly D, Andersen CY, Balen A, et al. The physiology and clinical utility of anti-Müllerian hormone in women. *Hum Reprod Update*. 2014;**20**(**3**):370–385.

16 Gracia CR, Sammel MD, Freeman E, et al. Impact of cancer therapies on ovarian reserve. *Fertil Steril*. 2012;**97**:134–140 e131.

17 Anderson RA, Cameron DA. Pre-treatment serum anti-Müllerian hormone predicts long term ovarian function and bone mass after chemotherapy for early breast cancer. *J Clin Endocrinol Metab*. 2011;**96**:1336–1339.

18 Shalet SM, Hann IM, Lendon M, et al. Testicular function after combination chemotherapy in childhood for acute lymphoblastic leukaemia. *Arch Dis Child*. 1981;**56**:275–278.

19 Whitehead E, Shalet SM, Jones PH, et al. Gonadal function after combination chemotherapy for Hodgkin's disease in childhood. *Arch Dis Child*. 1982;**47**:287–291.

24 Aubier F, Flamant F, Caillaud JM, et al. Male gonadal function after chemotherapy for solid tumors in childhood. *J Clin Oncol*. 1989;**7**:304–309.

26 Green DM, Liu W, Kutteh RW, et al. Cumulative alkylating agent exposure and semen parameters in adult survivors of childhood cancer: a report from the St Jude lifetime cohort study. *Lancet Oncol*. 2014;**15**:1215–1223.

34 Rueffer U, Breuer K, Josting A, et al. Male gonadal dysfunction in patients with Hodgkin's disease prior to treatment. *Ann Oncol*. 2001;**12**:1307–1311.

36 Viviani S, Santoro A, Ragni G, et al. Gonadal toxicity after combination chemotherapy for Hodgkin's disease: comparative results of MOPP vs ABVD. *Eur J Cancer Clin Oncol*. 1985;**21**:601–605.

43 Horning SJ, Hoppe RT, Breslin S, et al. Stanford V and radiotherapy for locally extensive and advanced Hodgkin's disease: mature results of a prospective clinical trial. *J Clin Oncol*. 2002;**20**:630–637.

44 Horning SJ, Hoppe RT, Kaplan HS, Rosenberg SA. Female reproductive potential

after treatment for Hodgkin's disease. *N Engl J Med*. 1981;**304**:1377–1382.

45 Sieniawski M, Reineke T, Josting A, et al. Assessment of male fertility in patients with Hodgkin's lymphoma treated in the German Hodgkin study group (GHSG) clinical trials. *Ann Oncol*. 2008;**19**:1795–1801.

48 Drasga RE, Einhorn LH, Williams SD, et al. Fertility after chemotherapy for testicular cancer. *J Clin Oncol*. 1983;**1**:179–183.

51 Hansen PV, Trykker H, Helkjaer PE, Andersen J. Testicular function in patients with testicular cancer treated with orchiectomy alone or orchiectomy plus cisplatin-based chemotherapy. *J Natl Cancer Inst*. 1989;**81**:1246–1250.

54 Shamberger RC, Rosenberg SA, Siepp CA, Sherins RJ. Effects of high-dose methotrexate and vincristine on ovarian and testicular functions in patients undergoing post-operative adjuvant treatment of osteosarcoma. *Cancer Treat Rep*. 1981;**65**:739–746.

64 Santoro A, Bonadonna G, Valagussa P, et al. Long-term results of combined chemotherapy-radiotherapy approach in Hodgkin's disease: superiority of ABVD plus radiotherapy versus MOPP plus radiotherapy. *J Clin Oncol*. 1987;5:27–37.

66 Meirow D. Reproduction post-chemotherapy in young cancer patients. *Mol Cell Endocrinol*. 2000;**169**:123–131.

70 Dominik B, Burkhard FC, Mills R, et al. Fertility and sexual function following orchiectomy and 2 cycles of chemotherapy for stage I high risk nonseminomatous germ cell cancer. *J Urol*. 2001;**165**:441–444.

73 Meinardi MT, Gietema JA, van der Graaf WTA, et al. Cardiovascular morbidity in long-term survivors of metastatic testicular cancer. *J Clin Oncol*. 2000;**18**:1725–1732.

75 Quigley C, Cowell C, Jimenez M, et al. Normal or early development of puberty despite gonadal damage in children treated for acute lymphocytic leukemia. *N Engl J Med*. 1989;**321**:143–151.

89 Elis A, Tevet A, Yerushalmi R, et al. Fertility status among women treated for aggressive non-Hodgkin's lymphoma. *Leuk Lymphoma*. 2006;**47**:623–627.

90 Marchetti M, Romagnolo C. Fertility after ovarian cancer treatment. *Eur J Gynaecol Oncol*. 1992;**13**:498–501.

93 Bines J, Oleske DM, Cobleigh MA. Ovarian function in premenopausal women treated with adjuvant chemotherapy for breast cancer. *J Clin Oncol*. 1996;**14**:1718–1729.

94 Martin M, Pienkowski T, Mackey J, et al. Adjuvant docetaxel for node-positive breast cancer. *N Engl J Med*. 2005;**352**:2302–2313.

96 Pfitzer C, Orawa H, Balcerek M, et al. Dynamics of fertility impairment and recovery after allogeneic hematopoietic stem cell transplantation in childhood and adolescence: results from a longitudinal study. *J Cancer Res Clin Oncol*. 2015;**141**(**1**):135–142.

109 Weickhardt AJ, Doebele RC, Purcell WT, et al. Symptomatic reduction in free testosterone levels secondary to crizotinib use in male cancer patients. *Cancer*. 2013;**119**:2383–2390.

111 McLaughlin M, Patrizio P, Kayisli U, et al. mTOR kinase inhibition results in oocyte loss characterized by empty follicles in human ovarian cortical strips cultured in vitro. *Fertil Steril*. 2011;**96**(**5**):1154–1159.

116 Hallak J, Kolettis PN, Sekhon VS, Thomas AJ, Agarwal A. Sperm cryopreservation in patients with testicular cancer. *Urology*. 1999;**54**:894–899.

124 Damani MN, Masters V, Meng MV, et al. Postchemotherapy ejaculatory azoospermia: fatherhood with sperm from testis tissue with intracytoplasmic sperm injection. *J Clin Oncol*. 2002;**20**:930–936.

127 Pacheco BP, Ribas JMM, Milone G, et al. Use of GnRH analogs for functional protection of the ovary and preservation of fertility during cancer treatment in adolescents: a preliminary report. *Gynecol Oncol*. 2001;**81**:391–397.

139 Martin JR, Kodaman P, Oktay K, Taylor HS. Ovarian cryopreservation with transposition of a contralateral ovary: a combined approach for fertility preservation in women receiving pelvic radiation. *Fertil Steril*. 2007;**87**:189.e5–189.e7.

150 Doll DC, Ringenberg S, Yarbro JW. Management of cancer during pregnancy. *Arch Intern Med*. 1988;**148**:2058–2064.

第 137 章 性功能障碍

Leslie R. Schover, PhD

概述

与癌症有关的性问题通常是由治疗导致的生理性损害引起的，但由于沟通不良、关系冲突或先前存在的性功能障碍等社会心理问题会使性问题加剧。据估计，美国约有 1 400 万癌症幸存者，其中有 2/3 的人受到性功能障碍的影响，其中超过 50% 的人接受盆腔或乳腺肿瘤的治疗，至少 25% 的人接受其他部位的治疗。最佳治疗是多学科的，解决身体损害和应对技能。如果存在一种承诺的关系，最好让伴侣参与到指导和干预中来。

历史的角度

自 20 世纪 50 年代以来，我们一直认为性功能障碍是癌症治疗一种并发症。早期的研究侧重于彻底清除乳房肿瘤的手术，会造成患者身体形象受损和女性特征的丧失[1]。后来研究表明，系统性治疗的作用要比乳腺局部治疗大得多[2]。

20 世纪 80 年代，学者们重新设计根治性盆腔手术方案，以保留阴茎血流和自主神经[3]。然而，保留神经的根治性前列腺切除术仅使不到 25% 的男性恢复勃起功能[4]。近期研究发现机器人辅助腹腔镜前列腺切除术（RALP）可以提高神经保留的精准性，并提高正常勃起恢复的能力。尽管 RALP 缩短了患者住院时间，减少了急性并发症发生，但两项使用医疗保险和监测、流行病学和最终结果（SEER）数据库的大型研究发现，与开放式手术相比，RALP 在保留性功能方面和减少尿失禁方面没有优势[5,6]。

为了将盆腔放射治疗的性功能并发症降到最低，研究者开始尝试引入近距离治疗[7]或用于外束治疗的计算机化的三维适形场[8]。但研究发现仍不能长期维持性功能，后来使用调强放射疗法或质子治疗也得到类似结果[8,9]。

从 20 世纪 80 年代，人们逐渐在妇科恶性肿瘤治疗过程中认识到性功能问题[10]。在手术或辅助放射治疗期间，人们也像对待男性患者一样试图保留影响性快感和产生性功能的神经和组织[9]。然而，越来越多的人认识到卵巢早衰和盆腔放疗引起的外阴阴道萎缩加重是造成性功能障碍的重要危险因素[11]。认知行为性疗法是一种短期的、以行动为导向的心理治疗方法[12]。研究人员对男性和女性癌症患者采用了这种疗法，包括努力提高互相关系的满意度和性沟通[13]。

然而，目前只有不到 20% 的癌症患者/幸存者有性功能问题时寻求帮助[14,15]。只有少数癌症治疗中心能为性功能问题提供治疗，因此性功能障碍仍然是癌症幸存者长期未得到解决的问题[16,17]。

尽管于 20 世纪 50 年代开始就对癌症相关的性问题开始关注，但大多数男、女患者仍然没有为他们的性功能问题寻求专业帮助，并且通过试图更改癌症治疗方案来避免性功能障碍发生的尝试也没有取得令人满意的结果。

发病率和流行病学-地方和全球

据估计，约 59% 美国 1 400 万男性肿瘤患者和 66% 接受盆腔或乳房肿瘤治疗的女性肿瘤患者中[18]，其中至少 50% 的患者发生严重的长期性功能障碍[19]。在非生殖系统肿瘤（包括血液恶性肿瘤[20]和儿童肿瘤）治疗的患者中，至少 25% 会出现性功能问题[21,22]。

在欧洲和其他工业化国家，癌症患者中性功能障碍的发生风险也类似[23]。在医疗资源较差的美国关于肿瘤患者性功能障碍发生的数据非常少，但在这些国家里发生人类免疫缺陷病毒（HIV）和人类乳头状病毒（HPV）引起的如宫颈癌，外阴、肛门和阴茎癌更常见，可能具有更高的性病的生[24]。在农村地区，患性相关疾病的诊断可能导致离婚和受到排挤[25]。

与癌症有关的性问题是严重和普遍的，包括对性的欲望或性唤起丧失和达到高潮的能力缺失，以及遭受疲劳、疼痛或尿失禁的影响[19]。没有接受专业的治疗，大多数问题不会随着时间而解决。大多数性功能障碍是由癌症治疗引起[19]，包括骨盆自主神经受损、性唤起期间生殖器血流减少[3,4]（尤其是男性）[26]以及骨盆放疗对生殖器官血管和组织的直接损伤[9]。男性勃起功能障碍也是由于手术或放疗导致生殖器官血流量减少所致[9]。如果没有正常的含氧血液流入，阴茎的勃起组织就会萎缩。结酚酞致血液从静脉系统流出，降低勃起的硬度[27]。

尽管女性的阴道会扩张，阴蒂会随着性唤起膨胀[28]，但对其中血流动力学的原理却知之甚少。雌激素缺乏在女性性功能问题中起着重要的作用[19,29,30]，减少了阴道黏膜在性唤起过程中产生润滑。随着外阴阴道萎缩，造成性交爱抚和插入疼痛，经常如此导致性欲丧失和性高潮困难[31]。

无论男性还是女性，性欲的丧失往往导致最终避免性接触[19]。低雄激素水平有时是导致男性性欲重要因素，例如在前列腺癌的抗雄激素治疗期间[32]，化疗后或[33]放疗对睾丸造成损伤[34]。

癌症治疗的毒副作用会导致严重和长期的性功能障碍，影响包括影响性欲、性唤起、性高潮和疼痛。

风险因素——发病前性功能、癌症治疗和行为特点

很多患者(尤其是男性)在癌症诊断之前就有性功能方面的问题。勃起功能障碍与年龄相关的心血管疾病、高血压、糖尿病、吸烟、久坐不动的生活方式和肥胖密切相关[35,36]。勃起功能障碍是也老年夫妇停止性生活的最常见原因[37]。在50岁以上的女性中,至少有一半因为缺少功能性的性伴侣而不再有性行为[38]。在癌症诊断时有活跃的性生活的男女患者会增加对新的性问题忧虑[39,40]。

癌症治疗相关性功能障碍的高危因素包括密集化疗,全身照射,同种异体移植后移植物抗宿主病[41],治疗导致绝经前妇女卵巢衰竭[30],盆腔放疗[9],男性根治性盆腔肿瘤的手术[4~6,42],盆腔肿瘤的放化疗[43],前列腺癌的抗雄治疗[32],乳腺癌芳香化酶的抑制剂[40]。虽然阴茎癌和外阴癌在西方国家很少见,但切除生殖组织主要部位的根治性手术显然也会造成此类问题[44,45]。晚期宫颈癌或直肠癌的阴道重建后常常不能恢复女性的性快感[46]。

社会心理或行为因素也会导致癌症相关的性功能障碍。有性虐待史或创伤史的患者可能难以应对癌症治疗,尤其是在生殖系统中存在恶性肿瘤的情况下[47]。人际关系冲突和沟通不良也与不良的结果有关。传统的男性观念和压抑的情绪可能会导致前列腺癌治疗后性功能的恶化[48]。神经质是一种涉及抑郁和焦虑的人格特征。无论是在神经质上评分高的男性还是女性,都有更高的患癌后性功能问题的发生[49,50]。

预防——手术、药物、行为治疗

为了预防性功能障碍,癌症手术方式的改进包括保留前列腺自主神经[3~6],不仅在根治性前列腺切除术中,而且在根治性膀胱切除术或结肠直肠癌手术中也保留自主神经[42,51]。虽然在盆腔手术中避免了对阴茎副动脉的损伤[52],但此治疗效果有限。动物研究和理论模型支持利用促进阴茎血流方法恢复阴茎的功能,但对人类勃起功能恢复的益处尚不明确。保留神经的根治性子宫切除术对女性性功能影响不大。保留组织的手术已经被用来代替阴茎局部切除术来治疗局限性阴茎癌或代替根治性手术来治疗女性外阴癌[45,53],但大多数患者仍然会发生性功能问题。在保持女性的性快感和性欲方面,保乳或乳房重建术相比乳房切除术也没有优势[2]。

采用保留年轻女性卵巢功能的治疗方法,如对低级别卵巢癌保守治疗[54]或仅局部治疗原位导管癌[55],能保持多数女性的正常性生活。化疗会增加男性[33]和女性[56]的性功能障碍,但毒性较低的方案很少能达到相同的生存获益。一个治疗例外是用非烷基类药物治疗早期霍奇金淋巴瘤[57]。个体化治疗和应用生物反应调节剂的治疗趋势可能最终会降低性功能障碍发病,但关于其副作用信息很少。

行为治疗措施可能有助于预防癌症相关的性问题。保持性活跃或使用真空勃起装置或阴道扩张器拉伸生殖器官可以防止发生萎缩[27,58,59]。促进更积极的性问题交流和持续的亲密行为,可以防止夫妻关系中满足感的减低或自尊的降低[60,61]。

> 癌症后性功能障碍的危险因素包括:
> - 强化化疗
> - 因癌症治疗导致的性腺功能减退
> - 生殖器组织部位的切除
> - 性创伤史
> - 关系冲突
> - 人格因素,如神经质或传统性别信仰
>
> 预防措施可能包括:
> - 更保守的癌症手术
> - 毒性更小的化疗
> - 使用行为策略来保护生殖器组织或增进亲密度

筛查

在癌症持续治疗过程中,应该关注和筛查患者性功能问题。在制订治疗方案期间,应对患者解释癌症治疗可能对性功能的潜在损害,包括告知其他保守治疗方式。尽管大多数患者将生存排在性功能之前,但也有少数患者为了保持性功能而选择一种肿瘤控制较差的治疗方式。在治疗和随访期间,应监测患者性功能,至少应定期提出问题,例如:"在一项针对姑息治疗患者的研究中,尽管性功能问题的发生率非常高,但约有一半的人想继续维持性生活"[62]。2013年,一项新的美国综合癌症网络生存指南建议通过访谈或问卷形式对患者性功能障碍进行系统筛查,然后进一步进行评估和推荐治疗方案。尽管该指南被归类为癌症幸存者名目,但它包括了医院的所有患者[63]。

一份简短的问卷可以用来筛查性功能障碍。美国国家癌症研究所(National Cancer Institute)赞助创建了"患者报告结果测量信息系统(Patient-reporting Outcomes Measurement Information System)。男女性功能调查。这些分别有8项和10项的多项调查问卷,只需要询问相关内容,就可以制作一个完整的量表或使用计算机自适应软件进行管理[64]。

诊断

因为性功能障碍最典型的诊断方法是自我报告,所以诊断术语一直存在争议[65]。许多术语并不能帮助临床医生基于循证的治疗方法。可以通过以方面下将性功能障碍归类:

- 渴望性和体验主观刺激的能力
- 性器官在性唤起时充血的能力(如男性勃起,女性阴道润滑和扩张)
- 体验令人满意的高潮的能力
- 疼痛干扰性快感的问题
- 性交时尿失禁或大便失禁

大多数接受癌症治疗的患者都有不止一个特定的性问题。例如,一名因局部宫颈癌而接受放化疗的妇女可能会出现外阴阴道萎缩和阴道狭窄,通过性爱抚或插入引起干涩和急性疼痛。因此,她对性的渴望和达到高潮的能力也受到了影响。前列腺根治性切除术后,男性可能无法获得或保持勃起功能。尿液也可能随性兴奋和高潮从阴茎中滴落。如果他使用药物治

疗勃起,他可能会意识到阴茎已经缩小或弯曲[66]。这些问题导致他避免性生活。

花时间全面描述患者的性功能问题仍然是诊断最重要方面。对女性来说,进行盆腔检查时注意外阴和阴道内的疼痛和萎缩是至关重要的。对于勃起功能障碍的男性患者,泌尿科医生可能会在阴茎勃起之前和之后注射药物以对阴茎进行彩色多普勒超声成像的检查[68]。这种检测可查明因勃起组织萎缩而引起的静脉功能障碍,这可能会限制口服药物或阴茎注射治疗的疗效。然而,许多泌尿科医生根据经验开出治疗勃起功能障碍的处方,从口服药物开始,必要时进行阴茎注射治疗、真空负压吸引或尿道栓剂,最后一步是使用阴茎假体[69]。在许多老年男性患者中,心血管疾病负担增加癌症相关的性问题的治疗复杂程度[70]。

> 性功能问题筛查和诊断应该是多学科的,使用简短的问卷调查、仔细的访谈和相关的重点检查,以全面了解问题的类型及其医学和社会心理原因。

预后因素

仅发现少数与性功能恢复相关的预后因素。在癌症确诊前没有性生活的男性或女性在癌症确诊后不太可能寻求帮助,除非他们之前曾为自己的问题寻求过治疗[37,40]。刚开始勃起正常的年轻男性在前列腺癌手术后更痛苦,更有可能寻求帮助[71]。有一个仍然享受性爱的伴侣也是至关重要的[72]。对女性来说,保持性关系是寻求帮助的关键[40]。

性沟通不良是认知行为治疗性功能问题的障碍[13]。事实上,有问题的夫妻更不可能进行性咨询的临床试验[73,74]。目前还没有针对单身或同性伴侣治疗的研究结果[75,76]。

> 由于研究的重点是短期的医疗或咨询治疗,所以治疗成功的障碍包括有性功能病史、缺乏有动力的伴侣和性沟通不良。

多学科治疗

研究表明,结合医学和社会心理护理的多学科治疗方法是治疗癌症相关的性问题最有效的办法[72,74]。表 137-1 列出了常见的性问题和建议的治疗方案。恢复令人满意的性生活需要良好的沟通[104,105],亲密关系可能包括非性交的性刺激[72,74,104],以及应对某些“表演”的限制能力。另一方面,在没有任何医疗治疗的情况下,通过简短的咨询服务可能会减少对性问题的困扰,或在一定程度上提高性满意度,但不能最终解决性功能障碍问题[72,105,106]。

表 137-1 男性和女性常见癌症相关性问题的多学科护理组成部分

性问题	患者教育	简短的性咨询	生理治疗
男性低欲望	问题往往是多因素的,而不仅仅是荷尔蒙(对勃起、疲劳、药物治疗、糟糕的形象感到羞愧)	帮助那些失去男性自尊,形象不佳,关系冲突的人	雄激素替代只有性腺功能减退[33,34],前列腺癌术后有争议[77],改变可能有作用的药物
勃起功能障碍	衰老,病前危险因素和癌症治疗都会损害勃起	帮助做出有关医疗保健的决策;包括合作伙伴;帮助进行性交流以提高依从性[14,78]	PDE5 抑制剂,真空勃起装置,阴茎注射疗法,尿道栓剂[78],阴茎假体手术[79]
性高潮快感的变化	癌症治疗可能导致性高潮没有勃起或射精,性高潮感觉减弱,无法达到性高潮(中枢神经系统受损)[66]	重新学习如何达到性高潮,或加强感觉,使用振动器或色情诱惑[80]	治疗性腺功能减退或高催乳素血症,改变可能干扰性高潮的药物[80,81]
早泄	如果需要长时间的刺激来勃起,然后快速射精,勃起功能障碍可以被误认为是早泄	性治疗方法,如停止开始或挤压[80]	口服药物,虽然不是很有效[80],治疗勃起功能障碍可能会纠正问题[80]
阴茎弯曲	癌症治疗可以产生阴茎弯曲,通过勃起和曲率变化了解疼痛的时间线[82]	关于抑郁和身体形象问题的咨询	使用医学治疗来减少弯曲;使用或不使用阴茎假体手术矫正曲率[82]
在性爱中疼痛	性生活中生殖器疼痛的原因及慢性非生殖器疼痛对性生活的干扰	感知焦点练习或正念,专注于性快感和远离疼痛[83]	用药物或其他方式治疗慢性非生殖器疼痛;高潮或睾丸疼痛的医学治疗[84,85]
在性行为中失禁	如果有造口,请咨询专业护士,尽量减少对性的干扰;根治性前列腺切除术后常见的尿失禁	关于应对失禁性行为,使用床垫和其他辅助工具的法律顾问	口服药物或阴茎紧张环以防止性交期间尿漏[86],注射胶原蛋白[87];次插入人工括约肌的手术[88],使用饮食和药物控制大便失禁[89]

续表

性问题	患者教育	简短的性咨询	生理治疗
女性低欲望	理解这个问题往往是多因素的，而不仅仅是荷尔蒙[90]	帮助身体形象不佳，关系冲突，应对创伤性经历的历史[47]，应对慢性疲劳和生活压力	治疗可能导致避免性生活的疼痛[67,74] 更改可能有作用的药物[90]；雄激素替代治疗很少有帮助，可能会增加患乳腺癌的风险[91]
外阴阴道干燥和性交疼痛	外阴阴道萎缩在正常绝经后很常见，在一些癌症治疗后更严重[67,74]	咨询医疗选择和更好的性刺激和沟通，以最大限度地提高性唤起，渗透的位置可能有助于避免疼痛[67,80,92]	在性活动期间经常使用阴道保湿剂和水或有机硅润滑剂[67,74]，使用渐变阴道扩张器[59,93]，如果癌症对激素不敏感，则使用低剂量阴道雌激素[94]，鱼精蛋白[95]
难以达到性高潮	女性通常通过阴蒂刺激更容易达到性高潮，遗传有助于达到性高潮[96]	通过自我刺激或振动器达到性高潮的训练；过渡到伴侣性交[37]	可能干扰性高潮的药物变化[81,97]
在性行为中失禁	如果有造口，请咨询专业护士，尽量减少对性的干扰；尿失禁通常会干扰性生活[98]，盆腔放射后大便失禁[99]	膀胱行为训练和骨盆底治疗[100]	使用口服药物[101]或填充剂[102]预防尿漏；神经源性过度活跃膀胱的骶神经调节[103]；使用饮食和药物控制大便失禁[89,99]

遗憾的是，即使在综合性癌症中心，包括心理学家和医生在内提供综合治疗的专业诊所也很少见。接受过心理肿瘤学培训的心理健康专业人士通常缺乏治疗性功能障碍的专业知识。大多数性治疗师对癌症及其治疗知之甚少。

心理社会因素与管理

除了已经提到的心理社会因素，临床医生还应该评估文化[25]、性取向[75,76]、种族[107~109]和宗教对性问题的影响。如果治疗措施与患者的性态度不相符，就不可能有良好的治疗结果。

生存和随访

在生存期间持续的评估性功能问题非常重要，特别是考虑到癌症相关性功能障碍的可能会长期存在。

未满足的需求、未来的方向和结论

虽然性问题经常被认为是一种不幸发生的癌症治疗产生的轻微副作用，却影响了25%~50%的癌症存活者，并对其生活质量产生了负面影响。在评估成本效益解决方案，患者教育和多学科治疗的方面仍需要改进。对于具有一定文化水平的患者，可以通过高质量的在线咨询提供教育和自助帮助[72,74]。来自医疗服务欠缺社区的患者可能需要寻求咨询师[108]或患者引导员的额外指导。当一线干预措施不能解决性功能问题时，可以使用分步护理方法来转介患者接受更高级的治疗。

（陈东 译 邢念增 校）

参考文献

The complete reference list can be found on the Wiley Companion Digital Edition of this title (see inside front cover for login instructions).

4 Salonia A, Burnett AL, Graefen M, et al. Prevention and management of post-prostatectomy sexual dysfunctions. Part 1: choosing the right patient at the right time for the right surgery. *Eur Urol*. 2012;**62**:261–272.

5 Hu JC, Gu X, Lipsitz SR, et al. Comparative effectiveness of minimally invasive vs open radical prostatectomy. *JAMA*. 2009;**302**:1557–1564.

9 Incrocci L, Jensen PT. Pelvic radiotherapy and sexual function in men and women. *J Sex Med*. 2013;**10(Suppl 1)**:53–64.

12 Schover LR, Evans RB, von Eschenbach AC. Sexual rehabilitation in a cancer center: diagnosis and outcome in 384 consultations. *Arch Sex Behav*. 1987;**16**:445–461.

14 Prasad MM, Prasad SM, Hevelone ND, et al. Utilization of pharmacotherapy for erectile dysfunction following treatment for prostate cancer. *J Sex Med*. 2010;**7**:1062–1073.

15 Hill EK, Sandbo S, Abramsohn E, et al. Assessing gynecologic and breast cancer survivors' sexual health care needs. *Cancer*. 2011;**117**:2643–2651.

17 Holm LV, Hansen DG, Johansen C, et al. Participation in cancer rehabilitation and unmet needs: a population-based cohort study. *Support Care Cancer*. 2012;**20(29)**:13–24.

19 Schover LR, van der Kaaij M, van Dorst E, Creutzberg C, Huyghe E, Kiserud CE. Sexual dysfunction and infertility as late effects of cancer treatment. *EJC Suppl*. 2014;**12**:41–53.

21 Bober SL, Zhou ES, Chen B, Manley PE, Kenney LB, Recklitis CJ. Sexual function in childhood cancer survivors: a report from Project REACH. *J Sex Med*. 2013;**10**:2084–2093.

26 Pieterse QD, Kenter GG, Maas CP, et al. Self-reported sexual, bowel and bladder function in cervical cancer patients following different treatment modalities: longitudinal prospective cohort study. *Int J Gynecol Cancer*. 2013;**23**:1717–1725.

27 Fode M, Ohl DA, Ralph D, Sønksen J. Penile rehabilitation after radical prostatectomy: what the evidence really says. *BJU Int*. 2013;**112**:998–1008.

31 Kingsberg SA, Wysocki S, Magnus L, Krychman ML. Vulvar and vaginal atrophy in postmenopausal women: findings from the REVIVE (REal Women's VIews of Treatment Options for Menopausal Vaginal ChangEs) survey. *J Sex Med*. 2013;**10**:1790–1799.

33 Kiserud CE, Schover LR, Dahl AA, et al. Do male lymphoma survivors have

impaired sexual function? *J Clin Oncol*. 2009;**27**:6019-6026.

38 Lutfey KE, Link CL, Rosen RC, Wiegel M, McKinlay JB. Prevalence and correlates of sexual activity and function in women: results from the Boston Area Community health (BACH) survey. *Arch Sex Beh*. 2009;**38**:514-527.

39 Steinsvik EA, Axcrona K, Dahl AA, Eri LM, Stensvold A, Fosså SD. Can sexual bother after radical prostatectomy be predicted preoperatively? Findings from a prospective national study of the relation between sexual function, activity and bother. *BJU Int*. 2012;**109**:1366-1374.

40 Schover LR, Baum GP, Fuson LA, Brewster A, Melhem-Bertrandt A. Sexual problems during the first 2 years of adjuvant treatment with aromatase inhibitors. *J Sex Med*. in press.

41 Wong FL, Francisco L, Togawa K, et al. Longitudinal trajectory of sexual functioning after hematopoietic cell transplantation: impact of chronic graft-versus-host disease and total body irradiation. *Blood*. 2013;**122**:3973-3981.

44 Kieffer JM, Djajadiningrat RS, van Muilekom EA, Graafland NM, Horenblas S, Aaronson NK. Quality of life in patients treated for penile cancer. *J Urol*. 2014;**192**:1105-1110.

46 Scott JR, Liu D, Mathes DW. Patient-reported outcomes and sexual function in vaginal reconstruction: a 17-year review, survey, and review of the literature. *Ann Plast Surg*. 2010;**64**:311-314.

55 Bober SL, Giobbie-Hurder A, Emmons KM, Winer E, Partridge A. Psychosexual functioning and body image following a diagnosis of ductal carcinoma in situ. *J Sex Med*. 2013;**10**:370-377.

56 Rosenberg SM, Tamimi RM, Gelber S, et al. Treatment-related amenorrhea and sexual functioning in young breast cancer survivors. *Cancer*. 2014;**120**:2264-2271.

57 Behringer K, Mueller H, Goergen H, et al. Sexual quality of life in Hodgkin lymphoma: a longitudinal analysis by the German Hodgkin Study Group. *Brit J Cancer*. 2013;**108**:49-57.

64 Flynn KE, Lin L, Cyranowski JM, et al. Development of the NIH PROMIS® Sexual Function and Satisfaction measures in patients with cancer. *J Sex Med*. 2013;**10(Suppl 1)**:43-52.

66 Frey A, Sønksen J, Jakobsen H, Fode M. Prevalence and predicting factors for commonly neglected sexual side effects to radical prostatectomies: results from a cross-sectional questionnaire-based study. *J Sex Med*. 2014;**11(9)**: 2318-2326.

67 Carter J, Goldfrank D, Schover LR. Simple strategies for vaginal health promotion in cancer survivors. *J Sex Med*. 2011;**8**:549-559.

69 Montorsi F, Adaikan G, Becher E, et al. Summary of the recommendations on sexual dysfunctions in men. *J Sex Med*. 2010;**7**:3572-3588.

72 Schover LR, Canada AL, Yuan Y, et al. A randomized trial of internet-based versus traditional sexual counseling for couples after localized prostate cancer treatment. *Cancer*. 2012;**118**:500-509.

74 Schover LR, Yuan Y, Fellman BM, Odensky E, Lewis PE, Martinetti P. Efficacy trial of an Internet-based intervention for cancer-related female sexual dysfunction. *J Natl Compr Canc Netw*. 2013;**11**:1389-1397.

79 Tal R, Jacks LM, Elkin E, Mulhall JP. Penile implant utilization following treatment for prostate cancer: analysis of the SEER-Medicare database. *J Sex Med*. 2011;**8**:1797-1804.

80 McMahon CG, Jannini E, Waldinger M, Rowland D. Standard operating procedures in the disorders of orgasm and ejaculation. *J Sex Med*. 2013;**10**:204-229.

81 Gitlin M. Sexual dysfunction with psychotropic drugs. *Expert Opin Pharmacother*. 2003;**4**:2259-2269.

82 Tal R, Heck M, Teloken P, Siegrist T, Nelson CJ, Mulhall JP. Peyronie's disease following radical prostatectomy: incidence and predictors. *J Sex Med*. 2010;**7**:1254-1261.

84 Seyam R. A systematic review of the correlates and management of nonpremature ejaculatory dysfunction in heterosexual men. *Ther Adv Urol*. 2013;**5**:254-297.

86 Mehta A, Deveci S, Mulhall JP. Efficacy of a penile variable tension loop for improving climacturia after radical prostatectomy. *BJU Int*. 2013;**111**: 500-504.

92 Kao A, Binik YM, Amsel R, Funaro D, Leroux N, Khalifé S. Biopsychosocial predictors of postmenopausal dyspareunia: the role of steroid hormones, vulvovaginal atrophy, cognitive-emotional factors, and dyadic adjustment. *J Sex Med*. 2012;**9**:2066-2076.

95 McLendon AN, Clinard VB, Woodis CB. Ospemifene for the treatment of vulvovaginal atrophy and dyspareunia in postmenopausal women. *Pharmacotherapy*. 2015;**34(10)**:1050-1060.

97 Meston CM, Hull E, Levin RJ, Sipski M. Disorders of orgasm in women. *J Sex Med*. 2004;**1**:66-68.

100 Rutledge TL, Rogers R, Lee SJ, Muller CY. A pilot randomized control trial to evaluate pelvic floor muscle training for urinary incontinence among gynecologic cancer survivors. *Gynecol Oncol*. 2014;**132**:154-158.

108 Schover LR, Rhodes MM, Baum G, et al. Sisters Peer Counseling in Reproductive Issues After Treatment (SPIRIT): a peer counseling program to improve reproductive health among African American breast cancer survivors. *Cancer*. 2011;**117**:4983-4992.

第 138 章 内分泌并发症和副肿瘤综合征

Sai-Ching Jim Yeung, MD, PhD, FACP ■ Robert F. Gagel, MD

概述

正常细胞的转化可导致多种激素活性基因的激活和/或抑制。本章节概述了数种临床内分泌副肿瘤综合征及其相应的治疗方法。癌症的治疗导致许多内分泌或代谢方面的并发症,其中大多数与激素分泌失调或药物毒性有关。与预期相反,干扰信号通路的靶向治疗和免疫治疗的引入,实际上增加了内分泌并发症的数量。本章节除了介绍既往观察到的传统化疗及放疗导致的细胞毒性并发症外,也会介绍新型治疗方式导致的内分泌毒性并发症。

介绍

本章分为两个主要部分。第一部分着重于介绍癌症患者的内分泌并发症,第二部分着重于介绍副肿瘤综合征。癌症及其治疗可导致内分泌功能紊乱、临床和实验室检查异常,从而掩盖或模仿内分泌疾病。副肿瘤综合征是一组表现多样化临床综合征,是由循环中生物体液因子(包括激素、免疫球蛋白、细胞因子和其他因子)刺激所引起。

内分泌并发症

下丘脑-垂体功能失调

放疗是肿瘤患者出现下丘脑-垂体功能失调的常见原因。尽管一些新的靶向治疗可能会影响垂体功能,但没有直接强有力的证据表明化疗是造成腺垂体永久性功能失调的原因之一。下丘脑区或垂体转移不常见[1],因为疾病转移至这些部位导致内分泌失调的临床表现十分罕见。然而,某些良性肿瘤比如垂体瘤和颅咽管瘤经常影响这个解剖部位导致内分泌功能失调。通过免疫检查点阻断剂(抗 CTLA4 抗体和抗 PD-1 抗体)引入的免疫治疗与自身免疫性垂体炎的发生有关,2%~3%接受免疫治疗的患者需要用到激素替代治疗(如皮质激素或甲状腺素)。

放疗引起的下丘脑功能异常进展隐匿,激素不足能在放疗结束后多年出现。一般而言,功能失调发生的速度和严重性取决于放疗总剂量及传递速率。下丘脑-垂体轴功能失调的顺序和频率多样化。促生长轴是最容易受影响的,而促甲状腺轴是最不易受影响的(图 138-1)[2~5]。诊断下丘脑-垂体功

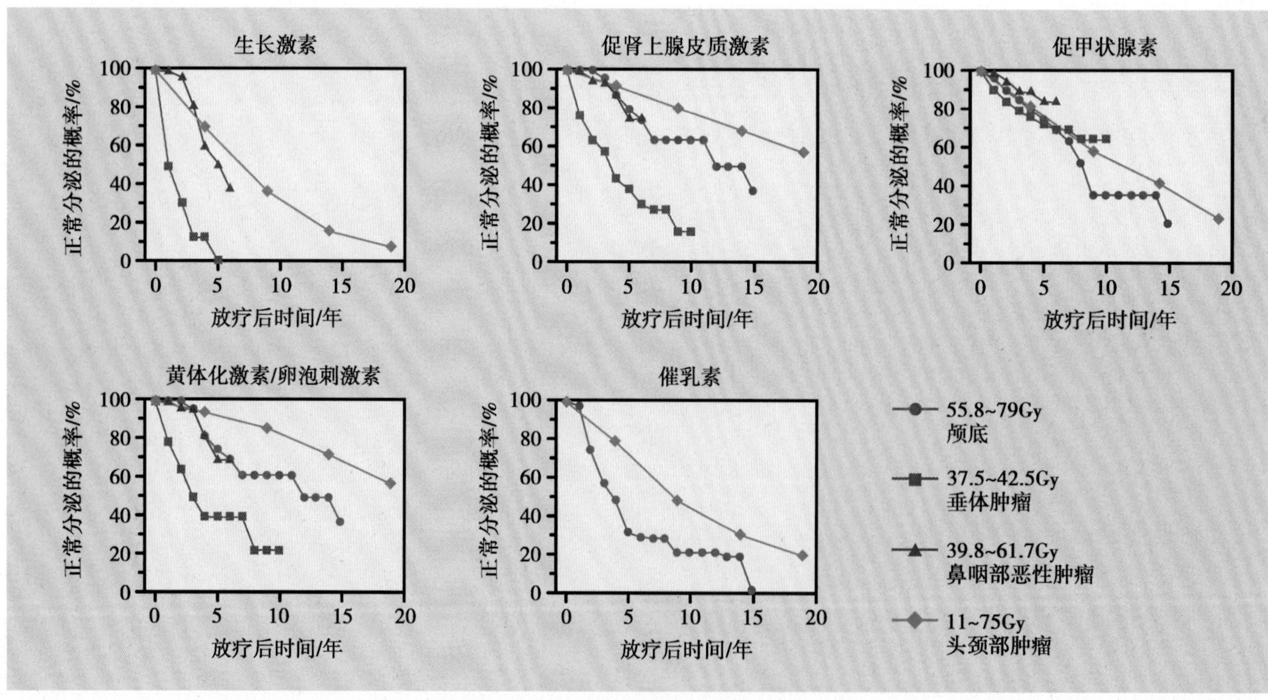

图 138-1 下丘脑-垂体区暴露于放射后随时间推移可能出现的正常垂体激素分泌。该图反映了四个研究的数据。第一套数值(封闭圆圈)来自 Pai 等[3]的研究,患者的颅底接受 55.8~79Gy 放疗。第二套数值(实心方形)来自 Shalet 等[3]的研究,垂体肿瘤的患者接受 37.5~42.5Gy 治疗。第三套数值(敞开三角形)来自 Lam 等[2]的研究,展示 39.8~61.7Gy 放疗对鼻咽癌患者的效果。最后的系列(敞开钻石形)代表来自 Samman 等[4]的数据,给予头颈肿瘤 11~75Gy 治疗

能失调需要依赖于医师的警觉性，因为大部分出现的症状是非特异性（如消瘦和虚弱），这些症状也可以归因于肿瘤患者常见的其他临床表现。下丘脑/垂体功能失调诊断筛选可能包括血清生长激素（GH）和胰岛素样生长因子-1（IGF-1）的测量及性腺衰竭的评价。垂体功能减退的明显标志包括低血糖、低血压和低体温。

在儿童和青少年，性发育的评估是一个有效的诊断工具。根据 Tanner 标准的性发育分期，应该评估女孩月经史和男孩阴茎/睾丸大小。对于接受过颅骨放射的儿童，应该每 6 个月测量一次身高、体重。接受过脊髓或颅脊柱放射的儿童，可能出现局部异常而不是全身生长异常，如果是这样，需进行特殊评估。脚的大小是一个容易测量的可靠生长指标。偏离正常生长曲线应考虑生长激素不足，甲状腺功能减退或者肾上腺功能不足。如果初步评估 GH，IGF-1，促甲状腺素（TSH）和游离甲状腺素（T_4）水平，及射线照相骨龄显示异常，则应进行详细动态检测来评估下丘脑/垂体轴的功能（表 138-1）。

表 138-1　下丘脑-垂体轴动态检测

检测	剂量/取样	禁忌证
生长激素轴		
胰岛素低血糖	正常胰岛素 0.075～0.1U/kg 静推达到血糖≤40mg/dl。在 0，30，45，60 和 90min 时取样检测血糖和生长激素	冠心病或癫痫
精氨酸	0.5g/kg（上限 30g）静推大于 30min。在 0，30，60，90 和 120min 时取样检测生长激素	肝病或肾病
左旋-多巴	500mg 口服。在 0，30，60，90 和 120min 时取样检测生长激素	收缩压<100mmHg 或年龄>60 岁
精氨酸和生长激素释放激素（GHRH）	精氨酸剂量同上。生长激素释放激素 1μg/kg 静推。在 0，30，60，90 和 120min 时取样检测生长激素	肝病或肾病
可乐定刺激方案	可乐定 0.15mg/m^2 口服。在 0，30，60，90 和 120min 取样检测生长激素	
生长激素释放激素（GHRH）刺激方案	GHRH1.0μg/kg 体重静推。在基线，15，30，45，60，90 和 120min 收集生长激素样本	
生长激素抑制试验	检测应该在患者保持卧床休息一晚后快速进行。患者应喝下 100g 葡萄糖溶液。在基线，60，120min 时收集生长激素样本	
肾上腺轴		
ACTH 刺激试验，1h	促肾上腺皮质激素 1 或 250μg 肌注或静推。在注射后 30 和 60min 抽血验皮质醇	
ACTH 刺激试验，48h	早上 9 点开始，获取 24h 尿液测 17-羟皮质醇（17-OHCS）和肌酐。第一天同前收集 24h。早上 9 点开始，给予 250μg 皮质素加入 250ml 生理盐水，输注 8h 以上，每 8h 一次，共 48h。另一种方法，使用 40IU 储存剂型提纯的凝胶牛 ACTH，每 12h 肌注一次，共 48h。第 1 和第 2 日重复收集 24h 尿，第 4 和第 5 日收集 24h 尿同前	
促肾上腺皮质激素释放激素（CRH）刺激试验	试验前至少禁食 4h。给予人 CRH 1.0μg/kg 静推大于 30s。血液取样应该在 CRH 给予前 15min、1min，以及给予后 15，30，45，60，90 和 120min 来测量皮质醇和 ACTH	
小剂量地塞米松试验，过夜	在夜晚 11～12 点钟之间口服地塞米松 1.0mg（成人）或 20μg/kg（儿童）。第 2 日早上 8～9 点钟收集血清皮质醇。皮质醇水平<1.8μg/dl 基本上排除库欣综合征	
小剂量地塞米松试验，48h	早上 8～9 点钟收集血清皮质醇。在抽取皮质醇后立即口服地塞米松 0.5mg（成人）或 10μg/kg（儿童），每 6h 重复一次，共 48h。第二次血浆皮质醇抽取在早上 9 点钟，最后一次予地塞米松后 6h。血清皮质醇水平<1.8μg/dl 基本上排除库欣综合征	

续表

检测	剂量/取样	禁忌证
大剂量地塞米松试验,48h	早上9点钟收集血清皮质醇。每6h给予(2.0mg;儿童50μg/kg)一次,共48h。第二次血浆皮质醇抽取在早上9点钟,最后一次予地塞米松后6h。有肾上腺瘤的患者48h样本中皮质醇水平与初始样本(基线)相比没有显示出抑制。过量ACTH来源于垂体的患者中大约78%显示血浆皮质醇抑制>50%,然而过量ACTH为异常来源的患者中只有11%显示抑制>50%	
全面的,6日,大/小剂量地塞米松试验	这个方案包含连续的小剂量和大剂量地塞米松试验。24h尿游离皮质醇和/或17-羟皮质醇(17-OHCS)测量能帮助证实血清皮质醇和ACTH的结果	
促性腺激素释放激素(GnRH)刺激试验	GnRH 100μg静推。血清LH样本应该在给予GnRH后40min收集	
甲吡酮刺激(过夜)试验	在晚上11点,甲吡酮30mg/kg(最大3g)与点心一起口服。第二天早上8点钟,测量血清皮质醇和11-脱氧皮质醇	

GHRH,生长激素释放激素。

在接受过颅脑或头颈放射的成年人,检测下丘脑-垂体功能失调更有挑战性。诊断成年人下丘脑-垂体功能失调的一个方法包括常规筛查GH不足及性腺衰竭。推荐每年测量男性的IGF-1和睾酮水平,记录女性月经史,共5年,然后在接下来10年里每5年检测一次。任何筛查试验中异常记录都应该进行追踪,用进一步动态试验评估所有下丘脑-垂体轴功能。

免疫疗法诱发的垂体炎

随着免疫治疗在黑色素瘤以及越来越多的其他肿瘤上应用的增加,已经产生了许多旁观者效应。这些副作用中最突出的是免疫治疗引起的垂体炎(IH)。在伊匹木单抗(易普利姆玛)的三期临床试验中,2.3%的患者出现垂体炎症状和包括糖皮质激素、甲状腺、性腺和GH缺乏的激素缺乏的表现,需要长期的激素替代治疗。1.9%的患者的垂体相关事件程度为3级或4级,需要紧急治疗或住院。在开始使用伊匹木单抗治疗后,脑垂体功能衰竭的发病时间为11~19周。患者常见的主诉包括头痛、精神状态改变、腹痛、排便习惯改变和低血压;只凭借症状,IH通常很难与脑转移或与广泛转移性疾病区分开来。该困难也表明,临床医生开始使用免疫治疗药物前,应获得患者基线甲状腺(游离T_4和TSH),肾上腺(促肾上腺皮质激素、促肾上腺皮质激素、上午8点血清皮质醇水平),性腺[促黄体素(LH)、卵泡刺激素、男性睾酮和女性雌二醇]和与生长有关的激素(GH和IGF-1)水平作为初始治疗前的基线参照。如果患者出现疑似内分泌缺乏的症状或垂体炎的急性症状(头痛和视力障碍),则应再次重复测量以上指标。对于症状或体格检查与垂体炎一致的患者,应进行垂体的磁共振成像(MRI)检查、重复激素测试以及肾上腺内分泌轴的动态测试(如低剂量的促皮质醇刺激测试)。最近的一份基于多中心大队列研究的报告指出[6],不仅在抗CTLA4药物(伊匹木单抗和替西利姆单抗)的治疗过程中观察到垂体炎,而且在抗PD1药物(尼沃鲁单抗)的治疗过程中也观察到了垂体炎。在此份报告中,描述了968名单中心用上述药物治疗黑色素瘤、前列腺癌和肾细胞癌的患者的情况,其中2.7%(27例患者)患有一到两种激素缺陷,同时伴有磁共振(MRI)扫描中脑垂体增大或出现头痛症状[6]。在这27例患者中,有77%出现中枢肾上腺皮质功能减退,有89%为中枢性甲状腺功能减退,有79%为中枢性腺功能减退,85%的患者在MRI检查发现垂体异常[6]。在随访过程中[中位随访期为17个月(范围:1~76个月)],所有患有肾上腺皮质功能减退的患者均未恢复,而患有甲状腺或性腺功能减退的患者则有12%~13%恢复。显而易见的是,这是一个重大的、不断演变的问题。目前尚不清楚的是,目前正在开发的两种或两种以上免疫治疗药物联合治疗是否会导致更高的相关疾病的发病率和或更严重的毒性反应。

甲状腺疾病

甲状腺疾病和甲状腺功能异常通常与癌症及其治疗相关联。

血清甲状腺素结合蛋白异常

甲状腺素结合蛋白[甲状腺素结合球蛋白(TBG),前白蛋白,及白蛋白]水平能被性激素水平和营养状态影响;两者均异常的情况常见于肿瘤患者中。数种化疗药能影响甲状腺功能。左旋天冬酰胺表现出可逆性抑制白蛋白和TBG,导致低的总甲状腺素(T_4)但游离T_4水平正常[7]。鬼臼脂和烷化剂联合也有报道能降低TBG[8]。氟尿嘧啶[9]和米托坦[10]均能增加总T_4和三碘甲腺原氨酸(T_3)水平,且不抑制TSH,此现象提示这些药物能增加血清中甲状腺素结合能力。

甲状腺功能正常病态综合征

甲状腺素代谢改变发生在癌症和其他严重系统疾病的患者中[11]。低水平血清T_3,能在70%中的重度癌症患者中发现,这是由于甲状腺外T_4转化为T_3减少所致。血清游离T_4水平一般正常或升高，然而游离 T_3 浓度低于正常或降低。这些患者临床甲状腺功能正常，即血清 TSH 水平及 TRH 刺激试验结果正常。

在大部分甲状腺功能正常的病态综合征的患者中，T_3、T_4、TSH 水平是正常的。一般不存在甲状腺功能减退（甲状腺功能减退）的临床表现，但评估可能会被伴随的严重症状如迟钝、水肿、低体温所混淆。在甲状腺功能正常病态综合征的情况下，低游离 T_4 水平预示较差的预后，死亡率大于 50%。虽然普遍公认甲状腺素治疗没有获益，有时很难去区分甲状腺功能正常病态综合征和继发性甲状腺功能减退。如果没有禁忌证（如活动的缺血性心脏病），在这些罕见的患者中审慎地补充生理水平甲状腺素可能是更合适的。

甲状腺功能减退

甲状腺切除术

在处理甲状腺癌、头颈癌或者甲状腺转移癌时，由于各种各样肿瘤的原因可能实施甲状腺切除术。在这组患者中需要甲状腺素替代。甲状腺癌患者调整高于生理剂量的甲状腺素，在没有明显甲状腺功能亢进下抑制 TSH。另外，甲状腺素剂量应该调整至保持 TSH 在正常范围内。

放疗

放射是一个引起甲状腺功能减退（原发性、继发性、三发性）的重要原因。放射诱导的原发性甲状腺功能减退是由于甲状腺细胞破坏，抑制细胞分化，血管破坏，以及可能的免疫介导现象。增加发生原发性甲状腺功能减退的危险因素包括对甲状腺附近组织的高放射剂量，治疗持续时间，治疗中缺乏对甲状腺保护，以及联合放射和手术治疗[12]。

放射治疗后各种癌和各种情况下甲状腺功能减退的发生率见表 138-2[4,12~22]。放射剂量和甲状腺功能减退患病率的关系是根据霍奇金淋巴瘤患者的研究得出[15,18]。通过长期随访低剂量放疗的患者发现引起临床显著甲状腺功能减退的阈值大概为 10Gy。对于接受>30Gy 的霍奇金病患者，放射 20 年后甲状腺功能减退的精确风险上升到 45%[15]。有明显或亚临床甲状腺功能减退的患者应接受甲状腺素替代治疗。

表 138-2　放疗后甲状腺功能减退发生率（包括代偿性甲状腺功能减退）[a]

恶性类型或情况	放疗剂量	%甲状腺功能减退
霍奇金病	30~60Gy	30~50
头颈癌	40~72Gy	25~50
淋巴瘤	20~40Gy（中位 36Gy）	30~42
乳腺癌	?	15~21
骨髓移植（BMT）全身照射	13.75~15Gy	15~43

[a] 数据来自参考文献[12~22]；缩写 BMT：骨髓移植。

化疗

接受过化疗但没接受过全身放射的骨髓移植患者有 14% 诊断为甲状腺功能减退[23]，这提示着甲状腺功能减退和高剂量细胞毒联合化疗之间存在因果关系。这个观点也被在用多种联合药物加或不加放疗治疗的患者中原发性甲状腺功能减退发生率增加的现象所证实[24,25]。左旋天冬酰胺酶（L-Asparaginase），除了之前讨论过的抑制 TBG 合成外，可能也抑制 TSH 可逆的合成，以及导致暂时降低游离 T_4 水平的甲状腺功能减退[26]。

甲状腺功能障碍是细胞因子治疗的一个可预见到的副作用。20%~35%的患者用重组人白介素-2（interleukin-2）治疗后产生甲状腺功能障碍[27]。这些患者有甲状腺功能亢进、甲状腺功能减退，或者甲状腺功能亢进后甲状腺功能减退[28]。大约 10%患者用干扰素（interferon）治疗后出现原发性甲状腺功能减退[29]。继发于干扰素引起甲状腺功能减退的垂体增大也有报道[30]。在治疗前有抗甲状腺抗体的患者存在更高的细胞因子引起甲状腺功能障碍的风险。

维 A 酸（retinoid）X 受体（RXR）的配体可能用在特定恶性肿瘤，例如皮肤 T 细胞淋巴瘤的治疗。贝沙罗汀（bexarotene，一种 RXR 选择性受体）引起剂量依赖型继发性甲状腺功能减退[31]。健康受试者中单次剂量能迅速抑制 TSH[32]。除了以 RXR 介导的甲状腺素依赖机制来抑制 TSH 转录，贝沙罗汀也以非去碘酶介导通路来增加甲状腺素代谢清除[33]。

酪氨酸激酶抑制剂

在过去的十年中，抑制激酶活性的小分子（酪氨酸激酶抑制剂，TKI）迅速被引入到癌症治疗中，我们发现这些药物对甲状腺功能有着深远的影响。第一个机制是这些药物对甲状腺功能的直接影响。TKI 目标受体酪氨酸激酶可以明确地影响甲状腺的功能，包括血管内皮生长因子受体、表皮生长因子受体、*RET* 基因、*KIT* 基因和 *MET* 基因。其他间接的影响是通过下游信号通路，如 RAF、PI3K 和 mTOR。这些信号通路可以影响甲状腺的功能和维持或促进正常甲状腺细胞生长。当这些通路的中断时，甲状腺细胞的生长、死亡和甲状腺素的合成显然会受到影响。的确，在接受酪氨酸激酶抑制剂的患者中，甲状腺功能减退的发生率很高，与多种药物有关：舒尼替尼，7%~85%；培唑帕尼，12%；尼洛替尼，22%；阿昔替尼，20%~100%；卡博替尼，15%；索拉非尼，8%~39%；达沙替尼，50%；和伊马替尼，0~25%[34]。在使用以上药物中的任何一种进行治疗的第一年期间，定期对患者甲状腺功能（游离 T_4 和 TSH）进行常规测量是明智的，因为通常我们很难将 TKI 治疗的非特异性副作用与原发性甲状腺功能减退或转移性癌症的临床表现鉴别开来。

对于已经接受全甲状腺切除术的转移性甲状腺癌的特定 TKI 治疗的患者，还有另一种导致甲状腺功能减退的机制。已被批准的特殊药物[凡德他尼、卡博替尼、索拉非尼和仑伐替尼（lenvatinib）]或已研究的[培唑帕尼、莫特沙芬（motesanib）和舒尼替尼]可用于治疗分化型或髓样甲状腺癌，这些药物有更高的概率导致血清 TSH 浓度升高，血清 T_4 水平低：凡德他尼，49%；卡博替尼，57%；索拉非尼，41%；仑伐替尼，57%。由于每一种药物都会引起腹泻和吸收不良，因此推测其作用机制是甲状腺素的吸收减少，尽管尚未排除其对甲状腺素代谢的影响。额外补充 1/3 的甲状腺素剂量通常可以解决这个问题。值得注意的是，在轻度甲状腺切除相关的甲状旁腺功能减退患者中，钙、镁和维生素 D 的吸收不良也可能导致低钙血症或低镁血症程度的恶化[35]。游离 T_4 和 TSH 的常规测量应纳入日常监测中，因为超过半数的患者需要甲状腺素的剂量调整(以及补充镁、钙和维生素 D)。值得注意的是，原发性甲状腺功能减退、低钙血症或低镁血症是很容易治疗的，如果及时处理，这些并发症不应成为限制 TKI 使用的原因。但是，对于使用 TKI 出现甲状腺功能低下，低血钙或低镁血症的患者，此类并发症还会导致 QT 间隔延长，比如凡德他尼[35]、仑伐替尼[36]和索拉非尼。当出现 QT 间隔延长时，需要停止使用 TKI，直至 QT 间隔恢复正常。

含^{131}I 化合物

使用^{131}I 治疗甲状腺癌要求较高的血清 TSH 水平。可以停止甲状腺素替代或给予重组人 TSH 来达到高的血清 TSH 水平。使用含^{131}I 化合物来治疗其他肿瘤可能导致甲状腺功能减退。例如，用高剂量(100~1 000mCi)^{131}I-间碘苄胍(metaiodobenzylguanidine)来治疗不可切除的嗜铬细胞瘤可能导致原发性甲状腺功能减退[37]。

甲状腺转移

甲状腺功能减退继发于甲状腺转移是极为罕见的。

筛查

接受过头颈或颅脑放射的儿童应该每年检测游离 T_4 和 TSH，共 5 年，之后每 2 年一次。早期检测 T_4 和 TSH 水平异常能进行医学干预，在甲状腺功能减退前逆转对身体和智力生长发育的影响。对于成年人，淋巴瘤和各种头颈部肿瘤的颈部放射治疗与原发性甲状腺功能减退的高发生率相关。接受过放射的患者应该每年检测游离 T_4 和 TSH 水平，共 5 年，然后每隔 1 年共 10 年，之后 10 年每 5 年一次。一旦诊断甲状腺功能减退，患者应该接受甲状腺素替代治疗。

甲状腺功能亢进

放疗引起的无痛性甲状腺炎伴高甲状腺素血症是一种头颈部外放疗少见的副作用。作为炎症和甲状腺组织破坏伴甲状腺球蛋白(包括甲状腺氨酸和三碘甲腺原氨酸)释放的结果，暂时的甲状腺功能亢进可能发生，通常紧接着甲状腺功能减退。在霍奇金病的患者覆盖放疗后有报道出现暂时性甲状腺功能亢进，而且通常在治疗 18 个月内发生[38]。大部分情况下患者表现为低摄入放射性碘，这表明应该诊断为静止性甲状腺炎，但一部分是格雷夫斯病(Graves disease)。放射治疗的一系列霍奇金病患者，患格雷夫斯病的风险估计至少是正常人群的 7.2 倍[15]。

眼病，与格雷夫斯病相似，有报道颈部淋巴瘤、乳腺癌、鼻咽癌或喉癌患者在接受高剂量放疗后 18~84 个月内出现眼病。眼病可能不伴有甲状腺功能亢进和人白细胞抗原-B8 缺乏[39]。这表示放疗诱导的甲状腺损伤可能引起自身免疫反应，与格雷夫斯病相似。

也有 TKI 相关的甲状腺功能亢进的例子，包括两例死亡案例(与索拉非尼和舒尼替尼相关)[40]。甲状腺功能亢进的可能的机制是甲状腺炎。甲状腺功能亢进患者应积极治疗甲状腺风暴；在这种情况下，应考虑保留 TKI 治疗，直到患者状态稳定[34]。

甲状腺结节和癌症

低剂量放疗增加甲状腺结节和癌症的发病风险。甲状腺癌和低剂量放射的联系被广泛地研究[41]，并已在第 80 章节中讨论。

能量平衡和葡萄糖代谢

肥胖和代谢综合征

肿瘤治疗可能导致肥胖和代谢综合征[42~44]。代谢综合征是一组增加 2 型糖尿病和心血管疾病风险的异常情况，包括向心性肥胖、血脂异常、高血糖和高血压。肥胖是影响肿瘤形成和肿瘤进展的危险因素。肥胖促进肿瘤的机制包括：由于胰岛素抵抗所致高胰岛素血症、高胰岛素样生长因子-1(IGF-1)、脂肪因子、低脂肪素、增加脂肪组织产生的雌激素以及增加炎症反应。肥胖在肿瘤存活者可能增加疾病不良预后的风险[42,45,46]。肥胖增加结直肠癌和生殖泌尿系统的风险[47]。虽然肿瘤存活者身体活动水平低可能导致肥胖的形成，体重增加的病理生理学原理仍不清楚。既然肥胖在许多肿瘤是一个不良的预后因素，并且它是一个可改变的危险因素，在肿瘤治疗后继发性肥胖需要进行处理。

糖尿病

2 型糖尿病(DM2)与胰腺癌、肝癌、结肠癌、胃癌、乳腺癌和子宫内膜癌的环保风险升高有关[48~53]。越来越多的流行病学数据认为糖尿病在肿瘤的发生、发展和肿瘤患者的预后中发挥重要作用[54]。相关性最强的可能是胰腺癌[55~59]。除了经常与肥胖共存外，糖尿病促进肿瘤的机制包括：高胰岛素血症、高 IGF-1 和高血糖。高血糖自身有对肿瘤增殖的促进作用。在男性中，肿瘤存活者空腹血糖浓度>126mg/dl 有更高患肝、胰腺、胆第二原发肿瘤的相关风险[47]。对肿瘤患者中 2 型糖尿病的处理使患者生存最佳化，缺少基于证据的指引。

使用糖皮质激素(如联合治疗方案、对脑转移水肿、预防移植排斥、对骨髓移植中移植物抗宿主病以及恶心/呕吐)可能是导致肿瘤患者患糖尿病的最常见原因。因此，接受糖皮质激素的患者必须在治疗期间对糖尿病定期筛查评估空腹血糖水平。用链佐星(streptozocin)[60]或左旋天冬酰胺酶(L-asparaginase)[61]治疗可能导致胰岛素不足的糖尿病。虽然没有证据表明链佐星治疗后发生延迟性糖尿病，然而随访受到限制并且是短期的。对于用链佐星治疗后的长期生存者，可能应指示患者定期筛查延迟性发展的糖尿病。糖尿病也可能由于左旋天冬酰胺酶治疗后的严重胰腺炎而进展。对肿瘤的免疫治疗，用细胞因子，例如重组人白介素-2 和干扰素可能引起对胰腺 β 细胞的毒性进而导致胰岛素依赖型糖尿病[62]。他克莫司(tacrolimus)，一种免疫抑制剂用于预防骨髓抑制中移植物抗宿主病，也会增加糖尿病发病率，可能通过破坏胰腺 β 细胞而发病[63]。接受同种异体骨髓移植的患者可能接受糖皮质激素、环孢素(cyclosporine A)和他克莫司治疗，特别容易发生糖尿病[64]。处理血糖水平依据血糖水平异常的严重程度以及基础血糖增加的病理生理机制。通常在胰岛素缺乏的患者需要使用胰岛素。

代谢性骨病

骨质疏松症

四种成年患者在加速骨丢失和骨质疏松方面特别危险：

①淋巴瘤、骨髓瘤、白血病的患者；②乳腺癌的妇女用细胞毒化疗治疗，经常处于早期更年期[65]以及不能接受雌激素替代治疗；③绝经后妇女患有雌激素受体阳性的乳腺癌；④前列腺癌男性患者使用抗雄激素治疗或进行去势治疗。正常的骨重建包括成骨细胞骨形成和破骨细胞骨吸收之间微妙的平衡。抗肿瘤治疗对成骨细胞功能有毒性，减少骨形成。肿瘤产生的类激素活性物质（如甲状旁腺激素相关蛋白[PTHrP]、淋巴毒素、白介素-1 和白介素-6）可能有助于临床照片的骨丢失。大部分情况下，不清楚骨丢失是否因为抗肿瘤治疗或潜在的疾病进展以及其他的影响（包括恶病质、营养不良、低钙、维生素 D 摄入或者综合因素）。在乳腺癌或前列腺癌的患者中，性类固醇激素不足是骨丢失最重要的原因。在有多种失调（骨髓瘤、白血病、淋巴瘤）影响造血细胞的患者中骨丢失是明显的，可能因为细胞因子的产生以及原始造血细胞与成骨细胞的关系，或使用高剂量或持续的糖皮质激素治疗。

许多药物能引起骨质疏松症[66]。在肿瘤患者中，引起肾脏丢失钙、镁或磷的糖皮质激素、甲氨蝶呤（methotraxate）和细胞毒药物[如铂类化合物、环磷酰胺（cyclophosphamide）、异环磷酰胺（ifosfamide）]对骨密度有显著的影响。在接受甲氨蝶呤治疗的急性淋巴细胞白血病（ALL）的儿童中有报道出现骨质疏松症[67]。骨质疏松症在停止甲氨蝶呤治疗后明显改善。对 ALL 患者的纵向研究表明白血病过程、高剂量糖皮质激素和低镁血症（由于使用循环的糖皮质激素和肾毒性化疗或抗感染药后肾损耗）可导致损伤钙和维生素 D 代谢，在治疗过程的不同阶段减少骨质[68]。乳腺癌辅助化疗[通常包括氟尿嘧啶、环磷酰胺和多柔比星（doxorubicin）或甲氨蝶呤]与绝经前期患者的低骨质相关[69]。化疗期间骨丢失是大量的，可能导致骨折风险增加。治疗后性腺功能减退是这些成年患者骨质疏松症的主要因素。尽管他莫昔芬（tamoxifen）有轻度的骨丢失保护作用，芳香酶抑制剂的作用却是相反。骨髓移植经常用细胞毒药物、糖皮质激素、免疫抑制剂治疗。在 24 个进行高剂量化疗骨髓移植的患者中，观察到骨密度减低[70]。

即时调查肿瘤存活者性腺功能障碍，推荐年轻性腺功能减退的男性或女性患者即时给予性腺类固醇激素（排除禁忌证）替代，能减少未来骨折的风险。对长期肿瘤存活者在患者大约 30 岁时应评估骨质，这个年龄大多数人达到骨质的最高峰[71]。如果骨质正常，不需要超过正常推荐的方法进一步防止骨质疏松症。如果是异常（低于超过 2 个标准差），应该推荐患者进行多个骨质疏松症可逆性因素的评估。

处理肿瘤患者骨质疏松综合征的一个关键点是监测骨矿物质密度（如双能谱 X 线吸光测定法）来评估骨折风险以及监测治疗效果。这种测量应该在处理恶性肿瘤早期就进行，因此能够实施适当的预防措施。在使用含有可能减少骨质药物的药物时，肿瘤医师应该考虑积极使用双膦酸盐类[如阿仑膦酸钠（alendronate）、利塞膦酸钠（risedronate）或伊班膦酸钠（ibandronate）]、降钙素（calcitonin）、选择性雌激素受体调节剂（SERM）或者特立帕肽（teriparatide），除此之外每日摄入 1 200～1 500mg 钙元素。双膦酸盐类对这些患者是有效的治疗方式。当白血病儿童出现骨质疏松症时经常可以逆转，因为儿童处于骨发育的形成期，对成年人有必要采取更积极的措施例如双膦酸盐类或特立帕肽治疗来预防骨丢失，不应该放任骨折综合征的发展。

另一个关键点是通过食物补充来纠正矿物质和维生素 D 代谢。在青少年和年轻成人中营养不足可导致骨密度低下。治疗低钙血症、低镁血症和维生素 D 不足是成功治疗肿瘤患者骨质疏松症的一部分。最近研究证明正常人群中有 50% 出现临床相关的维生素 D 不足；在接受肿瘤治疗的患者这个百分比肯定更高。

软骨病

软骨病，一种特点为骨基质未矿物化的状态，是一种罕见的化疗并发症，但在骨质减少以及有骨软化临床综合征（骨痛和近端肌病）的患者应该考虑该病的可能性。最常见的原因是营养不足以及肾丢失磷和钙引起的血清钙和/或磷浓度减少。患者接受化疗后出现低磷血症、低镁血症或低钙血症者发病的风险高。血清离子钙、磷、镁和维生素 D 代谢物水平的调查应该包括在最初的评估中。这些维生素和矿物质一旦发现不足就应该开始适当的替代疗法。其他影响因素包括系统性酸中毒和药物例如抗痉挛药和铝[66]。肿瘤引起的软骨病会放在讨论副肿瘤综合征后的章节。

异环磷酰胺引起的肾小管损害导致肾性磷丢失，低磷血症，佝偻病/软骨病[72]。异环磷酰胺对肾小管的毒性作用包括成人和儿童范科尼综合征（Fanconi syndrome）。当异环磷酰胺给予 $50g/m^2$ 剂量或更多时，肾小管损害最常见，或者当它与顺铂联用时[73]。佝偻病在儿童中最常报道。雌莫司汀（estramustine）用于治疗前列腺癌，被报道会增加骨吸收以及同时引起低钙血症、低磷血症和继发性甲状旁腺功能亢进的发生[74]。

肾上腺疾病

肾上腺转移

肿瘤血行转移至肾上腺是常见的，频率上只低于血行转移至肺、肝和骨[75]。尸检证明 9%～27% 死于恶性疾病的患者存在肾上腺转移，1/2～2/3 肾上腺转移的患者中双侧均涉及。

肾上腺转移的出现可能对诊断和治疗计划有重要的意义。当肿瘤患者有肾上腺肿块，但没有其他部位转移的证据时，判断这个肿块是否是转移病灶或是单独的不相关的肾上腺病变至关重要。作为肿瘤分期评估的一部分，最近在成像技术的进步能够分辨肾上腺病变性质。位于肾周脂肪的肾上腺允许探测几乎全部正常腺体以及小至 5～10mm 轮廓畸形的肿块。计算机断层扫描（CT）探测肾上腺肿块有敏感性和特异性。CT 检查提示肾上腺转移而不是原发性肾上腺疾病的特点包括不均匀性、对比增强、两侧对称以及直径大于 3cm[76]。

没有其他转移性疾病的证据，肾上腺肿块是否真的为转移性肿瘤是决定肿瘤正确治疗的关键信息。评价有恶性肾上腺肿块的患者应该包括病史和体格检查，来得出肾上腺功能不全、库欣综合征（Cushing syndrome）、盐皮质激素过量或嗜铬细胞瘤的证据。生物化学评估应该包括短期 ACTH 激发试验来排除肾上腺功能不足。应该获得 24h 收集的尿液来测定尿游离皮质醇、醛固酮、儿茶酚胺和甲基肾上腺素。必须排除嗜铬细胞瘤，特别是如果有高血压或者预期的任何类型的手术操作。曾经报道有临床上未预期嗜铬细胞瘤的患者，一半出现临床恶化甚至在非肾上腺相关的手术过程后立即死亡[77]。

如果生物化学方法评估嗜铬细胞瘤为阴性,应该考虑 CT 引导下细针穿刺。这种操作检测肿瘤有 85%的敏感性[78]。磁共振成像(MRI)可能有助于诊断嗜铬细胞瘤。用^{131}I-6-四甲基-19-非-胆固醇(^{131}I-6-iodomethyl-19-nor-cholesterol [NP-59])的功能闪烁扫描法可能用于联合 CT 和 MRI,来帮助诊断单侧大于 2cm 的肾上腺肿块[79]。

肾上腺功能不全

尽管肾上腺被多种常见的肿瘤侵犯的可能性高,但临床上明显的肾上腺功能减退很少发生,除非双侧肾上腺都有转移性疾病[80]。据估计在正常或应激状态下,糖皮质激素产生受损前必须有大于 80%的肾上腺组织受破坏[81]。因为肾上腺功能不全的临床表现是非特异性并且与肿瘤患者的其他症状存在交叉性,需要高度警惕来检测这种可治疗的情况。肾上腺功能不全患者的恶病质和虚弱与广泛转移患者常见的消耗症状相似。电解质异常能用摄入少、营养不良、化疗药物的副作用或副肿瘤综合征来解释。肾上腺功能不全可能逐步发展,因此与肿瘤相关的恶病质混淆。

有双侧肾上腺转移的患者 20%~30%会发生肾上腺功能不全[80]。这些患者全部应该用 ACTH 激发试验来评估,当怀疑肾上腺功能不全时应该接受糖皮质激素和盐皮质激素替代治疗,直到证明肾上腺功能正常。稳定的患者应该早上接受 20mg,下午接受 10mg 氢化可的松(hydrocortisone)。发生循环不稳定、败血症、紧急手术或者其他主要并发症时,应给予胃肠外应激剂量的糖皮质激素[如氢化可的松丁二酸(hydrocortisone succinate)应该每 8h 给予 100mg 静脉注射]。

肿瘤患者肾上腺功能不全的其他原因包括自身免疫性肾上腺炎、肾上腺出血和肉芽肿病。许多肿瘤患者可能存在免疫功能不全。例如,白血病或淋巴瘤的患者,或者经历骨髓移植的患者其免疫功能不全的。这些患者的肾上腺感染巨细胞病毒、分枝杆菌或真菌可能导致肾上腺功能不全。

肾上腺功能不全可能是由药物引起的。依托咪酯(etomidate)[81],一个常用的静脉内麻醉药,以及酮康唑(ketoconazole),一个抗真菌药,均会抑制糖皮质激素合成通路的细胞色素 P450-依赖酶的产生。氨鲁米特(aminoglutethimide)和美替拉酮(metyrapone)是抑制类固醇生成酶的药物,当用于治疗前列腺、乳腺和肾上腺皮质肿瘤时可能引起肾上腺功能不全。米托坦(mitotane),在结构上与杀虫剂二氯二苯二氯乙烷(DDT)有关联,对正常的和肿瘤性肾上腺皮质细胞有选择性毒性。当给予必要剂量治疗肾上腺皮质肿瘤的米托坦时,经常观察到肾上腺功能不全;在这些患者中糖皮质激素替代治疗是必须[10]。增加蛋白结合可能导致增加替代疗法中每日糖皮质激素需要量。苏拉明(suramin),基于它对肿瘤生长因子的活性,最近被提出作为一种抗肿瘤药物,可能也会引起肾上腺皮质功能不全。

垂体或下丘脑转移也可能发生继发性肾上腺功能不全。然而继发性肾上腺功能不全的最常见原因是外源性糖皮质激素治疗抑制下丘脑-垂体-肾上腺轴。一个持续的治疗过程可能导致下丘脑-垂体持续多个月的抑制。在白血病和淋巴瘤患者短期的类固醇治疗(如 1、2、4 周)后,大部分患者肾上腺功能会抑制 2~4 日,在一些患者中抑制时间更久。在接受糖皮质激素治疗超过 2 周的患者,应该考虑逐渐减量,共 10~14 日。这对包含高剂量糖皮质激素的化疗疗程尤其正确,例如那些用于治疗急性白血病和淋巴瘤的方案。此外,在过去几年接受持续糖皮质激素治疗的患者,如果发生急性内科或外科并发症(如中性粒细胞减少性发热伴低血压、急性阑尾炎)应该接受应激剂量的糖皮质激素。下丘脑-垂体区域放射治疗的患者有 19%~42%会引起 ACTH 缺乏和继发性肾上腺功能不全(图 138-1)。几种诊断方法被用于评估继发性肾上腺功能不全,包括基础 8am 血清皮质醇测定和 1μg 合成 ACTH 动态试验(1~24),胰岛素诱发低血糖,或者美替拉酮。免疫治疗对垂体 ACTH 的影响在本章前面已经讨论过。

生长激素(GH)分泌紊乱和生长

儿童期肿瘤或它的治疗经常会损害生长。髓母细胞瘤和 ALL 是常见的儿童期恶性肿瘤,经常会用颅脑或脑脊放射和/或化疗。接近 40%儿童期脑肿瘤的存活者,成年时身高低于人群 10%,低身高的风险因素是低年龄时诊断和影响下丘脑-垂体轴的放射治疗[82]。GH 缺乏和骨生长板破坏是生长迟缓的两个普遍机制。

颅脑放射可能引起下丘脑或垂体功能障碍。下丘脑似乎比脑垂体对放射更加敏感,可能会被低放疗剂量损害(<40Gy)。高剂量(>40Gy)很可能损害下丘脑和垂体功能。在下丘脑/垂体区域放射后 5 年,几乎 100%患者缺乏一种或多种垂体激素(图 138-1)。

GH 缺乏是最常见的缺乏,经常是在颅脑放射后首先出现的缺乏。单独的放射后 GH 缺乏是常见的,其效益是剂量依赖性的。在低剂量时(20~24Gy),唯一的影响可能是改变 GH 分泌模式和对胰岛素引起的低血糖的亚正常反应。中等或更高的剂量,GH 对精氨酸的反应受损,脉冲 GH 分泌的频率和幅度减少[5]。当剂量升高到 30Gy,35%的患者中观察到异常的 GH 分泌和生长迟缓,其必须接受 GH 治疗[83]。

除了生长激素缺乏引起生长迟缓外,血液恶性肿瘤或中枢神经系统的脑脊或脊髓放射,以及骨髓移植前全身放射可能造成两个其他的影响。第一,放射影响椎体和骨盆生长板,减慢椎体生长。第二,放射引起 GH 或胰岛素样因子抵抗。

儿童接受化疗治疗恶性肿瘤后经常在一段时期内生长速率减低,随后有一个生长“追赶”期。虽然化疗可能扮演一个重要角色,但系统性疾病似乎是这些儿童生长迟缓的最重要原因。接受高剂量化疗以及长期联合化疗治疗的儿童与那些接受正常治疗或低强度化疗的儿童相比,生长速率和身高都较低。如果 0.5~2 年后生长没有追赶上来,很有必要排除 GH 缺乏。

对于成年人,GH 缺乏被认为会降低骨和肌肉质量、降低运动能力、增加脂肪组织、疲劳、较差的幸福感、心肌功能受损以及增加心血管风险。GH 替代可能提高患者生活质量和幸福感[84],但在讨论时应该考虑 IGF-1 引起恶性疾病复发的可能性。

电解质/矿物质代谢紊乱

低钠血症

低钠血症的风险因素包括治疗引起的恶心呕吐、某些化疗药、低渗液脱水、疼痛、阿片制剂以及压力(生理和心理)。在一个肿瘤住院患者的前瞻性研究中,低钠血症发生率为 3.7%,钠消耗和抗利尿激素分泌失调综合征(SIADH)大约各占所有原因的 1/3[85]。SIADH 的特点是低血清渗透压和不适当的高尿液渗透压,不存在利尿剂、心力衰竭、肝硬化、肾上腺功能不全和甲状腺功能减退。在肿瘤患者,SIADH 可能是肿瘤分泌的抗利尿激素引起(如高达 15%的非小细胞肺癌),异常的分泌刺激(如胸内感染、正压通气)或者细胞毒性影响脑室旁和视上神经元。也可能是化疗引起含有抗利尿激素的肿瘤细胞溶解导致或恶化 SIADH。药物引起的肾脏盐丢失或肿瘤引起的盐丢失(心房钠尿肽介导)也能导致低钠血症、血清低渗透压,尿钠、尿渗透压升高[86]。当液体容量消耗的标志和症状不明显或缺乏时,这些 SIADH 样综合征很难与 SIADH 区分。尽管如此,有令人信服的报告提供证据认为化疗引起的下丘脑或垂体损害可导致 SIADH。至少 7 份报告认为长春新碱(vincristine)与 SIADH 相关,这些报告中有些记录着不适当的高水平血清抗利尿激素[87]。长春碱也被报道引起严重的低钠血症和 SIADH[87]。长春碱引起 SIADH 的假设机制是脑室旁或视上细胞微管损害。

环磷酰胺治疗与低钠血症和 SIADH 相关。尸体解剖发现在一例环磷酰胺(1 800mg/m^2)引起的致死性低钠血症中,环磷酰胺直接影响下丘脑[88]。那些发现包括漏斗的坏死、减少内轴突分泌颗粒以及耗尽后丘脑抗利尿激素。接受低剂量环磷酰胺治疗的患者也可发生低钠血症、低渗透压、尿液高渗透压以及增加血浆抗利尿激素水平。肾脏微管破坏致使盐和水转运缺陷,可能是低钠血症与低剂量环磷酰胺治疗相关的主要原因[89]。

有许多报告显示顺铂可造成肾脏盐丢失引起低钠血症[90]。几份报告声称顺铂引起 SIADH。顺铂引起 SIADH 的机制不明确,但有认为顺铂肾脏毒性作用,也就是,降低乳头溶质含量,最大化尿液浓度是主要原因而不是顺铂对抗利尿激素分泌的直接影响。在大多数抗利尿激素水平升高的患者中,纠正低血容量后出现抗利尿激素水平受抑制[90]。因此,在这些患者中很可能是肾脏盐丢失引起的低血容量刺激抗利尿激素释放。

图 138-2 概括了评估和治疗低钠血症的演示。对低血容量和钠丢失,水钠补充是主要的治疗。AVP 受体拮抗剂直接阻断 AVP 与其受体结合。在临床试验中,考尼伐坦、利希普坦、托伐普坦和萨特普坦有效地纠正与 SIADH、肝硬化或充血性心力衰竭相关的低钠血症,这类新药可能对肿瘤相关低钠血症有效[91]。

高钠血症

高钠血症继发于中枢性尿崩症,经常作为神经外科手术或肿瘤破坏腺垂体或相关下丘脑核的并发症。异环磷酰胺或链佐星对肾小管重吸收水分的影响能导致肾源性尿崩症。异环

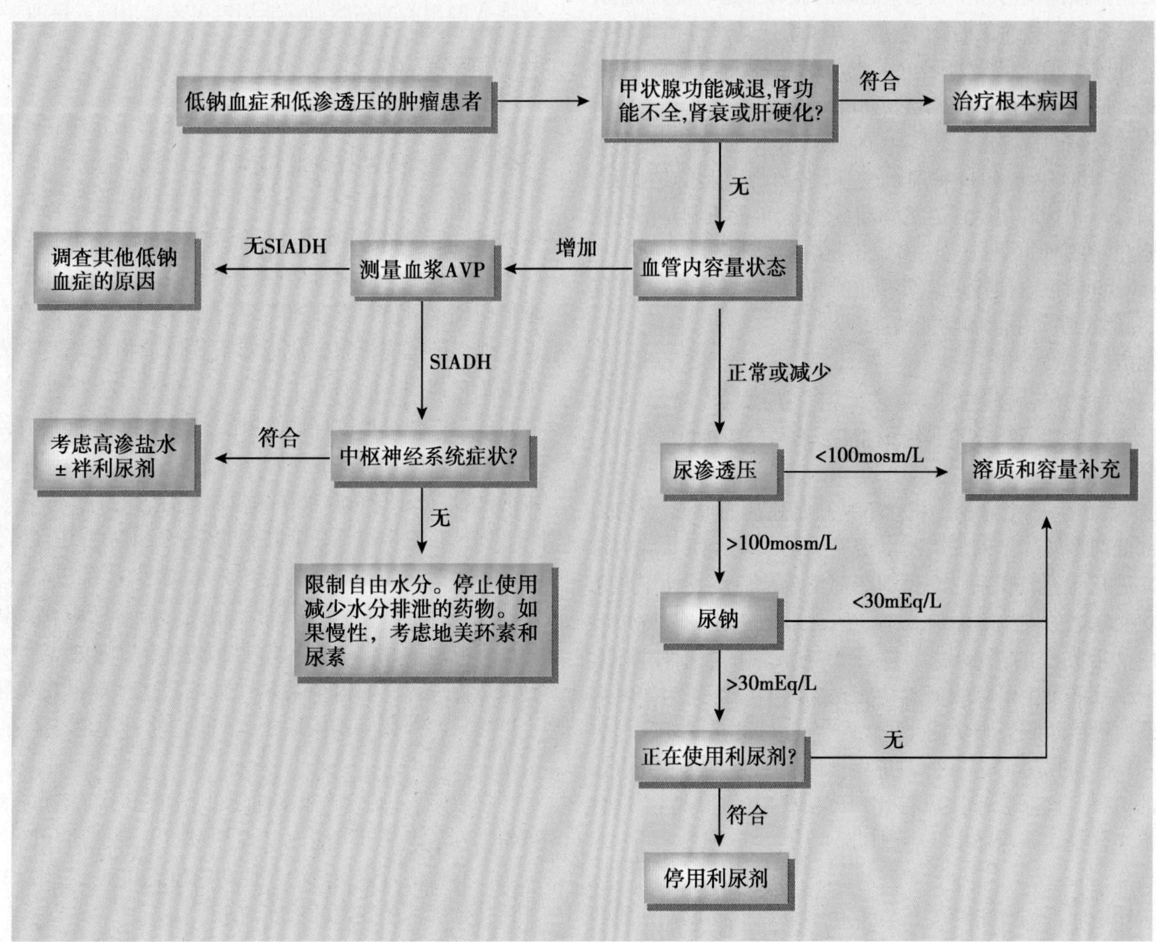

图 138-2　肿瘤患者评估低钠血症的方法

磷酰胺有广泛的肾毒性作用，以肾小管损害占主导。远端肾小管缺陷在大约一半异环磷酰胺治疗的患者中发生。然而，直接的肾源性尿崩症导致高钠血症不常见[92]。链佐星是另一种肾毒性药物；除了引起肾小球缺陷（蛋白尿）和肾小管缺陷（范可尼综合征）外，有报道称链佐星治疗能引起肾源性尿崩症[93]。

低钙血症

低钙血症可能是肿瘤溶解综合征的表现之一。低钙血症也能由以牺牲或损害了甲状旁腺（如全喉切除术，全甲状腺切除术）的颈部外科操作后原发性甲状旁腺功能减退所引起。低钙血症也是一个化疗常见的并发症[87]。有报道称在顺铂治疗的患者中有6%~20%出现低钙血症。顺铂对肾小管功能、镁代谢、骨重吸收以及维生素D代谢的影响可能可以解释低钙血症。低镁血症可能引起甲状旁腺激素分泌减少和甲状旁腺激素钙动员效应降低。低镁血症也抑制1,25-二羟维生素D_3（1,25-二羟胆钙化醇）的形成。顺铂可能抑制肾脏线粒体功能从而抑制25-羟胆钙化醇向1,25-二羟胆钙化醇的转化。此外，顺铂可能对骨重吸收有直接抑制作用。类似于顺铂治疗，卡铂（carboplatin）治疗，与16%~31%低钙血症发生率有关。普卡霉素（placamycin）[光神霉素（mithramycin）]是一种抗肿瘤的抗生素抑制脱氧核糖核酸（DNA）-依赖核糖核酸（RNA）聚合酶。这种药物主要影响钙代谢。在25mg/kg的剂量，低于抗肿瘤的需要剂量，它在24~48h内抑制骨重吸收和降低血清钙浓度。普卡霉素抑制基础的和甲状腺素刺激的破骨细胞功能，机制并不清楚。普卡霉素对破骨细胞功能的作用使其对骨佩吉特病和与恶性肿瘤相关破骨细胞介导的低钙血症的治疗很有用。普卡霉素的低血钙作用，以及它的肝、肾毒性，限制它作为抗肿瘤药物的有效性。放线菌素D（dactinomycin）是另一种阻断DNA指导RNA合成的抗肿瘤抗生素，在动物引起低钙血症。放线菌素D也废除甲状腺素的钙动员效应，可能机制是干扰破骨细胞介导的骨重吸收。在多柔比星（doxorubicin）和阿糖胞苷（cytarabine）联合治疗的患者中也有报道出现无症状的低镁血症、低钙血症和甲状腺功能减退。

高钙血症

高钙血症在肿瘤患者的发生率大约为1%[94]。高钙血症对于肿瘤患者是一个较差预后的指标，其与较短的生存相关。恶性肿瘤副肿瘤综合征之高钙血症在“内分泌副肿瘤综合征（异位激素产生）”中讨论。化疗不是高钙血症的原因。然而，头颈部低剂量外部光束放射与随后发生的原发性甲状腺旁腺功能亢进有明确的联系。在颈部低剂量放疗后原发性甲状腺旁腺功能亢进的发生率增加2.5~3倍[95]。在发生原发性甲状腺旁腺功能亢进的患者中，14%~30%有先前的放射暴露史。从放射治疗到发生甲状腺旁腺功能亢进的间隔区间为29~47年。原发性甲状腺旁腺功能亢进也发生在多种内分泌肿瘤（特别是MEN1）的情况下。手术是原发性甲状腺旁腺功能亢进最重要的治疗。摘除腺瘤一般有效，但在MEN1的情况下，选择的手术步骤是3.5-腺体甲状旁腺切除术[96]。

低镁血症

顺铂引起近端肾小管形态学改变和坏死，此部位是镁重吸收的一个重要位置。大约90%顺铂治疗的患者发生低镁血症[97]，10%的低镁血症患者有肌无力、颤动、头晕的症状。大量的水化和使用渗透性利尿剂例如甘露醇（mannitol）可能防止肾衰竭，但对肾脏镁丢失没有作用。低镁血症在停止顺铂治疗后可能持续很长时间。没有大型系列文献研究低镁血症的发生率，但制造商的资料表明60%用顺铂的患者可能受到影响。低镁血症也在接受环磷酰胺和卡铂的患者中发生。

脂肪代谢紊乱

肿瘤治疗引起的短期脂肪异常通常没有临床意义。然而，重要的异常能导致畸形并发症。干扰素和维生素A衍生物能引起甘油三酯显著的增加，导致胰腺炎。干扰素以增加肝脏和外周脂肪酸[98]和抑制肝脏甘油三酯脂肪酶[99]来引起高甘油三酯血症。长期用IFN-α_2在大约1/3的患者可引起高甘油三酯血症，这些患者大部分有早前的血清脂肪异常。血清甘油三酯水平大于1 000mg/dl并不常见。在一个例报告中，进行连续IFN-α治疗，观察饮食治疗效果和二甲苯氧庚酸（gemfibrozil）[100]。所有反式维A酸（retinoic acid/tretinoin）和其他衍生物，例如，13-顺式维A酸[异维A酸（isotretinoin）]，用于治疗几种恶性肿瘤，最显著的是头颈肿瘤和急性早幼粒细胞白血病。脂肪代谢的作用很有特点，虽然脂肪异常的机制暂不清楚。这些异常包括极低密度脂蛋白水平升高引起的高甘油三酯血症，以及低密度脂蛋白水平增加引起的高胆固醇血症。维A酸（retinoid）引起的高甘油三酯血症能导致脑卒中和胰腺炎。与维A酸相关的高脂血症能用二甲苯氧庚酸或鱼油来治疗。

性功能障碍

对头部的放射治疗可能引起广泛的下丘脑-垂体异常（图138-1）。合成的甲状腺素、GH或肾上腺素缺乏可能间接影响生殖功能。性功能直接受高泌乳素血症或促性腺激素缺乏所影响，这些现象经常在颅脑放射治疗>40Gy的患者中观察到。

高泌乳素血症通常（在2年内高达50%发生率）在下丘脑-垂体中位放射值暴露在50~57Gy的头颈放射后发生[4]。高泌乳素血症的可能机制是放射对下丘脑的损伤导致泌乳素分泌失去正常抑制。高泌乳素血症以减少垂体对促性腺激素释放激素的应答性来抑制促性腺激素分泌，因此引起继发性性腺功能减退。多巴胺治疗能逆转这一过程，如果其他腺垂体功能正常的话，进行一个治疗性试验可能是合理的。

促性腺激素缺乏在脑肿瘤的患者放射治疗中经常发生（高达61%）[101]。在儿童，延迟青春期，缺少月经初潮，以及不成熟的性发育是促性腺激素缺乏相关的显著问题。在联合化疗和颅脑放射治疗ALL[102]或颅脑放射治疗脑肿瘤[103]的患者，有报道出现青春期提早甚至性早熟。这种现象在女性患者发生更频繁。常伴随GH缺乏，虽然它对性早熟发生的作用不清楚。

在成年人，促性腺激素缺乏可能引起性激素缺乏和性功能障碍。性激素缺乏可能改变性欲及对骨和脂肪代谢有不利影响。需要评估及恰当地治疗性功能障碍和阳痿。图138-3概括了评估性腺功能减退的诊断演示。

抗肿瘤治疗引起的性腺并发症和功能障碍在之前的章节已被综述[87]。

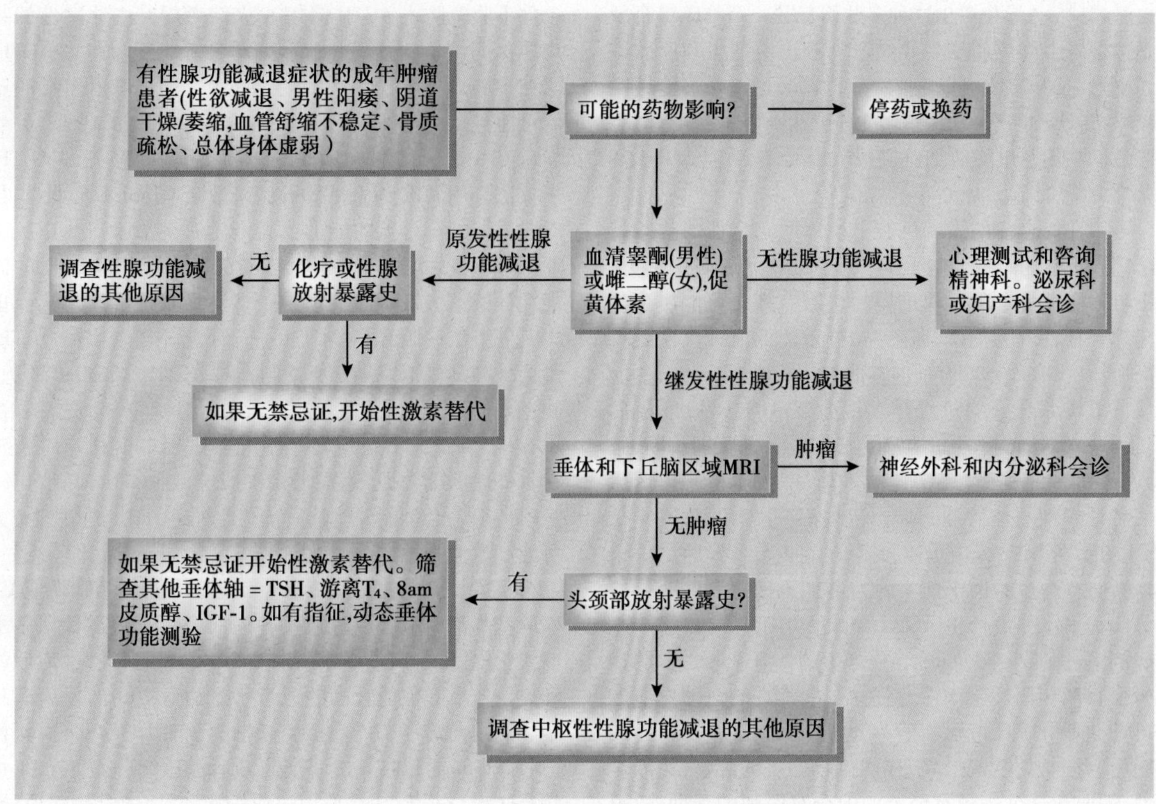

图 138-3　肿瘤患者评估性腺功能减退的方法

内分泌副肿瘤综合征(“异位”激素产生)

在各种肿瘤临床表现中,更加令人感兴趣和千变万化的是激素类物质的产生及其引起的特殊类型临床综合征。这些综合征被广义的分为几种不同类型。第一类是一种常规分泌激素的细胞类型所产生的激素物质。例子包括甲状旁腺癌产生的甲状旁腺激素,髓质甲状腺癌产生的降钙素,以及类癌产生的 5-羟色胺。在这种情况下,恶性肿瘤的分化细胞类型继续产生它的正常产品,但在某种意义上这极大地依赖于正常的调控过程。这些临床综合征在本文讨论恶性肿瘤的相关章节中讨论。第二类在这里详细讨论的“异位”激素是一种正常时不产生激素物质或正常时产生低水平激素物质的细胞类型。在一些例子中,它可能在细胞发育早期阶段产生激素产物。例子之一是鳞状细胞癌产生的甲状旁腺激素相关蛋白(PTHrP)。PTHrP 在分化好的鳞状细胞正常表达,但在未分化的鳞状上皮中不表达或低水平表达[104]。第二类“异位”激素产生模式发生在产生激素的细胞,是新增产生的另一种激素。例子之一是一种广谱的神经内分泌肿瘤类型产生 ACTH,小细胞肺癌是一个例子。

神经内分泌肿瘤产生多肽构成最常见的“异位”激素综合征。神经内分泌细胞分散遍及几乎所有器官,主要分布在肺、胃肠道、胰腺、甲状腺、肾上腺髓质、乳腺、前列腺以及皮肤。这些细胞最常从神经嵴分化,产生生命必需的有机胺和多肽激素。从这一组神经内分泌细胞成员中分化的肿瘤所产生的激素名单包括 ACTH、降钙素、血管活性肠肽(VIP)、铃蟾肽、生长激素释放激素、胰腺多肽、促肾上腺皮质激素释放激素(CRH)、神经降压素、生长激素释放抑制激素(SRIH),以及其他小多肽。

临床综合征的定义

有明确定义的临床异位激素综合征会以一定频率发生。它们的识别可能会帮助定义肿瘤类型以及引导合适的处理方法。此外,这些综合征是发病和死亡的主要原因;许多这些综合征的治疗方法是可行的,并通过治疗能提高生存质量和生存时间。

异位 ACTH 产生

过量的分泌 ACTH,虽然不常见,却是特定恶性肿瘤发病和死亡的重要原因。至少有 2 种不同的机制:异位 ACTH 产生或正常刺激 ACTH 合成和释放的下丘脑多肽所产生的异位 CRH。异位 ACTH 产生的最常见原因是肿瘤表达阿黑皮素原(proopiomelanocortin,POMC)。POMC 的后翻译过程通常在两个相互排斥的通路之一进行下去[105]。POMC 前体能分开成两个不同的路径用完全不同的生物学反应来产生多肽。导致 ACTH 产生和库欣综合征的是 POMC 分开产生大黑色素细胞刺激激素和 ACTH 通路之一。肿瘤患者幸运的是,使 POMC 产生 ACTH 的酶不常在正常垂体腺之外表达。大多数表达 *POMC* 基因的恶性肿瘤产生的多肽会引起不典型的临床综合征。与 ACTH 产生相关的最常见肿瘤是小细胞肺癌(SCLC),此外广谱的肿瘤类型包括肺类癌、髓质甲状腺癌、胰岛细胞恶性肿瘤、嗜铬细胞瘤以及偶尔的神经节瘤会产生这种激素。“异位”产生 ACTH 引起的库欣综合征的特点为肾上腺皮质增生和皮质醇增多症[106]。

过量 ACTH 产生的第二个原因是肿瘤产生促肾上腺皮质

激素释放激素[107]。异位产生这种多肽引起的一个临床综合征特点为垂体促肾上腺皮质增生导致肾上腺皮质增生和库欣综合征。识别过量的 CRH 产生需要临床医师考虑这个可能性和测量血液中 CRH。能产生 CRH 的肿瘤包括髓质甲状腺癌、副神经节瘤、前列腺癌和胰岛细胞肿瘤。其中有产生 ACTH 和 CRH 两者的肿瘤例子。

异位 ACTH 综合征的患者可能出现库欣综合征的临床特征-容易挫伤、向心性肥胖、肌肉消耗、高血压、糖尿病，并以代谢性碱中毒为主。另一种迅速进展的小细胞肺癌可能出现的一种临床综合征特点为消瘦、肌萎缩、严重的低血钾代谢性碱中毒和高血压，没有库欣综合征的其他临床发现。

异位 ACTH 综合征的特点是发现血浆 ACTH 浓度升高。然而，对血浆 ACTH 浓度升高的肾上腺功能亢进鉴别诊断，临床医师应该考虑一种产生 ACTH 的垂体肿瘤[108]。垂体产生 ACTH（一种原发性垂体肿瘤）和异位肿瘤产生 ACTH，或异位产生 CRH 的鉴别诊断，模仿垂体肿瘤，是在内分泌学科之中最困难的诊断。有许多的例子证实因为不能正确鉴别诊断异位产生 ACTH 和垂体肿瘤产生 ACTH 导致了不正确的治疗[109]。在这些病例中，例如小细胞肺癌异位产生的 ACTH，根据其临床综合征（低血钾、代谢性碱中毒、高血压、极其高的血清皮质醇水平和迅速进展的肿瘤）可以直接进行诊断[110]。在其他病例，尤其是那些与常见异位 ACTH 产生不相关的肿瘤，诊断会有挑战性，需要在这个领域有经验的内分泌医师的帮助，以及全面使用全光谱介入放射技术用于鉴别垂体和非垂体来源的 ACTH。

诊断评估基于测量肾上腺功能亢进患者的血浆 ACTH（图 138-4）。血清 ACTH 浓度大于 100pg/ml 提示应该调查异位来源的 ACTH[111]。对于 ACTH 值大于 10pg/ml 的患者（在合适的条件下收集防止 ACTH 降解），应该考虑是由原发性的肾上腺皮质疾病（肾上腺腺瘤或癌）所导致。大部分患者 ACTH 值会落在 10pg/ml 到 100pg/ml 的区间里。这些患者主要的鉴别诊断可能包括中枢（垂体）或外周（异位）来源的 ACTH，肿瘤产生异位 CRH 的可能性很小。鉴别中枢和外周来源的 ACTH 有几个方法。用 MRI 识别垂体肿瘤来诊断垂体来源的假设，虽然有时候垂体肿瘤是无功能的或者产生其他激素产物。基于这个原因经常使用岩部静脉窦取样[112]。异位产生 CRH 的诊断只能在怀疑这个诊断和测量这个多肽血浆浓度时作出。也可能用其他方法诊断异位 ACTH 综合征。肿瘤产生的 ACTH 一般不会被高剂量地塞米松所抑制。对 ACTH>10pg/ml 的患者，在晚上 11∶00 单独口服使用 8mg 剂量的地塞米松，之后在次日上午 8∶00 测量血清皮质醇水平能够区别中枢和外周来源[106]。在垂体库欣综合征，地塞米松一般会被 ACTH 抑制 50%；这个策略一般不会抑制非垂体肿瘤产生的 ACTH。这些检查方法都可能产生假阳性或假阴性结果。

手术切除或使用化疗药治疗肿瘤是产生 ACTH 或 CRH 肿瘤的基本治疗方法。有这些肿瘤的患者应该在计划手术操作前纠正电解质异常、糖尿病以及高血压。长期存在库欣综合征和血浆皮质醇数值升高的患者手术后有更高的发病率和死亡率。手术前治疗选择包括美替拉酮（口服 1～4g/d），氨鲁米特（口服 250mg，每日 4 次滴定），或者酮康唑（口服 200～400mg，每日 2 次）[113,114]。注射用的依托咪酯，用于镇静和诱导麻醉，在亚催眠浓度能快速抑制皮质醇合成[115]。它从 0.3～4mg/(kg·h)滴定至正常血清皮质醇测量值，曾在少数患者用于快速逆转肾上腺功能亢进。当使用皮质醇产物的药物学抑制剂时需要糖皮质激素替代治疗来防止肾上腺功能不全。如果不能或者不建议手术切除一个产生 ACTH 或者 CRH 的肿瘤时，

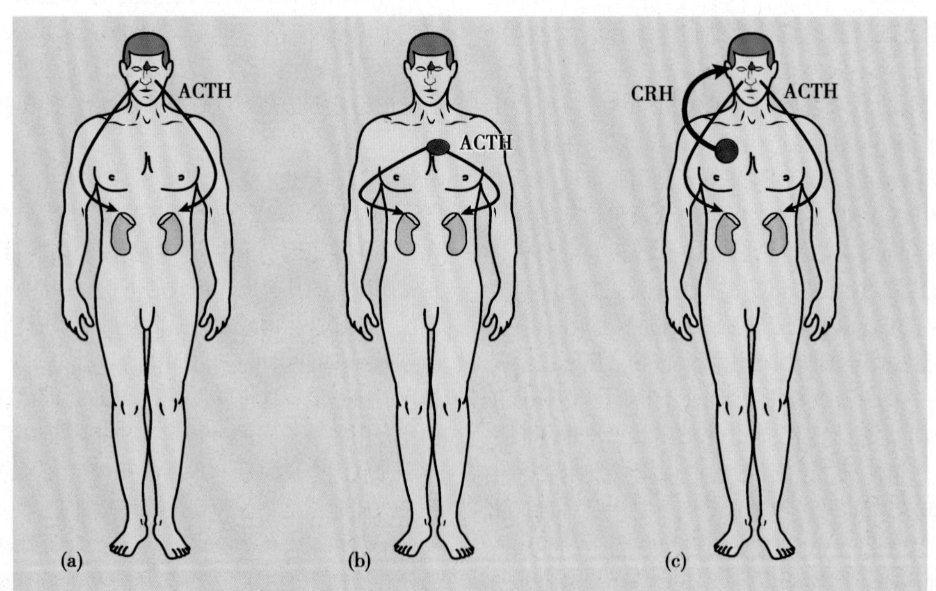

图 138-4　促肾上腺皮质激素（ACTH）依赖性库欣综合征的鉴别诊断。很难鉴别垂体（a）和异位（b）来源的 ACTH，两者都是 ACTH 依赖性库欣综合征的最常见原因。要准确地鉴别，放置抽取垂体腺（岩下窦）静脉的导管联合外源性促肾上腺皮质激素释放激素刺激能够准确地鉴别（在文章中讨论）。肿瘤产生的异位促肾上腺皮质激素释放激素（CRH）导致垂体腺产生 ACTH 增加（c）。很难鉴别产生异位 CRH 和垂体依赖性库欣综合征，必须测量外周血 CRH 来作出确定诊断。恶性肿瘤偶尔产生 CRH 和 ACTH，诊断评估会更加复杂（未显示）

可能需要长期使用皮质醇合成抑制剂来治疗。另一种方法是腹腔镜下肾上腺切除术及随后的类固醇替代来提供一个快速和比较安全的方法处理肾上腺功能亢进。作为一种处理异位 ACTH 综合征的治疗方法，该技术还没有得到充分地使用。

由于需要迅速开始化疗，迅速进展的 SCLC 和异位 ACTH 综合征的患者组成一个独特的患者群体。遗憾的是，这些患者也非常容易受到机会性感染以及开始化疗后经常导致死亡或严重的感染相关性发病[116]。这些患者治疗的困境在于用皮质醇合成抑制剂使血清皮质醇正常化可能需要 1～2 周的时间（可能需要更长的时期使免疫力正常化），而这从肿瘤科医师的角度来看，延迟化疗是不可接受的。在电解质和高血压正常后进行腹腔镜下肾上腺切除术是一个明确和耐受性好的技术，这可能是一个使过量皮质醇分泌快速正常化的策略。如果化疗在血清皮质醇正常化后不久开始，应该考虑预防性治疗卡氏肺孢子虫或真菌引起的机会性感染。

恶性肿瘤引起的高钙血症

高钙血症是引起肿瘤患者发病和死亡的常见和重要原因。

肿瘤患者引起高钙血症最常见的原因是 PTHrP 介导的高钙血症，增加维生素 D、骨化三醇或 1,25 二羟维生素 D_3 活性代谢产物的产生，以及局部的溶骨性高钙血症[117,118]。异位 PTH 产生是肿瘤相关性高钙血症的罕见原因。高钙血症的其他原因，最明显的是原发性甲状旁腺功能亢进，有高钙血症的肿瘤患者应该考虑到这个因素。测量血清完整的甲状旁腺激素（iPTH）能够鉴别高甲状旁腺血症和高钙血症的其他原因。高钙血症和血清甲状旁腺激素水平升高联合尿钙排泄增加为原发性甲状旁腺功能亢进提供了合理的证据。iPTH 受抑制低于正常范围见于 PTHrP 或骨化三醇介导的高钙血症。肿瘤其他高钙血症少见的原因会在下面讨论。

甲状旁腺激素相关蛋白

PTHrP 是起始 16 个氨基酸有 8 个和 PTH 完全相同的小分子多肽。这些小分子多肽以结合 PTH 受体和激活成骨细胞-特异性细胞表面蛋白，受体活化因子受体配体（RNAKL）来引起高钙血症。RANKL 和 RANK 受体在破骨细胞前体的相互作用下增加破骨细胞分化、骨吸收和高钙血症。其他 PTHrP 的 PTH 类似反应包括低磷酸血症和增加尿钙排泄。PTHrP 介导高钙血症的特征是抑制 iPTH 水平和低或正常的骨化三醇水平。这个与原发性甲状旁腺功能亢进升高的 iPTH 和骨化三醇水平相反。PTHrP 产生常见于鳞状细胞癌；产生它的其他肿瘤包括：乳腺、神经内分泌、肾、黑色素和前列腺肿瘤。

恶性肿瘤产生的骨化三醇

淋巴瘤经常产生骨化三醇，导致胃肠道的钙吸收增加。淋巴瘤组织，如同肉瘤、铍中毒、结核和真菌感染中的肉芽组织，表达 1α-羟化酶，是将 25-羟维生素 D 转化为骨化三醇的酶。临床研究表明淋巴瘤患者在诊断时有尿钙过高的比例很高；明显的高钙血症比例不高[119]。在淋巴瘤情况下典型高钙血症的临床特点包括抑制血清 iPTH、正常或轻微增加的磷水平（抑制 PTH 引起）、高尿钙、骨代谢缺乏，以及在大约一半高钙血症的患者中血清骨化三醇水平升高[119]。

局部溶骨性骨吸收引起高钙血症

某些恶性肿瘤经常转移至骨，一些引起高钙血症。与乳腺癌和骨髓瘤相关的高钙血症较常见。相反，前列腺癌，尽管它更经常出现在骨，很少产生高钙血症。引起高钙血症的恶性肿瘤产生细胞因子、PTHrP，或其他增加骨吸收的刺激因素[117,118]。最有特点的可能是乳腺癌细胞产生的 PTHrP。在动物模型中有强力的证据表明乳腺癌细胞产生的 PTHrP 刺激破骨细胞吸收和从正常骨骼释放转化生长因子-β（TGF-β）[120,121]。在这个动物模型中骨释放的 TGF-β 刺激乳腺癌生长增殖，进而建立一个循环，即 PTHrP 的产生不仅仅增加破骨细胞吸收，也加速相邻乳腺癌的生长。事实上，这种观点导致了双膦酸盐这类抑制破骨细胞骨吸收的药物，用来防止乳腺癌转移的药物相关的临床试验[122,123]。

在多发性骨髓瘤中几种因素促进了局部骨质溶解。增加 RANKL 的表达引起局部破骨细胞增殖看起来是最重要的原因。在骨髓瘤中可能有助于破骨细胞增殖的其他因素是白介素-6 和巨噬细胞炎性蛋白 1α，虽然他们看起来没有 RANKL 重要[118]。

恶性肿瘤相关高钙血症的影响

在恶性肿瘤中严重的高钙血症与较短的生存时间相关。严重和无应答高钙血症的患者其平均生存时间为数周到数月。死亡原因包括高钙血症的并发症（昏迷、肾衰竭）和肿瘤进展。高钙血症的发展经常是评估肿瘤治疗进展的指标。由于并不总能预测患者对肿瘤治疗的反应，在所有新诊断的肿瘤患者中治疗高钙血症是重要的。是否继续治疗复发和/或难治的高钙血症应该基于原发肿瘤对肿瘤治疗的反应及患者的整体预后来作出决定。严重的高钙血症经常引起大脑功能抑制或昏迷，可能减轻垂死患者的痛苦。

高钙血症的治疗

高钙血症患者经常发生脱水。增加尿液钙排泄引起浓缩缺陷导致液体丢失增加。最初的处理应该强调用输注 100～300ml/h 速率的生理盐水溶液来逆转脱水。在 6～12h 水化后常常会降低 10%～40%的血清钙离子。严重高钙血症的患者定义为血清钙离子浓度>13mg/dl（3.25mmol/L），出现精神状态改变，或由于高钙血症引起肾衰竭时应该用静脉注射帕米膦酸盐（pamidronate，60～90mg 大于 4h）或唑来膦酸（zoledronate，4mg 大于 30min）[124]，糖皮质激素（40～60mg/d，等量转换的泼尼松），或硝酸镓（gallium nitrate，200mg/m²・d，每日注射，共 7 日）来治疗[125,126]。鲑鱼降钙素在早期治疗过程可能降低 1～2mg/dl 的血清钙浓度，但很少长期有效。对于反应较差的患者，这些药物有时需要联合或序贯使用。糖皮质激素，能抑制钙的吸收，是最常用的淋巴瘤药物，然而双膦酸盐治疗在实体肿瘤相关的高钙血症中可能更有效。唑来膦酸通常比帕米膦酸盐更有效，因为它的效价增加了[127]。用双膦酸盐长期治疗骨转移后有 1%～2.5%的患者发生颌骨坏死。用双膦酸盐短期治疗肿瘤相关高钙血症的患者并不存在这个问题。

在高钙血症的早期发展阶段有几种新的治疗方法显示出希望。一种直接对抗 RANKL 的单克隆抗体在破骨细胞前体防止它与 RANK 受体的相互作用，因此降低破骨细胞介导的骨吸收[128]。这个抗体（地诺单抗，denosumab）的初步研究显示它是骨吸收的有效抑制剂，临床研究正在明确它在高钙血症和骨转移患者中的功效。

人绒促性素

人绒促性素（HCG）形成于单独基因编码的 2 种不同蛋白

亚基。第一种是 α 亚基被全部垂体类糖蛋白激素共享,包括HCG、促黄体素(LH)、卵泡刺激素(FSH)和促甲状腺素(TSH)。第二种是 β 亚基,在这些激素中都是独特的。产生HCG见于滋养层肿瘤(绒毛膜癌、睾丸胚胎癌、精原细胞瘤)以及,不常见的,肺和胰腺肿瘤。在幼年儿童,HCG刺激卵巢功能可引起青春期提前。在成年男性则经常发生男性乳房发育。甲状腺功能亢进可能在HCG与甲状腺刺激激素受体(TSHR)相互作用时进展,尤其是当β-HCG高水平表达时。

切除或有效治疗原发肿瘤是β-HCG产生过量所引起的临床综合征最有效的治疗。如果化疗或其他治疗基础恶性肿瘤的策略可能有效时,甲状腺功能亢进能短期用硫脲类治疗。在肿瘤低反应的患者,可能需要甲状腺切除术或放射性碘治疗。

低血糖

在肿瘤患者,肿瘤是诱导低血糖不常见,但有挑战性的病因。其临床综合征可分为三种。第一种,胰岛素能在胰岛细胞恶性肿瘤产生。胰岛细胞肿瘤通常产生低水平的胰岛素,临床表现常不显著直到肿瘤负荷变大,最常见于肝转移。第二种原因是葡萄糖异生作用缺乏,见于邻近肝实质被肿瘤完全替代的患者,干扰或消除葡萄糖的产生。第三种形式是胰岛素样生长因子-Ⅱ(IGH-Ⅱ)浓度增加所引起,IGH-Ⅱ是一个激活胰岛素受体的多肽。这个综合征常见于纤维肉瘤、血管外皮细胞瘤或肝癌的患者。在这些患者中,IGF-Ⅱ水平经常升高,IGF结合蛋白3(IGFBP3)不能和酸性不稳定亚组能够有效结合形成IGF-Ⅱ的复合物。升高的循环IGF-Ⅱ激活胰岛素受体,进而引起低血糖[129~131]。

这些临床综合征最通常出现的临床表现是空腹低血糖,在空腹时期患者最可能发生症状,尤其是在夜间。在低血糖期间测量血浆胰岛素、胰岛素原、C-肽是区分临床1型(胰岛素产生)和2型(肿瘤代替肝脏)以及3型(IGF-Ⅱ)最重要的诊断工具。在低血糖(缺乏可能刺激正常胰腺释放胰岛素的任何药物)时,胰岛素、胰岛素前体和C-肽升高,这是胰岛素生成上调导致低血糖的有力证据。与此相反,在肿瘤替代的肝脏或IGF-Ⅱ介导的低血糖中,胰岛素、胰岛素前体以及C-肽水平会较低。IGF-Ⅱ介导的低血糖,实验室检查结果包括血清IGF-Ⅱ升高,胰岛素、胰岛素前体和C-肽低或正常,IGF-Ⅰ水平低,以及在巨大肉瘤或腹膜后肿瘤中IGFBP3或酸性不稳定亚基一般正常。

通过手术切除或者抗肿瘤治疗来减少肿块对胰岛素或IGF-Ⅱ介导的低血糖是有效;当肝脏被肿瘤替代时,除了给予葡萄糖外没有其他有效的治疗。通过频繁的进餐治疗低血糖。在夜间时段叫醒患者摄取热量可能保持无症状。可能需要通过中心静脉通道连续输注20%葡萄糖来保持患者正常的血糖,尤其是那些肝脏被肿瘤替代的情况。予患者高血糖素输注(0.5~2mg/h)来刺激肝糖原异生作用也是产生胰岛素的肿瘤或那些IGF-Ⅱ介导的低血糖一个有效的治疗方法。重要的是在尝试这个治疗方法之前必须证明对高血糖素的反应(1mg皮下注射后在30和60min测量血糖)。高血糖素可以少量给药(1~5ml超过24h),这使其可能通过小的输液泵给药[132]。高血糖素治疗的患者可能发生典型的与高血糖素瘤相关的皮疹,迫使中止这个治疗方式。其他能周期性成功并被应用的治疗包括重组生长激素(每日3~6μg/kg,皮下)或糖皮质激素(每日20~40mg等量的泼尼松)。奥曲肽(octreotide)或兰瑞肽(lanreotide)被用于产生胰岛素的胰岛细胞肿瘤患者,通常不成功。治疗失败与目前可用的生长抑素类似物抑制高血糖素比抑制胰岛素分泌更有效的事实相关。二氮嗪(diazoxide,3~8mg/(kg·d),分成2~3个剂量)被成功用于抑制胰岛素分泌,但引起液体潴留,因此限制了有效剂量的运用。

在终末期白血病或淋巴瘤的情况下,低血糖也可能发生在乳酸酸中毒的患者。这个临床综合征发生在终末期或疾病广泛以及累及肝脏的白血病/淋巴瘤患者。有猜测显示肿瘤细胞产生的乳酸超过肝脏对它的清除能力。低血糖的病因学还不清楚,但可能是肝脏糖原异生作用受损的结果[133]。

抗利尿激素分泌失调综合征

抗利尿激素分泌失调综合征(SIADH)较早前作为肿瘤治疗的副作用被讨论(见"电解质/矿物质代谢紊乱:低钠血症")。此外,大约15%的小细胞肺癌(SCLC),1%其他肺癌和3%头颈鳞状细胞癌以不受调节的方式产生抗利尿激素,导致低钠血症、低渗透压、增加尿钠排泄,以及相对血浆张力不适当的高尿渗透压[134]。其他良性或恶性肿瘤包括原发性脑肿瘤、血液肿瘤、皮肤肿瘤,以及胃肠道、妇科、乳腺、前列腺癌和肉瘤,也能产生这个临床综合征。

大部分患者发生这个综合征是无症状的。在血清钠浓度下降至<120mEq/L的情况,可能发生精神状态的改变和癫痫。尤其是生育年龄的妇女发生低钠血症可能发生严重的大脑退化。限制液体在短期处理上是有效的。但用地美环素(demeclocycline,150~300mg/d)一种抑制抗利尿激素对肾脏作用的药物来治疗,其长期治疗效果更好。抗利尿激素受体拮抗剂,考尼伐坦(conivaptan)、利希普坦(lixivaptan)、托伐普坦(tolvaptan)和萨特普坦(satavaptan),在临床试验中表现出有效性,在美国,现在临床上可供使用的至少有考尼伐坦已经通过药物监督管理局的批准(静脉使用,20mg,输液时间30min;此后调整为20mg,输液时间超过24h)。托伐普坦可以口服(15~60mg/d)。这两种药物都是非常有效的,在开始治疗后仔细监测血清钠浓度是非常重要的。

长期使用去甲环素和V2受体拮抗剂的一个考虑因素是治疗费用。在血清钠浓度为120mEq/L的患者中,静脉使用考尼伐坦可在24h~48h内改善或使血清钠水平正常化,可能最适合于这种紧急情况;去甲环素效应持续数日。对于较长期的治疗,特别是当无法减少肿瘤体积时,应考虑使用较便宜的去甲环素,它的耐受性和有效性一般较好。

其他的异位激素综合征

肿瘤引起的软骨病

肾脏磷丢失引起的严重低磷血症是肿瘤引起软骨病的原因。这个临床综合征的特点是骨质软化,由类骨质矿化不足所引起,以及中到重度的近端肌病[135]。产生这个临床综合征的肿瘤包括:间叶细胞肿瘤(成骨细胞瘤、巨细胞骨肉瘤、血管外皮细胞瘤、血管瘤、非骨化纤维瘤)[136],罕见的恶性肿瘤例如前列腺癌或肺癌。有证据表明成纤维细胞生长因子-23,成纤维细胞生长因子家族成员之一在常染色体显性软骨病中突变[137],在一些肿瘤中过表达进而导致肿瘤引起软骨病[138]。口服或静脉补充磷联合维生素D治疗通常对根除或改善临床症状有效。完整的手术切除肿瘤可以达到根治的目的。

促红细胞生成素、促血小板生成素、促白细胞生成素或集落刺激因子产生

异位促红细胞生成素引起的红细胞增多症是一种罕见的临床综合征。它被发现于大脑血管母细胞瘤、子宫肌瘤、嗜铬细胞瘤，以及肾脏细胞、卵巢和肝癌中[139,140]。治疗可以包括手术或化疗缩小肿块或放血疗法。其他的还没有很好定义的综合征包括一些肿瘤产生的促血小板生成素、促白细胞生成素或集落刺激因子。这些情况可以通过适当的化疗来减少肿瘤的大小或手术切除来治疗。

肾素产生

肾脏（肾母细胞瘤、肾脏细胞癌或血管外皮细胞瘤）、肺（SCLC、腺癌）、肝、胰腺或卵巢恶性肿瘤产生的肾素能够引起一种以高血压、低血钾和醛固酮产生增加为特点的临床综合征[141]。对肿瘤不能被切除的患者用螺内酯（spironolactone）、血管紧张素转化酶抑制药或血管紧张素受体拮抗剂治疗可能降低血压和使异常电解质正常化。

生长激素和泌乳素

肢端肥大症是一种以生长激素和 IGF-1 值升高为特点的疾病，通常是由垂体肿瘤所引起，少见于肺和胃腺癌。在胰岛细胞瘤、支气管类癌和 SCLC 中发现异位产生的生长激素释放激素，一种调节垂体正常产生 GH 的下丘脑肽[142]。异位产生泌乳素罕见于性腺胚细胞瘤[143]、淋巴瘤[144]、白血病[145]和结直肠癌[146]。临床综合征包括女性溢乳、闭经以及男性性腺功能减退和男性乳房发育。多巴胺激动剂［溴隐亭（bromocriptine）、喹高利特（quinagolide）或卡麦角林（cabergoline）］，对治疗垂体泌乳素瘤有效，对治疗异位产生的泌乳素通常无效。

（郭威 译 毛友生 校）

参考文献

The complete reference list can be found on the Wiley Companion Digital Edition of this title (see inside front cover for login instructions).

1 Fassett DR, Couldwell WT. Metastases to the pituitary gland. *Neurosurg Focus*. 2004;**16**:E8.

2 Lam KS, Tse VK, Wang C, Yeung RT, Ho JH. Effects of cranial irradiation on hypothalamic-pituitary function—a 5-year longitudinal study in patients with nasopharyngeal carcinoma. *Q J Med*. 1991;**78**:165–176.

3 Pai HH, Thornton A, Katznelson L, et al. Hypothalamic/pituitary function following high-dose conformal radiotherapy to the base of skull: demonstration of a dose-effect relationship using dose-volume histogram analysis. *Int J Radiat Oncol Biol Phys*. 2001;**49**:1079–1092.

4 Samaan NA, Schultz PN, Yang KP, et al. Endocrine complications after radiotherapy for tumors of the head and neck. *J Lab Clin Med*. 1987;**109**:364–372.

5 Shalet SM. Disorders of the endocrine system due to radiation and cytotoxic chemotherapy. *Clin Endocrinol (Oxf)*. 1983;**19**:637–659.

11 Chopra IJ. Clinical review 86: euthyroid sick syndrome: is it a misnomer? *J Clin Endocrinol Metabol*. 1997;**82**:329–334.

13 Grande C. Hypothyroidism following radiotherapy for head and neck cancer: multivariate analysis of risk factors. *Radiother Oncol*. 1992;**25**:31–36.

16 Constine LS, Donaldson SS, McDougall IR, et al. Thyroid dysfunction after radiotherapy in children with Hodgkin's disease. *Cancer*. 1984;**53**:878–883.

30 Vecil GG, Papadopoulos NV, Vassilopoulou-Sellin R, McCutcheon IE. Interferon-induced hypothyroidism causing reversible pituitary enlargement. *Endocr Pract*. 2008;**14**:219–223.

31 Sherman SI. Etiology, diagnosis, and treatment recommendations for central hypothyroidism associated with bexarotene therapy for cutaneous T-cell lymphoma. *Clin Lymphoma*. 2003;**3**:249–252.

32 Golden WM, Weber KB, Hernandez TL, et al. Single-dose rexinoid rapidly and specifically suppresses serum thyrotropin in normal subjects. *J Clin Endocrinol Metab*. 2007;**92**:124–130.

34 Illouz F, Braun D, Briet C, Schweizer U, Rodien P. Endocrine side-effects of anti-cancer drugs: thyroid effects of tyrosine kinase inhibitors. *Eur J Endocrinol*. 2014;**171**:R91–R99.

35 Wells SA Jr, Gosnell JE, Gagel RF, et al. Vandetanib for the treatment of patients with locally advanced or metastatic hereditary medullary thyroid cancer. *J Clin Oncol*. 2010;**28**:767–772.

36 Schlumberger M, Tahara M, Wirth LJ, et al. Lenvatinib versus placebo in radioiodine-refractory thyroid cancer. *N Engl J Med*. 2015;**372**:621–630.

37 Quach A, Ji L, Mishra V, et al. Thyroid and hepatic function after high-dose 131 I-metaiodobenzylguanidine (131 I-MIBG) therapy for neuroblastoma. *Pediatr Blood Cancer*. 2011;**56**:191–201.

40 Haraldsdottir S, Li Q, Villalona-Calero MA, et al. Case of sorafenib-induced thyroid storm. *J Clin Oncol*. 2013;**31**:e262–e264.

43 Makari-Judson G, Judson CH, Mertens WC. Longitudinal patterns of weight gain after breast cancer diagnosis: observations beyond the first year. *Breast J*. 2007;**13**:258–265.

46 Kroenke CH, Chen WY, Rosner B, Holmes MD. Weight, weight gain, and survival after breast cancer diagnosis. *J Clin Oncol*. 2005;**23**:1370–1378.

48 Nilsen TI, Vatten LJ. Prospective study of colorectal cancer risk and physical activity, diabetes, blood glucose and BMI: exploring the hyperinsulinaemia hypothesis. *Br J Cancer*. 2001;**84**:417–422.

59 Everhart J, Wright D. Diabetes mellitus as a risk factor for pancreatic cancer. A meta-analysis. *JAMA*. 1995;**273**:1605–1609.

75 Abrams H, Spiro R, Goldstein N. Metastasis in carcinoma—one thousand autopsied cases. *Cancer*. 1950;**3**:74.

82 Gurney JG, Ness KK, Stovall M, et al. Final height and body mass index among adult survivors of childhood brain cancer: childhood cancer survivor study. *J Clin Endocrinol Metab*. 2003;**88**:4731–4739.

87 Yeung SC, Chiu AC, Vassilopoulou-Sellin R, Gagel RF. The endocrine effects of nonhormonal antineoplastic therapy. *Endocr Rev*. 1998;**19**:144–172.

95 Cohen J, Gierlowski TC, Schneider AB. A prospective study of hyperparathyroidism in individuals exposed to radiation in childhood. *JAMA*. 1990;**264**:581–584.

97 Stewart AF, Keating T, Schwartz PE. Magnesium homeostasis following chemotherapy with cisplatin: a prospective study. *Am J Obstet Gynecol*. 1985;**153**:660–665.

101 Constine LS, Woolf PD, Cann D, et al. Hypothalamic-pituitary dysfunction after radiation for brain tumors. *N Engl J Med*. 1993;**328**:87–94.

104 Maioli E, Fortino V. The complexity of parathyroid hormone-related protein signalling. *Cell Mol Life Sci*. 2004;**61**:257–262.

108 Newell-Price J. Cushing's syndrome. *Clin Med*. 2008;**8**:204–208.

114 Nieman LK, Ilias I. Evaluation and treatment of Cushing's syndrome. *Am J Med*. 2005;**118**:1340–1346.

116 Dimopoulos MA, Fernandez JF, Samaan NA, Holoye PY, Vassilopoulou-Sellin R. Paraneoplastic Cushing's syndrome as an adverse prognostic factor in patients who die early with small cell lung cancer. *Cancer*. 1992;**69**:66–71.

117 Stewart AF. Clinical practice. Hypercalcemia associated with cancer. *N Engl J Med*. 2005;**352**:373–379.

118 Roodman GD. Mechanisms of bone metastasis. *N Engl J Med*. 2004;**350**:1655–1664.

119 Seymour JF, Gagel RF, Hagemeister FB, Dimopoulos MA, Cabanillas F. Calcitriol production in hypercalcemic and normocalcemic patients with non-Hodgkin lymphoma. *Ann Intern Med*. 1994;**121**:633–640.

120 Guise TA, Yin JJ, Thomas RJ, et al. Parathyroid hormone-related protein (PTHrP)-(1-139) isoform is efficiently secreted in vitro and enhances breast cancer metastasis to bone in vivo. *Bone*. 2002;**30**:670–676.

122 Wang Z, Qiao D, Lu Y, et al. Systematic literature review and network meta-analysis comparing bone-targeted agents for the prevention of skeletal-related events in cancer patients with bone metastasis. *Oncologist*. 2015;**20**:440–449.

128 Hu MI, Glezerman IG, Leboulleux S, et al. Denosumab for treatment of hypercalcemia of malignancy. *J Clin Endocrinol Metab*. 2014;**99**:3144–3152.

129 Baxter RC, Holman SR, Corbould A, et al. Regulation of the insulin-like growth factors and their binding proteins by glucocorticoid and growth hormone in nonislet cell tumor hypoglycemia. *J Clin Endocrinol Metab*. 1995;**80**:2700–2708.

134 Flombaum CD. Metabolic emergencies in the cancer patient. *Semin Oncol*. 2000;**27**:322–334.

138 Jonsson KB, Zahradnik R, Larsson T, et al. Fibroblast growth factor 23 in oncogenic osteomalacia and X-linked hypophosphatemia. *N Engl J Med*. 2003;**348**:1656–1663.

第 139 章　肿瘤患者的感染

Lior Nesher, MD ■ Kenneth V. I. Rolston, MD, FACP

概述

由于潜在的疾病及其治疗，癌症患者发生感染的风险增加。血液恶性肿瘤患者和造血细胞移植受体发生这种风险的可能性是最大的。这主要是由于各种免疫缺陷，如中性粒细胞减少和细胞和/或体液免疫受损，每种缺陷都与一个独特的感染谱相关。较新的治疗癌症的方法正在改变感染谱，导尿管和其他医疗器械的使用也在增加感染的发生率。虽然目前报道的细菌感染最常见，但真菌和病毒的机会性感染也越来越频繁。癌症患者感染的发病率和死亡率通常高于一般人群。因此，早期诊断和及时给予适当的治疗至关重要。这些病原菌的耐药性已成为世界性的难题，只有开发出新的抗菌药物才能部分解决。因此，为了发现流行病学变化而进行频繁的流行病学监测以及感染预防、感染控制和抗生素管理的重要性怎么强调都不为过。癌症幸存者的数量正在稳步增加，许多患者在相当长的一段时间内需接受免疫抑制治疗。维持这些幸存者的健康和帮助他们免受感染仍将是未来几年的挑战。

在肿瘤患者中，感染一直是一种常见的问题。感染的发病率和肿瘤的类型有关[1]。多次感染并不罕见。中性粒细胞减少、细胞或体液免疫失调、使用导尿管或其他医疗器械、脾切除术、外科手术、放射治疗、营养状况不佳和局部因素如梗阻等都会增加这些患者对感染的易感性。每个危险因素都与其特异的感染相关，尽管有一些重叠。同一患者可能存在多重易感因素，表 139-1 列出了不同肿瘤类型的宿主防御机制的主要缺陷和该缺陷相关的感染。

表 139-1　与恶性疾病相关的常见感染和宿主防御机制缺陷

疾病	缺陷机制	主要感染
急性白血病、再生障碍性贫血	粒细胞减少	革兰阳性球菌、革兰阴性杆菌、白色念珠菌、曲霉菌、镰刀菌、毛孢子菌
毛细胞白血病	粒细胞减少、淋巴细胞功能受损	荚膜性病原体、肺炎链球菌、流感嗜血杆菌、脑膜炎奈瑟菌
慢性淋巴细胞白血病、多发性骨髓瘤	低球蛋白血症	荚膜性病原体、肺炎链球菌、流感嗜血杆菌、脑膜炎奈瑟菌
霍奇金病	T 淋巴细胞应答受损	肺炎肺囊虫、隐球菌、分枝杆菌、弓形虫、李斯特菌、隐孢子虫、白色念珠菌、巨细胞病毒
骨肿瘤、移植受体	粒细胞减少、细胞和体液免疫受损	革兰阳性球菌、革兰阴性杆菌、巨细胞病毒、白色念珠菌、曲霉菌、疱疹病毒
乳腺癌	组织坏死	革兰阳性球菌、革兰阴性杆菌、厌氧菌
肺癌	局部栓塞、组织坏死	革兰阳性球菌、革兰阴性杆菌、厌氧菌
妇科恶性疾病	局部栓塞、组织坏死	需氧和厌氧混合性肠道菌

中性粒细胞减少

发热的类型

在 20%～25%的中性粒细胞减少症患者发热病例中可发现特征性的致病病原体（微生物检查证实的感染）。另有 20%～25%的病例有特征性的感染部位（如肺炎、蜂窝织炎和小肠结肠炎），但培养物阴性（仅有临床证据的感染）。40%～45%的病例既没有明显的临床感染部位，也没有阳性培养结果，被称为不明原因的发热（图 139-1）。这些发热大多数被认为是由于隐匿性感染和对抗生素治疗有反应而产生的。少于 5%的发热是由非感染性原因引起的，如输血反应、肿瘤热或药物热[2,3]。

感染的部位

中性粒细胞减少症患者最常见的感染部位是呼吸道，其次是血液系统［包括导管相关血行感染（central line-associated bloodstream infection, CLABSI）］、泌尿道、皮肤、皮肤附属器感染

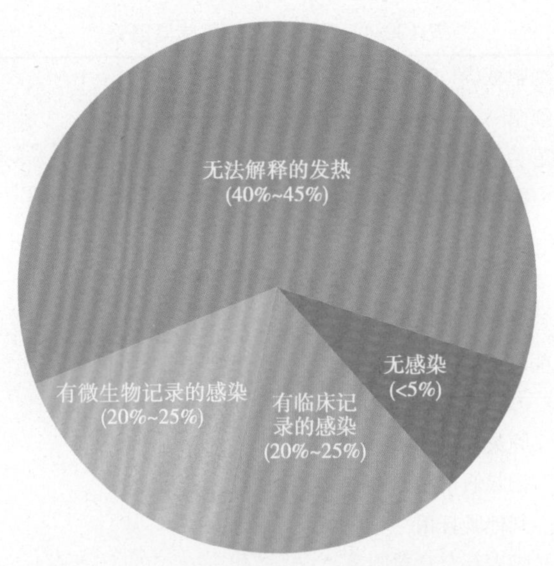

图 139-1　中性粒细胞减少症患者的发热类型

(SSSI)和口咽及胃肠道(图 139-2)。感染率低但临床上重要的部位包括中枢神经系统、骨骼、关节和终末器官如肝脏和脾脏。大多数感染是由患者自身的微生物菌群引起的,少数是通过外源性/环境暴露获得的。

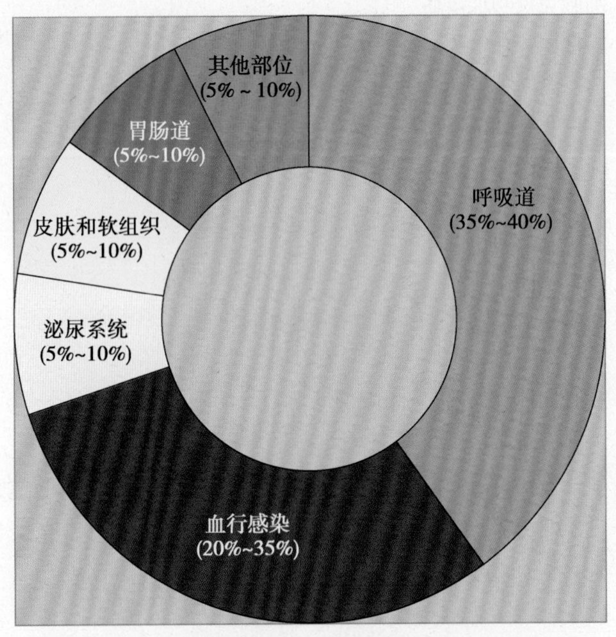

图 139-2　中性粒细胞减少症患者的常见感染部位

细胞免疫和体液免疫失调

恶性血液系统疾病患者常伴随细胞免疫缺陷,在同种异体造血细胞移植接受者(HCT),接受者的高剂量糖皮质激素治疗,以及接受新治疗模式的患者(核苷类似物、单克隆抗体和替莫唑胺)均可增加如感染军团菌、沙门菌、诺卡菌属、单核细胞增多性李斯特菌和红球菌属等细菌引起的感染[4~6]。支原体感染、结核分枝杆菌和非结核分枝杆菌在此类患者中也相对常见。大部分的真菌感染是由曲霉菌、肺孢子菌和地方真菌(新生隐球菌、荚膜组织胞浆菌和球孢子菌)引起的[7,8]。病毒感染以巨细胞病毒(CMV)为最常见的疱疹病毒群为主。社区呼吸道病毒是同种异体造血细胞移植接受者(HCT)发病和死亡的重要原因。弓形虫病、类圆线虫病和巴贝斯虫病等寄生虫感染在细胞免疫或体液免疫失调的患者中也更为常见[9~11]。在体液免疫失调的患者中,常见由肺炎链球菌和流感嗜血杆菌引起的感染。

实体瘤患者的感染

没有明显免疫失调的实体瘤患者也经常发生感染。危险因素包括通常短暂的中性粒细胞减少症、正常的防御屏障(皮肤和黏膜表面)的破坏、由体积庞大或迅速扩大的肿瘤引起的阻塞、辐射损伤、外科手术和各种医疗设备的存在。表 139-2 总结了各种实体瘤患者常见的感染部位。感染的部位取决于肿瘤的位置和大小,或医疗设备、辐射或外科手术的部位和性质。手术部位感染和导管相关感染最常是由皮肤上的微生物引起的,尽管条件致病菌如铜绿假单胞菌和其他革兰阴性杆菌也在这种情况下出现[12]。移除责任装置和完全或部分解除梗阻是处理实体瘤患者感染的重要方法。如果这是不可行的,延长抑制治疗可能是必要的。

表 139-2　实体瘤患者常见感染

肿瘤部位	感染部位或种类
乳腺	外科伤口感染、腋下淋巴结切除引起的蜂窝织炎或淋巴管炎、乳管炎、乳腺脓肿、菌血症
中枢神经系统(脑、脑膜)	外科伤口感染、硬膜外/下感染、脑脓肿、脑膜炎/脑室炎、近端和远端引流管末端感染、吸入性肺炎、尿道感染、菌血症
生殖系统和前列腺	膀胱炎、尿道炎、急慢性肾盂肾炎伴或不伴菌血症、导管相关性复杂尿道感染(肾造口术支架)、伤口感染、急慢性前列腺炎、附睾炎、睾丸炎、盆腔脓肿
肝胆-胰腺	外科伤口感染、腹膜炎、上行性胆管炎伴或不伴菌血症、肝炎、胰腺炎、膈下脓肿
头颈	蜂窝织炎、外科伤口感染、颜面深部感染、乳突炎、骨髓炎、鼻窦炎、吸入性/院内感染性肺炎、菌血症、化脓性颅内静脉炎、脑膜炎、脑脓肿、咽后和椎旁脓肿
骨骼肌肉系统(肌肉、骨骼、关节)	外科伤口感染、皮肤感染、脓性肌炎、淋巴管炎、软骨炎、淋巴结炎、滑囊炎、滑膜炎、化脓性关节炎、骨髓炎、伤口感染、假体相关性感染、菌血症
上消化道	食管炎、肺炎或肺脓肿引起的气管食管瘘、胃肠道穿孔和感染、进食管引起的感染、纵隔炎/骨髓炎
下消化道	外科伤口感染、腹内或盆腔脓肿、腹膜炎(穿孔引起)、小肠结肠炎、尿道感染、肛周感染、骶尾骨骨髓炎

感染分类

细菌感染

目前,约有50%的中性粒细胞减少患者会感染革兰氏阳性菌(表139-3)。革兰氏阴性杆菌引起的感染约占18%,其中相当大的比例(尤其是深部软组织感染)是由多种微生物引起的[13~16]。中性粒细胞减少症患者的常见感染细菌见表139-4。地理和机构间的确存在差异[17]。因此,临床医生在开始经验性抗生素治疗时,应考虑当地流行病学和耐药模式。

革兰氏阳性菌

凝血酶阴性葡萄球菌(CoNS)是最常被分离的CLABSI主要致病菌[18]。路邓葡萄球菌(*Staphylococcus lugdunensis*)是一种毒性更强的葡萄球菌,需要更积极的处理[19,20]。金黄色葡萄球菌常与深部感染(深部脓肿和心内膜炎)有关,所有金黄色葡萄球菌菌血症患者应评估此类病灶[21]。其他感染包括SSSI、肺炎、骨骼和关节感染以及感染性血栓性静脉炎。令人担忧的是,在很多肿瘤治疗中心耐甲氧西林的金黄色葡萄球菌上升的比例目前为50%[22]。这些分离株中有许多对万古霉素产生了耐药性或降低了敏感性,从而降低了该制剂的疗效[23~27]。替代治疗药物包括达托霉素(daptomycin)、特拉万星(telavancin)、达巴万星(dalbavancin)、奥利万星(oritavancin)、利奈唑胺(linezolid)、泰地唑胺(tedizolid)和头孢洛林(ceftaroline)[28~30]。

草绿色链球菌(VGS)对正接受化疗的急性白血病患者和异体骨髓移植接受者而言是重要的病原菌[31,32]。危险因素包括:用引起严重口腔黏膜损害的药物进行化疗,预防性使用氟喹诺酮类药物(可促进部分微生物的选择性过度生长),以及治疗化疗相关性胃炎使用抑酸剂或2型组胺拮抗剂[33,34]。链球菌为主要菌种。菌血症是其最常见的表现。一些患者会发生急速进展弥漫性感染,涉及血液、肺部、中枢神经系统和皮肤(图139-3)。尽管及时并有效地予抗生素治疗,发病率极高,死亡率为25%~30%。令人担忧的是,有报道称,在一些情况下,20%~60%的草绿色链球菌对青霉素耐药[31,36]。β-溶血性链球菌在中性粒细胞减少的患者中也会引起感染,但比VG要少[37]。

表139-3 中性粒细胞减少患者在2 223次热流行中细菌分布情况

感染类型	2002—2003		2012—2013	
	数量	百分比/%	数量	百分比/%
微生物记录	262	26	321	26
革兰阳性	134	51	163	51
革兰阴性	51	20	55	17
多种微生物	71	27	92	29
厌氧菌	6	2	11	3
临床记录	210	21	298	24
病因未明	521	53	611	50

表139-4 肿瘤患者常见感染因素

粒细胞减少
细菌
革兰阳性菌
凝血酶阴性的葡萄球菌
金黄色化脓性葡萄球菌
肠球菌(包括耐万古霉素的肠球菌)
草绿色链球菌
革兰阴性菌
大肠埃希菌
肺炎克雷伯菌
铜绿假单胞菌
其他肠杆菌
嗜麦芽窄食单胞菌
真菌
念珠菌属
曲霉属
酵母菌
镰刀菌属
细胞免疫功能障碍
细菌
李斯特菌
马红球菌
沙门菌
分枝杆菌
诺卡菌属
军团菌属
真菌
曲霉属
新型隐球菌
荚膜组织胞浆菌
粗球孢子(真菌)
耶氏肺孢子虫
原生动物
弓形虫
蠕虫
粪圆线虫
病毒
巨细胞病毒
Ⅰ和Ⅱ型单纯疱疹病毒
水痘-带状疱疹病毒
EB病毒
体液免疫功能障碍
肺炎链球菌
嗜血杆菌流感

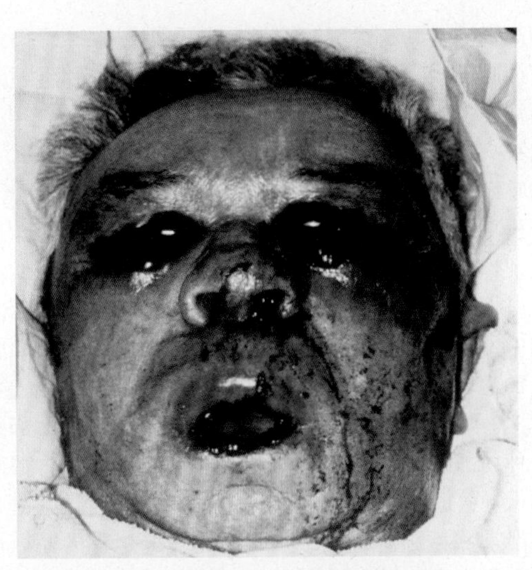

图139-3　由α-溶血性(草绿色)链球菌引起的浸润性感染。请留意这例血小板减少症患者的溶血性病变

肠球菌在肠道中定植[38,39]。最常见的感染源头为血液、尿道和腹部感染。粪肠球菌是临床分离出的主要的菌株,占到60%~70%。绝大部分粪肠球菌对一定药物浓度的青霉素、氨苄西林和万古霉素敏感,尽管有些药物不具备杀菌能力。故在严重肠球菌感染时推荐和氨基糖苷类抗生素联合应用,如庆大霉素。粪肠球菌和耐万古霉素肠球菌(VRE)对氨基糖苷类、氨苄西林表现出高水平的耐药性。感染VRE的危险因素包括肠道定植和使用对厌氧菌有效的抗生素(甲硝唑、克林霉素和亚胺培南)[40]。使用万古霉素(经口腔或胃肠外)也是一个危险因素。已知的治疗方案包括利奈唑胺、达托霉素、奥利万星和喹诺普生/达佛普生(quinupristin/dalforpristin)[41~43]。联合治疗可能是必要的。不太常见但重要的革兰氏阳性病原体包括芽孢杆菌、棒状杆菌、微球菌和黏液口球菌[44,45]。诺卡菌病是由几种诺卡菌引起的。最常见的感染部位是肺部(70%)和软组织(16%)[46]。由于鉴别诊断的范围很广,因此建立一个特定的微生物学诊断是至关重要的。虽然经常与碳青霉烯类、四环素类或氨基糖苷类药物联合使用,但甲氧苄啶/磺胺甲噁唑仍是治疗的主要药物。L-单核细胞增生主要是通过食用生牛奶或生牛奶制品(奶酪)获得的。菌血症(75%)和脑膜脑炎(20%)是最常见的症状[47]。

免疫球蛋白在免疫系统对各种感染的反应中起着重要的作用。体液免疫功能受损导致对肺炎链球菌和其他微生物感染的易感性增加[37]。结合肺炎球菌疫苗的广泛使用已使得肺炎链球菌感染发病率的降低,特别是在儿童中。

革兰氏阴性菌

中性粒细胞减少的患者感染革兰阴性杆菌的重要感染源之一是胃肠道。大肠埃希菌、克雷伯菌和铜绿假单胞菌仍然是三种主要的致病菌[48]。其他肠杆菌科(枸橼酸杆菌属、肠杆菌属、变形杆菌属和沙雷菌属)较少见。尽管由于预防性使用抗生素使得革兰氏阴性杆菌感染率下降,但由非发酵革兰氏阴性杆菌(NFGNB)引起的感染比例有所增加,如铜绿假单胞菌、嗜麦芽窄食单胞菌和不动杆菌[49]。铜绿假单胞菌是最常见的致病菌,也是毒性最强的NFGNB,15%~20%的革兰氏阴性菌感染与其相关。它也是从多种微生物感染中分离出来的最常见的革兰氏阴性菌。由嗜麦芽链球菌引起的感染在血液系统恶性肿瘤患者和HCT受者中越来越多地被发现[50,51]。菌血症是最常见的表现,其次是肺炎和尿路感染。发烧常常是感染的唯一表现。其他表现如坏疽性深脓疮病并不常见(图139-4)。多菌种感染和深部组织感染(肺炎、中性粒细胞小肠结肠炎(NEC)和直肠周围感染)与较高的发病率和死亡率相关[16,52]。耐药性的出现使得单环β-内酰胺类和碳青霉烯类得到关注[53~55]。有些微生物,特别是铜绿假单胞菌和不动杆菌,已经具有多重耐药性[56,57]。目前治疗这类微生物的方法很少(黏菌素、替加环素和联合疗法),而且很少有新的药物正在研发[58,59]。许多机构现在对高危患者进行监测研究,寻找耐万古霉素肠球菌、铜绿假单胞菌、ESBL菌群和碳青霉烯类耐药肠杆菌(CRE)患者的粪便定植,因为阳性者通常与随后的感染相关[60~63]。

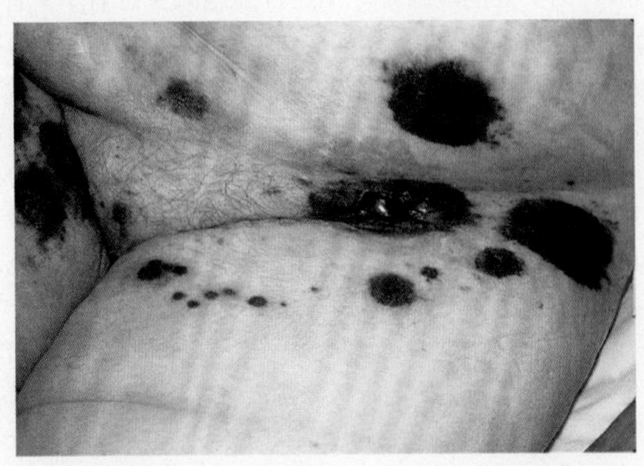

图139-4　铜绿假单胞菌感染引起的多发性皮肤病变(坏疽性深脓疱病)

细胞免疫功能受损是军团菌感染的危险因素。引起感染的最常见军团菌是嗜肺军团菌。医院的供水系统往往含有军团菌,而许多医院感染的军团菌感染病例都可以追溯到这些源头[64]。肺炎是最常见的症状。需要尿抗原的检测或军团菌在特殊培养基上的生长才可明确诊断。氟喹诺酮类和大环内酯类药物是治疗中最常用的药物,联合使用似乎没有优势。非伤寒沙门菌和弯曲杆菌感染在细胞免疫功能受损的患者中也有所增加[65]。

细胞免疫在控制分枝杆菌感染中起着至关重要的作用。结核病和霍奇金病及毛细胞白血病之间的联系已经得到很好的证实[66]。

肺结核可以发生于恶性肿瘤的诊断之前,或同时发生,或在治疗期间或之后发生。肺部感染引起发烧、咳嗽和体重减轻是常见的。弥漫性肺浸润伴或不伴纵隔扩大是最常见的影像学表现。非结核分枝杆菌感染不常见[67,68]。它们产生肺部感染、淋巴结炎、SSSI、导管相关感染和播散性疾病。感染菌的种类主要有胞内分枝杆菌、脓肿分枝杆菌、龟分枝杆菌、偶发分枝杆菌、堪萨斯分枝杆菌和海鱼分枝杆菌。对进展性感染通常采用延长的多药联合治疗[69]。

厌氧菌

厌氧菌常涉及深部组织、多种微生物感染,如腹部/盆腔脓肿、NEC、直肠周围感染、复杂性SSSI和肺炎[52,70]。艰难梭状芽孢杆菌感染(CDI)是导致癌症患者腹泻的主要感染原因[71]，患者的病情严重程度增加，死亡率升高，复发和并发症的风险增加。较新的诊断试验包括基于聚合酶链反应(PCR)的检测[72]。甲硝唑现在被认为在治疗 CDI 方面不如万古霉素[73]。利福昔明和硝唑胺(nitazoxamide)的治疗效果有限[74~76]。非达霉素(fidaxomycin)是一种口服大环内酯类抗生素，最近被 FDA 批准用于成人 CDI 的治疗，尤其是那些复发风险最高的人群[77,78]。粪便移植也在这种情况下被成功应用，而且前景看好[79]。预防措施包括严格执行感染控制措施、适当使用抗菌药物和改进环境清洁方法。

真菌感染

中性粒细胞减少时间延长(>7~10 日)是发生侵袭性真菌感染(IFI)的关键危险因素。中性粒细胞减少患者 IFI 最常见的真菌是念珠菌属和曲霉菌属[80,81]。在使用氟康唑等药物之前，侵袭性念珠菌病很常见，以白色念珠菌为主。唑类药物的常规应用降低了念珠菌病发生的频率，使得如口咽念珠菌病(鹅口疮)、食管炎和慢性全身性(肝源性)念珠菌病等的临床表现几乎成为历史。念珠菌病常与消化道有关，是目前最常见的表现，消化道是主要的入口。最近的研究表明了从白色念珠菌到非白色念珠菌的主要转变[82~84]。

播散性念珠菌病无特征性体征和症状。通常，唯一的症状是持续发热和患者的临床症状逐渐恶化。有些患者因眼部感染而导致视力模糊、疼痛、盲点或丧失视力。近 10%的患者出现特征性的红斑性大结节性皮肤病变(图 139-5)。患者持续发热和虚弱，体重明显下降。症状包括右上腹或肩部疼痛。碱性磷酸酶水平通常升高。肝脾肿大可被发现。肝脏和脾脏的影像显示有多个病变。大约 90%的患者对适当的抗真菌治疗有反应[62]。在预防性使用氟康唑的部位念珠菌感染已经消失。治疗应以体外抗真菌药敏数据为指导。在棘球菌素治疗过程中，可能会出现蕈状分枝杆菌菌病，而在唑类药物治疗过程中，可能会出现棉球菌感染。棘白菌分离株对棘白菌素的耐药性呈上升趋势[86]。克柔念珠菌对氟康唑耐药。与全身性念珠菌感染相关的死亡率高达 40%。治疗念珠菌病的指南已在社会各界广泛应用[87~90]。

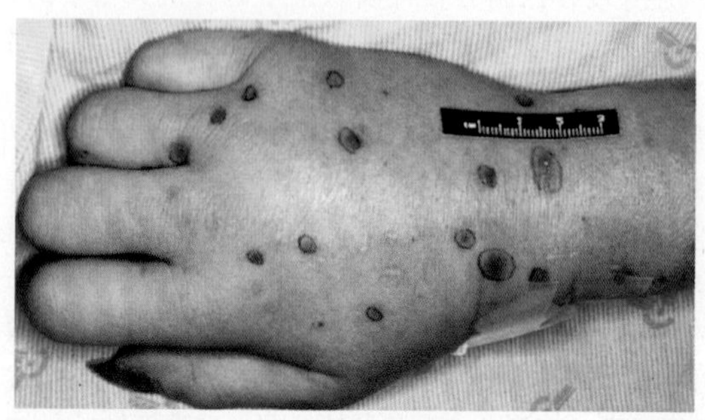

图 139-5 典型急性白血病患者的皮肤巨结节灶，播散性克鲁斯念珠菌感染

曲霉菌病在持续性中性粒细胞减少症患者中也很常见。其他危险因素包括长期接受高剂量糖皮质激素治疗、移植物抗宿主病(GVHD)、反复循环的中性粒细胞减少症、呼吸道病毒感染和高龄[91]。最常见的病原体是烟曲霉[92]。感染通常是由鼻窦或肺部吸入的孢子引起。与医院内部或邻近建筑有关的曲菌病暴发已经发生。超过 70%的感染涉及肺部(IPA，侵袭性肺曲霉病)，约 35%的患者血行播散到其他器官[93]。通常，感染的唯一证据是长时间发热，肺部浸润，对抗菌治疗无效。肺高分辨率 CT 扫描有助于曲菌病的早期诊断[94,95]。早期疾病的特征性表现为肺多发结节，周围有毛玻璃衰减晕，出血性肺梗死(图 139-6)[94~96]。愈合发生时，梗死组织出现坏死，从黑曲霉中留下一个空气半月征。在急性白血病患者和骨髓移植的受助患者中，达 15%的病例可能发生曲霉菌眼眶感染(图 139-7)。感染可能通过侵犯颅底造成眼部、鼻窦及面部结构破坏。一种局部的曲菌病与血管内导管置入有关。曲霉菌孢子可在插入导管时沉积，也可浸渍于导管敷料中。这些潜在感染可能很严重，因为它们可以传播[97,98]。大约 5%的播散性感染患者中会发生皮肤损害，如清晰的黑色焦痂。伏立康唑是治疗

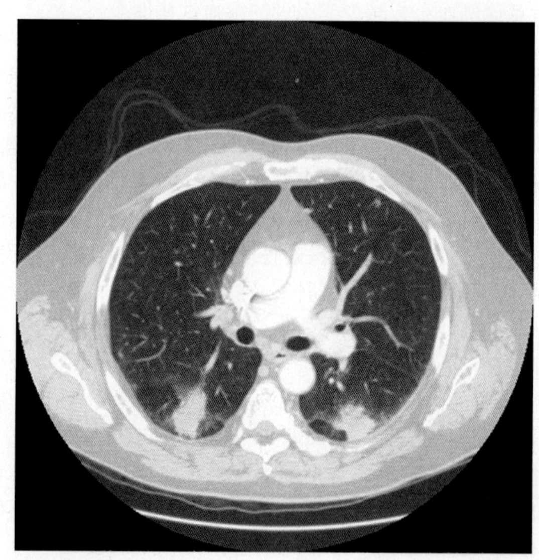

图 139-6 伴有环状的圆形肺部病变和侵袭性肺曲霉菌病共存

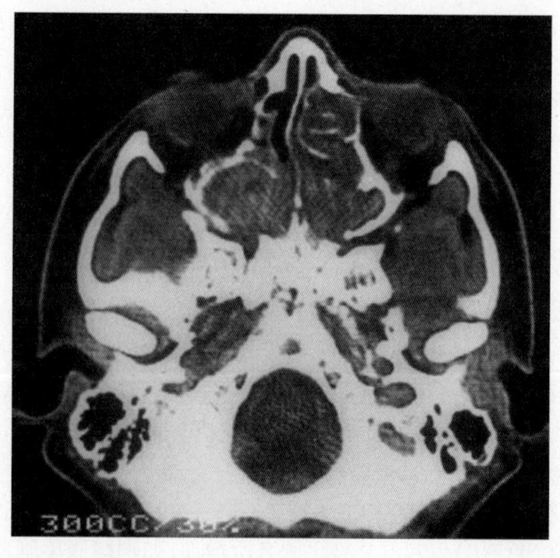

图 139-7 持续发热的异基因骨髓移植接受者中由曲霉菌引起的全鼻窦炎

侵袭性或播散性曲菌病的首选药物。两性霉素B、泊沙康唑常用于抢救治疗或当伏立康唑不耐受时。联合应用三唑和棘白菌素可能对侵袭性曲霉病的抢救治疗有一定的价值[85,90,99,100]。最近的一项随机试验显示,伏立康唑和阿尼杜阿芬净治疗的侵袭性曲菌病患者的存活率高于伏立康唑单药治疗的患者[101]。

隐球菌病是由两种同属的新生隐球菌和嘉地隐球菌引起的。吸入孢子之后感染的主要部位是肺部。传播通常涉及中枢神经系统(脑膜脑炎和隐球菌性肉瘤)。发烧和脑膜症状很常见。脑脊液(CSF)异常包括压力升高、淋巴细胞增多、蛋白升高和葡萄糖水平降低。大多数病例的脑脊液和血清中也检测到隐球菌抗原。目前的护理标准是使用两性霉素B或其脂质制剂加5-氟胞嘧啶诱导治疗,然后使用氟康唑维持治疗[102]。组织胞浆菌病和其他地方性真菌引起的感染不太常见[8]。它们通常引起肺部、中枢神经系统或播散性感染,在流行地区应将其作为鉴别诊断的依据。传统上认为,由肺孢子菌引起的肺炎与细胞免疫功能受损有关,从而导致休眠体的重新激活[103,104]。临床通常表现为亚急性。临床特征包括发热、无痛性咳嗽和进行性呼吸困难。最常见的CT表现为弥漫性双肺磨玻璃影,以肺尖为主,周围正常[105]。诊断通常是使用Gomori银或甲苯胺蓝对呼吸道标本活检组织染色以发现病原体(图139-8)。目前该方法被更敏感的分子技术包括半定量或定量PCR所替代[106,107]。大剂量TMP/SMX仍然是预防和治疗的首选。替代药物包括喷他脒、阿托伐醌、克林霉素联合伯氨喹、氨苯砜联合甲氧苄啶[108]。

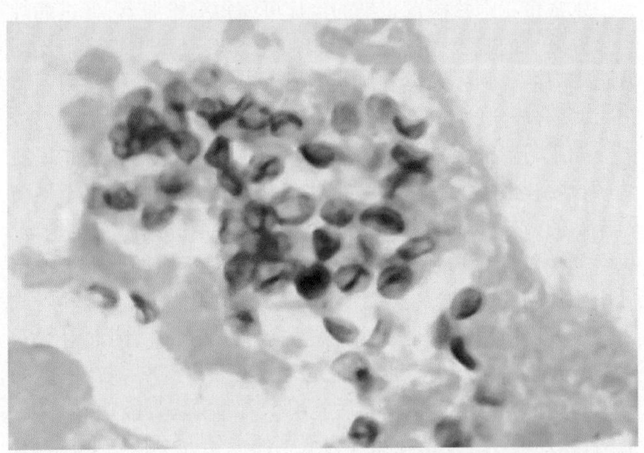

图139-8 一名感染卡氏肺孢子虫肺炎的AIDS患者的支气管肺泡灌洗液标本的Gomori六胺银染色

其他机会性真菌

毛霉病(接合菌病)是一种罕见的感染,最常见的病原体是毛霉、根霉、犁头霉和根毛霉属。侵入性肺部感染是最常见的感染形式。一些患者出现鼻旁窦支气管综合征、鼻、大脑、胃肠道、皮肤或传播性感染[109,110]。接合菌病的临床表现往往和曲霉菌病没有什么区别。在免疫抑制患者、鼻窦炎或有侵入性真菌感染、长期应用伏立康唑治疗效果不佳的患者,应考虑接合菌病[111~113]。随着感染组织的外科清创术,早期诊断和抗真菌治疗至关重要。控制潜在疾病和在可行时逆转危险因素也至关重要[85,114]。两性霉素B和泊沙康唑是唯一对黏膜真菌有可靠活性的抗真菌药物[115],艾沙康唑(isavuconazole)也刚刚被批准用于治疗黏膜真菌病。脂质制剂的两性霉素B是首选的初始治疗,有一些证据表明,这些制剂与棘白菌素联用可能是有益的[116]。在可行的情况下,治疗常改用泊沙康唑。皮状丝孢酵母可引起播散性感染,多发生在伴有严重中性粒细胞减少症的血液肿瘤患者。约30%的感染者出现前述的多种皮肤病变。包括胃肠道、呼吸道和静脉导管在内都是感染入侵的通道。镰刀菌,在过去十年里,已成为中性粒细胞减少患者重要的病原体[117]。肺部、鼻窦、皮肤常发生局限性感染,但大多数患者会发生播散性感染。皮肤和皮下组织是常见的播散性感染灶[118]。像曲霉菌属,这些病原体入侵血管,造成血栓形成和梗死。镰刀菌通常可以轻易地从血液培养或组织标本中分离[119,120]。应用组织病理学方法区分镰刀菌和其他真菌很困难[121]。感染的康复取决于中性粒细胞减少症的治愈程度,而目前可用的抗真菌药物也只能达到微弱的效果[122]。

病毒感染

病毒感染在中性粒细胞减少症患者中并不常见,除非他们是HCT接受者。最常见的是疱疹病毒感染,尤其是单纯疱疹病毒(HSV)、水痘-带状疱疹病毒(VZV)和巨细胞病毒(CMV)。大多数成年人是HSV血清阳性,对于血液系统恶性肿瘤进行HCT或强化化疗的患者,60%~80%可发生活化。通常情况下,当患者仍处于严重的中性粒细胞缺乏状态时,就会发生复发,最常见的表现是口腔黏膜炎/溃疡。食管炎与念珠菌性食管炎难以区分。脑炎和播散是不常见的。HSV预防被推荐用于白血病HCT患者或缓解诱导治疗[123]。社区呼吸道病毒,包括呼吸道合胞病毒RSV、甲型和乙型流感病毒、副流感病毒病毒、人类嗜肺病毒、人类冠状病毒和人类鼻病毒,是常见的HCT接受者和急性白血病患者上呼吸道感染的常见病毒,感染后可以发展成肺炎,且与大量的发病率和死亡率有关。建议对高危患者进行呼吸道病毒检测。标本包括鼻咽拭子、冲洗液或吸引物、气管吸引物和支气管肺泡灌洗标本。除流感病毒外,对大多数这些病毒感染的最佳治疗仍有待确定。利巴韦林治疗RSV上呼吸道感染可延缓肺炎的进展,并可能改善HCT受体的整体预后[124~127]。

骨髓干细胞抑制后嘌呤类似物如氟尿嘧啶化疗后的患者易于发生EBV的复活。慢性淋巴细胞白血病的患者发生EBV感染也许与Richter综合征或霍奇金病相关。在骨髓移植或其他器官移植患者,EBV可能感染B细胞,产生移植后淋巴细胞增生异常综合征(PTLD)。在年轻患者,PTLD表现常类似于单核细胞增多症,发热、咽痛、淋巴结肿大是典型症状。全身病变可以起于局部淋巴结病灶,也可以是暴发的、快速而致命的。利妥昔单抗被推荐用于PTLD的治疗[128,129]。

HHV-6被认为是移植患者相关的一种重要的病原菌。在骨髓移植、肾移植、肝脏移植的患者,血清学反应经常与临床表现同时出现,如发热、皮疹、肺部感染、肝炎、骨髓抑制、神经功能异常。HHV-6病毒血症不一定与死亡率增加有关,也不需要进行常规筛查。更昔洛韦和膦甲酸可抑制病毒复制,用这些药物治疗严重感染的患者可能有用。免疫治疗的预防和治疗策略正在制订中[130~135]。

CMV 感染常发生于免疫功能低下的患者，特别是细胞免疫功能受损的患者。这是异基因肝移植患者常见的并发症，对移植后的总生存率有负面影响[136]。CMV 在 HCT 受体中的阳性反应是一个重要的危险因素。如果不采取预防措施，50%~80%的血清阳性患者在接受 HCT 治疗后会重新激活潜伏感染。无论是受体还是供体，CMV 的血清阳性率都会影响 CMV 终末器官疾病的后续进展[137]。CMV 感染的其他危险因素包括全身照射、脐带血移植、使用 T 细胞衰竭的干细胞、接受嘌呤类似物（氟达拉滨和克拉屈滨）治疗、抗 CD20 单克隆抗体（利妥昔单抗）、CD52 单克隆抗体（阿伦珠单抗）、GVHD 和高龄[138]。CMV 肺炎是最常见的表现（图 139-9），其他表现包括视网膜炎、食管炎、肠炎、肝炎、心肌炎、脑炎。除了终末器官疾病外，CMV 感染还与 GVHD 和继发性细菌和真菌感染有关。为了提前预防，早期发现巨细胞病毒感染是至关重要的。提前治疗优于其他 CMV 感染的预防措施。提前治疗是指在 CMV PP65 抗原分析或 PCR 发现 CMV 感染即刻使用抗感染治疗（更昔洛韦和膦甲酸）。基于病毒载量、适应风险、先发制人的治疗策略成功地预防了 CMV 感染，降低了发病[139]。遗憾的是，对已确诊的终末器官疾病，尤其是肺炎的治疗不是很令人满意。目前可用的系统性抗病毒药物包括更昔洛韦（ganciclovir）、膦甲酸（foscarnet）、西多福韦（cidofovir）和来氟米特（leflunomide），此外还有一些正在开发的新型药物，如来特莫韦（letermovir）和布林西多福韦[140,141]。

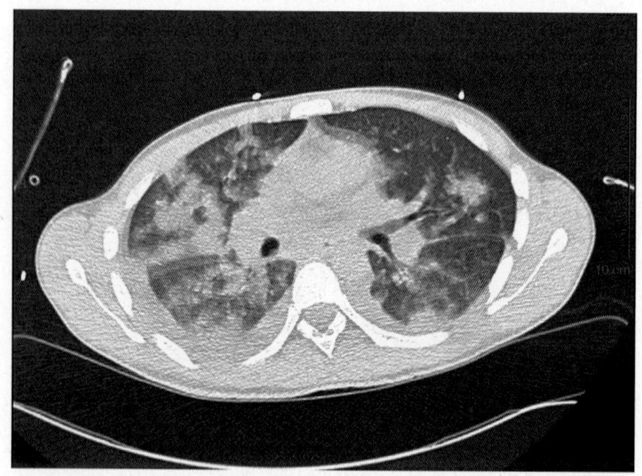

图 139-9 接受 HCT 治疗的 CMV 肺炎患者的计算机断层扫描图像，显示弥漫性双侧肺浸润

水痘（VZV）是正在接受化疗的儿童肿瘤患者的一种严重感染。近 30%接受化疗的儿童肿瘤患者感染 VZV 后发生严重并发症，病死率为 7%左右。水痘感染的临床特点为全身广泛的水疱、皮疹和发热。水疱皮疹最初出现在面部和头皮，随后蔓延到躯干和四肢。新的病灶出现时，老病灶开始结痂。肿瘤患者的感染期会延长，血小板减少症患者囊泡可能出血、坏死。大约 10%的儿童继发细菌感染。严重感染可导致肺炎以及肝脏，胰腺或肾上腺局灶性坏死。

带状疱疹通常发生在淋巴增殖异常患者。感染的特点是一个或两个相邻的感觉皮节区域的单侧水疱皮疹（图 139-10）。有时，患者会发生水痘样疱疹。皮疹伴有的疼痛（带状疱疹相关的疼痛）可持续数周或数月。大约 35%的肿瘤患者发生带状疱疹皮肤传播，而非肿瘤患者发生率仅 4%。肾上腺皮质激素、放疗、抗肿瘤药物治疗均促进传播。

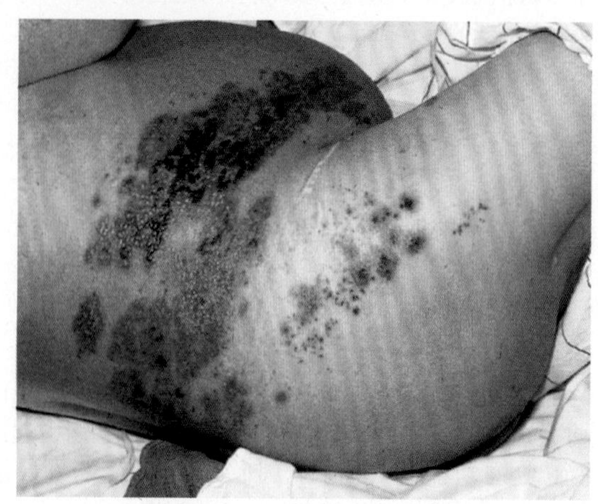

图 139-10 VZV 感染所致的典型的水疱疹。注意皮肤损害的表现，血小板减少的患者存在病灶出血的表现

大多数水痘患者不需要实验室确诊。水痘可以在暴发后数天随着水疱破裂流液消失，其他部位复发少见。培养的阳性率是 30%~60%。使用荧光水痘显微镜检测皮肤碎屑中水痘带状疱疹病毒抗原和利用 PCR 技术检测脑脊液或其他组织中水痘带状疱疹病毒 DNA 是比较快速，敏感的诊断技术。

水痘带状疱疹病毒感染的治疗可缩短病毒脱落，促进病灶愈合并减少内脏疾病的发生。口服泛昔洛韦和伐昔洛韦比阿昔洛韦有效。脑膜脑炎和肺炎等严重感染需要静脉使用阿昔洛韦，联合成熟的支持治疗。尽管采取这些治疗，死亡率仍较高。如果阿昔洛韦单药无效，应该考虑膦甲酸钠治疗或膦甲酸钠联合阿昔洛韦治疗。水痘带状疱疹免疫球蛋白可用于预防暴露后的高危个体感染，也可以缓解已经存在的感染。水痘带状疱疹免疫球蛋白在暴露后 96h 内使用是有效的。水痘疫苗可用于计划免疫和暴露后预防[142,143]。在化疗开始前一周或治疗后一周使用疫苗是安全的，且具有免疫原性，因而对严重感染的儿童白血病患者也可能是有效的。约 50%存在中度的皮疹。高危人群可以在暴露后使用 1 周的抗病毒治疗[144]。已证明，热处理过的疫苗在免疫力低下的成年人中是安全且具有免疫原性的[145]。

肝炎病毒

乙型肝炎病毒（hepatitis B virus，HBV）的激活主要发生在接受抗 CD20 药物（利妥昔单抗和奥法木单抗）的患者以及 HCT 接受者中，其临床表现可能为无症状肝酶升高，甚至暴发性肝衰竭和死亡。慢性 HBV 感染（阳性 HBsAg）的再激活风险高于感染缓解的患者（阳性 HBsAb 和阴性 HBsAg）。诸如定量 HBV-DNA 测量之类的诊断工具和新型抗病毒药物（恩替卡韦，拉米夫定和替诺福韦）已改善了 HBV 的检测和感染治疗。与基于风险的筛查相比，针对癌症患者的 HBV 普查仍存在争议。目前，包括 ASCO 和 NCCN 在内的许多指南都建议对将接受免疫抑制疗法（包括抗 CD20 疗法）的高风险患者进行筛查[146,147]。丙型肝炎病毒（hepatitis C virus，HCV）在美国引起超过 300 万人慢性感染，是肝癌发展的主要危险因素。HCV 的激活主要出现在血液系统恶性肿瘤患者和接受利妥昔单抗治疗的患者[148]。但其重新激活的发生频率低于 HBV，并且对肿瘤患者筛查 HCV 的意义尚无定论[149,150]。

其他感染

弓形虫病是人类最常见的寄生虫感染之一。播散性疾病通常发生在免疫受损的个体，其中中枢神经系统、心脏和肺部受累最频繁[151]。脑部的计算机断层扫描（CT）或磁共振成像（MRI）常表现为多个低密度病变，通常带有中等程度的环形强化。如果可行，可以通过血清学检查或活检确认诊断。具体治疗方法包括乙胺嘧啶加磺胺二嗪或螺旋霉素。替代药物如克林霉素、阿托伐醌以及 TMP/SMX 也已用于治疗和预防[152]。粪类圆线虫（*Strongyloides stercoralis*）是土壤传播的蠕虫，淋巴瘤是伴有粪类圆线虫的最常见恶性肿瘤。其在临床上常无症状，有些仅产生嗜酸性粒细胞增多症[153]。常见的临床特征包括发烧和胃肠道症状，例如腹泻和腹痛、痉挛。粪类圆线虫通常引起的免疫抑制可引起传播性过度感染的发生[10,154]。常会出现肺部出血和积液，继而出现呼吸功能不全甚至呼吸衰竭。肠杆菌革兰氏阴性杆菌和厌氧菌引起的多菌种菌血症也不少见。诊断测试包括粪便和呼吸道标本中微生物鉴定，以及血清酶联免疫吸附测定（enzyme-linked immunosorbent assay，ELISA）等方法。伊维菌素（ivermectin）是其治疗药物之一。建议对高危患者（同种接受 HCT 和糖皮质激素治疗的患者），尤其是在流行地区，进行筛查[155]。

特殊情况

腹部感染

癌症患者的急腹症是医师最难解决的问题之一[156]。急腹症的原因包括阑尾炎、胆囊炎、憩室炎、腹膜炎、腹腔脓肿、脾梗死、NEC、肿瘤溶解和穿孔。患者通常会出现腹痛、腹胀、压痛、反跳痛、肠鸣音减弱或消失。急腹症常常发生在化疗后伴中性粒细胞减少症和血小板减少症时。伴中性粒细胞减少症的患者不能够建立足够的炎症反应，因此，可能发生无症状的腹膜炎。急腹症的治疗和管理包括支持治疗、抗生素和必要的手术干预治疗。

中性粒细胞性小肠结肠炎（NEC）主要见于血液系统恶性肿瘤患者，但在使用紫杉烷等可引起严重肠黏膜炎的药物的实体瘤患者中 NEC 的发病率也正在增加[52]。其常见表现包括发烧、腹痛或绞痛、腹胀和腹泻。并发症包括多种细菌引起的菌血症、出血、肠壁穿孔和脓肿形成。病变可能局限在盲肠，也可累及整个下消化道。影像学检查（推荐 CT）通常显示出麻痹性肠梗阻的征象，即右下腹缺乏肠气、回肠末端张力减低以及肠壁增厚超过 4mm，这被认为是 NEC 的标志。起始治疗应以支持为主，包括胃肠减压、静脉补液和覆盖铜绿假单胞菌和厌氧菌的广谱抗生素。如出现出血或肠穿孔等并发症，可能需要手术干预来处理。

肛周感染

据估计，肛周感染在血液系统肿瘤的患者中发生率约为6%，其中一个常见的易感因素是中性粒细胞减少症，它在这些患者中的发生率超过 90%[157]。主要的症状是由排便引起的疼痛，多数患者会出现发热，病灶表现为红斑、硬结和溃疡。脓肿形成较少见，但可能会出现大面积坏死并破溃入直肠。感染常发生在有裂伤或痔疮的部位。这些感染多数由需氧革兰阴性菌引起，尤其是铜绿假单胞菌和大肠埃希菌。治疗包括一般措施，例如坐浴、温热敷、大便软化剂、止痛药以及广谱抗生素。不推荐使用经验性的抗真菌治疗。如果有脓肿，则应引流[158]。在中性粒细胞减少症的患者中，感染的治疗取决于中性粒细胞数量的恢复。血液病患者由痔疮或肛裂引起的肛周感染恢复后，应在原发病缓解期接受外科手术治疗；否则之后可能再次发生感染。

导管相关感染（CLABSI）

与导管相关的血液感染已变得相对普遍[159]。这些感染中的大多数是由葡萄球菌引起的，还可能由其他定植在皮肤上的革兰氏阳性生物，铜绿假单胞菌、肠杆菌、嗜麦芽孢杆菌和假丝酵母菌引起。定量的血培养和阳性反应时间有助于确立 CLABSI 的诊断，尽管这两种方法准确率都不是 100%[160~164]。出现阳性反应的时间也可以作为判断结果和预后的指标[165]。某些感染，尤其是由 CoNS 引起的感染，即使不移除导管也可能治愈[166]。然而，对于由金黄色葡萄球菌、不动杆菌、假单胞菌属、嗜麦芽孢杆菌、念珠菌属和非结核分枝杆菌引起的 CLABSI，通常必须拆除导管。此外，如果在导管插入部位有局部感染的迹象，或者尽管进行了充分的治疗但仍持续发烧或菌血症，则需拆除导管[160]。抗生素锁可能非常有用，尤其是在无法拆除导管的情况下。CLABSI 最严重的并发症是化脓性血栓性静脉炎和心内膜炎。近来有抗菌导管已被证明可以减少导管相关感染的发生率[159,167]。

伴中性粒细胞减少症患者感染的治疗

初始患者评估

中性粒细胞减少症的患者出现发热需尽快开始足量的经验性的广谱抗菌治疗[168]。患者治疗前应尽快进行治疗前评估，因为延迟开始经验性治疗可导致反应率降低[169]。必须要仔细地询问病史和完成体格检查。需特别注意常见的感染部位或感染传播的途径。包括口咽、肺、食管下段、会阴、鼻窦、指甲和血管导管插入部位。在经验性抗生素治疗开始前，至少要留取 2 次血培养和其他相应部位的培养（喉、尿、便）来获取细菌和真菌病原体。对有中心静脉导管的患者，需获得导管和外周的标本培养[170,171]。对中性粒细胞减少症合并肺炎的患者，还需行影像学检查。如胸部和鼻窦为可能的感染源时需行 CT 检查。其他的实验室检查还包括血细胞计数和反映肾和肝功能基础水平的检查。最后，应进行风险评估，以确定患者是否需要住院[172]。如果门诊基础医疗设施到位，低危发热性中性粒细胞减少症患者的可以采用门诊肠胃外或口服抗生素治疗[173~175]。其他所有患者均应接受医院治疗。门诊治疗可以在短期住院后或整个高热时期进行[176~179]。这种治疗已被证明对成人和儿童都是安全有效的[180~182]。门诊治疗可节省大量成本，降低耐药医院病原体的重感染发生率，改善患者的生活质量并为他们的家人和护理人员带来便利[173,183]。美国多个学会，包括美国传染病学会（Infectious Diseases Society of America）、美国国家综合癌症网络（National Comprehensive Cancer Network）和美国临床肿瘤学会（American Society of Clinical Oncology）已出版了有关癌症患者感染管理的最新指南，其中包括针对低危患者进行门诊治疗[168,184,185]。

起始抗生素治疗

经验性抗生素治疗方案需基于当地的流行病学和耐药特点，并需要能够覆盖足够多的革兰氏阴性菌，如铜绿假单胞菌和革兰氏阳性菌。这通常可以通过使用单一广谱抗生素（单一疗法）或抗生素组合来实现[168,185]。表 139-5 和表 139-6 列出了在这种情况下使用的常见抗生素和治疗方案。没有任何一种方案是最佳方案，在作出选择前都要仔细考虑上述的因素。对于高达 60%的发热性中性粒细胞减少症，尤其是在无法确定明显的感染灶时，采用 2 类碳青霉烯类、头孢吡肟或哌拉西林/他唑巴坦等药物进行单药治疗是较为合适的[168]。如果发现疑似耐药的革兰氏阳性菌感染（如耐甲氧西林的金黄色葡萄球菌（MRSA）或 VRE），将这些药物与万古霉素、利奈唑胺或达托霉素组合使用是适当的。然而，研究表明在确定在耐药革兰氏阳性感染后再增加这些药物与经验性使用同样有效。由于易感性的改变，万古霉素的疗效在某些医疗机构中可能不再足够，尽管对于中性粒细胞减少症患者的临床经验有限，但可以考虑使用其他药物如达托霉素、达巴万星（dalbavancin）和特拉万星（telavancin）等[23,27~29]。通常使用抗假单胞菌 β-内酰胺类和氨基糖苷类的组合来协同治疗革兰氏阴性病原体（如铜绿假单胞菌）。当可能发生厌氧菌感染时（如直肠周围感染和 NEC），应使用具有有效抗厌氧菌作用的药物。根据临床样本中分离出的微生物的易感性，细菌、真菌或病毒的感染进展，或在给药 3 日后缺乏明显的疗效，可能需要在高热发作期间改变初始方案。因此，需要仔细监测所有患者的治疗反应、毒性和其他并发症的发生，应根据临床或微生物情况进行适当的改变[186]。最初的经验疗法通常反应率为 65%~85%（低风险患者较高）[180]。很大一部分患者在更换初始方案后会出现效果，包括在 5~7 日后添加抗真菌治疗[168]。

表 139-5 中性粒细胞减少性发热患者的常见经验性抗生素治疗方案

方案
低风险患者方案
经口
喹诺酮类+阿莫西林/克拉维酸
喹诺酮类+克林霉素/阿奇霉素
莫西沙星或左氧氟沙星（单药疗法）
肠道外
头孢曲松/厄他培南+阿米卡星
氨曲南+克林霉素
喹诺酮类+克林霉素
头孢他啶/头孢吡肟
中-高风险患者方案
组合方案
氨基糖苷+抗假单胞菌青霉素/β-内酰胺酶抑制剂或头孢菌素或碳青霉烯（carbapenem）或喹诺酮（如果患者未接受喹诺酮预防）
万古霉素（或利奈唑胺或达托霉素）+抗假单胞菌青霉素，或头孢菌素，或碳青霉烯或喹诺酮（如果患者未接受喹诺酮预防）
单药治疗方案（单药治疗）
广谱头孢菌素（头孢吡肟）
碳青霉烯类（亚胺培南、美罗培南或多利培南（doripenem），但非厄他培南）
抗假单胞菌青霉素/β-内酰胺酶抑制剂（哌拉西林/他唑巴坦）

表 139-6 中性粒细胞减少症患者常用的抗生素

药物	剂量	药物	剂量
氨基糖苷类		单酰胺菌素	
阿米卡星	5mg/kg q8h 或 15~20g/(kg·d)（单日剂量）	氨曲南	1.5~2.0g q6~8h，iv
抗假单胞菌青霉素+β-内酰胺酶抑制剂		喹诺酮类	
哌拉西林+他唑巴坦	3.375g q6h，iv	环丙沙星	200~400mg q8h[a]，iv
广谱头孢菌素		左氧氟沙星	500mg 或 750mg，q24h[a]，iv
头孢吡肟	1~2g q8h，iv	莫西沙星	400mg q24h[a]，iv
碳青霉烯		其他	
亚胺培南/西司他丁	500mg q6h，iv	万古霉素	1g q12h，iv
美罗培南	1g q8h，iv	甲氧苄啶	2.0~20.0mg/(kg·d)（甲氧苄啶）iv q6h[a]
		甲硝唑	500mg iv q6~8h[a]

续表

利奈唑胺	600mg iv q12h[a]
达托霉素	4~6mg/kg·d iv
替加环素	初始剂量 100mg,此后 50mg iv,q12h
抗真菌药物	
唑类	
氟康唑	200~800mg q24h[a]
伊曲康唑	200mg q12h[a]
伏立康唑	6mg/kg q12h×2 次,然后 4mg/kg q12h[a]
泊沙康唑	悬浮液 200mg q8h 随餐服用片剂/静脉输注 300mg q12h × 2, 然后 300mg q24h[a]
异氟康唑	iv/po 200mg q8h×6 次,此后 200mg q24h
棘白菌素	
卡泊芬净	第一天 70mg,此后 50mg q24h
米卡芬净	100mg q24h
阿尼达芬净	第一天 200mg,之后 100mg q24h
多烯类	
两性霉素 B 脱氧胆酸盐	0.3~1mg/(kg·d),qd
两性霉素 B 脂质体(安必素)	1~10mg/(kg·d),qd
两性霉素 B 脂质复合物(abelcet)	5mg/(kg·d),qd
抗病毒药	
阿昔洛韦	5~12mg/kg q8h[a]
伐昔洛韦	1g q8h
更昔洛韦	5mg/kg q12h
口服缬更昔洛韦	900mg q12h
膦甲酸酯	90mg/kg q12h
西多福韦	5mg/kg,iv 每周一次,必须在输注前 3g 丙磺舒并且输注后 q2&8h 给予 1g 丙磺舒
口服利巴韦林	10~20mg/kg q8h,可吸入,注意药物具有细胞毒性和致畸性

iv,静脉注射。

[a]制剂可用于静脉和口服给药,检查每种特定制剂的剂量。

治疗时间

一些权威推荐对确定感染的患者给予持续抗生素治疗至中性粒细胞数值恢复正常(即连续两天中性粒细胞绝对计数超过 500 细胞/μl)。这个方法花费昂贵,因为它实际上是在预防感染解决后的感染,可能会增加超级感染的数量,需要更换大量的抗生素和/或加上抗真菌治疗。还有一个方法是持续应用抗生素直至所有感染部位均炎症消退,病原菌(如分离到)已根除,患者接受至少 7 日治疗并已没有明显的感染症状和体征至少 4 日。抗生素治疗在此时可停用,虽然仍然有持续的中性粒细胞减少症。这一方法可能复发率低且很少有超级感染。

持续发热

尽管进行了抗菌和抗真菌治疗,但仍有部分患者仍然持续发热。这些患者可能为耐药菌或其他病原体(病毒和寄生虫)感染,也有可能是药物相关发热或肿瘤热。侵入性(多是有创性)诊断操作有时对这些患者很必要。对不能耐受侵入性检查的患者,可能就需要持续抗生素治疗并加用经验性抗真菌、抗病毒或抗寄生虫治疗。

其他治疗方法

近 15%~25%发生于中性粒细胞减少症患者的感染对相应的抗微生物治疗无反应。在大多数病例中,有严重的中性粒细胞减少症。造血生长因子的出现使得获益再次增加,因为粒细胞集落刺激因子(G-CSF)使供体可收集的中性粒细胞数量增加[187~189]。初步的临床研究表明这个收集白细胞的治疗方法使得部分患者获益[190,191]。

给接收化疗的癌症患者使用造血生长因子可缓解中性粒细胞减少并缩短持续时间,进一步减少感染并发症的发生。美国临床肿瘤学会已经制订了使用这类药物的指南[192]。这些因子作为中性粒细胞减少症患者感染后抗生素的附加用药的有效性已经非常明确。应当将这类药物用于中性粒细胞计数低于 500 细胞/mm^3 并发生肺炎、感染性休克、脓毒病综合征或真菌感染的患者,因为这些患者如不能恢复中性粒细胞,预后将很差。这类药物还应考虑用于适当治疗 24~48h 后仍无反应的患者[193],IFN-γ 也可能对经适当治疗无反应的非病毒感染有益[194]。

预防感染

大部分感染往往来自内生微生物群,而抑制它们通常通过在危险期使用预防性抗菌(真菌、病毒和原生动物)药物来实现。预防新病原菌感染需要使用多种技术,包括严格的感染控制、仔细烹调食物,这些都能够减少革兰阴性菌的污染,以及各种隔离技术和环境保护措施。

预防性抗微生物

预防性抗微生物治疗是降低患者的微生物负荷的主要手段。喹诺酮类(环丙沙星、左氧氟沙星)是应用最广泛的预防性抗生素。这类药物的应用显著降低了革兰阴性菌感染的发生,但它们对革兰阳性菌的感染率影响较小[195,196]。预防性应用喹诺酮类已经导致了肠内革兰阴性菌喹诺酮耐药性的出现,其中包括大肠埃希菌[197~199]。因此不推荐中性粒细胞减少症的患者常规应用,而是仅考虑对细菌感染高风险患者(即过长时间中性粒细胞减少症的患者)应用[168,184,185]。必要时中止预防是至关重要的。监测耐药菌的出现也非常重要[200,201]。

预防真菌和病毒感染

由于高风险患者感染侵袭性真菌的增加,开始有预防性抗真菌治疗[202]。预防性应用氟康唑(和伊曲康唑)能够降低念珠菌的表面定植和全身感染。耐药菌(克柔假丝酵母和光滑念珠菌)是潜在的问题,虽然这些菌种在未应用唑类药物的患者中也可见到。虽然有抗霉活性更强的新药如米卡芬净、伏立康唑和泊沙康唑,预防性抗霉(包括曲霉)效果欠佳[203~205]。伏立康唑应用的增加已出现穿透性接合菌类感染,对此广泛应用的方法发出了警告。

预防应用阿昔洛韦能够预防 HCT 前密集化疗(伴或不伴放疗)或白血病或淋巴瘤诱导治疗患者 HSV 感染的再次激活。对 CMV 抗原血症阳性的高危患者应用更昔洛韦或膦甲酸提前治疗(而不是预防性治疗)是目前较为推荐的方法[139]。

分离

新病原菌获得的减少将患者置入逆向隔离的风险。需予患者以煮熟的食物,并被要求避免食用新鲜水果和蔬菜(如番茄、沙拉),因为这些食物天然有革兰阴性菌如铜绿假单胞菌、克雷伯肺炎杆菌和大肠埃希菌污染。更复杂的方法更昂贵且费时,并没有证明比严格遵守洗手方法更有效。

防护环境要联合两种方法,即使用隔离单元以保护患者免受院内污染,并且用抗生素减少患者内生微生物群。防护环境主要要有隔离单元,提供患者与医院环境的屏障,使用积极的净化技术和空气过滤。患者的食物要特别制备或灭菌减少污染。患者的消毒需要加强药物治疗,其中包括口服不吸收抗生素。患者要用杀菌皂洗澡、在微生物感染健康部位使用局部抗生素软膏或喷雾。

因为目前抑制内生微生物群和防止获得性感染的尝试还没有完全成功,所以需要开发其他防止感染的方法。造血刺激因子(GM-CSF 和 G-CSF)已经证明能够缩短中性粒细胞减少症的时间、减少发热的天数和伴中性粒细胞减少症患者可确定的感染。目前的指南建议对既往未经治疗和接受化疗的患者开始不予原则性应用这些药物。接下来在早期生长因子的应用能够降低中性粒细胞减少伴发热的可能性。它还能够缩短中性粒细胞减少症的时间和接受大剂量细胞毒治疗的自体骨髓移植患者感染并发症的频率。

抗生素管理

抗生素抵抗已经被证明导致发病率、死亡率和全世界医疗费用增加的原因。因此,适当的将抗微生物药物用于预防、经验性治疗、抢先治疗、靶向治疗或维持治疗是癌症患者管理的重要部分,尤其是在一个新的抗微生物药物开发停滞的时期。抗生素管理的主要目标是优化抗生素的应用,同时减少不良后果如毒性反应和耐药菌的产生[206,207]。有效的抗生素管理策略列在表 139-7。这些策略由一个独立、多学科、抗生素管理小组(MAST)严格执行[208~210]。

表 139-7 抗生素管理策略

持续对所有医务工作者进行教育
根据当地微生物学和敏感/耐药决定适当的抗生素使用指南/途径
严格规定特殊药物的使用
使用抗生素的审核需对处方进行反馈进行监控和治疗策略制订的研究
监测预后(发病率、死亡率和存活时间)和耐药方式综合感染控制方案

展望

对于许多癌症患者而言,感染仍然是严重的并发症。随着感染谱不断变化,特别是在新药开发相当有限的情况下,多重耐药病原体的出现为肿瘤患者感染治疗提出了严峻的挑战。播散性真菌感染已成为血液系统恶性肿瘤患者和接受 HCT 患者死亡的主要原因。尽管已取得一些改进,但许多 IFI 的早期诊断和适当治疗仍然不能令人满意。病毒感染带来了越来越大的威胁,尤其是在血液系统恶性肿瘤和接受 HCT 患者中。新出现的席卷全球的感染(如 MERS 和埃博拉病毒)可能会对处于免疫抑制状态的癌症患者产生毁灭性影响。仍需要开发用于快速诊断这些病毒感染的可靠方法,以及有效的预防和治疗手段。寄生虫感染在其流行地区外仍然相对少见。尽管目前对于抗寄生虫治疗具备有效疗法,但其毒性和长期维持治疗仍成问题。风险评估策略的发展使得我们可以从中性粒细胞减少症患者中筛选出"低风险"亚组。对于这些患者,门诊口服治疗等新的治疗策略已节省了大量成本,减少了院内感染,并改善了患者生活质量。受保护的环境、预防计划、感染控制策略和集落刺激因子降低了癌症患者感染的风险。抗生素管理可延迟耐药菌的发展,新技术的出现可进一步预防耐药。尽管如此,随着我们朝着消除癌症的更大目标努力,癌症患者感染的识别、预防、诊断和治疗将继续对我们提出更大挑战。

(刘嘉琦 张梦璐 译 王翔 王昕 校)

参考文献

The complete reference list can be found on the Wiley Companion Digital Edition of this title (see inside front cover for login instructions).

2 Bow EJ. Neutropenic fever syndromes in patients undergoing cytotoxic therapy for acute leukemia and myelodysplastic syndromes. *Semin Hematol.* 2009;**46**:259–268.

3 Zell JA, Chang JC. Neoplastic fever: a neglected paraneoplastic syndrome. *Support Care Cancer.* 2005;**13**:870–877.

7 Roblot F, Imbert S, Godet C, et al. Risk factors analysis for Pneumocystis jiroveci pneumonia (PCP) in patients with haematological malignancies and pneumonia. *Scand J Infect Dis.* 2004;**36**:848–854.

12 Rolston KV, Nesher L, Tarrand JT. Current microbiology of surgical site infections in patients with cancer: a retrospective review. *Infect Dis Ther.* 2014;**3(2)**:245–256.

13 Wisplinghoff H, Seifert H, Wenzel RP, et al. Current trends in the epidemiology

of nosocomial bloodstream infections in patients with hematological malignancies and solid neoplasms in hospitals in the United States. *Clin Infect Dis.* 2003;**36**:1103–1110.

14 Nesher L, Rolston KV. The current spectrum of infection in cancer patients with chemotherapy related neutropenia. *Infection.* 2014;**42**:5–13.

16 Rolston KV, Bodey GP, Safdar A. Polymicrobial infection in patients with cancer: an underappreciated and underreported entity. *Clin Infect Dis.* 2007;**45**: 228–233.

22 Liu C, Bayer A, Cosgrove SE, et al. Clinical practice guidelines by the infectious diseases society of america for the treatment of methicillin-resistant *Staphylococcus aureus* infections in adults and children. *Clin Infect Dis.* 2011;**52**:e18–e55.

34 Bochud PY, Eggiman P, Calandra T, et al. Bacteremia due to viridans streptococcus in neutropenic patients with cancer: clinical spectrum and risk factors. *Clin Infect Dis.* 1994;**18**:25–31.

37 Shelburne SA, Tarrand J, Rolston KV. Review of streptococcal bloodstream infections at a comprehensive cancer care center, 2000–2011. *J Infect.* 2013;**66**:136–146.

41 Dubberke ER, Hollands JM, Georgantopoulos P, et al. Vancomycin-resistant enterococcal bloodstream infections on a hematopoietic stem cell transplant unit: are the sick getting sicker? *Bone Marrow Transplant.* 2006;**38**:813–819.

50 Safdar A, Rolston KV. Stenotrophomonas maltophilia: changing spectrum of a serious bacterial pathogen in patients with cancer. *Clin Infect Dis.* 2007;**45**:1602–1609.

52 Nesher L, Rolston KVI. Neutropenic enterocolitis, a growing concern in the era of widespread use of aggressive chemotherapy. *Clin Infect Dis.* 2013;**56**:711–717.

53 Boucher HW, Talbot GH, Bradley JS, et al. Bad bugs, no drugs: no ESKAPE! An update from the Infectious Diseases Society of America. *Clin Infect Dis.* 2009;**48**:1–12.

54 Bushnell G, Mitrani-Gold F, Mundy LM. Emergence of New Delhi metallo-β-lactamase type 1-producing enterobacteriaceae and non-enterobacteriaceae: global case detection and bacterial surveillance. *Int J Infect Dis.* 2013;**17**:e325–e333.

58 Boucher HW, Talbot GH, Benjamin DK, et al. 10 x '20 progress—development of new drugs active against gram-negative bacilli: an update from the Infectious Diseases Society of America. *Clin Infect Dis.* 2013;**56**:1685–1694.

67 Chen CY, Sheng WH, Lai CC, et al. Mycobacterial infections in adult patients with hematological malignancy. *Eur J Clin Microbiol Infect Dis.* 2012;**31**:1059–1066.

72 Cohen SH, Gerding DN, Johnson S, et al. Clinical practice guidelines for Clostridium difficile infection in adults: 2010 update by the society for healthcare epidemiology of America (SHEA) and the infectious diseases society of America (IDSA). *Infect Control Hosp Epidemiol.* 2010;**31**:431–455.

80 Lewis RE, Cahyame-Zuniga L, Leventakos K, et al. Epidemiology and sites of involvement of invasive fungal infections in patients with haematological malignancies: a 20-year autopsy study. *Mycoses.* 2013;**56**:638–645.

87 Pappas PG, Kauffman CA, Andes D, et al. Clinical practice guidelines for the management of candidiasis: 2009 update by the Infectious Diseases Society of America. *Clin Infect Dis.* 2009;**48**:503–535.

89 Groll AH, Castagnola E, Cesaro S, et al. Fourth European Conference on Infections in Leukaemia (ECIL-4): guidelines for diagnosis, prevention, and treatment of invasive fungal diseases in paediatric patients with cancer or allogeneic haemopoietic stem-cell transplantation. *Lancet Oncol.* 2014;**15**:e327–e340.

90 Mousset S, Buchheidt D, Heinz W, et al. Treatment of invasive fungal infections in cancer patients-updated recommendations of the Infectious Diseases Working Party (AGIHO) of the German Society of Hematology and Oncology (DGHO). *Ann Hematol.* 2014;**93**:13–32.

94 Caillot D, Latrabe V, Thiébaut A, et al. Computer tomography in pulmonary invasive aspergillosis in hematological patients with neutropenia: an useful tool for diagnosis and assessment of outcome in clinical trials. *Eur J Radiol.* 2010;**74**:e172–e175.

101 Marr KA, Schlamm HT, Herbrecht R, et al. Combination antifungal therapy for invasive aspergillosis: a randomized trial. *Ann Intern Med.* 2015;**162**:81–89.

103 Kamel S, O'Connor S, Lee N, et al. High incidence of Pneumocystis jirovecii pneumonia in patients receiving biweekly rituximab and cyclophosphamide, adriamycin, vincristine, and prednisone. *Leuk Lymphoma.* 2010;**51**:797–801.

108 Cooley L, Dendle C, Wolf J, et al. Consensus guidelines for diagnosis, prophylaxis and management of Pneumocystis jirovecii pneumonia in patients with haematological and solid malignancies, 2014. *Intern Med J.* 2014;**44**:1350–1363.

123 Zaia J, Baden L, Boeckh MJ, et al. Viral disease prevention after hematopoietic cell transplantation. *Bone Marrow Transplant.* 2009;**44**:471–482.

126 Hirsch HH, Martino R, Ward KN, et al. Fourth European Conference on Infections in Leukaemia (ECIL-4): guidelines for diagnosis and treatment of human respiratory syncytial virus, parainfluenza virus, metapneumovirus, rhinovirus, and coronavirus. *Clin Infect Dis.* 2013;**56**:258–266.

134 Zerr DM, Boeckh M, Delaney C, et al. HHV-6 reactivation and associated sequelae after hematopoietic cell transplantation. *Biol Blood Marrow Transplant.* 2012;**18**:1700–1708.

136 Ljungman P, Griffiths P, Paya C. Definitions of cytomegalovirus infection and disease in transplant recipients. *Clin Infect Dis.* 2002;**34**:1094–1097.

139 Green ML, Leisenring W, Stachel D, et al. Efficacy of a viral load-based, risk-adapted, preemptive treatment strategy for prevention of cytomegalovirus disease after hematopoietic cell transplantation. *Biol Blood Marrow Transplant.* 2012;**18**:1687–1699.

145 Mullane KM, Winston DJ, Wertheim MS, et al. Safety and immunogenicity of heat-treated zoster vaccine (ZVHT) in immunocompromised adults. *J Infect Dis.* 2013;**208**:1375–1385.

160 Mermel LA, Allon M, Bouza E, et al. Clinical practice guidelines for the diagnosis and management of intravascular catheter-related infection: 2009 update by the Infectious Diseases Society of America. *Clin Infect Dis.* 2009;**49**:1–45.

168 Freifeld AG, Bow EJ, Sepkowitz KA, et al. Clinical practice guideline for the use of antimicrobial agents in neutropenic patients with cancer: 2010 update by the infectious diseases society of america. *Clin Infect Dis.* 2011;**52**:e56–e93.

172 Klastersky J, Paesmans M, Rubenstein EB, et al. The multinational association for supportive care in cancer risk index: a multinational scoring system for identifying low-risk febrile neutropenic cancer patients. *J Clin Oncol.* 2000;**18**:3038–3051.

184 Flowers CR, Seidenfeld J, Bow EJ, et al. Antimicrobial prophylaxis and outpatient management of fever and neutropenia in adults treated for malignancy: American Society of Clinical Oncology clinical practice guideline. *J Clin Oncol.* 2013;**31**:794–810.

185 Baden LR, Bensinger W, Angarone M, et al. Prevention and treatment of cancer-related infections. *J Natl Compr Canc Netw.* 2012;**10**:1412–1445.

192 Smith TJ, Khatcheressian J, Lyman GH, et al. 2006 update of recommendations for the use of white blood cell growth factors: an evidence-based clinical practice guideline. *J Clin Oncol.* 2006;**24**:3187–3205.

195 Bucaneve G, Micozzi A, Menichetti F, et al. Levofloxacin to prevent bacterial infection in patients with cancer and neutropenia. *N Engl J Med.* 2005;**353**:977–987.

196 Cullen M, Steven N, Billingham L, et al. Antibacterial prophylaxis after chemotherapy for solid tumors and lymphomas. *N Engl J Med.* 2005;**353**:988–998.

197 Gafter-Gvili A, Fraser A, Paul M, et al. Antibiotic prophylaxis for bacterial infections in afebrile neutropenic patients following chemotherapy. *Cochrane Database Syst Rev.* 2012;**1**:CD004386.

203 van Burik JA, Ratanatharathorn V, Stepan DE, et al. Micafungin versus fluconazole for prophylaxis against invasive fungal infections during neutropenia in patients undergoing hematopoietic stem cell transplantation. *Clin Infect Dis.* 2004;**39**:1407–1416.

205 Cornely OA, Maertens J, Winston DJ, et al. Posaconazole vs. fluconazole or itraconazole prophylaxis in patients with neutropenia. *N Engl J Med.* 2007;**356**:348–359.

206 Dellit TH, Owens RC, McGowan JE, et al. Infectious diseases society of America and the Society for Healthcare Epidemiology of America guidelines for developing an institutional program to enhance antimicrobial stewardship. *Clin Infect Dis.* 2007;**44**:159–177.

209 Tverdek FP, Rolston KV, Chemaly RF. Antimicrobial stewardship in patients with cancer. *Pharmacotherapy.* 2012;**32**:722–734.

第 140 章　肿瘤急症

Sai-Ching Jim Yeung, MD, PhD, FACP ■ Carmen P. Escalante, MD

概述

癌症及其治疗可能导致肿瘤急症发生。本章讨论了解决癌症患者发生急性紧急情况的方法。本章选择了一些癌症急症进行重点讨论。讨论了突发的心肺骤停以及癌症患者复苏中特殊情况的考虑。心律不齐，上腔静脉综合征，心脏压塞和急性出血是重要的心血管急症。肿瘤溶解综合征可能会迅速致死，因此早期识别和治疗对于预防灾难性的后果非常重要。肺部疾病包括气道阻塞、胸腔积液、咯血、气胸和肺栓塞。神经病学紧急情况包括脊压迫、脑疝和癫痫持续状态。中性粒细胞减少症可能是肿瘤急诊中最常讨论的重要话题。本章还讨论了其他重要问题，例如内脏穿孔、过敏反应和细胞因子释放综合征。肿瘤科医生和急诊医师必须意识到癌症患者的这些潜在的严重急性并发症，以便及时开始适当的治疗。

简介

肿瘤急症是由癌症或其治疗所引起的急性疾病，需要尽快干预以避免死亡或患者恶性发病。癌症患者比非癌症患者更有可能需要紧急护理。由于恶性肿瘤或其治疗而导致的身体虚弱，凝血改变和免疫力下降，也使癌症患者在日常生活中容易发生事故和不幸。由于癌症患者具有独特的心理关注点和生理状态的变化，因此急救人员需要适应他们的特殊需求。

癌症患者的急症正在发展成为一门综合学科，即肿瘤学和急诊医学之间的交叉学科。这里汇集了癌症患者向急诊医疗机构提出的许多类型的问题，并且这些问题需要进行深入的讨论[1~3]。由于页面的限制以及本书其他各章中某些相关主题的覆盖，本章将仅涵盖选定的几个主题。

急性Ⅲ期癌症患者的治疗方法

癌症患者常合并冠心病、糖尿病和慢性阻塞性肺疾病。其

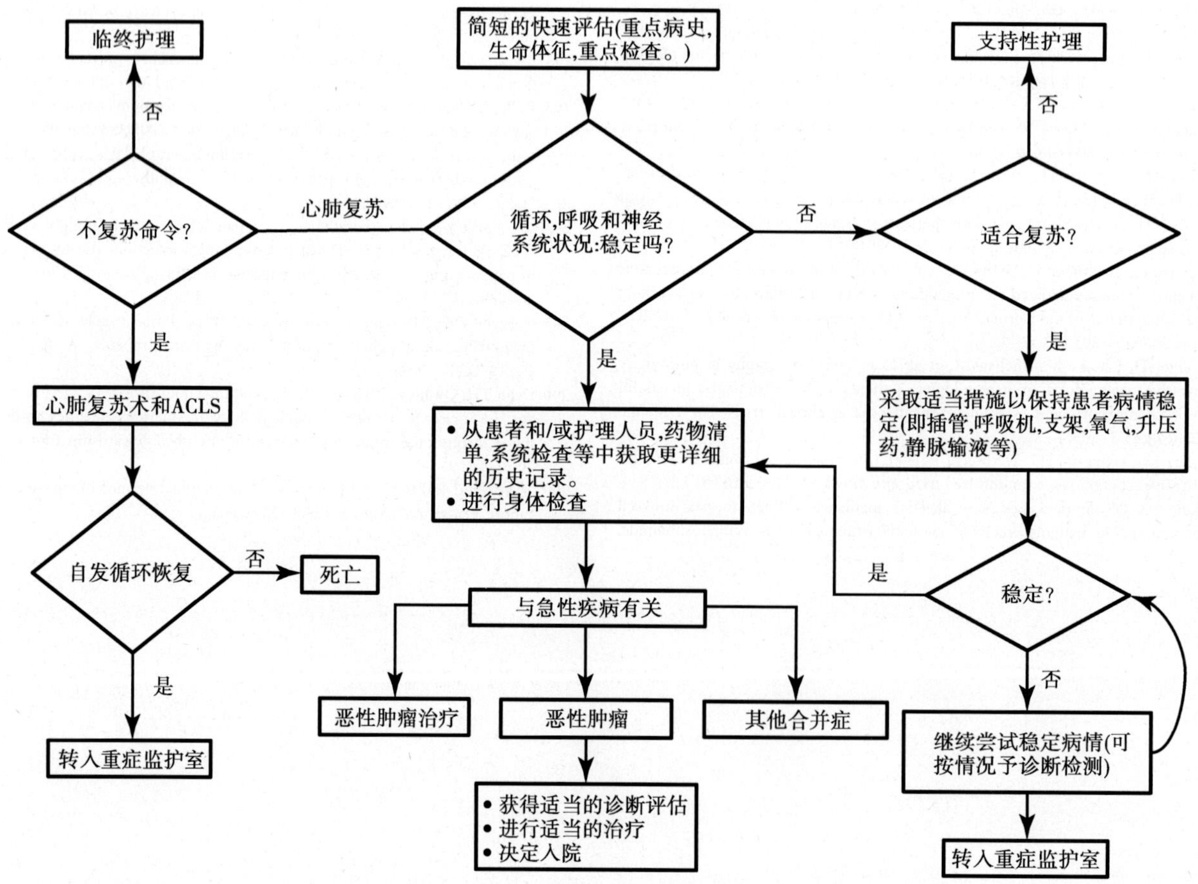

图 140-1　所有癌症患者的急症处理办法

中一些可归因于相同的致癌危险因素(即老年、饮食、吸烟或苯丙胺类)。急救护理人员必须评估疾病的严重程度、相应的治疗、总体预后以及患者和家庭的意愿,以便制订适当的治疗计划(图 140-1)。大多数接近生命终点的癌症患者不希望采取“英勇”措施,不及时处理预先指示和不复苏(DNR)命令,可能会提高临终前几周的生活质量[4]。

首先,应迅速评估患者。该评估应包括主诉、重点病史、生命体征和快速全面的身体评估。如果患者无法提供当前疾病的病史,家庭成员、同伴或照料者可以提供相关信息。对不稳定生命的干预应立即开始。在心肺骤停时,应遵循适当的指导原则(http://www.acls.net/aclsalg.htm)[5]。一旦患者病情稳定,应完成完整的病史和体格检查。对于大多数有急症的癌症患者,综合评价是必要的。紧急情况可能是由于癌症、癌症治疗或共病引起的,所有这些都应该在鉴别诊断中考虑。

肿瘤循环系统急症

心肺骤停

大多数死亡都是在心肺骤停之前。当心肺骤停是由急性可逆性损伤引起的,而不是由身体功能的持续不可逆性下降引起时,复苏更有可能成功。癌症患者和非癌症患者的复苏成功率和出院率相似[6]。对患者复苏(包括癌症患者)的荟萃分析估计,复苏成功率和出院率分别约为 30% 和 12%[7]。同样,对在癌症中心急诊室接受复苏的院外停药癌症患者,复苏成功率为 43%,存活出院率为 17%[8]。这与重病非癌症患者的情况相似[9]。如果癌症患者表现良好,预期不会很快死亡,那么不愿意让患者苏醒或接受重症监护是没有道理的。在心肺骤停的非终末期癌症患者应以与任何非癌症患者相同的强度进行复苏。然而,当心肺骤停作为预期的最终事件发生时,复苏通常是徒劳的。

肿瘤学家应确保与癌症患者及其家属讨论预先指令(医疗授权、生存意愿和院外 DNR 指令)。许多患者很容易签署生前遗嘱或指定医疗代理人。及时推荐 DNR 状态可以避免对患者造成不必要的创伤,对家庭造成不必要的徒劳的努力、浪费的资源和痛苦。这也为公开讨论解决患者和家庭成员之间的分歧提供了时间。

当癌症患者在急诊或完全心肺骤停时到医疗机构就诊时,急诊医生可能从未见过患者,而且评估预后是困难的,而且往往是不可能的。开始或继续接受治疗的决定应基于对患者生理状况的快速评估,停药前事件的简要历史,以及以下因素:①停药持续时间;②最初的心律;③尸僵或阿尔戈尸僵;④癌症的类型、阶段和预后;⑤癌症治疗的历史和成功的前景;⑥患者或家庭的明确指示;⑦并发症情况;⑧表现状况和营养状况;⑨患者生存的潜在生活质量;以及⑩高龄。

癌症患者复苏的特殊考虑

患者被送往急救中心的事实可能表明死亡是意外的,家属没有接受患者的严重预后,或者患者或家属在生命的最后时刻寻求症状或痛苦的缓解。对复苏的要求可能是由于拒绝接受最终条件。一项基于问卷调查的研究发现,尽管生存率很低,但大多数癌症患者仍希望得到复苏,他们希望自己和他们的近亲在决策过程中得到解决[10]。在知道“一切可能已经完成”的情况下,复苏可能需要给家庭“一个了结”。然而,晚期难治性疾病患者的复苏可能不合适,因为复苏只会延长疼痛和痛苦。

大多数医生和医疗保健提供者遵循高级心脏生命支持(ACLS)协议(http://www.acls.net/aclsalg.htm)中概述的恢复算法[5]。然而,识别心肺骤停的特定原因可能使医生能够针对逆转或控制特定原因的努力。类癌性危象是癌症患者心肺骤停少见但可预防和治疗的原因之一。危象可能是由麻醉、活检、手术、化疗或肾上腺素能药物(如多巴胺和肾上腺素)引起的。由于肿瘤中大量释放血管活性肽和血清素,受影响的患者可能会出现顽固性低血压、心律失常和支气管痉挛。癌症危象可以中止或用奥曲肽醋酸酯治疗,一种生长抑素类似物,150~500μg 静脉注射[11]。心脏压塞是另一个例子。如果患者因恶性心包积液导致心脏压塞而出现无脉冲电活动,在心包穿刺术解除对心腔的压力之前,复苏不会成功。

癌症患者心搏骤停的原因分析

在一般人群中,未确诊的肿瘤是一种罕见的猝死原因。对癌症患者死亡原因的回顾发现,4% 的患者死于心脏问题,90% 死于动脉粥样硬化相关的缺血性心脏病[12]。癌症患者心肺骤停的主要原因与癌症或抗肿瘤治疗有关,而不是原发性心脏病。

肿瘤相关的病因

肿瘤相关的心脏问题通常是心包受累(如肿瘤性心包炎和心脏压塞)的结果。肿瘤可通过分泌激素介质(如嗜铬细胞瘤引起的儿茶酚胺和类癌性肿瘤引起的 5-羟色胺)或直接机械刺激心脏或心包引起的儿茶酚胺。据报道,心律失常与心肌肿瘤、肿瘤引起的冠状动脉阻塞和大量肿瘤栓塞有关,可导致心肺骤停。心脏淀粉样变性也可导致顽固性充血性心力衰竭、心律失常、传导障碍和猝死[13]。其他与肿瘤相关的猝死原因包括出血、通气功能丧失和器官衰竭。

全身治疗相关原因

抗肿瘤药物可引起导致心肺骤停的并发症(心绞痛、心肌梗死、充血性心力衰竭、低血压、心律失常)[14]。多柔比星可引起约 30% 的患者心电图和心律变化(多数为良性),15% 的患者可导致心肺骤停[16]。一些药物(如伊马替尼、曲妥珠单抗)可干扰细胞毒性心肌损伤后的心肌重塑,引起心肌病和心力衰竭[15]。高剂量环磷酰胺可引起室性心律失常、心脏病、心包积液[17],氟尿嘧啶和卡培他滨与导致心绞痛和心肌梗死的急性冠状动脉痉挛有关;他们也被报道引起急性心源性休克。据报道,低血压、心律失常和猝死与细胞因子(重组人白介素-2(IL-2)、干扰素)和单克隆抗体有关。

放疗相关的原因

辐射可损伤心包和心脏[18]。心包炎可能发生在暴露于辐射后不久或数月至数年。放疗可导致瓣膜病、心包积液、心脏压塞、心包纤维化或限制性心肌病。辐射的直接毒性作用可引起心电图改变,包括 t 波异常和房性心律失常。心脏暴露在辐射下也与冠状动脉问题(加速粥样硬化、内膜炎、中层纤维化、内膜增生)有关,导致心肌梗死和猝死[19]。

心律失常

心律失常是癌症患者普遍存在的问题,需要加强护理。持续性心律失常可导致心跳停止和死亡;否则,间歇性心律失常的症状可能很微妙。这些症状主要是由于血流动力学的影响。重要的症状和体征包括意识丧失(晕厥)、头晕、心悸、胸痛、呼吸困难和急性神经功能减退。

持续性心律失常可用心电图诊断。然而,心律失常往往是暂时性或间歇性的,导致诊断困难。心电图节律短暂的连续监测并不排除晚期和潜在的严重节律紊乱。当症状提示有心律失常时,24~48h 动态心电图监测或事件记录器(连续循环、事件后或实时连续)可记录心律失常。癌症患者的心律分析可能很复杂,因为他们经常有电轴的过度呼吸变化和平均 QRS 电压的变化,这可能与心律不规则相混淆。这种改变可能是由于胸腔或心包积液、肺外科手术(肺切除或肺叶切除)或放射损伤引起的。

原发性心律失常

原发性心律失常是由心脏和心包结构引起的。所有患者原发性心律失常的常见原因包括心力衰竭;心内压和室壁应力增加;充血性、肥厚性和浸润性心肌病;纤维化。在癌症患者中,原发性心律失常的原因是原发性或转移性心内肿瘤、淀粉样蛋白浸润、心肌炎、心包炎、心包收缩,以及与抗肿瘤药物(特别是抗 HER2 疗法)有关的心脏病[14]。

继发性心律失常

继发性心律失常由药物毒性反应、交感神经状态增强(严重焦虑、甲状腺功能亢进、嗜铬细胞瘤、类癌肿瘤等)、异常电解质和辐射性心脏损伤引起。一些癌症药物具有致心律失常作用(表 140-1)[20~24],除了常用于治疗癌症患者感染性并发症的化疗、抗真菌药物、抗普罗托松和抗生素外,还可能延长 QT 间期[在 http://www.qtdeproces.org(亚利桑那州治疗学教育和研究中心)上列出],这可能导致心律失常。

表 140-1　抗肿瘤药物与心血管副作用

	肺性 HTN	系统性 HTN	缺血	LVEF 减少	QT 间期延长	VT/猝死	心动过缓	AF/SVT
酪氨酸激酶抑制剂								
伊马替尼	报道			0.5%~1.7%				
达沙替尼	报道			2%~4%	<1%~3%			
卡波替尼		33%			QTcF 平均增加 10~15 毫秒;无 QTcF>500 毫秒			
拉帕替尼				1.5%~4%	16%			
厄洛替尼			2.3%					
尼洛替尼	报道	10%~11%			1%~10% QTcF>500ms 在 1%	报道		
培唑帕尼		40%~42%		8%~11%	QTcF > 500ms 在 0.2%~2%	尖端扭转速度<1%		
索拉非尼		9%~43%	2.7%~3%	12%	没有大的变化(即<20 毫秒)			
舒尼替尼		5%~47%		2.7%~27%	剂量依赖	尖端扭转速度<1%		
万得他尼		33%			1%的患者 QTcF>500ms	报道		
抗体								
贝伐单抗		4%~35%	0.6%~1.5%	1.7%~3%				
曲妥珠单抗		4%		2%~28%				
烷基化剂								
顺铂		报道	报道	报道		报道		报道
异环磷酰胺				17%				报道
环磷酰胺			报道	7%~28%				报道

续表

	肺性 HTN	系统性 HTN	缺血	LVEF 减少	QT 间期延长	VT/猝死	心动过缓	AF/SVT
白消安				报道				
丝裂霉素				报道				
蒽环类/蒽醌类								
柔红霉素				报道				
多柔比星				3%~26% 累积剂量为 400~450mg/m^2 时为 5%		6%	报道	2.2%~10.3%
伊达比星				5%~18%				
表柔比星				0.9%~3.3%				
米托蒽醌				报道				
抗代谢物								
卡培他滨			3%~9%	报告心源性休克		2.1%		
氟尿嘧啶			1%~68%	报告心源性休克				4.2%~6.5%
吉西他滨								8.2%
阿糖胞苷				报道				
氯法拉滨				27%				
拓扑异构酶 I 抑制剂								
伊立替康								
紫杉烷类							报道	
紫杉醇			<1%~5%			0.26%	<0.1%~31%	0.18%
多西他赛			1.7%	2.3%~8%				
长春花生物碱								
长春新碱			报道					
长春碱			报道					
其他								
白介素 2				报道		0.2%		17.4%
三氧化二砷					26%			
伏林司他					3.5%~6%			
干扰素 α			1%	报道				1%
维 A 酸(视黄酸)				报道				
硼替佐米				2%~5%				
沙利度胺								
戊他汀				报道				

AF,房颤;HTN,高血压;LVEF,左室射血分数;QTcF,按 Fridericia 公式校正的 QT 间期;SVT,室上性心动过速;VT,室性心动过速。
摘自 Yeh[20]、Lenihan 和 Kowey[21]、Guglin 等人[22]、Yeh and Bickford[23]、Ewer and Ewer[24] 等人的数据。

心律失常的治疗

心律失常的治疗应以急迫性和病因学为基础。对于二级来源血流动力学稳定的心律失常,主要治疗应集中在纠正代谢障碍(特别是钾、钙和镁)和停止罪魁祸首药物。应给予特定的治疗来逆转诱发因素。当需要以控制心律为目的的治疗时,可遵循心律失常管理的标准指南[5]。表 140-2 中列出了常用的静脉注射抗心律失常药物。

阵发性室上性心动过速(SVT)可在相当大比例的迷走神经操作中逆转为窦性心律。在心电图监测下,腺苷作为一个或两个剂量的快速注射给药,经常有效地恢复窦性心律。腺苷也被用来确定心律失常的机制时,诊断不清楚的心电图。

稳定的继发性心律失常不可能恶化为致命的灾难。通常,继发性心律失常表现为室性异位(有时表现为二联律、三联律或其他偶合型)或室上异位(常为间歇性或持续性 SVT)。孤立的早发性脑室复合体不需要任何治疗。复杂的三叉静脉异位通常由 β-肾上腺素能阻滞剂控制。

表 140-2 常用静脉注射抗心律失常药物

名称	分类	剂量	适应证
腺苷	核苷	6mg 静脉注射<3s,然后注射生理盐水 20ml;需要第二次和第三次剂量为 12mg,间隔 2min	狭窄的复杂 PSVT;由于 AV 节点或窦房结折返导致的 PSVT
胺碘酮	三类抗心律失常药	心搏骤停:300mg 静脉注射;150mg 静脉注射每 3~5min 1 次,每日 2.2g。稳定的复杂性心动过速:在 10min 内静脉注 150mg;根据需要重复 q10min;维持输注 0.5mg/min;最高 2.2g/d	室上或室性快速性心律失常;地高辛无效时低 LVEF 患者快速心律失常的控制
阿托品	抗胆碱能	0.5~1mg IVP q3~5min(根据需要),最高 0.04mg/kg	有症状的窦性心动过缓;Mobitz 1 型 AV 区块;心搏停止
地高辛	洋地黄苷	负荷剂量:10~15μg/kg,分次服用	减慢房颤的心室反应。房扑或 PSVT
地尔硫䓬	钙通道阻滞剂	在 2min 内静脉注射 0.25mg/kg;15min 内 2min 内第二次注射 0.35mg/kg 静脉注射;维持:滴定 5~15mg/h	减慢房颤或房扑的心室反应,PSVT;终止房室结折返性心动过速
艾司洛尔	β 肾上腺素受体阻滞剂	1min 内为 0.5mg/kg;然后注入 0.05mg/kg/min;最高滴定至 0.3mg/kg/min	PSVT,房颤或房扑;或减少 MI 或 USA 的 VF 发生率
伊布利特	三类抗心律失常药	10min 内 1mg 静脉注射;在 10min 内重复	SVT 包括房颤、房扑;对房颤的转换有效。房扑持续时间相对短者
异丙肾上腺素	β 肾上腺素受体激动剂	注入 2~10μg/min;滴定	症状性心动过缓;指向性扭转性心动过速(mg);β 肾上腺素受体阻滞剂过量
利多卡因	局麻药	IVP 1~1.5mg/kg;重复 0.5~0.75mg/kg IVP q5~10min,直至总计 3mg/kg prn;维持:30~50μg/kg/min 静脉注射	VT 或 VF;复杂性心动过速明显的心室异位;尖端扭转
美托洛尔	β 肾上腺素受体阻滞剂	5mg 慢 IVP q5min,直至总剂量 15mg	PSVT,房颤或房扑;降低 MI 或 USA 心室纤颤的发生率
普鲁卡因胺	ⅠA 类抗心律失常药	20~50mg/min,最高剂量为 17mg/kg	复发性 VF 或 VT
盐酸盐普萘洛尔	β 肾上腺素受体阻滞剂	0.1mg/kg 缓慢 IVP,分 3 次服用 2~3min 分开	PSVT,房颤或房扑;减少 MI 或 USA 的 VF 发生率
葡萄糖酸奎尼丁	ⅠA 类抗心律失常药	每 5~10min 间歇性推注 80mg 或以 10mg/min 的速度静脉输注至 400mg	室上和室性心律失常
维拉帕米	钙通道阻滞剂	在 2min 内静脉注射 2.5~5mg;重复 q 15~30min;总剂量为 20mg	PSVT,房颤或房扑

AV,房室;IVP,静脉推注;LVEF,左室射血分数;MI,心肌梗死;ns,生理盐水;prn,根据需要;PSVT,阵发性室上性心动过速;USA,不稳定心绞痛;VF,心室纤颤;VT,室性心动过速。

摘自 ACLS 提供者手册[5]。

胺碘酮应考虑用于左心室射血分数较低的患者,但对于肝功能不全或潜在甲状腺疾病患者应谨慎。胺碘酮很少能引起低血压、心动过缓和 qt 延长,从而导致尖端扭转性心动过速。除了 β 肾上腺素受体阻滞剂,许多抗心律失常药物,特别是1A、1C 和 3 型,有潜在的促心律失常的作用[25]。在开始抗心律失常治疗期间,应考虑进行心脏监测,因为癌症患者可能因代谢紊乱和同时使用其他 qt 延长药物而对促心律失常 mic 效应的敏感性增加。

SVT 是癌症患者最常见的心律失常,虽然药物是用来维持SVT 稳定的血流动力学,但有意识镇静下选择性同步心动过速仍应及早考虑并适当计划。美国心脏学会推荐的同步复律初始能量水平为 100J,但最初的能量水平为 200J 的休克被其他人推荐为心房颤动的转换[26]。当癌症患者伴有积液或明显超重时,更高的能量水平用于心脏复律是合适的。如果在 48h 内SVT 可以恢复节律,则可以避免抗凝治疗。然而,心律失常发作的时间并不总是很清楚。经食管超声心动图可排除心内血栓形成。由于缺乏明确的起病时间证据,患者应在复律前抗凝。

癌症患者结构性心律失常比代谢性心律失常更难控制。在紧急情况下,治疗目标是稳定情绪和呼吸状态,发现可纠正的病理条件,控制症状。根据心律失常的病因,可能需要与心脏病学专家进行紧急会诊和紧急诊断或介入治疗。

不稳定心律失常患者应采用积极的药物或电干预治疗。干预措施应遵循美国心脏学会制订的算法[27]。这些干预措施包括给药加压素,如加压素或肾上腺素(如需要);给药抗心律失常药物,如胺碘酮、利多卡因和普鲁卡因胺;电复律或除颤;气道管理;氧气通气;静脉输液;胸部按压(如果需要)。尖端扭转型室性心动过速的急诊治疗不同于室性心动过速的标准治疗方法;它需要方便地使用硫酸镁、电超速起搏、异丙肾上腺素药物治疗或苯妥英钠或利多卡因。

肿瘤溶解综合征

肿瘤溶解综合征(TLS)由严重的高磷血症、高钾血症、高尿酸血症、氮质血症、低钙血症和代谢性酸中毒(与肾功能不全不成比例)组成,其原因是大量释放细胞内容物并将死亡的肿瘤细胞降解到血液中[28]。TLS 可以自发发生,但白血病和淋巴瘤患者化疗后 72h 内通常发生,但新的治疗方案可能会改变发病时间。TLS 也可发生在非血液系统恶性肿瘤的住院患者中,包括小细胞癌、非小细胞肺癌、乳腺癌和卵巢癌。

TLS 的症状是非特异性的。常见症状包括恶心、呕吐、尿混浊、虚弱、疲劳和关节痛。其他与代谢和电解质异常有关的症状和体征包括神经肌肉易怒、癫痫、肌肉无力和心律失常。心律失常可导致 TLS 患者猝死[29]。肾小管中尿酸的沉淀可导致肾病和急性肾衰竭[30]。TLS 死亡的急性原因是严重的电解质异常(尤其是高钾血症)和肾衰竭引起的心律失常。早期发现代谢异常和及时治疗可避免死亡。

与 TLS 风险增加相关的因素包括恶性肿瘤类型(如急性淋巴细胞白血病、白细胞计数>75 000/μl 的急性髓细胞性白血病、Burkitt 瘤)、对治疗的反应性、恶性细胞快速转换和巨大的肿瘤负担[31]。其他风险因素是先前存在的肾衰,治疗后不久发生急性肾衰竭,对水化反应差。治疗前血清乳酸脱氢酶水平与肿瘤体积、淋巴瘤或淋巴细胞白血病相关,可预测治疗后氮质血症的发展,但治疗前高尿酸血症不能预测。根据正在接受诱导治疗的急性粒细胞白血病患者的数据,提出了 TLS 的预测评分系统[32,33]。该评分可能用于 TLS 的风险预防。高危患者应及早采取预防措施。使用高达 3L/(m^2·d)的Ⅳ类晶体液体进行积极的水合作用,可在有或无利尿剂的情况下保持尿量>100ml/h。黄嘌呤氧化抑制物别嘌醇(100~300mg/d 口服)可以预防严重的高尿酸血症。作为一种黄嘌呤氧化抑制剂,罗非他汀还有待研究。

TLS 的诊断需要高度的怀疑,因为早期很少有迹象或症状。常规尿酸和电解质筛查(包括钙和磷水平的测量)适用于肿瘤占位大或血液恶性肿瘤患者。TLS 的诊断可能基于 Cairo-Bishop 的定义[31~34]。一旦确诊,重度 TLS 患者应持续监测强度的血流动力学和心电图参数。多柔比星剂量可增加至900mg/d。rasburicase 是一种重组尿酸氧化酶,可将尿酸转化为兰豆素,在降低尿酸水平方面非常有效。可以使用 rasburicase(每日 150~200μg/kg 静脉注射或一次性使用所需的抢救剂量)来预防或治疗尿毒症肾病[35]。增加静脉液体水合作用可与使用循环利尿剂(如呋塞米,每 4~6h 静脉注射 20~200mg)和乙酰唑胺(每日 250~500mg 静脉注射)的利尿相结合。只有在出现严重高尿酸血症而没有黑曲霉酶的情况下,才应考虑用碳酸氢钠或醋酸钠静脉输注来增加尿酸盐在尿液中的溶解度。可能需要经常测量电解液(每 4~6h 一次)。高钾血症应与口服钾离子交换树脂(聚磺苯乙烯)一起用胰岛素加葡萄糖、钙和碳酸氢盐静脉注射治疗。在高磷酸盐血症的低钙血症患者中,口服钙基复合物(如醋酸钙或碳酸钙)将减少叶酸的吸收并增强钙的吸收。静脉钙蛋白融合可能导致严重高磷血症时磷酸钙沉淀,应谨慎使用。有症状性低钙血症且血清磷水平>3. 3mmol/L(>10. 2mg/dl)的患者可能需要透析。透析的其他适应证包括持续性难治性氮质血症、高钾血症、高尿酸血症、少尿、尽管使用利尿剂仍无尿、酸血症和容量超负荷。应立即进行透析,并持续监测,直到生化异常得到解决。血液透析是最常见的透析方式;长时间的血液透析,持续的动静脉血液透析,持续的静脉-静脉血液滤过,以及在透析液或置换液流量高(>3L/h)的情况下持续的肾脏替代治疗。

心脏压塞

心包积液损害心包动力学时发生心脏压塞。癌症患者心包腔积液是由于淋巴引流阻塞和/或心包表面肿瘤结节分泌过多液体所致。间皮瘤是最常见的恶性肿瘤,起源于心包。肺癌和恶性胸腺瘤可直接累及心包。更常见的是,恶性肿瘤通过逆行淋巴管或血行播散到达心包。黑色素瘤是最有可能转移到心脏的恶性肿瘤。淋巴瘤、白血病和胃肠道肿瘤也有心包积液[36]。心包积液的细胞学检查显示,70%~80%的心包积液患者有转移性疾病。心脏压塞的非恶性原因包括心脏脓肿、念珠菌性心包炎和心静脉置管并发症。

恶性心包积液多发生于晚期恶性心包积液,预后差(中位生存时间约 6 个月,1 年生存率 28%)[37],2/3 以上的恶性心包积液无症状。症状性患者常见的症状是呼吸急促、劳累呼吸困难、胸痛、端坐呼吸和全身无力,体检结果可能从正常到血流动力学衰竭不等。心动过速、低血压、颈静脉扩张、器官肿大和水肿可能表明心脏输出受损。心脏压塞的典型表现是由心包积液量和积液速度决定的。对上型肺动脉压是一种典型但非特异性的心脏压塞表现，因为它也见于肺癌、严重肺病或肺心病的住院患者。

心脏压塞的诊断通常需要额外的检查。低 QRS 电压和电交替造影是提示性的发现。胸片可能显示纵隔和心脏轮廓的扩大（图 140-2a，b）。计算机断层扫描（CT）或磁共振（MR）检查经常发现心包积液作为偶然发现。这些研究提供了心包积液的位置（室化或非室化）和大小的信息，但没有充分评估血流动力学的意义。二维超声心动图是诊断心包积液和评价其血流动力学意义，即心内压塞的存在的最有效的方法。右心房的塌陷或压迫、右心室的舒张性塌陷和心脏的"摇摆"（侧对侧或前后运动）常被观察到是嵌顿性压塞。通过多普勒位移测量二尖瓣血流的呼吸变化也有助于评估血流动力学。恶性心包积液的初步治疗依赖于血流动力学的稳定性。评分系统可以指导紧急心包穿刺术的决定[38]。对于血流动力学正常的患者，超声引导下的心包穿刺术，在心包间隙放置药物导管（图 140-2c），可在急救中心或重症监护室紧急形成（图 140-2d）。并发症很少见，可能包括大量的心周出血和气胸。心包积液可以从导管中排出，直到每日排出的液体少于 50ml。纤溶剂可用于疏通导管，以便于引流，避免重复心包穿刺或更换导管[39]。然而，心包积液通常在导管取出后重新积聚。

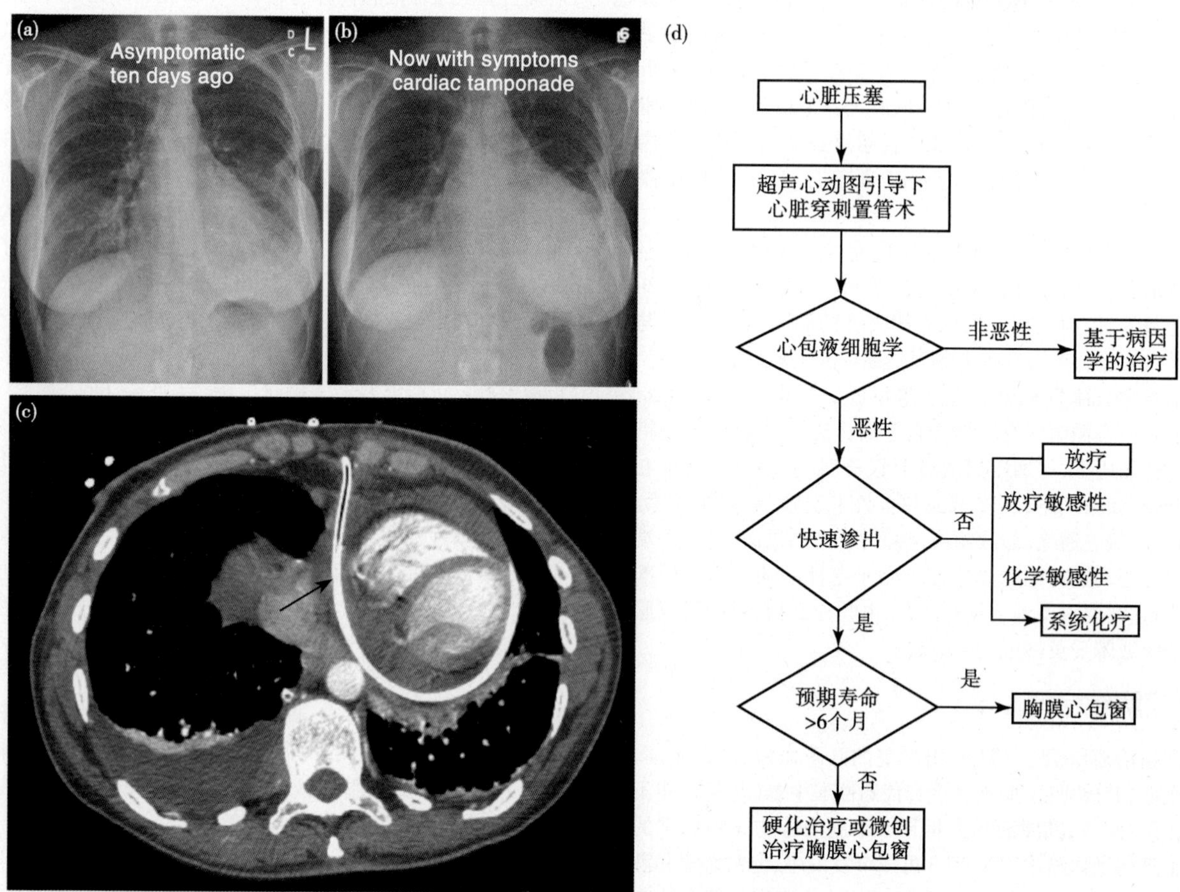

图 140-2　心脏压塞患者的 HEST 成像及处理算法。与先前的胸片相比（a），纵隔和心脏轮廓明显扩大（b）。另一例心脏压塞患者的胸部 CT 显示有留置引流导管（c）。一个心包积液的处理算法显示（d）

恶性心包积液病灶的长期治疗可防止积液的再积聚，50% 以上的患者出现积液。由于大多数恶性心包积液患者的长期生存受到限制，应采用对患者不适和风险有限的有效治疗。使用各种方法制作胸膜心包窗避免反复心包穿刺。这种手术通常在手术室进行，但在内科病房或重症监护室使用局部麻醉。使用经皮心包内球囊导管制造心包不全窗已经取得了一些成功[40]。也描述了 40 例经鼻翼镜横膈入路制造心包腹膜分流术[41]。在稳定的患者中，可以使用全身化疗、心包放射性胶体或胸外束照射。对这些治疗方式敏感的肿瘤。心脏暴露前应加强放疗，局部应用细胞毒剂或硬化剂可预防心包积液，42 例硬化治疗可能非常痛苦[42]。

急性出血

急性消化道出血和泌尿生殖道出血将在其他章节讨论。咯血，可以迅速压缩呼吸功能，将在本章后面讨论。本节将涵盖一些不太常见但严重的出血事件：颈动脉破裂、脾破裂和腹膜后出血。

急性出血的表现取决于出血率和出血部位。在大多数情况下，出血部位是明显的，但有时出血可能是内部的，很难诊断。低血容量和低灌注的体征和症状包括心动过速、低血压、少尿和精神状态低落。通常，诊断性影像学研究或程序，如 CT 扫描、超声、动脉造影或内镜检查，对诊断内出血是必要的。

急性出血的主要治疗目标是迅速确定出血源,达到止血的目的。在紧急情况下,只要可行,在迅速评估心肺功能状态的同时,应直接按压出血血管或部位。静脉液体复苏对维持血管内容量、心排出量和脑外器官灌注至关重要。等渗晶体液(生理盐水、乳酸林格溶液、血浆细胞等)应作为第一血缘,因为胶体(如明胶、葡萄糖酐、羟乙基淀粉、白蛋白)尚未被证明能提高生存率[43]。凝血病或血小板减少症应立即通过输注血液制品纠正。输注血细胞的决定取决于血细胞比容、血流动力学稳定性、出血持续性、估计失血量和并发症(如冠状动脉疾病和脑血管疾病)。首选血型和交叉配型红细胞,但非交叉配型特异性血或 O 型血可能必须用于危及生命的病例。控制出血的特殊治疗程序,如栓塞、球囊填塞或外科手术,应及时进行。

颈动脉破裂

颈动脉"爆裂"大多发生在头颈部肿瘤患者身上。颈动脉爆裂综合征可能是由肿瘤直接侵入或侵蚀颈动脉引起的,也可能是由于癌症治疗的复杂性引起的,例如术后伤口感染、放疗后坏死或口皮肤瘘。它通常发生在突然而大量的动脉喷射。偶尔,不祥的小出血和短暂出血(哨兵出血)预示着大规模井喷。在某些情况下,通过食管或气管瘘出血可能表现为大量吐血或咯血。如果不及时治疗,患者的病情会迅速恶化为低血压、低血容量性休克、意识丧失和死亡。

止血是最重要的。由于颈动脉可直接人工压迫,颈动脉破裂处应连续用力压迫,直至患者到达手术室接受手术治疗。对重要脏器的主要灌注,应进行静脉补液复苏及时输血和使用血管升压药。颈动脉破裂的手术选择是有限的,手术结扎出血的颈动脉可导致高发病率(25%的患者有神经科疾病)和高死亡率(40%)[44],血管阻断(栓塞或球囊闭塞)或支架置入(覆膜支架)已成为主要的治疗方法[45,46]。

脾脏破裂

脾脏脆弱,容易因外伤而破裂。癌症患者,自发性脾破裂相对少见,与急性白血病、非霍奇金淋巴瘤、慢性髓细胞性白血病、毛细胞白血病和霍奇金淋巴瘤有关。胃癌、前列腺癌、肺癌等实体瘤的脾转移也可导致破裂,自发性脾破裂的机制尚不清楚。脾脏小脓肿在某些情况下可能有作用。其他因素包括脾肿大、脾包膜木质细胞浸润、脾破裂、血小板减少、凝血作用、抗凝治疗和弥散性血管内凝血。脾脏破裂的典型临床表现包括左肩或腹部疼痛(左上象限)、心动过速和低血压。症状和体征的严重程度可能取决于出血的程度。诊断性腹腔灌洗广泛应用于非创伤性病例,因此,对脾破裂的确诊依赖于影像学研究。CT 增强扫描是首选的诊断方法;对血流动力学不稳定的脾破裂患者可在床边进行超声检查[47]。

对于脾脏破裂和血液系统恶性肿瘤的患者,由于未经手术的死亡率极高,必须立即进行脾切除术。在选择的有手术禁忌证的患者中,破裂部位的选择性动脉栓塞可以止血[48]。其他支持性治疗包括静脉输液、补充氧气、止痛药、输血、血小板减少症和凝血病的纠正。

腹膜后出血

致腹膜或组织结构损伤致急性腹腔出血。恶性肿瘤很少引起海绵状新生腹膜后出血;在这种情况下,罪魁祸首通常是肾细胞癌或肾上腺肿瘤(原发性)。抗凝、血小板减少和凝血因子。腹膜后或腹腔内的侵入性过程和经股动脉放置中心静脉导管也可导致严重的腹膜后出血。

腹膜后出血可引起非特异性征象和症状,这些征象和症状随出血率和继发疾病的不同而不同。患者可能会出现腹痛、腹部肿块、心动过速和低血压。如果血液以某种方式进入输尿管或胃肠道,有些人可能有血尿或便血。根据临床表现很难确定腹膜后出血的诊断,保持高度的临床怀疑和早期影像学检查是成功治疗腹膜后出血的关键。腹部和骨盆的 CT 是诊断腹膜后出血最常用的非侵入性研究(图 140-3)。床旁超声也可快速诊断腹膜后出血。

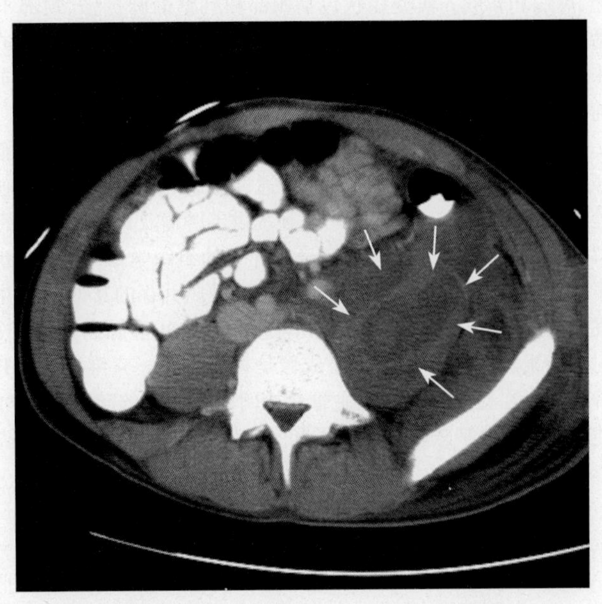

图 140-3　腹膜后出血。腹部和骨盆的 CT 扫描显示一个血小板减少性白血病患者的腹膜后巨大的不均匀集合(白色箭头)与血液系统相一致,左侧腰大肌向右侧移位肠管

腹膜后出血的处理取决于出血的严重性和根本原因。急性出血经初步稳定治疗后,应密切观察患者血流动力学的稳定性和失血的持续性。在危及生命的情况下,大多数患者需要紧急开腹切除出血的肿瘤或器官[49]。肾细胞癌常为高血管性,选择性动脉栓塞可控制肾损害的出血。对于血细胞比容相对稳定的血流动力学稳定的患者,外照射治疗出血性肿瘤是另一种选择[50]。

上腔静脉综合征

上腔静脉综合征(SVC)是指一组信号和症状,这些信号和症状是由于部分或完全阻断了通过 SVC 到右心房的血流而引起的。阻塞可能是由血管压迫、侵袭、血栓形成或纤维化引起的。肺癌是 SVC 综合征的主要病因;非霍奇金淋巴瘤是第二常见病因[51,52]。尽管霍奇金淋巴瘤通常累及纵隔,但很少引起 SVC 综合征。原发性纵隔恶性肿瘤如胸腺瘤和生殖细胞瘤占 SVC 综合征的 2%以下。乳腺癌是引起 SVC 综合征最常见的转移性疾病[53];其他转移性肿瘤包括胃肠腺癌、前列腺癌、肉瘤和黑色素瘤。SVC 综合征的非恶性原因包括胸骨后甲状腺肿、化脓性感染、结节病、畸胎瘤、胸膜钙化、硅沉着病、放射性后纤维化、化疗引起的纤维化、缩窄性心包炎[52]。癌症患者 SVC 综合征增加的原因是中心静脉导管引起血栓。

上腔静脉阻塞导致上腔静脉压升高。侧支静脉循环经常流经奇静脉系统。在奇静脉下方或入口处的阻塞迫使血液沿着髂骨和胸壁静脉的相反方向流动,到达下腔静脉。肿瘤引起的上腔静脉阻塞常在数周内发生,但血栓形成可导致阻塞的迅速发生。上腔静脉阻塞是一种真正的紧急情况,因为上腔静脉内压力的迅速升高会导致颅内压升高,导致脑水肿、颅内血栓形成或出血,以及死亡。

SVC 综合征的常见症状是头部有饱胀感和压迫感、咳嗽、呼吸困难、胸痛和咽痛。更显著的症状包括视觉障碍、沙哑、昏迷、癫痫和晕厥。典型症状包括颈部和胸壁静脉扩张、颈部不适性水肿、面部水肿、面部过胸、舌水肿、突眼、视网膜血管扩张、擦伤和上肢水肿。通过降低上身相对于心脏的位置(即向前弯腰、弯腰或躺下),症状和体征会加重。

CT,特别是增强螺旋 CT 是最有用的诊断方法。它不仅能显示梗阻部位和侧支循环,而且能通过肿瘤的外源性压迫和血栓形成来区分 SVC 综合征。CT 还提供了肿瘤及其周围结构的解剖学细节,如果之前还没有确定肿瘤的组织学诊断,则有助于指导活检程序。CT 还可检出与 SVC 梗阻并存的其他气道并发症,如气道近端阻塞和心包积液。如果禁止静脉碘造影,放射性核素静脉造影和磁共振成像是替代方法。三维增强 MR 静脉造影在检测和判断胸血管血栓闭塞性疾病的范围方面可能优于 CT、数字减影血管造影和多普勒超声[54]。对比血管造影对 SVC 综合征的诊断很少有指征。

SVC 综合征的算法是可获得的(http://www.factsoncancer-treatment.org.uk/index.php?option=com_alresource &keyword=S &catid=1& Itemid=107)。确定组织学癌症诊断的方法可能取决于工作诊断、肿瘤的位置、患者的身体状况、共病情况以及卫生保健机构的现有专业知识。CT 引导下穿刺活检可替代开胸或纵隔镜手术活检[55]。支气管镜检查可为多达 50% 的 SVC 综合征患者提供癌症诊断。如果淋巴结可触及,切除活检可确定诊断,发病率最低。如果怀疑淋巴瘤,切除活检是首选方法,因为淋巴结的组织学分类是以淋巴结结构为基础的。

在罕见的气道阻塞或颅内压升高的紧急情况下,应立即进行血管内介入治疗[56],包括血管成形术、SVC 支架置入术和药物代谢。支架置入术能迅速缓解大多数患者的症状,提高生活质量。这些支架通常在患者的余生中保持专利[57]。一些作者建议将支架作为 SVC 综合征的一线治疗[57,58]。支架可以缓解严重的症状,同时进行恶性肿瘤的组织学诊断,或者当放疗或化疗失败或无效时。

补充氧气、上半身抬高卧床休息和镇静可能有助于缓解静脉压和心排出量。利尿剂的使用可能会暂时减轻水肿,但利尿剂的疗效尚未得到证实,过量的尿会导致脱水,应避免脱水,以降低血栓形成的风险。糖皮质激素(如地塞米松)可用于气道损害或颅内压升高。尽管有高达 50% 的 SVC 综合征存在叠加血栓形成,抗凝治疗仍存在争议。抗凝和溶栓可能有助于将导管诱发的血栓或血栓转移到头臂或子臂系统。然而,抗凝增加了颅内出血的风险,尤其是颅内压升高时,抗凝可能会使活检程序复杂化或延迟;因此,除非明确的指征,否则抗凝应该无效。

放射治疗仍然是许多恶性 SVC 综合征患者的主要治疗方法,尤其是在化疗后复发的疾病或非小细胞肺癌等化疗不敏感肿瘤中[59]。一般来说,放射治疗耐受性良好,SVC 综合征症状在 1 周左右开始好转。如果组织学诊断不能及时确定,放射治疗也有正当理由。化疗是化疗敏感肿瘤如小细胞肺癌和淋巴瘤所致 SVC 综合征的首选初始治疗方法,大多数小细胞肺癌患者在几周内症状和体征部分或完全消失。尽管 SVC 障碍在约 25% 的病例中复发,但挽救性化疗和/或放射治疗可使症状得到缓解。大细胞淋巴瘤和纵隔大肿块患者化疗后局部强化放疗可能是有益的。SVC 造成的癌侵不再被认为是不可切除的[60]。对于某些肿瘤类型或选择的患者,可采用外科手术治疗并重建[61]。

呼吸系统肿瘤学急症

大咯血

咯血发作约 5% 被认为是大咯血。大咯血的定义是:咯血量 1 次超过 100ml 血液、24h 内超过 600ml 血液[62]。气道出血导致危及生命的呼吸道阻塞、低血压或贫血也被认为是大咯血。大咯血的死亡率约为 30%,根据咯血量和出血量的不同,死亡率为 5%~71%[63~67]。增加死亡风险的相关其他因素包括较低的基础肺储备,肺内残余较多血[64]。支气管及肺泡出血的死亡原因通常是窒息而不是出血。

癌症患者的大咯血的主要原因是恶性肿瘤、感染和凝血异常。支气管肺癌和其他恶性肿瘤的肺转移可能会引起大咯血。肺癌是 40 岁以上癌症患者的大咯血的最常见原因。约有 3% 的肺癌患者有致命性咯血[68]。坏死的肺鳞状细胞癌可能比其他亚型的肺癌患者更常见致命性咯血。导致咯血的肺转移瘤的原发癌中最常见的是黑色素瘤、乳腺癌、肾癌、喉癌和结肠癌。其他肿瘤,如食管肿瘤,可能引起直接延伸到气管、支气管树的大咯血[64]。那些恶性血液病患者和曾接受骨髓移植、中性粒细胞减少或免疫功能低下者出现大咯血会增加坏死性血管侵入性真菌感染(曲霉病,白真菌病)的风险。血液系统异常如恶性肿瘤或其治疗导致的严重的血小板减少和凝血止血异常可能会导致严重的肺出血。

除了大咯血,患者的症状可能包括低血压、心动过速、中央性发绀、皮肤湿冷、呼吸困难或胸痛。血流动力学不稳定的患者可能需要容量复苏。美国胸科医师协会(American College of Chest Physicians)的指导方针建议使用单腔管进行气管内插管和紧急支气管镜检查来确定出血部位,以便进行支气管内干预,如激光或等离子凝血和电烧术[69]。大咯血的支气管镜治疗包括外用药物(凝血酶,纤维蛋白原凝血酶)、冰盐水灌洗、支气管填塞、激光和电灼。气球导管可用于支气管内填塞,以减轻出血。硬质气管镜可改善气道,提供更大的吸力,而且在清除大血块方面比光纤镜有效。光纤镜的优点是提高了远端气道的可视范围。其他气道管理选择包括经支气管镜单侧插管或双腔气管内管隔离未受影响的肺。右肺大出血的患者,可进行左侧主支气管的气管插管。因为会增加右上肺叶阻塞的危险所以左肺大出血的患者不建议行右侧气管插管。在这种情况下,可选用双腔气管导管隔离健侧肺。对于单侧肺出血的患者,偏向患侧侧卧的体位会减少出血对健侧呼吸的影响。必须纠正潜在的口腔癌,抑制咳嗽可能会有帮助。

Noe 等人提出了一种处理大咯血的算法，其中 CT 血管造影发挥了重要作用[70]。支气管动脉栓塞正成为辅助或复发性咯血的一线治疗方法。除了支气管镜和胸透，CT 血管造影还提供了关于肿瘤、出血部位、支气管和支气管外动脉的解剖学信息，为血管内介入治疗提供参考。支气管动脉栓塞是安全有效的。出血血管栓塞可能使用聚乙烯醇酒精沫、Gianturco 钢卷、异丁基-2-氰基丙烯酸酯或可吸收明胶脱脂棉。其中栓塞失败患者可以从放射治疗中获益，因为放射治疗可引起血管血栓形成和促进血管坏死从而抑制出血。一般通过手术治疗其他治疗方法无效的顽固性咯血患者和危及生命的心血管病患者[71]。

大量胸腔积液

大量胸腔积液被描绘为几乎完全混浊的胸水。胸膜腔大量渗出的状况约 10%为渗出液。约 2/3 的患者考虑有癌症[72]（图 140-4）。大多数（约 80%）的恶性胸腔积液是源自肺癌（36%）、乳腺癌（25%）、淋巴瘤（10%）和卵巢癌（5%）[73]。79%肺腺癌会转移至胸膜[74]。在青壮年中，恶性淋巴瘤是最常见的导致胸腔积液的原因[75]。恶性胸腔积液可能会呈现出浆液性、血清性或血性。除了肺炎，导致渗出性胸腔积液的原因中恶性肿瘤占第二位，恶性肿瘤造成了 8%～20%的渗出性胸腔积液[76]。恶性肿瘤的相关状况也可能会导致积液，这些状况包括肿瘤的局部作用（肺门和纵隔淋巴结肿大造成的胸膜腔淋巴引流障碍）、肿瘤的全身作用、低蛋白血症和癌症治疗的并发症［放疗和化疗（如甲氨蝶呤、丙卡巴肼、环磷酰胺、丝裂霉素、博来霉素、IL-1）］，肺炎（如阻塞性肺炎）和充血性心力衰竭。

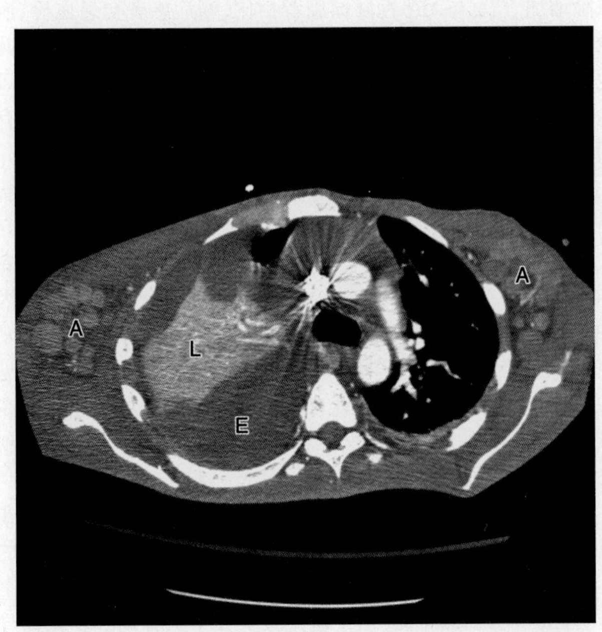

图 140-4　大量胸腔积液。患者的胸部 CT 扫描显示大量胸腔积液。L，肺崩溃；E，胸腔积液；A，广泛的腋窝淋巴结肿大

对于某些患者，胸腔积液可能是恶性肿瘤的首发症状。常见的症状有咳嗽、呼吸困难和端坐呼吸。这些症状的严重程度取决于胸腔积液的容量和液体的积聚速度。症状偶见发热，原因可能是感染或肺不张或肺炎。出现胸痛和胸膜摩擦音的症状并不常见，如果这两种症状出现通常表明肿瘤侵犯胸膜、肋骨和胸壁。

胸腔积液的诊断可通过临床查体与 X 线检查明确。查体发现，积液区叩诊为浊音，听诊呼吸音减低，膈肌移动度下降，患侧触诊语音震颤减弱。有时叩诊浊音区的上方可闻及语音震颤。患者大量积液（大于 1 500ml）可能有呼吸运动受限，气管移向健侧和肋间隙增宽。当胸腔积液是由肺癌引起的，一般积液为癌变的同侧[72]。胸腔积液的原因一般通过胸腔穿刺诊断。胸腔穿刺很容易操作，并且比较安全。对于有症状的患者，胸腔穿刺引流部分胸水可缓解症状。胸腔积液经分析可区分出积液为渗出液还是漏出液，对查明积液的原因可能很有帮助[76]。细胞学检查比经皮胸膜穿刺活检更敏感[74,77]。如果这两个微创手段未能明确诊断，其他诊断方法还包括支气管镜、胸膜镜、视频辅助胸腔镜手和开胸活检。

症状的严重程度、积液聚集的速度、整体预后、患者的一般状况以及对肿瘤治疗的反应综合决定了治疗方案。患者如有大量胸腔积液和血流动力学不稳定的状况，表现为呼吸困难、低氧血症或纵隔移位应立即行胸腔穿刺治疗。胸膜固定术可以防止再次出现积液。在近 70%未行胸膜固定术的症状性恶性胸腔积液引流的患者，除非行有效的全身化疗，否则 30 日内会再次出现胸腔积液。如果癌症患者的肺被脏胸膜包膜所困，经胸腔穿刺后没有任何症状改善，则不建议放置留置胸膜导管[78]。否则，留置胸膜导管将允许门诊患者定期引流胸膜液以改善症状[79,80]，尤其是呼吸困难，并提高生存质量[81]。随着时间的推移，一些患者也可能出现胸膜粘连。对于预期寿命超过一个月或胸腔镜术后出现症状的病，应考虑行化学胸膜固定术。有效硬化剂可达 72%～90%的成功率，包括多西环素、米诺环素、博来霉素和滑石粉[82,83]。根据临床和影像学检查结果和积液的生化特性来判断胸腔状况。胸腔积脓或由细菌培养或显微镜证实（如革兰氏染色）感染性胸腔积液和复杂肺旁积液患者建议行胸腔闭式引流[84]。

急性呼吸道梗阻

急性呼吸道阻塞，通常是指上呼吸道。上呼吸道阻塞，可能是由于恶性或者非恶性原因。头颈部（舌、喉、咽、甲状腺癌或气管）的原发肿瘤和纵隔肿瘤（肺癌，胸腺瘤）的直接蔓延可造成上呼吸道阻塞。乳腺癌、食管癌、肾癌、结肠癌、黑色素瘤、肉瘤和纵隔淋巴瘤的转移播散也会发生上呼吸道阻塞。肿瘤侵犯及与肿瘤相关的呼吸道水肿或出血也可能导致气道阻塞。肿瘤患者的气道阻塞的非肿瘤性原因包括食物或异物吸入、气道水肿、严重的气管软化、气管狭窄，及罕见的感染因素——真菌、病毒或细菌。严重的急性上呼吸道阻塞可引起血管性水肿（药源性：例如，血管紧张素转化酶抑制药，紫杉醇）。下呼吸道梗阻最常见的原因是原发性支气管癌。另外，下呼吸道阻塞的罕见的原因是结肠癌、乳腺癌、甲状腺癌、肾癌、黑色素瘤、淋巴瘤、肉瘤的转移。原发于胃肠道的类癌因释放激素介质可使患者患有严重呼吸道阻塞（支气管痉挛）。

呼吸困难可能是气道阻塞的唯一早期症状。当患者劳累时发生呼吸困难，气道直径通常减少到 8mm，而当患者休息时发生呼吸困难，气道直径通常下降到 5mm，而且这种直径的减

少通常与喘鸣的发展相吻合。当上呼吸道进行性阻塞时,还可能出现喘憋、端坐呼吸、心动过速、大汗、喘鸣和肋间肌收缩。喘鸣是一个不好的预兆,后面可能紧接着会是心动过缓、发绀、衰竭和死亡。

应该迅速检查口腔以排除异物。在大多数上呼吸道阻塞的情况下,临床查体可明确诊断。当检查气管内时可能需要喉镜或支气管镜。对于上呼吸道阻塞的患者,除了临床查体,往往还需根据病变部位决定进行直接的可视化喉镜或者支气管镜。对于较低的气道阻塞的患者,75%的阻塞病例可经胸部X线片明确。颈部或胸部CT在诊断肿瘤引起的梗阻时很有帮助。在一个明显狭窄的气道里由急性感染引起的水肿,应该被纳入鉴别诊断。

气道阻塞的处理是逆转或绕过阻塞部位。除了补充氧气外,支持性治疗可能包括其他辅助治疗包括糖皮质激素、支气管扩张剂和氦氧混合剂和抗生素(如果怀疑感染)。喉镜或支气管镜检查对于指导上呼吸道阻塞气管插管可能是必要的[85]。气管上1/3时可能需要下段气管切开术。当综合考虑疾病的进展、对肿瘤治疗的反应、患者的一般状况和其他并发症等因素后可以考虑外科手术干预。对于中央气道阻塞,介入治疗肺部可能使用硬性或软性气管镜[86],可能包括球性支气管成形术、支气管支架、激光支气管镜、支气管内氩离子凝固术、冷冻手术和近距离治疗。其他治疗选择包括引导射频消融术,外束放射治疗,外科去体积或切除术。

气胸

癌症患者的大部分气胸是医源性的或作为其他医疗条件的后果而自发形成的。大多数在医院接受治疗的气胸是医源性的[87]。导致气胸的操作包括经皮肺穿刺活检、支气管活检、中心静脉插入和肺动脉导管置入。即使放置鼻胃管也可能会偶尔引起气胸。继发性的自发性气胸最常见的原因是慢性阻塞性肺疾病。原发的和转移性肺肿瘤可能会导致气胸。化疗药物相关性气胸包括博来霉素、卡莫司汀和洛莫司汀。气胸相关传染病的药物包括金黄色葡萄球菌、肺炎克雷伯菌和假单胞菌属、卡氏肺囊虫和牛分枝杆菌的物种。足菌肿破裂进入胸膜腔可能导致气胸,并与烟曲霉感染、球孢子菌病、隐球菌和毛霉菌感染有关。

患者的临床表现和症状的严重程度与患者的基础肺部状况有关。患者的临床表现可能会有呼吸困难、呼吸急促、心动过速、发绀、大汗和情绪激动。有潜在肺疾病患者往往无法忍受肺活量减低或动脉氧分压降低,出现继发性气胸以致呼吸衰竭的风险较高。患者的临床表现和症状的严重程度与患者的基础肺部状况有关。患者的临床表现可能会有呼吸困难、呼吸急促、心动过速、发绀、大汗和情绪激动。有潜在肺疾病患者往往无法忍受肺活量减低或动脉氧分压降低,出现继发性气胸以致呼吸衰竭的风险较高。

小量气胸往往在查体时无法发现,查体通常会有心动过速、触觉震颤消失、叩诊鼓音、听诊患侧呼吸音减弱或消失。大量或张力气胸患者可能有对侧气管偏移,患者呼吸动度减弱。张力性气胸患者可能有中心静脉压升高,肺动脉和右心房压力升高。当中心静脉压升高、胸腔内压力阻碍静脉回流时会出现低血压、严重低氧血症、呼吸性酸中毒。

气胸的诊断依据是正位胸片显示肺纹理消失超出脏层胸膜。对于一个小量气胸的患者,胸膜线可能难以辨别。因此,诊断小量气胸时需要良好品质的X线和明亮的观赏光线。以往的工作表明,其中1/3的气胸因为照相时半直立和仰卧位所以未被发现[88]。在某些情况下,呼气相拍片可能会有帮助。胸膜超声检查诊断气胸可能比胸片检查更准确[89]。

小量气胸及轻微症状的患者可能需要密切观察和吸氧。在取得初始X线片后3~6h后应再行胸部X线片检查。如果没有张力性气胸,患者可密切观察,于12~48h后复查X线片并出院[90]。对于有症状的气胸,迅速扩大的气胸和超过同侧胸膜腔15%肺容量的气胸,应该做胸导管。胸部活检后出现医源性气胸需要置入胸导管的可在门诊安全地置入细导管和海姆利希阀门,成功率可达78%[91]。成功置入导管后复张失败或复发的气胸患者需要做胸腔闭式引流术。经常使用的是海姆利希阀。胸腔闭式引流术最初用于创伤性气胸和血胸的患者、气胸占据超过15%患侧肺容量的并有分泌物的患者、患侧肺部感染和机械通气患者。在患者行胸腔闭式引流术后由于支气管胸膜瘘导致持续漏气的患者和只有部分肺部扩张5~7日后,应考虑行开胸手术修补。胸膜固定术中用滑石粉或其他药物,可以预防再次发生[92]。

肺栓塞

肺栓塞的诊断是很困难的,因为癌症患者的症状和体征可能被肿瘤治疗过程或并发症所掩盖。总体来讲,深静脉血栓形成的高危人群是受到严重创伤的患者、接受整形外科手术的患者、接受过腹部手术的患者。患者高龄、近期得过心肌梗死、有过脑血管意外、制动、恶性肿瘤、肥胖或有血栓史则患肺栓塞的风险增加[93]。与无恶性肿瘤患者相比,癌症患者初患血栓、血栓复发、致命的肺栓塞的比率较高。患恶性肿瘤、但不伴有其他潜在并发症的患者有15%~20%发生血栓栓塞性疾病的风险。接受外科手术后,相较于非癌症患者而言,癌症患者会有两到三倍的术后静脉血栓形成的风险[94]。

在大多数情况下,肺栓塞的症状并不典型。最常见的症状是呼吸困难。有关肺动脉栓塞的诊断研究的前瞻性调查研究中的血管造影记录了97%的患者会有呼吸困难,胸膜炎性胸痛和呼吸急促[95,96]。大规模肺栓塞的患者可能有晕厥。患者因右心室缺血可能会出现心绞痛。咯血可能很少出现,如若发生,会与血栓栓塞事件12~36h后发生的肺梗死有关。最常见的,肺栓塞患者呼吸急促及心动过速。下肢深静脉血栓形成在只有不到一半的肺动脉栓塞患者中发生。有时候,可能会查到发烧和胸膜摩擦音。

疑似肺栓塞的患者应该测量血氧饱和度,并且可能需要在吸氧之前行动脉血气分析。胸部X线片对于排除肺部症状的其他原因最有帮助,并能根据Hampton hump(圆顶形胸膜肺不透明)或Westermark征(由于血流减少或中央肺动脉扩张而导致的外周放射通畅)提示肺动脉栓塞。

常见的心电图显示窦性心动过速,T波倒置,或者非特异性ST-T波异常。电轴右偏,房性心律失常,右束支传导阻滞及P-心病可能发生,但典型的S1-Q3-T3波形并不常见。在癌症患者中,对于肺栓塞来讲,D-二聚体有很高的阴性预测值和灵敏度,正常的D-二聚体数值可以排除肺栓塞[97]。在另一项包括癌症患者的研究中,一个中心肺栓塞的 D-二聚体浓度>3 000ng/ml 会在 15 日内死亡[98]。

高分辨率 CT 肺血管造影或螺旋 CT 是首选诊断手段(图 140-5);在碘造影剂过敏的情况下,磁共振血管造影是一种选择。对于肺动脉栓塞的诊断,CT 和 MR 血管造影的敏感性和特异性分别约为 80%和 90%[99,100]。CT 血管造影阴性预测值为 98%[101]。当因肾功能不全或超敏反应而禁止 CT 或 MR 血管造影时,放射性核素呼吸灌注(V/Q)扫描为次选。CT 或 MR 血管造影不能可靠地检测到远端肺血管中的血管栓子,高度怀疑有肺栓塞的患者但两种成像方式结果都为阴性时应考虑用肺血管造影,这是诊断的金标准。

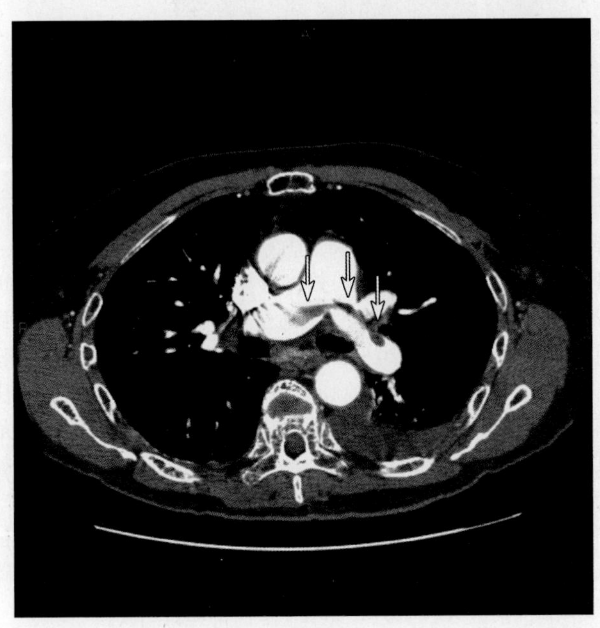

图 140-5　鞍栓子。CT 扫描显示,这在进入肺动脉分支鞍栓子(三个箭头下所指)

血流动力学不稳定的患者应使之稳定。使之稳定的干预措施可能包括输液和使用正性肌力药,通常由重症监护设置中心静脉监测。当巨大的肺栓塞发生时需要面罩吸氧或气管插管。溶栓治疗通常用于有大面积肺栓子及血流动力学不稳定的患者。溶栓质量的适应证是血栓超过 40%的肺血管阻塞、根据超声心动图判定的右心室功能不全和严重的低氧血症。在引起急性右心室功能障碍的肺栓塞中,尽管大出血和颅内出血增加,但溶栓治疗与全因死亡率降低相关[102]。溶栓需要特别注意与出血风险相关的禁忌证(特别是在存在脑转移的情况下)。由于大量出血和颅内出血的风险增加,但不能降低死亡率,因此不应将溶栓用于大多数正常血压的肺栓塞患者[103]。溶栓疗法已被证明可加速纤溶和血块溶解,能改善早期和晚期的心肺功能,但尚无大规模研究证实其能明确降低死亡率[104]。外科治疗和导管取栓术通常用于常规去除血栓方法失败的患者。

对于癌症患者的静脉血栓栓塞的处理,已有发表的指南[105,106]。低分子肝素(LMWH)被推荐用于新诊断为肺栓塞的癌症患者的抗凝 5~10 日,血肌酐清除率为>30ml/min。未分离的肝素(静脉注射 80 单位/公斤,然后持续输注 18 单位/公斤/小时)可以替代低分子肝素。低分子肝素的优点是不需要部分凝血活酶时间监测和静脉介入。单纯肝素的半衰期较短,可能需要介入治疗。静脉使用未分离的肝素,一次注射 5 000~10 000 单位,然后持续输注 1 000~1 500 单位/小时,并进行调整,以使激活的部分凝血活酶时间保持在控制值的 1.5~2.0 倍[107]。对于长期(≥6 个月)抗凝,低分子肝素优于维生素 K 拮抗剂(如华法林),因为它与其他药物和化疗相互作用的可能性较小,不需要监测,与静脉血栓栓塞的复发较少相关,而且可能延长癌症患者的生存期[108]。当低分子肝素不能长期治疗时,用维生素 K 拮抗剂按国际标准比例 2~3 进行治疗是可接受的替代方案。对于原发恶性肿瘤的患者,可考虑将抗凝时间延长至 6 个月以上,直至肿瘤治疗结束,恶性肿瘤消退[109]。目前正在研究一些新的抗凝血剂在癌症患者中的应用[110]。目前不推荐使用它们来预防或治疗癌症患者的肺栓塞。

抗凝禁忌在活跃的存在颅内出血,近期手术,血小板减少症(血小板<50 000/μl),或凝血功能障碍所引起。下腔静脉滤器可用于抗凝治疗、肺栓塞复发或已有血栓在低分子肝素最佳治疗下恶化,但终末期癌症患者获益甚微[111]。应定期复查抗凝的禁忌证,以便在安全时恢复抗凝。过滤器不推荐用于癌症患者的初级预防。

对于原发性脑恶性肿瘤患者,与其他癌症患者一样,推荐抗凝治疗。许多有肺栓塞的癌症患者可以作为门诊患者安全治疗,特别是偶然发生肺栓塞的病例,临床上未被怀疑,并在 CT 扫描中被发现用于治疗反应评估或分期[112]。由于偶发病例的复发率,发病率和死亡率可与有症状的病例相提并论,因此,对于有症状的肺栓塞,应采用初始和长期抗凝治疗方法对偶发的肺栓塞进行相同的治疗,但被判定为极可能的影像学表现的外周节段性栓塞除外[106,110,113]。

神经肿瘤学急诊情况

脊髓压迫

癌症患者中脊髓压迫发生率是 3%~5%,视为肿瘤急诊。延误治疗可能会导致不可逆转的后果,甚至截瘫[114]。脊髓压迫有 95%是由骨膜转移侵及脊髓造成。其中,70%侵及胸椎,20%侵及腰骶部脊椎,10%侵及颈椎。胸椎转移症状较轻。但应引起重视的是,胸椎区域血供脆弱,椎管狭窄。脊髓压迫常见于肺癌、乳腺癌、原发灶不明癌、前列腺癌和肾细胞癌。

背痛是脊髓压迫患者最典型的症状。通常在出现神经受损症状之前的数周到数月就可以出现疼痛。患者疼痛可局限在脊椎或由于神经受压出现根性疼痛。运动、咳嗽、打喷嚏可使疼痛加重。随着病情进展可出现瘫痪、感觉丧失。自主神经功能紊乱,可出现尿潴留和排便困难,并可很快出现不可逆性截瘫。截瘫和尿潴留提示病情预后差。可由疼痛和触痛部位判断受侵脊椎节段。临床查体还可发现肌力下降,异常肌肉伸展反射和伸跖反射,在所涉及的神经根分布区域感觉丧失。下肢共济失调可出现在肌力下降和疼痛之前。受侵脊椎节段以下出现感觉丧失。自主神经功能紊乱患者可出现尿潴留,排尿后残余尿尿量增加,听诊肠鸣音减弱。

准确的病史和查体对诊断脊髓压迫十分重要，神经系统功能检查可初步判断可疑病灶，以供影像学参考[115,116]。通常脊髓压迫患者脊椎的X线检查会发现异常。可表现为骨侵蚀、蒂损失，部分或全部椎体塌陷和脊椎旁软组织肿块。然而，即使脊椎片正常也不能排除转移。脊椎的MRI成像是诊断脊髓压迫的最佳方法（图140-6）。钆增强可用于怀疑硬膜外脓肿导致的脊髓压迫。钆使炎症组织强化，并确定解剖边界。需要一个有经验的医生进行脊髓造影。行CT脊髓造影可使患者的不适感最小。然而，当转移病灶完全压迫脊髓时，脊髓造影无法确定肿瘤上缘。

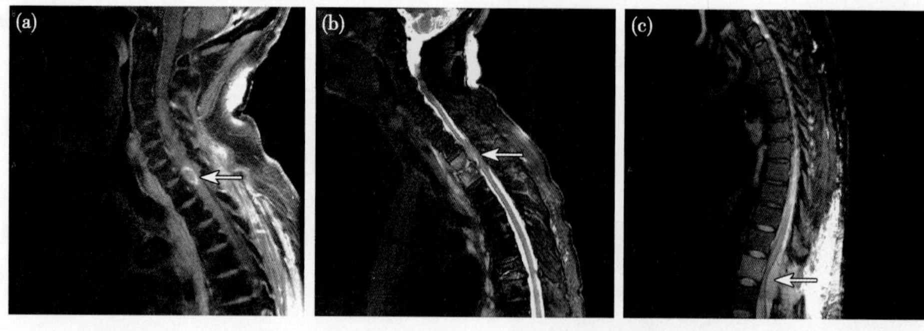

图140-6　脊髓受压。脊柱矢状面MRI图像从三个不同的患者表现出一种低位颈椎髓内病变（箭头）(a)，转移瘤所致胸椎压缩性骨折（箭头）(b)，硬膜外肿瘤所致腰椎压缩性骨折（箭头）(c)

治疗脊髓压迫的目的是维持正常的神经功能，改善神经功能，同时控制局部肿瘤，稳定脊椎及控制疼痛。骨转移会造成严重疼痛，应及时果断的给予镇痛药，尤其阿片类药物。如果疼痛控制不满意，应延迟体格检查和影像检查。对于可疑脊髓压迫患者，应给予糖皮质激素治疗。通常使用地塞米松，因其胃肠道吸收良好，半衰期较长，有36h。对于在高剂量（100mg）的静脉注射后是否有必要再给予维持剂量（通常为16mg/6h）还存在争议[117]。其他的研究表明，低剂量（4～10mg/6h）同样有效，而且副作用较少[116,118]。对于有脊髓压迫且放疗敏感的恶性肿瘤患者，单纯放疗是标准的首选治疗。患者现存的神经功能状态比恶性肿瘤的放疗敏感性对放射治疗的结果有更加直接的关系。手术也是一个治疗选择，尤其是对需要稳定脊椎、曾经放疗过的部位出现脊髓压迫、需要病理诊断及使用类固醇药物和放疗后病情仍进展的患者是恰当的选择。手术是否恰当也应考虑到患者的恶性肿瘤情况，不适合生存期有限的晚期恶性肿瘤患者。一项荟萃分析表明，手术切除后放疗可能比单纯放疗更好地改善行走能力和生存[119]。对于化疗敏感的恶性肿瘤患者可选择化疗。也可以联合治疗。患者手术风险增加或脊髓压迫区域曾经接受过放疗时，可选择化疗。

脑疝

应对可疑脑疝的患者迅速进行评估，血流动力学不稳定者，应予以紧急治疗[120]。以下症状和查体提示脑疝：意识变化，视乳头水肿，瞳孔和眼球运动异常，姿势异常，恶心，呕吐和假性脑膜炎水平。脑疝晚期的临床表现是高血压，心动过缓和库欣反射。如果提示有颅内压增高，需要进行影像学检查。首先行CT检查以排除脑出血。MRI是更好的检查脑疝的成像技术，但如果患者病情不稳定，因CT可以快速完成，此时是更安全的选择。

如果颅内压增高，病情不稳定，要在影像学确诊之前立即进行降颅压治疗。予以过度通气、甘露醇和类固醇预防或治疗脑疝。过度换气是降低颅内压最迅速的方法。必要时给予镇静、插管通气，使PCO_2达到25～30mmHg。这样可使血管收缩，降低脑血流量，使颅内压下降，但效果维持短暂。甘露醇，是一种高渗剂，数分钟内起效，药效可维持几个小时。在血脑之间形成渗透压梯度，使水分从大脑通过血脑屏障进入血液。但此机制是有争议的。在20～30min内静脉给予20%～25%甘露醇0.5～2.0g/kg。如果患者的临床状况继续恶化，需要加量。甘露醇可引起颅内压反弹，应谨慎使用。可使用类固醇药物，尤其对于血管性水肿[121]。地塞米松是最常用的，首次注射剂量为40～100mg/d静脉注射，然后每日维持使用此剂量。

重症监护的进一步治疗包括静脉滴注高渗盐水、丙泊酚和低体温[120]。如果患者神经系统功能恶化，必要时可神经外科干预。一旦颅内压控制，应针对根本原因进行治疗。

癫痫持续状态

癫痫持续状态定义为连续发作>5min或连续发作>2次发作而未完全恢复[122]。癫痫持续状态可损伤神经系统，如神经细胞损伤和细胞死亡、神经源性肺水肿、肾衰竭、横纹肌溶解综合征。大脑肿瘤导致7%的癫痫持续状态，这些病例的短期死亡率高于无肿瘤的癫痫持续状态[123]。

引起癌症患者癫痫发作的病因可能包括脑组织损伤、代谢、感染及治疗相关因素。在癫痫急救中心，对50个癌症患者调查，发现16%的癫痫发作是由于新出现的脑组织损伤，52%是由于中枢神经系统陈旧性病变所致[124]。癫痫发作通常见于脑转移瘤或原发性脑肿瘤患者。转移到脑的最常见肿瘤有肺癌、乳腺癌、黑色素瘤、泌尿生殖系统恶性肿瘤、胃肠道恶性肿瘤。

癫痫大发作之后，神经系统功能受到抑制（意识混乱或意识丧失）癫痫发作后的临床表现包括瘀伤、舌头咬伤，二便失禁，乳酸和肌肉中相关酶升高。要确定患者是否有发作史、发作类型及使用的控制药物。还应了解恶性肿瘤情况以及治疗过程。如果不能确定癫痫发作的诱因，应进行诊断性的检查，包括检测电解质、血糖、钙、镁，肝、肾功能，血液细胞计数、血培养、血气分析，心电图以及选择抗癫痫药物。必要时行CT或MRI检查[125]。如发现可疑的沉淀物，可行腰穿检查。

癫痫持续状态需要紧急处理，应立即进行气道，呼吸和循环的评估（图 140-7）。癫痫发作的原因是低血糖，必须首先排除、诊断和治疗。静脉给予短效苯二氮䓬类药物（劳拉西泮或地西泮）抗惊厥治疗终止癫痫发作。通常使用劳拉西泮（通常为 4～8mg 静脉注射），该药起效快和作用持续时间长。癫痫发作停止后，应将昏迷患者置于恢复体位上，以防止误吸。可能需要气道吸入和补充氧气。可逆的癫痫发作的医学原因应该被纠正。这些患者可能不需要长期的抗惊厥治疗。有其他原因的癫痫患者需要长期服用抗惊厥。一些临床医生更喜欢左乙拉西坦，因为它不会被肝脏代谢，而且与抗肿瘤治疗的药物相互作用极小。还可给予其他抗癫痫药，如苯妥英钠。苯妥英钠和苯巴比妥分别是二线和三线药物。新型的静脉注射用抗惊厥药物例如左乙拉西坦等尚未确定治疗癫痫持续状态的地位。对于持续癫痫患者，除给予抗惊厥治疗外，必要时还可给予镇静，重症监护设备监测下气管插管，以及行脑电图检查。

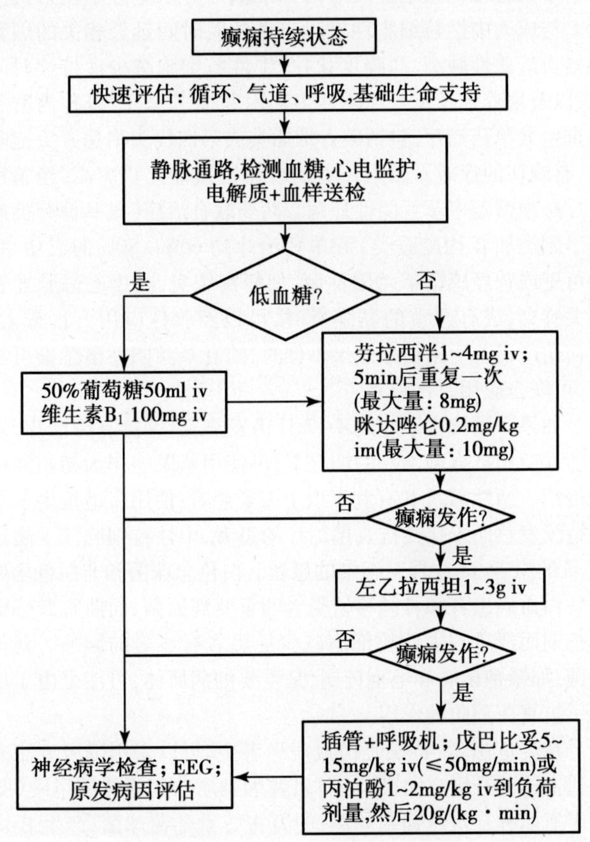

图 140-7 癫痫持续状态的处理

其他肿瘤急诊情况

肠穿孔

胃肠道穿孔也需要紧急处理。在癌症患者中，穿孔最常见的原因是继发于肿瘤（原发或转移）的自发性穿孔，和继发于内镜或癌症治疗的医源性穿孔。如果胃肠壁被肿瘤取代，那么放疗或化疗引起的肿瘤坏死可能导致肠穿孔。如抗血管生成抑制剂贝伐单抗和小分子抑制剂伊马替尼和索拉非尼与肠穿孔有关[126]。肠穿孔可由严重的感染引起，如斑疹伤寒和中性粒细胞肠炎[127]。由于放疗或化疗引起的严重肠胃炎可导致严重的肠扩张和随后的穿孔。常见的穿孔与癌症无关，包括阑尾炎、憩室炎和胃病。

通常情况下，发生胃肠道穿孔会引起急性或突发疼痛，需要紧急处理。颈段食管穿孔，会发生如下症状：颈部疼痛，吞咽困难，声音嘶哑，皮下气肿。胸段食管穿孔，会出现上腹部紧张，严重的胸骨后疼痛，吞咽疼痛和呕血。胃癌穿孔，急性剧烈腹痛通常是首发症状。疼痛可伴发恶心、呕吐，发生率约占15%，可同时发生消化道出血。由于隔膜受到刺激，腹痛可放射到肩膀。游离性穿孔可出现腹胀，腹膜炎体征（腹反跳痛、肌紧张、肠鸣音消失）。腹膜炎时，可出现腹韧和反跳痛。弥漫性腹膜炎时，腹部听诊肠鸣音减弱或消失。

腹膜炎患者可出现发热、白细胞左移、纵隔感染、脓肿。应注意最近是否应用了细胞毒性药物化疗或中性粒细胞刺激因子，影响白细胞计数。肠食管或胃穿孔时淀粉酶和脂肪酶水平可能升高。宫颈穿孔时，宫颈部侧位平片可显示宫颈深部组织中的气体。食管穿孔时胸部 X 线对于观察纵隔是有价值的。游离气体检测（位于立位或卧位的胸部 X 线或腹部 X 线片的上部）（图 140-8）可以作为急腹症肠穿孔的证据。十二指肠穿孔时，腹部 X 线片同时口服造影剂可显示腹膜后气体。其他影像学表现包括两侧肠壁和肝韧带的显现。如果临床高度怀疑肠穿孔，可口服造影剂。水溶性造影剂（如胃影葡胺）是一种钡剂，流入腹膜腔可引起严重炎症反应。CT 检查可确诊肠穿孔，并且可提供穿孔位置和周围结构的详细情况。

肠穿孔的治疗包括保守治疗，或保守治疗之后手术，或根据穿孔大小、部位而定是否急诊手术，还应考虑到穿孔的原因，穿孔是游离的或包裹的，临床进程（脓毒血症的发展情况），患者一般状况、穿孔前的生活质量，恶性肿瘤的预后以及增加围术期死亡风险的并发症情况。非手术治疗措施包括鼻胃管负压吸引，静脉用广谱抗生素，静脉营养和密切监测[128]。如果在保守治疗期间患者病情恶化，应进行手术。

中性粒细胞减少性发热

中性粒细胞是具吞噬作用的白细胞，抵御人体感染细菌和真菌。中性粒细胞减少定义为中性粒细胞计数≤1 000 个/μl，中性粒细胞缺乏定义为中性粒细胞计数≤500/μl，严重者中性粒细胞计数≤100 个/μl[129]。感染风险与中性粒细胞减少持续的时间有关。中性粒细胞减少症常发生在癌症患者身上，是密集化疗或恶性肿瘤的结果。感染是中性粒细胞减少症患者发病和死亡的主要原因。中性粒细胞减少性癌症患者的发烧［定义为单次口服＞38.3℃（101℉）或＞38.0℃（100.4℉），＞1h］通常在经验性全身广谱抗生素治疗后才会消退（约 60% 的病例）[130]。中性粒细胞缺乏症是一种真正的医学急症，及时使用抗生素可以预防败血症和死亡。

中性粒细胞缺乏患者免疫功能低下，缺乏对感染作出充分炎症反应的能力。因此，应充分检查任何感染症状或体征[131]。体格检查应包括仔细检查常见的感染部位，如口腔、咽、会阴、眼睛、血管通路、经皮导管和皮肤。初步的实验室评估应包括：血细胞计数、血清肌酐、血尿素氮、转氨酶、血培养（包括外周肺

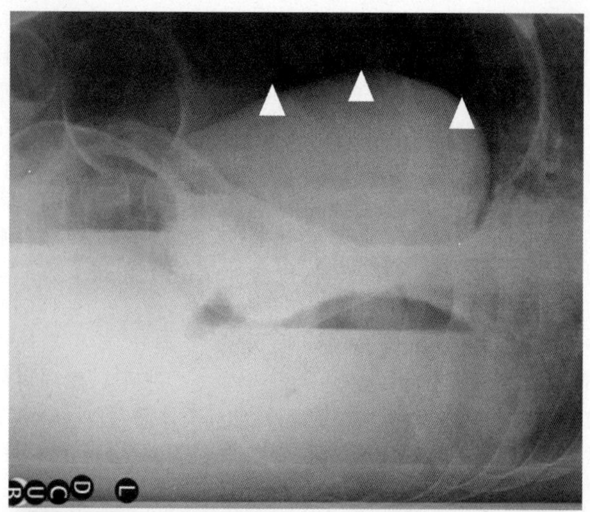

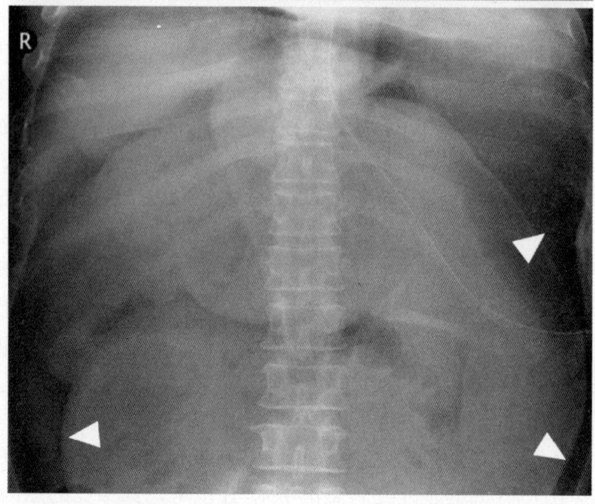

图 140-8 腹部平片。53 岁男性，多发性骨髓瘤，消化道淀粉样变性，接受沙利度胺和地塞米松的治疗，突发急性腹痛，腹胀。腹部 X 线片显示腹腔游离气体（箭头所指）。剖腹探查发现继发于大规模结肠扩张的肠穿孔

泡和血管、导尿管、尿液分析、尿培养）。对于有呼吸系统症状或体征的患者，应进行胸片检查。

应对这类患者进行全面检查。黏膜和皮肤损伤，可感染病毒（如单纯疱疹和水痘带状疱疹），细菌（如脓肿、坏疽），或真菌（如播散性念珠菌病，曲霉菌病或镰刀菌感染）。局部感染的任何部位都应进行抽吸或活检，以识别病原体，指导治疗。鼻窦症状可能是由于细菌或真菌感染，其中一些可能是侵入性的和致命的。当腹泻出现时，粪便标本应通过毒素检测或聚合酶链反应来评估梭状芽孢杆菌感染。腹痛、腹胀、便血、恶心、呕吐是中性粒细胞减少性肠炎的典型临床表现[132]。肛周症状表明可能存在肛周脓肿。在中性粒细胞减少性发热患者中，必须鉴别肺部疾病的其他情况：感染（病毒、细菌、真菌和原虫），放射性肺炎，化疗引起的副作用，肺出血，肺栓塞。中性粒细胞减少性发热患者胸部查体异常而胸部 X 线片正常，对于临床诊断是一种挑战。经典的微生物检测方法有标本染色、培养以及药敏试验，辅之以先进的分子方法检测微生物 DNA（尤其是聚合酶链反应）和体液或组织的微生物抗原检测。在 17%～25% 缺乏肺部体征的患者中，胸部 X 线可发现异常[133]，肺部 X 线浸润可预示复杂的临床过程[134]。因此，如果一个中性粒细胞减少的患者正在考虑抗生素治疗，即使没有迹象或症状也应进行 X 线检查排除肺部浸润[131]。

根据中性粒细胞缺乏症的治疗指南，80% 的临床医生会使用抗生素[135]。尽管指南和一般说明应被注意，但也应考虑到局部流行病学和临床实践[136]。中性粒细胞缺乏症发热的最初管理方法应基于风险，随后应根据临床反应进行修改。低危患者[130,137～139]（即跨国支持性 MASCC 得分≥21 或 Talcott4）与血流动力学稳定，没有疾病和低症状负担，门诊治疗口服氟喹诺酮+阿莫西林/克拉维酸（克林霉素，如果对青霉素过敏克林霉素）作为初始经验方案可能是合适的，除非氟喹诺酮已被用于预防发热出现之前[140]。患者应在分诊后 1h 内接受初始剂量的经验性抗生素治疗。接受门诊治疗的资格应通过至少 4h 的监测来确定。然而，成功的门诊管理依赖于初级护理、肿瘤科和急诊部门之间的协调，以确保在门诊治疗期间快速反应和密切跟进临床医生和患者以及他们的照顾者之间的有效沟通[141]。

中性粒细胞缺乏症发热的标准治疗方法是静脉注射抗生素。与成人中性粒细胞性发热患者住院时间延长相关的因素包括血液恶性肿瘤、高强度化疗、中性粒细胞减少症持续时间长，以及培养生长革兰氏阴性多药耐药菌[142]。广谱 β-内酰胺类抗生素单药治疗，包括碳青霉烯类或第四代头孢菌素头孢吡肟，有确切的疗效。因为革兰阴性菌败血症死亡率高，经验性治疗必须覆盖率革兰阴性杆菌。两药联合治疗（氨基糖苷类或喹诺酮类加 β-内酰胺类）和单药治疗均 60%～80% 的成功率。如可疑或曾经感染革兰阳性菌，如蜂窝织炎，或中心静脉导管相关感染，或有严重的黏膜炎时，可以经验性应用万古霉素。对初始广谱抗生素治疗效果不佳时，因有革兰阳性菌感染可能性，可联合应用万古霉素[135]。

如果广谱抗生素应用 4～7 日仍发热，建议抗真菌治疗，未预防性应用抗真菌治疗的情况下，可使用氟康唑作为初始经验性治疗。两性霉素 B 有利于以下三类患者：使用广谱抗生素期间持续发热而未接受抗真菌治疗的患者，中性粒细胞减少超过 15 日的患者，既往真菌感染的患者。白色念珠菌和非白色念珠菌是白血病患者和骨髓移植受者的重要病原菌，而曲霉菌感染对长期而严重的中性粒细胞减少症患者有显著的影响。其他真菌，如镰孢菌属和毛孢菌属，是重要的病原体，可能是由于增加了抗真菌预防的作用。

在高危患者，特别是白血病患者中，可以采用降级方法来替代上述的升级方法[138]。名患者感染耐药病原体的风险（如耐甲氧西林金黄色葡萄球菌，耐万古霉素葡萄球菌，产生 β-内酰胺酶革兰氏阴性细菌，和产生碳青霉烯酶的细菌）和不稳定的患者血流动力学应该与广谱抗生素治疗最初的组合。耐药病原体感染的主要危险因素包括以前的定殖或耐药微生物的感染，以及在中性粒细胞缺乏患者开始发热时在培养物中耐药病原体的高度局部流行。抗生素治疗的降级是基于抗生素治疗开始后 72～96h 的培养结果和临床反应。

在化疗引起的中性粒细胞减少症发热中，利用髓样集落刺激因子增加白细胞的辅助治疗并不能提高总死亡率，尽管这种治疗与较短的发热时间、中性粒细胞减少症和使用抗生素有关[143]。如果化疗引起的中性粒细胞缺乏症发热的风险为>20%，那么在中性粒细胞缺乏症患者一般不推荐在发热后开始

考虑这些预防性刺激因素[130]。

化疗药物过敏性反应

化疗药物的过敏性反应是癌症患者另一种紧急情况。荨麻疹和血管性水肿是最常见的过敏表现，占过敏反应的 90%。美国过敏研究所感染性疾病、食品过敏反应和过敏反应网络建立了过敏反应的诊断标准；根据接触过敏原的可能性，使用了不同数量的标准，这些标准基于急性发作和涉及的皮肤、呼吸系统、心血管系统或胃肠道系统[144]。速发型过敏反应治疗的重要因素是早期识别、气道维护和血流动力学支持（表 140-3）[145~149]。可能引起过敏反应的常见化疗药物包括：L-天冬酰胺酶、紫杉烷类（紫杉醇和多西他赛）、依托泊苷、替尼泊苷、丙卡巴肼、铂类化合物（顺铂和卡铂）、异环磷酰胺、环磷酰胺、蒽环类药物（柔红霉素、多柔比星、阿达霉素）。

表 140-3　成人过敏反应处理建议

1. 去除抗原或延缓抗原吸收
2. 评估气道；有喉头水肿或即将发生的严重呼吸道阻塞的证据时气管插管，在极端情况下，当经口气管插管或气囊/瓣膜/面罩通气无效时，可能需要环甲切开术或导管喷射通气
3. 评估血流动力学；将患者平卧（或半躺在舒适的位置，如果出现呼吸困难或呕吐），抬高双腿
4. 给予肾上腺素
• 轻度发作：0.3mg SQ，1mg/ml，间隔 10~20min 后重复给予
• 中度发作：0.3~0.5mg im，1mg/ml，间隔 5~10min 后重复给予
• 休克或呼吸道梗阻：1mg/100ml iv，0.01~0.02mg/min，直至总剂量 0.1mg/min
• 难治性休克：可重复剂量或持续滴入。加 1~500ml 生理盐水，2~10μg/min
• 患者大于 50 岁或有既往病史或心脏病史而存在危及生命的症状：则试验性予以 0.1~0.15mg SQ 或 im
5. 静脉给予晶体液（生理盐水或乳酸林格液）
• 低血压时，15min 1L，然后重新评估；依次重复，总量至 3L
6. 给予糖皮质激素
• 甲泼尼龙 125mg 静脉推注；如症状持续可 4h 重复（替代品：氢化可的松 500mg，地塞米松 20mg，或其他有效的糖皮质激素）
7. 给予抗组胺药物
• 苯海拉明 25~50mg iv 或 im，必要时每 2~4h 重复
• 西咪替丁 300mg iv 或法莫替丁 20mg iv
8. 雾化吸入肾上腺素可减轻喉肿胀；β-受体阻滞剂缓解支气管痉挛和喘息
9. 难治性休克
• 军用抗休克裤和头低脚高的体位可能会有所帮助
• 多巴胺 5~20μg/（kg · min）iv
• 纳洛酮 0.4~2.0mg 每 2min iv（最多 10mg）
• 西咪替丁 300mg iv 或法莫替丁 20mg iv
10. 应用 β 肾上腺素受体阻滞剂加剧抵抗肾上腺素抗过敏
• 高血糖素 1~5mg iv 2~5min 以上
• 特布他林 0.25mg SQ
• 异丙肾上腺素 2~10μg/min，iv

im，肌内注射；iv，静脉注射；SQ，皮下。

摘自 Simons et al[145]，Lieberman et al[146]，Boyce et al[147]，和 Muraro et al[149]。

细胞因子与单克隆抗体的全身反应

生物药物是利用生物技术生产的蛋白质药物，包括单克隆抗体、融合蛋白和细胞因子。一些细胞因子（干扰素和 ILs）和单克隆抗体已经被批准用于治疗特定的恶性肿瘤。一个新的生物制剂不良反应的分类区分五种类型：（α）反应由于大规模释放细胞因子，（β）过敏因为针对生物制剂的一种免疫反应，（γ）免疫或细胞因子失衡综合征表现为免疫抑制，自身免疫或炎性疾病，由于大（δ）和（ε）不直接涉及免疫系统[150]。细胞因子可引起严重的毒性反应。单克隆抗体可诱发大量细胞因子释放，而导致发热、呼吸困难、缺氧、低血压，甚至死亡。最近，这些生物制剂可诱发的一些反应已引起重视[151]。

干扰素

干扰素治疗可产生急性的不良反应，发生在给药后的最初 2~8h，但很少限制治疗。常见的副作用有类似流感的症状，低血压或高血压，心动过速，恶心和呕吐。长期给药，可使疲劳和厌食加重，并导致体重减轻[148]。在治疗后的第一周，可发生轻度粒细胞减少（约50%的细胞数减少），并迅速发展，但在停药后可恢复。自身免疫性疾病和免疫溶血性贫血，骨髓抑制，和血小板减少很少见。缺血性结肠炎、缺血性视神经病变和充血性心力衰竭也有报道。可用乙酰氨基酚或非甾体抗炎药处理流感样的副作用。根据症状可提供其他支持治疗措施。

重组人白介素-2

高剂量IL-2治疗可引起心血管和血流动力学不稳定，类似于感染性休克[152]。大剂量静脉注射IL-2导致低血压，血管渗漏综合征，和呼吸功能不全等副作用时，需要使用增加周围血管阻力的升压药物、气管插管以及液体复苏，因此需住院使用（有时需要重症监护）。高剂量IL-2治疗还可导致急性中枢神经系统疾病如精神病，神志不清和行为异常。一出现神经系统副作用应尽快停止IL-2治疗而进行观察。已建议制订高剂量IL-2应用指南[153]。低剂量静脉注射和皮下注射IL-2的方案可在日间病房进行，在注射后观察几个小时。常见的症状包括发热，寒战，恶心，呕吐，厌食，倦怠，疲劳，肌肉痛，关节痛，瘙痒。

预防措施包括治疗前1、4和8个小时后给予对乙酰氨基酚650~1 000mg，1型和2型组胺受体拮抗剂（如治疗1h前口服苯海拉明50mg，和治疗开始后4、8和12h口服25mg，治疗开始前口服西咪替丁800mg）。

单克隆抗体

抗体药物的种类越来越多（表140-4）。给药后的第一个小时内出现即时反应，其病因和表现各异（恶心、呕吐、皮肤反应、呼吸道症状和低血压）[151]。其机制有的涉及细胞因子（α型）的释放；其他涉及IgE相关过敏反应（β型）。过敏反应、荨麻疹和血管性水肿均可发生。患者相关的危险因素包括恶性肿瘤，伴随治疗，和当前的免疫状态；与药物相关的因素包括药物的个性化程度、生产方法、糖基化模式和辅料的过敏潜能。迟发性过敏可在输液[151]后2h至14日出现，常表现为血清性疾病样（如皮疹、血管炎和多型红斑）。

表140-4　获得美国食品药品管理局批准的抗体疗法

药物	抗原靶点	单克隆抗体类型	共轭聚合	适应证	急性副作用
阿伦珠单抗（campath-1H）	CD52	人类	—	B细胞慢性淋巴细胞白血病	血细胞减少、感染心肌病
贝伐单抗（阿伐他汀）	VEGF	人类	—	结直肠癌	鼻出血、头痛、高血压、鼻炎、背痛、剥脱性皮炎味觉改变、直肠出血
brentuximab vedotin（adcetris）	CD30	嵌合体	monomethyl auristatin E	间变性大细胞淋巴瘤	血细胞减少、周围感觉神经病变、疲劳、上呼吸道感染、腹泻、皮疹、咳嗽、恶心、呕吐
西妥昔单抗（爱必妥）	EGFR	嵌合体	—	结直肠癌头颈癌	皮肤毒性（痤疮皮疹）、肺间质病变、感染、腹泻、恶心、结膜炎、肺栓塞
地诺单抗（denosumab）	RANK ligand	人类	—	骨转移	低钙血症、低磷酸盐
吉姆单抗、奥佐米星（麦罗塔）	CD33	人类	calicheamicin	CD33+髓系白血病	血细胞减少、感染、出血、黏膜炎、肝毒性
替伊莫单抗（zevalin）	CD20	小鼠	放射性标记的（^{90}Y或^{111}In）	非霍奇金淋巴瘤	血细胞减少、疲劳、鼻咽炎、恶心、腹痛、咳嗽、腹泻
伊匹木单抗（yervoy）	CTLA-4	人类	—	黑色素瘤	疲劳、腹泻、瘙痒、皮疹、结肠炎
奥法木单抗（arzerra）	CD20	人类	—	慢性淋巴细胞白血病	中性粒细胞减少
帕尼单抗（vectibix）	EGFR	人类	—	结直肠癌	皮肤中毒、甲癣、疲劳、恶心、腹泻、肠梗阻
帕妥珠单抗（帕杰塔）	HER2	人类	—	HER-2阳性乳腺癌	腹泻、脱发、中性粒细胞减少、恶心、疲劳、皮疹、周围神经病变
美罗华（rituxan）	CD20	单克隆抗体	—	B细胞非霍奇金淋巴瘤	感染、血细胞减少、低丙球蛋白血症
tositumomab（bexxar）	CD20	小鼠	放射性^{131}I	非霍奇金淋巴瘤	血细胞减少、感染、甲状腺功能减退
曲妥珠单抗（赫赛汀）	HER2	人类	—	HER-2阳性乳腺癌	血细胞减少、腹泻、疲劳、口腔炎、上呼吸道、感染、黏膜炎症、鼻咽炎、味觉障碍

虽然这些药物不良反应的发生率可能不同，但一般的预防措施和治疗是相同的。均表现为一过性的恶心，头痛，乏力，发热，寒战，皮疹，气喘，低血压，心律失常，支气管痉挛和血管性水肿等免疫反应。可用乙酰氨基酚和苯海拉明预防性治疗减轻不良反应。一般的解决方法是放慢输液速度或停止输液。症状消失后，输液速度可按之前的 50%继续进行。

(冯轲昕　孟祥志　刘嘉琦 译　王翔　王昕 校)

参考文献

The complete reference list can be found on the Wiley Companion Digital Edition of this title (see inside front cover for login instructions).

1 Perkins JC, Davis JE (eds). *Hematology/Oncology Emergencies, An Issue of Emergency Medicine Clinics of North America*. Philadelphia, PA: Elsevier Health Sciences; 2014.

5 American Heart Association. *Advance Cardiovascular Life Support (ACLS) Provider Manual*. Dallas, TX: American Heart Association, Inc.; 2011.

8 Hwang JP, Patlan J, de Achaval S, Escalante CP. Survival in cancer patients after out-of-hospital cardiac arrest. *Support Care Cancer*. 2010;**18**:51-55.

9 Staudinger T, Stoiser B, Müllner M, et al. Outcome and prognostic factors in critically ill cancer patients admitted to the intensive care unit. *Crit Care Med*. 2000;**28**:1322-1328.

10 Ackroyd R, Russon L, Newell R. Views of oncology patients, their relatives and oncologists on cardiopulmonary resuscitation (CPR): questionnaire-based study. *Palliat Med*. 2007;**21**:139-144.

21 Lenihan DJ, Kowey PR. Overview and management of cardiac adverse events associated with tyrosine kinase inhibitors. *Oncologist*. 2013;**18**:900-908.

23 Yeh ET, Bickford CL. Cardiovascular complications of cancer therapy: incidence, pathogenesis, diagnosis, and management. *J Am Coll Cardiol*. 2009;**53**:2231-2247.

24 Ewer MS, Ewer SM. Cardiotoxicity of anticancer treatments: what the cardiologist needs to know. *Nat Rev Cardiol*. 2010;**7**:564-575.

27 Kern KB, Halperin HR, Field J. New guidelines for cardiopulmonary resuscitation and emergency cardiac care: changes in the management of cardiac arrest. *JAMA*. 2001;**285**:1267-1269.

28 Howard SC, Jones DP, Pui CH. The tumor lysis syndrome. *N Engl J Med*. 2011;**364**:1844-1854.

31 Wilson FP, Berns JS. Tumor lysis syndrome: new challenges and recent advances. *Adv Chronic Kidney Dis*. 2014;**21**:18-26.

38 Ristic AD, Imazio M, Adler Y, et al. Triage strategy for urgent management of cardiac tamponade: a position statement of the European Society of Cardiology Working Group on Myocardial and Pericardial Diseases. *Eur Heart J*. 2014;**35**:2279-2284.

43 Annane D, Siami S, Jaber S, et al. Effects of fluid resuscitation with colloids vs crystalloids on mortality in critically ill patients presenting with hypovolemic shock: the CRISTAL randomized trial. *JAMA*. 2013;**310**:1809-1817.

45 Haas RA, Ahn SH. Interventional management of head and neck emergencies: carotid blowout. *Semin Interv Radiol*. 2013;**30**:245-248.

58 Fagedet D, Thony F, Timsit JF, et al. Endovascular treatment of malignant superior vena cava syndrome: results and predictive factors of clinical efficacy. *Cardiovasc Intervent Radiol*. 2013;**36**:140-149.

69 Simoff MJ, Lally B, Slade MG, et al. Symptom management in patients with lung cancer: Diagnosis and management of lung cancer, 3rd ed: American College of Chest Physicians evidence-based clinical practice guidelines. *Chest*. 2013;**143**:e455S-e497S.

78 Sweatt AJ, Sung A. Interventional pulmonologist perspective: treatment of malignant pleural effusion. *Curr Treat Options in Oncol*. 2014;**15**:625-643.

81 Ost DE, Jimenez CA, Lei X, et al. Quality-adjusted survival following treatment of malignant pleural effusions with indwelling pleural catheters. *Chest*. 2014;**145**:1347-1356.

89 Alrajab S, Youssef AM, Akkus NI, Caldito G. Pleural ultrasonography versus chest radiography for the diagnosis of pneumothorax: review of the literature and meta-analysis. *Crit Care*. 2013;**17**:R208.

90 Baumann MH, Strange C, Heffner JE, et al. Management of spontaneous pneumothorax: an American College of Chest Physicians Delphi consensus statement. *Chest*. 2001;**119**:590-602.

97 King V, Vaze AA, Moskowitz CS, Smith LJ, Ginsberg MS. D-dimer assay to exclude pulmonary embolism in high-risk oncologic population: correlation with CT pulmonary angiography in an urgent care setting. *Radiology*. 2008;**247**:854-861.

98 Klok FA, Djurabi RK, Nijkeuter M, et al. High D-dimer level is associated with increased 15-d and 3 months mortality through a more central localization of pulmonary emboli and serious comorbidity. *Br J Haematol*. 2008;**140**:218-222.

102 Chatterjee S, Chakraborty A, Weinberg I, et al. Thrombolysis for pulmonary embolism and risk of all-cause mortality, major bleeding, and intracranial hemorrhage: a meta-analysis. *JAMA*. 2014;**311**:2414-2421.

103 Riera-Mestre A, Becattini C, Giustozzi M, Agnelli G. Thrombolysis in hemodynamically stable patients with acute pulmonary embolism: A meta-analysis. *Thromb Res*. 2014;**134**:1265-1271.

105 Farge D, Debourdeau P, Beckers M, et al. International clinical practice guidelines for the treatment and prophylaxis of venous thromboembolism in patients with cancer. *JTH*. 2013;**11**:56-70.

106 Lyman GH, Khorana AA, Kuderer NM, et al. Venous thromboembolism prophylaxis and treatment in patients with cancer: American Society of Clinical Oncology clinical practice guideline update. *J Clin Oncol*. 2013;**31**: 2189-2204.

113 van Es N, Bleker SM, Di Nisio M. Cancer-associated unsuspected pulmonary embolism. *Thromb Res*. 2014;**133(Suppl 2)**:S172-S178.

114 Robson P. Metastatic spinal cord compression: a rare but important complication of cancer. *Clin Med*. 2014;**14**:542-545.

116 O'Phelan KH, Bunney EB, Weingart SD, Smith WS. Emergency neurological life support: spinal cord compression (SCC). *Neurocrit Care*. 2012;**17(Suppl 1)**:S96-S101.

119 Lee CH, Kwon JW, Lee J, et al. Direct decompressive surgery followed by radiotherapy versus radiotherapy alone for metastatic epidural spinal cord compression: a meta-analysis. *Spine*. 2014;**39**:E587-E592.

120 Stevens RD, Huff JS, Duckworth J, et al. Emergency neurological life support: intracranial hypertension and herniation. *Neurocrit Care*. 2012;**17(Suppl 1)**:S60-S65.

122 Brophy GM, Bell R, Claassen J, et al. Guidelines for the evaluation and management of status epilepticus. *Neurocrit Care*. 2012;**17**:3-23.

123 Arik Y, Leijten FS, Seute T, Robe PA, Snijders TJ. Prognosis and therapy of tumor-related versus non-tumor-related status epilepticus: a systematic review and meta-analysis. *BMC Neurol*. 2014;**14**:152.

125 Claassen J, Silbergleit R, Weingart SD, Smith WS. Emergency neurological life support: status epilepticus. *Neurocrit Care*. 2012;**17(Suppl 1)**:S73-S78.

130 Freifeld AG, Bow EJ, Sepkowitz KA, et al. Clinical practice guideline for the use of antimicrobial agents in neutropenic patients with cancer: 2010 update by the infectious diseases society of america. *Clin Infect Dis*. 2011;**52**: e56-e93.

137 Alp S, Akova M. Management of febrile neutropenia in the era of bacterial resistance. *Ther Adv Infect Dis*. 2013;**1**:37-43.

138 Averbuch D, Orasch C, Cordonnier C, et al. European guidelines for empirical antibacterial therapy for febrile neutropenic patients in the era of growing resistance: summary of the 2011 4th European Conference on Infections in Leukemia. *Haematologica*. 2013;**98**:1826-1835.

145 Simons FE, Ardusso LR, Bilò MB, et al. World Allergy Organization anaphylaxis guidelines: summary. *J Allergy Clin Immunol*. 2011;**127**:587-593.e1-22.

148 Campbell RL, Li JT, Nicklas RA, Sadosty AT. Emergency department diagnosis and treatment of anaphylaxis: a practice parameter. *Ann Allergy, Asthma Immunol*. 2014;**113**:599-608.

151 Corominas M, Gastaminza G, Lobera T. Hypersensitivity reactions to biological drugs. *J Investig Allergol Clin Immunol*. 2014;**24**:212-225; quiz 211p following 225.

第十三篇

展　望

第 141 章　21 世纪医疗保健的愿景

Leroy Hood，MD，PhD ■ Kristin Brogaard，PhD ■ Nathan D. Price，PhD

概述

系统医学、大数据以及患者驱动的社交网络的融合，正引领一种可预测、可预防、个性化和可参与的医学模式（简称 P4 医疗）。P4 医疗有两个中心目标：优化健康和理解疾病。为了将 P4 医疗引入医疗保健系统，我们启动了一项纵向试点研究，为 108 位健康人生成个体数据云。个人数据云的集成为实现个性化优化健康或避免疾病的可操作性打下基础。我们相信，这种在一个新的医疗保健领域，即科学健康领域的尝试，可以降低成本、提高质量和促进创新，真正改变医疗保健。

医疗保健的愿景

医疗保健是我们这个时代最重大的挑战之一。世界范围内的医疗保健的成本正在迅速增长，但卫生状况并未得到相应的改善[1]。例如，尽管美国是世界上最大的医疗保健支出国，但在 50 岁及以上人群的存活率方面，它在前 17 个发达国家中几乎垫底[1~2]。此外，根据健康和疾病驱动因素的研究表明，约 30% 的疾病是由遗传因素引起的，60% 的疾病是由环境和行为因素引起的，只有约 10% 的疾病是由医疗保健本身引起的，而且这些因素之间存在相互作用[3]。因此，今天医疗保健的重点几乎完全集中在治疗疾病上，却忽视了疾病的真正重要的驱动因素。这种方式是有问题的，因为一旦生物体已经受到疾病的影响，它们往往无法再恢复到疾病前完全健康的状态。显然，医疗保健的模式需要进行系统性改革，以支持 21 世纪我们真正需要的医疗保健。

量化健康和揭开疾病的神秘面纱

为了改革当前的医疗体系，我们建议采用两大推动力，一是量化健康，二是通过研究疾病的起源来揭开疾病的神秘面纱。健康对于优化人类潜能（或资本）和提供疾病预防的基本洞见都至关重要，通过检查，我们识别最早期阶段的疾病，从而从可检测的起始点研究疾病，为研究疾病和预防疾病提供基本的见解。相反，目前的医疗保健一般只在患者生病后才对其进行分析和治疗。

这种转变的关键是采用系统生物学的方法来研究疾病，这自然决定未来的医疗保健模式隶属于系统性医疗，且具有可预测、可预防、个性化和可参与的特性-P4 医疗。摆在眼前的最基本的问题是如何将 P4 医疗应用于治疗患者，并将其引入当前的医疗保健领域。在本章中，我们概述了一种卓有成效的量化健康和减轻病患的新方法，它将作为医疗保健模式变革的一个模型。此模型源自一项对 10 万“健康人”进行的长期、数据完整的纵向研究。该模型旨在建立健康的定量指标和为研究从健康到最常见疾病的过渡状态提供基础。

P4 医疗的出现

作为背景介绍，我们也将从个人经验出发，说明过去 40 年来这种 P4 医疗的愿景是如何出现，以及它的实施将如何影响二十一世纪的医疗保健系统。

早期

让我们回顾一下过去五十年前的生物医学研究的现状。当我们研究者中的一人（李·胡德）于 1970 年开始在加州理工学院担任助理教授时，很明显，生物学和疾病远比当时大多数研究人员设想的要复杂得多。而且仅仅关注一种基因或一种蛋白质的各种研究，不可能破译这种生物学系统的复杂性[4]。大象与六个盲人的语言便很贴切：每个人感觉到的都只是大象身体的不同部分（如鼻子、腿、象牙等），并把所观察到的特征当作是大象。所以，对一个人来说，大象可能就像一条蛇（鼻子），而对另一个人来说，大象就像一把扇子（耳朵），以此类推。理解大象需要一种集成数据的整体方法。生物学和医学的研究也有类似的复杂性，我们测量一个或几个基因或蛋白质，却不能看到全部。我们需要整合不同的全球性或综合性的生物信息来解读疾病的复杂性。这个新的综合学科的出现，现在被称为系统科学，已经导致了生物学和医学的转变。

在 20 世纪 70 年代变得明显的是，科学家缺乏解决生物复杂性的方法（系统科学）、技术和系统驱动策略。在那段时间里，我阅读了托马斯·库恩（Tomas Kuhn）的《科学革命的结构》[5]，此书强调了由于科学家的保守主义以及不愿超越传统观念而跳出框框思考的问题，推动物理学范式变革的难度很大。对我来说，很明显，生物学领域需要范式的转变，从还原主义思维转向更广泛的系统方法。就在那时，我决定把我的职业生涯奉献给以各种方式解读生物复杂性。正如库恩预测的那样，这些努力最初都受到了相当大的怀疑。

面对这些挑战，在接下来的四十年里，我参与了五项范式变革，它们解决了生物学的复杂性，并导致了系统生物学、系统医学以及一种具有预测性、预防性、个性化和参与性的 P4 医学模式的出现[6,7]。这些范式变革包括：

1. 通过开发六种可以读取和写入 DNA 和蛋白质的仪器，将工程学引入生物学。这些仪器引入了高通量生物数据生成及其相关的大数据和分析的概念[8~10]。

2. 其中一种仪器，即自动 DNA 测序仪，使人类基因组计划成为可能。该计划产生了一个完整的基因列表，并借此通过推断蛋白质的部分列表，使系统科学成为可能[9,11,12]。

3. 跨学科生物学的出现使生物学家、化学家、计算机科学家、工程师、数学家、物理学家和医生聚集在一起，在一个屋檐下学习彼此的语言，组成有效的团队，高效地解决非常复杂的生物学问题。这种合作推动了生物发现驱动技术的循环，进而推动分析学理解生物学的机制。1992 年，比尔·盖茨(Bill Gates)邀请我在华盛顿大学医学院(University of Washington Medical School)成立了分子生物技术系，在推动生物学科向交叉学科转变方面发挥了关键作用。该系在基因组学、蛋白质组学、细胞分选和大规模 DNA 合成方面起到关键技术开发和引领先河的作用[13]。该部门还建立了涉及人类基因组测序的 16 个中心中的两个。

4. 在 2000 年，我和其他人共同基于系统科学创立了系统生物科学研究所以及其配套的必要的技术和分析方法[14,15]。这种全球性系统分析方法是解决生物复杂性难题的关键。它在疾病防诊治中的应用导致了第五种范式转移的发生。

5. 系统医学和 P4 医学都源自系统科学在疾病防诊治中的应用[16~18]。因此，前四个范式转移导致了研究疾病、健康和医学的革命性新方法。

回顾过去，这些经验产生了以下关于如何催化现代社会范式变化的有益见解：

- 新思想需要新的组织结构：这五个范式变化中的每一个都需要创建新的组织实体来充当它们的领导者。长期存在的官僚制度很少能采纳新思想，因为它们是由过时的需求和过去的经验磨砺出来的，因此往往难以适应现在，更不用说未来了。
- 如果你想说服组织采用新的想法，则必须聘请组织的领袖。中层管理人员经常陷入组织的日常运营中，因此往往无法理解范式的变化。
- 这些想法最初都受到了相当多的怀疑。面对广泛的阻力，坚定的乐观是推动思想向前发展的关键。
- 这些变化从根本上改变了我们看待和实践生物学和医学的方式。
- 至关重要的是为生物科学家带来新的，最广泛的社区，并最终向公众开放。在系统生物学研究所(ISB)，洛根教育中心(Logan Center for Education)致力于将现代科学带给这些受众，并在新的背景下促进 K-12 科学教育。

生命之书——生物信息的四个层次

这些范式的变化提供了概念性的框架和工具，让人类以前所未有的整体方式来理解生物学信息。这是四个离散水平的信息：DNA、RNA、蛋白质和生物网络或系统(图 141-1)。它们的存在也证明了我们需要倚赖生物信息集成和模型来解决生物复杂性的问题。

基因组可以被描述为一本包含生命数字指令的书[11]。基因组源于 DNA 的四字母碱基：G、C、A、T。它被包装在每个人 10^{13} 个细胞中的 23 对染色体中。人类基因组(二倍体)包含约 60 亿个碱基或约 6m 的 DNA。由于人类身体包含 10^{13} 个细胞，因此它含有的 DNA 排成行可以是地球和太阳之间距离的 600 倍。基因组被分为约 20 000 个信息单元，称为基因。

这些基因可以读取为 DNA 碱基的拷贝数(或转录本)，这些拷贝称为 RNA。这些基因可以进行化学修饰或通过它们与蛋白质的相互作用进行修饰，从而改变了他们的表达水平。这些被称为表观遗传修饰。个体基因的 RNA 转录本的产生允许根据它们的使用需要进行不同的扩增(每个细胞最多可复制数百万个 RNA)，并允许对转录本进行化学改变以改变其信息含量。例如，我们研究了一个名为 *neurexin* 的人类基因，它至少有 2 000 种不同的 RNA 转录本，有趣的问题是这些独特的转录本中到底有多少代表特殊的信息单位(其他的可能是噪音)[19]。

大多数 RNA 转录本可以被复杂的生物机器翻译成蛋白质，这代表了信息的第三个层次。20 个字母的语言对应 20 个氨基酸编码蛋白质。这种语言指导着每一个前体的折叠成一个独特的和复杂的三维结构，执行生命的特定功能。蛋白质可以单独发挥作用，也可以通过与其他蛋白质或信息分子的相互作用来创建复杂的分子机器或生物网络。

网络是 DNA、RNA 和蛋白质之外的第四个层次的信息，它

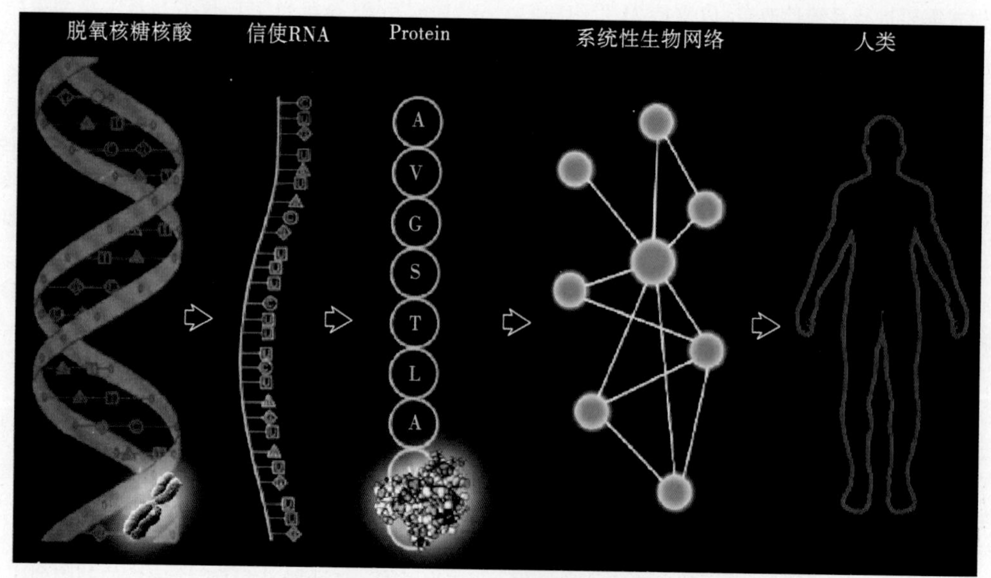

图 141-1 单个数据云中现实的不同类型数据的示意图

产生于各种生物网络(如基因调控网络、蛋白质相互作用网络、代谢网络等)中蛋白质与 DNA、RNA、其他蛋白质和生命小分子(代谢物)之间的相互作用。这些网络是动态的,随时间变化的,是由基因信息和环境信息共同形成的。生物网络调节关键的生命过程,包括发育、生理和衰老,而生物网络的错乱则会引起人类疾病。

经典分子生物学涉及对生命的研究,一次分析一个或几个基因或蛋白质。系统生物学包括对发育过程、生理反应和衰老的网络动力学的分析。为了促进对这些动态网络的系统分析,开发能够对基因组中所有基因进行序列分析的工具至关重要。所有基因修饰(表观基因组),所有的 RNA(转录组);一个细胞、器官或生物中的所有蛋白质(蛋白质组);以及存在于给定细胞,器官或生物中的代谢物(代谢组)。这些统称为“组学分析”。测量至少一些更高层次的生理和心理表型也很重要。

今天,有数种理解生物学和医学的方法。例如,基因组医学这个术语非常流行,它阐述了基因组在疾病中扮演的角色。相比之下,系统医学(疾病的系统方法)对生命和疾病的动力学采取整体和综合的方法,包括基因组,也包括转录组、表观基因组、蛋白质组、代谢组和更复杂的表型。系统医学侧重于理解基因组和环境变化在健康和疾病中所起的作用,部分是通过研究其动态生物网络来进行的。

系统医学:转折点

系统医学具有两个主要特征:

第一,每个个体将拥有一个由数十亿数据点组成的虚拟的、个性化的、动态的云(图 141-2)。这些数据在类型上是异质的,在维度上是多维的。它们的范围从分子、细胞和器官数据到将个体联系在一起的网络,同时它们也是动态的,因为它们会随着时间和环境的改变而变化。ISB 正在开发分析工具来整合和建模这些数据,以确定行动的可能性,使每个人能够对这些机会作出反应,以优化他们的健康和或最小化疾病的严重程度。

这些大数据云为噪音挑战提供了一个巨大的信号,而噪音来自与当前健康问题无关的生物信息中固有的可变性(噪音)。因此,系统方法对于挖掘这些大数据集以获取可操作的信息,从大量噪声中识别出潜在的小信号至关重要[20]。

第二,动态生物网络负责管理、整合和传输生物分子和生物有机体的相关信息,而这些信息反过来又可以调节正常发育和生理反应。这些网络在疾病中变得混乱[21,22],从而反过来改变他们处理的信息(图 141-3)。评估正常网络和受到疾病扰动后的网络之间的差异,可以深入了解疾病机制,发现新型的诊断方法和新的治疗靶标。

2008 年,ISB 与卢森堡政府启动了一项 1 亿美元的合作计划。它每年向 ISB 提供 2 000 万美元,为期 5 年,以发展促进系统医学所必需的战略和技术。这种资助是灵活的,因此研究所可以采取高风险、高回报的战略。这些努力是非常成功的,并导致了九项新技术和系统驱动的战略的发展,加速了转化医学的实现,如下三个例子所示:

- 第一,我们率先对整个家族进行了完整的基因组测序,这大大提高了我们鉴定疾病基因的能力[23]。迄今为止,我们已经分析了 23 种疾病,数百个家庭和 9 000 多个完整的人类基因组。最近,我们利用家族基因组测序来鉴定编码神经兴奋性的基因簇中的罕见变异,而这些变异会影响双相情感障碍的发病风险[24]。
- 第二,我们证明了一种由朊病毒引起的神经退行性疾病,在

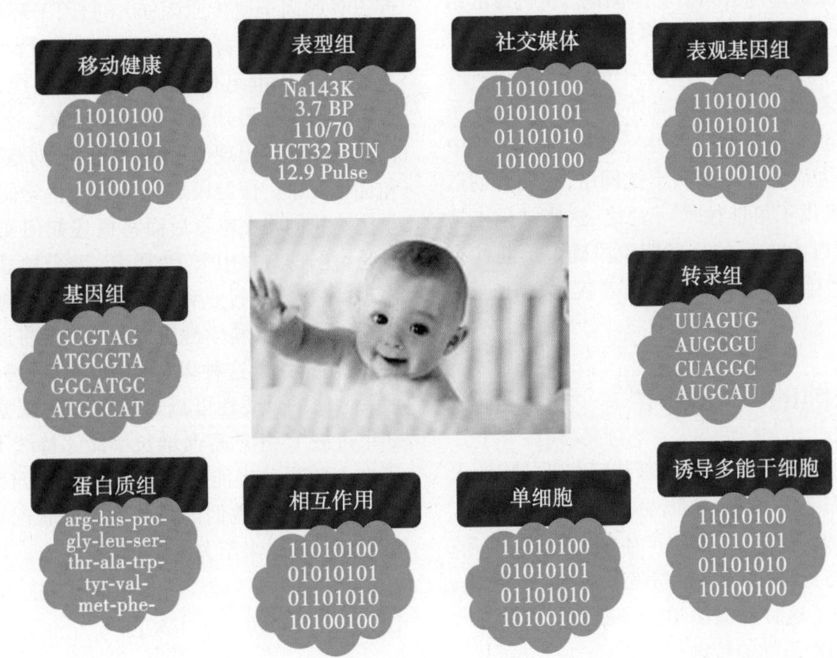

图 141-2　“网络的网络”一览表。生物网络可以在个体的基因,蛋白质和其他分子,细胞,器官甚至社会网络的水平上运行。在疾病中,这些网络中的一些信息被改变成为疾病困扰。正常和疾病干扰网络之间的差异为疾病机制、早期诊断和改进的候选药物靶点标志别提供了见解

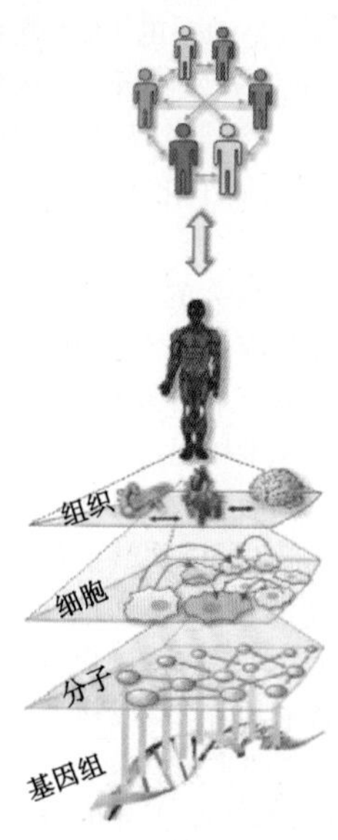

图 141-3 生物信息的四个层次的示意图:DNA、RNA、蛋白质、相互作用,网络和生物系统

小鼠体内 22 周的病程中出现了 10 个疾病扰动的生物网络[25]。我们发现这些网络在疾病发展的不同阶段都受到了疾病的干扰。因此,最早的变化网络提供了早期诊断的可能性,以及早期治疗靶点的识别。我们进一步证明了这 10 个不同网络的动态共同解释了这种疾病的病理生理学的几乎每一个方面。这些结果为早期疾病机制和疾病进展的后期阶段提供了基石般的见解。

- 第三,我们使用系统的血液蛋白诊断方法开发了 13 种血液蛋白,从而使我们能够区分良性肺结节和癌性肺结节[26]。通过 ISB 附属公司,集成诊断公司的临床测试。从确诊的结节过度诊断肺癌是一个大问题,导致多达 40% 的手术是在良性结节上进行的。因此,广泛实施这项检测,除了显著降低发病率和对患者健康的不必要风险外,还可以为医疗系统节省数十亿美元的不必要手术费用。这 13 种蛋白质中的 12 种可以映射到肺癌的 3 个疾病干扰网络,它们为创造新的鉴别诊断方法提供了可能性[25]。总之,这些结果支持这样一种观点,即可以为疾病的最早期阶段确定诊断性生物标志物,并且这些生物标志物可以随着疾病的进展而变化。

P4 医学:医疗保健的一场革命

ISB 与卢森堡伙伴关系的成功带来的新战略和新技术使人们认识到,新药物必须具有预测性、预防性、个性化和参与性。事实上,P4 医学是在三大科技的交汇中产生的,它们分别是:①系统医学;②大数据与分析;③患者消费者激活的社交网络。四个 P 分别准确地描述了这种新型医学的一般特征以及它与传统医学的显著区别。P4 医学的特点:

- 它是主动的,不是被动的
- 它关注的是个人,而不是平均人群
- 它把重点放在健康上,而不仅仅是疾病
- 它生成动态的个人数据云,可用于优化健康状况并避免或消除疾病
- 它赋予个人参与自身健康的权利

传统的以人群为基础的医学研究是传统医疗无法达到 P4 医学要求的典型例子。目前,药物研究包括,例如,多达 3 万名患者服用药物或安慰剂;他们的疗效反应被外推到曲线中,从而确定了总体的平均反应,并以此为基础确定药物是否有效。事实上,这种方法有很大的局限性,因为每个患者在遗传和环境暴露方面都是独一无二的。研究不应该只关注人群的平均结果。

我们必须研究个体而不是群体。因此,P4 医疗将对这 3 万人的个体数据云进行单独分析,然后根据医生感兴趣的特征(如对给定药物的反应、对给定药物的不良反应)将其聚合到相关组中。这一观点还认为,P4 医疗对单个患者($n=1$)的实验可能非常有用,特别是如果我们可以采取纵向措施,在疾病发生和进展时,能让处于“健康”状态的患者作为自身对照。

P4 医疗还利用了患者(消费者)激活的社交网络的力量。个人将通过沟通网络获得授权,并让他们参与到 P4 医学的机遇中。被授权的患者将是使医生了解新药物的动力,并将是改变临时医疗保健的主要推动者。这些患者驱动的社交网络还使患者能够参与众包过程,通过分享宝贵的经验和学习他人的经验来优化自己的健康。最终,这些网络将成为推动医生和保守的医疗保健系统接受变革的强大社会力量。

P4 医疗:量化健康和揭秘疾病

P4 药物有两个中心点:健康和疾病[27~29]。当今的医疗保健几乎全部集中于疾病,并且是目前社会上绝大多数医疗保健支出的来源。但是,有关健康和疾病驱动因素的研究表明,接近 30% 归因于遗传原因,60% 归因于环境和行为原因,只有大约 10% 归因于医疗保健,同时这些因素相互之间存在影响[3]。为了促进 21 世纪有效的卫生保健系统,我们需要更充分地理解影响健康的另外 90% 的驱动因素。这需要重新定位,我们不仅仅是在症状出现或变得严重时才对疾病做出反应,更要保持和优化健康。使健康成为可信的科学研究的关键是对其进行量化。我们将在本章后面将概述如何实现这一点。我们的观点是,在未来的 10 年和 15 年,两个独立的医疗保健行业将会出现,科学健康行业和疾病行业(即目前的医疗行业)。此外,在这段时间内,科学健康行业的市值将远远超过疾病行业。现在,我们正处于这种以科学为基础的健康产业转型的最早阶段。健康的重要性可以通过下面的观察得到进一步的阐述。如果过去 15 年的寿命增长率能够持续下去,2015 年出生的孩子中大约有一半能活到 100 岁[30]。问题是,在他们生命的最后二三十年里,他们的身体和智能状况将如何?显然,迈向健康对我们的未来至关重要。

健康先锋试点计划

一旦达到了系统医学的临界点,并划定了 P4 医学,就出现了如何将其引入当前医疗体系的问题。我们意识到,我们需要一个引人注目的试点计划,它包括四个 P 的所有原则,并且重点关注健康和疾病。我们之所以称其为科学健康,是因为它使

用了高密度的、动态化的个人数据云。

十万人健康计划

2013 年，我们提出了一个基于系统科学的项目，其中包括四个 P 原则，生成动态的患者数据云。项目的重点是关注与每个个体相关的科学健康和疾病状况，即在数十年的时间框架内对 10 万名健康人群进行的纵向、高密度数据的研究[27,31]。我们提出：①确定每个个体的完整基因组序列；②每 3 个月对血液、唾液、尿液进行研究，描绘临床化学反应、700 种代谢物、约 400 种蛋白质；③每 3 个月分析一次肠道菌群；④包括对过去的病史、当前的生理和心理状态的描述性评估，以及量化的自我测量（活动、脉搏、睡眠质量、血压和体重）。最重要的理念是分析个体的测量，并将这些数据类型的各种组合集成到每个个体的模型中，这些模型揭示了可操作的可能性，如果根据这些可能性采取行动，就可以改善他们的健康或让他们避免疾病（见下文）。

随着时间的推移，这些测量是评估可能很快成为可能先把人分成两组：一组是健康状况良好或得到改善的人群；另一组是转变为疾病的人群（图 141-4）。从那些仍远，或改进，我们可以识别度规板，应该允许我们量化健康。我们相信，这些指标将允许我们描绘健康的身体和心理方面。从那些保持健康或得到改善的人群中，我们可以确定指标面板，以使量化健康状况。我们坚信，这些指标将使我们能够描述健康的身体和心理方面。可能有人会想象每个人都有一个概念上的"健康之井"，而我们认为我们中的许多人都处于低谷。采取个性化可行的行动，使我们迈向井井有条，同时优化了我们的生理和心理健康状况。个人如何有效地优化自己的健康状况，取决于他们如何有效地制订和响应自己的个性化可行机会。

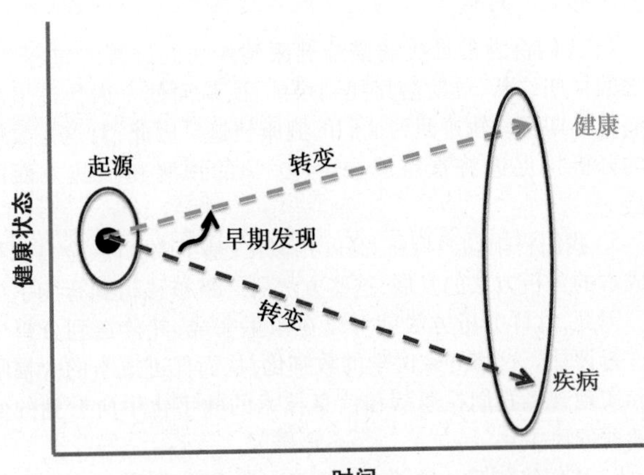

图 141-4　健康状况随时间而变化。个人可能会沿着某种轨迹运动从而导致维持健康状态，或者可能转变为身体不适并进入疾病状态。早期发现问题，付诸可行的措施可以帮助个人从疾病轨迹过渡到健康轨迹，并为每个人优化健康状况

对于那些已转变到疾病的人，我们可以分析纵向数据，以确定健康到疾病过渡点，从而使我们能够研究相关疾病干扰生物网络的最早干扰（图 141-4）。这些见解将导致有可能了解疾病最早阶段的发病机制，开发早诊制剂，并可能确定可用于预防医学的候选药物靶点，以避免最终导致疾病表现的下游级联不良事件。假以时日，这将使人们有可能在疾病发展的早期就改变个人健康的轨迹，从而为医疗保健系统节省大量资金。因此，这项健康研究不仅要研究健康，而且还要从疾病发生之初就对疾病进行研究。传统医学通常仅在疾病发生健康过渡后很长时间才研究患病的患者，这通常是无效的过程。许多系统，即使在疾病得到治疗之后，也无法恢复到疾病之前的效力水平。对健康的研究将使我们既能调整人力资本，又能确定健康到疾病的过渡，从而使我们能够及早终止疾病，并使个人迅速地从疾病的起始阶段回到健康的轨道。

可操作性是用于将数据连接到行为（即通过识别可操作的项）的中心概念。我们不仅提供了未来负面事件的风险（这种行为对行为的影响极小），而且还提供了有关个人体内当前正在发生的情况的深入信息，并提供了可以立即进行的操作的路线图（和在一段时间内保持一致）对他或她的身体产生实质性影响（确实会激发行为）。可操作的可能性将由教练提供给个人，教练可以清楚地解释可操作的可能性，以及个人如何根据自己的健康愿望适当地对这些可能性作出反应。这些教练将由医生通过现有的医疗保健系统提供临床建议。教练是这个过程中非常重要的一部分，帮助人们改善自己的健康。

纵向 10 万人健康研究项目提供数据可访问性的重要性

我们对数据可访问性的看法非常简单。至关重要的是，所有被剔除患者身份的数据都要提供给合格的调查人员，他们将挖掘这些数据，用于未来的预测和预防医学。

因此，我们每个人对自己的数据进行分析时，我们的子孙后代都将从中受益，因为未来的医学将改善我们孩子的健康状况，优化健康，避免疾病。我们认为，一个人的社会义务是允许他们的数据被用来发明未来的医学。乔治・丘奇（George Church）在他的个人基因组计划（PGP）[32] 中也提出了类似的请求。如果消费者和患者的数据要广泛提供给合格的研究者，必须考虑两个重要的问题：第一，必须具有强大的安全性来保护数据。可以使用诸如加密之类的适当方法来保护数据，并且必须采用这种方法。第二，有旨在保护个人免受遗传歧视的联邦和州法律，包括《遗传信息非歧视法》（GINA）。GINA 禁止健康保险公司仅基于遗传信息拒绝承保或收取更高的保费。GINA 还禁止雇主使用遗传信息进行雇用，解雇，晋升和其他雇用决定。但是，GINA 不能避免很多类型的歧视，包括人寿保险，长期护理保险和伤残保险的歧视。国会应通过扩大 GINA 并制订其他相关法律来解决这些问题，以确保不存在基于遗传数据的歧视。

按比例扩大

我们的主要目标之一是了解如何将健康计划扩展到 10 万人。我们最初的想法是分四个阶段，从 100 到 1 000 再到 10 000，最后在一年左右的时间里达到 10 万。然而，我们对这个策略有很多疑问：

- 我们应该测量什么？多久测一次？

- 我们如何开发所有的分析工具?
- 一个10万人的研究项目要花费多少?
- 我们怎样才能把这个项目的规模从100人扩大到10万人?

百人健康计划

这项研究需要一个成熟的团队来管理,涉及大量的科学、后勤、组织和参与者等各种问题。这些问题包括样本收集过程,决定适当的分析包括(发现以及临床实效),样本分布分析(供应商和ISB),开发分析工具来整合和模拟先驱者的数据,以揭示可操作的可能性,健康教练的招聘和培训,形成一个医学顾问小组来监督整个过程。在参与研究的108名先驱者中,所有人在整个研究期间都留在了研究中,大多数人表示有兴趣将研究继续到下一个阶段。我们的先驱者中有70%的人遵从教练对他们可采取行动可能性的建议。此项研究的高留存率和参与度受到三个因素的影响:①教练非常有效地解释了每个人的行动可能性,并鼓励每个人根据自己的健康目标采取行动;②了解自己的基因是如何与其他类型的数据相互作用并对其产生影响的,在鼓励人们改变行为方面尤其具有说服力;③观察一个人的数据云随时间的推移而发生的积极(和适当的)变化,以应对特定的生活方式变化,是一种有效的强化体验。

第一组临床化学数据显示,91%的先驱者有特定的营养缺乏,68%有炎症指标(均可纠正)。三位先驱者体内的汞含量极高。其中两个人吃了大量的金枪鱼寿司,而另一个人则因为补牙而摄入了汞。其中一个人用鲑鱼代替金枪鱼寿司,两个月后他体内的汞含量下降了一半,另外两个也有类似的处理汞源的经历。

我们发现了数个可能的疾病转归的征象。例如,两个先驱者是导致血红蛋白沉着症(C282Y)基因变异的纯合者。在一小部分这样的个体中,这种疾病会导致血液中铁和铁蛋白水平升高。高血铁水平可以攻击关节、胰腺、肝脏或心脏,潜在地导致关节炎,糖尿病,肝硬化/癌症,或心脏失代偿在内的各种组合并发症。由于该病常伴有心脏并发症,患者可能已经患有慢性糖尿病。

治疗方法很简单。将具有*C282Y*突变的个体送到医生那里进行诊断检查;如果有指示,则该人可以定期抽血,直到达到正常的铁水平。我们确定了这两个具有纯合*C282Y*基因型的个体,只有在发生任何严重的组织损伤之前,它们的变化最早,因此避免了慢性血红蛋白沉着病,从而随着时间的推移为医疗系统节省了大量资金。此外,这些个体的孩子正在接受基因测试进行诊断-阻止了无法诊断和可治疗的疾病传递到下一代。

使用空腹血糖的标准临界值,我们确定了108名空腹血糖处于基线糖尿病前期范围(如糖尿病前期)的参与者中的53人。在仅仅接受了5~6个月的健康指导后,其中7人恢复了正常血糖,总体血糖水平呈下降趋势。

两种或多种不同数据类型(如血液,微生物组,遗传学,活性)的整合分析也很有用。例如,使用全基因组关联研究(GWAS),我们可以根据108位先驱者对克罗恩病的遗传(GWAS)倾向将其分为五个低风险至高风险类别。当将肠道微生物组中的细菌种群与这些遗传倾向进行比较时,随着每组个体的遗传风险增加,两种更具"致病性"细菌的菌株也会增加。因此,克罗恩病易感性的遗传与肠道微生物组中微生物种群的变化之间存在关联。目前我们尚不清楚因果关系可能是什么,或者这里是否存在可采取行动的可能性。

很明显,107位开拓者中的每一位都有多种可操作的可能性。有70%以上的先驱者根据他们的行动能力采取行动,这是一种显著的服从。因此,这个项目可以优化健康和或减少每个人的疾病。

这些研究结果使许多参与者得出三个结论:

- 你的基因决定你的潜力,而不是你的命运。在许多情况下,行为的改变可以突破遗传的限制
- 个性化、全面、实时的数据支持。有了这些知识,一个人对自己的健康负起责任就变得更加容易和更有动力。这是控制医疗费用起步阶段的关键
- 许多先驱者对继续进行下一阶段的纵向研究感兴趣(我们将简要介绍)。这是一种评价方法,它表明大多数人是多么确信这项研究已经深刻地改变了他们的生活

10万人福利和107人健康先锋试点计划的健康研究

1. 我们将创建一系列可行的方法,以优化健康状况并最大限度地减少疾病,并帮助其他人开展类似的研究。这种以指数形式增加可操作可能性(分析新数据确定新可操作可能性)的目录将成为未来优化个人健康的重点。

2. 我们将生成动态的、个性化的数据云,允许提取个人可操作的可能性,如果采取行动,允许个人优化健康和最小化疾病。

3. 我们将生成一个多参数的健康生物标记面板,我们相信,随着时间的推移,将允许我们从血液中分离出健康的物理和心理成分。它将帮助个人提升他们的"健康井",以最大化他们自己的人类潜力。

4. 我们将为常见疾病描绘健康到疾病的过渡的过程,为疾病的早期诊断、早期治疗找到可能性,从而使个人快速地从他们的早期疾病轨迹回到他们的健康轨迹。因此,对这一数据集的分析将促进将重点放在P4医学的预测和预防方面的机会。

5. 我们将推动微型化、高度相似化、基于微流体、全自动和低成本的分析方法的发展,这些方法最终将被移植到智能手机上。因此,这样分析方法就可以在家里完成,并传送到分析中心进行评估。这将导致医学的数字化,从而促进成本的大幅降低和实现曾经我们在通信和信息技术的数字化中所看到的使用效益的民主化。

6. 我们将创建一个数据库,其中包含大量关于健康和疾病过渡的信息。这些数据将为健康和疾病过渡领域的创新和创建公司提供原材料。

7. 10万人健康项目将从三方面有助于促进P4医疗进入医疗保健系统:降低成本、引入更有效的医疗保健、加速创新和支持公司创建。

我们计划如何进行?

我们有两个主要的策略来推进10万健康计划:

1. ISB计划通过引入国内和国际合作伙伴来推进10万健康项目，这些合作伙伴将管理小规模的健康先锋项目，并雇佣易患某些疾病的患者，使我们能够更快地跟踪疾病的转变。我们在欧盟有几个潜在的合作伙伴，并正在与亚洲和中东美国探讨更多的可能性。这些将是学术努力，也可以推动发展新的化验试剂（见前文）和分析工具。

2. 我们已经成立了一家名为Arivale的公司，该公司将为消费者提供科学的健康之路。我们希望该公司能及时帮助降低成本并提高维持或增强健康的功效。通过确定如何有效地优化需要汇总的数据类型的过程，以及通过建立数据分析功能，以及从这些数据中提取可操作知识的过程，我们已经看到了医学的数字化。在成立的前六个月中，未经广告宣传的Arivale在西雅图地区吸引了1 000多名消费者。

系统医学和癌症：补充说明

本书的读者可能会问，究竟什么系统医学（和P4医学）可能为癌症诊治助力。很明显，系统方法对癌症有很多贡献，我们将简要概述几个例子：

1. 癌症将罕见的细胞转移到血液中，这些细胞可以被分离和鉴定，特别是通过新的单细胞分析技术。这些细胞可能为早期诊断提供新的机会，随着癌症的进展，确定癌症的复发，甚至可能定位远处转移的位置。

2. 可以评估小鼠模型系统中癌症进展的网络动力学（就像我们对病毒诱导的神经发生的研究一样），并且可以洞悉早期疾病扰动的网络，从而为开发癌症早期诊断方法和潜在的攻击性治疗靶点提供帮助。例如，我们正在进行胶质母细胞瘤小鼠模型的研究，其惊人的结果表明，受疾病困扰的网络可以解释许多癌症的基本特性。

3. 可以开发出针对癌症的血液诊断方法，跟踪其进展情况，跟踪对治疗的反应，确定复发情况，甚至确定可以为可能的治疗药物候选者提供见解的疾病扰动网络（请参阅我们之前对肺癌诊断方法的描述）。

4. 有一种形式的RNA，微小RNA（miRNA），在细胞调节中起着非常重要的作用。这些微小RNA与重要的调控网络相互作用，为识别可能成为药物靶点候选分子的分子识别提供了另一种系统驱动的方法。

5. 未来癌症治疗的一个关键将是在疾病治疗开始时开展三种药物疗法。癌症和人类免疫缺陷病毒获得性免疫缺陷综合征（HIV/AIDS）都是突变率过高的疾病。就像三联疗法将HIV/AIDS从一种致命的疾病转变为一种慢性疾病一样，三联疗法也将为癌症带来同样的机会。理解和分析癌症的疾病干扰网络是识别多种潜在药物靶点候选靶点协同作用的关键。

6. 如上所述，对健康人群的纵向研究将最终使我们能够确定癌症患者的健康状况，并开始研究疾病早期的干扰网络。对这些疾病早期转变的理解将为早期诊断和治疗开辟新的可能性。

7. 在这一艰难的过程中，我们可以应用纵向健康研究，对正在接受癌症治疗的个体进行研究，以优化他们的健康状况。如今，健康从未被严肃地视为癌症治疗的一部分。此外，我们也可以对那些已经成功接受了癌症治疗（细胞毒性、化疗）的患者进行同样的治疗，以再次优化他们的健康状况。

这些只是P4医疗如何治疗癌症的几个例子，而我们也只是在想象所有的P4医疗可能带来的优化癌症诊治的各种研究机会。关键是要将P4医疗迅速引入卫生保健系统，使医学能够开始利用这些机会。一个主要的挑战，很明显，是如何把这些机遇的理解带给那些难以接受新思想保守派医生。

健康和保健的民主化

我们对医疗保健未来的展望是，患者将通过对自己的健康负责，医疗实现数字化以及使用个性化数据云来优化健康和避免疾病。我们共同参与其中，将大大降低医疗成本，同时提高了医疗效果。我们相信，这目的将通过对健康的关注和疾病转变的早期识别来实现，这些疾病的转变可以被快速有效地识别和治疗。随着成本下降和模式落地，P4医疗不仅将被带到发达国家，而且也将被带到发展中国家。在1990年的时候，谁能想到印度农村的妇女可以利用手机养家糊口呢？然而，这正是通信数字化所带来的结果。以类似的方式，医学的数字化，连同上面提到的其他变化，将显著地降低医疗保健的成本，而这反过来又将使P4医疗保健大众化，无论对穷人还是富人。很难想象，在未来十年里，会有多少个人，无论贫富，能够通过优化健康和减少疾病，来改变他们的人类潜能。这确实是医学进步的激动人心的时刻。随着我们进入21世纪，医学将越来越具有预测性、预防性、个性化和参与性。它将关注我们每一个人，并根据我们每个人的个人和独特的特点优化我们的健康。

致谢

我们感谢健康先锋试点项目中的受试者的参与，以及许多出色的团队成员（不胜枚举），是他们使这个项目成为可能。我们感谢Gretchen Sorensen和Jennifer Lovejoy对手稿的许多宝贵评论。我们还感谢Institute for Systems Biology为该项目提供慈善支持，感谢Robert Wood Johnson Foundation和MJ Murdock Charitable Trust为该研究提供了部分资金。

（郭威 译　谭锋维　赫捷 校）

参考文献

1 de la Maisonneuve C, Martins JO. Public spending on health and long-term care: a new set of projections. OECD Economic Policy Papers; 2013.

2 Woolf S, Aron L (eds). *US Health in International Perspective: Shorter Lives, Poorer Health*. National Research Council and Institute of Medicine. Washington, DC: National Academies Press; 2013.

3 Schroeder SA. Shattuck Lecture. We can do better—improving the health of the American people. *N Engl J Med*. 2007;**357**(**12**):1221–1228.

4 Hood L. Biological Complexity under Attack. 2011: Genetic Engineering and Biotechnology News.

5 Kuhn T. *The Structure of Scientific Revolution*. **264**. 1962: University of Chicago Press, Chicago.

6 Hood L, Heath JR, Phelps ME, Lin B. Systems biology and new technologies enable predictive and preventative medicine. *Science*. 2004;**306**(**5696**):640–643.

7 Flores M, Glusman G, Brogaard K, Price ND, Hood L. P4 medicine: how systems medicine will transform the healthcare sector and society. *Per Med*. 2013;**10**(**6**):565–576.

8 Hood L. Systems biology: integrating technology, biology, and computation. *Mech Ageing Dev*. 2003;**124**(**1**):9–16.

9 Hood L. A personal view of molecular technology and how it has changed biology. *J Proteome Res*. 2002;**1**(**5**):399–409.

10 Hood L. Biotechnology and medicine of the future. *JAMA*. 1988;**259**(**12**): 1837–1844.

11 Hood L, Galas D. The digital code of DNA. *Nature*. 2003;**421**(**6921**):444–448.

12 Smith LM, Sanders JZ, Kaiser RJ, et al. Fluorescence detection in automated DNA sequence analysis. *Nature*. 1986;**321**(**6071**):674–679.

13 Hood L. A personal journey of discovery: developing technology and changing biology. *Annu Rev Anal Chem (Palo Alto Calif)*. 2008;**1**:1–43.

14 Hood L, Rowen L, Galas DJ, Aitchison JD. Systems biology at the Institute for Systems Biology. *Brief Funct Genomic Proteomic*. 2008;**7**(**4**):239–248.

15 Kitano H. Systems biology: a brief overview. *Science*. 2002;**295**(**5560**):1662–1664.

16 Hood L. Systems biology and p4 medicine: past, present, and future. *Rambam Maimonides Med J*. 2013;**4**(**2**):e0012.

17 Hood L, Friend SH. Predictive, personalized, preventive, participatory (P4) cancer medicine. *Nat Rev Clin Oncol*. 2011;**8**(**3**):184–187.

18 Tian Q, Price ND, Hood L. Systems cancer medicine: towards realization of predictive, preventive, personalized and participatory (P4) medicine. *J Intern Med*. 2012;**271**(**2**):111–121.

19 Rowen L, Young J, Birditt B, et al. Analysis of the human neurexin genes: alternative splicing and the generation of protein diversity. *Genomics*. 2002;**79**(**4**):587–597.

20 Sung J, Wang Y, Chandrasekaran S, Witten DM, Price ND. Molecular signatures from omics data: from chaos to consensus. *Biotechnol J*. 2012;**7**(**8**):946–957.

21 Ideker T, Galitski T, Hood L. A new approach to decoding life: systems biology. *Annu Rev Genomics Hum Genet*. 2001;**2**:343–372.

22 Ideker T Thorsson V, Ranish JA, et al. Integrated genomic and proteomic analyses of a systematically perturbed metabolic network. *Science*. 2001;**292**(**5518**):929–934.

23 Roach JC, Glusman G, Smit AFA, et al. Analysis of genetic inheritance in a family quartet by whole-genome sequencing. *Science*. 2010;**328**(**5978**):636–639.

24 Ament SA, Szelinger S, Glusman G, et al. Rare variants in neuronal excitability genes influence risk for bipolar disorder. *Proc Natl Acad Sci U S A*. 2015;**112**(**11**):3576–3581.

25 Hwang D, Lee IY, Yoo H, et al. A systems approach to prion disease. *Mol Syst Biol*. 2009;**5**:252.

26 Li X-J, Hayward C, Fong PY, et al. A blood-based proteomic classifier for the molecular characterization of pulmonary nodules. *Sci Transl Med*. 2013;**5**(**207**): 207ra142.

27 Hood L, Price ND. Demystifying disease, democratizing health care. *Sci Transl Med*. 2014;**6**(**225**):225ed5.

28 Hood L., Price ND. Promoting Wellness and Demystifying Disease: The 100K Project. Clinical Omics; 2014.

29 Hood L, Lovejoy JC, Price ND. Integrating big data and actionable health coaching to optimize wellness. *BMC Med*. 2015;**13**(**1**):4.

30 Office for National Statistics. *Historic and Projected Data from the Period and Cohort Life Tables, 2012-Based Revised*. UK: Office for National Statistics; 2014.

31 Gibbs WW. Medicine gets up close and personal. *Nature*. 2014;**506**(**7487**):144–145.

32 Church GM. The personal genome project. *Mol Syst Biol*. 2005;**1**:2005.0030.

索引

C

D

E

F

G

H

J

K

L

M

N

P

Q

R

S

T

W

X